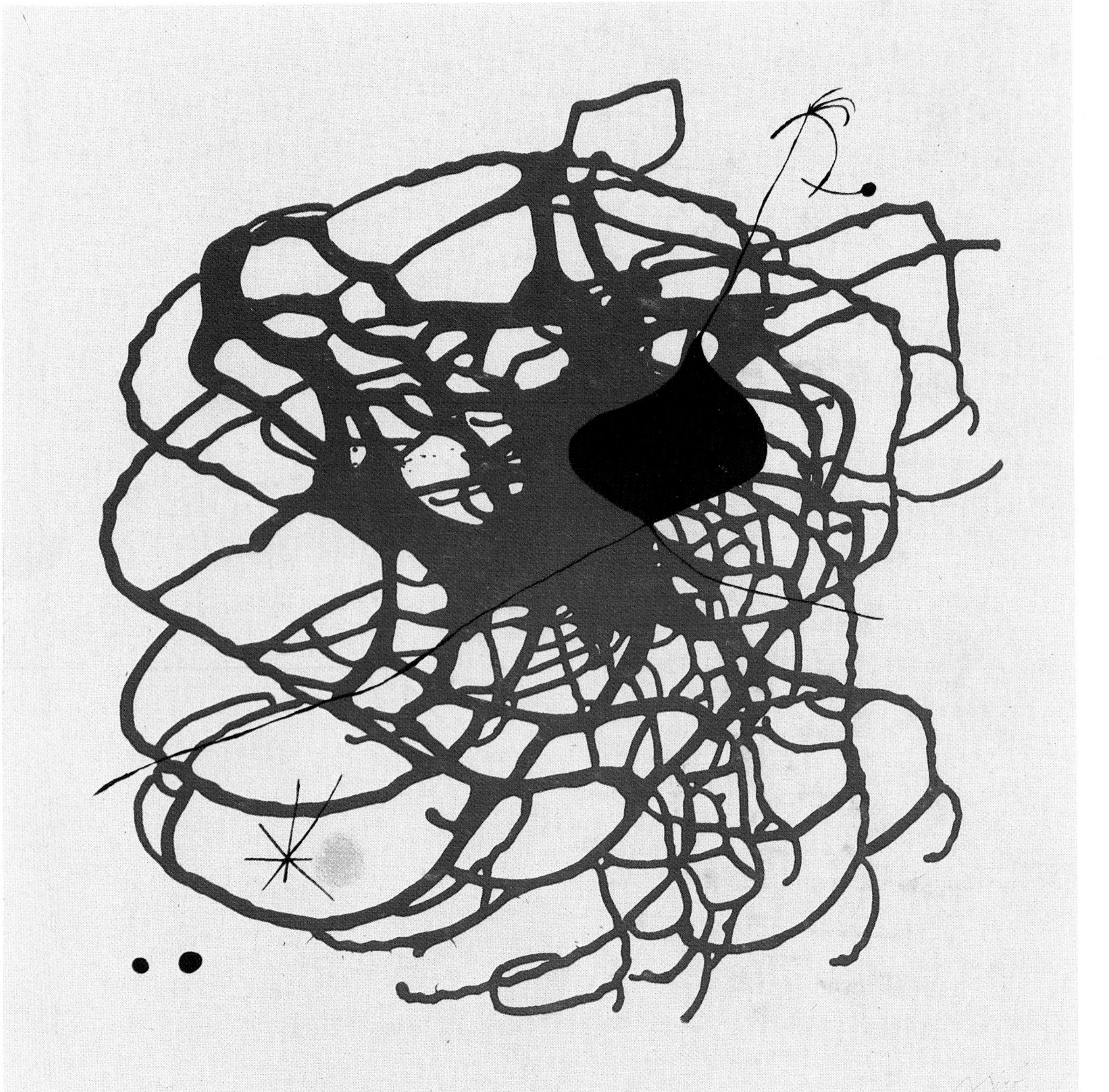

Miró
Courtesy of Galerie Maeght, Paris

HEART DISEASE

Third Edition

A TEXTBOOK OF CARDIOVASCULAR MEDICINE

Edited by

EUGENE BRAUNWALD A.B., M.D., M.S. (hon.), M.D. (hon.)

Hersey Professor of the Theory and Practice of Physic;
Herrman Ludwig Blumgart Professor of Medicine, Harvard Medical School;
Chairman, Department of Medicine,
Brigham and Women's and Beth Israel Hospitals, Boston

1988 W. B. SAUNDERS COMPANY
Harcourt Brace Jovanovich, Inc.
Philadelphia, London, Toronto, Montreal, Sydney, Tokyo

W. B. SAUNDERS COMPANY
Harcourt Brace Jovanovich, Inc.

West Washington Square
Philadelphia, PA 19105

Library of Congress Cataloging-in-Publication Data

Heart disease.

Includes bibliographies and indexes.

1. Heart—Diseases. 2. Cardiovascular system—Diseases. I. Braunwald, Eugene, 1929– . [DNLM: 1. Heart Diseases—complications. WG 200 H4364]

RC681.H362 1988 616.1′2 86–31445

ISBN 0–7216–1953–3 (single v.)
ISBN 0–7216–1956–8 (set)
ISBN 0–7216–1954–1 (v. 1)
ISBN 0–7216–1955–X (v. 2)

Manuscript Editor: Edna Dick
Production Manager: Frank Polizzano
Illustration Coordinator: Kenneth Green
Indexer: Ella Shapiro

HEART DISEASE

ISBN	Single Volume	0–7216–1953–3
ISBN	Set	0–7216–1956–8
ISBN	Volume 1	0–7216–1954–1
ISBN	Volume 2	0–7216–1955–X

Last digit is the print number: 9 8 7 6 5 4 3 2

Dedicated
to the memory of my father,

WILLIAM BRAUNWALD

CONTRIBUTORS

DONALD S. BAIM, M.D.

Assistant Professor of Medicine, Harvard Medical School. Director of Invasive Cardiology, Beth Israel Hospital, Boston, Massachusetts.

Interventional Catheterization Techniques: Percutaneous Transluminal Balloon Angioplasty, Valvuloplasty, and Related Procedures

MURRAY G. BARON, M.D.

Professor of Radiology and Vice Chairman, Department of Radiology, Emory University School of Medicine. Associate Chief, Radiology Service, Emory University Hospital and Grady Memorial Hospital, Atlanta, Georgia.

Radiological and Angiographic Examination of the Heart

WILLIAM H. BARRY, M.D.

Nora Eccles Harrison Professor of Cardiology, University of Utah School of Medicine. Attending Physician, University of Utah Medical Center, Salt Lake City, Utah.

Cardiac Catheterization

EUGENE H. BLACKSTONE, M.D.

Professor, Department of Surgery, University of Alabama at Birmingham School of Medicine. Professor of Surgery, University of Alabama Hospitals, Birmingham, Alabama.

Cardiac Surgery

KENNETH M. BOROW, M.D.

Associate Professor of Medicine (Cardiology), University of Chicago. Director, Cardiac Noninvasive Imaging Laboratories, University of Chicago Medical Center and Michael Reese Hospital and Medical Center, Chicago, Illinois.

Congenital Heart Disease in the Adult

EUGENE BRAUNWALD, M.D.

Hersey Professor of the Theory and Practice of Physic; Herrman Ludwig Blumgart Professor of Medicine, Harvard Medical School. Chairman, Department of Medicine, Brigham and Women's and Beth Israel Hospitals, Boston, Massachusetts.

The History; The Physical Examination; Mechanisms of Cardiac Contraction and Relaxation; Pathophysiology of Heart Failure; Assessment of Cardiac Function; Clinical Manifestations of Heart Failure; Management of Heart Failure; Pulmonary Edema: Cardiogenic and Noncardiogenic; High–Cardiac Output States; Pulmonary Hypertension; Congenital Heart Disease in the Adult; Valvular Heart Disease; Coronary Blood Flow and Myocardial Ischemia; Acute Myocardial Infarction; Chronic Ischemic Heart Disease; The Cardiomyopathies and Myocarditides; Primary Tumors of the Heart; Pericardial Disease; Traumatic Heart Disease; Pulmonary Embolism; Cor Pulmonale; General Anesthesia and Noncardiac Surgery in Patients with Heart Disease; Hematologic-Oncologic Disorders and Heart Disease; Endocrine and Nutritional Disorders and Heart Disease; Renal Disorders and Heart Disease

MICHAEL S. BROWN, M.D., D.Sc. (Hon.)

Professor, Department of Molecular Genetics, and Director, Center for Genetic Diseases, University of Texas Health Science Center at Dallas. Senior Attending Physician, Parkland Memorial Hospital, Dallas, Texas.

Genetics and Cardiovascular Disease

CONTRIBUTORS

AGUSTIN CASTELLANOS, M.D.

Professor of Medicine, School of Medicine, University of Miami. Director, Clinical Electrophysiology, Jackson Memorial/University of Miami Medical Center, Miami, Florida.

Cardiac Arrest and Sudden Cardiac Death

PETER F. COHN, M.D.

Professor of Medicine and Chief, Cardiology Division, State University of New York Health Sciences Center at Stony Brook, Stony Brook, New York.

Traumatic Heart Disease; Chronic Ischemic Heart Disease

WILSON S. COLUCCI, M.D.

Associate Professor of Medicine, Harvard Medical School. Associate Physician, Cardiovascular Division, Department of Medicine, Brigham and Women's Hospital, Boston, Massachusetts.

Primary Tumors of the Heart

ERNEST CRAIGE, M.D.

Henry A. Foscue Distinguished Professor of Cardiology, University of North Carolina School of Medicine, Chapel Hill, North Carolina.

Heart Sounds: Phonocardiography; Carotid, Apex, and Jugular Venous Pulse Tracings; and Systolic Time Intervals; Echophonocardiography and Other Noninvasive Techniques to Elucidate Heart Murmurs

ROMAN W. DE SANCTIS, M.D.

Professor of Medicine, Harvard Medical School. Physician and Director of Clinical Cardiology, Massachusetts General Hospital, Boston, Massachusetts.

Diseases of the Aorta

EDWIN G. DUFFIN, PH.D.

Bakken Fellow, Tachyarrhythmia Management Group, Medtronic, Inc., Minneapolis, Minnesota.

Cardiac Pacemakers

KIM A. EAGLE, M.D.

Instructor in Medicine, Harvard Medical School. Clinical Assistant, Massachusetts General Hospital. Assistant Director of Fellowship Training, Cardiac Unit, Massachusetts General Hospital, Boston, Massachusetts.

Diseases of the Aorta

JOHN A. FARMER, M.D.

Assistant Professor of Medicine, Baylor College of Medicine. Assistant Physician, The Methodist Hospital and Ben Taub General Hospital, Houston, Texas.

Risk Factor for Coronary Artery Disease

HARVEY FEIGENBAUM, M.D.

Distinguished Professor of Medicine, Indiana University School of Medicine, Director, Hemodynamic Laboratory, Indiana University School of Medicine, Indianapolis, Indiana.

Echocardiography

CHARLES FISCH, M.D.

Distinguished Professor of Medicine; Director, Krannert Institute of Cardiology and Cardiovascular Division, Indiana University School of Medicine, Indianapolis, Indiana.

Electrocardiography and Vectorcardiography

WILLIAM F. FRIEDMAN, M.D.

J. H. Nicholson Professor of Pediatrics (Cardiology) and Executive Chairman, Department of Pediatrics, University of California, Los Angeles School of Medicine, Pediatrician-in-Chief, UCLA Medical Center, Los Angeles, California.

Congenital Heart Disease in Infancy and Childhood; Acquired Heart Disease in Infancy and Childhood

GEOFFREY A. GARDINER, M.D.

Assistant Professor; Director, Cardiovascular Interventional Radiology Department, Thomas Jefferson University Hospital, Philadelphia, Pennsylvania.

Coronary Arteriography

GARY GERSTENBLITH, M.D.

Associate Professor of Medicine, Johns Hopkins School of Medicine. Full-time Medical Staff, Johns Hopkins Hospital, Baltimore, Maryland.

Aging and Cardiac Disease

SAMUEL Z. GOLDHABER, M.D.

Assistant Professor of Medicine, Harvard Medical School. Associate Physician, Brigham and Women's Hospital, Boston, Massachusetts.

Pulmonary Embolism

LEE GOLDMAN, M.D.

Associate Professor of Medicine, Harvard Medical School. Assistant Physician-in-Chief, Brigham and Women's Hospital, Boston, Massachusetts.

Cost-Effective Strategies in Cardiology; General Anesthesia and Noncardiac Surgery in Patients with Heart Disease

JOSEPH L. GOLDSTEIN, M.D., D.Sc. (Hon.)

Paul J. Thomas Professor and Chairman, Department of Molecular Genetics, University of Texas Health Science Center at Dallas. Senior Attending Physician, Parkland Memorial Hospital, Dallas, Texas.

Genetics and Cardiovascular Disease

ANTONIO M. GOTTO, Jr., M.D., D.Phil.

Chairman and Professor, Department of Medicine, and Distinguished Service Professor, J. S. Abercrombie Chair for Atherosclerosis and Lipoprotein Research, Baylor College of Medicine. The Bob and Vivian Smith Professor and Chairman, Department of Medicine, Baylor and The Methodist Hospital; Chief, Internal Medicine Service, The Methodist Hospital; Chief, Internal Medicine, Ben Taub General Hospital and the Harris County Hospital District, Houston, Texas.

Risk Factors for Coronary Artery Disease

WILLIAM GROSSMAN, M.D.

Herman Dana Professor of Medicine, Harvard Medical School. Chief, Cardiovascular Division, Beth Israel Hospital, Boston, Massachusetts.

Cardiac Catheterization; High–Cardiac Output States

THOMAS P. HACKETT, M.D.

Eben S. Draper Professor of Psychiatry, Harvard Medical School. Chief of Psychiatry, Massachusetts, General Hospital, Boston, Massachusetts.

Emotion, Psychiatric Disorders, and the Heart

ROBERT I. HANDIN, M.D.

Associate Professor of Medicine, Harvard Medical School. Chief, Hematology Division, Department of Medicine, Brigham and Women's Hospital, Boston, Massachusetts.

Hemostasis, Thrombosis, Fibrinolysis, and the Heart

CHARLES B. HIGGINS, M.D.

Professor of Radiology, University of California, San Francisco Medical School. Chief, Magnetic Resonance Imaging, University of California, San Francisco Medical Center, San Francisco, California.

Newer Cardiac Imaging Techniques: Digital Subtraction Angiography; Computed Tomography; Magnetic Resonance Imaging

B. LEONARD HOLMAN, M.D.

Professor of Radiology, Harvard Medical School. Acting Chairman, Department of Radiology, Brigham and Women's Hospital, Boston, Massachusetts.

Nuclear Cardiology

ROLAND H. INGRAM, Jr., M.D.

Parker B. Francis Professor of Medicine, Harvard Medical School. Senior Physician and Director, Respiratory Division, Brigham and Women's Hospital, Boston, Massachusetts.

Pulmonary Edema: Cardiogenic and Noncardiogenic

NORMAN M. KAPLAN, M.D.

Professor of Internal Medicine, University of Texas Southwestern Medical School. Head, Hypertension Service, Parkland Memorial Hospital, Dallas, Texas.

Systemic Hypertension: Mechanisms and Diagnosis; Systemic Hypertension: Therapy

RALPH A. KELLY, M.D.

Assistant Professor of Medicine, Harvard Medical School. Associate Physician, Brigham and Women's Hospital, Boston, Massachusetts.

Management of Heart Failure

JAMES K. KIRKLIN, M.D.

Associate Professor of Surgery, University of Alabama at Birmingham School of Medicine. Associate Professor of Surgery, Division of Cardiothoracic Surgery, University of Alabama Hospitals, Birmingham, Alabama.

Cardiac Surgery

JOHN W. KIRKLIN, M.D.

Professor of Surgery, University of Alabama at Birmingham School of Medicine. Professor of Surgery, Division of Cardiothoracic Surgery, University of Alabama Hospitals, Birmingham, Alabama.

Cardiac Surgery

EDWARD G. LAKATTA, M.D.

Chief, Laboratory of Cardiovascular Science, Gerontology Research Center, National Institute on Aging, National Institutes of Health. Associate Professor of Medicine, Johns Hopkins School of Medicine. Associate Professor of Physiology, University of Maryland School of Medicine, Baltimore, Maryland.

Aging and Cardiac Disease

DAVID C. LEVIN, M.D.

Professor of Radiology, Jefferson Medical College. Chairman, Department of Radiology, Thomas Jefferson University Hospital, Philadelphia, Pennsylvania.

Coronary Arteriography

BEVERLY H. LORELL, M.D.

Assistant Professor of Medicine, Harvard Medical School. Co-Director, Hemodynamic Research Laboratory, Beth Israel Hospital, Boston, Massachusetts.

Pericardial Disease

JOSEPH LOSCALZO, M.D., PH.D.

Assistant Professor of Medicine, Harvard Medical School. Associate Physician, Brigham and Women's Hospital, Boston, Massachusetts.

Hemostasis, Thrombosis, Fibrinolysis, and the Heart

E. REGIS MCFADDEN, JR., M.D.

Argyle J. Beams Professor of Medicine, Case Western Reserve University School of Medicine. Director, Airway Disease Center, University Hospitals, Cleveland, Ohio.

Cor Pulmonale; Relationship Between Diseases of the Heart and Lungs

ROBERT J. MYERBURG, M.D.

Professor of Medicine and Physiology, Director, Division of Cardiology, Department of Medicine, University of Miami School of Medicine, Miami, Florida.

Cardiac Arrest and Sudden Cardiac Death

ALBERT OBERMAN, M.D., M.P.H.

Professor of Medicine, University of Alabama at Birmingham School of Medicine. Director, Division of General and Preventive Medicine, University of Alabama Medical Center. Active Medical Staff, University of Alabama Hospitals, Birmingham, Alabama.

Rehabilitation of Patients with Coronary Artery Disease

STEPHEN O. PASTAN, M.D.

Clinical Fellow, Harvard Medical School. Clinical Fellow in Medicine, Beth Israel Hospital, Boston, Massachusetts.

Renal Disorders and Heart Disease

RICHARD C. PASTERNAK, M.D.

Assistant Professor of Medicine, Harvard Medical School. Director, Coronary Care Unit, Beth Israel Hospital, Boston, Massachusetts.

Acute Myocardial Infarction

JOSEPH K. PERLOFF, M.D.

Streisand/American Heart Association Professor of Medicine and Pediatrics, University of California, Los Angeles, School of Medicine. Divisions of Cardiology Departments of Medicine and Pediatrics, UCLA Center for the Health Sciences, Los Angeles, California.

Neurological Disorders and Heart Disease; Pregnancy and Cardiovascular Disease

ERIC C. RACKOW, M.D.

Professor and Vice Chairman, Department of Medicine, and Chief, Division of Critical Care Medicine/Center for Critical Care Medicine, University of Health Sciences/The Chicago Medical School. Consultant Physician, North Chicago Veterans Administration Medical Center, Hines Veterans Administration Medical Center, Naval Hospital Great Lakes, Cook County Hospital, and Jackson Park Hospital Center, Chicago, Illinois.

Acute Circulatory Failure (Shock)

ROBERT ROBERTS, M.D.

Professor of Medicine, Baylor College of Medicine. Chief of Cardiology, The Methodist Hospital, Houston, Texas.

Hypotension and Syncope

JERROLD F. ROSENBAUM, M.D.

Assistant Professor of Psychiatry, Harvard Medical School. Chief, Clinical Psychopharmacology Unit, Massachusetts General Hospital, Boston, Massachusetts.

Emotion, Psychiatric Disorders, and the Heart

DAVID S. ROSENTHAL, M.D.

Associate Professor of Medicine, Harvard Medical School. Clinical Director of Hematology, Brigham and Women's Hospital, Boston, Massachusetts.

Hematological-Oncological Disorders and Heart Disease

JOHN ROSS, JR., M.D.

Professor of Medicine and Head, Division of Cardiology, Department of Medicine, University of California, San Diego, School of Medicine. Attending Physician, University of California, San Diego, Medical Center, San Diego, California.

Mechanisms of Cardiac Contraction and Relaxation

RUSSELL ROSS, PH.D., D.D.S.

Professor and Chairman, Pathology, and Adjunct Professor, Biochemistry, University of Washington School of Medicine, Seattle, Washington.

The Pathogenesis of Atherosclerosis

JOHN D. RUTHERFORD, M.B., FRACP

Assistant Professor of Medicine, Harvard Medical School. Co-Director, Clinical Cardiology Service, Brigham and Women's Hospital, Boston, Massachusetts.

Chronic Ischemic Heart Disease

L. THOMAS SHEFFIELD, M.D.

Professor, Department of Medicine, University of Alabama School of Medicine, Birmingham, Alabama.

Exercise Stress Testing

DAMON SMITH, B.M.E.

Heart Sounds: Phonocardiography; Carotid, Apex, and Jugular Venous Tracings; and Systolic Time Intervals

THOMAS W. SMITH, M.D.

Professor of Medicine, Harvard Medical School–MIT Division of Health Sciences and Technology. Senior Physician and Chief, Cardiovascular Division, Brigham and Women's Hospital; Consultant in Cardiology, Children's Hospital Medical Center; Consultant in Medicine, Massachusetts General Hospital, Boston, Massachusetts.

Management of Heart Failure

BURTON E. SOBEL, M.D.

Lewin Professor of Medicine, and Director, Cardiovascular Division, Washington University School of Medicine. Cardiologist-in-Chief, Barnes Hospital, St. Louis, Missouri.

Hypotension and Syncope; Coronary Blood Flow and Myocardial Ischemia; Acute Myocardial Infarction

EDMUND H. SONNENBLICK, M.D.

Olson Professor of Medicine, The Albert Einstein College of Medicine. Chief, Division of Cardiology, Hospital of The Albert Einstein College of Medicine and the Bronx Municipal Hospital Center, Bronx, New York.

Cardiac Contraction and Relaxation

GENE H. STOLLERMAN, M.D.

Professor of Medicine, Boston University School of Medicine. VA Distinguished Physician, Edith Nourse Rogers Memorial Veterans Hospital, Bedford, Massachusetts.

Rheumatic and Heritable Connective Tissue Diseases of the Cardiovascular System

GEORGE E. TESAR, M.D.

Instructor in Psychiatry, Harvard Medical School. Director, Acute Psychiatric Service, Massachusetts General Hospital, Boston, Massachusetts.

Emotion, Psychiatric Disorders, and the Heart

MARTIN VON PLANTA, M.D.

Research Fellow, Divisions of Critical Care and Cardiology, Department of Medicine, University of Health Sciences/The Chicago Medical School, Chicago, Illinois.

Acute Circulatory Failure (Shock)

MAX HARRY WEIL, M.D., PH.D.

Professor and Chairman, Department of Medicine; Professor of Physiology and Biophysics; Chief, Division of Cardiology, University of Health Sciences/The Chicago Medical School. Consultant Physician, North Chicago Veterans Administration Medical Center, Hines Veterans Administration Medical Center, Naval Hospital Great Lakes, Cook County Hospital, and Jackson Park Hospital Center, Chicago, Illinois.

Acute Circulatory Failure (Shock)

LOUIS WEINSTEIN, M.D., PH.D.

Professor Emeritus of Medicine, Tufts University School of Medicine. Lecturer in Medicine, Harvard Medical School. Senior Consultant in Medicine, Brigham and Women's Hospital, Boston, Massachusetts.

Infective Endocarditis

MYRON L. WEISFELDT, M.D.

Professor of Medicine, Johns Hopkins University School of Medicine. Director of Cardiology, Johns Hopkins Hospital. Director of Cardiology, Francis Scott Key Medical Center, Baltimore, Maryland.

Aging and Cardiac Disease

GORDON H. WILLIAMS, M.D.

Professor of Medicine, Harvard Medical School. Director, Endocrine-Hypertension Division, Brigham and Women's Hospital, Boston, Massachusetts.

Endocrine and Nutritional Disorders and Heart Disease

MARSHALL A. WOLF, M.D.

Associate Professor of Medicine, Harvard Medical School. Associate Physician-in-Chief, Brigham and Women's Hospital, Boston, Massachusetts.

General Anesthesia and Noncardiac Surgery in Patients with Heart Disease

JOSHUA WYNNE, M.D.

Professor of Medicine, Wayne State University. Chief, Divsion of Cardiology, Harper Hospital, Detroit, Michigan.

The Cardiomyopathies and Myocarditides

DOUGLAS P. ZIPES, M.D.

Professor of Medicine, Senior Research Associate, Krannert Institute of Cardiology, Indiana University School of Medicine. Attending Physician, Roudebusch Veterans Administration Hospital, Wishard Memorial Hospital, and University Hospital, Indianapolis, Indiana.

Genesis of Cardiac Arrhythmias: Electrophysiological Considerations; Management of Cardiac Arrhythmias: Pharmacological, Electrical, and Surgical Techniques; Specific Arrhythmias: Diagnosis and Treatment; Cardiac Pacemakers

PREFACE TO THE THIRD EDITION

The rates at which the various branches of medicine progress are by no means uniform. To even the most casual observer of the medical scene, it is evident that cardiology is now moving ahead at an unprecedented velocity. Because of the enormous advances in clinical cardiology and cardiovascular science that have occurred in the 4 years since publication of the second edition of *Heart Disease*, preparation of the third edition has been a task that has been both more challenging and intellectually invigorating than I had anticipated.

Although the basic format of the book has remained the same, the new edition incorporates extensive changes. *Heart Disease* is now divided into 5 parts: Part I deals with the examination of the patient in the broadest sense, including clinical findings and the theory and application of modern invasive and noninvasive techniques used to elicit information about the heart and the circulation. Part II is concerned with the pathophysiology, diagnosis, and treatment of the principal abnormalities and circulatory function, including heart failure, shock, arrhythmias, and abnormalities of arterial pressure. Part III, the longest in the book, consists of descriptions of the principal congenital and acquired diseases affecting the heart, pericardium, aorta, and pulmonary vascular bed in adults and children. Part IV, new to this edition, deals with the interaction between broad fields such as genetics, aging, surgery, and heart disease. Part V deals with the manner in which diseases of other organ systems affect the circulation and vice versa. The third edition of *Heart Disease* is approximately 20 per cent longer than the second. This has been accomplished with little increase in the number of pages through a more efficient page layout, the use of somewhat smaller illustrations, and more liberal use of special type face.

Twelve new chapters have been added or substituted: Coronary Arteriography by David C. Levin and Geoffrey A. Gardiner, Jr.; Newer Cardiac Imaging Techniques by Charles B. Higgins; Acute Circulatory Failure (Shock) by Max Harry Weil, Martin von Planta, and Eric C. Rackow; Cardiac Arrest and Sudden Death by Robert J. Myerburg and Agustin Castellanos; The Pathogenesis of Atherosclerosis by Russell Ross; Risk Factors for Coronary Artery Disease by Antonio M. Gotto, Jr., and John A. Farmer; Acute Myocardial Infarction by Richard C. Pasternak, Eugene Braunwald, and Burton E. Sobel; Chronic Ischemic Heart Disease by John D. Rutherford, Eugene Braunwald, and Peter F. Cohen; Pulmonary Embolism by Samuel Z. Goldhaber and Eugene Braunwald; Aging and Cardiac Disease by Myron S. Weisfeldt, Edward G. Lakatta, and Gary Gerstenblith; Cost-Effective Strategies in Cardiology by Lee Goldman; Hemostasis, Thrombosis, Fibrinolysis, and Cardiovascular Disease by Robert I. Handin and Joseph Loscalzo. All of the other chapters have been extensively revised.

The influence of molecular and cellular biology on cardiology is growing rapidly and is discussed extensively in the third edition of *Heart Disease*, particularly in the chapters on Genetics and Cardiovascular Disease by Goldstein and Brown, on Mechanisms of Cardiac Contraction and Relaxation by Braunwald, Sonnenblick, and Ross, as well as in the new chapters on Pathogenesis of Arteriosclerosis by Ross and on Risk Factors for Coronary Artery Disease by Gotto and Farmer.

Many other important new areas are covered in detail. These include Doppler echocardiography; CT scanning and magnetic resonance imaging of the heart; thrombolytic therapy of acute myocardial infarction and pulmonary embolism; newer concepts regarding the pathogenesis, treatment, and prevention of atherosclerosis, cardiac arrhythmias, and congestive heart failure; percutaneous transluminal angioplasty and balloon valvuloplasty; the newly discovered atrial natriuretic peptide; the role of electrical and surgical techniques in the treatment of tachyarrhythmias; heart and heart-lung transplantation and artificial devices in the treatment of end-stage heart failure.

The modern practice of cardiology involves much more than the application of high technology to patients with heart disease. It requires the careful integration of findings on clinical and laboratory examination as well as the exercise of judgment and discretion in the selection of the growing number of diagnostic and therapeutic modalities which are now available. Accordingly, the chapter on Physical Examination has been thoroughly revised and expanded. Diagnostic and therapeutic options are discussed in detail in every chapter in Part III, Diseases of the Heart, Pericardium, Aorta and Pulmonary Vascular Bed. The new chapter on Cost-Effective Strategies in Cardiology by Goldman explains how cost-conscious practice need not impair the quality of care.

Considerable revisions have been made in both galley and page proofs to accommodate information about the most recent advances in the field. Particular emphasis has been placed on insuring a comprehensive and up-to-date bibliography, and a substantial number of references to pertinent publications that appeared in 1987 are included. There are 773 *new* figures and 228 *new* tables.

Despite these efforts, the rapid pace at which cardiology advances makes it ever more difficult to provide a timely picture of this field in a traditional textbook. Therefore, a new publication, *Updates to Heart Disease*, will be made available on a quarterly basis commencing in the Spring of 1988. The *Updates* will complement *Heart Disease* and describe new developments in the field which have occurred since the preparation of the textbook. Also, an electronic version of the third edition of *Heart Disease* will be made available by BRS-Colleague; this version should be particularly useful in frequent updating and revision. In addition, a Question and Answer Self-Assessment and Review Book will accompany the third edition of *Heart Disease*. It consists of 600 questions based on material discussed in the textbook and provides the answers as well as detailed explanations. These multiple efforts—the printed and electronic versions of the text, the printed *Updates*, the electronic revisions, and the Self-Assessment Book—all are attempts to assist the reader with the awesome task of learning and remaining current in this dynamic field.

It is hoped that this textbook will prove useful to those who wish to broaden their knowledge of cardiovascular medicine. To the extent that it achieves this goal and thereby aids in the care of patients afflicted with heart disease, credit must be given to the many talented and dedicated persons involved in its preparation. I offer my deepest appreciation to my fellow contributors for their professional expertise, knowledge, and devoted scholarship, which have so enriched this book. It has been a personal pleasure for me to deal with the W. B. Saunders Company. Ms. Carol Trumbold, the Executive Editor, and Ms. Lorraine Kilmer, Manager of the Editoral/Design/Production Team, have been particularly helpful, as have been the effective members of this team—especially Mr. Frank Polizzano and Ms. Edna Dick. Ms. Patricia DeLosh in my office rendered most capable editorial and secretarial services.

Without question, this edition could not have become a reality were it not for the skill and dedication of several individuals. My responsibilities to the Harvard Medical School and the Brigham and Women's and Beth Israel Hospitals during the leave of absence which I required for much of my own writing were shouldered most effectively by my colleagues, Drs. Marshall Wolf, Stephen Robinson, and Steven Come, who provided the Department of Medicine with exemplary leadership. My administrative assistants, Mrs. Mary Jackson at the Brigham and Women's Hospital and Ms. Carolyn Farley at the Beth Israel were enormously helpful in maintaining the orderly flow of activity essential to a busy Department of Medicine. I am also deeply indebted to Dr. Daniel C. Tosteson, Dean of the Harvard Medical School; Dr. H. Richard Nesson, President of the Brigham and Women's Hospital; and Dr. Mitchell T. Rabkin, President of the Beth Israel Hospital, for graciously allowing me the freedom to devote myself to this task. My wife, Dr. Nina S. Braunwald, my mother, Mrs. Clare Braunwald, and my children, Karen Gail, Denise Allison, and Adrienne Jill, provided the personal support, encouragement, and understanding so essential for one who adds a task of this magnitude to an already full professional life.

EUGENE BRAUNWALD

Adapted from the PREFACE TO THE FIRST EDITION

Cardiovascular disease is the greatest scourge afflicting the population of the industrialized nations. As with previous scourges—bubonic plague, yellow fever, and smallpox—cardiovascular disease not only strikes down a significant fraction of the population without warning but causes prolonged suffering and disability in an even larger number. In the United States alone, despite recent encouraging declines, cardiovascular disease is still responsible for almost one million fatalities each year and more than one half of all deaths; almost 5 million persons afflicted with cardiovascular disease are hospitalized each year. The cost of this disease in terms of human suffering and of material resources is almost incalculable.

Fortunately, research focusing on the causes, diagnosis, treatment, and prevention of heart disease is moving ahead rapidly. In the last 25 years in particular we have witnessed an explosive expansion of our understanding of the structure and function of the cardiovascular system—both normal and abnormal—and of our ability to evaluate these parameters in the living patient, sometimes by means of techniques that require penetration of the skin but also, with increasing accuracy, by noninvasive methods. Simultaneously, remarkable progress has been made in preventing and treating cardiovascular disease by medical and surgical means. Indeed, in the United States, the aforementioned steady reduction in mortality from cardiovascular disease during the past decade suggests that the effective application of this increased knowledge is beginning to prolong the human life span—the most valued resource on earth.

An attempt to summarize our present understanding of heart disease in a comprehensive textbook for the serious student of this subject is a formidable undertaking. Following the untimely death of Dr. Charles K. Friedberg, whose masterful text served as a bible to me and to a whole generation of cardiologists during the 1950's and 1960's, the W. B. Saunders Company invited me to accept this responsibility. Younger colleagues, particularly cardiology fellows and medical residents at the Brigham, convinced me of the need for such a book.

In order to provide a comprehensive, authoritative text in a field that has become as broad and deep as cardiovascular medicine, I chose to enlist the contributions from a number of able colleagues. However, I hoped that my personal involvement in the writing of about half the book would make it possible to minimize the fragmentation, gaps, inconsistencies, organizational difficulties, and impersonal tone that sometimes plague multiauthored texts. I also sought a compromise between a book that is too long as a result of excessive repetition and one in which all duplication is eliminated, resulting in fragmented coverage of certain subjects. To help achieve this objective, extensive cross references have been provided within the text.

Since the early part of this century, clinical cardiology has had a particularly strong foundation in the basic sciences of physiology and pharmacology. More recently, the disciplines of molecular biology, genetics, developmental biology, biophysics, biochemistry, experimental pathology, and bioengineering have also begun to provide critically important information about cardiac function and malfunction. Although *Heart Disease: A Textbook of Cardiovascular Medicine* is primarily a clinical treatise and not a textbook of fundamental cardiovascular science, an effort has been made to explain, in some detail, the scientific basis of cardiovascular diseases.

EUGENE BRAUNWALD

CONTENTS

PART I EXAMINATION OF THE PATIENT

PART V HEART DISEASE AND DISORDERS OF OTHER ORGAN SYSTEMS

PLATE 1

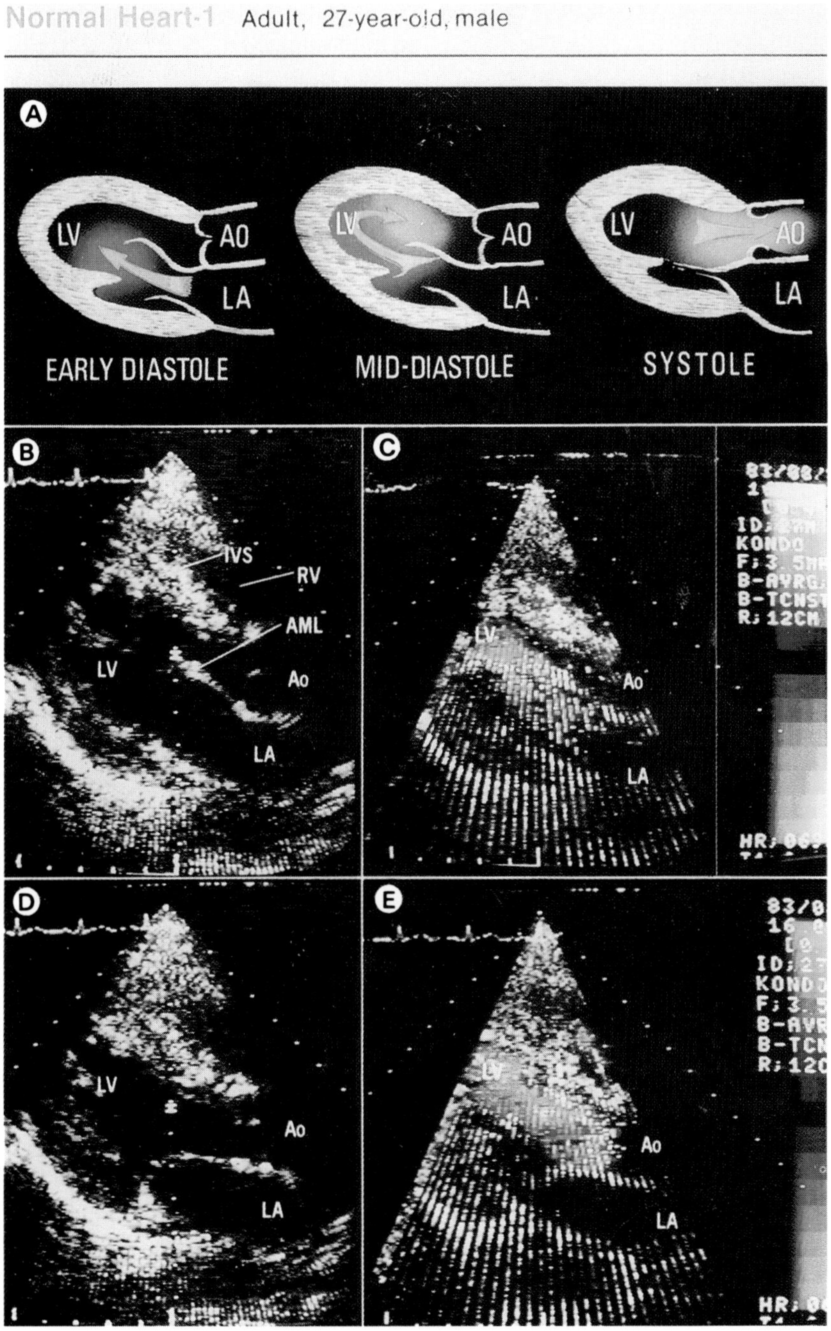

FIGURE 5-12 (See page 88).
Diagram *(A)* and echocardiograms *(B, C, D, E)* demonstrating the principles of color flow mapping of Doppler signals superimposed on two-dimensional echocardiograms. Flow moving toward the transducer is displayed in red, and flow away from the transducer is blue. This illustration demonstrates normal diastolic flow (red) through the mitral orifice into the left ventricle *(C)*. With systole *(E)*, blood flows from the left ventricle into the aorta (blue). LV = left ventricle, AO = aorta, LA = left atrium, IVS = interventricular septum, RV = right ventricle, AML = anterior mitral leaflet. (From Omoto, R.: Color Atlas of Real-time Two-dimensional Doppler Echocardiography. Tokyo, Shindan-To-Chiryo Co., 1984.)

PLATE 2

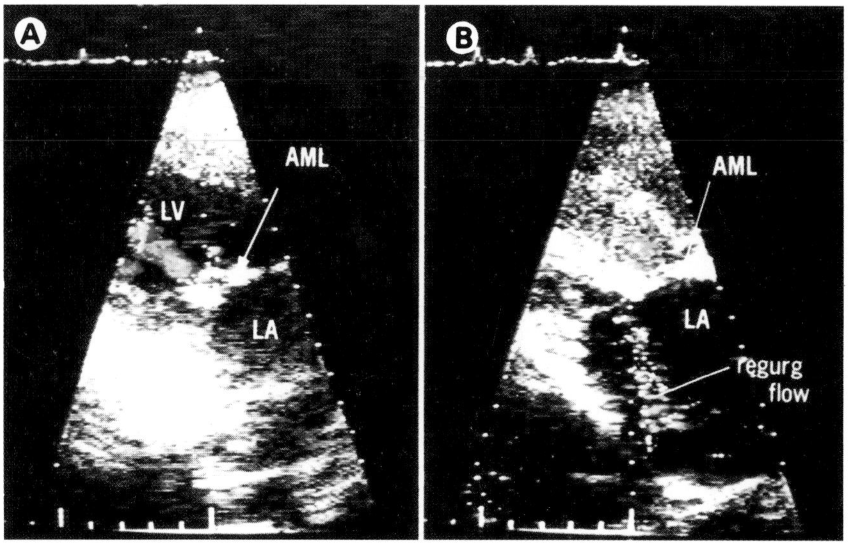

FIGURE 5–49 (See page 105).
Color flow two-dimensional Doppler recording in a patient with mitral stenosis and regurgitation. A multicolored regurgitant flow can be seen in the left atrium (LA) in systole *(B)*. In diastole *(A)*, an orange, flame-shaped jet of blood passes through the stenotic mitral valve into the left ventricle (LV). AML = anterior mitral leaflet. (From Omoto, R.: Color Atlas of Real-time Two-dimensional Doppler Echocardiography. Tokyo, Shindan-To-Chiryo Co., Ltd., 1984.)

FIGURE 5–83 (See page 83).
Apical four-chamber view recorded with real-time two-dimensional color Doppler echocardiography in a patient with a primum artrial septal defect. Forward flow toward the transducer is orange and flow away from the transducer is blue. Note the stream of blood from the left atrium (LA) through the primum atrial septal defect into the right atrium (RA) and right ventricle (RV). LV = left ventricle. (From Omoto, R.: Color Atlas of Real-Time Two Dimensional Doppler Echocardiography. Tokyo, Shindan-To-Chiryo Co., Ltd., 1984.)

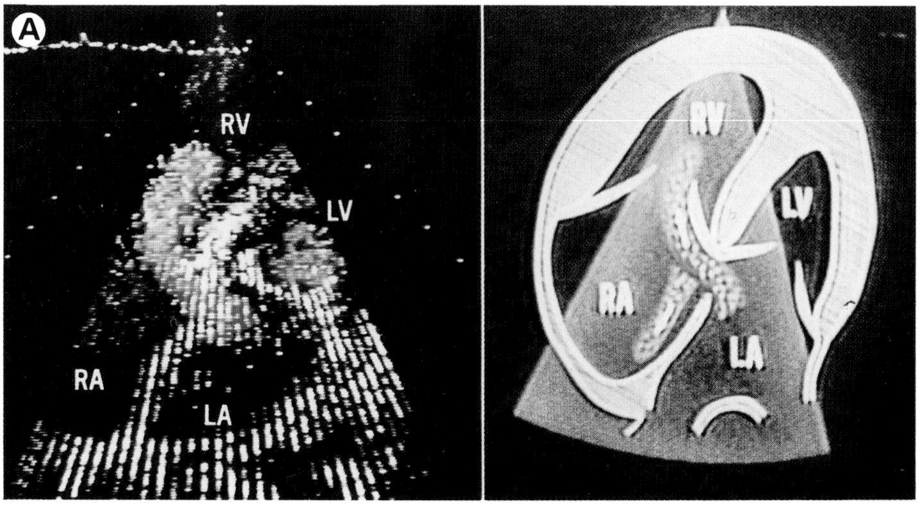

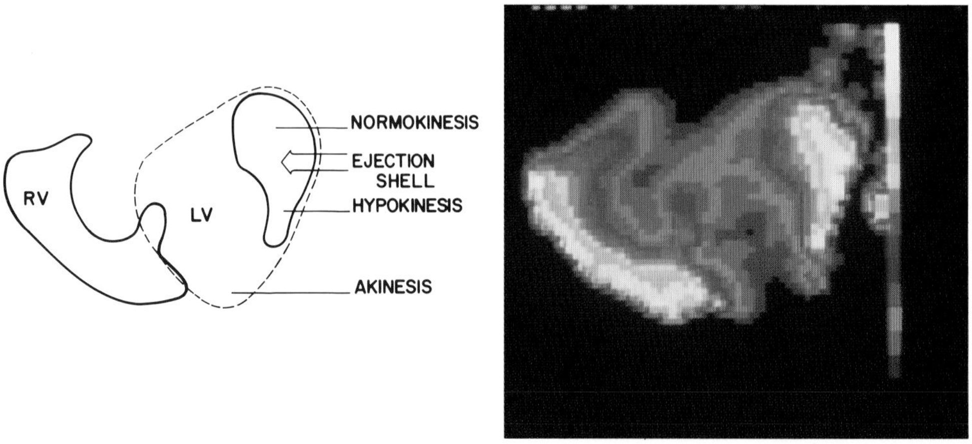

FIGURE 11–9 (See page 321).
A, Schematic representation of left ventricular ejection shell with thinning (hypokinesis) and fracture (akinesis). *B*, Corresponding ejection fraction image in a patient with a large akinetic segment (apical) and adjacent hypokinesis. (From Maddox, D.E., et al.: The ejection fraction image: A noninvasive index of regional left ventricular wall motion. Am. J. Cardiol. 41:1230, 1978.)

PLATE 3

FIGURE 11–22 (See page 335).
Bull's eye image displaying three-dimensional tomographic data acquired with SPECT and Tl-201 in a patient with severe exercise-induced ischemia of the ventricular septum and anterior wall. The immediate post-exercise bull's eye image *(top left)* demonstrates a marked abnormality involving the septum and anterior wall, extending from the base to the apex. In the redistribution image *(top right)* there is nearly complete tracer redistribution into this area. Bull's eye plots in which the patient's data are compared to the gender-matched normal files are displayed below. The immediate anteroseptal defect is noted to be quite marked with most pixels 5–7 standard deviations (coded blue) and even greater than 7 standard deviations (coded black) below normal. In the delayed image, nearly all pixels are within normal limits (coded white). (Courtesy of Gordon DePuey, M.D., Emory University Medical School and Hospitals.)

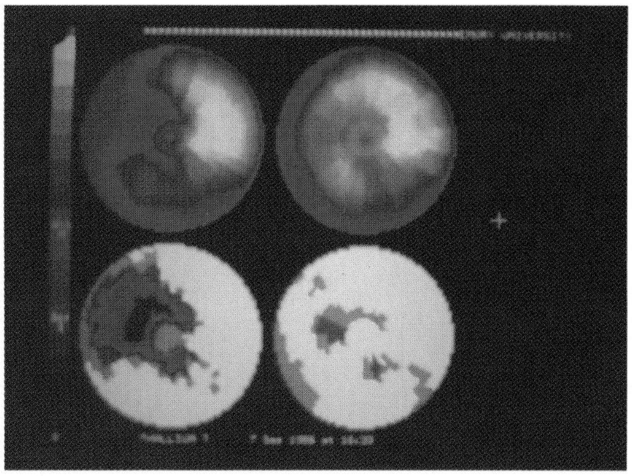

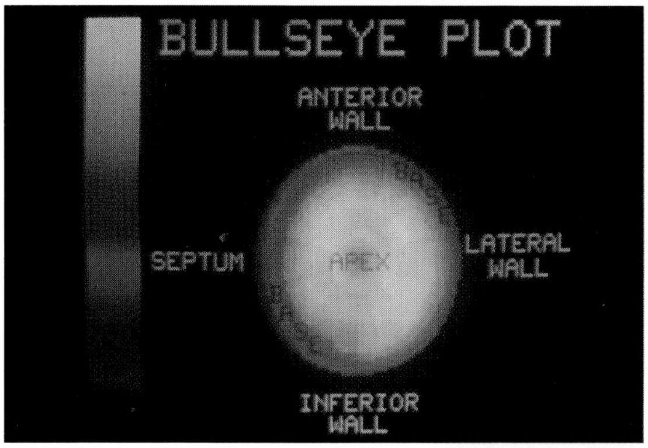

FIGURE 11–23 (See page 335).
Bull's eye image displaying three-dimensional tomographic data acquired with SPECT and T1-201. The apex of the left ventricle is at the center of the bull's eye plot with the base at the periphery. The anterior wall is above, the inferior wall below, the septum to the left, and the posterolateral wall to the right. (Courtesy of Gordon DePuey, M.D., Emory University Medical School and Hospitals.)

FIGURE 11–24 (See page 335).
Three-dimensional surface maps of myocardial perfusion using Tc-99m isonitrile and SPECT in a patient with coronary artery stenosis involving the left anterior descending coronary artery. The images on the left were obtained after injection during maximal exercise and demonstrate the geographical distribution of the ischemic zone (*upper left,* 30° left anterior oblique projection; *lower left,* 30° right anterior oblique projection). The images on the right were obtained after injection at rest and demonstrate uniform perfusion throughout the left ventricle (*upper right,* 30° left anterior oblique projection; *lower right,* 30° right anterior oblique projection).

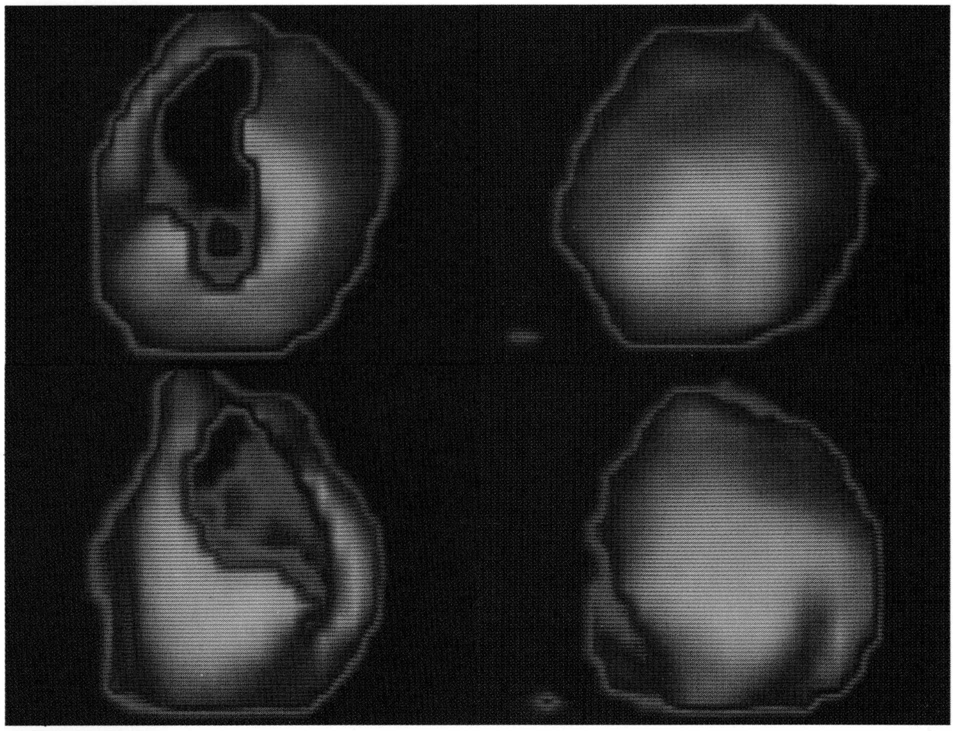

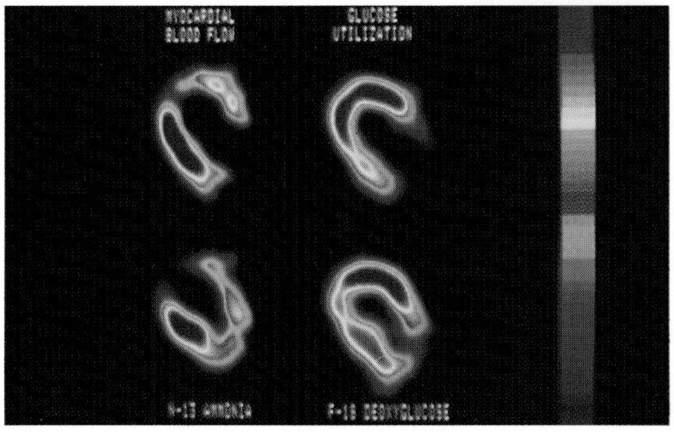

FIGURE 11–25 (See page 340).
Evaluation of blood flow and glucose metabolism using positron-emission tomography (PET) in a patient with ischemic heart disease. Wall motion was impaired in the anteroseptal and anterior walls. The patient was studied at rest, first with intravenous N-13 ammonia to evaluate regional myocardial blood flow and subsequently with intravenous F-18 2-deoxyglucose to examine exogenous glucose utilization. *Left,* Two contiguous cross-sectional images of regional myocardial blood flow with decreased blood flow in the anterior septum and the anterior wall, shown as the blue-black regions at 10–11 o'clock. *Right,* Glucose utilization is maintained or even elevated in these regions, shown as the yellow-red areas of increased activity, reflecting the presence of ischemic but viable tissue. (Courtesy of Heinrich R. Schelbert, M.D., UCLA School of Medicine.)

PLATE 4

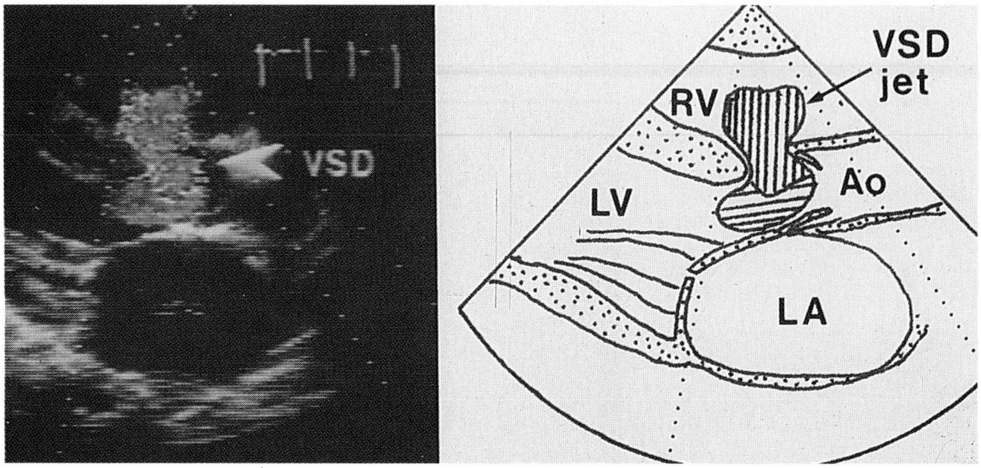

FIGURE 31–8 (See page 987).
Color flow Doppler mapping study performed from a parasternal long axis view in a 34-year-old woman with a moderately large membranous ventricular septal defect (VSD). Systolic flow through VSD is in a left-to-right direction. The change in color of the Doppler signal from red to blue represents aliasing due to increased velocity of blood as flow goes through the defect. RV = right ventricle, LV = left ventricle, LA = left atrium.

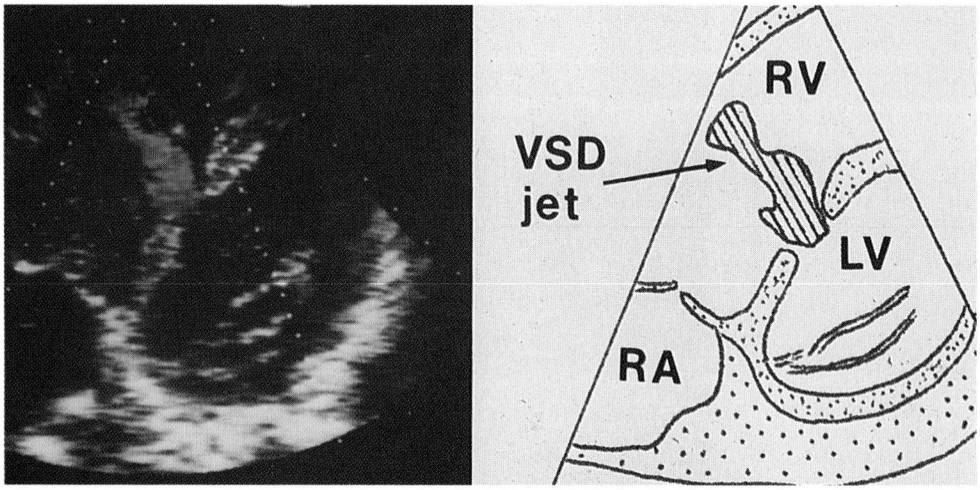

FIGURE 31–9 (See page 987).
Color flow Doppler mapping recorded from a somewhat angulated parasternal short axis view in a 38-year-old man with a VSD in the mid-portion of the interventricular septum. Flow across the VSD is left-to-right in direction. RV = right ventricle, LV = left ventricle, RA = right atrium.

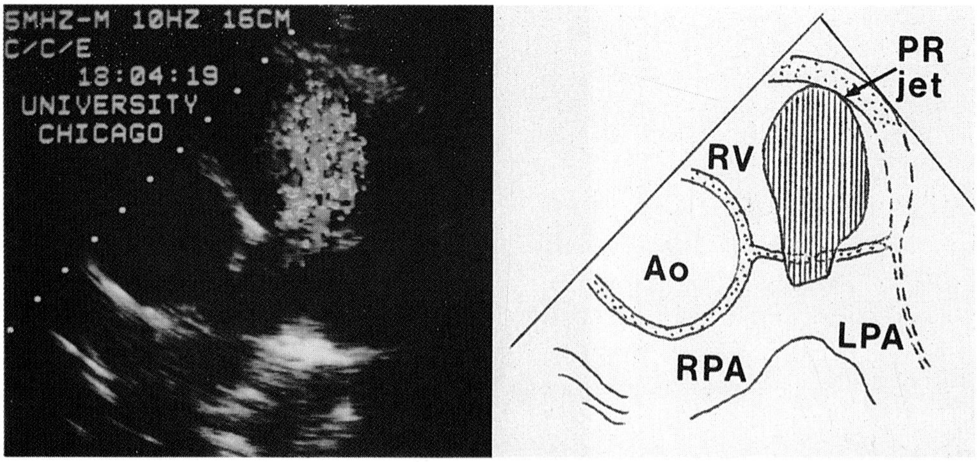

FIGURE 31–12 (See page 989).
Color flow Doppler mapping study from the 23-year-old woman who had previously undergone correction of tetralogy of Fallot and whose Doppler tracings are shown in Figure 31-11. In this mid-diastolic frame, moderately severe pulmonary regurgitation is present as demonstrated by the regurgitant jet in the outflow portion of the right ventricle (RV). A = aorta, PR = pulmonary regurgitation, RPA = right pulmonary artery, LPA = left pulmonary artery.

PART I EXAMINATION OF THE PATIENT

1 THE HISTORY

by EUGENE BRAUNWALD, M.D.

IMPORTANCE OF THE HISTORY: THE PHYSICIAN'S ROLE

Specialized examinations of the cardiovascular system, presented in Chapters 3 to 12, provide a large portion of the data base required to establish a specific anatomical diagnosis of cardiac disease and to determine the extent of functional impairment of the heart. Although the development of these methods represents one of the triumphs of modern medicine, their appropriate use is to *supplement but not to supplant* a careful clinical examination, which remains the cornerstone of the assessment of the patient with known or suspected cardiovascular disease. There is a temptation in cardiology, as in many other areas of medicine, to carry out expensive, uncomfortable, and occasionally even hazardous procedures to establish a diagnosis when a detailed and thoughtful history and physical examination may be sufficient. Obviously, it is undesirable to subject patients to the unnecessary risks and expenses inherent in many specialized tests when a diagnosis can be made on the basis of an adequate clinical examination or when their management will not be altered significantly as a result of these tests.[1] Intelligent selection of investigative procedures from the ever-increasing array of tests now available requires far more sophisticated decision-making than was necessary when the choices were limited to the electrocardiogram and chest roentgenogram (Chap. 52). The history and physical examination provide the critical information necessary for these decisions.

THE ROLE OF THE HISTORY. The overreliance on laboratory tests has increased as physicians attempt to utilize their time more efficiently by delegating responsibility for taking the history to a physician's assistant or nurse or even by limiting the history to a questionnaire—an approach that I consider to be an undesirable trend insofar as the patient with known or suspected heart disease is concerned.[2] First, it must be appreciated that the history remains the richest source of information concerning the patient's illness, and any practice that might diminish the quality of information provided by the history could ultimately impair the quality of care. Second, the physician's attentive and thoughtful taking of a history establishes a bond with the patient that may be valuable later in securing the patient's compliance in following a complex treatment plan, undergoing hospitalization for an intensive diagnostic work-up or a hazardous operation, and, in some instances, accepting that heart disease is not present at all. It is largely through the direct contact established between the patient and physician during the clinical examination that this confidence can best be established.

Taking a history also permits the physician to evaluate the results of diagnostic tests that have strong subjective components, such as the determination of exercise capacity (Chap. 8). Perhaps most importantly, a careful history allows the physician to evaluate the impact of the disease, or the fear of the disease, on the patient's total life and to assess the patient's personality, emotion, and stability; often it provides a glimpse of the patient's responsibilities, fears, aspirations, and threshold for discomfort as well as the likelihood of compliance with one or another therapeutic regimen. Whenever possible, the physician should question not only the patient but also relatives or close friends in order to obtain a clearer understanding of the extent of the patient's disability and a broader perspective concerning the impact of the disease on both the patient and the family. (For example, the patient's spouse is much more likely than the patient to provide a history of Cheyne-Stokes [periodic] respiration.)

In interpreting the history obtained from a patient with known or suspected heart disease, it must be appreciated that the combination of the widespread fear of cardiovascular disorders and the deep-seated emotional, symbolic, and sometimes even religious connotations concerning this organ's function may, on the one hand, provoke symptoms that mimic those of organic heart disease in persons with normal cardiovascular systems and, on the other, cause so much fear that serious symptoms are repressed or denied by patients with organic heart disease. Functional complaints referable to the cardiovascular system may also develop in patients with organic heart disease.

TECHNIQUE. Several approaches can be employed successfully in obtaining a medical history. I believe that patients should first be given the opportunity to relate their experiences and complaints in their own way. Although time-consuming and likely to include much seemingly irrelevant information, this technique has the advantage of providing considerable information concerning the patient's intelligence and emotional make-up, as well as providing the patient with the satisfaction that he or she has been "heard out" by the physician, rather than merely having been exposed to a series of laboratory examinations based on "high technology." After the patient has given an account of the illness, the physician should obtain information concerning the onset and chronology of symptoms; their location, quality, and intensity; the precipitating, aggravating, and relieving factors; and the details of response to therapy.

Of course, a detailed general medical history including the personal past history, occupational history, nutritional history, and review of systems must be obtained. Concern should focus on a past history of rheumatic fever, chorea, venereal disease or exposure to it, thyroid disease, recent dental extractions or manipulations, catheterization of the bladder, and earlier examinations that showed abnormalities of the cardiovascular system as reflected in restriction from physical activity at school and in rejection for life insurance, employment, or military service. Personal habits such as exercise, cigarette smoking, alcohol intake, and parenteral use of drugs—illicit and otherwise—should be ascertained, and the exact nature of the patient's work should be assessed. The increasing appreciation of the importance of genetic influences in many forms of heart disease (Chap. 49) underscores the importance of the family history. Details of obtaining the family history in a patient with a possible genetic disorder involving the heart are presented on p. 1622.

A wide variety of disorders including, but not limited to, neurological (Chap. 57), endocrine (Chap. 58), and rheumatological (Chap. 54) may have important effects on the cardiovascular system; it is vital to ascertain the presence of these and other conditions which are not *primarily* cardiological. A history of the risk factors for ischemic heart disease—the family history, cigarette smoking, hypertension, hypercholesterolemia, diabetes mellitus, artificial or early menopause, and long-term contraceptive pill ingestion (Chap. 36)—should always be sought.

A cardinal principle of cardiovascular evaluation is that myocardial or coronary function that may be adequate at rest may be inadequate during exertion; therefore, specific attention should be directed to the influence of activity on the patient's symptoms. Thus, a history of chest pain or discomfort and/or undue shortness of breath that appears only during activity is characteristic of heart disease, whereas the opposite pattern, i.e., the appearance of symptoms at rest and their remission during exertion is observed only rarely in patients with heart disease but is more characteristic of functional disorders. In attempting to assess the severity of functional impairment, both the *extent* of activity and the *rate* at which it is performed before symptoms develop should be determined and related to a detailed consideration of the therapeutic regimen. For example, the complaint of exertional dyspnea after walking slowly up a flight of stairs in a patient on maximal treatment for heart failure denotes far more severe functional disability than does a similar symptom occurring in an untreated patient who has run up a flight of stairs.

As the patient relates the history, important nonverbal clues are often provided. The physician should observe the patient's attitude, reactions, and gestures while being questioned, as well as his or her choice of words or emphasis. Tumulty has aptly likened obtaining a meaningful clinical history to playing a game of chess: "The patient makes a statement and based upon its content, and mode of expression, the physician asks a counter-question. One answer stimulates yet another question until the clinician is convinced that he understands precisely all of the circumstances of the patient's illness."

PRINCIPAL SYMPTOMS OF HEART DISEASE

The principal symptoms of heart disease include dyspnea, chest pain or discomfort, syncope, collapse, palpitation, edema, cough, hemoptysis, and excess fatigue. Cyanosis is more often a sign rather than a symptom, but it may be a key feature of the history, particularly of patients with congenital heart disease. Without doubt, history-taking is the most valuable technique available for determining whether or not these symptoms are caused by heart disease. Examples of the manner in which these symptoms may serve as a guide to diagnosis are given in the following pages, and reference is made to other portions of the book that contain more detailed information.

DYSPNEA

(See also pp. 475 and 1896)

Dyspnea is defined as an abnormally uncomfortable awareness of breathing; it is one of the principal symptoms of cardiac and pulmonary disease.[3] Since dyspnea is regularly caused by strenuous exertion in healthy, well-conditioned subjects and by only moderate exertion in those who are normal but unaccustomed to exercise, it should be regarded as abnormal only when it occurs at rest or at a level of physical activity not expected to cause this symptom. Dyspnea is associated with a wide variety of diseases of the heart and lungs, chest wall, and respiratory muscles as well as with anxiety[4]; the history is the most valuable means of establishing the etiology. Table 1–1 provides a list of the various syndromes which may cause dyspnea and the primary pathophysiological mechanisms that are responsible.[5] Borg and Noble have developed a scale which is useful in quantitating the severity of dyspnea.[6]

The *sudden* development of dyspnea suggests pulmonary embolism, pneumothorax, acute pulmonary edema, pneumonia, or obstruction of a major airway. In contrast, in most forms of *chronic* heart failure, dyspnea progresses slowly over weeks or months. Such a protracted course may also occur in a variety of unrelated conditions, including obesity, pregnancy, and bilateral pleural effusions. *Inspiratory dyspnea* suggests obstruction of the upper airways, whereas *expiratory dyspnea* characterizes obstruction of the lower airways. Exertional dyspnea suggests the presence of organic diseases, such as left ventricular failure (Chap. 16) or chronic obstructive lung disease (Chap. 48), whereas dyspnea developing at rest may occur in pneumothorax or pulmonary embolism (Chap. 47) or may be functional. Dyspnea that occurs *only* at rest and is absent on exertion is almost invariably functional. A functional

TABLE 1–1 DISORDERS CAUSING DYSPNEA AND LIMITING EXERCISE PERFORMANCE, PATHOPHYSIOLOGY, AND DISCRIMINATING MEASUREMENTS*

DISORDERS	PATHOPHYSIOLOGY	MEASUREMENTS THAT DEVIATE FROM NORMAL
Pulmonary		
Airflow limitation	Mechanical limitation to ventilation, mismatching of $\dot{V}A/\dot{Q}$, hypoxic stimulation to breathing	$\dot{V}E$ max/MVV, expiratory flow pattern, VD, VT; $\dot{V}O_2$ max, $\dot{V}E/\dot{V}O_2$, $\dot{V}E$ response to hyperoxia, (A-a)PO_2
Restrictive	Mismatching $\dot{V}A/\dot{Q}$, hypoxic stimulation to breathing	
Chest wall	Mechanical limitation to ventilation	$\dot{V}E$ max/MVV, $PACO_2$, $\dot{V}O_2$ max
Pulmonary circulation	Rise in physiological dead space as fraction of VT, exercise hypoxemia	VD/VT, work–rate-related hypoxemia $\dot{V}O_2$ max, $\dot{V}E/\dot{V}O_2$, (a-ET)PCO_2, O_2-pulse
Cardiac		
Coronary	Coronary insufficiency	ECG, $\dot{V}O_2$ max, anaerobic threshold $\dot{V}O_2$, $\dot{V}E/\dot{V}O_2$ O_2-pulse, BP (systolic, diastolic, pulse)
Valvular	Cardiac output limitation (decreased effective stroke volume)	
Myocardial	Cardiac output limitation (decreased ejection fraction and stroke volume)	
Anemia	Reduced O_2 carrying capacity	O_2-pulse, anaerobic threshold $\dot{V}O_2$, $\dot{V}O_2$ max, $\dot{V}E/\dot{V}O_2$
Peripheral circulation	Inadequate O_2 flow to metabolically active muscle	Anaerobic threshold $\dot{V}O_2$, $\dot{V}O_2$ max
Obesity	Increased work to move body; if severe, respiratory restriction and pulmonary insufficiency	$\dot{V}O_2$-work rate relationship, PAO_2, $PACO_2$, $\dot{V}O_2$ max
Psychogenic	Hyperventilation with precisely regular respiratory rate	Breathing pattern, PCO_2
Malingering	Hyperventilation and hypoventilation with irregular respiratory rate	Breathing pattern, PCO_2
Deconditioning	Inactivity or prolonged bed rest; loss of capability for effective redistribution of systemic blood flow	O_2-pulse, anaerobic threshold $\dot{V}O_2$, $\dot{V}O_2$ max

*$\dot{V}A$ indicates alveolar ventilation; $\dot{Q}$, pulmonary blood flow; $\dot{V}E$, minute ventilation; MVV, maximum voluntary ventilation; VD/VT, physiologic dead space/tidal volume ratio; O_2, oxygen; $\dot{V}O_2$, O_2 consumption; (A–a)PO_2, alveolar-arterial PO_2 difference; and (a–ET)PCO_2, arterial-end tidal PCO_2 difference.

Modified from Wasserman, D: Dyspnea on exertion: Is it the heart or the lungs? J.A.M.A. *248*:2042, 1982.

origin is suggested when dyspnea, or simply a heightened awareness of breathing, is accompanied by brief stabbing pain in the region of the cardiac apex or by prolonged (more than 2 hours) dull chest pain, and is associated with difficulty in getting enough air into the lungs, claustrophobia, or sighing respirations that are relieved by exertion, by taking a few deep breaths, or by sedation. A history of relief of dyspnea by bronchodilators and corticosteroids suggests asthma as the etiology, whereas relief of dyspnea by rest, diuretics, and digitalis suggest left heart failure.

In patients with *heart failure*, dyspnea is a clinical expression of pulmonary venous and capillary hypertension (p. 475). It occurs either during exertion or, in resting patients, in the recumbent position and is relieved promptly by sitting upright or standing (orthopnea). In patients with heart failure, dyspnea may be accompanied by edema (p. 476), upper abdominal pain (due to congestive hepatomegaly), and nocturia. The *sudden* occurrence of dyspnea in a patient with a history of mitral valve stenosis suggests the development of atrial fibrillation, rupture of chordae tendineae, or pulmonary embolism.

Paroxysmal nocturnal dyspnea is due to interstitial pulmonary edema secondary to left ventricular failure (p. 476). This condition, beginning usually 2 to 5 hours after the onset of sleep and often associated with sweating and wheezing, is frightening to the patient. Paroxysmal nocturnal dyspnea is relieved by the patient's sitting on the side of the bed or getting out of bed. Although paroxysmal nocturnal dyspnea secondary to left ventricular failure is usually accompanied by coughing, a careful history often discloses that the dyspnea *precedes* the cough, not vice versa. In contrast, patients with *chronic pulmonary disease*, may also awaken at night, but cough and expectoration often precede the dyspnea. These patients also often have a long history of smoking and a chronic cough with sputum production and wheezing and may be able to breathe more easily while leaning forward. Nocturnal dyspnea in patients with pulmonary disease is usually relieved after the patient rids himself of secretions rather than specifically by sitting up. Details of the value and limitations of the history of dyspnea in differentiating between primary diseases of the heart and lungs[7] are presented on pp. 477 and 1876.

Patients with *pulmonary embolism* usually experience sudden dyspnea that may be associated with apprehension, palpitation, hemoptysis, or pleuritic chest pain (Chap. 47). The development or intensification of dyspnea, sometimes associated with a feeling of faintness, may be the only complaint of the patient with pulmonary emboli. Dyspnea accompanying thoracic pain occurs in *acute myocardial infarction*. Occasionally dyspnea is an *"anginal equivalent"* (p. 1316), i.e., a symptom secondary to myocardial ischemia that occurs in place of typical anginal discomfort. This form of dyspnea may be closely associated with a sensation of tightness in the chest, is present on exertion or emotional stress, is relieved by rest (more often in the sitting than the recumbent position), has a duration similar to angina (i.e., 2 to 10 minutes), and is usually responsive to nitroglycerin but not to digitalis. The sudden development of severe dyspnea in the sitting rather than in the lying position, or whenever a particular position is assumed, suggests the possibility of a *myxoma* (p. 1480) or *ball-valve thrombus* in the left atrium. When dyspnea is relieved by squatting, it is caused most commonly by tetralogy of Fallot or a variant thereof (p. 946).

CHEST PAIN OR DISCOMFORT

(See also p. 1316)

Although chest pain or discomfort is one of the cardinal manifestations of cardiac disease, it is critical to recognize that it may originate not only in the heart but also in (1) a variety of noncardiac intrathoracic structures, such as the aorta, pulmonary artery, bronchopulmonary tree, pleura, mediastinum, esophagus, and diaphragm; (2) the tissues of the neck or thoracic wall, including the skin, thoracic muscles, cervicodorsal spine, costochondral junctions, breasts, sensory nerves, or spinal cord; and (3) subdiaphragmatic organs such as the stomach, duodenum, pancreas, and gallbladder[8–11] (Table 1–2). Factitious pain or pain of functional origin may also occur in the chest.

TABLE 1–2 DIFFERENTIAL DIAGNOSIS OF EPISODIC CHEST PAIN RESEMBLING ANGINA PECTORIS

	DURATION	QUALITY	PROVOCATION	RELIEF	LOCATION	COMMENT
Effort angina	5–15 minutes	Visceral (pressure)	During effort or emotion	Rest, nitroglycerin	Substernal radiates	First episode vivid
Rest angina	5–15 minutes	Visceral (pressure)	Spontaneous (? with exercise)	Nitroglycerin	Substernal radiates	Often nocturnal
Mitral prolapse	Minutes to hours	Superficial (rarely visceral)	Spontaneous (no pattern)	Time	Left anterior	No pattern, variable character
Esophageal reflux	10 minutes to 1 hour	Visceral	Recumbency, lack of food	Food, antacid	Substernal epigastric	Rarely radiates
Esophageal spasm	5–60 minutes	Visceral	Spontaneous, cold liquids, exercise	Nitroglycerin	Substernal radiates	Mimics angina
Peptic ulcer	Hours	Visceral, burning	Lack of food, "acid" foods	Foods, antacids	Epigastric substernal	
Biliary disease	Hours	Visceral (wax and wane)	Spontaneous, food	Time, analgesia	Epigastric ? radiates	Colic
Cervical disc	Variable (gradually subsides)	Superficial	Head and neck movement, palpation	Time, analgesia	Arm, neck	Not relieved by rest
Hyperventilation	2–3 minutes	Visceral	Emotion tachypnea	Stimulus removal	Substernal	Facial paresthesia
Musculoskeletal	Variable	Superficial	Movement, palpation	Time, analgesia	Multiple	Tenderness
Pulmonary	30 minutes +	Visceral (pressure)	Often spontaneous	Rest, time, bronchodilator	Substernal	Dyspneic

Reproduced with permission from Christie, L. G., Jr., and Conti, C. R.: Systemic approach to the evaluation of angina-like chest pain. Am. Heart J. *102*:897, 1981.

Although a wide variety of laboratory tests are available to aid in the differential diagnosis of chest pain, the history is without question the most valuable mode of examination. In obtaining the history of a patient with chest pain it is helpful to have a mental checklist and to ask the patient to describe the location, radiation, and character of the pain; what causes and relieves the pain; time relationships, including the duration, frequency, and pattern of recurrence of the pain; and associated symptoms. It is also particularly useful to observe the patient's gestures. Clenching the fist in front of the chest while describing the sensation (Levine's sign) is a strong indication of an ischemic orgin for the pain.

QUALITY. *Angina pectoris* may be defined as a discomfort in the chest or adjacent area associated with myocardial ischemia but without myocardial necrosis.[12] It is important to recognize that angina means *choking*, not pain. Thus, the discomfort of angina often is described not as pain at all but rather as an unpleasant sensation; "pressing," "squeezing," "strangling," "constricting," "bursting," and "burning" are some of the adjectives commonly used to describe this sensation (Table 1–3). "A band across the chest" and "a weight in the center of the chest" are other frequent descriptions. Often with severe attacks the discomfort may radiate from the chest to the shoulders, extremities, neck, jaws, and teeth. It is characteristic of angina that the intensity of effort required to incite it seems to vary from day to day and throughout the day in the same patient, but often a careful history will uncover explanations for this, such as meals ingested, weather, emotions, and the like. The anginal threshold is lower in the morning than at any other time of day; thus patients note frequently that activities that may cause angina in the morning or when first undertaken do not do so later in the day. When the threshold for angina is quite variable, defies any pattern, and is prominent at rest, the possibility that myocardial ischemia is caused by coronary spasm should be considered (p. 1317). Thus, a careful history may indicate not only the cause of the pain (i.e., myocardial ischemia) but can even provide a clue to the mechanism of the ischemia (spasm vs. organic obstruction).

When dyspnea is an "anginal equivalent," the patient may describe the midchest as the site of the shortness of breath, whereas true dyspnea is usually not as well localized. Other anginal equivalents are discomfort limited to areas that are ordinarily sites of secondary radiation, such as the ulnar aspect of the left arm and forearm, lower jaw, teeth, neck, or shoulders, and the development of gas and belching, nausea, "indigestion," dizziness, and diaphoresis. Anginal equivalents above the mandible or below the umbilicus are quite uncommon. In patients with either typical or atypical angina, it is useful to determine whether the patient has symptoms or complications caused by atherosclerosis of other vascular beds, e.g., intermittent claudication, transient ischemic attacks, and stroke. In patients with suspected angina, a history of one of these manifestations of extracardiac atherosclerosis lends weight to the diagnosis of myocardial ischemia. In those with typical angina, such a history may uncover important extracardiac disease.

The chest discomfort of *pulmonary hypertension* may be identical to that of typical angina; it is caused by dilatation

TABLE 1–3 SOME FEATURES DIFFERENTIATING CARDIAC FROM NONCARDIAC CHEST PAIN

FAVORING ISCHEMIC ORIGIN	AGAINST ISCHEMIC ORIGIN
1. CHARACTER OF PAIN	
Constricting	dull ache
Squeezing	"knife-like," sharp, stabbing
Burning	"jabs" aggravated by respiration
"Heaviness," "heavy feeling"	
2. LOCATION OF PAIN	
Substernal	in the left submammary area
Across mid-thorax, anteriorly	in the left hemithorax
In both arms, shoulders	
In the neck, cheeks, teeth	
In the forearms, fingers	
In the interscapular region	
3. FACTORS PROVOKING PAIN	
Exercise	pain *after* completion of exercise
Excitement	provoked by a specific body motion
Other forms of stress	
Cold weather	
After meals	

From Selzer, A.: Principles and Practice of Clinical Cardiology. 2nd ed. Philadelphia, W. B. Saunders Company, 1983, p. 17.

of the pulmonary arteries, most commonly acute pulmonary embolism, and/or by right ventricular ischemia. The chest discomfort of *unstable angina* and *acute myocardial infarction* (p. 1235) is similar in quality to that of angina pectoris in location and character; however, it usually radiates more widely than does angina and is more severe and therefore is generally referred to as true *pain* rather than *discomfort* by the patient. This pain generally develops unrelated to unusual effort or emotional stress, often with the patient at rest or even sleeping. Usually nitroglycerin does not provide complete or lasting relief.

Acute pericarditis (p. 1487) is frequently preceded by a history of a viral upper respiratory infection. The inflammation causes pain that is sharper than is anginal discomfort, is more left-sided than central, and is often referred to the neck or flank. The pain of pericarditis lasts for hours and is little affected by effort but often aggravated by breathing, turning in bed, swallowing, or twisting the body; unlike angina, the pain of acute pericarditis may lessen when the patient sits up and leans forward.

Aortic dissection (p. 1554) is suggested by persistent, severe pain with radiation to the back and into the lumbar region in an individual with a history of hypertension. An expanding *thoracic aortic aneurysm* may erode the vertebral bodies and cause localized, severe, boring pain that may be worse at night. An aneurysmally enlarged left atrium in patients with mitral valve disease rarely causes chest pain; instead, patients commonly complain of discomfort in the back or right side of the chest that intensifies on exertion.

Chest-wall pain due to *costochondritis* or *myositis* is common in patients who present with fear of heart disease.[13] It is associated with both local costochondral or muscle tenderness, which may be aggravated by moving or coughing. Chest wall pain may also accompany or follow herpes zoster, chest injury, or *Tietze syndrome* (i.e., discomfort localized in swelling of the costochondral and costosternal joints, which are painful on palpation). When herpes zoster affects the left chest it may mimic myocardial infarction. However, its persistence, its localization to a dermatome, and the appearance of the characteristic vesicles allow recognition of this condition.

Functional or *psychogenic chest pain* may be one feature of an anxiety state, also called Da Costa syndrome or neurocirculatory asthenia. It is localized typically to the area of the cardiac apex and consists of a dull, persistent ache that lasts for hours and is often accentuated by or alternates with attacks of sharp, lancinating stabs of inframammary pain of 1 or 2 seconds' duration. The condition may occur with emotional strain and fatigue, bears little relation to exertion, and may be accompanied by precordial tenderness. Attacks are usually associated with palpitation, hyperventilation, numbness and tingling in the extremities, sighing, dizziness,[14] dyspnea, generalized weakness, and a history of and other signs of emotional instability or depression. The pain may not be completely relieved by any medication other than analgesics, but it is partially attenuated by many types of interventions, including rest, exertion, tranquilizers, and placebos. Therefore, in contrast to ischemic discomfort, functional pain is more likely to show variable responses to interventions on different occasions. Since functional chest pain is often preceded by hyperventilation, which in turn may cause increased muscle tension and be responsible for diffuse chest tightness, some instances of so-called functional chest pain may, in fact, have an organic basis. Chest pain is common in patients with *prolapse of the mitral valve* (p. 1045). The pain varies considerably among patients with this condition; it may be similar to that of classic angina pectoris or may resemble the chest pain of neurocirculatory asthenia described above.

LOCATION. Embryonically the heart is a midline viscus; thus, cardiac ischemia produces anginal symptoms that are characteristically felt across both sides of the chest or chiefly substernally (Fig. 1–1). Occasional patients complain of discomfort only to the left or less commonly to the

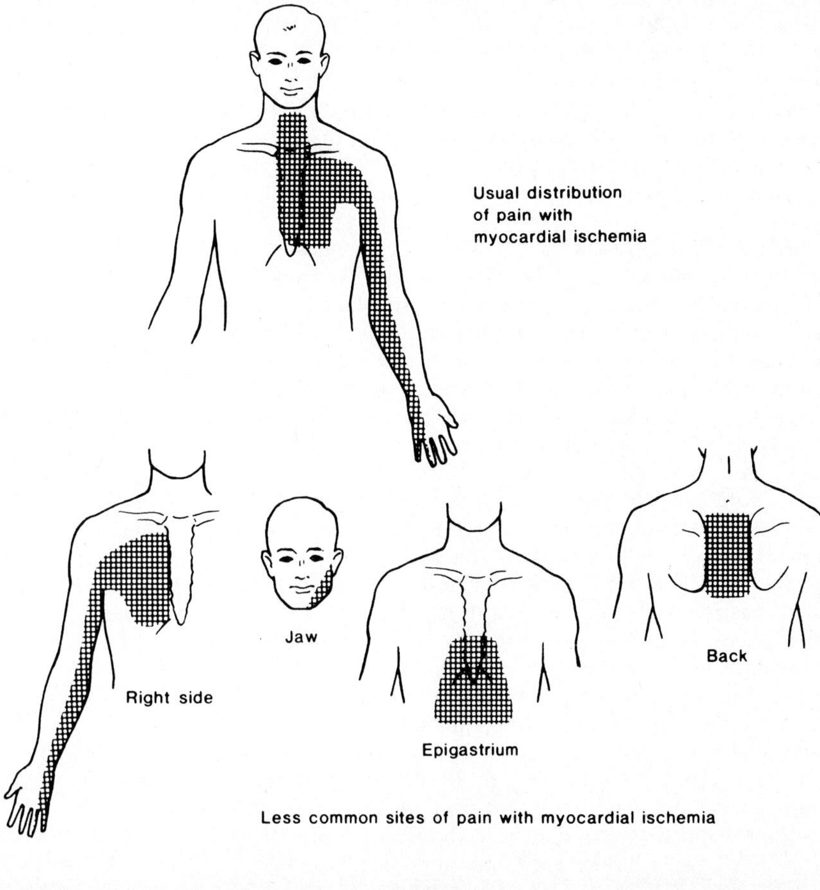

FIGURE 1–1. Pain patterns with myocardial ischemia. The usual distribution is referral to all or part of the sternal region, the left side of the chest, the neck, and down the ulnar side of the left forearm and hand. With severe ischemic pain, the right chest and right arm are often involved as well, although isolated involvement of these areas is rare. Other sites sometimes involved, either alone or together with pain in other sites, are the jaw, epigastrium, and back. (From Horwitz, L. D.: Chest pain. *In* Horwitz, L. D., and Groves, B. M. [eds.]: Signs and Symptoms in Cardiology. Philadelphia, J. B. Lippincott, 1985, p. 9.)

right of the midline. If the pain or discomfort can be localized to the skin or superficial structures, and can be reproduced by localized pressure, it generally arises from the chest wall. Thus, if the patient can point directly to the site of discomfort, it is usually not angina pectoris, which, like other symptoms arising in deeper structures, tends to be diffuse and eludes precise localization. Pain that is localized to the region of or under the left nipple or that radiates to the right lower chest[15] is usually noncardiac in origin and may be functional or due to osteoarthritis, gaseous distention of the stomach, or the splenic flexure syndrome. Although pain due to myocardial ischemia often radiates to the left arm or left shoulder, such radiation also occurs in pericarditis and disorders of the cervical spine. Chest pain that radiates to the neck and jaw occurs in pericarditis as well as in myocardial ischemia. Dissection of the aorta or enlargement of an aortic aneurysm produces pain in the *back* rather than in the front of the chest.

DURATION. The duration of the pain is important in determining its etiology. Angina pectoris is relatively short, usually lasting from 2 to 10 minutes. However, if the pain is very brief, i.e., a momentary, lancinating, sharp pain, "stitch" or other discomfort that lasts less than 30 seconds, angina can usually be excluded; such a short duration points instead to musculoskeletal pain, pain due to hiatal hernia, or functional pain. Chest pain lasting for hours may be seen with acute myocardial infarction, pericarditis, aortic dissection, musculoskeletal disease, herpes zoster, and anxiety.

PRECIPITATING AND AGGRAVATING FACTORS. Angina pectoris occurs characteristically on exertion, particularly when hurrying or walking on an upgrade. Thus, the development of chest discomfort or pain when walking, typically in the cold and against a wind, and after a heavy meal, is characteristic of angina pectoris. An exception is *Prinzmetal's (variant) angina*, which characteristically occurs at rest (p. 1360) and may or may not be affected by exertion; however, it must be remembered that classic (nonvariant) angina, although most often precipitated by effort, not uncommonly may be experienced at rest, as in unstable angina (p. 1353); in these patients exertion intensifies the discomfort. Emotional stress also may precipitate angina.

DIFFERENTIAL DIAGNOSIS. Chest pain that occurs after protracted vomiting may be due to the *Mallory-Weiss syndrome*, i.e., a tear in the lower portion of the esophagus. Pain that occurs while bending over is often radicular and may be associated with *osteoarthritis* of the cervical or upper thoracic spine. Chest pain occurring when moving the neck may be due to a *herniated intervertebral disk.*

Substernal and epigastric discomfort during swallowing may be due to *esophageal spasm.*[16] *Esophagitis*, often with acid reflux, with or without a hiatal hernia may also be associated with substernal or epigastric burning pain that is brought on by eating or lying down after meals and that may be relieved with antacids. Pain due to esophageal spasm has many of the features of and may be difficult to differentiate from angina pectoris[15]; the presence of acid reflux into the mouth (water brash) and/or dysphagia[17] may be a useful diagnostic clue pointing to esophageal disease.[18] The difficulty in distinguishing angina from esophageal disease is compounded by the frequent coexistence of these two common conditions and by the observations that esophageal reflux lowers the threshold for the development of angina[19] and that esophageal spasm may be precipitated by ergonovine and relieved by nitroglycerin. The discomfort produced by *peptic ulcer disease* may also resemble angina pectoris, but its characteristic relationship to food ingestion and its relief by antacids are important differentiating features. *Acute pancreatitis* may mimic acute myocardial infarction, but with the former there is usually a history of alcoholism or biliary tract disease. The pain of pancreatitis, like that of myocardial infarction, may be predominant in the epigastrium. However, unlike the pain of myocardial infarction, it is usually transmitted to the back, is position sensitive, and may be relieved in part by leaning forward.[15] Chest pain aggravated by swallowing may also be due to acute pericarditis, whereas pain intensified by coughing may be due to pericarditis, bronchitis, or pleurisy or may be of radicular origin. Pain that occurs when the patient is exhausted is often functional. *Congenital absence of the pericardium* (p. 1525) produces chest pain that is relieved by changing position in bed, is brought on by lying on the left side, and lasts a few seconds. Pain due to the *scalenus anticus (thoracic outlet) syndrome* may be confused with angina because it is often associated with paresthesias along the ulnar distribution of the arm and forearm. However, in contrast to angina, not only is it typically precipitated by abduction of the arm, lifting a weight, or working with the hands above the shoulders, but it is not brought on by walking.

RELIEF OF PAIN. Rest and nitroglycerin characteristically relieve the discomfort of angina in approximately 1 to 5 minutes. If more than 10 minutes transpire before relief, the diagnosis of chronic stable angina becomes questionable and instead suggests unstable angina, acute myocardial infarction, or pain not caused by myocardial ischemia at all. Although nitroglycerin commonly relieves the pain of angina pectoris, the discomfort of esophageal spasm and esophagitis may also be relieved by this drug. Angina pectoris is alleviated by quiet standing or sitting; the recumbent position may not relieve angina. Chest pain secondary to *acute pericarditis* is characteristically relieved by leaning forward, whereas pain that is relieved by food or antacids may be due to *peptic ulcer disease* or esophagitis. Pain that is alleviated by holding the breath in deep expiration is commonly due to pleurisy. Some patients with upper gastrointestinal disease or anxiety report relief of symptoms after belching.

ACCOMPANYING SYMPTOMS. The physician should always be respectful of the patient who reports the presence of chest pain and profuse sweating. This combination of symptoms frequently signals a serious disorder, often acute myocardial infarction. Severe chest pain accompanied by nausea and vomiting is also often due to myocardial infarction. The latter diagnosis, as well as pneumothorax or pulmonary embolism, is suggested when pain is associated with shortness of breath. Chest pain accompanied by palpitation may be due to the acute myocardial ischemia that results from a tachyarrhythmia-induced increase in myocardial oxygen consumption in the presence of coronary artery disease. Chest pain accompanied by hemoptysis suggests pulmonary embolism with infarction or lung tumor, whereas pain accompanied by fever occurs in pneumonia, pleurisy, and pericarditis. Functional pain is commonly accompanied by frequent sighing, anxiety, or depression.

CYANOSIS

(See also p. 909)

Cyanosis is a bluish discoloration of the skin and mucous membranes resulting from an increased amount of reduced hemoglobin or of abnormal hemoglobin pigments in the blood perfusing these areas. There are two principal forms of cyanosis: (1) *central cyanosis*, characterized by decreased arterial oxygen saturation due to right-to-left shunting of blood or impaired pulmonary function, and (2) *peripheral cyanosis*, most commonly secondary to cutaneous vasoconstriction due to a low cardiac output or exposure to cold air or water; if peripheral cyanosis is localized to an extremity, arterial or venous obstruction should be suspected. A history of cyanosis localized to the hands suggests *Raynaud's phenomenon.* Central cyanosis due to congenital heart disease or pulmonary disease characteristically worsens during exertion, whereas the resting peripheral cyanosis of congestive heart failure may be accentuated only slightly, if at all, during exertion.

Central cyanosis usually becomes apparent at a mean capillary concentration of 4 gm/dl reduced hemoglobin (or 0.5 gm/dl methemoglobin). In general, a history of cyanosis in Caucasians is rarely elicited unless arterial saturation is 85 per cent or less; in pigmented races arterial saturation has to drop far lower before cyanosis is perceptible. Cyanosis generally occurs in patients with *congenital heart disease* when the volume of a right-to-left shunt exceeds 25 per cent of the left ventricular output. Since it is the *absolute* quantity of reduced hemoglobin in the blood that is responsible for cyanosis, the higher the total hemoglobin content, the greater the tendency toward cyanosis; thus, patients with marked polycythemia become cyanotic at higher levels of arterial oxygen saturation than do patients with normal hematocrit values, and cyanosis may be absent in patients with severe anemia despite marked arterial desaturation. Patients with congenital heart disease often have a history of cyanosis which is intensified during exertion because of the lower saturation of blood returning to the right side of the heart and the augmented right-to-left shunt.

Although a history of cyanosis beginning in infancy suggests a congenital cardiac malformation with a right-to-left shunt, *hereditary methemoglobinemia* is another, albeit rare, cause of congenital cyanosis; the diagnosis of this condition is supported by a family history of cyanosis in the absence of heart disease.

A history of cyanosis limited to the neonatal period suggests the diagnosis of atrial septal defect with transient right-to-left shunting or, more commonly, pulmonary parenchymal disease or central nervous system depression. Cyanosis beginning at age 1 to 3 months may be reported when spontaneous closure of a patent ductus arteriosus causes a reduction of pulmonary blood flow in the presence of right-sided obstructive cardiac anomalies (p. 950). If cyanosis appears at age 6 months or later in childhood, it may be due to the development or progression of obstruction to right ventricular outflow in patients with ventricular septal defect. Development of cyanosis between ages 5 and 20 years suggests an Eisenmenger's reaction with right-to-left shunting as a consequence of a progressive increase in pulmonary vascular resistance (p. 921).

SYNCOPE

(See also p. 887)

Syncope, which may be defined as a loss of consciousness, results most commonly from reduced perfusion of the brain. The history is extremely valuable in the differential diagnosis of syncope (Tables 1–4 and 29–1, p. 885). Several daily attacks of loss of consciousness suggest (1) Stokes-Adams attacks, i.e., transient asystole or ventricular fibrillation in the presence of atrioventricular block; (2) other cardiac arrhythmias (Chap. 22); or (3) a seizure disorder, i.e., petit mal epilepsy. These diagnoses are suggested when the loss of consciousness is abrupt and occurs over 1 or 2 seconds; a more gradual onset suggests vasodepressor syncope (i.e., the common faint), syncope due to hyperventilation or, much less commonly, hypoglycemia. Cardiac syncope is usually of rapid onset without aura, and is usually *not* associated with convulsive movements, urinary incontinence, and a postictal confusional state. Syncope in aortic stenosis is usually precipitated by effort.[20] Patients with epilepsy often have a prodromal aura preceding the seizure. Injury from falling is common, as is urinary incontinence and a postictal confusional state, associated with headache and drowsiness. Unconsciousness, developing gradually and lasting for a few seconds, suggests vasodepressor syncope or syncope secondary to postural hypotension, whereas a longer period suggests aortic stenosis or hyperventilation. *Hysterical fainting* is usually not accompanied by any untoward display of anxiety or change in pulse, blood pressure, or skin color, and there may be a question about whether any true loss of consciousness occurred. It is often associated with paresthesias of the hands or face, hyperventilation, dyspnea, chest pain, and feelings of acute anxiety.

Syncope independent of body position suggests Stokes-Adams attacks, hyperventilation, or epilepsy, whereas syncope of other etiologies usually occurs in the upright position. Syncope occurring upon bending, leaning, or assuming a particular body position should raise the possibility of a left atrial myxoma (p. 1480) or a ball-valve thrombus. Since syncope is an unusual feature of mitral stenosis, when it does occur in a patient thought to have this condition, the possibility of left atrial *myxoma* or *ball-valve thrombus* should be considered. Syncope occurring during or immediately following exertion suggests *aortic stenosis, hypertrophic obstructive cardiomyopathy,* or *primary pulmonary hypertension.* Syncope is rare in patients with angina pectoris unless the latter is secondary to one

TABLE 1–4 CLUES FROM THE HISTORY IN ELUCIDATING THE CAUSE OF SYNCOPE

PRECEDING EVENTS	
Drugs:	Orthostatic hypotension (antihypertensives), hypoglycemia (insulin)
Severe pain, emotional stress:	Vasovagal syncope, hyperventilation
Movement of head and neck:	Carotid sinus hypersensitivity
Exertion:	Any form of obstruction to left ventricular outflow, Takayasu's arteritis
Upper extremity exertion:	Subclavian "steal"
TYPE OF ONSET	
Sudden:	Neurological (seizure disorder); arrhythmia (ventricular tachycardia or fibrillation, Stokes-Adams)
Rapid with premonition:	Vasovagal, neurological (aura)
Gradual:	Hyperventilation, hypoglycemia
POSITION AT ONSET	
Arising:	Orthostatic hypotension
Prolonged standing:	Vasovagal
Any position:	Arrhythmias, neurological, hypoglycemia, hyperventilation
POST SYNCOPAL CLEARING OF SENSORIUM	
Slow:	Neurological
Rapid:	All others
ASSOCIATED EVENTS	
Incontinence, tongue biting, injury:	Neurological

Modified from Lindenfeld, J. A.: Syncope. *In* Horwitz, L. D., and Groves, B. M. (eds.): Signs and Symptoms in Cardiology. Philadelphia, J. B. Lippincott, 1985, 506 pp.

of the aforementioned conditions. Syncope following insulin administration suggests a hypoglycemic etiology; syncope several hours after eating is characteristic of reactive hypoglycemia. Loss of consciousness following an emotional stress suggests that it is vasodepressor syncope or secondary to hyperventilation.

Patients with *vasodepressor syncope* often have a long history of fainting, commonly associated with emotional or painful stimuli. This, the most usual form of syncope, may be precipitated by the sight or loss of blood or by physical or emotional stress; it can be averted by promptly lying down, and it is characteristically preceded by symptoms of autonomic hyperactivity such as dim vision, giddiness, yawning, sweating, and nausea (p. 888). Syncope secondary to *cerebrovascular disturbance* is often preceded by aphasia, unilateral weakness, or confusion. A history of fainting following sudden movements of the head, shaving the neck, or wearing a tight collar suggests carotid sinus syncope (p. 888). Syncope associated with chest pain may be secondary to massive acute myocardial infarction or infarction associated with arrhythmias; occasionally, following recovery of consciousness, the associated chest pain may be forgotten, and the infarction may be recognized only by means of characteristic changes in serum enzymes and the electrocardiogram.

Consciousness is regained quite promptly in syncope of cardiovascular origin but more slowly with epilepsy. When consciousness is regained after vasodepressor syncope, the patient is usually pale and diaphoretic with a slow heart rate, whereas after a Stokes-Adams attack, the face is often flushed and there may be cardiac acceleration. Patients who sustain an injury when falling to the ground during a fainting spell usually have epilepsy or occasionally syncope of cardiac origin, but they rarely have sustained physical damage during reported unconsciousness related to emotional disturbance.

A *family history of syncope* or near syncope can often be elicited in patients with hypertrophic obstructive cardiomyopathy (p. 891) or ventricular tachyarrhythmias associated with Q-T prolongation (pp. 669 and 1635). A family history of epilepsy is positive in approximately 4 per cent of patients with convulsive disorders. Syncope associated with progressive intensification of cyanosis in an infant or child with cyanotic congenital heart disease is likely to be due to cerebral anoxia as a consequence of an increase in the right-to-left shunt, secondary to an increase in the obstruction to right ventricular outflow or a reduction in systemic vascular resistance (p. 911). A history of syncope during childhood suggests the possibility of a cardiovascular anomaly obstructing left ventricular outflow—valvular, supravalvular, or subvalvular aortic stenosis. In patients with hypertrophic obstructive cardiomyopathy, syncope is often post-tussive and occurs in the erect position, when arising suddenly, after standing erect for long periods, and during or immediately after cessation of exertion.

Patients with syncope secondary to *orthostatic hypotension* often have a history of drug therapy for hypertension or of abnormalities of autonomic function, such as impotence, disturbances of sphincter function, peripheral neuropathy, and anhidrosis (p. 885). When syncope is secondary to hypovolemia, there is often a history of melena, anemia, menorrhagia, or treatment with anticoagulants. Syncope associated with *cerebrovascular insufficiency* is frequently associated with a history of unilateral blindness, weakness, paresthesias, or memory defects.

PALPITATION

This common symptom is defined as an unpleasant awareness of the forceful or rapid beating of the heart. It may be brought about by a variety of disorders involving changes in cardiac rhythm or rate, including all forms of tachycardia, ectopic beats, compensatory pauses, augmented stroke volume due to valvular regurgitation, hyperkinetic (high cardiac output) states, and the sudden onset of bradycardia. In the case of premature contractions the patient is more commonly aware of the postextrasystolic beat than of the premature beat itself, and it appears that it is the increased motion of the heart within the chest that is perceived rather than the increase in cardiac contractility. This explains why palpitation is not a characteristic feature of aortic or pulmonic stenosis or of severe systemic or pulmonary hypertension, conditions characterized by an increased force of cardiac contraction.

When episodes of palpitation last for an instant, they are described as "skipped beats" or a "flopping sensation" in the chest and most commonly are due to extrasystoles. On the other hand, the sensation that the heart has "stopped beating" often correlates with the compensatory pause following a premature contraction. Palpitation characterized by a slow heart rate may be due to atrioventricular block or sinus node disease. When palpitation begins and ends abruptly, it is often due to a paroxysmal tachycardia such as paroxysmal atrial or junctional tachycardia, atrial flutter, or fibrillation, whereas a gradual onset and cessation of the attack suggest sinus tachycardia and/or an anxiety state. A history of chaotic rapid heart action suggests the diagnosis of atrial fibrillation; fleeting and repetitive palpitation suggests multiple ectopic beats. A history of multiple paroxysms of tachycardia followed by palpitation that occurs only with effort or excitement suggests paroxysmal atrial fibrillation that has become permanent—the palpitation being experienced only when the ventricular rate rises. Some patients have taken their pulse during palpitation or have asked a companion to do so. A rate between 100 and 140 beats/min suggests *sinus tachycardia*, a rate of approximately 150 beats/min suggests *atrial flutter*, and a rate exceeding 160 beats/min suggests *paroxysmal supraventricular tachycardia*.

A history of palpitation during or after strenuous physical activities is normal, whereas palpitation during mild exertion suggests the presence of heart failure, atrial fibrillation, anemia, or thyrotoxicosis, or that the individual is severely "out of condition." A feeling of forceful heart action accompanied by throbbing in the neck suggests aortic regurgitation. When palpitation can be relieved suddenly by stooping, breathholding, or induced gagging or vomiting, i.e., by vagal maneuvers, the diagnosis of paroxysmal supraventricular tachycardia is suggested. A history of syncope following an episode of palpitation suggests either asystole or severe bradycardia following the termination of a tachyarrhythmia or a Stokes-Adams attack. A history of palpitation associated with anxiety, a lump in the throat, dizziness, and tingling in the hands and face suggests sinus tachycardia accompanying an anxiety state with hyperventilation. Palpitation followed by angina suggests that myocardial ischemia has been precipitated by increased oxygen demands induced by the rapid heart rate.

As an adjunct to the history, it may be possible to ascertain the rhythm responsible for the palpitation by tapping the finger on the patient's chest in a variety of rhythms and asking the patient to identify the pattern which most closely resembles the abnormal feeling.

In many individuals no obvious cause for palpitation

emerges despite careful work-up, including a correlation between episodes of palpitation with a simultaneously recorded ambulatory electrocardiogram (p. 609) or an electrocardiogram recorded by transtelephonic transmission (p. 609). Anxiety is responsible for the symptom in many such patients, some of whom have known heart disease and may be receiving a vasodilator for the treatment of hypertension or nifedipine for the treatment of myocardial ischemia. In these patients palpitation may be due to postural hypotension resulting in reflex cardiac acceleration.

EDEMA

(See also p. 480)

Localization of edema is helpful in elucidating its etiology. Thus a history of edema of the legs that is most pronounced in the evening is characteristic of heart failure or bilateral chronic venous insufficiency. Inability to get the feet into shoes is a common early complaint. In most patients any visible edema of both lower extremities is preceded by a weight gain of at least 7 to 10 lb. Cardiac edema is generally symmetrical. As it progresses, it usually ascends to involve the legs, thighs, genitalia, and abdominal wall. In patients with heart failure who remain chiefly in bed, the edema localizes particularly in the sacral area. Edema located in both the abdomen and the legs is observed in heart failure and hepatic cirrhosis. Edema may be generalized (anasarca) in the nephrotic syndrome, severe heart failure, and hepatic cirrhosis. A history of edema around the eyes and face is characteristic of the nephrotic syndrome, acute glomerulonephritis, angioneurotic edema, hypoproteinemia, and myxedema. Edema limited to the face, neck, and upper arms may be associated with obstruction of the superior vena cava, most commonly by carcinoma of the lung, lymphoma, or aneurysm of the aortic arch. Edema restricted to one extremity is usually due to venous thrombosis or lymphatic blockage of that extremity.

ACCOMPANYING SYMPTOMS. A history of dyspnea associated with edema is most frequently due to heart failure but may also be observed in patients with large bilateral pleural effusions, elevation of the diaphragm due to ascites, angioneurotic edema with laryngeal involvement, and pulmonary embolism. When dyspnea precedes edema, left ventricular dysfunction, mitral stenosis, or chronic lung disease with cor pulmonale is usually responsible. A history of jaundice suggests that edema may be of hepatic origin, whereas edema associated with a history of ulceration and pigmentation of the skin of the legs is most commonly due to chronic venous insufficiency or postphlebitic syndrome. When cardiac edema is *not* associated with orthopnea, it may be due to tricuspid stenosis or regurgitation or constrictive pericarditis; in these conditions edema is not always most prominent in the lower extremities but may be generalized and may even involve the face.

The development of ascites *preceding* edema suggests cirrhosis, whereas a history of ascites *following* edema suggests cardiac or renal disease. *Angioneurotic edema* occurs intermittently, particularly after emotional stress or eating certain foods. *Idiopathic cyclic edema* is associated with menstruation. A history of edema on prolonged standing is observed in patients with chronic venous insufficiency.

COUGH

Cough, one of the most frequent of all cardiorespiratory symptoms, may be defined as an explosive expiration which provides a means of clearing the tracheobronchial tree of secretions and foreign bodies. It can be caused by a variety of infectious, neoplastic, or allergic disorders of the lungs and tracheobronchial tree. Cardiovascular disorders most frequently responsible for cough include those that lead to pulmonary venous hypertension, interstitial and alveolar pulmonary edema, pulmonary infarction, and compression of the tracheobronchial tree (aortic aneurysm). Cough due to pulmonary venous hypertension secondary to left ventricular failure or mitral stenosis tends to be dry, irritating, spasmodic, and nocturnal. When cough accompanies exertional dyspnea, it suggests either chronic obstructive lung disease or heart failure, whereas in a patient with a history of allergy and/or wheezing, cough is often a concomitant of bronchial asthma. A history of cough associated with expectoration for months or years occurs in chronic obstructive lung disease and/or chronic bronchitis.

The *character* of the sputum may be helpful in the differential diagnosis. Thus, a cough producing frothy, pink-tinged sputum occurs in pulmonary edema; clear, white, mucoid sputum suggests viral infection or longstanding bronchial irritation; thick, yellowish sputum suggests an infectious cause; rusty sputum suggests pneumococcal pneumonia; blood-streaked sputum suggests tuberculosis, bronchiectasis, carcinoma of the lung, and pulmonary infarction.

The combination of cough with *hoarseness* without upper respiratory disease may be due to pressure of a greatly enlarged left atrium on an enlarged pulmonary artery compressing the recurrent laryngeal nerve.

HEMOPTYSIS

The expectoration of blood or of sputum, either streaked or grossly contaminated with blood, may be due to (1) escape of red cells into the alveoli from congested vessels in the lungs (acute pulmonary edema); (2) rupture of dilated endobronchial vessels that form collateral channels between the pulmonary and bronchial venous systems (mitral stenosis); (3) necrosis and hemorrhage into the alveoli (pulmonary infarction); (4) ulceration of the bronchial mucosa or the slough of a caseous lesion (tuberculosis); minor damage to the tracheobronchial mucosa, produced by excessive coughing of any cause, can result in mild hemoptysis; (5) vascular invasion (carcinoma of the lung); (6) necrosis of the mucosa with rupture of pulmonary-bronchial venous connections (bronchiectasis).

The history is often decisive in pinpointing the etiology of hemoptysis. Recurrent episodes of minor bleeding are observed in patients with chronic bronchitis, bronchiectasis, tuberculosis, and mitral stenosis. Rarely, these conditions result in the expectoration of large quantities of blood, i.e., more than one-half cup. Massive hemoptysis may also be due to rupture of a pulmonary arteriovenous fistula; exsanguinating hemoptysis may occur with rupture of an aortic aneurysm into the bronchopulmonary tree. Hemoptysis associated with a history of expectoration of clear, gray sputum suggests chronic obstructive lung disease and of yellowish-green sputum, pulmonary infection. Hemoptysis associated with shortness of breath suggests mitral stenosis; in this condition the hemoptysis is often precipitated by sudden elevations in left atrial pressure during effort or pregnancy and is attributable to rupture of small pulmonary or bronchopulmonary anastomosing veins. Blood-tinged sputum in patients with mitral stenosis may also be due to transient pulmonary edema; in these circumstances it is usually associated with severe dyspnea.

A history of hemoptysis associated with acute pleuritic

chest pain suggests pulmonary embolism with infarction. Recurrent hemoptysis in a young, otherwise asymptomatic woman favors the diagnosis of bronchial adenoma. A history of recurrent hemoptysis with chronic marked sputum production suggests the diagnosis of bronchiectasis. Hemoptysis associated with the production of putrid sputum occurs in lung abscess, whereas hemoptysis associated with weight loss and anorexia in a male smoker suggests carcinoma of the lung. When blunt trauma to the chest is followed by hemoptysis, lung contusion is the probable cause. Hemoptysis associated with congenital heart disease and cyanosis suggests Eisenmenger syndrome (p. 999).

A history of drug ingestion may be helpful in elucidating the etiology of hemoptysis; e.g., anticoagulants and immunosuppressive drugs can cause bleeding. A history of ingestion of contraceptive pills may be a risk factor for the development of deep vein thrombosis and subsequent pulmonary embolism and infarction.

OTHER SYMPTOMS

Cardiovascular disorders can cause symptoms emanating from every organ system. Several of these are mentioned here primarily to point out how detailed the history should be in providing a comprehensive evaluation of a patient suspected of having cardiovascular disease; fuller discussions are found elsewhere in this text.

Fatigue is among the most common symptoms in patients with impaired cardiovascular function. However, it is also one of the most nonspecific of all symptoms in clinical medicine; in patients with an impaired systemic circulation as a consequence of a depressed cardiac output, it may be associated with muscular weakness. In other patients with heart disease, fatigue may be caused by drugs, such as beta-adrenoceptor blocking agents, by excessive blood pressure reduction in patients treated too vigorously for hypertension or heart failure, and in the latter it may also be caused by excessive diuresis and by diuretic-induced hypokalemia. *Nocturia* is a common early complaint in patients with congestive heart failure. *Anorexia*, abdominal fullness, right upper quadrant discomfort, weight loss, and cachexia are symptoms of advanced heart failure (p. 479). Anorexia, *nausea*, *vomiting*, and *visual changes* are important signs of digitalis intoxication (p. 504). Nausea and vomiting occur frequently in patients with acute myocardial infarction. *Hoarseness* may be caused by compression of the recurrent laryngeal nerve by an aortic aneurysm, a dilated pulmonary artery, or an enormously enlarged left atrium. A history of *fever* and *chills* is common in patients with infective endocarditis (p. 1103).

The aforementioned symptoms are examples of the wide variety not obviously associated with abnormalities of the cardiovascular system that can be of critical importance in differential diagnosis when they are elicited in patients known to have or suspected of having heart disease. They serve to reemphasize that the physician whose responsibility it is to care for patients with heart disease must be first and foremost a broadly based clinician.

THE HISTORY IN SPECIFIC FORMS OF HEART DISEASE

Just as the history is of central importance in determining whether or not a specific symptom is caused by heart disease, it is equally valuable in elucidating the *etiology* of recognized heart disease. A few examples are given below; considerably greater detail is provided in later chapters that deal with each specific disease entity.

HEART DISEASE IN INFANCY AND CHILDHOOD

The history is particularly helpful in establishing a diagnosis of *congenital heart disease*. In view of the familial incidence of certain congenital malformations (pp. 897 and 1635), a history of congenital heart disease, cyanosis, or heart murmur in the family should be ascertained. Rubella in the first 2 months of pregnancy is associated with a number of congenital cardiac malformations (patent ductus arteriosus, atrial and ventricular septal defect, tetralogy of Fallot, and supravalvular aortic stenosis). A maternal viral illness in the last trimester of pregnancy may be responsible for neonatal myocarditis. Syncope on exertion in a child with congenital heart disease suggests lesion in which the cardiac output is fixed, such as aortic or pulmonic stenosis. Exertional angina in a child suggests severe aortic stenosis, pulmonary stenosis, primary pulmonary hypertension, or anomalous origin of the left coronary artery. A history of syncope or faintness with straining and associated with cyanosis suggests tetralogy of Fallot.

In infants or children with cardiac murmurs, it is important to ascertain as precisely as possible when the murmur was first heard. Murmurs due to either aortic or pulmonic stenosis are usually audible within the first 48 hours of life, whereas those produced by a ventricular septal defect are usually apparent a few days or weeks later. On the other hand, the murmur produced by an atrial septal defect often is not heard until age 2 to 3 months.

Frequent pneumonias early in infancy suggest a large left-to-right shunt, and excessive diaphoresis occurs in left ventricular failure, most commonly due to ventricular septal defect in this age group. A history of squatting is most frequently associated with tetralogy of Fallot or tricuspid atresia (p. 946). Dysphagia suggests the presence of an aortic arch anomaly such as double aortic arch or an anomalous origin of the right subclavian artery passing behind the esophagus. A history of headaches, weakness of the legs, and intermittent claudication is compatible with the diagnosis of coarctation of the aorta (p. 994). Weakness or lack of coordination in a child with heart disease suggests cardiomyopathy associated with Friedreich's ataxia or muscular dystrophy (p. 1789). Recurrent bleeding from the nose, lips, or mouth, associated with dizziness and visual disturbances and a family history of bleeding in a cyanotic child suggest hereditary hemorrhagic telangiectasia (Osler-Weber-Rendu disease) with pulmonary arteriovenous fistula(s). A cerebrovascular accident in a cyanotic patient may be due to cerebral thrombosis or abscess or paradoxical embolization (p. 903).

MYOCARDITIS AND CARDIOMYOPATHY

Rheumatic fever (p. 1706) is suggested by a history of sore throat followed by symptoms including rash and chorea (St. Vitus dance), manifest as a period of twitching or clumsiness for a few months in childhood, as well as by frequent epistaxes and growing pains, i.e., nocturnal pains in the legs. In patients suspected of having myocarditis or cardiomyopathy, a history of Raynaud's phenomenon, dysphagia, or tight skin suggests scleroderma (p. 1723); a history of dyspnea following an influenza-like illness with myalgia suggests acute myocarditis. Pain in the hip or lower back that awakens the patient in the morning and is followed by morning back stiffness suggests rheumatoid spondylitis that is often associated with aortic valve disease

(p. 1717). *Carcinoid heart disease* is associated with a history of diarrhea, bronchospasm, and flushing of the upper chest and head (p. 1437). A history of diabetes, particularly if resistant to insulin and associated with bronzing of the skin, suggests *hemochromatosis* that may be associated with heart failure due to cardiac infiltration. *Amyloid heart disease* (p. 1431) is often associated with a history of postural hypotension and peripheral neuropathy. *Hypertrophic cardiomyopathy* (p. 1418) is often associated with a family history of this condition and sometimes with a family history of sudden death. The characteristic symptoms are angina, dyspnea, and syncope, which are often intensified paradoxically by digitalis and which occur during or immediately after exercise.

HIGH-OUTPUT HEART FAILURE AND COR PULMONALE

Patients with symptoms of heart failure (breathlessness and excess fluid accumulation) with warm extremities often have *high-output heart failure* (Chap. 25). They should be questioned about a history of anemia and of its common causes and accompaniments, such as menorrhagia, melena, peptic ulcer, hemorrhoids, sickle cell disease, and the neurological manifestations of vitamin B_{12} deficiency. Also, in such patients an attempt should be made to elicit a history of thyrotoxicosis (p. 1806) (weight loss, polyphagia, diarrhea, diaphoresis, heat intolerance, nervousness, breathlessness, muscle weakness, and goiter). Patients with beriberi heart disease responsible for high-output heart failure often present with a history characteristic of peripheral neuritis, alcoholism, poor eating habits, diet fads, or upper gastrointestinal surgery.

Patients with chronic *cor pulmonale* (see Chap. 48) frequently have a history of smoking, chronic cough and sputum production, dyspnea, and wheezing relieved by bronchodilators. Alternatively, they may present with a history of pulmonary emboli, phlebitis, and the sudden development of dyspnea at rest with palpitations, pleuritic chest pain, and, in the case of massive infarction, syncope.

PERICARDITIS AND ENDOCARDITIS

In patients in whom *pericarditis* or *cardiac tamponade* is suspected (Chap. 44), an attempt should be made to elicit a history of chest trauma, a recent viral infection, recent cardiac surgery, neoplastic disease of the chest with or without extensive radiation, myxedema, scleroderma, tuberculosis, or contact with tuberculous patients. The *sequence of development* of abdominal swelling, ankle edema, and dyspnea should be determined since, in patients with chronic constrictive pericarditis, ascites often precedes edema, which in turn usually precedes exertional dyspnea. A history of joint symptoms with a face rash suggests the possibility of systemic lupus erythematosus (SLE), an important cause of pericarditis, and it should be recalled that procainamide, hydralazine, and isoniazid can produce an SLE-like syndrome (p. 1720).

The diagnosis of *infective endocarditis* is suggested by a history of fever, severe night sweats, anorexia and weight loss, and embolic phenomena expressed as hematuria, back pain, petechiae, tender finger pads, and a cerebrovascular accident (p. 1113).

DRUG-INDUCED HEART DISEASE

The increasing appreciation that a wide variety of cardiac abnormalities can be induced by drugs makes a meticulous history of drug intake of great importance.[21] Catecholamines, whether administered exogenously or when secreted by a pheochromocytoma (p. 1812), may produce a myocarditis and arrhythmias. Digitalis glycosides can be responsible for a variety of tachy- and bradyarrhythmias as well as gastrointestinal, visual, and central nervous system disturbances (p. 504). Quinidine may cause Q-T prolongation, ventricular tachycardia of the torsades de pointes variety, syncope, and sudden death, presumably due to ventricular fibrillation (p. 701). Paradoxically the administration of antiarrhythmic drugs is one of the major causes of serious cardiac arrhythmias.[22]

Disopyramide (p. 631), beta-adrenoceptor blockers (p. 663), and the calcium channel blocker verapamil (p. 636) may depress ventricular performance, and in patients with ventricular dysfunction these drugs may intensify heart failure. Alcohol is also a potent myocardial depressant and may be responsible for the development of a cardiomyopathy (p. 1417), arrhythmias, and possibly sudden death. Tricyclic antidepressants may cause orthostatic hypotension and arrhythmias (p. 1894). Lithium, also used in the treatment of psychiatric disorders, can aggravate preexisting cardiac arrhythmias, particularly in patients with heart failure in whom the renal clearance of this ion is impaired.

The anthracycline compounds doxorubicin (Adriamycin) and daunorubicin, which are widely used because of their broad spectrum of activity against various tumors, may cause or intensify left ventricular failure, arrhythmias, myocarditis, and pericarditis (p. 1748). Cyclophosphamide, an antineoplastic alkylating agent, may also cause left ventricular dysfunction. Radiation therapy to the chest may cause acute and chronic pericarditis (p. 1517), a pancarditis (p. 1453), and coronary artery disease; further, it may enhance the aforementioned cardiotoxic effects of the anthracyclines.

ASSESSING CARDIOVASCULAR DISABILITY

(Table 1–5)

One of the greatest values of the history is in categorizing the *degree* of cardiovascular disability, so that a patient's status can be followed over time, the effects of a therapeutic intervention assessed, and patients compared with one another. The Criteria Committee of the New York Heart Association has provided a widely used classification that relates symptoms to "ordinary" activity.[23] The term "ordinary," of course, is subject to varying interpretation, as are terms such as "undue fatigue" that are used in this classification, and this has limited its accuracy and reproducibility. Somewhat more detailed and specific criteria were provided by the Canadian Cardiovascular Society,[24] but this classification and grading are limited to patients with angina pectoris. Goldman et al.[25] developed a specific activity scale in which classification is based on the estimated metabolic cost of various activities. This scale has not yet been widely used, but it appears to be more reproducible and to be a better predictor of exercise tolerance than either the New York Heart Association Classification or the Canadian Cardiovascular Society Criteria.

A key element of the history is to determine whether the patient's disability is stable or progressive. A useful way to accomplish this is to inquire whether a specific task which now causes symptoms, e.g., dyspnea after climbing two flights of stairs, did so 3, 6, and 12 months previously. Precise questioning on this point is important since a gradual reduction of ordinary activity as heart disease progresses may lead to an underestimation of the apparent degree of disability.[26]

TABLE 1–5 A COMPARISON OF THREE METHODS OF ASSESSING CARDIOVASCULAR DISABILITY

Class	New York Heart Association Functional Classification	Canadian Cardiovascular Society Functional Classification	Specific Activity Scale
I	Patients with cardiac disease but without resulting limitations of physical activity. Ordinary physical activity does not cause undue fatigue, palpitation, dyspnea, or anginal pain.	Ordinary physical activity, such as walking and climbing stairs, does not cause angina. Angina with strenuous or rapid or prolonged exertion at work or recreation.	Patients can perform to completion any activity requiring ≥ 7 metabolic equivalents, e.g., can carry 24 lb up eight steps; carry objects that weigh 80 lb; do outdoor work (shovel snow, spade soil); do recreational activities (skiing, basketball, squash, handball, jog/walk 5 mph).
II	Patients with cardiac disease resulting in slight limitation of physical activity. They are comfortable at rest. Ordinary physical activity results in fatigue, palpitation, dyspnea, or anginal pain.	Slight limitation of ordinary activity. Walking or climbing stairs rapidly, walking uphill, walking or stair climbing after meals, in cold, in wind, or when under emotional stress, or only during the few hours after awakening. Walking more than two blocks on the level and climbing more than one flight of ordinary stairs at a normal pace and in normal conditions.	Patients can perform to completion any activity requiring ≥ 5 metabolic equivalents but cannot and does not perform to completion activities requiring ≥ 7 metabolic equivalents, e.g., have sexual intercourse without stopping, garden, rake, weed, roller skate, dance fox trot, walk at 4 mph on level ground.
III	Patients with cardiac disease resulting in marked limitation of physical activity. They are comfortable at rest. Less than ordinary physical activity causes fatigue, palpitation, dyspnea, or anginal pain.	Marked limitation of ordinary physical activity. Walking one to two blocks on the level and climbing more than one flight in normal conditions.	Patients can perform to completion any activity requiring ≥ 2 metabolic equivalents but cannot and does not perform to completion any activities requiring ≥ 5 metabolic equivalents, e.g., shower without stopping, strip and make bed, clean windows, walk 2.5 mph, bowl, play golf, dress without stopping.
IV	Patient with cardiac disease resulting in inability to carry on any physical activity without discomfort. Symptoms of cardiac insufficiency or of the anginal syndrome may be present even at rest. If any physical activity is undertaken, discomfort is increased.	Inability to carry on any physical activity without discomfort—anginal syndrome *may be* present at rest.	Patient cannot or does not perform to completion activities requiring ≥ 2 metabolic equivalents. *Cannot* carry out activities listed above (Specific Activity Scale, Class III).

From Goldman L., et al.: Comparative reproducibility and validity of systems for assessing cardiovascular functional class: Advantages of a new specific activity scale. Circulation *64*:1227, 1981, by permission of the American Heart Association, Inc.

REFERENCES

1. Sandler, G.: The importance of the history in the medical clinic and the cost of unnecessary tests. Am. Heart J. *100*:928, 1980.
2. Hickam, D. H., Sox, H. C., Jr., and Sox, C. H.: Systematic bias in recording the history in patients with chest pain. J. Chronic Dis. *38*:91, 1985.
3. Fishman, A. P.: The first approach to the patient with respiratory signs and symptoms. *In* Fishman, A. P. (ed.): Pulmonary Diseases and Disorders. New York, McGraw-Hill Book Co., 1980, pp. 3–28.
4. Weber, K. T., and Szidon, J. P.: Exertional dyspnea. *In* Weber, K. T., and Janick, J. S. (eds.): Cardiopulmonary Exercise Testing. Philadelphia, W. B. Saunders Company, 1986, pp. 290–301.
5. Wasserman, K.: Dyspnea on exertion. Is it the heart or the lungs? J.A.M.A. *248*:2039, 1982.
6. Borg, G., and Noble, B.: Perceived exertion. *In* Wilmore, J. H. (ed.): Exercise and Sports. Science Reviews. New York, Academic Press, 1974, pp. 131–153.
7. Loke, J.: Distinguishing cardiac versus pulmonary limitation in exercise performance. Chest *83*:441, 1983.
8. Levene, D. L., Billings, R. F., Davies, G. M., Edmeads, J., and Saibil, F. G. (eds.): Chest Pain: An Integrated Diagnostic Approach. Philadelphia, Lea and Febiger, 1977.
9. Levine, H. J.: Difficult problems in the diagnosis of chest pain. Am. Heart J. *100*:108, 1980.
10. Christie, L. G., and Conti, C. R.: Systematic approach to the evaluation of angina-like chest pain. Am. Heart J. *102*:897, 1981.
11. Constant, J.: The clinical diagnosis of nonanginal chest pain: The differentiation of angina from nonanginal chest pain by history. Clin. Cardiol. 6:11, 1983.
12. Matthews, M. B., and Julian, D. G.: Angina pectoris: Definition and description. *In* Julian, D. G. (ed.): Angina Pectoris. New York, Churchill Livingstone, 1985, p. 2.
13. Peyton, F. W.: Unexpected frequency of idiopathic costochondral pain. Obstet. Gynecol. *62*:605, 1983.
14. Selzer, A.: Histology. *In* Principles and Practice of Clinical Cardiology 2nd ed. Philadelphia, W. B. Saunders Company, 1983, pp. 14–22.
15. Horwitz, L. D., and Groves, B. M. (eds.): Signs and Symptoms in Cardiology. Philadelphia, J. B. Lippincott, 1985, 506 pp.
16. Mellow, M. H.: A gastroenterologist's view of chest pain. Curr. Probl. Cardiol. 7:36, 1983.
17. Patterson, D. R.: Diffuse esophageal spasm in patients with undiagnosed chest pain. J. Clin. Gastroenterol. *4*:415, 1982.
18. DeMeester, T. R., O'Sullivan, G. C., Bermudez, G., Midell, A. I., Cimochowski, G. E., and O'Drobinak, J.: Esophageal function in patients with angina-type chest pain and normal coronary angiograms. Ann. Surg. *196*:488, 1982.
19. Davies, H. A., Rush, E. M., Lewis, M. J., Page, Z., Brown, A. L., and Petch, M. C.: Oesophageal stimulation lowers exertional angina threshold. Lancet *1*:1011, 1985.
20. Forssell, G., Jonasson, R., and Orinius, E.: Identifying severe aortic valvular stenosis by bedside examination. Acta Med. Scand. *218*:397, 1985.
21. Bristow, M. R. (ed.): Drug-Induced Heart Disease. Amsterdam, Elsevier, 1980, 476 pp.
22. Velebit, V., Podrid, P., Lown, B., Cohen, B. M., and Graboys, T. B.: Aggravation and provocation of ventricular arrhythmias by antiarrhythmic drugs. Circulation *65*:880, 1982.
23. The Criteria Committee of the New York Heart Association: Diseases of the Heart and Blood Vessels; Nomenclature and Criteria for Diagnosis, 6th ed. Boston, Little, Brown and Co., 1964
24. Campeau, L.: Grading of angina pectoris. Circulation *54*:522, 1975.
25. Goldman, L., Hashimoto, B., Cook, E. F., and Loscalzo, A.: Comparative reproducibility and validity of systems for assessing cardiovascular functional class: Advantages of a new specific activity scale. Circulation *64*:1227, 1981.
26. Goldman, L., Cook, E. F., Mitchell, N., Flatley, M., Sherman, H., and Cohn, P. F.: Pitfalls in the serial assessment of cardiac functional status. How a reduction in "ordinary" activity may reduce the apparent degree of cardiac compromise and give a misleading impression of improvement. J. Chronic Dis. *35*:763, 1982.

GENERAL REFERENCES

Braunwald, E.: Alterations in circulatory and respiratory function. *In* Braunwald, E., et al. (eds.): Harrison's Principles of Internal Medicine. 11th ed. New York, McGraw-Hill Book Co., 1987, pp. 138–162.

Constant, J.: The evolving check list in history-taking. *In* Bedside Cardiology. 3rd ed. Boston, Little, Brown and Co., 1985, pp. 1–22.

Dressler, W.: Clinical Aids in Cardiac Diagnosis. New York, Grune and Stratton, 1970.

Fowler, N. O.: The history in cardiac diagnosis. *In* Fowler, N. O. (ed.): Cardiac Diagnosis and Treatment. 3rd ed. Hagerstown, Md., Harper and Row, 1980, pp. 23–29.

Kraytman, J.: Cardiorespiratory system. *In* The Complete Patient History. New York, McGraw-Hill Book Co., 1979, pp. 11–112.

Oram, S.: Clinical examination. *In* Clinical Heart Disease. 2nd ed. London, William Heinemann, 1981, pp. 45–60.

Parkinson, J.: Cardiac symptoms. Ann. Intern. Med. 35:499, 1951.

Tumulty, P. A.: Obtaining the history. *In* The Effective Clinician. Philadelphia, W. B. Saunders Company, 1973, pp. 17–28.

White, P. D.: Clues in the Diagnosis and Treatment of Heart Disease. Springfield, Ill., Charles C Thomas, 1955.

Wood, P.: The chief symptoms of heart failure. *In* Diseases of the Heart and Circulation. 3rd ed. Philadelphia, J. B. Lippincott, 1968, pp. 1–25.

2 THE PHYSICAL EXAMINATION

by EUGENE BRAUNWALD, M.D.

Two of the most common pitfalls in cardiovascular medicine are the failure by the cardiologist to recognize the effects of systemic illnesses on the cardiovascular system and the failure by the noncardiologist to recognize the cardiac manifestations of systemic illnesses that have major effects on other organ systems. In order to avoid these pitfalls, patients known to have or suspected of having heart disease require not only a detailed examination of the cardiovascular system but a meticulous general physical examination as well. For example, the condition of patients with previously stable rheumatic valvular or coronary artery disease may suddenly deteriorate, not because of the progression of the underlying cardiac condition, but rather because of the development of an unrelated disease—such as a painless bleeding peptic ulcer or a malignant neoplasm—and a change in the patient's cardiac condition, such as the intensification of angina or dyspnea, may result from the anemia caused by the other disorder.

The presence of cardiac disease should prompt a careful search for frequent noncardiac concomitants such as arteriosclerosis of the cerebral vessels and of the arteries of the lower extremities and aorta in patients with ischemic heart disease. Conversely, the very high incidence (approximately 50 per cent) of coronary artery disease in patients with cerebrovascular disorders must be considered in dealing with patients who have these disorders. In some patients a cardiovascular abnormality may be responsible for a disorder involving another organ system; for example, retarded physical development and failure to thrive in infants may be secondary to congenital heart disease, and embolic strokes are important complications of rheumatic mitral stenosis and atrial fibrillation, of mitral valve prolapse, and of infective endocarditis.

Examples of disorders which have effects principally on other organs but which often also affect the heart include the following:[1]

1. *Muscular dystrophies* (Chap. 57) causing cardiomyopathies.
2. *Metabolic disorders,* such as hemochromatosis (p. 1434), glycogen storage disease (p. 1013), Gaucher's disease (p. 1434), and Fabry's disease (p. 1434) (myocardial infiltration, heart failure, and conduction defects).
3. *Chromosomal disorders,* such as the Turner syndrome (p. 1624) associated with a variety of congenital cardiac defects, particularly coarctation of the aorta.
4. *Endocrine disorders,* such as acromegaly (p. 1800) associated with accelerated coronary atherosclerosis and myocardial hypertrophy; hyperthyroidism (p. 1805) associated with heart failure and atrial fibrillation, and myxedema associated with pericardial effusion.
5. *Congenital deafness* (p. 1635) associated with Q-T interval prolongation and serious cardiac arrhythmias.
6. *Raynaud's disease* associated with primary pulmonary hypertension (p. 805), coronary spasm, and sclerodermatous involvement of the heart (p. 1723).
7. *Inherited connective tissue disorders* (Chap. 54), such as Marfan syndrome, osteogenesis imperfecta, Ehlers-Danlos syndrome, pseudoxanthoma elasticum, associated with aortic dilatation, dissection and regurgitation, mitral valve prolapse, coronary artery disease, and pericarditis; Hurler syndrome and related disorders of mucopolysaccharide metabolism (p. 1728) associated with arrhythmias, valvular disease, and heart failure.
8. *Collagen vascular diseases* (Chap. 54): systemic lupus erythematosus (valvulitis, myocarditis, coronary arteritis, and pericarditis), ankylosing spondylitis (diseases of the aorta and aortic valve), rheumatoid arthritis (pericarditis and valve disease), vasculitis (coronary arteritis and myocarditis), polymyositis (arrhythmias, pericarditis, and myocarditis).
9. *Sarcoidosis* (p. 1434) associated with restrictive cardiomyopathy and arrhythmias.
10. *Chronic hemolytic anemia* (p. 1736) causing cardiac

Editor's Note: Examination of the cardiovascular system includes inspection and palpation of the arterial and venous pulses and of the chest as well as auscultation of the heart. The findings elicited on physical examination can be aided enormously by graphic recordings. The details of carrying out the cardiovascular examination and the interpretation of the findings are presented in this chapter and in Chapters 3 and 4. This chapter focuses on the findings elicited by physical examination, while Chapters 3 and 4 deal primarily with the graphic recording of these findings. The three chapters should be considered as a unit, since the subjects covered are similar and the material does not lend itself well to a rigid separation between physical and graphic modes of examination; some degree of overlap in content among these chapters is therefore unavoidable.

dilatation and myocarditis secondary to transfusional hemosiderosis.

In patients in whom these and related systemic disorders are present or suspected, the physical examination should be conducted so as to allow recognition of the systemic disorder and evaluation of the presence and severity of cardiovascular involvement.

THE GENERAL PHYSICAL EXAMINATION

Although one can employ a variety of techniques in carrying out the physical examination, I favor commencing with an assessment of the general appearance of the patient and then utilizing the regional approach, starting with the head and ending with the lower extremities. It is desirable, whenever possible, to examine the patient on an examining table or bed whose head section may be raised. Examination in a quiet room at a comfortable temperature and in daylight is optimal.

GENERAL APPEARANCE

An assessment of the patient's general appearance is usually begun with a detailed inspection at the time when the history is being obtained.[1-3] The general build and appearance of the patient, the skin color, and the presence of pallor or cyanosis should be noted, as well as the presence of shortness of breath, orthopnea, periodic (Cheyne-Stokes) respiration (p. 481), and distention of the neck veins. If the patient is in pain, is he or she sitting quietly (typical of angina pectoris); moving about, trying to find a more comfortable position (characteristic of acute myocardial infarction); or most comfortable sitting upright (heart failure) or leaning forward (pericarditis)? Simple inspection will also reveal whether the patient's whole body shakes with each heart beat and whether Corrigan's pulses (bounding arterial pulsations, as occur with the large stroke volume of severe aortic regurgitation, arteriovenous fistula, or complete atrioventricular block) are present in the head, neck, and upper extremities. Marked weight loss, malnutrition, and cachexia, which occur in severe chronic heart failure (p. 481), may also be readily evident on inspection. The cold, sweaty palms and frequent sighing respirations typical of *neurocirculatory asthenia* may be detected, as well as the marked obesity, somnolence, and cyanosis suggestive of the *pickwickian syndrome* (p. 1610).

The distinctive general appearance of the *Marfan syndrome* (p. 1725) is often apparent, i.e., long extremities with an arm span that exceeds the height; a longer lower segment (pubis to foot) than upper segment (head to pubis); arachnodactyly (spider fingers); and a variety of thoracic deformities, including kyphoscoliosis, pectus carinatum, and pectus excavatum. Patients with *muscular dystrophy*—a cause of cardiomyopathy (Chap. 57)—may have difficulty rising from a chair or walking. The diagnosis of *hyperthyroidism,* which frequently causes cardiac disease (p. 1805), can often be suspected from simple inspection (exophthalmos, lid lag, perspiration, a fine tremor). In *Cushing's syndrome,* a cause of secondary hypertension (pp. 846 and 1810), there is truncal obesity and rounding of the face, with disproportionately thin extremities.

Many congenital somatic abnormalities such as cleft palate or harelip are frequently apparent on simple inspection and are observed in 25 per cent of infants with congenital heart disease; their presence should prompt a search for a cardiac malformation. In the *Ellis–van Creveld syndrome,* dwarfism, polydactyly, and ectodermal dysplasia frequently accompany congenital heart disease.[4] In patients with *coarctation of the aorta,* the lower extremities may be poorly developed, while the upper extremities are normal. Although heart failure may be associated with slight temperature elevation (p. 481), if it exceeds 38° C, it should not be attributed to heart failure alone; it is possible that a complication such as a respiratory or urinary tract infection, endocarditis, or pulmonary embolus is responsible.

HEAD AND FACE

Examination of the face often aids in the recognition of many disorders that can affect the cardiovascular system. *Myxedema* is characterized by a dull, expressionless face; periorbital puffiness; loss of the lateral eyebrows; a large tongue; and dry, sparse hair. An *earlobe crease* occurs more frequently in patients with coronary artery disease than in those without this condition.[5] The presence of an earlobe crease in a relatively young person (i.e., under 45 years), in particular should alert the examiner to the possibility of premature coronary artery disease.

Patients with *rheumatic heart disease* and severe mitral stenosis may exhibit a characteristic facies—a malar flush, cyanotic lips, and slight jaundice due to hepatic congestion. Bobbing of the head coincident with each heartbeat (de Musset's sign) is characteristic of severe aortic regurgitation. Facial edema may be present in patients with *tricuspid valve disease* and *constrictive pericarditis. Infective endocarditis* may result in a "café au lait" complexion. Anemia, cyanosis, and polycythemia may all be suspected from examination of the conjunctivae and oral mucosa. Telangiectasia of the lips and tongue may be associated with pulmonary arteriovenous fistula.

In *Down syndrome* (mongolism, trisomy 21), which is often associated with congenital heart disease (p. 1624), there is mental deficiency, a prominent medial epicanthus, and a large, often protruding tongue, low-set ears, a poorly formed nasal bridge, and hypoplastic mandible. Adenoma sebaceum of the face may be accompanied by a cardiac *rhabdomyoma* (p. 1475). Approximately 5 per cent of infants with congenital heart disease (most commonly ventricular septal defect) have the so-called cardiofacial syndrome, characterized by unilateral partial lower facial weakness, which may become apparent only when the patient cries.[6] In the so-called *velocardiofacial syndrome,*[7] a cleft of the secondary palate, a long vertical face, and deep overbite with retruded mandible accompany congenital heart disease, most commonly a ventricular septal defect.

Hypertelorism (widely set eyes) is observed in patients with *Noonan syndrome,*[8] who often have pulmonic stenosis (Fig. 49–1, p. 1625); *Turner syndrome,* often accompanied by coarctation of the aorta (p. 1624); the *multiple lentigines syndrome* (also termed LEOPARD syndrome) (Fig. 49–3, p. 1627), often associated with pulmonic stenosis and hypertrophic cardiomyopathy[9]; and *Hurler syndrome* (arrhythmias and valvular regurgitation) (p. 1728). The facies of one group of patients with a nonfamilial type of *supravalvular aortic stenosis* and mental retardation is quite characteristic (Fig. 30–37, p. 937) and includes hypertelorism; a broad, high forehead; strabismus and epicanthal folds; low-set ears; upturned nose; a long upper lip and wide mouth; and hypoplasia of the mandible, with a pointed chin, small teeth, and dental deformities.[10] Patients with *stenosis of the pulmonary artery* and/or its branches often have an unusual facial appearance characterized by a large mouth, a blunt upturned nose, wide-set eyes, internal strabismus, and malformed teeth.[2, 4]

Scleroderma, which can cause several forms of heart disease (p. 1723), can often be recognized in the face, where skin becomes firm, thickened, and leathery in texture and is tightly bound to the underlying subcutaneous tissues. In the late stages of this disease the skin is atrophic, and there is immobility, particularly around the mouth. Patients with *systemic lupus erythematosus* (which may cause pericarditis, myocarditis, and endocarditis) (p. 1720) may present with a butterfly rash on the face. *Acromegaly,* which may cause cardiomyopathy (p. 1800), is associated with enlargement of the head, coarse facial features, prognathism, and macroglossia. *Cushing's syndrome,* in which hypertension is often present (p. 1810), is characterized by moon facies, hirsutism, and acne. *Paget's disease* of bone, which may be associated with a high cardiac output state (p. 787), is characterized by enlargement of the skull. Episodic facial flushing occurs in patients with *carcinoid tumors* (p. 1439) and *pheochromocytoma* (p. 1812). A high, arched palate, prominent ears, and shimmering irides are characteristic of the *Marfan syndrome* (p. 1725).

The *muscular dystrophies,* the cardiac manifestations of which are described in Chapter 57, may also affect facial appearance profoundly. Patients with *myotonic dystrophy* (p. 1787) exhibit a dull, expressionless face, with ptosis due to weakness of the levator muscles; the forehead is furrowed, and the temporalis and sternocleidomastoid muscles are atrophied. In the *facioscapulohumeral type* of *muscular dystrophy* (Landouzy-Déjerine) (p. 1786), nearly all the facial muscles are weak, particularly the orbicularis oris, preventing the patients from puckering the mouth and whistling; weakness of the orbicularis oculi, diffuse fattening of the face, and facial asymmetry (particularly around the mouth) are also characteristic.

In patients with *Werner syndrome,* who are at high risk of developing premature coronary and arterial atherosclerosis, there is premature graying of the hair, frontal baldness, beaking of the nose, cataract formation, and proptosis. Myotonic muscular dystrophy (p. 1787) may also cause premature graying of the hair, frontal thinning or baldness, and early cataracts.

EYES

External ophthalmoplegia and ptosis due to muscular dystrophy of the extraocular muscles occur in the *Kearns-Sayre syndrome,* which may be associated with complete heart block and myocardial failure[11] (p. 792).

Exopthalmos and stare occur not only in hyperthyroidism, which can cause high-output cardiac failure (p. 783), but also in advanced congestive heart failure, in which there is severe pulmonary venous hypertension and weight loss (p. 479).[12] The stare is probably due to lid retraction caused by the increased adrenergic tone that accompanies heart failure. Severe tricuspid regurgitation[13] and a carotid artery–cavernous sinus fistula can also cause pulsation of the eyeballs (pulsatile exophthalmos).

Attention should be directed to the *iris* to look for an arcus, a circumferential light ring around the iris. When this ring begins inferiorly, leaving a rim peripherally, and occurs in a young person, it is frequently associated with hypercholesterolemia,[14] xanthelasma (small yellowish deposits of cholesterol on the eyelids), and premature atherosclerosis. (In blacks, an arcus often does not reflect hypercholesterolemia.) Iridodonesis (tremulous iris), in which the iris is not properly supported by the lens because of dislocation or weakness of the suspensory free ligament, occurs in Marfan syndrome. Gray-white spots (Brushfield's spots) in the iris occur in Down syndrome. Iridocyclitis and enlargement of the lacrimal glands are seen in sarcoidosis, which may be associated with cardiomyopathy (p. 1434).

Blue scleras may be seen in patients with Marfan syndrome, Ehlers-Danlos syndrome, and osteogenesis imperfecta—disorders that may be associated with aortic dilatation, regurgitation, and dissection and with prolapse of the mitral valve (Chap. 54). *Argyll Robertson pupils* (small, irregular, unequal pupils that do not dilate properly on administration of mydriatic drugs and that fail to react to light but constrict on accommodation) are diagnostic of central nervous system syphilis; this may be associated with cardiovascular syphilis, characterized by aneurysm of the ascending aorta, coronary ostial stenosis, and aortic regurgitation (p. 1566). The *cornea* may be clouded in the Hurler syndrome (p. 1728). *Cataracts* are associated with the so-called rubella syndrome, in which a variety of congenital cardiac malformations occur (p. 897); premature cataracts also occur in Refsum's disease and in myotonic muscular dystrophy, both of which may be associated with cardiomyopathy (p. 1787); *vitreous opacities* are frequent in patients with familial amyloidosis, in whom a restrictive cardiomyopathy may be present (p. 1431).

FUNDI. Examination of the *fundi* allows classification of arteriolar disease in patients with hypertension (Fig. 2–1*A*) and may be helpful in the recognition of arteriosclerosis. Beading of the retinal artery may be present in patients with hypercholesteremia (Fig. 2–1*B*), and wreathlike arteriovenous anastomoses around the disc are characteristic of Takayasu's disease (p. 1563) (Fig. 2–1*C*). Hemorrhages near the discs with white spots in the center (Roth's spots) occur in infective endocarditis (p. 1110) (Fig. 2–1*D*). Embolic retinal occlusions may occur in patients with rheumatic heart disease, left atrial myxoma, and atherosclerosis of the aorta or arch vessels. Papilledema is present not only in patients with malignant hypertension (Chap. 27) but also in cor pulmonale with severe hypoxia. In coarctation of the aorta, the retinal arteries are particularly tortuous but may not show other changes characteristic of hypertensive retinopathy.[15] In patients with cyanosis and polycythemia, the retinal veins are particularly dilated and edema and retinal papilledema are occasionally present.

SKIN AND MUCOUS MEMBRANES

Central cyanosis (due to intracardiac or intrapulmonary right-to-left shunting) involves the entire body, including warm, well perfused sites such as the conjunctivae and the mucous membranes of the oral cavity, while peripheral cyanosis (due to reduction of peripheral blood flow, such as occurs in heart failure and peripheral vascular disease) is characteristically most prominent in cool, exposed areas that may not be well perfused, such as the extremities, particularly the nailbeds and nose. Polycythemia can often be suspected from inspection of the conjunctivae, lips, and tongue, which in anemia are pale and in polycythemia are darkly congested. A blotchy cyanotic tinge to the skin associated with episodic flushing, particularly of the face, occurs in patients with *carcinoid tumors,* which may be associated with valvular heart disease (p. 1439).

Bronze pigmentation of the skin and loss of axillary and pubic hair occur in *hemochromatosis* (which may result in cardiomyopathy owing to iron deposits in the heart, p. 1434). Jaundice may be observed in patients following pulmonary infarction as well as in patients with congestive hepatomegaly or cardiac cirrhosis. *Lentigines,* i.e., small

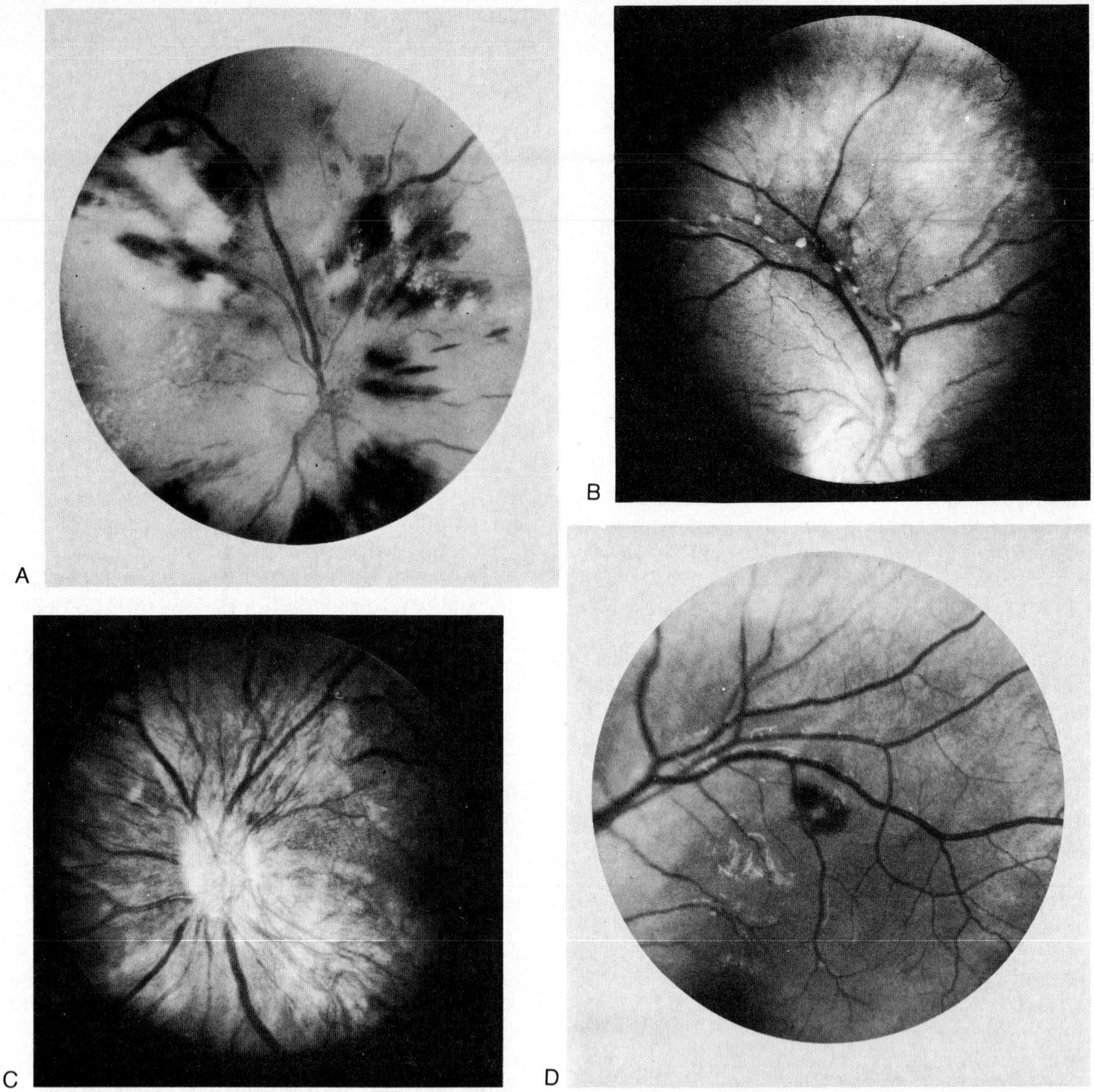

FIGURE 2–1. ***A,*** **Severe hypertensive retinopathy. The patient was a 43-year-old man with the symptoms of malignant hypertension. He subsequently died of massive cerebral hemorrhage.** ***B,*** **Beading of the retinal artery in a patient with hypercholesteremia. The patient was a 37-year-old man with a serum chlesterol level of 400 mg per 100 ml.** ***C,*** **Proliferative retinopathy of Takayasu-Ohnishi disease. The patient was a 27-year-old Oriental woman with postural amaurosis and hemiplegia. Brachial pulses unobtainable.** ***D,*** **Roth spots (hemorrhage with white center) in a patient with subacute bacterial endocarditis. (From Cogan, D. G.: Ophthalmic Manifestations of Systemic Vascular Disease. Philadelphia, W. B. Saunders Company, 1974, p. 52.)**

brown macular lesions on the neck and trunk that begin at about age 6 and do not increase in number with sunlight, are observed in patients with pulmonic stenosis and hypertrophic cardiomyopathy[9] (p. 1418).

The skin is ruddy in patients with polycythemia and Cushing's syndrome; sallow and yellowish in myxedema and in uremia; café au lait in late stages of infective endocarditis[16]; fine and silky in thyrotoxicosis; coarse and dry in myxedema and acromegaly; thickened and yellow (particularly in the neck and anticubital region) in pseudoxanthoma elasticum; smooth and glossy in longstanding Raynaud's syndrome; and warm and moist in anemia, beriberi, and other high-output states (Chap. 25). Increased sweating, most commonly a cold sweat in the palms, is observed in patients with neurocirculatory asthenia. *Erythema marginatum* (evanescent lesions confined primarily to the trunk) and *subcutaneous nodules* (which occur on the extensor surface of the elbows or over bony prominences such as the spine or skull) may be present in acute rheumatic fever (p. 1706). *Petechiae* occur in infective endocarditis; café-au-lait spots, freckles, and cutaneous neurofibromas occur in patients with pheochromocytoma (p. 1812), while *symmetric vitiligo* of the extremities is seen in patients with hyperthyroidism. Bluish pigmentation of the ear and nose cartilage is characteristic of *ochronosis*, which can produce serious valvular deformities (Chap. 33). Large areas of *psoriasis* or *exfoliative dermatitis* may be responsible for high-output heart failure (p. 790).

Several types of xanthomas, i.e., cholesterol-filled nodules, are found either subcutaneously or over tendons in patients with hyperlipoproteinemia (Chap. 36). Premature atherosclerosis frequently develops in these individuals. *Tuberoeruptive xanthomas*, present subcutaneously or on the extensor surfaces of the extremities, and *xanthoma striatum palmare*, which produces yellowish, orange, or pink discoloration of the palmar and digital creases, occur most commonly in patients with type III hyperlipoproteinemia (p. 1165). Patients with *xanthoma tendinosum* (Fig. 2–2), i.e., nodular swellings of the tendons, especially of the elbows, extensor surfaces of the hands, and Achilles'

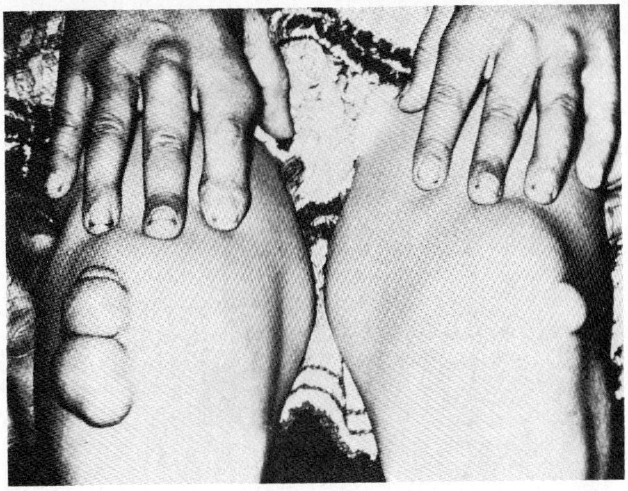

FIGURE 2–2. Tendinous xanthomas of the knees in a patient with familial hypercholesteremia. The patient was a 10-year-old girl with a serum cholesterol level of 665 mg/100 ml. Several other members of the family had a similar syndrome. (From Cogan, D. G.: Ophthalmic Manifestations of Systemic Vascular Disease. Philadelphia, W. B. Saunders Company, 1974, pp. 14 and 15.)

tendons, usually have type II hyperlipoproteinemia (p. 1164). *Xanthelasma* also occur in this condition but are less specific. *Eruptive xanthomas* are tiny, yellowish nodules, 1 to 2 mm in diameter on an erythematous base, which may occur anywhere on the body and are associated with hyperchylomicronemia and are therefore often found in patients with type I and type V hyperlipoproteinemia (pp. 1164 nd 1166).

Hereditary telangiectasia are multiple capillary hemangiomas occurring in the skin, lips (Fig. 2–3), nasal mucosa, and upper respiratory and gastrointestinal tracts that resemble the spider nevi seen in patients with liver disease. When present in the lung, they are associated with pulmonary arteriovenous fistulas and cause central cyanosis. Spider nevi on the face occur in patients with *chronic liver disease*, which may be associated with a high cardiac output state (p. 789). Nicotine staining of the fingers suggests excessive cigarette smoking, an important risk factor for the development of coronary artery and peripheral vascular disease (p. 1172).

EXTREMITIES

A variety of congenital and acquired cardiac malformations are associated with characteristic changes in the extremities. Among the congenital lesions, short stature, cubitus valgus, and medial deviation of the extended forearm is characteristic of *Turner syndrome* (p. 1624). Patients with the *Holt-Oram syndrome* (Table 30–2, p. 898), i.e., atrial septal defect with skeletal deformities, often have a thumb with an extra phalanx, a so-called "fingerized thumb," which lies in the same plane as the fingers, making it difficult to appose the thumb and fingers. In addition, they may exhibit deformities of the radius and ulna, causing difficulty in supination and pronation. There is often asymmetry of skeletal involvement, with the left side more severely affected. Polydactyly and hypoplastic fingernails are part of the *Ellis–van Creveld syndrome* (chondroectodermal dysplasia), a disorder frequently associated with atrial or ventricular septal defect (p. 1628). Arachnodactyly is characteristic of the *Marfan syndrome* (p. 1725). Normally, when a fist is made over a clenched thumb, the latter does not extend beyond the ulnar side of the hand, but it usually does so in Marfan syndrome (Fig. 2–4*A*). When the wrist is encircled by the thumb

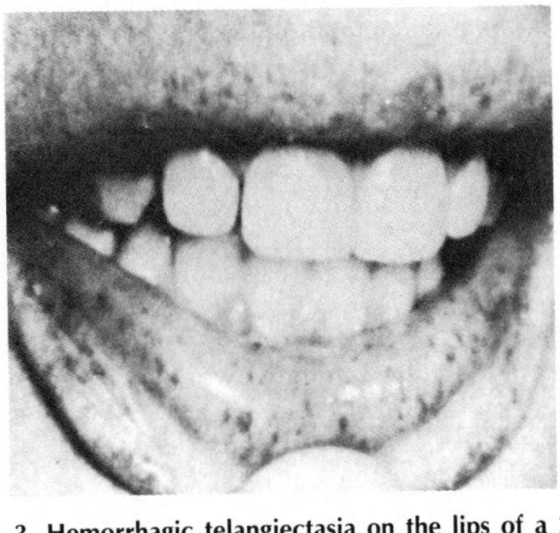

FIGURE 2–3. Hemorrhagic telangiectasia on the lips of a 25-year-old woman and pulmonary arteriovenous fistulas. (From Perloff, J. K.: The Clinical Recognition of Congenital Heart Disease. Philadelphia, W. B. Saunders Company, 1987, p. 645.)

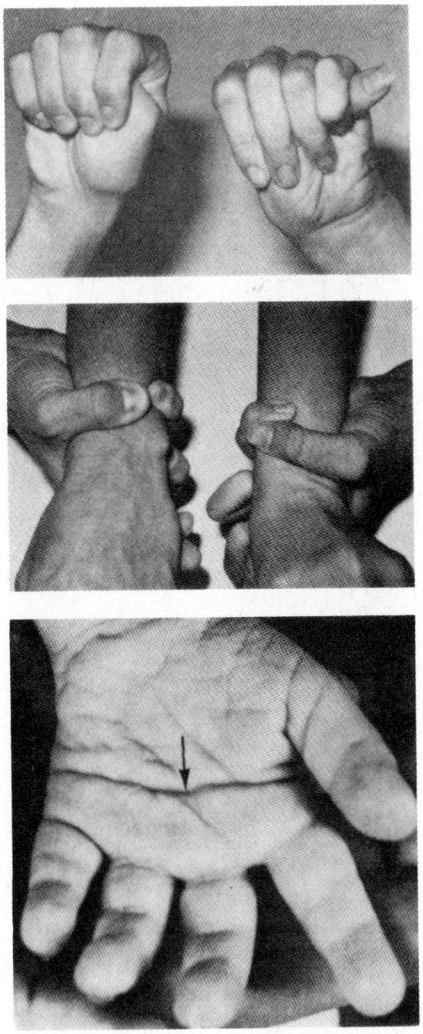

FIGURE 2–4. *Top,* At left is the hand of a normal subject, who is unable to protrude his thumb beyond his clenched fingers, as can the patient with Marfan syndrome at right, who can do this because of a long thumb and lax joints. *Center,* The normal patient at left cannot overlap his thumb and little finger around his wrist because, unlike the patient with Marfan syndrome at right, his fingers are not long relative to his wrist. *Bottom,* Transverse simian crease in a 6-month-old infant with Down syndrome. (Top and center from Constant, J.: Bedside Cardiology. 3rd ed. Boston, Little, Brown & Co., 1985, pp. 30 and 31. Bottom from Perloff, J. K.: The Clinical Recognition of Congenital Heart Disease, Philadelphia, W. B. Saunders Company, 1987, p. 328.)

and little finger of the opposite hand, the little finger will overlap the thumb by at least 1 cm in more than three-fourths of patients with Marfan syndrome but will rarely do so in individuals without this syndrome[17] (Fig. 2–4*B*). In *osteogenesis imperfecta*, hyperextensibility of the joints is common, but arachnodactyly is not.[18] In patients with *homocystinuria*, the extremities may be elongated and other skeletal abnormalities, such as kyphoscoliosis and pectus carinatum, may be present. Ulnar deviation of the fourth and fifth fingers and flexion at the metacarpophalangeal joints occur in *Jaccoud's arthritis*,[19] a rare concomitant of rheumatic heart disease. In *Down syndrome*, there is a simian palm crease (Fig. 2–4*C*) and sometimes increased space between the fourth and fifth fingers, and a short fifth finger that is curved inward, while in Turner syndrome the fingers tend to be short.

Raynaud's phenomenon, which sometimes occurs in association with primary pulmonary hypertension (p. 805), scleroderma (p. 1723), and coronary spasm (p. 1228), is characterized by intermittent pallor and/or cyanosis of the extremities precipitated by exposure to cold. With the passage of time, the skin overlying the fingers and under the nails becomes atrophic. Cold, pale, or blue hands accompanied by collapse of the forearm veins signifies peripheral vasoconstriction, which may be a normal response to cold, anxiety, or a low cardiac output. In patients with peripheral vascular disease, the ischemic foot typically exhibits paleness on elevation and rubor on dependency.

High cardiac output states (Chap. 25) produce warm, pink hands associated with distention of the forearm veins (signs of vasodilatation). Redness of the palmar eminences may be a sign of severe liver disease, while a fine tremor of the outstretched hands suggests thyrotoxicosis. Peripheral *arteriovenous fistula* or *Paget's disease* of bone may cause local warmth and excessive growth of the affected limb. Systolic flushing of the nailbeds, which can be readily detected by pressing a flashlight against the terminal digits (Quincke's sign), is a sign of aortic regurgitation and of other conditions characterized by a greatly widened pulse pressure. *Differential cyanosis*, in which the hands and fingers (especially on the right side) are pink and the feet and toes are cyanotic, is indicative of patent ductus arteriosus with reversed shunt due to pulmonary hypertension (p. 923); this finding can often be brought out by exercise. On the other hand, *reversed differential cyanosis*, in which cyanosis of the fingers exceeds that of the toes, suggests transposition of the great arteries, pulmonary hypertension, preductal narrowing of the aorta, and reversed flow through a patent ductus arteriosus.[20]

CLUBBING OF THE FINGERS AND TOES[21] (Fig. 2–5). Clubbing of the digits is characteristic of central cyanosis (cyanotic congenital heart disease or pulmonary disease with hypoxia). It may also appear within a few weeks of the development of infective endocarditis but usually develops after 2 or 3 years of central cyanosis. Clubbing is also observed in a variety of suppurative pulmonary lesions and carcinoma of the lung as well as in gastrointestinal disorders, including biliary cirrhosis and regional enteritis; occasionally, it is a harmless familial condition. The earliest forms of clubbing are characterized by increased glossiness and cyanosis of the skin at the root of the nail.[22] Following obliteration of the normal angle between the base of the nail and the skin, the soft tissue of the pulp becomes hypertrophied, the nail root floats freely, and its loose proximal end can be palpated. In the more severe forms of clubbing, bony changes occur, i.e., *hypertrophic pulmonary osteoarthropathy;* these changes involve the terminal digits and in rare instances even the wrists, ankles, elbows, and knees. *Unilateral clubbing* of the fingers is rare but can occur when an aortic aneurysm interferes with the arterial supply to one arm. Not to be confused with clubbing are the subungual fibromas of the fingers that occur in tuberous sclerosis, a condition often associated with cardiac rhabdomyoma.[23]

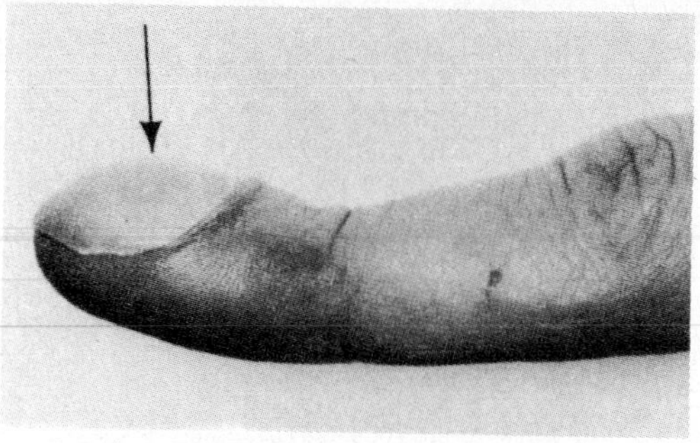

FIGURE 2–5. Typical cyanosis and clubbing, close-up, profile. (From Perloff, J. K.: The Clinical Recognition of Congenital Heart Disease, 3rd ed. Philadelphia, W. B. Saunders Company, 1987, p. 6.)

Osler's nodes are small, tender, erythematous skin lesions due to infected emboli and occurring most frequently in the pads of the fingers or toes and in the palms of the hands or soles of the feet, whereas *Janeway lesions* are slightly raised, nontender hemorrhagic lesions in the palms of hands and soles of the feet; both these lesions as well as petechiae occur in infective endocarditis (p. 1110). When the latter occur under the nailbeds, they are termed *splinter hemorrhages*. The terminal digits may also show, early in endocarditis, a mottled pink followed by a bluish discoloration which darkens as necrosis occurs; it is probably due to arteriolar embolism.[16]

Edema of the extremities is a common finding in congestive heart failure; however, if it is present in only one leg, it is more likely due to venous obstructive disease than to heart failure. Firm pressure on the pretibial region for 10 to 20 seconds may be necessary for the detection of edema in ambulatory patients. In patients confined to bed, edema appears first in the sacral region. Edema may involve the face in children with heart failure of any etiology and in adults with heart failure associated with marked elevation of systemic venous pressure (e.g., constrictive pericarditis and tricuspid valve disease).

CHEST AND ABDOMEN

Examination of the thorax should begin with observations of the respiratory rate, effort, and regularity. The shape of the chest is important as well; thus, a barrel-shaped chest with low diaphragms suggests emphysema, bronchitis, and possibly cor pulmonale. In chronic obstructive pulmonary disease, accessory muscles are used during inspiration, while expiration is prolonged and often accompanied by wheezing.

Inspection of the chest may reveal a bulging to the right of the upper sternum caused by an aortic aneurysm or a venous collateral pattern caused by obstruction of the superior vena cava, which may also be caused by aortic aneurysm. Pectus excavatum may occur in Marfan syndrome, with mitral valve prolapse or atrial septal defect; it is also seen in Noonan syndrome (often with pulmonic stenosis).

Painful enlargement of the *liver* may be due to venous congestion; the tenderness disappears in longstanding heart failure. Hepatic systolic expansile pulsations occur in

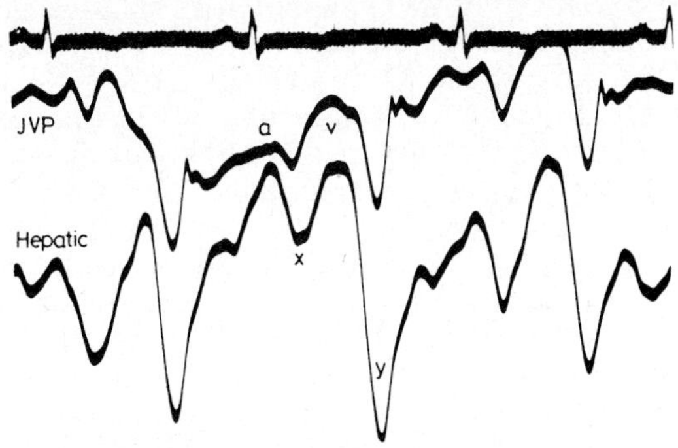

FIGURE 2–6. Simultaneous pressure tracings of externally recorded jugular venous (JVP) and hepatic pulsations in a patient with constrictive pericarditis. Note the almost identical phasic relation between the two tracings. Sharp *y* descents are the prominent waves in both tracings. (From Manga, P., Vythilingum, S., and Mitha, A. S.: Pulsatile hepatomegaly in constrictive pericarditis. Br. Heart J. *52*:466, 1984.)

patients with severe tricuspid regurgitation (Fig. 16–3, p. 480), and presystolic pulsations can be felt in patients with pure tricuspid stenosis and sinus rhythm. Patients with constrictive pericarditis often have pulsatile hepatomegaly, the contour of the pulsations resembling those of the jugular venous pulse in this condition[24, 25] (Fig. 2–6). Transmitted (as opposed to intrinsic) pulsations of the liver occur in patients with right ventricular enlargement, aneurysmal dilatation of the upper abdominal aorta, and a widened pulse pressure. When firm pressure over the abdomen causes cervical venous distention, i.e., when there is *abdominojugular reflux*, right heart failure is usually present. *Ascites* is also characteristic of heart failure, but is especially characteristic of tricuspid valve disease and chronic constrictive pericarditis.

Splenomegaly may occur in the presence of severe congestive hepatomegaly, most frequently in patients with constrictive pericarditis or tricuspid valve disease. The spleen may be enlarged and painful in infective endocarditis as well as following splenic embolization. Splenic infarction is frequently accompanied by an audible friction rub.

Both *kidneys* may be palpably enlarged in patients with hypertension secondary to polycystic disease. Auscultation of the abdomen should be carried out in all patients with hypertension; a systolic bruit secondary to renal artery stenosis may be audible near the umbilicus or in the flank (p. 843).

Atherosclerotic aneurysms of the abdominal aorta are usually readily detected on palpation (p. 1548), except in markedly obese patients. In patients with *coarctation of the aorta*, no abdominal pulsations are palpable despite the presence of prominent arterial pulses in the neck and upper extremities; arterial pulses in the lower extremities are reduced or absent.

THE JUGULAR VENOUS PULSE

Important information concerning the dynamics of the right side of the heart can be obtained by inspection of the jugular venous pulse.[2, 26–28] The *internal* jugular vein is ordinarily employed in the examination; the venous pulse can usually be analyzed more readily on the right than on the left side of the neck, because the right innominate and jugular veins extend cephalad in an almost straight line along with the superior vena cava, thus favoring transmission of hemodynamic changes from the right atrium, while the left innominate vein may be kinked or compressed by a variety of normal structures, by a dilated aorta, or by an aneurysm.

The patient should be lying comfortably during the examination; clothing should be removed from the neck and upper thorax, and although the head should rest on a pillow, it must not be elevated at a sharp angle from the trunk. The jugular venous pulse may be examined effectively by shining a light tangentially across the neck. Most patients with heart disease are examined most effectively in the 45-degree position, but in patients in whom venous pressure is high, a greater inclination (60 or even 90 degrees) is required to obtain visible pulsations, while in those in whom jugular venous pressure is low, a lesser inclination (30 degrees) is desirable. In order to amplify the pulsations of the jugular veins, it may be helpful to place the patient in the supine position and try to increase venous return by elevating the patient's legs.

The internal jugular vein is located deep within the neck, where it is covered by the sternocleidomastoid muscle and is therefore not usually visible as a discrete structure, except in the presence of severe venous hypertension. However, its pulsations are transmitted to the skin of the neck, where they are usually easily visible. Sometimes considerable difficulty may be experienced in differentiating between the carotid and jugular venous pulses in the neck, particularly when the latter exhibits prominent *v* waves, as occurs in patients with tricuspid regurgitation, in whom the valves in the internal jugular veins may be incompetent. However, there are several helpful clues: (1) The arterial pulse is a sharply localized rapid movement that may not be readily visible but that strikes the palpating fingers with considerable force; in contrast, the venous pulse, while more readily visible, often disappears when the palpating finger is placed lightly on or below the pulsating area. (2) The arterial pulsations do not change when the patient is in the upright position, whereas venous pulsations usually disappear or diminish greatly, unless the venous pressure is greatly elevated. (3) Compression of the root of the neck does not affect the arterial pulse but usually abolishes venous pulsations, except in the presence of extreme venous hypertension.

Two principal observations can usually be made from examination of the neck veins: the level of venous pressure and the type of venous wave pattern. In order to estimate jugular venous pressure, the height of the oscillating top of the distended proximal portion of the internal jugular vein, which reflects right atrial pressure, should be determined. The upper limit of normal is 4 cm above the sternal angle, which corresponds to a central venous pressure of approximately 9 cm H_2O, since the right atrium is approximately 5 cm below the sternal angle. When the veins in the neck collapse in a subject in the horizontal position, it is likely that the central venous pressure is subnormal. When obstruction of veins in the lower extremities is responsible for edema, pressure in the neck veins is not elevated and the abdominal-jugular reflex is negative.

The *abdominal-jugular reflux* can be tested by applying firm pressure to the periumbilical region for 30 to 60 seconds with the patient breathing quietly while the jugular veins are observed; increased respiratory excursions or strain should be avoided. In normal subjects jugular venous pressure rises only transiently, while pressure is continued, whereas in right ventricular failure and/or tricuspid regurgitation the jugular venous pressure remains elevated.

PATTERN OF THE VENOUS PULSE. The events of the cardic cycle, shown in Figure 13–26, p. 405, provide an explanation for the details of the jugular venous pulse pattern (Figs. 2–6, 2–7, and 3–34, p. 61). The *a* wave in

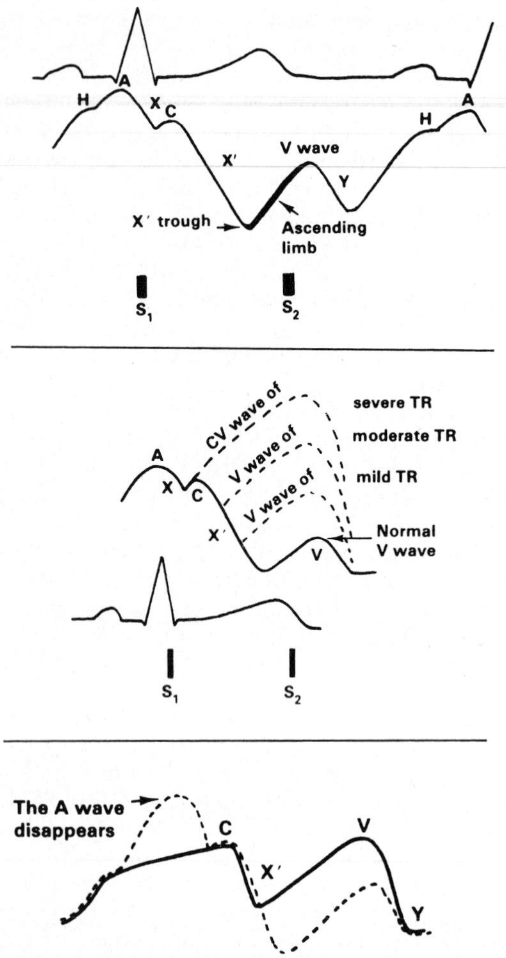

FIGURE 2–7. *Top,* Normal jugular venous pulse: the jugular *v* wave is built up during systole, and its height reflects the rate of filling and the elasticity of the right atrium. Between the bottom of the *y* descent (*y* trough) and beginning of the *a* wave is the period of relatively slow filling of the "atrioventricle" or diastasis period. The wave built up during diastasis is the *H* wave. The *H* wave height also reflects the stiffness of the right atrium. S_1 and S_2 refer to the first and second heart sounds, respectively. *Center,* As the degree of tricuspid regurgitation (TR) increases, the x^1 descent is increasingly encroached upon. With severe TR, no x^1 descent is seen, and the jugular pulse wave is said to be "ventricularized." *Bottom,* Effect of development of atrial fibrillation on the jugular venous pulse. The dominant descent in atrial fibrillation is almost always the *y* descent, i.e., it has the superficial appearance of the pulse wave of TR. (From Constant, J.: Bedside Cardiology. 3rd ed. Boston, Little, Brown & Co., 1985, pp. 95, 105, and 108.)

the venous pulse results from venous distention due to right atrial systole, while the *x* descent is due to atrial relaxation; the *c* wave, which occurs simultaneously with the carotid arterial pulse, is an inconstant wave in the jugular venous pulse and may be due in part to forceful closure of the tricuspid valve; sometimes it is an artifact produced by the adjacent carotid arterial pulse. It is followed by the x' descent or trough, caused by the pulling down of the floor of the atrium (descent of the base) by ventricular contraction. (Many investigators refer to this wave as the *x* descent.) The *v* wave results from the rise in right atrial pressure when blood flows into the right atrium during ventricular systole when the tricuspid valve is shut, and the *y* descent, i.e., the downslope of the *v* wave, is related to the decline in right atrial pressure when the tricuspid valve reopens. Following the bottom of the *y* descent (the *y* trough) and beginning of the *a* wave is a period of relatively slow filling of the atrium or ventricle, the diastasis period, a wave termed the *H* wave. While all or most of these events can usually be recorded, they are not readily distinguishable on inspection. The descents or downward collapsing movements of the jugular veins are more rapid, produce larger excursions, and are therefore more prominent to the eye than are the ascents (Figs. 2–7 and 3–34, p. 61). The normal dominant jugular venous descent, the x' descent, occurs just prior to the second heart sound, while the *y* descent ends after the second heart sound. With an increase in central venous pressure, the *v* wave becomes higher and the *y* collapse becomes more prominent. The *a* wave can be recognized when it is abnormally prominent; it occurs just before the first heart sound or carotid pulse and has a sharp rise and fall. The *v* wave occurs just after the arterial pulse and has a slower, undulating pattern.

ALTERATIONS IN DISEASE. Elevation of jugular venous pressure reflects an increase in right atrial pressure and occurs in heart failure, reduced compliance of the right ventricle, pericardial disease, hypervolemia, and obstruction of the superior vena cava. During inspiration, the jugular venous pressure normally declines but the *amplitude* of the pulsations increases. *Kussmaul's sign* is a paradoxical rise in the height of the jugular venous pressure during inspiration, which occurs frequently in patients with chronic constrictive pericarditis and sometimes in congestive heart failure and tricuspid stenosis. The *x* descent may be prominent in patients with enlarged *a* waves, as well as in patients with right ventricular volume overload (atrial septal defect). Constrictive pericarditis is characterized by a rapid and deep *y* descent followed by a rapid rise to a diastolic plateau (*H* wave) without a prominent *v* wave (Fig. 2–6, p. 61); occasionally, the x' descent is prominent in this condition as well. A prominent *v* wave or *cv* wave, i.e., fusion of the *c* and *v* waves in the absence or attenuation of an x' descent, occurs in tricuspid regurgitation (Figs. 2–7*B* and 3–37, p. 62 and Fig. 16–3, p. 480); a prominent *v* wave and *y* descent are also seen in atrial septal defect; the *y* descent is gradual in tricuspid stenosis and steep in tricuspid regurgitation. Tall *a* waves are present in patients with sinus rhythm and tricuspid stenosis or atresia, right atrial myxoma, or reduced compliance and/or marked hypertrophy of the right ventricle (Fig. 3–35, p. 61). Cannon (giant) *a* waves are noted in patients with atrioventricular dissociation when the right atrium contracts against a closed tricuspid valve (see Fig. 3–36, p. 62). In atrial fibrillation, the *a* wave and *x* descent disappear, and the x' descent becomes more prominent. In right ventricular failure and sinus rhythm, there may be increases in prominence of both the *a* and *v* waves. A steeply rising *H* wave is observed (or recorded) in restrictive cardiomyopathy, constrictive pericarditis, and right ventricular infarction. The *a* wave is absent in atrial fibrillation, accompanied by a diminished x' descent and a prominent *v* wave (Fig. 2–7*C*).

INDIRECT MEASUREMENT OF ARTERIAL PRESSURE

Systolic arterial pressure can be *estimated* without a sphygmomanometer cuff by gradually compressing the brachial artery while palpating the radial artery; the force required to obliterate the radial pulse represents the systolic blood pressure, and with practice, one can often estimate this level within 20 mm Hg. Ordinarily, however, a sphygmomanometer is used to obtain an indirect measurement of blood pressure. The cuff should fit snugly around the arm, with its lower edge at least 1 inch above the antecubital space, and the diaphragm of the stethoscope should be placed close to or under the edge of the sphygmomanometer cuff. The width of the cuff selected should be at least 40 per cent of the circumference of the limb to be used. The standard size, with a 5-inch-wide cuff, is designed for adults with an arm of average size. When this cuff is applied to a large upper arm or a normal adult thigh, arterial pressure will be overestimated, leading to spurious hypertension in the obese (arm circumference > 35 cm)[28, 29]; when it is applied to a small arm, the pressure will be underestimated. The cuff width should be approximately 1½ inches in infants and small children, 3 inches in young children (2 to 5 years), and 8 inches in obese adults. The bag should be long enough to extend at least halfway around the limb (10 inches in adults). In patients with rigid, sclerotic vessels the systolic pressure may also be overestimated, by as much as 30 mm Hg. Mercury manometers are, in general, more accurate and reliable than the aneroid type; the latter should be calibrated once yearly.

In order to measure arterial pressure in the upper extremity,[30] the patient should be seated or lying comfortably and relaxed, the arm should be slightly flexed and at heart level, and the arm muscles should be relaxed. The cuff should be inflated rapidly to approximately 30 mm Hg above the anticipated systolic pressure.[31] These maneuvers, which diminish the volume of blood in the venous bed, decrease the tissue pressure distal to the cuff and thereby increase the flow into the occluded brachial artery. The cuff is then deflated slowly, no faster than 3 mm Hg/sec; the pressure at which the brachial pulse can be palpated is close to the systolic pressure. The cuff should be deflated rapidly after the diastolic pressure is noted and a full minute allowed to elapse before pressure is remeasured in the same limb. Although excessive pressure on the stethoscope head does not affect systolic pressure, it does erroneously lower diastolic readings.[32] In one study, the anxiety associated with blood pressure measurement was shown to elevate arterial pressure by an average of 27/17 mm Hg.[33] It is desirable for the patient to reduce anxiety and bladder distension and to avoid exercise, caffeine, eating, and smoking for a half hour preceding the screening.

To measure pressure in the legs, the patient should lie on his or her abdomen, an 8-inch-wide cuff should be applied with the compression bag over the posterior aspect of the midthigh and should be rolled diagonally around the thigh to keep the edges snug against the skin, and auscultation should be carried out in the popliteal fossa. In order to measure pressure in the lower leg, an arm cuff is placed over the calf, and auscultation is carried out over the posterior tibial artery. Regardless of where the cuff is applied, care must be taken to avoid letting the rubber part of the balloon of the cuff extend beyond its covering and to avoid placing the cuff on so loosely that central ballooning occurs.

KOROTKOFF SOUNDS. There are five phases of Korotkoff sounds, i.e., sounds produced by the flow of blood as the constricting blood pressure cuff is gradually released. The first appearance of clear, tapping sounds (phase I) represents the systolic pressure. These sounds are replaced by soft murmurs during phase II and by louder murmurs during phase III, as the volume of blood flowing through the constricted artery increases. The sounds suddenly become muffled in phase IV, when constriction of the brachial artery diminishes as arterial diastolic pressure is approached. Korotkoff sounds disappear in phase V, which is usually within 10 mm Hg of phase IV. Diastolic pressure measured directly through an intraarterial needle and external manometer corresponds closely to phase V.[34] In severe aortic regurgitation, however, when the disappearance point is extremely low, sometimes 0 mm Hg, the sound of muffling (phase IV) is much closer to the intraarterial diastolic pressure than is the disappearance point (phase V). When there is a sizable difference between phases IV and V of the Korotkoff sounds (> 10 mm Hg), both pressures should be recorded (e.g., 142/54/10 mm Hg). Korotkoff sounds may be difficult to hear and arterial pressure difficult to measure when arterial pressure rises at a slow rate (as in aortic stenosis), when the vessels are markedly constricted (as in shock [Fig. 19–2, p. 562]), and when the stroke volume is reduced (as in severe heart failure). Very soft or inaudible Korotkoff sounds can often be accentuated by dilating the blood vessels of the upper extremities simply by opening and closing the fist repeatedly. In states of shock, the indirect method of measuring blood pressure is unreliable, and arterial pressure should be measured through an intraarterial needle.

The *auscultatory gap* is a silence that sometimes separates the first appearance of the Korotkoff sounds from their second appearance at a lower pressure. This phenomenon tends to occur when there is venous distention or reduced velocity of arterial flow into the arm, as occurs in severe aortic stenosis. If the first muffling of sounds is considered to be the diastolic pressure, it will be overestimated. If the second appearance is taken as the systolic pressure, it will be underestimated. On the other hand, sounds transmitted through the arterial tree from prosthetic aortic valves may be responsible for falsely high readings.

In order to determine arterial pressure in the basal condition, the patient should have rested in a quiet room for 15 minutes. It is desirable to record the arterial pressure in both arms at the time of the initial examination; differences in systolic pressure exceeding 10 mm Hg between the two arms when measurements are made in rapid sequence[35] suggest obstructive lesions involving the aorta or the origin of the innominate and subclavian arteries, or supravalvular aortic stenosis (p. 938). In patients with vertebral-basal artery insufficiency, a difference in pressure between the arms may signify that a subclavian steal is responsible for the cerebrovascular symptoms.[36] In order to determine whether orthostatic hypotension is present, arterial pressure should be determined with the patient in both the supine and the erect positions. However, regardless of the patient's posture, the brachial artery should be

TABLE 2–1 COMMON SOURCES OF ERROR IN THE INDIRECT MEASUREMENT OF BLOOD PRESSURE

1. Failure for the patient to be in the basal state
2. Failure to use the proper size cuff
3. Failure to apply the cuff snugly
4. Failure to center the cuff over the brachial artery
5. Failure to relax the arm muscle
6. Failure to position the arm at heart level
7. Failure to inflate the cuff rapidly
8. Pressing too hard with the stethoscope
9. Failure to use the stethoscope bell
10. Failure to record systolic blood pressure at the first tapping sound
11. Failure to record diastolic blood pressure at the point of complete disappearance of the sound (Korotkoff Phase V)
12. Failure to record the blood pressure in both arms
13. Failure to record the position of the patient
14. Overly rapid cuff deflation
15. Reliance on single blood pressure measurement in the diagnosis of hypertension
16. Inaccuracies in patients with irregular cardiac rhythms
17. Failure to consider that shock may lead to serious underestimation of the true intravascular pressure

Adapted with permission from Nelson, W. P., and Egbert, A. M.: How to measure blood pressure—accurately. Primary Cardiol. *10*:14, 1984.

at the level of the heart to avoid superimposition of the effects of gravity on the recorded pressure.

Normally, the systolic pressure in the legs is up to 20 mm Hg higher than in the arms, but the diastolic pressure is usually virtually identical. The recording of a higher diastolic pressure in the legs than in the arms suggests that the thigh cuff is too small. When systolic pressure in the popliteal artery exceeds that in the brachial artery by more than 20 mm Hg (Hill's sign), aortic regurgitation is usually present.[37] Blood pressure should be measured in the lower extremities in patients with hypertension to detect coarctation of the aorta or when obstructive disease of the aorta or its immediate branches is suspected.

The most common errors in the indirect measurement of blood pressure are listed in Table 2–1.

THE ARTERIAL PULSE

The volume and contour of the arterial pulse are determined by a combination of factors, including the left ventricular stroke volume, the ejection velocity, the relative compliance and capacity of the arterial system, and the pressure waves that result from the antegrade flow of blood and reflections of the arterial pressure pulse returning from the peripheral circulation.[38] Bilateral palpation of the carotid, radial, brachial, femoral, popliteal, dorsalis pedis, and posterior tibial pulses should be part of the examination of all cardiac patients. The frequency, regularity, and shape of the pulse wave and the character of the arterial wall should be determined.[39] The carotid pulse (Fig. 2–8*C*) provides the most accurate representation of the central aortic pulse.[40] The brachial artery is the vessel ordinarily most suitable for appreciating the rate of rise of the pulse and the contour, volume, and consistency of the peripheral vessels. This artery is located at the medial aspect of the elbow, and it may be helpful to flex the arm in order to palpate it; palpation of the artery should be carried out with the thumb exerting pressure on the artery until its maximal movement is detected (Fig. 2–8*B*). A normal rate of rise of the arterial pulse suggests that there is no obstruction to left ventricular outflow, whereas a pulse wave of small amplitude with normal configuration suggests a reduced stroke volume.

THE NORMAL PULSE. The pulse in the ascending aorta normally rises rapidly to a rounded dome; this initial rise reflects the peak velocity of blood ejected from the left ventricle. A slight anacrotic notch or pause is frequently recorded, but only occasionally felt, on the ascending limb of the pulse. The descending limb of the central aortic pulse is less steep than is the ascending limb, and it is interrupted by the incisura, a sharp downward deflection related to closure of the aortic valve (Fig. 3–21, p. 54 and Fig. 4–3, p. 66). Immediately thereafter, the pulse wave rises slightly and then declines gradually throughout diastole. As the pulse wave is transmitted to the periphery, its upstroke becomes steeper, the systolic peak becomes higher, the anacrotic shoulder disappears, and the sharp incisura is replaced by a smoother, later dicrotic notch followed by a dicrotic wave. Normally, the height of this dicrotic wave diminishes with age, hypertension, and arteriosclerosis. In the central arterial pulse (central aorta and innominate and carotid arteries), the rapidly transmitted shock of left ventricular ejection results in a peak in early systole, referred to as the *percussion wave;* a second, smaller peak, the *tidal wave,* presumed to represent a reflected wave from the periphery, can often be recorded

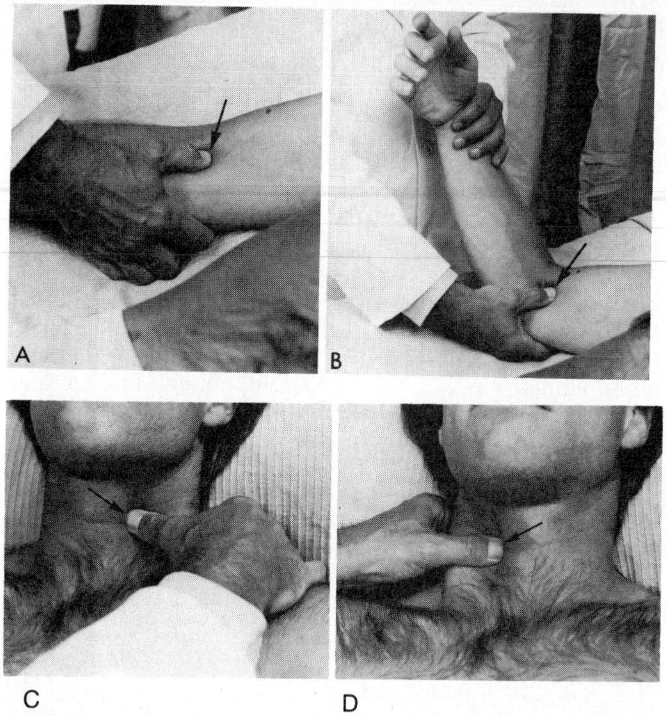

FIGURE 2–8. *A,* Palpation of the right brachial pulse with the thumb while the patient's arm lies at the side with the palm up. *B,* Palpation of the right brachial pulse with the patient's elbow resting in the palm of the examiner's hand. The thumb explores the antecubital fossa (*arrow*), while the patient's forearm is passively raised and lowered to achieve maximum relaxation of muscles around the elbow. *C* and *D,* Palpation of the carotid pulse. The examiner places the right thumb (*arrow*) on the patient's left carotoid artery (*C*). The left thumb (*arrow*) is then applied separately to the right carotid (*D*). (From Perloff, J. K. [ed.]: Physical Examination of the Heart and Circulation. Philadelphia, W. B. Saunders Company, 1982, pp. 58 and 60.)

but is not normally palpable. However, in older subjects, particularly those with increased peripheral resistance, as well as in patients with arteriosclerosis and diabetes, the tidal wave may be somewhat higher than the percussion wave; i.e., the pulse reaches a peak in late systole. In peripheral arteries, the pulse wave normally has a single sharp peak.

ABNORMAL PULSES. When vascular resistance and arterial stiffness are increased, as in hypertension, there is an elevation in pulse wave velocity, and the pulse contour has a more rapid upstroke and greater amplitude. Reduced or unequal carotid arterial pulsations occur in patients with carotid atherosclerosis and with diseases of the aortic arch, including aortic dissection, aneurysm, and Takayasu's disease (p. 1563). In *supravalvular aortic stenosis* there is a streaming of the jet toward the innominate artery, and the carotid and brachial arterial pulses are stronger on the right than on the left side, and pressures are higher in the right than in the left arm (Fig. 4–6, p. 68, and p. 938). The pulses of the upper extremity may be reduced or unequal in a variety of other conditions, including arterial embolus or thrombosis, anomalous origin or aberrant path of the major vessels, and cervical rib or scalenus anticus syndrome. Asymmetry of right and left popliteal pulses is characteristic of iliofemoral obstruction. Weakness or absence of radial, posterior tibial, or dorsalis pedis pulses on one side suggests arterial insufficiency. In *coarctation of the aorta* the carotid and brachial pulses are bounding, rise rapidly, and have large volumes, while in the lower extremities, the systolic and pulse pressures are reduced, their rate of rise is slow, and there is a late peak. This delay in the femoral arterial pulses can usually be readily detected by simultaneous palpation of the femoral and radial arterial pulses.

In patients with fixed obstruction to left ventricular outflow, the carotid pulse rises slowly (*pulsus tardus*); the upstroke is frequently characterized by a thrill (the *carotid shudder*); and the peak is reduced, occurs late in systole, and is sustained (Figs. 3–22, p. 56; 4–4, p. 67; and 4–7, p. 68). There is a notch on the upstroke of the carotid pulse (anacrotic notch) that is so distinct that two separate waves can be palpated in what is termed an *anacrotic pulse*. *Pulsus parvus* is a pulse of small amplitude, usually because of a reduction of stroke volume. *Pulsus parvus et tardus* refers to a small pulse with a delayed systolic peak, which is characteristic of severe aortic stenosis. This type of pulse is more readily appreciated by palpating the carotid rather than a more peripheral artery. Patients with severe aortic stenosis and heart failure usually exhibit simply a reduced pulse amplitude, i.e., *pulsus parvus*, and the delay in the upstroke is not readily apparent. However, this delay is readily recorded. In elderly patients with inelastic peripheral arteries, the pulse may rise normally despite the presence of aortic stenosis.

The carotid arterial pulse may be prominent or exaggerated in any condition in which pulse pressure is increased, including anxiety or other high cardiac output states (Chap. 25), as well as in bradycardia, and peripheral arteriosclerosis with loss of arterial distensibility. In patients with *mitral regurgitation* or *ventricular septal defect*, the forward stroke volume (from the left ventricle into the aorta) is usually normal, but the fraction ejected during early systole is greater than normal; hence, the arterial pulse is of normal volume (the pulse pressure is normal), but the pulse may rise abnormally rapidly.[41] Exaggerated or bounding arterial pulses may be observed in patients with an elevated stroke volume, with sympathetic hyperactivity, and in patients with a rigid, sclerotic aorta. In *aortic regurgitation*, there is a very brisk rate of rise with an increased pulse pressure[37] (Fig. 3–24, p. 56). The *Corrigan or water-hammer pulse* of aortic regurgitation consists of an abrupt upstroke (percussion wave) followed by rapid collapse later in systole, but no dicrotic notch. Corrigan's pulse reflects a low resistance in the reservoir into which the left ventricle rapidly discharges an abnormally elevated stroke volume, and it can be exaggerated by raising the patient's arm. In *acute* aortic regurgitation, the left ventricle may not be greatly dilated, and premature closure of the mitral valve may occur and limit the volume of aortic reflux[42]; therefore, the aortic diastolic pressure may *not* be very low, the arterial pulse *not* bounding, and the pulse pressure *not* widened despite a serious abnormality of valve function (p. 1063). "Pistol-shot" sounds heard over the femoral artery when the stethoscope is placed on it (*Traube's sign*), a systolic murmur heard over the femoral artery when it is gradually compressed proximally, and a diastolic murmur when the artery is compressed distally (*Duroziez's sign*[37, 43]) and Quincke's sign (p. 1064) are also characteristic of severe, chronic aortic regurgitation; of these, Duroziez's sign is the most predictive. Bounding arterial pulses are also present in patients with patent ductus arteriosus or large arteriovenous fistulas; in hyperkinetic states such as thyrotoxicosis, pregnancy, fever, and anemia; in severe bradycardia; and in vessels proximal to a coarctation of the aorta.

In the presence of atrioventricular dissociation, when atrial activity is irregularly transmitted to the ventricles, the strength of the peripheral arterial pulse depends on the time interval between atrial and ventricular contractions. In a patient with rapid heart action, the presence of such variations is suggestive of ventricular tachycardia; with an equally rapid rate, an absence of variation of pulse strength suggests a supraventricular mechanism.

BISFERIENS PULSE. A bisferiens pulse is characterized by two systolic peaks, the percussion and tidal waves, separated by a distinct midsystolic dip; the peaks may be equal or either may be larger. This type of pulse may be detected most readily by palpation of the carotid and less commonly of the radial arteries. It occurs in conditions in which a large stroke volume is ejected rapidly from the left ventricle[44] and is observed most commonly in patients with pure aortic regurgitation (Fig. 3–24, p. 56) and with a combination of aortic regurgitation and stenosis; it may disappear as heart failure supervenes.

A bisferiens pulse is also noted in patients with *hypertrophic obstructive cardiomyopathy*[45, 46] (Figs. 3–23, p. 56, and 4–9, p. 69), but the bifid nature may only be recorded, not palpated; on palpation there may merely be a rapid upstroke. In these patients the initial prominent percussion wave is associated with rapid ejection of blood into the aorta during early systole, followed by a rapid decline as obstruction becomes manifest in midsystole and by a tidal (reflected) wave. The bisferiens pulse of hypertrophic obstructive cardiomyopathy must be distinguished from the anacrotic pulse palpable in some patients with pure aortic stenosis; in both groups of patients with obstruction to left ventricular outflow a double pulse may be palpable. However, in patients with fixed obstruction the pulse rises slowly and the tidal (second) wave is the higher of the two, while in hypertrophic obstructive cardiomyopathy, the pulse rises rapidly and the percussion (first) wave is dominant. In some patients with hypertrophic cardiomyopathy with no or little obstruction to left ventricular outflow, the arterial pulse is normal in the basal state, but obstruction and a bisferiens pulse can be elicited by means of the Valsalva maneuver or inhalation of amyl nitrite. Occasionally, a bisferiens pulse is observed in hyperkinetic circulatory states, and very rarely it occurs in normal individuals.

DICROTIC PULSE. Not to be confused with a bisferiens pulse, in which both peaks occur in systole, is a dicrotic pulse, in which the normally small wave that follows aortic valve closure (i.e., the dicrotic notch) is exaggerated and measures more than 50 per cent of the pulse pressure on direct pressure recordings and in which the dicrotic notch is low (i.e., near the diastolic pressure) (Fig. 3–25, p. 56). It may be present in normal hypotensive subjects with reduced peripheral resistance, as occurs in fever, and it may be elicited or exaggerated by inspiration or the inhalation of amyl nitrite. Rarely, a dicrotic pulse may be noted in healthy adolescents or young adults, but it usually occurs in conditions such as cardiac tamponade, severe heart failure, and hypovolemic shock, in which a low stroke volume is ejected into a soft elastic aorta. In these conditions the dicrotic pulse is due to a shrinkage of the systolic wave with preservation of the incisura. A dicrotic pulse is rarely present when systolic pressure exceeds 130 mm Hg.

PULSUS ALTERNANS. Mechanical alternans is a sign of severe depression of myocardial function (p. 1496). Although more readily recognized on sphygmomanometry, when the systolic pressure alternates by more than 20 mm Hg it can be detected by palpation of a peripheral (femoral or radial) pulse or by the recording of an indirect carotid pulse tracing (Fig. 3–26, p. 57). Palpation should be carried out with light pressure and with the patient's breath held in midexpiration to avoid the superimposition of respiratory variation on the amplitude of the pulse. Pulsus alternans is generally accompanied by alternation in the intensity of the Korotkoff sounds and occasionally by alternation in intensity of the heart sounds. Rarely, alternans is so marked that the weak beat is not perceived at all. Aortic regurgitation, systemic hypertension, and reducing venous return by head-tilting or nitroglycerin all exaggerate pulsus alternans and assist in its detection. Pulsus alternans, which is frequently precipitated by a premature ventricular contraction, is characterized by a regular rhythm and must be distinguished from pulsus bigeminus (see below), which is usually regularly irregular.

PULSUS BIGEMINUS. A bigeminal rhythm is caused by the occurrence of premature contractions, usually ventricular, occurring after every other beat and results in alternation of the strength of the pulse, which can be confused with pulsus alternans. However, in contrast to the latter, in which the rhythm is regular, in pulsus bigeminus the weak beat always follows the shorter interval. In normal persons or in patients with fixed obstruction to left ventricular outflow, the compensatory pause following a premature beat is followed by a stronger-than-normal pulse. However, in patients with hypertrophic obstructive cardiomyopathy, the postpremature ventricular contraction beat is weaker than normal because of increased obstruction to left ventricular outflow[47] (p. 1427).

PULSUS PARADOXUS. This is a reduction in the strength of the arterial pulse during inspiration or an exaggerated inspiratory fall in systolic pressure (more than 10 mm Hg during quiet breathing). When marked, i.e., an inspiratory reduction of pressure greater than 20 mm Hg, it can be detected by careful palpation of the radial or brachial arterial pulse; in some instances there is inspiratory disappearance of the pulse. Milder degrees of a paradoxical pulse can be readily detected on sphygmomanometry: the cuff is inflated to suprasystolic levels and is deflated slowly at a rate of about 2 mm Hg per heartbeat; the peak systolic pressure during expiration is noted. The cuff is then deflated even more slowly, and the pressure is again noted when Korotkoff sounds become audible throughout the respiratory cycle. Normally, the difference between the two pressures should not exceed 8 mm Hg during quiet respiration. (Pulsus alternans can also be detected by this maneuver by noting whether peak systolic pressure or the intensity of the Korotkoff sounds alternates when respiration is held.)

Pulsus paradoxus represents an exaggeration of the normal decline in systolic arterial pressure with inspiration, which results from the reduced left ventricular stroke volume and the transmission of negative intrathoracic pressure to the aorta. It is a frequent, indeed characteristic, finding in patients with cardiac tamponade (p. 1493), occurs less frequently (in about half) in patients with chronic constrictive pericarditis (p. 1501), and is also observed in patients with emphysema and bronchial asthma (who have wide respiratory swings of intrapleural pressure),[48] as well as in hypovolemic shock, pulmonary embolus, pregnancy, and extreme obesity. Aortic regurgitation tends to prevent the development of pulsus paradoxus despite the presence of cardiac tamponade. *Reversed* pulsus paradoxus (an inspiratory rise in arterial pressure) may occur in hypertrophic obstructive cardiomyopathy.[49]

THE ARTERIAL PULSE IN VASCULAR DISEASE. Examination of the arterial pulses is helpful in the diagnosis of extracardiac obstructive arterial disease. Systematic bilateral palpation of the common carotid, brachial, radial, femoral, popliteal, dorsalis pedis, and posterior tibial vessels, as well as palpation of the abdominal aorta, should be part of every examination in patients suspected of having ischemic heart disease.[50] To diminish cold-induced vaso-

Anatomic Area(s)	Artery(s) Ausculted
Anterior Cervical	Internal/External Carotid
Supraclavicular	Subclavian
Infraclavicular	Axillary
Epigastrium	Celiac
Abdominal Upper Quadrants	Renal
Lumbar	
Umbilical	Aortoiliac Bifurcation
Inguinal	Common Femoral
Femoral Triangles	Superficial Femoral
Anteromedial Thighs	
Popliteal Fossae	Popliteal

FIGURE 2–9. Major anatomical regions for arterial bruit auscultation. (From Kurtz, K. J.: Dynamic vascular auscultation. Am. J. Med. *76*:1067, 1984.)

constriction, peripheral pulses should be palpated after the patient has been in a warm room for at least 20 minutes.[51] Absent or weak peripheral pulses usually signify obstruction, but the dorsalis pedis and posterior tibial arteries may be absent in approximately 2 per cent of normal persons because they pursue an abnormal course. Arterial bruits should be searched for by examination of specific anatomical sites (Fig. 2–9). When the lumen diameter is reduced by approximately 50 per cent, a soft early systolic bruit is heard; as the obstruction becomes more severe, the bruit becomes high-pitched, louder, and longer. With approximately 80 per cent diameter reduction it spills into early diastole, but it disappears with very severe stenosis or complete occlusion. Arterial bruits are augmented by elevations of cardiac output (e.g., as occurs in anemia), by poor development of collaterals, and augmented arterial outflow (as occurs in regional exercise).

EXAMINATION OF THE HEART

INSPECTION

The cardiac examination proper should commence with inspection of the chest, which can best be accomplished with the examiner standing at the foot of the bed or examining table. Respirations—their frequency, regularity, and depth—as well as the relative effort required during inspiration and expiration, should be noted (p. 479). Simultaneously, one should search for cutaneous abnormalities, such as spider nevi (seen in hepatic cirrhosis and Osler-Weber-Rendu disease). Dilation of veins on the anterior chest wall with caudal flow suggests obstruction of the superior vena cava, while cranial flow occurs in patients with obstruction of the inferior vena cava. Precordial prominence is most striking if cardiac enlargement developed before puberty, but it may also be present, although to a lesser extent, in patients in whom cardiomegaly developed in adult life, after the period of thoracic growth.[52, 53]

A heavy muscular thorax, contrasting with less developed lower extremities, suggests coarctation of the aorta, in which visible collateral arteries may be present in the axillae and along the lateral chest wall. The upper portion of the thorax exhibits symmetrical bulging in children with stiff lungs in whom the inspiratory effort is increased. An anterior bulge in the area of the manubrium in a child suggests pulmonary hypertension. A "shield chest" is a broad chest in which the angle between the manubrium and the body of the sternum is greater than normal and is associated with widely separated nipples; it is frequently observed in the Turner and Noonan syndromes. Careful note should be made of other deformities of the thoracic cage, such as *kyphoscoliosis,* which may be responsible for cor pulmonale (p. 1610); *ankylosing spondylitis,* sometimes associated with aortic regurgitation (p. 1717); and *pectus carinatum* (pigeon chest), which may be associated with Marfan syndrome but does not directly affect cardiovascular function.

Pectus excavatum, a condition in which the sternum is displaced posteriorly, is commonly observed in Marfan syndrome, homocystinuria, Ehlers-Danlos syndrome, Hunter-Hurler syndrome (Chap. 54), and a small fraction of patients with mitral valve prolapse (p. 1047). This thoracic deformity rarely compresses the heart or elevates the systemic and pulmonary venous pressures, and the signs of heart disease are more often apparent rather than real. Displacement of the heart into the left thorax, prominence of the pulmonary artery, and a parasternal midsystolic murmur all may falsely suggest the presence of organic heart disease. It may be associated with palpitation, tachycardia, fatigue, mild dyspnea, and some impairment of cardiac function.[54] Lack of normal thoracic kyphosis, i.e., the *straight back* syndrome,[1] is often associated with expiratory splitting of the second heart sound, a parasternal midsystolic murmur, and enlargement of the pulmonary artery on x-ray; therefore, it may be confused with atrial septal defect.[55] It is frequently associated with mitral valve prolapse and/or a bicuspid aortic valve.[56]

Cardiovascular pulsations should be looked for on the entire chest but specifically in the regions of the cardiac apex, the left parasternal region, and the third left and second right intercostal spaces. Prominent pulsations in these areas suggest enlargement of the left ventricle, right ventricle, pulmonary artery, and aorta, respectively. A thrusting apex exceeding 2 cm in diameter suggests left ventricular enlargement; systolic retraction of the apex may be visible in constrictive pericarditis. Normally, cardiac pulsations are not visible lateral to the midclavicular line; when present there, they signify cardiac enlargement unless there is thoracic deformity or congenital absence of the pericardium. Shaking of the entire precordium with each heartbeat may occur in patients with severe valvular regurgitation, large left-to-right shunts, complete AV block, hypertrophic obstructive cardiomyopathy, and various hyperkinetic states (Chap. 25). Aortic aneurysms may produce visible pulsations of one of the sternoclavicular joints of the right anterior thoracic wall.

PALPATION (Table 2–2)

Pulsations of the heart and great vessels that are transmitted to the chest wall are best appreciated when the examiner is positioned on the right side of a supine patient. In order to palpate the movements of the heart and great vessels, the examiner should utilize the fingertips or the area just proximal thereto. Precordial movements should be timed by using the simultaneously palpated carotid pulse or auscultated heart sounds.[57] The examination should be carried out with the chest completely exposed and elevated to 30 degrees, both with the patient supine and in the partial left lateral decubitus positions; the latter increases the amplitude of the left ventricular impulse. Rotating the patient into the left lateral decubitus position with the left arm elevated over the head causes the heart to move laterally and increases the palpability of both normal and pathological thrusts of the left ventricle. Indeed, it converts the normal systolic retraction of the apex to an outward expansion. Obese, muscular, emphysematous, and elderly persons may have weak or undetectable cardiac pulsations in the absence of cardiac abnormality, while thoracic deformities (e.g., kyphoscoliosis, pectus excavatum) can alter the pulsations transmitted to the chest wall. In the course of cardiac palpation, precordial tenderness may be detected; this important finding (p. 1319)

TABLE 2–2 CHARACTERISTICS OF PRECORDIAL MOTION IN VARIOUS CARDIAC ABNORMALITIES

Aortic Regurgitation	Atrial Septal Defect	Congestive Cardiomyopathy	Coronary Artery Disease
Apex impulse hyperdynamic in mild to moderate AR Severe AR: LV dilatation results in sustained impulse which is displaced laterally and downward (especially chronic AR) Systolic retraction medial to PMI Palpable *a* wave may be present	Hyperdynamic parasternal impulse PA impulse may be present RV impulse may be sustained if pulmonary hypertension is present and occasionally with large L to R shunt without elevated PA pressure	Sustained and displaced LV impulse, usually felt over 2 interspaces Palpable *a* wave (S_4) and S_3 common Parasternal lift, midsystolic bulge common	Usually normal at rest unless prior MI Palpable S_4 in left decubitus position Ectopic LV bulge thrust if dyssynergy or LV aneurysm. May have transient abnormalities (e.g., bulge, heave) during acute infarction or attack of angina
Hypertrophic Cardiomyopathy	**Mitral Regurgitation**	**Mitral Stenosis**	**Valvar Aortic Stenosis**
Systolic thrill superior, medial to apex impulse Vigorous LV apical impulse, often sustained Large palpable *a* wave, especially in left decubitus position Occasional mid- or late systolic bulge—"triple ripple"	Apical systolic thrill in severe MR Apex impulse hyperdynamic Severe and/or chronic MR: apex is displaced laterally, sustained with amplitude Can have late parasternal impulse with severe MR without pulmonary hypertension Parasternal (RV) heave if significant pulmonary hypertension S_3 visible and palpable if severe MR S_4 palpable with acute onset MR	Small or impalpable apex impulse but S_1 typically palpable Opening snap palpable medial to apex Apical diastolic thrill in left decubitus position Parasternal lift is common; suggests pulmonary hypertension at rest or with effort	Systolic thrill—aortic area, 2 LICS. Or occasionally at apex Sustained and forceful LV apical impulse Little lateral (leftward) displacement of apex unless LV dilatation has occurred Palpable *a* wave (S_4) is common and indicates severe aortic obstruction

AR = aortic regurgitation; LV = left ventricular; PA = pulmonary artery; RV = right ventricle; MI = myocardial infarction; MR = mitral regurgitation; L to R = left to right. (Reproduced with permission from Abrams, J.: Examination of the precordium. Primary Cardiol. 8:156–158, 1982.)

may result from trauma, costochondritis, or Tzietse's syndrome and may be an important indication that chest pain is not due to myocardial ischemia.

THE LEFT VENTRICLE. The *apex beat*, also referred to as the cardiac impulse and the apical thrust, is usually produced by left ventricular contraction and is the lowest and most lateral point on the chest at which the cardiac impulse can be appreciated; normally it is medial and superior to the intersection of the left midclavicular line and the fifth intercostal space. Although it may not be palpable in the supine position in as many as half of all normal subjects more than 50 years of age, it can usually be felt in the left lateral decubitus position. Displacement of the apex beat lateral to the midclavicular line or more than 10 cm lateral to the midsternal line is a sensitive but not specific indicator of left ventricular enlargement. However, when the patient is in the left lateral decubitus position a palpable apical impulse which has a diameter of more than 3 cm is an accurate sign of left ventricular enlargement.[58] Thoracic deformities—particularly scoliosis, straight back, and pectus excavatum—can result in the lateral displacement of a normal-sized heart. Although the apex beat is also often the point of maximal impulse (PMI), this is not always the case, since the pulsations produced by other structures, e.g., an enlarged right ventricle, a dilated pulmonary artery, or an aneurysm of the aorta, may be more powerful than the apex beat.

The apex cardiogram (p. 57), which traces the movement of the chest wall, often represents the pulsation of the entire left ventricle, not only the movement of the apex itself. Therefore, its contour differs from what is perceived on palpation of the apex or what is recorded by the kinetocardiogram, a device in which the motion of specific points on the chest wall are recorded relative to a fixed point in space,[59] and which therefore presents a more faithful graphic registration of the movements of the palpating finger on the chest wall.

Systolic Motion. During isovolumetric contraction, the heart normally rotates counterclockwise (as one faces the patient), and the lower anterior portion of the left ventricle strikes the anterior chest wall, causing a brief outward motion followed by retraction of the left ventricle and the adjacent chest wall during ejection (Fig. 2–10). The segment of the left ventricle responsible for the apex beat is usually medial to the actual cardiac apex, identified on radiological or angiographic examination. For timing purposes it is useful to correlate pulsations while simultaneously listening to heart sounds; a convenient way to do this is to correlate the observed motion of the stethoscope, placed lightly at the apex, with the auscultatory events.

The peak outward motion of the apex impulse is brief and occurs simultaneously with, or just after, aortic valve opening; then the left ventricular apex moves inward. In asthenic persons, in patients with mild left ventricular enlargement, and in subjects with a normal left ventricle but an augmented stroke volume, as occurs in anxiety and other hyperkinetic states, mild mitral or aortic regurgitation, the cardiac impulse may be overactive but with a normal contour; i.e., the outward thrust during systole is exaggerated in amplitude, but it is not sustained during ejection. With moderate or severe left ventricular enlargement and/or dysfunction, the outward systolic thrust persists throughout ejection, often lasting up to the second heart sound (Figs. 2–10, 2–11, and 2–12), and this motion may be accompanied by retraction of the left parasternal region. This rocking motion can often be appreciated by placing the index finger of one hand on the apex beat and that of the other hand in the parasternal region and by observing the simultaneous outward motion of the former with retraction of the latter. The left ventricular heave or lift, which is more prominent in left ventricular dilatation than in concentric hypertrophy, is characterized by a sustained outward movement of an area that is larger than the normal apex, i.e., more than 2 cm by 2 cm. In patients with ischemic heart disease a definitively sustained apex beat is usually associated with a reduced ejection fraction.[60] An *aneurysm of the left ventricle* also produces a larger-than-normal area of pulsation of the left ventricular apex. Alternatively, it may produce a sustained systolic bulge several centimeters superior to the left ventricular impulse. In left ventricular pressure overload with normal ventricular function the left ventricular impulse is prolonged and

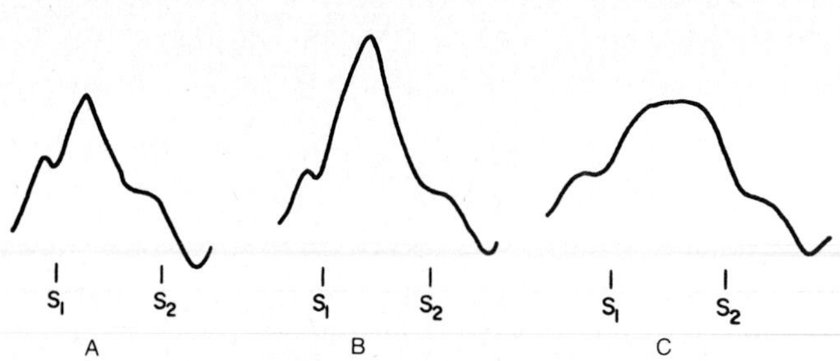

FIGURE 2–10. Major types of precordial motion: (*A*) Normal, (*B*) Hyperdynamic, and (*C*) Sustained. S_1 and S_2 represent the first and second heart sounds, respectively. (From Abrams, J.: Precordial palpation. *In* Horwitz, L. D., and Groves, B. M. [eds.]: Signs and Symptoms in Cardiology. Philadelphia, J. B. Lippincott, 1985, p. 158.)

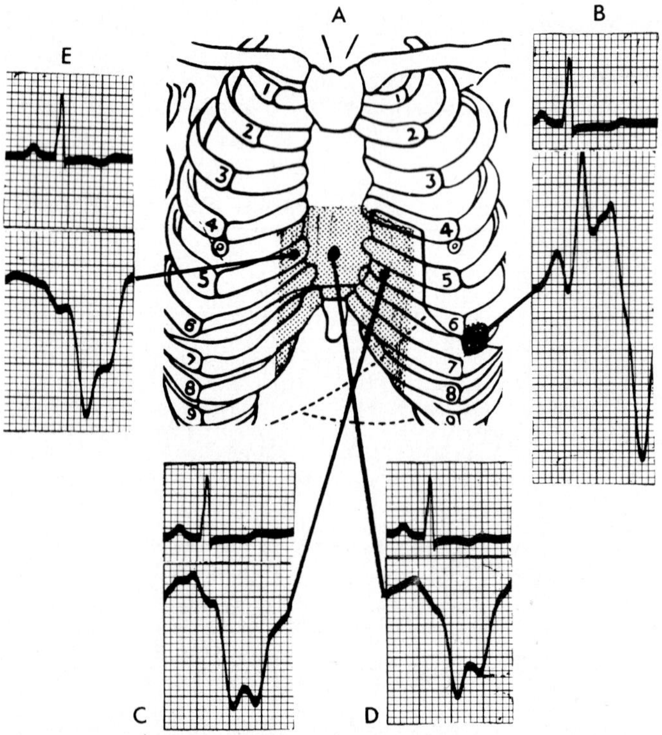

FIGURE 2–11. A large area of systolic retraction is indicated on the chest wall diagram (*A*) by light shading. Graphs taken from three points of this area (*C, D,* and *E*) show a sweeping downward movement during systole as evidence of retraction. The apex beat, felt in the 6th intercostal space, is indicated by an area of heavy shading. A graph of the apical thrust (*B*) shows a sustained upward movement, indicative of a left ventricular overload. The patient was a 40-year-old man with marked rheumatic aortic regurgitation. (From Dressler, W.: Clinical Aids in Cardiac Diagnosis. New York, 1970, p. 83, by permission of Grune and Stratton.)

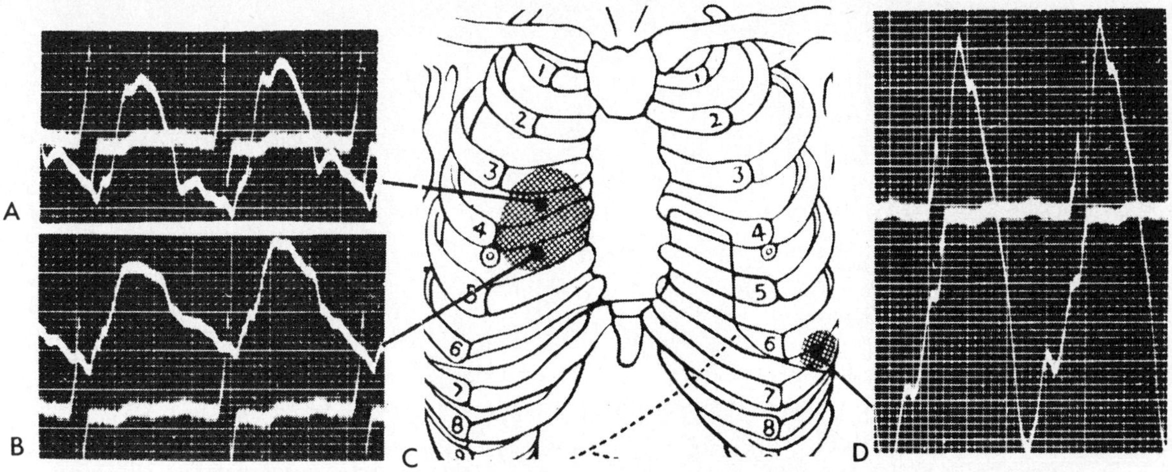

FIGURE 2–12. Diagram of the anterior wall (*C*) showing two areas of heaving pulsation (indicated by heavy shading). The area on the left side of the chest represents the apical thrust of a hypertrophied ventricle, as is shown on a graph (*D*). The curve rises 0.05 sec after onset of QRS and forms a broad, high peak during systole. Another area of systolic outward movement is present on the right side of the chest. Two recordings taken from this area (*A* and *B*) show curves that differ distinctly from that of the apical thrust. They rise 0.12 sec after QRS and resemble an arterial pulse. The pulsation on the right half of the chest was caused by a dissecting aneurysm of the ascending aorta. (From Dressler, W.: Clinical Aids in Cardiac Diagnosis. New York, 1970, p. 91, by permission of Grune and Stratton.)

forceful. In patients with *left ventricular dyskinesia,* as occurs in acute myocardial ischemia or following myocardial infarction, there may be two distinct impulses separated from each other by several centimeters; alternatively, a mid- or late systolic bulge may be palpated. In *mitral stenosis* there may be a brief prominent apical tap owing to an accentuated first sound, which must be distinguished from the apical thrust of an enlarged left ventricle.

A double systolic outward thrust of the left ventricle is occasionally present in patients with prolapse of the mitral valve (Fig. 3–31, p. 59) and is characteristic of patients with hypertrophic obstructive cardiomyopathy (Fig. 3–30, p. 59) who also often exhibit a typical presystolic cardiac expansion, thus resulting in three separate outward movements of the chest wall during each cardiac cycle.[45] In *aortic regurgitation* the apex exhibits a prominent outward thrust, but this may be followed by systolic retraction of the anterior chest wall as a consequence of the large stroke volume that evacuates the thorax during systole (Fig. 2–11). *Constrictive pericarditis* (as well as nonconstricting adherent pericarditis) is characterized by systolic retraction of the chest, particularly of the ribs in the left axilla (Broadbent's sign) (Fig. 3–33, p. 60). This inward movement results from interference with the descent of the base of the heart and the compensatory exaggerated motion of the free wall of the left ventricle during ventricular ejection.[61] When left ventricular filling is very rapid during early diastole, outward movement of the chest wall may be particularly prominent and mistaken for systole, but it is usually accompanied by a third heart sound (Fig. 3–28, p. 58). A hypokinetic apical impulse is associated with a variety of low cardiac output states, including those secondary to hypovolemia, constrictive pericarditis, and pericardial effusion.

Diastolic Motion. The outward motion of the apex characteristic of rapid left ventricular diastolic filling is accentuated when the inflow of blood into the left ventricle is accelerated, as occurs, for example, in mitral regurgitation (Fig. 3–28, p. 58), when the volume of the left ventricle is increased or its function is impaired.[57] This motion is the mechanical equivalent of and occurs simultaneously with a third heart sound. Prominent early diastolic left ventricular filling in constrictive pericarditis may be palpable.

When the atrial contribution to ventricular filling is augmented, as occurs in patients with reduced left ventricular compliance associated with concentric left ventricular hypertrophy, myocardial ischemia, and myocardial fibrosis, a presystolic pulsation (usually accompanying a fourth heart sound) is palpable, resulting in a double outward movement of the left ventricular impulse (Figs. 3–29, p. 59, and 4–4, p. 67). This presystolic expansion is most readily discernible during expiration, when the patient is in the left lateral decubitus position, and it can be confirmed by detecting the motion of the stethoscope placed over the left ventricular impulse or by observing the motion of the tip of a pencil or tongue depressor when the proximal portion is placed near the left ventricular impulse. It can be enhanced by sustained hand grip. Presystolic expansion of the left ventricle is usually associated with marked elevation of left ventricular enddiastolic (rather than early diastolic) pressure, and in contrast to prominence of early diastolic filling, in patients without ischemic heart disease it is usually associated with normal or almost normal left ventricular function.[57] In patients with ischemic heart disease presystolic pulsation is usually associated with moderate left ventricular dysfunction.[60] Presystolic expansion of the right ventricle occurs in right ventricular hypertrophy and pulmonary hypertension. It may be appreciated by subxiphoid palpation of the right ventricle during inspiration.

THE RIGHT VENTRICLE. A palpable anterior systolic movement (replacing systolic retraction) in the left parasternal region (Fig. 2–13*A*), best felt by the proximal palm, usually represents *right ventricular enlargement,* which, in the absence of associated left ventricular enlargement, may be accompanied by reciprocal systolic retraction of the apex. Exaggerated motion of the entire parasternal area i.e., a hyperdynamic impulse with normal contour, usually reflects increased right ventricular recoil due to augmented stroke volume, as occurs in patients with atrial septal defect or tricuspid regurgitation, while a sustained left parasternal outward thrust reflects right ventricular hypertrophy due to pressure overload, as occurs in pulmonic stenosis or pulmonary hypertension. With marked right ventricular enlargement, this chamber occupies the apex and the left ventricle is displaced posteriorly. When both ventricles are enlarged, both the left parasternal and

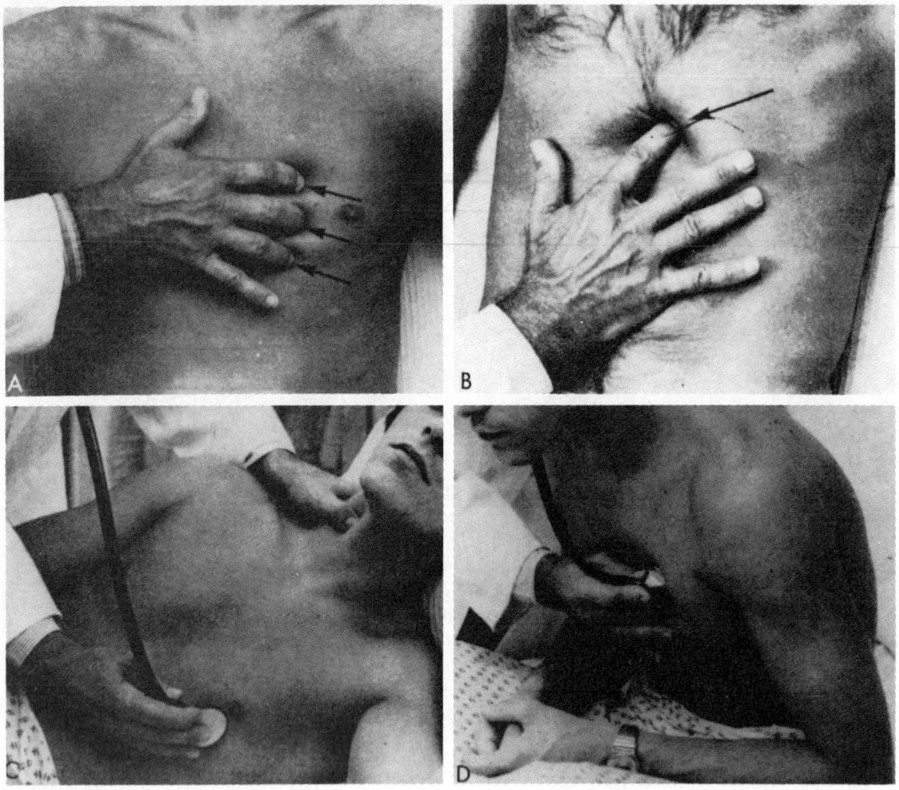

FIGURE 2–13. *A,* Palpation of the anterior wall of the right ventricle by applying the tips of three fingers in the third, fourth, and fifth interspaces, left sternal edge, during full held exhalation. Patient is supine with the trunk elevated 30 degrees. *B,* Palpation of the inferior wall of the right ventricle in the epigastrium. The flat of the hand is directed upward and toward the left shoulder. The tip of the index finger (arrow) palpates the right ventricle as it descends during full held inspiration. The patient is supine with trunk elevated 30 degrees. *C,* The stethoscope is applied to the cardiac apex while the patient lies in a partial left lateral decubitus position. The examiner's free left hand is used to palpate the carotid artery for timing purposes. *D,* The soft-high frequency early diastolic murmur of either aortic regurgitation or pulmonary hypertensive pulmonary regurgitation is best elicited by applying the stethoscopic diaphragm very firmly to the mid-left sternal edge. The patient leans forward with breath held in full exhalation. (From Perloff, J. K. [ed.]: Physical Examination of the Heart and Circulation. Philadelphia, W. B. Saunders Company, 1982.)

the apical areas may rise with systole, but an area of systolic retraction between them can sometimes be appreciated. In patients with emphysema or obesity, an enlarged right ventricle is sometimes detected most readily in the subxiphoid region by palpating the epigastrium and pointing the fingers upward (Fig. 2–13*B*). With marked isolated right ventricular enlargement, the heart may rotate in a clockwise manner, and the right ventricle may form the cardiac apex, producing findings that may be confused with those of left or biventricular enlargement. When acute myocardial ischemia or myocardial infarction causes dyskinetic movement of the ventricular septum, there may be a transient left parasternal impulse not caused by right ventricular enlargement.

Pulmonary hypertension and/or increased pulmonary blood flow frequently produces a prominent systolic pulsation of the pulmonary artery in the second intercostal space just to the left of the sternum. This pulsation is often associated with a prominent left parasternal impulse, reflecting right ventricular enlargement, and a palpable shock synchronous with the second heart sound, reflecting forceful closure of the pulmonic valve.

LEFT ATRIUM. An enlarged left atrium or a large posterior left ventricular aneurysm can make right ventricular pulsations more prominent by displacing the right ventricle anteriorly against the left parasternal area, and in severe mitral regurgitation an expanding left atrium may be responsible for marked left parasternal movement, even in the absence of right ventricular hypertrophy. The left atrial lift, which is transmitted through the right ventricle, commences and terminates after the left ventricular thrust. It can be appreciated by placing the index finger of one hand at the left ventricular apex and the index finger of the other in the left parasternal region; the movement of the latter finger begins and ends slightly later than that of the former. While this difference in timing may be difficult to appreciate on palpation, particularly when the heart rate is rapid, recordings of chest wall motion in severe chronic mitral regurgitation demonstrate a delayed fall in the left lower precordium compared to the cardiac apex (Fig. 4–16, p. 73). Outward movement of the chest wall that is more marked to the right than to the left of the sternum is usually due to aneurysm of the aorta (Fig. 2–8) or to marked enlargement of the right atrium.

AORTA. Enlargement or aneurysm of the ascending aorta or aortic arch may cause visible or palpable systolic pulsations of the right or left sternoclavicular joint; they may also cause a systolic impulse in the suprasternal notch or the first or second right ventricular space.[1]

PALPABLE SOUNDS. Valve closure, if abnormally forceful, can be appreciated as a tapping sensation. It occurs most prominently in the third left intercostal space in patients with pulmonary hypertension (pulmonic valve closure), in the second right intercostal space in patients with systemic hypertension (aortic valve closure), and at the cardiac apex in patients with mitral stenosis (mitral valve closure). Occasionally, in congenital aortic stenosis, aortic ejection sounds can be palpated at the cardiac apex; ejection sounds originating in a dilated aorta or pulmonary artery can sometimes be felt at the base of the heart.[61]

THRILLS. The flat of the hand or the fingertips usually best appreciate thrills, vibratory sensations which are palpable manifestations of loud, harsh murmurs having low-frequency components.[62] Since the vibrations must be quite intense before they are felt, far more information can be obtained from the auscultatory than from the palpatory features of heart murmurs. High-pitched murmurs such as those produced by valvular regurgitation, even when loud, are not usually associated with thrills.

PERCUSSION. Palpation is far more helpful than is percussion in determining cardiac size. However, in the absence of an apical beat, as occurs in patients with pericardial effusion, or in some patients with congestive cardiomyopathy, heart failure, and marked displacement of a hypokinetic apical beat, the left border of the heart can be outlined by means of percussion. Also, percussion of dullness in the right lower parasternal area may, in some instances, aid in the detection of a greatly enlarged right atrium. Percussion is of aid in determining visceral situs, i.e., in ascertaining the side on which the heart, stomach, and liver are located. When the heart is in the right chest, but the abdominal viscera are located normally, congenital heart disease is usually present. When both the heart and abdominal viscera are in the opposite side of the chest (situs inversus), congenital heart disease is uncommon.

CARDIAC AUSCULTATION

GENERAL PRINCIPLES. Vibrations on the surface of the chest set into motion a column of air that is collected and conducted to the ear by the stethoscope.[63–66] Since high frequencies are damped by a large volume of air between the chest and the ear, the most effective stethoscopes are made of plastic tubing 10 to 12 inches in length with an internal diameter of ⅛ inch; the thicker the tubing, the more room noise is eliminated. The stethoscope should have two chest pieces: a shallow bell and a stiff diaphragm. Since their ability to collect sound is proportional to their diameter, they should be as large as is practical, without impairing contact with the chest wall. A small bell and diaphragm are desirable for examining children and thin patients. The ear pieces should be large and comfortable, with their axes parallel to the long axes of the external auditory canals. Air leaks—anywhere between the patient's chest and the examiner's auditory canal—are the greatest source of auscultatory difficulties, and must be avoided.

High-frequency sounds, such as the first and second heart sounds, and systolic clicks and high-pitched murmurs, such as those of valvular regurgitation, are best appreciated by using the diaphragm, which has a relatively high natural frequency and damps out low frequencies ($<$ 300 Hz), particularly when firm pressure is applied to the stethoscope. In order to detect low frequencies (30 to 150 Hz), the bell of the stethoscope should be applied to the chest with slight pressure, just enough to prevent detection of room noise. When the bell is applied too tightly, the skin under the bell forms a diaphragm, defeating the purpose of the bell by damping out low-frequency sounds. Third and fourth heart sounds and diastolic murmurs originating from the mitral and tricuspid valves, which are usually low pitched, are best heard through the bell.

Cardiac auscultation should be carried out in a quiet room with the patient comfortable and the chest exposed.[67] Ordinarily the examiner should be on the patient's right side, and the patient should be examined routinely in three positions: supine, sitting, and left lateral decubitus (Figs. 2–13*C* and *D*). Occasionally, the effects of squatting, standing, or the prone position (p. 37) and other physiological and pharmacological interventions are studied (p. 38). Although the principal areas of cardiac auscultation (Fig. 2–14) are the second right interspace ("aortic" area), the second left interspace ("pulmonic" area), the fourth interspace adjacent to the left sternal border ("tricuspid" area), and the cardiac apex ("mitral" area), auscultation should not be limited to these sites, since important findings are sometimes present in other locations, such as the right parasternal region, axilla, neck, and interscapular regions. For example, auscultation just above the sternoclavicular joints is best for detecting a venous hum. Murmurs produced by pulmonary arteriovenous fistula, bronchial collateral vessels, and systemic arterial collaterals in patients with coarctation of the aorta as well as murmurs of pulmonary branch stenosis may be heard over the posterior chest. In some patients with pulmonary emphysema, heart sounds are best heard in the epigastrium.

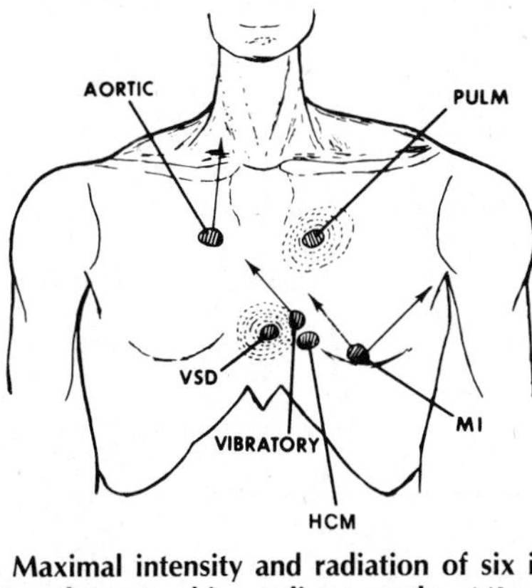

FIGURE 2–14. Maximal intensity and radiation of six isolated systolic murmurs. HCM = hypertrophic cardiomyopathy; MI = mitral incompetence; PULM = pulmonary; VSD = ventricular septal defect. (From Barlow, J B.: Perspectives on the Mitral Valve. Philadelphia, F. A. Davis, 1987, p. 140.)

When the heart rate is rapid, it may be difficult to identify the phase of the cardiac cycle and the resultant auscultatory events. Levine and Harvey have recommended the technique of first listening at the apex, where the first heart sound is normally the loudest sound audible and can usually be readily identified because it occurs just before the carotid arterial upstroke, and then "inching up" the chest along the left sternal border, using the diaphragm and bell alternately.[68] This allows correct identification of systole and diastole at other precordial sites. Auscultation should be carried out during normal quiet respiration, during normal held expiration, and during forced expiration; the effects of variations in respiration and posture on auscultatory findings should be determined.

It is desirable to employ a systematic plan for cardiac auscultation, listening in sequence and selectively to the first heart sound (S_1), the second heart sound (S_2), the systolic interval, and then the diastolic interval. An attempt should be made to listen to each component separately. The intensity, quality, and splitting of each of the sounds should be determined and the effects of respiration on the splitting of the second heart sound ascertained.[69–75]

Heart Sounds

(See also pp. 43 to 53)

FIRST AND SECOND HEART SOUNDS. S_1 occurs just before the palpable arterial upstroke in the carotid pulse and can be distinguished from S_2, which occurs immediately *after* the peak of the carotid pulse. S_1 is often heard best medial to the apex at the lower sternal border. Its intensity is increased in mitral stenosis, left atrial myxoma,[76] holosystolic mitral valve prolapse, short P-R interval, and any condition that causes tachycardia or unusually vigorous ventricular contraction. The loudness of S_1 is diminished or absent with P-R prolongation, fibrosis or calcification of the mitral valve, severe left ventricular failure, left bundle branch block, and mitral regurgitation (not due to prolapse). Wide splitting of S_1 with an audible delayed tricuspid component is best heard in inspiration and at the lower left sternal border. It may occur in tricuspid stenosis, Ebstein's anomaly, and right bundle branch block. Narrow splitting of S_1 is a normal finding, heard best at the lower left sternal border.

S_2 is ordinarily most readily audible in the second or third right and left intercostal spaces along the sternal borders. S_2 is higher pitched than S_1, heard best with the diaphragm of the stethoscope, and is split into two components, the aortic (A_2) and pulmonic (P_2) closure sounds, because of a synchronous closure of these two valves.[71] P_2 is normally softer than A_2 and is less widely transmitted. Splitting of S_2 is most readily assessed with the patient supine, first during normal respiration and then during slow, deep respiration (Figs. 2–15 and 2–16, Table 2–3). The intensity of A_2 is dependent on the anatomical relationship between the aorta and the anterior chest wall as well as on the level of the aortic pressure. It is loud in systemic hypertension, with a "tambour" quality, and in congenital malformations in which the aorta arises anteriorly. The intensity of P_2 varies directly with the level of pulmonary artery pressure and the degree of dilatation of the pulmonary artery. P_2 is not normally audible at the apex; when it is audible, pulmonary hypertension is usually present. Stenosis of the aortic and pulmonic valve causes decreased intensity of A_2 and P_2 respectively.

EJECTION SOUNDS. These usually coincide with the full opening of the semilunar valves, are high-pitched and clicking, and are heard best with the diaphragm of the stethoscope. They are caused by opening of the stenotic semilunar valves or from the ejection of blood into the aorta or pulmonary arteries. Aortic ejection sounds are heard best in the second right interspace and at the apex and are not notably affected by respiration, while pulmonic ejection sounds are heard best in the second left interspace and often diminish in intensity during inspiration. Mid- to

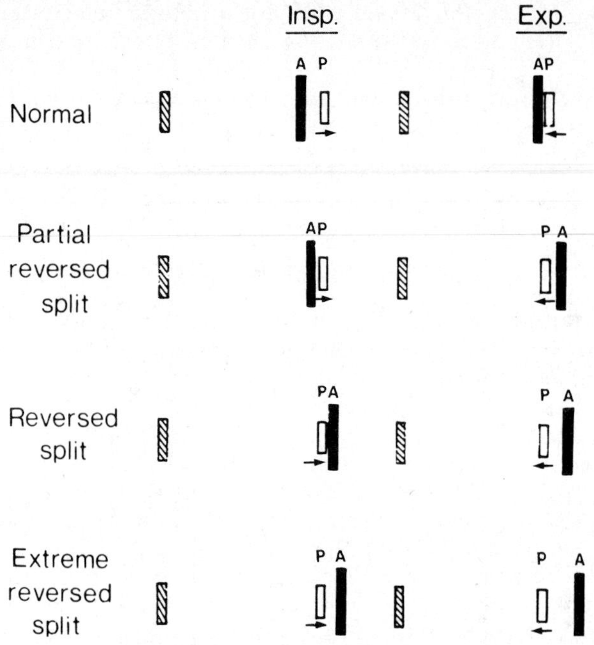

FIGURE 2–16. Reversed and partially reversed splitting of the second heart sound. Arrows indicate the direction of the movement of P during inspiration and expiration. (From Barlow, J. B.: Perspectives on the Mitral Valve. Philadelphia, F. A. Davis, 1987, p. 24.)

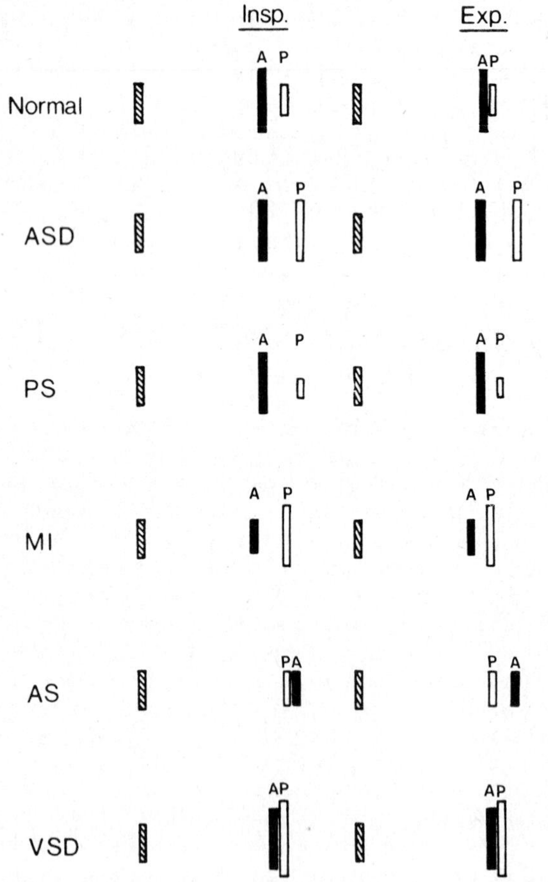

FIGURE 2–15. Diagrammatic representation of normal and abnormal patterns in the respiratory variation of the second heart sound. The height of the bars are proportional to the sound intensity. A = aortic component; P = pulmonary component; ASD = atrial septal defect; PS = pulmonary stenosis; MI = mitral incopetence; AS = aortic stenosis; VSD = ventricular septal defect. (From Barlow, J. B.: Perspectives on the Mitral Valve. Philadelphia, F. A. Davis, 1987, p. 23.)

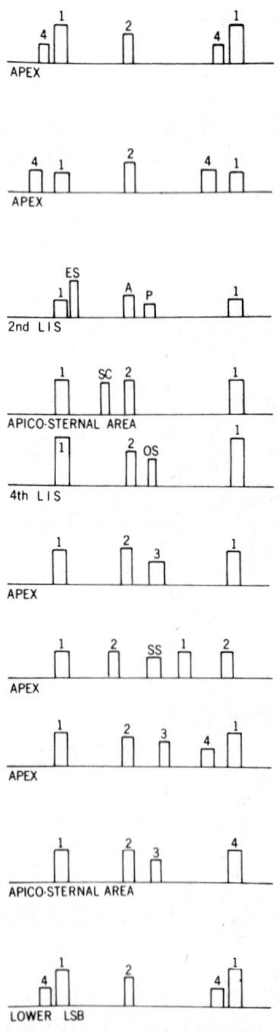

Left-sided fourth heart sound. Louder in expiration. Systemic hypertension, coronary artery disease, myocardiopathy, aortic stenosis.

Left-sided fourth heart sound with prolonged AV conduction. Faint first heart sound.

Pulmonic ejection sound (ES) in mild pulmonary valvular stenosis. Louder in expiration. Delayed pulmonic second heart sound.

Systolic click (SC).

Opening snap (OS) of the mitral valve in mitral stenosis.

Left-sided third heart sound (ventricular filling sound). Left ventricular failure. Mitral regurgitation.

Summation sound (SS) with ventricular failure plus rapid heart rate.

Fourth and third heart sound (quadruple rhythm).

Constrictive pericarditis. Third heart sound occupies a position between an opening snap and the usual third heart sound.

Right-sided fourth heart sound. Louder in inspiration. Pulmonary hypertension, large left-to-right shunt at atrial level.

FIGURE 2–17. Interpretation of extra sounds. 1, 2, 3, and 4, refer to the first, second, third, and fourth sounds. A and P refer to the aortic and pulmonic valve closure sounds, respectively. LIS = left intercostal space; LSB = left sternal border. (From Ravin, A., et al.: Auscultation of the Heart. Chicago, Year Book Medical Publishers, 1977, p. 80.)

TABLE 2–3 CAUSES OF SPLITTING OF THE SECOND HEART SOUND

Delayed Pulmonic Closure
Delayed electrical activation of the right ventricle
Complete RBBB (proximal type)
Left ventricular paced beats
Left ventricular ectopic beats
Prolonged right ventricular mechanical systole
Acute massive pulmonary embolus
Pulmonary hypertension with right heart failure
Pulmonic stenosis with intact septum (moderate to severe)
Decreased impedance of the pulmonary vascular bed (increased hang-out)
Normotensive atrial septal defect
Idiopathic dilatation of the pulmonary artery
Pulmonic stenosis (mild)
Atrial septal defect, postoperative (70%)
Early Aortic Closure
Shortened left ventricular mechanical systole (LVET)
Mitral regurgitation
Ventricular septal defect
Reversed Splitting
Delayed Aortic Closure
Delayed electrical activation of the left ventricle
Complete LBBB (proximal type)
Right ventricular paced beats
Right ventricular ectopic beats
Prolonged left ventricular mechanical systole
Complete LBBB (peripheral type)
Left ventricular outflow tract obstruction
Hypertensive cardiovascular disease
Arteriosclerotic heart disease
Chronic ischemic heart disease
Angina pectoris
Decreased impedance of the systemic vascular bed (increased hang-out)
Poststenotic dilatation of the aorta secondary to aortic stenosis or insufficiency
Patent ductus arteriosus
Early Pulmonic Closure
Early electrical activation of the right ventricle
Wolff-Parkinson-White syndrome, type B

RBBB = right bundle-branch block; AES = audible expiratory splitting; LVET = left ventricular ejection time; LBBB = left bundle-branch block.

(Modified from Shaver, J. A., O'Toole, J. D.: The second heart sound: Newer concepts. Parts 1 and 2. Mod. Concepts Cardiovasc. Dis. *46*:7 and 13, 1977.)

late systolic clicks are heard in mitral valve prolapse occasionally in aortic regurgitation,[77] are of high frequency, and are also heard best with the diaphragm.

If more than two heart sounds are heard, it must be determined whether the extra sound occurs in systole or diastole, whether it is early or late, and whether it is high-pitched (such as a systolic click) or low-pitched (such as a third or fourth heart sound, i.e., S_3 or S_4) (Fig. 2–17). When two heart sounds are heard at the time of S_1, it is often difficult to differentiate between a split S_1, a combination of S_4 and S_1, and a combination of S_1 and an ejection click.[73] The S_4 is usually audible only at the apex and often in the left lateral decubitus position; it is low-pitched, associated with palpable presystolic distention of the left ventricle, and attenuated by increased pressure on the bell of the stethoscope. It is rarely heard at the lower left sternal border, where splitting of S_1 is most easily detected. The ejection click is usually louder than the second (tricuspid) component of a split S_1 and is often audible at the base of the heart, while splitting of S_1 is rarely heard in this area.

OPENING SNAPS. These sounds usually occur with mitral or tricuspid valves that are stenotic but mobile. Opening snaps are high-pitched and heard best through the diaphragm. It may be difficult to differentiate an opening snap from P_2 by clinical examination. However, the former radiates more widely and is often heard both at the apex and in the aortic area; P_2 also usually changes its relationship to A_2 during respiration, while an opening snap does not. Finally, the A_2–opening snap interval is usually longer (> 40 msec) than the A_2-P_2 interval. Opening snaps originating from the tricuspid valve frequently increase in intensity during inspiration.

THIRD AND FOURTH HEART SOUNDS. The diastolic sound during passive filling which occurs during the *y* descent of the atrial pressure pulse is termed the *third heart sound* (S_3), while the sound which occurs during ventricular filling caused by atrial contraction is called the *fourth heart sound* (S_4).[78] When S_3 and S_4 are abnormal, they are referred to as third or fourth heart sound *gallops*. Third and fourth heart sounds are low-pitched sounds which are intensified by the recumbent position and by exercise, such as a few sit-ups or sustained handgrip. Inspiration enhances third or fourth heart sounds originating from the right ventricle but has little detectable effect on such sounds originating from the left ventricle. At heart rates above 100 beats/min, when both S_3 and S_4 gallops are present they may fuse, producing a loud sound, a so-called *summation gallop* (Fig. 3–18, p. 52).

S_3 occurs as active ventricular relaxation (reflected in the decline in ventricular pressure) ends and passive filling (reflected in a diastolic rise in ventricular pressure) commences.[79] It appears to be caused by an early diastolic impact of the ventricle on the chest wall; it is intensified by rapid early diastolic filling, by an elevated atrial pressure, and by increased or abnormal diastolic distensibility of the ventricle. Third heart sounds may be audible in normal children and young adults. However, when they are heard in men over the age of 40 and women over 50, they are generally abnormal. The disappearance of a normal S_3 with age appears to result from a decrease in the rate of early ventricular filling and resulting deceleration.[80] S_3 is usually maximally audible at the apex, with the patient in the left lateral recumbent position and during expiration, and with the bell of the stethoscope. An S_3 originating from the right ventricle, due to tricuspid regurgitation or right ventricular failure, is heard best along the lower left sternal border.

Conditions causing ventricular diastolic overload with atrial hypertension are often responsible for an S_3 which is audible in states of increased cardiac output,[81] such as during the third trimester of pregnancy, after exertion, and in anxiety-related tachycardia (Table 2–4). It also occurs with impaired left ventricular function of any cause.[81a] In the presence of coronary artery disease, an S_3 strongly suggests left ventricular dyskinesia or aneurysm. In patients with aortic regurgitation, a third heart sound usually signifies a reduced ejection fraction and elevated end-systolic volume.[82] In patients with reduced cardiac reserve it correlates well with the response to digitalis.[83]

Healthy older adults rarely may have an S_4, but when heard in the young, this sound is usually abnormal. S_4 is probably caused by vibrations of the ventricular wall during the rapid influx of blood during atrial contraction and is best heard with the patient in the left lateral recumbent position and with the bell of the stethoscope gently applied to the chest; it is generally associated with an elevated ventricular enddiastolic pressure and a high ratio of left ventricular wall thickness-to-cavity diameter. As left ventricular compliance decreases, atrial systole becomes responsible for more than 25 per cent of ventricular filling, and an S_4 may become prominent. Vigorous atrial contraction is necessary to produce an audible S_4, which can be recorded phonocardiographically in about 50 per cent of normal adults, but it is extremely low in intensity and

TABLE 2–4 PHYSIOLOGICAL AND PATHOLOGICAL STATES WITH A THIRD AND FOURTH HEART SOUND

THIRD HEART SOUND
Physiological
- Children and young adults (<40 yr)

Pathological
- Hyperdynamic states
  - High outputs
  - Anemia
  - Thyrotoxicosis
  - Arteriovenous fistula
- Hypertrophic cardiomyopathy
- Regurgitant atrioventricular valve lesions
  - Mitral regurgitation
  - Tricuspid regurgitation
- Increase in end-systolic volume
  - Ventricular dysfunction
  - Left ventricle:
    - Congenital heart disease
    - Valvular disease
    - Systemic hypertension
    - Ischemic heart disease
    - Cardiomyopathy
  - Right ventricle:
    - Congenital heart disease
    - Valvular disease
    - Pulmonary hypertension
    - Right ventricular infarct
    - Cardiomyopathy
- Constrictive pericarditis

FOURTH HEART SOUND
Physiological
- Recordable but not audible

Pathological
- Left ventricular hypertrophy
  - Left ventricular outflow tract obstruction
  - Systemic hypertrophic cardiomyopathy
- Right ventricular hypertrophy
  - Right ventricular outflow tract obstruction
  - Pulmonic hypertension
  - Idiopathic hypertrophic cardiomyopathy (rarely)
- Ischemic heart disease
  - Angina
  - Acute myocardial infarction
  - Left ventricular dysfunction
- Hyperkinetic states
  - Anemia
  - Thyrotoxicosis
  - Arteriovenous fistula
- Acute valvular regurgitation
  - Acute mitral regurgitation
  - Acute aortic regurgitation
  - Acute tricuspid regurgitation
- Arrhythmia
  - Heart block
  - Atrial flutter

From Reddy, P. S., Salerni, R., and Shaver, J. A.: Normal and abnormal heart sounds in cardiac diagnosis. Part II. Diastolic sounds. Cur. Probl. Cardiol. *10*(4):26 and 44, 1985.

usually not audible. A distinctly audible, palpable S_4 is usually abnormal (Table 2–4). The common denominators with which it is associated are left ventricular hypertrophy, increased left ventricular enddiastolic pressure, some restriction to diastolic filling, and a high ratio of left ventricular wall thickness-to-cavity diameter. An S_4 is characteristic of aortic stenosis with a significant left ventricular-aortic pressure gradient, systemic hypertension, hypertrophic cardiomyopathy, ischemic heart disease, and acute mitral regurgitation. Reduced left ventricular compliance following myocardial infarction often results in an audible S_4. A right ventricular S_4 is common in pulmonary hypertension and pulmonary stenosis.

MURMURS AND OTHER ADVENTITIOUS SOUNDS

(See also Chap. 4)

Cardiac murmurs should be timed, and their length in the cardiac cycle and their shape, i.e., their intensity (or loudness) as a function of time, should be determined. Murmurs are classified as systolic (between S_1 and S_2) or diastolic (between S_2 and S_1) and continuous (enveloping S_2). They are subclassified as early, mid, late or pan (systolic or diastolic). Their shape is characterized as crescendo, decrescendo, or crescendo-decrescendo. The *intensity* of a murmur is determined by the quantity and velocity of blood flow across the sound-producing area, by its distance from the stethoscope, and by the transmission qualities of the tissue between the origin of the murmur and the stethoscope.[84] Murmurs are accentuated in thin persons and diminished in patients who are obese, in emphysema, and in the presence of pleural or pericardial fluid.[63] They are accentuated in hyperdynamic and reduced in hypodynamic states.

It is helpful to grade the intensity of murmurs; six grades, as described by Freeman and Levine, are commonly distinguished.[85] A *Grade 1/6* murmur is the faintest that can be detected, often only after close concentration and adjustment of the stethoscope. A *Grade 2/6* murmur

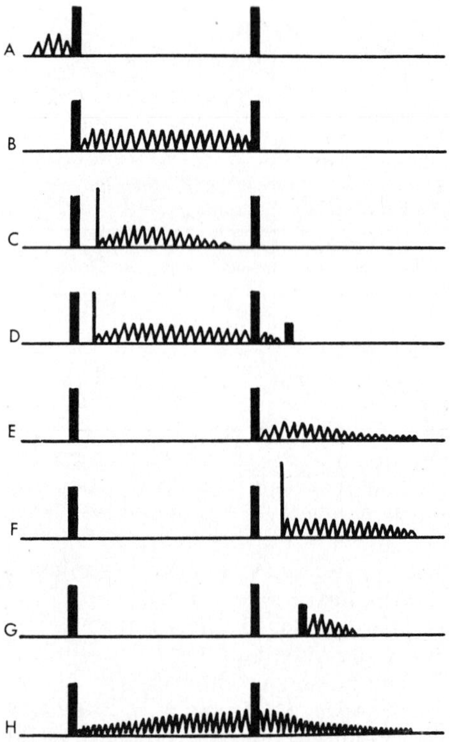

FIGURE 2–18. Diagram depicting principal heart murmurs:
A, Presystolic murmur of mitral or tricuspid stenosis.
B, Pansystolic murmur of mitral or tricuspid incompetence or of ventricular septal defect.
C, Aortic ejection murmur beginning with an ejection click and fading before the second heart sound.
D, Systolic murmur in pulmonic stenosis spilling through the aortic second sound, pulmonic valve closure being delayed.
E, Aortic pulmonary diastolic murmur.
F, Long diastolic murmur of mitral stenosis following the opening snap.
G, Short mid-diastolic inflow murmur following a third heart sound.
H, Continuous murmur of patent ductus arteriosus.
(From Wood, P.: Diseases of the Heart and Circulation. Philadelphia, J. B. Lippincott, 1968, p. 75.)

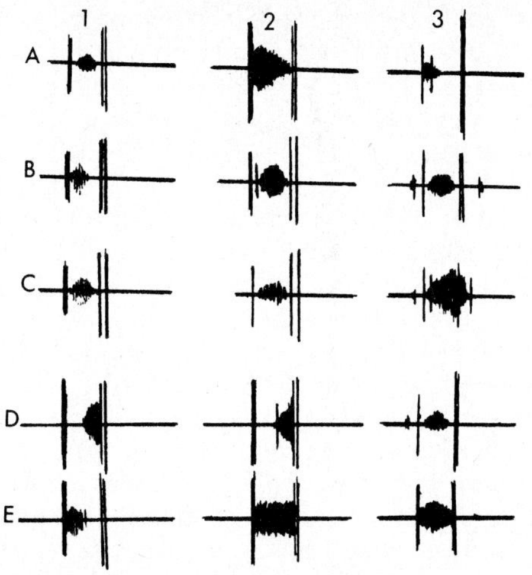

FIGURE 2–19. Sketches of various murmurs and heart sounds.

A–1, Short, midsystolic murmur, with normal aortic and pulmonic components of S_2—findings consistent with an innocent murmur.

A–2, Holosystolic murmur that decreases in the latter part of systole—a configuration observed in acute mitral regurgitation.

A–3, An ejection sound and a short early systolic murmur, plus accentuated, closely split S_2—consistent with pulmonary hypertension, as with Eisenmenger's ventricular septal defect.

B–1, Early to midsystolic murmur with vibratory component—typical of an innocent murmur.

B–2, An ejection sound followed by a diamond-shaped murmur and wide splitting of S_2 that may be present with atrial septal defect or mild pulmonic stenosis; an ejection sound is more likely with valvular pulmonic stenosis.

B–3, Crescendo-decrescendo systolic murmur, not holosystolic; S_3 and S_4 are present–findings consistent with mitral systolic murmur heard in congestive cardiomyopathy or coronary artery disease with papillary muscle dysfunction and cardic decompensation.

C–1, Longer, somewhat vibratory crescendo-decrescendo systolic murmur with wide splitting of S_2 sound. If S_2 becomes fused with expiration, atrial septal defect is less likely; if the remainder of the cardiovascular evaluation is normal, this finding is consistent with an innocent murmur.

C–2, Midsystolic murmur and wide splitting of S_2 that was "fixed"—findings typical of atrial septal defect.

C–3, Prolonged diamond-shaped systolic murmur masking A_2 with delayed P_2, S_4, and ejection sound—findings typical of valvular pulmonic stenosis of moderate severity.

D–1, Late apical systolic murmur of prolapsing mitral valve leaflet.

D–2, Systolic click-late apical systolic murmur of prolapsing mitral leaflet syndrome.

D–3, S_4 and midsystolic murmur consistent with mitral systolic murmur of cardiomyopathy or ischemic heart disease.

E–1, Early crescendo-decrescendo systolic murmur ending in midsystole consistent with innocent murmur and small ventricular septal defect.

E–2 and *E–3,* Holosystolic murmurs consistent with mitral or tricuspid regurgitation and ventricular septal defect. (From Harvey, W. P.: Innocent vs. significant murmurs. Curr. Probl. Cardiol. Vol. 1, No. 8, 1976.)

is a faint murmur but can be detected immediately by an experienced observer. A *Grade 3/6* murmur is moderately loud, and a *Grade 4/6* murmur is loud. A *Grade 5/6* murmur is a very loud murmur but requires placement of the stethoscope on the chest to be audible. A *Grade 6/6* murmur is so loud that it can be heard even without placing the stethoscope on the chest. The *duration* of a murmur depends upon the duration of the events, such as the pressure gradient which is responsible for it, while the *radiation* of a murmur is determined by its site of origin, its intensity, the direction of the blood flow responsible for the murmur (Fig. 2–14), and the physical characteristics of the chest.[84] The *quality* of murmurs should be described using adjectives such as blowing, harsh, rumbling, scratchy, musical, and high- or low-pitched. Murmurs with mixed high and medium frequencies sound harsh or rasping, while those with a narrow frequency range, often owing to vibration of an intracardiac structure such as a valve leaflet, are musical or honking in quality.[86]

The interpretation of heart murmurs is based equally on their characteristics (timing, shape intensity, duration, location, quality, and pitch) and the accompanying auscultatory features, such as the character of the splitting of S_2 as well as the presence of ejection sounds and of S_3 and S_4. The etiology of various murmurs is presented in Table 2–5, and Figures 2–18 and 2–19 illustrate a variety of murmurs and sounds. A discussion of the most important heart murmurs is presented in Chapter 4.

A *cervical venous hum* is a continuous murmur heard best with the stethoscopic bell placed lightly on the lateral portion of the right supraclavicular fossa with the patient sitting or standing, with the patient's head turned to the left. It can be confused with the murmur produced by a patent ductus arteriosus.[87] It is due to the rapid downward flow of blood through a jugular vein that becomes artificially stenosed when the patient is in the upright position, and it disappears when the jugular vein is compressed above or with the stethoscope or when the patient assumes the recumbent position. A venous hum can be intensified by tilting the chin upward and can be abolished by pressure over the upper part of the jugular vein (Fig. 2–20). It is common in normal children and in conditions in which the circulation is hyperkinetic such as anemia, thyrotoxicosis, or pregnancy.

A *mammary souffle* is a systolic or continuous murmur sometimes heard over the breasts of pregnant or lactating women[88] that can be confused with continuous murmurs produced by pulmonary arteriovenous fistula, patent ductus arteriosus, and other forms of congenital heart disease (Table 2–5*D*). It is presumably caused by the increased flow of blood through the engorged breast, generally commences just after the first heart sound, is best heard with the patient supine and may disappear in the upright position or with pressure from the stethoscope.

Pericardial friction rubs are the sounds made by two inflamed layers of the pericardium sliding over one an-

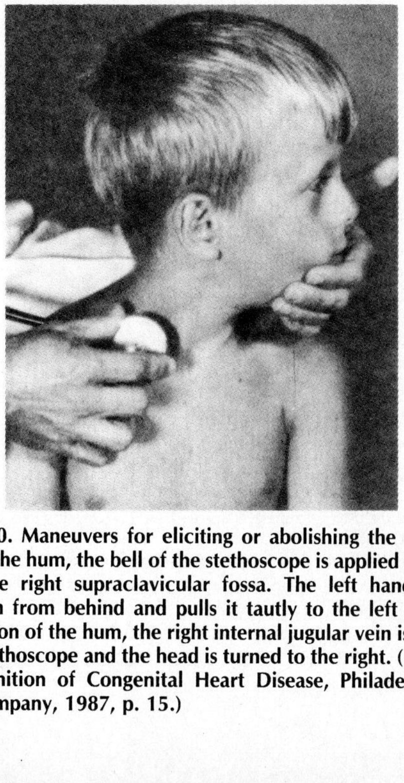

FIGURE 2–20. Maneuvers for eliciting or abolishing the venous hum: For eliciting the hum, the bell of the stethoscope is applied to the medial aspect of the right supraclavicular fossa. The left hand grasps the patient's chin from behind and pulls it tautly to the left and upward. For obliteration of the hum, the right internal jugular vein is compressed above the stethoscope and the head is turned to the right. (From Perloff, J. K.: Recognition of Congenital Heart Disease, Philadelphia, W. B. Saunders Company, 1987, p. 15.)

TABLE 2–5 PRINCIPAL CAUSES OF HEART MURMURS

A. Organic Systolic Murmurs
1. Midsystolic (Ejection)
   a. Aortic
      (1) Obstructive
         (a) Supravalvular—supraaortic stenosis, coarctation of the aorta
         (b) Valvular—AS and sclerosis
         (c) Infravalvular—HOCM
      (2) Increased flow, hyperkinetic states, AR, complete heart block
      (3) Dilatation of ascending aorta, atheroma, aortitis, aneurysm of aorta
   b. Pulmonary
      (1) Obstructive
         (a) Supravalvular—pulmonary arterial stenosis
         (b) Valvular—pulmonic valve stenosis
         (c) Infravalvular—infundibular stenosis
      (2) Increased flow, hyperkinetic states, left-to-right shunt (e.g., ASD, VSD)
      (3) Dilatation of pulmonary artery
2. Pansystolic (Regurgitant)
   a. Atrioventricular valve regurgitation (MR, TR)
   b. Left-to-right shunt to ventricular level

B. Early Diastolic Murmurs
1. Aortic regurgitation
   a. Valvular: rheumatic deformity; perforation post-endocarditis, post-traumatic, post-valvulotomy
   b. Dilatation of valve ring: aorta dissection, annuloectasia, cystic medial necrosis, hypertension
   c. Widening of commissures: syphilis
   d. Congenital: bicuspid valve, with ventricular septal defect
2. Pulmonic regurgitation
   a. Valvular: post-valvulotomy, endocarditis, rheumatic fever, carcinoid
   b. Dilatation of valve ring: pulmonary hypertension; Marfan syndrome
   c. Congenital: isolated or associated with tetralogy of Fallot, VSD, pulmonic stenosis

C. Middiastolic Murmurs
1. Mitral stenosis
2. Carey-Coombs murmur (middiastolic apical murmur in acute rheumatic fever)
3. Increased flow across nonstenotic mitral valve (e.g., MR, VSD, PDA, high-output states, and complete heart block)
4. Tricuspid stenosis
5. Increased flow across nonstenotic tricuspid valve (e.g., TR, ASD, and anomalous pulmonary venous return)
6. Left and right atrial tumors

D. Continuous Murmurs
1. Patent ductus arteriosus
2. Coronary AV fistula
3. Ruptured aneurysm of sinus of Valsalva
4. Aortic septal defect
5. Cervical venous hum
6. Anomalous left coronary artery
7. Proximal coronary artery stenosis
8. Mammary souffle
9. Pulmonary artery branch stenosis
10. Bronchial collateral circulation
11. Small (restrictive) ASD with MS
12. Intercostal AV fistula

AR = aortic regurgitation; AS = aortic stenosis; ASD = atrial septal defect; AV = arteriovenous; HOCM = hypertrophic obstructive cardiomyopathy; MR = mitral regurgitation; MS = mitral stenosis; PDA = patent ductus arteriosus; TR = tricuspid regurgitation; VSD = ventricular septal defect. (*A* and *C* modified from Oram, S. (ed.): Clinical Heart Disease. London, William Heinemann Medical Books, Ltd., 1981; *D* modified from Fowler, N. O. (ed.): Cardiac Diagnosis and Treatment. Hagerstown, Harper and Row, 1980.)

other, but they may be present even when there is considerable pericardial effusion. Friction rubs are generally described as scratching, grating, crunching, and creaking; they seem close to the ear and may vary in distribution from a site that is sharply localized to a small area of the precordium to the entire left hemithorax.[89] Usually they are most readily audible along the left sternal edge in the third and fourth intercostal spaces using the diaphragm with firm pressure and are often better heard during deep inspiration and with the patient leaning forward or in the prone position and propped up by the elbows.[90] They often exhibit nonrespiratory variations in intensity from beat to beat.[91] The sounds are commonly "to and fro" and have a systolic and either one or two diastolic components. In some patients, however, only a systolic component is audible. Friction rubs may be confused with the to-and-fro murmurs of combined aortic stenosis and regurgitation. Pleural-pericardial friction rubs are caused by the inflamed pleura against the parietal pericardium and are usually heard only during inspiration.

Acute mediastinal emphysema produces loud, bizarre, crunching sounds over the precordium, mainly during systole; these are audible most prominently near the apex and sometimes only with the patient in the left lateral recumbent position.[68] *Diaphragmatic flutter* produces regular sounds that are independent of the pulse and are audible over the entire thorax, even in the right axilla, far removed from the heart.[68]

Cardiorespiratory murmurs are systolic (rarely continuous) murmurs heard on inspiration but not when the breath is held or during expiration, and they may result from the movement of air in the bronchial tree during systole and inspiration.[89]

DYNAMIC AUSCULTATION

This is the technique of altering circulatory dynamics by means of a variety of physiological and pharmacological maneuvers and determining their effects on heart sounds and murmurs.[92–95] As outlined in Figures 2–15, 2–16, 2–21, and Tables 2–6, and 2–7, an appreciation of the effects of these interventions can be of great value in the interpretation of a variety of auscultatory findings. The interventions most commonly employed in dynamic auscultation include respiration, postural changes, the Valsalva maneuver, premature ventricular contractions, isometric exercise, and one of the vasoactive agents—amyl nitrite, methoxamine, or phenylephrine.

RESPIRATION

SPLITTING OF S_2. The splitting of S_2 is audible best along the left sternal border and can usually be appreciated when A_2 and P_2 are separated by more than 0.02 sec. During inspiration A_2 ordinarily becomes softer in part because of the increased volume of lung that becomes interposed between the heart and chest wall; P_2 becomes louder because of increased flow into the pulmonary artery. A_2 normally occurs less than 0.02 sec after the pressure in the left ventricle falls below that in the aorta, while P_2 occurs 0.03 to 0.09 sec after the decline of pressure in the right ventricle below that in the central pulmonary artery; these intervals have been termed the "hang-out" intervals, and their durations are inversely proportional to the impedance to blood flow in the aortic and pulmonic circuits.[96] The higher capacitance and lower resistance of the systemic compared to the pulmonary circulation result in a longer hang-out interval in the pulmonary artery than in the aorta and this difference contributes to the normal delay in P_2

TABLE 2–6 PHYSIOLOGICAL AND PHARMACOLOGICAL MANEUVERS USEFUL IN DIFFERENTIAL DIAGNOSIS OF SIMILAR AUSCULTATORY FINDINGS

Auscultatory Problems	Helpful Maneuvers*
Systolic murmur of valvular aortic stenosis vs. hypertrophic subaortic stenosis	Sudden squatting, Valsalva maneuver
Systolic murmur of valvular aortic stenosis vs. mid- to late systolic miral valve dysfunction	Sudden standing, amyl nitrite
Systolic murmur of valvular aortic stenosis vs. mitral regurgitation	Amyl nitrite, phenylephrine, variation in cycle length
Diastolic rumble of mitral stenosis vs. Austin Flint murmur	Amyl nitrite
Diastolic murmur of mitral stenosis vs. tricuspid stenosis	Respiration
Systolic murmur of mitral regurgitation vs. tricuspid regurgitation	Respiration
Supraclavicular bruit vs. aortic stenosis	Extension of shoulder, compression of subclavian artery
Ejection sound in pulmonic stenosis vs. aortic stenosis	Respiration
Small ventricular septal defect vs. pulmonic stenosis	Amyl nitrite, phenylephrine
Large ventricular septal defect with fixed vs. hyperkinetic pulmonary hypertension	Amyl nitrite
Systolic murmur of pulmonic stenosis vs. tetralogy of Fallot	Amyl nitrite
Continuous murmur of patent ductus arteriosus vs. cervical venous hum	Compression of neck veins
Fourth sound plus first sound vs. separation of two components of first heart sound	Respiration, sudden standing, lying with passive leg-raising
Second sound plus opening snap vs. wide separation of second heart sound components	Respiration, phenylephrine, sudden standing

*See Table 2–7 for typical response. (From Criscitiello, M. G.: Physiologic and pharmacologic aids in cardiac auscultation. *In* Fowler, N. O. (ed.): Cardiac Diagnosis and Treatment, Hagerstown, Harper and Row, 1980, p. 89.)

compared to A_2 and therefore to the splitting of S_2. As the impedance to pulmonary flow increases with progressive pulmonary hypertension, the hang-out interval in the pulmonary artery shortens, and there is a reduction in the width of splitting of S_2, so that in severe pulmonary hypertension S_2 may become fused. Several factors play a role in the normal widening of the separation between A_2 and P_2 during inspiration.

During inspiration, venous return to the right side of the heart is augmented, resulting in a higher right ventricular stroke volume and lengthening of the duration of right ventricular ejection. When the respiratory rate is normal, these changes are accompanied by a reduced return of blood to the left side of the heart and a lower left ventricular stroke volume and shorter ejection time. In part, the difference in the effects of respiration on the stroke volumes of the two ventricles is due to the delay in transmission of the augmented right ventricular stroke volume through the pulmonary vascular bed, so that it reaches the left ventricle three or four cardiac cycles later, i.e., during the following respiration.[97] The greater delay in P_2, which accounts for about three-fourths of the widening of the splitting,[70] results from the increased right ventricular stroke volume and ejection time and an inspiratory decline in pulmonary vascular impedance, with further prolongation of the hang-out interval. The pooling of blood in the lungs during inspiration, with decreased venous return to the left heart, is responsible for shortening of left ventricular systole; earlier occurrence of A_2 accounts for about one-fourth of the inspiratory augmentation of the width of splitting of S_2.

In normal adults, A_2 and P_2 are separated by 0.04 to 0.05 sec during inspiration, with a single S_2 heard during expiration (split $\leq$ 0.02 sec). Occasionally there may be residual audible splitting in expiration (0.03 to 0.04 sec) in the supine position, but in normal adults auditory expiratory splitting disappears in the sitting or standing position. Expiratory splitting heard in both the supine and upright positions is uncommon in normal subjects of any age. Expiratory splitting of $\geq$ 0.03 sec, with an increase of $\leq$ 0.015 sec in the width of splitting, is considered to be "fixed" splitting.

There are four types of abnormal splitting of S_2: (1) Absent splitting (single S_2), (2) splitting that is persistent during expiration, (3) fixed splitting, and (4) paradoxical splitting. Major causes are presented in Table 2–3, and further discussion of this subject can be found on p. 47.

S_3, S_4, AND EJECTION SOUNDS. When third and fourth sounds originate from the right ventricle, they are characteristically diminished during expiration and augmented during inspiration, whereas they exhibit the opposite response when they originate from the right side of the heart. Like other left-sided events, the opening snap of the mitral valve may become softer during inspiration and louder during expiration owing to respiratory alterations in venous return, whereas the opening snap of the tricuspid valve behaves in the opposite fashion. Inspiration also diminishes the intensity of valvular pulmonic ejection sounds, since the elevation of right ventricular diastolic pressure causes partial presystolic opening of the pulmonic valve and therefore less upward motion of the valve during systole. On the other hand, respiration does not affect the intensity of nonvalvular pulmonic ejection sounds or of aortic ejection sounds.

MURMURS. Respiration exerts more pronounced and consistent alterations on murmurs originating from the right than the left side of the heart. During inspiration, the diastolic murmurs of tricuspid stenosis and pulmonic regurgitation, the systolic murmurs of tricuspid regurgitation[98] (Carvallo's sign) and of mild or moderate pulmonic stenosis, the diastolic murmur of pulmonary regurgitation, and the pre-systolic murmur of Ebstein's anomaly may all be accentuated. During expiration, the increased venous return to the left side of the heart may result in mild accentuation of the diastolic murmur of mitral stenosis and the systolic murmurs of mitral regurgitation, ventricular septal defect, and valvular aortic stenosis. The inspiratory reduction in left ventricular size in patients with mitral valve prolapse increases the redundancy of the mitral valve and therefore the degree of valvular prolapse; consequently, the midsystolic click and the systolic murmurs occur earlier during systole and frequently become accentuated.[99] The effects of inspiration on auscultatory findings may be accentuated by the use of the Müller maneuver, i.e., forced inspiration against a closed glottis. Deep, maintained expiration tends to accentuate soft, early diastolic murmurs of aortic or pulmonic regurgitation.

TABLE 2–7 RESPONSE OF MURMURS AND HEART SOUNDS TO PHYSIOLOGICAL AND PHARMACOLOGICAL INTERVENTIONS

Clinical Disorder	Intervention and Response
Systolic Murmurs	
Aortic outflow obstruction	
Valvular aortic stenosis	Louder with passive leg-raising, with sudden squatting, with Valsalva release (after five to six beats), following a pause induced by a premature beat, or after amyl nitrite; fades during Valsalva strain and with isometric handgrip
Hypertrophic obstructive cardiomyopathy	Louder with standing, during Valsalva strain, or with amyl nitrite; fades with sudden squatting, recumbency, or isometric handgrip
Pulmonic stenosis	Midsystolic murmur increases with amyl nitrite except with marked right ventricular hypertrophy; also increases during first few beats after Valsalva release
Mitral regurgitation	
Rheumatic	Murmur louder with sudden squatting, isometric handgrip, or phenylephrine; softens with amyl nitrite
Mitral valve prolapse	Midsystolic click moves toward S_1 and late systolic murmur starts earlier with standing, Valsalva strain, and amyl nitrite; click may occur earlier on inspiration; murmur starts later and click moves toward S_2 during squatting, with recumbency, and often after pause induced by a premature beat
Papillary muscle dysfunction	Late systolic murmur generally softer after a pause induced by a premature beat; response to amyl nitrite variable, depending on acute or chronic nature of this disorder
Tricuspid regurgitation	Murmur increases during inspiration, with passive leg-raising, and with amyl nitrite
Ventricular septal defect	
Small defect with pulmonary hypertension	Fades with amyl nitrite; increases with isometric handgrip or phenylephrine
Large defect with hyperkinetic pulmonary hypertension	Louder with amyl nitrite; fades with phenylephrine
Large defect with severe pulmonary vascular disease	Little change with any of above interventions
Tetralogy of Fallot	Murmur softens with amyl nitrite
Supraclavicular bruit	Altered by compression of subclavian artery; may be eliminated by extension of ipsilateral shoulder
Diastolic Murmurs	
Aortic regurgitation	
Blowing diastolic murmur	Increases with sudden squatting, isometric handgrip, or phenylephrine
Austin Flint murmur	Fades with amyl nitrite
Pulmonary regurgitation	
Congenital	Early or mid-diastolic rumble increases on inspiration and with amyl nitrite
Pulmonary hypertension	High-frequency blowing murmur not altered by above interventions
Mitral stenosis	Mid-diastolic and presystolic murmurs louder with exercise, left lateral position, coughing, isometric handgrip, or amyl nitrite; phenylephrine widens A_2-OS interval; inspiration produces sequence of A_2-P_2-OS
Tricuspid stenosis	Mid-diastolic and presystolic murmurs increase during inspiration, with passive leg-raising, and with amyl nitrite
Continuous Murmurs	
Patent ductus arteriosus	Diastolic phase amplified with isometric handgrip or phenylephrine; diastolic phase fades with amyl nitrite
Cervical venous hum	Obliterated by direct compression of jugular veins or by Valsalva strain
Added Heart Sounds	
Gallop rhythm	
Ventricular gallop (S_3) and atrial gallop (S_4)	Accentuated by lying flat with passive leg-raising; decreased by standing or during Valsalva; right-sided gallop sounds usually increase during inspiration; left-sided during expiration
Summation gallop	Separates into ventricular gallop (S_3) and atrial gallop (S_4) sounds when heart rate slowed by carotid sinus massage
Ejection sounds	Ejection sound in pulmonary stenosis fades and occurs closer to the first sound during inspiration

From Criscitiello, M. G.: Physiologic and pharmacologic aids in cardiac auscultation. *In* Fowler, N. O. (ed.): Cardiac Diagnosis and Treatment. Hagerstown, Harper and Row, 1980.

POSTURAL CHANGES

Sudden assumption of the *lying* from the standing or sitting position results in an increase in venous return, which augments first right ventricular and, several cardiac cycles later, left ventricular stroke volume. The principal auscultatory changes include widening of the splitting of S_2 in all phases of respiration and augmentations of right-sided S_3 and S_4 and, several cardiac cycles later, left-sided S_3 and S_4.[100] The systolic murmurs of valvular pulmonic and aortic stenosis, the systolic murmurs of mitral and tricuspid regurgitation and ventricular septal defect, and most functional systolic murmurs are augmented. On the other hand, since left ventricular end-diastolic volume is increased, the systolic murmur of hypertrophic obstructive cardiomyopathy is diminished, and the midsystolic click and systolic murmur associated with mitral valve prolapse are delayed and sometimes attenuated.[93, 94, 99]

Rapid standing or sitting up from a lying position has the opposite effect; in patients in whom there is relatively wide splitting of S_2 during expiration—a finding that may be confused with fixed splitting—the width of the splitting is reduced, so that a normal pattern emerges during the respiratory cycle. No change in splitting occurs in patients with true fixed splitting. The decrease in venous return reduces stroke volume and the murmurs of semilunar valve stenosis and of atrioventricular valve regurgitation. The auscultatory changes in hypertrophic cardiomyopathy and mitral valve prolapse are opposite to those on assumption of the lying posture described above.

SQUATTING. A sudden change from standing to squatting increases venous return and systemic resistance simultaneously. Stroke volume and arterial pressure rise, and the latter may induce a transient reflex bradycardia. The auscultatory features include augmentation of S_3 and S_4 (from both ventricles) and as a consequence of an increase in stroke volume, the systolic murmurs of aortic and pulmonic stenosis and the diastolic murmurs of mitral and tricuspid stenosis become louder.[93] Squatting may make audible a previously inaudible murmur of aortic regurgitation and a pericardial knock.[91] The elevation of arterial pressure increases blood flow through the right ventricular outflow tract of patients with the tetralogy of Fallot and increases the volume of mitral regurgitation and of the left-to-right shunt through a ventricular septal defect, thereby increasing the intensity of the systolic murmur in these conditions. Also, the diastolic murmur of aortic regurgitation is augmented consequent to an increase in aortic reflux. The combination of elevated arterial pressure and increased venous return increases left ventricular size, which reduces the obstruction to outflow and therefore the intensity of the systolic murmur of hypertrophic obstructive cardiomyopathy[1]; the midsystolic click of mitral valve prolapse and the systolic murmur are delayed.

Assumption of the left lateral recumbent position accentuates the intensity of S_1, S_3, and S_4 originating from the left side of the heart; the opening snap and the murmurs associated with mitral stenosis and regurgitation; the midsystolic click and late systolic murmur of mitral valve prolapse; and the Austin Flint murmur associated with aortic regurgitation. Sitting up and leaning forward make the diastolic murmurs of aortic and pulmonic regurgitation more readily audible.

THE VALSALVA MANEUVER. During the initial phase of the Valsalva maneuver, phase I, intrathoracic pressure rises, producing a transient increase in left ventricular output. During the straining phase, phase II, systemic venous return declines; filling of the right and then of the left side of the heart is reduced; and the stroke volume and mean arterial and pulse pressures fall and heart rate increases. As a consequence, S_3 and S_4 become attenuated and the A_2–P_2 interval narrows.[70] As stroke volume and arterial pressure fall, the systolic murmurs of aortic and pulmonic stenosis and of mitral and tricuspid regurgitation, and the diastolic murmurs of aortic and pulmonic regurgitation and of tricuspid and mitral stenosis all diminish. However, as left ventricular volume is reduced, the systolic murmur of hypertrophic obstructive cardiomyopathy becomes louder,[101, 102] and the systolic click and murmur of mitral valve prolapse commence earlier. During the release of the Valsalva maneuver, phase III, the aortic and pulmonic components of S_2 normally become more widely separated.[70, 103] During the first two cycles following release of the Valsalva maneuver, murmurs and filling sounds (S_3 and S_4) originating from the right side of the heart return to normal and may be transiently accentuated. Filling sounds and murmurs originating from the left side of the heart also return to pre-Valsalva levels after six to eight beats and then may be transiently augmented during phase IV, the so-called overshoot phase.

An abnormal "square-wave" response to the Valsalva maneuver (see Fig. 16–4, p. 483) occurs in patients with atrial septal defect, mitral stenosis, and heart failure of any etiology. With such a response, the above-described changes in hemodynamics and therefore in the auscultatory findings do *not* occur.

POSTPREMATURE VENTRICULAR CONTRACTIONS. When a premature contraction is followed by a significant pause, both an increase in ventricular filling and an augmentation of cardiac contractility occur. Consequently, during the postpremature beat, the systolic murmurs of aortic and pulmonic stenosis and of hypertrophic obstructive cardiomyopathy are augmented,[47] while the systolic murmurs of rheumatic mitral regurgitation and of ventricular septal defect are not altered significantly. The systolic murmur of tricuspid regurgitation and the diastolic murmur of aortic regurgitation become louder consequent to increased right ventricular filling and an elevated arterial pressure, respectively. The increase in left ventricular size delays the systolic click and the systolic murmur of mitral valve prolapse. Similar auscultatory changes follow prolonged diastolic pauses in atrial fibrillation and sinus arrhythmia.

ISOMETRIC EXERCISE. This can be carried out simply and reproducibly using a calibrated handgrip device, but isometric exercise should be avoided in patients with ventricular arrhythmias and myocardial ischemia. Handgrip should be sustained for 20 to 30 seconds, but a Valsalva maneuver during the handgrip must be avoided. Isometric exercise results in significant increases in systemic vascular resistance, arterial pressure, heart rate, cardiac output, left ventricular filling pressure, and heart size. As a consequence, (1) S_3 and S_4 originating from the left side of the heart become accentuated, (2) the systolic murmur of aortic stenosis is diminished as a result of reduction of the pressure gradient across the aortic valve,[104] (3) the diastolic murmur of aortic regurgitation and the systolic murmurs of rheumatic mitral regurgitation and ventricular septal defect increase, (4) the diastolic murmur of mitral stenosis becomes louder consequent to the increase in cardiac output, and (5) the systolic murmur of hypertrophic obstructive cardiomyopathy and the systolic click and murmur secondary to mitral valve prolapse are delayed because of the increased left ventricular volume.

PHARMACOLOGICAL AGENTS

Inhalation of *amyl nitrite* for 10 to 15 seconds produces marked vasodilatation, resulting in the first 30 to 40 seconds in a reduction of systemic arterial pressure, and 30 to 60 seconds later in a reflex tachycardia, followed in turn by a reflex increase in cardiac output, velocity of blood flow, and heart rate.[2, 91, 94, 95] S_1 is augmented and A_2 is diminished. The opening snaps of the mitral and tricuspid valves become louder, and as arterial pressure falls, the A_2-opening snap interval shortens. An S_3 originating in either ventricle is augmented, owing to greater rapidity of ventricular filling, but since mitral regurgitation is reduced, the S_3 associated with this lesion is diminished. The systolic murmurs of valvular aortic stenosis, pulmonic stenosis, hypertrophic obstructive cardiomyopathy, tricuspid regurgitation, and functional systolic murmurs are all accentuated because of the increase in left ventricular contractility and stroke volume (Fig. 2–21). The reduction of arterial pressure increases the right-to-left shunt and decreases the blood flow from the right ventricle to the pulmonary artery and diminishes the systolic ejection murmur in patients with tetralogy of Fallot. The increase in cardiac output augments the diastolic murmurs of mitral and tricuspid stenosis and of pulmonary regurgitation and the systolic murmur of tricuspid regurgitation. However, as a result of the fall in systemic arterial pressure, the systolic murmurs of mitral regurgitation and ventricular septal defect, the diastolic murmurs of aortic regurgitation, and the Austin Flint murmur as well as the continuous

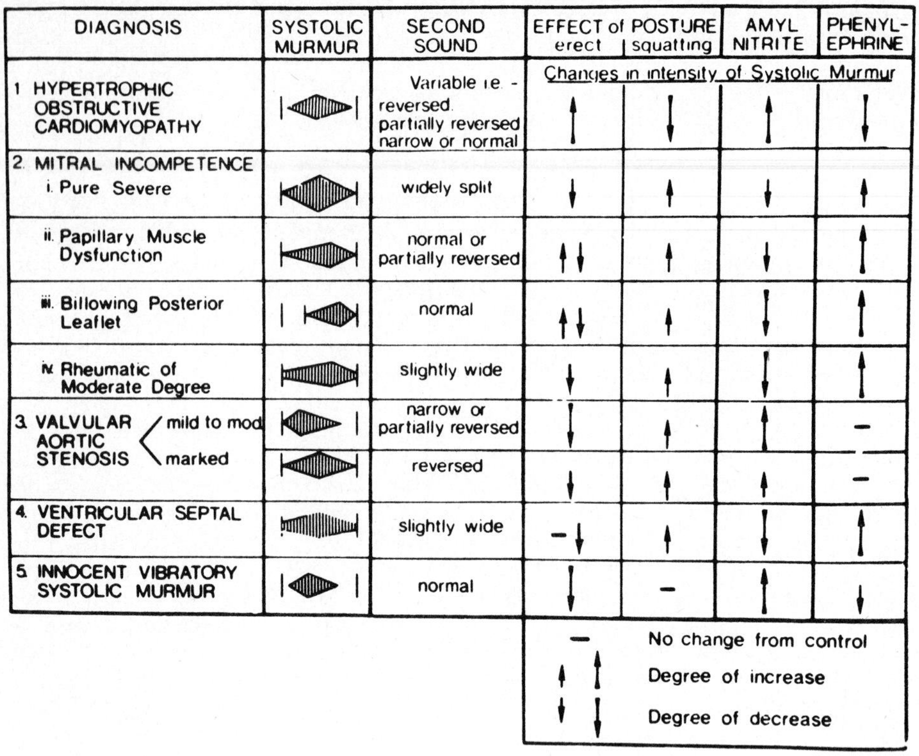
DIAGNOSIS
SYSTOLIC MURMUR
SECOND SOUND
EFFECT of POSTURE
erect
squatting
AMYL NITRITE
PHENYL-EPHRINE
Changes in intensity of Systolic Murmur
1 HYPERTROPHIC OBSTRUCTIVE CARDIOMYOPATHY
Variable ie. - reversed. partially reversed narrow or normal
2. MITRAL INCOMPETENCE
i. Pure Severe
widely split
ii. Papillary Muscle Dysfunction
normal or partially reversed
iii. Billowing Posterior Leaflet
normal
iv. Rheumatic of Moderate Degree
slightly wide
3. VALVULAR AORTIC STENOSIS
mild to mod
marked
narrow or partially reversed
reversed
4. VENTRICULAR SEPTAL DEFECT
slightly wide
5. INNOCENT VIBRATORY SYSTOLIC MURMUR
normal
No change from control
Degree of increase
Degree of decrease

FIGURE 2–21. Diagrammatic representation of the character of the systolic murmur and of the second heart sound in five conditions. The effects of posture, amyl nitrite inhalation, and phenylephrine injection on the intensity of the murmur are shown. (From Barlow, J. B.: Perspectives on the Mitral Valve. Philadelphia, F. A. Davis, 1987, p. 138.)

murmurs of patent ductus arteriosus and of systemic arteriovenous fistula are all diminished.[104] The reduction of cardiac size results in an earlier appearance of the midsystolic click and systolic murmur of mitral valve prolapse; the intensity of the systolic murmur exhibits a variable response.

The response to amyl nitrite is useful in distinguishing (1) the systolic murmur of aortic stenosis (which is augmented) from that of mitral regurgitation (which is diminished),[105] (2) the systolic murmur of tricuspid regurgitation (augmented) from that of mitral regurgitation (diminished), (3) the systolic murmur of isolated pulmonic stenosis (augmented) from that of tetralogy of Fallot (diminished), (4) the systolic murmur of isolated pulmonic stenosis (increased) from that of ventricular septal defect (diminished), (5) the diastolic rumbling murmur of mitral stenosis (augmented) from the Austin Flint murmur of aortic regurgitation (diminished), and (6) the early blowing diastolic murmur of pulmonic regurgitation (augmented) from that of aortic regurgitation (diminished).[82]

Methoxamine and *phenylephrine* increase systemic arterial pressure. In general, methoxamine, 3 to 5 mg intravenously, elevates arterial pressure by 20 to 40 mm Hg for 10 to 20 minutes, but phenylephrine is preferred because of its shorter duration of action; 0.5 mg of phenylephrine administered intravenously elevates systolic pressure by approximately 30 mm Hg for only 3 to 5 minutes. Both drugs cause a reflex bradycardia and decreased contractility and cardiac output. They should not be used in the presence of congestive heart failure and essential hypertension.

After administration the intensity of S_1 is usually reduced, A_2 becomes softer, and the A_2-mitral opening snap interval becomes prolonged. The responses of S_3 and S_4 are variable. As a result of the increased arterial pressure, the diastolic murmur of aortic regurgitation; the systolic murmurs of mitral regurgitation, ventricular septal defect, and tetralogy of Fallot; and the continuous murmur of patent ductus arteriosus and systemic arteriovenous fistula all become louder.[104] On the other hand, as a consequence of the increase in left ventricular size, the systolic murmur of hypertrophic obstructive cardiomyopathy becomes softer, and the click and murmur of mitral valve prolapse syndrome are delayed. The reduction in cardiac output diminishes the systolic murmur of valvular aortic stenosis,[93] functional systolic murmurs, and the diastolic murmur of mitral stenosis. On the other hand, the rumbling diastolic murmurs of mitral regurgitation and the Austin Flint murmur diminish.

REFERENCES

THE GENERAL PHYSICAL EXAMINATION

1. Abrams, J.: Essentials of Cardiac Physical Diagnosis. Philadelphia, Lea and Febiger, 1987.
2. Perloff, J. K.: Physical Examination of the Heart and Circulation. Philadelphia, W. B. Saunders Company, 1982.
3. Silverman, M. E.: Causes of valve disease: Visual clues. J. Cardiovasc. Med. 8:340, 1983.
4. Greenwood, R. D., Rosenthal, A., Parisi, L., Flyer, D. C., and Nadas, A. S.: Extracardiac abnormalities in infants with congenital heart disease. Pediatrics 55:485, 1975.
5. Elliott, W. J.: Ear lobe crease and coronary artery disease: 1,000 patients and review of the literature. Am. J. Med. 75:1024, 1983.
6. Cayler, G. G., Blumenfeld, C. M., and Anderson, R. L.: Further studies of patients with the cardiofacial syndrome. Chest *60*:161, 1971.
7. Young, D., Shprintzen, R. J., and Goldberg, R. B.: Cardiac malformations in the velocardiofacial syndrome. Am. J. Cardiol. *46*:643, 1980.
8. Noonan, J. A.: Hypertelorism with Turner phenotype. Am. J. Dis. Child. *116*:373, 1968.
9. St. John Sutton, M. G., Tajik, A. J., Giuliani, E. R., Gordon, H., and Su, W. P. D.: Hypertrophic obstructive cardiomyopathy and lentiginosis: A little known neural ectodermal syndrome. Am. J. Cardiol. *47*:214, 1981.
10. Beuren, A. J., Schultze, C., Eberle, P., Harmjanz, D., and Apitz, J.: The syndrome of supravalvular aortic stenosis, peripheral pulmonary stenosis, mental retardation and similar facial appearance. Am. J. Cardiol., *13*:471, 1964.
11. Clark, D. S., Myerburg, R. J., Morales, A. R., Befeler, B., Hernandez, F. A., and Gelband, H.: Heart block in Kearns-Sayre syndrome. Chest *68*:727, 1975.
12. Cogan, D. G.: Ophthalmic Manifestations of Systemic Vascular Disease. Philadelphia, W. B. Saunders Company, 1974.
13. Allen, S. J., and Naylor, D.: Pulsation of the eyeballs in tricuspid regurgitation. Can. Med. Assoc. J. *133*:119, 1985.
14. Winder, A. F.: Relationship between corneal arcus and hyperlipidemia is clarified by studies in familial hypercholesterolaemia. Br. J. Ophthalmol. *67*:789, 1983.

15. Walker, G. L., and Stanfield, T. F.: Retinal changes associated with coarctation of the aorta. Trans. Am. Ophthalmol. Soc. *50*:407, 1952.
16. Proudfit, W. L.: Skin signs of infective endocarditis. Am. Heart J. *106*:1451, 1983.
17. Walker, B. A., and Murdoch, J. L.: The wrist sign. Arch. Intern. Med. *126*:276, 1970.
18. Criscitiello, M. G., Ronan, J. A., Besterman, E. M., and Schoenwetter, W.: Cardiovascular abnormalities in osteogenesis imperfecta. Circulation *31*:255, 1965.
19. Zvaifler, N. J.: Chronic postrheumatic fever (Jaccoud's) arthritis. N. Engl. J. Med. *267*:10, 1962.
20. Buckley, M. J., Mason, D. T., Ross, J., Jr., and Braunwald, E.: Reversed differential cyanosis with equal desaturation of the upper limbs. Syndrome of complete transposition of the great vessels with complete interruption of the aortic arch. Am. J. Cardiol. *15*:111, 1965.
21. Finger clubbing. Lancet *1*:1285, 1975.
22. Lanken, P. N., and Fishman, A. P.: Clubbing and hypertrophic osteoarthropathy. *In* Fishman, A. P. (ed.): Pulmonary Diseases and Disorders. New York, McGraw-Hill Book Co., 1980, pp. 84–91.
23. Pomerleau, O. F., and Schwarz, H. J.: Tuberous sclerosis with unusual findings: A case report. J. Maine Med. Assoc. *60*:137, 1969.
24. Manga, P., Vythilingum, S., and Mitha, A. S.: Pulsatile hepatomegaly in constrictive pericarditis. Br. Heart J. 52:465, 1984.
25. Coralli, R. J., and Crawley, I. S.: Hepatic pulsations in constrictive pericarditis. Am. J. Cardiol. 58:370, 1986.
26. Swartz, M. H.: Jugular venous pressure pulse: Its value in cardiac diagnosis. Primary Cardiol. 8:197, 1982.
27. Constant, J.: Bedside Cardiology. 3rd ed. Boston, Little, Brown & Co., 1985.
28. Linfors, E. W., Feussner, J. R., Blessing, C. L., Starmer, C. F., Neelon, F. A., and McKee, P. A.: Spurious hypertension in the obese patient. Effect of sphygmomanometer cuff size on prevalence of hypertension. Arch. Intern. Med. *144*:1482, 1984.
29. Manning, D. M., Kuchirka, C., and Kaminski, J.: Miscuffing: Inappropriate blood pressure cuff application. Circulation *68*:763, 1983.
30. Nelson, W. P., and Egbert, A. M.: How to measure blood pressure—accurately. Prim. Cardiol. *10*:14, 1984.
31. Kirkendall, W. M., Burton, A. C., Epstein, F. H., and Freis, E. D.: Recommendations for human blood pressure determination by sphygmomanometers. Circulation *36*:980, 1967.
32. Londe, S., and Klitzner, T. S.: Auscultatory blood pressure measurement—Effect of pressure on the head of the stethoscope. West. J. Med. *141*:193, 1984.
33. Mancia, G., Grassi, G., Pomidossi, G., Gregorini, L., Bertinieri,G., Parati, G., Ferrari, A., and Zanchetti, A.: Effects of blood-pressure measurement by the doctor on patient's blood pressure and heart rate. Lancet *2*:695, 1983.
34. Finnie, K. J. C., Watts, D. G., and Armstrong, P. W.: Biases in the measurement of arterial pressure. Crit. Care Med. *12*:965, 1984.
35. Gould, B. A., Hornung, R. S., Kieso, H. A., Altman, D. G., and Raftery E. B.: Is the blood pressure the same in both arms? Clin. Cardiol. *8*:423, 1985.
36. Sproul, G.: Basilar artery insufficiency secondary to obstruction of left subclavian artery. Circulation *28*:259, 1963.
37. Sapira, J. D.: Quincke, de Musset, Duroziez, and Hill: Some aortic regurgitations. South Med. J. *74*:459, 1981.
38. Abrams, J.: The arterial pulse. Primary Cardiol. *8*:138, 1982.
39. Schlant, R. C., and Feiner, J. M.: The arterial pulse—clinical manifestations. Curr. Probl. Cardiol. Vol. 1, No. 5, 1976, 50 pp.
40. Perloff, J. K.: The physiologic mechanisms of cardiac and vascular physical signs. J. Am. Coll. Cardiol. *1*:184, 1983.
41. Elkins, R. C., Morrow, A. G., Vasko, J. S., and Braunwald, E.: The effects of mitral regurgitation on the pattern of instantaneous aortic blood flow. Clinical and experimental observations. Circulation *36*:45, 1967.
42. Kelly, E. R., Morrow, A. G., and Braunwald, E.: Catheterization of the left side of the heart: A key to the solution of some perplexing problems in cardiovascular diagnosis and management. N. Engl. J. Med. *262*:162, 1960.
43. Rowe, G. G., Afonso, S., Castillo, C. A., and McKenna, D. H.: The mechanism of the production of Duroziez's murmur. N. Engl. J. Med. *272*:1207, 1965.
44. Fleming, P.R.: The mechanism of the pulsus bisferiens. Br. Heart J. *19*:519, 1957.
45. Braunwald, E., Lambrew, C. T., Rockoff, S. D., Ross, J., Jr., and Morrow, A. G.: Idiopathic hypertrophic subaortic stenosis. I. A description of the disease based upon an analysis of 64 patients. Circulation *30*(Suppl. 4):3, 1964.
46. Bartall, M., Auber, S., Desser, K. B., and Benchimol, A.: Normalizaton of the external carotid pulse tracing of hypertrophic subaortic stenosis during Müller's maneuver. Chest *74*:77, 1978.
47. Brockenbrough, E. C., Braunwald, E., and Morrow, A. G.: A hemodynamic technic for the detection of hypertrophic subaortic stenosis. Circulation *23*:189, 1961.
48. Rebuck, A. S., and Pengelly, L. D.: Development of pulsus paradoxus in the presence of airways obstruction. N.Engl. J. Med. *288*:66, 1973.
49. Massumi, R. A., Mason, D. T., Zakauddin, V., Zelis, R., Otero, J., and Amsterdam, E. A.: Reversed pulsus paradoxus. N. Engl. J. Med. *289*:1272, 1973.
50. Kurtz, K. J.: Dynamic vascular auscultation. Am. J. Med. *76*:1066, 1984.
51. Linhart, J.: Bedside examination of peripheral vascular disease. Eur. Heart J. *4*:137, 1983.

EXAMINATION OF THE HEART

52. Davies, H.: Chest deformities in congenital heart disease. Br. J. Dis. Chest *53*:151, 1959.
53. Perloff, J. K.: Diagnostic inferences drawn from observation and palpation of the precordium with special reference to congenital heart disease. Adv. Cardiopulm. Dis. *4*:13, 1969.
54. Beiser, G. D., Epstein, S. E., Stampfer, M., Goldstein, R. E., Noland, S. P., and Levitsky, S.: Impairment of cardiac function in patients with pectus excavatum. N. Engl. J. Med. *287*:267, 1972.
55. Siegel, J. S., and Schechter, E.: The straight back syndrome. Am. J. Med. 42:309, 1967.
56. Ansari, A.: The "straight back" syndrome. Clin. Cardiol. *8*:290, 1985.
57. Abrams, J.: Precordial palpation. *In* Horwitz, L. D., and Groves, B. M. (eds): Signs and Symptoms in Cardiology. Philadelphia, J. B. Lippincott, 1985, pp. 156–177.
58. Eilen, S. D., Crawford, M. H., and O'Rourke, R. A.: Accuracy of precordial palpation for detecting increased left ventricular volume. Ann. Intern. Med. *99*:628, 1983.
59. Bancroft, W. H., Jr., Eddleman, E. E., Jr., and Larkin, L. N.: Methods and physical characteristics of the kineto-cardiographic and apex cardiographic systems for recording low-frequency precordial motion. Am. Heart J. *73*:756, 1967.
60. Ranganathaı., Juma, Z., and Sivaciyan, V.: The apical impulse in coronary heart disease. Clin. Cardiol. *8*:20, 1985.
61. Dressler, W.: Clinical Aids in Cardiac Diagnosis. New York, Grune and Stratton, 1970, 246 pp.
62. Counihan, T. B., Rappaport, M. B., and Sprague, H. B.: Physiologic and physical factors that govern the clinical appreciation of cardiac thrills. Circulation *4*:716, 1951.
63. Rappaport, M. B., and Sprague, H. B.: Physiologic and physical laws that govern auscultation, and their clinical application: The acoustic stethoscope and the eletrical amplifying stethoscope and stethograph. Am. Heart J. *21*:257, 1941.
64. Stein, P. D.: A Physical and Physiological Basis for the Interpretation of Cardiac Auscultation. Mt. Kisco, N.Y., Futura Publishing Co., 1981, 288 pp.
65. Kindig, J. R., Beeson, T. P., Campbell, R. W., Andries, F., and Tavel, M. E.: Acoustical performance of the stethoscope: A comparative analysis. Am. Heart J. *104*:269, 1982.
66. Selzer, A.: Principles and practice of clinical cardiology. Philadelphia, W. B. Saunders Company, 1983, pp. 23–43.
67. Leatham, A.: Auscultation of the Heart and Phonocardiography. Edinburgh, Churchill Livingstone, 1975, p. 181.
68. Levine, S. A., and Harvey, W. P.: Clinical Auscultation of the Heart. 2nd ed. Philadelphia, W. B. Saunders Company, 1959, 657 pp.
69. Luisada, A. A., and Portaluppi, F.: The Heart Sounds. New York, Praeger Publishers, 1982, 246 pp.
70. Aygen, M. M., and Braunwald, E.: The splitting of the second heart sound in normal subjects and in patients with congenital heart disease. Circulation 25:328, 1962.
71. Leatham, A.: The second heart sound: Key to auscultation of the heart. Acta Cardiol. *19*:395, 1964.
72. Leatham, A.: Auscultation of the heart since Laennec. Thorax *36*:95, 1981.
73. Abrams, J.: The first heart sound. Primary Cardiol. *8*:15, 1982.
74. Shaver, J. A., Salerni, R., and Reddy, P. S.: Normal and abnormal heart sounds in cardiac diagnosis. Part I. Systolic sounds. Cur. Probl. Cardiol *10*(3):1, 1985.
75. Reddy, P. S., Salerni, R., and Shaver, J. A.: Normal and abnormal heart sounds in cardiac diagnosis. Part II. Diastolic sounds. Cur. Probl. Cardiol. *10*(4):1, 1985.
76. Gershlick, A. H., Leech, G., Mills, P. G., and Leatham, A.: The loud first heart sound in left atrial myxoma. Br. Heart J. *52*:403, 1984.
77. Robertson, W. S., and Tavel, M. E.: Mid-systolic sound associated with aortic insufficiency and bisferiens pulse. Chest *83*:141, 1983.
78. Abrams, J.: The third and fourth heart sounds. Primary Cardiol. *8*:47, 1982.
79. Van de Werf, F., Minten, J., Carmeliet, P., De Geest, H., and Kesteloot, H.: The genesis of the third and fourth heart sounds. A pressure-flow study in dogs. J. Clin. Invest. *73*:1400, 1984.
80. Van de Werf, F., Geboers, J., Kesteloot, H., De Geest, H., and Barrios, L.: The mechanism of disappearance of the physiologic third heart sound with age. Circulation *73*:877, 1986.
81. Van de Werf, F., Boel, A. N., Geboers, J., Minten, J., Willems, J., De Geest, H., and Kesteloot, H.: Diastolic properties of the left ventricle in normal adults and in patients with third heart sounds. Circulation *69*:1070, 1984.
81a. Reddy, P. S.: The third heart sound. Int. J. Cardiol. *7*:213, 1985.
82. Abdulla, A. M., Frank, M. J., Erdin, R. A., Jr., and Canedo, M. I.: Clinical significance and hemodynamic correlates of the third heart sound gallop in aortic regurgitation: A guide to optimal timing of cardiac catheterization. Circulation *64*:463, 1981.
83. Lee, D. C-S., Johnson, R. A., Bingham, J. B., Leahy, M., Dinsmore, R. E., Goroll, A. H., Newell, J. B., Strauss, H. W., and Haber, E.: Heart failure in outpatients: A randomized trial of digoxin versus placebo. N. Engl. J. Med. *306*:699, 1982.
84. Rushmer, R. F., and Morgan, C.: Meaning of murmurs. Am. J. Cardiol. *21*:722, 1968.
85. Freeman, A. R., and Levine, S. A.: The clinical significance of the systolic murmur. A study of 1000 consecutive "noncardiac" cases. Ann. Intern, Med. 6:1371, 1933.
86. Sheikh, M. U., Lee, W. R., Mills, R. J., and Dais, K.: Musical murmurs: Clinical implications, long-term prognosis, and echo-phonocardiographic features. Am. Heart J. *108*:377, 1984.
87. Fowler, N. O., and Gause, R.: The cervical venous hum. Am. Heart J. *67*:135, 1964.

88. Tabatznik, R., Randall, T. W., and Hersch, C.: The mammary souffle of pregnancy and lactation. Circulation 22:1069, 1960.
89. Harvey, W. P.: Auscultatory findings in diseases of the pericardium. Am. J. Cardiol. 7:15, 1961.
90. Dressler, W.: Effect of respiration on the pericardial friction rub. Am. J. Cardiol. 7:130, 1961.

Dynamic Auscultation

91. Tavel, M. E.: Clinical Phonocardiography and External Pulse Recording. Chicago, Year Book Medical Publishers, 1985.
92. Harvey, W. P.: Innocent versus significant murmurs. Curr. Probl. Cardiol. Vol. 1., No. 8, 1976, 51 pp.
93. Delman, A. J., and Stein, E.: Dynamic Cardiac Auscultation and Phonocardiography: A Graphic Guide. Philadelphia, W. B. Saunders Company, 1979, pp. 559–792.
94. Baragan, J., Fernandez, F., and Thiron, J. M.: Dynamic Auscultation and Phonocardiography. *In* Tavel, M. E. (ed.): Maryland, Charles Press, 1979.
95. Rothman, A., and Goldberger, A. L.: Aids to cardiac auscultation. Ann. Intern. Med. 99:346, 1983.
96. Shaver, J. A.: Clinical implications of the hangout interval. Int. J. Cardiol. 5:391, 1984.
97. Goldblatt, A., Harrison, D. C., Glick, G., and Braunwald, E.: Studies on cardiac dimensions in intact, unanesthetized man. II. Effects of respiration. Circ. Res. *13*:455, 1963.
98. Cha, S. D., and Gooch, A. S.: Diagnosis of tricuspid regurgitation. Arch. Intern. Med. *143*:1763, 1983.
99. Barlow, J. B.: Perspectives on the Mitral Valve. Philadelphia, F. A. Davis 1987.
100. Rodin, P., and Tabatznik, B.: The effect of posture on added heart sounds. Br. Heart J. *25*:69, 1963.
101. Nishimura, R. A., and Tajik, A. J.: The Valsalva maneuver and response revisited. Mayo Clin. Proc. *61*:211, 1986.
102. Braunwald, E., Oldham, H. N., Jr., Ross, J., Jr., Linhart, J. W., Mason, D. T., and Fort, L., III: The circulatory response of patients with idiopathic hypertrophic subaortic stenosis to nitroglycerin and to the Valsalva maneuver. Circulation *29*:422, 1964.
103. van der Hauwaert, L. G.: The effect of the Valsalva maneuver on the splitting of the second sound. Acta Cardiol. *19*:518, 1964.
104. Criscitiello, M.: Physiologic and pharmacologic aids in cardiac auscultation. *In* Fowler, N. O. (ed.): Cardiac Diagnosis and Treatment. 3rd ed. Hagerstown, Harper and Row, 1980, pp. 77–90.
105. Barlow, J., and Shillingford, J.: The use of amyl nitrite in differentiating mitral and aortic systolic murmurs. Br. Heart J. *20*:162, 1958.

3

HEART SOUNDS: Phonocardiography; Carotid, Apex, and Jugular Venous Pulse Tracings; and Systolic Time Intervals

by ERNEST CRAIGE, M.D., and DAMON SMITH, B.M.E.

HEART SOUNDS

The invention of the stethoscope by Laennec in 1826[1] opened an era of intense excitement in the diagnostic possibilities afforded by auscultation. Details of the fascinating history of this technique may be found in the classic textbook of McKusick.[2] It is interesting to note that within 5 or 10 years of the introduction of the stethoscope there was already a lively controversy in England and France concerning the origin of heart sounds.[3] The view which prevailed from the early nineteenth century to the present has been called the "classic" or valvular theory; it was first enunciated by Rouanet.[4] He proposed that the first heart sound is associated with closure of the atrioventricular valves and the second sound with closure of the semilunar valves.

This view has been challenged in recent years by investigators who denigrate the importance of valves in sound production and ascribe a major role to ventricular events—the rise of pressure in the left ventricle and ejection of blood into the aortic root.[5] Similarly, the genesis of the third heart sound remains controversial, with conflicting arguments being offered by advocates of various mechanisms: valvular,[6] ventricular,[7] and impact of the heart against the chest wall.[8] The current views of the authors with respect to these problems are discussed below in paragraphs devoted to each of the respective heart sounds. We hope that these explanations may lead to a common meeting ground for previously polarized viewpoints.

Illustrations of the various heart sounds and murmurs discussed in Chapters 3 and 4 are provided by phonocardiograms. Phonocardiography as a diagnostic technique has declined in popularity in recent years; however, it remains a valuable, safe, and inexpensive method of displaying acoustic phenomena emanating from the heart. It is most informative when combined with other noninvasive methods such as echocardiography,[9] Doppler echo[10] (Chap. 5), or, for investigative purposes, intracardiac pressure monitoring via micromanometer-tipped catheters.[11] As commonly used, the term *phonocardiography* also embraces pulse tracings—carotid, apex, and jugular venous—so that a relatively complete graphic reproduction of auscultatory, visible, and palpable signs of cardiac origin can be given. Therefore, a brief description of the method that we employ in the Cardiac Graphics Laboratory is offered. In

Chapter 4, the role of echophonocardiography in studies of heart murmurs will be considered. Echocardiography is discussed in Chapter 5.

CARDIAC VIBRATIONS AND THEIR REGISTRATION BY GRAPHIC METHODS

Contraction and relaxation of the heart produces vibrations over the precordium which are perceived by auscultation and palpation, as discussed in Chapter 2. The spectrum of vibrations reaching the chest wall is dominated by the very low frequencies noted at the bedside as palpable phenomena.[2] A recording that would represent the cardiac vibrations exactly as received and without filtration would not be useful since the enormous size of the low-frequency vibrations would preclude an adequate representation of the less intense higher frequencies, appreciated acoustically as heart sounds and murmurs. Therefore the recording apparatus must be provided with a system of filters, so that the resulting graphic record may more nearly approximate the sound spectrum perceived by the ear.[12–14]

The lower threshold of audibility, although variable, is approximately at 30 cps and extends up to several thousand cycles per second. Most vibrations of cardiac origin that appear to be of diagnostic importance are in the spectrum of 30 to 1000 cps.[15] Thus, the phonocardiograph should be able to filter out the very low-frequency vibrations which can be represented as a displacement tracing or apexcardiogram. The remaining higher frequency vibrations can then be suitably amplified, so that the resulting graphic records may approximate the phenomena appreciated by auscultation. However, the true graphic analog of what is perceived on auscultation has yet to be developed and is perhaps unobtainable. By a selective filtration system, the lower frequencies in the audible range may be permitted to dominate the tracing, such as might be useful in recording third and fourth heart sounds and low-frequency rumbling murmurs. Alternatively, suppression of low frequencies and amplification of high-frequency vibrations result in optimal presentation of the first and second heart sounds, ejection sounds, opening snaps, and murmurs such as those of mitral and aortic regurgitation.[2]

PHONOCARDIOGRAPHIC TECHNIQUE

FACILITIES AND EQUIPMENT. The room must be quiet or sound-conditioned, with a sound-absorbent ceiling and wall covering, drapes over the windows, and a carpet. Mechanical noises must be eliminated in order to obtain tracings free of background noise. The bed should be comfortable, allow elevation of the patient's head, and be high enough so that the examiner can conveniently auscultate and apply the necessary transducers. Usually the patient is supine, with the head elevated for comfort or as required for optimal visualization or registration of venous or carotid pulsations. During recording of the carotid pulse, a pillow should be placed beneath the patient's shoulders in order to hyperextend the neck and thereby thrust the carotid artery forward, supported firmly by the transverse processes of the cervical spine. It may be necessary for the patient to assume the left lateral decubitus position to enhance auscultatory and palpable phenomena at the cardiac apex.

Paper speed is usually set at 100 mm/sec, which is optimal for measurement of systolic time intervals[16] as well as for observation of the relationship of heart sounds and valvular and ventricular events. However, slower paper speeds may be preferable for displaying the effects of respiration or other physiological or pharmacological maneuvers or in scanning the heart by means of the accompanying echocardiogram.

Although a variety of microphones for heart-sound registration is available, we prefer the air-coupled type, attached to the lightly lubricated chest wall by means of a rubber suction bulb.* Any excess hair that might interfere with the firm, air-tight attachment of the microphone should be removed. Smaller transducers are essential for infants and small children and are also useful when prominent ribs preclude adequate contact with the microphone rim.

Transducers for pulse tracings—carotid, apex, or venous—are commonly of the piezoelectric crystal type. A funnel or tambour is applied to the pulsation under study, and changes in air pressure are conducted via a rubber tube to the crystal device for conversion to electrical signals. The transducer-recording system must have an adequate time constant of 3.0 sec or more. With some of the older equipment, too short a time constant resulted in distortion of the curves and subtle temporal displacement of important landmarks in the carotid and apex tracings.[14, 17] A simple test of one's apparatus for the adequacy of the duration of the time constant consists merely of observing the effect on the oscilloscope of sustained pressure applied to the funnel or tambour of the transducer. If after a rapid rise of the signal on the oscilloscope there is an immediate (0.3 sec or so) fall to the baseline, despite continued pressure on the sensing head of the transducer, then obviously the apparatus will yield a systematic distortion of the pulsatile phenomena being recorded. This distortion is equivalent to a high-pass filtering of the signal. A plateau will appear as an inverted V, and a shallow trough may become a deep crevasse. Besides these morphological alterations, the timing of landmarks (which constitutes one of the principal uses of pulsatile records) may be disturbed, resulting in erroneous interpretations. A time constant of 3.0 sec or more is adequate for recording carotid, apex, and venous pulsations. An infinite time constant may be theoretically superior but is usually impractical, owing to the wide swings of the baseline associated with respiration that make interpretation difficult.

Respiration can be monitored by means of a nasal thermistor probe. This produces a satisfactory curve that can be superimposed on the other parameters of a multichannel tracing. The technique and equipment required for echocardiography and Doppler studies are described in Chapter 5.

RECORDING TECHNIQUE. In view of the many possible combinations of transducers and chest-wall locations, the registration of graphic tracings must be preceded by a bedside assessment of the problem. Ideally, the clinician should be present in the noninvasive laboratory to supervise application of the microphones to the most informative locations on the chest wall. If this is not possible, the areas best suited for registration can be designated with a mark, or at least the problem should be indicated clearly, so that laboratory personnel can make the most appropriate choices. Informative tracings cannot be provided by a technician applying transducers to the chest wall in a routine, unsupervised manner. Phonocardiograms recorded in this manner are more often misleading than helpful in cardiac diagnosis. In general, it is preferable to record from two microphones simultaneously in order to clarify the transmission of certain sounds such as P_2 and to separate such sounds from others occurring in close temporal proximity, such as opening snaps, third sounds, and the like (Fig. 3–1).[18]

The most commonly used sites for application of the microphones are those generally employed in auscultation: the second right interspace, often called the "aortic area"; the second left interspace, or the "pulmonary area"; the lower left sternal edge and xiphoid region, or the "tricuspid area"; and the cardiac apex, or the "mitral area." The designation of these anatomical locations on the thoracic wall as "valve areas" is an oversimplification that may be misleading, since there is no exclusive transmission of acoustical events from any particular valve to a certain area on the chest wall. Thus the designations "AA," "MA," and other similar symbols for second right interspace, cardiac apex, and so on are used in the illustrations in Chapters 3 and 4 simply for economy of space.

Occasionally, there may be a competition for chest-wall space between microphones and ultrasound transducers, especially in children. In such instances, some judgment regarding priorities for positions will have to be exercised. Following the application of the microphones, it is imperative to listen through an amplifying stethoscope plugged into the recorder in order to determine whether the auscultatory phenomena in question can be heard and adequately visualized on the oscilloscope. This precaution also helps to eliminate artifacts due to hair or poor contact with the chest wall and to identify artifacts due to bowel sounds or percussion noises from hyperdynamic chest-wall movement. All these extraneous sounds are more easily identified by means of auscultation than by means of a graphic record, in which their rhythmic recurrence with the heartbeat may simulate some important intracardiac manifestation.

DEFINITION OF HEART SOUNDS. Before we can discuss the individual sounds, we must arrive at a definition of heart sounds in general. This task is not as straightforward as it might seem. For instance, various electronic vibration sensors can detect "sounds" of cardiovascular origin which would not be heard with a conventional acoustic stethoscope. Whether these electronically perceived vibrations have clinical relevance is unclear. Lacking a better definition, we advocate that the term "heart sound" be reserved in its classic sense as that aspect of cardiac activity that can be heard on the precordium with a conventional acoustic stethoscope.

RELATIONSHIP BETWEEN GRAPHICALLY RECORDED VIBRATIONS AND HEART SOUNDS. Although in Chapters 3 and 4 extensive

*Leatham microphone, J & J Ultrasound, Ramsey, New Jersey.

use is made of phonocardiograms to illustrate heart sounds and murmurs, it must be admitted that the relationship between what is heard and what is graphically recorded is ambiguous. This ambiguity becomes especially important when researchers seek to determine the onset of a particular heart sound with extreme temporal resolution on the order of a few milliseconds. For instance, the onset of the second heart sound in a "low-filter" phonocardiogram can appear as much as 10 msec before it is seen in a "medium-filter" phonocardiogram. This can cause very different conclusions regarding the exact timing of the sound with respect to the closure of the aortic valve. Since there is no "gold standard" phonocardiogram, any signal which shows pressure or motion dynamics in the amplitude and frequency range of audibility should be considered as providing information pertinent to heart sounds.

INVOLVEMENT OF THE HEART WALL AS A PRIMARY SOURCE OF HEART SOUNDS TRIGGERED BY VALVE CLOSURE. There is widespread acceptance of the temporal relationship between mitral valve closure and the mitral component of the first heart sound (M_1) and aortic valve closure and the aortic component of the second heart sound (A_2).[19] These sounds are thus believed to originate from the valves. Some investigators, however, have pointed out that the vibration cannot be so distinctly localized and attributed exclusively to the valve, since the heart is a complex structure which responds as a vibrational system to the perturbation of valve closure.[20–25] Even with this awareness of the heart as a complex vibrational system, a persistent concept among cardiologists is that the structure which triggers an oscillation of the system must be the primordial generator of all the vibrations that result. Therein lies a fundamental misconception that greatly confuses the subject.

The heart has many vibrational modalities. The valves most certainly have the capability to vibrate as a result of their closing and tensing. However, because of the fluid continuity between the valve and the rest of the cardiac structure, and the essential incompressibility of the fluid, it is a great oversimplification to assume that the vibrations emanate from the valve as a point source. The hemodynamic transition which is triggered by the valve closure also has the capability of triggering other vibrations of the heart, with frequencies and amplitudes in many ways different from the oscillations of the valve. Thus it can be realized that factors which affect the intensity of the valvular vibration may also be manifest in a similar change in the amplitude of the vibrations of the wall. These considerations may narrow the conceptual gap between the "valvular" and "muscular" proponents of sound generation.

TRANSMISSION OF HEART SOUNDS. Clinicians have long been aware of the importance of transmission of heart sounds and murmurs from their source to various locations on the chest wall. It has been generally assumed that transmission is through the blood mass within the heart and great vessels.[26] Some have taken exception to this view, however, and attribute better transmissibility to bone.[27] Obviously transmission is diminished by obesity and emphysema, which place greater distance and inferior conducting tissue between the point of reception and its source. Smith et al. demonstrated in open-chest canine preparations the importance of the state of contraction or stiffness of the ventricular wall in the transmission of an artificial mechanical vibration from a source at the base of the heart to a sensor at the cardiac apex.[28] In a relatively healthy canine heart, transmission in their experiments was confined almost exclusively to systole. In a dilated failing heart, however, diastolic transmission became more prominent, surpassing that which occurred in systole.[28a]

The intracardiac phonocardiogram has long been considered the reference standard for detecting heart sounds at their presumed source. The studies of Smith et al. suggest, however, that phasic variations of vibration transmission play an important role in determining what is perceived with the stethoscope. Their comparison of simultaneously received intracardiac and heart surface phonocardiograms showed profound differences in the vibrations detected within the blood and at the apical heart surface. Furthermore, certain pathological conditions resulted in significant alterations of the phasic pattern such that diastolic transmission became relatively enhanced. If these observations are confirmed in humans, it would mean that events which occur in systole (S_1, A_2, and ejection sounds) would normally be better transmitted to the precordium than would diastolic events of comparable intensity. In a hypertrophied heart, moreover, a fourth sound gallop would have preferential transmission.

One of the implications of the purely valvular hypothesis of heart sound generation is the concept of the sound originating at a point source and radiating centrifugally to other locations, eventually reaching the precordium. However, the role of the wall of the heart as a primary generator of heart sounds necessitates the consideration of multiple sources and modalities so that no exploration, intracardiac or otherwise, will reveal a single point of origin.

THE FIRST HEART SOUND

The first heart sound (S_1) is best recorded at the cardiac apex and is identified by its relationship to the ECG and carotid upstroke (Fig. 3–1). It consists phonocardiographically of an initial inaudible low-frequency vibration, "M," occurring at the onset of ventricular systole, then two intense high-frequency bursts of vibrations at the time of atrioventricular valve closure, followed by a few variable low-intensity vibrations (Fig. 3–2).[29] The technique of echophonocardiography is particularly applicable to studies of the first heart sound,[30, 31] since valvular and acoustical events are transmitted with essentially no time delay (Fig. 3–3).

SPLITTING OF S_1. Normal. The two major components of S_1 are separated by a narrow interval of 0.02 to 0.03 sec in most normal subjects.[19] This degree of separation is difficult to perceive by means of auscultation; and phonocardiography may record the two elements of S_1 blurring into a continuum of vibrations. Normal splitting is recorded most satisfactorily in children. The mitral component, M_1, normally is the louder and is best recorded at the cardiac

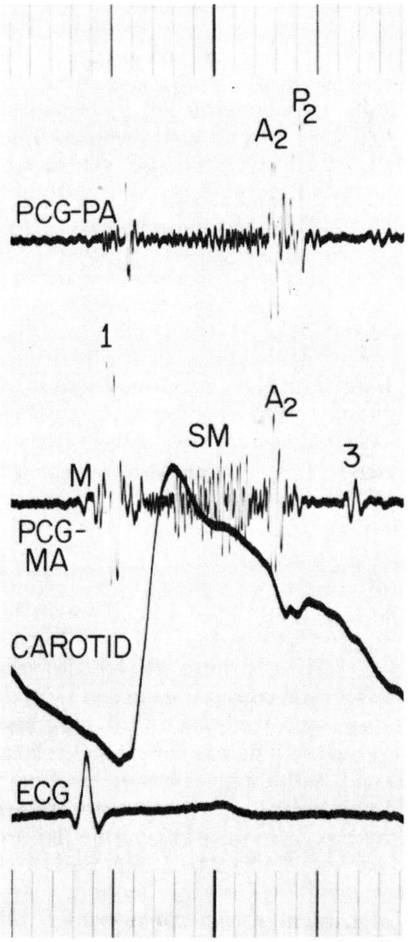

FIGURE 3–1. Phonocardiogram in mild mitral regurgitation. Two phonocardiograms are taken simultaneously, one at the second left intercostal space (PCG-PA) and one at the cardiac apex (PCG-MA). This demonstrates the wide transmission of the aortic component of the second heart sound (A_2) while the pulmonic component (P_2) is confined to the upper left sternal edge. A late systolic murmur (SM) and third sound (3) are best seen at the apex. Also, the initial low-frequency component (M) of the first sound (1) is seen at the same location. In the illustrations in this chapter, the following symbols will be used to indicate location of the microphones on the chest wall: AA = second right intercostal space; PA = second left intercostal space; LSE = lower left sternal edge (third or fourth left intercostal space); MA = cardiac apex. (Time lines = 0.04 sec.)

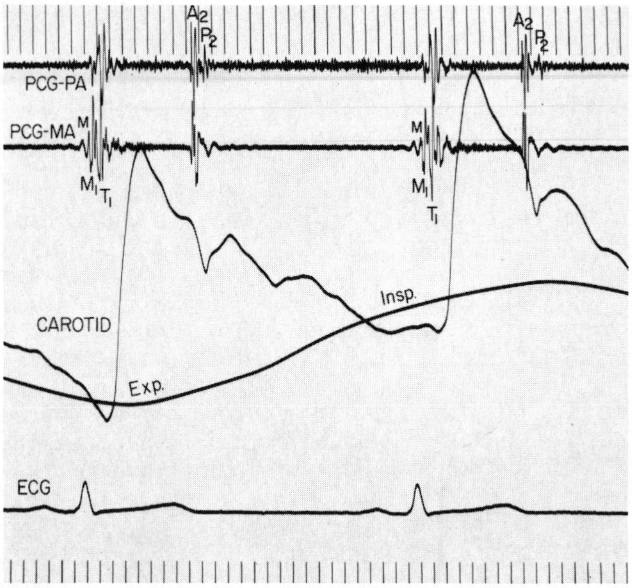

FIGURE 3–2. Normal phonocardiogram. The first heart sound is best seen at the cardiac apex (PCG-MA) and consists of a low-frequency component (M), followed by two high-frequency bursts of vibrations (M_1, T_1), and finally a few low-intensity, low-frequency vibrations in early systole. Normal widening of the A_2–P_2 interval with inspiration is demonstrated. A_2 is well recorded at the apex, but P_2 is not.

apex. The tricuspid component, T_1, that immediately follows is best recorded at the left lower sternal border.

Abnormal. Abnormal splitting of S_1 may result from either electrophysiological or hemodynamic changes that alter the timing of atrioventricular valve closure.

Electrical Factors. These include abnormalities associated with bundle branch block,[32, 33] ectopic ventricular beats, ventricular tachycardia, idioventricular rhythm, preexcitation, and ventricular pacing. Wide splitting with preservation of the normal sequence (M_1 to T_1) may be recorded in right bundle branch block, ectopic beats, or idioventricular rhythms originating in the left ventricle, pacing from the left ventricle, or preexcitation patterns that result in left ventricular contraction before right ventricular contraction.[34] Reversed splitting may occur with the opposite of these situations, i.e., ectopic rhythms and paced beats originating in the right ventricle. It does not follow, however, that reversed splitting necessarily occurs in left bundle branch block (LBBB), since the *onset* of the left ventricular pressure rise often starts on time despite the *delay* in the completion of depolarization of the left side, which causes the characteristic electrocardiographic pattern.[35] Burggraf has shown that in LBBB there may be a normal sequence (M_1 followed by T_1) or a simultaneous M_1T_1 or a reversal of the two elements.[36] Typically, the low amplitude of S_1 in LBBB makes identification of individual components more difficult.

Hemodynamic Factors. Hemodynamic abnormalities that result in alteration in the timing of M_1 and T_1 include mitral stenosis and left atrial myxoma. In mitral stenosis, pressure in the left ventricle must rise to higher than normal levels before pressure in the left atrium is exceeded and the mitral valve starts to close.[37] In severe cases the delay in the timing of mitral valve closure, and therefore of M_1, may result in reversed splitting of S_1 (Fig. 3–4). Similarly, in left atrial myxoma, M_1 is delayed as the result of a hemodynamic situation simulating that of mitral stenosis. With extrusion of the tumor from ventricle to atrium, a loud, late S_1 is audible and usually palpable.

Mixed Electrical and Hemodynamic Factors. In Ebstein's anomaly the combination of right bundle branch block (RBBB) and an unusually large, deformed tricuspid valve results in a greatly delayed T_1 (pp. 951 and 997).[38] Closure of the large anterior tricuspid leaflet in association with a loud, high-frequency sound as long as 0.14 sec after closure of the mitral valve provides a characteristic echophonocardiographic picture (Fig. 3–5).[38–40] The diagnostic specificity of these findings obviates cardiac catheterization in most instances.

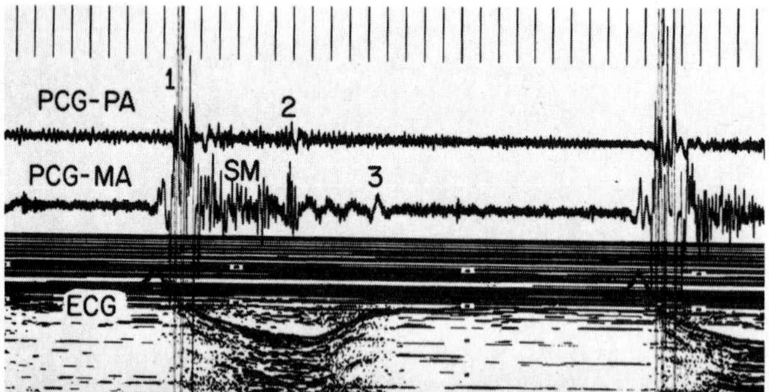

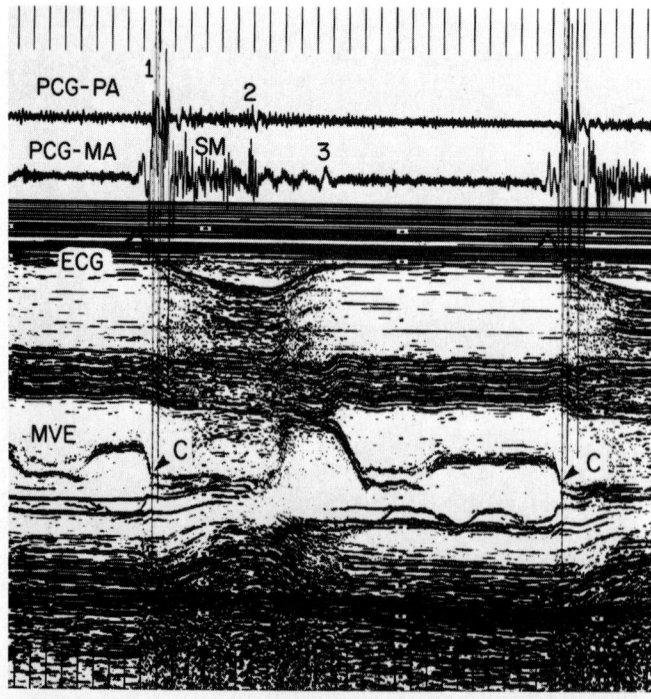

FIGURE 3–3. An echophonocardiogram showing the relationship between mitral valve closure and a very loud first heart sound (1). PCG at the cardiac apex (MA) shows a holosystolic murmur of mild mitral regurgitation. The C points indicate apposition of the leaflets of the mitral valve on the mitral valve echogram (MVE).

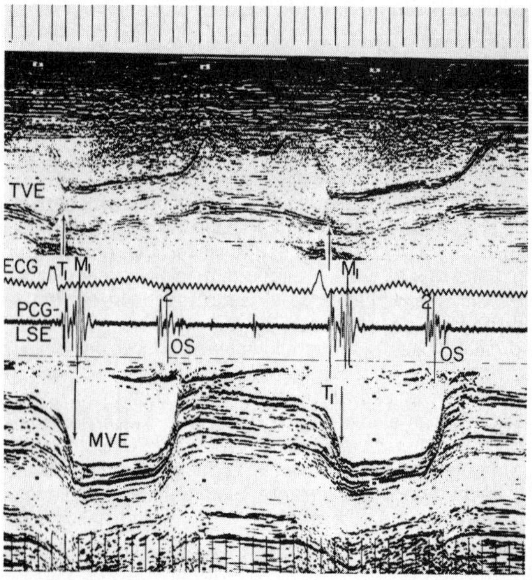

FIGURE 3–4. Reversed splitting of S_1 in mitral stenosis. A dual echophonocardiogram shows a widely split S_1 with T_1 identified by its coincidence with tricuspid valve closure (↑) preceding M_1, which occurs at the time of mitral valve closure (↓). An opening snap (OS) follows S_2 and is identified by its occurrence at the time of full opening of the mitral valve in early diastole.

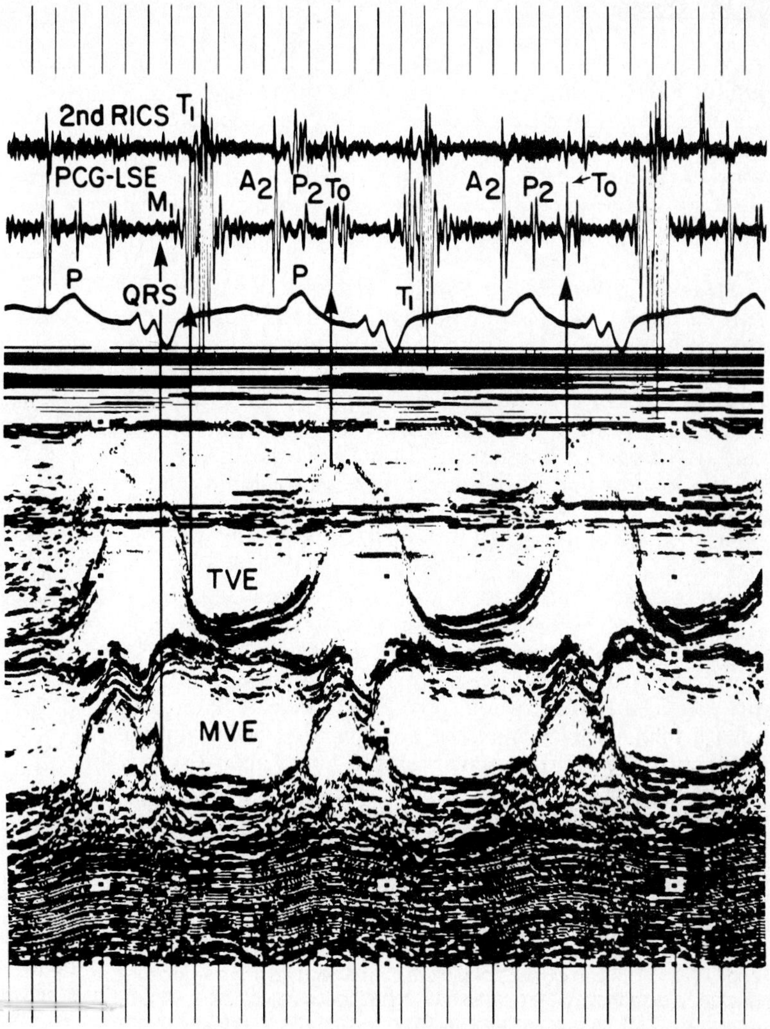

FIGURE 3–5. Ebstein's anomaly. Echophonocardiogram of the tricuspid valve (TVE) and mitral valve (MVE) showing delayed closure of the large tricuspid valve 0.12 sec from onset of the QRS complex. Closure of the tricuspid valve is associated with a very loud T_1 or "sail sound," which dwarfs the mitral component of S_1 (M_1). Additional sounds include tricuspid opening (T_0) synchronous with the E-point of the tricuspid echo.

Intensity of S_1. As pointed out earlier, the hemodynamic transition triggered by the closed and tensed AV valve is manifested as a vibration of the cardiohemic system, two specific components of which are the oscillation of the valve itself and the vibrations of the myocardium. The force which drives the various vibrational modalities is the result of the halting of momentum when the valve reaches its functionally closed position. The array of factors discussed below which have been shown to correlate with S_1 intensity can be understood through consideration of their role in determining the magnitude of the momentum which has developed and the abruptness with which it is halted by the closed and seated valve. These factors include the ability of the atrioventricular valves to close, their mobility, the velocity of their closing movement, and the strength of ventricular systole. Closure of the atrioventricular valves as perceived echocardiographically occurs at the "*c*-point," where the leaflets are seen to approximate each other in early systole. Echocardiography cannot distinguish between *apposition* of the leaflets and the *tension* on the bellies of the leaflets, which immediately follows. Presumably, it is the latter event that is associated with vibrations perceived as sound.

Ability of the AV Valves to Close. In mitral regurgitation, in which closure of the valve is ineffectual, S_1 may be soft (p. 1040). This is best illustrated in rheumatic valvular disease—in which shortening and thickening of the chordae tendineae preclude normal closure. In prolapse of the mitral valve, however, the valve may seat normally in early systole, an event associated with a loud S_1 (Fig. 3–1), although prolapse of the valve and regurgitation may occur later in systole.[41]

Mobility of the Valve. A calcified valve that is completely immobilized is associated with a soft or absent S_1.

Velocity of Closure. This is an important factor in determining the intensity of S_1. This statement is not meant to imply that the sound originates from the impact of leaflet coaptation. Since there is a fluid continuity between the valve and the intracardiac blood mass, the *velocity* of valve closure movement is indicative of the *momentum of the blood* contiguous with the leaflets. Clinical observations in patients with complete heart block[42, 43] and atrial fibrillation[9] have indicated that the velocity of closure of the mitral valve varies on a beat-to-beat basis. A high velocity of closure has been found to correlate with a loud S_1 and a slow velocity of closure with a soft S_1. When the valve is completely closed at the onset of ventricular systole, as with a long P-R interval[44] or with severe, acute aortic regurgitation,[45] S_1 may be silent. These observations support the clinical teaching of Wolferth and Margolies, who many years ago proposed that the intensity of S_1 depends on mitral (atrioventricular) valve position at the onset of systole.[46]

The loudness of T_1 in atrial septal defect may be explained by the same hypothesis, since the valve is held open by the augmented flow from right atrium to right ventricle, until final closure occurs with right ventricular systole.[47, 48] The loud M_1 characteristic of mitral stenosis may also be related to the fact that the valve is held open by the transvalvular pressure gradient until a very sharp, high-velocity closing movement of the valve apparatus is effected by ventricular systole (Fig. 3–4). If a loud M_1 is present in mitral stenosis, one may assume that some portion of the valve is capable of moving (bulging) in the direction of the atrium even though the mouth of the valve may be largely immobilized by fibrosis and even calcification.

Strength of Ventricular Systole. Although obviously closure of the AV valves is dependent on ventricular systole, the contribution of the *force of ventricular contraction* to the intensity of S_1 is less than that of the *velocity of valve closure.*[9, 49] Thus, in atrial fibrillation, the long diastoles which, according to the Starling principle, should lead to the most forceful contractions are not necessarily followed by the loudest first heart sounds.[9] In fact, a sound may at times be observed when the mitral valve closes precociously in diastole when no ventricular contraction at all has taken place.[50, 51] In left bundle branch block a variety of factors may contribute to the characteristic softness of S_1, including extracardiac abnormalities such as emphysema in older subjects, impaired ventricular contraction due to myocardial disease, and partial closure of the valve prior to ventricular systole owing to a long P-R interval plus a further delay between onset of the QRS complex and initiation of ventricular systole in some cases of LBBB.[33, 36]

THE SECOND HEART SOUND

The classic explanation of the origin of the two components of the second heart sound relates these events to closure of the aortic and pulmonic valves, respectively, thus warranting the designations "A_2" and "P_2".[4, 19] The coincidence of the onset of A_2 and aortic valve closure is clearly demonstrable in combined echophonocardiographic recordings (Fig. 3–6). In vitro studies of Stein and associate utilizing high-speed cinematographic techniques have confirmed and delineated in precise detail the movements of the aortic valve following leaflet coaptation. These studies clearly indicate the development of transient but significant retrograde movement as the flexible valve seats.[52] Furthermore, their results show a close correlation between A_2 intensity and the magnitude of this retrograde seating velocity. Because of the

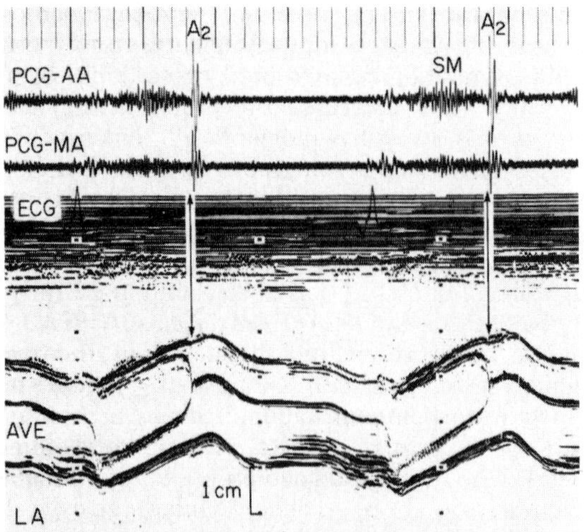

FIGURE 3–6. Echophonocardiogram illustrating the relationship between closure of the aortic valve and onset of the high-frequency vibrations of A_2. An ejection systolic murmur (SM) is noted in the phonocardiogram from the second right intercostal space. AVE = aortic valve echo; LA = left atrium.

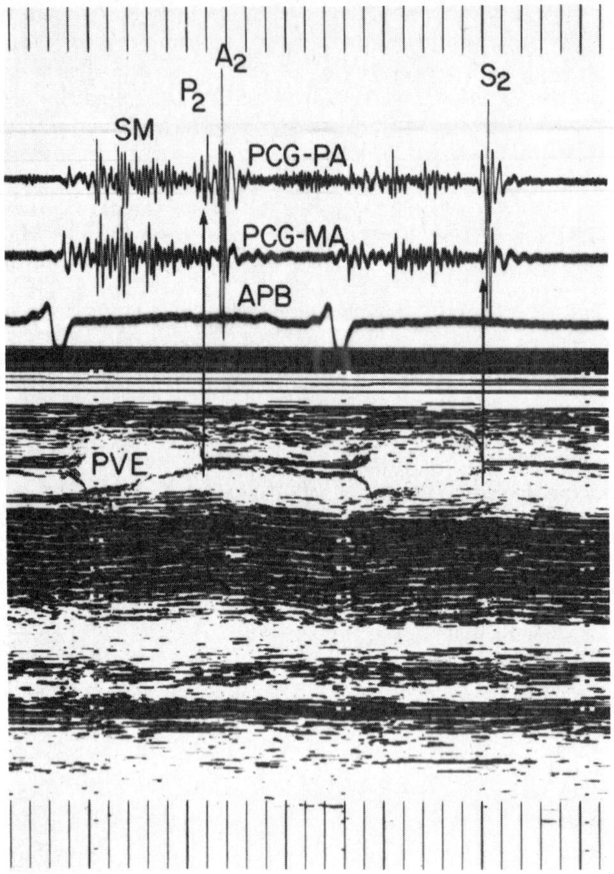

FIGURE 3–7. Echophonocardiogram from a patient with severe chronic rheumatic heart disease. There is reversed splitting of S_2 such that P_2 precedes A_2 in the first beat. In the second beat, which is premature (APB), the two elements of S_2 fuse. A simultaneous echo of the pulmonary valve (PVE) shows that P_2 occurs coincident with closure of the two visible cusps.

fluid continuity of the blood with the leaflets, the high-speed cinematography of Stein and associate documents the presence of retrograde blood momentum at the time of aortic valve seating. It is the abrupt halting of this momentum, at the instant that the semilunar valve reaches its functionally seated and tensed configuration, which drives the various vibrational modalities of the second heart sound. As is the case with S_1, factors which correlate with S_2 intensity are those which play a role in the determination of the magnitude of the developed momentum and the abruptness with which this momentum is halted.

Smith and Craige[53] have shown in open-chest canine experiments that the halting of retrograde blood momentum by the aortic valve generates an overall A_2 force vector. This results in a translational displacement type of oscillation of the entire left ventricle as a separate vibrational aspect of A_2 in many ways distinct from those of the valve, although it is valve closure which triggers it. This concept is consistent with the studies of Verburg and van Vollenhoven, in which the A_2 force vector was described as a mechanical dipole analogous to the electrical vector of the heart.[54]

The pulmonic component of the second heart sound (P_2) is generally attributed to closure and tensing of the pulmonic valve.[4, 19] This relationship is more difficult to demonstrate by echophonocardiography than the analogous events on the left side of the heart, because one can rarely visualize more than one cusp of the pulmonic valve and therefore the exact moment of closure cannot be accurately pinpointed. In Figure 3–7, however, from a patient with chronic rheumatic heart disease, the closing point of the valve cusps can be seen and is synchronous with P_2.

By auscultation or phonocardiography the two elements of the second heart sound are best appreciated in the pulmonary area or second left intercostal space where normal splitting is demonstrated on inspiration. The aortic component of S_2 can be identified by its occurrence just before the incisura of the carotid pulse tracing and by its transmission to the cardiac apex. P_2, on the other hand, is usually recorded only at the upper left sternal edge, unless it is of abnormal intensity.

Therefore the method of utilizing two sound transducers simultaneously is ideally suited for recording the timing, relative intensity, transmission, and behavior in conjunction with respiration of the two elements of S_2.[19] Quiet deep breathing with the mouth open is the best method of producing the desired physiological alterations, since it will be relatively free from obscuring artifacts.

SPLITTING OF S_2. Normal. In newborn infants S_2 is initially single.[55] However, during the first day of life, with falling resistance in the pulmonary circuit, the inspiratory separation of A_2 and P_2 becomes perceptible phonocardiographically. Normally thereafter, fusion of the elements of S_2 occurs with expiration, and separation varying from 0.02 to 0.06 sec occurs with inspiration.[56] In older subjects in whom auscultation and phonocardiographic observations may be obscured by emphysema, only one element of S_2 may be audible, giving the erroneous impression that splitting is no longer present.

Wide Splitting of S_2 with Respiratory Variation. As with splitting of S_1, wide splitting of S_2 may occur for either electrical or hemodynamic reasons.

Electrical Factors. Those factors contributing to prolongation of the interval between A_2 and P_2 include right bundle branch block, pacing of the left ventricle, preexcitation, and ventricular premature beats originating on the left side of the heart. Under these circumstances graphic records demonstrate a further prolongation of the A_2-P_2 interval with inspiration, even though this is usually difficult to perceive by means of auscultation.

Hemodynamic Factors. Those factors that increase the splitting of S_2 include the following:

Obstruction to Right Ventricular Outflow. Valvular pulmonic stenosis results in prolongation of right ventricular systole, with delay and diminution of P_2. The magnitude of the separation of A_2-P_2 can be used to estimate the severity of the stenosis, being greater with higher right ventricular pressures (Fig. 3–8).[57] With infundibular stenosis, a similar separation of the components of S_2 is seen.

Shortening of Left Ventricular Ejection Time. In severe mitral regurgitation, the left ventricular ejection time is abnormally short, and A_2 is early, resulting in a prolongation of the interval between A_2 and P_2 (p. 60). Respiratory variation is preserved.

Broad Fixed Splitting of S_2. In atrial septal defect there is, in most instances, broad and fixed splitting of S_2 (Fig. 3–9)[58] (p. 982). Fixed separation of A_2-P_2 is defined as a gap that varies no more than 0.01 sec with inspiration and expiration. This important diagnostic feature results from the presence of two inflow sources to the right atrium—the venae cavae and the septal defect. In the various phases of respiration, presumably the waxing and waning of inflow of blood into the right atrium from the systemic venous bed results in reciprocal fluctuations in flow across the septal defect, with consequent steady filling of the right ventricle throughout the respiratory cycle.

Paradoxical Splitting of S_2. Reversal in the normal sequences of A_2-P_2 can occur from either electrical or hemodynamic causes.

Electrical Factors. Electrical disturbances that alter the normal sequence of depolarization of the ventricles include left bundle branch block (Fig. 3–10) and ectopic beats, paced beats, or idioventricular rhythm originating on the right side of the heart. Preexcitation may also result in a precedence of right ventricular systole and reversal of S_2.

Hemodynamic Factors. Mechanical factors that are associated with prolongation of left ventricular ejection time include outflow obstruction of the left ventricle, as in aortic

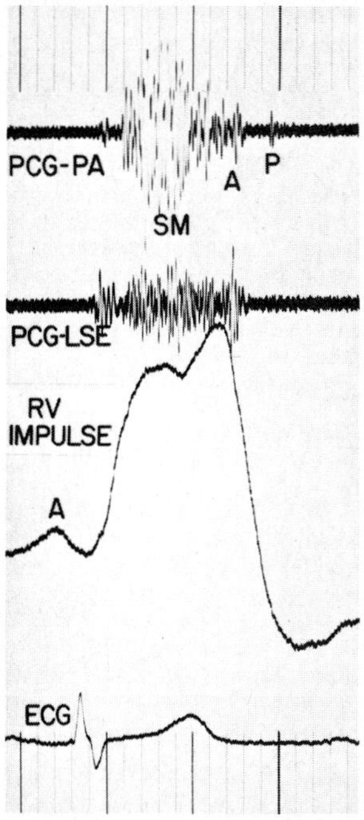

FIGURE 3–8. Wide splitting of S_2 in infundibular pulmonic stenosis. There is an associated ventricular septal defect with left-to-right shunting. The separation of A_2- P_2 is 0.08 sec, a figure consistent with the systemic pressures encountered in the right ventricle (RV).[57] There is an ejection murmur in the second left intercostal space (PA) from the RV outflow obstruction, whereas at the lower sternal edge (LSE), the murmur has a holosystolic configuration, suggesting that it is largely the result of the ventricular septal defect. The RV impulse recorded at LSE shows a prominent *a* wave (A) and a sustained systolic thrust consistent with right ventricular hypertrophy.

stenosis (Fig. 3–9) or hypertrophic obstructive cardiomyopathy (HOCM). Paradoxical splitting of S_2 is found only in the most severe cases. In patent ductus arteriosus, the increased stroke volume of the left ventricle may also

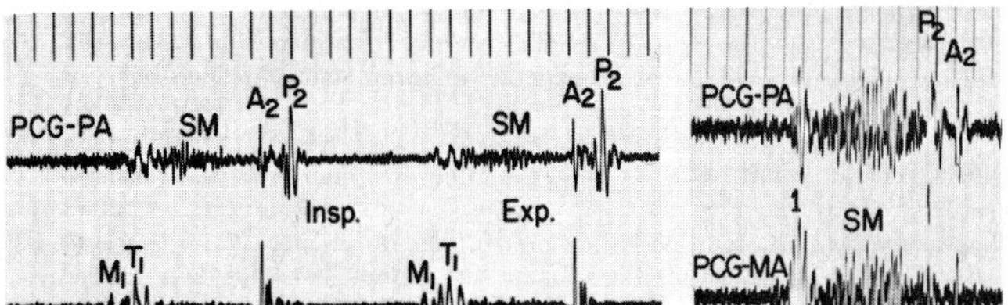

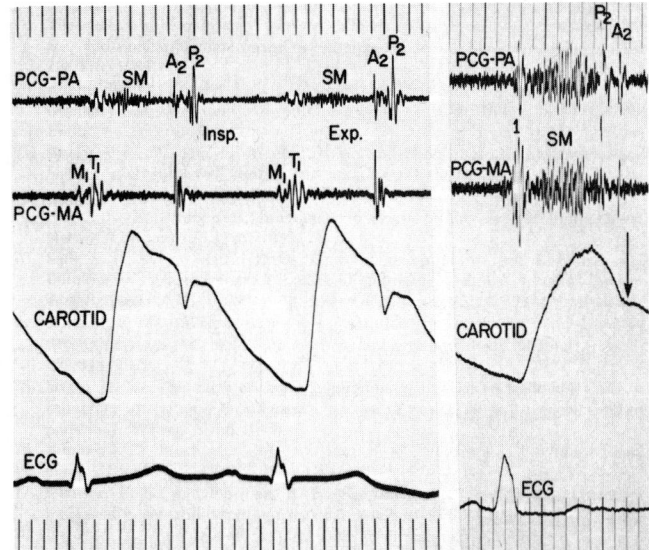

FIGURE 3–9. *Left,* Atrial septal defect showing a midsystolic murmur (SM) and "fixed" splitting of S_2 in the second left intercostal space (PCG-PA). The separation of A_2 and P_2 is 0.06 sec in inspiration and expiration. The first heart sound shows a relatively loud tricuspid component (T_1). *Right,* Aortic stenosis, with reversed splitting of S_2. There is a prominent midsystolic murmur. A_2 is identified by its occurrence immediately prior to the incisura (arrow) on the carotid pulse tracing. P_2 is seen to fall still earlier by 0.04 sec. The carotid upstroke is slow and is shattered by coarse vibrations.

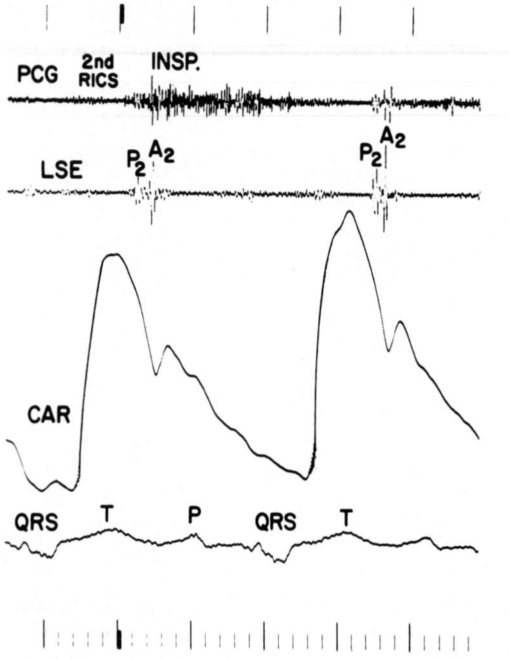

FIGURE 3–10. Reversed splitting of S_2 in left bundle branch block PCG at left sternal edge (LSE) shows P_2 before A_2, the latter being identified by its occurrence immediately before the incisura in the carotid pulse tracing. With inspiration the gap between P_2 and A_2 narrows, illustrating the physical sign that would permit the detection of reversed splitting by auscultation.

lengthen left ventricular ejection time, resulting in a reversal of A_2-P_2 (p. 923). However, the accentuation of the murmur at the time of S_2, which is characteristic of this defect, obscures the details of S_2 both on auscultation and on the phonocardiogram.

Single S_2. The second sound may seem to be single on auscultation or on the phonocardiogram because (1) it is indeed single, (2) one of its two elements is inaudible, or (3) both components occur simultaneously. The most common cause for an *apparently* single S_2 is inability to hear or record the fainter of the two elements of the sound (usually P_2) because of emphysema, obesity, or other technical problems. A truly single S_2, however, is seen in tetralogy of Fallot or pulmonary atresia, in which A_2 is loud and is usually easily recorded, whereas pulmonary closure is absent or so soft that it escapes detection. Fusion of the two elements of S_2 resulting in a very loud single S_2 occurs with ventricular septal defect with pulmonary hypertension.

Intensity of S_2. Recording the two elements of S_2 is best accomplished with the microphone at the upper left sternal border. Although P_2 is best appreciated in this location and is poorly transmitted elsewhere, it ordinarily does not exceed A_2 in intensity in normal subjects, even at the upper left sternal edge. When it is shown by graphic records to exceed A_2 in amplitude or to be unusually well transmitted, such as to the cardiac apex, one must suspect pulmonary hypertension or atrial septal defect.[59] An exaggerated P_2 is, however, only a crude indicator of pulmonary hypertension. In atrial septal defect, P_2 may be accentuated and widely transmitted even when the pulmonary arterial pressure is normal.

A *diminished P_2* is found in pulmonic stenosis (pp. 992 and 1076), either valvular or infundibular, since this obstructing lesion results in low pressure in the pulmonary artery and a diminished force effecting closure of the valve (Fig. 3–8).

Accentuation of A_2, like other phonocardiographic observations of heart-sound intensity, is usually a subjective assessment owing to variations in thickness of the chest wall and other technical factors that make quantitation virtually impossible. Nevertheless, an increase in A_2 is frequently present in systemic hypertension, coarctation of the aorta, and corrected transposition of the great arteries.

Reduction in intensity of A_2 occurs in aortic stenosis in adults, in whom the valve is often immobilized by calcification (p. 1055). The high-speed cinematographic studies of aortic valve motion of Stein have documented a reduced development of retrograde seating velocity in these valves.[60] In children with congenitally deformed but still mobile valve cusps, the intensity of A_2 is usually normal (p. 933). A soft A_2 is characteristic of aortic regurgitation, since the incompetent valve fails to halt effectively the retrograde blood momentum developed during valve seating.

EJECTION SOUNDS

Ejection sounds of *aortic origin* are of high frequency and occur early in systole, usually 0.12 to 0.14 sec after the Q wave of the electrocardiogram. These sounds are most prominent in association with a deformed aortic valve, as in congenital aortic stenosis bicuspid configuration (Fig. 3–11),[61–63] or rheumatic heart disease. A mobile valve is necessary for sound production, since with heavy calcification and immobilization of the valve the ejection sound disappears. Aortic ejection sounds from deformed valves are widely transmitted over the precordium and are well recorded at the cardiac apex. They also occur in association with systemic hypertension and other conditions in which the aortic root may be dilated. Such ejection sounds have a similar timing but are usually less prominent

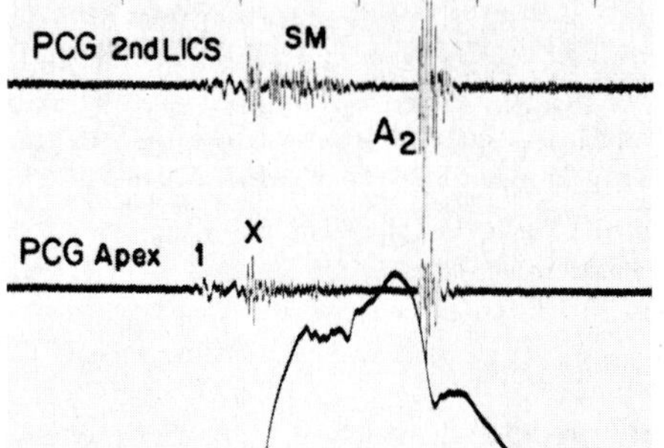

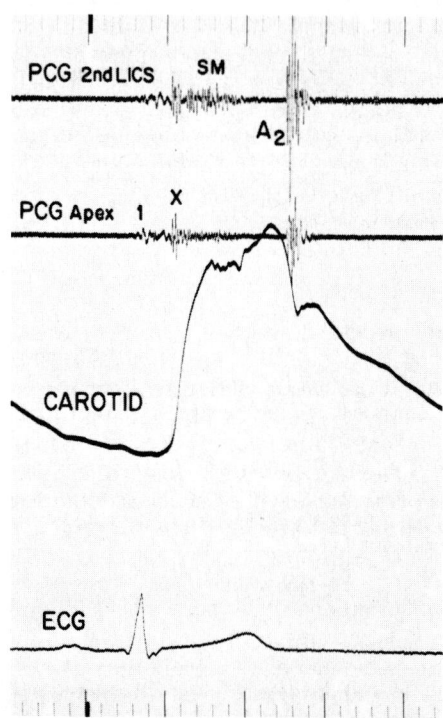

FIGURE 3–11. Aortic ejection sound of valvular origin in a 22-year-old man. The ejection sound (X) is widely transmitted over the precordium and is well seen at cardiac apex. An early to midsystolic murmur is recorded at the base of the heart (PCG 2nd LICS). The carotid tracing is deformed with a delayed peak. These findings are best explained by a bicuspid aortic valve with mild stenosis.

than those caused by valvular disease. Under these conditions the sound is not as widely transmitted as with a deformed valve and may be confined to the upper right sternal border (Fig. 3–12). The intensity of aortic ejection sounds does not vary with respiration.

The clinical conditions in which *pulmonic ejection sounds* occur are similar to those in which aortic ejection sounds are found—valve abnormalities, such as congenital pulmonic stenosis (p. 942), or pulmonary hypertension.[64, 65] These sounds are usually confined to the upper left sternal border. Their timing is earlier than that of aortic ejection sounds, usually occurring 0.09 to 0.11 sec after the Q wave. The pulmonic ejection sound associated with valve stenosis fluctuates with respiration, being loudest during expiration, and this fluctuation is attributed to the position of the valve at the onset of right ventricular systole.[65] With inspiration, blood is drawn into the right ventricle, augmenting the effect of atrial systole and resulting in partial opening of the pulmonic valve prior to ventricular systole. The consequently diminished additional movement of the valve imparted by ventricular systole is associated with a muted ejection sound. With expiration, on the other hand, the pulmonic valve opens swiftly from a fully closed

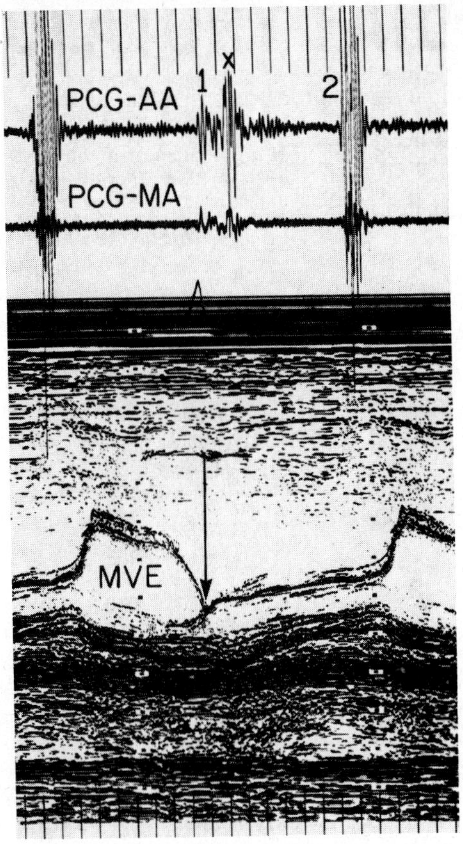

FIGURE 3–12. Aortic ejection sound of "vascular" origin in a patient with syphilitic aortitis and dilated aorta. An ejection sound (X) is seen to follow the first sound and mitral valve closure in the mitral valve echo (MVE = arrow) by 0.06 sec. It is coincident with full opening of the aortic valve (not illustrated) and is not widely transmitted, being clearly recorded only in the second right intercostal space (AA). The second sound is very prominent in the phonocardiogram and had a ringing "tambour" quality on auscultation.

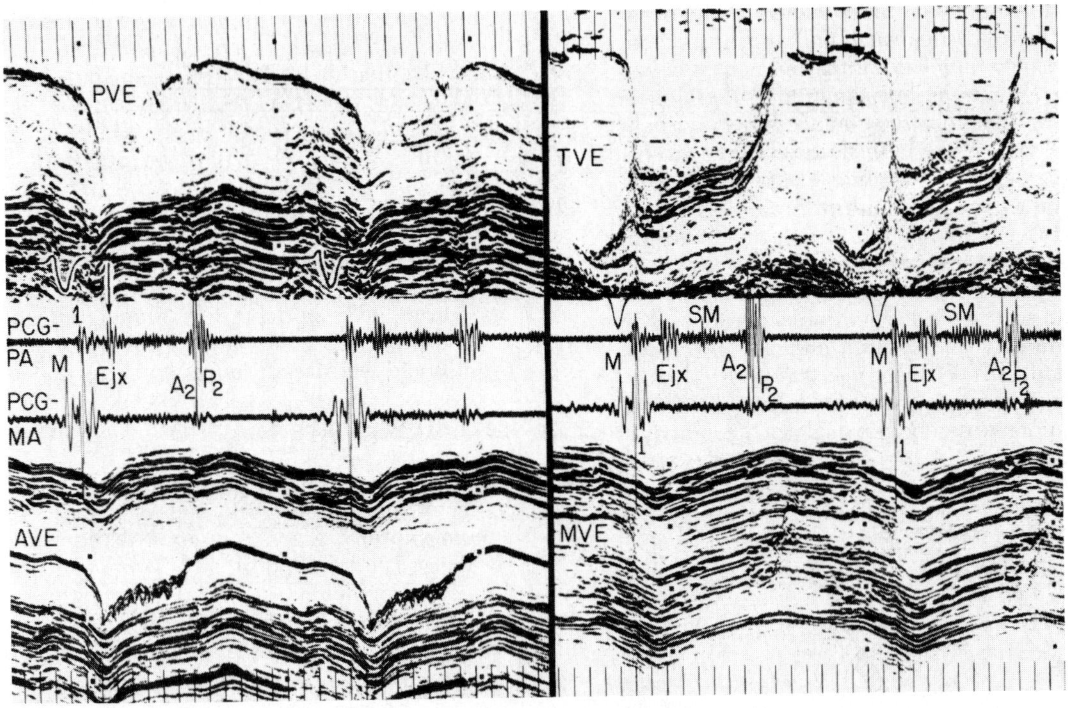

FIGURE 3–13. Ejection sound associated with pulmonary hypertension. The patient had mitral stenosis, and a Hancock porcine aortic valve had been inserted in the mitral position. Dual echophonocardiograms identify the various sounds occurring in early systole.

Left, **Dual echophonocardiogram of pulmonic valve (PVE) and of patient's own aortic valve (AVE). The pulmonic valve achieves a fully open position coincident with the ejection sound (Ejx), which is much delayed at 0.17 sec from the onset of QRS, consistent with the pulmonary hypertension.[66] The aortic valve (AVE) opens earlier and thus cannot be responsible for the Ejx. The low-frequency vibration M occurs before S_1 (1) and is attributed to ventricular muscular contraction.**

Right, **Dual echophonocardiogram of same patient showing the tricuspid valve (TVE) and prosthetic valve (MVE) closing simultaneously coincident with S_1. The echocardiographic representation of the valves has been magnified to facilitate examination of details of their movements. The QRS complex in the left-hand panel has been retouched to permit its identification within a mass of echoes.**

position, and at the sudden termination of its opening movement, a maximal ejection sound ensues. The *decrease* in intensity of the ejection sound in pulmonic valve stenosis with inspiration contrasts with the behavior of T_1, which *increases* with inspiration. Careful attention to this detail may be helpful in identifying auscultatory events in early systole. The ejection sound of pulmonic valve stenosis occurs slightly earlier with severe obstruction in contrast to the mild type. The ejection sound of pulmonary hypertension, however, is delayed slightly when the level of pressure in the pulmonary artery is high (Fig. 3–13).[66, 67]

Although some details of the controversies concerning the origin of the first and second sounds may seem merely "academic," the principles involved are of considerable clinical importance, especially in recognition of ejection sounds, which begin at the exact time of *maximal opening* of the semilunar valves (Fig. 3–13). Ejection sounds are called "valvular" when found in association with abnormal valves and "vascular" when valves are normal, but the physiology is otherwise disturbed. In either case it can be shown by echophonocardiography that the high-frequency ejection sound starts at the moment of full opening of the aortic or pulmonic valve.[68] Although it is generally accepted that the "valvular" ejection sound is caused by halting of the "doming" valve, the origin of the "vascular" sounds is not clear, and their presence is by no means invariable in systemic or pulmonary hypertension. It may be that "vascular" ejection sounds result from a distorted configuration of a normal valve situated in the root of a dilated great vessel. Under these circumstances, the valve may functionally resemble a bicuspid valve, with a similar vibrational mechanism.

OTHER HEART SOUNDS

OPENING SNAPS. *Mitral opening snaps* can best be recorded approximately midway between the pulmonary and mitral areas, i.e., over the midprecordium.[69] High-frequency settings of the recording apparatus are preferred for these sounds. *Tricuspid opening snaps* can occasionally be recorded at the lower left sternal edge in the presence of tricuspid stenosis, atrial septal defect, or Ebstein's anomaly (Fig. 3–5).[58] Echophonocardiographic studies show that opening snaps from either side of the heart occur at exactly the time of maximal opening of the respective atrioventricular valve in early diastole (Fig. 3–14).[70] Recognition of these relationships allows identification of sounds in this phase of the cardiac cycle with considerably more precision than has been possible with phonocardiography alone. The occurrence of mitral and tricuspid opening snaps, once a fully open position of the valve is achieved, is of importance in the establishment of general principles of the genesis of sound, since it parallels the situation described above in connection with ejection sounds and their relationship to full opening of the semilunar valves. Opening snaps are characteristic of a stenotic valve that is still pliable, but they are also seen in circumstances in which there is swift opening of a nonstenotic valve, such as occurs in severe mitral regurgitation or atrial septal defect.[71]

An acoustically similar sound is the tumor "plop" of a left atrial myxoma (p. 1471). This occurs when the tumor has moved in early diastole and comes to a sudden halt at the full extent of its excursion into the ventricle. The anatomical correlates of this sound can easily be demonstrated by echophonocardiography (Fig. 3–15).[9]

MITRAL VALVE PROLAPSE (see also p. 1045). The midsystolic click, which is one of the principal diagnostic features of prolapse of the mitral valve, has been shown to coincide with the time of maximal valve prolapse (Fig. 3–31.[72] This observation is consistent with the thesis advanced above that high-frequency sounds of cardiac origin occur when a valve has moved in response to hemodynamic forces and is suddenly checked in its course.

THIRD AND FOURTH HEART SOUNDS. In contrast to S_1, S_2, ejection sounds, and opening snaps, which are predominantly of *high frequency*, third (S_3) and fourth (S_4) sounds are of *low frequency*. The left-sided S_3 occurs in association with rapid filling of the ventricle, as in normal youthful

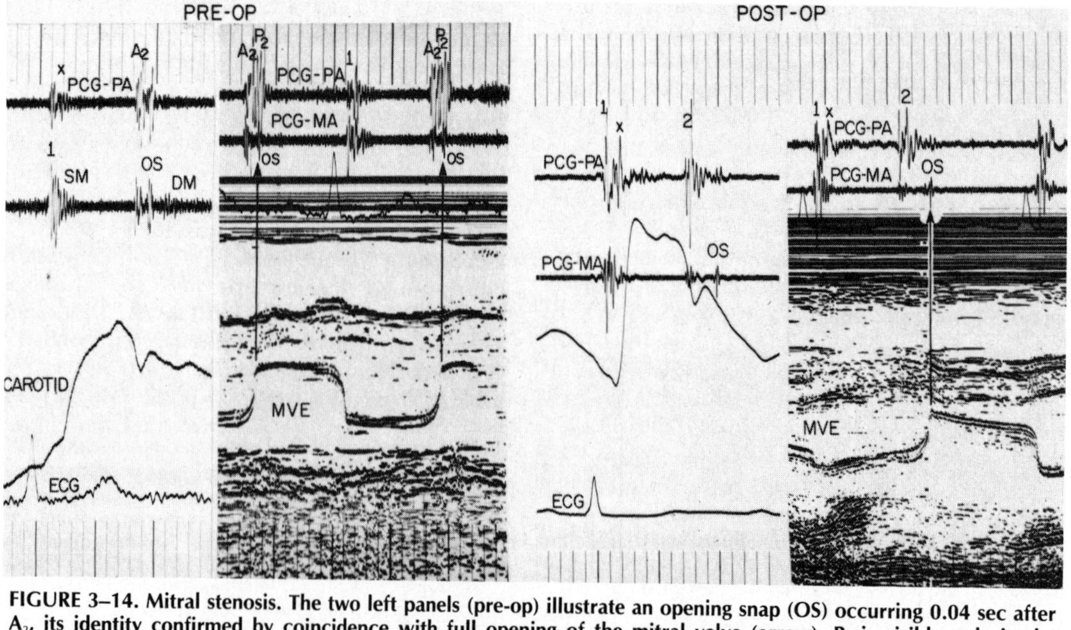

FIGURE 3–14. Mitral stenosis. The two left panels (pre-op) illustrate an opening snap (OS) occurring 0.04 sec after A_2, its identity confirmed by coincidence with full opening of the mitral valve (arrow). P_2 is visible only in the phonocardiogram of PA, occupying the space between A_2 and OS. An ejection sound (x) is seen in the tracing from the second left interspace (PA), reflecting pulmonary hypertension. Following successful valvulotomy (post-op), the OS moves out to 0.10 sec from A_2. The differences in carotid pulse wave contour in the two tracings are accounted for by technical imperfections in the pre-op record, since there was no evidence of aortic valve disease.

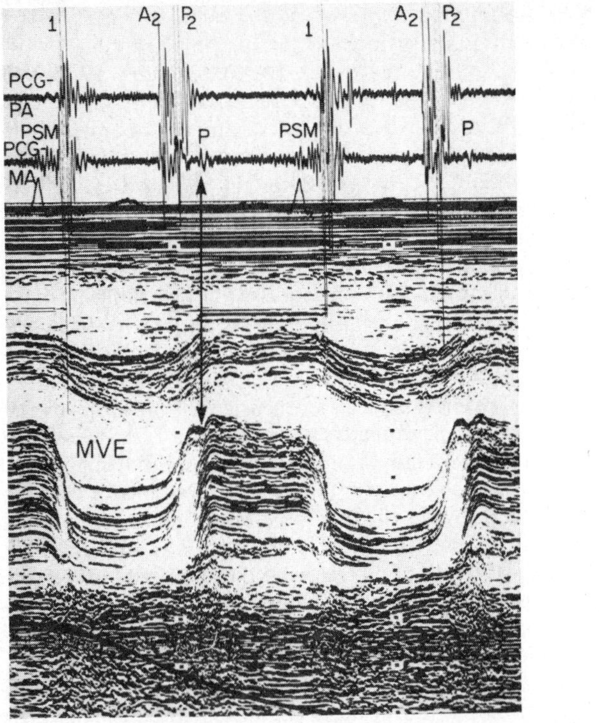

FIGURE 3–15. Left atrial myxoma. A young woman with a large myxoma resulting in symptoms of pulmonary congestion. S_1 is accentuated and delayed and is preceded by a brief "presystolic" crescendo murmur (PSM) occurring as the tumor mass (dense echoes in MVE) is thrust by ventricular contraction into the orifice of the mitral valve, thereby obstructing inflow from the atrium. P_2 is accentuated because of pulmonary hypertension and is widely transmitted to the cardiac apex (MA). It is followed by a tumor "plop" (P), which occurs 0.10 sec from A_2 and is coincident with completion of the ventricular excursion of the tumor mass (arrow).

subjects, mitral regurgitation (Fig. 3–1), and thyrotoxicosis.[73] In other pathological conditions, such as left ventricular failure, the term "gallop" is applied to the analogous sound,[74] but once again its pathogenesis is related to ventricular filling in early diastole. In pericardial constriction, ventricular filling is also confined to early diastole and terminates with a sharp S_3 or pericardial "knock" (p. 1503) (Fig. 3–16).[75] In all these situations, the phonocardiogram records a low-frequency vibration (S_3) simultaneously with the peak of the rapid filling wave of the apexcardiogram.

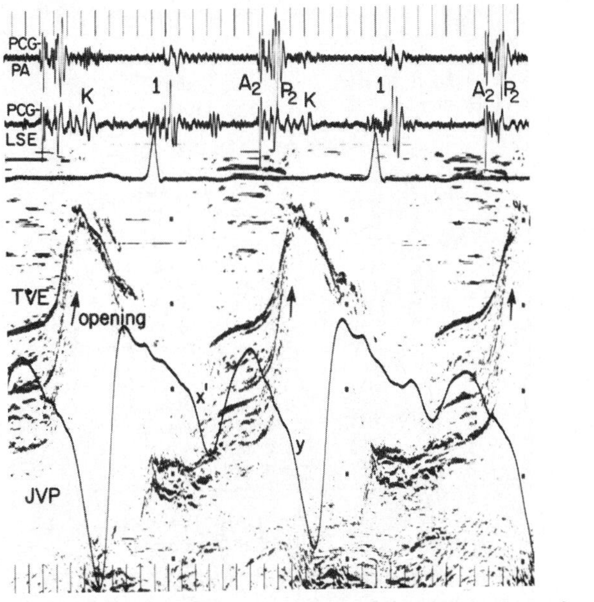

FIGURE 3–16. Pericardial knock. The relationship of the third sound or knock (K) associated with constrictive pericarditis to the jugular venous pulse (JVP) and movements of the tricuspid valve TVE is shown. The valve opens completely (arrows) before the knock. The latter, however, is closely related temporally to the nadir of the *y* descent of the JVP. P_2 is accentuated and widely transmitted, consistent with the pulmonary hypertension that was found at cardiac catheterization.

The exact mechanism of the genesis of the third sound has been controversial, there being proponents of valvular,[6] ventricular,[7, 76, 77] and impact of the left ventricle against the chest wall[8] mechanisms. Our own observations indicate the sound to be the result of a sudden inherent limitation in the long axis filling movement of the left ventricle,[7, 78, 79] a view consistent with traditional concepts dating from Potain in the 19th century. Studies in the authors' laboratory[79] have indicated the presence of exaggerated velocity of filling of the left ventricle in its long axis in both hyper- and hypodynamic global chamber filling conditions. We believe that this is a common feature explaining the presence of S_3 in a wide variety of conditions ranging from mitral regurgitation to cardiomyopathy and observed also in normal young people.

Fourth sounds, or atrial sounds, occur under circumstances of altered compliance of the ventricle, either left or right.[80] Thus, in coronary heart disease, HOCM, aortic stenosis, and systemic hypertension, a left-sided S_4 is a common feature (Fig. 3–17). A right-sided S_4 may be found under analogous circumstances, as in pulmonary hypertension or pulmonic valve stenosis.[81]

Identification of S_4 in a graphic tracing is best accomplished by noting its coincidence with the peak of the *a* wave in the accompanying apexcardiogram.[82] The combination of a long P-R interval and a rapid heart rate may result in a confluence of diastolic events in such a way that third and fourth sounds may merge to form a loud summation sound (Fig. 3–18).[83]

PROSTHETIC VALVE SOUNDS. Surgical implantation of prosthetic valves and pacemakers results in a whole array of auscultatory phenomena. The sounds produced by prostheses vary, depending on their location, their manner of opening and closing, and their constituents—plastic, steel, or biological tissues. In general, the metal balls used

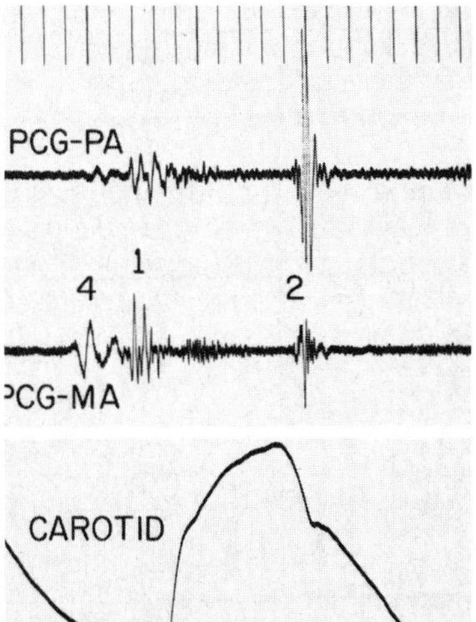

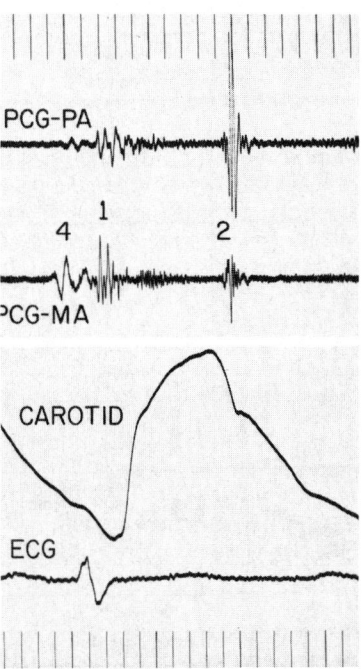

FIGURE 3–17. Fourth heart sound (4) in association with systemic hypertension and left ventricular hypertrophy. The low frequency of S_4 is apparent, compared with S_1 and S_2.

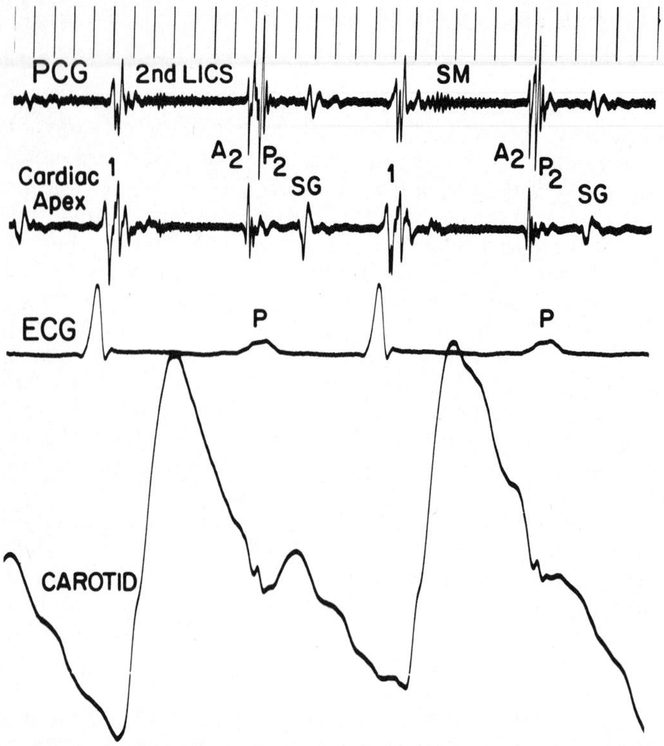

FIGURE 3–18. Summation sound, often called summation gallop (SG), in a young woman with second-degree AV block characterized by Wenckebach periods. Atrial systole occurs in early diastole owing to the long P-R interval, and the augmented left ventricular filling results in a summation sound.

in Starr-Edwards valves produce the loudest, most distinctive sounds on both opening and closing.[84] Tilting disk valves (e.g., Björk-Shiley or Lillehei-Kaster) produce loud, crisp sounds on closing but little or no sound on opening.[85] Porcine heterograft valves produce a sound similar to that of a normal valve on closing, and they may open silently.[86]

The timing of prosthetic valve movements may occasionally provide information regarding malfunction, since the movements of prostheses are in response to rapidly fluctuating pressures in adjacent heart chambers.

For example, the expected time of opening of most of the currently used prostheses in the mitral position is approximately 0.08 sec following the aortic component of S_2 (Figs. 3–19 and 3–20).[84–86] This period reflects the isovolumetric relaxation time of the left ventricle, and a major factor determining its length is left atrial pressure. Obstruction of the prosthesis by a thrombus or a paravalvular leak will produce elevation of left atrial pressure, and isovolumetric relaxation time will be abbreviated.[87]

PACEMAKER SOUNDS. A sharp, high-frequency sound of very brief duration is occasionally audible overlying a transvenous pacemaker placed in the right ventricle. This sound, which may be accompanied by a slight twitch of skeletal muscle in the underlying area of the chest wall, is coincident with the pacemaker spike and is believed to arise from the stimulation of intercostal muscle.[88]

FRICTION RUBS. The principal elements of a pericardial friction rub occur during those phases of the cardiac cycle in which there is maximal movement of the heart in the pericardial sac. These are atrial systole, ventricular systole, and passive ventricular filling in early diastole (p. 404). This timing of auscultatory events can be portrayed graphically if desired. Unfortunately, however, phonocardiography does not reproduce the unique auscultatory quality of a rub, and therefore it usually adds nothing to a bedside assessment made by a competent examiner.

ECHOPHONOCARDIOGRAPHY FOR THE IDENTIFICATION OF HEART SOUNDS.[89] The finding on auscultation of two discrete sounds in quick succession at the onset of systole presents a common auscultatory problem. This combination could be due to normal splitting of S_1, with both mitral (M_1) and tricuspid (T_1) elements being well heard, as in normal youthful subjects (Figs. 3–2, 3–4, and 3–5), atrial septal defect, or right bundle branch block. Alternatively, a somewhat similar combination of sounds could be produced by S_4-S_1 or by S_1 and an ejection sound, as with a bicuspid aortic valve or valvular pulmonic stenosis (Figs. 3–11 to 3–14, and 3–17). A sequence of S_1 and an

Prosthesis type	Mitral Prosthesis	Acoustic Characteristics	Aortic Prosthesis	Acoustic Characteristics
Ball Valves	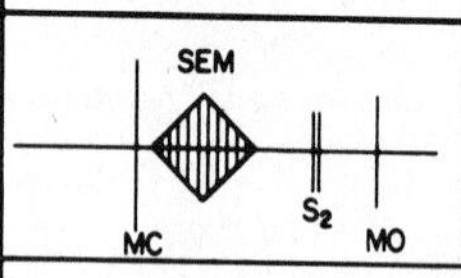 SEM; MC; S_2; MO	1) A_2–MO interval 0.07–0.11 sec. 2) MO > MC 3) II–III/VI Systolic ejection murmur (SEM) 4) No diastolic murmur	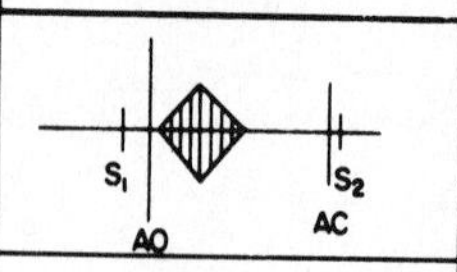 S_1; AO; S_2; AC	1) S_1–AO interval 0.07 sec. 2) AO > AC 3) II/VI harsh SEM 4) No diastolic murmur
Disc Valves	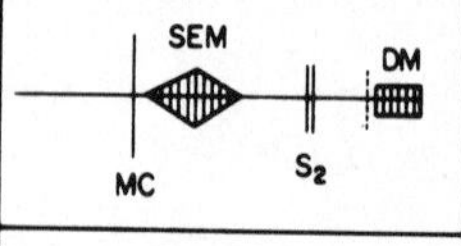 SEM; DM; MC; S_2	1) A_2–MO interval 0.05–0.09 sec. 2) MO is rarely heard 3) II/VI SEM is usually heard 4) I–II/VI diastolic rumble is usually heard	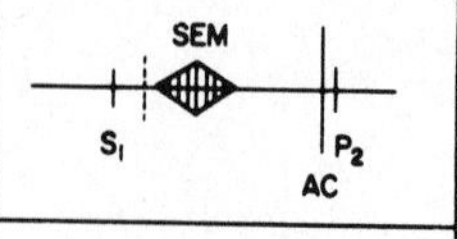 SEM; S_1; P_2; AC	1) S_1–AO interval 0.04 sec. 2) AO is uncommonly heard, AC is usually heard 3) II/VI SEM is usually heard 4) Occasional diastolic murmur
Porcine Valves	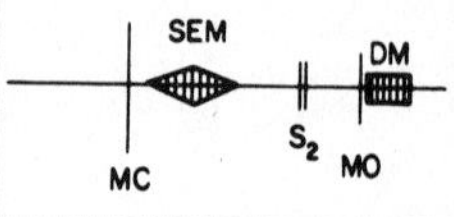 SEM; DM; MC; S_2; MO	1) A_2–MO interval 0.1 sec. 2) MO is audible 50% 3) I–II/VI apical SEM 50% 4) Diastolic rumble ½–⅔	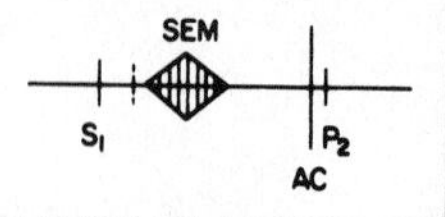 SEM; S_1; P_2; AC	1) S_1–AO interval 0.03–0.08 sec. 2) AO is uncommonly heard, AC is usually heard 3) II/VI SEM in most 4) No diastolic murmur
Bileaflet Valve (St. Jude)			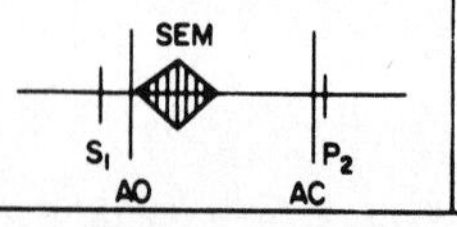 SEM; S_1; AO; P_2; AC	1) AO and AC commonly heard 2) A soft SEM is common

FIGURE 3–19. Summary of the acoustic characteristics of each valve prosthesis according to type and location. SEM = systolic ejection murmur; DM = diastolic murmur; S_1 = first heart sound; S_2 = second heart sound; P_2 = pulmonic second sound; A_2 = aortic second sound; AO = aortic valve opening sound; AC = aortic valve closure sound; MO = mitral valve opening sound; MC = mitral valve closure sound. (From Smith, N. D., Raizada, V., and Abrams, J.: Auscultation of the normally functioning prosthetic valve. Ann. Intern. Med. 95:594, 1981.)

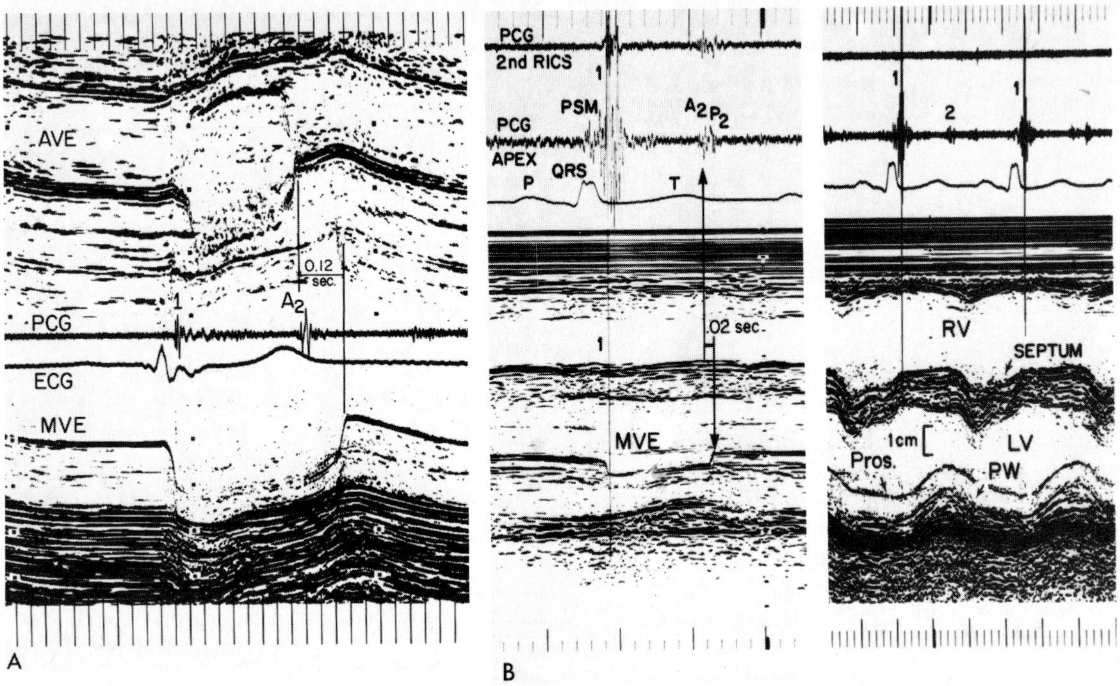

FIGURE 3–20. *A*, Echophonocardiogram from a patient with a normally functioning Lillehei-Kaster prosthesis in the mitral position. The dual echo shows the aortic valve above (AVE) and mitral prosthesis below (MVE). A_2 is coincident with aortic valve closure and is followed after 0.12 sec by full opening of the prosthesis.

B, Left, A Starr-Edwards prosthesis in the mitral position, malfunctioning due to thrombosis causing obstruction. The valve closes with a loud sound (1) preceded by a presystolic crescendo murmur (PSM) resembling that of mitral stenosis. The prosthesis opens only 0.02 sec after A_2, indicating an extremely short isovolumetric relaxation time, which in turn suggests a high left atrial pressure.

Right, In the same patient the echo shows a dilated right ventricle (RV) with paradoxical septal movement consistent with the clinically evident tricuspid regurgitation. The left ventricle (LV) is relatively small, a point discounting paravalvular leak and favoring obstruction at the valve level as an explanation for the suspected left atrial hypertension.

early systolic click of mitral origin can also present in this fashion. Although the associated findings on physical examination, x-ray, and electrocardiogram may clarify this problem, echophonocardiography usually provides a more certain solution. M_1 and T_1 can be identified by their coincidence with full closure of the mitral and tricuspid valves, respectively. Aortic and pulmonic ejection sounds occur with full opening of the respective semilunar valve. Fourth sounds, or atrial sounds, occur at the peak of the *a* wave of the apexcardiogram, whereas the click of mitral prolapse may be identified as occurring after the above-mentioned events. Mitral clicks sometimes coincide with prolapse of the valve on the echocardiogram, but this relationship is not invariable.

A similar problem often exists at the end of systole and in early diastole when various combinations of A_2, P_2, opening snaps, and third sounds from either side of the heart may lead to a confused interpretation of bedside physical signs (Figs. 3–14 to 3–16). Opening of a prosthetic valve in the mitral or tricuspid position also occurs in this phase of the cardiac cycle. A very early opening snap, indicative of a high left atrial pressure and a severe degree of stenosis of the mitral valve (p. 1027), may occur close to P_2, so that the accurate identification of these sounds is of more than academic importance. A_2 is most precisely identified as being synchronous with closure of the aortic valve on the echocardiogram as well as by its occurrence just prior to the incisura in the carotid artery tracing. Opening snaps and prosthetic valve sounds coincide with achievement of a fully open position of the respective valve; third sounds occur at the peak of the rapid filling wave on the apexcardiogram. P_2, then, is often identified by exclusion because of the difficulty in delineating closure of the pulmonic valve echocardiographically.

CAROTID PULSE TRACINGS AND SYSTOLIC TIME INTERVALS

The carotid pulse is recorded by placement of the transducer firmly over the arterial pulsation, previously identified by palpation. As noted above, its prominence can be enhanced by hyperextension of the neck.

NORMAL CAROTID PULSE. The normal carotid pulse tracing (Figs. 3–1 and 3–2) has a rapid, smooth upstroke, beginning approximately 0.12 to 0.15 sec from the onset of the QRS complex in adults; it reaches a peak within 0.12 sec. Following the period of rapid ejection of blood from the left ventricle, the pulse wave declines to the dicrotic notch, or incisura, which is caused by aortic valve closure. Owing to the transmission time of the pulse wave from the aortic root to the site of application of the transducer over the carotid artery, there is a variable delay from the aortic closure sound, A_2, to the incisura of approximately 0.02 to 0.03 sec (Figs. 3–1 and 3–2). During diastole, the carotid pulse wave usually falls gently until the next systolic pulse. The shape of carotid pulse curves varies widely among different normal individuals and even in the same subject, depending on the mode of application of the transducer.

The incisural notch occurs approximately 0.02 to 0.03 sec after aortic valve closure and A_2. Therefore the carotid pulse tracing is a reliable marker for this important auscultatory and phonocardiographic event (Figs. 3–1 and 3–2) and is a most valuable basic ingredient in the phonocardiographic examination.

SYSTOLIC TIME INTERVALS

Systolic time intervals (STI) have been used sporadically for a century as a measure of left ventricular performance.[90–93] It is only in recent years, however, that validation of the significance of STI has been obtained through comparative studies with various invasive indices of ventricular function (Chap. 15). This has led to widespread acceptance of STI as a simple, inexpensive, and nontraumatic method of estimating left ventricular performance and following the patient's progress over time. Many investigators have contributed to our rapidly increasing knowledge of the significance and utility of STI in clinical medicine. In particular, Weissler, Lewis, and associates have been responsible for popularization of this noninvasive method, and the reader is referred to their extensive publications for further details on the subject.[16, 94–97]

The three basic STI are the preejection period (PEP), the left ventricular ejection time (LVET), and the total electromechanical interval (QS_2) (Fig. 3–21). In order to avoid misleading errors, the technique of recording must be carried out with meticulous attention to detail. STI are obtained from simultaneous fast-speed (100 mm/sec) recordings of the electrocardiogram, the phonocardiogram, and the carotid pulsation.[16] The ECG lead that most clearly displays the onset of left ventricular depolarization is chosen. The phonocardiogram must provide a clear view of the initial high-frequency vibrations of the aortic component of the second heart sound (A_2). The carotid pulsation is generally recorded with a funnel-shaped pick-up attached by polyethylene tubing to a transducer with an adequate time constant, as discussed earlier in this chapter under Phonocardiographic Technique. For clear and accurate measurement of STI, one should employ tracings with the following characteristics: (1) a clear initial depolarization force departing acutely from a flat baseline on the electrocardiogram, to mark the beginning of QRS; (2) a sharp inscription of the initial high-frequency vibrations of A_2; and (3) a clearly discernible rapid upstroke and pointed single incisural notch on the carotid arterial pulse tracing. Amplification of the carotid signal should be adequate to provide a pulse wave of at least 5 cm in height on the recording paper.

TABLE 3–1 CALCULATION OF STI INDEX VALUES FROM RESTING REGRESSION EQUATIONS

Sex	Equation	Normal Index (msec)	SD
M	$QS_2I = 2.1\ hr + QS_2$	546	14
F	$QS_2I = 2.0\ hr + QS_2$	549	14
M	LVETI = 1.7 hr + LVET	413	10
F	LVETI = 1.6 hr + LVET	418	11
M	PEPI = 0.4 hr + PEP	131	10
F	PEPI = 0.4 hr + PEP	133	10

Key: I = index; SD = standard deviation; M = male; F = female; hr = heart rate.

From Weissler, A. M., et al.: Bedside technics for the evaluation of ventricular function in man. Am. J. Cardiol. 23:577, 1969.

The QS_2 is measured from the onset of the QRS to the earliest high-frequency vibrations of A_2. LVET is measured from the beginning upstroke to the trough of the incisural notch of the carotid pulse tracing (Fig. 3–21). The PEP is that interval from the beginning of ventricular depolarization to the beginning of ventricular ejection. PEP is derived by subtracting LVET from QS_2, this step being necessary in order to eliminate the delay in transmission of the arterial pulse from the aortic root to the position on the carotid artery of the transducer. The PEP is made up of the electromechanical interval plus the isovolumetric contraction time. The electromechanical interval is relatively constant in most individuals, except where there is left ventricular conduction delay, as in left bundle branch block. Therefore, variations in isovolumetric contraction time constitute the principal information of physiological significance in measurements of the PEP.

In applying STI measurements, correction must be made for differences in heart rate. When heart rate is derived from the R-R interval, a simple linear equation best describes the relationship of STI to rate. The regression equations of Weissler have been generally adopted for this purpose (Table 3–1).

In applying STI clinically, derivations from normal

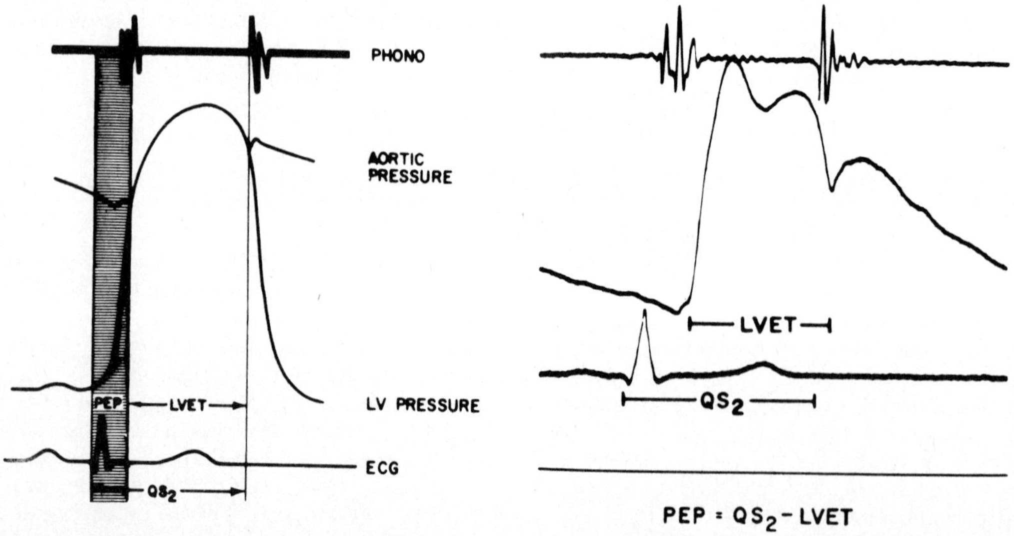

FIGURE 3–21. On the left is a diagram of the left ventricular events which constitute the STI. On the right is a recording of a phonocardiogram, external carotid pulse, and electrocardiogram at 100 mm/sec paper speed. The subintervals of the STI are indicated on both. (From Lewis, R. P., et al.: A critical review of the systolic time intervals. Circulation 56:146, 1977, by permission of the American Heart Association, Inc.)

regressions can be indicated by expressing each of the systolic time intervals as an "index" value, as shown in Table 3–1. By calculating the index value, one obtains an estimate of the deviation from normal that cannot be explained by the heart rate. Thus, for example, a QS_2 index (QS_2I) of 506 msec in a man is easily recognized as being 40 msec shorter than the expected normal value of 546 msec.

At rates below 110 beats/min, the PEP and LVET shorten proportionately as heart rate increases. Therefore, a simple and increasingly popular method of expressing variations in STI in the normal range of heart rates is by the ratio of PEP/LVET. This ratio may identify left ventricular dysfunction when either the PEPI or the LVETI or both are still within the limits of normal. Since in many types of left ventricular dysfunction PEP lengthens and LVET shortens, higher ratios for PEP/LVET are abnormal. The PEP/LVET ratio is normally approximately 0.34 to 1,[95] with the upper limit being 0.42 to 1.[94]

FACTORS INFLUENCING THE STI. Factors known to influence the PEP and LVET are listed in Table 3–2. With left ventricular failure, regardless of cause, PEPI lengthens and LVETI shortens. Prolongation of PEPI is principally due to a reduced rate of left ventricular pressure rise during isovolumetric systole (LV dP/dt).[16] PEPI can also be prolonged by delayed electrical activation, as in LBBB. Under these circumstances, obviously a prolongation of PEPI cannot be used as an indicator of diminished left ventricular performance, since the problem may be simply due to electrical delay.

The shortening of LVETI that occurs with heart failure is a complex result of alterations in the rate and extent of fiber shortening of the left ventricle as well as delay in the onset of ejection due to prolongation of PEPI. Of these several factors, probably the most influential is a diminished extent of fiber shortening.[98] Thus, a shortened LVETI or abnormally elevated PEP/LVET ratio may be found in the presence of a diminished stroke volume. The absolute stroke volume index does not appear to determine LVET but rather the size of the stroke volume relative to the end-diastolic volume.[98] Studies relating the PEP/LVET ratio to left ventricular ejection fraction determined by quantitative angiography have shown a close correlation.[96] The relationship has been obtained in patients having valvular and nonvalvular heart disease with a wide variation in functional impairment.

The duration of systole (QS_2I) is remarkably constant for any individual patient. Many types of heart disease result in directionally opposite changes in PEPI and LVETI. QS_2I may therefore be relatively unaffected.[97] However, with inotropic stimulation, such as with digitalis or catecholamines, QS_2I is shortened.[95]

TABLE 3–2 FACTORS INFLUENCING SYSTOLIC TIME INTERVALS

	INCREASE(↑)	DECREASE(↓)
PEP	LV muscle failure Left bundle branch block ↓ Preload Negative inotropic agents	Aortic valve disease ↓ LV isovolumic pressure Positive inotropic agents
LVET	Aortic valve disease ↓ Afterload	LV muscle failure ↓ Preload Positive inotropic agents Negative inotropic agents
QS_2	Left bundle branch block Aortic valve disease	Positive inotropic agents

From Lewis, R. P., et al.: A critical review of the systolic time intervals. Circulation *56*:146, 1977, by permission of the American Heart Association, Inc.

CLINICAL APPLICATIONS OF SYSTOLIC TIME INTERVALS

EVALUATION OF LEFT VENTRICULAR PERFORMANCE IN CHRONIC MYOCARDIAL DISEASE. In a wide variety of heart diseases involving the left ventricle, including myocarditis, cardiomyopathy, coronary artery disease, and hypertensive heart disease, a deterioration in left ventricular performance may be manifested in an elevated PEP/LVET ratio. As mentioned above, this ratio correlates best with the left ventricular ejection fraction.[94, 96] Frequently, when overt manifestations of heart failure have been eliminated with diuretics, the persisting severe left ventricular dysfunction continues to be reflected in an abnormal PEP/LVET ratio.[99] On the other hand, a fundamental change such as a subsidence of myocarditis or relief of a reversible cardiomyopathy can be monitored by means of a gradually falling PEP/LVET ratio in serial observations. The STI have been used to estimate prognosis in patients following healed myocardial infarction, with an abnormal PEP/LVET ratio being found to indicate a significantly worse prognosis over a 5-year period.[94] These results are consistent with the generally agreed-upon observation that left ventricular function is a major prognostic factor in coronary artery disease.

AORTIC VALVE DISEASE. In aortic valve disease, either stenosis or regurgitation, there is a shortening of PEPI and a lengthening of LVETI such that the PEP/LVET ratio tends to fall.[95] The PEPI is short in aortic stenosis owing to the rapid dP/dt and low aortic diastolic pressure. Significant outflow tract obstruction lengthens LVETI. This observation has led to the use of STI as an additional noninvasive parameter for estimating severity of aortic stenosis.[95] When left ventricular dysfunction has complicated the course of aortic stenosis, opposing trends are found, with PEPI lengthening and LVETI shortening. The net result is that PEP/LVET cannot be reliably used to assess left ventricular function in aortic stenosis.

In aortic regurgitation there is also a shortening of PEPI (because of the low diastolic pressure) and a lengthening of LVETI.[95] Although a tendency can be found for PEP/LVET to fall with severe aortic regurgitation, the quantitative value of such a measurement has not been established.

CAROTID PULSE CONTOUR PATTERNS

Variability in morphological and temporal details of the carotid pulse may result from technical aspects of the recording, including the choice and application of transducers.[16] In spite of these problems, however, a considerable amount of qualitative information can be derived from alterations in carotid pulse wave tracings in various disease states. A slowly rising carotid pulse deformed by a shudder—the graphic representation of a thrill—is characteristic of valvular or subvalvular diaphragmatic aortic stenosis (Fig. 3–22). Unfortunately, efforts to quantitate the severity of aortic stenosis by the contour of the carotid pulse, the rapidity of its upstroke, or the achievement of its peak[100] have been disappointing.[101] In elderly patients with arteriosclerotic and therefore inelastic peripheral vasculature, the upstroke of the carotid pulse may be relatively swift despite severe obstruction. Conversely, in some cases of severe aortic regurgitation without any systolic gradient across the valve, the physical and graphic signs during systole may nevertheless simulate those of aortic stenosis.

A spike-and-dome pattern characterizes the carotid pulse wave of HOCM (Fig. 3–23). A bisferiens pulse is characteristic of aortic regurgitation or mixed aortic stenosis and

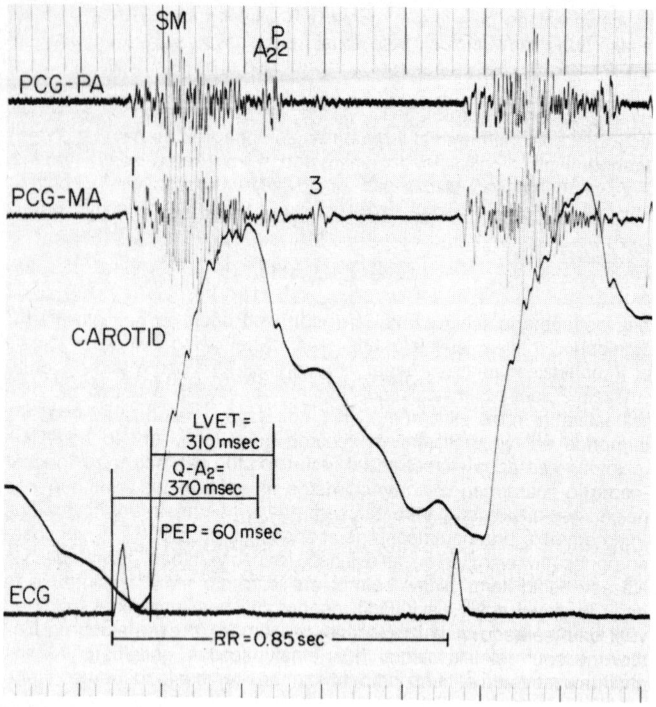

FIGURE 3–22. Valvular aortic stenosis in an 11-year-old boy with moderately severe obstruction (gradient = 50 to 60 mm Hg across the aortic valve). A loud midsystolic murmur is seen in all valve areas. The carotid upstroke is delayed and shattered by coarse vibrations. A_2 is well preserved. A third sound (3) is present, probably a normal finding in this youthful subject. The STI indicate a short PEP and prolonged LVET.[16]

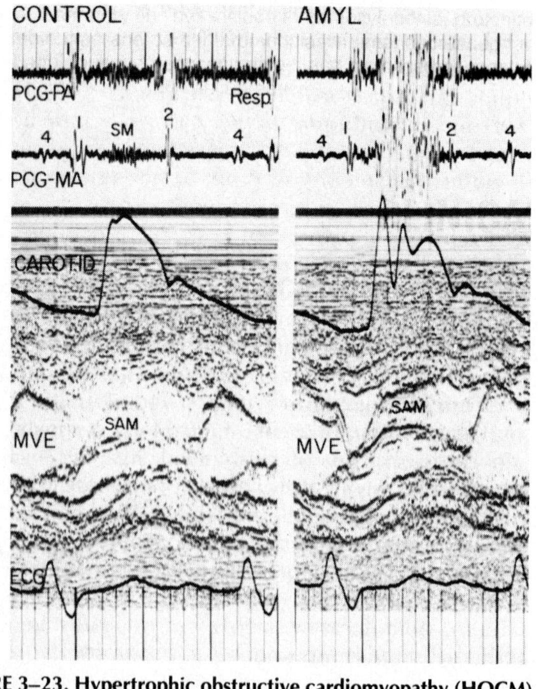

FIGURE 3–23. Hypertrophic obstructive cardiomyopathy (HOCM). *Left,* The control echophonocardiogram shows a fourth sound (4) at MA. The PCG-PA is obscured by a respiratory artifact (Resp). A midsystolic ejection murmur coincides with systolic anterior movement of the MVE (SAM). The carotid pulse contour is within normal limits. *Right,* Following inhalation of amyl nitrate (AMYL) the murmur becomes louder and the carotid pulse becomes deformed with a spike-and-dome pattern characteristic of HOCM. These changes are coincident with a more prominent SAM, which appears to be in contact with the interventricular septum.

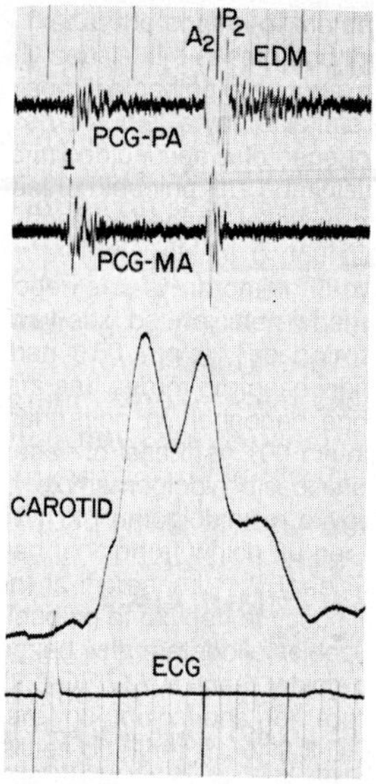

FIGURE 3–24. Pulsus bisferiens in aortic regurgitation. The carotid pulse is bifid, and there is a large excursion reflecting the wide pulse pressure. The phonocardiogram establishes that both humps of the carotid pulse are systolic in time (i.e., prior to A_2), thus separating the bisferiens pulse from a large dicrotic wave (Fig. 3–25), with which it may be confused at the bedside. There is no incisura, owing to aortic incompetence. EDM = early diastolic murmur.

regurgitation (Fig. 3–24). A dicrotic pulse is sometimes seen in cardiomyopathy (Fig. 3–25) and other low-output conditions such as postoperatively in valve replacement for aortic or mitral regurgitation.[102, 103] The dicrotic pulse is distinguished by two pulsations, the second of which is diastolic, immediately following the second heart sound. In the past cardiologists interpreted the dicrotic pulse as an exaggeration of the dicrotic wave. The actual basis of the unusual wave form appears to be a reduction of the overall pressure pulse in conjunction with an essentially normal magnitude of the incisural downslope and rebound.[103a] Further examples of the use of carotid pulse tracings in combination with other noninvasive techniques, including echocardiograms, are illustrated in Chapter 4.

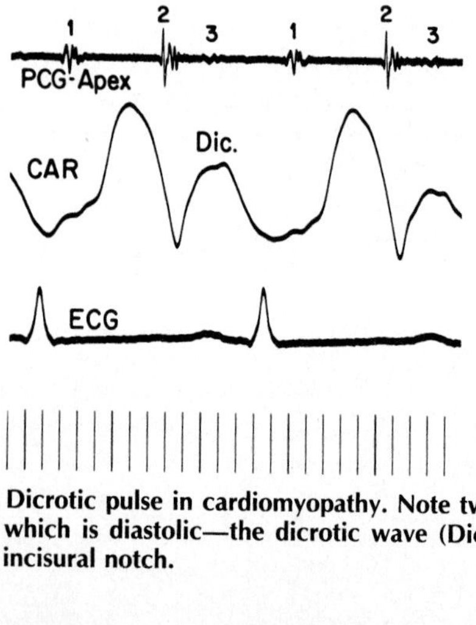

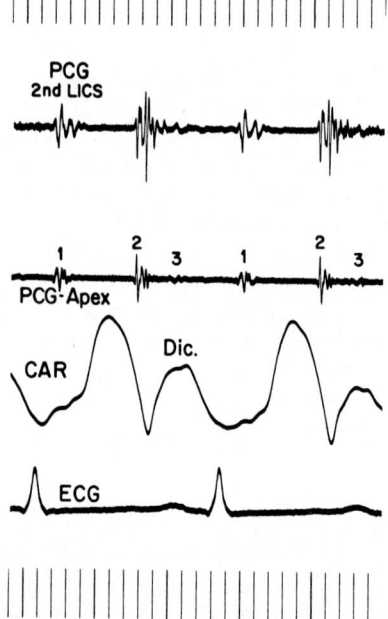

FIGURE 3–25. Dicrotic pulse in cardiomyopathy. Note two pulsations, the second of which is diastolic—the dicrotic wave (Dic.). Note also the prominent incisural notch.

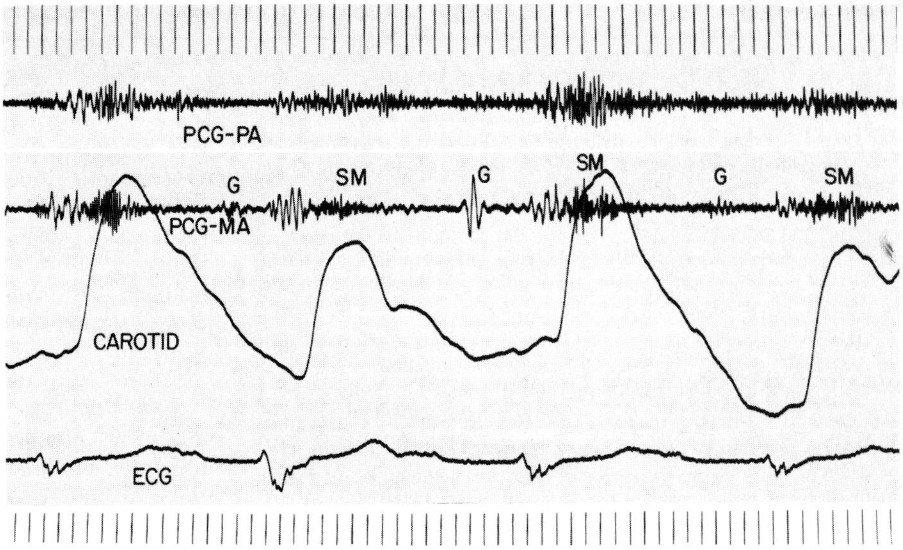

FIGURE 3–26. Pulsus alternans in a man with aortic stenosis and left ventricular failure. The first and third beats are of greater amplitude than are the second and fourth beats. The stronger beats are also marked by a louder murmur (SM) and less abnormality of STI. The diastolic sound (G) is louder after the second (weak) beat. It is a summation sound caused by merging of S_3 and S_4, resulting from the combined effect of a rapid heart rate and a prolonged P-R interval.

Abnormalities of Pulse Frequency, Regularity, and Amplitude

INEQUALITY OF PULSES. By using two pulse-sensitive transducers simultaneously, one can document inequality of the carotid pulses in arteriosclerotic occlusive disease, dissecting aneurysm, or supravalvular aortic stenosis. Diminished amplitude and delay in the femoral arterial pulse in coarctation of the aorta can be demonstrated by the simultaneous recording of the femoral and the brachial or carotid pulses.

CHANGES IN AMPLITUDE WITH NORMAL RHYTHM. The reduction in amplitude of the pulse on inspiration characteristic of *paradoxical pulse* is readily documented by carotid pulse recording performed in conjunction with a pneumogram. The patient should be instructed to breathe slowly and more deeply than usual during the registration of this phenomenon.

Pulsus alternans can also be confirmed by arterial pulse tracings and is often accentuated during the first few beats following a premature ventricular beat (Fig. 3–26). Since the peripheral pulses are more sensitive for the detection of pulsus alternans than is the carotid pulse, one may find it useful to apply the pulse transducer over the femoral artery. The graphic record demonstrates not only the alternating height of the pulse waves but also a beat-to-beat alteration in the rate of rise of the pulse wave as well as in systolic time intervals. The stronger beats display a shorter PEP and longer LVET and therefore a lower PEP/LVET ratio than do the weaker beats, reflecting the higher level of the contractile state in the former.[104]

ECTOPIC RHYTHMS. With ventricular tachycardia, variations in the amplitude of the pulse from beat to beat reflect the rapidly changing sequence of atrial and ventricular systole and the results of more effective ventricular contraction when fortuitously there is a properly timed atrial systole. The totally irregular rhythm and beat-to-beat changes in the amplitude of the pulse characteristic of atrial fibrillation can be documented by carotid pulse tracings. Similarly, the ineffective systoles occasioned by premature beats are easily demonstrable.

APEXCARDIOGRAPHY[105]

Since the middle of the 19th century, graphic records have been made of precordial movements resulting from cardiac activity. Despite the term *apexcardiography*, the method can be used to record pulsatile movements wherever they are perceived over the thorax. The curves obtained by this method resemble sensations derived by palpation but provide additional temporal correlations, since the apex tracing is usually made in conjunction with an ECG, phonocardiogram, and M-mode echocardiogram. It should be realized that the sensitive nerve endings of the palpating fingers appreciate primarily the pressure of indentation produced by outward movements of the chest wall but are less capable of detecting corresponding receding movements. Therefore the outward thrust of the cardiac apex is sensed by palpation as the "point of maximal impulse." It can be appreciated that the tactile sense as employed in palpation is frequency selective and has preferential sensitivity to frequencies extending into the range of heart sounds.[106]

TECHNIQUE. The apex impulse is best appreciated on palpation as well as for recording purposes by having the patient lie in a partial left lateral decubitus position. A triangular supporting pillow beneath the back promotes comfort and relaxation. The optimal registration of the apexcardiogram may require that the patient hold his breath in partial exhalation. The transducer funnel or tambour may be held by hand over the left ventricular apex. The transducer used in apexcardiography senses the *relative* position of the diaphragm of the transducer with respect to its rim. (With a funnel device, the skin serves as a diaphragm.) Thus, ordinarily the rim of the sensing head of the transducer rests on the ribs, and its diaphragm moves with the soft tissues in the intercostal space. Reproducibility in recording the apexcardiogram is adversely affected by differences in the patient's position, the pressure with which the transducer is applied, and, most of all, failure to place the transducer precisely, over the point of maximum impulse.

NORMAL APEXCARDIOGRAM

The physiological correlations of the major landmarks of the apexcardiogram have been carefully worked out by Willems et al.[107, 108] by means of simultaneous registration of the left ventricular apexcardiogram and high-fidelity left ventricular pressures in dogs. These studies showed a very precise synchronism in the upstroke of the systolic wave of the apexcardiogram and the rise in left ventricular pressure (Fig. 3–27). A similar relationship has been reported in humans.[109] The early diastolic nadir or "O"-point in the apexcardiogram and that in the left ventricular pressure are also practically simultaneous.[107] The rapid upstroke of the apexcardiogram therefore initiates the isovolumetric phase of systole and is largely completed during this portion of the cardiac cycle. During this phase the external circumference of the heart increases as the ventricle changes its shape and the intraventricular pressure rises. The upstroke terminates in normal subjects with the "E"-point, which occurs approximately at the onset of ejection. The E-point, however, is often obliterated in disease states that result in hypertrophy or dysfunction of the ventricle. During the remainder of systole in normal subjects, the apexcardiogram describes a declining plateau as the volume of the heart diminishes. A more abrupt decline begins to occur just before the second heart sound. A nadir or 0-point is reached in early diastole at approximately the time of opening of the mitral valve. This is followed by a rapid filling wave and a slow filling wave, reflecting analogous events in the left ventricular pressure curve. In late diastole, the *a* wave is recorded, reflecting movement of a small amount of blood into the left ventricle as a result of atrial systole. In normal subjects the *a* wave is of modest height, usually less than 15 per cent in amplitude with respect to the total height of the apexcardiogram.

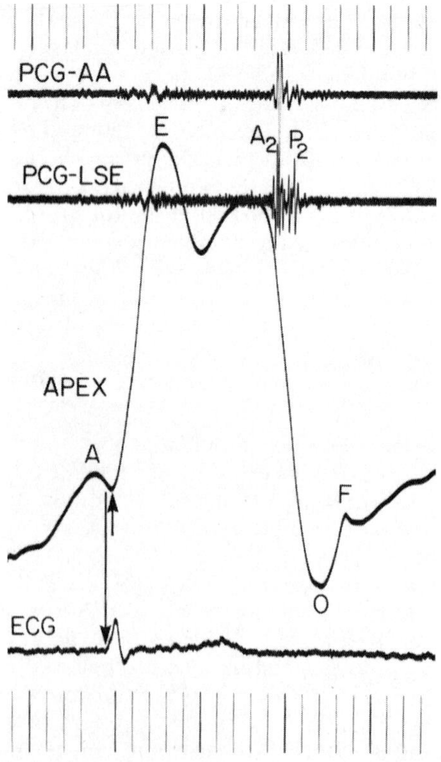

FIGURE 3–27. Normal apexcardiogram. A low-amplitude *a* wave (A) in presystole follows the P wave of the ECG, which is not visible in this lead. The onset of the QRS (downward arrow) is followed after a brief electromechanical interval (0.02 sec) by the onset of the swift upward movement of the apex tracing (upward arrow), culminating in the E point at approximately the time of beginning ejection into the aorta. A generally declining curve during systole ends with an abrupt downward fall at the time of A_2. The nadir (0) is reached at approximately the time of mitral valve opening. The rapid filling wave (F) occurs during early diastolic filling of the left ventricle.

APEXCARDIOGRAPHY IN DISEASE

The systolic portion of the apexcardiogram has only a limited number of patterns of diagnostic utility. These can be broadly classified as (1) *normal* (described above), (2) *hyperdynamic*, and (3) *sustained*.[110]

Hyperdynamic movement is perceived at the bedside as a thrust of exaggerated height but one which falls away immediately from the palpating fingers. It is found in conditions characterized by an increased stroke volume such as in normal subjects after exercise, in thyrotoxicosis, or in mitral regurgitation (Fig. 3–28).[111] The graphic tracing shows a systolic wave of normal shape but of increased amplitude (although this is difficult to measure) and a prominent rapid filling wave.

The *sustained* impulse is the graphic equivalent of a heave or thrust, as may be found in left ventricular hypertrophy, such as that associated with hypertension or aortic stenosis (Fig. 3–29). The systolic portion of a sustained apical impulse is characterized by a plateau or a dome-shaped or rising curve, in contrast to the gentle systolic decline seen in the normal or hyperdynamic tracing. An accompanying finding is a prominent *a* wave. A somewhat similar heave is found in cardiomyopathy or chronic ischemic heart disease. A variant of the sustained impulse occurs in HOCM, in which the systolic portion may be bifid in configuration preceded by a large *a* wave, thus giving a triple-humped appearance (Fig. 3–30).

In the mitral prolapse or click murmur syndrome, a

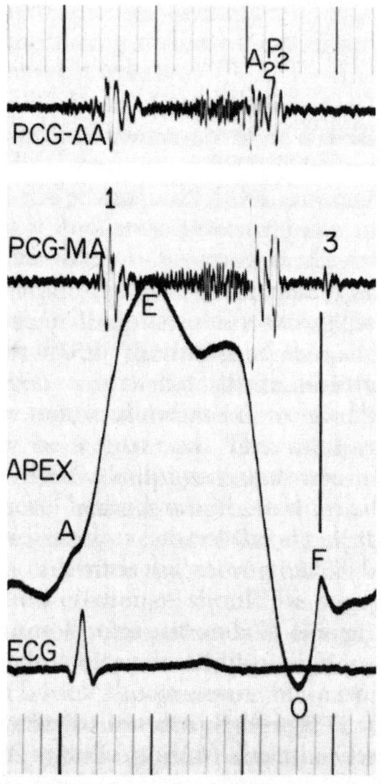

FIGURE 3–28. Hyperdynamic apexcardiogram in mitral regurgitation. The configuration of the tracing in systole is qualitatively similar to a normal curve, although the amplitude was clearly exaggerated by palpation. The rapid filling wave (F) is higher than normal and terminates in a sharp point coincident with its audible counterpart, the third heart sound (3).

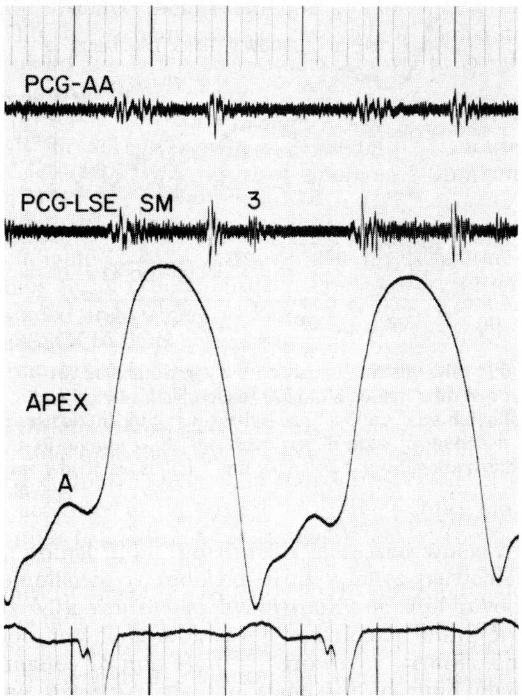

FIGURE 3–29. Sustained type of apexcardiogram in cardiomyopathy. The systolic portion of the tracing is dome-shaped, the graphic representation of a heave. It is preceded by a prominent *a* wave (A). The PCG shows a holosystolic murmur (SM) and a third sound (3).

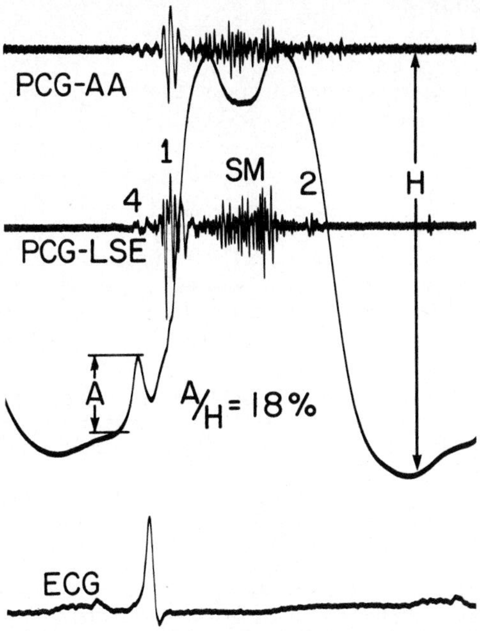

FIGURE 3–30. Apexcardiogram in HOCM. The *a* wave (A) is exaggerated in height, being 18 per cent of the entire amplitude of the apexcardiogram (H), and has an unusually rapid upstroke that culminates in a sharp peak, coinciding with the fourth heart sound (4). The systolic phase of the apexcardiogram has a bifid appearance with a prominent late systolic hump. The saddle-shaped decline in midsystole coincides in time with the systolic murmur and carotid pulse deformity, which, in turn, are related to the obstruction occasioned by the systolic anterior motion of the mitral valve, as illustrated in Figure 3–23.

collapse or deep notch in the apex impulse may occasionally be noted coinciding with the click as recorded on an accompanying phonocardiogram (Fig. 3–31).[112]

Exaggeration of the height of the rapid filling wave and assumption of a sharper configuration of its peak are characteristic of mitral regurgitation or left-to-right shunts such as patent ductus arteriosus and ventricular septal defect, which result in augmentation of ventricular filling in early diastole (Fig. 3–28). Unfortunately, owing to the wide range of normal findings, as well as the difficulty in

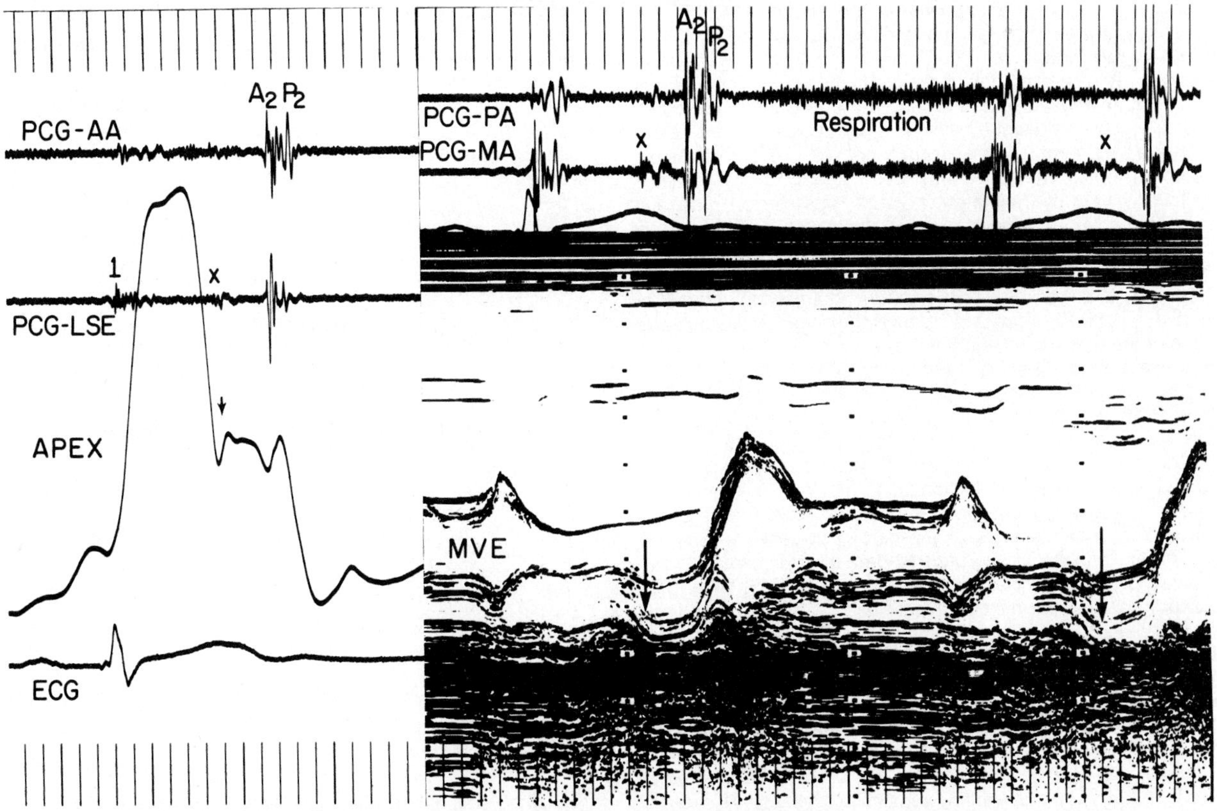

FIGURE 3–31. Mitral valve prolapse. The apexcardiogram (APEX) on the left shows a notch (arrow) in midsystole at the time of the click (X), followed by a plateau. In the echophonocardiogram on the right, X coincides with the downward movement or prolapse of the valve (arrow).

quantitating an apexcardiogram, there is no clear cut-off point between the pathological conditions listed above and the prominent rapid filling wave seen in a healthy young subject who might be expected to have a normal third heart sound. Similarly, a heightened *a* wave is found in a variety of conditions having in common diminished compliance of the left ventricle.[80, 113] These include left ventricular hypertrophy, as in systemic hypertension, aortic stenosis, and HOCM; or myocardial disease, as in ischemic heart disease and cardiomyopathy (Figs. 3–29 and 3–30).

PULSATILE MOVEMENTS IN OTHER PRECORDIAL LOCATIONS. Following preliminary examination by palpation, useful patterns of precordial movement may be obtained by placement of the transducer over locations other than the apex.

Normal Right Ventricular Movement. In normal children, a gentle thrust can usually be appreciated and recorded in the third and fourth interspaces at the left sternal edge. In older normal subjects it is usually impossible to feel or record a right ventricular impulse.

Right Ventricular Hypertrophy. In right ventricular hypertrophy, as with pulmonary hypertension or pulmonary valve stenosis, a heave at the left sternal edge can be perceived by palpation.[81, 114] This can usually be recorded with the patient supine and the sensing head of the transducer firmly applied to the interspace where the systolic impulse has been detected. Occasionally in emphysematous patients, the optimal site may be just beneath the xiphoid.

Tetralogy of Fallot (see also Chaps. 30 and 31). Although the degree of infundibular stenosis in this condition may be extreme, and right ventricular pressures are equal to those on the left, the precordial movement in cyanotic children with tetralogy of Fallot is remarkably quiet.[105] There is usually a brief shock or vibration that can be palpated and recorded at the time of S_1 and S_2. The systolic phase is marked by a plateau or even a concave pattern in the graphic record. There is no atrial sound and no exaggeration of the *a* waves in the right apexcardiogram or the jugular venous pulse tracing. In contrast, in pure valvular pulmonic stenosis one can usually palpate or record an outward (convex) movement at the left sternal edge, preceded by an enlarged *a* wave. These differences probably result from the escape route afforded by the right-to-left shunt through the septal defect, in the tetralogy, which may serve to decompress the right ventricle.

Tricuspid Regurgitation (see also Chap. 33). Tricuspid regurgitation usually appears as a complication of elevated right ventricular pressure as occurs in mitral stenosis with pulmonary hypertension. Under these circumstances a right ventricular heave may be appreciated on palpation and in graphic records, as described above.[115] In pure tricuspid regurgitation in which the valve has been destroyed by infective endocarditis or injured by trauma but in which hypertension is absent, a different precordial pulsatile pattern is encountered. The grossly evident precordial "heave" proves to be *diastolic* in time, whereas systole is marked by a retraction or inward movement (Fig. 3–32).[105, 115, 116] These events mirror the massive filling and emptying of the right ventricle and graphically appear as a mirror image of the pulsatile movements of the great veins and the liver.

Constrictive Pericarditis (see also Chap. 44). Although in some long-standing cases of constrictive pericarditis the precordium may be immobile, a little appreciated but frequently encountered sign is an inward systolic movement, as in pure tricuspid regurgitation (Fig. 3–33).[116] The outward heave is in early diastole and corresponds in time to the pericardial knock. Palpation alone may be misleading, with inadvertent inversion of the phases of the cardiac cycle, unless one is careful to use the heart sounds or the carotid pulse as a temporal landmark. An explanation for the unusual pattern of precordial movement in constrictive pericarditis has been provided by El-Sherif and El-Said, who propose that the pulsatile record is a reflection of filling and emptying of the heart, its usual outward thrust during the isovolumetric phase of systole being inhibited by the constriction.[117]

Left Ventricular Aneurysm (see also Chap. 39). A large anterior myocardial infarction may lead to formation of an aneurysm with a palpable systolic heave in an ectopic location, usually over the midprecordium. Graphic records over such a bulge made with the patient supine usually reveal a bifid impulse made up of a large *a* wave followed by a sustained plateau during ventricular systole.[118] This finding in association with a QS pattern in precordial electrocardiographic leads and persistent ST elevation is strongly suggestive of aneurysm. Regarding the physiological derangement, additional information obtained by noninvasive means is provided by systolic time intervals. Prolongation of PEP and shortening of LVET accurately predict a seriously disturbed state of left ventricular function.[94]

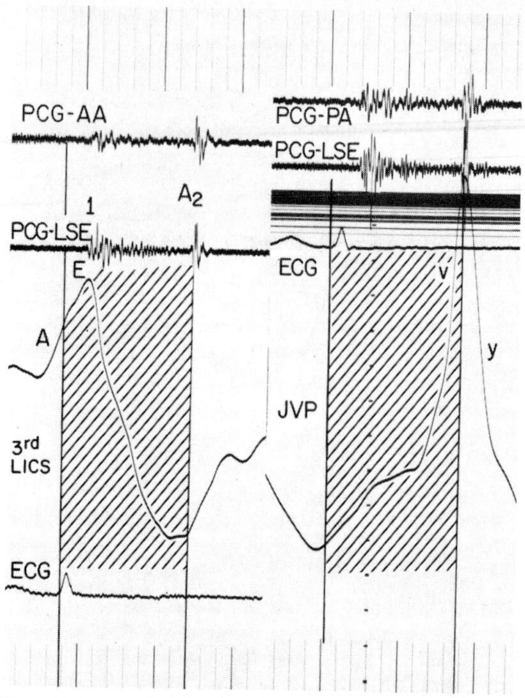

FIGURE 3–32. Precordial movement in pure tricuspid regurgitation in a young woman with infective endocarditis on the tricuspid valve due to heroin addiction. The right ventricular impulse tracing (left) taken at the left sternal edge shows a brief outward (upward) move during the isovolumetric phase of systole (E), merging with the preceding *a* wave. This is followed by a deep inward (downward) movement during the remainder of systole, reflecting reduction of right ventricular volume. Systole is shaded to facilitate comparison with JVP (right), which shows a reciprocal relationship to the precordial pattern, with a large late systolic *v* wave due to tricuspid regurgitation.

Mitral Regurgitation (see also Chap. 33). In severe mitral regurgitation, either acute or chronic, there may be a striking lift of the whole precordium in systole. This is attributed to expansion of the posteriorly located left atrium, causing the heart to push forward against the thoracic cage. This movement peaks late in systole coincident with the *v* wave in the left atrial pressure pulse and thus differs morphologically from the more localized heave of right ventricular hypertrophy, which reaches its maximal height earlier in systole.[119]

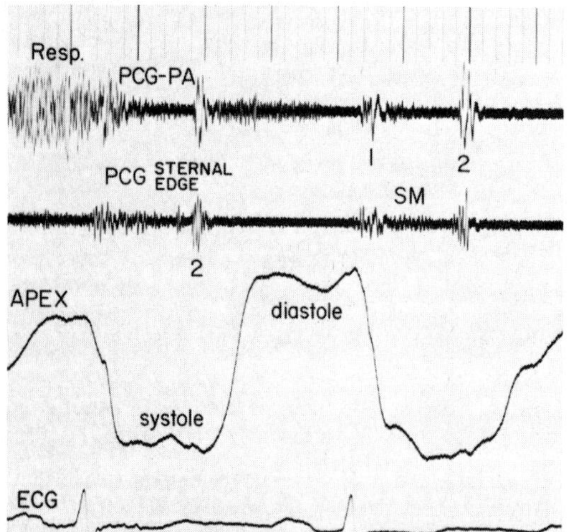

FIGURE 3–33. Precordial movement in constrictive pericarditis. The precordium moves inward (downward on graphic record) during systole and outward during diastole, probably resulting from volume changes in the right ventricle.[117]

JUGULAR VENOUS PULSE

TECHNIQUE. The jugular venous pulse (JVP) is recorded by pressing the funnel of the pulse transducer in the fossa above the clavicle between the attachments of the sterno-cleidomastoid muscle. Care must be taken to direct the transducer to exclude, if possible, the underlying arterial pulsation. The venous pulse obtained in this manner closely resembles the pressure curve of the right atrium.

NORMAL JVP

The normal JVP consists of three peaks (*a, c,* and *v*) and three descents (*x*, *x′*, and *y*) (Fig. 3–34).[120] The *a* wave is the result of right atrial systole, follows the P wave of the electrocardiogram, and is slightly delayed from its counterpart in the right atrial pressure pulse by transmission to the jugular venous system. Relaxation of the atrium results in an insignificant downward movement, the *x* descent. In patients with a normal P-R interval, the *x* descent is quickly interrupted by a second peak of minor dimension, the *c* wave. This occurs as a result of tricuspid valve closure and therefore accompanies T_1, or the tricuspid component of the first heart sound. The *c* wave is often confused in JVP recordings because of interference from the underlying carotid arterial pulse. Its identity as a separate and distinct wave can be clarified in circumstances in which the carotid pulse is delayed, as in left bundle branch block.[121]

Following the *c* wave, there is in normal subjects a prominent *x′* descent, a downward movement which usually dominates the venous pulse record. The *x′* descent occurs during ventricular systole and is attributed to the "descent of the base"—a movement of the atrial floor in the direction of the ventricle due to contraction of the latter chamber. A mass of blood is thus drawn in an antegrade direction from the venous system to the right atrium, with resulting collapse of the JVP.[122] There follows, during the latter portion of ventricular systole, a positive wave *v*, which results from passive accumulation of blood in the right atrium while the triscuspid valve remains closed. With opening of the tricuspid valve in early diastole and emptying of the atrium, the *v* wave collapses, providing in graphic tracings the *y* descent—a prominent negative wave. In normal subjects the *y* descent is not of the magnitude of the *x′* descent just described. In subjects with slow heart rates there may be another positive wave (*h*) later in diastole, resulting from passive distention of the venous system (Fig. 3–34).[120]

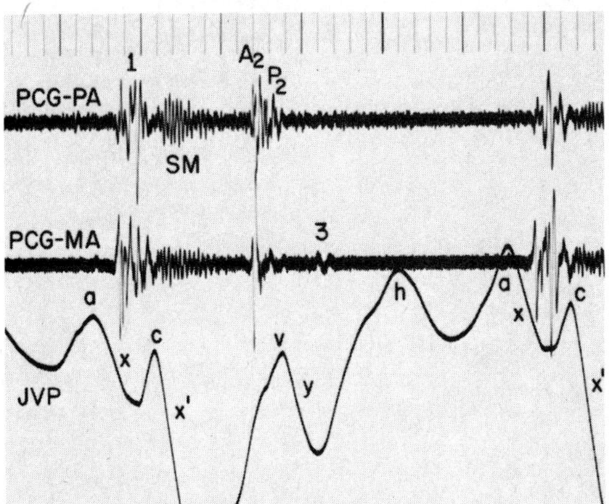

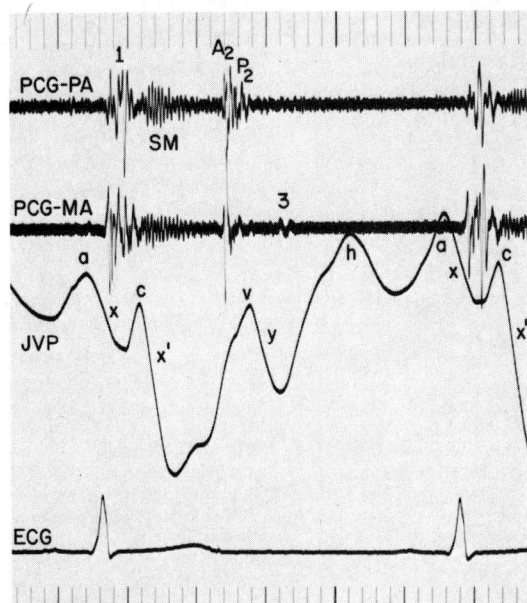

FIGURE 3–34. Normal jugular venous pulse (JVP) tracing in a young person with a functional systolic murmur (SM). The major features of the JVP are as follows: *a* wave, resulting from right atrial systole; *x* descent, atrial relaxation; *c* wave, tricuspid closure resulting from right ventricular contraction; *x′* descent, descent of the base plus continuing effect of atrial relaxation, associated with antegrade flow from the great veins; *v* wave, passive accumulation of blood in the right atrium while tricuspid valve is closed; *y* descent, filling of the right ventricle following opening of the tricuspid valve; *h* wave, a stasis wave in the venous system, apparent only at slower heart rates.

ABNORMALITIES OF THE JVP

In all efforts to use the JVP in cardiac diagnosis, the enormous variability of the pulse contour and relative height and depth of its constituents must be appreciated.[123] This is true among different subjects as well as in the same patient on successive occasions or with minor alterations in technique. Therefore only rather gross alterations in pulse morphology as described below can be utilized safely if one is to avoid overreading the tracings. Nevertheless, examination of the venous pulse either at the bedside or in graphic records has a long history of utility in assessing arrhythmias and in anticipating physiological derangements involving the right side of the heart. In circumstances in which there is some impediment to right atrial systole, as with tricuspid stenosis or right ventricular hypertrophy resulting from pulmonic valvular stenosis or pulmonary hypertension, the *a* wave may increase in amplitude (Fig. 3–35). Persistent or intermittent *exaggeration of the a wave* may also reflect contraction of the atrium against a closed tricuspid valve resulting from electrocardiographic

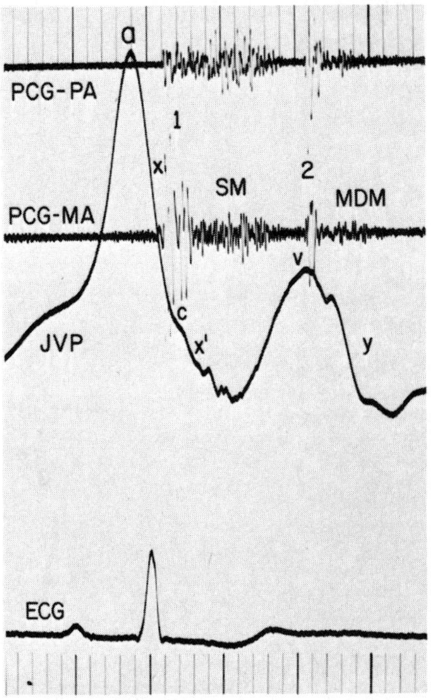

FIGURE 3–35. Jugular venous pressure (JVP) in mitral stenosis with pulmonary hypertension. The JVP is dominated by a very large *a* wave resulting from diminished compliance of the right ventricle associated with pulmonary hypertension. The peaked *a* wave represents a brief period of retrograde flow from right atrium to great veins.[121]

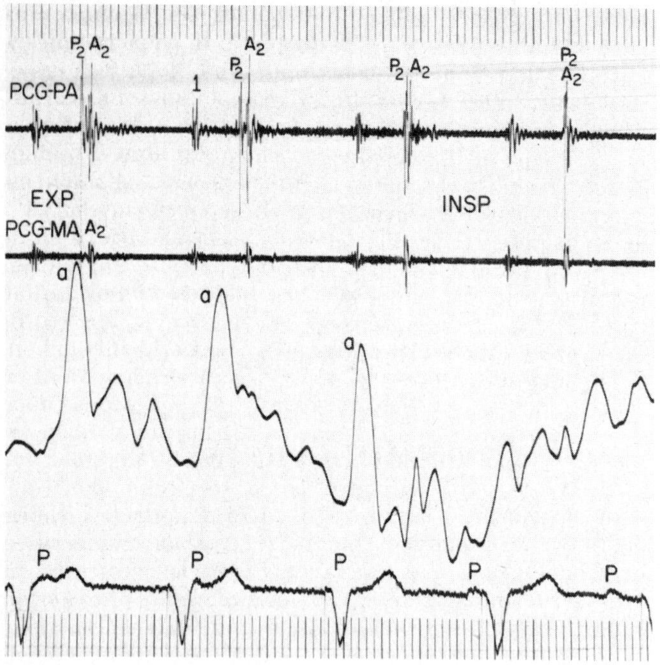

FIGURE 3–36. Jugular venous pressure (JVP) showing "cannon" *a* waves in a patient with a transvenous pacemaker in the right ventricle. In the first three cycles, atrial systole coincides with ventricular systole, so that the right atrium is contracting against a closed tricuspid valve. There is reversed splitting of S_2, with P_2 preceding A_2 in expiration (EXP), but narrowing of separation occurs with inspiration (INSP).

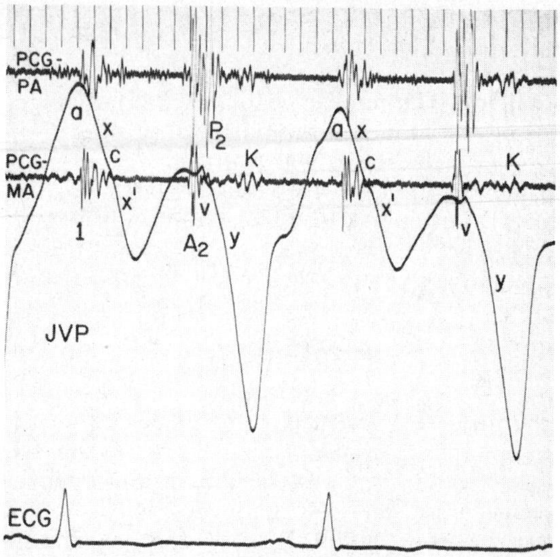

FIGURE 3–37. Jugular venous pressure (JVP) in constrictive pericarditis. In this severe and longstanding case, the *x'* descent has become very shallow and the *y* descent is the principal feature, indicating that antegrade flow from the venous system to the right heart is now limited to early diastole.[124] A pericardial knock (K) is seen at approximately the nadir of the *y* descent.

abnormalities that distort the usual sequence of atrioventricular (AV) contraction. These include AV nodal and ventricular tachycardia, premature ventricular beats, and atrioventricular dissociation (Fig. 3–36). An intermittent accentuation of the *a* wave in ventricular tachycardia indicates that atria and ventricles are out of phase, and it may therefore be of some help in certain clinical circumstances in distinguishing ventricular tachycardia from atrial tachycardia with bundle branch block. A prominent *a* wave may be found in association with *left* ventricular hypertrophy, presumably reflecting encroachment by the hypertrophied interventricular septum on the right ventricle—the Bernheim effect.

The *x* descent that results from atrial relaxation is seldom of any prominence and can reach significant proportions only when atrial and ventricular systoles are separated, as with a long P-R interval or in complete heart block.

The *x'* descent is normally one of the most prominent features of the JVP. It becomes shallow or is eliminated in tricuspid regurgitation. It may be deep in some cases of constrictive pericarditis.[124]

The *y* descent is less steep in tricuspid stenosis. Unfortunately, this assessment must be subjective, since the waves of the JVP cannot be quantitated and the relative swiftness of their movements is dependent on apparatus, technique, and paper speed. In constrictive pericarditis, however, a rapid, deep *y* descent interrupting an otherwise

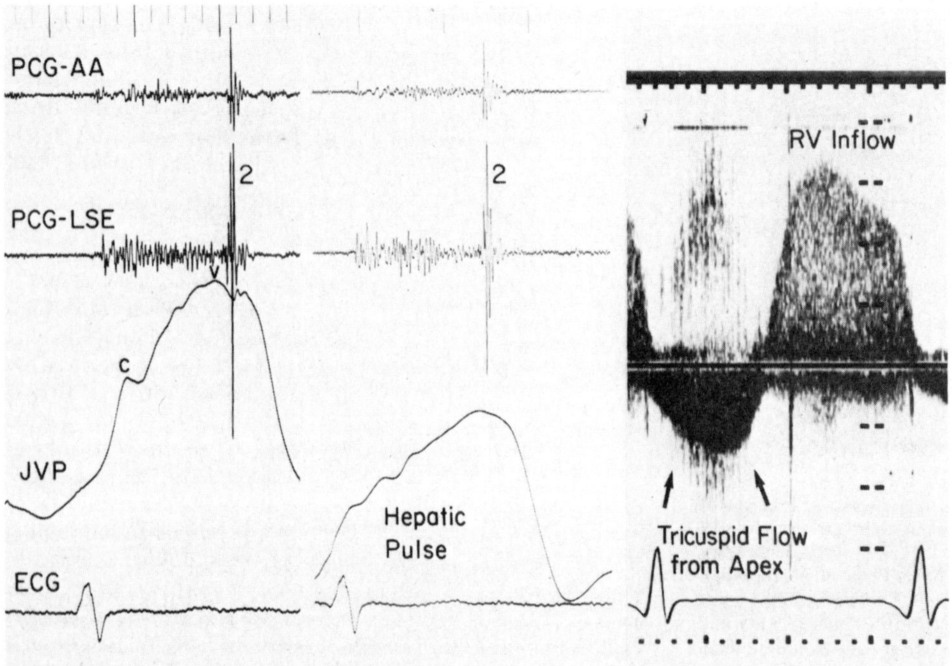

FIGURE 3–38. Tricuspid regurgitation. *Left,* A systolic murmur is recorded at left sternal edge (LSE). It coincides with the abnormal CV wave in the JVP and the expansile pulsation of the liver seen in the center panel. *Right,* A Doppler study of tricuspid flow reveals prominent regurgitant flow out of the right ventricle (RV) during systole and correspondingly augmented RV inflow during diastole.

high plateau of the venous pulse provides a pattern familiar to hemodynamicists, since it simulates the "square-root sign" recorded in diastolic pressure tracings from all the heart chambers (Fig. 3–37 and Fig. 2–6, p. 19).

In tricuspid regurgitation, the *v* wave is unusually prominent, the x' descent becomes shallower, and with increasing hemodynamic deterioration the *c* and *v* waves merge to form a prominent ascending plateau (Fig. 3–38). Under these circumstances, the *v* wave no longer reflects merely the normal passive accumulation of blood in the right atrium and venous system while the tricuspid valve is closed in systole; rather, it is due to a massive retrograde wave through an incompetent valve into the great veins. Unfortunately, the time-honored custom of using the letter *v* for both the normal systolic peak and the abnormal regurgitant wave when the valve is incompetent has interfered with understanding the genesis of these waves of the JVP in health and disease.

Acknowledgments

We are grateful for the technical assistance of Ms. Carla Pasi of the Cardiac Graphics Laboratory at North Carolina Memorial Hospital, Chapel Hill, North Carolina, who is responsible for the records used as illustrations in Chapters 3 and 4.

REFERENCES

HEART SOUNDS

1. Laennec, R. T. H.: Traité de l'auscultation médiate. 2nd ed. Paris, Brosson et Chaude, 1826.
2. McKusick, V. A.: Cardiovascular Sound in Health and Disease. Baltimore, Williams and Wilkins, 1958.
3. O'Farrell, P. T.: A famous cardiac controversy. Irish J. Med. Sci. *6*:278, 1957.
4. Rouanet, J.: Analyse des bruits du coeur. Thesis No. 252, Paris, 1832. (Reprinted in reference 2.)
5. Luisada, A. A., MacCanon, D. M., Kumar, S., and Feigen, L. P.: Changing views on the mechanism of the first and second heart sounds. Am. Heart J. *88*:503, 1974.
6. Dock, W., Grandell, F., and Taubman, F.: The physiologic third sound, its mechanism and relation to protodiastolic gallop. Am. Heart J. *50*:449, 1955.
7. Ozawa, Y., Smith, D., and Craige, E.: Origin of the third heart sound. I. Studies in dogs. Circulation *67*:393, 1983.
8. Reddy, P. S., Salerni, R., and Shaver, J. A.: Normal and abnormal heart sounds in cardiac diagnosis. Part 2. Diastolic sounds. Curr. Probl. Cardiol. *10*(4):1, 1985.
9. Mills, P., and Craige, E.: Echophonocardiography. Prog. Cardiovasc. Dis. *20*:337, 1978.
10. Hada, Y., Amano, K., Yamaguchi, T., Takenaka, K., Takahashi, H., Takikawa, R., Hasegawa, I., Takahashi, T., Suzuki, J., Sakamoto, T., and Sugimoto, T.: Noninvasive study of the presystolic component of the first heart sound in mitral stenosis. J. Am. Coll. Cardiol. *7*:43, 1986.
11. O'Toole, J. D., Reddy, P. S., Curtiss, E. L., Griff, F. W., and Shaver, J. A.: The contribution of tricuspid valve closure to the first heart sound. An intracardiac micromanometer study. Circulation *53*:752, 1976.
12. Lewis, D. H.: Phonocardiography. *In* Hamilton, W. F., and Dow, P. (eds.): Handbook of Physiology. Section 2, Circulation. Vol. 1. Washington, D.C., American Physiological Society, 1962, p. 685.
13. Zalter, R., Hodara, H., and Luisada, A. A.: Phonocardiography. I. General principles and problems of standardization. Am. J. Cardiol. *4*:3, 1959.
14. Kesteloot, H., Willems, J., and van Vollenhoven, E.: On the physical principles and methodology of mechanocardiography. Acta Cardiol. *24*:147, 1969.
15. Butterworth, J. S., Chassin, M. R., McGrath, R., and Reppert, E. H.: Cardiac Auscultation. New York, Grune and Stratton, 1960.
16. Lewis, R. P., Rittgers, S. E., Forester, W. F., and Boudoulas, H.: A critical review of the systolic time intervals. Circulation *56*:146, 1977.
17. Mashimo, K., Tanabe, T., Kinoshita, S., Sakamoto, S., and Tsushima, N.: An instrumental aspect of apexcardiography: Decay characteristic of transducers and its clinical implication. Jpn. Heart J. *7*:536, 1966.
18. Leatham, A.: Phonocardiography. Br. Med. Bull, *8*:333, 1952.
19. Leatham, A.: Splitting of the first and second heart sounds. Lancet *2*:607, 1954.
20. Rushmer, R. F.: Cardiovascular Dynamics. 4th ed. Philadelphia, W. B. Saunders Company, 1976, p. 421.
21. Kupari, M.: Aortic valve closure and cardiac vibrations in the genesis of the second heart sound. Am. J. Cardiol. *52*:152, 1983.
22. Drui, S., Brandt, C. M., and Fincker, J. L.: Origine valvulaire ou musculaire des bruits du coeur? Ann. Cardiol. Angeiol. (Paris) *32*:247, 1983.
23. Lim, K. O., Boughner, D. R., Hui, P. W., and Lee, M.: Frequency analysis of the first and second heart sounds of humans. Jpn. Heart J. *25*:293, 1984.
24. Shaver, J. A., Salerni, R., and Reddy, P. S.: Normal and abnormal heart sounds in cardiac diagnosis. Part 1. Systolic sounds. Curr. Probl. Cardiol. *10*(3):1, 1985.
25. Luisada, A. A., and Portaluppi, F.: Considerations on the mechanism of the systolic click of mitral valve prolapse. Acta Cardiol. (Brux.) *40*:301, 1985.
26. Leatham A., and Leech, G. J.: Auscultation of the heart. *In* Hurst, J. W. (ed.): The Heart. 5th ed. New York, McGraw-Hill, 1986, p. 207.
27. Levine, S. A., and Harvey, W. P.: Clinical Auscultation of the Heart. Philadelphia, W. B. Saunders Company, 1959, p. 219.
28. Smith, D., Ishimitsu, T., and Craige, E.: Mechanical vibration transmission characteristics of the left ventricle: Implications with regard to auscultation and phonocardiography. J. Am. Coll. Cardiol. *4*:517, 1984.

28a. Smith, D., Ishimitsu, T., and Craige, E.: Abnormal diastolic mechanical vibration transmission characteristics of the left ventricle. J. Cardiography *15*:507, 1985.

29. Rappaport, M. B., and Sprague, H. B.: The graphic registration of the normal heart sound. Am. Heart J. *23*:591, 1942.
30. Craige, E.: Echocardiography in studies of the genesis of heart sounds and murmurs (Chapter 2). *In* Yu, P., and Goodwin, J. (eds.): Progress in Cardiology. Vol. 4. Philadelphia, Lea and Febiger, 1975.
31. Waider, W., and Craige, E.: The first heart sound and ejection sounds: Echophonocardiographic correlation with valvular events. Am. J. Cardiol. *35*:346, 1975.
32. Brooks, N., Leech, G., and Leatham, A.: Complete right bundle branch block: Echophonocardiographic study of first heart sound and right ventricular contraction times. Br. Heart J. *41*:637, 1979.
33. Hultgren, H. N., Craige, E., Nakamura, T., and Bilisoly, J.: Left bundle branch block and mechanical events of the cardiac cycle. Am. J. Cardiol. *52*:755, 1983.
34. Haber, E., and Leatham, A.: Splitting of heart sounds from ventricular asynchrony in bundle-branch block, ventricular ectopic beats, and artificial pacing. Br. Heart J. *27*:691, 1965.
35. Braunwald, E., and Morrow, A. G.: Origin of heart sounds as elucidated by analysis of the sequence of cardiodynamic events. Circulation *18*:971, 1958.
36. Burggraf, G. W.: The first heart sound in left bundle branch block: An echophonocardiographic study. Circulation *63*:429, 1981.
37. Wooley, C. F.: Intracardiac phonocardiography; intracardiac sound and pressure in man. Circulation *57*:1039, 1978.
38. Crews, T. L., Pridie, R. B., Benham, R., and Leatham, A.: Auscultatory and phonocardiographic findings in Ebstein's anomaly. Correlation of first heart sound with ultrasonic records of tricuspid valve movement. Br. Heart J. *34*:681, 1972.
39. Tajik, A. J., Gau, G. T., Giuliani, E. R., Ritter, D. G., and Schattenberg, T. T.: Echocardiogram in Ebstein's anomaly with Wolff-Parkinson-White preexcitation syndrome, type B. Circulation *47*:813, 1973.
40. Willis, P. W. IV, and Craige, E.: First heart sound in Ebstein's anomaly: Observations on the cause of wide splitting by echophonocardiographic studies before and after operative repair. J. Am. Coll. Cardiol. *2*:1165, 1983.
41. Tei, C., Shah, P. M., Cherian, G., Wong, M., and Ormiston, J. A.: The correlates of an abnormal first heart sound in mitral valve prolapse syndromes. N. Engl. J. Med. *307*:334, 1982.
42. Shah, P. M., Kramer, D. H., and Gramiak, R.: Influence of the timing of atrial systole in mitral valve closure and on the first heart sound in man. Am. J. Cardiol. *26*:231, 1970.
43. Burggraf, G. W., and Craige, E.: The first heart sound in complete heart block. Circulation *50*:17, 1974.
44. Leech, G., Brooks, N., Green-Wilkinson, A., and Leatham, A.: Mechanism of influence of PR interval on loudness of first heart sound. Br. Heart J. *43*:138, 1980.
45. Mann, T., McLaurin, L., Grossman, W., and Craige, E.: Acute aortic regurgitation due to infective endocarditis. N. Engl. J. Med. *293*:108, 1975.
46. Wolferth, C. C., and Margolies, A.: Certain effects of auricular systole and prematurity of beat on the intensity of the first heart sound. Trans. Am. Assoc. Physicians *45*:44, 1930.
47. Leatham, A., and Gray, I.: Auscultatory and phonocardiographic signs of atrial septal defect. Br. Heart J. *18*:193, 1956.
48. Lopez, J. F., Linn, H., and Shaffer, A. B.: The apical first heart sound as an aid in the diagnosis of atrial septal defect. Circulation *26*:1296, 1962.
49. Stept, M. E., Heid, C. E., Shaver, J. A., Leon, D. F., and Leonard, J. J.: Effect of altering P-R interval on the amplitude of the first heart sound in the anesthetized dog. Circ. Res. *25*:255, 1969.
50. Mills, P. G., Chamusco, R. F., Moos, S., and Craige, E.: Echophonocardiographic studies of the contribution of the atrioventricular valves to the first heart sound. Circulation *54*:944, 1976.
51. Traill, T. A., and Fortuin, N. J.: Presystolic mitral closure sound in aortic regurgitation with left ventricular hypertrophy and first degree heart block. Br. Heart J. *48*:78, 1982.
52. Sabbah, H. N., and Stein, P. D.: Relation of the second sound to diastolic vibration of the closed aortic valve. Am. J. Physiol.: Heart Circ. Physiol. *3*:H696, 1978.
53. Smith, D., and Craige, E.: Influence of the aortic component of the second heart sound on left ventricular maximal negative dP/dt in the dog. Am. J. Cardiol. *55*:205, 1985.
54. Verburg, J., and van Vollenhoven, E.: Phonocardiography: Physical and technical aspects and clinical uses. *In* Rolfe, P. (ed.): Noninvasive physiological measurements. New York, Academic Press, 1979, pp. 213–259.
55. Craige, E., and Harned, H. S.: Phonocardiographic and electrocardiographic studies in normal newborn infants. Am. Heart J. *65*:180, 1963.
56. Harris, A., and Sutton, G. C.: Second heart sound in normal subjects. Br. Heart J. *30*:739, 1968.

57. Leatham, A., and Weitzman, D.: Auscultatory and phonocardiographic signs of pulmonary stenosis. Br. Heart J. *19*:303, 1957.
58. Leatham, A., and Gray, I.: Auscultatory and phonocardiographic signs of atrial septal defect. Br. Heart J. *18*:193, 1956.
59. Perloff, J. K.: Auscultatory and phonocardiographic manifestations of pulmonary hypertension. Prog. Cardiovasc. Dis. 9:303, 1967.
60. Stein, P. D.: A Physical and Physiological Basis for the Interpretation of Cardiac Auscultation: Evaluations Based Primarily on the Second Heart Sound and Ejection Murmurs. Mt. Kisco, N.Y., Futura Publishing Co., 1981, pp. 37–41.
61. Ross, R. S., and Criley, J. M.: Cineangiocardiographic studies of the origin of cardiovascular physical signs. Circulation *30*:255, 1964.
62. Hancock, E. W.: The ejection sound in aortic stenosis. Am. J. Med. *40*:569, 1966.
63. Leech, G., Mills, P., and Leatham, A.: The diagnosis of a non-stenotic bicuspid aortic valve. Br. Heart J. *40*:941, 1978.
64. Leatham, A., and Vogelpoel, L.: Early systolic sound in dilatation of the pulmonary artery. Br. Heart J. *16*:21, 1954.
65. Hultgren, H. N., Reeve, R., Cohn, K., and McLeod, R.: The ejection click of valvular pulmonic stenosis. Circulation *40*:631, 1969.
66. Mills, P., Amara, I., McLaurin, L. P., and Craige, E.: Noninvasive assessment of pulmonary hypertension from right ventricular isovolumic contraction time. Am. J. Cardiol. *46*:272, 1980.
67. Curtiss, E. I., Reddy, P. S., O'Toole, J. D., and Shaver, J. A.: Alterations of right ventricular systolic time intervals by chronic pressure and volume overloading. Circulation *53*:997, 1976.
68. Mills, P. G., Brodie, B., McLaurin, L. P., Schall, S., and Craige, E.: Echocardiographic and hemodynamic relationships of ejection sounds. Circulation *56*:430, 1977.
69. Margolies, A., and Wolferth, C. C.: The opening snap in mitral stenosis. Am. Heart J. 7:443, 1932.
70. Craige, E.: Editorial. On the genesis of heart sounds: Contribution made by echocardiographic studies. Circulation *53*:207, 1976.
71. Millward, D. K., McLaurin, L. P., and Craige, E.: Echocardiographic studies to explain opening snaps in presence of nonstenotic mitral valves. Am. J. Cardiol. *31*:64, 1973.
72. Criley, J. M., Lewis, K. B., Humphries, J. O., and Ross, R. S.: Prolapse of the mitral valve: Clinical and cine-angiocardiographic findings. Br. Heart J. 28:488, 1966.
73. Nixon, P. G. F.: The genesis of the third heart sound. Am. Heart J. *65*:712, 1963.
74. Harvey, W. P., and Stapleton, J.: Clinical aspects of gallop rhythm with particular reference to diastolic gallops. Circulation *18*:1017, 1958.
75. Tyberg, T. I., Goodyer, A. V. N., and Langou, R. A.: Genesis of pericardial knock in constrictive pericarditis. Am. J. Cardiol. *46*:570, 1980.
76. Van de Werf, F., Minten, J., Carmeliet, P., DeGeest, H., and Kesteloot, H.: The genesis of the third and fourth heart sounds: A pressure flow study in dogs. J. Clin. Invest. *73*:1400, 1984.
77. Van de Werf, F., Boel, A., Geboers, J., Minten, J., Willems, J., DeGeest, H., and Kesteloot, H.: Diastolic properties of the left ventricle in normal adults and in patients with third heart sounds. Circulation *69*:1070, 1984.
78. Ozawa, Y., Smith, D., and Craige, E.: Origin of the third heart sound. II. Studies in humans. Circulation *67*:399, 1983.
79. Ishimitsu, T., Smith, D., Berko, B., and Craige, E.: Origin of the third heart sound: Comparison of ventricular wall dynamics in hyperdynamic and hypodynamic types. J. Am. Coll. Cardiol. *5*:268, 1985.
80. Gibson, T. C., Madry, R., Grossman, W., McLaurin, L. P., and Craige, E.: The A wave of the apexcardiogram and left ventricular diastolic stiffness. Circulation *49*:441, 1974.
81. Kesteloot, H., and Willems, J.: Relationship between the right apexcardiogram and the right ventricular dynamics. Acta Cardiol. *22*:64, 1967.
82. Craige, E.: The fourth heart sound. *In* Leon, D. F., and Shaver, J. A. (eds.): Physiologic Principles of Heart Sounds and Murmurs. New York, American Heart Association Monograph, No. 46, 1975, p. 74.
83. Shah, P. M., and Jackson, D.: Third heart sound and summation gallop. *In* Leon, D. F., and Shaver, J. A. (eds.): Physiologic Principles of Heart Sounds and Murmurs. New York, American Heart Association Monograph, No. 46, 1975, p. 79.
84. Hultgren, H. N., and Hubis, H.: A phonocardiographic study of patients with the Starr-Edwards mitral valve prosthesis. Am. Heart J. *69*:306, 1965.
85. Gibson, T. C., Starek, P. J. K., Moos, S., and Craige, E.: Echocardiographic and phonocardiographic characteristics of the Lillehei-Kaster mitral valve prosthesis. Circulation *49*:434, 1974.
86. Smith, N. D., Raizada, V., and Abrams, J.: Auscultation of the normally functioning prosthetic valve. Ann. Intern. Med. *95*:594, 1981.
87. Brodie, B. R., Grossman, W., McLaurin, L. P., Starek, P. J. K., and Craige, E.: Diagnosis of prosthetic mitral valve malfunction with combined echophonocardiography. Circulation *53*:93, 1976.
88. Harris, A.: Pacemaker "heart sound." Br. Heart J. *29*:608, 1967.
89. Craige, E.: On the genesis of heart sounds: Contributions made by echocardiographic studies. Circulation *53*:207, 1976.

CAROTID PULSE TRACINGS AND SYSTOLIC TIME INTERVALS

90. Garrod, A. H.: On some points connected with the circulation of the blood, arrived at from a study of the sphygmograph trace. Proc. R. Soc. Lond. 23:140, 1874–1875.
91. Bowen, W. P.: Changes in heart rate, blood pressure and duration of systole resulting from bicycling. Am. J. Physiol. *11*:59, 1904.
92. Wiggers, C. J.: Studies on the consecutive phases of the cardiac cycle. II. The laws governing the relative durations of ventricular systole and diastole. Am. J. Physiol. *56*:439, 1921.
93. Lombard, W. P., and Cope, O. M.: The duration of the systole of the left ventricle of man. Am. J. Physiol. *77*:263, 1926.
94. Weissler, A. M., O'Neill, W. W., Shohn, Y. H., Stack, R. S., Chew, P. C., and Reed, A. H.: Prognostic significance of systolic time intervals after recovery from myocardial infarction. Am. J. Cardiol. *48*:995, 1981.
95. Weissler, A. M.: Systolic time intervals. *In* Cheng, T. O. (ed.): International Textbook of Cardiology. Elmsford, N.Y., Pergamon Press, 1986, Chapter 12.
96. Garrard, C. L., Jr., Weissler, S. M., and Doge, H. T.: The relationship of alterations in systolic time intervals to ejection fraction in patients with cardiac disease. Circulation *42*:455, 1970.
97. Weissler, A. M., Harris, W. S., and Schoenfeld, C. D.: Systolic time intervals in heart failure in man. Circulation *37*:149, 1968.
98. Lewis, R. P.: The use of systolic time intervals for evaluation of left ventricular function. *In* Fowler, N. O. (ed.): Noninvasive Diagnostic Methods in Cardiology. Philadelphia, F. A. Davis Co., 1983.
99. Unverferth, D. V., Lewis, R. P., Leier, C. V., Magorien, R. D., and Fulkerson, P. K.: The use of echocardiography and systolic time intervals in monitoring therapy of congestive heart failure. J. Clin. Ultrasound *8*:479, 1980.
100. Bonner, J. A., Sacks, H. N., and Tavel, M. E.: Assessing the severity of aortic stenosis by phonocardiography and external carotid pulse recordings. Circulation *48*:247, 1973.
101. Ichiyasu, H., and Craige, E.: Assessment of the severity of aortic stenosis from the carotid pulse tracing. Jpn. Heart J. *21*:465, 1980.
102. Orchard, R. C., and Craige, E.: Dicrotic pulse after open heart surgery. Circulation *62*:1107, 1980.
103. Ewy, G. A., Rios, J. C., and Marcus, F. I.: The dicrotic arterial pulse. Circulation *39*:655, 1969.
103a. Smith, D., and Craige, E.: Mechanism of the dicrotic pulse. Br. Heart J. (*In press*).
104. Hada, Y., Wolfe, C., and Craige, E.: Pulsus alternans determined by biventricular simultaneous systolic time intervals. Circulation *65*:617, 1982.
105. Craige, E.: Apexcardiography. *In* Weissler, A. M. (ed.): Noninvasive Cardiology. New York, Grune and Stratton, 1974, p. 1.
106. Smith, D., and Craige, E.: Enhancement of tactile perception in palpation. Circulation *62*:1114, 1980.
107. Willems, J. L., Kesteloot, H., and De Geest, H.: Influence of acute hemodynamic changes on the apexcardiogram in dogs. Am. J. Cardiol. *29*:504, 1972.
108. Willems, J. L., De Geest, H., and Kesteloot, H.: On the value of apexcardiography for timing intracardiac events. Am. J. Cardiol. *28*:59, 1971.
109. Bush, C. A., Lewis, R. P., Leighton, R. F., Fontana, M. E., and Weissler, A. M.: Verification of systolic time intervals and true isovolumic contraction time from the apexcardiogram by micromanometer catheterization of the left ventricle and aorta. Circulation *41*(Suppl. 3):121, 1970.
110. Sutton, G. C., Prewitt, T. A., and Craige, E.: Relationship between quantitated precordial movement and left ventricular function. Circulation *41*:179, 1970.
111. Sutton, G. C., Craige, E., and Grizzle, J. E.: Quantitation of precordial movement. II. Mitral regurgitation. Circulation *35*:483, 1967.
112. Lucardie, S. M., and Durrer, D.: The late systolic murmur. Arch. Kreislaufforsch. *53*:174, 1967.
113. Voigt, G. C., and Friesinger, G. C.: The use of apexcardiography in the assessment of left ventricular diastolic pressure. Circulation *41*:1015, 1970.
114. Schmidt, R. E., and Craige, E.: Precordial movements over the right ventricle in children with pulmonary stenosis. Circulation *32*:241, 1965.
115. Mounsey, J. P. D.: Inspection and palpation of the cardiac impulse. Prog. Cardiovasc. Dis. *10*:187, 1967.
116. Armstrong, T. G., and Gotsman, M. S.: The left parasternal life in tricuspid incompetence. Am. Heart J. *88*:183, 1974.
117. El-Sherif, A., and El-Said, G.: Jugular, hepatic, and praecordial pulsations in constrictive pericarditis. Br. Heart J. *33*:305, 1971.
118. Craige, E., and Fortuin, N. J.: Noninvasive measurement of ventricular function in chronic ischemic heart disease. *In* Likoff, W., Segal, B. L., Insull, W., and Moyer, J. H. (eds.): Atherosclerosis and Coronary Heart Disease. New York, Grune and Stratton, 1972, p. 221.
119. Basta, L. L., Wolfson, P., Eckbert, D. L., and Abboud, F. M.: The value of left parasternal impulse recordings in the assessment of mitral regurgitation. Circulation *48*:1055, 1973.

JUGULAR VENOUS PULSE

120. Constant, J.: The x′ descent in jugular contour nomenclature and recognition. Am. Heart J. *88*:372, 1974.
121. Rich, L. L., and Tavel, M. E.: The origin of the jugular C wave. N. Engl. J. Med. *284*:1309, 1971.
122. Sivaciyan, V., and Ranganathan, N.: Transcutaneous Doppler jugular venous flow velocity recording: Clinical and hemodynamic correlates. Circulation *57*:930, 1978.
123. Tavel, M. E.: Clinical Phonocardiography and External Pulse Recording, 4th ed. Chicago, Year Book Publishers, 1985.
124. Kesteloot, H., and Denef, B.: Value of reference tracings in the diagnosis and assessment of constrictive epi- and pericarditis. Br. Heart J. *32*:675, 1970.

4 ECHOPHONOCARDIOGRAPHY AND OTHER NONINVASIVE TECHNIQUES TO ELUCIDATE HEART MURMURS

by ERNEST CRAIGE, M.D.

Most cardiac murmurs are believed to arise from disturbances of blood flow that become manifest as turbulence. *Turbulence* is defined as an irregular condition of motion in which velocity and pressure show a random variation in relation to time and space coordinates.[1] Fluctuating velocities and pressures due to turbulence presumably produce local vibrations at the wall of the vessel or heart chamber, which then are transmitted to the chest wall and perceived as murmurs.[2] Maximum turbulence is found in the recipient vessel or chamber, such as, for example, the root of the great vessels in aortic or pulmonic stenosis, the left atrium in mitral regurgitation, and the cavity of the left ventricle in aortic regurgitation. The location of maximum intensity of murmurs over the chest and neck is generally over the site of the turbulence. Auscultation is favored by a slim body build and normal lungs and is made difficult by obesity and emphysema. An additional element in transmission is the phase of the cardiac cycle and the stiffness of the ventricular wall. The potential importance of these factors in murmur transmission has been recently demonstrated by Smith et al.[3] in canine preparations. In the normal ventricle, transmissibility of an artificial vibratory tone from base to apex was confined essentially to systole. In contrast, in the failing heart diastolic transmissibility became dominant.[3a] If confirmed in humans, these observations will have important implications regarding the intensity and distribution of acoustic phenomena reaching the chest surface. Noninvasive cardiac diagnostic methods—specifically echophonocardiography and Doppler echocardiography—can be used to illustrate the common types of heart murmurs encountered in clinical practice.

SYSTOLIC MURMURS[4, 5]

CLASSIFICATION. The convenient classification of systolic murmurs into two main categories—*ejection* and *regurgitant*—as popularized by Leatham has improved our understanding of pathogenetic mechanisms as well as facilitated communication among observers.[4] In general, "ejection murmurs" are midsystolic in timing and are the result of ejection of blood into the root of one of the great vessels. A classic example of an ejection murmur is that associated with stenosis of one of the semilunar valves (Fig. 4–1). The term "regurgitant murmur" has been used to describe a holosystolic murmur that may be found when the pressure relationships between the donor chamber (ventricle) and the recipient chamber (atrium, or lower pressure ventricle) favor retrograde flow *throughout* systole (Fig. 4–2). With improved understanding of variations in the hemodynamic patterns of mitral valve disease, it has become apparent that the physical signs associated with mitral regurgitation may also vary greatly (see Chapter 33). For instance, in acute mitral regurgitation, the murmur may be prominent in early and midsystole but may terminate before the second heart sound. In mitral valve prolapse, on the other hand, the murmur may be confined to late systole. These alterations from the classic pattern are readily explicable on the basis of known information

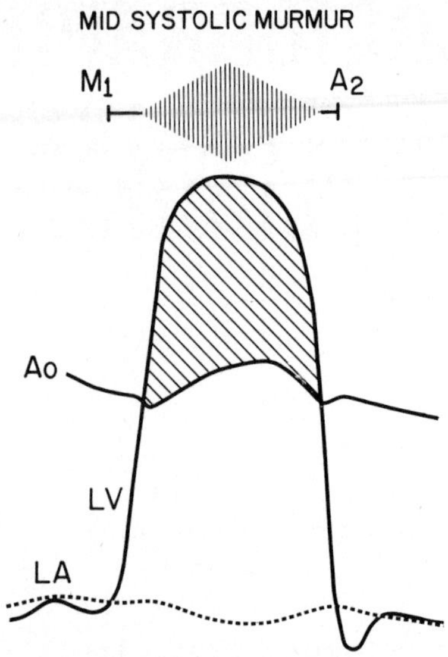

FIGURE 4–1. Midsystolic murmur in aortic stenosis, with pressure records from left ventricle (LV), left atrium (LA), and aorta (A_o). In early systole, LV pressure rises swiftly and opens the aortic valve, whereupon ejection into the root of the aorta can begin; only then does the midsystolic or ejection murmur start, peaking at the time of maximum gradient across the valve (shaded area). At the end of systole, the falling pressure in the LV results in diminishing flow across the aortic valve, and the murmur fades away before A_2.

concerning the anatomical and physiological derangements in these conditions. Thus, efforts to describe these abbreviated murmurs within the framework of the "ejection" and "regurgitant" terminology have led to a confusing misuse of terms, such as "ejection-type" murmur to describe a murmur that results from regurgitation but is less than holosystolic in duration.

Therefore, in this chapter simple descriptive terms, such as "early systolic," "late systolic," "holosystolic," and "midsystolic," will be used to indicate the position of systolic murmurs in the cardiac cycle. Murmurs that begin with the first heart sound and proceed to the second sound on their side of origin are called *holosystolic.* A murmur that begins with the first heart sound and finishes in either mid- or late systole but well before the second heart sound on its side of origin is designated an *early systolic* murmur.

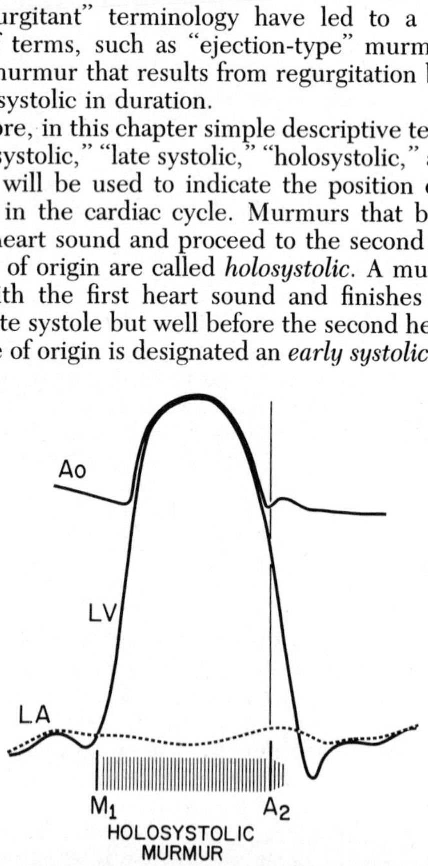

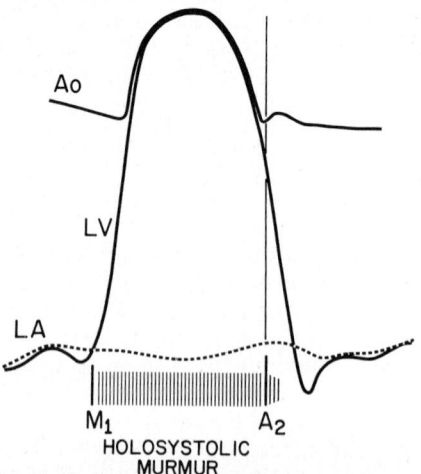

FIGURE 4–2. Holosystolic murmur. In mitral regurgitation LV pressure rises and immediately exceeds LA pressure. Thus the regurgitant murmur begins with M_1, continues throughout systole, and may continue even slightly beyond A_2, because the falling pressure in the LV still exceeds that of the LA, thus favoring continuing regurgitation.

Conversely, with a *late systolic* murmur, early systole is silent, the murmur generally beginning in mid- to late systole and proceeding to the second heart sound on its side of origin. If the murmur begins at an interval after the first heart sound and ends before the second, and both early and late systole are murmur-free, the murmur is designated "midsystolic."

MIDSYSTOLIC MURMURS

PHYSIOLOGICAL MURMURS. The commonest murmur is soft, midsystolic in time, and not associated with any cardiac abnormality. Such functional or innocent murmurs are usually best heard and recorded at the left sternal edge in either the second or the third left intercostal space. Most commonly they consist phonocardiographically of random noise, i.e., vibrations of various frequencies.[6] The intensity of physiological murmurs can be magnified by physical activity, excitement, pregnancy, anemia, thyrotoxicosis, fever, and so on, presumably owing to increases in the volume and velocity of ejection. In thin subjects or individuals with a depressed sternum, proximity of the stethoscope or microphone to the source of the murmur may result in even greater intensity. The source of physiological midsystolic murmurs is thought to be the right ventricular outflow tract and root of the pulmonary artery, because their area of maximal intensity is at the left sternal edge overlying these anatomical structures. The innocent murmurs which are maximal lower over the midprecordium are often more musical or even grunting in quality and appear on the phonocardiogram in crescendo-decrescendo silhouette, with vibrations of a constant frequency rather than random noise (Fig. 4–3). Appreciation of the innocent nature of the murmurs just described is facilitated by the absence of other evidence of heart disease by means of physical examination, electrocardiogram, and chest x-ray. From a phonocardiographic point of view, the midsystolic timing of the murmur is important in differentiating it from the holosystolic murmur of an interventricular

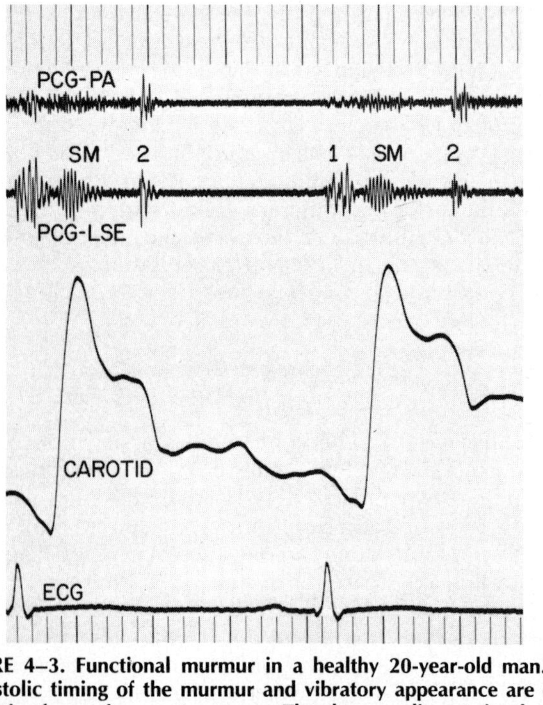

FIGURE 4–3. Functional murmur in a healthy 20-year-old man. The midsystolic timing of the murmur and vibratory appearance are characteristic of many innocent murmurs. The phonocardiogram is otherwise normal, as is the carotid pulse tracing. PCG-PA = phonocardiogram in second left intercostal space; PCG-LSE = phonocardiogram at left sternal edge.

septal defect. The basal systolic murmur of an atrial septal defect, however, represents an exaggerated flow murmur in midsystole resulting from augmentation of right ventricular stroke volume. It therefore resembles an innocent murmur. Attention to the details of the second heart sound, however, should clarify this problem, since the wide, fixed splitting of S_2, which is characteristic of atrial septal defect (Fig. 3–9, *left*, p. 47), would not be found with an innocent or physiological murmur. Other causes of midsystolic murmurs resulting from ejection across deformed or obstructing outflow tracts and semilunar valves are described in the following paragraphs.

OBSTRUCTION TO LEFT VENTRICULAR OUTFLOW.[7, 8] Midsystolic murmurs are characteristically found in patients with obstruction of the outflow tract. Combined Doppler, phono-, and echocardiographic studies are particularly useful in determining the underlying pathological condition in these cases, although conventional M-mode echocardiography alone may be of very limited value. Echophonocardiography may also provide valuable guidelines when difficult decisions regarding the timing of invasive studies must be made. It may also be useful in serial observations of patients in whom the obstruction is not critical.

Congenital Valvular Aortic Stenosis (See also pp. 932 and 978). This condition produces a characteristic midsystolic murmur best recorded in the second right interspace or aortic area (Fig. 4–4). In children and adolescents, this abnormality is almost invariably associated with an aortic ejection sound that initiates the murmur. The ejection sound is widely transmitted over the precordium and can be recorded at the mitral area. Its identity can be established echophonocardiographically by its coincidence with the achievement of a maximally open position by the aortic valve (see Fig. 3–11, p. 48). A_2 is well preserved in young individuals in whom the valve, although deformed, is capable of closing and being set into vibration at the onset of diastole.[9] With advancing age, the valve may become calcified and immobilized, with diminution or obliteration of both the ejection sound and A_2. The murmur itself is of little help in determining the severity of the valvular abnormality. There is a tendency for the murmur to peak later in systole with severe stenosis.[10] The loudness of the murmur is not proportional to the severity of the obstruction. A loud murmur may occur merely with sclerosis of the valve when there is no significant gradient across it. Conversely, in a moribund patient with the most severe stenosis, the murmur may become faint or disappear entirely as the left ventricular stroke volume declines.

Severe aortic stenosis results in prolongation of the left ventricular ejection time,[10] concentric hypertrophy of the left ventricle as manifested in the echocardiogram (Fig. 4–4), an audible S_4,[11, 12] and a large *a* wave in the jugular venous pulse. This latter sign reflects altered filling characteristics of the right ventricle possibly caused by encroachment by the hypertrophied interventricular septum—the so-called Bernheim syndrome. The most accurate noninvasive estimate of the severity of aortic stenosis is provided by the Doppler method[13, 14] (Fig. 4–5; see also Fig. 5–58, p. 109).

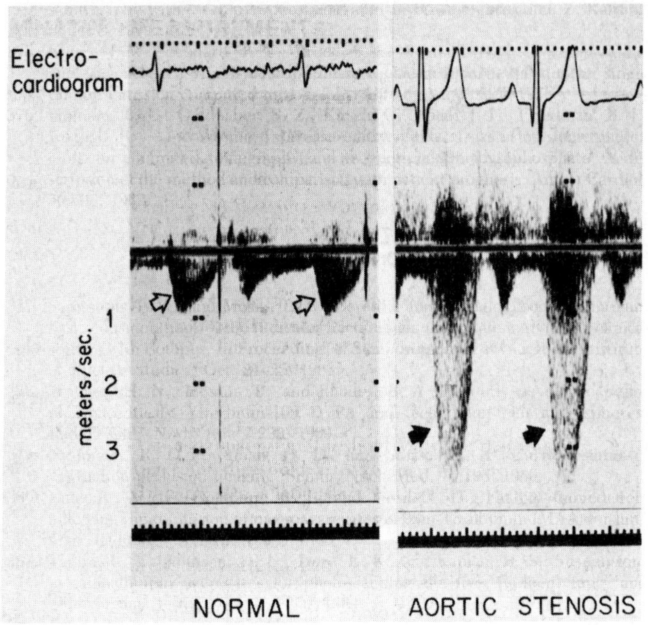

FIGURE 4–5. Valvular aortic stenosis. A Doppler study contrasts normal velocity (*left*) with aortic stenosis (*right*). The peak velocity of 3.5 msec indicates a peak gradient of approximately 50 mm Hg. (See Chapter 5 for details of Doppler method.)

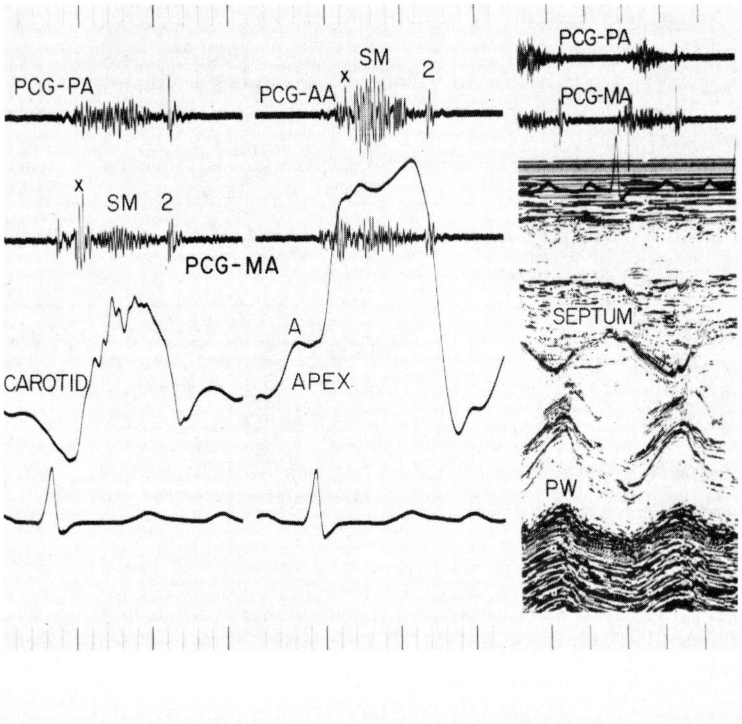

FIGURE 4–4. Congenital valvular aortic stenosis. An asymptomatic 10-year-old boy, successfully operated upon in infancy for coarctation of the aorta, had a residual murmur characteristic of valvular aortic stenosis presumably due to a bicuspid aortic valve. *Left*, Phonocardiogram at the cardiac apex (PCG-MA) shows a loud ejection sound (X) followed by a midsystolic murmur (SM) transmitted from the aortic area. The carotid pulse is shattered with coarse vibrations and peaks late in systole. *Center*, The "diamond shape" or prominent systolic murmur is best seen at the second right interspace (AA). The apexcardiogram is abnormal, with an exaggerated *a* wave followed by a systolic heave shown graphically by an upward slope. The findings are consistent with left ventricular hypertrophy. *Right*, Concentric hypertrophy of the left ventricle was verified by an echocardiogram which shows a small chamber but a thick septum and posterior wall (PW). The combined study indicated the presence of significant aortic stenosis despite absence of symptoms. At catheterization a systolic gradient of 80 mm Hg was demonstrated.

Fibrous Subaortic Stenosis (See also p. 936). This condition is congenital in origin and is associated with a murmur identical to that of valvular stenosis, although its focus of maximal intensity may be over the midprecordium rather than the aortic area. The carotid pulse is also similar to that in valvular stenosis. However, two observations are of value in differential diagnosis by echophonocardiographic methods: (1) the absence of an ejection sound at the time of full aortic valve opening in the patient with fibrous or diaphragmatic subaortic stenosis (Fig. 4–5),[15] and (2) partial closure and fluttering of the aortic valve in early systole (Fig. 4–5).[16] This curious behavior of the valve is not peculiar to fibrous subaortic stenosis but may occur in hypertrophic obstructive cardiomyopathy (HOCM) as well as in normal individuals, to a minor degree. However, the combination of the midsystolic murmur, absence of an ejection sound, partial closure and fluttering of the aortic valve in early systole, and absence of poststenotic dilatation on the x-ray should permit a reasonably confident diagnosis of fibrous or diaphragmatic subaortic stenosis. An early diastolic murmur of mild aortic regurgitation may be found in association with fibrous subvalvular stenosis. An estimate of severity may be provided by the Doppler method, as with congenital valvular aortic stenosis.

Supravalvular Aortic Stenosis (See also p. 937). The midsystolic murmur in this congenital abnormality is similar to that of valvular and subvalvular stenosis.[7, 15] It is usually of great intensity over the aortic area, to the right of the upper sternum, and is well transmitted over the vessels of the neck. Graphic tracings can be used to display the murmur, but such records are of little value in localizing the obstruction or determining its severity. A simultaneous recording of both carotid pulses, however, may disclose an inequality in amplitude and slope, apparently resulting from the direction of the jet of blood that has traversed the stenotic area (Fig. 4–6). This usually leads to inequality of the carotid and brachial pulses, which are more prominent on the right side (p. 57). An ejection sound is usually not present in supravalvular aortic stenosis,[17] and aortic regurgitation is most unusual.

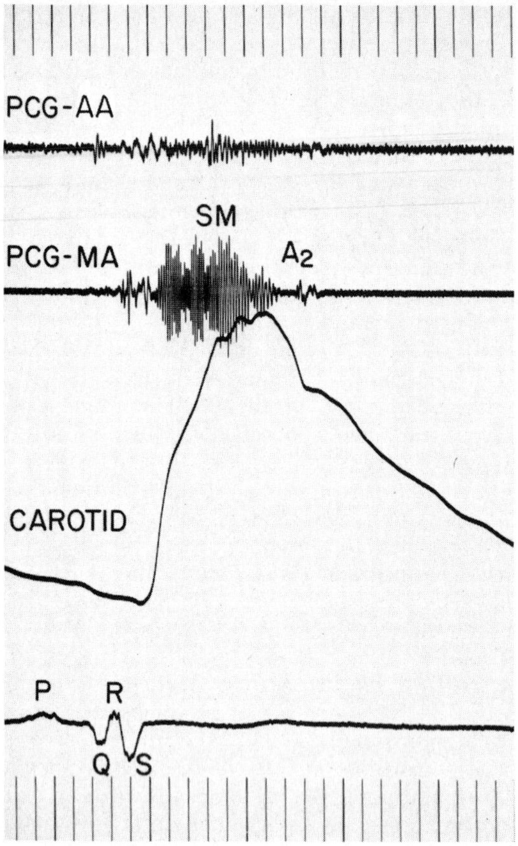

FIGURE 4–7. Aortic stenosis in an elderly man. The murmur is faint in the second right interspace (PCG-AA) but is prominent at the cardiac apex (MA). The carotid upstroke is delayed and demonstrates coarse vibrations.

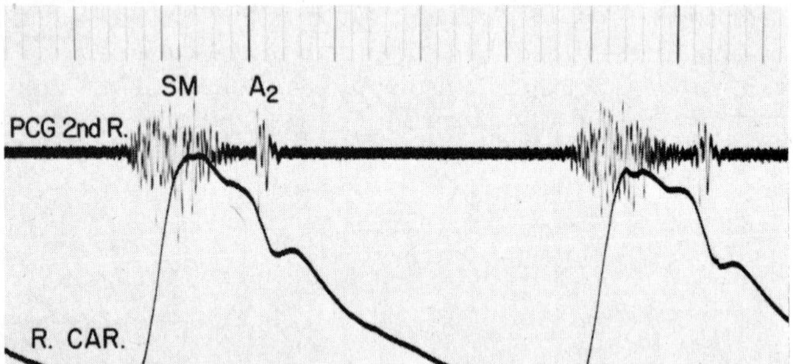

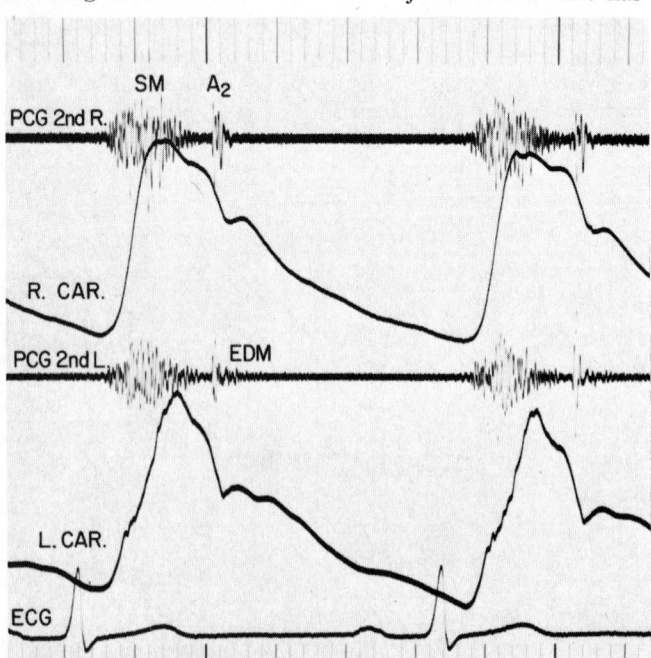

FIGURE 4–6. Supravalvular aortic stenosis. A loud midsystolic murmur was recorded in the right and left second intercostal spaces and was audible over the whole upper chest. Right and left carotid pulse tracings recorded simultaneously illustrate differences in their contours; note the more delayed upstroke in the left compared with the right carotid pulse. At catheterization a gradient of 95 mm Hg was recorded between left ventricle and aorta beyond the obstruction. The early diastolic murmur (EDM) of slight aortic regurgitation is unusual in this condition.

Valvular Aortic Stenosis of Rheumatic Origin (see also p. 1052). The findings here are similar to those found in the congenital variety, although the ejection sound is seen only rarely and when present is inconspicuous, especially later in the natural history when the valve has calcified. The presence of associated valvular lesions may be helpful in establishing the etiology.

Atypical Presentation of Aortic Stenosis. In older patients, particularly those suffering from complicating conditions such as emphysema, the presentation of aortic stenosis may differ markedly from that of congenital stenosis in childhood. In elderly patients, the murmur of valvular aortic stenosis, regardless of etiology, is sometimes heard best, if not exclusively, at the mitral area (Fig. 4–7).[18–20] Under these circumstances, identification of the murmur as being ejection in character and presumably of aortic origin may be made by an experienced auscultator by noting the midsystolic peaking of the murmur and its termination before S_2. This latter sign may be obscured, however, by the faintness or absence of the second sound. The ejection sound is also faint or usually absent because of the inevitable calcification of the valve. Clarification of this problem may be gained by noting the behavior of the murmur with an arrhythmia such as premature beats or atrial fibrillation, and confirmation by phonocardiography may be very helpful (Fig. 4–8). The ejection murmur of aortic stenosis fluctuates remarkably in intensity with the strength of left ventricular systole, whereas the murmur of mitral regurgitation is much less affected.[18] The problem

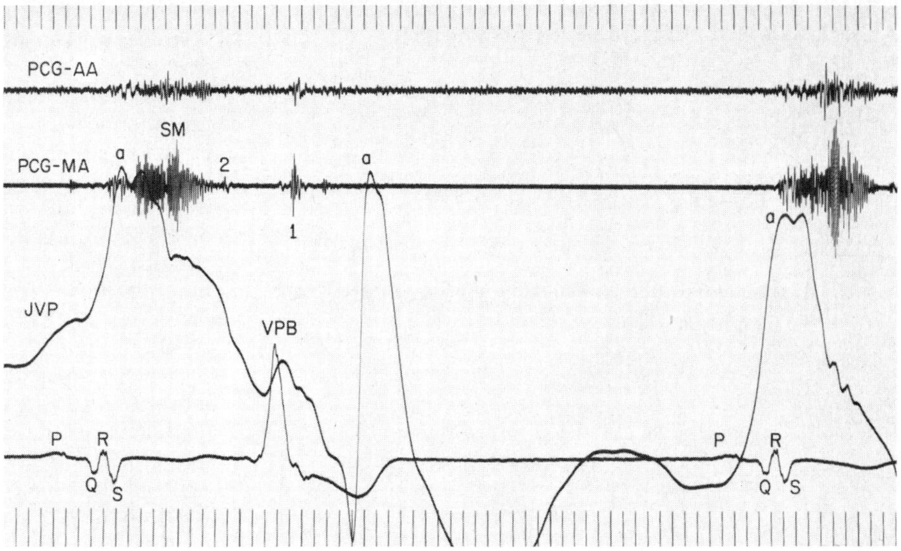

FIGURE 4–8. Aortic stenosis (same patient as in Figure 4–7). The weak ventricular premature beat (VPB) fails to produce a murmur, but the postextrasystolic beat results in accentuation of the murmur. The JVP demonstrates a prominent *a* wave in the conducted beats and a "cannon wave" with the VPB, owing to contraction of the right atrium against a closed tricuspid valve.

of deciding the origin of such a murmur may be easily settled by the Doppler method. Other graphic records which may be helpful in differentiating aortic stenosis from mitral regurgitation include the carotid pulse tracing and systolic time intervals. The carotid upstroke is characteristically sharp in mitral regurgitation, but it is slow rising and shattered in aortic stenosis (Fig. 3–22, p. 56, and Fig. 4–4). PEP is prolonged in mitral regurgitation and LVET is shortened, giving an abnormally high PEP/LVET ratio (see p. 55). In aortic stenosis, the reverse is found—PEP is abbreviated and LVET is prolonged.[21]

Hypertrophic Obstructive Cardiomyopathy (HOCM) (See also p. 1419). The presence or absence of left ventricular outflow obstruction in patients with HOCM was an early stimulus to the correlation of echo- and phonocardiographic abnormalities.[22, 23] It is now well established that systolic anterior motion of the mitral valve impinging on the grossly hypertrophied septum results in obstruction to left ventricular outflow (Chap. 5) and produces a midsystolic murmur resembling that of valvular obstruction except that its location of maximal intensity is at the left sternal edge. The murmur may be augmented by an element of mitral regurgitation, which is a frequent additional physiological derangement. However, it is seldom possible to distinguish a separate holosystolic murmur at the cardiac apex. The midsystolic murmur suggests the presence of outflow tract obstruction[24] but may occur when there is concentric hypertrophy without obstruction.[25] Other features of HOCM that can be documented in a noninvasive assessment include the characteristic deformity of the carotid pulse—the spike-and-dome pattern, as described in Chapter 3—and the apexcardiogram with its exaggerated *a* wave and bifid or saddle-shaped appearance in systole (see Fig. 3–30, p. 59). The cusps of the aortic valve can be seen, in an accompanying echo, to close partially at the time of the systolic anterior movement of the mitral leaflet and the onset of the murmur.[26] A combined study utilizing all these parameters with echocardiography is useful, therefore, in demonstrating the simultaneity and presumed physiological relationship of the systolic anterior movement of the mitral valve impinging on the hypertrophied septum and the dramatic array of auscultatory and pulsatile events that ensue (Fig. 4–9). In addition, the modifications in these signs produced by pharmacological and physical maneuvers, as described in Chapter 2, can be documented by echophonocardiography.

Ejection Through a Normal Valve into a Dilated Aortic Root. In hypertension, arteriosclerosis, and other conditions associated with aortic dilatation, a midsystolic murmur may be recorded over the aortic area. It is usually less intense than that associated with obstructive lesions and terminates earlier in systole. The upstroke of the carotid pulse is normal, and there is no prolongation of left ventricular systole manifest by lengthening of LVET.

OBSTRUCTION TO RIGHT VENTRICULAR OUTFLOW. The physiological principles underlying the echophonocardiographic findings in obstruction to left ventricular outflow also apply to the right side of the heart. On the right side, however, the effect of inspiration in augmenting ventricular filling represents an additional factor.

Pulmonic Valve Stenosis (See also p. 1075). The murmur of pulmonic valvular stenosis is intense and of a harsh quality. It is maximal in the second left interspace and diminishes in all directions from this point. The murmur is midsystolic. However, the timing of peak

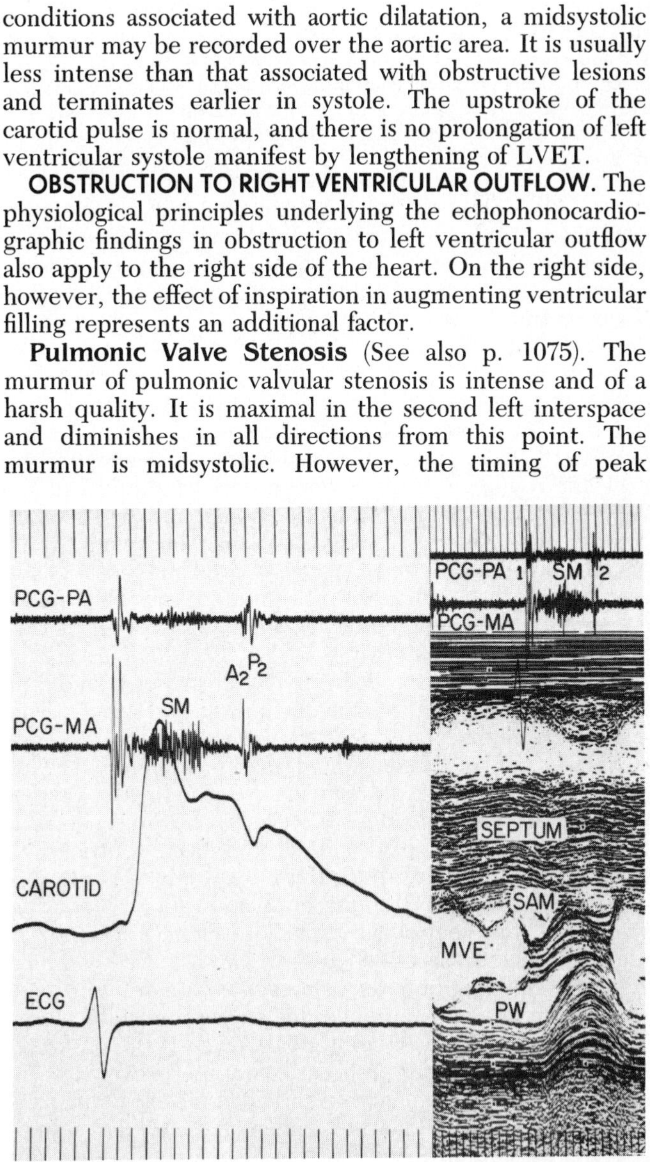

FIGURE 4–9. Hypertrophic obstructive cardiomyopathy (HOCM). *Left*, Carotid tracing illustrating a swift upstroke with a dip at the time of the midsystolic murmur, followed by a second hump during systole. *Right*, Echophonocardiogram showing the relationship between the murmur and the outflow tract obstruction resulting from the systolic anterior movement of the mitral valve (SAM), which appears to appose itself closely to the enormously hypertrophied septum.

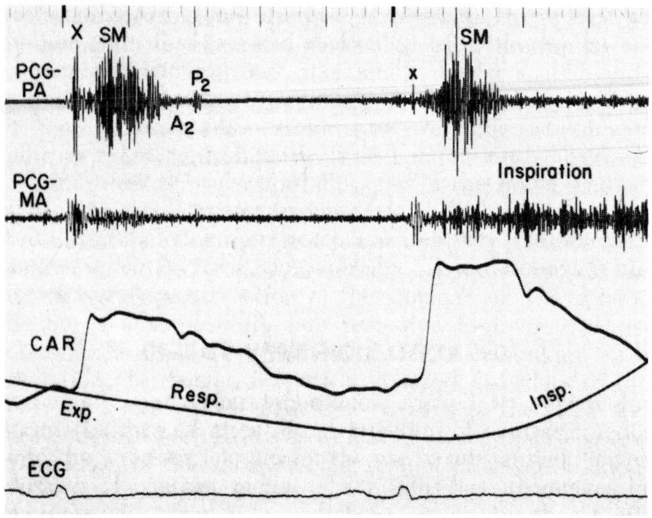

FIGURE 4–10. Valvular pulmonic stenosis. The first sound is not visible. The loud sound "X" at the beginning of systole is an ejection sound that is maximal in the second left interspace (PA). It is loud in expiration and diminishes with inspiration. The ejection sound is followed by a midsystolic murmur (SM). P_2 is diminutive and delayed.

intensity can be used as an indicator of severity, more than that of aortic stenosis, since it is delayed in those patients with more severe obstruction. In the most severe cases, the murmur may peak late in systole and continue to or even *through* A_2, thus appearing to be holosystolic. Under these circumstances, however, since P_2 becomes further delayed with prolongation of right ventricular systole, the murmur remains *midsystolic* with respect to *right*-sided events of the cardiac cycle[27] (see Chap. 3). The murmur is initiated by a pulmonary ejection sound which is also localized to the upper left sternal border and is loudest in *expiration* (Fig. 4–10).[28] Echophonocardiography can be very helpful in identifying an ejection sound by its exact coincidence with the achievement of a maximally open position by the pulmonary valve. The characteristic fluctuations of the sound with respiration can be readily documented. The phonocardiogram is also useful in displaying the increased separation of A_2-P_2, which is roughly proportional to the severity of the obstruction and the resultant rise in right ventricular systolic pressure.[27] The apexcardiographic transducer can be used to register the right ventricular heave, which marks the more severe examples of pulmonic valve stenosis.[29] The jugular venous pulse displays a prominent *a* wave in the presence of a thickened, hypertrophied, and noncompliant ventricle.

Subpulmonic (Infundibular) Stenosis. When this obstructive condition is found in isolation, i.e., without an associated interventricular septal defect, the murmur is identical to that described earlier for valvular pulmonic stenosis,[30] although the location of its maximal intensity is lower along the left sternal border, in the third interspace. The ejection sound is lacking, however, as is the poststenotic dilatation on x-ray. Echocardiography reveals an early partial closing movement and fluttering of the pulmonary valve.[31] More often than in isolation, infundibular pulmonary stenosis occurs in conjunction with an interventricular septal defect. In this situation a whole spectrum of combinations of murmurs and heart sounds can be recorded as determined by the relative severity of the two major pathophysiological factors—the outflow obstruction and the interventricular defect.[32] At the one extreme, when the infundibular stenosis is mild, the physical signs as recorded phonocardiographically are dominated by the loud holosystolic murmur of the interventricular septal defect, upon which is superimposed the ejection murmur resulting from the stenosis. Frequently the silhouette of the murmur in the phonocardiogram taken low along the left sternal edge is holosystolic with a more or less constant intensity, whereas in the pulmonary area there is a definite midsystolic peak reflecting the obstructive lesion. There is no ejection sound. S_2 is widely split, as in valvular pulmonic stenosis, but P_2 is louder, probably reflecting the augmented flow through the pulmonary artery and higher pressures in the pulmonary artery as a result of the left-to-right shunt.

In cases in which the degree of infundibular stenosis is more severe, right-to-left shunting occurs through the ventricular septal defect, i.e., the classic tetralogy of Fallot (p. 988). Under these circumstances, the murmur from the ventricular defect disappears. The midsystolic murmur in the pulmonary area, however, can still be recorded, but its duration and intensity are lessened.[32] P_2 becomes inaudible and can rarely be recorded, even under ideal conditions. Thus the second sound becomes single, being made up of A_2 alone. An ejection sound of aortic origin is frequently audible and can be recorded widely over the precordium.

In the most extreme cases, when pulmonary atresia is present, the right-sided systolic murmur disappears, but there may be a short, early to midsystolic murmur resulting from ejection into a dilated aortic root. S_2 is single, and an aortic ejection sound can usually be recorded. Elsewhere over the thorax one can occasionally hear and record the continuous murmur from the bronchial collateral circulation.

HOLOSYSTOLIC MURMURS

MITRAL REGURGITATION[4, 18, 33, 34] (See also p. 1034). Combined echo- and phonocardiographic studies are particularly important in assessing patients with mitral regurgitation. Although the presence of the characteristic holosystolic murmur suggests the diagnosis by noninvasive means, neither the etiology nor the hemodynamic importance of the condition is usually apparent from the phonocardiographic findings alone. The echocardiographic appearance of the valve leaflets may be most helpful in this regard. A useful index of the severity of the regurgitation is provided by the hyperdynamic left ventricular wall motion, left ventricular cavity dimensions, and left atrial enlargement (Chap. 5). Thus, whereas auscultation and phonocardiography establish the diagnosis of mitral regurgitation, echocardiography is used to assess the severity of the regurgitation and, on occasion, its pathogenesis.

Mitral Regurgitation due to Rheumatic Heart Disease. The holosystolic murmur is best recorded at the cardiac apex (Fig. 4–11). It immediately follows S_1, which may be of reduced intensity unless there is a mixed lesion of stenosis and regurgitation. The murmur continues to, or at times slightly beyond, A_2. The second sound is normally split or may be more widely split than normal. However, variation with respiration is preserved. A third sound is a common accompaniment of moderate to severe mitral regurgitation, and in the more severe cases a mid-diastolic rumble may be recorded in the mitral area.[35]

The echocardiographic appearance of rheumatic mitral regurgitation comprises a spectrum of mitral valve motion ranging from an apparently normal pattern to one in which the features of mitral stenosis are prominent. The combination of a holosystolic murmur and an echocardiogram

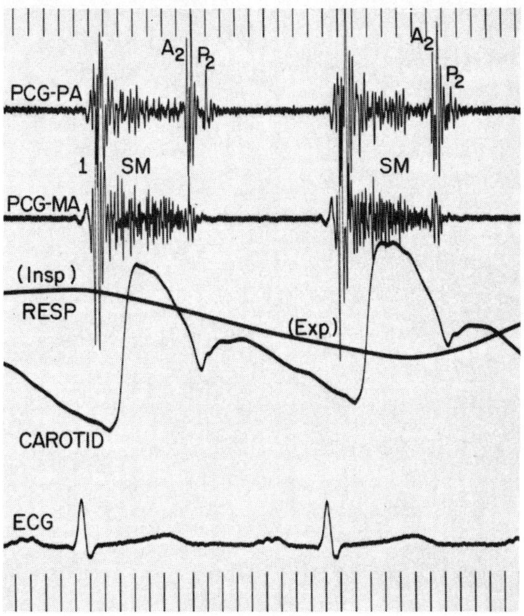

FIGURE 4–11. Mitral regurgitation due to rheumatic heart disease in a 25-year-old man with no symptoms and a small heart. The holosystolic murmur is most prominent at the cardiac apex (PCG-MA). S_1 is unusually loud, suggesting the possibility of early mitral stenosis, although there is no diastolic murmur.

consistent with mitral stenosis indicates the presence of mitral valvular disease with a rheumatic basis.

Mitral Regurgitation Secondary to Cardiomyopathy. Phonocardiography is of little help in the important differential diagnosis of severe diffuse cardiomyopathy as opposed to that of primary valvular disease. In cardiomyopathy, the murmur is holosystolic as in rheumatic heart disease, and there may be a prominent third sound that is also nonspecific, since it is a feature common to both cardiomyopathy and severe mitral regurgitation, regardless of pathogenesis. Systolic time intervals display similar abnormalities—prolongation of PEP and shortening of LVET, with a resulting increase in the PEP/LVET ratio (p. 55).[21] However, the echocardiogram may be most helpful in this differential diagnosis, since the dilated inert left ventricle of cardiomyopathy[36] contrasts sharply with the hyperdynamic movements of the septum and posterior wall in severe mitral regurgitation of rheumatic origin (Fig. 4–12).

TRICUSPID REGURGITATION SECONDARY TO PULMONARY HYPERTENSION[37] (see p. 1072). Although noninvasive methods are useful in the diagnosis of tricuspid regurgitation, the graphic registration of the murmur may be disappointing (Fig. 4–13). Even more than with mitral regurgitation, the intensity of the murmur fails to correlate with the severity of the hemodynamic abnormality.[38, 39] It is often overshadowed by the murmurs of accompanying valvular disease, since tricuspid regurgitation is most often a complication of left-sided disease that has resulted in pulmonary hypertension. The murmur is classically recorded best at the left lower sternal edge. With dilatation of the right ventricle, its point of maximal intensity may be shifted toward the left to the usual location of mitral murmurs. This can lead to an erroneous impression of *mitral* regurgitation, when tricuspid insufficiency has developed as a late result of severe mitral stenosis with pulmonary hypertension. Accentuation of the murmur with inspiration (Carvallo's sign) is a well-known feature of tricuspid regurgitation[40] that can be documented phonocardiographically. An accompanying venous pulse tracing will illustrate the parallel accentuation of *cv* waves with

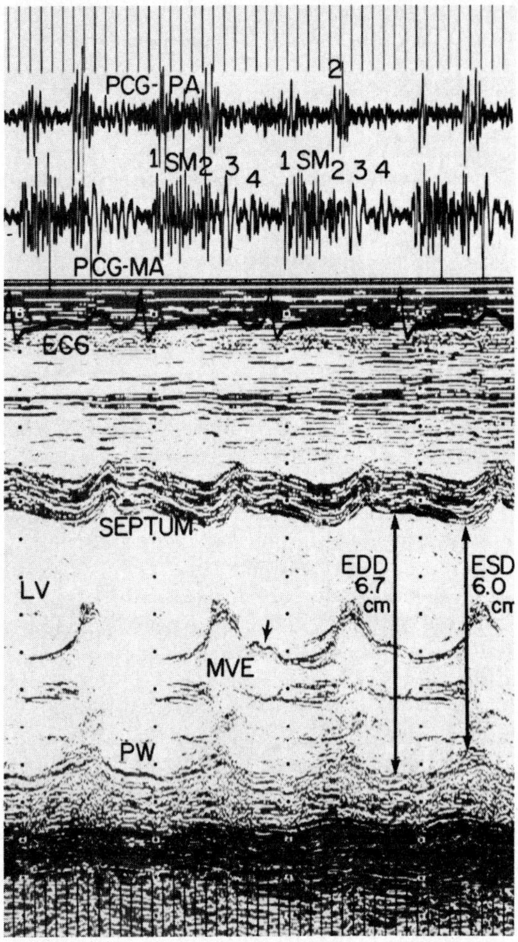

FIGURE 4–12. Systolic murmur with cardiomyopathy. The prominent holosystolic murmur at the cardiac apex (MA) is secondary to a severe diffuse alcoholic cardiomyopathy. There is very little difference between the left ventricular diameter in diastole (EDD) and that in systole (ESD). Additional phonocardiographic findings include gallop sounds (3 and 4). Arrow points to B notch on mitral valve echo, suggesting elevated left ventricular end-diastolic pressure. (Paper speed = 50 mm/sec.)

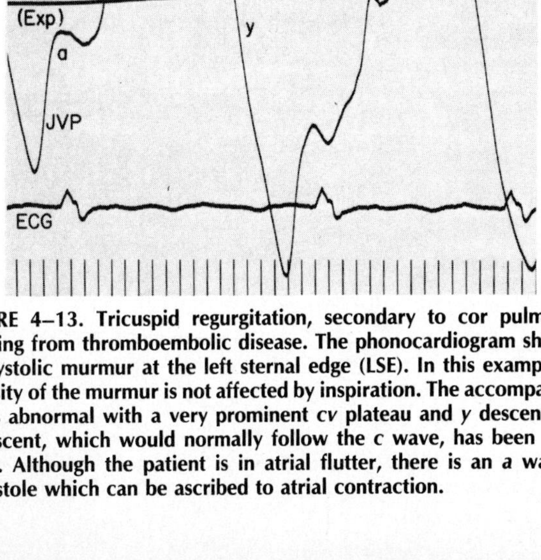

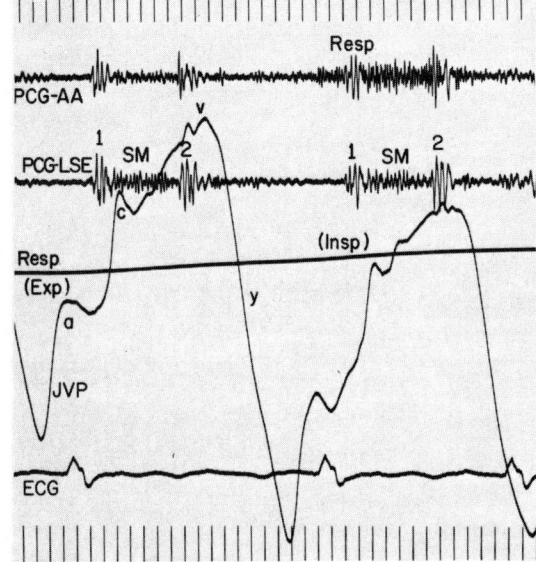

FIGURE 4–13. Tricuspid regurgitation, secondary to cor pulmonale resulting from thromboembolic disease. The phonocardiogram shows a holosystolic murmur at the left sternal edge (LSE). In this example the intensity of the murmur is not affected by inspiration. The accompanying JVP is abnormal with a very prominent *cv* plateau and *y* descent. The *x′* descent, which would normally follow the *c* wave, has been eliminated. Although the patient is in atrial flutter, there is an *a* wave in presystole which can be ascribed to atrial contraction.

inspiration. Carvallo's sign, however, is not invariably present[41] and can be abolished by the onset of right ventricular failure, which prevents the inspiratory augmentation of right ventricular stroke volume responsible for intensification of the murmur. A third sound and middiastolic flow rumble of right-sided origin occur with the more severe cases of tricuspid regurgitation,[37] as in the analogous situation on the left side of the heart. Precordial movement at the left sternal edge consists of a systolic heave of right ventricular hypertrophy when tricuspid regurgitation occurs as a consequence of right ventricular failure secondary to pulmonary hypertension.[42] The echocardiogram demonstrates a dilated right ventricular chamber and paradoxical movement of the interventricular septum. When tricuspid regurgitation occurs as a consequence of isolated damage to the valve itself rather than secondary to pulmonary hypertension, the physical signs and their graphic representation may be quite different (p. 73). The murmur may have a decrescendo configuration and be confined to early and midsystole.[43] This variant is discussed below, under Early Systolic Murmurs.

VENTRICULAR SEPTAL DEFECT (See also pp. 920 and 985). The murmur of a ventricular septal defect (VSD) is holosystolic, since in its typical expression (Roger's murmur)[44] it arises from the passage of blood throughout systole from the high-pressure left ventricle to the relatively low-pressure right ventricle through the defect. Thus the hemodynamic situation favors a holosystolic timing of the shunt as well as the murmur, which arises from the turbulence generated in the recipient chamber, the right ventricle. The murmur is quite intense and is located maximally in the third and fourth left interspaces, from which focus it diminishes centrifugally (Fig. 4–14).[45, 46] The second heart sound is usually normal, although the degree of splitting may be somewhat exaggerated. However, respiratory variation is maintained.

In the smaller defects that characterize the classic Roger type of ventricular septal defect, the volume of the shunt is determined by the size of the septal aperture. The variations in hemodynamic patterns, which are conditioned by the size of the defect and the level of pulmonary arterial pressure, are roughly reflected in modifications in the

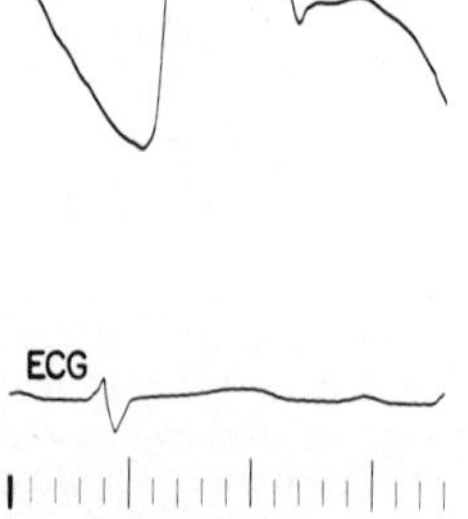

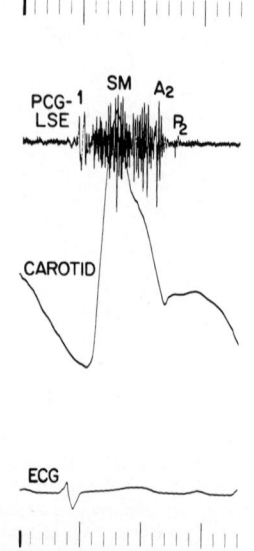

FIGURE 4–14. Ventricular septal defect with a large left-to-right shunt. A loud holosystolic murmur is seen, with accentuation in midsystole.

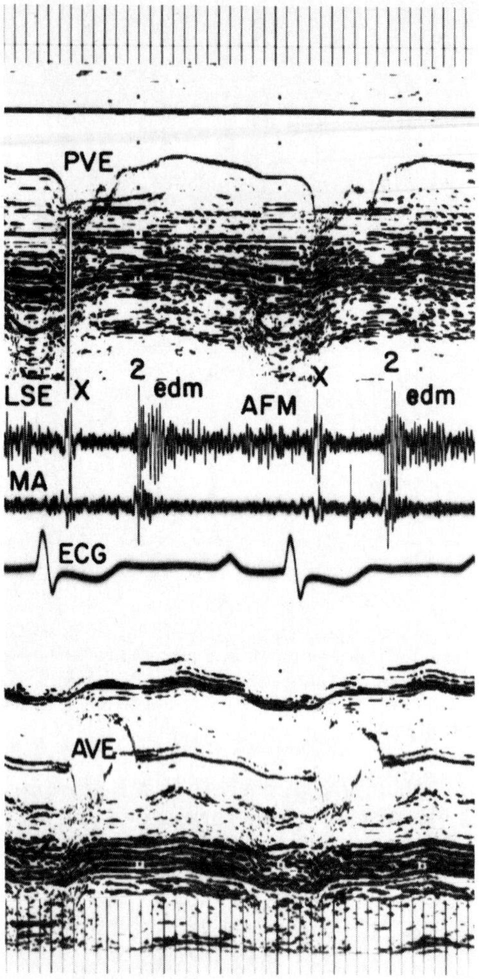

FIGURE 4–15. Dual echophonocardiogram in Eisenmenger syndrome. A loud second sound (2) is followed by a high-frequency decrescendo diastolic murmur (edm) of pulmonary regurgitation. In the latter part of diastole, this merges with a lower frequency right-sided Austin Flint murmur (AFM). The loud ejection sound (X) is of pulmonary valve origin, as shown by the vertical line. The simultaneous echo of the aortic valve shows a tendency to closure in the latter half of systole, reflecting a dwindling stroke volume in this very ill patient.

graphic signs.[45] With larger shunts, the auscultatory and phonocardiographic signs of increased diastolic flow across the mitral valve may be manifest in an S_3 and middiastolic rumbling murmur. It may be possible to visualize the defect in the septum by two-dimensional echocardiography, and one can detect indirect signs of the magnitude of the shunt in the size of the left-sided heart chambers and mobility of the left ventricular walls.

With pulmonary hypertension (the Eisenmenger type of VSD), the physical and graphic signs are remarkably altered (Fig. 4–15). The volume and direction of shunting are now regulated by the relative resistances of the pulmonary and systemic circuits. As pressures in the two ventricles equilibrate in systole and as bidirectional shunting ensues owing to the large size of the defect, the systolic murmur resulting from the shunt disappears.[45] There remains a brief early to midsystolic ejection murmur resulting from flow into the dilated root of the pulmonary artery. This murmur is initiated by an ejection sound occurring at the time of full opening of the cusps of the pulmonic valve. The timing of the ejection sound is delayed with pulmonary hypertension, owing to prolongation of the isovolumetric contraction time.[46] The second sound is very intense and is often palpable and results from the simultaneous closure of A_2 and an accentuated P_2. Accompanying murmurs that may be recorded in the more severe and longstanding cases of the Eisenmenger variant of ventricular septal defect include those of pulmonary regurgitation (Graham Steell), tricuspid regurgitation,[47] and, on occasion, a right-sided Austin Flint murmur.[48]

EARLY SYSTOLIC MURMURS

ACUTE MITRAL REGURGITATION (See also p. 1034). Acute mitral regurgitation constitutes a syndrome that has been increasingly identified in recent years. Although less common than the chronic variety, acute mitral regurgitation is important because of its severity and reversibility in many instances, if it is accurately and promptly diagnosed. It occurs in association with rupture of the chordae tendineae or papillary muscle, or with severe damage to the valve itself, such as from trauma or infective endocarditis. Acute mitral regurgitation requires special consideration, since its auscultatory and phonocardiographic manifestations are unusual for mitral regurgitation—often resembling those of aortic stenosis. The murmur is usually holosystolic but tapers in intensity in late systole and in extreme cases may terminate before A_2.[49] The reason for the decrescendo character of the murmur is the unusual hemodynamic situation resulting from regurgitation of a large volume of blood during systole into a small, previously normal left atrium. The impact of the regurgitant bolus on a relatively noncompliant atrium results in an extraordinarily high *v* wave in late systole. Thus ventricular and atrial pressures (Fig. 4–16)[50, 51] may equilibrate in late systole, with reduction of the regurgitant stream and suppression of the murmur. Despite its shortened duration, the murmur can be seen in a combined echophonocardiogram to be initiated at the time of mitral valve closure or well before the opening of the aortic valve, thus distinguishing it from a midsystolic murmur, which would

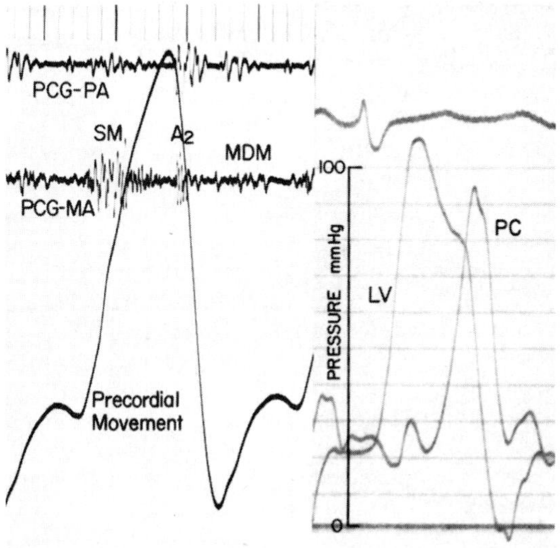

FIGURE 4–16. Acute mitral regurgitation in a young man with infective endocarditis. *Left*, Phonocardiogram at the cardiac apex (PCG-MA); an early systolic murmur (SM) begins with the onset of systole and terminates in mid- to late systole. *Right*, Pressure tracings from left ventricular (LV) and pulmonary capillary (PC) wedge positions. The high pressure (> 90 mm Hg) achieved in the left atrium in late systole results in equilibrium of pressures in LV and LA and termination of the systolic murmur. The unusual precordial movement pattern in the left-hand panel resembles the *v* wave in the PC wedge pressure and presumably reflects a forward thrust of the heart, resulting from massive left atrial expansion during systole. The mid-diastolic murmur (MDM) is a ventricular filling murmur or flow rumble.

also diminish in intensity in late systole but which would not start until after the aortic valve had opened. Other phonocardiographic signs include an S_3, as in the more usual types of mitral regurgitation. An S_4 may be recorded in acute mitral regurgitation[52] as well as its palpable counterpart, an *a* wave on the apexcardiogram. This is an important feature of the syndrome, which, like the unusual murmur just described, would not be expected in chronic mitral regurgitation. In the more severe cases, a precordial heave that peaks in late systole can be recorded (Fig. 4–16). Its graphic configuration is qualitatively similar to the *v* wave of the left atrial pressure pulse. It is thought to originate from the action of the whole heart being pushed against the chest wall, caused by sudden expansion during systole of the posteriorly located left atrium.[53]

TRICUSPID REGURGITATION DUE TO ISOLATED DISEASE OF THE VALVE (See also p. 1072). When tricuspid regurgitation occurs because of isolated disease of the valve itself rather than secondary to pulmonary hypertension, the phonocardiographic "silhouette" of the systolic murmur may be altered, so that it is decrescendo and terminates before the second heart sound. Isolated damage to the valve may occur from infective endocarditis or trauma. Under those circumstances, pressures in the right ventricle may be virtually normal. However, the high *v* wave generated in the right atrial pressure pulse by the regurgitant stream may lead to equalization of ventricular and atrial pressures in the latter part of systole, with diminution or suppression of the murmur. This occurs in a manner analogous to the alteration of the systolic murmur in acute mitral regurgitation, already described. Unfortunately, neither the timing nor the intensity of the murmur can be used to estimate the severity of the leak. Precordial movement in severe tricuspid regurgitation with normal right ventricular pressure may consist of an inward movement during systole and an expansion in diastole, reflecting massive volume changes in the underlying right ventricle.[54]

CONGENITAL HEART DISEASE WITH PULMONARY HYPERTENSION (see also Chaps. 30 and 31). Although the classic murmur of a ventricular septal defect is holosystolic, circumstances occur at both ends of the spectrum of severity of this condition that may drastically modify the physical signs and their graphic representation. The most minute of defects, consisting of a slit-like aperture through the muscular septum, may only momentarily provide a patent channel between the ventricles in early systole. Thus the murmur at the left sternal edge could terminate in midsystole. Physical examination is otherwise within normal limits, as are the electrocardiogram and chest roentgenogram. This type of minimal defect is likely to close spontaneously with the passage of time.

On the other hand, a very large defect results in free communication between the two ventricles, with equilibration of their peak systolic pressures at systemic levels. The direction of flow through the defect is determined by the relative resistance of the pulmonary and systemic vascular beds. Bidirectional shunting or predominantly right-to-left shunting may result (i.e., Eisenmenger complex). The systolic murmur becomes small in amplitude and is confined to early systole.[45] Accompanying signs of pulmonary hypertension include an ejection sound in the pulmonic area, a loud P_2, and, in severe cases, murmurs of regurgitation from the pulmonary and tricuspid valves.[47]

In similar fashion, other shunts, such as in patent ductus arteriosus and atrial septal defect, may be altered significantly both hemodynamically and in their physical manifestations by the presence of pulmonary hypertension of severe degree. The characteristic continuous murmur of patent ductus, which will be described in more detail below, becomes abbreviated when there is an elevation of pressure in the pulmonary arterial system to the effect that the aortic and pulmonary pressures become equal in diastole. The murmur remains loud throughout systole and continues through the second sound but terminates in early diastole.[55]

With even higher levels of pulmonary arterial pressure, shunting from right to left takes place through the ductus. Physical signs would then be indistinguishable from those of the Eisenmenger type of ventricular septal defect; namely, a brief early systolic murmur, a pulmonary ejection sound, a loud P_2, and frequently a prominent decrescendo diastolic murmur of pulmonary regurgitation.[56] A similar alteration in physical signs and their graphic registration occurs with atrial septal defect complicated by severe pulmonary hypertension and right-to-left shunting, although in this circumstance, splitting of S_2 is preserved to a greater extent than in the Eisenmenger type of ventricular septal defect or patent ductus.[57]

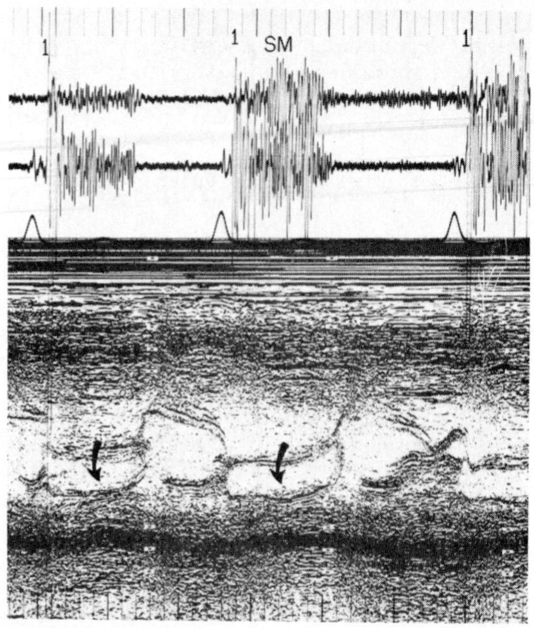

FIGURE 4–17. Mitral valve prolapse. Echophonocardiogram illustrating a holosystolic murmur associated with "hammock-shaped" prolapse of the valve of similar duration.

LATE SYSTOLIC MURMURS

MITRAL VALVE PROLAPSE (See also p. 1045). A wide spectrum of physical signs may be recorded in the mitral prolapse syndrome. In the milder cases a midsystolic click or clicks can be documented, with alterations in timing and intensity with various maneuvers. The click and late systolic murmur, the most characteristic features of the syndrome, can best be recorded at the cardiac apex. The click may coincide with prolapse of one or both cusps of the valve, as perceived in a simultaneous echocardiogram (see Figure 3–31, p. 59). The apexcardiogram in such cases may have an unusual configuration, with a notch at the time of the click and therefore a bifid configuration in systole. The murmur in most cases commences with the click and continues with increasing intensity to the second heart sound.[58] In some cases the murmur may be so intense as to be audible to the patient and others in the room. Under these circumstances the quality of the murmur is musical and is aptly described as a whoop or honk. Its high-intensity vibrations are of uniform frequency rather than the random frequencies which constitute most murmurs. Conversion of an ordinary late systolic murmur to a loud honk or whoop may occur transiently under the influence of changes of position.

In the presence of holosystolic prolapse (Fig. 4–17), the systolic murmur is also holosystolic and may achieve considerable intensity. A third heart sound and middiastolic flow rumble may be recorded as in mitral regurgitation of rheumatic origin; however, the first heart sound may be loud in contrast with its reduced intensity in pure mitral regurgitation of rheumatic origin.[59] Prolapse of the mitral valve is thought to occur because of a redundancy of valve tissue with respect to the ring in which it is located.[60] Thus, maneuvers which decrease ventricular volume result in an earlier and more pronounced prolapse of the mitral valve.[18]

Phonocardiography in combination with echocardiography can be used to document the effects of pharmacological agents and postural changes that alter preload, afterload, and left ventricular contractility. For example, the effect of amyl nitrite is to decrease left ventricular volume at the onset of systole, causing the click to occur earlier in systole as well as increasing the intensity and duration of the murmur. Similar effects may be noted with standing or the Valsalva maneuver (strain phase).[60] On the other hand, squatting or elevating the legs may cause the click to move later in systole and the murmur to become abbreviated and softer. A similar effect may be achieved with propranolol through the mechanism of increasing left ventricular volume.[60]

The diagnosis of mitral valve prolapse is relatively easy in the full-blown syndrome with characteristic auscultatory and echocardiographic findings. There are, however, borderline cases in which the manifestations are minimal or evanescent. In these cases, the echophonocardiographic technique emphasized in this chapter, specifically the parallel auscultatory and echocardiographic findings, combined with the pharmacological and physical maneuvers mentioned above, are extremely helpful.

DIASTOLIC MURMURS

VENTRICULAR FILLING MURMURS

These murmurs, which result from flow across the atrioventricular valves, are generally *middiastolic* in timing. Since they are dependent on flow across the mitral or tricuspid valve, they cannot begin until ventricular pressure has fallen below that in the atrium, and the atrioventricular valve has opened. Thus there is inevitably a slight delay between the second heart sound (closure of semilunar valves) and the initiation of ventricular filling murmurs.[61] The term *middiastolic* serves to differentiate those murmurs from the *early* diastolic murmurs of semilunar valve regurgitation. Actually, whether or not murmurs associated with ventricular filling do in fact occur in the first or middle third of diastole depends to a major extent on the heart rate. At slow heart rates, with long diastoles, a "middiastolic" ventricular filling murmur may actually have run its course during the first third of diastole. The low pitch, which accounts for the rumbling character of ventricular filling murmurs, is the result of the relatively low pressure gradient that exists across the atrioventricular valve. By intracardiac phonocardiography the location of maximal intensity of these murmurs can be determined as being in the recipient chamber, the ventricle.[62]

The common denominator in the generation of diastolic murmurs that result from flow across atrioventricular valves is a disproportion between the volume of flow and the size of the orifice between the donor and recipient chambers. This can occur from three types of anatomical and physiological derangements:

1. *Stenosis of atrioventricular valves.* In mitral stenosis, which provides the classic example of murmurs of this type, the passage from atrium to ventricle is narrowed as a consequence of rheumatic fever or, rarely, a congenital defect. Tricuspid stenosis, although rarely diagnosed, is the right-sided analog.
2. *Increased flow across the valve.* Mitral and tricuspid regurgitation and shunts that result in increased flow across the atrioventricular valves cause rumbling murmurs, owing to excessive flow across nonobstructing valves.
3. *Normal volume of flow across a normal valve that closes prematurely.* The Austin Flint murmur can be so classified, since it results from premature partial closure of the mitral valve in diastole, owing to the aortic leak that leads to rising left ventricular diastolic pressure. Thus there is a normal volume of atrioventricular flow through a valvular orifice of diminishing size.

These three categories of low-frequency diastolic murmurs will now be considered in further detail.

STENOSIS OF ATRIOVENTRICULAR VALVES

MITRAL STENOSIS (See also p. 1023). The murmur of mitral stenosis is dependent on turbulence resulting from flow across the narrowed mitral orifice. Therefore the duration and intensity of the murmur are affected by the severity of the obstruction and the volume of flow across the valve.[63] Thus in situations characterized by very low flow across the valve, the murmur may be of minimal intensity, despite severe valvular disease.[64] Conversely, the intensity and duration of the murmur may be increased by exercise or other maneuvers that augment diastolic flow.[65]

Echophonocardiography can graphically demonstrate the opening of the mitral valve in early diastole and the coincident opening snap.[66, 67] This event is followed by the diastolic murmur, which is often difficult to record away from its circumscribed zone of audibility. The patient should be tilted into a left lateral decubitus position, and the microphone should be placed at the point of the left ventricular apex impulse, as determined by palpation.[68] The early to middiastolic portion of the murmur occurs during the period of maximal ventricular filling. The duration of the murmur may be prolonged in the more severe cases, owing to persistence of a gradient across the mitral valve throughout a longer portion of diastole.[63]

Echophonocardiography has been very helpful in studies of the genesis of the presystolic crescendo phase of the diastolic murmur of mitral stenosis. This has traditionally been attributed to atrial systole.[69] In normal sinus rhythm, the characteristic crescendo murmur clearly follows the P wave of the ECG in a multichannel graphic record and is initiated by atrial systole. However, it has been pointed out that the crescendo murmur may be found in cases in which the rhythm is atrial fibrillation, and consequently there is no effective atrial systole.[70, 71] The suggestion has been made by Criley et al. that the final crescendo phase of the murmur is actually produced primarily by *ventricular* systole during the preisovolumetric phase of contraction.[72] Their studies based on phonocardiography and angiography indicate that the onset of the crescendo phase is at the time of the sharp closing movement of the valve apparatus by ventricular systole. Ventricular systole begins in the more severe cases while there is still antegrade flow across the valve orifice. Thus the rigid, scarred valve apparatus is thrust into the stream of blood that is still moving from atrium to ventricle, creating conditions for a high-velocity flow through a narrow orifice. The presystolic crescendo murmur terminates with a loud first heart sound as the valve apparatus reaches the full extent of its move toward the atrium and is checked. The theory advanced by Criley et al. to explain this crescendo murmur has been supported by echophonocardiographic studies relating valve movements and the generation of the murmur in atrial fibrillation (Fig. 4–18) as well as in normal sinus rhythm.[71–73]

The proposal of Criley and Matthews[74] that transmitral flow during the crescendo phase of the murmur has been challenged recently by Hada et al.[75] These investigators, using Doppler method combined with phonocardiography, found a falling velocity of flow consistent with the shrinking gradient across the valve with the onset of ventricular systole. A further complex feature of these kaleidoscopic hemodynamic-acoustic events is the observation of Smith et al.[3, 3a] that the transmission of mechanical vibrations through the heart is greatly enhanced by passage through a stiff, contracting ventricle. Thus the perception of the murmur at the chest surface will be expected to increase dramatically during the brief period of ventricular contraction prior to mitral valve closure, regardless of the actual intensity of the sound-producing turbulence at its intracardiac source.

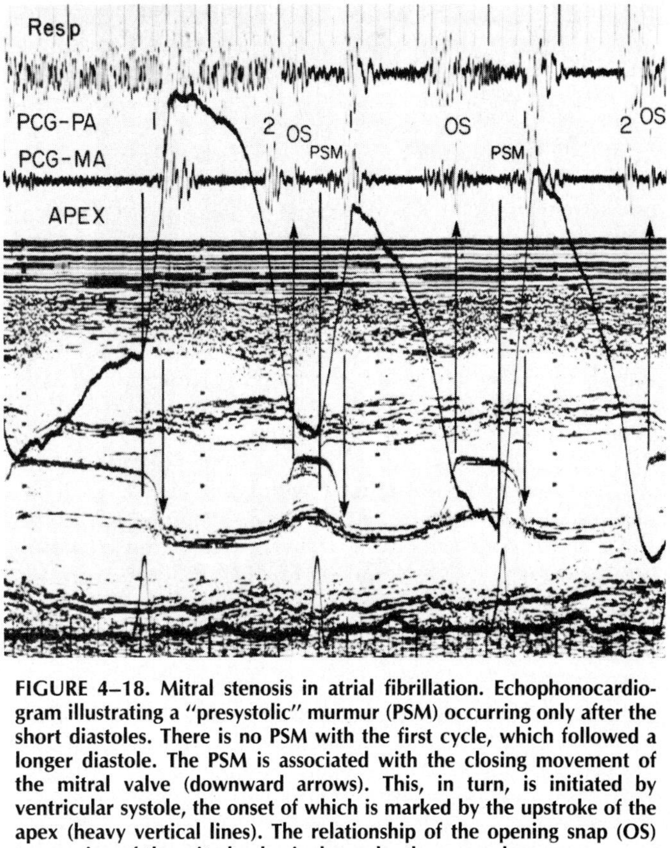

FIGURE 4–18. Mitral stenosis in atrial fibrillation. Echophonocardiogram illustrating a "presystolic" murmur (PSM) occurring only after the short diastoles. There is no PSM with the first cycle, which followed a longer diastole. The PSM is associated with the closing movement of the mitral valve (downward arrows). This, in turn, is initiated by ventricular systole, the onset of which is marked by the upstroke of the apex (heavy vertical lines). The relationship of the opening snap (OS) to opening of the mitral valve is shown by the upward arrows.

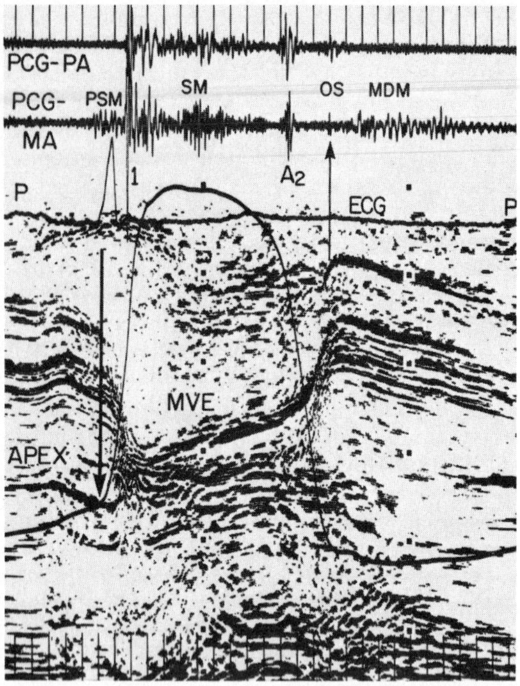

FIGURE 4–19. Mitral stenosis in a 49-year-old woman with a history of mitral commissurotomy 16 years previously with a good result. Sinus rhythm remains normal. An echophonocardiogram is combined with an apexcardiogram to show the relationship of the onset of LV systole to the presystolic crescendo murmur (PSM) (see text). The opening snap of the mitral valve (OS) occurs with full opening of the mitral valve (light arrow) and is followed by a middiastolic murmur (MDM). Mild accompanying aortic valve disease accounts for the crescendo-decrescendo systolic murmur transmitted to the mitral area (SM).

The importance of ventricular systole in precipitating the swift closing movement of the mitral valve and the acoustic events dependent on this event can be demonstrated using noninvasive methods by combining an apexcardiogram with echo- and phonocardiographic tracings. The upstroke of the apexcardiogram signals precisely the time of left ventricular pressure rise; this provides a useful marker for analysis of those events of the cardiac cycle that are responsible for the characteristic galaxy of physical signs found in mitral stenosis at the beginning of systole (Fig. 4–19).

TRICUSPID STENOSIS (See p. 1069). Tricuspid stenosis is a relatively rare condition occurring principally in association with far-advanced rheumatic heart disease with mitral stenosis. Therefore the phonocardiographic signs may be overshadowed by those of the accompanying valvular disease.[76] Since most patients in the later stages of rheumatic heart disease will be in atrial fibrillation, the murmur of tricuspid stenosis will be found in early to middiastole, when there is a maximal gradient across the valve and a high velocity flow.[77] In normal sinus rhythm, the murmur may be confined to presystole and can be attributed to flow across the obstructing valve resulting from right atrial systole.[76] Maximal intensity of the murmur is at the left lower sternal edge.

Since the graphic signs already described could easily be confused with those of mitral stenosis, it is necessary to observe and record the effects of respiration on the intensity of the murmur.[78] A dramatic increase in intensity of the murmur with inspiration is very helpful, since this occurs with tricuspid but not with mitral stenosis. Simultaneous registration of the jugular venous pulse usually demonstrates enormous *a* waves in patients in normal sinus rhythm,[78] owing to retrograde flow in the venous system while the right atrium is contracting against a stenotic valve.[79] The echocardiogram may disclose alterations in the movements of the tricuspid valve in diastole similar to those of mitral stenosis. However, this valve is considerably more difficult to record by echo than is the mitral.

LEFT ATRIAL MYXOMA (See p. 1473). Murmurs associated with left atrial myxoma simulate those of mitral valve disease, but both the character and the intensity of the murmurs may change profoundly on successive examinations or with alterations in position. The systolic murmur results from mitral regurgitation due to damage to the valve from trauma inflicted by the movable tumor mass[80] or from interference with apposition of the valve leaflets. A diastolic murmur is often present and is usually confined to late diastole or presystole. The pathogenesis of this murmur is probably analogous to that of the final crescendo phase of the presystolic murmur of mitral stenosis,[74] as can be demonstrated by combined echophonocardiographic observation (Fig. 4–20). Thus it can be shown that the "presystolic" crescendo actually occurs with the onset of ventricular systole at a time when the rising pressure in the ventricle is forcing the movable tumor back through the mitral orifice against the stream of blood that is still flowing from atrium to ventricle. The crescendo phase of the murmur culminates in the loud delayed first sound, related to the completed excursion of the tumor toward the atrium.[81]

Atrioventricular Flow Rumbling Murmurs

MITRAL REGURGITATION. Rapid flow across atrioventricular valves in early to middiastole often results in low-pitched rumbling murmurs simulating the physical sign of mitral stenosis. The most common example of this type of

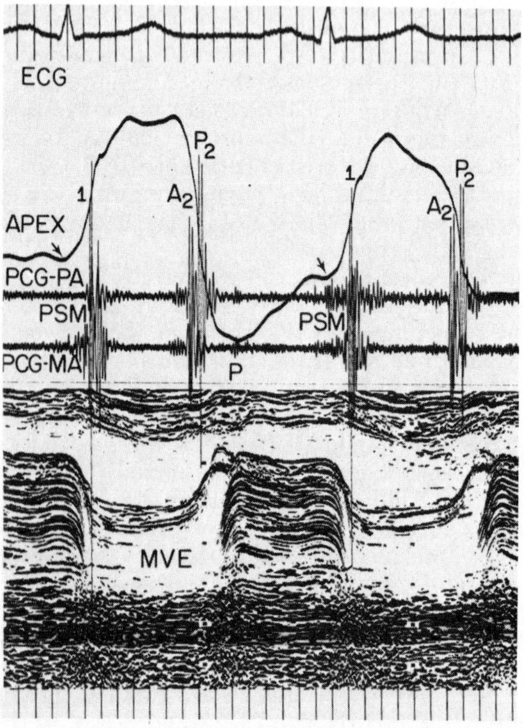

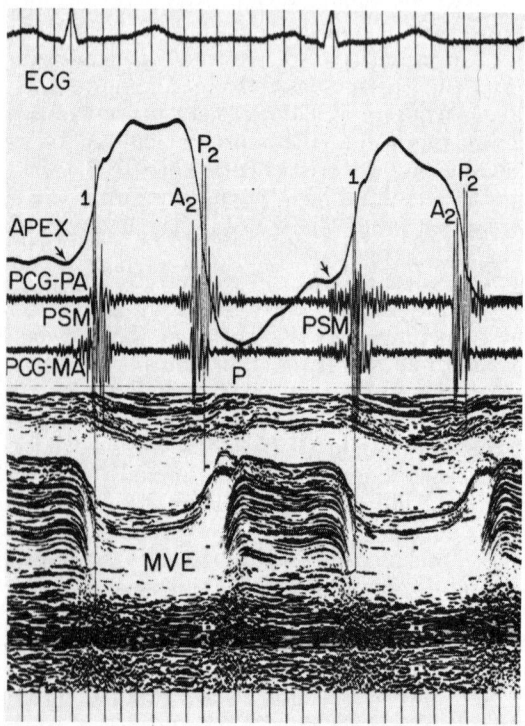

FIGURE 4–20. Left atrial myxoma. Echophonocardiogram illustrating the relationship between the presystolic murmur (PSM) and movement of the tumor mass through the mitral valve and into the atrium under the impact of ventricular systole. Timing of ventricular systole is provided by the apexcardiogram, the upstroke of which is indicated by an arrow.

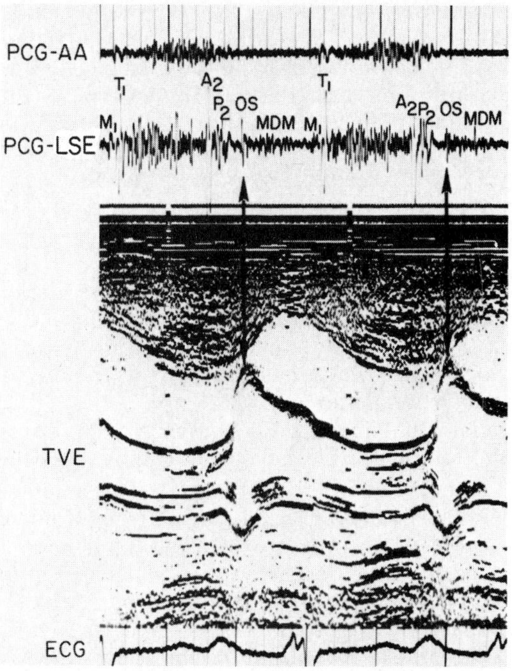

FIGURE 4–21. Middiastolic rumble in atrial septal defect. Echophonocardiogram demonstrating a middiastolic murmur (MDM) at the left sternal edge. The tricuspid valve is closing sharply during this phase of diastole while antegrade flow is occurring across it. Other phonocardiographic features of ASD include an accentuated T_1, an opening snap (OS) of tricuspid origin (arrow), and an ejection systolic murmur. The movements of the valve in systole are not well recorded.

murmur is in mitral regurgitation, in which an increased volume of blood is moving from atrium to ventricle during passive ventricular filling. It is interesting that the flow rumble does not occur when the mitral valve has first opened and is most widely open with presumably maximal flow.[82, 83] Rather it begins a few hundredths of a second later. Echophonocardiographic studies have clarified the relationship between valve motion and generation of the murmur.[73] These observations show that after opening widely in early diastole, the mitral valve makes a partial closing movement while presumably a high volume of blood is still moving antegrade across its closing orifice. This results, in effect, in a functional mitral stenosis, in which too large a volume of blood is moving across the valve for the dimensions of the aperture. A middiastolic pressure gradient may be demonstrated under these circumstances.[84, 85]

LEFT-TO-RIGHT SHUNTS. A similar pathogenetic mechanism probably occurs in left-to-right shunts, such as patent ductus arteriosus or ventricular septal defect, in which there is augmented flow across a normal mitral valve.[86] On the right side of the heart, diastolic flow rumbles occur with atrial septal defect or anomalous pulmonary venous drainage in a manner analogous to the left-sided murmurs noted above. In atrial septal defect, combined echophonocardiographic examination shows a closing movement of the tricuspid valve in early to middiastole at a time when a very large flow is taking place from atrium to ventricle (Fig. 4–21). The location of maximal intensity of the murmur by intracardiac phonocardiography is in the right ventricular inflow tract.[87]

AUSTIN FLINT MURMUR. The apical rumbling diastolic murmur occurring in pure aortic regurgitation (see p. 1060) was first described by the renowned American clinician Austin Flint.[88] He attributed the murmur to functional mitral stenosis resulting from impingement of the regurgitant stream on the anterior leaflet of the mitral valve. Although a number of alternative hypotheses to explain the genesis of the murmur have been advanced since Flint's time, modern studies combining echo- and phonocardiography support his original contention.[89] The mitral valve can be seen to effect a premature partial closing movement in early to middiastole and again following atrial systole while atrial contents are moving in an antegrade direction across the mitral orifice. Thus conditions exist for a functional type of mitral stenosis and the genesis of a murmur simulating organic obstruction. The murmur may be confined to late diastole (presystolic) in the milder cases, but in moderately severe aortic regurgitation there may be both middiastolic and late diastolic components, giving an hourglass configuration to the murmur on the phonocardiogram. The Flint murmur has been thought by some to be related to the vibrations of the anterior leaflet of the mitral valve, a characteristic echocardiographic feature of aortic regurgitation. These vibrations are the result, however, of the play on the leaflet of the regurgitating cascade of blood from the aortic root. The mitral valvular vibrations are therefore coincident in time with the early diastolic murmur of aortic regurgitation and *not* the Flint murmur, the timing of which is mid- and/or late diastolic.

In the most severe cases, such as in acute aortic regurgitation resulting from infective endocarditis, the Flint murmur may be confined to middiastole. This variant of the murmur is explained by the highly abnormal pressure relationships resulting from massive aortic regurgitation and generation of very high pressures in end diastole in

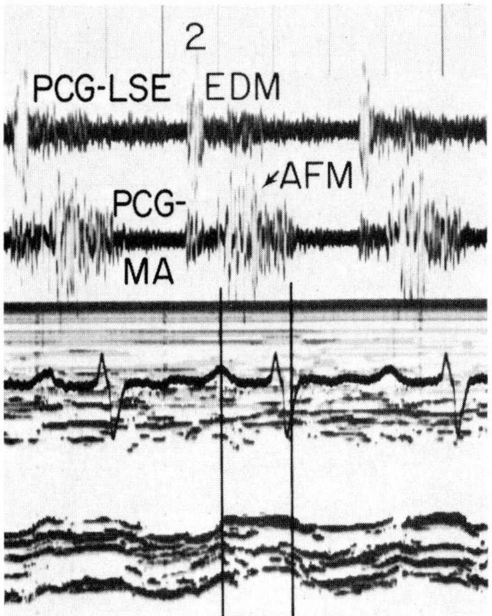

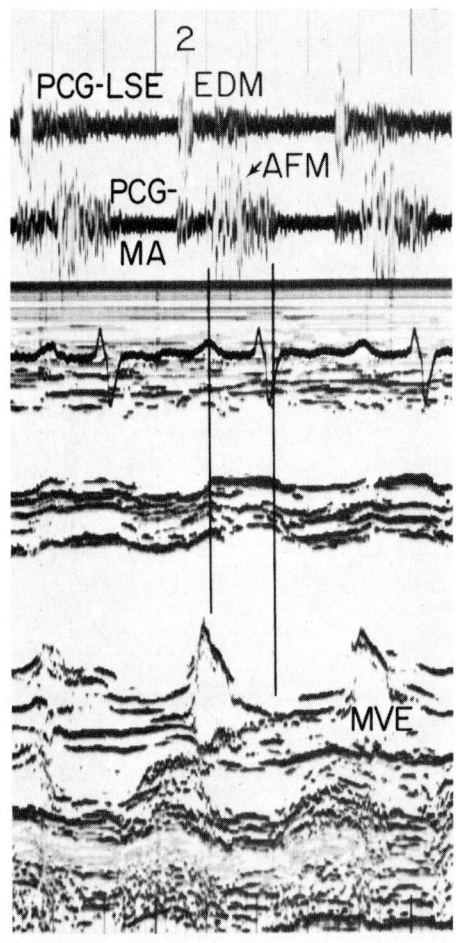

FIGURE 4–22. Austin Flint murmur in aortic regurgitation. An early diastolic murmur (EDM) is shown at top; in the lower phono channel, an Austin Flint murmur (AFM) is recorded at the cardiac apex (MA). It is associated with a rapid closing movement of the mitral valve, as seen in the echocardiogram (vertical arrows).

the left ventricle.[90, 91] Thus, when the left ventricular end-diastolic pressure exceeds the pressure in the left atrium, the mitral valve closes prematurely in diastole, preventing further antegrade movement of blood across the valve (Fig. 4–22). Under these circumstances the Flint murmur is seen to arise during the middiastolic closing phase of mitral valve movement (Fig. 4–22). Accompanying features of this hemodynamic situation, as revealed in noninvasive studies, are the absence of M_1 due to premature mitral valve closure[91, 92] and the disappearance of the *a* wave in the apexcardiogram, since antegrade flow can no longer take place in response to atrial systole.[93] In summary, the ventricular filling murmurs, such as those associated with atrioventricular valvular regurgitation or the Flint murmur as well as the presystolic murmur of mitral stenosis, can all be shown by means of echophonocardiography to arise from antegrade flow across an orifice of diminished or diminishing size.[74, 89]

SEMILUNAR VALVE REGURGITATION

AORTIC REGURGITATION (See p. 1060)

Chronic Aortic Regurgitation. The early diastolic murmur of aortic regurgitation is the prototype of this class of murmurs. It begins with the aortic component of the second heart sound and continues with decreasing intensity throughout most of diastole (Fig. 4–23).[94] Thus the murmur commences as the pressure within the left ventricle falls below that in the root of the aorta, allowing retrograde passage of blood across the incompetent valve, and it continues with lessening intensity as the volume and velocity of the regurgitant stream wane in the latter portion of diastole. By graphic techniques, the murmur of aortic regurgitation may be difficult to capture if it is faint because of its high frequency. Therefore phonocardiography is not useful as a means of determining the existence of a murmur that is doubtful on auscultation. The location of the murmur's maximal intensity should be determined by auscultation prior to application of the microphone for graphic registration. In *valvular* regurgitation, as with rheumatic heart disease, the location of maximal intensity is at the left sternal edge in the third or fourth interspace.[95] In aortic regurgitation associated with dilatation of the aortic root, the murmur may be maximal at the upper right sternal border.[95] In elderly or emphysematous individuals, one may have to record the murmur from unusual locations, since it may be perceptible only at the cardiac apex or in the subxiphoid area.

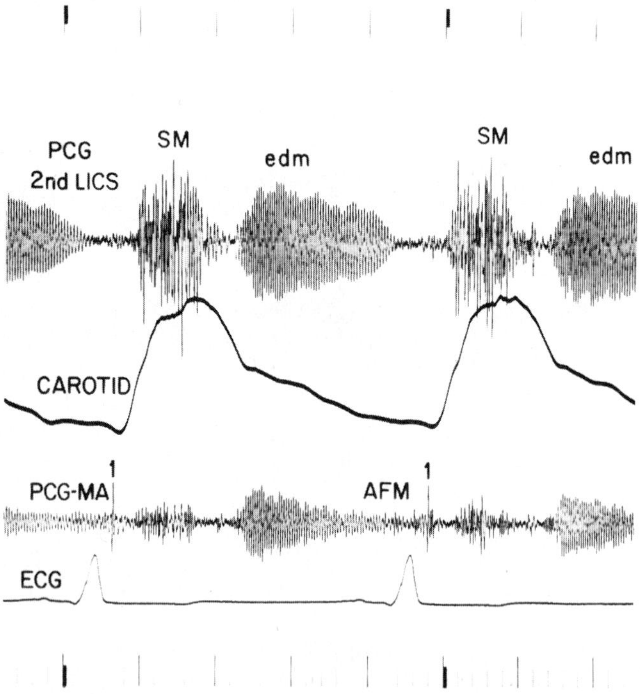

FIGURE 4–23. Aortic regurgitation. PCG at the second left intercostal space (2nd LICS) demonstrates a loud decrescendo diastolic murmur (edm) of unusual musical quality. There is a loud midsystolic murmur (SM) associated with the augmented stroke volume, although there was no stenosis of the aortic valve. At the cardiac apex (PCG-MA), the transmitted edm is seen, but in late diastole it merges with an Austin Flint murmur (AFM) of lower frequency. The incisural notch on the carotid tracing is poorly formed as a result of the valvular insufficiency.

Accompanying findings on noninvasive assessment include the alterations in the pulse contour noted on page 57. In the more severe cases, the pulse may assume a bifid (bisferiens) shape during systole, its high amplitude reflecting the wide pulse pressure. The incisural notch in the carotid tracing may disappear as the valve is unable to close and check the retrograde movement of blood at the onset of diastole (Fig. 4–23). The aortic component of S_2 is therefore diminished or absent.[96] The apexcardiogram verifies an increased amplitude representing hyperdynamic movements over the left ventricle associated with the increased stroke volume. The rapid filling wave is accentuated, and at the time of its peak, a third sound may be recorded as a result of the sudden massive filling of the left ventricle from two directions. Echocardiography supplies information regarding dilatation and hyperdynamic movements of the left ventricle, size of the aortic root, and vibrations of the anterior leaflet of the mitral valve. The Doppler technique has proved valuable in detecting the presence of aortic regurgitation and in estimating its severity[97, 98] (p. 109). However, the extreme sensitivity of the method may result in detection of aortic regurgitation of minor clinical significance. Therefore, despite the sophistication of these methods it is worth emphasizing that the stethoscope remains the best tool for detecting aortic regurgitation.

Acute Aortic Regurgitation (See p. 1063). In acute aortic regurgitation—an important syndrome that occurs with infective endocarditis, trauma, or aortic dissection—striking alterations in the graphic manifestations are found. In this situation the burden of massive regurgitation of sudden onset is placed on a ventricle that has not previously become dilated, as would be the case in the more common chronic form of aortic regurgitation. This results in dramatic elevations of left ventricular pressure in mid- to late diastole, so that left atrial pressure is exceeded, and the mitral valve is closed prematurely in diastole. Equilibration of pressure in the left ventricle and aortic root occurs in mid- to late diastole in this situation,[99] and this results in sudden cessation of the regurgitant flow across the aortic valve and therefore truncation of the murmur in middiastole.[91]

Other accompanying features of this syndrome have been described already and include the confinement of the Austin Flint murmur to middiastole, absence of the mitral component of S_1, and disappearance of the *a* wave in the apexcardiogram as a result of the inability of atrial systole to move blood into the left ventricle owing to the reversal of the atrioventricular pressure gradient.

PULMONIC REGURGITATION.

The murmur associated with regurgitation across the pulmonic valve occurs in two classes of physiological disturbances:[100]

1. When pulmonary hypertension results in dilatation

of both the main pulmonary artery and the valve ring. As a result, the valve cusps become incapable of closing competently, and a regurgitant murmur ensues, known as the Graham Steell murmur.[47, 101]

2. When the pressure in the pulmonary circuit is normal, but the valve is incompetent owing to a congenital malformation or surgical procedure.

These two pathogenetic mechanisms are manifested in different ways, as follows.

Pulmonary Hypertension (Graham Steell Murmur). The murmur associated with pulmonary hypertension (Graham Steell) is similar to that of aortic regurgitation, being high-pitched and decrescendo (Figs. 4–15 and 4–24), and follows the pulmonic component of S_2 in graphic records. It is unusual, however, to find a degree of separation of A_2P_2 that will allow one to ascribe with confidence a decrescendo, high-pitched murmur recorded at the upper left sternal edge to an aortic or pulmonic source on the basis of its inception with one or the other of the S_2 components. Rather, one must use the balance of clinical evidence and Doppler method data (p. 87) to make this differential assessment.[102] The same problems in recording a high-pitched murmur exist with pulmonic as with aortic regurgitation, since most modern commercial phonocardiographic equipment is not particularly sensitive in the upper frequency range. Accompanying graphic signs often include an ejection sound of pulmonic origin, recordable in the second left intercostal space, and an accentuated P_2. The movements of the bulging pulmonary artery can often be recorded in the same location by application of the transducer used for apexcardiography over the palpable pulsation which precedes the vibrations of P_2.[103, 104] Lower

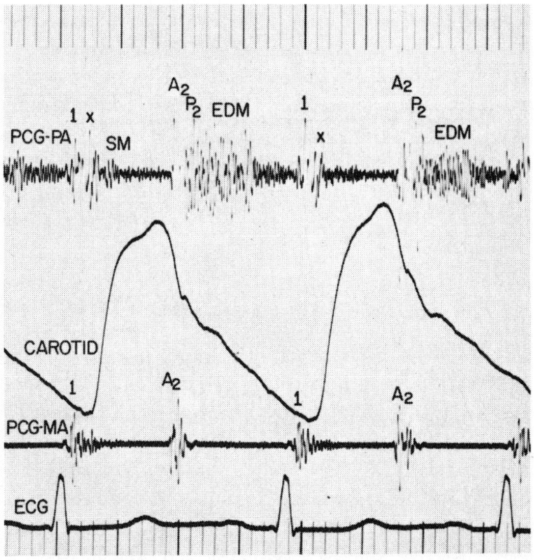

FIGURE 4–24. Patent ductus arteriosus, pulmonary hypertension, and pulmonary regurgitation in a 24-year-old woman known to have systemic pressure (140/70) in the pulmonary artery, with a bidirectional shunt. Phonocardiogram shows an ejection sound (X) in early systole and in the pulmonary area as well as a loud early diastolic murmur (EDM) of pulmonary regurgitation, which can be seen to follow immediately after P_2.

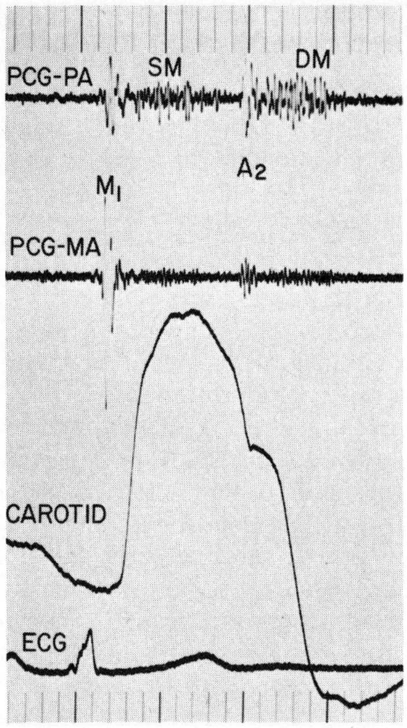

FIGURE 4–25. Pulmonary regurgitation due to organic valvular disease. Pulmonic valve stenosis had been relieved surgically, leaving a slight residual systolic murmur (SM) and a prominent early to middiastolic murmur of low frequency (DM). These murmurs are best seen in the second left interspace (PA).

along the left sternal edge, the heave of right ventricular hypertrophy can frequently be palpated and recorded, and there may be an associated *a* wave of right ventricular origin.[105] The venous pulse reflects the altered compliance of the right ventricle with exaggeration of the *a* wave. The echocardiogram, ideally performed in conjunction with the other graphic methods described, can provide an estimate of right ventricular size and can confirm the presence of a pulmonic ejection sound by showing its coincidence with full opening of the pulmonic valve.[104, 106] Doppler studies have been found useful in predicting the severity of pulmonary hypertension.[107]

Pulmonic Regurgitation with Normal Pulmonary Arterial Pressures (See p. 1075). The murmur of pulmonic regurgitation of valvular origin when pulmonary arterial pressure is normal differs from the Graham Steell murmur in that it is lower in pitch and located slightly later in diastole, so that its timing may be properly designated as middiastolic. These differences reflect the later onset and reduced velocity of retrograde flow when pressure in the pulmonary artery is not high. Regurgitation begins after the pressure in the right ventricle has fallen below that in the pulmonary artery and a significant regurgitant movement of blood exists. The murmur therefore begins a perceptible distance after P_2, builds in intensity, and then fades away in mid- to late diastole (Fig. 4–25). It forms a crescendo-decrescendo silhouette made up of low-frequency vibrations, in contrast to the high-frequency, pennant-shaped graphic representation of the Graham Steell murmur, which follows immediately after P_2.

CONTINUOUS MURMURS[108]

DEFINITION. Continuous murmurs may be defined as murmurs that begin in systole and persist without interruption through the second heart sound into diastole. They frequently terminate in the latter part of diastole and do not therefore necessarily continue throughout the cardiac cycle (Fig. 4–26). Graphic records may be useful in establishing the timing and duration of continuous murmurs, but the findings usually lack specificity.

CLASSIFICATION. Continuous murmurs generally result from four classes of hemodynamic conditions: (1) connections between the aorta and the pulmonary artery or its branches, (2) arteriovenous fistulas, (3) altered flow in arteries, and (4) altered flow in veins.

AORTOPULMONARY CONNECTIONS

PATENT DUCTUS ARTERIOSUS (See pp. 923 and 993). Patent ductus arteriosus is the most common example of this group of conditions.[109] Here, as in all fistulas, the magnitude, velocity, and duration of the abnormal flow and the resulting murmur are determined by the pressure relationships between the high-pressure aorta, which is the donor vessel, and the pulmonary artery or its branch, which is the recipient vessel. The murmur begins in systole when pressure in the aorta greatly exceeds that in the pulmonary artery and continues into diastole because of the persistence of a pressure gradient favoring the shunt. The peculiar quality and timing of the ductus murmur have been vividly described by Neill and Mounsey.[109]

". . .two opposing streams crash head-on within the pulmonary artery, one surging from the right ventricle upwards and backwards along its course, and the other, a narrower powerful jet, projected by the high aortic pressure through the ductus into the pulmonary artery, where it meets the on-coming stream from the right ventricle. Since the pulmonary orifice is larger than that of the ductus and since a different course is taken by the two streams, the greater flow into the pulmonary artery in early systole is from the right ventricle. Later as ventricular systole nears completion, the greater flow is from the ductus, and one may imagine turbulent eddies forming at the Waters meet of the main pulmonary artery until finally in diastole the flow is from the ductus alone. The typical patent ductus arteriosus murmur mirrors these events, since it continues and increases at end systole and beginning of diastole, and it is often punctuated by reverberations from beat to beat as eddies swirl within the pulmonary artery."

In graphic records, the ductus murmur is usually best recorded at the upper left sternal border (Fig. 4–26). It is best to use two phonocardiographic microphones simultaneously, with the second one located at the cardiac apex.[4]

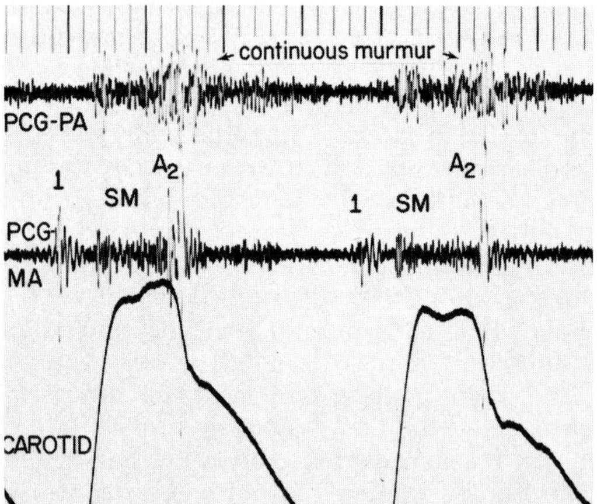

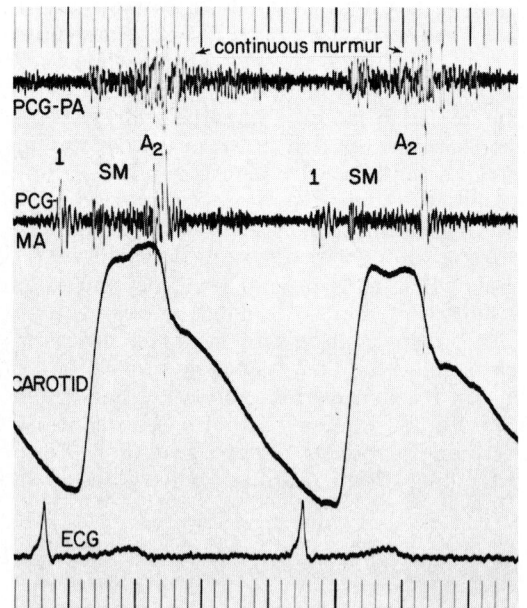

FIGURE 4–26. Patent ductus arteriosus. Phonocardiogram in the second left interspace (PA) demonstrates a prominent continuous murmur that is maximal at the time of S_2, obscuring the details of the latter. A_2 is well transmitted, however, to the cardiac apex (MA) and can be further identified by its position immediately before the incisural notch in the carotid tracing.

The details of the second heart sound are usually obscured at the upper left sternal border, since the intensity of the murmur is maximal at the time of S_2. Since A_2 is usually widely transmitted, however, the second microphone can be used to appreciate A_2 in a location such as the cardiac apex, sufficiently removed from the main focus of intensity of the murmur. At the cardiac apex additional signs may be recorded that are of significance in estimating the volume of the shunt. These are S_3 and a middiastolic rumble.[86] The third sound is less helpful, since it is a normal finding in a child, but a middiastolic flow rumble indicates a substantially increased flow across the mitral valve and therefore a truly significant shunt. An additional noninvasive manifestation is echocardiographic evidence of dilatation of the left-sided heart chambers where the shunt is of large dimensions.

In patent ductus with high pulmonary vascular resistance, there is equilibration of pressures in diastole, which results in abbreviation and finally elimination of the diastolic phase of the murmur.[55] In more severe cases the systolic portion of the murmur may be confined to early systole. The murmur then ceases to be the major graphic manifestation of the abnormality and is replaced by the stigmata of pulmonary hypertension, as described on p. 79, in some cases including a loud murmur of pulmonary regurgitation (Fig. 4–24).[47, 56]

An aortopulmonary window is associated with hemodynamic alterations similar to those of a patent ductus. Owing to the large size of the aperture between the great vessels, there is usually a significant degree of pulmonary hypertension, so that the murmur and other graphic findings are modified as in the case of patent ductus complicated by elevated pulmonary arterial pressure.

SYSTEMIC-PULMONARY SHUNTS CREATED SURGICALLY. Operations designed to create fistulas between the aorta and the pulmonary artery or its branches (e.g., Blalock, Potts) result in murmurs resembling those of patent ductus arteriosus (PDA). The site of maximal intensity depends on the location of the shunt in the chest. Accompanying signs of increased flow (middiastolic rumble) or pulmonary hypertension, when the size of the communication has been larger than optimal, are identical with those of PDA.

ARTERIOVENOUS CONNECTIONS

Shunts of this type may be congenital or acquired. Examples include congenital or traumatically acquired arteriovenous fistulas and the shunts created surgically for purposes of hemodialysis. An example of a congenital connection of this type is a *coronary arteriovenous fistula*[109, 110] (p. 927). This anomaly consists of a tortuous, elongated arterial communication that drains, in most instances, into the right atrium, coronary sinus, or right ventricle. The physician's attention is attracted to the possibility of a coronary arteriovenous fistula by the discovery of a continuous murmur resembling that of a patent ductus arteriosus. The location of the murmur, however, is usually lower over the precordium than in patent ductus, with the exact location to the right or left of the sternum being determined by the identity of the recipient chamber—right atrium or ventricle.

Traumatic fistulas may occur anywhere and must be discovered by searching with the stethoscope, especially in the region of scars from knife or bullet wounds.[111] Graphic records can serve to document the presence of such a murmur but seldom are of critical importance in making the diagnosis. The physiological consequences of the increase in systemic blood flow over a long period, however, may be manifested in echocardiograms showing dilatation and hyperdynamic movements of the left heart chambers.

Altered Flow in Arteries

When blood flow in major arteries, whether systemic or pulmonary, is altered by a significant constriction, a murmur may be generated. This is generally systolic in time, either exclusively or predominantly. However, when constriction has severely altered the pattern of blood flow, a continuous murmur may be produced. A systolic pressure gradient across the constricted segment is a prerequisite for the genesis of this type of continuous murmur.[112] In coarctation of the aorta, for instance, it has been shown that a very severe constriction (less than 2.5 mm in internal diameter) is required to produce the hemodynamic situation conducive to continuity of the murmur.[113] Lesser degrees of constriction result in a murmur confined to systole. An analogous situation may exist in the pulmonary arterial system with pulmonary branch stenosis[114, 115] or occasionally with incomplete arterial occlusion by pulmonary embolism.[116]

Altered Flow in Veins

The most common continuous murmur is the venous hum. Its loudness and location (usually over the great veins at the lower part of the neck)[117] occasionally are confused with those of a patent ductus arteriosus. The venous hum, however, is truly a continuous murmur, existing through the cardiac cycle. Its intensity may increase in diastole. Graphic records can be used to demonstrate its presence, its cyclical silhouette, and, more importantly, its obliteration with recumbency or pressure over the great vein from which it originates. Such documentation should not be necessary for the diagnosis of this ubiquitous and innocent physical sign.

REFERENCES

1. Hinze, J. O.: Turbulence. 2nd ed. New York, McGraw-Hill Book Co., 1975, pp. 1–4 and 534–535.
2. Rushmer, R. F., and Morgan, C.: Meaning of murmurs. Am. J. Cardiol. *21*: 722, 1968.
3. Smith, D., Ishimitsu, T., and Craige, E.: Mechanical vibration transmission characteristics of the left ventricle: Implications with regard to auscultation and phonocardiography. J. Am. Coll. Cardiol. *4*:517, 1984.

SYSTOLIC MURMURS

3a. Smith D., Ishimitsu, T., Craige, E.: Abnormal diastolic mechanical vibration transmission characteristics of the left ventricle. J. Cardiography *15*:507, 1985.
4. Leatham, A.: Auscultation of the Heart and Phonocardiography. 2nd ed. New York, Churchill Livingstone, 1975.
5. Reddy, P. S., Shaver, J. A., and Leonard, J. J.: Cardiac systolic murmurs: Pathophysiology and differential diagnosis. Prog. Cardiovasc. Dis. *14*:1, 1971.
6. Castle, R. F.: Clinical recognition of innocent cardiac murmurs in children. J.A.M.A. *177*:1, 1961.
7. Perloff, J. K.: Clinical recognition of aortic stenosis; the physical signs and differential diagnosis of the various forms of obstruction to the left ventricular outflow. Prog. Cardiovasc. Dis. *10*:323, 1968.
8. Paley, H. W.: Left ventricular outflow tract obstruction. *In* Leon, D. F., and Shaver, J. A. (eds.): Physiologic Principles of Heart Sounds and Murmurs. New York, American Heart Association Monograph, No. 46, 1975, p. 107.
9. Stein, P. D., and Sabbah, H. N.: Origin of the second heart sound: clinical relevance of new observations. Am. J. Cardiol. *41*:108, 1978.
10. Bonner, A. J., Sacks, H. N., and Tavel, M. E.: Assessing the severity of aortic stenosis by phonocardiography and external pulse recordings. Circulation *48*: 247, 1973
11. Goldblatt, A., Aygen, M. M., and Braunwald, E.: Hemodynamic-phonocardiographic correlations of the fourth heart sound in aortic stenosis. Circulation *26*: 92, 1962.
12. Gibson, T. C., Madry, R., Grossman, W., McLaurin, L. P., and Craige, E.: The A wave of the apexcardiogram and left ventricular diastolic stiffness. Circulation *49*:441, 1974.
13. Skajaerpe, T., Hegrenaes, L., and Hatle, L.: Noninvasive estimation of valve area in patients with aortic stenosis by Doppler ultrasound and two-dimensional echocardiography. Circulation *72*:810, 1985.
14. Currie, P. J., Hagler, D. J., Seward, J. B., Reeder, G. S., Fyfe, D. A., Bove, A. A., and Tajik, A. J.: Instantaneous pressure gradient: A simultaneous Doppler and dual catheter correlative study. J. Am. Coll. Cardiol. *7*:800, 1986.
15. Hancock, E. W.: Differentiation of valvar, subvalvar and supravalvar aortic stenosis. Guy's Hosp. Rep. *110*:1, 1961.
16. Davis, R. A., Feigenbaum, H., Chang, S., Konecke, L. L., and Dillon, J. C.: Echocardiographic manifestations of discrete subaortic stenosis. Am. J. Cardiol. *33*:277, 1974.
17. Vogel, J. H. K., and Blount, S. G., Jr.: Clinical evaluation in localizing level of obstruction to outflow from left ventricle. Importance of early systolic ejection click. Am. J. Cardiol. *15*:782, 1965.
18. O'Rourke, R. A., and Crawford, M. H.: Mitral valve regurgitation. Curr. Probl. Cardiol. *9*:1, 1984.
19. Burch, G. E., and Phillips, J. H.: Murmurs of aortic stenosis and mitral insufficiency masquerading as one another. Am. Heart J. *66*:439, 1963.
20. Roberts, W. C., Perloff, J. K., and Costantino, T.: Severe valvular aortic stenosis in patients over 65 years of age. Am. J. Cardiol. *27*:497, 1971.
21. Lewis, R. P., Rittgers, S. E., Forester, W. F., and Boudoulas, H.: A critical review of the systolic time intervals. Circulation *56*:146, 1977.
22. Shah, P. M., Gramiak, R., and Kramer, D. H.: Ultrasound localization of left ventricular outflow tract obstruction in hypertrophic obstructive cardiomyopathy. Circulation *40*:3, 1969.
23. Popp, R. L., and Harrison, D. C.: Ultrasound in the diagnosis and evaluation of therapy of idiopathic hypertrophic subaortic stenosis. Circulation *40*:905, 1969.
24. Sabbah, H. N., Marzilli, M., and Stein, P. D.: Intracardiac phonocardiography in experimental left ventricular cavity obstruction: Potential clinical applicability for the distinction of obliterating left ventricle from hypertrophic obstructive cardiomyopathy. Am. Heart J. *100*:77, 1980.
25. Come, P. C., Bulkley, B. H., Goodman, Z. D., Hutchins, G. M., Pitt, B., and Fortuin, N. J.: Hypercontractile cardiac states simulating hypertrophic cardiomyopathy. Circulation *55*:901, 1977.
26. Chahine, R. A., Raizner, A. E., Nelson, J., Winters, W. L., Miller, R. R., and Luchi, R. J.: Mid-systolic closure of the aortic valve in hypertrophic cardiomyopathy. Am. J. Cardiol. *43*:17, 1979.
27. Leatham, A., and Weitzman, D.: Auscultatory and phonocardiographic signs of pulmonary stenosis. Br. Heart J. *19*:303, 1957.
28. Hultgren, H. N., Reeve, R., Cohn, K., and McLeod, R.: The ejection click of valvular pulmonic stenosis. Circulation *40*:631, 1969.
29. Schmidt, R. E., and Craige, E.: Precordial movements over the right ventricle in children with pulmonary stenosis. Circulation *32*:241, 1965.
30. Vogelpoel, L., and Schrire, V.: Auscultatory and phonocardiographic assessment of pulmonary stenosis with intact ventricular septum. Circulation *22*:55, 1960.
31. Mills, P., Wolfe, C., Redwood, D., Leech, G., Craige, E., and Leatham, A.: Non-invasive diagnosis of subpulmonary outflow tract obstruction. Br. Heart J. *43*:276, 1980.
32. Vogelpoel, L., and Schrire, V.: Auscultatory and phonocardiographic assessment of Fallot's tetralogy. Circulation *22*:73, 1960.
33. Brigden, W., and Leatham, A.: Mitral incompetence. Br. Heart J. *15*:55, 1953.
34. Perloff, J. K., and Harvey, W. P.: Auscultatory and phonocardiographic manifestations of pure mitral regurgitation. Prog. Cardiovasc. Dis. *5*:172, 1962.
35. Nixon, P. G. F.: The third heart sound in mitral regurgitation. Br. Heart J. *23*: 677, 1961.
36. Corya, B. C., Feigenbaum, H., Rasmussen, S., and Black, M. J.: Echocardiographic features of congestive cardiomyopathy compared with normal subjects and patients with coronary artery disease. Circulation *49*:1153, 1974.
37. Wooley, C. F.: The spectrum of tricuspid regurgitation. *In* Leon, D. F., and Shaver, J. A. (eds.): Physiologic Principles of Heart Sounds and Murmurs. New York, American Heart Association Monograph, No. 46, 1975, p. 139.
38. Muller, O., and Shillingford, J.: Tricuspid incompetence. Br. Heart J. *16*:195, 1954.
39. Sepulveda, G., and Lukas, D. S.: The diagnosis of the tricuspid insufficiency—clinical features in 60 cases with associated mitral valve disease. Circulation *11*: 552, 1955.
40. Rivero-Carvallo, J. M.: Signo para el diagnóstico de las insufficiencias tricupídias. Arch. Inst. Cardiol. Méx. *16*:531, 1946.
41. Leon, D. F., Leonard, J. J., Lancaster, J. F., Kroetz, F. W., and Shaver, J. A.: Effect of respiration and pansystolic regurgitant murmurs as studied by biatrial intracardiac phonocardiography. Am. J. Med. *39*:429, 1965.
42. Mounsey, J. P. D.: Inspection and palpation of the cardiac impulse. Prog. Cardiovasc. Dis. *10*:187, 1967.
43. Rios, J. C., Massumi, R. A., Breesmen, W. T., and Sarin, R. K.: Auscultatory features of acute tricuspid regurgitation. Am. J. Cardiol. *23*:4, 1969.
44. Roger, H.: Recherches cliniques sur la communication congenitale des deux coeurs par inocclusion du septum interventriculaire. Bull. Acad. Méd. (Paris) *8*: 1074 and 1189, 1879.
45. Craige, E.: Phonocardiography in interventricular septal defects. Am. Heart J. *60*:51, 1960.
46. Leatham, A., and Segal, B. L.: Auscultatory and phonocardiographic findings in ventricular septal defect with left-to-right shunt. Circulation *25*:318, 1962.
47. Perloff, J. K.: Auscultatory and phonocardiographic manifestations of pulmonary hypertension. Prog. Cardiovasc. Dis. *9*:303, 1967.
48. Green, E. W., Arguss, N. S., and Adolph, R. J.: Right-sided Austin Flint murmur. Documentation by intracardiac phonocardiography, echocardiography and postmortem findings. Am. J. Cardiol. *32*:370, 1973.

49. Sanders, C. A., Scannell, J. G., Harthorne, J. W., and Austen, W. G.: Severe mitral regurgitation secondary to ruptured chordae tendineae. Circulation *31*: 506, 1965.
50. Raftery, E. B., Oakley, C. M., and Goodwin, J. F.: Acute subvalvar mitral incompetence. Lancet *2*:360, 1966.
51. Sutton, G. C., and Craige, E.: Clinical signs of acute severe mitral regurgitation. Am. J. Cardiol. *20*:141, 1967.
52. Cohen, L. S., Mason, D. T., and Braunwald, E.: Significance of an atrial gallop sound in mitral regurgitation: Clue to diagnosis of ruptured chordae tendineae. Circulation *35*:112, 1967.
53. Basta, L. L., Wolfson, P., Swain, L., Eckbert, D. L., and Abboud, F. M.: The value of left parasternal impulse recordings in the assessment of mitral regurgitation. Circulation *48*:1055, 1973.
54. Boicourt, O. W., Nagle, R. E., and Mounsey, J. P. D.: The clinical significance of systolic retraction of the apex impulse. Br. Heart J. *27*:379, 1965.
55. Myers, G. S., Scannell, J. G., Wyman, J. M., Dimond, E. G., and Hurst, J. W.: Atypical patent ductus arteriosus with absence of the usual aortic pressure gradient and the characteristic murmur. Am. Heart J. *41*:819, 1951.
56. Fishleder, B. L., Serra, C., Prati, P. L., and Friedland, C.: La persistencia del conducto arterial con hipertension pulmonar: Vareidad "diastolica ruda." Arch. Inst. Cardiol. Méx. *32*:610, 1962.
57. Sutton, G. C., Harris, A., and Leatham, A.: Second heart sound in pulmonary hypertension. Br. Heart J. *30*:743, 1968.
58. Barlow, J. B., Bosman, C. K., Pocock, W. A., and Marchand, P.: Late systolic murmur and non-ejection ('mid-late') systolic clicks. Br. Heart J. *30*:203, 1968.
59. Tei, C., Shah, P. M., Cherian, G., Wong, M., and Ormiston, J. A.: The correlates of an abnormal first heart sound in mitral valve prolapse syndromes. N. Engl. J. Med. *307*:334, 1982.
60. Fontana, M. E., Kissel, G. L., and Criley, J. M.: Functional anatomy of mitral valve prolapse. *In* Leon, D. F., and Shaver, J. A. (eds.): Physiologic Principles of Heart Sounds and Murmurs. American Heart Association Monograph, No. 46, 1975, p. 126.

DIASTOLIC MURMURS

61. Nixon, P. G. F., and Wooler, G. H.: Left ventricular filling pressure gradient in mitral incompetence. Br. Heart J. *25*:382, 1963.
62. Esper, R. J., and Madoery, R. J.: Progresos en Auscultació n y Fonomecanocardiografía. Buenos Aires, López Libreros, 1974, p. 301.
63. Wood, P.: An appreciation of mitral stenosis. Br. Med. J. *1*:1051 and 1113, 1954.
64. Ueda, H., Sakamoto, T., Kawai, N., Watanabe, H., Uozumi, Z., Okada, R., Kobayashi, T., and Kaito, G.: "Silent" mitral stenosis. Pathoanatomical basis of the absence of diastolic rumble. Jpn. Heart J. *6*:206, 1965.
65. Ota, S.: Quantitative studies on the apical diastolic murmur in the mitral stenosis. Jpn. Circ. J. *25*:410, 1961.
66. Joyner, C. R., Jr., and Dear, W. E.: The motion of the normal and abnormal mitral valve. A study of the opening snap. J. Clin. Invest. *45*:1029, 1966.
67. Craige, E.: Echocardiography in studies of the genesis of heart sounds and murmurs. *In* Yu, P. N., and Goodwin, J. F. (eds.): Progress in Cardiology. Philadelphia, Lea and Febiger, 1975.
68. Levine, S. A., and Harvey, W. P.: Clinical Auscultation of the Heart. Philadelphia, W. B. Saunders Company, 1959, p. 255.
69. Gairdner, W. T.: Further remarks on auricular systolic murmur. Med. Times Gaz. *2*:460, 1864.
70. Constant, J.: Bedside Cardiology. Boston, Little, Brown and Co., 1976, p. 346.
71. Criley, J. M., and Hermer, A. J.: Crescendo presystolic murmur of mitral stenosis with atrial fibrillation. N. Engl. J. Med. *285*:1284, 1971.
72. Criley, J. M., Feldman, J. M., and Meredith, T.: Mitral valve closure and the crescendo presystolic murmur. Am. J. Med. *51*:456, 1971.
73. Fortuin, N. J., and Craige, E.: Echocardiographic studies of genesis of mitral diastolic murmurs. Br. Heart J. *35*:75, 1973.
74. Criley, J. M., and Matthews, R. W.: The presystolic murmur of mitral stenosis. Letter to the editor. J. Am. Coll. Cardiol. (*In press*.)
75. Hada, Y., Amano, K., Yamaguchi, I., Takenaka, K., Takahashi, H., Takikawa, R., Hasegawa, I., Takahashi, T., Sakamoto, T., Suzuki, J., and Sugimoto, T.: Noninvasive study of the presystolic component of the first heart sound in mitral stenosis. J. Am. Coll. Cardiol. *7*:43, 1986.
76. Bousvaros, G. A., and Stubington, D.: Some auscultatory and phonocardiographic features of tricuspid stenosis. Circulation *29*:26, 1964.
77. Sanders, C. A., Hawthorne, J. W., DeSanctis, R. W., and Austen, W. G.: Tricuspid stenosis: A difficult diagnosis in the presence of atrial fibrillation. Circulation *33*:26, 1966.
78. Perloff, J. K., and Harvey, W. P.: Clinical recognition of tricuspid stenosis. Circulation *22*:346, 1960.
79. Sivaciyan, V., and Ranganathan, R.: Transcutaneous Doppler jugular venous flow velocity recording: Clinical and hemodynamic correlates. Circulation *57*: 930, 1978.
80. Nasser, W. K., Davis, R. H., Dillon, J. C., Tavel, M. E., Helmen, C. H., Feigenbaum, H., and Fisch, C.: Atrial myxoma. I. Clinical and pathologic features in nine cases. Am. Heart J. *83*:694, 1972.
81. Pitt, A., Pitt, B., Schaefer, J., and Criley, J. M.: Myxoma of the left atrium: Hemodynamic and phonocardiographic consequences of sudden tumor movement. Circulation *36*:408, 1967.
82. Nixon, P. G. F.: The third heart sound in mitral regurgitation. Br. Heart J. *23*: 677, 1961.
83. Silverman, B., and Fortuin, N.: Diastolic filling in cardiac disease. Clin. Res. *20*(Abst.):398, 1972.
84. Hubbard, T. F., Dunn, F. L., and Neis, D. D.: A phonocardiographic study of the apical diastolic murmurs in pure mitral insufficiency. Am. Heart J. *57*:223, 1959.
85. Nixon, P. G. F., and Wooler, G. H.: Left ventricular filling pressure gradient in mitral incompetence. Br. Heart J. *25*:382, 1963.
86. Ravin, A., and Darley, W.: Apical diastolic murmurs in patent ductus arteriosus. Ann. Intern. Med. *33*:903, 1950.
87. Wooley, C. F., Levin, H. S., Leighton, R. F., Goodwin, R. S., and Ryan, J. M.: Intracardiac sound and pressure events in man. Am. J. Med. *42*:248, 1967.
88. Flint, A.: On cardiac murmurs. Am. J. Med. Sci. *44*:29, 1862.
89. Fortuin, N. J., and Craige, E.: On the mechanism of the Austin Flint murmur. Circulation *45*:558, 1972.
90. Reddy, P. S., Curtiss, E. I., Salerni, R., O'Toole, J. D., Griff, F. W., Leon, D. F., and Shaver, J. A.: Sound pressure correlates of the Austin Flint murmur: An intracardiac sound study. Circulation *53*:210, 1976.
91. Mann, T., McLaurin, L., Grossman, W., and Craige, E.: Acute aortic regurgitation due to infective endocarditis. N. Engl. J. Med. *293*:108, 1975.
92. Meadows, W. R., Van Praagh, S., Indreika, M., and Sharp, J. T.: Premature mitral valve closure. A hemodynamic explanation for absence of the first sound in aortic insufficiency. Circulation *28*:251, 1963.
93. DiMattéo, J., LaFont, H., Hui Bon Hoa, F., et al.: La courbe méchanique ventriculaire dans l'insuffisance aortique. Arch. Mal. Coeur *60*:1320, 1967.
94. Wells, B. G., Rappaport, M. B., and Sprague, H. B.: The graphic registration of basal diastolic murmurs. Am. Heart J. *37*:586, 1949.
95. Harvey, W. P., and Perloff, J. K.: Some recent advances in clinical auscultation of the heart. Prog. Cardiovasc. Dis. *2*:97, 1959.
96. Sabbah, H. N., Khaja, F., Anbe, D. T., and Stein, P. D.: The aortic closure sound in pure aortic insufficiency. Circulation *56*:859, 1977.
97. Kitabatake, A., Ito, H., Inoue, M., Tanouchi, J., Ishihara, K., Morita, T., Fujii, K., Yoshida, Y., Masuyama, T., Yoshima, H., Hori, M., and Kamada, T.: A new approach to noninvasive evaluation of aortic regurgitant fraction by two-dimensional Doppler echocardiography. Circulation *72*:523, 1985.
98. Touche, T., Prasquier, R., Nitenberg, A., deZuttere, D., and Gourgon, R.: Assessment and followup of patients with aortic regurgitation by an updated Doppler echocardiographic measurement of the regurgitant fraction in the aortic arch. Circulation *72*:819, 1985.
99. Rees, J. R., Epstein, E. J., Criley, J. M., and Ross, R. S.: Hemodynamic effects of severe aortic regurgitation. Br. Heart J. *26*:412, 1964.
100. Runco, V., and Levin, H. S.: The spectrum of pulmonic regurgitation. *In* Leon, D. F., and Shaver, J. A. (eds.): Physiologic Principles of Heart Sounds and Murmurs. New York, American Heart Association Monograph, No. 46, 1975, p. 175.
101. Steell, G.: The murmur of high pressure in the pulmonary artery. Med. Chron. *9*:182, 1888.
102. Cohn, K. E., and Hultgren, H. N.: The Graham Steell murmur reevaluated. N. Engl. J. Med. *274*:486, 1966.
103. Sakamoto, T., Matsuhisa, M., Inoue, K., Hayashi, T., and Ito, U.: Clinical and hemodynamic observation of indirect pulmonary artery pulse tracing. Cardiovasc. Sound Bull. *3*:127, 1973.
104. Waider, W., and Craige, E.: First heart sound and ejection sounds. Am. J. Cardiol. *35*:346, 1975.
105. Kesteloot, H., and Willems, J.: Relationship between the right apexcardiogram and the right ventricular dynamics. Acta Cardiol. *22*:64, 1967.
106. Mills, P. G., Brodie, B., McLaurin, L., Schall, S., and Craige, E.: Echocardiographic and hemodynamic relationships of ejection sounds. Circulation *56*:430, 1977.
107. York, P. G., and Popp, R. L.: Noninvasive estimation of right ventricular pressure by Doppler ultrasound in patients with tricuspid regurgitation. Circulation *70*:657, 1984.

CONTINUOUS MURMURS

108. Craige, E., and Millward, D. K.: Diastolic and continuous murmurs. Prog. Cardiovasc. Dis. *14*:38, 1971.
109. Neill, C., and Mounsey, P.: Auscultation in patent ductus arteriosus, with a description of two fistulae simulating patent ductus. Br. Heart J. *20*:61, 1958.
110. Gasul, B. M., Arcilla, R. A., Fell, E. H., Lynfield, J., Bicoff, J. P., and Luan, L. I.: Congenital coronary arteriovenous fistula. Pediatrics *25*:531, 1960.
111. Muenster, J. J., Graettinger, J. S., and Campbell, J. A.: Correlation of clinical and hemodynamic findings in patients with systemic arteriovenous fistulas. Circulation: *20*:1079, 1959.
112. Myers, J. D.: The mechanisms and significance of continuous murmurs. *In* Leon, D. F., and Shaver, J. A. (eds.): Physiologic Principles of Heart Sounds and Murmurs. New York, American Heart Association Monograph, No. 46, 1975, p. 201.
113. Spencer, M. P., Johnston, F. R., and Meredith, J. H.: The origin and interpretation of murmurs in coarctation of the aorta. Am. Heart J. *56*:722, 1958.
114. Eldridge, F., Selzer, A., and Hultgren, H.: Stenosis of branch of pulmonary artery. An additional cause of continuous murmurs over the chest. Circulation *15*:865, 1957.
115. Franch, R. H., and Gay, B. B., Jr.: Congenital stenosis of pulmonary artery branches. Am. J. Med. *35*:512, 1963.
116. Levine, S. A., and Harvey, W. P.: Clinical Auscultation of the Heart. Philadelphia, W.B. Saunders Company, 1959, p. 613.
117. Palmer, R., and White, P. D.: Note on continuous humming murmur heard in supra- and infraclavicular fossae and over manubrium sterni in children. N. Engl. J. Med. *199*:1297, 1928.

5 ECHOCARDIOGRAPHY

by HARVEY FEIGENBAUM, M.D.

PRINCIPLES OF ECHOCARDIOGRAPHY

CREATION OF IMAGE USING PULSED REFLECTED ULTRASOUND

The term *echocardiography* refers to a group of tests that utilize ultrasound to examine the heart and record information in the form of echoes, i.e., reflected sonic waves.[1-3] The upper limit for audible sound is 20,000 cycles/second; or 20 kiloHertz (kHz = 1000 cycles/second).[1] The sonic frequency used for echocardiography ranges from 1 to 10 million cycles/second, or 1 to 10 megaHertz (MHz).[2] In adults the frequencies commonly employed are 2.0 to 5.0 MHz, while in children they are usually higher, ranging from 3.5 to 10.0 MHz. The *resolution* of the recording, which is the ability to distinguish two objects that are spatially close together, varies directly with the frequency and inversely with the wave length. High-frequency (short wave length) ultrasound can identify separate objects that are less than 1 mm apart. Beams having lower frequencies and longer wave lengths have poorer resolution. However, the degree of *penetration*, which is the ability to transmit sufficient ultrasonic energy into the chest to provide a satisfactory recording, is inversely proportional to the frequency of the signal. Since a high-frequency ultrasonic beam (i.e., 3 or 5 MHz) is unable to penetrate a thick chest wall, lower frequency ultrasonic beams are used in adults. While this permits penetration through the chest wall, it partially sacrifices resolution; however, even with a transducer producing a beam of 2.25 MHz, which is commonly used in adult echocardiography, it is still possible to resolve objects that are 1 to 2 mm apart.

PRINCIPLES OF ULTRASOUND IMAGING. The principles by which ultrasound creates an image are depicted in Figure 5–1. The transducer at the side of the beaker of water has a piezoelectric element that vibrates very rapidly and produces ultrasound when activated by an electrical field.[3] If a burst of electrical energy is imparted to the transducer, it will emit a burst of ultrasound, which travels through the beaker. As long as the medium through which the sound travels is homogeneous, the ultrasonic waves will travel in a straight line. When the ultrasound strikes an interface between two media which have different acoustical properties, the sound behaves according to the laws of reflection and refraction,[1,2] analogous to light. Whether or not ultrasound is reflected by an interface depends upon the difference in the acoustical impedances of the two media. Although acoustical impedance is the product of the density of the object and the velocity of sound through that object, for all practical purposes one can consider the acoustical impedance to be a function of density. Thus, if the interface is between a liquid and a solid, the ultrasonic wave will generally be reflected. If the interface is between two solids of different densities, the quantity of reflected ultrasound is usually less. Thus, the quantity of energy reflected is directly proportional to the difference in the acoustical impedances (or densities) of the object and its surrounding media.

The left panel of Figure 5–1 shows diagrammatically an ultrasonic beam, which consists of individual bursts of ultrasound that leave the transducer, travel through the fluid, strike the far side of the beaker, are reflected by this interface, retrace their original path, and again strike the transducer. The piezoelectric element in the transducer not only converts electrical energy into ultrasonic impulses but also converts ultrasound back to electrical energy. Thus, when the reflected ultrasound (echo) strikes the piezoelectric element in the transducer, an electrical signal is produced. If the time it takes for (a) the ultrasound to leave the transducer and return and (b) the velocity of sound through the medium are both known, the distance between the transducer and the reflected interface can be calculated. By calibrating the echograph (ultrasonoscope) for a velocity of sound in the medium under examination, the time that it takes for the ultrasound to leave and return as an echo can be automatically converted to distance. Thus, the far wall of the beaker is depicted on the oscilloscope as being 6 cm from the transducer.

If a rod is placed in the water so that it transects the ultrasonic beam, part of the energy will strike and be reflected by the rod before the beam strikes the far side of the beaker. Thus, the returning ultrasonic energy or echo from the rod will strike the transducer sooner than that returning from the far side of the beaker, and the corresponding electrical signal produced by the echo from the rod will be closer to the transducer than will that from the beaker. Also, since some of the ultrasonic energy is reflected by the rod, less energy will remain to strike the far wall of the beaker, and the magnitude of the echo (Fig. 5–1, center panel) will be reduced. There are adjustments in ultrasonic instrumentation which provide depth compensation and thereby correct for this loss of ultrasonic energy from distant or far objects. From examination of the A-mode echo ("A" refers to amplitude) in Figure 5–1 (center panel), one could deduce that the far wall of the beaker is 6 cm from the transducer and that an echo-reflecting object is present in the center of the beaker, 3 cm from the transducer.

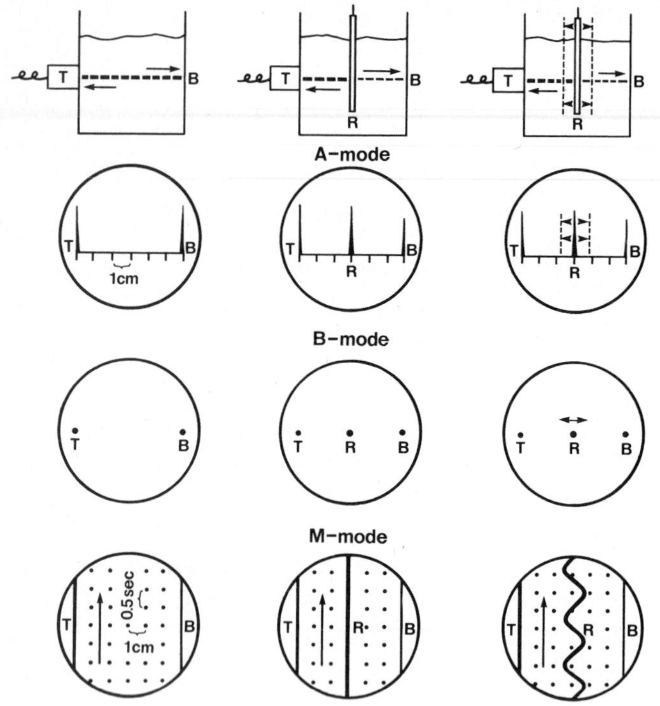

FIGURE 5–1. Diagrams illustrating the principles of acoustic imaging using pulsed reflected ultrasound (see text for details). T = transducer, B = beaker, R = rod. (Modified from Feigenbaum, H., and Zaky, A.: Use of diagnostic ultrasound in clinical cardiology. J. Indiana State Med. Assoc. *59*:140, 1966.)

IMAGING A MOVING OBJECT. If the rod were moving back and forth as in the right panel of Figure 5–1, the ultrasonic examination would differ. The transducer functions as a transmitter of ultrasound for a very short period of time, just over one μsec in commercial echocardiographs. During the remaining time the transducer functions as a receiver, waiting for echoes to be converted into electrical signals. The rapidity or the repetition rate with which the transducer fires the 1 μsec impulses varies depending upon the design of the instrument. Commercial M-mode instruments commonly pulse the transducer 1000 times/sec with 1 μsec impulses. Thus, the transducer functions as a receiver during approximately 999 μsec of each msec.

A-MODE, B-MODE, AND M-MODE PRESENTATIONS. In the left and center panels of Figure 5–1, the wall of the beaker and the rod are not moving. All the ultrasonic impulses firing at a rate of 1000/sec take the same time to leave the transducer and return as echoes. Therefore, the signals or echoes seen on the oscilloscope are static. In the right panel, the object moves constantly and therefore the time required for the ultrasound to leave the transducer and return as an echo varies correspondingly and the echo signal on the oscilloscope moves. In the A-mode presentation the echo from the rod moves back and forth within the center of the beaker. To record the motion of the rod, one converts the amplitude of the echo to brightness, which changes the display from the A-mode to the B-mode (the "B" refers to brightness), in which the returning echoes are displayed on the oscilloscope as dots rather than as spikes. Stronger signals are therefore taller on the A-mode and brighter on the B-mode presentation. On the M-mode presentation ("M" refers to motion) displayed in Figure 5–1, the oscilloscope sweeps from bottom to top. In the left and center panels the structures are fixed, and therefore the M-mode presentation shows simply a series of parallel lines. In the right panel the rod moves back and forth in a regular manner, its echo inscribing a sinusoidal curve on the M-mode oscilloscope.

Thus, the M-mode presentation permits recording of amplitude and of the rate of motion of moving objects with great accuracy; the sampling rate is essentially 1000 pulses/second, the repetition rate of the transducer. Since electrocardiograms and other cardiac parameters are conventionally displayed on the oscilloscope together with the echocardiograph, the oscilloscope usually sweeps from left to right rather than from bottom to top; therefore, the transducer is generally displayed at the top of the oscilloscopic image rather than on the left side, as depicted in Figure 5–1.

M-MODE ECHOCARDIOGRAPHY

TECHNIQUE. The ultrasonic transducer is ordinarily placed on the surface of the chest, usually along the left sternal border, and the ultrasonic beam is directed toward the part of the heart to be examined. In Figure 5–2 the ultrasound is depicted as passing through a small portion of the right ventricle, the interventricular septum, and the cavity and posterior wall of the left ventricle. Structures such as the chest wall which do not move with cardiac activity are depicted as horizontal lines. Moving cardiac walls and valves move with cardiac action and inscribe wavy signals. The blood-filled cavities are relatively echo-free.

THE M-MODE TRACING. An M-mode recording is sometimes called a one-dimensional or an "ice-pick" view of the heart. However, since time is the second dimension on M-mode tracings, this display is not truly one-dimensional. The information provided by an isolated M-mode view of the heart, such as in Figure 5–2, can be augmented by changing the direction of the ultrasonic beam, as in an arc or sector (Fig. 5–3). With the transducer placed along the left sternal border in approximately the third or fourth intercostal space, the ultrasonic beam can be swept in a sector between the apex (Fig. 5–3*A*, position 1) and the base of the heart (Fig. 5–3*A*, position 4). When the transducer is pointed toward the apex of the heart, the ultrasonic beam traverses the left ventricular cavity at the level of the papillary muscles and passes through a small portion of the right ventricular cavity (Fig. 5–3*B*, position 1). Tilting the transducer superiorly and medially causes the ultrasonic beam to traverse the left ventricular cavity at the level of the edges of the mitral valve leaflets or the chordae (position 2). The beam again passes through a small portion of the right ventricle. By directing the transducer more superiorly and medially (position 3), more

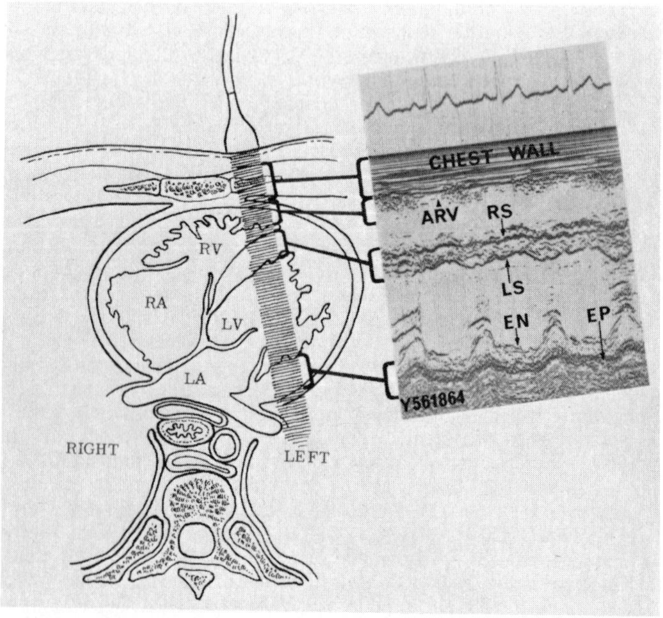

FIGURE 5–2. Diagrammatic cross-section of the heart and corresponding echocardiogram showing the cardiac structures transected by an ultrasonic beam directed toward the left ventricle. The ultrasound passes through the chest wall, the anterior right ventricular wall (ARV), a small portion of the right ventricular cavity, the interventricular septum, the cavity of the left ventricle, and the posterior left ventricular wall. RS = right side of interventricular septum, LS = left side of interventricular septum, EN = posterior left ventricular endocardium, EP = posterior left ventricular epicardium. (Modified from Popp, R. L., et al.: Estimation of right and left ventricular size by ultrasound. A study of the echoes from the interventricular septum. Am. J. Cardiol. *24*:523, 1969.)

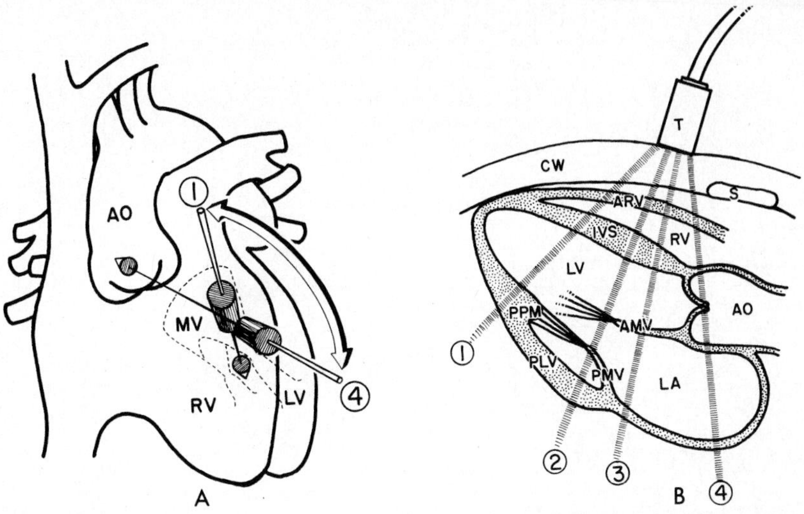

FIGURE 5–3. Diagram demonstrating how the ultrasonic transducer is commonly directed in an arc or sector between the base of the heart and the apex (*A*). *B*, Cross-section of the heart parallel to the long axis of the left ventricle showing the structures through which the ultrasound beam passes as it is directed from the apex toward the base of the heart, as shown in *A*. T = transducer, S = sternum, ARV = anterior right ventricular wall, RV = right ventricular cavity, IVS = interventricular septum, LV = left ventricle, PPM = posterior papillary muscle, PLV = posterior left ventricular wall, AMV = anterior mitral valve, PMV = posterior mitral valve, AO = aorta, LA = left atrium, MV = mitral valve. (From Feigenbaum, H.: Clinical applications of echocardiography. Progr. Cardiovasc. Dis. *14*:531, 1972, by permission of Grune and Stratton.)

of the anterior leaflet of the mitral valve can be recorded and the beam may traverse part of the left atrial cavity. Further tilting of the transducer superiorly and medially (position 4) directs the beam through the root of the aorta, the leaflets of the aortic valve, and the body of the left atrium.

Figure 5–4 is a diagram of an echocardiographic recording as the transducer is swept in a sector from the apex toward the base of the heart. An electrocardiogram helps to identify the events of the cardiac cycle. Beginning on the left side of Figure 5–4 (position 1), the chest wall echoes are recorded, followed by those of the anterior wall of the right ventricle. The right ventricular cavity is then recorded as an echo-free space. The next structure is the interventricular septum. Frequently, a mass of echoes originating from the posterior papillary muscle is evident posterior to the left ventricular cavity. Even further posterior is the posterior wall of the left ventricle. The intense echoes behind the heart originate from the lung. In transducer position 2 the principal change in the echogram is that parts of the mitral valve apparatus, either chordae or edges of the leaflets, are recorded within the left ventricular cavity. In this position the ultrasonic beam also traverses more of the body of the left ventricle, and the diameter of the left ventricular cavity, i.e., the distance between the left side of the interventricular septum and the posterior left ventricular endocardium, is greatest.

As the transducer is tilted slightly superiorly and medially, the anterior and posterior leaflets of the mitral valve are recorded. Tilting the transducer even further toward the base of the heart (position 3) causes the echoes produced by the posterior leaflet to drop out, and only the anterior leaflet of the mitral valve is recorded. The beam now passes through the posterior wall of the left atrium instead of that of the left ventricle. The posterior wall of the atrium moves posteriorly, i.e., away from the chest wall, during systole, while the posterior wall of the left ventricle moves anteriorly. When the transducer is directed toward the base of the heart (position 4), the beam passes through the anterior wall of the aorta (rather than the interventricular septum) and the posterior wall of the aortic root, which also constitutes the anterior wall of the left atrium (rather than the anterior leaflet of the mitral valve). Echoes from two or more leaflets of the aortic valve can frequently be recorded from between the two aortic walls. The leaflets separate and form a boxlike structure during systole and come together as a single line in diastole; the left atrial cavity lies behind the aorta.

Figure 5–5 shows echoes from the aorta and aortic valve; by tilting the transducer medially from the aortic valve, it is possible to record the anterior leaflet of the tricuspid valve, which is similar in appearance to the recording from the anterior leaflet of the mitral valve. When the transducer is directed superiorly and laterally from the aortic valve, a posterior leaflet of the pulmonary valve can be recorded (Fig. 5–5).

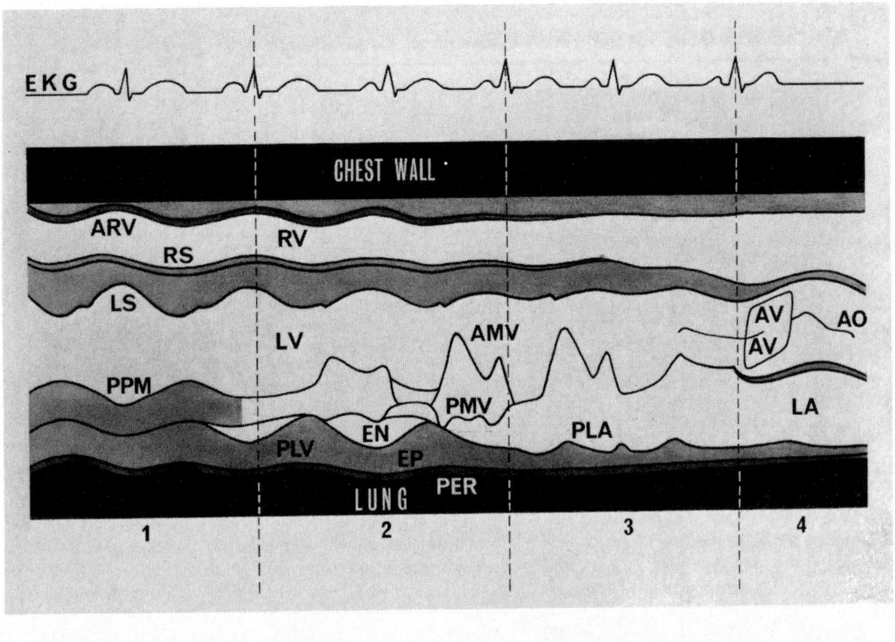

FIGURE 5–4. Diagrammatic presentation of an M-mode echocardiogram as the transducer is directed from the apex (position 1) to the base of the heart (position 4). Areas between the dotted lines correspond to the transducer position, as depicted in Figure 5–3. EN = endocardium of the left ventricle, EP = epicardium of the left ventricle, PER = pericardium, PLA = posterior left atrial wall. Other abbreviations as in Figure 5–3. (From Feigenbaum, H.: Clinical applications of echocardiography. Progr. Cardiovasc. Dis. *14*:531, 1972, by permission of Grune and Stratton.)

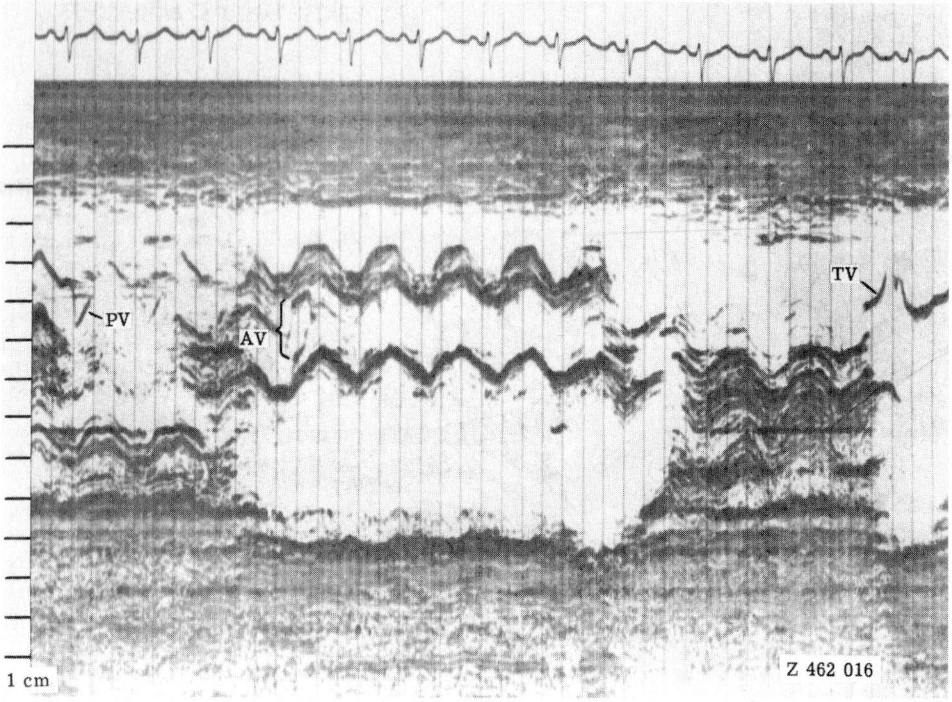

FIGURE 5–5. M-mode scan recording echoes from a pulmonic valve (PV), aortic valve (AV), and tricuspid valve (TV). (From Feigenbaum, H.: Echocardiography. 2nd ed. Philadelphia, Lea and Febiger, 1976.)

TWO-DIMENSIONAL ECHOCARDIOGRAPHY

The principle of two-dimensional echocardiography is depicted in Figure 5–6. The ultrasonic beam now moves in a sector so that a pie-shaped slice of the heart is interrogated. Most commercial two-dimensional echocardiographs move the ultrasonic beam so that approximately 30 slices per second are obtained. The ultrasonic beam can be moved mechanically by oscillating a single transducer or by rotating a series of transducers. The ultrasound can also be steered electronically using the so-called *phased array principles*,[4] in which multiple ultrasonic elements are utilized to make up the beam and in which the firing sequence of the elements is controlled. A computer or microprocessor is necessary to control the firing of the elements and the direction of the beam. Figure 5–7

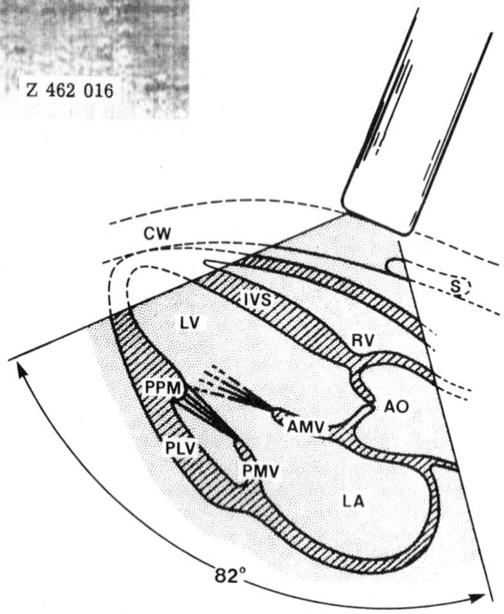

FIGURE 5–6. Diagram showing how to obtain a cross-sectional or two-dimensional image of the heart parallel to the long axis of the left ventricle. CW = chest wall. Other abbreviations as in Figure 5–3.

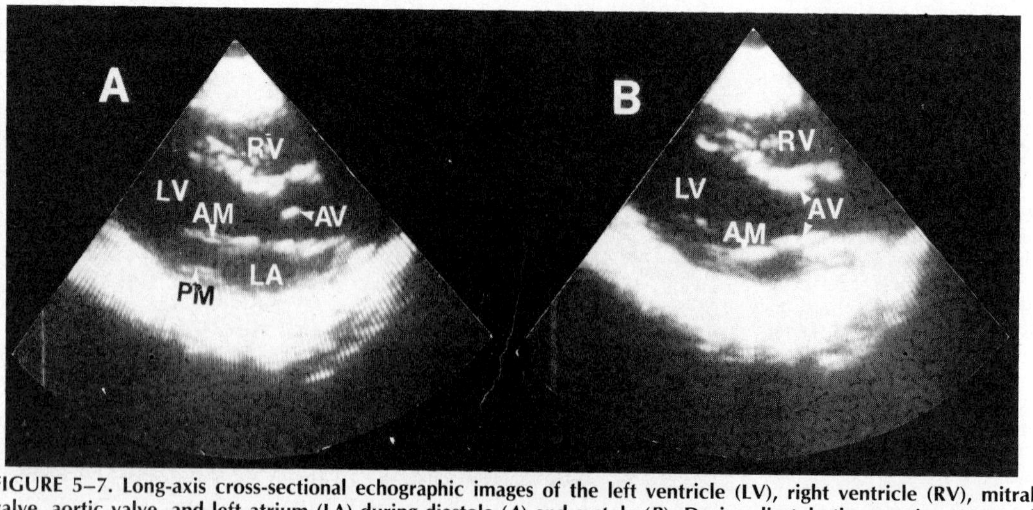

FIGURE 5–7. Long-axis cross-sectional echographic images of the left ventricle (LV), right ventricle (RV), mitral valve, aortic valve, and left atrium (LA) during diastole (*A*) and systole (*B*). During diastole the anterior (AM) and posterior (PM) mitral leaflets are apart and the aortic valve leaflets (AV) come together as a single echo in the midportion of the aorta (*A*). With systole, (*B*) the mitral leaflets come together and the aortic valve leaflets separate.

illustrates two individual frames representing stop-action sequences from a videotape recording of a normal heart in which the mitral and aortic valves and parts of the left ventricle, left atrium, and aorta are imaged. It must be recalled that all of these structures do not lie in the same plane. For example, it is not ordinarily possible to include both the long axis of the apex and the aorta in a single picture; this is not the case with angiography. Since these two-dimensional echocardiograms are displayed on videotape, they superficially resemble cineangiograms. However, they later display intracavitary contrast material, while the two-dimensional images represent individual "slices" of the heart.

DOPPLER ECHOCARDIOGRAPHY

M-mode and two-dimensional echocardiography essentially create ultrasonic images of the heart. Doppler echocardiography utilizes ultrasound to record blood flow within the cardiovascular system. The principle of the Doppler effect is noted in Figure 5–8.[5, 6] If the ultrasonic beam is reflected by a stationary object (Fig. 5–8*A*), the transmitted frequency (f_t) and the reflected frequency (f_r) are equal. However, if the target reflecting the ultrasonic energy is moving toward the transducers (Fig. 5–8*B*), the reflected frequency (f_r) is greater than the transmitted frequency. When the target is moving away from the transducer (Fig. 5–8*C*), the reflected frequency is less than the transmitted frequency. The difference between the reflected and transmitted frequencies represents the Doppler shift or Doppler frequency. By knowing the Doppler frequency it is possible to calculate the velocity of the moving target. Figure 5–9 shows the Doppler equations which relate Doppler frequency (f_d) and the velocity of the moving target (v). In order to determine the velocity of blood flow, it is necessary to know the Doppler frequency, the angle (θ) between the paths of the ultrasonic beam and moving target, and the velocity of sound in the medium being examined; in Doppler echocardiography the targets are the red blood cells.

Figure 5–8 demonstrates the principles of *continuous wave Doppler*. There are two transducers, one of which continuously transmits ultrasonic energy, and the other, which continuously records the reflected ultrasonic signals. One can also use *pulsed ultrasound* to obtain the Doppler information (Fig. 5–10). With pulsed Doppler only one

$$f_d = f_r - f_t$$

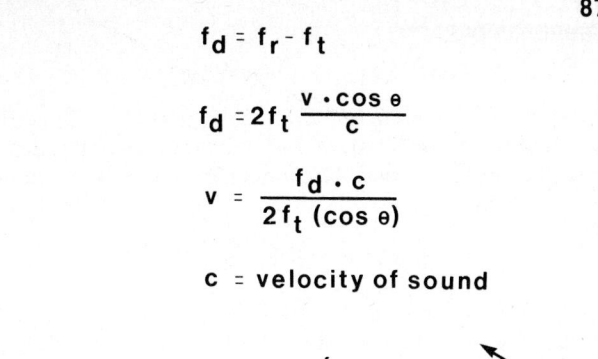

$$f_d = 2f_t \frac{v \cdot \cos\theta}{c}$$

$$v = \frac{f_d \cdot c}{2f_t(\cos\theta)}$$

c = velocity of sound

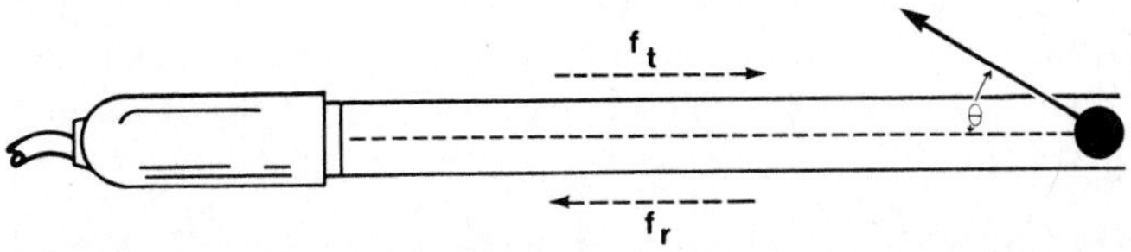

FIGURE 5–9. Doppler equations relating Doppler frequencies (f_d), received frequency (f_r), transmitted frequency (f_t), and the angle (θ) between the direction of the moving target and the path of the ultrasonic beam. (From Feigenbaum, H.: Echocardiography. 4th ed. Philadelphia, Lea and Febiger, 1986.)

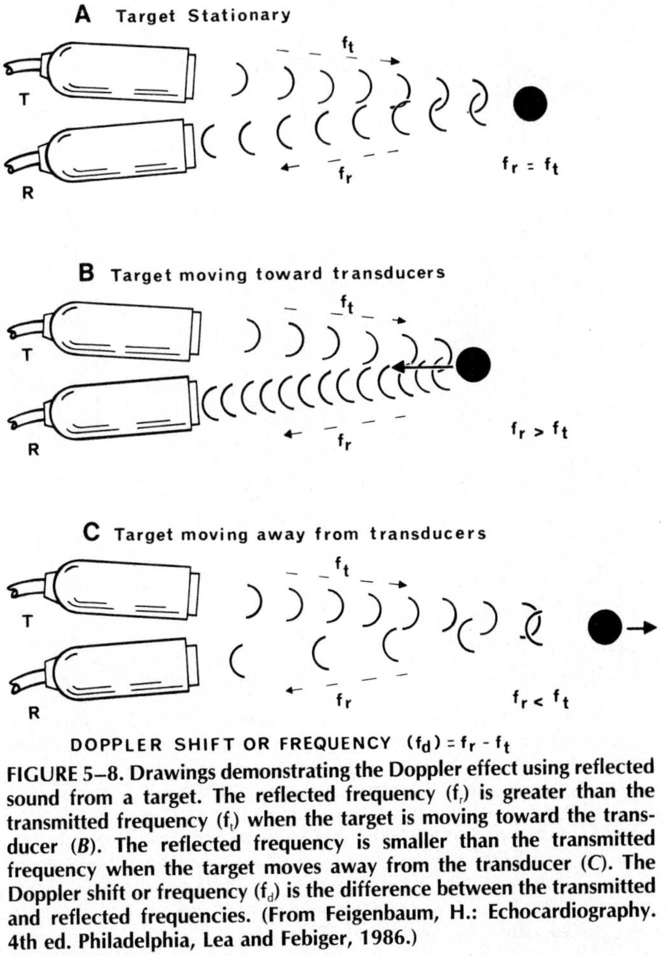

FIGURE 5–8. Drawings demonstrating the Doppler effect using reflected sound from a target. The reflected frequency (f_r) is greater than the transmitted frequency (f_t) when the target is moving toward the transducer (*B*). The reflected frequency is smaller than the transmitted frequency when the target moves away from the transducer (*C*). The Doppler shift or frequency (f_d) is the difference between the transmitted and reflected frequencies. (From Feigenbaum, H.: Echocardiography. 4th ed. Philadelphia, Lea and Febiger, 1986.)

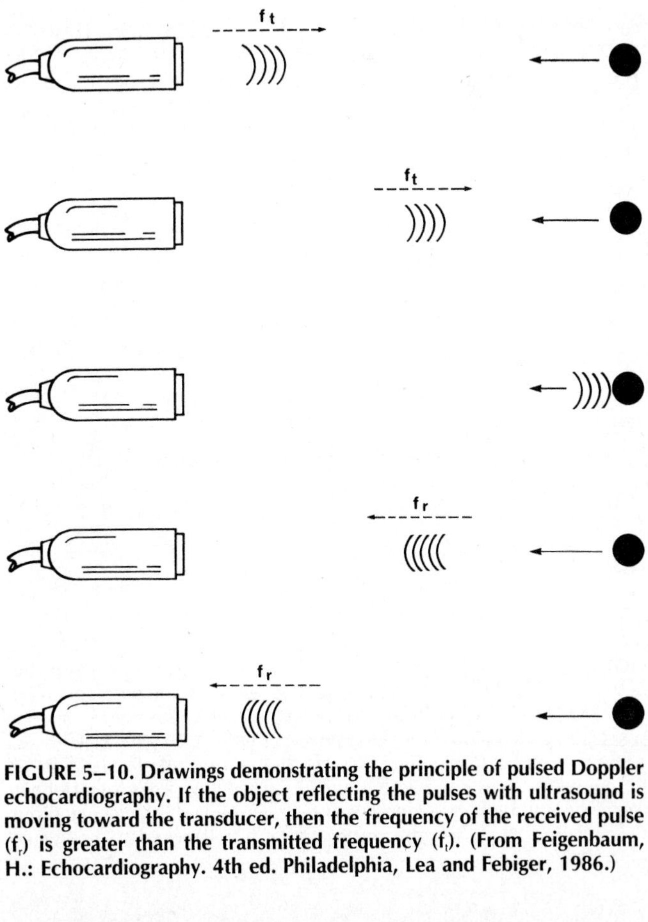

FIGURE 5–10. Drawings demonstrating the principle of pulsed Doppler echocardiography. If the object reflecting the pulses with ultrasound is moving toward the transducer, then the frequency of the received pulse (f_r) is greater than the transmitted frequency (f_t). (From Feigenbaum, H.: Echocardiography. 4th ed. Philadelphia, Lea and Febiger, 1986.)

transducer is needed. In addition, pulsed Doppler permits creation of a simultaneous M-mode or two-dimensional image.[7] To derive the Doppler frequency, the frequencies of the reflected and transmitted bursts of ultrasound are subtracted.

There are significant differences between continuous wave and *pulsed Doppler*. The velocity that can be recorded using pulsed Doppler is limited by the pulse repetition frequency of the system. Thus if the blood is moving very rapidly, as might occur when it is passing through a stenotic valve, then pulsed Doppler cannot sample rapidly enough to identify the Doppler frequency. This technical problem is known as *aliasing*.[8] As a result, continuous wave Doppler is necessary for recording very high velocities within the cardiovascular system. An alternative way is to use a multiple pulsed or high pulse repetition frequency (high PRF) Doppler system. High PRF allows simultaneous imaging and recording of high flow rates; however, it is technically more difficult. The continuous wave approach is the more commonly used technique for recording high frequency flows.[9]

The diagram in Figure 5–11 illustrates two types of flow that can be recorded using Doppler echocardiography. Laminar flow produces a Doppler signal consisting of fairly uniform frequencies all moving in the same direction. If blood flow is turbulent or disturbed, multiple frequencies will be recorded, some of which may be moving in opposite directions as depicted by signals below the baseline. The Doppler recording is a spectral display using fast Fourier analysis of the audible Doppler signal. The recording is usually on strip chart paper or videotape. The audio signal is helpful in interpreting the various types of flow and represents an important aspect of the Doppler examination.

Doppler information from the cardiovascular system can also be recorded in a spatially correct format superimposed on an M-mode or two-dimensional echocardiogram.[10] Doppler flow imaging is created by multiple Doppler gates that are spatially correct and display the moving blood within the two-dimensional or M-mode recording.[11–13] The direction of the blood is displayed in *color* as in Figure 5–12. With this particular instrument blood moving toward the transducer is depicted in shades of yellow and red, whereas blood moving away from the transducer is in shades of blue.

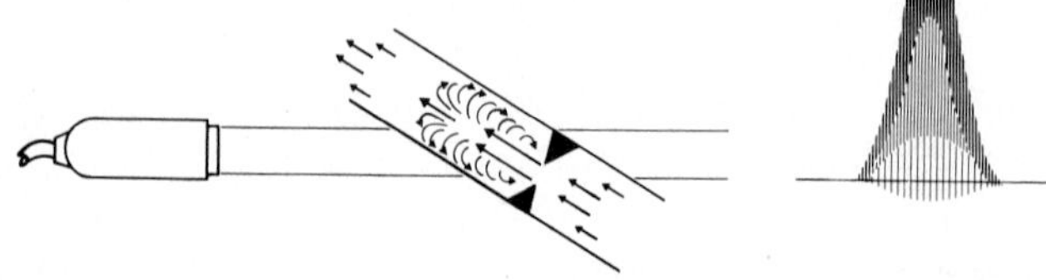

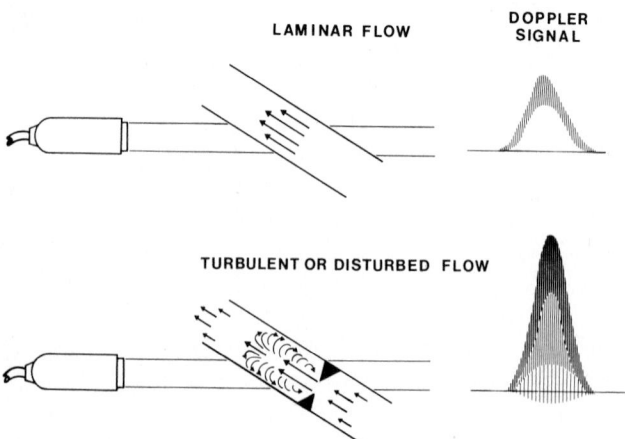

FIGURE 5–11. Doppler signals recorded from laminar flow and turbulent or disturbed flow. With laminar flow, all the velocities are similar. The Doppler signal produces a relatively thin wave form with minimal spectral broadening. When blood flows across an area with a significant change in the caliber of the vessel, flow with multiple velocities in different directions is produced. Such disturbed flow produces a Doppler signal with multiple frequencies and marked spectral broadening. (From Feigenbaum, H.: Echocardiography. 4th ed. Philadelphia, Lea and Febiger, 1986.)

FIGURE 5–12. See color plate 1.

CONTRAST ECHOCARDIOGRAPHY

Ultrasound is an extremely sensitive detector of intravascular bubbles. The injection of almost any liquid into the intravascular spaces will introduce many microbubbles that appear as a cloud of echoes on the echocardiogram. Figure 5–13 demonstrates an M-mode echocardiogram of a patient with a right-to-left shunt at the ventricular level. The contrast can be seen initially in the right ventricle. It then traverses the interventricular septum and appears in the left ventricle. This technique is obviously a sensitive method of detecting right-to-left shunts. The contrast agents that have been used include the patient's blood, saline, dextrose in water, and indocyanine green dye. In all cases the contrast effect originates from suspended microbubbles in the fluid. Injection of small quantities of carbon dioxide gas has also been used for contrast echocardiography.[14] Hydrogen peroxide will give a strong contrast effect by producing tiny intravascular bubbles of oxygen.[15, 16] Commercially manufactured microbubbles may be available soon.[17] The potential clinical uses for contrast echocardiography are numerous. There is much ongoing research in this area.

INVASIVE ECHOCARDIOGRAPHY

Although echocardiography is one of the most common noninvasive examinations, this ultrasonic examination need not be limited to merely placing the transducer on the surface of the chest. Esophageal echocardiography has been available for many years. With the technical advances in placing a two-dimensional transducer at the end of a flexible endoscope it is now possible to obtain high quality

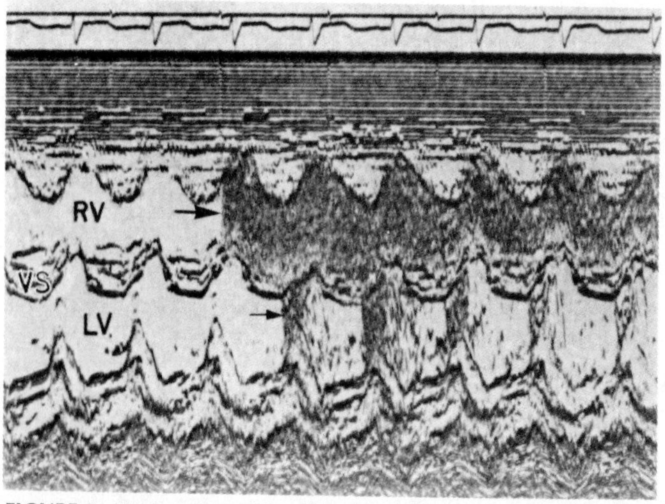

FIGURE 5–13. A contrast M-mode echocardiogram in a patient with a right-to-left shunt at the ventricular level. The dark mass of echoes from the injected contrast (large arrow) is initially seen in the right ventricular cavity (RV) and next is seen (small arrow) in the left ventricle (LV) above the mitral valve. Normally the contrast should not appear on the left side of the heart at all. If the shunt were at the atrial level, contrast would appear in the left and right ventricles simultaneously and would be seen posterior to the mitral valve. VS = ventricular septum. (From Seward, J. B., et al.: Echocardiographic contrast studies: Initial experience. Mayo Clin. Proc. *50*:163, 1975.)

two-dimensional images via the esophagus.[18] It is also possible to obtain Doppler information with this approach. This type of examination is useful in patients in whom examination from the usual positions is impossible technically. The other major application for esophageal echocardiography is in the patient undergoing cardiac surgery.[18, 19] The esophageal ultrasonic probe can be used to monitor cardiac function throughout the surgical procedure and into the postoperative state to observe any alterations in cardiac function.

Echocardiography is also being used in the operating room during open heart surgery.[20] Cardiac surgeons are finding echocardiography to be helpful in assessing cardiac morphology and function before and after surgical procedures.[21] Such an examination can be combined with contrast studies,[22] pulsed Doppler, or color Doppler.[23]

Echocardiography can also be used in conjunction with invasive procedures.[24, 25] Echocardiographic monitoring for pericardiocentesis has been done for some time.[26] A similar type of monitoring has been very useful to follow an endomyocardial biopsy,[27] especially from the right ventricle.[28] Therapeutic catheter techniques using balloon angioplasty or septostomy are also monitored effectively using echocardiography.[29]

Advantages and Limitations of Echocardiography

The advantages of echocardiography are numerous. The examination is painless, as best as can be determined it is virtually harmless,[30] and it is less costly than other sophisticated imaging techniques. However, some technical difficulties exist which require expertise on the part of the examiner and interpreter of the echocardiographic recordings. The principal problem is posed by the poor transmission of ultrasound through bony structures or air-containing lungs. The examiner must thus try to avoid these structures. A variety of techniques have been developed to circumvent this problem. The patient is commonly placed in the left recumbent position to move the heart from beneath the sternum. The subxiphoid or subcostal transducer position is frequently used in patients with hyperinflated lungs and a low diaphragm.[31] The apical examination with two-dimensional echocardiography has greatly increased the success rate in examining difficult patients.[32] The suprasternal notch approach[33] offers yet another useful echocardiographic window especially for Doppler studies. Thus many examining techniques have been developed to minimize the technical difficulties in performing an echocardiographic examination. With the increasing number of skilled individuals performing echocardiography and the introduction of echocardiographic instruments with better performance, the number of technically unsatisfactory echocardiographic recordings is diminishing dramatically. Unfortunately, however, in some patients the echocardiogram may not provide all of the desired clinical information. In a laboratory run by well-trained individuals the number of nondiagnostic echocardiograms should be less than 5 per cent.

EXAMINATION OF THE NORMAL HEART

M-MODE ECHOCARDIOGRAM

Figure 5–14*A* shows an M-mode scan that encompasses the full length of the *mitral valve apparatus*. The echoes from this structure are striking and are readily identified. The anterior leaflet of the mitral valve shows a downward motion in mid-diastole, and the characteristic "M" pattern is recorded. The posterior mitral leaflet is essentially a mirror-image of the anterior leaflet, except the amplitude of its motion is less.

Figure 5–14*B* is an M-mode examination of a normal mitral valve. The end of systole, just prior to the opening of the valve, is designated "D." The maximum excursion of the anterior leaflets is designated "E" and the nadir of the initial diastolic closing wave "F." The diastolic closing rate, or the "E to F slope," is indicated by the line drawn on Figure 5–14*B*. This slope is frequently not straight but curved. With atrial systole, blood is propelled through the mitral orifice and the leaflets reopen. The peak of this reopening of the mitral valve is designated "A"; with atrial relaxation, the valve begins to close again. Ventricular systole begins during the downward slope of the mitral leaflet and may produce a slight interruption of the closure wave, at point "B." (This is not always evident and is not so in Figure 5–14*B*.) Complete closure occurs following the onset of ventricular systole at "C."

The *left ventricular cavity* is bordered by the interventricular septum anteriorly and the posterior left ventricular wall posteriorly. Both walls move toward each other during systole, so that the diameter of the cavity decreases with systole. Both walls are approximately 1 cm thick in diastole, and the thickness increases during systole. A small portion of the right ventricular cavity lies anterior to the interventricular septum, and the anterior wall of the right ventricle is shown at the top of the tracing; the latter structure cannot always be imaged, especially in adults.

As the ultrasonic beam is swept superiorly and medially toward the base of the heart, the posterior leaflet of the mitral valve drops out and the posterior left atrial wall is seen to lie behind the anterior leaflet of the mitral valve. At the junction between the left atrium and ventricle the ultrasonic beam traverses both chambers during a given cardiac cycle. Because the atrioventricular junction moves in a superoinferior direction during each cycle, the stationary ultrasonic beam may record the left atrial wall during systole and the left ventricular wall during diastole. As the beam is directed more superiorly into the body of the left atrium, the relatively stationary posterior wall of the left atrium is imaged. The aorta, represented by two parallel moving echoes which move anteriorly during systole and posteriorly during diastole, lies anterior to the left atrium. The anterior wall of the aorta is in continuity with the echoes from the interventricular septum, and the posterior wall of the aorta is in continuity with the echoes of the anterior leaflet of the mitral valve. The aortic valve leaflets lie within the root of the aorta; only the anterior aortic valve leaflet is recorded in Figure 5–14. Two of the leaflets, probably the right coronary leaflet and the noncoronary leaflet, make up the boxlike configuration observed during systole as the aortic valve opens (Fig. 5–5). As the leaflets come together in diastole a *single* echo is commonly recorded.

M-Mode Echocardiographic Measurements

Numerous measurements have been suggested for M-mode echocardiography. Figure 5–15 demonstrates some of the measurements that can be obtained from an M-mode echocardiogram. Most of these measurements involve the left ventricle, the aortic root, and the left atrium. The American Society of Echocardiography has standardized the common measurements used in M-mode echocardiography.[34] A key consideration in these measurements is that the leading edge of an echo, i.e., that portion of the echo closest to the transducer, is more readily identified and precisely measured than is the trailing edge. The left ventricular dimension should be taken just beyond the mitral valve or at the chordae tendineae. In infants and young children, left ventric-

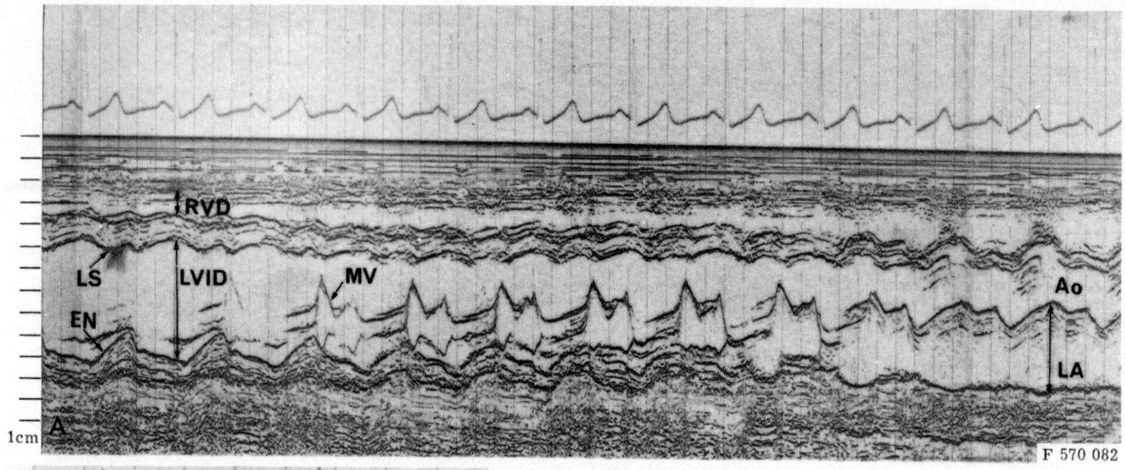

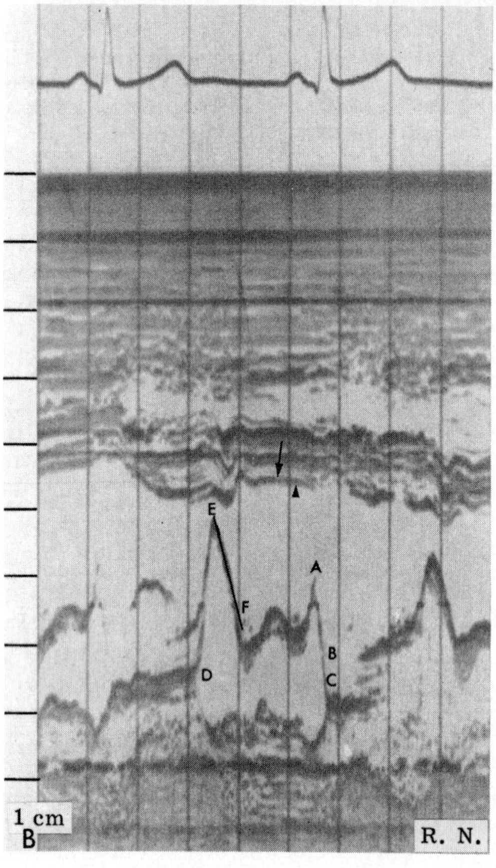

FIGURE 5–14. *A,* M-mode scan from the left ventricle to the aorta (AO) and left atrium (LA) in a normal subject. RVD = right ventricular dimension, LVID = left ventricular internal dimension, LS = left septal echoes, EN = posterior left ventricular endocardial echoes, MV = mitral valve. (From Chang, S.: M-mode Echocardiographic Techniques and Pattern Recognition. Philadelphia, Lea and Febiger, 1976.)

B, M-mode echocardiogram of a normal mitral valve. The letters A through F denote various portions of the anterior leaflet motion. The arrow indicates the leading edge of the echo from the left side of the interventricular septum; the arrowhead denotes the trailing edge of that echo. (From Feigenbaum, H.: Echocardiography. 2nd ed. Philadelphia, Lea and Febiger, 1976.)

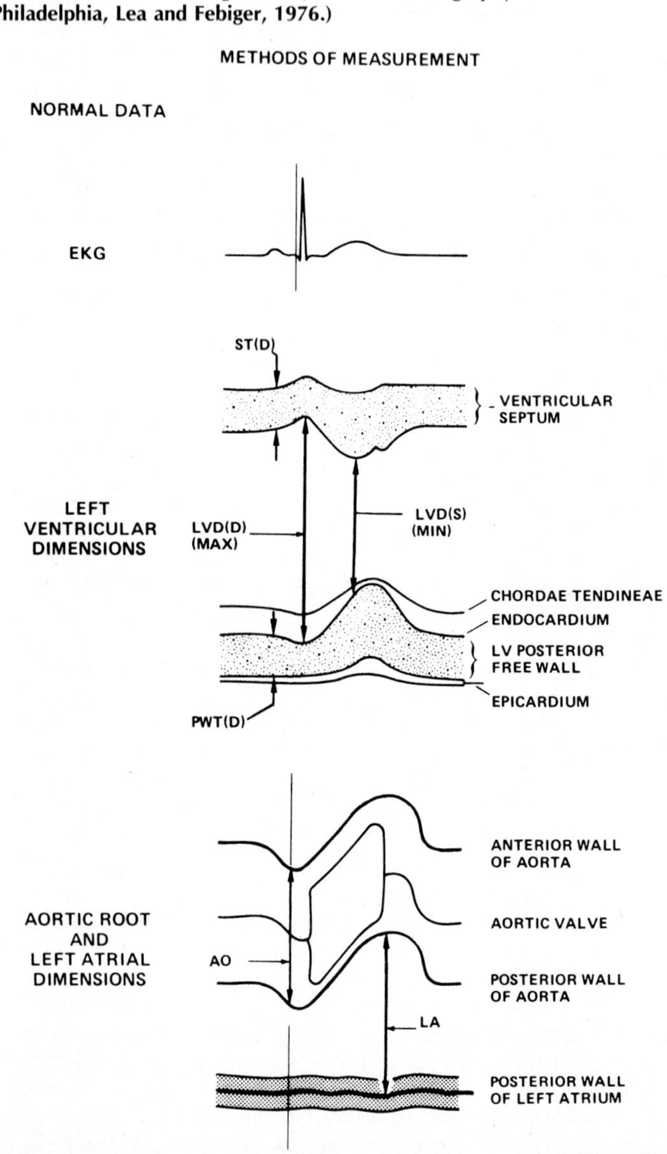

ular dimensions are probably best recorded at the level of the mitral valve. The end-diastolic dimension is taken at the onset of the QRS complex, while end-systolic measurement is obtained at the instant of maximum posterior (downward) position of the interventricular septum, which usually precedes the peak anterior (upward) position of the posterior left ventricular wall. When septal motion is abnormal, the instant of peak upward position of the posterior ventricular endocardium may be taken at end-systole. A true right ventricular dimension can be obtained only when the anterior right ventricular wall is well delineated; otherwise, only an estimate of this dimension can be made.

Wall thickness is also measured from leading edge to leading edge. The width of the interventricular septum is the distance from the anterior surface of the right to the anterior surface of the left septal echo. The thickness of the posterior left ventricular wall is measured from the

FIGURE 5–15. Methods for obtaining M-mode echocardiographic measurements. ST(D) = diastolic septal thickness; LVD(D) and LVD(S) = diastolic and systolic left ventricular diameter; PWT(D) = diastolic posterior wall thickness; AO = aorta; LA = left atrium. (From Henry, W. L., Gardin, J. M., and Ware, J. H.: Echocardiographic measurements in normal subjects from infancy to old age. Circulation *62*:1054, 1980, by permission of the American Heart Association, Inc.)

TABLE 5–1 NORMAL VALUES OF ECHOCARDIOGRAPHIC MEASUREMENTS IN ADULTS

	RANGE (CM)	MEAN (CM)	NUMBER OF SUBJECTS
Age (years)	13 to 54	26	134
Body surface area (M^2)	1.45 to 2.22	1.8	130
RVD—flat	0.7 to 2.3	1.5	84
RVD—left lateral	0.9 to 2.6	1.7	83
LVID—flat	3.7 to 5.6	4.7	82
LVID—left lateral	3.5 to 5.7	4.7	81
Posterior LV wall thickness	0.6 to 1.1	0.9	137
Posterior LV wall amplitude	0.9 to 1.4	1.2	48
IVS wall thickness	0.6 to 1.1	0.9	137
Mid IVS amplitude	0.3 to 0.8	0.5	10
Apical IVS amplitude	0.5 to 1.2	0.7	38
Left atrial dimension	1.9 to 4.0	2.9	133
Aortic root dimension	2.0 to 3.7	2.7	121
Aortic cusps' separation	1.5 to 2.6	2.9	93
Percentage of fractional shortening*	34% to 44%	36%	20%
Mean rate of circumferential shortening (Vcf),† or mean normalized shortening velocity	1.02 to 1.94 circ/sec	1.3 circ/sec	38

$$* \frac{LVIDd - LVIDs}{LVIDd}$$

$$\dagger \frac{LVIDd - LVIDs}{LVIDd \times \text{Ejection time}}$$

RVD = Right ventricular dimension
LVID = Left ventricular internal dimension; d = end diastole; s = end systole
LV = Left ventricle
IVS = Interventricular septum

anterior surface of the posterior left ventricular endocardial echo to that from the anterior surface of the posterior left ventricular epicardium.

Table 5–1 provides some normal values for commonly used M-mode echocardiographic measurements. These data represent approximations and do not conform in all instances to the criteria developed by the American Society of Echocardiography. Nor do they take into account that some changes in measurements occur during aging.[35] Normal values for children can be quite complex. The reader is encouraged to refer to some of the references, since more exhaustive normal values have been obtained.[2]

Although M-mode measurements have been made since the development of echocardiography in the 1950's, the role played by these measurements is decreasing. The closing velocity or E to F slope of the mitral valve is nonspecific and has relatively little diagnostic value. Even the left ventricular dimensions have significant limitations, especially in patients with regional wall motion abnormalities, such as with coronary artery disease or left bundle branch block. Thus, although M-mode measurements are still clinically helpful and are being used in many laboratories, they are gradually being replaced by quantitative two-dimensional and Doppler measurements. The rapid sampling rate inherent in M-mode echocardiography, however, makes the examination suitable for rate changes of cardiac dimensions. Many investigators and clinicians use a computer to trace the borders of the left ventricular cavity from the M-mode echocardiogram (Fig. 5–16).[36] In this way the rate of change of left ventricular dimensions can be obtained. This type of recording is particularly useful in identifying changes in left ventricular filling or diastolic compliance.

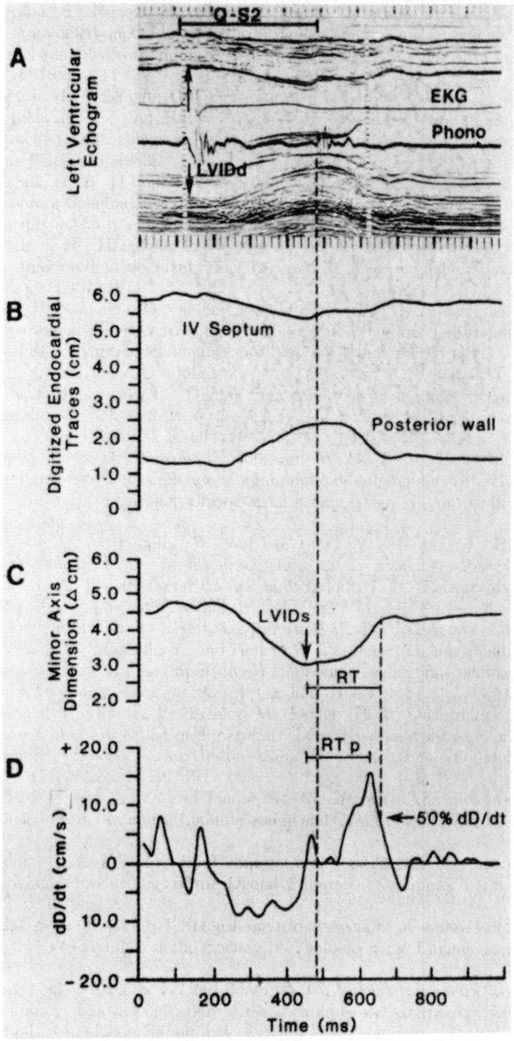

FIGURE 5–16. Digitized M-mode echocardiogram of the left ventricle demonstrating the unprocessed M-mode recording (*A*), the digitized tracing of the interventricular septum and posterior left ventricular walls (*B*), the minor axis dimension, which is the difference between the two opposing walls (*C*), and the rate of change of the minor axis (dD/dt). LVIDd = left ventricular diastolic diameter; LVIDs = left ventricular systolic diameter; RT = relaxation time; RTp = relaxation time to peak velocity of lengthening. (From Bahler, R. C., et al.: The relation of heart rate and shortening fraction to echocardiographic indexes of left ventricular relaxation in normal subjects. Reprinted by permission of the American College of Cardiology. J. Am. Coll. Cardiol. 2:926, 1983.)

TWO-DIMENSIONAL ECHOCARDIOGRAPHY

One could essentially obtain an infinite number of slices of the heart using two-dimensional echocardiography. The American Society of Echocardiography has attempted to standardize and simplify the many two-dimensional examinations.[37] The Society thought that all views could be categorized into three orthogonal planes, as illustrated in Figure 5–17. These planes are the long-axis, short-axis, and four-chamber. The long-axis plane is the imaging plane that transects the heart perpendicular to the dorsal and ventral surfaces of the body and parallel to the long axis of the heart. The plane transecting the heart perpendicular to the dorsal and ventral surfaces of the body, but perpendicular to the long axis of the heart, is defined as the short-axis plane. The plane that transects the heart approximately parallel to the dorsal and ventral surfaces of the body is referred to as the four-chamber plane. It should be emphasized that these views or planes are with reference to the heart and not to the thorax or body.

TRANSDUCER LOCATIONS. These ultrasonic planes or views can be obtained from more than one transducer location. Figure 5–18*A* demonstrates that one can obtain the long-axis view with the transducer in the apical position, in the parasternal position (left sternal border), or in the suprasternal notch. A short-axis view (Fig. 5–18*B*) cuts across the heart so that the left ventricle looks like a circle. The right ventricle can be seen curving around the left ventricle. Such an examination can be obtained with the transducer in the parasternal position or in the subcostal (subxiphoid) position. The four-chamber view is depicted in Figure 5–18*C*. Such a view permits the examination of all four cardiac chambers simultaneously. This type of examination can be obtained with the transducer over the cardiac apex or with the transducer in the subcostal position.

Table 5–2 lists the various two-dimensional echocardiographic examinations categorized according to the location of the transducer, the plane of the examination, and the cardiac structure being examined.

Figure 5–17 is an example of a *parasternal long-axis examination* through the left ventricle. The right ventricle, right atrium, and tricuspid valve can also be recorded with the transducer in the parasternal

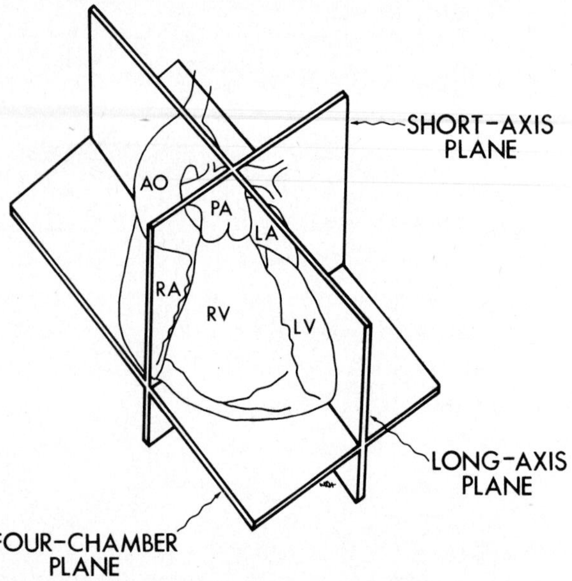

FIGURE 5–17. Diagram demonstrating the three orthogonal planes for two-dimensional echocardiographic imaging. AO = aorta; PA = pulmonary artery; LA = left atrium; RA = right atrium; RV = right ventricle; LV = left ventricle. (From Henry, W. L., et al.: Report of the American Society of Echocardiography Nomenclature and Standards in Two-dimensional Echocardiography. Circulation *62*:212, 1980, by permission of the American Heart Association, Inc.)

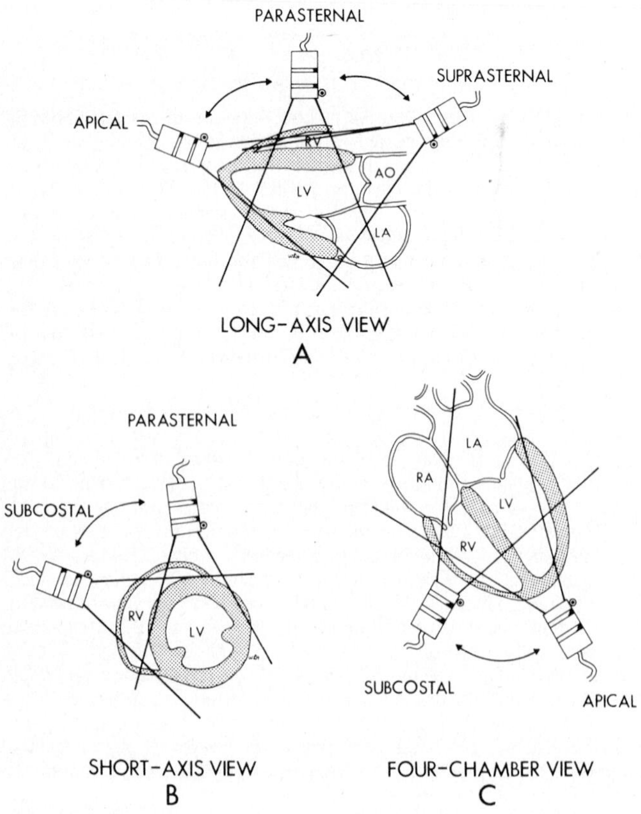

FIGURE 5–18. Diagrams demonstrating how one can obtain the various orthogonal planes from different transducer positions. (From Henry, W. L., et al.: Report of the American Society of Echocardiography Nomenclature and Standards in Two-dimensional Echocardiography. Circulation *62*:212, 1980, by permission of the American Heart Association, Inc.)

TABLE 5–2 TWO-DIMENSIONAL ECHOCARDIOGRAPHIC EXAMINATION

Parasternal Approach
Long-axis plane
Root of aorta–aortic valve, left atrium, left ventricular outflow tract
Body of left ventricle–mitral valve
Left ventricular apex
Right ventricular inflow tract–tricuspid valve
Short-axis plane
Root of the aorta–aortic valve, pulmonary valve, tricuspid valve, right ventricular outflow tract, left atrium, pulmonary artery, coronary arteries
Left ventricle–mitral valve
Left ventricle–papillary muscles
Left ventricle–apex
Apical Approach
Four-chamber plane
Four chamber
Four chamber with aorta
Long-axis plane
Two chamber–left ventricle, left atrium
Two chamber with aorta
Subcostal Approach
Four-chamber plane–all four chambers and both septa
Short-axis plane
Left ventricle
Right ventricle
Inferior vena cava
Suprasternal Approach
Four-chamber plane
Arch of aorta–descending aorta
Long-axis plane
Arch of aorta–pulmonary artery, left atrium

position (Fig. 5–19). The plane of the transducer does not exactly fit either the long axis or short axis. However, the plane is closer to that of the long axis than that of the short axis and thus is categorized as a long-axis study. Figure 5–20 shows the right ventricular inflow tract and right atrium by way of such a parasternal examination.

Various *short-axis examinations* are diagrammatically illustrated in Figure 5–21. The short-axis views are commonly obtained at the level of the apex, the papillary muscles, the mitral valve, and the base of the heart. With slight variation in angulation the short-axis examination of the base of the heart can also record the pulmonary valve and the pulmonary artery with its bifurcation. It is also possible to use this examination to record the origins of the coronary arteries and the left atrial appendage.

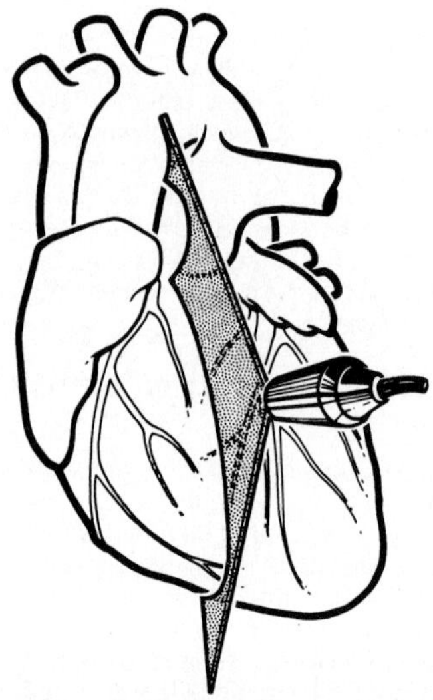

FIGURE 5–19. Transducer position for long-axis parasternal examination of the tricuspid valve, right atrium, and right ventricular inflow tract. (From Feigenbaum, H.: Echocardiography. 4th ed. Philadelphia, Lea and Febiger, 1986.)

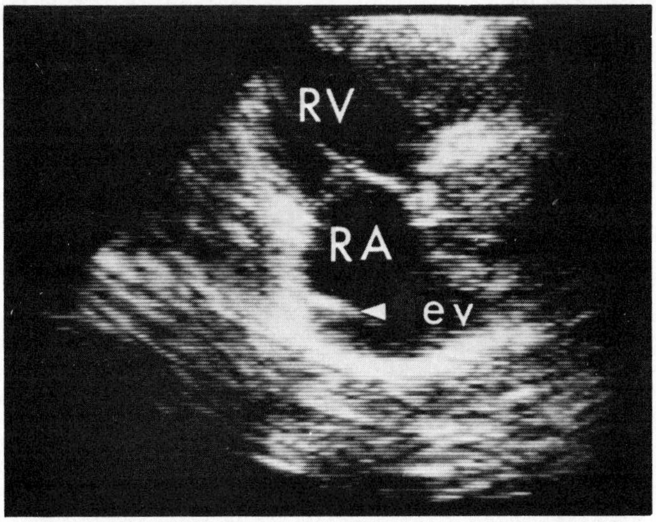

FIGURE 5–20. Two-dimensional echocardiogram of the right atrium (RA) and right ventricular inflow tract (RV). ev = eustachian valve. (From Feigenbaum, H.: Echocardiography. 4th ed. Philadelphia, Lea and Febiger, 1986.)

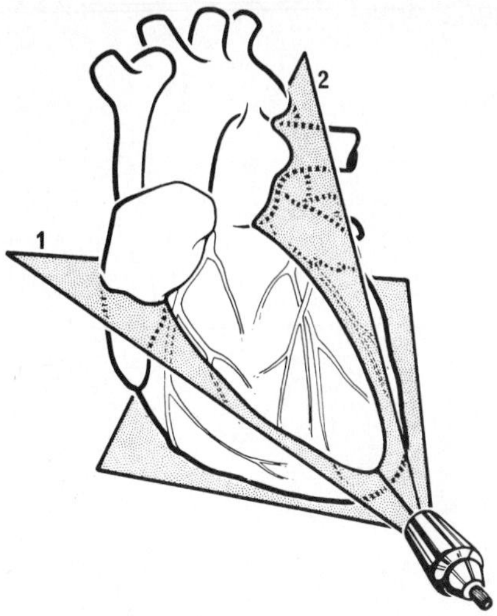

FIGURE 5–22. Transducer position and examining planes for apical two-dimensional echocardiograms. Plane 1 passes through the four chamber plane of the heart. Plane 2 represents the path of the ultrasonic beam for the two-chamber apical examination. (From Feigenbaum, H.: Echocardiography. 4th ed. Philadelphia, Lea and Febiger, 1986.)

Figure 5–22 diagrammatically illustrates the two commonly used two-dimensional echocardiographic views with the transducer placed at the *cardiac apex*. Plane 1 demonstrates the apical four-chamber view of the heart. Figure 5–23*A* shows an example of a four-chamber apical echocardiogram. It is possible to obtain an apical view of the long axis of the heart similar to that seen from the parasternal view. Such an examination would include portions of the right ventricle and the aorta. A more common examination is a so-called apical two-chamber view (Fig. 5–22, plane 2). This examination requires slight clockwise rotation of the transducer to avoid the right ventricle completely. Thus, one records only the left ventricle and the left atrium (Fig. 5–23*B*). This view can be considered a modification of an apical long-axis view.

The *subcostal transducer location* produces examinations roughly in the four-chamber and short-axis planes. The ultrasonic plane indicated in Figure 5–24*A* is similar to examining plane 1 in Figure 5–22. The resultant subcostal four-chamber echocardiogram appears in Figure 5–25*A*. Figures 5–24*B* and 5–25*B* show how the transducer can be rotated 90 degrees to provide a subcostal short-axis examination of the heart. The subcostal four-chamber view is particularly helpful in examining the interatrial and interventricular septa. By directing the transducer in a slightly modified short-axis examination, one can obtain an excellent view of the right side of the heart (Fig. 5–26*A*). The subcostal location also permits an opportunity to direct the ultrasonic beam through the inferior vena cava and hepatic vein (Figs. 5–26*B* and 5–27).

The two examining planes with the transducer in the suprasternal

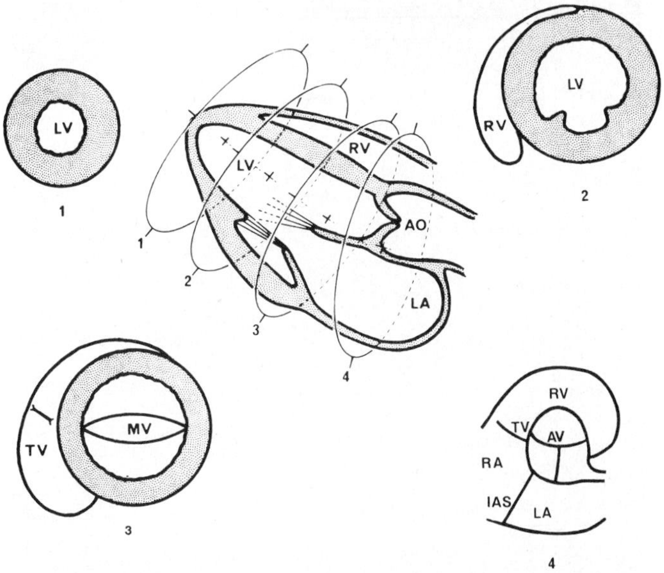

FIGURE 5–21. Diagrams showing how short-axis echographic cross-sectional images of the heart, which are perpendicular to the long axis of the left ventricle, are obtained. Diagram 1 shows a short-axis left ventricular echogram near the cardiac apex. Diagram 2 demonstrates part of the right ventricle (RV) and the circular left ventricular cavity (LV) at the level of the papillary muscles, which can be seen to bulge into the LV cavity. Diagram 3 is closer to the base of the heart and shows the left ventricle at the level of the mitral valve (MV). Diagram 4 shows a short-axis cross-section of the base of the heart with the aorta, aortic valve (AV), left atrium (LA), interatrial septum (IAS), right atrium (RA), tricuspid valve (TV), and right ventricular outflow tract (RV).

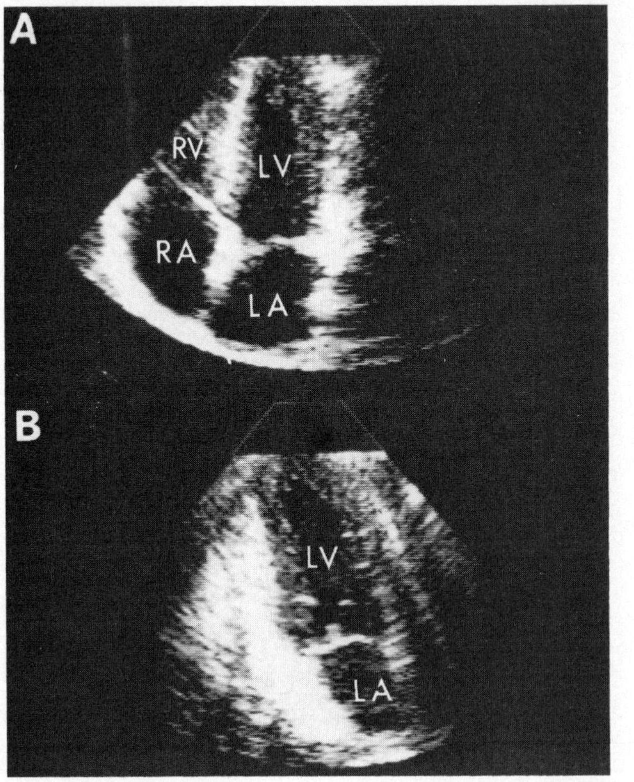

FIGURE 5–23. Four-chamber (*A*) and two-chamber (*B*) apical two-dimensional echocardiograms. RV = right ventricle; LV = left ventricle; RA = right atrium; and LA = left atrium. (From Feigenbaum, H.: Echocardiography. 4th ed. Philadelphia, Lea and Febiger, 1986.)

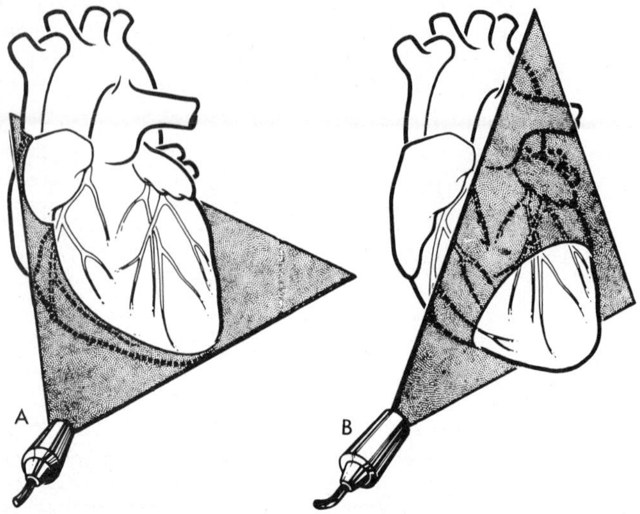

FIGURE 5–24. Diagrams showing the transducer position and examining planes for a subcostal four-chamber examination (*A*) and a subcostal short-axis examination (*B*). (From Feigenbaum, H.: Echocardiography. 4th ed. Philadelphia, Lea and Febiger, 1986.)

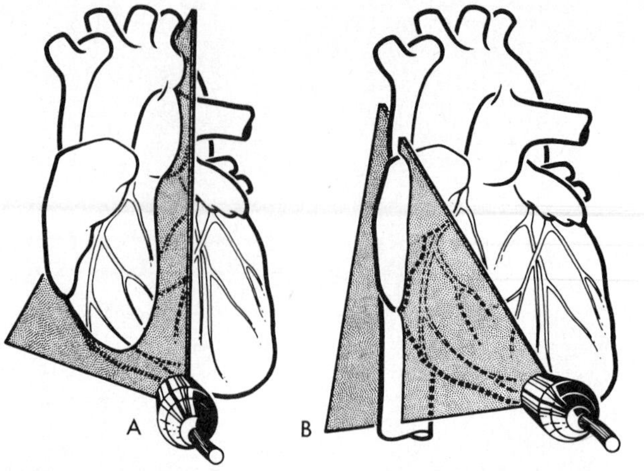

FIGURE 5–26. Diagram demonstrating the examining planes and transducer positions for the subcostal examination for the right side of the heart (*A*) and the inferior vena cava (*B*). (From Feigenbaum, H.: Echocardiography. 4th ed. Philadelphia, Lea and Febiger, 1986.)

notch are depicted in Figure 5–28. The ultrasonic view in Figure 5–28*A* is roughly equivalent to that of a four-chamber plane, and the view in Figure 5–28*B* is somewhat comparable to that of the long-axis plane. However, it is probably best to orient the ultrasonic beam with regard to the arch of the aorta rather than to the heart, since one does not record much of the heart with the transducer in this position, especially in the adult. In addition, the planes are different than with the transducer at the apex or subcostal region. Thus, better terminology with regard to the examining plane from the suprasternal location would be parallel or perpendicular to the arch of the aorta. Figure 5–29 shows a suprasternal examination parallel to the arch of the aorta.

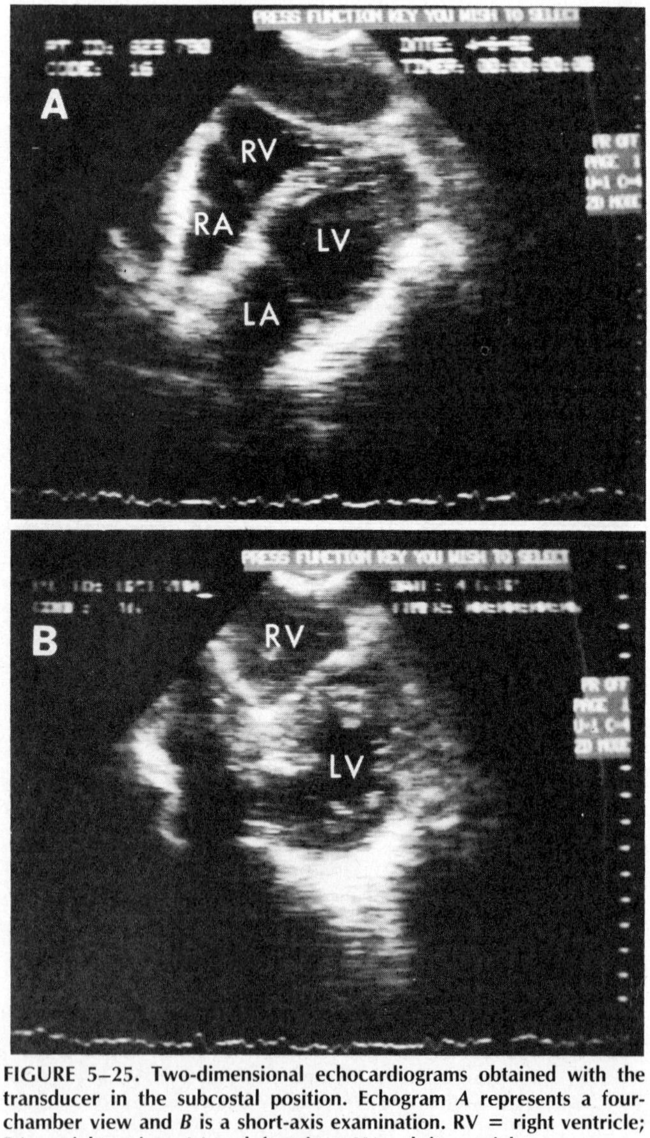

FIGURE 5–25. Two-dimensional echocardiograms obtained with the transducer in the subcostal position. Echogram *A* represents a four-chamber view and *B* is a short-axis examination. RV = right ventricle; RA = right atrium; LA = left atrium; LV = left ventricle.

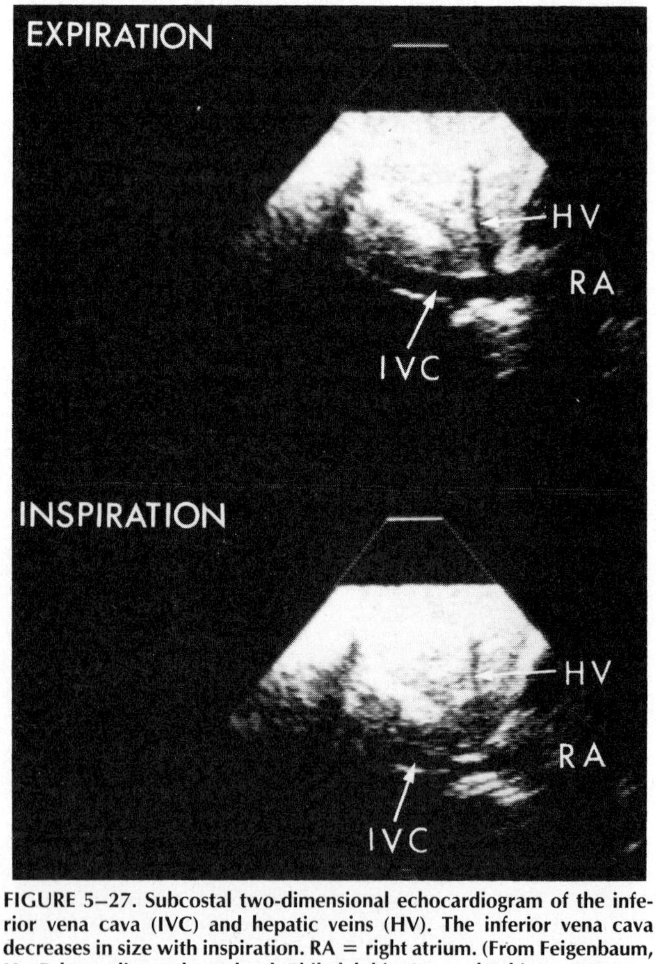

FIGURE 5–27. Subcostal two-dimensional echocardiogram of the inferior vena cava (IVC) and hepatic veins (HV). The inferior vena cava decreases in size with inspiration. RA = right atrium. (From Feigenbaum, H.: Echocardiography. 4th ed. Philadelphia, Lea and Febiger, 1986.)

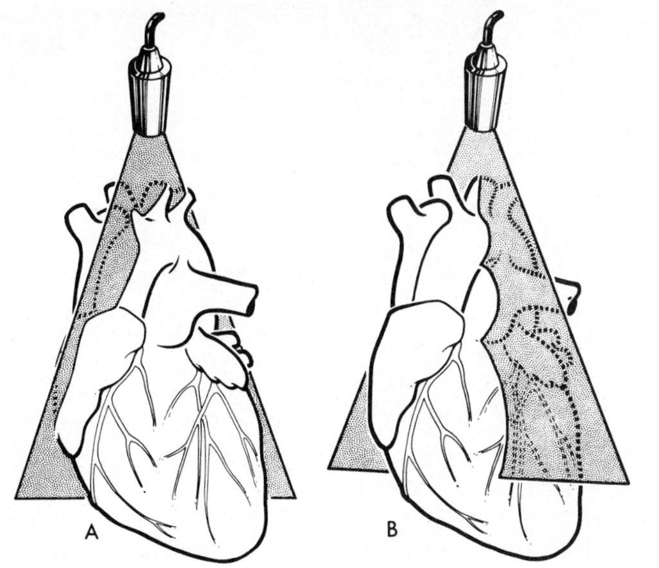

FIGURE 5–28. Transducer position in examining planes for the suprasternal examination parallel to the arch of the aorta (*A*) and perpendicular to the arch of the aorta (*B*). (From Feigenbaum, H.: Echocardiography. 4th ed. Philadelphia, Lea and Febiger, 1986.)

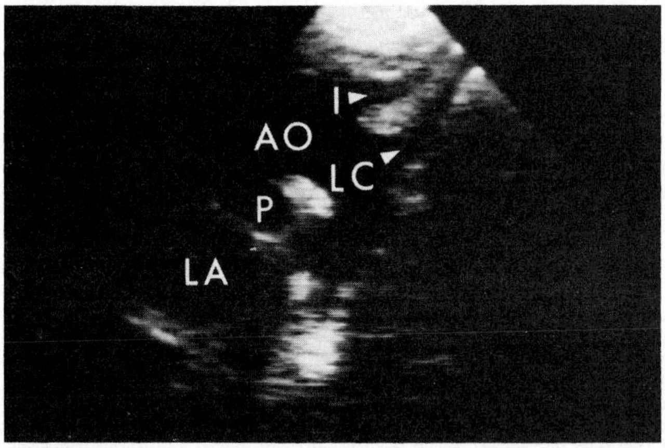

FIGURE 5–29. Suprasternal echocardiographic examination of the arch of the aorta (AO), pulmonary artery (P), and left atrium (LA). I = innominate artery; LC = left common carotid artery.

DOPPLER ECHOCARDIOGRAPHY

Doppler echocardiographic recordings of the normal heart consist primarily of two types of flow patterns. The two types of blood flow are ventricular outflow and ventricular inflow. Figure 5–30 shows Doppler recordings of left ventricular outflow in the ascending aorta, the descending aorta, and the left ventricular outflow tract. The only difference in the recordings is whether the flow is toward or away from the transducer. With the transducer in the suprasternal notch the normal systolic flow in the ascending aorta is toward the transducer. In the descending aorta systolic flow is away from the transducer and the Doppler signal is below the baseline. With the transducer at the cardiac apex and the Doppler sample in the left ventricular outflow tract, blood flow is again away from the transducer. A similar flow pattern is noted in the right ventricular outflow tract (Fig. 5–31). The peak velocity and acceleration are greater in the aorta than in the pulmonary artery.

Figure 5–32 demonstrates the Doppler flow pattern in the left ven-

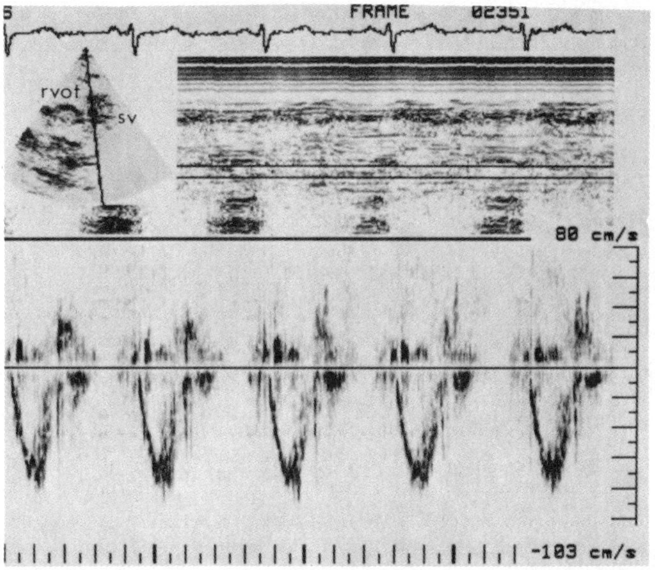

FIGURE 5–31. Pulsed Doppler recording of pulmonary artery flow. The two-dimensional scan is a parasternal short-axis examination through the base of the heart. rvot = right ventricular outflow tract; sv = sample volume. (From Feigenbaum, H.: Echocardiography. 4th ed. Philadelphia, Lea and Febiger, 1986.)

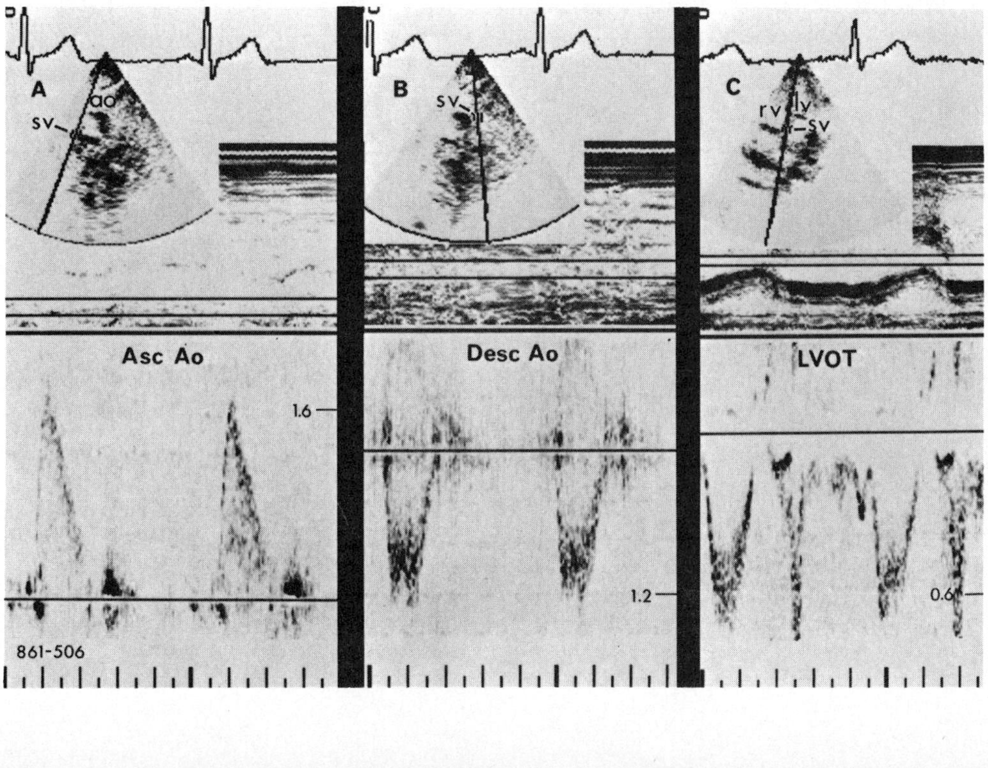

FIGURE 5–30. Pulsed Doppler echocardiogram of flow in the ascending aorta (Asc Ao) with the transducer in the suprasternal notch (A), flow in the descending aorta (Desc Ao) with the transducer in the suprasternal notch (B), and Doppler flow in the left ventricular outflow tract (LVOT) with the transducer at the apex (C). sv = sample volume; lv = left ventricle; ao = aortic root; rv = right ventricle. (From Feigenbaum, H.: Echocardiography. 4th ed. Philadelphia, Lea and Febiger, 1986.)

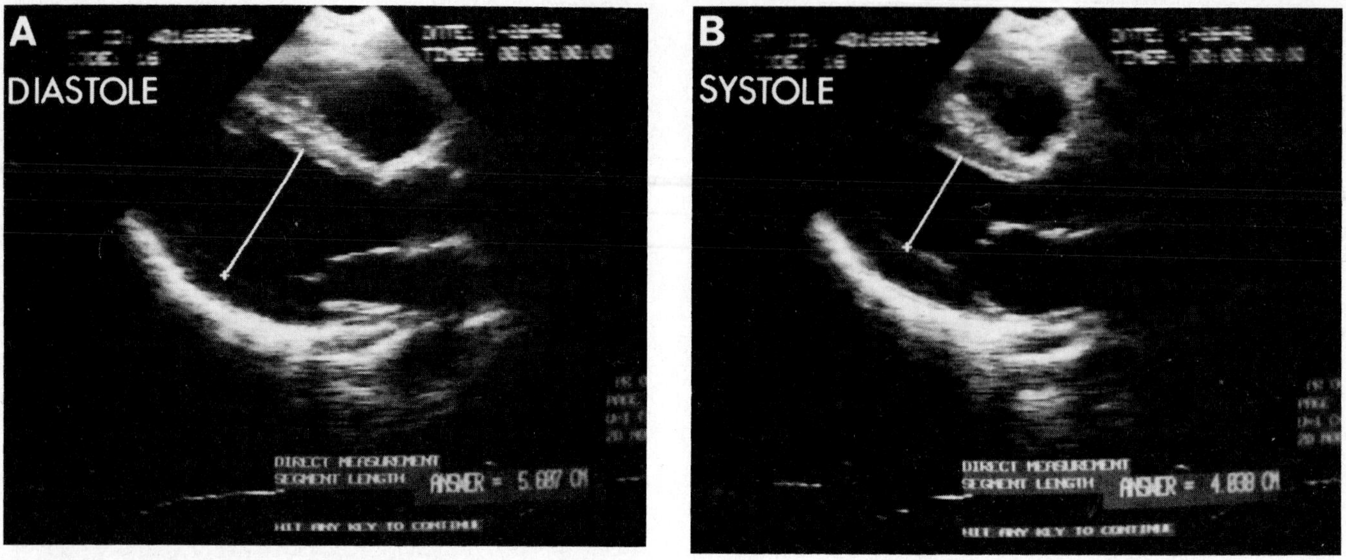

FIGURE 5–32. Parasternal long-axis examinations demonstrating how a minor dimension of the left ventricle can be measured in diastole and systole.

tricular inflow tract just past the mitral valve. The Doppler recording superficially resembles an M-mode tracing of the anterior mitral leaflet. There is rapid inflow in early diastole, decreasing flow in mid-diastole, and a subsequent increase in flow with atrial systole. Doppler tricuspid flow is almost identical to that of mitral flow except that the peak velocity is somewhat lower.

EVALUATION OF CARDIAC PERFORMANCE

(see Chap. 15)

M-MODE ECHOCARDIOGRAPHY

The ability to evaluate the function of the left ventricle by means of echocardiography has been one of the principal factors in the increasing application of this technique. The standard M-mode technique may be used to record a dimension of the left ventricle between the left side of the interventricular septum and the endocardial surface of the posterior left ventricular wall (Figs. 5–14 and 5–15).[38] Measurements of this dimension in end-diastole and end-systole may be made. Although these dimensions can be used to estimate ventricular volume, there are many potential errors in such calculations,[39, 40] since many assumptions that are not always valid are required to obtain the volume of a three-dimensional object from measurement of a single dimension. Irrespective of whether or not M-mode echocardiography can calculate true left ventricular volumes, simple dimensions of the left ventricle can provide an estimate of the overall size and performance of the left ventricle in many patients.[41] Fractional shortening, i.e., the difference between the end-diastolic and end-systolic dimensions divided by the end-diastolic dimension,[41] provides information about left ventricular systolic function. The quotient of fractional shortening and ejection time provides the mean fractional or circumferential shortening.[42] While these measurements are useful in judging left ventricular performance, it must be appreciated that the ventricle must be contracting uniformly for them to reflect global function. These echocardiographic measurements assess the status of only the basal portion of the chamber and must be interpreted with caution in patients with segmentally diseased left ventricles,[43] with left bundle branch block, with a dilated right ventricle, or with a low echocardiographic window so that the M-mode measurement is closer to the major axis rather than the minor axis.

Another M-mode echocardiographic technique for assessing the status of the left ventricle is to measure the distance between the E point of the mitral valve and the left side of the interventricular septum.[44, 45] Normally, the mitral E point and the left side of the septum are within a few millimeters of each other. The upper limits of normal of the mitral E point–septal separation (EPSS) is approximately 8 mm. As the left ventricular ejection fraction decreases, the EPSS increases. Although there are some limitations to the utility of this measurement, especially when there is regional left ventricular dysfunction, this measurement is useful and fairly popular. Even though the observation is principally empiric, there is some rationale behind the measurement. As the left ventricle dilates, the septum moves anteriorly. The opening of the mitral valve is largely dependent upon the volume of blood passing through that orifice. As the mitral valve flow or left ventricular stroke volume decreases, the amplitude of the E point is decreased. Thus, with a decreased stroke volume and/or left ventricular dilatation, the septum and anterior mitral leaflet would move in opposite directions. Therefore, with a decreased ejection fraction, which is stroke volume divided by diastolic volume, it is not unreasonable to expect an increase in the distance between the mitral valve E point and the interventricular septum. Naturally, if there is intrinsic valvular disease, such as mitral stenosis, then the excursion of the mitral valve is not a reliable indicator of flow through that orifice. In patients with aortic regurgitation, mitral valve flow is not an indicator of total left ventricular stroke volume, and one would not be able to provide an assessment of ejection fraction.

TWO-DIMENSIONAL ECHOCARDIOGRAPHY

The limited number of sampling sites for the M-mode dimensions and the lack of spatial orientation limits the clinical usefulness of these measurements. Thus, it is not surprising that there has been interest in using two-dimensional echocardiography for assessing the cardiac chambers. Hesitancy to use the two-dimensional approach has been caused by the inconvenience associated with analyzing a recording made on videotape. With the advent of newer videotape and video disc systems, electronic calipers, bit pads, light pens, and computers, it is becoming

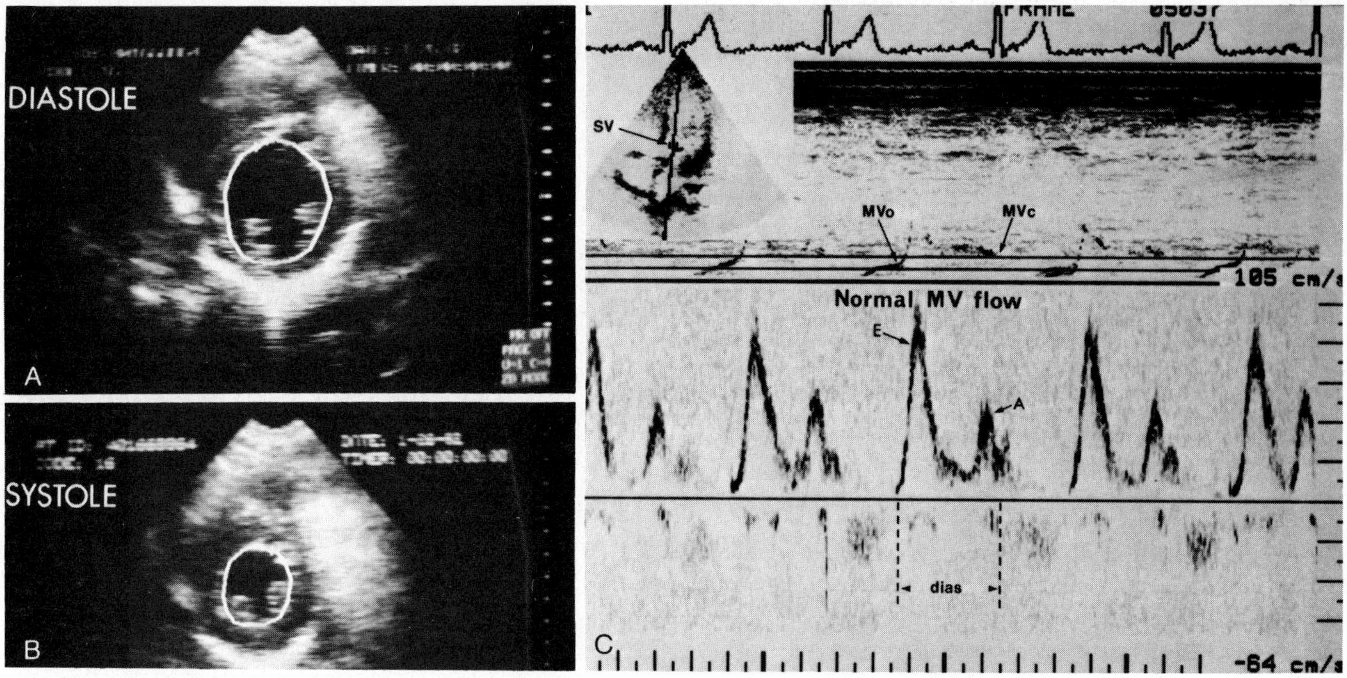

FIGURE 5–33. *A, B,* Short-axis two-dimensional echocardiograms demonstrating how the area of the left ventricle at the papillary muscle level can be measured in diastole and systole. *C,* Normal mitral valve (MV) flow with the transducer at the apex and the sample volume (sv) in the left ventricle. MVo = mitral valve opening; MVc = mitral valve closure. (From Feigenbaum, H.: Echocardiography. 4th ed. Philadelphia, Lea and Febiger, 1986.)

more convenient to make the necessary measurements from the two-dimensional examination.

There have been numerous attempts to use two-dimensional echocardiography to calculate left ventricular volumes.[46–49] Several geometric formulas have been suggested. These include the *area-length technique* commonly used for angiographic volumes. The *Simpson's rule* formula is attractive because it minimizes the effect of geometric shape for calculating volumes. An intriguing formula is that which describes the left ventricle as a bullet, which consists of a cylinder and a half of a prolate ellipse.[50] The formula for calculating left ventricular volume using the *bullet formula* is volume equals five-sixths the area of the left ventricle times the length of the left ventricle ($V = 5/6\ AL$). This formula is attractive because of its simplicity and because the area of the left ventricle and the length of the left ventricle can be easily obtained with two-dimensional echocardiography.

Another simplified approach to assessing the left ventricle with two-dimensional echocardiography is merely to obtain minor axis measurements using the parasternal long-axis and short-axis views.[2] It is possible to obtain a true minor dimension using the parasternal long-axis examination. One can also obtain a short-axis area at the level of the papillary muscles. Derived indices, such as fractional shortening or fractional area change, can be obtained with this approach. Figures 5–32 and 5–33 illustrate how one can obtain the minor dimension from the parasternal long-axis examination (Fig. 5–32) and how the short-axis area can be measured at the level of the papillary muscles (Fig. 5–33).

Doppler Echocardiography

This technique can be used to evaluate left ventricular systolic function with a recording of flow in the ascending aorta. Acceleration time, from the onset of flow to the time of peak acceleration (Fig. 5–34), and peak acceleration have been shown to be related to global left ventricular systolic function.[51, 52]

Diastolic Function

Echocardiography has been used to evaluate left ventricular diastolic function. M-mode techniques have been used to record the rate of relaxation of the left ventricular cavity. This technique utilizes digitization of the borders of the left ventricular cavity, with the rapidity being noted with which the left ventricular dimension increases in early diastole (Fig. 5–35). Doppler echocardiography is also being used for evaluating left ventricular diastolic function.[53, 54] It can be noticed that early diastolic flow is reduced and the velocity following atrial contraction is increased.[55] This phenomenon has been quantitated in several ways. The simple technique is to take a ratio of the peak velocity with early filling or E point and the peak velocity with atrial filling or A point. Normally the velocity at the E point is significantly higher than at the A point (Fig. 5–32). With reduced left ventricular compliance this ratio is reversed (Fig. 5–35).

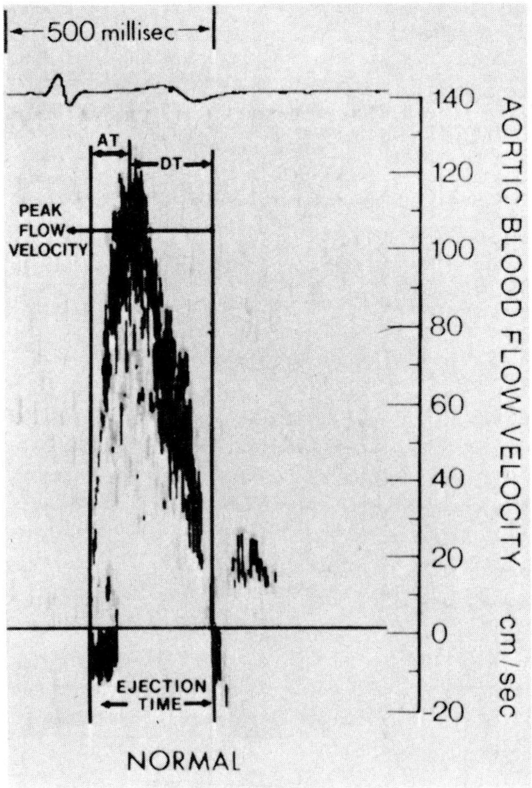

FIGURE 5–34. Pulsed Doppler recording of aortic blood flow velocity demonstrating how ejection time, peak flow velocity, acceleration time (AT), and deceleration time (DT) are measured. (From Gardin, J. M., et al.: Evaluation of blood flow velocity in the ascending aorta and main pulmonary artery of normal subjects by Doppler echocardiography. Am. Heart J. *107*:310, 1984.)

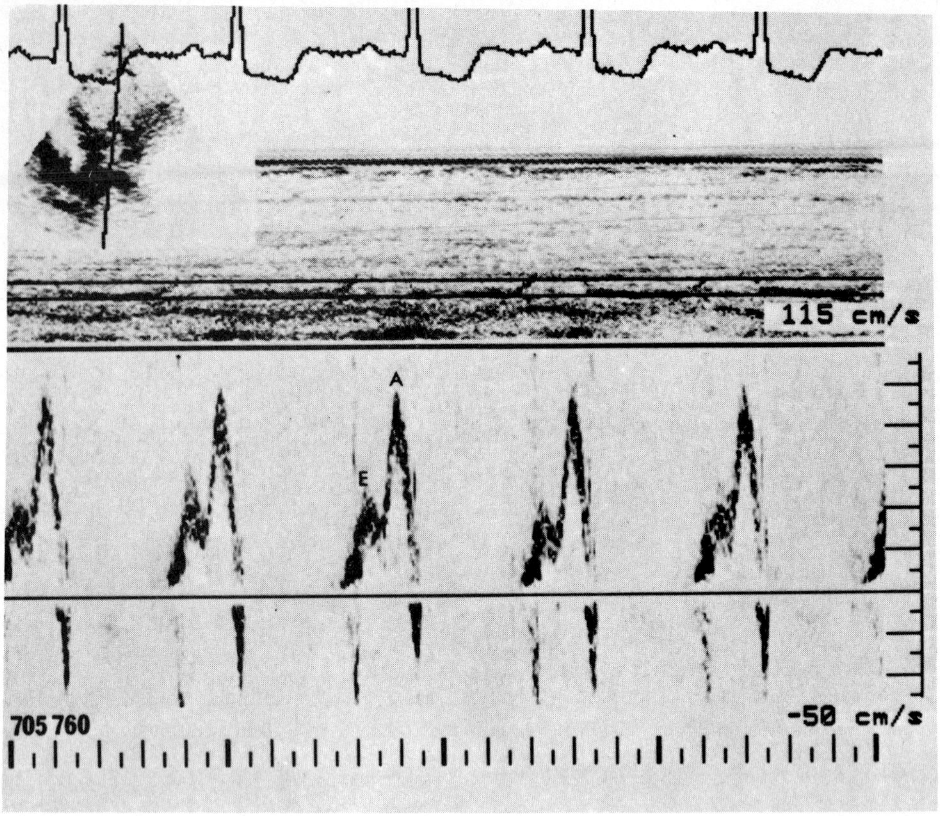

FIGURE 5–35. Mitral valve flow pattern in a patient with reduced left ventricular compliance. Early diastolic velocity (E) is reduced, and late velocity following atrial contraction (A) is increased. (From Feigenbaum, H.: Echocardiography. 4th ed. Philadelphia, Lea and Febiger, 1986.)

Exercise Echocardiography

Although echocardiography has been used primarily for evaluating the cardiac chambers at rest, there is increasing interest in performing the ultrasonic examination during or immediately after exercise. These studies have utilized supine or upright bicycle exercise,[56] immediate post-treadmill exercise, pharmacological stress, and atrial pacing.[57] Many of the technical difficulties involved in recording an echocardiogram while the patient is hyperventilating following exercise have been overcome by using digital techniques which record a single cardiac cycle in a continuous loop display.[58] This digital approach eliminates the respiratory artifact and permits the resting and exercise studies to be presented side by side for ease of interpretation. This type of examination is being done primarily for detecting exercise-induced regional wall motion abnormalities in patients with coronary artery disease. Exercise studies using Doppler measurements of ascending aortic flow have also been used to assess global changes in left ventricular function during exercise.[59]

Wall Thickness

Echocardiography may also be employed to measure the thickness of the walls of the ventricle.[60] The absolute thickness of the ventricle is important in determining the presence of left ventricular hypertrophy (Fig. 5–36), in estimating left ventricular mass,[61–63] and in calculating left ventricular end-systolic stress.[64] Echocardiography also permits measurement of changes in left ventricular thickness during the cardiac cycle.[65] Normally, the left ventricular wall thickens during systole, but in pathological conditions this thickening decreases and actual systolic thinning has been noted in acute ischemia or myocardial infarction.[66]

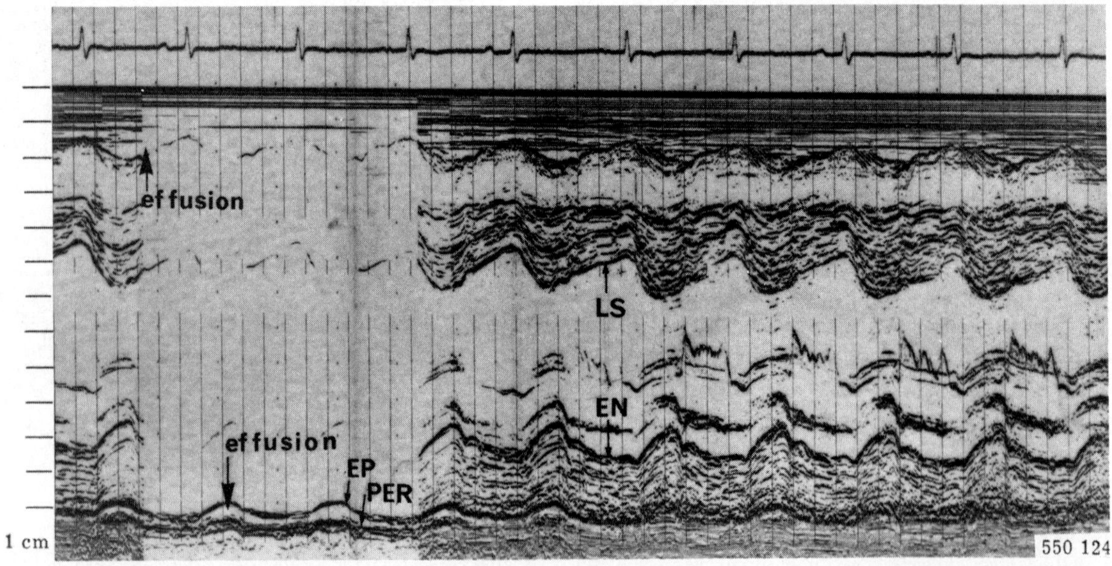

FIGURE 5–36. Left ventricular echocardiogram from a patient with left ventricular hypertrophy and a small pericardial effusion. The thickness of the interventricular septum and posterior left ventricular wall is markedly increased. LS = left septum, EN = posterior left ventricular endocardium, EP = posterior left ventricular epicardium, PER = posterior pericardium. (From Chang, S.: M-Mode Echocardiographic Techniques and Pattern Recognition. Philadelphia, Lea and Febiger, 1976.)

Other Chambers

LEFT ATRIUM. Echocardiography offers the opportunity to evaluate all four cardiac chambers and not just the left ventricle. Left atrial dilatation is readily recognized on the M-mode[67] or two-dimensional echocardiogram.[68, 69] A variety of quantitative measurements have been introduced. A simple anterior-posterior dimension of the chamber is usually sufficient for identifying patients with dilated left atria. Such measurements can be done with either the M-mode or parasternal long-axis two-dimensional view. In patients in whom the left atrium does not uniformly expand or if there is distortion by a dilated aorta,[70] other views including the suprasternal M-mode and the apical two-dimensional views can be used to assess the size of the left atrium.[71, 72]

RIGHT VENTRICLE AND ATRIUM. The right ventricle is more difficult to evaluate quantitatively because of its unusual shape.[73, 74] However, gross dilatation is easily assessed with M-mode[75] or two-dimensional examinations. Probably the most common technique is to use the relative size of the right and left ventricles in the apical four-chamber view. The thickness of the right ventricular walls can also be detected using either M-mode or two-dimensional echocardiography.[76] With right ventricular dilatation there is frequently distortion of the shape of the interventricular septum.[77] Whether the distortion in shape occurs primarily during diastole or systole will indicate whether or not there is primarily a pressure or volume overload of the right ventricle.[78] With a diastolic overload the septum is flat in diastole and assumes a more normal curvature in systole. With a pressure overload the flattened interventricular septum can be seen with systole.

The right atrium can also be evaluated with two-dimensional echocardiography, using the apical four-chamber view.

HEMODYNAMIC INFORMATION

DOPPLER ECHOCARDIOGRAPHY. This is now the principal ultrasonic technique for obtaining hemodynamic information. By recording the velocity of intracardiac blood flow, one can obtain quantitative data concerning both blood flow and intracardiac pressures. The principle is illustrated in Figure 5–37. To calculate flow the mean velocity passing through an orifice or vessel and the cross-sectional area of the orifice or vessel must be known. The mean velocity is acquired by measuring the velocity time integral of the Doppler signal which is the area under the recording. The cross-sectional area of the orifice through which the blood is flowing can be obtained directly with two-dimensional echocardiography or the diameter can be measured with either two-dimensional[79] or M-mode echocardiography and then the area can be calculated. Such flow determinations are feasible through any orifice or vessel.[80]

Blood flow in the ascending aorta is commonly used for cardiac output calculations.[81] The integrated velocity from the ascending aorta is combined with the calculated cross-sectional area determined at any of three locations: the aortic annulus, the separation of the aortic valve leaflets, or just past the sinus of Valsalva. All three approaches have been used with reasonable success. In a similar manner pulmonary blood flow can be measured by taking Doppler pulmonary artery velocity and multiplying it by the cross-sectional area of the pulmonary artery. Flow through the mitral[82] and tricuspid[83] valves has also been calculated. Atrioventricular valve flow is somewhat more complicated since the flow is phasic and early and late diastolic flow must be allowed for.[84] Although the measurements are more complex, they have been reasonably accurate.

The effectiveness of Doppler echocardiography for measuring flow has been validated.[85] There are many technical details in making such calculations. The biggest limitation is the calculation of the orifice or vessel area. It is difficult to obtain an accurate cross-sectional area of the various orifices. Since a measured diameter would be squared, any error would also be squared. For example, in many adult patients it is difficult to obtain an accurate orifice measurement of the pulmonary artery.

Although the Doppler technique for measuring blood flow is fairly new and is not routinely done in many laboratories, the potential clinical utility is readily apparent. It can be used to measure cardiac output or stroke volume.[81, 86] The technique is particularly useful for following directional changes in these variables in a given patient.[87] By calculating flow through different orifices, regurgitant fractions[88] and shunt ratios can be quantified.[89] For example, pulmonary to systemic flow ratios can be obtained by measuring aortic and pulmonary artery flows. Mitral regurgitant fraction can be calculated by measuring aortic flow and mitral valve flow. With the increasing availability of computer analysis, the technical difficulties of making these calculations have been resolved.

DOPPLER MEASUREMENT OF PRESSURE GRADIENTS. Possibly the most important development in Doppler echocardiography has been the utilization of a modified version of the Bernoulli equation to calculate the pressure drop or gradient across a narrowed part of the cardiovascular system;[5] the principle is shown in Figure 5–38. Although the Bernoulli equation is fairly complex and involves convective acceleration, flow acceleration, and viscous friction, the equation can be limited to convective acceleration alone since flow acceleration and viscous friction are probably not relevant in the clinical setting. Essentially the equation relates the difference in pressure across a stenosis with the differences in velocities. As blood flows through a narrowed orifice, the velocity increases proportionally. By making a few assumptions which seem to be clinically appropriate, a fairly complicated equation can be condensed to the difference in pressure (Δ P) equals 4 times the square of the velocity distal to the obstruction.

The accuracy and validity of this approach has been confirmed in numerous laboratories.[90–92] This observation is now the basis for many clinical applications of Doppler echocardiography.

CLINICAL APPLICATIONS: THE ESTIMATION OF INTRACARDIAC PRESSURES. The first application was calculating

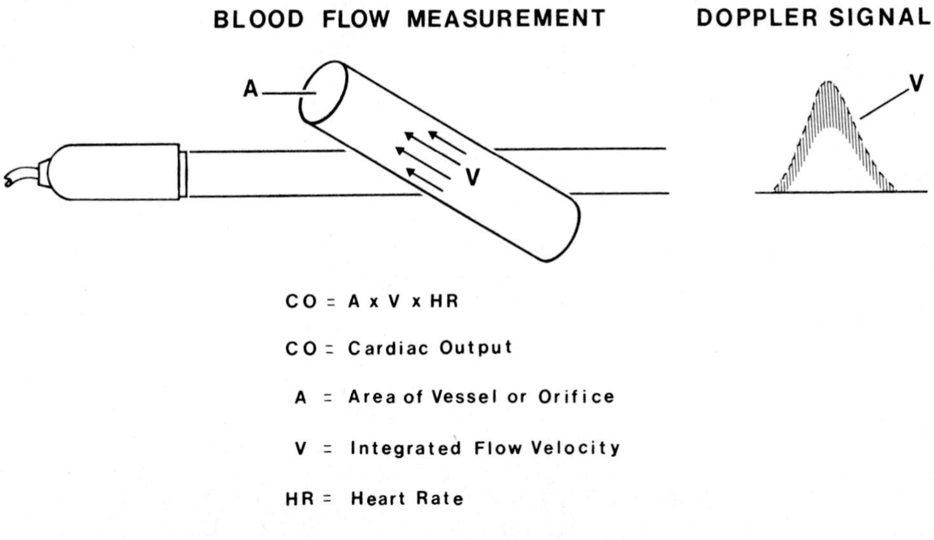

FIGURE 5–37. Principles of using Doppler echocardiography to measure blood flow. (From Feigenbaum, H.: Echocardiography. 4th ed. Philadelphia, Lea and Febiger, 1986.)

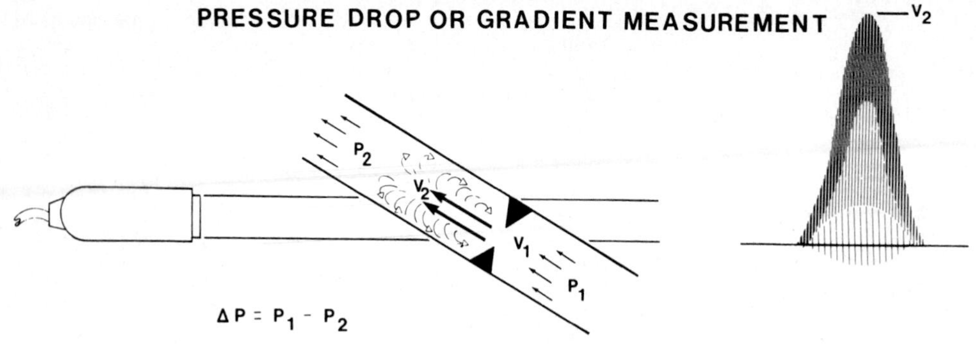

BERNOULLI EQUATION

$$P_1 - P_2 = \underbrace{\frac{1}{2}\rho(V_2^2 - V_1^2)}_{\text{CONVECTIVE ACCELERATION}} + \underbrace{\rho \int_1^2 \frac{\vec{DV}}{DT} DS}_{\text{FLOW ACCELERATION}} + \underbrace{R(\vec{V})}_{\text{VISCOUS FRICTION}}$$

$$P_1 - P_2 = \frac{1}{2}\rho(V_2^2 - V_1^2)$$

V_1 MUCH < V_2 ∴ IGNORE V_1

ρ = MASS DENSITY OF BLOOD = $1.06 \cdot 10^3$ KG/M^3

$$\therefore \Delta P = 4V_2^2$$

FIGURE 5–38. Principles of using Doppler echocardiography to measure a pressure drop or gradient across an obstruction. P_2 = pressure distal to an obstruction; V_2 = blood velocity distal to an obstruction; V_1 = velocity proximal to an obstruction; P_1 = pressure proximal to an obstruction. (From Feigenbaum, H.: Echocardiography. 4th ed. Philadelphia, Lea and Febiger, 1986.)

a pressure gradient across a stenotic mitral valve.[90] The approach was then used with stenotic semilunar valves.[91] This same technique can be used to assess the difference in pressure across a regurgitant valve as well as a stenotic valve. For example, in the presence of tricuspid regurgitation the difference in pressure can be assessed between the right ventricle and the right atrium in systole by noting the peak velocity of the regurgitant jet.[93, 94] Knowing the pressure differential between the right ventricle and right atrium and by adding an estimate of the right atrial pressure, one can calculate right ventricular systolic pressure. If there is no obstruction to right ventricular outflow, the pulmonary artery systolic pressure is also known. If the velocity of blood flow across a ventricular septal defect is measured, the difference in pressure between the left and right ventricles can also be calculated. By knowing the left ventricular systolic pressure and the gradient between that chamber and the right ventricle, one can calculate right ventricular systolic pressure.[95] A similar approach is possible with aortic-pulmonary shunts.[96] With the help of the modified Bernoulli equation Doppler echocardiography is playing an increasing role in determining intracardiac pressures.

The timing of the Doppler flow velocities can also provide hemodynamic information. For example, the flow pattern within the pulmonary artery can give clues to the presence of pulmonary hypertension.[97, 98] Figure 5–39 shows how the preejection period, acceleration time, and ejection time can be measured from the pulmonary artery Doppler recording. Acceleration time becomes short in the presence of pulmonary hypertension. The ratio of acceleration time to ejection time can also be used to make an assessment of pulmonary artery pressure. These measurements are better at identifying those patients with or without pulmonary hypertension than at providing a direct assessment of pulmonary artery pressure.

Since M-mode echocardiography has a sampling rate of 1000 impulses/second, the recording is virtually continuous and provides a very accurate assessment of cardiac motion. The motion of a valve is influenced by the flow of blood through its orifice and by alterations in the relative pressure on its two sides and thus provides considerable physiological information (Chaps. 3 and 4).

There have been many studies correlating echocardiographic *mitral valve* motion with hemodynamics. Figure 5–40, for example, demonstrates simultaneous recording of left ventricular pressure and a mitral valve echogram in a patient with atrial fibrillation and severe aortic regurgitation; the latter is reflected in the fluttering of the anterior

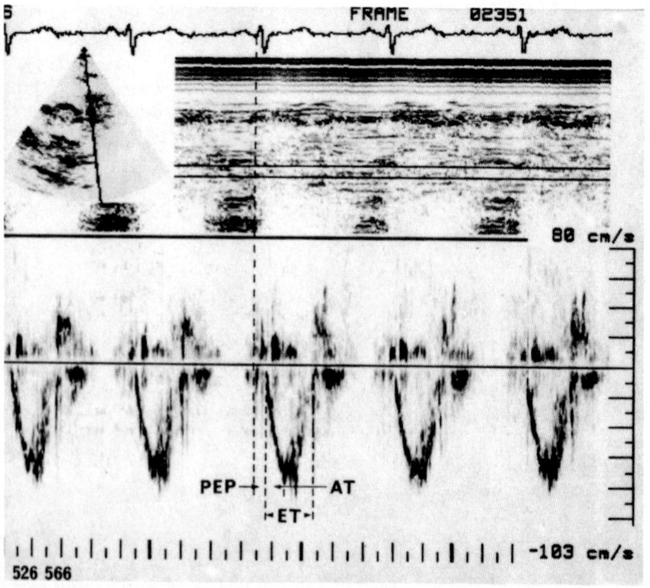

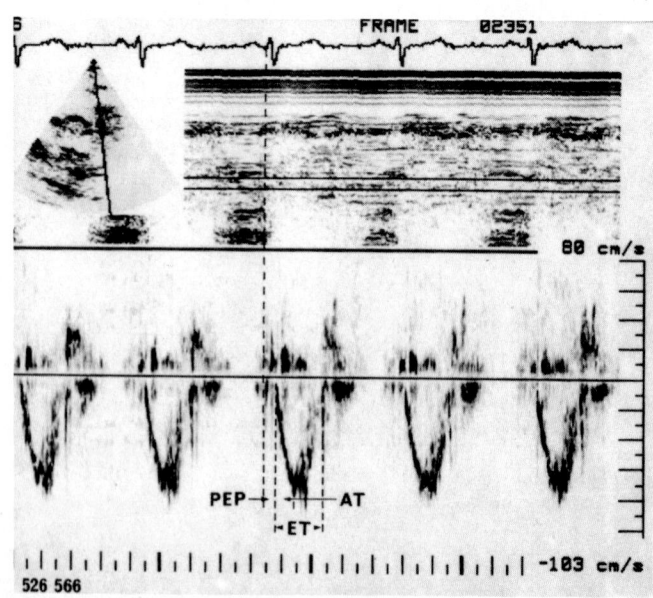

FIGURE 5–39. Measurements of pulmonary artery flow that can be used for estimating pulmonary artery pressure. PEP = pre-ejection period; AT = acceleration time; ET = ejection time. (From Feigenbaum, H.: Echocardiography. 4th ed. Philadelphia, Lea and Febiger, 1986.)

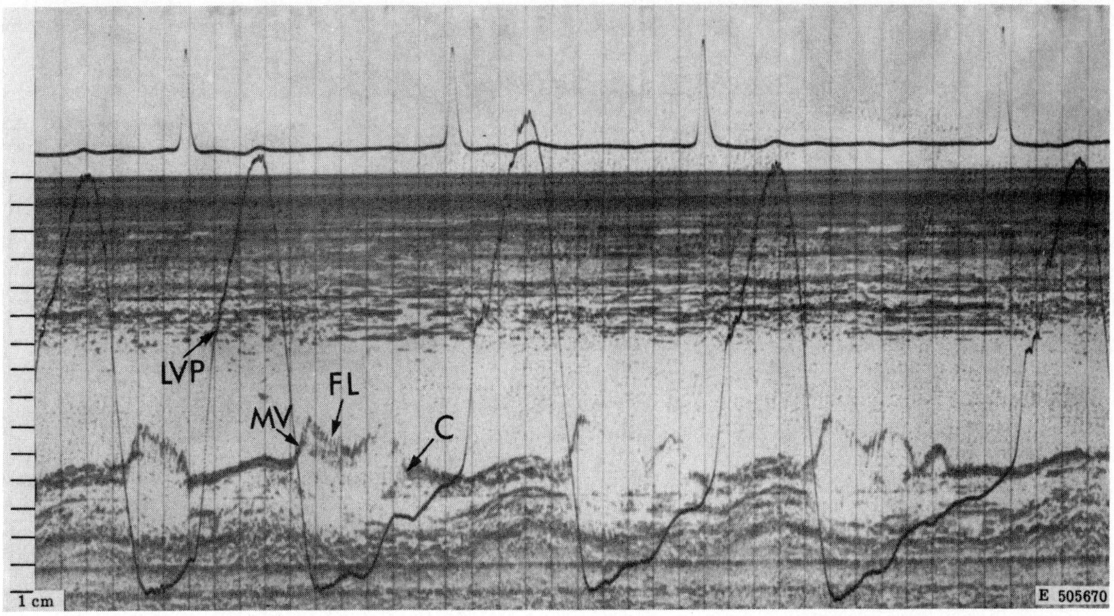

FIGURE 5–40. Simultaneous left ventricular pressure (LVP) and mitral valve echocardiogram (MV) from a patient with severe aortic regurgitation and atrial fibrillation. With a long diastolic internal pressure and a high left ventricular diastolic pressure, closure (C) of the valve occurs before the onset of electrical depolarization. Fluttering (FL) of the mitral valve can be noted. (From Feigenbaum, H.: Echocardiography. 2nd ed. Philadelphia, Lea and Febiger, 1976.)

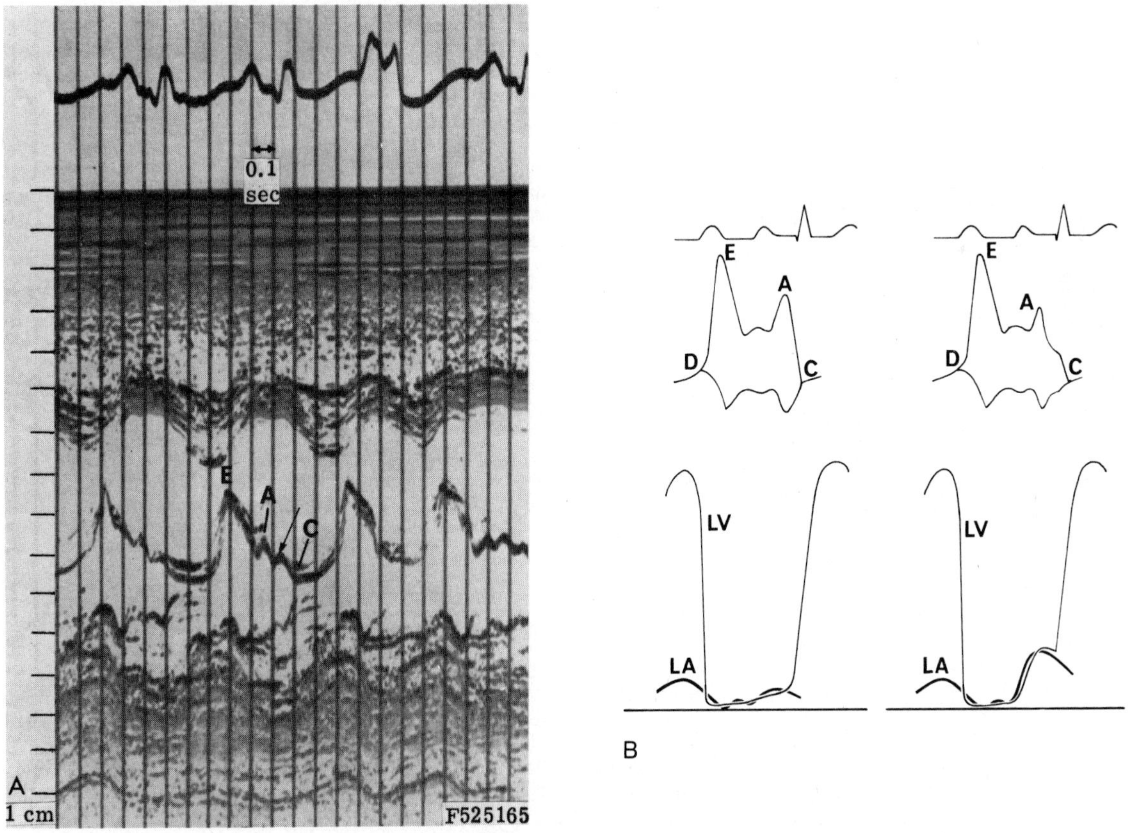

FIGURE 5–41. *A,* Mitral valve echocardiogram showing abnormal mitral valve closure in a patient with a high left ventricular end-diastolic pressure secondary to an elevated atrial component of the left ventricular pressure. Closure of the mitral valve (A to C) is prolonged and interrupted by a notch or plateau (arrow). (From Konecke, L. L., et al.: Abnormal mitral valve motion in patients with elevated left ventricular diastolic pressure. Circulation *47*:989, 1973, by permission of the American Heart Association, Inc.)

B, Diagrams illustrating how the mitral valve echogram relates to changes in left ventricular and left atrial diastolic pressures. With normally low left-heart pressures (*left*) mitral valve closure, from A to C, is smooth and uninterrupted. With an elevated left ventricular end-diastolic pressure secondary to an elevated atrial component (*right*), there is commonly interruption in the closure of the mitral valve with prolongation of the A-C interval. (From Feigenbaum, H.: Echocardiography. Philadelphia, Lea and Febiger, 1972.)

leaflet of the mitral valve, and the former is marked by variation in the duration of diastolic intervals and the left ventricular diastolic pressure. The first cardiac cycle has a low end-diastolic pressure, and the mitral valve closes with ventricular systole. The following diastolic intervals are longer, and the left ventricular diastolic pressure rises. With a high left ventricular diastolic pressure, as in the second cardiac cycle, the mitral valve is closed long before the onset of ventricular systole. Thus, in the setting of aortic regurgitation, premature closure of the mitral valve is a sign of a high left ventricular diastolic pressure.[99] This finding may be particularly helpful in the recognition of this hemodynamic abnormality in patients with acute aortic regurgitation secondary to infective endocarditis[100] (Ch. 34). The mitral valve M-mode echogram becomes distorted in patients who have tall and prominent *a* waves reflected in the left ventricular diastolic pressure.[101] Following atrial systole, closure of the valve is interrupted, and there is a plateau or notch between the A and C points just before the onset of ventricular systole (Fig. 5–41).[102]

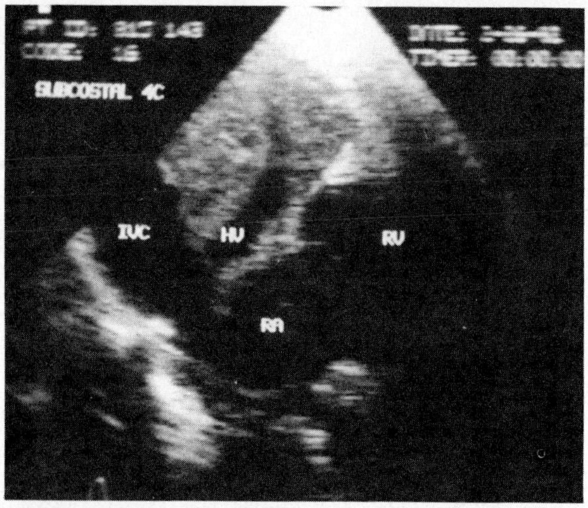

FIGURE 5–43. Subcostal two-dimensional echocardiogram of the right atrium (RA) and right ventricle (RV) in a patient with elevated right atrial pressure and a markedly dilated inferior vena cava (IVC) and hepatic vein (HV).

Analysis of *aortic valve* motion also provides useful hemodynamic information. In patients with obstructive hypertrophic cardiomyopathy, or discrete subaortic stenosis, closure of the aortic valve occurs during midsystole as the subaortic obstruction suddenly becomes manifested (Fig. 4–9, p. 69).[103] Patients with mitral regurgitation exhibit a gradual premature closure of the aortic valve late during systole as blood regurgitates into the left atrium and forward flow into the aorta diminishes.[2] This gradual late systolic closure of the aortic valve may also be seen in low cardiac output states in which the left ventricle may not be capable of sustaining a continuous flow of blood across the aortic valve. A correlation has been observed between the amplitude and duration of separation of the aortic leaflets and the left ventricular stroke volume.[104] In patients with severe aortic regurgitation and markedly elevated left ventricular diastolic pressure the aortic valve may open prior to ventricular systole.[105]

M-mode echograms of the *pulmonary valve* have proved to be useful in reflecting hemodynamic events as well. Although the pulmonary valve echogram is probably influenced in part by the movement of

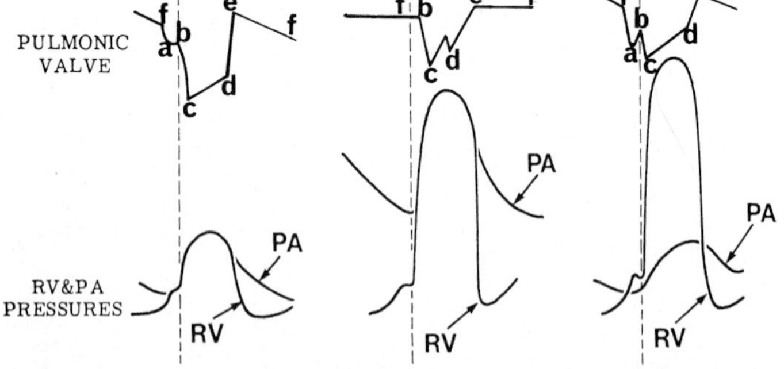

FIGURE 5–42. Diagrams demonstrating the relationship of the pulmonic valve echogram and right-heart pressure in the normal state, with pulmonary hypertension, and with pulmonic stenosis. PA = pulmonary artery pressure, RV = right ventricular pressure. (See text for details.) (From Feigenbaum, H.: Echocardiography. 2nd ed. Philadelphia, Lea and Febiger, 1976.)

structures to which it is attached,[106] the pressure relationship between the right ventricle and the pulmonary artery also influences the motion of the pulmonary valve (Fig. 5–42). Normally, atrial systole produces a slight downward motion of the pulmonary valve.[107] Whether at least part of this motion is due wholly or in part to the posterior motion of the entire base of the heart with atrial systole is not clear. However, there is evidence to suggest that the normal rise in right ventricular pressure occurring during atrial contraction may affect the position of the pulmonary valve. In pulmonic stenosis, the right ventricular systolic and end-diastolic pressures rise without any similar elevation in pulmonary artery pressure, and the atrial contribution to right ventricular pressure is exaggerated and usually sufficient to open the pulmonary valve prior to ventricular systole (Fig. 5–42).[108] In patients with elevated right ventricular diastolic pressure due to right ventricular failure, tricuspid regurgitation, constrictive pericarditis, or a communication between the aorta and right ventricle, the elevated pressure in the right ventricle in early diastole may cause opening of the pulmonic valve even prior to the onset of atrial systole.[109]

PULMONARY HYPERTENSION. An increase in pulmonary artery pressure has been shown to influence pulmonary valve motion in several ways (Fig. 5–42).[110] One of the most consistent changes is the elimination of atrial systolic motion, and the absence or marked reduction of the pulmonary valve *a* wave is one of the echocardiographic signs of pulmonary hypertension. As might be expected, when right ventricular failure occurs in pulmonary hypertension, right ventricular diastolic pressure may rise sufficiently so that a small *a* wave may again be recorded.[2] Another sign of pulmonary hypertension is midsystolic closure of the pulmonary valve.[110] Although this finding has not been explained, it is probably related to elevated pulmonary vascular resistance.[111]

The pulmonary valve echogram has been used to calculate systolic time intervals of the right side of the heart,[112] and these intervals, in turn, have been used to estimate pulmonary artery pressure and right ventricular performance.[113] Most of these measurements have now been replaced by calculations from Doppler echocardiography (p. 87).

With the two-dimensional echocardiographic examination of the inferior vena cava and hepatic vein, more information concerning right-sided hemodynamics is being obtained (Fig. 5–43).[114] This particular examination can be helpful in assessing the central venous pressure by noting the size of the veins[115] and the lack of the normal respiratory variation in the size of the inferior vena cava.

ACQUIRED VALVULAR HEART DISEASE (See also Chap. 33)

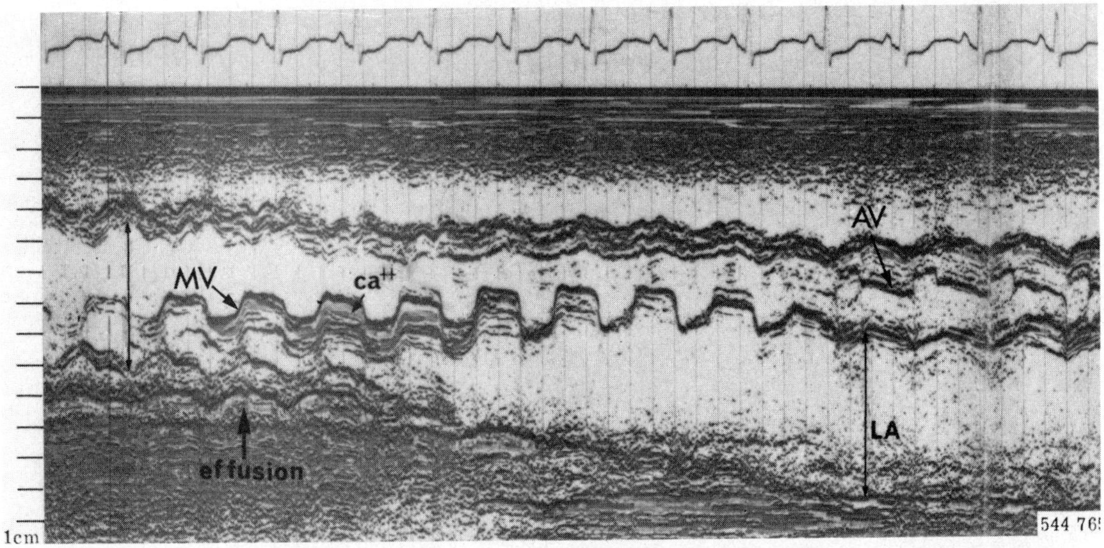

FIGURE 5–44. M-mode scan from a patient with mitral stenosis. The valve is calcified (ca^{++}) and immobile. The left atrium (LA) is dilated and there is moderate posterior pericardial effusion. AV = aortic valve. (From Chang, S.: M-Mode Echocardiographic Techniques and Pattern Recognition. Philadelphia, Lea and Febiger, 1976.)

MITRAL STENOSIS

The detection of mitral stenosis was the first clinical application of echocardiography[116] and remains an important technique in the evaluation of patients with suspected mitral valve disease since echocardiography can allow visualization of the mitral valve in a manner not possible with any other procedure. The M-mode examination provides a sensitive assessment of the motion and thickness of the valve leaflets, while the two-dimensional technique provides a spatial image of the valve and allows direct measurement of the valve orifice.[117] Doppler echocardiography provides a hemodynamic assessment of the stenotic orifice.

Figure 5–44 shows an M-mode echocardiogram of a patient with calcific mitral stenosis. The motion of the mitral valve is considerably altered from the normal pattern seen in Figure 5–14; the normal "M"-shaped configuration during diastole is no longer present, since the presence of a holodiastolic atrioventricular pressure gradient (diastasis) prevents rapid closure of the valve in mid-diastole. Although sinus rhythm was present, there was no reopening of the valve with atrial contraction and no *a* wave. Thus, the echocardiographic hallmark of mitral stenosis is the absence of valve closure in mid-diastole and of reopening in late diastole. Although this decreased (flat) diastolic (E-F) slope is characteristic of mitral stenosis, it is not specific. Other conditions such as decreased left ventricular compliance or a low cardiac output may also reduce the diastolic slope of mitral valve motion.[118]

In addition to the change in motion of the valve, the number of echoes originating from the valve is increased when the valve is fibrotic or calcified, and the second echocardiographic sign of mitral stenosis is increased thickness of the valve leaflets. (Note that the quantity of echoes originating from the mitral valve in Figure 5–44 is considerably greater than in Figure 5–14.) The third sign is inadequate separation of the anterior and posterior leaflets of the valve during diastole.[118] Normally, the two leaflets move in opposite directions during diastole, but when fused, as in mitral stenosis, they do not separate widely and may actually appear to move in the same direction (Fig. 5–44). The echocardiographic findings of reduced diastolic slope, increased thickness, and decreased separation of the valve leaflets provide a sensitive and accurate

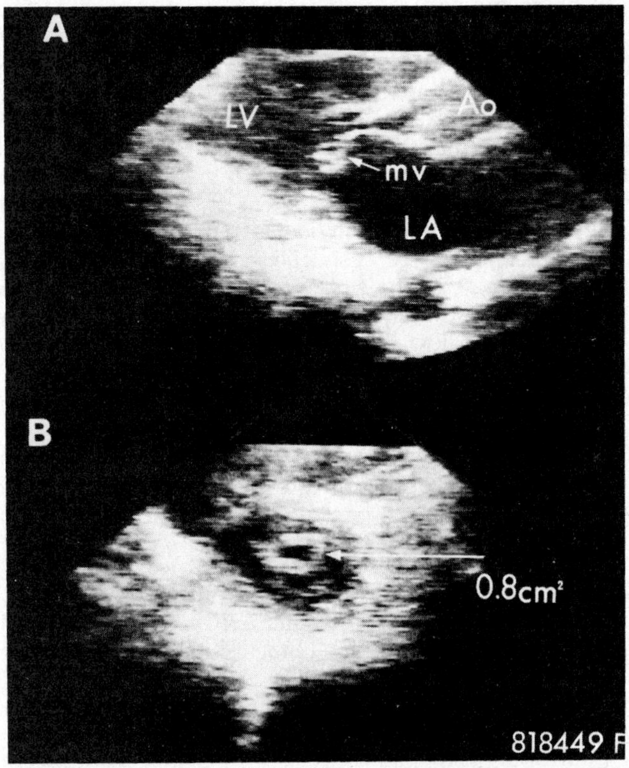

FIGURE 5–45. Two-dimensional echocardiograms of a patient with mitral stenosis. The domed mitral valve (mv) can be seen in the long-axis examination (*A*). The short-axis examination (*B*) demonstrates the orifice of the stenotic valve and provides the opportunity for determining the degree of stenosis.

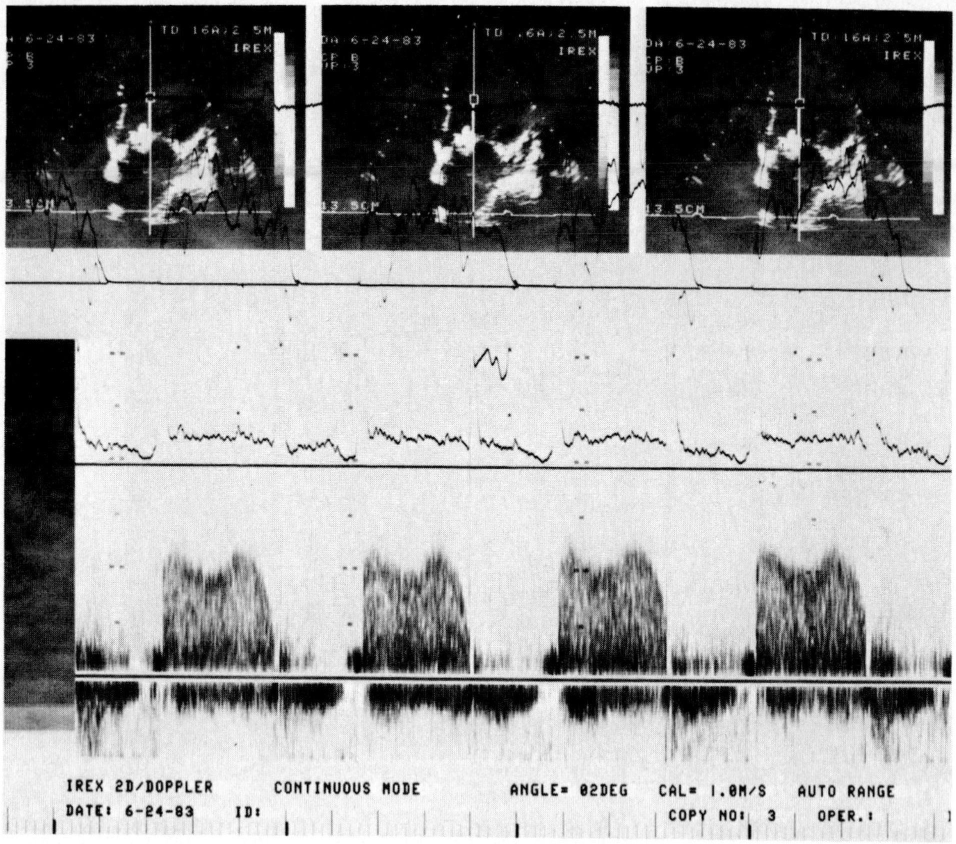

FIGURE 5–46. Continuous-wave Doppler recording of the left ventricular inflow tract in a patient with mitral stenosis. The velocity of flow in diastole is over 2 m/sec and the fall in velocity in early diastole is markedly reduced.

method for detection of mitral stenosis. There are relatively few conditions that can be confused with hemodynamically significant mitral stenosis echocardiographically; these include reduced compliance of the left ventricle as well as a combination of mild rheumatic mitral stenosis and a markedly reduced cardiac output.

Two-dimensional echocardiography assists in the qualitative diagnosis of mitral stenosis. When doming of the mitral leaflets is noted (Fig. 5–45*A*) restricted motion of the valve may be recognized. Doming of any valve on two-dimensional echocardiography is a characteristic sign of stenosis. The distortion in shape with opening of the valve indicates that the tips of the leaflets are restricted in their ability to open, whereas the bodies of the leaflets still wish to accommodate more blood flow; thus, the leaflets are curved, or domed. The presence of doming distinguishes a valve that is truly stenotic from one that opens poorly because of low flow. Two-dimensional echocardiography provides an opportunity to visualize and measure the flow-restricting orifice of the stenotic mitral valve directly (Fig. 5–45).[119]

Doppler echocardiography provides another means of quantitating the degree of mitral stenosis.[120] Figure 5–46 shows a continuous wave recording of mitral valve flow in a patient with mitral stenosis. The peak velocities are increased to over 200 cm/sec. (Normal peak velocity = 0.6–1.3 msec.) The rate of decline of the flow in early diastole is clearly diminished and the velocity with atrial systole is elevated. This type of recording is similar to that seen with an M-mode mitral valve examination except that the atrial velocity or A point is increased on the Doppler record while the A wave on the M-mode tracing is decreased. Figure 5–47 shows a pulsed Doppler recording of a patient with mitral stenosis and atrial fibrillation. There is no atrial contraction. The peak velocities are again increased and the fall in velocity in early diastole is decreased. The technique for quantitating the degree of stenosis depends on the rate of velocity decrease in early diastole. The time interval required for the peak velocity to reach half of its initial level is related directly to the severity of the obstruction of the mitral orifice.[90, 91] This pressure half-time has correlated reasonably well with the mitral valve area. The modified Bernoulli equation can also be used to calculate the mean gradient transmitral valve pressure gradient by calculating the instantaneous gradients periodically throughout diastole. Doppler quantitation of mitral stenosis is particularly helpful in patients with a previous commissurotomy in whom the two-dimensional echocardiographic measure of valve area could be inaccurate.[121]

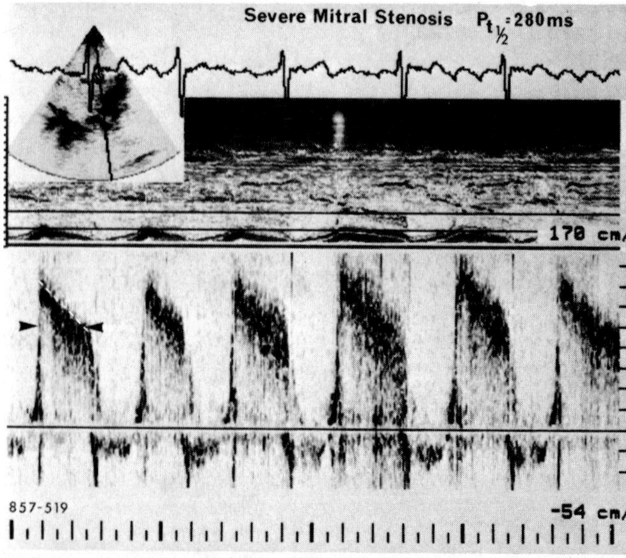

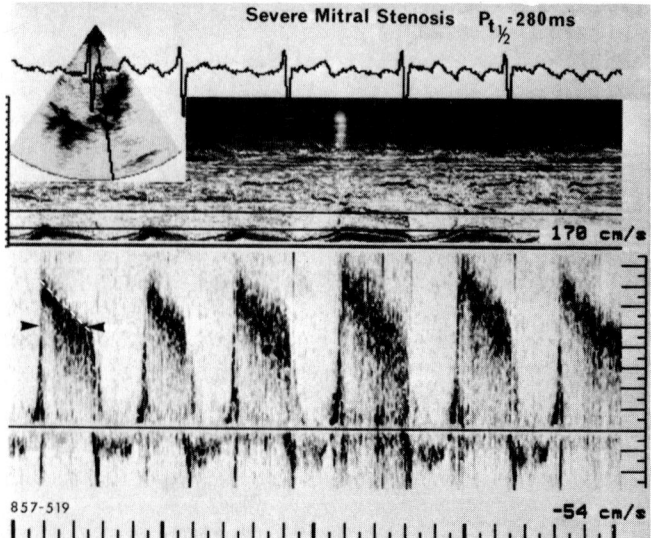

FIGURE 5–47. Pulsed Doppler echocardiogram of mitral flow in a patient with mitral stenosis. This echocardiogram demonstrates how the pressure half-time ($P_{1/2}$) (arrowheads) is measured. (From Feigenbaum, H.: Echocardiography. 4th ed. Philadelphia, Lea and Febiger, 1986.)

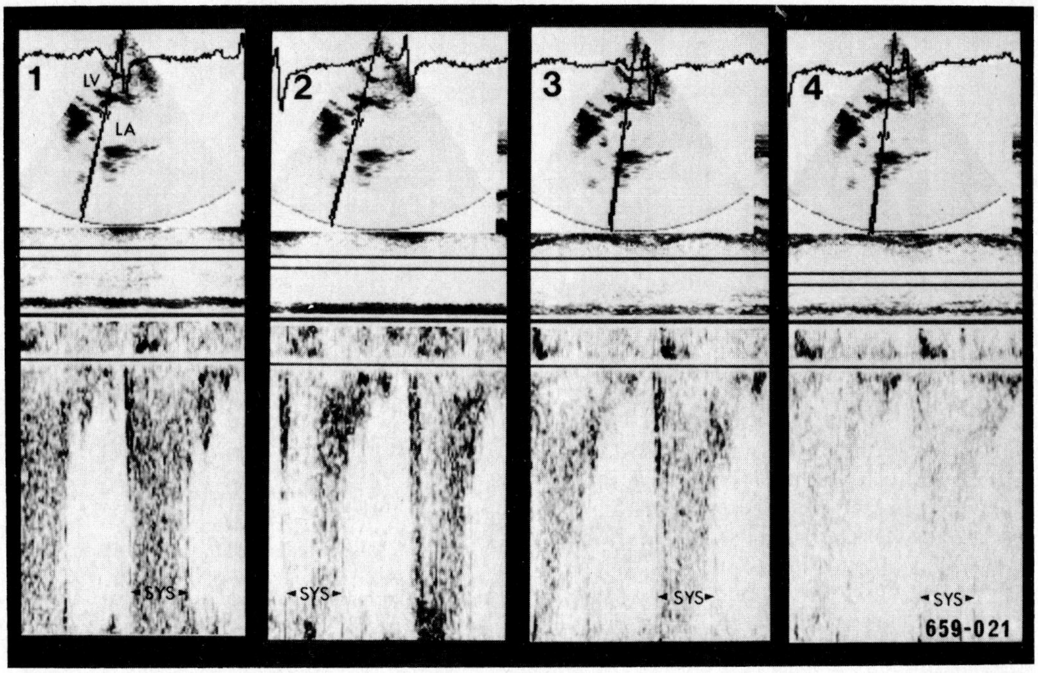

FIGURE 5–48. Serial Doppler examinations showing mapping from mitral regurgitation with the transducer in the parasternal long-axis position. SYS = systole. The regurgitant signal becomes progressively fainter as the sampling site is moved progressively from the mitral valve. (From Feigenbaum, H.: Echocardiography. 4th ed. Philadelphia, Lea and Febiger, 1986.)

Echocardiography can help determine whether or not a stenotic valve is suitable for commissurotomy by estimating its pliability and degree of calcification. Although the M-mode echocardiogram can be used to judge the amplitude of motion of the anterior leaflet, two-dimensional echocardiography is the procedure of choice for assessing the fibrosis and pliability of the mitral valve apparatus,[122] especially when subvalvular adhesions are present.[123] Secondary effects of mitral stenosis, such as left atrial dilatation and pulmonary hypertension, can be detected with various echocardiographic examinations.

MITRAL REGURGITATION

DOPPLER ECHOCARDIOGRAPHY. This is the ultrasonic procedure of choice for the detection of any valvular regurgitation.[124, 125] Figure 5–48 shows a pulsed Doppler recording with the Doppler sample (arrows) in the left atrium. With this type of examination one sees a high velocity recording during ventricular systole in the left atrium. The severity of the regurgitation is generally assessed by the distance from the valve orifice that the regurgitant jet can still be detected on the Doppler recording. For example, in Figure 5–48 the Doppler sample is in the mid portion of the left atrium and regurgitation is still detected. This finding would generally be interpreted as indicating a moderate degree of mitral regurgitation. If the jet were present only near the orifice, such as in Figure 5–48*A*, then a mild degree of regurgitation would be present. Detecting high velocity systolic flow with the sample volume near the back of the left atrial wall indicates a more severe form of valvular regurgitation.

COLOR FLOW DOPPLER. This is another technique for assessing the presence of valvular regurgitation.[13, 125] Figure 5–49 shows the color flow study in a patient with mitral stenosis and mitral regurgitation. The narrow, high velocity jet protruding into the left ventricle in diastole can be seen in Figure 5–49*A*. In Figure 5–49*B* the regurgitant blood flows into the left atrium during ventricular systole. The velocity is very high and a mosaic, multicolored pattern is recorded because of aliasing. The location, direction, and size of the regurgitant flow are readily depicted by the color flow system. There is a rough relationship between the size of the regurgitant flow and the extent of regurgitation.

Unfortunately, all flow mapping techniques either with color mapping or standard pulsed Doppler have only a limited relationship to the degree of valvular regurgitation. Many of the limitations are similar to those present with contrast ventriculography. The size of the chamber into which regurgitant blood is flowing influences both the contrast ventriculographic appearance of regurgitant dye and also the size of the regurgitant Doppler signal. Thus the quantitation of valvular regurgitation using Doppler flow mapping is at best semiquantitative. An alternative Doppler technique for quantifying mitral regurgitation is to calculate stroke volumes through two different orifices, one which reflects flow ejected from the left ventricle to the aorta and one measuring flow passing from the left atrium to the left ventricle.[126, 127] The difference is the regurgitant volume, and regurgitant fraction can be calculated. This approach requires accurate stroke volume measurements and may not be possible in all patients.

Echocardiography is also helpful in evaluating the hemodynamic consequences of the mitral regurgitation. The left atrium is invariably dilated and left ventricular stroke volume increases with frequent left ventricular dilatation.[128] All of these findings are detectable on the echocardiogram. Possibly one of the most important uses of echocardiography is in identifying the *etiology* of the mitral regurgitation. Rheumatic mitral regurgitation almost always produces some thickening of the mitral valve and at least minimal echocardiographic evidence of mitral stenosis. There are numerous other causes for mitral regurgita-

FIGURE 5–49. See color plate 2.

tion and echocardiography plays an important role in identifying these etiologies.

Nonrheumatic Mitral Regurgitation

MITRAL VALVE PROLAPSE (See p. 1045). Echocardiography is particularly useful in the diagnosis of prolapse of the mitral valve. Figure 5–50 demonstrates the principal M-mode finding in this condition—a fairly abrupt posterior (downward) motion of the mitral valve apparatus in mid- or late systole.[129] This motion often commences simultaneously with the mid- or late systolic click (Fig. 5–50), a typical auscultatory and phonocardiographic finding in this condition (p. 50). Although this mid- or late systolic posterior motion of the mitral valve is a reasonably *specific* sign of mitral valve prolapse, it is not a very *sensitive* sign. Many patients with this lesion fail to show it, while in others the prolapse is a holosystolic event, i.e., there is posterior displacement of the valve throughout systole (Fig. 33–20, p. 1047).[130] Minor degrees of posterior displacement of the mitral valve can occur normally, and there is a troublesome "gray zone" in which it is difficult to determine whether the prolapse is normal or not.[131] Late or holosystolic prolapse, as in Figure 5–50, in which the leaflets move posteriorly by at least 5 mm, is generally accepted as abnormal. However, when the holosystolic "hammocking" is less than 5 mm,[132] the diagnosis is not clear-cut.

Several findings on two-dimensional echocardiography have been suggested for the diagnosis of mitral valve prolapse,[133, 134] including the recording of buckling of one or both mitral leaflets into the left atrium during systole. Figure 5–51 demonstrates a parasternal long-axis examination of a patient with mitral valve prolapse. Both leaflets

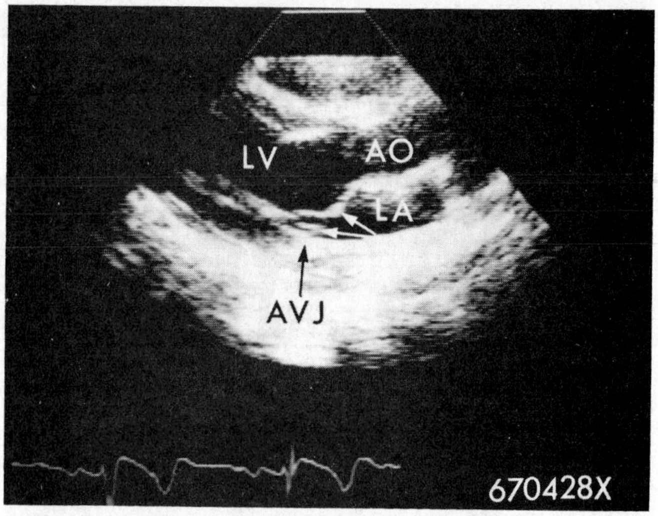

FIGURE 5–51. Two-dimensional long-axis echocardiogram of a patient with mitral valve prolapse. Both the anterior and posterior mitral leaflets (arrows) curve into the left atrium (LA). The posterior leaflet makes almost a hairpin turn as it moves to the atrial side of the atrioventricular junction (AVJ). LV = left ventricle; AO = aorta. (From Feigenbaum, H.: Echocardiography. 4th ed. Philadelphia, Lea and Febiger, 1986.)

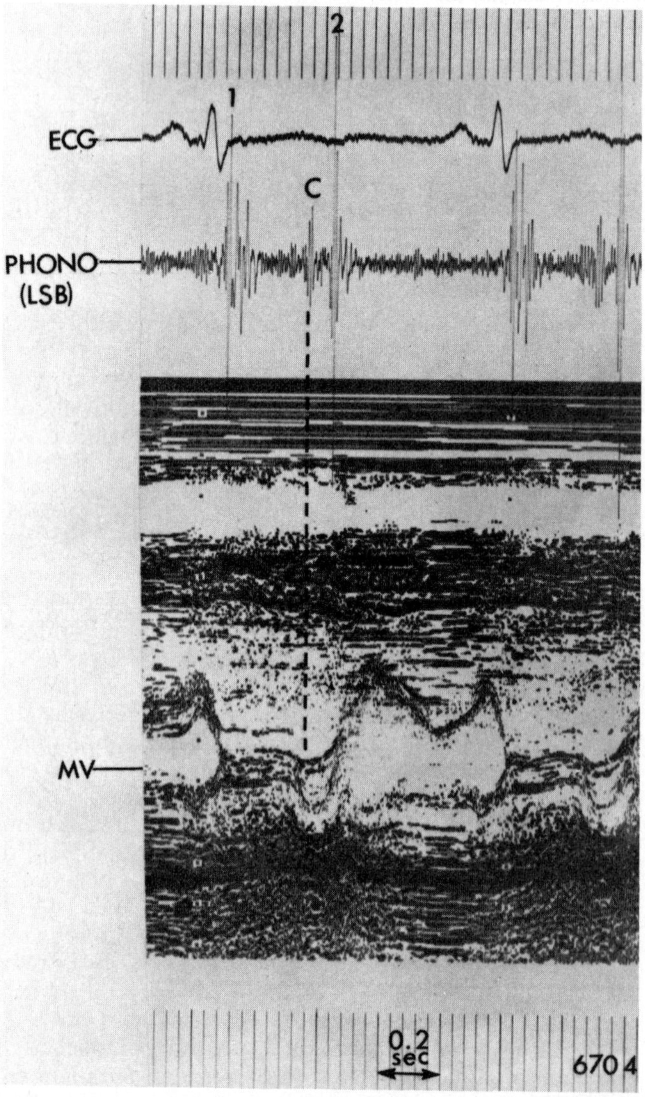

FIGURE 5–50. Phonocardiogram and M-mode echocardiogram from a patient with mitral valve prolapse. The late systolic click (C) on the phonocardiogram corresponds to late systolic posterior displacement of the mitral valve (MV). (From Tavel, M. E.: Clinical Phonocardiography and External Pulse Recordings. 3rd Ed. Chicago, Year Book Medical Publishers, 1978.)

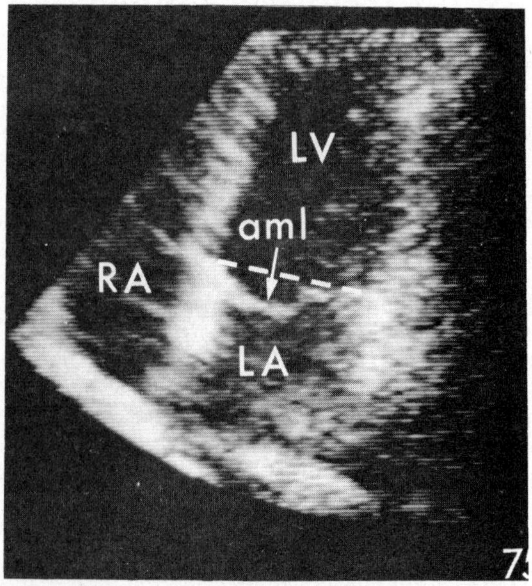

FIGURE 5–52. Apical four-chamber echocardiogram of a patient with mitral valve prolapse demonstrating a curved anterior mitral leaflet (aml) that extends beyond the plane of the mitral annulus (dashed line). LV = left ventricle; LA = left atrium; RA = right atrium. (From Feigenbaum, H.: Echocardiography. 4th ed. Philadelphia, Lea and Febiger, 1986.)

can be seen buckling or herniating into the left atrium in late systole. Figure 5–52 demonstrates an apical four-chamber view of a patient with mitral valve prolapse. The level of the mitral valve annulus is noted by the dashed line. The anterior or septal mitral leaflet bulges well into the left atrium on this echocardiogram. Unfortunately, the amount of systolic prolapse noted on the two-dimensional echocardiograms also exhibits a continuum from normal to abnormal, and there may still be a problem in differentiating between prolapse and a normal variant with this technique.[135]

Other echocardiographic findings in patients with mitral valve prolapse include excessive amplitude of motion of the valve during diastole which can be appreciated in both M-mode and two-dimensional examinations. Thickening of the leaflets is common and is presumably due to myxomatous degeneration.[136] The leaflets may also be redundant and seem to fold on themselves in diastole. When there is redundancy and thickening of the leaflets, the diagnosis of mitral valve prolapse is more secure than when the leaflets are seen to move into the left atrium in systole.[137] It must be emphasized that although echocardiography can frequently be used to make a positive diagnosis of mitral valve prolapse, it is also difficult to distinguish minor degrees of prolapse from a normal variant.

FLAIL MITRAL VALVE. In many patients with a flail mitral valve, i.e., with a leaflet that has lost its normal support and therefore flutters in the bloodstream, the mitral valve echogram presents an extreme form of mitral valve prolapse with marked posterior displacement of the mitral valve during systole.[138] In some patients flail valves are a consequence of infective endocarditis,[139] and vegetations can sometimes be imaged (Fig. 34–10, p. 1115). In Figure 5–53 a very coarsely fluttering anterior leaflet of the mitral valve is imaged, a motion which is characteristically chaotic, without a reproducible pattern from beat to beat.

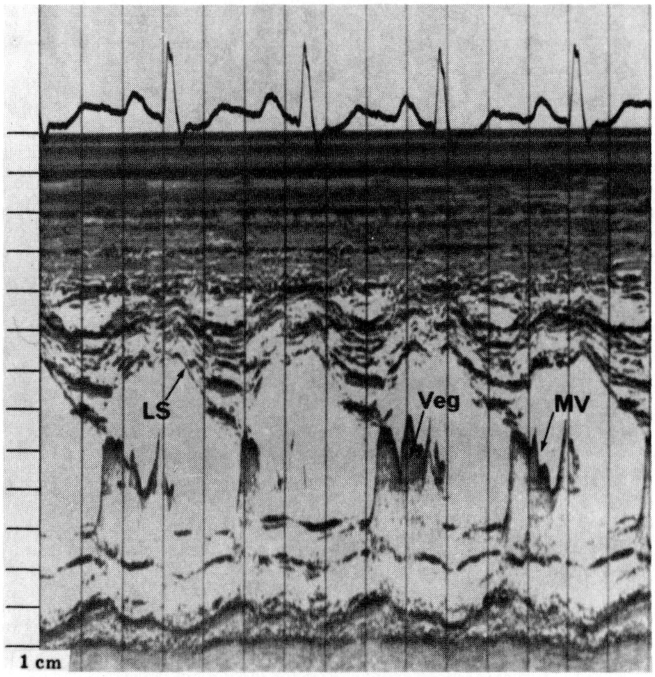

FIGURE 5–53. M-mode echocardiogram from a patient with torn chordae of the anterior mitral leaflet and vegetations (Veg) secondary to bacterial endocarditis. During diastole the anterior mitral leaflet (MV) exhibits chaotic coarse fluttering. LS = left septum. (From Feigenbaum, H.: Echocardiography. 4th ed. Philadelphia, Lea and Febiger, 1986.)

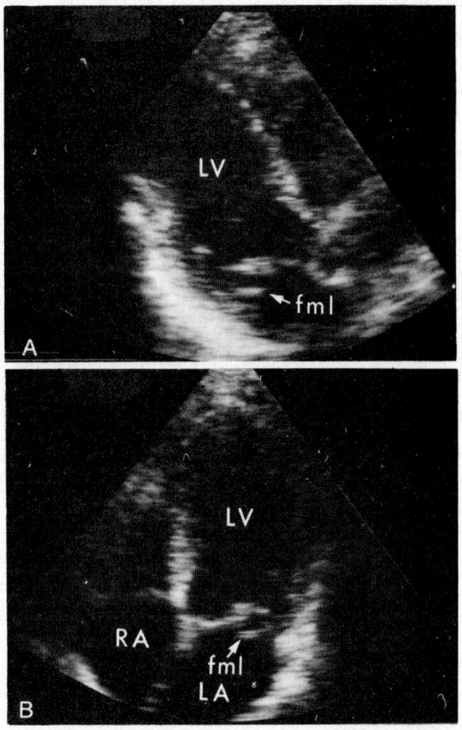

FIGURE 5–54. *A,* Apical two-chamber and *B,* four-chamber views of a patient with a flail mitral leaflet. The flail leaflet (fml) can be seen protruding into the left atrium (LA) during ventricular systole. LV = left ventricle; RA = right atrium. (From Feigenbaum, H.: Echocardiography. 4th ed. Philadelphia, Lea and Febiger, 1986.)

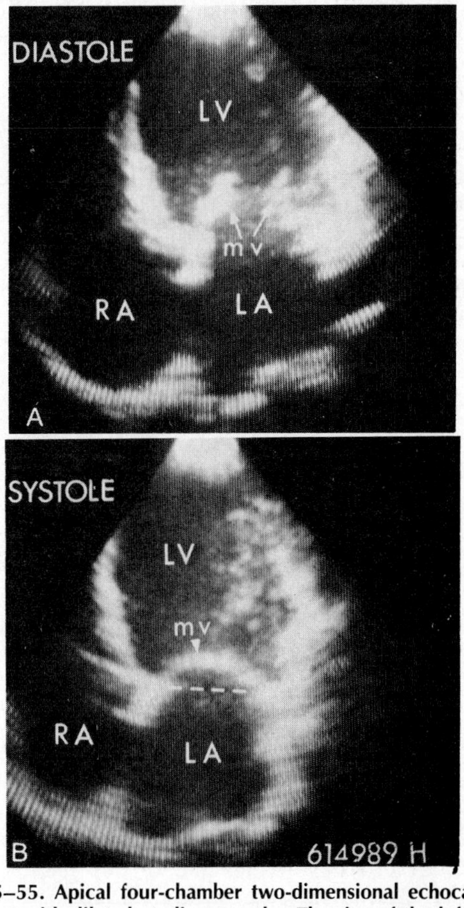

FIGURE 5–55. Apical four-chamber two-dimensional echocardiogram of a patient with dilated cardiomyopathy. The size of the left ventricle (LV) changes little from diastole (*A*) to systole (*B*). In addition, there is incomplete closure of the mitral valve (mv) in systole. The closed leaflets fail to reach the plane of the mitral annulus (dotted line). RA = right atrium; LA = left atrium. (From Feigenbaum, H.: Echocardiography. 4th ed. Philadelphia, Lea and Febiger, 1986.)

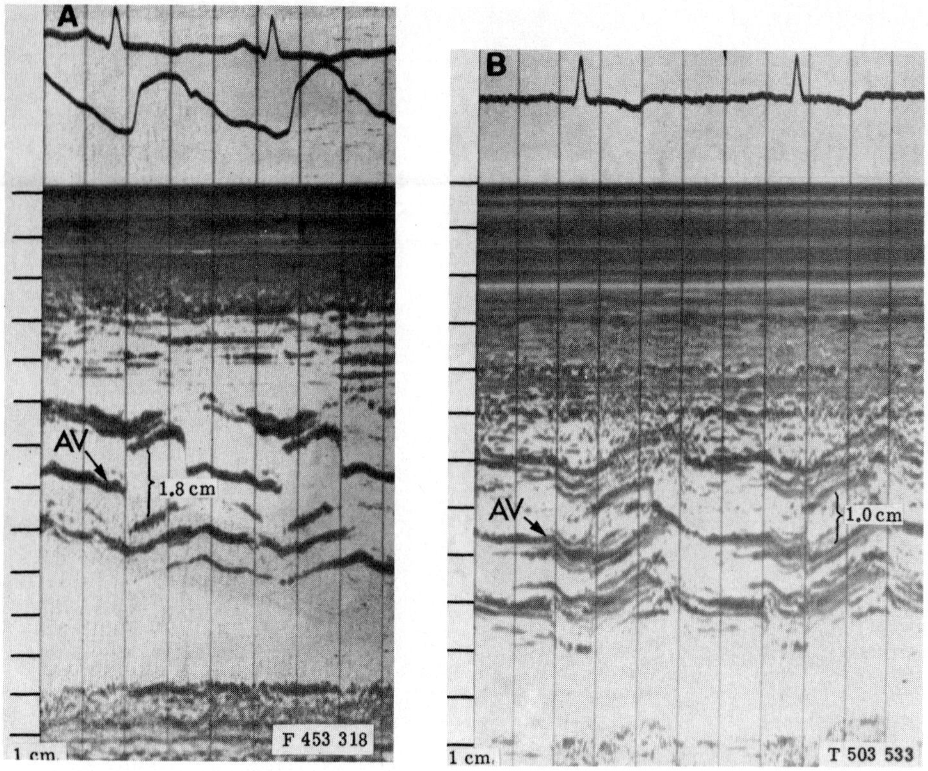

FIGURE 5–56. Aortic valve echocardiograms from a patient with a normal aortic valve (*A*) and from a patient with valvular aortic stenosis (*B*). The echoes are thinner and less echo-producing and separate more widely in the normal valve than in aortic stenosis. AV = aortic valve. (From Feigenbaum, H.: Echocardiography. 4th ed. Philadelphia, Lea and Febiger, 1986.)

This type of motion is suggestive of torn chordae tendineae inserting primarily into the anterior mitral leaflet.

Two-dimensional echocardiography is the examination of choice for establishing the presence of a flail mitral leaflet. With this abnormality the leaflets are seen to protrude into the left atrium (Fig. 5–54).[140] The differentiation between a flail mitral leaflet and mitral valve prolapse depends on whether the tips of the leaflet point toward the left atrium (flail valve) or curve back and point toward the left ventricle (prolapse).[141]

PAPILLARY MUSCLE DYSFUNCTION. Two-dimensional echocardiography provides an opportunity to detect incomplete closure of the mitral valve because of left ventricular dilatation or scarring of the papillary muscles. In this situation the leaflets in the four-chamber view fail to reach the level of the mitral annulus (Fig. 5–55).[142]

AORTIC STENOSIS

Doppler echocardiography has revolutionized the role of echocardiography in the management of patients with aortic stenosis. M-mode and two-dimensional echocardiography have always provided an excellent qualitative diagnosis of aortic stenosis. Doppler echocardiography now provides an opportunity for the quantitative diagnosis. With aortic stenosis M-mode echocardiography reveals a thickened aortic valve and reduced motion of the leaflets (Fig. 5–56).[143] The *two-dimensional* echocardiographic diagnosis of valvular aortic stenosis is doming of the leaflets (Fig. 5–57).[144] The valve may be heavily calcified and immobile, in which case only distorted, echo-producing, immobile valve leaflets are apparent.[145] Two-dimensional echocardiography is fairly specific for the qualitative diagnosis of valvular aortic stenosis and is superior to the M-mode technique, which can miss congenital aortic stenosis and thin leaflets. It is also possible to make a semiquantitative assessment of aortic stenosis with two-dimensional echocardiography by judging the mobility of the leaflets, especially in the short-axis view.

The best ultrasonic technique for quantifying aortic stenosis utilizes continuous-wave Doppler.[91, 146–148] Using the modified Bernoulli equation it is possible to measure the pressure gradient across the aortic valve. Figure 5–58 shows a composite of simultaneous Doppler recordings and intracardiac pressure measurements in four different patients with aortic stenosis. An increase in the Doppler velocity occurs as the gradient increases. There is an excellent relationship between the instantaneous gradient across the stenotic valve as measured by both catheterization and Doppler techniques.[149]

It should be recalled that in the cardiac catheterization laboratory it is customary to measure the difference between the peak left ventricular pressure and the peak aortic pressure (Fig. 5–59). This type of measurement is used because it is the easiest one to make in the catheterization laboratory. This measurement actually does not exist at any instant in time because the peak aortic pressure occurs later than the peak left ventricular pressure. Thus the hemodynamic pressure gradient commonly used is actually the "peak-to-peak" pressure gradient. The peak instantaneous pressure gradient measured by the Doppler technique is invariably larger. If one measures the more

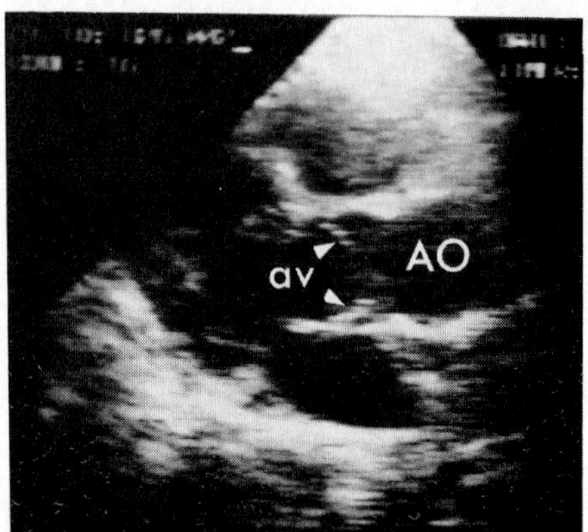

FIGURE 5–57. Two-dimensional echocardiogram of a patient with valvular aortic stenosis. The domed aortic valve (av) can be easily recognized in this systolic frame. AO = aorta.

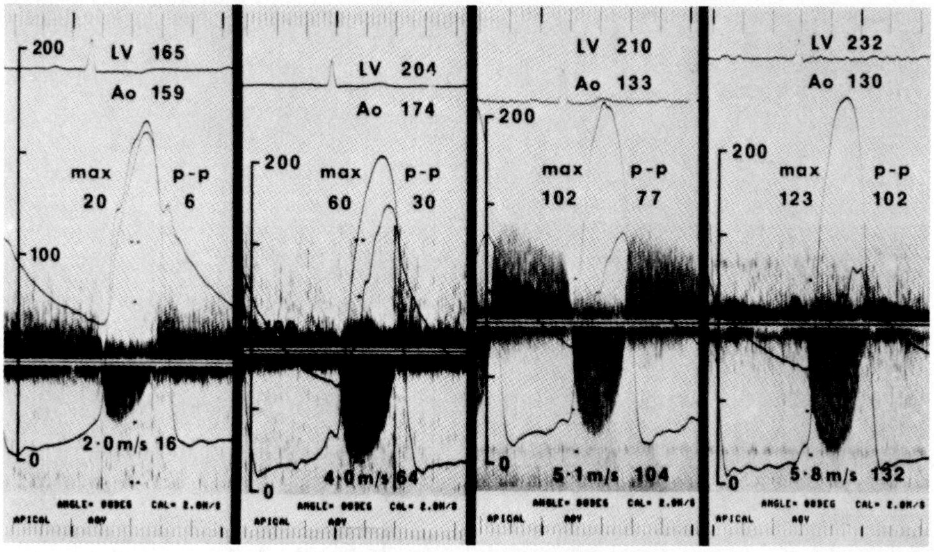

FIGURE 5–58. Simultaneous continuous-wave Doppler and hemodynamic measurements in four different patients with valvular aortic stenosis. The peak velocity increases as the gradient between the left ventricular and aortic pressure increases. (From Currie, P. J., et al.: Continuous wave Doppler echocardiographic assessment of severity of calcific aortic stenosis: A simultaneous Doppler-catheter correlative study in 100 adult patients. Circulation *71*:1162, 1985, by permission of the American Heart Association, Inc.)

accurate mean gradients both in the catheterization laboratory and with the Doppler examination, then the measurements are quite similar.

The Doppler technique thus gives a good estimate of the gradient across the aortic valve. Obviously the gradient can differ from aortic valve area depending upon the flow across the valve. With a reduced cardiac output one can have a small gradient in a patient with severe aortic stenosis. Cardiac output could be measured with a right heart catheter and thermodilution techniques[150] or by using one of the Doppler stroke volume measurements through an orifice that does not have a diseased valve. Another Doppler approach for calculating aortic valve area uses the "continuity equation," which is based on the principle that the amount of blood entering a chamber or orifice must equal the amount of blood leaving that chamber or orifice. By recording the velocity of blood flow in the left ventricular outflow tract and noting the cross-sectional area of the outflow tract, the stroke volume passing through the left ventricular outflow tract can be calculated. That blood in turn must pass through the stenotic aortic valve. Thus, if the stroke volume through a stenotic orifice and the mean velocity of flow through that orifice are known, the size of the orifice can be calculated.[151] This technique has been used in the clinical setting with reasonable accuracy in attempts to calculate the aortic valve orifice in patients with valvular aortic stenosis. A modification of the continuity equation uses blood

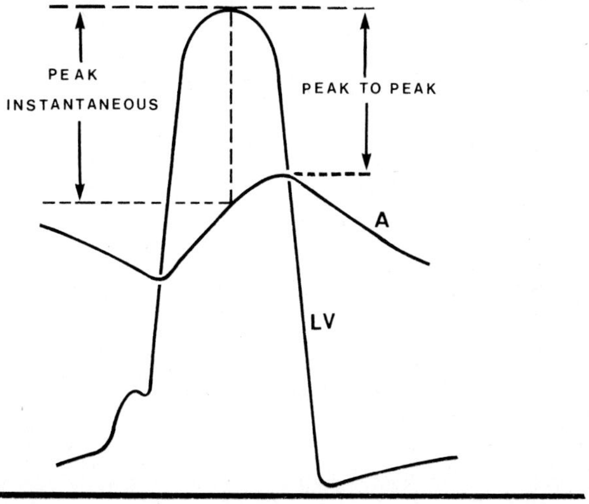

FIGURE 5–59. Diagram of left ventricular (LV) and aortic (A) pressures in aortic stenosis. The peak instantaneous pressure difference or gradient is greater than the peak-to-peak gradient because the peak aortic pressure occurs later than the peak left ventricular pressure. (From Feigenbaum, H.: Echocardiography. 4th ed. Philadelphia, Lea and Febiger, 1986.)

flow through the mitral orifice rather than the left ventricular outflow tract.[152]

The theoretical basis for using Doppler echocardiography for calculating valve gradient is well established. However, there are technical details which must be recognized. It is critical that the maximal velocity be recorded and that the ultrasonic beam is parallel to the aortic stenotic jet. This requirement can make the examination fairly lengthy. Various ultrasonic windows must be tried to make certain that the optimal jet is identified.

From a practical point of view, if a high-velocity jet (in excess of 4 m/sec) is identified, the probability of critical aortic stenosis is extremely high and the patient's condition can be managed accordingly. On the other hand, if the velocity is within normal limits or mildly elevated, the possibility of significant aortic stenosis can be excluded. When the velocity is in an intermediate zone, which would indicate a pressure gradient between 25 and 50 mm Hg, additional hemodynamic information may be necessary for proper management.[153]

There are secondary signs of aortic stenosis which can be noted on the echocardiogram. Both M-mode and two-dimensional echocardiography can detect left ventricular hypertrophy with increased thickness of the left ventricular walls. Although the degree of left ventricular hypertrophy has been used to assess the severity of aortic stenosis,[154] this technique is not nearly as reliable as using Doppler for valve gradients and valve area.

AORTIC REGURGITATION

As with all valvular regurgitation, Doppler echocardiography is the examination of choice for detecting the presence of aortic regurgitation.[155, 156] Figure 5–60 shows a Doppler sample in the left ventricular outflow tract and the recording of high-velocity flow during diastole. This type of examination is both sensitive and specific for the presence of aortic regurgitation. As with mitral regurgitation the magnitude of the regurgitation is assessed by mapping the regurgitant flow into the left ventricle.[155] Color-flow Doppler has also been used to judge the severity of aortic regurgitation.[15] However, the accuracy of Doppler flow mapping for quantitating aortic regurgitation is at best semiquantitative. The same limitations pertain to aortic regurgitation as were discussed with mitral regurgitation. Some investigators are using the width of the aortic jet at the valve orifice as judged by color flow Doppler to judge the severity of aortic regurgitation.[157, 157a] The validity of this observation has yet to be confirmed. The severity of aortic regurgitation can also be judged by

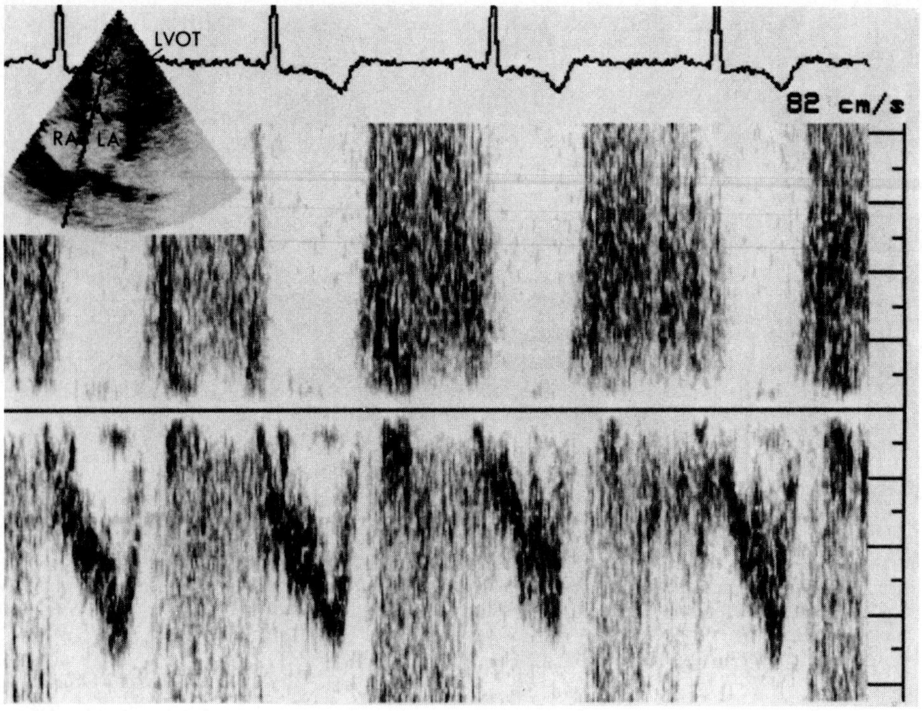

FIGURE 5–60. Pulsed Doppler echocardiogram with the sample volume (arrow) in the left ventricular outflow tract (LVOT) in a patient with aortic regurgitation. RA = right atrium; LA = left atrium. (From Feigenbaum, H.: Echocardiography. 4th ed. Philadelphia, Lea and Febiger, 1986.)

examining the flow pattern within the aorta. Normally, the retrograde flow in diastole in the descending aorta is minor. With severe aortic regurgitation retrograde flow is markedly increased (Fig. 5–61). The rate of decrease in velocity of the regurgitant blood as recorded in the left ventricle using continuous-wave Doppler has been used as a reflection of severity of the aortic valve leak.[158] Severe regurgitation produces a faster fall in velocity as the pressure difference between the aorta and left ventricle falls rapidly. Aortic regurgitation can also be judged by the difference between aortic flow and pulmonary artery flow[159] or mitral flow.[160]

There are several indirect echocardiographic signs for aortic regurgitation which have become obsolete with the advent of Doppler techniques. Fluttering of the mitral valve on the M-mode echocardiogram was the principal indication for the qualitative diagnosis of aortic regurgitation. The sign is not nearly as sensitive or specific for aortic regurgitation as is Doppler. The aortic regurgitant jet can distort the shape of the anterior mitral leaflet on the two-dimensional echocardiogram.[161] In diastole an indentation of the leaflet in the short-axis, four-chamber, and two-chamber views on a two-dimensional echocardiogram usually signifies at least a moderate amount of aortic regurgitation.

One M-mode sign of aortic regurgitation which remains very useful is the premature closure of the mitral valve in the presence of severe, usually acute, aortic regurgitation (Fig. 5–40).[99, 100] With an elevated left ventricular diastolic pressure there may even be early opening of the aortic valve on the M-mode recording.[105] Both of these signs represent severe aortic regurgitation and markedly elevated left ventricular diastolic pressures. The secondary effects of aortic regurgitation on the left ventricle can be detected with both M-mode and two-dimensional echocardiographic examinations. Serial measurements of left ventricular size and systolic function are important in following patients with chronic aortic regurgitation or judging the efficacy of surgery.[162, 163] Deterioration in left ventricular systolic function is one criterion for valve replacement[164] (p. 1068).

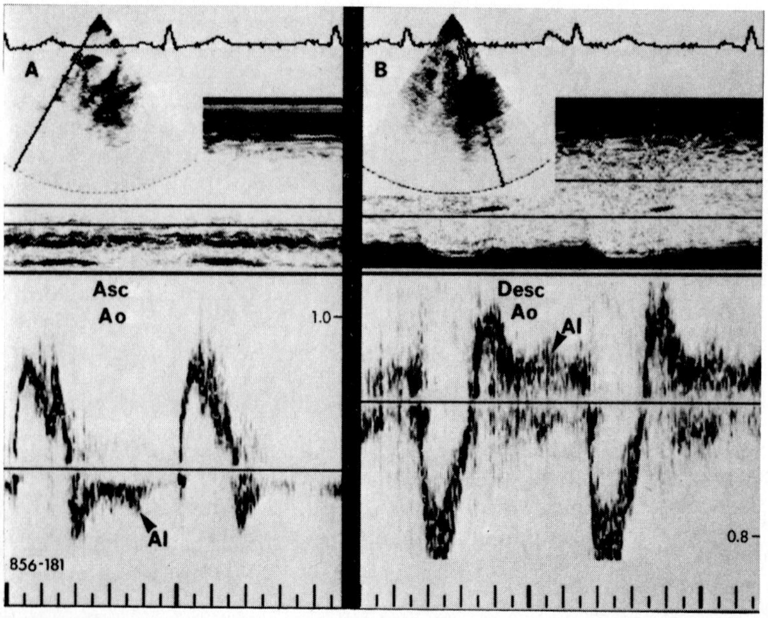

FIGURE 5–61. Pulsed Doppler echocardiograms of flow in the ascending aorta (*A*) and the descending aorta (*B*) of a patient with aortic regurgitation. The diastolic reverse flow from the aortic regurgitation (AI) is seen throughout diastole in both examinations. Ao = aorta; arrows indicate location of sample volumes. (From Feigenbaum, H.: Echocardiography. 4th ed. Philadelphia, Lea and Febiger, 1986.)

TRICUSPID VALVE DISEASE

TRICUSPID STENOSIS. The echocardiographic findings of tricuspid stenosis and regurgitation are very similar to those for mitral stenosis and mitral regurgitation. Two-dimensional and Doppler echocardiography are the procedures of choice for detecting tricuspid stenosis. Doming of the tricuspid valve is the hallmark of a tricuspid stenosis.[165] The Doppler findings of tricuspid stenosis are similar to those with mitral stenosis.[166] The velocities passing through the orifice are increased and the rate of diastolic decline in velocity is decreased. The pressure half-time can also be used to calculate the severity of the valvular obstruction.

TRICUSPID REGURGITATION. This abnormality is also best determined by Doppler echocardiography.[167, 168] With a sample volume in the right atrium a high velocity flow can be recorded at various locations within the right atrium. As noted previously the Doppler recording of tricuspid regurgitation can be used to estimate the pressure gradient across the tricuspid valve. This measurement provides an opportunity for estimating right ventricular systolic pressure by adding an estimate of right atrial pressure. Contrast echocardiography can be used for detecting tricuspid regurgitation but is being replaced by the Doppler approach.[167, 169]

Two-dimensional echocardiography can help determine the etiology of tricuspid regurgitation. *Rheumatic tricuspid regurgitation* usually has an element of tricuspid stenosis and invariably exhibits mitral stenosis. Pulmonary hypertension can be detected by estimating the right ventricular systolic pressure. *Tricuspid valve prolapse* gives an appearance similar to mitral valve prolapse (Fig. 5–62).[170] A *flail* tricuspid valve is noted by finding parts of the tricuspid valve protruding into the right atrium in ventricular systole.[171] *Carcinoid valve disease* produces stiff immobile tricuspid leaflets that are continuously open.[172] Valvular *vegetations* and *Ebstein's anomaly* are discussed on pp. 1094 and 997, respectively.

Secondary effects of tricuspid regurgitation can be noted on both M-mode and two-dimensional studies. Right ventricular and right atrial dilatation are invariably present. Abnormal motion of the interventricular septum indicates that a right ventricular volume overload may be present.

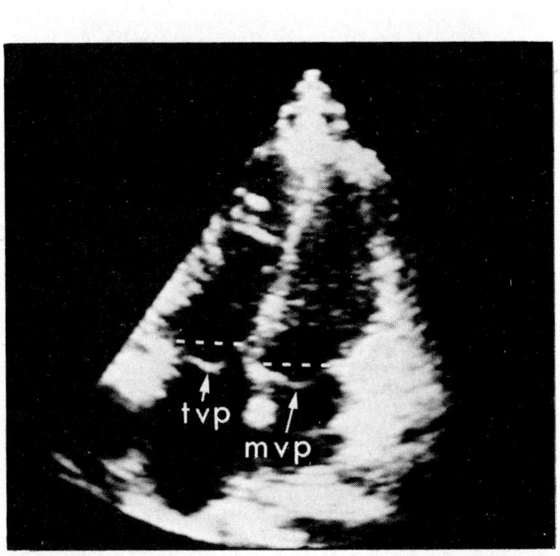

FIGURE 5–62. Apical four chamber two-dimensional echocardiogram of a patient with tricuspid valve prolapse (tvp) and mitral valve prolapse (mvp). (From Feigenbaum, H.: Echocardiography. 4th ed. Philadelphia, Lea and Febiger, 1986.)

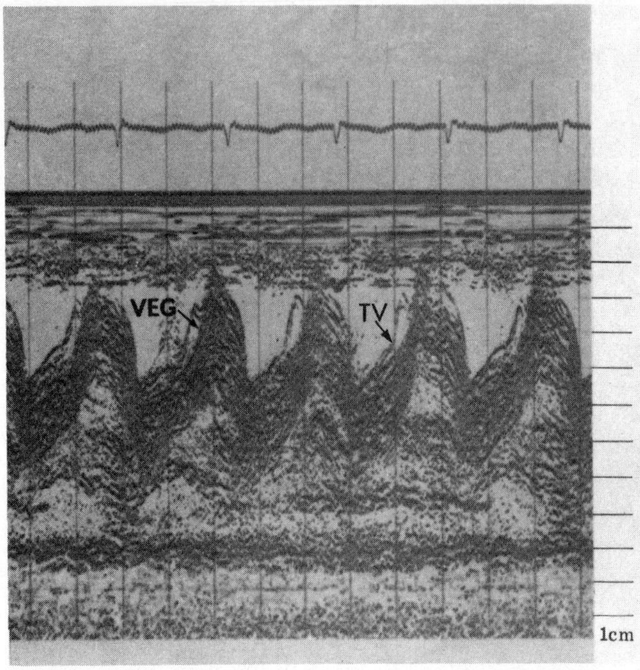

FIGURE 5–63. Echocardiogram demonstrating a large bacterial vegetation (VEG) on the tricuspid valve (TV). (From Feigenbaum, H.: Echocardiography. 4th ed. Philadelphia, Lea and Febiger, 1986.)

INFECTIVE ENDOCARDITIS (See Chap. 34)

Echocardiography provides a means for visualizing the vegetations of infective valvular endocarditis, which appear as echo-producing masses attached to the infected valve (Fig. 34–10, p. 1115).[173, 174] Vegetations must be approximately 3 to 4 mm in diameter before they can be appreciated on the echocardiogram;[175] they are usually asymmetrical, commonly involving one leaflet more than another, but may be present on more than one valve. If the vegetation is associated with destruction of the valve or if it is on a long "stalk," it can be readily imaged; its excessive motion can be appreciated on both M-mode[176, 177] and two-dimensional echocardiography.[177] Some very large vegetations have been described.[178] Often these seem to involve the tricuspid valve (Fig. 5–63)[2, 179] or may result from infection with *Candida albicans*.[180]

Many patients with clinically proven infective endocarditis do not have recognizable vegetations on the echocardiogram,[181] especially if the involved valves remain competent. In one study, only one-third of patients with proven endocarditis had vegetations that could be visualized on the echocardiogram.[181] In some studies, especially those in which two-dimensional echocardiography was used,[182] investigators have noted a much higher frequency of vegetations on the echocardiogram. However, the frequency is not 100 per cent,[183] so that a negative echocardiogram does not rule out endocarditis. When vegetations are evident, the valve frequently may be diseased to the point at which its function is significantly impaired and surgical replacement may be necessary.[181] However, with more sensitive echocardiographic methods for detecting vegetations, principally two-dimensional echocardiography, the finding of vegetations is not as ominous as first thought.

Vegetations visualized echocardiographically need not be bacterial[184] or even infected. Infected vegetations may be difficult to distinguish from myxomatous degeneration of the valve,[177] although this differentiation is usually readily accomplished clinically.

One of the major applications of echocardiography in

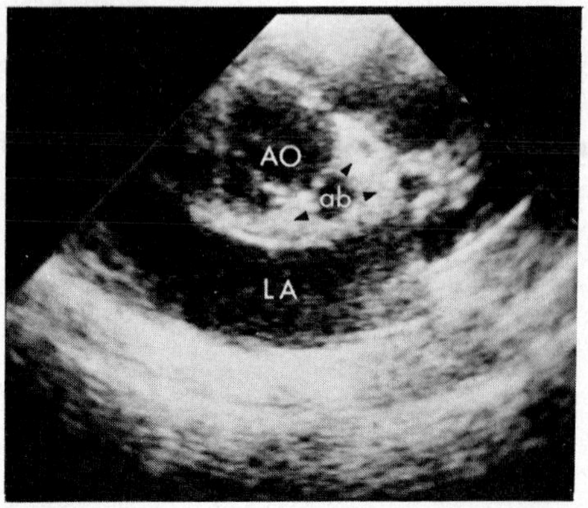

FIGURE 5–64. Short-axis two-dimensional echocardiogram through the root of the aorta in a patient with an abscess (ab) involving the aortic root (AO). LA = left atrium. (From Feigenbaum, H.: Echocardiography. 4th ed. Philadelphia, Lea and Febiger, 1986.)

patients with endocarditis is in the identification of complications. When the valve is damaged to the point that it is grossly incompetent, echocardiography can both detect and assess the hemodynamic importance of the valvular regurgitation. When the aortic valve is involved, premature closure of the mitral valve because of the very high left ventricular diastolic pressure may be evident. On rare occasion the left ventricular diastolic pressure may actually exceed the aortic pressure and premature opening of the aortic valve can be seen during late diastole. Another serious complication of aortic valve endocarditis is the development of an aortic abscess (Fig. 5–64).[185] This problem is seen as a relatively echo-free space adjacent to the aortic root. Mitral ring abscess can also be detected by means of echocardiography.[186]

Prosthetic Valves

Despite extensive attention to this problem, there are still no sensitive and specific echocardiographic signs of prosthetic valve malfunction. Most published reports of prosthetic valve malfunction represent isolated case studies, and the findings include large thrombi[187, 188] and balls or discs that adhere to the cage intermittently or permanently.[189, 190] Abnormal motion of a ball or disc usually results from a thrombus[191] or from ball variance.[190] A useful sign of a malfunctioning Björk-Shiley valve in the mitral position is a rounding of the E point on the M-mode echocardiogram.[192] An abnormal rocking motion of a prosthetic valve resulting from the sutures pulling loose from the annulus has been reported.[193] The significance of the "fine" intracavitary echoes originating from prosthetic valves in the mitral position is unclear.[194] Thickening of the porcine valve leaflets is useful in judging deterioration of this valve.[195] A flail porcine valve, especially in the mitral position, can be easily identified with two-dimensional echocardiography (Fig. 5–65).[196]

Doppler echocardiography is very helpful in evaluating prosthetic valves.[197, 198] Valvular regurgitation is detected readily with the Doppler technique.[199] Color Doppler has the advantage of locating some of these unusually located valvular regurgitations. Doppler echocardiography can also assist in judging stenotic prosthetic valves. The technique is most effective with valves which have a central orifice, such as a tissue valve[200] or St. Jude mechanical valve.[201] Ball valves or tilting disk valves present more difficulties in judging the flow characteristics through the valve.

Although echocardiography is still an imperfect technique for judging the status of prosthetic valves, the combined use of M-mode, with or without phonocardiography, two-dimensional, and Doppler echocardiography can lead to a correct assessment in the majority of cases. It is still somewhat difficult to evaluate the presence of a vegetation superimposed on a prosthetic valve because of its normally echogenic quality. However, if the vegetation protrudes into the cavity of the heart, the diagnosis can be made with more confidence.[202, 203]

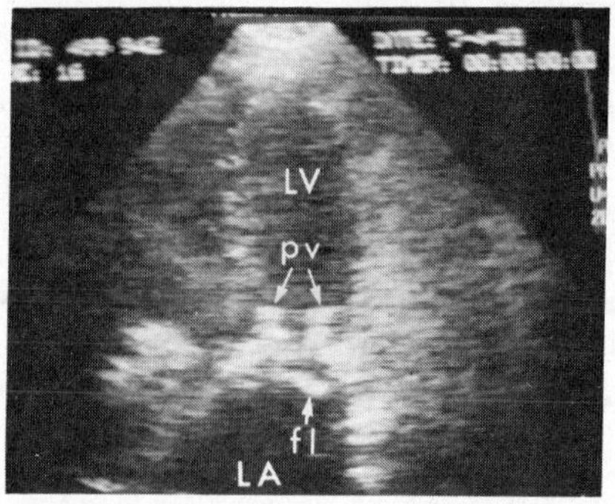

FIGURE 5–65. Apical four-chamber view of a patient with a degenerated flail porcine mitral prosthesis (pv). The flail leaflet (fl) can be seen protruding into the left atrium (LA) in systole. LV = left ventricle. (From Feigenbaum, H.: Echocardiography. 4th ed. Philadelphia, Lea and Febiger, 1986.)

Calcified Mitral Annulus (See p. 1042)

Calcification of a mitral annulus can be readily demonstrated by echocardiography.[204, 205] The principal finding is a band of dense echoes between the mitral valve and the posterior left ventricular wall (Fig. 5–66). Calcification can be extensive and involve the posterior mitral leaflet and much of the base of the heart.

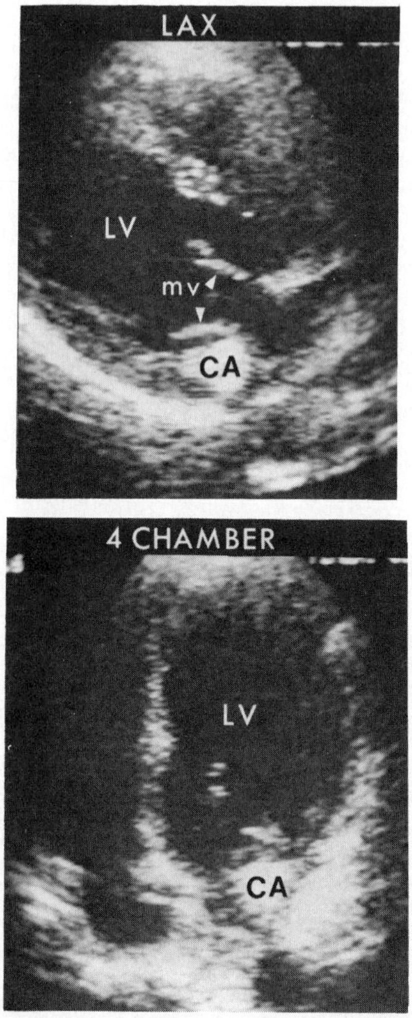

FIGURE 5–66. Long-axis (LAX) and four-chamber two-dimensional echocardiograms of a patient with a large echo producing abscess involving the mitral annulus (CA). LV = left ventricle; mv = mitral valve leaflet. (From Feigenbaum, H.: Echocardiography. 4th ed. Philadelphia, Lea and Febiger, 1986.)

CONGENITAL HEART DISEASE

(See also Chaps. 29 and 30)

DEDUCTIVE ECHOCARDIOGRAPHY

With the advent of two-dimensional echocardiography and Doppler techniques, echocardiography is rapidly becoming a definitive study for many patients with congenital heart disease.[206, 207] This type of study is providing critical morphological and functional information in the management of these patients. Even the most complex anomalies have been recognized with echocardiography. The question is now being raised as to how often these patients require cardiac catheterization following an adequate echocardiographic examination.

There are many ways in which echocardiography can be used to decipher a congenitally malformed heart. The term *deductive echocardiography* refers to a technique by which an attempt is made to deduce the anatomy of the heart by identifying the atria, atrioventricular valves, ventricles, semilunar valves, and great vessels. Initially this type of examination was done by combining the chest roentgenogram with the M-mode echocardiogram. Two-dimensional echocardiography alone can now recognize almost all of the cardiovascular components.[208, 209] Locating the vena cava identifies the right atrium. The pulmonary veins can be seen in the apical four-chamber view and signify the location of the left atrium. The pulmonary artery bifurcation distinguishes this vessel from the aorta and its arch branches.[210] The tricuspid valve is identified by the fact that it inserts into the interventricular septum closer to the apex than does the mitral valve.[211] Recognizing and distinguishing between the mitral and tricuspid valves help to identify the ventricles since they always accompany the appropriate atrioventricular valve. The semilunar valves are always a part of the appropriate great vessel. Thus these valves are identified once the aorta and pulmonary artery are recognized (Fig. 30–63, p. 955). This deductive approach can frequently unravel even the most complex malformation.

VALVULAR DISEASE

VALVULAR STENOSIS. A *bicuspid aortic valve* (p. 1052) is probably the most common congenital cardiac anomaly. The best echocardiographic criterion for making this diagnosis utilizes two-dimensional echocardiography. With this technique two cusps rather than the normal three cusps can be identified (Fig. 5–67). The aortic valve opening is frequently oval rather than circular. The diagnosis can be confusing since occasionally a fused commissure may resemble a third leaflet echocardiographically. In addition, if the commissure is in an anterior-posterior direction, it is sometimes difficult to record echocardiographically.[212] The M-mode technique of looking for eccentric closure of the aortic valve within the aorta[213] is less reliable.

In *aortic stenosis* the echocardiographic findings are similar whether the valve is congenitally deformed (p. 1057) or diseased as a result of rheumatic fever. In the adult the valve is frequently heavily calcified and the etiology is difficult to determine. The qualitative diagnosis is made by finding doming and/or restricted motion of the valve during systole. The quantitative diagnosis is now best obtained using continuous wave Doppler.

A host of congenitally deformed mitral valves can be detected echocardiographically.[214] *Congenital mitral stenosis* is rare but has been recognized by echocardiography. A *parachute mitral valve* has also a fairly characteristic echocardiographic appearance. Two-dimensional echocardiography can identify a *double orifice mitral valve*.[215] The domed *stenotic pulmonary valve* resembles the congenitally stenotic aortic valve on two-dimensional echocardiography.[216] Normally, the open leaflets are parallel to the wall of the pulmonary artery during systole, but when the valve is domed and stenotic, they curve away from the wall (Fig. 5–68). Though only a single leaflet of the

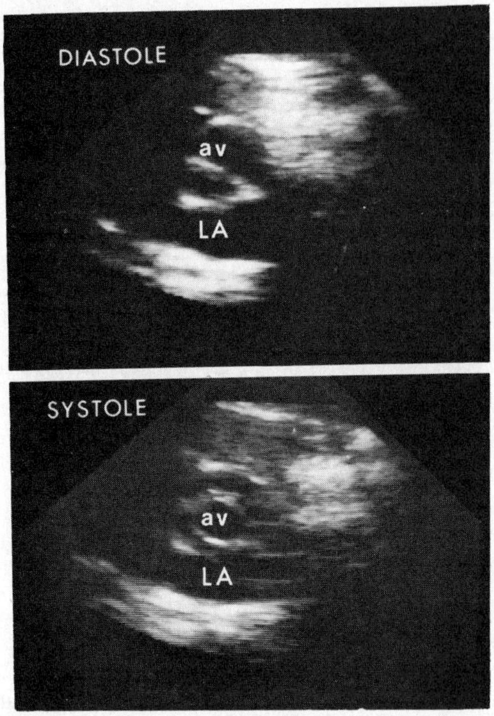

FIGURE 5–67. Short-axis echocardiograms of a bicuspid aortic valve. Note the relatively horizontal commissure of the aortic valve in diastole and oval orifice in systole. av = aortic valve; LA = left atrium. (From Feigenbaum, H.: Echocardiography. 4th ed. Philadelphia, Lea and Febiger, 1986.)

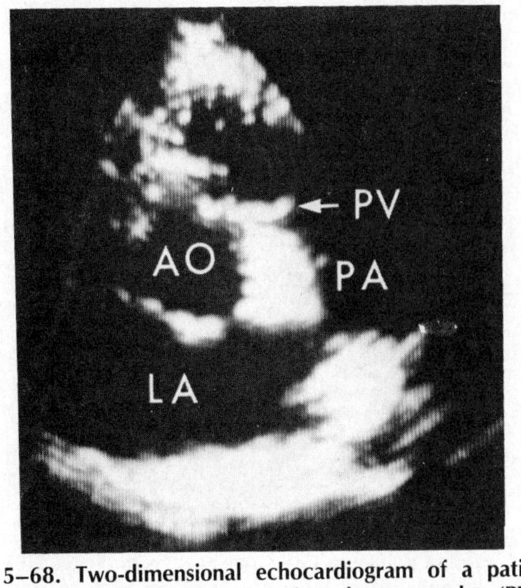

FIGURE 5–68. Two-dimensional echocardiogram of a patient with pulmonic stenosis. The domed, stenotic pulmonary valve (PV) curves into the pulmonary artery (PA) in the systolic frame. AO = aorta; LA = left atrium. (From Feigenbaum, H.: Echocardiography. 4th ed. Philadelphia, Lea and Febiger, 1986.)

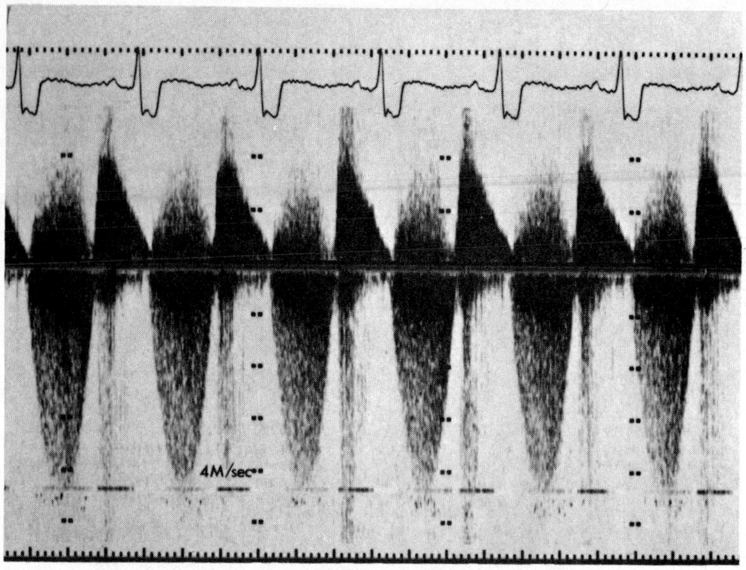

FIGURE 5–69. Continuous wave Doppler recording of a patient with pulmonic stenosis and pulmonary regurgitation. In systole downward deflection the velocity is very high and exceeds 4 m/sec. Diastolic reverse flow is noted from the pulmonic regurgitation.

pulmonary valve is ordinarily imaged, its domed appearance is sufficient to establish the diagnosis. The *severity* of pulmonic stenosis is assessed by Doppler echocardiography.[217, 218] Utilizing criteria similar to those for aortic stenosis (p. 108), the gradient across the stenotic pulmonary valve can be estimated using continuous-wave Doppler (Fig. 5–69). A common associated abnormality is the presence of pulmonic regurgitation. This abnormality is noted using Doppler recordings which reveal diastolic flow into the right ventricle.

EBSTEIN'S ANOMALY (See p. 997). The echocardiographic diagnosis of Ebstein's anomaly is based on the displacement of the tricuspid valve leaflets within the body of the right ventricle on the two-dimensional echocardiogram (Fig. 5–70).[219, 220] Normally the tricuspid valve inserts on the interventricular septum slightly above the insertion of the mitral valve. However, with Ebstein's anomaly this displacement is marked and much of the tricuspid valve lies within the body of the right ventricle. On M-mode echocardiography the diagnosis of Ebstein's anomaly was based on delayed closure of the tricuspid valve.[221] The two-dimensional echocardiogram is more specific and reliable for this diagnosis.

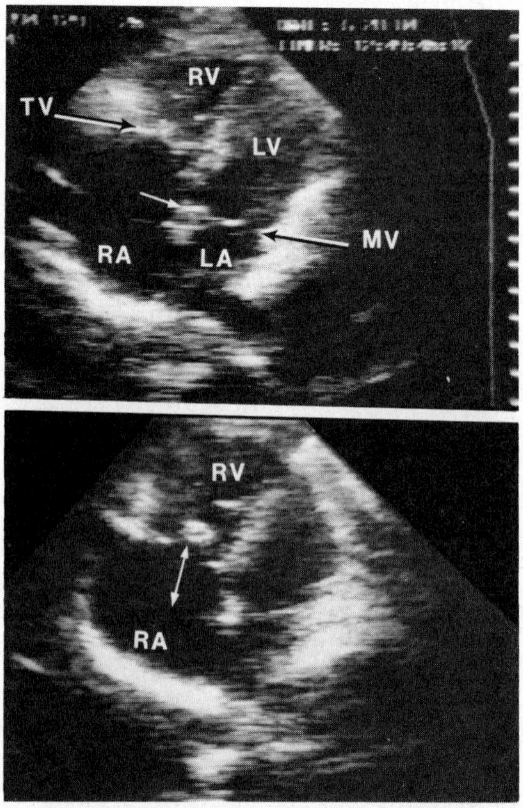

FIGURE 5–70. Apical four-chamber view in a patient with Ebstein's anomaly. The tricuspid valve (TV) is displaced from the tricuspid annulus (arrow). The effective right ventricular volume (RV) is decreased and the volume of the right atrium (RA) is increased. LV = left ventricle; LA = left atrium; MV = mitral valve. (From Feigenbaum, H.: Echocardiography. 4th ed. Philadelphia, Lea and Febiger, 1986.)

VALVULAR ATRESIA. Atresia of cardiac valves is generally associated with hypoplasia of the ipsilateral ventricle (Chap. 30). Thus, aortic or mitral atresia is associated with a hypoplastic left ventricle,[222] while tricuspid or pulmonary atresia is associated with hypoplasia of the right ventricle.[223] Diminutive ventricles and the atretic valves have been imaged with both M-mode[222] and two-dimensional techniques (Fig. 5–71).[224, 225]

SUBVALVULAR OBSTRUCTIONS. A variety of congenital subvalvular obstructions have been detected echocardiographically. Early systolic closure of the aortic valve has been observed in patients with both *discrete* (Fig. 5–72)[226] and *hypertrophic obstructive cardiomyopathy* (Fig. 42–4, p. 1419).[103] In addition, systolic fluttering of the aortic valve is often exaggerated, although some degree of aortic valve fluttering may be seen normally. Although midsystolic closure and fluttering of the aortic valve are not specific findings for subaortic stenosis, they can be very helpful in differentiating valvular from subvalvular obstruction, since they do not occur in the former condition.

Examination of the outflow tract is accomplished with two-dimensional echocardiography, and the subvalvular obstruction can be identified directly by this technique (Fig. 5–73).[227, 228] The two-dimensional technique also permits the classification of discrete obstruction into the discrete membranous and the diffuse types.[229] Distinguishing between them may be of considerable clinical importance, since their management may differ. The membranous form is frequently situated just below the aortic valve and may therefore be difficult to recognize at catheterization, since the short subvalvular chamber can be missed on a pull-out pressure recording. Indeed, the thin membrane can even be missed on the angiogram, so that its recognition by two-dimensional echocardiography can be very helpful. Doppler echocardiography can be used to

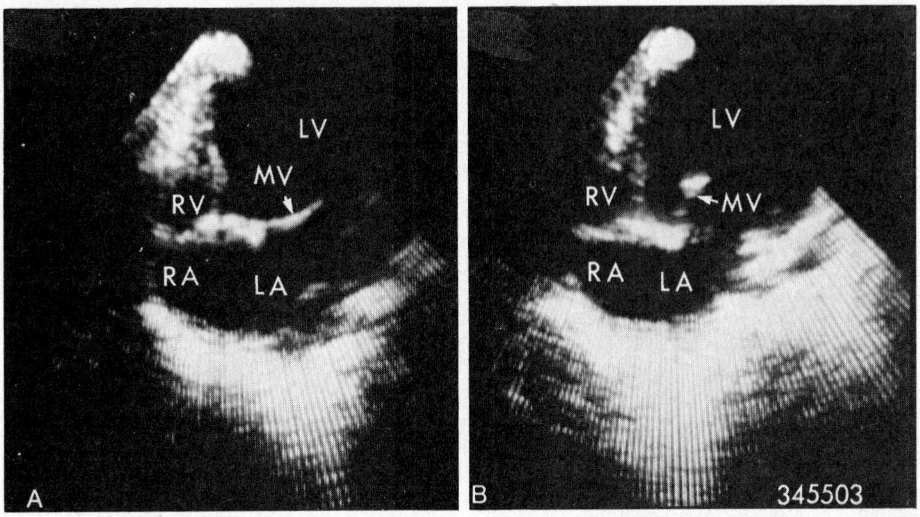

FIGURE 5–71. Apical four-chamber two-dimensional echocardiograms of a patient with tricuspid atresia. The mitral valve (MV) can be seen opening into a large left ventricular chamber (LV). The right ventricle (RV) is small and is separated from the right atrium (RA) by a dense band of linear echoes. No valvular structure could be identified in the region of the tricuspid valve. LA = left atrium. (From Feigenbaum, H.: Echocardiography. 3rd ed. Philadelphia, Lea and Febiger, 1981.)

assess the severity of subvalvular as well as valvular stenosis.[230]

In *subpulmonic obstruction* the M-mode tracing exhibits coarse fluttering of the pulmonary valve.[231] The actual subpulmonic obstruction can be detected and its severity quantified in patients with tetralogy of Fallot by means of two-dimensional examination of the right ventricular outflow tract and subpulmonic area.[232]

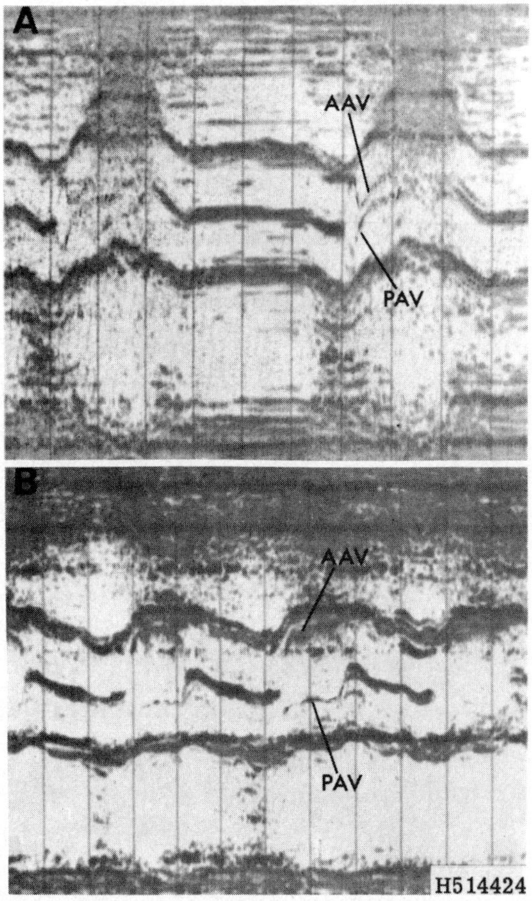

FIGURE 5–72. Aortic valve echograms from a patient with discrete subaortic stenosis before (*A*) and after (*B*) surgery for the subaortic obstruction. Prior to surgery the aortic valve anterior (AAV) and posterior (PAV) leaflets come together shortly after the onset of ventricular ejection and remain essentially closed throughout systole. This systolic closure of the valve leaflets is no longer present following surgery. (From Davis, R. A., et al.: Echocardiographic manifestations of discrete subaortic stenosis. Am. J. Cardiol. *33*:277, 1974.)

CARDIAC SHUNTS

Echocardiography can be helpful in the diagnosis of cardiac shunts by detecting the actual defect between the two sides of the heart, by evaluating the hemodynamic consequences of the shunt, and by recording the shunted blood using the contrast or Doppler methods.

Two-dimensional echocardiography is the technique of choice for visualizing intracardiac communications.[233, 234] Figure 5–74 demonstrates a small ventricular septal defect. Figure 5–75 demonstrates an apical four-chamber view in a patient with a single ventricle.[235]

The two-dimensional echocardiographic examination, especially from the subcostal position, provides an opportunity for direct examination of the interatrial septum (Fig.

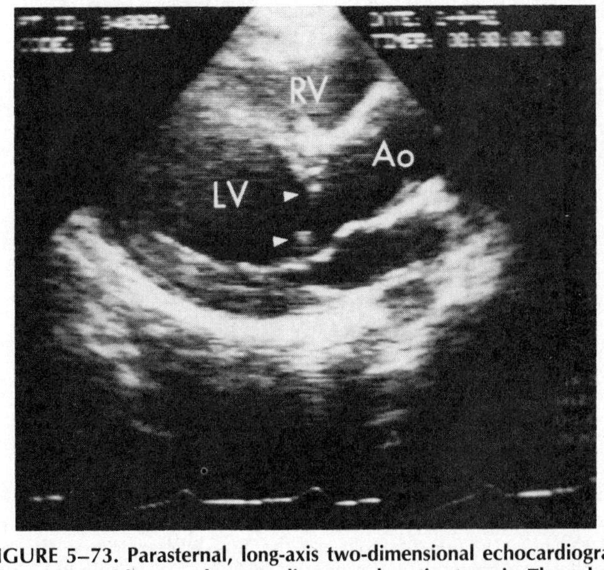

FIGURE 5–73. Parasternal, long-axis two-dimensional echocardiogram of a patient with a membranous discrete subaortic stenosis. The echoes from the subvalvular membrane (arrowheads) can be seen between the left ventricle (LV) and the aorta (AO). RV = right ventricle.

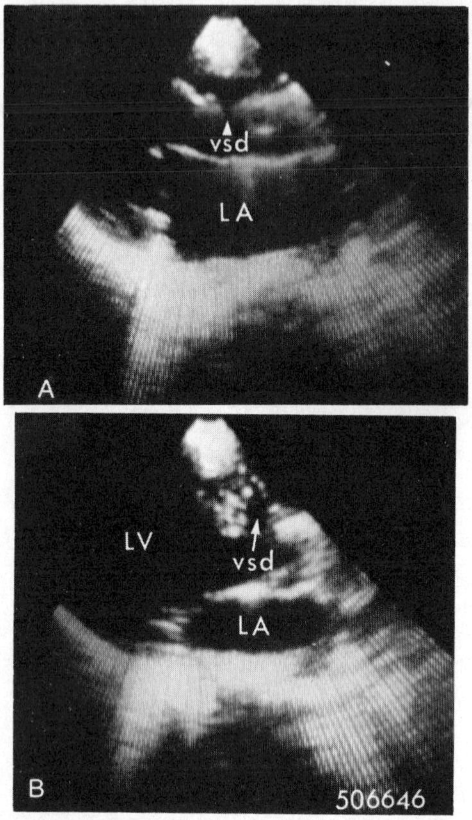

FIGURE 5–74. Two-dimensional long-axis echocardiograms of a patient with a membranous ventricular septal defect. *A*, The discontinuity of echoes from the ventricular septal defect (vsd) can be seen. *B*, A peripheral contrast injection fills the right ventricle, but an echo-free jet, i.e., negative contrast, can be seen anterior to the ventricular septal defect. LV = left ventricle; LA = left atrium. (From Feigenbaum, H.: Echocardiography. 4th ed. Philadelphia, Lea and Febiger, 1986.)

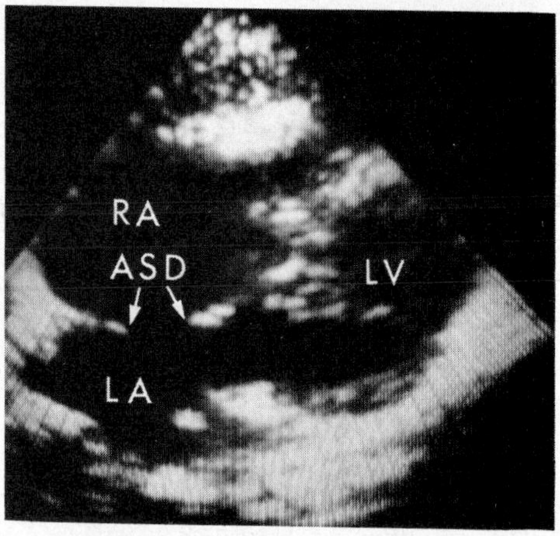

FIGURE 5–76. Subcostal two-dimensional echocardiogram of a patient with a secundum atrial septal defect. Remnants of the interatrial septum are visible on both sides of the defect (ASD). RA = right atrium; LA = left atrium; LV = left ventricle. (From Feigenbaum, H.: Echocardiography. 3rd ed. Philadelphia, Lea and Febiger, 1981.)

5–25*A*).[236] Figure 5–76 demonstrates findings in a patient with an ostium secundum atrial septal defect. A remnant of the interatrial septum can be seen attached to the ventricular septum. In contrast, Figure 5–77 demonstrates an atrial septal defect in a patient with an ostium primum defect. There is no residual septum attached to the ventricular septum. Thus, the two-dimensional technique not only helps identify the presence of an atrial septal defect, but is also an excellent means of differentiating a secundum from a primum type abnormality.[237] One can also identify more severe forms of endocardial cushion defect with a coexistent ventricular septal defect (Fig. 5–78). A sinus venosus type atrial septal defect is the most difficult type of atrial septal defect to detect echocardiographically.[238]

The usual criteria for the identification of shunts by M-mode echocardiography are indirect and depend on their hemodynamic effects on the various cardiac chambers. In patients with left-to-right shunts distal to the atrioventric-

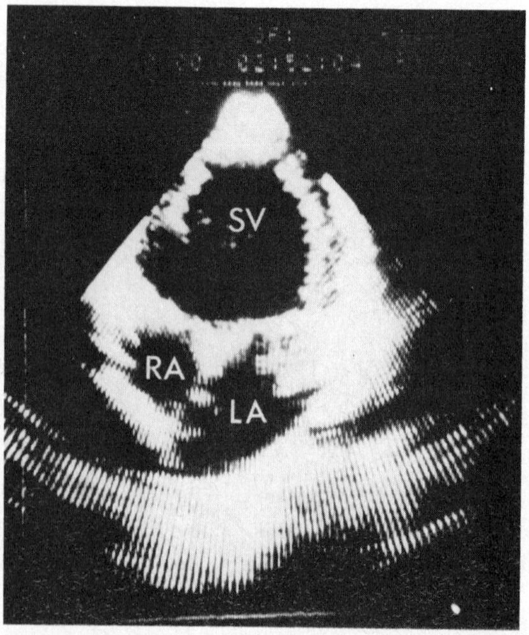

FIGURE 5–75. Cross-sectional echogram of a patient with a single ventricle (SV). The ultrasonic probe is placed at the apex of the heart, and the plane of the scan transects the interatrial septum so that all chambers can be seen simultaneously. This view is particularly helpful in demonstrating the absence of the interventricular septum. RA = right atrium, LA = left atrium.

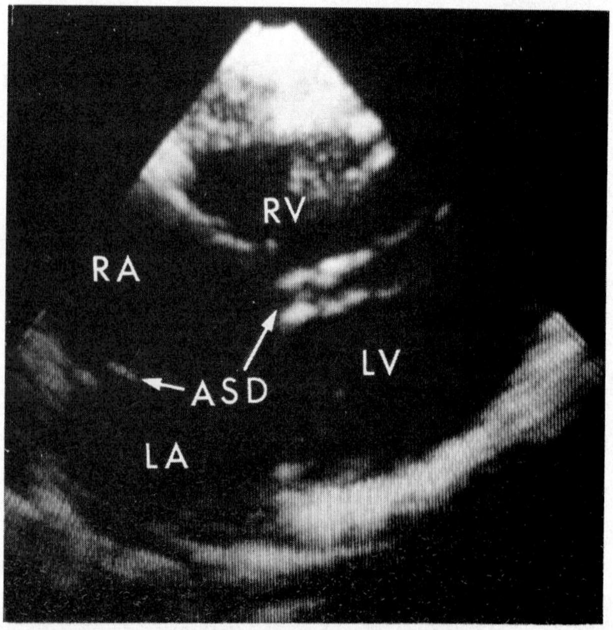

FIGURE 5–77. Subcostal two-dimensional echocardiogram of a patient with an ostium primum atrial septal defect. No residual septal tissue is apparent between the defect (ASD) and the interventricular septum. RA = right atrium; LA = left atrium; RV = right ventricle; LV = left ventricle. (From Feigenbaum, H.: Echocardiography. 4th ed. Philadelphia, Lea and Febiger, 1986.)

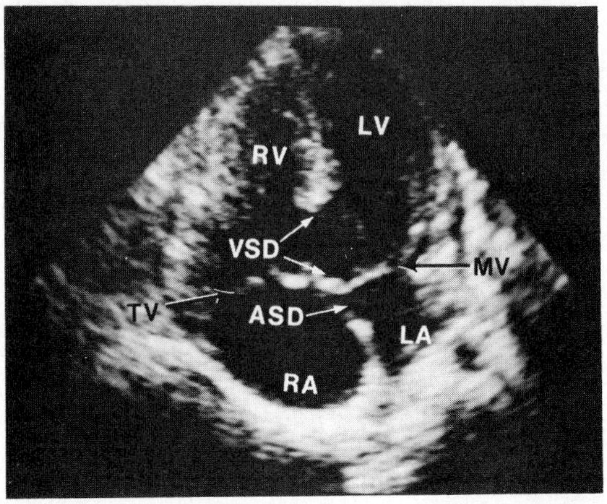

FIGURE 5–78. Apical four-chamber view of a patient with an endocardial cushion defect showing the perimembranous ventricular septal defect (VSD) and primum atrial septal defect (ASD). RA = right atrium; LA = left atrium; RV = right ventricle; LV = left ventricle; MV = mitral valve; TV = tricuspid valve. (From Feigenbaum, H.: Echocardiography. 4th ed. Philadelphia, Lea and Febiger, 1986.)

ular valve (i.e., patent ductus arteriosus, ventricular septal defect, and aortopulmonary window), the left atrium is enlarged because of the increased volume of blood flow that traverses it, and its dimension is the most critical measurement in judging the presence and severity of such a shunt.[71, 239] It is useful to follow the size of the left atrium very closely in infants with known or suspected patent ductus arteriosus or ventricular septal defect, and management of such patients may be aided substantially by this measurement.[240] Left ventricular volume overload, as reflected in the combination of a dilated left ventricle and increased systolic motion of the ventricular septum which accompanies these left-to-right shunts, is also useful in confirming the presence and estimating the size of the shunt.[71, 241] With left-to-right shunts at the atrial level (atrial septal defect or partial anomalous pulmonary venous return) the volume overload of the right ventricle is reflected in dilatation of the right ventricle and abnormal motion of the ventricular septum (Fig. 5–79).[75, 242] Small left-to-right shunts usually produce no abnormalities in the M-mode echocardiogram.

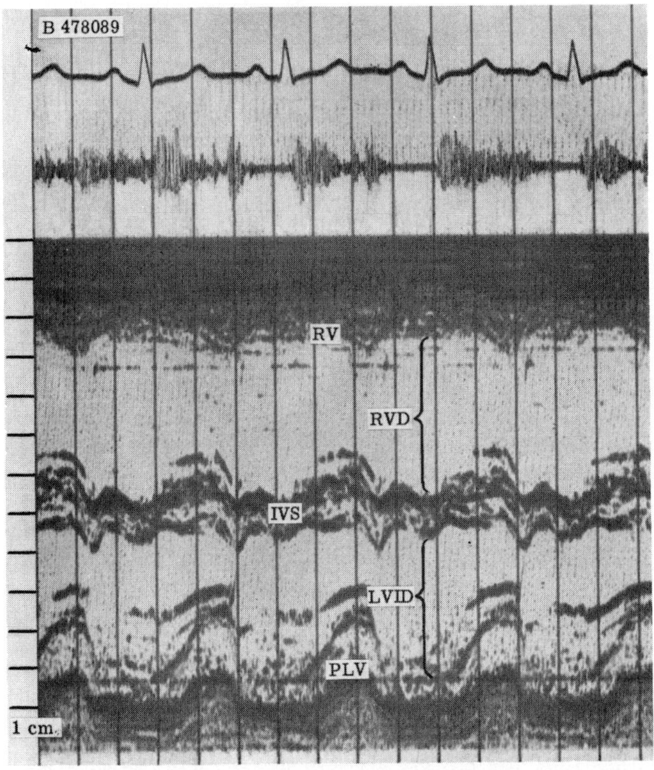

FIGURE 5–79. M-mode echocardiogram from a patient with atrial septal defect. The right ventricular dimension (RVD) is dilated and the right side of the interventricular septum (IVS) moves paradoxically. The left side of the interventricular septum shows a rapid upward motion with the onset of electrical depolarization and then flat motion during ventricular ejection. (From Feigenbaum, H.: Clinical applications of echocardiography. Progr. Cardiovasc. Dis. *14*:531, 1972, by permission of Grune and Stratton.)

In *total anomalous pulmonary venous return* all four pulmonary veins empty into a common pulmonary venous chamber behind the left atrium which produces additional echoes posterior to the left atrium.[243] From an echocardiographic viewpoint the recording is similar to that in *cor triatriatum,* in which the additional echoes are imaged in the left atrium.[222, 244]

Contrast echocardiography is useful in the detection of circulatory shunts. When injections are made into a peripheral vein, or through a central venous catheter, the echo-producing bubbles will traverse the right side of the heart. In the presence of a right-to-left shunt, however, some of these echoes will pass into and become apparent on the left side of the heart and aorta, the specific site depending on the location of the shunt[245, 246] (Fig. 5–13). If the right-to-left shunt is at the atrial level, the bubbles will be imaged in the left atrium and behind the mitral valve in the inflow tract of the left ventricle. If the shunt is at the ventricular level, the echo-producing bubbles will be imaged in the left ventricular outflow tract above the mitral valve (Fig. 5–13). *Negative contrast echocardiography* may be used for the detection of left-to-right shunts;[247] for example, in ventricular septal defect, contrast from a peripheral injection is diluted in the right ventricle by blood shunting from the left ventricle, producing a "negative jet" (Fig. 5–74*B*). The negative contrast technique is not as sensitive as the recording of right-to-left shunting. In the case of a left-to-right shunt at the atrial level there is frequently some small right-to-left shunting so that even in patients with a predominant left-to-right shunt, one may record a small right-to-left shunt with contrast echocardiography.[248]

Although contrast echocardiography usually involves injection into a peripheral vein, a central vein, or the right side of the heart, it is possible in the course of cardiac catheterization or even in the operating room at the time of cardiac surgery, to make the injection anywhere within the cardiovascular system.[249] Selective contrast echocardiography may reduce the need for angiography in the catheterization laboratory or for evaluating postoperative shunts or valvular regurgitation at the time of surgery.

Doppler echocardiography is a very effective technique in the detection of intracardiac shunts because of its ability to detect and localize abnormal flow patterns in the heart. It is particularly useful in the detection of ventricular septal defect[250] and patent ductus arteriosus,[251] anomalies which are rarely recognized using either M-mode or two-dimensional echocardiography. Left-to-right atrial shunts have also been detected with the Doppler technique.[252] An important use of Doppler echocardiography is the diagnosis of multiple shunts. Figure 5–80 demonstrates a Doppler echocardiographic study of a patient with a ventricular septal defect. The Doppler sample is obtained from the right ventricular side of the interventricular septum and demonstrates turbulent systolic flow toward the transducer.

The Doppler velocity across the ventricular septal defect can reflect the pressure difference between the right and left ventricles during systole.[253] Subtracting the pressure gradient from the left ventricular systolic pressure provides an estimate of the right ventricular systolic pressure.[254]

The Doppler technique is helpful in patients with *patent ductus arteriosus.*[255] Although two-dimensional echocardiography can occasionally visualize the patent ductus between the aorta and pulmonary artery, Doppler is more sensitive and reliable in detecting the abnormal communication. Although continuous flow within the ductus itself

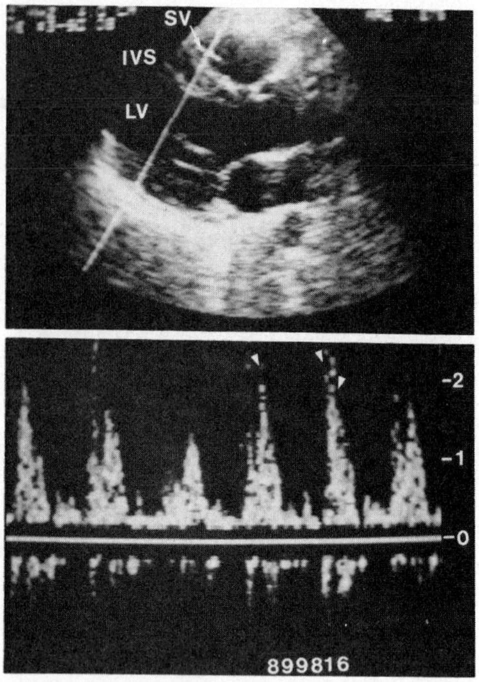

FIGURE 5–80. Parasternal long-axis examination and pulsed Doppler interrogation of a ventricular septum from a patient with a muscular ventricular septal defect. The Doppler sample volume (SV) is to the right of the interventricular septum and a high velocity jet consistent with a left-to-right shunt is seen flowing through the defect (white arrowheads). (From Feigenbaum, H.: Echocardiography. 4th ed. Philadelphia, Lea and Febiger, 1986.)

has been detected, since the ductus is frequently perpendicular to the sample volume the Doppler signal can be somewhat difficult to record. It is actually easier to make the diagnosis by obtaining Doppler recordings from the

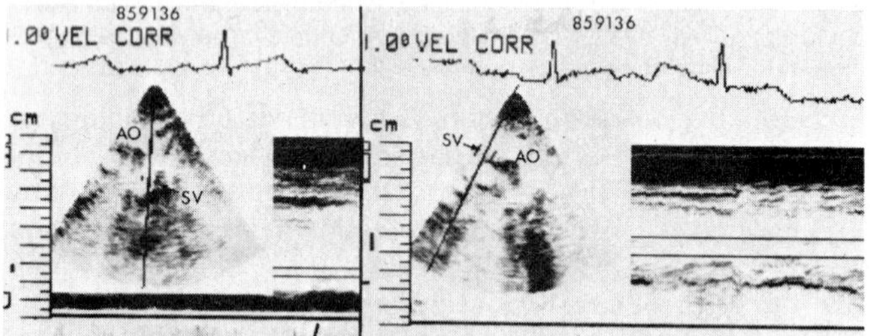

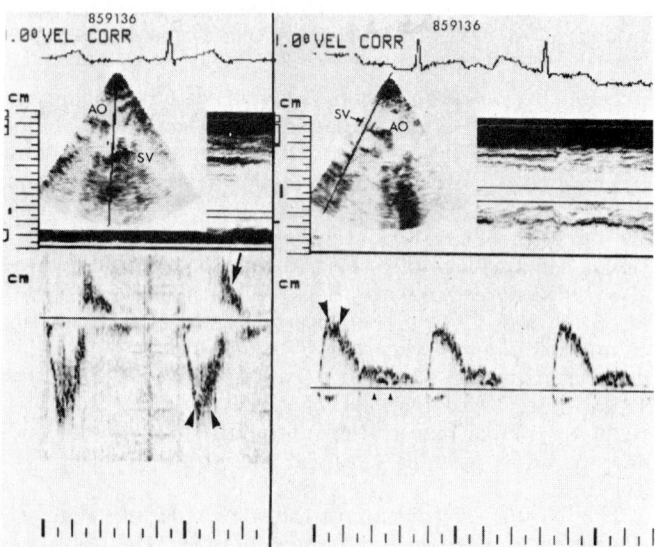

FIGURE 5–81. Composite pulsed Doppler tracings from the descending aorta (left) and ascending aorta (right) in a patient with a patent ductus arteriosus. The sample volume (SV) is placed distal to the great vessels in the left hand panel, and systolic flow away from the transducer (arrowheads) is recorded. There is also prominent retrograde flow in the aorta (arrow). With the sample volume in the ascending aorta (right) systolic flow towards the transducer is apparent; however there is no retrograde flow documenting the absence of aortic regurgitation. AO = aorta. (From Feigenbaum, H.: Echocardiography. 4th ed. Philadelphia, Lea and Febiger, 1986.)

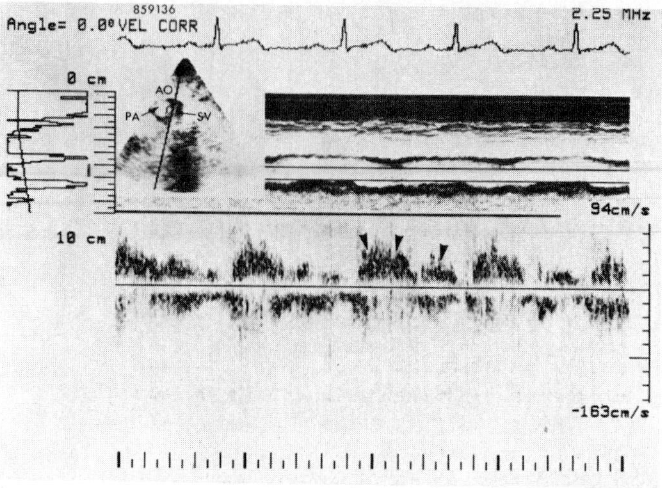

FIGURE 5–82. Pulsed Doppler examination with the sample volume (SV) placed in the wall of the pulmonary artery (PA) in the region of the presumed patent ductus. Note the presence of continuous flow in the region of the ductus (arrowheads). Ao = aorta. (From Feigenbaum, H.: Echocardiography. 4th ed. Philadelphia, Lea and Febiger, 1986.)

aorta and pulmonary artery. With the Doppler sample in the descending aorta systolic flow away from the transducer and reversed diastolic flow toward the transducer may be recorded (Fig. 5–81*A*). When the sample volume is placed in the ascending aorta, however, the reverse diastolic flow is not present (Fig. 5–81*B*). Whatever diastolic flow is recorded it is in the same direction as the systolic flow. By placing the sampling volume in the pulmonary artery, flow into the pulmonary artery can be noted in both systole and diastole as the shunted blood comes from the aorta (Fig. 5–82).

Color flow Doppler is an effective means of detecting intracardiac shunts.[256] Figure 5–83 shows a color flow recording of a patient with an ostium primum atrial septal defect. Blood flowing from the left atrium into the right atrium and right ventricle can be readily identified with this approach.

FIGURE 5–83. See color plate 2.

Besides septal defects one can also record septal aneurysms frequently associated with septal defects. The aneurysm involving the membranous portion of the interventricular septum can be imaged on the right side of the septum.[257] Atrial septal aneurysms can also be detected by two-dimensional echocardiography.[258, 259] These aneurysms are frequently quite mobile and may be seen moving between the two atria throughout the cardiac cycle.

Intracardiac shunts are frequently associated with other anomalies of the heart that can be recognized echocardiographically. For example, in patients with defects of the atrioventricular canal, anomalies of the mitral and/or tricuspid valves can be appreciated on the echocardiogram.[260] The mitral valve appears to be closer than normal to the interventricular septum, a finding consistent with the abnormal insertion of the mitral leaflet in this anomaly. Also, the tricuspid valve echo appears to traverse the interventricular septum as a result of its abnormal position. The cleft in the mitral valve commonly present with ostium primum atrial septal defect may be detected using two-dimensional echocardiography.[261]

Another valvular anomaly that may be associated with an intracardiac shunt is a tricuspid valve that overrides the ventricular septum, which can pose major problems in the repair of a ventricular septal defect and which is therefore important to recognize preoperatively. The echocardiographic findings in this condition resemble those in atrioventricular canal defects in that the tricuspid valve is recorded to the left of the interventricular septum.[262, 263]

Abnormalities of the Great Arteries

Supravalvular aortic stenosis can be detected using two-dimensional echocardiography.[224, 264, 265] The method of examination is similar to that used for the detection of valvular aortic stenosis, except that the scanning is carried out superior to the aortic valve.

Coarctation of the aorta (Fig. 31–15, p. 996) is detected with two-dimensional echocardiography by placing the probe in the suprasternal notch,[266] which allows imaging of both the narrowed segment of the aorta and the poststenotic dilation and detection of the excessive pulsation of the aorta proximal to the coarctation. Doppler echocardiography can be used to assess the hemodynamic obstruction across the coarctation.[267]

Tetralogy of Fallot is detected echocardiographically by noting a membranous ventricular septal defect and a dilated aorta which overrides the interventricular septum (Fig. 5–84 and Fig. 30–49, p. 946). The short-axis view also demonstrates a narrowing of the right ventricular outflow tract, usually at the subpulmonic level.[232] *Double-outlet right ventricle* (p. 960) is clinically similar to tetralogy of Fallot but can be differentiated echocardiographically from the more common anomaly by noting a mass of tissue between the anterior mitral leaflet and the aorta.[268] This tissue indicates that the aorta is communicating directly with the right ventricle and cannot be repaired surgically as is possible in tetralogy of Fallot. For the diagnosis of *truncus arteriosus* (p. 925), two-dimensional echocardiography helps establish the number of great arteries leaving the heart.[269] The definitive diagnosis is made by identifying the branch from the truncus that supplies the lungs.

Two-dimensional echocardiography has greatly improved the ultrasonic detection of *anomalies of the great arteries*.[269, 270] In the diagnosis

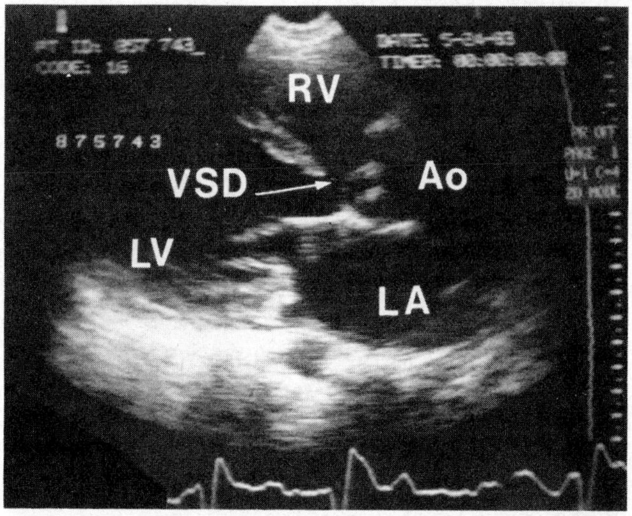

FIGURE 5–84. Parasternal long-axis examination of an adult with uncorrected tetralogy of Fallot. The ventricular septal defect (VSD) in the area of a membranous septum and overriding of the aorta (Ao) are apparent. LA = left atrium; LV = left ventricle; RV = right ventricle. (From Feigenbaum, H.: Echocardiography. 4th ed. Philadelphia, Lea and Febiger, 1986.)

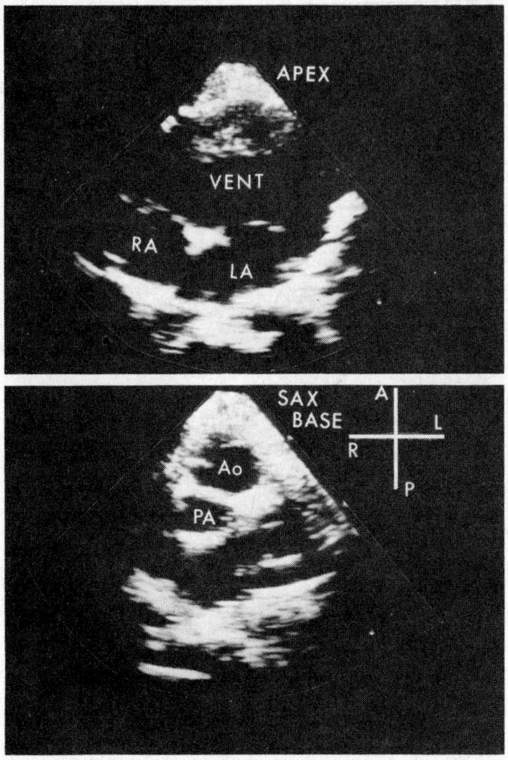

FIGURE 5–85. Apical four-chamber view (top) and short-axis (SAX) view (bottom) of the great vessels in a patient with a single ventricle and transposition of the great arteries. A single ventricular chamber (VENT) can be seen which receives blood from both the right and left atria (RA, LA). In the short-axis view two great vessels oriented in a parallel direction can be seen. The aorta (Ao) is anterior and to the left of the pulmonary artery (PA). (From Feigenbaum, H.: Echocardiography. 4th ed. Philadelphia, Lea and Febiger, 1986.)

of truncus arteriosus, two-dimensional echocardiography helps to establish the number of great arteries leaving the heart.[271] Normally, with a short-axis view of the great vessels, a circular aorta surrounded by a curved, tubular right ventricular outflow tract and pulmonary artery is recorded (Fig. 5–21, diagram 4); in truncus arteriosus only a single large circular vessel can be visualized. In addition, a new technique has been devised by actually recording the branch of the truncus that supplies the lungs in an effort to establish definitely the diagnosis of truncus arteriosus.

The two-dimensional technique for the detection of *transposition of the great arteries* (p. 957) is based on determining the relationship between the two great arteries[232, 272]; normally the pulmonary artery twists around the aorta as the latter passes posteriorly. With transposition of the great arteries, on the other hand, the two arteries run parallel to each other, and with a two-dimensional view parallel to the arteries it is possible to appreciate how the transposed arteries do not twist around each other.[273] A perpendicular or short-axis view of the great vessels demonstrates two circular structures (Fig. 5–85) rather than the pulmonary artery normally wrapping around the circular aorta (Fig. 5–21, diagram 4). Doppler examinations together with two-dimensional echocardiography helps in the recognition of corrected transposition.[274]

CORONARY ARTERY DISEASE

DETECTION OF MYOCARDIAL ISCHEMIA

Echocardiography can detect ischemic myocardium by allowing appreciation of the motion, thickening, and thickness of various segments of the heart.[275–278] Figure 5–86 shows long-axis and short-axis two-dimensional echocardiograms of a patient with an acute anterior myocardial infarction. The posterior left ventricular wall moves and thickens normally in systole (arrowheads). The anterior and septal walls fail to move or thicken from diastole to systole. This finding is characteristic of acute ischemia. The four-chamber view in Figure 5–87 shows the findings with chronic ischemia. The basal half of the left ventricle contracts normally (inward-pointing arrowheads, Fig. 5–87). The normal muscle moves toward the left ventricular cavity and increases in thickness during systole. The

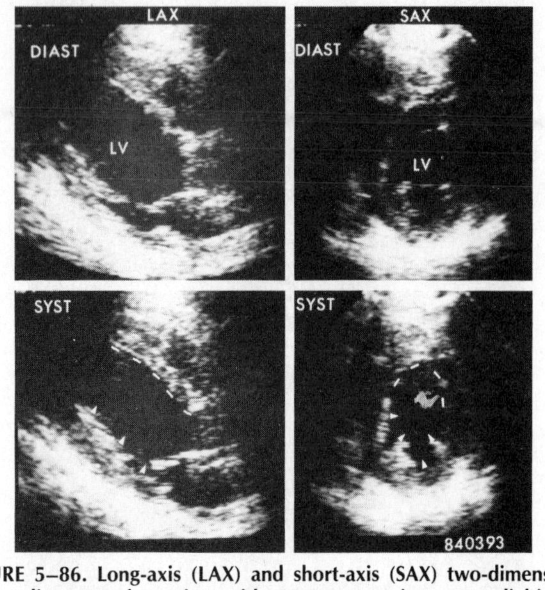

FIGURE 5–86. Long-axis (LAX) and short-axis (SAX) two-dimensional echocardiograms of a patient with an acute anterior myocardial infarction with an akinetic anterior interventricular septum and left ventricular free wall. In systole the non-ischemic walls move normally (arrowheads). The ischemic muscle fails to contract (dashed line). LV = left ventricle. (From Feigenbaum, H.: Echocardiography. 4th ed. Philadelphia, Lea and Febiger, 1986.)

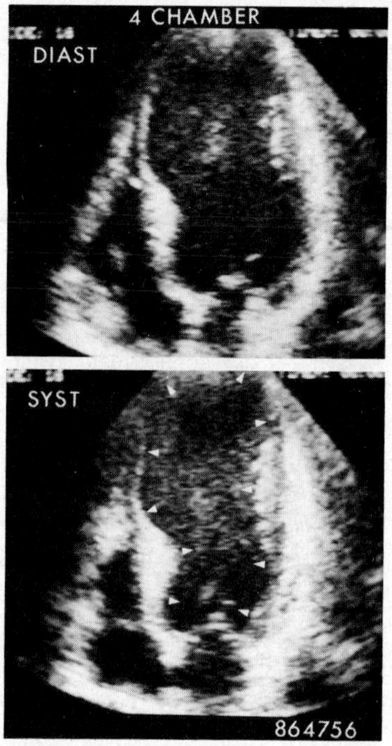

FIGURE 5–87. Apical four-chamber view of a patient with a scarred, dilated, aneurysmal apex and distal interventricular septum. The proximal half of the septum has normal thickness and contracts normally with systole. (From Feigenbaum, H.: Echocardiography. 4th ed. Philadelphia, Lea and Febiger, 1986.)

apical half of the septum and the apex is much thinner than the basal half and fails to move with systole. The loss of myocardial tissue is indicative of scar formation (outward pointing arrowheads).[279] When the myocardium decreases in total thickness, the muscle is irreversibly damaged. As long as the myocardium retains normal thickness (Fig. 5–86), the damage is potentially reversible.

Figure 5–88 shows an M-mode recording of a patient with reversible ischemia.[280] The control recording shows normal septal and posterior ventricular wall motion. With handgrip, ischemia is produced and septal motion and thickening are abolished. Total wall thickness remains normal. The posterior ventricular wall motion is unchanged. Following recovery from ischemia, septal motion and thickening return to normal. Because wall motion and thickening are excellent indicators of ischemia, exercise or stress echocardiography is becoming increasingly popular.[281–285] Many of the technical difficulties involved in performing echocardiograms during or immediately after exercise have been resolved with the use of computer

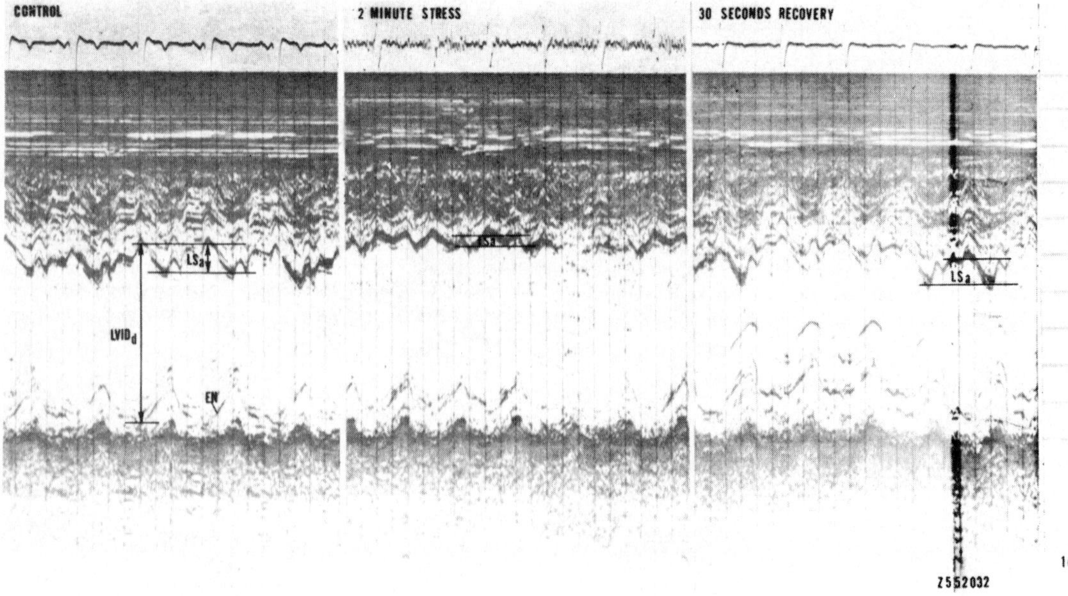

FIGURE 5–88. Serial M-mode echocardiograms from a patient with spasm of the left anterior descending coronary artery. At rest, the left septal echo amplitude (LS_a) is normal. During handgrip stress, the patient develops angina, and the amplitude of septal motion is markedly reduced. Following cessation of handgrip and the disappearance of pain, septal motion returns to normal. (From Widlansky, S., et al.: Coronary angiography, echocardiographic, and electrocardiographic studies on a patient with variant angina due to coronary artery spasm. Am. Heart J. *90*:631, 1975.)

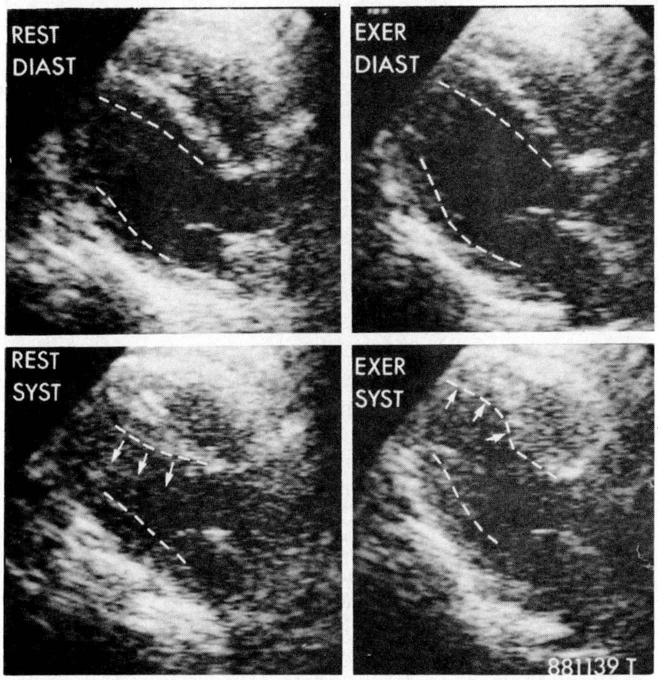

FIGURE 5–89. Resting and immediate postexercise echocardiograms of a patient with an obstruction in the left anterior descending coronary artery. At rest the septal motion is normal (arrows) (REST, SYST). Immediately following exercise the septum becomes dyskinetic (reverse arrows) (EXER, SYST). (From Feigenbaum, H.: Echocardiography. 4th ed. Philadelphia, Lea and Febiger, 1986.)

technology and the construction of continuous loop two-dimensional echocardiograms.[58] With these digital techniques the resting and exercise continuous loops can be placed side by side on a split screen or quad screen format. Thus, subtle changes in wall motion as a result of exercise-induced ischemia can be detected. Figure 5–89 shows a long-axis echocardiogram before and immediately after treadmill exercise. At rest systolic motion of the interventricular septum is normal; however, with exercise the distal half of the septum becomes ischemic and akinetic (reverse arrows).

ASSESSMENT OF LEFT VENTRICULAR PERFORMANCE

There are many echocardiographic techniques available for assessing left ventricular performance in patients with coronary artery disease. Although the M-mode left ventricular dimensions are of limited value in patients with regional heart disease, measurements such as mitral valve E point septal separation and abnormal closure of the mitral valve can give a reasonable assessment of altered left ventricular function in patients with coronary artery disease. The E point–septal separation increases when left ventricular ejection fraction decreases and abnormal closure of the mitral valve occurs in patients with elevated atrial components of the left ventricular diastolic pressure. Doppler echocardiography can also be used to evaluate global left ventricular function. Flow in the ascending aorta reflects global left ventricular systolic function. Acceleration and peak velocity are reduced as global left ventricular function deteriorates. Instantaneous mitral valve flow can reflect reduced left ventricular compliance.[286] With ischemia the early diastolic flow or E point is reduced and the velocity of flow with atrial systole (A point) is increased. As a result the E/A ratio turns from a normal positive value to a negative one.[287]

The best echocardiographic technique for evaluating left ventricular performance utilizes two-dimensional echocardiography and the assessment of regional wall motion.[288, 289] The left ventricle is divided into a number of segments. Determining the motion of each segment provides a *wall motion score* for the entire chamber.[290] A number of schemes have been suggested in the literature. Any or all of these techniques provides a reasonable assessment of both regional and global left ventricular function. Standard ejection fractions can also be calculated from the apical two-chamber or four-chamber views in patients with coronary artery disease.[291, 292] Because of the frequently distorted shape of the ventricle in these patients Simpson's rule technique (p. 97) is preferred. Minor axis measurements using parasternal long-axis or short-axis views can also be very helpful in patients with coronary artery disease by providing regional systolic function. Frequently the status of the base of the left ventricle is a better predictor of prognosis than is global ejection fraction, especially in patients who have apical aneurysms.[293, 294]

MYOCARDIAL INFARCTION

COMPLICATIONS. All of the common complications of myocardial infarction have been detected with echocardiographic techniques. Probably the most common problem is the development of a left ventricular aneurysm.[293–295] Figure 5–87 shows the echocardiographic findings characteristic of an aneurysm. There is a loss of myocardial thickness, scar formation, localized dilatation, and frequently dyskinesis. Figure 5–90 shows another patient with an apical aneurysm. The anterior septum is thin and scarred. The apex shows a characteristic distortion in shape and function.

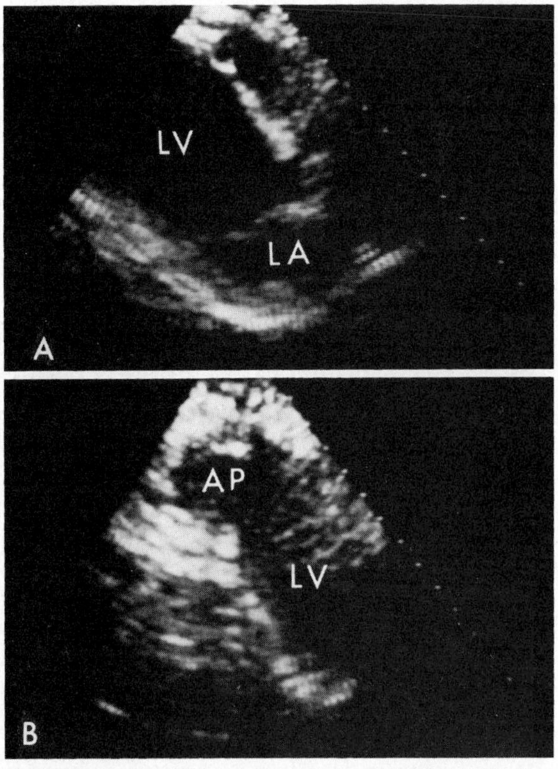

FIGURE 5–90. Parasternal long-axis two-dimensional echocardiograms of a patient with coronary artery disease, a scarred interventricular septum, and an apical aneurysm. *A* demonstrates the body of the left ventricle (LV) and left atrium (LA). Note the thin, relatively echo-dense septum. *B*, Apical examination reveals the aneurysm (AP). (From Feigenbaum, H.: Echocardiography. 3rd ed. Philadelphia, Lea and Febiger, 1981.)

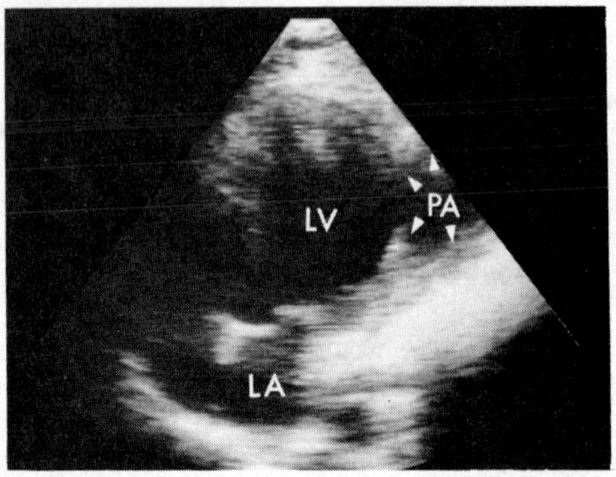

FIGURE 5–91. Four-chamber two-dimensional echocardiogram of a patient with a pseudoaneurysm (PA) adjacent to the posterior lateral free wall of the left ventricle (LV). LA = left atrium. (From Feigenbaum, H.: Echocardiography. 4th ed. Philadelphia, Lea and Febiger, 1986.)

A *pseudoaneurysm* (p. 1282) is a serious complication which represents rupture of the free wall. The blood leaving the cavity of the left ventricle is trapped in the pericardium, clot forms within the pericardial sac, and an aneurysmal wall consisting of clot and pericardium keeps the patient from exsanguinating. The echocardiographic appearance of this complication is fairly characteristic, with the neck of the aneurysm being smaller than the body (Fig. 5–91).[296] Doppler flow patterns within the aneurysm can help differentiate between a true and a false aneurysm.[297] Indications for surgery are more urgent with a pseudoaneurysm; therefore, the diagnosis is critical.

Aneurysmal dilatation and subsequent *perforation of the ventricular septum* (p. 1284) is another complication that can occur with myocardial infarction. The septal aneurysm is commonly seen on the two-dimensional echocardiogram.[298] On rare occasions the actual perforation can be visualized.[299] The echocardiographic diagnosis, however, is best made with Doppler echocardiography.[300] Putting the sample volume on the right ventricular side of the interventricular septum, one can record the high velocity systolic flow going from the left ventricle to the right ventricle through the ruptured septum (Fig. 5–92).

Right ventricular infarction (p. 1242) is an increasingly recognized complication of myocardial infarction and can have important clinical implications in the management of the patient. Figure 5–93 shows the common echocardiographic findings with right ventricular infarction.[301–303] These patients usually have evidence of an inferior infarction. The inferior-posterior wall of the left ventricle is akinetic in systole (dashes) as noted in the short-axis view. The evidence for right ventricular infarction is right ventricular dilatation and right ventricular free wall motion akinesis (dashes) (Fig. 5–93). Premature pulmonary valve opening may occur with right ventricular infarction.[304]

Mural thrombi (p. 1285) represent another common complication with myocardial infarction that can be detected with echocardiography.[305, 306] These clots occur most often with aneurysms, especially involving the anterior wall and apex. Figure 5–94 shows a thrombus in the apex of a patient with an apical aneurysm. The thrombi may have a variety of configurations; those which protrude into the cavity, such as in Figure 5–94, are easier to detect echocardiographically and may have a higher likelihood of producing systemic emboli.[307, 308] Other thrombi are layered along the wall and may not be as likely to break loose.

Other complications of acute myocardial infarction, such as mitral regurgitation[309] and pericardial effusion, are easily detected echocardiographically.

NATURAL HISTORY AND PROGNOSIS. Echocardiogra-

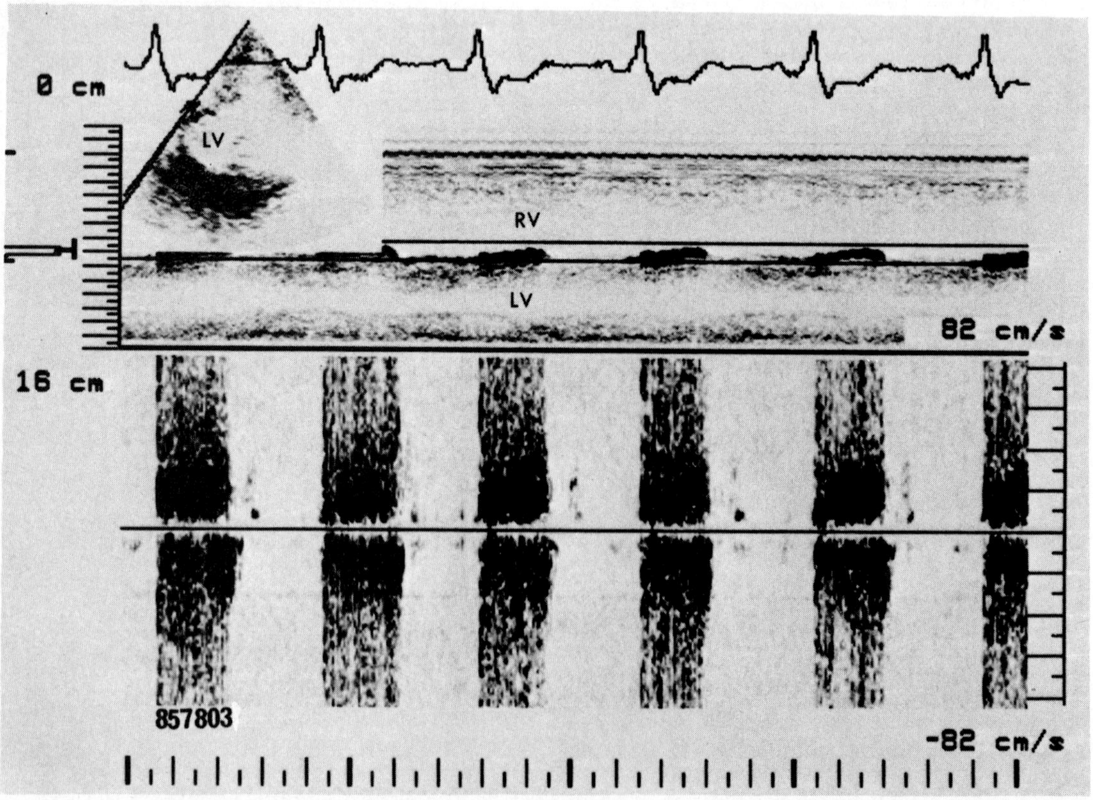

FIGURE 5–92. Pulsed Doppler echocardiogram of a patient with a ruptured ventricular septum following an acute myocardial infarction. With the sample volume to the right of the interventricular septum one records a high velocity systolic flow from the left-to-right shunt. RV = right ventricle; LV = left ventricle.

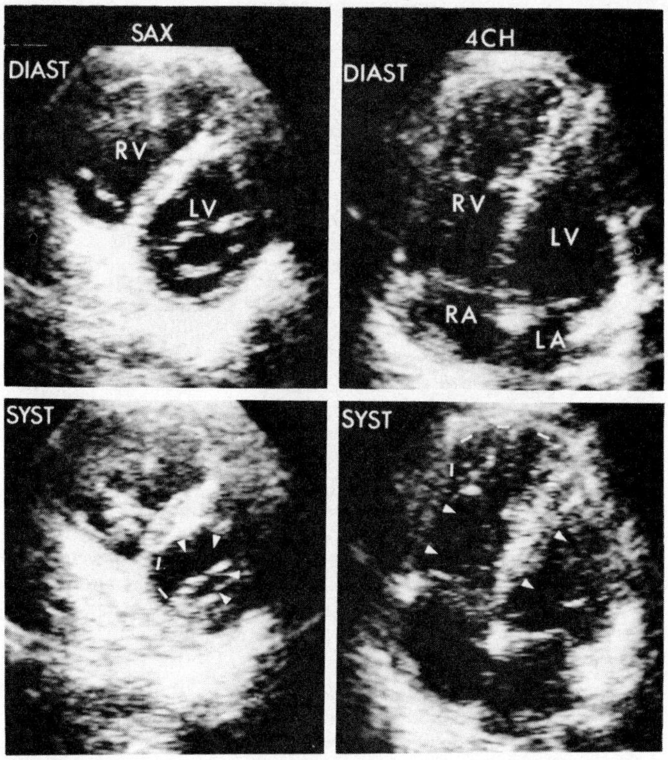

FIGURE 5–93. Short-axis (SAX) and four-chamber (4CH) two-dimensional echocardiograms of a patient with an inferior myocardial infarction complicated by right ventricular infarction. The posterior-inferior wall is akinetic (dashed line SAX SYST). In addition, the apical half of the right ventricular free wall is akinetic (arrows, 4CH SYST). The right ventricle (RV) is also dilated. RA = right atrium; LV = left ventricle; LA = left atrium. (From Feigenbaum, H.: Echocardiography. 4th ed. Philadelphia, Lea and Febiger, 1986.)

phy is ideal for serial studies in patients with myocardial infarction. Two-dimensional echocardiography carried out early in the course of an infarction is helpful in establishing the diagnosis,[310] but provides prognostic information as well.[311, 312] This examination is useful in the assessment of the status of the myocardium not involved in the current infarction; an unsuspected previous infarction may be discovered. An early echocardiographic study also can serve as a baseline for detecting future ischemic events or complications. The initial examination may even help identify the patients who are at high risk of experiencing complications.[313, 314] A two-dimensional echocardiogram prior to discharge can also provide long-term prognostic information.[315]

EXAMINATION OF THE CORONARY ARTERIES

Two-dimensional echocardiography can indirectly evaluate myocardial perfusion and can be helpful in predicting obstruction in specific coronary arteries because of the predictable relationship between certain myocardial segments and specific coronary arteries.[316] For example, the anterior interventricular septum and apex are invariably perfused by the left anterior descending coronary artery while the posterior septum and inferior wall are always supplied by the posterior descending coronary artery, which usually arises from the right coronary artery. Thus one can usually predict the vessel with severe obstruction from a two-dimensional echocardiogram showing impaired regional myocardial contraction.

Direct visualization of the proximal coronary arteries is also feasible.[317, 318] With improved technology, especially the development of annular array two-dimensional echocardiographic systems, the resolution required for visualizing the coronary arteries has been improved dramatically.[319] Figure 5–95 shows an annular array study of the left proximal coronary artery system in which it is possible to identify the left main, proximal circumflex, left anterior

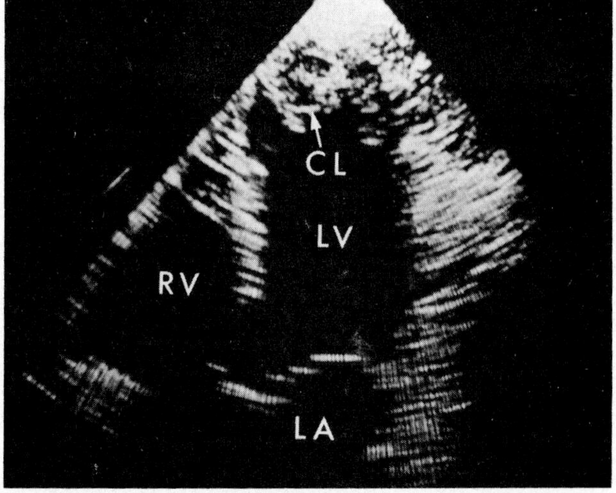

FIGURE 5–94. Apical four-chamber two-dimensional echocardiogram of a patient with an apical clot (CL). LV = left ventricle; RV = right ventricle; LA = left atrium. (From Feigenbaum, H.: Echocardiography. 3rd ed. Philadelphia, Lea and Febiger, 1981.)

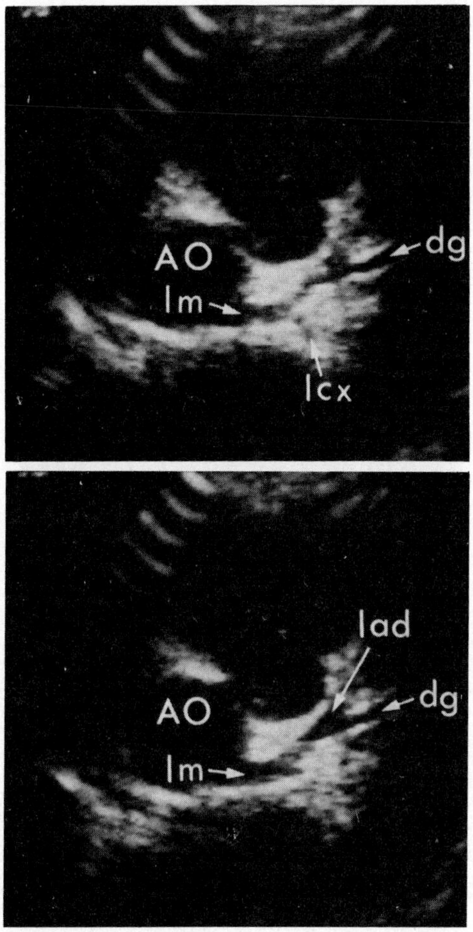

FIGURE 5–95. Short-axis two-dimensional echocardiogram of the left coronary artery using an annular phased array system. AO = aorta; lm = left main coronary artery; lcx = left circumflex; dg = diagonal; lad = left anterior descending.

descending, and diagonal arteries. The ultimate value of examining the coronary arteries echocardiographically has yet to be determined. Several investigators have noted the ability of echocardiography to detect atherosclerotic obstructions in the left main coronary artery.[320] It is also likely that obstructive lesions in the proximal left anterior descending coronary artery will also be detectable by echocardiographic examination.

Congenital anomalies of the coronary arteries (pp. 952 and 1000) can be detected by means of both two-dimensional, Doppler, and Doppler color echocardiography.[321, 322] The value of two-dimensional echocardiography in visualizing coronary artery aneurysms in Kawasaki disease has been well demonstrated (Fig. 32–7, p. 1016).[323]

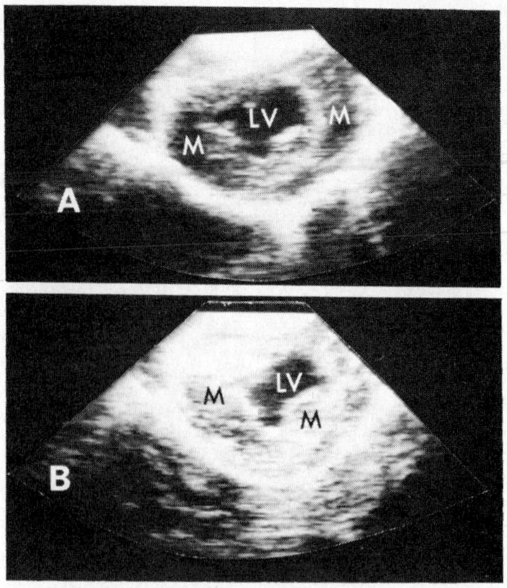

FIGURE 5–96. Short-axis two-dimensional echocardiogram of a dog before and after injection of contrast in the root of the aorta. Prior to contrast (A) the myocardium (M) is relatively echo-free. Following the injection of fluid containing tiny microbubbles (B) the myocardium becomes uniformly echogenic.

Myocardial Perfusion Using Contrast Echocardiography

Contrast echocardiography may also be employed to study myocardial perfusion.[324–326] If a fluid containing microbubbles is injected into the root of the aorta or directly into the coronary arteries, the echogenicity of the myocardium will be increased (Fig. 5–96), provided that the blood supply is intact. When blood flow is impeded, then the increase in echogenicity in that segment is reduced or absent. Such studies have been done extensively in animal models. One can determine infarct size and myocardial perfusion rather precisely with this technique. There is only limited experience in patients thus far. The examination is obviously invasive and requires injections into the aortic root or coronary artery; the clinical role for this procedure has yet to be determined.

CARDIOMYOPATHIES

(See also Chap. 42)

HYPERTROPHIC OBSTRUCTIVE CARDIOMYOPATHY (HOCM)

Echocardiography is an important diagnostic tool in patients with HOCM and has enriched our understanding of this abnormality. The first echocardiographic abnormality to be noted was systolic anterior motion of the mitral valve (termed "SAM") (Fig. 5–97, Fig. 42–8, p. 1422),[327] which appeared to be related to and was correlated with the presence of obstruction to left ventricular outflow.[328] The shorter the distance between the septum and the leaflet and the longer the duration of apposition between these two structures, the greater the degree of obstruction.[329] This echocardiographic finding not only provided another diagnostic sign of HOCM but also demonstrated the critical importance of involvement of the mitral valve apparatus in the obstruction.[330] More recently SAM has been noted in a variety of patients, some of whom had no evidence of left ventricular hypertrophy;[331, 332] it has been observed in patients with anemia and hypovolemia as well as in those with a hyperdynamic left ventricle.[331] It is possible that SAM is a nonspecific sign that occurs when-

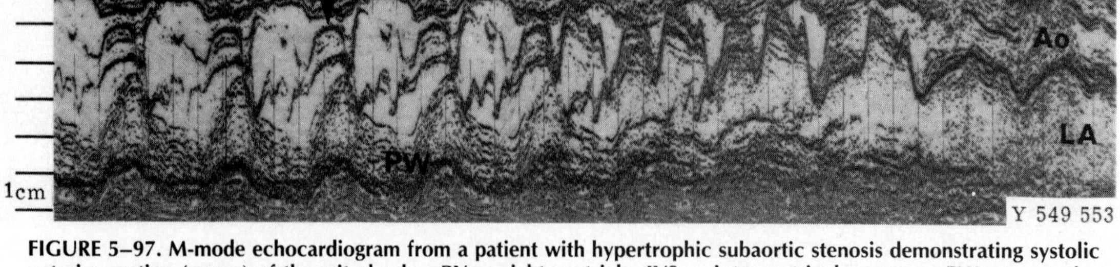

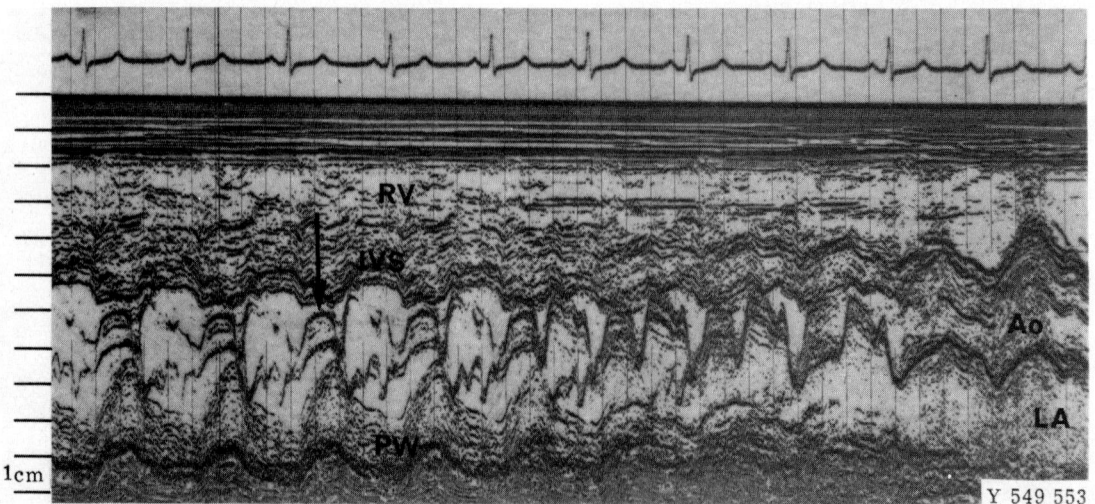

FIGURE 5–97. M-mode echocardiogram from a patient with hypertrophic subaortic stenosis demonstrating systolic anterior motion (arrow) of the mitral valve. RV = right ventricle, IVS = interventricular septum, PW = posterior left ventricular wall, Ao = aorta, LA = left atrium. (From Chang, S.: M-Mode Echocardiographic Technique and Pattern Recognition. Philadelphia, Lea and Febiger, 1976.)

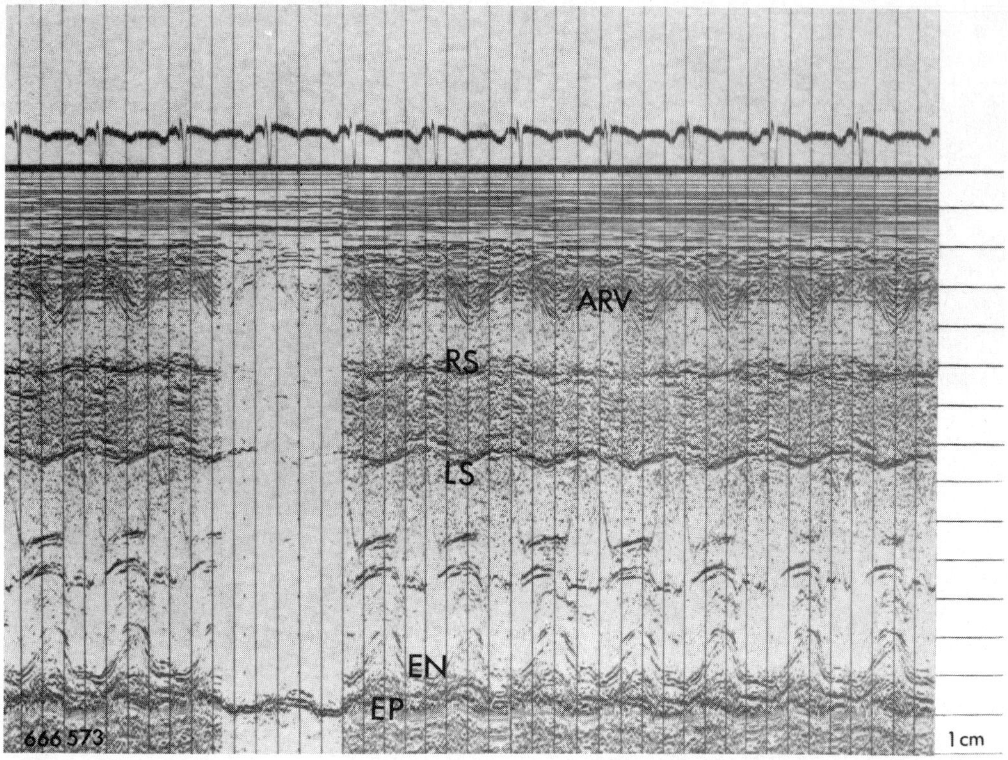

FIGURE 5–98. Echocardiogram from a patient with asymmetrical septal hypertrophy but no evidence of outflow obstruction. The distance between the right (RS) and left (LS) septal echoes is considerably greater than is the thickness of the posterior left ventricular myocardium between the endocardial (EN) and epicardial (EP) echoes.

ever the left ventricular systolic volume is reduced, either because of hypertrophy, as in HOCM, or in the presence of a hyperdynamic state.[333]

A second echocardiographic finding in patients with HOCM is midsystolic closure of the aortic valve. However, as noted earlier, this sign is not specific for HOCM and is also present in patients with discrete subaortic stenosis. While not sensitive, this finding, when present, usually indicates a significant amount of obstruction.

Hypertrophy of the septum with abnormal organization of myocardial cells may be one of the basic abnormalities of HOCM[334] (p. 1419), and key echocardiographic findings are disproportionate hypertrophy of the septum in relation to the posterior wall of the left ventricle, so that the ratio of thickness of the septum to the free wall exceeds 1.3/1.0 (Fig. 5–97),[334] and the motion of the hypertrophied septum is reduced.[335] It has also been shown that asymmetrical septal hypertrophy (ASH) is transmitted as an autosomal dominant trait and that there are patients with asymmetrical septal hypertrophy who do not show SAM and therefore do not have obstruction to left ventricular outflow (Fig. 5–98).[334, 336] These patients may be considered to have hypertrophic cardiomyopathy without obstruction. While the concept of recognizing ASH with or without obstruction to left ventricular outflow by echocardiography is an important one, there are limitations to echocardiographic diagnosis. First, the thickness of the septum may be difficult to measure precisely echocardiographically. (In Figure 5–97 the left side of the septum is clearly identified, but the right side is not as distinct.) Second, it must be appreciated that ASH is not pathognomonic for HOCM and related myopathies and can occur in a variety of other disease states (including right ventricular hypertrophy and coronary artery disease and even in patients on chronic hemodialysis) in a form which is indistinguishable echocardiographically from genetically determined ASH. In addition, some patients with HOCM may have concentric rather than asymmetrical hypertrophy, in which the septal and posterior left ventricular walls are equal in thickness (p. 1419).

Two-dimensional echocardiography provides additional information by indicating the shape and location of the hypertrophied septum in patients with known or suspected HOCM.[337] A variety of hypertrophied septal segments has been recorded by this technique. Figure 5–99 shows a hypertrophied septum limited to the basal two-thirds of the septum, while the apex is virtually free of muscular hypertrophy. Other patients exhibit an apical form of hypertrophy with the proximal septum being relatively

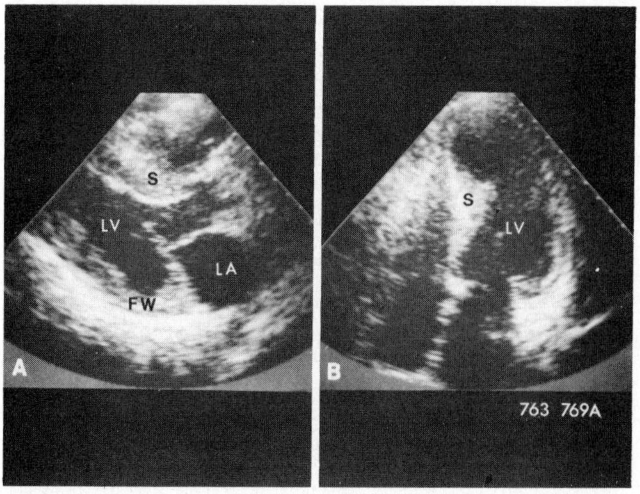

FIGURE 5–99. Long-axis (*A*) and apical four-chamber (*B*) echocardiograms of a patient with hypertrophic cardiomyopathy whose hypertrophy primarily involves the proximal two-thirds of the interventricular septum (S). The apex is spared from the hypertrophic process. LV = left ventricle; FW = left ventricular free wall; LA = left atrium. (From Feigenbaum, H.: Echocardiography. 4th ed. Philadelphia, Lea and Febiger, 1986.)

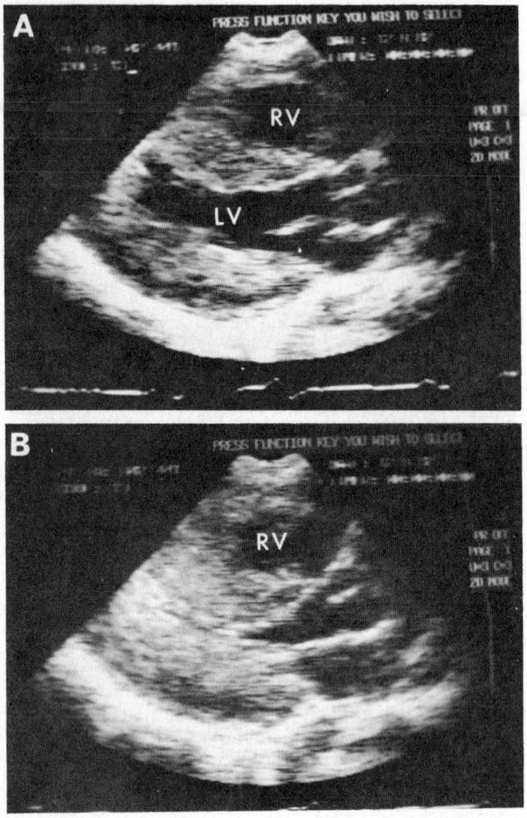

FIGURE 5–100. Long-axis two-dimensional echocardiogram of a patient with hypertrophic cardiomyopathy who exhibits uniform hypertrophy of the entire left ventricle (LV). RV = right ventricle; A = diastole; B = systole. (From Feigenbaum, H.: Echocardiography. 4th ed. Philadelphia, Lea and Febiger, 1986.)

thin.[338] Concentric hypertrophy is also a fairly common form of hypertrophic myopathy (Fig. 5–100). Cavity obliteration with ventricular systole is almost always present with this type of disease. Two-dimensional echocardiography is useful in assessing the effectiveness of myotomy and myectomy. An intriguing observation is that the echoes from the diseased septum in HOCM are more reflective or "speckled" than those from the free posterior wall.

Doppler echocardiography may also be helpful in evaluating patients with hypertrophic cardiomyopathy.[339] The Doppler recording of the left ventricular outflow may show an abnormal pattern with cessation of flow in mid systole. In addition, the systolic gradient can be estimated using the Doppler technique. The left ventricular hypertrophy and reduced left ventricular compliance alters the Doppler recording of mitral valve flow. The early diastolic velocity or E point is reduced and the late velocity with atrial systole is increased.[340] Altered diastolic function can also be recorded with digital M-mode recordings.[341]

CONGESTIVE (DILATED) CARDIOMYOPATHY

The echocardiogram characteristically reveals a dilated, poorly contracting left ventricle in patients with congestive cardiomyopathy (Fig. 42–13, p. 1425).[342, 343] Signs of reduced cardiac output include a poorly moving aorta, reduced opening of the mitral valve, and slow closure of the aortic valve. The left atrium is dilated, and the abnormal closure of the mitral valve indicative of elevated left diastolic pressure is frequently noted. The rate of left ventricular filling on the digitized M-mode tracing is reduced. It must be appreciated that these findings are nonspecific and may also occur in patients with ischemic heart disease. However, at least one portion of the left ventricle, usually the posterior wall, continues to exhibit normal motion in most, though not all, patients with severe coronary artery disease.[342] In patients with cardiomyopathy the impairment of left ventricular wall motion is diffuse and includes the posterior wall. If mitral regurgitation develops in patients with cardiomyopathy, septal motion may increase slightly in keeping with the left ventricular volume overload, although this increase in septal motion is certainly not as striking as that which occurs in primary mitral valve disease with secondary myocardial failure.

RESTRICTIVE (INFILTRATIVE) CARDIOMYOPATHY

The principal echocardiographic findings in patients with infiltrative cardiomyopathy are reduced wall motion and thickening of the left ventricular wall without dilatation;[344, 345] these changes are usually uniform throughout the ventricle. Obviously, these findings are not specific for infil-

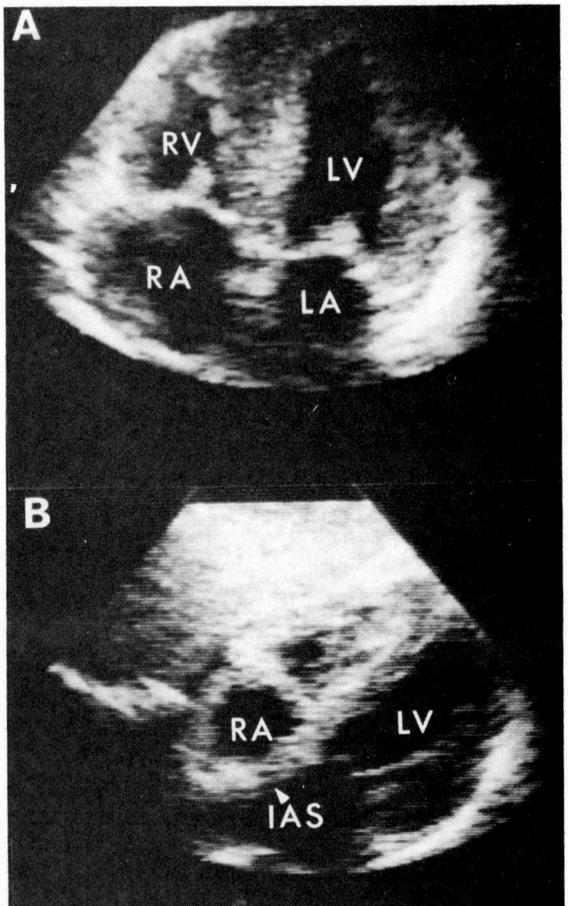

FIGURE 5–101. Four-chamber (*A*) and subcostal (*B*) two-dimensional echocardiograms of a patient with hereditary amyloidosis. The four-chamber view demonstrates markedly hypertrophied cardiac walls, especially the interventricular septum and free wall of the right ventricle. The tricuspid and mitral valve leaflets are also thickened. The left ventricle (LV) and right ventricle (RV) cavities are small. The subcostal examination demonstrates a thickened interatrial septum (IAS). RA = right atrium; LA = left atrium. (From Feigenbaum, H.: Echocardiography. 4th ed. Philadelphia, Lea and Febiger, 1986.)

trative cardiomyopathy and, like those obtained by means of electrocardiography, chest roentgenography, hemodynamics, and angiocardiography, must be interpreted in terms of the total clinical setting. In patients with amyloid heart disease (Fig. 5–101)[346, 347] the echocardiographic findings are usually nonspecific and show left ventricular hypertrophy. There are also frequently more specific findings in that the valves may be uniformly thickened in addition to the hypertrophy of the ventricular walls. The interatrial septum may also be unusually thick, and a peculiar speckled appearance of the myocardium may be noted, reflecting localized variations in echo density. Diastolic relaxation as judged by digitized M-mode recordings is impaired.[36]

PERICARDIAL DISEASE

(See Chap. 44)

PERICARDIAL EFFUSION

The theory underlying the use of ultrasound in the recognition of pericardial effusion is relatively simple; since the acoustical properties of fluid differ significantly from those of cardiac muscle, the effusion surrounding the heart is less echo-producing than is the myocardium. Accordingly, the detection of effusion was one of the first and has remained one of the most useful applications of echocardiography.[348, 349] Figure 5–36 shows the echocardiographic appearance of a relatively small pericardial effusion in a patient with left ventricular hypertrophy. There is a clear space between the posterior left ventricular epicardial echo and the surrounding pericardium, and on close inspection there is also a small echo-free space between the anterior wall of the right ventricle and the chest wall. This figure demonstrates the sensitivity of echocardiography in detecting a small amount (as little as 20 ml) of pericardial fluid,[350] an amount which would easily be missed by other techniques.

Figures 5–102 and 44–11 (p. 1497) are echograms from patients with large pericardial effusions; although there is a potential space behind the left atrium, it rarely fills with pericardial fluid. When it does,[351] the quantity is considerably less than that behind the posterior wall of the left ventricle. There is a large echo-free space anteriorly, and during much of the cardiac cycle, the anterior and posterior cardiac walls move in the same direction, rather than in opposite directions, and the amplitude of motion of the anterior wall of the right ventricle is excessive. This type of cardiac motion has been referred to as a "swinging heart"[352, 353]; as would be expected, the motion of all the cardiac structures is distorted by this excessive cardiac displacement, and any diagnosis based on this pattern of motion can be misleading. False-positive findings of prolapse of the mitral valve, of systolic anterior motion of the mitral valve, and of abnormal septal motion have all been reported in such patients.[354]

When the motion of the heart within the pericardial effusion is increased markedly and, in particular, when this is accompanied by tachycardia, the heart may not have returned to its previous position by the time the next cardiac cycle commences. Figure 5–103A demonstrates an echogram in such a patient; with each depolarization the heart is in a slightly different position, and the electrocardiographic QRS complex also varies[352] with alternating heights of R waves on the electrocardiogram, i.e., electrical alternans (p. 214). When, in the same patient, the cardiac motion becomes regular, as reflected in the echogram in Figure 5–103*B*, electrical alternation ceases. Parenthetically it should be pointed out that the manner in which echocardiography helped to explain the mechanism for electrical alternans in patients with pericardial effusion is an excellent example of how this technique has elucidated cardiac physiological and pathophysiological phenomena.

Two-dimensional echocardiography plays a dominant role in the assessment of pericardial effusion (p. 1492). Although M-mode echocardiography can make the qualitative diagnosis, there are many situations in which the fluid collects in a nonuniform fashion around the heart, and two-dimensional echocardiography is more reliable in identifying the location and amount of fluid.[355] Figure 5–104 demonstrates long-axis (*A*) and short-axis (*B*) views of a patient with both pericardial and pleural effusions. The pleural effusion can be identified since it is separated from the heart by the descending aorta.[356] Pericardial effusion, on the other hand, is between the aorta and the heart.

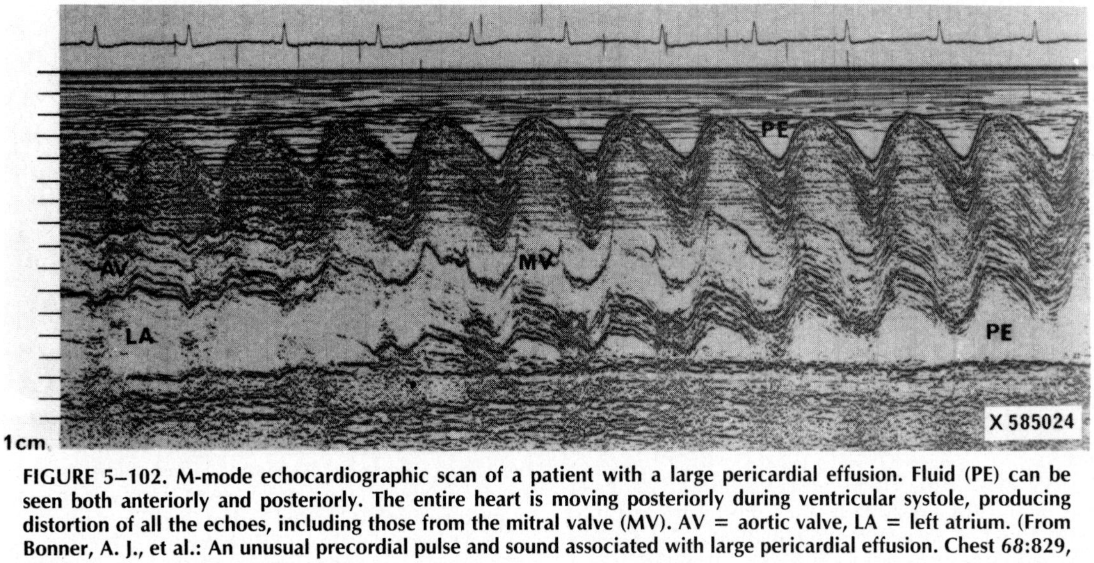

FIGURE 5–102. M-mode echocardiographic scan of a patient with a large pericardial effusion. Fluid (PE) can be seen both anteriorly and posteriorly. The entire heart is moving posteriorly during ventricular systole, producing distortion of all the echoes, including those from the mitral valve (MV). AV = aortic valve, LA = left atrium. (From Bonner, A. J., et al.: An unusual precordial pulse and sound associated with large pericardial effusion. Chest *68*:829, 1975.)

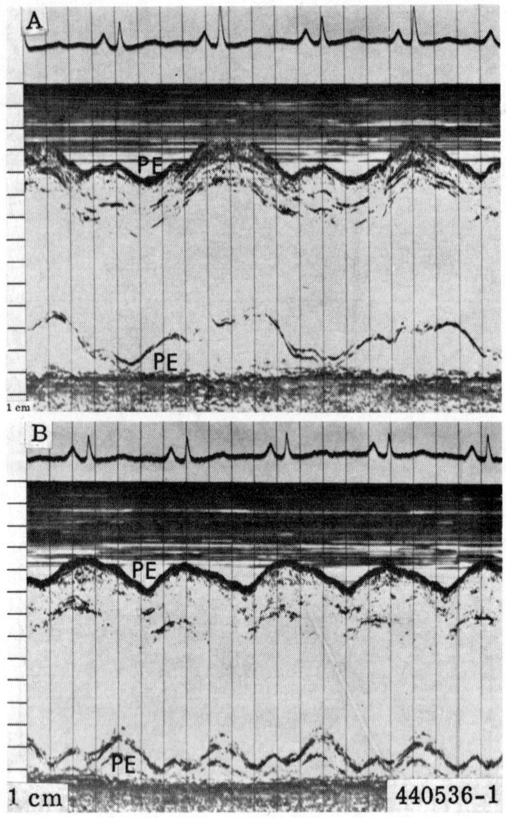

FIGURE 5–103. Echocardiograms from a patient with massive pericardial effusion (PE). *A*, Anterior right ventricular echo (ARV) and posterior left ventricular epicardial echoes move essentially in similar directions. The position of the heart differs slightly with each cardiac cycle. The corresponding electrocardiogram shows electrical alternation. Upon removal of some of the pericardial fluid (*B*), cardiac excursions are synchronous with each electrical depolarization, and electrical alternation is no longer present. (From Feigenbaum, H.: Echocardiography. 2nd ed. Philadelphia, Lea and Febiger, 1976.)

CARDIAC TAMPONADE. Once the diagnosis of pericardial effusion has been established, a number of echocardiographic findings which are characteristic of cardiac tamponade should be searched for.[357, 358] A reliable echocardiographic finding with tamponade is compression of the right ventricular free wall in early diastole. This finding is noted by posterior displacement of the anterior free wall on the M-mode echocardiogram (Fig. 5–105).[352] The free wall then moves anteriorly following atrial systole. This observation has been confirmed with two-dimensional echocardiography by noting a collapse of the right ventricular free wall (Fig. 5–106).[358, 359] Another finding is a diastolic indentation (collapse) of the right atrial free wall on the two-dimensional four-chamber view (Fig. 5–107).[360] Both of these signs (diastolic collapse of the right atrium and right ventricle) appear to be very sensitive for detecting hemodynamic impairment secondary to tamponade, and sometimes even antedate the clinical signs of tamponade. The other echocardiographic signs of tamponade, such as reduction of the size of the right ventricular cavity, flat diastolic motion of the left ventricular wall, and variations in the E to F slope of the mitral valve,[357] have not proved to be reliable.

CONSTRICTIVE PERICARDITIS. Echocardiography can be of some value in the diagnosis of a thickened pericardium with constrictive pericarditis.[361–363] However, the reliability of the technique is limited. Although a thickened pericar-

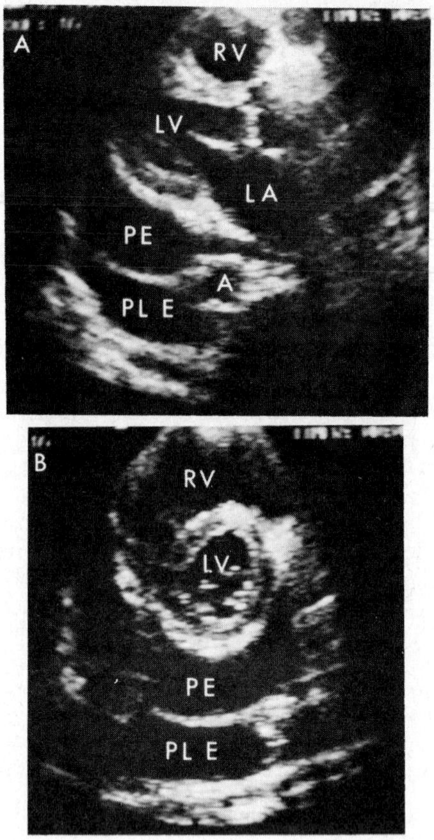

FIGURE 5–104. Long-axis (*A*) and short-axis (*B*) two-dimensional echocardiograms of a patient with pericardial effusion (PE) and pleural effusion (PL E). In the long-axis view the aorta (A) lies between the two bodies of fluid. RV = right ventricle; LV = left ventricle; LA = left atrium. (From Feigenbaum H.: Echocardiography. 4th ed. Philadelphia, Lea and Febiger, 1986.)

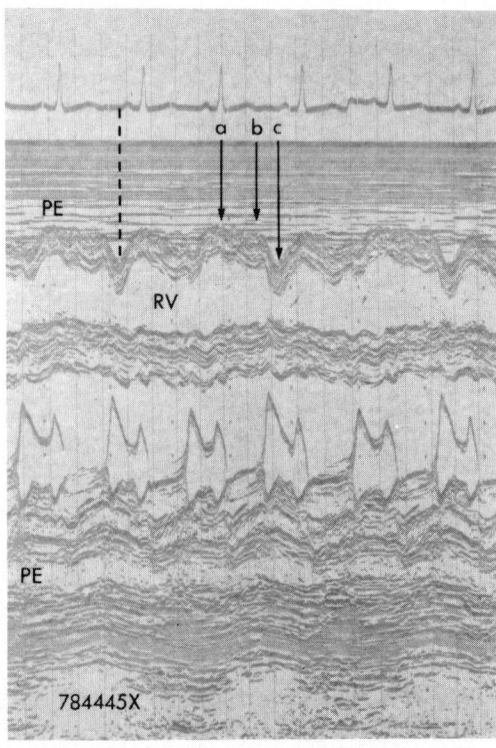

FIGURE 5–105. M-mode echocardiogram of a patient with pericardial effusion and clinical evidence of tamponade. The right ventricular free wall moves gradually posteriorly during systole (from a to b). In early diastole there is an abrupt downward or posterior motion of the right ventricular free wall (c and dashed line). PE = pericardial effusion; RV = right ventricle. (From Feigenbaum, H.: Echocardiography. 4th ed. Philadelphia, Lea and Febiger, 1986.)

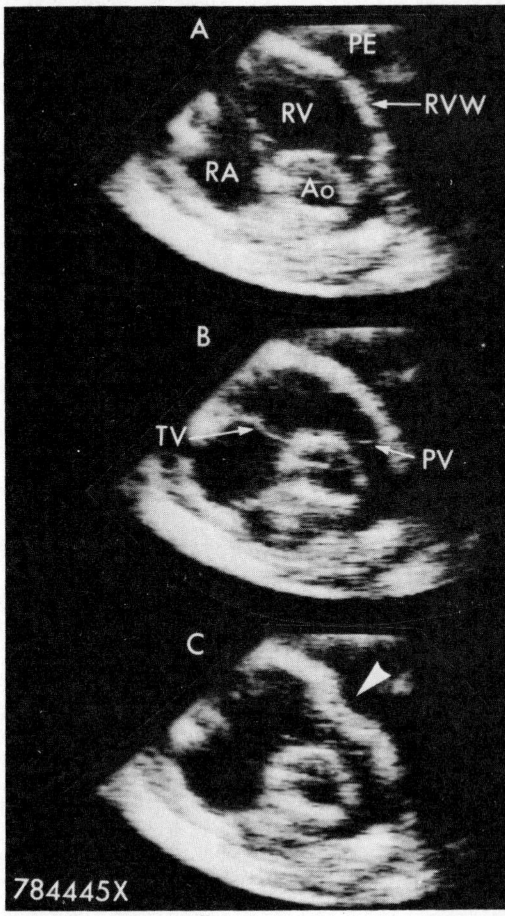

FIGURE 5–106. Parasternal short-axis two-dimensional echocardiograms in a patient with cardiac tamponade. *A* represents end-diastole. At end-systole (*B*), the right ventricle (RV) is smaller but normal in shape. Both the tricuspid valve (TV) and pulmonary valve (PV) are closed. With early diastole (*C*) the tricuspid valve has opened and the shape of the right ventricle has been distorted (large arrowhead) by collapse of the right ventricular wall (RVW). PE = pericardial effusion; RA = right atrium; Ao = aorta. (From Armstrong, W. F., Schilt, B. F., Helper, D. J., Dillon, J. C., and Feigenbaum, H.: Diastolic collapse of the right ventricle with cardiac tamponade: An echocardiographic study. Circulation *65*:1491, 1982, by permission of the American Heart Association, Inc.)

dium can be detected in many patients,[2, 363] particularly those who also have pericardial fluid, this finding by itself does not imply the presence of constriction. The echocardiographic signs of constriction include lack of diastolic motion, i.e., a flat diastolic slope of the posterior left

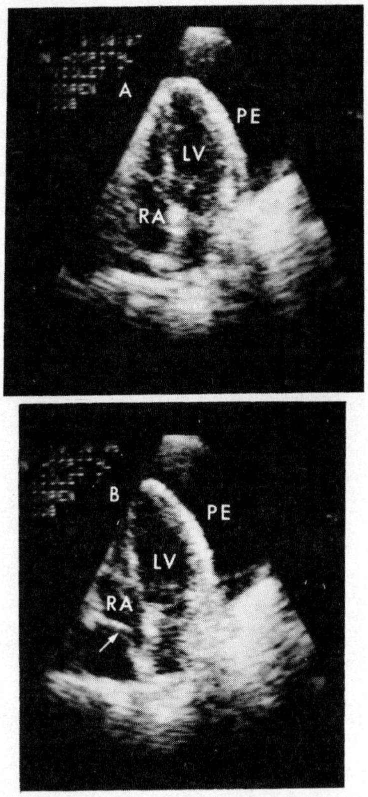

FIGURE 5–107. Apical four-chamber two-dimensional echocardiograms of a patient with a large pericardial effusion (PE) during systole (*A*). Collapse (arrow) of the right atrial (RA) free wall during diastole (*B*), LV = left ventricle. (From Feigenbaum, H.: Echocardiography. 4th ed. Philadelphia, Lea and Febiger, 1986.)

ventricular wall,[2, 364] abnormal motion of the interventricular septum,[364] a very short and steep E to F slope of the mitral valve,[2] and a dilated inferior vena cava that does not get smaller with inspiration. The echocardiographic signs of constriction are not very sensitive and are certainly not specific; at best they raise the suspicion of this condition.

CONGENITALLY ABSENT PERICARDIUM (p. 1525). Echocardiography can provide clues to the presence of a congenitally absent left pericardium. On the M-mode echocardiogram, the right ventricle is dilated and there is paradoxical septal motion similar to a right ventricular volume overload. Two-dimensional echocardiography reveals bulging or displacement of part of the left ventricle or left atrium in a distorted manner which suggests an absent pericardium.[365, 366]

CARDIAC TUMORS AND THROMBI

(See Chap. 43)

ATRIAL TUMORS. Left atrial myxoma (p. 1473) is by far the most common cardiac tumor, and echocardiography has proved to be an extremely important diagnostic technique for its recognition.[367–370] Figure 43–3 (p. 1475) is from a patient with such a tumor in whom the clinical diagnosis was mitral stenosis, as is commonly the case. The echocardiographic feature diagnostic of a left atrial tumor is the "mass" of extraneous echoes posterior to the mitral valve which almost fill the left atrial cavity during systole and which pass partly through the mitral orifice during diastole. The posterior leaflet of the mitral valve is virtually obscured by the echo-producing mass and only a faint trace of the anterior mitral leaflet can be imaged. An interesting echocardiographic sign in establishing the diagnosis of a mobile left atrial tumor is a slight echo-free gap between the anterior leaflet of the mitral valve and the extraneous echoes in early diastole,[370] a gap resulting from more rapid movement of the leaflets than of the tumor. However, it is difficult to distinguish left atrial tumor from thrombus. Although a large vegetation may also mimic a tumor, a vegetation is usually attached to the mitral valve while a tumor is continuous with the left atrium. Occasionally a dense homogeneous tumor may produce only the echo of a leading edge with relatively few echoes from the body of the tumor (less than those illustrated in Figure 5–108).[2] Two-dimensional echocar-

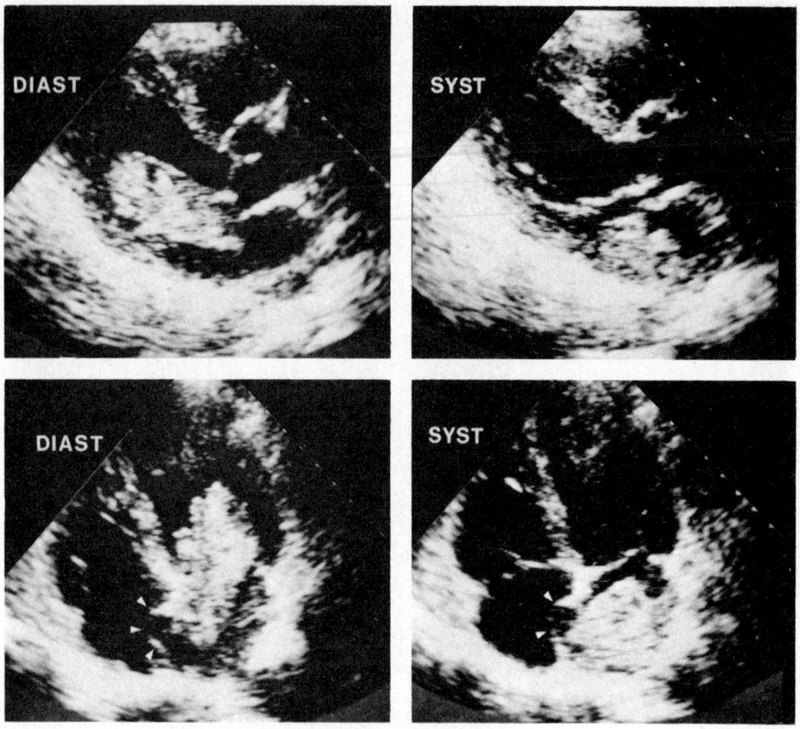

FIGURE 5–108. Long-axis (top) and apical four-chamber (bottom) two-dimensional echocardiograms in diastole and systole in a patient with a left atrial myxoma and an atrial septal aneurysm. The septal aneurysm (arrowheads) can be seen bulging towards the right atrium in both diastole and systole in the four-chamber view. (From Feigenbaum, H.: Echocardiography. 4th ed. Philadelphia, Lea and Febiger, 1986.)

diography is superior in the detection of cardiac masses, especially neoplasms.[370, 371] Figure 5–108 demonstrates a two-dimensional echocardiogram of a patient with left atrial myxoma. The spatial orientation inherent in this examination provides additional useful information, and the size and shape of the mass are apparent. In addition, one can frequently detect the site of attachment of the mass to the cardiac structure. On rare occasions a two-dimensional echocardiogram will detect a myxoma missed on the M-mode tracing.

LEFT ATRIAL THROMBI. Other space-occupying structures—atrial thrombi—have been identified in the left atrium by means of echocardiography (Fig. 5–109).[2, 372, 373] However, since most of them are located in or near the left atrial appendage, an area which is not well visualized echocardiographically, echocardiography is not a sensitive technique for their detection. Although transesophageal echocardiography may be superior to conventional echocardiography in visualizing left atrial appendage thrombi,[374] the detection of clots in this chamber by the latter technique is still not as reliable as detecting masses in other areas of the heart.[375]

RIGHT ATRIAL MYXOMA (p. 1472). These tumors are not as common as the left atrial variety. They can also be detected echocardiographically.[370, 376] Such tumors appear as extraneous echoes behind the *tricuspid* valve in the right atrium during systole and within the right ventricle during diastole. As on the left side of the heart, a large vegetation involving the tricuspid valve can simulate a right atrial myxoma (Fig. 5–63). Bilateral atrial myxomas have also been detected echocardiographically.[377]

OTHER INTRACARDIAC ECHOGENIC STRUCTURES. *Right atrial thrombi* which have the potential of producing massive pulmonary emboli have been detected with two-dimensional echocardiography.[378, 379] However, it should be kept in mind that not all echogenic structures in the right atrium are pathologic. It is possible to detect various structures in the right atrium which are possibly normal variants. The so-called Chiari network may produce mobile echoes within the right atrium which may not be pathologic.[380] In addition, the eustachian valve may be prominent and simulate a pathologic mass.[376, 381]

There are nonpathologic echo-producing structures on the left side of the heart as well.[382] Left ventricular bands or false tendons straddling the left ventricular chamber can frequently be imaged.[383, 384] Moderator bands are routinely seen in the right ventricle. Iatrogenic masses, such as various catheters, are also easily detected on the two-dimensional echocardiogram. Frequently this examination can help detect an incorrectly placed catheter or pacemaker catheter which may have perforated one of the cardiac walls.[385]

VENTRICULAR TUMORS. Myxomas can occur in the ventricles as well as in the atria[386, 387] (p. 1472) and have been imaged in both ventricles. When the tumors are mobile, they can produce very dramatic echograms on both M-mode and two-dimensional examinations; they may move above the mitral valve into the left ventricular outflow tract during systole.[388] Pedunculated right ventricular masses can prolapse into the pulmonary artery[389] or simulate pulmonic stenosis.[390] Rhabdomyomas[391] and fibromas[392] can also involve the ventricles and have been imaged successfully.[393]

VALVULAR TUMORS. Neoplasms may involve the cardiac valves. Cardiac papillary fibroelastoma represent small tumors on the edges of the valve leaflets, primarily the mitral valve.[394] Systemic emboli and stroke occur in patients with these neoplasms.[395] Other neoplasms,

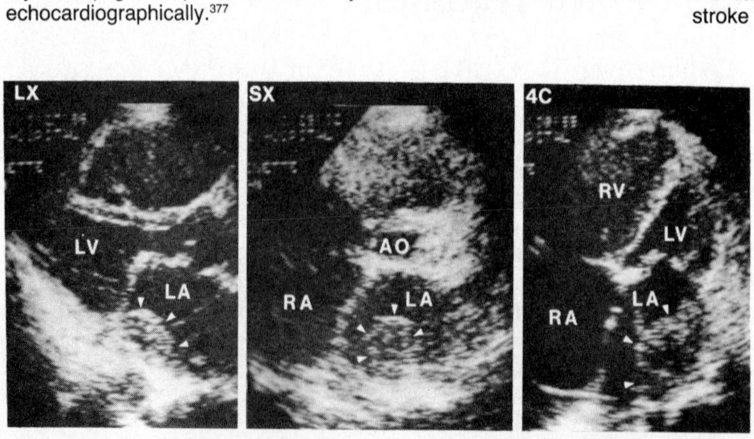

FIGURE 5–109. Long-axis (LX), short-axis (SX), and four-chamber (4C) two-dimensional echocardiograms of a patient with a large clot (arrowheads) in the left atrium (LA). LV = left ventricle; AO = aorta; RA = right atrium. (From Feigenbaum, H.: Echocardiography. 4th ed. Philadelphia, Lea and Febiger, 1986.)

such as a rhabdomyosarcoma, may also involve the mitral valve and can be detected echocardiographically.[396] Primary myxoma can also be attached to the mitral valve.[397]

INVASION AND METASTASIS TO THE HEART (p. 1476). Invasion of the walls of the heart[398] and compression of the heart[399, 400] by neoplasms arising elsewhere have been imaged echocardiographically. Seeding of the pericardium with metastases and the production of pericardial effusion (p. 1515) probably represent the most common types of cardiac involvement with malignant disease. Occasionally, a massively thickened pericardium is produced.[2] On echocardiography the position and configuration of the heart may be distorted by a large tumor mass in the mediastinum. Echocardiography has also been shown to be helpful in distinguishing between cystic and solid tumors involving the heart.[401, 402]

DISEASES OF THE AORTA

(See Chap. 46)

DILATATION AND ANEURYSM. It is possible to examine almost the entire aorta using echocardiography. The root of the aorta and proximal portion of the ascending aorta may be recorded with both M-mode and two-dimensional echocardiography. The two-dimensional technique utilizing the parasternal long-axis examination permits recording of the descending aorta posterior to the left atrium and left ventricle.[403] The suprasternal approach provides visualization of the arch of the aorta and the proximal portion of the descending aorta.[403] The abdominal aorta can then be imaged with the transducer in the subcostal position or over the abdomen itself.[404] In the adult it may still be difficult to record part of the ascending aorta because of the overlying sternum.

Supravalvular aortic stenosis can be detected echocardiographically using either two-dimensional or Doppler echocardiography. As might be expected, dilatation of the aorta, such as occurs in the Marfan syndrome and cystic medial necrosis, is imaged relatively easily (Fig. 5–110).[405] The echocardiographic detection of coarctation of the aorta has already been discussed (p. 119). Aneurysms of the abdominal aorta are routinely examined quite successfully by two-dimensional echocardiography (Fig. 46–1, p. 1547).

AORTIC DISSECTION. Two-dimensional echocardiography has been used extensively for the detection of aortic dissection (Fig. 5–111).[406–408] In addition to the usual transducer position, the right parasternal position may be useful in detecting dissection with its true and false lumina and noting systolic fluttering of the intimal flap.[409] Doppler

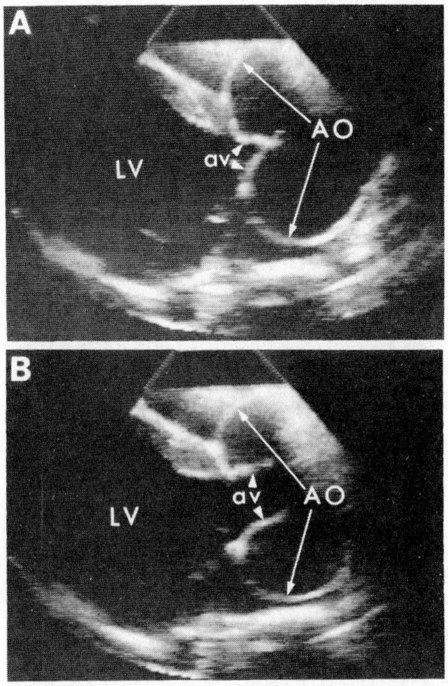

FIGURE 5–110. Diastolic (*A*) and systolic (*B*) long-axis, parasternal two-dimensional echocardiograms of a patient with Marfan syndrome. The aorta (AO) is markedly dilated. Note the marked discrepancy between the aortic valve (av) opening and the size of the aorta. LV = left ventricle. (From Feigenbaum, H.: Echocardiography. 3rd ed. Philadelphia, Lea and Febiger, 1981.)

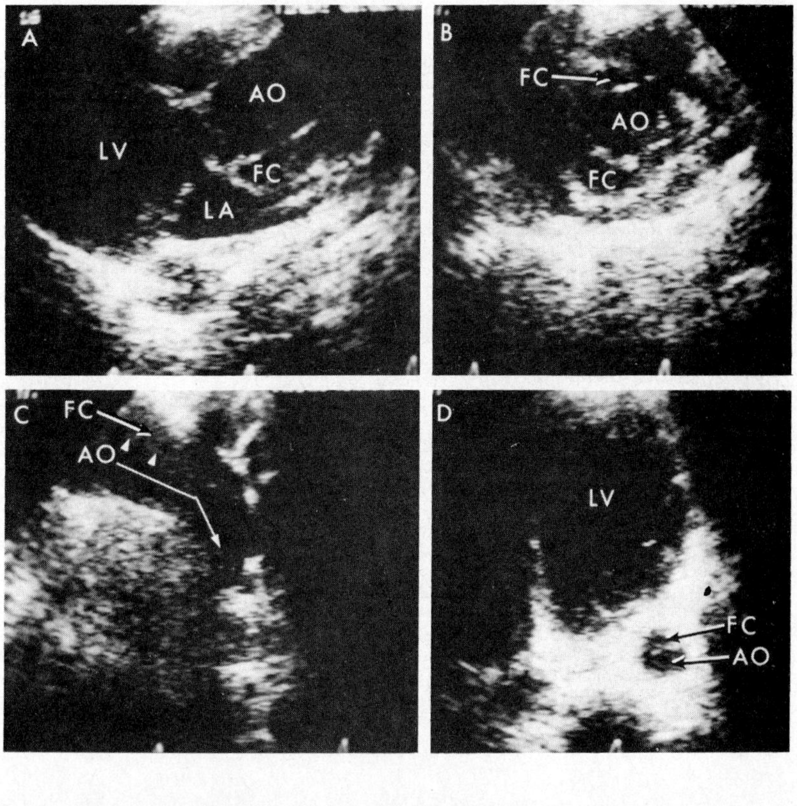

FIGURE 5–111. Parasternal long-axis (*A*), short-axis (*B*), suprasternal (*C*), and apical (*D*) views of a patient with aortic dissection. The false channel (FC) can be seen in every view. The intimal flap (arrowheads) is only faintly seen in the suprasternal examination (*C*). AO = true aortic lumen; LV = left ventricle; LA = left atrium. (From Feigenbaum, H.: Echocardiography. 4th ed. Philadelphia, Lea and Febiger, 1986.)

echocardiography has also been useful in the diagnosis of aortic dissection.[410] The flow characteristics in the false channel are distinctly different from those in the true channel. Color-flow Doppler may also help in establishing the correct diagnosis.[411]

ANEURYSM OF THE SINUS OF VALSALVA. Because examination of the root of the aorta is possible, two-dimensional echocardiography has been used to image the sinuses of Valsalva, allowing detection of aneurysms of these sinuses.[412] Bulging of the sinus, usually the anterior or right coronary sinus, into the right ventricular outflow tract[413] or interventricular septum[414, 415] has been recorded. With rupture there is discontinuity of the anterior wall of the sinus and mid-systolic closure and coarse fluttering of the right coronary cusp of the aortic valve.[416] With rupture of the sinus of Valsalva into the right side of the heart, fluttering of the tricuspid valve as well as premature opening of the pulmonary valve have been reported.[109] Doppler echocardiography can also assist in the diagnosis of sinus of Valsalva aneurysms. The flow pattern within the aneurysms helps identify aortic flow still present in these abnormal spaces.

REFERENCES

PRINCIPLES OF ECHOCARDIOGRAPHY

1. Carlsen, E. N.: Ultrasound physics for the physician: A brief review. J. Clin. Ultrasound *3*:69, 1975.
2. Feigenbaum, H.: Echocardiography. 4th ed. Philadelphia, Lea and Febiger, 1986.
3. Wells, P. N. T.: Ultrasonics in Clinical Diagnosis. 2nd ed. New York, Churchill Livingstone, 1977.
4. Von Ramm, O. T., and Thurstone, F. L.: Cardiac imaging using a phased array ultrasound system. Circulation *53*:258, 1976.
5. Hatle, L., and Angelsen, B.: Doppler Ultrasound in Cardiology: Physical Principles and Clinical Applications. 2nd ed. Philadelphia, Lea and Febiger, 1984.
6. Goldberg, S. J., Allen, H. D., Marx, G. R., and Flinn, C. J.: Doppler Echocardiography. Philadelphia, Lea and Febiger, 1985.
7. Baker, D. W., Rubenstein, S. A., and Lorch, G. S.: Pulsed Doppler echocardiography: Principles and applications. Am. J. Med. *63*:69, 1977.
8. Bom, K., deBoo, J., and Rijsterborgh, H.: On the aliasing problem in pulsed Doppler cardiac studies. J. Clin. Ultrasound *12*:559, 1984.
9. Stewart, W. J., Galvin, K. A., Gillam, L. D., Guyer, D. E., and Weyman, A. E.: Comparison of high pulse repetition frequency and continuous-wave Doppler echocardiography in the assessment of high flow velocity in patients with valvular stenosis and regurgitation. J. Am. Coll. Cardiol. *6*:565, 1985.
10. Sahn, D. J.: Real-time two-dimensional Doppler echocardiographic flow mapping, Circulation *71*:849, 1985.
11. Omoto, R.: Color Atlas of Real-Time Two-Dimensional Doppler Echocardiography. Tokyo, Shindan-to-Chiryo Co. Ltd., 1984.
12. Miyatake, K., Okamoto, M., Kinoshita, N., Izumi, S., Owa, M., Takao, S., Sakakibara, H., and Nimura, Y.: Clinical applications of a new type of real-time two-dimensional Doppler flow imaging system. Am. J. Cardiol. *54*:857, 1984.
13. Omoto, R., Yokote, Y., Takamoto S., Kyo, S., Ueda, K., Asano, H., Namekawa, K., Kasai, C., Kondo, Y., and Koyano, A.: The development of real-time two-dimensional Doppler echocardiography and its clinical significance in acquired valvular regurgitation. Jpn. Heart J. *25*:325, 1984.
14. Meltzer, R. S., Serruys, P. W., Hugenholtz, P. G. and Roelandt, J.: Intravenous carbon dioxide as an echocardiographic contrast agent. J. Clin. Ultrasound *9*:127, 1981.
15. Wang, X. F., Wang, J. E., Cao, L. S., Feng, Y. B., Cao, Z. S., Huang, Y. Z., Cai, C. D., Wu, Y., Chen, H. R., and Lu, C. F.: Left-sided heart contrast echocardiography by pulmonary wedge injection of hydrogen peroxide. Chin. Med. J. *98*:121, 1985.
16. Gaffney, F. A., Lin, J-C., Peshock, R. M., Bush, L., and Buja, M.: Hydrogen peroxide contrast echocardiography. Am. J. Cardiol. *52*:607, 1983.
17. Meltzer, R. S., Klig, V., and Teichholz, L. E.: Generating precision microbubbles for use as an echocardiographic contrast agent. J. Am. Coll. Cardiol. 5:978, 1985.
18. Aschenberg, W., Schluter, M., Kremer, P., Schroeder, E., Siglow, V., and Bleifeld, W.: Transesophageal two-dimensional echocardiography for the detection of left atrial appendage thrombus. J. Am. Coll. Cardiol. *7*:163, 1986
19. Smith, J. S., Cahalan, M. K., Benefiel, D. J., Byrd, B. F., Lurz, F. W., Shapiro, W. A., Roizen, M. F., Bouchard, A., and Schiller, N. B.: Intraoperative detection of myocardial ischemia in high-risk patients: Electrocardiography versus two-dimensional transesophageal echocardiography. Circulation *72*:1015, 1985.
20. Mindich, B. P., Goldman, M. E., Fuster, V., Burgess, N., and Litwak, R.: Improved intraoperative evaluation of mitral valve operations utilizing two-dimensional contrast echocardiography. J. Thorac. Cardiovasc. Surg. *90*:112, 1985.
21. Ren, J. F., Panidis, I. P., Kotler, M. N., Mintz, G. S., Goel, I., and Ross, J.: Effect of coronary bypass surgery and valve replacement on left ventricular function: Assessment by intraoperative two-dimensional echocardiography. Am. Heart J. *109*:281, 1985.
22. Goldman, M. E., Mindich, B. P., Teichholz, L. E., Burgess, N., Staville, K., and Fuster, V.: Intraoperative contrast echocardiography to evaluate mitral valve operations. J. Am. Coll. Cardiol. *4*:1035, 1984.
23. Goldman, M. E., and Mindich, B. P.: Intraoperative two-dimensional echocardiography: New application of an old technique. J. Am. Coll. Cardiol. 7:374, 1986.
24. Perry, L. W., Galioto, F. M., Jr., Blair, T., Shapiro, S. R., Ruckman, R. N., and Scott, L. P.: Two-dimensional echocardiography for catheter location and placement in infants and children. Pediatrics *67*:541, 1981.
25. Kronzon, I., Glassman, E., Cohen, M., and Winer, H.: Use of two-dimensional echocardiography during transseptal cardiac catheterization. J. Am. Coll. Cardiol. *4*:425, 1984.
26. Callahn, J. A., Seward, J. B., Nishimura, R. A., Miller, F. A., Reeder, G. S., Shub, C., Gallahan, M. J., Schattenberg, T. T., and Tajik, A. J.: Two-dimensional echocardiographically guided pericardiocentesis: Experience in 117 consecutive patients. Am. J. Cardiol. *55*:476, 1985.
27. Mortensen, M.: Endomyocardial biopsy guided by cross-sectional echocardiography. Br. Heart J. *50*:246, 1983.
28. Strachovsky, G., Zeldis, S. M., Katz, S., and McNulty-Mackey, M.: Two-dimensional echocardiographic monitoring during percutaneous endomyocardial biopsy. J. Am. Coll. Cardiol. *6*:609, 1985.
29. Lin, A. E., DiSessa, T. G., Williams, R. G., Leighton, J., Gross, K., and Wong, A. L.: Balloon and blade atrial septostomy facilitated by two-dimensional echocardiography. Am. J. Cardiol. *57*:273, 1986.
30. Stewart, H. D., Stewart, H. F., Moore, R. M., and Garry, J.: Compilation of reported biological effects data and ultrasound exposure levels. J. Clin. Ultrasound *13*:167, 1985.
31. Chang, S., and Feigenbaum, H.: Subxiphoid echocardiography. J. Clin. Ultrasound *1*:14, 1973.
32. Silverman, N. H., and Schiller, N. B.: Apex echocardiography. A two-dimensional technique for evaluating congenital heart disease. Circulation *57*:503, 1978.
33. Goldberg, B. B.: Suprasternal ultrasonography. J.A.M.A. *215*:245, 1971.

EXAMINATION OF THE NORMAL HEART

34. Sahn, D. J., DeMaria, A., Kisslo, J., and Weyman, A.: Recommendations regarding quantitation in M-mode echocardiography: Results of a survey of echocardiographic measurements. Circulation *58*:1072, 1978.
35. Henry, W. L., Gardin, J. M., and Ware, J. H.: Echocardiographic measurements in normal subjects from infancy to old age. Circulation *62*:1054, 1980.
36. St. John Sutton, M. G., Reichek, N., Kastor, J. A., and Guiliani, E. R.: Computerized M-mode echocardiographic analysis of left ventricular dysfunction in cardiac amyloid. Circulation *66*:790, 1982.
37. Henry, W. L., DeMaria, A., Gramiak, R., King, D. L., Kisslo, J. A., Popp, R. L., Sahn, D. J., Schiller, N. B., Tajik, A., Teichholz, L. E., and Weyman, A. E.: Report of the American Society of Echocardiography Nomenclature and Standards in Two-dimensional Echocardiography. Circulation *62*:212, 1980.

EVALUATION OF CARDIAC PERFORMANCE

38. Feigenbaum, H., Popp, R. L., Wolfe, S. B., Troy, B. L., Pombo, J. F., Haine, C. L., and Dodge, H. T.: Ultrasound measurements of the left ventricle: A correlative study with angiography. Arch. Intern. Med. *129*:461, 1972.
39. Teichholz, L. E., Kreulen, T., Herman, M. V., and Gorlin, R.: Problems in echocardiographic volume determinations: Echocardiographic-angiographic correlations in the presence or absence of asynergy. Am. J. Cardiol. *37*:7, 1976.
40. Rasmussen, S., Corya, B. C., Phillips, J. F., and Black, M. J.: Unreliability of M-mode left ventricular dimensions for calculating stroke volume and cardiac output in patients without heart disease. Chest *81*:614, 1982.
41. McDonald, I. G., Feigenbaum, H., and Change, S.: Analysis of left ventricular wall motion by reflected ultrasound: Application to assessment of myocardial function. Circulation *46*:14, 1972.
42. Quinones, M. A., Gaasch, W. H., and Alexander, J. K.: Echocardiographic assessment of left ventricular function: With special reference to normalized velocities. Circulation *50*:42, 1974.
43. Feigenbaum, H.: Echocardiographic examination of the left ventricle. Circulation *51*:1, 1975.
44. Rosoff, M. H., and Cohen, M. V.: Significance of E point-septal separation by M-mode echocardiography in patients with aortic regurgitation. Am. J. Cardiol. *56*:809, 1985.
45. Ahmadpour, H., Shah, A. A., Allen, J. W., Edmiston, W. A., Kim, S. J., and Haywood, L. J.: Mitral E point septal separation: A reliable index of left ventricular performance in coronary artery disease. Am. Heart J. *106*:21, 1983.
46. Shiller, N. B., Acquatella, H., Ports, T. A., Drew, D., Goerke, J., Ringertz,

H., Silverman, N. H., Carlsson, E., and Parmley, W. W.: Left ventricular volume from paired biplane two-dimensional echocardiography. Circulation *60*:547, 1979.
47. Gordon, E. P., Schnittger, I., Fitzgerald, P. J., Williams, P., and Popp,. R. L.: Reproducibility of left ventricular volumes by two-dimensional echocardiography. J. Am. Coll. Cardiol. 2:506, 1983.
48. Starling, M. R., Crawford, M. H., Sorensen, S. G., Levi, B., Richards, K. L., and O'Rourke, R. A.: Comparative accuracy of apical biplane cross-sectional echocardiography and gated equilibrium radionuclide angiography for estimating left ventricular size and performance. Circulation *63*:1075, 1981.
49. Erbel, R., Schweizer, P., Lambertz, H., Henn, G., Meyer, J., Krebs, W., and Effert, S.: Echoventriculography–a simultaneous analysis of two-dimensional echocardiography and cineventriculography. Circulation *67*:205, 1983.
50. Gueret, P., Meerbaum, S., Wyatt, S., Wyatt, H. L., Uchiyama T., Lang, T. W., and Corday, E.: Two-dimensional echocardiographic quantitation of left ventricular volumes and ejection fraction. Importance of accounting for dyssynergy in short-axis reconstruction models. Circulation *62*:1308, 1980.
51. Gardin, J. M., Iseri, L. T., Elkayam, U., Tobis, J., Childs, W., Burn, C. S., and Henry, W. L.: Evaluation of dilated cardiomyopathy by pulsed Doppler echocardiography. Am. Heart J. *106*:1057, 1983.
52. Elkayam, U., Gardin, J. M., Berkley, R., Highes, C. A., and Henry, W. L.: The use of Doppler flow velocity measurement to assess the hemodynamic response to vasodilators in patients with heart failure. Circulation *67*:377, 1983.
53. Rokey, R., Kuo, L. C., Zoghbi, W. A., Limacher, M. C., and Quinones, M. A.: Determination of parameters of left ventricular diastolic filling with pulsed Doppler echocardiography: Comparison with cineangiography. Circulation *71*:543, 1985.
54. Spirito, P., Maron, B. J., and Bonow, R. O.: Noninvasive assessment of left ventricular diastolic function: Comparative analysis of Doppler echocardiographic and radionuclide angiographic techniques. J. Am. Coll. Cardiol. 7:518, 1986.
55. Miyatake, K., Okamoto, M., Kinoshita, N., Owa, M., Nakasone, I., Sakakibara, H., and Nimura, Y.: Augmentation of atrial contribution to the left ventricular inflow with aging as assessed by intracardiac Doppler flowmeter. Am. J. Cardiol. *53*:586, 1984.
56. Ginzton, L. E., Conant, R., Brizendine, M., Thigpen, T., and Laks, M. M.: Quantitative analysis of segmental wall motion during maximal upright dynamic exercise: Variability in normal adults. Circulation *73*:268, 1986.
57. Iliceto, S., Sorino, M., D'Ambrosio, G., Papa, A., Favale, S., Biasco, G., and Risson, P.: Detection of coronary artery disease by two-dimensional echocardiography and transesophageal atrial pacing. J. Am. Coll. Cardiol. *5*:1188, 1985.
58. West, S. R., Feigenbaum, H., Armstrong, W. F., Green, D., and Dillon, J. C.: Split screen simultaneous digital imaging of rest and stress echocardiogram—a new method for evaluation of exercise-induced wall motion abnormalities. J. Am. Coll. Cardiol. *3*:563 (Abstract), 1984.
59. Gardin, J. M., Kozlowski, J., Dabestani, A., Murphy, M., Kusnick, C., Allfie, A., Russell, D., and Henry, W. L.: Studies of Doppler aortic flow velocity during supine bicycle exercise. Am. J. Cardiol. *57*:327, 1986.
60. Feigenbaum, H., Popp, R. L., Chip, J. N., and Haine, C. L.: Left ventricular wall thickness measured by ultrasound. Arch. Intern. Med. *121*:391, 1969.
61. Devereux, R. B., Alonso, D. R., Lutas, E. M., Gottlieb, G. J., Campo, E., Sachs, I., and Reichek, N.: Echocardiographic assessment of left ventricular hypertrophy: Comparison to necropsy findings. Am. J. Cardiol. *57*:450, 1986.
62. Byrd, III, B. F., Wahr, D., Wang, Y. S., Bouchard, A., and Shiller, N. B.: Left ventricular mass and volume/mass ratio determined by two-dimensional echocardiography in normal adults. J. Am. Coll. Cardiol. *6*:1021, 1985.
63. Reichek, N., Helak, J., Plappert, T. A., St. John Sutton, M. G., and Weber, K. T.: Anatomic validation of left ventricular mass estimates from clinical two-dimensional echocardiography: Initial results. Circulation *67*:348, 1983.
64. Reichek, N., Wilson, J., St. John Sutton, M., Plappert, T. A., Goldberg, S., and Hirshfeld, J. W.: Noninvasive determination of left ventricular end-systolic stress: Validation of the method and initial application. Circulation *65*:99, 1982.
65. Goldberg, S. J.: Analysis and interpretation of thickening and thinning phases of left ventricular wall dynamics. Ultrasound Med. Biol. *10*:797, 1984.
66. Corya, B. C., Rasmussen, S., Feigenbaum, H., Knoebel, S. B., and Black, M. J.: Systolic thickening and thinning of the septum and posterior wall in patients with coronary artery disease, congestive cardiomyopathy, and atrial septal defect. Circulation 55:109, 1977.
67. Feigenbaum, H.: Estimation of left atrial size using ultrasound. Am. Heart J. *78*:43, 1969.
68. Schabelman, S., Schiller, N. B., Silverman, N. H., and Ports, T. A.: Left atrial volume estimation by two-dimensional echocardiography. Cathet. Cardiovasc. Diagn. 7:165, 1981.
69. Hoglund, C., and Rosenhamer, G.: Echocardiographic left atrial dimension as a predictor of maintaining sinus rhythm after conversion of atrial fibrillation. Acta Med. Scand. *217*:411, 1985.
70. Lemire, F., Tajik, A. J., and Hagler, D. J.: Asymmetric left atrial enlargement: An echocardiographic observation. Chest *59*:779, 1976.
71. Gehl, L. G., Mintz, G. S., Kotler, M. N., and Segal, B. L.: Left atrial volume overload in mitral regurgitation: A two-dimensional echocardiographic study. Am. J. Cardiol. *49*:33, 1982.
72. Hiraishi, S., DiSessa, T. G., Jarmakani, J. M., Nakanishi, T., Isabel-Jones, J., and Friedman, W. F.: Two-dimensional echocardiographic assessment of left atrial size in children. Am. J. Cardiol. *52*:1249, 1983.
73. Gibson, T. C., Miller, S. W., Aretz, T., Hardin, N. J., and Weyman, A. E.: Method for estimating right ventricular volume by planes applicable to cross-sectional echocardiography: Correlation with angiographic formulas. Am. J. Cardiol. *55*:1584, 1985.
74. Silverman, N. H., and Hudson, S.: Evaluation of right ventricular volume and ejection fraction in children by two-dimensional echocardiography. Pediatr. Cardiol. *4*:197, 1983.
75. Popp, R. L., Wolfe, S. B., Hirato, T., and Feigenbaum, H.: Estimation of right and left ventricular size by ultrasound. A study of the echoes from the interventricular septum. Am. J. Cardiol. *24*:523, 1969.
76. Baker, B. J., Scovil, J. A., Kane, J. J., and Murphy, M. L.: Echocardiographic detection of right ventricular hypertrophy. Am. Heart J. *105*:611, 1983.
77. King, M. E., Braun, H., Goldblatt, A., Liberthson, R., and Weyman, A. E.: Interventricular septal configuration as a predictor of right ventricular systolic hypertension in children: A cross-sectional echocardiographic study. Circulation *68*:68, 1983.
78. Ryan, T., Petrovic, O., Dillon, J. C., Feigenbaum, H., Conley, M. J., and Armstrong, W. F.: An echocardiographic index for separation of right ventricular volume and pressure overload. J. Am. Coll. Cardiol. 5:918, 1985.
79. Gardin, J. M., Tobis, J. M., Dabestani, A., Smith, C., Elkayam, U., Castleman, E., White, D., Allfie, A., and Henry, W. L.: Superiority of two-dimensional measurement of aortic vessel diameter in Doppler echocardiographic measurement of aortic vessel diameter in Doppler echocardiographic estimates of left ventricular stroke volume. J. Am. Coll. Cardiol. *6*:66, 1985.
80. Sahn, D. J.: Determination of cardiac output by echocardiographic Doppler methods: Relative accuracy of various sites for measurement. J. Am. Coll. Cardiol. *6*:663, 1985.
81. Ihlen, H., Amlie, J. P., Dale, J., Forfang, K. Nitter-Hauge, S., Otterstad, J. E., Simonsen, S., and Myhre, E.: Determination of cardiac output by Doppler echocardiography. Br. Heart J. *51*:54, 1984.
82. Zhang, Y., Nitter-Hauge, N., Ihlen, H., and Myhre, E.: Doppler echocardiographic measurement of cardiac output using the mitral orifice method. Br. Heart J. *53*:130, 1985.
83. Meijboom, E. J., Horowitz, S., Valdes-Cruz, L. M., Sahn, D. J., Larson, D. F., and Lima, C. O.: A Doppler echocardiographic method for calculating volume flow across the tricuspid valve: Correlative laboratory and clinical studies. Circulation *71*:551, 1985.
84. Valdes-Cruz, L. M., Horowitz, S., Goldberg, S. J., and Allen, H. D.: The mitral valve orifice method for noninvasive two-dimensional echo Doppler determinations of cardiac output. Circulation *67*:872, 1983.
85. Alverson, D. C., Eldridge, M., Dillon, T., Yabek, S. M., and Berman, W., Jr.: Noninvasive pulsed Doppler determination of cardiac output in neonates and children. J. Pediatr. *101*:46, 1982.
86. Nishimura, R. A., Callahan, M. J., Schaff, H. V., Illstrup, D. M., Miller, F. A., and Tajik, A. J.: Non-invasive measurement of cardiac output by continuous-wave Doppler echocardiography: Initial experience and review of the literature. Mayo Clin. Proc. *59*:484, 1984.
87. Ihlen, H., Myhre, E., Amlie, J. P., Forfang, K., and Larsen, K.: Changes in left ventricular stroke volume measured by Doppler echocardiography. Br. Heart J. *54*:378, 1985.
88. Goldberg, S. J., and Allen, H. D.: Quantitative assessment by Doppler echocardiography of pulmonary or aortic regurgitation. Am. J. Cardiol. *56*:131, 1985.
89. Kitabatake, A., Inoue, M., Asao, M., Ito, H., Masuyama, T., Tanouchi, J., Morita, T., Hori, M., Yoshima, H., Ohnishi, K., and Abe, H.: Noninvasive evaluation of the ratio of pulmonary to systemic flow in atria septal defect by duplex Doppler echocardiography. Circulation *69*:73, 1984.
90. Hatle, L., Brubakk, A., Tromsdal, A., and Angelsen, B.: Noninvasive assessment of pressure drop in mitral stenosis by Doppler ultrasound. Br. Heart J. *40*:131, 1978.
91. Stamm, R. B., and Martin, R. P.: Quantification of pressure gradients across stenotic valves by Doppler ultrasound. J. Am. Coll. Cardiol. *2*:707, 1983.
92. Teirstein, P. S., Yock, P. G., and Popp, R. L.: The accuracy of Doppler ultrasound measurement of pressure gradients across irregular, duel, and tunnellike obstructions to blood flow. Circulation *72*:577, 1985.
93. Yock, P. G., and Popp, R. L.: Non-invasive estimation of right ventricular systolic pressure by Doppler ultrasound in patients with tricuspid regurgitation. Circulation *70*:657, 1984.
94. Berger, M., Haimowitz, A., Van Tosh, A., Berdoff, R. L., and Goldberg, E.: Quantitative assessment of pulmonary hypertension in patients with tricuspid regurgitation using continuous wave Doppler ultrasound. J. Am. Coll. Cardiol. *6*:359, 1985.
95. Marx, G. R., Allen, H. D., and Goldberg, S. J.: Doppler echocardiographic estimation of systolic pulmonary artery pressure in pediatric patients with interventricular communications. J. Am. Coll. Cardiol. *6*:1132, 1985.
96. Marx, G. R., Allen, H. D., and Goldberg, S. J.: Doppler echocardiographic estimation of systolic pulmonary artery pressure in patients with aortic-pulmonary shunts. J. Am. Coll. Cardiol. *7*:880, 1986.
97. Kosturakis, D., Goldberg, S. J., Allen, H. D., and Loeber, C.: Doppler echocardiographic prediction of pulmonary arterial hypertension in congenital heart disease. Am. J. Cardiol. *53*:1110, 1984.
98. Isobe, M., Yazaki, Y., Takaku, F., Koizumi, K., Hara, K., Tsuneyoshi, H., Yamaguchi, T., and Machii, K.: Prediction of pulmonary arterial pressure in adults by pulsed Doppler echocardiography. Am. J. Cardiol. *57*:316, 1986.
99. Pridie, R. B., Beham, R., and Oakley, C. M.: Echocardiography of the mitral valve in aortic valve disease. Br. Heart J. *33*:296, 1971.
100. Botvinick, E. H., Schiller, N. B., Wickramasekaran, R., Klausner, S. C., and Getz, E.: Echocardiographic demonstration of early mitral valve closure in severe aortic insufficiency. Its clinical implications. Circulation *51*:836, 1975.
101. Konecke, L. L., Feigenbaum, H., Chang, S., Corya, B. C., and Fischer, J. C.: Abnormal mitral valve motion in patients with elevated left ventricular diastolic pressures. Circulation *47*:989, 1973.

102. Lewis, J. R., Parker, J. O., and Burggraf, G. W.: Mitral valve motion and changes in left ventricular end-diastolic pressures: A correlative study of the PR-AC interval. Am. J. Cardiol. *42*:383, 1978.
103. Sabbah, H. N., and Stein, P. D.: Mechanism of early systolic closure of the aortic valve in discrete membranous subaortic stenosis. Circulation *65*:399, 1982.
104. Corya, B. C., Rasmussen, S., Phillips, J. F., and Black, M. J.: Forward stroke volume calculated from aortic valve echograms in normal subjects and patients with mitral regurgitation secondary to left ventricular dysfunction. Am. J. Cardiol. *47*:1215, 1981.
105. Nathan, M. P. R., Arora, R., and Rubenstein, H.: Mid-diastolic aortic valve opening in bacterial endocarditis of aortic valve. Clin. Cardiol. *5*:294, 1982.
106. Green, S. E., and Popp, R. L.: The relationship of pulmonary valve motion to the motion of surrounding cardiac structures: A two-dimensional and dual M-mode echocardiographic study. Circulation *64*:107, 1981.
107. Gramiak, R., Nanda, N. C., and Shah, P. M.: Echocardiographic detection of pulmonary valve. Radiology *102*:153, 1972.
108. Weyman, A. E., Dillon, J. C., Feigenbaum, H., and Change, S.: Echocardiographic patterns of pulmonic valve motion in pulmonic stenosis. Am. J. Cardiol. *34*:644, 1974.
109. Wann, L. S., Weyman, A. E., Dillon, J. C., and Feigenbaum, H.: Premature pulmonary valve opening. Circulation *55*:128, 1977.
110. Weyman, A. E., Dillon, J. C., Feigenbaum, H., and Chang, S.: Echocardiographic patterns of pulmonary valve motion with pulmonary hypertension. Circulation *50*:905, 1974.
111. Tahara, M., Tanaka, H., Nakao, S., Yoshimura, H., Sakurai, S., Tei, C., and Kashima, T.: Hemodynamic determinants of pulmonary valve motion during systole in experimental pulmonary hypertension. Circulation *64*:1249, 1981.
112. Hirschfeld, S., Meyer, R., Schwartz, D. C., Korfhagen, J., and Kaplan, S.: Measurement of right and left ventricular systolic time intervals by echocardiography. Circulation *51*:304, 1975.
113. Hirschfeld, S., Meyer, R., Schwartz, D. C., Korfhagen, J., and Kaplan, S.: The echocardiographic assessment of pulmonary artery pressure and pulmonary vascular resistance. Circulation *52*:642, 1975.
113a. Chan, K. L., Currie, P. J., Seward, J. B., Hagler, D. J., Mair, D. D., and Tajik, A. J.: Comparison of three Doppler ultrasound methods in the prediction of pulmonary artery pressure. J. Am. Coll. Cardiol. *9*:549, 1987.
114. Moreno, F. L. L., Hagan, A. D., Holman, J. R., Pryor, T. A., Strickland, R. D., and Castle, C. H.: Evaluation of size and dynamics of the inferior vena cava as an index of right-sided cardiac function. Am. J. Cardiol. *53*:579, 1984.
115. Reeves, W. C., Leaman, D. M., Bounocore, E., Babb, J. D., Dash, H., Schwiter, E. J., Ciotola, T. J., and Hallahan, W.: Detection of tricuspid regurgitation and estimation of central venous pressure by two-dimensional contrast echocardiography of the right superior hepatic vein. Am. Heart J. *102*:374, 1981.

ACQUIRED VALVULAR HEART DISEASE

116. Edler, I.: Ultrasound cardiogram in mitral valve disease. Acta Chir. Scand. *111*:230, 1956.
117. Wann, L. S., Weyman, A. E., Dillon, J. C., and Feigenbaum, H.: Determination of mitral valve area by cross-sectional echocardiography. Ann. Intern. Med. *88*:337, 1978.
118. Duchak, J. M., Jr., Chang, S., and Feigenbaum, H.: The posterior mitral valve echo and the echocardiographic diagnosis of mitral stenosis. Am. J. Cardiol. *29*:628, 1972.
119. Motro, M., Schneeweiss, A., Lehrer, E., Rath, S., and Neufeld, H. N.: Correlation between cardiac catheterization and echocardiography in assessing the severity of mitral stenosis. Int. J. Cardiol. *1*:25, 1981.
120. Diebold, B., Theroux, P., Bourassa, M. G., Thuillez, C., Peronneau, P., Guermonprez, J. L., Xhaard, M., and Waters, D. D.: Non-invasive pulsed Doppler study of mitral stenosis and mitral regurgitation: Preliminary study. Br. Heart J. *42*:168, 1979.
121. Smith, M. D., Handshoe, R., Handshoe, S., Kwan, O. L., and DeMaria, A. N.: Comparative accuracy of two-dimensional echocardiography and Doppler pressure half-time methods in assessing severity of mitral stenosis in patients with and without prior commissurotomy. Circulation *73*:100, 1986.
122. Zanolla, L. Marino, P., Nocolosi, G. L., Peranzoni, P. F., and Poppi, A.: Two-dimensional echocardiographic evaluation of mitral valve calcification. Sensitivity and specificity. Chest *82*:154, 1982.
123. Zaretskii, V. V., Kuznetsoa, L. M., Bobkov, V. V., and Aksiuk, M. A.: Diagnosis of subvalvular adhesion in mitral stenosis by two-dimensional echocardiography. Kardiologiia *225*:68, 1985.
124. Patel, A. K., Rowe, G. G., Thomsen, J. H., Dhanani, S. P., Kosolcharoen, P., and Lyle, L. E. W.: Detection and estimation of rheumatic mitral regurgitation in the presence of mitral stenosis by pulsed Doppler echocardiography. Am. J. Cardiol. *51*:986, 1983.
125. Miyatake, K., Izumi, S., Okamoto, M., Kinoshita, N., Asonuma, H., Nakagawa, H., Yamamoto, K., Takamiya, M., Sakakibara, H., and Nimura, Y.: Semiquantitative grading of severity of mitral regurgitation by real-time two-dimensional Doppler flow imaging technique. J. Am. Coll. Cardiol. *7*:82, 1986.
126. Zhang, Y., Ihlen, H., Myhre, E., Levorstad, K., and Nitter-Hauge, S.: Measurement of mitral regurgitation by Doppler echocardiography. Br. Heart J. *54*:384, 1985.
127. Ascah, K. J., Stewart, W. J., Jiang, L., Guerrero, J. L., Newell, J. B., Gillam, L. D., and Weyman, A. E.: A Doppler two-dimensional echocardiographic method for quantitation of mitral regurgitation. Circulation *72*:377, 1985.
128. Zile, M. R., Gaasch, W. H., Carroll, J. D., and Levine, H. J.: Chronic mitral regurgitation: Predictive value of preoperative echocardiographic indexes of left ventricular function and wall stress. J. Am. Coll. Cardiol. *3*:235, 1984.
129. Dillon, J. C., Haine, C. L., Chang, S., and Feigenbaum, H.: Use of echocardiography in patients with prolapsed mitral valve. Am. J. Cardiol. *43*:503, 1971.
130. DeMaria, A. N., King, J. F., Bogren, H. G., Lies, J. E., and Mason, D. T.: The variable spectrum of echocardiographic manifestations of the mitral valve prolapse syndrome. Circulation *50*:33, 1974.
131. Sahn, D. J., Wood, J., Allen, H. D., Peoples, W., and Goldberg, S. J.: Echocardiographic spectrum of mitral valve motion in children with and without mitral valve prolapse: The nature of false-positive diagnosis. Am. J. Cardiol. *39*:422, 1977.
132. Markiewicz, W., Stoner, J., London, E., Hunt, S. A., and Popp, R. L.: Mitral valve prolapse in one hundred presumably healthy young females. Circulation *53*:464, 1976.
133. Sahn, D. J., Allen, H. D., Goldberg, S. J., and Friedman, W. F.: Mitral valve prolapse in children. A problem defined by real-time cross-sectional echocardiography. Circulation *53*:651, 1976.
134. Morganroth, J., Jones, R. H., Chen, C. C., and Naito, M.: Two dimensional echocardiography in mitral, aortic and tricuspid valve prolapse. The clinical problem, cardiac nuclear imaging considerations and a proposed standard for diagnosis. Am. J. Cardiol. *46*:1164, 1980.
135. Wann, L. S., Gross, C. M., Wakefield, R. J., and Kalbfleisch, J. H.: Diagnostic precision of echocardiography in mitral valve prolapse. Am. Heart J. *109*:803, 1985.
136. Chun, P. K. C., and Sheehan, M. W.: Myxomatous degeneration of mitral valve M-mode and two-dimensional echocardiographic findings. Br. Heart J. *47*:404, 1982.
137. Ballester, M., Presbitero, P., Foale, R., Richards, A., and McDonald, L.: Prolapse of the mitral valve in secundum atrial septal defect: A functional mechanism. Eur. Heart J. *4*:472, 1983.
138. Sweatman, T., Selzer, A., Kamagaki, M., and Cohn, K.: Echocardiographic diagnosis of mitral regurgitation due to ruptured chordae tendineae. Circulation *46*:580, 1972.
139. Giles, T. D., Burch, G. E., and Martinez, E. C.: Value of exploratory "scanning" in the echocardiographic diagnosis of ruptured chordae tendineae. Circulation *49*:678, 1974.
140. Ballester, M., Foale, R., Presbitero, P., Yacoub, M., Richards, A., and McDonald, L.: Cross-sectional echocardiographic features of ruptured chordae tendineae. Eur. Heart J. *4*:795, 1983.
141. Mintz, G. S., Kotler, M. N., Segal, B. L., and Parry, W. R.: Two-dimensional echocardiographic recognition of ruptured chordae tendineae. Circulation *57*:244, 1978.
142. Godley, R. W., Wann, L. S., Rogers, E. W., Feigenbaum, H., and Weyman, A. E.: Incomplete mitral leaflet closure in patients with papillary muscle dysfunction. Circulation *63*:565, 1981.
143. Gramiak, R., and Shah, P. M.: Echocardiography of the normal and diseased aortic valve. Radiology *96*:1, 1970.
144. Weyman, A. E., Feigenbaum, H., Dillon, J. C., and Chang, S.: Cross-sectional echocardiography in assessing the severity of valvular aortic stenosis. Circulation *52*:828, 1975.
145. Godley, R. W., Green, D., Dillon, J. C., Rogers, E. W., Feigenbaum, H., and Weyman, A. E.: Reliability of two-dimensional echocardiography in assessing the severity of valvular aortic stenosis. Chest *79*:657, 1981.
146. Currie, P. J., Seward, J. B., Reeder, G. S., Vlietstra, R. E., Bresnahan, D. R., Bresnahan, J. F., Smith, H. C., Hagler, D. J., and Tajik, A. J.: Continuous-wave Doppler echocardiographic assessment of severity of calcific aortic stenosis: A simultaneous Doppler-catheter correlative study in 100 adult patients. Circulation *71*:1162, 1985.
147. Hegrenaes, L., and Hatle, L.: Aortic stenosis in adults. Non-invasive estimation of pressure differences by continuous wave Doppler echocardiography. Br. Heart J. *54*:396, 1985.
148. Teien, D., and Ericksson, P.: Quantification of transvalvular pressure differences in aortic stenosis by Doppler ultrasound. Int. J. Cardiol. *7*:121, 1985.
149. Currie, P. J., Seward, J. B., Reeder, G. S., Vliestra, R. E., Bresnahan, D. R, Bresnahan, J. F., Smith, H. L., Hagler, D. J., and Tajik, A. J.: Continuous-wave Doppler echocardiographic assessment of severity of calcific aortic stenosis: A simultaneous Doppler-catheter correlative study in 100 adult patients. Circulation *71*:1162, 1985.
150. Warth, D. C., Stewart, W. J., Block, P. C., and Weyman, A. E.: A new method to calculate aortic valve area without left heart catheterization. Circulation *70*:978, 1984.
151. Zoghbi, W. A., Farmer, K. L., Soto, J. G., Nelson, J. G., and Quinones, M. A.: Accurate noninvasive quantification of stenotic aortic valve area by Doppler echocardiography. Circulation *73*:452, 1986.
152. Richards, K. L., Cannon, S. R., Miller, J. F., and Crawford, M. H.: Calculation of aortic valve area by Doppler echocardiography: A direct application of the continuity equation. Circulation *73*:964, 1986.
153. Yeager, M., Yock, P. G., and Popp, R. L.: Comparison of Doppler-derived pressure gradient to that determined at cardiac cathetherization in adults with aortic valve stenosis: Implications for management. Am. J. Cardiol. *57*:644, 1986.
154. Reichek, N., and Devereux, R. B.: Reliable estimation of peak left ventricular systolic pressure by M-mode echographic-determined end-diastolic relative wall thickness: Identification of severe valvular aortic stenosis in adult patients. Am. Heart J. *103*:202, 1982.
155. Ciobanu, M., Abbasi, A. S., Allen, M., Hermer, A., and Spellberg, R.: Pulsed Doppler echocardiography in the diagnosis and estimation of severity of aortic insufficiency. Am. J. Cardiol. *49*:339, 1982.

156. Grayburn, P. A., Smith, M. D., Handshoe, R., Friedman, B. J., and DeMaria, A. N.: Detection of aortic insufficiency by standard echocardiography, pulse Doppler echocardiography, and auscultation. Ann. Intern. Med. *104*:599, 1986.
157. Byard, C. E., Perry, G. J., Roitman, D. I., and Nanda, N. C.: Quantitative assessment of aortic regurgitation by color Doppler. Circulation 72:III–146 (Abstract), 1986.
157a. Perry, G. J., Helmcke, F., Nanda, N. C., Byard, C., and Soto, B.: Evaluation of aortic insufficiency by Doppler color flow mapping. J. Am. Coll. Cardiol. 9:952, 1987.
158. Masuyama, T., Kodama, K., Kitabatake, A., Nanto, S., Sato, H., Uematsu, M., Inoue, M., and Kamada, T.: Noninvasive evaluation of aortic regurgitation by continuous-wave Doppler echocardiography. Circulation *73*:460, 1986.
159. Kitabatake, A., Ito, H., Inoue, M., Tanouchi, J., Ishihara, K., Morita, T., Fujii, K., Yoshida, Y., Masuyama, T., Yoshima, H., Hori, M., and Kamada, T.: A new approach to noninvasive evaluation of aortic regurgitant fraction by two-dimensional Doppler echocardiography. Circulation *72*:523, 1985.
160. Zhang, Y., Nitter-Hauge, S., Ihlen, H., Rootwelt, K., and Myhre, E.: Measurement of aortic regurgitation by Doppler echocardiography. Br. Heart J. *55*:32, 1986.
161. Robertson, W. S., Stewart, J., Armstrong, W. F., Dillon, J. C., and Feigenbaum, H.: Reverse doming of the anterior mitral leaflet with severe aortic regurgitation. J. Am. Coll. Cardiol. *3*:431, 1984.
162. Fioretti, P., Roelandt, J., Sclavo, M., Domenicucci, S., Haalebos, M., Bos, E., and Hugenholtz, P. G.: Postoperative regression of left ventricular dimensions in aortic insufficiency: A long-term echocardiographic study. J. Am. Coll. Cardiol. *5*:856, 1985.
163. Henry, W. L., Bonow, R. O., Borer, J. S., Ware, J. H., Kent, K. M., Redwood, D. R., McIntosh, C. L., Morrow, A. G., and Epstein, S. E.: Observations on the optimum time for operative intervention for aortic regurgitation. I. Evaluation of the results of aortic valve replacement in symptomatic patients. Circulation *61*:741, 1980.
164. Bonow, R. O., Rosing, D. R., Kent, K. M., and Epstein, S. E.: Timing of operation for chronic aortic regurgitation. Am. J. Cardiol. *50*:325, 1982.
165. Guyer, D. E., Gillam, L. D., Foale, R. A., Clark, M. C., Dinsmore, R., Palacios, I., Block, P., King, M. E., and Weyman, A. E.: Comparison of the echocardiographic and hemodynamic diagnosis of rheumatic tricuspid stenosis. J. Am. Coll. Cardiol. *3*:1135, 1984.
166. Veyrat, C., Kalmanson, D., Farjon, M., Manin, J. P., and Abitbol, G.: Noninvasive diagnosis and assessment of tricuspid regurgitation and stenosis using one and two dimensional echo-pulsed Doppler. Br. Heart J. *47*:596, 1982.
167. Skjaerpe, T., and Hatle, L.: Diagnosis of tricuspid regurgitation. Sensitivity of Doppler ultrasound compared with contrast echocardiography. Eur. Heart J. *6*:429, 1985.
168. Missri, J., Agnarsson, U., and Sverrisson, J.: The clinical spectrum of tricuspid regurgitation detected by pulsed Doppler echocardiography. Angiology *36*:746, 1985.
169. Curtius, M. M., Thyssen, M., Breuer, H. W. M., and Loogen, F.: Doppler versus contrast echocardiography for diagnosis of tricuspid regurgitation. Am. J. Cardiol. *56*:333, 1985.
170. Ogawa, S., Hayashi, J., Sasaki, H., Tani, M., Handa, S., and Nakamura, Y.: Evaluation of combined valvular prolapse syndrome by two-dimensional echocardiography. Circulation *65*:174, 1982.
171. Eckfeldt, J. H., Weir, E. K., and Chesler, E.: Echocardiographic findings in ruptured chordae tendineae of the tricuspid valve. Am. Heart J. *105*:1033, 1983.
172. Forman, M. B., Byrd, B. F., Oates, J. A., and Robertson, R. M.: Two-dimensional echocardiography in the diagnosis of carcinoid heart disease. Am. Heart J. *107*:492, 1984.
173. Sheikh, M. U., Covarrubias, E. A., Ali, N., Sheikh, N. M., Lee, W. R., and Roberts, W. C.: M-mode echocardiographic observations in active bacterial endocarditis limited to the aortic valve. Am. Heart J. *102*:66, 1981.
174. Berger, M., Gallerstein, P. E., Benhuri, P., Balla, R., and Goldberg, E.: Evaluation of aortic valve endocarditis by two-dimensional echocardiography. Chest *80*:61, 1981.
175. Dillon, J. C., Feigenbaum, H., Konecke, L. L., Davis, R. H., and Chang, S.: Echocardiographic manifestations of valvular vegetations. Am. Heart J. *86*:698, 1973.
176. Roy, P., Tajik, A. J., Giuliani, E. R., Schattenberg, T. T., Gau, G. T., and Frye, R. L.: Spectrum of echocardiographic findings in bacterial endocarditis. Circulation *53*:474, 1976.
177. Gallis, H. A., Johnson, M. L., and Kisslo, J. A.: Two-dimensional echocardiographic assessment of vegetative endocarditis. Circulation *55*:346, 1977.
178. Zee-cheng, C-S., Gibbs, H. R., Johnson, K. P., and Smith, J. C.: Giant vegetation due to *Staphylococcus aureus* endocarditis simulating left atrial myxoma. Am. Heart J. *111*:414, 1986.
179. Berger, M., Delfin, L. A., Jelveh, M., and Goldberg, E.: Two-dimensional echocardiographic findings in right-sided infective endocarditis. Circulation *61*:855, 1980.
180. Pruett, T. L., Rotstein, O. D., Anderson, R. W., and Simmons, R. L.: Tricuspid valve candida endocarditis. Am. J. Med. *80*:116, 1986.
181. Wann, L. S., Dillon, J. C., Weyman, A. E., and Feigenbaum, H.: Echocardiography in bacterial endocarditis. N. Engl. J. Med. *295*:135, 1976.
182. Rakowski, H., and Popp, R. L.: Clinical utility of two-dimensional echocardiography in infective endocarditis. Am. J. Cardiol. *46*:379, 1980.
183. Hickey, A. J., Wolfers, J., and Wilcken, D. E. L.: Reliability and clinical relevance of detection of vegetations by echocardiography in bacterial endocarditis. Br. Heart J. *46*:624, 1981.
184. Gomes, J. A., Calderon, J., Lajam, F., Sakural, H., Friedman, H. S., and Tatz, J. S.: Echocardiographic detection of fungal vegetations in *Candida parasilopsis* endocarditis. Am. J. Med. *61*:273, 1976.
185. Pollak, S. J., and Felner, J. M.: Echocardiographic identification of an aortic valve ring abscess. J. Am. Coll. Cardiol. *7*:1167, 1986.
186. Nakamura, K., Suzuki, S., Satomi, G., Hayashi, H., and Hirosawa, K.: Detection of mitral ring abscess by two-dimensional echocardiography. Circulation *65*:816, 1982.
187. Bloch, W. N., Jr., Felner, J. M., Wickliffe, C., and Symbas, P. N.: Echocardiographic diagnosis of thrombus on a heterograft aortic valve in the mitral position. Chest *70*:399, 1976.
188. Ben-Zvi, J., Hildner, F. J., Chandraratna, P. A., and Samet, P.: Thrombosis on Bjork-Shiley aortic valve prosthesis: Clinical, arteriographic, echocardiographic, and therapeutic observations in seven cases. Am. J. Cardiol. *34*:538, 1974.
189. Bernal-Ramirez, J. A., and Phillips, J. H.: Echocardiographic study of malfunction of the Bjork-Shiley prosthetic heart valve in the mitral position. Am. J. Cardiol. *40*:449, 1977.
190. Wann, L. S., Pyhel, H. J., Judson, W. E., Tavel, M. E., and Feigenbaum, H.: Ball variance in a Harken mitral prosthesis. Echocardiographic and phonocardiographic features. Chest *72*:785, 1977.
191. Pfeifer, J., Goldschlager, N., Sweatman, T., Gerbode, E., and Selzer, A.: Malfunction of mitral ball valve prosthesis due to thrombus. Am. J. Cardiol *29*:95, 1972.
192. Assad-Morell, J. L., Tajik, A. J., Anderson, M. W., Tancredi, R. G., Wallace, R. B., and Giuliani, E. R.: Malfunctioning tricuspid valve prosthesis: Clinical phonocardiographic, echocardiographic and surgical findings. Mayo Clin. Proc. *42*:443, 1974.
193. Mehta, A., Kessler, K. M., Tamer, D., Pefkaros, K., Kessler, R. M., and Myerburg, R. J.: Two-dimensional echographic observations in major detachment of a prosthetic aortic valve. Am. Heart J. *101*:231, 1981.
194. Schuchman, H., Feigenbaum, H., Dillon, J. C., and Chang, S.: Intracavitary echoes in patients with mitral prosthetic valves. J. Clin. Ultrasound *3*:111, 1975.
195. Alam, M., Goldstein, S., and Lakier, J. B.: Echocardiographic changes in the thickness of porcine valves with time. Chest *79*:663, 1981.
196. Bansal, R. C., Morrison, D. L., and Jacobsen, J. G.: Echocardiography of porcine aortic prostheses with flail leaflets due to degeneration and calcification. Am. Heart J. *107*:591, 1984.
197. Williams, G. A., and Labovitz, A. J.: Doppler hemodynamic evaluation of prosthetic (Starr-Edwards and Bjork-Shiley) and bioprosthetic (Hancock and Carpentier-Edwards) cardiac valves. Am. J. Cardiol. *56*:325, 1985.
198. Ryan, T., Armstrong, W. F., Dillon, J. C., and Feigenbaum, H.: Doppler echocardiographic evaluation of patients with porcine mitral valves. Am. Heart J. *111*:237, 1986.
199. Ferrara, R. P., Labovitz, A. J., Wiens, R. D., Kennedy, H. L., and Williams, G. A.: Prosthetic mitral regurgitation detected by Doppler echocardiography. Am. J. Cardiol. *55*:229, 1985.
200. Gross, C. M., and Wann, L. S.: Doppler echocardiographic diagnosis of porcine bioprosthetic cardiac valve malfunction. Am. J. Cardiol. *53*:1203, 1984.
201. Weinstein, I. R., Marbarger, J. P., and Perez, J. E.: Ultrasonic assessment of the St. Jude prosthetic valve: M-mode, two-dimensional and Doppler echocardiography. Circulation *68*:897, 1983.
202. Grenadier, E., Sahn, D. J., Roche, A. H. G., Valdes-Cruz, L. M., Copeland, J. G., Goldberg, S. J., and Allen, H. D.: Detection of deterioration or infection of homograft and porcine xenograft bioprosthetic valves in mitral and aortic positions by two-dimensional echocardiographic examination. J. Am. Coll. Cardiol. 2:452, 1983.
203. Nagata, S., Park, Y.-D., Nagae, K., Beppu, S., Kawazoe, K., Tujita, T., Sakakibara, H., and Nimura, Y.: Echocardiographic features of bioprosthetic valve endocarditis. Br. Heart J. *51*:263, 1984.
204. Nair, C. K., Aronow, W. S., Sketch, M. H., Mohiuddin, S. M., Pagano, T., Esterbrooks, D. J., and Hee, T. T.: Clinical and echocardiographic characteristics of patients with mitral annular calcification. Am. J. Cardiol. *51*:992, 1983.
205. Nestico, R. F., DePace, N. L., Morganroth, J., Kotler, M. N., and Ross, J.: Mitral annular calcification: Clinical, pathophysiologic, and echocardiographic review. Am. Heart J. *107*:989, 1984.

CONGENITAL HEART DISEASE

206. Gutgesell, H. P., Huhta, J. C., Latson, L. A., Huffines, D., and McNamara, D. G.: Accuracy of two-dimensional echocardiography in the diagnosis of congenital heart disease. Am. J. Cardiol. *55*:514, 1985.
207. Dickinson, D. F., Goldberg, S. J., and Wilson, N.: A comparison of information obtained by ultrasound examination and cardiac catheterization in paediatric patients with congenital heart disease. Int. J. Cardiol. *9*:275, 1985.
208. Foale, R., Stefanini, L., Rickards, A., and Somerville, J.: Left and right ventricular morphology in complex congenital heart disease defined by two-dimensional echocardiography. Am. J. Cardiol. *49*:93, 1982.
209. Silverman, N. H.: An ultrasonic approach to the diagnosis of cardiac situs, connections, and malpositions. Cardiol. Clin. *1*:473, 1983.
210. Houston, A. V., Gregory, N. L., and Coleman, E. N.: Echocardiographic identification of aorta and main pulmonary artery in complete transposition. Br. Heart J. *40*:377, 1978.
211. Hagler, D. J., Tajik, A. J., Seward, J. B., Edwards, W. D., Mair, D. D., and Ritter, D. G.: Atrioventricular and ventriculoarterial discordance (corrected transposition of the great arteries). Wide-angle two-dimensional echocardiographic assessment of ventricular morphology. Mayo Clin. Proc. *56*:591, 1981.

212. Lesbre, J. P., Scheuble, C., Kalisa, A., Lalau, J. D., and Andrejak, M. T.: Echocardiography in the diagnosis of severe aortic valve stenosis in adults. Arch. Mal. Coeur. *76*:1, 1983.
213. Nanda, N. C., Gramiak, R., Manning, J., Mahoney, E. B., Lipchik, E. O., and DeWeese, J. A.: Echocardiographic recognition of the congenital bicuspid aortic valve. Circulation *49*:870, 1974.
214. Smallhorn, J., Tommasini, G., Deanfield, J., Doublas, J., Gibson, D., and Macartney, F.: Congenital mitral stenosis. Anatomical and functional assessment by echocardiography. Br. Heart J. *45*:527, 1981.
215. Trowitzsch, E., Bano-Rodrigo, A., Burger, B. M., Colan, S. D., and Sanders, S. P.: Two-dimensional echocardiographic findings in double orifice mitral valve. J. Am. Coll. Cardiol. *6*:383, 1985.
216. Weyman, A. E., Hurwitz, R. A., Girod, D. A., Dillon, J. C., Feigenbaum, H., and Green, D.: Cross-sectional echocardiographic visualization of the stenotic pulmonary valve. Circulation *56*:769, 1977.
217. Johnson, G. L., Kwan, O. L., Handshoe, S., Noonan, J. A., and DeMaria, A. N.: Accuracy of combined two-dimensional echocardiography and continuous wave Doppler recordings in the estimation of pressure gradient in right ventricular outlet obstruction. J. Am. Coll. Cardiol. *3*:1013, 1984.
218. Hagler, D. J., Tajik, A. J., Seward, J. B., and Ritter, D. G.: Noninvasive assessment of pulmonary valve stenosis, aortic valve stenosis, and coarctation of the aorta in critically ill neonates. Am. J. Cardiol. *57*:369, 1986.
219. Shiina, A., Seward, J. B., Edwards, W. D., Hagler, D. J., and Tajik, A. J.: Two-dimensional echocardiographic spectrum of Ebstein's anomaly: Detailed anatomic assessment. J. Am. Coll. Cardiol. *3*:356, 1984.
220. Radford, D. J., Graff, R. F., and Neilson, G. H.: Diagnosis and natural history of Ebstein's anomaly. Br. Heart J. *54*:517, 1985.
221. Milner, S., Meyer, R. A., Venables, A. W., Korfhagen, J., and Kaplan, S.: Mitral and triscupid valve closure in congenital heart disease. Circulation *53*:513, 1976.
222. Lundstrom, N. R.: Ultrasound cardiographic studies of the mitral valve region in young infants with mitral atresia, mitral stenosis, hypoplasia of the left ventricle and cor triatriatum. Circulation *45*:324, 1972.
223. Meyer, R. A., and Kaplan, S.: Echocardiography in the diagnosis of hypoplasia of the left or right ventricle in the neonate. Circulation *46*:55, 1972.
224. Weyman, A. E., Caldwell, R. L., Hurwitz, R. A., Girod, D. A., Dillon, J. C., Feigenbaum, H., and Green, D.: Cross-sectional echocardiographic characterization of aortic obstruction. I. Supravalvular aortic stenosis and aortic hypoplasia. Circulation *57*:491, 1978.
225. Cabrera, A., Pastor, E., and Lekuona, I.: Congenital aortic atresia with intact ventricular septum and normal left ventricle. Diagnosis by cross-sectional echocardiography. Int. J. Cardiol. *8*:339, 1985.
226. Davis, R. A., Feigenbaum, H., Chang, S., Konecke, L. L., and Dillon, J. C.: Echocardiographic manifestations of discrete subaortic stenosis. Am. J. Cardiol. *33*:277, 1974.
227. DiSessa, T. G., Hagan, A. D. Isabel-Jones, J. B., Ti, C. C., Mercier, J. C., and Friedman, W. F.: Two-dimensional echocardiographic evaluation of discrete subaortic stenosis from the apical long axis view. Am. Heart J. *101*:774, 1981.
228. Isaaz, K., Cloez, J. L., Canchin, N., Marcon, F., Worms, A. M., and Pernot, C.: Assessment of right ventricular outflow tract in children by two-dimensional echocardiography using a new subcostal view. Am. J. Cardiol. *56*:539, 1985.
229. Motro, M., Schneeweiss, A., Shem-Tov, A., Vered, A., Hegesh, J., Neufeld, H. N., and Rath, S.: Two-dimensional echocardiography in discrete subaortic stenosis. Am. J. Cardiol. *53*:896, 1984.
230. Valdes-Cruz, L. M., Jones, M., Scagnelli, S., Sahn, D. J., Tomizuka, F. M., and Pierce, J. E.: Prediction of gradients in fibrous subaortic stenosis by continuous wave two-dimensional Doppler echocardiography: Animal studies. J. Am. Coll. Cardiol. *5*:1363, 1985.
231. Weyman, A. E., Dillon, J. C., Feigenbaum, H., and Chang, S.: Echocardiographic differentiation of infundibular from valvular pulmonary stenosis. Am. J. Cardiol. *36*:21, 1975.
232. Caldwell, R. L., Weyman, A. G., Hurwitz, R. A., Girod, D. A., and Feigenbaum, H.: Right ventricular outflow tract assessment by cross-sectional echocardiography in tetralogy of Fallot. Circulation *59*:395, 1979.
233. Piot, J. D., Lucet, P., Losay, J., Touchot, A., Petit, J., David, P., Piot, C., and Binet, J. P.: Diagnosis and localization of ventricular septal defects by two-dimensional echocardiography. 50 cases. Arch. Mal. Coeur. *74*:1001, 1981.
234. Capelli, H., Andrade, J. L., and Somerville, J.: Classification of the site of ventricular septal defect by two-dimensional echocardiography. Am. J. Cardiol. *51*:1474, 1983.
235. Ribgy, M. L., Anderson, R. H., Gibson, D., Jones, O. D. H., Joseph, M. C., and Shinebourne, E. A.: Two dimensional echocardiographic categorization of the univentricular heart. Br. Heart J. *46*:603, 1981.
236. Shub, C., Dimopoulos, I. N., Seward, J. B., Callahan, J. A., Tancredi, R. G., Schattenberg, T. T., Reeder, G. S., Hagler, D. J., and Tajik, A. J.: Sensitivity of two-dimensional echocardiography in the direct visualization of atrial septal defect utilizing the subcostal approach: Experience with 154 patients. J. Am. Coll. Cardiol. *2*:127, 1983.
237. Dillon, J. C., Weyman, A. E., Feigenbaum, H., Eggleton, R. C., and Johnston, K. W.: Cross-sectional echocardiographic examination of the interatrial septum. Circulation *55*:115, 1977.
238. Nasser, F. N., Tajik, A. J., Seward, J. B., and Hagler, D. J.: Diagnosis of sinus venosus atrial septal defect by two-dimensional echocardiography. Mayo Clin. Proc. *56*:568, 1981.
239. Goldberg, S. J., and Friedman, W. F.: Echocardiographic detection of large left to right shunts and cardiomyopathies in infants and children. Am. J. Cardiol. *38*:73, 1976.
240. Baylen, B. G., Meyer, R. A., Kaplan, S., Ringenburg, W. E., and Korfhagen, J.: The critically ill premature infant with patent ductus arteriosus and pulmonary disease—an echocardiographic assessment. J. Pediatr. *86*:423, 1975.
241. Baylen, B., Meyer, R. A., Korfhagen, J., Benzing, G., Bubb, M. E., and Kaplan, S.: Left ventricular performance in the critically ill premature infant with patent jductus arteriosus and pulmonary disease. Circulation *55*:182, 1977.
242. Chazal, R. A., Armstrong, W. F., Dillon, J. C., and Feigenbaum, H.: Diastolic ventricular septal motion in atrial septal defect: Analysis of M-mode echocardiograms in 31 patients. Am. J. Cardiol. *52*:1088, 1983.
243. Paquet, M., and Gutgesell, H.: Echocardiographic features of total anomalous pulmonary venous connection. Circulation *51*:599, 1975.
244. Ostman-Smith, I., Silverman, N. H., Oldershaw, P., Lincoln, C., and Shinebourne, E. A.: Cor triatriatum sinistrum. Diagnostic features on cross-sectional echocardiography. Br. Heart J. *51*:211, 1984.
245. Kerber, R. E., Kioschos, J. M., and Lauer, R. M.: Use of an ultrasonic contrast method in the diagnosis of valvular regurgitation and intracardiac shunts. Am. J. Cardiol. *34*:722, 1974.
246. Rose, G. C., Armstrong, W. F., Mahomed, Y., and Feigenbaum, H.: Atrial level right-to-left intracardiac shunt associated with postoperative hypoxemia: Demonstration with contrast two-dimensional echocardiography. J. Am. Coll. Cardiol. *6*:920, 1985.
247. Weyman, A. E., Wann, L. S., Hurwitz, R. A., Dillon, J. C., and Feigenbaum, H.: Negative contrast echocardiography: A new technique for detecting left-to-right shunts. Circulation *56*:II-89 (Abstract), 1977.
248, Kronik, G., and Mosslacher, H.: Positive contrast echocardiography in patients with patent foramen ovale and normal right hemodynamics. Am. J. Cardiol *49*:1806, 1982.
249. Seward, J. B., Tajik, A. J., Spangler, J. G., and Ritter, D. G.: Echocardiographic contrast studies: Initial experience. Mayo Clin. Proc. *50*:163, 1975.
250. Magherini, A., Azzolina, G., Weichmann, V., and Fantini, F.: Pulsed Doppler echocardiography for diagnosis of ventricular septal defects. Br. Heart J. *43*:143, 1980.
251. Stevenson, J. G., Kawabori, I., and Guntheroth, W. G.: Pulsed Doppler echocardiographic diagnosis of patent ductus arteriosus: Sensitivity, specificity, limitations, and technical features. Cathet. Cardiovasc. Diagn. *6*:255, 1980.
252. Minagoe, S., Tei, C., Kisanuki, A., Arikawa, K., Nakazono, Y., Yoshimura, H., Kashima, T., and Tanaka, H.: Noninvasive pulsed Doppler echocardiographic detection of the direction of shunt flow in patients with atrial septal defect: Usefulness of the right parasternal approach. Circulation *71*:745, 1985.
253. Murphy, D. J., Ludomirsky, A., and Huhta, J. C.: Continuous-wave Doppler in children with ventricular septal defect: Noninvasive estimation of interventricular pressure gradient. Am. J. Cardiol. *57*:428, 1986.
254. Marx, G. R., Allen, H. D., and Goldberg, S. J.: Doppler echocardiographic estimation of systolic pulmonary artery pressure in pediatric patients with interventricular communications. J. Am. Coll. Cardiol. *6*:1132, 1985.
255. Vick, G. W., III, Huhta, J. C., and Gutgesell, H. P.: Assessment of the ductus arteriosus in preterm infants utilizing suprasternal two-dimensional/Doppler echocardiography. J. Am. Coll. Cardiol. *5*:973, 1985.
256. Ortiz, E., Robinson, P. J., Deanfield, J. E., Franklin, R., Macartney, F. J., and Wyse, R. K. H.: Localisation of ventricular septal defects by simultaneous display of superimposed colour Doppler and cross sectional echocardiographic images. Br. Heart J. *54*:53, 1985.
257. Barron, J. V., Sahn, D. J., Valdes-Cruz, L. M., Grenadier, E., Allen, H. D., and Goldberg, S. J.: Two-dimensional echocardiographic features of ventricular septal aneurysm paradoxically bulging into the left ventricular outflow tract. Am. Heart J. *104*:156, 1982.
258. Arvan, S.: Incidental interatrial septal aneurysm associated with valve prolapse. Am. Heart J. *111*:603, 1986.
259. Belkin, R. N., Waugh, R. A., and Kisslo, J.: Interatrial shunting in atrial septal aneurysm. Am. J. Cardiol. *57*:310, 1986.
260. Beppu, S., Nimura, Y., Nagata, S., Tamai, M., Matsuo, H., Matsumoto, M., Kawashima, Y., Sakakibara, H., and Abe, H.: Diagnosis of endocardial cushion defect with cross-sectional and M-mode scanning of echocardiography. Differentiation from secundum atrial septal defect. Br. Heart J. *38*:911, 1976.
261. Beppu, S., Nimura, Y., Sakakibara, H., Nagata, S., Park, Y-D., Baba, K., Naito, Y., Ohta, M., Kamiya, T., Koyanagi, H., and Fujita, T.: Mitral cleft in ostium primum atrial septal defect assessed by cross-sectional echocardiography. Circulation *62*:1099, 1980.
262. Rice, M. J., Seward, J. B., Edwards, W. D., Hagler, D. J., Danielson, G. K., Puga, F. J., and Tajik, A. J.: Straddling atrioventricular valve: Two-dimensional echocardiographic diagnosis, classification and surgical implications. Am. J. Cardiol. *55*:505, 1985.
263. Smallhorn, J. F., Tommasini, G., and Macartney, F. J.: Detection and assessment of straddling and overriding atrioventricular valves by two-dimensional echocardiography. Br. Heart J. *46*:254, 1981.
264. Weyman, A. E., Feigenbaum, H., Dillon, J. C., Chang, S., Hurwitz, R. A., and Girod, D. A.: Localization of left ventricular outflow obstruction by cross-sectional echocardiography. Am. J. Med. *60*:33, 1976.
265. Vogt, J., Rupprath, G., Grimm, T., and Beuren, A. J.: Qualitative and quantitative evaluation of supravalvar aortic stenosis by cross-sectional echocardiography. Pediatr. Cardiol. *3*:13, 1982.
266. Snider, A. R., and Silverman, N. H.: Suprasternal notch echocardiography: A two-dimensional technique for evaluating congenital heart disease. Circulation *63*:165, 1981.
267. Shaddy, R. E., Snider, A. R., Silverman, N. H., and Lutin, W.: Pulsed Doppler findings in patients with coarctation of the aorta. Circulation *73*:82, 1986.
268. Hagler, D. J., Tajik, A. J., Seward, J. B., Mair, D. D., and Titter, D. G.: Double-outlet right ventricle: Wide-angle two dimensional echocardiographic observations. Circulation *63*:419, 1981.

269. Hagler, D. J., Tajik, A. J., Seward, J. B., Mair, D. D., and Ritter, D. G.: Wide-angle two-dimensional echocardiographic profiles of conotruncal abnormalities. Mayo Clin. Proc. 55:73, 1980.
270. Daskalopoulos, D. A., Edwards, W. D., Driscoll, D. J., Seward, J. B., Tajik, A. J., and Hagler, D. J.: Correlation of two-dimensional echocardiographic and autopsy findings in complete transposition of the great arteries. J. Am. Coll. Cardiol. 2:1151, 1983.
271. Marin-Garcia, J., and Tonkin, I. L. D.: Two-dimensional echocardiographic evaluation of persistent truncus arteriosus. Am. J. Cardiol. 50:1376, 1982.
272. Marino, B., DeSimone, G., Pasquini, L., Giannico, S., Marcelletti, C., Ammirati, A., Guccione, P., Boldrini, R., and Ballerini, L.: Complete transposition of the great arteries: Visualization of left and right outflow tract obstruction by oblique subcostal two-dimensional echocardiography. Am. J. Cardiol. 55:1140, 1985.
273. Sahn, D. J., Terry, R., O'Rourke, R., Leopold, G., and Friedman, S. F.: Multiple crystal cross-sectional echocardiography in the diagnosis of cyanotic congenital heart disease. Circulation 50:230, 1974.
274. Meissner, M. D., Panidis, I. P., Eshaghpour, E., Mintz, G. S., and Ross, J.: Corrected transposition of the great arteries: Evaluation by two-dimensional and Doppler echocardiography. Am. Heart J. 111:599, 1986.

CORONARY ARTERY DISEASE

275. Jacobs, J. J., Feigenbaum, H., Corya, B. C., and Phillips, J. F.: Detection of left ventricular asynergy by echocardiography. Circulation 48:263, 1973.
276. Lima, J. A., Becker, L. C., Melin, J. A., Lima, S., Kallman, C. A., Weisfeldt, M. L., and Weiss, J. L.: Impaired thickening of nonischemic myocardium during acute regional ischemia in the dog. Circulation 71:1048, 1985.
277. Buda, A. J., Zotz, R. J., Pace, D. P., and Krause, L. C.: Comparison of two-dimensional echocardiographic wall motion and wall thickening abnormalities in relation to the myocardium at risk. Am. Heart J. 111:587, 1986.
278. Heger, J. J., Weyman, A. E., Wann, L. S., Rogers, E. W., Dillon, J. C., and Feigenbaum, H.: Cross-sectional echocardiographic analysis of the extent of left ventricular asynergy in acute myocardial infarction. Circulation 61:1113, 1980.
279. Rasmussen, S., Corya, B. C., Feigenbaum, H., and Knoebel, S. B.: Detection of myocardial scar tissue by M-mode echocardiography. Circulation 57:230, 1978.
280. Distante, A., Picano, E., Moscarelli, E., Palombo, C., Benassi, A., and L'Abbate, A.: Echocardiographic versus hemodynamic monitoring during attacks of variant angina pectoris. Am. J. Cardiol. 55:1319, 1985.
281. Wann, L. S., Faris, J. V., Childress, R. H., Dillon, J. C., Weyman, A. E., and Feigenbaum, H.: Exercise cross-sectional echocardiography in ischemic heart disease. Circulation 60:1300, 1979.
282. Jaarsma, W., Visser, C. A., Kupper, A. J. F., Res, J. C. J., VanEenige, M. J., and Ross, J. P.: Usefulness of two-dimensional exercise echocardiography shortly after myocardial infarction. Am. J. Cardiol. 57:86, 1986.
283. Iliceto, S., D'Ambrosio, G., Sorino, M., Papa, A., Amico, A., Ricci, A., and Rizzon, P.: Comparison of postexercise and transesophageal atrial pacing two-dimensional echocardiography for detection of coronary artery disease. Am. J. Cardiol. 57:547, 1986.
284. Picano, E., Distante, A., Masini, M., Morales, M. A., Lattanzi, F., and L'Abbate, A.: Dipyridamole-echocardiography test in effort angina pectoris. Am. J. Cardiol. 56:452, 1985.
285. Crawford, M. H., Petru, M. A., Amon, W., Sorensen, S. G., and Vance, W. S.: Comparative value of two-dimensional echocardiography and radionuclide angiography for quantitating changes in left ventricular performance during exercise limited by angina pectoris. Am. J. Cardiol. 53:42, 1984.
286. Okamoto, M., Kajiyama, G., Beppu, S., Izumi, S., Miyatake, K., Kinoshita, N., Sakakibara, H., and Nimura, Y.: Relationship between extension of acute myocardial ischemia and mitral flow: A study with pulsed Doppler echocardiography. Jpn. J. Med. Ultrasonics 12:1, 1985.
287. Fujii, J., Yazaki, Y., Sawada, H., Aizawa, T., Watanabe, H., and Kato, K.: Noninvasive assessment of left and right ventricular filling in myocardial infarction with a two-dimensional Doppler echocardiographic method. J. Am. Coll. Cardiol. 5:1155, 1985.
288. Erbel, R., Schweizer, P., Meyer, J., Krebs, W., Yalkinoglu, O., and Effert, S.: Sensitivity of cross-sectional echocardiography in detection of impaired global and regional left ventricular function: Prospective study. Int. J. Cardiol. 7:375, 1985.
289. Ren, J-F., Kotler, M. N., Hakki, A-H., Panidis, I. P., Mintz, G. S., and Ross, J.: Quantitation of regional left ventricular function by two-dimensional echocardiography in normals and patients with coronary artery disease. Am. Heart J. 110:552, 1985.
290. Shiina, A., Tajik, A. J., Smith, H. C., Lengyel, M., and Seward, J. B.: Prognostic significance of regional wall motion abnormality in patients with prior myocardial infarction: A prospective correlative study of two-dimensional echocardiography and angiography. Mayo Clin. Proc. 61:254, 1986.
291. Van Reet, R. E., Quinones, M. A., Poliner, L. R., Nelson, J. G., Waggoner, A. D., Kanon, D., Lubetkin, S. J., Pratt, C. M., and Winters, W. L.: Comparison of two-dimensional echocardiography with gated radionuclide ventriculography in the evaluation of global and regional left ventricular function in acute myocardial infarction. J. Am. Coll. Cardiol. 3:243, 1984.
292. Iliceto, S., Ricci, A., Sorino, M., Gaglione, A., Chiddo, A., Biasco, G., and Rizzon, P.: Evaluation of the ejection fraction using two simplified echocardiographic methods in patients with ischemic heart disease and left ventricular asynergy. G. Ital. Cardiol. 15:142, 1985.
293. Ryan, T., Petrovic, O., Armstrong, W. F., Dillon, J. C., and Feigenbaum, H.: Quantitative two-dimensional echocardiographic assessment of patients undergoing left ventricular aneurysmectomy. Am. Heart J. 111:714, 1986.
294. Visser, C. A., Kan, G., Meltzer, R. S., Moulijn, A. C., David, G. K., and Dunning, A. J.: Assessment of left ventricular aneurysm resectability by two-dimensional echocardiography. Am. J. Cardiol. 56:857, 1985.
295. Matsumoto, M., Watanabe, F., Goto, A., Hamano, Y., Yasui, K., Minamino, T., and Abe, H.: Left ventricular aneurysm and the prediction of left ventricular enlargement studied by two-dimensional echocardiography: Quantitative assessment of aneurysm size in relation to clinical course. Circulation 72:280, 1985.
296. Hamilton, K., Ellenbogen, K., Lowe, J. E., and Kisslo, J.: Ultrasound diagnosis of pseudoaneurysm and contiguous ventricular septal defect complicating inferior myocardial infarction. J. Am. Coll. Cardiol. 6:1160, 1985.
297. Loperfido, F., Pennestri, F., Mazzari, M., Biasucci, L. M., Vigna, C., and Manzoli, U.: Diagnosis of left ventricular pseudoaneurysm by pulsed Doppler echocardiography. Am. Heart J. 110:1291, 1985.
298. Stephens, J. D., Giles, M. R., and Banim, S. O.: Ruptured postinfarction ventricular septal aneurysm causing chronic congestive cardiac failure. Detection by two-dimensional echocardiography. Br. Heart J. 46:216, 1981.
299. Smith, G., Endresen, K., Sivertssen, E., and Semb, G.: Ventricular septal rupture diagnosed by simultaneous cross-sectional echocardiography and Doppler ultrasound. Eur. Heart J. 6:631, 1985.
300. Panidis, I. P., Mintz, G. S., Goel, I., McAllister, M., and Ross, J.: Acquired ventricular septal defect after myocardial infarction: Detection by combined two-dimensional and Doppler echocardiography. Am. Heart J. 111:427, 1986.
301. Sharkey, S. W., Shelley, W., Carlyle, P. F., Rysavy, J., and Cohn, J. N.: M-mode and two-dimensional echocardiographic analysis of the septum in experimental right ventricular infarction: Correlation with hemodynamic alterations. Am. Heart J. 110:1210, 1985.
302. D'Arcy, B., and Nanda, N. C.: Two-dimensional echocardiographic features of right ventricular infarction. Circulation 65:167, 1982.
303. Jugdutt, B. I., Sussex, B. A., Sivaram, C. A., and Rossall, R. E.: Right ventricular infarction: Two dimensional echocardiographic evaluation. Am. Heart J. 107:505, 1984.
304. Doyle, T., Troup, P. J., and Wann, L. S.: Mid-diastolic opening of the pulmonary valve after right ventricular infarction. J. Am. Coll. Cardiol. 5:366, 1985.
305. Asinger, R. W., Mikell, F. L., Elsperger, J., and Hodges, M.: Incidence of left-ventricular thrombosis after acute transmural myocardial infarction. Serial evaluation by two-dimensional echocardiography. N. Engl. J. Med. 305:297, 1981.
306. Sharma, B., Carvalho, A., Wyeth, R., and Franciosa, J. A.: Left ventricular thrombi diagnosed by echocardiography in patients with acute myocardial infarction treated with intracoronary streptokinase followed by intravenous heparin. Am. J. Cardiol. 56:422, 1985.
307. Meltzer, R. S., Visser, C. A., and Fuster, V.: Intracardiac thrombi and systemic embolization. Ann. Intern. Med. 104:689, 1986.
308. Johannessen, K. A., Nordrehaug, J. E., and Von Der Lippe, G.: Left ventricular thrombosis and cerebrovascular accident in acute myocardial infarction. Br. Heart J. 51:553, 1984.
309. Come, P. C., Riley, M. F., Weintraub, R., Morgan, J. P., and Nakao, S.: Echocardiographic detection of complete and partial papillary muscle rupture during acute myocardial infarction. Am. J. Cardiol. 56:787, 1985.
310. Horowitz, R. S., Morganroth, J., Parrotto, C., Chen, C. C., Soffer, J., and Pauletto, F. J.: Immediate diagnosis of acute myocardial infarction by two-dimensional echocardiography. Circulation 65:323, 1982.
311. Stamm, R. B., Gibson, R. S., Bishop, H. L., Carabello, B. A., Beller, F. A., and Martin, R. P.: Echocardiographic detection of infarct-localized asynergy and remote asynergy during acute myocardial infarction: Correlation with the extent of angiographic coronary disease. Circulation 67:233:1983.
312. Erlebacher, J. A., Weiss, J. L., Weisfeldt, M. L., and Bulkley, B. H.: Early dilation of the infarcted segment in acute transmural myocardial infarction: Role of infarct expansion in acute left ventricular enlargement. J. Am. Coll. Cardiol. 4:201, 1984.
313. Nishimura, R. A., Tajik, A. J., Shib, C., Miller, F. A., Ilstrup, D. M., and Harrison, C. E.: Role of two-dimensional echocardiography in the prediction of in-hospital complications after acute myocardial infarction. J. Am. Coll. Cardiol. 4:1080, 1984.
314. Abrams, D. S., Starling, M. R., Crawford, M. H., and O'Rourke, R. A.: Value of noninvasive techniques for predicting early complications in patients with clinical class II acute myocardial infarction. J. Am. Coll. Cardiol. 2:818, 1983.
315. Bhatnagar, S. K., and Al-Yusuf, A. R.: The role of prehospital discharge two-dimensional echocardiography in determining the prognosis of survivors of first myocardial infarction. Am. Heart J. 109:472, 1985.
316. Stamm, R. B., Gibson, R. S., Bishop, H. L., Carabello, B. A., Beller, G. A., and Martin, R. P.: Echocardiographic detection of infarction: Correlation with the extent of angiographic coronary disease. Circulation 67:233, 1983.
317. Weyman, A. E., Feigenbaum, H., Dillon, J. C., Johnston, K. W., and Eggleton, R. C.: Noninvasive visualization of the left main coronary artery by cross-sectional echocardiography. Circulation 54:169, 1976.
318. Rink, L. D., Feigenbaum, H., Godley, R. W., Weyman, A. E., Dillon, J. C., Phillips, J. F., and Marshall, J. E.: Echocardiographic detection of left main coronary artery obstruction. Circulation 65:719, 1982.
319. Vasey, C. G., Ryan, T., Armstrong, W. F., and Feigenbaum, H.: Digital echocardiographic visualization of the left coronary arteries using an annular phased array system. J. Am. Coll. Cardiol. 7:147A (Abstract), 1986.
320. Block, P. J., and Popp, R. L.: Detecting and excluding significant left main coronary artery narrowing. Am. J. Cardiol. 55:937, 1985.

321. King, D. H., Danford, D. A., Huhta, J. C., and Gutgesell, H. P.: Noninvasive detection of anomalous origin of the left main coronary artery from the pulmonary trunk by pulsed Doppler echocardiography. Am. J. Cardiol. *55*:608, 1985.
322. Shah, R. M., Nanda, N. C., Hsiung, M. C., Moos, S., and Roitman, D.: Identification of anomalous origin of the right coronary artery from pulmonary trunk by Doppler color flow mapping. Am. J. Cardiol. *57*:366, 1986.
323. Capannari, T. E., Daniels, S. R., Meyer, R. A., Schwartz, D. C., and Kaplan, S.: Sensitivity, specificity, and predictive value of two-dimensional echocardiography in detecting coronary artery aneurysms in patients with Kawasaki disease. J. Am. Coll. Cardiol. *7*:355, 1986.
324. Armstrong, W. F., Mueller, T. M., Kinney, E. L., Tickner, E. G., Dillon, J. C., and Feigenbaum, H.: Assessment of myocardial perfusion abnormalities with contrast-enhanced two-dimensional echocardiography. Circulation *66*:166, 1982.
325. Kemper, A. J., Force, T., Kloner, R., Gilfoil, M., Perkins, L., Hale, S., Alker, K., and Parisi, A. F.: Contrast echocardiographic estimation of regional myocardial blood flow after acute coronary occlusion. Circulation *72*:1115, 1985.
326. Kaul, S., Pandian, N. G., Gillam, L. D., Newell, J. B., Okada, R. D., Weyman, A. E., and Lutrario, D.: Contrast echocardiography in acute myocardial ischemia. III. In vivo comparison of the extent of abnormal wall motion with the area at risk for necrosis. J. Am. Coll. Cardiol. *7*:383, 1986.
327. Shah, P. M., Taylor, R. D., and Wong, M.: Abnormal mitral valve coaptation in hypertrophic obstructive cardiomyopathy: Proposed role in systolic anterior motion of mitral valve. Am. J. Cardiol. *48*:258, 1981.

CARDIOMYOPATHIES

328. Henry, W. L., Clark, C. E., Glancy, D. L., and Epstein, S. E.: Echocardiographic measurement of the left ventricular outflow gradient in idiopathic hypertrophic subaortic stenosis. N. Engl. J. Med. *288*:989, 1973.
329. Pollick, C., Rakowski, H., and Wigle, E. D.: Muscular subaortic stenosis: The quantitative relationship between systolic anterior motion and the pressure gradient. Circulation *69*:43, 1984.
330. Henry, W. L., Clark, C. E., Griffith, J. M., and Epstein, S. E.: Mechanism of left ventricular outflow obstruction in patients with obstructive asymmetric septal hypertrophy (idiopathic hypertrophic subaortic stenosis). Am. J. Cardiol. *35*:337, 1975.
331. Mintz, G. S., Kotler, M. N., Segal, B. L., and Parry, W. R.: Systolic anterior motion of the mitral valve in the absence of asymmetric septal hypertrophy. Circulation *57*:256, 1978.
332. Maron, B. J., Epstein, S. E., Bonow, R. O., Wyngaarden, M. K., and Wesley, Y. E.: Obstructive hypertrophic cardiomyopathy associated with minimal left ventricular hypertrophy. Am. J. Cardiol. *53*:377, 1984.
333. Maron, B. J., Gottdiener, J. S., and Perry, L. W.: Specificity of systolic anterior motion of anterior mitral leaflet for hypertrophic cardiomyopathy. Br. Heart J. *45*:206, 1981.
334. Henry, W. L., Clark, C. E., Roberts, W. C., Morrow, A. G., and Epstein, S. E.: Difference in distributions of myocardial abnormalities in patients with obstructive and nonobstructive asymmetric septal hypertrophy (ASH): Echocardiographic and gross anatomic findings. Circulation *50*:447, 1974.
335. TenCate, F. J., Hugenholtz, P. G., and Roelandt, J.: Ultrasound study of dynamic behaviour of left ventricle in genetic asymmetric septal hypertrophy. Br. Heart J. *39*:627, 1977.
336. Clark, C. E., Henry, W. L., and Epstein, S. E.: Familial prevalence and genetic transmission of idiopathic hypertrophic subaortic stenosis. N. Engl. J. Med. *289*:709, 1973.
337. Maron, B. J., Gottdiener, J. S., and Epstein, S. E.: Patterns and significance of distribution of left ventricular hypertrophy in hypertrophic cardiomyopathy. A wide angle, two-dimensional echocardiographic study of 125 patients. Am. J. Cardiol. *48*:418, 1981.
338. Rovelli, E. G., Parenti, F., and Devizzi, S.: Apical hypertrophic cardiomyopathy of "Japanese type" in a Western European person. Am. J. Cardiol. *57*:358, 1986.
339. Maron, B. J., Gottdiener, J. S., Arce, J., Rosing, D. R., Wesler, Y. E., and Epstein, S. E.: Dynamic subaortic obstruction in hypertrophic cardiomyopathy: Pulsed Doppler echocardiography. J. Am. Coll. Cardiol. *6*:1, 1985.
340. Spirito, P., Maron, B. J., Chiarella, F., Bellotti, P., Tramarin, R., Pozzoli, M., and Vecchio, C.: Diastolic abnormalities in patients with hypertrophic cardiomyopathy: Relation to magnitude of left ventricular hypertrophy. Circulation *72*:310, 1985.
341. Shapiro, L. M., Zezulka, A., and Perrins, E. J.: Longitudinal changes in left ventricular diastolic function in hypertrophic cardiomyopathy. Int. J. Cardiol. *8*:261, 1985.
342. Corya, B. C., Feigenbaum, H., Rasmussen, S., and Black, M. J.: Echocardiographic features of congestive cardiomyopathy compared with normal subjects and patients with coronary artery disease. Circulation *49*:1153, 1974.
343. Goldberg, S. J., Valdes-Cruz, L. M., Sahn, D. J., and Allen, H. D.: Two-dimensional echocardiographic evaluation of dilated cardiomyopathy in children. Am. J. Cardiol. *52*:1244, 1983.
344. Borer, J. S., Henry, W. L., and Epstein, S. E.: Echocardiographic observations in patients with systemic infiltrative disease involving the heart. Am. J. Cardiol. *39*:184, 1977.
345. Siegel, R. J., Shah, P. K., and Fishbein, M. C.: Idiopathic restrictive cardiomyopathy. Circulation *70*:165, 1984.
346. Cueto-Garcia, L., Reeder, G. S., Kyle, R. A., Wood, D. L., Seward, J. B., Naessens, J., Offord, K. P., Greipp, P. R., Edwards, W. D., and Tajik, A. J.: Echocardiographic findings in systemic amyloidosis: Spectrum of cardiac involvement and relation to survival. J. Am. Coll. Cardiol. *6*:737, 1985.
347. Hongo, M., and Ikeda, S-I.: Echocardiographic assessment of the evolution of amyloid heart disease: A study with familial amyloid polyneuropathy. Circulation *73*:249, 1986.

PERICARDIAL DISEASE

348. Edler, I.: Diagnostic use of ultrasound in heart disease. Acta Med. Scand. *308*:32, 1955.
349. Feigenbaum, H., Waldhausen, J. A., and Hyde, L. P.: Ultrasound diagnosis of pericardial effusion. J.A.M.A. *191*:107, 1965.
350. Horowitz, M. S., Schultz, C. S., Stinson, E. B., Harrison, D. C., and Popp, R. L.: Sensitivity and specificity of echocardiographic diagnosis of pericardial effusion. Circulation *50*:239, 1974.
351. Nanda, N. C., Reeves, W., and Gramiak, R.: Echocardiographic demonstration of pericardial effusion behind the left atrium. Clin. Res. *24*:232A, 1976.
352. Feigenbaum, H., Zaky, A., and Grabhorn, L.: Cardiac motion in patients with pericardial effusion: A study using ultrasound cardiography. Circulation *34*:611, 1966.
353. Krueger, S. K., Zucker, R. P., Dzindzio, B. S., and Forker, A. D.: Swinging heart syndrome with predominant anterior pericardial effusion. J. Clin. Ultrasound. *4*:113, 1976.
354. Nanda, N. C., Gramiak, R., and Gross, C. M.: Echocardiography of cardiac valves in pericardial effusion. Circulation *54*:500, 1976.
355. Houppe, J. P., Villemot, J. P., Houppe-Nousse, M. P., Neimann, J. L., and Mathieu, P.: Compressive pericardial effusion after heart surgery in the adult. Contribution of bidimensional echocardiographic findings. Presse Med. *14*:1591, 1985.
356. Haaz, W. S., Mintz, G. S., Kotler, M. N., Parry, W., and Segal, B. L.: Two-dimensional echocardiographic recognition of the descending thoracic aorta: Value in differentiating pericardial from pleural effusions. Am. J. Cardiol. *46*:739, 1980.
357. Schiller, N. B., and Botvinick, E. H.: Right ventricular compression as a sign of cardiac tamponade. An analysis of echocardiographic ventricular dimensions and their clinical implications. Circulation *56*:774, 1977.
358. Armstrong, W. F., Schilt, B. F., Helper, D. J., Dillon, J. C., and Feigenbaum, H.: Diastolic collapse of the right ventricle with cardiac tamponade: An echocardiographic study. Circulation *65*:1491, 1982.
359. Singh, S., Wann, L. S., Klopfenstein, H. S., Hartz, A., and Brooks, H. L.: Usefulness of right ventricular diastolic collapse in diagnosing cardiac tamponade and comparison to pulsus paradoxus. Am. J. Cardiol. *57*:652, 1986.
360. Gillam, L. D., Guyer, D. E., Gibson, T. C., King, M. E., Marshall, J. E., and Weyman, A. E.: Hydrodynamic compression of the right atrium: A new echocardiographic sign of cardiac tamponade. Circulation *68*:294, 1983.
361. Lewis, B. S.: Real time two-dimensional echocardiography in constrictive pericarditis. Am. J. Cardiol. *49*:1789, 1982.
362. Engel, P. J., Fowler, N. O., Tei, C., Shah, P. M., Driedger, H. J., Shabetai, R., Harbin, A. D., and Franch, R. H.: M-mode echocardiography in constrictive pericarditis. J. Am. Coll. Cardiol. *6*:471, 1985.
363. Schnittger, I., Bowden, R. E., Abrams, J., and Popp, R. L.: Echocardiography: Pericardial thickening and constrictive pericarditis. Am. J. Cardiol. *42*:388, 1978.
364. Voelkel, A. G., Pietro, D. A., Folland, E. D., Fisher, M. C., and Parisi, A. F.: Echocardiographic features of constrictive pericarditis. Circulation *58*:871, 1978.
365. Ruys, F., Paulus, W., Stevens, C., and Brutsaert, D.: Expansion of the left atrial appendage is a distinctive cross-sectional echocardiographic feature of congenital defect of the pericardium. Eur. Heart J. *4*:738, 1983.
366. Kansal, S., Roitman, D., and Sheffield, L. T.: Two-dimensional echocardiography of congenital absence of pericardium. Am. Heart J. *109*:912, 1985.
367. Charuzi, Y., Bolger, A., Beeder, C., and Lew, A. S.: A new echocardiographic classification of left atrial myxoma. Am. J. Cardiol. *55*:614, 1985.
368. Markel, M. L., Armstrong, W. F., Waller, B. F., and Mahomed, Y.: Left atrial myxoma with multicentric recurrence and evidence of metastases. Am. Heart J. *111*:409, 1986.
369. Wolfe, S. B., Popp, R. L., and Feigenbaum, H.: Diagnosis of atrial tumors by ultrasound. Circulation *39*:615, 1969.

CARDIAC TUMORS

370. Perry, L. S., King, J. F., Zeft, H. J., Manley, J. C., Gross, C. M., and Wann, L. S.: Two-dimensional echocardiography in the diagnosis of left atrial myxoma. Br. Heart J. *45*:667, 1981.
371. Tway, K. P., Shah, A. A., and Rahimtoola, S. H.: Multiple bilateral myxomas demonstrated by two-dimensional echocardiography. Am. J. Med. *71*:896, 1981.
372. Schweizer, P., Bardos, P., Erbel, R., Meyer, J., Merx, W., Messmer, B. J., and Effert, S.: Detection of left atrial thrombi by echocardiography. Br. Heart J. *45*:148, 1981.
373. Hsu, T. L., Chen, C. C., Chen, C. Y., Hsiung, M. C., and Chiang, B. N.: Two-dimensional echocardiographic features of floating left atrial thrombus. Am. J. Cardiol. *57*:701, 1986.

374. Aschenberg, W., Schluter, M., Kremer, P., Schroder, E., Siglow, V., and Bleifeld, W.: Transesophageal two-dimensional echocardiography for the detection of left atrial appendage thrombus. J. Am. Coll. Cardiol. 7:163, 1986.
375. Come, P. C., Riley, M. F., Markis, J. E., and Malagold, M.: Limitations of echocardiographic techniques in evaluation of left atrial masses. Am. J. Cardiol. *48*:947, 1981.
376. Riggs, T., Paul, M. H., DeLeon, S., and Ilbawi, M.: Two-dimensional echocardiography in evaluation of right atrial masses: Five cases in pediatric patients. Am. J. Cardiol. *48*:961, 1981.
377. Gustafson, A. G., Edler, I. G., and Dahlback, O. K.: Bilateral atrial myxomas diagnosed by echocardiography. Acta Med. Scand. *201*:391, 1977.
378. Cameron, J., Pohlner, P. G., Stafford, E. G., O'Brien, M. F., Bett, J. H. N., and Murphy, A. L.: Right heart thrombus: Recognition and management. J. Am. Coll. Cardiol. *5*:1239, 1985.
379. Sans, P., Provansal, D., Balansard, P., and Gerard, R.: Large right intracardiac thrombus cause of recurrent pulmonary embolism. Arch. Mal. Coeur. *78*:650, 1985.
380. Cloez, J. L., Neimann, J. L., Chivoret, G., Danchin, N., Bruntz, J. F., Godenir, J. P., and Faivre, G.: Echocardiographic rediscovery of an anatomical structure: The Chiari network. Apropos of 16 cases. Arch. Mal. Coeur. *76*:1284, 1983.
381. Limacher, M. C., Gutgesell, H. P., Vick, G. W., Cohen, M. H., and Huhta, J. H.: Echocardiographic anatomy of the eustachian valve. Am. J. Cardiol. *57*:363, 1986.
382. Keren, A., Billingham, M. E., and Popp, R. L.: Echocardiographic recognition and implications of ventricular hypertrophic trabeculations and aberrant bands. Circulation *70*:836, 1984.
383. Glover, M. U., Bloor, C., and Vieweg, W. V. R.: Anomalous left ventricular band diagnosed by two-dimensional echocardiography. Am. Heart J. *111*:805, 1986.
384. Casta, A., and Wolf, W. J.: Left ventricular bands (false tendons): Echocardiographic and angiocardiographic delineation in children. Am. Heart J. *111*:321, 1986.
385. Chazal, R. A., and Feigenbaum, H.: Two-dimensional echocardiographic identification of epicardial pacemaker wire perforation. Am. Heart J. *107*:165, 1984.
386. Meller, J., Teichholz, L. E., Pichard, A. O., Matta, R., Litwak, R., Herman, M. V., and Massie, K. F.: Left ventricular myxoma. Echocardiographic diagnosis and review of the literature. Am. J. Med. *63*:816, 1977.
387. Roelandt, J., Bletter, W. B., Leuftink, E. W., vanDorp, W. G., tenCate, F., and Nauta, J.: Ultrasonic demonstration of right ventricular myxoma. J. Clin. Ultrasound *5*:191, 1977.
388. Levisman, J. A., MacAlpin, R. N., Abbasi, A. S., Ellis, N., and Eber, L. M.: Echocardiographic diagnosis of a mobile, predunculated tumor in the left ventricular cavity. Am. J. Cardiol. *36*:957, 1975.
389. Nanda, N. C., Barold, S. S., Gramiak, R., Ong, L. S., and Heinle, R. A.: Echocardiographic features of right ventricular outflow tumor prolapsing into the pulmonary artery. Am. J. Cardiol. *40*:272, 1977.
390. Grantham, N.: Echocardiographic, angiocardiographic, and surgical correlations in right ventricular myxoma simulating valvar pulmonic stenosis. Circulation *55*:619, 1977.
391. Bass, J. L., Breningstall, G. N., and Swaiman, K. F.: Echocardiographic incidence of cardiac rhabdomyoma in tuberous sclerosis. Am. J. Cardiol. *55*:1379, 1985.
392. Yabek, S. M., Isabel-Jones, J., Gyepes, M. T., and Jarmakani, J. M.: Cardiac fibroma in a neonate present with severe congestive heart failure. J. Pediatr. *91*:310, 1977.
393. Ports, T. A., Schiller, N. B., and Strunk, B. L.: Echocardiography of right ventricular tumors. Circulation *56*:439, 1977.
394. Topol, E. J., Biern, R. O., and Reitz, B. A.: Cardiac papillary fibroelastoma and stroke. Am. J. Med. *80*:129, 1986.
395. Fowles, R. E., Miller, D. C., Egbert, B. M., Fitzgerlad, J. W., and Popp, R. L.: Systemic embolization from mitral valve papillary endocardial fibroma detected by two-dimensional echocardiography. Am. Heart J. *102*:128, 1981.
396. Hajar, R., Roberts, W. C., and Folger, G. M.: Embryonal botryoid rhabdomyosarcoma of the mitral valve. Am. J. Cardiol. *57*:376, 1986.
397. Grosse, P., Herpin, D., Roudaut, R., Malergue, M.-C, Longy, M., Baudet, E., and Dallocchio, M.: Myxoma of the mitral valve diagnosed by echocardiography. Am. Heart J. *111*:803, 1986.
398. Weg, I. L., Mehra, S., Azueta, V., and Rosner, F.: Cardiac metastasis from adenocarcinoma of the lung. Am. J. Med. *80*:108, 1986.
399. Canedo, M. I., Otken, L., and Stefadouros, M. A.: Echocardiographic features of cardiac compression by a thymoma simulating cardiac tamponade and obstruction of the superior vena cava. Br. Heart J. *39*:1038, 1977.
400 Cueto-Garcia, L., Shub, C., Sheps, S. G., and Puga, F. J.: Two-dimensional echocardiographic detection of mediastinal pheochromocytoma. Chest *87*:834, 1985.
401. Farooki, Z. Q., Adelman, S., and Green, E. W.: Echocardiographic differentiation of a cystic and solid tumor of the heart. Am. J. Cardiol. *39*:107, 1977
402. Kruger, S. R., Michaud, J., and Cannom, D. S.: Spontaneous resolution of a pericardial cyst. Am. Heart J. *109*:1390, 1985.

DISEASES OF THE AORTA

403. Come, P. C., Sacks, B., Vine, H., McArdle, C., Koretsky, S., and Weintraub, R.: Ultrasonic visualization of the posterior thoracic aorta in long axis: Diagnosis of a saccular mycotic aneurysm. Chest *79*:470, 1981.
404. Goldberg, B. B.: Aortosonography. Int. Surg. *62*:294, 1977.
405. Lababidi, Z., and Monzon, C.: Early cardiac manifestations of Marfan's syndrome in the newborn. Am. Heart J. *102*:943, 1981.
406. Victor, M. F., Mintz, G. S., Kotler, M. N., Wilson, A. R., and Segal, B. L.: Two dimensional echocardiographic diagnosis of aortic dissection. Am. J. Cardiol. *48*:1155, 1981.
407. Diehl, J. T., Kaiser, L. R., Howard, R. J., and Salerno, T. A.: Two-dimensional echocardiography for diagnostic acute ascending aortic dissection. Can. J. Surg. *28*:345, 1985.
408. Granato, J. E., Dee, P., and Gibson, R. S.: Utility of two-dimensional echocardiography in suspected ascending aortic dissection. Am. J. Cardiol. *56*:123, 1985
409. D'Cruz, I. A., Jain, M., Campbell, C., and Goldberg, A. N.: Ultrasound visualization of aortic dissection by right parasternal scanning, including systolic flutter of the intimal flap. Chest *80*:239, 1981.
410. Mohri, M., Nagata, Y., Hisano, R., Koyanagi, S., Hirata, T., and Nakamura, M.: Detection of different blood flow patterns in the true and false lumen with aortic root dissection by pulsed Doppler echocardiography. Clin. Cardiol. *8*:225, 1985.
411. Dagli, S. V., Nanda, N. C., Roitman, D., Moos, S., Hsiung, M. C., Nath, P. H., and Soto, B.: Evaluation of aortic dissection by Doppler color flow mapping. Am. J. Cardiol. *56*:497, 1985.
412. Lewis, B. S.: Echocardiographic diagnosis of unruptured sinus of Valsalva aneurysm. Am. Heart J. *107*:1025, 1984.
413. Kiefaber, R. W., Tabakin, B. S., Coffin, L. H., and Gibson, T. C.: Unruptured sinus of Valsalva aneurysm with right ventricular outflow obstruction diagnosed by two-dimensional and Doppler echocardiography. J. Am. Coll. Cardiol. *7*:438, 1986.
414. Hands, M. E., Lloyd, B. L., and Hung, J.: Cross-sectional echocardiographic diagnosis of unruptured right sinus of Valsalva aneurysm dissecting into the interventricular septum. Int. J. Cardiol. *9*:380, 1985.
415. Chen, W. W. C., and Tai, Y. T.: Dissection of interventricular septum by aneurysm of sinus of Valsalva. Br. Heart J. *50*:293, 1983.
416. Terdjman, N., Bourdarias, J. P., Farcot, J. C., Gueret, P., Dubourg, O., Ferrier, A., and Hanania, G.: Aneurysms of sinus of Valsalva: Two dimensional echocardiographic diagnosis and recognition of rupture into the right heart cavities. J. Am. Coll. Cardiol. *3*:1227, 1984.

6 RADIOLOGICAL AND ANGIOGRAPHIC EXAMINATION OF THE HEART

by MURRAY G. BARON, M.D.

The radiological examination of the heart provides detailed information regarding cardiac structure and function that cannot be duplicated by any other diagnostic method. The appearance of the heart and lungs on ordinary chest roentgenograms often indicates the presence of heart disease and, at times, is diagnostic of a specific cardiac abnormality. Correct interpretation of the cardiac shadow in the frontal view is particularly important, because a chest roentgenogram in this projection is included as part of most routine medical examinations and provides a convenient survey method for the detection of otherwise unsuspected heart disease. In those patients with a known cardiac condition, the chest roentgenogram is of use in assessing its severity, in documenting the progress of the disease, in evaluating the presence and severity of secondary complications, and as an indicator of the efficacy of treatment. *Fluoroscopy* is of value in the detection of intracardiac and coronary arterial calcification and in the diagnosis of conditions such as pericardial effusion or atrial septal defect. Aside from such specific indications, fluoroscopy is of limited usefulness. Of all the imaging techniques, *angiocardiography* is the most comprehensive method for studying the intracardiac anatomy. Although it is an "invasive procedure" in that it is usually carried out in conjunction with cardiac catheterization (Chap. 9) (digital radiographic examinations can be carried out with intravenous injection of contrast medium [p. 356]), the risk to the patient is usually minimal, while the anatomical and hemodynamic information derived from angiocardiograms is often essential for establishing a correct diagnosis and planning a logical therapeutic approach. A special form of angiography, that of the coronary arteries (i.e., coronary arteriography), is considered in Chapter 10.

THE HEART ON THE CHEST ROENTGENOGRAM

The heart appears relatively homogeneous on a chest film because the myocardium, valves, and other cardiac structures have essentially the same radiodensity as blood, and their shadows blend imperceptibly with one another. Intracardiac lesions cannot be visualized unless they are calcified. The contours of the cardiac silhouette are clearly outlined because they contrast with the adjacent radiolucent air-containing lungs. Only those chambers and vessels that form a border on any particular view can be evaluated. However, the heart is a three-dimensional structure, and therefore multiple views are required in order to bring each of the chambers and great vessels into profile. Even then, the posterior border of the heart cannot be clearly identified unless the esophagus is filled with radiopaque material. A complete plain film study of the heart comprises four views of the chest: frontal, lateral, 60-degree right anterior oblique, and 45-degree left anterior oblique. On the first three views the patient swallows barium in order to opacify the esophagus.

Except in the more severe congenital anomalies, such as the transposition complexes or hypoplasia of the left ventricle, the chambers of the heart and great vessels always occupy the same relative position within the cardiac silhouette. *Dilatation* of each structure affects the contours of the heart in a fairly characteristic manner that is similar from case to case. However, this is not true with concentric cardiac *hypertrophy*. As the ventricular wall thickens, it tends to encroach on the cavity and may not increase the outer diameter of the chamber. Considerable myocardial hypertrophy can be present without causing a significant change in the shape of the cardiac silhouette. Even when the hypertrophy does result in cardiac enlargement, the appearance of the heart is often nonspecific.

FRONTAL VIEW (Fig. 6–1)

In this view, the upper half of the right cardiac border is formed by the superior vena cava and the lower half by the right atrium. The caval portion is relatively straight,

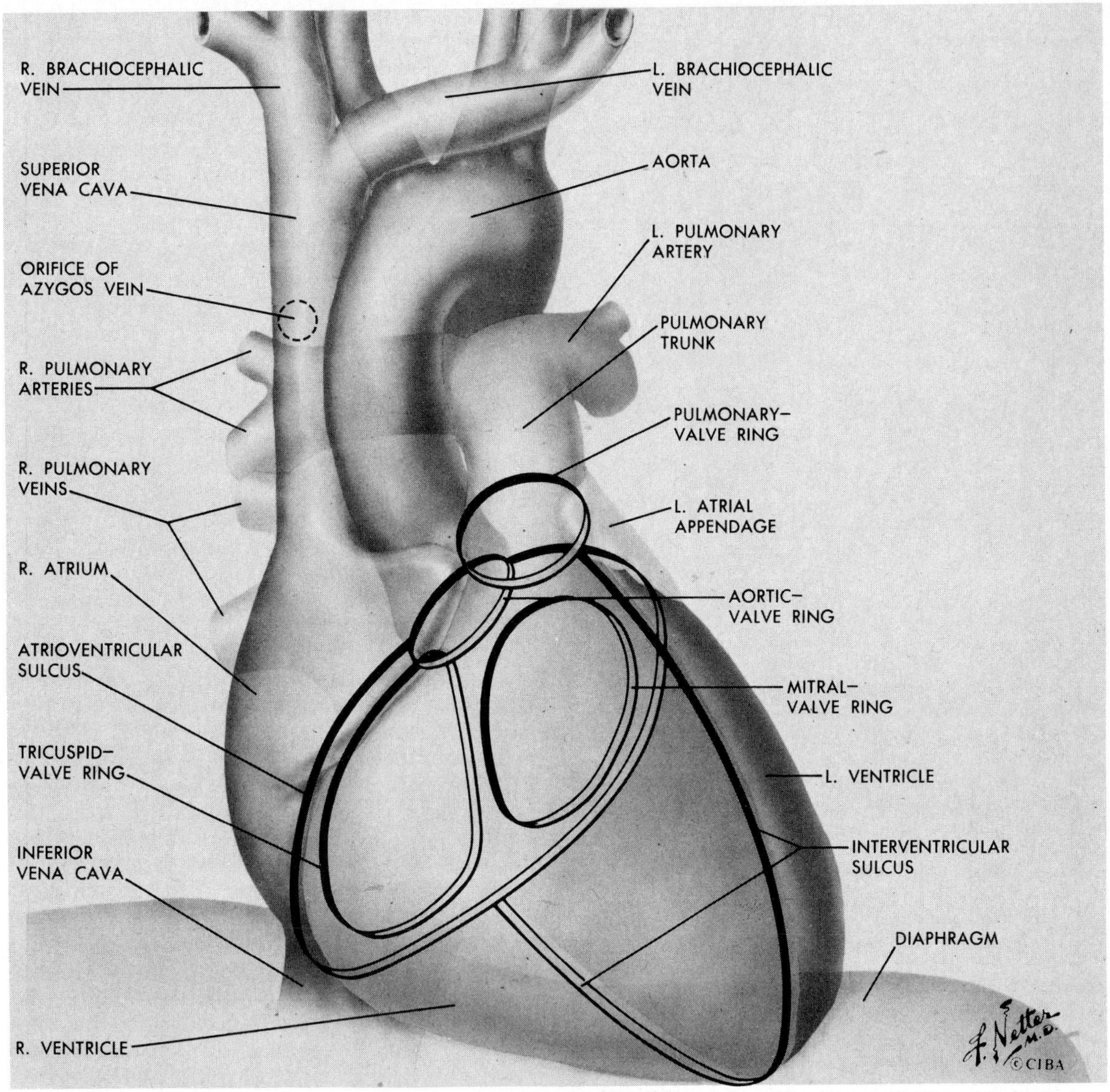

FIGURE 6–1. Frontal projection of the heart. (Reproduced with permission from The CIBA Collection of Medical Illustrations by Frank H. Netter, M.D. Vol. 5, The Heart, edited by F. Y. Yonkman. Copyright 1969, CIBA Pharmaceutical Co., Division of CIBA-GEIGY Corp. All rights reserved.)

while the lateral margin of the atrium forms a gentle, convex curve that extends to the diaphragm. The junction of the two structures is usually indicated by a shallow angle, where their contours meet. If the patient can take a sufficiently deep inspiration, a small portion of the inferior vena cava may become visible as a triangular shadow between the diaphragm and the border of the right atrium.

The left cardiac border is composed of three distinct curvatures: The uppermost bulge is formed by the aortic knob, below which is the curve of the main pulmonary artery and sometimes a portion of the left pulmonary artery; most of the remainder of the left cardiac contour represents the anterolateral margin of the left ventricle. The left atrial appendage reaches the left border of the heart and is seen in profile as a short, straight segment between the pulmonary artery and the left ventricle. If the atrium is not enlarged, this segment cannot be delimited on plain films; however, it is identifiable fluoroscopically, because its pulsations are not in phase with those of the ventricle.

THE ATRIA. Enlargement of the *right atrium* causes broadening of the cardiac silhouette to the right, with accentuation of the curvature of the atrial contour (Fig. 6–2). Normally, the *right ventricle* does not form a border in the frontal projection and cannot be viewed directly. As the ventricle dilates, it tends to push the left ventricle laterally and posteriorly, causing widening of the cardiac shadow to the left. Especially with congenital lesions, such as tetralogy of Fallot, the enlarged right ventricle may extend beyond the left ventricle and form the left cardiac border. The cardiac apex is then elevated and rounded (see Fig. 6–37, p. 162). As the *left atrium* increases in size, its appendage bulges from the left cardiac contour, the border of the atrium may form a second contour within the right part of the cardiac shadow, and the left bronchus may be displaced upward. The last two signs, although accurate, are relatively insensitive and are not present unless there is considerable dilatation of the atrium. Even then, they may be absent.

When the left atrium enlarges, it tends to project backward beyond the remainder of the heart. This localized increase in the thickness of the heart causes the central portion of the cardiac silhouette to be abnormally dense. The increased density ends suddenly at the margins of the left atrium, and its right border can be visualized as a

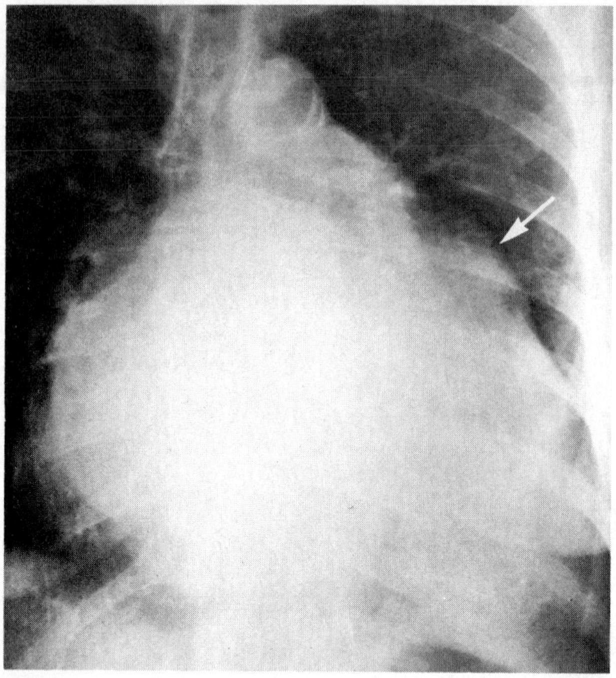

FIGURE 6–2. Enlargement of the atria, frontal view. The enlargement of the right portion of the cardiac silhouette and the increased curvature of its border are caused by dilatation of the right atrium. The left atrial appendage is dilated and forms a localized bulge (arrow) on the left cardiac border. The double contour on the right side, the increased density of the central portion of the heart, and the elevation of the left main bronchus are all signs of left atrial enlargement. The widening of the heart to the left indicates ventricular enlargement, in this case involving both ventricles. The patient had severe mitral valve disease with pulmonary hypertension and tricuspid regurgitation.

distinct contour through the cardiac silhouette (Fig. 6–2). However, if the atrium distends from side to side more than posteriorly, so that it does not form a localized bulge, its shadow blends in with the rest of the heart, and its borders may not be visualized. Furthermore, when the right atrium enlarges, it may also extend posteriorly, alongside the left atrium, obliterating the latter's right border. A double contour, even when present, is often difficult to visualize on standard films. Because the roentgen technique used for chest films is adjusted so that the exposure provides an optimal picture of the lungs, an enlarged heart is usually underpenetrated. The dense cardiac shadow then obscures the contour of the left atrium, although it may be quite obvious on an overexposed film or one made with a Bucky grid.

Occasionally, the confluence of the *right pulmonary veins* is visible through the right portion of the cardiac silhouette and can resemble the double density caused by left atrial enlargement. However, the lateral border of the venous shadow is relatively straight and not convex as is the contour of an enlarged left atrium. In addition, when the left atrium is enlarged, the entire central portion of the cardiac silhouette is abnormally dense. A giant left atrium can extend beyond the right atrium and form part, or all, of the right cardiac border, in which case the margin of the right atrium is seen within the cardiac silhouette. *Elevation of the left main bronchus* has some drawbacks as a sign of left atrial enlargement. Often, the bronchus is hidden by the hilar and mediastinal shadows. When the bronchus can be identified, it is difficult to be certain whether its course is normal or not if the displacement is not marked. Displacement of the bronchus must be interpreted with caution if the film was not made during full inspiration or if the patient was supine rather than erect. In both situations, the carinal angle is widened and the left bronchus elevated.

Abnormal *prominence of the left atrial appendage* is the most sensitive sign of left atrial enlargement in the frontal view. The appendage dilates along with the body of the atrium, and its segment on the left heart border, which is normally flat, becomes convex. As the appendage becomes larger, it forms a well-defined bulge immediately beneath the pulmonary artery segment. An aneurysm of the anterolateral wall of the left ventricle can cause a similar bulge but at a lower level on the cardiac contour, some distance below the pulmonary artery (Fig. 6–3).

THE LEFT VENTRICLE. The shape of an enlarged *left ventricle* depends, to some extent, on the underlying cause. When the dilatation results from a diastolic overload, particularly in aortic regurgitation, the chamber enlarges mainly along its long axis. The cardiac apex is displaced downward and to the left (Fig. 6–4*A*). Although this axis of the ventricle is elongated when the dilatation is due to myocardial disease, the width of the chamber is also significantly increased, so that the dilated ventricle assumes a more globular shape (Fig. 6–4*B*).

As the left ventricle enlarges, it becomes more difficult to evaluate the size of the left atrium on the frontal film. Widening of the cardiac silhouette to the left tends to minimize, or even mask, the prominence of a dilated left atrial appendage (see Figs. 6–8 and 6–11). In order to judge the size of the two chambers properly, it is usually necessary to obtain other views of the heart, particularly the left oblique projection (see Fig. 6–14*B*). When both the left atrium and the left ventricle are enlarged, the relative degrees of dilatation of the chambers have diagnostic importance. Left atrial enlargement does not necessarily indicate disease of the mitral valve but can occur in response to elevation of the left ventricular end-diastolic pressure. In the latter case, the degree of enlargement of the left atrium will be less than that of the left ventricle, while the opposite is usually true when the chambers are dilated because of mitral valve disease.

CARDIAC VALVES. The frontal view is of limited usefulness for the detection of *valve calcification.* The aortic valve is projected over the left border of the spine, and calcific deposits on the valve cusps are usually obscured by the vertebral bodies. The mitral valve lies below and to the left of the aortic valve within the densest portion of the cardiac shadow, and only relatively coarse calcific deposits can be visualized. Valve calcifications are easier to recognize by means of fluoroscopy. As the heart beats, the mitral valve describes a shallow, elliptical trajectory, with its long axis oriented to the left and slightly downward, while the aortic valve moves in a vertical direction.

LATERAL AND OBLIQUE VIEWS

(Fig. 6–5)

LATERAL VIEW. The anterior border of the cardiac shadow is formed by the body and the outflow tract of the right ventricle, the supravalvular portion of the main pulmonary artery, and the aorta. The normal ventricle abuts the lower third of the sternum. Because lung is interposed between the sternum and the cardiac structures, the upper retrosternal space is radiolucent. As the right ventricle dilates, its outflow portion extends anteriorly toward the sternum and encroaches on the retrosternal clear space. However, this is not always a reliable sign of right ventricular enlargement, because it depends upon the shape of the chest as well as upon the size of the

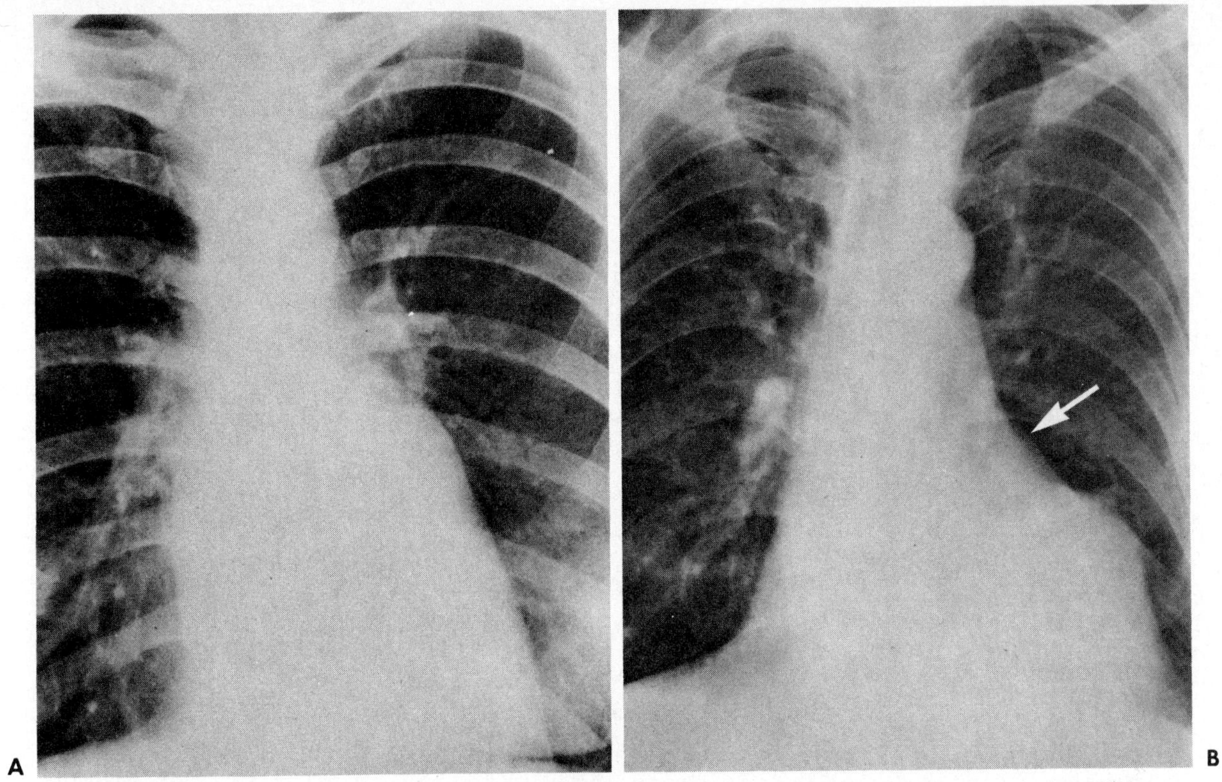

FIGURE 6–3. Dilatation of the left atrial appendage—differential diagnosis. *A*, Mitral stenosis. The only sign of left atrial enlargement is dilatation of its appendage, which forms a bulge on the left cardiac contour immediately beneath the pulmonary artery segment. *B*, Ventricular aneurysm. In this case, the bulge on the left cardiac contour is separated from the pulmonary artery segment. The intervening portion of the heart border is formed by the left atrial appendage (arrow) and the basal portion of the anterolateral left ventricular wall.

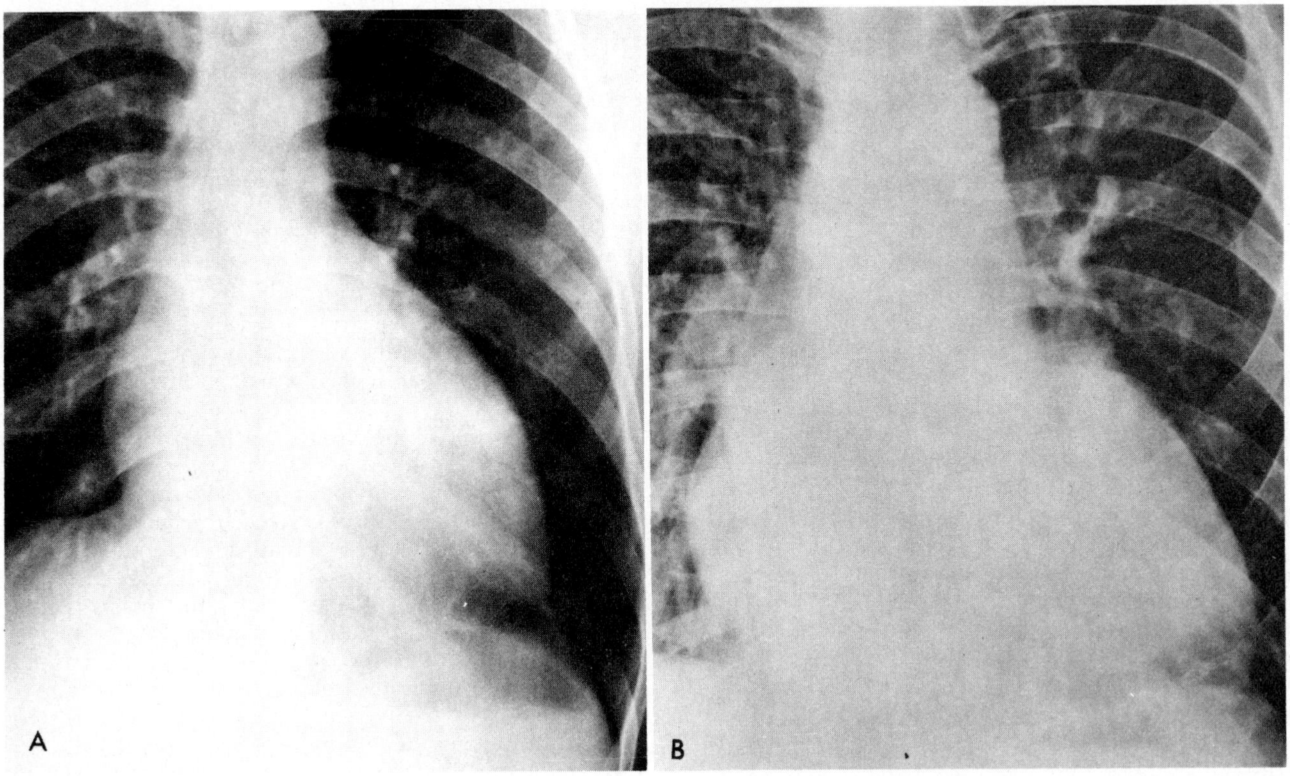

FIGURE 6–4. Enlargement of the left ventricle, frontal view. *A*, Aortic regurgitation. Enlargement of the left ventricle has occurred mainly along its long axis, so that the cardiac apex is displaced downward and to the left. This shape of the cardiac silhouette is characteristic of the type of ventricular dilatation associated with regurgitation of the aortic valve. (From Donoso, E., and Gorlin, R. [eds.]: Current Cardiovascular Topics. Vol. 3, Angina Pectoris. New York, Stratton Intercontinental Medical Book Co., 1977.) *B*, Ischemic heart disease with significant impairment of myocardial function. The long and short axes of the ventricle are more or less evenly elongated, causing the chamber to have a globular shape.

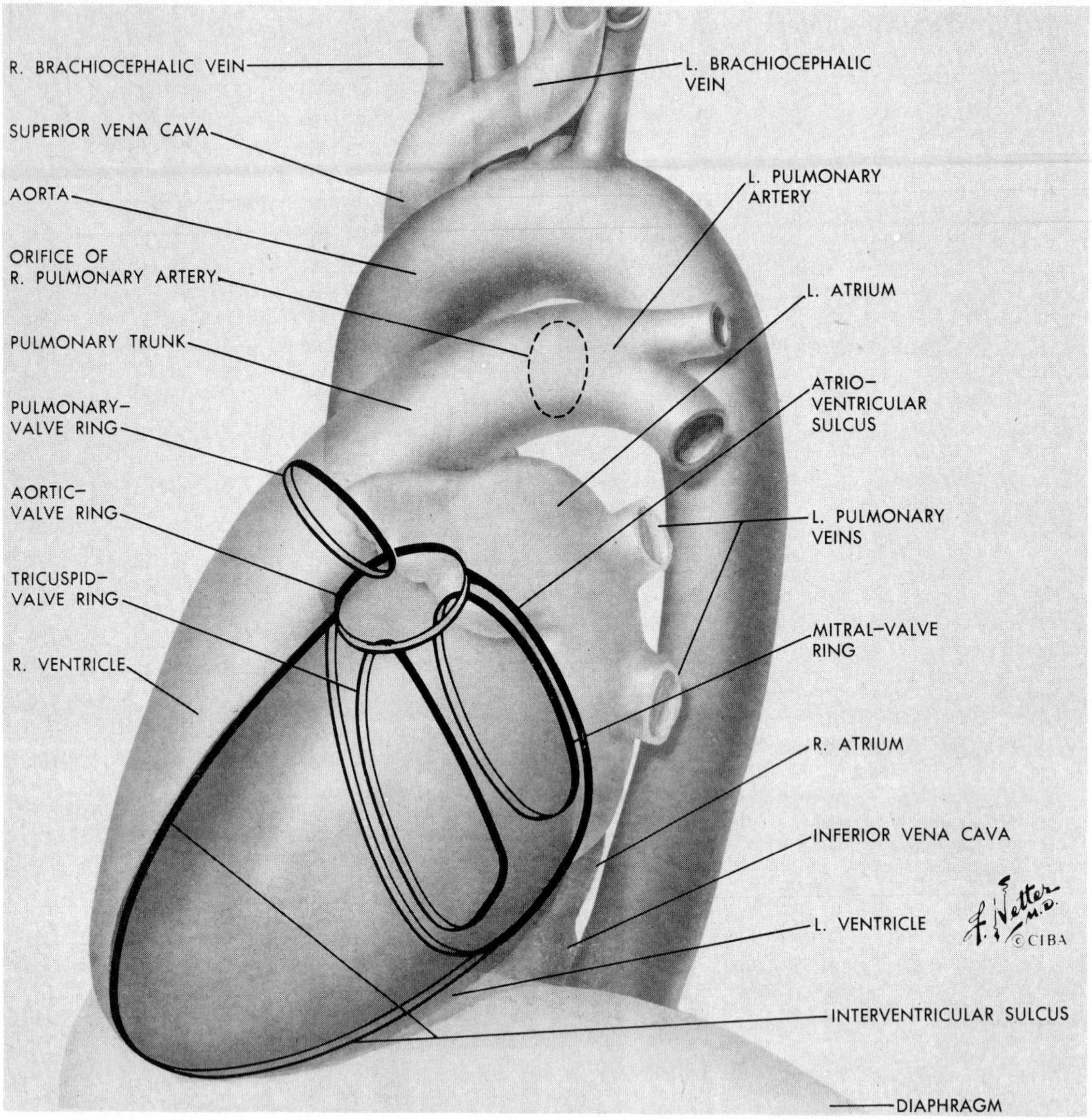

FIGURE 6–5. Lateral projection of the heart. (Reproduced with permission from The CIBA Collection of Medical illustrations by Frank H. Netter, M.D. Vol. 5, The Heart, edited by F. Y. Yonkman. Copyright 1969, CIBA Pharmaceutical Co., Division of CIBA-GEIGY Corp. All rights reserved.)

heart. In a patient with a narrow chest, as in the "straight back" syndrome, the retrosternal space is often obliterated by a normal-sized heart simply because there is no space for it in the thorax. Conversely, in a patient with pulmonary emphysema and a barrel-shaped chest, the heart can be considerably enlarged and still barely reach the sternum.

The posterior border of the heart is formed by the posterior aspect of the left atrium and the left ventricle. On a film made during deep inspiration, the supradiaphragmatic portion of the inferior vena cava and a small part of the right atrium may be uncovered. The ventricular border is usually clearly seen as it is outlined by adjacent air-containing lung. However, the left atrial component of the posterior cardiac border merges with the shadow of the mediastinum and is not well delineated. The esophagus lies directly behind the heart and, when filled with opaque material, can be used to evaluate left atrial size. The normal atrium, in the erect position, does not affect the esophagus, but as it enlarges, it indents the anterior wall of the esophagus and displaces it posteriorly (Fig. 6–6*A*). The indentation caused by an enlarged atrium begins immediately below the carina and involves the midportion of the esophagus. The lower esophagus lies below the atrium and is adjacent to the left ventricle. When only the atrium is enlarged, the supradiaphragmatic portion of the esophagus remains in its normal position and shows no indentation.

The portion of the esophagus immediately above the diaphragm may be indented by an enlarged left ventricle (Fig. 6–6*B*). More commonly, the dilated ventricle extends laterally as well as posteriorly and bypasses the esophagus (Fig. 6–7). When both the left atrium and the left ventricle are dilated, the esophagus is usually displaced posteriorly in one continuous sweep, beginning just below the carina and continuing down to the diaphragm (Fig. 6–8).

On occasion, the appearance of the esophagus in the lateral view can be misleading. If there are tertiary contractions of the esophagus or if it is not well distended with barium, no indentation or displacement will be seen even though the left atrium is of considerable size. Furthermore, because the esophagus is not fixed to the heart, it may slide medially as the heart enlarges and will not appear displaced when viewed from the side. On the other hand, the esophagus is loosely attached to the descending aorta and can be pulled backward when this vessel is tortuous, the displacement being almost identical to that

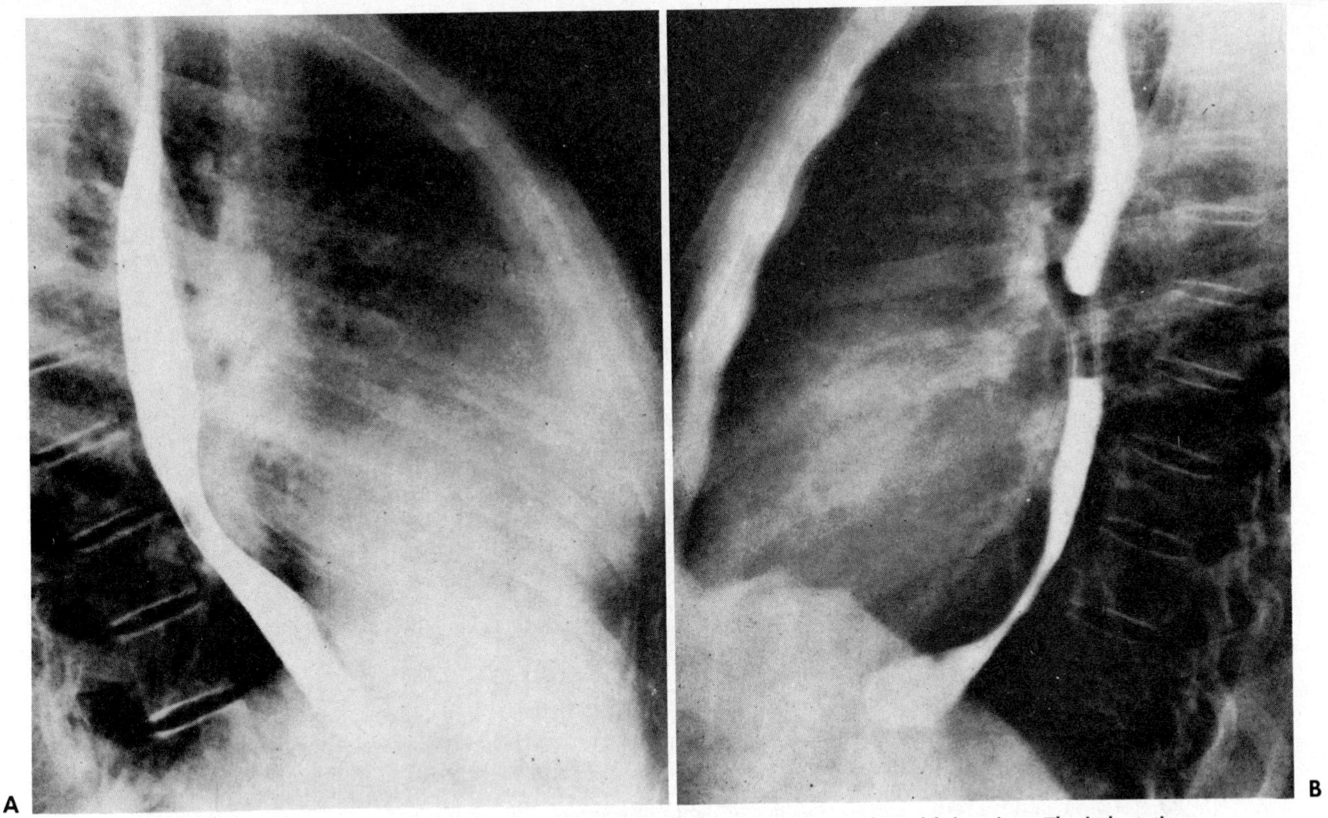

FIGURE 6–6. Indentation of the esophagus by the left cardiac chambers. *A*, Enlarged left atrium. The indentation on the anterior esophageal wall begins just below the level of the carina and involves only the midportion of the esophagus. The lower esophagus is in its normal position and shows no indentation. *B*, Enlarged left ventricle. The dilated ventricle extends posteriorly and impinges on the lowermost portion of the esophagus. The esophageal indentation continues to the diaphragm.

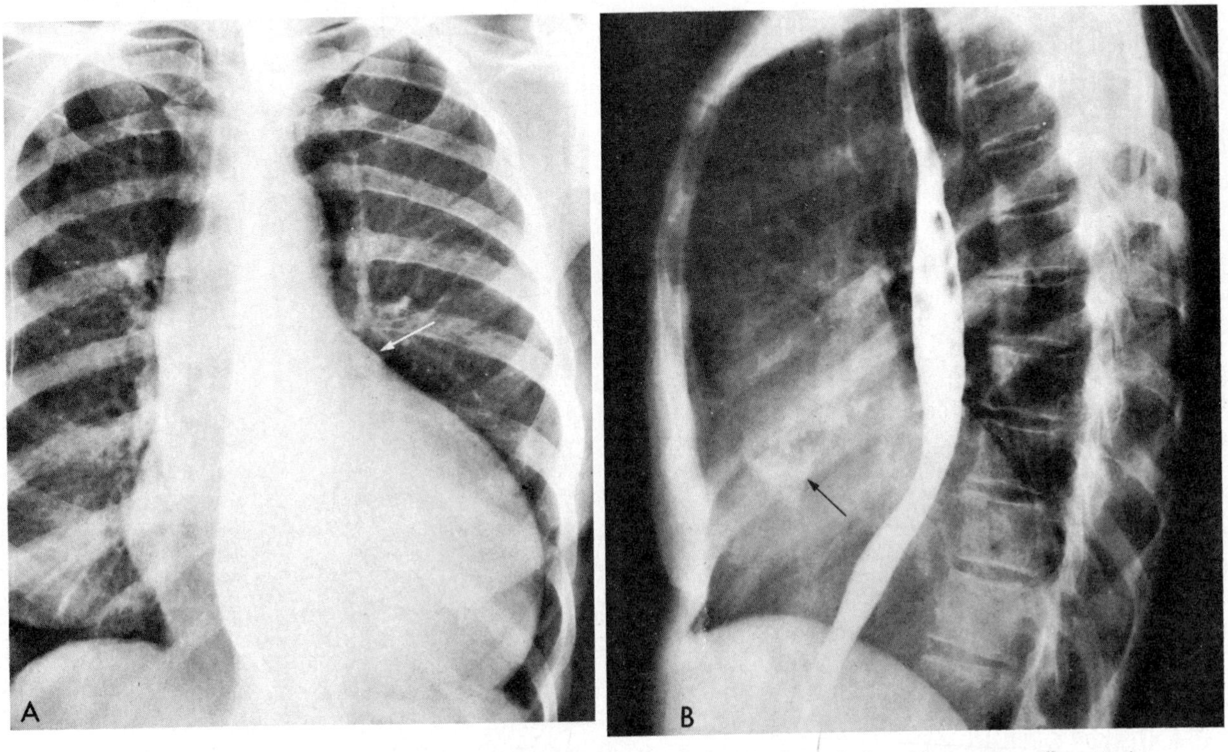

FIGURE 6–7. Dilatation of the left ventricle in aortic valve disease. *A*, Frontal view. The cardiac silhouette is elongated downward and to the left, indicating left ventricular enlargement. There is slight prominence of the left atrial appendage (arrow). The esophagus is displaced medially. *B*, Lateral view. The left ventricle is markedly enlarged and extends posterior to the esophagus. The aortic valve is densely calcified (arrow). The indentation on the anterior wall of the midesophagus is caused by the moderately dilated left atrium. There was no evidence of mitral valve disease.

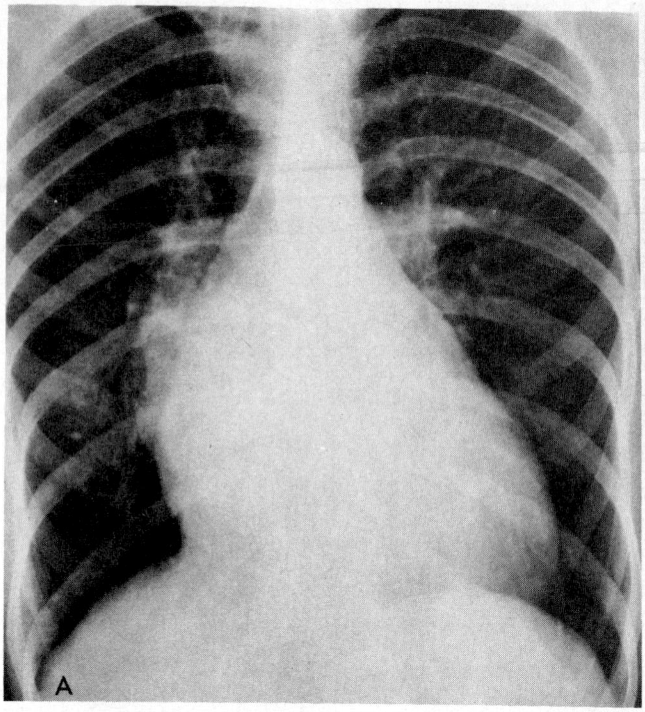

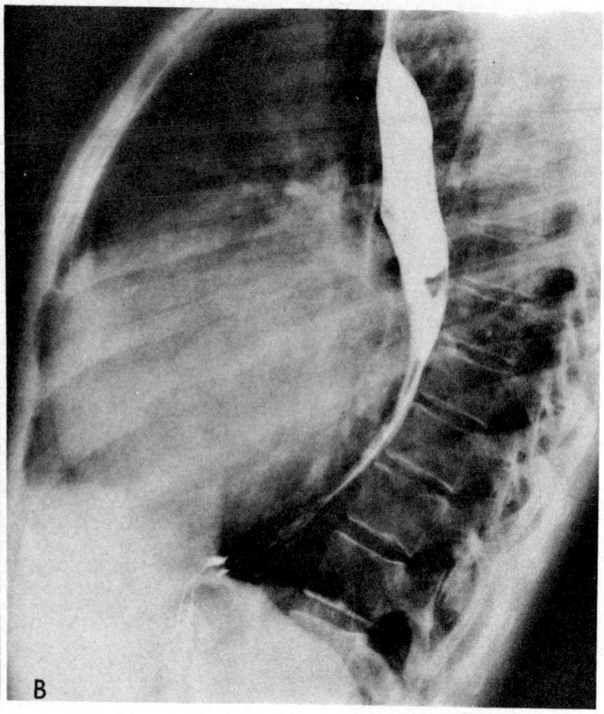

FIGURE 6–8. Enlargement of the left atrium and left ventricle. *A*, Frontal view. The abnormal density of the central portion of the cardiac silhouette and the double contour on the right side indicate enlargement of the left atrium. The bulge of the atrial appendage on the left cardiac border is less prominent than would be expected, considering the size of the atrium, because of the widening of the cardiac shadow. The displacement of the apex of the heart downward and to the left is caused by enlargement of the left ventricle. The increased size of the pulmonary vessels in the upper lungs and the narrowed vessels at the bases as well as the Kerley B lines in the costophrenic sulci reflect the presence of pulmonary venous hypertension. *B*, Lateral view. The esophagus is displaced backward in a continuous curve from the carina to the diaphragm. The posterior border of the heart crosses the shadow of the inferior vena cava almost at the level of the diaphragm, confirming the presence of left ventricular enlargement.

caused by an enlarged atrium. The correct cause of the displacement can be recognized because the curve of the esophagus exactly parallels that of the aorta.

The relationship between the shadow of the inferior vena cava and the posterior border of the heart in the lateral projection provides a fairly accurate indicator of left ventricular size. The cava can usually be identified as a curvilinear shadow that extends upward and forward from the right diaphragm (see Fig. 6–5). The lower part of the cardiac border is formed by the left ventricle and, as it curves forward, it crosses the posterior margin of the caval shadow about 2 cm above the left leaf of the diaphragm. As the left ventricle dilates, the apex of the chamber extends downward, and the point of intersection between the border of the ventricle and the cava moves closer to a diaphragm (Fig. 6–8).[1] However, the accuracy of this sign is considerably diminished if the patient is rotated slightly to either side and the film is not a true lateral projection.[2]

When valvular calcification is identified in the lateral view, fluoroscopy is usually not needed to determine whether the leaflets of the aortic valve or the mitral valve are involved. The two valves can be separated by a line drawn from the origin of the left main bronchus to the anterior costophrenic sulcus. (The bronchus can be recognized because it is projected on end and casts a round, lucent shadow at the lower end of the trachea.) The mitral valve almost always lies below this line, while the aortic valve lies more anteriorly, above the line (Figs. 6–7 and 6–9).[3]

RIGHT ANTERIOR OBLIQUE VIEW (Figs. 6–10 and 6–11). If the patient is properly positioned, the cardiac silhouette will be projected completely to the left of the shadow of the spine. The upper half of the right heart border is formed by the posterolateral wall of the left atrium and its lower half by the back of the right atrium. As in the lateral view, the left atrial contour cannot be satisfactorily delineated unless the esophagus is filled with barium. The ascending aorta forms the relatively straight, upper portion of the left cardiac contour. Beneath this segment, the

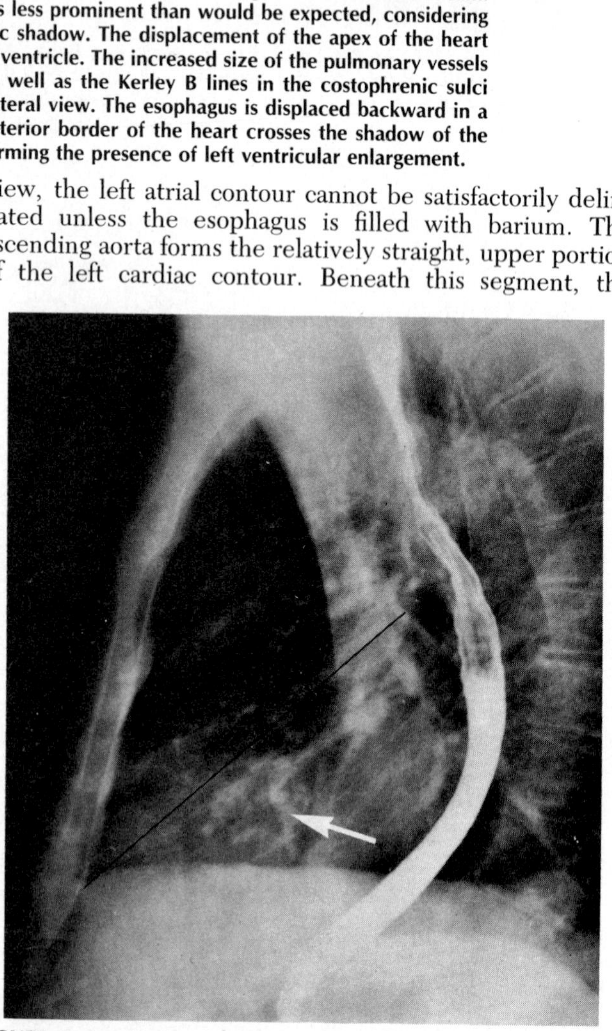

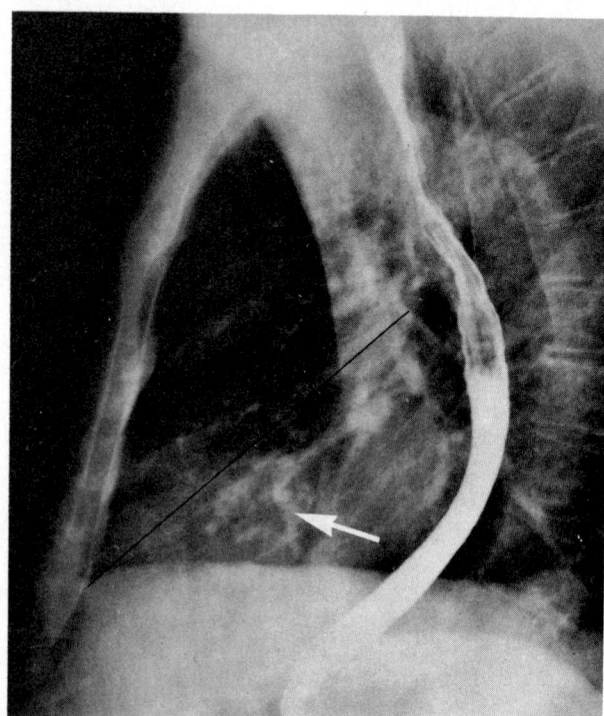

FIGURE 6–9. Mitral valve calcification, lateral view. The valvular calcification (arrow) lies below the line drawn from the left main bronchus to the anterior costophrenic sinus, localizing it to the mitral valve. The aortic valve, in this view, lies more anteriorly, above the line.

cardiac border slopes downward and to the left in a shallow curve formed by the margins of the outflow tract of the right ventricle and the main pulmonary artery. The inferior continuation of the curve represents the anterior border of the left ventricle.

The information provided by this view regarding left atrial size is essentially the same as that gained from the lateral projection. When the atrium is large, it indents or displaces the barium-filled esophagus. The lowermost portion of the esophagus will not be affected if the left ventricle is normal in size. When the ventricle is also enlarged, the esophagus is displaced backward in a continuous curve that extends from the carina to the diaphragm.

Dilatation of the outflow tract of the right ventricle and the main pulmonary artery produces a bulge on the left cardiac contour just beneath the straight aortic segment. This is a common finding when there is a sizable left-to-right shunt through an atrial or ventricular septal defect. In mitral valve disease, abnormal prominence of the right ventricular outflow tract usually signifies the presence of pulmonary hypertension (Fig. 6–10).

The right anterior oblique view is the best for detection of mitral valve calcification. The valve is seen within the midportion of the cardiac silhouette, free of the shadow of the spine (Fig. 6–10), and because it is projected tangentially, it exhibits its maximal range of motion between systole and diastole. The valve can be located fluoroscopically because it is aligned with the atrioventricular sulcus in this view. In adults, the sulcus usually contains an accumulation of fat and casts a lucent, vertical, linear shadow that moves from side to side with the heartbeat. If no calcific densities are identified in relation to the sulcus, one can assume that the mitral valve is free of significant calcification. The aortic valve is situated above and slightly to the right of the mitral valve and moves in a vertical direction.

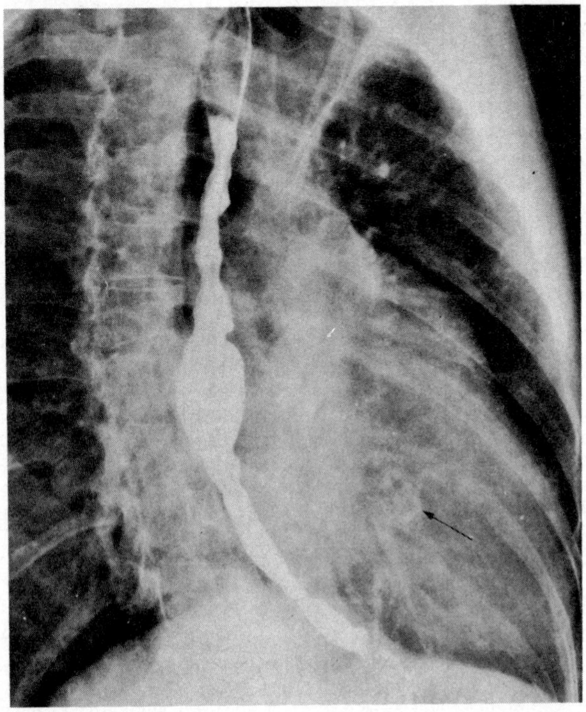

FIGURE 6–10. Mitral valve disease. Right anterior oblique view. The outflow tract of the right ventricle is dilated, indicating elevation of pulmonary artery pressure. The calcified mitral valve (arrow) is clearly visible within the midportion of the cardiac silhouette. The size of the left atrium cannot be evaluated because of esophageal spasm. There is prominence of the right ventricular outflow tract.

LEFT ANTERIOR OBLIQUE VIEW (Fig. 6–12). This is the only projection of the cardiac series in which the body of the left atrium can be visualized directly. The posterior atrial wall forms the upper third of the left cardiac contour, just beneath the left main bronchus. The lower two-thirds of this contour are formed by the left ventricle. The right border of the cardiac shadow represents mostly right atrium except for a short segment just above the diaphragm, where the right ventricle comes into profile. The arch of the aorta parallels the plane of the film in this view and is projected with a minimum of foreshortening. The origins of the great vessels are maximally separated. The atrioventricular valves are projected en face so that calcification of the mitral valve is more difficult to detect than in the right oblique view. The aortic valve is projected almost tangentially, and calcification of its cusps is easily seen.

Enlargement of the *right atrium* causes widening of the cardiac silhouette to the right and an increase in the curvature of the right cardiac contour (Fig. 6–13). In some instances, it may not be possible to separate the atrial and ventricular components of this border on plain films. This can be resolved by fluoroscopy, because the borders of the chambers move in opposite directions during the cardiac cycle.

Normally, the segment of the left cardiac contour formed by the left atrium is straight or slightly concave. As the chamber increases in size, this border becomes convex (Fig. 6–13) and encroaches on the "aortic window," the clear space beneath the aortic arch. Upward displacement of the left main bronchus is often better seen in this view than in the frontal projection. Because the barium-filled esophagus is often projected over the border of the heart, it may obscure the left atrial contour. The left anterior oblique view, therefore, should be obtained first when filming a cardiac series, before the patient is given barium to swallow.

When the left ventricle dilates, its long axis elongates in a posterior direction as well as downward and laterally. The ventricle is thus foreshortened in the frontal view, and its size can easily be underestimated. However, when the patient is in the left oblique position, the long axis of the ventricle is aligned parallel to the film. For this reason, this view is essential, in addition to the frontal view, for proper evaluation of left ventricular size (Fig. 6–14). Whether the ventricle is elongated (Fig. 6–15) is of considerably greater diagnostic significance than whether the cardiac silhouette is projected clear of the shadow of the spine or not. The latter sign depends to a large extent on the position of the patient.[4] The steeper the oblique angle, the more likely that the shadow of the ventricle—regardless of its size—will not overlap the spine. Even with a standard degree of obliquity, the ventricle that is elongated mainly to the left will tend to clear the spine, whereas the same size ventricle extending more posteriorly will not. In addition, this sign may be falsely positive if the right ventricle is significantly enlarged. An increase in the size of this chamber displaces the left ventricle to the left and posteriorly, and the heart may not clear the shadow of the spine in the left oblique view, even though the left ventricle is normal in size.

HEART SIZE

Although heart disease can be present without causing cardiomegaly, the converse is not true. Enlargement of the heart is indicative of cardiac disease and, at times, may

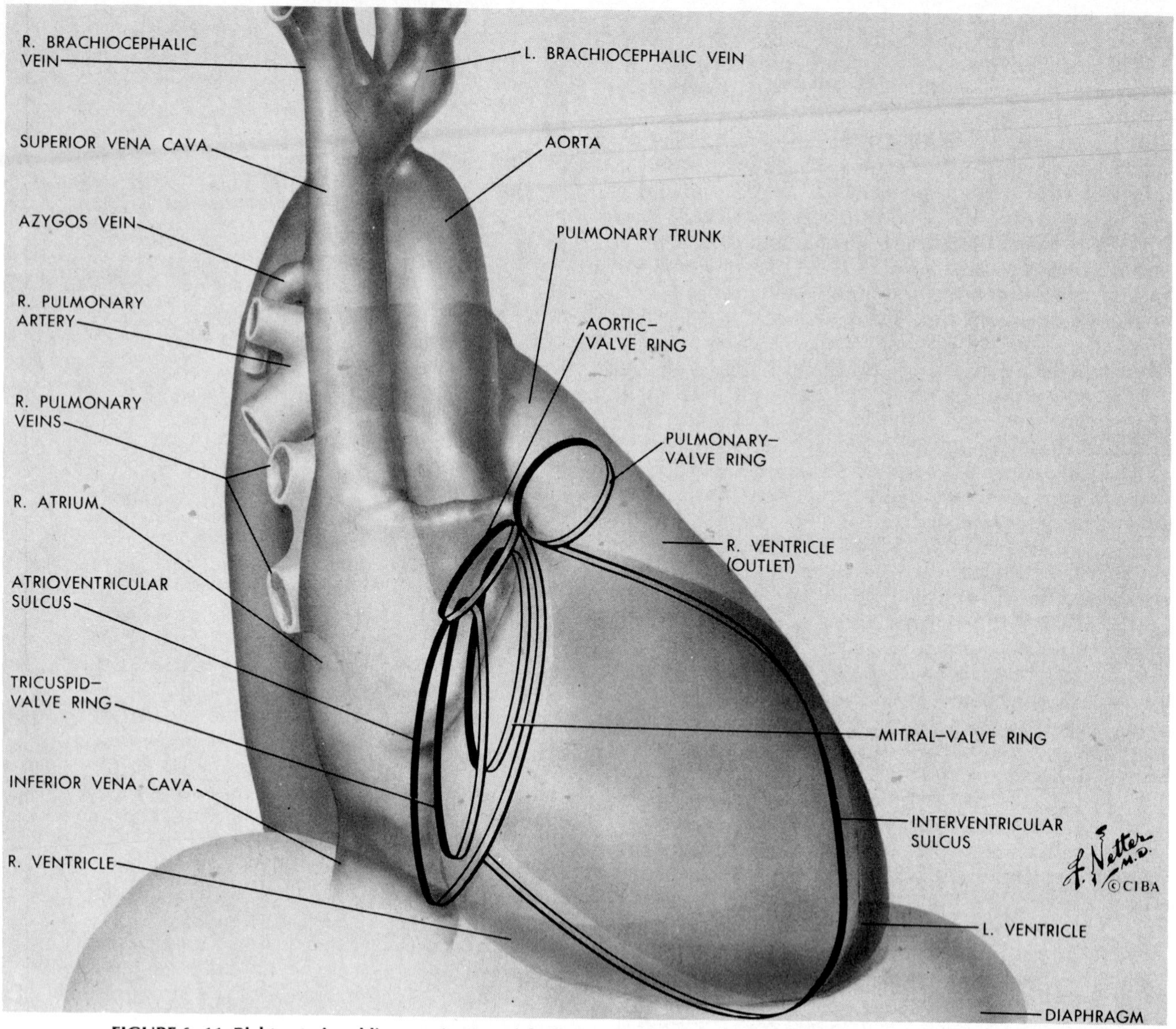

FIGURE 6–11. Right anterior oblique projection of the heart. (Reproduced with permission from The CIBA Collection of Medical Illustrations by Frank H. Netter, M.D. Vol. 5, The Heart, edited by F. Y. Yonkman. Copyright 1969, CIBA Pharmaceutical Co., Division of CIBA-GEIGY Corp. All rights reserved.)

be its first overt manifestation. When a patient is known to have heart disease, changes in cardiac size over a period of time can be used to evaluate the progress of the disease or the results of treatment.

Even though an experienced observer can estimate cardiac size with an acceptable degree of accuracy from the appearance of the cardiac silhouette, a more objective method of measurement is often desirable. A simple measurement of one or more diameters of the cardiac silhouette has little meaning, because normal heart size varies considerably with sex and body habitus. The *cardiothoracic ratio* was designed to compensate for these factors and uses the width of the chest as an indicator of body build. A vertical reference line is drawn on the frontal chest film through the spinous processes of the vertebrae. The sum of the maximum distances from this line to the right and to the left borders of the cardiac silhouette constitutes the transverse cardiac diameter (Fig. 6–16). This value is then divided by the greatest width of the thorax as measured from the inner margins of the ribs to give the cardiothoracic ratio. A value of 0.5 is generally considered to indicate the upper limit of normal heart size, but a figure of 0.6 is preferable, since it will decrease the number of false-positive results.[5, 6] Unfortunately, the maximum width of the chest is not a particularly accurate index of body build, and its use introduces a second variable that is independent of the presence or absence of cardiac disease. The transverse cardiac diameter alone is a better measure of heart size if it is compared with standard tables of cardiac diameters in adults of different height and weight.[7]

A more accurate determination of cardiac size can be achieved by calculating the relative cardiac volume.[8, 9] Three measurements are required: the long axis of the heart (L) is measured on the frontal film from the break in the right cardiac contour, where the superior vena cava joins the right atrium, to the cardiac apex; the short axis (S) is measured from the right cardiophrenic angle to the junction of the pulmonary artery and left atrial segments on the left heart border; the third dimension (D) represents the greatest anteroposterior diameter of the heart and is measured on the lateral chest film (Fig. 6–17). The final calculation is made from the formula

$$\frac{L \times S \times D \times K}{\text{Body surface area}} = \text{Relative cardiac volume}$$

K is a constant that is related to the distance between the x-ray tube and the film. For the usual 6-foot chest film, K equals 0.42. Figures for body surface area are obtained from the DuBois standards.[10]

A volume of less than 450 cc/m^2 for women and 500 cc/m^2 for men is considered to be normal. Values over 490 cc/m^2 for women and 540 cc/m^2 for men are definitely abnormal. Aside from the inherent mathematical accuracy of this method, it is of particular value because it is not significantly affected by the phase of the cardiac cycle. Even in patients with large stroke volumes and a considerable change in the

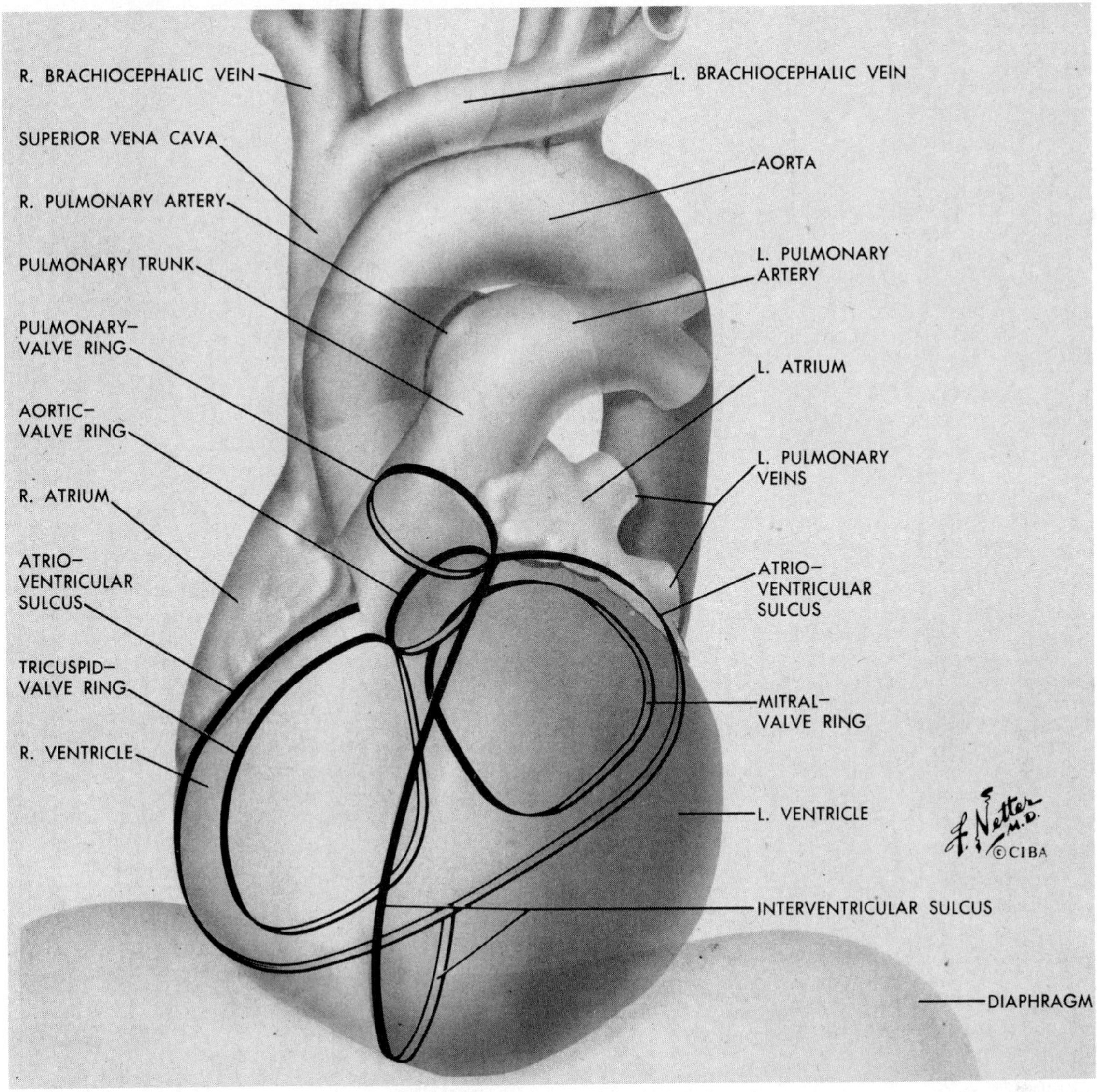

FIGURE 6–12. Left anterior oblique projection of the heart. (Reproduced with permission from The CIBA Collection of Medical Illustrations by Frank H. Netter, M.D. Vol. 5, The Heart, edited by F. Y. Yonkman. Copyright 1969, CIBA Pharmaceutical Co., Division of CIBA-GEIGY Corp. All rights reserved.)

apparent size of the heart between systole and diastole, the relative cardiac volume varies little because it is determined from the volumes of all four cardiac chambers. When the ventricles contract during systole, the atria become larger as they fill with blood, whereas in diastole the atria decrease in size and the ventricles distend. The measurement has definite prognostic significance in ischemic heart disease[11] but not in the presence of aortic regurgitation or mitral valve disease. The measurement will obviously be grossly incorrect if enlargement of the cardiac silhouette is due to a pericardial effusion.

In most instances, calculation of cardiac volume, or even measurement of the transverse cardiac diameter, is too time-consuming to be a routine procedure. A visual estimate of heart size from the frontal film is generally adequate for most clinical purposes. However, several possible pitfalls must be recognized if gross errors are to be avoided.

First, the degree of inspiration is the single factor with

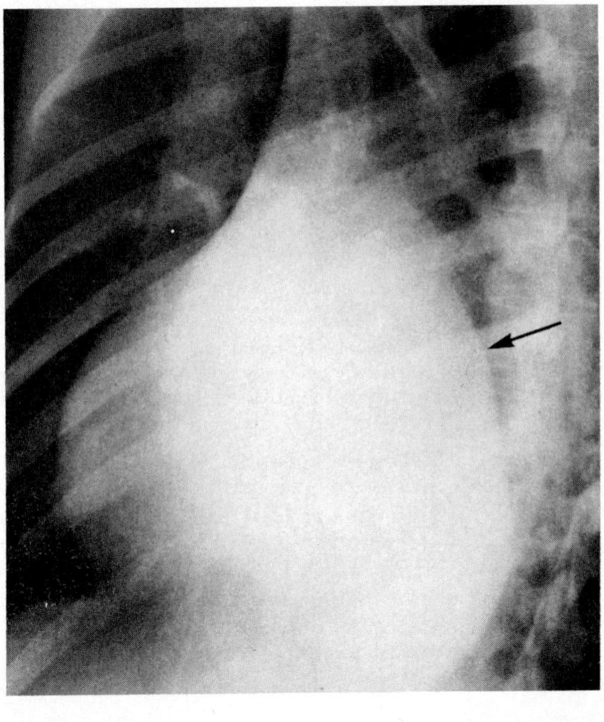

FIGURE 6–13. Left anterior oblique projection showing enlargement of both atria in mitral valve disease. The right side of the cardiac silhouette is enlarged and its curvature increased because of dilatation of the right atrium. The convexity of the upper left cardiac border (arrow) just beneath the left main bronchus indicates that the left atrium is also enlarged. (From Baron, M. G.: Left anterior oblique view for evaluation of left atrial size. Circulation *44*:926, 1971, by permission of the American Heart Association, Inc.)

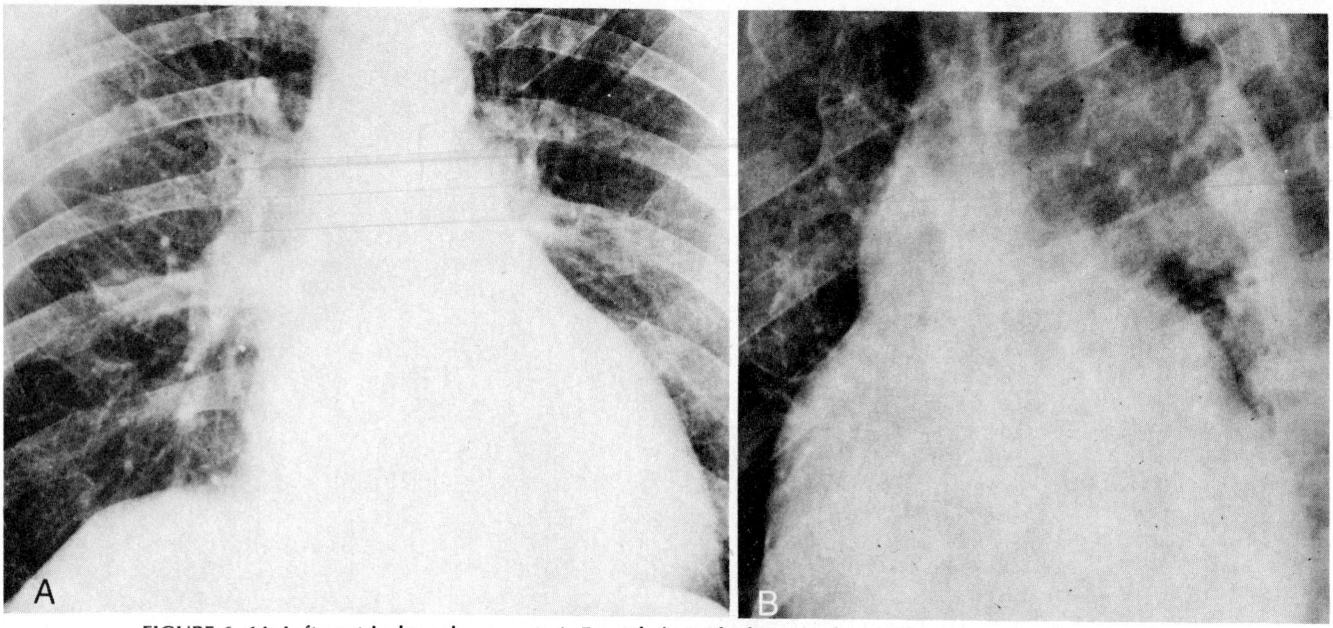

FIGURE 6–14. Left ventricular enlargement. *A*, Frontal view. The heart is elongated and has a configuration most suggestive of aortic regurgitation. *B*, Left anterior oblique view. The double bulge of the left cardiac contour reflects the considerable increase in size of the left atrium as well as of the left ventricle. Elevation of the left main bronchus is well visualized in this projection. The patient has both aortic and mitral valve disease.

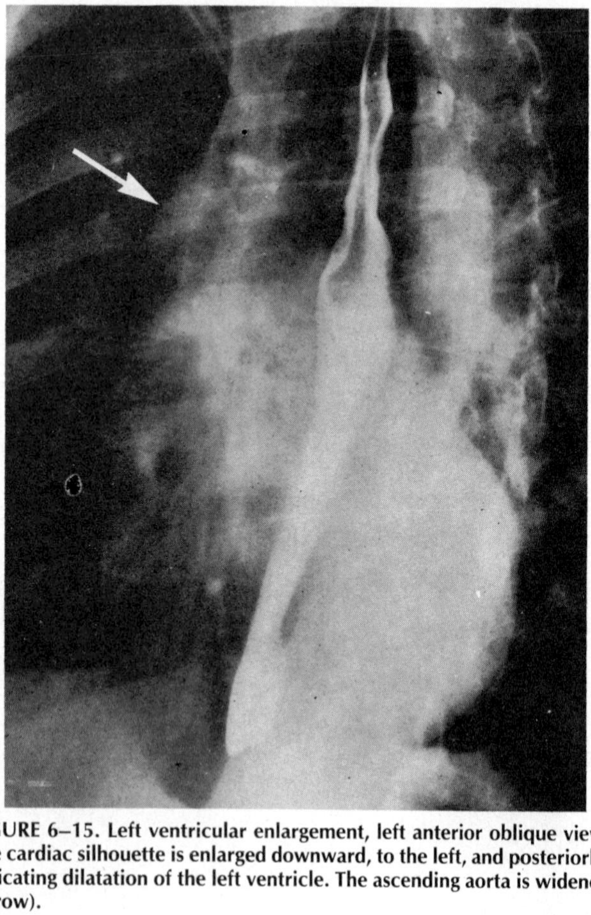

FIGURE 6–15. Left ventricular enlargement, left anterior oblique view. The cardiac silhouette is enlarged downward, to the left, and posteriorly, indicating dilatation of the left ventricle. The ascending aorta is widened (arrow).

the greatest effect on the apparent size of the heart. During a maximal inspiratory effort, patients should be able to lower their diaphragms at least to the level of the tenth rib posteriorly. If the diaphragm is at a higher level, the long axis of the heart lies more horizontally, and its transverse diameter is increased (Fig. 6–18). In addition, because lung volume is decreased, the heart, which does not change in size, occupies a relatively greater portion of the available thoracic space.

Second, because chest films are exposed at random, some are made during diastole and others during systole. In the great majority of patients, the difference in the transverse cardiac diameter between the two phases of the cardiac cycle is relatively small.[12] However, in patients with a slow heart rate and a large stroke volume, such as a trained athlete or a patient with complete atrioventricular block, the change in transverse diameter between systole and diastole may be as much as 2 cm. When two films of such a patient are compared, the differences in heart size

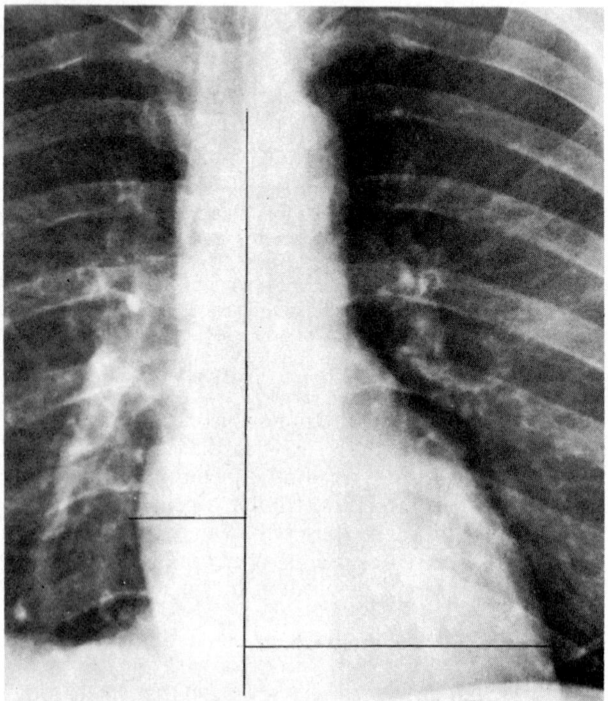

FIGURE 6–16. Measurement of the transverse cardiac diameter. A vertical reference line is first drawn through the spinous processes of the vertebrae. The greatest distances from this line to the right and to the left margins of the cardiac silhouette are then measured. Their sum constitutes the transverse cardiac diameter.

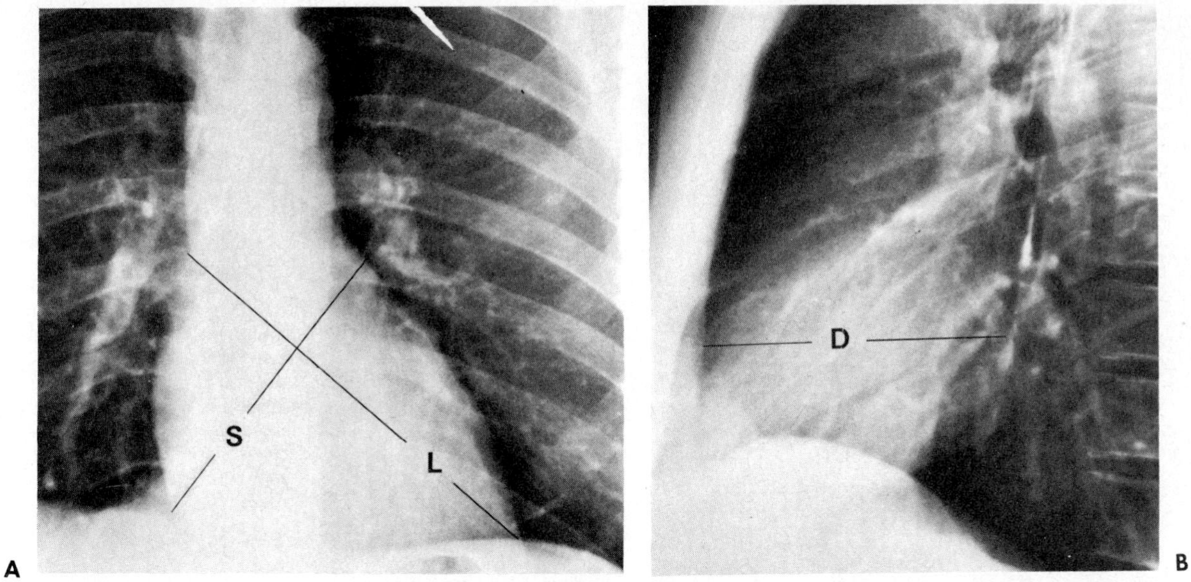

FIGURE 6–17. Measurement of relative cardiac volume. *A*, Frontal projection. The long axis of the heart (L) is measured from the break in the right cardiac contour, where the superior vena cava joins the right atrium, to the apex of the heart. The short diameter (S) extends from the right cardiophrenic angle to the junction of the left atrial and pulmonary artery segments. This line is roughly perpendicular to the long axis. *B*, Lateral view. The widest anteroposterior dimension of the cardiac silhouette constitutes the depth of the heart (D). If the posterior border of the heart cannot be clearly identified, the anterior margin of the barium-filled esophagus can be used as the boundary for this measurement.

can be misinterpreted to indicate an important change in the cardiac status. This error can be avoided by calculation of the relative cardiac volume.

Third, visualization of more of the cardiac apex than is usually seen can cause the heart to appear abnormally large. The heart lies anteriorly and is situated below the highest point of the curve of the diaphragm. In the frontal projection, the cardiac silhouette appears to end at the diaphragm because its lowermost portion is obscured by the shadows of the abdominal viscera. However, when there is a moderate quantity of air in the stomach, the "infradiaphragmatic portion" of the heart may be seen through the gastric air bubble. This causes the cardiac silhouette to appear larger than it really is. Mistakes can

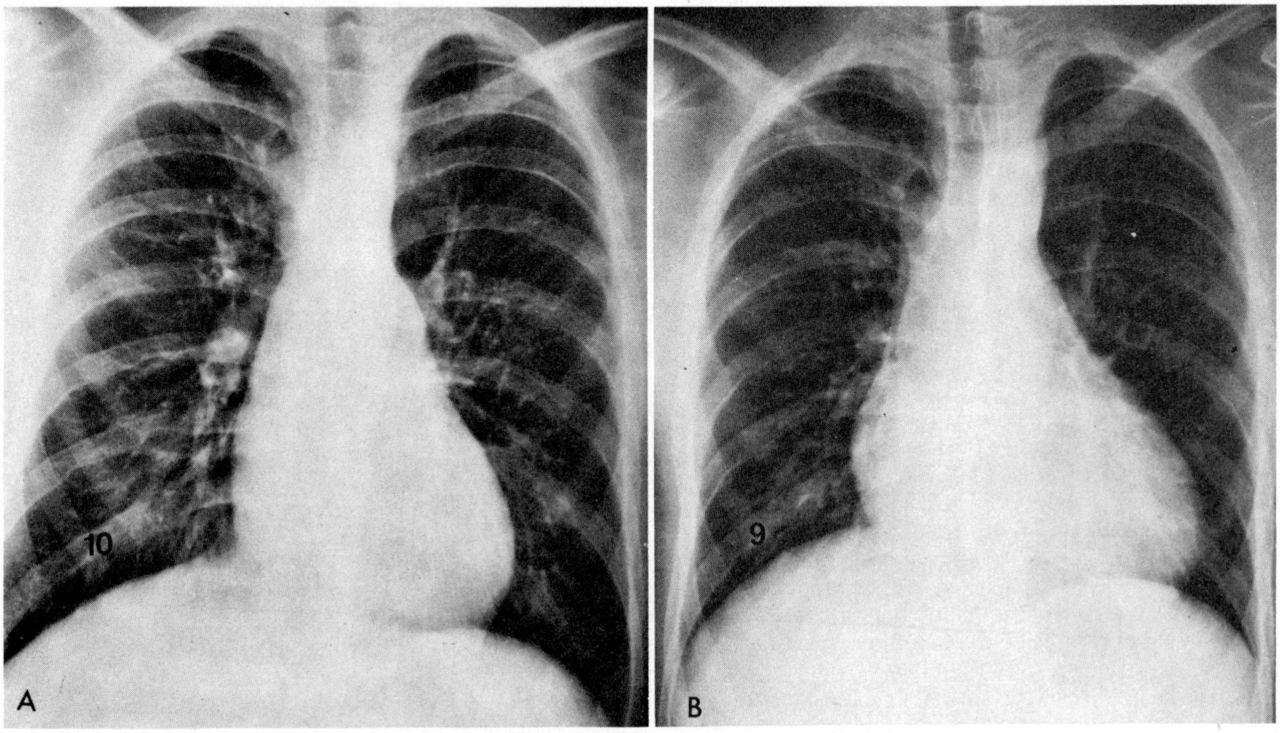

FIGURE 6–18. The effect of respiration on heart size in a patient with coarctation of the aorta. *A*, Deep inspiration. The aortic knob is obscured, and ribs 5 to 9 on the right side and 8 on the left show notching of the undersurface—an appearance pathognomonic of coarctation. The patient has taken a deep inspiration, lowering the diaphragm to the 10th posterior interspace. Although the heart is normal in size, elongation of its long axis indicates some enlargement of the left ventricle. *B*, With a lesser inspiratory effort, the diaphragm is at the level of the 9th posterior interspace. The long axis of the heart is displaced toward the horizontal, increasing the transverse cardiac diameter. The heart appears larger than in *A*.

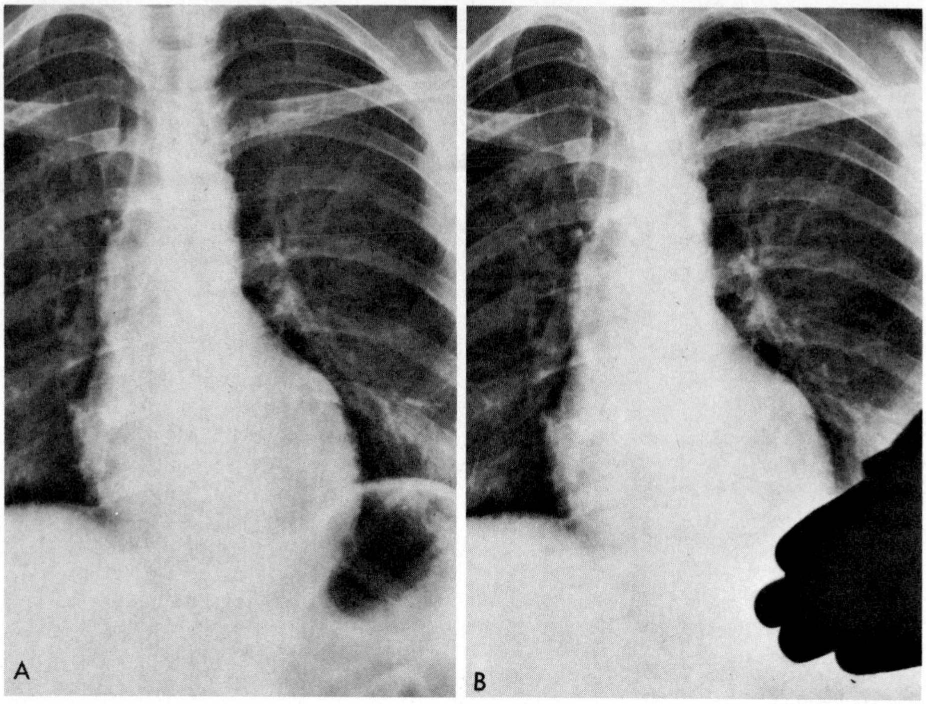

FIGURE 6–19. The "infradiaphragmatic" portion of the cardiac silhouette. *A*, A portion of the apical and diaphragmatic aspects of the heart, usually hidden by the diaphragm and the abdominal organs, is seen through the gastric air bubble. Visualization of this additional area of the heart causes the cardiac shadow to appear enlarged. *B*, Same film. Evaluation of heart size is simplified if the area beneath the diaphragm is covered. The heart is normal.

be avoided if the area beneath the left diaphragm is simply covered before the size of the heart is assessed (Fig. 6–19).

Fourth, when the anteroposterior diameter of the chest is abnormally narrow because of loss of the thoracic kyphotic curvature, or pectus excavatum, the heart may be compressed between the sternum and the spine and splayed to one or both sides. The transverse cardiac diameter is then abnormally large. The cause of the apparent cardiomegaly is obvious if a lateral film is available. However, the chest deformity can usually be recognized from the appearance of the ribs on the frontal film. The course of the posterior ribs tends to be horizontal or angled upward, while the downward slope of the anterior ends of the ribs is much steeper than normal. In addition, the cardiac silhouette is not as dense as expected for a heart with such a large transverse diameter, and the ribs and vascular markings in the left lower lobe are easily visible through it.

Finally, the size of the cardiac shadow is also determined by the degree to which the heart is magnified on the film. The farther the heart is from the film, or the nearer the x-ray tube to the film, the larger the cardiac silhouette. Most bedside examinations are made with a tube-to-film distance of 3 feet, with the cassette behind the patient. The shadow of the heart is therefore more magnified and appears larger than on a standard chest film made at a distance of 6 feet, with the patient facing the cassette. Thus it is extremely difficult to compare the size of the heart on a portable film with that on a standard chest film with any degree of accuracy.

ACQUIRED HEART DISEASE

CORONARY ARTERY DISEASE

(See also Chap. 39)

There is no direct relationship between the appearance of the heart and the presence or severity of coronary artery disease. So long as myocardial function is not significantly impaired, the heart size and contour are normal, even in a patient who may be totally incapacitated by angina. Similarly, if sufficient functioning muscle remains after a myocardial infarction, the heart can retain its normal configuration. On the other hand, the finding of an enlarged heart may at times be the first indication of coronary artery disease.[13, 14]

Ischemic heart disease, from a practical standpoint, is a disease of the left ventricle. Enlargement of the heart implies significant impairment of left ventricular function, and the degree of dilatation is roughly related to the degree of limitation of ventricular contractility. Since the size of the heart is an indicator of cardiac decompensation, the chest film is a simple means of following the course of ischemic heart disease.

Deterioration of left ventricular function results in an increase in left ventricular end-diastolic pressure. This, in turn, increases resistance to left atrial emptying, and the atrium tends to dilate. The appearance of the heart at this stage of left ventricular failure may be similar to that of mitral valve disease (Fig. 6–20). With further progression, the right heart chambers also enlarge, and the cardiac silhouette becomes rounded. The appearance may also resemble that caused by a pericardial effusion; the cardiac pulsations are markedly diminished in both conditions. The two can usually be differentiated by the appearance of the hilar vessels. Cardiac enlargement of this extent is associated with some degree of congestive failure, and the hilar vessels become engorged and unduly prominent. On the other hand, the dilated cardiac silhouette caused by a pericardial effusion tends to obscure the hilar vessels (Fig. 6–43, p. 166).[15]

A myocardial infarct cannot be identified on plain films unless it is calcified or forms an aneurysm. In some cases, the abnormal motion of the infarcted segment of the ventricular wall can be noted on fluoroscopic examination,

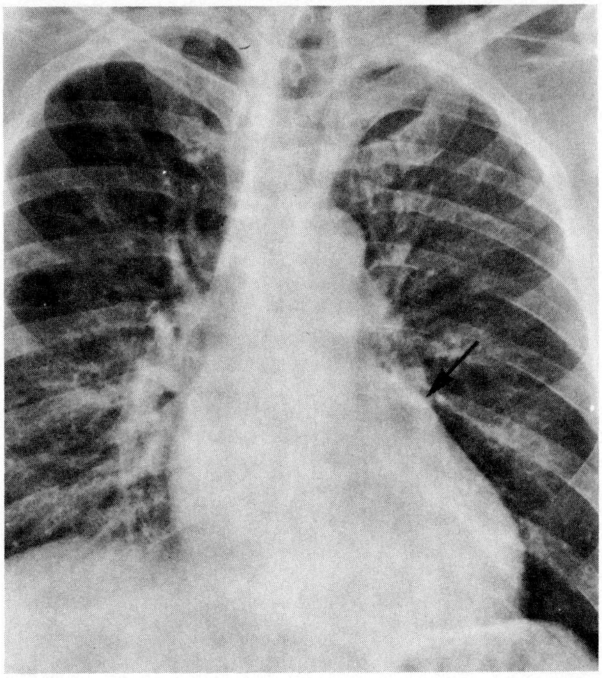

FIGURE 6–20. Mitral configuration in ischemic heart disease. The left ventricle is dilated because of myocardial ischemia. Ventricular end-diastolic pressure is elevated and is the cause of the left atrial dilatation (arrow).

but because the septal and diaphragmatic aspects of the ventricle are not adequately visualized, a large number of infarcts cannot be detected by this technique. When calcium is deposited within an infarct, it produces a fine shell that is seen as a dense, curvilinear line when viewed tangentially. However, when projected en face or obliquely, the calcific layer is often too thin to cast a recognizable shadow. Both the thinning of the ventricular wall and the calcification, if present, are more easily detected by computed tomography (p. 360).

A calcified infarct is almost always transmural in extent. Because the fibrotic scar is thin, the calcific rim lies close to, and parallels, the outer border of the heart (Fig. 6–21). The infarcts visualized in the frontal projection involve the anterolateral wall of the left ventricle or its apex, although on a well-penetrated film it may be possible to detect a calcified infarct of the interventricular septum. Because of its proximity to the outer border of the heart, the calcific rim of an infarct can be confused with calcification of the pericardium. However, calcific deposits on the pericardium are usually coarser and more irregular. In addition, they tend to accumulate over the atrioventricular sulci and the interventricular groove to a greater extent than over the free wall of the left ventricle (Fig. 6–22).

An *aneurysm* that is not calcified can be detected when it projects beyond the normal cardiac contour. Even when the left ventricle is markedly enlarged, the border of the chamber is made up of a single smooth curve. A localized bulge in this curve is presumptive evidence of a ventricular aneurysm (Fig. 6–3*B*). However, some aneurysms project from the cardiac contour only during systole and blend in with the curve of the distended ventricle during diastole. This type of aneurysm may be recognizable by means of fluoroscopy, but as a rule, fluoroscopy is not a very effective method for detection of a ventricular aneurysm. Considerably more than half of all aneurysms will be hidden within the cardiac silhouette and cannot be detected by fluoroscopy.[16] In the occasional case when an aneurysm is so large that it forms most of the left cardiac contour, the appearance of the heart can be almost identical to that of a failing ventricle due to diffuse, as opposed to localized, myocardial fibrosis (Fig. 6–23). Fluoroscopic examination is useful in this instance to determine the need for angiocardiography. In most cases, an aneurysm of this size will pulsate paradoxically, whereas the pulsations of a dilated, flabby ventricle will be in proper phase, although grossly diminished in amplitude.

Calcific deposits within the coronary arteries are usually thin and their shadows are not very dense. Because of the blurring caused by motion of the heart, they are almost never seen on plain films, and a careful fluoroscopic examination is required for their detection. Most commonly, calcification occurs first in the proximal portions of the coronary arteries near the base of the heart. When the calcification is more extensive, it may be seen more distally in the vessels in the atrioventricular sulci or the interventricular groove. Calcific plaques are too fine to be visible when viewed en face and are seen only where they are projected tangentially. Thus, coronary calcification appears as a single, sharp, linear shadow or, if the entire circumference of the vessel is involved, as two parallel linear densities. When the calcified vessel is projected on end, it casts a fine, ring-shaped shadow.

Coronary artery calcification is very common in patients with ischemic heart disease.[17, 18] However, it does not always indicate the presence of ischemic heart disease. The significance of calcification of the coronary arteries varies with the age of the patient, the incidence of coronary artery calcification not associated with stenosis increasing with age. It has little importance as an indicator of significant coronary artery narrowing in patients older than 65 or 70.[18, 19] On the other hand, there is an extremely high correlation between coronary artery calcification and coronary artery disease in patients under the age of 50. Because the search for coronary artery calcification is time-consuming and involves moderate radiation exposure, it is not a suitable screening procedure. There is little point in searching for such calcification in patients who have other evidence of coronary atherosclerosis or who are in the older age group. From a practical standpoint, such a study is best limited to younger patients who have chest pain of unknown etiology.[20]

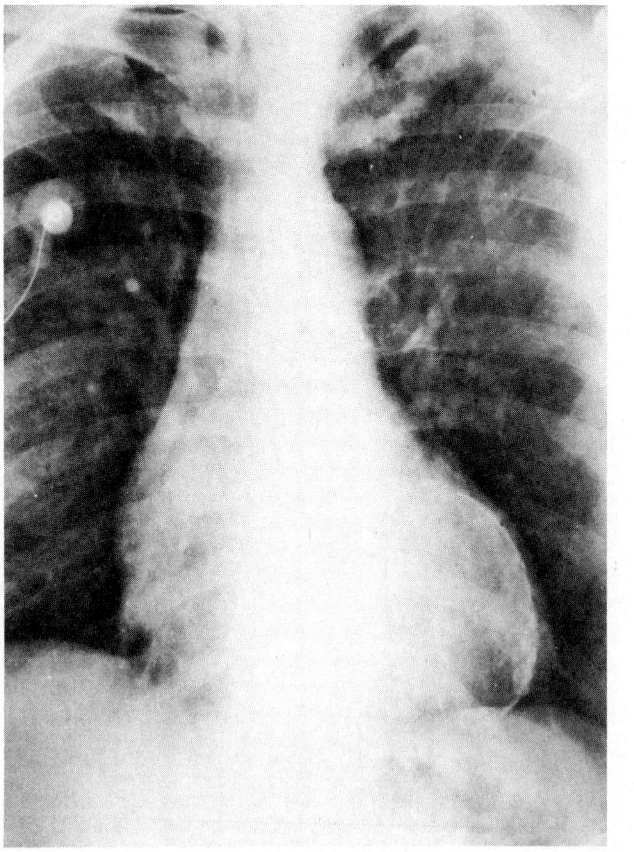

FIGURE 6–21. Calcified myocardial infarct. The rim of calcium paralleling the lateral border of the heart outlines an old infarct of the anterolateral left ventricular wall. Although the calcification extends around to the anterior and posterior surfaces of the ventricle, it is well visualized only where it is projected tangentially.

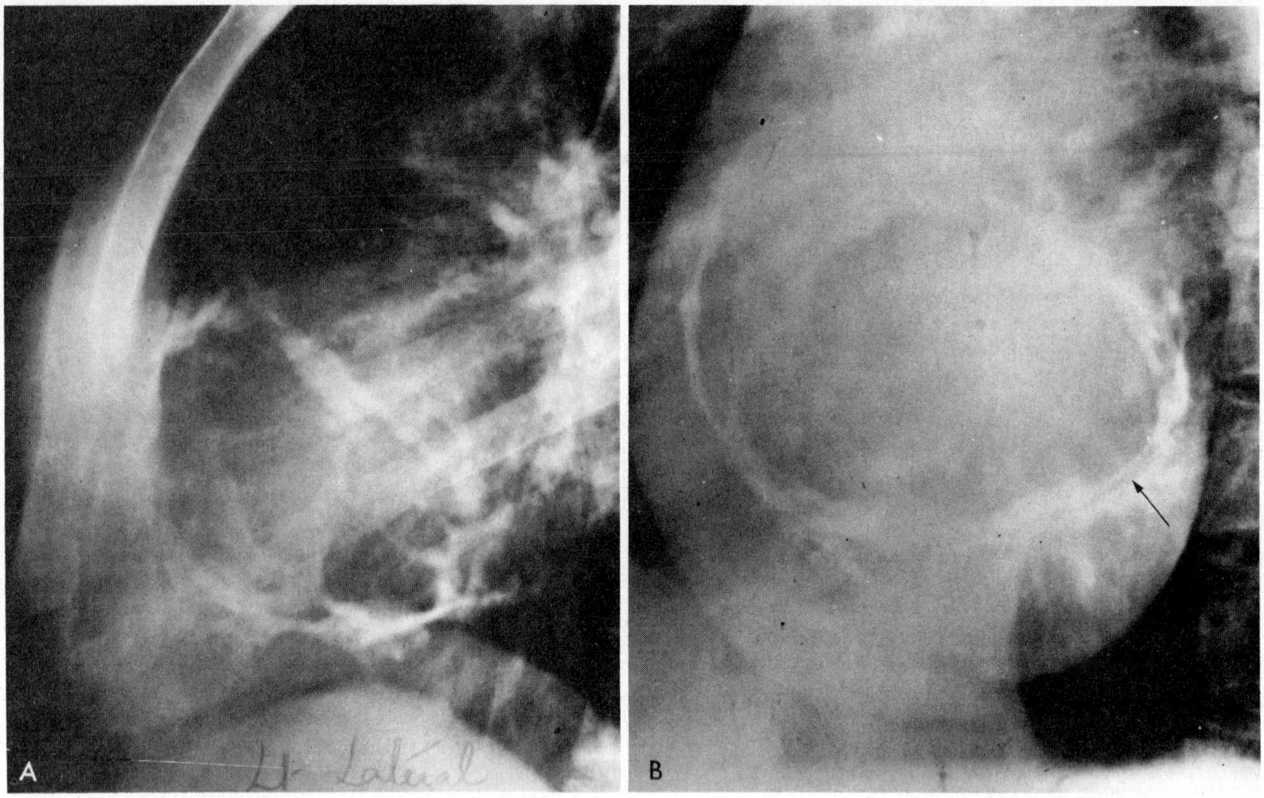

FIGURE 6–22. Pericardial calcification. *A*, Lateral chest film of a young woman showing dense, calcific patches distributed along the course of the atrioventricular sulcus and over the anterior portion of the right ventricle. *B*, Left anterior oblique view. The lucent line within the calcified sulcus (arrow) most likely represents the circumflex branch of the left coronary artery, which is not calcified. (Courtesy of S. Bharati, M.D.)

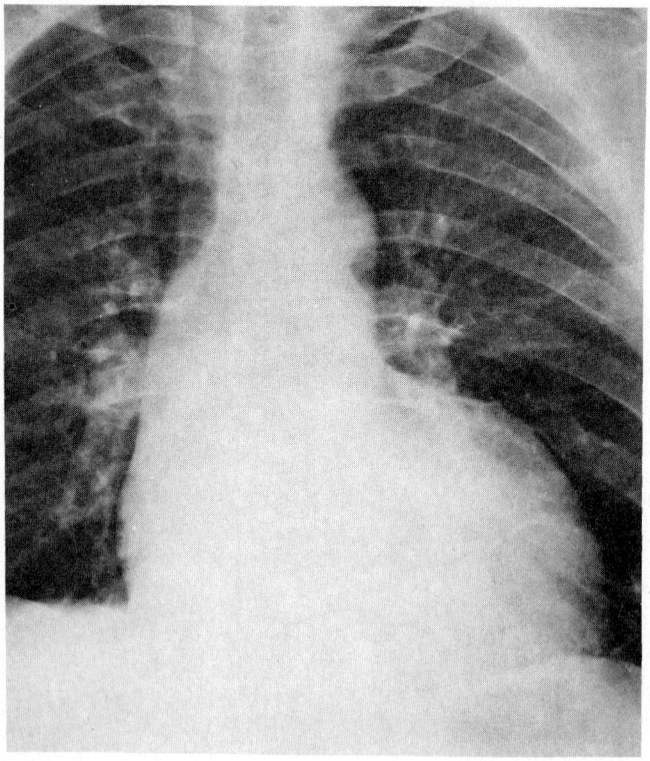

FIGURE 6–23. Left ventricular aneurysm. The aneurysm is so large that it forms almost the entire lateral profile of the left ventricle. A similar appearance can be caused by the dilated, failing ventricle that results from diffuse ischemic disease. The two can be distinguished by fluoroscopy, because the aneurysm will show paradoxical pulsations. (From Donoso, E., and Gorlin, R. [eds.]: Current Cardiovascular Topics. Vol. 3, Angina Pectoris. New York, Stratton Intercontinental Medical Book Co., 1977.)

VALVULAR HEART DISEASE

(See also Chap. 33)

MITRAL VALVE DISEASE (See also p. 1023) (Figs. 6–3, 6–6, 6–11, 6–13, 6–24, 6–25, and 6–26). Disease of the mitral valve, whether it causes stenosis or regurgitation, results in dilatation of the left atrium. When *mitral stenosis* predominates, the heart is usually normal in size, and the left atrium may be the only chamber that is enlarged. There is a poor correlation between the size of the left atrium and the severity of the mitral stenosis, but moderate to marked left atrial enlargement occurs more commonly in patients with atrial fibrillation than in those with normal sinus rhythm.[21, 22] In *mitral regurgitation*, diastolic overloading of the left ventricle causes the chamber to enlarge together with the left atrium. In practice, it is difficult to determine which of the two lesions is predominant.

Longstanding, moderate, or severe mitral stenosis is commonly associated with pulmonary arterial hypertension and dilatation of the right ventricle. As a result, the transverse diameter of the heart is widened, and the cardiac apex is displaced to the left. Dilatation of the left ventricle also widens the cardiac silhouette to the left, so that in many cases it is difficult to be sure whether the cardiac enlargement is due to the right ventricle alone or to both ventricles. This is further complicated by the fact that rheumatic heart disease often involves both the aortic and mitral valves. The combination of aortic regurgitation and mitral stenosis can produce a cardiac shape indistinguishable from that associated with mitral regurgitation. Conversely, a marked degree of mitral regurgitation may be present in the absence of significant enlargement of the left ventricle. This is most commonly seen following rup-

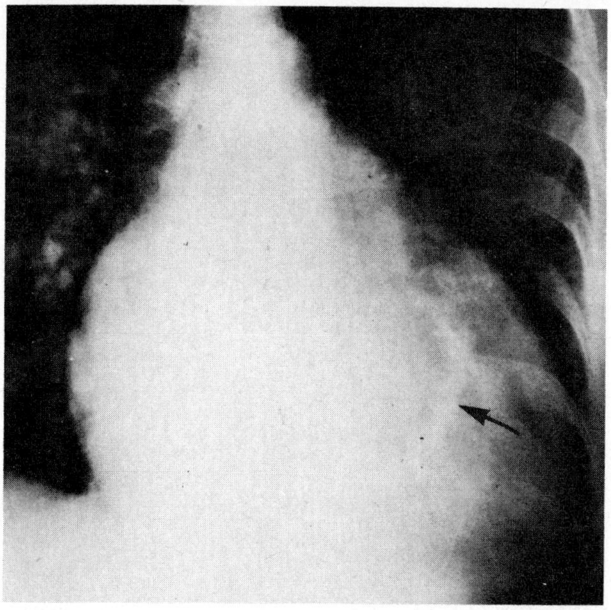

FIGURE 6–24. Calcification of the mitral annulus. The broad, curved density (arrow) in the mitral region represents calcification of the valve annulus. The arc of the calcific shadow is larger than that of the mitral orifice, distinguishing it from calcification of the leaflets, and it is too small for the calcium to be within the atrioventricular sulcus.

ture of a papillary muscle or a chorda tendineae, when regurgitation, although severe, is of recent onset.[23]

Calcification of the mitral valve (Fig. 6–9) is indicative of stenosis (although there may be some accompanying regurgitation). The calcium is usually deposited in clumps on the valve leaflets but may also involve the commissures.[24] Extensive calcification may be visible on chest films, but fluoroscopy is required to detect smaller depos-

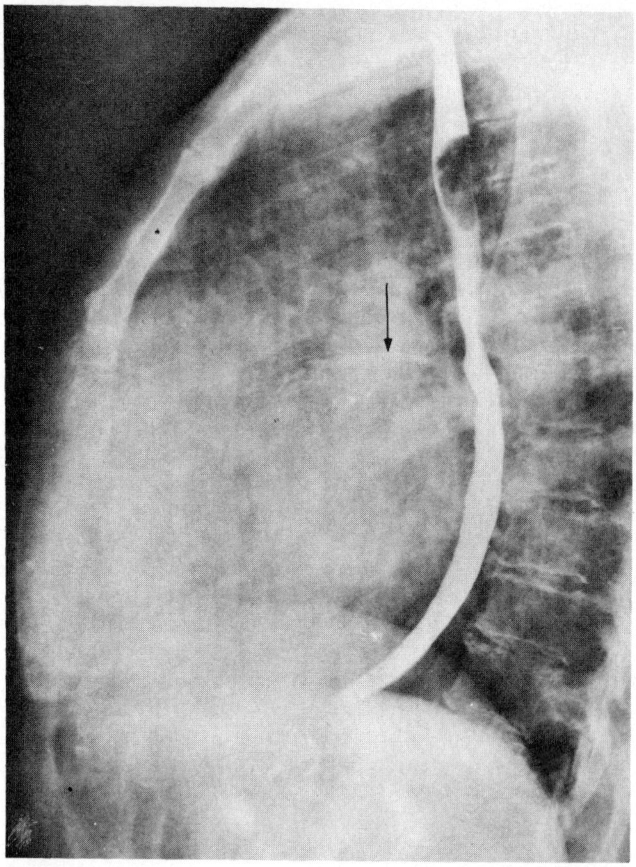

FIGURE 6–25. Calcification of the left atrium in rheumatic mitral disease. Lateral view. The calcified superior wall of the enlarged atrium is visualized (arrow) just below the level of the carina. The esophagus is displaced backward in a continuous curve that extends to the diaphragm, indicating dilatation of both left atrium and left ventricle.

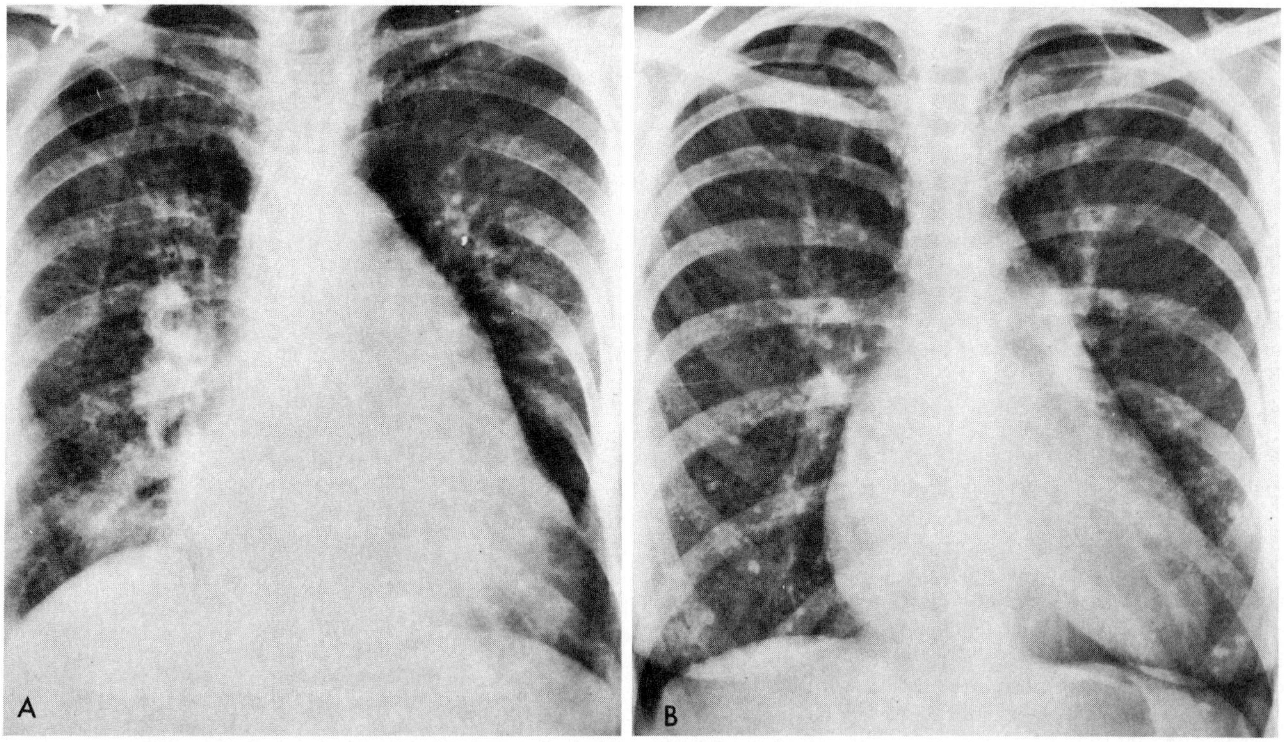

FIGURE 6–26. Lung changes in mitral stenosis. *A*, Pulmonary hemosiderosis. The lower lungs are studded with small nodules of moderate radiodensity. The left atrium and left ventricle are enlarged. Kerley B lines are present in the lateral basal portions of the lungs. *B*, Pulmonary ossifications. Scattered calcific nodules of differing size and shape are present in the lower lungs. They represent foci of organized bone within the alveoli. The left atrium is enlarged, and a double contour can be seen through the right side of the cardiac silhouette. The left atrial appendage is obscured by the dilated left ventricle.

its. Valvular calcification must be distinguished from *calcification of the mitral annulus*. The latter occurs in older patients, particularly women,[25] and as long as the calcification does not extend onto the valve leaflets, it does not signify the presence of mitral valve disease.[26] The calcified annulus appears as a broad, curved shadow that may form a complete ring or, if the entire annulus is not involved, a U-shaped or J-shaped density. The curve of a calcified annulus has a larger diameter than that of a calcified valve, and it tends to appear as one continuous deposit rather than as separate calcific clumps (Fig. 6–24).

Except for its rare occurrence in metabolic calcinosis, calcification of the left atrium signifies mitral stenosis. The calcification may appear as a thin shell completely outlining the atrial wall or as a curvilinear shadow involving only one portion of the atrial circumference. The posterior atrial wall is the area most commonly involved and is best seen in the lateral view, below the carina and just in front of the esophagus (Fig. 6–25). If the atrial appendage is calcified, it presents as a short, arcuate density along the left border of the heart below the pulmonary segment in the frontal view and within the midportion of the cardiac silhouette in the lateral view. In the great majority of cases, a mural thrombus is present when the left atrium is calcified.[27] The calcium is usually deposited within the wall of the atrium but on occasion is present only within the thrombus.[28]

Narrowing of the mitral orifice results in elevation of left atrial and pulmonary venous pressures. Eventually, pulmonary hypertension may result (Chap. 26). These changes are associated with a sequence of alterations in the appearance of the lungs and especially of the pulmonary vascular pattern. The resultant pictures are not specific for mitral stenosis but occur with any disease that causes an elevation of left atrial pressure (p. 163). *Pulmonary hemosiderosis* and pulmonary ossifications, however, are rarely encountered with any form of heart disease other than mitral stenosis. Because of the chronic pulmonary congestion and elevated capillary pressure caused by mitral stenosis, small intraalveolar hemorrhages are common. Hemosiderin from the broken-down red cells is picked up by phagocytes, and clusters of these iron-laden cells form small nodules that can be seen on the chest film.[29, 30] Their appearance is almost identical to that seen in idiopathic hemosiderosis or in some of the miliary lung diseases (Fig. 6–26*A*). Although in mitral stenosis the nodules are distributed mainly in the mid and lower lung fields, rather than evenly throughout the lungs, the main differential point is the association with a cardiac shadow that has a mitral configuration.

Pulmonary ossifications are probably also the result of intraalveolar hemorrhage. The nodules of bone lie within the alveoli, mostly in the lower portions of the lungs. They are larger and more dense than hemosiderotic nodules and are fewer in number (Fig. 6–26*B*). The nodules vary considerably in size and often have an irregular shape. This, together with their distribution, serves to differentiate them from other calcific nodules in the lungs, such as those caused by histoplasmosis or chickenpox pneumonia.[31] Both pulmonary hemosiderosis and ossifications occur in patients with longstanding mitral disease, often with pulmonary hypertension. However, the two are unrelated, and it is not uncommon for one to be present without the other. The bony nodules are pathognomonic of mitral stenosis but can occur when the valve is partially occluded by a myxoma of the left atrium.[32]

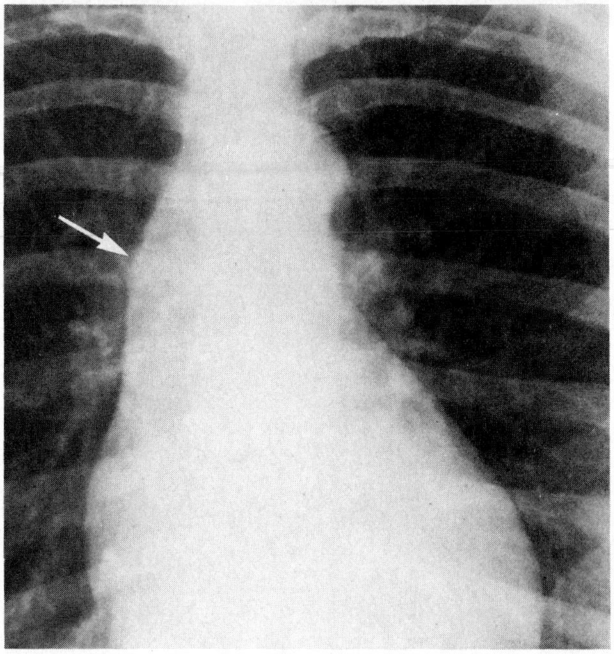

FIGURE 6–27. Aortic stenosis. The transverse diameter of the heart is slightly enlarged, and the curvature of the left cardiac contour is accentuated, suggesting left ventricular hypertrophy. The prominence of the midascending aorta (arrow) is due to poststenotic dilatation. A gradient of 90 mm Hg was measured across the aortic valve.

AORTIC VALVE DISEASE (See also p. 1052) (Figs. 6–4*A*, 6–7, 6–14, 6–15, 6–27). *Aortic regurgitation* causes elongation and dilatation of the left ventricle. The cardiac apex is displaced downward, to the left, and posteriorly (Fig. 6–4*A*). Often the entire ascending aorta is dilated, and fluoroscopic examination reveals an increase in the amplitude of its pulsations.

Aortic stenosis is more difficult to recognize on chest films. The heart is usually normal in size or only slightly enlarged, even with severe narrowing of the valve. However, the shape of the heart is often abnormal. Concentric hypertrophy of the left ventricle causes an increase in the curvature of the lower left cardiac contour and blunting of the cardiac apex (Fig. 6–27). Elongation of the long ventricular axis occurs occasionally in pure aortic stenosis but is never marked. Significant dilatation of the left ventricle in the absence of aortic regurgitation indicates failure of the myocardium and heralds the end stage of the disease.

Calcification of the aortic valve is common in congenital as well as acquired stenosis.[33, 34] Poststenotic dilatation involving the ascending aorta at the junction of its proximal and middle thirds also occurs with both types of aortic stenosis. The poststenotic bulge may protrude from the right side of the mediastinum in the frontal view but is best seen on the left anterior oblique projection.[35] There is no correlation between the degree of poststenotic dilatation and the severity of the stenosis.[36] A similar localized dilatation of the ascending aorta can occur when the stenosis is due to a membranous web in the subvalvular region, but it is not associated with the hypertrophic form of subaortic stenosis.

PRIMARY MYOCARDIAL DISEASE

(See also Chap. 42)

The roentgen manifestations depend on whether the main effect of the disease is impairment of myocardial contractility, as in congestive (dilated) cardiomyopathy, or thickening of the ventricular wall, as in restrictive or hypertrophic cardiomyopathy. In either case, the heart may appear normal in the early stages or when the disease is of limited severity. More extensive involvement usually results in cardiac enlargement.

Diminution of ventricular function is reflected in an increase in the size of the ventricles. The cardiac silhouette is enlarged and tends to have a globular shape. The transverse cardiac diameter is widened, the curves of the heart border are accentuated, and cardiac pulsations are diminished. The hilar vessels are often prominent because of elevated left ventricular end-diastolic pressure, and the overall appearance of the heart may be similar to that seen with extensive ischemic disease of the myocardium.

In general, the degree of cardiac dilatation is proportional to the impairment of myocardial function. This relationship does not hold with myocardial hypertrophy. Severe and incapacitating degrees of hypertrophy may be present with only minimal or moderate cardiac enlargement. Most commonly, only the left ventricle is hypertrophied, but both ventricles may be involved. As the wall of the left ventricle thickens, the transverse cardiac diameter increases and the curvature of the left heart border becomes accentuated (see Fig. 42–1, p. 3033). This configuration is suggestive of myocardial hypertrophy, but as a rule the chest film is of little value in establishing a definite diagnosis or in evaluating the extent of the disease.

CONGENITAL HEART DISEASE

(See also Chaps. 30 and 31)

As a general rule, the younger the patient with congenital heart disease, the more difficult it is to make an accurate diagnosis from films of the chest. Although some congenital lesions seen in infants are associated with a fairly characteristic cardiac silhouette, e.g., the egg-shaped heart of complete transposition of the great arteries (see Fig. 30–62, p. 954), or the "snowman" heart of total anomalous pulmonary venous drainage; in a significant number of cases these same lesions produce nonspecific changes. Furthermore, infants who attract clinical attention because of heart disease often have complex abnormalities that involve multiple lesions, each one producing some distortion of the cardiac silhouette and thus compounding the diagnostic difficulties. An additional problem is the inability to see the heart clearly in infants because it is obscured by the overlapping shadow of the thymus. Perhaps the most important information regarding the nature of heart disease in young children is gained from the appearance of the pulmonary vessels. A decrease in the vasculature indicates a right-to-left shunt, while an increase usually indicates a left-to-right shunt.

Actually, in the symptomatic child, the radiological appearance of the heart is not of major diagnostic importance, because these children will usually require further study with other imaging modalities such as echocardiography or angiocardiography in order to delineate the specific cardiac abnormalities accurately. Once the correct diagnosis is established, the course of the disease or the results of surgical correction can be followed with serial chest films. For these purposes, the pertinent parameters are changes in cardiac size and shape and the pulmonary vascular pattern. The routine chest film is considerably more important in the *detection* of congenital cardiac lesions that were overlooked in childhood.

ATRIAL SEPTAL DEFECT (See also pp. 915 and 982). With the exception of the bicuspid aortic valve, the secundum type of atrial septal defect is the most common congenital cardiac lesion of adult life.[37–39] A significant number of these patients are first recognized as having heart disease because of an abnormal chest film, while others have been considered to have rheumatic mitral stenosis.[40, 41] The characteristic picture of an atrial septal defect shows a generalized increase in pulmonary vascularity, dilatation of the main pulmonary artery, and enlargement of the right ventricle (Fig. 6–28). These findings are present in almost every patient in whom there is a significant shunt. The right atrium may be dilated, particularly in older patients. Enlargement of the left atrium is not uncommon and occurs in more than half of patients over the age of 40.[40, 42] Enlargement of the left atrium may be related to the presence of atrial fibrillation or, in older patients, can represent one of the effects of coronary artery disease. In other cases, the size of the atrium is referable to the regurgitation of left ventricular blood because of accompanying mitral valve prolapse [43, 44] (p. 1045). Also, as a general rule, for any given set of hemodynamic parameters, the older the patient, the larger the heart.[42, 45]

The left-to-right shunt through the atrial septal defect increases pulmonary blood flow and causes the vessels in the lungs to dilate. Although the pulmonary pressure may be considerably elevated because of the increased flow, it usually declines after the defect is closed. However, when the pulmonary hypertension is due to an elevation of vascular resistance rather than of pulmonary blood flow,[46] it may remain the same or may even progress following surgical correction. The two causes of pulmonary hypertension cannot always be differentiated from the chest film. Although in many cases the typical changes of

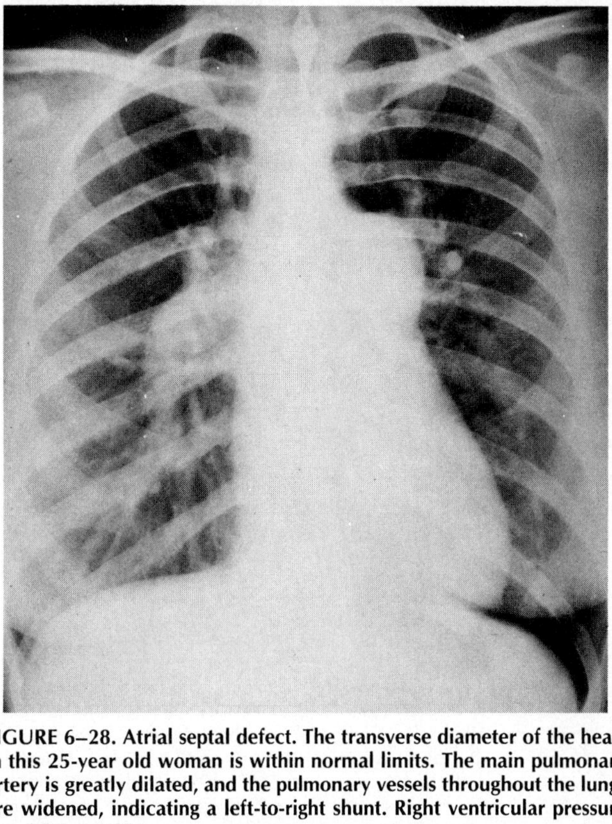

FIGURE 6–28. Atrial septal defect. The transverse diameter of the heart in this 25-year old woman is within normal limits. The main pulmonary artery is greatly dilated, and the pulmonary vessels throughout the lungs are widened, indicating a left-to-right shunt. Right ventricular pressure was 87/5 mm Hg.

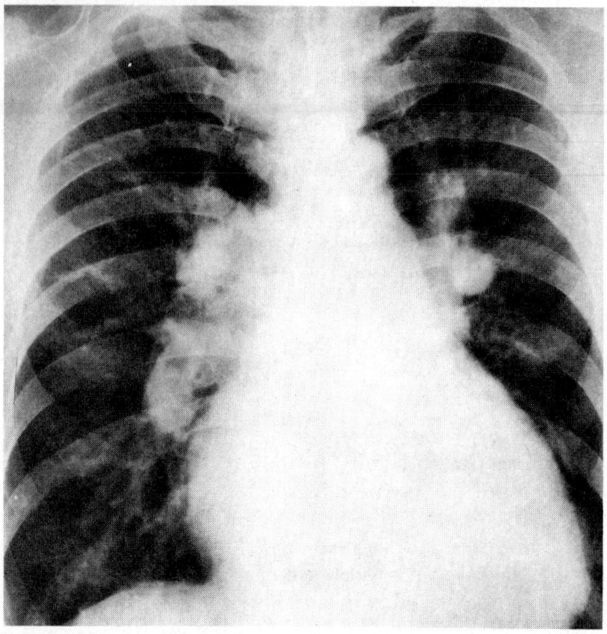

FIGURE 6–29. Atrial septal defect, with elevated pulmonary vascular resistance. Secundum atrial septal defect. There is a marked disparity between the size of the hilar arteries and the peripheral pulmonary vessels, indicating an increase in pulmonary vascular resistance. The right ventricular pressure was almost at systemic levels.

elevated pulmonary resistance are reflected in a marked disparity between the dilated central pulmonary arteries and the constricted peripheral vessels (Fig. 6–29), severe elevation of vascular resistance can be present while the peripheral pulmonary vessels still appear engorged.

Differentiation of an atrial septal defect from other left-to-right shunts is often possible if there is marked pulmonary plethora. The peripheral pulmonary vessels are usually constricted in adults with a large ventricular septal defect, and patent ductus arteriosus rarely causes such marked vascular dilatation. Distinction between a secundum type of atrial septal defect and an ostium primum lesion is usually not possible from the best roentgenogram, although the heart tends to be larger with the latter defect. Because of the presence of mitral regurgitation, dilatation of the left atrium is more common. A secundum atrial septal defect in which the left atrium is enlarged can present a cardiac configuration almost identical to that seen with mitral valve disease. The distinction between the two conditions can be made from the appearance of the pulmonary vessels. In mitral stenosis, there is a redistribution of pulmonary blood flow with constriction of the vessels at the lung bases and dilatation of the vessels in the upper lobes. When there is significant shunting through an atrial septal defect, all the pulmonary vessels, at the bases as well as at the apices, are dilated (Fig. 6–30*A*). However, once the characteristic vascular pattern of elevated pulmonary resistance appears, it often is not possible to differentiate an atrial septal defect from other causes of pulmonary hypertension.

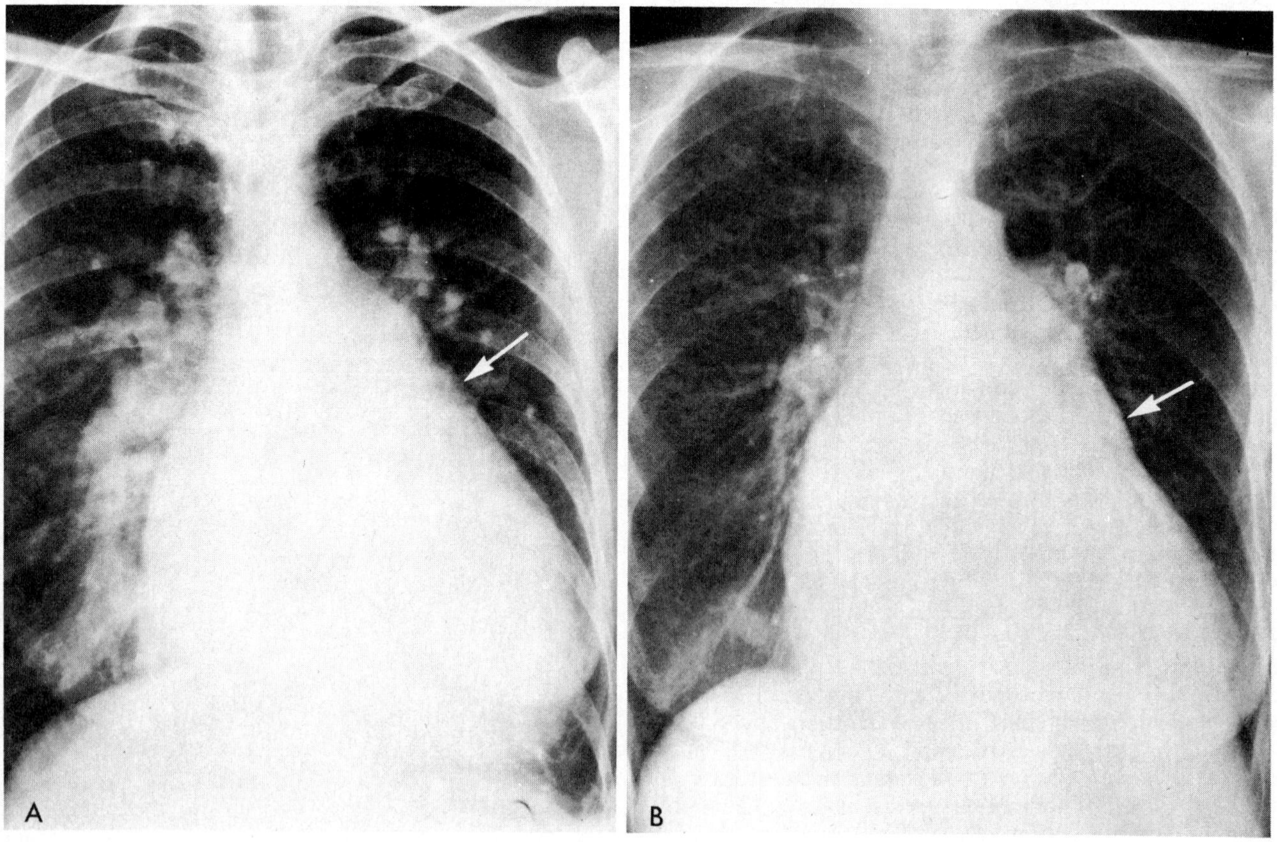

FIGURE 6–30. The diagnostic value of the pulmonary vascular pattern. *A*, Secundum atrial septal defect. The heart is large because of dilatation of the ventricles and the right atrium. The left atrium is also enlarged (arrow). Because of the left-to-right shunt, the pulmonary vessels throughout the lungs are dilated. *B*, Mitral stenosis. The shape of the heart is almost the same as in *A*. Both ventricles as well as the right atrium are dilated. The left atrium is enlarged (arrow) and extends to the right beyond the border of the right atrium. Pulmonary vessels in the lung bases are constricted, while vessels in the upper lobe are distended. The redistribution of pulmonary blood flow is characteristic of postcapillary pulmonary hypertension; this does not occur with a left-to-right shunt.

PATENT DUCTUS ARTERIOSUS (See also pp. 923 and 993). A small or moderate shunt through a patent ductus often produces no abnormalities in the radiological appearance of the heart or lungs. When the ductal flow is large, the pulmonary vessels become dilated, and the left atrium and left ventricle enlarge. The aorta is usually prominent in contrast to the rather diminutive aorta often seen with an atrial or a ventricular septal defect. However, this is not a strong differential point, particularly in adults. It is difficult to make an accurate diagnosis of a patent ductus from plain films unless the duct is calcified.

Calcification of the ductus is relatively uncommon, but when present it provides a pathognomonic x-ray picture. The calcified ductus is seen as a curvilinear density within the aortic shadow below the aortic knob,[47] slanting downward and to the right. It does not parallel the outer border of the descending aorta, which differentiates it from a calcific atheromatous plaque on the aortic wall. The ductus calcification often has an inverted Y-shape, with the lower limbs representing extension of the calcification onto the main pulmonary artery (Fig. 6–31). Although calcification of the ligamentum arteriosum has been observed on rare occasions at autopsy, it can be assumed that when a calcified ductus is identified on a chest film, it is patent. In most cases, the pulmonary artery pressure is elevated and there is reversal of the shunt.

PULMONIC VALVE STENOSIS (See also pp. 942 and 993). Because of the increased resistance to ventricular emptying, stenosis of the pulmonic valve is accompanied by hypertrophy of the right ventricle. This has little effect on the configuration of the cardiac silhouette, and significant enlargement of the heart is uncommon. Nevertheless, the heart often has a characteristic appearance because of poststenotic dilatation of the pulmonary artery. Dilatation of the main pulmonary artery is related to distortion of the pressure vectors within the vessel caused by the high-velocity jet of blood spurting through the stenotic valve.[48] Because the jet is usually directed toward the left, the left pulmonary artery tends to be dilated. In addition, the artery protrudes farther laterally than normal. In the frontal view, the shadow of the main pulmonary artery is increased in height and width and often is considerably larger than the normal-sized aortic knob. The left pulmonary artery, which usually courses almost directly posteriorly and is largely hidden by the main pulmonary artery, is abnormally prominent because it projects outward from the hilum (Fig. 6–32). These changes may not be evident in infants or young children.

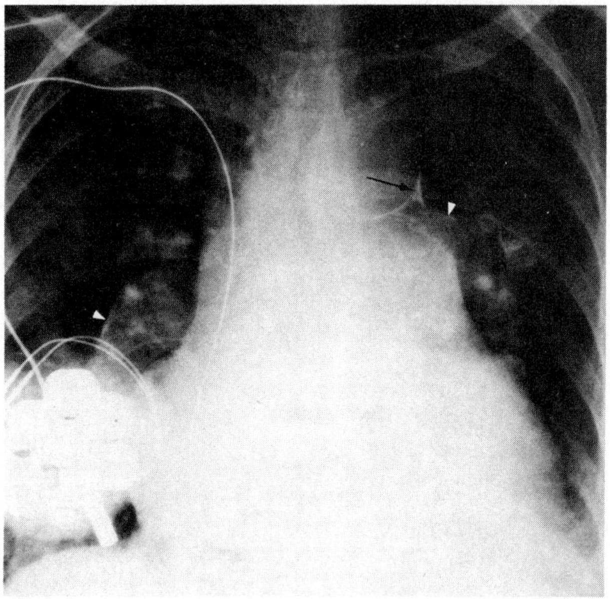

FIGURE 6–31. Calcification of the ductus arteriosus. The inverted Y-shaped calcific deposit (black arrow) is diagnostic of a patent ductus arteriosus. The calcified duct forms the vertical portion of the shadow, while the lower limbs represent calcification in the roof of the main pulmonary artery. Calcium has also been deposited in the walls of the hilar pulmonary arteries (white arrowheads). These vessels are markedly dilated, but the peripheral vessels are constricted, indicating the presence of elevated pulmonary resistance.

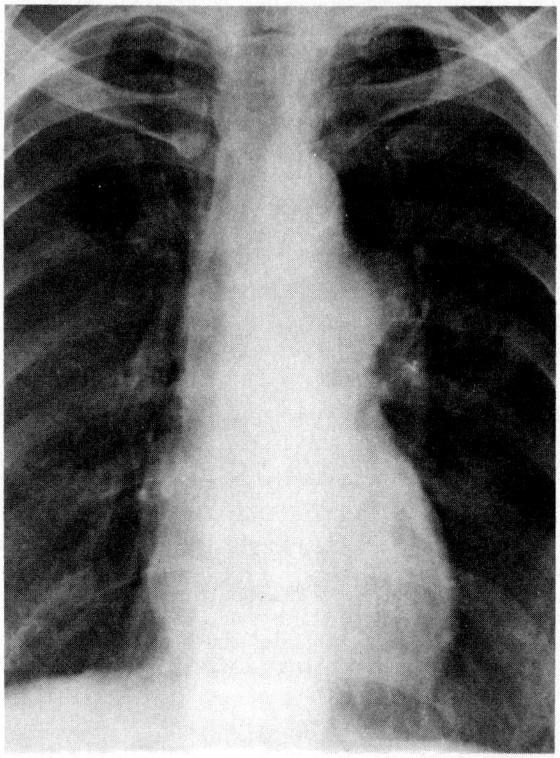

FIGURE 6–32. Pulmonic valvular stenosis. The heart is normal in size, but the main pulmonary artery is dilated. The left pulmonary artery is considerably wider than the right and protrudes outward from the cardiac shadow. The peripheral pulmonary vasculature is within the limits of normal.

The roentgen diagnosis of pulmonic valve stenosis is based on dilatation of the main pulmonary artery and prominence of the left pulmonary artery. If the latter is not dilated or displaced laterally, the diagnosis is much less certain. Dilatation of only the main pulmonary artery can be seen with pulmonic valve stenosis but also occurs with idiopathic dilatation of the pulmonary artery and in some cases of patent ductus. Prominence of the left pulmonary artery without dilatation of the main pulmonary artery is of little significance and most commonly is due to elevation of the hilum secondary to partial shrinkage of the left upper lobe because of previous inflammatory disease.

The cardiac output is usually within normal limits in isolated pulmonic stenosis. In the absence of an atrial or ventricular septal defect, all the blood ejected by the right ventricle must flow through the pulmonary circulation. The vascularity of the lungs is therefore not decreased. However, in the end stages of the disease, once the right ventricle fails, pulmonary blood flow may decrease considerably, and this is associated with marked dilatation of the right ventricle and right atrium (Fig. 6–33).

COARCTATION OF THE AORTA (See also pp. 929 and 994). In most cases, the diagnosis of coarctation of the aorta can be made from the frontal chest film.[49] The aortic knob and the uppermost portion of the descending aorta have a rather constant abnormal contour. Classically, this

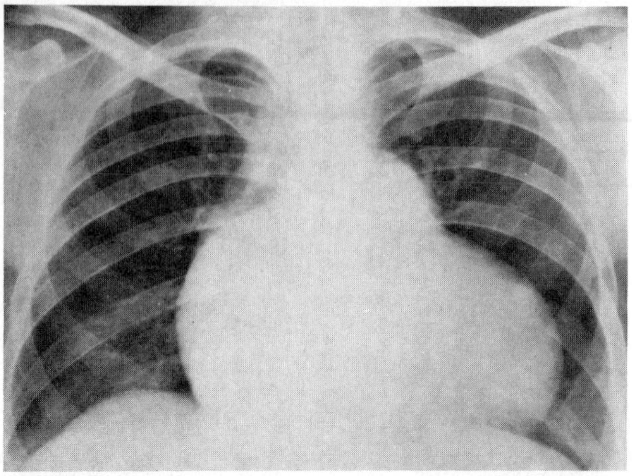

FIGURE 6–33. Pulmonic valvular stenosis with right heart failure. Congenital stenosis of the pulmonic valve in a 38-year-old woman. The shadow of the heart is widened to the left, and the cardiac apex is rounded and elevated because of dilatation of the right ventricle. The tricuspid valve was regurgitant, and the right atrium is markedly enlarged. The main pulmonary artery is dilated, and there is decreased vascularity of the lungs.

is described as having a "figure-three" configuration (Fig. 6–34). The upper convex arc is formed by the aortic knob and the left subclavian artery, while the lower arc represents the dilated portion of the aorta immediately beyond the stenotic area.[50] The indentation on the lateral aortic contour, between the two bulges, marks the site of the coarctation. The aorta also produces a double indentation on the left margin of the barium-filled esophagus, the curves being a mirror image of those on the lateral border of the aorta. In many cases, however, this pathognomonic appearance is not present. Obliteration of the aortic knob, although less specific, is a more constant sign of coarctation.

The aortic knob is not a discrete anatomical structure. It represents the most posterior portion of the aortic arch, distal to the origin of the left subclavian artery as it turns downward to become the descending aorta. Where the curve of the aorta is parallel to the x-ray beam, it is viewed on end and is projected as a circular shadow. The right portion of the shadow cannot be seen as it blends in with the mediastinum, but the remainder of the shadow forms a localized bulge on the left side of the mediastinum—the aortic knob.

When there is coarctation of the aorta, the aortic arch appears to be foreshortened,[51] and the left subclavian artery arises from its descending limb, near the coarcted segment and beyond the aortic knob. The subclavian artery is usually dilated and comes into profile along the left side of the mediastinum, thus overlying and obscuring the medial portion, or all, of the aortic knob (Figs. 6–18 and 6–35).[52] Although obscuration of the knob is suggestive of coarctation, a similar appearance can be caused by enlargement of the supraaortic lymph nodes or by obliteration of the pulmonary recess above the aorta, usually as a result of pleuritis.

Because of the increased resistance to blood flow offered by the coarcted segment, a collateral circulation usually develops between the internal mammary arteries, which arise above the coarctation and the intercostal arteries that join the aorta below the coarcted segment. The intercostal arteries become dilated and tortuous, and the amplitude of their pulsations increases. The constant pounding of the arteries on the undersurfaces of the ribs causes localized erosions of the bone and produces multiple, discrete notches. True rib notches can be distinguished from the normal irregularities of the inferior rib margins because each notch is outlined by a rim of sclerotic bone (Fig. 6–35).

Notching of the ribs, together with obscuration of the aortic knob, is diagnostic of coarctation of the aorta. Absence of rib notching, however, does not exclude the

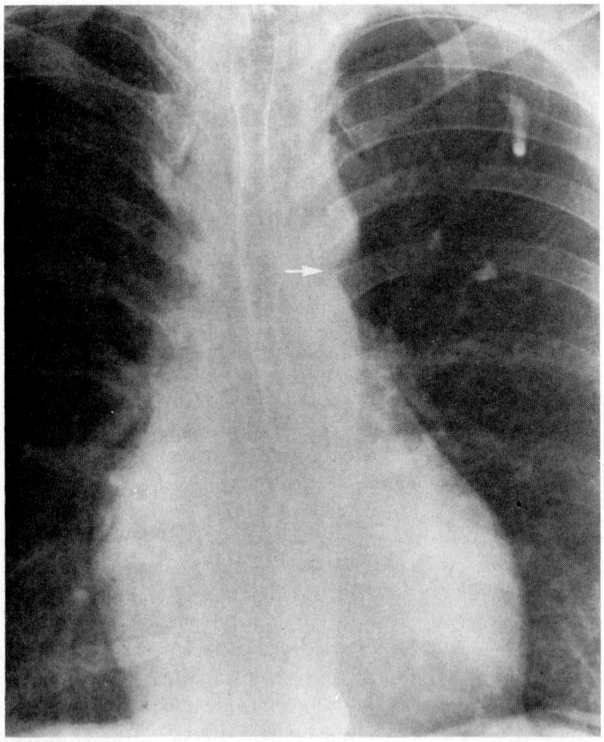

FIGURE 6–34. Coarctation of the aorta. The lateral border of the proximal descending aorta is composed of two arcs separated by a sharp indentation (arrow). The latter represents the site of coarctation. The upper bulge is formed by the dilated left subclavian artery, which obscures the aortic knob, and the lower bulge is caused by poststenotic dilatation of the aorta. The two bulges also indent the barium-coated esophagus. (From Baron, M. G.: Obscuration of the aortic knob in coarctation of the aorta. Circulation *43*:311, 1971, by permission of the American Heart Association, Inc.)

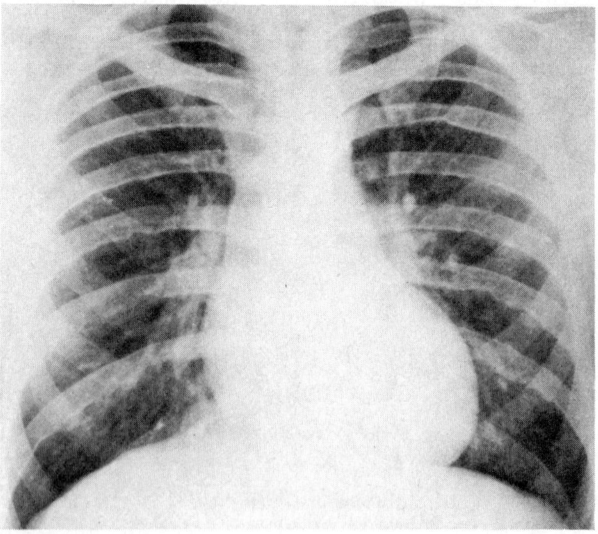

FIGURE 6–35. Coarctation of the aorta. The size of the heart in this young boy is within the limits of normal, but the rounding of the cardiac apex suggests left ventricular hypertrophy. The aortic knob is obscured, and there is notching of the ribs. Each indentation on the undersurface of a rib is outlined by a rim of sclerotic bone, characteristic of the notches that result from pressure atrophy of bone.

diagnosis, since this occurs in almost one-fourth of all adults with coarctation.[53] On the other hand, rib notching alone is not a specific finding. Although coarctation of the aorta is the most common cause, notching does occur in a number of other conditions.[54]

INDICATORS OF CONGENITAL HEART DISEASE

Certain extracardiac abnormalities are commonly associated with anomalies of the heart. Some of these are evident on the chest film and, although it may not be possible to deduce the presence of a specific cardiac lesion from their presence, they do indicate the likelihood of coexisting congenital heart disease.

ABNORMALITIES OF SITUS (See also p. 964). Normally, the apex of the heart is on the same side as the left atrium. Thus, the apex is on the left in situs solitus and on the right in situs inversus. However, in certain anomalies, the cardiac apex may lie on the opposite side and cannot be used as an indicator of situs. Nevertheless, the situs can usually be determined from the chest film. If the aortic knob and the stomach bubble are on the same side, the left atrium will also be on that side.[55] The position of the left atrium indicates the situs of the heart.

Discordance between the cardiac apex and the gastric air bubble—regardless of which side each is on and regardless of the situs of the patient—almost always signifies the presence of ventricular inversion or polysplenia. This does not hold if the abnormal position of the heart is secondary to pulmonary disease. Occasionally, the situs of the patient is indeterminate. The cardiac silhouette is usually abnormal, the apex often cannot be identified, the stomach may be on either side, and the liver shadow extends across the upper abdomen. This picture is diagnostic of asplenia, a syndrome associated with multiple, profound cardiac anomalies.[56–58]

RIGHT AORTIC ARCH. There are two major types of right aortic arch. In the first, the pattern of origin of the great vessels is a mirror image of the pattern found when there is a normal left arch. The first branch to arise from the proximal portion of the arch is a left innominate artery, which divides into the left common carotid artery and the left subclavian artery. The next branch is the right common carotid artery and, lastly, the right subclavian artery (Fig. 6–36*A*). All the vessels lie anterior to the trachea. In the second type of right arch, there is no innominate artery. The first vessel arising from the aorta is the left common carotid artery, followed by the right common carotid and then the right subclavian artery. The left subclavian arises independently as a fourth branch from the aorta. Actually, it does not come directly from the aorta but originates from a diverticulum of the distal arch, which extends to the left behind the esophagus (Fig. 6–36*B*). This last type of right arch is the one most commonly encountered in adults and is not associated with an increased incidence of congenital heart disease. On the other hand, a cardiac anomaly, most often tetralogy of Fallot, is present in over 90 per cent of those patients with a mirror-image type of right arch.[59, 60]

Both types of right aortic arch appear the same on the frontal chest film. The aortic knob is situated on the right side of the mediastinum and displaces the trachea to the left. If the esophagus is opacified, the aortic indentation is seen on its right border. Differentiation between the two types of right arch can be made from the appearance of the barium-filled esophagus in the lateral view. The posterior diverticulum commonly present in the "benign" type of right arch produces a marked, localized anterior bowing of the upper esophagus.[61] With a mirror-image right arch, all the great vessels course in front of the trachea, and the esophagus appears normal in the lateral view.

AZYGOS CONTINUATION OF THE INFERIOR VENA CAVA. When the suprarenal portion of the inferior vena cava fails to develop, blood from the lower extremities, the kidneys, and the retroperitoneum returns to the heart by way of the azygos venous system. Although this may exist as an isolated anomaly, it is often associated with congenital heart disease, particularly the polysplenia syndrome (p. 964). Because of the increased blood flow, the azygos vein is dilated and appears as a rounded mass in the right tracheobronchial angle. The true nature of the mass can often be recognized by means of fluoroscopic examination, since the vein will diminish in size when the patient performs the Valsalva maneuver. In addition, the upper portion of the dilated azygos

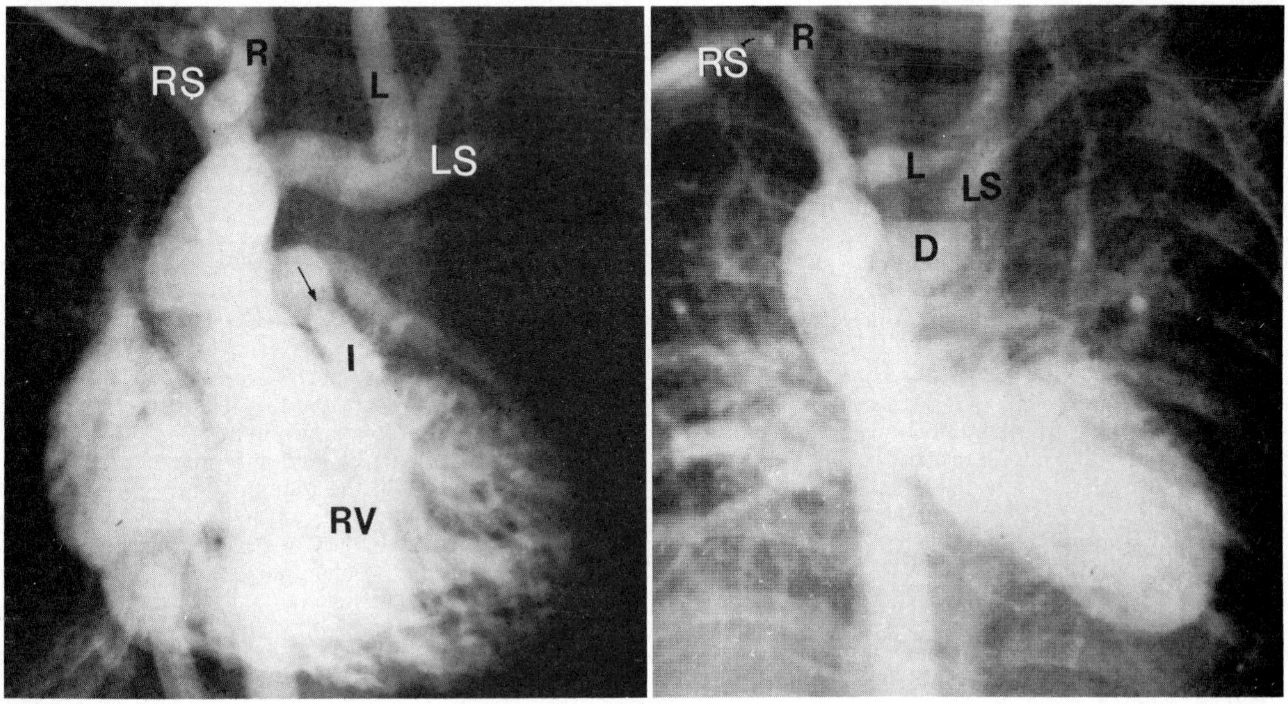

A B

FIGURE 6–36. The two types of right aortic arch. *A*, Mirror-image right arch in tetralogy of Fallot. Following a venous injection of contrast material, the aorta and pulmonary artery become opacified simultaneously. The right ventricle (RV) extends to the left border of the heart and obscures the left ventricle. The infundibulum (I) is narrowed. The pulmonic valve is stenotic (arrow). The first branch to arise from the right aortic arch is the left innominate artery, which gives rise to the left common carotid (L) and the left subclavian artery (LS). The second branch is the right common carotid artery (R) and, lastly, the right subclavian artery (RS). *B*, Right arch with posterior diverticulum. Levocardiogram phase of a venous angiogram. The first branch to arise from the right aortic arch is the left common carotid artery (L), followed by the right common carotid artery (R) and the right subclavian artery (RS). A large diverticulum (D) extends from the distal aortic arch to the left and gives rise to the left subclavian artery (LS). (*B* from Baron, M. G.: Right aortic arch. Circulation *44*:1137, 1971, by permission of the American Heart Association, Inc.)

trunk may be visible on adequately penetrated films along the right side of the vertebral bodies.[62]

Dilatation of the azygos vein does not necessarily signify an abnormality of the inferior vena cava. The vein may be enlarged as a result of congestive failure or portal hypertension. However, in the absence of a known cause for azygos vein dilatation, a femoral venogram may be required to determine whether there is an interruption of the inferior vena cava.

THE PULMONARY VASCULATURE

Almost all the linear shadows within the lung field are cast by the pulmonary arteries and veins. The normal vessels radiate outward from the hila and exhibit an orderly branching pattern as they extend peripherally. The vessels taper gradually, becoming progressively smaller with each successive division. An abrupt change in the caliber of a vessel is abnormal. Vessels at the lung bases are normally larger than those at the apices because they serve a greater volume of lung (Chap. 18). The terminal branches of the arteries and veins, in the outer third of the lungs, are so small that most cannot be visualized as individual structures. Nevertheless, the summation of their shadows imparts a slight overall density to the pulmonary fields. It is often possible to distinguish pulmonary veins from pulmonary arteries because the veins course toward the left atrium and converge to enter the cardiac silhouette at a lower level than do the arteries. In the upper lobes, the vessels follow parallel courses with the vein lateral to the artery.[63]

ALTERATIONS IN PULMONARY BLOOD FLOW

DECREASED PULMONARY BLOOD FLOW. The size of the pulmonary vessels conforms to the volume of blood within them. When flow is diminished, the vessels become narrow, and many of the small branches are no longer visible. Because of the paucity of vascular shadows in the peripheral pulmonary fields, the background density of the lung decreases and the lungs appear abnormally radiolucent.

A regional decrease in perfusion, which can involve as much as an entire lung, is commonly produced by an embolus of a pulmonary artery or one of its branches[64] (p. 1579). A similar change can result from partial obstruction of a vessel because of vasoconstriction or extrinsic compression. In any case, the increase in local vascular resistance causes a redistribution of blood flow to other portions of the lung, and the affected area becomes oligemic.

Diffuse diminution of pulmonary vascularity involving both lungs can occur with right heart failure or in the presence of a right-to-left shunt. In the former instance, the decreased blood flow reflects an abnormally low cardiac output, and the right heart chambers are dilated. When there is a right-to-left shunt, the lungs are oligemic because some of the blood from the right heart bypasses the pulmonary circulation. Usually the main pulmonary artery is small, and its segment on the left cardiac contour may lose its normal convexity or, as in the boot-shaped heart of the tetralogy of Fallot, become concave (Fig. 6–37).

A marked decrease in pulmonary blood flow is usually accompanied by an increase in the bronchial collateral circulation. Although it is possible for the bronchial vessels to become so prominent that the vascularity of the lung actually appears to be increased, the resulting vascular pattern is abnormal. Bronchial arteries arise from the descending aorta and do not radiate out from the pulmonary hilum. Because of the decreased pulmonary arterial flow, the hilar shadows are small. The bronchial vessels do not branch in a regular fashion, and there is little difference between their caliber in the central portions of the lung and in the periphery (Fig. 6–37). This imparts a reticular appearance to the peripheral pulmonary field. Frequently, as the large bronchial arteries leave the aorta, they produce one or more indentations on the anterior border of the barium-filled esophagus.

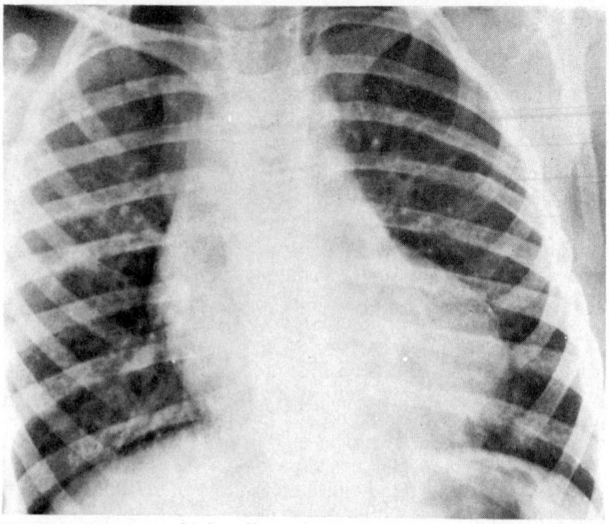

FIGURE 6–37. Bronchial collateral circulation in tetralogy of Fallot. The heart is slightly widened, the apex is rounded and elevated, the prominence of the normal main pulmonary artery is absent, and there is a right aortic arch. These findings are typical of tetralogy of Fallot. Although the pulmonary vasculature does not appear decreased, its pattern is definitely abnormal. The vessels do not radiate from the hilum, do not branch in an orderly fashion, and do not taper as they progress outward into the lungs. This pattern is characteristic of bronchial collateral vessels.

INCREASED PULMONARY BLOOD FLOW. As pulmonary blood flow increases, the vessels in the lungs become enlarged and abnormally prominent. Lesser degrees of overcirculation produce no apparent change in the pulmonary vasculature, and small left-to-right shunts usually cannot be detected on plain films. A moderate increase in pulmonary vascularity can be seen in high-output states such as severe anemia, hyperthyroidism, or pregnancy and with left-to-right shunts. More marked pulmonary plethora is almost always due to a large shunt.

Increased pulmonary blood flow results in dilatation and increasing tortuosity of the pulmonary arteries and veins. The vessels in the periphery of the lungs as well as those at the hila are affected (Fig. 6–28). All of the vessels are enlarged, so that the normal gradation in size between the vessels at the lung bases and those at the apices is maintained. There is nothing specific about the appearance of the pulmonary vessels or their pattern to indicate the cause of the increased blood flow. However, if the patient is cyanotic, the presence of an increased circulation strongly suggests the diagnosis of persistent truncus arteriosus, transposition of the great arteries, or total anomalous venous drainage (Fig. 30–72, p. 962).

PULMONARY HYPERTENSION (See also Chap. 26). A significant increase in pulmonary blood flow causes the pressure within the pulmonary arteries to rise. The roentgen picture reflects the overcirculation of blood through the lungs rather than the degree of elevation of the arterial pressure. On the other hand, when the hypertension results from an increase in pulmonary vascular resistance, the appearance of the lung parenchyma and the pulmonary vessels can provide a rather accurate indicator of pulmonary arterial and venous pressures.[65]

The pattern of vascular changes seen on the x-ray in pulmonary hypertension due to increased vascular resistance depends on the severity of the hypertension and the location of the lesions that impede blood flow through the lungs.[66, 67] Lesions downstream in relation to the pulmonary capillary bed, such as mitral stenosis, or left ventricular failure cause elevation of pulmonary venous pressure, which affects all of the pulmonary veins equally. However, the pressure in the veins at the bases of the lungs is higher than that at the apices in erect persons, because hydrostatic pressure is greatest in the dependent portions of the lungs. With relatively slight increases in venous pressure, the veins tend to dilate, but as the venous pressure increases further, the veins constrict. Venoconstriction occurs first in the higher pressured veins of the lower lungs,[68–70] causing an elevation in local vascular resistance. The pulmonary blood flow is then redistributed to the areas of lesser resistance, the upper portions of the lungs. Radiologically, this is manifested by a reversal of the relative sizes of the pulmonary vessels. The shadows of the vessels at the lung bases become attenuated, while the upper lobe vessels dilate (Fig. 6–30*B*). Further elevation of pulmonary venous pressure usually results in interstitial pulmonary edema and, eventually, alveolar edema.

Narrowing of the small pulmonary arteries, from spasm of their muscular coat or thickening of the medial and intimal layers of their walls, results in precapillary pulmonary hypertension (Chap. 26). Many of the terminal arterial branches are often occluded. The peripheral vessels that remain decrease in size and no longer appear as individual shadows on the film. The outer portions of the lungs then appear more radiolucent than normal, and vascular markings are hardly visible at all.[71] Because of the generalized increase in the peripheral arterial resistance, pressure in the central vessels is elevated, and their elastic walls stretch. Thus, the main pulmonary artery, the right and left pulmonary arteries, and their first- and sometimes second-order branches become dilated. The decrease in the caliber of the vessels beyond this point is abrupt, and many of the branches appear to be amputated (Fig. 6–29).

Although precapillary pulmonary hypertension often occurs without abnormalities on the venous side of the circuit, as in primary pulmonary hypertension (Chap. 26) or pulmonary embolization (Chap. 47), it can also develop as a response to longstanding elevation of pulmonary venous pressure. This is commonly seen with mitral stenosis. Initially, there is a redistribution of pulmonary blood flow and evidence of interstitial edema, but over a period of time the typical picture of precapillary hypertension develops (Chap. 26). Hypertrophy and dilatation of the right atrium and ventricle occur in response to the elevation of pulmonary arterial pressure.

PULMONARY EDEMA

(See also Chap. 18)

In the normal lung, there is a constant transudation of fluid from the pulmonary capillaries into the interstitial tissues. The fluid is drained by an extensive network of pulmonary lymphatics and eventually returns to the bloodstream. If fluid pours into the interstitium faster than it can be removed, the fluid content of the tissue increases. Although the patient may be severely tachypneic during this stage of interstitial edema, there are few, if any, abnormal auscultatory findings. Continued outpouring of fluid so overloads the interstitial tissues that the fluid leaks through the alveolar walls into the pulmonary air spaces.[72] As the alveoli fill, the characteristic bubbly rales of pulmonary edema appear, and the diagnosis becomes clinically obvious. However, the edematous thickening of the interstitial tissues that precedes the stage of alveolar edema produces changes in the roentgen appearance of the lungs that can be detected on the ordinary chest film. These films are a sensitive indicator of the development of pulmonary congestion.

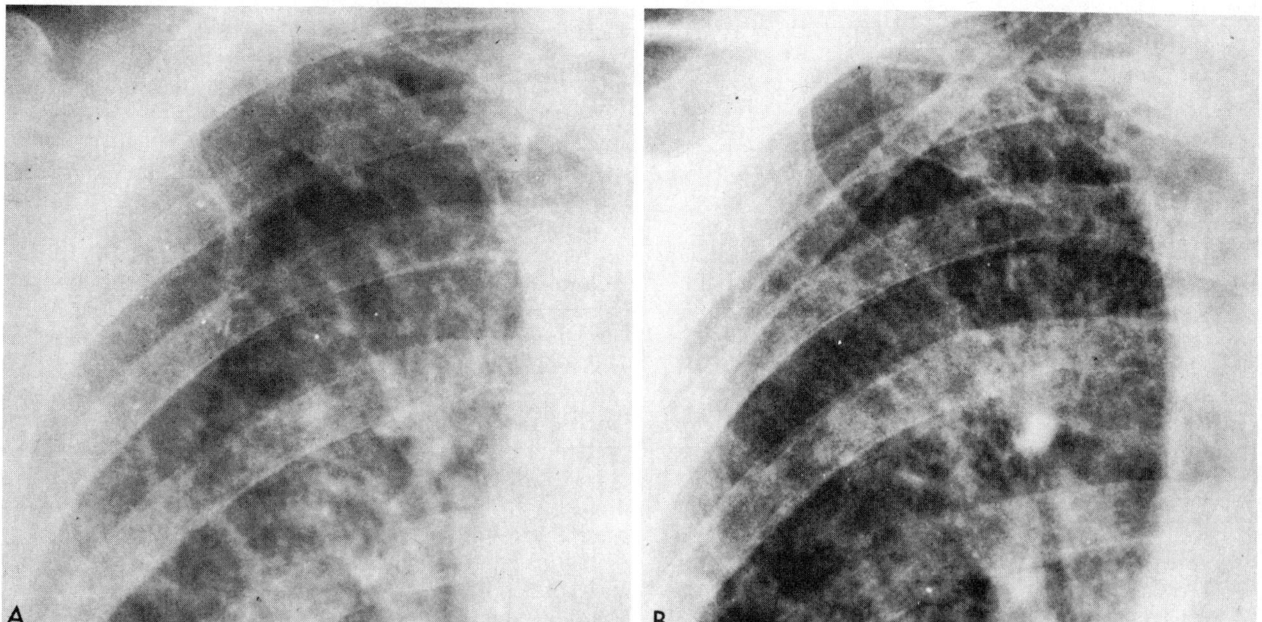

FIGURE 6–38. Interstitial pulmonary edema. *A*, Portable film made shortly after admission for an acute myocardial infarction. The vessels in the right upper lung are prominent and congested. However, their shadows can be delineated. At this time the patient was relatively asymptomatic. *B*, The following day the patient became tachypneic. The portable film shows an increase in the random shadows within the lung, obscuring the outlines of the pulmonary vessels. (From Rabin, C. B., and Baron, M. G.: Radiology of the Chest. Baltimore, Williams and Wilkins Co., 1979.)

INTERSTITIAL EDEMA. The interstitial connective tissues invest the bronchi and bronchioles as well as the pulmonary vessels, lymphatics, and nerves. They support the alveolar air spaces and form the septa that delimit the pulmonary lobules. This reticular interstitial network is too fine to cast recognizable individual shadows on the chest film, but the summation of all their superimposed shadows does contribute an overall, faint homogeneous density to the pulmonary fields.

Even when the interstitial tissues are thickened by edema, most are still too thin to cast discrete shadows. However, their summation now produces numerous, small linear shadows that are randomly distributed throughout the lungs. These overlap and distort the shadows of the pulmonary vessels so that they can no longer be clearly visualized (Fig. 6–38). In addition, where the vessels can be seen, their outlines are indistinct because of the edema of the connective tissue that surrounds them.[73] Convergence of the pulmonary septa in the region of the lung roots causes an accentuation of the background density in this region, producing a perihilar haze (Fig. 6–39).[74]

Where the thickened interlobular septa are viewed on end, they may cast discrete shadows. This occurs most commonly in the outer portions of the lung bases. The edematous septa cast short, horizontal linear shadows that are parallel to each other and perpendicular to the pleural surface and are called Kerley B lines (Fig. 6–40).[75, 76] Kerley A lines also appear when the interstitial tissues are swollen.[77, 78] They are longer than B lines, measuring as much as 4 to 6 cm in length, and are not limited to the basal areas of the lungs. They are situated deep within the lungs and do not extend to the pleural surface (Fig. 6–39).

Edema of the subpleural connective tissue causes an increase in the thickness and density of the interlobar fissures, and often their shadows first become visible with the onset of congestive failure.[79] However, from a practical standpoint this sign is of little value. If the x-ray tube is not aligned perpendicular to the patient, even a thickened fissure will not be visualized because it is projected obliquely rather than on end. Films in an intensive care unit are usually made with portable equipment, and the orientation of the x-ray tube and the patient is determined visually by the technologist. The appearance or disappearance of a pleural fissure most often represents an artifact of positioning rather than the presence or absence of pulmonary congestion (Fig. 6–41).

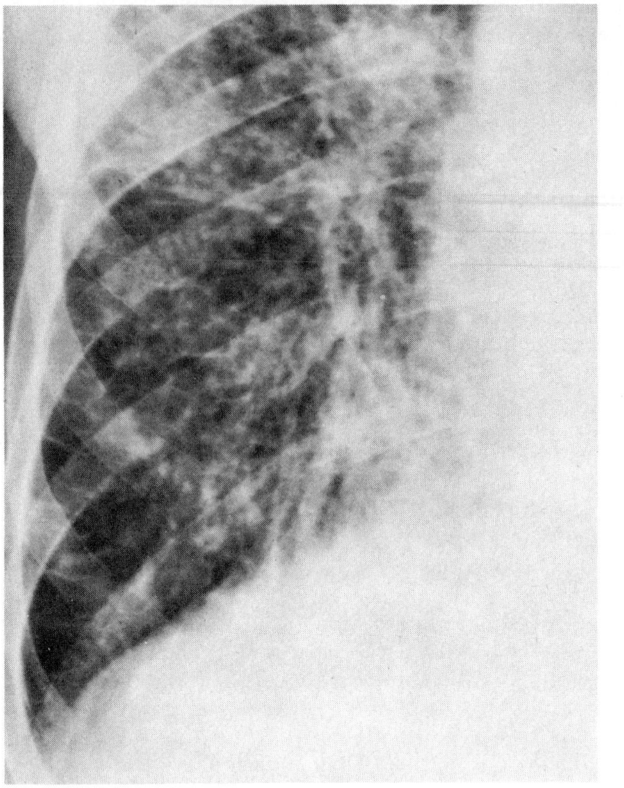

FIGURE 6–40. Interstitial pulmonary edema—Kerley B lines. The short, horizontal linear shadows in the periphery of the right lower lobe represent edematous interlobular septa projected on end. (From Rabin, C. B., and Baron, M. G.: Radiology of the Chest. Baltimore, Williams and Wilkins Co., 1979.)

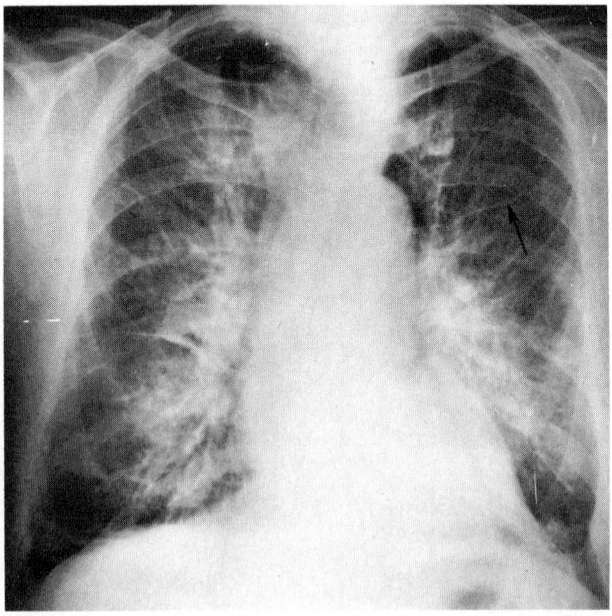

FIGURE 6–39. Interstitial pulmonary edema. There is an indistinct haze in the perihilar regions, and vascular shadows cannot be identified in the peripheral portions of the lungs. The short fissure on the right side is thickened because of subpleural edema, and the linear shadow in the left upper lobe (arrow) is a Kerley A line. (From Rabin, C. B., and Baron, M. G.: Radiology of the Chest. Baltimore, Williams and Wilkins Co., 1979.)

The appearance of peribronchial cuffing is caused by edematous swelling of the bronchial walls and the connective tissue around the bronchi.[80] At least one of the bronchi is usually projected on end near the upper part of the hilum and casts a thin, sharply outlined ring shadow. In the presence of interstitial edema, this shadow becomes broader and indistinct (Fig. 6–41). Vascular congestion is reflected by an increase in the thickness of the artery that accompanies the bronchus, but this is difficult to appreciate unless the diameter of the artery is accurately measured and compared with the diameter of the same vessel on previous films.

The roentgen picture of interstitial edema is not unique, and thickening of the interstitial tissues from almost any cause can produce a similar appearance. However, when thickening is due to fibrosis or lymphangitic carcinomatosis, for example, the shadows tend to be sharply outlined, whereas they are less distinct when due to edema. Magnetic resonance imaging (MRI) (Chap. 12) provides an accurate measure of the amount of lung water and its distribution, independent of perfusion and ventilation abnormalities.[81]

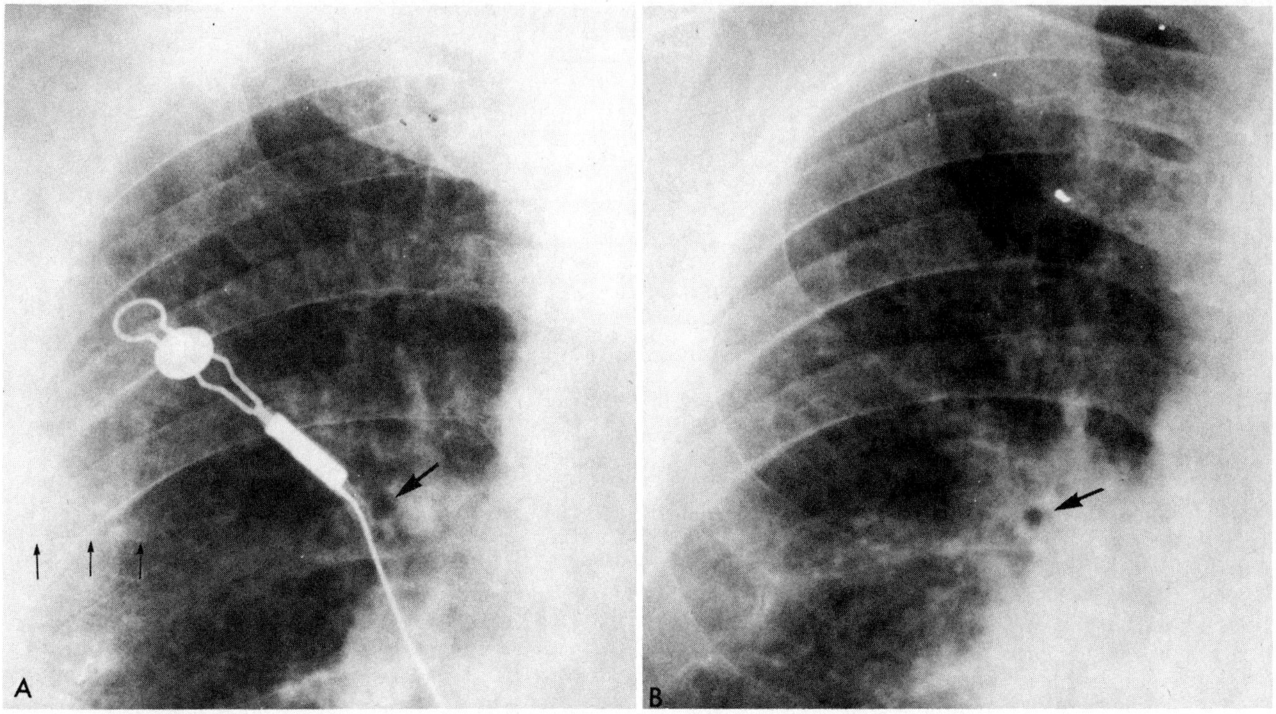

FIGURE 6–41. Interstitial pulmonary edema—peribronchial cuffing. *A*, At the time of this film, the patient was not in congestive heart failure. The vessels in the right upper lung are clearly outlined. The thin circular shadow (oblique arrow) represents a bronchus viewed on end. The outer part of the short fissure (vertical arrows) can be visualized. *B*, Several days later the patient became tachypneic. The pulmonary vessels are now poorly outlined because of edema of the interstitial tissues. The wall of the anterior segmental bronchus (arrow) is thick and hazy as a result of peribronchial edema. The short fissure cannot be identified even though the patient is in failure. This "disappearance" of the fissure is due to a change in the angulation of the x-ray tube in relation to the patient. (From Rabin, C. B., and Baron, M. G.: Radiology of the Chest. Baltimore, Williams and Wilkins Co., 1979.)

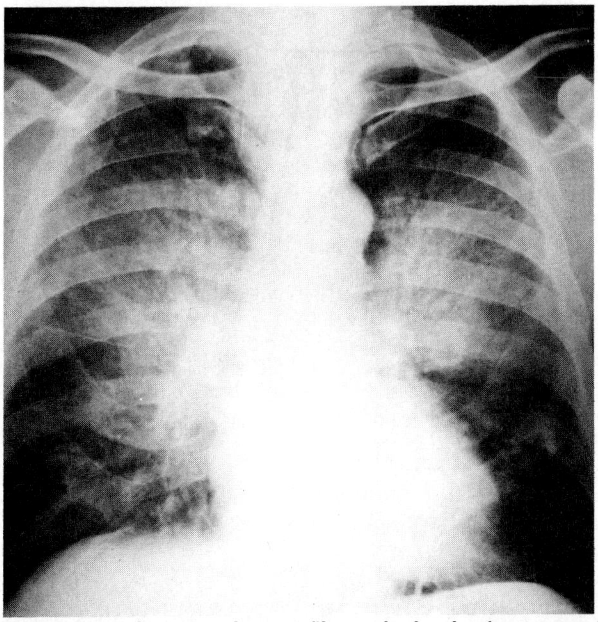

FIGURE 6–42. Pulmonary edema. A film made shortly after myocardial infarction shows hazy areas of increased density in the central portion of each lung. Air-filled bronchi are visualized within the density, indicating that it represents consolidation of lung. The appearance and pattern are characteristic of alveolar pulmonary edema. Because air-filled alveoli are intermingled with fluid-filled ones, the shadows are only moderately dense and are not homogeneous. (From Rabin, C. B., and Baron, M. G.: Radiology of the Chest. Baltimore, Williams and Wilkins Co., 1979.)

ALVEOLAR EDEMA. The shadows of alveolar edema appear when the air in the alveoli is replaced by fluid. The appearance differs from other causes of pulmonary consolidation mainly in the distribution of the opacities and in the rapidity with which their pattern can change. It is uncommon for all the alveoli in any area to be completely filled with fluid. The intermingling of alveoli partially filled with air and fluid-filled alveoli results in a less dense shadow than in many forms of pneumonia, in which the regional involvement tends to be more uniform. The confluent, patchy densities of pulmonary edema tend to involve the inner two-thirds of the lungs and create the appearance of wings extending outward from the mediastinum (Fig. 6–42).[82] Most often, both lungs are equally affected, but on occasion only one lung appears edematous.[83] This usually represents a transitory state, and within a day or two the typical hazy patchy shadows appear in the opposite lung.

Oxygen toxicity, acquired respiratory distress syndrome, or bronchopneumonia can produce a roentgen picture similar to that of pulmonary edema. In general, however, the shadows in these conditions are more stable, whereas those of pulmonary edema tend to change rapidly, clearing in one area and appearing in another. Such evanescent shadows are also characteristic of eosinophilic pneumonia, but this is asssociated with a peripheral eosinophilia not present in pulmonary edema.

THE PERICARDIUM

(See also Chap. 44)

The pericardium is a closed, invaginated sac that completely surrounds the heart except for a small area on its posterior surface where the pulmonary veins enter the left atrium. The visceral layer of pericardium is intimately applied to the heart and to the great arteries and veins. It is reflected from these vessels and doubles back to form the outer wall of the sac, the parietal pericardium. A small amount of fluid, 20 to 30 ml, is usually contained within the pericardial cavity.

PERICARDIAL EFFUSION

As fluid collects in the pericardial space, the parietal pericardium is pushed outward, increasing the size of the cardiac silhouette. The fluid fills in all the recesses between the cardiac structures and smoothes out the normal bulges and indentations of the cardiac contours. The end result is a smoothly distended, flask-shaped cardiac shadow. Even though there may be no tamponade, cardiac pulsations are diminished because of the damping effect of the fluid. These characteristics of a pericardial effusion are not specific, and almost identical findings can be caused by a failing heart with generalized dilatation of the cardiac chambers and decreased myocardial contractility.

The two conditions usually can be distinguished by the appearance of the pulmonary hila. The pericardial sac extends to the level of the bifurcation of the main pulmonary artery, or slightly above. Therefore, as it distends laterally, it tends to cover up the shadows of the hilar vessels.[15] On the other hand, the failing heart is associated with pulmonary congestion and abnormally prominent vessels. This distinction can be made from the frontal chest film and does not require fluoroscopy (Fig. 6–43).

A second, and pathognomonic, sign of a pericardial effusion is displacement of the epicardial fat line. A variable amount of fat is usually present beneath the epicardium, particularly around the coronary vessels in the atrioventricular and interventricular sulci. With increasing age, the accumulation of fatty tissue tends to increase and spreads between the epicardium and the walls of the ventricles. The layer of fat over the anterior surface of the heart is projected on end in the lateral view and appears as a relatively radiolucent band abutting the retrosternal soft tissues. The shadows of the pericardium and epicardium are not discrete, because they blend imperceptibly with the shadow of the retrosternal soft tissues. When the latter tissues contain a fair amount of fat, they form a second lucent band, immediately behind the sternum. The two layers of pericardium and the small amount of fluid can then be seen as a fine linear soft tissue shadow between the two bands (Fig. 6–44*B*). Their combined shadow is normally no thicker than 2 mm. The pericardial shadow can be identified in about 40 per cent of routine lateral chest films.[84]

As fluid collects between the layers of pericardium, the pericardial soft tissue stripe becomes progressively wider and displaces the epicardial fat line away from the sternum into the cardiac silhouette (Fig. 6–44*C*). This line is more easily identified by fluoroscopy than on plain films.[85] Absence of an identifiable fat line has no significance. Relatively small amounts of pericardial effusion can be detected by computed tomography (p. 364). In addition to indicating the volume of the effusion, the scan also provides an indication of the nature of the fluid. For example, a hemopericardium casts a denser shadow and therefore has a higher CT number than a simple serous effusion.[86]

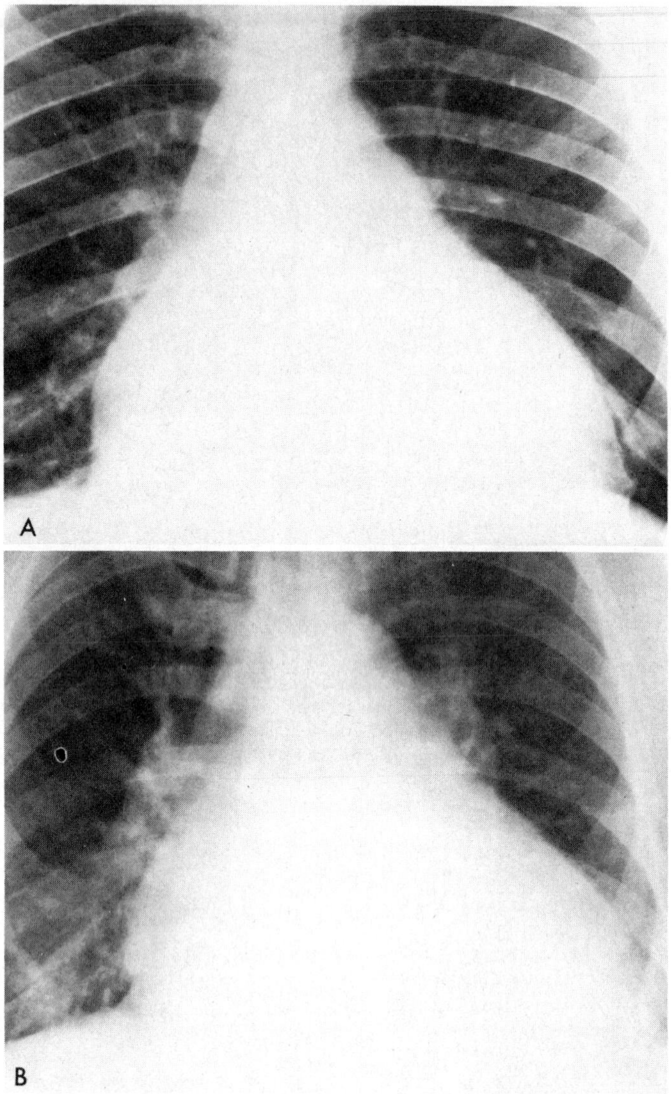

FIGURE 6–43. Differentiation between pericardial effusion and a dilated heart. *A*, Pericardial effusion. The cardiac silhouette is markedly enlarged, and its contours are smoothed out. Most of the right hilum and all of the left hilum are obscured by the shadow of the heart. *B*, Cardiac failure. The cardiac silhouette is enlarged, and its contours are smoothed out. However, in this case the hilar vessels are dilated, and both hilar shadows are abnormally prominent.

CONSTRICTIVE PERICARDITIS

In most cases of constrictive pericarditis the appearance of the heart is nonspecific. The heart is often small or normal in size but may be enlarged.[87] Cardiac pulsations are usually diminished but can be normal. Calcification of the pericardium (Figs. 6–22 and 6–44*A*) is the one finding that is suggestive of constrictive pericarditis. It is usually a sequel to tuberculous pericardial infection. Since this is a relatively rare cause of pericarditis at present, pericardial calcification is absent in almost 90 per cent of cases of constrictive pericarditis.[88] Conversely, the presence of

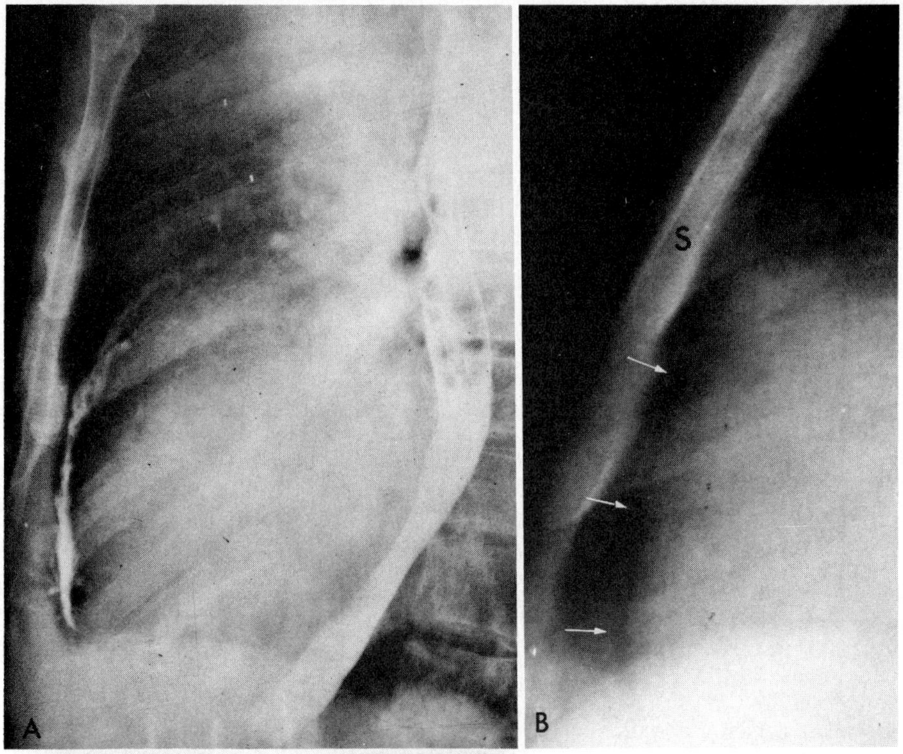

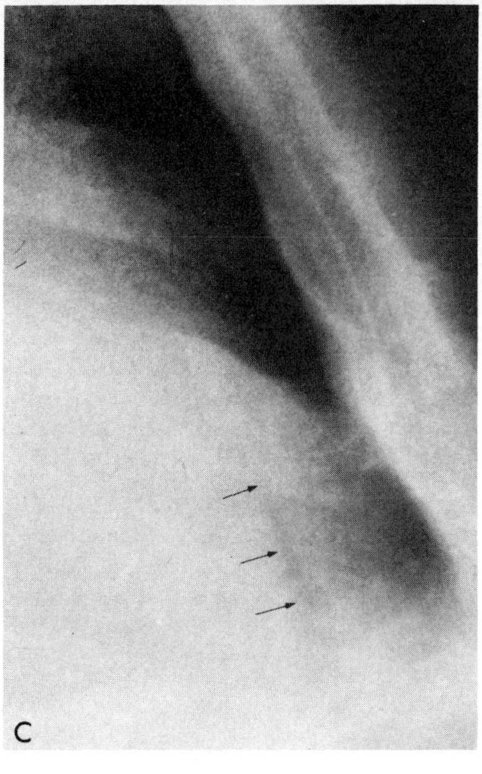

FIGURE 6–44. Pericardial shadows. *A*, pericardial calcification. The calcified pericardium casts a linear shadow behind the lucency of the retrosternal fat and in front of the lucency of the epicardial fat. The patient had tuberculous pericarditis many years previously. *B*, Routine lateral chest film of another patient shows a considerable accumulation of fat in the retrosternal region. The fine linear soft tissue density (arrows) represents the two layers of pericardium and the small amount of fluid normally between them. The lucency between the pericardium and the cardiac silhouette is caused by fat beneath the epicardium. S = sternum. *C*, Right lateral chest film. The epicardial fat line (arrows) is displaced backward. The broad band of density between the epicardial fat and the retrosternal fat represents the two layers of pericardium and a collection of fluid between them. (From Baron, M. G.: Interlobar effusion. Circulation *44*:475, 1971, by permission of the American Heart Association, Inc.)

pericardial calcification is not diagnostic of constrictive pericarditis and can occur without any evidence of restriction of the heart. A diagnosis of pericarditis can be made, in the absence of pericardial calcification, by computed tomography which demonstrates the thickening of the pericardium (p. 364).[89, 90]

CONGENITAL ABSENCE OF THE PERICARDIUM

The most common form of this anomaly is absence of the left pericardium. This is almost always associated with a defect in the mediastinal portion of the left parietal pleura, so that the pericardial space and the pleural space communicate with each other. The appearance of the heart on the frontal chest film is characteristic.[91] Although the trachea remains in the midline, the cardiac shadow is shifted into the left hemithorax. The pulmonary artery segment is abnormally prominent and is sharply demarcated from the shadow of the aortic knob. The left ventricle is elongated and has a broad area of contact with the diaphragm (Fig. 6–45). Fluoroscopic findings are unique. The mobility of the heart is markedly increased, and it appears to bounce around wildly with each beat. A similar type of hyperactivity may be seen with a pneumopericardium. Here, too, the restraining effect of the pericardium is absent. However, with pneumopericardium, the heart is not displaced from its normal position. If necessary, the

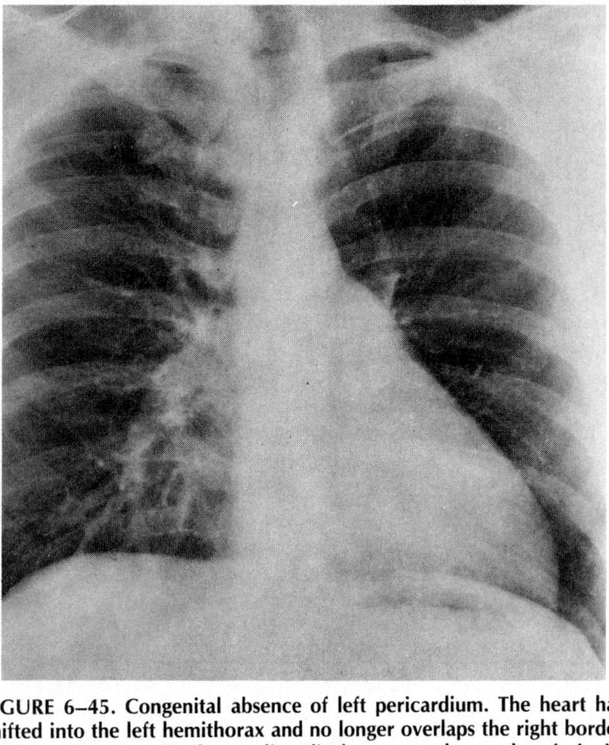

FIGURE 6–45. Congenital absence of left pericardium. The heart has shifted into the left hemithorax and no longer overlaps the right border of the spine. Despite the cardiac displacement, the trachea is in its normal position. The main pulmonary artery is prominent and is sharply demarcated from the aortic knob.

diagnosis of absent left pericardium can be confirmed by inducing left pneumothorax. Because the pleural and pericardial spaces are no longer separated, the injected air will appear between the diaphragm and the heart and beneath the intact right pericardium.

Partial absence of the pericardium is rare. It can occur on either side but is more common on the left. In some cases, the appearance of the heart is entirely normal, and the defect is found incidentally at surgery or at autopsy. If the left atrial appendage herniates through the defect, it will bulge from the left cardiac border,[92] and distinction from a mediastinal tumor or mitral valvular disease may be difficult on plain films. Fluoroscopy usually shows increased pulsation of the appendage if the pericardium is absent. A similar bulge on the right side of the heart can be caused by herniation of the right atrial appendage.[93]

ANGIOCARDIOGRAPHY

In order to visualize the internal anatomy of the heart, the radiodensity of the blood must be increased so that it will contrast with the cardiac soft tissue structures. Rapid serial films are required to record the passage of the opacified blood through the heart and provide information regarding the function of the cardiac chambers and the pattern of blood flow within the heart and great vessels.

TECHNIQUE

Opacification of the blood is accomplished by the intravascular injection of a radiopaque contrast material. All the angiographic media used currently are solutions of organic iodine compounds. The quantity of iodine delivered per unit time and the volume of blood into which it is delivered determine the degree of opacification of the blood on the angiocardiogram. This in turn depends on the concentration of the contrast material and the speed with which it is injected. As the concentration of iodine in the contrast agent is increased, the viscosity also increases, and it becomes more difficult to inject. Thus, a contrast material that is moderately concentrated but more liquid is usually preferable to a denser but thicker one. In order to minimize dilution of the radiopaque bolus by nonopacified blood, the contrast material must be introduced rapidly and as close to the point of interest as possible. This requires selective catheterization of the vessel or chamber and the use of a pressure injector[94] or the use of digital angiography (p. 356).

The radiological equipment used for angiocardiography must be able to provide sharply detailed pictures in rapid sequence. The image on the output screen of the image intensifier is photographed by a 35-mm cine camera, usually at the rate of 30 or 60 frames per second or on 100- to 105-mm film at a rate of 6 to 12 frames per second. As the images are recorded on the film, they can also be seen on the television monitor, so that the entire procedure is carried out under fluoroscopic control.

The internal structure of the heart is complex, and multiple views are usually needed in order to delineate the pertinent anatomy adequately. If only a single changer or image intensifier is available, a separate injection of contrast material is required for each view. Because the quantity of contrast material that can be given safely to a patient is limited, it is difficult, especially in children, to obtain a complete study during one catheterization without biplane equipment. A cardiac catheterization laboratory, unless designed solely for coronary arteriography, should have the capability of obtaining simultaneous biplane films.[95]

There is no one set of optimal views for all of angiocardiography. Projections are chosen depending on the nature of the cardiac lesion and the area of the heart to be visualized. Thus, frontal and lateral views will effectively demonstrate infundibular narrowing, ventricular septal defect, and stenosis of the pulmonic valve associated with tetralogy of Fallot. But, in order to visualize adequately the supravalvular region of the pulmonary artery in the same patient, it is necessary to angle the equipment or prop up the patient, so that the frontal x-ray beam is oriented toward the patient's head, anteriorly. Evaluation of left ventricular contractility is best accomplished from films made in the left and right oblique projections. Complex angled views, in which the x-ray tube is tilted in relation to the coronal, sagittal, and cross-sectional planes of the patient, were first used for delineation of the coronary arteries (Fig. 10–14, p. 280) but have proved to be of great value in the study of congenital cardiac lesions.[96–98] These angled views can be obtained by turning the patient and propping the patient partially upright, by rotating the patient and angling the x-ray tube, or by rotating and angling the x-ray tube while the patient remains supine. Each method requires specific types of equipment and has its own advantages and disadvantages.

COMPLICATIONS

The hazards of selective angiocardiography fall into two major groups: those due to mechanical trauma from the catheter and from the force of the injected stream of contrast material, and those due to the pharmacological effects of the contrast media.

CARDIAC PERFORATION. Mechanical trauma can result in perforation of the heart or dissection of the contrast material into the myocardium. *Perforation of a ventricle* usually has no serious sequelae.[99] The muscular wall contracts around the puncture site once the catheter is removed, and there is only minor leakage of blood into the pericardium. The perforation should be recognized before injection of the main bolus of contrast material if a small test injection is routinely made to confirm the position of the catheter. Contrast material injected into the pericardium may cause considerable pain, but this can be controlled with medication and usually abates within a day or so. Although the quantity of contrast material injected is usually not enough to produce cardiac tamponade, the solution is hypertonic and will increase in volume as it draws fluid into the pericardial cavity. Most of the contrast material can be withdrawn by pericardiocentesis, so that thoracotomy is usually not required.

Perforation of an atrium is a more serious consequence of catheterization. The thinner atrial wall does not seal off the puncture site as well as does the ventricular wall, and a greater outpouring of blood into the pericardium usually accompanies atrial perforation. Although this may cause cardiac tamponade, the bleeding often ceases spontaneously. Therefore, it is not necessary to rush the patient to the operating room once the perforation is discovered. The catheter should be removed and the patient's vital signs carefully monitored. Accumulation of blood in the pericardium can be detected and measured by echocardiography (Fig. 5–102, p. 127).

INTRAMURAL INJECTION. Intramural deposition of contrast material usually results when the catheter tip is trapped by muscular trabeculae and cannot recoil during the injection. The full force of the fluid jet issuing from the catheter is thus applied to the endocardium. Small intramural dissections are usually of no consequence; however, if a critical portion of the conduction system is involved, significant arrhythmias can result. A large intramural deposit is more serious because of the volume of myocardium that is injured. Rarely, a myocardial infarct results. The intramural location of the contrast material is easily recognized because it appears denser than the opacified blood within the cardiac lumen and because it persists for some time after the opacified blood is cleared from the heart.

Even though there is no evidence of intramural injection, the force of the jet of contrast material impinging on the ventricular wall can cause an episode of arrhythmia. Most often, this is simply a self-limited short run of extrasystoles. However, heart block or ventricular tachycardia is encountered on rare occasions and may require medication or cardioversion. The jet effect can be largely avoided through careful technique and proper catheter design. The velocity of the jet exiting from the tip of the catheter can be decreased if there are side holes near the tip.[100] The use of balloon-tipped catheters has almost completely solved this problem, since contrast material exiting from holes in the side of the catheter is kept away from the wall of the heart by means of the balloon at the catheter tip.

COMPLICATIONS OF CONTRAST AGENTS. All angiocardiographic contrast agents are relatively radiopaque because they contain iodine. Until recently, almost all were ionic solutions of meglumine and sodium salts of organic iodine compounds. They all cause similar hemodynamic changes and alterations in cardiac function. The newer, nonionic agents that are now generally available show the same side effects[101] but to a significantly lesser extent.[102] The exact mechanism of the changes is not completely understood; they probably are the result of multiple factors: the hyperosmolarity of the contrast solution,[103] the quantity injected, and the pharmacological effects and myocardial toxicity of the iodine and sodium. In addition, some of the additives in the contrast agents, such as EDTA and sodium citrate, may play a role because of their propensity to bind calcium.

Within a minute or two of the intravascular injection of contrast material, peripheral vasodilation occurs and results in systemic hypotension. At the same time there is a significant, transient expansion in plasma volume.[104, 105] After the first three or four heartbeats, hemodynamic evidences of reduced myocardial contractility begin to appear. There is a reduction in the left ventricular systolic pressure, an increase in heart rate, and an increase in the left ventricular endiastolic volume and endiastolic pressure[106, 107] together with elevation of pressure in the left atrium and pulmonary artery. These changes gradually revert to normal over a period of 10 to 20 minutes. The cardiac changes appear most rapidly following selective injections into the coronary arteries but the systemic effects are less marked. Reaction to the injection of contrast material in normal patients is different from that in patients with coronary artery disease, and this may be used as a rough test of ventricular function.[108]

All the contrast agents have a slight but definite toxicity, primarily to the kidneys[109] and central nervous system. Some patients exhibit a mild allergic reaction, usually in the form of hives, but anaphylactic reactions are extremely rare. Sensitivity testing is of no value in identifying those patients who will react adversely to the contrast material.[110] Patients with previous allergic history are more prone to develop a reaction, but this does not constitute an absolute contraindication to angiocardiography.[111] Most reactions can be avoided by premedication with antihistamines or steroids or both. Contrast material is not well tolerated and may prove fatal in patients with marked elevations of pulmonary vascular resistance. This is especially true with selective injections into the right ventricle or main pulmonary artery. Those patients with right ventricle end-diastolic pressure of over 20 mmHg are at the greatest risk. The cause of the reaction is not known but seems to be related to the osmolarity of the contrast material.[99]

Hives and other minor allergic reactions can be successfully managed with antihistaminics. More severe reactions, namely respiratory arrest or cardiac arrest, usually require intubation and assisted ventilation as well as vasopressor agents to maintain blood pressure. Convulsive seizures tend to be self-limited and can be controlled with barbiturates or diazepam. Because iodine compounds are excreted by the kidneys, mostly through glomerular filtration, the hypertonic effects of the contrast material can be increased and prolonged by dehydration, especially in the presence of renal disease. Therefore, patients should be well hydrated before an angiographic study.[112]

ANGIOCARDIOGRAPHIC INTERPRETATION

The multiple films of an angiocardiographic sequence contain considerable information regarding cardiac anatomy and function. Rather than attempting to comprehend everything at once, it is preferable to review the films in a systematic fashion. Films should be scanned several times, with a different aspect of the study being evaluated at each reading. Such an orderly approach lessens the chances of overlooking significant findings and simplifies their correct interpretation. Eventually, this structured type of approach becomes a habit, no longer requiring a conscious effort.

DIRECTION OF BLOOD FLOW. Except for the occasional artifact due to a ventricular arrhythmia or interference of a catheter with closure of a valve, the flow of the radiopaque bolus on an angiocardiogram can be assumed to represent the true pattern of blood flow in that heart. Normally, blood flows through the heart in only one direction, and the sequence of opacification of the cardiac chambers is always the same. Only those chambers and vessels downstream in relation to the site of injection of the contrast material will be visualized. The angiocardiogram is completed once the opacified blood flows through the major systemic arteries. The flow rate of blood through the various organs varies greatly, and the original bolus of contrast material returns to the great veins over a period of time and is too diluted to allow revisualization of the cardiac chambers. The occasional exception is seen in infants and young children in whom the right atrium and ventricle may be reopacified by the venous return from the cerebral circulation. In older children and adults such revisualization is almost never seen except in the presence of a large, peripheral arteriovenous fistula. Deviations from the normal pattern of blood flow fall into two groups: (1) opacification of a chamber or vessel before its proper turn, indicating that the direction of blood flow is normal but that one or more of the intermediate structures is bypassed; and (2) the direction of blood flow is reversed, and a chamber or vessel upstream to the point of injection becomes opacified.

RIGHT-TO-LEFT SHUNTS. Premature visualization of a chamber or vessel is the result of a right-to-left shunt and indicates the presence of an abnormal communication between the two sides of the heart. However, pressures in the left cardiac chambers are normally higher than those on the right side, so that the flow through an uncomplicated atrial septal defect, for example, should be from left to right. In order for the flow to travel in the opposite direction, there must be a reversal of the pressure differential between the two sides of the heart, and this implies the presence of a second lesion. Most often, the pressures on the right side are abnormally high because of either increased resistance to emptying, as in tricuspid atresia (Fig. 30–55, p. 950) or pulmonic stenosis, or diastolic overloading, as in total anomalous pulmonary venous drainage. Less commonly, the pressures in the left heart and aorta are lower than normal because of an upstream obstruction, as in mitral atresia or preductal coarctation of the aorta.

In either case, the obstruction must lie beyond the chamber from which the shunt originates but upstream in relation to the recipient chamber or vessel. Thus, if there is a right-to-left shunt through an atrial septal defect, and there is no diastolic overloading of the atrium, the cause of the increased resistance to flow can be present anywhere from the tricuspid valve to the point of entry of the pulmonary veins into the left atrium. Although a lesion beyond the left atrium, such as mitral or aortic stenosis, can result in elevation of the right atrial pressure, it causes an even greater elevation of left atrial pressure, so that the shunt would still be from left to right.

At times, two lesions can be localized from the sequence of opacification of the cardiac chambers. If contrast material injected into the right atrium first opacifies the left atrium, then the left ventricle, and finally the right ventricle, the presumptive diagnosis is tricuspid atresia with a right-to-left shunt through the atrial septum and a left-to-right shunt through a ventricular septal defect (Fig. 6–46).[113, 114] More often, the abnormal flow pattern simply indicates the general location of the lesions, and a definitive diagnosis depends upon identification of specific anatomical abnormalities. If the opacified blood flows from the right atrium into the right ventricle as well as into the left atrium, a second injection of contrast material into the right ventricle is usually required in order to study the infundibular region of the right ventricle, the pulmonic valve, and the pulmonary circulation (see Figs. 30–43, p. 942, 30–44, p. 943, and 30–45, p. 943).

Premature visualization of the descending aorta from an injection into the right side of the heart indicates reversed flow through a patent ductus arteriosus. This is most often due to preductal coarctation of the aorta.[115] The ascending aorta and the subclavian and carotid arteries are not visualized because they are filled by antegrade flow of nonopacified blood from the left ventricle. However, if the entire aorta is opacified through the ductus, the pressure in the ascending aorta must be similar to that in the descending aorta, and the possibility of a coarctation is excluded (Fig. 6–46). Usually, this pattern of flow is seen with hypoplasia of the left heart[116, 117] but is rarely caused by severe pulmonary hypertension.[118]

Rare exceptions to the rule that two lesions are needed to produce a right-to-left shunt are a pulmonary arteriovenous fistula and anomalous drainage of a systemic vein (such as a persistent left superior vena cava) into the left atrium.[119]

LEFT-TO-RIGHT SHUNTS. Opacification of a chamber or vessel upstream in relation to the site of injection of the contrast material results from a left-to-right shunt or when a cardiac valve is incompetent. Some retrograde filling of the inferior or superior vena cava from the right atrium or of the pulmonary veins from the left atrium is not abnormal because the orifices of these vessels are not guarded by valves.

Accurate localization of a left-to-right shunt is usually

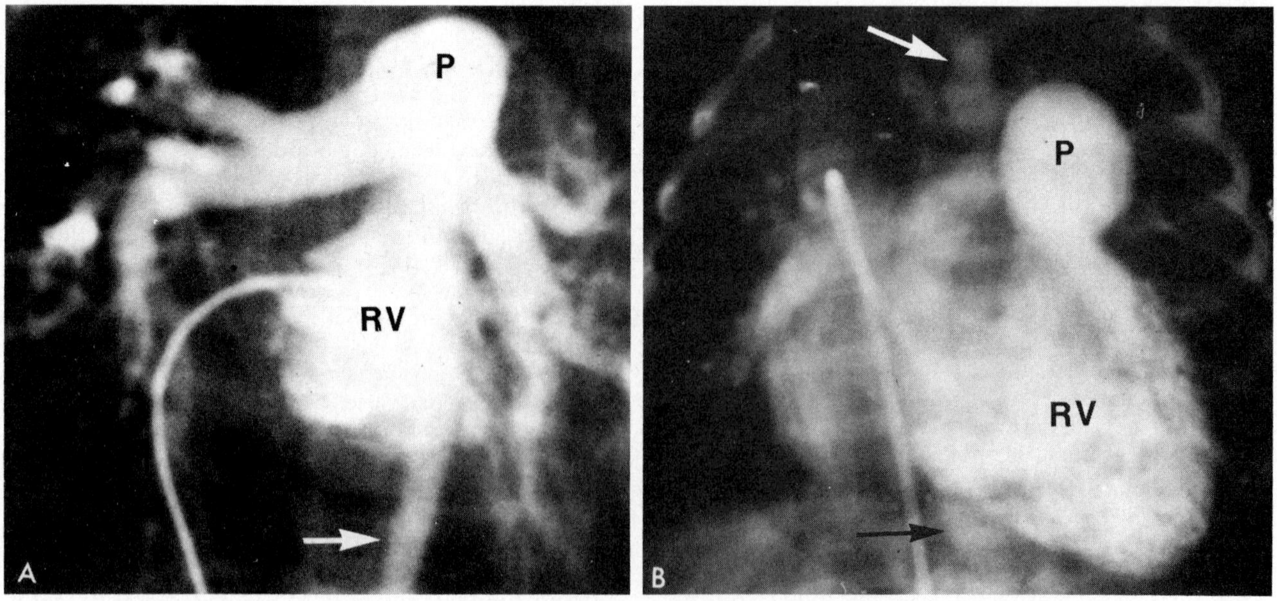

FIGURE 6–46. Patent ductus arteriosus and right-to-left shunt. *A*, Preductal coarctation. Contrast material has been injected selectively into the right ventricle (RV). The descending aorta (arrow) is filled through a patent ductus from the pulmonary artery (P). The ascending aorta and great vessels are not opacified. *B*, Hypoplastic left heart syndrome and interruption of the inferior vena cava. A catheter inserted into the femoral vein reaches the heart by way of the azygos vein, and contrast material is injected selectively into the right ventricle (RV). Both the ascending aorta (white arrow) and the descending aorta (black arrow) are filled from the pulmonary artery (P) by way of a patent ductus arteriosus.

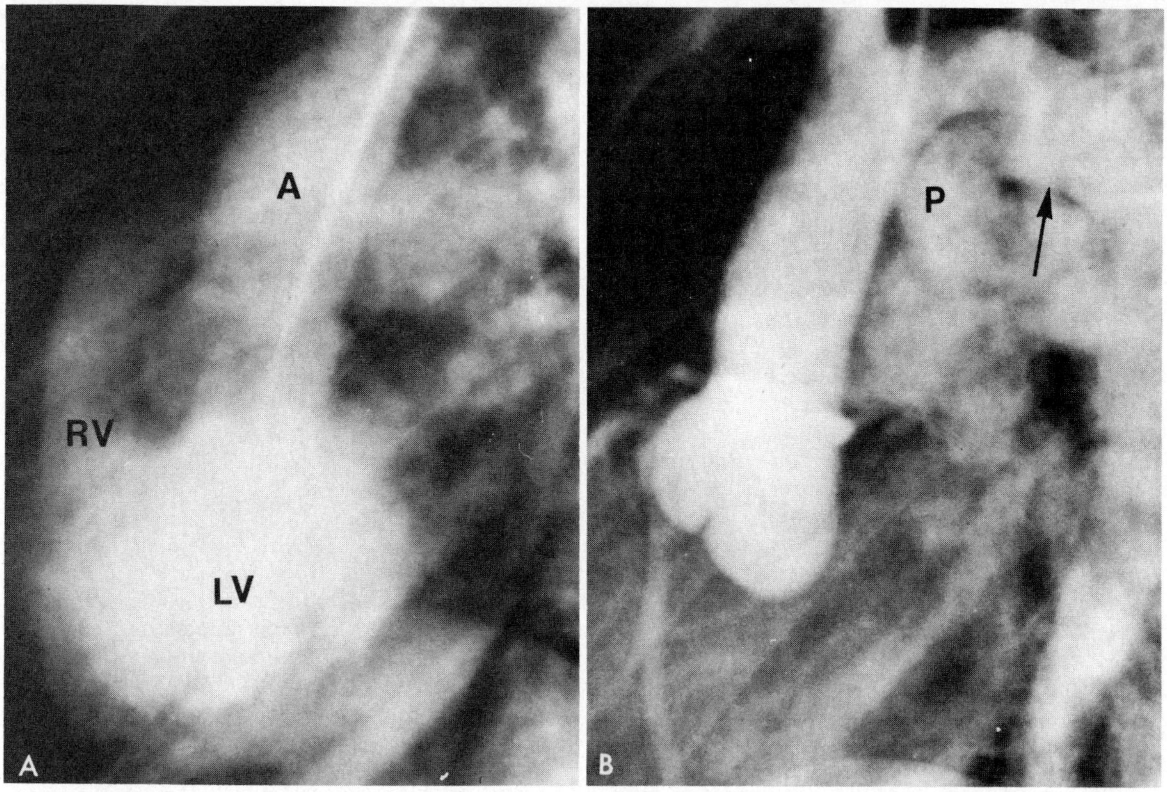

FIGURE 6–47. Multiple left-to-right shunts. *A*, Left ventriculogram, lateral view. Contrast material injected into the left ventricle (LV) flows rapidly across a large ventricular septal defect into the right ventricle (RV). The pulmonary artery is opacified by antegrade flow from the right ventricle. Although the aorta (A) is well opacified, it is not possible to identify a patent ductus arteriosus. *B*, The catheter was withdrawn into the ascending aorta, and a second injection was made. This time the pulmonary artery (P) is opacified by way of a patent ductus arteriosus (arrow). (From Angrissola, A. B., and Puddu, V. [eds.]: Cardiologia D'Oggia. Torino, C. B. Edizion Scientifiche, 1976.)

possible when the jet of opacified blood crossing the defect between the two sides of the heart can be identified.[120, 121] This usually requires selective injection of contrast material into the chamber from which the shunt arises. If the shunt itself is not visualized, it may be possible to establish the diagnosis by correlating the appearance of the opacified blood on the right side of the heart with the filling of the left-heart structures. For example, if, following a supraaortic injection of contrast material, the pulmonary artery does not become opacified until the proximal descending aorta is filled, a patent ductus is most likely. However, filling of the pulmonary artery when only the ascending aorta is opacified is indicative of an aorticopulmonary window.

In some instances, the defect cannot be localized with certainty without two or more selective angiograms. If the right atrium becomes opacified during the levocardiogram phase of a right ventriculogram, the presence of an atrial septal defect is most likely. However, the shunt could have originated in the left ventricle (atrioventricular septal defect) or in the aorta (ruptured sinus of Valsalva aneurysm). A left ventricular injection, and possibly an aortogram, is required to exclude these lesions. A similar picture can be caused by anomalous drainage of a pulmonary vein into the right atrium. The abnormal venous connection can be demonstrated by selective injections into the right and left pulmonary arteries. When there is more than one left-to-right shunt, only the most proximal one that is opacified can be identified with certainty. For example, opacification of the right ventricle from a left ventricular injection indicates the presence of a ventricular septal defect. Forward flow of the opacified blood from the right ventricle rapidly fills the pulmonary artery, and it is usually not possible to recognize the presence of an associated patent ductus arteriosus. A second injection above the aortic valve is needed to evaluate this possibility (Fig. 6–47) or the presence of aortic septal defect (Fig. 30–21, p. 925).

CARDIAC CHAMBERS

The size of a cardiac chamber has little diagnostic specificity. Although a chamber may be small because of malseptation, more commonly this is the result of a decreased volume load because of an anomaly that allows blood to bypass the chamber during embryonic life. Thus, tricuspid atresia (Fig. 30–55, p. 950) or pulmonary valve atresia with an intact ventricular septum (Fig. 30–47) is associated with a small right ventricle. A small left ventricle is often associated with a double-outlet right ventricle (Fig. 30–70, p. 961), and when the aortic or mitral valve is atretic, the ventricle may be represented only by an endocardium-lined slit.

When estimating chamber size from the angiogram, it is important to consider the size of the other cardiac chambers, a possible source of distortion. Enlargement of the right ventricle causes posterior displacement of the ventricular septum and the left ventricle. The left ventricle may be rotated medially, so that its lateral projection resembles that normally seen in the left anterior oblique view. The shadow of the ventricle is thus foreshortened, and the chamber, although normal in size, can appear small.

Dilatation of a chamber usually results from a volume overload, as in valvular regurgitation or a shunt, or from a decrease in the functional capacity of the myocardium. The underlying cause of such dilatation can be determined from a properly designed angiographic study. A right-sided angiocardiogram is usually inadequate when the cause of left ventricular enlargement is sought. A selective left ventriculogram is required in order to study contractility of the ventricular wall and to demonstrate regurgitation of the mitral valve. An aortogram is needed to evaluate the competency of the aortic valve and the possibility of an anomalous left coronary artery (see Fig. 30–26, p. 928).

Myocardial hypertrophy can be detected on the angiocardiogram. The distance between the edge of an opacified cardiac chamber and the outer border of the heart represents the combined thickness of the cardiac wall and the pericardium. A significant increase in this distance on an angiocardiogram can be due to hypertrophy of the myocardium or a pericardial effusion; however, hypertrophy rarely causes the thickness of the atrial wall to increase by more than a few millimeters. Atrial wall thickness of 8 mm or more is diagnostic of pericardial disease, almost always an effusion.[122]

Filling defects within the opacified atrium that occur early in the angiographic sequence, when contrast material is first injected into the chamber, usually result from incomplete mixing of the contrast material with the incoming nonopaque venous blood. The defects disappear after one or two cardiac cycles. A persistent defect that appears essentially the same from film to film indicates the presence of an intraluminal mass, either a thrombus or a tumor. A local dilution defect, such as that caused by nonopaque blood shunted through an atrial septal defect, can mimic the appearance of a mass. However, these dilution defects are never sharply outlined, and their appearance constantly changes during the cardiac cycle.

Ventricular filling defects are almost always due to hypertrophied musculature (Fig. 30–45, p. 943). In the right ventricle, the thickened myocardial bands and trabeculae cause scalloped indentations on the margins of the opacified chamber or round filling defects within it. Hypertrophy of the crista supraventricularis and the septal and parietal bands produce a narrowing of the infundibulum. Hypertrophic papillary muscles in the left ventricle are best seen in the frontal projection, since they encroach on the superior and inferior aspects of the ventricular cavity, narrowing the midbody of the chamber (Fig. 6–48). When the interventricular septum hypertrophies, it assumes a fusiform shape and bulges into the adjacent portions of both ventricular cavities.[123, 124]

A thin, lucent line stretching across the outflow portion of the left ventricle is usually due to a subaortic membrane. This lesion may be difficult to demonstrate, and multiple views of the opacified ventricle are often required. The subaortic membrane can be delineated without equivocation, if contrast material is injected selectively into the space between the membrane and the aortic valve.[125] A more jagged, V-shaped lucent line seen in the outflow portion of the left ventricle in the frontal view is characteristic of hypertrophic obstructive cardiomyopathy[126] (Fig. 42–15, p. 1427). The linear defect is present only in late systole, when the anterior mitral leaflet swings forward and makes contact with the ventricular septum.

If the minor intrusions of the muscular trabeculae are ignored, the overall shape of the ventricular cavities is regular. Local outpocketings of the lumen are abnormal. On the left side, they usually represent postmyocardial

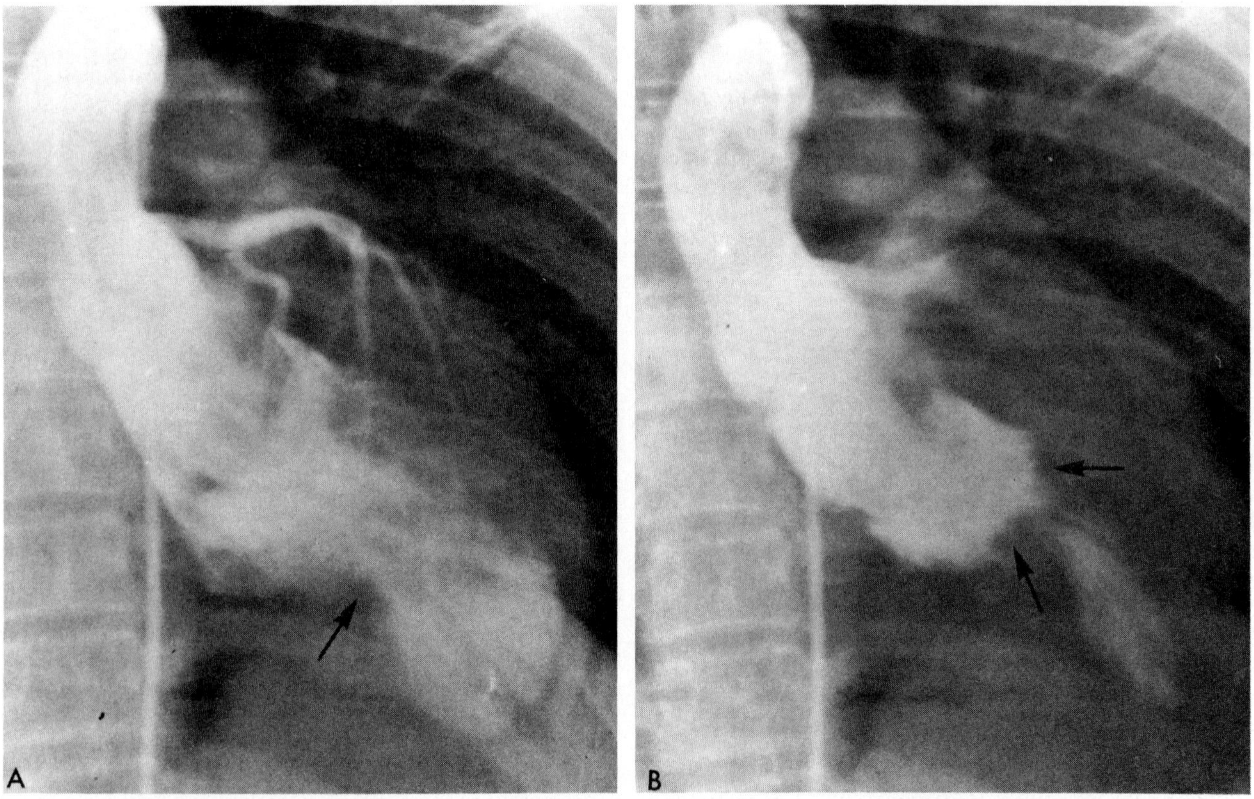

FIGURE 6–48. Left ventriculogram in hypertrophic obstructive cardiomyopathy. *A*, Diastole. The left ventricular wall is abnormally thickened because of muscular hypertrophy. The indentation on the medial aspect of the chamber (arrow) is caused by hypertrophy of the interventricular septum and the medial papillary muscle. *B*, Systole. As the heart contracts, the papillary muscles (arrows) constrict the midbody of the ventricle and sequester the apical region.

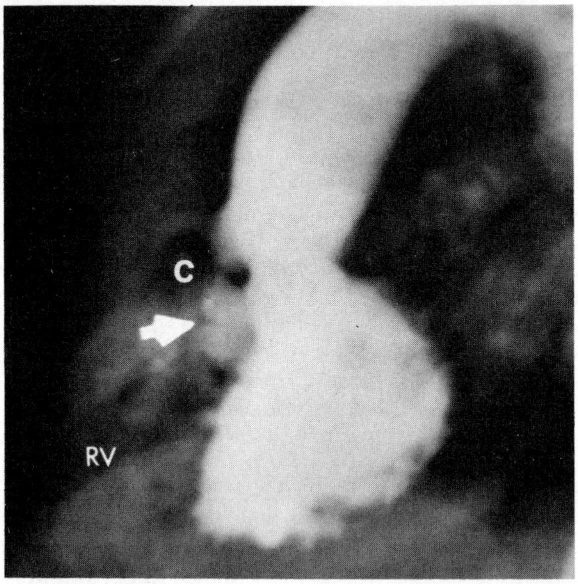

FIGURE 6–49. Aneurysm of the membranous septum. Left ventricular angiocardiogram, lateral view. The scalloped protrusion of the left ventricle (arrow) arises from the region of the membranous septum and extends anteriorly into the right ventricle beneath the crista supraventricularis (C). The right ventricle (RV) is opacified because of a small shunt through a defect in the aneurysm.

infarction aneurysm (Fig. 39–33, p. 1365) or, rarely, a congenital aneurysm or ventricular diverticulum. As the ventricle contracts, the aneurysm remains unchanged or bulges outward, and the contrast material pools within it. The opacified blood persists in the aneurysm, while it is washed away from the rest of the chamber. Aneurysms of the right ventricle are rare and are usually related to previous surgery.

An aneurysm of the membranous septum communicates with the left ventricular cavity and arises immediately beneath the commissure between the right coronary and noncoronary aortic cusps. The aneurysm usually has a trabeculated contour and extends anteriorly into the outflow tract of the right ventricle (Fig. 6–49). It is likely that most membranous septal aneurysms are misnamed and actually are formed by a portion of the tricuspid valve that has adhered to the margins of a membranous ventricular septal defect.[127, 128]

ASSESSMENT OF VENTRICULAR FUNCTION. Cineangiocardiography is ordinarily used for detailed study of ventricular function. End-diastolic and end-systolic volumes can be calculated from the size of the opacified ventricle in one or two projections and can be used to derive stroke volume, ejection fraction, and other measurements of myocardial performance (Chap. 15). The ventricular wall is usually divided into segments and the shortening of each during systole is determined to disclose abnormalities in regional wall motion that may not be apparent from simple observation of the contracting chamber.[129, 130]

Hypercontractility of the musculature is usually associated with hypertrophy and results in abnormal constriction of the ventricular lumen in end systole. In the right ventricle, this is most easily seen in the infundibular region. Normally, this area narrows slightly during systole. However, when the muscular contraction is abnormally forceful, the caliber of the infundibulum may be decreased by 80 per cent or more. Such systolic narrowing of the infundibulum is commonly seen with pulmonic valve stenosis.[131] If the infundibulum distends normally during diastole, the systolic narrowing was caused by hypercontraction of the hypertrophied musculature (Fig. 6–50). However, if the infundibulum is fibrotic, the narrowing is fixed, and it appears essentially the same in systole and diastole.

Hypercontraction of the left ventricle is manifested mainly in the body of the chamber. When there is a diffuse increase in contractility of the ventricular wall, the end-systolic volume of the chamber is decreased, and the cavity of the ventricle, except for its outflow portion, may be completely effaced. This can represent a response to obstruction in the aortic valve or the subaortic region but also occurs without known cause.[132] Eccentric hypertrophy and hypercontractility of the ventricle usually involves the septum and the papillary muscles and produces a pinching of the body of the ventricle that sequesters the apical region from the rest of the chamber (Fig. 6–48).[126, 133]

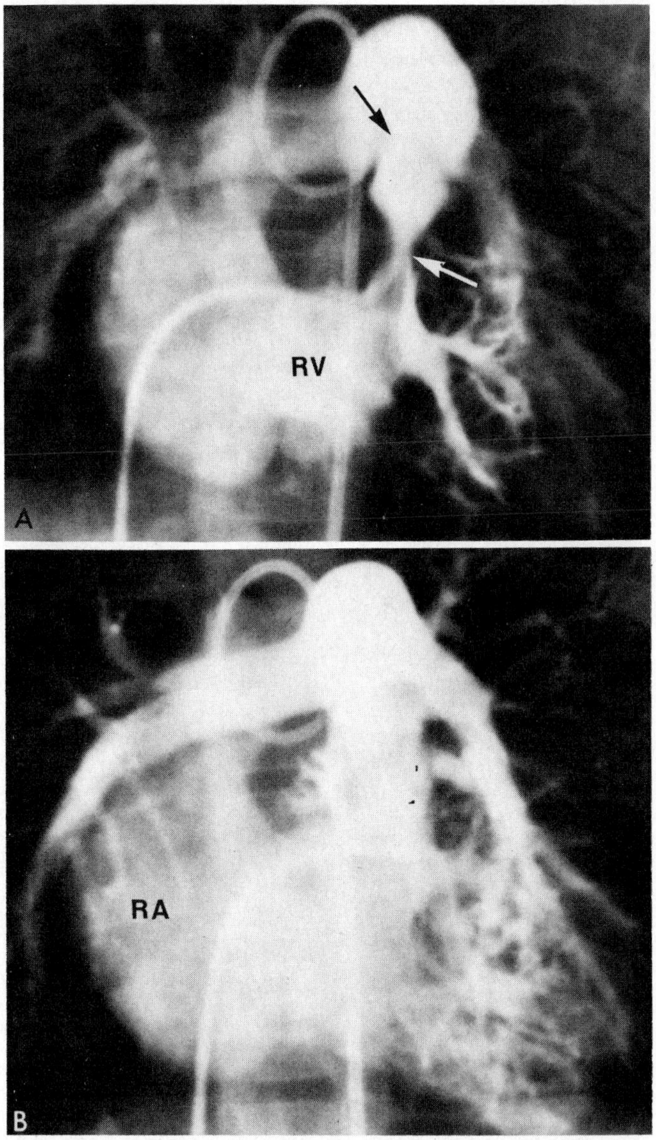

FIGURE 6–50. Pulmonary stenosis with hypercontraction of the infundibulum. *A*, Systole. A catheter has been advanced through the inferior vena cava to the right ventricle (RV). The stenotic pulmonic valve forms a dome (black arrow) bulging away from the ventricle. The infundibulum is markedly narrowed (white arrow). The multiple filling defects within the apical regions of the right ventricle are caused by hypertrophied trabeculae. The second catheter is positioned in the arch of the aorta. *B*, Diastole. The infundibulum appears of normal caliber, indicating that the narrowing was due to muscular contraction and does not represent fixed infundibular stenosis. The right atrium (RA) is opacified because of tricuspid regurgitation. (From Angrissola, A. B., and Puddu, V: [eds.]: Cardiologia D'Oggia. Torino, C. B. Edizion Scientifiche, 1976.)

CARDIAC VALVES

Angiocardiography is probably the best single method for evaluation of the structure of cardiac valves. It is an accurate and sensitive technique for the detection of stenosis of the aortic and pulmonic valves and, to a lesser extent, of the mitral valve. It is not very effective for evaluation of tricuspid stenosis. Regurgitation of all four valves, even of the slightest degree, can be routinely demonstrated.

When the blood on both sides of the valve is opacified and the valve is viewed tangentially, the cusps normally appear as thin, smooth, curvilinear lucencies. If the valve is projected obliquely or en face, the cusps usually cannot be identified. However, because the cusps are sheetlike structures, it is not necessary to visualize both surfaces in order to study their function. For example, on a supravalvular aortogram, the line of demarcation between the opacified blood in the aorta and the radiolucent blood in the ventricle actually represents the aortic surface of the valve cusps. The cusps are more easily seen on this type of examination, and in many instances their motion can be studied in detail (Fig. 6–51).

AORTIC AND PULMONIC STENOSIS.[134] The cusps of the normal aortic and pulmonic valves are rarely identified during systole because of their rapid motion. Even in the fully opened position, the cusps are not still, since their free margins are unsupported and tend to vibrate in the rapidly flowing arterial stream. However, during diastole, the cusps coapt and support each other so that they are relatively immobile for a considerable part of the cardiac cycle.

When the valve is stenotic, the cusps cannot separate from each other, and they form a membrane with a narrow orifice. During systole, the membrane, stretched taut by the stream of blood ejected from the ventricle, is relatively motionless. A dome-shaped curvilinear lucency, bulging away from the contracting chamber, is the angiographic hallmark of valvular stenosis (Figs. 6–51, 6–52, and 30–34, p. 935).[135, 136] If the cusps cannot be visualized during systole, it may be assumed that the valve is not stenotic. The aortic and pulmonic valves are so well visualized that mild degrees of stenosis may be detected on the angiogram before a pressure gradient is demonstrable. On the other hand, when a gradient across either valve is due to increased blood flow, the angiographic appearance of the valve will be normal. It should be noted that so long as the cusps are pliable, the valve will appear normal during diastole, no matter how narrow its orifice. A dysplastic valve is usually considerably thicker than a simple stenotic valve and has an irregular, nodular contour. Valve motion tends to be markedly limited.

MITRAL AND TRICUSPID STENOSIS. Both the mitral and tricuspid valves are best studied in the right anterior oblique projection. The *mitral valve* can be adequately delineated on a selective left ventriculogram. The interface between the opacified ventricle and the nonopacified left atrium represents the ventricular surface of the mitral leaflets. During systole, this interface is normally washed away by the incoming atrial blood. However, if the valve is stenotic, the interface persists and assumes a dome-shaped contour, convex toward the ventricle (Fig. 6–53). If the valve is fibrotic and rigid, the interface will be somewhat irregular and will move only slightly between systole and diastole.[137] The same information can be obtained from a selective pulmonary arteriogram. In this case, the valve leaflets will be seen as linear lucencies, separating the opacified left atrium from the opacified left ventricle.

The *tricuspid valve* is more difficult to visualize. On a selective right atrial injection, it may be seen as a curved interface between the opacified atrium and the radiolucent

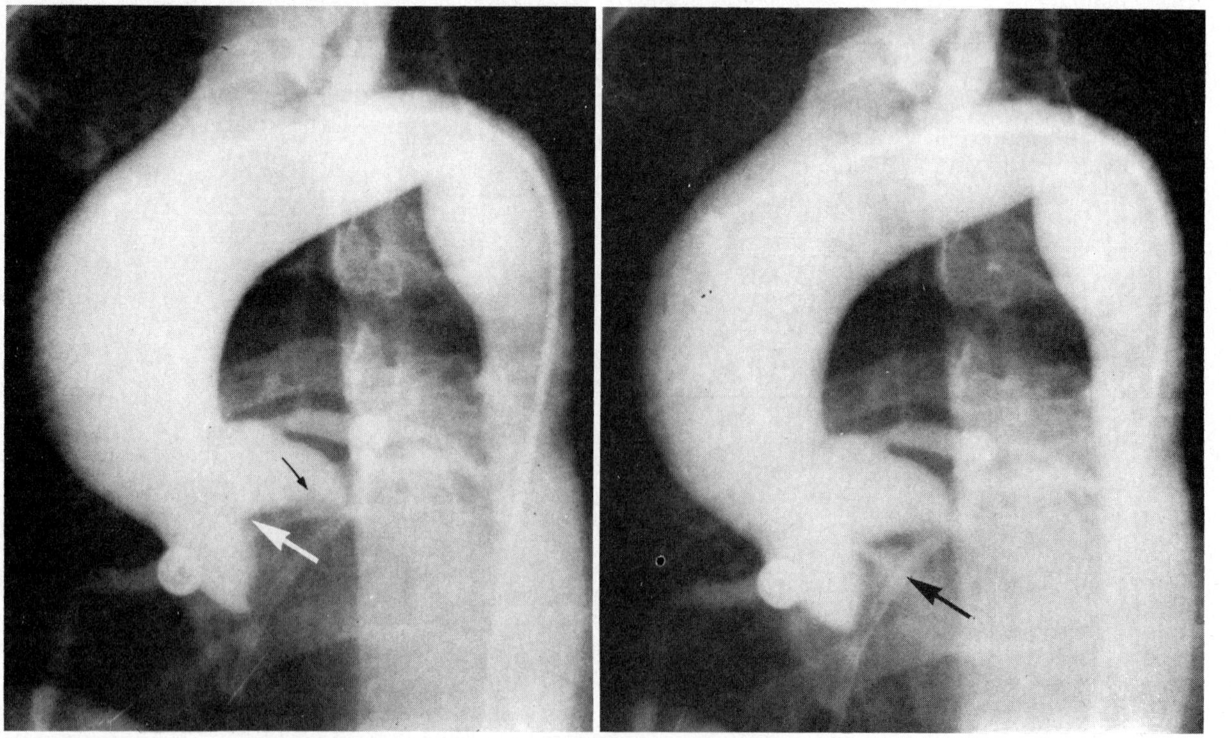

A B

FIGURE 6–51. Aortic stenosis, supravalvular aortogram. *A*, Systole. The aortic valve is rigid and cannot open. The narrow dilution defect (white arrow) represents radiolucent blood ejected from the left ventricle and indicates the diameter of the valve orifice. The irregularity of the left coronary cusp (black arrow) is caused by a vegetation on the valve. There is poststenotic dilatation of the ascending aorta. *B*, Diastole. The valve hardly moves at all, and there is a fine jet of aortic regurgitation (arrow).

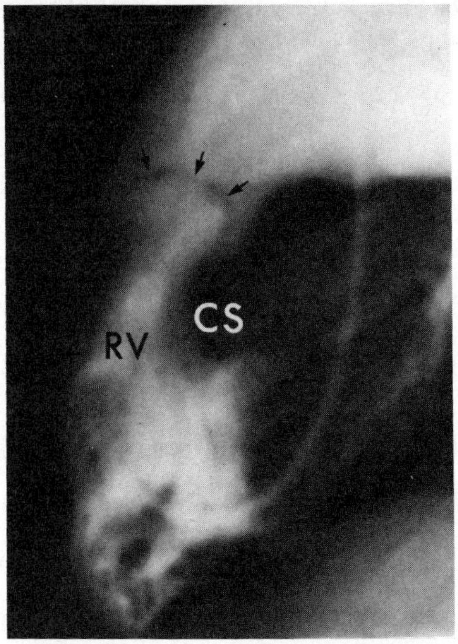

FIGURE 6–52. Pulmonic valve stenosis. Right ventriculogram, lateral view during stystole. The pulmonic valve (arrows) forms a dome, bulging away from the right ventricle (RV). The crista supraventricularis (CS) is hypertrophied. (From Baron, M. G.: The angiocardiographic diagnosis of valvular stenosis. Circulation *44*:143, 1971, by permission of the American Heart Association, Inc.)

right ventricle. However, after a few cardiac cycles, when the ventricle becomes opacified, it is difficult to identify the valve. As a general rule, pressure measurements across the tricuspid valve are more accurate for the detection of stenosis than is the angiocardiogram.

The angiocardiographic diagnosis of valvular atresia is made from the course of the blood flow and the associated anatomical abnormalities. When the tricuspid valve is atretic, blood flows directly from the right atrium into the left atrium (Fig. 30–50, p. 947). The right ventricle is abnormally small and fills through an interventricular communication.[138] A similar appearance can be seen with atresia of the pulmonic valve when the ventricular septum is intact. In this case, however, the diminutive right ventricle is opacified directly from the right atrium (Fig. 30–47, p. 945).[139] Aortic and mitral atresia is generally associated with hypoplasia of the left heart chambers. The ascending aorta is often no larger than a major visceral artery and fills from the right side of the heart through the ductus. The appearance of the aorta is so characteristic that the general diagnosis of hypoplasia of the left heart can often be made from a retrograde aortogram (Fig. 30–41, p. 939).

REGURGITATION.[140] In order to evaluate valvular competency, contrast material should be injected selectively into the chamber or vessel just beyond the valve. With normal flow, only those structures downstream in relation to the point of injection will be opacified. If the valve is incompetent, the contrast material will reflux into the upstream chamber. When studying the mitral and tricuspid valves, the patient should be placed in the right anterior oblique position. In this view, the valves are seen on end, separating the atrium from the ventricle, and there is no overlapping of the shadows of the two chambers.

Catheter position creates a possible source of error in evaluating insufficiency of the tricuspid and pulmonic valves. In order to reach their downstream side, the catheter must be passed through the valve. Most often, the catheter will lie in a commissure between the cusps and will not interfere with valve closure. Nevertheless, small amounts of regurgitation, probably due to the catheter, are sometimes seen. On occasion, the artifactual regurgitation may be of moderate degree,[141] but even then, it is rarely great enough to be of clinical importance. Free reflux of opacified blood is indicative of true valvular regurgitation. If there is any question as to the cause of the reflux, the catheter should be repositioned, and a second angiogram should be performed. It is unlikely that an artifact will be exactly duplicated.

Catheter position is of less concern with the left-sided cardiac valves, because the catheter can be passed retrograde through the aorta and reach the left ventricle without traversing the mitral valve. If the catheter is not positioned in the valve orifice, artifactual regurgitation is extremely rare unless the pressure injection triggers a run of extrasystoles. When the regurgitation is the result of a cardiac arrhythmia, the recipient chamber rapidly clears of contrast material once normal sinus rhythm has been restored. In true regurgitation, opacification of the chamber persists. A minimal amount of regurgitation may occur through the normal aortic valve, but this never opacifies more than a portion of the outflow tract of the left ventricle.

It is possible to gauge visually the severity of mitral

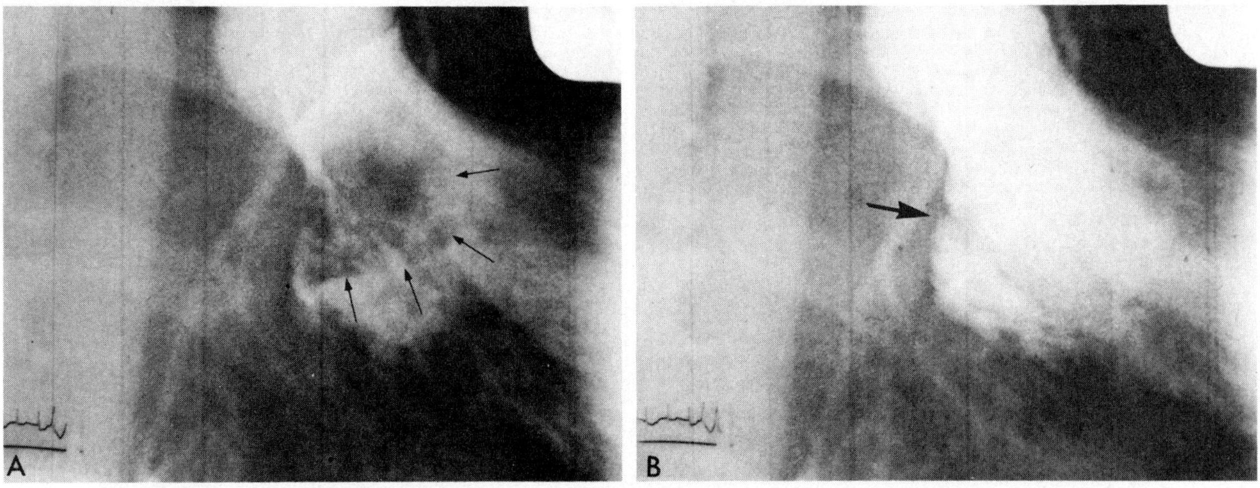

FIGURE 6–53. Mitral stenosis. Left ventricular angiogram, right anterior oblique view. *A*, Diastole. The mitral valve cannot open completely and forms a dome (arrows) that bulges into the left ventricle during atrial contraction. The leaflets are outlined by contrast material within the left ventricle and radiolucent blood in the atrium. *B*, Systole. The mitral valve (arrow) is closed. The wide excursion of the leaflets between the two phases of the cardiac cycle indicates that they are pliable.

valve regurgitation from a left ventriculogram by means of the relative densities of the left atrium and the aorta.[142] Equal opacification of the two structures indicates wide-open regurgitation, while a slight degree of reflux will produce only a minimum increase in the density of the left atrium. However, the size of the atrium must be taken into consideration. When the left atrium is very large, the regurgitant contrast material becomes so diluted by the blood already in the chamber that the amount of regurgitation will usually be underestimated.

The same principle can be used to measure aortic regurgitation. However, because of the rapid forward flow of blood within the aorta, the position of the catheter is very important. If the catheter tip is not adjacent to the valve, much of the contrast material will be washed away as it is injected, and the severity of the valvular regurgitation as judged by the opacity of the left ventricle will appear to be less than it actually is and may be overlooked completely.

SPECIFIC VALVULAR ABNORMALITIES. In the right anterior oblique projection, the subaortic portion of the right margin of the left ventricle is formed by the mitral valve. On a selective left ventriculogram, during systole, the mitral valve sharply delimits the opacified ventricle from the nonopacified left atrium. The line of demarcation is rather straight and almost vertical, extending from the aortic valve to the posteroinferior free wall of the ventricle (Fig. 6–53*B*). Protrusion of a portion of the valve beyond this line into the left atrium is indicative of *mitral prolapse*.[143, 144] Usually, the angiocardiographic diagnosis is substantiated by echocardiography (Fig. 33–20, p. 1047). However, the reverse is not true. In many instances, when the echocardiogram is positive, the roentgen appearance of the valve is normal. Whether this is because the echocardiographic criteria are not sufficiently specific or because the angiocardiogram is too insensitive a technique for detecting this abnormality is not certain.[145]

Ebstein's malformation of the tricuspid valve (Fig. 30–57, p. 951) is best demonstrated on a right atrial angiogram in the frontal projection. The tricuspid valve normally overlies the shadow of the spine or is projected slightly to the left of it. Because the valve is attached to the fibrous skeleton of the heart, its position is not affected by the size of the right atrium. Significant leftward displacement of the tricuspid valve into the right ventricle is diagnostic of Ebstein's anomaly.[146] The septal and posterior leaflets of the valve can often be seen as linear lucencies within the opacified right ventricle.

A cleft in the anterior leaflet of the mitral valve is the common denominator in all forms of *endocardial cushion defects of the atrioventricular canal type*. The mitral orifice, in these conditions, is rotated, so that the anterior mitral valve leaflet forms the right border of the left ventricle in the frontal projection. During systole, this border is scalloped rather than straight because of the abnormal valve tissue. During diastole, the two segments of the anterior leaflet swing open in different directions, causing an apparent narrowing of the outflow portion of the left ventricle (gooseneck deformity), and outline the upper margin of the defective ventricular septum (Figs. 6–54 and 30–16, p. 919).[147] The angiocardiographic manifestations of an endocardial cushion defect are so specific that the angiocardiogram is the most accurate means for establishing this diagnosis.

SPATIAL RELATIONSHIPS

The heart is composed of three pairs of structures: the atria, the ventricles, and the great vessels. In all normal hearts, the two members of each pair have a constant positional relationship to each other and to the other cardiac structures. Although minor variations can result

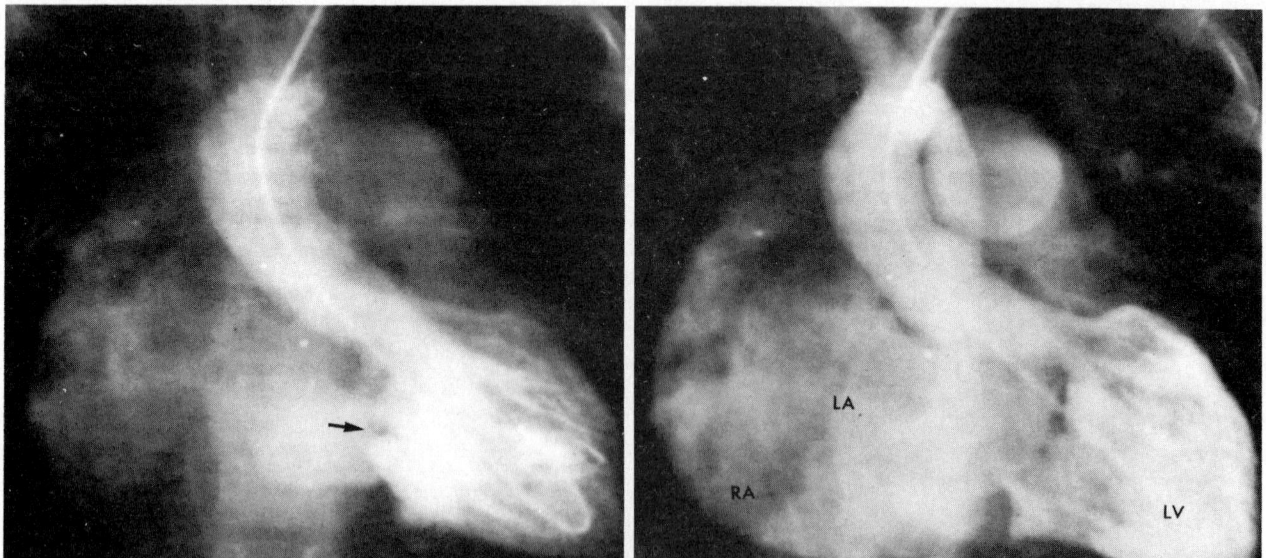

FIGURE 6–54. Endocardial cushion defect. Left ventriculogram, frontal view. *A*, Systole. The right border of the left ventricle is scalloped. The lucent niche (arrow) indicates a cleft in the anterior mitral valve leaflet. The valve is regurgitant, and contrast material refluxes into the left atrium. *B*, Diastole. The upper segment of the anterior mitral valve leaflet has swung into the outflow portion of the left ventricle, producing an apparent narrowing (arrow). This has been termed the "gooseneck" deformity. Contrast material has refluxed from the left ventricle (LV) into the left atrium (LA) and across the ostium primum defect into the right atrium (RA). Antegrade flow from the right atrium has filled the right ventricle and pulmonary artery. (From Baron, M. G., et al.: Endocardial cushion defects: Specific diagnosis by angiocardiography. Am. J. Cardiol. *13*:162, 1964.)

from dilatation of one or more of the chambers, a definite reversal of position is always due to a developmental fault.

Normally, the right atrium is situated to the right of the left atrium and slightly anteriorly. When the left atrium becomes very large, as it can in mitral disease, it may extend to the right, beyond the right atrium. However, the mitral valve and the left atrial appendage remain in their normal position to the left of the midline. The right ventricle lies anterior to and partly to the right of the left ventricle. When the right ventricle dilates, it may extend to the left, beyond the border of the left ventricle. Nevertheless, the tricuspid valve maintains its normal position, and part of the right ventricle still lies on the right side of the left ventricle. The pulmonic valve and main pulmonary artery are positioned to the left of the root of the aorta and in front of it. Although the pulmonary artery may be projected to the right of the aorta in a steep left anterior view, it is not possible to project the aortic valve in front of the pulmonic valve in any view.[148] When the aorta is large and overrides the ventricular septum, as in tetralogy of Fallot, it may extend farther anteriorly than the pulmonary artery, but its posterior margin, which is in contact with the mitral valve, is still behind the pulmonary artery (Fig. 30–51, p. 947).

In general, when the side-to-side relationship of one pair of cardiac structures is reversed, the downstream pairs will be similarly affected. If the right atrium is situated on the left side of the heart, the ventricles and the great vessels will also be reversed—a condition called situs inversus. When the ventricles are inverted, the atria are usually in their normal position, but the great vessels are transposed—a condition called ventricular inversion (corrected transposition) (p. 957). In isolated transposition of the great arteries, the atria and ventricles are positioned normally.

Identification of a cardiac chamber is usually based largely on its position and its relationship to the other chambers. In the presence of a rotational anomaly, this criterion is no longer valid. In general, the side-to-side relationship of the atria is concordant with the situs of the body. The right atrium usually receives the two venae cavae and the coronary sinus, while the pulmonary veins empty into the left atrium. On rare occasions, a left superior vena cava can enter the left atrium, or the inferior venae cava may be absent. However, anomalous drainage of the pulmonary veins is considerably more common. Pulmonary veins are therefore a less reliable indicator of atrial situs than are systemic veins. None of these is of any value in the asplenia syndrome because of the symmetrical development of the body and the indeterminate cardiac situs.

The ventricles can usually be identified because of their internal structure. The left ventricle tends to be oval in shape, while the right ventricle is trapezoidal. The trabeculation of the left ventricular wall is finer than that on the right, and the papillary muscles are often seen in the frontal view as two finger-like lucent defects within the opacified chamber. Of greater importance is the relationship between the inflow and outflow valves of each ventricle. In the left ventricle, the mitral valve and the aortic valves are in fibrous continuity. In contrast, the tricuspid valve and the pulmonic valve are separated by the muscular infundibulum of the right ventricle. This distinction does not hold when both great vessels arise from the right ventricle (Fig. 30–70, p. 961), because in this anomaly the mitral and aortic valves are also separated by a band of myocardium. The great vessels are identified primarily by the organs to which their branches are distributed.

The angiocardiogram of the heart in situs inversus in the frontal projection is a mirror image of the normal presentation. The right atrium and right ventricle lie on the left side of the heart. The aorta ascends along the left side of the mediastinum, and the aortic knob is on the right side. The anatomy of the bronchial tree is the reverse of normal, and there is almost always situs inversus of the abdominal viscera.

When the ventricles are inverted (Fig. 30–68, p. 959, congenitally corrected transposition), the two atria are in normal position. The right ventricle, the one with the muscular infundibulum, lies on the left side of the anatomical left ventricle. The aorta arises from the right ventricle, to the left of the pulmonary artery, and its ascending limb forms the left margin of the superior mediastinum. The arch of the aorta extends posteriorly and to the right, so that the aortic knob is completely hidden within the mediastinal shadow. The main pulmonary artery arises from the left ventricle within the cardiac silhouette and divides almost symmetrically into right and left main branches. The aorta and pulmonary artery often lie side by side and are superimposed on each other in the lateral view. The abnormal position of the pulmonary artery can be identified in the lateral view because it is set back on the ventricle and does not arise flush with its anterior wall. The appearance of a step between the ventricle and the pulmonary artery has not been encountered in any other cardiac anomaly.

In transposition of the great arteries, the aorta arises from the infundibular portion of the right ventricle. Usually, the aorta lies directly in front of the main pulmonary artery (Fig. 30–65, p. 956), but in a small percentage of patients the vessels lie alongside each other.[148, 149] The relationship of the great arteries therefore cannot be used as the sole criterion for differentiating transposition from ventricular inversion.[150, 151]

REFERENCES

1. Hoffman, R. B., and Rigler, L. G.: Evaluation of left ventricular enlargement in the lateral projection of the chest. Radiology *85*:93, 1965.
2. Bachman, D. M., Ellis, K., and Austin, J. H. M.: The effects of minor degrees of obliquity on the lateral chest radiograph. Radiol. Clin. North Am. *16*:465, 1978.
3. McGinnis, K. D., Eyler, W. R., and Alvarez, H., Jr.: Cardiac laminagraphy. Radiology *77*:553, 1961.
4. Ravin, A., and Nice, C. M.: The angle of clearance of the left ventricle. Ann. Intern. Med. *36*:1413, 1952.
5. Glover, L., Baxley, W. A., and Dodge, H. T.: A quantitative evaluation of heart size measurements from chest roentgenograms. Circulation *47*:1289, 1973.
6. Nickol, K., and Wade, A. J.: Radiographic heart size and cardiothoracic ratio in three ethnic groups: A basis for a simple screening test for cardiac enlargement in men. Br. J. Radiol. *55*:399, 1982.
7. Ungerleider, H. E., and Clark, C. P.: A study of the transverse diameter of the heart silhouette with prediction table based on the teleroentgenogram. Trans. Life Insur. Med. Dir. Am. 25:84, 1938.
8. Jonsell, S.: A method for determination of heart size by teleroentgenography (a heart volume index). Acta Radiol. *20*:325, 1939.
9. Keats, T. E., and Enge, I. P.: Cardiac mensuration by the cardiac volume method. Radiology 85:850, 1965.
10. DuBois, E. F.: Basal Metabolism in Health and Disease. 2nd ed. Philadelphia, Lea and Febiger, 1931, p. 119.
11. Oberman, A., Jones, W. B., Riley, C. P., Reeves, T. J., Sheffield, L. T., and Turner, M. E.: Natural history of coronary artery disease. Bull. N.Y. Acad. Med. *48*:1109, 1972.
12. Gammill, S. L., Krebs, C., Meyers, P., Nice, C. M., Jr., and Becker, H. C.: Cardiac measurements in systole and diastole. Radiology *94*:115, 1970.

ACQUIRED HEART DISEASE

13. Kannel, W. B., Castelli, W. P., and McNamara, P. M.: The coronary profile: 12-year follow-up in the Framingham study. J. Occup. Med. 9:613, 1967.
14. Sherman, R. S., Bertrand, C. A., and Duffy, J. C.: Roentgenographic detection of cardiomegaly in employees with normal electrocardiograms. Am. J. Roentgenol. *119*:493, 1973.
15. Felson, B.: More chest roentgen signs and how to teach them. Radiology *90*: 429, 1968.

16. Sos, T. A., Levin, D. C., Sniderman, K. W., and Beckmann, C. F.: Cinefluoroscopy in evaluating left ventricular contractility and aneurysms. Circulation *56* (Suppl.):III-18, 1977.
17. Bartel, A. G., Chen, J. T., Peter, R. H., Behar, V. S., Yihong, K., and Lester, R. G.: The significance of coronary calcification detected by fluoroscopy. A report of 360 patients. Circulation *49*:1247, 1974.
18. Hamby, R. I., Tabrah, F., Wisoff, B. G., and Hartenstein, M. L.: Coronary artery calcification: Clinical implications and angiographic correlates. Am. Heart J. *87*:565, 1974.
19. Frink, R. J., Achor, R. W. P., Brown, A. L., Jr., Kincaid, O. W., and Brandenburg, R. O.: Significance of calcification of the coronary arteries. Am. J. Cardiol. *26*:241, 1970.
20. Oliver, M. F.: The diagnostic value of detecting coronary calcification (Editorial). Circulation *42*:981, 1970.
21. Chen, J. T. T., Behar, V. S., Morris, J. J., Jr., McIntosh, H. D., and Lester, R. G.: Correlation of roentgen findings with hemodynamic data in pure mitral stenosis. Am. J. Roentgenol. *102*:280, 1968.
22. Probst, P., Goldschlager, N., and Selzer, A.: Left atrial size and atrial fibrillation in mitral stenosis. Factors influencing their relationship. Circulation *48*:1282, 1973.
23. Raphael, M. J., Steiner, R. E., and Raftery, E. B.: Acute mitral incompetence. Clin. Radiol. *18*:126, 1967.
24. Edwards, J. E.: An Atlas of Acquired Diseases of the Heart and Great Vessels. Philadelphia, W. B. Saunders Company, 1961, pp. 22–66.
25. Korn, D., De Sanctis, R. W., and Sell, S.: Massive calcification of the mitral annulus: A clinical pathological study of 14 cases. N. Engl. J. Med. *267*:900, 1962.
26. Hemley, S. D.: Mitral annulus calcification. Radiology *83*:464, 1964.
27. Seltzer, R. A., Harthorne, J. W., and Austen, W. G.: The appearance and significance of left atrial calcification. Am. J. Roentgenol. *100*:307, 1967.
28. Leonard, J. J., Katz, S., and Nelson, D.: Calcification of the left atrium: Its anatomic location, diagnostic significance, and roentgenologic demonstration. N. Engl. J. Med. *256*:629, 1957.
29. Lendrum, A. C., Scott, L. D. W., and Park, S. D. S.: Pulmonary changes due to cardiac disease with special reference to hemosiderosis. Q. J. Med. *19*:249, 1950.
30. Taylor, H. E., and Strong, G. F.: Pulmonary hemosiderosis in mitral stenosis. Ann. Intern. Med. *42*:26, 1965.
31. Kerley, P.: Lung changes in acquired heart disease. Am. J. Roentgenol. *80*: 256, 1958.
32. Galloway, R. W., Epstein, E. J., and Coulshed, N.: Pulmonary ossific nodules in mitral valve disease. Br. Heart J. *23*:297, 1961.
33. Lehman, J. S., Florence, H., Schimert, A. P., and Evans, G. C.: Acquired aortic valvular stenosis. Its diagnosis by conventional radiological study. Radiology *81*:24, 1963.
34. Spindolo-Franco, H., Fish, B. G., Dachman, A., Grose, R., and Attai, L.: Recognition of bicuspid aortic valve by plain film calcification. Am. J. Roentgenol. *139*:867, 1982.
35. Jarchow, B. H., and Kincaid, O. W.: Poststenotic dilatation of the ascending aorta: Its occurrence and significance as a roentgenologic sign of aortic stenosis. Proc. Mayo Clin. *36*:23, 1961.
36. Rockoff, S. D., and Austen, W. G.: The hemodynamic significance of the radiologic changes in acquired aortic stenosis. Am. Heart J. *65*:458, 1963.

CONGENITAL HEART DISEASE

37. Cooley, D. A., Hallman, G. L., and Hammam, A. S.: Congenital cardiovascular anomalies in adults: Results of surgical treatment in 167 patients over the age of 35. Am. J. Cardiol. *17*:303, 1966.
38. Mark, H., and Young, D.: Congenital heart disease in the adult. Am. J. Cardiol. *15*:293, 1965.
39. Fisher, J. M., Wilson, J. R., and Theilen, E. O.: Recognition of congenital heart disease in the fifth to eighth decades of life. Diagnostic criteria and natural history. Circulation *25*:831, 1962.
40. Novack, P., Segal, B., Kasparian, H., and Likoff, W.: Atrial septal defect in patients over 40. Geriatrics *18*:421, 1963.
41. Kuzman, W. J., and Yuskis, A. S.: Atrial septal defects in the older patient simulating acquired valvular heart disease. Am. J. Cardiol. *15*:303, 1965.
42. Siltanen, P.: Atrial septal defect of secundum type in adults. Clinical and hemodynamic studies of 129 cases before and after surgical correction under cardiopulmonary bypass. Acta Med. Scand. (Suppl.) 497, 1968.
43. Betriu, A., Wigle, E. D., Felderhof, C. H., and McLoughlin, M. J.: Prolapse of the posterior leaflet of the mitral valve associated with secundum atrial septal defect. Am. J. Cardiol. *35*:363, 1975.
44. Rippe, J. M., Sloss, L. J., Angoff, G., and Alpert, J. S.: Mitral valve prolapse in adults with congenital heart disease. Am. Heart J. *97*:561, 1979.
45. Markman, P., Hawitt, G., and Wade, E. G.: Atrial septal defect in the middle-aged and elderly. Q. J. Med. *34*:409, 1968.
46. Edwards, J. E.: The pathology of atrial septal defect. Semin. Roentgenol. *1*:24, 1966.
47. Ruskin, H., and Samuel, E.: Calcification in the patent ductus arteriosus. Br. J. Radiol. *23*:710, 1950.
48. Holman, E.: On circumscribed dilatation of an artery immediately distal to a partially occluding band: Poststenotic dilatation. Surgery *36*:3, 1954.
49. Martin, E. C., Stratford, M. A., and Gersony, W. M.: Initial detection of coarctation of the aorta: An opportunity for the radiologist. Am. J. Roentgenol. *137*:1015, 1981.
50. Figley, M. M.: Accessory roentgen signs of coarctation of the aorta. Radiology *62*:671, 1954.
51. Gladnikoff, H.: The roentgenological picture of coarctation of the aorta and its anatomical basis. Acta Radiol. *27*:8, 1946.
52. Baron, M. G.: Obscuration of the aortic knob in coarctation of the aorta. Circulation *43*:311, 1971.
53. Sloan, R. D., and Cooley, R. N.: Coarctation of the aorta. Radiology *61*:701, 1953.
54. Boone, M. L., Swenson, B. E., and Felson, B.: Rib notching: Its many causes. Am. J. Roentgenol. *91*:1075, 1964.
55. Elliott, L. P., and Schiebler, G. L.: X-ray Diagnosis of Congenital Cardiac Disease. Springfield, Ill., Charles C Thomas, 1968.
56. Ivemark, B. I.: Implication of agenesis of the spleen on the pathogenesis of conotruncus anomalies in childhood—An analysis of heart malformations in the splenic agenesis syndrome, with 14 new cases. Acta Paediatr. Upps. *44*(Suppl. 104):7, 1955.
57. Van Mierop, L. H. S., Patterson, P. R., and Reynolds, R. W.: Two cases of congenital asplenia with isomerism of the cardiac atria and the sinoatrial nodes. Am. J. Cardiol. *13*:407, 1964.
58. Ruttenberg, H. D., Neufeld, H. N., Lucas, R. V., Jr., Carey, L. S., Adams, P., Jr., Anderson, R. C., and Edwards, J. E.: Syndrome of congenital cardiac disease with asplenia. Distinction from other forms of congenital cyanotic cardiac disease. Am. J. Cardiol. *13*:387, 1964.
59. Stewart, J. R., Kincaid, O. W., and Titus, J. L.: Right aortic arch: Plain film diagnosis and significance. Am. J. Roentgenol. *97*:377, 1966.
60. Felson, B., and Palayew, M. J.: The two types of right aortic arch. Radiology *81*:745, 1963.
61. Baron, M. G.: Right aortic arch. Circulation *44*:1137, 1971.
62. Berdon, W. E., and Baker, D. H.: Plain film findings in azygos continuation of the inferior vena cava. Am. J. Roentgenol. *104*:452, 1968.
63. Michelson, E., and Salik, J. O.: Vascular pattern of lung as seen on routine and tomographic studies. Radiology *73*:511, 1959.
64. Westermark, N.: On the roentgen diagnosis of lung embolism. Acta Radiol. *19*:357, 1938.
65. Milne, E. N. C.: Physiological interpretation of the plain radiograph in mitral stenosis, including a review of criteria for the radiological estimation of pulmonary arterial and venous pressures. Br. J. Radiol. *36*:902, 1963.
66. Simon, M.: The pulmonary vessels: Their hemodynamic evaluation using routine radiographs. Radiol. Clin. North Am. *1*:363, 1963.
67. Steiner, R. E.: Radiology of pulmonary circulation. Chamberlain Lecture, 1963. Am. J. Roentgenol. *91*:249, 1964.
68. Simon, M.: The pulmonary veins in mitral stenosis. J. Fac. Radiol. *9*:25, 1958.
69. West, J. B., Dollery, C. T., and Heard, B. E.: Increased pulmonary vascular resistance in the dependent zone of the isolated dog lung caused by perivascular edema. Circ. Res. *17*:191, 1965.
70. Hughes, J. M. B., Glazier, J. B., Maloney, J. E., and West, J. B.: Effect of interstitial pressure on pulmonary blood flow. Lancet *1*:192, 1967.
71. Doyle, A. E., Goodwin, J. F., Harrison, C. V., and Steiner, R. E.: Pulmonary vascular patterns in pulmonary hypertension. Br. Heart J. *19*:353, 1957.
72. Fishman, A. P., and Renkin, E. M. (eds.): Pulmonary Edema. Bethesda, Md., American Physiological Society, 1979, 261 pp.
73. Harrison, M. O., Conte, P. J., and Heitzman, E. R.: Radiological detection of clinically occult cardiac failure following myocardial infarction. Br. J. Radiol. *44*:265, 1971.
74. Chait, A.: Interstitial pulmonary edema. Circulation *45*:1323, 1972.
75. Kerley, P. J.: Radiology in heart disease. Br. Med. J. *2*:594, 1933.
76. Fleischner, F. G., and Reiner, L.: Linear x-ray shadows in acquired pulmonary hemosiderosis and congestion. N. Engl. J. Med. *250*:900, 1954.
77. Grainger, R. G.: Interstitial pulmonary oedema and its radiological diagnosis. A sign of pulmonary venous and capillary hypertension. Br. J. Radiol. *31*:201, 1958.
78. Trapnell, D. H.: The peripheral lymphatics of the lung. Br. J. Radiol. *36*:660, 1963.
79. Meszaros, W. T.: Lung changes in left heart failure. Circulation *47*:859, 1973.
80. Don, C., and Johnson, R.: The nature and significance of peribronchial cuffing in pulmonary edema. Radiology *125*:577, 1977.
81. Hayes, C. E., Case, T. A., Ailion, D. C., Morris, A. H., Cutillo, A., Blackburn, C. W., Durney, C. H., and Johnson, S. A.: Lung water quantitation by nuclear magnetic resonance imaging. Science *216*:1313, 1982.
82. Fleischner, F. G.: The butterfly pattern of acute pulmonary edema. Am. J. Cardiol. *20*:39, 1967.
83. Richman, S. M., and Godar, T. J.: Unilateral pulmonary edema. N. Engl. J. Med. *264*:1148, 1961.

THE PERICARDIUM

84. Lane, E. J., Jr., and Carsky, E. W.: Epicardial fat: lateral plain film analysis in normals and in pericardial effusion. Radiology *91*:1, 1968.
85. Jorgens, J., Kundel, R., and Lieber, A.: The cinefluorographic approach to the diagnosis of pericardial effusion. Am. J. Roentgenol. *87*:911, 1962.
86. Tomoda, H., Hoshiai, M., Furuya, H., Matsumoto, S., Tanabe, T., Tamachi, H., Sasamoto, H., Koide, S., Kuribayashi, S., and Matsuyama, S.: Evaluation of pericardial effusion with computed tomography. Am. Heart J. *99*:701, 1980.
87. Heinz, R., and Abrams, H. L.: Radiologic aspects of operable heart disease. IV. The variable appearance of constrictive pericarditis. Radiology *69*:54, 1957.
88. Shanks, S. C., and Kerley, P. (eds.): A Textbook of X-ray Diagnosis. 4th ed. Philadelphia, W. B. Saunders Company, 1972, p. 353.

89. Moncada, R., Baker, M., Salinas, M., Demos, T. C., Churchill, R., Love, L., Reynes, C., Hale, D., Cardoso, M., Pifarre, R., and Gunnar, R.: Diagnostic role of computed tomography in pericardial heart disease: Congenital defects, thickening, neoplasms and effusions. Am. Heart J. *103*:263, 1982.
90. Doppman, J. L., Rienmuller, R., Lissner, J., Cyran, J., Bolte, H. D., Strauer, B. E., and Hellwig, H.: Computed tomography in constrictive pericardial disease. J. Comput. Assist. Tomogr. 5:1, 1981.
91. Ellis, K., Leeds, N. E., and Himmelstein, A.: Congenital deficiencies in the parietal pericardium. A review with 2 new cases including successful diagnosis by plain roentgenography. Am. J. Roentgenol. *82*:125, 1959.
92. Chang, C. H., and Leigh, T. F.: Congenital partial defect of the pericardium associated with herniation of the left atrial appendage. Am. J. Roentgenol. *86*: 517, 1961.
93. Chang, C. H., and Amory, H. I.: Congenital partial right pericardial defect associated with herniation of the right atrial appendage. Radiology *84*:660, 1965.

ANGIOGRAPHY

94. Williamson, D. E.: Experimental determination of flow equation in catheters for cardiology. Am. J. Roentgenol. *94*:704, 1965.
95. Inter-Society Commission for Heart Disease Resources: Optimal resources for examination of the chest and cardiovascular system. Catheterization—angiographic laboratories. Circulation *53*:A-1, 1976.
96. Bargeron, L. M., Jr., Elliott, L. P., Soto, B., Bream, P. R., and Curry, G. C.: Axial cineangiography in congenital heart disease. I. Concept, technical and anatomic considerations. Circulation *56*:1075, 1977.
97. Elliott, L. P., Bargeron, L. M., Jr., Bream, P. R., Soto, B., and Curry, G. C.: Axial cineangiography in congenital heart disease. II. Specific lesions. Circulation *56*:1048, 1977.
98. Elliott, L. P., Green, C. E., Rogers, W. J., Hood, W. P., Mantle, J. A., and Papapietro, S. E.: Advantages of the caudo-cranial left anterior oblique left ventriculogram in adult heart disease. Am. J. Cardiol. *49*:369, 1982.
99. Mills, S. R., Jackson, D. C., Older, R. A., Heaston, D. K., and Moore, A. V.: The incidence, etiologies and avoidance of complications of pulmonary angiography in a large series. Radiology *136*:295, 1980.
100. Susman, N., and Diboll, W. B., Jr.: Fluid dynamics in the tip of the multiholed angiographic catheter. Radiology 92:843, 1969.
101. Carlsson, E. C., Rudolph, A., Stanger, P., Teitel, D., Weber, W., and Yoshida, H.: Pediatric angiocardiography with iohexol. Invest. Radiol. *20*:S75, 1985.
102. Hanley, P. C., Holmes, D. R., Jr., Julsrud, P. R., and Smith, H. C.: Use of conventional and newer radiographic contrast agents in cardiac angiography. Prog. Cardiovasc. Dis. *28*:435, 1986.
103. Kozeny, G. A., Murdock, D. K., and Euler, D. E.: In vivo effects of acute changes in osmolality and sodium concentration on myocardial contractility. Am. Heart J. *109*:290, 1985.
104. Mullins, C. B., Leshin, S. J., Mierzwiak, D. S., Alsobrook, H. D., and Mitchell, J. H.: Changes in left ventricular function produced by the injection of contrast media. Am. Heart J. *83*:373, 1972.
105. Iseri, L. T., Kaplan, M. A., Evans, M. J., and Nickel, E. D.: Effect of concentrated contrast media during angiography on plasma volume and plasma osmolality. Am. Heart J. *69*:154, 1965.
106. Bettman, M. A., and Higgins, C. B.: Comparison of an ionic with a nonionic contrast agent for cardiac angiography. Results of a multicenter trial. Invest. Radiol. *20*:S70, 1985.
107. Tani, M., Handa, S., Noma, S., and Kojima, S.: Changes in left ventricular diastolic function after left ventriculography: A comparison of iopanidol and urografin. Am. Heart J. *110*:617, 1985.
108. Cohn, P. F., Horn, H. R., Teichholz, L. E., Kreulen, T. H., Herman, M. V., and Gorlin, R.: Effects of angiographic contrast medium on left ventricular function in coronary artery disease. Comparison with static and dynamic exercise. Am. J. Cardiol. *32*:21, 1973.
109. D'Elia, J. A., Gleason, R. E., Alday, M., Malarick, C., Godley, K., Warram, J., Kaldany, A., and Weinrauch, L. A.: Nephrotoxicity from angiographic contrast material. A prospective study. Am. J. Med. *72*:719, 1982.
110. Pendergrass, H. P., Tondreau, R. L., Pendergrass, E. P., Ritchie, D. J., Hildreth, E. A., and Askovitz, S. I.: Reactions associated with intravenous urography: Historical and statistical review. Radiology *71*:1, 1958.
111. Goldberg, M.: Systemic reactions to intravascular contrast media: A guide for the anaesthesiologist. Anaesthesiology *60*:46, 1984.
112. Giammona, S. T., Lurie, P. R., and Segar, W. E.: Hypertonicity following selective angiocardiography. Circulation *28*:1096, 1963.
113. Ellis, K., Griffiths, S. P., Bordiuk, J. M., Burris, J. O., and Baker, D. H.: Some congenital anomalies of the tricuspid valve: Angiocardiographic considerations. Radiol. Clin. North Am. *6*:383, 1968.
114. Kieffer, S. A., and Carey, L. S.: Tricuspid atresia with normal aortic root: Roentgen-anatomic correlation. Radiology *80*:605, 1963.
115. Chesler, E., Moller, J. H., and Edwards, J. E.: The congenital cardiovascular anomalies underlying "reversed coarctation." Am. Heart J. *75*:34, 1968.
116. Eliot, R. S., Shone, J. D., Kanjuh, V. I., Ruttenberg, H. B., Carey, L. S., and Edwards, J. E.: Mitral atresia. Am. Heart J. *75*:325, 1968.
117. Miller, G. A. H.: Aortic atresia. Diagnostic cardiac catheterization in first week of life. Br. Heart J. *33*:367, 1971.
118. Rudolph, A. M.: The changes in circulation after birth. Their importance in congenital heart disease. Circulation *41*:343, 1970.
119. Shumacker, H. B., Jr., King, H., and Waldhausen, J. A.: The persistent left superior vena cava. Ann. Surg. *155*:797, 1967.
120. Baron, M. G., Wolf, B. S., Steinfeld, L., and Gordon, A.: Left ventricular angiocardiography in the study of ventricular septal defects. Radiology *81*:223, 1963.
121. Baron, M. G., Wolf, B. S., Steinfeld, L., and Van Mierop, L. H. S.: Angiocardiographic diagnosis of subpulmonic ventricular septal defect. Am. J. Roentgenol. *103*:93, 1968.
122. Figley, M. M., and Bagshaw, M. A.: Angiocardiographic aspects of constrictive pericarditis. Radiology *69*:46, 1957.
123. Adelman, A. G., McLoughlin, M. J., Marquis, Y., Auger, P., and Wigle, E. D.: Left ventricular cineangiocardiographic observations in muscular subaortic stenosis. Am. J. Cardiol. *24*:689, 1969.
124. Bourdarias, J. P., Ourbak, P., Ferrane, J., Sozutek, Y., Scebat, L., and Lenegre, J.: Obstructive cardiomyopathy. Cineangiographic study of 50 cases. Am. J. Roentgenol. *102*:853, 1968.
125. Schaffer, A. I., Kania, H., Cucci, C. E., and DePasquale, N. P.: New technique for angiographic visualization of membranous subaortic stenosis. Br. Heart J. *34*:742, 1972.
126. Simon, A. L.: Angiographic diagnosis of idiopathic hypertrophic subaortic stenosis. Radiol. Clin. North Am. *6*:423, 1968.
127. Baron, M. G., Wolf, B. S., Grishman, A., and Van Mierop, L. H. S.: Aneurysm of the membranous septum. Am. J. Roentgenol. *191*:1303, 1964.
128. Freedom, R. M., White, R. D., Pieroni, D. R., Varghese, P. J., Krovetz, L. J., and Rowe, R. R.: The natural history of the so-called aneurysm of the membranous ventricular septum in childhood. Circulation *49*:375, 1974.
129. Herman, M. V., Heinle, R. A., Klein, M. D., and Gorlin, R.: Localized disorders in myocardial contraction. Asynergy and its role in congestive heart failure. N. Engl. J. Med. *277*:222, 1967.
130. Sniderman, A. D., Marpole, D., and Fallen, E. L.: Regional contraction patterns in normal and ischemic left ventricle in man. Am. J. Cardiol. *31*:484, 1973.
131. Lester, R. G., Osteen, R. T., and Robinson, A. F.: Infundibular obstruction secondary to pulmonary valvular stenosis. Am. J. Roentgenol. *94*:78, 1965.
132. Criley, J. M., Lewis, K. B., White, R. I., Jr., and Ross, R. S.: Pressure gradients without obstruction: A new concept of "hypertrophic subaortic stenosis." Circulation *32*:88, 1965.
133. Braunwald, E., Morrow, A. G., Cornell, W. P., Aygen, M. M., and Hilbish, T. F.: Idiopathic hypertrophic subaortic stenosis: Clinical, hemodynamic and angiographic manifestations. Am. J. Med. *29*:924, 1960.
134. Baron, M. G.: The angiocardiographic diagnosis of valvular stenosis. Circulation *44*:143, 1971.
135. Takekawa, S. D., Kincaid, O. W., Titus, J. L., and DuShane, J. W.: Congenital aortic stenosis. Am. J. Roentgenol. *98*:800, 1966.
136. Rudhe, U.: Angiocardiography in pulmonic stenosis. Radiol. Clin. North Am. *2*:395, 1964.
137. Demany, M. A., Kay, E. B., and Zimmerman, H. A.: An angiocardiographic sign for the evaluation of the stenotic mitral valve. Am. J. Cardiol. *18*:843, 1966.
138. Kieffer, S. A., and Carey, L. S.: Tricuspid atresia with normal aortic root: Roentgen-anatomic correlation. Radiology *80*:605, 1963.
139. Desilets, D. T., Marcano, B. A., Emmanouilides, G. C., and Gyepes, M. T.: Severe pulmonary valve stenosis and atresia. Radiol. Clin. North Am. *6*:367, 1968.
140. Baron, M. G.: Angiocardiographic evaluation of valvular insufficiency. Circulation *43*:599, 1971.
141. Cairns, K. B., Kloster, F. E., Bristow, J. D., Lees, M. H., and Griswold, H. E.: Problems in the hemodynamic diagnosis of tricuspid insufficiency. Am. Heart J. *75*:173, 1968.
142. Björk, V. O., Lodin, H., and Malers, E.: The evaluation of the degree of mitral insufficiency by selective left ventricular angiocardiography. Am. Heart J. *60*: 691, 1960.
143. Criley, J. M., Lewis, K. B., Humphries, J. O., and Ross, R. S.: Prolapse of the mitral valve: Clinical and cine-angiocardiographic findings. Br. Heart J. *28*:488, 1966.
144. Kittredge, R. D., Shimomura, S., Cameron, A., and Bell, A. L. L., Jr.: Prolapsing mitral leaflets. Cineangiographic determination. Am. J. Roentgenol. *109*:84, 1970.
145. Perloff, J. K.: Evolving concepts of mitral-valve prolapse. N. Engl. J. Med. *307*:369, 1982.
146. Ellis, K., Griffiths, S. P., Burris, J. O., Ramsay, G. C., and Fleming, R. J.: Ebstein's anomaly of the tricuspid valve; angiocardiographic considerations. Am. J. Roentgenol. *92*:1338, 1964.
147. Baron, M. G.: Endocardial cushion defects. Radiol. Clin. North Am. *6*:343, 1968.
148. Beuren, A.: Differential diagnosis of the Taussig-Bing heart from complete transposition of the great vessels with a posteriorly overriding pulmonary artery. Circulation *21*:1071, 1960.
149. Barcia, A., Kincaid, O. W., Davis, G. D., Kirklin, J. W., and Ongley, P. A.: Transposition of the great arteries. An angiocardiographic study. Am. J. Roentgenol. *100*:249, 1967.
150. Jackson, H.: The transposition complexes and other cardiovascular malalignments. Br. J. Radiol. *42*:721, 1969.
151. Anselmi, G., Munoz, S., Blanco, P., Machado, I., and de la Cruz, M. V.: Systematization and clinical study of dextroversion, mirror-image dextrocardia, and laevoversion. Br. Heart J. *34*:1085, 1972.

7 ELECTROCARDIOGRAPHY AND VECTORCARDIOGRAPHY

by CHARLES FISCH, M.D.

The clinical electrocardiogram (ECG) records the changing potentials of an electrical field imparted by the heart or, more precisely, at any instant an aggregate of cardiac cells. The ECG does not record directly the electrical activity of the source itself. Such activity is registered only when an electrode is in immediate contact with the tissue generating the current and at the moment when the electrode senses the edge of the wave of activation or recovery. In all other circumstances only potential differences in an electrical field are registered. It is important to appreciate that the ECG, while recording the changes of an electrical field, often provides only an approximation of the voltage generated by the heart. Efforts to predict surface potentials from the knowledge of behavior of the cardiac generator—the so-called electrocardiographic forward problem—or to predict the electrical behavior of the cardiac generator from the body surface potentials—the so-called electrocardiographic inverse problem—have to date been unsuccessful.[1]

Despite this basic limitation, the ECG has evolved into an extremely useful clinical laboratory tool and is the only practical means of recording the electrical behavior of the heart. Its usefulness as a diagnostic method is the result of careful, often purely deductive analysis of innumerable patient records and of studies correlating the ECG with basic electrophysiological properties of the heart; with clinical and laboratory findings; and with anatomical, pathological, and experimental observations.[2] The result has been that electrocardiography can be used, within limits, to identify anatomical, metabolic, ionic, and hemodynamic changes. It is often an independent marker of cardiac disease and occasionally the only indicator of a pathological process.[3–13]

Electrocardiography serves as a gold standard for the diagnosis of arrhythmias, which are discussed in detail in Chapters 20 to 23. Although arrhythmias have been studied by a variety of methods for centuries, none has approached the levels of sensitivity and specificity offered by the ECG. Free of the assumptions required for interpreting the electrocardiographic waveforms, arrhythmias recorded from the surface of the body, with rare exceptions, accurately reflect intracardiac events. However, while most arrhythmias are due to disordered impulse formation or conduction (or both) of the specialized tissue, the ECG reflects the electrical behavior of the myocardium and not of the specialized tissue. This limitation, once appreciated as inherent in the ECG, rarely interferes with proper analysis of even the most complex arrhythmias.

As with any other laboratory procedure, the sensitivity and specificity of the ECG and of its individual components are critical determinants of its clinical usefulness. This is far more complex for the ECG than for other laboratory techniques developed for any single purpose, since its multiple waveforms may be identically or differentially influenced by a wide spectrum of physiological, pathophysiological, or anatomical changes. Thus, it may be difficult—if not impossible—to identify a single cause for any given ECG abnormality.[12]

THE NORMAL ELECTROCARDIOGRAM AND VECTORCARDIOGRAM

THEORETICAL CONSIDERATIONS

Essential to an understanding of the derivation and interpretation of the clinical ECG is information about (1) the physical and electrophysiological events responsible for the electrical potential recorded as the transmembrane action potential, and the spread of excitation; (2) the role of the volume conductor; and (3) the theoretical basis of the lead systems.

ELECTRICAL BASES AND THEORY

At any instant, the cardiac generator can be viewed as a dipole consisting of a positive and a negative charge separated by a small distance. Since the dipole generates a force that has magnitude and direction, it can be expressed as a vector. By convention the arrowhead of the vector indicates the positive pole. When such a dipole is immersed in a volume conductor, an electrical field is generated.[14, 15] In a homogeneous volume conductor, the field is symmetrically distributed. The lines of the electrical field are symmetrical in relation to a line that is perpendicular to and transects the dipole at its midpoint.

At any instant, the magnitude of the potential at a given point (P) in the volume conductor can be estimated using the solid-angle concept, or the concept relating the potential to an angle formed by a line drawn from P to the midpoint of the dipole axis and the dipole axis itself (Fig. 7–1).

The electrical surface with its boundary projected to P results in a cone and defines the solid angle subtended by the area in question. The segment of a sphere inscribed by a radius of unity drawn about point P, with P as the center of the sphere, and its border delineated by the cone, is proportional to the area of electrical activity. With variables such as tissue resistance and geometry being constant, the voltage at P can be expressed as $Ep = \phi \cdot \Omega$, where ϕ is voltage per unit of the solid angle and Ω is the solid angle.[16, 17]

An alternative and perhaps clinically more applicable approach to estimating Ep considers the distance (r) of P from the source, the strength of the source (m), and the cosine of the angle formed by a line drawn from P to the midpoint of the dipole axis and the dipole axis

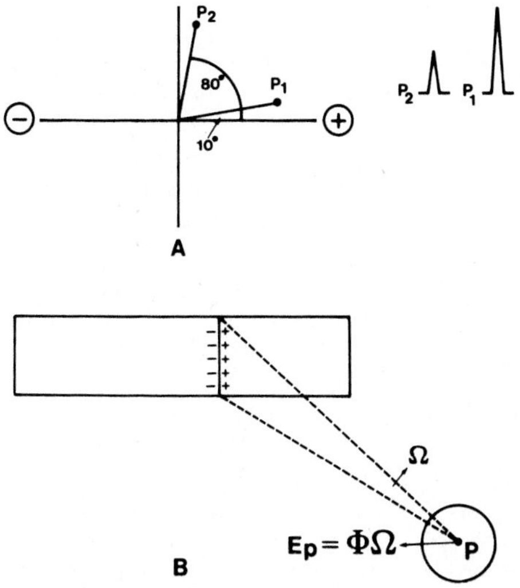

FIGURE 7–1. *A,* **The potentials at points P_1 and P_2 are inversely proportional to the square of the distance from the source and proportional to the cosine of angle formed by a line drawn from point P to the midpoint of the dipole axis and the axis itself.** *B,* **The potential E is proportional to the solid angle Ω and the strength of the charged surface subtending the angle ⇄. (Modified from Wolff, L.: Electrocardiography: Fundamentals and Clinical Application. 3rd ed. Philadelphia, W. B. Saunders Co., 1962, p. 15.)**

(Θ), with the magnitude of the angle estimated in reference to the positive pole of the dipole. This relationship can be expressed as

$$Ep = \frac{m \cos \Theta}{\gamma^2}$$

According to this formula, when the angle is 90°, the line drawn from P is perpendicular to the dipole axis and the Ep is zero. In the ECG the inscription would be isoelectric or equiphasic. On the other hand, with the angle becoming smaller, the P is closer to the positive pole of the dipole and the voltage becomes greater.[16, 17]

Assuming that the volume conductor is homogeneous and infinite and has a uniform boundary and that the generator is located in the center of the volume conductor, both approaches for estimation of Ep at P are correct. Such assumptions, however, are not entirely valid in man (see below).

The influence of polarity of the dipole, the distance of the electrode from the dipole, and the strength of the electrical field on waveform are important in analysis of the ECG. These relationships can be studied using a hypothetical dipole or tissue immersed in a homogeneous volume conductor. An electrode, located outside the electrical field, when moved into the negative field records a gradually increasing negativity. Halfway between the two poles, a sharp reversal of polarity is registered (intrinsic deflection) and the electrode enters the positive field. As the electrode is moved, positive voltage declines gradually until a potential difference is no longer registered. A similar sequence of events is registered with the electrode stationary and the electrical field moving relative to the electrode. When the positive field moves toward the electrode, a positive potential is recorded; when the electrode finds itself in the negative field, a negative potential is recorded.

ELECTROPHYSIOLOGICAL BASES AND THEORY

Transmembrane ionic fluxes are responsible for voltage differences between activated and resting tissue. These ionic fluxes are reflected as the transmembrane action potential, the cellular counterpart of the clinical ECG. The ECG counterparts of the phases 0, 1, 2, 3, and 4 of the transmembrane action potential are the QRS complex, the ST segment, the T wave, and the isoelectric baseline, respectively (Chap. 20).

DEPOLARIZATION AND REPOLARIZATION. To progress logically toward an understanding of the ECG, we will review the effect of a muscle strip immersed in a homogenous volume conductor on the electrical field generated by the muscle strip and on the electrode immersed in the field. A muscle strip, when uniformly positive on the outside, is in a resting or polarized state. Because it exhibits no difference of potential and fails to impart an electrical field, an electrode immersed in the volume conductor registers an isoelectric line. Stimulation of the muscle strip at any given point increases membrane permeability, and positive ions, largely sodium, enter the cell. The result is depolarized (relatively negative) muscle in apposition to polarized (relatively positive) muscle, with a potential difference across a boundary. In the surrounding medium the current flows from the positively (source) to the negatively (sink) charged muscle. The moving boundary between the polarized (positive) and the depolarized (negative) muscle can be represented by a dipole or vector. This dipole or vector moves along the muscle fiber from the point of excitation, leaving in its wake tissue that is electrically negative (depolarized) in relation to the still polarized (resting) muscle. When the wave of depolarization reaches the end of the muscle strip, the surface becomes uniformly negative and the strip is now completely depolarized. Since a difference of potential no longer exists, an isoelectric baseline is inscribed. The most intense difference of potential exists at the boundary between depolarized and resting tissue, and the recorded voltage changes reflect the events taking place at this boundary.[14, 15]

Restitution of membrane polarity, or *repolarization*, can be viewed as a "wave" of positivity enveloping the cells or tissue. As a result, the outside of the cell is again uniformly positive. Since the boundary moves in the direction of the depolarized, negative muscle, an electrode located at the point of origin of repolarization records a positive potential. An electrode placed at the opposite end records a negative potential. In a preparation of isolated myocardial tissue, the direction of repolarization is the same as that of depolarization but is preceded by the negative pole of the dipole. The repolarization inscribes an area equal to that inscribed by depolarization but of opposite polarity.

EFFECT OF THE BOUNDARY OF DEPOLARIZATION ON THE POLARITY OF THE RECORDED POTENTIAL. Three electrodes placed on a muscle strip will illustrate the effect of a boundary potential, which can be represented as a dipole or vector, on the recording electrode (Fig. 7–2). Electrode A is located at the point of excitation, electrode B at the midpoint of the muscle strip, and electrode C at the opposite end of the muscle strip. Immediately after excitation, electrode A finds itself in the most intensively negative field. As the dipole moves away, the potential becomes less negative, and at the end of depolarization the inscription returns to the baseline. Thus, the electrode at point A inscribes a negative deflection. At the moment of excitation, electrode B is located in the positive field of the dipole. As the dipole moves toward the recording electrode, the latter registers a gradually increasing positivity and records an upright deflection. When the dipole passes the electrode, there is a sudden reversal of polarity, termed the *intrinsic deflection*, and the electrode finds itself in a strongly negative field. A downward, negative deflection is recorded. With the dipole moving away, the electrode at point B registers a less negative potential, and finally, when the strip is completely depolarized, an isoelectric baseline is recorded. Thus, the electrode at point B registers a positive-negative deflection. Electrode C is

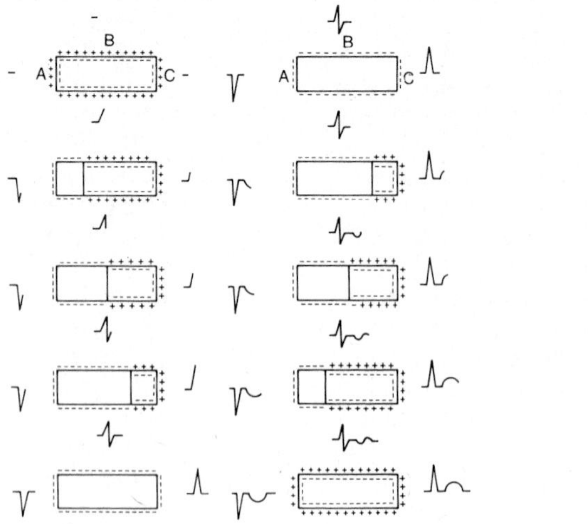

FIGURE 7–2. Potential generated during depolarization (*left vertical sequence of panels*) and repolarization (*right vertical sequence of panels*) recorded with an exploring electrode located at the endocardium (A), epicardium (C), and midway between the two (B). (Modified from Barker, J. M.: The Unipolar Electrocardiogram: A Clinical Interpretation. New York, Appleton-Century-Crofts, Inc., 1952.)

located in the positive field throughout the entire process of depolarization. As the dipole approaches the electrode, the field becomes more intensively positive, with the most intense positivity at the moment immediately prior to completion of depolarization. Thus, the electrode at point C records an upright deflection.

SEQUENCE OF CARDIAC ACTIVATION. The sequence of cardiac activation has been studied in animals, primarily in the dog and in the isolated perfused human heart.[18] The normal impulse originates in the sinoatrial (SA) node and traverses the atria in a wavelike front with a velocity of approximately 1000 mm/sec. The wave of atrial activation resembles a wavefront seen when a pebble is thrown into water. The sinoatrial node is located in the right atrium and initially activates the right atrium in a right and anterior direction, followed by excitation of the left atrium in a left and posterior direction. It has been suggested that preferential internodal pathways connect the SA node and the atrioventricular (AV) junctional tissue and that these specialized internodal pathways are capable of conducting an impulse in the presence of a quiescent atrium.[19] The concept has attracted considerable interest and is the subject of continued investigation.[20]

The impulse arrives at the AV node, where it is delayed, most probably because of decremental conduction (p. 600).[21] Study of the sequence of ventricular activation in the dog reveals an early (0 to 5 msec) and almost simultaneous activation of the central left side of the septum and the high anterior and apical posterior paraseptal areas of the left ventricle. At 5 to 10 msec after the onset of ventricular activation, the wave of activation envelops left and right ventricular walls and the remainder of the septum; the latter is completely activated at 12 msec. The earliest epicardial breakthrough occurs at the anterior right epicardial surface near the apex, followed by anterior and posterior paraseptal areas of the left ventricle. At 18 msec, activation of the central portion of the two ventricles is complete. Excitation continues along the lateral and basal aspects of the left ventricle, with the basal portion of the septum the last to become depolarized.[16]

Studies of perfused human heart indicate that its path of activation closely follows that of the canine heart (Fig. 7–3). The results obtained in the resuscitated human heart were validated by comparing the process of activation with that of a perfused and in situ dog heart. The only difference was that the activation proceeded more rapidly in the perfused dog preparation.[18] By means of intracardiac mapping during surgery it has also been shown that epicardial breakthrough occurred in the right ventricle followed by activation of the anterior and inferior left ventricle.[22]

Less information is available concerning the sequence of *repolarization* in the intact heart. For one thing, the electrodes used to plot the wave of repolarization may induce a current of injury and interfere with the recording of meaningful data. Human studies indicate that atrial repolarization follows approximately the same path as atrial depolarization, with the polarity of repolarization opposite to that of depolarization. Ventricular repolarization proceeds in a direction *opposite* to that of depolarization, and its polarity is therefore the *same* as that of depolarization. The process of repolarization recorded directly from the epicardium indicates that in the intact ventricle repolarization begins at the epicardium—a sequence opposite to that observed in isolated muscle strip. The reason for the in vivo reversal of the order of repolarization is not entirely clear. The presence of a transmural pressure gradient may be an important factor, since it prolongs the duration of the excited state of the endocardium and, consequently, recovery begins at the epicardium.

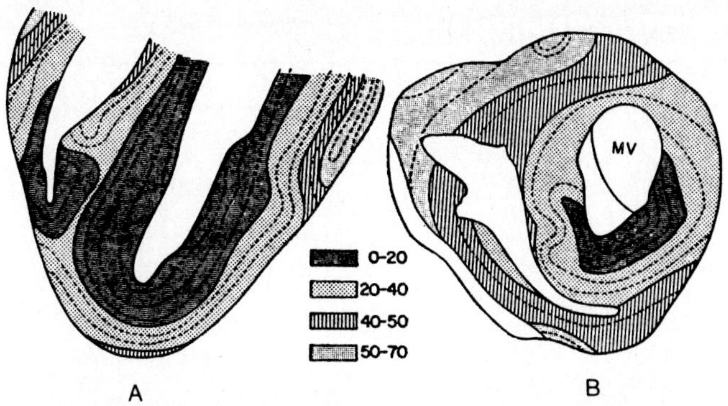

FIGURE 7–3. Sequence of ventricular activation of an isolated human heart. *A* and *B* represent sagittal and coronal sections, respectively. The dotted lines denote 5-msec sequences, while changes in pattern represent 20-msec intervals. (Durrer, D., et al.: Total excitation of the isolated human heart. Circulation *41*:899, 1970, by permission of the American Heart Association, Inc.)

VENTRICULAR GRADIENT. The ventricular gradient (G), introduced by Wilson, describes the relationships between depolarization (QRS) and repolarization (T).[23] In an isolated muscle strip depolarization and repolarization are equal in duration and follow the same path. The net areas of the QRS complex (AQRS) and the T wave (AT) are equal but of opposite polarity, so that their sum is zero and there is no gradient. In the intact heart, on the other hand, repolarization proceeds from the epicardium to endocardium, in a direction *opposite* to that of depolarization; the algebraic sum of their respective areas is no longer zero; and a gradient is said to exist. AQRS, AT, and G can be expressed as a vectorial quantity from any two of the three bipolar limb leads of the ECG. AQRS and AT are expressed in the form of vectors and are plotted using the Einthoven triangle or Bayley triaxial reference system. A parallelogram of the AQRS and the AT is constructed, with the resultant diagonal vector being the manifest AQRST vector or gradient (G). The G vector and the mean QRS vector are located in about the same plane. The G forms an angle of approximately 30° with the mean spatial QRS vector.

G is an index of variation in duration of the excited state and thus of the local rate of repolarization. Although it is of theoretical value in the study of T-wave abnormalities, the variations between individuals and in the same individual and the tedious calculations required, especially when small changes may prove important, limit its clinical usefulness. The electrocardiographer intuitively evaluates the ventricular gradient whenever reading the cardiogram.

THEORETICAL BASES OF SURFACE LEADS. At any instant the surface leads reflect projection of the electrical field of the equivalent or "net" dipole expressed as the mean instantaneous spatial vector. Orientation of a lead axis is defined as one that records a maximal voltage when its axis is parallel to that of the axis or vector of the equivalent dipole. The voltage registered in any lead, having magnitude and direction, can be expressed as a vector (lead vector), with the amplitude of deflection in any lead paralleling the magnitude of the vector. Since more than one dipole may exist at any instant, the net potential and consequently the resultant lead vector reflect the contribution of all such dipoles. Furthermore, because dipole vectors may vary in magnitude and direction, the equivalent or "net" dipole is an approximation of these forces and consequently its expression on a lead axis is also an approximation.

LEADS. *Bipolar limb leads,* introduced by Einthoven, register the direction, magnitude, and duration of voltage changes in the frontal plane. The three bipolar leads—I, II, and III—record the difference in potential between left arm (LA) and right arm (RA), left leg (LF) and RA, and LF and LA, respectively.

Unipolar limb leads are constructed by connecting all three extremities to a "central terminal" (Fig. 7–4A). Although in reality the central terminal registers a small voltage, for practical purposes it is considered to have a zero potential and serves as the *indifferent* or *reference electrode.* The potential differences recorded by the positive terminal, the *exploring electrode,* are dominated by local electrical events. When placed on the right arm, left arm, or left foot, the exploring electrode registers the potential from the respective limb. The letter V identifies a unipolar lead and the letters r, l, and f the respective extremities. If one disconnects the central terminal from the extremity from which the potential is being recorded, the amplitude registered by the respective unipolar limb lead is augmented; such leads are designated as aV_r, aV_l, and aV_f.

Locations of the exploring electrode for the *precordial leads* are as follows: V_1—fourth interspace to the right of the sternum; V_2—fourth interspace to the left of the sternum; V_3—midway between leads V_2 and V_4; V_4—fifth interspace at the midclavicular line; V_5—anterior axillary line at the level of lead V_4; and V_6—midaxillary line at the level of lead V_4 (Fig. 7–4A).[24]

Of the six precordial leads, it is assumed that in the absence of major thoracic deformity or cardiac malposition, leads V_1 and V_2, V_3 and V_4, and V_5 and V_6 face the right side of the septum, the septum itself, and the left side of the septum, respectively, and are referred to as right ventricular, septal or transitional, and left ventricular leads, respectively.

THE NORMAL ELECTROCARDIOGRAM

THE P WAVE

The cardiac impulse originating in the SA node activates the right and left atria in the general direction from right to left atrium, inferiorly and posteriorly. Initial activation

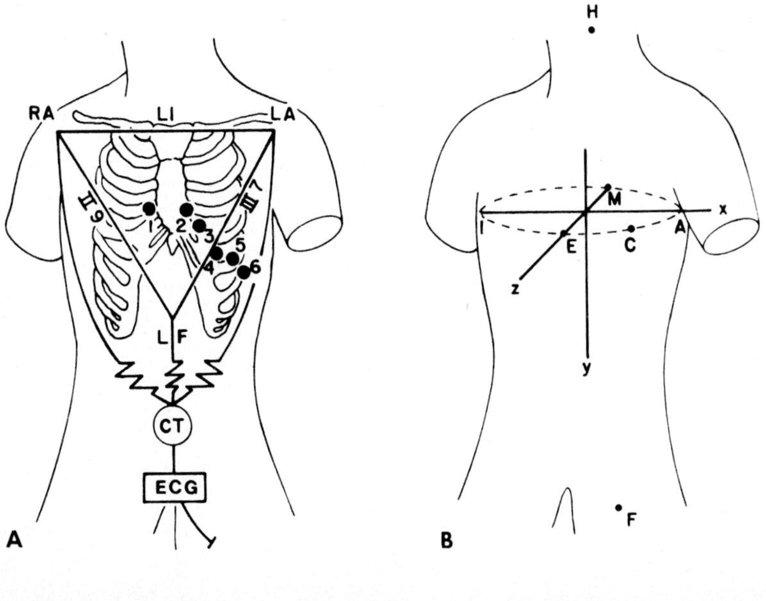

FIGURE 7–4. *A,* ECG lead system. Leads I, II, and III are formed by connecting RA-LA, RA-LF, and LA-LF respectively. The indifferent electrode of the unipolar system is obtained by connecting RA, LA, and LF through 50,000-ohm resistance into a central terminal (CT). (For details about positioning of the exploring unipolar electrode, see discussion under Leads.) *B,* Frank electrode system. Five horizontal electrodes are placed at the level where the fifth intercostal space intersects the sternal line. Specific locations include fifth intercostal space and sternum (E), the midaxillary line (A,I) and the vertebral column (M). Electrode C is located halfway between points E and A, while electrodes H and F are on the back of the neck and left lower extremity, respectively.

TABLE 7–1
P WAVE: AMPLITUDE AND DURATION IN NORMAL ADULTS

	LEAD I	LEAD II	LEAD III	LEAD V_1*
P Amplitude (mv)				
Mean	0.049	0.103	0.069	0.040
Range	0.02 to 0.10	0.03 to 0.20	0 to 0.20	0.005 to 0.080
P Duration (sec)				
Mean	0.08	0.09	0.16	0.05
Range	0.05 to 0.12	0.05 to 0.12	0.12 to 0.20	0 to 0.08
P-R Interval (sec)				
Mean	0.16	0.16		
Range	0.12 to 0.20	0.12 to 0.20		

AMPLITUDE OF Q, R, S, AND T WAVES IN SCALAR ELECTROCARDIOGRAM OF 100 NORMAL ADULTS†

	I	II	III	aV_r	aV_l	aV_f	V_1	V_5	V_6
Patients With Q Wave	38%	41%	50%	—	38%	40%	0%	60%	75%
Q Amplitude									
Mean	0.4	0.6	0.09	—	0.04	0.07	0	0.03	0.03
Range	0 to 0.1	0 to 0.16	0 to 0.23		0 to 0.11	0 to 0.17	0	0 to 0.18	0 to 0.18
R Amplitude									
Mean	0.56	0.89	0.45	0.13	0.34	0.6	0.19	1.2	1.0
Range	0.1 to 1.0	0.2 to 1.6	0.1 to 1.2	0 to 0.29	0 to 0.82	0 to 1.38	0.1 to 0.6	0.7 to 2.1	0.5 to 1.8
S Amplitude									
Mean	0.2	0.2	0.24	0.7	0.26	—	0.8	0.25	0.13
Range	0 to 0.5	0 to 0.37	0 to 0.64	0.22 to 1.18	0 to 0.58	—	0.3 to 1.3	0 to 0.5	0 to 0.2
T Amplitude									
Mean	0.19	0.23	0.1	—	0.03	0.17	0.1	0.33	0.1
Range	0.1 to 0.3	0.1 to 0.2	−0.2 to 0.2	—	−0.1 to 0.2	0 to 0.4	−0.2 to 0.2	0.2 to 0.7	0.1 to 0.4

*Twenty-five per cent of the series had a small terminal negative deflection of the P wave in lead V_1.
†Amplitude values are in millivolts (0.1 mV = 1 mm).
From Cooksey, J. D., et al.: Clinical Vectorcardiography and Electrocardiography, 2nd ed. Chicago, Year Book Medical Publishers, 1977.

of the right atrium, an anterior chamber, is directed anteriorly and inferiorly and is followed by activation of the left or posterior atrium, directed to the left, posteriorly, and inferiorly.

The P wave is rounded with a notch corresponding to the separation between right and left atrial activation. Amplitude of the P wave is normally less than 0.20 mV (2.0 mm) with a duration less than 0.12 sec (Table 7–1).

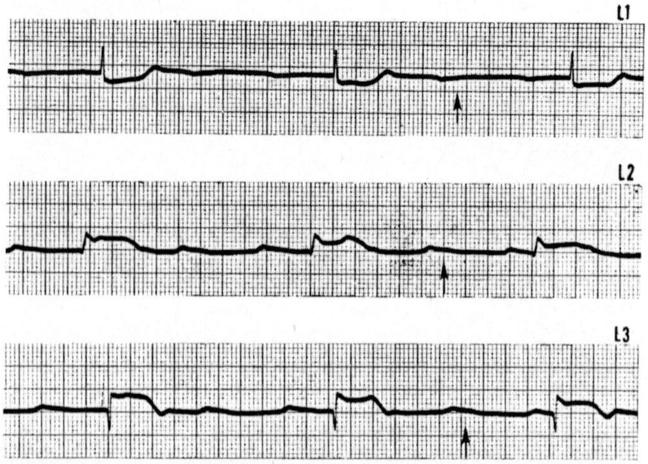

FIGURE 7–5. Atrial infarction. The tracing illustrates sinus rhythm, complete AV block, and an acute inferior myocardial infarction. The Ta segment indicative of atrial infarction is elevated in leads II and III (arrows) and depressed in lead I (arrow).

The P wave and the *Ta segment*, or atrial repolarization, define atrial electrical systole. The P vector varies from −50° to +60°. In the precordial leads the P wave is positive except in lead V_1, where the P wave may be upright, biphasic, or negative.

The Ta segment is inscribed during the QRS complex and the early part of the ST segment. It is best seen in the presence of AV block (Fig. 7–5). Duration of the Ta segment varies from 0.15 to 0.45 sec, and its amplitude is low, reaching 0.08 mV. The magnitude of the Ta is directionally related to the area of the P wave. The orientation of the Ta segment is opposite to that of the P wave. The P wave and Ta areas are equal and opposite in direction, and the resultant gradient is zero. In the presence of atrial enlargement, the Ta segment may result in displacement of the ST segment (p. 186).

P-R INTERVAL. The P-R interval includes the time for intraatrial, AV nodal, and His-Purkinje conduction, and its duration varies from 0.12 to 0.20 or 0.22 sec (Table 7–1; Chap. 20).

THE QRS COMPLEX

Ventricular activation proceeds chiefly symmetrically about the septum and from the endocardium to the epicardium. Consequently, much of its voltage is canceled; in fact, only 10 to 15 per cent of the potential generated by the heart is ultimately recorded on the surface ECG.

The normal QRS complex can be described by four vectors[11] (Fig. 7–6): (1) initial septal activation from left to

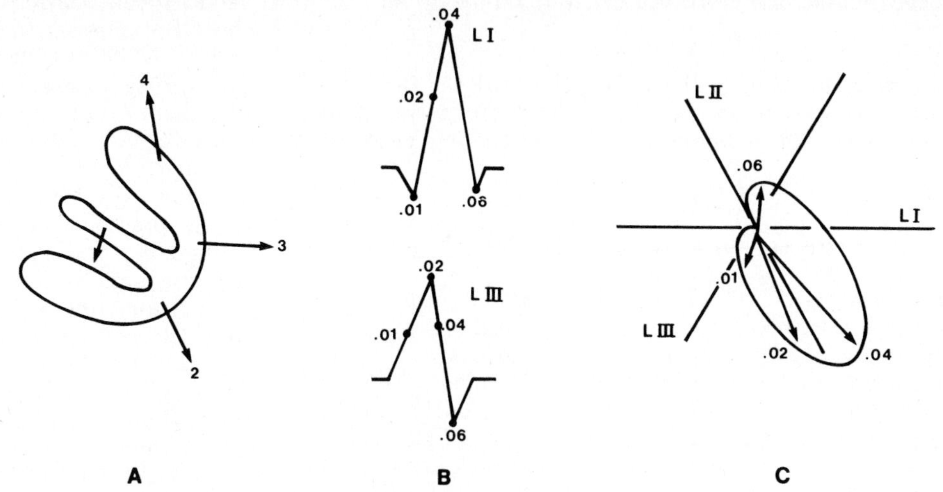

FIGURE 7–6. Correlation between the order of ventricular activation (*A*), scalar ECG (*B*), and vectorcardiogram (*C*). *A*, The sequence of ventricular activation is represented by four instantaneous frontal plane vectors. *B*, The four vectors plotted on leads I and III at the appropriate time during inscription of the QRS. *C*, Using the method of construction of vectors described in Figure 7–7, one can derive each of the four vectors in the frontal plane. A line joining the ends of the vectors results in a frontal plane QRS loop. The same method can be used to derive the orthogonal X, Y, and Z leads from the frontal, transverse, or sagittal planes. (Times given are in seconds.)

right, anteriorly, inferiorly, or superiorly, followed by further septal activation from left to right (0.01 sec); (2) an overlapping wave of excitation involving both ventricles, with the vector directed inferiorly and slightly to the left (0.02 sec); (3) unopposed activation of the apical and central portions of the left ventricle, the thin right ventricular wall having been depolarized, with a resultant vector directed posteriorly, inferiorly, and to the left (0.04 sec); and, finally, (4) activation of the posterior basal portion of the left ventricle and septum, with a vector directed superiorly and posteriorly (0.06 sec).

Septal activation from left to right and anteriorly results, normally, in an initial Q wave in leads I, II, III, aV_l, V_5, and V_6 and an R wave in the right precordial and septal leads V_1 to V_4. Lead aV_f registers an R or Q wave depending on whether the septal vector is directed superiorly or inferiorly. The ventricular vector directed inferiorly and to the left is reflected by an R wave in leads II and III and in the transitional or septal leads V_3 and V_4. The third vector, that of the unopposed force directed to the left, posteriorly, and somewhat inferiorly, gives rise to an R wave in leads I, II, III, aV_l, aV_f, V_5, V_6, and occasionally V_4, with an S wave in leads aV_r, V_1, V_2, V_3, and at times V_4. The terminal force directed superiorly and posteriorly and perhaps to the right may result in a terminal S wave in leads I, V_5, and V_6. A lead positioned in the right fourth interspace in the midclavicular line (V_{4r}) may record a terminal R wave (R′), which may also occasionally be recorded in lead V_1.[24]

The magnitude of the Q, R, and S waves is given in Table 7–1.

THE QRS AXIS, POSITION, AND ROTATION. The electrical position of the heart can be described by the QRS axis and the rotation of the heart on the anteroposterior and longitudinal (apex-to-base) axes. As the *order* of activation can be viewed as a sequence of instantaneous dipoles or vectors, *total* cardiac activation can be presented as a mean QRS vector. When such a vector is placed within the triangle formed by leads I, II, and III, which define the frontal plane, and assuming that this triangle is equilateral, that the heart is located in its center, and that the thorax is a homogeneous volume conductor with a uniform boundary, projection of the vector on the respective leads permits an estimate of the magnitude of voltage recorded in each lead. Similarly, if the voltage in each of the leads is known, the mean QRS vector can be reconstructed and the axis of the QRS complex can be estimated (Fig. 7–7).

The preceding assumptions—the Einthoven postulates—are applicable in the experimental setting. In the human, however, the heart is a large organ; it is not a point generator nor is it centrally located, and the thorax is not a homogeneous conductor within a uniform boundary. Burger, using a model of a human torso, with nonhomogeneous conduction to reflect the nature of human organs and an eccentrically located generator, found that the triangle formed by the axes of leads I, II, and III is not equilateral but is scalene, with lead I being shortest and lead III longest.[25] The scalene triangle configuration is more consistent with clinical electrocardiography.

The most accurate method for determining the QRS axis is based on estimation of the QRS area in each of the limb leads and a plot of these as vectors on the respective lead axis of a triaxial reference system. From the positive end of the vector, lines perpendicular to the lead axis are

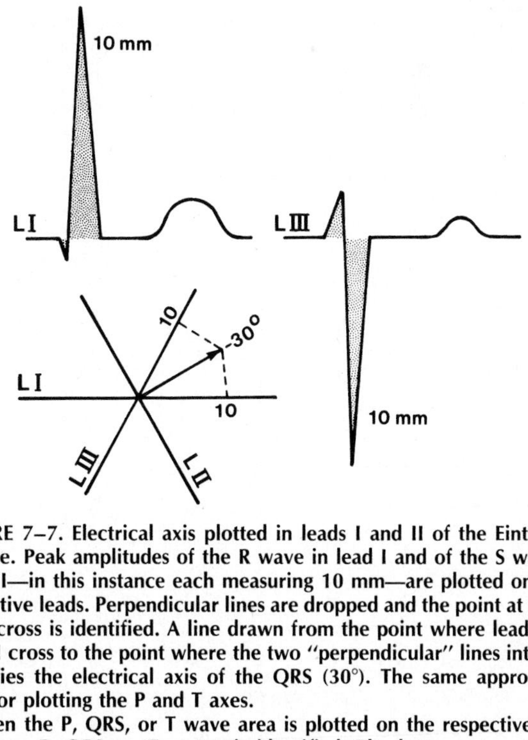

FIGURE 7–7. Electrical axis plotted in leads I and II of the Einthoven triangle. Peak amplitudes of the R wave in lead I and of the S wave in lead III—in this instance each measuring 10 mm—are plotted on their respective leads. Perpendicular lines are dropped and the point at which these cross is identified. A line drawn from the point where leads I, II, and III cross to the point where the two "perpendicular" lines intersect identifies the electrical axis of the QRS (30°). The same approach is used for plotting the P and T axes.

When the P, QRS, or T wave area is plotted on the respective lead, the mean P, QRS, or T vector is identified. The latter represents the mean magnitude, direction, and polarity of the entire period of depolarization. This is a more accurate but impractical method of estimating the electrical axis. Although the direction of the QRS axis and of the mean QRS vector differ, as a rule both lie in the same quadrant.

dropped. A vector is drawn from the center of the triaxial reference system to the point where the perpendicular lines cross. This vector defines the direction and magnitude of the mean QRS vector ($\overset{\Delta}{\text{AQRS}}$). The same method is used to estimate the T vector ($\overset{\Delta}{\text{AT}}$). Normally, the angle between $\overset{\Delta}{\text{AQRS}}$ and $\overset{\Delta}{\text{AT}}$ does not exceed 30°. For practical purposes, however, the assumption that the magnitude of the force projected on a given lead axis is directionally related to the cosine of the angle subtended by the lead vector and lead axis allows a rapid and reasonably accurate estimate of the QRS axis. Thus, if the mean QRS vector is perpendicular to a given lead axis, the angle between the two is 90°, the cosine of the angle is zero, and the QRS will be isoelectric, very small, or equiphasic. On the other hand, when the mean QRS vector is parallel to a lead axis, the angle between the two is zero, the cosine of the angle is one, and the amplitude of the QRS will be greatest in that lead.

Plotted on a hexaxial reference system, axes of −30° to +90°, −30° to −90°, +90° to 180°, and −90° to 180° are normal, left, right, and indeterminate, respectively (Fig. 7–8).[26]

An *anteroposterior axis* allows the apex to face either the left arm or the left foot or to assume a position between the two. Thus, when a QRS complex in aV_l resembles that in leads V_5 and V_6, the electrical position is said to be horizontal. On the other hand, when the QRS complex in aV_f reflects that in leads V_5 and V_6, the position is said to be vertical. Similarly, in the horizontal position the QRS complex in aV_f and in the vertical position the QRS complex in aV_r resemble the QRS complex in lead V_1. When the apex is approximately equidistant from the two extremities, both aV_l and aV_f exhibit QRS complexes resembling those in leads V_5 and V_6, and the position is said to be intermediate. If the position shifts more toward the left arm or the left foot, the position is said to be semihorizontal and semivertical, respectively. In the semihorizontal position, the QRS complex in lead aV_l resembles that of leads V_5 and V_6, while the QRS complex in lead aV_f is small. In the semivertical position, the QRS complex in lead aV_f resembles that of leads V_5 and V_6, while the QRS complex in aV_l is small.

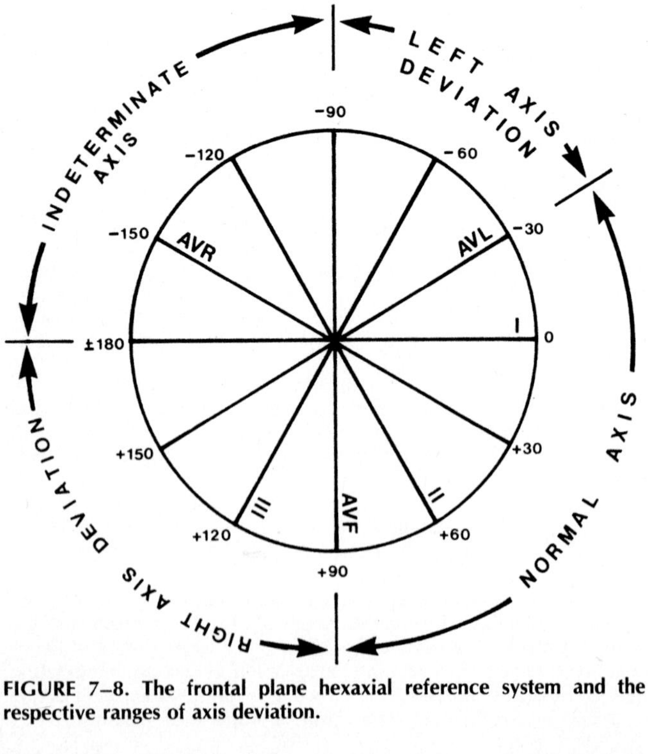

FIGURE 7–8. The frontal plane hexaxial reference system and the respective ranges of axis deviation.

Clockwise and counterclockwise rotation along the *longitudinal, apex-to-base axis* can be recognized by analysis of the precordial leads. The direction of rotation is described by viewing the heart from a position below the diaphragmatic surface. *Clockwise rotation* shifts the transitional zone (the position at which the rS complex changes to a qR complex) to the left and consequently the right ventricular QRS complex (rS) is displaced to the left and occasionally may be registered in all the precordial positions. *Counterclockwise rotation* results in a more anterior shift of the left ventricle and a more posterior displacement of the right ventricle. Consequently, the transitional zone is shifted to the right and the left precordial QRS (qR) pattern may be registered, for example, in the V_3 position.

THE ST SEGMENT

The ST segment reflects phase 2 of the transmembrane action potential (p. 181). Since there is little change in this potential during this phase, the ST segment is usually isoelectric in normal subjects.

THE T WAVE

The mechanism and sequence of ventricular repolarization were described on page 182. The right and left precordial T waves are upright in 75 and 50 per cent of newborns, respectively. After about 8 hours, and invariably after 60 to 90 hours, the left precordial T waves become upright. The right precordial T waves usually become upright after the age of 16 but occasionally the negative T waves persist into early adulthood—a normal variant—termed the *juvenile* T wave (Fig. 7–9A).[27]

In the adult, all the unipolar leads inscribe an upright T wave except for aV_r, and occasionally V_1. The amplitude of T waves is given in Table 7–1.

THE U WAVE

The genesis of the U wave, which follows the T wave, is not clear. It has been suggested that it represents a surface reflection of a negative afterpotential. The two prevailing concepts of the mechanism of the U wave include repolarization of the Purkinje fibers and a mechanical event, presumably ventricular relaxation.[28, 29]

The U wave is upright and its amplitude is 5 to 50 per cent that of the T wave. The tallest U wave is recorded in leads V_2 and V_3, where its amplitude may reach 0.2 mV (Fig. 7–9). Ordinarily the U and T waves are clearly separated. However, under conditions in which the U wave appears early, such as with abbreviated ventricular filling and ejection or when the Q-T interval is prolonged (as with hypocalcemia or after administration of drugs such as quinidine), the U wave may be difficult to separate from the T wave; on the other hand, when the Q-T interval is abbreviated, as with digitalis or hypercalcemia, the U wave is easily identifiable.

THE Q-T INTERVAL

The Q-T interval, measured from the beginning of the QRS complex to the end of the T wave, reflects, within

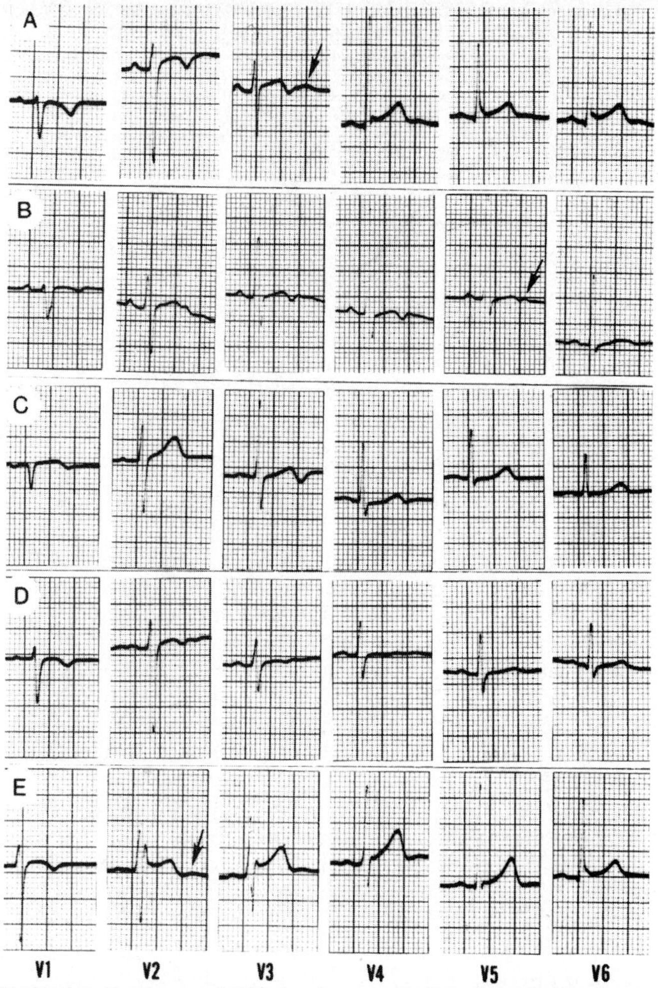

FIGURE 7–9. Abnormal ECG in absence of clinical heart disease. *A*, Persistence of juvenile T-wave inversion in leads V_1, V_2, and V_3 and ST-segment elevation in leads V_4, V_5, and V_6 due to early repolarization recorded in a 21-year-old man. *B*, Notched T waves and isolated T-wave inversion in leads V_3, V_4, and V_5 recorded in a 19-year-old man. *C*, Isolated midprecordial T-wave negativity recorded in a 24-year-old man. *D*, Abnormal T waves in leads V_1 to V_4 recorded in a 45-year-old woman. *E*, RR' pattern in leads V_2 andV_3 and ST-segment elevation in leads V_2 to V_6 due to early repolarization recorded in a 32-year-old man. A normal U wave follows the T wave.

limitations, the duration of depolarization and repolarization. Importantly, the Q-T interval may not always accurately reflect the recovery time of the ventricles. In some portions of the ventricles repolarization is complete before the end of the Q-T interval, while in other areas repolarization may continue after the end of the Q-T interval, but because of the small magnitude of the potential or because of cancellation, it cannot be identified in the surface tracing. In addition, because the onset of the QRS complex or the end of the T wave or both may be difficult to define, one cannot always obtain an accurate measurement of the Q-T interval. The point at which the line of maximal downslope of the T wave crosses the baseline helps to identify the end of the T wave.

Duration of the Q-T interval varies with cycle length, and numerous formulas have been suggested to correct for heart rate. Bazett proposed a formula for estimating the Q-T interval corrected for heart rate,[30] or the *Q-Tc interval:* $\frac{\text{Q-T}}{\sqrt{\text{R-R}}}$. The upper limit of the Q-Tc interval is 0.39 sec for men and 0.44 sec for women. Because of the variability of measurements and potential influences other than heart rate, different ranges of normal are accepted by different investigators.[31, 32] For practical purposes, therefore, minor deviations from the expected Q-Tc interval should be disregarded as being of questionable clinical significance.

THE NORMAL VECTORCARDIOGRAM

Vectorcardiography can be defined as registration of the time course of mean instantaneous spatial cardiac vectors.[11, 33] The concept of vectorcardiography was introduced in 1920 by Mann.[34] By plotting on a triaxial reference system a number of vectors derived simultaneously from leads I and III, and by connecting the ends of the derived vectors, Mann recorded a loop, which he termed a monocardiogram (Fig. 7–6*C*); the term vectorcardiogram (VCG) was coined by Wilson in 1938.[35] The advent of the cathode-ray oscilloscope allowed direct recording of the loop. The cathode-ray tube has two sets of plates controlling the horizontal and vertical displacement of an electronic beam. The *X (transverse) lead* is connected to the right and left plates, the *Y (vertical) lead* to the superior and inferior plates. The anterior and posterior connections of the *Z (sagittal) lead* are connected to the lower and upper plates. The X, Y, and Z leads constitute the *orthogonal lead system.*

The positive orientation indicated by the arrows is to the left for the X lead, to the foot (or inferior) for the Y lead, and to the back (or posterior) for the Z lead. A vector directed to the left, inferiorly, and posteriorly will inscribe a positive deflection in leads X, Y, and Z, respectively (Fig. 7–10).

VCG loops are recorded in three planes: frontal, transverse, and sagittal. Both right and left sagittal views are in use. Any two of the three leads of the orthogonal system will define a plane and will inscribe a loop in a given plane. The combination of X and Y, X and Z, or Y and Z will register the VCG loop in the frontal, transverse, or sagittal planes, respectively. To correct for nonuniformity of the conducting medium, eccentricity of the heart as a source,

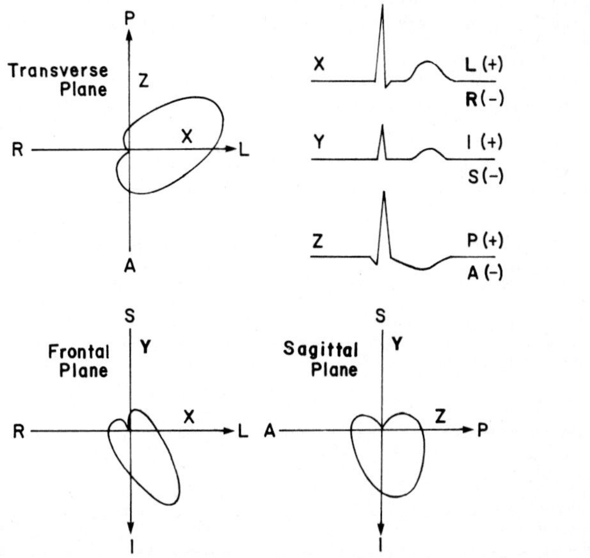

FIGURE 7–10. The transverse, frontal, and sagittal planes and the respective orthogonal leads XZ, XY, and YZ that define the planes. The arrow indicates the positive pole. Normal transverse, frontal, and right sagittal loops are diagrammed.

The right upper panel diagrams the orthogonal X, Y, and Z leads. When the vector points to the left (L), inferiorly (I), or posteriorly (P), a positive or upright deflection is recorded. Similarly, if the current flows to the right (R), superiorly (S), and anteriorly (A), a negative or downward deflection is recorded. In this instance the mean vector is oriented to the left, inferiorly, and posteriorly.

TABLE 7–2 DIRECTION AND MAGNITUDE OF MAXIMUM P VECTOR IN NORMAL SUBJECTS

Plane	Direction (degrees) Mean	Direction (degrees) 95% Range	Magnitude (mV) Mean	Magnitude (mV) 95% Range
Transverse	−5	−50 to 60	0.07	0.04 to 0.10
Right sagittal	85	50 to 110	0.12	0.04 to 0.18
Frontal	65	15 to 90	0.12	0.06 to 0.20

From Chou, T.-C., et al.: Clinical Vectorcardiography. 2nd ed. New York, Grune and Stratton, 1974, p. 50.

presence of a number of dipoles, and variation in vectorial expression of the magnitude of an electrical signal, and to assure that the three leads are perpendicular, a number of corrected orthogonal leads have been devised. Although none is ideal, the Frank system, because of its relative simplicity, is most widely used.[36] The values and recordings included in this chapter were derived using the Frank system (Fig. 7–4*B*).

The VCG differs from the ECG only in the method of display of the electrical field generated by the heart. *While the ECG reflects best the changes in time and amplitude, the VCG adds the important dimension of recognition of direction.* Despite the corrected nature of the orthogonal leads, the assumptions and limitations implicit in the ECG are also applicable to the VCG. The less than optimal sensitivity and specificity add a certain degree of empiricism, so that the findings on VCG must be correlated with clinical and laboratory information for proper interpretation.

Whether because of the relative complexity of recording the VCG compared to the ECG or because of its failure to routinely add information to that gained from the ECG, routine use of the VCG is a questionable practice in terms of cost effectiveness; therefore, the technique of vectorcardiography is not widely used. Unquestionably, the spatial VCG is without equal as a teaching tool, and an understanding of the VCG is essential for an intelligent appreciation of the ECG. It is for this reason that the VCG is discussed in detail in this chapter. In selected cases, the VCG may provide clinically useful information not otherwise obtainable. Because of differences of opinion, it is

TABLE 7–3 DIRECTION AND MAGNITUDE OF MAXIMUM T VECTOR IN NORMAL SUBJECTS (200)

Plane	Direction (degrees) Mean	Direction (degrees) 95% Range	Magnitude (mV) Mean	Magnitude (mV) 95% Range
Transverse	35	0 to 65	0.5	0.25 to 0.75
Right sagittal	45	20 to 90	0.4	0.20 to 0.70
Frontal	35	20 to 55	0.5	0.25 to 0.75

From Chou,T.-C., et al: Clinical Vectorcardiography. 2nd ed. New York, Grune and Stratton, 1974, p. 67.

difficult to list the specific clinical or pathological conditions in which the VCG is superior to the ECG.[37] It has been suggested that the VCG is particularly useful in detecting right ventricular hypertrophy (RVH), atrial enlargement, and myocardial infarction. While in myocardial infarction the VCG is perhaps more sensitive than the ECG, its specificity is not greater.[33]

The P loop of the VCG normally requires magnification for analysis. In the frontal plane, it is inscribed counterclockwise and is located in the left inferior quadrant. In the transverse plane, the usual inscription is counterclockwise, although a figure-of-eight may be encountered. The loop is located in the anterior and posterior left quadrants. In the right sagittal plane, the loop is inscribed clockwise and is positioned in the anterior and posterior inferior quadrants.

The order of activation and repolarization of the heart and the vectorial presentation—the basis of the clinical VCG—were described earlier. In a three-dimensional projection the major portion of the normal QRS loop is located in the left, inferior, and posterior octant[36] (Fig. 7-10). In the frontal plane, the loop is narrow and elongated, and in about one-third of subjects the inscription is clockwise; in the remaining two-thirds the inscription is counterclockwise or a figure-of-eight. The loop is most frequently located in the left inferior quadrant. In the transverse plane, the loop is inscribed counterclockwise and is oval in appearance, and the major portion is located in the left posterior quadrant. In the right sagittal plane, the loop is inscribed clockwise and is located in the anterior and posterior quadrants.

The VCG is most useful in analysis of the QRS complex. Although the QRS loop is routinely inscribed in the three orthogonal planes, with few exceptions, the characteristic

TABLE 7–4 SOME CHARACTERISTICS OF THE NORMAL QRSsÊ LOOP

Characteristic	Transverse Plane Mean	Transverse Plane 95% Range	Right Sagittal Plane Mean	Right Sagittal Plane 95% Range	Frontal Plane Mean	Frontal Plane 95% Range
Max QRS vector						
Direction (degrees)	−10	−80 to 20.0	100	50 to 165	35	10 to 65
Magnitude (mV)	1.30	0.85 to 1.95	1.00	0.3 to 1.9	1.50	0.9 to 2.2
0.02-sec vector						
Direction	55	0 to 120.0	15	−30 to 75	20	Widely scattered
Magnitude	0.40	0.15 to 0.75	0.30	0.10 to 0.55	0.25	0.05 to 0.7
0.04-sec vector						
Direction	−20	−90 to 25.0	110	60 to 170	35	−10 to 70
Magnitude	1.15	0.55 to 1.90	0.90	0.25 to 1.80	1.25	0.4 to 2.2
0.06-sec vector						
Direction	—90	−125 to −35	160	115 to 220	85	Widely scattered
Magnitude	0.45	0 to 0.9	0.55	0.1 to 1.0	0.25	0 to 0.6
Time of occurrence of max QRS vector (msec)	38	30 to 48	Same			Same
Direction of inscription	Counterclockwise		Clockwise		Clockwise 65% Figure-of-eight 25% Counterclockwise 10%	

From Chou, T.-C., et al: Clinical Vectorcardiography. 2nd ed. New York, Grune and Stratton, 1974, p. 60.

patterns can be recognized in the transverse plane. Patterns with a superior or inferior orientation require frontal projection for analysis. Of these, the most commonly encountered abnormalities include block of the divisions of the left bundle and inferior myocardial infarction.

Like the P loop, analysis of the T loop also ordinarily requires that the loop be magnified. In the frontal plane, its inscription is variable, with a maximal orientation similar to that of the QRS loop. In the transverse plane, the inscription is counterclockwise and the maximal T vector is located in the left anterior quadrant. In the right sagittal plane, the loop is inscribed clockwise and its maximal vector is located in the anterior and inferior quadrants.

The loops illustrated in this chapter are interrupted every 2.5 msec, each dot representing a 2.5-msec interval. The dot or line is comma shaped, with the thin end indicating the direction of the loop. The spacing of the dots reflects the speed of conduction, i.e., the closer the dots, the slower the conduction.

Normal values for the VCG are given in Tables 7–2 to 7–4.

BODY SURFACE POTENTIAL MAPPING

Body surface potential mapping may contribute information not available from the 12-lead ECG or the VCG, i.e., it provides regional electrophysiological information that cannot be extracted using these methods.[38] Analysis of surface potentials has been applied to the diagnosis of old inferior myocardial infarction, localization of the bypass pathway in the Wolff-Parkinson-White syndrome,[39] recognition of ventricular hypertrophy, estimation of the size of a myocardial infarction, and the effects of different interventions designed to reduce infarct size.[40, 41] The limiting factor at present is the complexity of the recording and analysis, which requires 100 or more electrodes, sophisticated instrumentation, and dedicated personnel. Initial efforts toward reducing the number of electrodes without loss of pertinent information are promising.[42] Once the technical obstacles are overcome, large numbers of patients can be studied and the ultimate utility of this procedure can be evaluated.

THE ABNORMAL ELECTROCARDIOGRAM AND VECTORCARDIOGRAM

ABNORMAL P WAVE AND THE Ta SEGMENT

Although an atrial abnormality usually implies atrial enlargement or hypertrophy, P-wave changes may reflect altered intraatrial pressure, volume, or conduction. Furthermore, shift of the site of origin of the P wave with an intraatrial conduction disturbance may simulate a pathological state. As stated earlier, initial atrial activation occurs in the right atrium and is directed anteriorly and inferiorly. As a result, right atrial enlargement or preponderance of the right atrium is manifested by an atrial vector that is increased in magnitude and shifted to the right. The P wave is normal in duration, low or isoelectric in lead I, and tall—but more importantly, peaked or pointed—in leads II, III, and aV_f (Fig. 7– 11*A*). P waves in leads V_{4r}, V_1, and V_2 may be upright and increased in amplitude. A P-wave axis greater than +90° with an isoelectric P wave in lead I is rarely, if ever, a normal finding (Fig. 7-11*A*). In the adult the most common cause of right atrial abnormality is chronic obstructive lung disease. The predictive value of P wave amplitude for detecting right atrial enlargement diagnosed with two-dimensional echocardiography is low.[43] P pulmonale pattern in the absence of right atrial enlargement, termed "pseudo-P pulmonale," has been found in association with a variety of disorders of the left heart, including coronary artery disease with angina pectoris, and less often in the absence of heart disease. It has been suggested that in the presence of left heart disease, "pseudo-P pulmonale" reflects an increase of the left atrial component of the P waves.[44]

Left atrial enlargement is manifested by prolongation of the P wave, shortening or absence of the P-R segment, and a shift of the P vector to the left and posteriorly (Fig. 7–11*B*). The duration of the P wave is 0.12 sec or longer, the prolongation is at the expense of the P-R segment, the P wave is notched, and its axis is shifted to the left. Because the vector is increased in magnitude and oriented posteriorly, lead V_1 registers a prominent negative P wave. A negative P wave in lead V_1, 0.04 sec in duration and 0.1

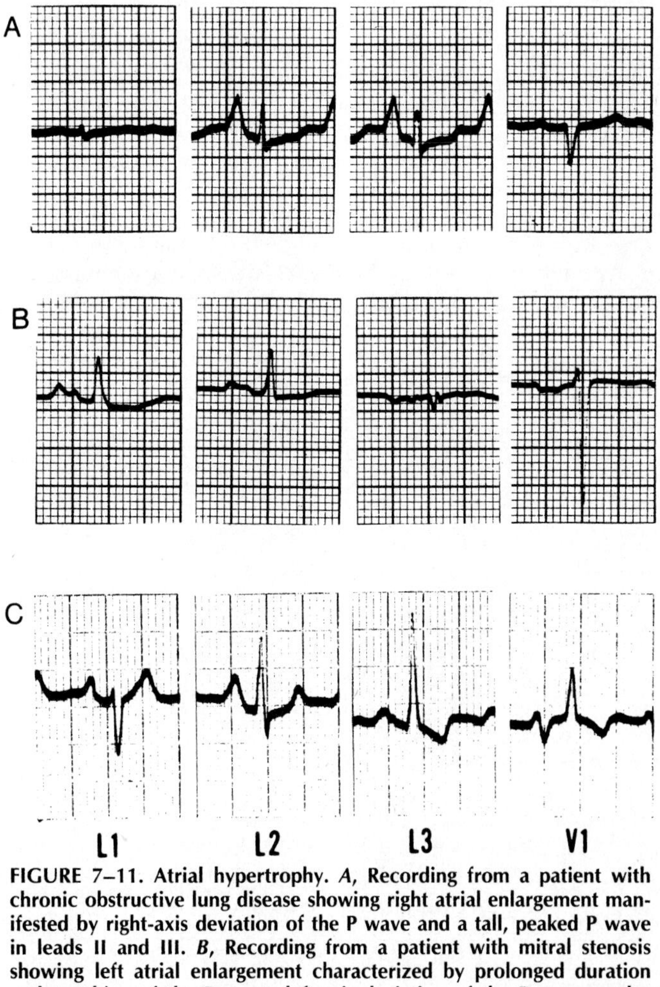

FIGURE 7–11. Atrial hypertrophy. *A*, Recording from a patient with chronic obstructive lung disease showing right atrial enlargement manifested by right-axis deviation of the P wave and a tall, peaked P wave in leads II and III. *B*, Recording from a patient with mitral stenosis showing left atrial enlargement characterized by prolonged duration and notching of the P wave, left-axis deviation of the P wave, and a negative orientation in lead V_1. A common feature not clearly visible in this tracing is loss of the P-R segment. *C*, Recording from a patient with mitral stenosis showing biatrial enlargement manifested by a tall P wave in lead II, a notched P wave in lead III, and a large biphasic P wave in lead V_1.

mV in depth, is consistent with left atrial preponderance, the so-called P mitrale. In a study of 57 patients with echocardiographically confirmed left atrial enlargement, the sensitivity of the various ECG criteria for left atrial enlargements varied from as low as 15 per cent for notched P wave with inter peak duration more than 0.04 sec, to as high as 83 for negative P wave of more than 0.04 sec in lead V_1. The specificity varied from 64 per cent for a foreshortened P-R segment to near 100 per cent for notched P wave with inter peak more than 0.04 sec.[45] Although P mitrale is common in mitral valve disease, the most frequent cause is left ventricular disease, with the increased left ventricular end-diastolic pressure reflected in the atrium.

In *biatrial* enlargement, both anterior and posterior forces are increased. The abnormality includes a prominent initial part of the P wave coupled with the left axis of the terminal portion of the P wave and a biphasic P wave in leads V_1 and occasionally in V_2 (Fig. 7–11*C*).

In the presence of atrial fibrillation, atrial disease can occasionally be suspected from an analysis of the QRS complex. With severe tricuspid regurgitation, right atrial enlargement displaces the tricuspid valve down and to the left. As a result, lead V_1 (and sometimes V_2), normally subtended by the right ventricle, now reflects the intracavitary (qR) right atrial potential as indicated by QR, qR, or qrS complexes in leads V_1 or V_1 and V_2 followed by a normal progression of R-wave amplitude from leads V_2 or V_3 to V_6 (Fig. 7–12). Atrial enlargement can also be suspected when coarse, relatively large fibrillatory waves are present, especially in lead V_1. This is in contrast to atrial fibrillation complicating arteriosclerotic and hypertensive heart disease, in which the fibrillatory waves are fine and frequently unidentifiable.

In the VCG, the P loop parallels the changing direction of the maximal P vector.[33] There is a significant increase of the spatial vector and of the loop. In the transverse plane, *right atrial enlargement* is recognized when a major portion of the loop is displaced anteriorly. The inscription is counterclockwise. In the right sagittal plane, the loop is inscribed counterclockwise and is displaced anteriorly and inferiorly; the posteriorly located component remains unaltered. In the frontal plane, the loop is narrow and has a vertical orientation.

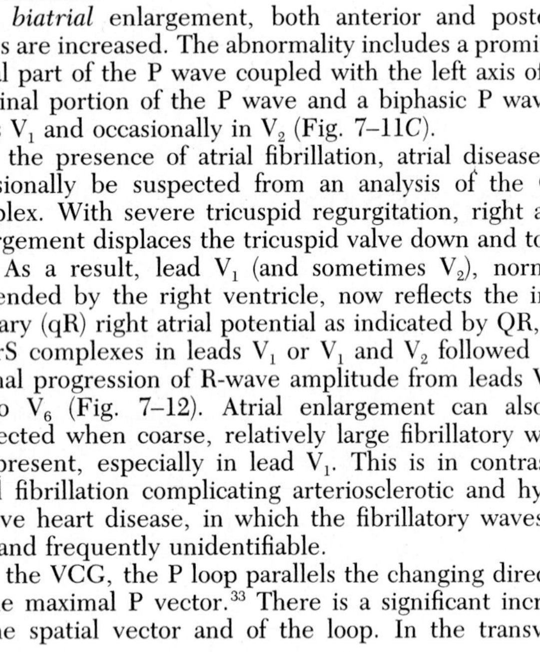

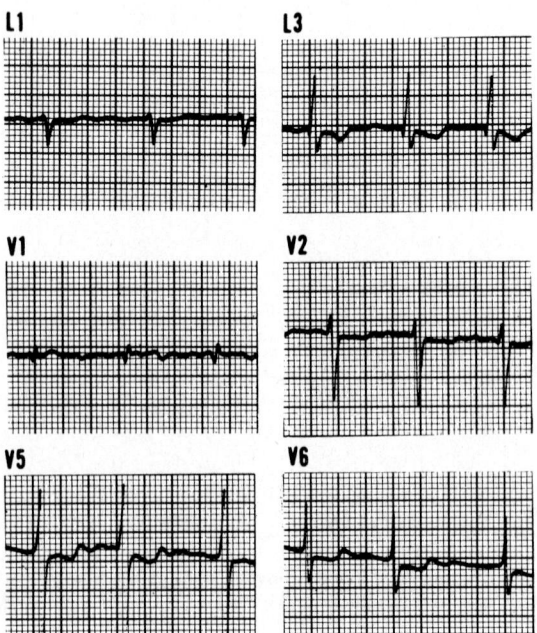

FIGURE 7–12. Rheumatic valvular heart disease with tricuspid regurgitation. The basic rhythm is atrial fibrillation. The right-axis deviation, "squatty" QRS in lead V_1, and clockwise rotation are consistent with mitral valve disease. The QR pattern in V_1 reflects the right atrial intracavitary potential and indicates right atrial enlargement with a regurgitant tricuspid valve.

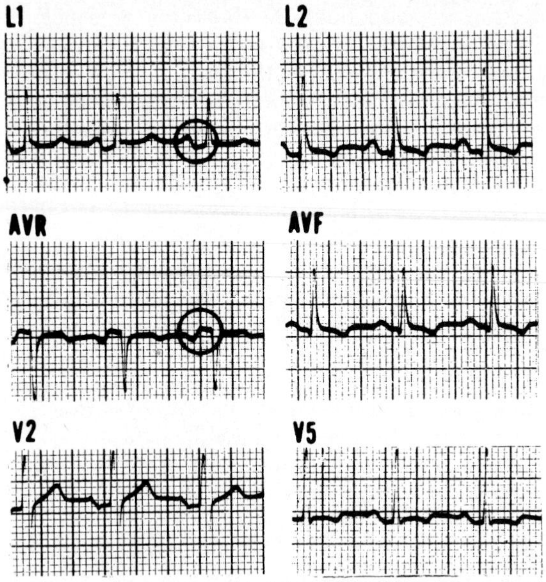

FIGURE 7–13. Acute pericarditis. The tracing shows sinus rhythm with nonspecific ST-segment and T-wave changes. The Ta segment is depressed in leads I, II, V_2, and V_5 and is elevated in lead aV_r. Ta displacement is the only change diagnostic of acute pericarditis in this tracing.

In the transverse plane, *left atrial enlargement* is inscribed in a counterclockwise direction or in the form of a figure-of-eight. Both the spatial vector and magnitude of the loop are increased. The increase is not as marked as in right atrial enlargement. With the exception of an initial component located anteriorly, the loop is shifted posteriorly and to the left. In the right sagittal plane, the loop is located more superiorly than normal and the major portion of the loop is located posteriorly; the inscription is clockwise. In the frontal plane, the loop is shifted to the left of normal; this is especially true for the left atrial component of the P wave.

In *biatrial enlargement*, the horizontal plane loop inscribes both the increased early anterior and the late posterior components of the loop. The size of the loop increases with large anterior and posterior components.

Intraatrial conduction abnormalities can result in enlargement of the loop in the absence of dilatation or hypertrophy. The loop displays localized conduction and anatomical abnormalities, the latter in the form of "notches" and "bites."[46]

Alteration of atrial repolarization (Ta), recognized by deviation from the T-P segment, can be either secondary or primary. Secondary changes appear in response to and are obligatory to atrial depolarization (Fig. 7–11*A*), while primary Ta changes are independent of atrial depolarization and indicate nonuniformity of atrial repolarization (Figs. 7–5 and 7–13). The usual pathological causes of secondary Ta-segment depression, which may exceed 1 mm (0.1 mV), include atrial dilation, hypertrophy, or intraatrial block. In chronic obstructive lung disease, for example, depression of the Ta segment may be exaggerated and mistaken for ST-segment displacement.

The usual causes of *primary* Ta-segment changes are pericarditis, atrial infarction, and atrial injury due to penetrating wounds. *Pericarditis* exaggerates the normally negative Ta-segment, and Ta-segment depression is recorded in all leads except aVR, in which it is elevated (Fig. 7–13).[47] Occasionally, a Ta-segment abnormality may be the only convincing evidence of acute pericarditis.

The incidence of *atrial infarction* in myocardial infarction is difficult to estimate and the reported numbers vary widely. Isolated atrial infarction in the absence of ventricular infarction is a most unlikely event. The manifestations of infarction may include elevation of the Ta segment in leads I, II, III, V_5, or V_6 or a depression that may exceed 0.15 mV in precordial leads and 0.1 mV in leads I, II, and III. Displacement of Ta segment in an opposite direction, a reciprocal change, may be recorded in "distal" leads, i.e., those facing noninfarcted areas of the atrium (Fig. 7–5). Attempts to localize the site of atrial infarction by ECG have been unsuccessful.[48] Supraventricular arrhythmias frequently accompany atrial infarction.

Penetrating injury of the atria due to gunshot wounds or perforation in the course of cardiac catheterization may be associated with diagnostic Ta-segment depression. Ta-segment displacement is also frequently observed following open heart surgery, and whether or not the displacement reflects mechanical injury, associated pericarditis, hemopericardium, or a combination of these factors is still unclear.

VENTRICULAR HYPERTROPHY

LEFT VENTRICULAR HYPERTROPHY (LVH)

ECG manifestations of LVH include an increase in voltage; shift of the mean QRS axis posteriorly, superiorly, and to the left; prolongation of depolarization (delayed intrinsicoid deflection); and gradual shift of the ST segment and T wave in a direction opposite to that of the QRS complex (Fig. 7–14). The exact mechanism of the voltage increase is not clear.[49] In addition to the muscle mass, other factors may play a role, such as intracavitary blood volume,[50] proximity to the chest wall, conducting properties of intrathoracic organs, location of the heart within the thorax, intraventricular and transmural pressures, and perhaps unopposed inscription of a portion of the QRS complex due to delayed activation.

The left superior and posterior orientation of the mean QRS vector in LVH is most likely related to hypertrophy of the basal portion of the left ventricle with delayed, and at times unopposed, activation. Variables that may be responsible for delayed depolarization include increased muscle mass, increased Purkinje activation, and localized intraventricular conduction delays. Marked superior orientation is noted in association with left anterior divisional block.

Prolongation of the excited state through the myocardium and prolongation of activation result in a change in the order of repolarization, which proceeds from endocardium to epicardium, resulting in a reversal of T-wave polarity. Of the mechanisms responsible for reversal of repolarization, increased muscle mass without a concomitant increase in the capillary bed—so-called relative coronary insufficiency—may be an important factor. It is also possible that as the muscle mass outgrows the Purkinje fiber mass, more of the activation proceeds through the myocardium, and this can contribute to a change in the T-wave vector. ST-segment depression may be due to the onset of repolarization prior to the completion of depolarization.

The mean QRS vector, increased in magnitude and oriented toward the left, posteriorly and superiorly, results in a positive deflection in leads I, II, aV_l, V_5, and V_6 and a positive or negative deflection in leads III and aV_f. The precordial transitional zone is shifted to the left. Leads V_1 and V_2 record an rS pattern, but in some instances the initial R wave may be absent for reasons that may remain obscure. Lack of the initial R wave may be erroneously interpreted as an anteroseptal myocardial infarction.

QRS voltage criteria for LVH include $R_I + S_{III} \geq 2.5$ mV, R in $aV_l > 1.2$ mV, R in $aV_f > 2.0$ mV, S in $V_1 \geq 2.4$ mV, R in V_5 or $V_6 > 2.6$ mV, R in V_5 or V_6 + S in $V_1 >$ 3.5 mV.[51] The following point system for diagnosing LVH has been suggested:[52] Amplitude of R or S wave in limb leads ≥ 2.0 mV *or* S_1 in V_1 or $V_2 \geq 3.0$ mV *or* R wave in V_5 or $V_6 \geq 3.0$ mV = 3 points. ST-segment changes with or without digitalis = 1 or 2 points, respectively. Left atrial enlargement = 3 points. Left-axis deviation of −30° or more = 2 points. QRS duration ≥ 0.09 sec and

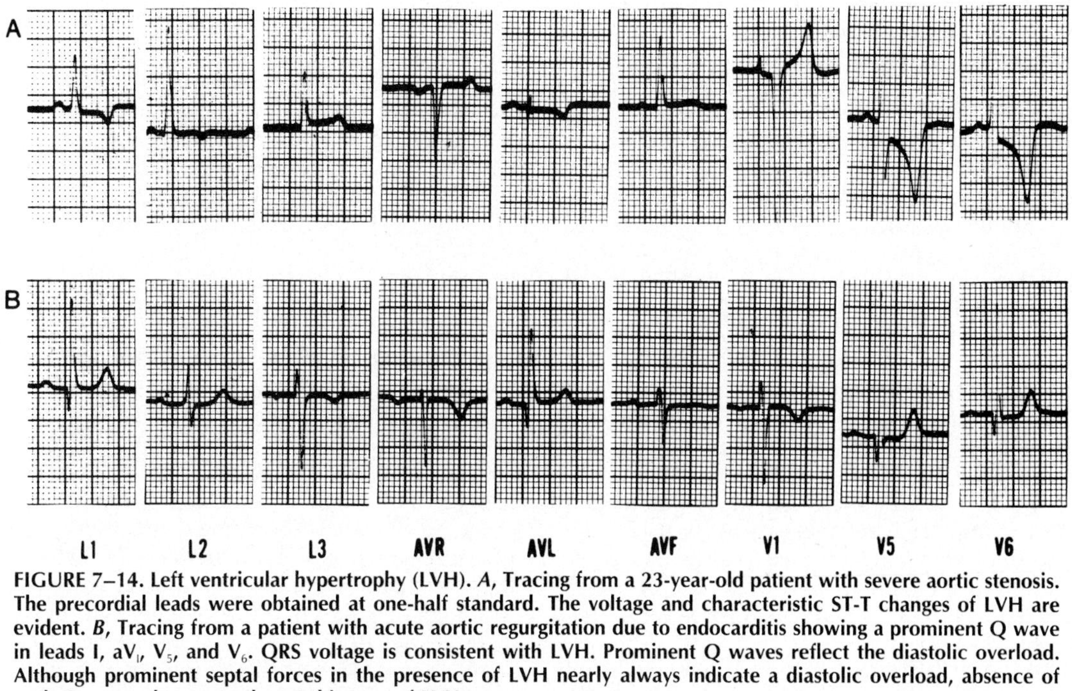

FIGURE 7–14. Left ventricular hypertrophy (LVH). ***A,*** **Tracing from a 23-year-old patient with severe aortic stenosis. The precordial leads were obtained at one-half standard. The voltage and characteristic ST-T changes of LVH are evident.** ***B,*** **Tracing from a patient with acute aortic regurgitation due to endocarditis showing a prominent Q wave in leads I, aV_l, V_5, and V_6. QRS voltage is consistent with LVH. Prominent Q waves reflect the diastolic overload. Although prominent septal forces in the presence of LVH nearly always indicate a diastolic overload, absence of such Q waves does not rule out this type of LVH.**

intrinsicoid deflection in V_5 and $V_6 \geq 0.05$ sec = 1 point each. Left ventricular hypertrophy is considered to be likely if the points total 4 and to be present if the total is 5 or more. The diagnosis of LVH is strengthened by a delayed intrinsicoid deflection in lead V_5 or V_6, measuring more than 0.05 sec in the adult. The *intrinsicoid deflection,* based on the concept of intrinsic deflection (p. 182) and applied to the indirect surface leads, is theoretically related to muscle mass. In the clinical ECG the time from the onset of the QRS to the peak of the R wave is an estimate of the intrinsicoid deflection. In the right (namely, V_1, V_2) and left (namely V_5, V_6) precordial leads, the time from onset of the QRS to appearance of the intrinsicoid deflection is 0.035 and 0.055 sec or less, respectively. For practical purposes in the study of conduction delays, the term "R peak time" is preferred.[26]

The direction of the ST segment and T wave is opposite to that of the QRS complex in LVH. Characteristically, the T wave is negative and asymmetrical, its ascending limb being steeper (Fig. 7–14*A*, leads V_5, V_6) with an occasional terminal positive inscription.[53] The J point and the ST segment are depressed in leads I, aV_l, V_5, and V_6. The T-wave inversion is greater in lead V_6 than in V_4. In the presence of a vertical position, these changes are recorded in leads II, III, and aV_f. It has been suggested that depression of the J point, asymmetry of the T wave with a more rapid return to the baseline, terminal positivity of the T wave ("overshoot"), T wave inversion in lead V_6 greater than 3 mm and T wave change greater in lead V_6 than V_4 help to distinguish LVH from coronary artery disease in the absence of voltage criteria for LVH.[54] Left atrial preponderance is common with LVH.

The limitations of the sensitivity of the ECG criteria for LVH are recognized. This is true for both the voltage criteria and the point system. Anatomical and echocardiographic studies suggest a sensitivity of about 25 per cent for Sokolow-Lyons voltage criteria[51] and approximately 50 per cent for Romhilt-Estes point score.[52] The specificity is approximately 95 per cent for both.[55] Sensitivity of the criteria for LVH varies depending on the etiology of the underlying heart disease, with the sensitivity lowest in the presence of coronary artery disease.[56]

In a population with a true prevalence of LVH of less than 10 per cent, there are more false-positive than true-positive diagnoses.[55] Similarly, autopsy data indicate that voltage changes consistent with LVH can be present in the absence of LVH.[57]

The concept of *diastolic overload* may be useful clinically.[58] It may point to such lesions as patent ductus arteriosus, ventricular septal defect, or aortic or mitral valve regurgitation, in which there is volume overload (Fig. 7–14*B*). The ECG pattern is one of LVH but with a prominent Q wave in the leads facing the left side of the septum, namely, I, aV_l, V_5, and V_6, and a reciprocal, prominent R wave in the leads facing the right side of the septum, namely, V_1 and V_2. As a rule, the Q wave is narrow, measuring 0.025 sec or less, and its depth is 0.2 mV or greater. Systolic or "pressure" overload is characterized by high-amplitude R waves and ST-segment and T-wave changes in the left ventricular leads and may be present in disorders with an increased resistance to left ventricular outflow (Fig. 7–14*A*). However, the accuracy of the pattern of LVH is not high in predicting the hemodynamic abnormality.

The VCG changes in LVH are due to an increase in and rotation of the forces further to the left and posteriorly.

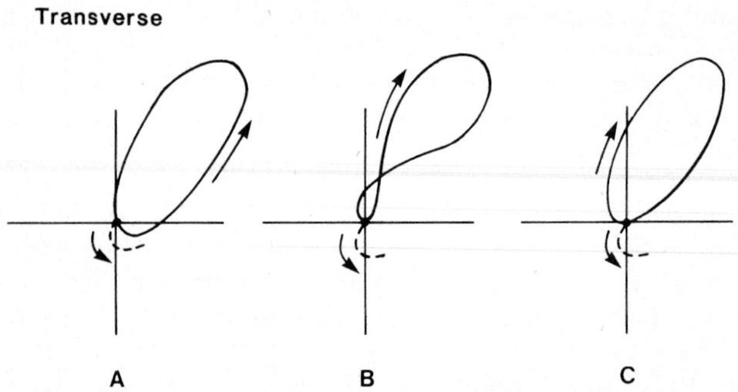

FIGURE 7–15. VCG loops in the transverse plane in left ventricular hypertrophy. The loops illustrate the occasional loss of the initial rightward force (*A*), rightward and anterior forces (*B, C*) as a result of LVH. Such changes are reflected in the precordial ECG by diminution or loss of the initial R wave in right precordial leads, which could mistakenly suggest myocardial infarction. The dashed lines represent the initial normal forces.

These events are best reflected in the transverse plane. The VCG loop is increased in magnitude, elongated, inscribed counterclockwise as a rule, and shifted posteriorly. The occasional posterior orientation of the initial part of the loop simulates anteroseptal myocardial infarction (Fig. 7–15). The termination of the loop is anterior, to the right, and superior to the origin of the loop. The loop is therefore open, and this displacement is reflected in the ECG by the ST-segment shift. *Secondary T-wave* changes, the result of alteration of timing and sequence, or both, of depolarization (p. 181), shift the T loop in a direction opposite to that of the QRS loop, namely, anteriorly, to the right, and superiorly.

RIGHT VENTRICULAR HYPERTROPHY (RVH)

In contrast to LVH, RVH is not simply an exaggeration of the normal. For RVH to become manifest, the right ventricular mass must be sufficiently large to overcome the left ventricular forces. For this reason, the specificity of the ECG pattern of RVH is much greater but the sensitivity is relatively low, varying from 25 to 40 per cent depending on the criteria used.[49, 59] While the ECG changes of RVH result largely from the chamber's anatomical dominance, the etiology of the heart disease and associated hemodynamic alterations often contribute to the abnormal ECG pattern. At times, the etiology of the cardiac disorder and the severity of right ventricular pressure can be estimated from an analysis of the ECG.

In RVH the axis shifts to the right, the degree of axis deviation varying with the clinical disorder, and this is accompanied by vertical position and clockwise rotation. Based on the QRS pattern in lead V_1, RVH can generally be separated into three groups, namely, a dominant R wave (qR rR, rsR′) (Fig. 7–16), RS (Rs, Rsr′), and rS or rsr′ complex. The different QRS patterns may provide a clue to the degree of elevation in right ventricular pressure. In general a qR complex, a prominent R wave with a slur on the upstroke, or an rsR′ complex (incomplete RBBB) suggest that right ventricular pressure exceeds (qR), is equal to (R or rR), or is lower than (rsR′) left ventricular pressure, respectively. Examples include severe pulmonary stenosis or primary pulmonary hypertension (qR), tetralogy of Fallot or Eisenmenger complex (R or rR), and atrial septal defect (rsR′), respectively. In the latter, hypertrophy of the outflow tract of the right ventricle is responsible for the r′ wave.[60]

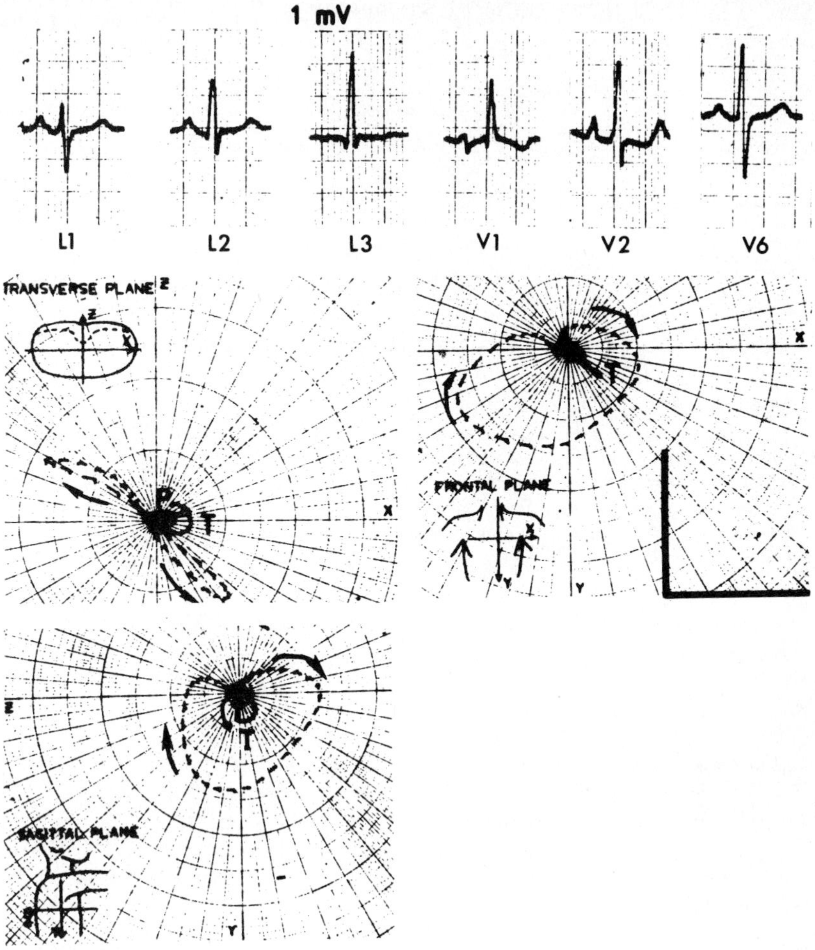

FIGURE 7–16. Right ventricular hypertrophy (RVH), Type A variant. In the transverse plane of the VCG there is anterior and rightward displacement of the mid and late portions of the QRS loop with a figure-of-eight inscription. In the frontal plane, the QRS loop is inscribed clockwise and displaced to the right. In the sagittal plane the loop is inscribed clockwise and displaced anteriorly. The T-wave loop is inscribed counterclockwise. The ECG illustrates the classic pattern of moderately severe to severe RVH (see text).

In the presence of RVH the delay of ventricular activation results in earlier recovery of the endocardium, and repolarization proceeds from endocardium to epicardium. The ST segment is thereby depressed and the T wave inverted in lead V_1 and occasionally in V_2. Significant ST-segment depression and T-wave inversion are, as a rule, indicative of moderate or severe right ventricular hypertension.

In the adult with acquired RVH the most commonly encountered ECG changes include right-axis deviation and an R/S ratio equal to or greater than 1 in V_1, with an R wave 0.5 mV or greater. Isolated right-axis deviation of $+100°$ to $-90°$ is considered by some to be indicative of RVH,[60] but this criterion alone is less sensitive. An R/S ratio greater than 1 in lead V_1 alone is not diagnostic of RVH, since it may be recorded in patients with a posterior infarction or occasionally in the absence of heart disease.

ACUTE PULMONARY EMBOLISM (ACUTE COR PULMONALE) (See Chap. 47). The most characteristic ECG feature of this disorder is probably the transient nature of the changes and for this reason serial tracings are most helpful. In the Urokinase–Pulmonary Embolism Trial,[61] the ECG was normal in 6 to 23 per cent of the patients depending on the severity of the embolism. The most common abnormalities were nonspecific T-wave changes and nonspecific ST-segment elevation or depression, the incidence being 42 and 41 per cent, respectively. The more classical changes—the S_1-Q_3T_3 pattern described by McGinn and White[62] (Fig. 7–17), RBBB, right axis deviation, and P pulmonale—were recorded in only 26 per cent of the patients. In this study the T-wave changes were more persistent, while QRS abnormalities were more transient. Other abnormalities included $S_1S_2S_3$ pattern, RVH, and right axis deviation with clockwise rotation.[63, 64] The ECG changes are most likely related to acute pulmonary hypertension with right atrial and ventricular dilation, hypoxia, and perhaps myocardial ischemia. Acute atrial dilation coupled with myocardial ischemia is probably responsible for the frequent atrial arrhythmias. Despite the high incidence of abnormal tracings the diagnosis is difficult because of the nonspecific nature of the ECG changes. While a single ECG is rarely helpful, a comparison with a tracing obtained before the acute episode and serial tracings after the episode increase significantly the sensitivity of the ECG.

CHRONIC OBSTRUCTIVE LUNG DISEASE (COLD) AND COR PULMONALE (See Chap. 48). The ECG pattern of COLD and COLD with pulmonary hypertension (cor pulmonale) can be ascribed to a combination of positional changes,

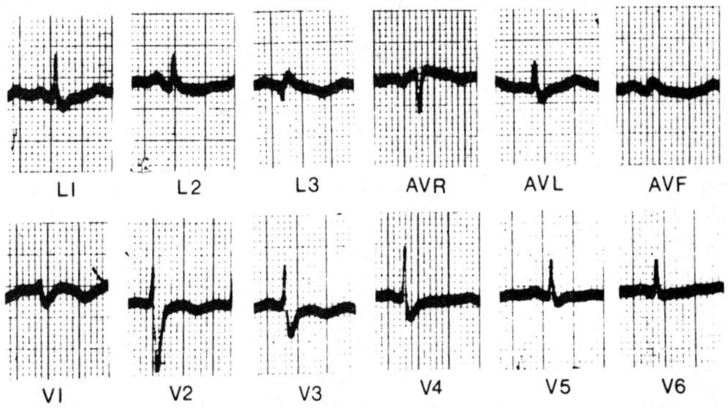

FIGURE 7–17. S_1Q_3 pattern of acute pulmonary embolism. In addition, some of the more common features of acute pulmonary embolism including inversion of T waves in leads V_1, V_2, and V_3, clockwise rotation, intraventricular conduction defect, and probable incomplete RBBB are also present.

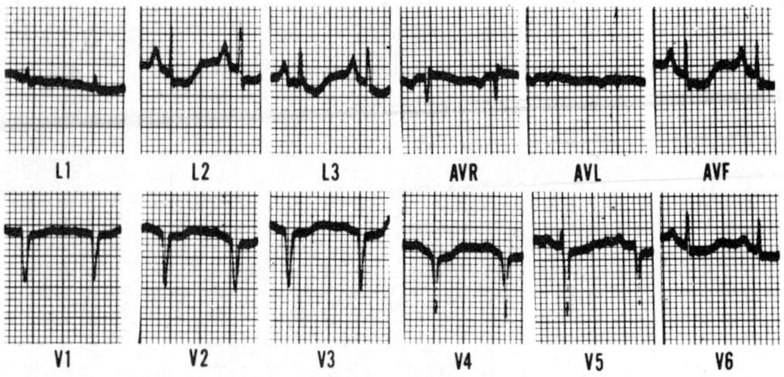

FIGURE 7–18. Chronic obstructive lung disease (COLD) simulating an anteroseptal myocardial infarction. The characteristic features of COLD include "pointed" tall P waves in leads II, III, AV_F with right axis deviation (+90°), tendency to right axis of the QRS, clockwise rotation, and "pseudo" ST segment depression. The latter reflects atrial repolarization. The clockwise rotation simulates anteroseptal myocardial infarction.

increased lung volume, and RVH. ECG changes include right-axis deviation of the P wave, increased amplitude and "peaked" appearance of the P wave in the limb leads, and "peaked" and biphasic morphology wave in lead V_1 (Figs. 7–11A and 7–18). A P-wave axis of +90° is highly suggestive of COLD. The shift of the P wave axis is most likely due to overinflation of the lungs. It is not seen with interstitial fibrosis.[65] Because of the large P-wave area, the Ta segment is exaggerated and occasionally interpreted as ST-segment depression. Right-axis deviation and clockwise rotation are characteristic findings. Occasionally, an S1, S2, S3 pattern may be present. Amplitude of the precordial R wave is reduced in leads V_5 and V_6, often measuring less than 0.7 mV. When the clockwise rotation is marked, absence of the R wave in precordial leads simulates an anterior myocardial infarction. With progression to pulmonary hypertension and RVH, prominent R waves may appear in leads V_1 and V_2. These changes are probably due to unopposed late activation of the crista terminalis and right ventricular free wall. Right atrial dilatation is probably responsible for the QR pattern in V_1, with the Q wave reflecting right atrial intracavitary potential (as occurs also in tricuspid regurgitation [Fig. 7–12]). As indicated, the sensitivity of the ECG for cor pulmonale is relatively low, the test being diagnostic in about 25 to 40 per cent of patients with confirmed RVH.[59]

In *biventricular hypertrophy*, the LV forces are dominant and often obscure the RVH.

In RVH, the characteristic VCG changes of the QRS loop are recorded in the transverse plane, and these fall into three general types (Fig. 7–19).[33] In type A, the configuration varies considerably. It may be oval, narrow, or figure-of-eight (Fig. 7–16). The major segment of the loops is located anteriorly and to the right. The loop is inscribed clockwise or, as in the case of the figure-of-eight loop, initially counterclockwise with the latter component recorded clockwise (Fig. 7–16). An oval loop is illustrated in Figure 7–19. In type B, the loop is inscribed clockwise, or counterclockwise, is often figure-of-eight, and is located primarily in the left anterior and to a lesser extent in the left and right posterior quadrants. In type C, the loop is inscribed counterclockwise, with 50 per cent of the loop located in posterior left and right quadrants. Of the three, type A usually reflects severe RVH, while type B is most often encountered in patients with atrial septal defect and mitral stenosis. Type C can be recorded with chronic obstructive lung disease.

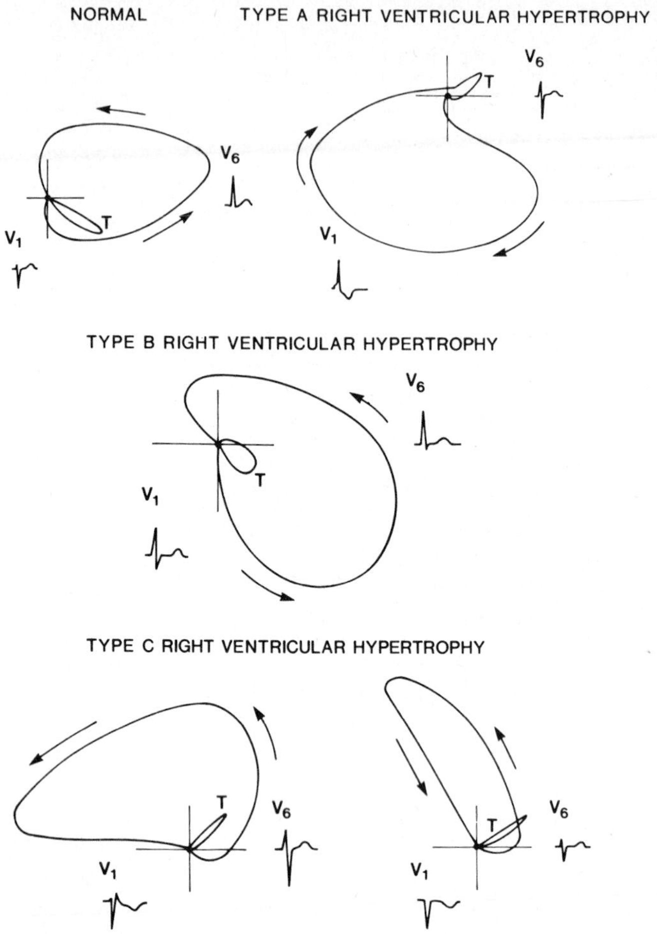

FIGURE 7–19. Diagrammatic representation of the three common, but not exclusive, VCG patterns of right ventricular hypertrophy recorded in the horizontal plane. When compared with the normal, the QRS loops are located in the right and left anterior quadrants in Type A and in the left anterior and to a lesser extent left and right posterior quadrants in Type B; a major portion of the loop is located in the left and right posterior quadrants in Type C. (Modified from Chou, T. C., Helm, R. A., and Kaplan, S.: Clinical Vectorcardiography. 2nd ed. New York, Grune and Stratton, 1974, pp. 87, 99, and 102.)

VENTRICULAR HYPERTROPHY IN THE PRESENCE OF CONDUCTION DEFECTS

The diagnosis of ventricular hypertrophy in the presence of BBB is difficult, if not impossible, owing in part to the fact that a portion of cardiac activation may be unopposed for a period of time, resulting in misleading voltage changes. It has been suggested that in the presence of RBBB, an R′ greater than 1.0 to 1.5 mV indicates associated RVH. However, it is not unusual to record preoperatively a normal QRS complex in lead V_1, only to register postoperatively an RBBB with an R′ wave greater than 1.0 or 1.5 mV, indicating that this criterion of RVH may not be valid in the presence of RBBB. LBBB makes a diagnosis of RVH and LVH essentially impossible. In the presence of RBBB, LVH may be suspected when the S wave in lead V_1 and the R wave in lead V_6 satisfy voltage criteria for LVH (p. 191). However, such an interpretation is subject to the limitations imposed by the relatively low sensitivity and specificity of the voltage criteria.

INTRAVENTRICULAR CONDUCTION DEFECTS

The bundle of His bifurcates into right and left bundles (see Fig. 20–2, p. 582). The ribbon-like right bundle descends subendocardially on the right side of the septum. At the base of the right ventricular anterior papillary muscle, it divides and supplies fibers to the free right ventricular wall and the right side of the septum. The left bundle divides into an anterior division (LAD) and posterior division (LPD), which supply the left ventricular wall and left side of the septum. Discrete anatomical lesions, asynchrony of conduction in the bundles or its branches, nonuniformity of refractoriness, changes in membrane responsiveness, and a decrease in the magnitude of phase 4 of the transmembrane action potential (p. 181) may, singly or in combination, cause block of conduction in the bundle branches (BBB) and the divisions of the left bundle. However, most commonly BBB is due to an anatomical lesion. In transient BBB, the specific underlying electrophysiological mechanism may be difficult to define.

LEFT BUNDLE BRANCH BLOCK

Interruption of the left bundle branch results in early activation of the right side of the septum and of the right ventricular myocardium. Transseptal activation from right to left is transmyocardial and thus slow, and probably a major cause of the prolonged ventricular activation. Initial activation of the ventricles proceeds from right to left, inferiorly, and more often anteriorly than posteriorly. This is followed by continued activation of the septum and of the adjacent free left ventricular wall, with the activation proceeding to the left, posteriorly, and inferiorly. This phase of activation is rapid, presumably because the impulse enters the Purkinje system below the site of the BBB. Last to be activated are the lateral wall and basal aspect of the left ventricle, with a vector oriented posteriorly, superiorly, and, less frequently, inferiorly.

In complete LBBB, the QRS complex is prolonged, measuring 0.12 to 0.18 sec (Fig. 7–20).[65a] An upright notched or slurred R wave reflecting the right-to-left myocardial activation is recorded in leads I and V_6. A small R wave followed by an S wave is present in aV_f, the R wave and the S wave reflect, respectively, the initial septal activation directed inferiorly and the superior orientation of the final vector. An rS or a QS complex, depending on whether the initial activation is oriented anteriorly or posteriorly, is recorded in lead V_1, with the S wave reflecting activation of the left ventricle from right to left. An initial R wave in lead V_1 is present in about 45 per cent of cases of LBBB. The precordial leads V_1 to V_4 may exhibit a small R wave, with the R waves in the midprecordial leads occasionally lower in amplitude than those in the right precordial leads. One clinically important feature of LBBB is an absence of a septal Q, owing to the initial right-to-left septal activation. Similarly, a Q wave fails to register when either myocardial infarction complicates preexisting LBBB or when LBBB complicates an acute myocardial infarction (p. 203). The frontal axis in LBBB may be either normal or directed to the left ($-30°$ to $-90°$), the prevalence of the two being about equal. Although it has been accepted that an abnormal left axis in excess of $-45°$ is nearly always due to a left anterior divisional block, LBBB per se may also result in pronounced left-axis deviation.

In LBBB, the direction of the ST-segment and T-wave vectors is opposite to that of the QRS vector. In the presence of an upright QRS complex in leads I, aV_l, and V_6 the ST segment is depressed and the T waves are inverted. The opposite is true in leads V_1, V_2, and V_3, where a predominantly negative QRS complex is recorded. The ST-segment and T-wave changes are secondary to the conduction disturbance, and the magnitude of the change parallels the magnitude of the QRS aberration. Occasionally LBBB is associated with an isoelectric ST segment and a T-wave vector concordant with the QRS vector. Such primary T-wave changes suggest a myocardial abnormality independent of the LBBB, which may be due, for example, to accompanying myocardial ischemia. However, this is not always a reliable sign of a primary myocardial disorder.

Incomplete LBBB implies a greater delay of conduction in the left than in the right bundle, with initial right-to-left septal activation and loss of the septal Q wave. In

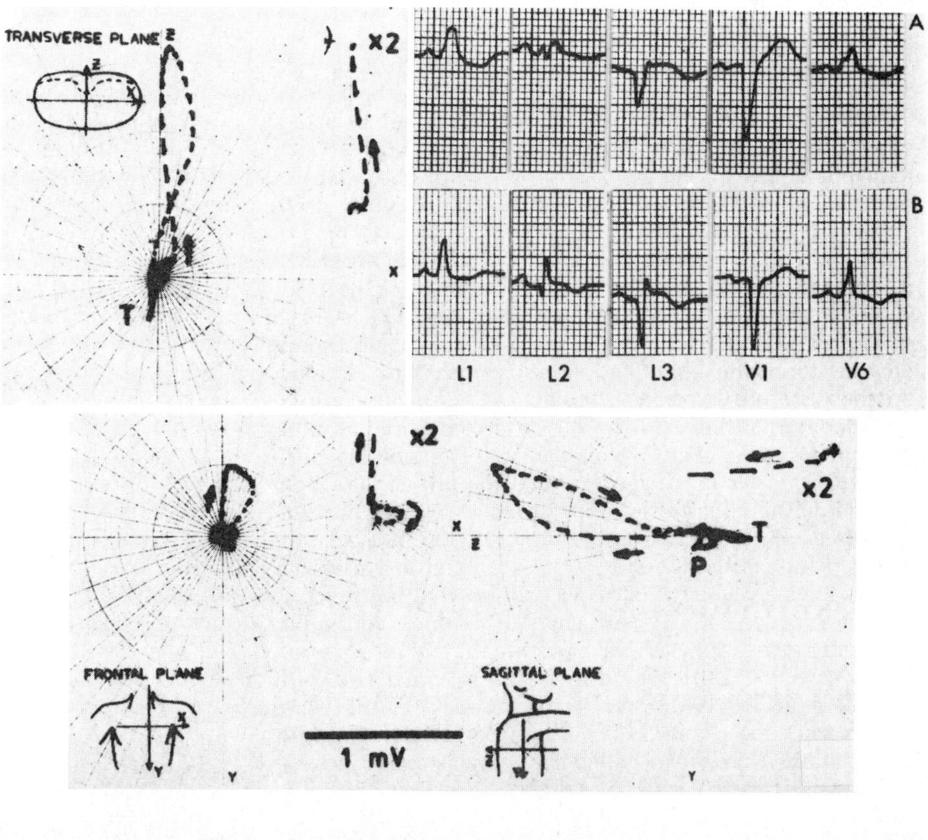

FIGURE 7–20. The ECG illustrates an intermittent LBBB (panel A) and an inferior myocardial infarction and normal intraventricular conduction in panel B. The VCG was recorded when LBBB was present. In the transverse plane, the initial anteriorly oriented portion of the QRS loop is decreased, and the entire loop shows a figure-of-eight inscription and is displaced posteriorly. There is a generalized slowing of inscription indicated by close spacing of the dots. This is particularly evident in the midportion of the QRS loop. (The duration of the loop is 120 msec.) A narrow T loop is directed anteriorly and slightly to the right. In the frontal plane, the QRS loop is displaced superiorly with the initial force directed inferiorly and to the left. The initial inscription is counterclockwise but clockwise during the remainder of the loop. A general slowing of inscription is present and is most pronounced in the midportion of the QRS loop. In the sagittal plane, there is posterior displacement of the QRS loop with a significant decrease of the initial anterior force. There is general slowing of inscription, which is most pronounced in the midportion of the QRS loop. The narrow T loop is directed opposite to the direction of the QRS loop. The initial portion of the QRS loop is displayed two times the standard (× 2).

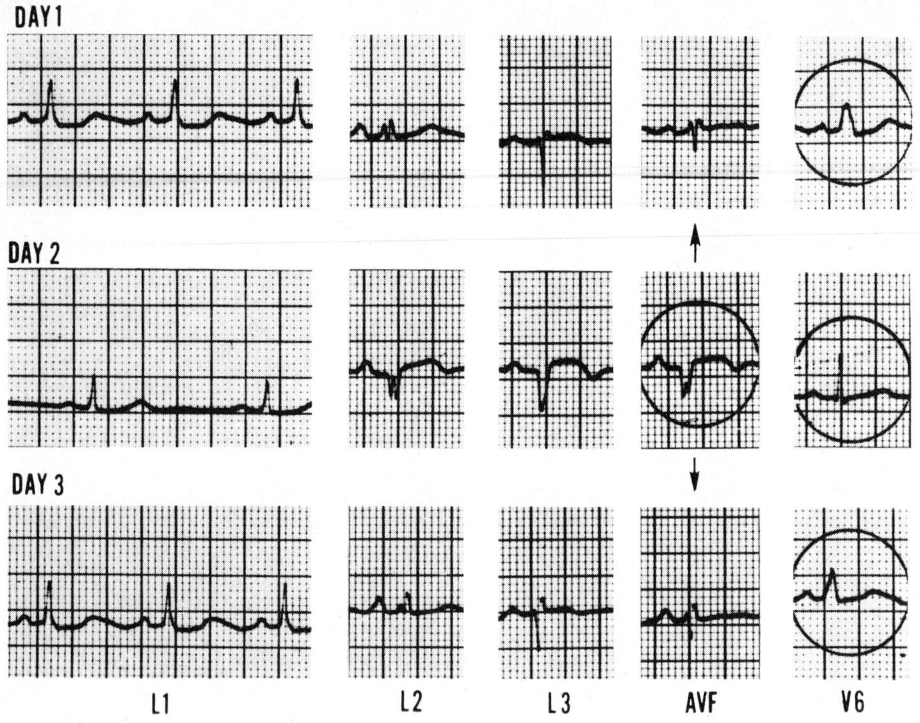

FIGURE 7–21. Inferior myocardial infarction obscured by incomplete LBBB due to acceleration of the heart rate. On day 1, the heart rate was 83 bpm with incomplete LBBB as reflected by loss of the septal Q wave in lead V_6 and prolongation of the QRS complex (circle). On day 2, the heart rate slowed to 60 bpm and incomplete LBBB is no longer evident (circle). Features of inferior myocardial infarction are now recorded in leads II, III, and aV_f (circle). On day 3, the heart rate accelerated to 88 bpm, and incomplete LBBB recurred, masking the inferior myocardial infarction (arrows).

contrast to complete LBBB, the left bundle ultimately contributes to activation of the septum and left ventricular wall. ECG criteria for incomplete LBBB include a QRS complex of 0.10 to 0.12 sec, loss of the initial septal Q wave, slurring or notching (Fig. 7–21), and often high voltage of the QRS complex.

In the transverse plane of the VCG, the QRS loop of LBBB is oriented to the left and posteriorly. The initial portion of the loop reflects septal activation and is inscribed slowly from right to left and anteriorly. The remainder of the loop is inscribed clockwise with slow inscription of the midportion, most likely reflecting slow intramyocardial conduction through the left ventricular wall. The T loop points in a direction opposite to that of the QRS (Fig. 7–20).

RIGHT BUNDLE BRANCH BLOCK

In RBBB the septum is activated normally, from left to right. While the left ventricle is activated normally, right ventricular depolarization is delayed, the right ventricle being last to be activated, and this terminal activation is unopposed. Prolongation of the QRS complex is largely due to delayed activation of the septum and right ventricular wall. The initial dominant septal force is directed from left to right, anteriorly and superiorly, followed by a vector dominated by the left ventricle, oriented to the left, inferiorly, and either somewhat anteriorly or posteriorly. The final vector representing activation of the right ventricle is directed to the right, anteriorly, and either superiorly, inferiorly, or horizontally.

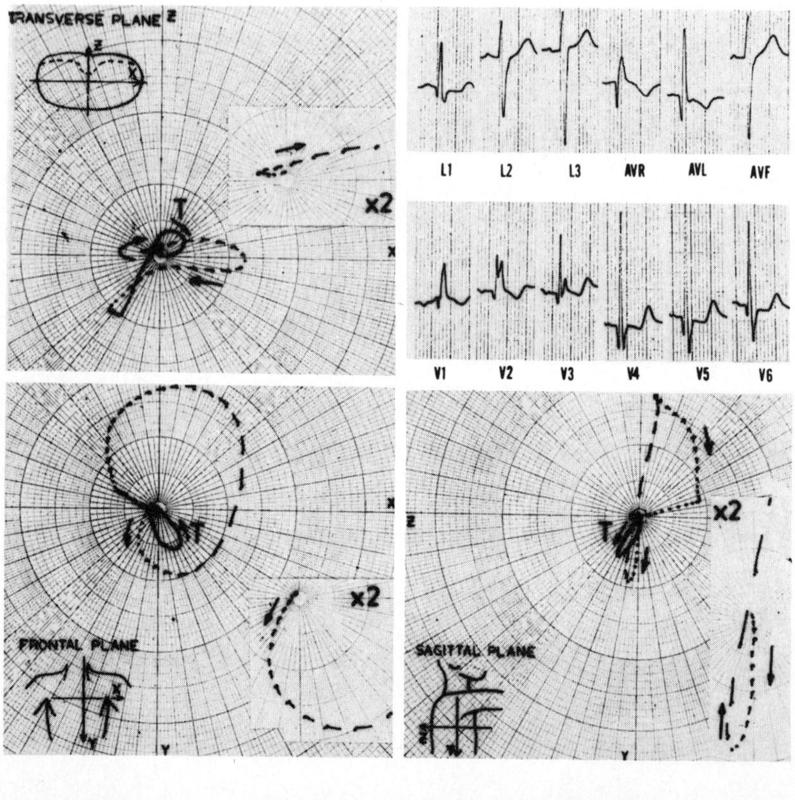

FIGURE 7–22. The ECG illustrates an anterior myocardial infarction, RBBB, and left anterior divisional block (LADB). In the transverse plane, the VCG displays an initial QRS force directed to the right and slightly anteriorly with a clockwise inscription. The decrease in the anteriorly directed initial QRS force is due to the infarction. A delayed terminal QRS loop exhibiting a figure-of-eight inscription is displaced anteriorly. The terminal, anteriorly directed, slowly inscribed part of the loop is due to RBBB. The clockwise-inscribed T-wave loop is oriented in a direction opposite to that of the main QRS force. In the frontal plane, the initial QRS is directed to the right and inferiorly. The loop is inscribed counterclockwise and is displaced superiorly and to the left. The superior and leftward displacement of the loop is due to LADB. The delayed terminal QRS forces are shifted superiorly and to the right. In the sagittal plane, the initial QRS loop is directed inferiorly and slightly anteriorly, with a decrease of the initial anteriorly directed QRS force. The delayed terminal loop is displaced anteriorly and superiorly. The initial portion of the QRS loop is displayed at two times the standard (× 2).

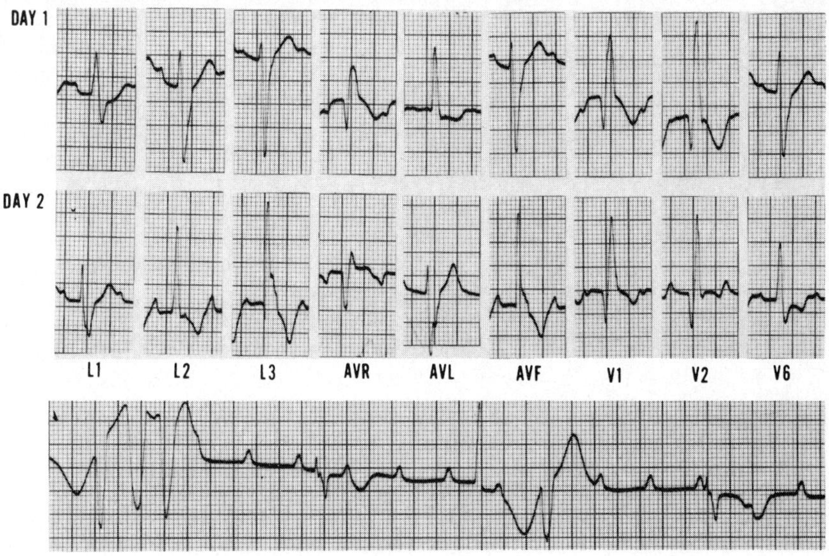

FIGURE 7–23. Acute anterior myocardial infarction complicated by RBBB, left anterior divisional block (LADB), left posterior divisional block (LPDB), and complete AV block. On day 1, the ECG records a sinus rhythm; LADB in leads I, II, and III; RBBB in leads V_1 and V_2; and anterior myocardial infarction manifest by a deep Q wave in leads V_1 and V_2. On day 2, the RBBB and anterior infarction are again noted, but with LPDB recorded in leads I, II, and III. The LPDB is indicated by shift of axis to the right, as estimated on the basis of the initial 0.08 sec of the QRS and the appearance of Q waves and tall R waves in leads II, III, and aV_f. Complete AV block, ventricular premature beats, prolonged Q-T interval, and deeply inverted T waves are recorded in row 3.

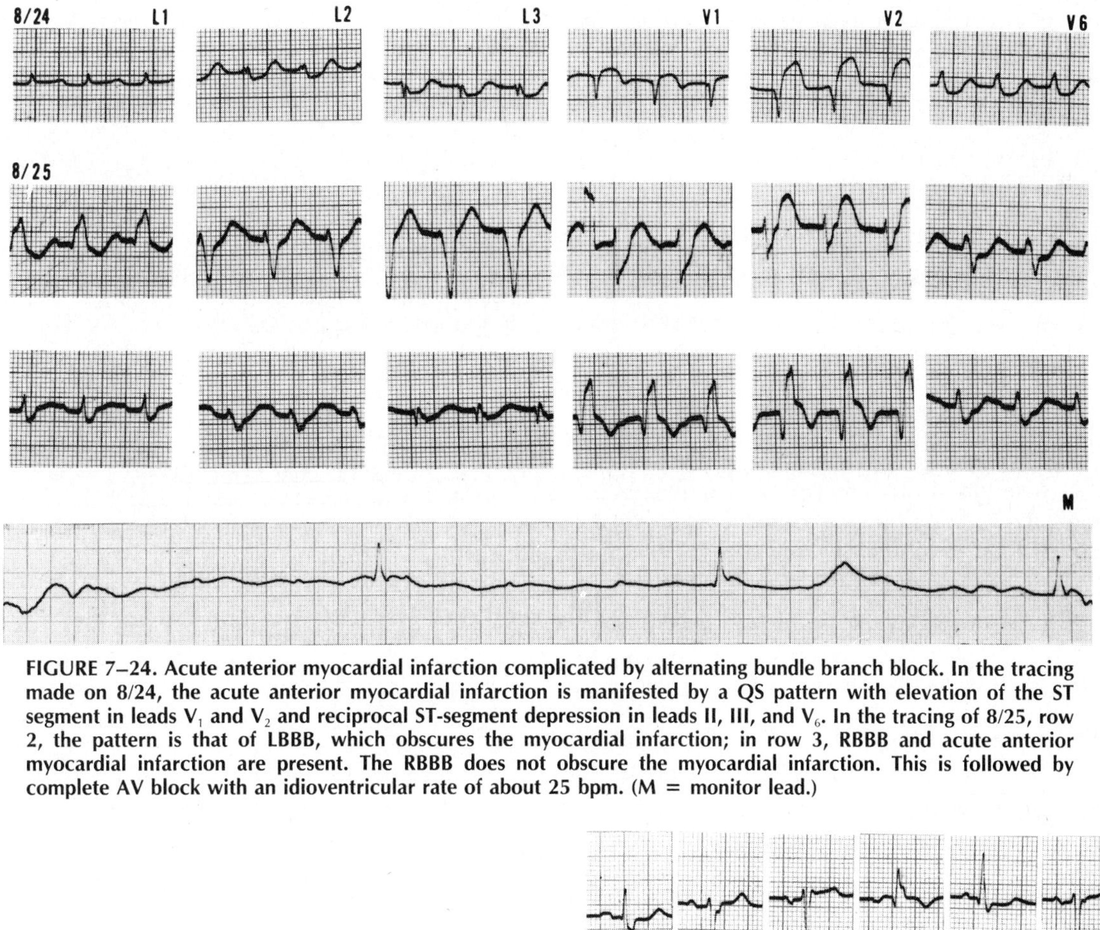

FIGURE 7–24. Acute anterior myocardial infarction complicated by alternating bundle branch block. In the tracing made on 8/24, the acute anterior myocardial infarction is manifested by a QS pattern with elevation of the ST segment in leads V_1 and V_2 and reciprocal ST-segment depression in leads II, III, and V_6. In the tracing of 8/25, row 2, the pattern is that of LBBB, which obscures the myocardial infarction; in row 3, RBBB and acute anterior myocardial infarction are present. The RBBB does not obscure the myocardial infarction. This is followed by complete AV block with an idioventricular rate of about 25 bpm. (M = monitor lead.)

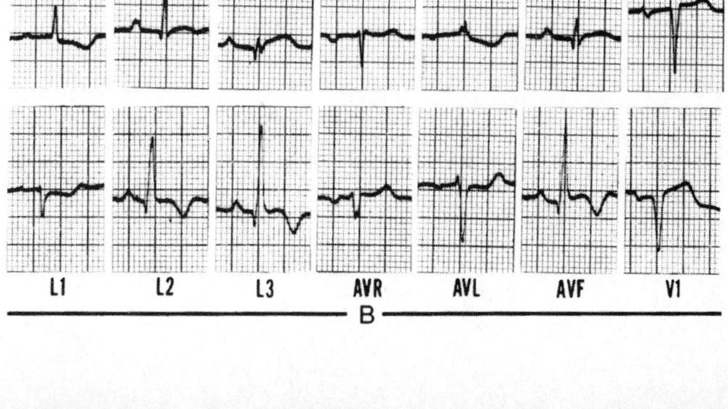

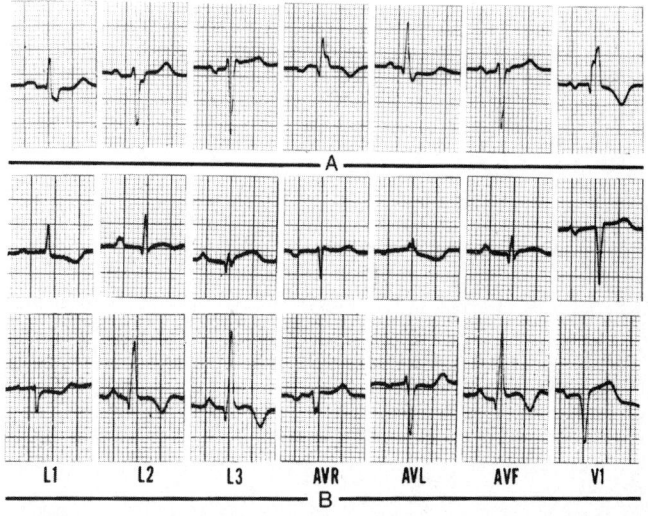

FIGURE 7–25. *A*, Right bundle branch block with left anterior divisional block. *B*, Upper trace, the control trace, illustrates an inferior myocardial infarction with a normal QRS axis. The bottom trace demonstrates left posterior divisional block (LPDB). Because the latter may be due to causes other than LPDB a diagnosis of LPDB requires evidence of normal conduction prior to appearance of LPDB such as illustrated in upper trace of panel B.

The characteristic ECG changes of RBBB are recorded in lead V_1. The initial normal septal activation inscribes an R wave, followed by an S wave reflecting left ventricular activation and a final R′ wave due to depolarization of the right ventricle from left to right and anteriorly. The depth of the S wave in lead V_1 varies depending on whether the left ventricular activation generates a more posteriorly or anteriorly oriented vector. In the former, a prominent S wave separates the R wave from the R′ wave, while in the latter, the S wave may be shallow or a slur or, indeed, may be absent. Leads facing the left side of the septum, namely, I, aV_l, V_5, and V_6, record an initial Q wave followed by an R wave of normal duration and a prolonged, relatively shallow S wave. The latter reflects delayed activation of the right ventricle (Figs. 7–22 to 7–25). Because the initial septal activation is normal, namely left to right, RBBB, in contrast to LBBB, does not obscure myocardial infarction.

The T wave is usually inverted in lead V_1 and occasionally in V_2, while it is upright in the remaining precordial and limb leads, a direction opposite to the *terminal* portion of the QRS complex.

The characteristic VCG feature is evident in the transverse plane and consists of a slowly inscribed terminal appendage directed to the right and anteriorly. The initial septal and left ventricular portion of the loop is normal (Fig. 7–22).

DIVISIONAL (FASCICULAR) BLOCKS

The ventricular conduction system, including the right bundle branch and the two divisions of the left bundle, can be considered for purposes of clinical electrocardiography to consist of three divisions (fascicles) (Fig. 7–26). Divisional blocks are, with rare exception, acquired.[66]

Although the evidence for the existence of anatomically discrete divisions of the left bundle branch is not convincing, experimental data support a functional divisional conduction system.[67–69] Furthermore, nearly simultaneous early endocardial activation at three sites—the middle anterior and posterior paraseptal areas—is consistent with the concept of functional divisions of the left bundle. This concept is also supported by distinctive and predictable ECG patterns. Thus, from the ECG standpoint, the concept of divisions of the left bundle is a useful one.[70]

BLOCK OF ANTERIOR DIVISION OF THE LEFT BUNDLE BRANCH (ANTERIOR FASCICULAR BLOCK). In the presence of left anterior divisional block, the initial septal activation proceeds inferiorly, anteriorly, to the right, and occasionally to the left. This is followed by activation of inferior and apical areas with the vector oriented inferiorly, to the left, and anteriorly. Final activation is that of the anterolateral and posterobasal left ventricular wall, the vector oriented superiorly, posteriorly, and to the left.

The resultant ECG pattern is characteristic (Figs. 7–25 and 7–26). Lead I records a dominant R wave, with or without an initial Q wave. The criterion of a small Q wave in leads I, aV_l is the subject of continued controversy.[26] The presence or absence of a Q wave depends on whether the initial septal activation is directed to the right or to the left. Since the initial activation is directed inferiorly, leads II, III, and aV_f inscribe an R wave followed by a deep S wave reflecting activation of the anterolateral and posterobasal segments of the left ventricle. The QRS axis varies from $-45°$ to $-90°$. The duration of the QRS is less than 0.12 sec[26] (Figs. 7–22, 7–23, 7–25, and 7–27).

The precordial transitional zone is frequently displaced to the left. The amplitude of the R wave is diminished, with a prominent S wave in V_5 and V_6 reflecting the superior orientation of the mean left ventricular vector. The S wave is exaggerated when the final order of activation is directed to the right. Because of the inferior orientation of the initial vector, the right and midprecordial leads may register an initial Q wave. Such patterns could be mistaken for anteroseptal myocardial infarction[71] were it not for the fact that an R wave is recorded when the leads are placed an interspace lower. The T waves are normally upright except in lead aV_r and occasionally in leads aV_l and V_1.

The frontal plane is the most useful for visualization of left anterior divisional block (Fig. 7–28). The inscription of the loop is counterclockwise, initially directed to the right and inferiorly, with the remaining major portion of the loop displaced superiorly. The superior orientation reflects activation of the anterior and lateral left ventricular wall. Left anterior divisional block is nearly always an acquired abnormality and thus a marker of organic disease.[33] Often, however, it is present without clinical evidence of heart disease. The prognosis depends on the underlying disease.

BLOCK OF POSTERIOR DIVISION OF THE LEFT BUNDLE BRANCH (POSTERIOR FASCICULAR BLOCK). Left posterior divisional block is a rare finding and its pattern is nonspecific. It can be recorded in asthenic individuals and patients with emphysema, RVH, and extensive lateral infarction.[70] Diagnosis is secure only if a normal ECG is recorded prior to appearance of the block.

In the presence of left posterior divisional block, acti-

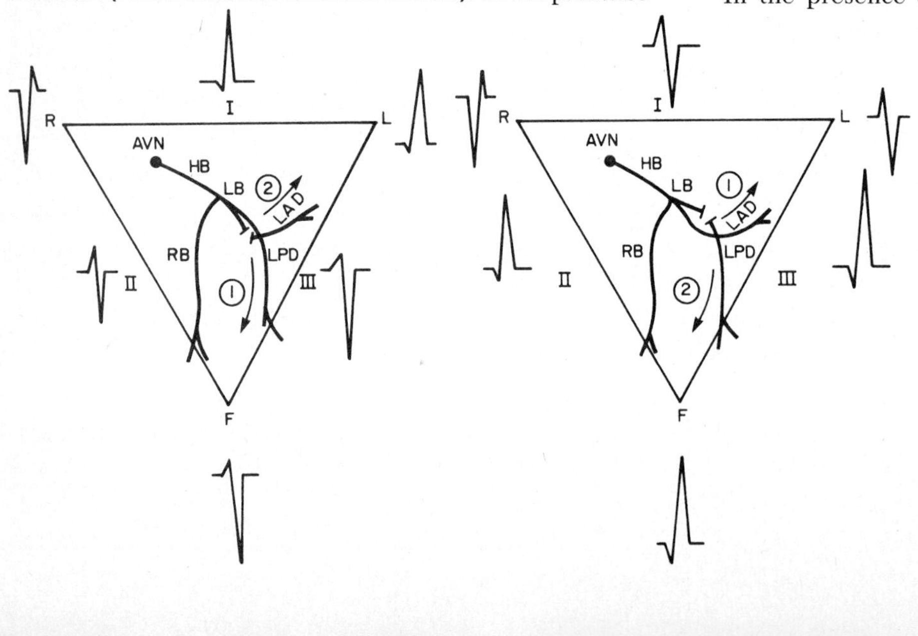

FIGURE 7–26. Diagrammatic representation of the conduction system. Interruption of the LAD (*left*) results in an initial inferior (*1*) followed by a dominant superior (*2*) direction of activation; interruption of the LPD (*right*) results in an initial superior (*1*) followed by a dominant inferior (*2*) direction of activation. AVN = atrioventricular node; HB = His bundle; LB = left bundle; RB = right bundle; LAD = left anterior division; LPD = left posterior division.

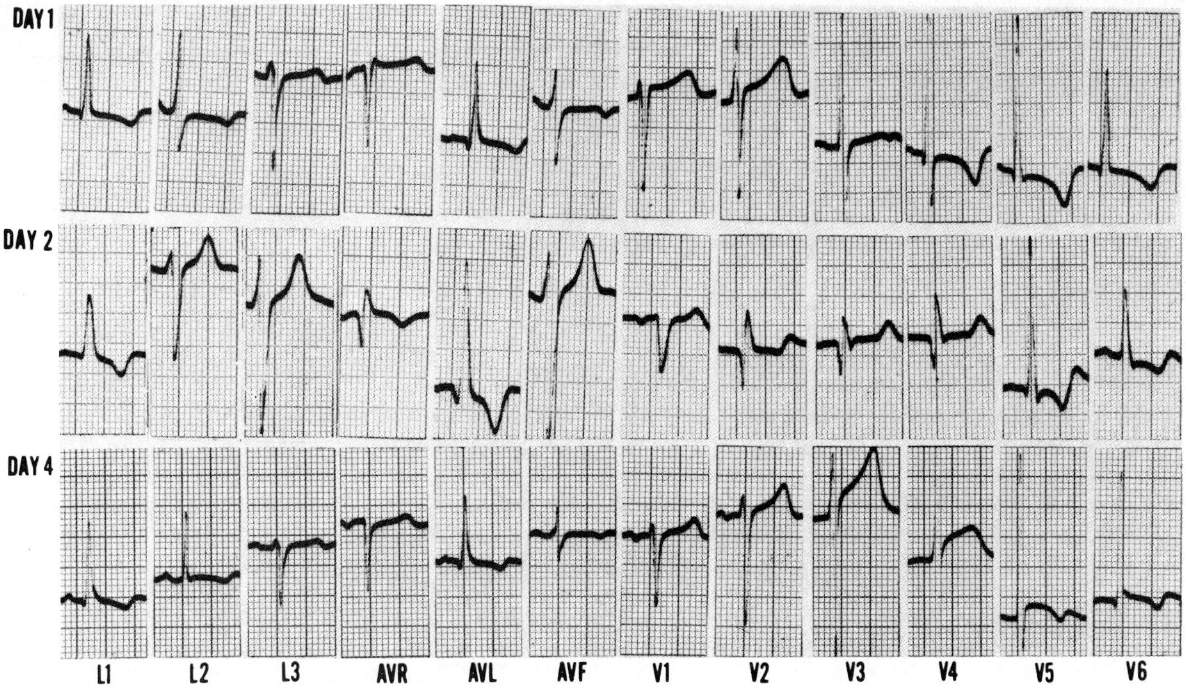

FIGURE 7–27. Transient Q waves and left anterior divisional block (LADB) recorded after aortic valve surgery. On day 1, nonspecific ST-segment and T-wave changes and voltage consistent with LVH are recorded. On day 2, LADB and prolongation of the QRS are accompanied by Q waves in leads V_1 to V_4. On day 4, the QRS duration is normal, and LADB and Q waves are no longer present.

vation begins in the midseptal and paraseptal areas, with the vector directed to the left, anteriorly, and superiorly. This is followed by activation of the left ventricular anterior and anterolateral walls, with the vector directed to the left and anteriorly. Final activation is of the inferior and posterior walls with the vector directed inferiorly, posteriorly, and to the right. The QRS duration is less than 0.12 sec.[26] In the limb leads, the initial superior and left orientation of septal vectors is reflected as R waves in leads I and aV_l and a narrow, 0.025-msec Q wave in leads II, III, I, and aV_f. The R waves in leads I and aV_l are small and followed by deep S waves reflecting the inferior, posterior, and right orientation of the wave of activation (Figs. 7–23, 7–25, and 7–26). The initial superior force and final inferior force result in a QR complex in leads II, III, and aV_f. The amplitude of the R wave in lead III exceeds the R wave in lead II. The frontal axis varies from about +90° to +120°, or perhaps +80° to +140°. The T wave is usually normal.

In the frontal plane of the VCG, the inscription is

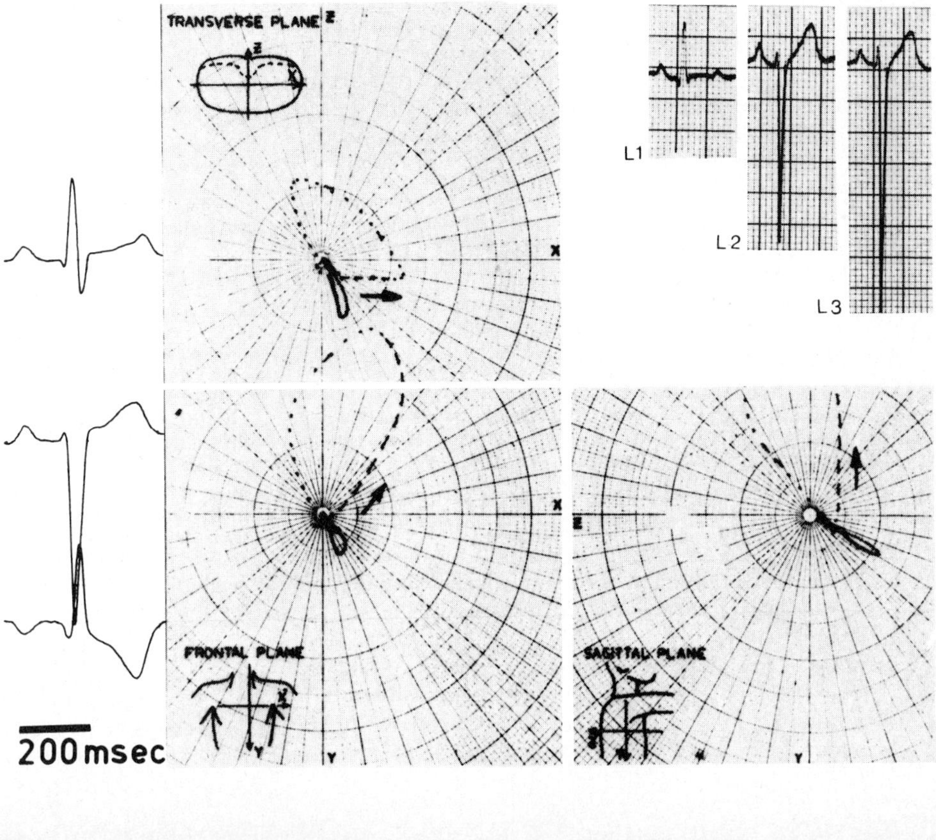

FIGURE 7–28. Left anterior divisional block and left ventricular hypertrophy (LVH). The ECG pattern of qR in lead I and rS in leads II and III indicates presence of left anterior divisional block. The diagnostic VCG features of left anterior divisional block are an initial small inferior deflection with rapid superior and counterclockwise displacement of the loop in the frontal plane, and the major area of the loop located in the left upper quadrant. LVH is suggested on ECG by the ST-T changes in lead I and the QRS voltage in leads II and III. On the VCG, LVH is indicated by posterior displacement of the loop in the transverse plane.

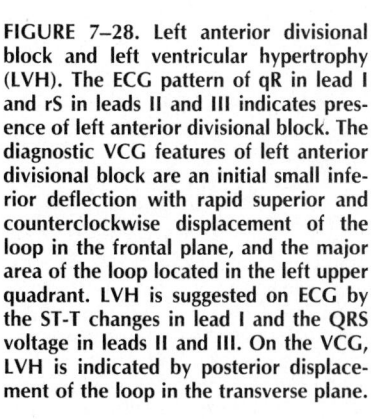

clockwise, initially superior and to the left, but with the major portion of the loop located in the right inferior quadrant.

RIGHT BUNDLE BRANCH BLOCK AND DIVISIONAL BLOCKS. RBBB with left anterior divisional block is the most common combination. The activation during the first 0.08 sec determines the axis and identifies the left anterior divisional block. The delay of depolarization due to RBBB results in a final activation of the right ventricle to the right and anteriorly (Figs. 7–23 and 7–25).

RBBB with left posterior divisional block is a rare combination. The initial 0.08 sec defines the axis and divisional block while the final delayed activation, oriented to the right and anteriorly, reflects RBBB (Fig. 7–23).

Block of the right bundle and both divisions of the left bundle (trifascicular block) can occur in the presence of RBBB with alternating left anterior and posterior divisional blocks. Such patterns are usually associated with Mobitz (type II) AV block. It has been suggested that RBBB with either hemiblock and a prolonged P-R interval may be a manifestation of trifascicular block. Although the prolonged P-R interval may be due to delayed conduction in the remaining division, the delay may also reflect AV nodal delay.[72]

The VCG records the characteristic terminal portion of the RBBB loop in the transverse plane, while the left anterior divisional block and left posterior hemiblock are best visualized in the frontal plane. The characteristic features of RBBB and left anterior divisional block with and without RBBB are shown in Figures 7–22 and 7–28. An initial inferior with rapid upward displacement of the loop or an initial superior with rapid inferior displacement in the frontal plane is recorded with left anterior or left posterior divisional block, respectively. A terminal and delayed activation to the right and anteriorly in the transverse plane is the characteristic finding in RBBB.

NONSPECIFIC INTRAVENTRICULAR CONDUCTION DEFECT (IVCD). The QRS complex may be abnormally prolonged but without the characteristic pattern of either RBBB or LBBB. Such conduction delays are referred to as "nonspecific" IVCD. These often resemble LBBB or LBBB with an abnormal left-axis deviation, a combination suggesting left anterior hemiblock with peripheral conduction delay. Presence of a normal Q wave supports peripheral delay as the cause of QRS prolongation. Although such a nonspecific prolongation may be due to drugs or electrolyte abnormalities, it is most often due to organic heart disease. An interesting form of right ventricular conduction delay has been described in patients with arrhythmogenic ventricular dysplasia. The delayed activation is inscribed in the form of a sharp deflection after termination of the QRS, during the ST segment or upstroke of the T wave.[73, 74]

BILATERAL BUNDLE BRANCH BLOCK. This diagnosis can be considered when alternating RBBB and LBBB are present (Fig. 7–24). Any other combination of conduction delays cannot be differentiated from block in the AV junction. For example, simultaneous block in both bundles results in complete AV block. Similarly, intermittent delay or block in one bundle and complete block of conduction in the contralateral bundle will manifest either as bundle branch block with a prolonged P-R interval or intermittent AV block. In the presence of BBB, a superimposed AV block due to failure of conduction in the contralateral bundle branch cannot be differentiated from block in the AV junction.

ABERRATION

Intraventricular aberration, a term introduced and defined by Lewis, describes a supraventricular impulse with abnormal, bizarre intraventricular conduction (Fig. 7–29).[75] It refers to intraventricular conduction abnormalities related to changing heart rate or other functional alterations in electrophysiological properties, anomalous AV conduction, metabolic and electrolyte abnormalities, and toxic effects of drugs. The term aberration, as used currently, does not include fixed organic conduction defects.

The mechanisms responsible for, or contributory to, aberration with changing cycle length include: (1) excitation prior to completion of repolarization (i.e., in the presence of a reduced transmembrane potential), (2) unequal refractoriness of conducting tissue resulting in local delay or block of conduction, (3) prolongation of the action potential due to prolongation of the preceding cycle length, (4) failure of restitution of transmembrane electrolyte concentration during diastole, (5) failure of the refractory period to shorten in response to acceleration of the heart rate, (6) a reduced take-off potential secondary to diastole depolarization, (7) concealed transseptal conduction with delay or block of bundle branch conduction, and (8) diffuse depression of intraventricular conduction including that of specialized as well as myocardial tissue.

Aberration may result when any of the above mechanisms alter conduction in the bundle branches or the divisions of the left bundle branch (or a combination of the two), the Purkinje fibers, or the myocardium. RBBB is the most common form of aberrancy and is frequently associated with left anterior divisional block. Aberrancy due to LBBB is much less common and in our experience often due to heart disease, although the heart disease may not be clinically evident.[76] An abnormality of intraventricular conduction due to diffuse depression of conduction in the Purkinje system and in the myocardium should be suspected when both the initial and terminal portions of the QRS complex are abnormal.

Of the mechanisms and manifestations of aberration, seven will be considered in further detail: (1) premature excitation, (2) the Ashman phenomenon, (3) acceleration-dependent aberrancy, (4) deceleration-dependent aberrancy, (5) concealed conduction, (6) diffuse myocardial depression of conduction, and (7) postextrasystolic aberrancy.

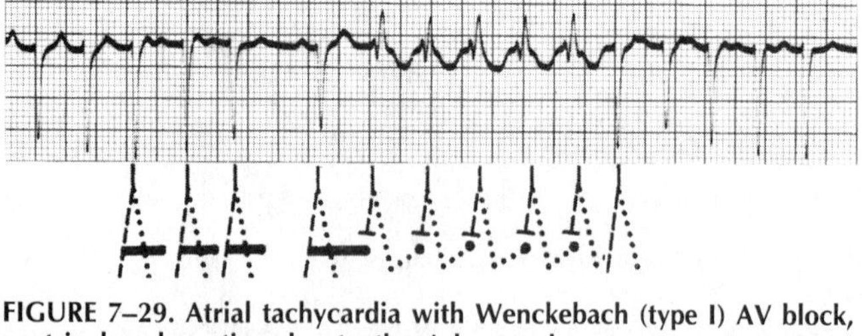

FIGURE 7–29. Atrial tachycardia with Wenckebach (type I) AV block, ventricular aberration due to the Ashman phenomenon (see p. 201), and probably concealed transseptal conduction. The long pause of the atrial tachycardia is followed by five QRS complexes with RBBB morphology. The RBBB of the first QRS reflects the Ashman phenomenon. The aberration is perpetuated by concealed transseptal activation from the left bundle into the right bundle with block of the anterograde conduction of the subsequent sinus impulse in the right bundle. Foreshortening of the R-R cycle, a manifestation of the Wenckebach structure, disturbs the relationship between transseptal and anterograde sinus conduction, and RBB conduction is normalized. In the ladder diagram below the tracing, the solid lines represent the His bundle, the dashes the RBB and the dots the LBB, while the solid horizontal bars denote the refractory period. Neither the P waves nor the AV node are identified in the diagram.

PREMATURE EXCITATION. Conduction will fail or be delayed if the stimulus falls during the effective or the relative refractory period of recovery.[5] When the impulse falls during the relative refractory period of a single bundle branch, the unilateral delay results in a bundle branch block. The duration of the refractory period may equal that of the transmembrane action potential, so-called voltage-dependent refractoriness, or it may exceed it, so-called time-dependent refractoriness. Duration of the refractory period depends to a great extent on the basic heart rate and on the duration of the immediately preceding cycle(s). Normally, the refractory period shortens with acceleration of the heart rate and lengthens with slowing of the heart rate.[77] With all variables affecting conduction being constant, the degree of aberration is usually a function of prematurity of excitation.

The site of conduction depression and thus the morphology of the aberrant QRS complex is determined by the length of the refractory period of the AV node, the bundle of His, and the bundle system itself. Normally, at slow heart rates, the right bundle branch has the longest refractory period, with the left bundle and the AV node somewhat shorter and the bundle of His the shortest. Only at very rapid rates may the duration of the refractory period of the left bundle exceed that of the right bundle.[78]

EFFECT OF CHANGING CYCLE LENGTH ON REFRACTORINESS (ASHMAN PHENOMENON). This form of aberrancy, also a function of premature excitation, differs from that due to early excitation just described in that the abnormal conduction is a function of an altered duration of the refractory period rather than of changing prematurity of stimulation. Since the duration of the refractory period is a function of the immediately preceding cycle length, the longer the preceding cycle, the longer the refractory period that follows. Consequently, with a relatively constant heart rate, sudden prolongation of the immediately preceding cycle length may result in aberration. This relationship of aberrancy to changes in the preceding cycle length is known as the Ashman phenomenon.[77] Aberrancy so initiated may persist for a number of cycles (Fig. 7–29), usually exhibits RBBB morphology, and may be associated with left anterior or rarely with left posterior divisional block.

In the presence of irregular supraventricular rhythms, such as atrial fibrillation, repetitive atrial tachycardia, or atrial tachycardia with Wenckebach (type I) AV block (Fig. 7–29), aberration due to the Ashman phenomenon is suggested by the following: (1) a relatively long cycle immediately preceding the cycle terminated by the aberrant QRS complex, (2) RBBB aberrancy with normal orientation of the initial QRS vector, (3) irregular coupling of the aberrant QRS complex, and (4) lack of a compensatory pause following the aberrant QRS complex.

ACCELERATION-DEPENDENT ABERRANCY (TACHYCARDIA-DEPENDENT ABERRANCY, PHASE 3 ABERRANCY). This form of aberration has been recognized since 1913.[79] At certain critical heart rates, impaired intraventricular conduction results in aberrancy (Figs. 7–30 and 7–31). This phenomenon has been described as tachycardia-dependent aberrancy or phase 3 aberrancy; however, the term *acceleration-dependent aberrancy* appears most appropriate. Aberration often appears at relatively slow rates, frequently below 75 bpm; similarly, because of the slow rate at which the conduction fails, one would have to postulate an extremely long transmembrane action potential in order to accept excitation during phase 3 as the cause of the impaired conduction. Finally, conduction will also fail with excitation during phase 2 of the action potential.

The appearance and disappearance of aberration often depends on very small changes in cycle length, a change frequently difficult if not impossible to detect in the ECG. Assuming that a reasonably long recording is available, a comparison of the earliest available cycle length terminated by a normal QRS complex with the cycle length terminated by the first aberrant QRS complex will aid in the diagnosis of acceleration-dependent aberrancy. The difference in the duration of two such cycles is often less than 0.04 sec.

Acceleration-dependent aberrancy differs in a number of respects from the physiological aberrancy observed in a normal heart. Differences include (1) appearance of aberrancy at relatively slow heart rates, (2) predominance of LBBB morphology, (3) independence from the immediately preceding cycle length, (4) occasional appearance without or with only a slight change in cycle length, and (5) association with heart disease.

QRS aberrancy may persist at an R-R interval considerably longer than the interval that initiated the aberrancy (Fig. 7–31). Three mechanisms have been suggested to explain this paradox: (1) concealed transseptal activation blocking conduction in the contralateral bundle; (2) "fatigue" of the bundle; and (3) concealed transseptal conduction coupled with suppression of conduction due to the increased heart rate, somewhat analogous to suppression of pacemakers by an ectopic tachycardia.[80] A discrepancy of as much as 210 msec between the

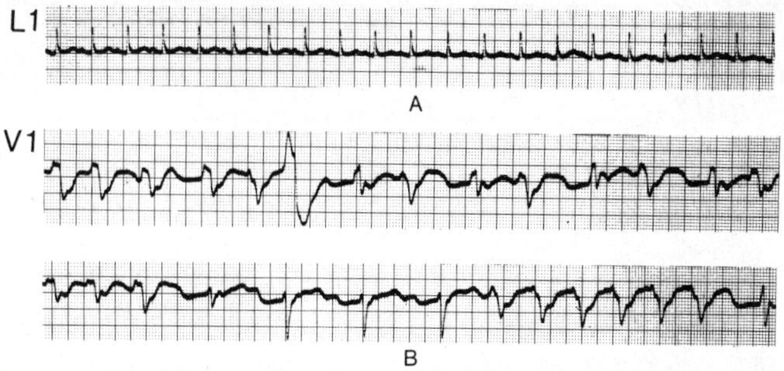

FIGURE 7–30. Intraventricular aberration due to quinidine and acceleration of the heart rate. In panel *A*, control tracing, the ECG is normal with a sinus rate of 130 bpm. After administration of quinidine (panel *B*), the heart rate is 120 bpm and the QRS widened to 0.20 sec with a 3:2 Wenckebach (type I) AV block interrupted by one VPC. P-wave duration is prolonged and the P-R interval is increased to 0.28 sec. The QRS complex which follows the longer pauses are narrower, probably owing to a longer period of recovery. In the bottom trace 1:1 AV conduction is interrupted by 2:1 AV conduction. P waves measure 0.20 sec in duration, the P-R interval is 0.40 sec, and the QRS complexes at onset of 2:1 AV block are foreshortened to 0.16 sec. The QRS prolongation to 0.16 sec is due to quinidine, while further widening of the QRS complexes to 0.20 sec in presence of 1:1 A-V conduction reflects both the effect of quinidine and the accelerated heart rate.

cycles initiating and terminating the aberration suggests that concealed transseptal conduction may not be the sole factor responsible for the unexpected persistence of aberrancy at the longer cycle lengths. The difference cannot be explained solely on the basis of time consumed by conduction along the contralateral bundle and across the septum.[81] Normal transseptal activation in the human heart is about 40 to 45 msec;[18] in the diseased heart, it may be prolonged to 115 msec.[82] It is likely, therefore, that a combination of mechanisms is operative.

One mechanism that would explain the unexpected delay in normalization of intraventricular conduction is "fatigue,"[76] a descriptive term that may reflect failure of restitution of transmembrane ionic gradients and lowering of the transmembrane resting potential and/or a shift of the membrane responsiveness to the right. The latter denotes a decrease in upstroke velocity of phase 0 for any given magnitude of transmembrane resting potential. A different mechanism, namely, concealed conduction, may explain the delayed normalization of bundle branch conduction in patients with atrial fibrillation. Concealed conduction of atrial fibrillatory impulses into the blocked bundle may result in a true bundle-to-bundle interval that is considerably shorter than the manifest QRS interval.

Occasionally, paradoxical normalization of the QRS complex without a change in heart rate—or, in fact, with acceleration of the heart rate—has been documented (Fig. 7–31). Mechanisms that may explain this phenomenon include physiological shortening of the refractory period in response to acceleration of the heart rate, equalization of conduction in the two bundles and conduction during the supernormal period, and the gap phenomenon.

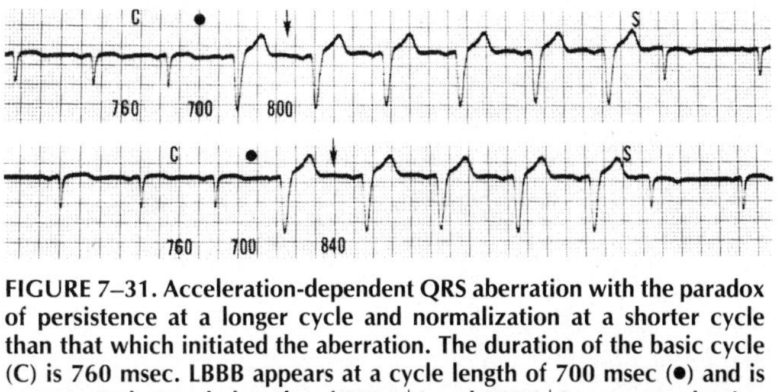

FIGURE 7–31. Acceleration-dependent QRS aberration with the paradox of persistence at a longer cycle and normalization at a shorter cycle than that which initiated the aberration. The duration of the basic cycle (C) is 760 msec. LBBB appears at a cycle length of 700 msec (●) and is perpetuated at cycle lengths of 800 (↓) and 840 (↓) msec; conduction normalizes after a cycle length of 600 msec (S). Perpetuation of LBBB at a cycle length of 800 and 840 (↓) msec is probably due to transseptal concealment, similar to that described in Figure 7–29. Unexpected normalization of the QRS (S) following the atrial premature contraction is probably due to equalization of conduction in the two bundles; however, supernormal conduction in the left bundle cannot be excluded. (From Fisch, C., et al.: Rate dependent aberrancy. Circulation *48*:714, 1973, by permission of the American Heart Association, Inc.)

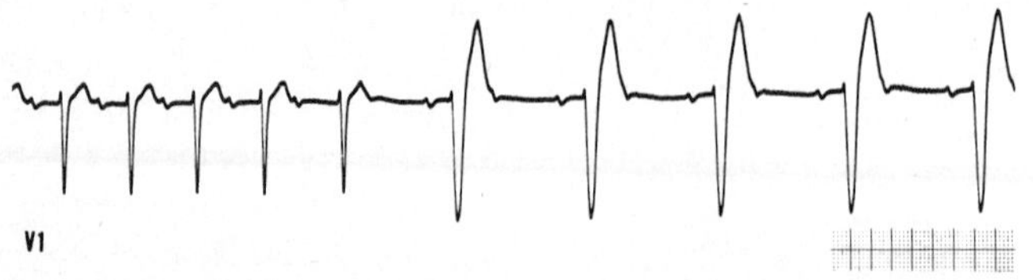

FIGURE 7–32. Deceleration-dependent aberration. The basic rhythm is sinus with Wenckebach (type I) AV block. With 1:1 AV conduction, the QRS complexes are normal in duration; with 2:1 AV block or after the longer pause of a Wenckebach sequence, LBBB appears. Slow diastolic depolarization (phase 4) of the transmembrane action potential during the prolonged cycle is implicated as the cause of the LBBB.

DECELERATION-DEPENDENT ABERRANCY (BRADYCARDIA-DEPENDENT ABERRANCY, PHASE 4 ABERRANCY). A prolonged cycle may be terminated by an aberrant QRS and foreshortening of the cycle may normalize the QRS (Fig. 7–32).[83] It has been suggested that this form of aberrancy is due to a gradual loss of transmembrane resting potential during a prolonged diastole with excitation from a less negative take-off potential.[84] Because a small change in resting potential may have a pronounced effect on the rate of rise of phase 0 of the action potential, deceleration aberrancy may be seen with a relatively small prolongation of the cycle length.[85]

CONCEALED CONDUCTION. Conduction in the bundle branches may be impaired by concealed penetration of a supraventricular impulse or by transseptal activation from the contralateral bundle (Fig. 7–29). In atrial fibrillation, concealed conduction into a bundle branch can be considered when acceleration-dependent aberrancy persists at a QRS cycle that is longer than a cycle terminated by a normal QRS. Transseptal concealed conduction into a bundle branch from the contralateral bundle should be suspected if aberrancy, once initiated, persists at rates slower than the rate that initiated the aberrancy (Fig. 7–31).

MYOCARDIAL DEPRESSION. Drugs and metabolic and electrolyte disorders are frequent causes of QRS aberrancy (Fig. 7–30). The severity of depression of conduction varies, and the QRS may exhibit RBBB or LBBB, divisional block, or the two combined. As indicated previously, aberrancy can be differentiated from ordinary BBB by the presence of distortion in the initial and terminal components of the QRS complex. The appearance of aberration is often rate related (Fig. 7–30).

POSTEXTRASYSTOLIC ABERRATION. Aberrant intraventricular conduction of a sinus impulse terminating a compensatory pause is rare and must be differentiated from an aberrant escape complex. The exact mechanism of the postpausal aberrancy is not clear. It may be due to slow diastolic depolarization, unequal recovery of conducting or myocardial tissue, or increased diastolic volume.

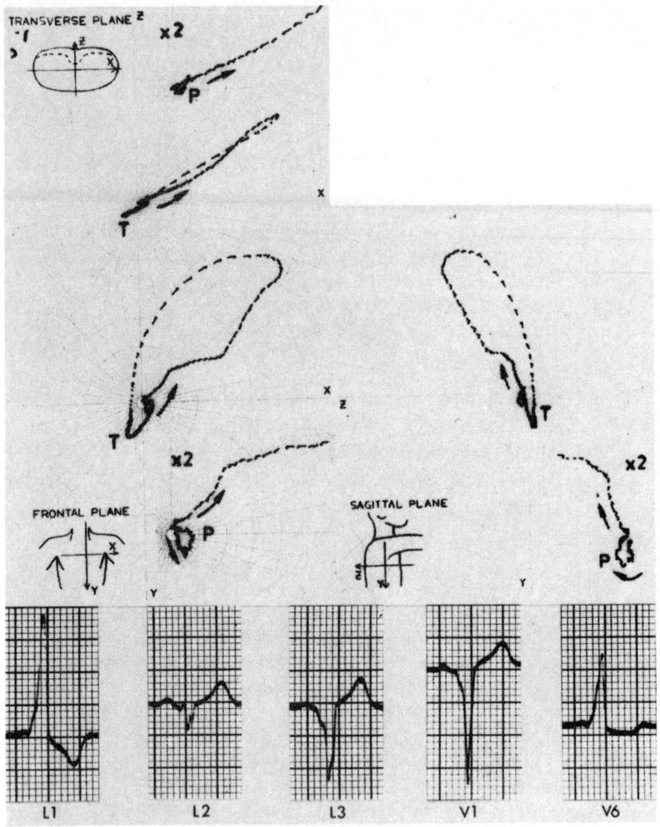

FIGURE 7–33. The ECG illustrates type B Wolff-Parkinson-White syndrome and simulates an inferior myocardial infarction. The VCG displays a delayed initial QRS force, indicated by close spacing of the dots. This initial force is directed to the left, posteriorly, and superiorly. The T-wave loop is oriented in a direction opposite to that of the initial QRS force. The initial portion of the QRS loop is also recorded at twice the standard (× 2).

WOLFF-PARKINSON-WHITE (WPW) SYNDROME (See pp. 604 and 685)

WPW, or preexcitation,[86] is an electrocardiographic syndrome characterized by a short P-R (≤0.12 sec) interval, prolonged QRS (≥0.12 sec) complex, a slur on the upstroke of the QRS (delta wave), and (as a rule) a normal P-J interval (Figs. 7–33 and 7–34). Secondary ST-segment and

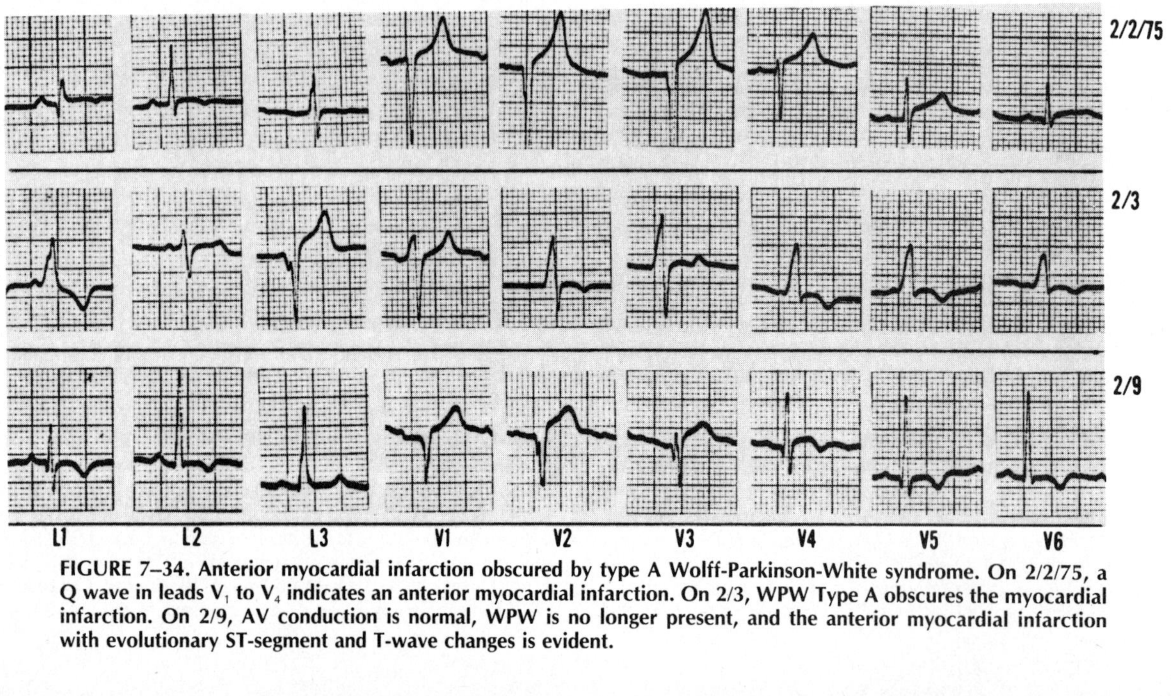

FIGURE 7–34. Anterior myocardial infarction obscured by type A Wolff-Parkinson-White syndrome. On 2/2/75, a Q wave in leads V_1 to V_4 indicates an anterior myocardial infarction. On 2/3, WPW Type A obscures the myocardial infarction. On 2/9, AV conduction is normal, WPW is no longer present, and the anterior myocardial infarction with evolutionary ST-segment and T-wave changes is evident.

T-wave changes are nearly always present. Paroxysmal supraventricular tachycardia is recorded in about 50 per cent of patients with WPW. The characteristic pattern of WPW can be altered by abnormalities of AV and intraventricular conduction. The prevalence of WPW in the general population is approximately 3 per thousand; the fact that this figure is identical for both the young and the aged supports a congenital origin for WPW.[66]

Although Wilson is credited with the initial report of WPW,[87] it was Cohn who brought the electrocardiograph to America and first described an ECG pattern to become known as WPW. His patient was described in 1913, and suffered from a supraventricular tachycardia.[88] In 1930, this pattern was recognized as a discrete ECG syndrome.[86] Shortly thereafter the bypass concept of WPW was proposed, and this concept has stood the test of time.[89] It is of interest to note that over the years a variety of mechanisms have been proposed to explain the ECG pattern of WPW, including an excitable focus within the ventricle mechanically triggered by contraction of the atrium, accelerated conduction over a segment of the normal AV pathway, and, most recently, AV nodal bypass coupled with conduction through the Mahaim fibers.[90]

In WPW the QRS complex is a fusion between the impulse traversing the bypass and the normal AV junction. The bypass component of the QRS complex, or *delta wave*, varies depending on the size of the ventricular muscle mass activated through the bypass. In some instances, especially in the presence of AV conduction delay, the entire ventricular mass may be activated by the impulse propagated through the bypass, and the entire QRS complex becomes essentially a delta wave.

Traditionally, WPW has been classified into types A and B. *Type A* is characterized by a prominent positive initial QRS deflection in leads V_1 and V_2 (Fig. 7–34) and *type B* by a predominantly negative deflection in leads V_1 and V_2 (Fig. 7–33).[91] In type A, the initial inscription of the QRS complex, the delta wave, reflects early activation of the posterior left ventricle and, in type B, early activation of the anterior superior right ventricle. *Type C WPW*, characterized by a negative delta wave in the left lateral leads, has also been described. Studies using surface potential mapping, epicardial mapping during surgery, and electrophysiological studies have identified a number of preexcitation sites.[39, 92, 92a] Presence of more than one QRS pattern in an individual patient suggests the possibility of multiple bypass tracts. A short P-R interval with a normal QRS complex accompanied by paroxysmal supraventricular tachycardia has been suggested as a variant of WPW (p. 685).[93]

First-, second-, and third-degree AV block have been reported with WPW.[94] Right and left BBB have been described in association with WPW. In the presence of a BBB, an ipsilateral bypass, by preexciting the ventricle normally activated by the blocked bundle branch, will obscure the BBB. Both supernormal and concealed conduction have been invoked to explain unexpected patterns of behavior of bypass conduction.[95]

WPW often complicates ECG interpretation because it may obscure or simulate a variety of patterns. It may mask (Fig. 7–34) or may simulate myocardial infarction. When the QRS vector is directed toward the left ventricular cavity, the cavity becomes initially positive and a Q wave will not be recorded. A diagnosis of ventricular hypertrophy in the presence of WPW (as in BBB) may be difficult, if not impossible. WPW has been mistaken for RBBB, LBBB, and RVH.[39] Supraventricular arrhythmias with aberration, resulting from conduction through the bypass, have been mistaken for ventricular tachycardia. Aberration due to WPW should be suspected when the ventricular rate is rapid, often approaching 300 bpm, or when the QRS morphology of the bizarre complexes is upright in leads V_1 and V_2 as well as in V_5 and V_6.

The characteristic VCG feature of WPW syndrome is a slowly inscribed initial portion of the loop, the delta wave of the ECG, which is best seen in the transverse plane.[33] The delta is defined as that portion of the loop which begins at point E, the resting or isoelectric point of the electronic beam, and ends with resumption of normal conduction speed. The direction of this initial portion of the loop classifies the WPW into type A, B, or C. Normally, the duration of the slow inscription varies from 0.02 to 0.08 sec, depending on how much of the ventricle is activated through the anomalous pathway.

In *type A WPW*, the slow portion of the loop is directed to the left or slightly to the right and anteriorly. The remainder of the QRS loop, usually inscribed counterclockwise, maintains the same direction as the delta wave and is located in the left anterior quadrant. In about 20 per cent of cases, the maximal vector of the loop points in the direction of the left posterior quadrant. In the ECG these changes are manifested by an upright QRS complex in leads V_1 and V_6.

Type B WPW is characterized by an initial slow inscription oriented to the left and posteriorly or slightly anteriorly. The major portion of the loop is located in the left posterior quadrant. In the ECG these are reflected as a QS complex in leads V_1 and V_2 and an R wave in leads V_5 and V_6 (Fig. 7–33).

Type C WPW is a rarely encountered variant characterized by a Q wave in leads V_5 and V_6. The slowly inscribed initial portion of the loop is directed anteriorly to the right, with the remainder of the loop inscribed normally.

MYOCARDIAL INFARCTION

The ECG changes of myocardial infarction, first described in man in 1920,[96] are those of ischemia, injury, and cellular death and are, within limits, reflected by T-wave changes, ST-segment displacement, and the appearance of Q waves, respectively. Such a clear-cut differentiation, although clinically useful, may be overly simplistic and artificial. For example, T-wave changes may be due to ischemia, injury, or death of muscle. Similarly, a Q wave may be due to impairment of transmembrane ionic fluxes and not necessarily cellular death. However, for the purpose of this discussion, T-wave changes, ST-segment displacement, and appearance of a Q wave are assumed to reflect ischemia, injury, and cell death, respectively.

ISCHEMIA

In the dog, the earliest change following ligation of a coronary artery is the almost immediate appearance of a primary, as a rule negative, T wave. After 60 to 90 seconds, there is a maximal shift of the ST segment. The T wave becomes positive and peaked, and the change is as a rule a primary change. The amplitude of the R wave decreases during the first 30 seconds after experimental occlusion. This is followed by an increase in the amplitude which peaks 20 to 30 seconds after the maximal increase of the left ventricular volume.[97] In man, unless an ECG is recorded at the moment of occlusion, the initial T-wave stage is usually missed. Occasionally, a giant R wave is recorded early during the ischemic episode.[98] Such changes in the QRS could contribute to the T-wave abnormality, and the abnormal T wave would reflect both primary and secondary changes in repolarization.

Normally the process of repolarization proceeds from the epicardium to the endocardium, and an upright T wave is recorded. Ischemia prolongs the regional duration of recovery, with the ischemic area being last to repolarize. If the ischemia is subendocardial, the direction of repolarization remains unchanged and the polarity of the T wave remains upright. In the presence of subepicardial ischemia,

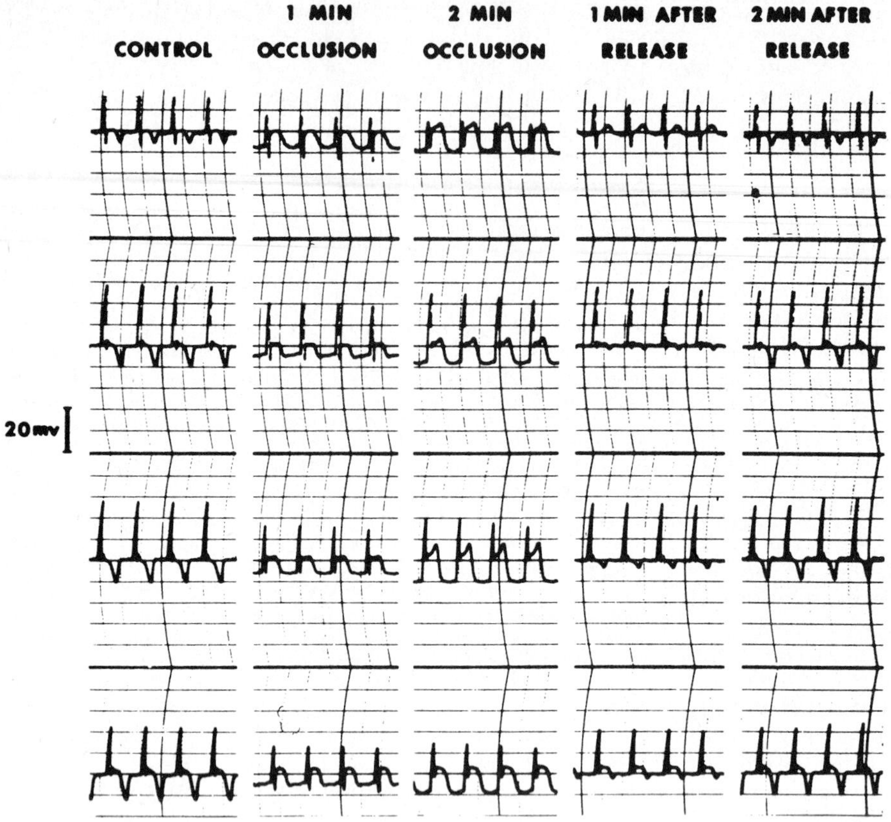

FIGURE 7–35. Simultaneous epicardial electrograms recorded from four sites. The electrodes were distributed randomly in the ischemic area, with some closer to the center of the ischemic area than others. After one minute of occlusion, TQ-segment depression is apparent in all recordings. After two minutes of occlusion, TQ-segment depression has increased. The ST-segment takeoff is slightly elevated or isoelectric in all recordings. The polarity of the T wave is changed from a negative during the control period to positive. These recordings emphasize that major changes in action potential downstroke, shape, and timing can occur without significant alteration of phase 2 and of the action potential. Similarly, T-wave changes can occur without a significant shift of the true ST segment. True TQ-segment depression appears to be the major cause of ST-segment displacement and the true ST-segment shift of lesser magnitude and variable. T waveform is markedly altered with occlusion. (From Vincent, G. M., et al.: Mechanisms of ischemic ST-segment displacement. Circulation *56*:559, 1977, by permission of the American Heart Association, Inc.)

the duration of the excited state is longer in the epicardium; the normal order of repolarization is reversed, proceeding from endocardium to epicardium; and an inverted T wave is inscribed. Because of local prolongation of recovery, the late phase of repolarization may be unopposed, and a large and prolonged T wave may be registered.[99]

INJURY

Two concepts based on systolic and diastolic phenomena have been suggested to explain the ST-segment displacement. One postulates local reduction or loss of resting potential, resulting in a *diastolic current of injury*. The second concept assumes an unopposed current flowing from the injured area during the isoelectric ST segment, resulting in a *systolic current of injury*. These systolic and diastolic phenomena cannot be differentiated with the ordinary clinical alternating-current (AC) electrocardiograph but can be recorded experimentally with direct-current (DC) equipment (Fig. 7–35).

The concept of the *diastolic current* of injury proposes that localized injury is associated with a flow of current from the uninjured to the injured area. As a result, the T-Q segment is displaced downward but is automatically shifted to control level by the capacitor-coupled amplifier of the ECG. When the entire heart (including the injured area) is depolarized, the ST segment is elevated with respect to the depressed but rectified (isoelectric) diastolic T-Q segment (Fig. 7–36).

The concept of the *systolic current* of injury proposes that during the ST segment, the normal heart is depolarized but the injured area undergoes early repolarization. The result is a current flow from the more positive injured area to a more negative or uninjured area. The result is true elevation of the ST segment. Similarly, if, rather than repolarizing early, the injured area fails to depolarize with the normal myocardium, a current of injury would exist and an elevated ST segment would be recorded (Fig. 7–36).

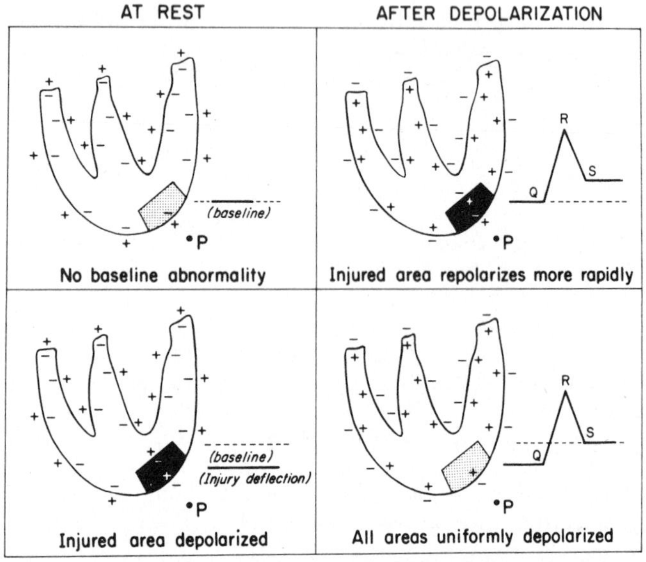

FIGURE 7–36. Systolic (*upper row*) and diastolic (*lower row*) currents of injury. *Upper row,* The ischemic area (shaded) is electrically identical to the nonischemic heart at rest, and there is no shift of the baseline potential. During repolarization, however, the ischemic area (black) has repolarized early and is positive relative to the depolarized heart, the baseline is shifted upward (positive), and the ECG records an elevated ST segment. Similarly, if the ischemic area fails to depolarize with the remainder of the heart, it would be positive relative to the remainder of the heart and a positive ST segment would be recorded. This latter mechanism may also be operative.

Lower row, The ischemic area (black) is depolarized at rest, thus negative relative to the remainder of the heart, and the baseline is shifted down (negative). This shift is not recognizable on ECG. However, with completion of depolarization the injured area is also depolarized; its potential becomes identical to that of the rest of the heart; and the ST segment, although isoelectric, is elevated relative to the depressed baseline; so that an elevated ST segment is registered.

These two mechanisms cannot be differentiated with the ECG, and although both contribute to the current of injury, the systolic is thought to dominate (Fig. 7–35). (From Scher, A. M.: Electrocardiogram. *In* Ruch, I. C., and Patton, H. D. (eds.): Physiology and Biophysics. Philadelphia, W. B. Saunders Company, 1974.)

Earlier experimental studies indicate that during injury both systolic and diastolic currents are present,[100] and at times the systolic precedes the diastolic current of injury. A more recent study suggests that the diastolic current predominates while the systolic current plays a lesser role and that the magnitude of the current is modified by the heart rate[101] (Fig. 7–35). As indicated, the clinical ECG does not differentiate between systolic and diastolic currents of injury. Furthermore, unless the onset of the injury is recorded, even a DC coupled ECG would not identify the mechanism of the ST-segment shift.

An electrode facing subendocardial injury registers an elevated ST segment, while an epicardial electrode subtended by the normal myocardium registers ST-segment depression. Similarly, an electrode facing epicardial injury registers elevation of the ST segment, while the endocardial electrode inscribes ST-segment depression.

INFARCTION

Infarction implies necrosis and an electrically inert myocardium. The diagnostic feature of infarction is the *Q wave*. Two concepts have been invoked to explain the appearance of the Q wave. The theory of proximity, the "window" theory, suggests that the electrically inert myocardium allows an electrode to record the intracavitary negativity.[102] There is ample evidence, however, to suggest that a Q wave can be recorded in the absence of a transmural infarction. Heterogeneity of electrophysiological changes associated with the dynamic events of ischemia and subsequent healing, with intermingling of fibrous and viable tissue, has been suggested as an explanation.[102]

According to the vectorial concept, the electrically inert myocardium fails to contribute to the normal electrical forces and the result is a vector that points away from the area of infarction, reflected by a Q wave. Theoretically, the infarction vector represents the force that alters the normal vector. It is equal to but opposite in direction from the vector generated by the infarcted myocardium prior to infarction.[33] If the net vector is directed normally but is reduced in magnitude, a Q wave will not be recorded, but the amplitude of the QRS complex will be reduced, indicating loss of myocardium. However, the specificity of such a change for infarction is low.

DIAGNOSIS OF MYOCARDIAL INFARCTION
(See Ch. 38)

One of the most valuable contributions of the ECG is in the diagnosis of myocardial infarction.[103] Usually it is the first laboratory test performed; the technique is reliable and reproducible, can be applied serially, and when properly interpreted is the cornerstone of the laboratory diagnosis of myocardial infarction.

Any discussion of the sensitivity, specificity, and diagnostic power of the ECG in myocardial infarction must consider that the ECG changes differ significantly depending on the stage and size of the infarction. Similarly, recognition of, and attention to, subtle and atypical changes, realization of the great importance of serial tracings, and an appreciation of the effect of coexisting conduction defects will enhance the diagnostic value of the ECG.

THE INITIAL ECG. The initial ECG is "diagnostic" of acute infarction in slightly more than half the patients. This statement should be accepted with the reservation that a single ECG may never be "diagnostic." However, a pattern of ST-segment displacement, especially with associated Q-wave and T-wave changes, and a clinical history suggestive of ischemic heart disease is highly suggestive—if not diagnostic—of acute myocardial infarction. In a study of all patients admitted to an emergency room and subsequently proven to have myocardial infarction, 65 per cent had an initial diagnostic ECG and 20 per cent were said to have a normal tracing.[104] In another study of 198 patients, the ECG recorded on the first day was diagnostic of infarction in 72 per cent of men and 61 per cent of the women. Serial tracings increased the sensitivity to 93 per cent.[105] In a series of 449 patients, the initial ECG was interpreted as diagnostic of myocardial infarction in 229 (51 per cent), probable myocardial infarction in 120 (27 per cent), doubtful in 30 (7 per cent), and no evidence of infarction in 70 (16 per cent). Serial cardiograms increased the sensitivity to 83 per cent.[106] In 150 patients with "slight or subacute infarction" treated at home, a pattern diagnostic of myocardial infarction was seen in 27 patients. Seventy-two patients showed significant but not diagnostic abnormalities. LVH was present in 10 patients and minor, 0.5-mm ST-segment depression and lowering of T waves were present in 24 patients. The ECG was borderline in seven and normal in 10 patients.[107]

CLASSIC PATTERN AND EVOLUTION OF INFARCTION. The sequence of ECG evolution of myocardial infarction in man is, in many respects, similar to that recorded in the experimental animal. If the ECG is inscribed at the onset of myocardial infarction, the characteristic early change—namely, an abnormal T wave—is often recorded. The T wave may be prolonged, increased in magnitude, and either upright or inverted.[98] This is followed by ST-segment elevation in leads facing the area of injury, with reciprocal depression in the "remote" opposite leads. The upright T wave may exhibit terminal inversion at a time when the ST segment is still elevated. A Q wave may be present in the first ECG or may not appear for hours or sometimes days. The amplitude of the QRS complex may diminish and may be replaced by a QS pattern. As the ST segment returns to the baseline, symmetrically inverted T waves evolve.[96] The time of appearance and the magnitude of the changes vary among patients[108] (Fig. 7–37).

The classic evolution of acute myocardial infarction is documented in approximately one-half to two-thirds of the patients (Fig. 7–38). In a prospective study of 230 patients, 66 per cent showed diagnostic changes characterized by typical evolution of ST segment and T waves with the appearance of Q waves, while in 34 per cent the infarct was manifested by ST-segment and T-wave changes only (Fig. 7–39).[109]

SUBTLE, ATYPICAL, NONSPECIFIC PATTERNS OF INFARCTION. Atypical features and characteristics of early infarction seen in about 40 to 50 per cent of the first ECG's include a normal ECG; subtle ST-segment and T-wave changes; isolated T-wave abnormality; transient normali-

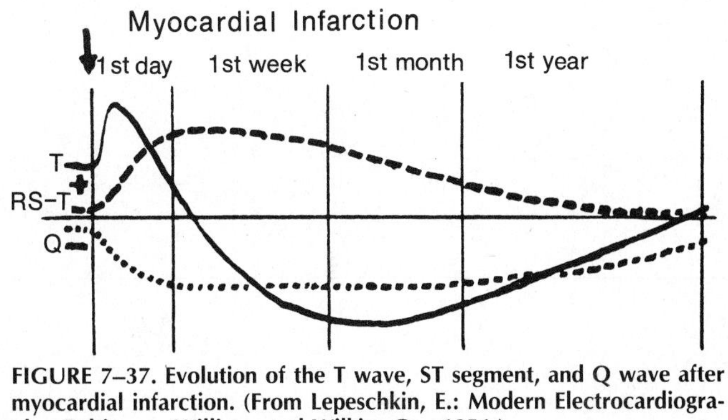

FIGURE 7–37. Evolution of the T wave, ST segment, and Q wave after myocardial infarction. (From Lepeschkin, E.: Modern Electrocardiography. Baltimore, Williams and Wilkins Co., 1951.)

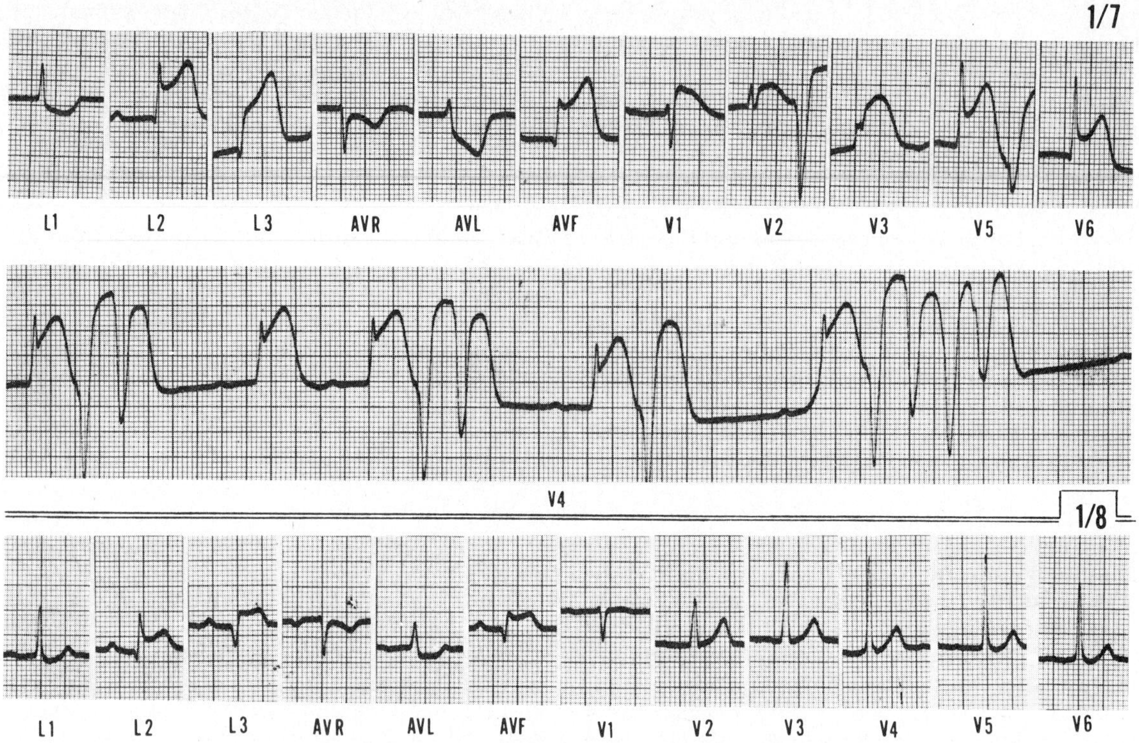

FIGURE 7–38. Acute inferior myocardial infarction and transient extensive anterior injury. Tracing made on 1/7 shows elevation of the ST segment in leads II, III, and aV_f, V_1 through V_6 with reciprocal depression of the ST segment in leads I and aV_l. In the second row the acute injury is accompanied by ventricular premature complexes (isolated and couplets) and a short run of ventricular tachycardia. In the tracing of 1/8, the anterior current of injury is no longer present, and the residual pattern is that of an acute inferior myocardial infarction manifest by a Q wave and ST-segment elevation in leads II, III, and aV_f. The tall R in lead V_2 and upright right precordial R waves suggest an associated posterior infarction.

zation of the ST segment, T wave, or QRS complex (Fig. 7–39); involvement of electrically "silent" areas (Fig. 7–40); or the masking effect of conduction defects (Figs. 7–21, 7–24, and 7–34). Awareness and recognition of the early, nondiagnostic, "atypical" or subtle abnormalities will improve the diagnostic sensitivity of the ECG.

Although ECG changes can be documented within seconds after experimental coronary occlusion and in man

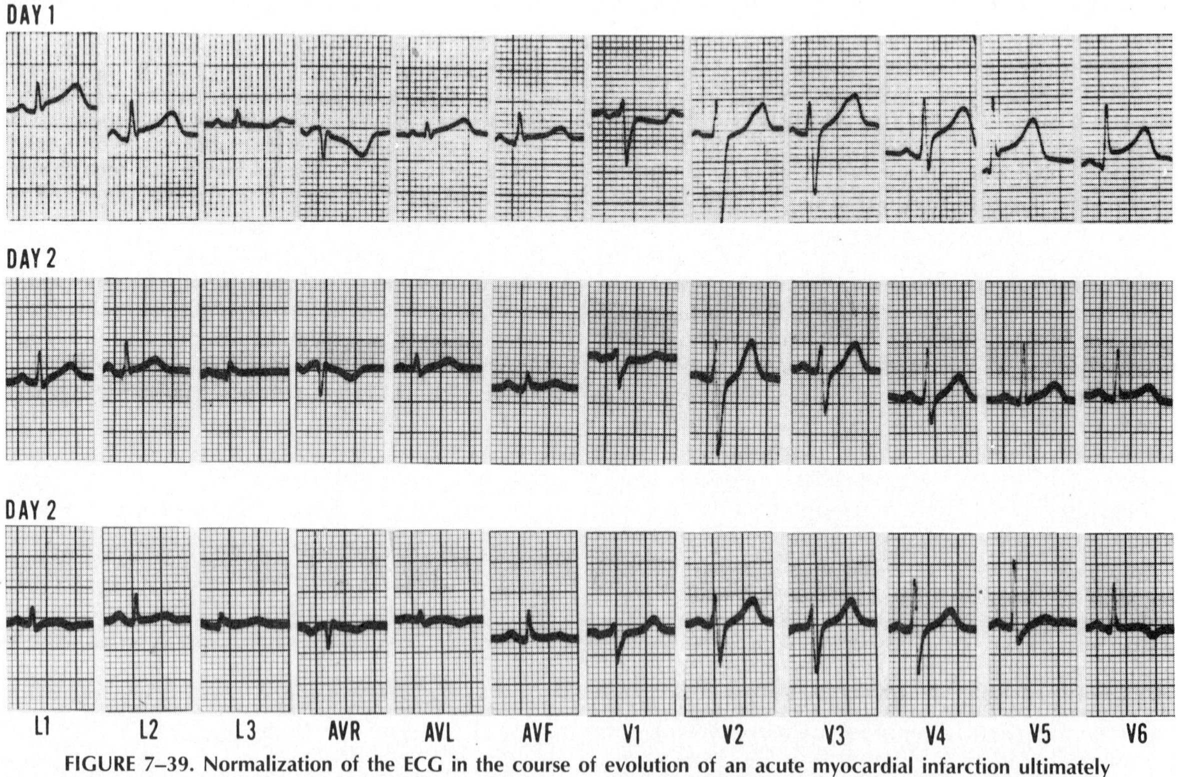

FIGURE 7–39. Normalization of the ECG in the course of evolution of an acute myocardial infarction ultimately manifest by T-wave changes only. Day 1, current of injury in leads I, II, aV_l, V_4, V_5, and V_6. Day 2, row 2, ECG is normal. Day 2, row 3, T waves are inverted in leads I, aV_l, V_5, and V_6. Inversion of the T wave is the only evidence of infarction.

during angioplasty,[109a] such changes may be delayed. A normal initial ECG in a patient with evolving clinical acute myocardial infarction may be due to absence of ischemia at the time of the initial tracing, a delay in evolution of the characteristic pattern, an initially small infarct that produces diagnostic ECG changes only after extension, transient normalization of the ECG in the course of evolution of acute myocardial infarction (Fig. 7–39), or infarction of an electrocardiographically silent area of the myocardium (Fig. 7–40).[106, 107]

Evolution of the characteristic ST-segment and T-wave changes coupled with appearance of Q waves is highly specific for acute myocardial infarction. In the first ECG, the sensitivity and specificity of the ST-segment change alone, especially when marked, is high. At times, however, *evolving* changes in the ST segment need to be demonstrated,[106] since conditions such as pericarditis, early repolarization, hyperkalemia, or ventricular aneurysm and Prinzmetal's angina may also manifest ST-segment elevation. Although subtle, minor ST-segment elevation can be easily overlooked, it is a relatively common, isolated early finding.

ST-segment depression may reflect subendocardial ischemia, infarction, or reciprocal changes secondary to infarction at a "remote" (opposite) site. It has also been suggested that depression of the ST segment in leads V_1 to V_4 in the presence of an inferior infarction may indicate ischemia secondary to significant obstruction of the left anterior descending coronary artery.[110] Strong evidence exists that the ST-segment depression is reciprocal to the inferior or posterolateral infarction[111–115] and that the severity of the anterior wall ST-segment depression is related to the severity and extent of the ischemic area rather than to anterior wall ischemia.[112, 116, 117] Minor, subtle ST-segment depression is a common early finding of acute myocardial infarction.[105, 118] However, ST-segment depression is often a nonspecific change and should be evaluated in light of other laboratory and clinical findings.

Tall, peaked T waves seen in experimental coronary occlusion are occasionally recorded in man and are thought to reflect subendocardial ischemia.[98] More often, the initial T wave may be isoelectric, negative, or biphasic. Subtle and nonspecific T-wave change is often the earliest recorded sign of infarction and is probably indicative of subepicardial ischemia. In about 20 to 30 per cent of patients with myocardial infarction, a T-wave abnormality is the only sign of acute infarction.

An *abnormal U wave* is a frequent marker of ischemic heart disease. Negative or biphasic U waves have been reported in up to 30 per cent of patients with chronic angina pectoris, either as a persistent finding or as a transient manifestation during an episode of angina. It is most often recorded in leads I, II, and V_4 to V_6. Appearance of a negative U wave during exercise-induced ischemia has been appreciated for some time and is highly specific for disease of the left anterior descending coronary artery.[119] A negative U wave is seen in 10 to 60 per cent of patients with anterior infarction and in up to 30 per cent of patients with inferior infarction.[28] Appearance of a negative U wave may precede other ECG changes of infarction by several hours (Fig. 7–41).

An abnormal QRS complex, ST segment, and T wave may normalize transiently in the course of evolution of acute myocardial infarction (Fig. 7–39), and this may be due to reversible ischemia or injury or conduction defects. Frequently, however, it represents a phase during progressive evolution of acute, irreversible myocardial infarction. Normalization of the ECG may be misleading and may suggest regression of the acute process or absence of myocardial infarction. Normalization and subsequent reappearance of ST-segment displacement alone in the presence of other unequivocal but stable ECG signs of infarction may be a manifestation of "reelevation"—a relatively frequent finding in acute infarction.[120]

A premature ventricular complex with a qR or QR morphology even in the absence of ECG findings of

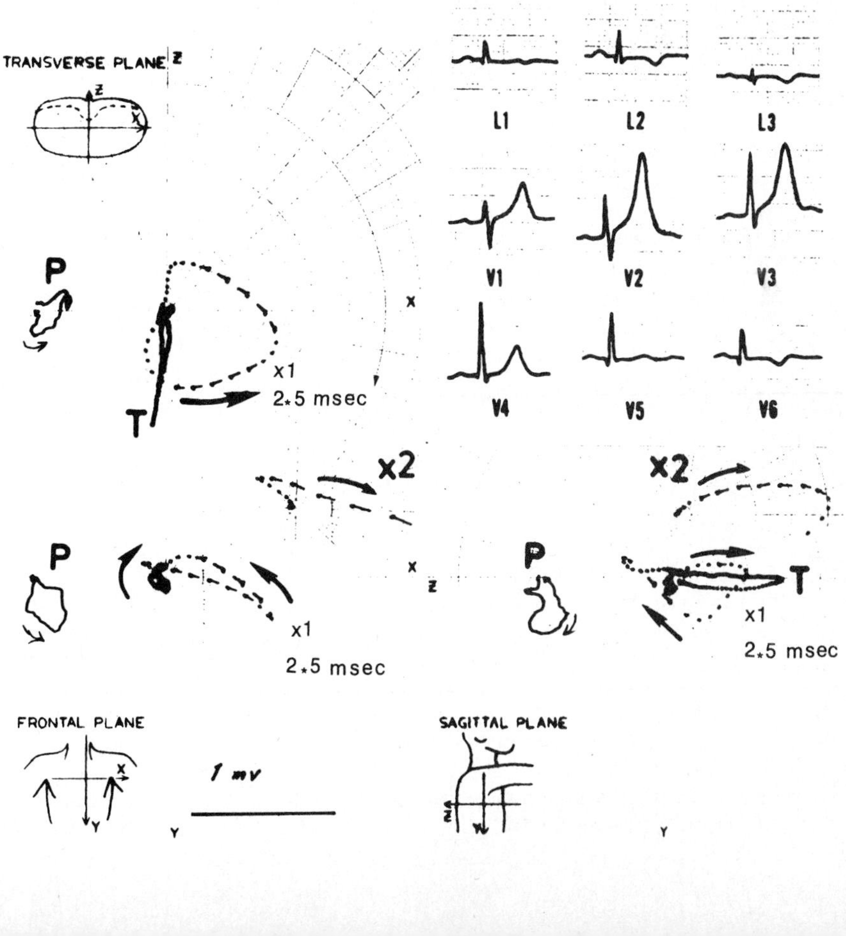

FIGURE 7–40. The ECG illustrates an inferior and posterior infarction. In the transverse plane, the VCG displays anterior displacement of the QRS loop with the anteriorly displaced area about 70 per cent of the entire loop owing to the posterior infarction. The large but narrow T loop is directed anteriorly and to the right and is inscribed counterclockwise at a uniform rate. In the frontal plane, the initial QRS force is directed superiorly and is inscribed clockwise with an inscription of 20 msec located superiorly. The initial leftward QRS magnitude, along the 0 to 180° axis, is 0.25 mV. In the sagittal plane, the initial QRS force is directed superiorly and anteriorly and is inscribed clockwise with a portion displaced superiorly. The entire QRS loop is also shifted anteriorly consistent with a posterior infarction. The large but narrow T-wave loop is directed anteriorly and is inscribed clockwise at an almost uniform rate. The initial QRS force in the frontal and sagittal planes is displayed at two times the standard (× 2), while the P-wave loop is displayed at four times the standard in each of the three planes. The Q waves in leads II, III, and V_6 and T-wave changes in leads I, II, III, V_5, and V_6 indicate an inferior apical infarction, while the tall R waves in leads V_1, V_2, and V_3 reflect the posterior infarction. The tall T waves in leads V_1, V_2, and V_3 may be due to the inferior or posterior infarction or both.

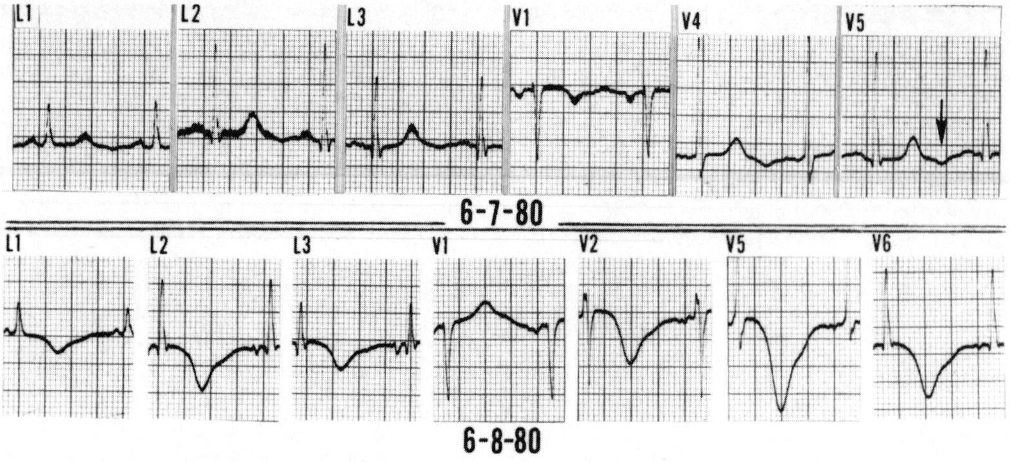

FIGURE 7–41. Negative U wave as the only marker of an acute ischemic episode. On 6/7/80 a negative U wave (↓) was recorded in leads I, II, III, V4, and V5, and an upright reciprocal U wave was present in lead V_1. In the tracing of 6/8/80 a prolonged Q-T interval and deeply inverted T waves are present in all the leads—evolutionary changes consistent with an acute myocardial infarction. At necropsy a subendocardial infarction was found.

infarction suggests the presence of myocardial infarction. This finding may prove particularly useful when the myocardial infarction is masked, for example, by LBBB or WPW. A recent study, however, questions the value of this finding in the absence of other ECG findings of myocardial infarction.[120a]

OLD INFARCTION. ECG diagnosis of an old infarction is often difficult and frequently impossible without the availability of tracings documenting the acute episode. A definitive diagnosis of old infarction depends on the presence of a pathological Q wave. Only rarely can it be based on T-wave changes alone. While a Q wave may be absent in transmural infarction[121] and present in nontransmural infarction, the sensitivity and specificity of the ECG for diagnosis of an old myocardial infarction still depend on the Q wave. The specificity of the Q wave is relatively high; its sensitivity is quite low. Within 6 to 12 months after an acute myocardial infarction, about 30 per cent of the tracings, although abnormal, are no longer diagnostic of infarction, because the Q wave is absent. Similarly, by the end of 10 years, or sooner, some 6 to 10 per cent of the cardiograms revert to normal.

In a series of 1184 tracings correlating myocardial infarction with postmortem findings, the specificity and sensitivity of the Q wave were 89 and 61 per cent, respectively, and varied with location of the infarction. Anteriorly located Q waves (leads V_1 to V_4) and inferiorly located Q waves (leads II, III, and aV_f) were falsely positive in 46 per cent. Q waves longer than 0.03 sec in lateral leads (V_5 and V_6) or Q waves in more than one "electrocardiographic zone," i.e., inferior and lateral, were false positive in only 4 per cent. The sensitivity of the Q wave was lowest for infarction located in the lateral basal portion of the left ventricle.[122] This anatomical area is usually reflected in leads I and aV_l.

MYOCARDIAL INFARCTION AND CONDUCTION DELAYS. Conduction defects may not interfere with, may mask, or may falsely suggest the diagnosis of myocardial infarction. In RBBB, the initial order of activation is normal and thus the pattern of infarction is unaltered (Figs. 7–22 to 7–24). Rarely, the development of RBBB will unmask an anteroseptal infarction.[123] In LBBB the sequence of early activation is altered, with the initial septal vector directed from right to left. As a result the earliest left ventricular intracavitary potential is positive. In keeping with the "window" concept of infarction, a Q wave cannot be registered except when there is extensive septal infarction. Restated in terms of the dipole or vector concept, since the free wall infarct is inscribed during the latter part of the QRS complex after the septal activation is complete, the direction of initial activation expressed as a dipole or vector is unaltered by the infarction, and the infarct is masked (Figs. 7–20, 7–21, and 7–24).

Numerous attempts at defining diagnostic criteria for myocardial infarction in the presence of LBBB have proved unsuccessful. The proposed criteria rarely correlate with autopsy findings. In a study of 52 patients with LBBB and autopsy findings of myocardial infarction, the following ECG findings were thought to correlate with myocardial infarction: (1) a Q wave 0.04 sec or greater in leads I, aV_l, V_5, or V_6; (2) rapid serial ST-segment and T-wave changes; (3) acute ST-segment elevation disproportionate to the area of the QRS complex; and (4) a Q wave of any size in lead V_6. Others suggest that a deep S wave in leads V_5 and V_6, a qRs complex with a slurred S wave in leads V_5 and V_6, loss of the R wave in the precordial leads, or a Q wave in leads II, III, and aV_f is consistent with myocardial infarction complicating LBBB. However, in another study of patients with LBBB, the significance of Q waves, broad R waves, notched mid and left precordial S waves, rsR′ complexes, ST-segment elevation, and T-wave changes was addressed and found to lack significant correlation with myocardial infarction.[124] A somewhat better correlation was noted between an ECG suggestive of acute inferior myocardial infarction and postmortem findings.

Studies of patients with intermittent LBBB and myocardial infarction provide additional evidence that LBBB masks myocardial infarction (Fig. 7–21).[125] It should be noted, however, that occasionally when acute infarction is evident during normal intraventricular conduction, acute changes are also recognizable in the presence of LBBB.

Block of divisions of the LBB may simulate[71] or obscure myocardial infarction.[70, 126–128] In addition, in WPW as in LBBB, the initial vector may be directed from right to left, precluding the appearance of a Q wave (Fig. 7–34). The ECG pattern of infarction masked by WPW is recognizable during normalization of intraventricular conduction and during preexcitation is suggested by ST-segment and T-wave changes.

Periinfarction block, as originally defined, is a specific conduction abnormality due to myocardial infarction.[129] The ECG changes include a Q wave of 0.04 sec and a QRS complex in the limb leads of 0.10 sec, with a slurred prolonged terminal component facing the site of infarction. Periinfarction block is not synonymous with left anterior divisional block. Periinfarction block may be of help in the

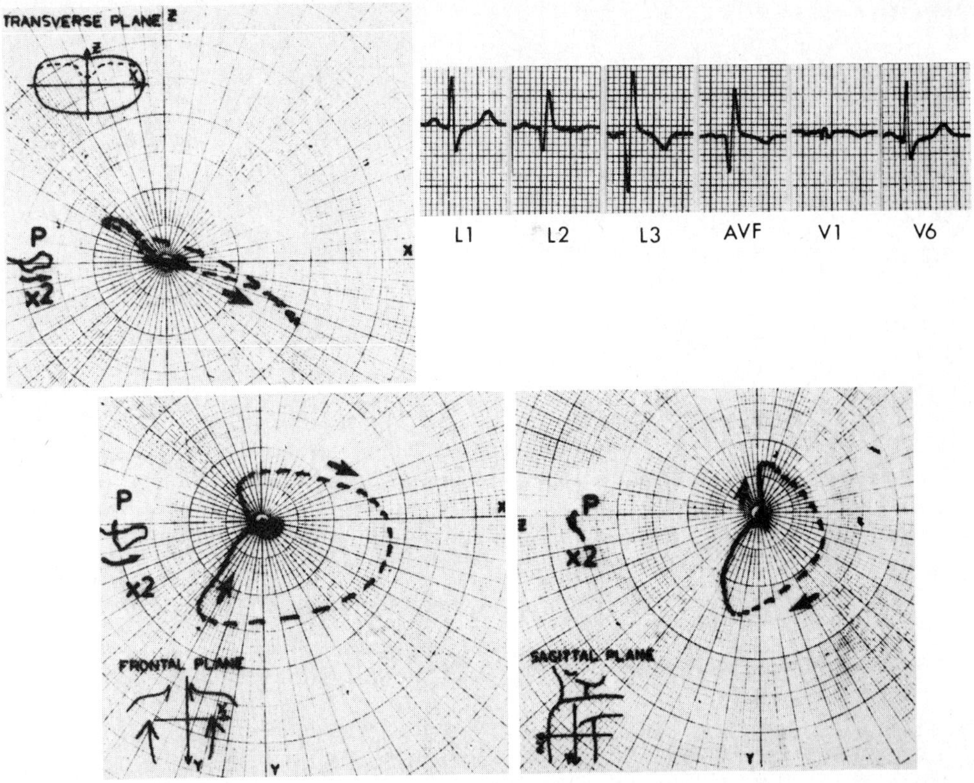

FIGURE 7–42. Inferior myocardial infarction and periinfarction block. Q waves in leads II, III, and aV_f coupled with T-wave changes are indicative of inferior myocardial infarction. QRS duration is 0.10 sec. S waves in leads I and V_6 and terminal positivity of QRS in leads II, III, and AVF suggest inferior periinfarction block.

In the VCG, superior displacement of the initial forces with clockwise rotation indicates an inferior myocardial infarction. In the sagittal plane, the superior displacement and clockwise rotation of the increased initial forces are consistent with inferior myocardial infarction. In the frontal plane terminal delay of the forces located inferiorly and to the right of the E point is indicated by close spacing of the dots and identifies periinfarction block. Total duration of the QRS is 10 msec. Slowing of conduction is also recorded in the transverse and sagittal planes.

diagnosis of old inferior infarction when the characteristic changes are no longer evident. Presence of terminal, somewhat delayed activation facing leads II, III, or aV_f and a terminal negative wave in leads I, V_5, and V_6—signs of periinfarction block—strengthen the diagnosis of inferior myocardial infarction (Fig. 7–42).

THE ECG AND SITE OF CORONARY ARTERY OBSTRUCTION. The correlation of ECG pattern and site of obstruction early in the course of myocardial infarction was investigated anteriographically in 152 patients. The sensitivity, specificity, and predictive value for (1) ECG indicative of anterior infarction and obstruction of left anterior descending coronary was 90, 95, and 96 per cent, respectively; (2) ECG indicative of inferior infarction and obstruction of right coronary was 56, 97, and 80 per cent, respectively; (3) ECG indicative of posterior or lateral infarction and obstruction of left circumflex coronary was 24, 98, and 75 per cent, respectively; (4) ECG indicative of inferior infarction and obstruction of right or left circumflex coronary was 53, 98, and 94 per cent, respectively; and (5) ECG indicative of posterior or lateral infarction and obstruction of right or left circumflex coronary was 53, 98, and 94 per cent, respectively.[130] Others have made similar observations.[131]

Presence of ST-segment elevation equal to or greater than 1 mm in lead V_4R has a sensitivity of 100 per cent and specificity of 87 per cent and a predictive accuracy of 92 per cent for occlusion of right coronary above the first right ventricular branch. The absence of ST-segment elevation of 1 mm excluded such lesions. Similarly, presence of ST-segment elevation in V_4R excluded isolated obstruction of left circumflex artery.[132]

THE ECG AND LOCATION OF INFARCTION. A precise anatomical location of anterior myocardial infarction based on ECG is not always possible. Accuracy of such localization is influenced, for example, by distance of the electrode from the heart, which varies considerably among individuals. The area subtending a given precordial electrode varies with the anteroposterior (AP) diameter of the chest and is greater in individuals with an increased diameter. Consequently, the same size anterior infarct would be recorded in more leads than in an individual with a normal AP diameter.

The diagnosis of transmural and nontransmural infarction when based on presence or absence of a Q wave shows a poor correlation with autopsy findings.[133] Experimental[134] and autopsy findings indicate that while nontransmural lesions may be accompanied by a Q wave, the Q wave may be absent in transmural infarction. It has been suggested that as many as 50 per cent of nontransmural myocardial infarctions manifest Q waves, making differentiation of nontransmural and transmural infarction based on the Q wave highly tenuous.[118, 133] It appears, therefore, that the terms Q and non-Q wave infarction (Fig. 7–41) may be preferable to transmural and nontransmural,[133] unless necropsy findings are available.

On the basis of the presence of the Q wave, an infarct is considered septal when a Q wave is present in leads V_1 and V_2;[135] anterior when it is present in leads V_3 and V_4 (Fig. 7–22); anteroseptal if present in V_1 to V_4 (Fig. 7–34); lateral when present in leads I, aV_l, and V_6; anterolateral when present in leads I, aV_l, and V_3 to V_6; extensive anterior when present in leads I, aV_l, and V_1 to V_6; high lateral when present in leads I and aV_l; inferior when present in leads II, III, and aV_f (Figs. 7–5, 7–20, 7–21, 7–34, 7–38); and anteroinferior, or apical, when present in leads II, III, aV_l, and in one or more of the V_1 to V_4 leads (Fig. 7–43). A posterior infarct is recognized by a prominent R wave in lead V_1 or V_2 (Fig. 7–40).

A right ventricular infarction is likely when an elevated right ventricular ST segment, especially in lead V_4R, complicates a Q wave inferior left ventricular septal infarction.[136] The sensitivity and specificity of ST-segment elevation in lead V_4R alone has been estimated between 82 to 100 and 68 to 77 per cent, respectively.[137, 138] ST-segment elevation equal to or greater than 1 mm in one or more leads V_4R to V_6R has been shown to have a sensitivity and specificity for infarction of the right ventricle of 90 and 91 per cent, respectively. It has been suggested that ST-segment elevation which is greater in lead V_4R

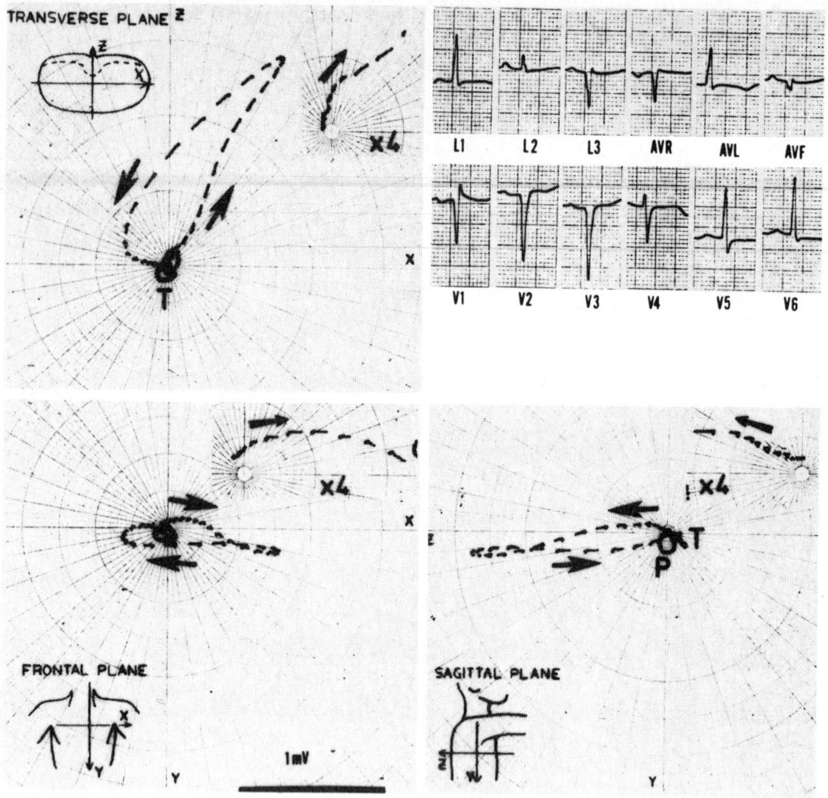

FIGURE 7–43. The ECG illustrates an anteroseptal and inferior myocardial infarction. On VCG, the transverse plane displays an initial QRS force directed to the left and posteriorly, with the entire QRS loop displaced posteriorly. The small oval T loop is situated anteriorly and to the right. In the frontal plane, the initial QRS force is directed to the right and superiorly and is inscribed clockwise. The duration of the superiorly displaced initial force is 22.5 msec and the amplitude of the superiorly displaced and leftward directed force along the 0 to 180° axis is 0.3 mV. In the sagittal plane, the initial QRS force is directed posteriorly and superiorly, with posterior displacement of the QRS loop. The small T-wave loop is located anteriorly. The initial QRS force is displayed four times the standard (× 4).

than in V_1, V_2, and V_3 reaches a specificity of 100 per cent but has a sensitivity somewhat lower (78 per cent) than when elevation of ST segment in V_4R is considered alone.[139]

Infarction isolated to the posterior left ventricular wall is rarely detected. This area of the left ventricle, the last to be depolarized, is inscribed during the terminal 0.04 to 0.06 sec of the QRS complex. Theoretically, therefore, it cannot be expressed as an initial positive wave in leads V_1 and V_2. In keeping with the dipole concept, however, the S wave may become smaller, a sign that lacks any degree of specificity. In a small number of patients, posterior myocardial infarction may be suspected when there is ST-segment depression in lead V_1 or V_2 or both, an R wave in lead V_1 of 0.04 sec, and an R/S ratio greater than 1.[140] The exact mechanism of the change in the initial QRS forces in leads V_1 and V_2 is not clear. Some have suggested that posterior myocardial infarction is not manifested in the ECG but that the findings in lead V_1 or V_2 or both reflect an associated lateral infarction. In patients with an inferior or lateral myocardial infarction, an R wave of increased amplitude 0.04 sec in duration in leads V_1 and V_2, and an upright R wave in lead V_1, suggest concomitant posterior wall involvement (Fig. 7–41).[141]

The terms subendocardial, nontransmural and non-Q wave infarction are frequently used interchangeably. If ST-segment depression and T-wave inversion are anterior, anterior subendocardial infarction is said to be present. If the T waves are inverted in the inferior leads, inferior subendocardial infarction is assumed to be present. However, in a small subset of isolated, pure nontransmural subendocardial infarction, the ECG findings include significant (0.2 mV) ST-segment depression in one or more leads, an upright T wave reflecting normal sequence of repolarization, and a decrease in R wave amplitude. The infarct usually involves the anterior wall and changes are recorded in leads I, II, aV_l and V_1 to V_6. Less frequently such a subendocardial infarction involves the inferior wall. Anatomical studies disclose large circumferential or nearly circumferential subendocardial infarcts.[133, 134] The mortality in this subset of nontransmural infarction is significantly greater than in those with T inversion alone (Fig. 7–41).[142]

In an effort to estimate the size of infarction a QRS scoring system based on duration of the Q and R waves and loss of R wave amplitude expressed in amplitude ratio of R/Q or R/S has been proposed.[143, 143a, 143b]

THE VCG IN MYOCARDIAL INFARCTION

The appearance of the loop in myocardial infarction depends on the site and size of the infarction. Deviation from normal reflects loss of forces normally generated by the infarcted area and resultant dominance of the noninfarcted myocardium. Anterior myocardial infarction is best visualized in the transverse plane, while an inferior infarction is best displayed in the frontal or sagittal plane (Figs. 7–44 and 7–45).

Anteroseptal myocardial infarction is recognized in the transverse plane by loss of the first 10- to 20-msec forces, with the initial position of the loop oriented posteriorly and to the left. The entire loop is displaced posteriorly with loss of the anterior convexity. In the vast majority of cases, the loop is inscribed in a counterclockwise direction. The initial posterior and leftward orientation of the loop is

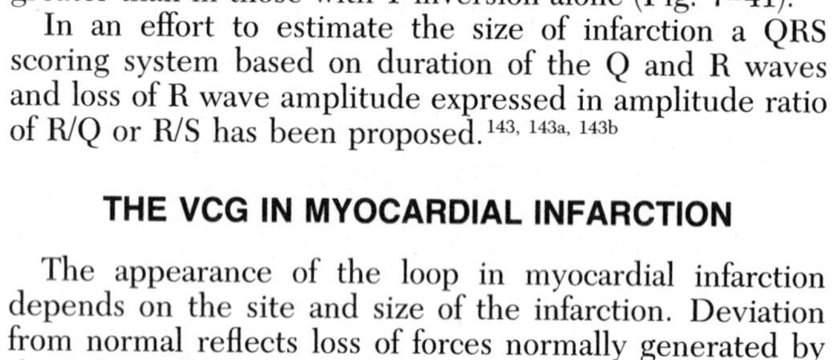

FIGURE 7–44. Vectorcardiogram (diagram) of anterior myocardial infarction. *A*, Anteroseptal; *B*, localized anterior; *C*, anterolateral; *D*, extensive anterior. (Modified from Chou, T. C., et al.: Clinical Vectorcardiography, 2nd ed. New York, Grune and Stratton, 1974, pp. 191, 196, 199.)

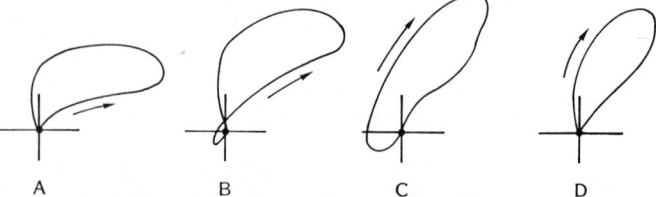

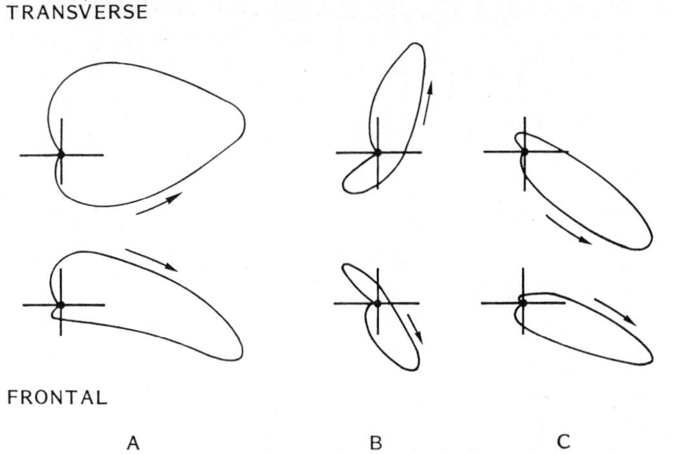

FIGURE 7–45. Vectorcardiogram of inferior and posterior myocardial infarction. *A*, Inferior; *B*, inferolateral; *C*, true posterior. (Modified from Chou, T. C., et al.: Clinical Vectorcardiography, 2nd ed. New York, Grune and Stratton, 1974, pp. 208, 220, 226.)

reflected in the ECG as a QS complex in leads V_1 to V_4 (Figs. 7–43 and 7–44).

In a *localized anterior infarction*, the transverse loop is similar in appearance to that present in anteroseptal myocardial infarction except for a normally inscribed initial force in a left and anterior direction. This initial inscription is displayed in the ECG as an R wave in lead V_1 and at times in V_2 (Figs. 7–22 and 7–44).

An *anterolateral infarction* is inscribed clockwise or as a figure-of-eight in the transverse plane. The initial normal part of the loop is followed by posterior and somewhat rightward displacement, reflecting the more extensive loss of left ventricular wall. Loss of the lateral wall may result in an increase in magnitude of the initial left-to-right portion of the loop, reflected in the ECG as a tall R wave inscribed in the right precordial leads (Fig. 7–44).

In an *extensive anterior infarction*, the transverse loop reflects loss of both the septal and free left ventricular walls. The initial normal anteriorly inscribed portion of the loop is lost, and the loop is shifted posteriorly and inscribed clockwise. The ECG shows a loss of R wave, at times, in all precordial leads.

TABLE 7–5 SUMMARY OF VECTORCARDIOGRAPHIC CRITERIA FOR DIAGNOSIS OF MYOCARDIAL INFARCTION (MI)

Anteroseptal MI (1 and 2)*
1. Initial anterior QRS forces absent
2. 0.02-sec QRS vector directed posteriorly

Localized Anterior MI (1, 2, and 3)
1. Initial anterior septal forces present
2. 0.02-sec QRS vector directed posteriorly
3. Voltage criteria for left ventricular hypertrophy absent

Anterolateral MI (1, 2, and 3)
1. Initial anterior septal forces normal
2. Initial rightward QRS forces > 0.022 sec
3. Efferent limb of transverse plane QRS loop inscribed clockwise
4. Initial rightward QRS forces > 0.16 mV
5. Maximum frontal plane QRS vector > 40°, QRS loop inscribed counterclockwise

Extensive Anterior MI (1 and 2)
1. Initial anterior QRS forces absent
2. Transverse plane QRS loop inscribed clockwise

Inferior MI (1 or more)
1. Initial superior QRS forces > 0.025 sec
2. Initial superior QRS forces ≥ 0.020 sec, maximum left superior force ≥ 0.25 mV
3. Maximum frontal plane QRS vector < 10°, efferent limb of frontal QRS loop inscribed clockwise
4. Bites in afferent limb of frontal QRS loop

Inferolateral MI (1 and 2)
1. Initial rightward QRS forces > 0.022 sec
2. Initial superior QRS forces > 0.025 sec

*Numbers in parentheses after each type of infarction indicate the minimum requirements for the diagnosis.

From Chou, T.-C., et al: Clinical Vectorcardiography. 2nd ed. New York, Grune and Stratton, 1974, p. 229.

Inferior myocardial infarction is best displayed in the frontal and sagittal planes (Figs. 7–40 and 7–45).[144] In the frontal plane, the loop is most often inscribed in a clockwise direction. The initial portion of the loop is directed superiorly, the superior displacement exceeding 25 to 30 msec. The loop crosses the X axis at 0.30 msec to the left of the point of origin.[144] It has been suggested that when the above diagnostic findings are absent, a shift to the left of the QRS loop combined with clockwise rotation is strongly indicative of an inferior infarction. Occasionally, when the inferior septum is spared, the initial loop may have a normal orientation, that is, to the right and inferiorly. This is followed by clockwise inscription and superior displacement of the remainder of the loop. In such instances the ECG will record a small initial R wave in leads II, III, and aV_f.

In a *posterior myocardial infarction*, the initial forces are normal in the transverse plane, but more than half the loop is ultimately displaced anteriorly. In the majority of cases, inscription of the loop is counterclockwise. The anterior displacement of the loop is reflected in the ECG by a prominent R wave in lead V_1 or V_2 that may exceed 0.04 sec in duration (Figs. 7–40 and 7–45).

A summary of VCG criteria for myocardial infarction is presented in Table 7–5 and Figures 7–44 and 7–45.

NONINFARCTION Q WAVES

While the vast majority of abnormal Q waves are due to myocardial infarction, a significant number is due to other causes.

Noninfarction Q waves may be transient or permanent. Transient Q waves have been produced experimentally in animals and observed in patients during anginal attacks.[145, 146] Such Q waves have been explained by a transient loss of electrophysiological function, but without irreversible cellular damage, a phenomenon referred to by some as "myocardial concussion"[147] or "stunned" myocardium.[148, 149] Q waves have been recorded with severe metabolic disturbances accompanying shock or pancreatitis. Similarly, transient Q waves have been noted during cardiac surgery and ascribed variously to transient ischemia and hypoxia, spasm, localized metabolic and electrolyte disturbances, and possible hypothermia (Fig. 7–27). Rarely a transient Q wave may result from tachycardia. The author has recorded transient Q waves and ST-segment and T-wave changes due to air embolism of the coronary artery complicating induction of a therapeutic pneumothorax.

The largest group of noninfarction Q waves is due to myocardial disease, including myocarditis, cardiac amyloidosis, neuromuscular disorders such as progressive muscular dystrophy, myotonia atrophica, Friedreich's ataxia, scleroderma, postpartum myopathy, myocardial replacement by tumor, sarcoidosis, idiopathic cardiomyopathy, and anomalous coronary artery.

Noninfarction Q waves are common in hypertrophic cardiomyopathy[150] and may simulate anterior or inferior myocardial infarction (Fig. 7–46). The exact mechanism of the Q wave in this condition is unclear. Increased septal mass or abnormal depolarization because of anomalous architecture of the septal myocardium, or both, has been proposed as the cause. The electrophysiological characteristics of septal muscle may differ from normal. For example, the refractory period of the myocardium responsible for the Q wave exceeds the refractory period of the

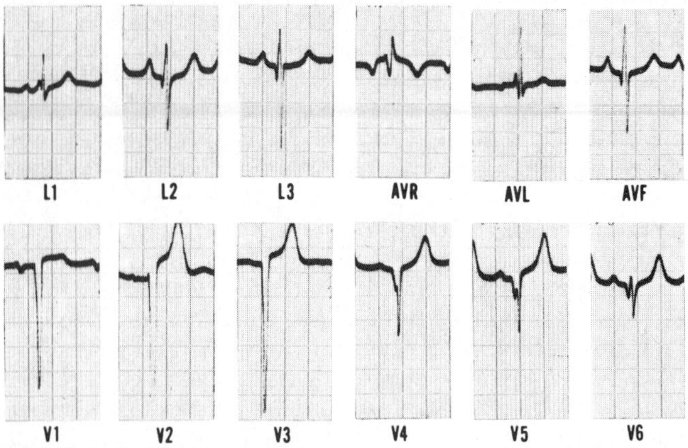

FIGURE 7–46. Noninfarction Q waves due to hypertrophic cardiomyopathy. This tracing recorded in a 16-year-old girl shows left axis deviation and Q waves in leads V_3 to V_6.

junctional tissue. This relationship may be altered by tachycardia with disappearance of the Q wave.[151]

A Q wave can be due to chronic obstructive lung disease (COLD) with or without cor pulmonale, pulmonary embolism, and pneumothorax. In COLD, findings in the precordial leads frequently simulate anterior myocardial infarction. The mechanism responsible for the QS complex is clockwise rotation and downward displacement of the diaphragm and of the heart. As a result, the electrodes are located superior to the initial vector; when this vector is directed inferiorly, a QS pattern results. By placing the electrode one interspace lower, it is often possible to record an R wave and thus provide strong evidence against myocardial infarction.[152] Occasionally in COLD the Q wave may simulate an inferior myocardial infarction. The positional origin of the anterior or inferior Q waves may be suspected when the Q wave is accompanied by other ECG findings of COLD. However, since both COLD and myocardial infarction frequently coexist, differential diagnosis may at times be difficult or impossible (Fig. 7–18).

Abnormal Q waves, especially in lead III and rarely in lead aV_f, with an S wave in lead I, can be recorded in acute cor pulmonale due to *pulmonary embolism* (see Fig. 7–17, p. 193). Clockwise rotation with superior orientation of the initial vector is most likely responsible for the Q wave in lead III. A Q wave in lead II is rarely recorded. Occasionally acute pulmonary embolus may simulate anterior myocardial infarction.

Spontaneous pneumothorax, particularly on the left, may result in a pattern simulating anterior myocardial infarction with occasional absence of the R wave in all the precordial leads.[153]

In LBBB the initial forces are directed from right to left and either superiorly or inferiorly. When the inferiorly directed forces dominate, a QS complex may be recorded in the precordial leads, simulating an anterior myocardial infarction. If the initial vector is oriented to the left and superiorly, a QS complex may be registered in the inferior leads, suggesting inferior myocardial infarction.

With left anterior divisional block, the transitional zone is shifted to the left, and an initial Q wave may appear in the right precordial leads. Loss of the forces normally contributed by the left anterior division results in a vector directed inferiorly, posteriorly, and to the right. Consequently, right precordial leads may register a qrS complex suggestive of an anteroseptal infarction. By placing the electrodes one interspace lower, an rS complex can be recorded attesting to the positional nature of the Q wave.[70]

Noninfarction Q waves are frequent in WPW (p. 604). WPW type B, with the initial forces directed from right to left, registers a QS complex in the right precordial leads and may be mistaken for anteroseptal or anterior myocardial infarction. Rarely, preexcitation of the left lateral wall, with the vector oriented anteriorly and to the right, simulates lateral infarction. Most often, however, WPW simulates inferior infarction (Fig. 7–33). The Q waves recorded in leads II, III, and aV_f are due to superior orientation of the initial vector and may be seen with either type A or type B WPW.

In LVH, failure to record an R wave in leads V_1 to V_4 may suggest an anteroseptal myocardial infarction (Fig. 7–15). Similarly, reciprocal elevation of the ST segments in these leads may contribute to an erroneous diagnosis of myocardial infarction. The exact mechanism of the initial negative deflection of the QRS is not clear, but it may be related to posterior rotation or inferior orientation of the initial vector.

ST-SEGMENT AND T-WAVE CHANGES

ST-SEGMENT ELEVATION. In addition to the three most common organic causes of ST segment elevations—acute myocardial infarction, pericarditis, and Prinzmetal's angina—ST-segment elevation is occasionally observed in acute cor pulmonale, hyperkalemia, cerebrovascular accidents, LVH, LBBB, hypertrophic cardiomyopathy, invasion of the heart by neoplastic tissue, and hypothermia. Elevation of the ST segment may also be an artifact caused by excessive inertia of the stylus of the electrocardiograph. In the normal heart the most common cause of ST-segment elevation is so-called *early repolarization*, a normal variant (Fig. 7–9*E*, p. 187).

T-WAVE ABNORMALITIES. A *primary T-wave change* indicates a regional alteration in the duration of the depolarized state. Some common clinical conditions associated with primary T-wave changes include myocardial ischemia, electrolyte abnormalities, effects of drugs, and a variety of primary myocardial and extracardiac disorders such as myocarditis and subarachnoid hemorrhage, respectively.

Giant negative or, at times, upright T waves, usually associated with a prolonged Q-T interval have been described with subarachnoid hemorrhage, complete heart block with marked bradycardia (Fig. 7–23), in myocardial ischemia (Fig. 7–41), and following cardiac resuscitation.

Secondary T-wave changes result from alterations of the timing or sequencing of depolarization, or both, with an obligatory change of the order of repolarization. For example, in LBBB, left ventricular epicardial activation is delayed because of slow conduction through the ventricular myocardium. As a result, repolarization begins in the subendocardium and an inverted T wave is recorded in precordial leads (Fig. 7–24). The change in the area of the QRS complex and T waves is identical but opposite in direction. Occasionally LBBB is associated with an upright T wave in the left ventricular leads, suggesting that in addition to altered activation due to LBBB, regional abnormalities of repolarization contribute to the T-wave morphology.

Rate-Related T-Wave Changes. Postextrasystolic T-wave change was first described in 1915.[154] Since then, a number of mechanisms have been proposed to explain this observation, including an abnormal pathway of repolarization, prolonged diastolic filling time,[155] and an abrupt change in the cycle length.

Minor T-wave changes following an abrupt cycle change

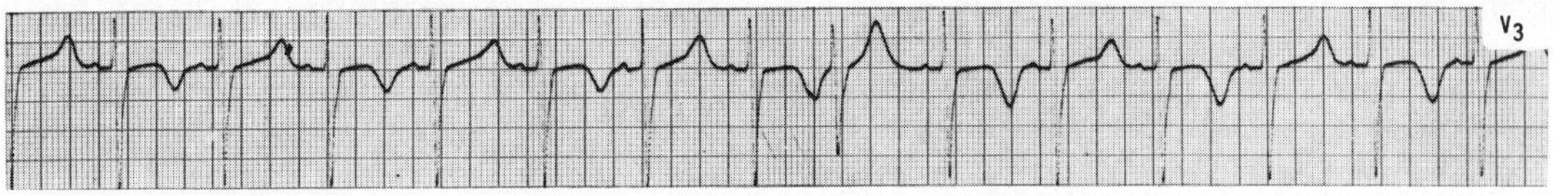

FIGURE 7–47. Isolated alternation of the T wave. The rhythm is sinus with occasional supraventricular premature complexes, probably atrial in origin. The QRS is normal in duration, with alternation of polarity of the T wave.

or after an interpolated ventricular premature complex may be recorded in normal tissue, while more pronounced T-wave alterations suggest an underlying myocardial disorder.

T-wave inversion is occasionally noted following supraventricular or ventricular tachycardia. The magnitude of the T-wave inversion varies, and when extreme, it may resemble the T-wave changes seen with cerebrovascular accidents or myocardial ischemia. The exact mechanism of the posttachycardia T wave is obscure.

T Wave Alternans. Isolated T wave alternans, i.e., without a change in either the QRS complex or the P wave, was first noted in the cat papillary muscle.[156] It is relatively rare and its mechanism not clear.[157] Alternans of phases 2 and 3 of the action potential of the T wave has been recorded without any demonstrable change in phase 0, supporting the concept that isolated alternation of repolarization reflected in the T wave is possible. T wave alternans of the type mentioned above is most often present during tachycardia or during a sudden change in cycle length. Isolated T wave alternans, independent of tachycardia or premature systole, is nearly always associated with advanced heart disease or severe electrolyte disturbance (Fig. 7–47)[158] or may follow cardiac resuscitation.

Notched, Bifid T Waves. Notched, bifid T waves are relatively common in the absence of heart disease, especially in the young.[159] They may also be present in congenital organic heart disease, the prolonged Q-T syndrome (Fig. 7–48), central nervous system disorders, alcoholic cardiomyopathy, and following the administration of drugs, especially the phenothiazines.[160] The mechanism of the bifid or notched T wave is unclear. It has been suggested that in some instances it is due to nonuniform repolarization secondary to differential innervation of the anterior and posterior ventricular walls.[161] It has also been proposed that in patients with left ventricular disease it may reflect regional delay of repolarization of the left ventricle.[159]

NONSPECIFIC ST-SEGMENT AND T-WAVE CHANGES. Although the ST segment and T wave represent different electrophysiological events and their respective changes may have different clinical connotations, the widespread practice among electrocardiographers is to refer to either one or both as *ST-T changes.* While it is more appropriate to discuss the two separately, it should be recognized that abnormalities of the ST segment and T wave frequently coexist.

Nondiagnostic ST-segment and T-wave changes are the most common ECG abnormality and account for about 50 per cent of the abnormal tracings recorded in a general medical hospital.[162] It has been estimated that nondiagnostic T-wave changes are present in 2.4 per cent[162] and 4.5 per cent[163] of all routine cardiograms. An abnormal T wave is extremely common because the wave is highly sensitive to a variety of abnormalities and interventions, and of all the ECG changes it is therefore least likely to suggest a specific diagnosis. This fact has been recognized since 1923, when Wilson first recorded inversion of the T wave following the ingestion of cold water.[164]

Although an abnormal T wave suggests the presence of an abnormal or, more appropriately, an altered state, it is recorded with relative frequency in the absence of any disorder (Fig. 7–9, p. 187) as a reflection of physiological influences, e.g., in highly trained athletes.[165, 166] For these reasons, an isolated T-wave change must be interpreted

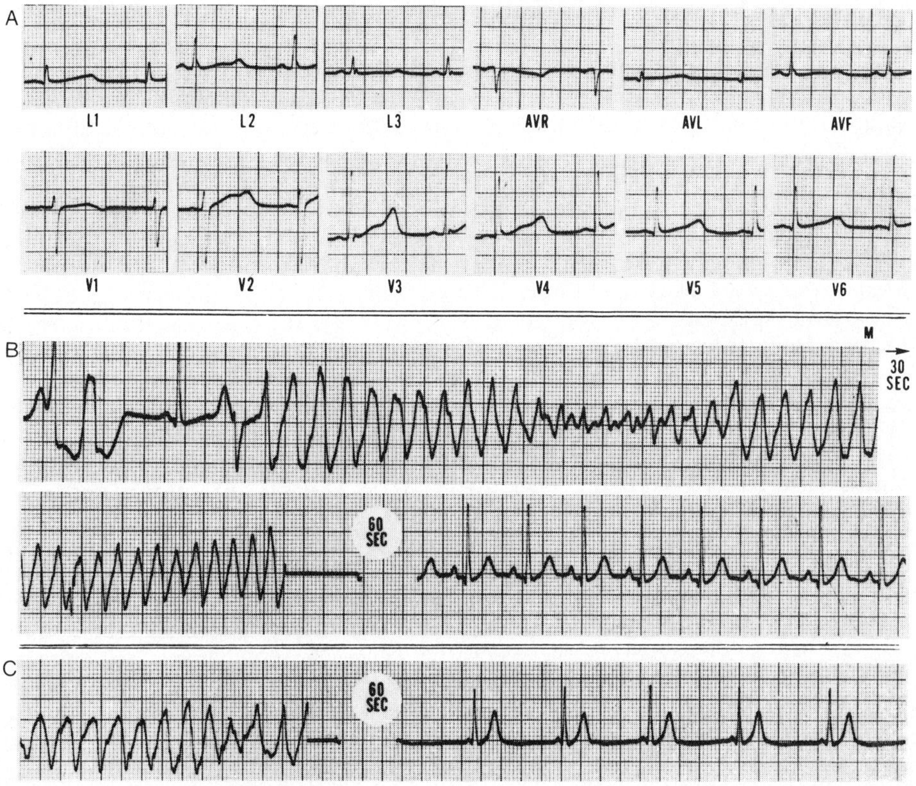

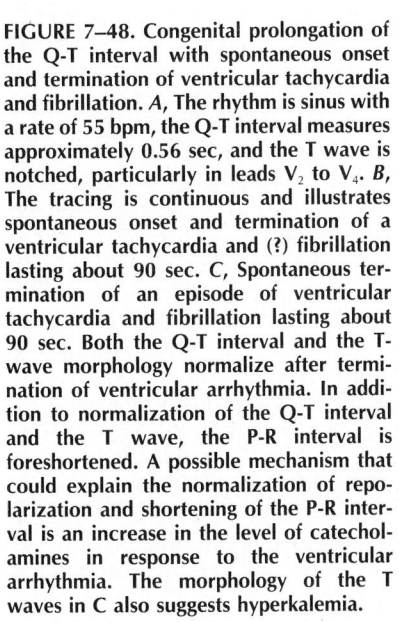

FIGURE 7–48. Congenital prolongation of the Q-T interval with spontaneous onset and termination of ventricular tachycardia and fibrillation. *A,* The rhythm is sinus with a rate of 55 bpm, the Q-T interval measures approximately 0.56 sec, and the T wave is notched, particularly in leads V_2 to V_4. *B,* The tracing is continuous and illustrates spontaneous onset and termination of a ventricular tachycardia and (?) fibrillation lasting about 90 sec. *C,* Spontaneous termination of an episode of ventricular tachycardia and fibrillation lasting about 90 sec. Both the Q-T interval and the T-wave morphology normalize after termination of ventricular arrhythmia. In addition to normalization of the Q-T interval and the T wave, the P-R interval is foreshortened. A possible mechanism that could explain the normalization of repolarization and shortening of the P-R interval is an increase in the level of catecholamines in response to the ventricular arrhythmia. The morphology of the T waves in C also suggests hyperkalemia.

with caution and must *always* be correlated with all available clinical and laboratory information. Misinterpretation of the significance of a T-wave abnormality is the most common cause of "iatrogenic ECG heart disease." Attempts to identify the etiology of an abnormal ST segment, T wave, or ST-T segment in isolation from clinical and other laboratory findings often fail.

The specificity of the purported "classic" ST-T changes, such as those seen with LVH, digitalis administration, and ischemic heart disease, is relatively low. For example, a negative wave reflecting persistence of a juvenile pattern cannot be differentiated from the symmetrically inverted T wave due to myocardial ischemia. The "classic" ST-T change of LVH may be due to ischemic heart disease or digitalis, while the marked ST-segment depression due to ischemia or subendocardial infarction may be simulated by the administration of digitalis in the presence of moderate or severe disease. When correlated with clinical and other laboratory data, ST-T changes assume a greater predictive value. In a series of 410 abnormal tracings analyzed without regard to clinical data, 70 per cent could be interpreted only as "nonspecific ST-T change." This number was reduced to 10 per cent when such changes were correlated with available clinical information.[162]

The nonspecific and labile nature of the ST segment and the T wave, especially the latter, is expected. Repolarization is a much more diverse process than depolarization. Depolarization is rapid, with a reasonably uniform potential difference across the boundary of activation and is reflected in the rate of rise of phase 0 and the amplitude of the action potential (p. 181). Repolarization, displayed as the ST segment and T wave, reflects phases 2 and 3 of the action potential, is considerably longer and is nonuniform, with many simultaneous boundaries and with differing potentials across various boundaries. It has been shown that shortening of the monophasic action potential by as little as 12 to 18 msec will alter the morphology of the T wave, and importantly, the change can be seen with involvement of 10 per cent or less of the myocardial mass. The magnitude of the T-wave changes, unlike that of the QRS complex, is not related to the mass of the myocardium. This condition has been ascribed to cancellation of repolarization voltages and to uneven contributions from the different regions of repolarization to the genesis of the T wave.[167] Such experimental findings explain, at least partially, the nonspecific character of ST-segment and T-wave changes.

A number of the clinical conditions which may alter the ST segment and T waves are listed in Table 7–6.

TABLE 7–6 CAUSES OF ST SEGMENT AND T WAVE CHANGES (SELECTED)

PHYSIOLOGICAL:
Position, temperature, hyperventilation, anxiety, food (glucose), tachycardia, neurogenic influences, physical training

PHARMACOLOGICAL:
Digitalis, antiarrhythmic and psychotrophic drugs (phenothiazines, tricyclics, lithium)

EXTRACARDIAC DISORDERS:
Electrolyte abnormalities, cerebrovascular accidents, shock, anemia, allergic reactions, infections, endocrine disorders, acute abdominal disorders, pulmonary embolism

PRIMARY MYOCARDIAL DISEASE:
Congestive, hypertrophic, postpartum cardiomyopathy, myocarditis

SECONDARY MYOCARDIAL DISEASE:
Amyloidosis, hemochromatosis, neoplasm, sarcoidosis, connective tissue, neuromuscular disorders

ISCHEMIC HEART DISEASE:
Myocardial infarction.

U-WAVE ABNORMALITIES. An abnormal U wave may be increased in amplitude, inverted or prolonged. A negative U wave is documented in about 1 per cent of cardiograms recorded in a general hospital. An exaggerated upright U wave may be due to hypokalemia, a variety of drugs (particularly digitalis), and some of the antiarrhythmic agents (e.g., amiodarone).

The most common causes of a *negative U wave* are hypertension, aortic and mitral valve disease, RVH, and myocardial ischemia (Fig. 7–41). The last was discussed in conjunction with myocardial infarction (p. 207). A negative U wave can occasionally be found in other metabolic or organic diseases. In hypertension, a negative U wave may be the earliest sign of myocardial involvement, appearing long before any change in the T wave, and has been reported in about 16 per cent of ECG's with an upright T wave and 45 per cent with negative T waves. It may revert to normal with control of the hypertension.[28] The majority of patients with aortic regurgitation and about 10 per cent of patients with aortic stenosis manifest a negative U wave. Approximately 5 and 80 per cent of patients with systolic and diastolic overload of the right ventricle, respectively, manifest a negative U wave in leads II, III, V_1, and V_2.[28] In essence, a negative U wave, even as an isolated finding in an otherwise normal ECG, is strongly indicative of a pathophysiological state.

Q-T INTERVAL ABNORMALITY (See also p. 187). *Shortening of the Q-T interval* may be recorded with hyperkalemia, digitalis, hypercalcemia, and acidosis. *Prolongation of the Q-T interval* may be primary and independent of the QRS, or it may reflect secondary changes of repolarization due to abnormal depolarization, or a combination of the two. Prolongation of the Q-T interval, independent of QRS duration, can be congenital (Fig. 7–48) or acquired.[168–170] Acquired disorders include ischemic heart disease, hypothermia, cardiomyopathy, mitral valve prolapse, complete heart block, a condition following cardiac resuscitation, electrolyte changes, and administration of drugs.[171] Q-T interval prolongation is a relatively frequent complication of acquired cerebral lesions, especially subarachnoid hemorrhage, and can also be present during and following neurosurgical procedures.

ELECTRICAL ALTERNANS. Alternation of amplitude and direction of the QRS complex was noted in the experimental animal and man as early as 1909 and 1910, respectively,[172, 173] followed by documentation of alternation of the P wave, ST segment, and T wave (Fig. 7–47). Isolated *alternation of the P wave* is seen frequently in the experimental setting but is rare in man. Most often it accompanies alternation of the QRS complex and occasionally the QRS complex and the T wave. The latter is referred to as *total alternans* and suggests pericardial effusion, usually due to malignancy and frequently associated with tamponade or impending tamponade.

Although pericardial effusion is the most common cause of alternation of the QRS complex, *QRS alternans* is also seen with myocardial ischemia and myocardial disease due to other causes. Two mechanisms of QRS alternans have been proposed: positional oscillation and aberrancy of intraventricular conduction. The early suggestion that oscillation or alternation of position is the mechanism of alternans of the QRS complex[174] was proved by means of echocardiography.[175] The concept of oscillation also explains the fact that P wave alternans is seen predominantly with massive pericardial effusion.

ST segment alternans has been described in dogs after ligation of the coronary artery, in severely ill infants with congenital heart disease, and in patients with Prinzmetal's

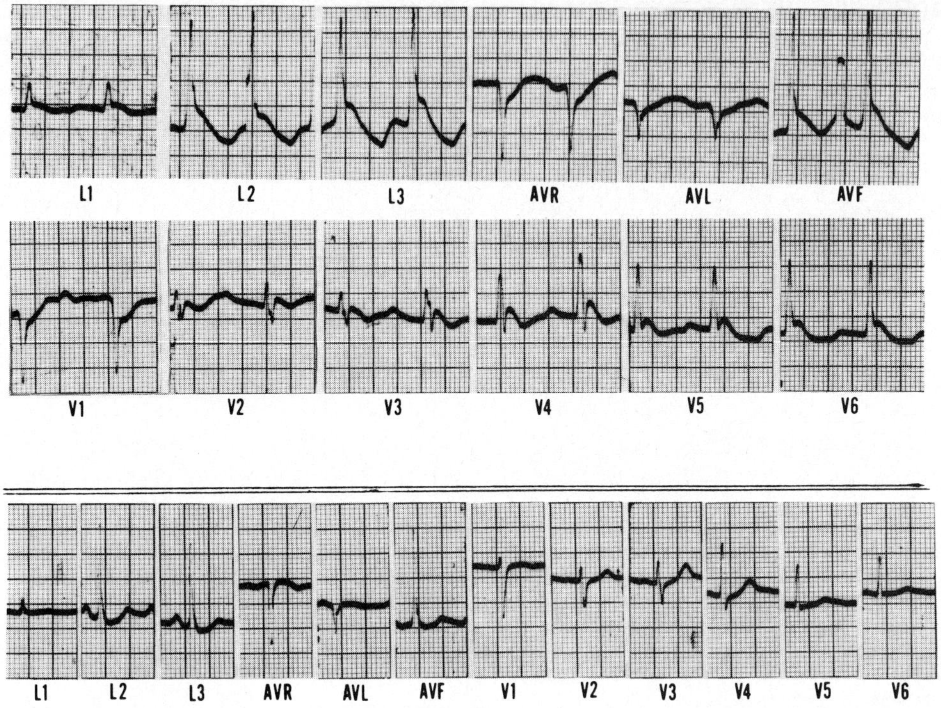

FIGURE 7–49. Osborne wave. Upper panel was recorded during hypothermia. The P-R interval is 0.28 sec; the QRS complex measures 0.10 sec and is followed by a wave (the Osborne wave) that merges with the ST segment: The T wave is inverted in leads I, II, III, aV_f, V_5, and V_6. It is difficult to separate the Osborne wave from the initial part of the ST segment. Bottom panel was recorded after the temperature returned to normal. The tracing is normal. The prolongation and increase in QRS amplitude noted during hypothermia, although within normal limits, are evident when compared with the normal ECG.

angina. *T wave alternans* is discussed on page 213. *U wave alternans* is least common; definitive diagnosis is most difficult.

The mechanism of alternans in severe myocardial disorders but in the absence of pericardial effusion is obscure. It has been ascribed to uneven duration of the excited state or to two alternating foci of impulse formation. However, the fact that alternation of depolarization, activation, and repolarization can be recorded in a single cell suggests that the mechanism is probably related to transmembrane ionic fluxes. Alternans of a human atrial monophasic action potential[176] adds further credence to the primary role of transmembrane ionic events.

THE OSBORNE WAVE. An Osborne wave, seen in hypothermia, is a deflection inscribed between the QRS complex and the beginning of the ST segment (Fig. 7–49).[177] It has been variously suggested that this wave reflects delay of depolarization, a current of injury, or early repolarization. In the left ventricular leads the polarity of the wave is positive and its amplitude is inversely related to body temperature. The electrophysiological mechanism of the Osborne wave remains unclear.

ABNORMAL ECG IN ABSENCE OF CLINICAL HEART DISEASE

Abnormal ECG may be recorded in patients with clinically normal hearts.[66, 178] The abnormalities may be those of the QRS, ST segment, or T wave. Abnormalities of the QRS include a QS complex in lead aV_l, or QS or QR complex in leads III and aV_f, a QS complex in leads V_1 and V_2, a tall R wave in leads V_1 and V_2,[179] and high voltage of the R wave over the left ventricle. A frequent "normal" alteration of the ST segment is an elevation, the so-called early repolarization, which may be recorded in the inferior, left precordial, and rarely right precordial leads. Abnormal T waves include persistence of juvenile T wave inversion over the right precordium (p. 186), isolated midprecordial T-wave inversion (Fig. 7–9), and terminal T wave inversion associated with ST-segment elevation due to early repolarization and right precordial T-wave inversion in middle-aged women (Fig. 7–9). A variety of physiological influences alter the T wave of a normal heart (Table 7–6).

An abnormal ECG in the absence of clinical signs of heart disease in the young should be evaluated carefully, because the prevalence of true heart disease in this setting is low and the chances are high that the tracing is false positive for disease.[180]

THE ECG AND ELECTROLYTE ABNORMALITIES

POTASSIUM

HYPERKALEMIA. In experimental hyperkalemia there is a good correlation between plasma K and the surface ECG. The earliest ECG change, at a plasma level of about 5.7 mEq/liter, is a tall, peaked, most often symmetrical T wave with a narrow base and a normal or decreased Q-Tc interval. The QRS complex widens uniformly at a level of 9 to 11 mEq/liter and an occasional acute current of injury resembling myocardial infarction may be present. Reduction in P-wave amplitude, intraatrial conduction delay, and P-R interval prolongation are recorded at a plasma level of about 7.0 mEq/liter. At plasma K levels of about 8.4 mEq/liter or higher, the P wave is no longer recognizable. When the plasma concentration exceeds 12 mEq/liter, either ventricular fibrillation or arrest follows. SA node fibers, being more resistant to the depressive action of K than is atrial myocardium, continue to generate impulses that are now delayed in their exit or may fail to propagate because of depressed intraatrial conduction. The result may be Wenckebach (type I) or Mobitz (type II) sinoatrial (SA) block (p. 702). Junctional escape and junctional rhythm are relatively common in experimental hyperkalemia.

In clinical hyperkalemia, abnormalities of impulse formation and conduction appear at K levels lower than those observed in the experimental animal, and the correlation between plasma K and the ECG is less reliable. A tall, peaked, symmetrical T wave with a narrow base, the so-called "tented" T wave, is the earliest ECG abnormality, usually best seen in leads II, III, V_2, V_3, and V_4. The

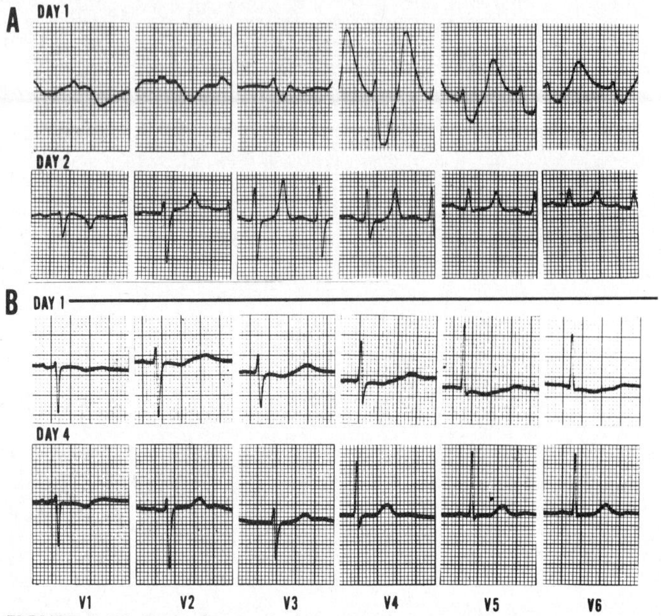

FIGURE 7–50. ECG changes in hyperkalemia (*A*) and hypokalemia (*B*). Panel *A*, On day 1, at a K^+ level of 8.6 mEq/liter the P wave is no longer recognizable and the QRS complex is diffusely prolonged. Initial and terminal QRS delay is characteristic of K^+ induced intraventricular conduction and is best illustrated in leads V_2 and V_6. On day 2, at a K^+ level of 5.8 mEq/liter, the P wave is recognizable with a P-R interval of 0.24 sec, the duration of the QRS complex is approximately 0.10 sec and the T waves are characteristically "tented." Panel *B*, On day 1, at a K^+ level of 1.5 mEq/liter the T and U waves are merged. The U wave is prominent and the Q-U interval prolonged. On day 4, at a K^+ level of 3.7 mEq/liter the tracing is normal.

pointed, symmetrical appearance and narrow base of the T wave help to differentiate the effect of hyperkalemia from other causes of tall T waves, often a normal variant. The tented appearance and the narrow base are probably more characteristic of hyperkalemia than is the amplitude of the T wave. A decrease in amplitude of the R wave, appearance of a prominent S wave, widening of the QRS complex, depression of the ST segment, and an occasional elevation of the ST segment evolve as plasma K continues to rise and approaches 8 to 9 mEq/liter (Fig. 7–50). A decrease in amplitude and prolongation of the P wave and lengthening of the P-R interval followed by disappearance of the P wave often makes recognition of arrhythmias in hyperkalemia difficult, if not impossible.

With hyperkalemia, depression of intraventricular conduction is characteristically diffuse and fairly uniform and results in prolongation of both the initial and terminal parts of the QRS complex. The resulting pattern may resemble RBBB, LBBB, left anterior or posterior divisional block, or a combination of the four. When the ECG resembles RBBB, the initial phase of the QRS complex is prolonged, in contrast to the conventional RBBB, in which only the terminal portion of the QRS complex is delayed. Similarly, when the ECG simulates LBBB, an S wave indicates slowing of the terminal portion of the QRS (Fig. 7–50). In conventional LBBB, on the other hand, prolongation involves only the initial component of the QRS complex.

In man, as in animals, SA block (p. 702), either Wenckebach (type I) or Mobitz (type II), passive or accelerated junctional or ventricular escape rhythms may be present. Potassium may normalize physiologically or functionally inverted T waves, but as a rule it has no effect on T-wave inversion due to organic disorders or drugs.

HYPOKALEMIA. The ECG in *hypokalemia* is characterized by gradual depression of the ST segment, decrease of T-wave amplitude, occasionally inversion of the T wave, and a prominent U wave but without a significant change in the Q-T interval (Fig. 7–50). In advanced hypokalemia the ST segment gradually fuses with the U wave, the latter greater in amplitude than the T wave. An increase in amplitude of the QRS complex may be present. There is reasonable correlation between ECG changes and K concentrations below 2.3 or 3.0 mEq/liter.[181] Prominent U waves with ST-segment and T-wave changes are not specific for hypokalemia, however. Such abnormalities can be the result of administration of digitalis and other drugs, ventricular hypertrophy, and bradycardia.

CALCIUM

The effects of calcium on the ECG were recognized in 1922.[182] In general, the ECG changes due to alteration in Ca levels correlate with the effect of Ca ion on the transmembrane action potential. Changes in duration of phase 2 parallel the altered duration of the ST segment and the Q-T interval.

Hypocalcemia prolongs phase 2, reflected by prolongation of the ST segment and Q-T interval (Fig. 7–51). The Q-aT (Q to the apex of the T wave) and Q-T intervals are prolonged, but the Q-Tc interval rarely exceeds 140 per cent of the normal. If longer, the U wave is likely to be included in the measurement. Hypocalcemia does not affect phase 3 of the action potential or the T wave.[181] Hypocalcemia with hyperkalemia, most often seen in patients with chronic renal disease, results in a prolonged ST segment and a "tented" T wave (Fig. 7–51). Hypocalcemia and hypokalemia exhibit a prolonged ST segment and a prominent terminal wave that includes both T and U waves.

Hypercalcemia shortens phase 2 of the action potential and the ST segment. The Q-T interval is shortened (Fig. 7–51), the ST segment occasionally depressed, and the T wave inverted.[183] A prominent J wave similar to that of hypothermia has been observed.[184]

The correlation between the Q-T interval and serum Ca concentration is unpredictable, largely because the Q-T

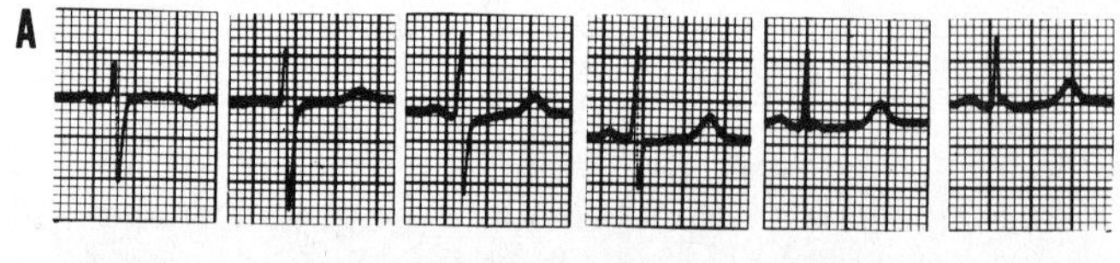

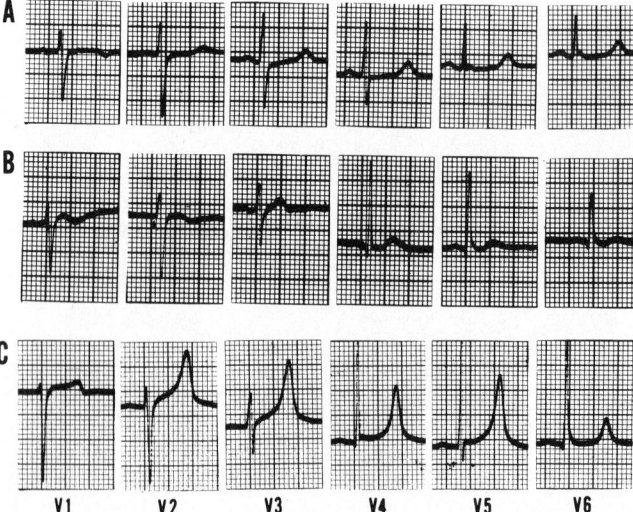

FIGURE 7–51. ECG changes of hypocalcemia, hypercalcemia, and hypocalcemia with hyperkalemia. *A*, At a Ca^{++} level of 5.7 mg/dl the QT interval is prolonged, characteristic of hypocalcemia. *B*, Tracing recorded at a Ca^{++} level of 16.0 mg/dl shows the short ST segment of hypercalcemia. *C*, Tracing recorded at a K^+ level of 6.0 mEq/liter, Ca^{++} of 5.5 mg/dl, and phosphorus of 12.0 mg/dl. The prolonged Q-T interval and the tented T wave reflect hypocalcemia and hyperkalemia often present in chronic renal disease.

duration is affected by factors other than calcium levels, such as age, sex, heart rate, myocardial disease, drugs, and other electrolytes. It has been suggested that when factors known to alter the Q-T interval are eliminated, a reasonably good correlation is found between the ECG and calcium levels. This assumption is supported by the fact that Ca levels in pure hypocalcemia induced by EDTA show a reasonably good correlation with the Q-T interval. Of the three intervals—Q-T, Q-oT (Q to the onset of the T wave), and Q-aT (Q to the apex of the T wave), the Q-aT interval can be measured with greatest accuracy and correlates best with the Ca level.[185]

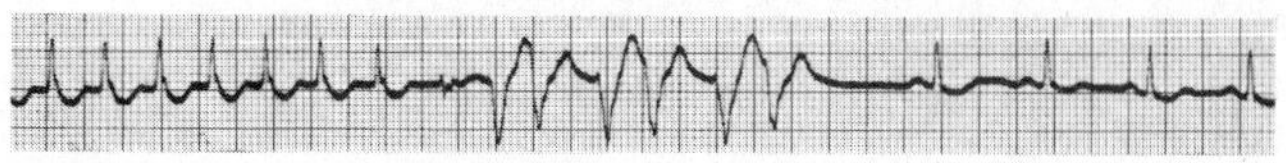

FIGURE 7–52. Supraventricular tachycardia treated with large doses of digitalis terminating with ventricular tachycardia with a 3:2 Wenckebach (type 1) exit block. Atrial tachycardia at a rate of 230 bpm is followed by a bigeminal rhythm, with ventricular complexes all of similar morphology. The longer cycles are less than twice the shorter cycle, suggesting a ventricular tachycardia with a 3:2 Wenckebach exit block. The interectopic ventricular cycle length is 0.22 sec. One possible mechanism of the ventricular tachycardia is delayed afterdepolarization, or "triggered" automaticity.

MAGNESIUM

Administration of magnesium may result in shortening of the Q-T interval. As a rule, however, abnormalities of the ST segment due to hypermagnesemia cannot be identified on the ECG because the changes are dominated by calcium. Hypomagnesemia cannot be recognized on the ECG.

EFFECTS OF DRUGS ON THE ECG

The effects of antiarrhythmic drugs on the ECG is considered in Chapter 22 and the effects of phenothiazines and other mood-altering agents in Chapter 61.

DIGITALIS

(See p. 489)

Alterations of the ST segment and T wave are the earliest recognizable changes due to the digitalis glycosides. The T-wave amplitude is lowered, and the ST segment is depressed and shortened, with occasional appearance of a prominent U wave.[186] While the "characteristic" digitalis-induced ST segment is described as sagging, it is often difficult if not impossible to differentiate it from ST-segment depression of other causes. When the ST segment is also shortened, digitalis is the likely cause of the depression. ST-segment displacement due to digitalis may be greatly exaggerated by myocardial disease, tachycardia, and high-amplitude QRS complexes. Rarely, digitalis causes symmetrical inversion of the T wave similar to that in pericarditis and ischemia, but there is usually associated shortening of the Q-T interval. A peaked, "tented" T wave, probably due to concomitant hyperkalemia, can also be present. Digitalis has no significant effect on depolarization of the atrium or ventricle. Consequently, prolongation of intraatrial and intraventricular conduction is rare.[187]

CLASSIFICATION OF DIGITALIS-INDUCED ARRHYTHMIAS. Digitalis has been known to induce nearly every known arrhythmia.[188–190]

1 Ectopic rhythms due to enhanced automaticity or reentry or both and, perhaps, to delayed diastolic afterdepolarizations (Fig. 7–52): atrial tachycardia with block (Fig. 22–13, p. 674), atrial fibrillation and flutter, nonparoxysmal junctional tachycardia (Fig. 22–17, p. 679), ventricular premature contractions, ventricular tachycardia (Fig. 7–52), ventricular flutter and fibrillation, multiple ectopic rhythms, bidirectional ventricular tachycardia (Fig. 7–53), or accelerated escape.

2. Depression of pacemaker: SA node arrest (p. 665).

3. Depression of conduction: SA block, AV block, exit block, or reciprocation.

4. AV dissociation: Suppression of the dominant pacemaker with passive escape of the lower junctional focus or inappropriate acceleration of a subsidiary pacemaker, or, rarely, dissociation within the AV junction (double junctional tachycardia).

Arrhythmias identical to those due to digitalis toxicity can be caused by heart disease, drugs other than digitalis, and a variety of extracardiac factors.

THERAPEUTIC AND TOXIC EFFECTS. Appearance of ectopic rhythms in the course of digitalis administration is nearly always a sign of toxicity. On the other hand, depression of AV conduction may at times be a desirable therapeutic endpoint. Acknowledging that some degree of overlap is unavoidable and that the clinical significance of an arrhythmia may differ depending on the setting, the effects of digitalis on the ECG can be divided into three general groups—therapeutic, excessive and/or toxic, and unequivocally toxic.

Clinically acceptable effects of digitalis include some prolongation of the P-R interval; slowing of the ventricular response in atrial flutter and fibrillation; and in atrial fibrillation, the appearance of isolated AV junctional escape impulses. Conversion of atrial arrhythmias to sinus

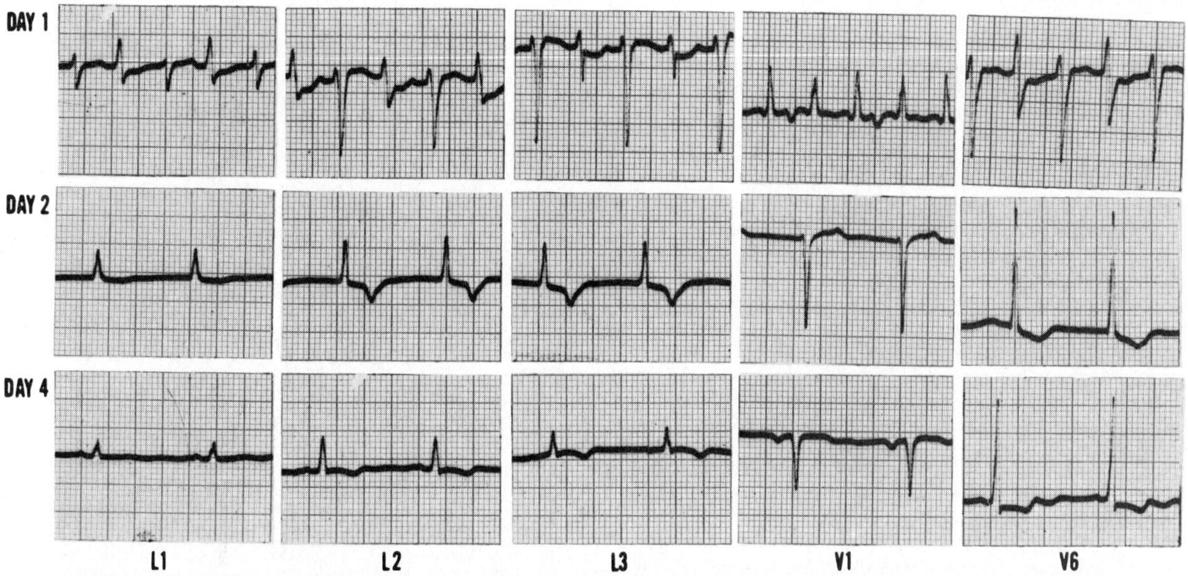

FIGURE 7–53. Bidirection ventricular tachycardia and junctional tachycardia due to digitalis. On day 1, the ECG shows bidirectional ventricular tachycardia with alternation of the axis and RBBB. The divisions of the left bundle are the site of the tachycardia. On day 2, after discontinuation of digitalis, the rhythm is junctional at a rate of 83 bpm, with retrograde P waves in leads II and III and an R-P interval of about 0.20 sec. On day 4, normal sinus rhythm is accompanied by nonspecific T-wave changes in leads II, III, and V_6.

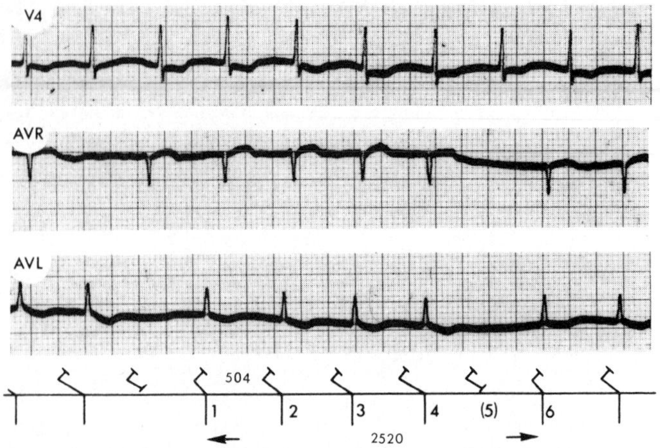

FIGURE 7–54. Atrial fibrillation and nonparoxysmal junctional tachycardia with Wenckebach (type 1) exit block due to digitalis intoxication. Lead V_4 illustrates a regular ventricular rhythm at a rate of 107 bpm, characteristic of this arrhythmia. In leads aV_r and aV_l the R-R cycle foreshortens gradually and the long pause is shorter than the length of two of the preceding R-R cycles. This is characteristic of a Wenckebach structure and identifies Wenckebach (type I) exit block from the junctional focus. Although at first glance leads aV_r and aV_l suggest atrial fibrillation, the repetitive Wenckebach structure indicates that there is, in addition, a regular junctional rhythm with a Wenckebach (type I) exit block.

The actual interectopic junctional interval and delay of conduction from the pacemaker to surrounding tissue can be calculated from the ECG with the aid of the Lewis diagram (bottom). The number of *manifest* QRS cycles of the Wenckebach sequence (QRS1 to QRS6) is four. To this number is added one additional pacemaker cycle to take into account the cycle that fails to manifest a QRS(5). The duration of the sequence from QRS1 to QRS6 is 2520 msec. The latter is divided by the five cycles, and the actual interectopic interval of the junctional pacemaker is calculated to be 504 msec. The increased distance between the junctional pacemaker and the manifest QRS is a measure of delay of conduction from the pacemaker to the myocardium. The same method is used to calculate the sinoatrial node (SAN) rate and conduction time to the atrium in the presence of Wenckebach type I exit block. The SAN and P wave are substituted for the junctional pacemaker and QRS, respectively.

rhythm, either directly or indirectly, is another desirable effect of the drug.

Excessive or toxic effects, or both, are heralded by the appearance of atrial tachycardia with block, nonparoxysmal junctional tachycardia (Fig. 7–54), AV dissociation, second- and third-degree AV block, SA block, AV junctional rhythm, and reciprocating rhythm. Ventricular arrhythmias due to digitalis are an unequivocal sign of toxicity. This group includes isolated ventricular premature complexes (VPC), ventricular bigeminy, multifocal or multiform VPC, ventricular tachycardia, and "bidirectional" ventricular tachycardia, flutter, and fibrillation.

The wide spectrum of arrhythmias induced by digitalis and the coexistence of a number of different arrhythmias in the same tracing can be explained by the effects of the interplay of digitalis and myocardial and extracardiac factors on the electrophysiological properties of cardiac tissues. The magnitude of the effect of the drug on specialized tissue, the SA node, specialized atrial tissue, AV junctional tissue, and the Purkinje fibers varies and, in fact, may have a different effect on the same tissue, i.e., it may depress conduction or enhance automaticity, or both. Furthermore, the electrocardiographic expression of electrophysiological effects of digitalis is a net result of altered automaticity, refractoriness, excitability, and conduction. Also, digitalis may act directly on the specialized tissue or its action may be mediated through the sympathetic or parasympathetic system or both.[191,192] In addition, the sensitivity of the tissues to digitalis may be altered by factors such as a changing acid-base balance, plasma and intracellular electrolyte levels, oxygen saturation, and mechanical stretch. Similarly, improvement of cardiac function with treatment may alter the variables affecting the electrophysiological properties of the cardiac tissue and consequently the tissue's response to digitalis.

Selected arrhythmias due to digitalis has been chosen for the following discussion here because of their frequency and relatively high specificity for digitalis toxicity.

ATRIAL TACHYCARDIA WITH BLOCK (see p. 674). The cause of this arrhythmia can be ascribed almost equally to severe heart disease and to digitalis toxicity. The diagnosis of atrial tachycardia with block may occasionally be difficult. At rapid rates it resembles atrial flutter. The amplitude of the atrial deflections may be low, and only careful attention to lead V_1 may disclose the true nature of the arrhythmia.

NONPAROXYSMAL JUNCTIONAL TACHYCARDIA (see also p. 678) (Fig. 7–54). In the proper setting, this arrhythmia is highly specific for digitalis excess or toxicity.[193] Other less common causes of nonparoxysmal junctional tachycardia—acute myocardial infarction, open heart surgery, myocarditis, and general anesthesia—must be ruled out. Nonparoxysmal junctional tachycardia differs from paroxysmal junctional or supraventricular tachycardia. It appears and disappears gradually and, when repetitive, the coupling, or relation of the first ectopic complex, to the dominant impulse varies. The rate is 70 to 130 bpm. AV dissociation resulting from acceleration of the AV junctional pacemaker is recorded in 85 per cent of patients. The ectopic junctional focus activates both atria and ventricles in the remaining 15 per cent. Rarely, two junctional foci coexist, one controlling the atria and the other the ventricles, resulting in a double junctional tachycardia.

In the absence of exit block, the rhythm in nonparoxysmal junctional tachycardia is generally perfectly regular and the diagnosis usually simple. Recognition becomes more difficult in the presence of exit block. A high degree of exit block may suggest a slow junctional rhythm or AV block. If the exit block is Mobitz (type II) (p. 703) with 3:2 exit block, a bigeminal rhythm appears, with longer cycles exact multiples of shorter cycles. If the exit block is Wenckebach (type I), the gradually shortening R-R interval and lack of the expected relationship of the long pause to the shorter cycles (i.e., the pause is not a multiple of the shorter cycle), atrial fibrillation may be suggested (Fig. 7–54). Only a careful search for the Wenckebach structure will reveal the true nature of the arrhythmia. Nonparoxysmal junctional tachycardia with an irregular ventricular response without conforming to the Wenckebach (type I) or Mobitz (type II) structure precludes the diagnosis, and nonparoxysmal junctional tachycardia cannot be differentiated from atrial fibrillation. Occasionally, this arrhythmia is masked and becomes evident with slowing of the dominant rhythm; it may appear as nonparoxysmal junctional tachycardia or as a single accelerated escape impulse.[194]

VENTRICULAR ARRHYTHMIAS. Ventricular premature contractions (VPC) are the most common manifestation of digitalis toxicity but, at the same time, are the least specific as a sign of glycoside toxicity. None of the morphological features of the QRS complex helps to differentiate VPC due to digitalis from those of other causes. The exception is ventricular bigeminy, with accurate coupling but varying morphology—a criterion that is suggestive of digitalis toxicity.

The problems of recognition associated with digitalis-induced VPC are also applicable to ventricular tachycardia. Ventricular tachycardia with exit block (Fig. 7–52) and bidirectional ventricular tachycardia (Fig. 7–53) strongly suggest digitalis intoxication. When the ventricular tachycardia originates in the divisions of the left bundle branch, the QRS complex may be normal in duration,[195] and the diagnosis rests on the presence of ventricular capture and fusion complexes. Studies in animals and man confirm that narrow QRS complex tachycardias may be ventricular in origin.

In rare instances, ventricular parasystole is due to digitalis. This is particularly the case when parasystole is accompanied by other arrhythmias known to be due to digitalis intoxication.

The presence of diverse ectopic rhythms, either simultaneously or serially, is strongly suggestive of digitalis toxicity as is the appearance of ectopic rhythms and AV conduction.[187]

Digitalis-induced ventricular fibrillation is seldom recorded in man. It is rarely, if ever, the initial manifestation of digitalis toxicity but is usually preceded by other digitalis-induced arrhythmias.

AV DISSOCIATION (See also p. 707). AV dissociation appearing in the course of digitalis administration is strongly indicative of digitalis intoxication.

AV CONDUCTION DELAY. Depression of AV conduction may be due to a vagal effect of the glycoside and can be reversed with atropine or catecholamines released during normal activities or during exercise. Such depression may also be due to a "direct" extravagal effect of the drug on the cell.[191, 192]

In contrast to ectopy which is a sign of toxicity, depression of conduction may be either a desirable therapeutic effect or a manifestation of digitalis toxicity. The differentiation of the two is a clinical decision. For example, in atrial fibrillation and atrial flutter depression of AV conduction is desirable. In the presence of sinus rhythm, however, AV delay, other than simple prolongation of the P-R interval, is, with rare exception, evidence of digitalis overdose. Although AV block in the presence of sinus rhythm is frequently mentioned as a sign of digitalis intoxication, third-degree AV block is a relatively rare manifestation of glycoside toxicity.

ACCELERATED JUNCTIONAL ESCAPE. This arrhythmia is seen in the same clinical conditions as is nonparoxysmal junctional tachycardia and its clinical significance is probably the same.[194] Accelerated junctional escape follows the rules set for cardiac arrhythmias induced by delayed afterdepolarization[196] and may be the clinical counterpart of the arrhythmias induced in the Purkinje fiber and the intact animal.

REFERENCES

THE NORMAL ELECTROCARDIOGRAM AND VECTORCARDIOGRAM

1. Scher, A. M., and Spach, M. S.: Cardiac depolarization and repolarization and the electrocardiogram. *In* Berne, R. M., Seperelakis, N., and Geiger, S. R. (eds.): Handbook of Physiology, The Cardiovascular System. Vol. I., Sect. 2. Bethesda, American Physiological Society, 1979, pp. 357–392.
2. Burch, G. E., and DePasquale, N. P.: A History of Electrocardiography. Chicago, Year Book Medical Publishers, 1964.
3. Waller, A. D.: A demonstration on man of electromotive changes accompanying the heart's beat. J. Physiol. 8:229, 1887.
4. Einthoven, W.: Selected Papers on Electrocardiography. Edited by A. Snellen. Leiden, University Press, 1977.
5. Lewis, T.: The Mechanism and Graphic Registration of the Heart Beat. London, Shaw and Sons, Ltd., 1920, p. 228.
6. Wilson, F. N.: Selected Papers, Edited by F. D. Johnston and E. Lepeschkin. Ann Arbor, Edward Brothers, Inc., 1954.
7. Pardee, H. E. B.: Clinical Aspects of the Electrocardiogram. New York, Paul B. Hoeber, Inc., 1924.
8. Chou, T. C.: Electrocardiography in clinical practice. 2nd ed. New York, Grune and Stratton, 1986.
9. Durrer, D.: Selected papers. Edited by F. L. Meijler and H. B. Burchell. Amsterdam, North Holland Publishing Co., 1986.
10. What's New in Electrocardiography. H. J. J. Wellens and H. E. Kulbertus (Eds.): The Hague, Martinus Nijhoff Publishers, 1981.
11. Cooksey, J. D., Dunn, M., and Massie, E.: Clinical Vectorcardiography and Electrocardiography. 2nd ed. Chicago, Year Book Medical Publishers, 1977.
12. Fisch, C.: The clinical electrocardiogram: A Classic American Heart Association. Lewis A. Connor Memorial Lecture. Circulation 62(Suppl. III):1, 1980.
13. Wellens, H. J. J.: The electrocardiogram 80 years after Einthoven. Bishop Lecture. J. Am. Coll. Cardiol. 7:484, 1986.
14. Craib, W. H.: A study of the electrical field surrounding active heart muscle. Heart *14*:71, 1927.
15. Wilson, F. N., MacLeod, A. G., and Barker, P. S.: The distribution of the action currents produced by the heart muscle and other excitable tissues immersed in extensive conducting media. J. Gen. Physiol. *16*:423, 1933.
16. Scher, A. M.: Electrocardiogram. *In* Ruch, T. C., and Patton, H. D. (eds.): Physiology and Biophysics. 20th ed. Philadelphia, W. B. Saunders Company, 1974, pp. 67–68.
17. Wolff, L.: Electrocardiography: Fundamentals and Clinical Application. 3rd ed. Philadelphia, W. B. Saunders Company, 1962, p. 15.
18. Durrer, D., VanDam, R. T., Freud, G. E., Janse, M. J., Meijler, F. L., and Arzbaecher, R. C.: Total excitation of the isolated human heart. Circulation *41*:899, 1970.
19. James, T. N., and Sherf, L.: Specialized tissues and preferential conduction in the atria of the heart. Am. J. Cardiol. *28*:414, 1971.
20. Spach, M. S., Miller, W. T., III, Dolber, P. D., Kootsey, J. M., Sommer, J. R., and Mosher, C. E., Jr.: The functional role of structural complexities in the propagation of depolarization in the atrium of the dog: Cardiac conduction disturbances due to discontinuities of effective atrial resistivity. Circ. Res. *50*:175, 1982.
21. Cardiac electrophysiology and arrhythmias. Zipes, D. P., and Jalife, F. (Eds.): New York, Grune and Stratton, 1985.
22. Wyndham, C. R., Meeran, M. K., Smith, T., Sazena, A., Engelman, R. M., Levitsky, S., and Rosen, K. M.: Epicardial activation of the intact human heart without conduction defect. Circulation *59*:161, 1979.
23. Wilson, F. N., MacLeod, A. G., Barker, P. S., and Johnston, F. D.: The determination and the significance of the areas of the ventricular deflections of the electrocardiogram. Am. Heart J. *10*:46, 1934.
24. Wilson, F. N., Johnston, F. D., Rosenbaum, F. F., Erlanger, H., Kossman, O.: The precordial electrocardiogram. Am. Heart J. *27*:19, 1944.

THE NORMAL ELECTROCARDIOGRAM

25. Burger, H. C., and Van Millaan, J. B.: Heart—Vector and leads. Br. Heart J. 9:154, 1947.
26. Willems, J. L., Robles de Medina, E., Bernard, R., Coumel, P., Fisch, C., Krikler, D., Mazur, N. A., Meijler, F. L., Mogensen, L., Moret, P., Pisa, Z., Rautaharju, P. M., Surawicz, B., Watanabe, Y., and Wellens, H. J. J.: WHO Task force on Criteria for Intraventricular Conduction Disturbances and Pre-excitation. J. Am. Coll. Cardiol. 5:1261, 1985.
27. Friedman, N. H.: Diagnostic Electrocardiography and Vectorcardiography. New York, McGraw-Hill Publishing Co., 1977.
28. Lepeschkin, E.: Physiological basis of the U wave. *In* Schlant, R. C., and Hurst, J. W. (eds.): Advances in Electrocardiography. New York, Grune and Stratton, 1972, pp. 431–477.
29. Kishida, H., Cole, J. S., and Surawicz, B.: Negative U wave: A highly specific but poorly understood sign of heart disease. Am. J. Cardiol. *49*:2030, 1982.
30. Bazett, H. C.: An analysis of the time-relations of electrocardiograms. Heart 7:353, 1920.
31. Bexton, R. S., Vallin, H. O., and Camm, A. J.: Diurnal variation of the QT interval—influence of the autonomic nervous system. Br. Heart J. *55*:253, 1986.
32. Mehta, D., Warwick, G. L., and Goldberg, M. J.: QT prolongation after ampicillin anaphylaxis. Br. Heart J. *55*:308, 1986.
33. Chou, T. C., Helm, R. A., and Kaplan, S.: Clinical Vectorcardiography. 2nd ed. New York, Grune and Stratton, 1974.
34. Mann, H.: A method of analyzing the electrocardiogram. Arch. Intern. Med. *25*:283, 1920.
35. Wilson, F. N., and Johnston, F. D.: The vectorcardiogram. Am. Heart J. *16*:14, 1938.
36. Frank, E.: An accurate clinically practical system for spatial vectorcardiography. Circulation *13*:737, 1956.
37. Chou, T. C.: When is the vectorcardiogram superior to the scalar electrocardiogram? J. Am. Coll. Cardiol. 8:791, 1986.
38. Abildskov, J. A., Burgess, M. J., Urie, P. M., Lux, R. L., and Wyatt, R. F.: The unidentified information content of the electrocardiogram. Circ. Res. *40*:3, 1977.
39. Giorgi, C., Ackaoui, A., Nadeau, R., Savard, P., Primeau, R., and Page, P.: Wolff-Parkinson-White VCG patterns that mimic other cardiac pathologies: A correlative study with the preexcitation pathway localization. Am. Heart J. *111*:891, 1986.
40. Maroko, P. R., Libby, P., Lovell, J. W., Sobel, B. E., Moss, J., and Braunwald, E.: Precordial S-T segment elevation mapping: An atraumatic method for assessing alterations in the extent of myocardial ischemic injury. Am. J. Cardiol. *29*:223, 1972.
41. Muller, J. E., Maroko, P. R., and Braunwald, E.: Precordial electrocardiographic mapping. A technique to assess the efficacy of intervention designed to limit infarct size. Circulation *57*:1, 1978.
42. Lux, R. L., Burgess, M. J., Wyatt, R. F., Evans, A. K., Vincent, G. M., and Abildskov, J. A.: Clinically practical lead systems for improved electrocardiography: Comparison with precordial grids and conventional lead systems. Circulation *59*:356, 1979.

THE ABNORMAL ELECTROCARDIOGRAM AND VECTORCARDIOGRAM

43. Reeves, W. C., Hallahan, W., Schwiter, E. J., Ciotola, T. J., Buonocore, E., and Davidson, W.: Two-dimensional echocardiographic assessment of electrocardiographic criteria or right atrial enlargement. Circulation *64*:387, 1981.

44. Chou, T. C., and Helm, R. A.: The pseudo-P pulmonale. Circulation *32*:96, 1965.
45. Munuswamy, K., Alpert, M. A., Martin, R. H., Whiting, R. B., and Mechlin, N. J.: Sensitivity and specificity of commonly used electrocardiographic criteria for left atrial enlargement determined by M-mode echocardiography. Am. J. Cardiol. 53:829, 1984.
46. Zoneraich, O., and Zoneraich, S.: Intraatrial conduction disturbances: Vectorcardiographic patterns. Am. J. Cardiol. *37*:736, 1976.
47. Spodick, D. H.: Diagnostic electrocardiographic sequences in acute pericarditis. Significance of PR segment and PR vector changes. Circulation *48*:575, 1973.

VENTRICULAR HYPERTROPHY

48. Gardin, J. M., and Singer, D. H.: Atrial infarction. Importance, diagnosis, and localization. Arch. Intern. Med. *141*:1345, 1981.
49. Surawicz, B.: Electrocardiographic diagnosis of chamber enlargement. J. Am. Coll. Cardiol. 8:714, 1986.
50. Brody, D. A.: A theoretical analysis of intracavitary blood mass influence on the heart-lead relationship. Circ. Res. *4*:731, 1956.
51. Sokolow, M., and Lyon, T. P.: The ventricular complex in left ventricular hypertrophy as obtained by unipolar precordial and limb leads. Am. Heart J. *37*:161, 1949.
52. Romhilt, D. W., Bove, K. E., and Norris, R. J.: A critical appraisal of the electrocardiographic criteria for the diagnosis of left ventricular hypertrophy. Circulation *40*:185, 1969.
53. Short, D., and Weir, J.: Significance of asymmetrically inverted T wave. Br. Heart J. *49*:564, 1983.
54. Beach, C., Kenmure, A. C. F., and Short, D.: Electrocardiogram of pure left ventricular hypertrophy and its differentiation from lateral ischemia. Br. Heart J. *46*:285, 1981.
55. Reichek, N., and Devereux, R. B.: Left ventricular hypertrophy: Relationship of anatomic, echocardiographic, and electrocardiographic findings. Circulation *63*:1391, 1981.
56. Murphy, M. L., Thenabadu, P. N., de Soyza, N., Meade, J., Doherty, J. E., and Baker, B. J.: Sensitivity of electrocardiographic criteria for left ventricular hypertrophy according to type of cardiac disease. Am. J. Cardiol. *55*:545, 1985.
57. Cumming, G. R., and Proudfit, W. L.: High-voltage QRS complexes in the absence of left ventricular hypertrophy. Circulation *19*:406, 1959.
58. Cabrera, E., and Gaxiola, A.: A critical re-evaluation of systolic and diastolic overloading patterns. Progr. Cardiovasc. Dis. *2*:219, 1959.
59. Scott, R. C.: The electrocardiographic diagnosis of right ventricular hypertrophy: Correlation with anatomic findings. Am. Heart J. *60*:659, 1960.
60. Burch, G. E., and DePasquale, N. P.: Electrocardiography in the Diagnosis of Congenital Heart Disease. Philadelphia, Lea and Febiger, 1967.
61. National Cooperative Study: The Urokinase–Pulmonary Embolism Trial. Circulation *47*(Suppl. II):1, 1973.
62. McGinn, S., and White, P. D.: Acute cor pulmonale resulting from pulmonary embolism: Its clinical recognition. J.A.M.A. *104*:1473, 1935.
63. Goldberger, A. L.: Myocardial Infarction. 3rd ed. St. Louis, The C. V. Mosby Co., 1984.
64. Brugada, P., Gorgels, A. P., and Wellens, H. J. J.: The electrocardiogram in pulmonary embolism. *In* Kulbertus, H. E., and Wellens, N. J. J. (eds.): What's New in Electrocardiography. Hingham, MA, Martinus Nijhoff, 1981, p. 366.
65. Ikeda, K., Kubota, I., Takahashi, K., and Yasui, S.: P-wave changes in obstructive and restrictive lung diseases. J. Electrocardiol. *18*:233, 1985.

INTRAVENTRICULAR CONDUCTION DEFECTS

65a. Flowers, N. C.: Left bundle branch block: A continuously evolving concept. J. Am. Coll. Cardiol. 9:684, 1987.
66. Fisch, C.: The electrocardiogram in the aged. Cardiovasc. Clin. *12*:65, 1981.
67. Watt, T. B., Murao, S., and Pruitt, R. D.: Left axis deviation induced experimentally in a primate heart. Am. Heart J. *70*:381, 1965.
68. Watt, T. B., Jr., Freud, G. E., Durrer, D., and Pruitt, R. D.: Left anterior arborization block combined with right bundle branch block in canine and primate hearts. An electrocardiographic study. Circ. Res. *22*:57, 1968.
69. Watt, T. W., and Pruitt, R. D.: Left posterior fascicular block in canine and primate hearts. An electrocardiographic study. Circulation. *40*:677, 1969.
70. Rosenbaum, M. B., Elizari, M. V., and Lazzari, J. O.: The Hemiblocks: New Concepts of Intraventricular Conduction Based on Human Anatomical, Physiological, and Clinical Studies. Oldsmar, FL, Tampa Tracings, 1970.
71. McHenry, P. L., Phillips, J. F., Fisch, C., and Corya, B. R.: Right precordial qrS pattern due to left anterior hemiblock. Am Heart J. *81*:498, 1971.
72. Rosenbaum, M. B., Elizari, M. V., Lazzari, J. O., Nau, G. J., Levi, R. J., and Halpern, M. S.: Intraventricular trifascicular blocks. The syndrome of right bundle branch block with intermittent left anterior and posterior hemiblock. Am. Heart J. 78:306, 1969.
73. Angelini, P., Springer, A., Sulbaran, T., and Livesay, W. R.: Right ventricular myopathy with an unusual intraventricular conduction defect (epsilon potential). Am. Heart J. *101*:680, 1981.
74. Marcus, F. I., Fontaine, G. H., Guiraudon, G., Frank, R., Laurenceau, J. L., Malergue, C., and Grosgogeat, Y.: Right ventricular dysplasia: A report of 24 adult cases. Circulation *65*:384, 1982.

ABERRATION

75. Lewis, T.: Observations upon disorders of the heart's action. Heart *3*:279, 1912.
76. Fisch, C., Zipes, D. P., and McHenry, P. L.: Rate-dependent aberrancy. Circulation *48*:714, 1973.
77. Gouaux, J. L., and Ashman, R.: Auricular fibrillation with aberration simulating ventricular paroxysmal tachycardia. Am. Heart J. *34*:366, 1947.
78. Mendez, C., Gruhzit, C. C., and Moe, G. K.: Influence of cycle length upon refractory period of auricles, ventricles, and A-V in the dog. Am. J. Physiol. *184*:287, 1956.
79. Lewis, T.: Certain physical signs of myocardial involvement. Br. Med. J. *1*:484, 1913.
80. Fisch, C.: Bundle branch block after ventricular tachycardia: A manifestation of "fatigue" or "overdrive suppression." J. Am. Coll. Cardiol. 3:1562, 1984.
81. Moe, G. K., Mendez, C., and Han, J.: Aberrant A-V impulse propagation in the dog heart: A study of functional bundle branch block. Circ. Res. *16*:261, 1965.
82. Katz, A., and Pick, A.: The transseptal conduction time in the human heart. Circulation 27:1061, 1963.
83. Dressler, W.: Transient bundle branch block occurring during slowing of the heart beat and following gagging. Am. Heart J. *58*:760, 1959.
84. Singer, D. H., Lazzarra, R., and Hoffman, B. F.: Interrelationship between automaticity and conduction in Purkinje fibers. Circ. Res. *21*:537, 1967.
85. Fisch, C., and Miles, W. M.: Deceleration ("bradycardia") dependent left bundle branch block: A spectrum of bundle branch conduction delay. Circulation *65*:1029, 1982.

WOLFF-PARKINSON-WHITE SYNDROME

86. Wolff, L., Parkinson, J., and White, P. D.: Bundle branch block with short P-R interval in healthy young people prone to paroxysmal tachycardia. Am. Heart J. *5*:685, 1930.
87. Wilson, F. N.: A case in which the vagus influenced the form of the ventricular complex of the electrocardiogram. Arch. Intern. Med. *16*:1008, 1915.
88. Cohn, A. E., and Fraser, F. R.: Paroxysmal tachycardia and the effect of stimulation of the vagus nerves by pressure. Heart *5*:93, 1913.
89. Holzmann, N., and Scherf, D.: Ueber Elektrokardiogramme mit verkuerzter Vorhof-Kammer-Distanz und positiven P-Zacken. Z. Klin. Med. *121*:404, 1932.
90. Lev, M., Fox, S. M., Bharati, S., and Greenfield, S. L., Jr.: Mahaim and James Fibers as a basis for a unique variety of ventricular preexcitation. Am. J. Cardiol. *36*:880, 1975.
91. Rosenbaum, F. F., Hecht, H. H., Wilson, F. N., and Johnston, F. D.: The potential variations of the thorax and the esophagus in anomalous atrioventricular excitation (Wolff-Parkinson-White syndrome). Am. Heart J. *29*:281, 1945.
92. Benson, D. W., Sterba, R., Gallagher, J. J., Waltson, II, A., and Spach, M. S.: Localization of the site of ventricular preexcitation with body surface maps in patients with W-P-W syndrome. Circulation *65*:1259, 1982.
92a. Kamakura, S., Shimomura, K., Ohe, T., Matsuhisa, M., and Toyoshima, H.: The role of initial minimum potentials on body surface maps in predicting the site of accessory pathways in patients with W-P-W syndrome. Circulation *74*:89, 1986.
93. Lown, B., Ganong, W. F., and Levine, S. A.: The syndrome of short P-R interval, normal QRS complex, and paroxysmal rapid heart action. Circulation *5*:693, 1952.
94. Fisch, C., Pinsky, S. T., and Shields, J. P.: Wolff-Parkinson-White syndrome. Report of a case associated with wandering pacemaker, atrial tachycardia, atrial fibrillation, and incomplete A-V dissociation with interference. Circulation *16*:1004, 1957.
95. McHenry, P. L., Knoebel, S. B., and Fisch, C.: The Wolff-Parkinson-White (WPW) syndrome with supernormal conduction through the anomalous bypass. Circulation *34*:734, 1966.

MYOCARDIAL INFARCTION

96. Pardee, H. E. B.: An electrocardiographic sign of coronary artery obstruction. Arch. Intern. Med. *26*:244, 1920.
97. David, D., Naito, M., Michelson, E., Watanabe, Y., Chen, C. C., Morganroth, J., Shaffenburg, M., and Blenko, T.: Intramyocardial conduction: A major determinant of R-wave amplitude during acute myocardial ischemia. Circulation *65*:161, 1982.
98. Madias, J. E.: The earliest electrocardiographic signs of acute transmural myocardial infarction. J. Electrocardiol. *10*:193, 1977.
99. Surawicz, B.: The pathogenesis and clinical significance of primary T-wave abnormalities. *In* Schlant, R. C., and Hurst, J. W. (eds.): Advances in Electrocardiography. New York, Grune and Stratton, 1972, pp. 377–421.
100. Samson, W. E., and Scher, A. N.: Mechanism of S-T segment alteration during acute myocardial injury. Circ. Res. *8*:780, 1960.
101. Vincent, G. M., Abildskov, J. A., and Burgess, M. J.: Mechanisms of ischemic ST-segment displacement. Evaluation by direct current recordings. Circulation *56*:559, 1977.
102. Wilson, F. N., Johnston, F. D., and Hill, I. G. W.: The form of the electrocardiogram in experimental myocardial infarction. IV. Additional observations on the later effects produced by ligation of the anterior descending branch of the left coronary artery. Am. Heart J. *10*:1025, 1935.
103. Wilson, F. N., MacLeod, A. G., Barker, P. S., Johnston, F. D., and

Klostermeyer, L. L.: The electrocardiogram in myocardial infarction with particular reference to the initial deflection of the ventricular complex. Heart *16*:155, 1933.
104. Behar, S., Schor, S., Kariv, L., Barrell, V., and Modan, B.: Evaluation of electrocardiogram in emergency room as a decision-making tool. Chest *71*:486, 1977.
105. Gunraj, D. R., and Rajapakse, D. A.: Daily ECG confirmation in acute myocardial infarction. Practitioner *213*:361, 1974.
106. McGuinness, J. B., Begg, T. B., and Semple, T.: First electrocardiogram in recent myocardial infarction. Br. Med. J. 2:449, 1976.
107. Short, D.: The earliest electrocardiographic evidence of myocardial infarction. Br. Heart J. *32*:6, 1970.
108. Thygesen, K., Horder, M., Lyager Nielsen, B., and Hyltoft Petersen, P.: Evolution of ST segment and Q and R waves during early phase of inferior myocardial infarction. Acta Med. Scand. *205*:25, 1979.
109. Abbott, J. A., and Scheinman, M. M.: Nondiagnostic electrocardiogram in patients with acute myocardial infarction: Clinical and anatomic correlations. Am. J. Med. *55*:608, 1973.
109a. Wohlgelernter, D., Cleman, M., Higman, H. A., Fetterman, R. C., Duncan, J. S., Zaret, B., and Jaffe, C. C.: Regional myocardial dysfunction during coronary angioplasty: Evaluation by two-dimensional echocardiography and 12 lead electrocardiography. J. Am. Coll. Cardiol. *7*:1245, 1986.
110. Salcedo, J. R., Baird, M. G., Chambers, R. D., and Beanlands, D. S.: Significance of reciprocal ST segment depression in anterior precordial leads in acute inferior myocardial infarction: Concominant left anterior descending coronary artery disease? Am. J. Cardiol. *48*:1003, 1981.
111. Odemuyiwa, O., Peart, I., Albers, C., and Hall, R.: Reciprocal ST depression in acute myocardial infarction. Br. Heart J. *54*:479, 1985.
112. Wasserman, A. G., Ross, A. M., Bogaty, D., Richardson, D. W., Hutchinson, R. G., and Rios, J. C.: Anterior ST segment depression during acute inferior myocardial infarction: Evidence for the reciprocal change theory. Am. Heart J. *106*:516, 1983.
113. Tzivoni, D., Chenzbraun, A., Keren, A., Benhorn, J., Gottlieb, S., Lonn, E., and Stern, S.: Reciprocal electrocardiographic changes in acute myocardial infarction. Am. J. Cardiol. *56*:23, 1986.
114. Pierard, L. A., Sprynger, M., Gilis, F., and Carlier, J.: Significance of precordial ST-segment depression in inferior acute myocardial infarction as determined by echocardiography. Am. J. Cardiol. *57*:82, 1986.
115. Quyyumi, A. A., Rubens, M. B., Rickards, A. F., Crake, T., Levy, R. D., and Fox, K. M.: Importance of "reciprocal" electrocardiographic changes during occlusion of left anterior descending coronary artery. Lancet *1*:347, 1986.
116. Goldberg, H. L., Borer, J. S., Jacobstein, J. G., Kluger, J., Scheidt, S. S., and Alonsto, D. R.: Anterior S-T segment depression in acute inferior myocardial infarction: Indicator of posterolateral infarction. Am. J. Cardiol. *48*:1009, 1981.
117. Berland, J., Cribier, A., Behar, P., and Letac, B.: Anterior ST depression in inferior myocardial infarction: Correlation with results of intracoronary thrombolysis. Am. Heart J. *111*:481, 1986.
118. Raunio, H., Rissanen, V., Romppanen, T., Jokinen, Y., Rehnberg, S., Helin, M., and Pyorala, K.: Changes in the QRS complex and ST segment in transmural and subendocardial myocardial infarctions. A clinicopathologic study. Am. Heart J. *98*:176, 1979.
119. Gerson, M. C., Phillips, J. F., Morris, S. N., and McHenry, P. L.: Exercise-induced U wave inversion as a marker of stenosis of the left anterior descending coronary artery. Circulation *60*:1014, 1979.
120. Nakagaki, O., Yano, H., Mitsutake, A., Kikuchi, Y., Takeshita, A., Kanaide, H., and Nakamura, M.: Reelevation of ST segment on precordial mapping in natural time course following acute anterior myocardial infarction. Jpn. Circ. J. *45*:562, 1981.
120a. Wahl, J. M., Hakki, A. H., Iskadrian, A. S., and Segal, B. L.: Limitations of ventricular complex morphology in the diagnosis of myocardial infarction. J. Electrocardiology *19*:131, 1986.
121. Durrer, D., Van Lier, A. A. W., and Boller, J.: Epicardial and intramural excitation in chronic myocardial infarction. Am. Heart J. *68*:765, 1964.
122. Horan, L. G., Flowers, N. C., and Johnson, J. C.: Significance of the diagnostic Q wave of myocardial infarction. Circulation *43*:428, 1971.
123. Rosenbaum, M. B., Girotti, L. A., Lazzari, J. O., Halpern, M. S., and Elizari, M. V.: Abnormal Q waves in right sided chest leads provoked by onset of right bundle-branch block in patients with anteroseptal infarction. Br. Heart J. *47*:227, 1982.
124. Horan, L. G., Flowers, N. C., Tolleson, W. J., and Thomas, J. R.: The significance of diagnostic Q waves in the presence of bundle branch block. Chest *58*:214, 1970.
125. Luy, G., Bahl, O. P., and Massie, E.: Intermittent left bundle branch block. A study of the effects of left bundle branch block on the electrocardiographic patterns of myocardial infarction and ischemia. Am. Heart J. *85*:332, 1973.
126. Altieri, P., and Schaal, S. F.: Inferior and anteroseptal myocardial infarction concealed by transient left anterior hemiblock. J. Electrocardiol. *6*:257, 1973.
127. Dhingra, R. C., Wyndhan, C., Ehsani, A. A., and Rosen, K. M.: Left anterior hemiblock concealing diaphragmatic infarction and simulating anterioseptal infarction. Chest *67*:716, 1975.
128. Warner, R. A., Hill, N. E., Mookherjee, S., and Smulyan, H.: Electrocardiographic criteria for the diagnosis of combined inferior myocardial infarction and left anterior hemiblock. Am. J. Cardiol. *51*:718, 1983.
129. First, S. R., Bayley, R. H., and Bedford, D. R.: Peri-infarction block electrocardiographic abnormality occasionally resembling bundle branch block and local ventricular block of other types. Circulation 2:31, 1950.
130. Blanke, H., Cohen, M., Schlueter, G. V., Karsch, K. R., and Rentrop, K. P.: Electrocardiographic and coronary arteriographic correlations during acute myocardial inarction. Am. J. Cardiol. *54*:249, 1984.
131. Fuchs, R. M., Achuff, S. C., Grunwald, B. A., Yin, F. C. P., and Griffith, L. S. C.: Electrocardiographic localization of coronary artery narrowings: Studies during myocardial ischemia and infarction in patients with one-vessel disease. Circulation *66*:1168, 1982.
132. Braat, S. H., Brugada, P., Dulk, K., Ommen, V., and Wellens, H. J. J.: Value of lead V_4R for recognition of the infarct coronary artery in acute inferior myocardial infarction. Am. J. Cardiol. *53*:1538, 1984.
133. Qgawa, J., Hiramoro, K., Haze, K., Saito, M., Sumiyoshi, T., Fukami, K., Goto, Y., and Ikeda, M.: Classification of non-Q wave myocardial infarction according to electrocardiographic changes. Br. Heart J. *54*:473, 1985.
134. Mirvis, D. M., Ingram, L., Holly, M. K., Wilson, J. L. and Ramanthan, K. B.: Electrocardiographic effects of experimental nontransmural myocardial infarction. Circulation *71*:1206, 1985.
135. Surawicz, B., Uhley, H., Borun, R., Laks, M., Crevasse, L., Rosen, K., Nelson,W., Mandel, W., Lawrence, P., Jackson, L., Flowers, N., Clifton, J., Greenfield, J., Jr., and Robles de Medina, E.: Tenth Bethesda Conference: Optimal electrocardiography. Am. J. Cardiol. *41*:130, 1978.
136. Chou, T. C., Van Der Bei-Kahn, J., Allen, J., Brockmeier, L., and Fowler, N. O.: Electrocardiographic diagnosis of right ventricular infarction. Am. J. Med. *70*:1175, 1981.
137. Klein, H. O., Tordjman, T., Ninio, R., Sareli, P., Oren, V., Lang, R., Gefen, J., Pauzner, C., Di Segni, E., David, D., and Kaplinsky, E.: The early recognition of right ventricular infarction: Diagnostic accuracy of the electrocardiographic V_4R lead. Circulation *67*:558, 1983.
138. Braat, S. H., Brugada, P., DeZwan, C., Coenegracht, J. M., and Wellens, H. J. J.: Value of electrocardiogram in diagnosing right ventricular involvement in patients with an acute inferior wall myocardial infarction. Br. Heart J. *49*:368, 1983.
139. Lopez-Sendon, J., Coma-Canella, I., Alcasena, S., Seoane, J., and Gamallo, C.: Electrocardiographic findings in acute right ventricular infarction: Sensitivity and specificity of electrocardiographic alterations in right precordial leads V_4R, V_3R, V_1, V_2, and V_3. J. Am. Coll. Cardiol. *6*:1273, 1985.
140. Benchimol, A., and Desser, K. B.: The electrovector cardiographic diagnosis of posterior wall myocardial infarction. *In* Fisch, C. (ed.): Complex Electrocardiography. Philadelphia, F. A. Davis Co., 1973, pp. 182–197.
141. Nestico, P. F., Hakki, A., Iskandrian, A. S., and Anderson, G. J.: Electrocardiographic diagnosis of posterior myocardial infarction revisited: A new approach using a multivariate discriminant analysis and thallium-201 myocardial scintigraphy. J. Electrocardiol. *19*:33, 1986.
142. Varat, M. A.: Non-transmural infarction: Clinical distinction between patients with ST depression and those with T wave inversion. J. Electrocardiol. *18*:15, 1985.
143. Ward, R. M., White, R. D., Ideker, R. E., Hindman, M. B., Alonso, D. R., Bishop, S. P., Bloor, C., Fallon, T., Gottlieb, G. J., Hackel, D. B., Hutchins, G. M., Phillips, H. R., Reimer, K. A., Roark, S. F., Rochlani, S. P., Rogers, W. J., Ruth, W. K., Savage, R. M., Weiss, J. L., Selvester, R. H., and Wagner, G. S.: Evaluation of QRS scoring system for estimating myocardial infarct size. IV. Correlation with the quantitative anatomic findings for posterolateral infarcts. Am. J. Cardiol. *53*:70, 1984.
143a. Hindman, N., Grande, P., Harrell, F. E., Anderson, C., Harrison, D., Ideker, R. E., and Sylvester, R. H.: Relation between electrocardiographic and enzymatic methods of estimating acute myocardial infarct size. Am. J. Cardiol. *58*:31, 1986.
143b. Mikell, F. L., Petrovich, J., Snyder, M. C., Taylor, G. J., Moses, H. W., Dove, J. T., Batchelder, J. E., Schneider, J. A., and Wellons, H. A.: Reliability of Q-wave formation and QRS score in predicting regional and global left ventricular performance in acute myocardial infarction with successful reperfusion. Am. J. Cardiol. *57*:923, 1986.
144. Starr, J. W., Wagner, G. S., Behar, V. S., Walston, A., II, and Greenfield, C., Jr.: Vectorcardiographic criteria for the diagnosis of inferior myocardial infarction. Circulation *49*:829, 1974.
145. Rubin, I. L., Gross, H., and Vigliano, E. M.: Transient abnormal Q waves during coronary insufficiency. Am. Heart J. *71*:254, 1966.
146. Meller, J., Conde, C. A., Donoso, E., and Dack, S.: Transient Q waves in Prinzmetal's angina. Am. J. Cardiol. *35*:691, 1975.
147. DePasquale, N. P., Burch, G. E., and Phillips, J. H.: Electrocardiograph alterations associated with electrically "silent" areas of myocardium. Am. Heart J. *68*:697, 1964.
148. Braunwald, E., and Kloner, R. A.: The stunned myocardium: Prolonged postischemic ventricular dysfunction. Circulation *66*:1146, 1982.
149. Bateman, T. M., Czer, L. S. C., Gray, R. J., Maddahi, J., Raymond, M. J., Geft, I. L., Ganz, W., Shah, P. K., and Berman, D. S.: Transient pathologic Q waves during acute ischemia events: An electrographic correlate of stunned but viable myocardium. Am. Heart J. *106*:1421, 1983.
150. Frank, S., and Braunwald, E.: Idiopathic hypertrophic subaortic stenosis: Clinical analysis of 126 patients with emphasis on the natural history. Circulation *37*:759, 1968.
151. Cosio, F. G., Moro, C., Alonso, M., de la Calzada, C. S., and Llovet, A.: The Q waves of hypertrophic cardiomyopathy. An electrophysiologic study. N. Engl. J. Med. *302*:96, 1980.
152. Hart, J. G., Barrett, P. A., Barnaby, P. F., Clark, E. H., Lyons, N. R., and Burke, J. J.: Diagnosis of old anterior myocardial infarction in emphysema with poor R wave progression in anterior chest leads. Br. Heart J. *45*:522, 1981.
153. Diamond, J. R., and Estes, M. N.: ECG changes associated with iatrogenic left pneumothorax simulating anterior myocardial infarction. Am. Heart J. *103*:303, 1982.

ST-SEGMENT AND T-WAVE CHANGES

154. White, P. D.: Alternation of the pulse: A common clinical condition. Am. J. Med. Sci. *150*:82, 1915.
155. Edmands, R. E., Greenspan, K., and Fisch, C.: Effect of cycle-length alteration upon the configuration of the canine ventricular action potential. Circ. Res. 9:602, 1966.
156. Taussig, H. B.: Electrograms taken from isolated strips of mammalian ventricular cardiac muscle. Bull. Johns Hopkins Hosp. *43*:81, 1928.
157. Fisch, C., Edmands, R. E., and Greenspan, K.: T wave alternans: An association with abrupt rate change. Am. Heart J. *81*:817, 1971.
158. Wellens, H. J. J.: Isolated electrical alternans of the T wave. Chest *62*:319, 1972.
159. Watanabe, Y., Toda, H., and Nishimura, M.: Clinical electrographic study of bifid T waves. Br. Heart J. *52*:207, 1984.
160. Surawicz, B., and Lasseter, K. C.: Effect of drugs on the electrocardiogram. Progr. Cardiovasc. Dis. *13*:26, 1970.
161. Abildskov, J. A.: Central nervous system influence upon electrocardiographic waveforms. *In* Schlant, R. C., and Hurst, J. W. (eds.): Advances in electrocardiography. New York, Grune and Stratton, 1976.
162. Friedberg, C. K., and Zager, A.: "Nonspecific" ST and T-wave changes. Circulation *23*:655, 1961.
163. Sleeper, J. C., and Orgain, E. S.: Differentiation of benign from pathologic T waves in the electrocardiogram. Am. J. Cardiol. *11*:338, 1963.
164. Wilson, F. N., and Finch, R.: The effect of drinking iced-water upon the form of the T deflection of the electrocardiogram. Heart *10*:275, 1923.
165. Oakley, D. G., and Oakley, C. M.: Significance of abnormal electrocardiograms in highly trained athletes. Am. J. Cardiol. *50*:985, 1982.
166. Balady, G. J., Cadigan, J. G., and Ryan, T. J.: Electrocardiogram of the athlete: An analysis of 289 professional football players. Am. J. Cardiol. *53*:1339, 1984.
167. Autenrieth, G., Surawicz, B., Kuo, C. S., and Arita, M.: Primary T wave abnormalities caused by uniform and regional shortening of ventricular monophasic action potential in dog. Circulation *51*:668, 1975.
168. Ward, O. C.: New familial cardiac syndrome in children. J. Ir. Med. Assoc. *54*:103, 1964.
169. Abildskov, J. A.: The prolonged QT interval. Ann. Rev. Med. *30*:171, 1979.
170. Burchell, H. B.: The QT interval historically treated. Pediatr. Cardiol. *4*:138, 1983.
171. Surawicz, B., and Knoebel, S. B.: Long QT: Good, bad or indifferent? J. Am. Coll. Cardiol. *4*:138, 1983.
172. Hering, H. E.: Experimentalle studien an Saugetieren uber das Electrocardiogramme. Z. Exp. Pathol. Ther. 7:363, 1909.
173. Lewis, T.: Notes upon alternation of the heart. Quart. J. Med. *4*:141, 1910.
174. McGregor, M., and Baskind, E.: Electric alternans in pericardial effusion. Circulation *11*:837, 1955.
175. Feigenbaum, H., Zaky, A., and Grabhor, L. L.: Cardiac motion in patients with pericardial effusion. A study using reflected ultrasound. Circulation *34*:611, 1966.
176. Pop, T., and Fleischmann, D.: Alternans in human atrial monophasic action potential. Br. Heart J. *39*:1273, 1977.
177. Osborn, J. J.: Experimental hypothermia. Respiratory and blood pH changes in relation to cardiac function. Am. J. Physiol. *175*:389, 1953.

ABNORMAL ECG IN ABSENCE OF CLINICAL HEART DISEASE

178. Fisch, C.: Abnormal ECG in clinically normal individuals. J.A.M.A. *250*:1321, 1983.
179. Zema, M. J., and Kligfield, P.: Electrocardiographic tall R waves in the right precordial leads. J. Electrocardiol. *17*:129, 1984.

THE ECG AND ELECTROLYTE ABNORMALITIES

180. Selzer, A.: The Bayes theorem and clinical electrocardiography. Am. Heart J. *101*:360, 1981.
181. Surawicz, B.: Relationship between electrocardiogram and electrolytes. Am. Heart J. *73*:814, 1967.
182. Carter, E. P., and Andrus, E. C.: Q-T interval in human electrocardiogram in absence of cardiac disease. J.A.M.A., *78*:1922, 1922.
183. Douglas, P. S., Carmichael, K. A., and Palevsky, P. M.: Extreme hypercalcemia and electrocardiographic changes. Am. J. Cardiol. *54*:674, 1984.
184. Sridharan, M. R., and Horan, L. G.: Electrocardiographic T wave of hypercalcemia. Am. J. Cardiol. *54*:672, 1984.
185. Nierenberg, D. W., and Ransil, B. J.: Q-at_c interval as a clinical indicator of hypercalcemia. Am. J. Cardiol. *44*:243, 1979.

EFFECTS OF DRUGS ON THE ECG

186. Cohn, A. E., Fraser, F. R., and Jamieson, A.: The influence of digitalis on the T wave of the human electrocardiogram. J. Exp. Med. *21*:593, 1915.
187. Fisch, C., Greenspan, K., Knoebel, S. B., and Feigenbaum, H.: Effect of digitalis on conduction of the heart. Progr. Cardiovasc. Dis. *6*:343, 1964.
188. Fisch, C., and Knoebel, S. B.: Digitalis cardiotoxicity. J. Am. Coll. Cardiol. *5*:92a, 1985.
189. Smith, T. W., Antman, E. M., Friedman, P. L., Blatt, C. M., and Marsh, J. D.: Digitalis glycosides: Mechanisms and manifestations of toxicity. Prog. Cardiovasc. Dis. *26*:413, 495, 1984.
190. Fisch, C., Zipes, D. P., and Noble, R. J.: Digitalis toxicity: Mechanism and recognition. *In* Yu, P., and Goodwin, R. (eds.): Progress in Cardiology. Philadelphia, Lea and Febiger, 1975, pp. 37–70.
191. Gold, H., Kwit, N. T., Otto, H., and Fox, T.: On vagal and extravagal factors in cardiac slowing by digitalis in patients with auricular fibrillation. J. Clin. Invest. *18*:429, 1939.
192. Mendez, C., Aceves, J., and Mendez, R. J.: The anti-adrenergic action of digitalis on the refractory period of the A-V transmission system. J. Pharmacol. Exp. Ther. *131*:199, 1961.
193. Pick, A., and Dominquez, P.: Nonparoxysmal A-V nodal tachycardia. Circulation *16*:1022, 1957.
194. Knoebel, S. B., and Fisch, C.: Accelerated junctional escape. A clinical and electrocardiographic study. Circulation *50*:151, 1974.
195. Cohen, H. C., Gozo, E. G., Jr., and Pick, A.: Ventricular tachycardia with narrow QRS complexes (left posterior fascicular tachycardia). Circulation *45*:1035, 1972.
196. Rosen, M. R., Fisch, C., Hoffman, B. F., Danilo, P., Jr., Lovelace, D. E., and Knoebel, S. B.: Can accelerated atrioventricular junctional escape rhythms be explained by delayed afterdepolarization? Am. J. Cardiol. *45*:1272, 1983.

Additional references in this field for the period prior to 1980 can be found in E. Braunwald, *Heart Disease.* 2nd ed. W. B. Saunders Company, 1984, pp. 252–257.

8 EXERCISE STRESS TESTING

by L. THOMAS SHEFFIELD, M.D.

EXERCISE STRESS TESTING FOR CORONARY ARTERY DISEASE

Although the incidence of coronary artery disease has been diminishing in the last 20 years, it is still a problem of epidemic proportion. It is the one frequently fatal disease that most often causes recurrent episodes of chest discomfort. Therefore, patients who have experienced chest pain should have significant coronary artery disease excluded or confirmed in order to allow for development of an appropriate management plan. Since exertion typically provokes attacks of angina pectoris, Goldhammer and Scherf introduced individualized exercise testing for coronary artery disease in 1931.[1] Master and colleagues adapted electrocardiographic recording to his standardized two-step fitness test. This test became the first popular objective aid to the diagnosis of angina pectoris.[2] When it was found to be safe to have patients exercise strenuously for improved test sensitivity, treadmills and cycle ergometers proved more practical than the step box.[3]

INDICATIONS FOR NONINVASIVE EXERCISE STRESS TESTING. Standardized treadmill or cycle ergometer testing is medically useful in several specific ways. It aids the evaluation of chest pain in adults, especially when the patient's description of the discomfort is not typical of angina pectoris (Table 8–1). In a patient known to have coronary artery disease, an exercise test is useful for estimating the patient's potential problem and prognosis and thus assists in the choice of therapy.[4] The patient categorized as being at high risk may be a candidate for consideration of prompt revascularization, whereas a low-risk patient may often be treated more conservatively. Exercise testing is useful in evaluating the degree of benefit received from antianginal and antiarrhythmic regimens. Exercise testing after myocardial infarction aids in identifying patients who may safely pursue increased activity to accelerate rehabilitation[1, 7, 13, 16] (see Table 8–6), and also identifies others who may be candidates for catheterization to evaluate ventricular function, coronary anatomy, and possibly their response to electrophysiological stimulation.

Stress testing is also recommended for sedentary individuals before beginning a physical fitness program, both to minimize the potential of provoking a coronary event and to provide data for developing an individualized exercise prescription.[5, 6] Exercise testing can measure the benefit provided by medical therapy for coronary artery disease, percutaneous transluminal coronary angioplasty, as well as surgical procedures such as coronary revascularization, femoral bypass, correction of congenital cardiovascular malformations, and valve replacement.[7, 8]

Most controversial is the question of use of exercise stress testing in the asymptomatic general public. Because the prevalence of coronary artery disease is low in this group, an ischemic type of response in such persons is much more likely to be a false-positive result than a true one. For that reason the test probably should not be used to seek out preclinical coronary heart disease in the asymptomatic public. However, it can be used effectively as part of a risk factor assessment program in which measurements of serum total cholesterol, high-density lipoprotein cholesterol, glucose, and blood pressure, and smoking history, age, and sex are combined with results of the exercise test in order to evaluate an asymptomatic individual's risk of developing coronary heart disease in the future. Considered as a *risk factor*, the abnormal test result offers an otherwise unavailable opportunity to prevent disease. When positive, it is far more predictive of a coronary event than are the "classical" risk factors, which are discussed in Chap. 36. Several large studies including the Coronary Primary Prevention Study and the Prevalence Study Mortality Follow-up of the National Lipid Research Clinics Program have shown that the exercise test contributes predictive data that is independent of and more powerful than the other risk factors listed above.[9–12]

CONTROVERSIES CONCERNING THE APPLICATION OF STRESS TESTING. These include: (1) the correlation between exercise electrocardiograms and coronary angiograms has been poorer than expected in spite of the good agreement between exercise tests and clinical follow-up.[13, 14] (An important reason for this discrepancy has been the wide range of methodological variation among the reported studies.[15–18]) (2) Epidemiological concepts have been introduced to explain why the test cannot be as accurate in the screening of asymptomatic subjects as it is in that of persons with chest pain. (3) The exercise test has been extended to include observations on heart rate, blood pressure, and

TABLE 8–1 INDICATIONS FOR NONINVASIVE EXERCISE STRESS TESTING

Aid in diagnosis of the cause of chest discomfort
Assess the prognosis of coronary heart disease
Assess the efficacy of therapy of coronary heart disease
Guide rehabilitation following myocardial infarction
Aid in the development of an exercise prescription and provide a safety check before a fitness program
Screen high-risk professionals
Assess a risk of development of clinical coronary artery disease in asymptomatic persons

endurance in addition to the electrocardiogram. These three issues are discussed below.

PHYSIOLOGY OF EXERCISE TESTING

(See also p. 466)

CORONARY ARTERIAL RESERVE. All systems of the body (including the cardiovascular systems) have substantial reserve capacity. Most measurements of cardiovascular function during the resting state are poor predictors of circulatory performance during vigorous exercise. During exercise, the flow in intracardiac shunts that at rest is from left to right may reverse and become predominantly right to left. Pulmonary artery pressures and transvalvular pressure gradients that are unimpressive at rest may become critical during heavy exercise. Regional left ventricular wall motion that is normal at rest may diminish during vigorous work, simulating an aneurysm. Advanced degrees of coronary arterial obstruction may exist without myocardial ischemia at rest (p. 1201). Exercise is currently the most convenient means of stimulating the myocardium to demand maximal blood flow and is the only way of stimulating such a rigorous demand for oxygen delivery that even moderate impairment of coronary blood flow capacity becomes detectable.

CARDIAC OUTPUT INCREASES IN EXERCISE. As an adult exercises maximally, cardiac output may rise from 5 to 25 liters/min.[19] Vasodilation in the skeletal muscular bed aids this increase in flow (p. 417), but an increase in mean arterial pressure also occurs. Pressure increases of 50 per cent are typical, producing corresponding increases in the contractile force of myocardial fibers, a major determinant of myocardial oxygen consumption. There is a variable increase in stroke volume during exercise, depending on the severity of exercise and the posture in which it is carried out[20] (p. 418). Since adaptation of stroke volume to increasing cardiac output demand is limited, the primary mechanism of increasing cardiac output is by raising the heart rate. With an increasing heart rate, the duration of systolic ejection per beat diminishes. Attainment of normal systolic emptying in shorter periods requires increasing the rate of tension development and shortening the myocardial fibers, a valuable adaptive mechanism that parallels increases in contractility but also exacts a price, i.e., an increase of the oxygen consumption with each contraction.

MYOCARDIAL OXYGEN CONSUMPTION IN EXERCISE. Myocardial oxygen consumption ($M\dot{V}O_2$) per contraction is determined mainly by the tension developed by the myofibrils and by the inotropic (contractile) state. The latter is reflected in the rapidity with which tension is generated and shortening occurs (p. 1192). Both of these determinants of $M\dot{V}O_2$ are increased by exercise, resulting in a net increase in oxygen consumption per contraction. $M\dot{V}O_2$ per minute is the product of $M\dot{V}O_2$ per beat and heart rate; the latter increases in proportion to the intensity of exercise. In the normotensive person the increase in heart rate accounts for the greatest increment in coronary blood flow during exercise. Measurements of contractility and heart wall tension are not practical in the intact human; fortunately, there is excellent correlation between $M\dot{V}O_2$ and the easily derived product of heart rate and systolic blood pressure.[21] The rate-pressure product is a reliable index of the myocardial perfusion requirement in normal persons as well as in patients with coronary artery disease,[21] and many patients with chronic stable angina pectoris tend to experience chest pain at a repeatable rate-pressure product.[22]

Because of these changes involved in vigorous exercise, the $M\dot{V}O_2$ increases from about 1.2×10^{-3} ml/100 gm to about 1.9×10^{-3} ml/100 gm per beat. At a normal arterial oxygen content of about 19 ml/dl, and when the fraction of oxygen taken up by the myocardium is essentially unchanged, coronary blood flow must increase from about 60 ml/100 gm at rest to about 240 ml/100 gm during vigorous aerobic exercise.[23] It is apparent that this degree of coronary flow increase may not take place if there is severe or moderately severe obstructive disease of major coronary arteries, and regions of the heart that are adequately perfused at rest may therefore become ischemic during exercise. Exercise stress testing is based on the premise that exercise-induced ischemia may be detected by both subjective and objective means and can be used to make diagnostic inferences.

ISCHEMIA NOT CAUSED BY CORONARY ATHEROSCLEROSIS. In view of the importance of coronary atherosclerosis as a cause of myocardial ischemia, it is easy to overlook other potential causes. Theoretically, pulmonary insufficiency, by inadequately oxygenating the blood, can cause myocardial ischemia. However, the remarkable vasodilating capability of the normal coronary circulation allows precapillary resistance to drop as a means of compensation. The resulting increase in coronary blood flow and the high myocardial capacity for oxygen extraction compared with other tissues explain why this rarely becomes clinically significant. Reduced oxygen transport capacity of the blood, due either to anemia or to carbon monoxide exposure, may occasionally cause myocardial ischemia. More frequently, a marked chronic increase in cardiac loading and secondary cardiac hypertrophy, as in severe aortic valve stenosis or prolonged hypertension, may result in oxygen requirements that exceed the perfusion capacity of even a normal coronary vascular bed. Although none of these conditions is common compared with coronary atherosclerosis, frequently the degree of myocardial hypoperfusion from one of these causes is aggravated by coexisting coronary atherosclerosis.

During maximal or near-maximal exercise, at least as performed in currently employed exercise protocols, myocardial ischemia does not develop if the heart and its coronary arteries are normal and if there is no disorder of oxygen transport.[24] However, these exercise protocols employ progressively increasing levels of exercise, so that each level serves as a warm-up period for the level to come. There is some evidence that normal individuals engaging in sprint-type exercise without adequate warm-up may indeed develop myocardial ischemia.[25] On the other hand, when exercise intensity is increased gradually, not only does the large coronary reserve prevent the development of ischemia when these vessels are normal, but this reserve probably also prevents ischemia when mild or moderate degrees of atherosclerotic obstruction are present. In most studies, correlations of exercise tests with angiograms show that there is a moderately severe or far-advanced degree of coronary atherosclerosis when exertional ischemia is demonstrated.[26–29]

MYOCARDIAL ISCHEMIA DUE TO INSUFFICIENT CORONARY BLOOD FLOW INCREASE. Patients with uncomplicated angina pectoris undertaking treadmill tests usually make the transition from normal function to ischemia in the course of an increase of one stage in the exercise protocol. Since these stages usually produce an increase in the rate-pressure product of approximately 40 per cent, the threshold for manifestation of detectable ischemia probably lies in this range as well.[30] This finding has practical implications with regard to the design of exercise stress protocols, since the incorporation of greater increases in work from one stage to the next would tend to reduce the precision with which one can estimate ischemic threshold. This threshold has important predictive value for appreciating the severity of coronary artery disease and is discussed later in this chapter.

Relationship Between Degree of Coronary Atherosclerosis and Degree of Blood Flow Restriction. Both clinical and laboratory studies confirm the high degree of reserve in normal coronary artery blood flow capacity.[31–33] They indicate that degrees of coronary atherosclerosis that obstruct the lumen up to 50 per cent are unlikely to be responsible for ischemia, even during ordinary (nonmaximal) exertion. The relative insensitivity of physiological tests such as the exercise test for detecting moderate coronary atherosclerosis makes it all the more important to enhance test sensitivity in any way possible. This requires that the degree of exercise stress be of a high order, either maximal or nearly so, and that the means of detecting ischemia be enhanced by the use of multiple modes of observation and multiple high-quality electrocardiographic leads.

CONSEQUENCES OF MYOCARDIAL ISCHEMIA

CHEST DISCOMFORT. This is not as sensitive an indicator of myocardial ischemia as some of the objective indices used,[34, 35] since it occurs only about half as frequently as ST-segment depression.[27] However, when angina pectoris does occur during testing, it is a valuable finding and increases the likelihood that significant coronary artery disease is present.

Accurate differentiation of angina pectoris from chest pain of other origin during the exercise test depends upon careful evaluation of the symptom. True angina is a deep visceral discomfort (pp. 4 and 1316). Patients frequently use the terms "pressure," "squeezing sensation," or "a bursting feeling." They may deny that the sensation is actual pain, preferring to call it an unpleasant or disagreeable feeling. Conversely, a sharp, clearly painful sensation is unlikely to be angina pectoris, especially if it is superficial in location. The classic locations of spontaneous angina pectoris—substernal, interscapular, and anterior cervical—are the same when ischemia is induced by stress testing. Radiation of discomfort to the shoulders, medial aspects of the arms, elbows, and (less commonly) forearms and hands, and up the neck into the mandible is also found in stress testing. Nonanginal pain is usually located elsewhere, in the right hemithorax or in the left midclavicular line at the level of the 4th through the 6th interspaces without any central component. The time-intensity course of discomfort helps in its identification. Angina that occurs during diagnostic exercise testing with progressively increasing workload will increase in severity until termination of exercise. "Walk-through angina" may occur with steady mild exercise but is most unlikely during stress testing. Nonanginal chest pain frequently fails to increase and may even improve or disappear with continued exercise. Hot, or sometimes cold, discomfort in a bandlike pattern across the sternum is likely to be an angina equivalent if the time-intensity characteristic is appropriate. A full description of any chest discomfort and its distinguishing characteristics should be recorded and evaluated as part of every exercise test.

ST-SEGMENT DISPLACEMENT. Occurrence and disappearance of negative displacement of a flat or downward-sloping ST segment corresponding to the application and termination of exercise stress has been a hallmark of ischemia since introduction of the exercise test (p. 229). Positive, or upward, displacement of the ST segment occurs less commonly. Negative ST-segment displacement is probably the result of subendocardial ischemia (p. 203), and ST-segment elevation is probably due to subepicardial or transmural ischemia (p. 203). In both cases the ST-segment deviation has a specific vector direction in contrast with the ST-segment elevation of acute pericarditis (p. 229), which is found in most leads of the ECG and is present at rest and usually not altered by exercise. It is not always appreciated that coronary atherosclerosis is not the only cause of subendocardial ischemia. Poor oxygen delivery for any reason, coronary arterial spasm (p. 1228), and high left ventricular pressure from any cause may also result in myocardial ischemia and displacement of the ST segment. Nearly all of these causes may be readily detected. Unfortunately, displacement of the ST segment sometimes occurs in the absence of any known cause of ischemia and behaves equivocally when certain drugs such as digitalis are present.[36]

ARRHYTHMIAS. An additional diagnostic problem is the interpretation of cardiac arrhythmias, particularly ventricular extrasystoles, which occur or increase during exercise. Ischemia is one cause of arrhythmias, yet the nonspecific nature of this finding, if it occurs without any other clear evidence of ischemia, has made the presence or absence of exertional arrhythmias almost useless in diagnostic stress testing. It is true that the statistical probability of developing coronary heart disease is approximately three times greater in otherwise healthy men with exertional ventricular arrhythmias, but how this should affect management of the individual patient is by no means clear.[37] On the other hand, ventricular arrhythmias accompanying ST-segment depression or in the post-myocardial infarction patient carry a much more serious prognosis than ST-segment depression occurring as an isolated finding.[38]

REDUCTION IN MAXIMAL CARDIAC PUMP FUNCTION. In patients without orthopedic deformity or a systemic illness which may limit exercise capacity and without valvular heart disease, myocarditis, or cardiomyopathy, the inability to sustain a normal peak level of cardiac work, as reflected in the heart rate–systolic pressure product, suggests significant coronary artery obstruction.[39] Also, patients who develop transient pump failure, as reflected in a drop in blood pressure at a low or moderate level of exercise, usually have advanced coronary obstruction.[40] Lastly, inability to continue the progressively increasing exercise of a graded treadmill or bicycle test protocol for a normal time is an important sign of myocardial ischemia when other possible causes have been excluded.[41]

When exercise induces ischemia that is "global," i.e., when the entire left ventricle or a large portion of it becomes ischemic as a result of widespread coronary atherosclerosis, many aspects of cardiac function are compromised. But the issue becomes more complex when ischemia is regional and affects primarily a single portion of the left ventricle. In this case, nonischemic portions of myocardium may have the contractility to compensate for local deterioration of function, and external measurement of blood pressure and heart rate, the electrocardiogram, and the degree of work endurance may not reflect the abnormality. This may occur in the presence of localized stenosis of a minority of the coronary vessels and branches and in the presence of localized and well-healed infarction.

TYPES OF EXERCISE TESTS

Exercise tests are used in two distinctly different settings: the noninvasive cardiovascular laboratory in the

TABLE 8–2 USES OF EXERCISE TESTING

IN THE NONINVASIVE LABORATORY
Detect and evaluate ischemia by ECG and other means
Measure aerobic capacity to estimate prognosis of coronary heart disease
Evaluate left ventricular performance during exercise by echocardiography, gated blood pool scintigraphy, or other indirect techniques
Detect and measure ischemia by ^{201}Tl scintigraphy
Evaluate functional capacity as a guide to timing surgical replacement of diseased valves
Evaluate effects of surgical treatment of congenital heart disease and coronary heart disease
Measure physical fitness and effects of athletic training in normal individuals and diseased patients
IN THE CATHETERIZATION LABORATORY
Evaluate valve gradients at high flow rates
Determine the effects of exercise on:
cardiac shunts, intravascular and intracardiac pressures, global and regional ventricular function, coronary blood flow, myocardial metabolism

hospital or physician's office and the one in the cardiac catheterization laboratory. The objectives of exercise testing in these two settings differ considerably (Table 8–2).

In the catheterization laboratory, a major constraint is the necessity of having the subject lie on an x-ray–equipped catheterization table. Surgical drapes and other practical considerations usually prohibit use of the patient's arms for exercise, leaving leg-pedaling ergometer exercise in the supine position as the most practical means of stressing the circulation. Circulatory stress is proportional to the mass of exercising muscle, so use of the legs, involving the large hamstring and quadriceps femoris muscle groups, is desirable. On the other hand, maximal body $\dot{V}O_2$ and cardiac output in the supine position are lower than those attainable in the erect position.[42] Although absence of the restraint of gravity on venous return improves venous inflow to the heart and results in larger stroke volumes than in the erect position, ventilation is less efficient in augmenting venous return because the diaphragm is more cephalad in the recumbent position. Fortunately, most research and diagnostic studies that employ exercise in the catheterization laboratory do not require maximal or near-maximal exercise. Measurements made at rest and at two or more progressive levels of exercise allow the construction of a work-response relationship. Whether this involves regulation of coronary blood flow or the hydrodynamic resistance of a valve, useful information can be obtained at submaximal exercise levels.

RELATIONSHIP OF WORKING MUSCLE MASS TO CIRCULATORY STRESS. The distribution of work among skeletal muscles affects hemodynamic performance. Any specified amount of work is done most efficiently when the largest muscle mass is employed. Thus 300 kpm/min of pedaling work can be performed with the least rise in the rate-pressure product when it is performed by both legs. If performed by a single leg, the rate-pressure product will be higher and even higher when the work is performed by both arms or a single arm.[42] This relationship also holds true for isometric work. The lowest rate-pressure product for any level of work is obtained when a weight is carried on the back, and the greatest rise in rate-pressure product occurs when the same weight is carried in one hand.[43]

CHOICE OF EXERCISE MODE. Factors determining the choice of exercise mode are the type of data to be collected, the type of subjects or patients to be studied, the familiarity of the subjects with the various exercise devices, and the intensity of cardiovascular stress intended. When measurement of *maximal exercise capacity* is intended, a motor-driven treadmill or bicycle ergometer in the upright position should be chosen.

Treadmill. The motor-driven treadmill permits the highest oxygen consumption rate of any common exercise device, since it involves both legs, the torso, and both arms. In contrast to electronically controlled bicycle ergometers, treadmills can be calibrated without resort to any special instrumentation. External control of the work rate can be attained with a minimum of subject cooperation. Conversely, the work rate in the step test and with the mechanical bicycle ergometer is controlled almost entirely by the subject; when the subject becomes tired, adherence to a standard work rate with the latter devices becomes progressively more difficult. Although the controlled bicycle ergometer maintains work rate by increasing its resistance in proportion to decreasing pedal velocity, this may produce a surprising and threatening aspect to the subject, who may thus discontinue exercise short of the work rate attainable with a more familiar device.

With the treadmill, active persons and sedentary ones can attain their maximal oxygen consumption even with untrained legs and knees. The only disadvantages of the treadmill are that it is expensive, noisy, and demanding of space. Electrocardiographic recordings during treadmill exercise are moderately distorted, owing to both myographic artifact and the bouncing effect of soft tissues with each step. Finally, treadmill exercise is *not* suitable for studies requiring a relatively immobile thorax, such as those involving indwelling vascular catheters or sensitive precordial detectors such as echocardiographs or scintillation cameras. Often measurements are made immediately *after* rather than *during* exercise.

Bicycle Ergometer. The upright bicycle ergometer excels in providing undistorted ECG's. With this it is possible for the subject to maintain the thorax immobile long enough for sensitive precordial measurements—even phonocardiograms—to be recorded during exercise. Intravascular catheters may be kept in place, expired air may be collected easily, and with perseverance both echocardiographic and scintigraphic observations may be made. Mechanical bicycle ergometers cost much less than do electronically regulated ones. All types are quieter than treadmills and require only one-third to one-half the space. Their main disadvantages are that they are unfamiliar to many adults (a situation which is now improving) and that they depend on subject cooperation in order to maintain a constant work rate in following a specific protocol.

TIME COURSE OF EXERCISE INTENSITY. The pattern of exercise intensity should be determined by the purpose of testing and the characteristics of the population to be tested. If the testing is to determine minimal qualification standards for some activity, such as participation in a school sports program or qualification for a certain industrial task, the test may be limited to a fixed duration of exercise, with the intensity chosen appropriately.

Single-Level vs. Multilevel Tests. If the group to be tested is fairly homogeneous in exercise capacity, the exercise test may consist of a single level of exercise suitable for that group. In selecting an exercise test suitable for a wide range of subjects—from sedentary elderly subjects to vigorous younger ones—it is apparent that no single level of exercise would provide suitable stress in each case. For this reason in the setting of industrial or sports medicine the ability to attain and maintain a certain arbitrary level of work intensity may be important to measure, but in clinical cardiology the aim most often is

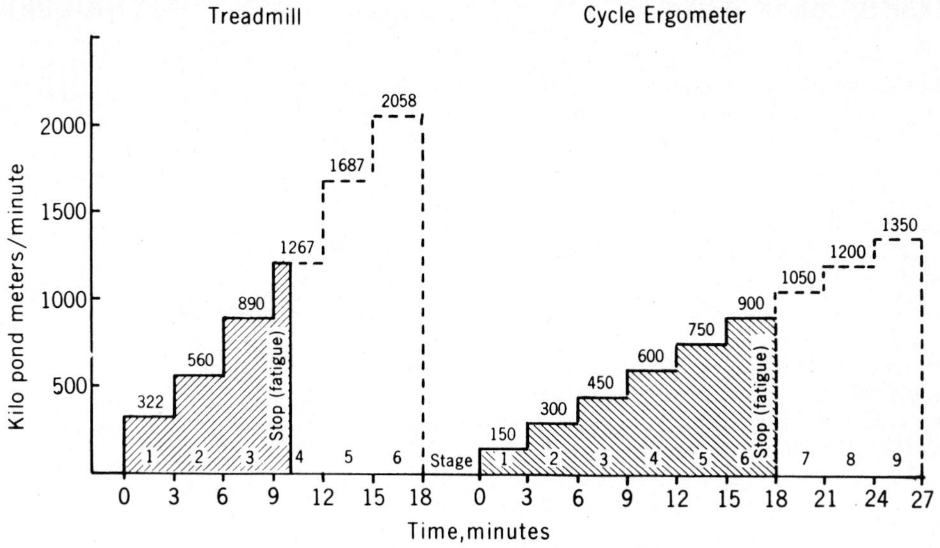

FIGURE 8–1. Comparison of external work performed by a 70-kg man in two stress test protocols. Rate of energy output in kilopond-meters/minute developed by a 50-year-old 70-kg man performing a graded exercise test on a treadmill (*left*) and on a cycle ergometer (*right*). The ergometer is calibrated as the product of distance traversed and resistance. External treadmill work is somewhat more complicated: 70-kg (body weight) = treadmill speed (meters/min) = treadmill grade (%) = body mass = rate of climb (kpm/min). Maximal work intensity is reached in about half the time on the treadmill compared with the ergometer, and the maximal work output is slightly higher on the treadmill as are the maximal oxygen consumption and maximal heart rates.

to detect and quantitate the ischemic threshold and maximal exercise capacity. In the physiology laboratory these levels may be identified by a progressive series of fixed level tests, with rest and recovery after each one.[42] However, this is neither practical nor necessary in the clinical setting, where exercise test protocols are dominated by graded or progressive increases in work rate with time. The initial work rate is low enough for the least able subject, and the progression continues until work rates suitable for the most vigorous subject have been reached (Fig. 8–1). In such a progressive test the highest stage completed gives an indication of that subject's functional capacity. The duration of each interval depends upon whether it is intended that the subject reach a circulatory and respiratory steady state in each stage before going on to the next. This requires about 5 or 6 minutes for most subjects. Since exercise tests that last longer than about 20 minutes introduce the possibility of fatigue and internal heat burden, thereby complicating the measurement of functional capacity, the use of stages of 6 minutes' duration would permit only three or four different levels of exercise. A practical compromise involves using stages of 3 minutes' duration, permitting five different exercise intensity levels which may be spaced more closely in terms of work rate and thus may be more precise in measuring maximal functional capacity. The widely used Bruce treadmill protocol is an example of such a test.[44]

Another approach is to employ small increases in work intensity in stages so brief that the rate of work increase is virtually continuous, and the concept of circulatory steady state is set aside entirely. Although such protocols are not well adapted for time-consuming measurements such as oxygen consumption or cardiac output, they can offer a precise measurement of maximal functional capacity. The Balke-Ware test, with stages only 1 minute in duration, is an example of this approach.[45]

Termination of Exercise: Open-Ended vs. Closed-Ended Tests. Regardless of which exercise protocol is used, exercise should always be terminated upon recognition of any evidence that further exercise may be harmful to the subject. This evidence includes certain arrhythmias and other electrocardiographic changes, a drop in blood pressure, and incoordination of gait. Other such safety considerations are discussed on p. 238. Tests that are terminated, usually by the subject, before a scheduled endpoint is arrived at or before diagnostic evidence of disease is apparent should be reported as incomplete. For terminating exercise, tests may be considered open ended (symptom limited) or close ended (fixed level). In open-ended tests, the duration of the test is determined by the reaction of the subject to exercise, and work is continued until a certain degree of reaction has taken place. Close-ended tests, generally milder in intensity, are continued for a certain fixed period (for example, the 3-minute double two-step test). Of the open-ended tests, three distinct choices are in common use for termination of exercise: (1) exercise to a variable heart rate, such as 90 per cent of predicted maximal,[46] (2) exercise to symptom-limited maximum tolerance,[44] and (3) exercise to physiologically documented maximal aerobic capacity.[47]

Exercise to an Individualized Heart Rate. Exercise to 90 per cent (or some other relatively high percentage) of estimated maximal heart rate has the advantage of avoiding the discomfort of all-out maximal exercise while retaining test sensitivity by presenting nearly maximal stress to persons of all ages. The highest heart rate anyone can attain during exercise gradually decreases with age. There is a moderate amount of individual variation, one standard deviation of maximal heart rate being about 10 beats/min[48, 49] (Table 8–3). Additionally, it has been found that persons actively engaged in athletics have maximal heart rates that are about 7 beats/min lower than physically untrained subjects of the same age.[48] Finally, the regression of maximal heart rate with age differs slightly between the sexes.[49] Thus by taking age, sex, and physical training into account, it is possible to arrive at a target heart rate that is approximately 90 per cent of maximal for that subject. Unfortunately, there are many drugs now in common use which alter heart rate response to exercise and render the target heart rate endpoint useless. Also, some patients have degenerative disease of the sinoatrial node, which restricts its cardioaccelerative response to exercise ("chronotropic incompetence"). For these reasons

TABLE 8–3 PREDICTED MAXIMAL HEART RATE RANGES DURING GRADED EXERCISE TESTING*

AGE (YEARS)	35	45	55	65
Predicted maximal heart rate range				
Men	167–191	163–187	158–182	154–178
Women	161–185	153–177	144–168	135–159

*Applicable only in the absence of beta-adrenoceptor blockers or other heart rate–altering drugs.

the target heart rate endpoint can no longer be considered the choice for general application.

Post-Myocardial Infarction Exercise Testing. Exercise testing is frequently performed just before the discharge from the hospital of acute myocardial infarction patients, in order to identify those who are at increased risk and thus who may need additional treatment (p. 236). Such testing can also identify low-risk patients who may safely follow an accelerated convalescence and return to work early. Early testing is indicated when this information can be applied beneficially to the patient's management. Predischarge exercise testing is *contraindicated* in the patient with persistent ventricular arrhythmias, any evidence of cardiac failure, or recurrent ischemia.

In the recent post-myocardial infarction patient, the modified treadmill stages zero and one-half (or similarly low work levels in other protocols) are employed, and exercise is usually terminated at 70 or 75 per cent of predicted maximal heart rate or at the onset of effort intolerance. Test interpretation is based upon evidence of ischemia and degree of exercise tolerance. The very low-risk category consists of patients able to exercise to the specified heart rate or to the point of normal fatigue and breathlessness without manifesting either ST-segment depression or angina pectoris. Intermediate-risk patients are those demonstrating transient ischemia but normal exercise tolerance; high-risk patients are those showing evidence of ischemia at a low heart rate or exercise level.[50, 51]

Subjective Maximal Exercise. Subjective maximal exercise testing is easiest to define. The person simply exercises in a standardized work pattern until unable to continue because of intolerable fatigue, dyspnea, or pain. The high level of circulatory stress provided by maximal exercise makes it possible to demonstrate exertional cardiac ischemia in some cases in patients in whom lower levels of exercise would have been insufficient to expose it. At any unaccustomed level of exercise there is some slight danger of precipitating circulatory arrest or myocardial infarction. On the basis of reported instances, however, the frequency of this complication is reassuringly low.[52, 53]

The subjective nature of the endpoint for this test naturally raises the question of whether all subjects stress themselves to the same degree or whether the more timid ones may tolerate appreciably less fatigue or discomfort than more determined subjects. However, the added predictive value of documenting the subjective maximal exercise capacity far outweighs any disadvantage of added exercise time or test variability. This variability may be reduced by close observation of the subject for evidence of vigorous consistent effort, and use of encouragement and reassurance in order to attain a convincingly high exercise peak.

DOCUMENTED MAXIMAL AEROBIC CAPACITY. Exercise to physiologically documented maximal aerobic capacity is a highly valuable investigative tool in work physiology. Typically, interrupted tests of fixed duration are employed with measurement of oxygen uptake at each stage. A level of work will finally be found at which the oxygen uptake reaches a plateau, and the least amount of exercise that clearly demonstrates such a plateau represents maximal aerobic exercise. Any exercise greater than this represents supramaximal or sprint-type exercise which can be supported only briefly on an anaerobic basis. This type of testing and its application to the study of patients with possible impaired pump function is discussed on p. 234.

TECHNIQUES OF EXERCISE TESTING

An appropriate cardiovascular history and physical examination should be performed prior to the exercise test. The subject should be tested either after an overnight fast or no earlier than 2 hours after a light meal. The patient should be informed of the indications for the test, the details of its procedure, and the potential hazards of testing, and should sign a consent form. The sites for the four "limb-lead" electrodes and the six precordial electrodes should be marked and prepared with acetone and mild dermabrasion. The Mason-Likar limb lead modification is recommended[54] (Fig. 8–2). Care should be taken to locate arm electrodes properly near the shoulders and not near the sternum in order to obtain accurate "limb" leads.[55] A 12-lead resting electrocardiogram must be recorded and examined for possible exercise contraindications, such as ischemia and serious ventricular arrhythmias, and the interpretation should be recorded before exercise is begun. A demonstration of appropriate treadmill walking gait should be given, and if the subject has never walked on a treadmill, a brief trial of walking should be undertaken. During and after exercise, leads V_2, V_5, and aVF should be displayed continuously on a monitor scope, and once every minute a 12-lead ECG should be recorded. Blood pressure should be measured before exercise, at least once near the end of each exercise stage, and every 2 minutes after exercise until stable.

SPECIFIC PROTOCOLS. Exercise is carried out on a motor-driven treadmill following a standardized protocol. For general diagnostic testing of ambulatory individuals, the Bruce[44] and Naughton[56] protocols are the most popular. For early post-myocardial infarction testing, the *modified* Bruce and the Naughton tests are preferred (Table 8–4). During exercise the patient is carefully and continuously observed, noting facial expression, tone of voice, manner of walking, and use of handrails (lightly touching with the fingertips or not touching at all). The subject is questioned frequently concerning the development and intensity of symptoms, and the time of appearance of chest pain or other important symptoms is recorded. The Borg scale of perceived exercise intensity may be useful for approximate quantitation of the subject's tolerance of each stage of exercise. A poster with a scale of numbers ranging from 6 (mildest degree of exercise) to 20 (absolute maximal severity of exercise) is displayed in front of the treadmill, and near the end of each stage the subject is asked to select a

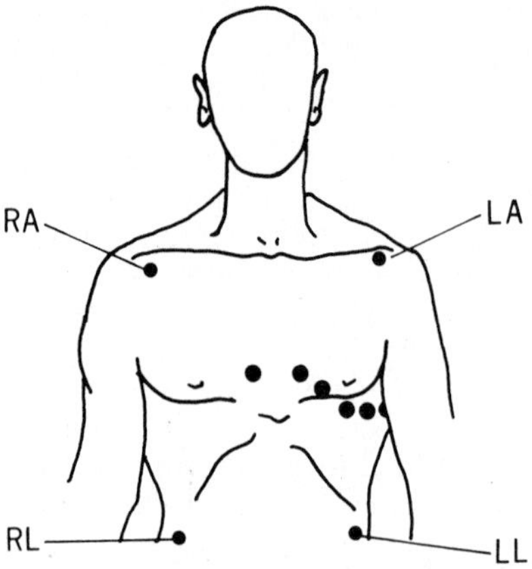

FIGURE 8–2. Locations of electrodes for the Mason-Likar modification for obtaining the 12-lead electrocardiogram during exercise. In order to achieve diagnostic quality of limb leads, the right arm and left arm electrodes must be located in the lateralmost aspects of the infraclavicular fossae. Locations of the precordial electrodes are conventional.

TABLE 8–4 TREADMILL EXERCISE TEST PROTOCOLS

Stage	Duration (min)	Speed (mph)	Grade %	Approx. $\dot{V}o_2$ (ml/kg/min)	Mets
		Bruce Protocol*			
0*	3	1.7	0	8	2.0
½*	3	1.7	5	12	3.1
1	3	1.7	10	18	4.8
2	3	2.5	12	25	6.8
3	3	3.4	14	34	9.6
4	3	4.2	16	46	13.2
5	3	5.0	18	55	16.1
6	3	5.5	20		
7	3	6.0	22		
		Naughton Protocol			
1	2	3	0	10	2.5
2	2	3	2.5	14	3.5
3	2	3	5	18	4.7
4	2	3	7.5	21	5.6
5	2	3	10	24	6.4
6	2	3	12.5	28	7.5
7	2	3	15	32	8.7
8	2	3	17.5	35	9.5
9	2	3	20	38	10.7
10	2	3	22.5	42	11.9

*Sheffield modification: begin at stage 0. Original Bruce: begin at stage 1.

number which represents the intensity of that stage.[57] This is useful in cardiac rehabilitation programs involving periodic retesting, but the author has not found it to be helpful in the diagnostic stress testing laboratory. Exercise is continued by the subject until terminated because of the appearance and excessive progression of symptoms, exhaustion, or development of marked ST-segment deviation or significant ventricular arrhythmia. Nonischemic responses are classified "incomplete" if the subject did not put forth a convincingly vigorous effort. Ischemic responses are deemed valid at any degree of effort.

In the postexercise period, the sitting position is employed because of the discomfort often caused by lying supine and still after maximal exercise. Cardiac auscultation should be carried out as quickly as possible in order to detect exercise-induced mitral regurgitation, atrial or ventricular gallops, or rales. Brief pulmonary auscultation for rales and wheezes is also worthwhile. Observation after exercise should continue for 6 minutes or until all exercise-induced abnormalities have disappeared. Exercise testing should be supervised by a physician trained in the procedure, and the exercise laboratory should be equipped and organized for patient safety, as described on p. 238. If significant ST-segment depression develops during or after testing, it must be determined whether this is attributable to hyperventilation or is probably due to myocardial ischemia. After the subject's heart rate, blood pressure, and respiratory rate have fully recovered from the exercise, the subject is requested to hyperventilate maximally for 2 minutes, after which the 12-lead ECG is repeated. If this maneuver reproduces the ST-segment depression, the exertional ST-segment depression may not be classed ischemic. In such a case one would expect blood pressure response and treadmill endurance time to be approximately normal. The authors prefer not to perform hyperventilation testing on all subjects before exercise because of its possible effect on the exercise test and because most test results are nonischemic and do not require the maneuver.

EXERCISE ELECTROCARDIOGRAPHY

TYPES OF ST-SEGMENT DISPLACEMENT. When myocardial perfusion is inadequate to meet the increased oxygen requirements during exercise, it is the subendocardium that becomes ischemic, since its perfusion is most precarious. As a consequence, a diastolic injury potential is produced characterized by a vector that is opposite in direction to the major QRS vector; hence there is ST-segment depression in leads with dominant R waves. Displacement of the ST segment caused by exercise, like that produced by angina at rest, is generally of three types. The most common type is a displacement beginning at the QRS-ST junction which is downward or negative in polarity and which is followed by an initially upsloping ST segment as it merges into the T wave.[58] As exercise progresses and presumably as ischemia also progresses, the degree of J-point depression increases and the ST segment becomes less and less upsloping. In its most characteristic form the ST segment becomes entirely flat for the first 80 msec of its duration and with further change may actually become negative or downsloping.

As an interpretive criterion, the development of 0.10 mv (1 mm) or more of flat ST-segment displacement in a standard electrocardiographic lead which persists 1 minute or longer after exercise is commonly considered indicative of ischemia. This is a conservative balance between sensitivity to detect ischemia and specificity to avoid false-positive results. At one time 0.05 mv (0.5 mm) ST displacement was used as a criterion of ischemia, and although the number of patients with obstructive coronary artery disease who were missed was small, the number of normal persons who shared this response was excessive, i.e., there were few false-negatives but many false-positives (high sensitivity, low specificity). Others have required 0.20 mv (2 mm) ST displacement for an ischemic response. This reduces the number of patients with positive tests who do not have ischemic heart disease but misses many patients with documented coronary obstruction; there were few false-positives but many false-negatives (low sensitivity, high specificity).

Other types of electrocardiographic leads (bipolar leads or Frank leads) have sensitivities different from the standard leads, warranting different criteria of ischemia. ST displacement of 0.20 mv (2 mm) is a logical and frequently used criterion for bipolar leads. The corresponding value for Frank leads would lie between 0.05 and 0.10 mv (0.5 to 1 mm) and in practice has not been defined adequately. Hollenberg has found that a diagnostic treadmill score is improved when ST segment amplitude is multiplied by 12/R wave amplitude (mm).[59]

When we consider that the spectrum of ischemic ST-segment displacement varies from zero to nearly the amplitude of the QRS in some patients, it is apparent that any criterion used is arbitrary, dictated partly by the recording format and partly by the desire for an optimal compromise between the ability to detect disease and to reject nondisease. The nature of the ST segment displacement has been categorized into several types.

An important feature of the first type of ischemic response is its quick disappearance early in the postexercise period (Fig. 8–3, Type I). The brevity of this response makes it almost impossible to detect unless electrocardiographic recording and display are carried out during exercise and continued without interruption into the immediate postexercise period.

The second most frequent ST-displacement response begins during exercise, but instead of immediate improvement with termination of exercise, the response becomes progressively more abnormal for several seconds or minutes following exercise (Fig. 8–3, Type II). During the postexercise period there is additional negative displacement of the flat or downsloping ST, which is frequently but not always associated with chest discomfort. In most

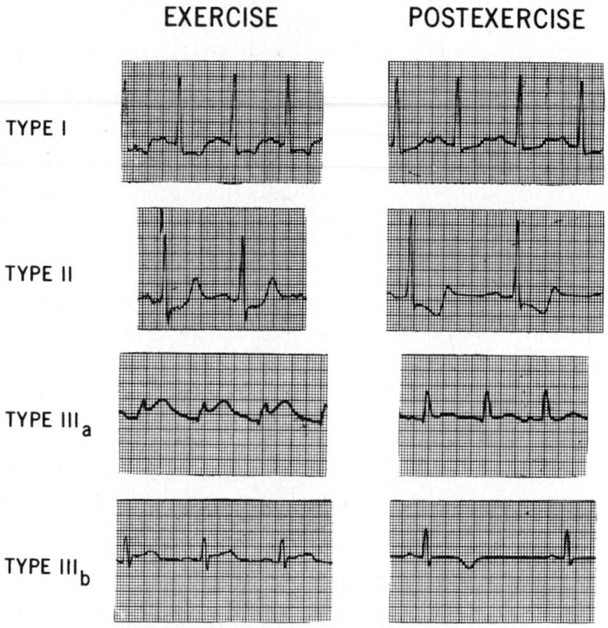

FIGURE 8–3. Types of exertional ST-segment displacement:
I: Transient depression during exercise that has virtually disappeared 1 minute after exercise.
II: Depression during exercise that becomes more pronounced after exercise before belatedly returning to normal.
IIIa: ST elevation characteristic of Prinzmetal's angina.
IIIb: ST elevation of modest degree usually caused by dyskinesis or scarring of the left ventricle.

cases this protracted response shows an evolutionary pattern in the course of returning to normal, developing a downsloping ST segment with upward convexity and merging into an inverted T wave. Usually from 5 to 20 minutes is required for the T wave to become fully upright thereafter and for the ST segment to return fully to its preexercise isoelectric contour. It is thought that the degree of ST-segment shift reflects the severity of myocardial ischemia, whereas the degree of coronary obstruction responsible for ischemia is inversely related to the amount of exercise stress required to provoke ischemia and directly related to the duration of ST-segment depression after exercise, once ischemia is provoked. Thus transient ST depression (Type I) occurring only with vigorous exercise would represent a minor deviation in prognosis from normal, whereas protracted ST depression (Type II) provoked only by mild exercise would constitute a major prognostic abnormality, such as usually caused by severe multivessel or left main coronary artery disease.

The least common positive ST-segment response, occurring in only 3 to 5 per cent of most series, consists of ST-segment elevation rather than depression. At least two mechanisms can be responsible for ST-segment elevation. Intense, localized transmural ischemia may be produced in Prinzmetal's variant angina by spastic occlusion of a single major coronary vessel. Although transmural ischemia caused by coronary spasm characteristically occurs at rest, there is now substantial evidence that it can be provoked by exercise as well[60] (p. 1197). Similar intense localized ischemia may be provoked by exercise (Fig. 8–3, Type IIIa). This type of response, when severe, usually distorts the QRS complex as well, causing the QRST configuration to resemble temporarily a directly recorded monophasic action potential. This response usually goes through a phase of T-wave inversion in the process of disappearing.

A second kind of ST-segment elevation response has been described (Fig. 8–3, Type IIIb). This is most frequently found in leads II, III, and aVf, reflecting the diaphragmatic surface of the left ventricle. This type of ST-segment elevation does not distort the QRS complex, is not followed by the evolutionary pattern of T-wave inversion during its improvement and disappearance, and has been related to the presence of scarring or dyskinesia due to preexisting disease rather than to temporary ischemia of otherwise normal myocardium.[61] Alternatively, it is possible that during exercise, as a greater quantity of myocardium becomes ischemic and akinetic, the larger noncontractile mass of myocardium behaves like a ventricular aneurysm, producing ST-segment elevation.

Junctional ST Depression. Depression of the QRS-ST junction (J) during exercise occurs in normal persons, although usually not more than 0.20 mv (2 mm). When this occurs, an upsloping depression of the ST segment results. Unfortunately, the ischemic ST-segment response goes through this phase in the process of approaching flat or downsloping ST-segment depression. In order to differentiate this reaction from normal, the exercise should, if possible, be continued to a higher level so a clearly ischemic response may evolve in patients with ischemia, while the ST segment remains steeply upsloping in the normal person. Thus, with respect to the ST-segment slope with exercise, there are three levels of prognostic significance: a steeply upsloping ST segment (normal), a gently upsloping one (probably abnormal), and a flat or downsloping ST segment (definitely abnormal).[62] As with ST-displacement criteria, any division between these levels will be arbitrary, but the authors have found it useful to consider slopes greater than 1 mv/sec (40 per cent slope when paper speed is 25 mm/sec) normal and those 0 to 1 mv/sec probably abnormal. Another useful rule of thumb is that an upsloping ST segment may be considered abnormal when the ST segment is depressed by 1.5 mm or more at 0.06 sec after the J-point.[63]

The possibility that exertional R wave amplitude changes could aid in the detection of ischemia has been suggested,[64] but extensive study has established the lack of diagnostic utility of this finding.[65, 66]

RECORDING ELECTROCARDIOGRAPHIC EFFECTS OF ISCHEMIA. As discussed on p. 203, subendocardial ischemia ordinarily produces not ST-segment depression but rather T-P-QRS elevation.[61, 67] Since clinical electrocardiographs are not direct-coupled and thus are insensitive to direct-current voltages, it is not possible to distinguish between true depression of one portion of the electrocardiogram, such as the ST segment, and true elevation of every other portion of the electrocardiogram, such as the T-P-Q segment. It is only by means of direct-coupled recorders connected to the exposed heart that the true nature of an ST displacement can be established. Although it is helpful to understand the true electrical alteration caused by ischemia, it continues to be impractical (if not impossible) to record and measure true shifts in the T-P-Q segment "baseline" by body surface recordings with conventional instruments. *Ischemic ST-segment depression* is a term widely used in this chapter even though it may be technically incorrect or only partially correct.

THE ELECTRODE-SKIN INTERFACE. It has long been recognized by electrocardiographers and electroencephalographers that a nonmetallic electrolyte interface must be interposed between the skin and the metal recording electrode in order to minimize recording artifacts.[68]

In 1959 a quick, painless, and effective means of reducing skin impedance for recording purposes was described.[69] The author's adaptation of this method involves the use of a No. 6 spherical dental burr inserted into a variable-speed hobby grinding tool.* When rotating at an intermediate speed and touched lightly to the skin (2 to 5 gm pressure) for 1 second, a pinhead-sized area of cornified epithelium is abraded without pain or bleeding. An exercise electrocardiographic electrode applied over this spot, or alternatively over an area prepared

*Such as a Dremel Moto-tool, model 380.

by lightly rubbing with fine sandpaper and scrubbing with acetone, will have a contact impedance of 1 to 5 kilohms instead of the 10 to 50 kilohms usually obtained without any kind of dermabrasion.

Disposable silver–silver chloride electrodes are best, but stainless steel electrodes are satisfactory if the active surface is maintained properly. The cable that connects the electrodes to the recorder should be shielded, preferably all the way to the electrode, to reduce power-line artifact. The cable should be thin, light, and compliant and should introduce no electrical potential of its own when flexed or agitated. Some exercise electrocardiographic systems contain preamplifier circuits located at the patient end of the cable. This virtually eliminates the problem of power-line artifact while only slightly increasing the bulk of the cable system carried by the subject.

ELECTROCARDIOGRAPHIC LEADS FOR DETECTION OF ISCHEMIA. There is not uniform agreement on the number of electrocardiographic leads required for optimal exercise electrocardiography. The ready availability of automatic three-channel electrocardiographs makes it easier to record a 12-lead sequence than it would be to select any lesser number of leads individually. A combination of 12 conventional leads and 2 bipolar leads gives greater sensitivity than 12 leads alone.[70]

Bipolar electrocardiographic leads were popularized during the era when it was thought that radiotelemetry was necessary to overcome the technical problems of recording the exercise electrocardiogram. The miniature radio transmitters used for this purpose could accept only a bipolar input signal, so this was derived by placing an active electrode over the V_5 position, where the electrocardiographic signal is strongest, and a reference electrode somewhere on the right side of the chest. Various positions for the reference electrode became standardized (Fig. 8–4). On the basis of current evidence the recommended choice of exercise electrocardiographic leads is the conventional 12-lead set using torso (Mason-Likar) locations for limb leads (Fig. 8–2). This procedure is easy to follow using an unmodified automatic three-channel electrocardiographic recorder, and the same leads used during and after exercise may be used for the resting control electrocardiogram.

BIOLOGICAL AND PHARMACOLOGICAL EFFECTS. As already noted, ischemic heart disease is only one of several causes of ST-segment depression. The subendocardial region is the most distal tissue perfused by the coronary vasculature, and thus has the lowest perfusion pressure. Yet it is this tissue which is subjected to direct ventricular pressure and thus has the greatest intramural force resisting coronary flow. Therefore any disparity between perfusion requirement and supply, short of total arterial occlusion, will affect the subendocardium first and most profoundly and with increasingly severe hypoperfusion will spread outward.

Pressure Overload. Pressure overload of the left ventricle due to either arterial hypertension or obstruction of

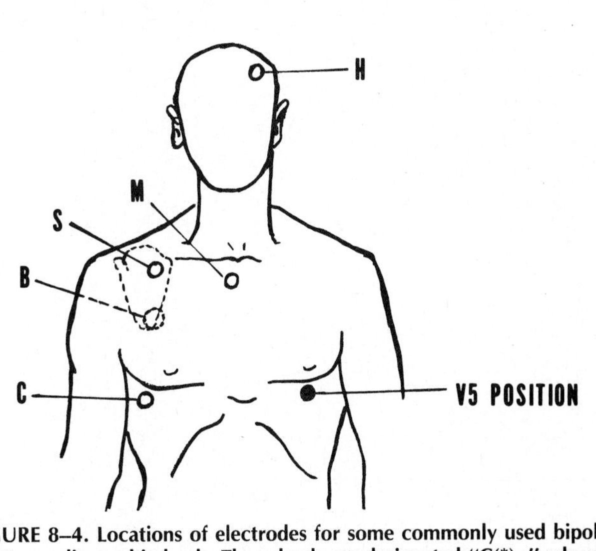

FIGURE 8–4. Locations of electrodes for some commonly used bipolar electrocardiographic leads. These leads are designated "C(*)$_5$," where * is replaced by the letter denoting the negative or reference electrode (e.g., CH_5 indicates that the active electrode is at V_5 and the reference electrode is on the head).

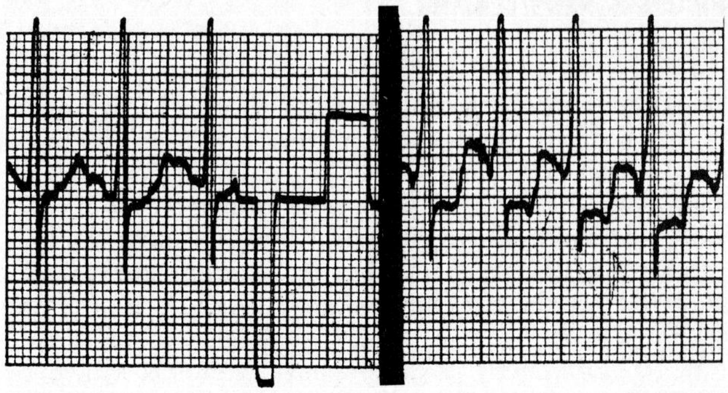

FIGURE 8–5. Wolff-Parkinson-White syndrome conduction disturbance developing during exercise and mimicking ischemic type of ST depression. *Left panel,* Recording immediately prior to disturbance. (Courtesy of I. Martin Grais, M.D.)

ventricular outflow may be expected to interfere with subendocardial perfusion and cause ST depression in the absence of atherosclerosis. In addition, diuretics administered as antihypertensive therapy may lower the serum potassium concentration sufficiently to cause equivocal changes in the exercise ECG. The ability of hypokalemia to confound interpretation of the exercise electrocardiogram has been established.[71] Therefore, when an exercise test is conducted, the operator should be sure that the potassium concentration is normal.

The mechanisms producing the various clinical manifestations of mitral valve prolapse (p. 1048), be they premature beats, chest discomfort, or ST-segment changes, are not fully understood. It is known, however, that patients with this disorder may develop exertional ST-segment depression in the absence of coronary atherosclerosis.[72]

Abnormal Activation Sequence of Ventricles. Abnormal activation sequence of the ventricles, especially the left, alters repolarization and prohibits interpretation of ST-segment changes.[73] This includes not only left bundle branch block but also the Wolff-Parkinson-White syndrome (a subtle cause of a false-positive test if it occurs only during exercise) (Fig. 8–5). Left ventricular ischemia may be recognized in the lateral electrocardiographic leads when right bundle branch block is present, although perhaps with somewhat less sensitivity.[74, 75]

Digitalis Effect. Digitalis is notorious for its effect on the ST segment.[76, 77] Even when the digitalis effect is not apparent in the resting ECG, it still may be responsible for exertional ST-segment depression. This effect persists longer than the half-life of the glycoside in the blood would suggest.[76] Therefore, a conservative policy would be to discontinue digoxin therapy a week before exercise electrocardiography. If glycoside therapy is necessary for its inotropic effect, one should question seriously whether an exercise test is even indicated. No dependable upper limit of digitalis-induced ST-segment displacement has been defined. On the other hand, digitalis does not cause falsely negative responses. Therefore, absence of ST-segment deviation at peak exercise or thereafter in a patient receiving a cardiac glycoside may be considered a valid negative response.

Psychoactive Drugs. Tricyclic and other antidepressant drugs are said to cause false-positive and false-negative responses, especially in women.[14, 78] This effect is not understood and needs additional study. More false-positive exercise electrocardiographic responses are seen in women than in men;[79] this is explained at least in part by the lower incidence of coronary artery disease in women than in men.[14] The author has found that asymptomatic women show exertional ST depression with the same frequency as do asymptomatic men.[48]

Antihypertensives and Vasodilators. Most antihypertensive drugs are not known to have any effect on the exercise ECG, although one study implicated methyldopa,[14] and the effect of kaliuretic diuretics has already been mentioned. Nitroglycerin, nifedipine, and other vasodilators will permit a higher level of exercise performance before the effects of ischemia become apparent. For this reason exercise testing is an objective means of assessing the degree of benefit of a therapeutic regimen. However, drugs will rarely prevent ischemia altogether in a progressive exercise test, and thus they are not a significant source of false-negative exercise results.

Beta-adrenoceptor Blockers. These agents, which are at once antiarrhythmic, antianginal, and antihypertensive, prevent angina by reducing two principal components of the myocardial oxygen requirement: heart rate and contractility. A compensatory increase in stroke volume, a more "oxygen-efficient" means of achieving an increase in cardiac output and an increase in peripheral oxygen extraction combine to permit an increased level of exercise performance. As with nitrate therapy, exercise testing can measure therapeutic benefits. However, if the diagnosis of angina pectoris is in doubt, the beta blocker may be tapered and discontinued and short-acting antianginal therapy (sublingual nitroglycerine) substituted for about 2 days.

EVALUATION OF ELECTROCARDIOGRAPHIC DATA

CONVENTIONAL CRITERIA OF ISCHEMIA. Three important considerations affect clinical interpretation of the electrocardiogram: the time course of ST-segment changes, the effect of lead choice, and the work threshold of ischemia.

Time Course of ST-Segment Changes (Fig. 8–6). The accumulated experience in interpreting the postexercise ECG, indicating that 0.10 mV of ST-segment depression is a critical index of ischemia, does not necessarily apply to tracings recorded during exercise. J-point depression with an upsloping ST segment is a normal response to exercise, and the area overlying the J-ST segment increases in proportion to the tachycardia.[80] However, a J-point depression of sufficient magnitude (≥ 2 mm), during exercise, usually signifies ischemia.[81] Lozner and Morganroth found the specificity of exercise ECG's much improved when a requirement was that 0.20 mv ST depression, appearing in exercise, persist for at least 1 minute after exercise in order to qualify as an ischemic response.[82] Thus a Type I ST-segment response (Fig. 8–3) with depression that persists less than 1 minute after exercise is less specific for coronary artery disease than a Type II response with ST segment depression that persists for 20 minutes. (When disease is present, it is more likely to be single-vessel or mild two-vessel disease.) These findings suggest that 0.10 mV of ST-segment depression may be a sufficient criterion of ischemia *after* exercise, but a larger degree of change—proportional to heart rate—should be required for the tracing recorded during exercise. If the resting 12-lead electrocardiogram shows ST-segment elevation of the "early repolarization" type in the course of exercise, the ST segment normally flattens out and becomes isoelectric. Any postexercise ST-segment depression should be measured from the PR-segment baseline without making any allowance for the preexercise ST-segment elevation.[18]

Effect of Electrocardiographic Lead Choice. Different electrocardiographic leads, which have differing sensitivities for the electrocardiographic waveform, require appropriately different amplitude criteria of ST-segment change. Bipolar leads—CM_5, for instance—show greater QRS amplitude, greater T amplitude, and greater ST-shift amplitude than are found in Wilson lead V_5. Conversely, Frank lead X shows slightly lower waveform amplitude than V_5. These differences in "scale factor," or amplitude sensitivity, should be taken into account in the interpretation. Investigators usually use a 0.20 mV ST-segment shift as a criterion for positivity for bipolar leads. The corresponding ST-segment criterion for Frank lead X would be about 0.08 mV.

Work Threshold of Ischemia. Finally, the intensity of cardiac work at which ischemia occurs is of critical importance.[41, 83] In subjects in whom the ischemia occurs only at normal peak exercise levels, the coronary blood flow is adequate at rest and during most levels of submaximal stress and becomes inadequate only when maximal or near-maximal exercise is undertaken. The high work threshold of ischemia usually reflects moderate coronary obstruction; in contrast, the development of ischemia at a low level of

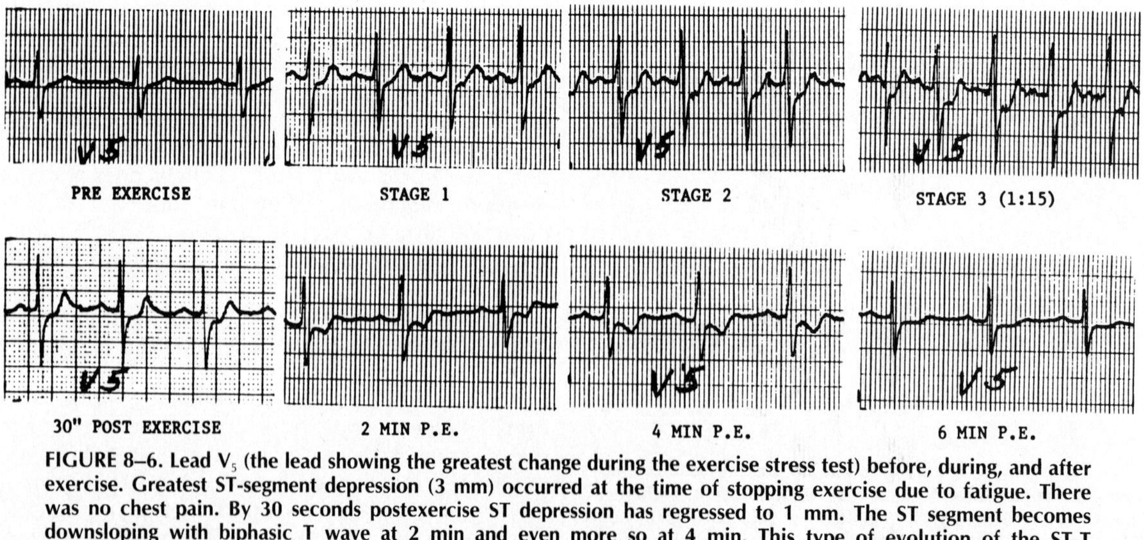

FIGURE 8–6. Lead V_5 (the lead showing the greatest change during the exercise stress test) before, during, and after exercise. Greatest ST-segment depression (3 mm) occurred at the time of stopping exercise due to fatigue. There was no chest pain. By 30 seconds postexercise ST depression has regressed to 1 mm. The ST segment becomes downsloping with biphasic T wave at 2 min and even more so at 4 min. This type of evolution of the ST-T abnormality greatly increases the specificity of the response for ischemia.

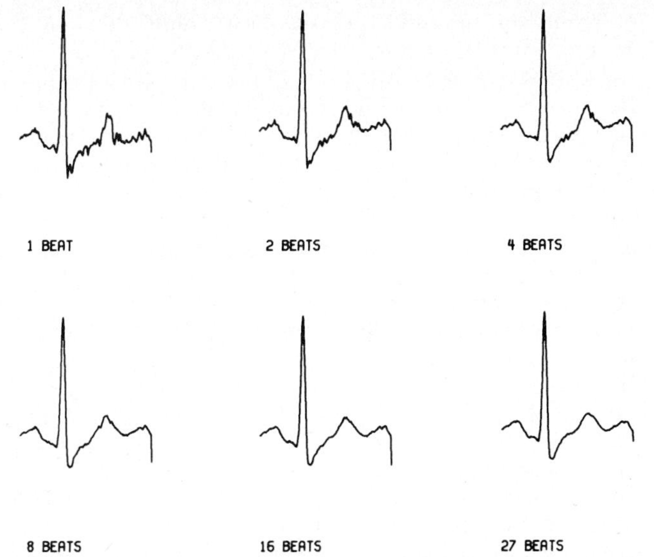

FIGURE 8–7. Reduction of distortion generated by exercise through averaging multiple electrocardiographic complexes by computer. Increasing the number of beats averaged decreases the amount of distortion.

exertion usually reflects severe coronary obstructive disease and indicates a poor prognosis.

Sex Differences in Electrocardiographic Response. Exercise electrocardiographic responses in men correspond more closely than in women with the presence or absence of coronary artery disease.[79] The influence of tranquilizers and other psychoactive drugs in women was mentioned earlier. Perhaps the most important factor explaining the sex difference in test accuracy is the different prevalence of coronary disease in men and women. It is well recognized that the accuracy of any (less than perfect) test is lower in test populations having lower disease prevalence. This effect has been documented in the Coronary Artery Surgery Study, involving tests on 3153 patients.[84] When allowance was made for disease prevalence, men and women demonstrated the same rate of false-positive responses and false-negative ones.

Computer Analysis. Development of ST-segment criteria other than exactly one or two divisions of the chart paper and problems with exercise artifact distortion of the ECG have set the stage for computer enhancement of electrocardiogram interpretation. By computerized averaging of electrocardiographic complexes, myographic and other artifacts are eliminated or reduced (Fig. 8–7). Recognition algorithms identify the points on the electrocardiogram to be measured (Fig. 8–8). Measurements made by computer have the capacity of much greater precision than is possible by visual measurement of conventionally recorded ECG's, and they adapt readily to variations in diagnostic criteria, depending on the phase of the test (control, exercise, or postexercise) and the leads employed. Precise measurement of QRS-duration changes with exercise permitted Ahnve and coworkers to detect prolongation of QRS with exercise in coronary artery disease patients but not in normal subjects.[85] Computerized exercise ECG systems are employed increasingly.

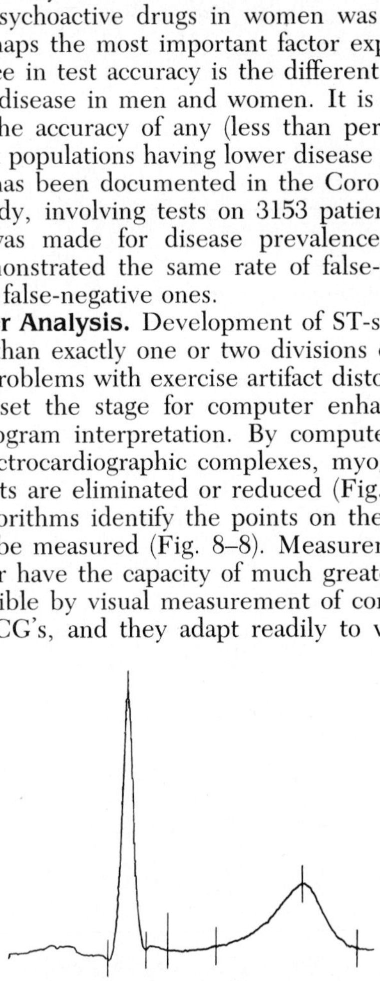

FIGURE 8–8. Fiducial points (V_5 lead) identification and measurements in exercise by EKAP computer program. Note absence of myographic artifact. Vertical recognition lines, from left to right, indicate QRS onset, R peak, S nadir, J point, J point + 80 msec, T peak, and T end.

NONELECTROCARDIOGRAPHIC OBSERVATIONS

Nonelectrocardiographic events in the course of exercise stress testing have been increasingly recognized as equal in importance to, if not more important than, ST-segment changes.[86]

BLOOD PRESSURE. The normal blood pressure response to exercise is a progressive rise in systolic pressure with increase in exercise intensity and very little change in the diastolic pressure. The systolic pressure at peak exercise ranges from 162 to 216 mm Hg. In younger individuals the diastolic pressure may fall slightly, whereas in middle-aged and older adults it is likely to rise.[87] Any rise or fall of diastolic pressure in normal persons is not likely to exceed 10 mm Hg. The resultant rise in mean arterial pressure with exercise reflects the fact that fall of the systemic resistance with exercise is insufficient in itself to allow for the rise in cardiac output. In most exercise protocols the systolic blood pressure rises about 8 to 10 mm Hg per stage (Fig. 8–9). Although in the interest of safety it is reasonable to specify a level of resting blood pressure, such as 180/110 mm Hg, above which exercise testing will not be carried out, in fact there are no reported instances of stroke or other hypertensive complication during diagnostic exercise testing.

A pathological fall in blood pressure during exercise is encountered occasionally, and although an insensitive sign, it is highly specific for severe coronary artery disease.[39, 88] Failure of arterial pressure to rise during exercise reflects an inadequate elevation of cardiac output in the face of vasodilation in exercising muscle. Any condition that severely limits the normal exercise-induced rise in cardiac output—cardiomyopathy, valvular heart disease, or coronary artery disease—is the most common cause of failure of arterial pressure to rise during exercise. In patients with

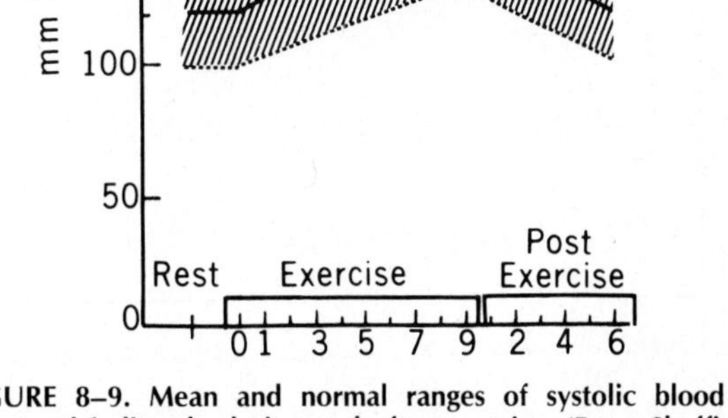

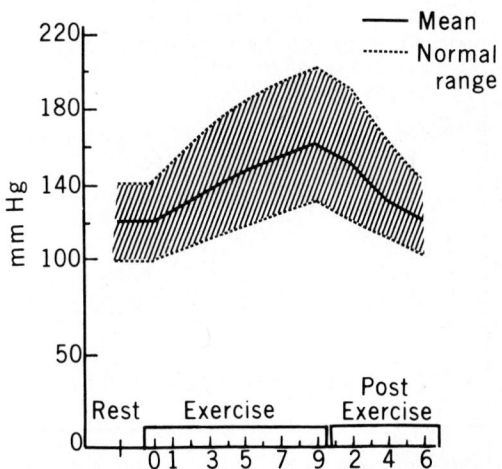

FIGURE 8–9. Mean and normal ranges of systolic blood pressure measured indirectly during and after exercise. (From Sheffield, L. T.: Electrocardiographic stress testing. *In* Chung, E. K. (ed.): Non-invasive Cardiac Diagnosis. Philadelphia, Lea and Febiger, 1976, p. 86.)

coronary artery disease, a large portion of the left ventricle must exhibit impaired function, due to ischemia or infarction or both, for arterial pressure to decline. In the absence of old infarction, this finding often denotes the development of widespread ischemia during exercise, as in patients with disease of the left main coronary artery, a left main equivalent lesion, or three-vessel disease.

HEART RATE. After an initial overreaction to the beginning of exercise and subsequent stabilization requiring only a minute or so, the sinus rate increases progressively with each increase in exercise intensity. This is expected, since cardiac output is linearly related to exercise intensity, and heart rate is the chief determinant of cardiac output in exercise. As maximal aerobic exercise capacity is approached, heart rate reaches a plateau just as oxygen consumption does.[89] Maximal exercise heart rate is highest in childhood and becomes lower with age (Fig. 8–10).[48, 49] The maximal level of exercise tachycardia is slightly less in trained athletes, averaging 7 beats/min lower than that of sedentary individuals in each age range. This description of normal heart rate response assumes normal sinus rhythm, of course. Abnormal rhythms may cause unpredictable rate responses.

There are two types of abnormal heart rate responses to exercise. First, the heart rate increment per stage of exercise may be lower than normal, and the heart rate may demonstrate a plateau at a distinctly subnormal intensity of work. This may be due to disease of the sinoatrial node and may also be the result of use of adrenoceptor blocking agents, such as propranolol. Second, occasionally a very high heart rate response at low levels of work is seen as a result of either physical deconditioning or marginal circulatory compensation.

The heart rate–systolic blood pressure product, which is an externally derived indicator of myocardial oxygen needs, rises progressively during exercise stress testing, and its peak value serves to characterize the normal cardiovascular performance. Normal individuals usually develop a peak rate-pressure product of 20 to 35 mm Hg × beats/min × 10^{-3}. On the other hand, most patients with overt ischemic heart disease will not be able to generate rate-pressure products exceeding 25 mm Hg × beats/min × 10^{-3}. Although on the average the peak rate-pressure products of normal persons are higher than those of ischemic heart disease patients, there is sufficient overlap between the two groups to prevent this product from being a useful single criterion of disease.[30] As one factor in a multivariate interpretation method, however, it contributes to increased test accuracy.[90]

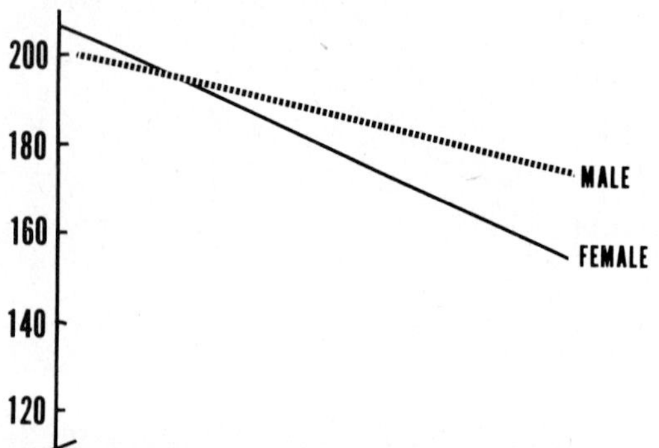

FIGURE 8–10. Maximal exercise heart rates of men and women in relation to age. Standard deviation from the mean is 10 beats/min for both sexes.

MAXIMAL WORK CAPACITY. This parameter is probably the most important measurement that can be gained from an exercise stress test. On a treadmill exercise protocol calling for increments of about 12 ml of oxygen/kg body weight/minute/3-minute stage, the exercise endurance of adult men is about 11.5 minutes and that of women 7.6 minutes.[48, 49] With the bicycle ergometer, average maximal aerobic exercise capacity of men is about 1200 kpm/min.* Average maximal bicycle ergometer capacity for adult women is about 800 kpm/min.[47] The length of time a subject is able to continue exercise by any of the progressive, continuous protocols correlates with the subject's maximal oxygen consumption ($\dot{V}O_{2\ max}$). It is tempting, therefore, to predict $\dot{V}O_{2\ max}$ from treadmill endurance time or to estimate "functional aerobic impairment,"[91] i.e., the difference between the predicted $\dot{V}O_2$ and the peak estimated $\dot{V}O_2$ divided by the predicted peak $\dot{V}O_2$. Such estimates should be used with caution, since the results vary significantly from protocol to protocol and from one test to another on the same protocol.[92]

The work capacity of normal sedentary individuals may be increased dramatically with regular training. More than doubling may be attained in young persons, and about a 50 per cent increase is possible in middle-aged individuals. In spite of the wide normal variability of work capacity, the measurement of exercise protocol endurance has great value in the study of patients with chest pain. It has been found that in patients with evidence of ischemia only after 7 minutes (about 10 METS) of exercise, 5-year prognosis is virtually as good as in patients who show no evidence of ischemia at all, whereas patients demonstrating ischemia after only 3 minutes (about 5 METS) of exercise or less have 4 times as high an incidence of disease progression or cardiovascular death.[93]

In view of the great importance of accurate assessment of exercise capacity, care should be taken that the subject is acquainted with the exercise device and not intimidated by it. A pretest familiarization visit to the exercise laboratory is worthwhile. Exercise should be begun at a sufficiently low level to serve as an unstressful warm-up for later stages. If the treadmill is used, subjects must be coached to walk properly, neither pushing on the front handrail and increasing their work rate ("lawn mower effect") nor partially supporting themselves on the side rails. When the exercise test is being used to measure maximal heart rate for the purpose of preparing an exercise prescription for training, a training heart rate of 60 to 80 per cent of the individual's maximum is prescribed. The training heart rate can be selected much more precisely if ventilatory gas measurements are made during the test, and the heart rate at which the slope of ventilation becomes steeper is identified. This heart rate corresponds closely to the increased slope of CO_2 production. Both of these changes are attributed to the onset of a rise in blood lactate concentration, which continues with progressive steepness until maximal exercise intensity has been reached. This point in exercise is termed the lactate or "anaerobic" threshold, and measures the peak level of exercise a person can continue for a fairly long time.[94] In marathon runners it corresponds with the running speed at which they compete and represents a very efficient level for physical training.

When a subject is unable to maintain position on the treadmill without grasping and pulling on the handrails,

*Kilopond-meters per minute = kilogram-weight force x meters per minute.

exercise should be terminated, since work rate drops when the handrails provide assistance. In using the bicycle ergometer, exercise should be terminated as soon as the subject becomes unable to maintain the set pedaling speed. If there are any limitations to maximal exercise capacity other than cardiovascular ones, these should be carefully noted, since psychological, musculoskeletal, or other non-cardiovascular limitations do not have the prognostic implications mentioned above.

EFFORT ANGINA. Although numerous kinds of chest discomfort are encountered during exercise testing, the finding of symptoms distinguished clearly as anginal may improve the sensitivity of exercise electrocardiographic testing considerably. Amsterdam and coworkers report that whereas ST-segment changes alone detect 67 per cent of patients with angina and significant coronary artery disease, when characteristic chest discomfort was also considered a positive finding, the detection rate rose to 100 per cent.[35]

INTERPRETATION OF STRESS TESTS

(See also p 1321)

Few diseases manifest a wider spectrum of morbidity and length of survival than coronary artery disease. Therefore, it is essential to determine not just whether or not a patient has the disease but also how it is likely to affect the prognosis. While exercise stress testing can help determine this, in order to make the best use of this procedure the dimensions of the test results should be familiar. Terms used in evaluating stress test results are found in Table 8–5.

SENSITIVITY. This provides an index of the capability of a test to detect an abnormality. The value is given as a percentage or decimal fraction. Although one would wish every test to have a sensitivity of 100 per cent, medical tests with high sensitivity frequently have the disadvantage of yielding some abnormal results erroneously. The sensitivity of maximal exercise tests for coronary artery disease is generally between 55 and 70 per cent when only the behavior of the ST segment is considered; however, when combined with other exercise test observations, test sensitivity increases to over 85 per cent.[35, 86]

SPECIFICITY. This indicates the ability of a test to recognize a normal subject. This is a very important characteristic because of the potential harm should diagnosis of a serious disease be applied to a subject in error. Because of this concern, tests are not usually considered for clinical application unless they have high specificity. Specificity of the maximal exercise electrocardiographic test usually ranges from 85 to 95 per cent.[35, 86]

ACCURACY. This is the measure of the capability of a test to yield correct results. It gives a general figure-of-merit for a test, since it includes the ability of the test to recognize true-positives as well as true-negatives.

TRUE-POSITIVE. This is the most clinically useful test result because of the avenue it opens for primary or secondary prevention of overt disease. In a predictive sense the true-positive result would identify the individual who, although healthy at present, is destined to have angina pectoris, myocardial infarction, or sudden death in the foreseeable future. False-positive, true-negative, and false-negative results do not require elaboration.

PREDICTIVE VALUE. This indicates the clinical significance of a positive test result. It is the percentage of likelihood that a positive result reflects the presence of the abnormality being tested. This term takes into consideration the prevalence of the disease in the population tested. If the prevalence is high, such as the prevalence of coronary atherosclerosis in a population of adults consulting a physician for chest pain, the number of true-positive results will be high and the number of false-positive results will be low, yielding a high predictive value. On the other hand, if the same test is conducted in the adult population at large in which the prevalence of coronary artery disease is probably between 1 and 2 per cent, the yield of true-positives will be overwhelmed by the large number of false-positives, and the predictive value will be quite low.

RELATIVE RISK. This indicates how a subject's statistical prognosis can be altered when tests results are taken into account. Most studies have shown very close agreement on relative risk, indicating that persons with abnormal test results have about 13 times greater incidence of coronary disease than those with a negative test result.

When exercise test results are thought of in terms of relative risk instead of clinical diagnosis, justification can be seen for screening selected asymptomatic subjects. Those having abnormal responses qualify for special attention to reduce risk factors, not to diagnose a disease. Kattus and coworkers showed the value of this approach in screening 309 asymptomatic executives.[95] Half of those with abnormal responses then participated in a remedial exercise program; all improved their functional capacity, and in one-third electrocardiographic responses converted to normal compared with this response in one-seventh of the nonexercising controls.

TABLE 8–5 TERMS USEFUL IN EVALUATION OF TEST RESULTS

Sensitivity	=	$\frac{\text{Number of true-positive detections}}{\text{Total number of positives in the group tested}}$
Specificity	=	$\frac{\text{Number of true normals detected}}{\text{Total number of normals in the group tested}}$
Accuracy	=	$\frac{\text{Number of true test results (true-positives + true-negatives)}}{\text{Total number of tests performed}}$
True-positive	=	Abnormal test result in individual who has (or will have) the disease*
False-positive	=	Abnormal test result in one who does not (and will not) have the disease
True-negative	=	Normal test result in one who does not (and will not) have the disease
False-negative	=	Normal test result in one who has (or will have) the disease
Predictive value	=	$\frac{\text{True-positives}}{\text{True-positives + false-positives}}$
Relative risk (risk ratio)	=	$\frac{\text{Disease rate† in persons with a positive test result}}{\text{Disease rate in persons with a negative test result}}$

*Whatever disease the test aims to detect.

†This may be in terms of current prevalence, future incidence, or both, and should be specified when the term is used.

Bayes' Theorem

In 1763 the English philosopher Thomas Bayes demonstrated the way in which the predictive value of a test is influenced not only by the sensitivity of the test but by the "prior probability" that an individual has the disease for which he is tested, i.e., the prevalence of the disease in the population being tested. This relationship is described by the following formula:

$$P[C/A] = \frac{P[A/C]}{P[A]} = \frac{P[A/C] \cdot P[C]}{P[A/C] \cdot P[C] + P[A_1/C_1] \cdot P[C_1]}$$

where

P [C/A] = probability that a person with a positive test has the disease tested for

C = sensitivity of test

C_1 = 1 − specificity of test

A = prevalence of disease

A_1 = rarity of disease (complement of A)

Applying this formula to some realistic approximations and assuming that exercise test sensitivity for ischemic heart disease is 70 per cent, that specificity is 85 per cent, and that in a population of United States adults complaining of chest pain the prevalence of ischemic heart disease is 50 per cent, Bayes' theorem would then determine that a patient with a positive exercise test would have an 82 per cent probability of having ischemic heart disease.

If sensitivity = 0.70, specificity = 0.85, and prevalence = 0.50

$$P = \frac{0.50 \times 0.70}{(0.50 \times 0.70) + (0.50 \times 0.15)} = 0.82$$

On the other hand, if the test with unchanged sensitivity and specificity is applied to a group of asymptomatic adults with a disease prevalence of 3 per cent, the probability that an individual with a positive test has ischemic heart disease is only 13 per cent! Of 100 such positive tests, 87 of them would be false-positives.

If sensitivity = 0.70, specificity = 0.85, and prevalence = 0.03

$$P = \frac{0.03 \times 0.70}{(0.03 \times 0.70) + (0.97 \times 0.15)} = 0.13$$

Thus in assessing the meaning of an exercise test result, Bayes' theorem emphasizes the importance of considering the identifiable risk group from which an individual is derived.[96] The patient with typical chest pain and positive exercise electrocardiogram, who has an 82 per cent likelihood of having significant coronary artery disease, presents justification for accepting this diagnosis and commencing treatment. However, a patient with atypical chest pain and thus only about a 20 per cent pretest likelihood of having coronary artery disease, after being tested and found positive will have a 54 per cent probability of having coronary disease. That is, there is about equal chance that such a person does not have it. In this case additional evidence for the presence of disease would be desirable before a potentially dangerous or difficult course of treatment is prescribed. In the asymptomatic person whose positive test raises the disease probability from 3 to 13 per cent, only moderate preventive measures that would be unlikely to be harmful or burdensome are justified; however, more intense measures might reduce the likelihood of future coronary events still further.

PROGNOSTIC SIGNIFICANCE OF EXERCISE TEST RESULTS

Exercise tests for ischemia, insensitive as they are for predicting exact coronary anatomy, correspond well with follow-up observations of actual coronary heart disease.[97] In a follow-up study of 2700 patients, Ellestad and colleagues found that 1067 normal responders had only a 7 per cent incidence of progression to angina, myocardial infarction, or death in 4 years, whereas 609 patients with abnormal ("positive") responses had a 46 per cent incidence of combined events in the same period.[97] McNeer and colleagues, combining observations of ST segment, exercise endurance, and maximal heart rate from exercise testing of 1472 patients, were able to define 876 patients with chest pain at low risk who had a 7 per cent mortality during 4 years of observation, whereas 134 patients who were classified to be at high risk according to the exercise test demonstrated a 37 per cent mortality during the same interval.[41]

The greatest change to have taken place in the field of stress testing currently is in the usage being made of test results. Originally the primary use was to aid in determining *whether* an individual had coronary artery disease or not—an either-or question with little or no emphasis on severity of disease or prospect for survival. Now it is known that typical anginal symptoms in combination with coronary artery disease risk factors make the diagnosis nearly certain. However, now there are multiple choices among effective modes of treatment, and stress testing is perhaps the best aid in selecting treatment. For example, if it was known that a given patient was in a group that was twice as likely to die while undergoing nonsurgical treatment than if operated upon, the choice would be clear. The NHLBI-sponsored Coronary Artery Surgery Study (p. 1320) found just that prospect for patients who were unable to exercise past Bruce Stage I and who developed 1.0 mm or greater ST depression on exercise testing, whereas patients with angiographically documented coronary artery disease who were able to exercise at Stage III or higher, and who did not develop as much as 1.0 mm ST segment depression, had the same expectancy of survival whether they were operated upon or not[12] (Fig. 8–11).

The ability to categorize patients permits continual improvement in choices of therapy. The Coronary Artery Surgery Study mentioned above showed that patients with one- and two-vessel coronary artery disease taken as a group had the same survival whether treated medically or surgically. Yet exercise testing showed that medical patients who had normal exercise capacity demonstrated by treadmill testing had survivals equal to or better than patients undergoing coronary artery bypass grafting. Even more striking was the finding that some medical patients with three-vessel coronary artery disease could exercise into the fifth stage of the Bruce protocol, and these patients exhibited 100 per cent survival over the 4-year period of observation.[12]

POSTINFARCTION ASSESSMENT OF PROGNOSIS. It is clinically valuable to predict postinfarction risk of mortality. In the MILIS study patients were offered maximal treadmill exercise testing 6 months after myocardial infarction. The offer alone had predictive value: those who declined

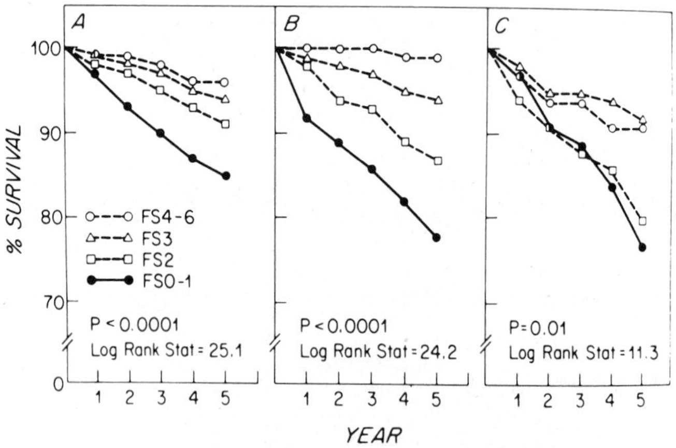

FIGURE 8–11. Five-year survival rates of patients participating in the Coronary Artery Surgery Study according to treadmill exercise capacity. Survival is plotted according to the final stage (FS) reached during exercise testing. The four identified categories begin with attainment of final stage 0 to 1 followed by a final stage of 2, final stage of 3, and final stages 4, 5, or 6. *Panel A* shows results for patients with less than 1 mm ST segment depression. *Panel B*, patients with 1 to 2 mm, and *Panel C*, patients with more than 2 mm ST segment depression. The figures show that best exercise capacity corresponds with best survival and vice versa. Least ST-segment depression also corresponds with improved survival and vice versa. (From Weiner, D. A., et al.: Prognostic importance of a clinical profile and exercise test in medically treated patients with coronary artery disease. J. Am. Col. Cardiol. *3*:772, 1984. Reprinted with permission from Elsevier Science Publishing Co., Inc.)

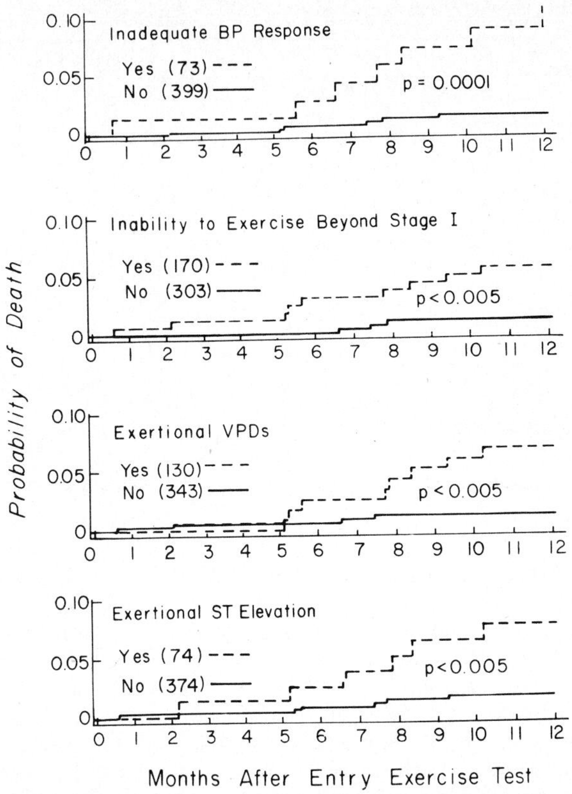

FIGURE 8–12. Cumulative probability of mortality 12 months after exercise testing performed 6 months post-myocardial infarction. Results are plotted according to presence or absence of four different types of exercise test abnormality. The marked increase in mortality associated with the presence of any of these exercise test findings is shown by the distance between the solid and dotted lines. (From Stone, P. H., et al.: Prognostic significance of the treadmill exercise test performance 6 months after myocardial infarction. J. Am. Col. Cardiol. *8*:1007, 1986. Reprinted with permission from Elsevier Science Publishing Co., Inc.)

or were deemed unable to take the test had a fivefold increase in mortality compared with those who did. Analysis of test results showed that the following were predictors of mortality: 1 mm or greater ST-segment depression, inadequate blood pressure response, development of ventricular premature complexes, and inability to exercise past Bruce Stage I. Patients who demonstrated no more than one of these findings had no mortality in the subsequent year, whereas patients with 2 findings had 8 per cent mortality and those with 3 or 4 findings had 15 per cent mortality. The investigators state that "the exercise performance characteristics were much more powerful in estimating prognosis than were clinical features obtained at the same time in the convalescent phase"[98] (Fig. 8–12). At a time when nearly all complications of coronary artery disease are treatable, identification of high-risk patients is likely to stimulate selection of appropriately preventive and therapeutic measures. Conversely, among those low-risk individuals with no more than one exercise test abnormality the assurance this categoric evaluation brings will be welcome news and the basis for a less strict regimen.

ASSESSMENT OF PROGNOSIS IN ASYMPTOMATIC PERSONS. The means to prevent at least some cases of coronary artery disease among those patients at increased risk has been demonstrated,[8] and further means of prevention are likely to be developed. The corollary of this is the need for early identification of patients with coronary artery disease or the risk of developing it, before heart damage occurs and while atherosclerotic deposits are still amenable to arrest (or regression). What is needed to accomplish this goal is a safe, noninvasive screening test to identify among asymptomatic subjects those at high risk of developing clinical evidence of coronary artery disease. Between 1970 and 1986 a formidable experience in the treadmill exercise testing of apparently healthy, asymptomatic individuals has accumulated.[10, 16, 99–104] In Table 8–6 are listed the results of 8 such studies in which volunteers were tested and followed up for 3 to 14 years to relate the incidence of coronary artery disease and development of angina, infarction, and sudden death to the initial result. In all, these studies represent 86,882 person-years of follow-up. All of the studies show a significant increase in coronary artery disease events in individuals who manifested an ischemic type response on exercise testing. (The LRC mortality follow-up study determined coronary artery disease only; the other seven reported total coronary artery disease events.) This increase in risk varied from a low of twofold in the relatively small VA study by Allen et al.[101] (2 per cent of the tabulated experience) to a high of twentyfold in the 1970 report by Doyle and Kinch.[104] The mean risk ratio for the entire table is 8.3. Results are skewed upward because of the large contribution (14 per cent) of the oldest study which employed less than near-maximal exercise, and therefore ischemic responses probably represented more advanced disease than did other studies. If only the last 7 studies are considered, the risk ratio becomes 6:3. That this risk ratio is almost surely valid is attested to by the fact that the 2 most recent studies, which account for 50 per cent of the total experience, yielded values very closely bracketing the mean value (Fig. 8–13).

These studies lead to two important conclusions: First, the exercise test clearly identifies among asymptomatic persons a subgroup at higher risk of developing coronary artery disease, providing the opportunity to take preventive measurements in an attempt to reduce their risk. Second, the studies show that exercise testing misses an appreciable fraction (about one-sixth in these studies) of patients who develop coronary artery disease after a normal exercise test. While the exercise test is highly effective for risk detection, additional improvements or directions in testing are needed to improve the detection rate. There is an even greater need to improve the application of preventive measures in those identified as being at high risk.

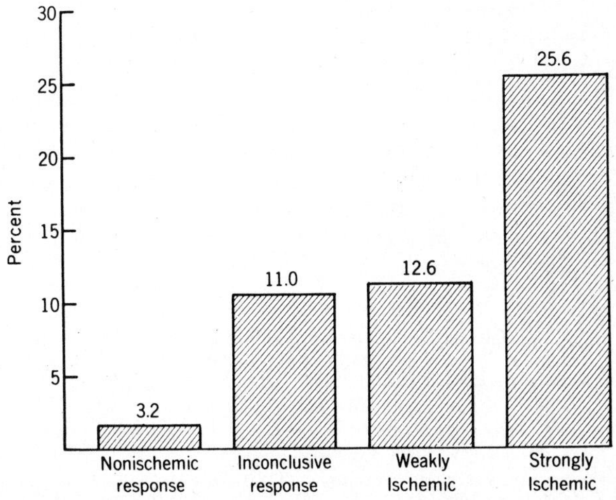

FIGURE 8–13. Eight-year follow-up study of asymptomatic men in the Lipid Research Clinic who performed a treadmill test at entry. The normal survival of those with nonischemic responses is contrasted with the high mortality among persons who developed 2 mm or more of ST-segment depression or developed ST-segment depression in stages I or II of the modified Bruce test. Mortality of persons with less ECG abnormality and better exercise endurance and persons with inconclusive responses ranked between the two extremes.

TABLE 8–6 FOLLOW-UP STUDIES AFTER EXERCISE TESTING OF ASYMPTOMATIC PERSONS

					All Positive Tests			Negative Tests	
Study	No. Subjects	Age	Follow-up (years)	Follow-up (person-years)	No.	% Developing Disease	Relative Risk	No.	% Developing Disease
Lipid Research Clinics[10]	3640	30–79	8.4	30,576	185	18%	5.6	2993	3.2%
McHenry[16]	916	27–55	14	12,824	23	39%	7.4	833	5.3%
Bruce[99]	2365	>25	6	14,190	260	18%	3.0	2105	2.0%
Milan[100]	10,723	18–65	10	5,040	135	16%	5.6	369 of 10,588*	3.5%
Allen[101]	356	>40	5	1,780	82	14%	2	274	7 %
Cumming[102]	510	40–65	3	1,530	66	25%	10	444	2 %
Froelicher[103]	1390	20–54	6.3	8,757	179	12%	14	1211	0.9%
Doyle[104]	2437	40–69	5	12,185	28	61%	20	1928	3 %
Total	22,337			86,882			mean = 8.3†		

*Of 10,588 negative tests, 369 case matched controls were followed up.
†If Doyle study subtracted, mean relative risk becomes 6.3.
Note: Studies 1, 2, and 8 had a category of inconclusive test result that is not tabulated. This caused the number of positive and negative test results to be less than the total number of subjects.

SAFETY AND RISKS OF EXERCISE TESTING

The primary requirements of any elective test are that it be as safe as possible and that the ratio of benefit to risk be favorable. Exercise stress testing has an excellent safety record. Maintenance of a high order of patient safety in testing depends on continual attention to three important factors: contraindications to testing, indications for terminating exercise, and incidence and management of complications.

CONTRAINDICATIONS TO TESTING. It is necessary that the subject considered for exercise stress testing understand the nature of the procedure, the importance of cooperation with the supervising physician, the necessity for reporting all symptoms promptly, and the realization of the very slight but definite risk which the procedure entails in an individual with preexisting cardiovascular disease. Although informed consent may be given verbally to the supervising physician after a discussion of the procedure, use of a written and signed informed consent form is more likely to avoid omission of important details, will emphasize the importance of the procedure, and will communicate the concern which the supervising physician has for the subject's well-being.

True contraindications of testing are conditions that are likely to be aggravated by vigorous exercise (Table 8–7). Such a list is headed by unhealed myocardial infarction. Breach of this contraindication is known to have been the result of misinterpretation or omission of the resting control 12-lead electrocardiogram. This emphasizes that the supervising physician must be expert in the interpretation of symptoms of coronary heart disease and of resting and exercise electrocardiograms.

TABLE 8–7 CONTRAINDICATIONS TO EXERCISE TESTING

Myocardial infarction—impending or acute
Unstable angina pectoris
Acute myocarditis or pericarditis
Known ominous coronary artery disease pattern (e.g., left main coronary artery stenosis)
Severe aortic stenosis
Congestive heart failure
Severe hypertension
Uncontrolled cardiac arrhythmias
Intracardiac conduction block greater than first degree
Acute systemic illness
Unwillingness to give informed consent

Another important contraindication is unstable angina pectoris (p. 1353), often defined as angina pectoris at rest, angina which is newly developed or has definitely become worse in frequency, ease of provocation, and severity (including rest angina) within the preceding 4 weeks.

Exercise may safely be conducted in the presence of mild to moderate aortic stenosis, with careful attention to blood pressure, the patient's symptoms, and electrocardiogram. Only severe aortic stenosis with palpably prolonged left ventricular ejection time and with clear-cut electrocardiographic left ventricular hypertrophy is a contraindication. The AMA Council on Scientific Affairs has determined the indications and contraindications for exercise testing,[105] and a joint committee of the American Heart Association and the American College of Cardiology has issued recommendations on this issue.[4] The recommendations of these groups are consistent with those proposed herein. Relative contraindications include known left main coronary disease or the equivalent, severe hypertension, and hypertrophic obstructive cardiomyopathy.

In addition to clinical contraindications, there are conditions which do not compromise safety but which in one way or another limit the usefulness of test results. These include confounding variables such as left ventricular hypertrophy, left bundle branch block, digitalis effect, and others, described above. When one or more of these conditions are present, one should reconsider whether the expected benefit of the test fully justifies its use.

TERMINATION OF EXERCISE. Termination of exercise has two aspects. (1) As a voluntary maximal test it should be terminated when subjects have a degree of fatigue or discomfort beyond which they are unwilling or unable to persist. (2) On the other hand, indications that continued exercise may be deleterious to the subject take precedence over maximal exercise (Table 8–8). Chest pain should convincingly simulate angina pectoris and should be tolerated until it is clear that it is definitely progressing and not stabilizing or regressing in the face of increasing exercise. One of the most difficult objective reasons to terminate exercise is "excessive ST-segment deviation." This certainly exceeds 2 mm (0.2 mV) deviation, but there is no general agreement on the precise level.

INCIDENCE OF COMPLICATIONS. The safety of exercise stress testing is well documented. Reports from nine groups, ranging from 500 to 170,000 tests, represent a cumulative experience of about 260,000 tests from about 80 medical centers. The largest single reported experience (170,000 tests) resulted from Rochmis and Blackburn's questionnaire survey of 73 medical centers.[52] They found

TABLE 8–8 INDICATIONS FOR TERMINATING GRADED EXERCISE TESTING

Physical exhaustion
Excessive dyspnea or leg fatigue
Excessive chest pain or other exercise induced symptom
Excessive ST segment deviation*
Ventricular tachycardia
Ventricular premature beats precipitated or aggravated by exercise (over 25% of beats)
Ectopic supraventricular tachycardia
Any intracardiac block precipitated by exercise
Peripheral circulatory insufficiency (pallor, clammy skin, drop in blood pressure)
Subject wishes to stop exercise

*See text for explanation.

a mortality rate of 10 per 100,000 tests and a morbidity rate of 24 per 100,000. Eight of the reports include a total of greater than 90,000 tests, among which there were 13 nonfatal myocardial infarctions and 3 deaths.[3, 106] This yields a mortality rate of 3.3 per 100,000 while maintaining a complication rate comparable to that found in the larger survey. The Lipid Research Clinics experience included no mortality or morbidity in over 3600 tests.[53] As skill in recognizing contraindications and reasons for stopping exercise increase, the risk of exercise testing approaches the baseline risk of the mere presence of coronary artery disease.

It is not possible to anticipate and prevent the rare instance when a small coronary arterial plaque, insufficient to provide detectable ischemia during even maximal exercise, may be the site of subintimal hemorrhage, resulting in dislodgment, occlusion of the vessel, and infarction or death. Such an occurrence is less likely to happen than the risk-producing events that patients face every day. The more common risks of exercise testing can be detected by careful, attentive search for contraindications prior to testing; meticulous observation of the patient during exercise with monitoring of the electrocardiogram and the blood pressure as well as the subject's symptoms and appearance; and close attention to the patient after exercise, including auscultation and palpation of the heart and inspection of the cervical veins, skin, and general appearance.

MANAGEMENT OF COMPLICATIONS. Appropriate management of exercise test complications depends primarily on the prior establishment of a protocol to be followed by everyone involved in the testing. This includes knowledge of what persons or services to employ immediately such as anesthesia or airway therapy, emergency patient transport service, and so on, depending on the local setting. A preselected set of equipment and medications in a specific location and arranged in an established pattern is necessary (Table 8–9). A previously specified treatment routine is essential and should include arranging for transfer of the patient and admission to a coronary care unit.

Rare complications of exercise stress testing include supraventricular tachycardias, such as paroxysmal atrial tachycardia or atrial fibrillation, and ominous multifocal ventricular premature complexes with excessively close coupling to preceding beats or occurring repetitively.

TABLE 8–9 EQUIPMENT AND SUPPLIES FOR MANAGEMENT OF COMPLICATIONS

1. Defibrillator with full tube of electrode paste
2. Assorted airways, ventilation bag, oxygen, and laryngoscope
3. Intravenous fluid (5% dextrose) with tubing, needles, and assorted syringes
4. Assorted drugs, including lidocaine, quinidine, disopyramide, procainamide, propranolol, atropine, isoproterenol, norepinephrine, metaraminol, digoxin, furosemide, dopamine, nifedipine, verapamil

Established ventricular tachycardia occurs infrequently, and in our experience has always been self-limiting upon cessation of exercise except when paroxysmal ventricular tachycardia was a preexisting problem in the patient tested. We have not encountered an episode of primary ventricular fibrillation in the course of approximately 35,000 exercise tests. Other complications include atrioventricular block, vasovagal syncope that has progressed through sinus bradycardia to several seconds of complete cardiac arrest before reverting to normal rhythm, prolonged postexercise angina pectoris, and rare instances of myocardial infarction.

REFERENCES

EXERCISE STRESS TESTING FOR CORONARY ARTERY DISEASE

1. Goldhammer, S., and Scherf, D.: Elektrokardiographische Untersuchungen bei Kranker mit Angina Pectoris ("ambulatorischer Typus"). Z. Klin. Med. *122*:134, 1933.
2. Master, A. M., Friedman, R., and Dack, S.: The electrocardiogram after standard exercise as a functional test of the heart. Am. Heart J. *24*:777, 1942.
3. Blomqvist, C. G.: Use of exercise testing for diagnostic and functional evaluation of patients with arteriosclerotic heart disease. Circulation *44*:1120, 1971.
4. Schlant, R. C., Blomqvist, C. G., Brandenburg, R. O., DeBusk, R., Ellestad, M. H., Fletcher, G. F., Froelicher, V. F., Hall, R. J., McCallister, B. D., McHenry, P. L., Ryan, T. J., and Sheffield, L. T.: Guidelines for exercise testing. A report of the American College of Cardiology/American Heart Association Task Force on Assessment of Cardiovascular Procedures. (Subcommittee on Exercise Testing.) J. Am. Col. Cardiol. 8:725, 1986.
5. Beljan, J. R., Cooper, T., Dolan, W. D., Dudrick, S. J., Gifford, R. W., Jr., Kuffner, M., Moxley, J. H., III., Murray, S. S., Schmidt, R. T. F., Smith, R. J., Snow, J. B., Jr., Tupper, C. J., and Jones, R. J.: Indications and contraindications for exercise testing. Council on Scientific Affairs. J.A.M.A. *246*:1015, 1981.
6. Cobb, L. A., and Weaver, W. D.: Exercise: A risk of sudden death in patients with coronary heart disease. J. Am. Col. Cardiol. 7:215, 1986.
7. James, F. W., Kaplan, S., Schwartz, D. C., Chou, T., Sandker, M. J., and Naylor, V.: Response to exercise in patients after total surgical correction of tetralogy of Fallot. Circulation *54*:671, 1976.
8. Weber, K. T., and Janicki, J. S.: Valvular heart disease. *In* Weber, K. T., and Janicki, J. S. (eds.): Cardiopulmonary Exercise Testing. Philadelphia, W. B. Saunders Company, 1986.
9. Lipid Research Clinics Program: The Lipid Research Clinics Coronary Primary Prevention Trial Results. I. Reduction in incidence of coronary heart disease. J.A.M.A. *251*:351, 1984.
10. Gordon, D. J., Ekelund, L. G., Karon, J. M., Probstfield, J. L., Rubenstin, C., Sheffield, L. T., and Weissfeld, L.: Predictive value of the exercise tolerance test for mortality in North American men. The Lipid Research Clinics mortality follow-up study. Circulation *74*:252, 1986.
11. Ellestad, M. H.: Stress Testing. Principles and Practice. 3rd ed. Philadelphia, F. A. Davis Co., 1986, pp. 317–323.
12. Weiner, D. A., Ryan, T. J., McCabe, C. H., Chaitman, B. R., Sheffield, L. T., Ferguson, J. C., Fisher, L. D., and Tristani, F.: Prognostic importance of a clinical profile and exercise test in medically treated patients with coronary artery disease. J.A.C.C. *3*:772, 1984.
13. Weiner, D. A., McCabe, C. H., and Ryan, T. J.: Identification of patients with left main and three vessel coronary disease with clinical and exercise test variables. Am. J. Cardiol. *46*:21, 1980.
14. Melin, J. A., Wijns, W., Vanbutsele, R. J., Robert, A., De Coster, P., Brasseur, L. A., Beckers, C., and Detry, J. R.: Alternative diagnostic strategies for coronary artery disease in women: Demonstration of the usefulness and efficiency of probability analysis. Circulation *71*:535, 1985.
15. Ahnve, S, Savvides, M., Abouantoun, S., Atwood, J. E., and Froelicher, V.: Can myocardial ischemia be recognized by the exercise electrocardiogram in coronary disease patients with abnormal resting Q waves? Am. Heart J. *111*:909, 1986.
16. McHenry, P.L., O'Donnell, J., Morris, S. N., and Jordan, J. J.: The abnormal exercise electrocardiogram in apparently healthy men: A predictor of angina pectoris as an initial coronary event during long-term follow-up. Circulation *70*:547, 1984.
17. Silverton, N. P., Elamin, M. S., Smith, D. R., Ionescu, M. I., Kardash, M., Whitaker, W, Mary, D. A. S. G., and Linden, R. J.: Use of the exercise maximal ST segment/heart rate slope in assessing the results of coronary angioplasty. Br. Heart J. *51*:379, 1984.
18. Alimurung, B. N., Gilbert, C. A., Felner, J. M., and Schlant, R. C.: The influence of early repolarization variant on the exercise electrocardiogram: A correlation with coronary arteriograms. Am. Heart J. 99:739, 1980.

PHYSIOLOGY OF EXERCISE TESTING

19. Epstein, S. E., Beiser, G. D., Stampfer, M., Robinson, B. F., and Braunwald, E.: Characterization of the circulatory response to maximal upright exercise in normal subjects and patients with heart disease. Circulation 35:1049, 1967.

20. Astrand, P., and Rodahl, K.: Evaluation of physical work capacity on the basis of tests. *In* Textbook of Work Physiology. New York, McGraw-Hill Book Co., 1970.
21. Gobel, F. L., Nordstrom, L. A., Nelson, R. R., Jorgensen, C. R., and Wang, Y.: The rate-pressure product as an index of myocardial oxygen consumption during exercise in patients with angina pectoris. Circulation *57*:549, 1978.
22. Robinson, B. F.: Relation of heart rate and systolic blood pressure to the onset of pain in angina pectoris. Circulation *35*:1073, 1967.
23. Cannon, P. J., Weiss, M. D., and Sciacca, R. R.: Myocardial blood flow in coronary artery disease: Studies at rest and during stress with inert gas washout techniques. Prog. Cardiovasc. Dis. *22*:95, 1977.
24. Ellestad, M. H.: Stress Testing. Principles and Practice. 3rd ed. Philadelphia, F. A. Davis Co., 1986, pp. 76–80.
25. Barnard, R. J., MacAlpin, R., Kattus, A. A., and Buckberg, G. D.: Ischemic response to sudden strenuous exercise in healthy men. Circulation *48*:936, 1973.
26. Hlatky, M. A., Pryor, D. B., Harrell, F. E., Jr., Califf, R. M., Mark, D. B., and Rosati, R. A.: Factors affecting sensitivity and specificity of exercise electrocardiography. Am. J. Med. *77*:64, 1984.
27. Singh, B. N.: A Symposium: Detection, quantification and clinical significance of silent myocardial ischemia in coronary artery disease. Am. J. Cardiol. *58*:1B, 1986.
28. Rozanski, A., Diamond, G. A., Forrester, J. S., Berman, D. S., Morris, D., Jones, R. H., Okada, R., Freeman, M., and Swan, H. J. C.: Should the intent of testing influence its interpretation? J. Am. Col. Cardiol. *7*:17, 1986.
29. Elamin, M. S., Boyle, R., Kardash, M. M., Smith, D. R., Stoker, J. B., Whitaker, W., Mary, D. A. S. G., and Linden, J. R.: Accurate detection of coronary heart disease by new exercise test. Br. Heart J. *48*:311, 1982.
30. Sheffield, L. T., and Roitman, D.: Systolic blood pressure, heart rate, and treadmill work at anginal threshold. Chest *63*:327, 1973.
31. Gould, K. L., Hamilton, G. W., Lipscomb, K., Ritchie, J. L., and Kennedy, J. W.: Method for assessing stress-induced regional malperfusion during coronary arteriography. Experimental validation and clinical application. Am. J. Cardiol. *34*:557, 1974.
32. Logan, S. E.: On the fluid mechanics of human coronary artery stenosis. IEEE Trans. Biomed. Eng. *22*:327, 1975.
33. Feldman, R. L., Nichols, W. W., and Pepine, C. J.: What is the coronary hemodynamic significance of the length of a coronary artery obstruction? Clin. Res. *24*:216A, 1976.
34. Singh, B. N., Nademanee, K., Figueras, J., and Josephson, M. A.: Hemodynamic and electrocardiographic correlates of symptomatic and silent myocardial ischemia: Pathophysiologic and therapeutic implications. Am. J. Cardiol. *58*:3B, 1986.
35. Amsterdam, E. A., Martschinske, R., Laslett, L. J., Rutledge, J. C., and Vera, Z.: Symptomatic and silent myocardial ischemia during exercise testing in coronary artery disease. Am. J. Cardiol. *58*:43B, 1986.
36. Varnauskas, E.: The ECG and exercise testing. *In* Julian, D. G. (ed.): Angina Pectoris. 2nd ed. New York, Churchill Livingstone, 1985, pp. 96–127.
37. Koppes, G., McKiernan, T., Bassan, M., and Froelicher, V. F.: Treadmill exercise testing. Part II. Curr. Prob. Cardiol. *7*:1, 1977.
38. Udall, J. A., and Ellestad, M. H.: Predictive implications of ventricular premature contractions associated with treadmill stress testing. Circulation *56*:985, 1977.
39. Robinson, B. F.: Relation of heart rate and systolic blood pressure to the onset of pain in angina pectoris. Circulation *35*:1073, 1967.
40. Thomson, P. D., and Kelleman, M. H.: Hypotension accompanying the onset of exertional angina. Circulation *52*:28, 1975.

TYPES OF EXERCISE TESTING

41. McNeer, J. F., Margolis, J. R., Lee, K.L., Kisslo, J. A., Peter, R. H., Kong, Y., Behar, V. S., Wallace, A. G., McCants, C. B., and Rosati, R. A.: The role of the exercise test in the evaluation of patients for ischemic heart disease. Circulation *57*:64, 1978.
42. Astrand, P., and Saltin, B.: Maximal oxygen uptake and heart rate in various types of muscular activity. J. Appl. Physiol. *16*:977, 1961.
43. Jackson, D. H., Reeves, T. J., Sheffield, L. T., and Burdeshaw, J.: Isometric effects on treadmill exercise response in healthy young men. Am. J. Cardiol. *31*:344, 1973.
44. Bruce, R. A., Blackmon, J. R., Jones, J. W., and Strait, G.: Exercising testing in adult normal subjects and cardiac patients. Pediatrics *32*:742, 1963.
45. Balke, B., and Ware, R. W.: An experimental study of "physical fitness" of Air Force personnel. U.S. Armed Forces Med. J. *10*:675, 1959.
46. Kansal, S., Roitman, D., Bradley, E. L., Jr., and Sheffield, L. T.: Enhanced evaluation of treadmill tests by means of scoring based on multivariate analysis and its clinical application: A study of 608 patients. Am. J. Cardiol. *52*:1155, 1983.
47. Weber, K. T., and Janicki, J. S.: Cardiopulmonary exercise testing. *In* Weber, K. T., and Janicki, J. S. (eds): Cardiopulmonary Exercise Testing. Philadelphia, W. B. Saunders Company, 1986.
48. Lester, F. M., Sheffield, L. T., and Reeves, T. J.: Electrocardiographic changes in clinically normal older men following near maximal and maximal exercise. Circulation *36*:5, 1967.
49. Sheffield, L. T., Maloof, J. A., Sawyer, J. A., and Roitman, D.: Maximal heart rate and treadmill performance of healthy women in relation to age. Circulation *57*:79, 1978.
50. DeBusk, R. F., Blomqvist, C. G., Kouchoukos, N. T., Luepker, R. V., Miller, H. S., Moss, A. J., Pollock, M. L., Reeves, T. J., Selvester, R. H., Stason, W. B., Wagner, G. S., and Willman, V. L.: Identification and treatment of low-risk patients after acute myocardial infarction and coronary-artery bypass graft surgery. N. Engl. J. Med. *314*:161, 1986.
51. Schaer, D. H., Leiboff, R. H., Wasserman, A. G., Katz, R. J., Schwartz, H., Schmidt, S. B., Bren, G. B., Varghese, P. J., and Ross, A. M.: Exercise testing after infarction/thrombolysis identifies patent vessels and residually ischemic myocardium. Circulation *72*(Suppl III):462, 1985.
52. Rochmis, P., and Blackburn, H.: Exercise tests. A survey of procedures, safety and litigation experience in approximately 170,000 tests. J.A.M.A. *217*:1061, 1971.
53. Sheffield, L. T., Haskell, W., Heiss, G., Kioschos, M., Leon, A., Roitman, D., and Schrott, H.: Safety of exercise-testing volunteer subjects: The Lipid Research Clinics' Prevalence Study Experience. J. Cardiol. Rehab. *2*:395, 1982.

TECHNIQUES OF EXERCISE TESTING

54. Mason, R. E., and Likar, I.: A new system of multiple-lead exercise electrocardiography. Am. Heart J. *71*:196, 1966.
55. Gamble, P., McManus, H., Jensen, D., and Froelicher, V.: A comparison of the standard 12-lead electrocardiogram to exercise electrode placements. Chest *85*:616, 1984.
56. Patterson, J. A., Naughton, J., Pietras, R. J., and Gunnar, R. M.: Treadmill exercise in assessment of the functional capacity of patients with cardiac disease. Am. J. Cardiol. *30*:757, 1972.
57. Borg, G.: Perceived exertion as an indicator of somatic stress. Scand. Rehab. Med. *2*:92, 1970.
58. Feil, H., and Siegel, M. L.: Electrocardiographic changes during attacks of angina pectoris. Am. J. Med. Sci. *175*:255, 1928.
59. Hollenberg, M., Zoltick, J. M., Go, M., Yaney, S. F., Daniels, W., Davis, R. C., Jr., and Bedynek, J. L.: Comparison of a quantitative treadmill exercise score with standard electrocardiographic criteria in screening asymptomatic young men for coronary artery disease. N. Engl. J. Med. *313*:600, 1985.
60. Prinzmetal, M., Kennamer, R., Merliss, R., Wada, T., and Bor, N.: Angina pectoris. I. A variant form of angina pectoris. Am. J. Med. *27*:375, 1959.
61. Chahine, R. A., Raizner, A. E., and Ishimori, T.: The clinical significance of exercise-induced ST-segment elevation. Circulation *54*:209, 1976.
62. Rijneke, R. D., Ascoop, C. A., and Talmon, J. L.: Clinical significance of upsloping ST segments in exercise electrocardiography. Circulation *61*:671, 1980.
63. Ellestad, M. H.: Stress Testing. Principles and Practice. 3rd ed. Philadelphia, F. A. Davis Co., 1986, pp. 233–235.
64. Bonoris, P. E., Greenberg, P. S., Castellanet, M. J., and Ellestad, M. H.: Significance of changes in R wave amplitude changes versus ST-segment depression in stress testing. Circulation *57*:904, 1978.
65. Wagner, S., Cohn, K., and Selyer, A.: Unreliability of exercise-induced R wave changes as indexes of coronary artery disease. Am. J. Cardiol. *44*:1241, 1979.
66. Myers, J., Ahnve, S., Froelicher, V., and Sullivan, M.: Spatial R wave amplitude changes during exercise: Relation with left ventricular ischemia and function. J. Am. Col. Cardiol. *6*:603, 1985.
67. Vincent, G. M., Abildskov, J. A., and Burgess, M. J.: Mechanisms of ischemic ST-segment displacement. Evaluation by direct current recordings. Circulation *56*:559, 1977.
68. Abarquez, R. F., Freiman, A. H., Reichel, F., and LaDue, J. S.: The precordial electrocardiogram during exercise. Circulation *22*:1060, 1960.
69. Shackel, B.: Skin drilling. A method of diminishing galvanic skin potentials. Am. J. Psychol. *72*:114, 1959.
70. Tubau, J. F., Chaitman, B. R., Bourassa, M. G., and Waters, D. D.: Detection of multivessel coronary disease after myocardial infarction using exercise stress testing and multiple ECG lead systems. Circulation *61*:44,1980.
71. Riley, C. P., Oberman, A., and Sheffield, L. T.: Electrocardiographic effects of glucose ingestion. Arch. Intern. Med. *130*:703, 1972.
72. Greenspan, M., Iskandrian, A. S., Mintz, G. S., Croll, M. N., Segal, B. L., Kimbiris, D., and Bemis, C. E.: Exercise myocardial scintigraphy with ^{201}thallium. Chest *77*:47,1980.
73. Whinnery, J. E., Froelicher, V. F., Jr., Stewart, A. J., Longo, M. R., Jr., Triebwasser, J. H., and Lancaster, M. C.: The electrocardiographic response to maximal treadmill exercise of asymptomatic men in left bundle branch block. Am. Heart J. *94*:316, 1977.
74. Whinnery, J. E., Froelicher, V. F., Jr., Stewart, A. J., Longo, M. R., Jr., and Triebwasser, J. H.: The electrocardiographic response to maximal treadmill exercise of asymptomatic men with right bundle branch block. Chest *71*:335,1977.
75. Johnson, S., O'Connel, J., Becker, P., Moran, J. F., and Gunnar, R.: The diagnostic accuracy of exercise ECG testing in the presence of complete right bundle branch block. Circulation *52*(Suppl II):48, 1975.
76. Kawai, C., and Hultgren, H. N.: The effect of digitalis upon the exercise electrocardiogram. Am. Heart J. *68*:409, 1964.
77. Yu, P. N. G., Lovejoy, F. W., Hulfish, B., Howell, M. M., Joos, H. A., Tenney, S. M., Haroutunian, L. M., and Evans, H. W.: Cardiorespiratory responses and electrocardiographic changes during exercise before and after intravenous digoxin in normal subjects. Am. J. Med. Sci. *224*:146, 1952.
78. Hung, J., Chaitman, B. R., Lam, J., Lesperance, J., Dupras, G., Fines, P., and Bourassa, M. G.: Noninvasive diagnostic test choices for the evaluation of coronary artery disease in women: A multivariate comparison of cardiac fluoroscopy, exercise electrocardiography and exercise thallium myocardial perfusion scintigraphy. J. Am. Col. Cardiol. *4*:8, 1984.

79. Cumming, G. R., Dufresne, C., Kich, L., and Samm, J.: Exercise electrocardiogram patterns in normal women. Br. Heart J. *35*:1055, 1973.
80. Sheffield, L. T., Holt, J. H., Lester, F. M., Conroy, D. V., and Reeves, T. J.: On-line analysis of the exercise electrocardiogram. Circulation *40*:935, 1969.
81. Kurita, A., Chaitman, B. R., and Bourassa, M. G.: Significance of exercise-induced junctional ST depression in evaluation of coronary artery disease. Am. J. Cardiol. *40*:492, 1977.
82. Lozner, E. C., and Morganroth, J.: New criteria for evaluation "positive" exercise tests in asymptomatic patients. Am. J. Cardiol. *39*:288, 1977.
83. Ellestad, M. H., and Wan, M. K. C.: Predictive implications of stress testing. Follow-up of 2700 subjects after maximum treadmill stress testing. Circulation *51*:363, 1975.
84. Weiner, D. A., McCabe, C. H., Fisher, L. D., Chaitman, B. R., and Ryan, T. J.: Similar rates of false positive and false negative exercise tests in matched males and females (CASS). Circulation 58(Suppl. II):140, 1978.
85. Ahnve, S., Sullivan, M., Myers, J., and Froelicher, V.: Computer analysis of exercise-induced changes in QRS duration in patients with angina pectoris and in normal subjects. Am. Heart J. *111*:903, 1986.
86. Hlatky, A. M., Pryor, D. B., Harrell, F. E., Jr., Califf, R. M., Mark, D. B., and Rosati, R. A.: Factors affecting sensitivity and specificity of exercise electrocardiography. Am. J. Med. 77:64, 1984.
87. Weber, K. T., and Janicki, J. S.: *In* Weber, K. T., and Janicki, J. S., (eds.): Cardiopulmonary Exercise Testing. Philadelphia, W. B. Saunders Company, 1986, p. 156.
88. Morris, S. N., Phillips, J. F., Jordan, J. W., and McHenry, P. L.: Incidence and significance of decreases in systolic blood pressure during graded treadmill exercise testing. Am. J. Cardiol. *41*:221, 1978.
89. Froelicher, V. F.: Exercise Testing and Training. New York, Le Jacq Publishing, Inc., 1983, p. 41.
90. Berman, J. L., Wynne, J., and Cohn, P. F.: Value of a multivariate approach for interpreting treadmill exercise tests in coronary artery disease. Am. J. Cardiol. *41*:375, 1978.
91. Bruce, R. A.: Exercise testing of patients with coronary heart disease. Principles and normal standards for evaluation. Ann. Clin. Res. *3*:323, 1971.
92. Froelicher, V. F., and Lancaster, M. C.: The prediction of maximal oxygen consumption from a continuous exercise treadmill protocol. Am. Heart J. 87:445, 1974.
93. Ellestad, M. H.: Stress Testing. Principles and Practice. 3rd ed. Philadelphia, F. A. Davis Co., 1986.
94. Davis, J. A.: Anaerobic threshold review of the concept and directions for future research. Med. Sci. Sports Exerc. *17*:6, 1985.
95. Kattus, A. A., Jorgensen, C. R., Worden, R. E., and Alvaro, A. B.: ST segment depression with near-maximal exercise: Its modification by physical conditioning. Chest *62*:678, 1972.
96. Detrano, R., Yiannikas, J., Salcedo, E. E., Rincon, G., Go, R. T., Williams, G., and Leatherman, J.: Bayesian probability analysis: A prospective demonstration of its clinical utility in diagnosing coronary disease. Circulation *69*:541,1984.

PROGNOSTIC SIGNIFICANCE OF EXERCISE TEST RESULTS

97. Ellestad, M. H.: Stress Testing. Principles and practice. 3rd ed. Philadelphia, F. A. Davis Co., 1986, pp. 316–334.
98. Stone, P. H., Turi, Z. G., Muller, J. E., Parker, C., Hartwell, T., Rutherford, J. D., Jaffe, A. S., Raabe, D. S., Passamani, E. R., Willerson, J. T., Sobel, B. E., Robertson, T. L., Braunwald, E., and The MILIS Study Group: Prognostic significance of the treadmill exercise test performance 6 months after myocardial infarction. J. Am. Col. Cardiol. *8*:1007, 1986.
99. Bruce, R. A., DeRouen, T. A., and Hossack, K. F.: Value of maximal exercise tests in risk assessment of primary heart disease events in healthy men. 5-years' experience of the Seattle Heart Watch Study. Am. J. Cardiol. *46*:371, 1980.
100. Giagnoni, E., Secchi, M. B., Wu, S. C., Morabito, A., Oltrona, L., Mancarella, S., Volpin, N., Fossa, L., Bettazzi, L., Arangio, G., Sachero, A., and Folli, G.: Prognostic value of exercise EKG testing in asymptomatic normotensive subjects. N. Engl. J. Med. *309*:1085, 1983.
101. Allen, W. H., Aronow, W. S., Goodman, P., and Stinson, P.: Five-year follow-up of maximal treadmill stress test in asymptomatic men and women. Circulation *62*:522, 1980.
102. Cumming, G. R., Samm, J., Borysyk, L., and Kich, L.: Electrocardiographic changes during exercise in asymptomatic men: Three-year follow-up. Can. Med. Assoc. J. *112*:578, 1975.
103. Froelicher, V. F., Jr., Thomas, M. M., Pillow, C., and Lancaster, M. C.: Epidemiologic study of asymptomatic men screened by maximal treadmill testing for latent coronary artery disease. Am. J. Cardiol. *34*:770, 1974.
104. Doyle, J. T., and Kinch, S. H.: The prognosis of an abnormal electrocardiographic stress test. Circulation *41*:545, 1970.

SAFETY OF EXERCISE TESTING

105. Council on Scientific Affairs, American Medical Association: Indications and contraindications for exercise testing. J.A.M.A. *246*:1015, 1981.
106. Atterhog, J. H., Jonsson, B., and Samuelsson, R.: Exercise testing. A prospective study of complication rates. Am. Heart J. *98*:572, 1979.

9 CARDIAC CATHETERIZATION

by WILLIAM GROSSMAN, M.D., and
WILLIAM H. BARRY, M.D.

HISTORICAL ASPECTS

THE EARLY PERIOD. According to André Cournand, cardiac catheterization was first performed (and so named) in 1844 by Claude Bernard,[1] who catheterized both the right and the left ventricles of a horse by means of a retrograde approach from the jugular vein and carotid artery. There followed an era of investigation of cardiovascular physiology in animals that resulted in the development of many important techniques and principles—including pressure manometry and the application of the Fick principle for measuring cardiac output—subsequently applied to the study of patients with heart disease.

Although others had previously passed catheters into the great veins, Werner Forssmann is generally credited as the first to pass a catheter into the heart of a living human being.[2] At age 25, he exposed a vein in his own left arm, introduced a ureteral catheter into the venous system, and advanced it under fluoroscopic control into the right atrium. He then walked to the Radiology Department, where the catheter position was documented by a chest x-ray. During the next 2 years, Forssmann continued to perform catheterization studies, including six additional attempts to catheterize himself.

The potential of Forssmann's technique was appreciated by other investigators. In 1930, Klein reported on catheterization of the right ventricle in 11 patients and measurement of cardiac output using the Fick principle.[3] The cardiac outputs were 4.5 and 5.6 liter/min in two patients without heart disease.[1] Except for these and several other studies, application of cardiac catheterization to evaluate the circulation in normal and disease states was limited and fragmentary until the work of Cournand and Richards, who in 1941 began a remarkable series of investigations of right-heart physiology in humans.[4–6] In 1947, Dexter and his colleagues at the Peter Bent Brigham Hospital reported their studies of congenital heart disease and mentioned some observations on "the oxygen saturation and source of pulmonary capillary blood" obtained from a catheter in the pulmonary artery "wedge" position.[7] Subsequent work from Dexter's laboratory[8] showed that the pressure measured in the pulmonary artery "wedge" position was an accurate estimate of pulmonary venous and left atrial pressure. During this exciting early period, catheterization was used to investigate problems in cardiovascular physiology by McMichael in England,[9] Lenegre in Paris,[10] and Cournand, Dexter, Warren, Stead, Bing, Burchell, Wood, and their respective coworkers in this country.[11–14]

THE 1950's AND BEYOND. Further developments came rapidly. Some of the highlights include the following: Retrograde left-heart catheterization was first introduced by Zimmerman[15] and Limon Lason[16] and their respective coworkers in 1950. The percutaneous technique developed by Seldinger in 1953 was soon applied to cardiac catheterization of both the left and right heart chambers.[17] Transseptal left-heart catheterization was developed[18] and applied clinically by Ross, Braunwald, and Morrow,[19] and it quickly became accepted as a standard technique. Selective coronary arteriography was developed by Sones et al. in 1959[20, 21] and was perfected in the ensuing years. In 1970, a practical balloon-tipped flow-guided catheter technique was introduced by Swan, Ganz, and their collaborators, making possible the applicability of catheterization outside the conventional catheterization laboratory.[22]

Many other landmark events could be mentioned and the contributions of many individuals could be recognized, but these have been detailed elsewhere.[23]

In this chapter, we discuss current methods of cardiac catheterization, including technical aspects important for optimal use of these methods and accurate interpretation of the data obtained. The development of these techniques and their application to the study of normal and abnormal human cardiac physiology have played a decisive role in improving the diagnosis and treatment of patients with cardiac disease.

TECHNICAL ASPECTS OF CARDIAC CATHETERIZATION

THE CARDIAC CATHETERIZATION FACILITY

A modern cardiac catheterization laboratory should be housed in a room of 500 to 700 square feet. A report by the Intersociety Commission for Heart Disease Resources on Optimal Resources for Cardiac Catheterization Facilities[24] dealt with a number of critical issues concerning the cardiac catheterization facility. These included the location of a catheterization laboratory (within a hospital as opposed to free standing); outpatient catheterization; administration, staff organization, and criteria for professional privileges; optimal annual caseload for physicians and for the laboratory; radiation safety and radiological techniques; and physiological measurements and patient safety.

Outpatient catheterization has been demonstrated to be safe, practical, and cost efficient by a variety of groups. In properly selected cases, outpatient catheterization should be encouraged as part of an overall effort to use hospital facilities more efficiently and to contain costs of medical

TABLE 9–1 INTERSOCIETY RECOMMENDATIONS FOR CATHETERIZATION LABORATORY AND PHYSICIAN CASELOAD

1. Adult catheterization laboratories	≥300 cases/year
2. Pediatric catheterization laboratories	≥150 cases/year
3. Physician caseload:	
a. Adult catheterizations	≥150 but ≤600
b. Pediatric catheterizations	≥50

From Friesinger, G. C., et al.: Optimal resources for evaluation of the heart and lungs: Cardiac catheterization and radiologic facilities. Circulation 68:893A, 1983.

Note: The report indicates that physicians with extensive experience (e.g., more than 1000 independently performed catheterizations) can perform fewer catheterizations to maintain their skill levels.

care. In most laboratories experienced with outpatient catheterization[25] the brachial arterial approach has been utilized; this technique allows the patient to be ambulatory shortly following the completion of the procedure.

A second issue addressed in the Intersociety Report concerns the proximity and availability of *cardiac surgical facilities*. As stated in the report, optimally, catheterization laboratories should be located only in institutions with well-organized and closely related programs of cardiovascular surgery. Exceptions will exist, but they should be uncommon.[24] Immediately available cardiac surgical back-up is particularly critical for laboratories performing coronary angioplasty, endomyocardial biopsy, and transseptal catheterization studies on patients suspected to have left main coronary artery disease, severe aortic stenosis, or other conditions that increase the risk of the catheterization procedure.

Utilization levels as well as optimal *physician caseload* are additional issues of importance in the operation of a cardiac catheterization facility, and current recommendations are given in Table 9–1.

RADIOGRAPHIC EQUIPMENT

Radiographic equipment must be capable of extremely high-quality image resolution and it must include a system for permanent recording. Usually, the system consists of three components: an x-ray generating system, an image intensifier, and an image recording system consisting of a video camera, video tape recorder, and 35 mm cine camera. Many laboratories are now switching to all-electronic techniques for permanent recording, eliminating the need for the 35 mm cine camera.

Details concerning radiographic principles and practice are beyond the scope of this text, and the reader is referred elsewhere[23] for further information. The radiographic equipment must be mounted on an appropriate support stand to allow multiple complex angulation. Cardiac catheterization and angiography should only be carried out in a room where complex angulation (including right and left anterior oblique angulation as well as cranial and caudal angulation) can be accomplished. A strict quality assurance program must be implemented, with regular checks on performance of the apparatus.

RADIATION SAFETY

It is essential that details of radiation safety be considered in the operation of any facility. A radiation safety officer must be appointed, with the proper credentials to interpret and enforce existing laws and regulations. Units of x-ray exposure are the roentgen (R), rad, and rem. The roentgen unit is defined in terms of the amount of ionization created per unit volume of air. The rad (radiation absorbed dose) is a unit of absorbed dose defined as the amount of energy deposited per unit mass of a radiation material. The relationship between radiation exposure expressed in R to the absorbed dose expressed in rads varies with the type of tissue exposed. An exposure of soft tissue to 1 R by either direct beam or scatter results in an absorbed dose of approximately 0.99 rad. Bone, which absorbs more, would receive a dose of 4 rads. Rem (roentgen equivalent, man) is the unit of dose used in state and federal radiation control regulations. The rem is intended to account for different types of radiation that produce varying damage for the same absorbed dose. For example, radiation due to alpha particles and neutrons produces a different number of rems than the number of rads; however, for x-rays and gamma rays, rem and rad are practically identical.

RECOMMENDED RADIATION LIMITS. It is not known whether there exists a lower limit for radiation exposure, below which there is no risk of biological damage. However, for regulatory purposes the recommended limits for the general population is 0.5 rem per person per year; for individuals involved in professions where radiation exposure is necessary (e.g., radiology technicians, physicians in cardiac catheterization laboratories) the maximal permissible dose is 5.0 rem per year. Obviously, these limits cannot guarantee complete elimination of any hazard.

Individuals working in a cardiac catheterization facility must wear film badges which monitor radiation exposure. No dose higher than 3 rems should be allowed within any 3-month period. Protection against radiation is achieved by wearing lead aprons and using lead neck wraps to protect the thyroid and leaded eyeglasses to protect the lens. Most important, however, is to minimize the use of fluoroscopy and cineangiography during the procedure. The operator must avoid the temptation to fluoroscope continuously. Guidelines for radiation protection in the cardiac catheterization laboratory have been issued by the Society for Cardiac Angiography.[26]

TECHNIQUE OF CARDIAC CATHETERIZATION

The majority of catheterizations performed today utilize either of two approaches: catheterization by direct exposure of an artery and a vein (e.g., brachial vessels, umbilical vessels in neonates) and catheterization by the percutaneous approach (including transseptal catheterization). Each method has its advantages and disadvantages, and it is our belief that the physician performing cardiac catheterization should be well versed in both techniques. The methods employed in the authors' laboratories are described below.

BRACHIAL ARTERIAL APPROACH

This approach usually involves surgical exposure of the brachial artery and brachial or basilic vein in the antecubital fossa and insertion of the catheters directly following vessel incision. The percutaneous approach of Seldinger may also be used in adults via the brachial vessels if catheters of small size (No. 5 French) are used.[27] The brachial approach has advantages in patients with obstructive and/or thrombotic arterial disease involving the abdominal aorta, iliac artery, or femoral artery; suspected thrombosis of the femoral vein or inferior vena cava; defective hemostatic mechanisms (e.g., marked thrombocytopenia); or coarctation of the aorta. It may also be advantageous in obese patients, in whom the percutaneous femoral technique may be technically quite difficult and in whom bleeding may be hard to control after removal of the catheter.

PROCEDURE. After the brachial artery is localized by means of palpation in the right antecubital fossa, local anesthesia is induced with 5 to 15 ml of 1 to 2 per cent lidocaine, and a single transverse incision is made just proximal to the flexor crease. Tissues are separated by blunt dissection, and a medial vein is isolated and encircled proximally and distally with 3–0 or 4–0 silk. The brachial artery is isolated from adjacent nerves and fascia and is encircled proximally and distally with moistened umbilical tape or silicone Elastomer surgical tape.

Right-heart catheterization is accomplished by means of antegrade passage of an appropriate catheter (e.g., Cournand, Goodale-Lubin, Swan-Ganz) via the basilic or brachial vein to the right atrium, right ventricle, pulmonary artery, and pulmonary capillary "wedge" positions under fluoroscopic guidance. In the wedge position, the catheter occludes the distal pulmonary artery segment, and thus the catheter tip is exposed to only the pulmonary venous pressure. Pressure recorded from the wedge position is accepted as a true wedge pressure only if a characteristic left atrial waveform is exhibited and if completely oxygenated blood (> 95 per cent oxygen saturation) can be aspirated from the catheter.[23] Left-heart catheterization is then accomplished by means of retrograde passage of an appropriate catheter (e.g., Sones, NIH) through a transverse brachial arteriotomy to the ascending aorta and left ventricle.

Systemic administration of heparin (5000 units) at the time of left-heart catheterization and coronary arteriography is indicated to prevent thrombotic complications. In case of difficulty in passing catheters from the brachial artery around the shoulder, an end-hole catheter with a flexible guidewire protruding beyond the tip should be used. As catheters with or without the aid of guidewires are advanced in the vascular system, their passage should be monitored fluoroscopically; if progress of the catheter is difficult, or if the patient complains of pain, caution should be exercised to avoid dissection or perforation of the vessel wall. Occasionally, spasm of the vessel around the catheter may occur, owing to the relatively small size of vessels in the upper extremities. In this case administration of small amounts of morphine should promptly facilitate catheter manipulation; if not, a catheter of smaller diameter should be used.

Termination of the Procedure. Following completion of hemodynamic and angiographic studies, the catheters are withdrawn, and the artery is repaired. In our laboratory, a Fogarty balloon catheter is routinely passed proximally and distally to remove any thrombi that may have formed within the arterial lumen during the catheterization. After proximal and distal flow is deemed adequate, 15 ml of heparinized solution (1500 units in 15 ml of 5 per cent dextrose in water) are infused into the artery proximally and distally through a small polyethylene catheter. The artery is immediately occluded with vascular clamps proximal and distal to the arteriotomy site. A stay suture is placed at each end of the arteriotomy, which is then closed using a continuous stitch of 6–0 Tevdek. It is important not to raise an intimal flap nor to penetrate the posterior intima with the needle. After suturing, first the distal and then the proximal clamp is removed. Minor leaks usually respond to gentle pressure applied directly with a finger over the site of the arteriotomy repair. The radial pulse should be palpable and as strong as it was prior to catheterization. If it is absent or markedly reduced, the artery should be reopened, a Fogarty balloon catheter passed again, and the vessel repaired. If this does not result in return of the pulse, an experienced vascular surgeon should be consulted. The vein may be tied off or repaired directly.

The wound is then flushed with sterile saline and a 1 per cent povidone-iodine solution, and the skin incision is closed. For skin closure, the authors use a subcuticular stitch with 4–0 Dexon, an absorbable polyglycolic acid suture material which makes a return visit for suture removal unnecessary. Antibiotic ointment (10 per cent povidone-iodine) is applied to the suture line, and the area should be covered with a dressing.

Postcatheterization orders should include the following:

1. Resume all previous medications.
2. Measure blood pressure and pulse and inspect dressing every 15 minutes for 1 hour, every hour for 4 hours, then every 4 hours for 12 hours.
3. Call a house officer or attending physician *and* a member of the catheterization laboratory staff in the event of bleeding, loss of pulse, hypotension, or chest pain.
4. Encourage oral fluid intake of 2 to 3 liters over 6 to 8 hours (if an angiographic contrast agent has been administered).
5. Administer analgesic medication, as needed.

FEMORAL ARTERIAL APPROACH

Right- and left-heart catheterization via the femoral approach is usually performed from the right groin, although the left groin may be used if necessary. The major landmarks of the femoral area are the anterior superior iliac spine, the pubic tubercle, and the inguinal ligament running between them. The femoral nerve, artery, and vein are located in the femoral triangle below the inguinal ligament. Proceeding from lateral to medial, the relationship of these structures may be remembered with the aid of the mnemonic NAVY (*n*erve, *a*rtery, *v*ein, empt*y* space).

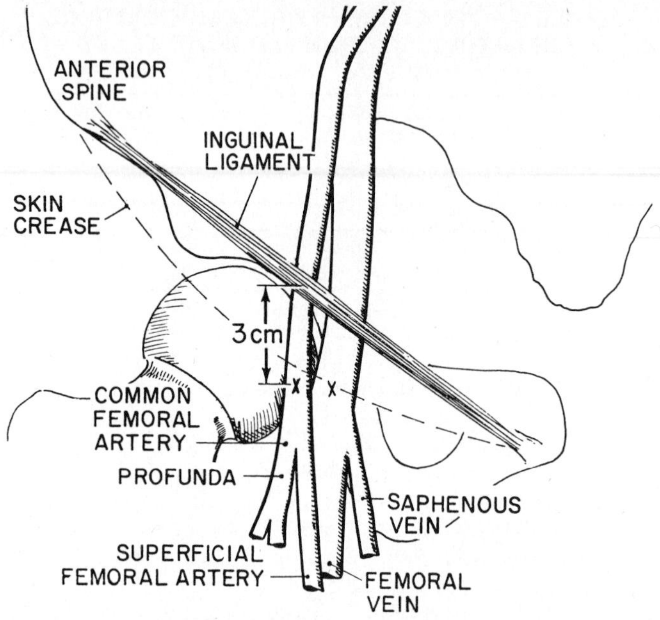

FIGURE 9–1. Anatomy relevant to percutaneous catheterization of femoral artery and vein: the right femoral artery and vein run underneath the inguinal ligament, which connects the anterior-superior iliac spine and pubic tubercle. The arterial skin nick (indicated by X) should be placed approximately 1½ to 2 fingerbreadths (3 cm) below the inguinal ligament and directly over the femoral artery pulsation. The venous skin nick should be placed at the same level, but approximately 1 fingerbreadth medial. (From Baim, D. S., and Grossman, W.: Percutaneous approach. *In* Grossman, W. [ed.]: Cardiac Catheterization and Angiography. 3rd ed. Philadelphia, Lea and Febiger, 1986.)

PROCEDURE. The femoral artery is located by means of palpation at a point approximately 1½ to 2 fingerbreadths below the inguinal ligament (Fig. 9–1). The skin and subcutaneous tissue over the artery and vein are anesthetized with 10 to 15 ml of 1 per cent lidocaine. The anesthetic must be given carefully and must not be injected directly into a vessel. It is important that percutaneous puncture of the femoral vessels be a correct distance below the inguinal ligament; if it is too high, hemostasis may be impaired, owing to the posterior course of the vessels in the pelvic cavity; if it is too low, the vein may run behind the artery, and the artery may be entered after it bifurcates into the profunda and superficial femoral branches. Although the inguinal crease is usually just below the inguinal ligament, this relationship is not constant, and the use of the inguinal ligament as the primary landmark is therefore advised.

When performing right-heart and left-heart catheterization via the femoral approach, the authors prefer to enter the femoral vein first. This is accomplished using an 18-gauge Seldinger needle, which consists of a blunt, tapered external cannula with a sharp obturator. After a one-fourth-inch skin incision has been made at the correct distance below the inguinal ligament and medial to the arterial pulse, the needle and obturator are inserted with a smooth motion at a 45-degree angle (Fig. 9–2). If the patient has discomfort as the needle penetrates the deeper femoral tissues, additional lidocaine can be infiltrated through the needle, after the obturator is removed and it is confirmed that the needle is extravascular. A small syringe is then attached to the needle, which is slowly withdrawn while continuous gentle aspiration is performed. When the vein is entered, blood is easily aspirated. The syringe is removed without moving the needle, and a Telfon-coated guidewire (preferably a J tip) is inserted into the needle and is advanced into the vein. The guidewire should pass easily, with its course checked fluoroscopically. The needle is then withdrawn over the guide, and a venous sheath of appropriate size with obturator is placed into the vein over the guidewire. The sheath should be inserted with a twisting, forward pressure. The obturator and guidewire are then removed, and the sheath is flushed via a stopcock.

Catheter Insertions. The femoral artery may then be punctured at a 45-degree angle with the Seldinger needle, once a skin incision one-fourth-inch long and deep has been made directly over the arterial pulse. The obturator is removed, and the needle is slowly withdrawn until the tip enters the artery lumen and a pulsatile flow of arterial blood exits from the needle hub. A Teflon-coated J guidewire is inserted into the needle and advanced into the artery. The guidewire should advance

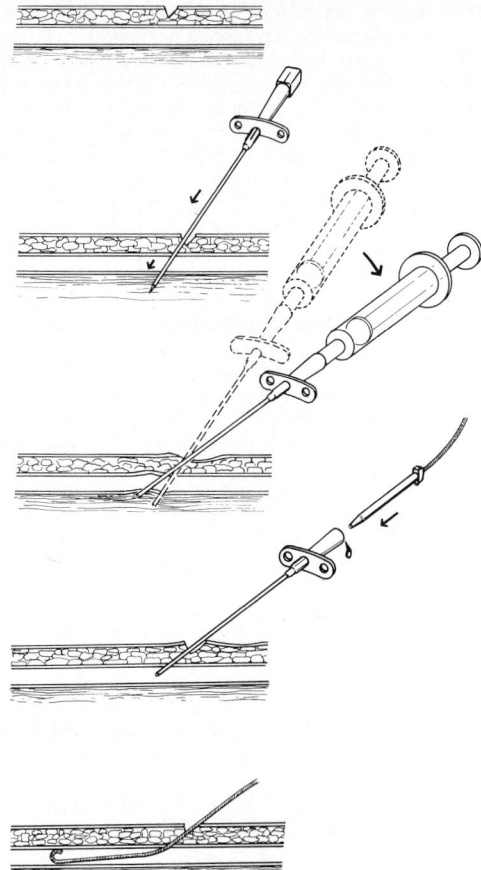

FIGURE 9–2. Seldinger technique for venous puncture and catheterization. In the top panel, a skin nick has been made overlying the desired vein, which is then transfixed through and through by Seldinger needle with obturator in place. The center panel shows the obturator removed and the needle cannula attached to a syringe. Lowering of the syringe toward the skin surface facilitates proper alignment of the needle tip at the moment that withdrawal brings the tip into the vessel lumen. Entry into the vessel lumen during withdrawal is recognized by sudden appearance of free-flowing blood in the syringe, which is held under gentle negative pressure. The syringe is then removed and a J guidewire (shown with plastic guide in place) is advanced into the vessel; following this, the needle cannula is removed and replaced with a catheter. A similar technique is used for arterial puncture, except that a syringe is unnecessary since arterial pressure will cause blood to spurt backward through the needle once the needle tip is in the vessel lumen. (From Baim, D. S., and Grossman, W.: Percutaneous approach. *In* Grossman, W. [ed.]: Cardiac Catheterization and Angiography. 3rd ed. Philadelphia, Lea and Febiger, 1986.)

easily, with its position observed on fluoroscopy as it passes into the abdominal aorta. The needle is then withdrawn over the guidewire, and the artery is compressed firmly at the puncture site. A No. 8 French arterial sheath with a proximal hemostasis valve and a side-port extension tube is inserted into the artery over the guidewire. The sheath obturator and guidewire are removed, and the sheath is flushed via the side-arm extension tube, which is connected to a pressure transducer for continuous monitoring of femoral arterial pressure. It is, of course, possible to insert an end-hole catheter into the artery directly over the guidewire without use of a sheath. This would be appropriate if only one arterial catheter were to be used. However, use of the arterial sheath greatly facilitates catheter changes, permits use of a greater variety of catheters, and allows continuous monitoring of femoral artery pressure during left-heart catheterization.[28] With sheaths in the femoral artery and vein, and the femoral artery pressure recorded for monitoring purposes, it is possible to proceed to right- and left-heart catheterization.

Right-Heart Catheterization. The right-heart catheters used with the femoral approach are the same as those described for the brachial approach (i.e., Cournand, Goodale-Lubin, or Swan-Ganz) (Fig. 9–3). The first two of these catheters have an elbow bend, which facilitates passage from the right ventricle into the pulmonary artery. As the catheter is advanced through the sheath and into the inferior vena cava, its motion should be observed on fluoroscopy. The movement of the catheter should be gentle and the passage effortless; catheter advancement should never be forced. While the right-heart catheter is passed from the groin, it frequently enters the renal or hepatic veins. If this occurs, the catheter should be withdrawn and rotated before it is advanced farther. A guidewire may be used if a tortuous venous system makes catheter passage difficult.

Once the right atrium has been entered, a pressure tracing from this chamber should be recorded, and a sample of blood should be obtained from the superior vena cava for measurement of oxygen saturation. The catheter is then advanced through the right ventricle and into the pulmonary artery. Blood pressure and oxygen saturation should then be measured in the pulmonary artery. A difference between superior vena caval and pulmonary artery oxygen saturation of greater than 7 per cent should indicate the possibility of a left-to-right shunt,[29] as discussed on p. 254. Occasionally it is difficult to maneuver a Cournand or a Goodale-Lubin catheter from the right ventricle to the pulmonary artery from the groin, in which case it is best to remove the right-heart catheter and use a balloon-tipped, flow-directed catheter for the right-heart study. In addition, in patients with left bundle branch block, a balloon catheter is preferred because of the reduced likelihood of trauma to the right bundle branch during right-heart catheterization with this type of catheter. Catheter-induced right bundle branch block in a patient with complete left bundle branch block results in complete heart block and can cause asystole. A Gorlin or Cournand right-heart pacing catheter may also be used in this situation to initiate emergency pacing, if necessary.

The right-heart catheter is then used to record pulmonary artery wedge pressure; it is advanced under fluoroscopic guidance into a peripheral pulmonary artery branch during a deep inspiration. To record a wedge pressure with a balloon-type catheter, the balloon is inflated while the catheter tip is in a proximal pulmonary artery. The catheter is then advanced until the pressure configuration changes to that of a wedge pressure. Deflation of the balloon at this point should result in reappearance of pulmonary artery pressure. To re-obtain wedge pressure, the balloon is *slowly* inflated while catheter pressure is monitored until the pressure waveform changes to a wedge contour. Overinflation of the balloon, or inflation of the balloon in a distal vessel, carries the risk of pulmonary artery rupture. Also, to reduce the likelihood of pulmonary infarction and/or pulmonary artery rupture, the balloon should not be left inflated for longer than the time required to record pressure and obtain a sample of blood to determine oxygen saturation. Positioning of the Cournand or balloon-tipped catheter during right-heart catheterization may be facilitated by the use of guidewires, but catheters should not be advanced into the wedge position with a guidewire protruding beyond the catheter tip.

Left-Heart Catheterization. When using a right femoral artery sheath, this procedure may be performed with a variety of catheters

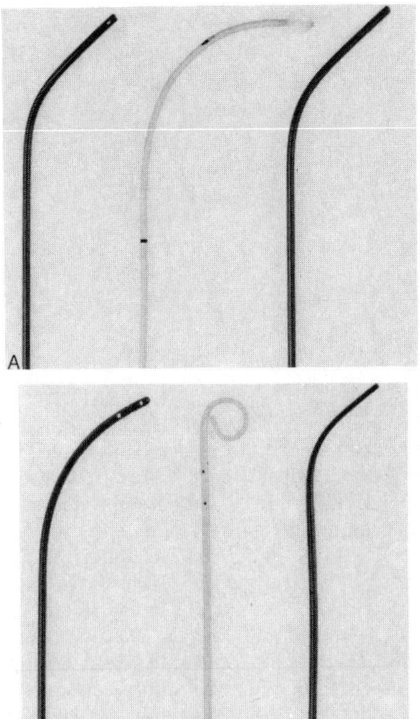

FIGURE 9–3. Various cardiac catheters. *A*, From left to right: Goodale-Lubin, balloon-flotation Swan-Ganz, and Cournand. *B*, From left to right: NIH, Nycore-pigtail, and Sones.

(Fig. 9–3). Closed-end hole catheters (NIH, Eppendorf) similar to those used in the direct brachial approach may be introduced through the sheath and advanced into the aorta and left ventricle. However, passage of catheters through the frequently tortuous iliofemoral system is facilitated by the use of end-hole catheters with J guidewires. In our laboratories the most commonly used catheter for this purpose is the "pigtail" catheter, which has multiple side holes and an end hole and can be used for angiography as well as pressure measurement. After introduction of the left-heart catheter, 5000 units of heparin are administered intravenously for anticoagulation.

When preformed catheters are used (pigtail, Judkins, or Amplatz), a J-shaped guidewire is inserted into the catheter prior to introducing the catheter into the sheath. Then, when the catheter tip is within the sheath, the J guide is advanced beyond the tip and into the femoral artery for several centimeters. Under fluoroscopic observation, the catheter is then advanced into the aorta, with the guidewire tip preceding it. Again, the catheter passage should be effortless. When the catheter is in the abdominal aorta, the guidewire is removed, and the catheter and sheath are aspirated and then flushed with heparinized saline. The catheter and sheath should be flushed every 5 minutes after heparin administration and every 2 to 3 minutes if heparin is not used.

The catheter is advanced carefully around the aortic arch to avoid inadvertently entering the aortic arch vessels. The pressure just above the aortic valve is recorded along with simultaneous femoral artery pressure via the side arm of the sheath. As will be discussed later, the peak femoral artery pressure is frequently slightly higher than the peak central aortic pressure; however, mean systolic pressures are usually identical. The catheter is then passed across the aortic valve into the left ventricle (Fig. 9–4). If the aortic valve is abnormal, a guidewire may be required to stiffen the catheter to permit crossing of the aortic valve. In aortic stenosis, the valve is best traversed with a straight-tip guidewire, and the catheter is then advanced over the wire into the ventricle for pressure measurement (Fig. 9–4). Other catheters, such as the Sones, right Judkins, and Gensini, may be preferable in selected patients. Not more than 15 minutes or so should be expended in attempting to cross an aortic valve with a single type of catheter before trying another.

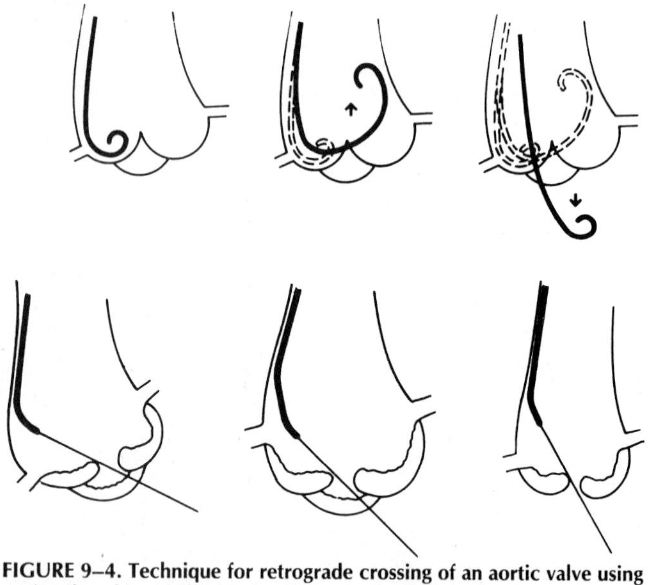

FIGURE 9–4. Technique for retrograde crossing of an aortic valve using a pigtail catheter. The upper three panels illustrate the technique for crossing a normal aortic valve. In the bottom row, the use of a straight guidewire and pigtail catheter in combination is illustrated. Increasing the length of protruding guidewire straightens the catheter curve and causes the wire to point more toward the right coronary ostium; reducing the length of protruding wire restores the pigtail contour and deflects the guidewire tip toward the left coronary artery. Once the correct length of wire and the correct rotational orientation of the catheter have been found, repeated advancement and withdrawal of catheter and guidewire together will allow retrograde passage across the valve. In a dilated aortic root, the angled pigtail catheter is preferable. In a small aortic root (bottom row, right) a right coronary Judkins catheter may have advantages. (From Baim, D. S., and Grossman, W.: Percutaneous approach. *In* Grossman, W. [ed.]: Cardiac Catheterization and Angiography. 3rd ed. Philadelphia, Lea and Febiger, 1986.)

When the catheter enters the left ventricle, the left ventricular and femoral artery pressures are recorded to evaluate aortic valve function, and the left ventricular and pulmonary artery wedge pressures are recorded to evaluate mitral valve function. Cardiac output is measured, and a right-heart pullback is performed to evaluate the pulmonic and tricuspid valves by recording, in close time sequence, pulmonary artery, right ventricular, and right atrial pressures. If left ventricular angiography is planned, and the aortic valve was not crossed with a pigtail or other catheter suitable for ventricular angiography, an exchange guidewire may be introduced into the left ventricle, the catheter may be removed over the guidewire, and a pigtail catheter then advanced over the exchange guidewire back into the left ventricle.

Termination of the Procedure. Following completion of the hemodynamic and angiographic studies (coronary arteriography is discussed in Chapter 10), the catheters are removed. Preformed arterial catheters should be withdrawn from the artery into the sheath with several centimeters of guidewire protruding from the catheter tip to avoid trauma to the arterial intima. Following administration of protamine to reverse the heparin effect, the arterial and venous sheaths are removed, and the vessels are compressed firmly by hand or a mechanical compressor for 15 to 20 minutes, with control of bleeding during this time. With this technique significant hematoma formation occurs in fewer than 2 per cent of patients. In patients with hypertension, or wide pulse pressure (aortic regurgitation), longer groin compression times may be required to achieve hemostasis.

The patient should rest in bed and keep the right leg immobile following a right femoral catheterization. However, most patients find it uncomfortable to be supine for several hours, and this is *not* necessary unless there is a problem with hypotension. Elevation of the head of the bed to 30 to 45 degrees does not increase the risk of femoral bleeding as long as the leg is kept immobile and Valsalva maneuver is avoided.

TRANSSEPTAL LEFT-HEART CATHETERIZATION

When the aortic valve cannot be crossed by the retrograde approach from either the brachial or the femoral artery, and it is essential that the left ventricular pressure be measured, transseptal catheterization of the left ventricle may be performed. In our experience, approximately 5 per cent of severely stenotic valves cannot be crossed in a retrograde manner within a reasonable period of time, and these patients, as well as those with tilting-disc prosthetic aortic valves, are candidates for this procedure. Patients with porcine heterograft valves and ball-cage prosthetic aortic valves can safely undergo retrograde left ventricular catheterization.[30] Transseptal left-heart catheterization is also indicated in patients with suspected mitral valve obstruction in whom a pulmonary artery wedge pressure cannot be measured. There has been a revival of interest in transseptal catheterization in recent years,[31, 32] and newer techniques involving the combination of an introducer and a sheath increase the safety and versatility of the procedure.[33] In addition, the transseptal technique is essential for some of the newer interventional techniques, such as balloon mitral valvuloplasty (Chap. 40).

PROCEDURE. Transseptal catheterization is performed in our laboratories using the Teflon 70-cm No. 8 French catheter developed by Brockenbrough and Braunwald.[34] Prior to insertion of the catheter into the right femoral vein, a Brockenbrough needle is inserted into the catheter, with a Bing stylet protruding 1 cm or so beyond the needle tip to prevent penetration of the catheter wall by the needle (Fig. 9–5).

With the patient positioned for a straight frontal projection, the Brockenbrough catheter is advanced to the junction of the right atrium and the superior vena cava by means of a guidewire. The guidewire is removed, the catheter is flushed, and right atrial pressure is recorded. The transseptal needle with its stylet is inserted and then gently advanced through the transseptal catheter under fluoroscopic observation. It is important to allow free rotation of the needle as it is advanced by holding the needle itself (not the direction indicator) between the fingertips. When the tip of the stylet is near the tip of the catheter, the stylet is removed, and the needle is advanced until the needle tip is just within the catheter. The needle is held firmly in this position, with the direction indicator pointing up, to prevent inadvertent extension of the needle tip out of the catheter. The needle is flushed

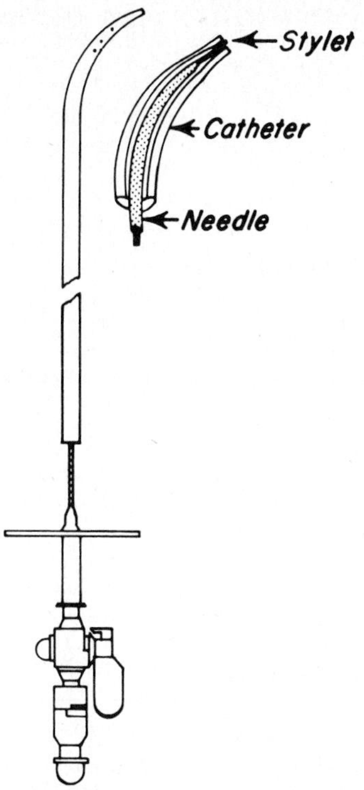

FIGURE 9–5. The Brockenbrough transseptal needle, catheter, and stylet. Use of the stylet prevents inadvertent puncture of the catheter by the needle tip during insertion of the needle into the catheter. The wide flange near the needle hub is pointed on one side to indicate the direction of the needle tip. (From Grossman, W.: Cardiac Catheterization and Angiography. 2nd ed. Philadelphia, Lea and Febiger, 1980.)

and connected to a pressure transducer, so that a phasic right atrial pressure and a mean pressure can be recorded through the needle and can be verified as similar to that recorded through the catheter prior to insertion of the needle. It is important not to use soft or excessively long lengths of connecting tubing for this purpose, since it is possible to overdamp the pressure recorded through the 21-gauge needle tip.

Puncture of Atrial Septum. After right atrial pressure has been recorded, the catheter and needle are slowly withdrawn as a unit while the direction indicator is rotated clockwise to the 4 o'clock position with fluoroscopic and pressure monitoring. The catheter will move over the aortic root in a sudden leftward motion; further inferior pull will usually result in a second, smaller leftward motion, as the catheter tip enters the fossa ovalis. Right atrial phasic pressure should be monitored during this time. The catheter and needle (with the needle tip still within the catheter) are then advanced, and the catheter tip will move superiorly, sliding up the interatrial septum. It will usually "hang up" on the lip of the fossa ovalis, at the level of or slightly superior to the plane of the aortic valve. Occasionally, the catheter will pass easily into the left atrium through a patent foramen ovale and will be manifest as leftward motion of the catheter tip and by the appearance of a left atrial phasic waveform. If this occurs, the oxygen saturation of blood aspirated through the needle should be checked and the pressure recorded to document entry into the left atrium. The catheter is then gently advanced 1 or 2 cm over the needle, and the needle is removed. More commonly, the foramen ovale is not patent and must be punctured with the needle tip. This is done during pressure and fluoroscopic monitoring by advancing the needle 1 cm beyond the catheter tip, when the tip is firmly wedged in the fossa ovalis.

After the needle penetrates the interatrial septum, a left atrial pressure waveform (usually a higher mean pressure than in the right atrium) will be evident. Entry into the left atrium should be confirmed by measurement of oxygen saturation. The needle and catheter are then slowly advanced into the left atrium, with the needle position indicator maintained in the 4 o'clock position. Resistance is usually encountered as the catheter tip punctures the septum, and it is important to stabilize the catheter position by holding the catheter in the groin with the left hand while advancing the catheter and needle with the right hand. When the catheter traverses the septum and enters the left atrium (a 1- to 2-cm leftward motion), the needle is withdrawn, the catheter is flushed, left atrial pressure is recorded, and blood is withdrawn for measurement of oxygen saturation through the catheter. Passage of the catheter from the left atrium into the left ventricle is achieved by advancing the catheter tip through the mitral valve. The transseptal catheter may enter a pulmonary vein or left atrial appendage. In this case, the left ventricle may be entered by withdrawing the catheter slowly while rotating it counterclockwise and/or by inserting a coiled-tip occluder to increase the bend in the catheter tip. An improved technique more widely used today is to place a Mullins' sheath in the left atrium at the time of the initial transseptal puncture, and advance a balloon-flotation catheter through this sheath into the left atrium and left ventricle.[33] It is important to emphasize that transseptal catheterization—as indeed all cardiac catheterization procedures—should be done only by or under the supervision of physicians experienced in the technique. The transseptal needle may perforate the right atrial wall, enter the coronary sinus or the aorta, or perforate the left atrial wall. The small needle tip itself (21-gauge) is not likely to cause a major problem unless an atrial wall is torn; however, passage of the catheter through these structures may result in tamponade and death. Thus, the emphasis placed on pressure monitoring through the needle is important.

PEDIATRIC CARDIAC CATHETERIZATION

The methods described above are broadly applicable to the cardiac catheterization of children, but *special considerations for the newborn* should be emphasized. In such patients, meticulous attention must be given to maintenance of body temperature by means of heating pads, an infrared lamp, or other devices designed for this purpose. In addition, precise attention must be paid to fluid balance, with care being taken to replace exactly the volume of fluid and blood removed, so as to cause neither hypovolemia and hypotension nor hypervolemia with pulmonary edema. In the newborn, the umbilical artery and vein may be used for catheterization for about 72 hours after birth. Of course, catheters should be of small diameters and lengths in procedures involving neonates, infants, and children. The reader is referred to texts and reviews detailing special technical considerations in cardiac catheterization on newborns.[23]

CATHETER SIZES AND CONSTRUCTION

In addition to the above-mentioned considerations, it is important that individuals involved in cardiac catheterization understand the sizing of catheters, needles, and guidewires and that they have a knowledge of different methods and materials used in their construction. Cardiac catheters differ in size, length, shape, and material of construction. The last factor determines the friction coefficient, hardness, curve retention, moisture absorption, and autoclavability. In addition, it is clear that different catheter materials have varying degrees of thrombogenicity.[35] Cardiac catheters are usually constructed of woven Dacron, polyethylene, or polyurethane. Some catheter walls are reinforced with stainless steel braids to increase torque control and to enable the catheter to withstand high intraluminal pressures during the injection of angiographic contrast material. In addition, the walls of most cardiac catheters are impregnated with lead or barium salts to render them radiopaque.

The outside diameter (OD) of a catheter is indicated in French units: one French (F) unit = 0.33 mm (0.013 inches). Thus a No. 7 French (7F) catheter has an OD of 2.33 mm. The internal diameter (ID) of a catheter is always, of course, less than the OD, the exact relationship between OD and ID depending on the thickness of the catheter wall. The ID of the catheter determines the thickness of the guidewire that can be passed through the catheter. The guidewire must in turn be small enough to fit through the lumen of the needle used for vessel puncture in percutaneous catheterization techniques. The diameter of the guidewire is usually expressed in inches (0.032, 0.035, 0.038, and so on), whereas needle size is expressed in "gauge," indicating the OD of the needle. An 18-gauge thin-walled needle has an OD of 0.086 inches. The cardiologist beginning to use these techniques must be familiar with these units. In addition, it is wise to check that catheter, guidewire, and needle are all compatible in size and length before the vessel is punctured.

HEMODYNAMIC MEASUREMENTS

MEASUREMENT OF INTRAVASCULAR AND INTRACARDIAC PRESSURES

THEORETICAL CONSIDERATIONS. Myocardial contractile force is transmitted through the fluid medium of blood as a pressure wave. An important objective of the cardiac catheterization procedure is to assess accurately the forces, and therefore the pressure waves, generated by various cardiac chambers. *A pressure wave may be considered a complex periodic fluctuation in force per unit area*, with one cycle consisting of the time interval from the onset of one wave to the onset of the next. The number of cycles within 1 second is termed the *fundamental frequency* of the waveform. Thus, for a left ventricular pressure waveform at a heart rate of 120 beats/min, the fundamental frequency would be 2 sec^{-1}, or 2 Hz.

Considered as a complex periodic waveform, the pressure wave may be subjected to a type of analysis developed by the French physicist Fourier, whereby any complex waveform may be considered to be the mathematical summation of a series of simple sine waves of differing frequencies and amplitudes.[36] The practical consequence of this analysis is that in order to record pressure accurately a system must respond in such a way that output amplitude is directly proportional to input throughout the range of frequencies contained within the pressure wave. If components in a given frequency range are either suppressed or exaggerated by the transducer system, the recorded signal will be a grossly distorted version of the original physiological waveform. For example, the incisura of the aortic pressure wave contains frequencies above 10 cycles/sec; if the pressure measurement system were unable to respond to these, the incisura would be slurred or absent.

The *frequency response* of a pressure measurement system may be defined as the ratio of output amplitude/input amplitude over a range of frequencies of the input or pressure wave. An ideal pressure measurement system would have an output/input ratio of one over an infinite range of input frequencies. In practice this is never the case, and the frequency response characteristics reflect the interaction of the *natural frequency* of the system and the degree of *damping*. If the sensing membrane in a pressure measurement system were shock-excited, in the absence of friction it would oscillate for an indefinite period of time in simple harmonic motion. The frequency of this motion would be the *natural frequency* of the system. The amplitude of the output signal tends to be augmented as the frequency of that signal approaches the natural frequency of the system (Fig. 9–6*A*). Optimal damping dissipates the energy of the oscillating system gradually, thereby maintaining the frequency response curve nearly flat (constant input/output ratio) as it approaches the region of the pressure measurement system's natural frequency. An extensive literature on the question of what frequency response is desirable and on the testing, construction, and evaluation of different pressure measurement systems is available.[23, 37]

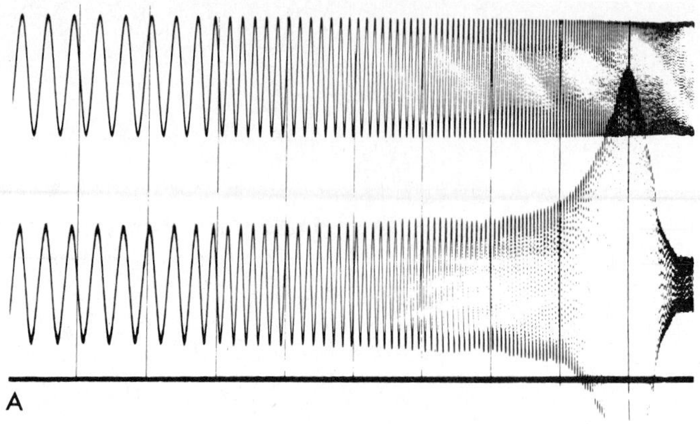

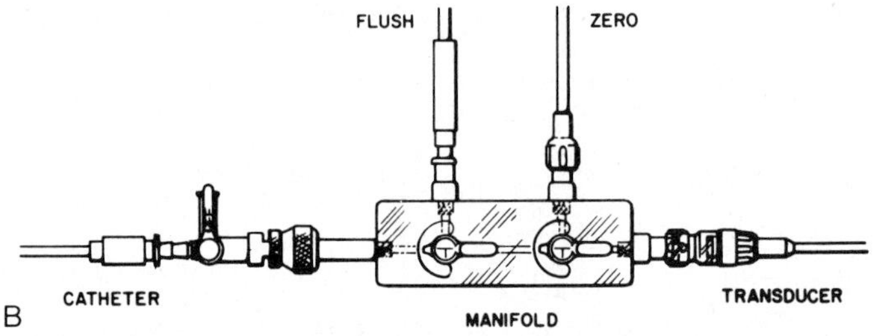

FIGURE 9–6. Recording of phasic pressures with a fluid-filled catheter system.

***A*, The upper trace shows a "true" phasic pressure of 20 mm Hg (sine wave of increasing frequency) generated within a closed chamber. The lower trace shows the same pressure recorded with a fluid-filled 110-cm catheter–external transducer system. Note that the pressures are equal in amplitude up to a frequency of about 15 Hz. As the frequency of the pressure sine wave increases above this point, an increase in amplitude occurs owing to resonance in the catheter-transducer system. The "resonant frequency" is about 40 Hz, and above this frequency, the amplitude of the signal falls rapidly. In this case, since the resonant frequency is well above most frequencies contained in the intracardiac pressure waveforms, little distortion of intracardiac pressure by the catheter-transducer recording system will be present. (The vertical lines are 1 sec apart.)**

***B*, The system used to record the pressure in *A*. A small volume-displacement transducer is attached directly to the back end of a two-side-arm manifold. Fluid-filled tubings are attached to the side arms for "zero" pressure reference and catheter flushing, and the front end of the manifold is connected directly to the catheter. Care must be taken during filling of the transducer and manifold to remove all air bubbles, which can markedly lower the resonant frequency of the system.**

FLUID-FILLED CATHETER SYSTEMS. With fluid-filled catheters, an external pressure transducer is used to detect changes in pressure at the catheter tip that are transmitted to the transducer by the fluid column in the catheter. A pressure transducer consists basically of a diaphragm that is deformed in a linear fashion by the application of pressure within the physiological range. Deformation of the diaphragm produces a proportional change in electrical resistance within the transducer. By use of a Wheatstone bridge-type circuit, this change in transducer resistance is converted into an electrical potential, which is then amplified and recorded as an analog signal that represents pressure applied to the transducer. Operation of the bridge requires an excitation voltage, usually supplied by the pressure amplifier. A variable resistance control, by means of which the electrical potential can be adjusted to zero when no pressure is applied, permits balancing of the transducer. Calibration of the system is performed by applying known pressures to the transducer by means of a mercury manometer and observing the analog voltage output. The sensitivity of the amplifiers used in pressure recording systems is adjustable, so that a given pressure may be made to correspond to a precise deflection of the recorder.

Because movement of the transducer diaphragm is necessary to produce a voltage output for a given pressure, a certain volume of fluid must move through the catheter-connector tubing system to the transducer to produce a pressure recording. This tends to cause low-frequency resonance in the system. The resonant frequency of a fluid-filled system should be above the frequencies contained in intracardiac pressure waveforms (see above). For usual clinical purposes, a system with frequency response that is flat to 10 or 12 Hz with a resonant frequency above this level is adequate. This can be achieved most easily by use of small volume-displacement transducers, with imposition of as few stopcocks and connecting tubings as possible between the catheter hub and the transducer. The system used in our cardiac catheterization laboratories is shown in Figure 9–6*B*.

With an aqueous fluid–filled catheter attached to a transducer, the transducer will indicate zero pressure when the catheter tip is at the same height as the transducer. If the catheter tip is elevated above the transducer, a positive pressure of 1 mm Hg will be indicated for every 1.36 cm of height difference; if the catheter tip is below the transducer level, a negative pressure of the same magnitude will be indicated. These effects are due simply to gravitational force acting on the fluid column in the catheter and the specific gravity of mercury of 13.6. The transducer is therefore positioned at a level approximately the same as that of the heart, usually the midchest. If the transducer is placed at

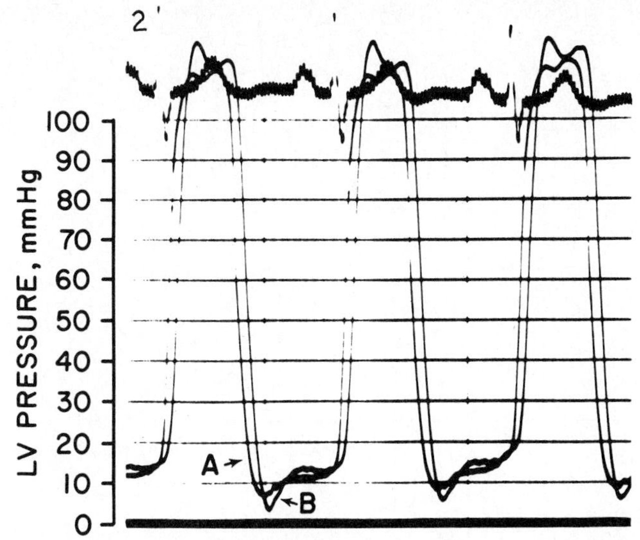

FIGURE 9–7. Left ventricular pressures recorded with a manometer-tipped catheter (*A*) and a fluid-filled catheter–extended transducer system with a low resonant frequency (*B*). Note undershoot of pressure in early diastole, overshoot of pressure in early systole, and delay of fluid-filled catheter pressure relative to the "true" pressure. (From Grossman, W.: Cardiac Catheterization and Angiography. 3rd ed. Philadelphia, Lea and Febiger, 1986.)

a different height, attaching a second fluid-filled catheter to the transducer and positioning the tip of that catheter at the zero (midchest) level permit proper zeroing of the transducer relative to the catheter tip position within the heart (Fig. 9–6*B*). It is important to note that pressures measured inside the heart chambers do not necessarily equal the true transmural pressures, because of the normal intrathoracic negative pressure, which ranges between 0 and −8 mm Hg during normal respiration.

Even when a pressure measurement system has a high degree of sensitivity, uniform frequency response, and optimal damping and is properly zeroed and balanced, distortions and inaccuracies in the pressure waveform may occur. Motion of the catheter within the heart and great vessels accelerates the fluid contained within the catheter, and such *catheter whip* artifacts may produce superimposed waves of ± 10 mm Hg. Catheter whip artifacts are particularly common in tracings from the pulmonary arteries and are difficult to avoid.

MANOMETER-TIPPED CATHETERS. In order to minimize artifacts associated with low resonant frequency systems, catheter whip, and excessive damping, some laboratories employ micromanometer-tipped catheters, with which the pressure transducer is actually placed in the cardiac chamber in which pressure is being measured. As is evident in Figure 9–7, there may be a distinct difference in waveform between "true" left ventricular pressure (as recorded using an intracardiac micromanometer) and that recorded through a standard fluid-filled catheter system. Low resonant frequency and inadequate damping of the fluid-filled system in this example resulted in exaggeration of the high-frequency components in the left ventricular pressure rise and fall, with corresponding artifactual overshoot of the pressures in early diastole and early systole. More optimal damping and natural frequency characteristics of the fluid-filled system can minimize these artifacts but cannot eliminate them. In addition, a 30- to 40-msec delay in the pressure waveform occurs with fluid-filled catheter systems, necessitating the use of manometer-tipped catheters in situations in which recording of simultaneous pressure and angiographic volume, echocardiographic, phonocardiographic, or electrocardiographic data is required. The high-frequency response of manometer-tipped catheter transducers (resonant frequency = 25 to 40 kHz) permits their application for the detection and recording of intracardiac sounds.

Some manometer-tipped catheters do not have an end-hold and must therefore be inserted via arteriotomy or a vascular sheath. Millar* manufactures several No. 8 French end-hole manometer-tipped angiocatheters that can be used with a guidewire. Since the zero level of the manometer-tipped catheter may drift, it is most useful to have a fluid-filled lumen in the catheter by means of which a true zero pressure reference level can be established.

*Millar Instruments, Inc., Houston, Texas.

Representative Pressure Tracings

In evaluating pressure tracings, specific phasic and mean pressure values should be measured, the phasic pressure waveform contours noted, and pressures in different chambers compared. Analysis of these data, interpreted in the light of cardiac output and angiographic measurement, permits detection and quantitation of valvular, myocardial, and pericardial abnormalities.

NORMAL PRESSURE WAVEFORMS. An understanding of pressure waveforms, both under normal conditions and in various disease states, is predicated on a thorough comprehension of the events of the cardiac cycle (Fig. 13–26, p. 405). Shown in Figure 9–8 are normal pressure waveforms obtained with fluid-filled catheters.

The *right atrial pressure waveform* consists of two major positive deflections—the *a* and *v* waves. The *a* wave is due to atrial systole and follows the P wave of the electrocardiogram. As the pressure declines from the peak of the *a* wave (the *x* descent), a small positive deflection, the *c* wave, occurs concomitant with tricuspid valve closure. After the "*c*" wave, right atrial pressure continues to fall (*x* descent) even though the atrium is filling with blood (the tricuspid valve is closed), owing to atrial relaxation. After full atrial relaxation occurs, at the nadir of the *x* descent, the pressure in the atrium starts to rise as atrial filling continues from peripheral venous return. This rise in the right atrial pressure during right ventricular systole is termed the *v* wave, and it reaches a peak just before the opening of the tricuspid valve. Following opening of the tricuspid valve, the right atrium empties into the right ventricle, and pressure in the atrium falls, constituting the *y* descent. Following the *y* descent, pressure in the atrium is equal to ventricular diastolic pressure and slowly increases as the ventricle fills. Peak *a* and *v* wave pressures are measured, and the mean pressure is obtained electronically. Normal values are shown in Table 9–2.

The *diastolic phase of the right ventricular pressure pulse* consists of an early rapid filling wave, during which approximately 60 per cent of ventricular filling occurs; a slow filling period, accounting for approximately 25 per cent of ventricular filling; and an atrial systolic wave (*a*), accounting for approximately 15 per cent of ventricular filling. During diastole, right atrial and right ventricular pressures are nearly equal, because of the low resistance to flow across the tricuspid valve. Two pressures are usually measured: the peak systolic right ventricular pressure and the end-diastolic right ventricular pressure immediately following the *a* wave. The normal range of values for the pressures is shown in Table 9–2.

The *pulmonary artery pressure waveform* contains a systolic pressure owing to flow of blood into the pulmonary artery from the right ventricle. As right ventricular ejection ends, pressure in the pulmonary artery falls, and when right ventricular pressure drops below the pulmonary pressure, the pulmonary valve closes, resulting in the incisura on the pressure waveform. Pressure in the pulmonary artery then falls gradually as blood flows through the pulmonary arteries and veins into the left atrium and ventricle. The nadir of this pressure in late diastole is termed the end-diastolic pulmonary artery pressure. This pressure, together with the peak systolic pressure and the mean pulmonary artery pressure, are the parameters usually measured. It is not unusual to observe a small (≤ 5 mm Hg) gradient in peak systolic pressure between the right ventricle and the pulmonary artery.

The *pulmonary artery wedge pressure* (also termed *pulmonary capillary wedge pressure*) has a waveform similar to that of the left atrial pressure but is both damped

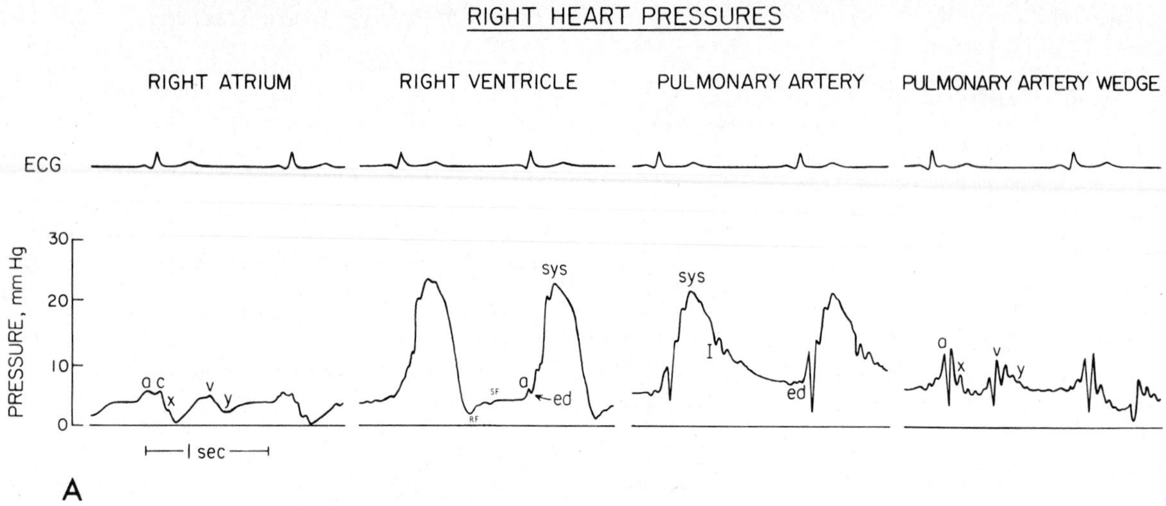

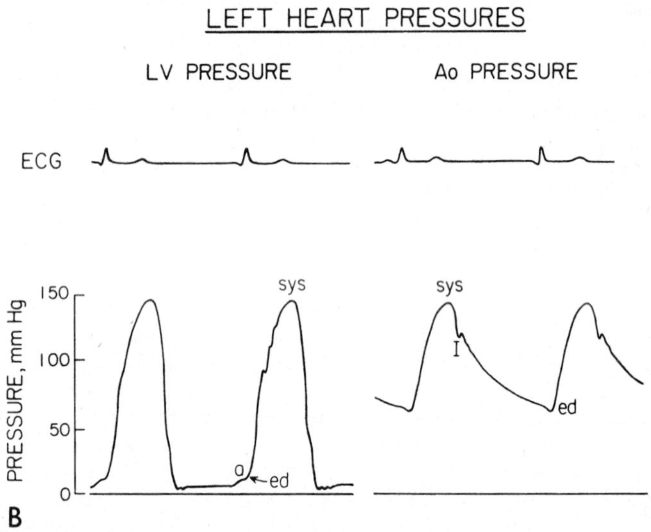

FIGURE 9–8. *A,* **Representative normal pressure tracings from the right side of the heart; sys = systolic, ed = end-diastolic.** *B,* **Representative normal pressures from the left ventricle (LV) and aorta (Ao).**

and delayed by transmission through the capillary vessels. A normal wedge pressure should show *a* and *v* waves, which reflect, respectively, left atrial systole and left atrial filling during left ventricular systole (see discussion of right atrial pressure above). However, *c* waves may not be apparent on the wedge pressure tracing. The *x* and *y* descents should be distinct in a wedge pressure tracing if it is not overdamped. The peak *a* and *v* wave pressures are usually measured, as is the mean wedge pressure. In a normal pulmonary circulation of low vascular resistance, the pulmonary artery flow is diminished at end diastole, so that end-diastolic pulmonary artery and mean pulmonary artery wedge pressures are approximately equal. Mean pulmonary artery pressure is always higher than mean wedge pressure (Table 9–2).

Normal left heart pressure waveforms are shown in Figure 9–8. The *left atrial pressure waveform* was discussed in the description of the pulmonary artery wedge pressure. Unless a transseptal catheterization is performed, pulmonary artery wedge pressure is recorded as an acceptable substitute for the actual left atrial pressure. It is important to recognize that this can be a source of error, unless a properly damped wedge pressure is observed and confirmed by determination of oxygen saturation.

The components of the *left ventricular waveform* are similar to those already described for that of the right ventricle. The pressures in the left ventricle in diastole (as well as systole) are normally higher than those in the right ventricle, owing in part to the greater wall thickness of the left ventricle, which results in greater chamber stiffness.

TABLE 9–2 RANGE OF NORMAL RESTING HEMODYNAMIC VALUES

	a Wave	*v* Wave	Mean	Systolic	End-Diastolic	Mean
Pressures						
Right atrium	2–10	2–10	0–8			
Right ventricle				15–30	0–8	
Pulmonary artery				15–30	3–12	9–16
Pulmonary artery wedge and left atrium	3–15	3–12	1–10			
Left ventricle				100–140	3–12	
Systemic arteries				100–140	60–90	70–105
Oxygen consumption index (ml/min/m²)		110–150				
Arteriovenous oxygen difference (ml/liter)		30–50				
Cardiac output index (liter/min/m²)		2.6–4.2				
Resistances (dynes-sec-cm^{-5})						
Pulmonary vascular		20–130				
Systemic vascular		700–1600				

The *central aortic pressure tracing* consists of a systolic wave, followed by the incisura, which denotes closure of the aortic valve, and then a gradual fall in pressure as the blood flows from the aorta through the peripheral arterial capillary and venous vessels. Pressure is normally measured at peak systole and at end diastole, and the mean pressure is determined electronically.

The *peripheral arterial pressure,* commonly measured during cardiac catheterization in the radial or femoral artery, has a waveform similar to that described for the central aorta. However, because of reflected waves within the arterial system, the peripheral arterial pressure may show a wider pulse pressure with a higher peak systolic pressure that that seen in the central aorta. The mean pressure is usually identical to or up to 5 mm Hg lower than the central aortic pressure. Thus, the peak systolic pressure gradients measured between the left ventricle and the systemic arterial system may vary depending on whether the central aortic pressure or a peripheral arterial pressure is measured.

ABNORMAL PRESSURE TRACINGS. As discussed in greater detail in subsequent chapters, pressure tracings may be virtually diagnostic of certain conditions. In *valvular aortic stenosis* (p. 1052), there is a pressure gradient between the left ventricle and the aorta; however, in addition, the rise in aortic pressure is slow and delayed compared with that of the left ventricle (Fig. 9–9). In contrast, hypertrophic obstructive cardiomyopathy (p. 1418) may also result in a large systolic pressure gradient but will show near identity of the slopes and timing of the left ventricular and aortic pressure increases. Both conditions are associated with increased ventricular stiffness and therefore may show prominent atrial systolic (*a*) waves transmitted into the left ventricular pressure tracing in late diastole.[38] *Aortic regurgitation* is characterized by near equalization of aortic and left ventricular pressures at end diastole, marked widening of the aortic pulse pressure, and slurring of the aortic incisura. *Mitral stenosis* is associated with a diastolic pressure gradient (pulmonary artery wedge or left atrium vs. left ventricle) across the mitral valve, which increases substantially with exercise (Fig. 9–10). If the patient is in sinus rhythm, there is a marked discrepancy between the large left atrial systolic wave (*a* wave) and the small or absent *a* wave in the left ventricular tracing.

A large *v* wave in the pulmonary artery wedge tracing may be present in patients with *mitral regurgitation* (p. 1034). The amplitude of the *v* wave is increased because the left atrium is being filled during systole not only with blood entering from the pulmonary veins but also with blood leaking across the mitral valve. Accurate evaluation of mitral valve function by measuring simultaneous pulmonary artery wedge and left ventricular pressure is based on the assumption that the wedge pressure accurately reflects both phasic and mean left atrial pressure (Fig. 9–11). If the wedge pressure is overdamped, it is possible, because the *v* wave height is reduced and the decline of the *v* wave delayed to overestimate the severity of mitral stenosis and underestimate the severity of mitral regurgitation.

Detection of *stenosis and regurgitation of the tricuspid* (p. 1069) and *pulmonic valves* (p. 1075) during right-heart catheterization is usually assessed by pullback of the catheters from the pulmonary artery to the right ventricle to the right atrium. However, more precise measurement of simultaneous pressures can be performed using a double-lumen right-heart catheter, in which the lumen tips are separated at the end of the catheter by a distance sufficient to permit monitoring pressures on opposite sides of the tricuspid valve or pulmonary outflow tract and valve.

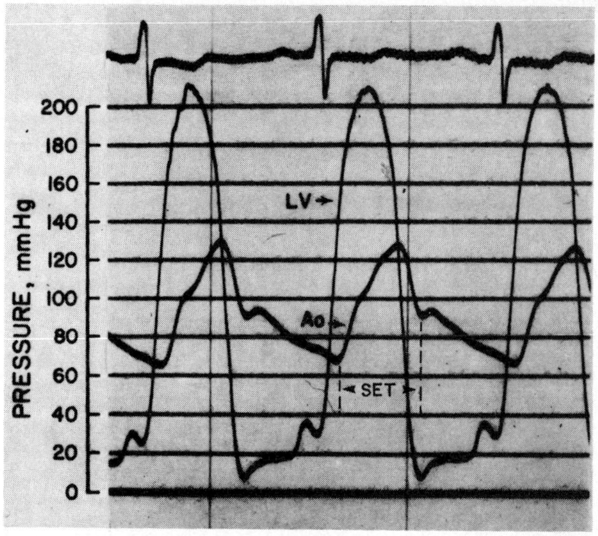

FIGURE 9–9. Left ventricle (LV) and aortic (Ao) pressure tracings in aortic stenosis. During systole, there is a large pressure gradient between LV and Ao, and the rate of rise of the aortic pressure is slow. The systolic ejection time (SET) is the period of time in each cycle during which blood is being ejected from the left ventricle into the aorta. The vertical time lines are 1 sec apart. (From Grossman, W.: Cardiac Catheterization and Angiography. 3rd ed. Philadelphia, Lea and Febiger, 1986.)

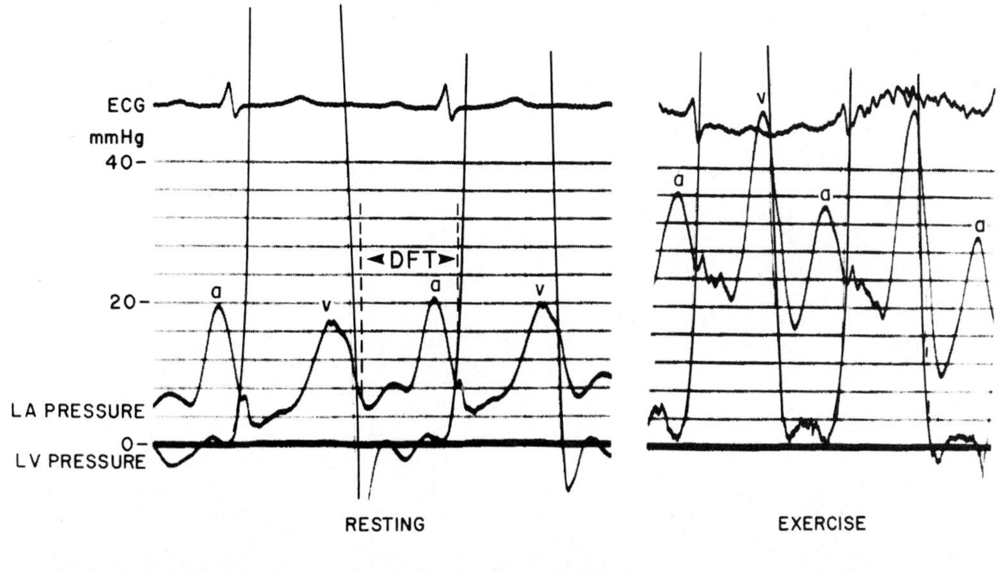

FIGURE 9–10. Left atrial (LA) and left ventricular (LV) pressures in a patient with mitral stenosis at rest (*left*) and during exercise (*right*). During diastole, there is a gradient of pressure between LA and LV. The diastolic filling time (DFT) is the period of time in each cycle when the mitral valve is open. The gradient is greater during exercise as flow across the stenotic valvular orifice increases. (From Grossman, W.: Cardiac Catheterization and Angiography. 3rd ed. Philadelphia, Lea and Febiger, 1986.)

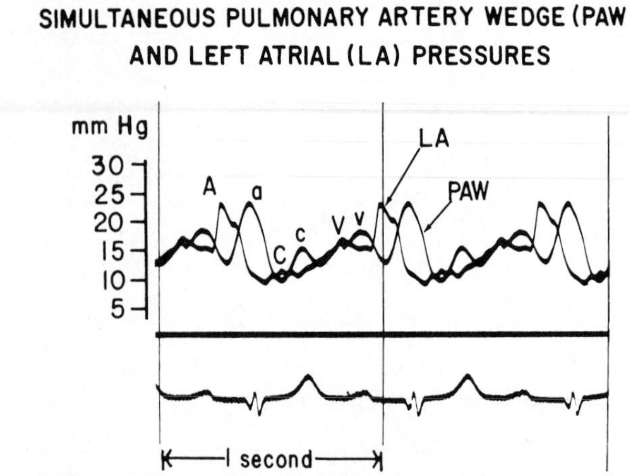

FIGURE 9–11. Simultaneous pulmonary artery wedge (PAW) and left atrial (LA) pressures. *a, c,* and *v* refer to the PAW and *A, C,* and *V* to the LA pressure pulses, respectively. The PAW pressure wave is delayed relative to the LA pressure because of the time required for retrograde propagation of the pressure wave through the pulmonary capillary bed. (From Kory, R. C., et al.: A Primer of Cardiac Catheterization. Springfield, Ill. Courtesy of Charles C Thomas, 1965.)

MEASUREMENT OF CARDIAC OUTPUT

FICK OXYGEN METHOD. Of the numerous techniques devised over the years to measure cardiac output,[39] two have won general acceptance in cardiac catheterization laboratories: the Fick oxygen method and the indicator-dilution technique. These methods resemble each other in that they are based on the theoretical principle enunciated by Adolph Fick in 1870.[40] The principle, which was never actually applied by Fick, states that total uptake or release of any substance by an organ is the product of blood flow to the organ and the arteriovenous concentration difference of the substance. For the lungs, the substance released to the blood is oxygen, and the pulmonary blood flow can be determined by measurement of the *arteriovenous difference of oxygen* across the lungs and the *oxygen consumption* per minute. If there is no intracardiac shunt, pulmonary blood flow is virtually equal to systemic blood flow, and this application of the Fick principle thus provides a measure of systemic blood flow.

Oxygen consumption is commonly estimated by measurement of oxygen extracted by the lungs over a given time period. A "steady state" is required in which oxygen consumption and cardiac output are constant over the time period of measurement.

Two different methods are used commonly for measurement of oxygen consumption: the polarographic method and the Douglas bag method.

The polarographic method is easily employed using an instrument such as the metabolic rate meter (MRM).* This instrument consists of a polarographic oxygen sensor cell, a hood or face mask, and a blower of variable speed connected with the oxygen sensor by a servocontrol loop (Fig. 9–12). This device is convenient and accurate, and represents a significant advance over the older, standard procedure of collecting expired air for 3 minutes in a Douglas bag and measuring volume (Tissot spirometer) and oxygen content. The principle of the polarographic method involves using a variable-speed blower to maintain a unidirectional flow of air from the room through the hood and via a connecting hose to the polarographic oxygen sensing cell. As illustrated in Figure 9–12, room air enters the hood at a rate, V_R (ml/min), which is determined by blower's discharge rate V_M (ml/min) as well as the patient's ventilatory rate (V_I, inhaled air in ml/min; V_E, exhaled air). The blower's speed, V_M, is controlled by a servo-loop designed to maintain the oxygen content of air flowing past the polarographic cell constant at a predetermined value. In a steady state, the patient's oxygen consumption, $\dot{V}_{O_2}$, can be calculated as follows:

$$\dot{V}_{O_2} = (F_RO_2 \cdot V_R) - (F_MO_2 \cdot V_M) \qquad (1)$$

where F_RO_2 and F_MO_2 are fractional contents of oxygen in room air and in the air flowing past the polarographic cell, respectively. As is apparent from Figure 9–12, $V_M = V_R - V_I + V_E$, which can be rewritten as $V_R = V_M + V_I - V_E$. Substituting this in equation 1 gives:

$$\dot{V}_{O_2} = V_M(F_RO_2 - F_MO_2) + F_RO_2(V_I - V_E). \qquad (2)$$

Since the fractional content of oxygen in room air (F_RO_2) is 0.209, oxygen consumption is given by $V_{O_2} = V_M(0.209 - F_MO_2) + 0.209(V_I - V_E)$. Thus, in a steady state (where $V_I - V_E$ is constant), oxygen consumption can be determined by measurement of the volume rate of air moved

*Waters Instruments, Rochester, Minnesota.

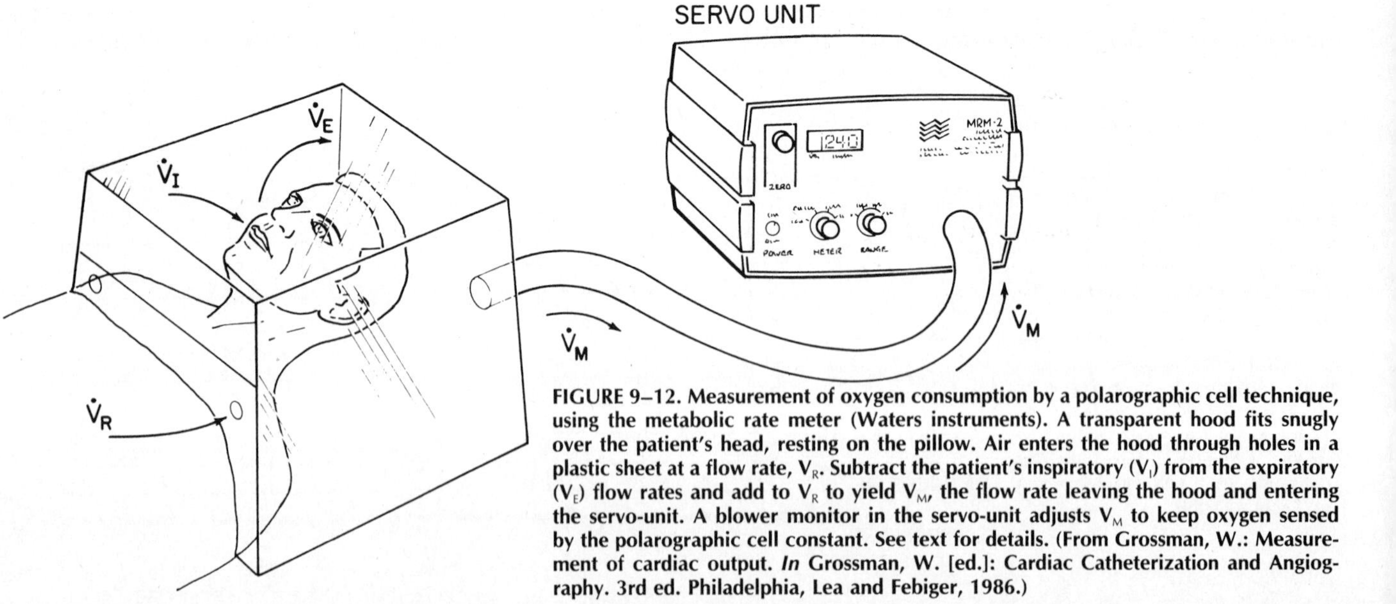

FIGURE 9–12. Measurement of oxygen consumption by a polarographic cell technique, using the metabolic rate meter (Waters instruments). A transparent hood fits snugly over the patient's head, resting on the pillow. Air enters the hood through holes in a plastic sheet at a flow rate, V_R. Subtract the patient's inspiratory (V_I) from the expiratory (V_E) flow rates and add to V_R to yield V_M, the flow rate leaving the hood and entering the servo-unit. A blower monitor in the servo-unit adjusts V_M to keep oxygen sensed by the polarographic cell constant. See text for details. (From Grossman, W.: Measurement of cardiac output. *In* Grossman, W. [ed.]: Cardiac Catheterization and Angiography. 3rd ed. Philadelphia, Lea and Febiger, 1986.)

by the blower motor (V_M) and the fractional O_2 content of air moving past the polarographic sensor. For practical purposes, the respiratory quotient (RQ) is assumed to be 1.0; accordingly, $V_I = V_E$. If the RQ is actually 0.9 (i.e., the patient releases 0.9 liters of carbon dioxide for each liter of oxygen consumed), the error in V_{O_2} resulting from the assumption of an RQ of 1.0 is 1.6 per cent; if RQ is 0.8, the error would be 3.2 per cent. Further details of this method, and the older Douglas bag method, are given elsewhere.[23]

The O_2 consumption in ml/min is usually divided by body surface area to correct for differences in O_2 consumption rate due to differences in size among patients. The normal basal oxygen consumption index is between 110 and 150 ml O_2/min/m^2 body surface area.

The arteriovenous oxygen difference across the lungs is determined as the difference between the oxygen content of pulmonary artery blood and that of left ventricular or systemic arterial blood, since pulmonary venous blood is not generally sampled. Actually, because of bronchial venous and thebesian venous drainage, the oxygen content of systemic arterial blood is commonly 2 to 5 ml/liter lower than that of pulmonary venous blood as it leaves the alveoli, and a small overestimation of cardiac output, of little clinical significance, results.

The pulmonary arterial blood is used for determination of mixed venous blood oxygen content, which can be measured by a variety of methods. The most widely used methods measure the O_2 saturation of hemoglobin by reflectance oximetry. Oxygen content (ml O_2/liter blood) is then calculated by multiplying the fraction of O_2 saturation by the theoretical oxygen-carrying capacity ([hemoglobin, gm/100 ml] × 1.36 [ml O_2/gm Hb]) × 10. The arteriovenous oxygen content difference is then simply calculated as the arterial minus the venous blood O_2 content.

Cardiac output/m^2 (cardiac index) is calculated as

$$\frac{O_2 \text{ consumption (ml/min/m}^2)}{\text{Arteriovenous } O_2 \text{ difference (ml/liter)}}$$

and is expressed in liters/min/m^2.

The normal range is 2.6 to 4.2 liters/min/m^2. The average error in determining oxygen consumption is approximately 6 per cent. The error for arteriovenous oxygen difference determination is approximately 5 per cent, and the total error in measurement of cardiac output by this method is probably about 10 per cent.[39, 41–44] The Fick oxygen method is most accurate in patients with low cardiac output, in whom the arteriovenous oxygen difference is wide.

INDICATOR-DILUTION METHOD. The Fick method is merely a specific application of the indicator-dilution method, in which O_2 being continuously infused by the lungs is the indicator and is diluted in the pulmonary blood flow. Stewart was the first to use a dye indicator-dilution method to measure cardiac output; he used the continuous infusion technique and reported his first studies in 1897.[45] Numerous indicators have since been successfully employed.[46–48] Indocyanine green dye has been used extensively in clinical practice, although currently thermodilution (in which cold saline is the indicator) has become the most widely used indicator-dilution method.[50–52]

Thermodilution Method. A thermal indicator method for measuring cardiac output is employed widely in clinical practice today.[51, 52, 57] In the initial report by Ganz et al.,[51] two thermistors were used—one in the superior cava at the site where the cold indicator was injected into the bloodstream and a second "downstream" thermistor located in the proximal pulmonary artery. This permitted accurate measurement of the temperature of the injectate as well as the temperature of blood downstream from the injectate. These parameters, together with knowledge of the specific heat of blood and injectate, permit calculation of cardiac output. Mathematical details of indicator dilution theory, as well as calculation of cardiac output using thermodilution method, are given elsewhere.[23, 51]

The thermodilution method for measuring cardiac output has several advantages over the indocyanine green dye method. These include: (1) It does not require withdrawal of blood; (2) it does not require an arterial puncture; (3) an inert and inexpensive indicator is used; (4) there is virtually no recirculation, making computer analysis of the primary curves simple.

Indocyanine Green Dye Method. When indocyanine green dye is used, a bolus is injected rapidly into the pulmonary artery, and its appearance and concentration in arterial blood are recorded from a peripheral systemic artery (e.g., brachial, femoral, or radial). A time-concentration curve is thus recorded that exhibits a rapid rise to

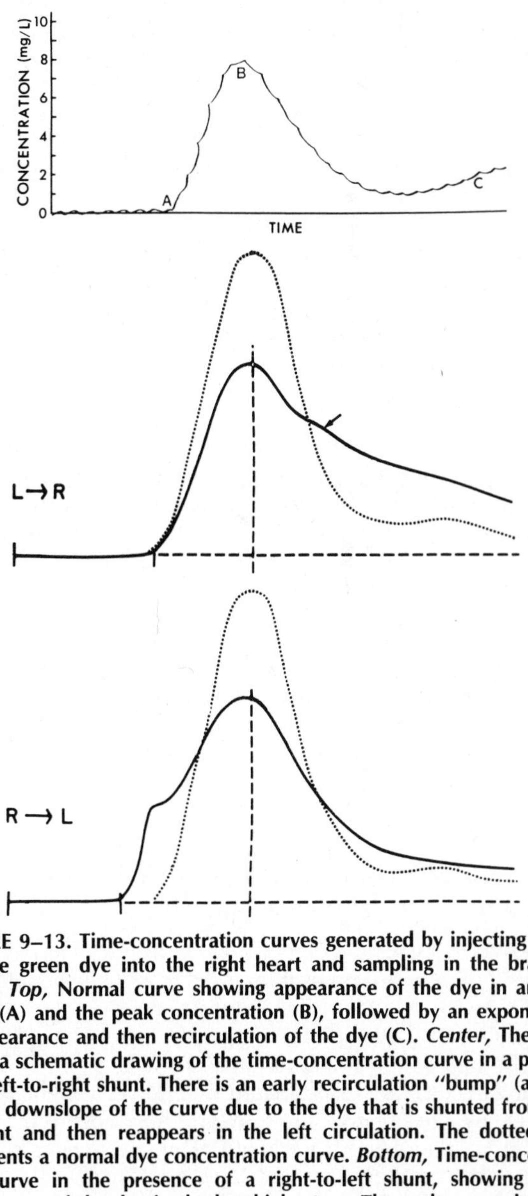

FIGURE 9–13. Time-concentration curves generated by injecting indocyanine green dye into the right heart and sampling in the brachial artery. *Top,* Normal curve showing appearance of the dye in arterial blood (A) and the peak concentration (B), followed by an exponential disappearance and then recirculation of the dye (C). *Center,* The solid line is a schematic drawing of the time-concentration curve in a patient with left-to-right shunt. There is an early recirculation "bump" (arrow) on the downslope of the curve due to the dye that is shunted from left to right and then reappears in the left circulation. The dotted line represents a normal dye concentration curve. *Bottom,* Time-concentration curve in the presence of a right-to-left shunt, showing early appearance of the dye in the brachial artery. The early appearing dye passes through the shunt and thus does not traverse the pulmonary circulation. The dotted line represents a normal dye concentration curve. (Top panel from Grossman, W.: Cardiac Catheterization and Angiography. 3rd ed. Philadelphia, Lea and Febiger, 1986. Center and lower panels from Kory, R. C., et al.: A Primary of Cardiac Catheterization. Springfield, Ill. Courtesy of Charles C Thomas, 1965.)

a peak and then a gradual decline in concentration that is interrupted by a secondary rise due to recirculation of the dye (Fig. 9–13, *top*). The problem of isolating those data that relate only to the first pass of the indicator has been approached by several investigators, but the method originally proposed by Kinsman, Moore, and Hamilton[53] is the one still used most widely today. Kinsman and coworkers showed mathematically that the true "first-pass" curve will be given by plotting the concentration decline on semilogarithmic paper and extrapolating the early linear part of the plot.

The cardiac output (CO) is then calculated as $CO = i/(\bar{c} \times t)$, where i is the quantity of indicator injected, $\bar{c}$ is the average concentration of the indicator during its first pass, and t is the total duration of the curve. The product of $\bar{c}$ and t is easily measured as the area under the first-pass curve, determined by planimetry. This may be simplified further by the use of any number of available computer methods in which the semilogarithmic replotting, area computation, and cardiac output calculation are all accomplished electronically. More precise methodological details, as well as a discussion of sources of error, can be found elsewhere.[23, 39]

Most laboratories,[46, 54–56] but not all,[49, 57] have found that there is excellent agreement between the indicator-dilution methods (either thermodilution or green dye) and independent methods for measuring cardiac output, particularly when the cardiac output is normal or elevated. The error of the indicator-dilution method is greatest in patients with extremely low outputs,[57] severe mitral or aortic regurgitation, or intracardiac shunts. Therefore it complements the Fick method of cardiac output determination, in which the accuracy is greatest in patients having low cardiac output with wide arteriovenous oxygen differences.

It is important to note that indocyanine green dye can cause interference when oxygen content is determined by spectrophotometric methods. Therefore, if cardiac output is to be determined by both the Fick and the indocyanine green dye indicator-dilution methods *in the same patient*, the former measurement should be done first. Not only does the use of cold saline (thermodilution) as an indicator avoid this problem, but also this technique can be performed repeatedly without buildup of indicator or recirculation problems. For these reasons, the thermodilution method has become the most commonly used indicator-dilution technique for measuring cardiac output.

ANGIOGRAPHIC MEASUREMENT OF CARDIAC OUTPUT

Measurement of left ventricular end-diastolic and end-systolic volumes by quantitative left ventricular angiography, described on p. 452, permits calculation of left ventricular stroke volume. In the absence of atrial fibrillation or significant mitral or aortic regurgitation, systemic cardiac output may be estimated by multiplying the stroke volume by the heart rate during the angiogram. This method is a less accurate method of measuring cardiac output than either the indicator-dilution or the Fick method.

REGIONAL BLOOD FLOWS. The principles discussed above may be applied to measure regional blood flows. Three common examples are intracardiac shunt flow as measured by the Fick principle, coronary sinus flow by thermodilution, and regurgitant valve flow by a combination of angiographic and Fick measurements of cardiac output.

INTRACARDIAC SHUNTS

Detection, localization, and quantification of intracardiac shunts can generally be accomplished with precision at cardiac catheterization. Although intracardiac shunts are usually suspected prior to catheterization, this is not always the case. Therefore, the operator must always be alert to the possibility of an intracardiac shunt and must search for one when unexpected arterial oxygen desaturation is detected or an inappropriately high pulmonary artery oxygen saturation is observed.

DETECTION AND LOCALIZATION OF SHUNTS. In a patient with a *left-to-right shunt* (atrial septal defect, ventricular septal defect, patent ductus arteriosus) pulmonary blood flow is higher than systemic blood flow, and the pulmonary artery oxygen saturation is greater than the true mixed venous blood saturation. The anatomical location of the shunt is determined by obtaining multiple samples for oxygen saturation. In the traditional "oximetry run"[7, 23, 58] duplicate samples are drawn in rapid succession from the left, right, and main pulmonary arteries; the outflow tract, body, and inflow area of the right ventricle; the low, mid, and high right atrium; the low and high superior vena cava; and the inferior vena cava at the level of the diaphragm.

The technique of the oximetry run is based on the work of Dexter et al.,[7] who reported in 1947 that multiple samples drawn from the right atrium of normal subjects could vary in oxygen content by as much as 2 volumes per cent (20 ml O_2/liter), reflecting the fact that the right atrium receives its blood from three sources: the superior vena cava, the inferior vena cava, and the coronary sinus. Maximal normal variation within the right ventricle was found to be 10 ml O_2/liter, while maximal variation within the pulmonary artery was 5 ml O_2/liter. Using these criteria, a significant oxygen "step-up" is present at the atrial level when the highest oxygen content in blood samples drawn from the right atrium exceeds the highest content in the venae cavae by 20 ml O_2/liter. Similarly, a significant step-up at the ventricular level is present if the highest right ventricular sample is 10 ml O_2/liter higher than the highest right atrial sample, and a significant step-up at the level of the pulmonary artery requires a pulmonary artery oxygen content more than 5 ml O_2/liter greater than the highest right ventricular sample. Few laboratories currently measure oxygen content of blood directly but rather measure blood oxygen saturation using reflectance oximetry.

The findings in a study in which normal variation of both oxygen content and oxygen saturation of blood in the right heart chambers in a large number of patients undergoing diagnostic cardiac catheterization were analyzed are summarized in Table 9–3. As can be seen, different criteria exist depending on whether an average of oxygen saturation (or oxygen content) values obtained for multiple samples is used, or whether only the highest value for oxygen saturation of content in a particular chamber is utilized. Using averaged samples, an oxygen saturation step-up of $\geq$ 7 per cent is necessary to diagnose a left-to-right shunt at the atrial level, while $\geq$ 5 per cent suffices at the ventricular or great vessel level. Thus, for a patient in whom average right ventricular oxygen saturation (three samples) is 72 per cent and average pulmonary artery saturation (again, three samples) is 79 per cent, the diagnosis of left-to-right shunt at the pulmonary artery level is suggested. The anatomical defect causing this shunt could

Table 9–3 DETECTION OF LEFT TO RIGHT SHUNT BY OXIMETRY

Level of Shunt	Criteria for Significant Step: [Mean of Distal Chamber Samples − Mean of Proximal Chamber Samples] O₂ Vol%	O₂% Sat	[Highest Value in Distal Chamber − Highest Value in Proximal Chamber] O₂ Vol%	O₂% Sat	Approximate Minimal Q_p/Q_s Required for Detection (Assuming SBFI = 3 liters/min/M²)	Possible Causes of Step-Up
Atrial (SVC/IVC to RA)	≥1.3	≥7	≥2.0	≥11	1.5–1.9	Atrial septal defect; anomalous pulmonary venous drainage; ruptured sinus of Valsalva; VSD with TR; coronary fistula to RA
Ventricular (RA to RV)	≥1.0	≥5	≥1.7	≥10	1.3–1.5	VSD; PDA with PR; primum ASD; coronary fistula to RV
Great Vessel (RV to PA)	≥1.0	≥5	≥1.0	≥5	1.3	PDA; aorta-pulmonic window; aberrant coronary artery origin

Abbreviations: SVC and IVC, superior and inferior vena cavae; RA, right atrium; RV, right ventricle; PA, pulmonary artery; VSD, ventricular septal defect; TR, tricuspid regurgitation; PDA, patent ductus arteriosus; PR, pulmonic regurgitation; ASD, atrial septal defect; SBFI, systemic blood flow index; Q_p/Q_s, pulmonary to systemic flow ratio.

From Grossman, W. (ed.): Cardiac Catheterization and Angiography. 3rd ed. Philadelphia, Lea and Febiger, 1986.

be a patent ductus arteriosus, an aortic-pulmonary window, or rarely of aberrant coronary artery origin (e.g., left anterior descending artery originating from the pulmonary artery) with left-to-right shunt.

One limitation of the oxygen method of detecting intracardiac shunts is its low degree of sensitivity. Small shunts ($\dot{Q}p/\dot{Q}s \leq 1.3$) at the level of the pulmonary artery or right ventricle and shunts at the atrial level with $\dot{Q}_p/\dot{Q}s < 1.5$ are not detected consistently by this technique alone because of the normal variability in O_2 saturation described above.[58] A more sensitive technique for the detection of small left-to-right intracardiac shunts involves detection of the early appearance of hydrogen in the right heart after inhalation of hydrogen gas using a right-heart hydrogen-sensitive platinum-tipped electrode catheter to measure direct-current voltage changes. In addition, in the presence of a left-to-right shunt, injection of indocyanine green dye into the pulmonary artery with sampling from the femoral artery will demonstrate early recirculation on the downslope of the dye curve.[23, 58, 59] These techniques are easily performed and can sometimes detect left-to-right shunts too small to be detected by the oxygen step-up method (Fig. 9–13, *center*).

In patients with *right-to-left shunts*, arterial blood is unsaturated, and cyanosis is commonly present. Clinically, the site of entry of a right-to-left intracardiac shunt may be localized by noting which of the left-heart chambers is the first to show desaturation. However, it is usually difficult to enter the pulmonary veins and left atrium in the adult, as discussed previously. Small right-to-left shunts may be detected by injecting indocyanine dye into a vena cava and detecting the early appearance of the dye in arterial blood prior to the primary peak (Fig. 9–13, *bottom*). The site of origin of the shunt can then be localized by injecting dye at a more distal site in the right heart until its early appearance disappears.

It should be remembered that an abnormal catheter position can also be useful in detecting an abnormal communication. This is particularly true for atrial septal defects and for anomalous pulmonary veins emptying into the right atrium. In addition, angiographic methods may be used to detect and localize intracardiac shunts (Chap. 10).

SHUNT QUANTIFICATION. The usefulness of the oximetry run method of shunt detection is enhanced by the fact that the data obtained are also used in quantification of the shunt. When the shunt is unidirectional (e.g., left-to-right), its magnitude is calculated simply as the difference between the pulmonary and systemic blood flows. Pulmonary blood flow ($\dot{Q}_p$) in liters/min is given as:

$$\dot{Q}_p = \frac{O_2 \text{ consumption (ml/min)}}{\underset{\text{(ml/liter)}}{\text{PV } O_2 \text{ content}} - \underset{\text{(ml/liter)}}{\text{PA } O_2 \text{ content}}}$$

where PV and PA refer to pulmonary venous and pulmonary arterial blood, respectively. If a pulmonary vein has not been entered, systemic arterial oxygen content may be used in lieu of PV O_2 content, as long as the systemic arterial oxygen saturation is 95 per cent or more. If systemic oxygen saturation is less than 95 per cent, one must determine whether a right-to-left shunt is present. If such a shunt exists, then a value of PV O_2 content is calculated from the assumption that it is 98 per cent of blood oxygen-carrying capacity, and this is used in calculating $\dot{Q}_p$. If arterial desaturation is present but is not due to a right-to-left intracardiac shunt, the observed systemic arterial oxygen content is used to calculate $\dot{Q}_p$.

Systemic blood flow ($\dot{Q}s$) in liters/min is calculated as

$$\dot{Q}_s = \frac{O_2 \text{ consumption (ml/min)}}{\left[\begin{array}{c}\text{Systemic arterial}\\ O_2 \text{ content (ml/liter)}\end{array}\right] - \left[\begin{array}{c}\text{Mixed venous}\\ O_2 \text{ content (ml/liter)}\end{array}\right]}$$

Mixed venous oxygen content is obtained as the average oxygen content of blood in the chamber immediately upstream in relation to the shunt, as defined by the level of the O_2 step-up in the oximetry run. The formula used to calculate mixed venous oxygen content when the shunt is at the level of the right atrium, as in atrial septal defect was derived by Flamm and coworkers.[60] They found that $\dot{Q}_s$ calculated from mixed venous oxygen content derived as

$$\frac{3 \text{ SVC } O_2 \text{ content} + 1 \text{ IVC } O_2 \text{ content}}{4}$$

most closely approximated $\dot{Q}_s$ measured by left ventricular to brachial artery indicator-dilution curves in patients with atrial septal defect.

Calculation of the shunt flow itself is then given as $\dot{Q}_p - \dot{Q}_s$. If the shunt is wholly left-to-right, this value is positive, whereas a negative value is observed in patients with pure right-to-left shunts (e.g., tetralogy of Fallot). When there is *bidirectional shunting*, the more complicated formula on the following page must be used.

$$L \rightarrow R = \frac{\text{PBF (PA } O_2 \text{ content } - \text{ Mixed venous } O_2 \text{ content)}}{\text{(PV* } O_2 \text{ content } - \text{ Mixed venous } O_2 \text{ content)}}$$

$$R \rightarrow L = \frac{\text{PBF (PV* } O_2 \text{ content } - \text{ BA } O_2 \text{ content) (PV* } O_2 \text{ content } - \text{ PA } O_2 \text{ content)}}{\text{(Ba } O_2 \text{ content } - \text{ Mixed venous } O_2 \text{ content) (PV* } O_2 \text{ content } - \text{ Mixed venous } O_2 \text{ content)}}$$

REGURGITANT FLOWS

In aortic or mitral valve regurgitation, left ventricular stroke volume measured angiographically is greater than the forward stroke volume (calculated by dividing the Fick cardiac output by the heart rate), and the difference is the volume of regurgitant blood that leaks across the abnormal valve(s) during each cardiac cycle. Calculation of this regurgitant flow from data obtained during cardiac catheterization can be helpful in evaluating the severity of regurgitant lesions. The regurgitant fraction (RF) is defined as

$$RF = \frac{\left[\begin{array}{c}\text{Angiographic}\\ \text{stroke volume}\end{array}\right] - \left[\begin{array}{c}\text{Fick stroke}\\ \text{volume}\end{array}\right]}{\text{Angiographic stroke volume}}$$

As a general rule, the correspondence of calculated regurgitant fraction to subjectively estimated severity of regurgitation from cineangiography is as follows: 1 + regurgitation corresponds to an RF of $\leq$ 20 per cent; 2 + regurgitation, RF 21 to 40 per cent; 3 + regurgitation, RF 41 to 60 per cent; 4 + regurgitation, RF $\geq$ 60 per cent. Thus, regurgitant fractions exceeding 30 to 40 per cent are considered hemodynamically important. However, because of potential errors of measurement of both the angiographic and Fick stroke volume, this measurement must be interpreted in light of other hemodynamic, angiographic, and clinical data.

CORONARY SINUS FLOW

Coronary sinus blood flow may be measured during cardiac catheterization by the thermodilution technique.[61–63] A thermodilution catheter is inserted into the coronary sinus via the right internal jugular vein or a left antecubital vein. Saline or 5 per cent dextrose solution at room temperature is infused continuously, and the temperature of the blood-saline mixture downstream in the coronary sinus is monitored by an external thermistor on the catheter. The temperature of the injected saline is monitored by an internal thermistor near the catheter injection orifice. The theoretical aspects of coronary venous thermodilution are summarized in Figure 9–14.

$$F_B = F_I \times 1.19 \times \left(\frac{T_B - T_I}{T_B - T_M} - 1\right) \text{ ml/min}$$

*If actual PV is not measured, assume 98 per cent blood O_2 capacity in a patient whose pulmonary function is normal or presumed to be so.

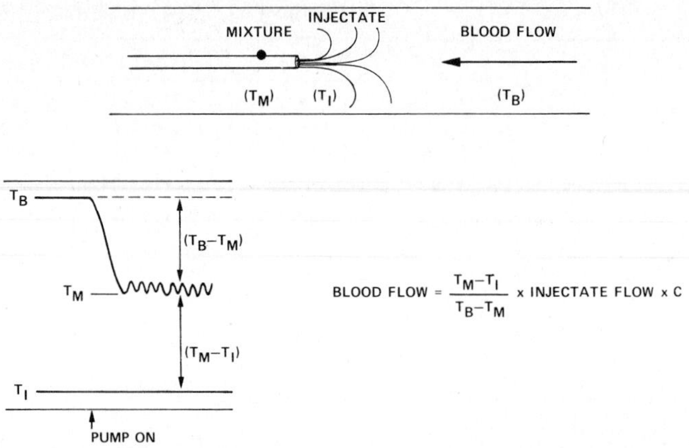

FIGURE 9–14. Schematic illustration of coronary venous thermodilution. The thermal indicator (injectate) at temperature T_I is infused at a constant rate (e.g., 15 ml/min). Turbulence causes mixing of the injectate with coronary venous blood at temperature T_B, resulting in a blood-injectate mixture at temperature T_M. The catheter tip thermistor monitors T_B and T_M, while an internal thermistor monitors T_I, and these are recorded continuously on a uniform temperature scale (*lower left*). Since heat loss by blood is gained by injectate, coronary venous flow is calculated using the measured temperatures, the rate of indicator injection, and the constant derived from the specific heats of blood and injectate. (From Bradley, A. B., and Baim, D. S.: Measurement of coronary blood flow in man. Methods and implications for clinical practice. Cardiovasc. Clin. *14*:67, 1984.)

where F_B = coronary sinus blood flow
F_I = flow of room temperature saline injectate (ml/min)
T_B = body temperature (°C)
T_I = injectate temperature (°C)
T_M = temperature of blood-injectate mixture (°C)

Other techniques may also be used to estimate coronary blood flow.[23] For example, a small amount of the inert gas isotope xenon-133 may be injected selectively into a coronary artery, and the initial washout of radioactivity from the heart can be recorded with a scintillation camera (p. 339). The regional myocardial blood flow in the distribution of that coronary artery can be estimated from the rate constant (k) derived from a semilogarithmic plot of the radioactivity washout curve, the partition coefficient of the tracer in myocardial tissue (λ), and the specific gravity of myocardial tissue (ρ). The formula used is

$$\text{Myocardial blood flow (cm}^3\text{/100 gm tissue} \times \text{min)} = \frac{k\ (\text{min}^{-1})\ \lambda\ 100}{\rho\ (\text{gm/cm}^3)}$$

Inaccuracies in the measurement of coronary blood flow with this method may occur because of recirculation of the isotope, deposition of xenon in myocardial fat, and the local inhomogeneity of flow.

Adaptation of Doppler methodology to the measurement of coronary artery blood flow velocity has been developed to a point of practical applicability.[64] A piezoelectric crystal is mounted into the wall of a woven Dacron catheter and passed into the coronary arteries selectively through a No. 8 French coronary guiding catheter. Measurement of a Doppler coronary blood flow velocity signal can be obtained continuously, and the measured signal can be shown to reflect instantaneous changes in coronary blood flow. Striking increases in coronary blood flow velocity (e.g., fivefold increases) have been noted using the Doppler technique in normal coronary arteries after an infusion of intravenous dipyridamole. This technique seems well suited to the selective measurement of coronary vasodilator reserve in the catheterization laboratory.

CALCULATION OF VASCULAR RESISTANCE

THEORETICAL CONSIDERATIONS. Hydraulic resistance (R) is defined by analogy to Ohm's law as the ratio of the mean pressure drop (ΔP) to flow (Q) between two points in a liquid flowing in a tube. The applicability of this simple equation to pulsatile flow in vascular beds is dubious. Nevertheless, vascular resistance calculated in this fashion has become standard practice in hemodynamic laboratories, and the calculated resistances so obtained often yield important clinical information. Poiseuille's studies of laminar steady-state flow in rigid glass tubes showed that

$$Q = \frac{\pi(\Delta P)r^4}{8\,\eta l}$$

where r = radius of the tube, l = length of the tube, and η = viscosity of the fluid.[36] By rearrangement, it can be seen that resistance (R) is given by

$$R = \frac{\Delta P}{Q} = \frac{8\,\eta l}{\pi r^4}$$

Thus, under the ideal conditions of laminar fluid flow in rigid tubes, resistance is directly proportional to the length of the tube and to the viscosity of the fluid and *inversely proportional to the fourth power of the tube's radius.* It is clear from this that reduction in cross-sectional area of a vessel lumen is the most powerful determinant of resistance to flow. It was observed by Reynolds in 1883 that the pressure drop across a length of tubing exceeded that predicted by the Poiseuille equation at a critical flow rate, dependent on the diameter of the tube and the viscosity of the fluid. He defined the Reynold's number (R_e) as being equal to $\frac{\bar{V}D\rho}{\mu}$, where $\bar{V}$ = average velocity of flow, D = diameter of the tube, ρ = density of the fluid, and μ = its viscosity.[36] When this number is exceeded, flow becomes turbulent, and the pressure drop exceeds that predicted by the Poiseuille equation, which assumes laminar flows. For blood, R_e = 2000, and it appears likely that during normal blood flow in arteries, R_e is not exceeded and that flow remains laminar. However, across severely stenotic valves or in areas of severe luminal arterial narrowing, this may not be the case. This will be considered further in the subsequent discussion of calculation of stenotic valve areas.

CALCULATIONS OF VASCULAR RESISTANCE. Vascular resistance for the systemic and pulmonary vascular beds (SVR and PVR, respectively) is usually calculated as

$$SVR = \frac{80\,(AO_m - RA_m)}{Q_s}$$

and

$$PVR = \frac{80\,(PA_m - LA_m)}{Q_p}$$

where AO_m, RA_m, and LA_m are the aortic, right atrial, pulmonary artery, and left atrial mean pressures in mm Hg; Q_s and Q_p are the systemic and pulmonary blood flows in liters/min (which are equal to the cardiac output in the absence of a shunt); and 80 is the factor used to convert resistance from "hybrid" units (mm Hg/liter/min) to metric units (dynes-sec-cm^{-5}). (See also Chap. 26.) These values can be corrected for body size by multiplying (not dividing) them by body surface area—an important factor in evaluating vascular resistance in infants and adolescents.

Cardiac output, usually measured by the Fick or indicator-dilution method, is used in the calculation of blood flow. It is important to appreciate that in the presence of an intracardiac shunt, in which pulmonary and systemic blood flows are not equal, the respective blood flows through each circuit must be measured and used in the calculation of resistance. Often, the mean pulmonary artery wedge pressure is used as an approximation of mean left atrial pressure, since there is ample evidence that these two measurements, when properly obtained, closely approximate each other.[65, 66]

The normal value for systemic vascular resistance in the author's laboratory is 1170 ± 270 dynes-sec-cm^{-5} (mean ± standard deviation),[23] or 2130 ± 450 dynes-sec-cm^{-5} · m^2. Thus values for systemic vascular resistance less than 1700 dynes-sec-cm^{-5} are probably normal. The normal pulmonary vascular resistance in the author's laboratory is 67 ± 30 dynes-sec-cm^{-5} or 123 ± 54 dynes-sec-cm^{-5} · m^2. Therefore, values of pulmonary vascular resistance less than 130 dynes-sec-cm^{-5} are probably normal.

Abnormal increases of systemic and pulmonary vascular resistance may be seen in a variety of conditions (Chaps. 26 and 27). It may be important to determine whether the increased resistance is fixed (i.e., due to chronic anatomical and pathological changes) or functional (i.e., due to increased tone in small muscular arteries and arterioles), since this finding can have important clinical implications. For example, major elevations in vascular resistance in the systemic bed may lead to a low cardiac output and left ventricular failure, particularly in the presence of mitral regurgitation. Lowering systemic resistance with specific agents (e.g., nitroprusside, hydralazine, prazosin, erythrityl tetranitrate) at the time of cardiac catheterization may yield important information about the potential therapeutic usefulness of such reduction of afterload in chronic therapy (Chap. 17). Marked fixed increases in pulmonary vascular resistance in patients with congenital heart disease and abnormal communication between the pulmonary and systemic circuits (e.g., ventricular septal defect, atrial septal defect, patent ductus arteriosus) may contraindicate corrective surgery. Therefore, a demonstration that the increased resistance is not fixed may be of considerable importance in the individual patient. In the catheterization laboratory various agents and manipulations have been utilized to assess the reversibility of high pulmonary vascular resistance, including infusions of acetylcholine,[67, 68] infusions of tolazoline hydrochloride,[69, 70] oxygen inhalation (Chap. 26), and exercise.

Since blood flow is pulsatile, and the vascular beds have nonlinear elastic and capacitative properties, the concept of *vascular impedance* has been employed. Resistance varies continuously with pressure, and blood flow is influenced by many factors, such as inertia, reflected waves, and the phase angle between pulse and flow velocities.[36, 71, 72] The impedance modulus is calculated to express the spectrum of impedance versus the frequency of a pressure wave.[36]

Stenotic Valves: Calculations of Orifice Area

The evaluation of valvular stenosis in the catheterization laboratory includes a calculation of orifice size based on measurement of the pressure gradient and flow across a valve. The equations used for the aortic and mitral valves were derived and validated by Gorlin.[23, 73, 74]

The following equations are used when valvular gradients are measured directly:

$$\text{Aortic Valve area (cm}^2) = \frac{F}{44.3\sqrt{\Delta P}}$$

$$\text{Mitral valve area (cm}^2) = \frac{F}{37.7\sqrt{\Delta P}}$$

where F = flow across the orifice in ml/sec and ΔP = mean pressure gradient in mm Hg across the orifice. A pressure drop across a stenotic valve occurs because of viscous resistance to flow (Poiseuille) and turbulent flow (Reynolds). The empirical constants 44.3 and 37.7 relate these factors to valve area and differ between aortic and mitral valves because of variations in flow pattern.

For specific application to cardiac valves, F is derived as:

$$\text{Flow (F) (ml/sec)} = \frac{\text{Cardiac output (ml/min)}}{\text{DFP (sec/min) or SEP (sec/min)}}$$

The diastolic filling period (DFP) and systolic ejection period (SEP) are derived by measuring the diastolic filling time (mitral valve opening to closure, Fig. 9–10) or systolic ejection time (aortic valve opening to closure, Fig. 9–9) per beat and multiplying by the heart rate.

In a typical patient, cardiac output might be 4300 ml/min, mean transmitral diastolic pressure gradient = 14 mm Hg, diastolic filling time per beat directly measured from the pressure tracings = 0.42 sec/beat, and heart rate = 72 beats/min. Thus, the mitral valve area will be

$$\frac{(4300\ \text{ml/min}) \div (0.42\ \text{sec/beat} \times 72\ \text{beats/min})}{37.7\sqrt{14\ \text{mm Hg}}} = 1.0\ \text{cm}^2$$

It is important to remember that variations in flow patterns may alter the relationship between orifice area and pressure gradient. In addition, stiff valve leaflets may be more widely opened at high flow velocities (and higher pressure gradients). Therefore, estimation of valve areas, particularly at low flow rates, may be in error and should be considered measurements of functional orifice size. In addition, the presence of valvular regurgitation will result in a falsely low valve area calculation, since the actual valve flow per beat is greater than the flow calculated from the systemic cardiac output. Stenotic valve areas calculated in patients with regurgitation across the stenotic valve should therefore be considered to be the lower limits of the true valve area. In general, errors in estimation of valve flow cause greater inaccuracies in calculations of valve area than do errors in measurement of the pressure gradient across the valve. Nevertheless, hemodynamic measurement of valve area, corrected for body surface area (valve area index), has proved very useful in the clinical management of patients.

There are many pitfalls in the calculation of valve areas. For calculation of mitral valve area, pulmonary capillary wedge pressure is commonly substituted for left atrial pressure under the assumption that a properly confirmed wedge pressure reflects left atrial pressure accurately. The weight of evidence and experience supports this assumption as correct, except in some patients with pulmonary veno-occlusive disease or cor triatriatum. However, failure to wedge the catheter properly may cause inappropriate comparison of a damped pulmonary artery pressure to left ventricular pressure, yielding a falsely high gradient. In order to insure that the right heart catheter is wedged properly, one should verify that: (1) the mean wedge pressure is lower than the mean pulmonary artery pressure, and (2) blood withdrawn from the wedged catheter is ≥ 95 per cent saturated with oxygen, or at least equal in saturation to arterial blood. If these two criteria are not fulfilled, serious error may result from acceptance of pulmonary capillary wedge pressure as accurately reflective of left atrial pressure.

Failure to calibrate pressure transducers properly and to adjust them to the same zero reference point may also yield erroneous gradient measurements. A quick way to check the validity of an unsuspected mitral or aortic pressure gradient is to switch catheters to opposite transducers, which if calibrated equally and adjusted to the same zero reference will yield the same gradient.

Inaccurate cardiac output determination may induce significant error in valve area calculation. Even in the absence of significant regurgitation across the valve whose area is being calculated, small errors in cardiac output measurement will substantially affect valve area determination. Cardiac output measurement should be carried out simultaneously with gradient determination.

Substitution of peripheral arterial pressure for central aortic pressure is commonly done during the measurement of gradients in patients with aortic stenosis. Since the peripheral arterial pressure is delayed temporally compared to central aortic pressure, appropriate realignment of pressure tracings is required prior to planimetry of gradients. However, in addition to distortion from temporal delay, peripheral arterial pressure waveforms are distorted by systolic amplification and spreading out of the pressure waveforms. Errors introduced as a result of this substitution have been recently discussed.[75]

Certain modifications and simplifications of the Gorlin formula have been introduced.[76–78] The reader is referred elsewhere for details.[23]

HEMODYNAMICS DURING EXERCISE

In many patients with heart disease, hemodynamics may be only slightly disturbed or normal at rest but become markedly abnormal during the stress of exercise. Exercise of a patient during cardiac catheterization (p. 226) can therefore provide very important information regarding the cause of symptoms that are exercise-related. Most commonly, bicycle ergometry in the supine position is used during catheterization; upright bicycle exercise, upper extremity exercise, or straight leg-raising may also be used, if appropriate.

In supine bicycle ergometry, the patient's feet are attached by straps to the pedals of the bicycle ergometer which is attached to the catheterization table or suspended from the ceiling. The workload may be adjusted by varying the speed of and resistance to turning of the pedals. When the subject's feet are upon the pedals, intracardiac pressures normally increase slightly (i.e., by 2 to 4 mm Hg), owing to increased venous return by gravity from the legs and elevation of the diaphragm. As the exercise load is increased, oxygen consumption is increased. Exercise level is frequently expressed as metabolic equivalents of resting O_2 consumption (METS), a level of 2 METS corresponding to a doubling of O_2 consumption and usually achieved at a workload of about 75 kg-meter/min. During exercise, increased O_2 consumption by skeletal muscles is supplied by increased cardiac output and a widened arteriovenous O_2 content difference. When exercise is carried out in the supine position, cardiac output is normally increased mainly by an increase in heart rate, with only slight increases in stroke volume. Patients with cardiac disease may be unable to increase cardiac output normally with exercise because of their inability to maintain stroke volume with increased heart rate and thus will supply most of the increased O_2 required by exercising tissue by means of an increase in the arteriovenous O_2 difference. The "exercise factor" expressed as ΔCO during exercise (ml/min)/ΔO_2 consumption (ml/min) is a measure of this response. It is normally greater than or equal to 6.0, since cardiac output normally increases linearly with increasing O_2 consumption. If the exercise factor is less than 6.0, the increase in cardiac output in response to exercise is impaired.

Changes in intracardiac pressures during exercise are also important. The left ventricular end-diastolic pressure does not normally increase above 16 mm Hg during exercise, but in ischemic, myocardial, and valvular disease it may rise to considerably higher levels. In some patients, exercise may exacerbate mitral or tricuspid regurgitation and usually markedly increases the left atrial–left ventricular pressure gradient in mitral stenosis (Fig. 9–10) (Chap. 3). Thus, an abnormal increase in pressures, an inadequate rise in the cardiac output, or both in response to the stress provided by mild to moderate exercise in the supine position can be a very important finding at catheterization (p. 465). In practice, it is important to maintain a given exercise load for at least 3 to 4 minutes before measuring cardiac output and pressures in order to insure a steady state of O_2 consumption and cardiac output. Pressures and the electrocardiogram, as well as the patient's symptoms, should be carefully monitored during exercise to avoid complications.

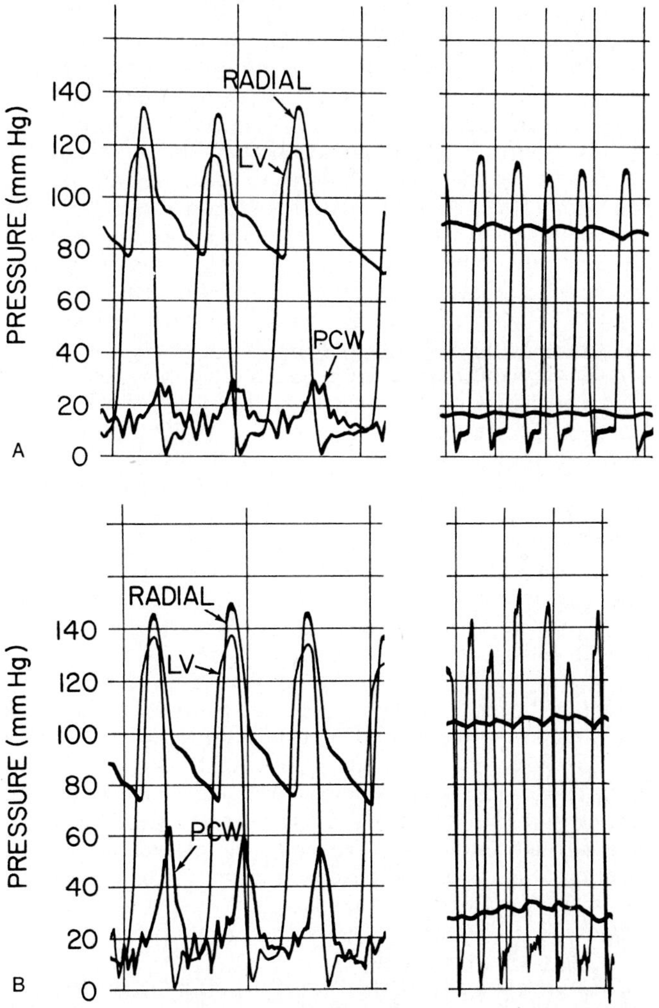

FIGURE 9–15. Hemodynamic findings during exercise in a 55-year-old man with mitral regurgitation. Left ventricular (LV), pulmonary capillary wedge (PCW), and radial artery pressure tracings are shown before (A) and during (B) the sixth minute of supine bicycle exercise. The peak systolic pressure normally is higher in the radial artery than in the left ventricle. (From Lorell, B. H., and Grossman, W.: Dynamic and isometric exercise during cardiac catheterization. *In* Grossman, W. [ed.]: Cardiac Catheterization and Angiography. 3rd ed. Philadelphia, Lea and Febiger, 1986.)

TABLE 9–4 RESPONSE TO SUPINE BICYCLE EXERCISE IN A 60-YEAR-OLD MAN WITH DILATED CARDIOMYOPATHY

	Resting	Exercise (6 minutes)
O_2 consumption index (ml/min/m^2)	128	469
AV O_2 difference (ml/liter)	40	96
Cardiac index (liter/min/m^2)	3.2	4.9
Heart rate (beats/min)	90	141
Systemic arterial pressure (mm Hg), systolic/diastolic (mean)	91/62 (73)	107/67 (88)
Right atrial mean pressure (mm Hg)	5	20
Pulmonary capillary wedge mean pressure (mm Hg)	12	34
Left ventricular pressure (mm Hg)	91/16	107/34
Exercise factor	—	4.9

From Grossman, W. (ed.): Cardiac Catheterization and Angiography. 3rd ed. Philadelphia, Lea and Febiger, 1986.

Figure 9–15 illustrates the hemodynamic findings during exercise in a 55-year-old man with mitral regurgitation. Pressures are recorded on a scale chosen so that all pressures may be visualized simultaneously, with the same baseline and sensitivity. After a brief recording of all three pressures in phasic mode at a paper speed of 25 to 50 mm/sec, the paper speed is slowed to 5 to 10 mm/sec and systemic arterial and pulmonary capillary pressures are recorded as "mean" pressures. The continuous observation and recording of pressures is quite important during exercise, since it permits accurate monitoring of any rise in filling pressure or fall in arterial pressure and insures that the catheters remain in correct position for the measurements during exercise. After the patient had achieved a steady-state level of exercise for 4 minutes, simultaneous left ventricular and systemic arterial, left ventricular and pulmonary capillary wedge pressure, and pulmonary capillary wedge pressure pull-back to pulmonary artery were recorded during minutes 4 through 6 of continued exercise. During exercise there was a substantial rise in pulmonary capillary mean pressure, as well as the development of tall "v" waves in the pulmonary capillary wedge tracing.

Dynamic bicycle exercise can be helpful in the evaluation of symptoms. Table 9–4 illustrates the response to supine exercise in a 60-year-old man with cardiomegaly, fatigue, and marked dyspnea with exertion. The right atrial mean pressure and cardiac index were normal at rest. Pulmonary capillary wedge pressure and left ventricular end-diastolic pressure are only minimally elevated. Interestingly, with exercise the patient failed to increase his forward cardiac output appropriately and achieved an exercise factor of 4.9 (less than the normal of ≥ 6.0). Simultaneously, marked elevations occurred in both right and left heart filling pressures. Coronary angiography was normal, and a diagnosis of dilated cardiomyopathy was suggested.

APPLICATIONS OF CARDIAC CATHETERIZATION

INDICATIONS. As with any diagnostic procedure, the decision to perform cardiac catheterization must be based upon a careful balance betwen the risk of the procedure and the anticipated value of the information obtained. Cardiac catheterization is generally recommended when there is a need to confirm the presence of a clinically suspected condition, define its anatomical and physiological severity, and determine the presence of associated conditions. This need most commonly arises when clinical assessment suggests that the patient may benefit from a *cardiac operation*. Cardiac catheterization is usually coupled with angiographic and/or arteriographic examination and may yield information that will be crucial in defining the need for cardiac operation as well as its risks and anticipated benefit for a given patient.

Although few would disagree that consideration of heart surgery is an adequate reason for performance of catheterization, there are differences of opinion about whether *all* patients being considered for such procedures should undergo preoperative cardiac catheterization.[79–81] In this regard, it should be emphasized that the risks of catheterization are small compared with those of operation in patients in whom (1) an incorrect diagnosis was made, (2) the presence of an unsuspected additional condition prolongs and complicates the planned surgical approach, or (3) the hemodynamic assessment by clinical means was inaccurate. The operating room is not a good place for surprises; preoperative cardiac catheterization can provide the surgical team with a precise and complete road map of the course ahead and thereby permit a carefully reasoned and maximally efficient operative procedure. Furthermore, information obtained by cardiac catheterization may be invaluable in the assessment of the crucial determinants of prognosis, such as left ventricular function and patency of the coronary arteries. For these reasons, we recommend that cardiac catheterization be carried out on almost all adult patients for whom a cardiac operation is contemplated. Of course, it is possible that in time noninvasive techniques may be further perfected and shown to be acceptable substitutes for catheterization data.[81] Following operation, catheterization may be necessary to evaluate the results of operation (graft patency, prosthetic valve function, and so forth).

A second broad indication for performing cardiac catheterization combined with coronary arteriography (Chap. 10) is to clarify the diagnosis in patients with *chest pain of uncertain etiology*, in whom there is confusion regarding the presence of obstructive coronary disease. The data obtained will help relieve the anxiety of patients and aid the physician in advising them concerning the appropriateness of their future personal or professional plans. Another example within this category might be the symptomatic patient with a suspected *cardiomyopathy*. Although some may be satisfied with a clinical diagnosis of this condition, the implications of such a diagnosis in terms of therapy and prognosis are so important that cardiac catheterization is usually recommended in such patients in order to rule out potentially correctible conditions (e.g., occult valvular or pericardial disease), even though the likelihood of their presence may appear remote on clinical grounds.

A third important indication for cardiac catheterization is the need to define the response of a patient to *specific pharmacological therapy*. This may be necessary during treatment of an unstable condition (e.g., following acute myocardial infarction) or in an intensive care unit setting, when monitoring of right and left atrial pressures, systemic pressures, and cardiac output is essential to patient management. In addition, the response of patients with chronic heart failure to afterload reduction or to changes in ventricular preload may be most precisely determined by cardiac catheterization. Pharmacological intervention with vasodilators in the treatment of pulmonary hypertension,[82] or with anticoagulation in suspected acute pulmonary embolism (Chap. 47), might well be considered of sufficient potential risk to warrant cardiac catheterization and/or angiography.

TABLE 9–5 RELATIVE CONTRAINDICATIONS TO CARDIAC CATHETERIZATION AND ANGIOGRAPHY

1. Uncontrolled ventricular irritability (increases the risk of ventricular tachycardia/fibrillation during catheterization)
2. Uncorrected hypokalemia or digitalis toxicity
3. Uncorrected hypertension (predisposes to myocardial ischemia and/or heart failure during angiography)
4. Intercurrent febrile illness
5. Decompensated heart failure (especially acute pulmonary edema, unless the catheterization can be done with patient sitting up)
6. Anticoagulated state (prothrombin time >18 seconds)
7. Severe allergy to radiographic contrast agent
8. Severe renal insufficiency and/or anuria (unless dialysis is planned to remove fluid and radiographic contrast fluid or if contrast radiography is not planned)

Finally, a major indication for cardiac catheterization today is the need for what has been called "interventional therapy" (e.g., balloon angioplasty, valvuloplasty, electrophysiologic ablation, and lasers). These techniques are discussed separately in Chapter 40.

CONTRAINDICATIONS. If it is important to consider the *indications* for cardiac catheterization in each patient, it is equally important to ascertain whether there are any *contraindications*. Over the past several years, our concept of contraindications has been modified, because patients previously considered too ill for this procedure with serious conditions such as acute myocardial infarction, intractable ventricular tachycardia, and cardiogenic shock have tolerated catheterization and coronary arteriography surprisingly well. A long list of relative contraindications (Table 9–5) must be kept in mind, however, and these include all intercurrent conditions that can be corrected and whose correction would improve the safety of the procedure. Ventricular irritability may greatly increase the risk of left-heart catheterization and can interfere with the interpretation of ventriculography. Hypertension should be controlled prior to and during cardiac catheterization. Other conditions that should be corrected prior to elective cardiac catheterization if at all possible include febrile illness, decompensated left-heart failure, anemia, digitalis toxicity, and electrolyte disturbance. Infective endocarditis and pregnancy are relative though not absolute contraindications to cardiac catheterization.

Anticoagulant therapy may increase the risk of serious bleeding during or following cardiac catheterization. It is our policy to maintain the prothrombin time less than 18 seconds and to avoid heparin administration for 4 to 6 hours prior to the procedure. If anticoagulant therapy cannot be interrupted, we prefer heparin because it can be easily and immediately reversed by intravenous administration of protamine sulfate should uncontrollable bleeding or cardiac perforation occur in the course of catheterization. If transseptal catheterization is planned, it is mandatory that coagulation be normal.

DESIGN OF CATHETERIZATION PROTOCOL. Every cardiac catheterization should have a protocol, that is, a carefully reasoned sequential plan designed specifically for the individual patient being studied. Certain general principles should be considered in the design of a protocol. First, hemodynamic measurements should precede angiographic studies, whenever possible, so that the physiological state may be as basal as possible at the time of pressure and flow measurements. Second, pressure and blood oxygen saturation should be measured and recorded for each chamber immediately after entry and before passing on to the next chamber. If problems should develop during the later stages of a catheterization procedure (atrial fibrillation or other arrhythmia, pyrogen reaction, hypotension, or reaction to contrast material), the physician will wish that pressures and saturations had been measured initially rather than waiting for the time the catheter is being withdrawn. A third principle is that pressure and cardiac output measurements should be made simultaneously insofar as this is possible. Beyond these general guidelines, the protocol will reflect individual differences from patient to patient. With regard to angiography, it is important to give the contrast injections in sequence, so that the most important diagnostic study is performed first in a given patient.

PREPARATION AND PREMEDICATION OF THE PATIENT. The emotional as well as the "medical" preparation of the patient for cardiac catheterization is the responsibility of the operator. It is proper practice always to inform patients and their families that there are some risks involved, and to be specific as to what those risks are (e.g., death, heart attack, stroke). When appropriate, patients and their families may be reasonably reassured that special problems are unlikely. However, the discomfort and duration of the procedure should not be understated.

Usually patients scheduled for catheterization are admitted to the hospital 24 hours prior to the procedure. However, as mentioned earlier, some centers are now performing cardiac catheterization on an outpatient basis for selected patients whose conditions are stable.[25, 83]

A wide variety of sedatives has been employed for premedication. The authors routinely use diazepam (Valium), 5 to 10 mg orally, and diphenhydramine (Benadryl), 25 to 50 mg orally, one-half hour prior to starting the procedure. When coronary arteriography is to be part of the procedure, some operators favor the addition of 0.4 mg atropine subcutaneously in order to avoid excessive bradycardia.[84] It is the authors' practice to have the patient fasting (except for oral medications) after midnight. A light breakfast is allowed if the patient is not scheduled for catheterization until late in the morning or afternoon.

Prior to catheterization the skin overlying the vessels to be entered (femoral areas or antecubital fossa) should be prepared by shaving and thorough cleansing with iodine or Zephiran chloride solution. This procedure as well as careful sterile technique during the catheterization procedure minimizes the incidence of infection.

COMPLICATIONS OF CARDIAC CATHETERIZATION

There is an extensive literature describing a wide array of complications associated with cardiac catheterization.[84–111] The incidence of various complications has been reported by the Registry of the Society for Cardiac Angiography.[111] A total of 53,581 patients underwent catheterization and angiography in 66 laboratories over a period of 14 months, beginning in October 1979. There were 75 deaths (0.14 per cent), 40 myocardial infarctions (0.07 per cent), and 35 cerebrovascular accidents (0.07 per cent). The incidence of death was greater in patients under 1 year of age (1.75 per cent) and over age 60 (0.25 per cent) than in patients between 1 and 60. In patients undergoing coronary angiography, the mortality ranged from 0.86 per cent in patients with significant left main coronary artery disease to 0 per cent in patients with normal coronary arteries or only minimal coronary disease. Vascular complications occurred in 291 patients (0.57 per cent).

These data indicate that the incidence of complications of cardiac catheterization as currently practiced is low, although careful attention to detail and meticulous technique are required to achieve this standard of performance.

RISK FACTORS. Characteristics of patients who have an increased risk of dying from cardiac catheterization are summarized in Table 9–6. Although the reported mortality rate of 0.14 per cent from the Registry of the Society for Cardiac Angiography[111] indicates a low risk of death associated with cardiac catheterization and angiography, certain caveats should be noted. The Registry report, based on self-reporting from a combination of academic and private laboratories, indicated that at least 28 per cent of the patients studied had either minimal or no cardiac disease.[111] Laboratories at which the percentage of normal or nearly normal studies is quite high might well be expected to have a lower rate of death and other major complications associated with cardiac catheterization and angiography. As indicated in Table 9–6, mortality in Class IV patients is more than 10 times greater than in Classes I and II patients. Similarly, the mortality for patients with left main coronary disease is more than 10 times greater than for patients with one- or two-vessel disease. Patients with substantial left ventricular dysfunction (left ventricular ejection fraction < 30 per cent) also have a risk of dying during cardiac catheterization more than ten times that in patients with normal ejection fractions. Thus the risk of serious complication from cardiac catheterization and angiography, although small, is not insignificant, especially in patients who are seriously ill.

Prevention of a fatal outcome in patients with one or more of the risk factors listed in Table 9–6 requires attention to many issues. During the cardiac catheterization procedure itself, keeping the volume of radiographic contrast to a minimum (especially in patients known to have depressed left ventricular contractile function) is important. If physiological measurements (e.g., measurement of pulmonary capillary wedge pressure, cardiac output) routinely precede angiography, such high-risk patients will be identified more easily and can be "pre-treated" with intravenous furosemide, oxygen, and a vasodilator

TABLE 9–6 PATIENT CHARACTERISTICS ASSOCIATED WITH INCREASED MORTALITY FROM CARDIAC CATHETERIZATION

1. *Age:* Infants (<1 year old) and the elderly (>65 years old) are at increased risk of death during cardiac catheterization. Elderly women appear to be at higher risk than elderly men.
2. *Functional Class:* Mortality in Class IV patients is more than 10 times greater than in Class I–II patients.
3. *Severity of Coronary Obstruction:* Mortality for patients with left main disease is more than 10 times greater than for patients with 1 or 2 vessel disease.
4. *Valvular Heart Disease:* Especially when combined with coronary disease is associated with a higher risk of death at cardiac catheterization than coronary artery disease alone.
5. *Left Ventricular Dysfunction:* Mortality for patients with LV ejection <30% is more than 10 times greater than in patients with ejection fraction ≥50%.
6. *Severe Non-Cardiac Disease:* Patients with renal insufficiency, insulin-requiring diabetes, advanced cerebrovascular and/or peripheral vascular disease, and severe pulmonary insufficiency appear to have an increased incidence of death and other major complications from cardiac catheterization.

From Grossman, W.: Complications of cardiac catheterization: Incidence, causes and prevention. *In* Grossman, W. (ed.): Cardiac Catheterization and Angiography, 3rd ed. Philadelphia, Lea and Febiger, 1986.

(e.g., nitroglycerin, sodium nitroprusside) prior to angiographic studies. The authors have found that a tilting cardiac catheterization table, which allows rapid transition to Trendelenburg position (for hypotension) or reverse Trendelenburg (for pulmonary congestion and edema), is valuable in helping very sick patients get through cardiac catheterization and angiography. Meticulous attention to the details of technique is important in preventing deaths in the cardiac catheterization laboratory, since even a minor complication such as vasovagal reaction or arrhythmia may be fatal in a patient with severely limited cardiac reserve. Despite all such measures, it seems likely that a certain irreducible mortality rate will be associated with cardiac catheterization in patients with the characteristics listed in Table 9–6.

Factors predisposing to *myocardial infarction* during or immediately following cardiac catheterization are unstable angina, recent subendocardial infarction, and insulin-requiring diabetes mellitus. Documentation of a small myocardial infarction may be difficult following cardiac catheterization, since intramuscular injections (e.g., lidocaine) and soft tissue trauma of the catheterization procedure itself may lead to increases in serum enzymes (LDH, SGOT, total CPK) often used to assess the presence or absence of myocardial infarction. Such elevations of enzyme levels may be seen with either brachial or femoral approaches. However, an increase in serum CPK-MB activity is not to be expected following routine cardiac catheterization and angiography, and ordinarily indicates the presence of myocardial necrosis.[102]

CEREBROVASCULAR COMPLICATIONS. These are rare events during cardiac catheterization. Prevention of cerebral emboli can be accomplished by using systemic anticoagulation, paying meticulous attention to proper technique of catheter flushing, wiping guidewires free of blood or clot prior to insertion, and restricting time for the use of guidewires to 2 to 3 minutes at a time (after which the guidewire is removed and the catheter aspirated and flushed before reentry of the wire).

ARTERIAL THROMBOSIS. This problem deserves special attention. Brachial artery thrombosis can be avoided by use of heparin during catheterization and by appropriate attention to the details of arterial repair.[23] It is generally acknowledged that the incidence of thrombosis is related to the duration of the procedure, the number of catheters used, the presence of underlying arterial disease, and the technique of arterial repair. With regard to the percutaneous femoral approach, local complications include thrombosis, distal embolization, false aneurysm, and delayed hemorrhage.[91, 97, 103, 104] Serious complications involving the femoral artery are usually related to the presence of preexisting iliofemoral disease, and in such patients it is preferable to avoid a percutaneous femoral approach.

PERFORATION OF THE HEART OR INTRATHORACIC GREAT VESSELS. This complication can occur with any approach but most commonly involves the right ventricular outflow tract and apex.[85] These areas are subject to perforation during right ventricular angiography or pacemaker placement. Perforations of the aorta, iliac artery, subclavian artery, or great veins have all been reported and are generally associated with excessive catheter manipulation. In many such instances, catheter manipulation was continued despite resistance to passage or complaints by the patient of pain related to the catheter passage. Since transseptal left-heart catheterization entails controlled perforation of the interatrial septum, perforation of the heart is its main hazard. Unintentional perforation of the aorta, atrial wall, coronary sinus, or right atrial appendage may occur, leading to cardiac tamponade.

OTHER COMPLICATIONS. *Vagal reactions* are common and may be quite serious. They are frequently, but not always, incited by pain in a tense anxious patient and consist of nausea, hypotension, and bradycardia. In older patients, the entire picture of a vagal reaction may be present without bradycardia. If promptly recognized, vagal reactions usually respond dramatically to cessation of catheter manipulation, intravenous atropine (0.5 to 1.0 mg), and tilting of the patient or elevation of the legs to increase venous return. If the hypotension and bradycardia persist for any period of time, serious arrhythmias and/or irreversible shock may develop, particularly in patients with ischemic heart disease or aortic stenosis.

Electrical hazards have been reported in association with cardiac catheterization.[106–108] Currents of only a few microamperes transmitted to a small area of myocardium by the wires of electrode catheters, catheters filled with saline, thermistor catheters, or manometer-tipped catheters may produce ventricular fibrillation. This occurrence is now rare, because of the use of common grounding of all electrical equipment, transformer isolation of electrical equipment from the power line by means of current-limiting devices, and establishment of an equal potential environment.

Contamination of catheters or fluids administered during cardiac catheterization with sterile bacterial products or other foreign substances can result in a *pyrogen reaction*, characterized by rigors followed by temperature elevation. If this occurs during catheterization, catheters and fluids should be set aside for subsequent culture; the reaction itself usually responds to small amounts of morphine sulfate (2 mg) administered intravenously. Pyrogen reactions are best treated by prevention. Careful cleaning and sterilization of catheters are essential in this regard.

OTHER PROCEDURES INVOLVING CARDIAC CATHETERIZATION

Cardiac catheterization techniques are now being employed in an increasing number of procedures for purposes other than hemodynamic or angiographic study. In many instances the approaches and catheters used and the indications and complications for these procedures differ, and they will therefore be discussed separately.

INTRACARDIAC ELECTROCARDIOGRAPHY AND PACING. Electrodes mounted on the tips of cardiac catheters can be used to record intracardiac electrical activity and to stimulate the heart at selected sites. This technique is of great value in elucidating the mechanism and treating a variety of arrhythmias, as discussed in Chapters 20–22. Both temporary and permanent pacing are also carried out, most commonly, through pacing catheters, as described in Chapter 23.

TRANSVENOUS ENDOMYOCARDIAL BIOPSY. Nonoperative cardiac biopsy was initially developed as a needle biopsy technique similar to needle biopsy of the kidney or liver.[112–114] In 1962, Japanese workers reported a method for transvenous endomyocardial biopsy of the right ventricle[115]; this has subsequently been modified and applied to endomyocardial biopsy of both right and left ventricles by a number of investigators.[116–121] This method is illustrated in Figure 9–16. A No. 9 French venous sheath is placed in the internal jugular vein via a percutaneous approach. The bioptome is inserted into the sheath and advanced to the right atrium and across the tricuspid valve. After

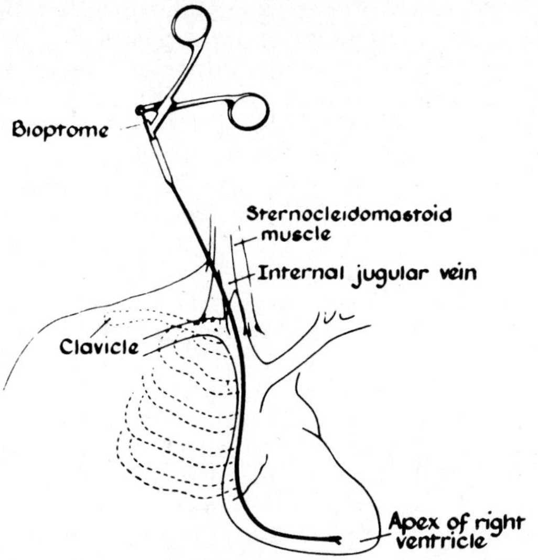

FIGURE 9–16. Endomyocardial biopsy. The bioptome is introduced via the right internal jugular vein and is passed across the tricuspid valve into the right ventricle. With the biotome a small segment of right ventricular endocardium is removed from the interventricular septum for microscopic examination. (From Mason, J. W., et al.: Myocardial biopsy. *In* Willerson, J. T., and Sanders, C. A. [eds.]: Clinical Cardiology. New York, Grune and Stratton, 1977.)

positioning the end of the bioptome against the endocardium of the interventricular septum, using fluoroscopic guidance, the bioptome is opened, gently advanced against the endocardium, and then closed. On withdrawal of the bioptome, a small (1 to 2 mm in diameter) portion of right ventricular myocardium with attached endocardium is obtained. This maneuver is repeated three times, and specimens are processed for light and electron microscopic study. This technique is useful in the diagnoses of myocarditis, hypertrophic and dilated cardiomyopathies (Chap. 42), amyloid and other infiltrative cardiomyopathies (p. 1431), and immunological rejection in cardiac transplant recipients (p. 1453).[116, 117, 119, 122] Serial endomyocardial biopsies have been used to evaluate cardiac toxicity in patients receiving high-dose systemic Adriamycin therapy for carcinoma (p. 1748).[123] A particularly promising application of this technique may be in detection of inflammatory myocarditis. In a report of clinicopathological correlates in 100 consecutive patients undergoing right ventricular endomyocardial biopsy at the Mayo Clinic,[124] myocarditis was detected in 15 per cent of patients with unexplained congestive heart failure and in 15 per cent of patients with unexplained dysrhythmia or syncope. Similar clinical utility for endomyocardial biospy was found by Parillo et al.[125] In their study, pathological information obtained was judged useful to the clinician in 54 of 100 consecutive patients undergoing biopsy[125] (Table 9–7). In some cases, inflammatory myocarditis and associated congestive heart failure may respond to immunosuppressive drugs.[126] Complications, which have been rare, include cardiac perforation and tamponade, pericarditis, and atrial and ventricular tachyarrhythmias.

PERCUTANEOUS INTRAAORTIC BALLOON PUMP INSERTION.[127–130] Intraaortic balloon pump (IABP) counterpulsation provides mechanical circulatory assistance by lowering aortic pressure in systole and increasing aortic pressure in diastole. Cardiac output is increased and left ventricular filling pressure is decreased by the reduction in afterload; myocardial ischemia is alleviated by reduction in oxygen demand while oxygen supply is increased. Therefore, this technique can have a dramatic beneficial effect in patients with cardiogenic shock (p. 1279) and severe, acute myocardial ischemia (p. 1353). It has become a well-accepted method of providing temporary circulatory support for critically ill patients, tiding them over during a stressful procedure, such as cardiac catheterization and angiography, and/or until cardiac surgery can be performed.[127] In the past, IABP catheters have been inserted via a direct surgical approach, requiring a cutdown on the femoral artery and surgical repair of the artery after the balloon pump has been removed. With this method, however, the incidence of complications was not inconsiderable. For example, in the series reported by Pace et al.[128] from the

TABLE 9–7 INDICATIONS AND FINDINGS OF ENDOMYOCARDIAL BIOPSY IN 100 PATIENTS

Clinical Indication for Transvenous Endomyocardial Biopsy	Pathologic Findings	Usefulness of Biopsy
Congestive heart failure of unknown etiology with a dilated heart (n = 74)[A]	Myocarditis (n = 19)[B]	Useful (n = 54)
	Vasculitis (n = 1)	Useful (n = 54)
	Doxorubicin cardiomyopathy (n = 2)	Useful (n = 54)
	Congestive cardiomyopathy (n = 16)	Useful (n = 54)
	Cardiac involvement with sarcoidosis (n = 1) or scleroderma (n = 1)	Useful (n = 54)
Elevated ventricular filling pressures, normal or mildly dilated heart, and constrictive or restrictive physiology (n = 26)	Radiation-induced cardiomyopathy (n = 5)	Useful (n = 54)
	Endomyocardial fibrosis (n = 3)	Useful (n = 54)
	Cardiac amyloidosis (n = 6)	Useful (n = 54)
	Normal transvenous endomyocardial biopsy leading to exploratory thoracotomy and finding constrictive pericarditis (n = 3)	Useful (n = 54)
Both indications	No pathologic diagnosis or nonspecific changes (n = 46)	Not useful (n = 46)

[A]Numbers in parentheses refer to the number of patients.

[B]Three patients had two diagnoses; one patient had amyloidosis and myocarditis, one patient had endomyocardial fibrosis with eosinophilic myocarditis, and one patient had vasculitis and myocarditis, so that the number of patients or indications totals 100 and the number of pathologic findings totals 103.

From Parillo, J. E., et al. (ed.): The results of intravenous endomyocardial biopsy care frequently can be used to diagnose myocardial disease in patients with heart failure. Circulation 69:93, 1984, by permission of the American Heart Association, Inc.

Brigham and Women's Hospital, thrombotic or embolic occlusion of the femoral artery occurred in 29 per cent of the patients, and there was a significant incidence of more severe problems, including dissection of the aorta or iliac artery, contributing to an overall mortality associated with the use of the balloon pump of 4.8 per cent.

Because of the widespread applicability of IABP, there has been great interest in developing techniques for percutaneous insertion[129, 130] and removal of the balloon catheter, in hopes of reducing the complication rate. There are several manufacturers of intraaortic balloon catheters that may be inserted percutaneously through a guiding sheath. Most of these catheters have a central lumen which allows insertion of a guidewire and provides the extra safety associated with guidewire-directed advancement of the catheter through potentially tortuous iliofemoral arterial systems. The central lumen may also be used for arterial pressure monitoring to adjust the timing of balloon counterpulsation. For details of the technique for balloon placement, the reader is referred elsewhere.[23] Once inserted, the adjustment of balloon timing is critical. Timing is adjusted with the balloon control console so that balloon inflation occurs at the time of the central aortic dicrotic notch (aortic valve closure), while deflation occurs immediately prior to aortic valve opening.

An example of the effectiveness of intraaortic balloon counterpulsation in a patient with cardiogenic shock caused by mitral regurgitation is illustrated in Figure 9–17. The patient was a 45-year-old woman who developed cardiogenic shock and pulmonary edema from acute ruptured chordae and massive mitral regurgitation. As seen in panel A, the patient's left ventricular systolic pressure is approximately 80 mm Hg with *v* waves in the pulmonary capillary wedge tracing of 50 to 60 mm Hg. Panel B shows that with intraaortic balloon counterpulsation of the pulmonary capillary wedge *v* waves are greatly reduced. However, left ventricular systolic pressure is lower than in panel A. Panel C shows the unusual tracing obtained when the left ventricular catheter was pulled back into the aorta. Close inspection demonstrates that the pressure waves to 100 mm Hg in the aorta are *diastolic* waves, resulting from expansion of the intraaortic balloon. The small systolic waves preceding each diastolic wave represent left ventricular systolic ejection. The patient's condition stabilized sufficiently to permit cardiac surgery and successful mitral valve replacement.

Successful percutaneous insertion of intraaortic balloon catheters can be achieved in over 90 per cent of patients. However, complications remain a significant problem. A report from Johns Hopkins of 206 consecutive patients undergoing intraaortic balloon placement between 1980 and 1982 noted vascular complications in 20 per cent of patients, half of whom required operation for these complications. Multivariate analysis demonstrated that preexisting peripheral vascular disease (evidenced by history of claudication, presence of femoral bruit, or absence of foot pulses) and the use of percutaneous approach were risk factors for major complications. In patients with previous peripheral vascular disease, the risk for a major vascular complication was 31 per cent in the patients having implantation of intraaortic balloon by percutaneous technique, and 16 per cent in patients having intraaortic balloon implantation surgically. In addition, the risk of a major vascular complication in patients *without* peripheral vascular disease was four times higher in women than in men. Specific complications include vascular injury and perforation, thrombosis, emboli, aortic dissection, limb is-

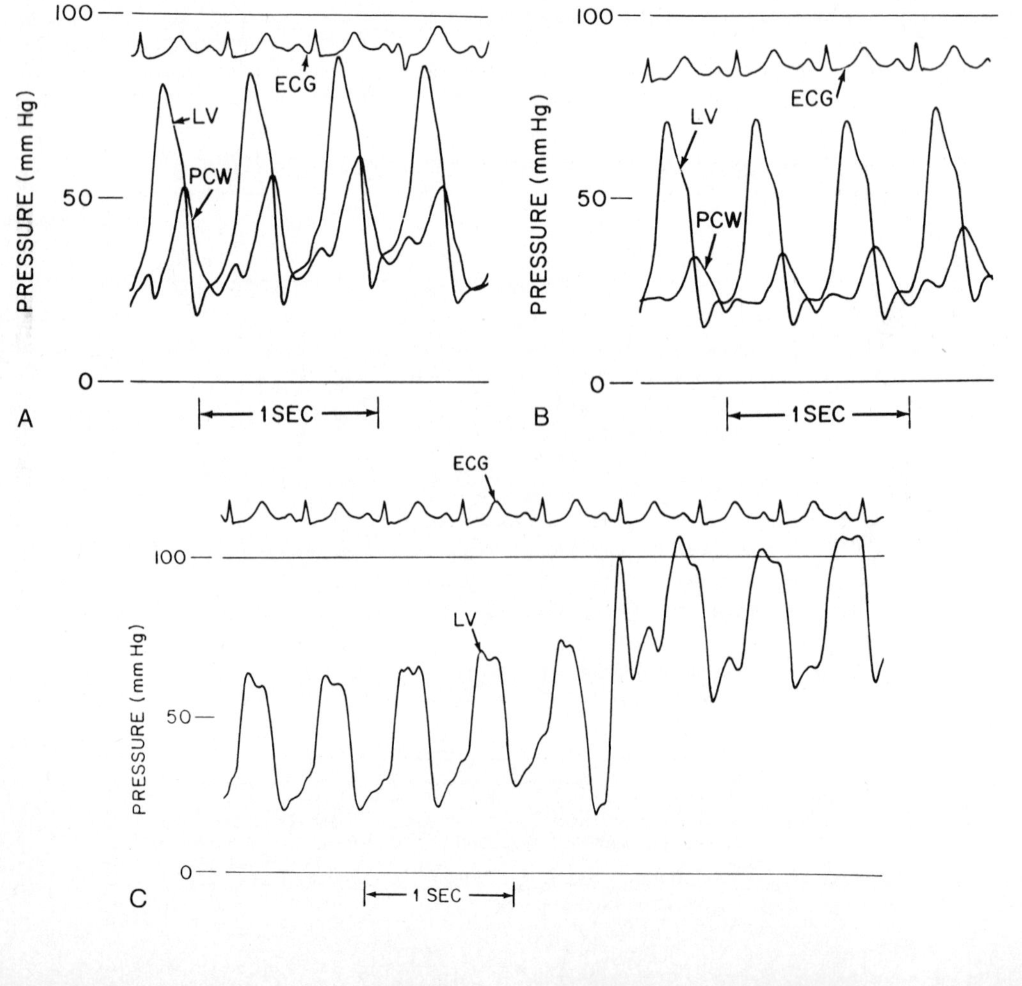

FIGURE 9–17. Left ventricular (LV) and pulmonary capillary wedge (PCW) tracings in a patient with cardiogenic shock from ruptured chordae tendineae. *A,* The pressure tracings prior to counterpulsation. *B,* Left ventricular and pulmonary capillary wedge pressure during counterpulsation. *C,* Left ventricle to aorta pullback during counterpulsation. See text for details. (From Aroesty, J. M., and Grossman, W.: Percutaneous intraaortic balloon insertion. *In* Grossman, W. [ed.]: Cardiac Catheterization and Angiography. 3rd ed. Philadelphia, Lea and Febiger, 1986.)

chemia, infection, renal failure, cerebrovascular accident, mesenteric infarction, balloon rupture, and death.[129] Advances in catheter design and insertion technique may reduce the complication rates.

THERAPEUTIC PROCEDURES. Coronary angioplasty, intracoronary thrombolysis balloon valvuloplasty, and balloon dilatation of stenotic pulmonary and systemic arteries are described in Chapter 40.

The technique of *balloon atrial septostomy*, developed by Rashkind, has become a standard procedure to improve mixing between systemic and pulmonary circulations in neonates with transposition of the great arteries and in patients with intact atrial septum or inadequate interatrial communication (Chap. 30).[131, 132]

There has been extensive experience primarily in Japan and Germany with *nonoperative closure of patent ductus arteriosus* (Chap. 31).[132–135] This has been accomplished by insertion of a plug, mounted on the tip of a catheter, into the patent ductus. Extension of this approach to *closure of an atrial septal defect* using a transvenous umbrella technique has been reported.[132, 136, 137]

A technique for *transvenous pulmonary embolectomy* has been devised that utilizes a catheter with a suction-cupped tip.[138, 139] This catheter is advanced to the pulmonary artery, and its tip is manipulated by externally controlled, braided wires within its wall until the suction cup makes contact with the embolus. The application of suction by syringe produces adherence of the end of the embolus to the suction cup, and the catheter and suction cup are then withdrawn together with the embolus.

In another interesting therapeutic application of cardiac catheterization, Taylor and colleagues have reported therapeutic *embolization of the pulmonary artery* in pulmonary arteriovenous fistulas.[140]

Special "snare" catheters have been designed to *retrieve from within the heart catheter fragments* introduced iatrogenically.[141, 142] Use of these techniques can obviate thoracotomy and cardiotomy.

This is by no means an exhaustive description or list of all the therapeutic uses of cardiac catheterization but should serve to illustrate how techniques originally developed to perform hemodynamic measurements have evolved into the therapeutic procedures. Thus, it is clear that cardiac catheterization can no longer be considered solely a diagnostic procedure.

REFERENCES

HISTORICAL ASPECTS

1. Cournand, A.: Cardiac catheterization. Development of the technique, its contributions to experimental medicine, and its initial application in man. Acta Med. Scand. 579 (Suppl.):1, 1975.
2. Forssmann, W.: Die Sondierung des rechten Herzens. Klin. Woenschr. 8:2085, 1929.
3. Klein, O.: Zur Bestimmung des zirkulatorischen Minutensvohumen nach dem Fickschen Prinzip, Münch. Med. Woenschr. 77:1311, 1930.
4. Cournand, A. F., and Ranges, H. S.: Catheterization of the right auricle in man. Proc. Soc. Exp. Biol. Med. 46:462, 1941.
5. Richards, D. W.: Cardiac output by the catheterization technique in various clinical conditions. Fed. Proc. 4:215, 1945.
6. Cournand, A. F., Riley, R. L., Breed, E. S., Baldwin, E. F., and Richards, D. W.: Measurement of cardiac output in man using the technique of catheterization of the right auricle. J. Clin. Invest. 24:106, 1945.
7. Dexter, L., Haynes, F. W., Burwell, C. S., Eppinger, E. C., Sagerson, R. P., and Evans, J. M.: Studies of congenital heart disease. II. The pressure and oxygen content of blood in the right auricle, right ventricle, and pulmonary artery in control patients, with observations on the oxygen saturation and source of pulmonary "capillary" blood. J. Clin. Invest. 26:554, 1947.
8. Hellems, H. K., Haynes, F. W., and Dexter, L.: Pulmonary "capillary" pressure in man. J. Appl. Physiol. 2:24, 1949.
9. McMichael, J., and Sharpey-Schafer, E. P.: The action of intravenous digoxin in man. Q. J. Med. 13:1123, 1944.
10. Lenègre, J., and Maurice, P.: Premiers recherches sur la pression ventriculaire droite. Bull. Mem. Soc. Med. Hop. Paris 80:239, 1944.
11. Stead, E. A., Jr., Warren, J. V., and Brannon, E. S.: Cardiac output in congestive heart failure: Analysis of reasons for lack of close correlation between symptoms of heart failure and resting cardiac output. Am. Heart J. 35:529, 1948.
12. Bing, R. J., Vandam, L. D., Gregoire, F., Handelsman, J. C., Goodale, W. T., and Echenhoff, J. E.: Measurement of coronary blood flow, oxygen consumption and efficiency of the left ventricle in man. Am. Heart J. 38:1, 1949.
13. Burchell, H. B.: Cardiac catheterization in diagnosis of various cardiac malformations and diseases. Proc. Mayo Clin. 23:481, 1948.
14. Wood, E. H., Geraci, J. E., Pollack, A. A., Groom, D., Taylor, B. D., Pender, J. W., and Puch, D. G.: General and special techniques in cardiac catheterization. Proc. Mayo Clin. 23:494, 1948.
15. Zimmerman, H. A., Scott, R. W., and Becker, N. D.: Catheterization of the left side of the heart in man. Circulation 1:357, 1950.
16. Limon Lason, R., and Bouchard, A.: El cateterismo intracardico; cateterization de las cavidades izquierdas en el hombre. Registro simultaneo depresion y electrocardiograma intracavetarios. Arch. Inst. Cardiol. Mexico 21:271, 1950.
17. Seldinger, S. I.: Catheter replacement of the needle in percutaneous arteriography: A new technique. Acta Radiol. 39:368, 1953.
18. Ross, J., Jr.: Transseptal left heart catheterization: A new method of left atrial puncture. Ann. Surg. 149:395, 1959.
19. Ross, J., Jr., Braunwald, E., and Morrow, A. G.: Transseptal left atrial puncture: A new method for the measurement of left atrial pressure in man. Am. J. Cardiol. 3:653, 1959.
20. Sones, F. M., Jr., Shirey, E. K., Proudfit, W. L., and Westcott, R. N.: Cine coronary arteriography. Circulation 20:773, 1959.
21. Sones, F. M., Jr., and Shirey, E. K.: Cine coronary arteriography. Mod. Concepts Cardiovasc. Dis. 31:735, 1962.
22. Swan, H. J. C., Ganz, W., Forrester, J., Marcus, H., Diamond, G., and Chonette, D.: Catheterization of the heart in man with use of a flow directed balloon-tipped catheter. N. Engl. J. Med. 283:447, 1970.

TECHNICAL ASPECTS

23. Grossman, W.: Cardiac Catheterization and Angiography. 3rd ed. Philadelphia, Lea and Febiger, 1986.
24. Friesinger, G. C., Adams, D. F., Bourassa, M. G., Carlsson, E., Elliott, L. P., Gessner, I. H., Greenspan, R. H., Grossman, W., Judkins, M. P., Kennedy, J. W., and Sheldon, W. C.: Optimal resources for evaluation of the heart and lungs: Cardiac catheterization and radiographic facilities. Circulation 68:893A, 1983.
25. Fierens, E.: Outpatient coronary arteriography. Cathet. Cardiovasc. Diagn. 10:27, 1984.
26. Guidelines for Radiation Protection in the Cardiac Catheterization Laboratory. Cath. Cardiovasc. Diagn. 10:87, 1984.
27. Fergusson, D. J. G., and Karnada, R. O.: Percutaneous entry of the brachial artery for left heart catheterization using a sheath: Further experience. Cath. Cardiovasc. Diagn. 12:209, 1986.
28. Barry, W. H., Levin, D. C., Green, L. H., Bettman, M. A., Mudge, G. H., Jr., and Phillips, D.: Left heart catheterization and angiography via the percutaneous femoral approach using an arterial sheath. Cathet. Cardiovasc. Diagn. 5:401, 1979.
29. Antman, E. M., Marsh, J. D., Green, L. H., and Grossman, W.: Blood oxygen measurement in the assessment of intracardiac left to right shunts: A critical appraisal of methodology. Am. J. Cardiol. 46:265, 1980.
30. Karsh, D. L., Michaelson, S. P., Langon, R. A., Cohen, L. S., and Wolfson, S.: Retrograde left ventricular catheterization in patients with an aortic valve prosthesis. Am. J. Cardiol. 41:893, 1978.
31. O'Keefe, J. H., Jr., Vliestra, R. E., Hanley, P. C., and Seward, J. C.: Revival of the transseptal approach for catheterization of the left atrium and ventricle. Mayo Clin. Proc. 60:790, 1985.
32. Schoenfeld, M. H., Palacios, I. F., Hutter, A. M., Jr., Jacoby, S. S., and Block, P. C.: Underestimation of prosthetic mitral valve areas: Role of transseptal catheterization in avoiding unnecessary repeat mitral valve surgery. J. Am. Coll. Cardiol. 5:1387, 1985.
33. Mullins, C. E.: Transseptal left heart catheterization: Experience with a new technique in 520 pediatric and adult patients. Ped. Cardiol. 4:239, 1983.
34. Brockenbrough, E. C., and Braunwald, E.: A new technique for left ventricular angiocardiography and transseptal left heart catheterization. Am. J. Cardiol. 6:1062, 1960.
35. Nachnani, G. H., Lessin, L. S., Motomiya, T., and Leusen, W. N.: Scanning electron microscopy of thrombogenesis on vascular catheter surfaces. N. Engl. J. Med. 286:139, 1972.
36. McDonald, D. A.: Blood flow in Arteries. 2nd ed. Baltimore, Williams and Wilkins Co., 1974.
37. Wood, E. H., Leusen, I. R., Warner, H. R., and Wright, J. L.: Measurement of pressures in man by cardiac catheters. Circ. Res. 2:294, 1954.
38. Grossman, W., McLaurin, L. P., and Stefadouros, M. A.: Left ventricular stiffness associated with chronic pressure and volume overloads in man. Circ. Res. 35:793, 1974.
39. Guyton, A. C., Jones, C. E., and Coleman, T. G.: Circulatory Physiology: Cardiac Output and Its Regulation. 2nd ed. Philadelphia, W. B. Saunders Company, 1973.
40. Fick, A.: Über die Messung des Blutquantums in den Herzventrikeln. Sitz der Physik. Med. Ges. Wurzburg 1870, p. 16.
41. Barratt-Boyes, B. G., and Wood, E. H.: The oxygen saturation of blood in the venae cavae, right heart chambers, and pulmonary vessels of healthy subjects. J. Lab. Clin. Med. 50:93, 1957.
42. Selzer, A., and Sudrann, R. B.: Reliability of the determination of cardiac output in man by means of the Fick principle. Circ. Res. 6:485, 1958.

43. Thomassen, B.: Cardiac output in normal subjects under standard conditions. The repeatability of measurements by the Fick method. Scand. J. Clin. Lab. Invest. 9:365, 1957.
44. Visscher, M. B., and Johnson, J. A.: The Fick principle: Analysis of potential errors and its conventional application. J. Appl. Physiol. 5:635, 1953.
45. Stewart, G. N.: Researches on the circulation time and on the influences which affect it. IV. The output of the heart. J. Physiol. 22:159, 1897.
46. Hamilton, W. F., Riley, R. L., Attyah, A. M., Cournand, A., Fowell, D. M., Himmelstein, A., Noble, R. P., Remington, J. W., Richards, D. W., Wheeler, N. C., and Witham, A. C.: Comparison of Fick and dye injection methods of measuring cardiac output in man. Am. J. Physiol. *153*:309, 1948.
47. Rahimtoola, S. H., and Swan, H. J. C.: Calculation of cardiac output from indicator dilution curves in the presence of mitral regurgitation. Circulation *31*:711, 1965.
48. Shepherd, R. L., Higgs, L. M., and Glancy, D. L.: Comparison of left ventricular and pulmonary arterial injection sites in determination of cardiac output by the indicator dilution technique. Chest *62*:175, 1972.
49. Reddy, P. S., Curtiss, E. I., Bell, B., O'Toole, J. D., Salerni, R., Leon, D. F., and Shaver, J. A.: Determinants of variation between Fick and indicator dilution estimates of cardiac output during diagnostic catheterization. Fick vs. dye outputs. J. Lab. Clin. Med. *87*:568, 1976.
50. Branthwaite, M. A., and Bradley, R. D.: Measurement of cardiac output by thermodilution in man. J. Appl. Physiol. *24*:434, 1968.
51. Ganz, W., Donoso, R., Marcus, H. S., Forrester, J. S., and Swan, H. J. C.: A new technique for measurements of cardiac output by thermodilution in man. Am. J. Cardiol. *27*:392, 1971.
52. Weisel, R. D., Berger, R. L., and Hechtman, H. B.: Measurement of cardiac output by thermodilution. N. Engl. J. Med. *292*:682, 1975.
53. Kinsman, J. M., Moore, J. W., and Hamilton, W. F.: Studies on the circulation. I. Injection method. Physical and mathematical considerations. Am. J. Physiol. *89*:322, 1929.
54. Moore, J. W., Kinsman, J. M., Hamilton, W. G., and Spurling, R. G.: Studies on the circulation. II. Cardiac output determinations; comparison of the injection method with the direct Fick procedure. Am. J. Physiol. *89*:331, 1929.
55. Doyle, J. T., Wilson, J. S., Lepine, C., and Warren, J. V.: An evaluation of the measurement of the cardiac output and of the so-called pulmonary blood volume by the dye-dilution method. J. Lab. Clin. Med. *41*:29, 1953.
56. Eliasch, H., Lagerlof, H., Bucht, H., Ek, J., Eriksson, K., Bergstrom, J., and Werkö, L.: Comparison of the dye dilution and the direct Fick methods for the measurement of cardiac output in man. Scand. J. Lab. Clin. Invest. 7 (Suppl. 20):73, 1955.
57. Van Grondelle, A., Ditchey, R. V., Groves, B. M., Wagner, W. W., and Reaves, J. T.: Thermodilution method overestimates low cardiac output in humans. Am. J. Physiol. *245*:H690, 1983.
58. Swan, H. J. C., and Wood, E. H.: Localization of cardiac defects by dye dilution curves recorded after injection of T-1824 at multiple sites in the heart and great vessels during cardiac catheterization. Proc. Staff Meet. Mayo Clin. *28*:95, 1953.
59. Castillo, C. A., Kyle, J. C., Gilson, W. E., and Rowe, G. G.: Simulated shunt curves. Am. J. Cardiol. *17*:691, 1966.
60. Flamm, M. D., Cohn, K. E., and Hancock, E. W.: Measurement of systemic cardiac output at rest and exercise in patients with atrial septal defect. Am. J. Cardiol. *23*:258, 1969.
61. Ganz, W., Tamura, K., Marcus, H. S., Donose, R., Yoshida, S., and Swan, H. J. C.: Measurement of coronary sinus blood flow by continuous thermodilution in man. Circulation *44*:181, 1971.
62. Baim, D. S., Rothman, M. T., and Harrison, D. C.: Improved catheter for regional coronary sinus blood flow and metabolic studies. Am. J. Cardiol. *46*:997, 1980.
63. Baim, D. S., Rothman, M. T., and Harrison, D. C.: Simultaneous measurement of coronary venous flow and oxygen saturation during transient alterations in myocardial oxygen supply and demand. Am. J. Cardiol. *49*:743, 1982.
64. Wilson, R. F., Laughlin, D. E., Ackell, P. H., Chilian, W. M., Holida, M. D., Hartley, C. J., Armstrong, M. L., Marcus, M. L., and White, C. W.: Transluminal, subselective measurement of coronary artery blood flow velocity and vasodilator reserve in man. Circulation *72*:82, 1985.
65. Rapaport, E., and Dexter, L.: Pulmonary "capillary" pressure. *In* Methods in Medical Research. Chicago, Year Book Medical Publishers, 7:85, 1958.
66. Connolly, D. C., Kirklin, J. W., and Wood, E. H.: The relationship between pulmonary artery pressure and left atrial pressure in man. Circ. Res. *2*:434, 1954.
67. Fritts, H. W., Harris, P., Clauss, R. H., Odell, J. E., and Cournand, A.: The effect of acetylcholine on the human pulmonary circulation under normal and hypoxic conditions. J. Clin. Invest. *37*:99, 1958.
68. Wood, P., Besterman, E. M., Towers, M. K., and McIlroy, M. B.: The effect of acetylcholine on pulmonary vascular resistance and left atrial pressure in mitral stenosis. Br. Heart J. *19*:279, 1957.
69. Rudolph, A. M., Paul, M. H., Sommer, L. S., and Nadas, A. S.: Effects of tolazoline hydrochloride (Priscoline) on circulatory dynamics of patients with pulmonary hypertension. Am. Heart J. *55*:424, 1958.
70. Grover, R. F., Reeves, T. J., and Blount, S. G., Jr.: Tolazoline hydrochloride (Priscoline): An effective pulmonary vasodilator. Am. Heart J. *61*:5, 1961.
71. Milnor, W. R.: Pulsatile blood flow. N. Engl. J. Med. *287*:27, 1972.
72. Nichols, W. W., Conti, C. R., Walker, W. E., and Milnor, W. R.: Input impedance of the systemic circulation in man. Circ. Res. *40*:421, 1977.
73. Gorlin, R., and Gorlin, G.: Hydraulic formula for calculation of area of stenotic mitral valve, other valves, and central circulatory shunts. Am. Heart J. *41*:1, 1951.
74. Cohen, M. V., and Gorlin, R.: Modified orifice equation for the calculation of mitral valve area. Am. Heart J. *84*:839, 1972.
75. Folland, E. D., Parisi, A. F., and Carbone, C.: Is peripheral arterial pressure a satisfactory substitute for ascending aortic pressure when measuring aortic valve gradients? J. Am. Coll. Cardiol. *4*:1207, 1984.
76. Hakki, A. H., Iskandrian, A. S., Bemis, C. E., Kimbiris, D., Mintz, G. S., Segal, B. L., and Brice, C.: A simplified formula for the calculation of stenotic cardiac valves. Circulation *63*:1050, 1981.
77. Angel, J., Soler-Soler, J., Anivarro, I., and Domingo, E.: Hemodynamic evaluation of stenotic cardiac valves: Modification of the simplified formula and aortic valve area calculation. Cathet. Cardiovasc. Diagn. *11*:127, 1985.
78. Cannon, S. R., Richards, K. L., and Crawford, M.: Hydraulic estimation of stenotic orifice area: A correction of the Gorlin formula. Circulation *71*:1170, 1985.

APPLICATIONS

79. St. John Sutton, M. G., St. John Sutton, M., Aldershaw, P., Sachetti, R., Paneth, M., Lennox, S. C., Gibson, R. V., and Gibson, D. G.: Valve replacement without preoperative cardiac catheterization. N. Engl. J. Med. *305*:1233, 1981.
80. Roberts, W. C.: Reasons for cardiac catheterization before cardiac valve replacement. N. Engl. J. Med. *306*:1291, 1982.
81. Alpert, J. S., Sloss, L. J., Cohn, P. F., and Grossman, W.: The diagnostic accuracy of combined clinical and noninvasive cardiac evaluation: Comparison with findings at cardiac catheterization. Cathet. Cardiovasc. Diagn. *6*:359, 1980.
82. Lupi-Herrera, E., Sandoval, J., Seoane, M., and Bialostozky, D.: The role of hydralazine therapy for pulmonary arterial hypertension of unknown cause. Circulation *65*:648, 1982.
83. Mahrer, P. R., and Eshoo, N.: Outpatient cardiac catheterization and coronary angiography. Cathet. Cardiovasc. Diagn. *7*:355, 1981.
84. Green, G. S., McKinnon, C. M., Rosch, J., and Judkins, M. P.: Complications of selective percutaneous transfemoral coronary arteriography and their prevention. Circulation *45*:552, 1972.
85. Braunwald, E., and Swan, H. J. C. (eds.): Cooperative study on cardiac catheterization. Circulation 37 (Suppl. 111):1, 1968.
86. Kloster, F. E., Bristow, J. D., and Seaman, A. J.: Cardiac catheterization during anticoagulant therapy. Am. J. Cardiol. *28*:675, 1971.
87. Campion, B. C., Frye, R. L., Pluth, J. R., Fairbairn, J. F., and Davis, G. D.: Arterial complications of retrograde brachial arterial catheterization. Mayo Clin. Proc. *46*:589, 1971.
88. Jeresaty, R. M., and Liss, J. P.: Effects of brachial artery catheterization on arterial pulse and blood pressure in 203 patients. Am. Heart J. *76*:481, 1968.
89. Machleder, H. I., Sweeney, J. P., and Barker, J. F.: Pulseless arm after brachial artery catheterization. Lancet *1*:407, 1972.
90. Bristow, J. D., Seaman, A. J., Kloster, F. E., Herr, R. H., and Griswold, H. E.: Late, heparin-induced bleeding after retrograde arterial catheterization. Circulation *37*:393, 1968.
91. Kloster, F. E., Bristow, J. D., and Griswold, H. E.: Femoral artery occlusion following percutaneous catheterization. Am. Heart J. *79*:175, 1970.
92. Gupta, P. K., and Haft, J. I.: Complete heart block complicating cardiac catheterization. Chest *61*:185, 1972.
93. Chahine, R. A., Herman, M. V., and Gorlin, R.: Complications of coronary arteriography: Comparison of the brachial to the femoral approach. Ann. Intern. Med. *76*:862, 1972.
94. Eshagy, B., Loeb, H. S., Miller, S. E., Scanlon, P. J., Towne, W. D., and Gunnar, R. M.: Mediastinal and retropharyngeal hemorrhage: A complication of cardiac catheterization. J. A. M. A. *226*:427, 1973.
95. Hey, E. G., Jr., Dyrda, I., and Joyner, C. R.: Entanglement of a cardiac catheter on a heart valve prosthesis. N. Engl. J. Med. *275*:434, 1966.
96. Goodman, D. J., Rider, A. K., Billingham, M. E., and Schroeder, J. S.: Thromboembolic complications with the indwelling balloon tipped pulmonary arterial catheter. N. Engl. J. Med. *291*:777, 1974.
97. Stanger, P., Heymann, M. A., Tarnoff, H., Hoffman, J. I. E., and Rudolph, A. M.: Complications of cardiac catheterization of neonates, infants and children. Circulation *50*:595, 1974.
98. Price, H. P., and Takaro, T.: Unusual coronary emboli associated with coronary arteriography. Chest *63*:698, 1973.
99. Walson, W. J., Lee, G. B., and Amplatz, K.: Biplane selective coronary arteriography via percutaneous transfemoral approach. A.J.R. *100*:332, 1967.
100. Nicholas, G. G., and DeMuth, W. E.: Long term results of brachial thrombectomy following cardiac catheterization. Ann. Surg. *183*:436, 1976.
101. Smith, W. R., Glauser, F. L., and Jemison, P.: Ruptured chordae of the tricuspid valve: The consequence of flow directed Swan-Ganz catheterization. Chest *70*:790, 1976.
102. Roberts, R., Ludbrook, P. A., Weiss, E. S., and Sobel, B. E.: Serum CPK isoenzymes after cardiac catheterization. Br. Heart J. *37*:1144, 1975.
103. Takahashi, O., Zakheim, R., Park, M. K., Mattioli, L., and Diehl, A. M.: The effects of transfemoral cardiac catheterization on limb blood flow in children. Chest *71*:159, 1977.
104. Rosengart, R., Nelson, R. J. and Emmanoulides, G. C.: Anterior tibial compartment syndrome in a child. An unusual complication of cardiac catheterization. Pediatrics *58*:456, 1967.
105. Dawson, D. M., and Fisher, E. G.: Neurologic complications of cardiac catherization. Neurology *27*:496, 1977.

106. Starmer, C. F., Whalen, R. E., and McIntosh, H. D.: Hazards of electric shock in cardiology. Am. J. Cardiol. 14:537, 1964.
107. Mody, S. M., and Richings. M.: Ventricular fibrillation resulting from electrocution during cardiac catheterization. Lancet 2:698, 1962.
108. Starmer, C. F., McIntosh, H. D., and Whalen, R. E.: Electrical hazards and cardiovascular function. N. Engl J. Med. *284*:181, 1971.
109. Adrouny, Z. A., Stephenson, M. J., Straube, K. R., Dotter, C. T., and Griswold, H. E.: Effect of cardiac catheterization and angiocardiography on the serum glutamic oxaloacetic transaminase. Circulation 27:565, 1963.
110. Burckhardt, D., Vera, C. A., LaDue, J. S., and Steinberg, I.: Enzyme activity following angiography. Am. J. Roentgenol. *102*:406, 1968.
111. Kennedy, J. W.: Complications associated with cardiac catheterization and angiography. Cathet. Cardiovasc. Diagn. *8*:5, 1982.
112. Sutton, D. C., and Sutton, G. C.: Needle biopsy of the human ventricular myocardium. Review of 54 consecutive cases. Am. Heart J. *60*:364, 1960.
113. Bulloch, R. T., Murphy, M. L., Pearce, M. B.: Intracardiac needle biopsy of the ventricular septum. Am. J. Cardiol. *16*:227, 1965.
114. Hirose, T., and Bailey, C. P.: New myocardial biopsy needle. Angiology *16*:288, 1965.
115. Sakakibara, S., and Konno, S.: Endomyocardial biopsy. Jpn. Heart J. *3*:537, 1962.
116. Caves, P., Billingham, M. B., Coltart, J., Rider, A., and Stinson, E.: Transvenous endomyocardial biopsy—application of a method for diagnosing heart disease. Postgrad. Med. J. *51*:286, 1975.
117. Hess, O. M., Schneider, J., Turina, M., Heeb, S., Grob, P., and Krayenbuehl, K. P.: Die transvenose Endomyokardbiopsie in der Bewiteilung der kongestivan Kardiomyopathie. Schweiz. Med. Woenschr. *109*:293, 1977.
118. Mason, J. W.: Technique for right and left ventricular endomyocardial biopsy. Am. J. Cardiol. *41*:887, 1978.
119. Olsen, E. G. J.: Results of endomyocardial biopsy—histological, histochemical and ultrastructural analysis. Postgrad Med. J. *51*:295, 1975.
120. Mason, J. W.: Endomyocardial biopsy: Balance of success and failure. Circulation *71*:185, 1985.
121. Kawai, C., and Kitaura, Y.: New endomyocardial biopsy catheter for the left ventricle. Am. J. Cardiol. *40*:63, 1977.
122. Colucci, W. S., Lorell, B. H., Schoen, F. J., Warhol, M. J., and Grossman, W.: Hypertrophic obstruction due to Fabry's disease. N. Engl. J. Med. *307*:926, 1982.
123. Bristow, M. R., Mason, J. W., Billingham, M. E., and Daniels, J. R.: Doxorubicin cardiomyopathy: Evaluation by phonocardiography, endomyocardial biopsy, and cardiac catheterization. Ann. Intern. Med. *88*:168, 1978.
124. Nippoldt, T. B., Edwards, W. D., Holmes, D. R., Relder, G. S., Hartzler, G. O., and Smith, H. C.: Right ventricular endomyocardial biopsy. Clinicopathologic correlates in 100 consecutive patients. Mayo Clin. Proc. *57*:407, 1982.
125. Parillo, J. E., Aretz, H. T., Palacios, I., Fallon, J. T., and Block, P. C.: The results of transvenous endomyocardial biopsy frequently can be used to diagnose myocardial diseases in patients with heart failure. Circulation *69*:93, 1984.
126. Mason, J. W., Billingham, M. E., and Ricci, D. R.: Treatment of acute inflammatory myocarditis assisted by endomyocardial biopsy. Am. J. Cardiol. *45*:1037, 1980.
127. Weintraub, R. M., Aroesty, J. M., Paulins, S., Levine, F. H., Markis, J. E., LaPraia, P. J., Cohen, S. I., and Kurland, G. F.: Medically refractory unstable angina pectoris. I. Long-term follow-up of patients undergoing intraaortic balloon counterpulsation and operation. Am. J. Cardiol. *43*:887, 1979.
128. Pace, P. D., Tilney, N. L., Lesch, M., and Couch, N. P.: Peripheral arterial complications of intra-aortic balloon counterpulsation. Surgery *88*:685, 1977.
129. Gottlieb, S. O., Brinker, A., Borkon, A. M., Kallman, C. H., Potter, A., Gott, V. L., and Baughman, K. L.: Identification of patients at high risk for complications of intraaortic balloon counterpulsation: A multivariate risk factor analysis. Am. J. Cardiol. *53*:1135, 1984.
130. Bregman, D., Nichols, A. B., Weiss, M. B., Powers, E. R., Martin, E. C., and Casarella, W. J.: Percutaneous intraaortic balloon insertion. Am. J. Cardiol. *46*:261, 1980.
131. Rashkind, W. J., and Miller, W. W.: Creation of an atrial septal defect without thoracotomy: A palliative approach to complete transposition of the great vessels. J.A.M.A. *196*:991, 1966.
132. Rashkind, W. J.: Transcatheter treatment of congenital heart disease. Circulation *67*:711, 1983.
133. Porstmann, W., Wierny, L., and Warnke, H.: Der Verschluss des Ductus Arteriosus Persistens ohne Thorakotomie. Fortschr. Roentgenstr. *109*:133, 1968.
134. Porstmann, W., Wierny, L., Warnke, H., Gertsberger, G., and Romaniuk, P. A.: Catheter closure of patent ductus arteriosus: 62 cases treated without thoractomy. Radiol. Clin. North Am. 9:203, 1971.
135. Sato, K., Fiyino, M., Kozuka, T., Naito, Y., Kitamura, S., Nakano, S., Ohyama, C., and Kawashima, Y.: Transfemoral plug closure of patent ductus arteriosus: Experience in 61 consecutive cases treated without thoractomy. Circulation *51*:1337, 1975.
136. Mills, N. L., and King, T. D.: Nonoperative closure of left to right shunts. J. Thorac. Cardiovasc. Surg. 72:371, 1976.
137. King, T. D., Thompson, S. L., Steiner, C., and Mills, N. L.: Secundum atrial septal defect. Nonoperative closure during cardiac catheterization. J.A.M.A. *235*:2506, 1976.
138. Scoggins, W. G., and Greenfield, L. J.: Transvenous pulmonary embolectomy for acute massive pulmonary embolism. Chest *71*:213, 1977.
139. Greenfield, L. J., Reif, M., and Guenter, C. A.: Hemodynamic and respiratory response to transvenous pulmonary embolectomy. J. Thorac. Cardiovasc. Surg. 62:890, 1971.
140. Taylor, B. G., Cockerill, E. M., Manfredi, F., and Klatte, E.: Therapeutic embolization of the pulmonary artery in pulmonary arterio-venous fistula. Ann. J. Med. *64*:360, 1978.
141. Massumi, R. A., and Ross, A. M.: Atraumatic non-surgical techniques for removal of broken catheters from cardiac cavities. N. Engl. J. Med. *277*:195, 1967.
142. Bloomfield, A.: Techniques of non-surgical retrieval of iatrogenic foreign bodies from the heart. Ann. J. Cardiol. *27*:538, 1971.

10 CORONARY ARTERIOGRAPHY

by DAVID C. LEVIN, M.D., and
GEOFFREY A. GARDINER, Jr., M.D.

Sporadic attempts to visualize the coronary arteries by angiography were reported in the mid 1940's and early 1950's.[1] However, the era of modern coronary arteriography began in earnest in 1959 with the development by Sones of a technique for selectively catheterizing the coronary arteries via a brachial artery cutdown and recording the images by cineangiography.[2] A detailed and delightful account of the first (and inadvertent) selective coronary arteriogram has been recorded by Hurst in an interview with Sones.[3] Another major landmark in the field occurred in 1967 with the development by Judkins of preformed catheters which could be used to cannulate selectively the coronary arteries via a percutaneous femoral approach.[4] Sones and Judkins, both of whom died in 1985, will be linked together in medical history as the two major pioneers in this most important diagnostic technique. Because of its ease, rapidity, and a somewhat lower complication rate, the Judkins technique has become the most widely used approach for coronary arteriography throughout the world. In the authors' laboratory at the Brigham and Women's Hospital it is used in the vast majority of cases, and it is therefore described in some detail.

TECHNIQUE OF CORONARY ARTERIOGRAPHY

JUDKINS' TECHNIQUE

EQUIPMENT FOR CORONARY ARTERIOGRAPHY. Although a wide variety of different guidewires is available, the standard wire for percutaneous transfemoral coronary arteriography is the 0.035-inch or 0.038-inch guidewire with a 3 mm J-shaped tip. The J configuration and flexible tip allow the wire to be passed safely through most iliac arteries, even those with considerable tortuosity and atherosclerotic irregularity.

The Judkins coronary catheters are shaped as shown in Figure 10–1*A*. The catheters contain a fine wire braid within the wall for stability and directional control and are fabricated of either polyethylene or polyurethane. They are available in different sizes; the appropriate size selected depends on the size of the aortic arch. In some cases, depending upon the body habitus of the patient and the size of the aortic root, additional alterations may be necessary, such as reshaping of the catheter in a steam jet or cutting off the tip with a blade to shorten it.

In most laboratories the coronary catheter is attached to a three-stopcock manifold (Fig. 10–1*B*), which enables the angiographer to switch rapidly between pressure monitoring, flushing the catheter with saline, and performing contrast injections, all in a closed system that allows for speed and maintenance of sterility. In addition to the three side ports, one end of the manifold has a rotating adapter for attachment to the catheter itself, while the other end has a Luer-Lok fitting to which a syringe is attached.

Some angiographers now use a side arm arterial sheath (Fig. 10–1*C*) for performing coronary arteriography. This sheath is inserted into the femoral artery percutaneously over a Teflon introducer which is then withdrawn, leaving only the sheath itself in place. It has a rubber check valve at its external end to maintain hemostasis and also to provide access for the catheter. It also has a side arm through which femoral artery pressure can be monitored. The inner diameter of the sheath is somewhat larger than the outer diameter of the angiographic catheter, and it is the column of blood between them which transmits pressure through the side arm to the transducer. Other advantages of the sheath are that it allows multiple catheter exchanges to be performed without compression of the groin and that it lessens patient discomfort caused by catheter manipulation. Although the sheath has the potential disadvantage of creating a larger hole in the arterial wall than if only a catheter is used, it has been the authors' experience that the use of this technique does not create an increased risk of local arterial complications.[5]

CATHETERIZATION TECHNIQUE. The groin area is palpated to ascertain the point of maximal impulse of the femoral artery. This is usually at or just below the level of the inguinal crease and is always several centimeters below the inguinal ligament. The skin area 1 to 2 cm below and slightly lateral to the point of maximal impulse is anesthetized locally. The artery is then punctured with a Seldinger type of needle using a relatively shallow approach (i.e., the needle direction is more parallel to the artery than

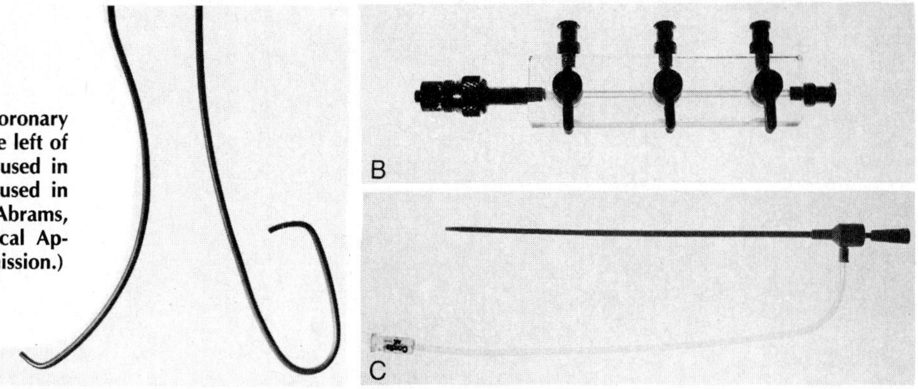

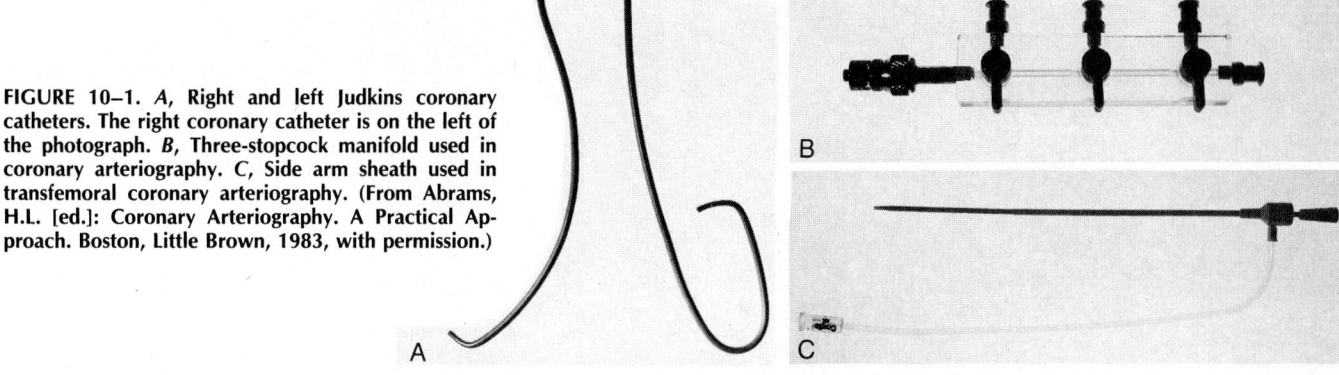

FIGURE 10–1. *A*, Right and left Judkins coronary catheters. The right coronary catheter is on the left of the photograph. *B*, Three-stopcock manifold used in coronary arteriography. *C*, Side arm sheath used in transfemoral coronary arteriography. (From Abrams, H.L. [ed.]: Coronary Arteriography. A Practical Approach. Boston, Little Brown, 1983, with permission.)

perpendicular to it). The operator should always be sure that the actual level of arterial entry is distal to the inguinal ligament. If the needle enters the femoral artery proximal to this ligament, it may be impossible by manual compression to control bleeding at the end of the procedure.

The guidewire is then passed through the needle into the aorta. The needle is removed over the guidewire and the introducer and sheath combination is inserted over the wire. Once the sheath is properly positioned in the artery, both the guidewire and introducer are removed, leaving only the sheath in place. Careful flushing of the side arm of the sheath is performed to extract any small clots that may have formed during this maneuver, and the side arm is then connected to a pressure transducer for continuous monitoring of femoral artery pressure.

A pigtail catheter is then loaded onto a 3 mm J-shaped guidewire, so that the flexible tip of the wire protrudes beyond the tip of the catheter. This combination is then inserted through the check valve of the sheath and into the aorta, using fluoroscopic control. The guidewire and catheter combination is passed up to the descending thoracic aorta, the wire is removed, and the catheter is connected to the rotating adapter of the three-stopcock manifold. The catheter is carefully flushed and central aortic pressure is recorded through one of the side ports of the manifold which has been connected to a second transducer. At this point, the operator should check both pressure tracings: one from the catheter tip (monitored through the manifold) and the other from the femoral artery (monitored through the side arm of the arterial sheath). If the pressure tracings are satisfactory, the catheter is advanced over the aortic arch and through the aortic valve into the left ventricle. Left ventricular pressure measurements, particularly left ventricular end-diastolic pressure (LVEDP), are recorded and left ventriculography is performed as described on page 305.

After left ventriculography, LVEDP should again be measured. Usually the contrast injection results in at least some degree of elevation of LVEDP. This is well tolerated as long as it remains below 25 to 30 mm Hg. The pigtail catheter is then removed over a guidewire and a selective coronary catheter is inserted in its place. To catheterize either coronary artery, the image intensifier should be positioned so that the angiographer views the patient's heart in the left anterior oblique (LAO) projection. When viewed in this projection, the left coronary artery (LCA) originates from the left side of the aorta, while the right coronary artery (RCA) originates from the right side of the aorta (from a true anatomical point of view, the LCA originates from the left posterolateral aspect of the aorta, while the RCA originates from its anterior aspect).

The technique for catheterizing the LCA is shown in Figure 10–2. In advancing the left Judkins catheter toward the left coronary ostium, the most important rules are to advance it slowly and to keep it positioned so that it remains in full profile (i.e., so that both curves of the catheter are clearly visible). If the catheter begins to turn out of profile, it should be gently rotated with the rotating adapter as it is advanced slowly. If the catheter is advanced too rapidly, it may snap forcefully into the left coronary ostium and cause dissection.

After the left coronary ostium is entered, the pressure at the catheter tip should be checked immediately to be sure that it still coincides with femoral artery pressure. If so, it can be safely assumed that the catheter tip is free within the lumen of the LCA, a fact which can be verified by a small test injection of contrast medium. However, if the pressure tracing shows significant damping or "ventricularization" (normal systolic pressure but a low diastolic pressure), this may indicate the presence of significant stenosis of the LCA. Sometimes these pressure changes can occur merely from abutment of the catheter tip upon the arterial wall. However, it should be assumed that left main coronary stenosis is present until proven otherwise. Whenever ventricularization

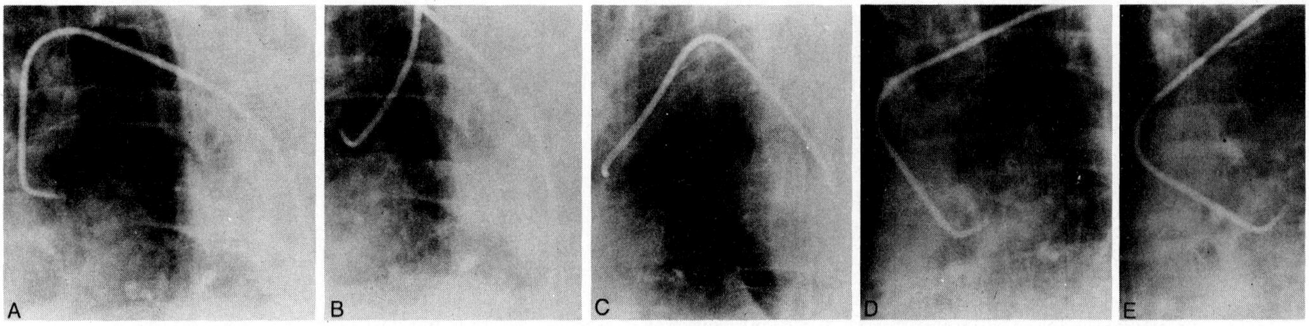

FIGURE 10–2. Technique for catheterizing the left coronary artery (LCA) while the patient is viewed in the left anterior oblique (LAO) projection. *A*, The catheter is seen in full profile as it is advanced around the aortic arch. Note that both curves of the catheter are clearly seen. *B*, The catheter is rotated too far in one direction. The curves are distorted. *C*, The tip is now rotated too far in the other direction, resulting again in loss of visualization of the tip curve. *D*, After proper rotation of the catheter, both curves are again seen in profile as it is advanced toward the aortic root. *E*, The tip of the catheter has now passed into the left coronary ostium. (From Abrams, H.L. [ed.]: Coronary Arteriography. A Practical Approach. Boston, Little Brown, 1983, with permission.)

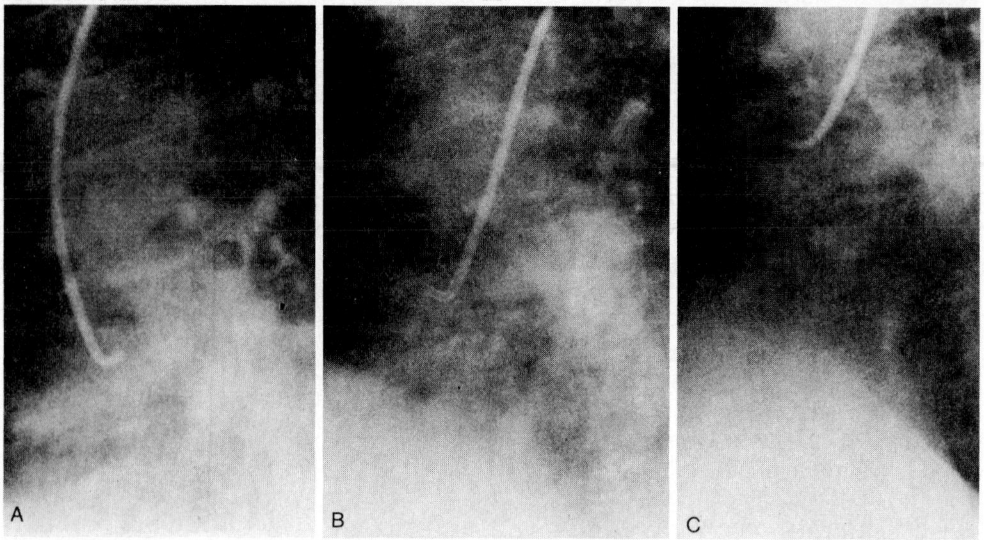

FIGURE 10–3. Catheterization of the right coronary artery (RCA) while viewing the patient in the LAO projection. *A*, The catheter tip is advanced to the root of the aorta with its tip directed to the left. *B*, The catheter is rotated in a clockwise direction as it is withdrawn. *C*, Further clockwise rotation and withdrawal results in passage of the tip into the right coronary ostium. (From Abrams, H.L. [ed.]: Coronary Arteriography. A Practical Approach. Boston, Little Brown, 1983, with permission.)

or damping occurs, the catheter should be removed from the left coronary ostium and an attempt at repositioning should be made. If the pressure abnormality persists, it is wise to withdraw the catheter slightly and perform a nonselective injection of contrast material with the catheter tip in the left aortic cusp just outside the ostium of the vessel. This will often allow demonstration of left main coronary stenosis if it is present.

If the catheter tip pressure is instead normal and a small test injection of contrast material shows that the main LCA is not stenotic, left coronary arteriography is then performed using multiple projections, as discussed below. A forceful hand injection of 6 to 9 ml of contrast material is usually required to fill the left coronary system; in some laboratories these injections are now performed with a power injector to provide complete opacification.

Catheterization of the RCA is also performed in the LAO position, but this requires different maneuvers than does catheterization of the LCA. Whereas the left coronary catheter tends to seek out the left coronary ostium almost automatically, the right coronary catheter must always be rotated by the angiographer to engage the vessel. Usually this is accomplished by passing the catheter to a point just above the aortic valve, then rotating it clockwise while slowly withdrawing it (Fig. 10–3). Entry into the RCA is generally signified by a sudden rightward movement of the catheter tip. Here again, the catheter tip pressure should be checked to be sure that damping or ventricularization has not occurred. If it has, this may signify ostial stenosis. However, these pressure changes can also result from a small RCA, inadvertent superselective entry of the catheter tip into the conus branch, presence of total obstruction shortly beyond the right coronary ostium, or spasm of the RCA. Catheter-induced spasm of the RCA is relatively common, but it is extremely rare in the left coronary system, for reasons which are not entirely clear. Generally, right coronary spasm can be alleviated by administration of sublingual nitroglycerin. If persistent damping or ventricularization of the pressure tracing is seen after use of nitroglycerin, a cusp injection should be performed to attempt to visualize a possible stenosis of the right coronary ostium. Alternatively, a very small injection of contrast medium into the RCA itself can be performed with immediate withdrawal of the catheter tip at the end of the injection (sometimes referred to as the "shoot and run" technique).

If the pressure tracing is normal upon entry of the catheter tip, the RCA should be visualized in at least two projections using hand injections of 3 to 6 ml of contrast material. The actual quantity of contrast used should be judged by the angiographer depending upon the size of the vessel.

OTHER TECHNIQUES OF CORONARY ARTERIOGRAPHY

SONES TECHNIQUE. The Sones catheter, shown in Figure 10–4, is constructed of either woven Dacron or polyurethane and has an end hole and four small side holes close to the catheter tip. The most commonly used catheters are size 7 or 8 French, with a tip that tapers to 5 French. The brachial artery cutdown is performed by blunt dissection and a small incision is made in the vessel.[6] A catheter is first introduced into the distal segment of the brachial artery and heparinized saline is injected to prevent clotting during the remainder of the procedure when there is no blood flow. The Sones catheter is then advanced into the ascending aorta. The technique most commonly used to enter the left coronary ostium with this catheter is to form an open loop on the right aortic cusp so that the shaft of the catheter and its tip form a 45-degree angle pointed toward the left coronary cusp. Alternate advancement and withdrawal of the catheter then often results in entry of the tip into the left coronary ostium. Stable seating of the catheter tip can be accomplished in some patients by advancing the catheter, while in other cases slight retraction is necessary. To enter the right coronary ostium, a slightly smaller open loop is formed, once again pointing toward the left coronary cusp. The catheter is then slowly withdrawn during clockwise rotation. This maneuver will often cause the tip to rotate and pass into the RCA.

AMPLATZ TECHNIQUE. During the same year the Judkins catheters were developed, Amplatz et al.[7] developed another set of catheters for percutaneous coronary arteriography via the femoral approach (Fig. 10–5). While the Amplatz catheters are much less commonly used than those devised by Judkins, they are an excellent alternative in the occasional cases in which the Judkins catheters are not appropriately shaped to enter the coronary arteries. To catheterize the LCA, the broad secondary curve of the appropriately sized left Amplatz catheter is positioned so it rests on the right aortic cusp with its tip pointing toward

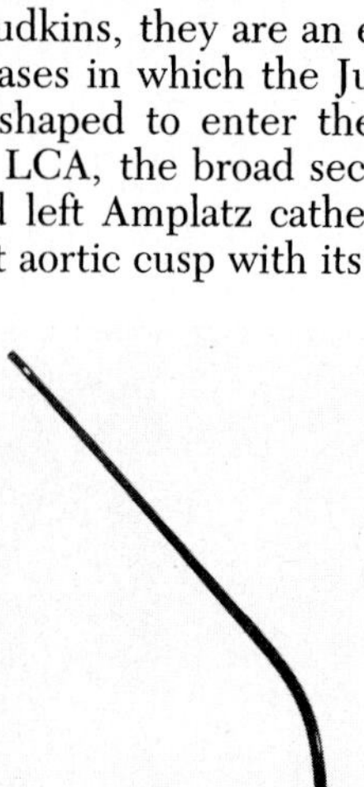

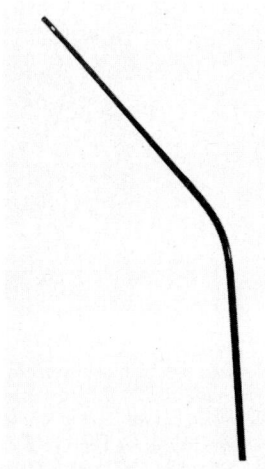

FIGURE 10–4. Sones coronary catheter.

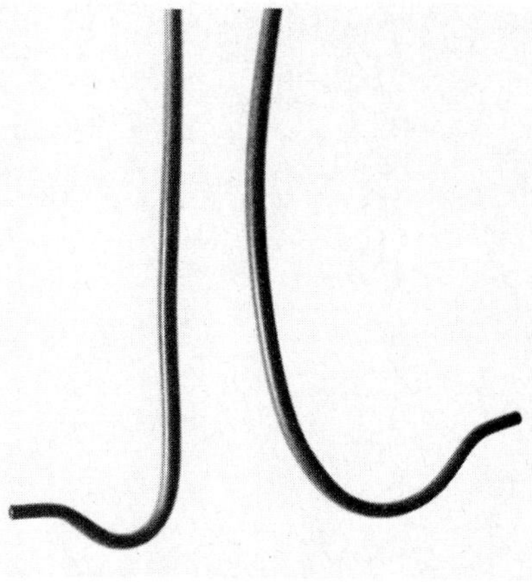

FIGURE 10–5. Amplatz right and left coronary catheters. The right coronary catheter is on the left of the photograph. (From Abrams, H.L. [ed.]: Coronary Arteriography. A Practical Approach. Boston, Little Brown, 1983, with permission.)

the left aortic cusp. Alternating advancement and retraction of the catheter in a slow and gentle manner will usually produce entry of the tip into the left coronary ostium. Once the tip enters the ostium, the position of the catheter can usually be stabilized by slight retraction. Catheterizing the RCA with the right Amplatz catheter requires a technique similar to that used with the right Judkins catheter.

MULTIPURPOSE CATHETER TECHNIQUE. A single catheter which can be inserted percutaneously via the femoral approach and used to catheterize both the right and left coronary arteries was originally described by Schoonmaker and King[8] and described in greater detail by King and Douglas.[9] The catheter has a configuration somewhat similar to that of the Sones catheter, although the tip is shorter. The maneuvers used to seat the catheter are also similar to those used in the Sones technique.

TECHNICAL FEATURES

CINEANGIOGRAPHIC EQUIPMENT. Cineangiographic equipment is expensive and complex.[10–12] In brief, the following types of equipment are needed: (1) A three-phase, 12-pulse, or constant-potential x-ray generator with cine pulsing, output of 100 kilowatts or more, and an automatic brightness control with very rapid response. (2) A high-heat–capacity x-ray tube capable of rotating at 10,000 RPM with a target angle of 10° or less. Dual focal spots should be available, with a small focal spot size of approximately 0.6 mm and a large focal spot size of approximately 1.2 mm. (3) Carbon fiber grids with a grid ratio of 8:1 and approximately 100 lines per inch. (4) A dual- or triple-mode cesium iodide image intensifier with a resolution capability of approximately 5 line pairs/mm, a contrast ratio of greater than 15:1, and conversion factor of greater than 50 for the small mode. The intensifier should have at least two modes with the large mode approximating 9 inches to be able to image large ventricles, and a small mode (magnified mode) of 6 inches or less. (5) An optical system consisting of an objective lens, an image-distributing mirror, and a cine camera lens. The focal length of the camera lens should allow the proper degree of overframing. A diaphragm should be interposed in front of the cine camera lens and, ideally, the entire system should be set up so that the lens can operate at two f-stops above maximum aperture. (6) A cine camera capable of operating at either 30 or 60 frames per second with low vibration levels. (7) Cine film should be chosen carefully with a speed and average gradient appropriate for the system and a low level of "base + fog."[8] (8) A cine film processor is needed which can maintain highly stable developer temperature and immersion time; it must also provide adequate replenishment of chemical solutions, proper agitation, and recirculation.

DRUGS USED DURING CORONARY ARTERIOGRAPHY. Adequate premedication is very important for efficient operation of the catheterization laboratory and the welfare of the patient. A variety of regimens is used in different laboratories. Gensini has recommended secobarbital, 100 mg, and diazepam, 5 mg, given orally 1 hour before the procedure.[6] King and Douglas recommend diazepam in 2.5 to 5 mg increments and 0.6 mg atropine, both given intravenously.[9] Atropine is avoided in patients whose condition is unstable, those with a rapid heart rate, or those in whom ergonovine provocation is contemplated. In the authors' laboratory, diazepam, 5 to 10 mg, and benadryl, 25 to 50 mg, are given orally approximately 1 hour before the procedure.

Heparin is used routinely in all patients in the authors' laboratory, and in most others as well. This is done despite the fact that heparin has not been clearly shown to exert a beneficial effect in the prevention of complications.[13] It is administered intravenously at a dose of 5000 units at the time the first arterial catheter is inserted.

Nitroglycerin has several effects upon the cardiovascular system (p. 1327) but from the point of view of the angiographer, its principal effect is to diminish vascular tone in the epicardial coronary arteries. It is given shortly before the procedure, at a dosage of 0.3 mg sublingually, to prevent catheter-induced spasm. This dose may not be sufficient to obviate spasm completely, so that additional doses may well be necessary during the procedure. Nitroglycerin can also be administered intravenously or directly into a coronary artery. The authors use this drug routinely except in patients with suspected variant angina. In these individuals, nitroglycerin might mask the demonstration of spasm.

The use of *atropine* is more controversial. Some laboratories avoid it in most cases. Atropine diminishes the likelihood of vasovagal reactions and the sinus bradycardia that frequently occurs after selective coronary injections. A drawback to its use is that it generally increases heart rate, which leads to increased myocardial oxygen demand and may make adequate opacification of the coronary arteries more difficult. In the authors' laboratory, atropine, 0.6 mg, is given intravenously at the start of the procedure provided that the patient has a heart rate below 80 beats/min.

The most commonly used contrast material in coronary arteriography is *Renografin-76*, an aqueous solution of 66 per cent *N*-methylglucamine diatrizoate and 10 per cent sodium diatrizoate. The sodium content of this agent is 0.19 mEq/ml. If the sodium content of contrast material injected into the coronary arteries is significantly lower than this, there is an increased incidence of ventricular fibrillation.[11, 14, 15] Other contrast agents with formulations similar to that of Renografin-76 are now also in use. Within the last several years, nonionic contrast agents have been developed and tested in cardiac catheterization laboratories.[16] These agents have less than half the osmolality of Renografin-76 and appear to cause less of a decrease in heart rate and arterial pressure following selective coronary injection. The major drawback to their routine use is their expense; nonionic contrast agents currently are more than 10 times as costly as standard agents.

ELECTROCARDIOGRAPHIC AND HEMODYNAMIC CHANGES IN CORONARY ARTERIOGRAPHY. The selective injection of Renografin-76 or other contrast agents into coronary arteries results in a variety of electrocardiographic and hemodynamic changes. Right coronary arteriography often produces T-wave inversion in leads II, III, and aVF. Sinus bradycardia and systemic hypotension also occur frequently, and sometimes can be quite severe. Left coronary arteriography generally results in peaking of the T wave in leads II, III, and aVF. Sinus bradycardia and hypotension may occur, but are usually less pronounced than during right coronary arteriography. If the patient has total right coronary occlusion, a biphasic response can occur during left coronary arteriography. The left coronary injection will first produce T-wave elevation, but as the contrast passes through collaterals to the distal right coronary tree, the characteristic T-wave inversion usually seen with right coronary arteriography will occur.

ANATOMY AND VARIATIONS OF THE CORONARY ARTERIES

Angiography visualizes only a small portion of the coronary circulation—the major epicardial branches and their second-, third-, and perhaps fourth-order branches. The myriad of small intramyocardial branches is not visualized because of their small size, cardiac motion, and limitations in resolution of cine imaging systems. Although these small "resistance" vessels play a major role in regulation of coronary blood flow, they are not thought to be important in human coronary artery disease (CAD).

In viewing the coronary arteries by cineangiography, the direct frontal and lateral views are used less commonly than the right anterior oblique (RAO) and left anterior oblique (LAO) views. This is because the heart is oriented obliquely in the thoracic cavity. Since the major coronary arteries traverse the atrioventricular and interventricular grooves, which in turn are aligned with the long and short axes of the heart, it follows that the best angiographic projections to visualize these vessels in profile are the oblique views. In the following discussion, most of the anatomical descriptions will refer to the RAO or LAO projections.

The concept of RCA or LCA preponderance was proposed by Schlesinger in 1940.[17] The preponderant, or "dominant," vessel is the one which supplies the posterior diaphragmatic portion of the interventricular septum and the diaphragmatic surface of the left ventricle. The RCA is dominant in 77 to 90 per cent of humans.[18, 19] The use of the term "dominance" is somewhat misleading, because it suggests that in most patients, the RCA is the more important vessel. Since human CAD is primarily the result of interruption of blood supply to left ventricular myocardium, the nondominant LCA is almost always more important than the dominant RCA. With this understanding, the term "dominance" will nevertheless be used because it is a commonly accepted anatomical concept.

Figure 10–6 is a diagram of the coronary anatomy in a typical patient with RCA dominance. The anatomy is demonstrated in the standard LAO and RAO projections for both the right and left coronary systems. In addition, an LAO view of the left coronary system with cranial angulation is shown, since this is the most commonly used sagittal-angulation view.

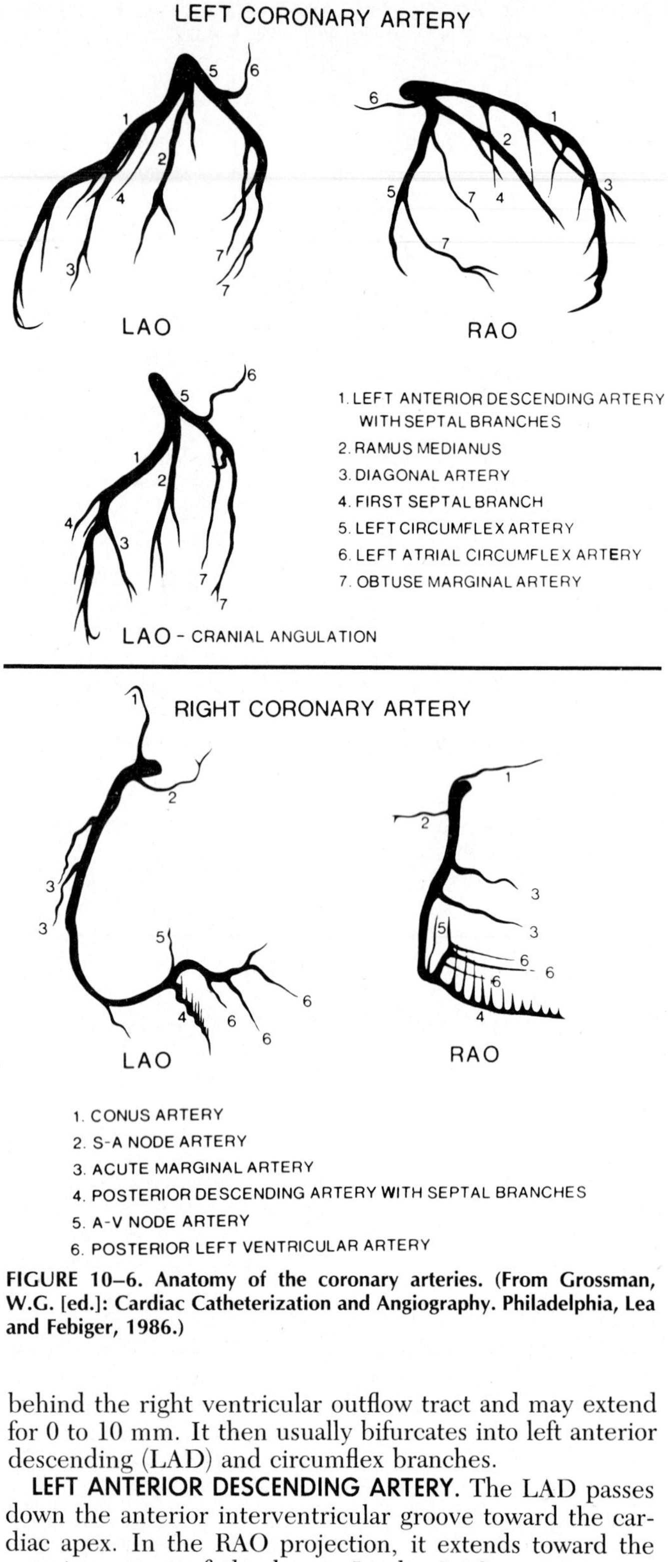

FIGURE 10–6. Anatomy of the coronary arteries. (From Grossman, W.G. [ed.]: Cardiac Catheterization and Angiography. Philadelphia, Lea and Febiger, 1986.)

LEFT CORONARY ARTERY
(Figs. 10–7*A* and *B*, 10–8*A*)

The main LCA arises from the upper portion of the left aortic sinus, just below the sinotubular ridge. It passes behind the right ventricular outflow tract and may extend for 0 to 10 mm. It then usually bifurcates into left anterior descending (LAD) and circumflex branches.

LEFT ANTERIOR DESCENDING ARTERY. The LAD passes down the anterior interventricular groove toward the cardiac apex. In the RAO projection, it extends toward the anterior aspect of the heart. In the LAO projection, it passes down the cardiac midline, between the right and left ventricles. Its major branches are the *septal* and *diagonal* branches.

The *septal* branches pass downward into the interventricular septum. They vary in size, number, and distribution. In some cases there is a large first septal branch which is vertically oriented and breaks up into a number of secondary branches which ramify throughout the septum. In other cases a more horizontally oriented large first septal branch is present, which passes parallel to and below the LAD itself. In still others there are a number of septal arteries, all of which are roughly comparable in size. These

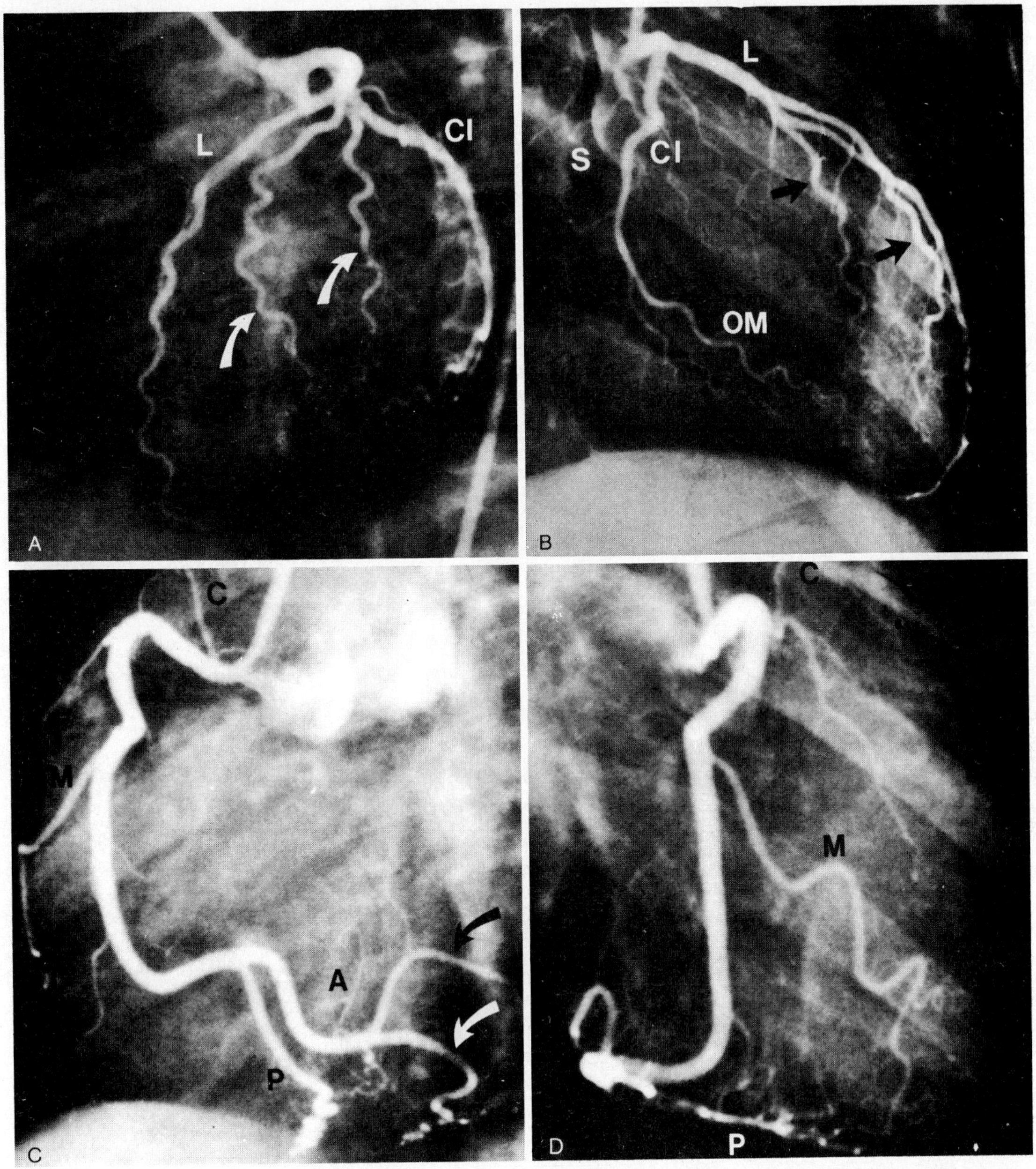

FIGURE 10–7. *A*, LCA in the LAO projection. *B*, LCA in the RAO projection. L = Left anterior descending artery (LAD); CI = Circumflex artery; OM = Obtuse marginal branch of the circumflex; S = Sinoatrial node artery; arrows point to two diagonal branches of the LAD. The small branches originating from the LAD and passing downward are the septal branches. *C*, RCA in the LAO projection. *D*, RCA in the right anterior oblique (RAO) projection. C = Conus branch; M = Acute marginal branch; P = Posterior descending artery; A = Atrioventricular node artery; arrows point to posterior left ventricular branches.

septal branches interconnect with similar septal branches passing upward from the posterior descending branch of the RCA to produce a network of potential collateral channels. The interventricular septum is the most densely vascularized area of the heart, and the first septal branch is its most important potential collateral channel.

The *diagonal* branches of the LAD pass over the anterolateral aspect of the heart, and it is usually one of these branches which supplies the apex itself. While virtually all patients have a single LAD in the anterior interventricular groove, there is wide variability in the number and size of diagonal branches. Over 90 per cent have one to three such branches.[20] Less than 1 per cent of patients have no diagonal branches at all. Thus, if none are seen, the angiographer should suspect the possibility that a diagonal branch might have originally been present but become totally occluded at its origin from the LAD. This is particularly true in cases in which there are unexplained contraction abnormalities of the anterior left ventricle.

In 37 per cent of patients, the LCA has a trifurcation instead of a bifurcation.[20] In these cases, a *ramus medianus* arises between the LAD and circumflex arteries—this vessel is analogous to a diagonal branch and generally supplies the free wall along the lateral aspect of the left ventricle.

In 78 per cent of patients, the LAD passes all the way around the apex and terminates along the diaphragmatic aspect of the left ventricle. However, in 22 per cent of patients, the LAD fails to reach the diaphragmatic surface, instead terminating either at or even before the cardiac apex.[21] In these cases, the posterior descending branch of the RCA is larger and longer than usual and supplies the apex. Correspondingly, since the LAD does not supply the cardiac apex in such cases, its distal segment is smaller

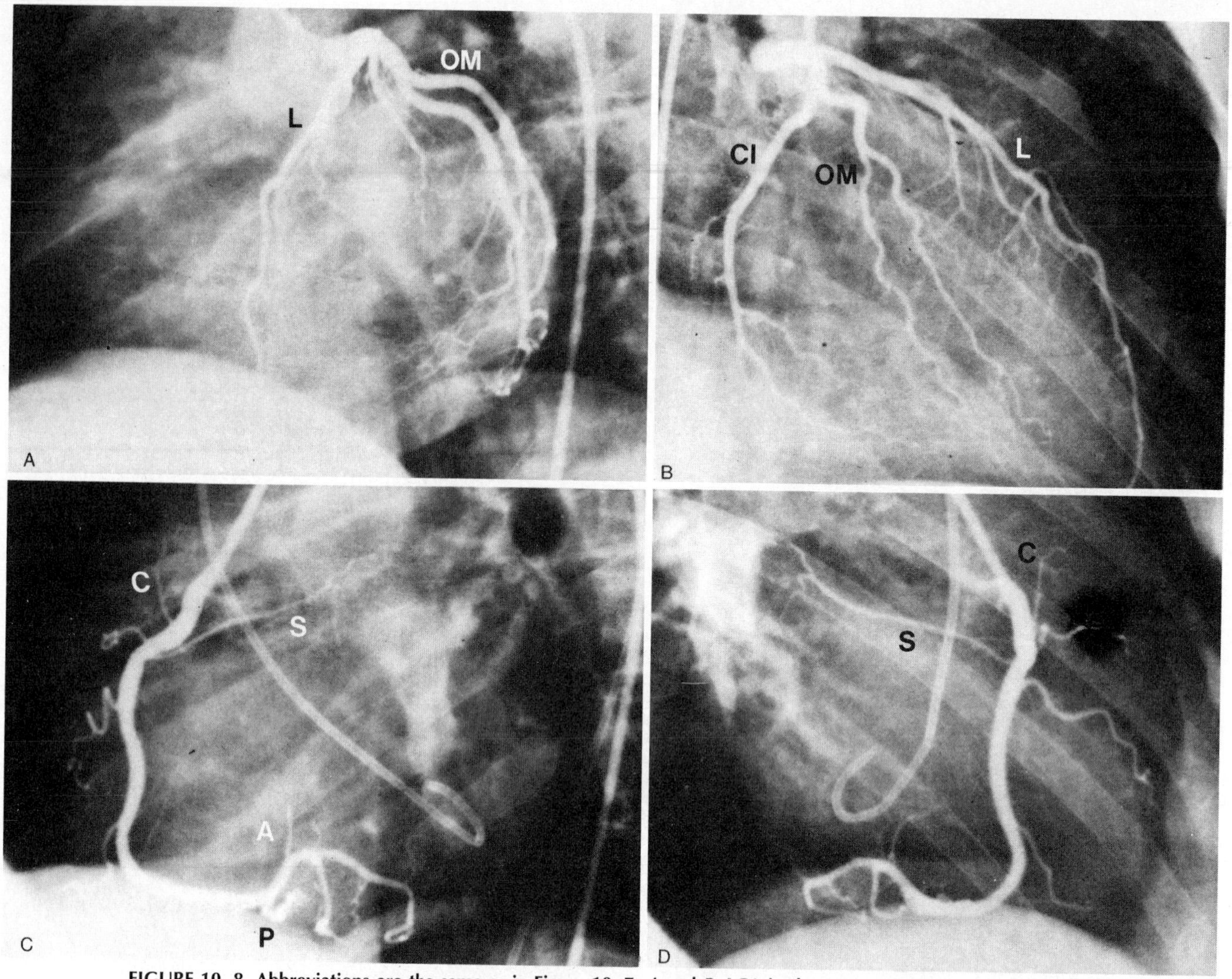

FIGURE 10–8. Abbreviations are the same as in Figure 10–7. *A* and *B*, LCA in the LAO and RAO projections. The LAD has only two small diagonal branches. This is compensated for by the presence of a large obtuse marginal branch which supplies the lateral wall of the left ventricle. *C* and *D*, RCA in the LAO and RAO projections. Both the conus and sinoatrial node branches arise from the RCA.

and shorter than usual. Early attentuation and a narrow distal caliber does not necessarily signify LAD disease if some or all of the cardiac apex is supplied by the posterior descending artery.

CIRCUMFLEX ARTERY. The left circumflex artery originates at the bifurcation (or trifurcation) of the main LCA and passes down the left atrioventricular groove. In 77 to 90 per cent of human hearts, the left circumflex artery is the nondominant vessel[18, 19] and varies in size and length, depending upon the actual degree of right coronary dominance. Generally, the left circumflex artery gives off one to three large *obtuse marginal branches* as it passes down the atrioventricular groove. These are the principal branches of the circumflex, since they supply the free wall of the left ventricle along its lateral aspect. Beyond the origins of these obtuse marginal branches, the distal left circumflex tends to be quite small. The actual position of the circumflex artery can best be determined on the late phase of a left coronary injection, when the coronary sinus becomes opacified with diluted contrast material. The position of the coronary sinus identifies the position of the left atrioventricular groove and the proper circumflex artery which runs in or near it. In the LAO projection, the obtuse marginal branches and the proper circumflex artery may be directly superimposed or nearly so. Therefore, it is best to try and localize lesions of these vessels on either frontal or RAO projections.

The circumflex artery may also give rise to one or two *left atrial circumflex branches*. These branches supply the lateral and posterior aspects of the left atrium.

RIGHT CORONARY ARTERY

(Fig. 10–7*C*, *D* and 8*C*, *D*)

The RCA originates from the right aortic sinus at a point somewhat lower than the origin of the LCA from the left aortic sinus. It passes down the right atrioventricular groove toward the crux (a point on the diaphragmatic surface of the heart where the right atrioventricular groove, the left atrioventricular groove, and the posterior interventricular groove come together).

The first branch of the RCA is generally considered to be the *conus artery*. In approximately 50 per cent of hearts, this vessel arises at the right coronary ostium or within the first few millimeters of the RCA. It passes upward and anteriorly over the right ventricular outflow tract toward the LAD. Its primary importance is to serve as a source of collateral circulation in patients with LAD occlusion. In the other 50 per cent, the conus artery is not actually a branch of the RCA, but instead arises from a small separate ostium in the right aortic sinus just above the right coronary ostium.[19] In this group of patients, selective right coronary arteriography may fail to opacify the conus artery unless sufficient reflux of contrast medium occurs to fill the separate ostium. In a series from the authors' laboratory, it was found that opacification of the right coronary artery failed to visualize adequately the conus artery in 20 per cent of cases.[22] Presumably this group came from the half of the population in which the conus artery has a separate origin.

The second branch of the RCA is usually the *sinoatrial node artery*. Kyriakidis et al.[23] found that this vessel originated from the RCA in 59 per cent, from the left circumflex in 38 per cent, and had a dual supply in the remaining 3 per cent. When it originates from the RCA, it passes obliquely backward through the upper portion of the atrial septum and the anteromedial wall of the right atrium. It sends branches to the sinus node and usually to the right atrium or both atria as well. When it originates from the left circumflex artery, it may pass backward in the atrial septum or around the posterolateral wall of the left atrium to reach the sinus node area.

The midportion of the RCA generally gives rise to one or several medium-sized *right ventricular* (or acute marginal) *branches*. These branches supply the anterior wall of the right ventricle and are relatively unimportant, except insofar as they also may serve as sources of collateral circulation in patients with LAD occlusion.

The next important branch of the RCA is the *posterior descending* (PD) *artery*. As indicated earlier, 77 to 90 per cent of patients have a dominant RCA. The dominant artery is considered to be that vessel (either the RCA or circumflex artery) which supplies the diaphragmatic aspect of the left ventricle and the lower portion of the interventricular septum. When the RCA is dominant, the PD originates at or shortly before the crux and passes forward in the posterior interventricular groove. During its course along this groove, it gives rise to a number of small *inferior septal branches* which pass upward to supply the lower portion of the interventricular septum and interdigitate with superior septal branches passing down from the LAD. After giving rise to the PD, a dominant RCA continues beyond the crux and begins to pass upward along the distal portion of the left atrioventricular groove. Here it usually terminates by giving rise to one or several *posterior left ventricular (PLV) branches* which supply the diaphragmatic surface of the left ventricle.

A minority of patients (10 to 23 per cent) do not have RCA dominance. About half of these have LCA dominance. With this anatomical pattern, the left circumflex artery is large and continues down to the diaphragmatic surface of the left ventricle, where it gives rise to the PLV branches and then reaches the crux and turns forward to become the PD. In these cases the RCA is very small, terminates before reaching the crux, and therefore does not supply any blood to left ventricular myocardium. The other half have a mixed or "balanced" circulation, wherein the RCA gives rise to the PD, while the left circumflex artery gives rise to the PLV branches. At or near the crux, the dominant artery gives rise to a small *atrioventricular node artery*, which passes upward to supply this node.

In approximately one-fourth of patients with right coronary dominance, there are significant anatomical variations in the origin of the PD artery.[24] These variations include partial supply of the PD territory by right ventricular branches, double PD, and early origin of the PD proximal to the crux.

ARTERIOGRAPHIC EXAMPLES

Figures 10–7 and 10–8 are examples of two different patients with dominant RCAs. The patient whose arteriogram is shown in Figure 10–7 has two diagonal branches of the LAD, one of which closely parallels the LAD itself in the RAO projection. In this projection it is still possible to differentiate the two, because the LAD is the longer of the two vessels, passes all the way around the cardiac apex, and gives rise to septal branches. This patient's sinoatrial node artery arises from the left circumflex artery. In the patient whose arteriogram is shown in Figure 10–8, both the conus and sinoatrial node arteries arise from the RCA. There are two diagonal branches of the LAD but both are quite small. Instead, a large obtuse marginal branch of the left circumflex artery supplies most of the lateral wall of the left ventricle. Minor variations such as those illustrated by these examples are seen in virtually every patient.

Figure 10–9 is an example of an arteriogram in a patient with a dominant left coronary system. Note that the PD and PLV branches all arise from the left circumflex artery. In patients with this type of anatomy, the RCA usually

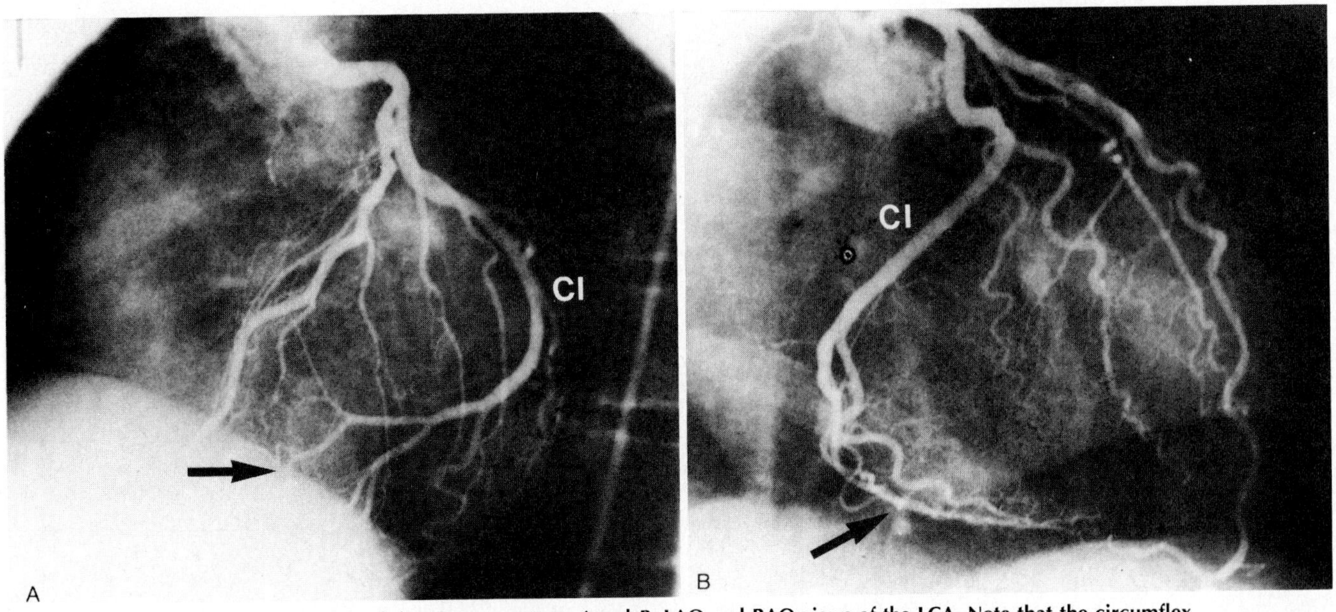

FIGURE 10–9. Dominant left coronary system. *A* and *B*, LAO and RAO views of the LCA. Note that the circumflex artery is large and extends all the way down to the crux of the heart where it turns forward to become the posterior descending artery (arrow). Proximal to this point, it gives rise to two large posterior left ventricular branches.

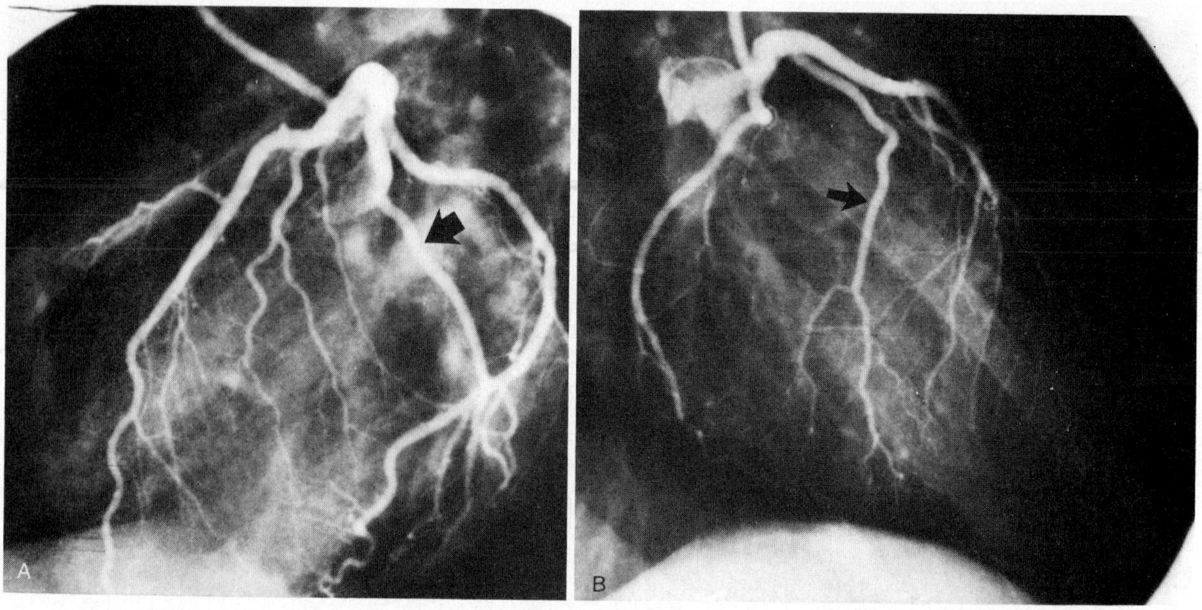

FIGURE 10–10. Left coronary arteriogram in a patient with a dominant left coronary system and a ramus medianus. *A* and *B*, LAO and RAO views. The LCA has a trifurcation instead of the usual bifurcation. Arrows mark the large ramus medianus arising between the LAD and circumflex arteries. (From Levin, D.C., Harrington, D.P., Bettmann, M.A., Garnic, J.D., Davidoff, A., and Lois, J.: Anatomic variations of the coronary arteries supplying the anterolateral aspect of the left ventricle. Possible explanation for the "unexplained" anterior aneurysm. Invest. Radiol. *17*:458, 1982.)

terminates before ever reaching the crux. Figure 10–10 shows an example of a ramus medianus in a patient with a dominant left coronary system.

Figure 10–11 illustrates the coronary arteriogram of a patient with a short LAD that terminates before reaching the cardiac apex. Instead, the apex is supplied by the PD branch of the RCA. Figure 10–12*A*, *B* is an example of extremely strong dominance of the RCA. In this patient the distal RCA passes almost all the way up the left atrioventricular groove and supplies most of the obtuse marginal branches. The left circumflex system consists only of a single high obtuse marginal branch.

Figure 10–12*C–E* shows three different variations in origin of the PD artery. Figure 10–12*C* is an instance of early origin of the PD, which then closely parallels the distal RCA itself prior to turning forward in the posterior interventricular groove. Figure 10–12*D* is an example of origin of the PD from a right ventricular branch of the RCA. Figure 10–12*E* is an example of double PD artery in a patient with multiple obstructive lesions in the RCA system.

ANGULATED VIEWS OF THE CORONARY ARTERIES

In the mid 1970's, several groups of investigators called attention to the fact that the routine RAO and LAO projections of the coronary arteries had serious shortcomings.[25–28] Foreshortening and superimposition of branches

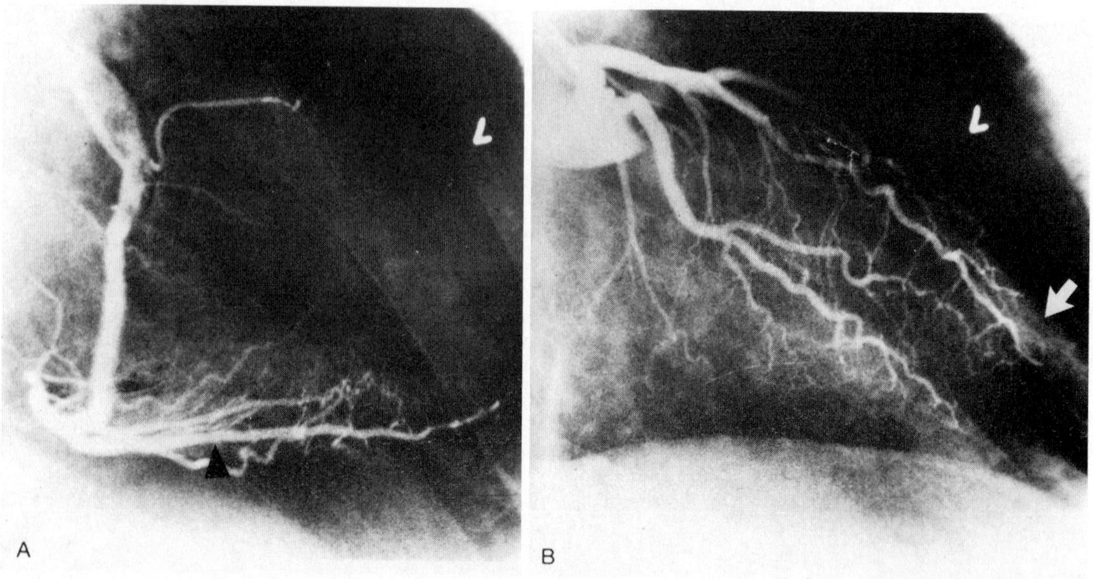

FIGURE 10–11. Short LAD. *A*, RAO right coronary arteriogram shows that the posterior descending branch (arrowhead) is longer than usual and supplies the apex. *B*, RAO left coronary arteriogram shows that the LAD terminates (arrow) before reaching the cardiac apex.

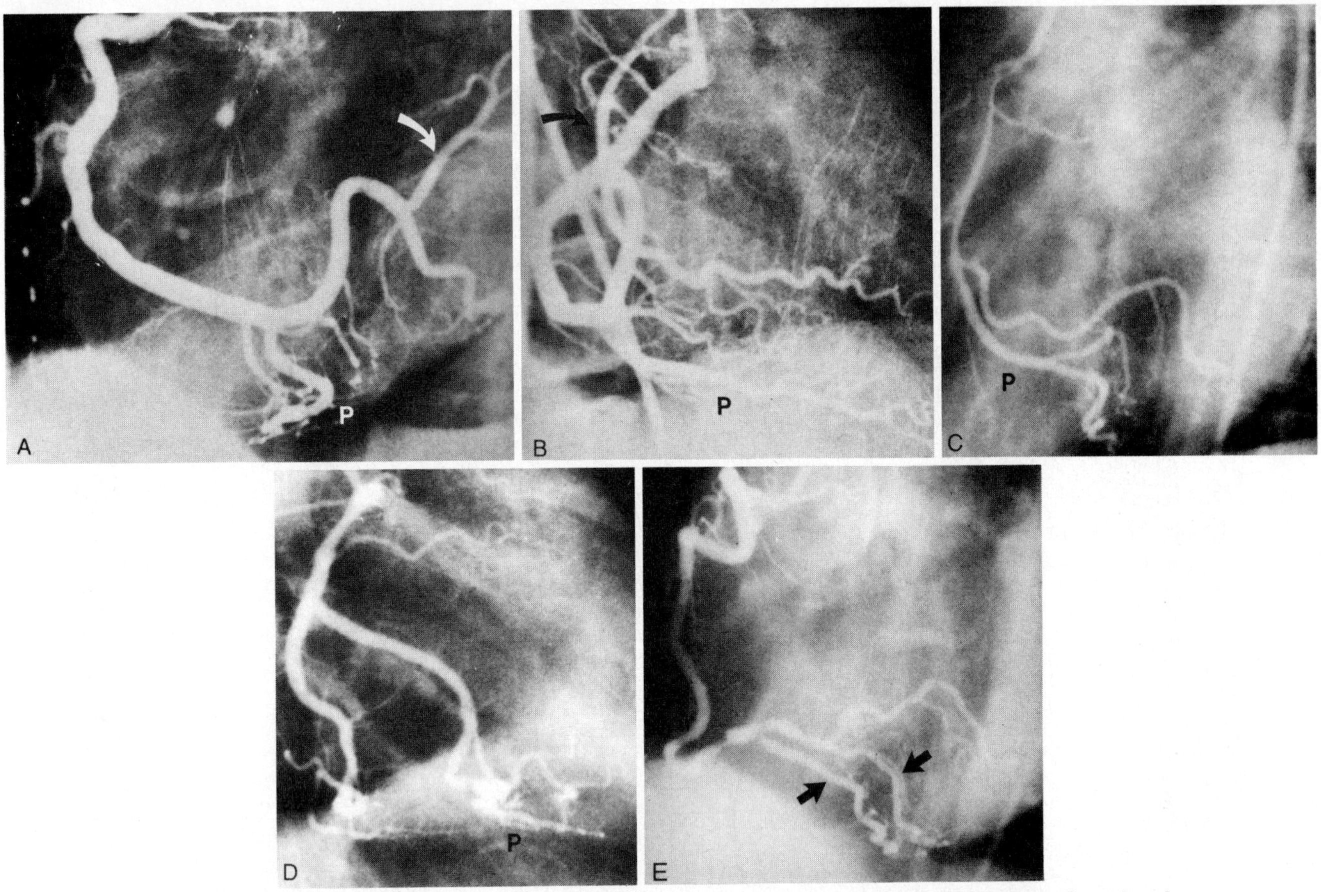

FIGURE 10–12. Unusually strong dominance of the RCA. *A* and *B*, LAO and RAO views of the RCA show that the distal segment of this vessel (arrows) extends all the way up the left atrioventricular groove. After giving rise to the posterior descending artery (P), it gives rise to multiple posterior left ventricular and obtuse marginal branches. *C*, Variations in origin of the posterior descending artery. LAO view of a dominant RCA. The posterior descending artery (P) originates early, then parallels the distal RCA before turning forward in the posterior interventricular groove. (From Levin, D.C., and Baltaxe, H.A.: Angiographic demonstration of important anatomic variations of the posterior descending coronary artery. A.J.R. *116*:41, 1972.) *D*, RAO right coronary arteriogram showing the posterior descending artery (P) arising from a right ventricular branch of the RCA. *E*, LAO right coronary arteriogram showing duplicated posterior descending arteries (arrows). (From Levin, D.C., and Baltaxe, H.A.: Angiographic demonstration of important anatomic variations of the posterior descending coronary artery. A. J. R. *116*:41, 1972.)

occurred in these projections, which frequently resulted in failure to detect significant lesions. In addition to rotation of the x-ray beam about the patient in the transverse plane, these investigators proposed rotation of the beam in the sagittal plane. Their studies revealed that lesions often missed on the standard LAO and RAO projections could be detected when a combination of both sagittal and transverse angulation of the x-ray beam was utilized. Sagittal angulation is most useful in evaluation of the left coronary system but can also aid in right coronary arteriography.[29]

The terminology originally employed to describe these views was somewhat confusing, in that a variety of different terms was used by different authors. A simple designation of these views has been proposed by Paulin,[30] as shown in Figure 10–14. In most modern cardiac catheterization laboratories, the x-ray tube is under the patient table and the image intensifier with its coupled video and cine cameras are over the patient table. If this over-table image intensifier is tilted up toward the head of the patient, this is referred to as the "cranial" view. The resulting images appear as if the angiographer were looking down at the heart from the patient's head. Conversely, if the image intensifier is tilted down toward the feet of the patient, this is referred to as the "caudal" view and provides images as if the angiographer were looking up at the heart from the patient's feet. Cranial and caudal angulation have now become a standard part of coronary arteriography and are routinely used in most laboratories having the necessary U or C arm mounting units for their cine systems.

Figure 10–13 shows a series of radiographs of a paraffin-imbedded human heart specimen in which the coronary arteries are filled with a barium mixture. They graphically demonstrate the advantages of the cranial and caudal views. In Figure 10–13*A*, the heart was filmed in a standard LAO projection. The left main coronary artery cannot be seen well because of overlap by the LAD. Also, the proximal portions of the LAD, its large diagonal branch, and the left circumflex artery are not visualized well. In Figure 10–13*B*, the same degree of LAO rotation is used, but cranial angulation has now been added; this view clearly demonstrates the main LCA and its bifurcation, the proximal portion of the LAD, and the origin of its large diagonal branch. Figure 10–13*C* is an LAO caudal view which also demonstrates the main LCA and proximal LAD well and is the best view for demonstrating the proximal portion of the left circumflex artery, which is often obscured in other views.

Figures 10–13*D–F* are three RAO views of the same specimen. Figure 10–13*D* shows a standard RAO projection, in which there is considerable overlap of the LAD and its diagonal branch. There is also foreshortening of the entire proximal portion of the left circumflex artery. The cranial angulation in Figure 10–13*D* displaces the LAD

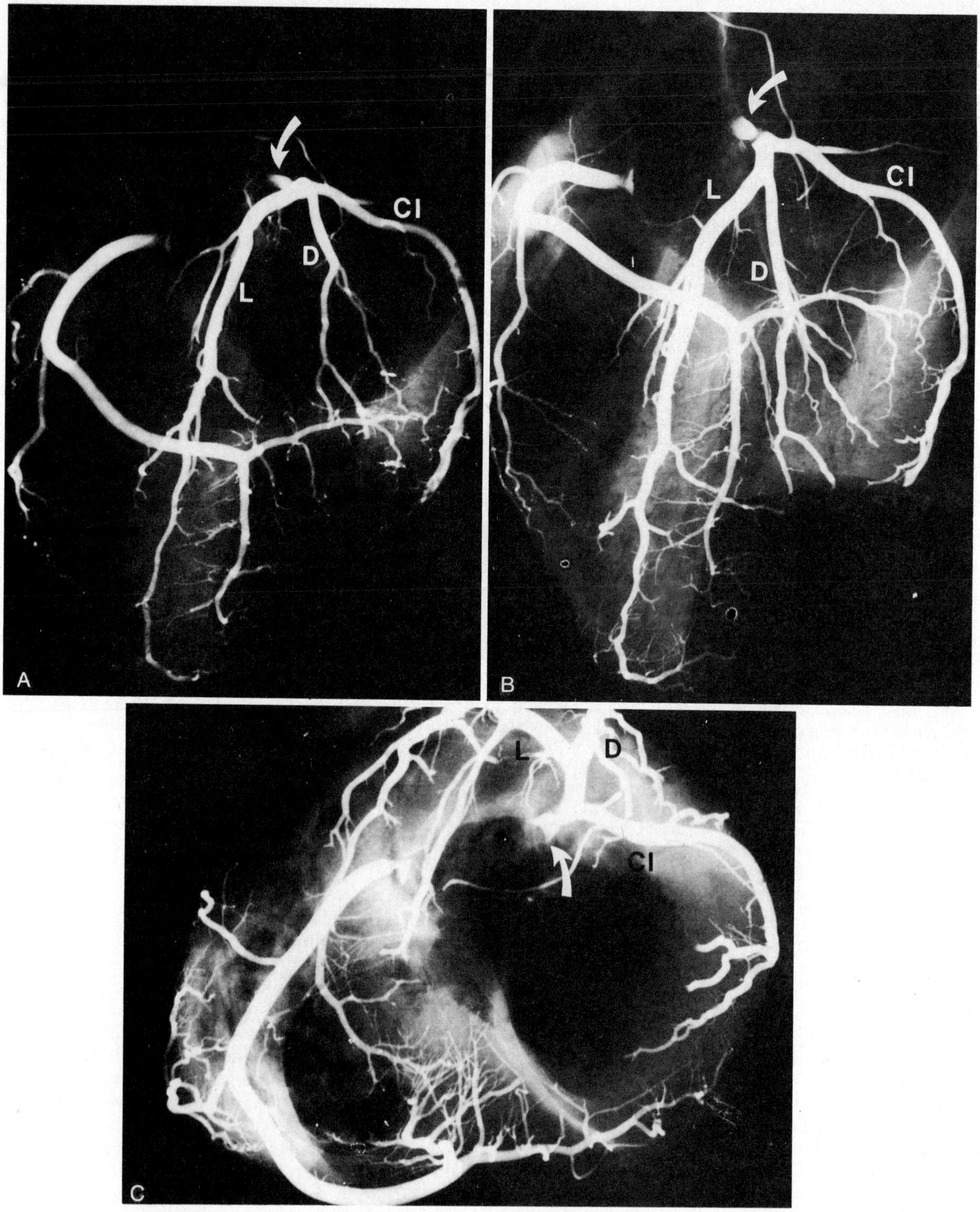

Figure 10–13. *See legend on opposite page*

downward and the first diagonal branch upward, so that these two vessels are no longer superimposed. The LAD can be seen along its entire length without any overlap. Figure 10–13*F* is an RAO caudal view which displaces the LAD upward and the diagonal branch downward, thereby providing another unobstructed view of both vessels. The origin of the diagonal branch is better demonstated in this view than in the RAO cranial view. The RAO caudal view is also particularly helpful in demonstrating the entire length of the left circumflex artery, which is foreshortened in both the standard and cranial RAO projections.

Figure 10–15*A* is a clinical example of a standard RAO projection of a left coronary arteriogram, in which there is marked overlap of the LAD with its diagonal branches and the proximal left circumflex artery. Figure 10–15*B* is an RAO cranial view in the same case in which the overlap has been completely alleviated. The LAD can be seen along its entire length without superimposition of the other branches, and the latter are themselves well visualized. Figure 10–16 is an arteriogram in which a severe proximal LAD stenosis is clearly visualized in the standard RAO projections. A second more distal LAD lesion was visual-

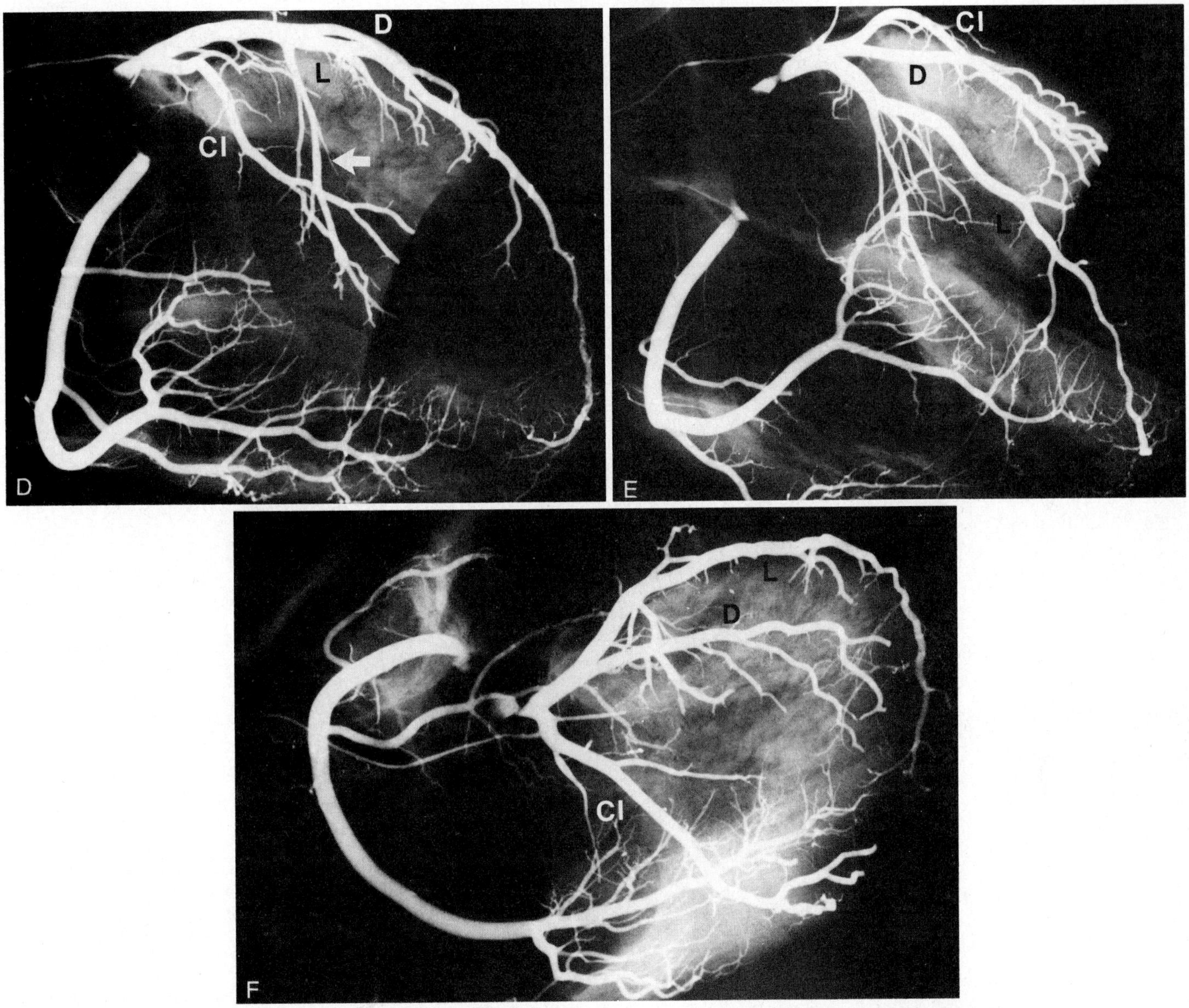

FIGURE 10–13. Views of an injected heart specimen in which a constricting ligature was placed around the main LCA to simulate an obstructing lesion. *A*, Standard LAO view. The main LCA (arrow) is not well seen. The proximal portions of both the LAD (L) and its diagonal branch (D) are not well seen because of foreshortening. The origin of the circumflex artery (CI) is obscured by the diagonal branch. *B*, LAO cranial view. The LCA is seen clearly and the bandlike narrowing created by the ligature can now be visualized. The proximal portions of the LAD and its diagonal branch are well seen. *C*, LAO caudal view. The main LCA is again well visualized, as is the origin of the LAD. This view is especially good for visualizing the origin of the circumflex artery. *D*, Standard RAO view. The LAD and its diagonal branch are almost completely superimposed. The circumflex artery is foreshortened. The arrow points to the first septal branch. *E*, RAO cranial view. The LAD is thrown downward and can now be seen along its entire length without superimposition. The diagonal and circumflex branches are thrown upward. *F*, RAO caudal view. The LAD is now thrown upward and its diagonal branch is thrown downward. Both vessels are well seen without superimposition. The circumflex artery is elongated in this view and is seen well along its entire length. (From Abrams, H.L. [ed.]: Coronary Arteriography. A Practical Approach. Boston, Little Brown, 1983, with permission.)

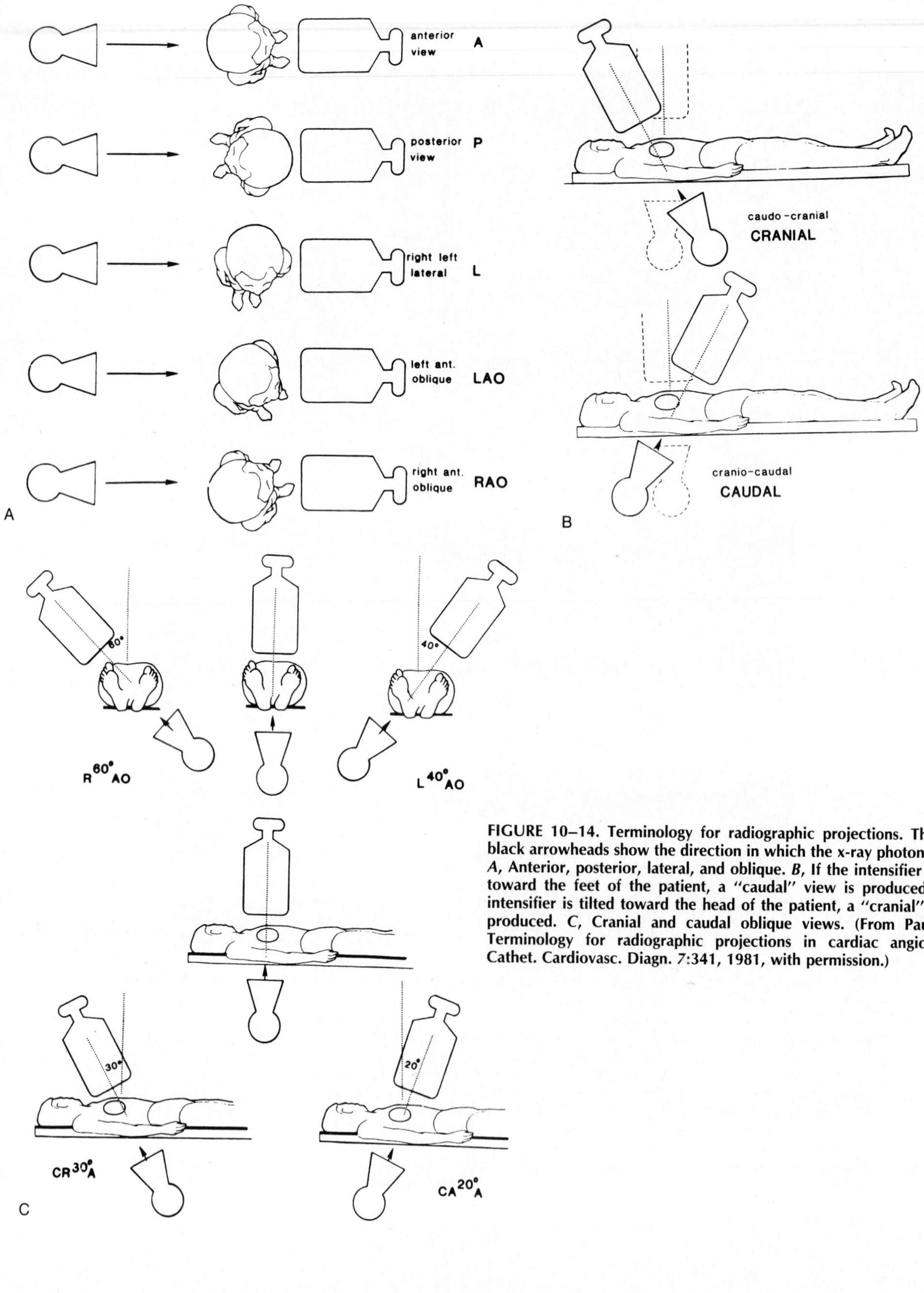

FIGURE 10–14. Terminology for radiographic projections. The small black arrowheads show the direction in which the x-ray photons travel. *A*, Anterior, posterior, lateral, and oblique. *B*, If the intensifier is tilted toward the feet of the patient, a "caudal" view is produced. If the intensifier is tilted toward the head of the patient, a "cranial" view is produced. *C*, Cranial and caudal oblique views. (From Paulin, S.: Terminology for radiographic projections in cardiac angiography. Cathet. Cardiovasc. Diagn. *7*:341, 1981, with permission.)

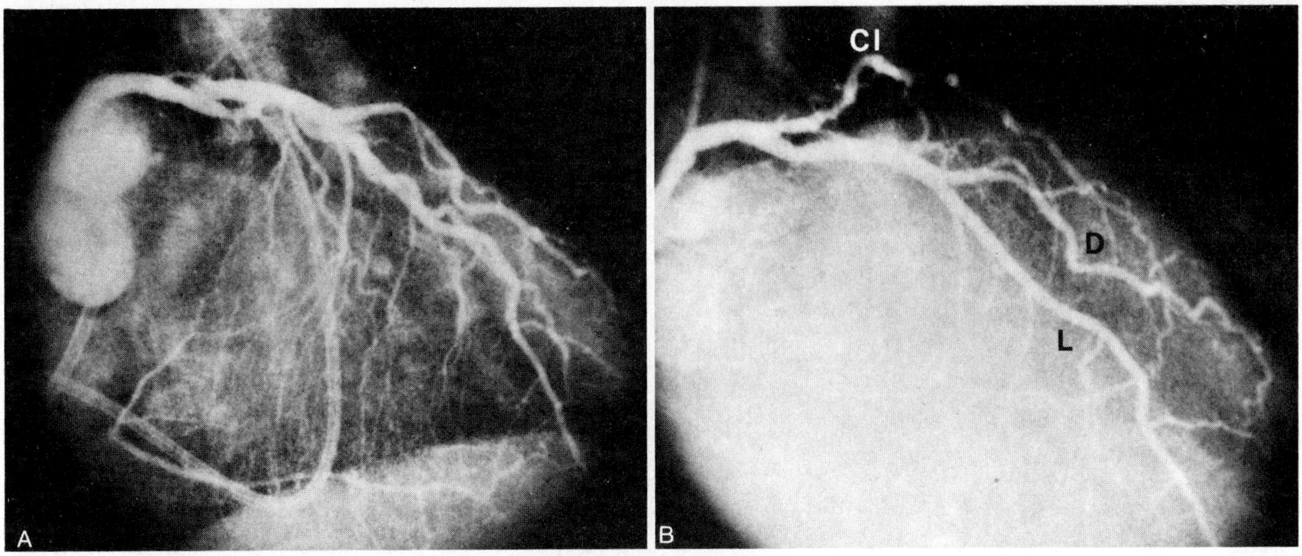

FIGURE 10–15. *A*, Standard RAO left coronary arteriogram, showing extensive superimposition of the circumflex and diagonal arteries upon the LAD. *B*, RAO cranial view throws the circumflex (CI) and diagonal (D) arteries upward and the LAD (L) downward. The LAD is now seen well along its entire length without superimposition.

ized only on the RAO cranial view, and not on the RAO caudal or LAO cranial projections.

It is difficult to predict which angulated views will be most useful in any given patient. This depends largely upon body habitus, variations in coronary anatomy, and location of lesions. The authors routinely employ cranial and caudal angulation views in both the LAO and RAO projections of the left coronary system. They employ them on occasion during examination of the right coronary system, though much less frequently.

PITFALLS OF CORONARY ARTERIOGRAPHY

MAIN LEFT CORONARY ARTERY STENOSIS. Stenosis of the main LCA is the most serious of all coronary lesions, and is generally considered an indication for immediate bypass surgery (Chap. 51). The likelihood of angiographic complications is also increased with this condition, because the tip of the catheter may dissect the plaque upon entry into the left coronary ostium or may totally occlude the already narrowed orifice. At times, ostial stenosis of the LCA may be unrecognized, particularly if careful attention is not paid to catheter and filming technique. On the standard LAO and RAO views, the LCA may be inadequately visualized because of superimposition by the LAD and circumflex branches. The LCA is best visualized on a direct frontal projection or by use of the sagittal-angulation views. LCA stenosis can also escape detection if the catheter tip passes across it, so that the injected contrast material passes entirely in the antegrade direction and fails to opacify the narrowed orifice. In still other cases, a forceful injection can result in filling of the LCA to such a degree that an eccentric plaque is obscured by overlying contrast material, at least in some cine frames.

Figure 10–17 is an angiogram of a patient with ostial stenosis of the LCA. Figure 10–17*A* shows a cine frame in which an intraluminal filling defect caused by an eccentric plaque is clearly visible adjacent to the catheter tip. Figure 10–17*B* is another frame from the same run in which rapidly injected contrast material obscures this lesion.

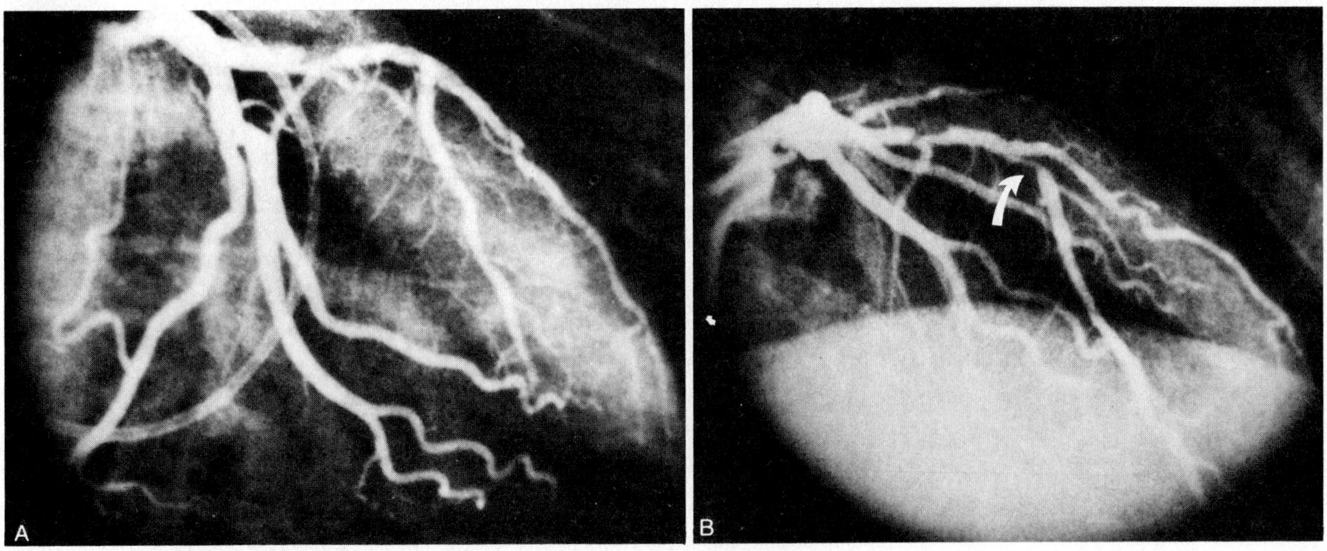

FIGURE 10–16. Left coronary arteriogram in a patient with a clearly visible proximal LAD stenosis. A second lesion is present 2 cm further distally but cannot be seen in most views. *A*, Standard RAO projection. *B*, RAO cranial view. The latter was the only one of many views to show the second LAD lesion (arrow).

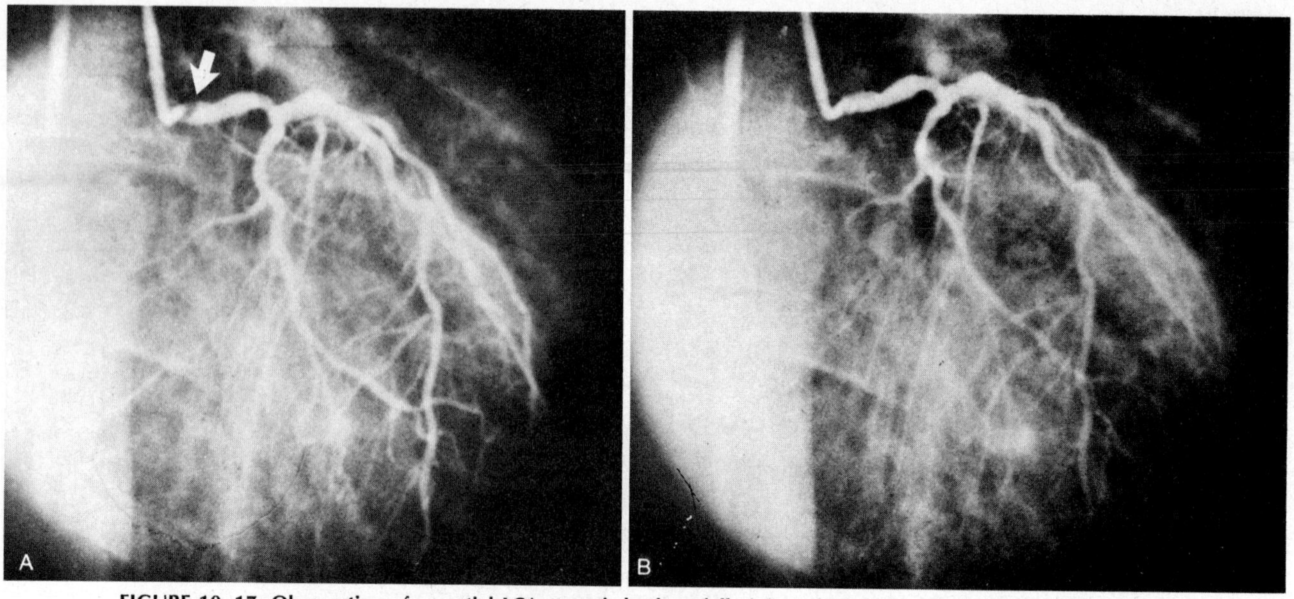

FIGURE 10–17. Obscuration of an ostial LCA stenosis by forcefully injected contrast material. *A*, A filling defect caused by the ostial stenosis is clearly seen adjacent to the catheter tip (arrow). *B*, On another cine frame from the same injection, contrast material obscures the lesion.

These two images taken less than 1 second apart illustrate how a life-threatening lesion could be overlooked purely as a result of angiographic technique. Figure 10–18*A* is a cine frame from a left coronary injection in another patient, which also shows an apparent intraluminal filling defect adjacent to the catheter tip in the LCA. However, multiple other frames from the same cine run and from views in other projections (Fig. 10–18*B*) showed that there was in fact no LCA lesion present. The apparent filling defect seen in Figure 10–18*A* was an artifact of injection, which was caused by streaming of contrast material and mixing with inflow of unopacified blood through the left coronary ostium.

In most cases, a forceful injection of contrast into the LCA produces sufficient reflux back through the left coronary ostium to provide satisfactory visualization of the proximal portion of the LCA. If no reflux occurs, and the ostium is therefore not seen, this may signify a stenotic lesion. Another clue to the presence of main LCA stenosis is the demonstration of damping or ventricularization of catheter tip pressure when the catheter passes from the aorta into the left coronary ostium. Under either of these circumstances, the catheter should be withdrawn into a nonselective position in the left aortic sinus. Contrast injections with the catheter in this position may satisfactorily demonstrate ostial or proximal LCA stenosis.

EARLY BIFURCATION OF THE LEFT CORONARY ARTERY. In 1 to 2 per cent of human hearts, the LCA is either absent or bifurcates immediately beyond the ostium.[19, 31] If the LCA is completely absent, there are instead two separate ostia in the left aortic sinus, one for the LAD and the other just below it for the left circumflex artery (Fig. 10–19). Alternatively, there may be a single ostium with immediate bifurcation into LAD and circumflex branches. In either case, catheterization of what is thought to be the LCA will invariably result in passage of the catheter tip

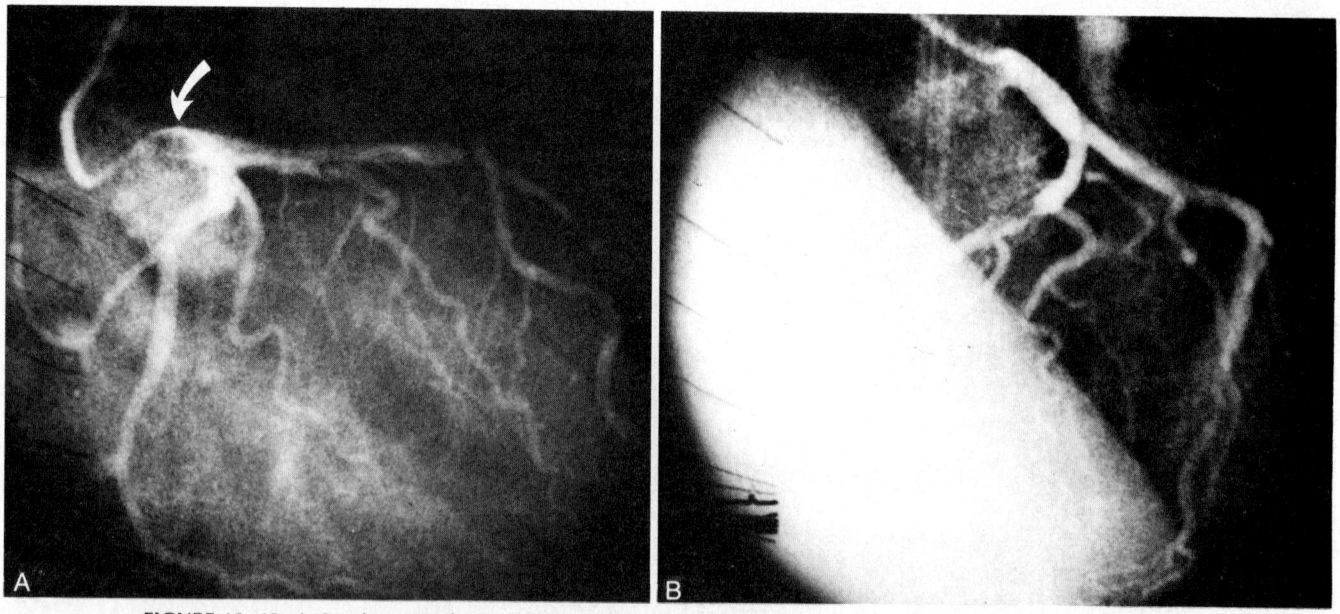

FIGURE 10–18. *A*, Spurious LCA lesion. Apparent filling defect in the LCA seen on this cine frame (arrow). Other frames from the same injection failed to show this defect, which probably was caused by streaming of contrast material. *B*, Other views of the LCA, such as this LAO cranial view, failed to confirm the presence of main LCA stenosis.

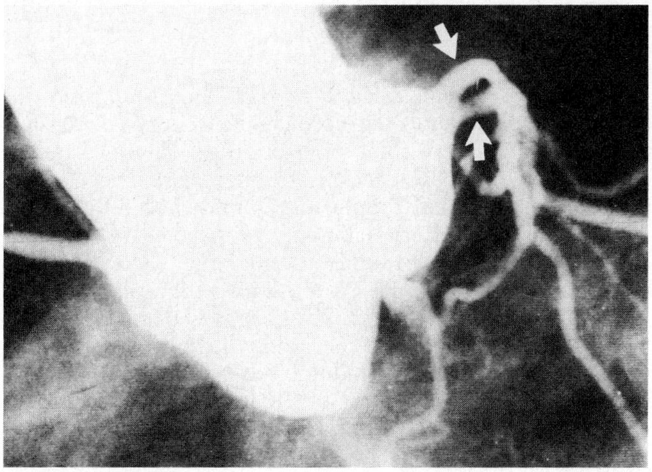

FIGURE 10–19. Aortic root angiogram, LAO projection. The LCA is absent. Instead, there are two adjacent ostia for the LAD and circumflex arteries (arrows) in the left aortic sinus. (Courtesy of Sven Paulin, M.D.)

into either the LAD or circumflex branch. Subsequent contrast injection may demonstrate only that branch, thereby creating the erroneous impression that the other branch is totally occluded. In some cases, there may be enough reflux of contrast material back into the left aortic sinus to opacify partially the other vessel. Whenever separate origin of the LAD and circumflex arteries is suspected, the catheter should be withdrawn to a nonselective position in the left aortic sinus and the arteriogram repeated, using forceful contrast injections. Often this will result in some degree of visualization of the second vessel.

CATHETER-INDUCED SPASM. Insertion of a catheter into the RCA can trigger pronounced spasm adjacent to the catheter tip. For reasons which are not entirely clear, this phenomenon is much less common in the LCA. Whenever right coronary arteriography reveals narrowing of the proximal portion of the RCA, the angiographer must rule out the possibility of catheter-induced spasm. The catheter should be removed, nitroglycerin should be administered sublingually or intravenously, and arteriography repeated shortly thereafter. Nitroglycerin reduces vasomotor tone in large coronary arteries[32, 33] and in most cases should be given prophylactically to prevent spasm from occurring during selective arteriography. However, the duration of action of this drug is relatively short (20 to 30 minutes) and it may have a variable effect in different patients. Thus, even if it is given prophylactically at the start of the procedure, by the time right coronary arteriography is performed its effect may have largely abated. Figure 10–20 is an example of catheter-induced spasm of the proximal RCA, relieved by sublingual nitroglycerin. Because of the rarity of this occurrence in the main LCA, angiographically demonstrated narrowing of this vessel is much more likely to represent organic disease than catheter-induced spasm.

FLOW ARTIFACTS DURING ARTERIOGRAPHY. It has been generally assumed that the pattern of flow of contrast material during arteriography accurately portrays blood flow under normal physiological circumstances. The assumption was that as long as the caliber of a catheter tip is somewhat smaller than the caliber of the artery into which it has been inserted, the force of the contrast injection would be dissipated out into the aorta. Therefore the injection itself would not alter flow and pressure in the catheterized vessel. Experimental studies have shown, however, that this assumption is incorrect. Injection of contrast material or other fluids through standard, nonoccluding catheters positioned selectively will significantly raise both flow and pressure in the vessel for the duration of the injection.[34] In effect, contrast is forced through the arterial tree, and artifactual flow patterns or accentuated filling of branch vessels and collateral circulation may result. The degree to which this occurs is largely related to the force of the injection itself, and to the relative sizes of the catheter tip and the artery into which it has been inserted. The smaller the size of the artery relative to that of the catheter tip, the greater the rise in flow and pressure during contrast injection. Thus, in a given patient, the speed and direction of flow seen on arteriography, the degree of opacification of distal branches, and the degree of filling of collateral vessels may not accurately reflect blood flow that occurs under physiological conditions.

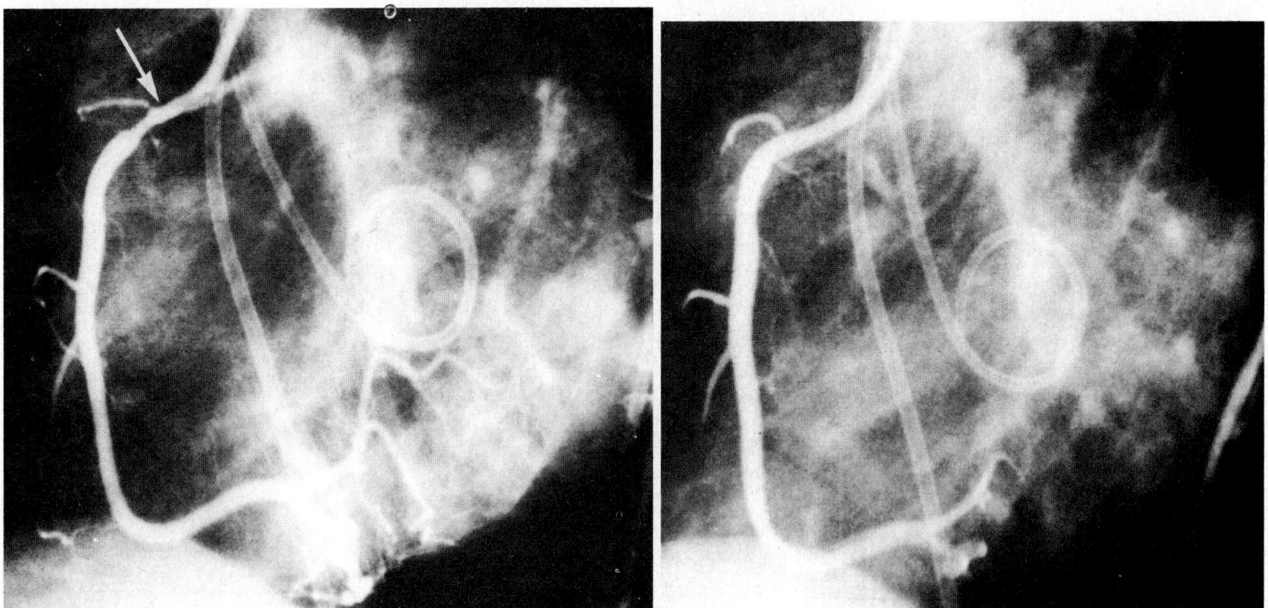

FIGURE 10–20. Catheter-induced spasm of the proximal RCA. *A*, LAO right coronary arteriogram showing apparent stenosis at the origin of the RCA (arrow). *B*, Repeat arteriogram several minutes after nitroglycerin administration. The proximal RCA is normal. (From Levin, D.C., Baltaxe, H.A., Lee, J.G., and Sos, T.A.: Potential sources of error in coronary arteriography. I. In performance of the study. A. J. R. 124:378, 1975.)

ECCENTRIC STENOSES. Eccentric or slit-like atherosclerotic narrowings of the coronary arteries are more common than circumferential lesions producing a central lumen.[31, 35] If, in such cases, the x-ray beam passes through the lesion perpendicular to the long axis of the lumen, the vessel may actually appear to have a normal or near-normal caliber. Only if the beam passes parallel to the long axis of the stenotic lumen will the narrowing be visible. In Figure 10–21*A*, a right coronary arteriogram in the LAO projection shows only a very minor narrowing of the proximal RCA. However, when this region is viewed in the RAO projection (Figure 10–21*B*), the lesion is seen to be considerably more severe. This is the result of the eccentric position of the atherosclerotic plaque within the coronary artery. For this reason, *coronary arteries must be viewed in at least two projections 90 degrees apart.*

A related problem is that of the bandlike or membranous stenosis. Lesions such as this may be exceedingly difficult to detect. The authors have seen cases in which such lesions could be seen on only one single view of a left coronary arteriogram, while multiple other views of the same vessel failed to demonstrate it (Bunnell, I., personal communication). It is not clear whether these peculiar lesions represent pure atherosclerotic stenosis or are caused in some instances by congenital membranous bands.[36] Aside from the difficulty in detecting these lesions, it is also difficult to ascertain their hemodynamic significance. Measurement of the pressure gradient across the lesion through a polyethylene catheter inserted through the angiographic catheter may be useful in this regard.

UNRECOGNIZED OCCLUSIONS. Occlusions of major coronary arteries often occur at branch points. Because of this, and the fact that there are anatomical variations in the number and distribution of branches, it is possible for occlusions at branch origins to go undetected. In some cases, occlusion of a branch can be recognized only by late filling of the distal segment of this branch via collateral circulation (Fig. 10–22).

SUPERIMPOSITION OF BRANCHES. Superimposition of major branches of the left coronary tree in the LAO and RAO projections can sometimes result in failure to detect stenoses or total obstructions of these branches.[37] This problem is particularly applicable to branches of the LAD. As indicated earlier, the anatomy of diagonal branches of the LAD is variable. In some cases, a large diagonal branch is present which closely parallels the LAD in both the LAO and RAO projections. If either this diagonal branch or the LAD itself is totally occluded at their branch point, the obstruction could go undetected. An illustration of this type of anatomy is shown in Figure 10–23. Because of overlapping of the LAD and diagonal branches in RAO projections, stenoses may be obscured. This problem can often be alleviated by the use of cranial or caudal angulation (p. 277). Septal branches can sometimes mimic the LAD in the LAO projection. In this projection, the LAD and septal branches occupy the same plane. When the LAD is totally occluded beyond the origin of the first septal branch, this branch often becomes quite enlarged, in an attempt to provide collateral circulation to the vascular bed of the distal LAD. In the case shown in Figure 10–24, the LAD is completely obstructed just beyond the origin of the first septal branch. The latter has become considerably enlarged and could be confused with the LAD itself on the LAO projection.

MYOCARDIAL BRIDGING. The major coronary arteries pass over the epicardial surface of the heart. In some cases, however, short segments descend into the myocardium for a variable distance. This occurs in 5 to 12 per cent of humans and is almost exclusively confined to the LAD.[38, 39] Because a "bridge" of myocardial fibers passes over the involved segment of the LAD, each systolic contraction of these fibers can cause narrowing of the artery. Myocardial bridging has a characteristic appearance on cineangiogra

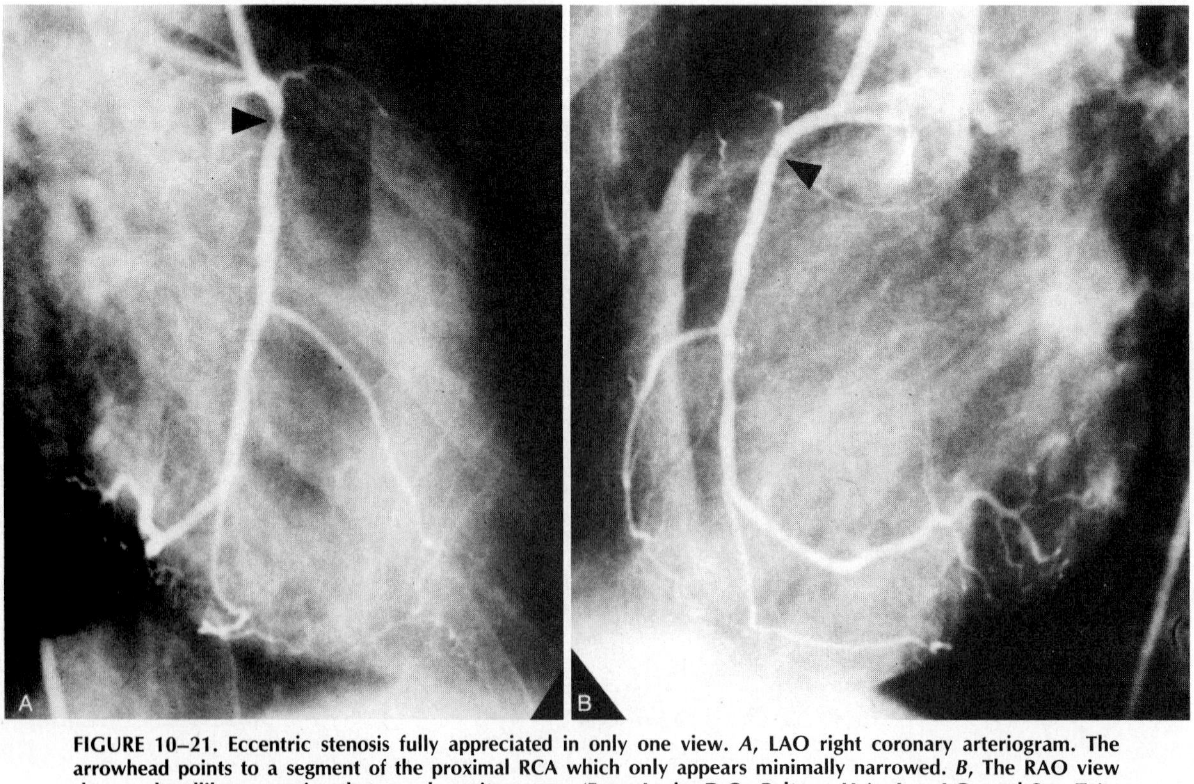

FIGURE 10–21. Eccentric stenosis fully appreciated in only one view. *A*, LAO right coronary arteriogram. The arrowhead points to a segment of the proximal RCA which only appears minimally narrowed. *B*, The RAO view shows a bandlike narrowing that may be quite severe. (From Levin, D.C., Baltaxe, H.A., Lee, J.G., and Sos, T.A.: Potential sources of error in coronary arteriography. I. In performance of the study. A. J. R. 124:378, 1975.)

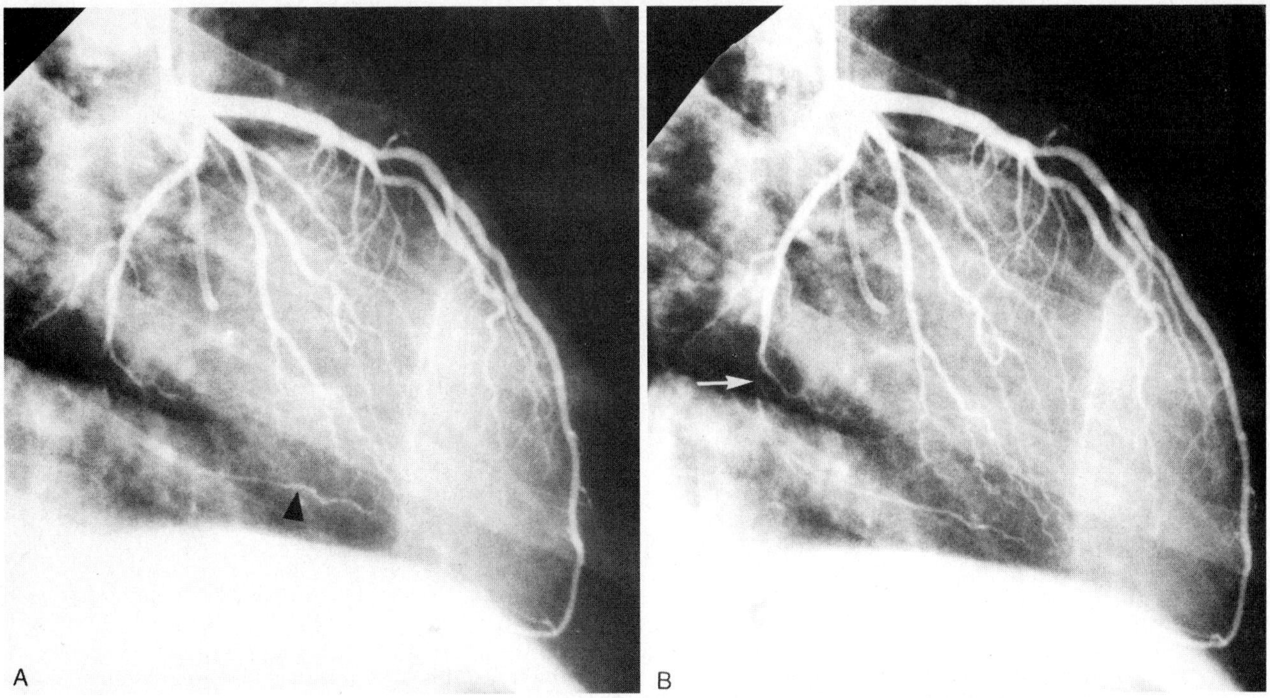

FIGURE 10–22. Distal circumflex occlusion which could only be recognized by late filling through collaterals. *A*, RAO left coronary arteriogram. Retrograde filling of a distal obtuse marginal branch (arrowhead) is seen. *B*, Later film shows further retrograde filling of this branch back to the point of occlusion of the distal circumflex (arrow). This occlusion would probably have gone unrecognized except for the collateral filling of the distal branch. (From Levin, D.C., Baltaxe, H.A., and Sos, T.A.: Potential sources of error in coronary arteriography. II. In interpretation of the study. A. J. R. *124*:386, 1975.)

phy. The bridged segment is of normal caliber during diastole but abruptly narrows with each systole. Systolic narrowing caused by myocardial bridging should not be confused with an atherosclerotic plaque. While bridging is not thought to have any hemodynamic significance in most cases, there have been several reports suggesting that when it produces severe systolic narrowing, myocardial ischemia can result.[40, 41] An example of pronounced bridging is shown in Figure 10–25.

RECANALIZATION. A narrowed segment of a coronary artery seen on arteriography is usually considered a "stenosis." However, such lesions may actually be segments which once were totally occluded but which have recanalized. Pathological studies have shown that as many as one-third of totally occluded coronary arteries ultimately recanalize.[42] The cineangiographic appearances of stenosis and recanalization may be indistinguishable.[37] Figure 10–26 shows a *postmortem* injection specimen of a recanalized

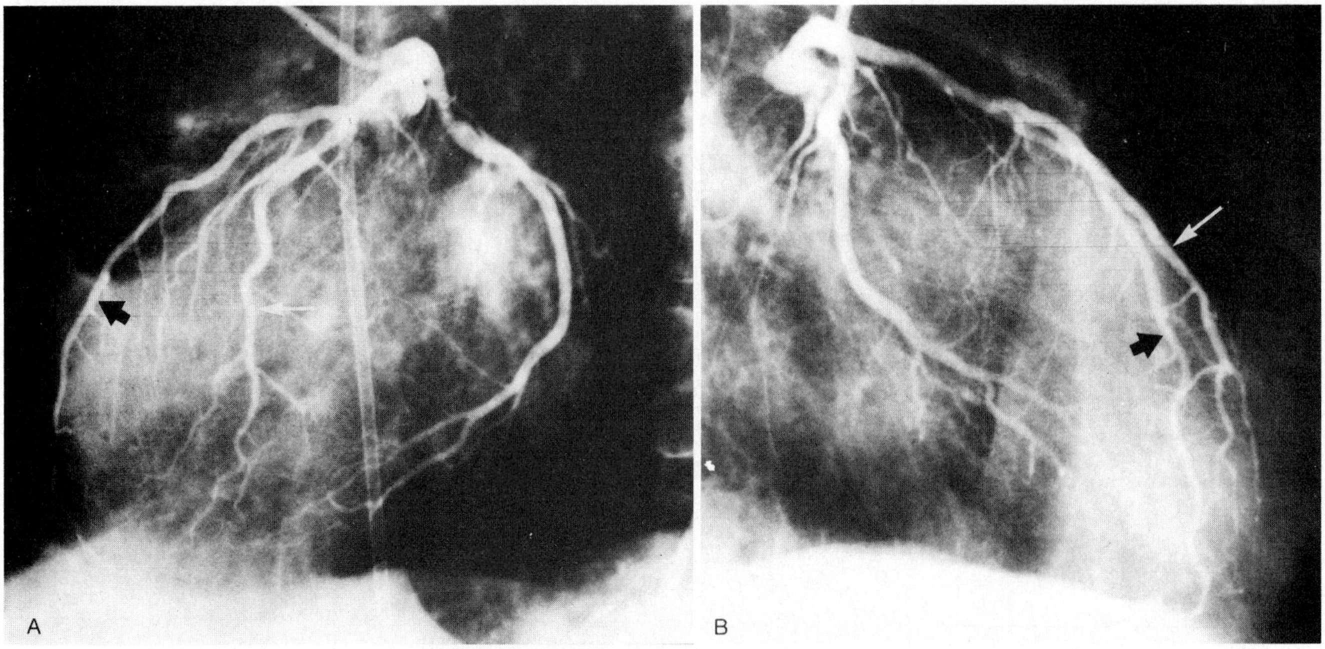

FIGURE 10–23. *A* and *B*, RAO and LAO views of a left coronary arteriogram. The LAD (black arrow) is normal in size and position. It has a large diagonal branch (white arrow) which closely parallels it. In either projection, if the LAD had become totally occluded at the origin of this diagonal branch, the latter might have then been mistaken for the LAD itself. (From Levin, D.C., Baltaxe, H.A., and Sos, T.A.: Potential sources of error in coronary arteriography. II. In interpretation of the study. A. J. R. *124*:386, 1975.)

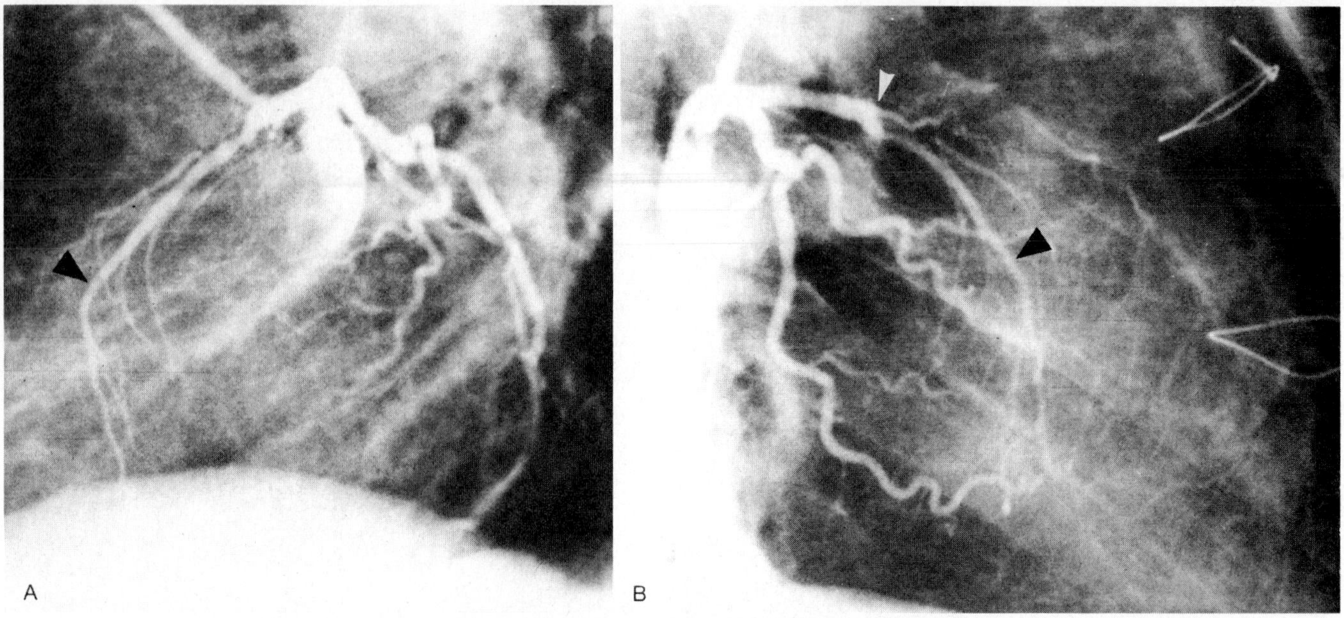

FIGURE 10–24. *A*, Septal branch mimicking the LAD. LAO left coronary arteriogram. The arrowhead points to an enlarged first septal branch which occupies the same course as the LAD and could be mistaken for the LAD. *B*, The RAO view shows that the LAD is totally obstructed (white arrowhead). The septal branch (black arrowhead) occupies a course roughly parallel to the normal position of the LAD but is below it and lies within the interventricular septum. (From Levin, D.C., Baltaxe, H.A., and Sos, T.A.: Potential sources of error in coronary arteriography. II. In interpretation of the study. A. J. R. *124*:386, 1975.)

segment of an RCA, along with the corresponding histologic section. Recanalization usually results in the development of multiple tortuous channels which are quite small and close to one another, creating an impression on cineangiography of a single, slightly irregular channel. The fine detail of the postmortem angiogram in Figure 10–26 shows the multiple tortuous and irregular channels, but it is unlikely that the spatial resolution of cineangiography would be sufficient to demonstrate this degree of detail in living patients.

COMPLICATIONS OF CORONARY ARTERIOGRAPHY

Considerable data have now been accumulated from a variety of sources on the incidence of complications of coronary arteriography. An early study, based on retrospectively collected data during 1970 and 1971 demonstrated a significantly higher mortality rate with the percutaneous femoral (Judkins) technique than with the brachial (Sones) technique.[43] Data from more recent experiences, collected prospectively, have indicated that this discrepancy has largely disappeared. If anything, the percutaneous femoral technique now seems to be associated with a slightly lower incidence of complications. This change may be related to greater experience, routine use of heparin, shortening of procedure times, or more accurate prospective data collection.

Bourassa and Noble[44] prospectively evaluated the complications in 5250 coronary arteriograms performed by the percutaneous femoral technique, using catheters shaped somewhat differently from the Judkins catheters. Mortality in their series was 0.23 per cent. Nonfatal

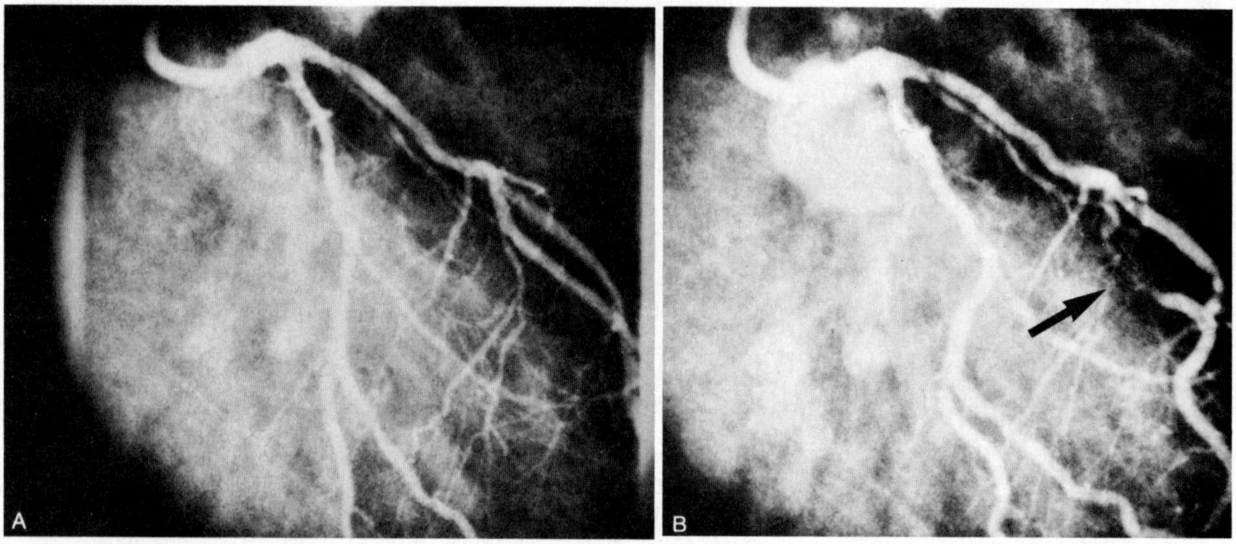

FIGURE 10–25. Myocardial bridging. *A*, RAO left coronary arteriogram, showing a normal LAD during diastole. *B*, During systole, there is pronounced narrowing of the LAD (arrow) at a point where it passes down into the myocardium.

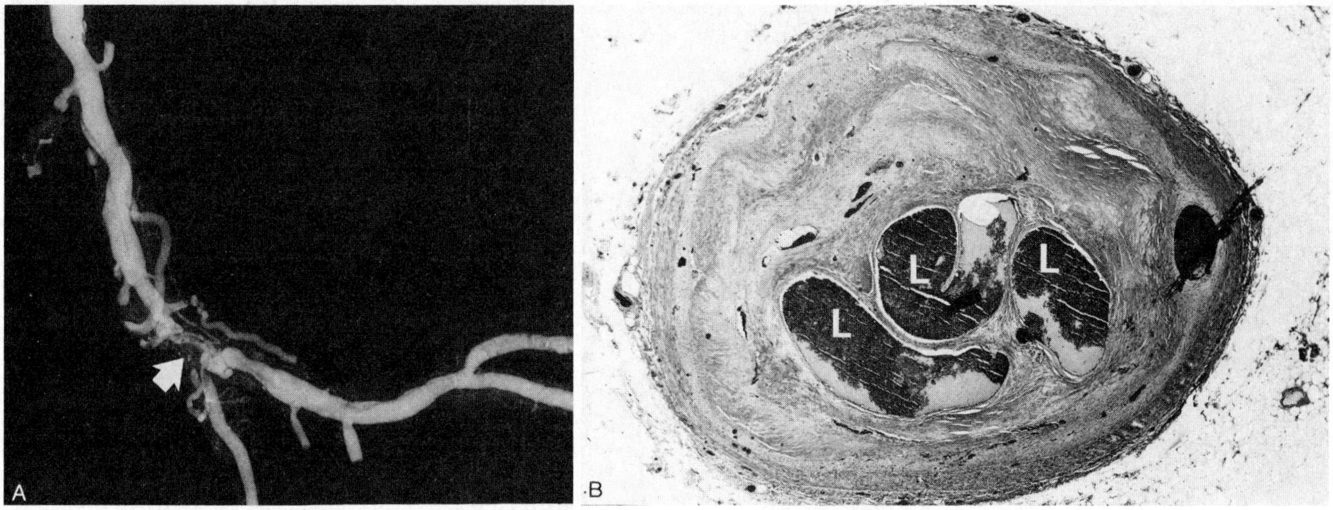

FIGURE 10–26. Recanalized segment of a totally occluded RCA. *A*, Postmortem injection specimen. The RCA was injected with a barium-gelatin mixture and then dissected off the epicardial surface of the heart. The recanalized segment (arrow) demonstrates several irregular channels. It is likely that angiography of such a segment in a living patient would not have sufficiently high spatial resolution to demonstrate these channels and that the lesion would instead appear simply as a localized stenosis. *B*, Histologic section of the recanalized segment. L = Recanalized lumina filled with the barium-gelatin mixture.

myocardial infarction occurred in 0.09 per cent. Potentially serious arrhythmias (ventricular fibrillation, ventricular tachycardia, and transient ventricular asystole) occurred in 0.80 per cent of cases. Local arterial puncture site complications (thrombosis and false aneurysm formation) occurred in 0.85 per cent, while cerebral ischemic events occurred in 0.13 per cent. All five patients with transient cerebral ischemia recovered within 24 hours.

In 1979, Davis et al.[45] reported upon the complications occurring in 7553 consecutive patients undergoing coronary arteriography at 13 different institutions participating in the Collaborative Study of Coronary Artery Surgery (CASS). They compared the complications in 1087 patients studied by the brachial approach and 6328 patients studied by the percutaneous femoral approach. Death occurred in 0.51 per cent of patients in the brachial group and 0.14 per cent of the femoral group. Nonfatal myocardial infarction occurred in 0.42 per cent in the brachial group compared with 0.22 per cent in the femoral group. Ventricular fibrillation unrelated to myocardial infarction occurred in 0.63 per cent of the entire population. Cerebral ischemia occurred in 0.17 per cent of the brachial group compared with 0.08 per cent of the femoral group. Local vascular complications were considerably higher in the brachial group, with arterial thrombosis occurring in 1.85 per cent of this group, as opposed to 0.24 per cent in the femoral group. Arterial dissection occurred in 0.93 per cent of the brachial group compared with 0.13 per cent in the femoral group.

In 1982, Kennedy[46] reported on the complications among 53,581 patients studied over a 14-month period in 66 laboratories staffed by members of the Society for Cardiac Angiography. Cases were not classified by the type of approach used. The overall mortality rate in this large series was 0.14 per cent. Nonfatal myocardial infarction occurred in 0.07 per cent. Arrhythmias occurred in 0.56 per cent. Among the noncardiac complications, cerebral ischemia occurred in 0.07 per cent and local vascular complications in 0.57 per cent. In 1985, Klinke et al.[47] discussed the complications occurring in 3071 outpatient coronary arteriograms, almost all of which were performed by the percutaneous femoral approach. The mortality rate was 0.13 per cent, while nonfatal myocardial infarction occurred in 0.07 per cent and arrhythmias in 0.42 per cent. Central nervous system complications occurred in 0.14 per cent and local vascular complications in 0.35 per cent.

While the overall incidence of death and serious complications has been shown to be acceptably low in these studies, certain groups of patients remain at significantly higher risks of mortality. In Kennedy's study[46] it was noted that among patients with an ejection fraction greater than 50 per cent, mortality was 0.05 per cent, whereas in those with an ejection fraction less than 30 per cent the mortality rate was 0.76 per cent. Patients with left main coronary artery disease are also at higher risk. In Kennedy's study[46] death occurred in 0.86 per cent of patients with LCA disease. Mortality in this category was 0.76 per cent in CASS.[45]

An interesting observation was made by Hildner et al.[48] regarding "pseudo complications" of coronary arteriography. They noted that the rate of complications during a 24-hour period immediately prior to scheduled cardiac catheterization was identical to that of procedure-related complications. This emphasizes the fact that a small but finite percentage of patients with coronary disease will experience complications on any given day, particularly under the emotional stress of a scheduled catheterization procedure. Therefore, the complication rate for this procedure may have reached an irreducible minimum in experienced hands.

ABNORMALITIES OF THE CORONARY CIRCULATION

CONGENITAL ANOMALIES OF THE CORONARY ARTERIES

(See also pp. 927 and 1000)

Congenital anomalies of the coronary arteries can be divided into two broad categories: those that alter myocardial perfusion and those that do not.[37]

ANOMALIES THAT ALTER MYOCARDIAL PERFUSION

CORONARY ARTERY FISTULAS (p. 1000). A review of a large series of patients with congenital anomalies of the coronary arteries revealed that coronary artery fistula is by far the most common.[49] While approximately half the patients with these lesions remain asymptomatic, the other half develop congestive heart failure, infective endocardi-

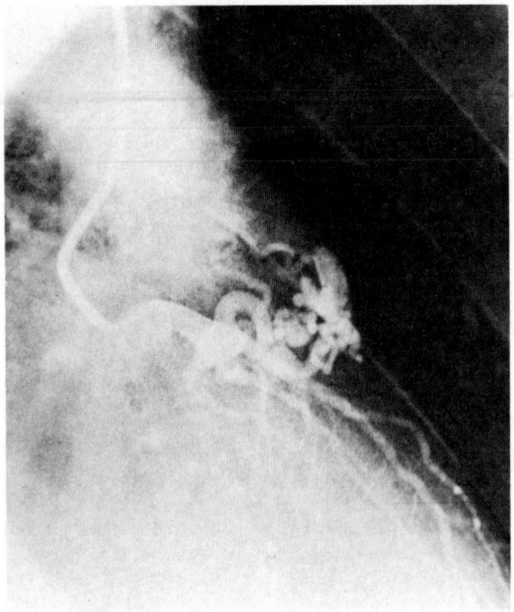

FIGURE 10–27. Left coronary arteriogram, RAO projection, showing a congenital fistula (consisting of multiple tortuous channels) from the LAD to the pulmonary artery. (From Levin, D.C., Fellows, K.E., and Abrams, H.L.: Hemodynamically significant primary anomalies of the coronary arteries. Angiographic aspects. Circulation *58*:25, 1978, by permission of the American Heart Association, Inc.)

tis, myocardial ischemia, or rupture of an aneurysmal fistula. Approximately half of these fistulas arise from the RCA or its branches; slightly fewer than half arise from the LAD or circumflex arteries or their branches; and in occasional cases there are multiple origins. Drainage occurs into the right ventricle in 41 per cent, the right atrium in 26 per cent, the pulmonary artery in 17 per cent, the coronary sinus in 7 per cent, the left atrium in 5 per cent, the left ventricle in 3 per cent, and the superior vena cava in 1 per cent.[49] Thus, a left-to-right shunt exists in over 90 per cent of cases. Selective coronary arteriography is the only way to demonstrate the origin of these fistulas. Figure 10–27 is an example of a fistula from the LAD to the main pulmonary artery.

ORIGIN OF THE LEFT CORONARY ARTERY FROM THE PULMONARY ARTERY (p. 927). Most patients with origin of the LCA from the main pulmonary artery develop myocardial ischemia early in life. Approximately 25 per cent survive to adolescence or adulthood but frequently experience mitral regurgitation, angina, or congestive heart failure.[50] Aortography (Fig. 10–28) typically shows a large RCA with absence of a left coronary ostium in the left aortic sinus. During the late phase of the aortogram, the LAD and circumflex branches fill via collateral circulation from RCA branches. Still later in the filming sequence, retrograde flow from the LAD and circumflex opacifies the LCA and its origin from the main pulmonary artery. The clinical course of the patient tends to be more favorable if extensive collateral circulation exists. In rare instances, the RCA rather than the LCA may arise from the main pulmonary artery.

CONGENITAL CORONARY STENOSIS OR ATRESIA. Congenital stenosis or atresia of a coronary artery can occur as an isolated lesion, or in association with other congenital diseases such as calcific coronary sclerosis, supravalvular aortic stenosis, homocystinuria, Friedreich's ataxia, Hurler's syndrome, progeria, and rubella syndrome.[49] In these cases, the atretic vessel usually fills via collateral circulation from the contralateral side.

ORIGIN OF EITHER CORONARY ARTERY FROM THE CONTRALATERAL SINUS WITH PASSAGE BETWEEN THE AORTA AND THE RIGHT VENTRICULAR OUTFLOW TRACT. Origin of the LCA from the proximal RCA or the right aortic sinus with subsequent passage between the aorta and the right ventricular outflow tract has been clearly shown to be a dangerous lesion, associated with sudden death in 27 to 33 per cent of patients.[51, 52] After its aberrant origin, the LCA takes an abrupt leftward turn and tunnels between the aorta and right ventricular outflow tract (Fig. 10–29). Sudden death usually occurs during exercise in these patients, and is thought to result from an increase in blood flow through the aorta and pulmonary artery that creates either a kink at the sharp leftward bend or a pinchcock mechanism in the tunnel. Origin of the RCA from the LCA or left aortic sinus with passage between the aorta and right ventricular outflow tract is less common and somewhat less dangerous. However, this anomaly has also been associated with myocardial ischemia or sudden death in several instances.[53, 54] Presumably, the mechanism is the same. In rare cases of anomalous origin of the LCA from the right aortic sinus, myocardial ischemia may occur even if the LCA passes anterior to the right ventricular outflow tract or posterior to the aorta (i.e., not through a tunnel between the two great vessels).[55] The case of the perfusion deficit is not clear in these cases.

CORONARY ANOMALIES NOT ALTERING MYOCARDIAL PERFUSION

In this category of anomalies, the coronary arteries originate from the aorta but their origins are in unusual positions. Although myocardial perfusion is normal, the angiographer may have trouble locating them. These anomalies occur in approximately 1 per cent of adult patients undergoing coronary arteriography.[56, 57]

ORIGIN OF THE CIRCUMFLEX ARTERY FROM THE RIGHT AORTIC SINUS. Anomalous origin of the circumflex artery from the right aortic sinus is by far the most common of these anomalies. In a series of almost 3000 patients, this anomaly was found in 0.67 per cent.[58] In these cases, the circumflex artery originates from the right aortic sinus via a common ostium with the RCA or a separate ostium of its own. It then passes posteriorly around the noncoronary aortic sinus toward the left atrioventricular groove (Fig. 10–30). Left coronary arteriography shows only the LAD arising from the left aortic sinus.

ORIGIN OF THE LEFT ANTERIOR DESCENDING ARTERY FROM THE RIGHT AORTIC SINUS. In these cases the LAD arises via a common ostium with the RCA or has a separate ostium in the right aortic sinus. It generally passes anterior to the right ventricular outflow tract on its way to the anterior interventricular groove.[59]

When either the LCA or the LAD arise from the right aortic sinus, it may be difficult to determine angiographically whether the aberrant vessel passes in front of the right ventricular outflow tract or behind it in a tunnel between the outflow tract and the aorta. This can be an important consideration, in view of the potential for acute occlusion posed by the latter type of anomaly. In the authors' experience, the best way to determine this is to pass a catheter into the main pulmonary artery, then perform an arteriogram of the aberrant coronary artery in the direct lateral projection. The catheter localizes the position of the pulmonary artery, and it is then usually possible to determine whether the course of the aberrant vessel is anterior or posterior to it.

SINGLE CORONARY ARTERY. There are numerous variations of this anomaly. Perhaps the best classification system is that of Lipton et al.,[60] which divided them into nine different categories. However, there are occasional cases of this anomaly which do not fall into any of these categories. Single coronary artery can be hemodynamically significant when a major branch passes between the aorta and the right ventricular outflow tract, as described earlier.

ORIGIN OF ALL THREE CORONARY ARTERIES FROM EITHER RIGHT OR LEFT AORTIC SINUSES VIA MULTIPLE SEPARATE OSTIA. This rare anomaly is similar to single coronary artery. There is absence of a coronary ostium in either the left or right aortic sinus. The missing vessels arise in the contralateral aortic sinus, but instead of arising as a single coronary artery, they arise through two or even three separate ostia.

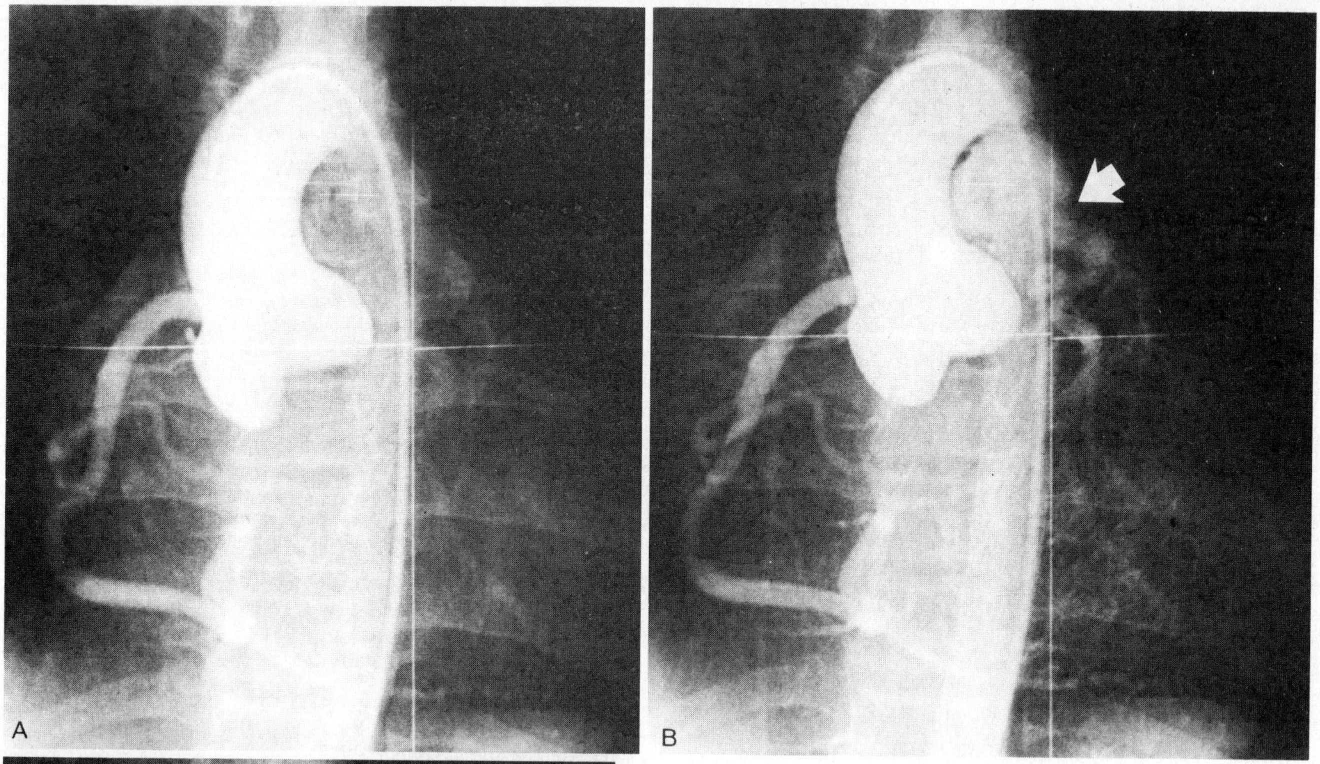

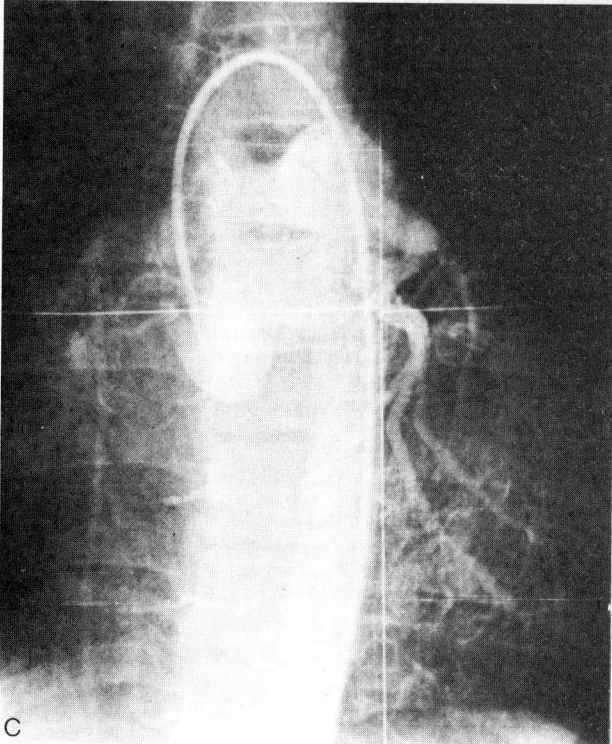

FIGURE 10–28. Origin of the LCA from the pulmonary artery. *A*, Aortic root angiogram in the early phase shows a large RCA and absence of the LCA. *B*, Later phase. The LAD and circumflex arteries have opacified as a result of collateral circulation from the RCA. There is retrograde flow with demonstration of the anomalous origin of the LCA from the pulmonary artery (arrow). *C*, Late phase film shows better opacification of the pulmonary artery.

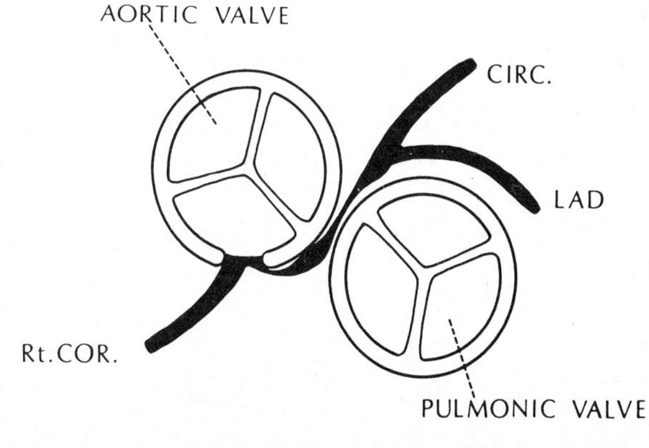

FIGURE 10–29. Diagram of origin of the LCA from the right aortic sinus with passage between the aorta and right ventricular outflow tract, viewed from above with the anterior chest wall facing downward. (From Levin, D.C., Fellows, K.E., and Abrams, H.L.: Hemodynamically significant primary anomalies of the coronary arteries. Angiographic aspects. Circulation *58*:25, 1978, by permission of the American Heart Association, Inc.)

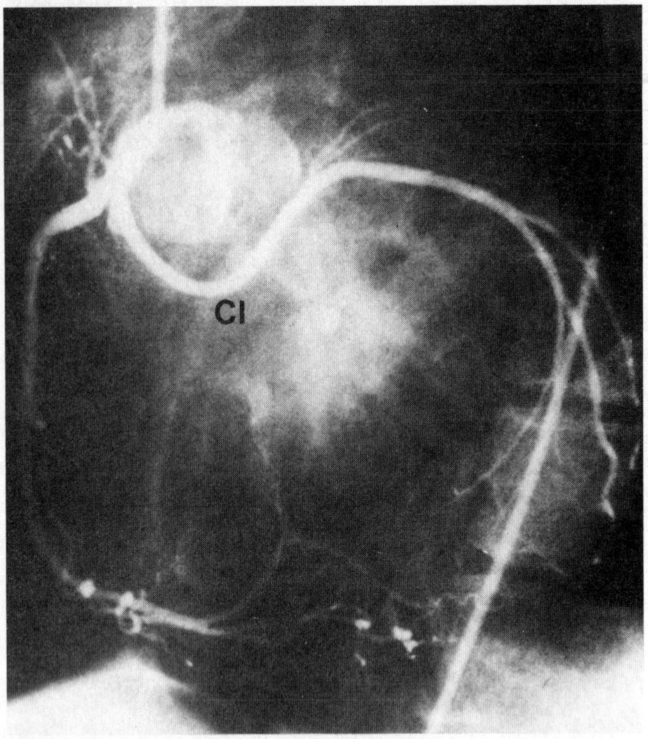

FIGURE 10–30. Origin of the circumflex artery from the right aortic sinus. LAO view of the RCA. The circumflex artery (CI) originates from the proximal RCA just beyond its origin, then passes posteriorly around the root of the aorta to reach the left atrioventricular groove. (From Abrams, H.L. [ed.]: Coronary Arteriography. A Practical Approach. Boston, Little Brown, 1983, with permission.)

HIGH ORIGIN OF THE CORONARY ARTERIES. The right and left coronary arteries generally arise in the upper portion of the aortic sinuses, just below the sinotubular ridges. On occasion, however, one or both coronary arteries may originate farther up the ascending aorta above this ridge.[59]

ANGIOGRAPHIC ASPECTS

EFFECT OF STENOSIS ON CORONARY BLOOD FLOW (See also Chap. 39)

Important concepts regarding the relationship between arterial stenosis and blood flow (Fig. 10–31) have resulted from the studies of Shipley and Gregg[61] and Gould et al.[62] Under resting conditions, progressive narrowing of a major artery does not cause a corresponding reduction in flow. Instead, flow remains relatively constant until the luminal area has been markedly reduced, at which time an abrupt decrease occurs. Under hyperemic conditions in the same artery, a considerably milder degree of stenosis will reduce peak blood flow. In the human heart, it has been noted that peak hyperemia such as can occur during exercise is approximately six times normal resting blood flow.[63] The hyperemic state is mediated by dilatation of the distal arteriolar bed, which is often referred to as *vasodilator reserve*. The point at which reduction in flow begins to occur can be called the *point of critical stenosis* (PCS). Expressed in different terms, Figure 10–31 shows that in a major artery under resting conditions the PCS is not reached until very severe stenosis (approximately 90 per cent of the luminal diameter) exists. In the same artery under hyperemic conditions, the PCS occurs with much less severe stenosis (approximately 50 per cent).

Some authors have postulated that the maintenance of resting blood flow in the face of progressively severe proximal stenosis results from compensatory vasodilation of the arteriolar bed distal to the lesion.[63, 64] Presumably, when the arterial lumen is approximately 90 per cent narrowed, the maximum vasodilatory capacity of the small arterioles is reached and they cannot compensate any further. Additional narrowing of the major artery beyond this PCS then leads to the rapid falloff in flow. It is further assumed that during hyperemia some of the vasodilator reserve has already been encroached upon to accommodate the demand for increased flow, so that the maximum vasodilatory capacity of the arteriolar bed is reached with lesser degrees of arterial stenosis. Therefore, according to this theory, the PCS during a hyperemic state is reduced to only 40 to 60 per cent stenosis.

Experiments in the authors' laboratory and in others[65, 66] and the earlier study by Shipley and Gregg[61] have provided alternative explanations for the relationship shown in Figure 10–31. In these studies, measurements of arterial pressure distal to progressive stenoses failed to show a pressure drop as the degree of stenosis increased. Instead, both pressure and flow remained constant until the PCS was reached. This meant that peripheral resistance was being maintained as stenosis increased. It further suggested that compensatory peripheral arteriolar dilation is not the explanation for the maintenance of resting blood flow. A more likely explanation for this phenomenon has been discussed by Logan.[66] The rate of flow through a vessel equals the driving pressure divided by the total resistance in its vascular bed. Total resistance (R_t) is the sum of stenosis resistance (R_s) in the proximal artery and peripheral resistance in the arteriolar bed (R_p). Under resting conditions, when flow is relatively low and R_p is high, R_t is high but consists almost entirely of R_p. As major arterial stenosis increases, R_s begins to increase but is initially of very small magnitude compared to R_p and therefore has little overall effect upon the magnitude of R_t of the entire system. Only when proximal arterial stenosis becomes severe does R_s begin to approach R_p. At this point further increase in R_s significantly elevates R_t, which in turn causes flow through the entire system to drop off rapidly. During hyperemic states induced by exercise or other vasodilator stimuli, R_p and therefore R_t are much lower to begin with. A given degree of arterial stenosis will create a level of R_s which is more significant relative to R_p. Any increase in the severity of that stenosis will begin to raise R_t by significant increments at an earlier stage, and the PCS accordingly is also reached at an earlier stage.

These concepts indicate why resting blood flow may be entirely normal even when a significant proximal stenosis is present, and why ischemic symptoms develop during exercise when they are not present at rest. They also explain why a very minor increase in degree of an already-existing stenosis can cause a profound decrease in blood flow and lead to the abrupt onset of severe ischemia.

Other important aspects of the flow-stenosis relationship relate to the effects of sequential arterial stenoses and length of the lesion. Gould and colleagues[67] showed that the resistances of coronary stenoses in series are additive. The effects of such sequential lesions are not determined solely by the most severe lesion. Feldman et al.[68] showed that the hemodynamic effects of coronary stenoses increased significantly as their length increased.

White et al.[69] have called into question the reliability of coronary arteriography in predicting the hemodynamic significance of a coronary

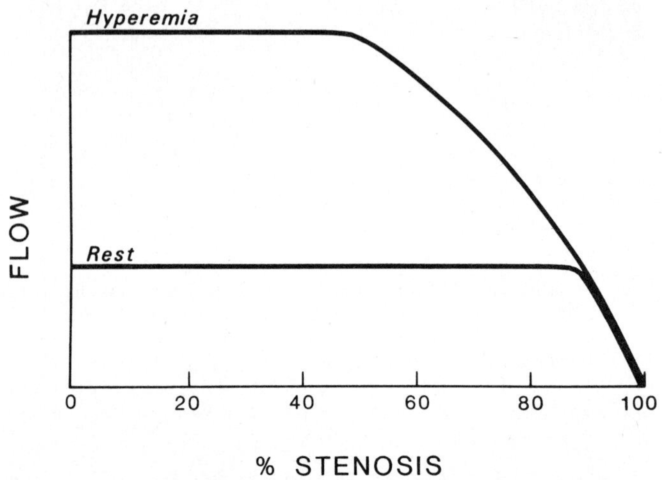

FIGURE 10–31. Relationship between arterial stenosis and blood flow under resting and hyperemic conditions.

stenosis. They compared the degree of coronary stenosis measured by arteriography with the reactive hyperemic response measured during coronary bypass surgery by a Doppler probe after 20 seconds of arterial occlusion. In each case, the ratio of peak to resting flow velocity was measured. It would be expected that if arteriography is an accurate way of assessing the hemodynamic significance of stenoses, the ratio of peak to resting flow would consistently be lower for severe stenoses than for minor stenoses. However, the study revealed lack of significant correlation between this ratio and the degree of stenosis as measured by arteriography. They suggested that the lack of correlation could be explained by a variety of factors, including interobserver and intraobserver variability, technical problems relating to radiographic magnification and distortion, and the diffuse nature of coronary atherosclerosis (which makes it difficult to establish an accurate denominator for the expression of percentage of stenosis). The nonphysiological circumstances of the measurements could also play a role. Their findings emphasize the importance of high-quality cineangiography with visualization of coronary lesions in multiple projections if any degree of accuracy is to be achieved.

The accuracy of angiographic assessment of coronary lesions which appear to be of borderline significance can be enhanced by the measurement of pressure gradients across the stenoses at the time of diagnostic coronary arteriography.[70] This can be accomplished by passing a small (2.0 French) catheter coaxially through the diagnostic arteriographic catheter and through the stenosis, then recording pressure measurements during pullback both at rest and under hyperemic conditions induced by the injection of contrast material.

CORONARY COLLATERAL CIRCULATION

(See also p. 1193)

In the normal human heart, a myriad of tiny anastomotic branches interconnect the major coronary arteries.[18, 19] These anastomotic vessels are generally less than 200 μ in diameter, and they are the precursors of the collateral circulation. In coronary arteriograms of patients with normal or mildly diseased coronary arteries, they cannot be visualized because they carry only minimal flow and their small caliber is well beyond the spatial resolution capabilities of cine imaging systems. If, however, obstruction of a major coronary artery occurs, a pressure gradient is created in the anastomotic vessels connecting the distal segment of the involved artery with either its proximal segment or the nearby segments of other vessels. With the creation of this gradient, an increased volume of blood is propelled through the anastomotic vessels, which progressively dilate and eventually become visible angiographically as collateral channels. The reason why this process seems to occur effectively in some patients and ineffectively in others is not entirely clear, but it may well have to do with the rate at which the obstruction develops. In any event, collateral circulation does not represent the formation of new vessels but rather the utilization of vessels which already exist but carry very little blood flow until the need arises. Collaterals cannot be demonstrated at coronary arteriography unless the recipient vessel has developed at least 90 per cent diameter stenosis.[71, 72]

A wide variety of collateral pathways exist in patients with severe coronary artery disease. These pathways are shown in Figures 10–32, 10–33 and 10–34. Figure 10–35 is an example of early collateral circulation to a stenotic LAD seen on right coronary arteriography. Figure 10–36 is an example of the small network of short channels which is often seen bridging a localized obstruction of a major coronary artery. James has suggested[19] that these do not represent preexisting anastomotic vessels but instead are enlarged vasa vasorum or adventitial arteries which form a cuff around the obstructed segment. Figures 10–37 to 10–41 are examples of collateral pathways in patients with complete occlusions of major coronary arteries.

The functional role of coronary collateral circulation has been the subject of debate for many years. An early study[73] suggested that collateral circulation did not protect against development of regional left ventricular contraction abnormalities. This study included patients both with and without total occlusions of coronary arteries, and some patients in the latter group undoubtedly had no demonstrable collaterals because

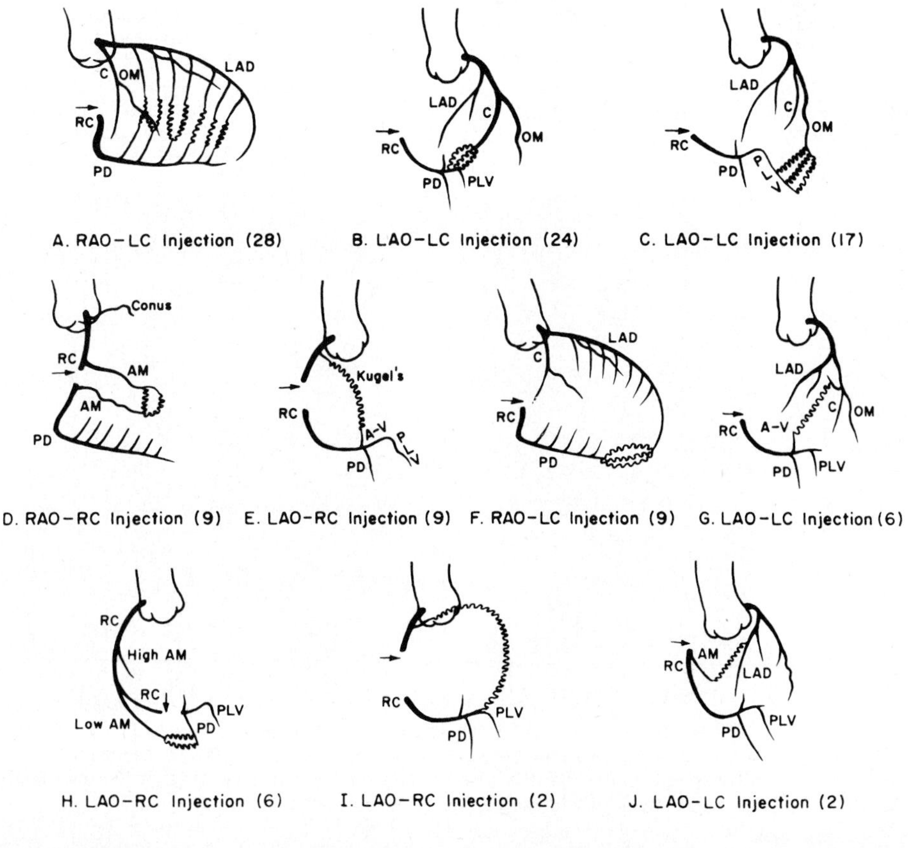

FIGURE 10–32. Common collateral pathways seen with RCA occlusion. The arrows point to the site of obstruction. The small tortuous channels represent the collateral connections. Numbers in parentheses refer to the frequency with which each pathway was visualized in a series of 200 patients with significant coronary disease. (From Levin, D.C.: Pathways and functional significance of the coronary collateral circulation. Circulation *50*:831, 1974, by permission of the American Heart Association, Inc.)

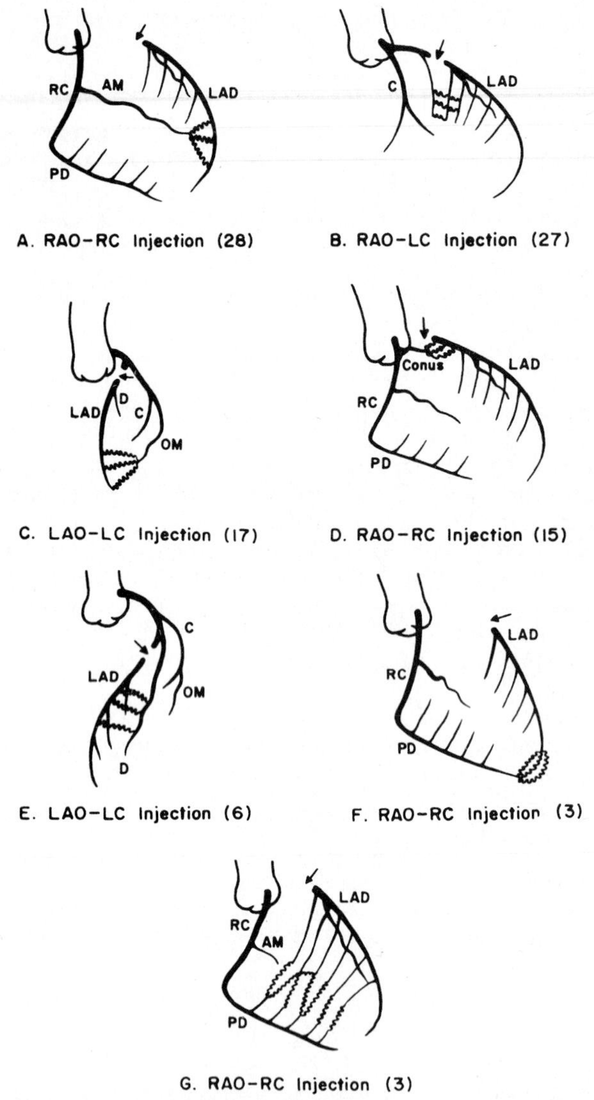

FIGURE 10–33. Common collateral pathways seen with LAD occlusion. (From Levin, D.C.: Pathways and functional significance of the coronary collateral circulation. Circulation 50:831, 1974, by permission of the American Heart Association, Inc.)

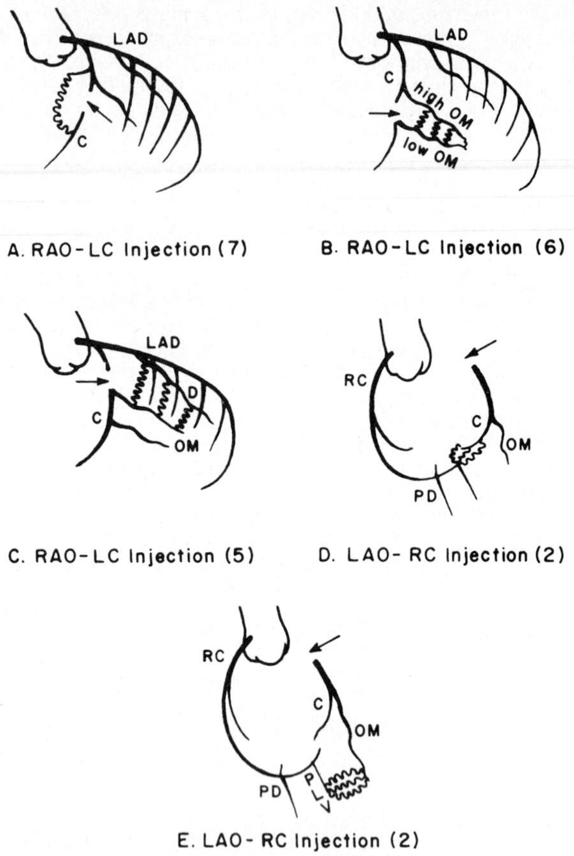

FIGURE 10–34. Common collateral pathways seen with left circumflex occlusion. (From Levin, D.C.: Pathways and functional significance of the coronary collateral circulation. Circulation *50*:831, 1974, by permission of the American Heart Association, Inc.)

their stenoses were not severe enough. A subsequent study of one of the authors[71] (D.C.L.) addressed the same issue but included only patients in whom total occlusion of a coronary artery was present, thereby insuring that the degree of obstruction was absolutely identical in all cases. This study revealed that regional left ventricular contraction was significantly better in segments supplied by adequate collateral circulation than in those segments supplied by inadequate or no collateral circulation.

A number of other studies have supported the concept that collateral circulation preserves distal perfusion and regional left ventricular contractility and may improve clinical prognosis. Thus, in patients with effective coronary collateral circulation, there was a significantly higher

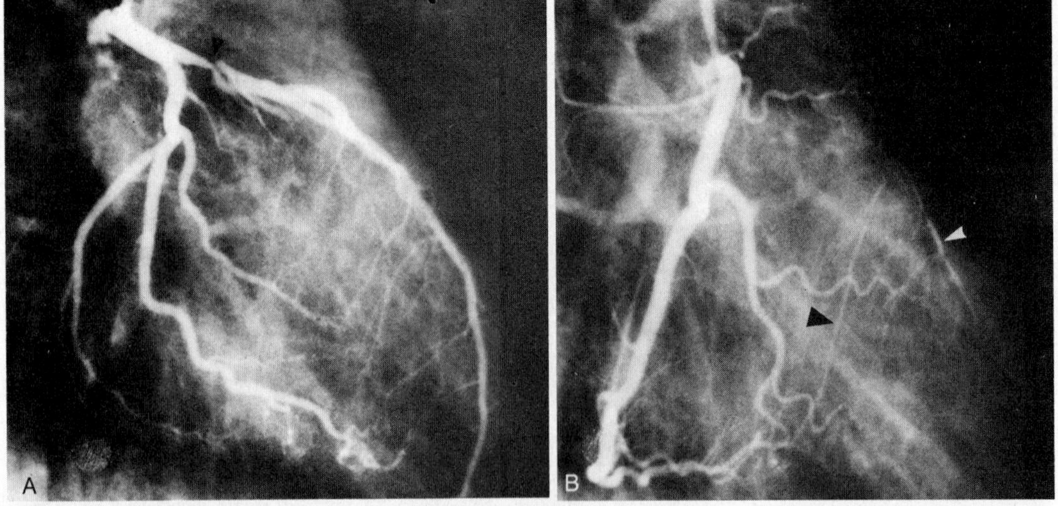

FIGURE 10–35. Early collateralization in a patient with severe LAD stenosis. *A*, RAO left coronary arteriogram, showing severe proximal LAD stenosis (arrowhead). *B*, RAO right coronary arteriogram. Early collateral circulation is seen extending from the posterior descending artery up through the interventricular septum (black arrowhead) and partially filling the distal LAD (white arrowhead).

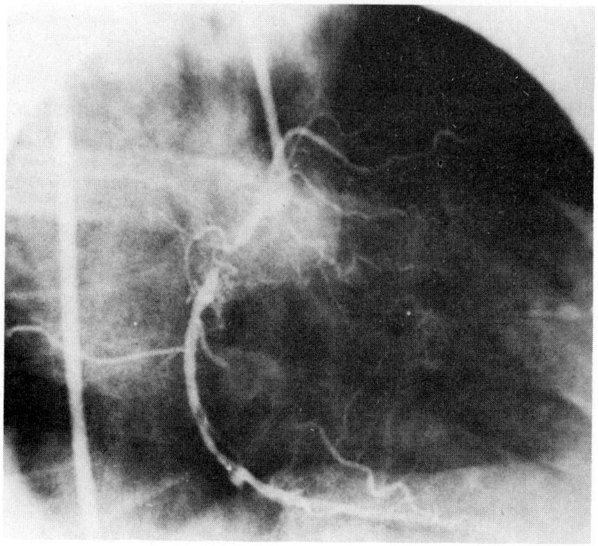

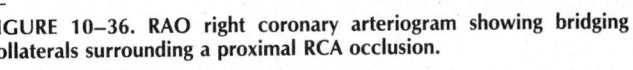

←
FIGURE 10–36. RAO right coronary arteriogram showing bridging collaterals surrounding a proximal RCA occlusion.

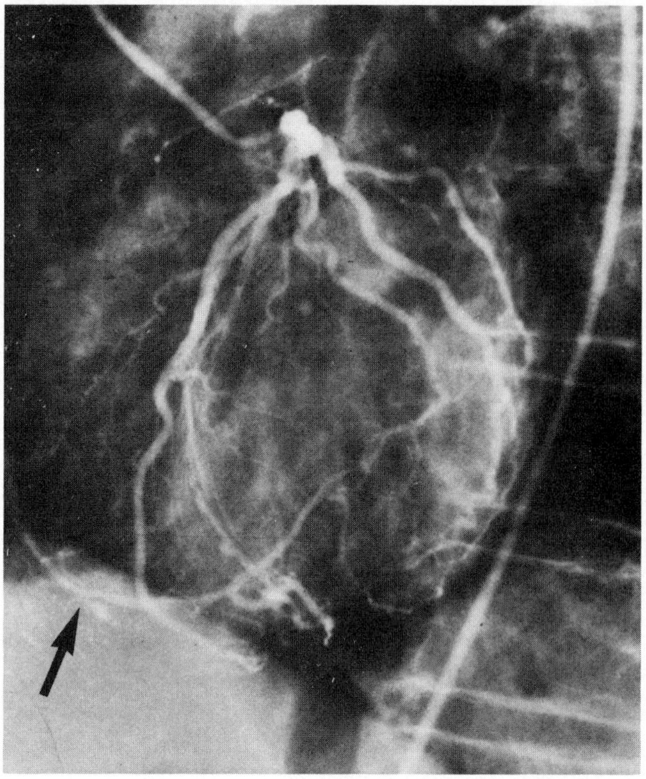

→
FIGURE 10–37. LAO left coronary arteriogram. The RCA is totally obstructed and fills distally (arrow) via collaterals from the LCA.

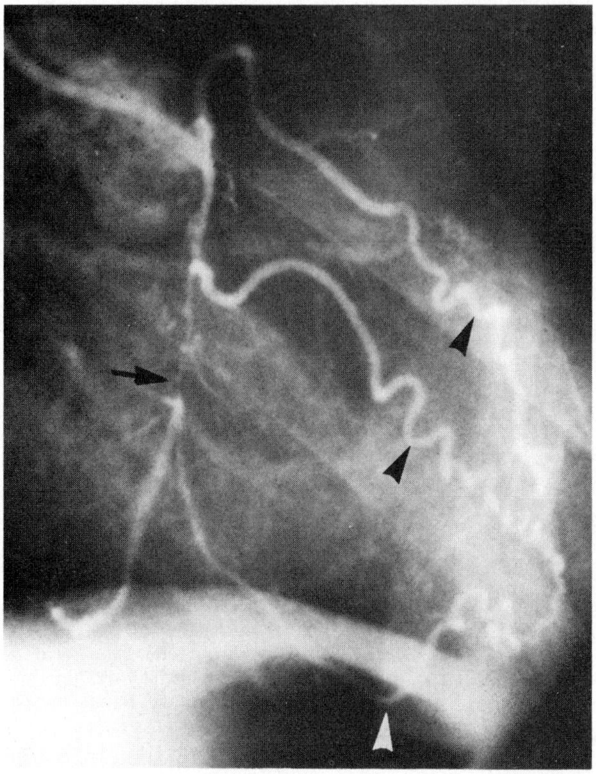

←
FIGURE 10–38. RAO right coronary arteriogram showing complete obstruction of the mid RCA (arrow). Collaterals extend from the conus branch and a high acute marginal branch (black arrowheads) to fill a more distal acute marginal branch (white arrowhead) and then the distal RCA itself. (From Levin, D.C., Kauff, M., and Baltaxe, H.A.: Coronary collateral circulation. A. J. R. *119*:463, 1973.)

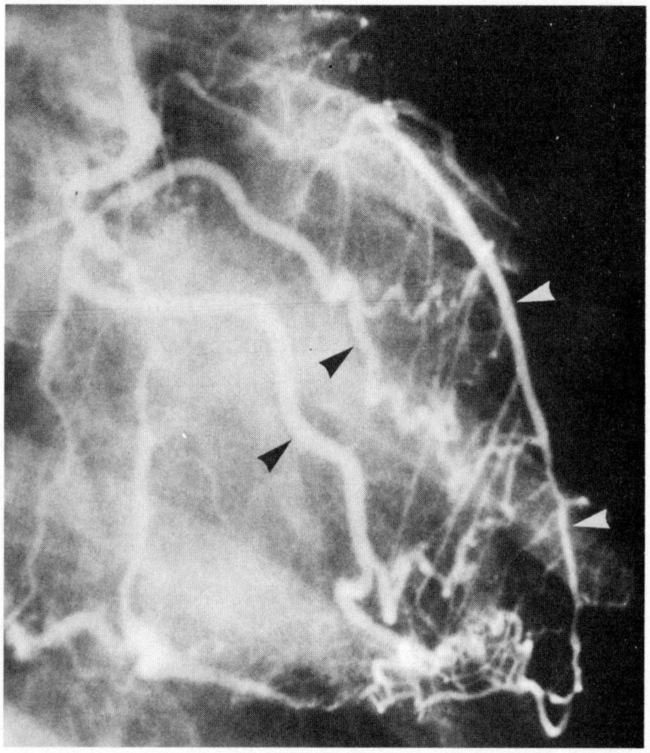

→
FIGURE 10–39. RAO right coronary arteriogram in a patient with total occlusions of the LAD and mid RCA. Extensive collaterals are seen originating from acute marginal branches (black arrowheads) of the RCA and filling the distal LAD (white arrowheads). (From Levin, D.C., Kauff, M., and Baltaxe, H.A.: Coronary collateral circulation. A. J. R. *119*:463, 1973).

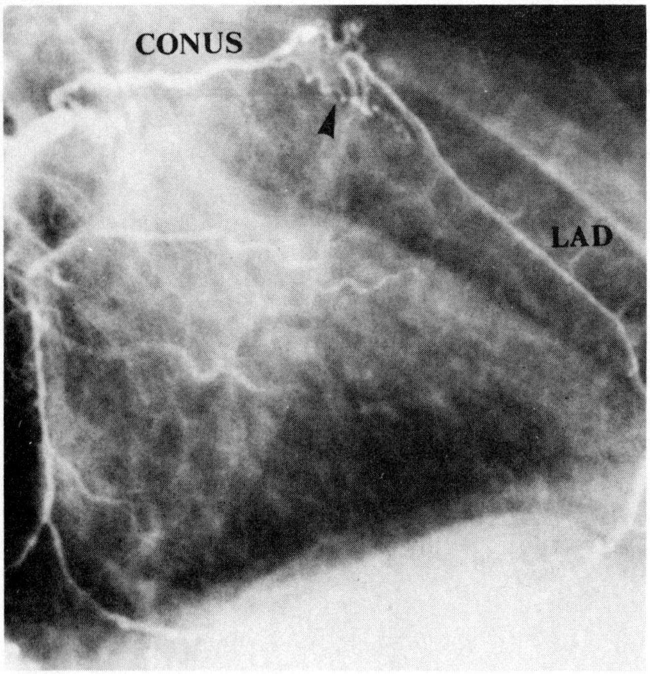

FIGURE 10–40. RAO right coronary arteriogram in a patient with LAD and RCA occlusions. Collaterals extend from the conus branch of the proximal RCA to the LAD. (From Abrams, H.L. [ed.]: Coronary Arteriography. A Practical Approach. Boston, Little Brown, 1983, with permission.)

incidence of normal left ventricular wall motion in the territory subserved by those collaterals.[74] In another study patients with acute myocardial infarction undergoing emergency cardiac catheterization were divided into those with adequate collateral circulation to the infarct vessel and those with inadequate or no collateral circulation to the infarct vessel.[75] The group with adequate collaterals had significantly lower left ventricular end-diastolic pressure, higher cardiac index, higher ejection fraction, and lower percentage of area dyssynergy. None of the patients with adequate collaterals died, whereas the majority with inadequate or no collaterals died. It has also been demonstrated that global and regional left ventricular function were better in patients with well-collateralized total coronary artery occlusions than in those with poorly collateralized occlusions.[76] Patients with severe coronary obstruction without collateral circulation were found to have a significantly higher incidence of thallium-201 myocardial perfusion defects than those with collateral circulation.[77] This suggests that collaterals may improve myocardial perfusion in the ischemic zone. Frequent absence of thallium-201 perfusion defects has also been reported in noninfarcted, collateralized myocardial regions with totally occluded coronary arteries.[78] The advent of coronary angioplasty has provided the opportunity to compare distal coronary artery pressure measurements in patients with varying degrees of collateral circulation. In patients with extensive collateral circulation, distal coronary pressure is higher than in those without collateral circulation.[79]

CORONARY ARTERY SPASM

(See also p. 1228)

Nearly three decades have elapsed since Prinzmetal et al.[80] described an unusual or variant form of angina in which the onset of chest pain was not provoked by the usual factors such as exercise, emotional upset, cold, and ingestion of a meal. According to currently accepted theories,[81] patients considered to have variant angina are those in whom chest pain commences at rest or both at rest and during exertion. The pain often occurs in a cyclical pattern at the same time every day, generally the morning, and is usually noted to be accompanied by ST-segment elevation if an electrocardiogram is recorded. Symptoms may occur many times daily and then cease for weeks or months, then recur again. Although the ST elevation is often striking, it reverts rapidly to normal when the pain disappears spontaneously or is terminated by the administration of nitroglycerin. Ischemic episodes may be accompanied by atrioventricular block, ventricular ectopic activity, ventricular tachycardia, or ventricular fibrillation. Although the original description of this syndrome emphasized its transient nature and its onset at rest, it has become apparent through further studies[81] that coronary spasm can also play a role in exercise-induced angina, unstable angina, acute myocardial infarction, and sudden death.

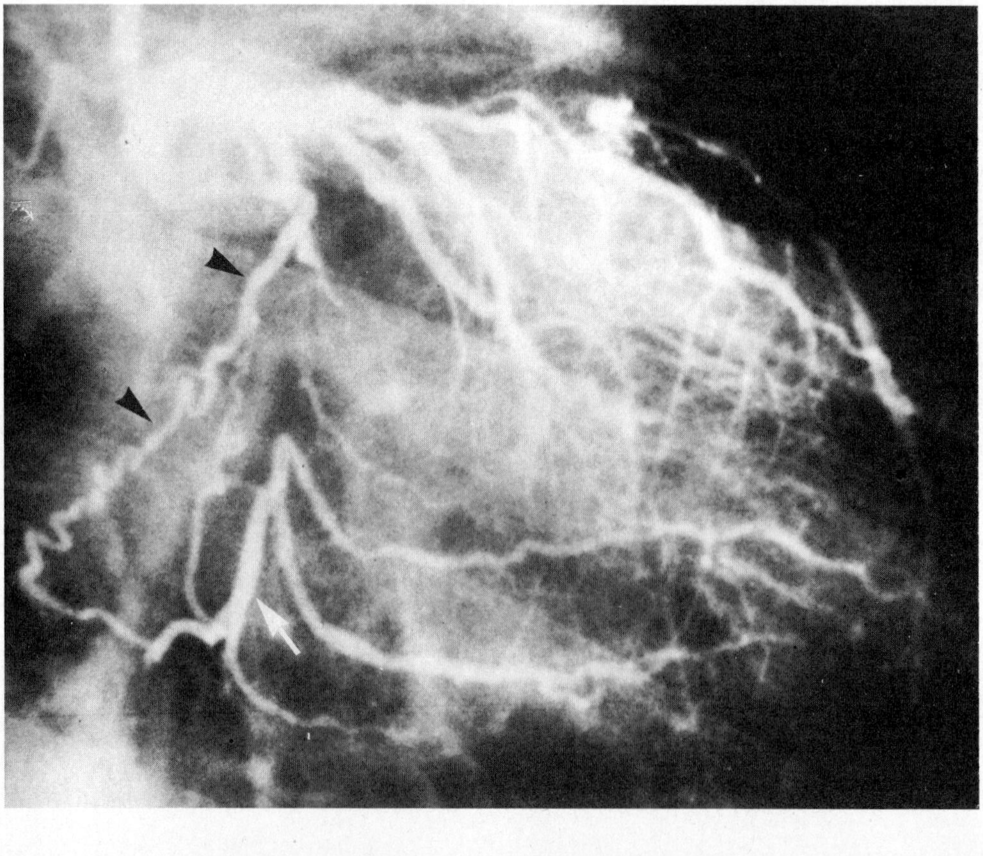

FIGURE 10–41. RAO left coronary arteriogram in a patient with total occlusions of the LAD and circumflex arteries. Collateral flow originates from the proximal circumflex artery, passes through a left atrial circumflex branch (black arrowheads), and fills the distal circumflex artery (white arrow). (From Levin, D.C., Kauff, M., and Baltaxe, H.A.: Coronary collateral circulation. A. J. R. *119*:463, 1973.)

Coronary arteriography has played an important role in understanding the pathophysiology and clinical consequences of coronary artery spasm. In the early 1970's, several studies angiographically demonstrated spasm in patients with clinical variant angina.[82–84] These studies showed that while spasm was generally superimposed upon areas of stenosis, in some cases it occurred in segments of coronary arteries that appeared normal. In the late 1970's, intravenous ergonovine maleate was used to provoke spasm in patients with suspected variant angina who were undergoing coronary arteriography.[85–87] These studies revealed that the vast majority of patients with this syndrome will demonstrate spasm on arteriograms performed immediately after the administration of ergonovine.

Ergonovine-induced provocation of coronary artery spasm entails intravenous administration of the drug in progressively increasing doses, usually starting with an initial dose of 0.05 mg. After each dose, the patient is observed for several minutes for the detection of ST-segment elevation or the onset of chest pain. If neither occurs, the next dose is administered and the cycle is repeated. Freedman et al.[88] recommend a cumulative dose of ergonovine as high as 0.65 mg, but many laboratories terminate the study at 0.50 mg. If no chest pain or ST-segment elevation occurs and the patient's systemic blood pressure rises by 10 per cent, it can be assumed that the ergonovine has had a physiological effect. When any of these endpoints is reached, repeat arteriography is performed to determine if coronary spasm has occurred. While the ergonovine provocative test is widely used and generally safe, it should be borne in mind that serious complications, including irreversible occlusion, can occur on rare occasions.[88–90] Figure 10–42 is an example of ergonovine-induced spasm in a vessel which appeared normal arteriographically.

CORONARY ATHEROSCLEROTIC PLAQUE MORPHOLOGY AND ITS CONSEQUENCES

(See also p. 1141)

There is abundant evidence that acute thrombosis in stenotic coronary arteries occurs in association with plaques which have undergone rupture, ulceration, or subintimal hemorrhage (p. 1142). By contrast, it seems less likely to occur with uncomplicated fatty or fibrous plaques having intact luminal surfaces. In a study of 19 coronary artery segments obstructed by recent thrombi,[91] it was found that in every single instance the thrombus was adherent to an area of rupture of the intimal surface of the plaque. Intramural hemorrhage and nonocclusive organizing thrombi were also frequently noted at these sites of acute thrombosis. Similarly, among 40 coronary artery segments containing occluding thrombi, the thrombus overlay a plaque rupture in 39.[92] Intraplaque hemorrhage was frequently noted, as was partial recanalization. Thrombi were found in 67 of 69 coronary arteries supplying zones of recently infarcted myocardium.[93] In 64 of these 67 vessels, ulcers or ruptures in the plaque surface underlay the thrombus. Horie et al.[94] reported that 91 per cent of occlusive coronary artery thrombi formed at sites of rupture of atheromatous plaques. In a pathological study of 51 recent coronary thrombi, 40 were associated with underlying ruptured atherosclerotic plaques and 2 others had rethrombosis of old recanalized occlusions.[95]

Willerson et al.[96] have discussed the mechanism by which atherosclerotic plaque rupture can lead to acute thrombosis. They postulate that at the site of coronary stenosis there is decreased local prostacyclin concentration to begin with. Plaque fissuring and hemorrhage lead to platelet aggregation and the release of vasoactive substances and activators of further platelet aggregation, including thromboxane A_2, serotonin, histamine, and platelet-activating factor. As circulating platelets become activated and adhere to this nidus, a vicious cycle is initiated, leading rapidly to occlusive thrombosis. Fuster et al.[97] have discussed additional factors causing plaque surface damage to be thrombogenic. First, when a plaque ruptures and hemorrhage enters it, ADP released from the red blood cells probably contributes to the process of platelet aggregation. In addition, the damaged vascular wall can generate tissue thromboplastin and thus promote thrombosis.

An attempt was made in the laboratory of one of the authors (D.C.L.) to determine whether "complicated" coronary atherosclerotic plaques (those characterized by plaque rupture, subintimal hemorrhage within the plaque, superimposed partially occluding thrombi, or recanalized thrombi) could be differentiated on postmortem angiography from "uncomplicated" fatty or fibrous plaques having intact luminal surfaces.[98] Postmortem coronary angiograms were studied and angiographic morphology was correlated with histological sections of 73 significant coronary stenoses to ascertain whether complicated and uncomplicated atherosclerotic lesions could be differentiated angiographically. Lesions were angiographically classified as type I if they had smooth borders and no intraluminal lucencies. Type II stenoses had irregular borders, intraluminal lucencies, or both. Only 4 of the 35 lesions (11 per cent) with type I angiographic morphology were complicated stenoses

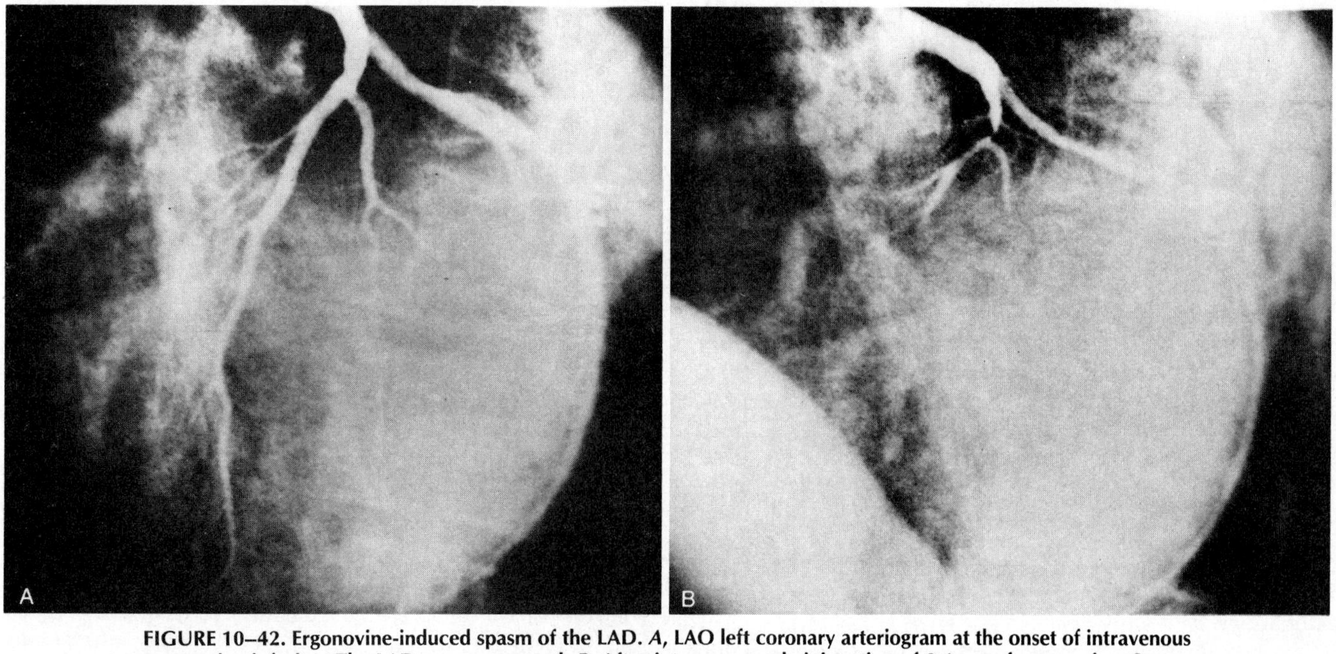

FIGURE 10–42. Ergonovine-induced spasm of the LAD. *A*, LAO left coronary arteriogram at the onset of intravenous ergonovine infusion. The LAD appears normal. *B*, After intravenous administration of 0.1 mg of ergonovine. Severe spasm has developed, causing nearly total occlusion of the LAD. The patient was experiencing mild chest pain and had pronounced ST-segment elevation. Spasm was quickly relieved with sublingual nitroglycerin.

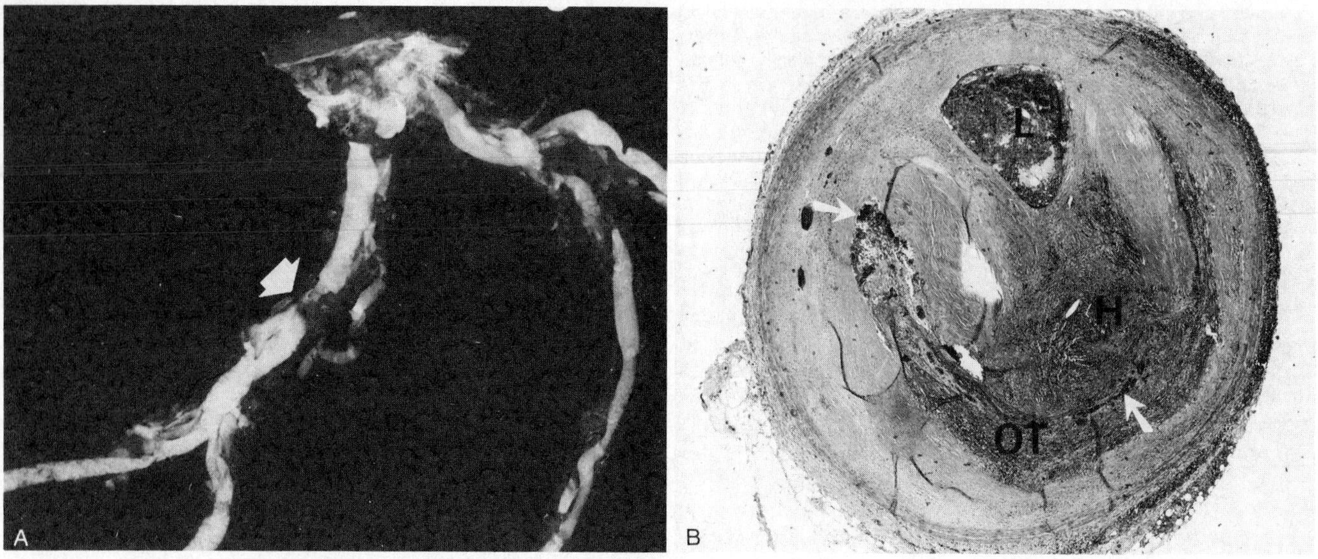

FIGURE 10–43. Complicated atherosclerotic plaque of the LAD. ***A,*** **Postmortem injection specimen, in which the left coronary system has been dissected from the epicardial surface of the heart. A severe irregular stenosis of the proximal LAD is present (arrow).** ***B,*** **Corresponding histological section. L = residual lumen; H = large area of hemorrhage within the plaque; OT = organizing thrombus within the plaque; arrows point to small recanalized channels within the organizing thrombus.**

on histological examination. However, 30 of the 38 (79 per cent) lesions characterized by type II angiographic morphology were complicated stenoses. Postmortem angiography had a sensitivity of 88 per cent and a specificity of 79 per cent in detecting complicated coronary artery stenoses on the basis of the presence of irregular borders or intraluminal lucencies. Figure 10–43 shows a postmortem coronary arteriogram of a complicated LAD stenosis, along with its corresponding histological section. It was postulated that since it was possible to detect complicated atherosclerotic plaques by postmortem angiography, it might also be possible (though undoubtedly more difficult) to detect such lesions in living patients by observing irregular borders or intraluminal lucencies on coronary angiograms. If present, they could create a greater danger to the patient because of their propensity to lead to acute thrombosis. Revascularization by means of angioplasty or bypass surgery might be more urgently needed in such cases.

Although the clinical question just posed has not yet been definitively answered, a number of subsequent studies have suggested that angiographic plaque morphology *can* be evaluated on coronary angiograms in living patients, and that it can be correlated with the clinical status of the patient. In a study of 110 patients with stable or unstable angina, Ambrose et al.[99] classified their lesions angiographically into four categories (Fig. 10–44). The first category included those with concentric stenoses and smooth borders. The second category was referred to as type I eccentric stenoses—lesions which were eccentric but which had smooth borders and a broad neck. The third category was designated type II eccentric stenoses—eccentric lesions usually in the form of a convex intraluminal obstruction with a narrow base or neck caused by overhanging edges, or borders that were irregularly scalloped. The fourth category included those lesions having multiple irregularities. The latter two categories (type II eccentric stenoses and lesions with multiple irregularities) probably correspond to lesions that would have been categorized as complicated stenoses on the authors' postmortem angiograms. Among Ambrose's patients with stable angina, type II eccentric stenoses or lesions with multiple irregularities were present in 18 per cent of coronary arteries. However, among the patients with unstable angina, 56 per cent had lesions in these categories, especially type II eccentric stenoses. Ambrose further identified a group of patients in whom the "angina-producing" artery could be clearly identified by angiographic, electrocardiographic, or radionuclide techniques. In this subgroup, lesions producing stable angina showed a 20 per cent incidence of type II eccentric stenoses or multiple irregularities. By comparison, 71 per cent of the lesions producing unstable angina were type II eccentric stenoses. These data show that in patients with unstable angina, lesions characterized by overhanging edges, scalloped borders,

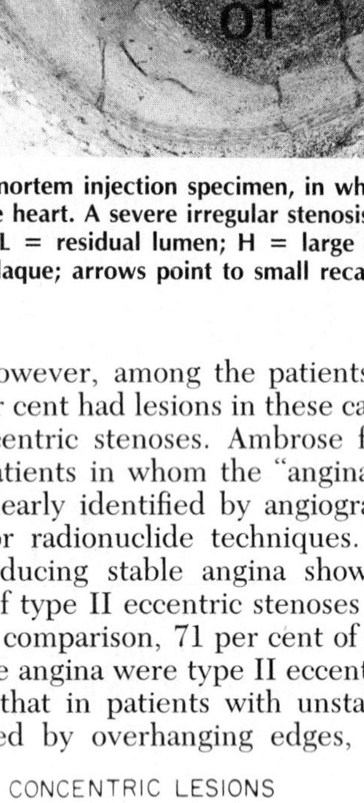

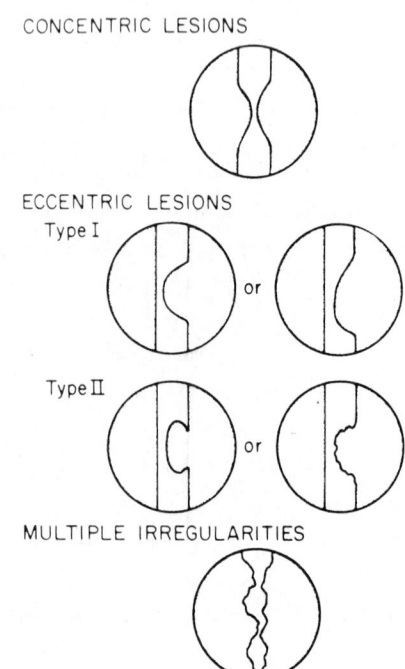

FIGURE 10–44. Method of Ambrose et al. of angiographically classifying coronary stenoses. See text for explanation. (From Ambrose, J.A., Winters, S.L., Arora, R.R., Haft, J.I., Goldstein, J., Rentrop, K.P., Gorlin, R., and Fuster, V.: Coronary angiographic morphology in myocardial infarction: A link between the pathogenesis of unstable angina and myocardial infarction. J. Am. Coll. Cardiol. 6:1233, 1985. Reprinted with permission of the American College of Cardiology.)

irregular borders, or multiple irregularities were more than three times as common as in patients with stable angina. They postulated that such lesions represent ruptured plaques or partially occlusive thrombi or a combination of the two.

A subsequent study by the same investigators[100] extended this angiographic classification to 41 patients with recent myocardial infarction who at angiography were found to have subtotally occluded infarct-related vessels. Twenty-seven of the 41 infarct vessels (66 per cent) were found to have a type II eccentric stenoses. Among 18 other noninfarct-related lesions in this group of patients, only 2 (11 per cent) had type II eccentric lesions. Another group of 23 patients were studied during acute myocardial infarction. All either had received intracoronary streptokinase and had reperfused (17 cases) or had subtotal occlusion before the streptokinase infusion (6 cases). Fourteen of the 23 infarct vessels (61 per cent) contained a type II eccentric stenosis, whereas only 1 of 11 (9 per cent) other noninfarct-related vessels with significant lesions had type II eccentric stenoses.

Wilson et al.[101] quantitatively assessed coronary stenoses at angiography in 40 patients falling into three clinical categories: recent myocardial infarction, recent onset of unstable angina in the presence of single vessel coronary disease, or stable angina. Lesions associated with unstable angina or recent myocardial infarction showed significantly greater degrees of ulceration than lesions not related to previous myocardial infarction or those associated with stable angina.

Bresnahan et al.[102] and Capone et al.[103] used somewhat different angiographic criteria in studying patients with unstable angina. Their studies, which produced similar results, addressed the question of the relative frequency with which intracoronary thrombi are found in patients with unstable and stable angina. Thrombi were considered to be present if the lesion contained an intraluminal filling defect surrounded largely by contrast material. Using this criterion, Bresnahan and colleagues noted the presence of intracoronary thrombi in 35 per cent of their patients with unstable angina, but in only 2.5 per cent of patients with stable angina. Capone et al. detected intracoronary thrombi in 37 per cent of patients with unstable angina but did not find them in any patients with stable angina.

In the authors' experience at the Brigham and Women's Hospital,[104] actual intraluminal thrombus was seen in 13 per cent of patients with unstable angina. However, the overall incidence of complicated atherosclerotic plaques (those with irregular or abruptly marginated borders or intraluminal filling defects) was 55 per cent. Thus, while our overall incidence of complicated plaques in unstable angina patients was similar to that found in the patients of Ambrose et al.,[99] our incidence of intraluminal thrombi was lower than that found by Bresnahan et al.[102] and Capone et al.[103] These differences undoubtedly reflect differences in interpretation of the angiographic findings among various authors.

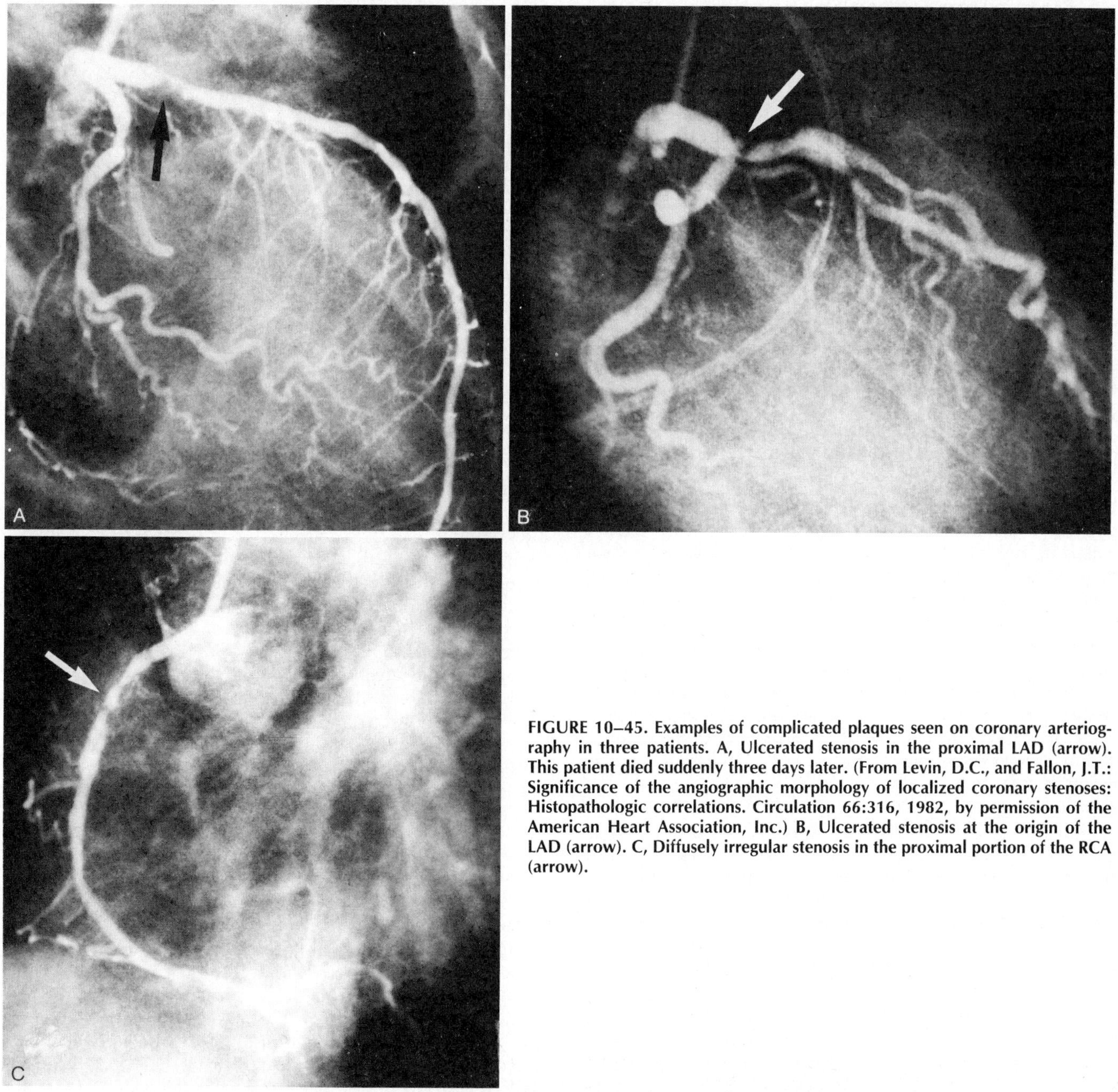

FIGURE 10–45. Examples of complicated plaques seen on coronary arteriography in three patients. A, Ulcerated stenosis in the proximal LAD (arrow). This patient died suddenly three days later. (From Levin, D.C., and Fallon, J.T.: Significance of the angiographic morphology of localized coronary stenoses: Histopathologic correlations. Circulation 66:316, 1982, by permission of the American Heart Association, Inc.) B, Ulcerated stenosis at the origin of the LAD (arrow). C, Diffusely irregular stenosis in the proximal portion of the RCA (arrow).

Figure 10–45 shows three examples of coronary arteriograms with what we would consider to be complicated plaques. All three patients had unstable angina and one died suddenly 3 days after the angiogram.

What seems clear from these correlative studies[99–104] is that while the severity of luminal narrowing appears to be similar in patients with stable or unstable angina, plaque morphology differs considerably between the two groups. Patients with unstable angina have a much higher incidence of lesions which are probably complicated atherosclerotic plaques. Such lesions include those with plaque rupture, intraplaque hemorrhage, or partially occluding thrombi. The prognostic significance of the detection of such lesions at coronary arteriography is not yet entirely clear. They may well place the patient at greater risk of myocardial infarction or sudden death. However, this hypothesis remains to be proven by additional clinical studies.

ARTERIOGRAPHIC ASSESSMENT OF RISK OF CORONARY ARTERIAL DISEASE

In addition to the possible role of plaque morphology in determining risk, there are several more traditional criteria which have been applied previously. The simplest method is to categorize patients by the number of diseased vessels.[105] The most comprehensive study of survival using this approach is that of the Coronary Artery Surgery Study (CASS) registry.[106] This study analyzed 4-year survival of 20,088 patients enrolled between 1975 and 1979 and treated medically thereafter. The 4-year survival rate for patients with more than 70 per cent diameter reduction of one coronary artery was 92 per cent. For patients with two vessel disease survival was 84 per cent, and for three-vessel disease it was 68 per cent. The CASS investigators found, however, that left ventricular ejection fraction (EF) was a more important predictor of survival. Thus, patients with one-vessel disease and an EF of over 50 per cent had 95 per cent 4-year survival. If EF ranged from 35 to 49 per cent, survival was 91 per cent, and if EF was less than 35 per cent, it dropped to 74 per cent. In patients with two-vessel disease, survival rates at 4 years were 93 per cent, 83 per cent, and 57 per cent in these three EF categories. In patients with three-vessel disease, survival rates at 4 years were 82 per cent, 71 per cent, and 50 per cent, respectively.

More recently, Califf et al.[107] described a useful "jeopardy score" to assess the prognostic significance of the arteriographic findings in 462 consecutive nonsurgically treated patients with at least 75 per cent diameter stenosis of at least one coronary artery. Patients with main LCA stenosis were excluded. To determine jeopardy score, the coronary circulation was considered as six arterial segments: the LAD, its major diagonal branch, its first major septal branch, the left circumflex artery, its major obtuse marginal branch, and the posterior descending branch of the RCA. Each segment with a 75 per cent or greater diameter reduction was given a score of 2 points, and each additional segment distal to such a stenosis was also given a score of 2 points. Thus, for example, a patient with 75 per cent stenosis of the LAD proximal to both the first septal and major diagonal branches would be assigned a score of 6–2 points for the LAD, 2 points for the septal branch, and 2 points for the diagonal branch. Thus, the maximal jeopardy score in any patient was 12. The results, according to both number of diseased vessels and jeopardy score, are shown in Table 10–1. By taking into account the quantity of myocardium at risk, the jeopardy score appears to provide a more reliable estimate of prognosis than does simply the number of diseased vessels. Other scoring systems for assessing prognosis based upon arteriographic findings are those of Gensini[108] and Friesinger et al.[109]

TABLE 10–1 FIVE-YEAR SURVIVAL BASED ON NUMBER OF DISEASED VESSELS AND JEOPARDY SCORE

	Jeopardy Score					
	2	4	6	8	10	12
One-vessel disease	0.97	1.0	0.84			
Two-vessel disease		0.86	0.82	0.80	0.72	
Three-vessel disease			1.0	0.77	0.75	0.55
All patients	0.97	0.95	0.85	0.78	0.75	0.56

From Califf, R. M., et al.: Prognostic value of a coronary artery jeopardy score. J. Am. Coll. Cardiol. 5:1055, 1985. Reprinted by permission of the American College of Cardiology.

Patients with significant stenosis of the main LCA are clearly in a higher risk category. Conley et al.[110] found that cumulative survival among a group of medically treated patients with more than 70 per cent diameter stenosis of the LCA was 72 per cent at 1 year and only 41 per cent at 3 years. The prognosis in patients with LCA stenosis of between 50 and 70 per cent was somewhat more favorable (91 per cent survival at 1 year and 66 per cent survival at 3 years). Takaro et al.[111] documented a cumulative survival at 42 months of 48 per cent in patients with at least 75 per cent main LCA stenosis on medical therapy, compared with 83 per cent survival in patients undergoing coronary bypass surgery. Campeau et al.[112] have also documented improved survival at 7 years in patients with LCA stenosis undergoing bypass surgery, compared with medical therapy. As a result of these and other similar studies, it is now widely accepted that the presence of main LCA stenosis is an indication for immediate bypass surgery.

Coronary arteriography and left ventriculography also help identify risk in patients who have survived recent myocardial infarction. Sanz et al.[113] studied 259 consecutive male survivors under age 60 who were catheterized a month after infarction and then followed for an extended period of time. They found that in patients with a normal ejection fraction (EF), survival was uniformly high (over 95 per cent), regardless of the number of diseased vessels. It remained high in patients with EF's between 21 to 49 per cent who had one-vessel and two-vessel disease. In patients with three-vessel disease and EF from 21 to 49 per cent, and in all patients with an EF of 20 per cent or less, 4-year survival was significantly reduced. DeFeyter et al.[114] evaluated 179 patients in a similar manner. During a mean follow-up period of 28 months, the mortality rate was 22 per cent in patients with an EF less than 30 per cent or three-vessel disease, but was only 1 per cent in patients with an EF greater than 30 per cent and either one or two diseased vessels.

CORONARY BYPASS ANGIOGRAPHY

Angiography following coronary bypass surgery is commonly performed to evaluate patients with recurrent angina. Since it is not possible to determine clinically whether symptoms are the result of compromise of the grafts or progression of disease in the native coronary arteries, careful angiographic evaluation of both is necessary.

TECHNIQUE OF CORONARY BYPASS ANGIOGRAPHY. Catheterization of coronary bypass grafts may be techni-

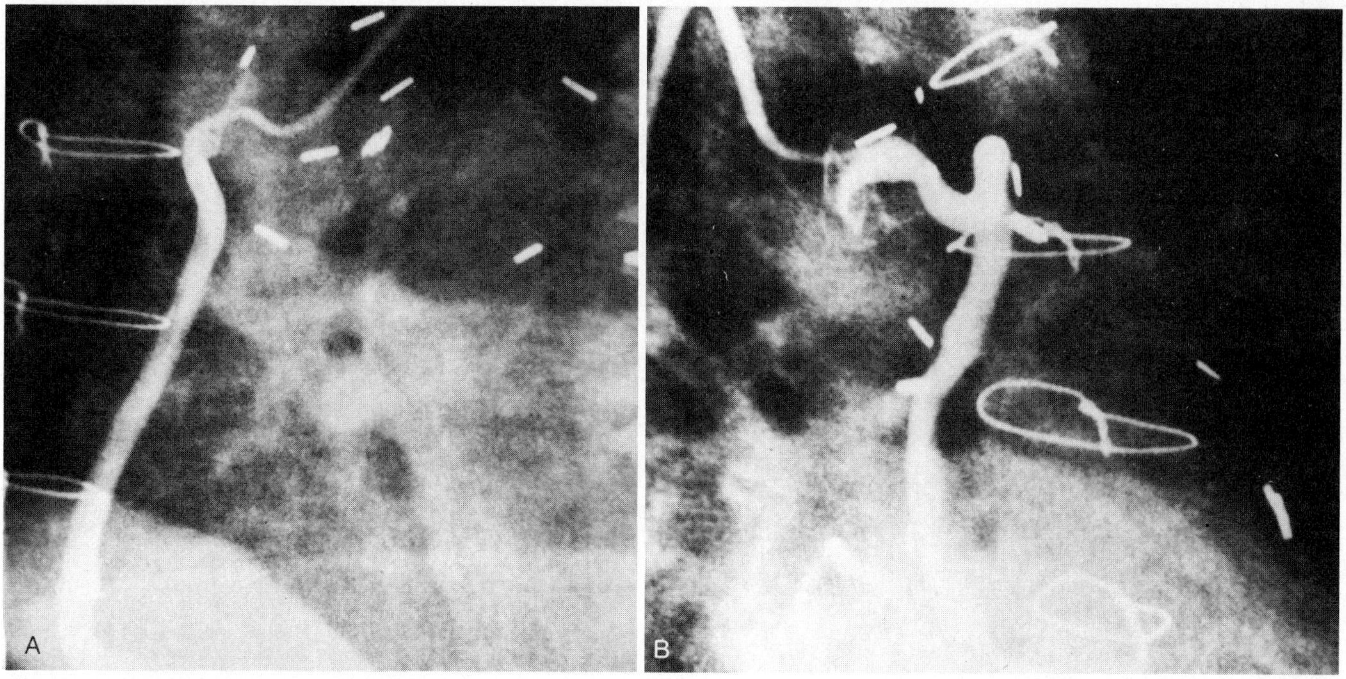

FIGURE 10–46. *A*, LAO angiogram of a saphenous vein bypass from the aorta to the distal RCA. *B*, RAO angiogram of a saphenous vein bypass from the aorta to the obtuse marginal branch of the circumflex artery. Both these angiograms utilized a No. 2 right Amplatz catheter.

cally more difficult than catheterization of the native coronary arteries because the locations of graft ostia are not totally predictable unless they are marked with surgical clips. However, even if clips are not used, or if they migrate, the experienced angiographer can usually successfully locate the ostia.

Saphenous vein grafts (SVG) from the aorta to the distal RCA are usually placed so they originate from the right anterolateral aspect of the aorta, whereas SVG's to the LAD and circumflex arteries are usually attached to the anterior aspect of the aorta. To catheterize SVG's, the authors routinely use No. 1 or 2 right Amplatz catheters via a percutaneous femoral approach. To enter right coronary SVG's, the patient is positioned in the LAO projection (Fig. 10–46*A*). To enter SVG's to either the LAD or circumflex arteries, the patient is positioned in the RAO projection (Fig. 10–46*B*). With the patient in the appropriate position, slow movement of the catheter tip up and down the aorta with varying degrees of rotation will usually result in entry into the graft, which is usually signified by an abrupt outward movement of the tip. When this occurs, a small test injection of contrast material will verify that the catheter is in the SVG. Even if the graft is occluded, the occlusion generally does not extend all the way back to the ostium itself. Usually a small stump remains into which the catheter tip can pass. The stump can be demonstrated by injection of a small amount of contrast (Fig. 10–47) and invariably indicates total graft occlusion. If neither a patent graft nor a stump can be located, it may be necessary to perform an ascending aortogram (preferably using biplane cineangiography) in an attempt at visualization.

Internal mammary arteries (IMA) are now being used for coronary bypass with increasing frequency, as a result of evidence that they have significantly higher patency rates than SVG's.[115, 116] To catheterize the IMA, a specially designed J-shaped catheter, usually referred to simply as the "femoral-internal mammary artery catheter" by the commercial manufacturers, is used via the percutaneous femoral approach. Rotation of the catheter tip in the aortic arch usually results in entry into the innominate artery or left subclavian artery. A guidewire is then passed through the catheter to a point in the subclavian artery distal to the expected origin of the IMA. The catheter is then advanced to this point, then slowly withdrawn and rotated anteriorly until it enters the IMA. Figure 10–48

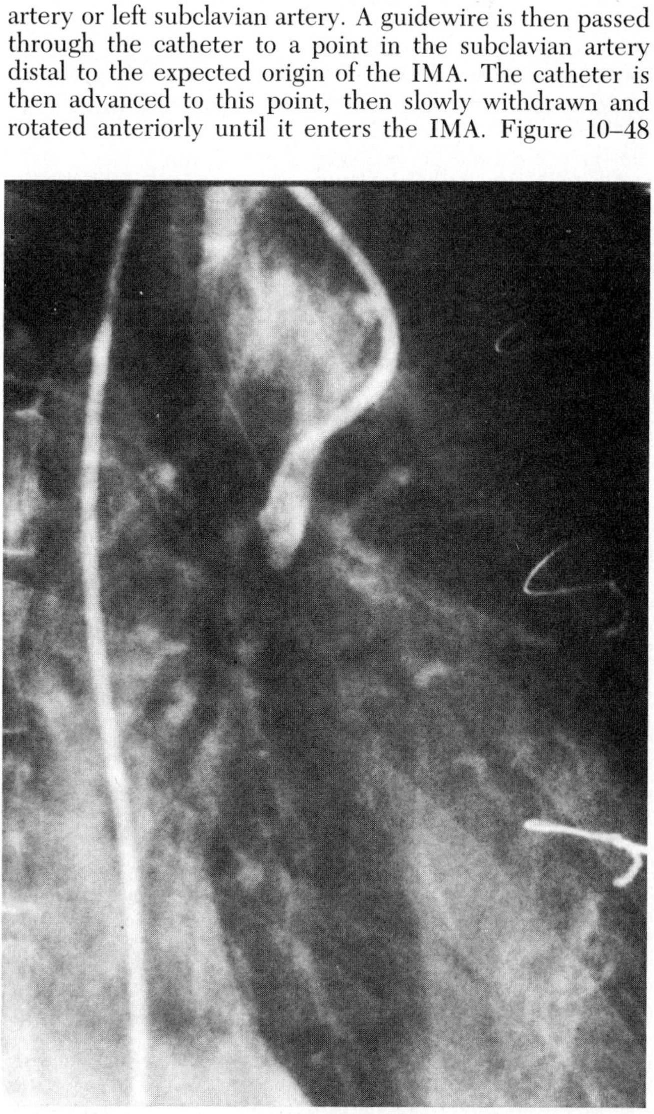

FIGURE 10–47. Stump of an occluded right coronary bypass.

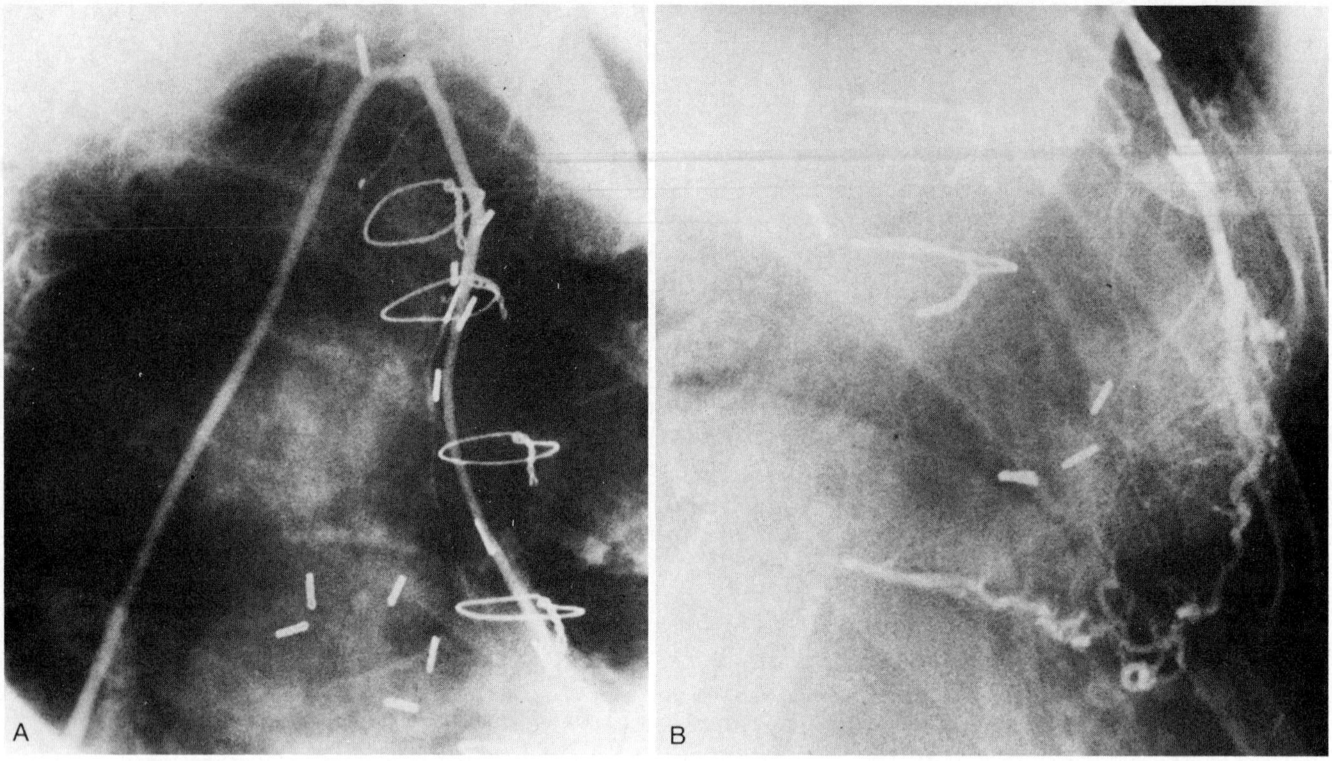

FIGURE 10–48. Angiogram of an internal mammary artery-to-LAD bypass. *A*, Proximal portion of the graft, seen in the RAO projection. *B*, Distal anastomosis of the internal mammary artery with the LAD.

shows an angiogram of a left IMA to LAD graft. Internal mammary arteriograms can be quite painful because contrast enters branches leading to thoracic wall muscles, and the patient should be forewarned about this.

Angiographic studies of grafts must not only assess their patency, but also the status of the distal anastomoses. It has been shown that approximately 10 per cent of patent grafts are compromised by significant stenoses[117]; these stenoses are most likely to occur at the distal anastomosis (Fig. 10–49).

GRAFT PATENCY. Considerable data from several large clinical trials regarding the short- and long-term patency rates of saphenous vein coronary bypass grafts have been reported. In the CASS trial, patency of SVG's was 90 per cent within 60 days after surgery; this decreased to 82 per cent at approximately 18 months after surgery, and then appeared to remain stable over the next 3 years.[117] Similar results were obtained in the European Coronary Surgery Study, in which SVG's were noted to have a 77 per cent patency rate on studies performed from 9 to 18 months after surgery.[118] Among a larger series of patients at the Montreal Heart Institute, SVG patency at one year was approximately 80 per cent and there was no further reduction in patency between 1 and 6 years after operation.[117] The most comprehensive longer term experience comes from the same group. By the time 10 to 12 years had elapsed after surgery, the patency rate of SVG's had dropped to 63 per cent.[117] Moreover, almost half the grafts still patent showed significant atherosclerotic changes.

The Cleveland Clinic group[115] compared patency rates of SVG's and IMA grafts. After a mean follow-up period of 36 months, the patency rate for IMA grafts was 96 per cent. The patency rate for SVG's at a mean follow-up period of 39 months was 77 per cent. At 7 to 10 years after surgery, IMA graft patency has been shown to range from 85 to 95 per cent.[115, 119] Furthermore, IMA grafts are only rarely involved by atherosclerosis. For these reasons, there is an increasing tendency among surgeons to choose the IMA for coronary bypass.[116]

SVG occlusion occurring within one month of surgery is almost invariably due to thrombosis.[117] Occlusions that occur between 1 month and 1 year following operation are primarily the result of intimal smooth muscle cell proliferation, which probably follows early platelet deposition on the walls of the graft. Figure 10–50 is an example of fibrous initimal proliferation developing within 10 months after surgery. Chesebro et al.[120] have shown that this process can be favorably altered by the early and continued administration of dipyridamole and aspirin, with significant reduction in late SVG occlusion rates. Late graft occlusions more than 1 year following operation appear to be caused by atherosclerosis, which in turn probably results from lipid incorporation in areas of initimal proliferation. Graft atherosclerosis therefore seems to be a continuum from early platelet deposition to intimal smooth muscle cell proliferation to late incorporation of lipid into a fully developed atherosclerotic plaque.

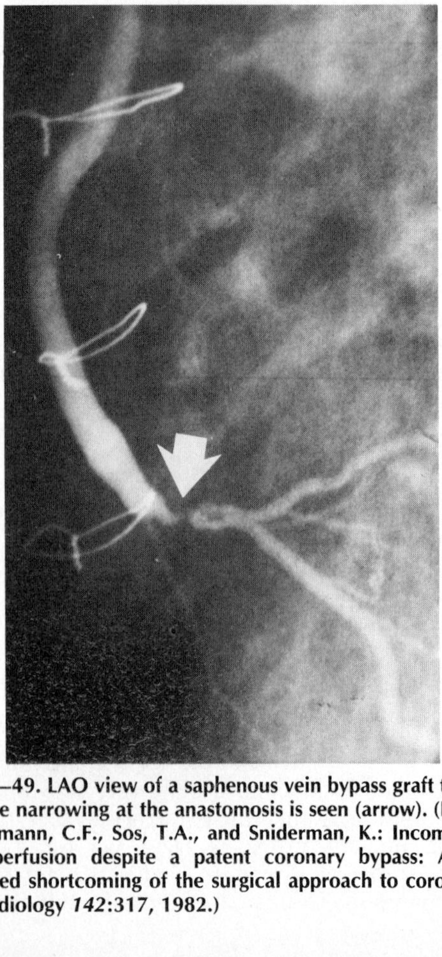

FIGURE 10–49. LAO view of a saphenous vein bypass graft to the distal RCA. Severe narrowing at the anastomosis is seen (arrow). (From Levin, D.C., Beckmann, C.F., Sos, T.A., and Sniderman, K.: Incomplete myocardial reperfusion despite a patent coronary bypass: A generally unrecognized shortcoming of the surgical approach to coronary artery disease. Radiology *142*:317, 1982.)

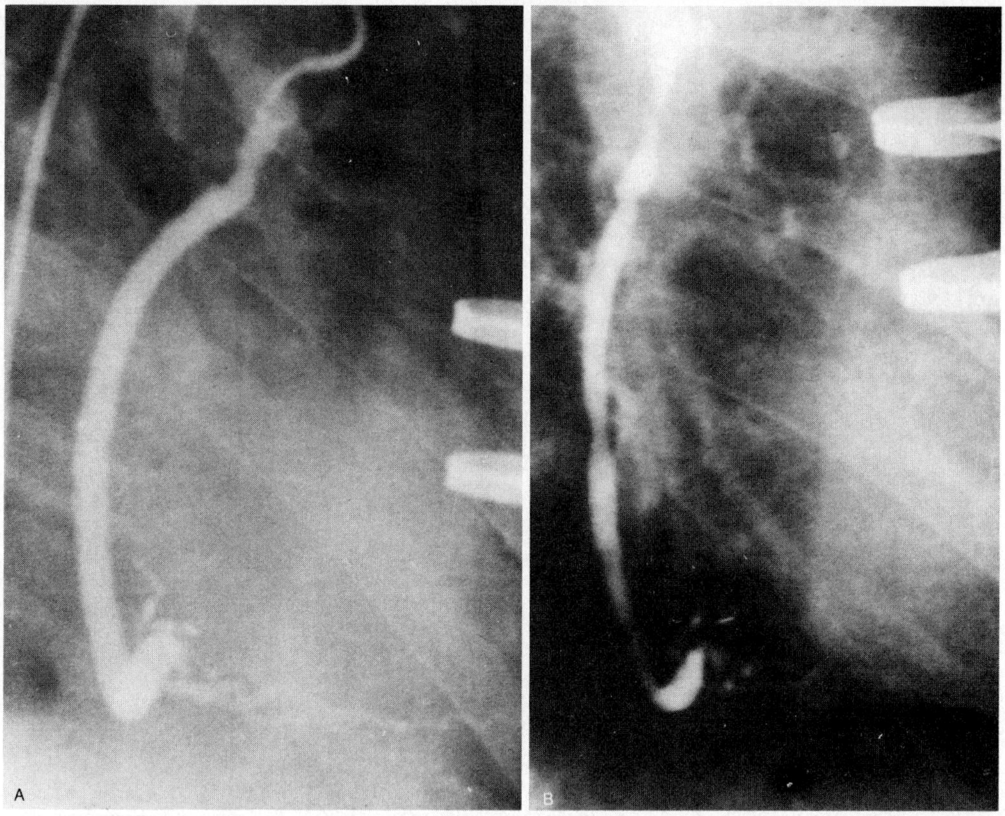

FIGURE 10–50. Fibrous intimal proliferation developing in a saphenous vein bypass graft to the RCA within ten months following operation. *A*, Graft angiogram four weeks after operation. No significant narrowing is seen. *B*, Graft angiogram ten months after surgery. Multiple areas of diffuse narrowing are seen along the course of the graft. (From Levin, D.C., Beckmann, C.F., Sos, T.A., and Sniderman, K.: Incomplete myocardial reperfusion despite a patent coronary bypass: A generally unrecognized shortcoming of the surgical approach to coronary artery disease. Radiology *142*:317, 1982.)

THROMBOLYSIS IN ACUTE MYOCARDIAL INFARCTION: ANGIOGRAPHIC ASPECTS

(See also p. 1253)

One of the most dramatic developments in the treatment of heart disease during the last decade has been the transformation of coronary arteriography from a strictly diagnostic to a therapeutic modality as well. Percutaneous transluminal coronary angioplasty (PTCA) and the delivery of thrombolytic agents directly into coronary arteries are now widely used methods of treating chronic and acute myocardial ischemia. PTCA is discussed in Chapter 40; the indications for thrombolysis and its effects on ventricular function and survival are discussed in Chapter 38. In this section, we will briefly review the technique and certain angiographic aspects of intracoronary and intravenous administration of thrombolytic agents in acute myocardial infarction.

Although preliminary work had been done in Europe and the Soviet Union on streptokinase (SK) therapy of myocardial infarction, the technique of intracoronary SK administration did not come into widespread use in this country until 1981. In that year, Rentrop et al.,[121] Mathey et al.,[122] and Ganz et al.[123] demonstrated the efficacy of this approach. The techniques used by these three groups have formed the basis for that used in most subsequent studies.

TECHNIQUE OF INTRACORONARY STREPTOKINASE ADMINISTRATION. Standard coronary arteriography is performed to identify the infarct vessel. This is usually readily apparent as an abrupt total thrombotic occlusion of a major coronary artery, or less commonly a subtotal occlusion. The patient is heparinized at the start of the procedure and is given a corticosteroid preparation to offset possible allergic reactions to SK, if that is the thrombolytic agent to be used. Nitroglycerin is administered through the coronary artery catheter in doses of 100 to 500 μg; these may be repeated frequently during the procedure. In a small minority of cases, nitroglycerin alone relieves the total occlusion and results in successful reperfusion. In the large majority of cases this does not occur, and SK is then administered through the coronary catheter in doses ranging from 2000 to 5000 units per minute. The infusion is usually continued for between 1 and 2 hours, with the total dose ranging from 125,000 to 250,000 units. Mathey et al.[122] also attempted to recanalize the infarct vessel by passing a guidewire through the thrombus to mechanically disrupt it. Others have used this technique on occasion, but it has not become a routine part of the procedure in most institutions. Ganz et al.[123] passed a small 2 French catheter through the outer coronary artery catheter and attempted to imbed it directly into the thrombus for superselective infusion of SK. This technique likewise is used in some laboratories but is not routine practice. Some investigators inject an initial bolus of 10,000 to 15,000 units of SK prior to starting the continuous infusion; others do not. If reperfusion is successfully achieved, the patient is generally maintained on heparin for the duration of hospitalization, and is then switched to oral anticoagulation.

ARTERIOGRAPHIC FINDINGS BEFORE AND AFTER STREPTOKINASE INFUSION. Rentrop[124] has reviewed his own material and that from 10 other centers to determine the frequency of total as opposed to subtotal occlusion of the infarct artery at initial arteriography. The aggregate data

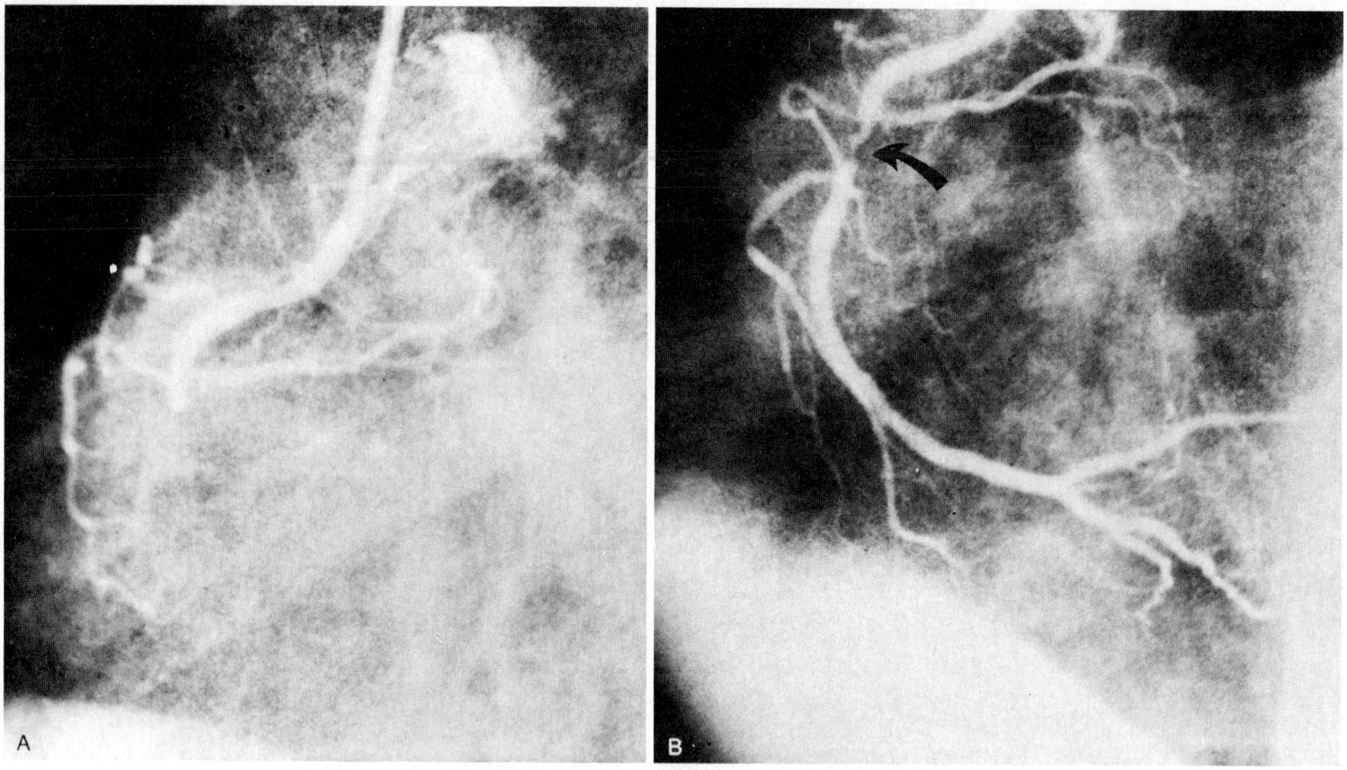

FIGURE 10–51. Intracoronary streptokinase therapy in a patient with acute inferior myocardial infarction. *A*, LAO right coronary arteriogram showing abrupt total occlusion of the proximal RCA. *B*, After a one-hour infusion of streptokinase into the RCA at 2000 units/min, thrombolysis has occurred and antegrade flow has been restored. However, a severe ulcerated stenosis remains at the site of previous occlusion (arrow).

in 847 patients revealed that total occlusion was present in 78 per cent and subtotal occlusion in 22 per cent. In a very small minority of the latter group, the degree of obstruction is only mild or moderate. Presumably, in these cases, the cause of infarction is either spasm or a thrombus which has lysed rapidly prior to the angiographic procedure.

Recanalization rates with intracoronary SK administration have varied considerably. Pooled data from 10 studies[124] demonstrated that recanalization occurred in 314 of 426 patients (74 per cent) and that the rates in individual studies varied from 60 to 94 per cent. In the vast majority of patients in whom successful reperfusion can be achieved, a high-grade residual stenosis is present at the end of the procedure. The spectrum of results is illustrated in Figures 10–51 and 10–52. In the first of these patients, successful

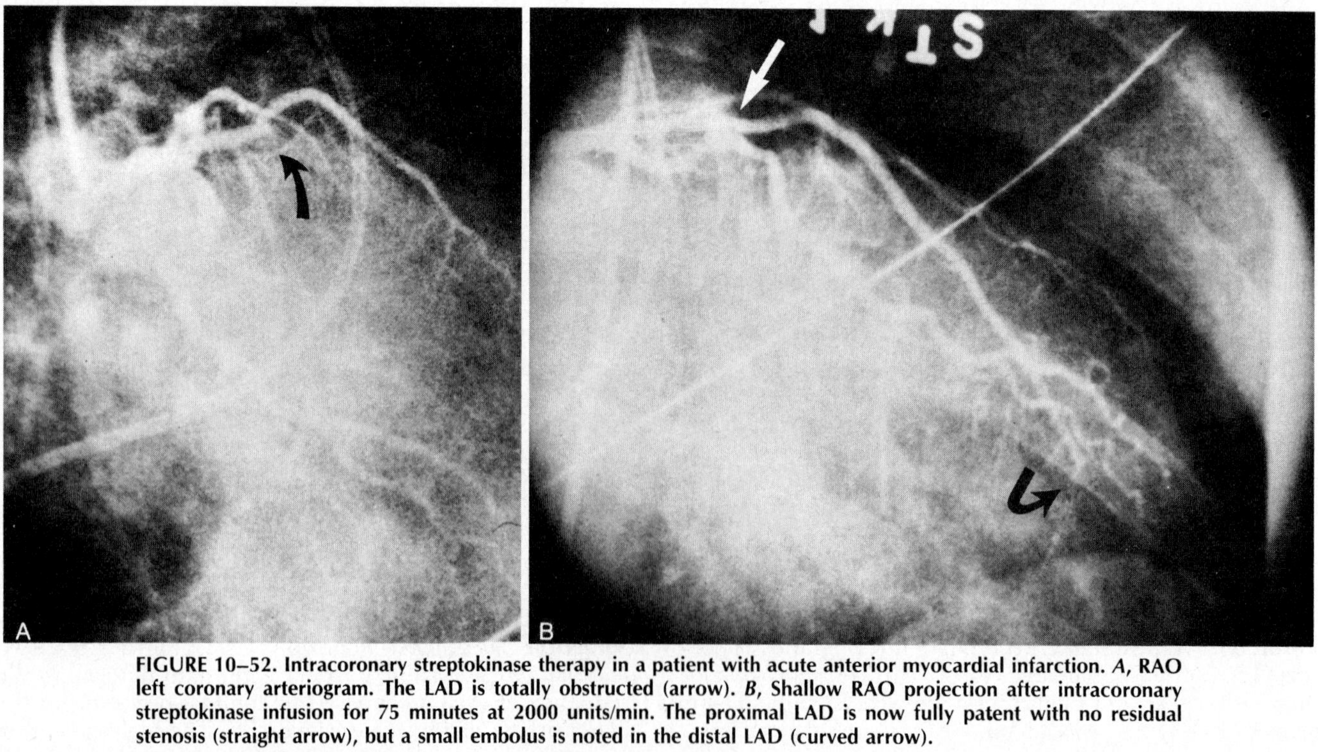

FIGURE 10–52. Intracoronary streptokinase therapy in a patient with acute anterior myocardial infarction. *A*, RAO left coronary arteriogram. The LAD is totally obstructed (arrow). *B*, Shallow RAO projection after intracoronary streptokinase infusion for 75 minutes at 2000 units/min. The proximal LAD is now fully patent with no residual stenosis (straight arrow), but a small embolus is noted in the distal LAD (curved arrow).

reperfusion of a totally obstructed RCA was achieved, leaving a severe and probably ulcerated stenosis at the conclusion of the procedure. In the second, although total obstruction of the LAD was present initially, by the end of the procedure there was no apparent residual narrowing at all. Complete absence of underlying stenosis, as in the latter case, is highly unusual.

NATURAL HISTORY OF CORONARY LESIONS AFTER SUCCESSFUL THROMBOLYSIS. In assessing the efficacy of thrombolytic therapy, a crucial question relates to the natural history of the residual lesions following successful thrombolysis. Several studies have shown[125, 126] that approximately one-third of recanalized vessels reocclude within the first 10 days after therapy. Gash et al.[126] reported that early reocclusion occurred only if the vessel contained some residual thrombus after therapy, and was twice as likely to occur if the residual stenosis was greater than 75 per cent than if it was less severe. Longer term follow-up of these lesions was provided by Schröder et al.[127] Sixty-three patients who had a patent infarct-related artery 4 weeks after intravenous SK for acute myocardial infarction were followed up for a mean of 34 ± 10 months. Approximately one-third of these patients had clinical courses complicated by death or the need for either coronary bypass surgery or PTCA. The incidence of reocclusion in this group was not known. Among patients with clinically uncomplicated long-term courses, repeat coronary arteriography 26 ± 9 months later showed that reocclusion occurred in approximately half the group. Only a small minority of these experienced reinfarction. Lesions in the other half remained stable or decreased in severity.

INTRAVENOUS VERSUS INTRACORONARY THROMBOLYTIC THERAPY. There is an obvious logistic advantage in administering the thrombolytic agent by the intravenous route in patients with acute myocardial infarction. Treatment does not hinge upon the ready availability of a cardiac catheterization laboratory, and the delay necessitated by the procedure can be avoided. A number of studies comparing intracoronary and intravenous SK administration have been carried out, and the results are somewhat conflicting. In the experience of Valentine et al.,[128] efficacy of the two methods was approximately equal. However, Rogers et al.[129] found that successful thrombolysis was achieved in significantly fewer patients receiving intravenous SK administration. A recent multicenter trial of high-dose (1.5 million units) intravenous SK demonstrated that successful reperfusion occurred only in approximately 40 per cent of patients and that one-quarter of them had reocclusion during the subsequent 10 days.[130]

Streptokinase has certain drawbacks as a thrombolytic agent.[131] The most important of these are that it is antigenic and induces a systemic lytic state. As a result, efforts have been made to develop newer, more fibrin-specific agents. The one most widely used in this country is tissue-type plasminogen activator (tPA). A recent clinical trial compared intravenous SK with intravenous tPA in acute myocardial infarction.[132] This study utilized careful angiographic grading of the degree of perfusion before and after therapy. Grade 0 indicated no flow beyond the occlusion. Grade 1 indicated a slow trickle of contrast agent past the occlusion with incomplete distal opacification. Grade 2 signified complete distal opacification beyond the obstruction but delayed filling and clearance from the distal bed. Grade 3 indicated prompt and complete distal filling and clearance of contrast agent. Reperfusion was considered successful only if the patient demonstrated grade 2 or grade 3 perfusion after treatment. Sixty-two per cent of patients with initially occluded vessels (Grade 0 to 1) treated with tPA had successful reperfusion, while only 31 per cent of SK-treated patients had reperfusion. The study concluded that intravenous tPA can lead to recanalization at rates similar to those achieved with intracoronary SK, without the inconvenience, risk, cost, or delay associated with acute catheterization.

It is likely that thrombolytic therapy for most patients with early infarction will involve intravenous injection of a relatively fibrin-specific thrombolytic agent. Intracoronary administration of thrombolytic agents will probably be limited to patients who develop infarction in the catheterization laboratory or elsewhere in the hospital, as well as in patients in whom acute myocardial infarction is treated by means of primary PTCA and in whom residual thrombus is apparent.

DIGITAL SUBTRACTION CORONARY ARTERIOGRAPHY

(See also p. 356)

Until the early 1980's, cine and sheet films were the standard methods of recording and archiving radiographic images. More recently, digital subtraction angiography (DSA) has been developed. This video-based, computer-assisted method of imaging, which avoids the use of film, is being evaluated as a possible replacement for standard cineangiography of the coronary arteries. This complex technology has been described in considerable detail elsewhere[133–135]; here some of the technological aspects and potential advantages of coronary DSA will be briefly summarized.

At the output phosphor of the image intensifier, a light image is created. The image is focused upon the target plate of the video camera pickup tube, where it is converted to a charge pattern. The charge at each point is proportional to the amount of incident light. The charge pattern of the entire target plate is "read out" every one-thirtieth of a second by a scanning electron beam. The readout is accomplished on a line-by-line basis, analogous to reading a book on a line-by-line basis. At each successive point along each of the so-called raster lines, electrical current flows with a voltage proportional to the charge at that point. This rapid temporal variation in voltage creates the analog video image seen with standard fluoroscopy and also serves as the input to the digital system. An analog-to-digital converter samples the voltage at specified intervals along the raster line and assigns a binary digit according to the analog voltage level at each point. The number of samplings along each raster line determines the number of horizontal pixels (picture elements). In the DSA systems most commonly used currently, 512 samples are collected along each line. These systems utilize video cameras having 525 raster lines, 512 of which are used as pixels in the vertical dimension. This creates a 512 × 512 matrix. DSA resolution in the horizontal direction is therefore determined by the sampling frequency of the analog-to-digital converter and the band width of the video camera. Resolution in the vertical dimension is determined by the number of raster lines. Commercial manufacturers have recently attempted to improve spatial resolution of DSA systems by creating 1024 × 1024 matrices, in which 1024 samples are taken along each line and there are 1024 raster lines.

The binary digit assigned to each pixel is entered into the image processor memory at the specific site for that pixel. A mask image is created just before the injection of contrast material and stored in memory. This mask image contains bone, gas, and soft tissue image information. Several seconds later, a contrast image is created in which the arteries are filled with dilute contrast agent but which contains the same bone, gas, and soft tissue information as the mask. For each pixel, the computer then subtracts the binary digit of the mask image from that of the contrast image. The difference is the subtracted image containing only the opacified arteries. The optical density of these arteries can be enhanced by changing the window and level settings. Images can be processed in other ways as well. For example, edges of blood vessels can be enhanced by low-frequency suppression filtering, and alternate masks can be chosen to improve the match with the contrast image. Some systems are now available which utilize only the raw video information, without subtraction. Figure 10–53 shows two digital coronary angiograms from the same patient, one (prior to angioplasty) utilizing only the unsubtracted video image, and the other (after angioplasty) utilizing subtraction.

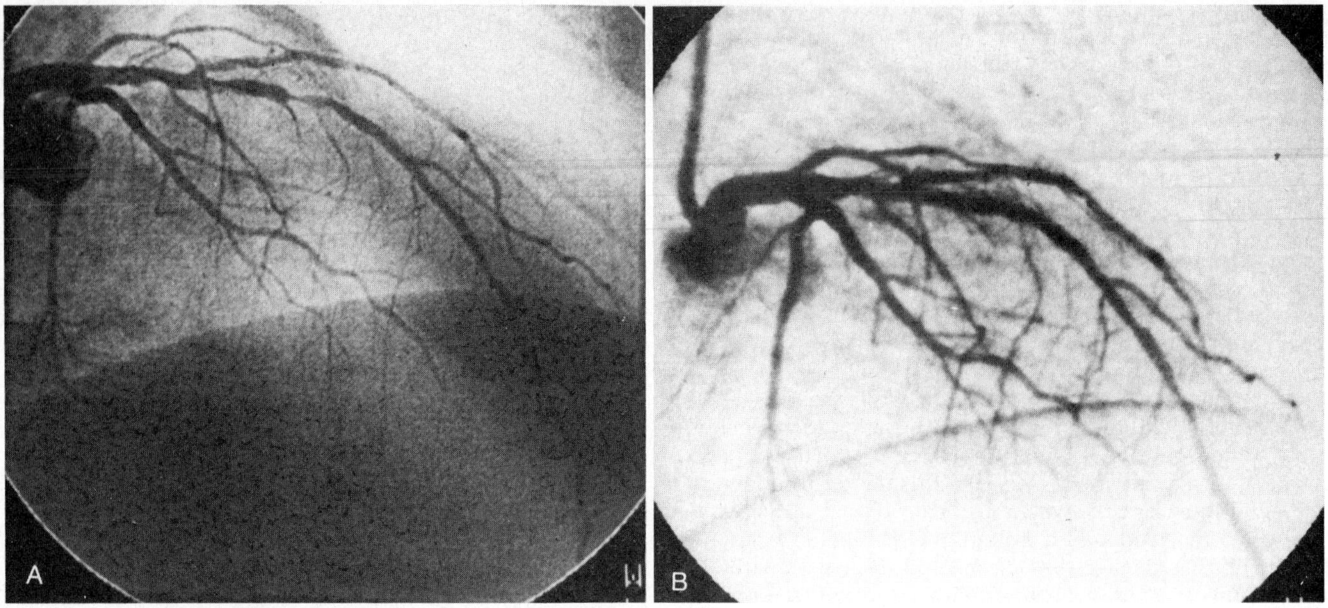

FIGURE 10–53. RAO cranial digital coronary arteriograms of the LCA. *A*, Unsubtracted video image prior to LAD angioplasty. *B*, Subtracted image in the same projection, following LAD angioplasty.

There are a number of potential and actual advantages to using DSA for coronary artery imaging: (1) It allows automated or semiautomated detection of the edges of blood vessels for improved quantification of the degree of coronary stenosis.[136, 137] (2) It has the potential to quantify coronary blood flow by analyzing temporal variations of optical density in myocardial or coronary artery pixels.[138, 139] (3) It helps alleviate the problem of undesirable background variations in optical density. (4) It has the ability to vary the window and level settings and thereby helps differentiate overlapped vessels and visualize lesions that might otherwise be obscured. (5) It can be used as a "road map" during PTCA.[140] These images are also available almost instantaneously, thus allowing the angiographer to ascertain the result of the procedure without delay. (6) It allows hard copy images to be made using a multiformat camera. These images can then be taken to the operating room to guide the surgeon during bypass operations, it can be sent to referring physicians, or it can be placed in the patient's medical record.

Digital subtraction left ventriculography can be performed by either venous or direct left ventricular injection of contrast. If venous injection is used, there are certain advantages. Premature ventricular contractions are avoided. Determination of chamber volume can be accomplished without the fluid volume artifacts produced by the injection of contrast material directly into the left ventricle. Right-sided injection facilitates mixing of contrast and blood and allows for more complete opacification of the left ventricle. Studies can easily be repeated periodically on outpatients to track the natural history or to monitor the effect of therapeutic regimens on left ventricular function. With either venous or direct left ventricular injection, automated analysis of ventricular volumes and function can be accomplished using computer technology.[141, 142] With direct left ventricular injection, a fourfold dilution in contrast material can be used. This reduction in contrast dose lessens the risk of the procedure, especially in patients with compromised cardiac or renal function.

DSA has certain important disadvantages as well. Spatial resolution is decreased, compared with cineangiography. Hardware and software are expensive and add significantly to the cost of catheterization laboratory equipment. Finally, storage and transfer of images is at present less convenient than with cine, although this may be alleviated as electronic archival and communications systems become more common in hospitals.

QUANTITATIVE CORONARY ARTERIOGRAPHY

The need for a reliable and accurate method of grading coronary stenoses has been demonstrated by numerous studies showing significant intra- and interobserver variation in grading severity of coronary stenoses[143–146] and poor correlation of angiographic and pathological findings.[147–149] A quantitative method for evaluation of coronary stenoses was introduced in 1977 by Brown et al.,[150] who used computerized analysis of hand-traced coronary artery images to assess the degree of vessel narrowing. Since that time considerable effort has been expended to develop a more consistent and effective method of quantitatively evaluating coronary arteriograms. Two important techniques have been developed. The first depends on computerized measurement of luminal dimensions using edge-detecting algorithms, and comparing "normal" vessel diameter to the diameter of a stenosis.[151, 152] Several steps are required for application of this technique. Initially a digital image must be obtained either directly or by digitizing a cine frame. Once digitized, the image may be adjusted to compensate for distortion and magnification produced by standard radiographic techniques. Semiautomatic or automatic edge-tracking techniques (Fig. 10–54) are then applied, and finally the computer measures the distance between vessel walls to determine the vessel diameter. The degree of stenosis is determined by comparing the diameter of the stenosis to that of the adjacent "normal" vessel. Most systems use the angiographic catheter as the scaling device to obtain actual luminal dimensions. Many obstacles to accurate measurements must be overcome. These include branching or crossing vessels in the area of the stenosis, variable background densities, poorly defined vessel edges caused by factors such as slow contrast injections and motion, and lesions which are not imaged in profile. Two orthogonal views are required to determine the area of an eccentric lesion.

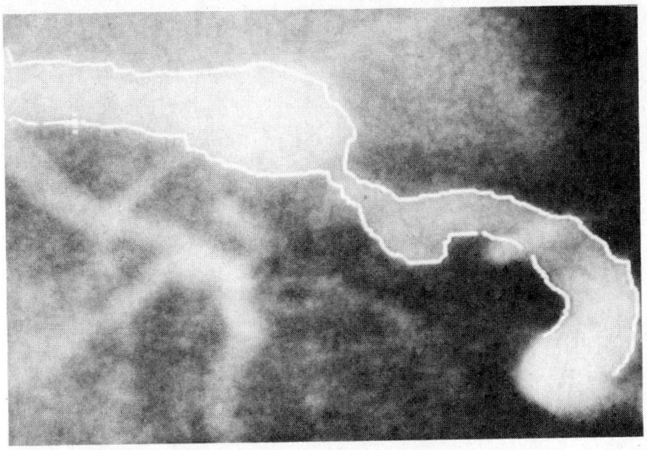

FIGURE 10–54. Coronary artery outline traced by an automatic edge-detecting program for quantitative arteriography.

The second approach to estimate the degree of arterial narrowing uses videodensitometry (computerized analysis of changes in contrast density caused by arterial stenoses).[153, 154] Changes in optical density produced by variable amounts of contrast within the vessel lumen are determined. The relative amount of contrast is less in stenotic regions since the cross-sectional area of the lumen is less, and this decrease is detected by a computer as a region of greater optical density (or greater degree of film blackening). Computer techniques are then utilized to estimate the degree of narrowing from this change in density. Although this technique is subject to most of the limitations of the edge-detecting method, it does have several advantages, including the necessity for only one view to determine the relative area of an eccentric stenosis. A constant rate of contrast injection is required as well as a homogeneous background, although nonuniform background densities can sometimes be subtracted by the computer before evaluation of vessel density.

These techniques are useful in studying the natural history as well as the short- and long-term effects of interventions on the coronary lumen. Their major limitations are cost, time required, and possible inaccuracies which may result if images are not obtained under optimal circumstances.

LEFT VENTRICULOGRAPHY AS AN ADJUNCT TO CORONARY ARTERIOGRAPHY

(See also Chap. 9)

Left ventriculography is an essential part of cardiac catheterization in most patients with known or suspected CAD because it allows evaluation of segmental and global myocardial function, and also demonstrates anatomical details of the ventricular chamber and associated valves. In patients with CAD, ventriculography provides evidence of the effect of coronary obstruction on myocardial contractility and it can reliably demonstrate complications resulting from myocardial infarction. In patients with cardiomyopathies and congenital or valvular heart disease, ventriculography is often helpful in establishing an accurate diagnosis and in classifying the disease properly. (See Chap. 6.)

Left ventriculography is performed from an arterial approach by passing a catheter across the aortic valve into the left ventricle. Ideally, it should be performed before coronary arteriography because of the depressant effect of radiographic contrast medium on myocardial function, which may last up to an hour following injection.[155] The average injection rate for ventriculography is 12 to 15 ml/sec for a total volume of 40 to 50 ml; however, this may be increased or decreased depending on the size of the left ventricle and the clinical status of the patient. The ventriculogram is imaged using the 9-inch mode of the image intensifier and 35-mm cine film at a rate of at least 30 frame/sec in the 30-degree RAO and 45- to 60-degree LAO projections. If only one view is possible, the RAO view is preferred. The LAO view may be angled 20 to 40 degrees cranially to profile optimally the ventricular cavity. This improves visualization of the septum and especially the ventricular outflow tract.

Ventricular injections of contrast medium adversely affect myocardial contractility and produce several hemodynamic changes.[156–158] In addition, there is rapid expansion of intravascular volume as water moves into the vascular system from the extravascular space due to the hypertonicity of most contrast media.[159, 160] These effects of contrast present some risk to patients with severely compromised myocardial function or with severe aortic stenosis. The hemodynamic effects of ventriculography can be minimized by using digital imaging with very small quantities of contrast material[161] or by using the newer nonionic agents (p. 271). Although injection of nonionic agents produces similar responses, the degree of hemodynamic change and myocardial toxicity is much less severe compared to the standard hypertonic agents.[16, 162–164]

Complications such as embolization from mural thrombus or valvular vegetations are possible, but a far more common cause of peripheral embolization is inadvertent injection of thrombus formed in or on the catheter. Routine heparinization may lower the incidence of this complication, especially if the procedure is prolonged, but careful technique is essential, and is probably the most important factor in avoiding this complication.

ABNORMALITIES OF VENTRICULAR CONTOUR. The ventricular contour can be divided into segments for purposes of analyzing myocardial motion (Fig. 10–55). Normally the left ventricular cavity is oval or ellipsoid in shape. The septum is free of trabeculations and is generally concave to the left ventricular cavity. The papillary muscles are best visualized during systole and appear as elongated filling defects on the diaphragmatic and anterior ventricular borders in the RAO view.

Localized abnormalities of ventricular contour include filling defects which usually represent thrombus. In most cases, ventricular thrombus is associated with severely hypokinetic, akinetic, or dyskinetic myocardial segments along the anterior wall or apex. At ventriculography, mural thrombus can range in appearance from a smooth defect following the contour of the left ventricle to an irregular polypoid mass extending into the left ventricular cavity. Thrombi which are pedunculated may be more prone to peripheral embolization.[165, 166] There are many causes for more generalized abnormalities of the ventricular contour.[167]

ABNORMALITIES OF VENTRICULAR FUNCTION. Considerable intra- and interobserver variability have been documented in the interpretation of segmental wall motion.[168–170] Several factors may be responsible for this variability, including cardiac rotation and positional changes during the cardiac cycle. Improved accuracy and consistency have been demonstrated when more objective methods are used than with visual assessment and qualitative grading.[169–172] However, segmental wall motion is not always an accurate predictor of coronary disease. Patients with severe CAD often have normal ventriculograms. On the other hand, patients may have segmental

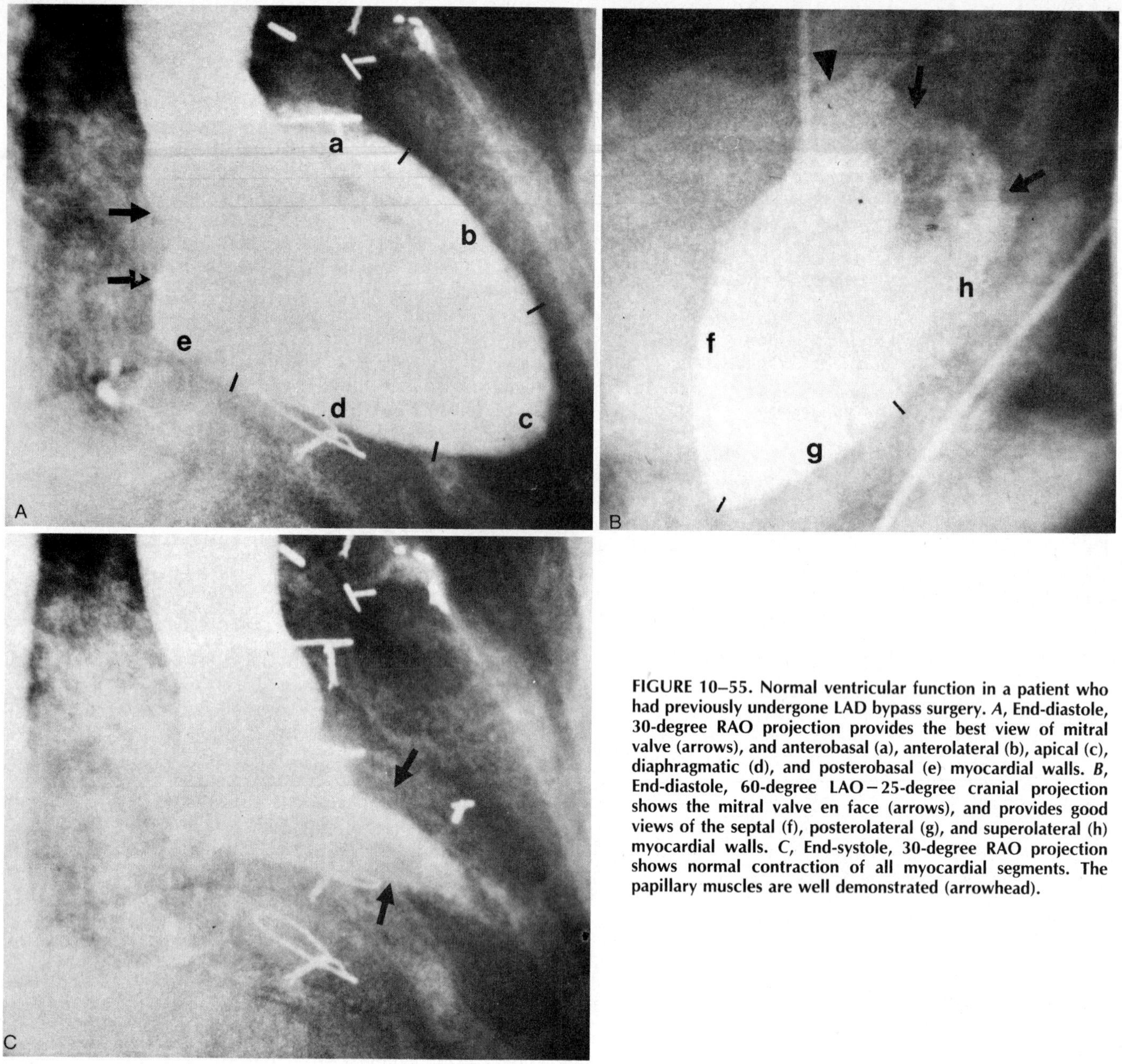

FIGURE 10–55. Normal ventricular function in a patient who had previously undergone LAD bypass surgery. *A*, End-diastole, 30-degree RAO projection provides the best view of mitral valve (arrows), and anterobasal (a), anterolateral (b), apical (c), diaphragmatic (d), and posterobasal (e) myocardial walls. *B*, End-diastole, 60-degree LAO – 25-degree cranial projection shows the mitral valve en face (arrows), and provides good views of the septal (f), posterolateral (g), and superolateral (h) myocardial walls. *C*, End-systole, 30-degree RAO projection shows normal contraction of all myocardial segments. The papillary muscles are well demonstrated (arrowhead).

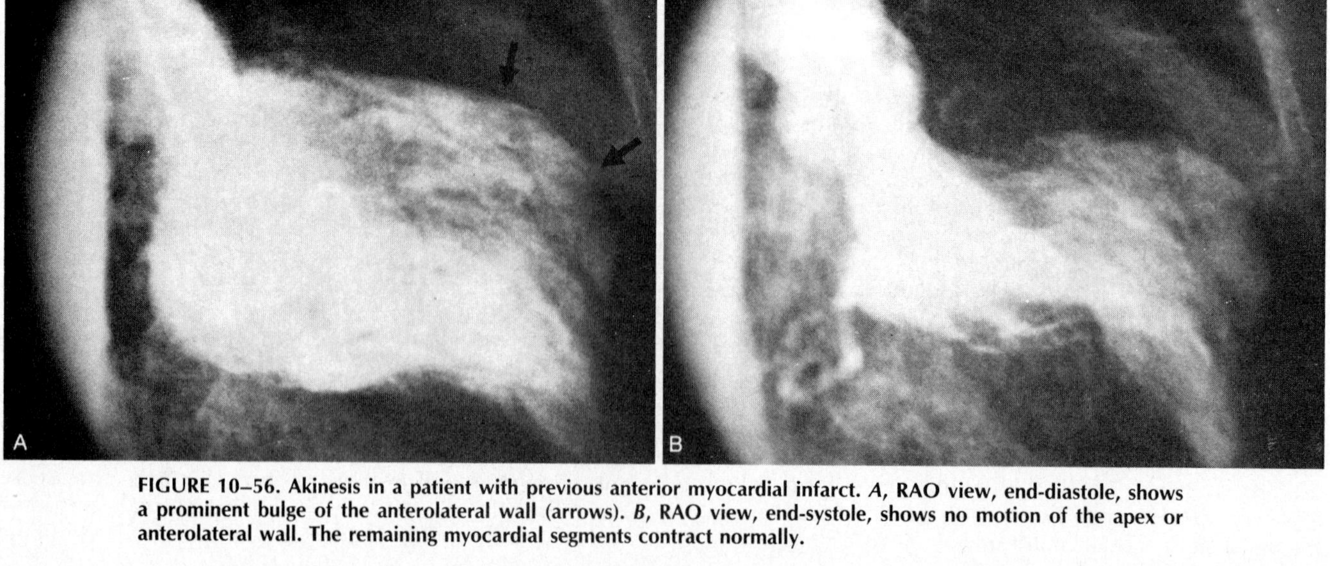

FIGURE 10–56. Akinesis in a patient with previous anterior myocardial infarct. *A*, RAO view, end-diastole, shows a prominent bulge of the anterolateral wall (arrows). *B*, RAO view, end-systole, shows no motion of the apex or anterolateral wall. The remaining myocardial segments contract normally.

abnormalities in a wide variety of conditions, in the presence of normal coronary arteries.[173–175]

Global myocardial function is an important indicator of CAD severity and prognosis. Accurate calculation of ventricular volumes is essential for reliable determination of stroke volume and ejection fraction.[176, 177]

Regional myocardial dysfunction (hypokinesia, akinesia, or dyskinesia) is the hallmark of CAD on ventriculography (Fig. 10–56). *Hypokinesia* is defined as reduced contractility during systole. *Akinesia* is defined as absence of contraction during systole. *Dyskinesia* means paradoxical outward bulging during systole and is usually associated with ventricular aneurysm. Hypokinesis may occur in ischemia without infarction, as well as in myocardial infarction producing varying degrees of myocardial fibrosis. Differentiation of these two conditions is an important factor in treatment and prognosis. Areas of dyskinesis are rarely if ever associated with significant quantities of viable myocardium.

Although not all patients with significant coronary obstruction demonstrate wall motion abnormalities, there is generally good correlation between the presence of CAD and myocardial dysfunction.[178] Demonstration of the reversibility of wall motion abnormalities is an important way of differentiating underperfused but viable myocardium from myocardial scar. Methods such as nitroglycerin administration, postextrasystolic potentiation, and epinephrine infusion have been used successfully to determine the viability of myocardium in areas of compromised myocardial function.[179, 180] There is good correlation between improvement in ventricular function using these methods and improvement following reperfusion by coronary bypass.[181, 182] In some patients with normal myocardial contractility associated with CAD, myocardial dysfunction may be induced by ischemia resulting from tachycardia produced by atrial pacing. Segmental wall motion abnormalities produced by this method signify hemodynamically significant stenoses.[183]

The sequelae of myocardial infarction may produce complications which are more serious than loss of myocardial function per se. These include ruptures of the ventricular septum, free wall, or papillary muscle (pp. 1281 to 1284) resulting in acquired ventricular septal defect, pseudoaneurysm, or severe mitral valve incompetence, respectively. These may be life-threatening situations requiring immediate surgical attention. A more common complication is the formation of ventricular aneurysm (p. 1284). Recognition of such lesions is important because of their long-term hemodynamic and thromboembolic consequences.

REFERENCES

TECHNIQUE OF CORONARY ARTERIOGRAPHY

1. Baltaxe, H. A., Amplatz, K., and Levin, D. C.: Coronary Angiography. Springfield, Charles C Thomas, 1973.
2. Sones, F. M., and Shirey, E. K.: Cine coronary arteriography. Mod. Concepts Cardiovasc. Dis. *31*:735, 1962.
3. Hurst, J. W.: History of cardiac catheterization. *In* King, S. B., III, and Douglas, J. S., Jr. (eds.): Coronary Arteriography and Angioplasty. New York, McGraw-Hill Book Co., 1985, p. 1.
4. Judkins, M. P.: Selective coronary arteriography: I. A percutaneous transfemoral technique. Radiology *89*:815, 1967.
5. Barry, W. H., Levin, D. C., Green, L. H., Bettmann, M. A., Mudge, G. H., Jr., and Phillips, D.: Left heart catheterization and angiography via the percutaneous femoral approach using an arterial sheath. Cathet. Cardiovasc. Diagn. *5*:401, 1979.
6. Gensini, G. G.: Coronary arteriography. *In* Braunwald, E. (ed.): Heart Disease. 2nd ed. Philadelphia, W. B. Saunders Company, 1984, p. 304.
7. Amplatz, K., Formanek, G., Stanger, P., and Wilson, W.: Mechanics of selective coronary artery catheterization via femoral approach. Radiology *89*:1040, 1967.
8. Schoonmaker, F. W., and King, S. B., III: Coronary arteriography by the single catheter percutaneous femoral technique. Circulation *50*:735, 1974.
9. King, S. B., III, and Douglas, J. S., Jr.: Coronary arteriography and left ventriculography: Multipurpose technique. *In* King, S. B., III, and Douglas, J. S., Jr. (eds.): Coronary Arteriography and Angioplasty. New York, McGraw-Hill Book Co., 1985, p. 239.
10. Friesinger, G. C., Adams, D. F., Bourassa, M. G., Carlsson, E., Elliott, L. P., Gessner, I. H., Greenspan, R. H., Grossman, W., Judkins, M. P., Kennedy, J. W., and Sheldon, W.: Report of the Inter-Society Commission for Heart Disease Resources: Optimal resources for examination of the heart and lungs: Cardiac catheterization and radiographic facilities. Circulation *68*:891A, 1983.
11. Judkins, M. P.: Angiographic equipment: The cardiac catheterization laboratory. *In* Abrams, H. L. (ed.): Coronary Arteriography: A Practical Approach. Boston, Little, Brown, 1983, p. 1.
12. Levin, D. C., Dunham, L. R., and Stueve, R.: Causes of cine image quality deterioration in cardiac catheterization laboratories. Am. J. Cardiol. *52*:881, 1983.
13. Davis, K., Kennedy, J. W., Kemp, H. G., Jr., Judkins, M. P., Gosselin, A. J., and Killip, T.: Complications of coronary arteriography. Circulation *59*:1105, 1979.
14. Paulin, S., and Adams, D. F.: Increased ventricular fibrillation during coronary arteriography with a new contrast medium preparation. Radiology *101*:45, 1971.
15. Synder, C. F., Formanek, A., Frech, R. S., and Amplatz, K.: The role of sodium in promoting ventricular arrhythmia during coronary arteriography. A. J. R. *113*:567, 1971.
16. Bettmann, M. A., Bourdillon, P. D., Barry, W. H., Brush, K. A., and Levin, D. C.: Contrast agents for cardiac angiography: Effects of a nonionic agent vs. a standard ionic agent. Radiology *153*:583, 1984.
17. Schlesinger, M. J.: Relation of anatomic pattern to pathologic conditions of coronary arteries. Arch. Pathol. *30*:403, 1940.
18. Baroldi, G., and Scomazzoni, G.: Coronary circulation in the normal and the pathologic heart. Washington, Office of the Surgeon General, 1967.
19. James, T. N.: Anatomy of the Coronary Arteries. New York, Paul B. Hoeber, 1961.
20. Levin, D. C., Harrington, D. P., Bettmann, M. A., Garnic, J. D., Davidoff, A., and Lois, J.: Anatomic variations of the coronary arteries supplying the anterolateral aspect of the left ventricle. Possible explanation for the "unexplained" anterior aneurysm. Invest. Radiol. *17*:458, 1982.
21. Perlmutt, L. M., Jay, M. E., and Levin, D. C.: Variations in the blood supply of the left ventricular apex. Invest. Radiol. *18*:138, 1983.
22. Levin, D. C., Beckmann, C. F., Garnic, J. D., Carey, P., and Bettmann, M. A.: Frequency and clinical significance of failure to visualize the conus artery during coronary arteriography. Circulation *63*:833, 1981.
23. Kyriakidis, M. K., Kourouklis, C. B., Papaioannou, J. T., Christakos, S. G., Spanos, G. T., and Avgoustakis, D. G.: Sinus node coronary arteries studied with angiography. Am. J. Cardiol. *51*:749, 1983.
24. Levin, D. C., and Baltaxe, H. A.: Angiographic demonstration of important anatomic variations of the posterior descending coronary artery. A. J. R. *116*:41, 1972.
25. Bunnell, I. L., Greene, D. G., Tandon, R. N., and Arani, D. T.: The half axial projection. A new look at the proximal left coronary artery. Circulation *48*:1151, 1973.
26. Sos, T. A., Lee, J. G., Levin, D. C., and Baltaxe, H. A.: New lordotic projection for improved visualization of the left coronary artery and its branches. A. J. R. *121*:575, 1974.
27. Aldridge, H. E., McLoughlin, M. J., and Taylor, K. W.: Improved diagnosis in coronary cinearteriography with routine use of 110° oblique views and cranial and caudal angulation. Comparison with standard tranverse oblique views in 100 patients. Am. J. Cardiol. *36*:468, 1975.
28. Arani, D. T., Bunnell, I. L., and Greene, D. G.: Lordotic right posterior oblique projection of the left coronary artery. A special view for special anatomy. Circulation *52*:504, 1975.
29. Gomes, A. S., Esposito, V. A., Grollman, J. H., Jr., and O'Reilly, R. J.: Angled views in the evaluation of the right coronary artery. Cathet. Cardiovasc. Diagn. *8*:71, 1982.
30. Paulin, S.: Terminology for radiographic projections in cardiac angiography. Cathet. Cardiovasc. Diagn. *7*:341, 1981.
31. Vlodaver, Z., Neufeld, H. N., and Edwards, J. E.: Pathology of coronary disease. Semin. Roentgenol. *7*:376, 1972.
32. Feldman, R. L., Pepine, C. J., Curry, R. C., and Conti, C. R.: Coronary arterial responses to graded doses of nitroglycerin. Am. J. Cardiol. *43*:91, 1979.
33. Brown, B. G., Bolson, E., Petersen, R. B., Pierce, C. D., and Dodge, H. T.: The mechanisms of nitroglycerin action: Stenosis vasodilatation as a major component of the drug response. Circulation *64*:1089, 1981.
34. Levin, D. C., Phillips, D. A., Lee-Son, S., and Maroko, P. R.: Hemodynamic changes distal to selective arterial injection. Invest. Radiol. *12*:116, 1977.
35. Levin, D. C., Baltaxe, H. A., Lee, J. G., and Sos, T. A.: Potential sources of error in coronary arteriography. I. In performance of the study. A. J. R. *124*:378, 1975.
36. Haraphongse, M., and Rossall, R. E.: Diaphragmatic coronary lesion mimics significant coronary stenosis: Report of 4 cases. Cathet. Cardiovasc. Diagn. *11*:173, 1985.
37. Levin, D. C., Baltaxe, H. A., and Sos, T. A.: Potential sources of error in coronary arteriography. II. In interpretation of the study. A. J. R. *124*:386, 1975.
38. Edwards, J. E., Burnsides, C., Swarm, R. L., and Lansing, A. I.: Arteriosclerosis in intramural and extramural portions of coronary arteries in the human heart. Circulation *13*:235, 1956.

39. Kramer, J. R., Kitazume, H., Proudfit, W. L., and Sones, F. M., Jr.: Clinical significance of isolated coronary bridges: Benign and frequent condition involving the left anterior descending artery. Am. Heart J. *103*:283, 1982.
40. Noble, J., Bourassa, M. G., Petitclerc, R., and Dyrda, I.: Myocardial bridging and milking effect of the left anterior descending coronary artery: Normal variant or obstruction? Am. J. Cardiol. *37*:993, 1976.
41. Faruqui, A. M. A., Maloy, W. C., Felner, J. M., Schlant, R. C., Logan, W. D., and Symbas, P.: Symptomatic myocardial bridging of coronary artery. Am. J. Cardiol. *41*:1305, 1978.
42. Friedman, M.: The coronary canalized thrombus: Provenance, structure, function and relationship to death due to coronary artery disease. Br. J. Exp. Pathol. *48*:556, 1967.
43. Adams, D. F., Fraser, D. B., and Abrams, H. L.: The complications of coronary arteriography. Circulation *48*:609, 1973.
44. Bourassa, M. G., and Noble, J.: Complication rate of coronary arteriography. A review of 5250 cases studied by a percutaneous femoral technique. Circulation *53*:106, 1976.
45. Davis, K., Kennedy, J. W., Kemp, H. G., Jr., Judkins, M. P., Gosselin, A. J., and Killip, T.: Complications of coronary arteriography from the Collaborative Study of Coronary Artery Surgery (CASS). Circulation *59*:1105, 1979.
46. Kennedy, J. W.: Complications associated with cardiac catheterization and angiography. Cathet. Cardiovasc. Diagn. *8*:5, 1982.
47. Klinke, W. P., Kubac, G., Talibi, T., and Lee, S. J. K.: Safety of outpatient catheterizations. Am. J. Cardiol. *56*:639, 1985.
48. Hildner, F. J., Javier, R. P., Tolentino, A., and Samet, P.: Pseudo complications of cardiac catheterization: Update. Cathet. Cardiovasc. Diagn. *8*:43, 1982.

ABNORMALITIES OF THE CORONARY CIRCULATION

49. Levin, D. C., Fellows, K. E., and Abrams, H. L.: Hemodynamically significant primary anomalies of the coronary arteries. Angiographic aspects. Circulation *58*:25, 1978.
50. Wilson, C. L., Dlabal, P. W., Holeyfield, R. W., Akins, C. W., and Knauf, D. G.: Anomalous origin of left coronary artery from pulmonary artery. Case reports and review of literature concerning teenagers and adults. J. Thorac. Cardiovasc. Surg. *73*:887, 1977.
51. Cheitlin, M. D., De Castro, C. M., and McAllister, H. A.: Sudden death as a complication of anomalous left coronary origin from the anterior sinus of Valsalva. A not-so-minor congenital anomaly. Circulation *50*:780, 1974.
52. Liberthson, R. R., Dinsmore, R. E., and Fallon, J. T.: Aberrant coronary artery origin from the aorta. Report of 18 patients, review of literature, and delineation of natural history and management. Circulation *59*:748, 1979.
53. Roberts, W. C., Siegel, R. J., and Zipes, D. P.: Origin of the right coronary artery from the left sinus of Valsalva and its functional consequences: Analysis of 10 necropsy patients. Am. J. Cardiol. *49*:863, 1982.
54. Brandt, B., III, Martins, J. B., and Marcus, M. L.: Anomalous origin of the right coronary artery from the left sinus of Valsalva. N. Engl. J. Med. *309*:596, 1983.
55. Kimbiris, D., Iskandrian, A. S., Segal, B. L., and Bemis, C. E.: Anomalous aortic origin of coronary arteries. Circulation *58*:606, 1978.
56. Engel, H. J., Torres, C., and Page, H. L., Jr.: Major variations in anatomical origin of the coronary arteries: Angiographic observations in 4250 patients without associated congenital heart disease. Cathet. Cardiovasc. Diagn. *1*:157, 1975.
57. Chaitman, B. R., Lesperance, J., Saltiel, J., and Bourassa, M. G.: Clinical, angiographic, and hemodynamic findings in patients with anomalous origin of the coronary arteries. Circulation *53*:122, 1976.
58. Page, H. L., Jr., Engel, H. J., Campbell, W. B., and Thomas, C. S., Jr.: Anomalous origin of the left circumflex coronary artery. Recognition, angiographic demonstration and clinical significance. Circulation *50*:768, 1974.
59. Ogden, J. A., and Stansel, H. C., Jr.: Roentgenographic manifestations of congenital coronary artery disease. A. J. R. *113*:538, 1971.
60. Lipton, M. J., Barry, W. H., Obrez, I., Silverman, J. F., and Wexler, L.: Isolated single coronary artery: Diagnosis, angiographic classification, and clinical significance. Radiology *130*:39, 1979.
61. Shipley, R. E., and Gregg, D. E.: The effect of external constriction of a blood vessel on blood flow. Am. J. Physiol. *141*:289, 1944.
62. Gould, K. L., Lipscomb, K., and Hamilton, G. W.: Physiologic basis for assessing critical coronary stenosis. Instantaneous flow response and regional distribution during coronary hyperemia as measures of coronary flow reserve. Am. J. Cardiol. *33*:87, 1974.
63. Klocke, F. J.: Measurements of coronary blood flow and degree of stenosis: Current clinical implications and continuing uncertainties. J. Am. Coll. Cardiol. *1*:31, 1983.
64. Neill, W. A., and Fluri-Lundeen, J. H.: Myocardial oxygen supply in left ventricular hypertrophy and coronary heart disease. Am. J. Cardiol. *44*:747, 1979.
65. Levin, D. C., Beckmann, C. F., and Serur, J. R.: Vascular resistance changes distal to progressive arterial stenosis: A critical re-evaluation of the concept of vasodilator reserve. Invest. Radiol. *15*:120, 1980.
66. Logan, S. E.: On the fluid mechanics of human coronary artery stenosis. IEEE Trans. Biomed. Eng. *22*:327, 1975.
67. Gould, K. L., and Lipscomb, K.: Effects of coronary stenoses on coronary flow reserve and resistance. Am. J. Cardiol. *34*:48, 1974.
68. Feldman, R. L., Nichols, W. W., Pepine, C. J., and Conti, C. R.: Hemodynamic significance of the length of a coronary arterial narrowing. Am. J. Cardiol. *41*:865, 1978.
69. White, C. W., Wright, C. B., Doty, D. B., Hiratza, L. F., Eastham, C. L., Harrison, D. G., and Marcus, M. L.: Does visual interpretation of the coronary arteriogram predict the physiologic importance of a coronary stenosis? N. Engl. J. Med. *310*:819, 1984.
70. Ganz, P., Abben, R., Friedman, P. L., Garnic, J. D., Barry, W. H., and Levin, D. C.: Usefulness of transstenotic coronary pressure gradient measurements during diagnostic catherization. Am. J. Cardiol. *55*:910, 1985.
71. Levin, D. C.: Pathways and functional significance of the coronary collateral circulation. Circulation *50*:831, 1974.
72. Freedman, S. B., Dunn, R. F., Bernstein, L., Morris, J., and Kelly, D. T.: Influence of coronary collateral blood flow on the development of exertional ischemia and Q wave infarction in patients with severe single-vessel disease. Circulation *71*:681, 1985.
73. Helfant, R. H., Kemp, H. G., and Gorlin, R.: Coronary atherosclerosis, coronary collaterals and their relation to cardiac function. Ann. Intern. Med. *73*:189, 1970.
74. Hecht, H. S., Aroesty, J. M., Morkin, E., Laraia, P. H., and Paulin, S.: Role of the coronary collateral circulation in the preservation of left ventricular function. Radiology *114*:305, 1975.
75. Williams, D. O., Amsterdam, E. A., Miller, R. R., and Mason, D. T.: Functional significance of coronary collateral vessels in patients with acute myocardial infarction: Relation to pump performance, cardiogenic shock, and survival. Am. J. Cardiol. *37*:345, 1976.
76. Schwarz, F., Flameng, W., Enssler, R., Sesto, M., and Thormann, J.: Effect of coronary collaterals on left ventricular function at rest and during stress. Am. Heart J. *95*:570, 1978.
77. Tubau, J. F., Chaitman, B. R., Bourassa, M. G., Lesperance, J., and Dupras, G.: Importance of coronary collateral circulation in interpreting exercise test results. Am. J. Cardiol. *47*:27, 1981.
78. Eng, C., Patterson, R. E., Horowitz, S. F., Halgash, D. A., Pichard, A. D., Midwall, J., Herman, M. V., and Gorlin R.: Coronary collateral function during exercise. Circulation *66*:309, 1982.
79. Probst, P., Zangl, W., and Pachinger, O.: Relation of coronary arterial occlusion pressure during percutaneous transluminal coronary angioplasty to presence of collaterals. Am. J. Cardiol. *55*:1264, 1985.
80. Prinzmetal, M., Kennamer, R., Merliss, R., Wada, T., and Bor, N.: Angina pectoris: I. Variant form of angina pectoris. Am. J. Med. *27*:375, 1959.
81. Braunwald, E.: Coronary artery spasm. Mechanisms and clinical relevance. J.A.M.A. *256*:1957, 1981.
82. Dhurandhar, R. W., Watt, D. L., Silver, M. D., Trimble, A. S., and Adelman, A. G.: Prinzmetal's variant form of angina with arteriographic evidence of coronary arterial spasm. Am. J. Cardiol. *30*:902, 1972.
83. Cheng, T. O., Bashour, T., Kelser, G. A., Weiss, L., and Bacos, J.: Variant angina of Prinzmetal with normal coronary arteriogram: Variant of the variant. Circulation *47*:476, 1973.
84. Oliva, P. B., Potts, D. E., and Pluss, R. G.: Coronary arterial spasm in Prinzmetal angina. Documentation by coronary arteriography. N. Engl. J. Med. *288*:745, 1973.
85. Schroeder, J. S., Bolen, J. L., Quint, R. A., Clark, D. A., Hayden, W. G., Higgins, C. B., and Wexler, L.: Provocation of coronary spasm with ergonovine maleate. New test with results in 57 patients undergoing coronary arteriography. Am. J. Cardiol. *40*:487, 1977.
86. Curry, R. C., Jr., Pepine, C. J., Varnell, J. H., Sabom, M. B., and Conti, C. R.: Clinical usefulness and safety of the ergonovine test in patients with chest pain. Am. J. Cardiol. *41*:369, 1978.
87. Heupler, F. A., Jr., Proudfit, W. L., Razavi, M., Shirey, E. K., Greenstreet, R., and Sheldon, W. C.: Ergonovine maleate provocative test for coronary arterial spasm. Am. J. Cardiol. *41*:631, 1978.
88. Freedman, S. B., Richmond, D. R., and Kelly, D. T.: Clinical studies of patients with coronary spasm. Am J. Cardiol. *52*:67A, 1983.
89. Crevey, B. J., Owen, S. F., Pitt, B.: Irreversible coronary occlusion related to administration of ergonovine. Circulation *64*:853, 1981.
90. Bertrand, M. E., LaBlanche, J. M., Tilmant, P. Y., Thieuleux, F. A., Delforge, M. R., Carre, A. G., Asseman, P., Berzin, B., Libersa, C., and Laurent, J. M.: Frequency of provoked coronary arterial spasm in 1089 consecutive patients undergoing coronary arteriography. Circulation *65*:1299, 1982.
91. Chapman, I.: Morphogenesis of occluding coronary artery thrombosis. Arch. Pathol. *80*:256, 1965.
92. Friedman, M., and van den Bovenkamp, G. J.: Pathogenesis of coronary thrombus. Am. J. Pathol. *48*:19, 1966.
93. Ridolfi, R. L., and Hutchins, G. M.: Relationships between coronary artery lesions and myocardial infarcts: Ulceration of atherosclerotic plaques precipitating coronary artery thrombosis. Am. Heart J. *93*:468, 1977.
94. Horie, T., Sekiguchi, M., and Hirosawa, K.: Relation between myocardial infarction and preinfarction angina. A histopathological study of coronary arteries in two sudden death cases employing serial section. Am. Heart J. *95*:81, 1978.
95. Falk, E.: Plaque rupture with severe pre-existing stenosis precipitating coronary thrombosis: Characteristics of coronary atherosclerotic plaques underlying fatal occlusive thrombi. Br. Heart J. *50*:127, 1983.
96. Willerson, J. T., Campbell, W. B., Winniford, M. D., Schmitz, J., Apprill, P., Firth, B. G., Ashton, J., Smitherman, T., Bush, L., and Buja, L. M.: Conversion from chronic to acute coronary artery disease: Speculation regarding mechanisms. Am. J. Cardiol. *54*:1349, 1984.
97. Fuster, V., Steele, P. M., and Chesebro, J. H.: Role of platelets and thrombosis in coronary atherosclerotic disease and sudden death. J. Am. Coll. Cardiol. *5*:175*B*, 1985.

98. Levin, D. C., and Fallon, J. T.: Significance of the angiographic morphology of localized coronary stenoses: Histopathologic correlations. Circulation *66*:316, 1982.
99. Ambrose, J. A., Winters, S. L., Stern A., Eng, A., Teichholz, L. E., Gorlin, R., and Fuster, V.: Angiographic morphology and the pathogenesis of unstable angina pectoris. J. Am. Coll. Cardiol. *5*:609, 1985.
100. Ambrose, J. A., Winters, S. L., Arora, R. R., Haft, J. I., Goldstein, J., Rentrop, K. P., Gorlin, R., and Fuster, V.: Coronary angiographic morphology in myocardial infarction: A link between the pathogenesis of unstable angina and myocardial infarction. J. Am. Coll. Cardiol. *6*:1233, 1985.
101. Wilson, R. F., Holida, M. D., and White, C. W.: Quantitative angiographic morphology of coronary stenoses leading to myocardial infarction or unstable angina. Circulation *73*:286, 1986.
102. Bresnahan, D. R., Davis, J. L., Holmes, D. R., and Smith, H. C.: Angiographic occurrence and clinical correlates of intraluminal coronary artery thrombus: Role of unstable angina. J. Am. Coll. Cardiol. *6*:285, 1985.
103. Capone, G., Wolf, N. M., Meyer, B., and Meister, S. G.: Frequency of intracoronary filling defects by angiography in angina pectoris at rest. Am. J. Cardiol. *56*:403, 1985.
104. Taus, R. H., Levin, D. C., Boxt, L. M., Meyerovitz, M. F., and Harrington, D. P.: Angiographic stenosis morphology: A new way to interpret coronary arteriograms. Radiology *157P*:67, 1985.
105. Burggraf, G. W., and Parker, J. O.: Prognosis in coronary artery disease. Angiographic, hemodynamic, and clinical factors. Circulation *51*:146, 1975.
106. Mock, M. B., Ringqvist, I., Fisher, L. D., Davis, K. B., Chaitman, B. R., Kouchoukos, N. T., Kaiser, G. C,, Alderman, E., Ryan, T. J., Russell, R. O., Jr., Mullin, S., Fray, D., and Killip, T., III.: Survival of medically treated patients in the Coronary Artery Surgery Study (CASS) registry. Circulation *66*:562, 1982.
107. Califf, R. M., Phillips, H. R., II, Hindman, M. C., Mark, D. B., Lee, K. L., Behar, V. S., Johnson, R. A., Pryor, D. B., Rosati, R. A., Wagner, G. S., and Harrell, F. E., Jr.: Prognostic value of a coronary artery jeopardy score. J. Am. Coll. Cardiol. *5*:1055, 1985.
108. Gensini, G. G.: Coronary arteriography. Mount Kisco, N.Y., Futura Publishing Co., 1975, p. 261.
109. Friesinger, G. C., Humphries, J. O., and Ross, R. C.: Prognostic significance of coronary arteriography. *In* Kaltenbach, M., Lichtlen, P., and Friesinger, G. C. (eds.): Coronary heart disease. Stuttgart, George Thieme Verlag, 1973.
110. Conley, M. J., Ely, R. L., Kisslo, J., Lee, K. L., McNeer, J. F., and Rosati, R. A.: The prognostic spectrum of left main stenosis. Circulation *57*:947, 1978.
111. Takaro, T., Peduzzi, P., Detre, K. M., Hultgren, H. N., Murphy, M. L., van der Bel-Kahn, J., Thomsen, J., and Meadows, W. R.: Survival in subgroups of patients with left main coronary artery disease. Veterans Administration Cooperative Study of Surgery for Coronary Arterial Occlusive Disease. Circulation *66*:14, 1982.
112. Campeau, L., Corbara, F., Crochet, D., and Peticlerc, R.: Left main coronary artery stenosis. The influence of aortocoronary bypass surgery on survival. Circulation *57*:1111, 1978.
113. Sanz, G., Castaner, A., Betriu, A., Magrina, J., Roig, E., Coll, S., Pare, J. C., and Navarro-Lopez, F.: Determinants of prognosis in survivors of myocardial infarction. A prospective clinical angiographic study. N. Engl. J. Med. *306*:1065, 1982.
114. DeFeyter, P. J., van Eenige, M. J., Dighton, D. H., Visser, F. C., DeJong, J., and Roos, J. P.: Prognostic value of exercise testing, coronary angiography and left ventriculography 6–8 weeks after myocardial infarction. Circulation *66*:527, 1982.
115. Loop, F. D., Lytle, B. W., Cosgrove, D. M., Stewart, R. W., Goormastic, M., Williams, G. W., Golding, L. A. R., Gill, C. C., Taylor, P. C., Sheldon, W. C., and Proudfit, W. L.: Influence of the internal-mammary-artery graft on 10-year survival and other cardiac events. N. Engl. J. Med. *314*:1, 1986.
116. Spencer, F. C.: The internal mammary artery: The ideal coronary bypass graft? N. Engl. J. Med. *314*:50, 1986.
117. Bourassa, M. G., Fisher, L. D., Campeau, L., Gillespie, M. J., McConney, M., and Lesperance, J.: Long-term fate of bypass grafts: The Coronary Artery Surgery Study (CASS) and the Montreal Heart Institute experiences. Circulation *72* (Suppl.V):V-71, 1985.
118. European Coronary Surgery Study Group: Long term results of prospective randomized study of coronary artery bypass surgery in stable angina pectoris. Lancet *2*:1173, 1982.
119. Tector, A. J., Schmahl, T. M., and Canino, V. R.: The internal mammary artery graft: The best choice for bypass of the diseased left anterior descending coronary artery. Circulation *68* (Suppl. II):II-214, 1983.
120. Chesebro, J. H., Clements, I. P., Fuster, V., Elveback, L. R., Smith, H. C., Holmes, D. R., Bardsley, W. T., Pluth, J. R., Wallace, R. B., Puga, F. J., Orszulak, T. A., Piehler, J. M., Danielson, G. K., Schaff, H. V., and Frye, R. L.: Effect of dipyridamole and aspirin on late vein-graft patency after coronary bypass operations. N. Engl. J. Med. *310*:209, 1984.
121. Rentrop, P., Blanke, H., Karsch, K. R., Kaiser, H., Kostering,H., and Leitz, K.: Selective intracoronary thrombolysis in acute myocardial infarction and unstable angina pectoris. Circulation *63*:307, 1981.
122. Mathey, D. G., Kuck, K-H., Tilsner, V., Krebber, H-J., and Bleifeld, W.: Nonsurgical coronary artery recanalization in acute transmural myocardial infarction. Circulation *63*:489, 1981.
123. Ganz, W., Buchbinder, N., Marcus, H., Mondkar, A., Maddahi, J., Charuzi, Y., O'Connor, L., Shell, W., Fishbein, M. C., Kass, R., Miyamoto, A., and Swan, H. J. C.: Intracoronary thrombolysis in evolving myocardial infarction. Am. Heart J. *101*:4, 1981.
124. Rentrop, K. P.: Thrombolytic therapy in patients with acute myocardial infarction. Circulation *71*:627, 1985.
125. Williams, D. O., Borer, J., Braunwald, E., Chesebro, J. H., Cohen, L. S., Dalen, J., Dodge, H. T., Francis, C. K., Knatterud, G., Ludbrook, P., Markis, J. E., Mueller, H., Desvigne-Nickens, P., Passamani, E. R., Powers, E. R., Rao, A. K., Roberts, R., Ross, A., Ryan, T. J., Sobel, B. E., Winniford, M., Zaret, B., and co-investigators: Intravenous recombinant tissue-type plasminogen activator in patients with acute myocardial infarction: A report from the NHLBI thrombolysis in myocardial infarction trial. Circulation *73*:338, 1986.
126. Gash, A. K., Spann, J. F., Sherry, S., Belber, A. D., Carabello, B. A., McDonough, M. T., Mann, R. H., McCann, W. D., Gault, J. H., Gentzler, R. D., and Kent, R. L.: Factors influencing reocclusion after coronary thrombolysis for acute myocardial infarction. Am. J. Cardiol. *57*:175, 1986.
127. Schröder, R., Vöhringer, H., Lindler, T., Biamino, G., Brüggemann, T., and Leiter, E. R.: Follow-up after coronary arterial reperfusion with intravenous streptokinase in relation to residual myocardial infarct artery narrowings. Am. J. Cardiol. *55*:313, 1985.
128. Valentine, R. P., Pitts, D. E., Brooks-Brun, J. A., Williams, J. G., Van Hove, E., and Schmidt, P. E.: Intravenous versus intracoronary streptokinase in acute myocardial infarction. Am. J. Cardiol. *55*:309, 1985.
129. Rogers, W. J., Mantle, J. A., Hood, W. P., Jr., Baxley, W. A., Whitlow, P. L., Reeves, R. C., and Soto, B.: Prospective randomized trial of intravenous and intracoronary streptokinase in acute myocardial infarction. Circulation *68*:1051, 1983.
130. Hillis, L. D., Borer, J., Braunwald, E., Chesebro, J. H., Cohen L. S., Dalen, J., Dodge, H. T., Francis, C. K., Knatterud, G., Ludbrook, P., Markis, J. E., Mueller, H., Desvigne-Nickens, P., Passamani, E. R., Powers, E. R., Rao, A. K., Roberts, R., Roberts, W. C., Ross, A., Ryan, T. J., Sobel, B. E., Williams, D. O., Zaret, B. L., and co-investigators: High-dose intravenous streptokinase for acute myocardial infarction: Preliminary results of a multicenter trial. J. Am. Coll. Cardiol. *6*:957, 1985.
131. Relman, A. S.: Intravenous thrombolysis in acute myocardial infarction. A progress report. N. Engl. J. Med. *312*:915, 1985.
132. TIMI Study Group: The thrombolysis in myocardial infarction (TIMI) trial. N. Engl. J. Med. *312*:932, 1985.
133. Kruger, R. A., and Riederer, S. J.: Digital subtraction angiography. Boston, G. K. Hall Medical Publishers, 1984.
134. Brody, W. R.: Digital radiography. New York, Raven Press, 1984.
135. Levin, D. C., Schapiro, R. M., Boxt, L. M., Dunham, L., Harrington, D. P., and Ergun, D. L.: Digital subtraction angiography: Principles and pitfalls of image improvement techniques. A. J. R. *143*:447, 1984.
136. Tobis, J., Nalcioglu, O., Iseri, L., Johnston, W. D., Roeck, W., Castlemen, E., Bauer, B., Montelli, S., and Henry, W. L.: Detection and quantification of coronary artery stenoses from digital subtraction angiograms compared with 35-millimeter film cineangiograms. Am. J. Cardiol. *54*:489, 1984.
137. Vas, R., Eigler, N., Miyazono, C., Pfaff, J. M., Resser, K. J., Weiss, M., Nivatpumin, T., Whiting, J., and Forrester, J.: Digital quantification eliminates intraobserver and interobserver variability in the evaluation of coronary artery stenosis. Am. J. Cardiol. *56*:718, 1985.
138. Vogel, R. A.: The radiographic assessment of coronary blood flow parameters. Circulation *72*:460, 1985.
139. Bates, E. R., Aueron, F. M., Legrand, V., LeFree, M. T., Mancini, G. B. J., Hodgson, J. M., and Vogel, R. A.: Comparative long-term effects of coronary angioplasty on regional coronary flow reserve. Circulation *72*:833, 1985.
140. Tobis, J., Johnston, W. D., Montelli, S., Henderson, E., Roeck, W., Bauer, B., Nalcioglu, O., and Henry, W.: Digital coronary roadmapping as an aid for performing coronary angioplasty. Am. J. Cardiol. *56*:237, 1985.
141. Nissen, S. E., Booth D., Waters, J., Fassas, T., and DeMaria, A. N.: Evaluation of left ventricular contractile pattern by intravenous digital subtraction ventriculography: Comparison with cineangiography and assessment of interobserver variability. Am. J. Cardiol. *52*:1293, 1983.
142. Tobis, J., Nalcioglu, O., Seibert, A., Johnston, W. D., and Henry, W. L.: Measurement of left ventricular ejection fraction by videodensitometric analysis of digital subtraction angiograms. Am. J. Cardiol. *52*:871, 1983.
143. Zir, L. M., Miller, S. W., Dinsmore, R. E., Gilbert, J. P., and Harthorne, J. W.: Interobserver variability in coronary angiography. Circulation *53*:627, 1976.
144. Detre, K. M., Wright, E., Murphy, M. L., and Takaro, T.: Observer agreement in evaluating coronary angiograms. Circulation *52*:979, 1975.
145. DeRouen, T. A., Murray, J. A., and Owen, W.: Variability in the analysis of coronary arteriograms. Circulation *55*:324, 1977.
146. Myers, M. G., Shulman, H. S., Saibil, E. A., and Naqvi, S. Z.: Variation in measurement of coronary lesions on 35 and 70 mm angiograms. A. J. R. *130*:913, 1978.
147. Grondin, C. M., Dyrda, I., Pasternac, A., Campeau, L., Bourassa, M. G., and Lesperance, J.: Discrepancies between cineangiographic and postmortem findings in patients with coronary artery disease and recent myocardial revascularization. Circulation *49*:703, 1974.
148. Hutchins, G. M., Bulkley, B. H., Ridolfi, R. L., Griffith, L. S. C., Lohr, F. T., and Piasio, M. A.: Correlation of coronary arteriograms and left ventriculograms with postmortem studies. Circulation *56*:32, 1977.
149. Vlodaver, Z., Frech, R., Van Tassel, R. A., and Edwards, J. E.: Correlation of the antemortem coronary arteriogram and the postmortem specimen. Circulation *67*:162, 1973.
150. Brown, B. G., Bolson, E., Frimer, M., and Dodge, H. T.: Quantitative coronary arteriography: Estimation of dimensions, hemodynamic resistance, and atheroma mass of coronary artery lesions using the arteriogram and digital computation. Circulation *55*:329, 1977.
151. Reiber, J. H. C., Serruys, P. W., Kooijman, C. J., Wijns, W., Slager, C. J., Gerbrands, J. J., Schuurbiers, J. C. H., Boer, A. D., and Hugenholtz, P. G.: Assessment of short-, medium-, and long-term variations in arterial dimensions

from computer-assisted quantitation of coronary cineangiograms. Circulation *71*:280, 1985.
152. Spears, J. R., Sandor, T., Als, A. V., Malagold, M., Markis, J. E., Grossman, W., Serur, J. R., and Paulin, S.: Computerized image analysis for quantitative measurement of vessel diameter from cineangiograms. Circulation *68*:453, 1983.
153. Nichols, A. B., Gabrieli, C. F. O., Fenoglio, J. J., Jr., and Esser, P. D.: Quantification of relative coronary arterial stenosis by cinevideodensitometric analysis of coronary arteriograms. Circulation *69*:512, 1984.
154. Jaques, P., DiBianca, F., Pizer, S., Kohout, F., Lifshitz, L., and Delany, D.: Quantitative digital fluorography: Computer vs. human estimation of vascular stenoses. Invest. Radiol. *20*:45, 1985.
155. Mattleman, S., Hakki, A-H., Iskandrian, A. S., and Kane, S. A.: Effects of angiographic contrast medium on left ventricular function: Evaluation by contrast angiography and radionuclide angiography. Cathet. Cardiovasc. Diagn. *10*:129, 1984.
156. Amundsen, A. K., Amundsen, P., and Muller, O.: Blood pressure and heart rate during angiocardiography, abdominal aortography, and arteriography of the lower extremities. Acta Radiol. (Stockh.) *45*:452, 1956.
157. Rowe, G. G., Huston, J. H., Tuchman, H., Maxwell, G. M., Weinstein, A. B., and Crumpton, C. W.: The physiologic effect of contrast media used for angiocardiography. Circulation *13*:896, 1956.
158. Brown, R., Rahimtoola, S. H., Davis, G. D., and Swan, H. J. C.: The effect of angiocardiographic contrast medium on circulatory dynamics in man. Circulation *31*:234, 1965.
159. Bristow, J. D., Porter, G. A., Kloster, F. F., and Griswold, H. E.: Hemodynamic changes attending angiocardiography. Radiology *88*:939, 1976.
160. Morris, T. W., Harnish, P. P., Reece, K., and Katzberg, R. W.: Tissue fluid shifts during renal arteriography with conventional and low osmolality agents. Invest. Radiol. *18*:335, 1983.
161. Mancini, G. B. J., and Higgins, C. B.: Digital subtraction angiography: A review of cardiac applications. Prog. Cardiovasc. Dis. *17*:111, 1985.
162. Almën, T., and Aspelin, P.: Cardiovascular effects of ionic monomeric, ionic dimeric and non-ionic contrast media: Effects in animals on myocardial contractile force, pulmonary and aortic blood pressure and aortic endothelium. Invest. Radiol. *10*:557, 1984.
163. Bettmann, M. A., and Higgins, C. B.: Comparison of an ionic with a nonionic contrast agent for cardiac angiography: Results of a multicenter trial. Invest. Radiol. *20*:570, 1985.
164. Gerber, K. H., Higgins, C. B., Yuk, Y-S., and Koziol, J. A.: Regional myocardial hemodynamic and metabolic effects of ionic and nonionic contrast media in normal and ischemic states. Circulation *65*:1307, 1982.
165. Hartman, R. B., Harrison, E. E., Pupello, D. F., Vijayanagar, R., and Sbar, S. S.: Characteristics of left ventricular thrombus resulting in perioperative embolism: A complication of coronary artery bypass grafting. J. Thorac. Cardiovasc. Surg. *86*:706, 1983.
166. Cabin, H. S., and Roberts, W. C.: Left ventricular aneurysm, intra-aneurysmal thrombus and systemic embolus in coronary heart disease. Chest *77*:586, 1980.
167. Baltaxe, H. A., Wilson, W. J., and Amiel, M.: Diverticulosis of the left ventricle. A. J. R. *133*:257, 1979.
168. Sheehan, F. H., Stewart, D. K., Dodge, H. T., Mitten, S., Bolson, E. L., and Brown, B. G.: Variability in the measurement of regional left ventricular wall motion from contrast angiograms. Circulation *68*:550, 1983.
169. Chaitman, B. R., DeMots, H., Bristow, D., Rösch, J., and Rahimtoola, S. H.: Objective and subjective analysis of left ventricular angiograms. Circulation *52*:420, 1975.
170. Vas, R., Diamond, G. A., Forrester, J. S., Whiting, J. S., Pfaff, M. J., Levisman, J. A., Nakano, F. S., and Swan, H. J. C.: Computer-enhanced digital angiography: Correlation of clinical assessment of left ventricular ejection fraction and regional wall motion. Am. Heart J. *104*:732, 1982.
171. Leighton, R. F., Wilt, S. M., and Lewis, R. P.: Detection of hypokinesis by a quantitative analysis of left ventricular cineangiograms. Circulation *50*:121, 1974.
172. Nissen, S. E., Booth, D., Waters, J., Fassas, T., and DeMaria, A. N.: Evaluation of left ventricular contractile pattern by intravenous digital subtraction ventriculography: Comparison with cineangiography and assessment of interobserver variability. Am. J. Cardiol. *52*:1293, 1983.
173. Simon, A. L., Ross, J., Jr., and Gault, J. H.: Angiographic anatomy of the left ventricle and mitral valve in idiopathic hypertrophic subaortic stenosis. Circulation *36*:852, 1967.
174. Williams, R. S., Behar, V. S., and Peter, R. H.: Left bundle branch block: Angiographic segmental wall motion abnormalities. Am. J. Cardiol. *44*:1046, 1979.
175. Cohn, P. F., Herman, M. V., and Gorlin, R.: Ventricular dysfunction in coronary artery disease. Am. J. Cardiol. *33*:307, 1974.
176. Dodge, H. T., Sandler, H., Ballew, D. W., and Lord, J. D., Jr.: Use of biplane angiocardiography for the measurement of left ventricular volume in man. Am. Heart J. *60*:762, 1960.
177. Wynne, J., Green, L. H., Mann, T., Levin, D. C., and Grossman, W.: Estimation of left ventricular volumes in man from biplane cineangiograms filmed in oblique projections. Am. J. Cardiol. *41*:726, 1978.
178. Banka, V. S., Bodenheimer, M. M., and Helfant, R. H.: Determinants of reversible asynergy: The native coronary circulation. Circulation *52*:810, 1975.
179. Banka, V. S., Bodenheimer, M. M., Shah, R., and Helfant, R. H.: Intervention ventriculography: Comparative value of nitroglycerin, post-extrasystolic potentiation and nitroglycerin plus post-extrasystolic potentiation. Circulation *53*:632, 1976.
180. McAnulty, J. H., Hattenhauer, M. T., Rösch, J., Kloster, F. E., and Rahimtoola, S. H.: Improvement in left ventricular wall motion following nitroglycerin. Circulation *51*:140, 1975.
181. Helfant, R. H., Pine, R., Meister, S. G., Feldman, M. S., Trout, R. G., and Banka, V. S.: Nitroglycerin to unmask reversible asynergy: Correlation with post-coronary bypass ventriculography. Circulation *50*:108, 1974.
182. Popio, K. A., Gorlin, R., Bechtel, D., and Levine, J. A.: Postextrasystolic potentiation as a predictor of potential myocardial viability: Preoperative analyses compared with studies after coronary bypass surgery. Am. J. Cardiol. *39*:944, 1977.
183. Hood, W. P., Jr., Rackley, C. E., and Grossman, W.: Cardiac ventriculography: *In* Grossman, W. (ed.): Cardiac Catheterization and Angiography. 2nd ed. Philadelphia, Lea and Febiger, 1980, p. 170.

11 NUCLEAR CARDIOLOGY

by B. LEONARD HOLMAN, M.D.

GLOSSARY

absorbed dose The energy absorbed by the patient from the decay of the **radionuclide**; expressed in rads or millirads (1 rad = 100 ergs/gm).

analog-to-digital conversion (ADC) Conversion of continuous analog signals (voltages) to discrete digital information.

annihilation photons The two 511-kev **photons** emitted during **positron** decay; these photons are released in opposite directions (180-degree angle between photons).

background Any radiation coming from an undesired location, including radioactivity emanating from structures surrounding the organ of interest (target organ).

beta rays Nonpenetrating radiation (electrons) emitted during beta decay; ^{3}H is a **radionuclide** that undergoes beta decay.

characteristic x-rays Low-energy photons released after electron capture (a type of radioactive decay); thallium-201 is an example of a **radionuclide** that decays by electron capture, and its characteristic x-rays are used for scintigraphic imaging.

coincidence detection Simultaneous detection of the two **annihilation photons** emitted during positron decay.

collimator The lens of the imaging system, absorbing photons traveling in inappropriate directions and originating from parts of the body other than the region under investigation; collimators are usually made of lead with holes to allow desired photons to pass through to the **crystal.**

- **(a) parallel-hole** A collimator with thousands of holes in a lead-absorbing sheet. The holes are parallel to each other and perpendicular to the crystal (straight-bore) or at some other angle to the crystal (for example, at a 30-degree slant). Standard high-sensitivity and high-resolution collimators are types of parallel-hole collimators.
- **(b) high-sensitivity** A collimator designed to achieve high count rates by using large, short holes.
- **(c) high-resolution** A collimator designed to maximize spatial resolution by using small, long holes; as a result, sensitivity is reduced.
- **(d) converging** A multihole collimator with holes that converge toward the center of the collimator; the field of view is compressed to encompass a small organ on a large crystal; allows for high resolution and high sensitivity.

Compton scatter A change in the direction of travel of a photon due to an interaction between the photon and matter (the patient or the crystal); a major cause of loss of spatial resolution; presents most difficulty at lower photon energies.

count(s) The disintegrations that the detector records. Counts/disintegrations represents the efficiency of the detector.

count rate The number of counts recorded per unit of time (counts/min).

crystal (sodium iodide scintillation) A high-density photon absorber that converts the energy of the incident photon to a number of light photons.

cycle-length window The range of cardiac cycle times (R-R interval times) that will be accepted in a gated radionuclide ventriculogram.

dead time The time required for the camera-computer system to recover after an interaction between a photon and the crystal; counts will not be recorded during this time; the dead time determines the maximum count rate that can be accurately recorded.

disintegration The radioactive decay of one atom.

disintegration rate Number of disintegrations per unit of time (disintegrations/sec). The standard units are the curie (2.22×10^{12} disintegrations/min) and the millicurie (1 Ci = 1000 mCi).

electron volts The unit of energy for the photon; usually expressed in thousands (kev) or millions (Mev) of electron volts (1 Mev = 1.6×10^{-6} erg).

electronic cursor An electronic device for selecting **a region of interest** by manually defining the region on an oscilloscope or video display; light pens and joysticks are examples.

emission tomography See **Tomography, emission.**

frames The division of a dynamic study into discrete temporal units; for example, a radionuclide angiocardiogram can be collected at a rate of 32 frames per second.

functional image, parametric image An image in which intensity reflects a physiological parameter rather than activity; for example, intensity may be proportional to blood flow or to ejection fraction.

gamma rays Electromagnetic waves with short wavelengths that originate from nuclear transitions; made up of photons capable of giving up energy in discrete interactions with matter.

gating (physiological) Acquisition of data only during some physiological event. In cardiovascular applications, acquisition is usually gated to the cardiac cycle. Data may be acquired from the entire cardiac cycle by dividing the R-R interval into frames that represent counts acquired at preset time intervals after the R wave; prospective selection of frame intervals is termed **matrix mode**; retrospective selection is termed **list mode.**

generator, radionuclide A device (usually an inorganic resin) through which a short-lived nuclide (the daughter) can be eluted (separated) from a long-lived parent ($^{99}Mo \rightarrow {}^{99m}Tc$).

half-life, physical The time necessary for the activity of a nuclide to decay to one-half its original activity (^{99m}Tc = 6 hours, ^{201}Tl = 73.1 hours).

half-life, biological The time necessary for the concentration of the tracer to fall to one-half its original concentration.

isotope Different nuclides of the same element, having the same proton number but different mass numbers; for example, $^{11}_{6}C$, $^{12}_{6}C$, $^{13}_{6}C$, $^{14}_{6}C$ are isotopes of carbon.

kev See **Electron volts.**

list mode Acquisition of data from a dynamic study in the form of a sequence of individual scintillation events which can then be reformatted retrospectively into a variable number of **frames**.

matrix The two-dimensional array into which positional data from the gamma camera are pigeonholed (32 × 32, 64 × 64, 128 × 128).

matrix (histogram) mode Acquisition of data from a dynamic study such as a radionuclide angiocardiogram which can be reformatted into a predefined number of **frames** and framing rate.

Mev See **Electron volts.**

parametric image See **Functional image**.

photon A packet of energy associated with electromagnetic radiation (gamma rays, x-rays, or light); the energy units are **electron volts** or kiloelectron volts (kev).

photopeak The energy of the predominant photons released during decay of the **radionuclide** (^{99m}Tc = 140 kev, ^{201}Tl = 69 to 83 kev).

pixel A single picture element in a digitized image; one of the **matrix** elements.

positron A positively charged electron released during positron decay of a nucleus; interacts with an electron, transforming the mass of the electron and the positron into two 511-kev **annihilation photons.**

pulse-height analyzer An electronic discriminator that selects those pulses arising from photons with energies approximating that of the **photopeak** and rejects pulses due to scattered radiation above and below the **photopeak**; the range of energies that are accepted constitutes the "window" of the analyzer.

radionuclide An atom or species of atom with an unstable nucleus that will spontaneously decay to a more stable form, emitting radiation in the process; examples include thallium-201 (^{201}Tl), tantalum-178 (^{178}Ta), and technetium-99m (^{99m}Tc, where "Tc" is the abbreviation for the element technetium, "99" is its atomic mass, and "m" indicates the metastable state).

reformat To rearrange retrospectively the parameters of a study; to convert **list mode** data to **matrix mode** data.

region of interest The **pixels** or matrix elements of a digitized image (or series of images in a dynamic study) that outline a desired structure, organ, or region within the image; may be defined manually with an **electronic cursor**.

resolution

- **(a) spatial** The ability of the detector to separate adjacent sources of activity
- **(b) temporal** The maximum combination of framing rate and number of **frames** that can be acquired.
- **(c) energy** The ability of the detector to discriminate between photons of adjacent energies.

scintigram An image of the distribution of radioactivity obtained with a **scintillation camera** after the internal administration of a **radionuclide.**

scintigraphy The process of acquiring a **scintigram.**

scintillation camera

- **(a) single-crystal, Anger-type** An imaging device with a single sodium iodide crystal with a 10- to 15-inch diameter and ¼- to ½-inch thickness; the detector records the spatial distribution of the internally administered radiotracer.
- **(b) multicrystal** An imaging with multiple crystals and a high count rate capability.

time-activity curve A histogram (in the **matrix mode**) of the change in the count rate as a function of time.

tomography, emission Computed cross-sectional reconstruction of the radionuclide distribution obtained by acquiring images or "slices" (about 1 to 2 cm in thickness) of the head or body; uses **coincidence detection** (positrons) or **single-photon detection** (nuclides such as ^{99m}Tc or ^{201}Tl).

Radionuclide methods provide a safe, relatively atraumatic, often quantitative approach to assessing a variety of cardiac functions. Their popularity can be attributed to the fact that they can be applied during exercise and other physiological and pharmacological interventions; they can be applied to very ill patients; they can provide a direct measure of cardiac function, myocardial blood flow, and metabolism; and they can provide quantitative landmarks to help evaluate the temporal progress of cardiac disease.

In this chapter, we will describe these methods, discussing first the required instrumentation and then the techniques used to assess cardiac wall motion and hemodynamics, myocardial perfusion, myocardial metabolism, and acute infarction and to detect pulmonary emboli.

INSTRUMENTATION

THE SCINTILLATION (ANGER, GAMMA) CAMERA

The scintillation camera provides a pictorial representation of the distribution of radioactivity. This device consists of a collimator, a position-sensitive detector (a large, flat sodium iodide crystal), and 37 to 91 photomultiplier tubes closely packed against the crystal. When gamma rays interact with the crystal, a portion of the gamma-ray energy is converted to light. The light is then converted into an electrical signal by the photomultiplier tubes. Electronically, the detector then calculates the position of the interaction and the energy of the gamma rays.

The *collimator* is analogous to a lens (Fig. 11–1). It is made from material that readily absorbs gamma rays, usually lead. The gamma rays can reach the crystal only by passing through the holes or channels of the collimator. The most common collimator is the *parallel-hole* collimator. Only gamma rays emitted from the patient in a direction perpendicular to the crystal can enter the detector. The diameter and length of the channels (holes) strongly affect the spatial resolution and sensitivity of the system. *High-resolution* parallel-hole collimators result in high spatial resolution at the expense of sensitivity, while *high-sensitivity* collimators result in an increase in count rate by a factor of two or three over high-resolution collimators but with a loss of resolution of about 25 per cent. A *general-purpose* collimator represents a compromise with regard to both resolution and sensitivity.

Multiple-hole collimators that diverge toward the patient are sometimes used to increase the field of view of the system (*diverging* collimators). Conversely, holes that con-

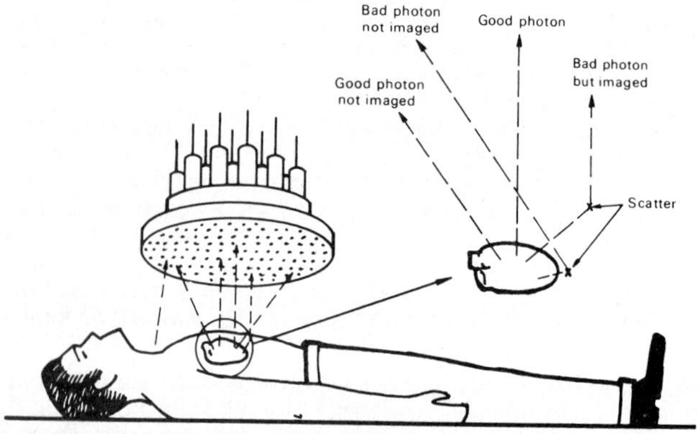

FIGURE 11–1. The multi-channel collimator acts as a lens for photon detection. (From Budinger, T. F., and Rollo, F. D.: Physics and instrumentation. Progr. Cardiovasc. Dis. *20*:19, 1977, by permission of Grune and Stratton, Inc.)

verge toward the camera increase sensitivity with a smaller field of view (*converging* collimators). In a *slant-hole* collimator the holes are angled with respect to the detector, and the camera can obtain an oblique view with the detector flat against the chest.

For nuclear cardiology, a *general-purpose* collimator is used for time-dependent studies such as exercise thallium-201 and gated blood pool imaging. *High-resolution* collimators are generally used for studies obtained at rest. A high-resolution, square-hole collimator has been introduced with increased sensitivity so that it may be used in time-dependent studies, such as during or after exercise. *High-sensitivity* collimators are used when the photon number is limited, as in first-pass radionuclide angiocardiography. *Slant-hole* collimators are used to maximize separation between atria and ventricles and to permit imaging along the long axis of the ventricles.

The important performance parameters of the Anger scintillation camera are sensitivity, spatial resolution, field uniformity, energy resolution, and count-rate linearity. *Sensitivity* is defined as the number of recorded counts per gamma-ray emitted from a radioactive tracer. The sensitivity of a gamma camera will depend on three principal factors: the gamma-ray energy, the thickness of the crystal, and the collimator employed. *Spatial resolution* is a measure of the imaging system's ability to resolve small structural details in an object. One measure of resolution is the camera's response to a line source, expressed as the line spread function. Spatial resolution can be described in terms of the full-width at half-maximum, the width of the line spread function at 50 per cent of the maximum value. State-of-the-art systems have spatial resolutions of at least 3.5 mm (FWHM) for technetium-99m and 4.5 mm for thallium-201 for sources measured at the collimator surface.

The characteristics of the Anger camera, such as the thickness of the sodium iodide crystal, represent a compromise between sensitivity and spatial resolution. For example, a 12-mm (½ inch-thick) crystal will absorb 98 per cent of the 140 kev photons of technetium-99m and 100 per cent of the 68 to 82 kev photons of thallium-201. A 6-mm (¼ inch-thick) crystal will absorb 84 per cent of the 140 kev photons of technetium-99m and 100 per cent of the 68 to 82 kev photons of thallium-201. The intrinsic resolution of thallium-201 is better with a thinner crystal, although the improvement in resolution drops with distance from the collimator. A ⅜-inch thick crystal is therefore a good compromise if both thallium-201 and technetium-99m are to be imaged with the same camera.

The *standard field of view* of most mobile cameras is 25 cm. Smaller diameters are used on some special-purpose cameras. The diameter should be large enough to encompass the entire heart within the field of view using parallel-hole collimators (20 cm for circular fields of view). Detectors with a large field of view (35 to 50 cm) are useful for pulmonary scintigraphy (see later).

The Anger camera should have a uniform response across its field so that a photon will produce an electrical signal of the same size wherever the photon is absorbed in the crystal. Variations should be less than 5 per cent across the field, and computer-assisted correction programs should reduce the variations to 1 to 2 per cent.

Count-rate linearity refers to a linear increase in the detected count rate as the activity increases. The count-rate loss should be less than 10 per cent of count rates at 75,000 counts per second, but this loss increases rapidly at higher counting rates. Other effects may also be seen at higher counting rates. For example, spurious counts can be recorded due to the coincidence of two low-energy photons. Finally, the uniformity of the camera can change at higher count rates. Improvements in camera design based on digital electronics have substantially increased the range of count-rate linearity.

THE MULTICRYSTAL CAMERA

The multicrystal scintillation camera has 294 separate sodium iodide scintillation crystals arranged in a matrix of 14 × 21 crystals. The crystals are 9.5 mm square and 2.5 mm thick. There are 35 photomultiplier tubes connected to the crystal array. An event is located in a particular crystal through detection of the simultaneous pulse from both a row and a column photomultiplier tube. A digital computer, which is an integral part of the camera, accumulates the image in its memory for display and processing.

The camera has good sensitivity, even at energies above 200 kev, because of its thick crystals. The constant picture element size means that, except for the effects of scattered radiation, image resolution is constant over the full energy range of 50 to 500 kev. The electronics have been designed for very fast processing of scintillation events leading to a short resolving time and a maximum count rate of 400,000 to 500,000 events per second—three to four times faster than the Anger camera. This is an advantage for rapid, dynamic studies, such as first-transit radionuclide angiocardiography.

Disadvantages of the matrix detector are related mainly to the light lost in the complex light guides and the coarse nature of the matrix itself. Approximately 50 per cent of the light from the crystals is lost in the light pipe arrangement. The energy resolution for technetium-99m is therefore about 50 per cent full-width at half-maximum compared to the Anger camera's resolution of 13 per cent. This means that in imaging studies with thick sources at energies from 50 to 200 kev, significant scattered radiation will lead to loss of image contrast. The coarse spatial resolution is determined by the size of the individual crystals (9.5 mm × 9.5 mm).

Recently, a mobile digital gamma camera has been introduced with a single sodium iodide crystal divided into 400 detector elements in a 20 × 20 matrix. Each individual detector element is surrounded by reflective material with every other row of detectors only partially cut through the crystal, creating a scintillation bridge between two adjacent elements and eliminating the need for the light pipe array. This camera has a maximum count rate capacity of 1×10^6 counts per second and a 20 per cent data loss at 4.5×10^5 counts/sec with no energy discrimination. With energy discrimination (80 to 200 kev), the count rate during radionuclide angiocardiography using 10 mCi of technetium-99m is 2×10^5 counts/sec. Improvement in digital electronics and the recent availability of ultrashort-lived radiotracers will increase the use of first-pass radionuclide angiocardiography, particularly for rapid sequential studies.

NONIMAGING PROBE

The scintillation probe offers the advantage of portability and enables the measurement of cardiac function in settings where it might be difficult to bring in an Anger scintillation camera (such as the operating room, the recovery room, and the intensive care unit). While cardiac studies performed with the scintillation probe provide reasonably accurate measurements of left ventricular ejection fraction and other measures of global left ventricular function, they do require considerable training to obtain accurate results, particularly in patients with very poor function, when it may be difficult to determine the edge of the ventricle and to determine background.

The standard sodium iodide scintillation probe is 1 to 3 inches in diameter and between 1 and 2 inches in depth. The crystal may be housed in a cylindrical collimator, a parallel-hole collimator similar to the low-resolution, high-efficiency collimators used with scintillation cameras, or a converging collimator. The sodium iodide crystal is used with a high temporal resolution rate meter (10 to 50 msec). Information is acquired after the intravenous injection of an intravascular tracer, such as technetium-99m–labeled red blood cells, and the studies are gated to the patient's electrocardiogram as in the equilibrium radionuclide angiocardiogram (see below). Although the data can be displayed directly on a strip chart recorder, most systems now use a microprocessor for data acquisition and analysis. The time-activity curves are displayed on an oscilloscope, and the processed data are read out through a teleprinter or a console.

Recently, substantially smaller probes have been constructed using *cadmium telluride* or *mercuric iodide* crystals. With these smaller systems, it is possible to monitor patients sequentially over prolonged periods with probes permanently positioned over the chest.[2, 3] Sequential monitoring may be particularly useful in patients with acute myocardial infarction and others in the intensive care setting.

TOMOGRAPHIC IMAGING SYSTEMS

Tomography is used in an attempt to solve one of the major constraints of standard two-dimensional imaging: the overlap of adjacent structures and background on the organ or tissue of interest. Both single-photon and positron-emission tomography are now in use.

SINGLE-PHOTON EMISSION COMPUTED TOMOGRAPHY (SPECT) (see also pp. 334 and 345). Using a rotating gamma camera, this technique is finding expanded clinical applications in nuclear cardiology because of the better contrast, edge definition, and separation of target from background compared with planar imaging. The technique is superior to planar imaging for quantification of source distributions.

The essence of SPECT is reconstruction from projections. There are several ways to form an image from projections gathered from many angles around the object. Back projection is the most commonly used method. The image is formed by adding all ray sums (a *ray sum* or *line integral* is the total activity along a line perpendicular to the detector and will include activity in the organ of interest as well as overlying activity) that intersect with each pixel to that pixel. In other words, the ray sum values are projected back along the line of the ray into each pixel that the ray intersects. If 64 images are obtained during the rotation of the detector around the patient, there will be 64 ray sums intersecting each point or pixel within the field of view. If the pixel contains high activity, more ray sums along rays intersecting that pixel will have high values, and the sum of these values will be greater than the sums surrounding the low-activity pixels. The method is imperfect, as some smearing occurs because some high ray sum values are projected into pixels which may contain little activity. To correct for this, the back projection is filtered. This filtering is an exact mathematical adjustment of pixel values on the basis of the values in surrounding pixels. Filtering is performed using either convolution or Fourier transform techniques.

The idealized method of data gathering ignores two major effects which distort the exact reconstruction of the source distribution. The first of these is a solid-angle problem. Because collimation is not ideal, information is gathered not from an ideal ray but from a cone extending from the camera. This means that the greater the distance of the collimator, the larger the volume for which the data are gathered. A second problem is attenuation of the source distribution. It is difficult to estimate the attenuation of the activity along the ray since real attenuating media are not uniform and the attenuation coefficients are not known. Myocardial SPECT incorporates data from the lung (low attenuation), the heart and other soft tissues (medium attenuation), and the bone (high attenuation). Attenuation corrections have not met with a great deal of success for the myocardium.

Spatial resolution for the rotating gamma camera in the tomographic mode is approximately 15 mm (full-width at half-maximum) in the plane of the slice and 19 mm along the long axis of the table, substantially lower resolution than can be obtained in the planar mode. The problems of solid-angle, attenuation, and spatial resolution are balanced by the high-contrast resolution and the potential for quantitative measurements.

THE COMPUTER

A computer is necessary for nearly all procedures in nuclear cardiology. It may be an integral part of the imaging system or may be separate from the scintillation camera as either a mobile or stationary system. The computer should be adequate for first-pass and equilibrium (gated) radionuclide angiocardiography; this requires high temporal resolution (a minimum of 30 to 40 frames/sec) and a matrix capability of at least 64 × 64 picture elements (pixels). Two basic types of computers are used in nuclear medicine: general-purpose (programmable) and special-purpose (hard-wire) units. The general-purpose systems are more flexible and programs can be developed and changed by the users. Special-purpose systems have fixed programs and are more limited in capability. The size and configuration of the computer system will vary with the types of procedures to be performed and local factors in a given department.

EXERCISE TESTING

An exercise table and bicycle are used for supine exercise testing during radionuclide angiocardiography. This equipment must not move during the study. The patient should be adequately stabilized on the table and the table itself must not move while the patient is exercising. The bicycle should permit the application of variable workloads, variable positions for the pedals to facilitate patient comfort, and variable positions for the patient. Some prefer a 45-degree angle for the patient's upper body. With equilibrium angiocardiography, exercise testing in the 45-degree upright position is particularly helpful for patients with pulmonary disease or heart failure and is used routinely in many departments. Equipment for upright exercise should also be available, since this is commonly used for first-pass radionuclide angiocardiography and thallium exercise studies. The most common method for upright exercise with ^{201}Tl-imaging is treadmill ergometry, which is superior to the bicycle because it is more likely to stress the patient maximally.

ASSESSMENT OF CARDIAC PERFORMANCE

Cardiac performance is a prime factor in determining appropriate medical and surgical management for patients with coronary heart disease.[4, 5] Ventricular ejection fraction and regional wall motion are directly related to clinical prognosis in patients with chronic coronary heart disease[6] and after myocardial infarction.[7] Although invasive techniques involving left ventricular catheterization and contrast angiography provide reliable measurements of ejection fraction and regional wall motion (p. 327), they have limited application in critically ill patients. Radionuclide techniques are noninvasive, requiring only a peripheral intravenous injection, and thus offer distinct advantages over more conventional, invasive methods. The radionuclide techniques are safe and repeatable and do not induce measurable hemodynamic alterations. In addition, cardiac performance can be studied during a variety of physiological or pharmaceutical interventions.

RADIOPHARMACEUTICALS

The requirements of a radiopharmaceutical for first-pass radionuclide angiocardiography (p. 315) are that it remain intravascular during its first passage through the right and left heart and that the physical properties of the radionuclide be satisfactory with respect to the instrumentation being used.

The radionuclide that is used for virtually all phases of radionuclide angiocardiography is technetium-99m. It has a 6-hour half-life, a photon energy of 140 kev, and minimal nonpenetrating radiation, and it effectively labels a large number of pharmaceuticals—a requirement that is particularly important for equilibrium studies. While pertechnetate leaks out rapidly into the extracellular space with an intravascular half-life of approximately one hour, it does remain intravascular during the first intravascular transit. Because the tracer must remain intravascular only during its first transit, technetium-99m pertechnetate can be used for first-pass studies. Since ^{99m}Tc-pertechnetate ($^{99m}TcO_4^-$) is the chemical form of ^{99m}Tc after elution from the ^{99}Mo*→ ^{99m}Tc generator, it is the most readily available and the least expensive of the technetium-99m pharmaceuticals.

The major disadvantage of ^{99m}Tc is its long half-life relative to the duration of the procedure. After intravenous injection, the material persists in the intravascular and extracellular space, precluding serial studies, and only two or three first-pass studies are possible within a 6-hour period. As a result, evaluation in multiple projections or after multiple physiological or pharmacological interventions is not possible.

One approach to increasing the number of serial studies is the use of ^{99m}Tc-sulfur colloid, a radiopharmaceutical extracted by the reticuloendothelial system, thereby radically shortening the biological half-life. The pharmaceutical is extracted primarily by the liver and spleen within several

*Mo = molybdenum.

minutes after intravenous injection.[8] The disadvantage of this approach is the relatively high radiation dose to the bone marrow. Approximately 5 per cent of the dose is sequestered by the bone marrow, the most radiosensitive of the body's tissues. ^{99m}Tc-pyrophosphate is an attractive alternative in the coronary care unit. Acute infarct scintigraphy can be performed 3 hours after the initial first-pass study. Thus, two studies can be performed after the injection of a single radiopharmaceutical. ^{99m}Tc-DTPA (diethylenetriaminepentaacetic acid) is commonly used for first-pass studies. Its blood clearance is more rapid than that of ^{99m}Tc-pertechnetate, reducing the whole-body radiation dosage and, more importantly, shortening the time between sequential studies.[9]

ULTRASHORT-LIVED NUCLIDES. The development of such nuclides has increased the flexibility of this technique. Gold-195m has a 30-second half-life and an acceptable gamma energy of 262 kev for use with multicrystal cameras and with Anger cameras using medium-energy collimators and adequate shielding.[10] It is obtained from a ^{195}Hg→ ^{195m}Au generator system. Its parent, mercury-195m, has a sufficiently long half-life (41.6 hours) so that each generator will last up to 3 or 4 days.

The advantages of gold-195m are that multiple views can be obtained and serial responses to exercise or drug interventions can be studied by repeating the injection at frequent intervals without build-up of significant background activity and with minimal patient radiation dosage. Also, because of the reduced patient dose relative to ^{99m}Tc, larger doses can be injected, taking full advantage of the higher count-rate capacities of multicrystal cameras and digital Anger cameras. Limitations of this tracer are that the parent, ^{195m}Hg, may be present as a contaminant in the injected dose; the half-life of the tracer is too short to permit measurement of the parent prior to each injection; high-energy photons result in scattered radiation; and the high cost of the generator will make it practical only in hospitals that carry out a large number of first-pass studies.

Other ultrashort half-life tracers have been introduced, including tantalum-178, with a half-life of 9 minutes,[11] iridium-191m, with a half-life of 4.9 seconds,[12] and krypton-81m, with a half-life of 75 seconds.[13, 14] Tantalum-178 is used with low-energy imaging systems such as the multiwire proportional camera. Iridium-191m is used for children, in whom the 4.9-second half-life is tolerable. Krypton-81m is particularly useful for studying right ventricular performance because of its ultrashort half-life and because it is completely extracted from the blood into the lungs during the first transient of the tracer through the circulation. It is particularly useful in acute settings when rapid serial assessments of right ventricular function are required.[13, 14] All three tracers are obtained from long-lived parents by elution through generator systems.

The radiopharmaceutical for equilibrium (ECG-gated) studies (p. 317) must remain within the intravascular space throughout the course of the study. If continual monitoring is anticipated, the radiopharmaceutical must remain within the intravascular space for at least one or two half-lives. Technetium-99m–labeled red blood cells (RBC's) are the tracers of choice for equilibrium imaging.

Once the initial equilibration of the tracer has been reached, ^{99m}Tc-RBC's are cleared from the blood very slowly. The red cells can be tagged in vivo by injecting 300 to 400 μg of stannous iron intravenously and injecting ^{99m}Tc-pertechnetate 15 minutes later. Approximately 60 to 80 per cent of the pertechnetate attaches to and labels the red blood cells; the remainder is excreted through the kidneys or labels iodine traps, such as the kidney and stomach. Equilibration is reached after 5 minutes. Since rapid renal clearance is a precondition for optimal studies, this technique is less satisfactory in patients with poor renal clearance and results in high background activity and poor target-to-background ratios. The primary advantage of this technique is the ease with which the red cells can be labeled. The labeling efficiency can be improved by withdrawing 5 to 10 cc of the patient's blood into the syringe containing the ^{99m}Tc-pertechnetate and gently agitating the syringe for the 30 seconds before reinjection. Kits have been developed for in vitro labeling of the patient's own red cells. The major advantage of this approach is the high labeling efficiency (greater than or equal to 98 per cent). This technique does take more time than in vivo labeling, but with the kits, labeling can be performed in 15 to 30 minutes.

TECHNIQUES

Radionuclide angiocardiography can be used to measure (1) left and right ventricular *ejection fraction*; (2) indices of *regional ventricular performance*; (3) left ventricular *cardiac output*; (4) end-diastolic and end-systolic *ventricular volumes*; (5) indices of early *systolic* and *diastolic function*; (6) indices of aortic, mitral, and tricuspid *regurgitation*; (7) indices of *asynchrony*; (8) *transit times* within the central circulation; and (9) *intracardiac shunts*. In addition, visual assessment of the cardiac chambers and the great vessels is also a routine part of the examination. All these indices can be assessed with either first-pass or equilibrium studies except for transit time measurements and shunt detection, which can be achieved only with first-pass methods.

FIRST-PASS STUDIES

First-pass radionuclide angiocardiography measures indices of cardiac performance from the initial transit of the radiotracer through the heart.[15, 16] For accurate quantitation of first-pass studies, it is important that the radiopharmaceutical be injected in as small a volume as possible, that it be injected rapidly, and that it not be delayed in the venous structures. While in some validation studies a central venous catheter or a Swan-Ganz catheter was used to administer the radiopharmaceutical, satisfactory results have been obtained using a 19-gauge butterfly-type needle inserted into a prominent medial antecubital vein or, in children, into an external jugular vein. Approximately 25 to 30 mCi of ^{99m}Tc-DTPA (or correspondingly less if several studies are going to be obtained in rapid sequence) should be injected rapidly in a volume of less than 1 ml and flushed immediately. Several techniques have been suggested for intravenous delivery.[17–20]

DATA COLLECTION. Computer acquisition is usually performed in frame mode with a framing rate of 10 to 50 msec depending on the heart rate and the temporal resolution desired. Imaging is performed in the right anterior oblique (RAO) or anterior projections since the right and left ventricles contain the radioactive bolus at different times after injection. The RAO projection is optimal for the separation of the left atrium and the left ventricle and the anterior view is best suited for separating cardiac and pulmonary activity (which is important in shunt quantitation). Like the equilibrium technique, the first-pass study can be gated using the electrocardiogram (ECG).

Ventricular Performance

The most frequent application of radionuclide angiocardiography is to evaluate ventricular performance, both subjectively and quantitatively.

ANATOMY. By observing the passage of the bolus during the first transit, it is possible to make a subjective analysis of cardiac anatomy. This is particularly useful for detecting intracardiac shunts but may also be of use in evaluating patients with valvular and congenital abnormalities (see p. 317). Gross changes can be observed, such as the large left atrium and the small, normally functioning left ventricle of mitral stenosis; the large left atrium and ventricle of mitral or aortic regurgitation; or the greatly enlarged right atrium of tricuspid regurgitation. Knowledge of the fine anatomy required for defining valvular lesions cannot be obtained with this technique, and thus its clinical application is not widespread.

Much more useful has been the definition of segmental wall motion. A radionuclide angiocardiogram with high temporal resolution is constructed from the left ventricular time-activity curve corrected for background. Each of two to four successive cardiac cycles is divided into 16 frames, and the corresponding frames of each cycle are added together to yield one summed or composite cardiac cycle.[21]

The composite image is played back repetitively, producing a cine display for subjective analysis of regional wall motion abnormalities. Quantitative measurements of hemiaxis shortening can be determined from the superimposed end-diastolic and end-systolic images.

QUANTITATIVE MEASUREMENTS. When the entire heart is considered to be the region of interest, a time-activity curve of combined right and left ventricular activity is generated (Fig. 11–2). To obtain meaningful hemodynamic information, the activity of the left ventricle must be isolated from that of the surrounding anatomical structures. Separation between the two ventricles is achieved temporally, since the activity enters the left ventricle after it has been cleared from the right ventricle. Frames corresponding to the left ventricular phase are determined and summed. From the composite image of the left ventricular blood pool, the contour of the left ventricle can be determined using either an electronic cursor or an edge-detection algorithm.

Background Correction. Even when the left ventricle is accurately delineated, the resultant activity is not entirely due to blood in its cavity. Background activity emanates from lung tissue behind and adjacent to the heart and from scattered radioactivity from other structures. A second region must be assigned for the correction of background. The ejection fraction can be underestimated by as much as 25 per cent if background correction is not made.

Best results are obtained when a semiannular background region is placed around the left ventricle but not overlying the aorta.[8] An alternative approach to background correction determines the count rate occurring from the left ventricle just prior to the left ventricular phase and uses this activity for background correction.[22, 23]

Left Ventricular Ejection Fraction. Time-activity curves of left ventricular and background activity are generated. The curve is made up of a series of oscillations with the greatest amplitude of these oscillations occurring at the greatest height of the curve itself. The count rates at the peaks in the oscillation are proportional to end-diastolic volume. If ejection fraction were determined from only one oscillation, the statistical reliability of the information would be poor; therefore, at least three or, if possible, five cardiac cycles should be averaged, beginning at the peak of the left ventricular time-activity curve (Fig. 11–3). The difference in count rate between end-diastole and end-systole is proportional to stroke volume. Ejection fraction (EF) is obtained by dividing that number by the

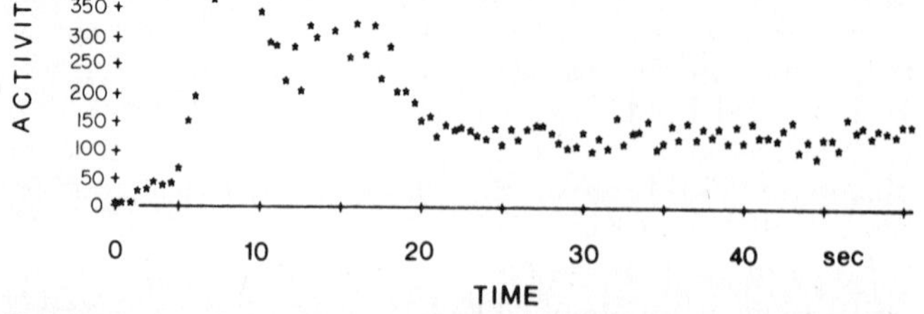

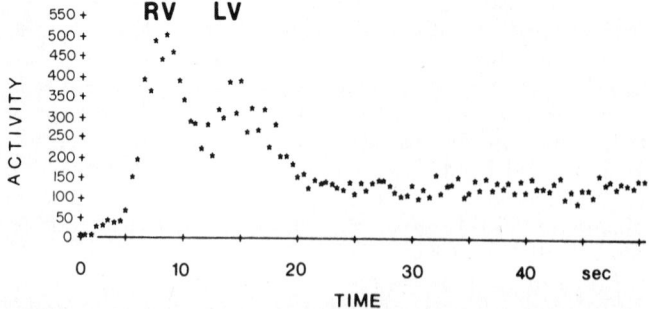

FIGURE 11–2. Time-activity curve resulting from the first transit of the radiotracer through the right ventricle (RV) and left ventricle (LV). (From Ashburn, W. L., et al.: Left ventricular ejection fraction—a review of several radionuclide angiographic approaches using the scintillation camera. Progr. Cardiovasc. Dis. *20*:267, 1978, by permission of Grune and Stratton, Inc.)

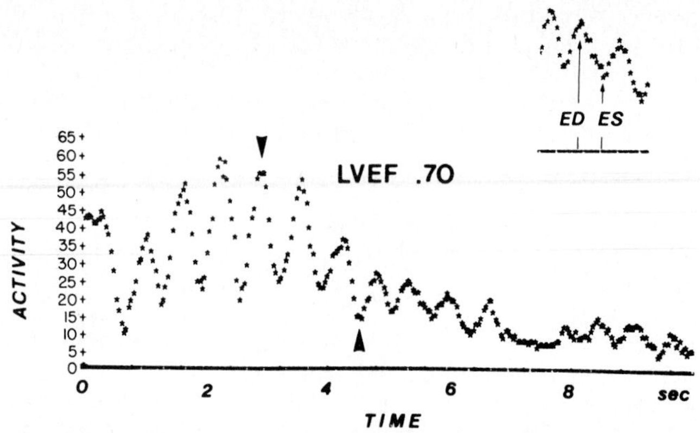

FIGURE 11–3. Time-activity curve from left ventricular region. Each point represents total counts for 40 msec. The highest value (peak) for each cycle corresponds to end-diastole (ED) and the subsequent low value (valley) to end-systole (ES). An average left ventricular ejection fraction (LVEF) of 0.70 was calculated for the three cycles between the arrows. (From Ashburn, W. L., et al.: Left ventricular ejection fraction—a review of several radionuclide angiographic approaches using the scintillation camera. Progr. Cardiovasc. Dis. *20*:267, 1978, by permission of Grune and Stratton, Inc.)

end-diastolic count rate minus background:

$$EF = \frac{\text{Diastolic counts} - \text{Systolic counts}}{\text{Diastolic counts} - \text{Background counts}} \quad (1)$$

Techniques for determining ejection fraction have been validated by comparison with values obtained using single-plane and biplane contrast ventriculography. Correlation coefficients ranging from $r = 0.94$ to $r = 0.97$ have been reported by a number of groups who have compared the two techniques.[8, 22, 24]

Right Ventricular Ejection Fraction. Right ventricular performance is difficult to quantitate, since the geometry of the right ventricle is complex, making calculation of the right ventricular ejection fraction by standard geometrical methods extremely difficult. A radionuclide method for this measurement has been developed and is similar in many respects to that for left ventricular ejection fraction.[25] The radiotracer is injected intravenously, through either a large medial antecubital vein or the jugular vein, in a volume of less than 2 ml. The first pass of the radioactive bolus through the central circulation is recorded in the 30-degree right anterior oblique projection. The ejection fraction is measured from the time-activity curve derived from the right ventricular blood pool. A region of interest is assigned to this pool, carefully excluding the right atrium and the pulmonary artery. A second semiannular region of interest is placed outside the right ventricle adjacent to the apical anterior and inferior walls. A high-frequency time-activity curve (25 frames/sec) is generated from both the right ventricular and the background regions of interest. Right ventricular ejection fraction is calculated by dividing the difference in counts between end-diastole and end-systole by the number of counts at end-diastole after correcting for background. Three to five beats from the downslope of the right ventricular time-activity curve are used for the calculation.

Background correction of the right ventricular ejection fraction measurement appears necessary only when serial studies are performed, since background activity alters right ventricular ejection fraction by less than 5 per cent.[25] Because the activity is high and the background is low during transit through the right ventricle, single-crystal cameras can be used for this purpose, although multi-crystal cameras provide significantly higher counting rates and therefore improve the statistical reliability of the measurement.[26] Using the first-pass method, investigators

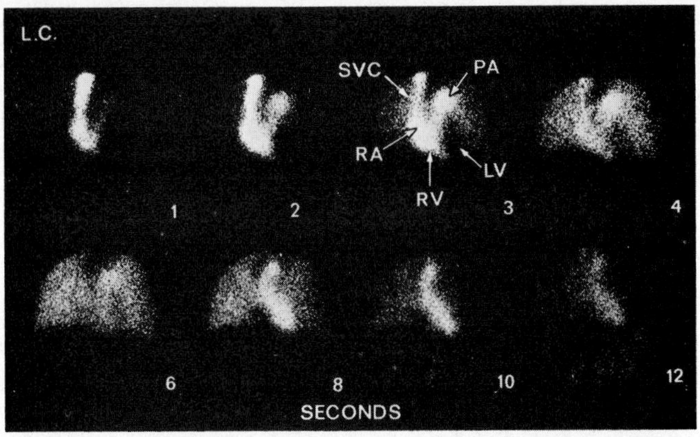

FIGURE 11–4. First-transit radionuclide angiogram. At 1 second, the tracer is in the superior vena cava, right atrium, and right ventricle. By 3 seconds, the radioactivity is entering the lungs through the pulmonary arteries. By 8 seconds, the radioactivity has returned to the left side of the heart. The left ventricle and aorta are clearly seen, and the lung background is rapidly diminishing. Numbers represent time of frames in seconds following the injection. (SVC = superior vena cava; RA = right atrium; RV = right ventricle; LV = left ventricle; PA = pulmonary artery.)

have found the mean right ventricular ejection fraction normally to be between 0.52 and 0.57.[25–27]

Shunt Detection

In normal patients, the lung time-activity curve has a characteristic appearance after intravenous injection of a first-pass tracer. There is an early peak due to the appearance of radiotracer in the lungs. This is followed by rapid clearance as the tracer moves into the systemic circulation. Eventually some recirculation will occur as the tracer returns from the systemic circulation to the right side of the heart and the lungs (Fig. 11–4). In patients with *left-to-right shunts,* the tracer passes from the left to the right side of the heart, short-circuiting the systemic circulation and resulting in rapid recirculation to the lungs. On first-pass radionuclide angiocardiography, the three distinct phases (right heart, lungs, and left heart) merge owing to rapid recirculation, and a clear definition of the left ventricle is not possible because of the high level of radioactivity in the lungs (Fig. 11–5).

The most satisfactory method for quantification of left-to-right shunts is to calculate the ratio of pulmonary flow to systemic flow ($\dot{Q}_p/\dot{Q}_s$).[28] ^{99m}Tc-pertechnetate is injected intravenously as a bolus (200 μCi/kg or 2 mCi, whichever is greater) into the right external jugular vein to ensure that the tracer enters the right side of the heart as a discrete bolus. The degree to which the bolus disperses can be assessed by obtaining a time-activity curve over the superior vena cava; its duration should be 2 seconds or less. The patient is positioned to obtain an anterior view, so that the right lung can be separated from the heart. Recording is begun immediately after injection and continued for 30 to 60 seconds. Since high temporal resolution is not required for evaluation of the pulmonary dilution curve, frames of 0.5-second duration can be used.

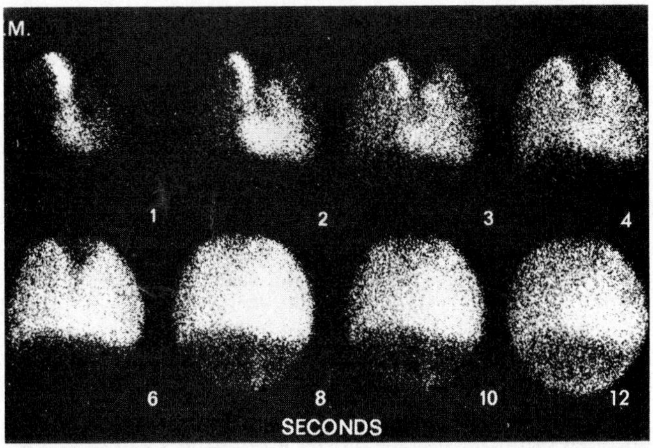

FIGURE 11–5. Left-to-right shunt at atrial level. Recirculation of radioactivity is seen in the lungs. In addition, radioactivity reappears in the right atrium, right ventricle, and pulmonary artery at 8, 10, and 12 seconds (bottom right). (From Treves, S., et al.: Intracardiac shunts. *In* James, A. E., et al. [eds.]: Pediatric Nuclear Medicine. Philadelphia, W. B. Saunders Company, 1974, p. 231.)

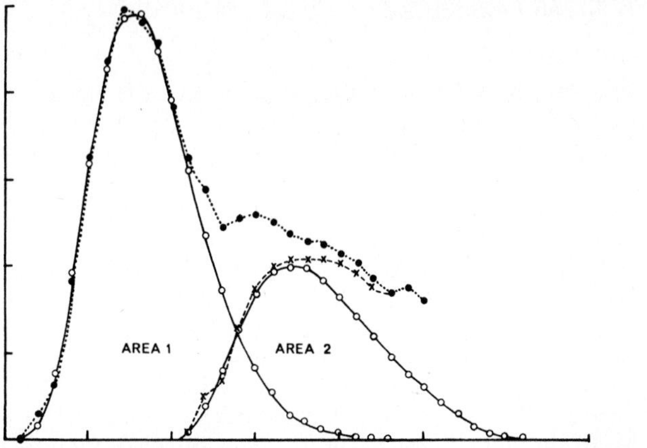

FIGURE 11–6. Quantitation of the left-to-right shunt by gamma variate analysis. For details, see the text. (From Maltz, D. L., et al.: Quantitative radionuclide angiocardiography: Determination of Q_p:Q_s in children. Circulation *47*:1049, 1973, by permission of the American Heart Association, Inc.)

The time-activity curve is generated by creating a region of interest over the right lung (Fig. 11–6). The component of the wash-out curve due to recirculation (Area 2 in Figure 11–6) is extracted from the curve using gamma variate analysis. After extracting the systemic flow component and determining its area, the portion of the curve due to pulmonary blood flow ($\dot{Q}_p$) (Area 1 in Figure 11–6) is extracted, and its area is measured. The size of the left-to-right shunt can then be determined from the formula

$$\dot{Q}_p/\dot{Q}_s = \frac{\text{Area 1}}{\text{Area 1} - \text{Area 2}} \qquad (2)$$

More sophisticated algorithms have been suggested using deconvolution analysis to correct for variations in the rate of injection and factor analysis for curve generation.[29, 30] Using either gamma variate or deconvolution analysis, the correlation with oximetric measurement of the pulmonary-to-systemic flow ratio has been excellent.[28] However, the technique cannot distinguish between poor ventricular performance and left-to-right shunting and should be used only when left ventricular performance is adequate.

Right-to-left shunts can be detected from inspection of the radionuclide angiocardiogram and by early visualization of either the left heart chambers or the aorta.[31, 32] An alternative approach is intravenous injection of a radioactive inert gas (xenon-133 or krypton-81m). Since the inert gas is extracted with very high efficiency from the lungs, significant systemic activity indicates a right-to-left shunt.[33, 34]

EQUILIBRIUM STUDIES

First-pass dynamic radionuclide studies are limited to the counts acquired during a few cardiac cycles. To increase the total number of counts and, hence, the resolution of the radionuclide angiocardiogram, a tracer that remains in the intravascular system can be imaged at equilibrium. To achieve high temporal resolution, count acquisition is gated to a physiological marker, usually the R wave of the electrocardiogram.

Unlike the first-pass study, the radionuclide must reach equilibration within the intravascular space prior to imaging. This means that all four cardiac chambers as well as the great vessels and surrounding organs, such as liver and spleen, will be visualized at the same time. As a result, special attention must be paid to separation of the right from the left side of the heart and separation of the surrounding organs from the heart. This can be accomplished by obtaining views in multiple projections and with specially designed collimators, since imaging is not restricted to one or two positions as in first-pass studies.

Since a large number of counts can be obtained by constructing one average cardiac cycle as a composite of many cycles, a high-resolution collimator can be used. The most informative projection is the modified left anterior oblique (MLAO), with the detector angled so that the right and left ventricles are completely separated. This usually occurs between 35 and 45 degrees in the left anterior oblique (LAO) projection. An additional 30-degree caudal tilt is required to separate the left atrium from the left ventricle and to enable imaging parallel to the long axis of the left ventricle. Since caudal angulation of this magnitude is difficult to achieve with standard collimators, the angulation should be built into the collimator. The 30-degree slant-hole collimator can then be placed flat against the patient's chest.

While global left ventricular hemodynamic information and much information concerning regional wall motion can be obtained from the modified left anterior oblique projection, other views—particularly the shallow (30-degree) right anterior oblique (RAO), anterior, and 70-degree left anterior oblique projections—are useful for providing information concerning the anterior, inferior, and lateral walls of the left ventricle, which are not imaged tangentially in the MLAO projection.

GATING. In gated studies, a "gate" is opened by a control signal. When the gate is closed, the signals are not passed on, and it appears that there are no scintillations. The control signal is usually based on some cyclic physiological process, such as the cardiac cycle. Two general methods are used for collecting all phases of the cardiac cycle simultaneously—*in-memory gating* and *gated list mode* collection. When in-memory gating is used, the main memory is divided into a large number of image matrices (Fig. 11–7). With the occurrence of the R wave, which is the control signal, the scintillation data are directed to the first frame. After a predefined time, usually 25 msec (or a predefined fraction of the R-R interval, usually 1/32 of the duration of the cardiac cycle), the data are directed to the second frame. After each subsequent 25 msec (or after each fraction of the R-R interval), data are directed sequentially to each of the remaining frames until the next R wave, when data are redirected to the first frame. Each matrix is a map of the two-dimensional distribution of the tracer during a specific portion of the cardiac cycle.

With this technique, the data can be viewed while being acquired, so that it can be determined immediately whether the data collection is adequate. In-memory gating requires a constant heart rate and cannot be applied effectively in the presence of an arrhythmia. It also requires

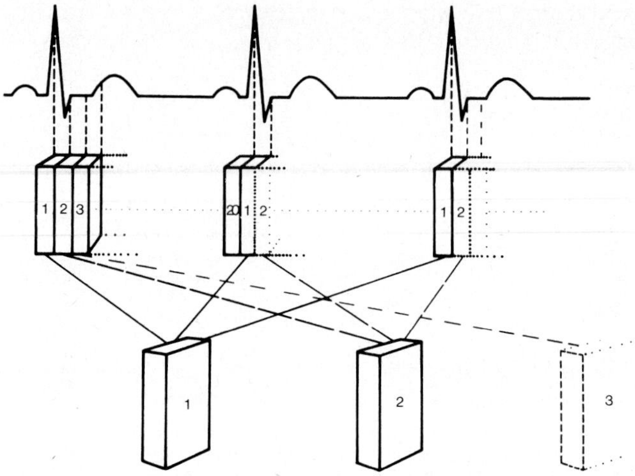

FIGURE 11–7. Camera acquisition is gated to the patient's electrocardiogram. Counts are stored in frames, where frame 1 represents the total counts obtained during the first portion (twentieth second) of all cardiac cycles recorded.

considerable main computer memory if adequate temporal and spatial resolution is to be achieved.

In the gated list mode, scintigraphic data are collected in a list mode along with samples of the electrocardiogram. In other words, the data are recorded as a list or table as they are received by the computer. After the collection period is over, the data are reformatted by sorting the list. With this method, the number of frames per second and the size of the image matrix can be determined *after* the data have been collected. Also, frames having a predefined R-R interval time can be analyzed, so that patients with arrhythmia can be studied.[35,36] This method uses a very large amount of auxiliary memory. Reformatting times may be long without the aid of array processors or large computers.

DATA COLLECTION. Between 2 million and 10 million counts are collected in 30 to 60 frames of 64 × 64 elements. More counts are collected when the patient is at rest and high resolution studies are required; fewer counts are collected during transient periods of steady-state heart rate, such as during exercise. For measurements of ejection fraction, a temporal resolution of 50 msec (20 frames/sec) is necessary at rest and 40 msec (25 frames/sec) with exercise. To obtain peak ejection rates and peak filling rates, 40 msec/frame at rest and 20 msec with exercise are required.[37]

RADIONUCLIDE CINEANGIOCARDIOGRAPHY. The cinematic display is an endless loop of the sequential frames that make up the equilibrium study. Data from the angiocardiogram can be interpolated to produce a continuous, flicker-free cinematic display. Overall anatomy, such as size and position of the great vessels, can be evaluated subjectively as can global and regional left and right ventricular size and function (Fig. 11–8). Criteria for the subjective interpretation of regional ventricular performance are derived from contrast ventriculography. Using similar criteria, radionuclide angiocardiography is almost as accurate as contrast ventriculography for assessing regional ventricular function.[38] The left ventricle is divided into anatomical segments, usually the anterior wall (best seen on the 30-degree RAO and 70-degree LAO views), anteroseptum (best seen on the 45-degree LAO or MLAO view), apex (seen on all views), and inferoposterior wall (best seen on the 45-degree MLAO and 70-degree LAO views). Each segment is interpreted as normal, mildly hypokinetic, severely hypokinetic, akinetic, or dyskinetic.

NUMERICAL ANALYSIS. Quantitative measurements of

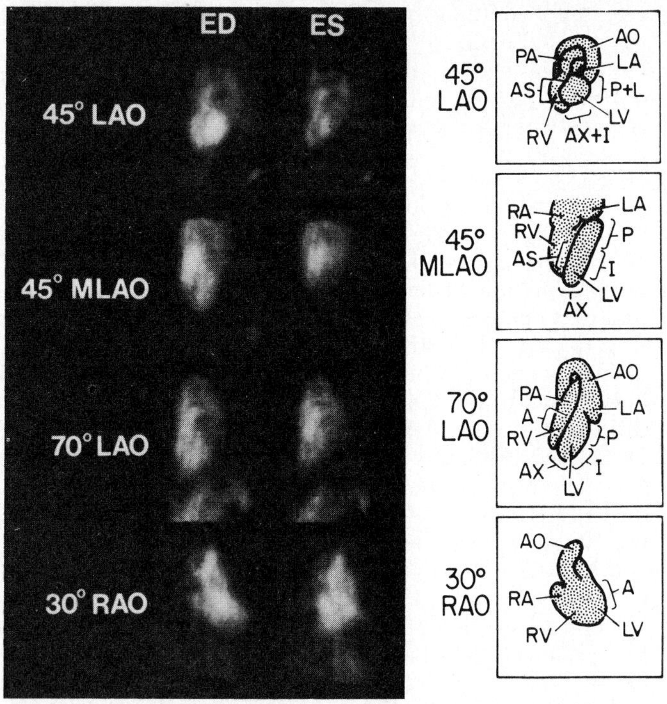

FIGURE 11–8. **Normal equilibrium (gated) radionuclide angiocardiogram. LAO = left anterior oblique projection; MLAO = modified left anterior oblique; RAO = right anterior oblique; ED = end-diastole; ES = end-systole; PA = pulmonary artery; AS = anteroseptal; RV = right ventricle; AX = apex; I = inferior; LV = left ventricle; P = posterior; L = lateral; LA = left atrium; AO = aorta; RA = right atrium.**

global and regional ventricular function can be obtained from the time-activity curves derived from the left and right ventricles and from regions of the ventricles. Since the radiopharmaceutical is uniformly mixed in the blood at equilibrium, a time-activity curve over the ventricles will represent the changes in ventricular volume occurring during the cardiac cycle. However, because activity is distributed throughout the intravascular space, including tissue in front of and behind the heart, accurate background correction is essential.

Wall motion can be assessed by radionuclide methods either from the geometrical approaches used in the standard contrast angiographic method or from analysis of changes in count rate. Background-corrected activity recorded from the region of the left ventricle is directly proportional to this chamber's blood volume. Although the radionuclide method provides limited spatial resolution and edge definition, it does offer an accurate measure of the activity viewed by the detector or a region of the detector. Therefore, assessment of global and regional ventricular function based on changing count rates has two inherent advantages over the geometrical approaches borrowed from contrast angiography: (1) The geometrical approaches assess only that part of the ventricular wall which is tangential to the detector. Techniques based on left ventricular activity assess the three-dimensional space viewed by the corresponding region of the detector, assessing ventricular function regardless of its orientation to the detector. Techniques based on activity do not require assumptions concerning left ventricular shape—a consideration that is particularly important in patients with asynergy, in whom such geometrical assumptions may not be valid. (2) The need to define the margins of the left ventricle during end-systole is eliminated with the count-rate method. During end-systole, the difference between ventricular and background activity may be small and edge resolution particularly poor.

Numerical analysis requires careful attention to quality control. Each of the indices that will be used on a routine clinical basis should be validated in the nuclear cardiology laboratory where it will be applied. Each laboratory should have a carefully supervised program which periodically assesses performance of the instrumentation, data collection, and data processing. Careful attention should be directed to standardization of the procedures so that serial assessments in the same patient will be reliable. All of the indices depend on accurate data collection and processing and on the patient's physiological state (supine or erect, fasting or postprandial, relaxed or psychologically stressed).[39]

SMOOTHING AND FILTERING. Noise in the image can be reduced by either increasing imaging time, increasing the dose, or smoothing the data. Smoothing can reduce the effects of noise that result from variations in radioactive decay. Noise interferes with both visual analysis and with data quantification by making edge detection more difficult and by increasing statistical uncertainties. Spatial smoothing is used to reduce the noise in static images, and temporal smoothing decreases the noise between the same region on consecutive images. After smoothing, the value of a pixel (picture element) is a weighted average of its original value with those regions surrounding it.

Filtering is a general term for smoothing and refers to an operation that suppresses or enhances certain frequencies of an image. Reducing the high frequencies (noise) of an image is equivalent to smoothing; decreasing the low frequencies results in background subtraction. Filters can also enhance those frequencies which define structures, such as edges. Finally, because of the cosine shape of the ventricular time-volume curve, Fourier filtering can be used to describe the shape of the curve while minimizing random fluctuations and improving the accuracy of the quantitative parameters.

BACKGROUND CORRECTION. The left ventricular time-activity curve is generated after the left ventricular outline and background regions have been defined either using an automated program or manually using a light pen or an electronic cursor and after subtraction of background. Automated programs for outlining the left ventricle and the background regions reduce operator variance and may improve the accuracy of the numerical analysis. Automated methods require that the position of the left ventricle be localized and that it be separated from surrounding structures. The ejection fraction, phase, or amplitude images are used for localization to delineate the contours of end-diastole because they clearly separate the left ventricle and left atrium. With these methods difficulty is experienced in regions of poor left ventricular function. Other factors which affect automated programs include poor image statistics because of the limited acquisition times and the injected doses, poor image resolution, and cross-contamination from surrounding chambers. Image filtering techniques to improve the signal-to-noise ratio result in accurate definition of a left ventricular outline in 80 to 90 per cent of patients.[40, 41]

As with first-pass studies, background correction is critical, since approximately 33 to 50 per cent of the activity emanating from the area of the left ventricle is due to background. The background regions, usually representing areas just lateral and inferior to the heart and including a portion of the interventricular septum, can be defined manually or automatically using predefined computer algorithms.

Several general approaches have been suggested for background correction: (1) fixed ventricular and background regions can be defined from the end-diastolic frame; and (2) a variable left ventricular region, shrinking during systole and expanding during diastole, can be defined. Background regions may be continuous or interrupted and may extend into the septum. Background regions never abut the base of the ventricle. However, each of these approaches can result in accurate measures of ejection fraction if applied carefully and if adequately controlled comparisons are made regularly with measurements derived at cardiac catheterization.

LEFT VENTRICULAR EJECTION FRACTION. Once background activity is known with reasonable accuracy, ejection fraction can be determined from changes in count rate rather than from geometrical analysis,[38, 42, 43] since changes in left ventricular activity are directly proportional to changes in ventricular blood volume. Ejection fraction is calculated from the formula

$$\mathrm{LVEF} = \frac{\mathrm{EDC} - \mathrm{ESC}}{\mathrm{EDC} - \mathrm{BC}} \quad (3)$$

where LVEF is left ventricular ejection fraction; EDC, or "end-diastolic counts," represents the activity emanating from the region of the left ventricle during the frame corresponding to end-diastole; and ESC, or "end-systolic counts," represents left ventricular activity during the end-systolic frame; BC stands for background counts. These two frames can be determined from the time-activity curve and correspond to the maximum and minimum points, respectively. Ejection fraction obtained using this algorithm correlates very well with ejection fractions derived by means of contrast ventriculography ($r = 0.92$).[37] While the count-based method for determination of left ventricular ejection fraction has been the most reliable and most useful of the global indices derived from the radionuclide angiocardiogram, the method does underestimate left ventricular ejection fraction in patients with dilated left ventricles and particularly with regional asynergy involving the anterior wall.[44]

VENTRICULAR VOLUME AND CARDIAC OUTPUT. Left ventricular volume can be measured using geometrical or count-rate principles. End-diastolic left ventricular volume can be measured using techniques originally developed for contrast ventriculography. A left ventricular end-diastolic contour is determined by means of an electronic cursor or an edge detection algorithm. A grid of known dimensions is then placed between the radioactive source and the detector for size correction, and the volume is determined using the technique of Sandler and Dodge.[45] Since the ventricular edges are not as well defined on radionuclide angiocardiography as with contrast left ventriculography, and because only one projection is used for the measurement (30-degree LAO), it would not be expected that the resulting measurement would be as accurate as biplane contrast ventriculography or count-based methods. The geometric method has the compelling advantage of simplicity and ease of performance, however. Gated emission computed tomography improves the accuracy of the geometric method by providing three-dimensional information on the shape of the left ventricle and eliminating the need for background correction but at the expense of substantially increasing the time and complexity of the study.[46, 47]

The count-rate method compares the background-corrected left ventricular activity with the activity in a known volume of the patient's blood. To obtain volumes in milliliters and output in liters/min, attenuation corrections must be introduced.[48] This is the most difficult of the numerical analyses to measure accurately because of the varying attenuation among patients, particularly between men and women, and the careful attention to detail that is required. Attenuation corrections are also dependent on the distance to the center of the ventricle from the chest wall; therefore, attenuation corrections are patient-dependent.[49]

Left ventricular ejection fraction and end-diastolic volume have been the most useful indices of global function in clinical practice. These measurements and end-systolic volume are of limited value, however, and are affected by changes in loading conditions independent of changes in muscle function (p. 316).[50] Therefore, left ventricular ejection fraction provides information concerning overall performance of the ventricle but is an unreliable indicator of *intrinsic* contractile performance. For clinical purposes, the end-systolic pressure-volume relationship constructed from several points obtained under varying loading conditions is the preferred means for assessing muscle function.

The count rate method for determining the left ventricular volume is well suited for the measurement of pressure-volume relations during gradual changes in the afterload conditions. While the changes in left ventricular volume are small from one measurement to the next, the patient serves as his own control, eliminating the problem of tissue attenuation and the distance of the left ventricle from the detector. Animal studies have shown an excellent correlation between these small changes in end-systolic volume as measured by the radionuclide technique and contrast ventriculography.[51]

Contrast ventriculography is unsuitable for serial assessment of left ventricular pressure volume relations with altered loading conditions. Radionuclide methods for assessing left ventricular ejection fraction and left ventricular end-diastolic volume are useful complements to the determination of left ventricular pressure at the time of cardiac catheterization when left ventricular pressure-volume curves are being constructed during altered loading conditions to evaluate left ventricular contractility.[52]

LEFT VENTRICULAR EJECTION-PHASE INDICES. A number of ejection-phase performance indices (p. 316) can be measured from the left ventricular time-activity curve. *Left ventricular ejection rate* can be measured from either the equilibrium or the first-pass radionuclide angiocardiogram. A weighted least-square analysis can be used to fit the ejection phase data (four to nine data points per ejection phase) to a straight line.[8] The slope of this line, representing the change in counts with time, dC/dT, is determined and normalized to the average number of counts over the ejection phase ($dC/dT/C_{ave}$). This measurement, unlike the left ventricular ejection fraction, appears to be sensitive to changes in the inotropic state in patients with cardiac disease. The normal value for the normalized left ventricular ejection rate is 3.40 ± 0.17 $dC/dT/C_{ave}$. In patients who have coronary artery disease, this value is 1.22 ± 0.11 $dC/dT/C_{ave}$.

LEFT VENTRICULAR DIASTOLIC PHASE INDICES. Indices of diastolic function are more sensitive for detecting the effects of myocardial ischemia than are systolic indices such as ejection fraction[53] (p. 321). These changes in the diastolic properties of the ventricle are seen in acute myocardial ischemia and may be present even at rest in patients with coronary artery disease.[54, 55] Both first-pass and equilibrium methods can be used to derive indices of diastolic function (as well as the other phase indices described in this section) from the left ventricular volume curve. The *first third filling fraction* is the difference between the ejection fraction measured at end-systole and at a time in the cardiac cycle one-third of the way between end-systole and peak filling. The difference is normalized by the ejection fraction at end-systole so that the index reflects the efficiency of left ventricular filling during the early phase of diastole.[56] The *isovolumic relaxation period* can be measured automatically from the high temporal resolution (10 to 20 msec) left ventricular time activity curve and represents the interval between minimal volume and onset of rapid filling.[57] The *peak diastolic filling rate* expresses diastolic filling as a fraction of the end-diastolic volume per second. It is calculated from the diastolic portion of the left ventricular volume curve by fitting a third-order polynomial to the first 400 msec of diastole.[58] The point of maximum filling is determined by setting the second derivative of the polynomial to zero. The third-order polynomial is then differentiated to yield the maximum filling rate, which is normalized to the total end-diastolic counts. With this method, the peak diastolic filling rate has been found to be 2.14 ± 0.63 end-diastolic volume/sec in normals and is reduced in about 90 per cent of patients with previous myocardial infarction when they are studied at rest. Patients with coronary artery disease but without previous infarction also have a high incidence of abnormal filling rates at rest.[58, 59] Abnormalities in both peak diastolic filling rates and first third filling fractions are also present in patients with systemic hypertension even in its mild to moderate stages.[56] While diastolic indices may be a nonspecific method for identifying patients with coronary artery disease, noninvasive assessment of diastolic function may be quite useful for identifying the underlying abnormality in patients with increased cardiac output or pulmonary vascular congestion who may have normal end-systolic cardiac function.

FUNCTIONAL IMAGES. It is important for the physician who is accustomed to using contrast ventriculography to keep in mind the differences between contrast and radionuclide studies. The contrast ventriculogram represents volume information relatively poorly because mixing of the contrast is not complete and because there are difficulties with film linearity. However, because it has excellent resolution, it defines the edges of the ventricle well; therefore, volume can be calculated from the two-dimensional silhouette of the ventricle, and edge motion is used to evaluate wall motion. By comparison, the radionuclide angiocardiogram has poor spatial resolution, but the image data are directly proportional to ventricular volume after background correction. For this reason, techniques such as functional imaging have been very useful aids in the interpretation of the radionuclide angiocardiogram. Subjective assessment of the cineangiocardiogram must rely on catching the wall motion abnormality on target, hence the need for multiple views. With functional imaging, we take advantage of the count-rate changes that occur throughout the ventricle and result in intensity changes in the image rather than alterations on the edges of the image.

Functional images are physiological maps. After certain arithmetic operations have been performed on a group of images, the resultant image(s) is no longer representative of the basic activity distribution but is representative of some physiological function, such as regional ejection fraction or onset of contraction. In such an image the intensities are proportional to a function rather than to the original activity distributions.

Ejection-Fraction Image. The ejection-fraction image makes use of the proportionality between background-corrected left ventricular count rate and blood volume. By subtracting the end-systolic image from the end-diastolic image, an image of regional stroke volume can be obtained. The stroke-volume image is divided by the background-corrected end-diastolic image to produce an ejection-fraction image, a map of regional ejection fractions throughout the left ventricle.[60]

In the ejection-fraction image, the intensity of each of the matrix areas is directly proportional to the regional ejection fraction. The normal ejection-fraction image is characterized by a peripheral ejection shell comprising matrices with greater than 50 per cent ejection—i.e., a reduction in blood volume of 50 per cent between diastole and systole in any given matrix area within the end-diastolic perimeter of the left ventricle. The width of the normal ejection shell exceeds one-third of the left ventricular transverse diameter throughout its inferoposterior and apical extent. Thinning of the ejection shell corresponds to hypokinesis, and absence of the shell corresponds to akinesis (Fig. 11–9). The accuracy of this technique compares favorably with contrast ventriculography for the detection of ventricular asynergy.[60]

Paradox Image. If the end-diastolic frame is subtracted from the end-systolic frame, the resultant image will show areas of left ventricular paradox. The presence and extent of paradox in each picture element is determined from the end-diastolic (ED) and end-systolic (ES) counts within that picture element according to the equation

$$\text{Paradox} = \text{ES} - \text{ED} \qquad (4)$$

The extent of paradox may be determined in terms of both the number of picture elements (pixels) within the left ventricle demonstrating paradox and the number of counts within those pixels. Both the number of pixels and the number of counts are normalized by dividing the number of pixels demonstrating paradox by the number of picture elements within the entire left ventricle during end-diastole and the number of counts within the left ventricle during end-diastole, respectively. There is an excellent correlation between this technique and contrast ventriculography for detecting dyskinetic wall motion.[61]

Phase and Amplitude Images. The radionuclide angiocardiogram can be used to assess regional ventricular performance quantitatively at different intervals during the cardiac cycle and to characterize regional asynchrony (Fig. 11–10). For example, the most sensitive components of

FIGURE 11–9. See Color Plate 2.

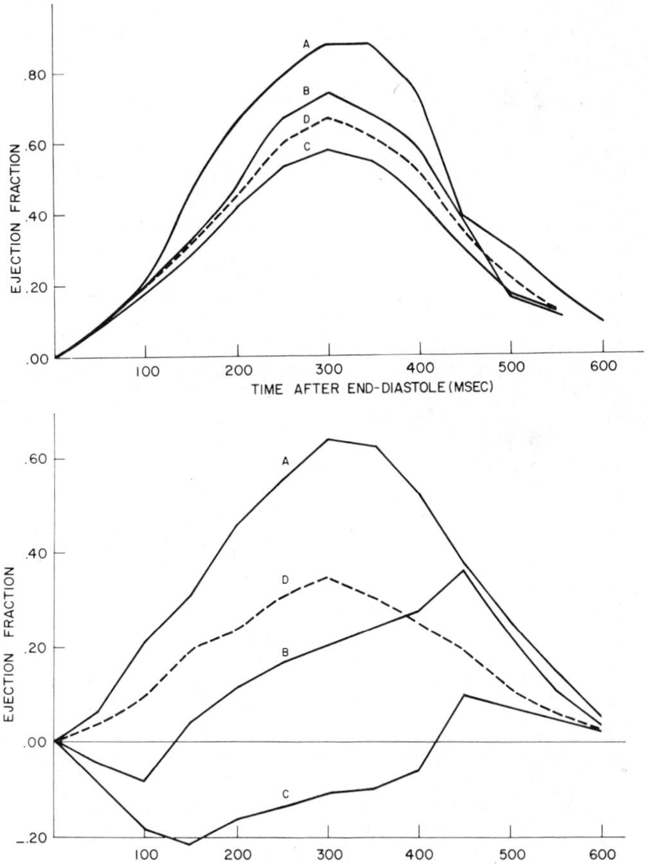

FIGURE 11–10. *Top*, Regional ejection fractions calculated at various times after the R-wave in a patient with normal cardiac performance. Ejection fractions were calculated regionally over the septum (A), inferoposterior left ventricular wall (B), and apex (C), as well as globally over the entire left ventricle (D). Note that contraction is uniform throughout the left ventricle. *Bottom*, Similar calculations were performed in a patient with previous myocardial infarction. At the apex of the left ventricle (C), there is early paradox which persists through end-systole (300 msec after the R wave) with contraction occurring only in the late stages of the cycle. In the border region (B) paradox occurs in early systole and peak contraction occurs well after global end-systole. These abnormalities in the temporal sequence of contraction are encoded in phase images. (From Holman, B. L., et al.: Disruption in the temporal sequence of regional ventricular contraction. Circulation *61*:1075, 1980, by permission of the American Heart Association.)

the cardiac cycle may be during early systole and during relaxation rather than at end-systole. Furthermore, delayed regional contraction and early systolic paradox characterize ventricular contraction in zones bordering on previous infarction.[62] Assessment of regional asynchrony is also useful to detect the foci of ventricular activation in patients with altered patterns of contraction due to pacemakers and to arrhythmias.[64]

Phase images pictorially describe the pattern of cardiac contraction. The first Fourier harmonic is used to fit a cosine wave to the time-activity curve for each pixel in the image. This approach therefore assumes that the ventricular volume curve is similar to one cycle or period of a cosine wave. The number of counts in each frame of the study is determined, and terminal frames containing less than 95 per cent of the average counts (determined over the first half of the study) are excluded. The remaining frames are temporally and spatially smoothed. A first Fourier harmonic phase image is generated so that each pixel in the image is coded to a color or gray scale to reflect the phase angle or regional phase delay. A phase histogram is compiled for the left and right ventricle (or regions of the ventricle) so that the number of pixels with a given phase angle is plotted against that phase angle.[63] An amplitude image is created from the set of cosine wave amplitudes derived from the pixels encompassing the right and left ventricles.

The resulting phase image has a homogeneous appearance with all ventricular pixels having approximately the same phase. Differences in phases are expressed in degrees (0 to 360); 0 degrees or 360 degrees indicates a perfect synchrony, while 180 degrees indicates a complete asynchrony of contraction (atrium versus ventricle, paradox during end-systole). A histogram of the phase angles versus their frequency characterizes and quantifies ventricular contraction. The normal histogram demonstrates a single and relatively narrow ventricular peak. In patients with ventricular contraction abnormalities, the distribution may be broadened, skewed, or bimodal. Mathematical characterization of the histogram is helpful for differentiating wall motion abnormalities. Statistical uncertainties must be taken into account because of their influence on these quantitative parameters. An "error image" representing the absolute or the relative error in each pixel can be computed and displayed alongside parametric images to help in determining the significance of the anomalies.

In *normal subjects,* the onset of contraction is fairly homogeneous throughout the right and left ventricles and begins soon after the R wave. Contraction begins at the base of the interventricular septum and spreads to the body of the septum, the apex, and then laterally throughout the ventricles. In patients with foci of premature ventricular activation, the focus corresponds to the region with an abnormally early onset of ventricular contraction on the phase image.[64] Phase imaging may be used to localize accurately the site of bypass tracts in patients with Wolff-Parkinson-White syndrome.[65] To localize the accessory conduction pathways visually, a two-dimensional projection of each of the 10 AV ring bypass tract sites in the Duke classification[65a] is superimposed onto three standard gated blood pool views. The region with the earliest phase angles on all three projections is considered to be the bypass tract site. The LAO view is the best for separating left- and right-sided tracts and for determining whether the tract is lateral or medial. The left lateral view separates the anterior from the posterior tracts while the anterior view differentiates lateral from medial tracts.

Phase imaging should be an attractive method for localizing the site of origin of spontaneous ventricular ectopy but would require data acquisition using list mode with reformatting of the ectopic beat. Since most ventricular ectopic beats arise at the periphery of severe wall motion abnormalities, the phase pattern resulting from ventricular ectopy must be distinguishable from the underlying phase pattern of the contraction abnormality itself. Only preliminary evidence is available to suggest that this is possible.[66]

REGIONAL EJECTION FRACTION AND REGIONAL VENTRICULAR FUNCTION. Several methods have been suggested for measuring regional ejection fraction. Basically, one method divides the ventricle into radial sectors while the other divides it into rectangular segments bordering the major and minor axes of the left ventricle.[67, 73] Background is subtracted regionally, using areas adjacent to the various regions. Regional ejection fraction is then calculated from the count-rate changes in each segment using Equation 3 (p. 319). Both methods yield similar results. With the rectangular method, normal regional ejection fraction is 0.66 ± 0.13 in the anteroseptum, 0.85 ± 0.12 in the apex, and 0.74 ± 0.16 in the inferoposterior segment. Regional ejection fraction has been validated as an index of ventricular function both at rest[68] and during exercise.[69]

This method is not as sensitive as functional imaging because normal and abnormal ventricular segments are mixed in the much larger region of interest that must be used for quantification. On the other hand, regional ejection fraction measurements are reproducible and useful in studies that require quantitative measures of wall motion, such as before and during drug therapy.

Regional left ventricular function can also be assessed by measuring the distance that regions of the left ventricle move between end-systole and end-diastole (sector shortening). In one method, the left ventricle is divided into 28 sectors radiating from its center of gravity. Time-activity curves are generated for the sectors and the ejection fraction and Fourier phase are computed for each curve. The area difference between the rest and exercise sector ejection fraction curves are taken as an index of regional contraction and sector phase differences are used as an index of wall motion asynchrony.[70]

RIGHT VENTRICULAR EJECTION FRACTION. Although equilibrium (ECG-gated) radionuclide ventriculography can be used for the sequential assessment of global and regional left ventricular performance, there are anatomical differences between the left and right sides of the heart that make assessment of right ventricular ejection fraction using count-rate techniques and the equilibrium radionuclide angiocardiogram more difficult. The right atrium lies behind the right ventricle to a greater extent than the left atrium overlies the left ventricle. This interference is solved in first-pass radionuclide angiocardiography by imaging in the right anterior oblique projection, thus spatially separating the right atrium from the right ventricle. This cannot be done easily using equilibrium radionuclide ventriculography because the right ventricle is superimposed on the left in that projection. Thus, initial attempts at measuring the ejection fraction by equilibrium methods have necessitated the use of either multiple regions of interest in an effort to define the right ventricular perimeter throughout the cardiac cycle[71] or a background region of interest extending into the right atrium and pulmonary outflow tract.[72]

An alternative method for assessing right ventricular ejection fraction from the equilibrium radionuclide angiocardiogram involves use of the slant-hole collimator, which provides a 30-degree caudal tilt that more effectively separates the right atrium from the right ventricle.[73] A fixed background correction region is defined in the usual manner for measurement of the global left ventricular ejection fraction. The same regions are also used for the right ventricle. Background is then subtracted from each pixel of the end-diastolic and end-systolic frames. The end-diastolic right ventricular perimeter is defined manually from the ejection fraction image and the end-diastolic frame. The ejection fraction image separates the right atrium from the right ventricle since the atrium moves paradoxically in relation to the right ventricle. Time-activity curves are then generated from the right ventricular region of interest to determine the frames corresponding to right ventricular end-systole and end-diastole.

Right ventricular ejection fraction is then calculated from the formula

$$RVEF = \frac{EDC - ESC}{EDC - BC} \quad (5)$$

where RVEF is right ventricular ejection fraction, EDC represents the counts within the right ventricular region of interest in the frame corresponding to right ventricular end-diastole, ESC represents the counts within the right ventricular region of interest in the right ventricular end-systolic frame, and BC represents the background counts.

With this method, right ventricular ejection fraction in patients without cardiopulmonary disease averages 0.59 ± 0.08 (S.D.). The correlation between right ventricular ejection fraction measured by both first-pass and equilibrium techniques is excellent.[73]

VALVULAR REGURGITATION. The severity of aortic and mitral regurgitation can be measured from the radionuclide angiocardiogram.[74–76] While first-pass techniques have been described for assessing left-sided regurgitation, the greatest experience has been derived from equilibrium (gated) studies. Radionuclide angiocardiography is performed as described above. Regions of interest are drawn over the left and right ventricles by visual inspection, taking care to include the entire right ventricular or left ventricular area, while excluding as much of the atria, pulmonary artery, and aorta as possible. This is best accomplished with the 30-degree slant-hole collimator and the stroke-volume image for outlining the ventricles. Changes in the counts in each ventricular area between systole and diastole are then determined. End-systole may not occur at the same time for the two ventricles and may have to be determined on separate frames. Since the same regions of interest are used for both systole and diastole, and since only the absolute change in counts is recorded, background activity is not subtracted. The results are expressed as a ratio of the change in counts in the left ventricular area over the change in counts in the right ventricular area (LV/RV stroke-index ratio).

In patients without aortic or mitral regurgitation, the left-to-right ventricular stroke-index is 1.15 ± 0.15. The ratio is greater than one in normal patients because the right ventricular stroke volume is underestimated owing to overlapping of the right atrium on the right ventricle. In patients with mitral or aortic regurgitation, the ratio is greater than 1.35. There is good agreement between the stroke-volume index and qualitative angiographic estimates of regurgitation. An alternate method, the Fourier amplitude ratio (the ratio of the summed amplitudes in the two ventricles), can also be used for evaluating aortic regurgitation. Fourier phase analysis is performed as described above and the phase image is used to define the free walls of the ventricles and the borders between the atria, aorta, and pulmonary artery.[77] The sum of the Fourier amplitudes in each ventricle represents the stroke counts and the ratio of the summed amplitudes in the two ventricles is equivalent to the stroke-count ratio. Correlation between the stroke-index ratio and the Fourier amplitude ratio is excellent.

Some constraints that must be considered when applying these techniques are that (1) right-sided regurgitation should not be present, (2) global left ventricular ejection fraction should be greater than 0.30, and (3) there should be good separation of the right atrium from the right ventricle. There is always some overlap of the right atrium on the right ventricle, even with a slant-hole collimator, and this problem may be more severe with significant right atrial enlargement.

Tricuspid regurgitation can be diagnosed and assessed by evaluating the change in liver blood volume during the cardiac cycle.[78] Normally there is no change in liver blood volume; however, with tricuspid regurgitation, liver blood volume increases by 1 per cent or more soon after ventricular end-systole.

EXERCISE

The advantage of radionuclide angiocardiography over other methods for assessing ventricular performance is that it can be performed during physiological stresses and during pharmacological interventions. This is particularly helpful in the evaluation of patients with suspected cardiopulmonary disease because diagnostic and management decisions often cannot be based on resting ventricular performance alone but require additional information about coronary and cardiac reserves.

Exercise is the most frequently applied stress and is particularly useful in evaluating patients suspected of having coronary artery disease[79, 80] (p. 324). With equilibrium radionuclide angiocardiography, a resting study is performed with the patient in the same position as will be used later during exercise. This is usually the 45-degree left anterior oblique projection, so that the right and left ventricles can be viewed separately, and with the patient supine or 45 degrees upright. The 45-degree upright position increases the likelihood that the patient will achieve an adequate exercise level but requires an appropriately designed table and camera mount. A high-sensitivity collimator is used because the acquisition time is short. A restraining harness is used to minimize patient motion under the camera during exercise. The imaging table should be secure, with minimal motion. Exercise loads are increased stepwise by 25-watt increments at 3-minute intervals until the patient experiences symptoms of angina, dyspnea, or fatigue of sufficient severity to limit further exercise or until the patient develops hypertension, arrhythmia, or marked ST-segment changes. Electrocardiographic leads are recorded and monitored continuously throughout the study. Multigated blood pool imaging is performed during the final 2 minutes of each exercise period.

This technique requires patient cooperation, since significant movement during the exercise test will substantially reduce spatial resolution and because patients must maintain their maximal level of exercise for at least 2 minutes so that adequate counting statistics can be acquired. This may be particularly difficult for many patients who are not accustomed to supine bicycle exercising or who have peripheral vascular disease. As a result, many patients will become fatigued well below their maximum predicted heart rate response.

Exercise radionuclide angiocardiography can also be performed with the first-pass technique. Only resting and peak exercise studies are obtained with ^{99m}Tc tracers; studies can be obtained at each stage of exercise with ^{195m}Au. This method has several advantages in that upright bicycle exercising can be employed. As a result, more patients will achieve maximum levels of stress. The first-pass study also requires that patients maintain their maximum exercise level for a considerably shorter time than with equilibrium radionuclide angiocardiography and does not require a steady-state heart rate for as long a period as equilibrium imaging.

Other forms of stress, such as isometric handgrip, atrial pacing, and the cold pressor test, have been suggested as alternative methods, particularly for patients who cannot use the bicycle ergometer.[81, 82] With *isometric handgrip*, an abnormal response in patients with coronary artery disease is based on impaired regional left ventricular performance. Left ventricular end-diastolic volume, stroke volume, and global ejection fraction will fall in most patients with coronary artery disease as the pacing rate is increased from 100 beats/min to 160.[83] While some reports have suggested that regional dysfunction occurs in most patients with coronary artery disease,[81] this method is not as sensitive as dynamic exercise.[84] The *cold pressor test* is performed by having the patient place a hand in a bucket of ice water for several minutes. This response to cold results in systemic vasoconstriction mediated through alpha-adrenoceptors.[85] The increase in the pressure-rate double product may be used to stress patients with coronary disease, resulting in a depression in left ventricular performance.[82] This test appears to be fairly sensitive for the detection of coronary artery disease, provided that the patient is not receiving beta-adrenoceptor blocker therapy.[85]

COMPARISON OF FIRST-PASS AND EQUILIBRIUM ANGIOCARDIOGRAPHY

Both the first-pass and equilibrium radionuclide angiocardiogram provide accurate measurement of global left ventricular ejection fraction. Correlation between the two methods is high (0.83), with a better correlation in patients with an ejection fraction below 0.5 than in patients with normal or high-normal values. In general, first-pass values for ejection fraction are lower than those obtained with the equilibrium method. Patients who are being followed serially should be studied with one method to avoid errors introduced by differences in technique.[86]

Other hemodynamic indices (such as the peak ejection rate) that depend on high temporal resolution of the left ventricular time-activity curve cannot be obtained as accurately from first-pass studies; they require the high counts obtained with gated studies. Regional wall motion can be assessed with either method, although, again, the high counting rate obtained with the gated studies provides superior spatial resolution and improved accuracy, particularly when indices of regional wall motion, such as regional ejection fraction, are measured.

Background is a greater problem with equilibrium studies than with first-pass studies and accounts for as much as half the activity from the left ventricular region of interest with the former method. As a result, it may be easier to detect the edges of the left ventricle with first-pass studies despite the lower intrinsic resolution. However, equilibrium studies are superior for patient monitoring and for sequential studies. Imaging can be continued for up to 4 hours after injection of the radiopharmaceutical, allowing imaging in multiple projections and during physiological or pharmacological interventions. With first-pass studies, a radiopharmaceutical must be administered each time imaging is to be performed. Background activity precludes more than two or three studies during the effective half-life of the tracer, thus limiting the number of sequential studies possible with ^{99m}Tc, for example. On the other hand, physiological or pharmacological interventions with concomitant rapid changes in heart rate may be studied best with the first-pass technique. For both techniques, a steady-state heart rate is necessary, but only five or six heartbeats are required for first-pass studies compared to at least 2 minutes of heartbeats for the gated studies.

CLINICAL APPLICATIONS

DETECTION AND EVALUATION OF CORONARY ARTERY DISEASE. In patients with coronary artery disease who have not yet sustained an acute myocardial infarction, resting ventricular performance is usually normal because the myocardium is not ischemic (Fig. 11–11). When these patients are stressed, an imbalance between oxygen supply and demand develops, resulting in ischemia. This, in turn, causes a fall in global left ventricular ejection fraction and the development of regional wall motion abnormalities. When radionuclide angiocardiography is applied during exercise in normal patients, left ventricular ejection fraction rises significantly compared to levels at rest, with no left ventricular wall motion abnormalities.[79, 80] In patients with coronary artery disease and angina, left ventricular ejection fraction falls during exercise and new regional wall motion abnormalities may develop. The normal increase in ejection fraction with exercise is due primarily to a decrease in end-systolic volume, while the exercise-induced decrease in ejection fraction in patients with angina is due to an increase in end-systolic volume. In patients with coronary artery disease without angina there is usually no change in ejection fraction during exercise, since there is no significant change in end-systolic volume.

The criteria for an abnormal left ventricular ejection fraction response with exercise vary considerably from laboratory to laboratory. Most groups, however, require at least a 5 or 10 per cent increase in ejection fraction to consider the result normal. In normal patients with high resting ejection fractions (> 75 per cent), there may be no change in ejection fraction with exercise. In addition to the measurement of global left ventricular function, the cineangiocardiograms obtained at rest and during exercise are evaluated to detect any new wall motion abnormalities. The numerical analyses described previously can also be applied to assess regional and global ventricular performance during exercise.

The accuracy of exercise radionuclide angiocardiography for the detection of coronary artery disease depends on the criteria used to diagnose it. Most laboratories use the

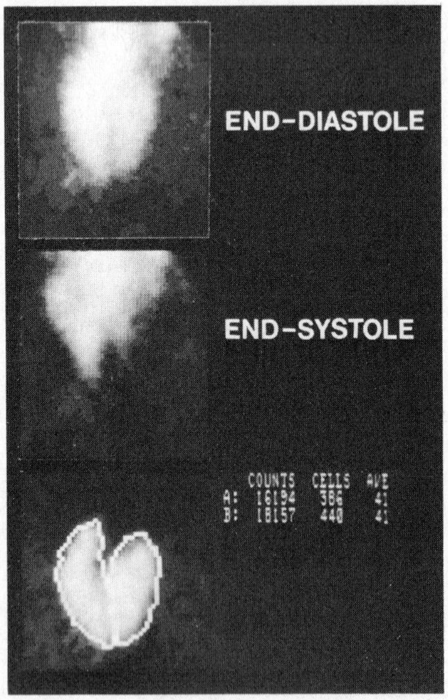

FIGURE 11–11. Equilibrium (gated) radionuclide angiocardiogram of a patient with coronary artery disease and normal ventricular performance at rest. Images were obtained in the 45-degree modified left anterior oblique projection. The end-systolic image demonstrates vigorous and uniform contraction of the left and right ventricles, which are at the right and left sides of each image, respectively. The stroke volume image (lower panel) has uniformly high activity throughout the right and left ventricle indicating normal ejection of blood from both ventricular cavities.

ejection fraction response as the sole criterion, in which case the test is highly sensitive (greater than 90 per cent) but has poor specificity.[87] When the presence of a wall motion abnormality during exercise is included in the criteria, the specificity of the test is very high. Unfortunately, the sensitivity of the test is markedly reduced. The sensitivity for detecting wall motion abnormalities is not high with this method because only one projection is obtained and the image has poor resolution because of the short acquisition time.

Other factors will play a major role in determining left ventricular response with exercise. For example, inadequate stress due to peripheral vascular disease or the concurrent administration of beta-adrenoceptor blocking drugs may result in normal responses in spite of coronary artery disease.[88] The ejection fraction response is greater with upright exercise than with supine exercise.[89] Small reductions in workload after an ischemic response to symptom-limited exercise are often associated with a rapid rise in ejection fraction and with improved regional wall motion. The workload must therefore be maintained during symptom-limited exercise to achieve optimal sensitivity for detecting myocardial ischemia.[90]

Most important in determining the specificity of the test is the definition of the control population.[91] Exercise response is dependent on the patient's sex, resting ejection fraction, and systemic blood pressure.[92–94] The number of false-positive tests is unacceptably high in patients with diastolic blood pressures higher than 100 mm Hg.[95] Age is another important factor. Most studies have involved control patients who were usually young individuals without cardiopulmonary disease. Patients over the age of 60, however, may demonstrate no increase in ejection fraction with exercise and may in fact demonstrate a decrease in ejection fraction due to aging rather than to coronary artery disease.[93]

In fact, an abnormal ejection fraction response to exercise is expected in any condition in which there is reduced left ventricular reserve, such as volume- or pressure-overload states and states of decreased left ventricular compliance. As a result, abnormal responses have been reported in patients with aortic stenosis,[96] aortic regurgitation,[97] mitral regurgitation,[98] mitral valve prolapse,[99] hypertrophic obstructive cardiomyopathy,[100] chronic obstructive pulmonary disease,[101] beta-thalassemia and chronic iron overload,[102] cystic fibrosis,[103] elderly patients,[104] female patients,[105] and patients receiving propranolol.[106]

In interpretation of the exercise radionuclide angiocardiogram, it is clear that additional information should be incorporated into the decision-making process. For example, almost three-fourths of patients suspected of having coronary artery disease without a high pretest probability of the disease (i.e., no previous infarction or typical anginal symptoms) can be diagnosed with an 85 per cent certainty by a combination of the results of exercise radionuclide angiocardiography and clinical variables such as the presence of chest pain and ST-segment changes with exercise.[107] Thus, the radionuclide angiocardiogram is most useful in the noninvasive diagnosis of coronary artery disease when it is coupled with additional clinical information.

In the diagnostic evaluation of patients with suspected coronary artery disease, the exercise electrocardiogram may provide the necessary diagnostic information without resorting to additional noninvasive or invasive methods. If the exercise electrocardiogram is nondiagnostic, an exercise radionuclide study may be useful. As of this writing exercise myocardial perfusion scintigraphy (p. 331) appears clearly to be the procedure of choice. Radionuclide angiocardiography provides higher sensitivity but poorer specificity in patients with valvular heart disease, primary myocardial disease, or severe lung disease. Furthermore, particularly with supine bicycle ergometry, many patients may not achieve an adequate chronotropic response. The exercise radionuclide angiocardiogram does provide more complete information, particularly when imaging is performed at each stage of exercise, which allows cardiac performance to be assessed at various levels of submaximal exercise.

On the other hand, thallium scintigraphy can be performed in multiple projections immediately after exercise and provides a more reliable map of the pattern and location of the regional abnormality. Furthermore, it is more likely that the patient will achieve an adequate exercise response with thallium scintigraphy, since ordinarily the exercise is performed upright and on a treadmill. The choice between the two procedures may depend heavily on the experience of the nuclear cardiology personnel, however.

The most important role of exercise radionuclide angiocardiography may lie in the physiological and functional information that it provides, supplementing the morphological information extracted from the coronary arteriogram. For example, a subset of patients with three-vessel disease who are at high risk can be identified on the basis of an abnormal left ventricular ejection fraction response during exercise coupled with the presence of ST depression and an abbreviated exercise tolerance.[108] Patient stratification on the basis of noninvasive physiological data will likely play an increasingly important role even in the treatment of patients who have already undergone coronary angiography.

Also, the ejection fraction response during exercise is an excellent predictor of outcome for those patients who achieve an adequate level of exercise.[6] Patients with a normal ejection fraction response to exercise have an excellent prognosis. In medically treated patients with stable coronary artery disease and with left ventricular ejection fractions during exercise of greater than 0.45, the mortality rate is less than 1 per cent within 2 years of initial evaluation.

ACUTE MYOCARDIAL INFARCTION. Ventricular performance is a major factor affecting patient prognosis after acute myocardial infarction. The equilibrium radionuclide angiocardiogram provides information concerning global left ventricular function, the extent and location of regional abnormalities, and the presence and extent of right ventricular involvement. As a result, it provides prognostic information, since the left ventricular ejection fraction is a predictor of early mortality and the development of congestive heart failure or sudden death.[109, 110]

Right ventricular infarction or extension of an inferior infarct to the right ventricle often cannot easily be detected at the bedside.[111] The equilibrium radionuclide angiocardiogram is a reliable method for detecting and assessing right ventricular infarction.[112, 113] Approximately half of the patients with inferior infarction will exhibit abnormalities in right ventricular performance and a small number of patients may have predominantly right ventricular infarction. Since there is a high correlation between ST-segment elevation in lead V4R and right coronary occlusion, this electrocardiographic finding could be used to select those patients who require radionuclide assessment of right ventricular function.[114] Right ventricular infarction causes reduced right ventricular ejection fraction and, in a large proportion of patients, regional wall motion abnormalities.[115] Regional wall motion abnormalities involving the right ventricle are highly specific indicators of right ventricular infarction. While an abnormal right ventricular ejection fraction is a highly sensitive marker of right ventricular infarction, it is nonspecific and is seen in other abnormalities which affect ventricular loading.

The radionuclide angiocardiogram plays its most important role in the determination of patient prognosis. It can also be used to assess patient recovery. Global and regional ventricular performance improves gradually over the first 2 weeks after infarction but improves significantly by 2 to 4 months if uninterrupted by complications such as reinfarction. The most valuable prognostic information is gained from submaximal exercise testing of patients prior to discharge from the hospital, since the ventricular response to exercise appears useful in selecting patients at high risk for subsequent complications.[110, 116] Left ventricular ejection fraction during both rest and exercise is a predictor of subsequent mortality and recurrent infarction. The changes in ejection fractions from rest to exercise and exercise-induced wall motion abnormalities provide highly useful information about the presence of exercise-induced ischemia.[117] It is frequently employed to identify patients who should undergo coronary arteriography and, depending on the findings, revascularization.

Development of a functional left ventricular aneurysm after myocardial infarction is another adverse prognostic factor and an indication for aggressive management.[118] In patients resuscitated after ventricular fibrillation, the radionuclide angiocardiogram provides useful information concerning outcome; a markedly abnormal left ventricular ejection fraction indicates a poor prognosis and the need for aggressive medical or surgical management.[119]

VALVULAR HEART DISEASE. Radionuclide angiography provides a useful, noninvasive means for quantifying the degree of left-sided valvular regurgitation.[76] While echocardiography offers excellent visualization of valve motion, assesses aortic dilatation, and measures the degree of mitral stenosis, the severity of regurgitation can be estimated only qualitatively, even with Doppler methods. In addition to its ability to detect and measure left-sided regurgitation, radionuclide angiocardiography may play a role in the management of patients with aortic valve regurgitation. In these patients, the decision to intervene surgically depends on the degree of left ventricular dysfunction (p. 1068). The dysfunction may not be apparent at rest and may be apparent only during exercise. It has been suggested that by the time symptoms develop in these patients, irreversible myocardial dysfunction has occurred and that functional abnormalities may appear during stress even in the asymptomatic patient.[120, 121] As a result, radionuclide assessment of left ventricular function during exercise has been suggested as a means of following patients with aortic regurgitation to determine the optimal time for valve replacement. The anaerobic threshold may represent a physiological endpoint for exercise in patients with aortic regurgitation, however.[122] If this is the case, only changes in ejection fraction occurring before the anaerobic threshold will be diagnostically significant, and they are in part related to the resting ejection fraction. The changes in left ventricular ejection fraction occurring between anaerobic threshold and peak exercise would be of less certain diagnostic value.

ASSESSMENT OF LEFT AND RIGHT VENTRICULAR DYSFUNCTION. Radionuclide angiocardiography is most useful in patients with symptoms suggesting ventricular dysfunction because it can (1) detect ventricular aneurysm, (2) distinguish regional from global dysfunction, (3) evaluate myocardial viability, (4) evaluate right and left ventricular function, and (5) evaluate the effectiveness of therapeutic interventions. It provides a noninvasive method for accurate quantitation of ventricular hemodynamics and regional wall motion in patients too ill to undergo invasive cardiac catheterization. In addition, the technique can be performed sequentially to evaluate the natural history of heart disease and the effectiveness of medical or surgical management.

The technique is comparable in sensitivity to contrast ventriculography in detecting and assessing *aneurysm* and in determining the location and extent of dyskinetic segments and the status of the remaining ventricle. These factors are particularly important in patients with coronary artery disease in whom aneurysmectomy is being considered (p. 1365). As a result, the radionuclide method can be used to screen patients to separate those with diffuse hypokinesis, who are poor candidates for surgery (Fig. 11–12) from those with localized akinesis or aneurysm (Fig. 11–13), who may then undergo cardiac catheterization prior to surgery.

Assessment of global and regional ventricular function is useful in patients with clinical evidence of congestive heart failure. The extent and intensity of regional left ventricular disease and the contribution of *right ventricular asynergy* have important therapeutic implications. Furthermore, congestive heart failure may be present with normal systolic function but with abnormal diastolic indices indicating abnormalities in ventricular compliance.[123, 124]

The technique is less useful for distinguishing the *etiology* of reduced left ventricular function. Both idiopathic dilated cardiomyopathy and ischemic cardiomyopathy produce regional wall motion abnormalities which are frequently indistinguishable. Regional wall motion abnormalities may occur in patients with acute inflammatory processes as well. While right ventricular ejection fraction is generally lower in patients with ischemic cardiomyopathies, there is a good deal of overlap between the two groups.[125]

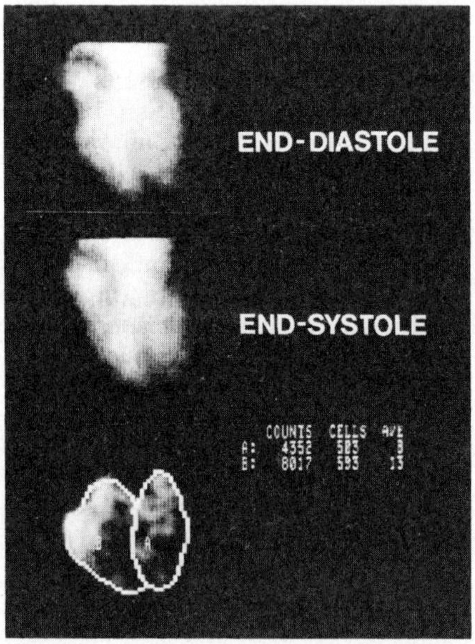

FIGURE 11–12. Equilibrium (gated) radionuclide angiocardiogram of a patient with ischemic cardiomyopathy. There is global asynergy of the markedly dilated left and right ventricles. Note the small difference in size and intensity of ventricular activity between diastole and systole. The stroke volume image (lower panel) shows a marked decrease in stroke volume throughout most of the right and left ventricles. Images were obtained in the 45-degree modified left anterior oblique projection. The left ventricle is on the right side of the image and the right ventricle is on the left side.

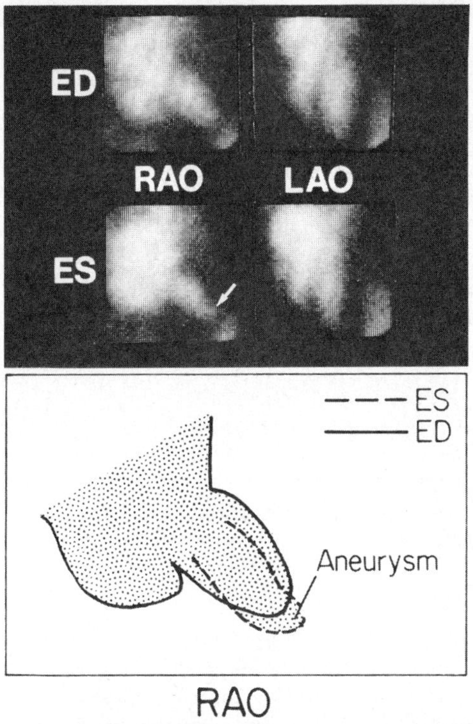

FIGURE 11–13. Equilibrium (gated) radionuclide angiocardiogram of a patient with an apical aneurysm. Note the apical dyskinesis seen best on the RAO projection (arrow). Performance is normal in the other ventricular segments. ED = end-diastolic frame; ES = end-systolic frame; RAO = 30-degree right anterior oblique projection; LAO = 45-degree modified left anterior oblique projection.

Regional wall motion abnormalities present at rest may be due to scar from previous myocardial infarction or to reversible ischemia of viable tissue. Since revascularization may improve regional function if the tissue is viable, it is important to differentiate between reversible ischemia and scar. Postextrasystolic potentiation and nitroglycerin have been used to help make this distinction, usually at the time of catheterization.[126–132] The radionuclide angiocardiogram can also be used to evaluate the change in regional wall motion after exercise.[126,132] In most patients with surgically reversible regional ventricular dysfunction during preoperative study, function in that region improves immediately after exercise compared to function at rest. The sensitivity of this test is controversial, however, since the number of patients whose regional function does not improve after exercise but does improve after surgery ranges from 16[126] to 50 per cent.[132]

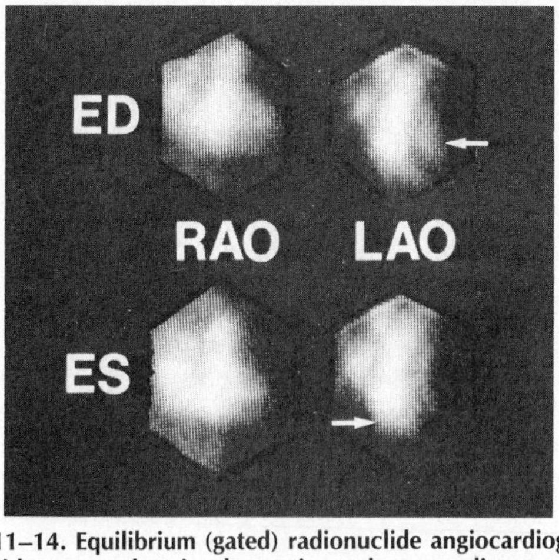

FIGURE 11–14. Equilibrium (gated) radionuclide angiocardiogram of a patient with severe chronic obstructive pulmonary disease and right-sided heart failure. Note the dilated, poorly contracting right ventricle (upper arrow) and dilated right atrium. The left ventricle is normal in size and performance (lower arrow). ED = end-diastolic frame; ES = end-systolic frame; RAO = 30-degree right anterior oblique projection; and LAO = 45-degree modified left anterior oblique projection.

Right Ventricular Function. This may be seriously compromised in patients with chronic obstructive pulmonary disease who have pulmonary artery hypertension or pulmonary vasoconstriction (Fig. 11–14). There is a direct relationship between right ventricular dysfunction and prognosis; right ventricular performance is also related to the magnitude of arterial hypoxemia and ventilatory impairment. Abnormal right ventricular function is a warning sign of subsequent cardiopulmonary decompensation.[133] During exercise, the majority of patients with chronic obstructive lung disease will have abnormal right ventricular reserve, as manifested by reduction in the ejection fraction.[134] This response is not necessarily due to intrinsic

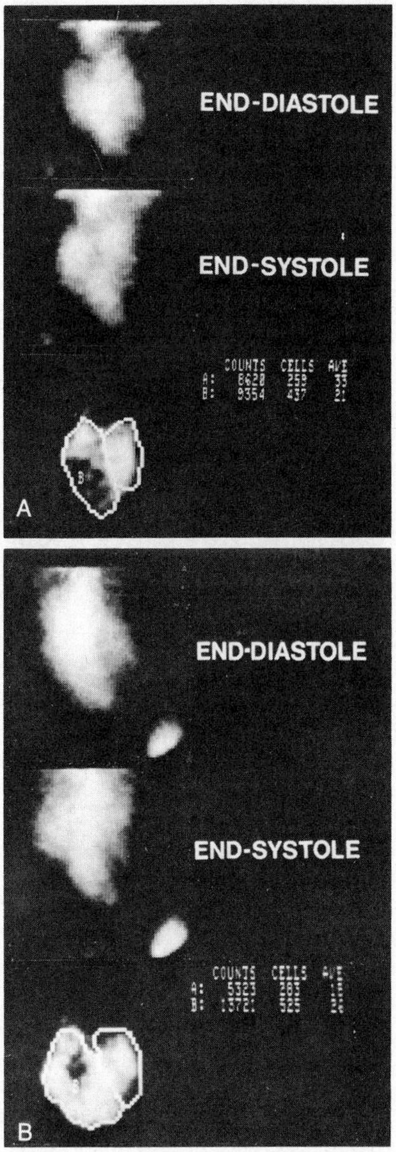

FIGURE 11–15. *A*, Equilibrium (gated) radionuclide angiocardiogram of a patient with recent right ventricular infarction. The right ventricle and right atrium (which appear at the left of the image) are markedly dilated with very little change in appearance between end-diastole and end-systole. The stroke volume image (lower panel) demonstrates markedly reduced stroke volume from the lower two-thirds of the right ventricle. Left ventricular volume and contraction are normal. *B*, End-diastolic and end-systolic images in a patient with atrial septal defect and pulmonary hypertension with right atrial and ventricular enlargement. The stroke volume image (lower panel) shows a high right ventricular stroke volume with more than twice the volume of blood ejected by the right ventricle compared to the left. Images were obtained in the 45-degree modified left anterior oblique projection.

myocardial dysfunction but is the result of a normal response to elevated pulmonary artery (and right ventricular systolic) pressure during exercise. Left ventricular response in these patients is generally normal.[135]

Right ventricular function can be affected in acute myocardial infarction (see above) and other conditions as well (Fig. 11–15). In patients in septic shock, right ventricular asynergy may be responsible for myocardial decompensation. Radionuclide angiocardiography plays an important role in these patients because right ventricular asynergy can have important therapeutic implications.[136]

Right ventricular performance is a highly predictive indicator of mortality in patients with chronic congestive cardiomyopathy secondary to coronary artery disease (Tables 11–1 and 11–2). In fact, right ventricular ejection fraction correlates more closely with mortality than does left ventricular ejection fraction in patients with left ventricular asynergy.[137] In patients with chronic left ventricular failure—particularly in those with underlying coronary artery disease—right ventricular ejection fraction correlates with maximal oxygen consumption and correlates better with exercise capacity than does left ventricular ejection fraction.[138] With the observation that afterload-reducing agents such as prazosin can improve right ventricular performance in these patients, the radionuclide angiocardiogram should play an increasingly important role not only in determining the extent of right and left ventricular dysfunction but also for defining prognosis and, potentially, proper therapy.[139, 140]

Radionuclide angiocardiography provides a noninvasive method for *monitoring the acute and chronic effects of drugs* on ventricular performance. A wide variety of drugs has been studied, including inotropic agents such as digitalis and amrinone,[116, 141] bronchodilators such as aminophylline,[142] beta-adrenoceptor blockers such as propranolol,[143] antiarrhythmics such as disopyramide, and calcium antagonists such as verapamil or nifedipine.[144] Individual patient responses can be studied as well. Ventricular performance can be used as a guide to determine when a particular therapeutic agent has lost its effectiveness and when replacement or combination therapy may be necessary.

Ventricular performance is an important indicator of cardiotoxicity with drugs, such as doxorubicin, that have a potentially detrimental effect on the heart[145] (p. 1748). By sequentially assessing patients who are receiving these agents at rest, it is possible to predict when irreversible cardiac failure might develop in an individual patient. As a result, medication can be continued as long as possible and discontinued before cardiac failure becomes irreversible. Doxorubicin probably should not be given to patients with baseline left ventricular ejection fraction of less than 30 per cent. Patients with values of 30 to 54 per cent should be studied at frequent intervals. Doxorubicin should be discontinued when the left ventricular ejection fraction decreases by 10 per cent or more.[146] Exercise radionuclide angiocardiography may also play a role, since the development of a reduction in ejection fraction during exercise is helpful in identifying patients at high risk for developing cardiac toxicity, who need to be followed more frequently.[147]

TABLE 11–1 FACTORS RELATING TO SURVIVAL IN CHRONIC CONGESTIVE CARDIOMYOPATHY

	SURVIVORS	NONSURVIVORS	*P* VALUE
LVEF	18.7 ± 6.8%	18.1 ± 10.3%	NS
RVEF	41.4 ± 23.0%	23.9 ± 10.2%	<.01
LV dyskinesia	20.9 ± 11.8%	29.7 ± 15.0%	<.05
Ventricular arrhythmia	50%	44%	NS
Functional class (NYHA)	3.0 ± 0.7	3.6 ± 0.5	<.01
Diabetes	19%	22%	NS
Hypertension	19%	33%	NS
Previous inferior infarction	17%	42%	NS
COPD	6%	33%	NS

LVEF = left ventricular ejection fraction; NS = not significant; RVEF = right ventricular ejection fraction; NYHA = New York Heart Association; COPD = chronic obstructive pulmonary disease.

(From Polak, J. F., et al.: Right ventricular ejection fraction: An indicator of increased mortality in patients with congestive heart failure associated with coronary artery disease. J. Am. Col. Cardiol. 2:217, 1983.)

TABLE 11–2 CORRELATES OF DEPRESSED RIGHT VENTRICULAR FUNCTION

	RVEF (<35%)	RVEF (≥35%)	*P* VALUE
LVEF	15.8 ± 8.6%	22.5 ± 7.4%	<.025
LV dyskinesia	30.1 ± 13.5%	18.2 ± 12.3%	<.025
Deaths	71%	23%	<.02
Ventricular arrhythmia	43%	54%	NS
Previous inferior infarction	35%	17%	NS
Functional stage (NYHA)	3.5 ± 0.6	3.0 ± 0.7	<.01
Right-sided failure*	38%	31%	NS
COPD	24%	15%	NS
Smoker (pack-years)	42.3 ± 32.4	41.5 ± 21.0	NS
Diabetes	24%	15%	NS
Hypertension	24%	31%	NS

Abbreviations as in Table 11–1.

*Either jugular venous distention, peripheral edema, or both.

(From Polak, J. F., et al.: Right ventricular ejection fraction: An indicator of increased mortality in patients with congestive heart failure associated with coronary artery disease. J. Am. Col. Cardiol. 2:217, 1983.)

MYOCARDIAL PERFUSION AND METABOLISM

The development of newer surgical and medical techniques for the treatment of coronary artery disease has emphasized the need for an objective measure of regional myocardial perfusion. Although the coronary arteriogram can precisely define vessel morphology (Chap. 10), the effect of a coronary artery lesion on tissue perfusion cannot be determined accurately by means of roentgenographic procedures.[148] Furthermore, objective screening procedures are needed to evaluate patients during the early stages of their disease, well before symptoms become severe enough to warrant catheterization. Silent ischemia occurs more frequently than ischemia accompanied by angina[149] and may be an important initial sign in those patients with acute myocardial infarction without antecedent symptoms.[150] Radionuclide techniques that assess regional myocardial perfusion provide information useful in the detection and evaluation of coronary artery disease and in the assessment of therapies aimed at limiting the degree of ischemia and the extent of tissue necrosis.[151] It is critical to obtain *regional* information, since coronary heart disease is usually a regional disease with areas of normal myocardium often adjacent to severely diseased tissue. It is also critical to measure perfusion both at rest and during exercise, pacing, or some other stress, since perfusion may be normal at rest even in patients with severe coronary artery disease.

RADIOPHARMACEUTICALS FOR PERFUSION SCINTIGRAPHY

The first radioactive *potassium analogs* available for human use emitted photons that were too energetic for scintillation imaging.[152–154] Potassium-43 was the first of a number of potassium analog with physical characteristics that were compatible with external imaging techniques.[155] Other potassium analogs have been used for myocardial scintigraphy, including cesium-129,[156] rubidium-81,[157] and thallium-201.[158] While all these radionuclides have limitations because of their long physical half-life, unsatisfactory gamma energies, or limited availability, thallium-201 has emerged clearly as the radiotracer of choice for myocardial perfusion scintigraphy.

THALLIUM-201. This radiopharmaceutical has a physical half-life of 73.1 hours and is a metallic element with properties similar to potassium.[159, 160] Its physical characteristics are reasonably well suited for imaging with scintillation camera systems.[161] Characteristic x-rays are emitted in a range from 69 to 83 kev, and these photons are routinely used for external imaging. In addition, gamma emissions of 135 and 167 kev are produced during 10 per cent of the disintegrations. In routine imaging, the pulse height analyzer is centered over the lower energy characteristic x-rays with a second window centered over the gamma ray peaks. The low-energy photons result in some loss of spatial resolution because the scattered radiation cannot be separated completely from the primary photopeak.

Thallium-201 has a number of biological characteristics that make it particularly attractive for perfusion scintigraphy. Clearance of thallium from the blood is almost as rapid as that of potassium or rubidium, and wash-out from the myocardium is slower. A maximum heart-to-blood ratio is reached within 6 to 10 minutes after injection. Distribution of thallium and rubidium is similar throughout the left ventricle, but thallium appears to concentrate in myocardial tissue to a somewhat greater degree than potassium or rubidium.[158, 161]

While thallium-201 has performed well, it has some disadvantages. For example, while its myocardial redistribution has been used to distinguish infarction from ischemia (p. 332), rapid tracer redistribution may occur following injection during stress, particularly if hyperemia occurs during reperfusion in areas of transient ischemia. The rate of redistribution may be rapid and is variable so that the myocardial distribution of thallium-201 may reflect blood flow for only a short time after injection. While standard imaging techniques have been particularly successful in identifying coronary artery disease, the redistribution phenomenon may result in underestimation of the total extent and severity of ischemia.

The physical characteristics of thallium-201 are also less than ideal. Its low-energy characteristic x-rays are not entirely appropriate for Anger camera imaging. Their attenuation by soft tissue is high, markedly reducing the efficiency with which activity in deep structures is measured. The long half-life of thallium-201 coupled with its long biological half-life in the myocardium limits serial studies to frequencies of a day or more.

TECHNETIUM-99m. This is the ideal radionuclide for Anger camera scintigraphy because of its gamma energy of 140 kev, its relatively short physical half-life (6 hours), its low-radiation dosage to the patient, and its general availability from a long-lived parent via a relatively inexpensive generator system. Several members of the hexakis (isonitrile) technetium family demonstrate high myocardial uptake in the human, enabling high-quality planar, tomographic, and gated images.[162] These isonitrile analogs distribute proportionally to myocardial blood flow and are not inhibited by ouabain.[163] Myocardial uptake appears passive and is not affected by calcium channel blockers or pH.

Two of these isonitriles, ^{99m}Tc CPI (carbomethoxyisopropyl isonitrile) and ^{99m}Tc MIBI (methoxyisobutyl isonitrile), have high initial myocardial uptake with no evidence of myocardial redistribution into zones of transient ischemia for several hours after exercise.[164] Only after reinjection during rest do the transiently ischemic areas appear normal. The myocardial activity clears slowly from the heart with ^{99m}Tc CPI so that repeat imaging is possible by 3 or 4 hours after the stress injection. ^{99m}Tc MIBI does not clear from the myocardium and behaves like a chemical microsphere. Both agents clear promptly from the lung and accumulate in the heart and liver. ^{99m}Tc MIBI is cleared rapidly from the liver through the hepatobiliary system (^{99m}Tc CPI clears more slowly), resulting in minimal interference from the liver on myocardial images

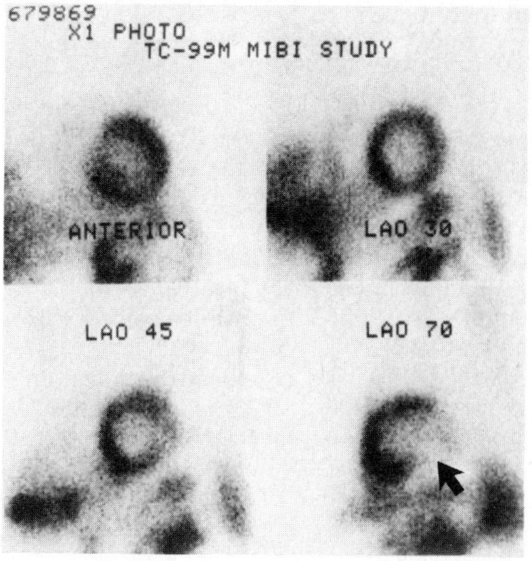

FIGURE 11–16. Planar gamma camera images of a patient with previous inferoposterior myocardial infarction obtained after injection of ^{99m}Tc MIBI isonitrile. Note high myocardial uptake with very little activity in the surrounding lung and liver. There is markedly decreased tracer uptake in the inferior posterior wall seen best on the 70-degree left anterior oblique projection (arrow).

obtained even 10 minutes after injection. Both radiotracers correlate well with thallium-201 with regard to the identification of segmental transient ischemia and infarction (Fig. 11–16).

The major advantages of this family of radiotracers arise from the physical characteristics of technetium-99m. Its gamma emission is better suited to standard imaging equipment than is thallium-201, resulting in better image quality with less attenuation of photons from deeper tissues. The higher photon flux from the 140-kev photons and the administered dose (10 to 15 mCi) result in improved SPECT (see p. 334) imaging and high-quality gated and first-past studies to assess global and regional ventricular performance. Because ^{99m}Tc is obtained from a generator system, these tracers can be prepared on site so that myocardial imaging can be applied to emergency situations such as acute myocardial infarction. Analogs that clear from the myocardium such as ^{99m}Tc CPI are useful in the serial assessment of patients undergoing procedures such as angioplasty or with unstable angina, myocardial infarction, or spontaneous angina. Analogs which remain fixed in the myocardium for hours after injection can be satisfactorily imaged hours after injection during stress or pharmacological intervention and may become an important complement to coronary angiography.

Until technetium-99m–labeled tracers become commercially available, thallium-201 will remain the most widely applied tracer of myocardial perfusion.

POSITRON-EMITTING TRACERS. When cyclotron-produced positron-emitting potassium analogs and positron imaging devices are used in perfusion scintigraphy, three-dimensional reconstruction of the heart is possible. The very short half-life of these agents also permits multiple studies under various stress states as well as frequent sequential examinations to follow the course of ischemia or infarction. One of these promising tracers is *rubidium-82*, a positron emitter with a 75-second half-life.[165] Aside from the obvious advantage that results from its short half-life, this potassium analog is the daughter of strontium-82, with a 25-day half-life. Since strontium-82/rubidium-82 generator systems have been developed,[166] the parent can be stored for considerable periods of time and eluted whenever rubidium-82 is needed for injection.

Another positron emitter, *nitrogen-13 ammonium*, has also been used as a marker of myocardial perfusion, and there has been a close correlation between changes in the size of the resultant perfusion defect and the clinical course of patients with acute infarction.[167] Because of the short half-life of this tracer, an on-site cyclotron is necessary for radiotracer production, markedly limiting its availability.

KINETICS OF THALLIUM-201

Regional alterations in myocardial perfusion can be measured when myocardial scintigraphy is performed after the intravenous injection of potassium analogs such as thallium-201. This approach is based on the indicator fractionation principle, which postulates that the uptake of these tracers by heart muscle equals the fraction of cardiac output perfusing the myocardium after the intravenous injection of the tracer.[168] Since approximately 5 per cent of the cardiac output supplies the myocardium at rest and since the myocardial extraction of thallium-201 is high, there is sufficient uptake of the tracer by the heart relative to surrounding structures to permit imaging with external detecting systems.

INITIAL DISTRIBUTION. After intravenous injection of thallium-201, the initial distribution of the tracer is equal to the product of regional myocardial blood flow times the extraction fraction, i.e., the percentage of the tracer extracted by the myocardium during a single passage through its circulation. Thus, the degree to which the distribution of thallium-201 reflects myocardial blood flow depends on an unchanging extraction fraction at different flows. The extraction fraction is high (85 to 90 per cent) when the patient is at rest, somewhat higher than the extraction fraction for the rest of the body. Approximately 3.5 per cent of the injected dose localizes in the myocardium.[169] At high flow rates, if the increase in flow is greater than the metabolic needs of the myocardium, the extraction fraction is reduced, and thallium-201 uptake consequently increases at a lower rate than the increase in coronary blood flow.[170] At peak exercise, 4.4 per cent of the total injected dose localizes in the myocardium. When thallium-201 is injected during coronary vasodilation using dipyridamole, 8 to 10 per cent of the dose concentrates in the heart. Thallium extraction is not affected by ouabain-induced inhibition of Na^+, K^+-ATPase,[169] and thallium influx is not dependent on the sodium-potassium pump.

Regional myocardial uptake of thallium-201 correlates linearly with regional myocardial blood flow from very low flow rates to normal resting levels.[171] At very low flows, there is slightly more thallium in the myocardium than would be predicted by flow alone.[169] At flow rates above the resting level, thallium uptake increases proportionately when the augmented flow levels are associated with increases in myocardial oxygen demand[172] and less than proportionately when the increases in flow exceed the metabolic needs of the heart.[170, 173, 174]

Exercise or other forms of stress are essential to detect coronary stenoses accurately by myocardial perfusion scintigraphy. Regions that are perfused normally at rest but exhibit reduced perfusion during exercise represent ischemic zones, while perfusion defects seen both at rest and during exercise usually represent zones of scar, most commonly previous infarction. Abnormal perfusion during stress in patients with transient ischemia is due to a heterogeneous increase in myocardial blood flow. In normal individuals, blood flow increases uniformly throughout the left ventricle during exercise or other forms of stress-simulating interventions. In patients with coronary artery disease, the increase in blood flow to the myocardium distal to a hemodynamically significant arterial stenosis is less than normal and may in fact be absent. There is an inverse relationship between the increase in flow and the percentage of coronary artery stenosis once the lumen is narrowed by approximately 30 to 50 per cent.[175] Thus, the difference between the absolute quantity of radiotracer available for uptake by myocardial cells beyond arterial obstructions and the quantity available in beds supplied by normal coronary arteries is maximal during exercise. Since myocardial thallium clearance is high, the relative differences in regional myocardial blood flow will be reflected in disproportionate concentrations of regional myocardial radioactivity on the scintiscan.[176]

REDISTRIBUTION. The indicator fractionation principle assumes that the tracer will remain trapped in the organ during the period of observation. This is true for microspheres injected intravenously or intra-arterially, but it is not true for thallium-201, particularly when it is injected during exercise. Redistribution of the tracer begins within 10 minutes after injection.[177] The thallium wash-out rate has a half-life of 4 hours after intravenous injection.[178] It is prolonged in regions of hypoperfusion[179] and is related to the rate of thallium clearance from the blood.[180]

Redistribution of thallium-201 has important implications for patients with coronary artery disease, especially when tracer is injected during exercise. When myocardial perfusion scintigraphy is performed during stress, transiently ischemic myocardium can be detected.[181, 182] By taking advantage of the redistribution phenomenon, one can detect exercise-induced ischemia by imaging after the exercise injection of thallium and by repeat delayed imaging. In regions of transient ischemia, the initial perfusion defect will no longer be present on delayed imaging.[183] In zones of ischemia where the initial uptake of thallium is low, the gradient between the extracellular and intracellular spaces is lower than in normal tissue and the clearance is therefore much slower.[184] The slow net clearance is partly due to reperfusion which results in entry (wash-in) of thallium into the previously ischemic tissue and partly to the initial low blood flow. The net effect in patients with transient ischemia is normalization of the image 2 to 3 hours after exercise. In zones of infarction and chronic ischemia where thallium clearance is similar to that of normal tissue and where there is no reperfusion between the initial and the delayed images, the defect persists and appears fixed between initial and delayed images.

Other factors affect the rate of thallium clearance from the myocardium. Glucose and insulin cause an accelerated loss from both normal and ischemic zones of myocardium.[185] This rapid clearance can cause regions of ischemia to appear as fixed lesions. Also, the heart rate achieved during exercise is inversely proportional to the rates of thallium clearance. As heart rate increases, there is redistribution of cardiac output from the splanchnic bed to skeletal muscle with an increase in gradient between the myocardial intra- and extracellular spaces resulting in a more rapid clearance. Myocardial clearance is 8 hours when thallium is injected at a heart rate of 100, accelerating to 4 hours with heart rates greater than 160 beats/min.

The *disadvantage* of the redistribution phenomenon is that the time during which the thallium distribution reflects myocardial blood flow is limited, lasting for only a short time after the tracer has cleared from the blood following intravenous injection. Consequently, it is essential that imaging begin very soon after injection and that imaging be performed as rapidly as possible.[186] Furthermore, in the face of transient ischemia, the time required for concentrations in the ischemic and normal zones to equalize may vary considerably among patients. While the use of a set time (e.g., 3 to 4 hours after injection) for redistribution imaging will differentiate transient ischemia from infarction in the majority of patients, in others redistribution will occur more slowly and further delayed imaging will be necessary to differentiate the two conditions. In some patients with ischemia, redistribution does not occur. These patients may not exhibit redistribution because they have chronic ischemia and thus either reduced capacity to trap thallium-201 or ischemia persisting well into the post-exercise period. After revascularization, these areas appear normal; this indicates that the previous fixed defect represented viable tissue.

TECHNIQUE

EXERCISE SCINTIGRAPHY. For exercise myocardial perfusion scintigraphy, thallium-201 is injected at the time of maximal stress during a multistage treadmill test according to the Bruce protocol. The patient should not eat for at least 4 hours before the exercise test so that splanchnic uptake of the tracer is reduced to a minimum. For the detection and evaluation of coronary artery disease, drugs that protect the myocardium, such as beta-adrenoceptor blockers, should be discontinued for a long enough time before the study to allow the amount of drug in the blood to decrease to less than pharmacologically significant levels. (For propranolol, this would be approximately 48 hours before the test.) If the protective effect of the drug is being studied specifically, the dosage regimen should be maintained at the levels administered prior to the test.

A 12-lead electrocardiogram is obtained prior to the test, and an intravenous line is inserted for rapid injection of the radiotracer and for emergency use if necessary. Exercise should be graded and the injection made at the time of maximal exercise, which should be maintained for at least 60 to 90 seconds following the injection to allow the tracer to be cleared from the blood. A near-maximum exercise level ($\geq$ 85 per cent of predicted maximal heart rate) should be achieved to assess the extent of the disease.[187] The heart rate response may be less critical for accurate diagnosis of coronary artery disease, although the incidence of false-negative examinations is high when the patient fails to achieve a heart rate of at least 110 beats/min. Electrocardiographic monitoring should continue throughout the test and during the immediate post-test period. The exercise test should be stopped if hypotension, marked electrocardiographic evidence of ischemia, serious arrhythmias, or significant pain develops.

Imaging may begin 6 to 8 minutes after injecting 2 to 3 mCi of thallium-201, allowing sufficient time for the thallium to be cleared from the blood but prior to significant redistribution. A camera and collimator with a system spatial resolution of at least 4.5 mm (full-width at half-maximum) for thallium-201 should be used for imaging. Because imaging must be performed as quickly as possible, the low-energy, all-purpose collimator is usually used, although the recently introduced high-resolution parallel square-hole collimator offers better spatial resolution with sensitivity comparable to that of the standard all-purpose collimators. With the latter collimator, care must be taken to keep the amount of the thallium-202 contaminant, with its high-energy emissions, to a minimum at the time of injection. The pulse height analyzer energy window is peaked over the low-energy (69 to 81 kev) thallium-201 photopeak. In cameras with multiple pulse height analyzer energy windows for data collection, the counts resulting from the higher energy gamma rays (135 and 165 kev) should also be collected, substantially increasing camera sensitivity and improving spatial resolution.

Projections obtained during myocardial perfusion scintigraphy include the 30- and 45-degree left anterior oblique, anterior, and 70-degree left anterior oblique, or left lateral views. Since the plane of the septum can vary, patient positioning should be tailored to the cardiac anatomy of the individual patient. Care must be taken in interpreting the 70-degree LAO and the left lateral views, particularly when the patient is imaged in the supine position. Increased attenuation of the diaphragm superimposed on the inferior wall of the left ventricle may cause apparent inferior perfusion defects in patients with normal blood flow.[188] Perfusion defects seen only on these views should be confirmed with additional imaging in the 70-degree LAO or left lateral view with the patient lying left side up. At least 3×10^5 counts are acquired per view; when computer acquisition is used, counts on each view can be collected for a preset time, usually 6 to 10 minutes per view. With a preset time, quantitative comparisons of thallium-201 activity can be made between serial images. These projections are repeated during redistribution imaging 3 to 4 hours after injection. The patient should not eat between initial and delayed imaging because carbohydrates increase the myocardial clearance of thallium-201; a greater number of false-positive studies can result.[189] In addition, if perfusion defects persist and the distinction between infarction and transient ischemia is critical, repeat imaging can be performed 24 hours after injection. Images may be acquired on Polaroid film or x-ray film for hard copy; however, the analog data should be converted to digital format by computer acquisition using a 128×128 matrix and, with large-field-of-view cameras, a zoom mode with a magnification of at least twofold. Image interpretation should be performed at the computer console so that the observer can adjust contrast and brightness.

Other forms of stress can be employed, including upright and supine bicycle ergometry, handgrip exercise, and atrial pacing. Treadmill ergometry is preferable, unless patients are physically unable to run. Treadmill testing is the most likely method to force patients to adequate exercise levels and to increase coronary flow sufficiently to permit accurate interpretations of the thallium-201 images.

DIPYRIDAMOLE. This drug may also be used to increase coronary blood flow; it has several advantages over exercise. Patients can be routinely and reproducibly stressed to a predefined endpoint, and the method can be used in patients who cannot exercise to maximum levels. Perfusion imaging can be performed after the intravenous injection of dipyridamole, a potent coronary vasodilator that produces little if any myocardial ischemia. Accuracy in detecting coronary artery disease is comparable to that of standard exercise testing,[190–192] with an improvement in image quality. While imaging is probably safer with dipyridamole than with exercise, patients have experienced severe headaches and postural hypotension after administration of this drug. Furthermore, the relationship between increases in flow and thallium activity are probably not linear in the face of a falling extraction fraction due to increasing flow without corresponding increases in metabolic needs.

Thallium-201 dipyridamole myocardial imaging is performed after overnight fasting.[193] The patient must avoid coffee and tea (which contain theophylline, a dipyridamole antagonist). Dipyridamole is infused at a rate of 0.15 mg/kg/min over 4 minutes with the patient supine and vital signs and electrocardiogram recorded every minute. After the infusion, the patient walks in place for 2 to 3 minutes. At that point, 2.0 mCi of thallium-201 is injected intravenously and the patient continues walking in place for 2 additional minutes. Imaging begins immediately thereafter with the patient supine. Aminophylline (125 mg) is available to reverse the adverse affects of dipyridamole if necessary. Oral dipyridamole (400 mg) may be an alternative if the intravenous pharmaceutical is not available.[193]

INTERPRETATION

In the normal scintigram there is uniform distribution of the tracer throughout the left ventricular wall, with a decrease in concentration in the region of the apex in

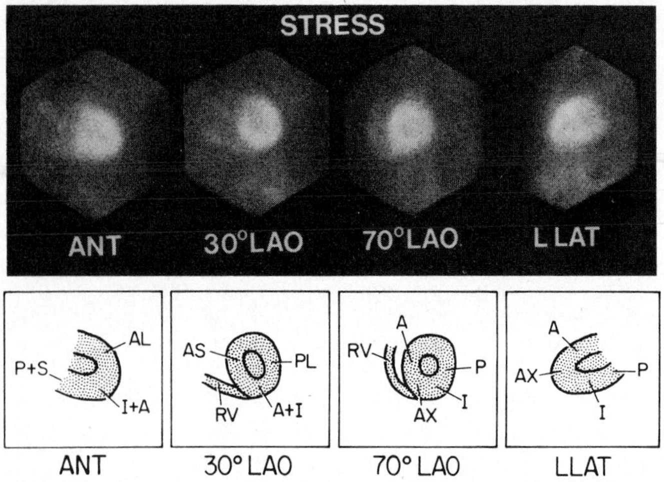

FIGURE 11–17. Normal myocardial perfusion scintigraphy with thallium-201 after stress in four different projections. Notice the uniform uptake of radiotracer throughout the left ventricular wall and the central defect due to the left ventricular cavity. ANT = anterior; 30° LAO = 30-degree left anterior oblique; 70° LAO = 70-degree left anterior oblique; LLAT = left lateral; P = posterior; S = septum; AL = anterolateral; I = inferior; A = anterior; PL = posterolateral; AX = apex; RV = right ventricle.

about half of the patients (Fig. 11–17).[194] The ventricle has a horseshoe appearance, with its long axis oriented anywhere from horizontal to vertical. Activity tapers near the base of the heart. In the majority of normal subjects, the inferior wall appears thicker than the anterolateral surface. In the central zone, a region of decreased or absent activity is noted and represents the left ventricular cavity. The right ventricular myocardium is not visualized in normal subjects at rest but may be seen as a thin wall extending from the apex when the injection is made at peak stress during redistribution imaging.

Multiple oblique projections are required, since perfusion defects are seen best on a tangent. In the anterior view, the apical, inferior, and anterolateral walls are well seen. The septum and posterolateral walls are seen best on the 30- to 45-degree LAO views. The anterior free wall, inferior and posterior walls are seen best on the 70-degree LAO and left lateral views. Right ventricular activity is seen when imaging is performed after stress but is less intense than left ventricular activity.

When stress (exercise or dipyridamole)[195] and redistribution imaging are performed, it is essential that each of the views obtained during redistribution be acquired in exactly the same position relative to the detector as the corresponding stress image. If proper technique is followed during stress and redistribution imaging, corresponding images can be evaluated for (1) reversible perfusion defects (those that appear on stress imaging but disappear after redistribution and are due to transient ischemia) (Fig. 11–18), (2) nonreversible perfusion defects (abnormalities that persist with equivalent intensity during redistribution imaging and are usually due to scar or infarction) (Fig. 11–19), and (3) normal anatomical variations (such as apical thinning and normally decreased perfusion at the base due to the aortic and mitral valves).

The greatest accuracy is achieved when perfusion defects are seen in the same segment on several views. Stenoses involving the left anterior descending coronary artery result in perfusion defects involving the anterior, septal, and lateral segments. Both the right coronary artery and the left circumflex artery perfuse the inferior and posterior segments; hence, perfusion defects in these segments may be due to stenoses involving either coronary arteries. The apex may be supplied by all three major coronary vessels.

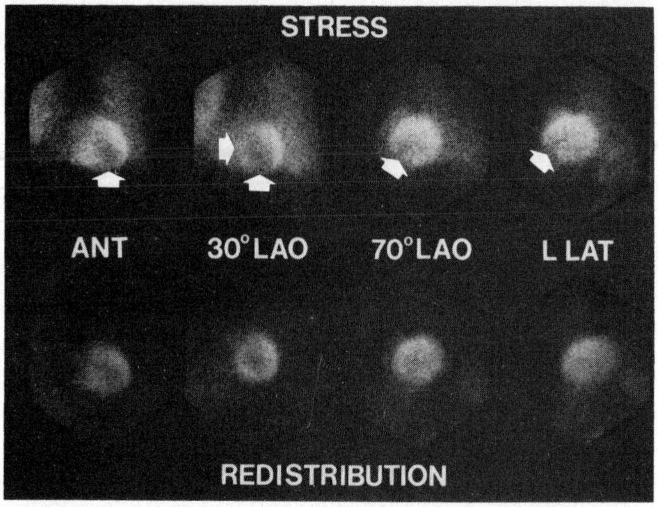

FIGURE 11–18. Myocardial perfusion scintigraphy with thallium-201 in a patient with 90 per cent stenosis of the left anterior descending artery along with less severe stenoses involving the left circumflex system. A large reversible perfusion defect involving the anteroseptal and apical segments of the left ventricle is seen best on the 30-degree LAO immediate postexercise image (arrows). The defect is not present on redistribution imaging four hours later (lower panel) because it is due to transient ischemia. Note the transiently increased lung uptake on the immediate postexercise images (upper panel). (ANT = anterior; 30° LAO = 30-degree left anterior oblique; 70° LAO = 70-degree left anterior oblique; LLAT = left lateral.)

In addition to interpretation of myocardial thallium-201 activity, attention should also be directed to the size of the cardiac chamber, wall thickness, and pulmonary uptake of thallium-201. An enlarged cardiac chamber may be seen at rest, indicating ventricular dilation. Cardiac chamber enlargement may be seen only during the exercise phase of the study and indicates a transient increase in end-diastolic volume, an index of diminished cardiac reserve in patients with a variety of cardiac diseases including, but not limited to, coronary artery disease. A transient increase in lung activity during exercise results from a transient increase in pulmonary blood volume and is associated with an elevated pulmonary capillary wedge pressure. The increase in pulmonary thallium-201 activity is probably

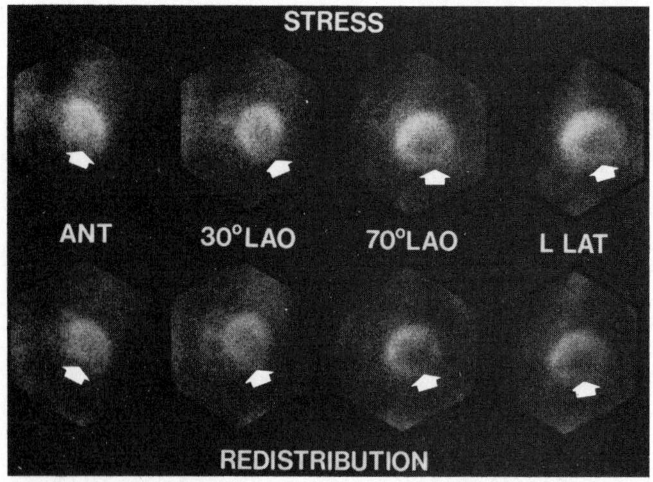

FIGURE 11–19. Myocardium perfusion scintigraphy with thallium-201 in a patient with a previous inferoposterior myocardial infarction. A large nonreversible perfusion defect involving the inferior and posterior segments of the left ventricle is seen best in the 70-degree LAO and LLAT projections. The defect is seen on the immediate poststress images (upper arrows) and involves the same area of the left ventricle on the redistribution images obtained four hours later (lower arrows). The defect is due to nonviable myocardium or to scar tissue. (ANT = anterior; 30° LAO = 30-degree left anterior oblique; 70° LAO = 70-degree left anterior oblique; LLAT = left lateral.)

due to an increase in capillary surface area and a resultant increase in tracer extraction. The ratio between lung and heart activity has been quantitated and found to be fairly specific and only moderately sensitive for coronary artery disease.[196, 197] On the other hand, the presence of transiently increased lung uptake and transiently increased left ventricular end-diastolic volume correlates strongly with the presence of multivessel disease even in patients in whom the perfusion abnormalities lead to underestimation of the extent of disease.[198]

QUANTIFICATION

Visual interpretation of unprocessed thallium-201 myocardial images leads to a significant degree of disagreement among observers and makes sequential assessment of regional myocardial perfusion difficult.[199] Thallium images have a relatively high level of background activity, which interferes with evaluation of the images. Computer processing is especially useful in thallium imaging because it affords the observer the capability for interactive image processing. This technique is very helpful in visualizing the subtle differences involved if the operator can raise the lower and upper thresholds while viewing the images. Overlaying of images is also helpful in comparing initial images with images after redistribution. In addition to simple threshold subtraction, several interpolative methods for background subtraction have been suggested. These take into account the nonuniformity of background that may result in excessive background subtraction.[200, 201] Image interpretation should not depend on background-corrected images alone and must take into account the unprocessed image as well.

Quantitative computer analysis of the thallium image has been suggested as a means for standardizing the interpretation of images and eliminating the high degree of subjectivity in visual analysis.[202, 203] In general, this technique evaluates the relative concentrations of thallium in the various segments of the left ventricle.[178, 201, 204–206] Regional activity is assessed quantitatively by breaking up the thallium myocardial image into anatomically defined left ventricular regions. Thallium-201 uptake in these segments is considered to be pathologically reduced if count rates are less than 75 to 80 per cent of maximum left ventricular thallium-201 uptake.

THALLIUM-201 DISTRIBUTION. This may also be analyzed as a function of time, measuring the net rate of thallium wash-in or wash-out from the myocardium during the redistribution phase of the study.[178, 207, 208] Both thallium wash-in to the myocardium and the rate of clearance in the myocardium are related to myocardial blood flow.[209] Well-perfused myocardium has the most thallium delivered initially, the largest myocardial-blood gradient, and the most rapid clearance. Zones with less perfusion have less thallium delivered initially and it clears from them more slowly. While these temporal changes in the myocardial distribution of thallium activity can be assessed by subjective assessment of the images, quantitative techniques provide a more reproducible and more objective basis on which to judge abnormalities in thallium kinetics.

Measurement of myocardial clearance of thallium is difficult, however, because the information is obtained from only two sets of images. There is a large statistical error in the measurement of the clearance and background (even with background subtraction techniques) that may significantly affect the slope of the clearance curve. The amount of thallium in the myocardium may vary with differences in the coronary flow response to exercise. As a result, thallium clearance data should be used cautiously in the interpretation and assessment of coronary artery disease.[209]

TECHNIQUE FOR OBTAINING QUANTITATIVE STUDIES. For quantitative studies, imaging is begun immediately after exercise in the 30-degree LAO projection to separate the myocardial territories of the left anterior descending coronary artery and left circumflex and right coronary arteries.[208] This image is followed by the left lateral view, which also separates the territories of the left anterior descending artery and the left circumflex and right coronary arteries. Finally, an anterior view is obtained. In this view, the territories of the left anterior descending and right coronary arteries are superimposed except along the anterolateral wall, which is supplied by the left anterior descending artery.

Count density is critical for satisfactory quantitative analysis. While 3.5×10^5 counts is adequate for standard planar imaging, a count density of between 5 and 6×10^5 counts (with 3.5×10^4 counts from the background corrected left ventricular region of interest) is needed for quantitation. Since the imaging time must be kept as short as possible because myocardial activity is continuously changing, the counting rate must be maximized either by use of a general purpose collimator or by use of dual energy peaking over the 80-kev and 167-kev photo peaks of thallium-201 so that images may be obtained within 8 to 10 minutes per view.

While standard planar thallium-201 visual interpretation is accurate even at submaximal levels of exercise, maximal exercise is essential for quantitative analysis. After injection of thallium-201 with the patient at rest, the myocardial concentration of the tracer increases gradually. After strenuous exercise, normal myocardium peaks quickly (within 5 minutes) and subsequently washes out. Without adequate exercise, thallium-201 wash-out may be slow even from normal myocardium.

Delayed imaging is performed between 2 and 4 hours after exercise. In some laboratories 2 hours is preferred to optimize the count rate during delayed imaging. In other laboratories it is argued that redistribution may be incomplete at that point, reducing the accuracy with which transient ischemia is detected by visual inspection of the images. Accurate repositioning of the patient is crucial because data derived from the delayed images will be compared with that from the corresponding initial images.

Data processing is performed after background subtraction, usually using a weighted bilinear interpolative correction. The background corrected post-exercise and delayed myocardial images are divided into segments. The left ventricle is divided into pie-shaped segments.[208] The activity in each segment is displayed as circumferential profiles which display (1) the distribution of thallium-201 activity in the ventricle during the post-exercise study and during the delayed study and (2) the wash-out of thallium-201 from the ventricle (obtained by subtracting the delayed from the post-exercise thallium activity for each segment) (Fig. 11–20).

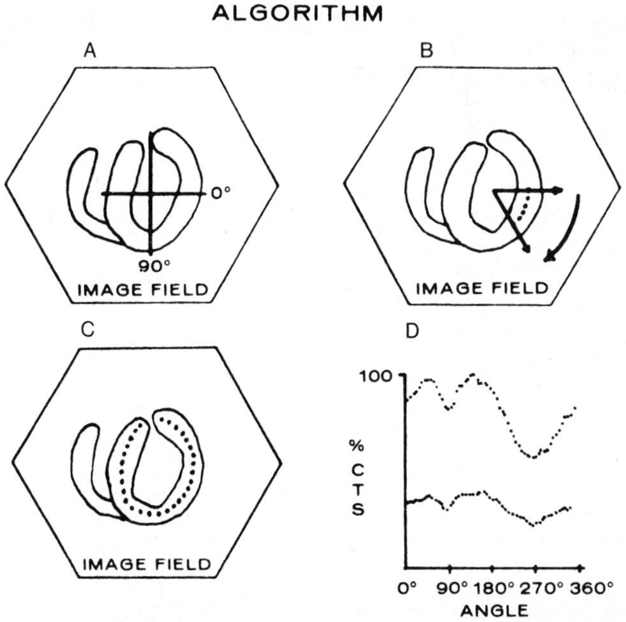

FIGURE 11–20. Diagrammatic representation of method for obtaining circumferential profiles from the myocardium. Polar coordinate reference axis is shown in *A*. Image pixels for circumferential profile analysis are found by performing a radial search for maximum tracer activity at 6-degree intervals throughout the 360-degree circumference, *B*. Activities in *B* and *C* are then replotted in *D* for each angle as a percentage of the maximum value for the circumferential profile. Top curve in *D* represents circumferential profile from stress thallium-201 image and bottom curve represents the profile from the 4-hour delayed image. (From Garcia, E., et al.: Space/time quantitation of thallium-201 myocardial scintigraphy. J. Nucl. Med. *22*:309, 1981, by permission of the Society of Nuclear Medicine.)

To interpret properly the distribution and wash-out profiles, data must first be obtained in a group of patients without cardiovascular disease. At the present time, it is necessary to develop such normal profiles in the user's nuclear cardiology laboratory. Eventually such data will become available from the commercial software vendors.

When care is taken to achieve adequate exercise, adequate count density, and careful and reproducible patient positioning, high predictive accuracy for the detection of coronary artery disease can be obtained. Defining a defect on the distribution and wash-out profiles as at least five adjacent segments (50-degree angle) below the lower limit of normal, one laboratory has achieved an excellent sensitivity (89 per cent) and specificity (95 per cent) for the detection of coronary artery disease.[208] The greatest improvement over visual assessment is in patients with single-vessel coronary artery disease. The predictive accuracy for detecting involvement of the left anterior descending artery is high but is considerably less for the right coronary artery and for the left circumflex artery. The accuracy with which triple-vessel and left main coronary artery disease is identified is also increased by quantitation.[210]

Quantitative analysis has become a standard adjunct to the interpretation of thallium-201 images. It requires substantially greater quality control than does standard visual assessment and does not replace the need for visual inspection of the images. Coronary artery disease usually is not detected by quantitative analysis alone[209, 211]; more commonly, subtle abnormalities noted on visual analysis of the images are confirmed by quantitative assessment.

TOMOGRAPHY

Many of the problems associated with conventional scintigraphy, such as superimposition of one portion of myocardium on another and the heterogeneity of background activities, are overcome by tomography.

SINGLE-PHOTON EMISSION COMPUTED TOMOGRAPHY. This technique, also known as SPECT (p. 313), is performed with a rotating gamma camera system.[212–215] The detector rotates 180 or 360 degrees around the patient. The camera detector makes between 32 and 64 stops; during each of these 20- to 40-second stops, the camera acquires a two-dimensional image. Data from all 32 to 64 images are summed and reconstructed into tomographic images. Quality control is critical with SPECT. If noise and reconstruction artifacts are to be minimized, uniformity of response across the gamma camera field is necessary. A flat field correction of at least 30×10^6 counts is necessary to obtain less than a 1 per cent flatfield variation.[216] Nonuniformity in the response of the gamma camera is amplified greatly by the reconstruction technique. A planar nonuniformity of 3 per cent at the center of rotation becomes a 60 per cent nonuniformity on the tomographic reconstruction. The center of rotation must be known to within 1 mm because the center of rotation offset is added to the full-width at half-maximum of the resolution of the tomographic reconstruction.

Once quality control is assured, there are several options for data collection. Most systems use low-energy all-purpose or high-resolution collimators, but this may vary depending on the isotope being imaged. Most data collection techniques use multiple views over a 180° rotation. Data are collected using a noncircular camera orbit, which results in the reduction of uniformity artifacts. The elliptical orbit reduces the distance between the camera and the patient to a minimum throughout the 180-degree rotation. The patient is studied in a supine position with the left arm above the head. The left ventricle is placed in the center of rotation and 180-degree acquisition begins from the 30-degree RAO to the 60-degree LPO positions. Thirty-two or 64 projections are obtained during the rotation, acquiring data from two photopeaks, the 69- to 83-kev photopeak resulting from the mercury characteristic x-rays and the 167-kev photopeak resulting from the thallium-201 gamma rays. A variety of filtered back projection reconstruction algorithms are available for data reconstruction.

A number of options are available for data formatting following reconstruction. For example, the short-axis projection views the left ventricle in planes perpendicular to its long axis, preventing overlap of the base of the heart and the valve plane on other aspects of the left ventricle. Similarly, horizontal and vertical long-axis reconstructions of the heart reorient the image for more accurate and easier anatomical localization.

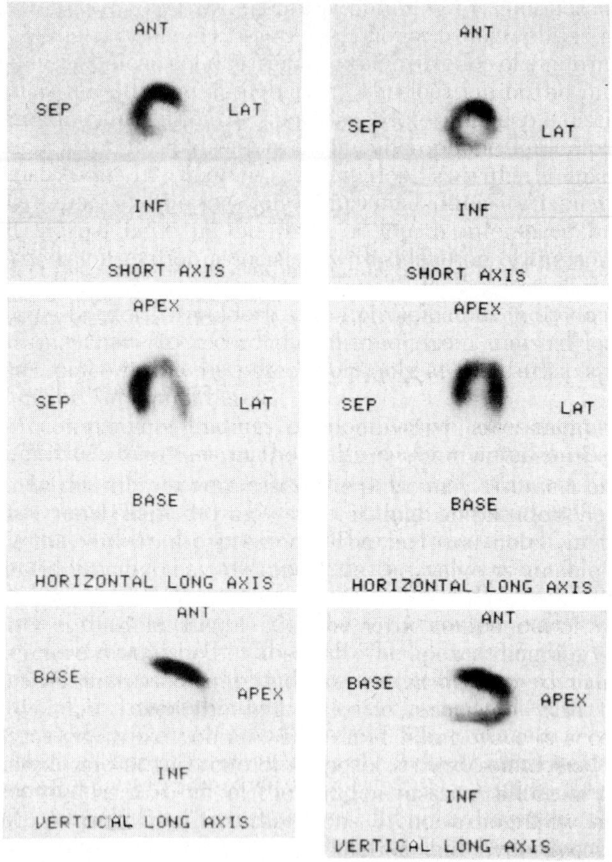

FIGURE 11–21. Myocardial single-photon emission computed tomography (SPECT) using thallium-201 in a patient with transient myocardial ischemia. The short axis (upper panel), horizontal long axis (middle panel), and vertical long axis (lower panel) tomographic reconstructions demonstrate markedly decreased perfusion to the inferolateral wall of the left ventricle immediately after maximal exercise (*left*). Redistribution imaging 4 hours later shows substantial redistribution of the radiotracer into the previously ischemic region (*right*).

SPECT has a characteristic appearance in the normal patient. In the short-axis view (with the myocardial image planes perpendicular to the long axis of the left ventricle), thallium activity is uniform throughout the left ventricular wall and appears doughnut shaped due to the central left ventricular cavity. The horizontal and vertical long-axis views are obtained parallel to the long axis of the left ventricle. The horizontal long-axis view highlights activity in the septum, apex, and lateral wall while the vertical long-axis view highlights the anterior and inferior walls of the left ventricle. Criteria for transient ischemia and infarction are the same as with planar imaging except that the extent of the perfusion defect is usually greater on emission tomography (Fig. 11–21). Similarly, the border between the normally perfused myocardium and perfusion defect is sharper and more clearly defined on tomography, since perfused myocardium is not superimposed on the ischemic tissue as it is with conventional imaging. Tomography also improves the contrast between the myocardium and surrounding structures such as the lung and liver.

Tomography is particularly promising for accurate delineation of the extent and localization of coronary artery disease and identification of the stenosed coronary vessels.[217] The technique is useful in identification of myocardial infarction, determination of the quantity of myocardium at risk of infarction, and identification of multivessel disease.[216, 218] Tomography is also useful for determining the mass of perfused myocardium.[219] Also, by subtraction of the remainder estimated from the exercise study, the mass of transiently ischemic myocardium as a percentage of the total perfused myocardial mass at rest can be determined.

New quantitative methods have been applied to tomographic thallium-201 imaging. Circumferential profile algorithms similar to those used with planar imaging have been applied to the short-axis tomographic data.[217] By superimposing each of the concentric circles—each representing one profile—and with the apex at the center of the circle and the base of the heart at the periphery, a bull's-eye polar coordinate map can be created (Fig. 11–22). The advantage of this approach is that all the tomographic data from the study can be displayed in a single functional image. Initial experience with this method suggests an accuracy of 85 per cent for detecting individual coronary lesions (Fig. 11–23). Another attractive quantitative scheme is the three-dimensional reconstruction of the tomographic slices using surface mapping techniques. The three-dimensional representation of the left ventricle permits geographical mapping of the extent and location of the ischemic lesion within the left ventricular wall (Fig. 11–24). As of this writing, all quantitative SPECT techniques require further validation before they can be used routinely.

FIGURE 11–22. See Color Plate 3.

FIGURE 11–23. See Color Plate 3.

FIGURE 11–24. See Color Plate 3.

APPLICATION IN THE DIAGNOSIS OF CORONARY ARTERY DISEASE

The diagnosis of coronary artery disease is the most important application of myocardial perfusion scintigraphy with thallium-201. It is significantly more accurate for the detection of coronary artery disease than the exercise electrocardiogram[220–225] (p. 323). In a review summarizing the results in over 1800 patients, overall sensitivity for detecting coronary artery disease using thallium-201 was 82 per cent and specificity was 91 per cent. Sensitivity for the exercise electrocardiogram was 60 per cent and specificity was 81 per cent.[87] The accuracy of the test is lower in patients who are on beta-blocker therapy and who fail to achieve a maximum heart rate of at least 110 beats/min. The specificity of the test is lower in women because of breast attenuation.

Myocardial perfusion scintigraphy with thallium-201 should be used as a complement to exercise electrocardiography. The exercise ECG should be obtained first, prior to perfusion scintigraphy. Thallium-201 scintigraphy should then be carried out when the exercise ECG is nondiagnostic or is abnormal in an asymptomatic patient or when there is a moderate probability of coronary artery disease.[226]

Nondiagnostic electrocardiograms may result when the resting electrocardiogram is abnormal but ischemic ST-segment changes cannot be defined. This may occur in patients with left bundle branch block or in those receiving digitalis. In this group of patients, the accuracy of thallium-201 perfusion scintigraphy remains high and is therefore extremely helpful. Another cause for uninterpretable exercise electrocardiograms is failure to achieve 85 per cent of predicted maximal heart rate with no ST-segment changes. The sensitivity and specificity of thallium-201 imaging in patients who achieve a maximum heart rate of only 100 to 110 beats/min are approximately the same as for patients who are able to achieve an adequate heart rate response.[187, 227, 228] These results suggest that the mechanisms underlying an abnormal stress electrocardiogram and an abnormal myocardial scintigram are different and help to explain why the sensitivities of these tests are additive. When the diagnosis of coronary artery disease is based on both an abnormal stress electrocardiogram and an abnormal thallium-201 test, the diagnostic sensitivity is substantially greater than when either test is used alone. However, it must be remembered that when the two tests are used additively, the diagnostic specificity for coronary artery disease falls substantially, i.e., in many patients with coronary artery disease, one of the tests is negative.

Patients with *atypical angina pectoris* are reasonable candidates for myocardial perfusion scintigraphy. The likelihood of these patients having coronary artery disease is between 30 and 50 per cent.[229] Perfusion scintigraphy is useful in this group of patients. The accuracy of the exercise electrocardiogram may be too low to affect substantially the likelihood of coronary artery disease, regardless of the outcome of the test (p. 235). The accuracy of myocardial perfusion scintigraphy is higher, so that in patients who are moderately likely to have coronary artery disease, the results of the test can be used to guide management. This is not true for patients with *typical angina pectoris*, in whom the likelihood of having the disease is so high prior to diagnostic testing that a normal perfusion test cannot be accepted as strong evidence that the patient does not have coronary artery disease. Similarly, in *asymptomatic* patients, the likelihood of disease is so small prior to testing that this likelihood will change little after the test.[230] Furthermore, if large numbers of asymptomatic patients are studied, a sizable number of false-positive results will occur even when the test's specificity is 90 per cent.

While the test has limited usefulness for asymptomatic patients in general, it is of value in asymptomatic patients with positive stress electrocardiograms. The prevalence of coronary artery disease in this population is approximately 30 per cent. A positive thallium perfusion scintigram raises the likelihood of disease to greater than 80 per cent, while a negative test reduces it to less than 10 per cent.

PREDICTION OF FUTURE CARDIAC EVENTS. Normal exercise myocardial scintigraphy has important predictive value. In patients who have a normal exercise thallium test and who experience chest pain, mortality due to cardiac disease and the rate of nonfatal myocardial infarction is low (1.1 per cent/year) and is comparable to that reported for patients with chest pain and normal coronary arteries on arteriography.[231–233] Even in patients with typical angina pectoris and with a high pretest probability of disease, a normal thallium exercise study is associated with a good prognosis.[234]

Exercise thallium-201 scintigraphy plays an important role in predicting cardiac events in patients with abnormal tests as well.[235] Thus, in patients with chest pain and no evidence of previous myocardial infarction, the number of myocardial segments with transient thallium-201 defects is an excellent predictor of future cardiac events.[236] Thallium-201 imaging is equally useful as a predictive index in patients with acute infarction (see below).

Detection of coronary artery disease may have important predictive value in patients who cannot undergo maximal treadmill exercise. In patients scheduled for peripheral vascular surgery, thallium myocardial imaging with a dipyridamole stress is useful in identifying those patients who are high surgical risks. Patients with transient perfusion defects on myocardial scintigraphy should be considered candidates for coronary angiography and myocardial revascularization before the peripheral vascular surgery is performed.[236]

DIAGNOSING THE EXTENT OF CORONARY ARTERY DISEASE. Thallium-201 perfusion scintigraphy has been most useful in providing the clinician with an objective guide to the severity of a patient's coronary artery disease and the effectiveness of medical therapy. For example, patients with coronary artery disease can be studied while receiving a beta blocker to determine whether they are adequately protected from ischemia at the maximum exercise levels they can achieve while on the drug.

Standard planar thallium-201 perfusion scintigraphy has not been particularly useful in determining the number of stenotic coronary arteries or in identifying which vessels are diseased. The sensitivity is approximately 60 to 80 per cent for identifying obstruction of the left anterior coronary artery, 50 to 60 per cent for the right coronary artery, and only 20 to 50 per cent for the left circumflex coronary artery.[237, 238] Sensitivity is affected by the severity of the stenosis,[239] with an increasing sensitivity as the degree of stenosis increases. Specific patterns of extensive coronary artery disease that involve either three vessels or the left main coronary artery are helpful when present.[240] More than 95 per cent of patients with left main coronary artery disease have abnormal thallium-201 exercise scintigrams with two-thirds of the patients having defects involving multiple vascular regions and 42 per cent with abnormal lung uptake.[241]

The accuracy with which exercise myocardial scintigraphy measures the extent of coronary artery disease and identifies the number and location of the diseased vessels is improved by the addition of the quantitative measurement of thallium-201 wash-out kinetics[242, 243] and by the use of single-photon emission computed tomography (see above). Regardless of the methodology applied, accurate estimation of the extent of the disease is highly dependent upon the patient achieving maximal levels of exercise.[188]

Exercise myocardial scintigraphy plays an important role in defining the *hemodynamic significance of coronary artery lesions* and is an important complement to coronary arteriography. Contrast studies provide highly useful information concerning the anatomy and morphology of the coronary vessels but only indirect information about the hemodynamic significance of coronary artery lesions. Only limited hemodynamic information can be derived from the degree of stenosis.[235] Furthermore, the measurement of coronary stenoses is prone to error because stenoses tend to be asymmetric and difficult to measure from only one or two projections.

Exercise thallium scintigraphy may provide information about hemodynamic abnormalities in the face of normal anatomy. Patients with normal coronary arteriograms and abnormal thallium exercise scintigrams will often have evidence of low coronary flow reserve, indicating an underlying hemodynamic abnormality.[232]

Perfusion scintigraphy may also be useful as an adjunct to coronary angiography by *differentiating viable from nonviable myocardium.* There is an inverse relationship between the degree of redistribution into regions of transient ischemia and the degree of asynergy in that myocardial segment.[244] Furthermore, the better the redistribution, the more likely the segment will contract normally after bypass surgery.[245]

STUDIES FOLLOWING MYOCARDIAL REPERFUSION. After coronary revascularization surgery, thallium uptake and wash-out is normal in almost all segments with total redistribution before surgery but in only three-fourths of areas that demonstrate partial redistribution preoperatively.[246] Almost half of the areas with persistent defects thought to represent myocardial scarring are normal after operation. Normalization of perfusion is seen far more often when the initial persistent defect is mild than when it is profound (greater than 50 per cent reduction in myocardial activity). The presence of a fixed defect, particularly if it is mild to moderate in intensity, may not represent myocardial scarring or fibrosis but rather viable ischemic tissue that will respond to revascularization surgery.

Thallium-201 perfusion scintigraphy has been used to study patients after coronary bypass surgery in whom the question of *graft patency* has arisen. In patients with exercise-induced perfusion defects that become normal after operation, the likelihood of bypass graft patency is high.[247, 248] If the segment was normal prior to operation, the postoperative development of transient ischemia indicates that the graft is probably occluded. If perfusion during exercise is normal after operation, the graft is probably patent. If there is no change in perfusion to the segment after surgery, graft patency cannot be predicted accurately.

Exercise myocardial scintigraphy is particularly useful in evaluating restenosis after *percutaneous transluminal coronary angioplasty,* which may occur in up to one-third of patients within 6 months of the procedure[249] (p. 1387). Perfusion scintigraphy has a high predictive value for detecting restenosis and recurrent angina in patients who have had a technically successful procedure. Myocardial scintigraphy may be performed in either of two time frames: (1) 2 to 3 weeks after angioplasty when it may be useful in predicting restenosis or, more commonly, (2) after 5 to 6 months when the procedure will detect the greatest number of restenosed coronary arteries.

OTHER CAUSES OF TRANSIENT PERFUSION DEFECTS. Many patients with transient perfusion defects on thallium-201 imaging but considered false-positives in reported studies have coronary stenoses of between 20 and 50 per cent of the vessel diameter.[250] That these patients have a higher incidence of transient ischemia than patients with less severe stenoses may indicate both the difficulty in defining accurately the severity of stenosis using coronary angiography and the possibility that what has traditionally been characterized as subcritical stenosis may result in myocardial hypoperfusion during maximal stress.

Abnormal results may also be seen in patients with *muscular myocardial bridges* without evidence of coronary atherosclerosis[251] (p. 284) and in patients with evidence of *diffuse myocardial disease.*[252] In patients with *aortic stenosis* and normal coronary arteries, exercise-induced subendocardial ischemia[253] or changes in left ventricular wall thickness may develop.[254] This ischemia will result in perfusion defects on thallium-201 imaging. While perfusion defects have been reported in patients with mitral valve prolapse, most studies have not substantiated this observation and have suggested that this test may be used for identifying underlying coronary artery disease in patients with prolapse.[255–257]

CORONARY ARTERY SPASM. This may occur in patients with or without detectable coronary artery stenoses (p. 1228). These patients will have transient perfusion defects on thallium-201 imaging if they have injection during or immediately after spasm.[258–260] Spasm has been demonstrated during exercise in some patients with exertional chest pain and ST-wave elevation who have normal coronary arteries at angiography. Spasm may occur at rest; in this case, transient perfusion defects are observed even without exercise. In the absence of spasm and fixed obstruction, the scintigram is normal.

FIXED DEFECTS. Nonreversible defects, i.e., perfusion defects that are present both at rest and during exercise, may be due to previous myocardial infarction, hypertrophic obstructive cardiomyopathy,[261] sarcoid heart disease,[262] idiopathic congestive cardiomyopathy,[263] amyloidosis, metastatic disease to the heart, and other infiltrative heart diseases. Most patients with diffuse scleroderma have clinically detectable myocardial involvement on thallium-201 scintigraphy with both fixed defects and reversible exercise-induced defects. This suggests that the myocardial dysfunction in this disease is secondary to ischemic injury resulting from abnormal intramyocardial circulation.[264]

Other causes of an abnormal test result from *technical factors*. For example, among patients with normal electrocardiographic exercise tests, the specificity of thallium-201 exercise testing is lower in women than in men and is due to attenuation of myocardial activity by overlying breast resulting in an apparent perfusion defect in the myocardial segment underlying the breast.[265] As mentioned previously, perfusion defects may appear on the lateral or 70-degree LAO projection in patients studied supine because of attenuation caused by abdominal organs and the diaphragm. Because camera nonuniformity may also result in apparent defects, it is critical to pay close attention to quality control. Probably the single most common cause of apparent perfusion abnormalities is heterogeneous background lung activity, especially when lung activity is high owing to increased pulmonary blood volume. This will result in apparently decreased activity in myocardium that does not overlie the lung and is only partially corrected by interpolative background-correction programs. Emission tomography will alleviate these background problems but may introduce additional problems due to inadequate correction of attenuation.

MYOCARDIAL INFARCTION (Ch. 38). Perfusion scintigraphy at rest has been used to detect the presence of acute myocardial infarction. Wackers et al. showed defects in 165 of 200 patients (82 per cent).[266] This technique is most sensitive soon after infarction. Thus, 90 of 96 patients had abnormal scintiscans within 24 hours of infarction, while only 75 of 104 had abnormalities after 24 hours. Defects also appear to decrease in size with time, particularly when the initial study is performed within 24 hours of infarction. Since perfusion defects can be seen at rest in some patients with unstable angina and during spasm in patients with Prinzmetal's angina, perfusion scintigraphy cannot always distinguish between myocardial infarction and these conditions. The greatest value of this technique lies in obtaining a normal scintigram within 24 hours of suspected infarction, greatly lowering the probability that the patient has sustained acute infarction. In acute infarction the perfusion defect will decrease in size during the first week, while the defect produced by scar tissue will not change in size. Consequently, serial imaging will be necessary to distinguish old from new infarction.

Patients with unstable angina pectoris have abnormal perfusion at the time of chest pain, but they may also have abnormal scintigrams after the pain has subsided.[267] Abnormal scintigrams occur more frequently in patients with a complicated course.

Perfusion scintigraphy may provide prognostic information, since it correlates well with estimates of infarct size made by serum creatine kinase curve analysis[268–270] and by pathological studies.[271–273] Initially, the thallium perfusion defect is larger than the acute infarct because of ischemia in the area around the infarct and it may remain larger if the patient has sustained previous infarctions and has myocardial scar in addition to necrosis.

Thallium perfusion scintigraphy may be useful as a prognostic indicator if it is obtained early after the onset of symptoms.[274] Patients with large defects have a higher mortality rate than patients with smaller defects. To use this test in a predictive way, it is essential that imaging be obtained early or at a predefined time after the onset of symptoms. Since the perfusion defect will shrink with time unless the patient sustains reinfarction or extension of the infarct, it will not be possible to compare the results obtained at variable times after infarction. The predictive value of this test is enhanced when the test is combined with technetium-99m-pyrophosphate scintigraphy (see Infarct-Avid Scintigraphy), particularly with emission computed tomography.

As already indicated, exercise radionuclide angiocardiography provides important predictive information in patients with acute myocardial infarction when performed prior to hospital discharge (see above). Comparable information can be obtained from predischarge exercise thallium-201 scintigraphy. When quantitative submaximal thallium-201 imaging is performed in patients with uncomplicated acute myocardial infarction before discharge from the hospital, 90 per cent of high-risk patients are identified (compared with 56 per cent by exercise electrocardiography testing alone).[275] High-risk patients are identified by scintigraphic defects in more than one vascular region, redistribution (evidence of transient ischemia), and/or increased lung uptake. Dipyridamole–thallium-201 scintigraphy may be used as an alternative to submaximal exercise.[276] With dipyridamole, thallium redistribution is highly predictive of subsequent cardiac events (33 per cent incidence in patients with thallium redistribution and 6 per cent in other patients).

THE RIGHT VENTRICLE. Right ventricular uptake on the resting thallium-201 images correlates with right ventricular overload (Fig. 11–25) and may be seen in either volume overload (atrial septal defect or pulmonic or tricus-

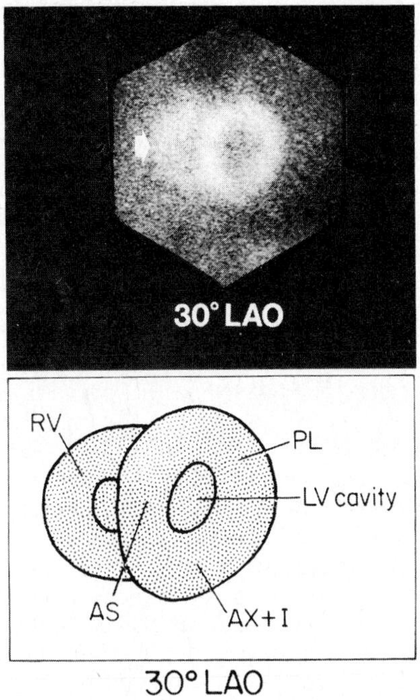

FIGURE 11–25. Myocardial perfusion scintigram in a patient with right ventricular hypertrophy. Note increased thallium-201 uptake in the right ventricle (arrow). 30° LAO = 30-degree left anterior oblique projection; RV = right ventricle; AS = anteroseptal; AX = apex; I = inferior; LV = left ventricular; and PL = posterolateral.

pid regurgitation) or pressure overload (mitral stenosis, primary pulmonary hypertension, ventricular septal defect, or Eisenmenger's syndrome). There is a direct relationship between the intensity of right ventricular uptake and the hemodynamic measurement of right ventricular work.

The appearance of the right ventricle on exercise thallium scintigraphy may be useful in the evaluation of patients with suspected coronary artery disease. The presence of perfusion defects involving the right ventricle correlates with proximal right coronary artery stenosis.[277] The sensitivity of this finding for detecting right coronary artery disease is low (59 per cent), possibly because of collateral vessels to the right coronary artery.[278]

THROMBOLYTIC THERAPY (See also p. 1257). The administration of thrombolytic agents or percutaneous transluminal angioplasty may reduce the extent of irreversible myocardial damage in patients with acute infarction.[279, 280] Since a coronary artery catheter is sometimes already in place in the vessel, coronary arteriography can be performed to demonstrate the degree to which the vessel has been reopened. In addition, thallium-201 can be injected directly into the coronary artery both before and after reperfusion therapy.

Thallium-201 (0.3 to 0.5 mCi) is injected into both coronary arteries immediately after the occlusion is located by coronary angiography. After imaging and treatment in the coronary catheterization laboratory, thallium-201 is reinjected into the coronary artery to evaluate recanalization. Intracoronary thallium-201 scintigraphy provides complementary information to the coronary arteriogram on the salvageability of the myocardium after thrombolysis.[281] Failure of thallium-201 uptake in previously ischemic tissue indicates a lack of capillary reperfusion and myocardial necrosis.[282] On the other hand, thallium-201 uptake during the reperfusion phase indicates reconstitution of the blood supply but does *not necessarily indicate either viability or survival* of the myocardial tissue.[283–285]

Successful reperfusion has also been reported after the intravenous administration of thrombolytic agents such as streptokinase. The effect of reperfusion in these patients can be assessed following the intravenous administration of thallium-201. Restoration of thallium uptake is seen after reperfusion of the infarct vessel whether or not recanalization occurs spontaneously or after successful thrombolysis.[286] Imaging must be performed before thrombolysis therapy to obtain a baseline study and may then be obtained serially after thrombolysis to determine the success of therapy either by reinjection of thallium-201 or, preferably, by assessing the degree of redistribution of the tracer injected for the baseline study into the reperfused tissue.

Since time is crucial in the salvage of myocardium, the initial scan may be dispensed with and the post-treatment scan used to evaluate efficacy of lysis of the occluding thrombus. A stress (exercise or dipyridamole) thallium-201 scintigram obtained prior to hospital discharge may reveal stress-induced ischemia. This often reflects persistent narrowing of the treated but infarct-related coronary artery; ordinarily this should be followed by coronary arteriography, and, depending on the findings, mechanical reperfusion (p. 1252).

POSITRON-EMISSION TOMOGRAPHY (PET) FOR ASSESSMENT OF REGIONAL MYOCARDIAL PERFUSION

A number of substances have been labeled with positron-emitting radionuclides and proposed as indicators for measuring myocardial blood flow. These indicators must meet several requirements: (1) They must remain in the tissue long enough for acquisition of statistically adequate images, (2) the kinetics of the indicator must be known, and (3) the kinetics must be suitable for tracer kinetic modeling so that blood flow can be determined from tracer distribution data. Microspheres have been labeled with gallium-68, carbon-11, and copper-62 and have resulted in accurate measurements of regional blood flow (see below).[287, 288] The technique requires the direct injection of the radioindicator into the left atrium or ventricle and is therefore highly invasive. Oxygen-15, a positron-emitting isotope of oxygen, has been labeled to water and has the potential for quantification of myocardial blood flow.[289] Measurement of blood flow using oxygen-15–labeled water requires either the direct injection of the radiotracer into the coronary artery or exponential infusion techniques, limiting the applicability of the method.

RUBIDIUM. Rubidium-82 is produced from a generator system, eliminating the need for on-site cyclotron production. It has a two-minute physical half-life with a marked reduction in the radiation dose and enables rapid sequential assessments of myocardial perfusion. A disadvantage of rubidium-82 use is that highly sensitive detection equipment is required for data acquisition because of the short half-life of the tracer.

Myocardial blood flow can be measured by relating the myocardial concentration of rubidium-82 to the arterial input function which can be derived from serial PET scans and external measurement of the arterial rubidium-82 concentration determined from the left ventricular blood pool activity.[290] Thirty to 50 mCi of rubidium-82 are eluted from a strontium-82/rubidium-82 generator and injected intravenously in a 10-ml saline solution over 20 to 25 seconds.[291] Because the physical half-life of rubidium-82 is so short (75 seconds), only one-half to two-thirds of the initial activity reaches the arterial circulation. To image rubidium-82, high-sensitivity imaging devices such as the multislice University of Texas positron-emission tomograph are used. These instruments have relatively high spatial resolution (8.1 mm full-width at half-maximum) and very high sensitivity (2×10^4 counts/sec/slice/μc/ml).

Absolute blood flow in units of ml/min/gm can be calculated using the integrated arterial input function derived from the blood pool images.[292] It may be possible to determine the viability of injured myocardium by following rubidium kinetics since there is some evidence that the first post-extraction fraction of rubidium-82 decreases in irreversibly ischemic myocardium independent of blood flow.[293, 294]

As with thallium-201 myocardial scintigraphy, coronary reserve can be assessed only during stress or pharmacological intervention. Because rubidium-82 has such a short physical half-life, standard exercise testing is very difficult to carry out using this tracer. Imaging must be done *during* the stress protocol and cannot be delayed until after the stress has been completed. For this reason, the technique has been coupled with pharmacological coronary vasodilatation (dipyridamole) and, to assess ischemia, with stress studies that can be carried out during imaging (handgrip stress).

NITROGEN-13-AMMONIA. Nitrogen-13-ammonia can be used as a marker of myocardial perfusion because it has a high extraction fraction through the myocardial microcirculation and its distribution is therefore flow dependent.[295] Changes in blood flow are associated with changes in nitrogen-13-ammonia tissue concentrations within the myocardium over a wide range of flows.[296] As with thallium-201, the extraction fraction is approximately 90 per cent at rest and falls gradually as blood flow increases. Unlike thallium-201, nitrogen-13-ammonia is trapped metabolically, and the extraction fraction is reduced when pH falls and in acute myocardial ischemia. These deviations from true flow dependence affect the flow-uptake relationship and limit the use of this agent as an indicator of myocardial blood flow.[296, 297] To date, nitrogen-13-ammonia has been used primarily as a qualitative index of the relative distribution of perfusion in the myocardium, although quantitative techniques to measure absolute myocardial blood flow are possible.

QUANTITATION OF MYOCARDIAL BLOOD FLOW USING THE INERT GAS WASH-OUT METHOD

The inert gas wash-out method provides a quantitative measure of tissue blood flow expressed in ml/min/100 gm. The inert gas dissolved in saline is injected directly and rapidly into the coronary artery. Once the tracer has diffused into the tissue, the organ is perfused by tracer-free blood, setting up a concentration gradient between tissue and blood. Since the tracer is not diffusion limited, the rate at which it diffuses back into the blood depends on blood flow through the tissue and the solubility partition coefficient between blood and tissue. The more rapid the flow rate, the more rapid the clearance (or wash-out) from the tissue.

Xenon-133 is the tracer most frequently used for quantifying perfusion. Because the energy of its photon emission is low (81 kev), scattered radiation cannot be easily eliminated from the photopeak by pulse height analysis, reducing the spatial resolution of the resultant data. Blood flow measurements are weighted more heavily toward superficial tissue lying close to the external detector since the attenuation of the 81-kev photons is greatest from deep structures. Other isotopes of xenon, such as xenon-127, reduce these problems because their photon energies are substantially higher than those of xenon-133. Krypton-81m has been suggested as a tracer to enable quantification of blood flow.[298] Rubidium-81 is injected into the coronary arteries and serves as an in vivo generator, continually producing krypton-81m (190 kev), which has a 13-second half-life. The technique provides quantitative measurement of transient changes in coronary blood flow following a single injection of rubidium-81.

Although the limitations of specific flow techniques must be taken into account, correlation between flow measurements obtained with electromagnetic flow meters and with the inert gas wash-out technique has been excellent.[299, 300] Also, regional flow values obtained in the clinic have been quite reproducible and have correlated with the extent of coronary artery disease, particularly during pharmacological or physiological stress.[301–306]

PERFUSION SCINTIGRAPHY WITH MICROPARTICLES

Myocardial perfusion can also be assessed following the intracoronary injection of either macroaggregated albumin[307, 308] or radiolabeled microspheres. However, single-photon applications of the microsphere method have been largely replaced by thallium-201– and technetium-99m–labeled myocardial imaging agents.

Organ blood flow can be measured following the intraventricular injection of carbon-11–labeled microspheres. Regional myocardial blood flow is measured in ml/min/100 gm by determining the regional activity from positron-emission tomograms. Blood flow in each region (RBF) is calculated from the equation

$$\text{RBF} = \frac{F_a \times C_m \times 100}{C_b} \text{ ml/min/100 gm} \tag{6}$$

Where F_a is the withdrawal rate of arterial blood (ml/min), C_m is the activity in each tomographic region corrected for attenuation, and C_b is the total activity in the arterial sample (counts/min).[309] While a quantitative technique is useful for assessing blood flow in ischemic tissue and for predicting viability of that tissue, the microsphere method is limited because of its invasiveness and the relatively poor resolution of the positron method, which limits the accuracy of quantitation.

MYOCARDIAL METABOLISM

Adequate cardiac function requires a sufficient supply of blood to meet the metabolic demands of the myocardium. With conventional radionuclide studies, perfusion of the myocardium and cardiac performance can be assessed. Recently, techniques have been developed to allow measurement of metabolism using the radiotracer method. Direct measurement of the uptake and utilization of fuel substrates may provide a more direct indication of the severity of myocardial ischemia, since ischemia results from a combination of inadequate blood supply and excessive demand for mechanical work. It may also be possible to better understand intrinsic disturbances in myocardial metabolism as might occur in cardiomyopathies and other diseases in which the primary etiology is alteration of biochemical pathways.

Perhaps the greatest impetus to the study of regional myocardial metabolism has been the development of PET. Three-dimensional reconstruction using positron emitters is based on coincidence detection. After a positron is formed through positron decay, it travels a short distance within the tissue, giving up its kinetic energy, and then interacts with an electron. Both particles are converted into annihilation photons, each with an energy of 511 kev. The photons leave the site of interaction in opposite directions, at an angle of 180 degrees. If two scintillation detectors are placed opposite one another, they will detect the annihilation photons simultaneously (coincidence detection). Scattered photons that reach only one of the detectors are rejected.

A number of approaches have been advocated for PET. In most cases, a ring of detectors is used in which each detector operates in coincidence with one or more detectors in the opposite bank. The patient is positioned within the detector ring. After imaging, the data are reconstructed into an image representing the transaxial distribution of the tracer using principles similar to those described for SPECT (p. 334).

PET has a number of advantages: (1) the field of view of the coincidence detectors is highly uniform over a large distance; (2) the coincidence counting rate remains virtually constant, regardless of the position of the radiation source within the absorber; (3) tissue attenuation is less with annihilation photons than with lower energy photon emissions of radionuclides such as technetium-99m and thallium-201; and (4) the short-lived positron-emitting radionuclides such as oxygen-15, nitrogen-13, and carbon-11 offer fundamental advantages in the study of metabolic processes. These last elements are ubiquitous in naturally occurring metabolic processes, and these nuclides are the only isotopes of these elements suitable for imaging. Thus, ^{15}O, ^{13}N, and ^{11}C can be incorporated into radiopharmaceuticals that are true metabolic substrates and consequently can be tailored to the investigation of selected metabolic pathways.

MYOCARDIAL GLUCOSE UPTAKE

Regional myocardial glucose uptake can be measured using ^{18}F 2-fluoro-2-deoxyglucose (FDG).[310] Fluorine-18 is a positron emitter with a 2-hour half-life. FDG exchanges rapidly across the capillary and cellular membranes in direct proportion to glucose transport. It competes for hexokinase and is phosphorylated to FDG-6-phosphate. Since it is not a substrate for glycolysis, it undergoes no further metabolism and therefore remains in the heart. As a result, the amount of tracer in the heart at the time of equilibrium is directly proportional to the rate of uptake of exogenous glucose.[311, 312]

While the initial tissue uptake of the tracer is a function of blood flow and the concentration of tracer in the blood, at the time of equilibrium—approximately 60 to 90 minutes after injection—the tissue activity represents primarily FDG-6-phosphate.[311–314] To measure *exogenous* glucose uptake, PET is performed 60 minutes after injection to determine the tissue concentration of the tracer. Arterial glucose and FDG plasma concentrations are also determined, and the information is fitted into a three-compartment model consisting of vascular, tissue, and metabolic components.

While this technique is a satisfactory measure of exogenous glucose uptake in man, it measures the glycolytic rate only when all the extracted glucose is used for glycolysis. This occurs only when glycogen stores are depleted, as in ischemia.[315] This technique has a number of technical limitations as well, in that it requires arterial or arterialized blood sampling; a knowledge of the rate constants required for application of the three-compartment model (since these rate constants may change during disease and during ischemia); and correction for wash-out of the tracer from the myocardium, which occurs late after injection.

With absolute quantification of myocardial glucose uptake, the same practical problems have been encountered as in other quantitative methods using PET. Cardiac wall motion, poor spatial resolution of the tomographs relative to the thickness of the left ventricular wall, and propagation of errors from the fairly complex mathematical models needed for quantification have resulted in measurements with wide ranges of uncertainty. As a result, qualitative and relative measures of regional metabolism are currently used by most workers in this field. For example, the UCLA group performs glucose metabolism studies without absolute quantification and therefore without the need for arterial blood sampling, increasing the clinical acceptance of the procedure.[316] Fifty grams of glucose is given by mouth 60 to 90 min before administration of the tracer. Uptake of the tracer depends on adequate levels of glucose in the blood and predosing with unlabeled glucose insures adequate uptake of the tracer for imaging. Transmission images are used to correct for photon attenuation. Ten millicuries of F-18-DG is injected intravenously; six cross-sectional images 1.0 to 1.5 cm apart are obtained 45 min after injection. Image analysis is performed after dividing the left ventricular cross-sectional image into 12 30-degree sectors. Activity is normalized to the maximum count in all planes and the activity/region is compared sector by sector. Sectors are interpreted as infarcted myocardium if the activity level deviates by more than two standard deviations below the normal range in each of three or more contiguous sectors; sectors are interpreted as ischemic myocardium if the FDG activity deviates by more than two standard deviations above the normal value; the latter reflects the increased uptake of glucose by viable ischemic myocardium.

When these studies are applied to patients, they provide insights into the biochemical pathways initiated during ischemia (p. 1316). In patients with unstable angina, there is a regional increase in glucose uptake in the ischemic segment despite a reduction in perfusion.[317, 318] Even when normal myocardium is primarily metabolizing free fatty acids and has low glucose uptake, regions of ischemia may show excessive glucose uptake, indicating the primary reliance on glycolysis for energy in ischemic myocardium.

Perhaps the most important clinical application of this approach is in predicting viability of ischemic myocardium.[316] Abnormal wall motion in regions in which FDG imaging shows preserved glucose uptake is highly predictive of reversible myocardial ischemia, while abnormal motion in regions with depressed glucose uptake is highly predictive of irreversible injury (Fig. 11–26). In regions with resting regional wall motion abnormalities, tissue can be classified as reversible with a predictive accuracy of 85 per cent if glucose utilization is normal or increased on the basis of the outcome of subsequent bypass surgery. The predictive accuracy for detection of irreversibly damaged myocardium is greater than 90 per cent. Similarly, most regions of infarction, with chronic Q-waves on the ECG, take up F-18-DG, indicating persistent tissue metabolism and the presence of viable tissue within the region. These chronically ischemic but viable zones might well benefit from revascularization or other aggressive forms of therapy (p. 1252).

FIGURE 11–26. See Color Plate 3.

FATTY ACID METABOLISM

(See also p. 1209)

Under normal, aerobic conditions, most of the energy requirements of the heart are met by oxidation of free fatty acids.[317–319] Free fatty acid metabolism has been studied in man using ^{11}C-labeled palmitic acid combined with PET.[320, 321] The initial distribution of this tracer in the myocardium is directly proportional to myocardial blood flow.[322] Free fatty acids are extracted by the myocardial cell and activated to FFA-CoA by way of thiokinase. FFA-CoA is either oxidized or sterified. Myocardial clearance of fatty acids depends on the oxygen demand and the availability of alternative substrates. In normal hearts, the slope of the early component of the wash-out curve corresponds to the rate of oxidation of ^{11}C-palmitic acid.[323–325] The early phase of the time-activity curve is associated with release of C-11-CO_2, while the sterified pathway is identified by a slow clearance phase. The preferred pathway depends on myocardial oxygen consumption and substrate availability in the plasma. With high myocardial oxygen consumption, more FFA-CoA is oxidized and the clearance rate of C-11 activity is therefore inversely related to myocardial oxygen consumption. As a result, the half-time of the early phase of the C-11 time-activity curve represents a measure of myocardial free fatty acid oxidation and provides a noninvasive assessment of regional myocardial free fatty acid metabolism.[326]

Abnormalities in initial clearance may be due to metabolic abnormalities in free fatty acid utilization or to alternative metabolic pathways, as may occur if free fatty acid plasma levels are low and the heart is using primarily glucose and lactic acid.[327] While this method provides a semiquantitative measure of free fatty acid utilization by the heart, accurate measurement is limited by wash-out of ^{11}C-palmitic acid when oxygen availability is restricted, because of reduced availability of the tracer in regions of markedly reduced flow and because other fatty acids are utilized by the heart.

PET using ^{11}C-palmitate has been utilized to identify the size and extent of myocardial infarction.[328] In normal subjects tomography shows uniform distribution of the tracer throughout the left ventricle. Tomograms from patients with previous myocardial infarction show diminished accumulation of ^{11}C-palmitate, delineating regions corresponding to the electrocardiographic focus of infarction (Fig. 37–26, p. 1210).

Since ischemia alters the myocardial metabolism of free fatty acid by decreasing oxidation and increasing conversion to triglycerides, fatty acids labeled with positron-emitting nuclides such as ^{11}C-palmitate may be used to localize zones of transient ischemia. Because of the very short half-life of the tracer, transient changes can be documented by serial injections of the tracer. Thus, regions that are transiently ischemic will show augmented accumulation of the tracer with reperfusion, while zones of infarction will show no change in uptake on sequential studies obtained over a relatively short period of time (up to 6 hours). It has therefore been suggested that this method may be a useful indicator of cell viability, and since its accumulation is related to blood flow, it may be used as a marker of the severity and extent of tissue infarction.

^{11}C-lactic acid and pyruvic acid may be useful markers for identifying acutely ischemic tissue.[329] Tracer clearance from the myocardium is extremely prolonged in areas of ischemia resulting in zones of increased tracer activity. This method may also prove useful in distinguishing reversible from irreversible ischemia. The underlying metabolic pathways involved in tracer retention are so far unknown.

IODINE-123 FATTY ACIDS

PET is very expensive, requiring an on-site production facility for most of the short-lived radiopharmaceuticals; even ^{18}F-FDG must be produced nearby. As a result, this method will be used primarily to improve our understanding of the pathophysiology of cardiac disease and may eventually lead to less expensive diagnostic tools, using single photon-emitting radiotracers.

^{123}I-hexadecanoic acid and ^{123}I-heptadecanoic acid have been used for measuring myocardial perfusion and fatty acid metabolism using standard single-photon imaging equipment such as Anger scintillation cameras. These tracers are extracted avidly from the blood and cleared quickly from the myocardial tissue with a half-time of approximately 25 minutes.[330] They are esterified and then undergo beta-oxidation.[331–333] The pattern of uptake and wash-out in the heart is similar to that for unlabeled free fatty acids.[334, 335]

A limitation of this technique is that the iodide label dissociates rather quickly from the free fatty acid. Subsequent wash-out of free iodide results in progressively higher blood levels of the contaminant. This ^{123}I wash-out added to the clearance of the free fatty acid makes quantification difficult. Furthermore, the increasing background activity interferes with quantification using two-dimensional imaging or limited-angle tomography. This may explain the discordance in clearance results obtained in ischemic myocardium between ^{11}C-labeled fatty acids and ^{123}I-labeled fatty acids.[336] Corrections have been proposed for this contamination.[337] The major drawback of ^{123}I-heptadecanoic acid is that its kinetics are different from those of ^{11}C-labeled palmitic acid. The half-time of the early phase of its wash-out does not provide quantitative information about free fatty acid oxidation.[326]

^{123}I-labeled fatty acids may also be used to measure myocardial perfusion, since their initial distribution is proportional to blood flow. The rapid wash-out of the ^{123}I-hexadecanoic and heptadecanoic acids makes high-quality imaging difficult and limits imaging to two-dimensional techniques and to limited-angle tomography. Other fatty acids that are more readily retained by the myocardium are more suitable for this purpose but still have three disadvantages: (1) the low dose of tracer that can be administered to the patient; (2) the high cost of the pharmaceutical; and (3) the high-energy photons associated with the tracer and with its contaminant, ^{124}I, which degrades spatial resolution. As a perfusion agent, the ^{123}I label offers no advantages over thallium-201 and would be clearly inferior to technetium-99m–labeled perfusion agents that localize in the human heart.

INFARCT-AVID MYOCARDIAL SCINTIGRAPHY

In infarct-avid scintigraphy, radiopharmaceuticals are sequestered by acutely infarcted myocardium, resulting in regions of increased myocardial uptake. This procedure has emerged as a useful noninvasive technique to aid in the detection, localization, and quantification of myocardial necrosis when other less direct methods are inconclusive. These indirect techniques—including serum enzyme tests, electrocardiography, and vectorcardiography—are usually satisfactory for detecting infarction, particularly during its early stages, but may be less useful in its later stages (p. 1239).

RADIOPHARMACEUTICALS

^{99m}Tc-Pyrophosphate

As of this writing, ^{99m}Tc-pyrophosphate is the most commonly used radiotracer for imaging acute myocardial infarction in man.[338–340] Fifty per cent of the injected dose is extracted by bone and the remainder is rapidly excreted through the kidneys in normal subjects. At 90 minutes, less than 5 per cent of the injected dose remains in the blood.

^{99m}Tc-pyrophosphate uptake in acute myocardial infarction depends on a number of factors: (1) regional blood flow, (2) myocardial calcium concentration, (3) irreversible myocardial injury, and (4) time after infarction.

BLOOD FLOW. While the uptake of ^{99m}Tc-pyrophosphate is directly related to the degree of tissue damage, the pharmaceutical must reach the damaged tissue before it can be extracted. Following acute coronary occlusion, increased concentrations of ^{99m}Tc-pyrophosphate are found in regions with only minimally reduced blood flow.[341] In animal studies, tissue concentrations have been found to be about 20 times the concentration in normal myocardium. The highest concentration ratio between damaged and normal myocardium occurs when normal local blood flow is reduced by 20 to 40 per cent. As flow is reduced further, the concentration ratios begin to fall until, in regions of minimal flow (0 to 5 per cent of normal levels), ^{99m}Tc-pyrophosphate concentrations may be normal. Furthermore, there is a greater concentration of the tracer in epicardial than in endocardial segments at the same blood flow.

MYOCARDIAL CALCIUM. This ion probably plays a key role in technetium-99m–pyrophosphate binding in acute infarction.[342–347] Approximately 50 per cent of the radiopharmaceutical is absorbed by bone in the normal patient.

The binding site in bone is probably low-density amorphous calcium phosphate. While binding is possible at both the crystalline and the amorphous calcium phosphate sites, the concentration is twice as high in amorphous calcium phosphate. Furthermore, there is a direct relationship between the number of moles of bone-seeking radiopharmaceutical and the number of moles of calcium.

IRREVERSIBLE TISSUE DAMAGE. In patients, ^{99m}Tc-pyrophosphate labels acutely necrotic myocardium. The concentration ratio between infarcted and normal myocardium may be as high as 18:1, and the distribution—even in large circumferential infarcts—may be homogeneous throughout the infarct,[348] although the central zones of tissue necrosis may have reduced tracer concentration if blood flow is very low. In the zone immediately bordering the infarct, the concentration of pyrophosphate is greater than in normal myocardium; however, the increase is less than 50 per cent higher than normal myocardium. Furthermore, this border zone of slightly increased radiotracer concentration extends only a small distance from the necrotic region.

Technetium-99m–pyrophosphate uptake may be increased in patients with unstable angina pectoris, although histopathological examination of several of these patients has indicated multifocal lesions of coagulation necrosis, myocytolysis, and replacement fibrosis.[349] Increased uptake has also been noted in patients with ventricular aneurysm and regions of ventricular dyskinesis.

TIME AFTER INFARCTION. Uptake of the radiopharmaceutical begins to increase after 4 hours of permanent coronary artery occlusion.[350] In most patients with transmural myocardial infarction, faint uptake will be seen shortly after this time and will increase in intensity over the next 36 to 48 hours. Intensity will reach a peak by 48 hours and will gradually diminish over the next 5 to 7 days.

Other Infarct-Avid Tracers

RADIOLABELED ANTIBODY AGAINST CARDIAC MYOSIN. Purified radiolabeled antibody against cardiac myosin has also been demonstrated in regions of acute infarction. After intravenous injection of radio-labeled $(FAB')_2$ fragments of antibodies specific for cardiac myosin, concentration ratios of up to 6:1 between infarcted and normal myocardium may be found in the animal model. There is an inverse relationship between regional myocardial blood flow and uptake of the tracer even in areas of low flow.[351] After intravenous injection, well-defined areas of increased myocardial activity are found by 72 hours after permanent occlusion of a coronary artery in animals.

This technique is based on the assumption that these antibodies are highly specific for myocardium and that as capillary and cellular membrane integrity is disrupted by myocardial ischemia, the antibodies attach themselves to the contractile proteins of the myocardium. Initial results demonstrate very slow blood clearance because of the relatively large size of the antibody molecules. When fragments of antimyosin antibody are used, blood clearance is significantly improved without loss of antibody specificity.

The tissue activity of the radiolabeled cardiac myosin antibody fragments is inversely related to blood flow. The radioconcentration is highest in segments of maximal flow reduction and tissue necrosis, unlike ^{99m}Tc-pyrophosphate, which concentrates most in myocardial segments with flow reductions of 20 to 40 per cent of normal. Thus, the radiolabeled antibodies are similar to ^{99m}Tc-tetracycline in distribution. The high uptake in low-flow areas results from prolonged intravascular transit, which allows the radiotracer time to reach poorly perfused tissue.

Detection of Q-wave acute myocardial infarcts is high (90 per cent), with ^{99m}Tc-labeled antimyosin FAB (fragments of the antimyosin antibody) when the tracer is injected intravenously within 24 hours of onset of symptoms, provided that imaging is delayed 15 to 24 hours after injection.[352] Inferior wall infarcts are most difficult to detect because of overlapping liver activity. Infarct sizing correlates with that performed with ^{99m}Tc-pyrophosphate imaging, although infarcts measure larger with the latter technique. The clinical applicability of this method will depend on the results of large-scale clinical testing and evaluation in patients with non Q-wave infarcts and conditions such as unstable angina which masquerade as acute infarction.

INDIUM-111–LABELED WHITE BLOOD CELLS. By labeling blood cell components, physiological parameters other than tissue necrosis can be measured. Acute coronary artery thrombosis and experimental infective endocarditis, and left atrial thrombi have been detected using indium-111–labeled platelets.[353–355] Although this technique is promising for evaluating coronary artery bypass graft patency and for assessing the inflammatory component of acute infarction, it is currently limited by the difficulty encountered in routine labeling of platelets.

Indium-111–labeled white blood cells provide an additional tool for visualizing acute myocardial infarctions, particularly for studying their pathophysiology.[356] Migration of polymorphous leukocytes into acutely infarcted myocardium is known to occur, and use of these labeled cells can provide useful information when the inflammatory response is being monitored in acutely infarcted myocardium as well as the effects of therapeutic intervention.

TECHNIQUE

Patients suspected of having sustained an acute myocardial infarction are usually admitted directly to the coronary care unit. Usually they are at risk for developing either electrophysiological or hemodynamic complications; if so, imaging must be performed at the bedside using a portable scintillation camera. The camera should be a 37-photomultiplier tube, high-resolution instrument used in conjunction with a high-resolution collimator.

Patients in clinically stable condition may be brought to the nuclear medicine clinical unit. In this case, the suite used for imaging should contain monitoring equipment, including an electrocardiographic monitor, defibrillator, and emergency drugs. Standard infarct imaging does not require additional equipment. Computer processing has been suggested to subtract uptake by overlying ribs in patients in whom costochondral cartilage uptake obscures the myocardial field. The author has found this to be a problem in less than 1 per cent of patients. More sophisticated equipment, such as transaxial tomographic imaging systems with a rotating gamma camera or a multidetector scanning tomograph, are necessary for sizing the acute infarction.

Imaging should be performed at least 3 hours after the intravenous injection of 10 to 15 mCi of the tracer. When imaging is performed at 90 minutes after injection, there is a high incidence of diffuse blood pool activity, which can lead to a false-positive test for acute infarction. By delaying the imaging time from 90 minutes to 3 hours, the probability of acute infarction with moderately intense diffuse uptake (greater than or equal to the ribs in intensity) increases from 40 to 75 per cent.[357]

Images are obtained in the anterior, left anterior oblique, and left lateral projections, with at least 400,000 counts collected in each projection. Multiple projections permit accurate localization of the infarct uptake as distinguished from that in overlying bone.

A number of other techniques have also been suggested to improve the specificity of a diffuse pattern. Since the initial distribution of the radiotracer is intravascular, images obtained shortly after injection represent the extent of myocardial blood flow. It may be useful to subtract the initial blood pool image from the final image obtained 3 hours later. If focal myocardial uptake is present, myocardial uptake will involve a smaller area of the myocardium than on the initial blood pool image. Several techniques have been suggested for this purpose, including subjective assessment and computer subtraction.[358, 359]

IMAGE INTERPRETATION

THE NORMAL IMAGE. Technetium-99m–pyrophosphate is a bone-seeking radiopharmaceutical. After injection, about half the tracer is extracted by bone and the remainder is excreted through the kidneys. In the normal image, myocardial uptake will be equal to that over the right hemithorax and there will be no identification of a discrete cardiac silhouette. The threshold for abnormal myocardial uptake is controversial, however (see below). Bone uptake is usually prominent, with activity in the sternum and anterior ribs seen on all three views. Activity from the thoracolumbar spine is seen superimposed on the sternum in the anterior view, extending to the left of the sternum on the LAO projection, and forming the border opposite the sternum on the left lateral view. Activity in the scapula may be seen as shine-through on the anterior projection; the inferior tip of the scapula frequently shows disproportionately increased activity compared to the rest of the bone, and this should not be confused with uptake in the lateral wall of the myocardium.

THE ABNORMAL IMAGE. A number of grading systems have been suggested for interpreting the abnormal image.[340, 360, 361] Because the specificity of the diffuse pattern depends on the time after injection and the intensity of the pattern, the authors suggest the following grading system:

Normal. (No identification of the discrete cardiac silhouette): Myocardial uptake that is equal to that over the right hemithorax.

Mild Diffuse. (Low probability of acute myocardial infarction): Myocardial uptake exceeding that over the right hemithorax but less intense than that over the ribs and distributed over most or all of the myocardium.

Moderate Diffuse. (Indeterminate for the diagnosis of acute infarction): Myocardial uptake equally or more intense than that over the ribs but less intense than that over the sternum.

Focal. (High probability of acute infarction): Discrete myocardial uptake.

Massive. (High probability of acute infarction): An increase in myocardial uptake that involves 50 per cent or more of the cardiac silhouette and is equally or more intense than uptake over the sternum. Most often there is a focal central area of decreased activity due either to the left ventricular cavity or to central necrosis.

When myocardial uptake is focal, it can be localized to one or more segments of the myocardial wall from an analysis of the scintigrams obtained in multiple projections. In patients with *anterior myocardial infarcts*, uptake involves much of the left ventricular silhouette on the anterior view; in the left lateral view, the uptake appears as a thin band directly behind the sternum, since the anterior free wall of the left ventricle is being viewed tangentially in this projection (Fig. 11–27). In patients with *inferior myocardial infarction*, the radiotracer appears curvilinear, usually extending from the lower portion of the sternum laterally toward the ribs on the anterior projection and from the lower portion of the sternum approximately two-thirds of the way toward the vertebrae on the left lateral view. *Inferior infarcts* are always imaged perpendicular to the collimator. The true extent of an inferior infarct can be appreciated only with the aid of single-photon transaxial tomography. *Lateral infarcts* are seen perpendicular to the collimator on the anterior view, usually lying directly under the anterior rib ends and well away from the sternum. Lateral infarcts are seen in their greatest extent on the left lateral or left anterior oblique projections. *Apical infarcts* usually result from uptake in several adjacent walls, usually the inferior and lateral or distal anterior and lateral walls. *Posterior infarction* is usually seen in conjunction with inferior wall uptake and is seen best in the left lateral projection extending superiorly and posteriorly from the inferior wall. Occasionally posterior uptake may be seen in isolation. *Right ventricular uptake* is most often seen in conjunction with inferior left ventricular activity and is appreciated best when there is also uptake in the inferior portion of the left ventricular septum. In this case, the right ventricular activity appears to the right of the septum and inferior wall. The activity may extend horizontally or at various angles from the inferior wall from a horizontal to an almost vertical orientation, depending on the anatomical position of the right ventricle and of the right ventricular free wall (Fig. 11–28).

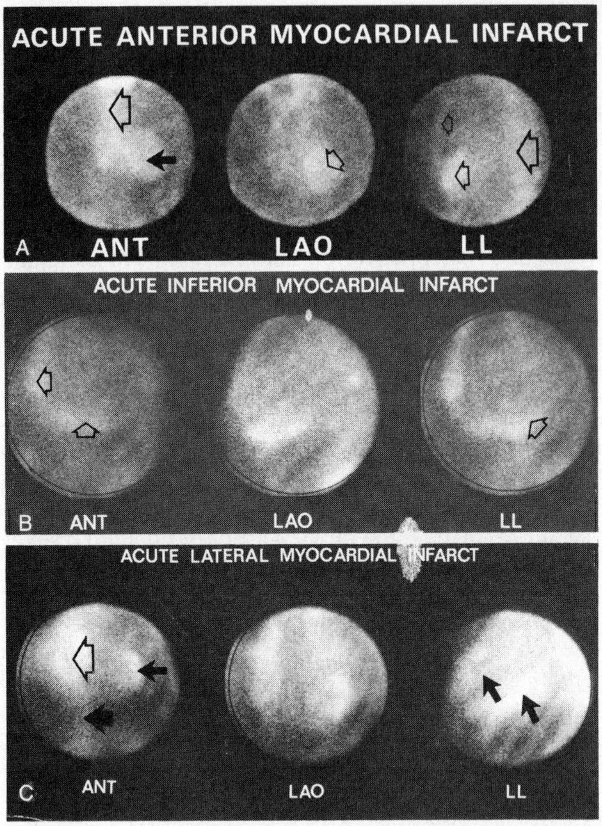

FIGURE 11–27. *A*, Myocardial scintigraphy with ^{99m}Tc-pyrophosphate in patients with acute anterior myocardial infarct. *Anterior*: Open arrow = sternum; arrow = myocardial uptake. *Left anterior oblique*: Arrow = myocardial activity. *Left lateral*: Upper arrow = sternum; lower arrow = myocardial activity; large arrow = vertebrae. *B*, Scintigrams of a patient with acute inferior myocardial infarction. *Anterior*: Upper arrow = sternum; lower arrow = myocardial activity. *Left lateral*: Note posterior wall extension (arrow). *C*, Myocardial scintigraphy in a patient with acute lateral myocardial infarct. *Anterior*: Open arrow = sternum; lower arrow = vertebrae; upper arrow = myocardial activity. *Left lateral*: Upper arrow = ribs; lower arrow = myocardial activity.

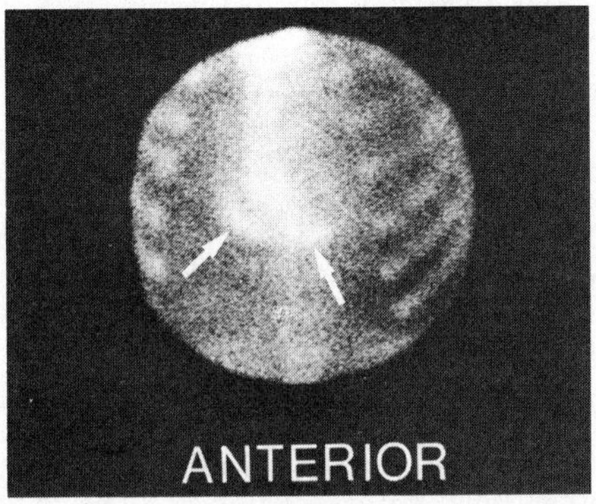

FIGURE 11–28. Infarct-avid scintigraphy with ^{99m}Tc-pyrophosphate in a patient with an acute inferior wall infarct (right arrow) with extensive right ventricular extension (left arrow).

In patients with large anteroseptal or anterolateral or circumferential left ventricular infarcts, the pattern of uptake is massive, and in most of these patients, the scintigraphic appearance has been described as a *doughnut pattern* with intense uptake along the borders and relatively diminished intensity in the center.

While most subendocardial and many transmural infarcts will appear normal on infarct-avid scintigraphy after the first week, many transmural infarcts will show persistent accumulation of the radiotracer for considerable periods of time after the initial episode, even when extension or reinfarction has not been documented. In approximately 40 per cent of patients with acute myocardial infarction, activity will persist beyond the first several weeks, the intensity of uptake will gradually diminish, and the appearance and the distribution of the radiotracer will appear more diffuse than on the initial scintigrams obtained several days after infarction.

Focal uptake may also be seen in patients with valvular calcifications,[362] repeated high-energy direct-current (DC) cardioversions,[363] ventricular aneurysms,[364] myocardial contusion,[365] and metastatic carcinoma to the heart (Table 11–3).

ASSESSMENT OF THE METHOD

Infarct scintigraphy with ^{99m}Tc-pyrophosphate is most sensitive in patients with transmural infarction. However, these patients can usually be diagnosed without the aid of infarct scintigraphy. It is in patients with nontransmural infarction that the diagnosis is frequently in doubt at the time of admission. The diagnosis of nontransmural infarction may be difficult to confirm because the accompanying electrocardiographic changes may be nonspecific. Nontransmural infarction frequently occurs during surgery or in other clinical settings characterized by hemodynamic instability. Furthermore, when patients present with nonspecific ST-segment or T-wave abnormalities several days after a prolonged episode of pain, it may be impossible to establish the diagnosis of acute myocardial infarction using currently available cardiac enzyme techniques.

The sensitivity of the technique is high in patients with nontransmural infarction if a correspondingly low specificity is accepted, since approximately 50 per cent of these patients show diffuse uptake that is indistinguishable from that seen in many patients with unstable angina pectoris but without clinical evidence of infarction. When rigid criteria are used and faint diffuse uptake is considered to be a normal finding, the sensitivity for the detection of nontransmural infarction has been low (40 to 60 per cent).[361, 366, 367]

CLINICAL APPLICATIONS

Myocardial scintigraphy with ^{99m}Tc-pyrophosphate is useful in patients with *suspected acute infarction* in whom other clinical and laboratory evidence is nondiagnostic. Thus, scintigraphy is helpful in patients who present more than 24 hours after the onset of symptoms when very sensitive serum enzyme tests such as MB-band CK may have returned to normal. The probability of acute infarction is high in patients with focal uptake, provided that an infarction has not occurred within 6 to 12 months of the acute event. The size and persistence of uptake may provide predictive information as well. Usefulness of the test in the presence of moderately intense diffuse uptake is limited, however. Myocardial scintigraphy can be used to diagnose *right ventricular infarction*. Although an elevation in right ventricular filling pressure may indicate right ventricular involvement, it may also occur in the presence of cor pulmonale. Myocardial scintigraphy with ^{99m}Tc-pyrophosphate provides more direct evidence of acute infarction of the right ventricle.[368]

This technique is also of value in evaluating patients following coronary bypass surgery. The diagnosis of myocardial infarction after cardiac surgery is complicated because chest pain, elevated enzyme levels, and electrocardiographic changes may result from the operation itself.[369] ^{99m}Tc-pyrophosphate scintigraphy is accurate in the postoperative patient provided that the patient has not sustained a myocardial infarction within the previous year.[370, 371]

Infarct-avid scintigraphy is useful in patients who develop symptoms suggestive of acute myocardial infarction after heavy exercise. For example, serum creatine kinase activity, including that of the MB isoenzyme fraction, is elevated in marathon runners because of skeletal muscle necrosis. Imaging with ^{99m}Tc-pyrophosphate may be useful to exclude myocardial infarction and to localize the site of tissue necrosis.[372] Similarly, scintigraphic imaging may define the extent of muscle necrosis after electrical injury.

The scintigraphic pattern of myocardial uptake provides clues to the patient's future course, both in the hospital and over the long term.[361] The complication rate, particularly during hospitalization, is directly related to the extent of uptake of pyrophosphate in patients with acute infarction. A number of other observations that reflect the extent and intensity of pyrophosphate uptake also have prognostic value. Patients with a doughnut pattern are likely to develop left ventricular failure.[373] Persistently positive ^{99m}Tc-pyrophosphate scintigrams are also associated with mortality and morbidity and with elevated pulmonary artery pressure.[374]

Accurate sizing of the acute infarction by measuring the extent of radiotracer uptake is limited by the geometrical constraints of standard two-dimensional imaging. Single-photon–emission computed tomography (SPECT) provides a three-dimensional map of radionuclide distribution and

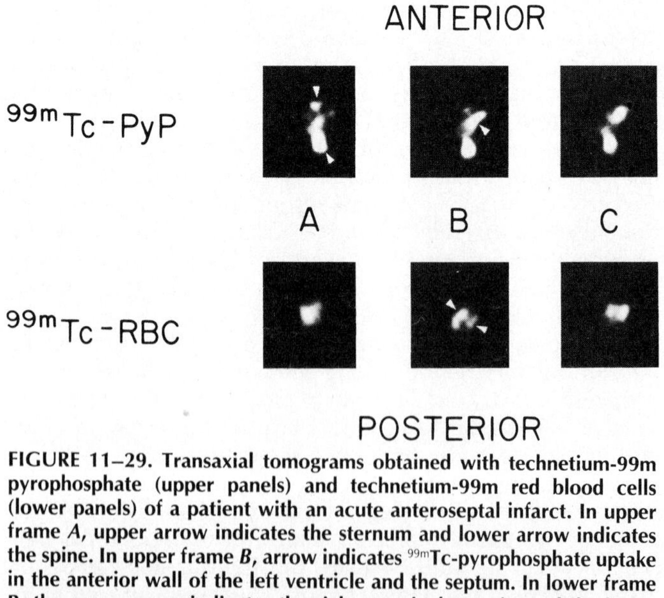

FIGURE 11–29. Transaxial tomograms obtained with technetium-99m pyrophosphate (upper panels) and technetium-99m red blood cells (lower panels) of a patient with an acute anteroseptal infarct. In upper frame *A*, upper arrow indicates the sternum and lower arrow indicates the spine. In upper frame *B*, arrow indicates ^{99m}Tc-pyrophosphate uptake in the anterior wall of the left ventricle and the septum. In lower frame B, the upper arrow indicates the right ventricular cavity and the lower arrow indicates the left ventricular cavity. A = transaxial plane corresponding to base of left ventricle; B = midventricle; C = apex.

may yield more accurate assessments of infarct size. Studies in an animal model have demonstrated a good correlation between infarct size and measured uptake of ^{99m}Tc-pyrophosphate.[375]

SINGLE PHOTON-EMISSION COMPUTED TOMOGRAPHY (SPECT)

SPECT (p. 313) can be performed in patients and provides a three-dimensional map of ^{99m}Tc-pyrophosphate uptake within the heart.[376] Rotating Anger camera imaging is performed 2 to 3 hours after the intravenous injection of ^{99m}Tc-pyrophosphate using a method similar to the one described on p. 338 for thallium-201 SPECT. Immediately after infarct imaging, the patient is injected with 20 mCi of ^{99m}Tc-pertechnetate. Red blood cell labeling occurs because of the presence of stannous ion in the tin pyrophosphate complex. Blood pool tomograms are acquired without a change in the patient's position, along the same tomographic slice planes as those used for ^{99m}Tc-pyrophosphate. The blood pool images are used to localize the left ventricular cavities facilitating localization of pyrophosphate uptake and distinguishing blood pool from myocardial wall activity.

The weight of the myocardial infarct can also be estimated from SPECT images. In patients with acute anterior infarction, uptake is seen within the anterior wall of the left ventricle, frequently involving the septum (Fig. 11–29). In patients with acute inferior infarction, uptake may occur in the posterior wall of the right ventricle, posterior septum, and posterolateral wall of the left ventricle as well. One of the advantages of tomography over other methods for infarct sizing is that imaging need be performed only once between 1 and 10 days after infarction. Furthermore, double-tracer emission tomography improves the specificity of the diffuse pattern by localizing the activity to the blood pool. Also, the size of the infarct can be measured directly. The volume of acutely infarcted myocardium as measured by ^{99m}Tc-pyrophosphate SPECT correlates well with patient prognosis. A high proportion of patients with infarcts greater than 40 gm (85 per cent) will die or develop serious complications in the 1 to 2 years after the acute event; the proportion of patients with smaller infarcts suffering serious complications is substantially less (30 per cent).[376]

PULMONARY SCINTIGRAPHY

PERFUSION SCINTIGRAPHY

Pulmonary perfusion scintigraphy is based on the principles developed by Sapirstein: regional blood flow is directly proportional to the quantity of the radiotracer in that region provided that (1) the radiotracer is completely extracted by the tissue, (2) complete mixing of the tracer has taken place within the blood, and (3) the radiotracer remains in the tissue and is not metabolized or released from the tissue.[377] When radioactive particles larger in size than the diameter of a pulmonary capillary are injected intravenously, they are mixed in the right side of the heart and are then trapped by the capillary and precapillary vasculature. As a result, the quantity of radioactivity in any region of the lung—and hence the activity emanating from that region—is directly proportional to blood flow to that region.

As of this writing, either ^{99m}Tc–macroaggregated albumin or ^{99m}Tc–human albumin microspheres are the tracers of choice for perfusion imaging. ^{99m}Tc-microspheres provide a more uniform particle size than other ^{99m}Tc-labeled particles[378]; on the other hand, macroaggregated albumin has been associated with fewer instances of allergic reactions than have the microspheres.[379] The aggregated albumin particles are between 10 and 40 microns in diameter; the albumin microspheres are more uniform in size and are between 20 and 40 microns in diameter. The particles break up slowly after entrapment in the lung; their biological half-life is approximately 7 hours in normal patients and somewhat longer in patients with pulmonary embolism or parenchymal lung disease. The fragments are then removed from the circulation by the reticuloendothelial system.

Perfusion scintigraphy is a safe procedure with a very low incidence of side effects.[380] It has been estimated that less than 0.1 per cent of the pulmonary capillaries are occluded when 200,000 to 500,000 particles are injected. Iatrogenic impairment of lung function is unlikely, even when the organ is severely compromised by disease, because of the sparsity of occlusion and rich collateral circulation.[381, 382] No change is observed in pulmonary diffusing capacity after injection of the radiopharmaceutical,[383] although fatal reactions have been reported to occur after the labeled particles were administered to patients with severe pulmonary hypertension.[384]

Routinely, 2 to 3 mCi of macroaggregated albumin (MAA) is injected slowly intravenously while the patient is supine. (To minimize the dosage in pregnant women, 1 mCi of high-specific-activity MAA is injected, minimizing the radiation exposure to the fetus. The risk of pulmonary embolism in the clinically symptomatic mother substantially outweighs the risk of radiation exposure to the fetus.[385]) Images are obtained, using a standard high-resolution gamma camera, in the right and left lateral, right and left posterior oblique, and anterior and posterior positions. The posterior oblique views have been recently incorporated into the imaging regimen because they provide better delineation of the posterior and lateral basal segments of the lower lobes and eliminate much of the overlapping radioactivity seen from the opposite lung on lateral views.[386] At least 4 to 6 $\times$ 10^5 counts should be obtained in each view. The two lateral views should be imaged for the same time rather than for the same counts; similarly, the two oblique views should be imaged for the same time.

In the normal perfusion lung scintiscan there is uniform distribution of activity throughout the lung, with increasing radioactivity seen from the anterior to the posterior projection if the patient is injected while supine (Fig. 11–30). The margins of the lung's radioactivity are smooth and correspond to the lung outline seen on the chest radiograph. The heart and mediastinal structures produce a midline defect extending to the left, particularly on the anterior view. The heart is usually not seen on the posterior view unless it is enlarged. Occasionally, the aortic notch produces a defect in the midline, particularly when it is tortuous. Diminished perfusion may be seen in the region of an azygous lobe.[387] More subtle changes occur with

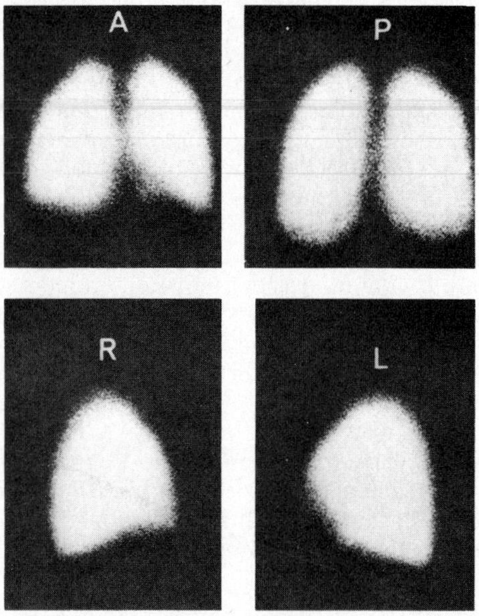

FIGURE 11–30. Normal pulmonary perfusion scintiscan. The distribution of tracer is relatively homogeneous but with a decreasing gradient toward the apex due to decreasing lung volume, an increasing gradient toward the dependent portion of the lung (posterior if injected supine) due to gravitational effects on perfusion, and no radioactivity in the mediastinum. (A = anterior view; P = posterior view; R = right lateral view; L = left lateral view.)

changes in the position of the diaphragm, particularly if there is central eventration. In patients with diaphragmatic paralysis and those who are very obese, basilar defects in the perfusion scan may cause confusion at times.

Of the pathological conditions that can interfere with regional lung perfusion, the most important are those involving the pulmonary arterial vasculature. These include primary diseases of the pulmonary arteries, either congenital (atresia) or acquired (arteritis); extraluminal compression by interstitial fluid, tumors, lymph nodes, or other mediastinal structures; and intraluminal filling by tumor, fat, air, parasites, amniotic fluid, or blood clots.

Parenchymal diseases (inflammatory, malignant) and extrapulmonic displacement of lung tissue due to pleural effusion or cardiomegaly also compromise regional lung perfusion. Intrapulmonary shunting caused by regional hypoxia diverts blood flow and therefore radioactive particles away from that portion of the lung. Shunts from the bronchial to the pulmonary arteries in bronchiectasis and some bronchogenic carcinomas also keep the particles away from the affected areas.[388] Although clinical attention has focused primarily on the value of pulmonary scintigraphy in detecting thromboembolic disease, it is important to remember that other conditions can interfere with regional perfusion, leading to abnormal scans.

VENTILATION SCINTIGRAPHY

Ventilation scintigraphy is a helpful maneuver in distinguishing between primary perfusion abnormalities and those secondary to regional hypoxia.[389, 390] Regional ventilation is usually assessed using the inert gas xenon-133. The maneuver can be performed before perfusion scintigraphy, in which case imaging is performed in the posterior projection. Alternatively, ventilation imaging can be performed after perfusion scintigraphy, in which case the physician has the flexibility to choose the projection to be used for imaging. If ventilation is assessed after perfusion scintigraphy, there is substantial scattered radiation within the xenon-133 energy window due to the higher energy technetium-99m. This interference must be overcome by using higher doses of xenon-133.

Areas of poor ventilation represent deficits in activity on the initial breathholding scintiscan, while regions of relatively increased activity indicate abnormal ventilation during the wash-out phase. The abnormal retention of xenon during the washout phase is due to air-trapping. The initial breathholding study alone is insufficient because patients with parenchymal disease may have normal ventilation in areas of reduced perfusion on the single-breath image but will trap xenon during the wash-out phase.[391] When initial breathholding imaging is used alone, without the wash-out phase of the study, the specificity for detection of pulmonary embolism is only 80 per cent; however, when the additional information obtained from the wash-out phase of the study is added, the specificity increases to over 90 per cent.

A number of other radiopharmaceuticals have been used for ventilation scintigraphy. Xenon-127 has a photon energy higher than that of technetium-99m. Ventilation scintigraphy can therefore be performed after perfusion imaging with far less interference from technetium-99m. At the present time, xenon-127 is not widely available; it is expensive and requires recycling because of its costs and long half-life.

An alternative approach uses the rubidium-81/krypton-81m generator. The patient inhales krypton-81m during normal respiration.[392, 393] Because the primary photopeak of krypton-81m is 190 kev, higher spatial resolution can be obtained than with xenon-133, and imaging can be performed following the perfusion study with little scattered radiation from technetium-99m. The primary disadvantage of this radiotracer—one that will severely limit its implementation in the community hospital—is the short half-life of its parent compound, rubidium-81 (4 hours). Since the physical half-life of this radiotracer is very short (13 seconds), the continual inhalation of krypton-81m results in images that depict the balance between regional ventilation and radioactive decay of the tracer. After about 30 seconds of inhalation, a steady state is reached, and the activity represents the distribution of tidal ventilation.[393] Thus, information contained in a single krypton-81m ventilation scan is only a crude representation of regional ventilation. The short time required for imaging, its simplicity, and the low absorbed radiation dose enable serial high-resolution images of ventilatory flow to be obtained in multiple views. However, because of the short half-life, wash-out studies cannot be obtained.

LABELED AEROSOLS. ^{99m}Tc-DTPA–labeled aerosols may be used as an alternative for ventilation imaging. Patients breathe the radiolabeled aerosol for 5 minutes followed by Anger camera planar imaging in six views (anterior, posterior, right and left posterior oblique, and right and left anterior oblique) collecting 1×10^5 counts per views.[394] Standard perfusion imaging is performed following the radioaerosol study after injecting 3 to 4 mCi of technetium-99m macroaggregated albumin. The advantages of radioaerosols over xenon-133 for ventilation imaging is that multiple projections can be obtained, the radiation dosage to the patient is reduced, and problems related to trapping and venting radioactive gases are eliminated. On the other hand, radioaerosols do not have a wash-out component which is helpful in identifying chronic obstructive pulmonary disease. Radioaerosols also tend to clump in airways proximal to parenchymal disease. Nevertheless, xenon-133 and radiolabeled aerosols provide similar information. Regions of discordance are usually associated with smaller perfusion defects that do not change the scintigraphic probability for pulmonary embolism.

PULMONARY EMBOLISM

(See also p. 1582)

The single most important application of pulmonary scintigraphy is in the diagnosis of pulmonary embolism. The clinical manifestations of pulmonary embolism are frequently vague and nonspecific.[395] The most frequent signs and symptoms are tachypnea (92 per cent), dyspnea (81 per cent), pleuritic chest pain (72 per cent), apprehension (59 per cent), cough (54 per cent), and rales (53 per cent). Signs and symptoms more specific for the diagnosis of pulmonary embolism occur much less frequently. For example, hemoptysis is seen in only 34 per cent of patients, cyanosis in 18 per cent, and thrombophlebitis in 33 per cent.

The value of pulmonary scintigraphy in detecting acute pulmonary emboli is based, in part, on its high sensitivity, since a normal lung scan virtually rules out clinically significant pulmonary emboli within the previous 48 hours.[396] Theoretically, microemboli might produce perfusion defects beyond the resolution of present instrumentation, or clots in the central pulmonary artery that only partially occlude the lumen might not affect regional blood flow. Nevertheless, a well-documented case of acute pulmonary embolism with a technically adequate normal perfusion scan obtained within 48 hours of the onset of symptoms has yet to be recorded.

The abnormal scintigram presents more of a problem. Diagnostic information must be garnered from clues derived from the anatomical distribution of the perfusion defects, the relationship between the degree of impairment in regional perfusion and ventilation, and the stability of the perfusion defects over time. In general, acute pulmonary emboli produce sharply delineated polysegmental or lobar defects (Fig. 11–31).[397] These are unlike the anatomically less well-defined defects seen in chronic lung disease. A large proportion of patients with lobar defects have pulmonary embolism, for example.[398, 399] On the other hand, subsegmental defects are the predominant perfusion abnormality in only a small fraction of patients with clinically apparent pulmonary embolism. Unilateral absence of perfusion is not pathognomonic of pulmonary embolism; it is also seen in bronchogenic carcinoma, the hyperlucent emphysematous lung, and pulmonary artery atresia.

Most patients with pulmonary emboli have multiple perfusion defects. In one series, for example, only 16 of 104 patients with abnormal lung scintigrams had single perfusion defects.[398] Of these, only three were present in patients with pulmonary embolism. Thus, 93 per cent of

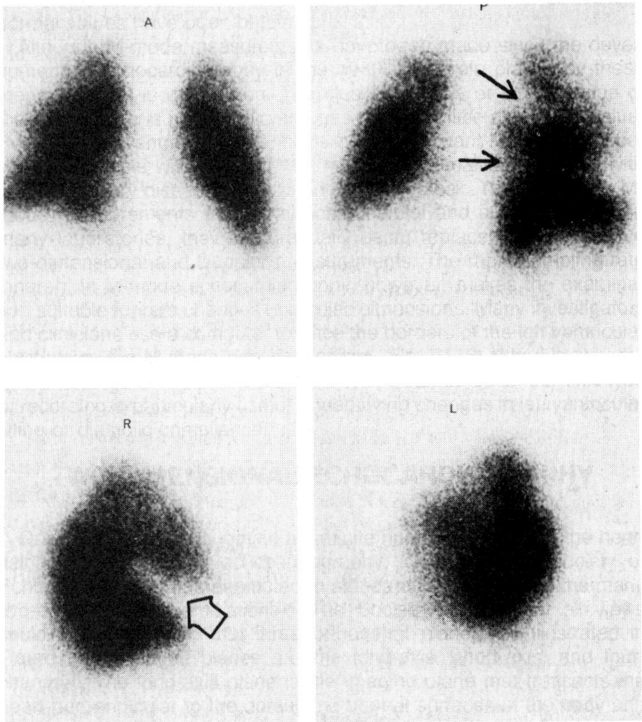

FIGURE 11–31. Perfusion scintiscan demonstrating absent perfusion to a segment of the right middle lobe (open arrow) with additional subsegmental perfusion defects (arrows).

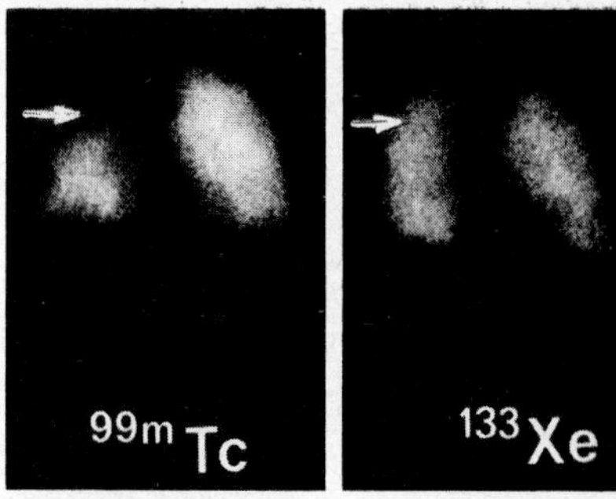

FIGURE 11–32. Perfusion scintiscan demonstrating that perfusion to the right upper lung field is absent (left, arrow). Single-breath ventilation scintiscan demonstrating normal ventilation in this region (right, arrow). Ventilation-perfusion mismatch is consistent with pulmonary embolism.

patients with pulmonary emboli have multiple perfusion defects. In patients with multiple perfusion defects, 52 per cent of patients with pulmonary embolism have perfusion defects involving lobar areas. Only 8 per cent of patients without pulmonary emboli had similar findings. Segmental defects occurred with about equal frequency (22 to 33 per cent) in patients with pulmonary embolism and in patients with chronic lung disease. Patients with pulmonary emboli rarely have small subsegmental defects as their largest perfusion defects (2 to 8 per cent).[400] Nevertheless, the pattern of perfusion abnormalities is only a fair discriminator of pulmonary embolism and, if possible, should not constitute the only radiodiagnostic criterion.

Ventilation scintigraphy is a helpful maneuver in distinguishing between primary perfusion abnormalities and those secondary to regional hypoxia.[389–391] In patients with pulmonary emboli, the perfusion abnormality clearly exceeds any abnormality in ventilation (Fig. 11–32). In patients with acute bronchospasm or chronic lung disease, the compromise of regional ventilation usually matches or exceeds that of perfusion. In patients with normal or near-normal chest x-rays, this comparison between perfusion and ventilation is particularly useful in differentiating pulmonary lung disease from pulmonary emboli.

Interpretation becomes more difficult when the chest x-ray is abnormal in the region of the perfusion defect. The pulmonary density seen on the x-ray may represent parenchymal pulmonary disease or may be secondary to pulmonary infarction. Since ventilation will be affected in either case, ventilation scintigraphy is of limited value unless other perfusion defects are present. The size relationship of the perfusion defect and the density on chest x-ray may be helpful, however.[401] If the perfusion defect is small relative to the density on the x-ray, the probability of pulmonary embolism is low (7 per cent). When the perfusion defect is substantially larger than the roentgenographic abnormality, the probability of pulmonary embolism is increased (89 per cent). The perfusion defect must be substantially larger or smaller than the corresponding radiographic abnormalities for these diagnostic criteria to apply. Otherwise, a scintigram with a perfusion defect and accompanying chest x-ray density with no other diagnostic clues is indeterminate for the diagnosis of pulmonary embolism.

Natural evolution of the appearance on perfusion scans after an acute episode is also a useful indicator of pulmonary embolism (Fig. 11–33).[402–404] In general, perfusion scintigraphy returns to normal soon after the embolic event. The rapidity of improvement seems to depend on the patient's age and cardiovascular status and the amount of lung involved. In the absence of heart failure, even major occlusions may revert to normal within weeks. Recurrent

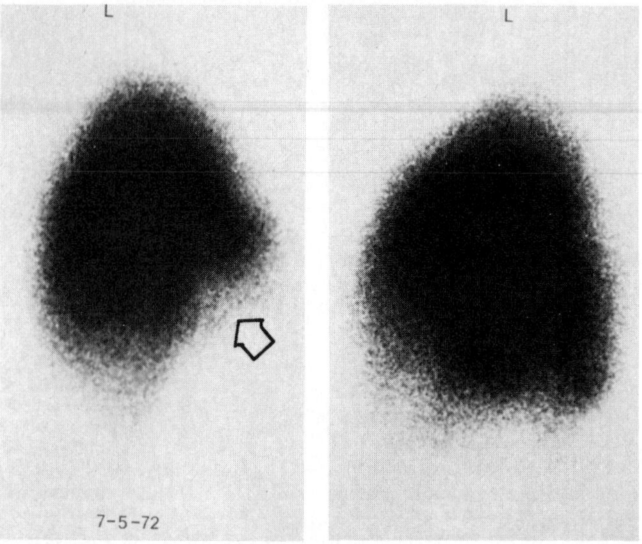

FIGURE 11–33. Initial scintiscan demonstrates that perfusion to most of left lower lobe is absent (*left*, arrow). Repeat scintigraphy (*right*) demonstrates markedly improved perfusion to this region six days later. This rapid resolution in the face of a normal chest x-ray is consistent with pulmonary embolism.

embolism is often characterized by the appearance of new regions of involvement as old ones disappear. Fragmentation of large central thromboemboli can produce new subsegmental defects, however. Because of this natural evolution, it is often difficult to document reembolization in patients already receiving therapy for previous pulmonary emboli.

Conditions other than acute pulmonary embolism can result in ventilation/perfusion mismatches (normal ventilation in regions of decreased or absent perfusion).[405] The ventilation/perfusion mismatch is, after all, evidence only of a vascular rather than a parenchymal etiology. In parenchymal disease, regional hypoxia results in a reflex reduction in decreased pulmonary blood flow to that region. Vascular diseases, such as previous pulmonary embolism, pulmonary artery agenesis or stenosis, vasculitis (polyarteritis nodosa), tuberculosis, pulmonary artery sarcoma, hemangioendotheliomatosis, and pulmonary venoocclusive disease would be expected to result in ventilation/perfusion mismatches. There are sporadic reports of parenchymal lung disease, including emphysema, radiation therapy, intravenous drug abuse, bronchogenic carcinoma, lymphangitic carcinomatosis, and pneumonia that result in ventilation/perfusion mismatch. Despite this extensive differential diagnosis, ventilation/perfusion mismatches and perfusion defects involving large subsegments, segments, and lobes are due to acute pulmonary embolism in over 90 per cent of the cases.

REFERENCES

INSTRUMENTATION

1. McCarthy, D. M., and Makler, P. T., Jr.: Accuracy of left ventricular ejection fraction using the nuclear stethoscope in left ventricular aneurysm. Am. J. Cardiol. 55:177, 1985.
2. Wilson, R. A., Sullivan, P. J., Moore, R. H., Zielonka, J. S., Alpert, N. M., Boucher, C. A., McJusick, K. A., and Strauss, H. W.: Ambulatory ventricular function monitor: validation and preliminary clinical results. Am. J. Cardiol. 52:601, 1983.
3. Lahiri, A., Crawley, J. C. W., Jones, R. I., Bowles, M. J., and Raftery, E. B.: Noninvasive techniques for continuous monitoring of left ventricular function using a new solid-state mercuric iodide radiation detector. Clin. Sci. 66:551, 1984.

ASSESSMENT OF CARDIAC PERFORMANCE

4. Ong, L., Green, S., Reiser, P., and Morrison, J.: Early prediction of mortality in patients with acute myocardial infarction: A prospective study of clinical and radionuclide factors. Am. J. Cardiol. 57:33, 1986.
5. Greenberg, H., McMaster, P., and Dwyer, E. M., Jr.: Left ventricular dysfunction after acute myocardial infarction: Results of a prospective multicenter study. J. Am. Coll. Cardiol. 4:867, 1984.
6. Pryor, D. B., Harrell, F. E., Jr., Lee, K. L., Rosati, R. A., Coleman, R. E., Cobb, F. R., Califf, R. M., and Jones, R. H.: Prognostic indicators from radionuclide angiography in medically treated patients with coronary artery disease. Am. J. Cardiol. 53:18, 1984.
7. Morris, K. G., Palmeri, S. T., Califf, R. M., McKinnis, R. A., Higginbotham, M. B., Coleman, R. E., and Cobb, F. A.: Value of radionuclide angiography for predicting specific cardiac events after acute myocardial infarction. Am. J. Cardiol. 55:318, 1985.
8. Marshall, R. C., Berger, H. J., Costin, J. C., Freedman, G. S., Wolberg, J., Cohen, L. S., Gottschalk, A., and Zaret, B. L.: Assessment of cardiac performance with quantitative radionuclide angiocardiography. Circulation 56:820, 1977.
9. Thrall, J. H., Rabinovitch, M. A., Pitt, B., and Buda, A.: Cardiac dynamics. *In* Harbert, J., and DaRocha, A. F. G. (eds.): Textbook of Nuclear Medicine. Vol. II. Philadelphia, Lea and Febiger, 1984, p. 406.
10. Wackers, F. J., Giles, R. W., Hoffer, P. B., Lange, R. C., Berger, H. J., and Zaret, B. L.: Gold-195m, a new generator-produced short-lived radionuclide for sequential assessment of ventricular performance by first pass radionuclide angiocardiography. Am. J. Cardiol. 50:89, 1982.
11. Holman, B. L., Neirinckx, R. D., Treves, S., and Tow, D. E.: Cardiac imaging with tantalum-178. Radiology 131:525, 1979.
12. Treves, S., Cheng, C., Samuel, A., Lambrecht, R., Babchyck, B., Zimmerman, R., and Norwood, W.: Iridium-191 angiocardiography for the detection and quantitation of left-to-right shunting. J. Nucl. Med. 21:1151, 1980.
13. Nienaber, C. A., Spielmann, R. P., Wasmus, G., Mathey, D. G., Montz, R., and Bleifeld, W. H.: Clinical use of ultrashort-lived radionuclide krypton-81m for noninvasive analysis of right ventricular performance in normal subjects and patients with right ventricular dysfunction. J. Am. Coll. Cardiol. 5:687, 1985.
14. Horn, M., Witztum, K., Neveu, C., Perkins, G., and Walsh, B.: Krypton-81m imaging of the right ventricle. J. Nucl. Med. 26:33, 1985.
15. Schiller, N. B., and Botvinick, E. H.: Noninvasive quantitation of the left heart by echocardiography and scintigraphy. *In* Kotler, M. M., and Steiner, R. M. (eds): Cardiac Imaging. Cardiovascular Clinics. Philadelphia, F. A. Davis, 1986, pp. 45–94.
16. Dymond, D. S., Elliott, A., and Stone, D.: Factors that affect the reproducibility of measurements of left ventricular function from first-pass radionuclide ventriculograms. Circulation 65:311, 1982.
17. Parker, J. A., and Treves, S.: Radionuclide detection, localization and quantitation of intracardiac shunts and shunts between the great arteries. Progr. Cardiovasc. Dis. 20:121, 1977.
18. Lane, S. D., Patton, D. D., Staab, E. V., and Baglan, R. J.: Simple technique for rapid bolus injection. J. Nucl. Med. 13:118, 1972.
19. Oldendorf, W. H.: Measurement of the mean transit time of cerebral circulation by external detection of an intravenously injected radioisotope. J. Nucl. Med. 3:382, 1962.
20. Treves, S., Maltz, D. L., and Adlestein, S. J.: Intracardiac shunts. *In* James, A. E., Wagner, H. N., and Cooke, R. E. (eds.): Pediatric Nuclear Medicine. Philadelphia, W. B. Saunders Company, 1974, p. 231.
21. Berger, H. J., Gottschalk, A., and Zaret, B. L.: Radionuclide assessment of left and right ventricular performance. Radiol. Clin. North Am. 18:441, 1980.
22. Schelbert, H. R., Verba, J. W., Johnson, A. D., Brock, G. W., Alazraki, N. P., Rose, F. J., and Ashburn, W. L.: Nontraumatic determination of left ventricular ejection fraction by radionuclide angiocardiography. Circulation 51:902, 1975.
23. Gal, R., Grenier, R. P., Schmidt, D. H., and Port, S. C.: Background correction in first-pass radionuclide angiography: Comparison of several approaches. J. Nucl. Med. 27:1480, 1986.
24. Jengo, J. A., Mena, I., Blaufuss, A., and Criley, J. M.: Evaluation of left ventricular function (ejection fraction and segmental wall motion) by single pass radioisotope angiography. Circulation 57:326, 1978.
25. Tobinick, E., Schelbert, H. R., Henning, H., LeWinter, M., Taylor, A., Ashburn, W. L., and Karliner, J. S.: Right ventricular ejection fraction in patients with acute anterior and inferior myocardial infarction assessed by radionuclide angiography. Circulation 57:1078, 1978.
26. Berger, H. J., Matthay, R. A., Pytlik, L. M., Gottschalk, A., and Zaret, B. L.: First-pass radionuclide assessment of right and left ventricular performance in patients with cardiac and pulmonary disease. Semin. Nucl. Med. 9:275, 1979.
27. Berger, H. J., Matthay, R. A., Loke, J., Marshall, R. C., Gottschalk, A., and Zaret, B. L.: Assessment of cardiac performance with quantitative radionuclide angiocardiography: Right ventricular ejection fraction with reference to findings in chronic obstructive pulmonary disease. Am. J. Cardiol. 51:897, 1978.
28. Maltz, D. L., and Treves, S.: Quantitative radionuclide angiocardiography: Determination of $Q_p:Q_s$ in children. Circulation 47: 1040, 1973.
29. Kuruc, A., Treves, S., and Parker, J. A.: Accuracy of deconvolution algorithms assessed by simulation studies. J. Nucl. Med. 24:258, 1983.
30. Villanueva-Meyer, J., Philippe, L., Cordero, S., Marcus, E. S., Mena, I.: Use of factor analysis in the evaluation of left to right cardiac shunts. J. Nucl. Med. 27:1442, 1986.
31. Treves, S.: Detection and quantitation of cardiovascular shunts with commonly available radionuclides. Semin. Nucl. Med. 10:16, 1980.

32. Greenfield, L. D., Vincent, W. R., Graham, L. S., and Bennett, L. R.: Evaluation of intracardiac shunts. CRC Crit. Rev. Clin. Radiol. Nucl. Med. *6*:217, 1975.
33. Braunwald, E., Long, R. T. L., and Morrow, A. G.: Injections of radioactive krypton (Kr^{85}) solution in the detection and localization of cardiac shunts. J. Clin. Invest. *38*:990, 1959.
34. Watson, D. D.: Shunt detection with the short-lived radioactive gases. Semin. Nucl. Med. *10*:27, 1980.
35. Polak, J. F., Holman, B. L., Podrid, P. J., and Lown, B.: Postextrasystolic potentiation during spontaneous ventricular ectopy in man. Associated left ventricular changes determined by list mode radionuclide ventriculography. Invest. Radiol. *19*:380, 1984.
36. Rabinovitch, M. A., Stewart, J., Chan, W., Dunlap, T. E., Kalff, V., Clare, J., Thrall, J. H., and Pitt, B.: Scintigraphic demonstration of ventriculoatrial conduction in the ventricular pacemaker syndrome. J. Nucl. Med. *23*:795, 1982.
37. Bacharach, S. L., Green, M. V., Borer, J. S., Hyde, J. E., Farkas, S. P., and Johnson, G. S.: Left-ventricular peak ejection rate, filling rate, and ejection fraction—frame rate requirements at rest and exercise. J. Nucl. Med. *20*:189, 1979.
38. Sinusas, A. J., Hardin, N. J., Clements, J. P., and Wackers, F. J.: Pathoanatomical correlates of regional left ventricular wall motion assessed by equilibrium radionuclide angiocardiography: A postmortem correlation. Am. J. Cardiol. *54*:975, 1984.
39. Brown, J. M., White, C. J., Sobol, S. M., and Lull, R. J.: Increased left ventricular ejection fraction after a meal: Potential source of error in performance of radionuclide angiography. Am. J. Cardiol. *51*:1709, 1983.
40. Hosoba, M., Wani, Hidenobu., Hiroe, M., and Kusakabe, K.: Clinical validation of fully automated contour detection for gated radionuclide ventriculography with slant-hole collimator. Eur. J. Nucl. Med. *12*:53, 1986.
41. Balachandran, S., Eason, S., McGuire, L., Bernard, S., and Boyd, C.: Ejection fraction by combined inverse Fourier analysis and second-derivative technique: Correlation with isocontour method. Eur. J. Nucl. Med. *12*:69, 1986.
42. Maddox, D. E., Holman, B. L., Wynne, J., Idoine, J., Parker, J. A., Uren, R., Neill, J. M., and Cohn, P. F.: The ejection fraction image: A noninvasive index of regional left ventricular wall motion. Am. J. Cardiol. *41*:1230, 1978.
43. Wackers, F. J., Berger, H. J., Johnstone, D. E., Goldman, L., Reduto, L. A., Langou, R. A., Gottschalk, A., and Zaret, B. L.: Multiple gated cardiac blood pool imaging for left ventricular ejection fraction: Validation of the technique and assessment of variability. Am. J. Cardiol. *43*:1159, 1979.
44. Schneider, R. M., Jaszczak, R. J., Coleman, R. E., and Cobb, F. R.: Disproportionate effects of regional hypokinesia on radionuclide ejection fraction: Compensation using attenuation-corrected ventricular volumes. J. Nucl. Med. *25*:747, 1984.
45. Sandler, H., and Dodge, H. T.: Use of single pace cineangiograms for the calculation of left ventricular volume in man. Am. Heart J. *75*:325, 1968.
46. Stadius, M. L., Williams, D. L., Harp, G., Cerqueira, M., Caldwell, J. H., Stratton, J. R., and Ritchie, J. L.: Left ventricular volume determination using single-photon emission computed tomography. Am. J. Cardiol. *55*:1185, 1985.
47. Massie, B. M., Kramer, B. L., Gertz, E. W., and Henderson, S. G.: Radionuclide measurement of left ventricular volume: Comparison of geometric and count-based methods. Circulation *65*:725, 1982.
48. Konstam, M. A., Wynne, J., Holman, B. L., Brown, E. J., Neill, J. M., and Kozlowski, J.: Use of equilibrium (gated) radionuclide ventriculography to quantitate left ventricular output in patients with and without left-sided valvular regurgitation. Circulation *64*:578, 1981.
49. McKay, R. G., Aroesty, J. M., Heller, G. V., Royal, H., Parker, J. A., Silverman, K. J., Kolodny, G. M., and Grossman, W.: Left ventricular pressure-volume diagrams and end-systolic pressure-volume relations in human beings. J. Am. Coll. Cardiol. *3*:301, 1984.
50. Nickoloff, E. L., Perman, W. H., Esser, P. D., Bashist, B., and Alderson, P. O.: Left ventricular volume: Physical basis for attenuation corrections in radionuclide determinations. Radiology *152*:511, 1984.
51. Kronenberg, M. W., Parrish, M. D., Jenkins, D. W. Jr., Sandler, M. P., and Friesinger, G. C.: Accuracy of radionuclide ventriculography for estimation of left ventricular volume changes and end-systolic pressure-volume relations. J. Am. Coll. Cardiol. *6*:1064, 1985.
52. Carabello, B. A., and Spann, J. F.: Uses and limitations of end-systolic indices of left ventricular function. Circulation *69*:1058, 1984.
53. Mann, T., Goldberg, S., Mudge, G. H., and Grossman, W.: Factors contributing to altered left ventricular diastolic properties during angina pectoris. Circulation *59*:14, 1979.
54. Hirota, Y.: A clinical study of left ventricular relaxation. Circulation *62*:756, 1980.
55. Bonow, R. O., Bacharach, S. L., Green, M. V., Kent, K. M., Rosing, D. R., Lipson, L. C., Leon, M. B., and Epstein, S. E.: Impaired left ventricular diastolic filling in patients with coronary artery disease: Assessment with radionuclide angiography. Circulation *64*:315, 1981.
56. Inouye, I., Massie, B., Loge, D., Topic, N., Silverstein, D., Simpson, P., and Tubau, J.: Abnormal left ventricular filling: An early finding in mild to moderate systemic hypertension. Am. J. Cardiol. *53*:120, 1984.
57. Betocchi, S., Bonow, R. O., Bacharach, S. L., Rosing, D. R., Maron, B. J., and Green, M. V.: Isovolumic relaxation period in hypertrophic cardiomyopathy: Assessment by radionuclide angiography. J. Am. Coll. Cardiol. *7*:74, 1986.
58. Polak, J. F., Kemper, A. J., Bianco, J. A., Parisi, A. F., and Tow, D. E.: Resting early peak diastolic filling rate: A sensitive index of myocardial dysfunction in patients with coronary artery disease. J. Nucl. Med. *23*:471, 1982.
59. Yamagishi, T., Ozaki, M., Kumada, T., Ikezono, T., Shimizu, T., Furutani, Y., Yamaoka, H., Ogawa, H., Matsuzaki, M., Matsuda, Y., Arima, A., and Kusukawa, R.: Asynchronous left ventricular diastolic filling in patients with isolated disease of the left anterior descending coronary artery: Assessment with radionuclide ventriculography. Circulation *69*:933, 1984.
60. Maddox, D. E., Holman, B. L., Wynne, J., Idoine, J., Parker, J. A., Uren, R., Neill, J. M., and Cohn, P. F.: Ejection fraction image: A noninvasive index of regional left ventricular wall motion. Am. J. Cardiol. *41*:1230, 1978.
61. Holman, B. L., Wynne, J., Idoine, J., Zielonka, J., and Neill, J.: The paradox image: A noninvasive index of regional left ventricular dyskinesis. J. Nucl. Med. *20*:1237, 1979.
62. Holman, B. L., Wynne, J., Idoine, J., and Neill, J.: Disruption in the temporal sequence of regional ventricular contraction. Circulation *61*:1075, 1980.
63. Frais, M., Botvinick, E., Shosa, D., O'Connell, W., Alvarez, J. P., Dae, M., Hattner, R., and Faulkner, D.: Phase image characterization of localized and generalized left ventricular contraction abnormalities. J. Am. Coll. Cardiol. *4*:987, 1984.
64. Botvinick, E. H., Frais, M. A., Shosa, D. W., O'Connell, J. W., Pacheco-Alvarez, J. A., Scheinman, M., Hattner, R. S., Morady, F., and Faulkner, D. B.: An accurate means of detecting and characterizing abnormal patterns of ventricular activation by phase image analysis. Am. J. Cardiol. *50*:289, 1982.
65. Johnson, L. L., Seldin, D. W., Yeh, H-L., Spotnitz, H. M., and Reiffel, J. A.: Phase analysis of gated blood pool scintigraphic images to localize bypass tracts in Wolff-Parkinson-White syndrome. J. Am. Coll. Cardiol. *8*:67, 1986.
66. Bashore, T. M., Stine, R. A., Shaffer, P. B., Bush, C. A., Leier, C. V., and Schaal, S. F.: The noninvasive localization of ventricular pacing sites by radionuclide phase imaging. Circulation *70*(Suppl IV):681, 1984.
67. Steckley, R. A., Kronenberg, M. W., Born, M. L., Rhea, T. C., Bateman, J. E., Rollo, F. D., and Friesinger, G. C.: Radionuclide ventriculography: Evaluation of automated and visual methods for regional wall motion analysis. Radiology *142*:179, 1982.
68. Maddox, D. E., Wynne, J., Uren, R., Parker, J. A., Idoine, J., Siegel, L. C., Neill, J. M., Cohn, P. F., and Holman, B. L.: Regional ejection fraction: A quantitative radionuclide index of regional left ventricular performance. Circulation *59*:1001, 1979.
69. Gibbons, R. J., Morris, K. G., Lee, K., Coleman, R. E., and Cobb, F. R.: Assessment of regional life ventricular function using gated radionuclide angiography. Am. J. Cardiol. *54*:294, 1984.
70. Vitale, D. F., Green, M. V., Bacharach, S. L., Bonow, R. O., Watson, R. M., Findley, S. L., and Jones, A. E.: Assessment of regional left ventricular function by sector analysis: Method for objective evaluation of radionuclide blood pool studies. Am. J. Cardiol. *52*:1112, 1983.
71. Silber, S., Schwaiger, M., Klein, U., and Rudolph, W.: Quantitative Beurteilung der linksventrikulären Funktion mit der Radionuklid-Ven trikulographie. Herz *5*:146, 1980.
72. Manno, B. V., Iskandrian, A. S., and Hakki, A. H.: Right ventricular function: methodologic and clinical considerations in noninvasive scintigraphic assessment. J. Am. Coll. Cardiol. *3*:1072, 1984.
73. Holman, B. L., Wynne, J., Zielonka, J. S., and Idoine, J.: A simplified technique for measuring right ventricular ejection fraction using the equilibrium radionuclide angiocardiogram and the slant-hole collimator. Radiology *138*: 429, 1981.
74. Morrison, D., Marshall, J., Wright, A. L., Daly, M., and Henry, R.: An improved method of right ventricular gated equilibrium blood pool radionuclide ventriculography. Chest *82*:607, 1982.
75. Nicod, P., Corbett, J. R., Firth, B. G., Dehmer, G. J., Izquierdo, C., Markham, R. V., Jr., Hillis, L. D., Willerson, J. T., and Lewis, S. E.: Radionuclide techniques for valvular regurgitant index: Comparison in patients with normal and depressed ventricular function. J. Nucl. Med. *23*:763, 1982.
76. Alderson, P. O.: Radionuclide quantification of valvular regurgitation. J. Nucl. Med. *23*:851, 1982.
77. Ormerod, O. J. M., Barber, R. W., Stone, D. L., Wraight, E. P., and Petch, M. C.: A comparison of radionuclide methods of evaluating aortic regurgitation with observations on the effect of exercise symptoms. Eur. J. Nucl. Med. *12*:72, 1986.
78. Tu'meh, S. S., Tracy, D., Wynne, J., Konstam, M. A., Kozlowski, J. F., Neumann, A. L., and Holman, B. L.: Scintigraphic diagnosis of tricuspid regurgitation. Radiology *145*:463, 1982.
79. Borer, J., Bacharach, S. L., Green, M. V., Kent, K. M., Epstein, S. E., and Johnston, G. S.: Real-time radionuclide cineangiography in the noninvasive evaluation of global and regional left ventricular function at rest and during exercise in patients with coronary-artery disease. N. Engl. J. Med. *296*:839, 1977.
80. Borer, J., Bacharach, S. L., and Green, M. V.: Radionuclide cineangiography in the clinical assessment of patients with coronary and valvular heart diseases. Progr. Nucl. Med. *6*:151, 1980.
81. Bodenheimer, M. M., Banka, V. S., Fooshee, C. M., Gillespie, J. A., and Helfant, R. H.: Detection of coronary heart disease using radionuclide determined regional ejection fraction at rest and during handgrip exercise: Correlation with coronary arteriography. Circulation *58*:640, 1980.
82. Wainwright, R. J., Brennand-Roper, D. A., Cueni, T. A., Sowton, E., Hilson, A. J. W., and Maisey, M. N.: Cold pressor test in detection of coronary heart-disease and cardiomyopathy using technetium-99m gated blood-pool imaging. Lancet *2*:320, 1979.
83. Rozenman, Y., Weiss, A. T., Atlan, H., and Gotsman, M. S.: Left ventricular volumes and function during atrial pacing in coronary artery disease: Radionuclide angiographic study. Am. J. Cardiol. *53*:497, 1984.
84. Peter, C. A., and Jones, R. H.: Effects of isometric handgrip and dynamic exercise on left-ventricular function. J. Nucl. Med. *21*:1131, 1980.

85. Holman, B. L.: Practical nuclear cardiology. Diagn. Nucl. Med. *1*:2, 1984.
86. Kaul, S., Boucher, C. A., Okada, R. D., Newell, J. B., Strauss, H. W., and Pohost, G. M.: Sources of variability in the radionuclide angiographic assessment of ejection fraction: Comparison of first-pass and gated equilibrium techniques. Am. J. Cardiol. *53*:823, 1984.
87. Okada, R. D., Boucher, C. A., Strauss, H. W., and Pohost, G. M.: Exercise radionuclide imaging approaches to coronary artery disease. Am. J. Cardiol. *46*:1188, 1980.
88. Marshall, R. C., Wisenberg, G., Schelbert, H. R., and Henze, E.: Effect of oral propranolol on rest, exercise and postexercise left ventricular performance in normal subjects and patients with coronary artery disease. Circulation *63*:572, 1981.
89. Poliner, L. R., Dehmer, G. J., Lewis, S. E., Parkey, R. W., Blomqvist, C. G., and Willerson, J. T.: Left ventricular performance in normal subjects: A comparison of the responses to exercise in the upright and supine positions. Circulation *62*:528, 1980.
90. Seaworth, J. F., Higginbotham, M. B., Coleman, R. E., and Cobb, F. R.: Effect of partial decreases in exercise workload on radionuclide indices of ischemia. J. Am. Coll. Cardiol. *2*:522, 1983.
91. Rozanski, A., Diamond, G. A., Berman, D., Forrester, J. S., Morris, D., and Swan, H. J. C.: Declining specificity of exercise radionuclide ventriculography. N. Engl. J. Med. *309*:518, 1983.
92. Jones, R. H., McEwan, P., Newman, G. E., Port, S., Rerych, S. K., Scholz, P. M., Upton, M. T., Peter, C. A., Austin, E. H., Leong, K., Gibbons, R. J., Cobb, F. R., Coleman, R. E., and Sabiston, D. C.: Accuracy of diagnosis of coronary artery disease by radionuclide measurements of left ventricular function during rest and exercise. Circulation *64*:586, 1981.
93. Port, S., Cobb, F. R., Coleman, R. E., and Jones, R. H.: Effect of age on the response of the left ventricular ejection fraction to exercise. N. Engl. J. Med. *303*:1133, 1980.
94. Gibbons, R. J., Lee, J. L., Cobb, F. R., Coleman, R. E., and Jones, R. H.: Ejection fraction response to exercise in patients with chest pain, coronary artery disease, and normal coronary arteriograms. Circulation *66*:643, 1982.
95. Wasserman, A. G., Katz, R. J., Varghese, P. J., Leiboff, R. H., Bren, G. G., Schlesselman, S., Varma, V. M., Reba, R. C., and Ross, A. M.: Exercise radionuclide ventriculographic responses in hypertensive patients with chest pain. N. Engl. J. Med. *311*:1276, 1984.
96. Borer, J. S., Bacharach, S. L., Green, M. V., Kent, K. M., Rosing, D. R., Seides, S. F., McIntosh, C. L., Conkle, D., Morrow, A. G., and Epstein, S. E.: Left ventricular function in aortic stenosis: Response to exercise and effects of operation (abstr). Am. J. Cardiol. *41*:382, 1978.
97. Greenberg, B., Massie, B., Thomas, D., Bristow, J. D., Cheitlin, M., Broudy, D., Szlachcic, J., and Krishnamurthy, G.: Association between the exercise ejection fraction response and systolic wall stress in patients with chronic aortic insufficiency. Circulation *71*:458, 1985.
98. Borer, J. S., Gottdiener, J. S., Rosing, D. R., Kent, K. M., Bacharach, S. L., Green, M. V., and Epstein, S. E.: Left ventricular function in mitral regurgitation: Determination during exercise (abstr). Circulation *60*(Suppl. II):38, 1979.
99. Ahmad, M., and Haibach, H.: Left ventricular function in patients with mitral valve prolapse: A radionuclide evaluation. Clin. Nucl. Med. *7*:562, 1982.
100. Bonow, R. O., Leon, M. B., Rosing, D. R., Kent, K. M., Lipson, L. C., Bacharach, S. L., Green, M. V., and Epstein, S. E.: Effects of verapamil and propranolol on left ventricular systolic function and diastolic filling in patients with coronary artery disease: Radionuclide angiographic studies at rest and during exercise. Circulation *65*:1342, 1981.
101. Matthay, R. A., Berger, H. J., Davies, R. A., Loke, J., Mahler, D. A., Gottschalk, A., and Zaret, B. L.: Right and left ventricular exercise performance in chronic obstructive pulmonary disease: Radionuclide assessment. Ann. Intern. Med. *93*:234, 1981.
102. Leon, M. B., Borer, J. S., Bacharach, S. L., Green, M. V., Benz, E. J., Griffith, P., and Nienhuis, A. W.: Detection of early cardiac dysfunction in patients with severe beta-thalassemia and chronic iron overload. N. Engl. J. Med. *301*: 1143, 1979.
103. Matthay, R. A., Berger, H. J., Loke, J., Dolan, T. F., Fagenholz, S. A., Gottschalk, A., and Zaret, B. L.: Right and left ventricular performance in ambulatory young adults with cystic fibrosis. Br. Heart J. *43*:474, 1980.
104. Hitzhusen, J. C., Hickler, R. B., Alpert, J. S., and Doherty, P. W.: Exercise testing and hemodynamic performance in healthy elderly persons. Am. J. Cardiol. *54*:1082, 1984.
105. Higginbotham, M. B., Morris, K. G., Coleman, R. E., and Cobb, F. R.: Sex-related differences in the normal cardiac response to upright exercise. Circulation *70*:357, 1984.
106. Ponto, J. A., and Holmes, K. A.: Discontinuation of beta blockers before exercise radionuclide ventriculograms. J. Nucl. Med. *23*:456, 1982.
107. Gibbons, R. J., Lee, K. L., Pryor, D., Harrell, F. E., Jr., Coleman, R. E., Cobb, F. R., Rosati, R. A., and Jones, R. H.: The use of radionuclide angiography in the diagnosis of coronary artery disease: A logistic regression analysis. Circulation *68*:740, 1983.
108. Bonow, R. O., Kent, K. M., Rosing, D. R., Gordon Lan, K. K., Lakatos, E., Borer, J. S., Bacharach, S. L., Green, M. V., and Epstein, S. E.: Exercise-induced ischemia in mildly symptomatic patients with coronary artery disease and preserved left ventricular function: Identification of subgroups at risk of death during medical therapy. N. Engl. J. Med. *311*:1339, 1984.
109. Nesto, R. W., Cohn, L. H., Collins, J. J., Wynne, J., Holman, L., and Cohn, P. F.: Inotropic contractile reserve: A useful predictor of increased 5 year survival and improved postoperative left ventricular function in patients with coronary artery disease and reduced ejection fraction. Am. J. Cardiol. *50*:39, 1982.
110. Borer, J. S., Rosing, D. R., Miller, R. H., Stark, R. M., Kent, K. M., Bacharach, S. L., Green, M. V., Lake, C. R., Cohen, H., Holmes, D., Donohue, D., Baker, W., and Epstein, S. E.: Natural history of left ventricular function during 1 year after acute myocardial infarction: Comparison with clinical, electrocardiographic and biochemical determinations. Am. J. Cardiol. *46*:1, 1980.
111. Shah, P. K., Maddahi, J., Berman, D. S., Pichler, M., and Swan, H. J. C.: Scintigraphically detected predominant right ventricular dysfunction in acute myocardial infarction: Clinical and hemodynamic correlates and implications for therapy and prognosis. J. Am. Coll. Cardiol. *6*:1264, 1985.
112. Reduto, L. A., Berger, H. J., Gottschalk, A., and Zaret, B. L.: Sequential radionuclide assessment of left and right ventricular performance after acute transmural myocardial infarction. Ann. Intern. Med. *89*:441, 1978.
113. Shah, P. K., Pichler, M., Berman, D. S., Singh, B. N., and Swan, H. J. C.: Left ventricular ejection fraction and first third ejection fraction determined by radionuclide ventriculography in early stages of first transmural myocardial infarction: Relation to short-term prognosis. Am. J. Cardiol. *45*:542, 1980.
114. Braat, S. H., Brugada, P., De Zwaan, C., Den Dulk, K., and Wellens, H. J. J.: Right and left ventricular ejection fraction in acute inferior wall infarction with or without S-T segment elevation in lead V_4R. J. Am. Coll. Cardiol. *4*:940, 1984.
115. Starling, M. R., Dell'Italia, L. J., Chaudhuri, T. K., Boros, B. L., and O'Rourke, R. A.: First-transit and equilibrium radionuclide angiography in patients with inferior transmural myocardial infarction: Criteria for the diagnosis of associated hemodynamically significant right ventricular infarction. J. Am. Coll. Cardiol. *4*:923, 1984.
116. Pulido, J. I., Doss, J., Twieg, D., Blomqvist, G. C., Faulkner, D., Horn, V., DeBates, D., Tobey, M., Parkey, R. W., and Willerson, J. T.: Submaximal exercise testing after acute myocardial infarction: Myocardial scintigraphic and electrocardiographic observations. Am. J. Cardiol. *42*:19, 1978.
117. Nicod, P., Corbett, J. R., Firth, B. G., Lewis, S. E., Rude, R. E., Huxley, R., and Willerson, J. T.: Prognostic value of resting and submaximal exercise radionuclide ventriculography after acute myocardial infarction in high-risk patients with single- and multivessel disease. Am. J. Cardiol. *52*:30, 1983.
118. Meizlish, J. L., Berger, H. J., Plankey, M., Errico, D., Levy, W., and Zaret, B. L.: Functional left ventricular aneurysm formation after acute anterior transmural myocardial infarction: Incidence, natural history, and prognostic implications. N. Engl. J. Med. *311*:1001, 1984.
119. Ritchie, J. L., Hallstrom, A. P., Troubaugh, G. B., Caldwell, J. H., and Cobb, L. A.: Out-of-hospital sudden coronary death: Rest and exercise radionuclide left ventricular function in survivors. Am. J. Cardiol. *55*:645, 1985.
120. Borer, J. S., Bacharach, S. L., Green, M. V., Kent, K. M., Henry, W. L., Rosing, D. R., Seides, S. F., Johnston, G. S., and Epstein, S. E.: Exercise-induced left and right ventricular dysfunction in symptomatic and asymptomatic patients with aortic regurgitation: Assessment with radionuclide cineangiography. Am. J. Cardiol. *42*:351, 1978.
121. Borer, J. S., Rosing, D. R., Kent, K. M., Bacharach, S. L., Green, M. V., McIntosh, C. J., Morrow, A. G., and Epstein, S. E.: Left ventricular function at rest and during exercise after aortic valve replacement in patients with aortic regurgitation. Am. J. Cardiol. *44*:1297, 1979.
122. Boucher, C. A., Kanarek, D. J., Okada, R. D., Hutter, A. M., Jr., Strauss, H. W., and Pohost, G. M.: Exercise testing in aortic regurgitation: Comparison of radionuclide left ventricular ejection fraction with exercise performance at the anaerobic threshold and peak exercise. Am. J. Cardiol. *52*:801, 1983.
123. Dougherty, A. H., Naccarelli, G. V., Gray, E. L., Hicks, C. H., and Goldstein, R. A.: Congestive heart failure with normal systolic function. Am. J. Cardiol. *54*:778, 1984.
124. Soufer, R., Wohlgelernter, D., Vita, N. A., Amuchestegui, M., Sostman, H. D., Berger, H. J., and Zaret, B. L.: Intact systolic left ventricular function in clinical congestive heart failure. Am. J. Cardiol. *55*:1032, 1985.
125. Greenberg, J. M., Murphy, J. H., Okada, R. D., Pohost, G. M., Strauss, H. W., and Boucher, C. A.: Value and limitations of radionuclide angiography in determining the cause of reduced left ventricular ejection fraction: Comparison of idiopathic dilated cardiomyopathy and coronary artery disease. Am. J. Cardiol. *55*:541, 1985.
126. Rozanski, A., Berman, D., Gray, R., Diamond, G., Raymond, M., Prause, J., Maddahi, J., Swan, H. J. C., and Matloff, J.: Preoperative prediction of reversible myocardial asynergy by postexercise radionuclide ventriculography. N. Engl. J. Med. *307*:212, 1982.
127. Bodenheimer, M. M., Banka, V. S., Hermann, G. A., Trout, R. G., Pasdar, H., and Helfant, R. H.: Reversible asynergy. Circulation *53*:792, 1976.
128. Chatterjee, K., Swan, H. J. C., Parmley, W. W., Sustaita, H., Marcus, H. S., and Matloff, J.: Influence of direct myocardial revascularization on left ventricular asynergy and function in patients with coronary heart disease: With and without previous myocardial infarction. Circulation *47*:276, 1973.
129. Popio, K. A., Gorlin, R., Bechtel, D., and Levine, J. A.: Postextrasystolic potentiation as a predictor of potential myocardial viability. Am. J. Cardiol. *39*: 944, 1977.
130. Righetti, A., Crawford, M. H., O'Rourke, R. A., Schelbert, H., Daily, P. O., and Ross, J., Jr.: Intraventricular septal motion and left ventricular function after coronary bypass surgery: Evaluation with echocardiography and radionuclide angiography. Am. J. Cardiol. *39*:372, 1977.
131. Helfant, R. H., Pine, R., Meister, S. G., Feldman, M. S., Trout, R. G., and Banka, V. S.: Nitroglycerin to unmask reversible asynergy: Correlation with post coronary bypass surgery. Circulation *50*:108, 1974.
132. DePuey, E. G., Mammen, G. P., Rivas, A. H., Thompson, W. L., Sonnemaker, R. E., Mathur, V., Burdine, J. A., Garcia, E., and Hall, R. J.: Postexercise potentiation of wall motion to identify myocardial viability. Texas Heart Inst. J. *9*:127, 1982.
133. Berger, H. J., Matthay, R. A., Loke, J., Marshall, R. C., Gottschalk, A., and

Zaret, B. L.: Assessment of cardiac performance with quantitative radionuclide angiocardiography: Right ventricular ejection fraction with reference to findings in chronic obstructive pulmonary disease. Am. J. Cardiol. *41*:897, 1978.

134. Berger, H. J., and Matthay, R. A.: Noninvasive radiographic assessment of cardiovascular function in acute and chronic respiratory failure. Am. J. Cardiol. *47*:950, 1981.

135. Matthay, R. A., Berger, J. H., Davies, R. A., Loke, J., Mahler, D. A., Gottschalk, A., and Zaret, B. L.: Right and left ventricular exercise performance in chronic obstructive pulmonary disease: Radionuclide assessment. Ann. Intern. Med. *93*:234, 1980.

136. Kimchi, A., Ellrodt, A. G., Berman, D. S., Riedinger, M. S., Swan, H. J. C., and Murata, G. H.: Right ventricular performance in septic shock: A combined radionuclide and hemodynamic study. J. Am. Coll. Cardiol. *4*:945, 1984.

137. Polak, J. F., Holman, B. L., Wynn, E. J., Colucci, W. S.: Right ventricular ejection fraction: An indicator of increased mortality in patients with congestive heart failure associated with coronary artery disease. J. Am. Col. Cardiol. *2*:217, 1983.

138. Baker, B. J., Wilen, M. M., Boyd, C. M., Dinh, H., and Franciosa, J. A.: Relation of right ventricular ejection fraction to exercise capacity in chronic left ventricular failure. Am. J. Cardiol. *54*:596, 1984.

139. Wynne, J., Malacoff, R. F., Benotti, J. R., Curfman, G. D., Grossman, W., Holman, B. L., Smith, T. W., and Braunwald, E.: Oral amrinone in refractory congestive heart failure. Am. J. Cardiol. *45*:1245, 1980.

140. Goldman, S. A., Johnson, L. L., Escala, E., Cannon, P. J., and Weiss, M. B.: Improved exercise ejection fraction with long-term prazosin therapy in patients with heart failure. Am. J. Med. *68*:36, 1980.

141. Colucci, W. S., Wynne, J., Holman, B. L., and Braunwald, E.: Long-term therapy of heart failure with prazosin: A randomized double blind trial. Am. J. Cardiol. *45*:337, 1980.

142. Matthay, R. A., Berger, H. J., Loke, J., Gottschalk, A., and Zaret, B. L.: Effects of aminophylline upon right and left ventricular performance in chronic obstructive pulmonary disease: Noninvasive assessment by radionuclide angiocardiography. Am. J. Med. *65*:903, 1978.

143. Marshall, R. C., Wisenberg, G., Schelbert, H. R., and Henze, E.: Effect of oral propranolol on rest, exercise, and postexercise left ventricular performance in normal subjects and patients with coronary artery disease. Circulation *63*:572, 1981.

144. Malacoff, R. F., Lorell, B. H., Mudge, G. H., Jr., Holman, B. L., Idoine, J., Bifolck, L., and Cohn, P. F.: Beneficial effects of nifedipine on regional myocardial blood flow in patients with coronary artery disease. Circulation *65*(Suppl. I):32, 1982.

145. Alexander, J., Dainiak, N., Berger, H. J., Goldman, L., Johnstone, D., Reduto, L., Duffy, T., Schwartz, P., Gottschalk, A., and Zaret, B. L.: Serial assessment of doxorubicin cardiotoxicity with quantitative radionuclide angiocardiography. N. Engl. J. Med. *300*:278, 1979.

146. Choi, B. W., Berger, H. J., Schwartz, P. E., Alexander, J., Wackers, F. J. Th., Gottschalk, A., and Zaret, B. L.: Serial radionuclide assessment of doxorubicin cardiotoxicity in cancer patients with abnormal baseline resting left ventricular performance. Am. Heart J. *106*(Pt. 1):638, 1983.

147. Druck, M. N., Gulenchyn, K. Y., Evans, W. K., Gotlieb, A., Srigley, J. R., Bar-Shlomo, B. Z., Feiglin, D. H., McEwan, P., Silver, M. D., Millband, L., Winter, K., Hilton, J. D., Jablonsky, G., Morch, J. E., and McLaughlin, P.: Radionuclide angiography and endomyocardial biopsy in assessment of doxorubicin cardiotoxicity. Cancer *53*:1667, 1984.

MYOCARDIAL PERFUSION AND METABOLISM

148. Abrams, H. L., and Adams, D. F.: The coronary arteriogram. Structural and functional aspects. N. Engl. J. Med. *281*:1276, 1969.

149. Gottlieb, S. O., Weisfeldt, M. L., Ouyang, P., Mellits, E. D., and Gerstenblith, G.: Silent ischemia as a marker for early unfavorable outcomes in patients with unstable angina. N. Engl. J. Med. *314*:1214, 1986.

150. Svensson, S. E., Lomsky, M., Olsson, L., Persson, S., Strauss, H. W., and Westling, H.: Noninvasive determination of the distribution of cardiac output in man at rest and during exercise. Clin. Physiol. *2*:467, 1982.

151. Bodenheimer, M. M., Banka, V. S., and Helfant, R. H.: Nuclear cardiology. II. The role of myocardial perfusion imaging using thallium-201 in diagnosis of coronary heart disease. Am. J. Cardiol. *45*:674, 1980.

152. Bennett, K. R., Smith, R. O., Lehan, P. H., and Hellems, H. K.: Correlation of myocardial ^{42} K uptake with coronary arteriography. Radiology *102*:117, 1972.

153. Carr, E. A., Jr., Beierwaltes, W. H., Wegst, A. V., and Bartlett, J. D., Jr.: Myocardial scanning with rubidium-86. J. Nucl. Med. 3:76, 1962.

154. Carr, E. A., Jr., Walker, B. J., and Bartlett, J., Jr.: The diagnosis of myocardial infarcts by photoscanning after administration of cesium^{131}. J. Clin. Invest. *42*:922, 1963.

155. Hurley, P. J., Cooper, M., Reba, R. C., Poggenburg, K. J., and Wagner, H. N., Jr.: ^{143} KCl: A new radiopharmaceutical for imaging the heart. J. Nucl. Med. *12*:516, 1971.

156. Romhilt, D. W., Adolph, R. J., Sodd, V. C., Levenson, N. I., August, L. S., Nishiyama, H., and Berke, R. A.: Cesium-129 myocardial scintigraphy to detect myocardial infarction. Circulation *48*:1242, 1973.

157. Martin, N. D., Zaret, B. L., McGowan, R. L., Wells, H. P., Jr., and Flamm, M. D.: Rubidium-81: A new myocardial scanning agent. Radiology *111*:651, 1974.

158. Lebowitz, E., Greene, M. W., Bradley-Moore, P., Atkins, H., Ansari, A., Richards, P., and Belgrave, E.: ^{201}Tl for medical use. J. Nucl. Med. *14*: 421, 1973.

159. Gehring, P. J., and Hammond, P. B.: The interrelationship between thallium and potassium in animals. J. Pharmacol. Exp. Ther. 55:187, 1967.

160. Britten, J. S., and Blank, M.: Thallium activation of the (Na^+-K^+)-activated ATPase of rabbit kidney. Biochim. Biophys. Acta *159*:160, 1968.

161. Strauss, H. W., Harrison, K., Langan, J. K., Lebowitz, E., and Pitt, B.: Thallium-201 for myocardial imaging. Relation of thallium-201 to regional myocardial perfusion. Circulation *51*:641, 1975.

162. Holman, B. L., Jones, A. G., Lister-James, J., Davis, A., Abrams, M. J., Kirshenbaum, J. M., Tumeh, S. S., and English, R. J.: A new Tc-99m-labeled myocardial imaging agent, hexakis (T-butylisonitrile)-technetium (I) (Tc-99m TBI): Initial experience in the human. J. Nucl. Med. *25*:1350, 1984.

163. Holman, B. L., Campbell, C. A., Lister-James, J., Jones, A. G., Davison, A., and Kloner, R. A.: Effect of reperfusion and hyperemia on the myocardial distribution of technetium-99m t-butylisonitrile. J. Nucl. Med. *27*:1172, 1986.

164. Holman, B. L., Sporn, V., Jones, A. G., Sia, S. T. B., Perez-Balino, N., Davison, A., Lister-James, J., Kronauge, J. F., Mitta, A. E. A., Camine, L. L., Campbell, S., Williams, S. J., and Carpenter, A. T.: Myocardial imaging with Tc-99m CPI: Initial experience in the human. J. Nucl. Med. *28*:13, 1987.

165. Budinger, T. F., Yano, Y., and Hoop, B.: A comparison of $^{82}Rb^+$ and $^{13}NH_3$ for myocardial positron scintigraphy. J. Nucl. Med. *16*:429, 1975.

166. Yano, Y., and Anger, H. O.: Visualization of heart and kidneys in animals with ultrashort-lived ^{82}Rb and the positron scintillation camera. J. Nucl. Med. *9*:413, 1968.

167. Walsh, W. F., Fill, H. R., and Harper, P. V.: Nitrogen-13–labeled ammonia for myocardial imaging. Semin. Nucl. Med. *7*:59, 1977.

168. Sapirstein, L. A.: Fractionation of the cardiac output of rats with isotopic potassium. Circ. Res. *4*:689, 1956.

169. Melin, J. A., and Becker, L. C.: Quantitative relationship between global left ventricular thallium uptake and blood flow: Effects of propranolol, ouabain, dipyridamole, and coronary artery occlusion. J. Nucl. Med. *27*:641, 1986.

170. Weich, H. F., Strauss, H. W., and Pitt, B.: The extraction of Tl-201 by the myocardium. Circulation *56*:188, 1977.

171. Mueller, T. M., Marcus, M. L., Ehrhardt, J. C., Kerber, R. E., Brown, D. D., and Abboud, F. M.: Limitations of thallium-201 myocardial perfusion scintigrams. Circulation *54*:640, 1976.

172. Chu, A., Murdock, R. H., and Cobb, F. R.: Relation between regional distribution of thallium-201 and myocardial blood flow in normal, acutely ischemic, and infarcted myocardium. Am. J. Cardiol. *50*:1141, 1982.

173. Strauss, H. W., and Pitt, B.: Noninvasive detection of subcritical coronary arterial narrowings with a coronary vasodilator and myocardial perfusion imaging. Am. J. Cardiol. *39*:403, 1977.

174. Gould, K. L.: Noninvasive assessment of coronary stenoses by myocardial perfusion imaging during pharmacologic coronary vasodilatation. I. Physiological basis and experimental validation. Am. J. Cardiol. *41*:267, 1978.

175. Holman, B. L., Cohn, P. F., Adams, D. F., See, J. R., Roberts, B. H., Idoine, J., and Gorlin, R.: Regional myocardial blood flow during hyperemia induced by contrast agent in patients with coronary artery disease. Am. J. Cardiol. *38*: 416, 1976.

176. Zaret, B. L., Strauss, H. W., Martin, N. D., Wells, H. P., Jr., and Flamm, M. D., Jr.: Noninvasive regional myocardial perfusion with radioactive potassium. Study of patients at rest, with exercise, and during angina pectoris. N. Engl. J. Med. *288*:809, 1973.

177. Schwartz, J. S., Ponto, R., Carlyle, P., Forstrom, L., and Cohn, J. N.: Early distribution of thallium-201 after temporary ischemia. Circulation *57*:332, 1978.

178. Garcia, E., Maddahi, J., Berman, D., and Waxman, A: Space/time quantitation of thallium-201 myocardial scintigraphy. J. Nucl. Med. *22*:309, 1981.

179. Grunwald, A., Watson, D., Holzgrefe, H., Irving, J., and Beller, G. A.: Myocardial thallium-201 kinetics in normal and ischemic myocardium. Circulation *64*:610, 1981.

180. Okada, R., Jacobs, M., Daggett, W., Leppo, J., Strauss, H. W., Newell, J. B., Moore, R., Boucher, C. A., O'Keefe, D., and Pohost, G. M.: Thallium-201 kinetics in nonischemic canine myocardium. Circulation *65*:70, 1982.

181. Berger, H. J., and Zaret, B. L.: Nuclear cardiology. N. Engl. J. Med. *305*:799 and 855, 1981.

182. Jengo, J. A., Freeman, R., Brizendine, M., and Mena, I.: Detection of coronary artery disease: Comparison of exercise stress radionuclide angiocardiography and thallium stress perfusion scanning. Am. J. Cardiol. *45*:535, 1980.

183. Pohost, G. M., Zir, L. M., Moore, R. H., McKusick, K. A., Guinep, T. E., and Beller, G. A.: Differentiation of transiently ischemic from infarct myocardium by serial imaging after a single dose of thallium-201. Circulation *55*:294, 1977.

184. Pohost, G. M., Alpert, N. M., Ingwall, J. S., and Strauss, H. W.: Thallium redistribution: Mechanism and clinical utility. Semin. Nucl. Med. *10*:70, 1980.

185. Strauss, H. W., and Boucher, C. A.: Myocardial perfusion studies: Lessons from a decade of clinical use. Radiology *160*:577, 1986.

186. Rothendler, J. A., Okada, R. D., Wilson, R. A., Brown, K. A., Boucher, C. A., Strauss, H. W., and Pohost, G. M.: Effect of delay in commencing imaging on the ability to detect transient thallium defects. J. Nucl. Med. *26*:880, 1985.

187. McLaughlin, P. R., Martin, R. P., Doherty, P., Daspit, S., Goris, M., Haskell, W., Lewis, S., Kriss, J. P., and Harrison, D. C.: Reproducibility of thallium-201 myocardial imaging. Circulation *55*:497, 1977.

188. Johnstone, D. E., Wackers, F. J., Berger, H. J., Hoffer, P. B., Kelley, M. J., Gottschalk, A., and Zaret, B. L.: Effect of patient positioning on left lateral thallium-201 myocardial images. J. Nucl. Med. *20*:183, 1979.

189. Wilson, R. A., Sullivan, P. J., Okada, R. D., Boucher, C. A., Morris, C., Pohost, G. M., and Strauss, H. W.: The effect of eating on thallium myocardial imaging. Chest *89*:195, 1986.

190. Francisco, D. A., Collins, S. M., Go, R. T., Ehrhardt, J. C., Van Kirk, O. C., and Marcus, M. L.: Tomographic thallium-201 myocardial perfusion scintigrams after maximal coronary artery vasodilation with intravenous dipyridamole. Circulation *66*:370, 1982.

191. Heiss, H. W.: Coronary blood flow at rest and during exercise. *In* Rackman, H., and Hahn, C. H. (eds.): Ventricular Function at Rest and During Exercise. Berlin, Springer-Verlag, 1976, p. 17.
192. Josephson, M. A., Brown, B. G., Hecht, H. S., Hopkins, J., Pierce, C. D., and Petersen, R. B.: Noninvasive detection and localization of coronary stenoses in patients: Comparison of resting dipyridamole and exercise thallium-201 myocardial perfusion imaging. Am. Heart J. *103*:1008, 1982.
193. Taillefer, R., Lette, J., Phaneuf, D-C., Leveille, J., Lemire, F., and Essiambre, R.: Thallium-201 myocardial imaging during pharmacologic coronary vasodilation: Comparison of oral and intravenous administration of dipyridamole. J. Am. Coll. Cardiol. *8*:76, 1986.
194. Verani, M. S.: Thallium-201 myocardial scintigraphy: An overview. Clin. Nucl. Med. *6*:276, 1983.
195. Wackers, F. J., Klay, J. W., Laks, H., Schnitzer, J., Zaret, B. L., and Geha, A. S.: Pathophysiological correlations of right ventricular thallium-201 uptake in a canine model. Circulation *64*:1256, 1981.
196. Boucher, C. A., Zir, L. M., Beller, G. A., Okada, R. D., McKusick, K. A., Strauss, H. W., and Pohost, G. M.: Increased lung uptake of thallium-201 during exercise myocardial imaging: Hemodynamic and angiographic implications of patients with coronary artery disease. Am. J. Cardiol. *46*:189, 1980.
197. Wahl, R. L., Kumar, B., Biello, D. R., and Miller, T. R.: The futility of thallium-201 quantitative lung/myocardial ratio in the detection of coronary artery disease. Eur. J. Nucl. Med. *12*:5, 1986.
198. Canhasi, B., Dae, M., Botvinick, E., Lanzer, P., Schechtmann, N., Faulkner, D., O'Connell, W., and Schiller, N.: Interaction of "supplementary" scintigraphic indicators of ischemia and stress electrocardiography in the diagnosis of multivessel coronary disease. J. Am. Coll. Cardiol. *6*:581, 1985.
199. Okada, R. D., Boucher, C. A., Kirshenbaum, H. K., Kushner, F. G., Strauss, H. W., Block, P. C., McKusick, K. A., and Pohost, G. M.: Improved diagnostic accuracy of thallium-201 stress test using multiple observers and criteria derived from interobserver analysis of variance. Am. J. Cardiol. *46*:619, 1980.
200. Goris, M. L., Daspit, S. G., McLaughlin, P., and Kriss, J. P.: Interpolative background subtraction. J. Nucl. Med. *17*:744, 1976.
201. Narahara, K. A., Hamilton, G. W., Williams, D. L., and Gould, K. L.: Myocardial imaging with thallium-201: An experimental model for analysis of the true myocardial and background image components. J. Nucl. Med. *18*:781, 1977.
202. Cantez, S., Harper, P. V., Atkins, F., Sbarboro, J., and Karunaratne, H.: Tomography in cardiac imaging. J. Nucl. Med. *18*:642, 1977.
203. Atwood, E., Jensen, D., Froelicher, V., Witztum, K., Gerber, K., Gilpin, E., and Ashburn, W.: Agreement in human interpretation of analog thallium myocardial perfusion images. Circulation *64*:601, 1981.
204. Meade, R. C., Bamrah, V. S., Horgan, J. D., Ruetz, P. P., Kronenwetter, C., and Yeh, E.: Quantitative methods in the evaluation of thallium-201 myocardial perfusion images. J. Nucl. Med. *19*:1175, 1978.
205. Koral, K. F., Rogers, W. L., and Knoll, G. F.: Digital tomographic imaging with time-modulated pseudorandom coded aperture and Anger camera. J. Nucl. Med. *16*:402, 1975.
206. Burow, R. D., Pond, M., Schafer, A. W., and Becker, L.: "Circumferential profiles:" A new method for computer analysis of thallium-201 myocardial perfusion images. J. Nucl. Med. *20*:771, 1979.
207. Smart, R. C., Burke, J. J., and Lyons, N. R.: Thallium circumferential profiles in the detection of coronary artery disease—assessment by receiver operating characteristic curve analysis. Eur. J. Nucl. Med. *12*:9, 1986.
208. Wackers, F. J. T. H., Fetterman, R. C., Mattera, J. A., and Clements, J. P.: Quantitative planar thallium-201 stress scintigraphy: A critical evaluation of the method. Semin. Nucl. Med. *15*:46, 1985.
209. Kaul, S., Chesler, D. A., Newell, J. B., Pohost, G. M., Okada, R. D., and Boucher, C. A.: Regional variability in the myocardial clearance of thallium-201 and its importance in determining the presence or absence of coronary artery disease. J. Am. Coll. Cardiol. *8*:95, 1986.
210. Maddahi, J., Abdulla, A., Garcia, E. V., Swan, H. J. C., and Berman, D. S.: Noninvasive identification of left main and triple vessel coronary artery disease: Improved accuracy using quantitative analysis of regional myocardial stress distribution and washout of thallium-201. J. Am. Coll. Cardiol. 7:53, 1986.
211. Kaul, S., Boucher, C. A., Newell, J. B., Chesler, D. A., Greenberg, J. M., Okada, R. D., Strauss, H. W., Dinsmore, R. E., and Pohost, G. M.: Determination of the quantitative thallium imaging variables that optimize detection of coronary artery disease. J. Am. Coll. Cardiol. 7:527, 1986.
212. Ritchie, J. L., Williams, D. L., Harp, G., Statton, J. L., and Caldwell, J. H.: Transaxial tomography with thallium-201 for detecting remote myocardial infarction: Comparison with planar imaging. Am. J. Cardiol. *50*:1236, 1982.
213. Coleman, R. E., Jaszczak, R. J., and Cobb, F. R.: Comparison of 180° and 360° data collection in thallium-201 imaging using single-photon emission computerized tomography (SPECT): Concise communication. J. Nucl. Med. 23:655, 1982.
214. Tamaki, N., Muaki, T., Ishii, Y., Fujita, T., Yamamoto, K., Minato, K., Yonekura, Y., Tamaki, S., Kambara, H., Kawai, C., and Torizuka, K.: Comparative study of thallium emission myocardial tomography with 180° and 360° data collection. J. Nucl. Med. *23*:661, 1982.
215. Borello, J. A., Clinthorne, N. H., Rogers, W. L., Thrall, J. H., and Keyes, J. W., Jr.: Oblique-angle tomography: A restructuring algorithm for transaxial tomographic data. J. Nucl. Med. *22*:471, 1981.
216. Caldwell, J. H., Williams, D. L., Harp, G. D., Stratton, J. R., and Ritchie, J. L.: Quantitation of size of relative myocardial perfusion defect by single-photon emission computed tomography. Circulation *70*(Suppl VI):1048, 1984.
217. Berger, H. J., McClees, E. C., Eisner, R., Malko, J., and Fajman, W. A.: New advances in tomographic cardiac imaging. Curr. Concepts Diagn. Nucl. Med. *1*:10, 1986.
218. Tamaki, S., Nakajima, H., Murakami, T., Yui, Y., Kambara, H., Katodota, K., Yoshida, A., Kawai, C., Tamaki, N., Mukai, T., Issii, Y., and Torizuka, K.: Estimation of infarct size by myocardial emission computed tomography with thallium-201 and its relation to creatine kinase-MB release after myocardial infarction in man. Circulation *66*:994, 1982.
219. Holman, B. L., Moore, S. C., Shulkin, P. M., Kirsch, C. M., English, J. J., and Hill, T. C.: Quantitation of perfused myocardial mass using Tl-201 and emission computed tomography. Invest. Radiol. *18*:322, 1983.
220. Ritchie, J. L., Zaret, B. L., Strauss, H. W., Pitt, B., Berman, D. S., Schelbert, H. R., Ashburn, W. L., Berger, H. J., and Hamilton, G. W.: Myocardial imaging with thallium-201: A multicenter study in patients with angina pectoris or acute myocardial infarction. Am. J. Cardiol. *42*:345, 1978.
221. Verani, M. S., Marcus, M. L., Razzak, M. A., and Ehrhardt, J. C.: Sensitivity and specificity of thallium-201 perfusion scintigrams under exercise in the diagnosis of coronary artery disease. J. Nucl. Med. *19*:773, 1978.
222. Blood, D. K., McCarthy, D. M., Sciacca, R. R., and Cannon, P. J.: Comparison of single-dose and double-dose thallium-201 myocardial perfusion scintigraphy for the detection of coronary artery disease and prior myocardial infarction. Circulation *58*:777, 1978.
223. Ritchie, J. L., Trobaugh, G. B., Hamilton, G. W., Gould, K. L., Narahara, K. A., Murray, J. A., and Williams, D. L.: Myocardial imaging with thallium-201 at rest and during exercise: Comparison with coronary arteriography and resting and stress electrocardiography. Circulation *56*:66, 1977.
224. Botvinick, E. H., Taradash, M. R., Shames, D. M., and Parmley, W. W.: Thallium-201 myocardial perfusion scintigraphy for the clinical clarification of normal, abnormal and equivocal electrocardiographic stress tests. Am. J. Cardiol. *41*:43, 1978.
225. Bailey, I. K., Griffith, L. S. C., Rouleau, J., Strauss, H. W., and Pitt, W.: Thallium-201 myocardial perfusion imaging at rest and during exercise. Comparative sensitivity to electrocardiography in coronary artery disease. Circulation *55*:79, 1977.
226. McCarthy, D. M., Blood, D. K., Sciacca, R. R., and Cannon, P. J.: Single dose myocardial perfusion imaging with thallium-201: Application in patients with nondiagnostic electrocardiographic stress tests. Am. J. Cardiol. *43*:899, 1979.
227. Berger, B. C., Watson, D. D., Taylor, G. T., Craddock, G. B., Martin, R. P., and Beller, G. A.: Sensitivity of quantitative thallium-201 scintigraphy following nondiagnostic exercise stress. Circulation *60*:II-72, 1979.
228. Iskandrian, A. S., and Segal, B. I.: Value of exercise thallium-201 imaging in patients with diagnostic and nondiagnostic exercise electrocardiograms. Am. J. Cardiol. *48*:233, 1981.
229. Diamond, G. A., and Forrester, J. S.: Analysis of probability as an aid in the clinical diagnosis of coronary-artery disease. N. Engl. J. Med. *300*:1350, 1979.
230. Ritchie, J. L.: Myocardial perfusion imaging. Am. J. Cardiol. *49*:1341, 1982.
231. Koss, J. H., Kobren, S. M., Grunwald, A. M., and Bodenheimer, M. M.: Role of exercise thallium-201 myocardial perfusion scintigraphy in predicting prognosis in suspected coronary artery disease. Am. J. Cardiol. *59*:531, 1987.
232. Pamelia, F. X., Gibson, R. S., Watson, D. D., Craddock, G. B., Sirowatka, J., and Beller, G. A.: Prognosis with chest pain and normal thallium-201 exercise scintigrams. Am. J. Cardiol. *55*:920, 1985.
233. Wackers, F. J. Th., Russo, D. J., Russo, D., and Clements, J. P.: Prognostic significance of normal quantitative planar thallium-201 stress scintigraphy in patients with chest pain. J. Am. Coll. Cardiol. *6*:27, 1985.
234. Legrand, V., Hodgson, J. M., Bates, E. R., Aueron, F. M., Mancini, J., Smith, J., Gross, M. D., and Vogel, R. A.: Abnormal coronary flow reserve and abnormal radionuclide exercise test results in patients with normal coronary angiograms. J. Am. Coll. Cardiol. *6*:1245, 1985.
235. Kalff, V., Kelly, M. J., Soward, A., Harper, R. W., Currie, P. J., Lim, Y. L., and Pitt, A.: Assessment of hemodynamic significance of isolated stenoses of the left anterior descending coronary artery using thallium-201 myocardial scintigraphy. Am. J. Cardiol. *55*:342, 1985.
236. Boucher, C. A., Brewster, D. C., Darling, R. C., Okada, R. D., Strauss, H. W., and Pohost, G. M.: Determination of cardiac risk by dipyridamole-thallium imaging before peripheral vascular surgery. N. Engl. J. Med. *312*:389, 1985.
237. Rigo, P., Bailey, I. K., Griffith, L. S. C., Pitt, B., Burow, R. D., Wagner, H. N., Jr., and Becker, L. C.: Value and limitations of segmental analysis of stress thallium myocardial imaging for localization of coronary artery disease. Circulation *61*:973, 1980.
238. Rigo, P., Bailey, I. K., Griffith, L. S. C., Pitt, B., Burow, R. D., Wagner, H. N., Jr., and Becker, L. C.: Value and limitations of segmental analysis of stress thallium myocardial imaging for localization of coronary artery disease. Circulation *61*:973, 1980.
239. Massie, B. M., Botvinick, E. H., and Brundage, B. H.: Correlation of thallium-201 scintigrams with coronary anatomy: Factors affecting region-by-region sensitivity. Am. J. Cardiol. *44*:616, 1979.
240. Dash, H., Massie, B. M., Botvinick, E. H., and Brundage, B. H.: The noninvasive identification of left main and three-vessel coronary artery disease by myocardial stress perfusion scintigraphy and treadmill exercise electrocardiography. Circulation *60*:276, 1979.
241. Nygaard, T. W., Gibson, R. S., Ryan, J. M., Gascho, J. A., Watson, D. D., and Beller, G. A.: Prevalence of high-risk thallium-201 scintigraphic findings in left main coronary artery stenosis: Comparison with patients with multiple- and single-vessel coronary artery disease. Am. J. Cardiol. 53:462, 1984.
242. Beller, G. A., Watson, D. D., Berger, B. C., Martin, R. D., and Taylor, G. J.: Detection of multivessel disease by exercise thallium-201 scintigraphy. Am. J. Cardiol. *45*:482, 1980.
243. Maddahi, J., Garcia, E. V., Berman, D. S., Waxman, A., Swan, H. J., and Forrester, J.: Improved noninvasive assessment of coronary artery disease by quantitative analysis of regional stress myocardial distribution and washout of thallium-201. Circulation *64*:924, 1981.

244. Leppo, J., Boucher, C. A., Okada, R. D., Newell, J. B., Strauss, H. W., and Pohost, G. M.: Serial thallium-201 imaging after dipyridamole infusion: Diagnostic utility in detecting coronary stenoses and relationship to regional wall motion. Circulation *66*:649, 1982.
245. Rozanski, A., Berman, D., Gray, R., Levy, R., Raymond, M., Maddahi, J., Pantaleo, N., Waxman, A. D., Swan, H. J. C., and Matloff, G.: Use of thallium-201 redistribution scintigraphy in the preoperative differentiation of reversible and nonreversible myocardial asynergy. Circulation *64*:936, 1981.
246. Gibson, R. S., Watson, D. D., Taylor, G. J., Crosby, I. K., Wellons, H. L., Holt, N. D., and Beller, G. A.: Prospective assessment of regional myocardial perfusion before and after coronary revascularization surgery by quantitative thallium-201 scintigraphy. J. Am. Coll. Cardiol. *3*:804, 1983.
247. Pfisterer, M., Emmenegger, H., Schmitt, H. E., Muller-Brand, J., Hasse, J., Gradel, E., Laver, M. B., Burckhardt, D., and Burkart, F.: Accuracy of serial myocardial perfusion scintigraphy with thallium-201 for prediction of graft patency early and late after coronary artery bypass surgery. A controlled prospective study. Circulation *66*:1017, 1982.
248. Rehn, T., Griffith, L., Achuff, S., Pond, M., and Becker, L.: Value and limitations of thallium-201 imaging to detect bypass graft patency. Am. J. Cardiol. *43*:434, 1979.
249. Wijns, W., Serruys, P. W., Reiber, J. H. C., de Feyter, P. J., van den Brand, M., Simoons, M. L., and Hugenholtz, P. G.: Early detection of restenosis after successful percutaneous transluminal coronary angioplasty by exercise-redistribution thallium scintigraphy. Am. J. Cardiol. *55*:357, 1985.
250. Brown, K. A., Osbakken, M., Boucher, C. A., Strauss, H. W., Pohost, G. M., and Okada, R. D.: Positive exercise thallium-201 test responses in patients with less than 50% maximal coronary stenosis: Angiographic and clinical predictors. Am. J. Cardiol. *55*:54, 1985.
251. Ahmad, M., Merry, S. L., and Harbach, H.: Thallium-201 scintigraphic evidence of ischemia in patients with myocardial bridges. Am. J. Cardiol. *45*:482, 1980.
252. Makler, P. T., Lavine, S. J., Denenberg, B. S., Bove, A. A., and Idell, S.: Redistribution on the thallium scan in myocardial sarcoidosis: Concise communication. J. Nucl. Med. *22*:428, 1981.
253. Bailey, I. K., Come, P. C., Kelly, D. T., Burow, R. D., Griffith, L. S. C., Strauss, H. W., and Pitt, B.: Thallium-201 myocardial perfusion imaging in aortic valve stenosis. Am. J. Cardiol. *40*:889, 1977.
254. Keyes, J. W., Orlandea, N., Heetderks, W. J., Leonard, P. F., and Rogers, W. L.: The humongotron—a scintillation camera transaxial tomograph. J. Nucl. Med. *18*:381, 1977.
255. Gaffney, F. A., Wohl, A. J., Blomqvist, C. G., Parkey, R. W., and Willerson, J. T.: Thallium-201 myocardial perfusion studies in patients with mitral valve prolapse syndrome. Am. J. Med. *64*:21, 1978.
256. Klein, G. J., Kostuk, W. J., Boughner, D. R., and Chamberlain, M. J.: Stress myocardial imaging in mitral leaflet prolapse syndrome. Am. J. Cardiol. *42*: 746, 1978.
257. Massie, B., Botvinick, E. H., Shames, D., Taradash, M., Werner, J., and Schiller, N.: Myocardial perfusion scintigraphy in patients with mitral valve prolapse. Circulation *57*:19, 1978.
258. Maseri, A., Parodi, O., Severi, S., and Pesola, A.: Transient transmural reduction of myocardial blood flow, demonstrated by thallium-201 scintigraphy, as a cause of variant angina. Circulation *54*:280, 1976.
259. Ricci, D. R., Orlick, A. E., Doherty, P. W., Cipriano, P. R., and Harrison, D. C.: Reduction of coronary blood flow during coronary artery spasm occurring spontaneously and after provocation by ergonovine maleate. Circulation *57*: 392, 1978.
260. Waters, D. D., Chaitman, B. R., Dupras, G., Theroux, P., and Mizgala, M. D.: Coronary artery spasm during exercise in patients with variant angina. Circulation *59*:580, 1979.
261. Bulkley, B. H., Rouleau, J., Strauss, W., and Pitt, B.: Idiopathic hypertrophic subaortic stenosis: Detection by thallium-201 myocardial perfusion imaging. N. Engl. J. Med. *293*:1113, 1975.
262. Bulkley, B. H., Rouleau, J. R., Whitaker, J. Q., Strauss, H. W., and Pitt, B.: The use of ^{201}thallium for myocardial perfusion imaging in sarcoid heart disease. Chest *72*:27, 1977.
263. Bulkley, B. H., Hutchins, G. M., Bailey, I., Strauss, H. W., and Pitt, B.: Thallium-201 imaging and gated cardiac blood pool scans in patients with ischemic and idiopathic congestive cardiomyopathy: A clinical and pathologic study. Circulation *55*:753, 1977.
264. Follansbee, W. P., Curtiss, E. I., Medsger, T. A. Jr., Steen, V. D., Uretsky, B. F., Ownes, G. R., and Rodnan, G. P.: Physiologic abnormalities of cardiac function in progressive systemic sclerosis with diffuse scleroderma. N. Engl. J. Med. *310*:142, 1984.
265. Dunn, R. F., Wolff, L., Wagner, S., and Botvinick, E. H.: The inconsistent pattern of thallium defects: A clue to the false positive perfusion scintigram. Am. J. Cardiol. *48*:224, 1981.
266. Wackers, F. J. T., Sokole, E. B., Samson, G., van der Schoot, J. B., Lie, K. I., Liem, K. L., and Wellens, H. J. J.: Value and limitations of thallium-201 scintigraphy in the acute phase of myocardial infarction. N. Engl. J. Med. *295*:1, 1976.
267. Wackers, F. J. T., Lie, K. I., Liem, K. L., Sokole, E. B., Samson, G., van der Schoot, J. B., and Durrer, D.: Thallium-201 scintigraphy in unstable angina pectoris. Circulation *57*:738, 1978.
268. DiCola, V. C., Downing, S. F., Donabedian, R. K., and Zaret, B. L.: Pathophysiological correlates of thallium-201 myocardial uptake in experimental infarction. Cardiovasc. Res. *11*:141, 1977.
269. Henning, H., Schelbert, H. R., Righetti, A., Ashburn, W. L., and O'Rourke, R. A.: Dual myocardial imaging with technetium-99m pyrophosphate and thallium-201 for detecting, localizing and sizing acute myocardial infarction. Am. J. Cardiol. *40*:147, 1977.
270. Mueller, H. S., Fletcher, J. W., and Ayres, S. M.: 201-Thallium image and creatine kinase MB infarct size—evaluation of variable treatment responses (abstr). Circulation *60*(Suppl. II):163, 1979.
271. Buja, L. M., Parkey, R. W., Stokely, E. M., Bonte, F. J., and Willerson, J. T.: Pathophysiology of technetium-99m stannous pyrophosphate and thallium-201 scintigraphy of acute anterior myocardial infarct in dogs. J. Clin. Invest. *57*:1508, 1976.
272. Wackers, F. J., Becker, A. E., Samson, G., Sokole, E. B., van der Schoot, J. B., Vet, A. J. T. M., Lie, K. I., Durrer, D., and Wellens, H.: Location and size of acute transmural myocardial infarction estimated from thallium-201 scintiscans: A clinicopathological study. Circulation *56*:72, 1977.
273. Smitherman, T. C., Osborn, R. C., and Narahara, K. A.: Serial myocardial scintigraphy after a single dose of thallium-201 in men after acute myocardial infarction. Am. J. Cardiol. *42*:177, 1978.
274. Silverman, K. J., Becker, L. C., Bulkley, B. H., Burow, R. D., Mellits, E. D., Kallman, C. H. and Weisfeldt, M. L.: Value of early thallium-201 scintigraphy for predicting mortality in patients with acute myocardial infarction. Circulation *61*:996, 1980.
275. Gutman, J., Brachman, M., Rozanski, A., Maddahi, J., Waxman, A., and Berman, D. S.: Enhanced detection of proximal right coronary artery stenosis with the additional analysis of right ventricular thallium-201 uptake in stress scintigrams. Am. J. Cardiol. *51*:1256, 1983.
276. Brown, K. A., Boucher, C. A., Okada, R. D., Strauss, H. W., McKusick, K. A., and Pohost, G. M.: Serial right ventricular thallium-201 imaging after exercise: Relation to anatomy of the right coronary artery. Am. J. Cardiol. *50*:1217, 1982.
277. Gibson, R. S., Watson, D. D., Craddock, G. B., Crampton, R. S., Kaiser, D. L., Denny, M. J., and Beller, G. A.: Prediction of cardiac events after uncomplicated myocardial infarction: Prospective study comparing predischarge exercise thallium-201 scintigraphy and coronary angiography. Circulation *68*:321, 1983.
278. Leppo, J. A., O'Brien, J., Rothendler, J. A., Getchell, J. D., and Lee, V. W.: Dipyridamole-thallium-201 scintigraphy in the prediction of future cardiac events after acute myocardial infarction. N. Engl. J. Med. *310*:1014, 1984.
279. Markis, J. E., Malagold, M., Parker, J. A., Silverman, K. F., Barry, W. H., Als, A. V., Paulin, J. S., Grossman, W., and Braunwald, E.: Myocardial salvage after intracoronary thrombolysis with streptokinase in acute myocardial infarction: Assessment of intracoronary thallium-201. N. Engl. J. Med. *305*:777, 1981.
280. Maddahi, J., Ganz, W., Ninomiya, K., Hashida, J., Fishbein, M. C., Mondkar, A., Buchbinder, N., Marcus, H., Geft, I., Shah, P. S., Rozanski, A., Swan, H. J. C., and Berman, D. S.: Myocardial salvage by intracoronary thrombolysis in evolving acute myocardial infarction: Evaluation using intracoronary injection of thallium-201. Am. Heart J. *102*:664, 1981.
281. Krebber, H. J., Schofer, J., Mathey, D., Montz, R., Kalmar, P., and Rodewald, G.: Intracoronary thallium-201 scintigraphy as an immediate predictor of salvaged myocardium following intracoronary lysis. J. Thorac. Cardiovasc. Surg. *87*:27, 1984.
282. Schofer, J., Montz, R., and Mathey, D. G.: Scintigraphic evidence of the "no-reflow" phenomenon in human beings after coronary thrombolysis. J. Am. Coll. Cardiol. *5*:593, 1985.
283. Melin, J. A., Becker, L. C., and Bulkley, B. H.: Differences in thallium-201 uptake in reperfused and nonreperfused myocardial infarction. Cir. Res. *53*:414, 1983.
284. Forman, R., and Kirk, E. S.: Thallium-201 accumulation during reperfusion of ischemic myocardium: Dependence on regional blood flow rather than viability. Am. J. Cardiol. *54*:659, 1984.
285. Granato, J. E., Watson, D. D., Flanagan, T. L., Gascho, J. A., and Beller, G. A.: Myocardial thallium-201 kinetics during coronary occlusion and reperfusion: Influence of method of reflow and timing of thallium-201 administration. Circulation *73*:150, 1986.
286. De Coster, P. M., Melin, J. A., Detry, J-M. R., Braseur, L. A., Beckers, C., and Col, J.: Coronary artery reperfusion in acute myocardial infarction: Assessment by pre- and postintervention thallium-201 myocardial perfusion imaging. Am. J. Cardiol. *55*:889, 1985.
287. Wisenberg, G., Schelbert, H., Hoffman, E., Huang, S. C., Phelps, M. E., and Kuhl, D.: Assessment of regional myocardial function by positron emission computed tomography. J. Nucl. Med. *21*:69, 1980.
288. Robinson, J. D.: Copper 62: A short-lived generator–produced, positron-emitting radionuclide. J. Nucl. Med. *17*:559, 1976.
289. Hack, S. N., Eichling, J. O., Bergmann, S. R., Welch, M. J., and Sobel, B. E.: External quantification of myocardial perfusion by exponential infusion of positron-emitting radionuclides. J. Clin. Invest. *66*:918, 1980.
290. Budinger, T. F., Yanoy Derenzose, Huseman, R. H., Yenc Myoer, B. R., and Sherman, L. G.: Infarction sizing and myocardial perfusion measurements using rubidium-82 and positron emission tomography. Am. J. Cardiol. *45*:39, 1980.
291. Gould, K. L., Goldstein, R. A., Mullani, N. A., Kirkeeide, R. L., Wong, W-H., Tewson, T. J., Berridge, M. C., Bolomey, L. A., Hearts, R. K., Smalling, R. W., Fuentes, F., and Nishikawa, A.: Noninvasive assessment of coronary stenoses by myocardial perfusion imaging during pharmacologic coronary vasodilation. VII. Clinical feasibility of positron cardiac imaging without a cyclotron using generator-produced rubidium-82. J. Am. Coll. Cardiol. *7*:775, 1986.
292. Mullani, N. A., Goldstein, R. A., Gould, K. L., Fisher, D. J., Marani, S. K., and O'Brien, H. A.: Myocardial perfusion with rubidium-82. I. Measurement of extraction fraction and flow with external detectors. J. Nucl. Med. *24*:898, 1983.
293. Goldstein, R. A.: Kinetics of rubidium-82 after coronary occlusion and reperfusion. Assessment of patency and viability in open-chest dog. J. Clin. Invest. *75*:1131, 1985.

294. Goldstein, R. A.: Rubidium-82 kinetics after coronary occlusion: Temporary relation of net myocardial accumulation and viability in open-chested dogs. J. Nucl. Med. *27*:1456, 1986.
295. Phelps, M. E., Huang, S. C., and Raybaud, C.: Factors which effect cerebral uptake and retention of $^{13}NH_3$. Stroke *8*:694, 1977.
296. Schelbert, H. R., Phelps, M. E., Hoffman, E. J., Wang, S. C., Selin, C. B., and Kuhl, D. E.: Regional myocardial perfusion assessed with N-13 labeled ammonia and positron emission computerized axial tomography. Am. J. Cardiol. *43*:209, 1979.
297. Rauch, B., Helus, F., Grunze, M., Braunwald, E., Mall, G., Hasselbach, W., Kubler, W.: Kinetics of N-13-ammonia uptake in myocardial single cells indicating potential limitations in its applicability as a marker of myocardial blood flow. Circulation *71*:387, 1985.
298. Idoine, J. D., Holman, B. L., Jones, A. G., Schneider, R. J., Schroeder, K. L., and Zimmerman, R. E.: Quantification of flow in a dynamic phantom using ^{81}Rb-^{81m}Kr and a sodium iodide detector. J. Nucl. Med. *18*:570, 1977.
299. Bassingthwaighte, J. B., Strandell, T., and Donald, D. E.: Estimation of coronary blood flow by washout of diffusible indicators. Circ. Res. *23*:259, 1968.
300. Shaw, D. J., Pitt, A., and Friesinger, G. C.: Autoradiographic study of the ^{133} xenon disappearance method for measurement of myocardial blood flow. Cardiovasc. Res. *6*:268, 1972.
301. Cannon, P. J., Weiss, M. B., and Casarella, W. J.: Studies of regional myocardial blood flow: Results in patients with left anterior descending coronary artery disease. Semin. Nucl. Med. *6*:279, 1976.
302. Holman, B. L., Adams, D. F., Jewitt, D., Eldh, P., Idoine, J., Cohn, P. F., Gorlin, R., and Adelstein, S. J.: Measuring regional myocardial blood flow with ^{133}Xe and the Anger camera. Radiology *112*:99, 1974.
303. Cannon, P. J., Dell, R. B., and Dwyer, E. M., Jr.: Measurement of regional myocardial perfusion in man with ^{133}xenon and a scintillation camera. J. Clin. Invest. *51*:964, 1972.
304. Cannon, P. J., Dell, R. B., and Dwyer, E. M., Jr.: Regional myocardial perfusion rates in patients with coronary artery disease. J. Clin. Invest. *51*:978, 1972.
305. Cohn, P. F., Maddox, D., Holman, B. L., Markis, J. E., Adams, D. F., and See, J. R.: Effect of sublingually administered nitroglycerin on regional myocardial blood flow in patients with coronary artery disease. Am. J. Cardiol. *39*: 672, 1977.
306. Mann, T., Cohn, P. F., Holman, B. L., Green, L. H., Markis, J. E., and Philips, D. A.: Effect of nitroprusside on regional myocardial blood flow in coronary artery disease. Results in 25 patients and comparison with nitroglycerin. Circulation *57*:732, 1978.
307. Ashburn, W. L., Braunwald, E., Simon, A. L., Peterson, K. L., and Gault, J. H.: Myocardial perfusion imaging with radioactive-labeled particles injected directly into the coronary circulation of patients with coronary artery disease. Circulation *44*:851, 1971.
308. Jansen, C., Judkins, M. P., Grames, G. M., Gander, M., and Adams, R.: Myocardial perfusion color scintigraphy with MAA. Radiology *109*:369, 1973.
309. Selwyn, A. P., Shea, M. J., Foale, R., Deanfield, J. E., Wilson, R., DeLandsheere, C. M., Turton, D. L., Brady, F., Pike, V. W., and Brookes, D. I.: Regional myocardial blood flow after myocardial infarction: Application of the microsphere principle in man. Circulation *73*:433, 1986.
310. Marshall, R. C., Tillisch, J. H., Phelps, M. E., Huang, S-C., Carson, R., Henze, E., and Schelbert, H. R.: Identification and differentiation of resting myocardial ischemia and infarction in man with positron computed tomography, ^{18}F-labeled fluorodeoxyglucose and N-13 ammonia. Circulation *67*:766, 1983.
311. Phelps, M. E., Hoffman, E. J., Selin, C., Huang, S. C., Robinson, G., MacDonald, O., Schelbert, H., and Kuhl, D. E.: Investigation of [^{18}F] 2-fluoro-2-deoxyglucose for the measure of myocardial glucose metabolism. J. Nucl. Med. *19*:1311, 1978.
312. Ratib, O., Phelps, M. E., Huang, S. C., Henze, E., Selin, C., and Schelbert, H. R.: Determination of myocardial metabolic rate (MRGlc) by positron computed tomography (PCT) and fluoro-18 deoxyglucose (FDG) (abstr). J. Nucl. Med. *22*:P11, 1981.
313. Huang, S. C., Phelps, M. E., Hoffman, E. J., Sideris, K., Selin, C. J., and Kuhl, D. E.: Noninvasive determination of local cerebral metabolic rate of glucose in man. Am. J. Physiol. *238*:E69, 1980.
314. Phelps, M. E., Huang, S. C., Hoffman, E. J., Selin, C., Sokoloff, L., and Kuhl, D. E.: Tomographic measurement of local cerebral glucose metabolic rate in man with (F-18)2-fluoro-2-deoxy-D-glucose: Validation of method. Ann. Neurol. *6*:371, 1979.
315. Opie, L. H., Owen, P., and Riemersma, R. A.: Relative rates of oxidation of glucose and free fatty acids by ischemic and nonischemic myocardium after coronary ligation in the dog. Eur. J. Clin. Invest. *3*:419, 1973.
316. Tillisch, J., Brunken, R., Marshall, R., Schwaiger, M., Mandelkern, M., Phelps, M., and Schelbert, H.: Reversibility of cardiac wall motion abnormalities predicted by positron tomography. N. Engl. J. Med. *314*:884, 1986.
317. Neely, J. R., Rovetto, M. J., and Oram, J. F.: Myocardial utilization of carbohydrate and lipids. Progr. Cardiovasc. Dis. *15*:289, 1972.
318. Neely, J. R., and Morgan, H. E.: Relationship between carbohydrates and lipid metabolism and the energy balance of heart muscle. Ann. Rev. Physiol. *36*: 413, 1974.
319. Schelbert, H. R.: The heart. *In* Ell, P. J., and Holman, B. L. (eds.): Computed Emission Tomography. Oxford, Oxford University Press, 1982, p. 91.
320. Padgett, H. C., Robinson, G. D., Barrio, J. R.: [1-^{11}C] palmitic acid: Improved radiopharmaceutical preparation. Int. J. Appl. Radiat. Isot. *33*:1471, 1982.
321. Geltman, E. M., Smith, J. L., Beecher, D., Ludbrook, P. A., Ter-Pogossian, M. M., and Sobel, B. E.: Altered regional myocardial metabolism in congestive cardiomyopathy detected by positron tomography. Am. J. Med. *74*:773, 1983.
322. Schelbert, H. R., Henze, E., Phelps, M. E., and Kuhl, D. E.: Assessment of regional myocardial ischemia by positron-emission computed tomography. Am. Heart J. *103*:588, 1982.
323. Schon, H. R., Schelbert, H. R., Robinson, G., Barrio, J., and Phelps, M.: C-11 palmitic acid for the noninvasive evaluation of regional myocardial fatty acid metabolism with positron computed tomography. I. Kinetics of C-11 palmitic acid in normal myocardium. Am. Heart J. *103*:532, 1982.
324. Schon, H. R., Schelbert, H. R., Najafi, A., Robinson, G., and Barrio, J. R.: C-11 labeled palmitic acid for the evaluation of regional myocardial fatty acid metabolism with positron computed tomography. II. Kinetics of C-11 palmitic acid in acute ischemic myocardium. Am. Heart J. *103*:548, 1982.
325. Hillis, L. D., and Braunwald, E.: Myocardial ischemia. N. Engl. J. Med. *296*:971, 1034, and 1093, 1977.
326. Schon, H. R., Senekowitsch, R., Berg, D., Schneidereit, M., Reidel, G., Kriegel, H., Pabsth, W., and Blomer, H.: Measurement of myocardial fatty acid metabolism: Kinetics of iodine-123 heptadecanoic acid in normal dog hearts. J. Nucl. Med. *27*:1449, 1986.
327. Klein, M. S., Goldstein, R. A., Welch, M. J., and Sobel, B. E.: External assessment of myocardial metabolism with [^{11}C] palmitate in rabbit hearts. Am. J. Physiol. *237*:H51, 1979.
328. Goldstein, R. A., Klein, M. S., Welch, M. J., and Sobel, B. E.: External assessment of myocardial metabolism with C-11 palmitate in vivo. J. Nucl. Med. *21*:342, 1980.
329. Goldstein, R. A., Klein, M. S., and Sobel, B. E.: Detection of myocardial ischemia before infarction, based on accumulation of labeled pyruvate. J. Nucl. Med. *21*:1101, 1980.
330. Poe, N. D., Robinson, G. D., Jr., and MacDonald, N. S.: Myocardial extraction of labeled long-chain fatty acid analogs. Proc. Soc. Exp. Biol. Med. *148*:215, 1975.
331. Reske, S. N., Machulla, H.-J., Biersack, H. J., Lackner, K., Knopp, R., and Winkler, C.: Nicht-invasive Erfassung des regionalen myocardialen Stoffwechsels von J-123-para-Phenylpentadecansaure durch single photon tomography. Nucklearmedizin *19*:258, 1982.
332. Chanusssot, F., and Debry, G.: Incorporation d'acid heptadé canoï que dans les lipides hé patiques du rat Wistar. J. Physiol. (Paris) *76*:831, 1980.
333. Knust, E. J., Kupfernagel, C. H., and Stocklin, G.: Long-chain F-18 fatty acids for the study of regional metabolism in heart and liver: Odd-even effects of metabolism in mice. J. Nucl. Med. *20*:1170, 1979.
334. van der Wall, E. E., Westera, G., den Hollander, W., and Visser, F. C.: External detection of regional myocardial metabolism with radioiodinated hexadecanoic acid in the dog heart. Eur. J. Nucl. Med. *6*:147, 1981.
335. van der Wall, E. E., Heidendal, G. A. K., den Hollander, W., Westera, G., and Roos, J. P.: Metabolic myocardial imaging with I-123 labeled heptadecanoic acid in patients with stable angina pectoris. Eur. J. Nucl. Med. *6*:391, 1981.
336. Okada, R. D., Strauss, H. W., Elmaleh, D., Yasuda, T., Werre, G., and Boucher, C. A.: Myocardial kinetics of I-123 labeled-16-hexadecanoic acid (abstr). Circulation *64*(Suppl. IV):235, 1981.
337. van der Wall, E. E., den Hollander, W., Heidendal, G. A. K., Westera, G., Majid, P. A., and Roos, J. P.: Dynamic myocardial scintigraphy with ^{123}I-labeled free fatty acids in patients with myocardial infarction. Eur. J. Nucl. Med. *6*:383, 1981.

INFARCT-AVID MYOCARDIAL SCINTIGRAPHY

338. Holman, B. L., Tanaka, T. T., and Lesch, M.: Evaluation of radiopharmaceuticals for the detection of acute myocardial infarction in man. Radiology *121*:427, 1976.
339. Bonte, F. J., Parkey, R. W., Graham, K. D., Moore, J., and Stokely, E. M.: A new method for radionuclide imaging of myocardial infarcts. Radiology *110*:473, 1974.
340. Parkey, R. W., Bonte, F. J., Meyer, S. L., Atkins, J. M., Curry, G. L., Stokely, E. M., and Willerson, J. T.: A new method for radionuclide imaging of acute myocardial infarction in humans. Circulation *50*:540, 1974.
341. Zaret, B. L., DiCola, V. C., Donabedian, R. K., Puri, S., Wolfson, S., Freedman, G. S., and Cohen, L. S.: Dual radionuclide study of myocardial infarction. Relationships between myocardial uptake of potassium-43, technetium-99m stannous pyrophosphate, regional myocardial blood flow and creatine phosphokinase depletion. Circulation *53*:422, 1976.
342. Jennings, R. B., Herson, P. B., and Sommers, H. M.: Structural and functional abnormalities in mitochondria isolated from ischemic dog myocardium. Lab. Invest. *20*:548, 1969.
343. Shen, A. C., and Jennings, R. B.: Myocardial calcium and magnesium in acute ischemic injury. Am. J. Pathol. *67*:417, 1972.
344. Sommers, H. M., and Jennings, R. B.: Experimental acute myocardial infarction: Histologic and histochemical studies of early myocardial infarct induced by temporary or permanent occlusion of a coronary artery. Lab. Invest. *13*:1491, 1964.
345. D'Agostino, A. N., and Chiga, M.: Mitochondrial mineralization in human myocardium. Am. J. Clin. Pathol. *53*:820, 1970.
346. Willerson, J. T., Parkey, R. W., Bonte, F. J., Lewis, S. E., Corbett, J., and Buja, L. M.: Pathophysiologic considerations and clinicopathological correlates of technetium-99m stannous pyrophosphate myocardial scintigraphy. Semin. Nucl. Med. *10*:54, 1980.
347. Buja, L. M., Parkey, R. W., Stokely, E. M., Bonte, F. J., and Willerson, J. T.: Pathophysiology of technetium-99m stannous pyrophosphate and thallium-201 scintigraphy of acute anterior myocardial infarcts in dogs. J. Clin. Invest. *57*:1508, 1976.
348. Holman, B. L., Ehrie, M., and Lesch, M.: Correlation of acute myocardial infarct scintigraphy with postmortem studies. Am. J. Cardiol. *37*:311, 1976.

349. Buja, L. M., Poliner, L. R., Parkey, R. W., Pulido, J. I., Hutcheson, D., Platt, M. R., Mills, L. J., Bonte, F. J., and Willerson, J. T.: Clinicopathologic study of persistently positive technetium-99m stannous pyrophosphate myocardial scintigrams and myocytolytic degeneration after myocardial infarction. Circulation *56*:1016, 1977.
350. Holman, B. L., Lesch, M., and Alpert, J. S.: Myocardial scintigraphy with technetium-99m pyrophosphate during the early phase of acute infarction. Am. J. Cardiol. *41*:39, 1978.
351. Khaw, B. A., Gold, H. K., Leinback, R. C., Fallon, J. T., Strauss, W., Pohost, G. M., and Haber, E.: Early imaging of experimental myocardial infarction by intracoronary administration of ^{131}I-labeled anticardiac myosin $(Fab')_2$ fragments. Circulation 58:1137, 1978.
352. Khaw, B. A., Gold, H. K., Yasuda, T., Leinbach, R. C., Kanke, N., Fallon, J. T., Barlai-Kovach, M., Strauss, H. W., Sheehan, F., and Haber, E.: Scintigraphic quantification of myocardial necrosis in patients after intravenous injection of myosin-specific antibody. Circulation *74*:501, 1986.
353. Riba, A. L., Thakur, M. L., Gottschalk, A., and Zaret, B. L.: Imaging experimental coronary artery thrombosis with indium-111 platelets. Circulation *60*: 767, 1979.
354. Yamada, M., Hoki, N., Ishikawa, K., Yoshima, H., Hata, S., Ohkubo, N., Matsuwaka, R., Furubayashi, K., Fukushima, M., Onishi, K., and Kobayashi, Y.: Detection of left atrial thrombi in man using indium-111 labeled autologous platelets. Br. Heart J. *51*:298, 1984.
355. Fox, K. A. A., Bergmann, S. R., Mathias, C. J., Powers, W. J., Siegel, B. A., Welch, M. J., and Sobel, B. E.: Scintigraphic detecting of coronary artery thrombi in patients with acute myocardial infarction. J. Am. Coll. Cardiol. *4*:975, 1984.
356. Riba, A. L., Thakur, M. L., Gottschalk, A., Andriole, V. T., and Zaret, B. L.: Imaging experimental infective endocarditis with indium-111–labeled blood cellular components. Circulation *59*:336, 1979.
357. Holman, B. L., and Wynne, J.: Infarct avid (hot spot) myocardial scintigraphy. Radiol. Clin. North Am. *18*:487, 1980.
358. Berman, D. S., Amsterdam, E. A., Hines, H. H., Denaro, G. L., Salel, A. F., Ikeda, R., Jansholt, H. A., and Mason, D. T.: Problem of diffuse cardiac uptake of technetium-99m pyrophosphate in the diagnosis of acute myocardial infarction: Enhanced scintigraphy accuracy by computerized selective blood pool subtraction. Am. J. Cardiol. *40*:768, 1977.
359. Cowley, M. J., Mantle, J. A., Rogers, W. J., Russell, R. O., Jr., Rackley, C. E., and Logic, J. R.: Technetium-99m stannous pyrophosphate myocardial scintigraphy. Reliability and limitations in assessment of acute myocardial infarction. Circulation *56*:192, 1977.
360. Berman, D. S., Amsterdam, E. A., Hines, H. H., Salel, A. F., Bailey, G. J., DeNardo, G. L., and Mason, D. T.: New approach to interpretation of technetium-99m pyrophosphate scintigraphy in detection of acute myocardial infarction. Am. J. Cardiol. *39*:341, 1977.
361. Holman, B. L., Chisholm, R. J., and Braunwald, E.: The prognostic implications of acute myocardial infarct scintigraphy with ^{99m}Tc-pyrophosphate. Circulation *57*:320, 1978.
362. Jengo, J. A., Mena, I., Joe, S. H., and Criley, J. M.: The significance of calcific valvular heart disease in Tc-99m pyrophosphate myocardial infarction scanning: Radiographic, scintigraphic, and pathological correlation. J. Nucl. Med. *18*:776, 1977.
363. Pugh, B. R., Buja, L. M., Parkey, R. W., Poliner, L. R., Stokely, E. M., Bonte, F. J., and Willerson, J. T.: Cardioversion and "false positive" technetium-99m stannous pyrophosphate myocardial scintigrams. Circulation *54*:399, 1976.
364. Ahmad, M., Dubiel, J. P., and Verdon, T. A.: Technetium-99m stannous pyrophosphate myocardial imaging in patients with and without left ventricular aneurysm. Circulation *58*:833, 1979.
365. Go, R. T., Chiu, C. L., Doty, D. B., Cheng, H. F., and Christie, J. H.: Radionuclide imaging of experimental myocardial contusion. J. Nucl. Med. *15*:1174, 1974.
366. Massie, B. M., Botvinick, E. H., Werner, J. A., Chatterjee, K., and Parmley, W. W.: Myocardial scintigraphy with technetium-99m stannous pyrophosphate: An insensitive test for nontransmural myocardial infarction. Am. J. Cardiol. *43*:186, 1979.
367. Malin, F. R., Rollo, D., and Gertz, E. W.: Sequential myocardial scintigraphy with technetium-99m stannous pyrophosphate following myocardial infarction. J. Nucl. Med. *19*:1111, 1978.
368. Sharpe, D. N., Botvinick, E. H., Shames, D. M., Schiller, N. B., Massie, B. M., Chatterjee, K., and Parmley, W. W.: The noninvasive diagnosis of right ventricular infarction. Circulation *57*:483, 1978.
369. Dailey, P. O., Ashburn, W., and Ross, J., Jr.: Usefulness of preoperative and postoperative Tc-99m(Sn) pyrophosphate scans in patients with ischemic and valvular heart disease. Am. J. Cardiol. *39*:43, 1977.
370. Burdine, J. A., DePuey, E. G., Orzan, F., Mathur, V. S., and Hall, R. J.: Scintigraphic, electrocardiographic, and enzymatic diagnosis of perioperative myocardial infarction in patients undergoing myocardial revascularization. J. Nucl. Med. *20*:711, 1979.
371. Platt, M. R., Parkey, R. W., Willerson, J. T., Bonte, F. J., Shapiro, W., and Sugg, W. L.: Technetium stannous pyrophosphate myocardial scintigrams in the recognition of myocardial infarction in patients undergoing coronary artery revascularization. Ann. Thorac. Surg. *21*:311, 1976.
372. Siegel, A. J., Silverman, L. M., and Holman, B. L.: Elevated creatine kinase MB isoenzyme levels in marathon runners. J.A.M.A. *246*:2049, 1981.
373. Rude, R. E., Parkey, R. W., Bonte, F. J., Lewis, S. E., Twieg, D., Buja, L. M., and Willerson, J. T.: Clinical implications of the technetium-99m stannous pyrophosphate myocardial scintigraphy "doughnut" pattern in patients with acute myocardial infarcts. Circulation *59*:721, 1979.
374. Aldor, E., Heeger, H., Kahn, P., and Kainz, W.: Long-time follow-up scintigraphy with ^{99m}Tc-pyrophosphate after myocardial infarction. Z. Kardiol. *68*: 461, 1979.
375. Keyes, J. W., Leonard, P. F., Brody, S. L., Svetkoff, D. J., Rogers, W. L., and Lucchesi, B. R.: Myocardial infarct quantification in the dog by single photon emission computed tomography. Circulation *58*:227, 1978.
376. Holman, B. L., Goldhaber, S. Z., Kirsch, C., Polak, J. F., Friedman, B. J., English, R. J., and Wynne, J.: Measurement of infarct size using single photon emission computed tomography and technetium-99m pyrophosphate: A description of the method and comparison with patient prognosis. Am. J. Cardiol. *50*:503, 1982.

PULMONARY SCINTIGRAPHY

377. Sapirstein, L. A., and Moses, L. E.: Cerebral and cephalic blood flow in man; basic considerations of the indicator fractionation technique in dynamic clinical studies with isotopes. *In* Proceedings of Symposium held at Oak Ridge Institute of Nuclear Studies, Oct. 21–25, 1963.
378. Wagner, H. N., Hosain, T., and Rhodes, B. A.: Recently developed radiopharmaceuticals: Ytterbium-169 DTPA and technetium-99m microspheres. Radiol. Clin. North Am. *7*:233, 1969.
379. Neumann, R. D., Sostman, H. D., and Gottschalk, A.: Current status of ventilation-perfusion imaging. Semin. Nucl. Med. *10*:198, 1980.
380. Vincent, W. R., Goldberg, S. J., and Desilets, D.: Fatality immediately following rapid infusion of macroaggregates of 99m-Tc albumin (MAA) for lung scan. Radiology *91*:1181, 1968.
381. Taplin, G. V., Johnson, D. E., Dore, E. K., and Kaplan, H. S.: Suspensions of radioalbumin aggregates for photoscanning the liver, spleen, lung, and other organs. J. Nucl. Med. *5*:259, 1964.
382. Tow, D. E., Wagner, H. N., Jr., Lopez-Majano, V., Smith, E. M., and Migita, T.: Validity of measuring regional pulmonary arterial blood flow with macroaggregates of human serum albumin. Am. J. Roentgenol. Rad. Ther. Nucl. Med. *96*:664, 1966.
383. Rootwelt, K., and Vale, J. R.: Pulmonary gas exchange after intravenous injection of ^{99m}Tc-sulphur-colloid albumin macroaggregates for lung perfusion scintigraphy. Scand. J. Clin. Lab. Invest. *30*:14, 1972.
384. Vincent, W. R., Goldberg, S. J., and Desilets, D.: Fatality immediately following rapid infusion of macroaggregates of ^{99m}Tc-albumin (MAA) for lung scan. Radiology *91*:1181, 1968.
385. Marcus, C. S., Mason, G. R., Kuperus, J. H., and Mena, I.: Pulmonary imaging in pregnancy: Maternal risk and fetal dosimetry. Clin. Nucl. Med. *10*:1, 1985.
386. Caride, V. J., Puri, S., Slavin, J. D., Lange, R. C., and Gottschalk, A.: The usefulness of posterior oblique views in perfusion lung imaging. Radiology *121*:669, 1976.
387. Polga, J. P., and Drum, D. E.: Abnormal perfusion and ventilation scintigrams in patients with azygos fissures. J. Nucl. Med. *13*:633, 1972.
388. Potchen, E. J.: Lung scintiscanning. J.A.M.A. *204*:907, 1968.
389. DeNardo, G. L., Goodwin, D. A., Ravasini, R., and Dietrich, P. A.: The ventilatory lung scan in the diagnosis of pulmonary embolism. N. Engl. J. Med. 282:1334, 1970.
390. Farmelant, M. H., and Trainor, J. C.: Evaluation of a ^{133}Xe technique for diagnosis of pulmonary disorders. J. Nucl. Med. *12*:586, 1971.
391. Alderson, P. O., and Line, B. R.: Scintigraphic evaluation of regional pulmonary ventilation. Semin. Nucl. Med. *10*:218, 1980.
392. Li, D. K., Treves, S., Heyman, S., Kirkpatrick, J. A., Jr., Lambrecht, R. M., Ruth, T. J., and Wolf, A. P.: Krypton-81m: A better radiopharmaceutical for assessment of regional lung function in children. Radiology *130*:741, 1979.
393. Fazio, F., and Jones, T.: Assessment of regional ventilation by continuous inhalation of radioactive krypton-81m. Br. J. Med. *1*:673, 1975.
394. Ramanna, L., Alderson, P. O., Waxman, A. D., Berman, D. S., Brachman, M. B., Kroop, S. A., Goldsmith, M., and Tanaseescu, D. E.: Regional comparison of technetium-99m DTPA aerosol and radioactive gas ventilation (xenon and krypton) studies in patients with suspected pulmonary embolism. J. Nucl. Med. 27:1391, 1986.
395. The Urokinase Pulmonary Embolism Trial: A national cooperative study. Circulation *47*:II-66, 1973.
396. Cook, D. J., and Lander, H.: The diagnosis of pulmonary embolism. A review with particular reference to the use of radionuclides. Postgrad. Med. J. *47*:214, 1971.
397. Sostman, H. D., Rapoport, S., Gottschalk, A., and Greenspan, R. H.: Imaging of pulmonary embolism. Invest. Radiol. *21*:443, 1986.
398. McNeil, B. J.: A diagnostic strategy using ventilation-perfusion studies in patients suspect for pulmonary embolism. J. Nucl. Med. *17*:613, 1976.
399. McNeil, B. J., Holman, B. L., and Adelstein, S. J.: The scintigraphic diagnosis of pulmonary embolism. J.A.M.A. *227*:753, 1974.
400. Biello, D. R., Mattar, A. G., McKnight, R. C., and Siegel, B. A.: Ventilation-perfusion studies in suspected pulmonary embolism. A. J. R. *133*: 1033, 1979.
401. Biello, D. R., Mattar, A. G., Osei-Wusu, A., Alderson, P. O., McNeil, B. J., and Siegel, B. A.: Interpretation of indeterminate lung scintigrams. Radiology *133*:189, 1979.
402. Tow, D. E., and Wagner, H. N., Jr.: Recovery of pulmonary arterial blood flow in patients with pulmonary embolism. N. Engl. J. Med. *276*:1053, 1967.
403. McCartney, W. H.: Ventilation-perfusion lung scanning in pulmonary embolus. Clin. Nucl. Med. *6*:P27, 1981.
404. Grossman, W., Dexter, L., and Dalen, J.: The late prognosis of acute pulmonary embolism. N. Engl. J. Med. *289*:55, 1973.
405. Siddiqui, A. R., Wellman, H. N., Klatte, E. C., and Faris, J. V.: Wedged Swan-Ganz catheter causing ventilation-perfusion mismatch: Case report and review of the literature. Clin. Nucl. Med. *8*:597, 1983.

12 NEWER CARDIAC IMAGING TECHNIQUES: Digital Subtraction Angiography; Computed Tomography; Magnetic Resonance Imaging

by CHARLES B. HIGGINS, M.D.

Definitive diagnosis and assessment of the severity of many cardiac diseases is accomplished by imaging techniques. The trend in recent years has been toward the development of less invasive or noninvasive imaging methods. Echocardiography (Chap. 5) and radionuclide imaging (Chap. 11) were early noninvasive techniques that have now matured and become central to cardiovascular diagnosis. During the past several years four new cardiac imaging modalities have been introduced: digital subtraction angiography, ultrafast computed x-ray tomography (cine CT), magnetic resonance (MR), and positron-emission tomography (PET). These techniques, with unique and impressive capabilities, are becoming increasingly important in cardiac diagnosis and assessment. This chapter describes the salient technical features of the first three and reviews the application of each in cardiovascular diseases. Positron-emission tomography is described in Chapter 11.

DIGITAL SUBTRACTION ANGIOGRAPHY

Digital angiography provides at least two advantages for cardiac imaging: enhancement of contrast opacification of the blood pool and facilitation of quantitative analysis of x-ray data. Cardiovascular structures can be evaluated with lower doses of contrast media, enabling the performance of multiple angiograms. Registration of x-ray data in a digital form permits quantitation of ventricular and coronary dimensional and functional parameters.

Upon the introduction of digital angiography in the late 1970's, initial attention focused on this technique as a method to achieve angiography following intravenous injection of contrast media.[1–3] For cardiac diagnosis, this use has not provided distinct advantages over radionuclide methods; instead, digital angiography has evolved as a technique for enhancing contrast of angiograms performed with direct ventricular or coronary injection of low dosages of contrast media and for novel and sophisticated analysis of angiograms.

TECHNICAL FEATURES

Digital angiography is an imaging technique in which the fluoroscopic image is directly converted into digital format by an analog to the digital converter. The various gradations of light (gray scale) on the image intensifier or video screen are converted into numbers. A number is assigned to the intensity of light at each of the picture elements (pixels) composing the video screen. The spatial density of pixels determines the spatial resolution of the system. Most systems currently in use have pixel densities of 256 × 256 or 512 × 512. The density of pixels required for a specific study is dictated by the size of the structure

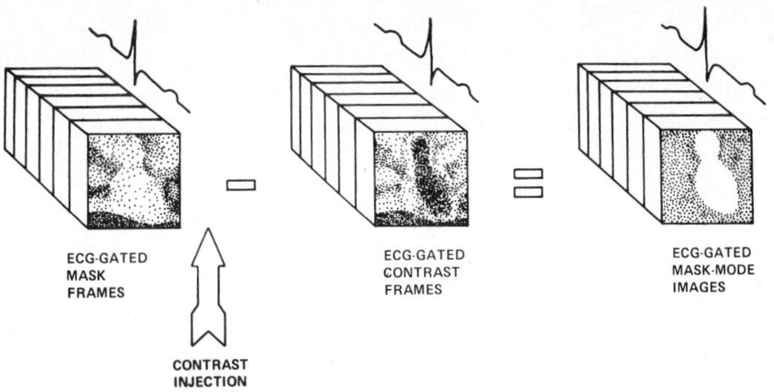

FIGURE 12–1. Schematic representation of mask-mode cardiac imaging. Single or averaged frames before contrast injection are used as the mask from which frames are subtracted during maximal cardiac opacification after contrast injection. In the resultant image, nonopacified structures are removed, leaving behind the contrast-containing heart chambers and vessels. (From Mancini, G. B. J., and Higgins, C. B.: Digital subtraction angiography: A review of cardiac applications. Prog. Cardiovasc. Dis. *52*:1112, 1986.)

to be imaged. A 256 × 256 matrix is adequate for ventriculography, while a 512 × 512 or even 1024 × 1024 matrix is required for coronary angiography. Matrix density has two practical limitations: with increasing density, the signal-to-noise ratio of each pixel decreases and the requirement for computer memory increases.

Contrast enhancement of the images is accomplished by several techniques, such as logarithmic amplification, mask mode subtraction, time interval difference subtraction, and energy subtraction. Only the first two techniques are now regularly utilized. With *mask mode subtraction*, a digitized image obtained prior to arrival of contrast medium is subtracted from the digitized images obtained during contrast opacification, yielding an image containing only the opacified cardiac chambers (mask mode image) (Fig. 12–1). Motion between the mask and opacified images causes misregistration artifacts which can be removed or reduced by using a later mask image or a mask averaged from several unopacified images. Because of cardiac motion, an averaged mask is usually better for mask mode subtraction images of the heart. The mask and opacified images can also be acquired in relation to the electrocardiogram (ECG) so that the end-diastolic mask image is subtracted from the end-diastolic opacified image. A type of time interval difference subtraction important for cardiac image has been called *functional subtraction*, which is useful for assessing left ventricular contraction. This is accomplished by subtracting the end-systolic mask mode image from the end-diastolic mask image to yield an *ejection shell image*, which shows the extent of contraction of the walls of the left ventricle, a technique useful for displaying abnormalities of regional wall motion.[4]

Because of the motion of the heart and the need for a high sampling rate in order to capture end systole, images of the heart must be acquired at 30 frames per second. Only recently have improvements in computer memory allowed direct digital storage of 512 × 512 images acquired in real time at 30 frames per second.

Volumetric analysis of digital ventriculograms has been accomplished using both geometric and videodensitometric methods. The latter method is similar to the count-based techniques applied to radionuclide studies (p. 315). However, videodensitometric measurements are limited by nonuniform x-ray beam, x-ray scatter, and other physical factors.

INTRAVENOUS VENTRICULOGRAPHY

Mask mode subtraction after intravenous injection of contrast media yields images of the left ventricle equivalent to direct left ventriculography for the purposes of quantitating volumes, ejection fraction, and regional wall motion. In several studies comparing intravenous subtracted and direct contrast ventriculography good correlation has been shown between these two techniques for the quantitation of left ventricular volumes and ejection fractions.[4–12] The frequency of arrhythmias during opacification of the left ventricle was considerably less for the intravenous subtraction angiograms.

Intravenous left ventriculograms have been used to evaluate regional left ventricular wall motion in patients with known or suspected coronary artery disease. The agreement between intravenous and direct angiography for detecting wall motion abnormalities is approximately 90 per cent.[10, 12–15] The analysis of regional left ventricular contraction from digital angiographic studies is improved by acquiring the data in a digital form upon which post-processing programs can be applied (Fig. 12–2). Regional contraction can be analyzed by measurements of geometric wall motion, wall thickness, regional ejection fraction from regional ejection shell images[16] and by amplitude and phase analysis of parametric images.[4, 17]

The sensitivity of intravenous ventriculography for detecting wall motion abnormalities has been increased by interventions which raise myocardial oxygen demands.[13–15, 18–20] Digital intravenous ventriculography with atrial pacing has increased considerably the sensitivity for identifying regional wall motion abnormalities compared with the resting study.[13–15] In normal subjects ventricular volumes either increase slightly or do not change, while ejection fraction declines slightly. Patients with ischemic heart disease exhibit a greater reduction in ejection fraction and increase of end-systolic volume during pacing-induced tachycardia.

Intravenous ventriculography has also been carried out during supine bicycle exercise.[18–20] Wall motion abnormalities and decline in global left ventricular function have been documented on exercise compared with resting ventriculograms. However, the quality of the images during exercise is degraded by motion artifacts caused by movement of the patient and greater respiratory excursion and

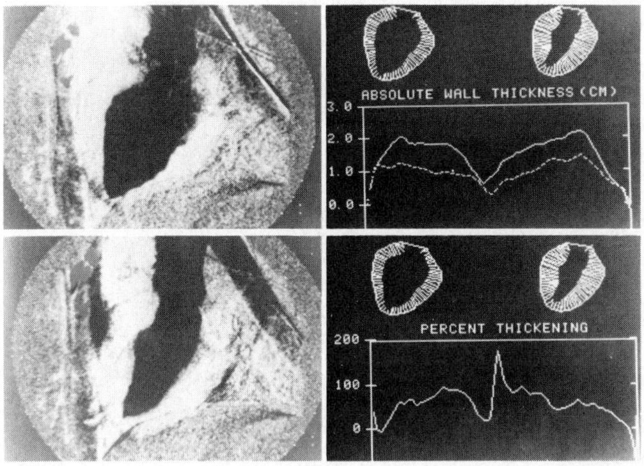

FIGURE 12–2. End-diastolic (*upper left*) and end-systolic (*lower left*) digital ventriculograms obtained in a dog in the left posterior oblique projection. Differential enhancement of the early (ventricular) and later (myocardial) phases of contrast injection allows excellent edge definition of both endocardial and epicardial edges, thereby allowing quantitative measurements of relative wall thickness (upper right) and estimates of wall thickening (lower right). The lower line represents the diastolic thickness around the ventricular circumference and the upper line the systolic thickness. Both systolic and diastolic endocardial edges are clearly visible on the insert. (From Mancini, G. B. J., and Higgins, C. B.: Digital subtraction angiography: A review of cardiac applications. Progr. Cardiovasc. Dis. *52*:1112, 1986.)

frequency during the exercise angiogram. In contrast to radionuclide rest-exercise studies (p. 314), the digital intravenous angiogram has considerably better spatial resolution, which improves regional wall motion analysis, but it is a far more cumbersome procedure for patient and physician and consequently is still infrequently used for routine clinical evaluation. Because of the lower patient acceptance and greater expense and complexity of digital intravenous angiography in comparison with radionuclide angiography, digital angiography by the intravenous route is not widely used.

DIRECT VENTRICULOGRAPHY

Digital subtraction techniques applied to ventriculograms performed after direct injection of contrast media into the left ventricle permit the use of substantially lower dosages of contrast media.[7, 9, 21–23] This has advantages in patients with renal failure, diabetes, congestive heart failure, aortic stenosis, unstable angina, and others at greater risk for complications from the contrast media. Lower dosages also permit several ventriculograms to be done with the same volume of contrast medium; this may be important when multiple ventriculograms are required to evaluate interventions such as atrial pacing and use of pharmacological agents (Fig. 12–3).

Studies with low doses of contrast medium comparing ventriculograms enhanced by digital subtraction with standard-dosage cineangiograms showed close agreement between the left ventricular volumes for the two techniques but a considerably lower incidence of ventricular arrhythmias and less of a rise in end-diastolic pressure accompanying the low-dosage digital study.[7, 9, 21, 22] Recording the study in the digital format also facilitates detailed, quantitative analysis of the imaged data (Figs. 12–2 and 12–3). Videodensitometric analysis of digital subtraction ventriculograms has provided an accurate, objective, and reproducible method for determining right and left ventricular ejection fraction.[24, 25] Left ventricular ejection fraction determined by videodensitometry and geometric (area-length) methods showed a correlation coefficient of 0.88.[25] Geometric assumptions needed for the standard area-length measurements are not needed for videodensitometric analysis so that changes in ventricular shape which are associated with some cardiac diseases are not a potential error. However, *absolute* ventricular volumes are difficult to determine since the concentration of contrast medium in the arterial circulation must be known for this calculation.

Low-dosage ventriculography has permitted multiple ventriculograms to be done without increasing unduly the total load of contrast medium.[26] Tobis et al.[27] compared low-dose ventriculograms at rest and during the peak phase of rapid atrial pacing (Fig. 12–4); 93 per cent of patients with anatomically significant coronary arterial stenoses showed a decrease or no change in ejection during pacing while four of five subjects with anatomically normal coronary arteries experienced an increase of 5 per cent or more.

Digital Coronary Arteriography (See also p. 303)

ANATOMY. Recording of coronary arteriograms with digital techniques has several potential benefits: contrast enhancement, digital size enhancement, application of objective edge detection methods, quantitation of severity of coronary arterial stenoses, estimation of coronary arterial flow velocity, semiquantitation of coronary flow reserve, and immediate availability of the images for examination. The availability of the data in the digital form provides the opportunity for post-processing of the images and application of several mensuration programs (Fig. 12–5). However, the most ambitious hope for digital angiography, the capability of performing coronary angiography by the intravenous injection of contrast media, has not been realized. Because of several unsolvable problems,[28] it is unlikely that the technique in its current configuration will accomplish this goal. The three major problems have been (1) difficulty in subtracting the large contrast pool within the left ventricle and pulmonary veins from the image, (2) low level of contrast enhancement of the coronary arteries, and (3) severe overlapping of some coronary vessels with only one or a few views.

The computer memory required for digital coronary arteriography is

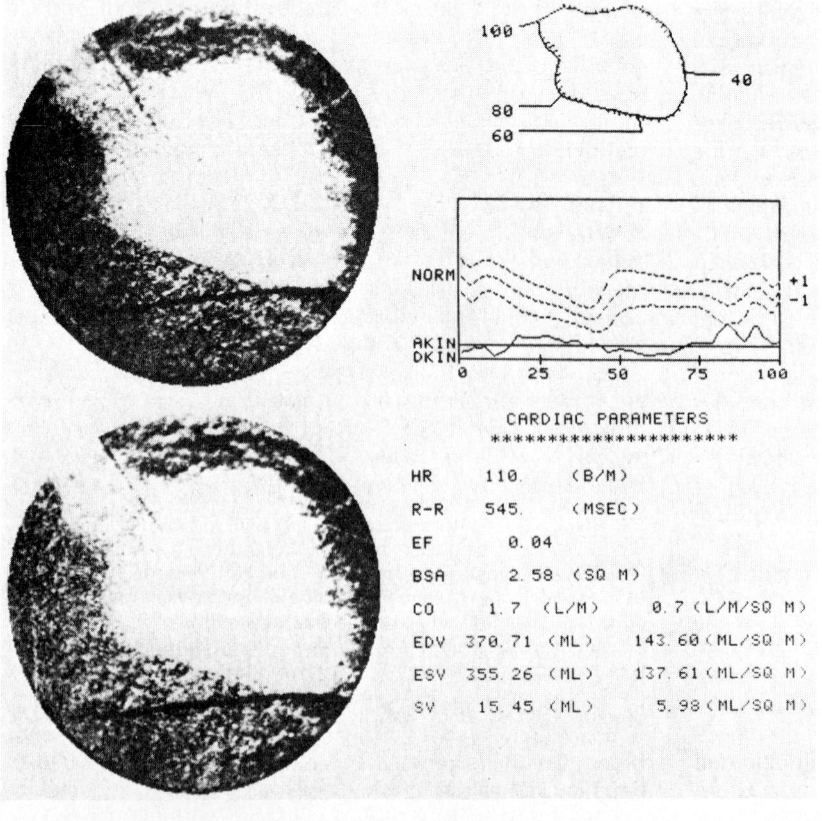

FIGURE 12–3. A direct left ventriculogram obtained with 10 ml of contrast medium diluted in 10 ml of saline and injected over 2 seconds in a young diabetic patient with post-viral cardiomyopathy. The end-diastolic frame is shown in the upper left panel and the end-systolic frame in the lower left. Quantitative parameters in the right panels demonstrate severe global dysfunction, an ejection fraction of less than 10 per cent, and markedly increased ventricular volumes. Despite a resting pulmonary wedge pressure of 40 mm Hg, this diagnostic ventriculogram was obtained without any major hemodynamic perturbations or patient discomfort. (From Mancini, G. B. J., and Higgins, C. B.: Digital subtraction angiography: A review of cardiac applications. Progr. Cardiovasc. Dis. *52*:1112, 1986.)

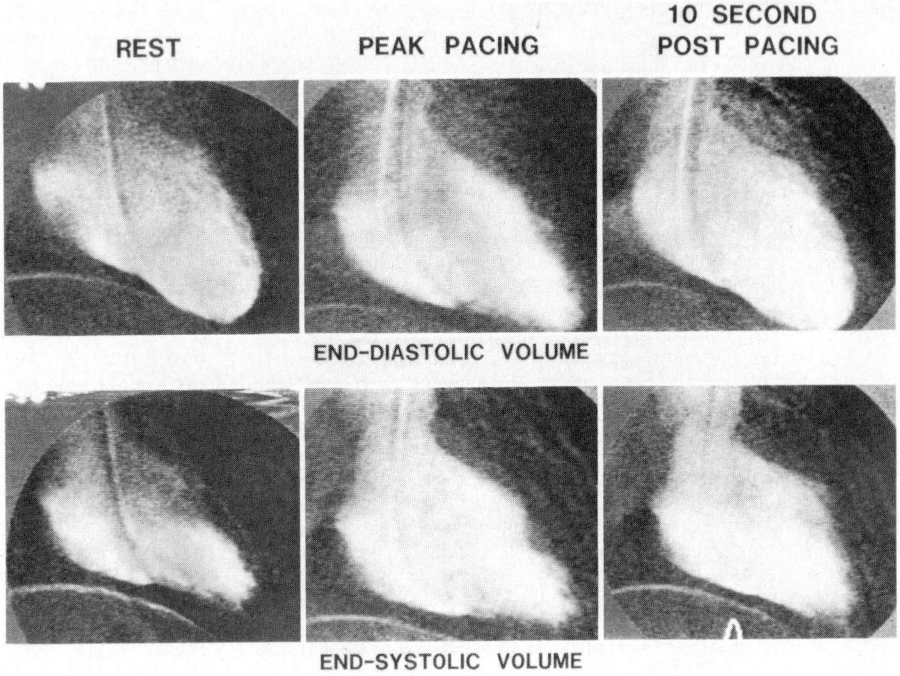

FIGURE 12–4. End-diastolic and end-systolic frames from low-dose direct ventriculogram with digital subtraction. Ventriculograms performed in the basal state at rest (*left*), during peak atrial pacing (*center*), and 10 seconds after cessation of pacing (*right*). Resting ventriculogram showed an ejection fraction of 40 per cent and inferior hypokinesis. At peak pacing, ventriculogram showed inferior akinesis and anterior, apical hypokinesis, and ejection fraction of 16 per cent. Ten seconds after pacing ejection fraction rose to 34 per cent. (From Sato, et al.: Re-evaluation of the role of digital angiography in cardiac diagnosis. *In* New Concepts in Cardiac Imaging. Vol. 3. Boston, G. K. Hall & Co., 1986.)

usually greater than that needed for ventriculography. Spatial resolution for coronary arteriography necessitates a denser matrix such as 1024 × 1024 pixels. Subjective interpretation and manual measurements of the severity of coronary stenosis on arteriograms recorded in the digital mode and subtracted were found to be similar to those defined from film-based cineangiograms.[29] Digital angiography facilitates rapid quantitation of a stenosis. Manual placement of a cursor onto the edges of the stenosis with calibration to the known size of the catheter provides a rapid measurement of the cross-sectional diameter. Recent studies have revealed that absolute lumen diameter or area correlates best with the loss of coronary vasodilation reserve and may be the most precise manner for defining stenosis severity.[30] Brown et al.[30] described and validated a procedure for the biplane outline and digitization of coronary stenoses on cineangiographic film in order to quantitate percentage of diameter stenosis, percentage of area stenosis, minimum diameter, and length of stenosis from which resistance to flow and pressure drop across the stenosis are estimated. With the images already in the digital form, such processing can be readily applied.

Videodensitometry can also be used to quantitate the severity of stenosis.[31–37] With this technique, density of contrast in a stenotic region is compared with density in a normal region, thereby providing an objective estimate of per cent stenosis.

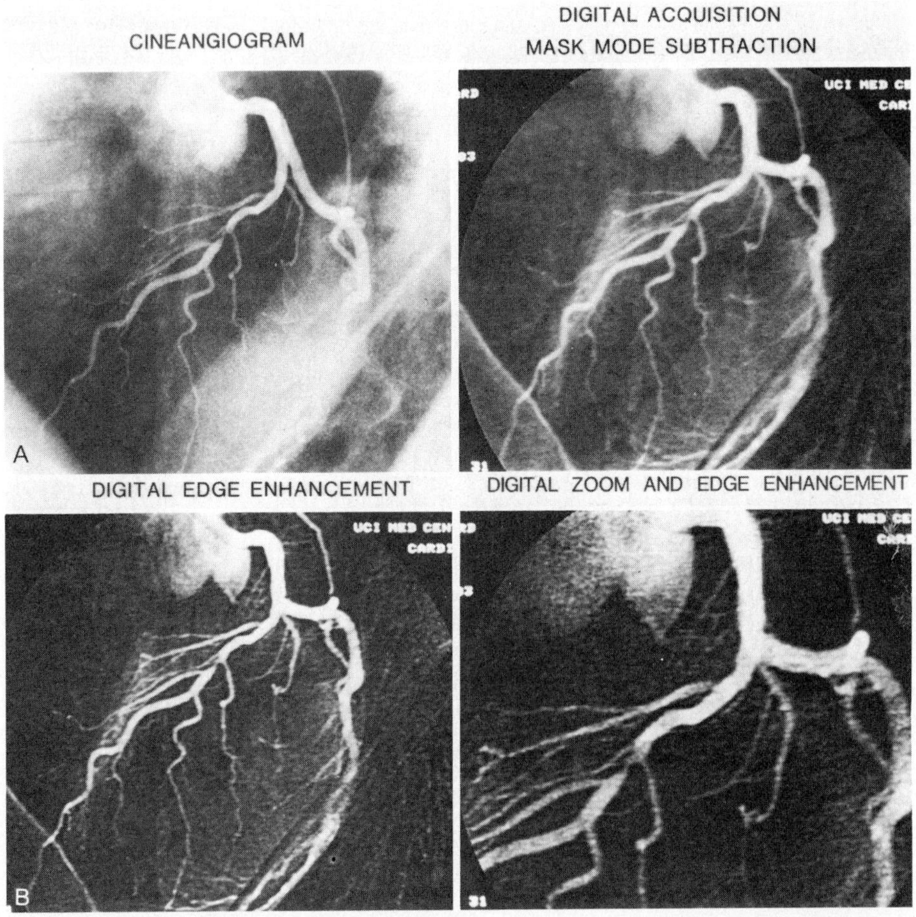

FIGURE 12–5. *A, Left,* Standard 35-mm film-based cineangiographic frame demonstrating high-grade stenosis of the left anterior descending artery (LAD). *Right,* Corresponding digital angiogram with mask-mode subtraction. *B, Left,* Digital angiogram after post-processing with digital-edge enhancement algorithm for increasing sharpness of boundaries. *Right,* region of interest on angiogram magnified fourfold. (From Sato, et al.: Re-evaluation of the role of digital angiography in cardiac diagnosis. *In* New Concepts in Cardiac Imaging. Vol. 3. Boston, G. K. Hall & Co., 1986.)

CORONARY ANATOMY AND MYOCARDIAL PERFUSION

Coronary blood flow and myocardial perfusion have been estimated by several new post-processing image analysis programs.[34–48] Physiological significance of coronary arterial stenoses is documented by demonstrating a decrease in flow in the jeopardized vessel compared with normal vessels. While blood flow at rest is reduced only when the reduction in luminal diameter reaches 85 to 90 per cent, 35 to 40 per cent reduction in luminal diameter has been shown experimentally to cause a decrease in maximal flow augmented by vasodilators.[48] Several post-processing computer algorithms have been used to estimate relative coronary flow and perfusion.[42–47] The input for these algorithms is the x-ray density of a region of interest in relation to time after injection of contrast medium. The flow estimate is generally based on the transit time of a contrast bolus from one site to another or on the rate of wash-out of contrast from a region. Specific measurements include coronary transit time, videodensitometric density-time curves of myocardial opacification (blush), and analysis of videodilution curves acquired from regions of interest placed on the coronary arteries.[45]

Vogel et al.[47] have used a color-coded expression of the transit time of contrast medium in the basal and vasodilated states. This method utilizes ECG-gated acquisition of a mask frame and contrast-enhanced frames of sequential heartbeats at the same phase of the cardiac cycle to depict the time of arrival of contrast medium in various arterial segments and the myocardium. The appearance times of contrast medium in various myocardial regions are determined in basal and dilated states; the appearance times in the basal state divided by hyperemic state is expressed as a reactive hyperemic ration. When the vessel is normal, appearance time decreases in the vasodilated state. The loss of hyperemic flow response caused by a significant stenosis reduces the reactive hyperemic ratio. The movement of the contrast medium into an arterial segment or myocardium on successive cardiac cycles has been recorded on a color-coded composite image called a *myocardial contrast appearance picture*. Somewhat similar semiquantitative estimates of regional flow have also been utilized. Whiting et al.[49] have estimated coronary flow from time-density curves generated from groups of pixels in regions of interest placed over coronary arteries or myocardium during the wash-in and wash-out of contrast media.

Rutishauser et al.,[38] as early as 1970, and more recently Spiller et al.[44] have used videodensitometry to measure transit time (reciprocal of velocity) of the bolus of contrast medium between reference points in the epicardial coronary arteries. Velocity measurements are converted to flow estimates by determining the length and width of the arterial segment between the reference sites. Good correlations have been described between videodensitometric flow and electromagnetic flow measurements in dogs[45, 49, 50] and in man.[44]

While many of the above-described radiographic methods for estimating severity of stenoses and coronary blood flow can be applied to film-based cineangiography, these analyses are facilitated by the presence of the image data in digital form. The image processing computers of digital radiographic units promote the sophisticated analysis of coronary angiograms.

Digital fluoroscopic units, with their imaging processing computer, are becoming adjuncts to catheterization laboratories. Since the majority of catheterizations are done for diagnosis of coronary artery disease, these units will have their most important use for recording coronary angiograms. Subtraction can be used to enhance contrast of low doses of contrast medium injected into the coronary arteries. However, usually unsubtracted standard dose angiograms are digitally acquired and stored for visualization immediately upon conclusion of the study and for further analysis by an expanding number of post-processing programs. Since comparative studies have shown equal capability of digital coronary angiograms and standard film-based angiograms for the diagnosis and assignment of severity of coronary artery stenoses, the advantages of digital storage—including economic considerations—suggest that it could replace cine films for routine coronary angiography.

Digital fluoroscopic units are also used as adjuncts to noncardiac angiographic laboratories. While the examination of peripheral arteries after intravenous injection is now done infrequently, direct angiography is recorded and stored in digital format. Digital intravenous angiography can serve as an alternative, although less than optimal, method to visualize large vessels (aorta, carotid, and renal arteries) in patients with poor arterial access owing to obstructive peripheral vascular disease.

COMPUTED TOMOGRAPHY (CT)

TECHNICAL ASPECTS

CT scanning of the heart usually requires modification of the standard CT techniques used for investigating other parts of the body. For some purposes, such as evaluation of pericardial disease[51–53] and patency of coronary arterial bypass grafts,[52–54] standard CT techniques are usually adequate. However, assessment of cardiac function and precise definition of intracardiac anatomy necessitate either electrocardiographic (ECG) gating of standard CT scanners[52, 53, 55] or preferably, the use of millisecond CT scanners.[56, 57]

GATED CT SCANNING. One method of overcoming the problem of cardiac motion is critical in obtaining quantitative dimensional data and ejection fractions when standard CT scanners are employed. It can also be used to measure the extent of wall thickening during the cardiac cycle.[55] Two gating techniques have been used: retrospective and prospective gating. With *retrospective gating* the CT scan data and the ECG are recorded simultaneously, but the ECG signal does not guide the acquisition of x-ray data in any manner. Subsequently, the image is reconstructed from data obtained within a select time-window (biological window), bracketing the desired portion of the ECG signal, such as the QRS complex at end-diastole.

The *prospective gating system* allows preselection of a fraction of the R-R interval to be monitored. The biological window width sets the fraction of the cardiac cycle to be represented by each image. Prospective gating insures the even distribution of R waves throughout the scanning circle in the minimal number of scans. This is accomplished by launching of the x-ray tube at the appropriate time relative to the R wave of the ECG input, so that one of the R waves falls into the largest gap in the already-acquired angular x-ray data.

Many of the limitations of the standard CT scanner in cardiac applications have been overcome by the successful construction of CT scanners specifically designed to evaluate central cardiovascular anatomy and function. The *fast CT scanner*, developed by Boyd and colleagues[56] and Ritman and his colleagues,[57] obtains scans at exposure times of 50 msec or less and can generate CT scans at multiple anatomical levels. The fast (cine) CT scanner with electronic scanning methods, which provides complete cardiac imaging in real time without the need for ECG gating, is being used at several centers (Fig. 12–6A).

The fast CT scanner is not limited by the inertia associated with moving mechanical parts. It uses a focused electron beam that is successively swept across four cadmium tungstate target arcs at the

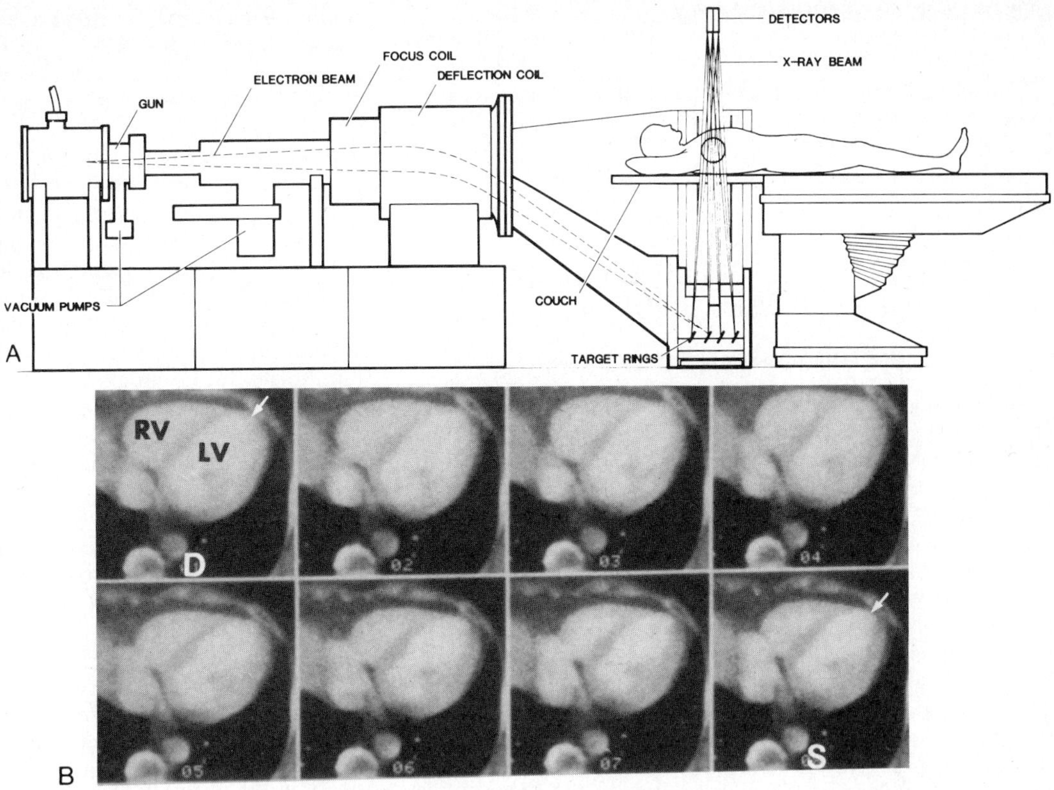

FIGURE 12–6. *A,* Diagram of cine CT scanner. Electron gun produces a stream of electrons that are magnetically focused and directed onto four tungsten target rings. Each target ring emits two fan beams of x-ray. Transmission of x-rays through the subject is registered by detectors arranged over a 180° arc. *B,* Cine CT scan (cine mode) of a patient with an anteroseptal myocardial infarction. Each frame is a 50-msec scan at a different phase of the cardiac cycle; scans done at the rate of 17 scans/sec. Note the thinning of the anterior segment (arrow) on late diastolic (D) frame and failure to thicken on late systolic (S) frame.

speed of light. Each of the four targets generates a fan beam of photons that pass from beneath the patient to a bank of photon detectors arranged in a semicircle above the patient. The cine CT scanner can be operated in three different modes: (1) the *cine mode* is used to assess global and regional myocardial function. The scans are obtained at an exposure time of 50 msec and at a rate of 17 scans/sec (Fig. 12–6*B*). (2) The *triggered mode,* used for flow analysis, employs a series of 20 to 40 successive scans in which each 50-msec exposure is triggered at a specific phase of the cardiac cycle of successive heart beats. From such a series of scans, time-density curves can be constructed for specific regions of interest in the cardiac chamber or myocardium, providing an estimate of transit time, perfusion, or blood flow. (3) The *volume mode* provides eight scans by the use of all four target arcs in an imaging period of approximately 200 msec. These eight transverse scans (1 cm thick) can frequently encompass the entire left ventricular chamber and thereby provide an estimate of left ventricular volume and mass.

For nearly all purposes, intravenous injection of iodinated contrast medium is used to delineate the blood pool on CT scans. The contrast medium can be given as an intravenous bolus injection or a rapid infusion. For evaluation of the heart and great vessels, contrast medium is usually delivered in a bolus over several seconds and in a volume of approximately 25 to 50 ml. Scans are exposed at the estimated time of peak enhancement of the structure of interest. Infrequently, scans are obtained without contrast medium in order to identify calcification of cardiac structures.

EVALUATION OF CARDIAC DIMENSIONS AND FUNCTION

CT scans have the capability of identifying not only the inner endocardial wall but also the epicardial surface. Wall thickness and myocardial mass have been estimated accurately both on standard[58] and ECG-gated CT scans.[55, 59] A recent report has also shown close agreement between mass estimated from fast CT scans and the postmortem measurement of mass (Fig. 12–7).[60]

CT scanning can be used in the assessment of the dynamics of regional myocardial wall-thickening.[55, 61, 62] The method of (1) objective edge detection of the endocardium and epicardium and (2) realignment of end-diastolic and end-systolic images has been used with fast CT scans to quantitate wall thickening dynamics during pharmacological intervention.[61] ECG-gated CT data acquisition with conventional body CT scanners[55] and cine CT[62] in an animal model of regional ischemia have identified the region of ischemia by demonstrating loss of wall thickening during the cardiac cycle. A close correlation has been found between CT measurements and postmortem anatomical measurements of wall thickness and mass.[55, 58, 59]

Left ventricular volumes and ejection fraction can be estimated by contrast angiography (p. 142), echocardiography (p. 89), and gated blood pool nuclear images (p. 317). While the quantitation of ventricular volumes and ejection fraction by CT is not a unique capability, the accuracy of CT can potentially exceed that of the other techniques.[63] It has been demonstrated that left ventricular volume, ejection fraction and stroke volume can be acquired by fast (cine) CT with accuracy and ease.[64–66] Since

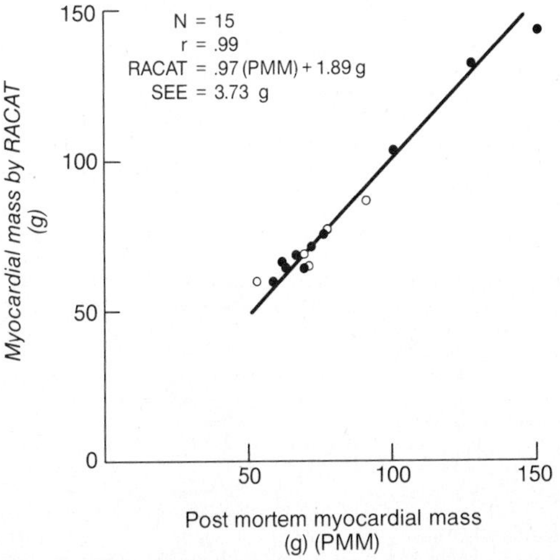

FIGURE 12–7. Graph plots mass determined by rapid-acquisition computer assisted tomography (RACAT) vs. postmortem measurement of left ventricular mass. RACAT is another denotation for cine CT. This study was done in anesthetized dogs. (From Feiring, A., et al.: Determination of left ventricular mass in dogs with rapid-acquisition cardiac CT scanning. Circulation, 72:1355, 1985, by permission of the American Heart Association, Inc.)

CT measures total ventricular stroke volume, the measurement of forward stroke volume by an independent method or the simultaneous quantitation of the right and left ventricular stroke volumes should permit quantification of regurgitant volume.

EVALUATION OF SPECIFIC CARDIAC DISEASES BY CT

ISCHEMIC HEART DISEASE

After myocardial infarction, CT can be used to demonstrate regional wall thinning[67] (Fig. 12–6) and complications of infarction, such as left ventricular aneurysm and mural thrombus (Fig. 12–8). Gated CT or cine CT can also demonstrate left ventricular segmental dysfunction, such as reduced wall thickening and wall motion. In one large series in which standard CT with gating and cineangiography CT were compared with left ventricular cineangiography, a sensitivity of 94 per cent and specificity of 87 per cent were shown for the detection of a regional wall abnormality.[52] The accuracy of detecting the anatomical and functional sequelae of infarction is substantially better for the anterior wall compared with the posterior and diaphragmatic walls of the left ventricle because of the orientation of the heart in relation to the fixed transverse imaging. In one study, all 13 anterior infarcts were detected as either wall thinning or decreased mural density on contrast-enhanced CT scans. However, the infarction site was not identified in three of six patients with inferior infarction.[68]

CT provides unequivocal spatial separation between various regions of the left ventricle, enabling better localization and estimation of the extent of wall thinning after infarction compared with projectional techniques such as left ventriculography and most scintigraphic techniques. Likewise, the site and extent of anterior (Fig. 12–8) and posterior aneurysms of the left ventricle can be well demonstrated. The differentiation by CT between true aneurysm and pseudoaneurysm depends on the identification of the small ostium connecting the left ventricular cavity and the aneurysm (Fig 39–33, p. 1365). False aneurysms are usually substantially larger than true aneurysms and frequently arise from the posterior or inferior wall of the left ventricle.

REGIONAL WALL MOTION. Quantitation of systolic myocardial wall thickening appears to be a particularly useful technique for evaluating regional myocardial contractile function in patients with ischemic heart disease. Gated CT scans[55] and fast CT[61] have been effective in identifying the region of ischemia by demonstrating loss of regional wall thickening during acute coronary occlusion in the canine model. In order to define the capability of the technique of fast CT scanning with contrast enhancement for demonstrating regional contraction abnormalities,[69] a 91 per cent correlation with left ventriculography was found in a group of patients with previous myocardial infarction. Regional wall thickening and inward motion were used as the parameters of regional function; they correlated well with wall motion abnormalities demonstrated on left ventriculography and critical coronary stenoses shown by coronary angiography. Using the cine mode in which 17 frames per second are obtained, wall thickening can be monitored during the course of a single cardiac cycle during peak opacification of the left ventricle (Fig. 12–6).

MYOCARDIAL PERFUSION. Fast CT may also be able to provide an indication of *regional myocardial perfusion.*[61] Estimates of myocardial perfusion are obtained by drawing regions of interest over various sites of the myocardium displayed on the transverse CT scans. The density of the myocardial regions is measured on sequential 50-msec scans acquired during an appropriate duration of the myocardial contrast enhancement phase. From these measurements, time-density curves are constructed; analyses of these curves in regard to contrast appearance and washout are used to estimate regional myocardial perfusion. Thus, fast CT has the potential of providing both regional function and perfusion in a single study. Further study is needed to confirm that flow can be reliably estimated under variable physiological (vasodilatation) and pathological (stenosis) conditions and with equal accuracy at various myocardial sites.

CT has been found to be as accurate as two-dimensional echocardiography for identifying left ventricular *mural thrombus* (p. 123).[70, 71] Indeed, comparative studies have shown greater accuracy of CT compared with two-dimensional echocardiography in demonstration of thrombus in the left atrium.[72]

MYOCARDIAL INFARCTION. Computed tomography with contrast enhancement provides direct visualization of the infarction because of differences between normal and infarcted myocardium in the distribution kinetics of iodinated contrast media.[73–77] The intravenous[74] or intracoronary[78] administration of contrast material produces temporally distinct phases of enhancement of normal and ischemically damaged myocardium. During the perfusion phase, normal myocardium is maximally enhanced (maximum increase in x-ray attenuation value), whereas the area of damage is nonenhanced or minimally enhanced (Fig. 12–9). Several minutes after administration of contrast material, enhancement of normal myocardium has declined and the damaged myocardium is nearly maximally enhanced. In the perfusion phase, the ischemically damaged

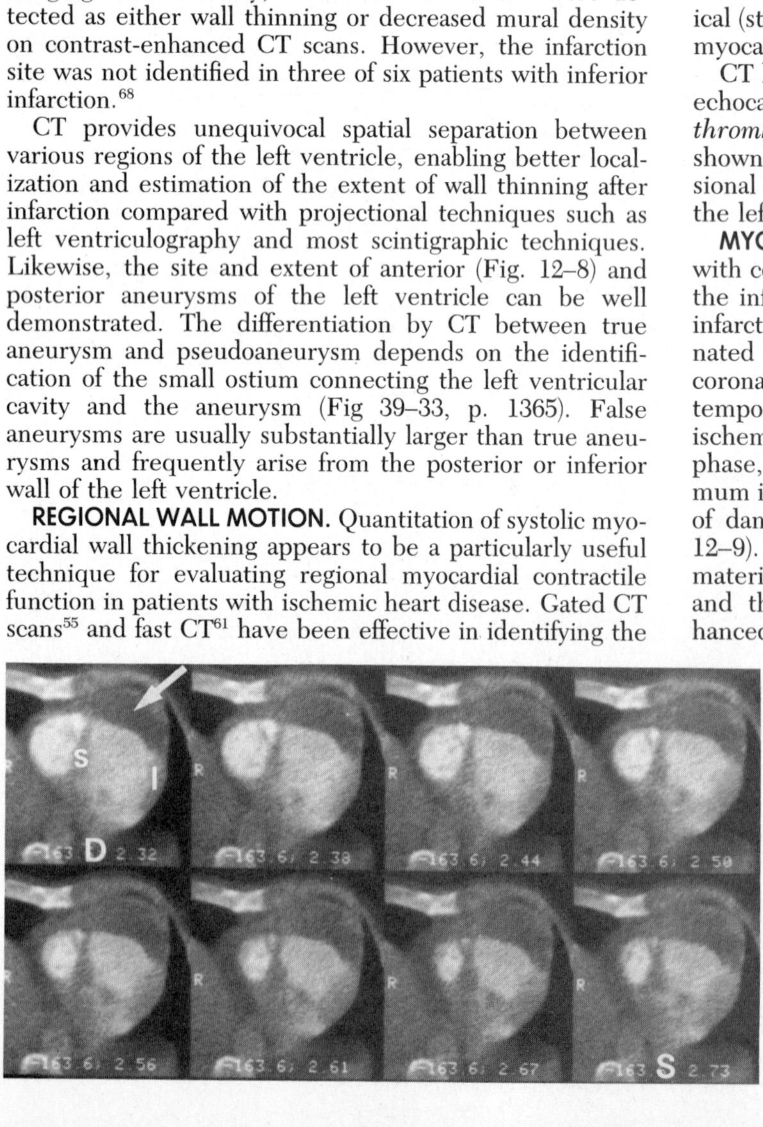

FIGURE 12–8. Cine CT scan shows anteroapical aneurysm filled with low-density thrombus (arrow). Note thickening of the septum (S) and lateral (L) walls from late diastole (D), *top, left frame,* to late systole (S), *bottom, right frame.*

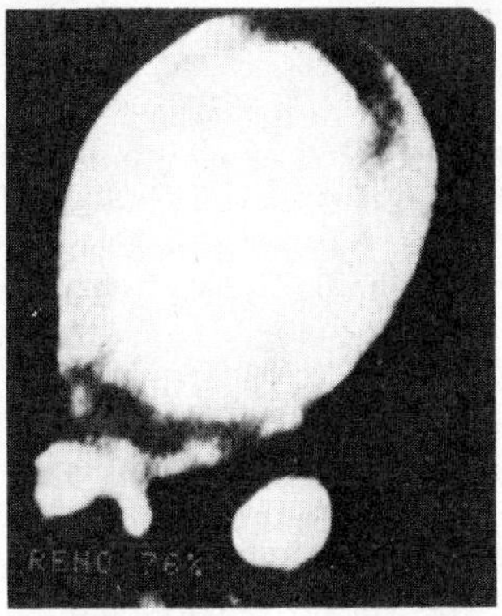

FIGURE 12–9. Contrast-enhanced CT scan of a dog with acute myocardial infarction. The scan was obtained during the myocardial enhancement (perfusion phase) after intravenous injection. Normal myocardium and chamber are enhanced while infarcted region is not enhanced.

area appears as a negative image within the myocardium, whereas in the later phase it appears as a positive image.

The delayed enhancement of the ischemic area after the intravenous administration of contrast material has been associated with a much higher concentration of iodine in infarcted compared with normal myocardium.[74, 79–81] The concentration of iodinated contrast material in the center, periphery, and margin of the infarct and in normal myocardium demonstrated a close linear relationship to the distribution of technetium-99m–pyrophosphate (^{99m}Tc-PYP)[76, 81] (p. 341). Both iodinated contrast material and ^{99m}Tc-PYP are markers of myocardial necrosis. Measurement of regional myocardial blood flow with indium-111–labeled microspheres indicated that both contrast material and ^{99m}Tc-PYP accumulated in the center of the infarct when residual blood flow was at least 5 per cent of normal.[81] These studies suggest that contrast enhancement of ischemically damaged tissue is a marker of myocardial necrosis, but its occurrence depends on the presence of a threshold level of residual myocardial perfusion. After intravenous administration, iodine-containing contrast material does not enter normal myocardial cells but does accumulate in ischemically damaged cells.[82]

In animal studies quantitation of infarct volume or mass from a series of transverse CT scans encompassing the full extent of the left ventricle has been found to correlate closely with postmortem measurements.[59, 76, 77, 83] In a canine model sequential CT scans have been utilized to monitor the mass of the infarct and of the remaining normal myocardium during the initial month after coronary occlusion.[59] Infarct size was shown to increase beginning shortly after occlusion and continuing to four days postocclusion and then to decrease progressively. The noninfarcted myocardial mass in animals with infarcts was found to increase 27 per cent during the initial month after occlusion, presumably representing compensatory hypertrophy. CT scans have also been used to document the beneficial effects of reperfusion 2 hours after occlusion in the dog.[83]

CORONARY ARTERY BYPASS GRAFTS. The patency of coronary artery bypass grafts can be assessed by sequential CT scans during the transit of intravenously administered contrast medium through the arterial side of the circulation. An early study[54] showed a 93 per cent sensitivity and 95 per cent specificity for defining graft patency using coronary angiography as the standard of reference. Subsequent reports in larger numbers of patients have shown somewhat lower diagnostic accuracy of CT in defining graft patency[84–86] and in one study only fair accuracy of the technique.[87] While all reports show high diagnostic accuracy for evaluation of grafts to the left anterior descending coronary artery system, the accuracy for assessing grafts to the circumflex and the right coronary arterial systems is poorer.[54, 84–87] Another limitation of the technique is the inability to identify grafts with significant stenoses.[85] It is possible that stenoses might be detected in grafts by time-density analysis or contrast transit time techniques applied to sequential scans of the same anatomical level acquired before and after pharmacological flow augmentation using the fast (cine) CT scanner.[88]

CT scanning may be used to assess graft patency within the first several days after bypass surgery with a view to reoperation in the event of documented early occlusion.[89, 90] CT revealed 70 per cent graft patency rate in patients with perioperative infarction compared with 95 per cent patency in those without infarction.[90]

The accuracy of CT for defining patency depends on the contrast enhancement technique and the criteria used to judge patency of the graft. The optimal CT scan level is free of metallic clips and situated at approximately the level of the pulmonary artery bifurcation. The site of the bypass graft on contrast-enhanced CT scans can be related to a clock viewed from the feet looking upward. The grafts

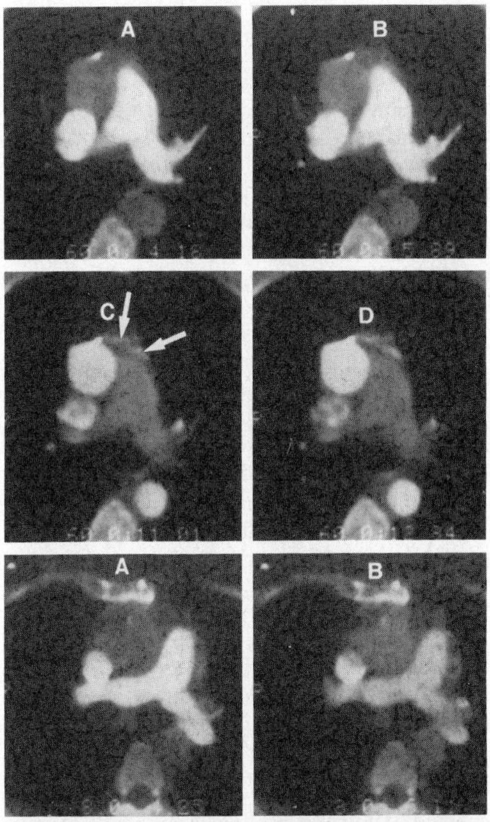

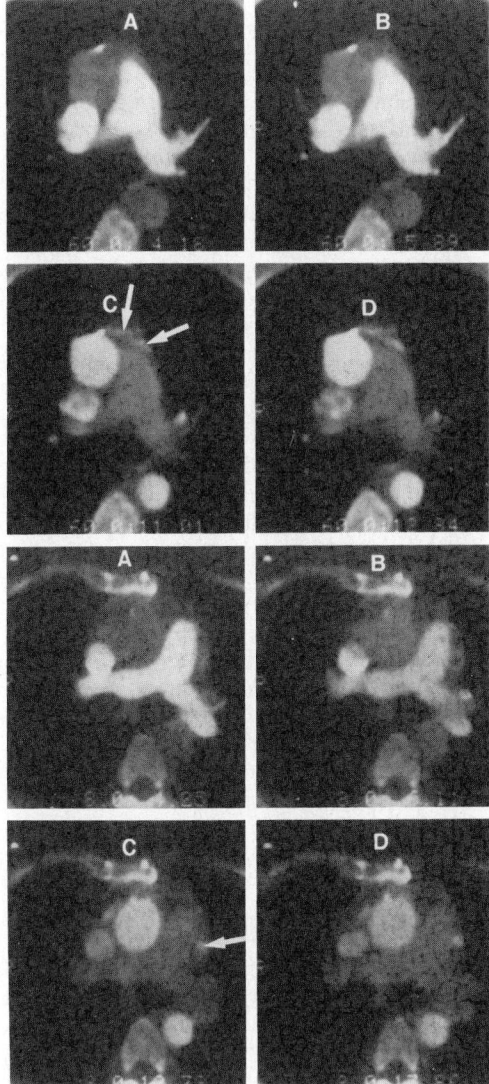

FIGURE 12–10. ***Top,*** **sequential cine CT scans show two patent bypass grafts (arrows) to the left anterior descending artery and acute diagonal.** ***Bottom,*** **graft to the obtuse marginal branch of the circumflex artery (arrow). Note in both cases the grafts opacify simultaneously with the ascending aorta. Each set of four images was obtained at the same anatomical level. The images were done with the passage of contrast medium through the central circulation. Early images (A,B) show contrast in the pulmonary artery and later images (C,D) show contrast in the aorta and bypass grafts.**

to the right coronary artery are situated between 9 and 11 o'clock; grafts to the left anterior descending artery system are situated at 12 to 2 o'clock, and the graft to the circumflex coronary system is located at 2 to 4 o'clock (Fig. 12–10). Diagnostic confidence is enhanced by visualizing the grafts at two adjacent anatomical levels and by showing contrast enhancement of the graft simultaneously with aortic opacification. Dynamic CT scanning (multiple segmental CT scans at the same level) demonstrates opacification and wash-out of contrast from the grafts. Sequential CT scans during the opacification and clearance of contrast medium from the grafts can be used to generate x-ray attenuation versus time curves for regions of interest over the grafts. Thereby it is possible to assess, at least roughly, the adequacy of blood flow in the graft.

PERICARDIAL DISEASE

Computed tomography provides distinct visualization of the pericardium in most patients. Discrimination of the pericardial line from the myocardium depends upon the presence of some epicardial and pericardial fat; it has been reported to be visible on CT scans of 95 per cent of normal subjects.[91] The mean width of the line in normal subjects is 2.2 mm at its thinnest portion and is always less than 4 mm. However, frequently it is visible only anteriorly over the right ventricle and near its diaphragmatic attachment, where it may be focally thickened. CT also frequently demonstrates the superior recesses of the pericardium extending over the ascending aorta and lateral to the main pulmonary artery. These recesses may be distended in the presence of a pericardial effusion.

Two-dimensional echocardiography is an extremely effective technique for the diagnosis of pericardial abnormalities and is the primary modality for evaluation of suspected pericardial disease (pp. 1490 and 1492). Although it is extremely sensitive for the detection of pericardial effusion, it has some limitations in defining loculated effusions, hemorrhagic effusions, and especially pericardial thickening. CT is especially effective in depicting these entities.[92–94] Consequently it is complementary to echocardiography in the diagnosis and assessment of pericardial disease.

CONGENITAL ABNORMALITIES AND CYSTS. Congenital abnormalities, such as absence of the pericardium[95] (p. 167) and pericardial cyst[92, 93, 96, 97] (p. 1524) can be well demonstrated by CT; other techniques are usually not definitive for diagnosis of these abnormalities. Pericardial defect (usually partial or complete absence of left-sided pericardium) is recognized on CT by the discontinuity of the pericardial line over the left aspect of the heart, with shift of the heart leftward or bulging of the left atrial appendage through the defect. CT demonstrates direct continuity of the heart and the left lung without intervening pericardium or pericardial fat.

PERICARDIAL CYST. This appears as a paracardiac mass with a thin capsule which is occasionally partially or completely calcified, and which has a homogeneous internal density nearly equivalent to that of water. However, rarely the cyst contains mucoid material, causing the density to be higher than water; such a cyst usually cannot be reliably distinguished from a solid mass. *Thymic cysts,* which may be adjacent to the pericardium, also may show homogeneous water density on CT densitometry and be indistinguishable from pericardial cysts.

PERICARDIAL FLUID. Fluid in the pericardial space may be reliably detected by CT.[92–94, 97] This technique can also provide an accurate estimate of the volume of this fluid.[98] Although two-dimensional echocardiography is sufficient and, for economic and logistic reasons, more clinically efficacious for the primary evaluation of most pericardial effusions, CT is indicated in some special situations. Loculated effusions (especially anterior loculations), which may pose difficulty for echocardiography, are readily demonstrated on CT[93] because of the wide field of view provided and the potentially three-dimensional nature of the technique. CT can be effective not only for diagnosing loculated effusions but also for guiding pericardiocentesis.[99] CT density measurements provide some degree of characterization of pericardial fluid.[92–94, 98] Density numbers (Hounsfield numbers) exceeding water density (water density = 0–12 units) are suggestive of hemopericardium, purulent exudate, or effusions associated with hypothyroidism. In one report[94] acute hemorrhage produced Hounsfield numbers between 40 and 50 units, while in another[93] hemopericardium of unspecified age had numbers ranging from 18 to 35 units. Low-density pericardial effusions have been reported in the presence of chylopericardium.[98]

CONSTRICTIVE PERICARDITIS. The establishment of the diagnosis of constrictive pericarditis can be substantially aided by CT. Since CT shows the pericardium, it can document pericardial thickening, defined as thickness greater than 4 mm. Focal plaques of thickening or the greater thickness of the pericardium near the diaphragm should not be confused with the more extensive pericardial thickening associated with constrictive pericarditis. However, the pericardial thickening may be limited to the right side of the heart, a form which appears to be more prevalent in patients who have undergone coronary arterial bypass surgery.

The documentation of pericardial thickening is the major discriminatory feature between constrictive pericarditis and restrictive cardiomyopathy[90] (p. 1506) (Fig. 12–11). However, thickened pericardium per se is not indicative of constrictive disease. Pericardial thickening without constriction is frequently observed in the early postoperative period and may persist for several months following operation in patients with the postpericardiotomy syndrome[92] (p. 1522). Thickened pericardium without constriction has also been observed in association with inflammation of the pericardium caused by a variety of conditions including

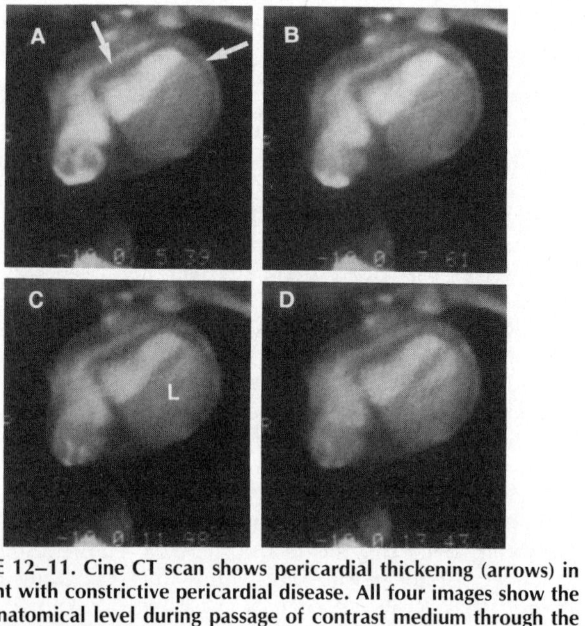

FIGURE 12–11. Cine CT scan shows pericardial thickening (arrows) in a patient with constrictive pericardial disease. All four images show the same anatomical level during passage of contrast medium through the central circulation. In panels A and B contrast is in the right-sided chambers and appears in the left ventricle (L) in panels C and D.

rheumatic heart disease, rheumatoid arthritis, sarcoidosis, and postmediastinal irradiation.[100] Pericardial thickening may also be caused by metastatic carcinoma, thymoma,[101] and lymphoma.[92, 94] These conditions are usually associated with effusion.[94]

EFFUSIVE-CONSTRICTIVE PERICARDITIS. This condition is demonstrated by an effusion in association with thickened pericardium; however, it may not always be possible to distinguish a small effusion from thickened pericardium.[92] Pericardial thickening alone usually measures between 5 to 20 mm, while greater thickening generally indicates associated effusion or effusion alone. Contrast enhancement of the thickened pericardium is indicative of pericardial inflammation.[102]

Additional CT findings in constrictive pericarditis often reflect the anatomical and physiological consequences of the thickened pericardium on the cardiac chambers.[103, 104] CT shows substantial dilatation of the inferior vena cava and some enlargement of the atria, especially the right atrium. The ventricles tend to have a small volume and a narrow tubular configuration.[103] In some cases, a sigmoid-shaped ventricular septum or prominent leftward convexity of the septum has been observed. Unusual contours, such as straightening or focal indentation of the free wall of either the right or left ventricle, have been noted on CT scans.[103]

The density resolution of CT makes it the most sensitive technique for identifying cardiac calcification (Fig. 12–12). Pericardial calcific deposits are usually residua of pericardial inflammation and are most commonly found in the visceral layer along the atrioventricular and interventricular grooves. Extensive calcification of the pericardium suggests but does not prove the presence of cardiac constriction.

PARACARDIAC AND CARDIAC MASSES

CT is useful for the evaluation of pericardial and paracardiac masses. CT and more recently MRI (p. 374) have emerged as the preferential techniques for defining the site and extent of such masses and in some cases even indicate their nature.[92, 93, 96, 97, 105, 106] CT may show the water density of pericardial cysts; this is an especially useful finding when the cyst is located in an unusual mediastinal location[96] or when it protrudes inwardly, displacing the thin atrial wall.[107] In one series CT detected eight of eight intrapericardial masses compared with echocardiography, which identified only one of them.[106] CT and MRI are currently the best techniques for defining the extension of mediastinal neoplasms (including lymphoma)

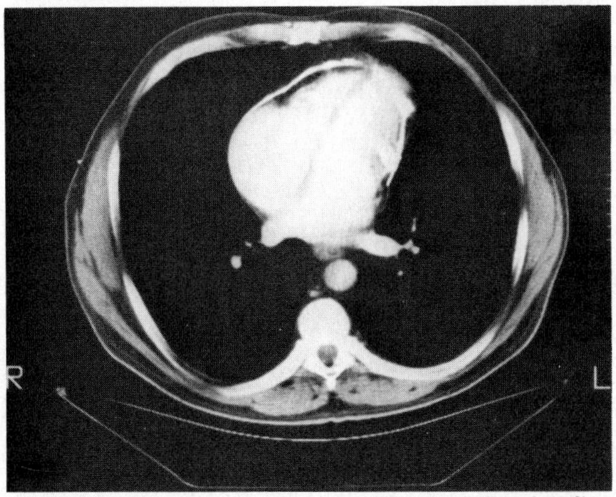

FIGURE 12–12. Cine CT scan shows calcification of pericardium extending into the myocardial wall and marked pericardial thickening in a patient with constrictive pericardial disease.

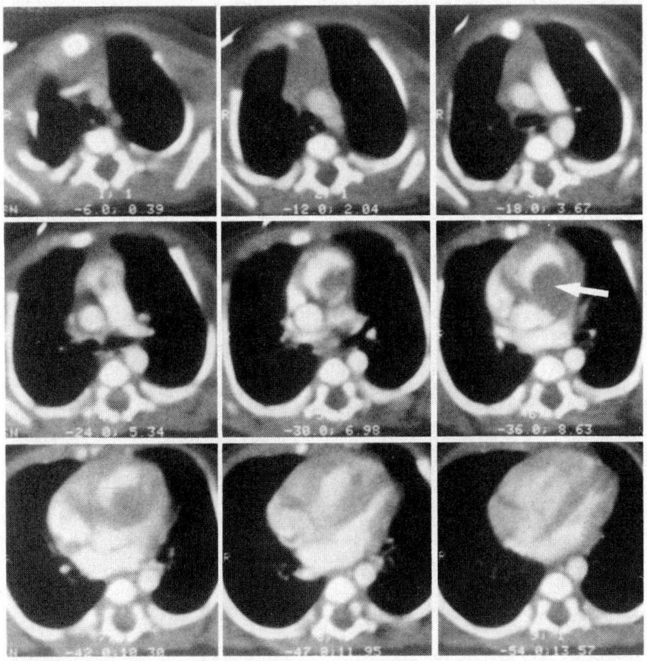

FIGURE 12–13. Cine CT scan at multiple levels extending through the mediastinum in an infant shows a large mass (arrow) in the right ventricle and protruding into and narrowing the right ventricular outflow tract. After a single intravenous injection of contrast media, four levels can be scanned simultaneously. These multiple levels defined the extent of the intracardiac mass.

and of carcinoma of the lung into the pericardium. Metastatic involvement of the pericardium is suggested by the CT findings of effusion with an irregularly thickened pericardium or the actual demonstration of a mass involving the pericardium.[92, 93, 106] An effusion with high CT density along with pericardial thickening also suggests metastatic pericardial involvement.[93, 98]

CT sometimes provides insight into the nature of the mass by demonstrating the shape, defining the density measurements, or showing multiple masses. The CT demonstration of multiple pericardial nodules suggests metastatic tumor or, rarely, multicentric mesothelioma. Pericardial cysts are regular, while lipomas have a very low density value (−55 or fewer Hounsfield units). Demonstration of calcium or bone and fat in a paracardiac mass by CT suggests teratoma.

Intracardiac masses can be detected very well by echocardiography and angiography (Chap. 43). However, CT not only can detect masses within the cardiac chambers but also can define fully their extent (Fig. 12–13). CT can demonstrate components of the mass within the myocardial wall and extending outside of the heart. The contrast resolution of CT may provide some insight into the composition of the mass, such as demonstrating the presence of fat or calcium. CT has detected simple intracardiac masses such as atrial myxoma[52, 108, 109] (Fig. 43–4, p. 1478) and complex masses involving the myocardial wall with extracardiac extension.[52] Finally, by defining clearly the myocardial wall, CT allows distinguishing of the extracardiac location of tumors which produce compression and invagination of cardiac walls, simulating an intracardiac origin.[107]

The identification of *intracardiac thrombi* by CT (Fig. 12–8) has been discussed (p. 362).

CONGENITAL HEART DISEASE

Standard CT, fast CT (cine CT), and MRI are useful noninvasive techniques for the visualization of cardiovas-

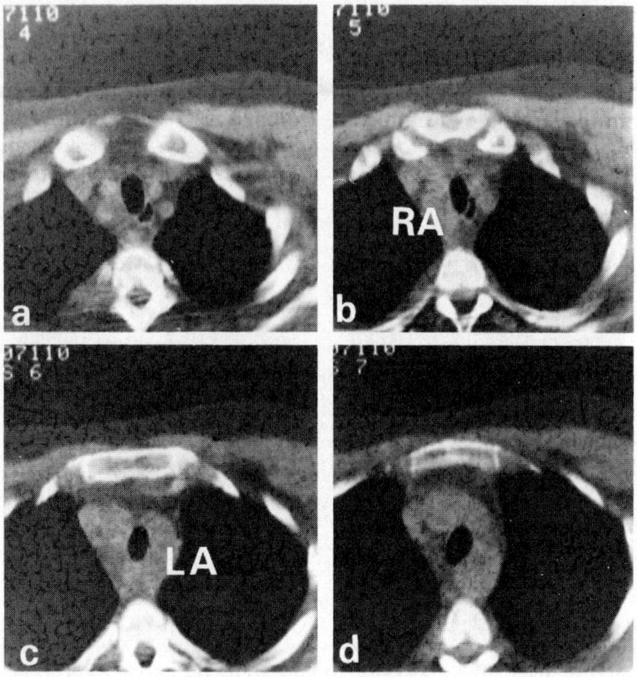

FIGURE 12–14. Standard cine CT scan of double aortic arch. *Top left,* Scan at level of arch vessels. *Top right,* Scan at top of the right arch (RA). *Bottom left,* Scan at top of left arch (LA). *Bottom right,* Scan through the left arch. Note the symmetrical arrangement of four-arch vessel. (From Farmer, D. W., et al.: Computed tomography in congenital heart disease. J. Comput. Assist. Tomogr. *8*:677, 1984.)

cular anatomy in patients with congenital heart disease. Fast CT and MRI can also provide assessment of cardiovascular function in these patients. MRI appears to be the most suitable of these techniques for defining the problem, while fast CT seems most effective for evaluating ventricular function and estimating the volume of cardiac shunts.

STANDARD CT. This technique has been found to be useful for evaluation of suspected *anomalies of the aortic arch*[110–112] (p. 994). Contrast-enhanced CT is usually required to show the vascular tissue surrounding the trachea in the presence of double aortic arch and the retroesophageal vascular structure indicating anomalous origin of the subclavian artery. Double arch is also suggested by the presence of four paratracheal vessels arranged symmetrically[110] (Fig. 12–14).

Standard CT is also effective for demonstrating abnormalities of the origin of the great vessels, such as *transposition and malposition.*[111, 112] Transaxial images at the level of the great vessels display the anterior with either leftward (levo-transposition or levo-malposition) or rightward (dextro-transposition or dextro-malposition) position of the aorta relative to the pulmonary artery. Reformatted images in the sagittal plane can be used to provide a composite view of anomalies of the great vessels and ventricles; however, such images have considerably reduced resolution. Although many intracardiac anomalies such as septal defects, tetralogy of Fallot, Ebstein's anomaly, and others have been demonstrated by standard CT, the technique has not found widespread use due to the ease and the usual diagnostic superiority of two-dimensional echocardiography (p. 113). An exception is the definitive demonstration of systemic veins, liver, and spleen possible with CT; this information is important for the complete evaluation of the situs-splenic syndrome.[113]

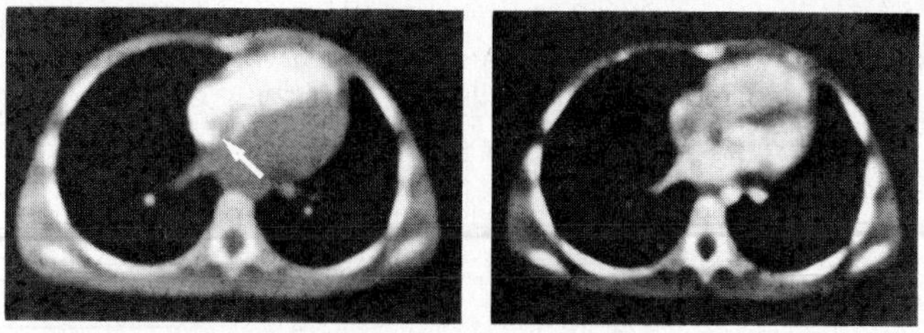

FIGURE 12–15. Cine CT scans of a patient with secundum atrial septal defect (ASD) after intravenous injection of contrast media. Sequential scans at same level obtained at time of the passage of contrast bolus through right heart (*left*) and left heart (*right*). Unopacified blood crosses ASD into RA early (arrow) and on levophase, contrast-enhanced blood is observed crossing the ASD. (Courtesy of J. Eldridge, M.D., Deborah Heart Institute.)

CINE CT. This technique has also been employed for the evaluation of congenital heart disease.[113, 114] Cine CT has been found to be accurate in defining systemic and pulmonary venous connections. Likewise, it has demonstrated atrial (Fig. 12–15) and ventricular septal defects (Fig. 12–16). The ostium primum atrial septal defect (p. 982) is characterized by a defect abutting the atrioventricular valve and shortening of the inflow ventricular septum. Because of the absence of overlying structures defined on CT scans and the three-dimensional nature of cine CT, the size of the ventricles can be measured.

Normal and abnormal atrioventricular valves can be demonstrated by cine CT,[114] which can be used to diagnose both tricuspid and mitral atresia. It can also demonstrate the size of the atrium above the atretic valve. A common atrioventricular valve spanning both ventricles can be identified on the transverse image. In Ebstein's anomaly (p. 951) the anterior displacement of tricuspid valve leaflets and the extent of thinning of the right ventricular wall can be demonstrated.

Transverse tomograms provide clear spatial separation of the inflow and outflow portions of the ventricular septum. This permits localization of defects and facilitates the detection of multiple ventricular septal defects.[114] In addition, an assessment of the hemodynamic effects of septal defects (and of other lesions) can be made by evaluation of chamber dimension and wall thickness.

Cine CT has been effective for defining abnormalities of the great vessels, including transposition complexes and double-outlet right ventricle[114] (Fig. 12–17). Abnormalities of the pulmonary arteries, such as congenital absence, peripheral coarctations, and hypoplasia, have been demonstrated by this technique.[114]

Cine CT appears to be an excellent technique for the evaluation of patients with surgically corrected congenital heart disease. Since ventricular volumes[64–66] and mass[60] can be measured accurately by CT, this technique can be used to evaluate the expected regression of ventricular dilatation and hypertrophy after corrective procedures.

EVALUATION OF CARDIAC FUNCTION. This can be accomplished in patients with congenital heart disease by

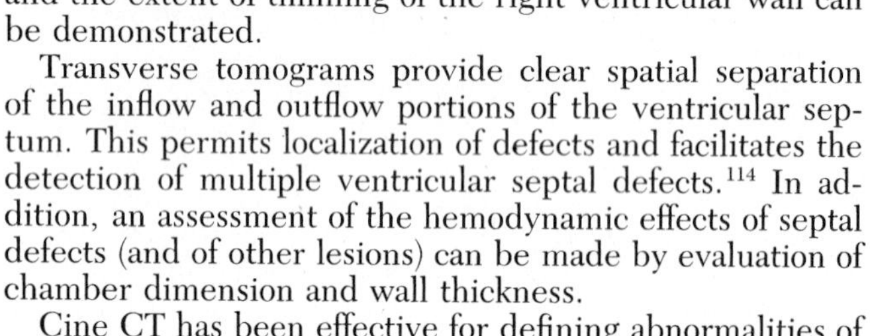

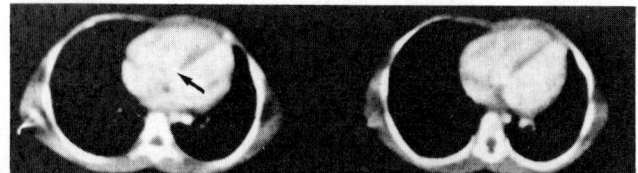

FIGURE 12–16. Cine CT scans of patient with ventricular septal defect. During the period of enhancement of both ventricles the ventricular septal defect is evident (arrow). (Courtesy of J. Eldridge, M.D., Deborah Heart Institute.)

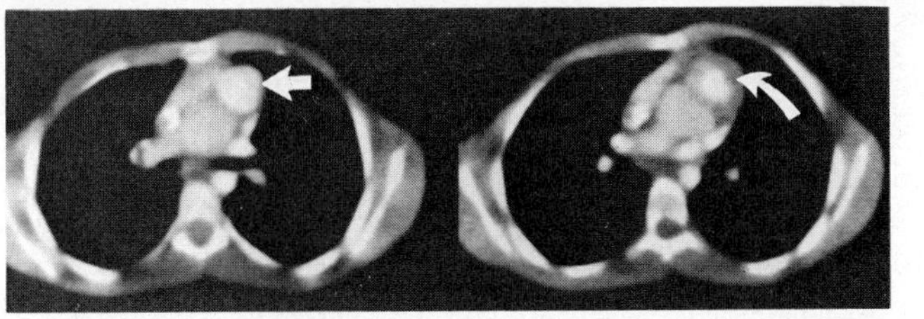

FIGURE 12–17. Cine CT scans of patient with levo-transposition. The aorta (arrow) is positioned anterior and to the left of the pulmonary artery. Scan at base of heart (*right*) shows that the aorta arises from the infundibulum (curved arrow).

cine CT, which, along with multiphasic ECG-gated MRI (p. 370), may be the best techniques for quantitating right ventricular volumes and ejection fraction. In addition, cine CT can be used to estimate the volume of shunts; its accuracy has been documented in an experimental right-to-left shunt model in the dog.[115] This is accomplished by measuring density of contrast medium within a cardiac chamber receiving shunt flow on sequential CT scans obtained during passage of contrast medium through the central circulation. A density versus time curve can be generated for such a region of interest. The normal curve is unimodal as contrast medium enters and leaves a cardiac chamber. A bimodal time-density curve may be generated from the region of interest cursor placed over any chamber involved in a shunt (Fig. 12–18). Using a gamma variate fit method, the areas under the primary and secondary portions of the curve can be measured in order to calculate pulmonary to systemic flow ratios. A close correlation has been found for the measurement of pulmonary to systemic flow ratio by cine CT and oximetry in experimental animals[115] (Fig. 12–19) and in patients.[114]

Another method for calculating the net shunt is to compare the difference in stroke volume between the two ventricles. For a left-to-right shunt at the ventricular level, the difference between the larger left ventricular stroke volume and right ventricular stroke volume indicates the net shunt value. Such an approach can be used also to calculate net volume and fraction of the regurgitant lesion.

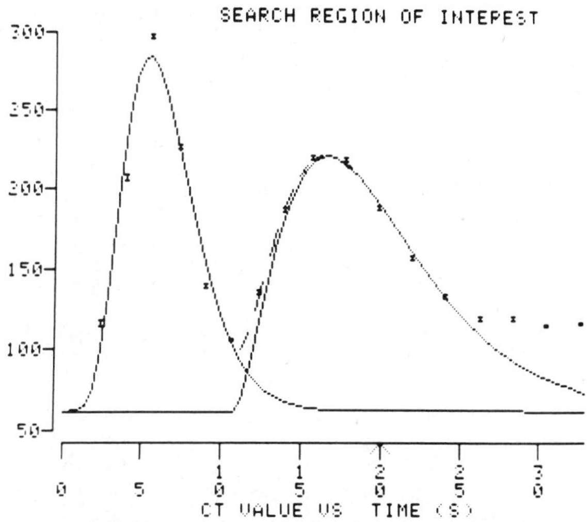

FIGURE 12–18. Density vs. time curves derived from measurements on sequential cine CT scans acquired during passage of contrast media through central circulation. A bimodal curve such as this indicates the presence of a central shunt occurring at or upstream from the chamber or great vessel where measurements are made. Bimodal curves were obtained from dogs with a shunt constructed between the pulmonary artery and left atrium. Analysis of the area of each curve provides an estimate of the volume of the shunt.

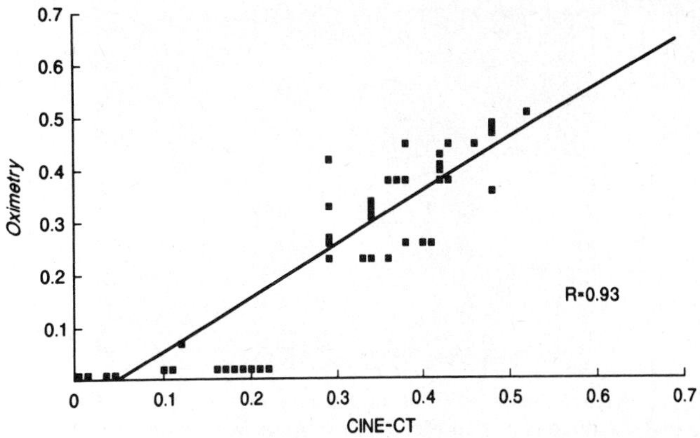

FIGURE 12–19. The shunt volume determined by cine CT is plotted against volume calculated from oximetry in an experimental model of right-to-left shunt. These canine models had shunts constructed between the pulmonary artery and left atrium. There is a close correlation between the two measurements.

DISEASE OF THE THORACIC AORTA

(See also Chap. 46)

CT has been shown to be extremely accurate for the diagnosis of thoracic aortic aneurysm and dissection.[116–121]

AORTIC DISSECTION. In one prospective study in 26 patients with suspected aortic dissection there were no false-negative or false-positive CT scans for this diagnosis.[120] In this study CT correctly indicated the true extent of dissection in patients in whom it was underestimated by angiography. In general, CT has an accuracy of approximately 90 per cent and is equivalent to angiography for the diagnosis of a variety of diseases of the thoracic aorta.[121] However, some instances of false-negative CT examination in aortic dissection have been reported.[114–121] Diagnosis of dissection requires the demonstration of the intimal flap, appearing as a lucency within the lumen of the contrast-enhanced aortic lumen on CT scans (Figs. 12–20 and 46–5, p. 1550). Supportive diagnostic findings are differential temporal enhancement of the true and false aortic channels or compression of the opacified true lumen by a thrombosed false channel. Inward displacement of calcium in the aortic wall is also a sign of aortic dissection. CT can effectively distinguish between dissections which involve the ascending aorta and those that are limited to the descending aorta. In the former, the intimal flap can be demonstrated in the ascending aorta. It may be difficult to

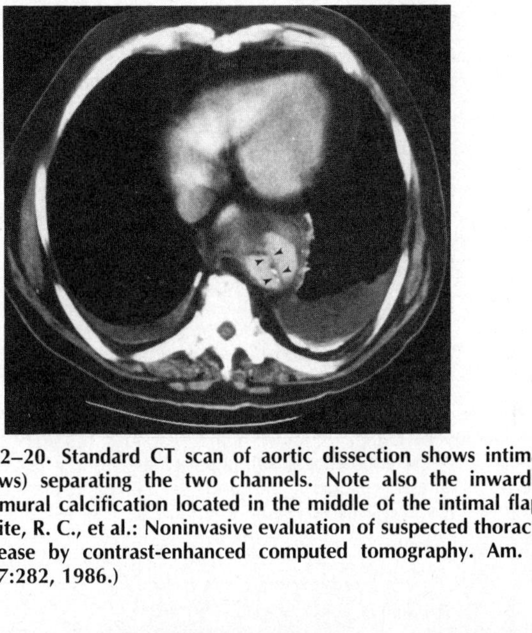

FIGURE 12–20. Standard CT scan of aortic dissection shows intimal flap (arrows) separating the two channels. Note also the inwardly displaced mural calcification located in the middle of the intimal flap. (From White, R. C., et al.: Noninvasive evaluation of suspected thoracic aortic disease by contrast-enhanced computed tomography. Am. J. Cardiol. *57*:282, 1986.)

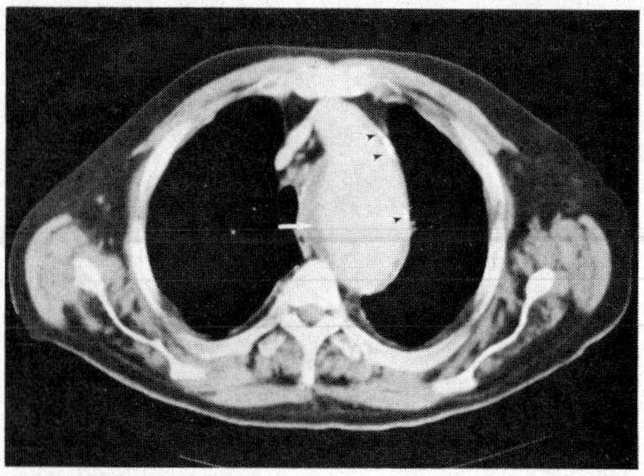

FIGURE 12–21. Standard CT scan of aneurysm of the aortic arch. There is marked dilatation of posterior aortic arch with mural calcification (arrowheads). Thrombus lines the wall of the aneurysm (arrow). (From White, R. C., et al.: Noninvasive evaluation of suspected thoracic aortic disease by contrast-enhanced computed tomography. Am. J. Cardiol. *57*:282, 1986.)

differentiate a dissection with thrombus of the false channel from an aortic aneurysm with mural thrombus (Fig. 12–21). A dissection is more likely when CT scans at multiple levels show the thrombus extending for more than 10 cm longitudinally. Also, dissection usually results in a compressed true aortic lumen while aneurysm has a normal or increased lumen.

CT may also be used for following the course of thoracic aortic dissections after initial treatment.[119, 122, 123] After surgical placement of an ascending aortic graft, the false channel beyond the distal anastomosis of the graft usually remains patent. Sequential CT studies have also revealed persistent patency of the false channel after medical as well as surgical therapy, but thrombosis of the false channel or even its disappearance is seen in some patients.

AORTIC ANEURYSM. These are characterized by an increase in aortic diameter and by outward displacement of calcium of the aortic wall.

MAGNETIC RESONANCE IMAGING

MAGNETIC RESONANCE GLOSSARY

Free Induction Decay. The signal produced by the release of energy absorbed by the nuclei from a previously applied radiofrequency pulse. The free induction decay is the signal analyzed in MR imaging and spectroscopy.

Hydrogen Density (Spin Density, Proton Density). Density of protons at a site in a sample which are resonating as part of the magnetic resonance process. From the point of view of quantum mechanics, these are the protons making transitions from high-energy states to lower ones and vice versa, when energy just equal to the difference between these two states is applied.

Magnetic Moment. Intensity and direction of the net magnetic field of spinning nuclei. In a magnetic field, nuclei align to produce a net magnetic moment parallel to the field.

Magnetic Resonance Imaging (MRI). Spatial two- or three-dimensional map of nuclei resonating at a characteristic frequency when placed in a magnetic field and subjected to intermittently applied radiofrequency pulses.

Proton MRI. Imaging dependent upon the concentration and relaxation time of hydrogen nuclei.

Multinuclear MRI. Imaging using nuclei other than hydrogen, such as sodium 23 and phosphorus 31.

Magnetic Resonance Signal. During relaxation after cessation of a radiofrequency pulse, energy absorbed from this pulse is released and provides a radiofrequency signal.

Relaxation. Return of nuclei into the original state of alignment with a magnetic field after having been tilted by a radiofrequency pulse.

Magnetic Resonance Spectroscopy. Spectrum of resonant frequencies of a specific nucleus contained within a sample. This spectrum results from the chemical shift of a nucleus caused by the influence of the local chemical environment. Consequently, the resonant frequency of phosphorus in the inorganic state is slightly different from its frequency in creatine phosphate. Magnetic resonance spectroscopy detects and maps these chemical shifts of a nucleus.

Proton Spectroscopy. Spectrum of resonant frequencies of hydrogen nuclei (protons) in relation to the chemical environment. Proton spectroscopy can define chemical peaks representative of substances such as fats, water, lactic acid, choline, and carnitine.

Paramagnetic Substances. Substances that alter the natural relaxation times of nuclei undergoing the magnetic resonance process. These are usually molecules with unpaired electrons which reduce the relaxation times of resonating nuclei. These substances are being used and developed as contrast media for magnetic resonance imaging.

Relaxation Times. Relaxation of nuclei undergoing the magnetic resonance process has two components called T1 and T2 relaxation times. These relaxation times are time-constant, measured as the magnetization vector precesses into alignment with the magnetic field after perturbation by a radiofrequency pulse.

Resonant Frequency. Each nucleus which is sensitive to the magnetic resonance process must be tilted in the magnetic field by a specific frequency (resonant frequency) in order to induce resonance. When this frequency is applied, the nucleus is rotated away from its equilibrium alignment with the magnetic field. When the radiofrequency pulse ceases, the nucleus realigns with the magnetic field through a process of magnetic relaxation.

Spin-Echo Imaging Sequence. Images are produced by sampling signal after an initial 90° radiofrequency pulse, followed by one or more 180° pulses. The 180° pulse refocuses spins and thereby enhances the signal from them. Signal is sampled some time after the 180° pulse.

Surface Coils. Radiofrequency receiver coils placed upon the surface of the subject or upon an organ of interest in order to detect the magnetic resonance signal. These coils increase the efficiency and signal strength for both MR imaging and spectroscopy.

T1 Relaxation Time. Also called spin-lattice or longitudinal relaxation time. T1 relaxation is a measure of the exponential rate of growth of the magnetization vector along the direction of the external magnetic field after the nuclei have been tilted (flipped) by a radiofrequency pulse.

T1 Weighted Image. Image in which the intensity of image voxels is heavily dependent upon the T1 relaxation time of tissues. For the spin echo technique, this is done with a short TR and TE.

T2 Relaxation Time. Also called spin-spin or transverse relaxation time. Immediately after cessation of a 90° radiofrequency pulse, the nuclei process in phase, resulting in a magnetization vector in the transverse plane. There is gradual dephasing of nuclei, leading to cancellation of the magnetization vector in the transverse plane.

T2 Weighted Image. Image in which the intensity of image voxels is heavily dependent upon the T2 relaxation time of tissues. For the spin echo technique, this is done with a long TR and TE.

TE. Echo delay time. Time between the initiation of a pulse sequence (90° pulse) and the sampling of the spin-echo signal. For the spin-echo sequence, this sampling is done after the 180° pulse. For example, the first spin-echo signal is sampled at a time which is twice the duration between the initial 90° pulse and the 180° refocusing pulse.

Tesla. A unit of magnetic field strength. One tesla is equal to 10,000 gauss.

TR. Repetition time. Time between sets of radiofrequency pulses. For the spin-echo sequence, each set of pulses consists of a 90° and usually one or more 180° pulses. This is the time between the 90° pulses initiating each set.

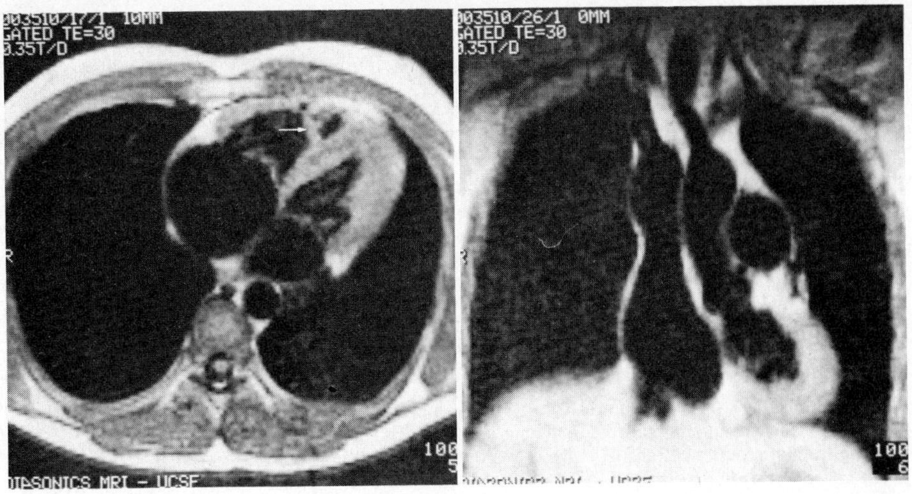

FIGURE 12–22. Gated transverse (*left*) and coronal (*right*) images display normal cardiac anatomy. Internal morphology of the ventricles, such as the moderator band (arrow) of the right ventricle and papillary muscle of the left ventricle (LV) are demonstrated. Interface between blood (no signal) and endocardium is sharply defined. Coronal image provides direct visualization of the diaphragmatic surface of the LV. Note also the sinuses of Valsalva.

Magnetic resonance (MR) imaging has two important attributes that make it intrinsically advantageous for cardiovascular diagnosis. First, a high natural contrast exists between the blood pool and the cardiovascular structures because of the lack of signal from flowing blood with standard MR pulse sequences. When the spin-echo technique is used, blood appears black on images; therefore, internal structures of the heart can be visualized within the signal void of the cardiac chambers (Fig. 12–22). Consequently, contrast medium is not required for discrimination of the blood pool. Second, a wide range of soft tissue contrast provides the potential for the characterization of myocardial tissue. This contrast among tissues is dependent upon proton (hydrogen nuclei) density and magnetic relaxation times of the protons. Brief descriptions of the MR process, general imaging techniques, and specific image techniques for the heart are given below, and some useful terminology for MR imaging and spectroscopy is presented as a glossary. A more detailed description of the principles underlying MRI is given elsewhere.[124]

TECHNICAL ASPECTS

Atomic nuclei with a net charge have a magnetic moment. A net charge exists when a nucleus contains unpaired (an odd number) of protons, neutrons, or both. The hydrogen nucleus contains only a proton; it is positively charged and has a strong magnetic moment. The magnetic properties of nuclei are expressed when they are placed in an external magnetic field. When protons or other nuclei with magnetic moment lie within a magnetic field and are then exposed to electromagnetic radiation (radiofrequency waves), energy is absorbed and subsequently emitted. This absorption and release of energy causes resonance—nuclear magnetic resonance. The radiofrequency (RF) necessary to induce resonance has to be proportional to the local magnetic field (H_L) and a constant (magnetogyric ratio) related to the specific nucleus involved. The relationship between frequency (f) and magnetic field is expressed by the following equation:

$$f = \delta H_L / 2\pi$$

When nuclei at equilibrium in a magnetic field are irradiated at the resonant frequency, they attain a higher energy state. When they return to equilibrium, they emit energy at the same frequency, if the magnetic field remains constant. If the magnetic field changes, between the time of excitation and emission, then the emission occurs at a frequency corresponding to the new field strength as expressed by this equation.

LOCALIZATION OF MAGNETIC RESONANCE SIGNAL. Magnetic resonance imaging depends on the reception of the emitted radiofrequency signal from resonating nuclei and on the capability of locating these nuclei in space. Location of the resonating nuclei can be achieved by spatially varying the field strength in a known manner. Since resonance frequency of a nucleus at a specific site is related to local field strength, the emitted frequency will characterize the spatial location of the nucleus when a magnetic gradient exists in one or more planes.

Selection of a transverse section for imaging is done by applying a magnetic gradient along the Z axis (long axis of the body). In such a gradient each transverse plane (XY plane) has a specific and different resonant frequency. If the body is irradiated with a 90° RF pulse consisting of a narrow range of frequencies corresponding to the resonance frequency of a single plane, only the nuclei in this plane will resonate. By this means, called *selection irradiation*, the image plane is delineated.

Once a plane is excited by selective irradiation, spatial localization is attained in this plane by another gradient oriented parallel to this plane. After the selective 90° radiofrequency pulse is applied, a magnetic field gradient is produced in the X or Y direction. Nuclei at the stronger end of the field gradient will resonate at a higher frequency than those at the weaker end of the gradient. This provides spatial localization within the selected plane.

The magnetic signal from a sample undergoing MR imaging is detected by an RF receiver coil. The intensity of the signal at foci in

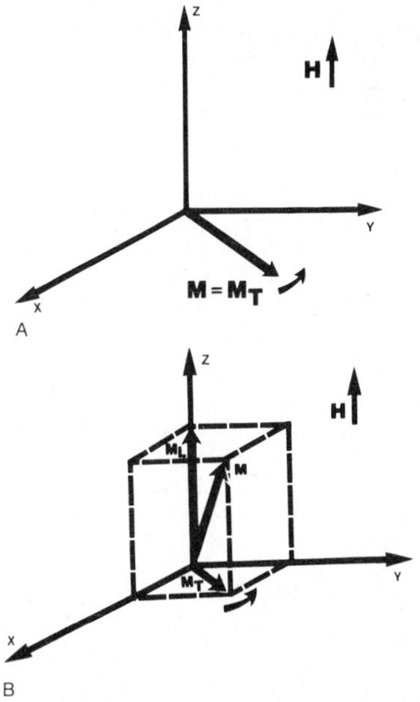

FIGURE 12–23. Behavior of nuclei undergoing magnetic resonance. Strong magnetic field (H) is present along the Z axis. After application of a 90° radiofrequency pulse the net magnetic moment of the nuclei are rotated into the transverse (XY) plane, causing the net magnetization to be equal to transverse magnetization (M_T). Subsequently, M_T decays as longitudinal magnetization (M_L) grows. The net magnetization vector (M) at any instant is the result of the instantaneous values of M_L and M_T. Since M_T decays more rapidly than M_L grows, the length of the vector changes as it returns to equilibrium. (From Margulis, A. R., et al.: Clinical Magnetic Resonance Imaging. San Francisco, Radiology Research and Education Foundation, 1983.)

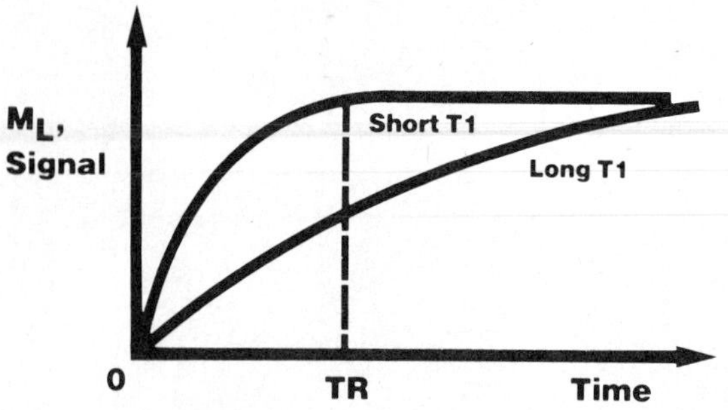

FIGURE 12–24. After perturbation of magnetic resonance–sensitive nuclei by a radiofrequency pulse, the magnetic resonance signal, owing to longitudinal magnetization (M_L), grows exponentially to the equilibrium value at a rate determined by T1. If the system is allowed a time TR to recover, contrast between tissues with different T1 values is produced. In general, there will be greater T1 contrast for shorter TR values and lower contrast for longer TR values. (From Margulis, A. R., et al.: Clinical Magnetic Resonance Imaging. San Francisco, Radiology Research and Education Foundation, 1983.)

the imaging plane depends on the concentration of resonating nuclei at the site and the magnetic relaxation times of the nuclei. The relaxation times are measures of the interaction of the resonating protons with the static magnetic field and the intermittently applied RF pulses.

The net magnetic moment of nuclei at any site can be expressed as a vector with length (intensity) and direction. At equilibrium, the vector points along the main static magnetic field. The vector can be tipped 90° by the application of a radiofrequency pulse. The component of the net magnetic moment that points along the main magnetic field is called *longitudinal magnetization*. The component at 90° to the main field is the *transverse magnetization*. After completion and before attainment of full alignment with magnetic field (equilibrium), the vector varies continuously between longitudinal and transverse magnetization and gradually approaches full longitudinal magnetization (Fig. 12–23).

MAGNETIC RELAXATION TIMES. After the application of a 90° radiofrequency pulse, net magnetization is rotated from the longitudinal direction (ZY plane) into the transverse direction (XY plane). At this instant, transverse magnetization is maximum and longitudinal magnetization is zero. Immediately after this, longitudinal magnetization gradually recovers toward its equilibrium value. This exponential growth has a time constant called *T1* (Fig. 12–24). Likewise, after the 90° pulse, transverse magnetization exponentially decays, the time constant is called *T2* (Fig. 12–25). In tissues, T2 is much shorter than T1. These relaxation times are related to several characteristics of tissues, including temperature. Tissues have different relaxation times and these differences contribute to contrast among tissues during imaging. Contrast between two tissues can be accentuated by sampling signal at an instant when there is maximum difference between the relaxation times of the two tissues (Figs. 12–24 and 12–25).

IMAGING, TR, AND TE. The MR image is produced by applying the sets of radiofrequency pulses many times over several minutes; generally, 256 to 512 pulse sequences are used. The time between application of sets of radiofrequency pulses is called the *repetition time* (TR). Depending on the technique employed for imaging, each set consists of one or more radiofrequency pulses. The time between the initial pulse in a sequence and the instance when signal is acquired from the sample is called the *echo delay time* (TE). It is possible to alter the pulse sequences in such a way that differences in T1 and T2 relaxation times among tissues can be accentuated to produce contrast among these tissues. This is referred to as *T1* or *T2 weighting of the images*. T1-weighted images have short TR and TE intervals, while T2-weighted images have long TR and TE intervals when using the spin-echo technique. T1 and T2 weighting for new fast imaging techniques is achieved to some extent by variations in the flip angles induced in the nuclei by the initial RF pulse.

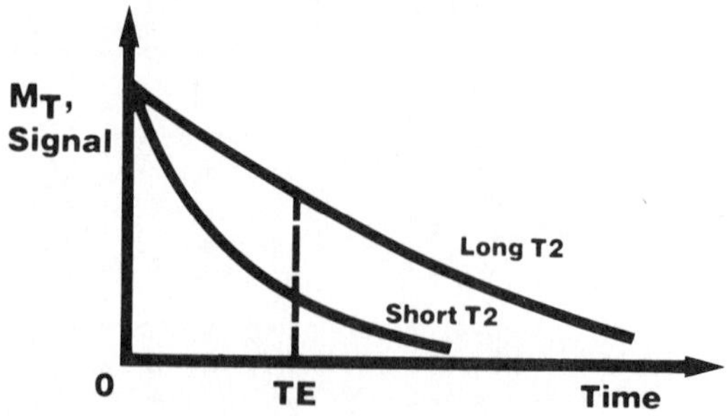

FIGURE 12–25. After perturbation of magnetic resonance sensitive nuclei by a radiofrequency pulse, transverse magnetization (M_T) exponentially decays at a rate determined by T2. The TE determines contrast between two tissues with different values of T2. In general, there is greater T2 contrast for longer TE values up to a maximum point at which signal declines severely. (From Margulis, A. R., et al.: Clinical Magnetic Resonance Imaging. San Francisco, Radiology Research and Education Foundation, 1983.)

As described above, MR imaging depends upon radiofrequency, (RF, radiowave) signals which result from the interaction of protons (hydrogen nuclei) with a strong magnetic field (0.15 to 2.0 Tesla) and intermittent applied RF pulses. Although imaging could possibly be carried out for other atoms which have a magnetic moment, imaging is now carried out almost exclusively with hydrogen nuclei (protons). The combined effect of the magnetic field and the RF pulses causes protons to resonate at a characteristic frequency. Spatial identification of the resonating protons is achieved by an intermittently applied weak magnetic gradient. This causes slight variations in resonant frequency, depending upon the site of the proton within the magnetic gradient, because of the proportionality between resonant frequency and magnetic field strength.

EFFECTS OF MOVING BLOOD. During an imaging sequence, the motion of nuclei through the region that is being imaged greatly influences signal intensity. Although the influence of blood flow on magnetic resonance images is complex, motion of the excited nuclei during the MR sequence generally causes a loss of signal intensity. Consequently, moving blood in the lumina of vessels appears dark (no signal), providing considerable natural contrast for visualization of the internal surfaces of the blood vessels and walls of the cardiac chambers. Since contrast medium is not required to mark the blood pool, MRI is a totally noninvasive technique for cardiovascular diagnosis. When blood velocity is such that protons move through the thickness of the tomogram (usually 5 to 10 mm) in the time between the 90° and 180° pulses of the spin-echo sequence, signal is lost from the blood. Using standard spin-echo sequences, this time (TE/2) is usually 15 msec for the first such image. On the other hand, with the fast imaging techniques recently introduced, the TE is greatly reduced (TE/2 = 5 msec) and consequently signal is received from blood flowing at normal velocities in the cardiac chambers and all blood vessels. In this circumstance, blood appears substantially brighter (white) than the cardiac walls (Fig. 12–26). High-velocity jets produced by flow across stenotic or regurgitant valves can be recognized as a signal void within the signal-filled cardiac chambers (Fig. 12–26).

Techniques for MR Imaging of the Heart

Cardiac imaging requires some form of physiological gating of the imaging sequence. Acquisition of MR signals of the thorax without gating results in poor cardiac images owing to loss of the signal from moving structures and to the variable position of the cardiac structure relative to imaging pixels when data are acquired indiscriminately throughout the cardiac cycle.

GATING WITH MRI. This is associated with unique problems. Sensors, wire leads, and transducers are usually composed of ferromagnetic materials, which can generate noise or may grossly distort the images within the radiofrequency-shielded room containing the MRI device. Consequently, gating with MRI requires the use of a nonferro-

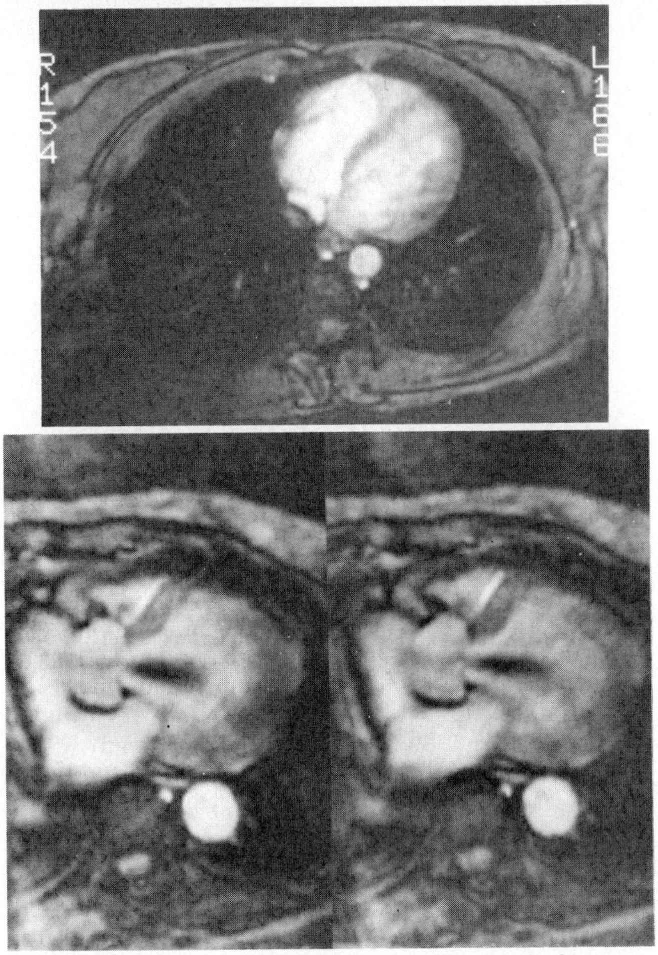

FIGURE 12–26. Transverse MR tomograms from a normal subject (*top*) and a patient with aortic regurgitation (*bottom*) obtained using an ECG-gated fast MR imaging technique with TR (repetition time) and TE (echo delay time) values of 21 and 12 msecs, respectively. With this fast imaging technique (short TR and TE), the blood pool has high MR signal intensity (appears white on images). The high-velocity regurgitant jet appears as a flame-shaped area of signal void located just beneath the aortic valve.

magnetic physiological signal-sensing circuit. An electronically isolated ECG electrode-lead circuit containing very little metal has been used for repetitive synchronization, i.e., ECG gating, of pulse sequences to fixed segments of the cardiac cycle. The uses and results of gating for the acquisition of MR images have been described in detail.[125, 126]

MULTISLICE TECHNIQUES. Several imaging strategies have been employed depending upon the information desired.[127] For anatomical diagnosis, the *ECG-gated multislice technique* is used. This technique is economical in time, requiring less than 10 minutes for the acquisition of tomograms (1 cm thickness) at 10 anatomical levels, which usually encompasses the entire heart and root of the great vessels. A difference of 50 to 100 msec exists between each adjacent level, so the images are obtained at different phases of the cardiac cycle. The reason why images can be obtained at multiple anatomical levels during a single imaging sequence is that the time required to complete a set of RF pulses and sample the emitted signal for each line on that image is usually 30 to 60 msec (T-E interval), while the time duration between the application of repetitive sets of pulses is approximately 500 to 1000 msec (T-R interval). Consequently, the inactive time for each cycle is long, frequently greater than 90 per cent of the cycle. Efficiency is improved by applying the set of spin-echo pulses at other levels during the magnetization recovery period. Therefore, upon completion of a 50-msec duty cycle at one level, the full set of pulses is selectively applied at the next adjacent tomographic level and then the next, and so forth. With this multislice technique, the total number of tomographic levels that can be imaged is approximately TR/TE. As indicated earlier, TR equals the length of the cardiac cycle (R-R interval) when using ECG gating.

For imaging small anatomical structures such as the coronary arteries, thin slices (0.25 to 0.5 cm thickness) are acquired. Each anatomical level is also imaged at multiple phases of the cardiac cycle in order to minimize the effect of movement of the structures into and out of the imaging plane during the cardiac cycle. In this manner, each adjacent tomogram is acquired at the same phase of the cardiac cycle during both systole and diastole. The gating window for such images is less than 30 msec using the spin echo technique; thus the time is minimized for coronary motion during image acquisitions.

The *multiphasic multislice technique* is also used for the evaluation of cardiac dimensions and function.[128] With this technique, each anatomical section is imaged at five phases of the cardiac cycle. From end-diastolic and end (late) systolic images of each anatomical level, measurement can be made of diastolic and systolic volumes, stroke volume, ejection fraction, myocardial mass, and extent of left ventricular regional wall thickening. With this technique, wall thickening dynamics have been measured for various regions of the left ventricle in normal subjects and patients with global and regional myocardial dysfunction and in patients with focal and generalized hypertrophy.[129]

CINE MR IMAGING. This can be accomplished by ECG referencing of fast imaging sequences. This approach can produce approximately 30 images (20 to 30 msec in duration) during the cardiac cycle. These images are laced together in a cinematic display so that a wall motion of the ventricles, valve motion, and blood flow patterns in the heart and great vessels can be visualized.

Volume or three-dimensional data acquisition has also been achieved with an ECG-gated sequence. With this technique, images of any desired plane can be reconstructed later, and all reconstructed planes are in the same phase of the cardiac cycle (in contrast to the multislice technique). The time cost of volume imaging is considerable; the acquisition time for volume imaging of an equal portion of the heart is longer for this technique than for the multislice technique.

INTERPRETATION OF MR IMAGES

Information on morphology, function, and tissue characteristics can be derived from MR images. Most abnormalities are evident from alterations in morphology, such as regional wall thinning in patients with ischemic heart disease. However, occasionally no morphological changes are evident but the disease process can be diagnosed because of abnormal tissue characteristics. Abnormal myocardial tissue may be manifested as a regional difference in myocardial intensity, such as the increased intensity of acutely infarcted myocardium compared with normal myocardium. Tissue characterization by MR is achieved by measurements of relative signal intensity and relaxation times of the tissue.[130–133] It is still imprecise due to motion-related artifactual variations in magnetic relaxation times of myocardial tissue currently relied upon for such characterization. Signal intensity increases with increases in hydrogen density and T2 relaxation time and decreases with T1 relaxation time. The contrast in intensity between tissues can be augmented by varying the technical factors used to acquire the MR images. Decreasing the TR (repetition time) and TE (echo delay time) factors produces greater contrast related to differences in T1 magnetic relaxation times among tissues (T1 weighted images) and increasing TR and TE causes greater contrast primarily on the basis of difference in T2 relaxation times among tissues (T2 weighted image).

EVALUATION OF SPECIFIC CARDIAC DISEASES BY MRI

The clinical use of MR imaging has been primarily for the demonstration of pathological anatomy. Precise demonstration of anatomical abnormalities has been useful for the evaluation of patients with ischemic heart disease, cardiomyopathies, pericardial disease, neoplastic disease, congenital heart disease, and thoracic aortic disease.

ISCHEMIC HEART DISEASE

MRI provides direct visualization of the myocardium with excellent delineation of the epicardial and endocardial

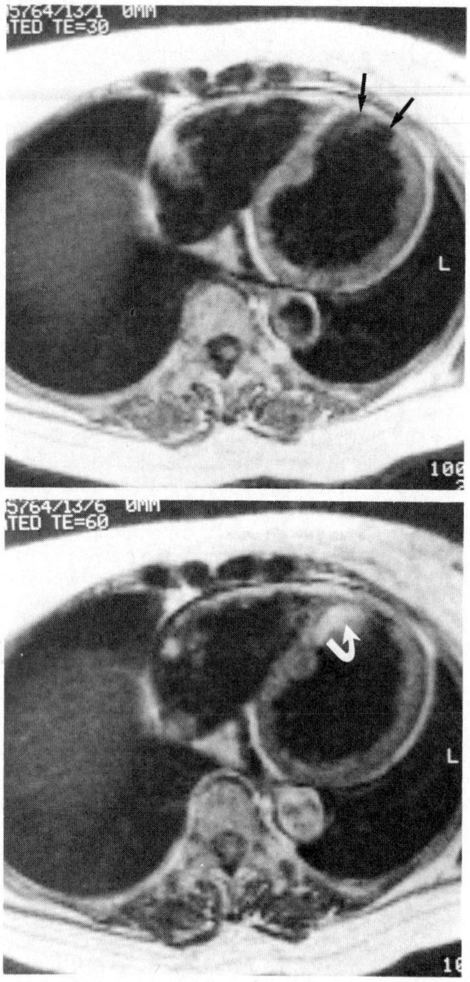

FIGURE 12–27. Chronic anterior myocardial infarction. First (*top*) and second (*bottom*) (spin echo) images show absence of myocardium in the anterior wall of the LV (arrows). Second echo image detects high signal from blood stasis (curved arrow) at the site of the old infarction, presumably due to segmental contractile dysfunction. (From Higgins, C. B.: MRI of the heart: Update 1986. Am. J. Roentgenol. *146*:931, 1986.)

interfaces. Consequently, it can define accurately segmental wall thinning that is indicative of previous myocardial infarction.[134, 135, 135a] In some patients with a history of transmural infarction, residual myocardium can be demonstrated at the site of the infarction. In others, MRI shows virtually complete absence of remnant muscle. Direct visualization of the myocardium could be used to determine whether there is sufficient residual myocardium in the region jeopardized by a coronary arterial lesion to warrant a bypass graft (Fig. 12–27). Regional wall thickening can also be assessed.[135b]

The recognition of decreased signal intensity of the myocardial wall at the site of old myocardial infarction suggests that MRI can identify the replacement of myocardium by fibrous scar.[135] Gated MR has also demonstrated complications of myocardial infarctions, such as left ventricular thrombus and aneurysms[134, 135] (Fig. 12–28).

Acute myocardial infarctions have been demonstrated by gated MRI. The region of ischemically damaged myocardium displays increased signal intensity compared with normal myocardium[130, 131] (Fig. 12–29). Contrast between infarcted and normal myocardium increases on images with greater T2 contribution to signal intensity.

CORONARY ARTERY BYPASS GRAFTS. Gated MRI has been used to evaluate the patency of coronary artery bypass

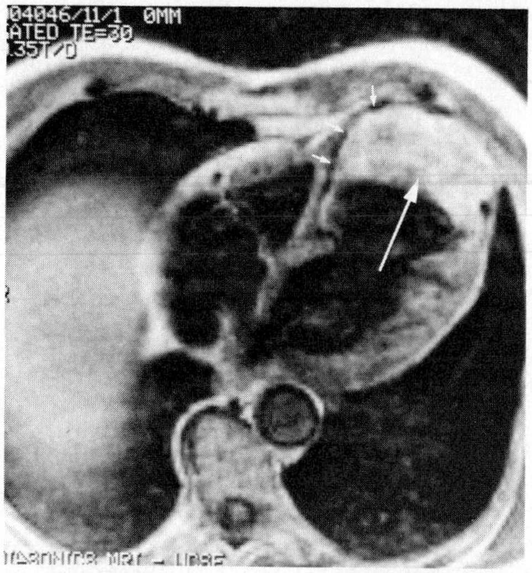

FIGURE 12–28. Anteroapical aneurysm and thrombus of the left ventricle. There is bulging of the anterior wall. The wall of the aneurysm shows lower intensity (small arrows) than the adjacent myocardial wall; the decreased intensity is consistent with fibrous replacement of the myocardium. The large thrombus has high signal intensity (arrow). (From Higgins, C. B.: MRI of the heart: Update 1986. Am. J. Roentgenol. *146*:931, 1986.)

grafts. Since blood usually flows rapidly through the grafts, they appear as small circular structures with absence of a luminal signal (Fig. 12–30). For visualization of grafts, ECG-gated images are acquired in order to minimize the effect of motion of the grafts. Generally, images are acquired at each anatomical level during multiple phases of the cardiac cycle to ensure that an image is acquired at a phase when there is a rapid rate of flow through the graft. High flow rate in the graft produces a flow void in the lumen of the graft using spin echo MR imaging and thus indicates patency of the graft. With the newer rapid MR imaging techniques, flowing blood causes bright signal intensity; therefore, bright signal rather than flow void would indicate graft patency with this technique. In order to achieve specificity in establishing patency, it is necessary to visualize absence of a luminal signal on at least two

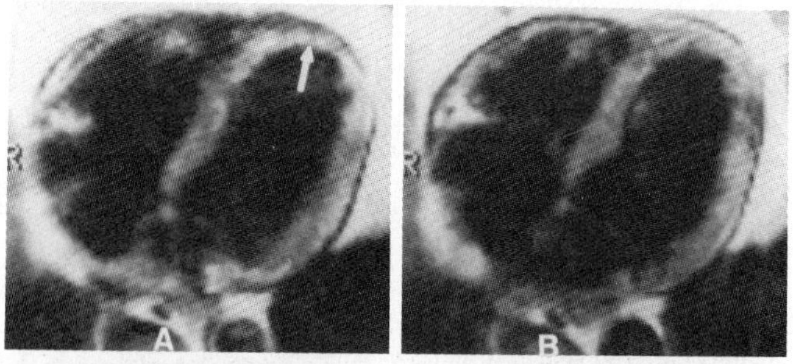

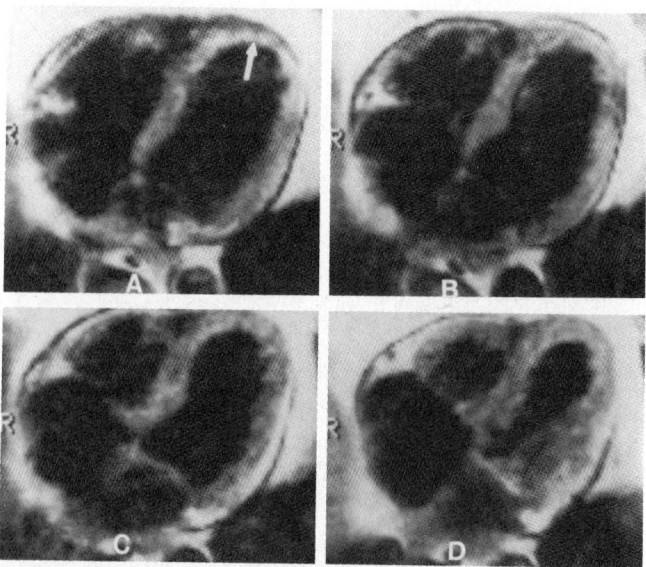

FIGURE 12–29. Anterior acute myocardial infarction. Images at four anatomical levels extending from cranial (*upper left*) to caudal (*lower right*) levels of the LV. Note the higher signal intensity (arrow) of the myocardium of the anterior wall of the LV at the site of the acute infarction. (From Higgins, C. B.: MRI of the heart: Update 1986. Am. J. Roentgenol. *146*:931, 1986.)

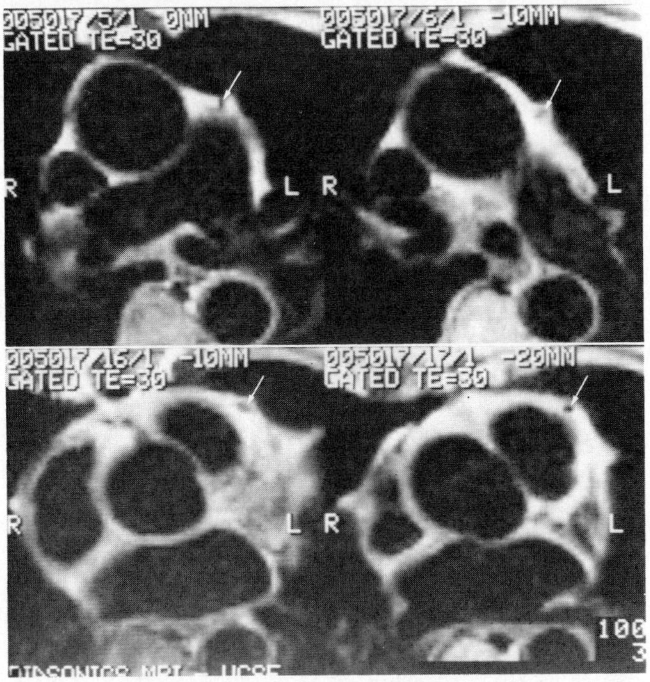

FIGURE 12–30. Multislice gated images extending from cranial (*upper left*) to caudal (*lower right*). A graft to the left anterior descending coronary artery is visible at each level (arrow). Absence of luminal signal indicates patency of the graft.

transverse images. Early results indicate an accuracy of 80 to 90 per cent for MRI in defining graft patency.

CARDIOMYOPATHIES

Gated MR sharply delineates the endocardial and epicardial surfaces of the myocardial walls. Consequently, it can accurately define the presence, distribution, and severity of hypertrophic cardiomyopathies.[136, 137] Gated MR imaging has revealed the extent of septal involvement (Fig. 12–31) and has been particularly useful for identifying the unusual distribution of hypertrophy in the variant forms of hypertrophic cardiomyopathy. Likewise, it has demonstrated the degree of ventricular dilatation in patients with congestive cardiomyopathies.[136] Since MR provides excellent discrimination of the edges of the myocardium, it can also be used to assess myocardial mass and wall thickness in patients with dilated cardiomyopathy; such information may prove useful prognostically in this condition.

Two-dimensional echocardiography provides excellent evaluation of the cardiomyopathies (p. 1424); it is unlikely that it will be supplanted by MR for the routine evaluation of these conditions. However, MR has proved valuable in the evaluation of variant types of hypertrophic cardiomyopathy, such as the midventricular and apical forms.[132, 136, 137] It has also demonstrated abnormal signal intensity of the myocardium due to nonocclusive infarction of the apical region of the left ventricle as a complication of hypertrophic cardiomyopathy.[132] In amyloid heart disease (p. 1431), MR has demonstrated thickened myocardial walls and diminished wall thickening during the cardiac cycle.[129, 138, 138a]

The MR findings in cardiomyopathies have thus far been limited to *anatomical* abnormalities. No consistent changes in MR relaxation times have been found for the myocardium in hypertrophic or congestive cardiomyopathies[133] or in amyloid heart disease.[139]

PERICARDIAL DISEASE

Gated MR provides direct visualization of the pericardium.[140–142] This technique is proving to be especially useful for the assessment of patients with known or suspected pericardial disease (Fig. 12–32). Normal pericardium is composed primarily of fibrous tissue and has low MR signal intensity. The thickness of pericardial line measured in normal subjects is 1.6 ± 0.4 mm (S.D.) with a range from 0.8 to 2.6 mm.[141] A variation in thickness of the low-intensity line has been observed during the cardiac cycle in normal subjects. These latter observations, along with information from postmortem studies, indicate that the normal pericardium measures less than 2.0 mm, and suggest that the low-intensity pericardial line consists of pericardium and some adherent pericardial fluid.[143] This is probably responsible for the pericardial line observed on CT as well, since normal CT measurements of pericardial thickness are similar to MR measurements.[84]

Gated MR has been useful for demonstrating pericardial thickness in patients with suspected constrictive pericarditis.[140, 144, 143] The signal intensity of the thickened pericardium is variable. The purely fibrous or calcified pericardium in chronic constrictive pericardial disease has low signal intensity (Fig. 12–32). However, in subacute forms of constrictive pericarditis caused by irradiation, surgical trauma, or uremia (Fig. 12–33), the thickened pericardium has moderate to high intensity on spin-echo images.[140, 141] The effusive-constrictive form of pericardial disease (p. 1507) has thickened pericardium and pericardial effusion (Fig. 12–33).

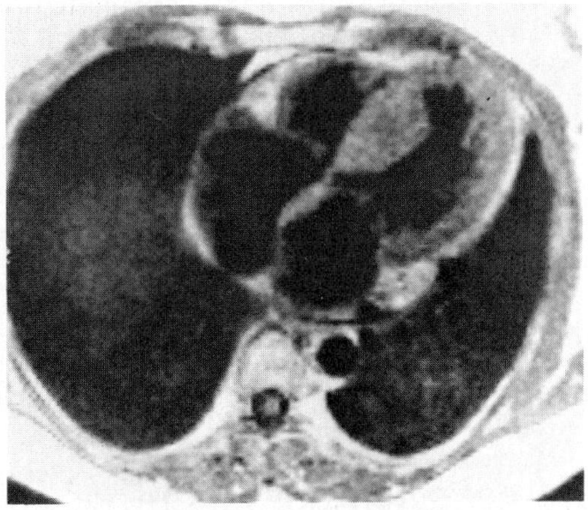

FIGURE 12–31. Hypertrophic cardiomyopathy. MR image displays severe hypertrophy of the entire septum and normal thickness of the lateral wall.

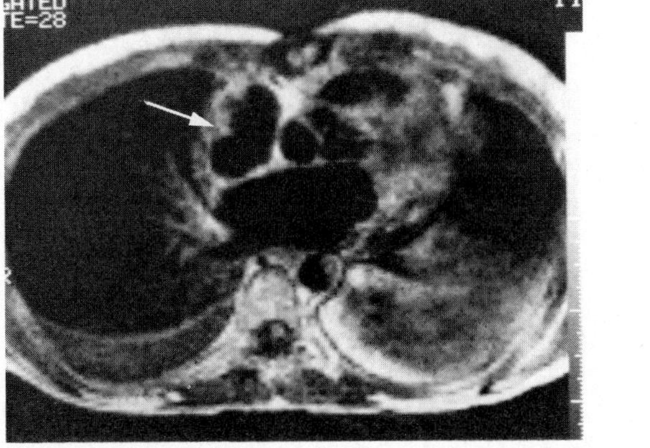

FIGURE 12–32. Transverse image in a patient with constrictive pericarditis caused by prior irradiation. Markedly thickened pericardium is present over the right atrium (arrow). There are bilateral pleural effusions.

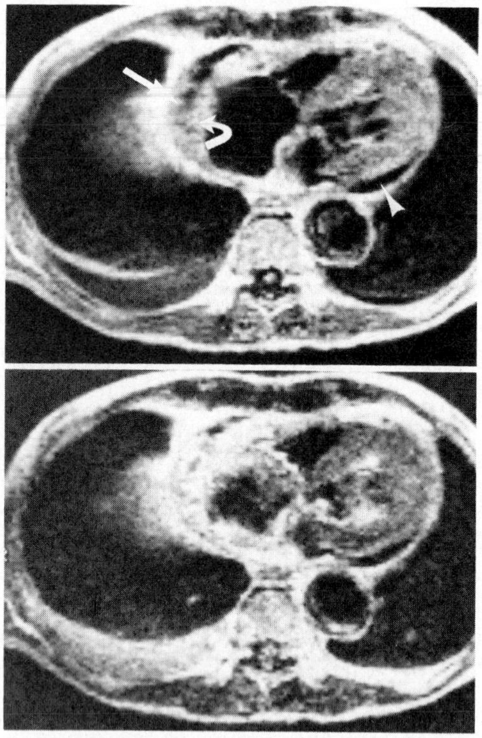

FIGURE 12–33. Effusive-constrictive pericarditis due to uremia. First (*top*) and second (*bottom*) echo images. Thickening of the visceral (curved arrow) and parietal pericardium (arrow) with inflammatory adhesions between them is evident. Pericardial fluid has low signal intensity. Both the thickened pericardium and fluid show a relative increase of intensity of the second echo image. Note the small posterior pericardial effusion (arrowhead).

Gated MR, like echocardiography, can be used to detect even very small pericardial effusions.[141] An advantage of MR over echocardiography is the capability to differentiate pericardial hematoma from other types of effusions. Determination of pericardial thickening seems to be a clear indication for use of gated MR.

NEOPLASTIC DISEASE

Several reports have documented the clinical utility of gated MR for the evaluation of cardiac[136, 145–147] and paracardiac masses.[140, 145, 148, 149] Because of the unequivocal delineation of the pericardium, myocardial walls, and chambers of the heart on MR images, the precise relationship of tumors to cardiovascular structures can be defined.

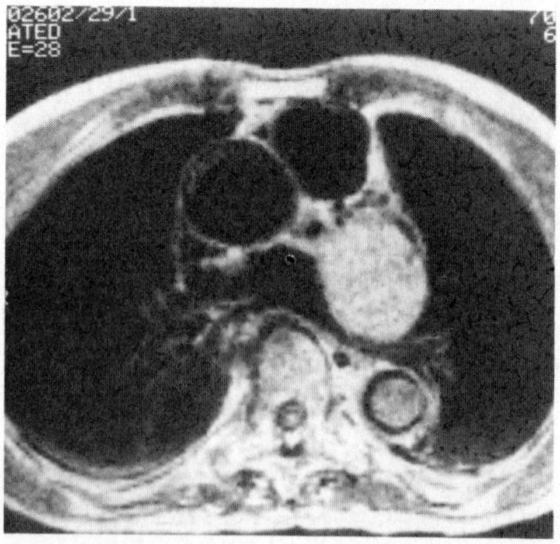

FIGURE 12–34. MR image shows an intrapericardial pheochromocytoma located adjacent to the left atrium. There is clear discrimination of the solid mass from the left atrial chamber so that the extrinsic compression of the atrium is evident.

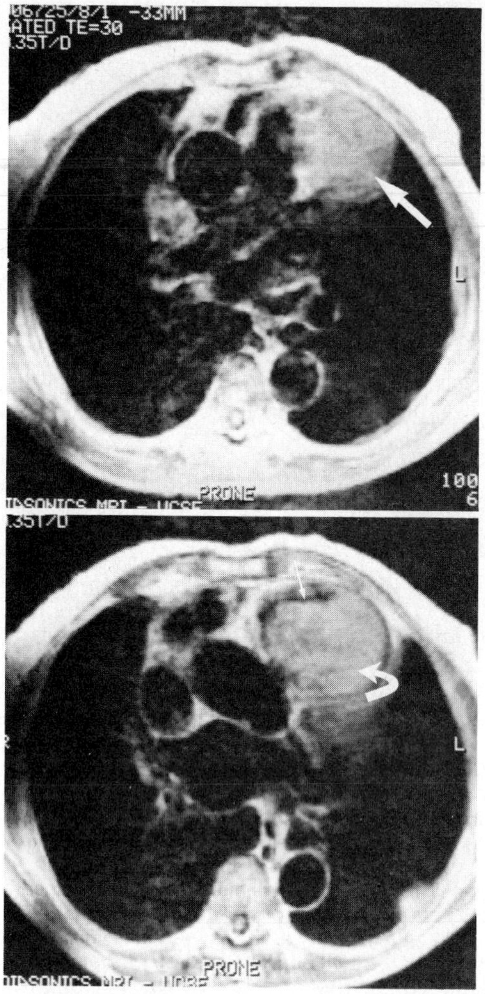

FIGURE 12–35. Dumbbell-shaped tumor of the right ventricle in a patient with neurofibromatosis. Transverse images at the level of the main pulmonary artery (*left*) and RV outflow tract (*bottom*). A portion of the mass is extracardiac (arrow) and rightwardly displaces the pulmonary artery, while the immense intracardiac portion (curved arrow) almost completely obstructs the RV outflow region. There is a very narrow residual channel (small arrow).

MR appears to be superior to CT for assessing the extent and effect of mediastinal masses adjacent to cardiovascular structures (Fig. 12–34). Gated MR is the imaging procedure of choice for identifying paracardiac masses, defining their nature and determining invasion of the pericardium. The intensity on spin-echo images can be used to differentiate such masses from innocuous lipomas, the pericardial fat pad, pericardial cysts, loculated pericardial effusions, and unusual enlargement or displacement of cardiac chambers. Gated MR has been extremely useful for demonstrating invasion of cardiac chambers by pulmonary and mediastinal malignancies. Metastases to the pericardium and the possibility of pericardial effusion can be readily established by gated MRI.

Intracardiac tumors can be clearly identified within the signal void of the cardiac blood pool. Because of its wide field of view, MR is ideal for defining both the intracardiac and extracardiac extent of masses (Fig. 12–35).

CONGENITAL HEART DISEASE

Reports from several centers indicate encouraging results with MRI for the evaluation of patients with congen-

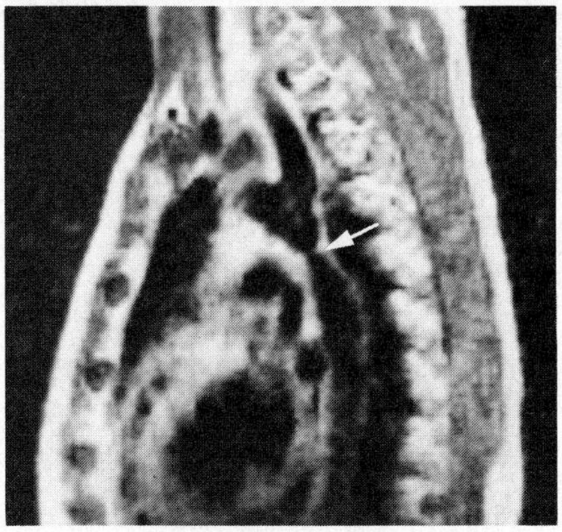

FIGURE 12–36. Coarctation of the aorta. Sagittal MR image shows discrete juxtaductal coarctation of the aorta (arrow).

ital heart disease.[149a–156] In a study from the author's institution, in which the results of MRI were corroborated by angiography and two-dimensional echocardiography, accurate anatomical diagnosis of anomalies was achieved by MRI in over 90 per cent of the patients.[151]

Visceroatrial situs, the type of ventricular loop, and the relationship of the great vessels could be identified in all patients in whom studies encompassing the entire heart were done. Forty-four of 47 abnormalities at the level of the great vessels, including coarctation of the aorta (Fig. 12–36) and vascular rings (p. 966), were correctly identified. MRI showed 30 of 33 ventricular abnormalities; two small ventricular septal defects and one Ebstein's anomaly were not demonstrated. All the abnormalities at the atrial level and those of systemic and pulmonary venous return were also shown. Complex cardiac anomalies (such as single ventricle) and the status of the pulmonary arteries were clearly demonstrated, and a good assessment of the postoperative anatomy after total and palliative surgery was attained. An especially useful contribution of MRI is the demonstration of the status of the pulmonary arteries in patients with pulmonary atresia; the central pulmonary vessels can be demonstrated without the need for opacification by contrast medium (Fig. 12–37).

Blinded analysis of MR images has shown a sensitivity and specificity of over 90 per cent for the identification of atrial level abnormalities (Fig. 12–38), including ostium secundum and primum atrial septal defects as well as

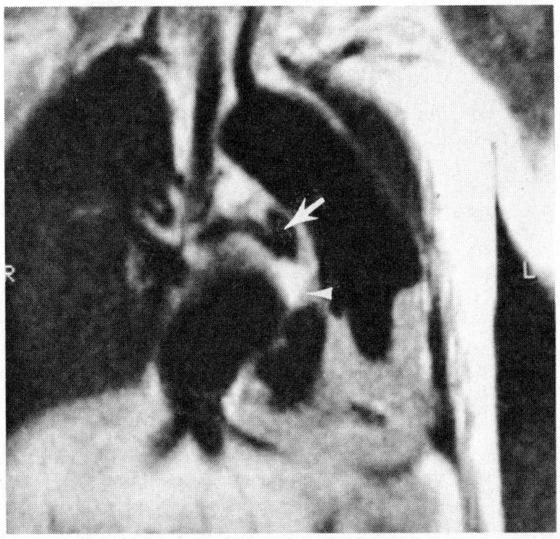

FIGURE 12–37. Single ventricle with levo-transposition and pulmonary atresia. Coronal MR image shows the large aorta in the levo-transposed position. Note the atresia of the pulmonary valve (arrowhead). Central confluence of the pulmonary arteries is demonstrated (arrow). (From Higgins, C. B.: MRI of the heart: Update 1986. Am. J. Roentgenol. *146*:931, 1986.)

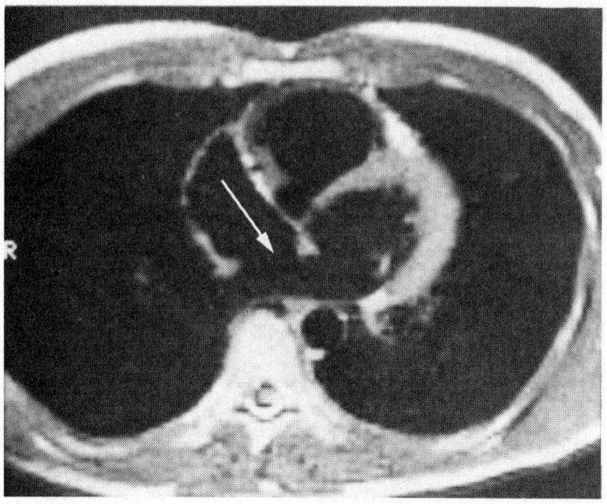

FIGURE 12–38. Secundum atrial septal defect. Transverse MR image shows a defect in the middle of the atrial septum (arrow).

anomalous pulmonary venous connection.[143] However, another report had been less encouraging in this regard.[144] It is recognized that a thin fossa ovalis can be confused with an atrial septal defect on static MR images. It may be possible to avoid this misinterpretation using cine MR techniques.

MRI is a completely noninvasive technique for the preoperative and postoperative evaluation of cardiac anatomy to congenital heart disease. Both simple and complex anomalies are often depicted as definitively by gated MRI as they are by angiography. However, at the time of this writing, large prospective comparative studies have not been carried out to determine the accuracy of MRI in relationship to angiography for the evaluation of the vast array of individual congenital cardiovascular anomalies. Two limitations of MRI have been recognized: the thickness of the MR tomogram in relationship to the heart size of infants and the difficulty of imaging perpendicular to the semilunar valves.

Much of the diagnostic information provided by MRI can also be shown by two-dimensional echocardiography (p. 86). The unique capabilities of MRI in congenital heart disease are visualization of the central pulmonary arteries in cases of pulmonary atresia (Fig. 12–37), and assessment of anomalies of the thoracic aorta (Fig. 12–36), and of complex anomalies involving both the great vessels and ventricles. In this regard, coronal images are particularly useful in providing a composite view of the ventricles and great vessels in complex anomalies such as single ventricle (Fig. 12–37).

Although the ultimate role of MRI in congenital heart disease is not yet clear, the necessity for catheterization and angiography for preoperative assessment will have to be reevaluated in the light of the extensive information available using the combination of two-dimensional echocardiography and gated MRI.

DISEASE OF THE THORACIC AORTA

MR imaging of the thoracic aorta is considerably improved by ECG gating. For imaging of the thoracic aorta, MR appears to be superior to echocardiography and CT. A number of reports attest to its effectiveness for the evaluation of aortic dissection, true and false aneurysms, periaortic abscess and hematoma, aortic arch anomalies, and coarctation of the aorta.[153, 157–159c] In aortic dissection, MRI can depict the intimal flap, and the proximal extent of the dissection, and it can distinguish true from false channel (Fig. 12–39 and Fig. 46–3, p. 1548). Intraluminal signal is usually seen in the false channel due to thrombus, slow blood flow, or both.

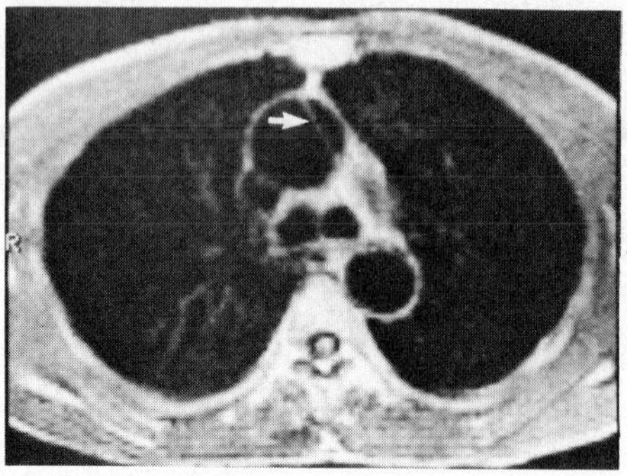

FIGURE 12–39. Aortic dissection. Transverse MRI scan of the upper thorax shows an intimal flap (arrow) in the ascending aorta. The descending aorta, just anterior and to the right of the spine, is normal. (From Amparo, E. G., et al.: Aortic dissection: Magnetic resonance imaging. Radiology *155*:399, 1985.)

MRI has been used to monitor the size of the thoracic aorta in patients with the Marfan syndrome and to exclude the presence of an occult dissection.[160] Dimensions at various segments of the thoracic aorta have been defined for normal subjects and patients with aneurysmal dilatation due to Marfan syndrome and other causes (Table 12–1). Since MRI is a completely noninvasive technique, it is ideal for monitoring patients with aortic diseases and patients who have undergone surgical or medical treatment of aortic dissection. MRI is also the most logical technique for the study of patients whose chest roentgenogram suggests a substantial increase in the size of the thoracic aorta.

MRI has been used to detect periaortic abscess complicating bacterial endocarditis.[159] The three-dimensional tomographic nature of the technique permits precise localization of these abscesses (Fig. 12–40).

Although MR can identify the presence and extent of aortic coarctation[153] (Fig. 12–36), it cannot define the severity of the stenosis. As further experience confirms the early results of MR for the diagnosis of thoracic aortic disease, it will be necessary to reconsider the traditional reliance upon angiography for identifying intimal flap, mural thrombus, and periaortic hematoma abscess.

EVALUATION OF CARDIOVASCULAR FUNCTION

Since MRI is a three-dimensional imaging technique it can provide most of the measurements upon which the

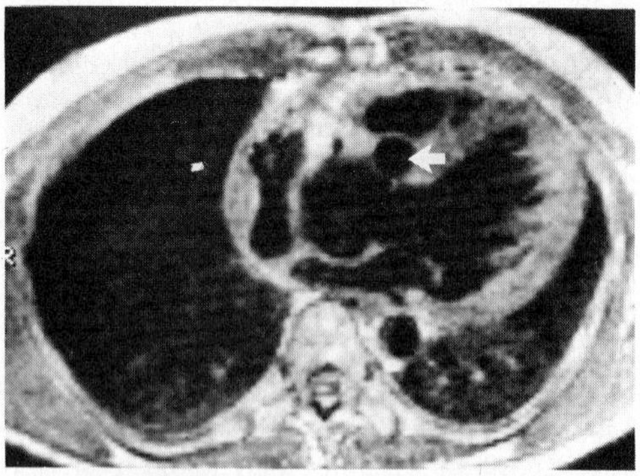

FIGURE 12–40. Periaortic pseudoaneurysm complicating bacterial endocarditis. Transverse MRI scan shows a cavity (arrow) in the ventricular septum representing a pseudoaneurysm originating from the aortic root. The absence of signal in the cavity indicates free communication with blood in the aorta. (From Winkler, M. L., and Higgins, C. B.: Magnetic resonance imaging of perivalvular infectious pseudoaneurysms. Am. J. Roentgenol. *147*:253, 1986.)

TABLE 12–1 MRI DIMENSIONS OF THORACIC AORTA IN NORMAL SUBJECTS AND MARFAN SYNDROME

	NORMAL	MARFAN
Sinus	33 ± 4 (30–38)	48 ± 7 (40–63)
Asc Ao proximal	30 ± 4 (19–37)	45 ± 10 (34–64)
Asc Ao distal	30 ± 4 (19–37)	31 ± 7 (25–37)
Desc Ao	24 ± 4 (16–29)	22 ± 6 (18–27)

± = SD

clinical evaluation of global left ventricular function has been based. Using sets of images encompassing the left ventricle, it is possible to calculate end-diastolic, end-systolic, and stroke volumes, and ejection fraction. This can be done directly and not depend upon the geometric assumptions used for such measurements from angiograms. Even more important, MR provides a three-dimensional direct visualization of the myocardium with excellent mural edge discrimination, thereby allowing quantitation of left ventricular mass. MR measurements have correlated closely with anatomical measurements of left ventricular mass[161, 162] and the mass of acute myocardial infarctions[162] (Fig. 12–41).

Since MR also defines the right ventricular myocardium, it may serve as the preferred technique for the accurate determination of right ventricular mass; reasonable accuracy has been shown for the measurement of right ventricular end-diastolic, end-systolic, and stroke volumes as well as ejection fraction.[163, 164] Moreover, comparison of right and left ventricular stroke volumes has been used to estimate the regurgitant fraction in patients with aortic and mitral regurgitation.

LEFT VENTRICULAR REGIONAL FUNCTION. Acquisition of MR images at various phases of the cardiac cycle

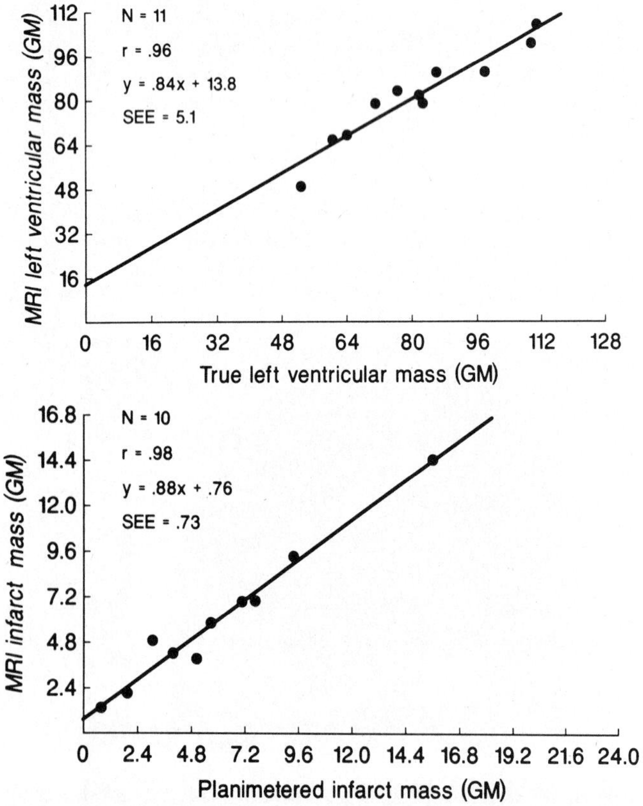

FIGURE 12–41. Graph (*top*) shows the relationship between left ventricular mass calculated from MRI scans (ordinate) and that measured at postmortem (abscissa). Graph (*bottom*) shows relationship between mass of infarcted myocardium measured from MRI and at postmortem. Correlations were done in a group of dogs with recent myocardial infarctions. Postmortem was done within hours after the MR study.

provides a noninvasive method of assessing regional myocardial function.[128, 129] Using a technique termed *rotating gated acquisition*, 10 transverse levels through the left ventricle are imaged at five sequential phases of the cardiac cycle. The 10 transverse levels (each approximately 10 mm in thickness) encompass the left ventricle; the five images at each transverse level start at end-diastole and then proceed in 100-msec intervals through the cardiac cycle (Fig. 12–42). Thereby, the maximum extent of wall thickening may be calculated from the following formula:

$$\% \text{ wall thickening} = \frac{\text{WTes} = \text{WTed}}{\text{WTed}} \times 100 \text{ per cent}$$

where WTes = wall thickness at end-systole, and
WTed = wall thickness at end-diastole

Using this technique, the extent of regional wall thickening in normal subjects has been defined.[128, 129] Diminished regional wall thickening has been demonstrated in patients with acute myocardial infarction, and generalized wall-thickening abnormalities have been demonstrated in patients with congestive cardiomyopathy and concentric left ventricular hypertrophy.[129] The unusual pattern consisting of increased end-diastolic wall thickness and diminished wall thickening was shown in amyloid heart disease (Fig. 12–42). Wall thickening measurements in normal subjects and in various disease states are shown in Tables 12–2 and 12–3.

Accuracy of measurement of wall thickness can be improved with the use of an imaging plane perpendicular to the long axis of the left ventricle.[165] Such short-axis views vitiate the problem of overestimation of wall thickness resulting from oblique sectioning of the heart on the standard transverse tomograms. Measurement of wall thickness on the transverse section through the middle of the left ventricle (equatorial plane) minimizes these potential mensuration errors.

BLOOD FLOW. The MR signal produced by flowing blood is variable and is determined by many factors, including the velocity and acceleration of blood flow, the flow profile (laminar or turbulent), the direction of flow in relation to the imaging plane, even or odd spin-echo image, type of image, and the pulse sequence being applied.[166–170] Disregarding the complex interplay of these mechanisms, intracavitary signals during various phases of the cardiac cycle have been described, and empirical observations have been made in normal subjects and in patients with various forms of cardiac disease.[171] In normal subjects, signals within the left ventricle or spin-echo images usually occur only in late diastole and are most prominent in the presence of a slow heart rate; in normal subjects with heart rates over 80, intracavitary signal may not be discernible at any time in the cardiac cycle. Signal is more prominent on second (even) echo images compared with first (odd) echo images. On the other hand, signal within the left ventricular chamber is frequently visualized during systole and diastole in patients with global and regional left ventricular dysfunction. Prominent intracavitary signal is observed in the left atrium in patients with elevated left ventricular end-diastolic pressure.[138] Visualization of intracavitary signal is consistent with momentary stasis of blood or slowly moving blood.

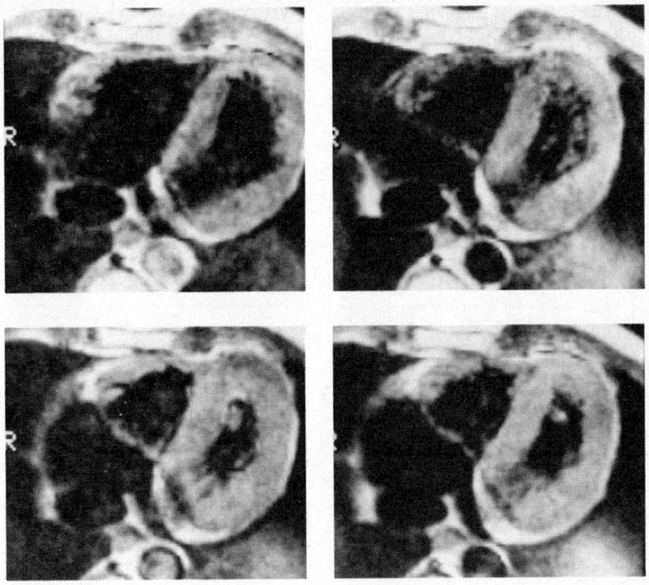

FIGURE 12–42. Image from a single anatomical level of a patient with cardiac amyloidosis is shown at four phases of the cardiac cycle. *Upper left*, end-diastole; *upper right*, early systole; *lower left*, mid-systole; *lower right*, late systole. There is symmetric increase in wall thickness at end-diastole. End-diastolic wall thickness is increased and wall thickening during systole is decreased in all regions. (From Higgins, C. B.: MRI of the heart: Update 1986. Am. J. Roentgenol. *146*:931, 1986.)

Abnormal flow patterns in the pulmonary arteries have also been observed on MR images in patients with pulmonary arterial hypertension and elevated pulmonary vascular resistance.[172] Using the rotated gated sequence, the normal pattern is to observe signal in the aorta and pulmonary artery at end-diastole, when flow velocity is low or when flow nearly ceases. During systole, there is no signal from blood in these vessels in normal subjects. On the other hand, patients with severe pulmonary arterial hypertension have signal in the pulmonary artery in systole (Fig. 12–43). This finding is consistent with slow flow in the pulmonary circulation and appears to be indicative of a marked increase in pulmonary vascular resistance. Indeed, a good direct linear relationship between signal intensity during systole in the central pulmonary arteries and pulmonary vascular resistance has been observed in patients with primary pulmonary hypertension.[172] A similar relationship has also been shown for patients with left-to-right shunts complicated by pulmonary hypertension.[173]

CHARACTERIZATION OF MYOCARDIAL TISSUE

Characterization of myocardial tissue depends upon estimation of signal intensity on images with varying TR and

TABLE 12–2 SYSTOLIC WALL THICKENING IN NORMAL SUBJECTS DETERMINED BY MRI

	Segments						
	PS	AS	AN	AL	PL	P	AP
Diastolic wall thickness (mm)	9 ± 1	9 ± 1	10 ± 2	9 ± 2	10 ± 1	10 ± 1	6 ± 2
Systolic wall thickness (mm)	12 ± 2	13 ± 1	14 ± 2	14 ± 2	14 ± 2	13 ± 1	8 ± 2
Absolute SWT (mm)	3 ± 1	4 ± 1	4 ± 1	4 ± 2	4 ± 1	4 ± 2	3 ± 1
Percent SWT (%)	35 ± 15	42 ± 10	43 ± 15	48 ± 28	43 ± 10	37 ± 9	46 ± 17

AL = anterolateral; AN = anterior; AP = apical; AS = anteroseptal; I = inferior; P = posterior; PL = posterolateral; SWT = systolic wall thickening; ± = SD

TABLE 12–3 ABSOLUTE AND PERCENTAGE WALL THICKENING IN PATIENTS WITH VARIOUS TYPES OF HEART DISEASE

No. Patients	Diagnosis	Normal Myocardium ASWT* (mm)	Normal Myocardium PSWT‡ (%)	Abnormal Myocardium ASWT (mm)	Abnormal Myocardium PSWT (%)
13	CAD† with wall motion abnormalities	5 ± 1	54 ± 13	1 ± 1	8 ± 14
4	CAD without wall motion abnormalities	5 ± 2	46 ± 16	——	——
4	Left ventricular hypertrophy	4 ± 0	41 ± 4	——	——
3	Hypertrophic cardiomyopathy	10 ± 2	73 ± 14	6 ± 3	28 ± 7
2	Dilated cardiomyopathy	——	——	1 ± 0	8 ± 3
1	Amyloidosis	——	——	4	33
4	Constrictive pericarditis§	4 ± 2	41 ± 9	——	——

*Absolute systolic wall thickening, † Coronary artery disease, ‡Percentage systolic wall thickening, §One patient with constrictive pericarditis and paradoxical septal motion on the echocardiogram is not included. ± = SD

TE values, hydrogen density, and T1 and T2 relaxation times. The measurements of relaxation times from gated images are approximations rendered inexact by cardiac and respiratory motion.[174] Despite these limitations, the T2 relaxation times have been found to discriminate between normal and pathological myocardium of the in situ beating heart.

Ex vivo measurements have revealed that several myocardial diseases, including ischemic myocardial injury,[175–177] cardiac transplant rejection,[177–179] and Adriamycin cardiomyopathy,[180] produce significant alteration of relaxation time. A number of experiments in the author's laboratory have been directed toward the identification and characterization of abnormal myocardium by MR imaging in vivo.

Experimental canine models of myocardial infarctions with and without reperfusion, cardiac transplant rejection, and Adriamycin cardiomyopathy have been produced and evaluated by MR.

ACUTE MYOCARDIAL INFARCTION. This is characterized in vivo by increased signal intensity and prolonged T2 relaxation time.[181–183] Animals imaged before and during the first 5 hours after coronary occlusion showed regional increase in MR signal intensity (prolongation of T2 relaxation time) in the jeopardized region by 3 hours after occlusion[181, 182] (Fig. 12–44). In some animals, increased signal intensity was noted in the jeopardized region within the first hour after occlusion. Gated MR of dogs with reperfused myocardial infarctions (1 hour of occlusion followed by reperfusion) showed significant alterations in regional signal intensity and T2 relaxation times by 30 minutes after reperfusion.[183] These studies show that MR can potentially detect ischemically injured myocardium soon after coronary occlusion.

MRI obtained in patients within 10 days after sustaining acute myocardial infarction has also shown that acutely infarcted myocardium is characterized by increased signal intensity and prolonged T2 relaxation time.[131, 184] However, variations in signal intensity are observed through the myocardial wall of normal subjects; this probably reflects an artifact due to cardiac and respiratory motion. It may be possible to distinguish between an artifactual increase in regional intensity and that caused by a change in T2 by comparing the contrast between the two regions on first and second echo images. Contrast between infarcted and normal myocardium has been greater on the second echo image, while the contrast has been similar or decreased between various regions in normal subjects. Good sensitivity and specificity of MR for the demonstration of acute myocardial infarctions in patients has been reported.[184] A regional decrease in signal intensity and decreased T2 relaxation time at the infarct site have been noted in some, but not all, patients with old myocardial infarctions.[135] These observations are consistent with fibrous replacement of myocardium.

CARDIAC TRANSPLANT REJECTION. Another model of myocardial disease is provided by cardiac transplant rejection; this process mimics acute myocarditis. In dogs that underwent heterotropic cardiac transplantation, serial ECG-gated MR imaging and histological examination of allograft biopsies were obtained at intervals after transplantation.[185] Since the transplant was placed in the circulation in parallel with the native heart, relaxation times in the two hearts could be compared. Some of the animals received therapy in order to prevent rejection. Untreated allografts showed an increase in T2 relaxation time and intensity of the myocardium compared with the native hearts. Rejecting allografts showed significant alterations in T2 relaxation time

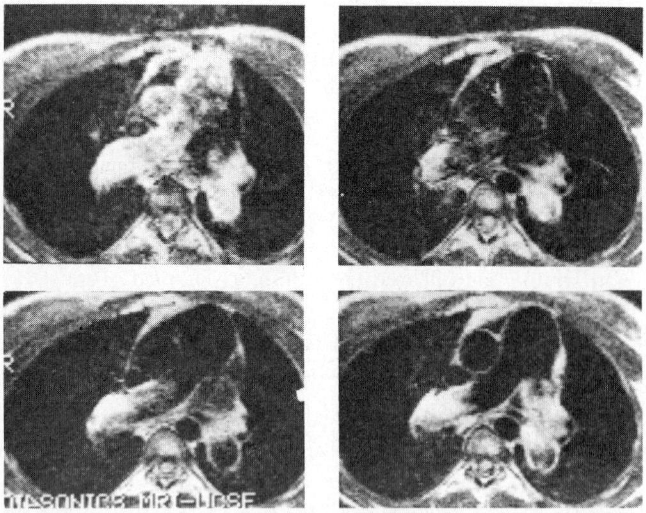

FIGURE 12–43. Rotated gated series of MR images at the level of the central pulmonary arteries of a patient with severe pulmonary arterial hypertension. Image on the upper left is obtained at end-diastole, while subsequent images are done at 100 msec intervals proceeding into systole (lower right image is approximately 300 msec after the R wave). Signal appears in the ascending and descending aorta only at end-diastole. There is signal in the pulmonary artery at end-diastole and on the images during systole, consistent with slow flow in the pulmonary circulation. (From Higgins, C. B.: MRI of the heart: Update 1986. Am. J. Roentgenol. *146*:931, 1986.)

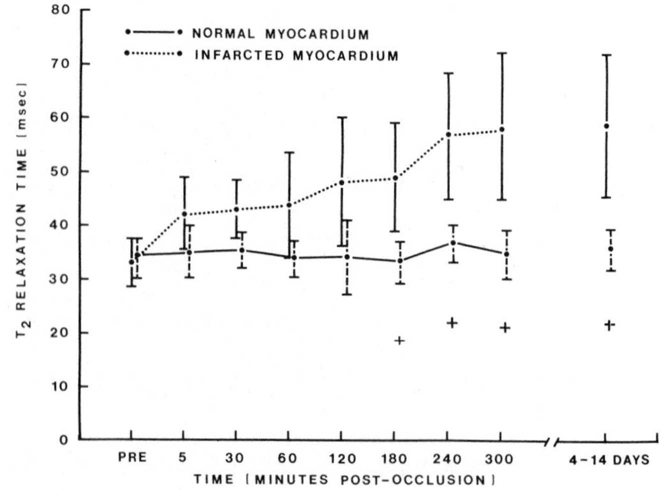

FIGURE 12–44. Graph displays the mean T2 relaxation times for normal and infarcted myocardium during the first six hours and at several days after acute occlusion of the left anterior descending coronary artery. Significant increases in T2 relaxation time of infarcted myocardium were present by three hours after occlusion. Crosses indicate the time intervals at which there were significant differences between normal and infarcted myocardium. (From Higgins, C. B.: MRI of the heart: Update 1986. Am. J. Roentgenol. *146*:931, 1986.)

and signal intensity compared with normal myocardium as early as one week after transplant. There was no significant difference in T1, T2, or intensity values between successfully immunosuppressed allografts and native hearts. Thus, in vivo gated MR imaging may be a sensitive noninvasive technique for detecting acute cardiac transplant rejection.

The wide range of MR signal intensities among soft tissue present with MRI and the numerous parameters that can potentially be monitored from tissue protons during the MR process suggest that this technique should be able to provide useful tissue characterization. Tissue characterization specific to disease processes is likely to depend on the recognition of new parameters for this purpose. Many features of the tissue appear to be evident in the proton MR spectrum. In vivo proton spectroscopy is currently under study in several laboratories, and it will be of great interest to determine whether it can provide new parameters for the characterization of myocardial tissue.

REFERENCES

DIGITAL SUBTRACTION ANGIOGRAPHY

1. Kruger, R. A., Mistretta, C. A., Houk, T. L., Riederer, S. J., Shaw, C. G., Goodsitt, M. M., Crummy, A. B., Zwiebel, W., Lancester, J., Roe, C. G., and Flemming, D.: Computerized fluoroscopy in real time for noninvasive visualization of the cardiovascular system. Radiology *130*:49, 1979.
2. Christenson, P. C., Ovitt, T. W., Fisher, H. D., Frost, M. M., Nudelman, S., and Roehrig, H.: Intravenous angiography using digital video subtraction: Intravenous cervicocerebrovascular angiography. Am. J. Radiol. *135*:1145, 1980.
3. Brennecke, R., Braun, T. K., and Bursch, J. H.: Digital processing of videoangiographic image series using a mini computer. *In* Proceedings of Computers in Cardiology. IEEE Computer Society, 1976, p. 255.
4. Mancini, G. B. J., and Higgins, C. B.: Digital subtraction angiography: A review of cardiac applications. Progr. Cardiovasc. Dis. 28:111, 1985.
5. Tobis, J., Nacioglu, O., Johnston, W. D., Siebert, A., Iseri, L. T., Roeck, W., Ekayama, U., and Henry, W. L.: Left ventricular imaging with digital subtraction angiography using intravenous contrast injection and fluoroscopic exposure levels. Am. Heart J. *104*:20, 1982.
6. Sato, D. A., Tobis, J., Nalcioglu, O., and Henry, W. L.: Re-evaluation of the role of digital angiography in cardiac diagnosis. *In*: Pohost, G. M., et al. (eds.): New Concepts in Cardiac Imaging 1987. Chicago, Year Book Medical Publishers, 1987.
7. Nichols, A. B., Martin, E. C., Fles, T. P., Stugensky, K. M., Balancio, L. A., Casarella, W. J., and Weiss, M. B.: Validation of the angiographic accuracy of digital left ventriculography. Am. J. Cardiol. *51*:224, 1983.
8. Goldberg, H. L., Borer, J. S., and Moses, J. W.: Digital subtraction intravenous left ventricular angiography: Comparison with conventional intraventricular angiography. J. Am. Coll. Cardiol. *1*:858, 1983.
9. Kronenberg, M. W., Price, R. R., Smith, C. W., Robertson, R. M., Perry, J. M., Pickens, D. R., Domanski, M. J., Partain, C. L., and Friesinger, G. C.: Evaluation of left ventricular performance using digital subtraction angiography. Am. J. Cardiol. *51*:837, 1983.
10. Nissen, S. E., Booth, D., Waters, J., Fassas, T., and DeMara, A. N.: Evaluation of left ventricular contractile pattern by intravenous digital subtraction ventriculography: Comparison of cineangiography and assessment of interobserver variability. Am. J. Cardiol. 52:1293, 1983.
11. Engels, P. H. C., Ludwig, J. W., and Verhoeven, L. A. J.: Left ventricular evaluation by digital video subtraction angiography. Radiology *144*:471, 1982.
12. Vas, R., Diamond, G. A., Forrester, J. S., Whiting, J. S., Pfaff, M. J., Levisman, J. A., Nakano, F. S., and Swan, H. J. C.: Computer-enhanced digital angiography: correlation of clinical assessment of left ventricular ejection fraction and regional wall motion. Am. Heart J. *104*:732, 1982.
13. Mancini, G. B. J., Norris, S. L., Peterson, K. L., and Higgins, C. B.: Quantitative assessment of segmental wall motion abnormalities at rest and after atrial pacing using digital intravenous ventriculography. J. Am. Coll. Cardiol. 2:70, 1983.
14. Johnson, R. A., Wasserman, A. G., and Leiboff, R. H.: Intravenous digital left ventriculography at rest and with atrial pacing as a screening procedure for coronary artery disease. J. Am. Coll. Cardiol. 2:905, 1983.
15. Mancini, G. B. J., Peterson, K. L., Gregoratos, G., and Higgins, C. B.: Effects of atrial pacing on global and regional left ventricular function in coronary heart disease assessed by digital intravenous ventriculography. Am. J. Cardiol. 53:456, 1984.
16. Mancini, G. B. J., Higgins, C. B., and Norris, S. L.: Cardiac imaging with digital subtraction angiography. Cardiovasc. Intervent. Rad. *6*:252–262, 1983.
17. Widmann, T. F., Ashburn, W. L., Higgins, C. B., and Peterson, K. L.: Assessment of left ventricular wall motion by regional phase analysis of digital intravenous contrast fluoroangiography. *In* Proceedings of Computers in Cardiology. IEEE Computer Society, 1982, pp. 105–108.
18. Yiannikis, J., Simpfendorfer, C., Detrano, K., Salcedo, E. E., and Sheldon, W. C.: Stress digital subtraction angiography to assess presence of coronary artery disease in patients without myocardial infarction. Circulation *68*(Suppl IV):41, 1983.
19. Goldberg, H. L., Moses, J. W., and Borer, J. S.: Exercise left ventriculography utilizing intravenous digital angiography. J. Am. Coll. Cardiol. 2:1092, 1983.
20. Tobis, J., Nalcioglu, O., Johnston, W. D., Seibert, J. A., and Henry, W. L.: Exercise digital subtraction angiograms in patients with coronary artery disease. Circulation *66*(Suppl II):229, 1982.
21. Sasayama, S., Nonogi, H., Kawai, C., Fujita, M., Eiho, S., and Kuwahara, M.: Automated method for left ventricular volume measurement by cineventriculography with minimal doses of contrast medium. Am. J. Cardiol. *48*:746, 1981.
22. Tobis, J. M., Nalcioglu, O., Johnston, W. D., Seibert, A., Roeck, W., Iseri, T., Elkayam, U., and Henry, W. L.: Correlation of 10 millimeter digital subtraction ventriculograms compared with standard cineangiograms. Am. Heart J. *105*:946, 1983.
23. Mancini, G. B. J., and Higgins, C. B.: The evaluation of left ventricular function in ischemic heart disease by digital subtraction angiography. *In* New Concepts in Cardiac Imaging. Boston, G. K. Hall & Co., 1983.
24. Bursch, J. H., Heintzen, P. H., and Simon, R.: Videodensitometric studies by a new method of quantitating the amount of contrast medium. Eur. J. Cardiol. *14*:437, 1974.
25. Tobis, J., Nalcioglu, O., Seibert, A., Johnston, W. D., and Henry, W. L.: Measurement of left ventricular ejection fraction by videodensitometric analysis of digital subtraction angiograms. Am. J. Cardiol. *52*:871, 1983.
26. Tobis, J., Nalcioglu, O., Johnston, W. D., Seibert, A., Isera, L. T., Roeck, W., and Henry, W. L.: Digital angiography in assessment of ventricular function and wall motion during pacing in patients with coronary artery disease. Am. J. Cardiol. *51*:668, 1983.
27. Tobis, J., Sato, D., Warren, D., Johnston, W. D., Resse, T., Nalcioglu, O., and Henry, W. L.: Correlation of minimum lumen diameter with left ventricular functional impairment during atrial pacing (abstr). J. Am. Coll. Cardiol. 7:216, 1986.
28. Mistretta, C. A., Peppler, W. W., Van Lysel, M., Dobbins, J., Hasegawa, B., Myerowitz, P. D., Swanson, D., Lee, C. S., Shaik, N., Zarnstorff, N., Crummy, A. B., Strothers, C. M., and Sackett, J. F.: Recent advances in digital angiography. Ann. Radiol. *26*:537, 1983.
29. Tobis, J., Nalcioglu, O., Iseri, L., Johnston, W. D., Roeck, W., Castleman, E., Bauer, B., Montelli, S., and Henry, W. L.: Detection and quantitation of coronary artery stenoses from digital subtraction angiograms compared with 35 mm film cineangiograms. Am. J. Cardiol. *54*:489, 1984.
30. Brown, B. G., Bolson, E., Frimer, M., Dodge, H. T.: Quantitative coronary arteriography: estimation of dimensions, hemodynamic resistance, and atheroma mass of coronary artery lesions using the arteriogram and digital computation. Circulation *55*:329, 1977.
31. Sandor, T., Als, A. V., and Paulin, S.: Cinedensitometric measurement of coronary arterial stenoses. Catheterization and Cardiovascular Diagnosis *5*:229, 1979.
32. Sandor, T., and Paulin, S.: Computer-aided evaluation of coronary cineangiograms. Proceedings of the Digital Equipment Computer Users Society, 1977, p. 1279
33. Paulin, S., and Sandor, T.: Densitometric assessment of stenoses in coronary arteries. Proceedings of the Society of Photoelectrical Engineering *70*:337, 1975.
34. Elion, J. L., Nissen, S. E., and Booth, D. C.: Videodensitometric assessment of coronary stenosis: validation of the technique and comparison with visual methods. Circulation *70*(Suppl II):30, 1984.
35. Collins, S. M., Johnson, M. R., and Ericksen, E. E.: Videodensitometric analysis of coronary stenosis: Methodologic considerations and geometric and functional validation. Circulation *70*:30, 1984.
36. Johnston, W. D., Tobis, J., and Nalcioglu, O.: Computer quantitation of coronary stenoses. Circulation *70*(Suppl II):32, 1984.
37. Nichols, A. B., Gabrieli, C. F. O., and Fenoglio, J. J.: Quantification of relative coronary arterial stenosis by cinevideodensitometric analysis of coronary arteriograms. Circulation *69*:512, 1984.
38. Rutishauser, W., Bussman, W. D., and Naseda, G.: Blood flow measurement through single coronary arteries by roentgen densitometry. Part I. Am. J. Roentgenol. *109*:12, 1970.
39. Rutishauser, W., Noseda, G., and Bussmann, W. D.: Blood flow measurement through single coronary arteries by roentgen densitometry. Part II. Am. J. Roentgenol. *109*:21, 1970.
40. Smith, H. C., Frye, R. L., and Donald, D. E.: Roentgen videodensitometric measure of coronary blood flow. Mayo Clin. Proc. *46*:800, 1971.
41. Smith, H. C., Sturm, R. E., and Wood, E. H.: Videodensitometric system for measurement of vessel blood flow, particularly in the coronary arteries in man. Am. J. Cardiol. *32*:144, 1973.
42. Foerster, J. M., Lantz, B. M. T., and Holcroft, J. W.: Angiographic measurement of coronary blood flow in video dilution technique. Acta Radiol. *22*:121, 1981.
43. Foerster, J. M., Link, D. P., and Lantz, B. M. T.: Measurement of coronary reactive hyperemia during clinical angiography by video dilution technique. Acta Radiol. *22*:209, 1981.
44. Spiller, P., Schmiel, F. K., Politz, B., Block, M., Fermor, U., Hackbarth, W., Jehle, J., Korfer, R., and Pannek, H.: Measurement of systolic and diastolic flow rates in the coronary artery system by x-ray densitometry. Circulation *68*:337, 1983.
45. Drury, J. K., Whiting, J. S., and Pfaff, J. M.: Validation of myocardial blood flow measurements using digital subtraction angiography (abstr). J. Am. Coll. Cardiol. *3*:588, 1984.
46. Johnson, R. A., Wasserman, A. G., and Katz, R. J.: Correlation of coronary stenosis and contrast density decay curves by on line subtracted digital fluoroscopy (abstr). J. Am. Coll. Cardiol. 3:588, 1984.
47. Vogel, R., LeFree, M., Bates, E., O'Neill, W., Foster, R., Kirlin, P., Smith, D., and Pitt, B.: Application of digital techniques to selective coronary arteriography: Use of myocardial contrast appearance time to measure coronary flow reserve. Am. Heart J. *107*:153, 1984.
48. Higgins, C. B., Kelley, M. J., Green, C. E., Newell, J. D., Gerber, K. H., and Haigler, F. H.: Physiologic angiographic correlates of coronary arterial

stenosis in resting and intensely vasodilated states. Invest. Radiol. *17*:444, 1982.
49. Whiting, J. S., Nivatypumin, T. L., Pfaff, M., Vas, R., Drury, K., Diamond, G., Swan, H. J. C., and Forrester, J. S.: Assessing the coronary circulation by digital angiography: Bypass graft and myocardial perfusion imaging. *In* Heintzen, P. H., and Brennecke, R., (eds.): Digital Imaging in Cardiovascular Radiology. New York, George Thieme Verlag, 1983, p. 205.

COMPUTED TOMOGRAPHY

50. Hodgson, JMcB, LeGrand, V., Bates, E. R., Mancini, G. B. J., Aueron, F. M., O'Neill, W. W., Simon, S. B., Beauman, G. J., LeFree, M. T., and Vogel, R. A.: Validation in dogs of a rapid digital angiographic technique to measure relative coronary blood flow during routine cardiac catheterization. Am. J. Cardiol. 55:188, 1985.
51. Moncada, R., Baker, M., Salinas, M., Demos, T. C., Churchill, R., Love, L., Reynes, C., Hale, D., Cardoso, M., Pifarre, R., and Gunnar, R. M.: Diagnostic role of computed tomography in pericardial heart disease. Am. Heart J. *103*:263, 1982.
52. Lackner, K., and Thurn, P.: Computed tomography of the heart: ECG gated and continuous scans. Radiology *140*:413, 1981.
53. Higgins, C. B., Carlsson, E., and Lipton, M. J. (eds.): CT of the Heart and Great Vessels. Mt. Kisco, N.Y., Futura Publishing Co., 1983, p. 167.
54. Brundage, B., Lipton, M. J., Herfkens, R. J., Berninger, W. H., Redington, R. W., Chatterjee, K., and Carlsson, E.: Detection of patent coronary artery bypass grafts by computed tomography. A preliminary report. Circulation *61*:826, 1980.
55. Mattrey, R. F., Long, S. A., and Higgins, C. B.: In vivo assessment of left ventricular wall and chamber dynamics during transmission tomography. Circulation *67*:1245, 1983.
56. Lipton, M. J., Higgins, C. B., Farmer, D., and Boyd, D. P.: Cardiac imaging with a high-speed cine-CT scanner: Preliminary results. Radiology *152*:579, 1983.
57. Sinak, L. J., and Ritman, E. L.: Dynamic spatial reconstructor. *In* CT of the Heart and Great Vessels. Mt. Kisco, N.Y., Futura Publishing Co., 1983, p. 61.
58. Skioldebrand, C. G., Lipton, M. J., Mavroudis, C., and Hayashi, T. T.: Determination of left ventricular mass by computed tomography. Am. J. Cardiol. 9:63, 1983.
59. Peck, W. A., Mancini, G. B. J., Mattrey, R. F., and Higgins, C. B.: In vivo assessment by CT of natural progression of infarct size, left ventricular mass, and function after myocardial infarction in the dog. Am. J. Cardiol. 53:929, 1984.
60. Feiring, A., Rumberger, J. A., Reiter, S. J., Skorton, D. J., Collins, S. M., Higgins, C. B., Lipton, M. J., Ell, S., and Marcas, M. L.: Determination of left ventricular mass in dogs with rapid-acquisition cardiac CT scanning. Circulation 72:1355, 1985.
61. Lanzer, P., Garrett, J., Sievers, R., Gould, R., Botvinick, E., Lipton, M., and Higgins, C. B.: Wall thickening dynamics: Assessment by cine CT (abstr). Circulation 72:III–180, 1985.
61a. Rumberger, J. A., Feiring, A. J., Lipton, M. J., Higgins, C. B., Ell, S. R., and Marcus, M. L.: Use of ultrafast computed tomography to quantitate regional myocardial perfusion: A preliminary report. J. Am. Coll. Cardiol. 9:59, 1987.
62. Farmer, D. W., Lipton, M. J., Higgins, C. B., Ringerts, H., Dean, P. H., Sievers, R., and Boyd, D. P.: In vivo assessment of left ventricular wall and chamber dynamics during transient myocardial ischemia using cine CT. Am. J. Cardiol. 55:560, 1985.
63. Lipton, M. J., Hayashi, T. T., Boyd, D., and Carlsson, E.: Measurement of left ventricular cast volume by computed tomography. Radiology *127*:419, 1978.
64. Rich, S., Chamka, E.V., Stagl, R., Kondos, G. T., Shanes, T. G., and Brundage, B. H.: Ultra-fast computed tomography to determine left ventricular ejection fraction (abstr). Circulation 72:III–180, 1985.
65. Bateman, T., Whiting, J., Pfaff, M., Raymond, M., Aronson, A., Forrester, J., and Berman, D.: Cine, C. T.: An accurate precise and rapid method for LVRF determination (abstr). Circulation 72:III–180, 1985.
66. Reiter, S. J., Rumberger, J. A., Feiring, A. J., Ell, S. R., Stanford, W., and Marcus, M. C.: Precise determination of left and right ventricular stroke volume with cine CT (abstr). Circulation 72:III–179, 1985.
66a. Rumberger, T. A., Feiring, A. J., Lipton, M. J., Higgins, C. B., Ell, S. R., and Marcus, M. L.: Use of ultrafast CT to quantitate regional myocardial perfusion: A preliminary report. Circulation 72:1355, 1985.
67. Lackner, K.: Clinical application of CTT for evaluation of ischemic heart disease—comparison with other imaging methods. *In* Higgins, C. B. (ed.): CTT of the Heart and Great Vessels. Mt. Kisco, N.Y., Futura Publishing Co., 1982, p. 267.
68. Kramer, P., Goldstein, J., Herfkens, R., Lipton, M. J., and Brundage, B.: Imaging of acute myocardial infarction in man with contrast enhanced computed transmission tomography. Am. Heart J. *108*:1514, 1984.
69. Lipton, M. J., Farmer, D. W., Killebrew, E. J., Bouchard, A., Dean, P. B., Ringertz, H. G., and Higgins, C. B.: Regional myocardial dysfunction: Evaluation of patients with prior myocardial infarction with fast CT. Radiology *157*:735, 1985.
70. Tomoda, H., Hoshiai, M., Furuya, H., Kuribayashi, S., Ootaki, M., Matsuyama, S., Koide, S., Kawada, S., and Shotsu, A.: Evaluation of intracardiac thrombus with computed tomography. Am. J. Cardiol. *51*:843, 1983.
71. Tomoda, H., Hoshiai, M., Furuya, H., Shotsu, A., Ootaki, M., and Matsuyama, S.: Evaluation of left ventricular thrombus with computed tomography. Am. J. Cardiol. *48*:573, 1981.
72. Tomoda, H., Hoshiai, M., Tozawa, R., Koide, S., Kawada, S., Shotsu, A., and Matsuyama, S.: Evaluation of left atrial thrombus with computed tomography. Am. Heart J. *100*:306, 1980.
73. Lipton, M. J., and Higgins, C. B.: Evaluation of ischemic heart disease by computerized transmission tomography. Radiol. Clin. North Am. *18*:557, 1980.
74. Higgins, C. B., Siemers, P. T., and Schmidt, W.: Evaluation of myocardial ischemic damage of various ages by computed transmission tomography. Circulation *60*:284, 1979.
75. Siemers, P. T., Higgins, C. B., Schmidt, W., Ashburn, W., and Hagan, P.: Detection, quantitation and contrast enhancement of myocardial infarction utilizing computerized axial tomography: Comparison with histochemical staining. Invest. Radiol. *13*:103, 1978.
76. Doherty, P. W., Lipton, M. J., Berninger, W. H., Skioldebrand, C. G., Carlsson, E., and Redington, R. W.: The detection and quantitation of myocardial infarction in vivo using transmission tomography. Circulation *63*:597, 1981.
77. Huber, D. J., Lupray, J. F., and Hessel, S. J.: In vivo evaluation of experimental infarcts by ungated computed tomography. Am. J. Roentgenol. *136*:469, 1981.
78. Carlsson, E., Lipton, M. J., Berninger, W. H., Doherty, P., and Redington, R. W.: Selective left coronary myocardiography by computed tomography in living dogs. Invest. Radiol. *12*:559, 1977.
79. Higgins, C. B., Sovak, M., Schmidt, W., and Siemers, P. T.: Differential accumulation of radiopaque contrast material in acute myocardial infarction. Am. J. Cardiol. *43*:47, 1979.
80. Higgins, C. B., Sovak, M., Schmidt, W., and Siemers, P. T.: Uptake of contrast material by experimental acute myocardial infarctions: A preliminary report. Invest. Radiol. *13*:337, 1978.
81. Higgins, C. B., Hagan, P. L., Newell, J. D., Schmidt, W., and Haigler, F. H.: Contrast enhancement of myocardial infarction: Dependence on ischemic necrosis, residual blood flow, and relationship to scintigraphic imaging agents. Circulation *65*:739, 1982.
82. Abraham, J.L., Higgins, C. B., and Newell, J. D.: Uptake of iodinated contrast material in ischemic myocardium as an indicator of loss of cellular membrane integrity. Am. J. Pathol. *101*:319, 1980.
83. Mancini, G. B. J., Peck, W. W., Ross, J., Jr., and Higgins, C. B.: Use of computerized tomography to assess myocardial infarct size and ventricular function in dogs during acute coronary occlusion and reperfusion. Am. J. Cardiol. *53*:282, 1984.
84. Moncada, R., Salinas, M., Churchill, R., Love, L., Reynes, C., Demos, T. C., Hale, D., and Schreiber, R.: Patency of saphenous aortocoronary grafts demonstrated by computed tomography. N. Engl. J. Med. *303*:503, 1980.
85. Daniel, W. G., Doring, W., Stender, H. S., and Lichten, P. R.: Value and limitations of computed tomography in assessing aortocoronary bypass graft patency. Circulation *67*:983, 1983.
86. Kohl, F. C., Wolfman, N. T., and Watts, L. E.: Evaluation of aortocoronary bypass graft status by computed tomography. Am. J. Cardiol. *48*:304, 1981.
87. Guthaner, D. F., Brody, W. R., Ricci, M., Oyer, P. E., and Wexler, L.: The use of computed tomography in the diagnosis of coronary artery bypass graft patency. Cardiovasc. Intervent. Radiol. *3*:3, 1980.
88. Bateman, T. M., Whiting, J. S., Forrester, J. S., Aronson, A. L., Schauer, S. V., Gray, R. J., Matloff, J. M., Berman, D. S., and Swan, H. J. C.: Noninvasive evaluation of aortocoronary bypass grafts using cine CT. J. Am. Coll. Cardiol. 7:154A, 1986.
89. Ullyot, D. J., Turley, K., McKay, C. R., Brundage, B. H., Lipton, M. J., and Ebert, P. A.: Assessment of saphenous vein graft patency by contrast enhanced computed tomography. J. Thorac. Cardiovasc. Surg. *83*:512, 1982.
90. McKay, C. R., Brundage, B. H., Ullyot, D. J., Turley, K., Lipton, M. J., and Ebert, P. A.: Evaluation of early postoperative coronary artery bypass graft patency by contrast enhanced computed tomography. J. Am. Coll. Cardiol. 2:312, 1983.
91. Silverman, P. M. and Harell, G. S.: Computed tomography of the normal pericardium. Invest. Radiol. *18*:141, 1983.
92. Moncada, R., Baker, M., Salinas, M., Demos, D. C., Churchill, R., Love, L., Reynes, C., Hale, D., Cardosa, H., Pifarre, R., and Gunnar, R. M.: Diagnostic role of computed tomography in pericardial heart disease: Congenital defects, thickening, neoplasms and effusions. Am. Heart J. *103*:263, 1981.
93. Isner, J. M., Carter, B. L., Bankoff, M. S., Konstum, M. A., and Salem, D. N.: Computed tomography in the diagnosis of pericardial heart disease. Ann. Intern. Med. 97:473, 1982.
94. Zerhouni, E. A., Scott, W. W., Baker, R. R., Whoram, W. D., and Siegelman, S.S.: Invasive thymomas: diagnosis and evaluation by computed tomography. J. Comput. Assist. Tomogr. *6*:92, 1982.
95. Baim, R. S., MacDonald, I. L., Wise, D. J., and Lenkei, S. C.: Computed tomography of absent left pericardium. Radiology *135*:127, 1980.
96. Roger, C. I., Seymour, Q., and Brock, G. I.: Atypical pericardial cysts location: the value of computed tomography. J. Comput. Assist. Tomogr. *4*:683, 1980.
97. Pugatch, R. D., Braver, J. H., Robbins, A. H., and Foling, L. F.: CT diagnosis of pericardial cysts. Am. J. Roentgenol. *131*:515, 1978.
98. Tomoda, H., Hoshiai, M., Furuya, H., Oeda, Y., Matsumoto, S., Tanabe, T., Tamachi, H., Sasamoto, H., Koide, S., Kuribayashi, S., and Matsuyama, S.: Evaluation of pericardial effusion with computed tomography. Am. Heart J. 99:701, 1980.
99. Higgins, C. B., Mattrey, R. F., and Shea, P.: CT localization and aspiration of postoperative pericardial fluid collection. J. Comput. Assist. Tomogr. *7*:734, 1983.

100. Conti, C. R. and Freisinger, G. C.: Chronic constrictive pericarditis. Clinical and laboratory findings in 11 patients. Johns Hopkins Med. J. *120*:262, 1967.
101. Zerhonni, E. A., Scott, W. W., Baker, R. R., Whoram, W. D., and Siegelman, S. S.: Invasive thymomas: Diagnosis and evaluation by computed tomography. J. Comput. Assist. Tomogr. *6*:92, 1982.
102. Hackney, D., Mattrey, R., Peck, W. W., Abraham, J. L., Shabetai, R., and Higgins, C. B.: Experimental pericardial inflammation evaluated by computed tomography. Radiology *151*:145,1984.
103. Doppman, J. C., Reinmuller, R., Lissner, J., Cyran, J., Bolto, H. D., Strauss, B. E., and Hellwig, H.: Computed tomography in constrictive pericardial disease. J. Comput. Assist. Tomogr. *5*:1, 1981.
104. Isner, J. M., Carter, B. L., Bankoff, M. S., Pastore, J. O., Ramaswamy, R., McAdam, K., and Salem, D. N.: Differentiation of constrictive pericarditis from restrictive cardiomyopathy by computed tomographic imaging. Am. Heart J. *105*:1019, 1983.
105. Handler, J. B., Higgins, C. B., Warrent, S. E., Gibbons, J. A., and Vieweg, W. V. R.: Computerized tomographic diagnosis of paracardiac masses. West. J. Med. *135*:271, 1981.
106. Glazer, G. M., Gross, B. H., Oringer, M. B., Buda, A. J., Francis, I. R., and Shapero, B.: Computed tomography of pericardial masses. J. Comput. Assist. Tomogr. *8*:895, 1984.
107. Patel, B. K., Markivee, C. R., and George, E. A.: Pericardial cyst simulating intracardiac mass. Am. J. Roentgenol. *141*:292, 1983.
108. Norlindh, T., Lilja, B., Nyman, U., and Hellekant, C.: Left atrial myxoma demonstrated by CT. Am. J. Roentgenol. *137*:153, 1981.
109. Huggins, T. J., Huggins, M. J., Schnopf, D. J., Brott, W. H., Simot, R. C., and Showl, F. A.: Left atrial myxoma: Computed tomography as a diagnostic modality. Invest. Radiol. *12*:559, 1977.
110. Baron, R. L., Guitterez, F. R., and McKnight, R. C.: Computed tomographic evaluation of the great arteries and aortic arch anomalies. In Freedman, W. F., Higgins, C. B. (eds.): Pediatric Cardiac Imaging. Philadelphia, W. B. Saunders Company, 1984, pp. 135–156.
111. Farmer, D. W., Lipton, M. J., Webb, W. R., Rigertz, H., and Higgins, C. B.: Computed tomography in congenital heart disease. J. Comput. Assist. Tomogr. *8*:677, 1984.
112. Webb, W. R., Gamsu, G., Speckman, G., Kaiser, J., Federle, M., and Lipton, M. J.: CT demonstration of mediastinal aortic arch anomalies. J. Comput. Assist. Tomogr. *6*:445, 1982.
113. Eldridge, W. J., Rees, M. R., and Flicker, S.: Cine CT scanning in the diagnosis of congenital heart disease. Analysis of the first 42 cases. *In* Doyle, F. F. et al. (ed.): Pediatric Cardiology. New York, Springer-Verlag, 1985, pp. 404–405.
114. Eldridge, W. J., Flicker, S., and Steiner, R. M.: Cine CT in the anatomical evaluation of congenital heart disease. *In* Pohost, G., Higgins, C. B., Morgenroth, J., et al. (eds.): New Concept in Cardiac Imaging, vol. 3, Chicago, Year Book Medical Publishers, 1986.
115. Garrett, J. S., Jaschke, W., Aherne, T., Botvinick, E. H., Higgins, C. B., and Lipton, M. J.: Quantitation of intracardiac shunts by cine CT. Radiology (Submitted).
116. Godwin, J. D., Herfkens, R. L., Skioldebrand, C. G., Federle, M. P., and Lipton, M. J.: Evaluation of dissections and aneurysms of the thoracic aorta by conventional and dynamic CT scanning. Radiology *136*:125, 1980.
117. Larde, D., Belloir, C., Vasile, N., Frija, J., and Ferrane, J.: Computed tomography of aortic dissection. Radiology *136*:147, 1980.
118. Heiberg, E., Wolverson, M., Sundaram, M., Connors, J., and Susman, N.: CT finding in thoracic aortic dissection. Am. J. Roentgenol. *136*:13, 1981.
119. Thorsten, M. K., San Drelto, M. A., Lawson, T. L., Foley, W. D., Smith, D. F., and Berland, L. L.: Dissecting aortic aneurysms: Accuracy of computed tomographic diagnosis. Radiology *148*:773, 1983.
120. Dudkerk, M., Overbosch, E., and Dee, P.: CT recognition of acute aortic dissection. Am. J. Roentgenol. *141*:671, 1983.
121. White, R. C., Lipton, M. J., Higgins, C. B., Federle, M. R., Pogany, A. C., Kerlan, R. K., Thaxton, T. S., and Turley, K.: Noninvasive evaluation of suspected thoracic aortic disease by contrast-enhanced computed tomography. Am. J. Cardiol. *57*:282, 1986.
122. Guthaner, D. F., Miller, D. C., Silverman, J. F., Stinson, E. B., and Wexler, L.: Fate of the false lumen following surgical repair of aortic dissection: An angiographic study. Radiology *133*:1, 1979.
123. Yamaguchi, T., Naito, H., Ohta, M., Sugahara, T., Takamija, M., Kozuka, T., and Nakajima, N.: False lumens in type III aortic dissection: progress in CT study. Radiology *156*:757, 1985.

MAGNETIC RESONANCE IMAGING

124. Crooks, L. E. and Kaufman, L.: Basic physical principles. *In* Margulis, A. R., Higgins, C. B., Kaufman, L., Crook, L. E. (eds.): Clinical Magnetic Resonance Imaging. San Francisco, Radiology Research and Education Foundation, 1983, pp. 13–24.
125. Lanzer, P., Botvinick, E. H., Schiller, N. B., Crooks, L. E., Arakawa, M., Kaufman, L., Davis, P. L., Lipton, M. J., and Higgins, C. B.: Cardiac imaging using gated magnetic resonance. Radiology *150*:121, 1984.
126. Lanzer, P., Barta, C., Botvinick, E. H., Weisindinger, H. U., Modin, G., and Higgins, C. B.: ECG synchronized cardiac MR imaging: Method and evaluation. Radiology *155*:681, 1985.
127. Crooks, L. E., Baker, B., Chang, H., Feinberg, D., Hoenning, J., Watts, J., Arakawa, M., Kaufman, L., Sheldon, P. E., Botvinick, E. H., and Higgins, C. B.: Magnetic resonance imaging strategies for heart studies. Radiology *153*:459, 1984.
128. Fisher, M. R., von Schulthess, G. K., and Higgins, C. B.: Quantitation of regional left ventricular wall thickness using rotated gated magnetic resonance imaging. Am. J. Roentgenol. *142*:661, 1984.
129. Sechtem, U., Sommerhoff, B. A., Markiewicz, W., White, R. D., Cheitlin, M. D., and Higgins, C. B.: Assessment of regional left ventricular wall thickening by MRI. Am. J. Cardiol. *59*:149, 1987.
130. Wesbey, G., Higgins, C. B., Lanzer, P., Botvinick, E., and Lipton, M. J.: In vivo imaging and characterization of acute myocardial infarction using gated nuclear magnetic resonance. Circulation *69*:125, 1984.
131. McNamara, M. T., Higgins, C. B., Schechtmann, N., Botvinick, E., Amparo, E. G., and Chatterjee, K.: Detection and characterization of acute myocardial infarctions in man using gated magnetic resonance imaging. Circulation *71*:717, 1985.
132. Farmer, D., Higgins, C. B., Yee, E., Wahr, D., and Ports, T.: Tissue characterization by magnetic resonance imaging in an unusual case of hypertrophic cardiomyopathy. Am. J. Cardiol. *55*:230, 1985.
133. Caputo, G., Fisher, M. R., McNamara, M. T., Lipton, M. J., and Higgins, C. B.: Myocardial tissue characterization with the use of magnetic resonance imaging (abstr). Circulation 72(Suppl III:III–23), 1985.
134. Higgins, C. B., Lanzer, P., Stark, D., Botvinick, E., Schiller, N. B., Crooks, L. E., Kaufman, L., and Lipton, M. J.: Imaging by nuclear magnetic resonance in patients with chronic ischemic heart disease. Circulation *69*:523, 1984.
135. McNamara, M. T. and Higgins, C. B.: Magnetic resonance imaging of chronic myocardial infarctions in man. Am. J. Roentgenol. *146*:315, 1986.
135a. Akins, E. W., Hill, J. A., Sievers, K. W., and Conti, C. R.: Assessment of left ventricular wall thickness in healed myocardial infarction by magnetic resonance imaging. Am. J. Cardiol. *59*:24, 1987.
135b. Sechtem, U., Sommerhoff, B. A., Mafrkiewicz, W., White, R. D., Cheitlin, M. D., and Higgins, C. B.: Assessment of regional left ventricular wall thickening by magnetic resonance imaging: Evaluation in normal persons and patients with global and regional dysfunction. Am. J. Cardiol. *59*:145, 1987.
136. Higgins, C. B., Byrd, B. F., McNamara, M. T., Lanzer, P., Lipton, M. J., Botvinick, E., Schiller, N. B., Crooks, L. E., and Kaufman, L.: Magnetic resonance imaging of the heart: A review of the experience in 172 subjects. Radiology *155*:671, 1985.
137. Higgins, C. B., Byrd, B. F., and Stark, D.: Magnetic resonance imaging of hypertrophic cardiomyopathy. Am. J. Cardiol. *55*:1121, 1985.
138. Sechtem, U., Higgins, C. B., Sommerhoff, B. A., Lipton, M. J., and Huycke, E. C.: Magnetic resonance imaging of restrictive cardiomyopathy: A report of 3 cases. Am. J. Cardiol. *59*:480, 1987.
138a. Sechtem, U., Higgins, C. B., Sommerhoff, B. A., Lipton, M. J., and Huycke, E. C.: Magnetic resonance imaging of restrictive cardiomyopathy. Am. J. Cardiol. *59*:480, 1987.
139. O'Donnell, J. K., Go, R. T., Bolt-Silverman, C., Feiglin, D. H. I., Salcedo, E.E., and MacIntyre, W. J.: Cardiac amyloidosis: comparison of MR imaging and echocardiography (abstr). Radiology *153*:261, 1984.
140. Stark, D. D., Higgins, C. B., Lanzer, P., Lipton, M. J., Schiller, N., Crooks, L., Botvinick, E., and Kaufman, L.: Magnetic resonance imaging of the pericardium: normal and pathologic findings. Radiology *150*:469, 1984.
141. Sechtem, U., Tscholakoff, D., and Higgins, C. B.: MRI of normal epicardium. Am. J. Roentgenol. *147*:239, 1986.
142. Sechtem, U., Tscholakoff, D., and Higgins, C. B.: Pericardial disease. Diagnosis by MRI. Am. J. Roentgenol. *147*:245, 1986.
143. Diethelm, L., Dery, R., Lipton, M. J., and Higgins, C. B.: Atrial level shunts: Sensitivity and specificity of MR in diagnosis. Radiology *162*:181, 1987.
144. Soulen R. L., Stark, D. D., and Higgins, C. B.: Magnetic resonance imaging of constrictive pericardial disease. Am. J. Cardiol. *55*:480, 1985.
145. Amparo, E. G., Higgins, C. B., Farmer, D., Gamsu, G., and McNamara, M. T.: Gated MRI of cardiac and paracardiac masses: Initial experiment. Am. J. Roentgenol. *143*:1151, 1984.
146. Go, R. T., O'Donnell, J. K., Underwood, D. A., Feiglin, D. H., Salcedo, E. E., Pantoja, M., MacIntyre, W. J., and Meaney, T. F.: Comparison of gated cardiac MRI and 2D echocardiography of intracardiac neoplasms. Am. J. Roentgenol. *145*:21, 1985.
147. Conces, D. J., Vox, V. A., and Klatte, E. C.: Gated MR imaging of left atrial myxomas. Radiology *156*:445, 1985.
148. Fisher, M. R., Higgins, C. B., and Andereck, W.: Magnetic resonance imaging of an intrapericardial pheochromocytoma. J. Comput. Assist. Tomogr. 9:1103, 1985.
149. Gamsu, G. and Higgins, C. B.: Magnetic resonance imaging of mediastinal masses. Radiology *158*:289, 1986.
149. Higgins, C. B., Byrd, B. F., III, Farmer, D., Silverman, N., and Cheitlin, M.: Magnetic resonance imaging in patients congenital heart disease. Circulation 70:851, 1984.
150. Fletcher, B. D., Jacobstein, M. D., Nelson, A. D., Riemenschneider, T. A., and Alfidi, R. J.: Gated magnetic resonance imaging of congenital cardiac malformations. Radiology *150*:137, 1984.
151. Didier, D., Higgins, C. B., Fisher, M. R., Osaki, L., Silverman, N., and Cheitlin, M.: Congenital heart disease: Imaging in 72 patients. Radiology *158*:227, 1986.
152. Didier, D., and Higgins, C. B.: Identification and localization of ventricular septal defects by gated magnetic resonance imaging. Am. J. Coll. Cardiol. *57*:1363, 1986.
153. von Schulthess, G. K., Higashino, S. M., Higgins, S. S., Didier, D., Fisher, M. R., and Higgins, C. B.: Coarctation of the aorta: MR imaging. Radiology *158*:474, 1986.
154. Peshock, R. M., Parrish, M., Fixler, D., Cohen, J. M., and Parkey, R. W.: MR imaging in the evaluation of single ventricle. Radiology *157*:355, 1985.
155. Jacobstein, M. D., Fletcher, B. D., Goldstein, S., and Rumenschneider, T. A.: Evaluation of atrioventricular septal defect by magnetic resonance imaging. Am. J. Cardiol. 55:1158, 1985.

156. Lowell, D. G., Turner, D. A., Smith, S. M., Buchelview, G. H., Santucci, B. A., Gresick, R. J., and Monson, D. O.: The detection of atrial and ventricular septal defects with electrocardiographically synchronized MRI. Circulation *73*:89, 1986.
157. Amparo, E. G., Higgins, C. B., Hoddick, W., Hricak, H., Kerlan, R. K., Ring, E. J., Kaufman, L., and Hedgecock, M. W.: Magnetic resonance imaging (MRI) of aortic disease. Am. J. Roentgenol. *143*:1203, 1984.
158. Amparo, E. G., Higgins, C. B., Hricak, H., and Sollitto, R.: Aortic dissection: Magnetic resonance imaging. Radiology *155*:399, 1985.
159. Winkler, M. L. and Higgins, C. B.: Magnetic resonance imaging of perivalvular infectious pseudoaneurysms. Am. J. Roentgenol. *147*:253, 1986.
159a. Dooms, G. C. and Higgins, C. B.: The potential of MRI for the evaluation of thoracic arterial disease. J. Thorac. Cardiovasc. Surg. *92*:1088, 1986.
159b. White, R. D., Dooms, G. C., and Higgins, C. B.: Advances in imaging thoracic aortic disease: progress in clinical radiology. Invest. Radiol. *21*:761, 1986.
159c. Amparo, E. G., Higgins, C. B., Hricak, H., and Sollitto, R.: Aortic dissection: Magnetic resonance imaging. Radiology *155*:399, 1985.
160. Sommerhoff, B. A., Sechtem, U. P., Schiller, N. B., Lipton, M. J., and Higgins, C. B.: MRI of thoracic aorta in Marfan patients. J. Comput. Assist. Tomogr., 1986.
161. Caputo, G. R., Tscholakoff, D., Sechtem, U., and Higgins, C. B.: Measurement of canine left ventricular mass using gated magnetic resonance imaging. Am. J. Roentgenol. *148*:33, 1987.
162. Caputo, G. R., Sechtem, U., Tscholakoff, D., and Higgins, C. B.: Measurement of canine myocardial infarct size at early and late time intervals using MRI. A. J. R. *148*:33, 1987.
163. Markiewicz, W., Sechtem, U., Kirby, R., Derugin, N., Caputo, G. R., and Higgins, C. B.: Measurement of ventricular volumes in the dog by MRI. J. Am. Coll. Cardiol. *10*:170, 1987.
164. Underwood, S. R., Firmin, D. N., Klipstein, H., Fox, K. M., and Poole-Wilson, P. A., Ress, R. S. O., and Langmore, D. B.: Rapid measurement of left ventricular volume from single oblique MR images. Radiology *157*:309, 1986.
165. Dinsmore, R. E., Wisner, G. L., Levine, R. A., Okada, R. D., and Brady, T. J.: Magnetic resonance imaging of the heart: Positioning and gradient angle selection for optimal imaging planes. Am. J. Roentgenol. *143*:1135, 1984.
166. von Schulthess, G. K. and Higgins, C. B.: Blood flow imaging with MR: spin phase phenomenon. Radiology *157*:687, 1985.
167. George, C. R., Jacobs, G., MacIntyre, W. J., Lorig, R. J., Go, R. T., Nose, Y., and Meaney, T. F.: Magnetic resonance signal intensity from continuous and pulsative flow models. Radiology *151*:421, 1984.
168. Bradley, W. G. and Waluch, V.: Blood flow: Magnetic resonance imaging. Radiology *154*:443, 1985.
169. Moran, P. R., Moran, R. D., and Karstardt, N. A.: Verification and evaluation of internal flow and motion. Radiology *154*:433, 1985.
170. Bradley, W. G. and Waluch, V.: NMR even echo rephasing in slow laminar flow. J. Comput. Assist. Tomogr. *8*:594, 1984.
171. von Schulthess, G. K., Fisher, M. R., Crooks, L. E., and Higgins, C. B.: The nature of intracardiac signal on gated NMR images in normals and patients with abnormal left ventricular function. Radiology *157*:687, 1985.
172. von Schulthess, G. D., Fisher, M. R., and Higgins, C. B.: Detection of abnormal pulmonary flow pattern by magnetic resonance imaging in pulmonary atrial hypertension. Ann. Intern. Med. *103*:125, 1985.
173. Didier, D., and Higgins, C. B.: Estimation of pulmonary vascular resistance by MRI in patients with congenital cardiovascular shunt lesions. Am. J. Roentgenol. *146*:919, 1986.
174. Ehman, R. L., McNamara, M. T., Brasch, R. C., Felmlee, J. P., Gray, J. E., and Higgins, C. B.: Influence of physiologic motion on the appearance of tissue in MR images. Radiology *159*:777, 1986.
175. Williams, E. S., Kaplan, J. L., Thatcher, F., Zimmerman, G., and Knoebel, S. B.: Prolongation of proton spin lattice relaxation times in regionally ischemic tissue from dog hearts. J. Nucl. Med. *21*:449, 1980.
176. Higgins, C. B, Herfkens, R., Lipton, M. J., Sievers, R., Sheldon, P., Kaufman, L., and Crooks, L. E.: Nuclear magnetic resonance imaging of acute myocardial infarction in dogs: Alterations in magnetic relaxation times. Am. J. Cardiol. *52*:184, 1983.
177. Johnston, D. L., Brady, T. J., Ratner, A. V., Rosen, B. R., Newell, J. B., Pohost, G. M., and Okada, R. D.: Assessment of myocardial ischemia with proton magnetic resonance: Effects of a three hour coronary occlusion with and without perfusion. Circulation *71*:595, 1985.
178. Ratner, A. V., Barrett, L. V., Okada, R. D., and Gang, D. L.: Alterations of the proton nuclear magnetic resonance spin-lattice relaxation time (T1) in rejecting cardiac allografts. J. Am. Coll. Cardiol. 3:538, 1984 (abstract).
179. Tscholakoff, D., Aherne, T., Yee, E. S., Derugin, N., and Higgins, C. B.: Cardiac transplantation in dogs: Evaluation with MRI. Radiology *157*:697, 1985.
180. Ratner, A. V., Okada, R. D., Thompson, R. D., Goldman, M. D., and Pohost, G. M.: Characterization of myocardium using proton NMR relaxation times (abstr). Proc. Scientific Progr. New York, MR Med, August, p. 291, 1983.
181. Tscholakoff, D., Higgins, C. B., McNamara, M. T., and Derugin, N.: Early phase myocardial infarction: Evaluation by magnetic resonance imaging. Radiology *159*:667, 1986.
182. Pflugfelder, P. W., Wisenberg, G., Prato, F. S., Carroll, E. S., and Turner, K. L.: Early detection of canine myocardial infarction by magnetic resonance imaging in vivo. Circulation *71*:587, 1985.
183. Tscholakoff, D., Higgins, C. B., Sechtem, U., Caputo, G., and Derugin, N.: MRI of reperfused myocardial infarctions. Am. J. Roentgenol. *146*:925, 1986.
184. Dinsmore, R. E., John, J. A., Yasuda, T., Wismer, G. L., Johnston, D. L., Gold, H. K., and Leinbach, R. C.: Characterization of myocardial signal intensity in normal and infarcted left ventricular segments of MR imaging. Radiology *157*(P):147, 1985.
185. Aherne, T., Tscholakoff, D., Finkbeiner, W., Sechtem, U., Yee, E., and Higgins, C. B.: MRI of cardiac transplants: Experimental study for evaluation of cardiac allograft rejection with and without treatment. Circulation *74*:145, 1986.

PART II NORMAL AND ABNORMAL CIRCULATORY FUNCTION

13 MECHANISMS OF CARDIAC CONTRACTION AND RELAXATION

by EUGENE BRAUNWALD, M.D.,
EDMUND H. SONNENBLICK, M.D.,
and JOHN ROSS, Jr., M.D.

The function of the heart is to propel unoxygenated blood to the lungs and oxygenated blood to the peripheral tissues in accordance with their metabolic requirements. Heart failure may therefore be defined as the pathophysiological state in which an abnormality of cardiac function is responsible for the failure of the heart to pump blood at a rate commensurate with these requirements. To understand the disturbances in cardiac contraction that characterize heart failure, described in Chapter 14, it is necessary to understand the structure and function of the normal cardiac cell and of the normal contractile process, described in this chapter.

CELLULAR MECHANISMS

STRUCTURE OF THE MYOCYTE

MYOCYTES, MYOFIBRILS, AND SARCOMERES (Table 13–1). *Ventricular myocytes* (myocardial cells or fibers) are normally 50 to 100 μ in length and 10 to 25 μ in diameter (Fig. 13–1). Atrial myocytes are smaller while myocytes from the conduction system (Purkinje cells) are larger in both dimensions (p. 385). Numerous cross-banded strands or bundles, termed *myofibrils*, traverse the length of the fibers and, unlike the case for skeletal muscle, are incompletely separated by clefts of cytoplasm that contain mitochondria and membranous tubules (Fig. 13–1*B*).[1–6]

Myofibrils are composed of longitudinally repeating *sarcomeres* separated by two adjacent dark lines—the Z lines (Fig. 13–1*B* and *C*).[6] Sarcomeres occupy about 50 per cent of the mass of the cardiac cells[7] and are aligned so that the ends of adjacent myofibrils are in register, giving the fiber its striated appearance.[1–3] The length of the sarcomere ranges from 1.6 to 2.2 μ, depending on muscle length. The center of the sarcomere is occupied by a dark band, the A band (the anisotropic or birefringent band that rotates polarized light), and is 1.5 μ in length. The A band is flanked by two lighter bands, termed I (isotropic) bands, which are variable in length depending on the length of the sarcomere. The bands of the sarcomere reflect the disposition of interdigitating myofilaments made up of contractile proteins (Figs. 13–1*C* and 13–2). Thin filaments composed of actin are attached to each Z line and project longitudinally into the middle of the sarcomere, where they interdigitate with an array of thicker filaments com-

TABLE 13–1 CHARACTERISTICS OF CARDIAC CELLS, ORGANELLES, AND CONTRACTILE PROTEINS

A. MICROANATOMY OF HEART CELLS

	Ventricular myocyte[1, 2]	Atrial myocyte[1, 3]	Purkinje cells[1, 4]
Shape	Long and narrow	Elliptical	Long and broad
Length, μm	50–100	About 20	150–200
Diameter, μm	10–25	5–6	35–40
T tubules	Plentiful	Rare or none	Absent
Intercalated disc	Prominent end-to-end transmission	Side-to-side as well as end-to-end transmission	Very prominent; abundant gap functions; fast end-to-end transmission
General appearance	Mitochondria and sarcomeres very abundant; rectangular, branching bundles with little interstitial collagen	Bundles of atrial tissue separated by wide areas of collagen	Fewer sarcomeres, more glycogen

B. COMPOSITION AND FUNCTION OF RAT VENTRICULAR CELL

Organelle	Percentage of cell volume	Function
Myofibril	About 50%[5]	Interaction of thick and thin filaments during contraction cycle
Mitochondria	16% in neonate[5] 33% in adult[5]	Provide ATP chiefly for contraction
T system	1%[6]	Transmission of electrical signal from sarcolemma to cell interior
Sarcoplasmic reticulum	33% in neonate[5] 2% in adult[5]	Takes up and releases Ca^{++} during contraction cycle
Terminal cisternae	0.33% in adult[6]	? site of calcium storage and release[7] ? site of calcium uptake en route to cisternae
Rest of network	Rest of volume	
Sarcolemma	Very low	Control of ionic gradients; channels for ions (action potential); maintenance of cell integrity; receptors for drugs and hormones
Nucleus	5%	Protein synthesis
Lysosomes	Very low	Intracellular digestion and proteolysis
Sarcoplasmic (= cytoplasm) (+ nuclei + other structures)	12%[6]	Provides cytosol in which rise and fall of ionized calcium occurs; contains other ions and small molecules

C. THE PROTEINS OF MYOFIBRILS

Function	Location	% of myofibrillar protein	Molecular weight
Contractile			
Myosin	Thick filaments	55–60	500,000
Actin	Thin filaments	20	43,000
Regulatory			
Tropomyosin	Thin filaments	5	70,000
Troponin I	Thin filaments		
Troponin C	Thin filaments	7	86,000
Troponin T	Thin filaments		
Structural			
C protein	Thick filaments		
apha-actinin	Thick filaments and Z lines		
beta-actinin	Thin filaments	8–13	40,000–750,000
M line proteins	M lines		
Other proteins	Various		

There are about 7 actins: 2 myosins: 1 tropomyosin: 1 troponin in the myofibrils, but their different molecular weights account for the different picture given by the percentage contributions each makes to the total myofibrillar mass (third column). Part C partly from Perry, S.V.: Biochem. Soc. Trans. 7:593, 1979.

[1]Legato: The Myocardial Cell for the Clinical Cardiologist, 1973.
[2]Laks et al.: Circ. Res. *21*:671, 1967.
[3]McNutt and Fawcett: J. Cell. Biol. *42*:46, 1969.
[4]Sommer: J. Mol. Cell. Cardiol. 14 Suppl 3:77, 1982.
[5]David et al.: J. Mol. Cell. Cardiol. *11*:631, 1979.
[6]Page and McCallister: Am. J. Cardiol. *31*:172, 1973.
[7]Page and Surdyk-Droske: Circ. Res. *45*:260, 1979.
Part B modified from Page and McCallister, 1973.
(From Opie, L.: The Heart. New York, Grune and Stratton, 1984, pp. 16 and 98.)

posed of myosin molecules.[2, 3, 6] Interactions between the thick and thin myofilaments in the A band generate force and shortening of the myocardium, with the myofilaments sliding past one another while maintaining a fixed length.

The *nucleus* is centrally placed within the myocardial cell. *Mitochondria,* which make up about 20 per cent of the volume of the cell,[7] are elliptically shaped, approximately 2 to 5 μ by 0.5 μ, and are situated between and in close apposition to the myofibrils as well as just beneath the sarcolemma.[6] Their platelike foldings, or cristae, which contain the enzymes of the tricarboxylic acid cycle, project inward from the surface membrane. The close proximity

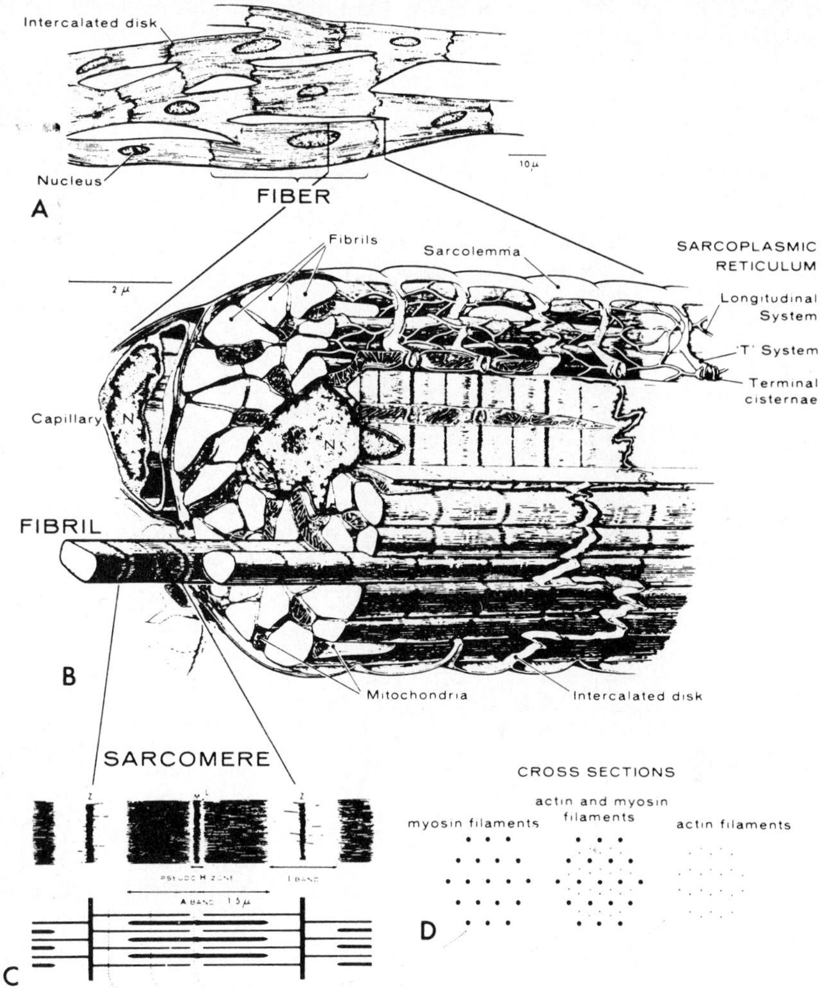

FIGURE 13–1. Schematic diagram of the microscopic structure of heart muscle.

A, Myocardium as seen under the light microscope. Branching of fibers is evident, with each containing a centrally located nucleus. Fibers or cells are connected across intercalated disks.

B, A myocardial cell or fiber reconstructed from electron micrographs, showing the arrangement of multiple parallel fibrils that compose the cell and of serially connected sarcomeres that compose the individual fibril. N = nucleus. The sarcotubular system, which mediates activation, includes the sarcolemma and sarcoplasmic reticulum. An intercalated disk in the center of the reconstruction serves to separate two cells.

C, An individual sarcomere from a myofibril. Diagrammatic representation of the arrangement of myofilaments that make up the sarcomere. Thick filaments, approximately 1.5 microns in length, composed of myosin, are localized to the A band, while thin filaments, 1.0 micron in length, composed primarily of actin, extend from the Z line through the I band into the A band, ending at the edges of the central H zone. The H zone is the central area of the A band where thin filaments are absent. Thick and thin filaments overlap only in the A band.

D, Diagrammatic cross section of the sarcomere showing the specific lattice arrangements of the myofilaments. In the center of the sarcomere (left), only the thick (myosin) filaments arranged in a hexagonal array are seen. In the distal portions of the A band (center), both thick and thin (actin) filaments are found, each thick filament surrounded by six thin filaments. In the I band, only thin filaments are present. (From Braunwald, E., et al.: Mechanisms of Contraction of the Normal and Failing Heart. 2nd ed. Boston, Little, Brown, 1976.)

of the mitochondria, the organelles in which ATP is produced, to the contractile filaments may facilitate the transfer of ATP from its site of production to its size of utilization during the contractile process. *Lysosomes*, membrane-limited vesicles about 0.1 μ in diameter and located near the pole of the nucleus, contain latent hydrolytic enzymes capable of lysing cellular membranes as well as other cellular components.[2]

Myocardial cells that initiate intrinsic activity in the heart, i.e., *pacemaker or automatic cells*, are somewhat smaller than ventricular fibers[6] (Table 13–1A). Those which are specialized for conduction and the spread of excitation, i.e., Purkinje fibers, are very large when compared to contractile fibers; they contain fewer myofibrils and greater quantities of clear cytoplasm, fine intracellular noncontractile filaments, and glycogen in addition to having a rich external investment of capillaries and small nerves.[8]

Myocardial fibers are surrounded by a rich capillary network, and small, nonmyelinated nerves are found lying free in the extracellular space.[5] These nerves have no specific junctions with cardiac cells but do exhibit bulbous ends bearing granules that contain neurotransmitter substances. These substances are *acetylcholine*, located primarily in the atria and in automatic and conduction tissues, and *norepinephrine*, found in these tissues but also in the ventricles; both can be released to act on membrane surface receptors of adjacent cells.

The atrial myocytes, but not the ventricular ones, also contain specific dense granules[2, 9] (Fig. 59–5, p. 1831), the source of atrial natriuretic hormone,[10] which may play an important role in salt and water metabolism and thus in the control of blood pressure.[11]

SARCOLEMMA, INTERCALATED DISCS, AND SARCOPLASMIC RETICULUM. A surface membrane, the *sarcolemma*, surrounds the myocardial cells and invaginates at the Z lines of the sarcomere.[1, 2, 12, 13] It is composed of a thin (7 to 9 nm), bimolecular phospholipid layer, the *plasmalemma*, which is the site of electrical polarization (Fig. 20–5, p. 585). Just exterior to the plasmalemma is the glycocalyx, i.e., the basement membrane, approximately 50 nm in thickness (Fig. 13–3), which in turn is composed of an inner and an outer coat. The plasmalemma is the major semipermeable membrane between the intracellular cytoplasm and the negatively charged glycocalyx to which Ca^{++} may be bound and which separates the cell from the extracellular matrix. Adjacent myocardial cells are connected end-to-end by a thickened portion of the sarcolemma, termed the *intercalated disc*,[1–5] a segment of which—the gap junction—represents a low-resistance pathway to the propagation of electrical activity between cells.[1, 2]

Myocardial fibers are also interconnected by an extensive network of collagen fibers, fine microfibrils, and microthreads,[14] which play an important role in cell orientation, tissue compliance, and intercellular force transmission. The elastic fibers are composed of microfilaments of glycoprotein and amorphous elastin.[15] This "skeleton" contributes importantly to the diastolic properties of the ventricle and limits the extent to which the heart can be dilated by a volume overload.

The hydrophobic phospholipid bilayer of the plasmalemma acts as an ionic barrier and maintains higher intracellular than extracellular potassium [K^+] concentrations and lower intracellular than extracellular sodium [Na^+] and

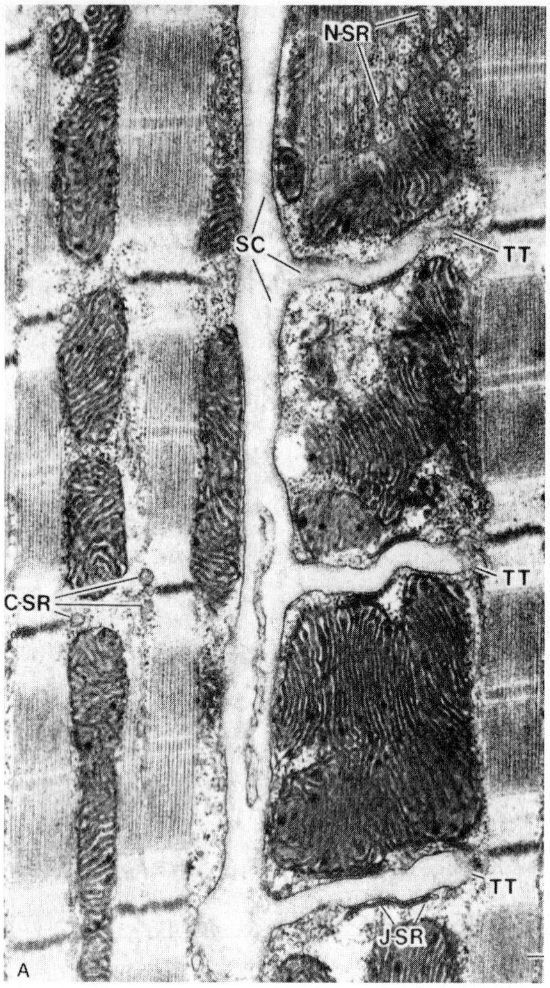

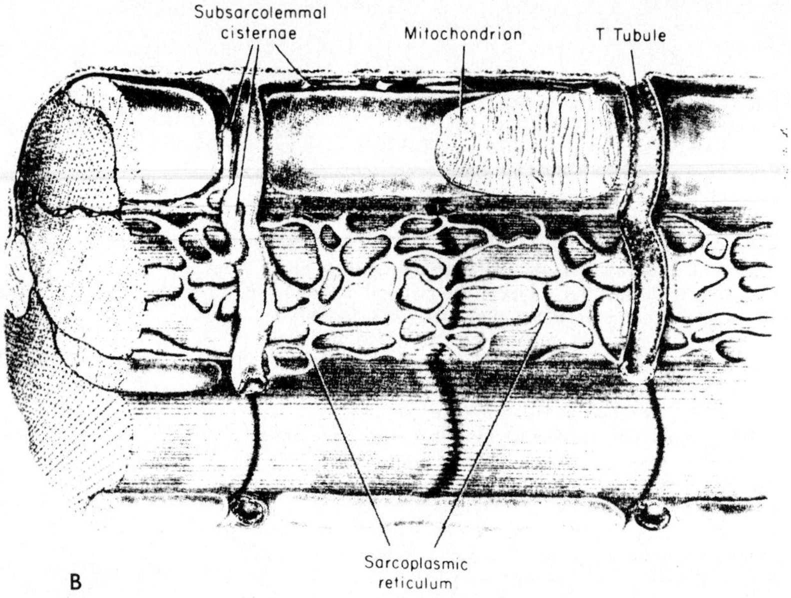

FIGURE 13–2. ***A,*** **Ventricular myocardial cells from dog right ventricular wall. The sarcolemma of the right-hand cell forms three transverse tubules (TT) oriented in register with Z bands of the nearest myofibrils. The substance of the myocardial surface coat (SC) can be seen both in association with the surface sarcolemma and within the T tubules' lamina. Three categories of sarcoplasmic reticulum can be discerned: network SR (N-SR) on the face of one myofibril; junctional SR (J-SR), flattened saccules apposed to the T tubules; and corbular SR (C-SR). Note mitochondria, either arranged in intermyofibrillar row or located just beneath the surface sarcolemma. Scale bar represents 0.5 μm. (From Forbes, M. S., and Sperelakis, N.: *In* Physiology and Pathophysiology of the Heart. Boston, Martinus Nijhoff, 1984, p. 21.)**

B, **Schematic of T tubules and sarcoplasmic reticulum of mammalian cardiac muscle. Note how the diffuse tubular network of the sarcoplasmic reticulum forms saccular expansions, the subsarcolemmal cisternae, which are in close apposition to the sarcolemma and T tubules. (From Fawcett, D. W., and McNutt, N. S.: The ultrastructure of the cat myocardium. I. Ventricular papillary muscle. J. Cell Biol. *42*:1, 1969.)**

calcium [Ca^{++}] concentrations. (Cytoplasmic [Ca^{++}] is of the order of 10^{-7} M; extracellular [Ca^{++}] is 10^{-3} M. The sarcolemma possesses enzyme systems that utilize ATP for energy in order to maintain these differences in ion concentrations.[16, 17] Na^+, K^+-stimulated ATPase (p. 390) are responsible for the active transport of Na^+ and Ca^{++} out of the cardiac cell and for the uptake of K^+. Near the Z lines the sarcolemma contains wide invaginations, the *T system,* which branch, both longitudinally and transversely, through the cell (Fig. 13–2). Closely coupled to but not continuous with the T system is the *sarcoplasmic reticulum* (SR),[18] a complex network of anastomosing, membrane-limited tubular intracellular channels, approximately 30 nm in diameter, which surround each myofibril and play a critical role in excitation of the muscle.[4, 19] Unlike the T system, the SR is not continuous with the

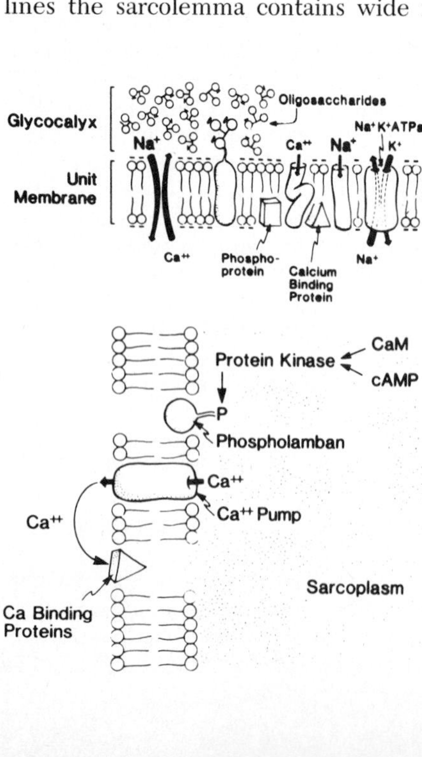

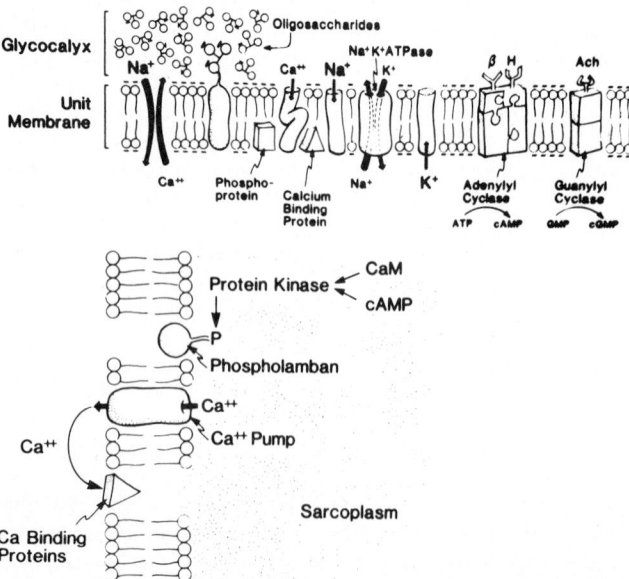

FIGURE 13–3. Schematic of the ultrastructure of the sarcolemma (*top*) and sarcoplasmic reticulum (*bottom*) of ventricular muscle cells. Both membrane systems have a lamina consisting of a sheet of lipids forming the matrix of the membrane and acting as a hydrophobic barrier. The outer surface of the sarcolemma is covered by a negatively charged glycocalyx that appears as a fuzzy layer in electron micrographs. Embedded in the sarcolemma are receptors for hormones and neurotransmitters along with the enzymes that transduce receptor binding to an alteration in intracellular concentrations of cyclic nucleotides. Major proteins in the sarcoplasmic reticulum (SR) are a calcium pump protein; calcium binding proteins that store transported calcium ions; and phospholamban, which, when phosphorylated by cAMP- or calmodulin-dependent protein kinases, alters the calcium pump and induces an increase in the rate of calcium transport into the lumen of the SR. (From Solaro, R. J.: The role of calcium in the contraction of the heart. *In* Flaim, S. F., and Zelis, R. [eds.]: Calcium Blockers: Mechanisms of Action and Clinical Applications. Baltimore, Urban and Schwarzenberg, 1982, p. 25.)

extracellular space. Where the SR approaches the T tubules or the sarcolemma, it widens into flattened saclike enlargements (cisternae). At their junction, the SR and T tubules are separated by gaps of 10 to 12 nm.[1, 2, 6] Depolarization of the sarcolemma may be channeled through the T system to release Ca^{++} from the SR, which mediates myofibrillar activation (see below). Like the sarcolemma, the SR has a bilayer matrix consisting principally of phospholipids.

Contractile Proteins

The contractile apparatus consists of partially overlapping, rodlike myofilaments that are fixed in length, both at rest and during contraction (Table 13–1*C*).[1, 20, 21]

MYOSIN. The thicker filaments, composed of *myosin* molecules, are limited to the A band, are about 100 to 150 nm in diameter with tapered ends, and measure 1.5 to 1.6 μ in length.[1, 22] They are created by an orderly aggregation of 300 longitudinally stacked molecules of myosin proteins with a molecular weight of approximately 500,000 daltons and are held parallel and in register by centrally located connections at the M line. A rodlike tail, approximately 1300 nm in length, lies along the filament, and a globular bilobed head forms bridgelike outcroppings from the filament in groups of 3, each group 14.3 nm from the next. Thus, there are 50 such sets on each half of the thick filament, rotating so that a head appears in line every 43 nm, and with activation of the muscle, can form attachments or cross bridges with actin filaments[23–26] to generate force and shortage (Fig. 13–4). Myosin by itself exhibits the ability to split ATP, i.e., it acts as an ATPase that is inhibited by Mg^{++} but activated by small amounts of Ca^{++}.[27] When myosin combines with actin, it forms an

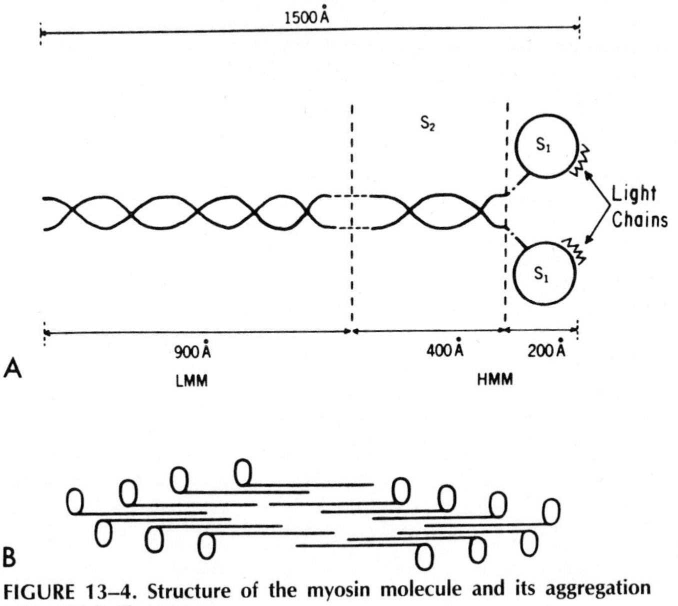

FIGURE 13–4. Structure of the myosin molecule and its aggregation into a thick filament.

A, The myosin molecule. The two-stranded portion of the molecule shows a point of cleavage between light meromyosin (LMM) and heavy meromyosin (HMM). Heavy meromyosin can be cleaved into two portions—an S_2 fragment, which is similar to the LMM portion of the molecule, and an S_1 fragment, which contains the ATPase portion of the molecule. Light chains are associated with the S_1 fragment. (From Lowey, S., et al.: Substructure of the myosin molecule. I. Subfragments of myosin by enzymatic degradation. J. Mol. Biol. *42*:1, 1969.)

B, Diagram of the aggregation of myosin filaments into a thick filament. The long portion of the molecule tends to be oriented toward the center of the filament, with the enzymatically active heads of the molecule oriented laterally. Thus, the center of this aggregation will contain no active enzyme sites.

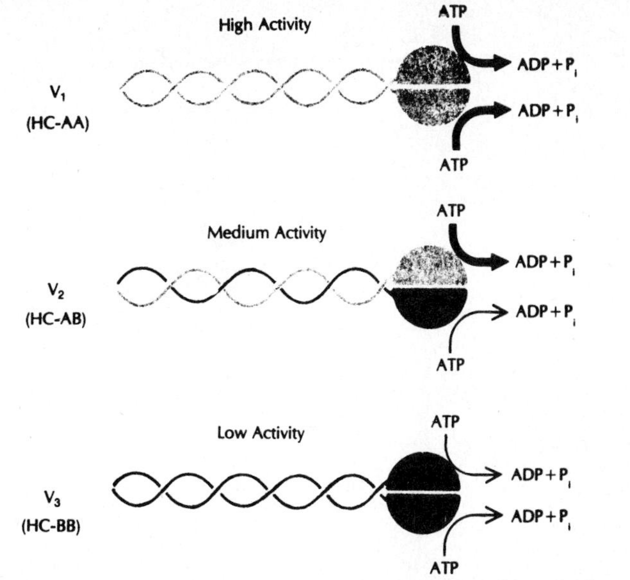

FIGURE 13–5. The three ventricular myosin isoenzymes, designated V_1, V_2, and V_3, originate from combinations of two heavy-chain subunits (HC-A and HC-B), which differ in amino acid sequence. Functionally, these differences are expressed in the level of myosin ATPase activity and contractile performance. Thus, hydrolysis of ATP and release of reaction products are most rapid for V_1 and slowest for V_3; V_3 is intermediate. (From Morkin, E.: Contractile proteins of the heart. Hosp. Pract. *18*:107, 1983.)

actomyosin complex that is enzymatically even more active in its ability to split ATP and is stimulated primarily by Mg^{++}. This actomyosin constitutes the enzyme which is physiologically active in force development. The myosin molecule can be broken down by the proteolytic enzyme trypsin into two fragments, *light meromyosin* and *heavy meromyosin*. The latter contains the bilobed globular heads (Fig. 13–4A) and is the site of ATPase activity.[23]

Myosin itself can be separated into three *isoenzyme* components—V_1, V_2, and V_3—which have a different heavy-chain composition.[28, 29] Only two chemically distinct heavy-chain subunits exist, α and β.[30] V_1 and V_3 comprise αα and ββ while V_2 is a heterodimer, αβ. Myosin ATPase and intrinsic muscle speed (V_{max}) depend on the proportions of these isoenzymes that are present, V_1 being fast and V_3 being slow[31] (Fig. 13–5). As noted later, hypertrophied heart muscle in animal models has a lowered V_{max} and a greater proportion of V_3.[30] Similar shifts in the V_1/V_3 ratio occur in experimental diabetics[32] and with aging.[27]

ACTIN. The thin filament, 1.0 μ in length in ventricular myocardium, is a double alpha-helix that consists of two strands of *actin* and has a molecular weight of 47,000 daltons and a diameter of 55 nm.[32] Actin filaments course from the Z line through the I band and into the A band (Fig. 13–1*C*). The A band is the region of the sarcomere where there is overlapping of thick and thin filaments, while the I band contains only thin filaments.

TROPONIN AND TROPOMYOSIN. These are regulatory proteins that constitute about 10 per cent of total myofibrillar protein and are associated with the thin filament.[32, 33] Tropomyosin is a rodlike protein, 400 nm in length and 20 to 30 nm in width, with a molecular weight of 70,000 daltons.[21] It comprises two helices, each of which lies slightly off the groove between the actin chains. Tropomyosin forms a continuing strand through the center of the thin filament while the troponin complex is located at intervals of 365 nm. *Troponin* can be separated into three components:[34] (1) troponin C, a "calcium-sensitizing factor" that binds Ca^{++}; (2) troponin I, an "inhibitory factor" that

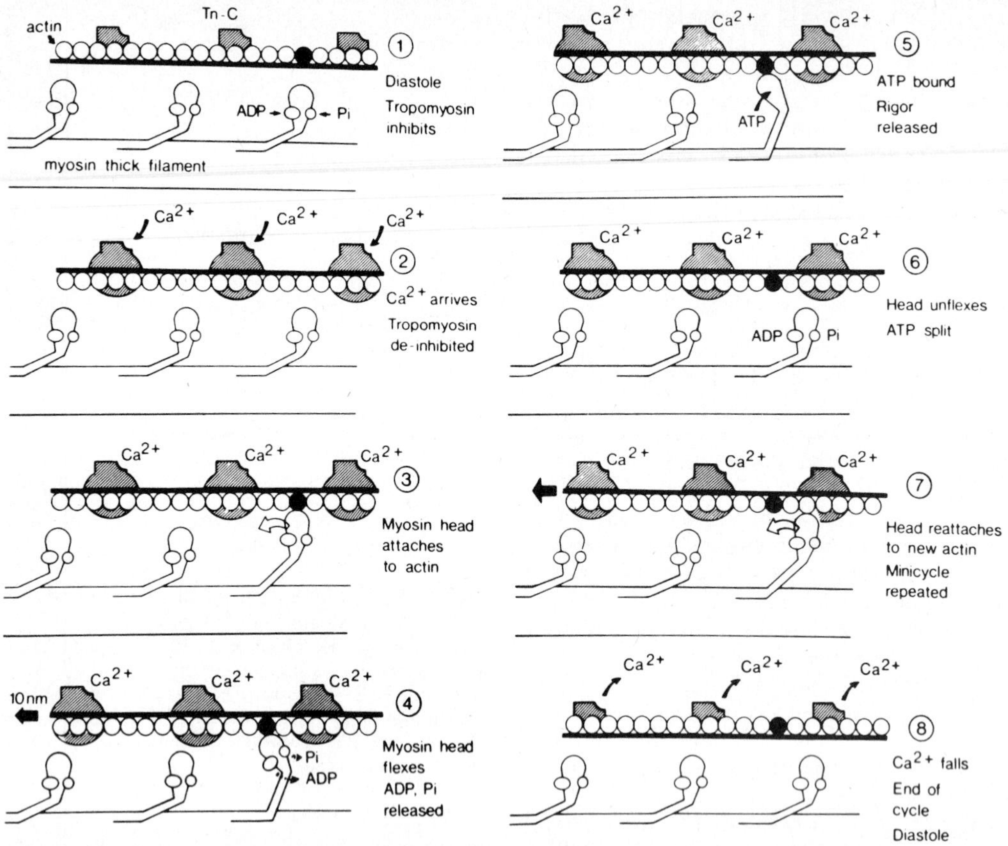

FIGURE 13–6. Contractile events in heart muscle. The cross-bridge cycle starts with relaxation in diastole (Step 1) when tropomyosin (Tm), the solid black horizontal line, "blocks" the myosin heads from binding to actin. At the start of systole (Step 2), Ca^{++} combines with troponin C (Tn-C) so that Tm no longer blocks the actin and so that myosin heads can bind and then "flex," whereupon ADP and inorganic phosphate (P_i) are released (Step 3). The "rigor state" develops transiently (Step 4). ATP moves in to the same binding site on the myosin head vacated by ADP, to "release" the myosin head (Step 5). After ATP has been split to ADP and P_i by the myosin ATPase, the head extends (Step 6) to rebind to another actin 2 to 4 units "downstream" (Step 7). Steps 1 to 7 are repeated until $[Ca^{++}]$ at the myofiber decreases at the start of diastole (Step 8). (From Opie, L.: The Heart. New York, Grune and Stratton, 1984, p. 101.)

inhibits the Mg^{++}-stimulated ATPase of actomyosin; and (3) troponin T, which is necessary for the entire complex to function and serves to allow attachment of the troponin complex to actin and tropomyosin.[35–37]

In the absence of troponin and tropomyosin, the contractile proteins actin and myosin interact and are fully activated, requiring the presence of only Mg^{++} and ATP to initiate the reaction leading to muscular contraction. When these regulatory proteins are present, however, cross-bridge formation between myosin and actin is inhibited[38] (Fig. 13–6). When Ca^{++} is bound to troponin C, the binding of troponin I to actin is inhibited, which in turn causes a conformational change in tropomyosin, so that the latter, instead of inhibiting, now enhances cross-bridge formation. Ca^{++} may thus be considered to be a "derepressor," since it inactivates an inhibitor of the reaction between actin and myosin. Inhibition of the interaction between actin and myosin is mediated by the ability of the Ca^{++}-troponin complex to alter the configuration of tropomyosin, which in turn changes the exposure of active sites all along the thin filaments. In relaxed muscle, tropomyosin blocks the active sites of actin that react to form cross bridges with myosin.[37, 38] With cellular depolarization, the myoplasmic $[Ca^{++}]$ rises from 10^{-7} to about 10^{-5} M. Ca^{++} is bound to troponin, and the actin rods are drawn toward the center of the sarcomere.[26] Once such a "stroke" is completed, an attached myosin head ejects its ATP hydrolysis products, binds another ATP molecule, and detaches from the actin site. The myosin head then returns to its original orientation and the cycle is repeated, the head attaching to a different actin monome farther along the thin filament[24, 39] (Fig. 13–5). Thus, shortening of cardiac muscle involves a relative change in position of these two sets of filaments, i.e., actin filaments are displaced by the force-generating process at many cross-bridge sites.[33] If the muscle is not permitted to shorten, i.e., during isometric contraction (in the presence of Ca^{++}), the heavy meromyosin does not undergo a conformational change, the cross bridges between actin and myosin are maintained, and ADP rather than ATP remains bound to myosin.[26] The force that is developed is related to the quantity of Ca^{++} which is bound to troponin C, which in turn is related to the intracellular $[Ca^{++}]$.[16] Subsequent removal of Ca^{++} from troponin results in relaxation.

Smaller proteins, termed "light chains," are located on the heads of myosin and can be phosphorylated to produce as yet controversial changes in the enzymatic activity of myosin.[33] It has also been suggested that the actomyosin ATPase activity can be increased by increments in ultracellular cyclic adenosine monophosphate (cyclic AMP),[40, 41] a possible mechanism by which beta-adrenergic stimulation exerts a positive inotropic effect. Such a change would be consonant with the mechanical response of heart muscle to catecholamines to produce increments in the unloaded velocity of shortening (V_{max}) (p. 396).

EXCITATION-CONTRACTION COUPLING: THE ROLE OF CALCIUM

Since the classic experiments of Ringer in 1882, it has been appreciated that cardiac contraction depends on the presence of Ca^{++}.[42] Heart muscle contains 2.5 mmol of Ca^{++} per liter of water, which is several hundred times higher than the concentration required for activation. However, the higher $[Ca^{++}]$ within the relaxed cell is not directly available to initiate contraction but is bound to many structures, including the nucleus, mitochondria, sarcolemma, T system, and particularly the SR. Ca^{++} is required to trigger the contractile process by repressing troponin, the inhibitor of the actin-myosin interaction. The key event in the initiation of contraction then is the rise in sarcoplasmic $[Ca^{++}]$.[19, 43, 44] This had been suspected for many years, but there was no *direct* evidence for it in cardiac muscle until Allen and Blinks succeeded in the difficult task of using the photoprotein aequorin as an intracellular indicator of $[Ca^{++}]$ in cardiac muscle[45–47] (Fig. 13–7).

The source of activating Ca^{++} is not certain and may differ in the myocardium of different species.[48] Extracellular Ca^{++} can enter via voltage-dependent gated "slow channels" or via a Na^{+}-Ca^{++} exchange mechanism.[16] Depolarization of the membrane associated with the upstroke of the action potential opens the ion channels that carry the Ca^{++} current. The Ca^{++} that flows into the cell through the Ca^{++} channels does not activate the contractile system directly but rather is stored in the membrane sites within the cell, i.e., the T system and the SR (Fig. 13–8). The Ca^{++} that actually activates the contractile system appears to be stored in the cisternae of the SR, which have the capacity to bind Ca^{++} actively and to store it in a bound form within their lumina.[46] Although the amount of Ca^{++} that enters the cell via the Ca^{++} current during the plateau of the action potential may not be sufficient to stimulate the contractile apparatus, it may, however, release a much larger quantity of Ca^{++} from the SR, allowing activation of the contractile system.

This release of Ca^{++} by the SR has been termed "calcium-induced" calcium release.[48–50] According to this concept, depolarization of the cell membrane causes release of Ca^{++} from a store, SR_1 (the terminal cisternae of the SR), into the cytoplasm; Ca^{++} binding by troponin molecules results in contractile activity; relaxation is brought about by the active uptake of Ca^{++} into the temporary store, SR_2 (area of the SR adjacent to the contractile proteins), and from there the Ca^{++} eventually returns to SR_1. Thus SR_1 is considered to be a labile store, the Ca^{++} content of which determines the inotropic state of the muscle.[50, 51] The Ca^{++} current in cardiac fibers is composed of an initial fast component followed by a slow component. Fabiato[48] used repeated microinjection-aspiration sequences to simulate the time course of the Ca^{++} current in cardiac fibers from which the sarcolemma had been removed (skinned fibers). This technique mimicked the changes in myoplasmic $[Ca^{++}]$ that would be produced by the native Ca^{++} current in fibers with intact sarcolemmas. The fast component of the simulated Ca^{++} current triggered a tension transient mediated by Ca^{++}-induced release of Ca^{++} from the SR. In contrast, the slow component of the simulated Ca^{++} current did not affect the first tension transient provoked by the fast component but did potentiate the subsequent tension transients. Thus, the fast initial component of the Ca^{++} current triggers release of Ca^{++}, whereas the slow component loads the SR with Ca^{++} that becomes available for release during subsequent beats.

Studies with the aequorin technique in atrial and ventricular muscle have shown that changes in the rate or pattern of stimulation, in extracellular $[Ca^{++}]$, and in catecholamines all produce a greater increase in cytoplasmic $[Ca^{++}]$.[45, 47] Catecholamines differ from the other inotropic interventions in that they produce a smaller increase in tension production than would be expected from the increase in the cytoplasmic $[Ca^{++}]$, presumably by reducing the sensitivity of the contractile system to Ca^{++}. This decrease in sensitivity may result from an increase in the degree of phosphorylation of troponin that is brought about by the cyclic AMP–induced activation of a protein kinase,[46] but this is controversial.[52]

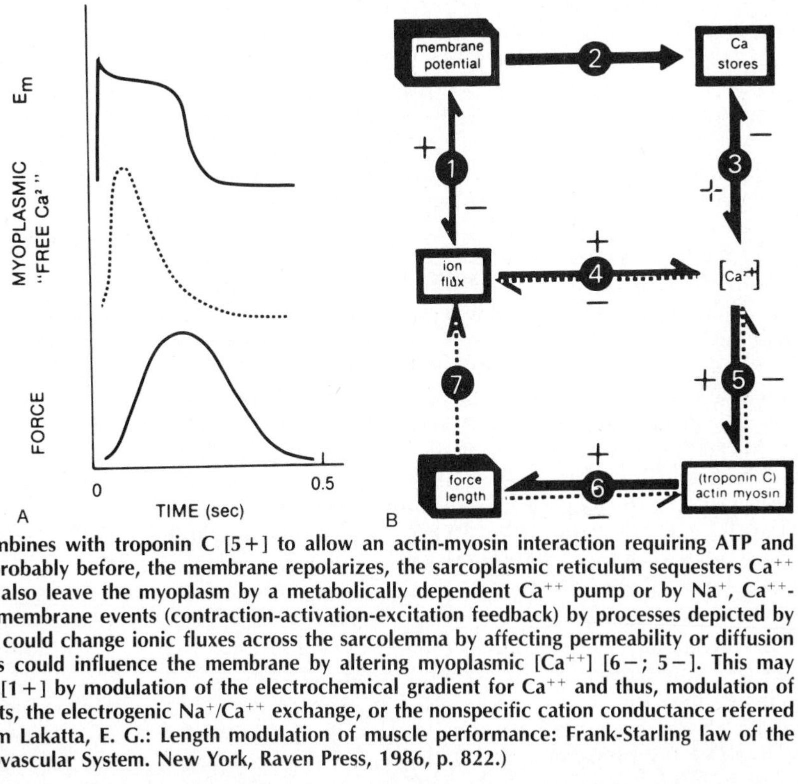

FIGURE 13–7. *A*, Schematic illustration of the approximate time course of excitation-activation-contraction coupling. From top to bottom, the transients are the cell membrane action potential, the myoplasmic $[Ca^{++}]$ as measured by the photoprotein aequorin, and myocardial force developed during an isometric contraction. Note the sequence of events: the action potential precedes the rise in myoplasmic free $[Ca^{++}]$, which in turn precedes the onset of force development. The decline in myoplasmic $[Ca^{++}]$ precedes the fall-off in force. *B*, Schematic diagram of some interactions between membrane potential and contraction in the heart. The sequence in excitation-activation-contraction coupling may be followed via the heavy black arrows (mainly clockwise). Ion fluxes across the sarcolemma [arrow 1+] determine the membrane potential, which itself can provide a driving force for ion movements [arrow 1−]. The changes in membrane potential are a function of the ionic equilibrium potentials and conductances. The depolarization [2] causes a rise in myoplasmic $[Ca^{++}]$ derived from intracellular stores [3+]. This results directly from the depolarization or possibly from Ca^{++}-induced Ca^{++} release. The Ca^{++} within the myoplasm combines with troponin C [5+] to allow an actin-myosin interaction requiring ATP and resulting in force development [6+]. At the time that, or probably before, the membrane repolarizes, the sarcoplasmic reticulum sequesters Ca^{++} [5−; 3−] permitting relaxation to occur [6−]. Ca^{++} can also leave the myoplasm by a metabolically dependent Ca^{++} pump or by Na^{+}, Ca^{++}-exchange [4−]. Force and length changes could influence membrane events (contraction-activation-excitation feedback) by processes depicted by the dotted lines. For example, these mechanical alterations could change ionic fluxes across the sarcolemma by affecting permeability or diffusion gradients directly [7]. Indirectly, force and length changes could influence the membrane by altering myoplasmic $[Ca^{++}]$ [6−; 5−]. This may influence ionic flux [4−], and hence, membrane potential [1+] by modulation of the electrochemical gradient for Ca^{++} and thus, modulation of the slow Ca^{++} channel, outward K^{+} currents, "leak" currents, the electrogenic Na^{+}/Ca^{++} exchange, or the nonspecific cation conductance referred to as the *oscillatory* or *transient inward* (TI) *current*. (From Lakatta, E. G.: Length modulation of muscle performance: Frank-Starling law of the heart. *In* Fozzard, H. A., et al. [eds.]: The Heart and Cardiovascular System. New York, Raven Press, 1986, p. 822.)

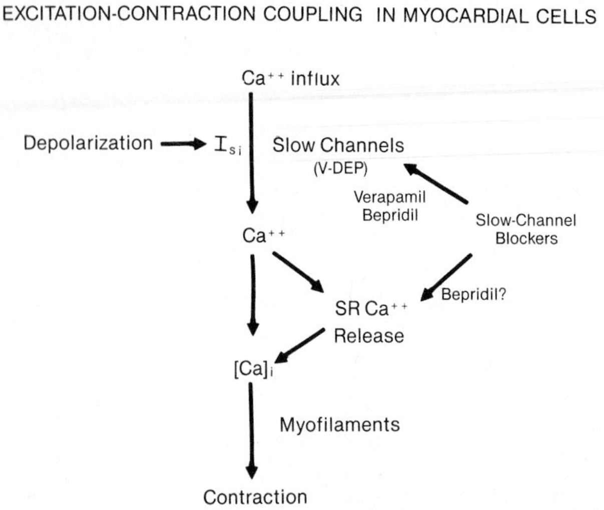

FIGURE 13–8. Summary diagram for excitation-contraction coupling in myocardial cells. Ca^{++} influx during excitation occurs through the voltage-dependent (V-DEP) and time-dependent gated slow channels. This entering Ca^{++} helps to raise the myoplasmic Ca^{++} concentration ($[Ca]_i$) to the level necessary to activate the contractile proteins (e.g., 10^{-5} M), and acts to bring about the release of additional Ca^{++} from the sarcoplasmic reticulum (SR) by the mechanism described by Fabiato and Fabiato. (From Sperelakis, N.: The slow action potential and properties of the myocardial slow channels. *In* Physiology and Pathophysiology of the Heart. Boston, Martinus Nijhoff, 1984, p. 160.)

THE CARDIAC ACTION POTENTIAL. As presented in detail on pages 585 to 595 and in Figure 20–7, p. 588, the action potential for cardiac cells is generated by the movement of ions across the cell membrane, which in turn is controlled by variations in membrane permeability and ion concentration gradient in a manner similar to that occurring in nerve cells.[53, 54] The action potential of ventricular myocardium has two components, the spike and the plateau; a large fast inward Na^+ current passing through "fast Na^+ channels" is responsible for the early spike,[55] while Ca^{++} influx into the myocardial cell occurs during the plateau phase of the action potential through a separate set of "slow channels" that are permeable primarily to Ca^{++}.[56, 57] The latter are blocked by the organic Ca^{++} antagonists such as verapamil, nifedipine, diltiazem, and their analogs[56–60] (p. 393) and by manganese ion, lanthanum ion, and acidosis; additional Ca^{++} channels are recruited by beta-adrenergic stimulation[52] (Fig. 13–8).

SODIUM-CHANNEL EXCHANGE. Total Ca^{++} within the cell is also affected by an exchange of more than 3 Na^+ for each Ca^{++} across the sarcolemma, the energy for which is supplied by the Na^+ gradient generated by the sodium pump.[61–63] Ca^{++} removal from the cell is enhanced when the Na^+ gradient is increased, and it is reduced (leading to intracellular Ca^{++} accumulation) when the gradient diminishes. The latter effect may explain the positive inotropic effect of lowering extracellular $[Na^+]$ or of inhibiting the Na^+, K^+-stimulated ATPase with digitalis, which elevates intracellular $[Na^+]$; both these interventions alter the transmembrane Na^+ gradient and elevate intracellular $[Ca^{++}]$.

As has already been pointed out, the absolute quantity of Ca^{++} that crosses the sarcolemma during the plateau (phase 2) of the action potential, i.e., during the slow inward current, is relatively small and is incapable in and of itself of bringing about full activation of the contractile apparatus.[64] Instead, the major portion of the Ca^{++} used to activate concentration is stored within the cell, largely in the SR, in its subsarcolemmal cisternae, or on the inner surface of the sarcolemma itself.[65, 66] This Ca^{++} diffuses toward the myofibrils and binds to troponin, which, together with tropomyosin but in the absence of Ca^{++}, prevents the interaction between heavy meromyosin and actin. The number of contractile sites activated and therefore the resultant force generated are directly related to the quantity of Ca^{++} present in the vicinity of the myofibrils, which in turn ultimately depends on the influx of Ca^{++} that accompanied the action potential.[67] This influx, in turn, is a function of the extracellular $[Ca^{++}]$, the duration of the action potential, and the number of action potentials per unit time.[66]

CARDIAC RELAXATION. This results from a cessation of the inward slow Ca^{++} current coupled with the uptake and storage of Ca^{++} by the SR, in which is embedded a 100,000-dalton membrane-bound protein, *phospholamban*, which spans the lipid bilayer (Fig. 13–3). This protein, a Ca^{++}-stimulated Mg-ATPase, has a very high affinity for Ca^{++} and is responsible for the active transport of Ca^{++} from the cytoplasm into the lumen of the SR. Thus, during repolarization, the SR in the presence of ATP avidly accumulates myoplasmic Ca^{++} against a concentration gradient, so that intracellular $[Ca^{++}]$ falls to below 10^{-7} M and Ca^{++} detaches from the troponin, resulting in inhibition of the interactions between actin and myosin and hence in relaxation.[57] Further, the process of shortening itself reduces Ca^{++} binding to the contractile protein (troponin C).[68, 69]

INOTROPIC EFFECTS AND CALCIUM KINETICS. There is evidence that (1) the total tension developed, (2) the rate of tension development, and (3) the rate of tension decline during relaxation are related, respectively, to (1) the quantity of Ca^{++} available for binding to troponin, (2) the rate of Ca^{++} delivery to troponin, and (3) the rate at which Ca^{++} is removed from troponin.[56, 68] Many interventions that augment or depress the contractile state of heart muscle are associated with—and indeed are caused by—alterations in Ca^{++} movement and concentrations in heart muscle.[57, 69] These include the force-frequency relation,[70] i.e, the increase in contractility resulting from an increase in the frequency of contraction[71, 72]; postextrasystolic potentiation (a special instance of the force-frequency relation)[73–76]; and pharmacological agents such as the cardiac glycosides (p. 489), sympathomimetic amines[77, 78] (p. 524), and xanthines[77]—all of which improve contractility—and agents such as beta-adrenoceptor blockers, Ca^{++} antagonists, quinidine and other Type I antiarrhythmic agents, and barbiturates—all of which depress it. Experiments on skinned muscle cells suggest that even moderate acidosis causes a reduction in the quantity of Ca^{++} released from the SR of cardiac muscle, accounting in part for the negative inotropic effect of acidosis.[79]

MECHANISM OF ACTION OF BETA-ADRENOCEPTOR AGONISTS. A proposed mechanism of action of *sympathomimetic amines* is shown in Figure 13–9, and involves cyclic AMP.[80] These drugs are thought to act on beta receptors on the cardiac sarcolemma; this process leads to the activation of a membrane-bound enzyme, adenylate cyclase, that catalyzes the production of cyclic AMP from ATP in the presence of Ca^{++}. Adenylate cyclase is modulated by both inhibitory and stimulatory subunits which are heterodimer proteins in the cell membrane modulated by guanine nucleotides (e.g., guanosine triphosphate).[81, 82] The stimulating subunit is inactive as a heterodimer, but in the presence of a guanine nucleotide, the stimulating subunit dissociates from its "repressor" subunit to activate

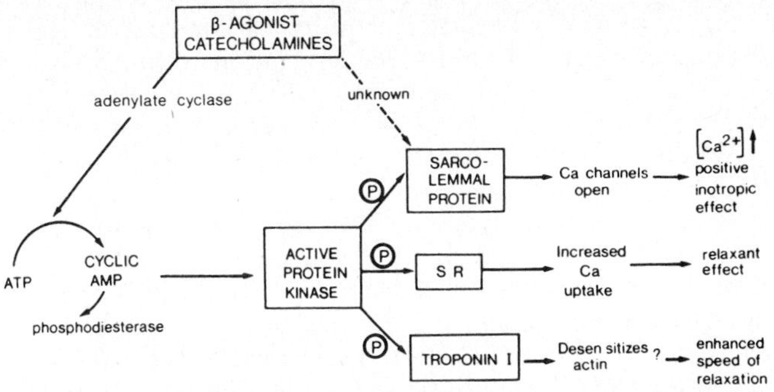

FIGURE 13–9. The major intracellular effects of beta-agonist catecholamines is by formation of cyclic AMP, which in turn increases the activity of protein kinases which phosphorylate (P) various proteins. SR = sarcoplasmic reticulum. It is proposed that phosphorylation of sarcolemmal proteins increases the number of open Ca^{++} channels, and that phosphorylation of a protein (phospholamban) in the SR increases the rate of Ca^{++} uptake by the SR and thereby enhances the rate of relaxation. Phosphorylation of troponin I may desensitize actin and also enhance the speed of relaxation. (From Opie, L.: The Heart. New York, Grune and Stratton, 1984, p. 80.)

adenyl cyclase. Multiple receptors on the sarcolemma can interact with the regulatory proteins of adenyl cyclase. The beta-adrenoceptor with a molecular weight of 60,000 to 69,000 dissociates by a $beta_1$-agonist occupying the receptor in the presence of a guanine nucleotide (Fig. 13–10). This stimulatory subunit, when thus activated, interacts with adenylate cyclase to increase its activity.[83]

Cyclic AMP, in turn, activates a class of enzymes, the cyclic AMP–dependent protein kinases, which phosphorylate a number of intracellular proteins.[84–86] This results in an increase in the transsarcolemmal influx of calcium through so-called depolarization-dependent "slow-calcium channels."[64, 87] At the same time, activity of the SR is enhanced, as characterized by accelerated release and more rapid uptake of Ca^{++}.[88] Activation of a protein kinase by an increase in cyclic AMP resulting from beta-adrenergic stimulation of the heart may induce phosphorylation of a protein located near the Ca^{++} channel and thus enhance its open state. Such Ca^{++} channels, which are recruited by beta-adrenergic agonists, are termed "receptor-operated channels." Another protein, phospholamban, when phosphorylated by cyclic AMP–dependent protein kinase, stimulates the rate of Ca^{++} uptake by increasing the ATP-dependent calcium pump in the SR.[84] There is also some evidence that beta-adrenergic agonists decrease the sensitivity of the contractile system to Ca^{++} as a consequence of phosphorylation of troponin-I by a cyclic AMP–activated protein kinase.[10, 78, 89] The reactions summarized in Figure 13–9, resulting from myocardial beta-receptor stimulation, increase the rate of Ca^{++} transport by the SR, which in turn is responsible for both enhancement of tension development and an increased rate of relaxation.

In *summary*, beta-adrenergic agonists augment Ca^{++} influx across the sarcolemma by recruiting additional (receptor-activated) slow channels. These substances do not appear to affect the *rate* at which the Ca^{++} channels open but rather they increase the *number* of open channels.[58] The increase in the rate of relaxation of tension produced by cyclic AMP appears to be caused by enhancement of Ca^{++} accumulation by the SR.[90] Theophylline and related compounds inhibit phosphodiesterase, an enzyme responsible for the breakdown of cyclic AMP, which has an effect similar to that of catecholamines. In addition, xanthines may increase the sensitivity of the contractile system to a given amount of Ca^{++}.[45]

Another cyclic nucleotide, cyclic 3′,5′-guanosine monophosphate (GMP) (Fig. 13–3), has been identified in the myocardium.[91] The reduction of the contractile state induced by acetylcholine is accompanied by significant *increases* in cyclic GMP, which appears to mediate effects opposing those of cyclic AMP.[92]

CONTROL OF CYTOPLASMIC [Ca^{++}]. As already indicated, cytoplasmic [Ca^{++}] is critical to the contractile state of the heart. Therefore, it is useful to recapitulate the determinants of myoplasmic [Ca^{++}].[59] At least seven mechanisms have been identified, and these are shown diagrammatically in Figure 13–11.

1. The inward movement of Ca^{++} along its concentration gradient, across the sarcolema, i.e., the slow inward current through the Ca^{++} channels (Fig. 13–11, Mechanism 1A and 1B).[64, 93] Ca^{++} antagonists act at these sites.[64]

2. Since small quantities of Ca^{++} enter the cardiac cell with each contraction, there must be some mechanism for removal of Ca^{++} from the cell so that [Ca^{++}] remains constant in a steady state. A bidirectional Na^+-Ca^{++} exchange system mediates Ca^{++} movement across the sarcolemma.[57] Energy required by this system for moving Ca^{++} out of the cell against a concentration gradient may be provided by the downhill movement of Na^{++} into the cell along its electrochemical gradient. The direction of this exchange depends upon the relative concentrations of extracellular and intracellular Na^+ and Ca^{++}. Thus, when cardiac glycosides inhibit Na^+, K^+-ATPase and thereby inhibit the pump responsible

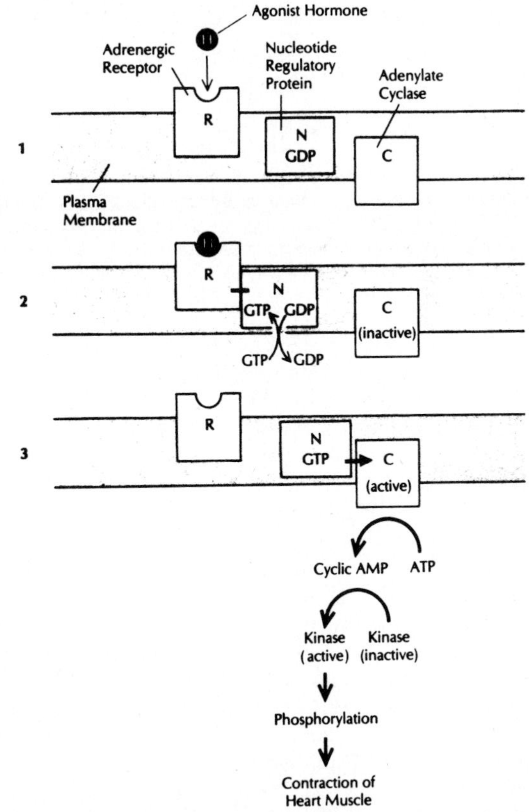

FIGURE 13–10. The receptor-effector model for beta-adrenoceptor activity postulates (1) the binding of the agonist (or hormone, H) to the beta-adrenoceptor, inducing formation of a ternary complex of hormone (H), receptor (R), and nucleotide regulatory protein (N). (2) Guanosine diphosphate (GDP), bound to N, can then be replaced by stimulatory guanosine triphosphate (GTP). (3) N-GTP activates the catalytic unit of the enzyme adenylate cyclase, leading to increased concentration of intracellular cyclic AMP, which, as seen in Figure 13–9, increases the activity of protein kinase, which in turn influences contraction of heart muscle. (From Heinsimer, J. A., and Lefkowitz, R. J.: The beta-adrenergic receptor in heart failure. Hosp. Pract. *18*:115, November, 1983.)

CONTROL OF [Ca^{++}] IN MYOCARDIUM

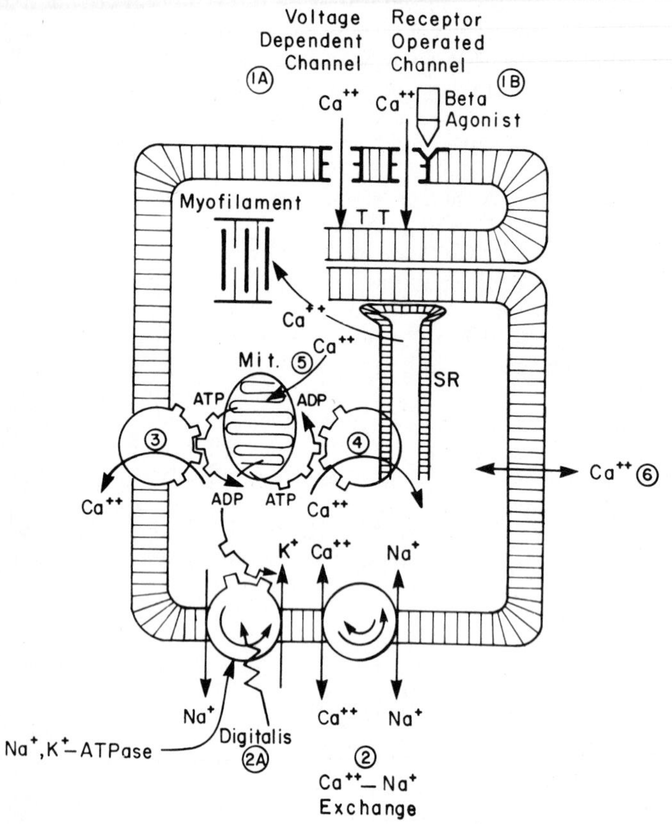

FIGURE 13–11. Determinants of [Ca^{++}] in myocardium. Numbers in circles denote the mechanisms affecting intracellular [Ca^{++}] described in the text. TT = transverse tubule; SR = sarcolemmic reticulum; Mit = mitochondrion. (Reprinted by permission, Braunwald, E.: Mechanisms of action of calcium channel blocking agents. N. Engl. J. Med. *307*:1618, 1982.)

for Na^+-K^+ exchange (Fig. 13–11, Mechanism 2A), intracellular [Na^+] is elevated. Ca^{++} enters the cell as a consequence of Na^+-Ca^{++} exchange, and this brings about a positive inotropic effect.[61, 94, 95]

3. The sarcolemma possesses a Ca^{++}-ATPase that extrudes Ca^{++} from the cell in an energy-requiring process (Fig. 13–11, Mechanism 3).[17, 96]

4. A Ca^{++}-stimulated Mg-ATPase in the membrane of the SR (Fig. 13–11, Mechanism 4) transports Ca^{++} into the lumen of the SR and sequesters it there through an energy-requiring process.[84]

5. Ca^{++} can also be taken up and released by other intracellular structures, particularly the mitochondria (Fig. 13–11, Mechanism 5), an internal aspect of the sarcolemma. When intracellular [Ca^{++}] rises, ATP, generated by the mitochondria, is involved in the uptake of Ca^{++} by these organelles; excess uptake of mitochondrial Ca^{++} in turn interferes with mitochondrial function.[97] This mechanism is relatively slow and its relation to activating Ca^{++} is unclear.

6. A variety of ionophores can effect the selective movement of Ca^{++} along its concentration gradient directly across the sarcolemma, i.e., not through the slow channels (Fig. 13–11, Mechanism 6).

7. The buffering of Ca^{++} by intracellular proteins such as calmodulin, troponin C, and myosin-P light chains also regulates myoplasmic [Ca^{++}].

Since cardiac contraction and relaxation are critically dependent on precisely timed modulations of myoplasmic [Ca^{++}], it is evident that abnormalities of *any* of the systems just described can affect myocardial performance.[57]

While an increase in the myoplasmic [Ca^{++}] is necessary to activate contraction in myocardial cells and the force of contraction is modulated by the myoplasmic [Ca^{++}], increases in myoplasmic [Ca^{++}] above a certain level can lead to deterioration of muscle function. This excessive increase in myoplasmic Ca^{++} has been called "calcium overload." For example, in skinned cardiac cells the level of tension development decreases under certain conditions when the myoplasmic [Ca^{++}] is raised above pCa 5.5 and that increasing free [Ca^{++}] above the optimal level can inactivate Ca^{++}-induced release of Ca^{++}. Digitalis intoxication can be associated with a decrease in force to values below the control level.[98] In this study aequorin was used to measure myoplasmic [Ca^{++}]; a high (18 mM) extracellular [Ca^{++}] could induce a state in which a persistently increased aequorin signal was associated with a decrease in an initially enhanced force of contraction.[98] Another important pathophysiological consequence of raising myoplasmic [Ca^{++}] beyond a certain level is the development of spontaneous mechanical and electrical oscillations, which could lead to arrhythmias through the development of delayed afterdepolarizations and triggered activity. The question of whether Ca^{++} overload can lead to temporary or permanent cardiac cell dysfunction and damage has yet to be answered.

CALCIUM CHANNELS

Although relatively little is known of the actual structure of ion channels in the sarcolemma, since these channels are highly specific for a given ion species, it can be assumed that the aqueous "pore" within the channel is provided with a selectivity filter that defines the type of ion that can pass through a given type of channel (Fig. 13–12). Because ion channels can be open or shut depending on the intracellular voltage, the channel also has voltage sensors, i.e., charged regions of the channel proteins that determine the state of channel "gates" as open or shut.[99, 100]

VOLTAGE-DEPENDENT CHANNELS. When a propagated wave of depolarization approaches the membrane region containing the Ca^{++} channel, a reduction of membrane potential (i.e., a decrease in the electronegativity of the cell interior) causes the activation gate to open, permitting Ca^{++} to cross the membrane and pass into the cell (Fig. 13–12). The gate closes when the interior of the cell has again become electronegative, i.e., when the resting level of transmembrane potential has been restored. Since the movement of Ca^{++} through these channels is controlled by electrical potentials, they have been termed voltage-dependent channels (Fig. 13–11, Mechanism 1A).

RECEPTOR-OPERATED CHANNELS. An important feature of many Ca^{++} channels is their sensitivity to control by sarcolemmal receptors. $Beta_1$-agonists in cardiac muscle (and alpha-adrenoceptor agonists in vascular smooth muscle) increase Ca^{++} influx via the slow inward current, thereby enhancing contractility, frequency, and conduction velocity in the heart in the case of $beta_1$ receptors, and the degree of contraction of arterioles in the case of alpha receptors on vascular smooth muscle. Activation of adrenoceptors does not appear to increase Ca^{++} influx by increasing the size of the Ca^{++} channels or the rates at which their gates open or close but rather appears to recruit an additional number of active channels[101, 102] (Fig. 13–13). The transfer of charge phosphate groups from ATP to the

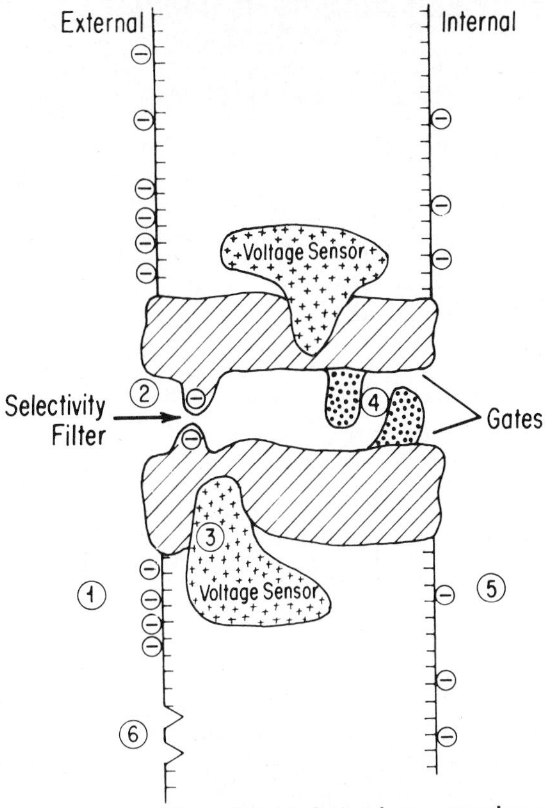

FIGURE 13–12. A calcium channel depicted as a membrane pore containing within it a negatively charged site (2) of dimensions and charge density appropriate to act as a "selectivity filter" to distinguish between different cations. Voltage sensor components (3) confer voltage-dependence on channel opening and closing and channel gates (4) determine the open or shut character of the channel. Negatively charged sites on the external (1) and internal (5) membrane surfaces serve as cation binding sites, particularly for divalent cations, by which transmembrane potential detected by voltage sensor components may be modulated. A receptor site (6) is shown adjacent to the channel. (From Triggle, D. J.: *In* Flaim, S. F., and Zelis, R. [eds.]: Calcium Channel Blockers: Mechanism of Action and Clinical Applications. Baltimore, Urban and Schwarzenberg, 1982.)

calcium channel produces a change in molecular configuration which increases the likelihood that the channels will open during depolarization. It has been proposed that when endogenous adrenergic nervous activity is low or is blocked by an adrenoceptor blocker, a certain proportion of the Ca^{++} channels is unable to open in response to a depolarizing stimulus. According to this theory, physiological stimuli or drugs that activate adrenoceptors elevate cyclic AMP levels in the myocardium, which in turn facilitates transfer of a phosphate in ATP to form a phosphoester bond with one of the proteins in an inactive Ca^{++} channel, permitting the channel to participate in Ca^{++} entry into the cell. As a consequence, adrenergic influences increase Ca^{++} influx across the sarcolemma; the channels acted upon by receptor-mediated events are termed receptor-operated channels (Fig. 13–11, Mechanism 1B).

CALCIUM ANTAGONISTS

A number of inorganic cations such as manganese, cobalt, and lanthanum can function as general Ca^{++} antagonists and are effective in blocking a wide variety of Ca^{++}-dependent processes.[100] This nonselectivity of action probably arises from the ability of these cations to substitute for Ca^{++} at a variety of Ca^{++}-binding sites.[96] They probably block the function of all Ca^{++}-channels or actually enter the cell, where they substitute for Ca^{++} at the intracellular Ca^{++} receptors. Of far more significance to clinical medicine are the organic Ca^{++} agonists. The pioneering work of Fleckenstein[103] revealed that these compounds can produce selective blockade of the slow inward current and produce electromechanical uncoupling in heart muscle.

Since organic Ca^{++} antagonists exert their actions at nanomolar concentrations and exhibit stereospecificity, it appears likely that they are recognized by specific structures of the Ca^{++} channel.[58, 104–106] However, the diversity of molecular structures of Ca^{++} antagonists is consistent with differing modes and sites of action[9, 100] rather than with the tight binding of these drugs to a specific receptor, analogous to the receptor that binds beta-adrenoceptor blockers.[105]

The action of nifedipine is consistent with the drug actually "plugging" Ca^{++} and decreasing the number of functional Ca^{++} channels that open.[99] In contrast, verapamil, and to a lesser extent diltiazem, are "use-dependent," i.e., their Ca^{++}-blocking activities are a function of the frequency of contraction so that they cause an inversion of the myocardium's normal force-frequency relationship, an

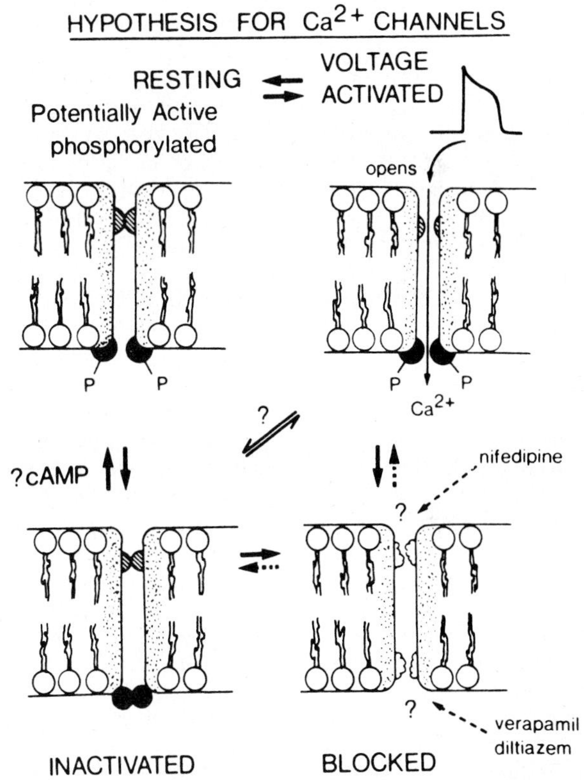

FIGURE 13–13. Postulated arrangement of calcium channel, modified from Sperelakis[1] and Bean et al.[2] Note the proposed role for phosphorylation (P) of Ca channel in changing inoperative channels to operative channels. Operative channels can change from the resting (*top left*) to the activated state (*top right*) in which the depolarization of the cell membrane has opened the outer (activation) gate and Ca^{++} enters the cell and then reverts spontaneously to the inactivated state (*bottom left*) when the inner (inactivation) gate is closed. During recovery, i.e., repolarization, the activation gate closes and the inactivation gate opens, returning the channel to the resting state and once again available for activation (*top left*). It is postulated that beta-adrenergic stimulation acts by its second messenger cyclic AMP (cAMP) to transfer charged phosphate groups (P) from ATP to the Ca channel so that there is a molecular change which allows a greater probability of the channels being open during depolarization. Ca^{++} antagonists interfere with the passage of Ca^{++} through the channel by causing a change in molecular configuration of the channel and/or gates (*bottom right*). (From Opie L: The Heart. New York, Grune and Stratton, 1984, p. 45.)

[1]Sperelakis, N.: *In* Opie, L. H. (ed.): Antagonists and Cardiovascular Disease. New York, Raven Press, 1984, pp. 277–291.

[2]Bean, B. P., et al.: Beta-adrenergic modulation of calcium channels in frog ventricular heart cells. Nature *307*:371, 1984.

increase in contraction frequency causing a reduction rather than an augmentation of contraction.[105] This situation is analogous to the better investigated, frequency-dependent inhibition of Na^+ (channels by local anesthetics and Type I antiarrhythmic drugs and suggests that verapamil interacts preferentially with the depolarized, inactivated state of the Ca^{++} channel.

The clinical use of calcium antagonists is discussed on pp. 636, 877, and 1332.

CARDIAC ADRENOCEPTORS

In 1967 Lands et al. demonstrated that beta-adrenoceptors could be classified into two types: $beta_1$ receptors, which mediate cardiac stimulation and lipolysis, and $beta_2$ receptors, which mediate relaxation of vascular and bronchial smooth muscle.[107] The effects of catecholamines on the contractile and electrical properties of the heart are mediated predominantly by the beta-adrenoceptors, embedded in the sarcolemma (Fig. 13–3 and Fig. 17–22, p. 527). As determined by physiological and radioligand-binding studies, the large majority of myocardial beta receptors are of the $beta_1$ subtype; likewise, the inotropic effects of beta-adrenoceptor agonists are mediated predominantly, if not exclusively, by $beta_1$ receptors.[83, 108, 109] However, it has been suggested that chronotropy, i.e., sinoatrial rate, may be mediated by $beta_2$ receptors located in the sinoatrial node.[110] $Beta_1$-adrenoceptors are located on effector cells in proximity to adrenergic synapses, while $beta_2$ receptors are located at some distance from the synapses.[111] $Beta_1$ receptors appear to respond primarily to neuronally released norepinephrine, whereas $beta_2$ receptors respond preferentially to circulating epinephrine from the adrenal medulla (and to exogenously injected beta agonists). Also, as in the case of alpha-adrenoceptors, beta-adrenoceptors located presynaptically on the nerve fiber regulate norepinephrine release. However, as opposed to presynaptic alpha receptors, which have an inhibitory role, stimulation of presynaptic beta receptors stimulates release of norepinephrine.[112] Whereas ventricular receptors are exclusively $beta_1$,[113] approximately 25 per cent of atrial receptors are of the $beta_2$ subtype. Atrial $beta_2$ receptors, presumably located within the sinoatrial node, contribute to mediating the chronotropic effects of catecholamines on the heart.

Catecholamines appear to exert at least some of their effects through myocardial alpha-adrenoceptors.[114] As with myocardial beta-adrenoceptors, stimulation of myocardial alpha receptors augments myocardial contractility.[115, 116] The subtype of myocardial alpha-adrenoceptors is somewhat controversial, although most evidence favors the presence of only $alpha_1$ receptors. A number of observations suggest that the molecular mechanism by which alpha-adrenoceptors exert a positive inotropic effect is different from that of beta receptors. Whereas stimulation of beta-adrenoceptors increases intracellular cyclic AMP, which is thought to mediate subsequent events, stimulation of alpha-adrenoceptors appears to have no effect on cyclic AMP production in myocardium. Also, alpha receptor–mediated effects on inotropy are more sensitive to the extracellular concentration of Ca^{++} or blockade of Ca^{++} influx by Ca antagonists than are beta-mediated effects. Based on these observations, it has been suggested that alpha-adrenoceptors mediate an increase in inotropy almost exclusively by means of an increase in Ca^{++} influx.[117]

MECHANICS OF CARDIAC CONTRACTION

ISOMETRIC CONTRACTION

Cardiac contraction can be readily studied in vitro by mounting a mammalian papillary muscle, trabeculae carneae, or strip of atrial myocardium in an oxygenated, physiological salt solution.[118–121] When the ends of the muscle are fixed and the muscle is activated by electrical stimulation, the strength of individual isometric cardiac contractions is modified by two major influences: (1) a *change in initial muscle length*, or preload, induced by a change in the passive stretch of the muscle; and (2) a *change in contractility or inotropic state at any given length.*[119]

The relationship between the actively developed tension (the total tension minus resting tension) during the isometric contraction and the initial muscle length at which contraction occurred constitutes the *length–active tension curve* (Fig. 13–14). When contractility is altered by an *inotropic intervention*, such as the addition of Ca^{++}, digitalis, or norepinephrine to the medium, the rate of force development rises, the peak force developed increases, and the time to reach peak force shortens; these changes in contractile activity occur at a constant preload. Inotropic interventions do not generally alter the relationship between the preload (the tension placed on the resting muscle) and the length of the muscle, i.e., the *length–resting tension relation*, an expression of the resting

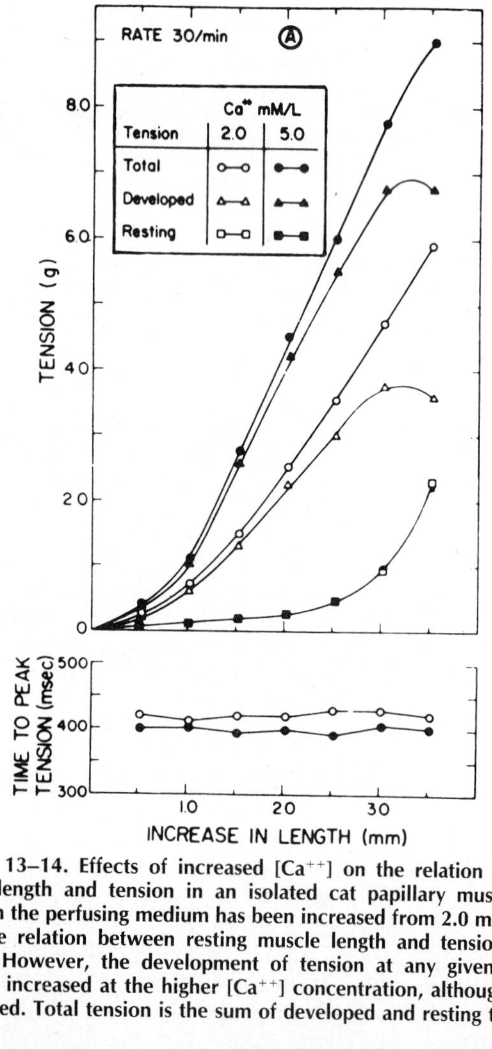

FIGURE 13–14. Effects of increased $[Ca^{++}]$ on the relation between muscle length and tension in an isolated cat papillary muscle. The $[Ca^{++}]$ in the perfusing medium has been increased from 2.0 mM to 5.0 mM. The relation between resting muscle length and tension is not altered. However, the development of tension at any given muscle length is increased at the higher $[Ca^{++}]$ concentration, although L_{max} is not altered. Total tension is the sum of developed and resting tension.

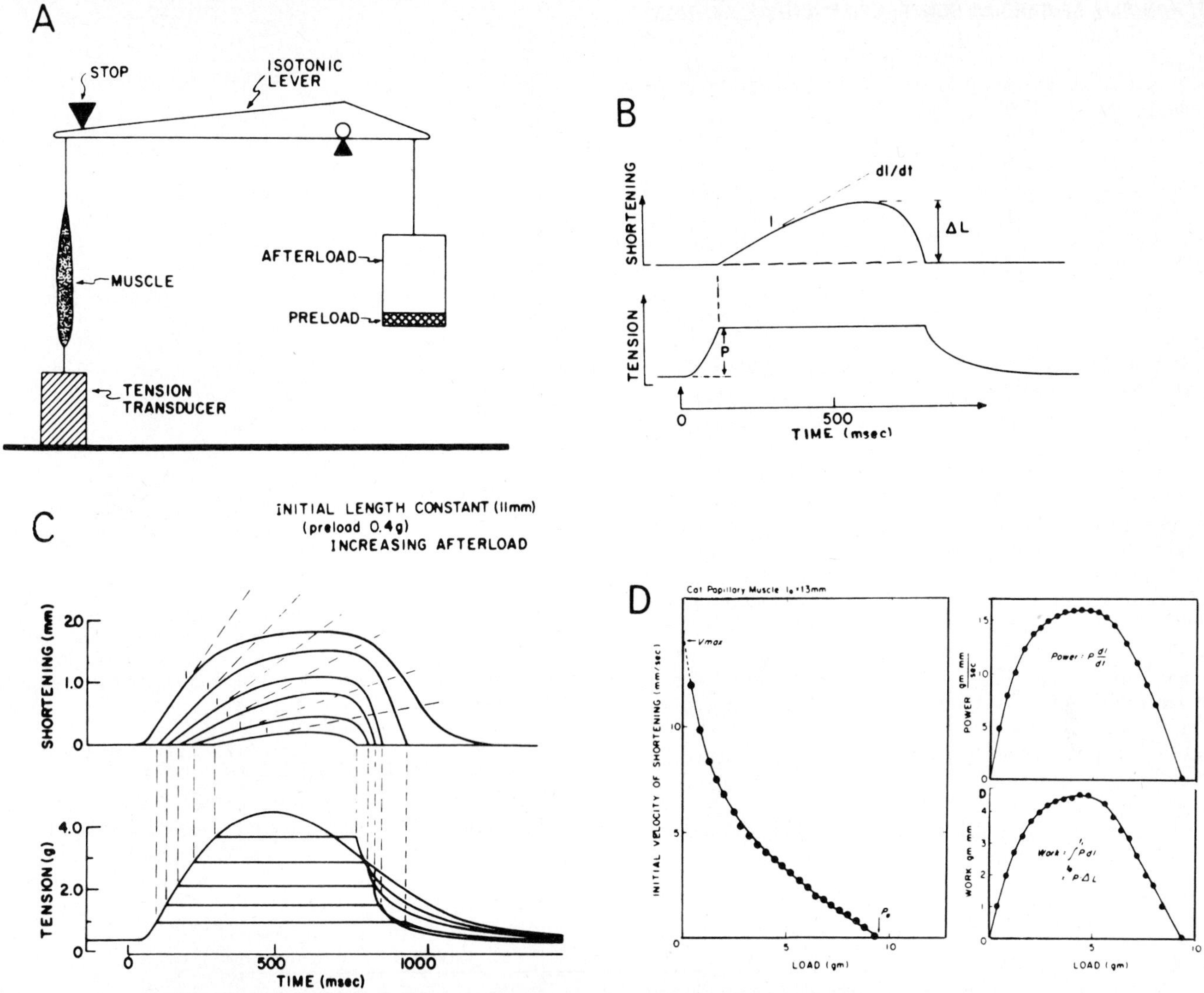

FIGURE 13–15. Use of afterloaded isotonic contractions to obtain force-velocity relations.

A, Diagrammatic representation of an isotonic lever system. A papillary muscle is placed in a bath (not shown) of Krebs-Ringer solution and stimulated by electrodes along its lateral aspect. The lower end of the muscle is attached to an extension from a tension transducer while the upper, free end is attached to the end of a lever system that is free to move. The fulcrum of the lever system is shown toward the right. Initially the stop is not above the tip of the lever, which is above the muscle. A small weight, termed a "preload," is placed on the opposite end of the lever; this preload will stretch the muscle to a length consistent with its resting length-tension relation. The stop is then fixed above the tip of the lever, so that any added weight above the preload will not be sensed by the muscle until it attempts to contract. Additional loads can be added to the preload (i.e., afterloads). Total load equals the sum of the preload and the afterload.

B, Tracings of an afterloaded isotonic contraction. The contraction is shown as a function of time, plotted along the abscissa. After stimulation at time zero, there is a short latent period followed by the generation of isometric force. When the force (P) equals the load, shortening begins, as shown in the upper half of the panel. Maximum velocity is reached shortly after shortening commences, and the tangent to this slope (dl/dt) approximates the maximum velocity of shortening with this particular load. ΔL denotes the extent of shortening. Subsequently the muscle elongates and then relaxes isometrically.

C, Effects of increasing afterloads on the course of tension development and subsequent shortening. Several superimposed contractions are displayed. The muscle develops a force equal to the afterload and thereafter shortens. As the afterload is increased, the velocity of shortening (dashed lines) and the extent of shortening decline.

D, Velocity of shortening plotted as a function of load: the force-velocity relation. As the load is increased, the velocity of shortening decreases. When the load is so high that no external shortening is recorded, velocity is zero, and the force is equivalent to the isometric contraction (P_0). When the curve is extrapolated back to zero load, V_{max} is obtained. Also shown at right are power (*top*) and work (*bottom*) curves as a function of increasing afterloads. Both power and work are zero when the load is zero or with isometric contractions, and both curves peak at an intermediate load. (From Braunwald, E., et al.: Mechanisms of Contraction of the Normal and Failing Heart. 2nd ed. Boston, Little, Brown, 1976.)

stiffness of the cardiac muscle.[120] When frequency of stimulation is altered, contractility is also changed, the pattern of which depends on conditions and species. In the cat, dog, and human, increased rate, within limits, increases the rate of force development and developed force, and shortens the time to peak tension with accelerated relaxation. This response is termed the *force-frequency relation*; this positive inotropic action of frequency presumably results from the increased intramyocardial [Ca^{++}] resulting from the increased number of depolarizations.

As the nonstimulated muscle is stretched, the resting tension rises progressively and a point is reached at which resting tension rises very rapidly while actively developed tension is maximal; this length is termed L_{max}.

By definition, the length-active tension relation at lengths below L_{max} is termed the *ascending limb* of the curve and the portion above L_{max}, the *descending limb* of the curve. When initial muscle length is altered slightly on either side of L_{max}, active tension is altered substantially; a 10 per cent reduction in muscle length below L_{max} may be responsible for a 30 per cent decrease in actively developed tension.[122] Lengths beyond L_{max} are poorly tolerated and associated with very high resting tensions.

ISOTONIC CONTRACTION: THE FORCE-LENGTH AND THE FORCE-VELOCITY RELATION. In order to analyze not only isometric contractions but also the physiologically pertinent shortening characteristics of the muscle, one end of the muscle is attached to a lever system and its degree of shortening is measured (Fig. 13–15*A*). The preload, a small weight placed on the opposite end of the lever, stretches the passive muscle; a stop is then adjusted above the tip of the lever and any weight added to the lever over and above the preload, termed the *afterload*, may be sensed by the muscle *after* the onset of contraction (Fig. 13–15*B*). The extent and maximum velocity of shortening for each contraction depend on the load (Fig. 13–15*C*), and the inverse relation between the tension (force) developed and the velocity of contraction constitutes the *force-velocity curve* (Fig. 13–15*D*). When the load is greatest, there is no shortening, i.e., the muscle develops maximal force during isometric contraction (P_0). Conversely, when the load is smallest, the velocity of shortening is greatest. Although the velocity of shortening with zero load cannot be measured directly, since the preload provides for initial length, extrapolation of the curve back to zero load allows approximation of this maximum velocity of unloaded shortening, termed V_{max}.[118–120, 123–125]

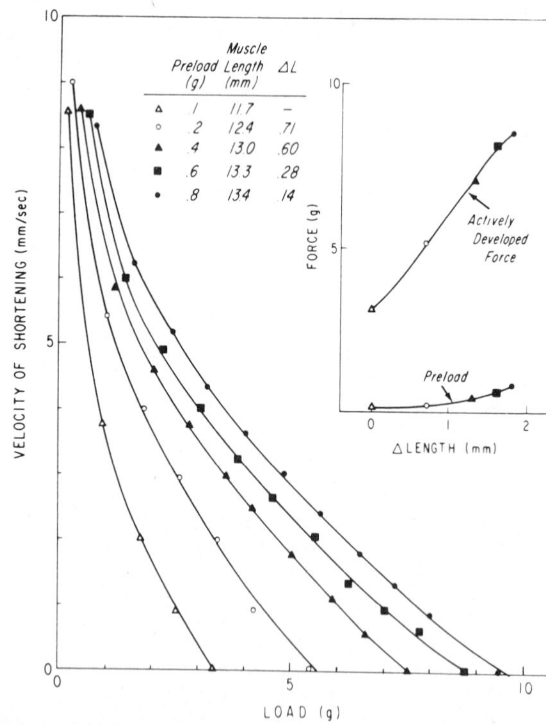

FIGURE 13–16. Relation between peak velocity of afterloaded, isotonic shortening and total load at several initial muscle lengths in a cat papillary muscle. The inset at the right shows the resting and developed active force at these various lengths. When initial muscle length is increased, the actively developed force is augmented, as is the velocity of shortening at any individual load. The maximum velocity of shortening with the preload alone is little altered. Moreover, if these curves were to be extrapolated back to zero load (V_{max}), this value would also show little or no change.

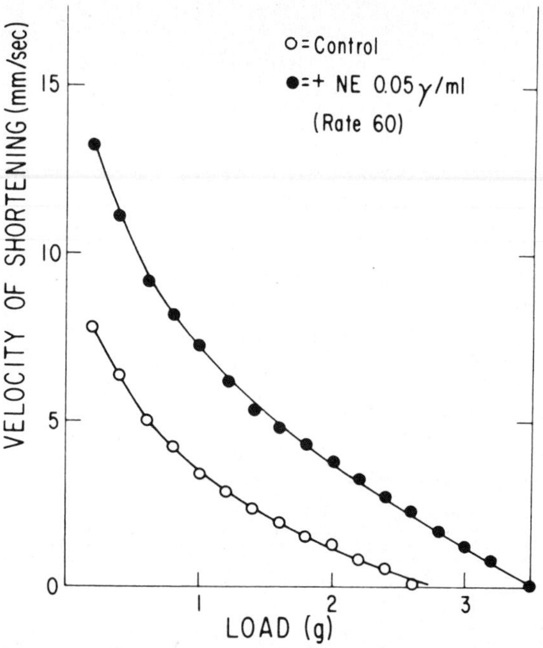

FIGURE 13–17. Effects of the addition of norepinephrine on the force-velocity relation of the cat papillary muscle. Norepinephrine induces an increase in the velocity of shortening at any load, in the maximum force and isometric contraction (P_0), and in the maximum velocity of zero load shortening (V_{max}).

When the *initial muscle length* is altered by increasing the preload, the force-velocity curve is shifted characteristically (Fig. 13–16); the velocity of shortening at any given load is increased as is P_0. However, V_{max} is little altered by a change in initial muscle length. In contrast, when the *contractility* is augmented (Fig. 13–17), the rate of tension development is increased, as are the velocity and extent of shortening with a given load.[126] The entire force-velocity curve is shifted upward and to the right with increases in *both* P_0 and V_{max}.

The length-active tension curve can also be constructed from isotonic contraction with increasing afterloads. The preload represents one point on the resting length-tension curve. With a given afterload, the muscle will develop an isometric force equal to the afterload and then shorten isotonically to a length that corresponds to the length–active tension curve for that given state of contractility. As the afterload is increased, shortening decreases until only isometric force is generated (see Fig. 13–27, left, point E). The same length–active tension curve is generated whether developed isotonically or isometrically, except under some conditions in which the muscle is very depressed and the isotonic points may fall to the right of the isometric ones.[124, 125]

When contractility is increased the length–active tension curve is moved to the left and once again a unique curve is created whether reached isometrically or isotonically.[123, 125]

MUSCLE MODELS

Models of muscle contraction provide a method for analyzing contraction of heart muscle[127] as well as some insight into the complexities of ventricular function. Current working models include a *contractile element* (CE), which represents the actively contracting portion of the muscle, arranged in series with a passive elastic component, the *series elastic element* (SE). At rest, CE is considered to be freely extensible, so that resting tension is sustained by another elastic component arranged in parallel, the *parallel elastic component* (PE). Depending on the model chosen, PE spans both CE and SE (Maxwell model) or CE alone (Voight model).

The resting stiffness of cardiac muscle is greater than that of skeletal muscle, but the reasons for this difference are not clear.[122, 128] Myocardial cells are smaller than skeletal muscle cells and therefore possess a relatively greater proportion of stiff sarcolemma per unit weight of tissue; intercellular collagen is also more abundant in heart muscle. The sarcomeres of cardiac muscle resist stretching beyond 2.2 μ, which may also be a factor in the stiffness of PE of heart muscle.[129] Minute intermediate filaments in the sarcomere of heart muscle may also contribute to its resting stiffness.[130]

The characteristics of muscular contraction are determined by the time course of activation of CE, its force-generating and shortening properties, and the stiffness of SE. The SE is a "lumped" elasticity, most of it being in elastic connections of the muscle to its points of fixation. In an isolated muscle, this would comprise the damaged ends of the muscle, while in the intact heart it would be any extraneous extensile tissue including the atrioventricular valves.

In the simplest model of an *isometric* contraction, with activation of the muscle, the CE shortens, stretching the springlike SE, and the force builds up at the ends of the system in a manner dependent upon the interaction of the shortening properties of the CE and compliance of the SE. On the other hand, in an *afterloaded isotonic* contraction, force is developed as shortening of the CE stretches the SE, until the force equals the load, and the load is then lifted. Muscle shortening occurs with the SE at a fixed length, and the subsequent course of shortening reflects shortening of the CE alone. Viscous elements are identified in the PE of resting heart muscle by the presence of stress relaxation, i.e., a fall in resting tension following a sustained stretch to a long length.

The mechanical activity of the CE reflects the summated contribution of cross bridges between myosin and actin and some form of conformational changes in the heads of the cross bridges, which then generate displacement of the actin filaments[33] (see Fig. 13–6). *Active state*, a term adapted from skeletal muscle physiology, has been used to describe the capacity of the CE to shorten in accordance with the force-velocity relation.[124, 131, 132] It is a mechanical measure of the chemical processes in the CE that generate both force and shortening.

Resting Length-Tension Relations

When relaxed heart muscle is stretched progressively, its resting tension increases slightly at first and then rises more markedly (Fig. 13–14). The stiffness of the resting muscle is represented by the slope of the curve relating the change in resting tension (ΔP) to the change in length (ΔL), which is approximately exponential. The resting length-tension relation is not generally altered by interventions that acutely alter the length–active tension curve or the force-velocity-length relation except that ischemia increases the apparent stiffness of the resting muscle, presumably by interfering with relaxation. Marked tachycardia also tends to increase the resting length-tension relation, because relaxation is not complete at the termination of diastole.[133] Aging also causes a significant increase in stiffness; less stress relaxation is exhibited by muscles from old compared to young adult rats, which may account, at least in part, for the age-associated changes in the resting length-tension curve.[134]

Force-Velocity-Length Relations

The interdependence between force, velocity, and muscle length is demonstrated as a *force-velocity-length diagram*.[124] The projection on the left of each of the panels of Figure 13–18 forms the *force-velocity* relation, the projection to the rear forms the *length-velocity* relation, and the base of this diagram represents the *length-tension* relation. During contraction, the muscle moves in a predictable manner across the surface, describing this relation between force, length, and velocity. With activation, the contractile elements rise onto a hypothetical force-velocity curve, with force increasing and the velocity of the contractile element decreasing until the afterload is reached, after which shortening

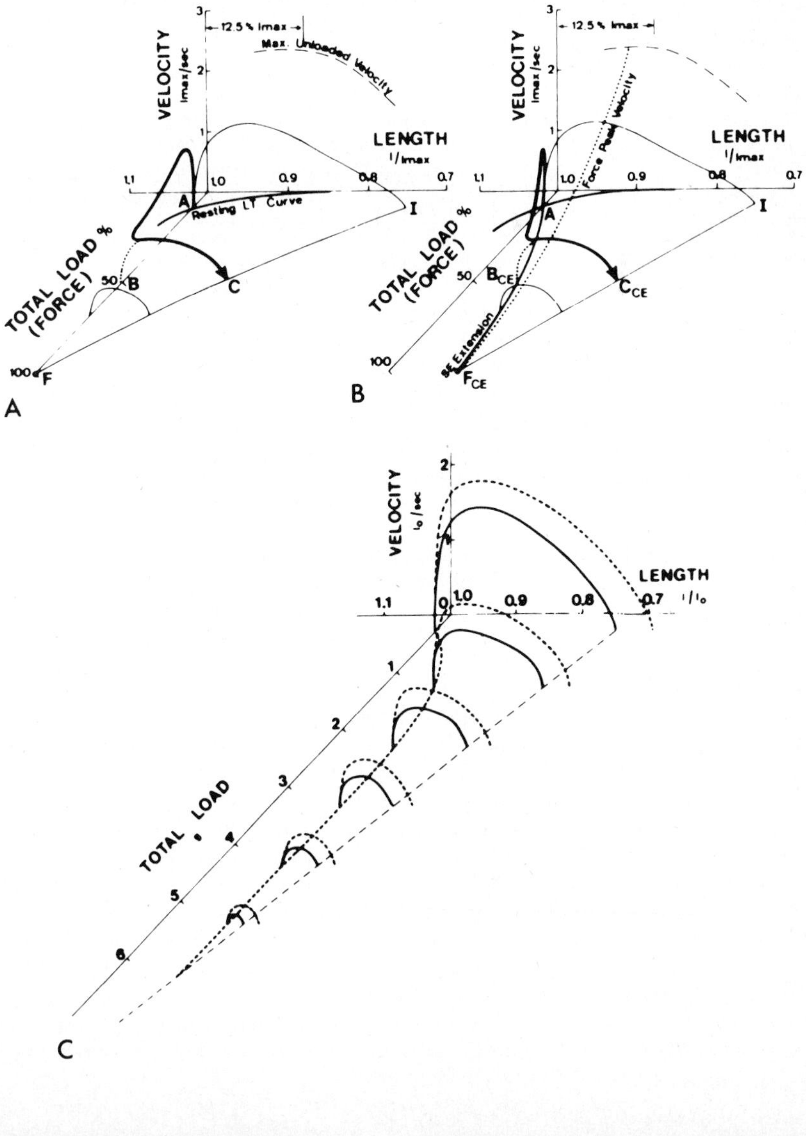

FIGURE 13–18. Three-dimensional representation of the force-velocity-length relations in the cat papillary muscle.

A, The velocity-length relations of isotonic contractions obtained at L_{max} have been replotted as a function of total load. The course of velocity of a hypothetical afterloaded isotonic contraction is superimposed (thick line). The velocity of shortening during the isometric phase of the contractions has been theoretically derived from a two-component muscle model. Velocity rises rapidly to the level appropriate for the plane of this three-dimensional composite. During isometric contraction the velocity of the contractile element falls as force rises. This velocity is not seen but is expressed in terms of the rate of force development, i.e., dP/dt. At point B, the force development equals the load, and external shortening can then proceed between points B and C. Velocity of shortening between B and C depends on the level of the force-velocity-length plane. The velocity-length relation and the maximum unloaded velocity of shortening (V_{max}) is shown on the right. Projection to the right of the plane of the force-velocity-length relation provides the force-velocity relation, while the length-tension curve is reflected on the base.

B, The force-velocity-length relations of the same muscle as shown in *A* after correction for extension of the series elastic component. The entire curve is moved to the right. The dashed line shown on the plane created by the force-velocity-length relation represents the force-velocity curve as obtained from afterloaded contractions.

C, Effect of a positive inotropic intervention (dashed line) on the force-velocity-length relation. The velocity of shortening at any given muscle length is augmented, so that the entire surface relating force-velocity and length is increased, and the extent of shortening is augmented. The projection of this surface to the right would be characterized by an increase in V_{max}. (From Brutsaert, D. L., and Sonnenblick, E. H.: Cardiac muscle mechanics in the evaluation of myocardial contractility and pump function: Problems, concepts and directions. Progr. Cardiovasc. Dis. *16*:337, 1973, by permission of Grune and Stratton.)

proceeds across the surface, ending at the length–active tension curve. The force-velocity-length relation is relatively independent of time during a major portion of the shortening phase of contraction.[120, 135] However, late in the course of contraction, shortening diverges from the velocity-length phase planes, indicating that the active state is declining.

Myocardial contractility can be described by the surface of the plane describing the force-velocity-length relation (Fig. 13–18).[124] The full activity of cardiac muscle commences rapidly after stimulation. The surface of the plane describing the force-velocity-length relation is reached rapidly, and its position may be considered to be a definition of the contractile state, since the position of this surface is essentially independent of preload and afterload. The duration of the active state is generally sufficient to allow shortening to occur to the same end-systolic length, regardless of the initial length if afterload and contractility remain constant.[125] This property of cardiac muscle is crucial to the use of end-systolic cardiac dimensions or volume in the assessment of cardiac contractility.[136, 137]

While force-velocity curves (Figs. 13–16 and 13–17) appear to provide valid descriptors of the contractile state in a wide variety of circumstances, an important theoretical limitation of such curves must be appreciated; the measurements to obtain each point in the curve are not made at the same time during contraction, so that the intensity of the active state might differ for each point. Thus, when the afterload is increased, velocity is measured later in time after the stimulus for contraction, and these measurements may occur at differing lengths of CE, thus distorting the enscribed curve from the "true" force-velocity curve.[124] The extrapolated V_{max} therefore could have been misleading. However, when the effects of these variables have been considered carefully, with unloading of the muscle to near zero external load once contraction has begun, the conclusions previously reached from simple afterloaded contractions have been supported.[135] Since initial length and end-systolic length can often be measured, indices of the end-systolic length allow one to approach the three-dimensional force-velocity-length relation. The assumption is made that the force-velocity-length relation moves symmetrically when contractility is altered.

When initial muscle length is reduced by 10 per cent, actively developed tension falls about 30 per cent, but unloaded velocity does not change. In intact muscle, this dependency of force development on the length of heart muscle is related to the compliance of SE.[125] When cardiac muscle is activated and made to contract isometrically, the development of force is accompanied by an internal shortening, so that when maximal isometric force is reached, the CE (sarcomeres) is actually substantially shorter and SE is longer than prior to activation. Indeed, sarcomeres actually do shorten substantially during "apparent" isometric contraction.[138–141] In contrast, isotonic contractions against very small loads do not involve the development of force, stretching of SE, and shortening of CE at the expense of SE; hence, shortening of CE is translated directly into shortening of the muscle, and velocities are measured at longer sarcomere lengths.[138] In studies in which sarcomere dynamics have been measured directly,[139] it appears that only a minor proportion of the SE is associated with the contractile machinery and cross bridges in heart muscle and that the effective SE largely reflects external elastic connections.

LENGTH-DEPENDENT ACTIVATION AND THE LENGTH-TENSION RELATION

In the foregoing discussion of the mechanics of muscular contraction, it has been generally assumed that inotropic interventions and changes in muscle length are independent regulators of myocardial performance. However, it is now clear that both inotropic interventions and changes of muscle length may act primarily through mechanisms that involve Ca^{++} activation,[142–147] although the mechanism and resultant mechanical correlate may differ. The traditional view that length and inotropic state are independent regulators of myocardial performance was based on the observation that a decline of tension production occurs at short muscle lengths; this would be expected, because tension is lost as a consequence of the double overlap of the thin filaments in the central region of each sarcomere, resulting in interference with normal cross-bridge formation. However, tension production in cardiac muscle falls off much more steeply at muscle lengths below L_{max} than would be expected according to the sliding filament hypothesis.[122, 144]

The inotropic effect of changes in extracellular $[Ca^{++}]$ depends on muscle length[142]; the mechanical performance of cardiac muscle is more sensitive to changes in extracellular $[Ca^{++}]$ at longer than at shorter muscle lengths.[46, 144, 147] There is evidence in skeletal muscle too that the affinity of troponin for Ca^{++} is length-dependent, and the same situation may well exist in cardiac muscle. It has been suggested that the same quantity of Ca^{++} released may thus be more actively bound at longer than at shorter sarcomere lengths and that an increase in muscle length (1) does not change or actually decreases the transsarcolemmal influx of Ca^{++}, (2) increases the release of Ca^{++}

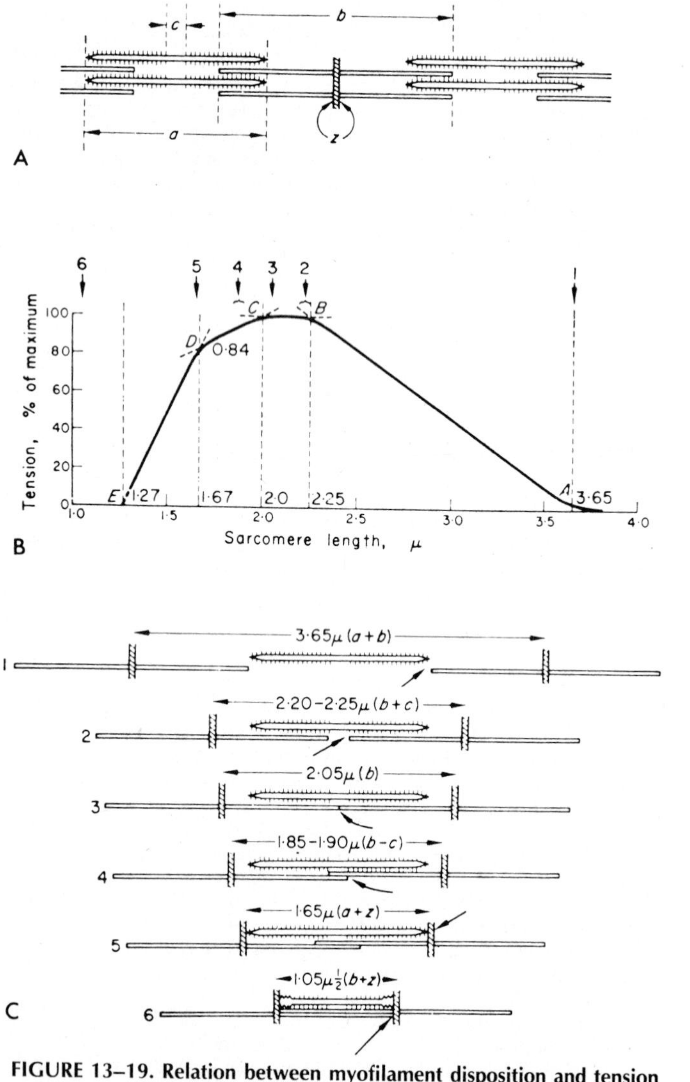

FIGURE 13–19. Relation between myofilament disposition and tension development in striated muscle. *A*, Diagram of myofilaments of the sarcomere drawn to scale. Thin filaments are 1.0 μ and thick filaments 1.6 μ in length. *B*, Relation between the tension development as percentage of maximum and the sarcomere length in single fibers of skeletal muscle. Numbers shown with arrows at top denote break points on the curve and correspond to the sarcomere lengths depicted diagrammatically in *C*. *C*, Myofilament overlap shown as a function of sarcomere length. At 3.65 μ (1) there is no overlap of myofilaments. The optimal overlap of myofilaments occurs at a sarcomere length of 2.05 to 2.25 μ (between 2 and 3). At a sarcomere length shorter than 2.0 μ (4), thin filaments pass into the opposite half of the sarcomere, and a double overlap occurs (5 and 6). Note that the central 0.2 μ of the thick filament is devoid of cross-bridges that could interact with sites on the thin filaments. (Adapted from Gordon, A. M., et al.: The variation in isometric tension with sarcomere length in vertebrate muscle fibers. J. Physiol. (Lond.) *184*:170, 1966.)

triggered by the transsarcolemmal Ca^{++} influx,[144] and/or (3) increases the sensitivity of the myofilaments to Ca^{++}.[147]

Thus, all changes in contractile behavior may result primarily from alterations in the degree of activation of the contractile system, and therefore contractility and muscle length (preload) should not be regarded as totally independent regulators of myocardial performance. While a change in contractility relates to changes in *quantity and rate* of Ca^{++} made available to troponin C, a change in muscle length appears to alter the *sensitivity* of the sarcomere to Ca^{++}.[147] However, the distinct differences in the effects of changes in preload and of contractility on V_{max} (Figs. 13–16 and 13–17), on the duration of the active state, and on the rate of tension development and decline all indicate that, regardless of the similarity in the fundamental molecular mechanism, consideration of preload and contractility as separate determinants of cardiac performance remains an extremely useful working model. Although a change in initial length may alter the binding of Ca^{++} to the regulatory protein troponin I and thus alter the number of contractile bridges, one would expect that the maximum velocity of cross-bridge interactions, V_{max}, to remain constant, while force altered; indeed, this is the case. However, when contractility is altered by inotropic interventions such as catecholamines, V_{max} rises.[119] It is notable that beta-adrenoceptor activation, acting through cyclic AMP, can apparently stimulate the enzymatic activity of actin-activated ATPase acutely in heart muscle.[41]

THE ULTRASTRUCTURAL BASIS OF STARLING'S LAW OF THE HEART

The capacity of the intact ventricle to vary its force of contraction on a beat-to-beat basis as a function of its preload, reflected in the initial (end-diastolic) size, constitutes one of the major principles of cardiac function and is generally referred to as the *Frank-Starling phenomenon*, or *Starling's Law of the Heart*.[148, 149] This fundamental property of the heart is based on the myocardial *length–active tension relation*, in which force of contraction and/or extent of shortening depends on initial muscle length, which in turn is dependent on the ultrastructural disposition of thick and thin myofilaments within the sarcomeres.[150] As has already been pointed out (p. 383), the sarcomere is composed of an array of partially overlapping thick and thin filaments. A change in the length of the sarcomeres is striated muscle, whether skeletal or cardiac, creates a predictable change in the extent of overlapping between the two sets of filaments. The critical relation between sarcomere length and isometric tension development was defined for skeletal muscle by A.F. Huxley and associates[150, 151] (Fig. 13–19), who found that developed tension was constant with a sarcomere length between 2.0 and 2.2 μ but that when sarcomeres were shortened to less than 2.0 μ, the developed force fell. These changes in force development were explained by the relative position of the two sets of myofilaments within the sarcomere. The thick filaments are about 1.5 μ in length while the thin filaments measure 1.0 μ.[20]

THE SLIDING FILAMENT THEORY. According to this theory, the length of both sets remains constant, both at rest and during contraction. The central region of the thick filaments contains an area approximately 0.2 μ in width that is devoid of cross bridges for the formation of force-generating cross links between myosin heads and actin (Fig. 13–19). The optimal overlap of the 1.0 μ thin filaments with thick filaments occurs in sarcomeres between 2.0 and 2.2 μ. In this range of sarcomere lengths, the number of force-generating cross links that can be formed and the resultant developed force are maximal and constant. With sarcomeres longer than 2.2 μ, the fall in developed force may be directly related to the widening H zone and the resultant decrease in overlap between thick and thin filaments, thereby reducing the potential for cross bridge formation. At 3.65 μ, no overlap of filaments remains, and force generation ceases.[151]

When sarcomere lengths are progressively reduced below 2.0 μ, a reduction in tension development also occurs, presumably because, as pointed out earlier, thin filaments of 1.0 μ meet in the center of the sarcomere and bypass one another as sarcomere length is decreased further, resulting in a double overlap of filaments. This may interfere with the formation of cross bridges, may alter the ability of the filaments to bind Ca^{++} for activation, may reduce the sensitivity of the overlapping filaments to Ca^{++},[144] and/or may generate significant internal loads that might impair shortening of the sarcomere.[142, 147] Also, thin filaments may actually be repelled from the opposite half of the A band. All these factors may contribute to the fall in force development with shorter sarcomere lengths.

Although it has been suggested that thin filaments may be pulled by electrostatic forces rather than attaching physically to the thick filaments,[140] the concept of cross bridges between thick and thin filaments provides a useful working model that satisfactorily explains most of the observations of a variety of interventions involving cardiac contraction.

Relation Between Sarcomere Length and the Length-Active Tension Curve of Heart Muscle

At L_{max}, the length of sarcomeres in mammalian ventricular myocardium fixed for electronmicroscopy averages 2.2 μ[152] (Fig. 13–20). Fixation results in about 5 per cent shrinkage so that measurements made during life need to be scaled upward somewhat.[142] As the resting muscle is shortened to about 85 per cent of L_{max}, sarcomere lengths decrease as a linear function of muscle length.[142, 152–154] With further passive shortening of myocardium, however, the tissue becomes slack and little additional passive shortening of sarcomeres occurs, with diastolic sarcomere length remaining at 1.9 μ.

DIFFERENCES BETWEEN CARDIAC AND SKELETAL MUSCLE. Although the structure of the sarcomere is similar in cardiac and skeletal muscle, important specialized differences permit cardiac muscle to function on the ascending portion of the length–active tension curve and maintain a length-dependent relation between sarcomere length and force development. First, the greater stiffness of the pas-

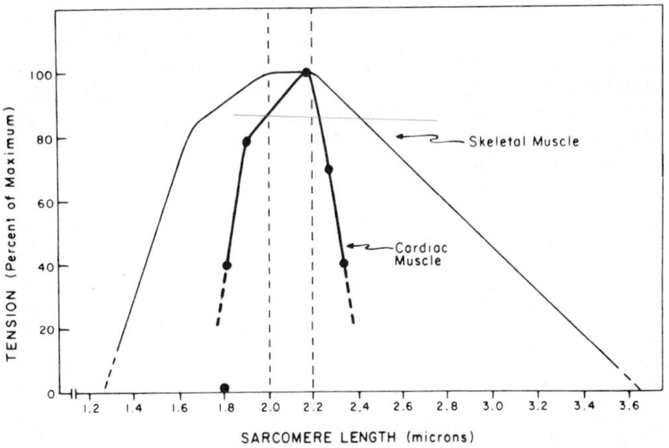

FIGURE 13–20. Relation between tension development and sarcomere length for cardiac muscle. Data were obtained by fixing cat papillary muscles with glutaraldehyde at various diastolic lengths relative to the length-tension curve and determining the average sarcomere length within the tissue using electron microscopic methods. The relation between tension development and sarcomere length obtained with skeletal fibers has been superimposed for comparison. In cardiac muscle, peak tension occurs with a diastolic sarcomere length of 2.2 μ. In skeletal muscle, there is a plateau of developed tension between sarcomere lengths of 2.2 and 2.0 μ, whereas in cardiac muscle this is not the case, and developed tension falls as sarcomere length is decreased below 2.2 μ. Furthermore, the shortest diastolic sarcomere length obtained in cardiac muscle in the absence of activation is 1.8 μ. As the papillary muscle is stretched beyond 2.2 μ, resting tension rises substantially (not shown; see Figure 13–22, p. 400) while actively developed tension falls precipitously. In contrast, in skeletal muscle, actively developed tension falls in a linear fashion between a sarcomere length of 2.2 and 3.6 μ. (From Sonnenblick, E. H., and Skelton, C. L.: Reconsideration of the ultrastructural basis of cardiac length-tension relations. Circ. Res. *35*:517, 1974, by permission of the American Heart Association, Inc.)

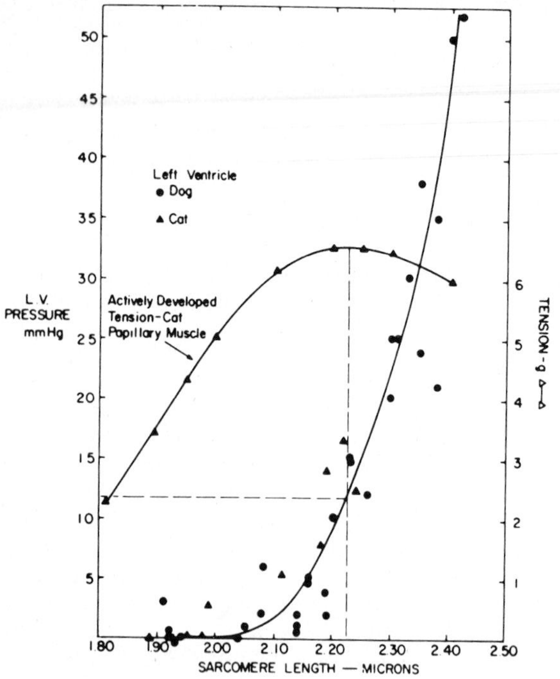

FIGURE 13–21. Relation between left ventricular pressure and average sarcomere length in the midwall of a canine left ventricle. The upper curve represents the relation between tension development and sarcomere length, as obtained from studies of cat papillary muscle. The lower curve relates left ventricular filling pressure to midwall sarcomere length for both dog and cat. At a left ventricular filling pressure of 12 mm Hg, which approximates the upper limit of normal filling pressure in the intact animal, average midwall sarcomere length is about 2.2 μ. This sarcomere length is also associated with the upper limits of the length–active tension curve, as shown by the vertical dashed line. Further increments in filling pressure yield only minor further increments in sarcomere length for very large increments in filling pressure. (From Spotnitz, J. H., et al.: Relation of ultrastructure to function in the intact heart: Sarcomere structure relative to pressure-volume curves of the intact left ventricles of dog and cat. Circ. Res. *18*:49, 1966, by permission of the American Heart Association, Inc.)

sive elastic component of cardiac muscle compared to skeletal muscle is such that diastolic sarcomere length is prevented from exceeding 2.3 μ,[155] thus preventing disengagement of the myofilaments[156] (Fig. 13–21). Second, the series elastic component is so compliant that during isometric contraction of cardiac muscle, substantial shortening of the sarcomeres occurs on the steep portion of their length-active tension curve.[142, 154]

When cardiac muscle is stretched beyond L_{max}, resting tension rises to very high levels (Fig. 13–21), while, by definition, actively developed tension rises no further. However, in contrast to skeletal muscle, sarcomeres in cardiac muscle resist overstretching. With extension of the muscle to 20 per cent beyond L_{max}, sarcomeres elongate only slightly beyond 2.2 μ, but developed tension falls substantially. A decrease in overlap between thick and thin filaments, i.e., disengagement of myofilaments, cannot explain the substantial decrements in developed force observed under these conditions; cellular damage occurs in cardiac muscle with this degree of overstretching and presumably is responsible, at least in part, for the reduction of tension development.[155]

SARCOMERE LENGTH-VENTRICULAR PERFORMANCE RELATION. Figure 13–21 shows the relation between average midwall sarcomere length and filling pressure for the left ventricles of the dog and cat.[156] When the left ventricle is empty, sarcomere length averages 1.9 μ, but as the left ventricle is filled, sarcomere lengths increase, so that at a filling pressure of 12 mm Hg the sarcomere length reaches 2.2 μ. With further ventricular distention, filling pressure rises markedly for small increments in ventricular volume, and only small increases in sarcomere length accompany large increases in intraventricular pressure. The same relation holds for the right ventricle but is scaled to lower filling pressures.[157] The relation between tension developed by the cat papillary muscle over a range of sarcomere lengths has been superimposed on the sarcomere resting length-tension relation in Figure 13–21. The optimal sarcomere length for maximum tension development (i.e., 2.2 μ) corresponds to the upper limits of normal ventricular filling pressure. When diastolic sarcomere length is related simultaneously to ventricular filling pressure and to active tension development, it becomes apparent that the apex of the sarcomere length–active tension curve and the normal upper limit of ventricular filling pressure coincide. Thus, the ventricle normally starts to contract when end-diastolic sarcomere lengths are along the upper half of the ascending portion of the sarcomere length–active tension curve. At any given sarcomere length, the developed tension is modified by the Ca^{++} available for activation[158]

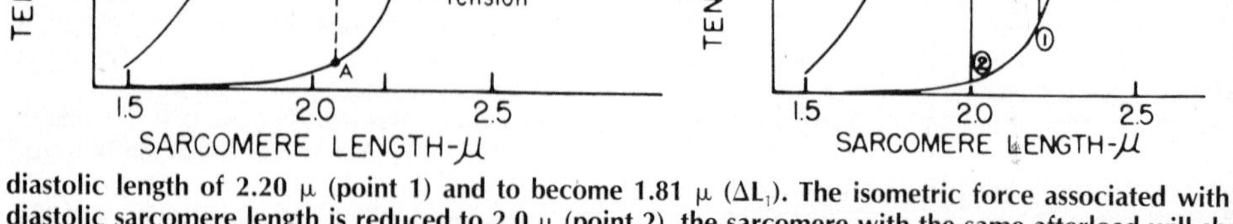

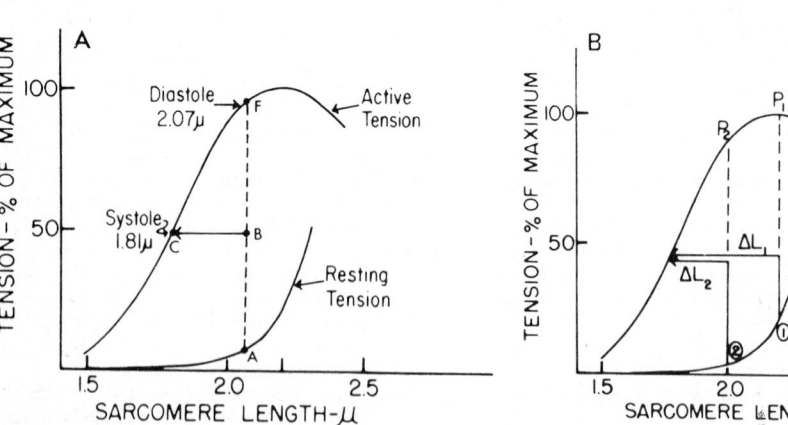

FIGURE 13–22. *A*, Relation between average diastolic sarcomere lengths as noted in the midwall of the normal diastolic and systolic left ventricle of the dog and the sarcomere length-tension curve of the isolated cat papillary muscle. In the intact dog, normal diastole is associated with a diastolic sarcomere length of 2.07 μ. During systole, sarcomeres in the intact heart shorten to an average of 1.81 μ. This provides for a 13 per cent change in sarcomere length, which would produce an ejection fraction of 55 per cent when considered in terms of a thick-walled model of the left ventricle.

B, Effects of altering initial muscle lengths on shortening of afterloaded sarcomeres. During an afterloaded isotonic contraction (1), the sarcomere begins to shorten from a diastolic length of 2.20 μ (point 1) and to become 1.81 μ (ΔL_1). The isometric force associated with this sarcomere length is noted at P_1. When diastolic sarcomere length is reduced to 2.0 μ (point 2), the sarcomere with the same afterload will shorten to the same point on the length–active tension curve (ΔL_2). This will result in a shortening from 2.00 to 1.81 μ. In this instance the associated isometric force occurs at P_2. Note that despite a minor change in peak developed isometric force, a substantial change in afterloaded isotonic shortening occurs at the same afterload. This would produce a substantial change in the stroke volume when extrapolated to the intact heart; e.g., in a 100-gram canine left ventricle, a change in diastolic sarcomere length from 2.0 to 2.2 μ in the midwall would increase stroke volume from 17 to 42 ml, with end-diastolic volume increasing from 40 to 65 ml. (From Ross, J., Jr., et al.: Architecture of the heart in systole and diastole: Technique of rapid fixation and analysis of left ventricular geometry. Circ. Res. *21*:409, 1967, by permission of the American Heart Association, Inc.)

In studies of the relation between sarcomere length and ventricular performance in the intact ejecting heart, the canine left ventricle has been fixed in situ during end diastole and end systole.[159, 160] Diastolic sarcomere lengths in the midwall of the left ventricle averaged 2.07 μ when filling pressure ranged from 6 to 8 mm Hg.[160] At end systole, when the ventricle had ejected about two-thirds of its end-diastolic volume, the average sarcomere length shortened to 1.8 μ (Fig. 13–22), and when contractility of the ventricle was augmented by postextrasystolic potentiation, maximum systolic emptying was increased substantially and end-systolic sarcomere lengths were 1.6 μ. During relaxation, these sarcomeres will elongate to 1.9 to 2.0 μ, generating a restoring force that provides "suction" in early diastole to enhance early ventricular filling.

Sarcomeres tend to be longest in the midwall of the ventricle and reach a maximal length (2.25 μ) at filling pressures of about 10 mm Hg, when subendocardial and subepicardial sarcomeres are shorter. As filling pressure is raised further, sarcomere length increases across the entire wall; this recruitment of shorter sarcomeres from across the wall may constitute a further functional reserve of the Frank-Starling mechanism.[161]

The relative degree of sarcomere shortening cannot be the same across the ventricular wall during ejection; geometrical considerations dictate that epicardial fibers must shorten relatively less than endocardial fibers. Nevertheless, when sarcomere lengths obtained from the intact heart are superimposed on the initial sarcomere length-tension curve (Fig. 13–22*A*), the normal sarcomere might be considered to start to contract at point A. Were the ends of the muscle fixed, the isometric force at point F would be developed. With an afterload, force is developed to point B, after which shortening occurs between points B and C from a sarcomere length of 2.07 μ to 1.81 μ. As diastolic sarcomere length is altered along the ascending limb of the sarcomere length–active tension curve, both peak isometric force development and the extent of shortening at any given load are changed (Fig. 13–22*B*). The extent of this shortening is of great physiological importance, since it ultimately determines the quantity of blood ejected by the intact ventricle at any given diastolic fiber length. The basis for the Frank-Starling mechanism in the intact heart (discussed in the next section) is apparent in Figure 13–22*B*, in which it is clear that small changes in diastolic sarcomere length can mediate relatively large changes in the extent of sarcomere shortening at any afterload.

DETERMINANTS OF CONTRACTION OF THE INTACT HEART

Although the geometry of the intact ventricle is far more complex than that of papillary muscle, with its parallel, longitudinally disposed fibers, if certain analogies are drawn and assumptions made, it becomes apparent that the basic mechanisms that influence the contraction of isolated cardiac muscle (described above) affect the performance of the whole heart in a similar manner.[161–165]

CHANGES IN VENTRICULAR SIZE AND SHAPE DURING THE CARDIAC CYCLE

The dimensions of the ventricular cavities, thickness of the ventricular walls, and intrinsic mechanical properties of cardiac tissue are the determinants of passive elasticity or stiffness of the ventricle and therefore of diastolic tension. In this manner they determine the filling of the ventricles, ultimately affecting the length of the sarcomeres at the onset of systole and as already described, the contractile events. The shape of the ventricles, the angles of adjacent muscle fibers, and the thickness of the ventricular walls also determine the distribution of active forces within the ventricular myocardium throughout systole and hence affect the extent and speed of muscle shortening. In addition to the changes that occur normally during the cardiac cycle and that are produced by acute physiological stresses, the shape of the ventricle often undergoes major alterations consequent to chronic cardiac disorders, such as valvular abnormalities, or local scarring due to coronary heart disease. The model often applied when one is considering the left ventricle as a thick-walled ellipsoid of revolution, which has practical utility in the calculation of left ventricular volume (p. 453).

The myocardial fibers are arranged in a spiral fashion around the central cavity of the left ventricle. The subendocardial and the subepicardial fibers run largely parallel to the long axis of the cavity, and the midwall fibers are mostly circumferential, i.e., perpendicular to the long axis. All the fibers tend to be perpendicular to the radius of the cavity. During contraction, the myocardial fibers shorten and thicken (Fig. 13–23), and the left ventricular cavity decreases circumferentially and longitudinally and the wall thickens. The generation of intraventricular pressure and the displacement of blood from the left ventricular cavity are produced by a combination of fiber shortening and wall thickening.

During isovolumetric left ventricular contraction, the chordae tendineae become tense, the mitral valve closes, and the ellipsoidal left ventricle becomes more spherical, with slight apex-to-base shortening and a small increase in the minor ventricular diameter.[166] The tendency toward sphericalization and wall thickening during isovolumetric contraction and toward ellipticalization and wall thinning during isovolumetric relaxation is more pronounced when ventricular size is reduced, as occurs during thoracotomy (i.e., in the absence of a negative intrapleural pressure) or with occlusion of venous inflow into the heart.[167] During ejection, the internal major (longitudinal) axis shortens by only 9 per cent.[167] Thus, shortening of the internal minor axis diameter accounts for approximately 85 to 90 per cent of the stroke volume.

Similar changes in shape occur in the human left ventricle studied by means of angiography. As the left ventricle empties during systole, the inner surface decreases proportionately more than the external surface, as dictated by the geometry of the heart. Since muscle mass remains constant, an increase in wall thickness must occur; direct measurements of the left ventricular wall in intact animals[168] as well as cineangiography in patients[169] have confirmed that left ventricular wall thickness increases by 25 and 35 per cent during systole.

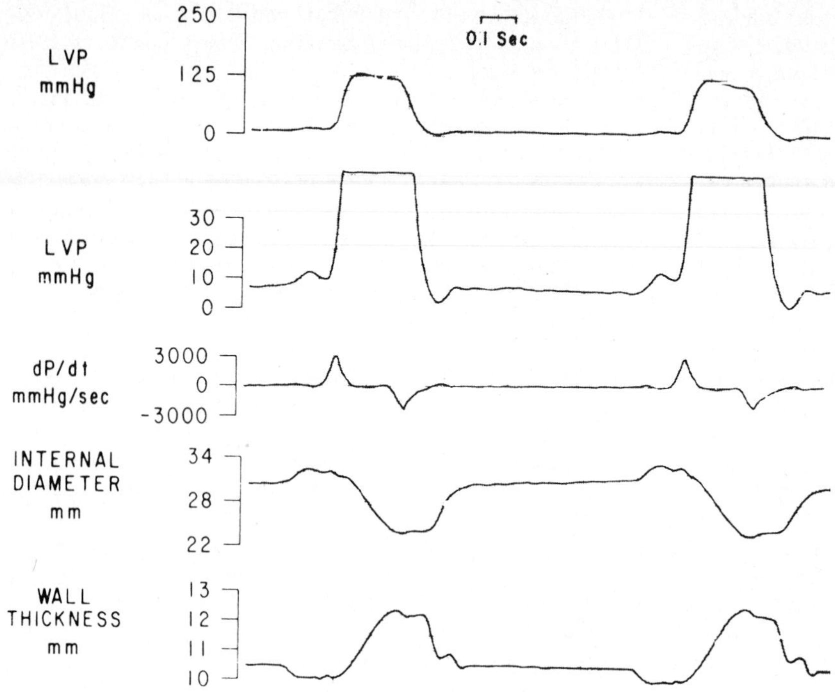

FIGURE 13–23. High-speed tracings obtained in a normal conscious, chronically instrumented dog with sinus arrhythmia. LVP = left ventricular pressure (in the top two tracings, at high and low amplification). dP/dt = the first derivative of left ventricular pressure. The internal diameter of the left ventricle was measured by means of a pair of ultrasonic crystals placed on the endocardium near the minor equator. The wall thickness of the left ventricle was measured by means of a pair of miniature ultrasonic crystals juxtaposed across the free wall near the minor equator. Note presystolic wall thinning with atrial systole, followed by wall thickening during ejection, with mirror image changes of the internal diameter. (From Theroux, P., Ross, J., Jr., et al.: Unpublished observations.)

DIASTOLIC PROPERTIES OF THE VENTRICLES

Certain terms are commonly used to describe the mechanical properties of cardiac muscle.[170, 171] Since there has been confusion about their meaning, they will be defined explicitly here. *Stress* is the force per unit of cross-sectional area, frequently expressed as gm/cm^2; *strain* is the fractional (or percentage of) change in dimension or size from the unstressed dimension that results from the application of stress; *elasticity* is the property of recovery of a deformed material after removal of the stress; *creep* is the time-dependent strain of tissue maintained at a constant level of stress after a rapid change in stress; *stress relaxation* is the time-dependent reduction of stress when tissue is maintained at a constant level of strain after a rapid change in strain. Like most biological materials, cardiac muscle exhibits a curvilinear relation between passive (diastolic) stress and strain (Fig. 13–14); this property is responsible for the nonlinear pressure-volume curve (Fig. 13–24) and stress-strain relation of the intact ventricle. *Elastic stiffness* defines the ratio of stress to strain at any defined point of the curve relating these two variables. The *elastic stiffness constant* is the slope of the straight line relating elastic stiffness to the corresponding stress. The term elastic stiffness, sometimes called *volume stiffness* or *chamber stiffness*, has also been used to refer to the stiffness of the ventricular chamber and, by simplification, has been defined as the ratio of the change in pressure (dP) to the change in volume (dV). When the stress-strain relation is analyzed, the term *myocardial stiffness* has been employed to differentiate those effects due to changes in the stiffness properties of each unit of muscle as opposed to those due to increased muscle mass alone, which can affect *chamber stiffness;* thus, in some patients with concentric left ventricular hypertrophy, chamber stiffness is increased and myocardial stiffness is normal, whereas in others, both are elevated.[170] The terms *compliance* and *distensibility* represent the inverse of elastic stiffness, i.e., in referring to isolated muscle it is the ratio of a change in strain relative to a change in stress (d_e/d_s). In the ventricle these terms have been used to refer to the ratio dV/dP. The term *specific compliance* introduces a correction for the initial volume. Efforts to correct this value for ventricles of different sizes have also led to such expressions as $\frac{dV/dP}{V}$ where V in the denominator represents end-diastolic volume.

The diastolic pressure-volume relation of the normal mammalian left ventricle is curvilinear (Fig. 13–24).[171] At a low ventricular end-diastolic pressure there is a relatively gentle slope, with large changes in volume being accompanied by small changes in pressure. At the upper limits

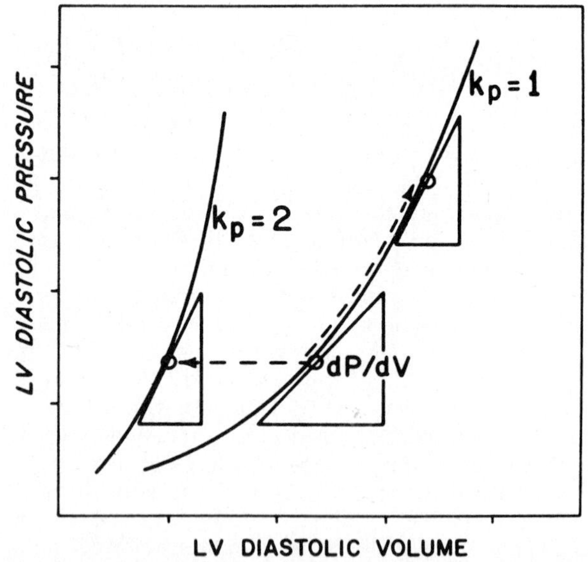

FIGURE 13–24. Diagrammatic representation of left ventricular (LV) diastolic pressure-volume relationships. *Right,* An increase in operative chamber stiffness (dP/dV) occurs in the absence of any change in the modulus of chamber stiffness (K_p). *Left,* An increase in operative chamber stiffness (relative to the curve on the right). Because operative chamber stiffness depends on the modulus of stiffness and the level of operative filling pressure, this comparison is made at equivalent levels of pressure. (From Gaasch, W. H., et al.: Left ventricular compliance: Mechanisms and clinical implications. Am. J. Cardiol. *38*:645, 1976.)

of normal end-diastolic pressure, the curve becomes steeper[172] and approximates an exponential relation, so that as the chamber becomes progressively filled during each diastole, instantaneous ventricular compliance (dV/dP) decreases; the inverse of compliance, i.e., elastic stiffness (dP/dV) bears a linear relation to the pressure in the normal dog left ventricle at diastolic pressures exceeding 3 mm Hg.[170] The slope of the line relating dP/dV to P represents the elastic stiffness constant of the chamber; it is relatively independent of ventricular shape and therefore may be useful for detecting changes in wall stiffness.[170, 170a] However, caution must be used in drawing conclusions from measuring these variables in one ventricle when the effects of changes in the volume of the other ventricle and the elastic limits of the pericardium cannot be excluded. Also, in comparing a normal chamber with a dilated one, identical chamber elastic stiffness constants might be obtained, and a definition of volume elasticity at a common pressure in which the different volumes are taken into account is needed to describe the properties of the two chambers.[173]

Although by definition, and as is apparent from Figure 13–24, the compliance of the ventricle changes as it fills an alteration of the compliance of the chamber as a whole can be identified by a change in the shape and position of the curve relating ventricular diastolic volume or dimensions to pressure.[171] Excluding the incomplete relaxation that occurs in tachycardia and myocardial ischemia, interventions that alter myocardial contractility acutely do not cause significant shifts in the ventricle's diastolic pressure-volume relation. The small changes in the relation reported in some studies may be secondary to effects on time-dependent, inertial, and viscous properties and to the influence of filling of the opposite ventricle. Since the diastolic pressure-volume relation is curvilinear, left ventricular diastolic compliance is determined by both the diastolic pressure-volume relation and the level of diastolic pressure at any instant, the so-called operating diastolic pressure (Fig. 13–24).[174] Therefore, ventricular compliance declines, i.e., the chamber elastic stiffness increases as it fills. Increased diastolic filling, for example, as occurs with acute aortic regurgitation, and, conversely, reduced ventricular preload, for example, as occurs after administration of nitroglycerin, result in increased and reduced stiffness, respectively, as the ventricle moves up or down its pressure-volume curve.[174]

Ventricular (chamber) stiffness is a function of muscle stiffness as well as of the thickness and geometry of the ventricle. If the stiffness of cardiac tissue (muscle stiffness) is increased, as may occur with a fibrous scar or with infiltration of amyloid, but the thickness of the ventricular wall remains normal, ventricular (chamber) stiffness will be increased. An increase in chamber stiffness will also occur if the stiffness of each individual unit of muscle (muscle stiffness) is normal but the ventricular wall becomes thicker.

In the intact heart, *stress relaxation* is of significance only when large increases in ventricular diastolic pressure and volume occur abruptly. For example, there is a small drop in ventricular end-diastolic pressure (about 1 mm Hg) when systolic pressure is suddenly elevated by 70 to 80 per cent in the isovolumetrically contracting left ventricle, which is held at a constant volume. This suggests the presence of viscous elements, but these changes are of relatively minor significance in the intact heart.[175] *Creep*, a time-dependent shift of the left ventricular diastolic pressure-volume relation, has also been documented in the conscious dog after large increases in systolic and diastolic pressures (ventricular diastolic volume being larger at the same levels of diastolic pressure).[176]

The normal *right ventricle is more compliant than the left,* not because of any intrinsic difference in muscle stiffness but because of its thinner wall.[157] In the isolated, nonbeating normal dog heart, when the left and right ventricles are filled simultaneously to a pressure of 10 mm Hg, the volume of the right ventricle is about 35 per cent greater than that of the left,[172] and the upper limit of normal for right ventricular end-diastolic pressure in humans is about one-half (6 mm Hg) that of the left ventricle (12 mm Hg). In humans, the end-diastolic volumes of the two ventricles are approximately equal,[177] and therefore the ejection fractions of the two ventricles are normally similar as well.

ROLE OF THE PERICARDIUM

(See also p. 1485)

Experimental data indicate that the normal pericardium has an important effect on the diastolic properties of the ventricles during acute volume overload and therefore could be important during acute heart failure. During acute volume loading in the dog, intrapericardial pressure rises when overall cardiac volume (both right and left heart chambers) is increased beyond the limit of pericardial distensibility, i.e., when the pericardium becomes restrictive. This factor may also play a role in the large decreases in left ventricular filling pressures that are observed during nitroprusside vasodilator therapy in human heart failure (p. 1486) when heart size decreases within the pericardial sac, which is no longer restrictive.

EFFECT OF PERICARDIUM ON VENTRICULAR LENGTH-PRESSURE RELATIONS. Figure 13–25 shows data from a conscious experimental animal instrumented for the measurement of left ventricular segment dimensions and left ventricular end-diastolic pressure; with the pericardium intact, overtransfusion produced a marked shift upward and to the left of the entire diastolic pressure-dimension curve of the left ventricle.[178] Infusion of nitroprusside under these conditions caused a partial shift downward of the entire curve, the degree of the shift being equal to the fall of intrapericardial pressure. Thus, although a portion of the drop in cardiac filling pressure produced by nitroprusside was due to a reduction of cardiac volume, a portion of the fall resulted from the shift of the entire curve due to lowering of the elevated intrapericardial pressure. In contrast, when the pericardium was removed and the same animal was studied several days later, acute volume overloading, followed by the administration of nitroprusside, moved the left ventricle upward and downward on a single diastolic pressure-dimension curve.[178] In a chronic volume overload model in the dog (arteriovenous fistula), little effect of the pericardium on the left ventricular diastolic pressure-volume relation was noted, since the pericardial sac gradually enlarged to accommodate the dilated heart.[179] However, in a similar model studied at an earlier time (average 2½ weeks after operation), a mild upward shift of the left ventricular diastolic pressure-volume relation was demonstrated using nitroprusside infusion, indicating a restrictive effect of the pericardium. This effect was absent after pericardiectomy.[180]

THE PERICARDIUM IN CHANGES IN CARDIAC COMPLIANCE. A reduction of left ventricular compliance occurs during angina pectoris (p. 1204), presumably as a consequence of impaired ventricular relaxation,[181] but whether or not the pericardium can contribute to the elevated left ventricular diastolic pressures and upward shift of the left ventricular diastolic pressure-volume curve under these conditions is not yet clear. Evidence suggests that during ischemia developing after pacing, changes in right heart diastolic pressures are not sufficient to account for such a shift.[182] Also, in animals a shift is seen during postpacing ischemia when the pericardium is absent.[183] Experimental work in hearts with the pericardium intact in which both the right atrium and the right ventricle were distended, while the left heart volume was constant at a relatively normal level, indicates that a 50 per cent increase in right heart volume accounts for an approximately 5 mm upward shift of the left ventricular diastolic pressure-volume relation.[184] When intrapericardial pressures were subtracted to yield transmural pressures, no such shifts were evident. Thus, substantial increases in right heart volume, as in the overtransfusion studies cited above,[178] appear to be required to affect the left ventricular diastolic pressure. The degree of filling of the atria at end diastole, which depends on

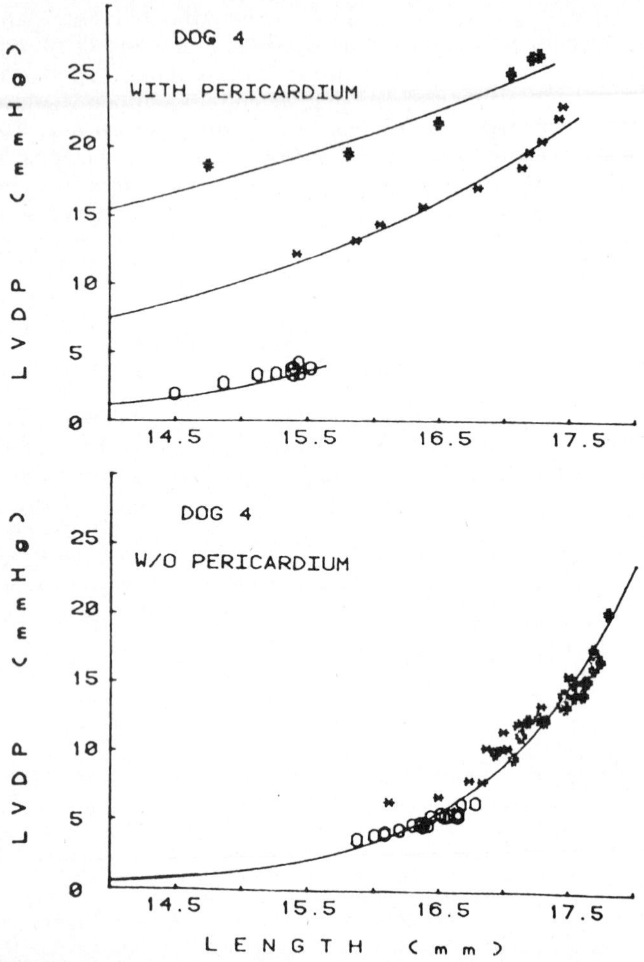

FIGURE 13–25. Relations between the length of a segment of left ventricle and left ventricular diastolic pressure (LVDP) in a conscious dog. Points were obtained during slow cardiac filling (diastasis). *Upper panel*, Relation with the *pericardium intact* before (open symbols) and after intravenous infusion of dextran to produce acute cardiac dilatation (asterisks, upper curve); the middle curve (x's) shows the effect of an intravenous infusion of nitroprusside in the presence of such acute cardiac dilatation. *Lower panel*, the same dog studied *without (W/O) the pericardium* (after its surgical removal). The same interventions, volume loading and nitroprusside, are carried out. The ventricle now appears to be operating on a single diastolic pressure–length relation. (Adapted from Shirato, K., et al.: Alteration of the left ventricular diastolic pressure–segment length relation produced by the pericardium: Effects of cardiac distention and afterload reduction in conscious dogs. Circulation *57*:1191, 1978, by permission of the American Heart Association, Inc.)

whether or not atrial contraction occurs (e.g., atrial fibrillation) or the timing of atrial systole, can affect the left ventricular end-diastolic pressure-volume relation (and hence shift the standard ventricular function curve) by affecting intrapericardial pressure.[185] Further research is needed to establish the importance of the pericardium in human subjects. There is evidence, however, that acute right ventricular infarction can lead to elevated intrapericardial pressure, with increased right ventricular and left ventricular diastolic pressure.[186]

Controversy exists as to whether intrapericardial pressure should be measured as a hydrostatic force (with a catheter-manometer system) or as a compressive force per unit surface area.[187] The latter has been measured experimentally using a flat, fluid-filled balloon, and higher intrapericardial pressures have been recorded under some circumstances than have been recorded with the more traditional approach.[188]

VENTRICULAR INTERACTION. Studies in isolated hearts (without the pericardium) in which the two ventricles were filled separately have shown that the filling of one chamber affects the properties of the other.[172] Other experiments in intact animals with the pericardium in place have shown that increased right ventricular filling not only can increase the left ventricular diastolic pressure but also can change the shape of the left ventricle, with displacement of the interventricular septum to the left[189] (Fig. 61–10, p. 1880). Conversely, with alterations in left ventricular loading, changes in the right ventricular diastolic pressure-volume relation may not reflect an alteration of the right ventricular myocardial or chamber stiffness but rather may be secondary to left ventricular volume changes with elevation of the intrapericardial pressure in a pericardial sac that restrains changes in volume of the entire heart.[190, 191]

In conscious dogs, changes in left ventricular shape and septal position appear to have only minor effects on the function of the left ventricle.[192] Thus, average fiber length rather than left ventricular shape or diastolic pressure was found to be the main determinant of performance. As might be expected, however, changes in the volume of the right ventricle importantly affect stroke output of the left ventricle in the same direction, as the two ventricles function in series.[192]

PERFORMANCE OF THE INTACT VENTRICLE

The three determinants of performance of isolated cardiac muscle—preload, afterload, and contractility—also affect the performance of the intact ventricle. In addition, heart rate represents a fourth determinant of performance per unit time.

THE CARDIAC CYCLE. The relations between left ventricular pressure, the diameter of the minor equator at the endocardial surface of the left ventricular wall, and the wall thickness in a conscious dog are shown in Figure 13–23, and the events of the cardiac cycle are shown diagrammatically in Figure 13–26. Ventricular end diastole is followed by a brief period of isovolumetric left ventricular contraction, the maximum rate of pressure change (peak dP/dt) occurring just before the onset of ejection.[162] The onset of inward motion of the ventricular wall then commences as blood is ejected into the aorta, and the rate of wall shortening becomes maximal near the middle of ejection. Wall thickness increases during shortening, becoming maximal at the end of ejection. Following isovolumetric relaxation, during which peak negative dP/dt is reached, a rapid increase in the diameter of the ventricle occurs during early diastole, followed by a slow phase of filling in mid-diastole (diastasis); a second, rapid increase in diameter takes place in late diastole, as a consequence of atrial contraction. The time course of changes in ventricular volume closely parallel those shown for ventricular internal diameter during each cardiac cycle. This relation between ventricular pressure and volume can also be plotted as a pressure-volume loop (Fig. 13–27) in a manner analogous to the sarcomere length-pressure (Fig. 13–21) and length-tension (Fig. 13–22) relations. This provides a convenient framework for understanding the responses of individual left ventricular contractions to alterations in preload, afterload, and contractility.

THE PRESSURE-VOLUME DIAGRAM. The pressure-volume loop of the left ventricle can be related to the performance of isolated cardiac muscle, in which the active isometric length-tension curve provides the limit of shortening for isotonic contractions (Fig. 13–22). The linear relation between the end-systolic volume and the end-systolic pressure of the left ventricle is analogous to this length-tension relation and has been well defined in the isolated heart preparation[193, 194] (Fig. 13–27, left). The end-systolic pressure–volume relation of the left ventricle (defined near end-ejection as the maximum ratio of pressure to volume) has been studied in detail in the isolated heart.[195, 196] It falls close to the active isovolumetric pressure-volume relation; it has been shown to be linear and

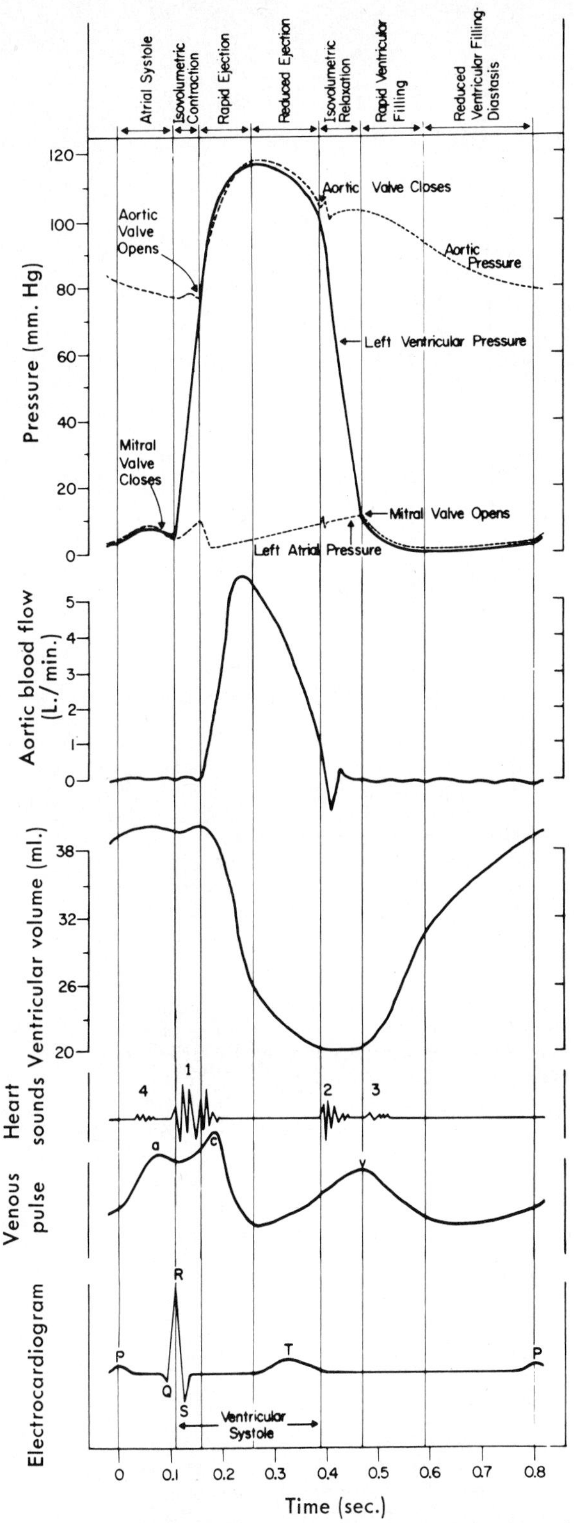

FIGURE 13–26. Events of the cardiac cycle. Left atrial, aortic, and left ventricular pressure pulses are correlated in time with aortic flow, ventricular volume, heart sounds, venous pulse, and electrocardiogram to provide a complete cardiac cycle in the dog. (From Berne, R. M., and Levy, M. N.: Cardiovascular Physiology. 3rd ed. St. Louis, The C. V. Mosby Co., 1977.)

shifted by inotropic influences without a change in the volume intercept, thereby providing a load-independent measure of contractility.[196] With major changes in characteristic impedance or resistance, slight changes in the position of the end-systolic pressure-volume relation also occur.[197]

THE END-SYSTOLIC PRESSURE-VOLUME RELATION. In the intact animal, linear end-systolic pressure-volume relations can be produced by altering loading conditions with infusion of a vasopressor which has no appreciable inotropic effects, such as angiotensin (Fig. 13–28),[198] or by vena caval obstruction.[199] In humans, the end-systolic ventricular volume can be determined by obtaining two or more angiocardiograms during infusion of phenylephrine, and the end-systolic values are then related to the corresponding ventricular or aortic pressure at the end of ventricular ejection.[200] Noninvasive techniques for measuring ventricular dimensions or volume (echocardiography and radionuclide methods)[201] can also be employed. The linear end-systolic pressure-volume relation of the left ventricle has been found to shift downward and to the right in the presence of myocardial disease (Fig. 13–27, right) and to shift upward and to the left (with steepening of its slope) during acute positive inotropic interventions (Fig. 13–27, right).

This relation is of particular importance because it defines the level of inotropic state under acutely changing conditions *independent* of the end-diastolic volume (preload) and the systolic pressure (as a measure of afterload). It is analogous to the length–active tension curve of isolated muscle. Thus, a given cardiac cycle arrives at end ejection and falls in this linear relation, regardless of the starting point for end-diastolic volume and the level of aortic pressure encountered during ejection, and the entire end-systolic pressure-volume relation is shifted acutely only by a change in inotropic state (Fig. 13–27). Use of the end-systolic pressure-volume relation for comparing one ventricle with another still has not been standardized,[202] although experimental work indicates that both the slope of the relation and its volume intercept are functions of body and left ventricular weight.[203]

It should be recognized that under conditions in which there are *chronic* changes in the shape and size of the ventricle or in the thickness of its wall, systolic pressure is not indicative of the level of afterload; under these conditions the end-systolic pressure-volume relation does not define the level of inotropic state, and the wall force must be calculated in order to determine the linear relations between end-systolic volume and end-systolic wall force (Fig. 13–28*B*) which does identify the status of contractility.[204]

LAPLACE'S LAW. In comparing the whole heart to isolated muscle, heart volume and pressure are analogous to muscle length and tension. More complex formulations have also been developed; thus, the average circumferential wall stress (force per unit of cross-sectional area of wall) is related directly to the product of intraventricular pressure and internal radius and inversely to wall thickness. In the simplest versions of Laplace's law for a spherical ventricle, $\sigma = Pa/2h$ and for an ellipsoidal ventricle, $\sigma = \frac{Pb}{h} \cdot \frac{1 - b^2}{2c^2}$ where σ = average circumferential wall stress, a = radius at the endocardial surface, P = intraventricular pressure, h = wall thickness; and b and c = the semiminor and semimajor axes at the endocardial surface.[170] In the ejecting ventricle, the extent and rate of wall shortening—and thus indirectly the stroke volume—are analogous to the extent and velocity of shortening of isolated muscle. The ventricular pressure during ventricular ejection is closely related to the afterload, although geometrical factors must be considered in order to calculate wall forces in the heart.

PRELOAD

Starling's Law of the Heart, which states that "the mechanical energy set free on passage from the resting to

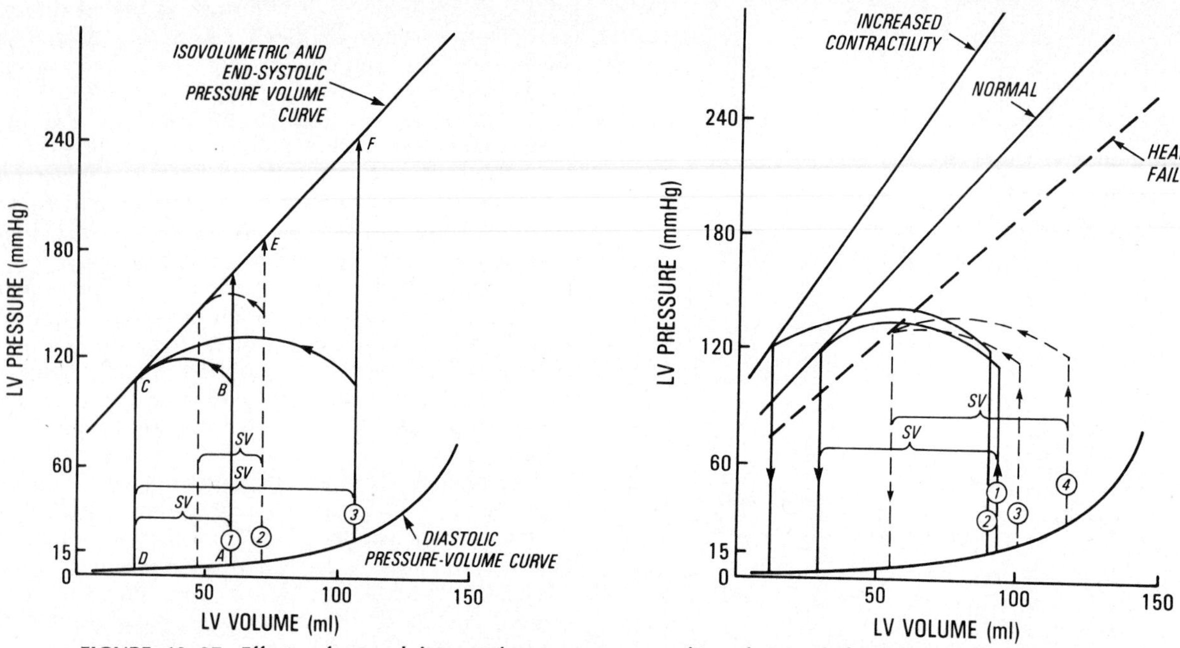

FIGURE 13–27. Effects of several interventions on pressure-volume loops of the left ventricle (LV) shown diagrammatically. *Left,* Effects of varying preload and afterload (with level of contractility remaining constant). Contraction 1 commences at end diastole (A) and is isovolumetric (arrow A to B) until the onset of ejection (B); the end of ejection or end-systolic volume (C) is followed by isovolumetric relaxation (C to D), and then filling of the ventricle occurs along the diastolic pressure-volume curve (from D to A). When a contraction originating from the same diastolic volume as contraction 1 is forced to contract isovolumetrically (top arrows), a point on the volume-isovolumetric systolic pressure curve is generated; if beats originating at larger end-diastolic volumes (contractions 2 and 3) are forced to contract isovolumetrically, points E and F are generated on that curve. This active pressure-volume curve provides the limit for the end-systolic volume of ejecting contractions. Ejecting contraction 3 shows that increasing end-diastolic volume causes an increase in stroke volume (SV) when aortic pressure is relatively constant. Ejecting contraction 2 (dashed lines) shows the effect of increasing systolic aortic pressure; when compared with contraction 1, SV is actually less, despite an increased end-diastolic volume, because of the higher level of aortic pressure or afterload. *Right,* Effects of increasing contractility (positive inotropic agent) and decreasing contractility (heart failure) on left ventricular pressure-volume loops. Contraction 1 is a normal pressure-volume loop, at a normal level of contractility. Contraction 2 shows that when contractility is increased, a larger stroke volume is generated from a similar or even slightly reduced end-diastolic volume, aortic pressure being relatively constant. In the presence of heart failure, SV may be diminished despite a slightly larger end-diastolic volume at a comparable level of aortic pressure (dashed line, contraction 3); however, SV may be restored if end-diastolic volume is further increased (contraction 4).

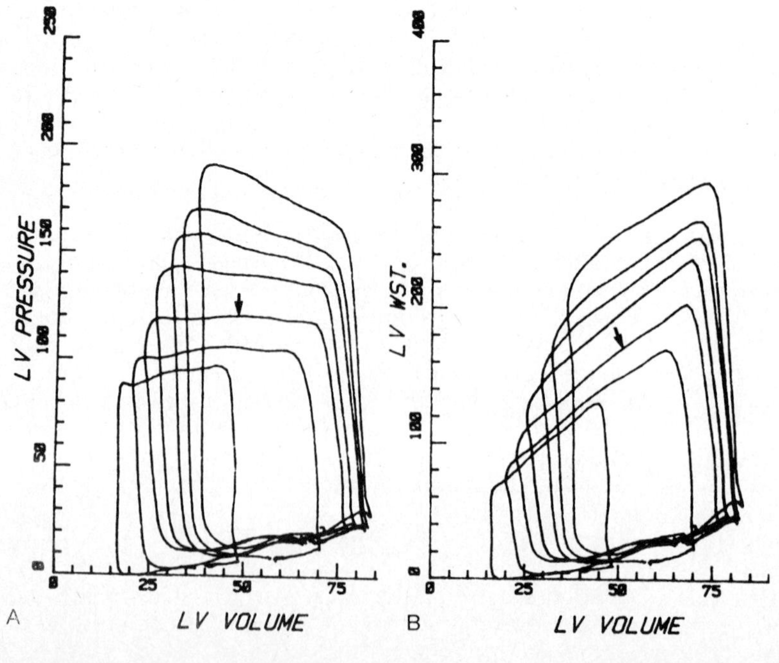

FIGURE 13–28. *A,* Pressure-volume loops (each loop being generated from the average of several cardiac cycles) showing left ventricular (LV) volume (ml) and pressure (mm Hg) at resting control (vertical arrow), after progressive infusions of angiotensin to increase LV pressure, and after brief inferior vena caval obstructions to decrease LV pressure. Note that the points at the end of LV ejection appear to form a straight line, which is independent of the LV end-diastolic volume and the systolic pressure during ejection. *B,* Wall stress (WST) volume loops of the left ventricle (LV) computed from the pressure-volume loops shown in *A.* Again, note the independence to loading conditions of the linear end-systolic points relating wall-stress to volume (From Ross, J., Jr.: Applications and limitations of end-systolic measures of ventricular performance. Fed. Proc. *43*:2418, 1984.)

the contracted state is a function of the length of the muscle fiber, i.e., of the area of chemically active surfaces,[149] is an expression of the length–active tension curve, reflecting the functional consequences of variations in preload. In the intact heart, ventricular end-diastolic wall stress or tension is analogous to the preload of isolated muscle and ultimately determines the resting length of the sarcomeres (Fig. 13–21).

PRELOAD RESERVE. As a consequence of the exponential shape of the left ventricular diastolic pressure-volume curve, there is considerably less preload reserve beyond the upper limit of normal for ventricular filling pressure than below it. However, studies in conscious resting dogs (without the pericardium) under basal conditions indicate that with volume loading alone, which is associated with little change in heart rate or systolic pressure, a stroke volume reserve of approximately 13 per cent exists.[205] With further volume loading, the left ventricular end-diastolic volume increases by an additional 3 or 4 per cent, and a theoretical stroke volume reserve of 31 per cent was calculated assuming an unchanged left ventricular systolic pressure.[205] Other experiments in conscious dogs suggest that less available preload reserve exists, although tachycardia and increased systolic pressure could have limited stroke volume increases due to use of preload reserve.[206] Studies of left ventricular volume by radionuclide techniques during supine and upright exercise suggest that considerable preload reserve is utilized during stress in humans.[207] Preload reserve is especially great in human subjects, in whom the basal resting end-diastolic volume is reduced by the pooling of blood in the lower extremities. Of course, a considerable further stroke volume reserve can be made available by enhanced inotropic state, which increases the ejection fraction and ventricular emptying.

In addition to some preload reserve available during stress, variations in the performance of both ventricles due to alterations in preload occur in a beat-to-beat basis in maintaining balanced outputs from the right and left heart during normal respiration, with abrupt changes in body position, as well as during other changing physiological conditions.

INFLUENCE OF PRELOAD ON VENTRICULAR CONTRACTION. The effect of alterations in preload independent of alterations in frequency, afterload, and inotropic state for the left ventricle are shown diagrammatically in Figure 13–27, left. Increases in preload augment the stroke volume as well as the extent and velocity of wall shortening.[208] This preload effect is operative at all levels of systolic pressure or afterload. From Figure 13–29, it can be seen that an inverse relation between systolic wall stress and stroke volume applies if the preload is constant, and that this entire relation is shifted upward by an increase in preload (Fig. 13–29, right panel)[209] and downward by diminished preload. If ejection is prevented and the ventricle contracts isovolumetrically, a direct correlation between preload, as reflected in the end-diastolic volume, and peak left ventricular systolic pressure or calculated wall stress can also be shown (analogous to the length–active tension curve of isolated muscle).

These relationships constitute expressions of the Frank-Starling mechanism and provide the basis for ventricular function curves in the normally ejecting heart, which relate ventricular end-diastolic volume or pressure to stroke volume and stroke work.[210] Any of the curves discussed above can, of course, be shifted up or down by positive and negative inotropic influences, respectively.

ATRIAL CONTRIBUTION TO PRELOAD. Like ventricular muscle, atrial muscle behaves in accord with Starling's law, with increasing stretch resulting in a more forceful contraction.[211] When properly timed, atrial contraction augments ventricular filling and preload. Rapid ventricular filling induced by atrial contraction at the end of diastole abruptly elevates ventricular end-diastolic pressure and volume. This allows a lower mean right or left atrial

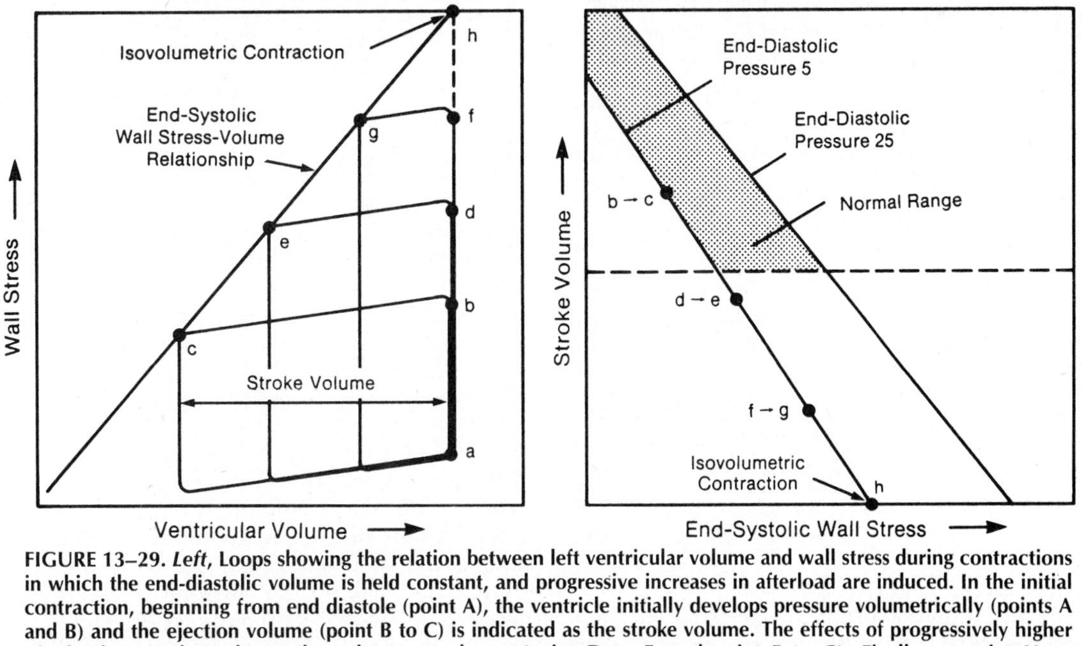

FIGURE 13–29. ***Left,*** **Loops showing the relation between left ventricular volume and wall stress during contractions in which the end-diastolic volume is held constant, and progressive increases in afterload are induced. In the initial contraction, beginning from end diastole (point A), the ventricle initially develops pressure volumetrically (points A and B) and the ejection volume (point B to C) is indicated as the stroke volume. The effects of progressively higher afterloads to reduce the stroke volume are shown (point D to E, and point F to G). Finally, at point H an isovolumetric contraction results at the same end-diastolic volume. *Right,* Inverse relation between end-systolic wall stress and stroke volume showing that progressively increased systolic wall stress causes a drop in stroke volume and vice versa, with zero stroke volume at point H. The left-hand inverse relation originates from a normal left ventricular end-diastolic pressure of 5 mm Hg, whereas the right-hand relation originates from an elevated end-diastolic pressure of 25 mm Hg, showing the effect of increased preload to shift the inverse end-systolic wall stress-stroke volume relation. Within the shaded range, the preload reserve can maintain the stroke-volume at a normal level, despite increasing end-systolic wall stress. (Modified from Weber, K. T., et al.: The mechanics of ventricular function. Hosp. Pract. *18*:113, 1983.)**

pressure to exist throughout most of diastole than would be the case if atrial contraction were ineffective (as in atrial fibrillation) or ill-timed (as in nodal rhythm or atrioventricular dissociation).[212] The atrial contribution to ventricular filling is of particular importance in the presence of ventricular hypertrophy and other states of reduced ventricular compliance. In these conditions, the loss of atrial systole reduces ventricular end-diastolic pressure and volume, ultimately impairing ventricular performance.[213]

DESCENDING LIMB OF STARLING'S CURVE. The question of whether a descending limb of cardiac function due to excessive increase in ventricular diastolic volume exists in the whole left ventricle has been of great interest.[214] In the isovolumetrically contracting isolated canine left ventricle, no reduction of developed wall stress or systolic pressure occurred until the ventricular end-diastolic pressure exceeded 60 mm Hg; when diastolic ventricular pressure was further elevated to 100 mm Hg, developed pressure declined by only 7.5 per cent. At these extremely high end-diastolic pressures, sarcomere lengths averaged 2.27 to 2.30 μ.[215] Based on this and other work showing that midwall sarcomere lengths did not exceed 2.27 μ at left ventricular end-diastolic pressure up to 40 mm Hg,[216] it may be postulated that the descending limb of ventricular performance, when observed in the ejecting ventricle, is not caused by operation of the heart on a descending limb of the sarcomere length-tension relation,[217, 218] i.e., it is not a consequence of overstretch with the disengagement of actin and myosin myofilaments.

APPARENT DESCENDING LIMB. However, a descending limb of curves that relate left ventricular end-diastolic pressure to stroke work, was demonstrated in dogs when volume loading was carried out to achieve end-diastolic pressures exceeding 30 mm Hg, after mean aortic pressure had initially been elevated.[218] Under these circumstances, slight further increases in aortic pressure occurred during the volume loading, which elevated left ventricular filling pressures above 30 mm Hg. It was concluded that the descending limb of function in the ejecting ventricle is only apparent and actually results from reduced myocardial wall shortening due to an increased afterload, when the ventricle is unable to compensate by further increases in sarcomere length.[218] It has also been proposed that the descending limb of function induced in the failing human heart by infusion of a vasopressor agent[219] is due to such an effect of augmented afterload, when preload reserve is absent.[208, 220] The development of mitral regurgitation consequent to ventricular dilatation can also depress forward stroke volume and result in an *apparent* depression of ventricular performance as preload is elevated to very high levels.

Another cause for an *apparent* descending limb of the relationship between left ventricular end-diastolic pressure (or volume) and the stroke volume has also been described. Excessive afterload produced by angiotensin infusion in the normal, conscious dog resulted in an inability of the ventricle to maintain the stroke volume despite an increase in the ventricular end-diastolic pressure and volume (Fig. 13–30, curve 1).[205] If volume loading was then produced by fluid infusion and the angiotensin infusion repeated, such a descending of function occurred at higher levels of stroke volume (Fig. 13–30, curve 2). Thus, originating from the basic Frank-Starling curve relating left ventricular end-diastolic volume to stroke volume, a series of descending limbs can be demonstrated when pressure loading is carried out at various levels of left ventricular end-diastolic volume. Such responses explain how the entire function curve can be shifted downward by increased afterload and upward by reduced afterload, as with a vasodilator. Such *apparent* descending limbs of left ventricular function due to pressure loading are due to insufficient venous return. This inadequate venous return prevents the left ventricle from compensating and increasing left ventricular end-diastolic volume to the level required to meet the increased afterload.[205]

In *summary*, alterations in preload, operating through changes in end-diastolic fiber length, serve as an important determinant of the performance of the intact ventricle and provide the basis for the function curves of the intact ventricle. The ability to augment preload provides a functional reserve to the heart in situations of acute stress and operates on a beat-to-beat basis in maintaining balanced outputs of the two ventricles during such normal maneuvers as respiration.[210] The possibility of increasing preload provides a reserve mechanism and allows some augmentation of cardiac performance during severe stresses such as maximum exercise performed in the upright position.[207, 221]

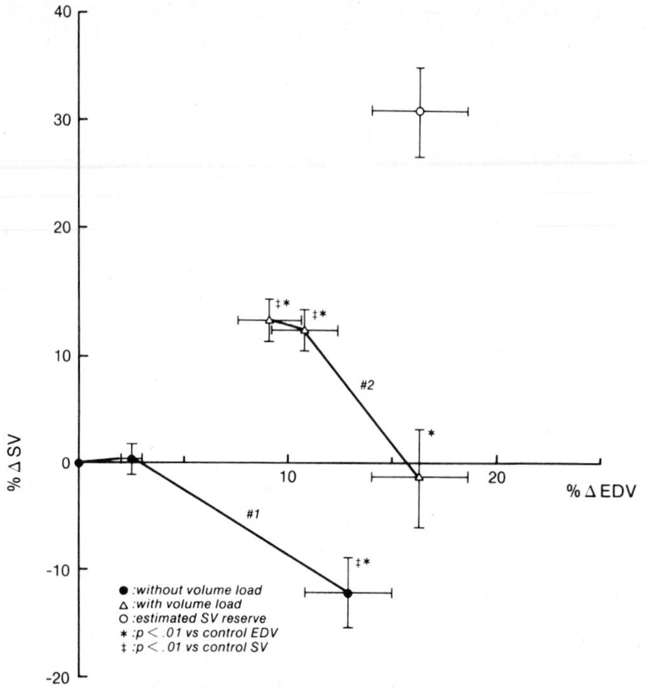

FIGURE 13–30. Relations between the percentage change in left ventricular end-diastolic volume (% Δ EDV) and the percentage change in stroke volume (% Δ SV) from the values before angiotensin infusion without (closed circles), and after volume loading (open triangles). The relationship during volume loading (curve 2) is shifted upward and to the right of that before volume loading (curve 1). The calculated maximum end-diastolic volume and stroke volume reserve are also shown (open circle) (± SEM). (From Lee, J. D., et al.: Preload reserve and mechanisms of afterload mismatch in the normal conscious dog. Am. J. Physiol. *19*:H464, 1986.)

Control of Preload in the Intact Organism

In the intact organism, preload is determined largely by venous return and total blood volume and its distribution (Fig. 13–31)[222, 223] as well as by the activity of the atrium.

VENOUS RETURN. In the absence of heart failure in the intact organism, most changes in cardiac output can be accounted for largely by changes in the *return* of blood to the heart, which in turn alters the preload. In the absence of heart failure, simple augmentation of myocardial contractility, as occurs with administration of a cardiac glycoside or institution of sustained postextrasystolic potentiation (paired electrical stimulation), has little effect on cardiac output.[224] In contrast, relatively major changes in output occur during maneuvers that alter venous return, such as lower body positive or negative pressure, positive-pressure respiration, a sudden change in posture, and rapid changes in blood volume.

Conditions that lower peripheral vascular resistance are among the most important of those augmenting venous return and include the opening of arteriovenous fistulas and conditions that mimic the latter, such as patent ductus arteriosus, fever, beriberi, pregnancy, and Paget's disease. (These and other chronic high-output states are discussed in Chapter 25.) A reduction in vascular resistance also occurs during *exercise*, when the arterioles supplying the exercising muscle dilate; in severe *anoxia*, when generalized vascular dilation occurs; and in the presence of *anemia*, when blood viscosity and hence resistance to flow in the vascular bed are reduced.

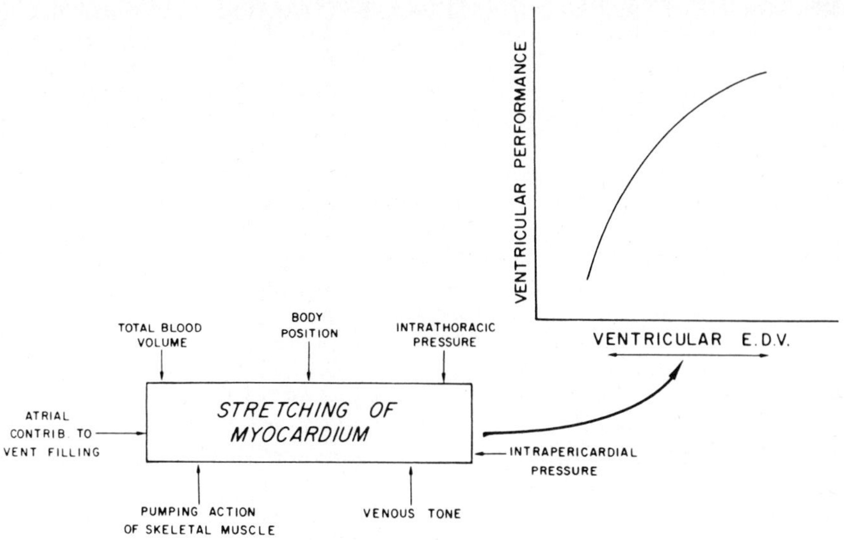

FIGURE 13–31. *Bottom left,* Major influences that determine the degree of stretching of the myocardium, i.e., the magnitude of end-diastolic volume (E.D.V.). *Top right,* Diagram of a Frank-Starling curve, relating ventricular E.D.V. to ventricular performance. (From Braunwald, E., et al.: Mechanisms of Contraction of the Normal and Failing Heart, 2nd ed. Boston, Little, Brown, 1976.)

VENOUS RETURN CURVES. The importance of venous return is illustrated by the opposite effects of a vasodilator drug on the stroke volume and cardiac output in the normal circulation and in heart failure. In the framework for describing overall heart and circulatory function described by Guyton[222] (Fig. 13–32), the venous return curve, an inverse relation between venous return and atrial pressure, is influenced by peripheral circulatory factors including the blood volume, venous tone (and to a much lesser extent arterial tone), and the venous resistance. For example, the entire venous return curve is shifted upward by increased peripheral blood volume, and vice versa. The cardiac output curve represents a positive relationship between the atrial pressure and the cardiac output (reflecting the influence of increased preload), and this curve can be shifted upward by positive inotropic effects or decreased afterload and downward by negative inotropic influences or increased afterload.[222] The cardiac output and venous return curves can be represented on the same diagram with right atrial pressure on the abscissa and the cardiac output or venous return on the ordinate (Fig. 13–32). Any steady-state condition can then be represented by the intercept of these two curves.[222]

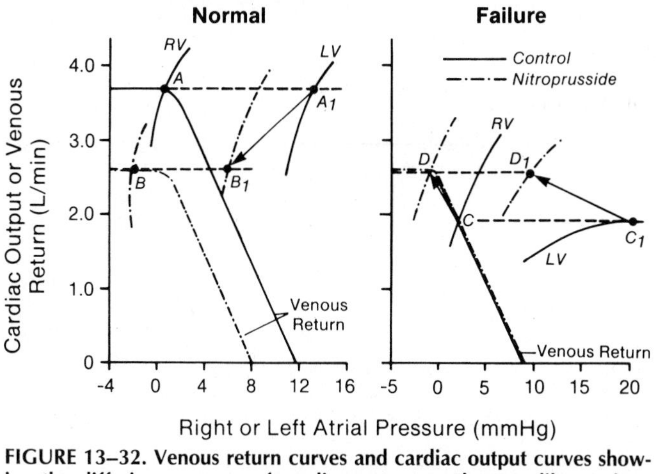

FIGURE 13–32. Venous return curves and cardiac output curves showing the differing response of cardiac output to the vasodilator nitroprusside of the normal and failing heart. *Left,* Responses in the normal heart of the anesthetized dog. Following nitroprusside, the venous return curve is shifted downward (dashed line). Since the cardiac output is limited by the venous return under these conditions, the right ventricular output will fall (point A to point B) despite the leftward shift of the right ventricular cardiac output curve due to decreased afterload. Likewise, despite the shift to the left of its cardiac output curve due to the lowered arterial impedance, the left ventricular output must also fall (point A_1 to B_1). *Right,* In the presence of left ventricular failure, a shift downward of the venous return curve does not occur during nitroprusside infusion (see text). The depressed left ventricular output, rather than the venous return, limits the cardiac output under these conditions, and the reduced afterload on the left ventricle produced by the vasodilator causes a marked shift upward of the left ventricular cardiac output curve and the cardiac output (point C_1 to D_1). The improved left ventricular output is also expressed as an increased right ventricular output (points C to D), as the right ventricular cardiac output curve is also displaced upward and to the left by reduced afterload in the pulmonary circuit. (Modified from Pouleur, H., et al.: Effects of nitroprusside on venous return and central blood volume in the presence of acute heart failure. Circulation *61*:328, 1980, by permission of the American Heart Association, Inc.)

Effects of Venodilation. If nitroprusside is administered intravenously in the relatively normal circulation of the anesthetized dog, the cardiac output falls, despite lowered vascular resistance and hence more favorable loading conditions on the normal left ventricle. This response takes place because nitroprusside induces dilation of the venous bed as well as arteriolar dilation, and the venodilation is only partially compensated for by a modest shift of blood volume from the central to the peripheral circulation.[225] Therefore, the venous return curve is displaced downward because of a decrease in the effective systemic blood volume (Fig. 13–32, left). The ensuing reduction of venous return to the right heart produces a reduction in right ventricular output and hence in left ventricular output via the Frank-Starling mechanism. Thus, a fall in cardiac output occurs because of the limited venous return, despite a reduction of the afterload on the left ventricle (Fig. 13–32, left).[225]

If nitroprusside is administered in the presence of acute experimental left ventricular failure (produced by multiple coronary artery ligations), in which the left ventricular end-diastolic pressure is elevated to more than 20 mm Hg, an *opposite* effect occurs and the cardiac output increases. Again, nitroprusside produces venodilation in the peripheral circulation, but in the setting of heart failure there is a more than threefold greater shift of blood volume from the distended central circulation to the peripheral bed.[225] This presumably occurs because the failing left ventricle is able to unload more effectively against the lowered systemic arteriolar resistance, thereby allowing a release of blood stored within the heart and lungs. Under these conditions, nitroprusside did not shift the venous return curve downward (Fig. 13–32, right), indicating that the shift of blood volume from the central circulation exactly counterbalanced the effect of nitroprusside to reduce the effective systemic blood volume. The marked shift upward of the cardiac output curve caused by correction of excessive afterload (afterload mismatch) on the failing left ventricle could then be expressed as an increase in the cardiac output. Under these conditions the failing left ventricle (not the venous return) became the limiting factor for cardiac output (Fig. 13–32, right).[225]

TOTAL BLOOD VOLUME. When blood volume is rapidly reduced, cardiac output and particularly stroke volume decline. However, in the intact organism, small (less than 15 per cent of control) or gradual reductions in blood volume can be tolerated with barely perceptible changes in cardiac output, as a consequence of a number of compensatory mechanisms resulting from activation of the adrenergic nervous system.

DISTRIBUTION OF BLOOD VOLUME. At any given total blood volume, the ventricular end-diastolic volume is a function of the distribution of blood between the intra-

and extrathoracic compartments. The principal determinants of this distribution are given in the following paragraphs.

Body Position. Gravitational forces pool blood in the dependent portions of the body; therefore, assumption of the upright posture increases extrathoracic blood volume at the expense of intrathoracic and ventricular end-diastolic volumes, thereby reducing preload and cardiac output. The effects of negative pressure (suction) applied to the lower extremities and trunk with the subject supine mimic those of assumption of the upright posture, while inflation of a lower-body positive-pressure suit, immersion of the lower extremities and trunk into water, or the absence of gravitational force during space flight increases intrathoracic blood volume and preload.

Intrathoracic Pressure. The negative intrathoracic pressure normally increases thoracic blood volume, improving cardiac filling and augmenting preload and thereby cardiac performance. The intrathoracic pressure becomes most negative during inspiration and approximates atmospheric pressure during expiration. Accordingly, the gradient for venous return (and therefore right ventricular stroke volume) rises during inspiration when the intrathoracic pressure declines. Elevation of mean intrathoracic pressure, as occurs with the application of positive-pressure respiration or the development of pneumothorax, tends to impede total venous return to the heart, diminishes intrathoracic blood volume, and ultimately reduces ventricular performance.[226]

Intrapericardial Pressure (See also Chapter 44). When pericardial pressure is elevated, as occurs in pericardial effusion, there is interference with cardiac filling, and the resultant reduction in ventricular diastolic volume (preload) reduces ventricular performance. With marked elevations of intrapericardial pressure, cardiac tamponade may occur, which is characterized by marked lowering of stroke volume and arterial pressure with circulatory collapse. Chronic constrictive pericarditis also impedes ventricular filling and thereby lowers stroke volume.[227]

Venous Tone. Smooth muscle in the walls of the veins responds to a variety of neural and humoral stimuli; venoconstriction occurs during exercise, anxiety, deep respiration, or marked hypotension, tending to augment intrathoracic blood volume.[228] A variety of drugs act on venous smooth muscle. Thus, sympathomimetic agents produce venoconstriction, while ganglionic blocking agents and sympatholytic and norepinephrine-depleting drugs or agents such as nitroglycerin that are direct venodilators[229] produce extrathoracic pooling and thereby ultimately reduce preload and cardiac output. Extravascular compression of the veins by skeletal muscle plays an important role in augmenting venous return by exercising skeletal muscle.[230]

ATRIAL CONTRIBUTION TO VENTRICULAR FILLING. A vigorous, appropriately timed atrial contraction augments ventricular filling and end-diastolic volume.[212]

AFTERLOAD

When applied to the intact ventricle, afterload may be defined as the tension, force, or stress (force per unit of cross-sectional area) acting on the fibers in the ventricular wall *after* the onset of shortening. It is importantly influenced by the arterial pressure and is a key determinant of the quantity of blood ejected by the ventricle.[231] In the intact heart, abrupt alterations in the impedance to left ventricular ejection when the preload is constant cause reciprocal changes in wall shortening and the stroke volume of the left ventricle[231–233] (Fig. 13–27, left).

VENTRICULOARTERIAL COUPLING. The coupling between the left ventricle and the arterial system depends on the independent properties of each (Fig. 13–33). At any equilibrium point, the inverse linear relation between the left ventricular systolic pressure and stroke volume or cardiac output resulting from the effect of afterload on shortening will intersect with the positive linear relation between stroke volume and the systolic arterial pressure.[197, 209] This reflects the increased arterial pressure as flow through the arteries is increased. If vascular resistance is increased, for example, the slope of the relation between cardiac output and arterial pressure will decrease (i.e., pressure will be higher at any cardiac output). At equilibrium, the capability of the heart of generating systolic pressure just balances the pressure needed to push blood through the arterial system.[209]

The influence of variations in afterload on the systolic performance of the intact ventricle also can be studied using the isotonically contracting heart preparation in which the other two determinants of ventricular performance (preload and contractility) are held constant. Increasing the afterload reduces both stroke volume and the extent and velocity of wall shortening. Curves showing inverse relationships between afterload (systolic pressure or wall stress) and stroke volume, extent of wall shortening (Fig. 13–29, right panel), and velocity of shortening can be constructed.[193, 194, 209, 234]

BASIS FOR USE OF AFTERLOAD REDUCTION. The low impedance to left ventricular ejection (reduction in afterload) produced by mitral regurgitation,[235] patent ductus arteriosus, ventricular septal defect, or arteriovenous fistula can increase the extent of shortening and the ejection fraction. In the acutely pressure- and/or volume-overloaded ventricle, when sarcomere length is optimal and there is no preload reserve, any alteration in afterload causes a reciprocal change in stroke volume.[220] It is clear that the more severely depressed the inotropic state of the heart, the greater the influence of a change in afterload on the extent of myocardial fiber shortening, as evidenced by the decreased slope of the end-systolic pressure-volume relation in heart failure (Fig. 13–27, right). These considerations are relevant to the use of vasodilating agents to augment cardiac output in patients with left ventricular failure (Fig. 17–17, p. 519) and the use of pressor agents in the assessment of left ventricular function.

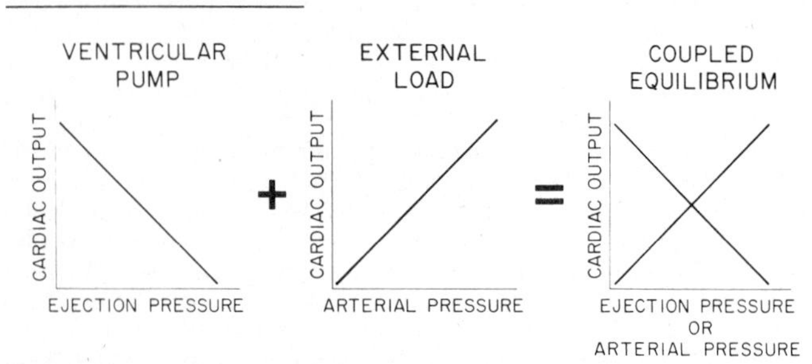

FIGURE 13–33. The functional coupling of the left ventricular pump to the arterial system. *Left,* The ventricular pump responds to an increase in ejection pressure (afterload) with a reciprocal reduction of cardiac output. *Center,* The arterial pressure rises directly with an increase in cardiac output. *Right,* The intersection of these two relations leads to unique values for arterial pressure and cardiac output (at any level of preload and myocardial contractility). (From Weber, K. T.: The contractile behavior of the heart and its functional coupling to the circulation. Prog. Cardiovasc. Dis. *24*:389, 1982, by permission of Grune and Stratton.)

When the ventricle is not operating along the steep portion of its diastolic pressure-volume curve, i.e., when there is still some preload reserve, an elevation of afterload often results in a compensatory elevation of ventricular end-diastolic volume, i.e, a rise in ventricular preload, which enhances myocardial contraction. However, as a consequence of the operation of Laplace's law (p. 405), this compensatory elevation of preload elevates myocardial tension development (afterload) further, and this in turn reduces myocardial fiber shortening. However, geometrical considerations dictate that the relative extent of myocardial fiber shortening required to maintain stroke volume constant is less in the larger ventricle. Hence, stroke volume may remain constant even though myocardial fiber shortening declines. If afterload rises, and if inflow into the ventricle is not restricted and preload can also rise, stroke volume can be maintained. In accord with these considerations, the normal subject responds to a modest rise in arterial pressure by maintaining stroke volume and increasing stroke work while augmenting left ventricular end-diastolic pressure and volume, i.e, the increase in afterload is met by an increase in preload (Fig. 13–27, left), whereas in the diseased heart stroke volume and stroke work tend to fall because there is little, if any, preload reserve.[219, 220] Thus, the response to increased aortic pressure is dependent in significant measure both on the level of myocardial contractility and on the preload, in that a moderate pressor stress will ordinarily produce little change in stroke volume in the normal heart but will diminish stroke volume in heart failure. When there is relative hypovolemia or the pressor stress is substantial, and preload cannot rise appropriately, an increase in afterload will reduce the stroke volume in the normal heart (Fig. 13–27, left, beat 2).

EFFECTS OF AFTERLOAD ON VENTRICULAR RELAXATION. In isolated muscle, an increase in afterload applied during the first two-thirds of contraction delays the onset and slows the rate of relaxation, whereas loading late in the cycle ("relaxation loading") induces premature relaxation and increases its rate.[236] Such load dependence of relaxation depends on the degree of muscle activation by calcium, and in one study load dependence diminished when the calcium reuptake mechanism was depressed, as in hypoxemia.[236] The load dependence of relaxation has recently been demonstrated in the whole heart by rapid, single-beat volume loading of the left ventricle at various phases of the cardiac cycle.[237] Late systolic loading after approximately the first third of ejection caused abbreviation of ejection and a more rapid relaxation rate, whereas early systolic loading prolonged the ejection-relaxation time.[237] Mixed early and late systolic loading which is more gradual (occurring over several beats, such as with descending aortic compression), even when the predominant loading is late during ejection, does not appear to cause enhanced relaxation but rather an abbreviated ejection time with reduced relaxation rate.[238, 239] The mechanism of the responses to sudden loading at different times of the cardiac cycle may relate to the availability of free Ca^{++} with stretch or loading early in the cycle (when Ca^{++} concentration is high) leading to increased cross-bridge formation, whereas later in the cycle (when Ca^{++} is being rapidly removed by the sarcoplasmic reticulum) the sudden load breaks cross bridges, which cannot re-form because of reduced Ca^{++} availability. The precise contribution of such load-dependent relaxation during the normal cardiac cycle, or in chronic states of abnormal loading such as valvular heart disease, remains to be elucidated. Such effects, together with the important influence on relaxation of catecholamines[239] (which increase the rate of Ca^{++} reuptake) and nonuniformity of contraction, constitute three intrinsic factors that can regulate ventricular relaxation.[236]

The influence of nonuniformity of relaxation[236] is illustrated by epicardial pacing, which slows isovolumetric ventricular relaxation rate compared with normal electrical activation.[239] Also, delayed early cardiac filling has also been demonstrated when nonuniformity of left ventricular contraction was produced by right ventricular pacing.[240] Studies on the rate of early rapid ventricular filling in animals appear to show changes directionally similar to those in the isovolumetric relaxation rate, during alterations in cardiac loading and infusion of pharmacological agents.[240]

Normally, left ventricular relaxation, reflecting active relaxation and/or viscous factors, usually continues beyond the isovolumetric period into the phase of rapid ventricular filling, so that a substantial deviation upward of this portion of the diastolic pressure-volume relation of the left ventricle can be seen compared to the static pressure-volume relation (as measured during long periods of diastasis, or at end-diastole).[241, 242] Such deviations can be enhanced by increases in the velocity of filling and by increased volume (or muscle length), reflecting viscous components in heart muscle.[243] Under conditions of tachycardia, incomplete relaxation has long been known to occur and to shift the diastolic pressure-volume relation upward. Under these circumstances,[242] as well as in certain disease states (e.g., ischemia, hypertrophic cardiomyopathy), incomplete relaxation may affect the diastolic pressure-volume relation during most of diastole. In addition to ventricular relaxation, other influences (including the pressure difference between the left atrium and the left ventricle[244]), fibrotic changes in the myocardium, or pericardial restraint can also affect the rate of early diastolic ventricular filling.

ROLE OF NONUNIFORMITY DURING ACTIVE CONTRACTION. In addition to significant effects on relaxation, asynchronous or nonuniform activation of the left ventricle can affect systolic performance. Such an effect on performance when normal electrical activation is replaced by ventricular activation (epicardial pacing) under resting conditions is relatively small.[245] However, during inotropic stimulation of the heart, as with treadmill exercise, the exercise-induced increase of left ventricular dP/dt was markedly less with ventricular pacing than with atrial pacing, indicating the importance of synchronous contraction under stress conditions.[246] The myocardial oxygen consumption was also higher at the same systolic pressure during ventricular pacing, suggesting a less efficient contraction.[246]

HOMEOMETRIC AUTOREGULATION, OR THE "ANREP EFFECT." A positive inotropic effect has been said to follow abrupt elevation of systolic aortic and left ventricular pressure.[210, 247–249] This response was first described by Von Anrep in 1912[250] and has been termed the "Anrep effect," or homeometric autoregulation. This effect occurs during the first minutes after aortic pressure is abruptly elevated, with end-diastolic pressure and circumference then tending to fall as stroke volume and stroke work recover. Force-velocity analyses of the left ventricle in anesthetized dogs suggest that it constitutes a small net positive inotropic effect.[248]

Homeometric autoregulation is most marked in the anesthetized state, and studies in conscious animals show that the initial increases in end-diastolic pressure and dimension are minimal at slow heart rates; however, during tachycardia greater initial increases in end-diastolic pressure and dimensions observed during aortic pressure elevation were followed by a much more marked Anrep effect.[251] These observations, together with the finding that reactive hyperemia in the myocardium occurs if aortic

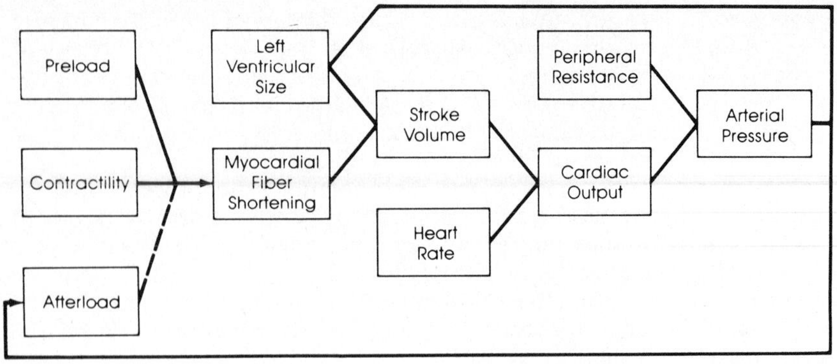

FIGURE 13–34. Schema showing interactions between various components regulating cardiac activity. Solid lines indicate an increasing effect; broken line represents a depressing effect. Note that left ventricular (L.V.) size is a determinant of both stroke volume and afterload. (Reprinted by permission from Braunwald, E.: Regulation of the circulation. N. Engl. J. Med. *290*:1124, 1974.)

pressure is lower early during the Anrep effect but not after the effect is complete, support the concept that the phenomenon is related to recovery from transient subendocardial ischemia.[251]

RIGHT VENTRICULAR FUNCTION. The right ventricle responds to the same determinants of contraction as the left ventricle (preload, afterload, contractility), and it can exhibit a normal ventricular function curve when the left ventricular function curve is depressed, or vice versa. Under normal conditions, the right ventricle is not required for maintenance of pulmonary blood flow, arterial pressure, and cardiac output, as demonstrated by right ventricular bypass models.[252] Although there is a mild increase in the venous pressure at rest when the right ventricle is excluded, the left ventricle is capable of maintaining the circulation. Normally, however, the right ventricle serves to maintain a low pressure in the systemic veins so that edema does not occur,[252] and its function becomes highly important during exercise, hypovolemia, or when the pulmonary vascular resistance is elevated.[253] Also, the right ventricle undergoes hypertrophy in chronic pulmonary hypertension, an adaptation which allows maintenance of a normal stroke volume.[253]

CONTROL OF AFTERLOAD IN THE INTACT ORGANISM. In the intact organism, afterload is determined largely by peripheral vascular resistance, the physical characteristics of the arterial tree, and the volume of blood that it contains at the onset of ejection. The critical role played by ventricular afterload in cardiovascular regulation is summarized in Figure 13–34. While increases in both preload and contractility increase myocardial fiber shortening, increases in afterload reduce it; the extent of myocardial fiber shortening and of left ventricular size determines stroke volume. Arterial pressure, in turn, is related to the product of cardiac output and systemic vascular resistance, while afterload is a function of left ventricular size and arterial pressure. For example, when vasoconstriction raises arterial pressure, afterload is also augmented, which, through a negative feedback mechanism, tends to depress myocardial fiber shortening, stroke volume, and cardiac output; the fall of the latter, in turn, acts to restore arterial pressure to its previous level.

When ventricular function is impaired, afterload becomes an increasingly important determinant of cardiac performance. In the case of the left ventricle, afterload may rise as a consequence of vasoconstriction resulting from the influence on the arterial bed of neural, humoral, and structural changes that occur in response to a fall in cardiac output. This increased afterload may reduce cardiac output further; on the other hand, pharmacological reductions of afterload may be beneficial in elevating cardiac output.

In *summary*, when acute changes in arterial pressure occur, the resultant alteration in afterload has an important effect on cardiac performance. An understanding of the effects of changes in afterload is central to an appreciation of the effects of conditions such as systemic or pulmonary arterial hypertension and obstruction to ventricular ejection by valvular disease (aortic and pulmonic stenosis), which increase afterload, and of mitral regurgitation and ventricular septal defect, which reduce it. Adaptation to a chronic increase in afterload by means of wall hypertrophy, in which a gradual increase in wall thickness occurs and tends to return wall stress and wall shortening characteristics toward normal,[254] is discussed in Chapter 14.

CONTRACTILITY (Inotropic State)

The term "contractility," or "inotropic state," has a different connotation from the term "performance." For practical purposes, it is useful to regard a *change in contractility as an alteration in cardiac performance that is independent of changes resulting from variations in preload or afterload.* When loading conditions remain constant, an improvement in contractility augments cardiac performance (a positive inotropic effect) while a depression in contractility lowers cardiac performance (a negative inotropic effect).

The effects of an increase in contractility induced by a positive inotropic agent such as a catecholamine have been studied in the isotonically contracting heart preparation in which the other determinants of performance (preload, afterload, and contraction frequency) can be held constant. As in isolated muscle, increases in the velocity and extent of wall shortening and increased stroke volume occur while the duration of contraction is shortened and the rate of relaxation increases.[255] The force-velocity relation is shifted upward, P_o and V_{max} both increase (Fig. 13–17), and curves relating diastolic volume to active peak isovolumetric pressure and ventricular function curves are shifted upward (Fig. 13–27, right). Acute administration of negative inotropic agents produces the opposite effects.[256]

THE INTERVAL-STRENGTH RELATION. In the intact ventricle, as in isolated cardiac muscle, premature depolarization results in a reduced mechanical contraction, the extent of the reduction being directly proportional to the degree of prematurity. However, the ensuing contraction is then more forceful than normal, a phenomenon termed "postextrasystolic potentiation".[73, 75] When studied in the isovolumetrically beating heart with preload held constant to exclude loading effects, the degree of augmentation of the postextrasystolic beat (increased contractility, manifested by increased dP/dt) is related in a positive exponential manner to the prematurity (coupling interval) of the extra electrical stimulus (within limits, the earlier the stimulus the greater the potentiation), and in an inverse exponential manner to the delay in the occurrence of the next (postextrasystolic) beat. The effect is related to the quantity of Ca^{++} released from an internal store during the postextrasystolic beat.[257] In the intact organism, when the premature beat is followed by a compensatory pause, the ventricular end-diastolic volume may be augmented, and this increased preload may contribute along with the greater contractility to the enhanced performance that characterizes the postextrasystolic contraction. Postextrasystolic potentiation can be sustained and results in a striking augmentation of myocardial contractility when pairs of stimuli are delivered repetitively to the intact ventricle. In this technique, termed "paired electrical stimulation," the second stimulus is placed immediately after the electrical refractory period and results in only a small secondary contraction.[74, 75, 258]

Pulsus alternans (alternating weak and strong beats) sometimes is observed experimentally when cardiac contractility has deteriorated and the heart rate is rapid, and can be noted in patients with severe myocardial disease. Its basic cause is unknown, but experimental studies indicate that alternating changes in contractility occur in addition to accompanying alterations of preload and afterload.[259]

Control of Contractility in the Intact Organism

The factors that modify the contractility of the myocardium may be considered to operate by modifying the level of ventricular performance at any given ventricular end-diastolic volume, i.e., the relative position of the entire Frank-Starling curve (Fig. 13–35).

Sympathetic Nerve Activity. The quantity of norepinephrine (NE) released by sympathetic nerve endings in the heart is probably the most important factor regulating myocardial contractility under physiological conditions. Rapid changes in contractility in the intact organism are effected by variations in the impulse traffic in the cardiac adrenergic nerves. Beta-adrenoceptor blocking agents and NE-depleting drugs interfere with the myocardial response to sympathetic nerve stimuli.

Circulating Catecholamines. When stimulated by nerve impulses, the adrenal medulla releases epinephrine, which is carried by the bloodstream to the myocardium, where it acts upon beta receptors to augment contractility. This mechanism is slower than the response to NE release by cardiac nerves but may be of physiological importance in conditions such as hypovolemia and a variety of chronic stresses, including congestive heart failure.

Interval-Strength Relation. As described above, myocardial contractility may be influenced profoundly by the rate and rhythm of cardiac contraction. For example, a ventricular extrasystole augments contractility, although to a decreasing extent, for several cardiac cycles. A simple increase in frequency in the physiological range also augments cardiac contractility, but this effect is more prominent in isolated heart muscle or in the intact heart with depressed function than it is in the normal heart of the intact organism.

Exogenous Inotropic Agents. The cardiac glycosides, sympathomimetic agents, Ca^{++}, caffeine, theophylline, amrinone, and their derivatives (Chap. 17) all augment cardiac contractility.

Physiological and Pharmacological Depressants. These include anoxia,[260] ischemia (Chap. 37),[261] acidosis,[262] and local anesthetics (Chap. 21), barbiturates, and most general anesthetics.

Loss of Contractile Mass. When a portion of the ventricle becomes necrotic, as occurs in ischemic heart disease, the overall performance of the ventricle at any given end-diastolic volume is reduced, even though the contractility of the remaining myocardium may be normal (Chap. 38).

Intrinsic Myocardial Depression. Although, as indicated in Chapter 14, the fundamental mechanism responsible for depression of myocardial contractility in heart failure still remains to be elucidated, it is now apparent that the contractile state of each unit of myocardium is depressed in this condition.

HEART RATE

Accelerating the frequency of contraction generally does not induce a shift of the ventricular function curve, i.e., the relation between ventricular end-diastolic pressure and stroke work, in the open-chest anesthetized dog; however, it does increase stroke power (rate of performance of stroke work) at any given level of filling pressure,[263] a finding consistent with improvement of myocardial contractility and with observations on the effects of increases in the frequency of contraction in isolated cardiac muscle. Pacing-induced increases in contraction frequency, unaccompanied by sympathetic stimulation of the ventricle, also increase the calculated V_{max} and elevate the force-velocity relation of the ventricle in the anesthetized open-chest dog, and augment the relaxation rate.[71]

The positive inotropic effect resulting from an increase in the frequency of contraction is more prominent in the anesthetized animal, in the depressed heart, and in isolated cardiac muscle than in the normal heart of the intact, conscious dog.[72] In the conscious state at rest, venous

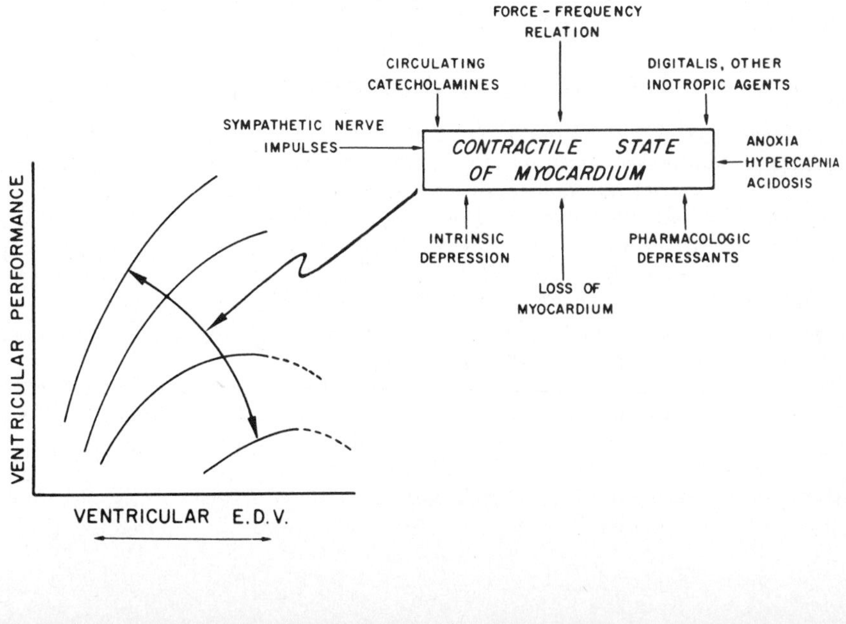

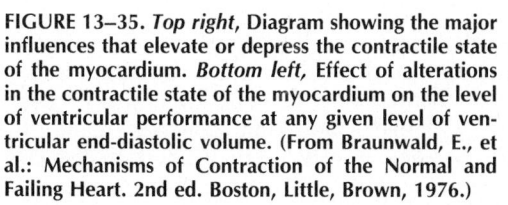

FIGURE 13–35. *Top right,* **Diagram showing the major influences that elevate or depress the contractile state of the myocardium.** *Bottom left,* **Effect of alterations in the contractile state of the myocardium on the level of ventricular performance at any given level of ventricular end-diastolic volume. (From Braunwald, E., et al.: Mechanisms of Contraction of the Normal and Failing Heart. 2nd ed. Boston, Little, Brown, 1976.)**

return to the heart is reflexly and metabolically stabilized, so that artificially varying heart rate between about 60 and 160 beats/min has little effect on cardiac output, despite the above-mentioned modest changes in contractility that accompany changes in heart rate.[263] However, if the diastolic volume of the heart is maintained, by increasing venous return as heart rate is increased, an elevation of frequency will augment cardiac output, and during exercise, tachycardia normally plays the major role in increasing cardiac output. Under these circumstances, the speed of ventricular contraction and relaxation are markedly augmented, atrial contraction is enhanced, and the increased venous return can be accommodated, despite the rapid heart rate and reduced diastolic filling time. However, when the heart is paced at a very rapid rate by electrical stimulation of the atrium, with the subject or experimental animal at rest, there is much less inotropic effect on contraction velocity and the duration of contraction, so that diastolic filling time per minute is much less. Therefore, with rapid pacing (and with tachyarrhythmias) the short duration of diastole can lead to interference with the ventricular filling, with a fall in cardiac output when rates approach 180 to 200 min.[264]

Since, at a constant stroke volume, cardiac output is a linear function of heart rate, the ability to alter the latter is a critically important mechanism in the adjustment of cardiac output.[207, 265] The importance of heart rate in the maintenance of cardiac output is reflected in the inability of patients or experimental animals with fixed heart rates to elevate cardiac output appropriately, even when myocardial function is entirely normal. Under normal circumstances, heart rate is determined largely by the slope of phase 4 (spontaneous depolarization) of the sinoatrial node; the intrinsic rhythmicity may be altered by a variety of influences, such as temperature and metabolism, rising with fever and thyrotoxicosis and falling with hypothermia and hypothyroidism. The two neurotransmitters released by autonomic nerves innervating the sinoatrial node play a critical role in the control of heart rate; acetylcholine slows while NE accelerates the slope of diastolic depolarization.

NEURAL CONTROL OF CARDIAC CONTRACTION

The autonomic nervous system is of critical importance in the moment-to-moment regulation of heart rate and contractility and of the capacitance and resistance of the vascular bed, thereby controlling cardiac output, blood flow distribution, and arterial pressure.[265] Neural regulation is capable of producing considerable changes in cardiocirculatory function within seconds, before more slowly acting mechanisms, such as those mediated by metabolic stimuli, circulating catecholamines, and the renin-angiotensin system, exert any effect. The basic function of cardiovascular reflexes is to integrate the function of the heart with the physiological demands of the peripheral circulation in the rest of the body.

Studies of control mechanisms have been greatly aided by observations of instrumented, conscious animals. Many of their responses are substantially different, even opposite, from those observed during study of anesthetized open-chest animals.[266] One major difference is that conscious animals (and humans) in the basal state have reduced sympathetic and augmented parasympathetic tone compared to that seen in the study of anesthetized and particularly anesthetized, open-chest animals.

ANATOMICAL CONSIDERATIONS
(Fig. 13–36)

Sympathetic and parasympathetic preganglionic cells represent the final common pathways of neural impulses to the cardiovascular system. These cells receive both excitatory and inhibitory impulses from all levels of the central nervous system but most importantly from the cardiovascular center in the medulla and from spinal neurons. The medullary cardiovascular centers, operating independently of higher structures, are capable of regulating cardiac contractility and rate, arterial pressure, and even blood flow distribution, but under normal conditions their activity is regulated by influences from higher centers, notably the cerebral cortex, especially its cingulate gyrus, the hypothalamus, and the reticular substance in the pons and the mesencephalon. The impulse traffic from the vasomotor center is heightened by wakefulness, pain, mental and muscular effort, or emotional stress. Tonic activity in the medullary cardiovascular-excitatory center is constantly inhibited by impulses from the cardiovascular mechanoreceptors (both the high-pressure receptors in the carotid sinuses, aorta, and left ventricle and the low-pressure receptors in the atria, pulmonary vascular bed, and ventricles), but the medullary centers also receive input from chemoreceptors in skeletal muscle, skin, the viscera, and the special senses. An increased activity of nerve impulse traffic in the carotid sinus and aortic nerves as well as in vagal afferent fibers from the heart reflexly reduces neural activity in efferent sympathetic fibers and augments efferent vagal discharges. As a result, vasomotor tone in resistance and capacitance vessels and heart rate are reduced, AV conduction is prolonged, and contractility of the atria and ventricles is reduced.

The cell bodies of the sympathetic preganglionic neurons lie in the intermediolateral horns of the spinal cord; most of their axons leave the spinal cord through the anterior roots of the thoracic and first two lumbar spinal nerves, synapse with postganglionic neurons in the chains of ganglia on each side of the spinal cord or in the peripheral sympathetic ganglia, and then traverse peripheral sympathetic nerves or spinal nerves to the heart and blood vessels. Some preganglionic sympathetic nerve fibers pass directly through the sympathetic chains, through the splanchnic nerves, and into the adrenal medulla where they synapse with secretory cells, which are analogous to postganglionic neurons. Catecholamines (predominantly epinephrine) may be released thereby from the adrenal medulla into the bloodstream at times when sympathetic efferent activity involving other organs is heightened. These two means of sympathetic stimulation (neural and humoral) supplement each other, the former acting rapidly but often briefly and the latter acting slowly but in a more sustained fashion.

While considerable overlap of autonomic innervation exists within most portions of the heart, certain regions receive their major supply from restricted sources. The

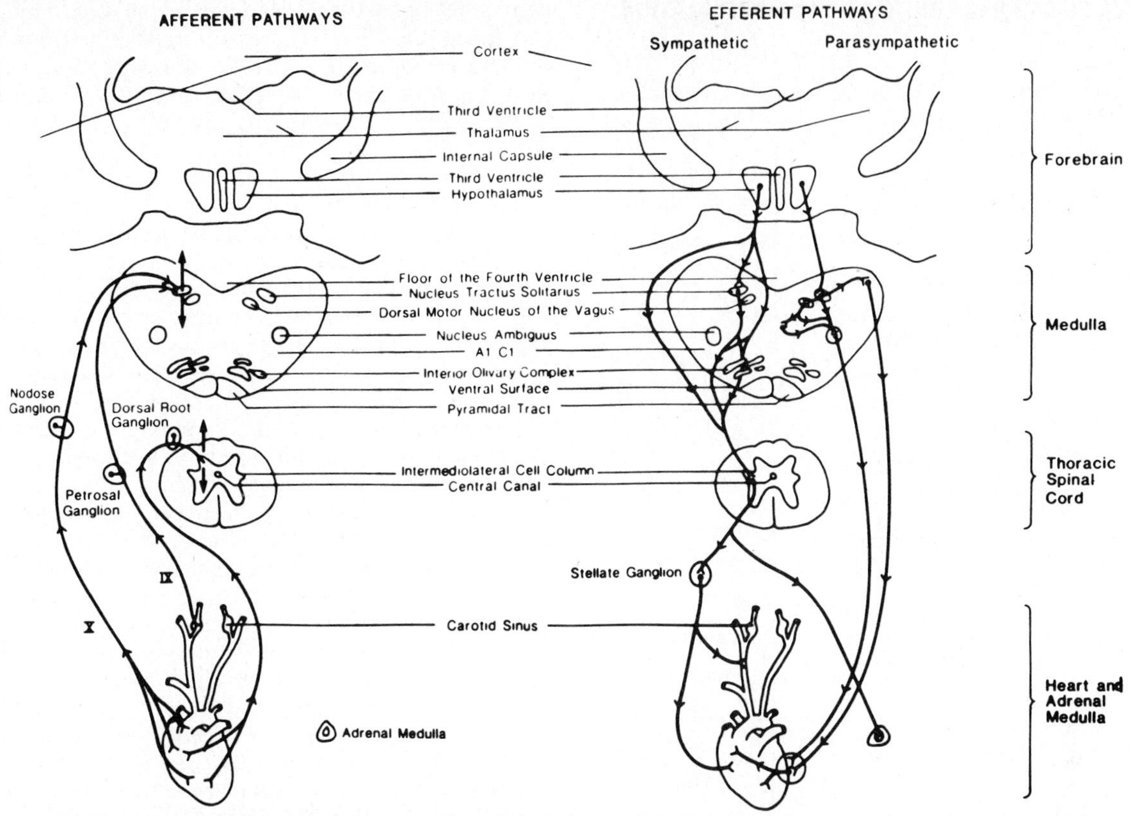

FIGURE 13–36. Schematic diagram of cardiovascular reflex pathways through the central nervous system. *Left,* Afferent limb of the supraspinal and spinal reflex arcs originating from the sensory receptors of the heart and vasculature. The site of the first synapse in the supraspinal arc is at the nucleus tractus solitarius (NTS). *Right,* Efferent sympathetic (left side of diagram) and parasympathetic (right side) pathways. The sympathetic pathway between NTS and the intermediolateral cell column of the spinal cord, which contains the cell bodies of the proganglionic sympathetic efferent fibers, may include synapses at a variety of medullary sites. The medulla depicted here is a composite diagram, because all of the structures, as drawn here, do not exist together in any one given section of the brain stem. The parasympathetic pathway between NTS and nucleus ambiguus, which contains the cell bodies of the preganglionic parasympathetic efferent fibers, may include synapses at a variety of sites, including the dorsal motor nucleus of the vagus, the midline raphe nuclei, or the external cuneate nucleus. Forebrain areas, such as the hypothalamus, may influence autonomic outflow. (From Corr, P. B., Yamada, K. A., and Witkowski, F. X.: Mechanisms controlling cardiac autonomic function and their relation to arrhythmogenesis. *In* Fozzard, H. A., et al. [eds.]: The Heart and Cardiovascular System. New York, Raven Press, 1986, p. 1357.)

sympathetic nerves originating from the right stellate ganglion are distributed primarily to the sinoatrial node and the right atrium, while the left ventrolateral cardiac nerve provides the primary supply to the posterolateral surfaces of the left atrium and ventricle; the central representation of these nerves may allow selective and rapid regulation of cardiac function. Contractility of both the epicardial and endocardial surfaces of the left ventricle can be independently altered, and it is now clear that certain nerves preferentially supply nodal tissues while others innervate contractile tissues.[267] The sympathetic nerve endings in the atria and ventricles are interposed between muscle bundles. The terminal sympathetic innervation of the heart is a plexiform structure, the so-called *perimuscular* or *perimysial plexus,* which extends around the muscle cells in close apposition to, but without penetrating, the myocardial cells. The cardiac muscle cells and innervating fibers might be considered to be analogous to a neuromuscular unit in skeletal muscle. When the rate of liberation of the neurotransmitter exceeds the capacity of the enclosed units to utilize or metabolize it, it may overflow into vascular channels.[268]

NOREPINEPHRINE, THE ADRENERGIC NEUROTRANSMITTER (Fig. 13–37)

The norepinephrine (NE) present in the heart is synthesized and then stored in the sympathetic nerve fibers rather than in the myocardial cells per se. Chemical sympathectomy with 6-hydroxydopamine, cardiac denervation, and treatment with catecholamine-depleting drugs such as reserpine all result in a striking reduction in NE content of the heart as well as in the disappearance of histochemical fluorescence. Sympathetic nerve endings contain neurosecretory granules ranging in size from 400 to 700 nm, and the depolarization of the neurons causes release of intraneuronal Ca^{++}, which in turn causes the NE-containing granules to migrate to the cell membrane of the neuron, there to liberate NE.

The effects of released NE are terminated by three mechanisms[269]: (1) approximately 75 per cent is taken back into the adrenergic neuron (reuptake) by means of an energy-dependent pump; once inside the neuron, much of the transmitter is again taken up into the neurosecretory granules and is available for subsequent re-release; (2) escape of NE into the circulation is metabolized by catechol-O-methyltransferase (COMT) to normetanephrine, some of which is further converted into vanillylmandelic acid (VMA) via the action of monoamine oxidase (MAO); and finally (3) conversion of NE intraneuronally to 3,4-dihydroxymandelic acid by MAO and then to VMA by COMT. The heart and other organs exhibit supersensitivity to NE after surgical denervation or the administration of cocaine and tricyclic antidepressants. These interventions prevent the neuronal uptake of NE, thus making a larger quantity of neurotransmitter available for binding to the

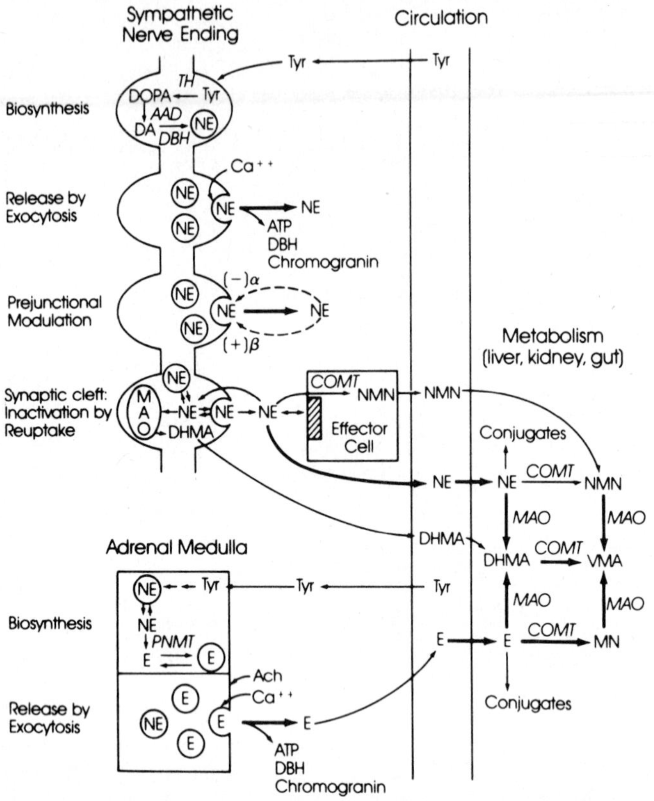

FIGURE 13–37. Catecholamine biosynthesis, release, and metabolism. Schematic representation of a peripheral sympathetic nerve ending is shown at the top; the bulbous areas on the terminal fiber represent varicosities identified by histochemical fluorescence techniques as areas of high neurotransmitter concentration. The processes of biosynthesis, release, modulation, and reuptake are shown sequentially for demonstration purposes only; in vivo they proceed concurrently. Adrenal medullary chromaffin cells are shown at the bottom of the diagram. TH = tyrosine hydroxylase, AAD = aromatic-L-amino acid decarboxylase, DA = dopamine, DBH = dopamine-beta-hydroxylase, NE = norepinephrine, PNMT = phenylethanolamine-N-methyltransferase, E = epinephrine, COMT = catechol-O-methyltransferase, NMN = normetanephrine, MAO = monoamine oxidase, DHMA = 3,4-dihydroxymandelic acid, VMA = 3-methoxy-4-hydroxymandelic acid. (From Landsberg, L., and Young, J. B.: Physiology and pharmacology of the autonomic nervous system. *In* Braunwald, E., Isselbacher, K., Petersdorf, R. G., Wilson, J. D., and Fauci, A. S. [eds.]: Harrison's Principles of Internal Medicine. 11th ed. New York, McGraw-Hill, 1987, p. 358.)

receptor sites, and augment the response to NE. The denervated heart also exhibits hyperresponsiveness to circulating catecholamines, principally epinephrine, because of an increase in beta-adrenoceptor density.[270]

The peripheral effects mediated by NE and epinephrine have been classified as alpha or beta. An important effect of NE is to cause vasoconstriction, an action on postsynaptic alpha$_1$ receptors on vascular smooth muscle. The mechanisms by which NE acts upon cardiac beta and alpha receptors is discussed on page 394. Adrenergic neurons contain a variety of presynaptic receptors (Fig. 13–37); acetylcholine (released from vagal nerve endings) acts on muscarinic receptors on adrenergic neurons, inhibiting the release of NE. Circulating epinephrine acts on presynaptic beta receptors, enhancing the release of NE. On the other hand, the released NE acts on presynaptic alpha$_2$ receptors, thereby inhibiting its own release (feedback inhibition).

As we have seen, NE, the natural transmitter for sympathetic neurons, has both alpha and beta receptor–stimulating properties. When NE is given systemically, the alpha vasoconstrictor action predominates, and the elevation of arterial pressure results in reflex bradycardia and an increase in stroke volume and coronary blood flow but no change in cardiac output. *Epinephrine*, synthesized only in the adrenal medulla, also has combined alpha and beta actions, but its beta effects are more striking than those of NE, especially in low doses; therefore, it produces tachycardia and an elevation of cardiac output. *Dopamine* is the third naturally occurring catecholamine that subserves a transmitter function in the central nervous system. When infused, it has both alpha and beta effects and in addition acts on what appear to be specific dopamine receptors. At low doses (1 to 5 μg/kg/min, administered intravenously), it dilates mesenteric and renal vessels, producing increased renal blood flow and sodium excretion by its action on dopamine receptors. At slightly higher doses (5 to 10 μg/kg/min), beta stimulation increases cardiac output with relatively little tachycardia. At even higher doses (> 10 μg/kg), tachycardia and alpha stimulation occur. *Isoproterenol* is a synthetic compound with pure beta-agonist activity, causing a reduction in peripheral vascular resistance with an increase in heart rate and contractility and thus an increase in cardiac output.

When sympathetic nerves to the heart are stimulated, arterial NE concentrations rise, proportional to the workload and heart rate achieved during exercise. Also, coronary sinus catecholamine concentrations exceed those in arterial blood, indicating that the heart liberates large quantities of NE consequent to activation of sympathetic fibers, and that this NE exceeds the capacity for reuptake and local metabolism, resulting in a "spillover" into the circulation.[271]

THE PARASYMPATHETIC SYSTEM. The vagi provide rich parasympathetic innervation of the sinoatrial and A-V nodes, and, to a slightly lesser extent, of the myocardium. The parasympathetic neurotransmitter acetylcholine has a very brief duration of action, since it is rapidly hydrolyzed by the large quantities of acetylcholinesterase in the heart. The ventricular myocardium is only sparsely innervated by parasympathetic efferent nerves. There is some functional parasympathetic innervation of the ventricles, because when heart rate, preload, afterload, atrial function, and coronary perfusion pressure are all held constant, vagal stimulation depresses ventricular contractility. In the basal state, sympathetic activity is low and parasympathetic restraint is dominant. For this reason, beta-adrenoceptor blockade has relatively little effect on sinoatrial automaticity or A-V conduction of a human or animal in the basal state, while cholinergic blockade with atropine causes an increase in heart rate and acceleration of A-V conduction. In addition, cholinergic blockade does not alter the left ventricular inotropic response during exercise, consistent with the hypothesis that there is little if any parasympathetic tone during exercise.[270]

CARDIAC CONTROL IN THE INTACT ORGANISM (Fig. 13–38)

In the normal state, there are several redundant mechanisms that contribute to cardiac performance, and interference with one or even more of them may not influence the resting cardiac output. For example, a moderate reduction of blood volume or loss of the atrial contribution to ventricular contraction can ordinarily be sustained without a reduction of cardiac output in the resting state. Presumably, other factors such as an increase in adrenergic nerve impulse traffic, which augments contractility, and

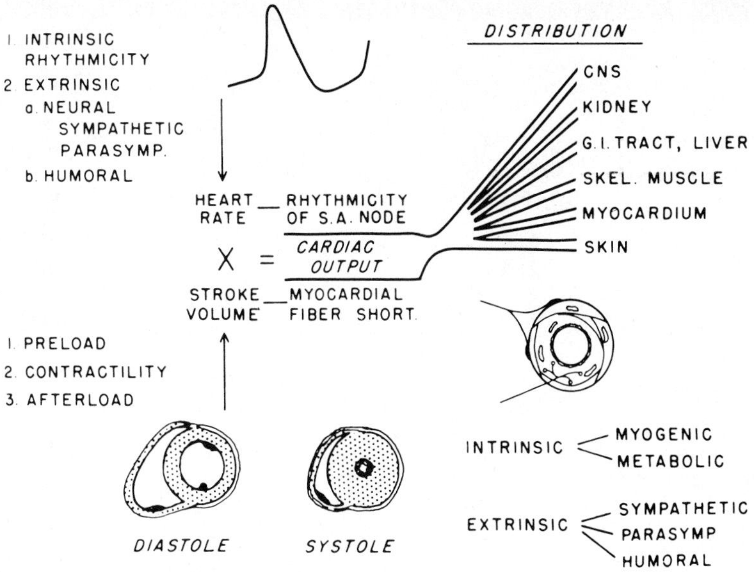

FIGURE 13–38. Schema of factors affecting systemic circulation. In the center, cardiac output is shown with its two determinants, heart rate and stroke volume; the former is a function of the automaticity of the sinoatrial (S.A.) node, while the latter is dependent on the extent of myocardial fiber shortening. The principal determinants of heart rate and stroke volume are listed at the extreme left. Distribution of cardiac output through various vascular beds is shown at the upper right (CNS = central nervous system). The two principal influences (intrinsic and extrinsic) on the lumen of the peripheral resistance vessels and their major determinants are shown at the lower right. (Reprinted by permission from Braunwald, E.: Regulation of the circulation. N. Engl. J. Med. *290*:1124, 1974.)

venoconstriction, which increases ventricular filling, can compensate for this depression.[272] Mechanisms are also available to prevent unnecessary elevation of cardiac output. For example, in normal subjects, expansion of blood volume, a simple increase in heart rate induced by atropine or electrical pacing, or augmentation of myocardial contractility by means of cardiac glycosides does not increase cardiac output.[273, 274] Some of these stimuli may reduce the frequency of adrenergic nerve impulses to the heart, thereby tending to oppose the direct inotropic effect.[275] More importantly, since the normal heart is capable of expelling all of the blood returned to it under most physiological conditions, cardiac output is ordinarily a function of venous return, not of the level of contractility. Since the latter does not limit the volume of blood ejected by the heart in the normal subject except perhaps under severe stress, stimulation of myocardial contractility would not be expected to elevate cardiac output in a normal subject at rest or during mild activity unless there is a simultaneous reduction in peripheral arterial resistance (as occurs with isoproterenol administration),[276] or when this increased contractility is accompanied by an augmentation of venous return. In the presence of congestive heart failure, on the other hand, cardiac output is usually limited by the contractile state of the myocardium, and a positive inotropic influence or reduction of afterload raises cardiac output.[258]

CIRCULATORY ADJUSTMENT DURING EXERCISE

During maximal exercise, total body oxygen consumption may increase ten- to twelvefold, cardiac output four- to fivefold, and the arteriovenous–mixed venous oxygen difference may rise more than twofold. There is a redistribution of blood flow from nonexercising areas such as the splanchnic bed, with an enormous increase in flow to the exercising muscles.

PERIPHERAL CIRCULATORY RESPONSES. As important as the heart may be in mediating the body's response to isotonic exercise, alterations in the peripheral circulation are of at least equal significance. Indeed, the elevation of cardiac output achieved in the resting state through infusion of a maximal dose of isoproterenol, which greatly augments cardiac rate and contractility, does not approach the level commonly observed during exercise. Changes in the peripheral circulation act in concert to augment the capacity of the vascular bed to return blood to the heart.[277] Perhaps the most important of these is the vasodilation that takes place in the blood vessels supplying the exercising muscles, resulting primarily from metabolic stimuli, but perhaps also through the activation of cholinergic nerves innervating arterioles that supply skeletal muscle. The marked reduction in systemic vascular resistance acts in a manner analogous to the opening of multiple arteriovenous fistulas and greatly reduces the resistance to the return of blood ejected from the left ventricle back to the right atrium. Despite profound vasodilation in the metabolizing muscles during exercise, arterial pressure tends to rise in normal subjects, primarily as a consequence of the marked elevation of cardiac output but also as a result of vasoconstriction, which occurs in many vascular beds other than in the heart and the exercising limbs.[278] This elevation of arterial pressure enhances perfusion of the exercising muscle. Failure of arterial pressure to rise during exercise usually signifies severe impairment of left ventricular function and reflects an inadequate rise of cardiac output (p. 403). Other factors that facilitate venous return during exercise include the rhythmic tensing of the skeletal muscles, not only of the exercising limbs but of the abdomen and thorax as well, which compresses the veins and displaces blood centrally.[277] In addition, during exercise, sympathetic impulses to capacitance vessels further augment venous return.[279]

VENTRICULAR VOLUMES AND DIMENSION. The cardiac response to exercise is complex and involves the interaction of changes in heart rate, contractility, preload, and afterload. In humans, the elevation of cardiac output that occurs during mild exercise in the supine position results almost exclusively from an increase in heart rate, with stroke volume and end-systolic volume showing little change.[280] During maximal exercise in the supine position, stroke volume and end-diastolic volume increase slightly.[281, 282] In contrast, in individuals at rest in the erect position blood pooling below the heart reduces ventricular end-diastolic and stroke volumes at rest. These variables increase markedly during strenuous exertion; these increases in stroke volume contribute substantially to the elevation of cardiac output. Indeed, during maximal treadmill exercise, stroke volume increases to approximately twice the levels present at rest in the upright position.[283, 284] Radionuclide ventriculography obtained at rest and during exercise in normal subjects (Fig. 13–39) has shown increases in ejection fraction, stroke volume, left ventricular end-diastolic vol-

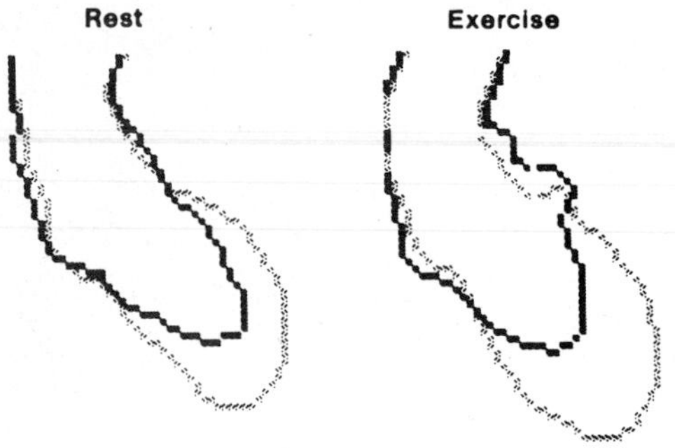

	Rest	Exercise
EF (%)	64	76
EDV (ML)	147	185
ESV (ML)	53	44
SV (ML)	94	140
CO (L/Min)	8.1	21.7
CI (L/Min/M²)	4.0	10.9
HR (Beats/Min)	86	155
PTT (Sec)	10.2	3.1
PBV (L)	1.37	0.56

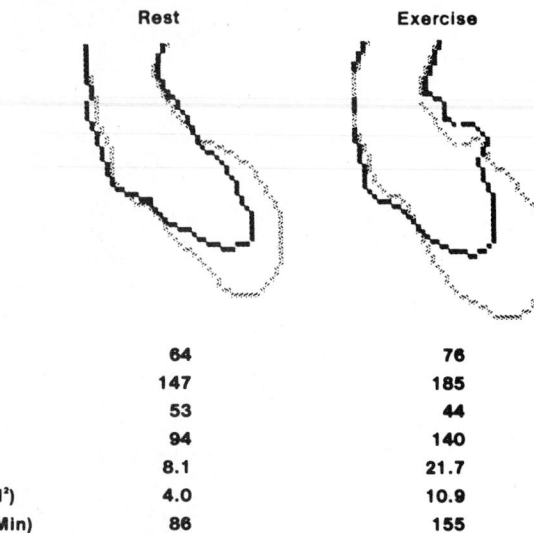

FIGURE 13–39. First-pass radionuclide ventriculograms obtained at rest and during exercise in a normal subject. The images show superimposed end-diastolic (light) and end-systolic (dark) perimeters. CI = cardiac index; CO = cardiac output; EDV = end-diastolic volume; EF = ejection fraction; ESV = end-systolic volume; HR = heart rate; PBV = pulmonary blood volume; PTT = mean pulmonary transit time; SV = stroke volume. (From Iskandrian, A. S., et al.: Evaluation of left ventricular function by radionuclide angiography during exercise in normal subjects and in patients with chronic coronary heart disease. Reprinted with permission from the American College of Cardiology. J. Am. Coll. Cardiol. *1*:1518, 1983.)

ume, and cardiac output, with a reduction of end-systolic volume.

The effects of *light* muscular exercise in the supine position on ventricular dimensions have been studied in patients by determining the distances between radiopaque markers sewn onto the epicardium[285] during light exercise in the supine position. End-diastolic dimensions in both ventricles decreased slightly[286, 287] while myocardial contractility rose, as attested to by a shift of the force-velocity relation.[287] Maximal exercise in the dog[221, 270] also results in an increase in end-diastolic dimensions.

HEART RATE. The ability to alter heart rate is an extremely important mechanism for the adjustment of cardiac output during exercise. Indeed, changes in heart rate account in large measure for changes in cardiac output occurring in many circumstances. The increase in cardiac output that occurs in humans during light to moderate exercise in the supine position is accompanied by a parallel augmentation of heart rate, while, as just noted, the stroke volume remains essentially unchanged. The tachycardia of exercise contributes to augmentation of cardiac contractility through operation of the interval-strength relation (p. 413). When heart rate fails to rise normally, as in patients with heart block, the maximal cardiac output that can be achieved during exercise is reduced. As already noted, an increase in heart rate alone in a resting subject does not augment cardiac output.

THE ADRENERGIC NERVOUS SYSTEM. The effects of adrenergic blockade have been studied in an effort to elucidate the role of adrenergic nervous activity in the cardiovascular response to exercise. Beta blockade reduces the endurance for maximal activity, cardiac output, mean arterial pressure, left ventricular minute work, and maximal oxygen uptake and increases the arteriovenous oxygen difference and central venous pressure in normal human subjects during maximal exercise in the upright position.[283] This intervention has no significant effect on ventricular dimensions recorded at rest in the supine position, indicating that there is little tonic adrenergic support under these circumstances. However, after beta blockade, little augmentation of the contractile state occurs during exercise; despite some elevations of heart rate, ventricular end-diastolic dimensions during submaximal exercise are greater than in the unblocked state.[287]

THE FRANK-STARLING MECHANISM. The finding that with light exercise, performed in the supine position, ventricular end-diastolic and stroke volume fail to rise has been used to support the view that the Frank-Starling mechanism is *not* involved in the cardiac response to exercise. However, it is more likely that the increase in end-diastolic volume that occurs during light exercise may not be evident because of the opposing effects of the tachycardia per se and the increased sympathetic activity normally occurring during exercise, both of which contribute to the reduction of end-diastolic cardiac volume; indeed, in the presence of beta blockade, exercise no longer reduces end-diastolic size. This finding is consonant with studies on denervated dogs[288] in which exercise results in greater increases in ventricular end-diastolic dimensions and stroke volume.

There is considerable evidence that the *intensity* of exercise also conditions the cardiac response to this stimulus. Indeed, since, as already noted, stroke volume may double in normal human subjects during maximal exercise in the erect posture,[283, 284] and since the ratio between stroke volume and end-diastolic volume (i.e., the ejection fraction) is normally in the range of 0.67, ventricular end-diastolic volume *must* increase during maximal exercise. The extent to which the Frank-Starling mechanism is utilized during heavy exercise in normal, healthy dogs has been investigated against this background.[221] Profound increases in heart rate (often exceeding 300 beats/min) occur while cardiac output rises four- to fivefold and stroke volume increases by 50 per cent; increases in contractility are also profound. These values probably represent *physiological maxima* in conscious dogs, since the increases in contractility exceed those resulting from maximally tolerable doses of isoproterenol or norepinephrine. Reductions in end-systolic diameter occur, and in contrast to the findings in supine human subjects carrying out mild exercise, small *increases* in end-diastolic diameter and pressure are consistently noted. Thus, an augmentation of preload clearly remains a mechanism by which the heart can augment its performance during severe exertion. Greater increases in end-diastolic size are observed during exercise when heart rate is held constant, indicating again that the tachycardia occurring during exercise counteracts the increase in dimensions that would otherwise occur and that might be considered to mask the contribution of the Frank-Starling mechanism.

Beta-adrenoceptor blockade imposes significant limitations on normal dogs' performance during maximal exercise. The increases in contractility are largely prevented, and the tachycardia and increases in stroke volume and cardiac output are blunted. While slightly greater increases in end-diastolic size occur during exercise after beta blockade, these are not sufficient to augment stroke volume normally.[221] Thus, in the normal dog, activation of beta receptors is responsible for approximately half the increment in heart rate during severe exercise and for an even greater fraction of the augmentation of contractility.

INTEGRATED RESPONSES. The concept that emerges from these observations is that simple tachycardia and adrenergic stimulation of the myocardium are complementary influences, both resulting in improvement of myocardial contractility during isotonic exercise, the latter to a greater extent than the former. Adrenergic stimulation of the heart also shortens the duration of systole, thereby providing more time for diastolic filling at any heart rate, further favoring an augmentation of cardiac output. Since the tachycardia that normally occurs during exercise is dependent only in part on sympathetic nerve stimuli and circulating catecholamines but is also due to withdrawal of vagal restraint, elevations of cardiac output and heart rate can still occur despite adrenergic blockade. However, the degree of improvement of contractility occurring during exercise is reduced during sympathetic blockade, and, as a consequence, the elevation of cardiac output that can occur under these circumstances is limited.[283]

Thus, the normal cardiac response to supine exercise involves the integrated effects on the myocardium of an increase in heart rate, adrenergic stimulation, and the operation of the Frank-Starling mechanism, through an increase in preload consequent to a marked augmentation of venous return. During submaximal exertion, cardiac output can rise when one or even two of these influences are inhibited. However, during maximal levels of muscular exercise, the ventricular myocardium requires all three influences to sustain a level of activity sufficient to satisfy the greatly augmented oxygen requirements of the exercising skeletal muscles.

OTHER ADJUSTMENTS TO EXERCISE. Several other systems aid in the augmented delivery of oxygen to the metabolizing tissues during exercise. Among these are (1) a large increase (up to threefold) in the extraction of oxygen from blood perfusing skeletal muscle; (2) sympathetic stimulation of venous capacitance in beds in the limbs, other muscular beds, and the splanchnic viscera, which displaces blood into the thorax[279]; (3) the augmented activity of thoracic and abdominal respiratory muscles during exercise, which aids substantially in displacing blood from the peripheral venous system to the heart; (4) augmentation of the oxygen-carrying capacity of the arterial blood, a phenomenon particularly prominent in species such as the dog and cat, in which splenic contraction can contribute a substantial quantity of red cell mass to the circulation; (5) rightward displacement of the oxygen-hemoglobin dissociation curve, which facilitates the unloading of oxygen from red cells to the peripheral tissues; and (6) in highly trained endurance athletes, the development of cardiac dilatation and eccentric hypertrophy with enlargement of the ventricular chambers, resembling those occurring in volume overload. This last adaptation, together with a slower than normal heart rate at rest and during exertion, appears to allow higher and more sustained levels of stroke volume and cardiac output.

Although so-called *athlete's heart* was at one time considered to represent an abnormal state, it is now thought that the cardiac enlargement and hypertrophy that occur during this type of physiological conditioning represent a useful adaptive mechanism, undoubtedly important to the elevated maximal oxygen uptake achieved by such individuals.[289] Thus, increased left ventricular dimensions and wall thickness[290] are associated with elevations of stroke volume and right ventricular end-diastolic dimensions at rest; however, the ejection fraction and normalized mean velocity of wall shortening of the left ventricle in the endurance athlete are normal.[291] Many such individuals show electrocardiographic evidence of ventricular hypertrophy as well.[291] Biochemical changes also occur in the trained heart. Hearts removed from rats which had undergone running training showed enhanced Ca-ATPase activities which could exhibit enhanced Ca-dependent myosin light-chain phosphorylation.[292]

During *isometric exercise*, arterial pressure rises even more profoundly than during isotonic exercise. Peripheral vascular resistance rises as a result of the activation of sensory receptors in muscles that cause reflex arteriolar constriction.[293]

OTHER CIRCULATORY ADJUSTMENTS

HYPOVOLEMIA. In contrast to dynamic exercise, causes of hypovolemia such as hemorrhage, dehydration, and others do not appear to induce a major increase in sympathetic stimulation of the heart in conscious dogs.[294] Rather, hypovolemia appears to cause nonuniform activation of the sympathetic nervous system with intense sympathetic activity to the peripheral vascular bed, inducing vasoconstriction in the mesenteric and iliac beds with some reduction in renal sympathetic nerve activity.[270] There is reflex increase in sympathetic stimulation of capacitance beds (and of the spleen in certain animal species), causing displacement of blood into the central circulation and thereby defending cardiac output.[279] The circulatory response to hemorrhage (and other forms of shock) is described in Chapter 19.

THE STARLING MECHANISM. The role of the Starling mechanism, i.e., control of ventricular performance by preload during exercise, is somewhat obscured, as described above. However, it is readily evident in the intact organism when filling pressures are low, as during hypovolemia. The Starling mechanism is also evident in the intact organism when changes in ventricular filling are brought about during respiration and with alterations in the duration of diastole. The Starling relationship also plays a critical role in maintaining equal output between the two ventricles in the steady state.

BAINBRIDGE REFLEX. An increase in heart rate with expansion of blood volume was first described in anesthetized animals early in this century.[295] Vatner and Boettcher studied the relation between blood volume and heart rate in conscious dogs. With volume loading, heart rate increased in proportion to cardiac output, even though the elevation of arterial pressure would tend to oppose it by activation of the carotid sinus reflex, affirming the importance of the Bainbridge reflex under these conditions.[296] On the other hand, volume depletion[297] also caused tachycardia, presumably as a consequence of reflex activation with reduced stimulation of arterial and low pressure receptors.

CHEMORECEPTOR REFLEXES. Chemoreceptors in the aortic arch and carotid bodies are stimulated by reductions in arterial pO_2 and pH, by elevations of arterial pCO_2, by hemorrhage, and by sympathetic efferents. The results are complex and represent the combined effects of the chemoreceptor reflex, which causes bradycardia, vasoconstriction and an increase in contractility, and hyperventilation (the pulmonary inflation reflex), which causes tachycardia and inhibits the positive inotropic response.[270, 298] The net observed effect of chemoreceptor stimulation depends on the balance between the direct reflex changes and those operating through the induced hyperventilation.

Cerebral hypocapnia causes peripheral venous constriction, and cerebral ischemia (the Cushing reflex) causes an increase in peripheral vascular resistance, constriction of the capacitance vessels, and bradycardia.

INTERACTIONS BETWEEN THE SYMPATHETIC AND PARASYMPATHETIC NERVOUS SYSTEMS. Under most physiological circumstances, sympathetic and vagal activity have opposing actions on various cardiac structures and their activity varies reciprocally.[299] For instance, during exercise and even during the anticipation of exercise, there is augmentation of sympathetic activity and inhibition of vagal restraint, causing tachycardia. Sympathetic stimulation increases, while parasympathetic activity inhibits atrial contractility, as reflected in the height of the *a* wave of the atrial pressure causing augmentation and depression of ventricular filling and preload, respectively.

A number of differences and interactions between these two limbs of the autonomic nervous system appear to exist. Thus, the latent period in cardiac activity following the onset of sympathetic stimulation is approximately 2 sec, but it is only about 200 msec following parasympathetic stimulation. Thus, the virtually instantaneous tachycardia induced by a sudden frightening event (the unexpected sound of gunfire at close range) is mediated almost entirely by sudden cessation of parasympathetic restraint on the sinoatrial node, with the effects of sympathetic stimulation to this frightening stimulus developing slightly later. Similarly, the dissipation of the offset are much more rapid for parasympathetic than for sympathetic stimulation.

Antagonism between the two limbs of the autonomic nervous system occurs at higher levels; activation of supramedullary centers cause reciprocal stimulation and depression. Antagonism also occurs both at the postganglionic sympathetic nerve ending (prejunctionally) and at the cardiac effector cell itself (postjunctionally). The vagus terminates in intracardiac ganglions, which are stimulated by acetylcholine released by preganglionic neurons. However, the ganglionic receptors are nicotinic, not muscarinic, and therefore not subject to blockade by atropine. These parasympathetic ganglia, through short interneurons, release acethylcholine, which acts on muscarinic receptors (and therefore can be blocked by atropine) on postganglionic *sympathetic* neurons and on cardiac cells. The action of acetylcholine released by these postganglionic nerve fibers inhibits the release of NE from the former.[299] Indeed, the rate of release of NE into the coronary sinus blood induced by cardiac sympathetic nerve stimulation is greatly diminished by simultaneous vagal stimulation.

Acetylcholine has a number of actions on muscarinic receptors of cardiac cells[300]: (1) It inhibits adenylate cyclase via an inhibitory guanine regulatory protein and thereby reduces the concentration of cardiac cyclic AMP. There are two guanine-nucleotide regulatory units: N_s, which couples sympathetic stimulation to the activation of adenylate cyclase, and N_i, which couples parasympathetic inhibition to depression of adenylate cyclase production (Fig. 17–22, p. 527). (2) Activation of muscarinic cardiac receptors stimulates sarcolemmal permeability of K^+, causing hyperpolarization and a negative chronotropic effect. (3) Stimulation of cardiac muscarinic receptors augments the concentration of cyclic GMP which (analogous to cyclic AMP) phosphorylates specific protein kinases, whose functions differ from those phosphorylated by cyclic AMP and which appear to depress cardiac contractility. (4) Cardiac muscarinic receptors also appear to be coupled through guanylate cyclase to sarcolemmal ion channels. (5) Activation of cardiac muscarinic receptors may also regulate membrane phospholipid turnover and the release of inositol triphosphate, which appears to be involved in the release of membrane-bound Ca^{++} in some tissues.

In conclusion, the manner in which the nervous system modulates cardiac performance is complex (Fig. 13–40). First, both the sympathetic and parasympathetic neurotransmitters affect the performance of working muscle cells

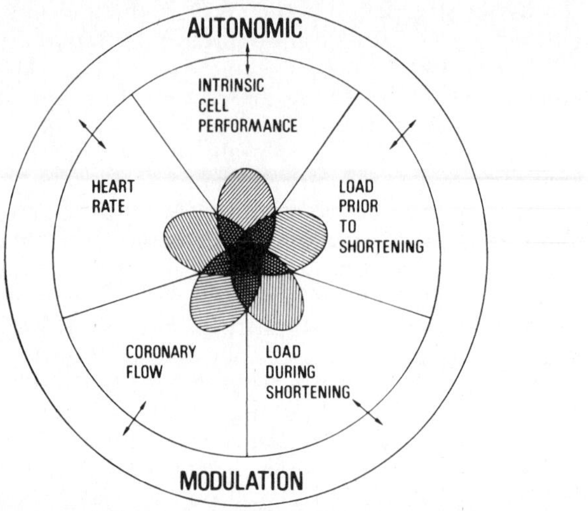

FIGURE 13–40. Multiple interdependent factors that modulate cardiac function. (From Lakatta, E. G.: Determinants of cardiovascular performance; modification due to aging. J. Chron. Dis. *36*:15, 1983.)

and specialized conduction tissue. They also modify heart rate, and by innervation of coronary vessels, myocardial perfusion (Chap. 37). Finally, by modifying nervous system influences they affect the load prior to shortening (preload) and during shortening (afterload).

More complex interactions between the sympathetic and parasympathetic systems also exist. For example, the inhibitory effect on heart rate of a given level of vagal activity is more pronounced the greater the prevailing level of sympathetic activity; this interaction is termed *accentuated antagonism*.

CLINICAL CORRELATIONS

A few examples will serve to demonstrate that the principles of circulatory regulation described above are readily applicable to a variety of clinical situations. For instance, the mechanical lesions characteristic of congenital and rheumatic valvular disease result in abnormalities of ventricular preload or afterload or both. In obstruction to left ventricular outflow, for example, the increase in afterload tends, in the absence of compensatory features, to depress stroke volume and hence cardiac output. Increased afterload imposed by the aorta, which becomes stiffer with age, limits the stroke volume response to exercise.[301] The development of left ventricular hypertrophy reduces the stress on each unit of myocardium, despite an elevated intraventricular pressure. In this manner hypertrophy tends to maintain the afterload of each myocardial cell at or close to normal, although there is, of course, a limit to the compensation that can be provided by this mechanism.

Of the many congenital and valvular abnormalities that produce alterations in ventricular preload, perhaps the most straightforward to consider is atrial septal defect (pp. 915 and 982); as a result of the interatrial communication and the greater compliance of the right ventricle than the left, the preload placed on the right ventricle is greatly augmented and the stroke volume of the right ventricle greatly exceeds that of the left. This congenital lesion is usually well tolerated unless pulmonary artery pressure rises, thereby elevating right ventricular afterload. Lesions such as ventricular septal defect, patent ductus arteriosus, and mitral regurgitation are more complex in that a measure of compensation for the increased preload that is placed on the left ventricle is provided by the lowered afterload that results from unloading of the ventricle through the regurgitant mitral valve, the septal defect, or the aorta–pulmonary artery communication.

REFERENCES

CELLULAR MECHANISMS

1. Sommer, J. R., and Waugh, R. A.: The ultrastructure of the mammalian cardiac muscle cell—with special emphasis on the tubular membrane systems. Am. J. Pathol. *82*:192, 1976.
2. Sommer, J. R.: Ultrastructural considerations concerning cardiac muscle. J. Mol. Cell. Cardiol. *14*: (Suppl. 3):77, 1982.
3. Forbes, M. J., and Sperelakis, N.: Ultrastructure of mammalian cardiac muscle. *In* Sperelakis, N. (ed.): Physiology and Pathophysiology of the Heart. Boston, Martinus Nijhoff, 1984, pp. 3–42.
4. Sommer, J. R., and Jennings, R. B.: Ultrastructure of cardiac muscle. *In* Fozzard, H. A., Haber, E., Jennings, R. B., Katz, A. M., Morgan, H. E. (eds.): The Heart and Cardiovascular System. New York, Raven Press, 1986, p. 61.
5. Fawcett, D. W., and McNutt, N. S.: The ultrastructure of the cat myocardium. I. Ventricular papillary muscle. J. Cell Biol. *42*:1, 1969.
6. Sommer, J. R., and Johnson, E. A.: Ultrastructure of cardiac muscle. *In* Berne, R. M. (ed.): Handbook of Physiology. Section 2, The Cardiovascular System. Vol. I, The Heart. Bethesda, American Physiological Society, 1979, pp. 113–186.
7. Schaper, J., Meiser, E., and Stammler, G.: Ultrastructural morphometric analysis of myocardium from dogs, rats, hamsters, mice and from human hearts. Circ. Res. *56*:377, 1985.
8. Thornell, L., and Erickson, A.: Filament systems in the Purkinje fibers of the heart. Am. J. Physiol. *241:H*-291, 1981.
9. Jamieson, J. D., and Palade, G. E.: Specific granules in atrial muscle cells. J. Cell Biol. *23*:151, 1964.
10. deBold, A. J., Borenstein, H. B., Veress, A. T., and Sonnenberg, H.: A rapid and potent natriuretic response to intravenous injection of atrial myocardial abstract in rats. Life Sci. *28*:89, 1981.
11. Laragh, J.: Atrial natriuretic hormone, the renin-aldosterone axis and blood-pressure-electrolyte homeostasis. N. Engl. J. Med. *313*:1329, 1985.
12. Langer, G. A.: The structure and function of the myocardial cell surface. *In* Levy, M. N., and Vassalle, M. (eds.): Excitation and Neural Control of the Heart. Baltimore, Williams and Wilkins, 1982, pp. 79–92.
13. Katz, A. M.: Membrane structure. *In* Fozzard, H. A., Haber, E., Jennings, R. B., Katz, A. M., and Morgan, H. E. (eds.): The Heart and Cardiovascular System. New York, Raven Press, 1986, p. 101.
14. Robinson, T. F., Cohen-Gould, L., Remily, R., Capasso, J. M., and Factor, S. M.: Extracellular structures in heart muscle. *In* Harris, P., and Poole-Wilson, P. A. (eds.): Advances in Myocardiology. New York, Plenum Publishing, 1985, pp. 243–255.
15. Sato, S., Ashrof, M., Millard, R. W., Fujwara, H., and Schwartz, A.: Connective tissue changes in early ischemia of porcine myocardium: An ultrastructural study. J. Mol. Cell. Cardiol. *15*:261, 1983.
16. Langer, G. A.: Calcium at the sarcolemma. J. Mol. Cell. Cardiol. *16*:147, 1984.
17. Caroni, P., and Carafoli, E.: An ATP-dependent Ca^{2+}-pumping system in dog heart sarcolemma. Nature *283*:765, 1980.
18. Jones, L. R.: Subcellular fractionation of cardiac sarcolemma and sarcoplasmic reticulum. *In* Fozzard, H. A., Haber, E., Jennings, R. B., Katz, A. M., and Morgan, H. E. (eds.): The Heart and Cardiovascular System. New York, Raven Press, 1986, p. 253.
19. Fabiato, A.: Calcium-induced release of calcium from the cardiac sarcoplasmic reticulum. Am. J. Physiol. *245*:Cl, 1983.
20. Huxley, H. E.: The double array of filament in cross-striated muscle. J. Biophys. Biochem. Cytol. *3*:631, 1957.
21. Warber, K. D., and Potter, J. D.: Contractile proteins and phosphorylation. *In* Fozzard, H. A., Haber, E., Jennings, R. B., Katz, A. M., and Morgan, H. E. (eds.): The Heart and Cardiovascular System. New York, Raven Press, 1986, p. 779.
22. Page, S.: Management of structural parameters in cardiac muscle. CIBA Foundation Symposium 24 (New Series), Amsterdam, Elsevier, 1974, p. 13.
23. Lowey, S., Slayter, H. S., Weeds, A. G., and Baker, H.: Substructure of the myosin molecule. I. Subfragments of myosin by enzymic degradation. J. Mol. Biol. *42*:1, 1969.
24. Gevers, W.: The mechanism of myocardial contraction. *In* Opie, L. (ed.): The Heart. New York, Grune and Stratton, 1986, pp. 98–107.
25. Murphy, R. A.: Contraction of muscle cells. *In* Berne, R. M., and Levy M. N. (eds.): Physiology. St. Louis, C. V. Mosby, 1983, pp. 359–386.
26. Eisenberg, E., and Hill, J. L.: Muscle contraction and free energy transduction in biological systems. Science *277*:999, 1985.
27. Scheuer, J., and Bhan, A. K.: Cardiac contractile proteins. Adenosine triphosphatase activity and physiological function. Circ. Res. *45*:1, 1979.
28. Hoh, J. F. Y., McGrath, P. A., and Hale, P. T.: Electrophoretic analysis of multiple forms of rat cardiac myosin: Effect of hypophysectomy and thyroxine replacement. J. Molec. Cell Cardiol. *10*:1053, 1978.
29. Samuel, J-L., Rappaport, L., Mercadier, J.-J., Lompre, A.-M., Sartore, S., Triban, C., Schiaffino, S., and Schwartz, K.: Distribution of myosin isozymes within single cardiac cells. An immunohistochemical study. Circ. Res. *52*:200, 1983.
30. Mercadier, J. J., Lompre, A. M., Wisnewsky, C., Samuel, J. L., Bercovici, J., Swynghedauw, B., and Schwartz, K.: Myosin isoenzymic changes in several models of rat cardiac hypertrophy. Circ. Res. *49*:525, 1981.
31. Schwartz, K., Lecarpentier, Y., Martin, J. L., Lompre, A. M., Mercadier, J. J., and Swynghedauw, B.: Myosin isoenzymic distribution correlates with speed of myocardial contraction. J. Mol. Cell. Cardiol. *13*:1071, 1981.
32. Malhotra, A., Penpargkus, S., Fein, F. S., Sonnenblick, E. H., and Schener, J.: The effect of streptozotocin-induced diabetes in rats on cardiac contractile proteins. Circ. Res. *49*:1243, 1981.
33. Eisenberg, E., and Greene, L. E.: The relation of muscle biochemistry to muscle physiology. Ann. Rev. Physiol. *42*:293, 1980.
34. Ebashi, S.: Regulatory mechanism of muscle contraction with special reference to Ca-troponin-tropomyosin system. Essays Biochem. *10*:1, 1974.
35. Potter, J. D., and Gergely, J.: Troponin, tropomyosin and actin interactions in the Ca^{++} regulation of muscle contraction. Biochemistry *13*:2697, 1974.
36. Greaser, M. L., Yamaguchi, M., Brekke, C., Potter, J., and Gergely, J.: Troponin subunits and their interactions. Cold Spring Harbor Symp. Quant. Biol. *37*:235, 1973.
37. Spudich, J. A., Huxley, H. E., and Finch, J. F.: Regulation of skeletal muscle contraction. II. Structural studies of the interaction of the tropomyosin-troponin complex with actin. J. Mol. Biol. *72*:619, 1972.
38. Perry, S. V.: The regulation of contractile activity in muscle. Biochem. Soc. Trans. *7*:593, 1979.
39. Julian, F. J., Moss, R. L., and Sollins, M. R.: The mechanism for verebrate striated muscle contraction. Circ. Res. *42*:2, 1978.
40. Winegrad. S.: Regulation of cardiac contractile proteins. Circ. Res. *55*:565, 1984.
41. Winegrad, S., Weisberg, A., Lin, E. L., and McClellan, G.: Adrenergic regulation of myosin adenosine triphosphatase activity. Circ. Res. *58*:83, 1986.
42. Ringer, S.: A further contribution regarding the influence of the different constituents of the blood on the contraction of the heart. J. Physiol. (Lond.) *4*:30, 1982.
43. Fabiato, A., and Fabiato, F.: Calcium and cardiac excitation muscle. Mayo Clin. Proc. *57* (Suppl.):6, 1982.
44. McDonald, T. F.: Excitation-contraction coupling: Relationship of the slow inward current to contraction. *In* Sperelakis, N. (ed.): The Physiology and Pathophysiology of the Heart. Boston, Martinus Nijhoff, 1984, p. 187.
45. Blinks, J. R.: Intracellular $[Ca^{2+}]$ measurements. *In* Fozzard, H. A., Haber, E., Jennings, R. B., Katz, A. M., and Morgan, H. E. (eds.): The Heart and Cardiovascular System. New York, Raven Press, 1986, p. 671.
46. Jewell, B. R.: Activation of contraction in cardiac muscle. Mayo Clin. Proc. *57* (Suppl.):6, 1982.
47. Morgan, J. P., Chesebro, J. H., Pluth, J. R., Puga, F. J., and Schaff, H. V.: Intracellular calcium transients in human working myocardium as detected with aequorin. J. Am. Coll. Cardiol *3*:410, 1984.
48. Fabiato, A., and Baumgarten, C. M.: Methods for detecting calcium release from the sarcoplasmic reticulum of skinned cardiac cells and the relationships between calculated transsarcolemmal calcium movements and calcium release. *In* Sperelakis, N. (ed.): Physiology and Pathophysiology of the Heart. Boston, Martinus Nijhoff, 1984, p. 215.
49. Tada, M., Shigekawa, M., and Nimura, Y.: Uptake of calcium by the sarcoplasmic reticulum and its regulation and functional consequences. *In* Sperelakis, N. (ed.): Physiology and Pathophysiology of the Heart. Boston, Martinus Nijhoff, 1984, p. 255.
50. Fabiato, A.: Simulated calcium current can both cause calcium loading in and trigger calcium release from the sarcoplasmic reticulum of a skinned canine cardiac Purkinje cell. J. Gen. Physiol. *85*:291, 1985.
51. Fabiato, A.: Time and calcium dependence of activation and inactivation of calcium-induced release of calcium from the sarcoplasmic reticulum of a skinned canine cardiac Purkinje cell. J. Gen. Physiol. *85*:247, 1985.
52. Watanabe, A. M., and Lindemann, J. P.: Mechanisms of adrenergic and cholinergic regulation of myocardial contractility. J. Gen. Physiol. *85*:377, 1985.
53. Baker, P. F., Hodgkin, A. L., and Ridgeway, E. B.: Depolarization and calcium entry in squid giant axon. J. Physiol. (Lond.) *218*:709, 1971.
54. Coraboeuf, E.: Ionic basis of electrical activity in cardiac tissue. *In* Levy, M. N., and Vassalle, M. (eds.): Excitation and Neural Control of the Heart. Baltimore, Williams and Wilkins, 1982, pp. 1–36.
55. Glitsch, H. G.: Characteristics of active sodium transport in intact cardiac cells. *In* Levy, M. N., and Vassalle, M. (eds.): Excitation and Neural Control of the Heart. Baltimore, Williams and Wilkins, 1982, pp 36–58.
56. Reuter, H., and Scholz, H.: A study of the ion selectivity and the kinetic properties of the calcium dependent slow inward current in mammalian cardiac muscle. J. Physiol. (Lond.) *264*:12, 1977.
57. Chapman, R. A.: Control of cardiac contractility at the cellular level. Am. J. Physiol. *245*:H535, 1983.
58. Flaim, S. F., and Zelis, R. (eds.): Calcium Blockers. Baltimore, Urban and Schwartzenberg, 1982, 303 pp.
59. Braunwald, E.: Mechanisms of action of calcium channel blocking agents. N. Engl. J. Med. *307*:1618, 1982.
60. Keung, E. C. H., and Aronson, R. S.: Physiology of calcium current in cardiac muscle. Prog. Cardiovasc. Dis. *25*:279, 1983.
61. Langer, G. A.: Sodium-calcium exchange in the heart. Ann. Rev. Physiol. *44*:435, 1982.
62. Sheu, S.-S., Sharma, V. K., and Uglesity, A.: Na^{+}-Ca^{2+} exchange contributes to increase of cytosolic Ca^{2+} concentration during depolarization in heart muscle. Am. J. Physiol. *250*:C651, 1986.
63. Sutko, J. L., Bers, D. M., and Reeves, J. P.: Postrest inotropy in rabbit ventricle: Na^{+}-Ca^{2+} exchange determines sarcoplasmic reticulum Ca^{2+} content. Am. J.Physiol. *250*:H654, 1986.
64. Speralakis, N.: The slow action potential and properties of the myocardial slow channels. J. Gen. Physiol. *85*:159, 1985.
65. Philipson, K. D., Bers, D. M., Nishimoto, A. Y., and Langer, G. A.: Binding of Ca^{2+} and Na^{2+} to sarcolemmal membranes: Relation to control of myocardial contractility. Am. J. Physiol. *238*:H373, 1980.
66. McDonald, T.: Excitation-contraction coupling: Relation of the slow inward current to contraction. J. Gen. Physiol. *85*:187, 1985.

67. McDonald, T. F., Pelzer, D., and Trautwein, W.: Does the calcium current modulate the contraction of the accompanying beat? A study of E-C coupling in mammalian ventricular muscle using cobalt ions. Circ. Res. *49*:576, 1981.
68. Maughan, D. W., Low, E. S., and Alpert, N. R.: Isometric force development, isotonic shortening, and elasticity measurements from Ca^{++} -activated ventricular muscle of the guinea pig. J. Gen. Physiol. *71*:431, 1978.
69. Lab, M. J., Allen, D. G., and Orchard, C. H.: The effects of shortening on myoplasmic calcium concentration and on the action potential in mammalian ventricular muscle. Circ. Res. *55*:825, 1984.
70. Johnson, E. A.: Force-interval relationship of cardiac muscle. *In* Berne, R. M. (ed.): Handbook of Physiology. Section 2, The Cardiovascular System. Vol. I, The Heart. Bethesda. American Physiological Society, 1979, pp. 475–496.
71. Covell, J. W., Ross, J., Jr., Taylor, R., Sonnenblick, E. H., and Braunwald, E.: Effects of increasing frequency of contraction of force-velocity relation of left ventricle. Cardiovasc. Res. *1*:2, 1967.
72. Higgins, C. B., Vatner, S. F., Franklin, D., and Braunwald, E.: Extent of regulation of the heart's contractile state in the conscious dog by alteration in the frequency of contraction. J. Clin. Invest. *52*:1187, 1973.
73. Hoffman, B. F., Bindler, E., and Suckling, E. E.: Postextrasystolic potentiation of contraction in cardiac muscle. Am. J. Physiol. *185*:95, 1956.
74. Ross, J., Jr., Sonnenblick, E. H., Kaiser, G. A., Frommer, P. L., and Braunwald, E.: Electroaugmentation of ventricular performance and oxygen consumption by repetitive application of paired electrical stimuli. Circ. Res. *16*:332, 1965.
75. Braunwald, E., Sonnenblick, E. H., Frommer, P. L., and Ross, J., Jr.: Paired electric stimulation of the heart: Physiologic observations and clinical implications. Adv. Intern. Med. *13*:61, 1967.
76. Cranefield, P. F.: The force of contraction of extrasystoles and the potentiation of force of the post-extrasystolic contraction: A historical review. Bull. N. Y. Acad. Med. *41*:419, 1965.
77. Colucci, W. S., Wright, B. F., and Braunwald, E.: New positive inotropic agents in the treatment of congestive heart failure. N. Engl. J. Med. *314*:290, 349, 1986.
78. Hicks, M. J., Shigekawa, M., and Katz, A. M.: Mechanism by which cyclic adenosine 3′:5′-monophosphate–dependent protein kinase stimulates calcium transport in cardiac sarcoplasmic reticulum. Circ. Res. *44*:384, 1979.
79. Fabiato, A., and Fabiato, F.: Effects of pH on the myofilaments and sarcoplasmic reticulum of skinned cells from cardiac and skeletal muscles. J. Physiol. *276*:233, 1978.
80. Katz, A. M.: Cyclic adenosine monophosphate effects on the myocardium: A man who blows hot and cold with one breath. J. Am. Coll. Cardiol *2*:143, 1983.
81. Ross, E. M., and Gilman, A. G.: Biochemical properties of hormone-sensitive adenylate cyclase. Ann. Rev. Biochem. *49*:533, 1980.
82. Gilman, A. G.: Guanine nucleotide-binding regulatory proteins and dual control of adenylate cyclase. J. Clin. Invest. *73*:1, 1984.
83. Lefkowitz, R. J., Stadel, J. M., and Caron, M. G.: Adenylate cyclase-coupled beta-adrenergic receptors: Structure and mechanisms of activation and desensitization. Ann. Rev. Biochem. *52*:159, 1983.
84. Tada, M., and Katz, A.: Phosphorylation of the sarcoplasmic reticulum and sarcolemma. Ann. Rev. *44*:401, 1982.
85. Barany, K., Barany, M., Hager, S., and Sayers, S. T.: Myosin, light chain and membrane protein phosphorylation in various muscles. Fed. Proc. *42*:27, 1983.
86. Winegrad, S., McClellan, G., Horowitz, R., Tucker, M., Lin, L.-E., and Weisberg, A.: Regulation of cardiac contractile proteins by phosphorylation. Fed. Proc. *42*:39, 1983.
87. Sperelakis, N.: Cyclic AMP and phosphorylation in regulation of Ca^{++} influx into myocardial cells and blockade by calcium antagonistic drugs. Am. Heart J. *107*:347, 1984.
88. Kranias, E. G., and Solaro, J.: Coordination of cardiac sarcoplasmic reticulum and myofibrillar function by protein phosphorylation. Fed. Proc. *42*:33, 1983.
89. Ray, K. P., and England, P. J.: Phosphorylation of the inhibitory subunit of troponin and its effect on the calcium dependence of cardiac myofibril adenosine triphosphatase. FEBS Lett. *70*:11, 1976.
90. Fabiato, A., and Fabiato, F.: Cyclic AMP-induced enhancement of calcium accumulation by the sarcoplasmic reticulum with no modification of the sensitivity of the myofilaments to calcium in skinned fibres from a fast skeletal muscle. Biochim. Biophys. Acta *539*:253, 1978.
91. Goldberg, N. D.: Cyclic nucleotides and cell function. Hosp. Pract. *9*:127, 1974.
92. Nawrath, H: Does cyclic GMP mediate the negative inotropic effect of acetylcholine in the heart? Nature *267*:72, 1977.
93. Carmeliet, E.: The slow inward current: Nonvoltage-clamp studies. *In* Zipes, D. P., Bailey, J. C., and Elharrar, V. (eds.): The Slow Inward Current and Cardiac Arrhythmias. The Hague. Martinus Nijhoff, 1980.
94. Barry, W. H., Biedert, S., Miura, D. S., and Smith, T. W.: Changes in cellular Na, K, and Ca contents, monovalent cation transport rate, and contractile state during washout of cardiac glycosides from cultured chick heart cells. Circ. Res. *49*:141, 1981.
95. Mullins, L. J.: The role of Na-Ca exchange in heart. *In* Sperelakis, N. (ed.): Physiology and Pathophysiology of the Heart. Boston, Martinus Nijhoff, 1984, p. 199.
96. Dhalla, N. S., Smith, C. I., Pierce, G. N., Elimban, V., Makimo, N., and Khatter, J. C.: Heart sarcolemmal cation pumps and binding sites. *In* Rupp, H. (ed.): The Regulation of Heart Function. New York, Thieme Inc., 1986, p. 121.
97. Solaro, R. J.: The role of calcium in the contraction of the heart. *In* Flaim, S. F., and Zelis, R. (eds.): Calcium Blockers. Baltimore, Urban and Schwarzenberg, 1982, pp. 21–36.
98. Wier, W. G., and Hess, P.: Excitation-contraction coupling in cardiac Purkinje fibers. Effects of cardiotonic steroids of intracellular $[Ca^{++}]$ transient membrane potential and contraction. J. Gen. Physiol. *83*:395, 1984.
99. Hess, P., Lansman, J. B., and Tsiem, R. W.: Different modes of calcium gating behavior favored by dihydropyridine Ca agonists and antagonists. Nature *311*:338, 1984.
100. Reuter, H.: Ion channels in cardiac cell membrane. Ann. Rev. Physiol. *46*:473, 1984.
101. van Breemen, C., Aaronson, P., and Loutzenhiser, R.: Na-Ca interactions in mammalian smooth muscle. Pharmacol. Rev. *30*:167, 1979.
102. Trautwein, W., and Cavalie, A.: Cardiac calcium channels and their control by neurotransmitters and drugs. J. Am. Coll. Cardiol. *6*:1409, 1985.
103. Fleckenstein, A.: Calcium Antagonism in Heart and Smooth Muscle. New York, John Wiley and Sons, 1983.
104. Braunwald, E.: Calcium-channel blockers: Pharmacologic considerations. Am. Heart J. *104*:665, 1982.
105. Hondeghem, L. M., and Katzung, B. G.: Control of vascular smooth muscle contractility and the action of calcium channel blockers. *In* Rupp, H. (ed.): The Regulation of Heart Function. New York, Thieme Inc., 1986, pp. 38–52.
106. Stone, P. H., Antman, E. M., Muller, J. E., and Braunwald, E.: Calcium channel blocking agents in the treatment of cardiovascular disorders. Part II. Hemodynamic effects and clinical applications. Ann. Intern. Med. *93*:886, 1980.
107. Lands, A. M., Arnold, A., McAuliff, J. P., Ludena, R. P., and Brown, T. G.: Differentiation of receptor systems activated by sympathomimetic amines. Nature *214*:597, 1967.
108. Watanabe, A. M.: Recent advances in knowledge about beta-adrenergic receptors: Application to clinical cardiology. J. Am. Coll. Cardiol. *1*:82, 1983.
109. Homcy, C. J., and Graham, R. M.: Molecular characterization of adrenergic receptors. Circ. Res. *56*:635, 1985.
110. Carlsson, E., Dahlot, C. G., Hedberg, A., Persson, H., and Tangstrand, B.: Differentiation of cardiac chronotropic and inotropic effects of beta adrenoceptor agonists. Naunyn-Schmiedeberg's Arch. Pharmacol. *300*:101, 1977.
111. Wilffart, B., Tummermans, P. B. M. W. M., and van Zwieten, P. A.: Extrasynaptic location of alpha-2 and non-innervated beta-2 adrenoceptors in the vascular system in the pithed normotensive rat. J. Pharmacol. Exp. Ther. *221*:762, 1982.
112. Langer, S. Z.: Presynaptic regulation of catecholamines. Pharmacol. Rev. *32*:337, 1981.
113. Hedberg, A., Minneman, K. P., and Molinoff, P. B.: Differential distribution of beta-1 and beta-2 adrenergic receptors in cat and guinea-pig heart. J. Pharmacol. Exp. Ther. *213*:503, 1980.
114. Schumann, H. J.: What role do alpha and beta adrenoceptors play in the regulation of the heart. Eur. Heart J. *4*(Suppl. A):55, 1983.
115. Lee, J. C., Fripp, R. R., and Downing, S. E.: Myocardial responses to alpha adrenoceptor stimulation with methoxamine hydrochloride in lambs. Am. J. Physiol. *242*:H405, 1982.
116. Colucci, W. S., and Braunwald, E.: Adrenergic receptors: New concepts and implications for cardiovascular therapeutics. *In* Conti, C. R. (ed.): Cardiac Clinics. Philadelphia, F. A. Davis, 1983.
117. Wagner, J., and Schumann, H.-J.: Different mechanisms underlying the stimulation of myocardial alpha- and beta-adrenoceptors. Life Sci. *24*:2045, 1979.
118. Abbott, B. C., and Mommaerts, W. F. H. M.: A study of inotropic mechanisms in the papillary muscle preparation. J. Gen. Physiol. *42*:533, 1959.
119. Sonnenblick, E. H.: Force-velocity relations in mammalian heart muscle. Am. J. Physiol. *202*:931, 1962.
120. Brutsaert, D. L., and Sonnenblick, E. H.: Force-velocity length-time relations of the contractile elements in heart muscle of the cat. Circ. Res. *24*:137, 1969.
121. Brady, A. J.: Contractile and mechanical properties of the myocardium. *In* Sperelakis, N. (ed.): Physiology and Pathophysiology of the Heart. Boston, Martinus Nijhoff, 1984, p. 279.
122. Sonnenblick, E. H., and Skelton, C. L.: Reconsideration of the ultrastructural basis of the cardiac length-tension relation. Circ. Res. *35*:517, 1974.
123. Ross, J.: Mechanical performance of isolated cardiac muscle. *In* West, J. B. (ed.): Best and Taylor's Physiological Basics of Medical Practice. 11th ed. Baltimore, Williams and Wilkins, 1985, pp. 197–206.
124. Brutsaert, D. L., and Sonnenblick, E. H.: Cardiac muscle mechanics in the evaluation of myocardial contractility and pump function: Problems, concepts and directions. Prog. Cardiovasc. Dis. *16*:337, 1973.
125. Strobeck, J. E., Krueger, J. W., and Sonnenblick, E. H.: Load and time considerations in the force-length relation of cardiac muscle. Fed. Proc. *39*:175, 1980.
126. Brady, A. J.: Mechanical properties of cardiac fibers. *In* Berne, R. M. (ed.): Handbook of Physiology. Section 2, The Cardiovascular System. Vol. I, The Heart. Bethesda, American Physiological Society, 1979, pp. 461–474.
127. Parmley, W. W., and Sonnenblick, E. H.: Series elasticity: In relation to contractile element velocity and proposed muscle models. Circ. Res. *20*:112, 1967.
128. Grimm, A. F., and Whitehorn, W. V.: Characteristics of resting tension of myocardium and localization of its elements. Am. J. Physiol. *210*:1362, 1966.
129. Robinson, T. F., Cohen-Gould, F., and Factor, S. M.: Skeletal framework of mammalian heart muscle. Lab. Invest. *49*:482, 1983.
130. Price, M. G.: Molecular analysis of intermediate filament cytoskeleton: A putative load-bearing structure. Am. J. Physiol. *246*:4566, 1984.
131. Edman, K. A. P., and Nilsson, L.: Time course of the active state in relation to muscle length and movement: A comparative study on skeletal muscle and myocardium. Cardiovasc. Res. 5(Suppl. 1):3, 1971.

132. ter Keurs, H. E. D. J., Rijnsburger, W. H., van Heuningen, R., and Negelsmit, M. J.: Tension development and sarcomere length in rat cardiac trabeculae. Circ. Res. *46*:703, 1980.
133. Braunwald, E., Frye, R. L., and Ross, J., Jr.: Studies on Starling's law of the heart: Determinants of the relationship between end-diastolic pressure and circumference. Circ. Res. *8*:1254, 1960.
134. Weisfeldt, M. L., Loeven, W. A., and Shock, N. W.: Resting and active mechanical properties of trabeculae carneae from aged male rats. Am. J. Physiol. *220*:1921, 1971.
135. Henderson, A. H., Van Ocken, E., and Brutsaert, D. L.: A reappraisal of force-velocity measurements in isolated heart muscle preparation. Europ. J. Cardiol. *1*:105, 1973.
136. Grossman, W., Braunwald, E., Mann, T., McLaurin, L. P., and Green, L. H.: Contractile state of the left ventricle in man as evaluated from endsystolic pressure-volume relations. Circulation *56*:845, 1977.
137. Suga, H., and Yamakoshi, K.: Effects of stroke volume and velocity of ejection on end-systolic pressure on canine left ventricle. Circ. Res. *40*:445, 1977.
138. Krueger, J. W., and Pollack, G. H.: Myocardial sarcomere dynamics during isometric contraction. J. Physiol. *251*:627, 1973.
139. Pollack, G. H., and Huntsman, L. L.: Sarcomere length-active force relations in living mammalian cardiac muscle. Am. J. Physiol. *227*:383, 1974.
140. Vassale, D. V., and Pollack, G. H.: The force-velocity relation and stepwise shortening in cardiac muscle. Cir. Res. *51*:37, 1982.
141. Van Henningen, R., Rijnsburger, W. H., and ter Keurs, H. E. D. J.: Sarcomere length control in striated muscle. Am. J. Physiol. *242*:H411, 1982.
142. Krueger, J. W., and Tsujioka, K.: Sarcomere mechanics: Towards a physical basis for cardiac contraction. *In* Mura, R. (ed.): Some Mathematical Questions in Biology. Lectures on Mathematics in the Life Sciences. Vol. 16. 1986, p. 1.
143. Jewell, B. R.: A reexamination of the influence of muscle length on myocardial performance. Circ. Res. *40*:221, 1977.
144. Fabiato, A., and Fabiato, F.: Dependence of calcium release, tension generation, and restoring forces on sarcomere length in skinned cardiac cells. Europ. J. Cardiol. *4*(Suppl.): 13, 1976.
145. Tarr, M., Trank, J. W., Goertz, K. K., and Leiffer, P.: Effect of initial sarcomere length on sarcomere kinetics and force development in single frog atrial cardiac cells. Circ. Res. *49*:767, 1981.
146. Gordon, A. M., and Pollack, G. H.: Effects of calcium on the sarcomere length-tension relation in rat cardiac muscle. Circ. Res. *47*:610, 1980.
147. Allen, D. G., and Kentish, J. C.: The cellular basis of the length-tension relation in cardiac muscle. J. Mol. Cell. Cardiol. *17*:821, 1985.
148. Frank, O.: On the dynamics of cardiac muscle. (Transl. by C. B. Chapman and E. Wasserman.) Am. Heart J. *58*:282 and 467, 1959.
149. Starling, E. H.: Linacre Lecture on the Law of the Heart (1915). London, Longmans, Green and Co., Ltd., 1918.
150. Gordon, A. M., Huxley, A. F., and Julian, F. J.: The variation in isometric tension with sarcomere length in vertebrate muscle fibers. J. Physiol. (Lond.) *184*:170, 1966.
151. Gordon, A. M., Huxley, A. F., and Julian, F. J.: Tension development in highly stretched vertebrate muscle fibers. J. Physiol. *184*:143, 1966.
152. Sonnenblick, E. H., Spiro, D., and Cottrell, J. S.: Fine structural changes in heart muscle in relation to the length-tension curve. Proc. Natl. Acad. Sci. (USA) *49*:193, 1963.
153. Grimm, A. F., Katele, K. V., Kubota, R., and Whitehorn, W. V.: Relation of sarcomere length and muscle length in resting myocardium. Am. J. Physiol. *218*:1412, 1970.
154. Pollack, G. H., and Krueger, J. W.: Sarcomere dynamics in intact cardiac muscle. Eur. J. Cardiol. *4*:53, 1976.
155. Sonnenblick, E. H., Skelton, C. L., Spotnitz, W. D., and Feldman, D.: Redefinition of the ultrastructural basis of cardiac length-tension relations. Circulation *48*(Suppl. 4):65, 1973.
156. Spotnitz, H. M., Sonnenblick, E. H., and Spiro, D.: Relation of ultrastructure to function in the intact heart: Sarcomere structure relative to pressure-volume curves of the intact left ventricles of dog and cat. Circ. Res. *18*:49, 1966.
157. Leyton, R. A., Spotnitz, H. M., and Sonnenblick, E. H.: Cardiac ultrastructure and function: Sarcomeres in the right ventricle. Am. J. Physiol. *221*:902, 1971.
158. Gordon, A. M., and Pollack, G. H.: Effects of calcium on the sarcomere length-tension relation in rat cardiac muscle. Circ. Res. *47*:610, 1980.
159. Ross, J., Jr., Sonnenblick, E. H., Covell, J. W., Kaiser, G. A., and Spiro, D.: Architecture of the heart in systole and diastole: Technique of rapid fixation and analysis of left ventricular geometry. Circ. Res. *21*:409, 1967.
160. Sonnenblick, E. H., Ross, J., Jr., Covell, J. W., Spotnitz, H. M., and Spiro, D.: Ultrastructure of the heart in systole and diastole. Circ. Res. *21*:423, 1967.

DETERMINANTS OF CONTRACTION OF THE INTACT HEART

161. Yoran, C., Covell, J. W., and Ross, J., Jr.: Structural basis for ascending limb of left ventricular function. Circ. Res. *32*:297, 1973.
162. Strobeck, J. E., and Sonnenblick, E. H.: Myocardial and ventricular function. Cardiovasc. Rev. Rep. *4*:568, 1983.
163. Weber, K. T., Janicki, J. S., Hunter, W. C., Shroff, S., Pearlman, E. S., and Fishman, A. P.: The contractile behavior of the heart and its functional coupling to the circulation. Prog. Cardiovasc. Dis. *4*:375, 1982.
164. Ross, J., Jr.: Cardiac function and myocardial contractility: A perspective. J. Am. Coll. Cardiol. *1*:52, 1983.
165. Braunwald, E., and Ross, J., Jr.: Control of cardiac performance. *In* Berne, R. M. (ed.): Handbook of Physiology. Section 2, The Cardiovascular System. Vol. I, The Heart. Bethesda, American Physiological Society, 1979, pp. 533–580.
166. Karliner, J. S., Bouchard, R. J., and Gault, J. H.: Dimensional changes of the human left ventricle prior to aortic valve opening: A cineangiographic study in patients with and without left heart disease. Circulation *44*:312, 1971.
167. Rankin, J. S., McHale, P. A., Arentzen, C. E., Ling, D., Greenfield, J. C., Jr., and Anderson, R. W.: The three dimensional dynamic geometry of the left ventricle in the conscious dog. Circ. Res. *39*:304, 1976.
168. Sasayama, S., Franklin, D., Ross, J., Jr., Kemper, W. S., and McKown, D.: Dynamic changes in left ventricular wall thickness and their use in analyzing cardiac function in the conscious dog. Am. J. Cardiol. *38*:870, 1976.
169. Sandler, H., and Alderman, E.: Determination of left ventricular size and shape. Circ. Res. *34*:1, 1974.
170. Mirsky, I.: Elastic properties of the myocardium: A quantitative approach with physiological and clinical applications. *In* Berne, R. M. (ed.): Handbook of Physiology. Section 2, The Cardiovascular System. Vol. I, The Heart. Bethesda, Md., American Physiological Society, 1979, pp. 497–532.
170a. Kurnik, M. S., Courtois, M. A., and Ludbrook, P. A.: Effects of nifedipine on intrinsic myocardial stiffness in man. Circulation *74*:126, 1986.
171. Grossman, W., and McLaurin, L. P.: Diastolic properties of the left ventricle. Ann. Intern. Med. *84*:316, 1976.
172. Taylor, R. R., Covell, J. W., Sonnenblick, E. H., and Ross, J., Jr.: The independence of ventricular distensibility in the filling of the opposite ventricle. Am. J. Physiol. *213*:711, 1967.
173. Mirsky, I.: Assessment of diastolic function: Suggested methods and future considerations. Circulation *69*:836, 1984.
174. Gaasch, W. H., Levine, H. J., Quinones, M. A., and Alexander, J. K.: Left ventricular compliance: Mechanisms and clinical implications. Am. J. Cardiol. *38*:645, 1976.
175. Pouleur, H., Karliner, J. S., LeWinter, M. M., and Covell, J. W.: Diastolic viscous properties of the intact canine left ventricle. Circ. Res. *45*:410, 1979.
176. LeWinter, M. M., Engler, R., and Pavelec, R. S.: Time-dependent shifts of the left ventricular diastolic filling relationship in conscious dogs. Circ. Res. *45*:641, 1979.
177. Gentzler, R. D., II, Briselli, M. F., and Gault, J. H.: Angiographic estimation of right ventricular volume in man. Circulation *50*:324, 1974.
178. Shirato, K., Shabetai, R., Bhargava, V., Franklin, D., and Ross, J., Jr.: Alteration of the left ventricular diastolic pressure-segment length relation produced by the pericardium: Effects of cardiac distention and afterload reduction in conscious dogs. Circulation *57*:1191, 1978.
179. LeWinter, M. M., and Porsche, R.: Influence of the pericardium on left ventricular end-diastolic pressure-segment relations during early and late stages of experimental chronic volume overloads in dogs. Circ. Res. *50*:501, 1981.
180. Bhargava, V., Shabetai, R., Ross, J., Jr., Shirato, K., Pavelec, R. C., and Mason, P. A.: Influence of the pericardium on left ventricular diastolic pressure-volume curves in dogs with sustained volume overload. Am. Heart. J. *105*:95, 1983.
181. Bourdillon, P. D., Lorell, B. H., Mirsky, I., Paulus, W. J., Wynne, J., and Grossman, W.: Increased regional myocardial stiffness of the left ventricle during pacing-induced angina in man. Circulation *67*:316, 1983.
182. Mann, T., Goldberg, S., Mudge, G. A., Jr., and Grossman, W.: Factors contributing to altered left ventricular diastolic properties during angina pectoris. Circulation *59*:14, 1979.
183. Serizawa, T., Carabello, B. A., and Grossman, W.: Effect of pacing-induced ischemia on left ventricular diastolic pressure-volume relations in dogs with coronary stenosis. Circ. Res. *46*:430, 1980.
184. Hess, O. M., Bhargava, V., Ross, J., Jr., and Shabetai, R.: The role of pericardium in interactions between the cardiac chambers. Am. Heart. J. *106*:1377, 1983.
185. Linderer, T., Chatterjee, K., Parmley, W. W., Sievers, R. E., Glantz, S. A., and Tyberg, J. V.: Influence of atrial systole on the Frank-Starling relation and the end-diastolic pressure-diameter relation of the left ventricle. Circulation *67*:1045, 1983.
186. Jensen, D. P., Goolsby, J. P., Jr., and Oliva, P. B.: Hemodynamic pattern resembling pericardial constriction after acute myocardial infarction with right ventricular infarction. Am. J. Cardiol. *42*:858, 1978.
187. Shabetai, R.: Measuring pericardial constraint. J. Am. Coll. Cardiol. *7*:315, 1986.
188. Smiseth, O. A., Frais, M. A., Kingma, I., Smith, E. R., and Tyberg, J. V.: Assessment of pericardial constraint in dogs. Circulation *71*:158, 1985.
189. Bemis, C. E., Serur, J. R., Korkenhagen, D., Sonnenblick, E. H., and Urschel, C. W.: Influence of right ventricular filling pressure on left ventricular pressure and dimension. Circ. Res. *34*:498, 1974.
190. Glantz, S. A., and Parmley, W. W.: Factors which affect the diastolic pressure volume curve. Circ. Res. *42*:171, 1978.
191. Ross, J., Jr.: Acute displacement of the diastolic pressure-volume curve of the left ventricle. Role of the pericardium and the right ventricle. Circulation *59*:32, 1979.
192. Olsen, G. O., Tyson, G. S., Maier, G. W., Spratt, J. A., Davis, J. W., and Rankin, J. S.: Dynamic ventricular interaction in the conscious dog. Circ. Res. *52*:85, 1983.
193. Burns, J. W., Covell, J. W., and Ross, J., Jr.: Mechanics of isotonic left ventricular contractions. Am. J. Physiol. *224*:725, 1973.
194. Weber, K. T., and Janicki, K. T.: The dynamics of ventricular contraction: Force, lengthening and shortening. Fed. Proc. 39:188, 1980.
195. Suga, H., Sagawa, K., and Shoukas, A. A.: Load independence of the instantaneous pressure-volume ratio of the canine left ventricle and effects of epinephrine and heart rate on the ratio. Circ. Res. *32*:214, 1973.
196. Sagawa, K.: The end systolic pressure-volume relation of the ventricle: Definition, modifications and clinical use. Circulation 63:1223, 1981.
197. Maughan, W. L., Sunagawa, K., Burkhoff, D., and Sagawa, K.: Effect of

arterial impedance changes on end-systolic pressure-volume relation. Circ. Res. *54*:595, 1984.
198. Lee, J., Tajimi, T., Widmann, T. F., and Ross, J., Jr.: Application of end-systolic pressure-volume and pressure-wall thickness relations in conscious dogs. J. Am. Coll. Cardiol. 9:136, 1987.
199. Kaseda, S., Tomoike, H., Ogaa, I., and Nakamura, M.: End-systolic pressure-volume, pressure-length, and stress-strain relations in canine hearts. Am. J. Physiol. *18*:H648, 1985.
200. Mehmel, H. C., Stocking, B., Ruffmann, K., Olhausen, K. V., Schuler, G., and Kubler, W.: The linearity of the end-systolic pressure-volume relationship in man and its sensitivity for assessment of left ventricular function. Circulation *63*:1216, 1981.
201. McKay, R. G., Aroesty, J. M., Heller, G. V., Royal, H., Parker, J. A., Silverman, K. J., Kolodny, G. M., and Grossman, W.: Left ventricular pressure-volume diagrams and end-systolic pressure-volume relations in human beings. J. Am. Coll. Cardiol. *3*:301, 1984.
202. Sagawa, K.: End-systolic pressure-volume relationship in retrospect and prospect. Fed. Proc. *43*:2399, 1984.
203. Belcher, P., Boerboom, L. E., and Olinger, G. N.: Standardization of end-systolic pressure-volume relation in the dog. Am. J. Physiol *18*:H547, 1985.
204. Ross, J., Jr.: Applications and limitations of end-systolic measures of ventricular performance. Fed. Proc. *43*:2418, 1984.
205. Lee, J. D., Tajimi, T., Patritta, J., and Ross, J., Jr.: Preload reserve and mechanisms of afterload mismatch in the normal conscious dog. Am. J. Physiol. *19*:H464, 1986.
206. Boettcher, D. H., Vatner, S. F., Heyndrikx, G. R., and Braunwald, E.: Extent of utilization of the Frank-Starling mechanisms in conscious dogs. Am. J. Physiol. *3*:338, 1978.
207. Poliner, L. R., Dehmer, G. J., Lewis, S. E., Parkey, R. W., Blomqvist, C. G., and Willerson, J. T.: Left ventricular performance in normal subjects: A comparison of the responses to exercise in the upright and supine positions. Circulation *62*:528, 1980.
208. Ross, J., Jr.: Mechanisms of cardiac contraction. What roles for preload, afterload and inotropic state in heart failure? Eur. Heart. J. (Suppl A): *19*, 1983.
209. Weber, K. T., Janicki, J. S., Shroff, S. G., and Laskey, W.: The mechanics of ventricular function. Hosp. Pract. *18*:113, 1983.
210. Sarnoff, S. J., and Mitchell, J. H.: Control of the function of heart. *In* Hamilton, W. F., and Dow, P. (eds.): Handbook of Physiology. Section 2, Circulation 2:489, Bethesda, American Physiology Society, 1962.
211. Williams, J. F., Jr., Sonnenblick, E. H., and Braunwald, E.: Determinants of atrial contractile force in intact heart. Am. J. Physiol. *209*:1061, 1965.
212. Braunwald, E., and Frahm, C. J.: Studies on Starling's law of the heart. IV. Observations on hemodynamic functions of left atrium in man. Circulation *24*:633, 1961.
213. Linderer, T., Chatterjee, K., Parmley, W. W., Sievers, R. E., Glantz, S. A., and Tyberg, J. V.: Influence of atrial systole on the Frank-Starling relation and the end-diastolic pressure-diameter relation of the left ventricle. Circulation *67*:1045, 1983.
214. Katz, A. M.: Editorial—The descending limb of the Starling curve and the failing heart. Circulation *32*:871, 1965.
215. Monroe, R. G., Gamble, W. J., LaFarge, C. G., Kumar, A. E., and Manasek, F. J.: Left ventricular performance at high-end diastolic pressures in isolated, perfused dog hearts. Circ. Res. *26*:85, 1970.
216. Ross, J., Jr., Sonnenblick, E. H., Taylor, R. R., Spotnitz, H. M., and Covell, J. W.: Diastolic geometry and sarcomere lengths in the chronically dilated canine left ventricle. Circ. Res. *28*:49, 1971.
217. Grimm, A. F., Lin, H. L., and Grimm, B. R.: Left ventricular free wall and intraventricular pressure-sarcomere length distributions. Am. J. Physiol. *239*:H101, 1980.
218. MacGregor, D. C., Covell, J. W., Mahler, F., Dilley, R. B., and Ross, J., Jr.: Relations between afterload, stroke volume, and the descending limb of Starling's curve. Am. J. Physiol. *227*:884, 1974.
219. Ross, J., Jr., and Braunwald, E.: The study of left ventricular function in man by increasing resistance to ventricular ejection with angiotensin. Circulation *29*:739, 1964.
220. Ross, J., Jr.: Afterload mismatch and preload reserve: a conceptual framework for the analysis of ventricular function. Progr. Cardiovasc. Dis. *18*:255, 1976.
221. Vatner, S. F., Franklin, D., Higgins, C. B., Patrick, T., and Braunwald, E.: Left ventricular response to severe exertion in untethered dogs. J. Clin. Invest. *51*:3052, 1972.
222. Guyton, A. C., Jones, C. E., and Coleman, T. G.: Graphical analysis of cardiac output regulation. *In* Circulatory Physiology: Cardiac Output and Its Regulation. 2nd ed. Philadelphia, W. B. Saunders Company, 1973, p. 237.
223. Braunwald, E.: Regulation of the circulation. N. Engl. J. Med. *290*:1124 and 1420, 1974.
224. Braunwald, E.: Editorial—On the difference between the heart's output and its contractile state. Circulation *43*:171, 1971.
225. Pouleur, H., Covell, J. W., and Ross, J., Jr.: Effects of nitroprusside on venous return and central blood volume in the absence and presence of acute heart failure. Circulation *61*:328, 1980.
226. Braunwald, E., Binion, J. T., Morgan, W. L., Jr., and Sarnoff, S. J.: Alterations in central blood volume and cardiac output induced by positive pressure breathing and counteracted by metaraminol (Aramine). Circ. Res. *5*:670, 1957.
227. Shabetai, R.: The Pericardium. New York, Grune & Stratton, 1981, p. 154.
228. Shepherd, J. T., and Vanhoutte, P. M.: Veins and Their Control. Philadelphia, W. B. Saunders Company, 1975, 269 pp.
229. Mason, D. T., and Braunwald, E.: The effects of nitroglycerin and amyl nitrite on arteriolar and venous tone in the human forearm. Circulation *32*:755, 1965.
230. Guyton, A. C., Douglas, B. H., Langston, J. B., and Richardson, T. Q.: Instantaneous increase in mean circulatory pressure and cardiac output at onset of muscular activity. Circ. Res. *11*:431, 1962.
231. Sonnenblick, E. H., and Downing, J. E.: Afterload as a primary determinant of ventricular performance. Am. J. Physiol. *24*:604, 1962.
232. Wilcken, D. E. L., Charlier, A. A., Hoffman, J. I. E., and Guz, A.: Effects of alterations in aortic impedance on the performance of the ventricles. Circ. Res. *14*:283, 1964.
233. Ross, J., Jr., Covell, J. W., Sonnenblick, E. H., and Braunwald, E.: Contractile state of heart characterized by force-velocity relations in variably afterloaded and isovolumic beats. Circ. Res. *18*:149, 1966.
234. Piene, H., and Covell, J. W.: A force-length-time relationship describes the mechanics of canine left ventricular wall segments during auxotonic contractions. Circ. Res. *49*:70, 1981.
235. Urschel, C. W., Covell, J. W., Sonnenblick, E. H., Ross, J., Jr., and Braunwald, E.: Myocardial mechanics in aortic and mitral valvular regurgitation: The concept of instantaneous impedance as a determinant of the performance of the intact heart. J. Clin. Invest. *47*:867, 1968.
236. Brutsaert, D. L., Rademakers, F. E., and Sys, S. U.: Triple control of relaxation: Implications in cardiac disease. Circulation *69*:190, 1984.
237. Gaasch, W. H., Ariel, Y., and McMahon, T. A.: Dynamics of left ventricular diastolic filling. J. Am. Coll. Cardiol. *7*:243A, 1986.
238. Hori, M., Inoue, M., Kitakaze, M., Tsujioka, K., Ishida, Y., Fukunami, M., Makajima, S., Kitabatake, A., and Abe, H.: Loading sequence is a major determinant of afterload-dependent relaxation in intact canine heart. Am. J. Physiol. *249*:H747, 1985.
239. Blaustein, A. S., and Gaasch, W. H.: Myocardial relaxation. VI. Effects of adrenergic tone and asynchrony on LV relaxation rate. Am. J. Physiol. *244*:H417, 1983.
240. Bahler, R. C., and Martin, P.: Effects of loading conditions and inotropic state on rapid filling phase of left ventricle. Am. J. Physiol. *248*:H523, 1985.
241. Rankin, J. S., Arentzen, C. E., McHale, P. A., Ling, D., and Anderson, R. W.: Viscoelastic properties of the diastolic left ventricle in the conscious dog. Circ. Res. *41*:37, 1977.
242. Weisfeldt, M. L., Frederiksen, J. W., Yin, F., and Weiss, J. L.: Evidence of incomplete left ventricular relaxation in the dog: Prediction from the time constant for isovolumic pressure fall. J. Clin. Invest. *62*:1296, 1978.
243. Pouleur, H., Karliner, J. S., LeWinter, M. M., and Covel, J. W.: Diastolic viscous properties of the intact canine left ventricle. Circ. Res. *45*:41, 1979.
244. Ishida, Y., Meisner, J. S., Tsujioka, K., Gallo, J. I., Yoran, C., Frater, R. W. M., and Yellin, E. L.: Left ventricular filling dynamics: Influence of left ventricular relaxation and left atrial pressure. Circulation *74*:187, 1986.
245. Wong, B., Rinkenberger, R., Dunn, M., and Goodyer, A.: Effect of intermittent left bundle branch block on left ventricular performance in the normal heart. Am. J. Cardiol. *39*:459, 1977.
246. Heyndricks, G. R., Vilaine, J., Knight, D. R., and Vatner, S. F.: Effects of altered site of electrical activation on myocardial performance during inotropic stimulation. Circulation *71*:1010, 1985.
247. Sarnoff, S. J., Mitchell, J. H., Gilmore, J. P., and Remensnyder, J. P.: Homeometric autoregulation of the heart. Circ. Res. *8*:1077, 1960.
248. Clancy, R. L., Graham, T. P., Jr., Ross, J., Jr., Sonnenblick, E. H., and Braunwald, E.: The influence of aortic pressure-induced homeometric autoregulation on myocardial performance. Am. J. Physiol. *214*:1186, 1968.
249. LaFarge, C. G., Monroe, R. G., Gamble, W. J., Rosenthal, A., and Hammond, R. P.: Left ventricular pressure and norepinephrine effux from the innervated heart. Am. J. Physiol. *219*:519, 1970.
250. Von Anrep, G.: On the part played by the suprarenals in the normal vascular reactions of the body. J. Physiol. (Lond.) *45*:307, 1912.
251. Vatner, S. F., Monroe, R. G., and McRitchie, R. J.: Effects of anesthesia, tachycardia, and autonomic blockade on the Anrep effect in intact dogs. Am. J. Physiol. *226*:1450, 1974.
252. Furey, S. A., III., Zieske, H. A., and Levy, M. N.: The essential function of the right ventricle. Am. Heart J. *107*:404, 1984.
253. Weber, K. T., Janicki, J. S., Shroff, S. G., Likoff, M. J., and Sutton, M. G. S.: The right ventricle: Physiologic and pathophysiologic considerations. Crit. Care Med. *11*:323, 1983.
254. Peterson, K. L., and Ross, J., Jr.: Application of cardiac muscle mechanisms to clinical heart disease. *In* Baan, J., Noordergraaf, D., Raines, J. (eds): Cardiovascular Systems. Cambridge, MIT Press, 1978.
255. Katz, A. M.: Regulation of myocardial contractility 1958–1983. J. Am. Coll. Cardiol. *1*:126, 1983.
256. Ross, J., Jr., Covell, J. W., and Sonnenblick, E. H.: The mechanics of left ventricular contraction in acute experimental cardiac failure. J. Clin. Invest. *46*:299, 1967.
257. Yue, D. T., Burkhoff, D., Franz, M. R., Hunter, W. C., and Sagawa, K.: Postextrasystolic potential of the isolated canine left ventricle: Relationship to mechanical restitution. Circ. Res. *56*:340, 1985.
258. Frommer, P. L., Robinson, B. F., and Braunwald, E.: Paired electrical stimulation. A comparison of the effects on performance of the failing and nonfailing heart. Am. J. Cardiol. *18*:738, 1966.
259. McGaughey, M. D., Maughan, W. L., Sunagawa, K., and Sagawa, K.: Alternating contractility in pulsus alternans studied in the isolated canine heart. Circulation *71*:357, 1985.
260. Beierholm, E. A., Grantham, R. N., O'Keefe, D. D., Laver, M. B., and Daggett, W. M.: Effects of acid-base changes, hypoxia, and catecholamines on ventricular performance. Am. J. Physiol. *228*:1555, 1975.
261. Braunwald, E.: Symposium on protection of the ischemic myocardium. Circulation *53*(Suppl. 1):217, 1976.

262. Williamson, J. R., Schaffer, S. W., Ford, C., and Safen, B.: Contribution of tissue acidosis to ischemic injury in the perfused rat heart. Circulation *53*(Suppl. 1):3, 1976.
263. Mitchell, J. H., Wallace, A. G., and Skinner, N. S., Jr.: Intrinsic effects of heart rate on left ventricular performance. Am. J. Physiol. *205*:41, 1963.
264. Ross, J., Jr., Linhart, J. W., and Braunwald, E.: Effects of changing heart rate in man by electrical stimulation of the right atrium: Studies at rest, during exercise and with isoproterenol. Circulation *32*:549, 1965.
265. Narahara, K. A., and Blettel, M. L.: Effect of rate on left ventricular volumes and ejection fraction during chronic ventricular pacing. Circulation *67*:323, 1983.

NEURAL CONTROL OF CARDIAC CONTRACTION

266. Vatner, S. F., and Braunwald, E.: Cardiovascular control mechanisms in the conscious state. N. Engl. J. Med. *293*:970, 1975.
267. Randall, W. C. (ed.): Neural Regulation of the Heart. New York, Oxford University Press, 1977, 440 pp.
268. Yamaguchie, N., de Champlain, J., and Nadeau, R.: Correlation between the response of the heart to sympathetic stimulation and the release of endogenous catecholamines into the coronary sinus of the dog. Circ. Res. *36*:662, 1975.
269. Landsberg, L., and Young, J. B.: Catecholamines and the adrenal medulla. *In* Wilson, J. D., Foster, D. W. (eds.): Williams' Textbook of Endocrinology. Philadelphia, W. B. Saunders, 1985, p. 891.
270. Fujii, I., and Vatner, S. F.: Sympathetic mechanisms regulating myocardial contractility in conscious animals. *In* Fozzard, H. A., et al. (eds.): The Heart and Cardiovascular System. New York, Raven Press, 1986, pp. 1119–1132.
271. Cousineau, D., Ferguson, R. J., DeChamplain, J., Gauthier, P., Cote, P., and Bourassa, M.: Catecholamines in coronary sinus during exercise in man before and after training. J. Appl. Physiol. *43*:801, 1977.
272. Martin, R. H., Lim, S. T., and VanCitters, R. L.: Atrial fibrillation in the intact anesthetized dog: Hemodynamic effects during rest, exercise, and beta-adrenergic blockade. J. Clin. Invest. *46*:205, 1967.
273. Frye, R. L., and Braunwald, E.: Studies on Starling's law of the heart. I. The circulatory response to acute hypervolemia and its modification by ganglionic blockade. J. Clin. Invest. *39*:1043, 1960.
274. Sonnenblick, E. H., Williams, J. F., Jr., Glick, G., Mason, D. T., and Braunwald, E.: Studies on digitalis. XV. Effects of cardiac glycosides on myocardial force-velocity relations in nonfailing human heart. Circulation *34*:532, 1966.
275. Daggett, W. M., and Weisfeldt, M. L.: Influence of sympathetic nervous system on response of normal heart to digitalis. Am. J. Cardiol. *16*:394, 1965.
276. Liedtke, A. M., Buoncristiani, J. F., Kirk, E. S., Sonnenblick, E. H., and Urschel, C. W.: Regulation of cardiac output after administration of isoproterenol and ouabain. Cardiovasc. Res. *6*:325, 1972.
277. Guyton, A. C.: The relationship of cardiac output and arterial pressure control. Circulation *64*:1079, 1981.
278. Vatner, S. F., Higgins, C. B., White, S., Patrick, T., and Franklin, D.: The peripheral vascular response to severe exercise in untethered dogs before and after complete heart block. J. Clin. Invest. *50*:1950, 1971.
279. Rothe, C. F.: Physiology of venous return: An unappreciated boost to the heart. Arch. Intern. Med. *146*:977, 1986.
280. Ross, J., Jr., Gault, J. H., Mason, D. T., Linhart, J. W., and Braunwald, E.: Left ventricular performance during muscular exercise in patients with and without cardiac dysfunction. Circulation *34*:597, 1966.
281. Poliner, L. R., Dehmer, G. J., Lewis, S. E., Parkey, R. W., Blomqvist, C. G., and Willerson, J. T.: Left ventricular performance in normal subjects: A comparison of the responses to exercise in the upright and supine positions. Circulation *62*:528, 1980.
282. Iskandrian, A. S., Hakki, A. H., DePace, N. L., Manno, B., and Segal, B. L.: Evaluation of left ventricular function by radionuclide angiography during exercise in normal subjects and in patients with chronic coronary heart disease. J. Am. Coll. Cardiol. *1*:1518, 1983.
283. Epstein, S. E., Robinson, B. F., Kahler, R. L., and Braunwald, E.: Effects of beta-adrenergic blockade on the cardiac response to maximal and submaximal exercise in man. J. Clin. Invest. *44*:1745, 1965.
284. Robinson, B. F., Epstein, S. E., Kahler, R. L., and Braunwald, E.: Circulatory effects of acute expansion of blood volume: Studies during maximal exercise and at rest. Circ. Res. *19*:26, 1966.
285. Braunwald, E., Goldblatt, A., Harrison, D. C., and Mason, D. T.: Studies on cardiac dimensions in intact, unanesthetized man. III. Effects of muscular exercise. Circ. Res. *13*:460, 1963.
286. Caldwell, J. H., Stewart, D. K., Dodge, H. T., Frimer, M., and Kennedy, J. W.: Left ventricular volume during maximal supine exercise. A study using metallic epicardial markers. Circulation *58*:732, 1978.
287. Sonnenblick, E. H., Braunwald, E., Williams, J. F., Jr., and Glick, G.: Effects of exercise on myocardial force-velocity relations in intact unanesthetized man: Relative roles of changes in heart rate, sympathetic activity, and ventricular dimensions. J. Clin. Invest. *44*:2051, 1965.
288. Bruce, T. A., Chapman, C. P., Baker, O., and Fisher, J. N.: Role of autonomic and myocardial factors in cardiac control. J. Clin. Invest. *42*:721, 1963.
289. Saltin, B., and Astrand, P. O.: Maximal oxygen uptake in the athlete. J. Appl. Physiol. *23*:353, 1967.
290. Morganroth, J., Maron, B. J., Henry, W. L., and Epstein, S. E.: Comparative left ventricular dimensions in trained athletes. Ann. Intern. Med. *82*:521, 1975.
291. Roeske, W. R., O'Rourke, R. A., Klein, A., Leopold, G., and Karliner, J. S.: Noninvasive evaluation of ventricular hypertrophy in professional athletes. Circulation *53*:286, 1976.
292. Resink, T. J., Gevers, W., Noakes, T. D., and Opie, L. H.: Increased cardiac myosin ATPase activity as biochemical adaptation to running training: Enhanced response to catecholamines and a role for myosin phosphorylation. J. Mol. Cell. Cardiol. *13*:679, 1981.
293. Mitchell, J. H., Payne, F. C., Saltin, B., and Schibye, B.: The role of muscle mass in the cardiovascular response to static conditions. J. Physiol. *309*:45, 1980.
294. Hintze, T. H., and Vatner, S. F.: Cardiac dynamics during hemorrhage: Relative unimportance of adrenergic inotropic responses. Circ. Res. *50*:705, 1982.
295. Bainbridge, F. A.: The influence of venous filling upon the rate of the heart. J. Physiol. (Lond.) *50*:65, 1915.
296. Vatner, S. F., Boettcher, D. H., Heyndricks, G. R., and McRitchie, R. J.: Reduced baroreflex sensitivity with volume loading in conscious dogs. Circulation Res. *37*:236, 1975.
297. Vatner, S. F., and Boettcher, D. H.: Regulation of cardiac output by stroke volume and heart rate in conscious dogs. Circ. Res. *42*:557, 1978.
298. Vatner, S. F., and Rutherford, J. D.: Control of the myocardial contractile state by carotid chemo- and baroreceptor and pulmonary inflation reflexes in conscious dogs. J. Clin. Invest. *61*:1593, 1978.
299. Levy, M. N., and Martin, P. J.: Neurol control of the heart. *In* Sperelakis, N. (ed.): Physiology and Pathophysiology of the Heart. Boston, Martinus Nijhoff, 1984, pp. 337–354.
300. Watanabe, A. M., and Lindemann, J. P.: Mechanism of adrenergic and cholinergic regulation of myocardial contractility. *In* Sperelakis, N. (ed.): Physiology and Pathophysiology of the Heart. Boston, Martinus Nijhoff, 1984, pp. 337–404.
301. Yin, F. C. P., Weisfeldt, M. L., and Milnor, W. R.: Role of aortic input impedance in the decreased cardiovascular response to exercise with aging in dogs. J. Clin. Invest. *68*:28, 1981.

14 PATHOPHYSIOLOGY OF HEART FAILURE

by EUGENE BRAUNWALD, M.D.

Heart (or cardiac) failure (the pathophysiological state in which an abnormality of *cardiac* function is responsible for failure of the heart to pump blood at a rate commensurate with the requirements of the metabolizing tissues, or can do so only from an elevated filling pressure) is frequently, but not always, caused by a defect in myocardial contraction, i.e., by *myocardial failure*. However, in some patients with heart failure, a similar clinical syndrome is present, but there is no detectable abnormality of *myocardial* function; in many such cases heart failure may be brought about by conditions in which the normal heart is suddenly presented with a load that exceeds its capacity or in which ventricular filling is impaired.[1] Heart failure must be distinguished from conditions in which there is circulatory congestion consequent to abnormal salt and water retention (the so-called congested state) but in which there is no disturbance of cardiac function per se.[2] A distinction must also be made between heart failure and *circulatory failure*, in which an abnormality of some component of the circulation—the heart, the blood volume, the concentration of oxygenated hemoglobin in the arterial blood, or the vascular bed—is responsible for inadequate cardiac output.

Thus, myocardial failure, heart failure, and circulatory failure are not synonymous but refer to progressively broader entities. Myocardial failure, when sufficiently severe, always produces heart failure, but the converse is not necessarily the case, since a number of conditions in which the heart is suddenly overloaded (e.g., acute aortic regurgitation secondary to acute infective endocarditis) can produce heart failure in the presence of normal myocardial function. Also, conditions such as tricuspid stenosis and constrictive pericarditis, which interfere with cardiac filling, can produce heart failure without myocardial failure. Heart failure, in turn, always produces circulatory failure, but again the converse is not necessarily the case, since a variety of noncardiac conditions, e.g., hypovolemic shock (Chap. 19) or extremely severe anemia, beriberi, and other high-output states (Chap. 25), can produce circulatory failure at a time when cardiac function is normal or only modestly impaired.

Hemodynamic, contractile, and wall motion disorders are discussed in the chapters on cardiac catheterization (Chap. 9), echocardiography (Chap. 5), exercise (Chap. 8), radionuclide imaging (Chap. 12), and assessment of cardiac function (Chap. 15). In this chapter, we focus on the anatomical, biochemical, cellular, and neurohumoral changes characteristic of heart failure.

COMPENSATORY MECHANISMS

In the presence of a disturbance in myocardial contraction or an excessive hemodynamic burden placed on the ventricle or both, the heart depends upon three principal compensatory mechanisms for maintenance of its pumping function: (1) the Frank-Starling mechanism, in which an increased preload (i.e., lengthening of sarcomeres to provide optimal overlap between thick and thin myofilaments and to increase activation) acts to sustain cardiac performance (p. 399); (2) increased release of catecholamines by adrenergic cardiac nerves and the adrenal medulla, which augment myocardial contractility (p. 415); and (3) myocardial hypertrophy with or without cardiac chamber dilatation, in which the mass of contractile tissue is augmented. Initially, these three compensatory mechanisms may be adequate to maintain the overall pumping performance of the heart at a relatively normal level at submaximal workloads, and the maximum workload may be supranormal, normal, or reduced. However, each of these three compensatory mechanisms has a limited potential, and if the disturbance in myocardial contraction and/or the excessive hemodynamic burden persists, the heart ultimately fails. The clinical syndrome of heart failure occurs as a consequence of the limitations and/or the ultimate failure of these compensatory mechanisms.[3]

Cardiac output is often depressed in the basal state in patients with the common forms of heart failure secondary to ischemic heart disease, hypertension, primary myocardial disease, valvular disease, and pericardial disease (so-called low-output heart failure). It tends to be elevated in patients with heart failure associated with conditions of reduced afterload and/or hypermetabolism, such as hyperthyroidism, anemia, arteriovenous fistula, beriberi, and Paget's disease (so-called high-output heart failure, Chap. 25). The mechanisms responsible for the development of heart failure in patients whose cardiac output is initially high are complex and depend on the specific underlying disease process and its effect on the myocardium. In most of these conditions, the heart is called upon to pump an abnormally large volume of blood in order to deliver an adequate quantity of oxygen to the metabolizing tissues. This increased volume load exerts an effect on the myocardium resembling that produced by regurgitant valvular lesions or cardiac left-to-right shunts. In some patients with high-output heart failure, severe anemia or thiamine deficiency also impairs myocardial function.

In the absence of the shunting of blood in the periphery, the inadequate delivery of oxygen to the metabolizing tissues characteristic of heart failure is reflected in an abnormally widened arterial–mixed venous oxygen difference. In mild cases this abnormality may not be present in the basal state and may become evident only during the stress of increased activity. In the presence of the peripheral arteriovenous shunting of blood and heart failure (as occurs, for example, in beriberi heart disease), although the arterial–mixed venous oxygen difference may be normal or even narrowed, the venous oxygen content proximal to the shunt—if it could be measured—would be reduced, reflecting an augmented extraction of oxygen by inadequately perfused tissues, and a reduced partial pressure of oxygen in the tissue.

When the volume of blood delivered into the systemic vascular bed is chronically reduced, and when one or both ventricles fail to expel the normal fraction of its end-diastolic volume, a complex sequence of adjustments occurs that ultimately results in an abnormal accumulation of fluid. These adjustments are described on pages 1828 to 1834. Although many of the clinical manifestations of heart failure are secondary to this excessive retention of fluid, the expansion of blood volume also constitutes an important compensatory mechanism that tends to maintain cardiac output by elevating ventricular preload, since the myocardium operates on an ascending limb of a depressed function curve[4–7] (Fig. 13–35, p. 413), and the augmented ventricular end-diastolic volume must be regarded as helping to maintain cardiac output, except in the terminal stages of heart failure. Elevation of ventricular end-diastolic volume and pressure, in accordance with the Frank-Starling mechanism, raises ventricular performance but at the same time causes pulmonary or systemic venous congestion and promotes the formation of pulmonary or peripheral edema.

REDISTRIBUTION OF LEFT VENTRICULAR OUTPUT. This is an important peripheral mechanism brought into play to conserve the limited cardiac output. Vasoconstriction, mediated largely by the adrenergic nervous system, is primarily responsible for this redistribution of peripheral blood flow, which occurs when an additional burden (such as exercise, fever, or anemia) is imposed on the circulation in the presence of impaired myocardial function, preventing cardiac output from rising normally. As heart failure advances, redistribution of left ventricular output ultimately occurs even in the basal state.[8–11] This redistribution maintains the delivery of oxygen to vital organs such as the heart and brain, whereas blood flow to less critical areas such as the skin is reduced. Occasionally, serious complications can result from the redistribution and the resulting severe reduction of blood flow. These include marked sodium and nitrogen retention as a consequence of diminished renal perfusion and, very rarely, gangrene of the tips of the phalanges and mesenteric infarction.

AUTONOMIC CONTROL OF THE HEART AND PERIPHERAL CIRCULATION. This control varies with the etiology of heart failure, as well as with the nature and severity of the inciting stimulus. In general, in the initial stages of heart failure, activation of the adrenergic limb of the autonomic nervous system acts to maintain cardiac output by increasing myocardial contractility and raising heart rate; in severe heart failure, vasoconstriction mediated by the sympathetic nervous system and circulating angiotensin II tends to sustain arterial pressure and diverts blood flow from the cutaneous, splanchnic, and renal beds to preserve perfusion of the coronary and cerebral beds.[12] In patients with moderate heart failure, these changes occur primarily during exercise, whereas in patients with severe heart failure they are present at rest. Sometimes in advanced stages of heart failure this compensatory mechanism may, however, have deleterious consequences, as discussed on page 442.

OTHER ADJUSTMENTS. *Increased vascular sodium content and raised interstitial pressure* resulting from sodium and water retention lead to stiffening, thickening, and compression of the blood vessel walls, which prevents a normal vasodilator response during exercise. Inadequate perfusion of skeletal muscle, in turn, leads to earlier dependence on anaerobic metabolism, lactic acidemia, an excessive oxygen debt, weakness, and fatigue. The veins in the extremities of patients with heart failure are constricted, apparently as a consequence of compression by pressure from increased interstitial volume, by circulating venoconstrictors (norepinephrine and angiotensin II), and, to a lesser extent, by the activity of the sympathetic nervous system. Venoconstriction in the extremities results in displacement of blood to the heart and lungs.

A progressive *decline in the affinity of hemoglobin for oxygen* due to an increase in 2,3-diphosphoglycerate (DPG) also occurs in heart failure.[13] This rightward shift in the oxygen-hemoglobin dissociation curve represents a compensatory mechanism which facilitates oxygen transport; increased DPG, tissue acidosis, and the slow circulation time characteristic of heart failure act synergistically to maintain the delivery of oxygen to the metabolizing tissues in the face of a reduced cardiac output.

CONTRACTILITY OF HYPERTROPHIED AND FAILING MYOCARDIUM

When an excessive pressure or volume load is imposed on a ventricle, myocardial hypertrophy develops, providing a fundamental compensatory mechanism that permits the ventricle to sustain this burden.[14] A ventricle subjected to an abnormally elevated load for a prolonged period, however, may fail to maintain compensation despite the presence of ventricular hypertrophy, and pump failure may ultimately occur, as discussed on page 429.

STUDIES ON ISOLATED MUSCLE. There has been substantial interest in the analysis of the behavior of isolated muscle removed from animals in which the heart was subjected to a controlled major stress. A convenient experimental model of ventricular pressure overload is the cat with pulmonary artery constriction. Papillary muscles are removed from the right ventricles in which either hypertrophy or overt failure has developed, and the excised muscle is then studied in vitro.[15, 16] Right ventricular hypertrophy and failure both reduce the maximum velocity of unloaded shortening (V_{max}) below the values observed in muscles obtained from normal cats; the changes are more marked in muscles obtained from animals in which heart failure was present than in those with hypertrophy alone (Figs. 14–1 and 14–2). Heart failure depresses the

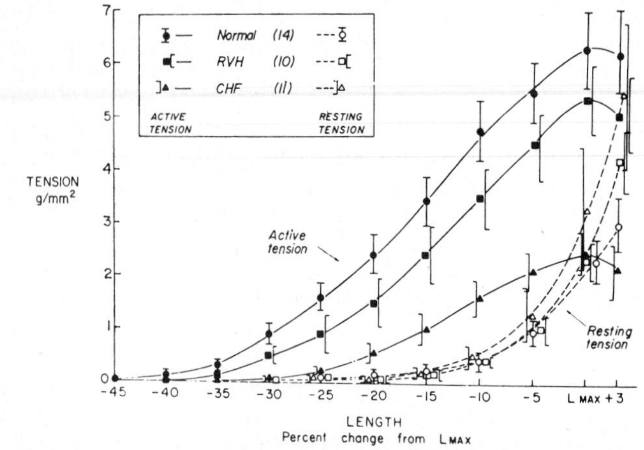

FIGURE 14–1. Relation between muscle length and tension of papillary muscles from normal (circles), hypertrophied (squares), and failing (triangles) right ventricles. Open symbols = resting tension; filled symbols = actively developed tension. Each value is the average of the group; vertical lines with cross bars = ± 1 SEM. Tension is corrected for cross-sectional area (g/mm²). Numbers in parentheses = number of animals. (From Spann, J. F., Jr., Buccino, R. A., Sonnenblick, E. H., and Braunwald, E.: Contractile state of cardiac muscle obtained from cats with experimentally produced ventricular hypertrophy and heart failure. Circ. Res. *21*:341, 1967, by permission of the American Heart Association, Inc.)

maximal isometric tension, but hypertrophy without failure produces only borderline depression of this variable. These changes are often accompanied by spontaneous electrical activity of isolated muscle.[17]

The findings summarized above are, in general, consonant with those of a number of other investigations on cardiac muscle isolated from animals with experimentally produced pressure overload.[18] For example, the trabecular or papillary muscles removed from the left ventricles of the rat in which left ventricular hypertrophy has been created by aortic constriction or by renovascular hypertension also exhibit a depression in the velocity of isotonic shortening, a prolongation of the action potential and of the duration of isometric contraction and of the time-to-peak tension even in the absence of a reduction in the

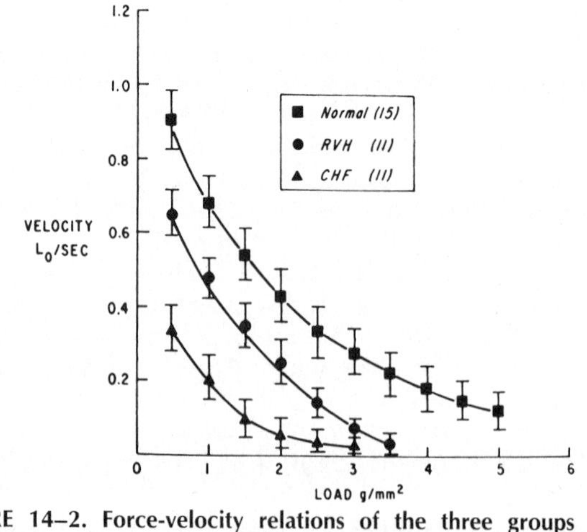

FIGURE 14–2. Force-velocity relations of the three groups of cat papillary muscles. Average values ± SEM are given for each point. Velocity has been corrected to muscle lengths per second (L_0/sec). Numbers in parentheses = number of animals. (From Spann, J. F., Jr., Buccino, R. A., Sonnenblick, E. H., and Braunwald, E.: Contractile state of cardiac muscle obtained from cats with experimentally produced ventricular hypertrophy and heart failure. Circ. Res. *21*:341, 1967, by permission of the American Heart Association, Inc.)

development of isometric tension.[19] The force and rate of force development are also depressed in muscles obtained from hearts with totally different forms of heart failure, i.e., from Syrian hamsters with hereditary cardiomyopathy,[20] as well as in papillary muscles removed from the left ventricles of patients with heart failure due to chronic valvular disease.[21]

In contrast to the depressed performance of cardiac muscle removed from cardiomyopathic or pressure-overloaded hearts, contractility is normal in papillary muscles removed from cats with a volume overload resulting from an experimentally produced atrial septal defect.[22] It should also be noted that although the length–active tension curve, the maximal rate of isometric force development, and force-velocity relations are all significantly depressed in cat papillary muscles removed 6 weeks after pulmonary artery banding, in some,[23] but not all,[16] studies these variables returned to normal when the elevated pressure was maintained for prolonged periods. With even longer periods of pressure overload, isometric force declined a second time.[24] These observations emphasize the important temporal relationships between the imposition of a load, its nature (volume or pressure), severity, time, and the resultant depression of the contractile state. However, the available data are consonant with Meerson's concept of three stages of hypertrophy in response to an acutely induced pressure overload.[25] The first stage reflects the initial myocardial damage as a consequence of the imposition of the load; then during the second stage there is a recovery period of stable hyperfunction, followed by late deterioration during the stage of "exhaustion."[24]

Electron microscopic studies of myocardium removed from overloaded, dilated hearts fixed at the elevated filling pressures that existed during life have revealed sarcomere lengths averaging 2.2 μm—no longer than those at the apex of the length–active tension curve of normal cardiac muscle.[26] This indicates that the depressed contractility of failing heart muscle is *not* due to an enlarging H zone, i.e., the disengagement of actin and myosin filaments. Thus, the depression of contractility in failing heart muscle appears to be related to an *intrinsic defect of the muscle* rather than to its operation on the descending limb of the Frank-Starling curve.[5]

STUDIES ON INTACT HEARTS. Immediately after imposition of a volume overload (such as an aortocaval fistula), contractility—as reflected in the slope of the end-systolic stress-circumference relationship—may increase. However, it then declines, while overall hemodynamic performance is sustained.[27] Changes in performance of the intact heart are, in general, similar to those observed in isolated cardiac tissue obtained from hearts subjected to abnormal hemodynamic loads. Thus, the contractile performance of the intact right ventricles of cats with pulmonary artery constriction reveals a marked depression paralleling that observed in the isolated papillary muscles removed from these ventricles.[28] When compared with normal values, the active tension developed by the right ventricle at equivalent end-diastolic fiber lengths is markedly reduced in cats with heart failure (Fig. 14–3). Studies involving manipulations of end-diastolic volume revealed that these failing hearts ordinarily function on the *ascending* limb of a *depressed* length–active tension curve rather than on the descending limb of a normal curve. Thus, as the ventricle fails, it moves to the right along a depressed length–active tension curve, so that it requires an abnormally elevated end-diastolic volume (and often an elevation of end-diastolic pressure as well) to generate a level of tension equal to that achieved by the normal heart at a normal end-diastolic volume. The similar level of active tension at

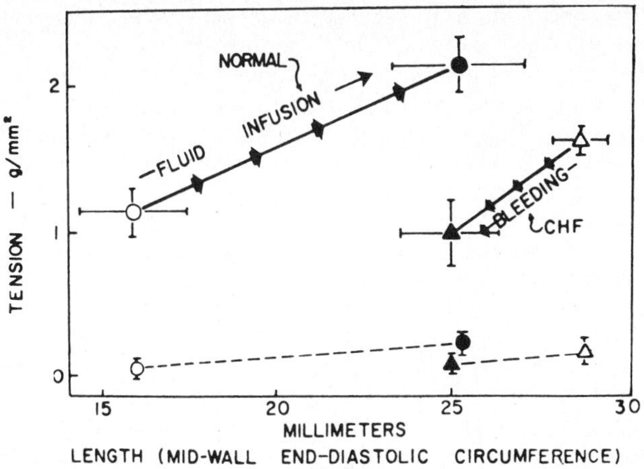

FIGURE 14–3. Length-tension relationships in the intact ventricle. Acute manipulation of end-diastolic volume to obtain ventricular Frank-Starling curves. Lines represent segments of active and resting length-tension curves (Frank-Starling relationship) of five normal (circles) and five failing (triangles) ventricles. Solid lines represent active tension, whereas dashed lines refer to resting or diastolic tension. Open symbols refer to values obtained at spontaneously occurring end-diastolic volume, whereas solid symbols refer to values obtained after volume infusion in normal cats and bleeding of cats with heart failure. Average values ± SEM are shown. Active and resting tensions are expressed on the ordinate, and normalized end-diastolic circumference, or muscle length, on the abscissa. (From Spann, J. F., Jr., Covell, J. W., Eckberg, D. L., Sonnenblick, E. H., Ross, J., Jr., and Braunwald, E.: Contractile performance of the hypertrophied and chronically failing cat ventricle. Am. J. Physiol. *223*:1150, 1972.)

spontaneously occurring end-diastolic volumes in normal and failing cat hearts is evidence of the compensation afforded the depressed myocardium by cardiac dilatation. Contractile tension is thus preserved, but at the expense of an increased end-diastolic pressure and volume. However, the velocity of myocardial fiber shortening and the velocity of contraction at any given load are depressed despite the normal levels of tension development.

Although cardiac output and left ventricular end-diastolic pressure are normal at rest in spontaneously hypertensive rats with chronic pressure overload, the left ventricular ejection fraction is depressed.[29–31] When such rats are stressed with infusions of fluid, the stroke volume and cardiac output rise subnormally. A depression of contractility, as reflected in the relationship between ejection fraction and afterload, occurs before the deterioration of ventricular performance as reflected in baseline and maximal cardiac indices.[31] Chronic left ventricular volume overload, produced by creating a large arteriovenous fistula, causes depression of a variety of indices of contractility.[32] Thus, there is substantial evidence that both chronic pressure and volume overload depress contractility and performance of the intact heart. In addition, left ventricular function has also been found to be depressed in isolated but intact hearts removed from rats with experimentally induced diabetes mellitus.[33]

MANIFESTATIONS OF DEPRESSED CONTRACTILITY. When all of the studies on isolated muscle and intact hearts are taken together, it may be concluded that the depression of the cardiac contractile state observed in the hypertrophied and failing ventricle, however caused, represents an *intrinsic* property of the muscle. Since this depression is evident in vitro, when the muscle's physical and chemical milieu is controlled, it is therefore not dependent on any altered humoral or other environmental factors existing in vivo. Although contractility is depressed in the intact ventricle and in isolated muscles of many preparations subjected to pressure overload, the cardiac index and stroke volume in the basal state are often maintained despite markedly depressed levels of contractility.

It appears, then, that when the ventricle is stressed, by either a pressure or a volume overload, the initial response is an increase in the length of sarcomeres, so that the overlap between myofilaments is optimal, i.e., approximately 2.2 μm (p. 400). This is followed by an increase in the total muscle mass, although the pattern of hypertrophy differs depending on whether the stress is a pressure load or a volume load (p. 432). If the overload is not extreme, this adaptation at first can allow maintenance of a high systolic pressure (in the case of a pressure overload) or augmented cardiac output (in the case of a volume overload) without a depression of contractility. If the intrinsic contractile state of each unit of myocardium becomes depressed, the increased muscle mass, operating in conjunction with increased sympathetic stimulation, maintains overall circulatory compensation. If the overload persists, Meerson has proposed that some of the hypertrophied cells become necrotic,[25] which places an additional load on the surviving cells and may thereby result in a vicious circle, ultimately causing heart failure.

In its mildest form, the depression of contractility is manifested by a reduction in the maximal velocity of shortening of unloaded myocardium (V_{max}) or by a reduction in the rate of force development in isometric contraction,[19] but by little, if any, decrease in the development of maximal isometric force (P_0). As the intrinsic contractile state of each unit of myocardium becomes further depressed, a more extensive reduction in V_{max} occurs, and this is now accompanied by a decline in P_0. At this point, circulatory compensation may still be provided by an increase in muscle mass and cardiac dilatation, which tend to maintain wall stress at normal levels. Cardiac output and stroke volume are maintained in the basal state, but ejection fraction is depressed, as are the maximal levels of cardiac output and/or left ventricular systolic pressure that can be attained during stress. As contractility declines further, overt congestive heart failure, as indicated by a depression of cardiac output and work and/or an elevation of ventricular end-diastolic volume and pressure, becomes manifested. In addition, although an improvement in function can occur in failing muscle in response to positive inotropic stimuli such as digitalis or sympathomimetic amines, the *degree* of augmentation falls, and at a late stage, the contractility of even the stimulated heart is subnormal.

Reversibility of Cardiac Depression. The depression of myocardial contractility in papillary muscles removed from cats with pressure overload–induced hypertrophy is reversible when the hypertrophy is reversed by unbanding the pulmonary artery.[24, 34] Sustained treatment of hypertension also reverses the impairment of contractility caused by that condition.[29, 30]

CAUSES OF HYPERTROPHY

The character of the stress (increased preload, increased afterload, loss of myocytes, as in myocardial infarction, or primary depression of contractility) responsible for inciting the hypertrophy appears to play a critical role in determining the nature of the response.[30a] After the neonatal period, an increase in myocardial mass is associated with a proportional increase in the size of individual cells, i.e., hypertrophy, without an increase in the number of cells, i.e., without hyperplasia.

One of the first cellular changes that occurs after the stimulus for hypertrophy is applied is a preferential synthesis of mitochondria; presumably the expanded mito-

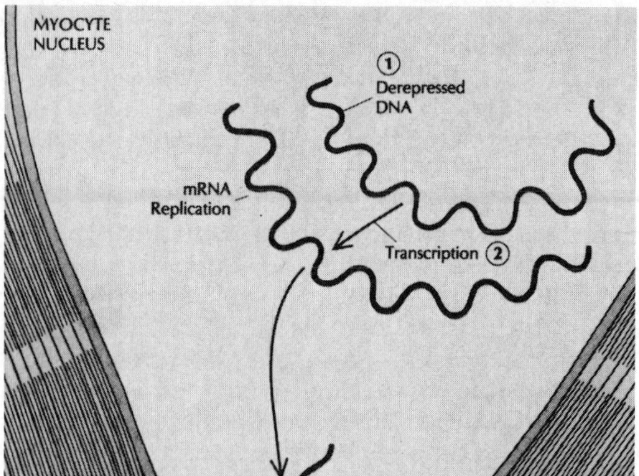

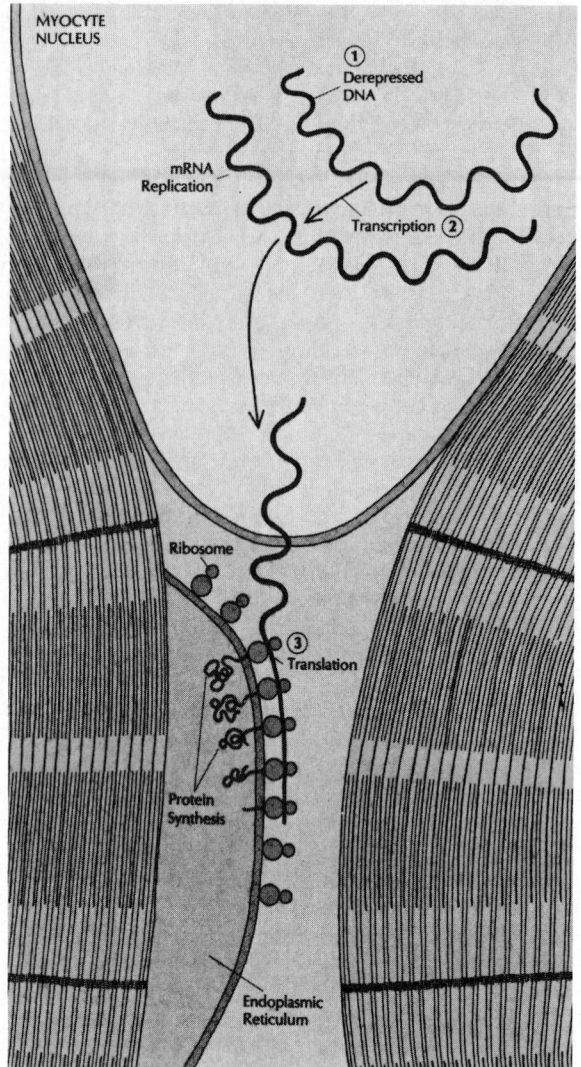

FIGURE 14–4. In order for cardiac hypertrophy to occur, biosynthetic pathways must first be derepressed so that DNA replication can take place (1). The nature of the signal that leads to activation of the repressed DNA remains elusive. The critical regulator may be acting at the stage of transcription (2), when RNA polynucleotides are synthesized on the DNA template or, alternatively, in the final process of translation (3) of the genetic code into protein assembly. (From Zak, R.: Cardiac hypertrophy: Biochemical and cellular relationships. Hosp. Pract. *18*:92, 1983.)

chondrial mass provides sufficient adenosine triphosphate (ATP) to meet the increased energy demands of the hypertrophying cell. Later, the myofibrillar mass increases, and it is possible that the mitochondrial/myofibrillar mass relationship becomes inadequate, ultimately interfering with myocardial function.[35] Cardiac hypertrophy can take place only when the DNA in the myocyte nucleus is derepressed, allowing DNA replication to occur (Fig. 14–4).[35a] There has been much debate about the nature of the stimulus that activates the DNA.[36] The following possible stimuli have been suggested:[35] (1) depletion of ATP; (2) stretch of myocytes caused by a sustained increase in preload or afterload; (3) accumulation of products of cell degeneration caused by "wear and tear"; and (4) humoral stimuli, such as thyroid hormone. While the specific stimulus (or stimuli) for derepression of DNA has not yet been identified, it could operate at various levels, including mRNA transcription, translation, or protein formation.

VOLUME OVERLOAD. When volume overload is produced by the creation of an aortocaval fistula, sarcomere length initially rises to the optimal level of 2.2 μm. Then progressive left ventricular dilatation and moderate left ventricular hypertrophy occur without clinical evidence of heart failure, and the length–active tension relations of the dilated, hypertrophied ventricle remain essentially normal.[37] Within one week of the creation of such a fistula, left ventricular end-diastolic pressure rises and then remains constant, whereas the left ventricular end-diastolic diameter continues to increase progressively. Following chronic adjustment to the shunt, the end-diastolic volume increases at any given end-diastolic pressure (Fig. 14–5); left ventricular function, as reflected in the velocity of circumferential fiber shortening, may be normal or depressed. The performance of the chronically volume-overloaded ventricle is characterized by normal or nearly normal performance of each unit of myocardium, allowing delivery of a stroke volume greater than normal. The chronic ventricular dilatation is associated with diastolic sarcomere lengths that are optimal (2.2 μm). Thus, despite the augmented volumes and filling pressures, there is *no* disengagement of thick and thin myofilaments.

Following the initial increase in stroke volume, mediated by increased sarcomere length during the acute phase of volume overloading, progressive cardiac dilatation subsequently occurs, whereas end-diastolic sarcomere lengths remain relatively constant. Cardiac dilatation presumably results from an increase in the size of myocardial cells or from a greater number of sarcomeres developing in series during the process of hypertrophy causing a lengthening of myocytes and perhaps slippage between adjacent fibers and fibrils.[38] In addition, the myocardial capillary network may not increase in proportion to myocardial mass. These changes may be irreversible[32] and may impair further contractile performance.[38] Thus, in summary, the ventricle ordinarily compensates for a volume overload with both a change in ventricular geometry and an increase in the number of sarcomeres, resulting in an augmented stroke volume. In the compensated state of chronic volume overloading, the combination of ventricular dilatation and

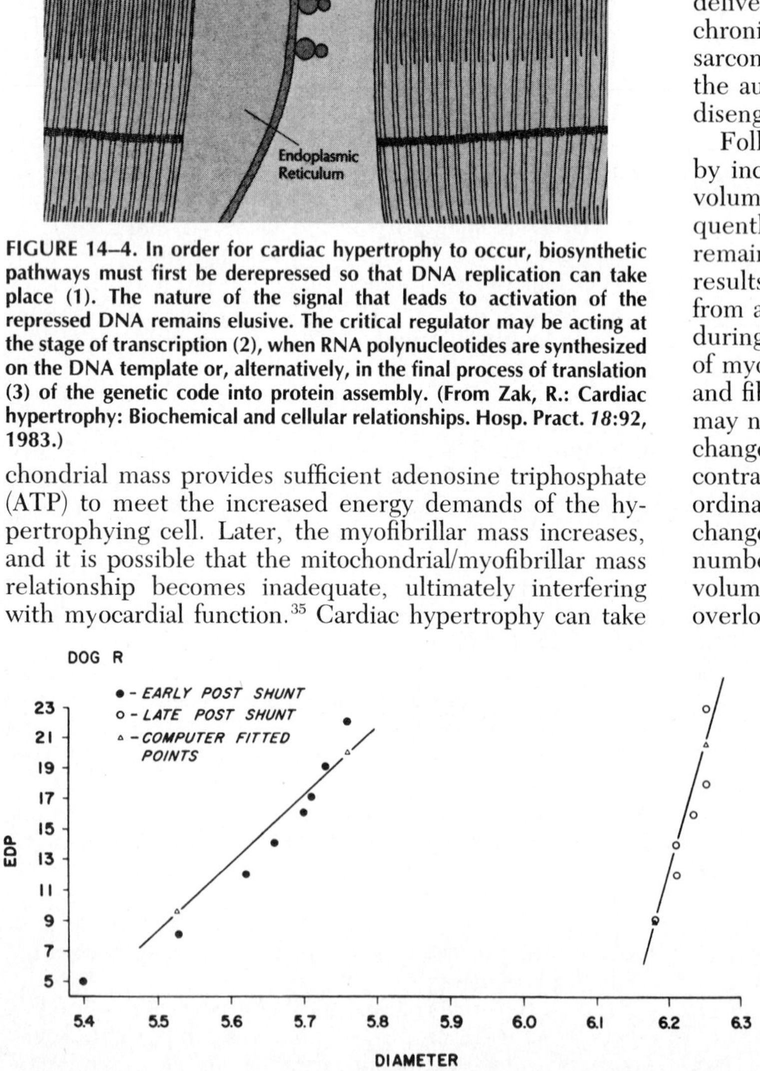

FIGURE 14–5. Relations between left ventricular end-diastolic pressure (EDP, mm Hg) and left ventricular diameter at end diastole (cm) in one dog studied early and late during the course of chronic volume overloading by means of an arteriovenous fistula. Each curve relating end-diastolic pressure to end-diastolic diameter was obtained by acute transfusion and bleeding. The shift to the right and increase in the slope of the pressure-diameter relation between the early postshunt study (closed circles) and the study many weeks after the occurrence of chronic cardiac dilatation (closed triangles) are apparent; the slope change reflects a reduction in diastolic compliance. (From McCullagh, W. H., et al.: Left ventricular dilatation and diastolic compliance changes during chronic volume overloading. Circulation *45*:943, 1972, by permission of the American Heart Association, Inc.)

hypertrophy allows enhancement of overall cardiac performance, with normal function of each unit of an enlarged ventricle operating at an optimal sarcomere length. However, in the presence of a very large volume overload and clinical evidence of congestive heart failure, myocardial contractility does become seriously depressed.[32]

PRESSURE OVERLOAD. More is known about this form of overload, especially in animal models in which the aorta or pulmonary artery is abruptly constricted. As described by Meerson,[25] the increase in work initially exceeds the augmentation of cardiac mass, the heart dilates, and contractility may be depressed. As a consequence, hypertrophy develops,[32a] a compensatory phase sets in, and the contractile function returns to approximately normal. Myofibrils are laid down in parellel so that the cross-sectional diameter of myocytes is increased.[38] Later, alterations in cellular organization take place, and during the "exhaustion" phase there is lysis of myofibrils, the sarcoplasmic reticulum becomes distorted, the surface densities of the key tubular system are reduced,[40] and fibrous tissue takes the place of the cardiac cells.[41, 41a] In addition, capillary density is reduced and coronary reserve, as reflected in the increase in coronary blood flow during adenosine reperfusion, is reduced.[40] The resulting ischemia might contribute to the impairment of cardiac function. Myocardial failure occurs in the stage of "exhaustion" when cellular function deteriorates. Some cells drop out and the remainder function abnormally and are forced to sustain an even greater burden, leading to a vicious circle (Fig. 14–6).

OTHER FORMS OF HYPERTROPHY. A mild form of cardiac hypertrophy is seen in athletes[41b, 41c] (Table 14–1). Prolonged athletic training causes a moderate increase in myocardial mass. Isotonic exercise, such as running or swimming, resembles volume overload and causes an increase in left ventricular diastolic volume; isometric exercise, such as weightlifting or wrestling, resembles pressure overload and causes an increase in wall thickness. Neither form of hypertrophy appears to be deleterious and rapidly disappears when training is discontinued.

Following myocardial infarction, there is hypertrophy of the spared myocytes with an increase of both myocyte diameter, as in pressure overload, and in myocyte length, as in volume overload.[38]

TABLE 14–1 ECHOCARDIOGRAPHIC CHANGES IN ISOTONIC AND ISOMETRIC ATHLETES*

	Isotonic	Isometric
Left ventricular end-diastolic diameter	↑	↑, no Δ
Left ventricular end-diastolic diameter per square meter or per kilogram	↑	no Δ
Left ventricular end-systolic diameter	↑, ↓, no Δ	↑, ↓, no Δ
Left ventricular end-diastolic volume	↑	no Δ
Left ventricular posterior wall thickness	↑	↑
Left ventricular mass	↑	↑
Left ventricular mass, per square meter or per kilogram	↑	no Δ
Interventricular septal thickness	↑	↑
Interventricular-septum/posterior wall ratio	↑, no Δ	↑, no Δ
Right ventricular diameter	↑	–
Left atrial diameter	↑	–
Ejection fraction	no Δ	no Δ
Cardiac output (resting)	no Δ	no Δ
Stroke volume	↑	↑, no Δ
Velocity of circumferential fiber shortening	↑, ↓, no Δ	no Δ

*↑ = increase, ↓ = decrease, and no Δ = no change. (From Huston, T. P., Puffer, J. C., and Rodney, W. M.: The athletic heart syndrome. N. Engl. J. Med. 313:29, 1985.)

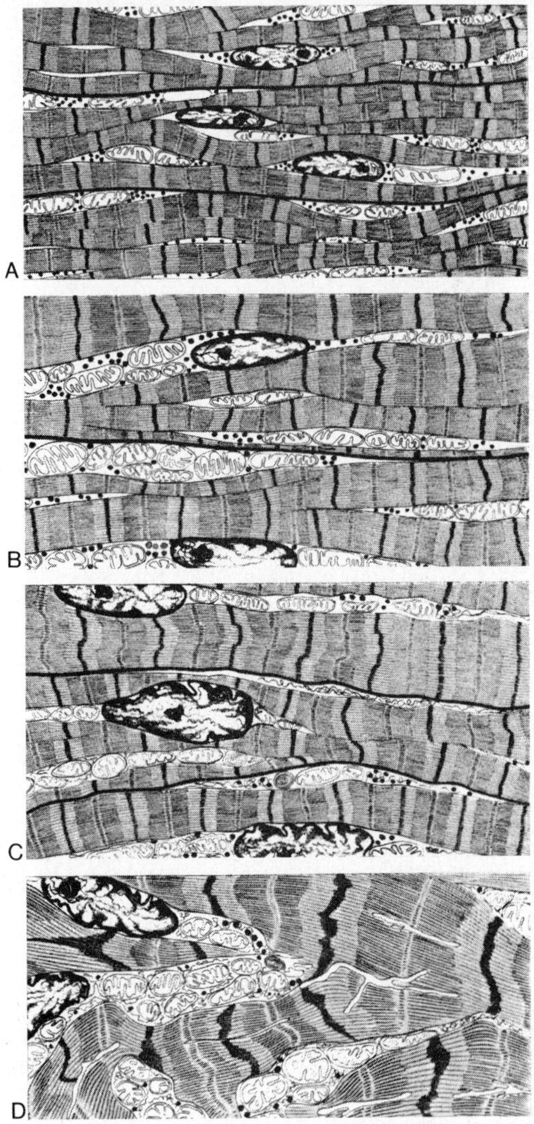

FIGURE 14–6. The early stage of cardiac hypertrophy (A) is characterized morphologically by increases in the number of myofibrils and mitochondria as well as enlargement of mitochondria and nuclei. Muscle cells are larger than normal, but cellular organization is largely preserved. At a more advanced stage of hypertrophy (B), preferential increases in the size or number of specific organelles, such as mitochondria, as well as irregular addition of new contractile elements in localized areas of the cell, result in subtle abnormalities of cellular organization and contour. Adjacent cells may vary in their degree of enlargement. Cells subjected to longstanding hypertrophy (C) show more obvious disruptions in cellular organization, such as markedly enlarged nuclei with highly lobulated membranes, which displace adjacent myofibrils and cause breakdown of normal Z-band registration. The early preferential increase in mitochondria is supplanted by a predominance by volume of myofibrils. The late stage of hypertrophy (D) is characterized by loss of contractile elements with marked disruption of Z bands, severe disruption of the normal parallel arrangement of the sarcomeres, deposition of fibrous tissue, and dilation and increased tortuosity of T tubules. (From Ferrans, V. J.: Morphology of the heart in hypertrophy. Hosp. Pract. *18*:69, 1983.)

Endomyocardial biopsies in patients with heart failure of diverse etiologies are consistent with the formulation presented above. Myocyte hypertrophy and fibrosis tend to be worse in patients with more severe forms of heart failure.[41d] Conversely, patients in whom myocytes are composed of a reduced fraction of myofibrils appear to exhibit a particularly poor prognosis.[42]

EFFECTS OF DEPRESSED CONTRACTILITY. The effects of

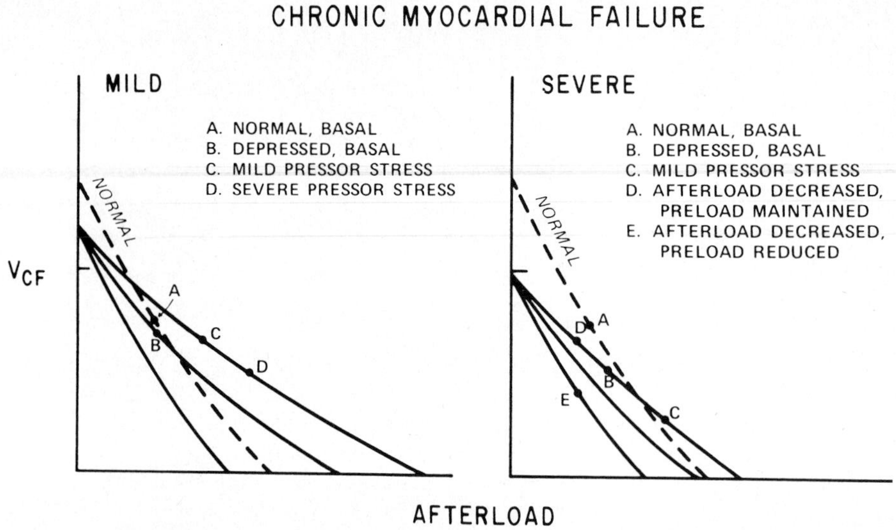

FIGURE 14–7. Alterations of force-velocity relations during afterload changes in the presence of left ventricular failure. *Left panel,* A normal force-velocity curve is indicated by the dashed line, and the normal basal state by point A. With mild depression of the inotropic activity in the basal state, through some encroachment on the Frank-Starling reserve, V_{CF} can be maintained near normal (point B). Some preload reserve may remain, and a mild pressor stress produced by infusion of a peripheral vasoconstrictor may cause little reduction in V_{CF} (point C). However, a more marked increase in afterload will result in a substantial drop in V_{CF} and stroke volume (point D). *Right panel,* With severe depression of the myocardial inotropic activity under basal conditions, V_{CF} is depressed to below the normal range (point B). Since the preload reserve has been fully utilized in the basal state, any afterload increase of even moderate degree will result in a marked drop in V_{CF} and stroke volume (point C). A reduction in afterload with preload maintained constant results in restoration of V_{CF} or stroke volume to near normal (point D), but if preload is allowed to fall substantially, such an afterload reduction may result in no change or even a fall in V_{CF} and stroke volume (point E). (From Ross, J., Jr.: Afterload mismatch and preload reserve: A conceptual framework for the analysis of ventricular function. Prog. Cardiovasc. Dis. *18*:255, 1976, by permission of Grune and Stratton.)

depression of myocardial contractility on the myocardial force-velocity relations are shown schematically in Figure 14–7.[39] Mild depression of contractility permits a normal extent and velocity of shortening of cardiac muscle through operation of the Frank-Starling mechanism, i.e., from an augmented end-diastolic fiber length, and the stress of any augmentation of afterload can be met only with even further augmentation of preload. When contractility is markedly depressed, no preload reserve is available, and any augmentation of afterload results in a marked reduction in the extent and velocity of shortening, a condition that Ross has referred to as "afterload mismatch." Under these circumstances, a reduction of afterload will improve ventricular performance but a reduction of preload will depress ventricular performance, although it may be helpful clinically by reducing ventricular filling pressure and thereby reducing the symptoms of pulmonary congestion (Fig. 17–13, p. 517).

CARDIAC RESPONSE IN VARIOUS FORMS OF VOLUME AND PRESSURE OVERLOADING

Since alterations in preload and afterload are important determinants of the dynamics of cardiac contraction (Fig. 13–27, p. 406), it is not surprising that cardiac performance differs in various cardiac abnormalities depending on the precise alterations in pressure and volume overloading. For example, with equivalent total and effective stroke volumes, left ventricular function is more severely stressed, with greater end-diastolic pressure and volume, in aortic than in mitral regurgitation.[43–45] In the former, the regurgitant volume is delivered into the high-pressure aorta whereas in the latter it must be ejected into the low-pressure left atrium. For similar reasons, left ventricular function appears to be less impaired in ventricular septal defect than in patent ductus arteriosus with similar degrees of left-to-right shunt.[46] Ventricular septal defect resembles mitral regurgitation in that the shunted flow is ejected directly into the low-pressure right ventricle, and there is a rapid fall in tension during systole as the result of a greater reduction in instantaneous impedance to left ventricular emptying, whereas patent ductus arteriosus is similar to aortic regurgitation in that the entire left ventricular stroke volume, including the shunted blood, is ejected into the high-pressure aorta. Furthermore, conditions in which the impedance to ejection is considerably reduced, such as mitral regurgitation and ventricular septal defect, impose a smaller demand on myocardial oxygen requirements than those such as patent ductus arteriosus and aortic regurgitation in which it is not.[47]

PATTERNS OF VENTRICULAR HYPERTROPHY

The development of ventricular hypertrophy constitutes one of the principal mechanisms by which the heart compensates for an increased load. Grossman et al. examined systolic and diastolic wall stresses in normal subjects and in well-compensated patients with chronically pressure-overloaded and volume-overloaded left ventricles.[48]

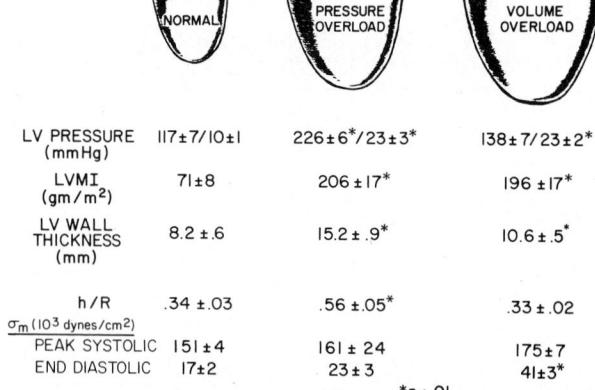

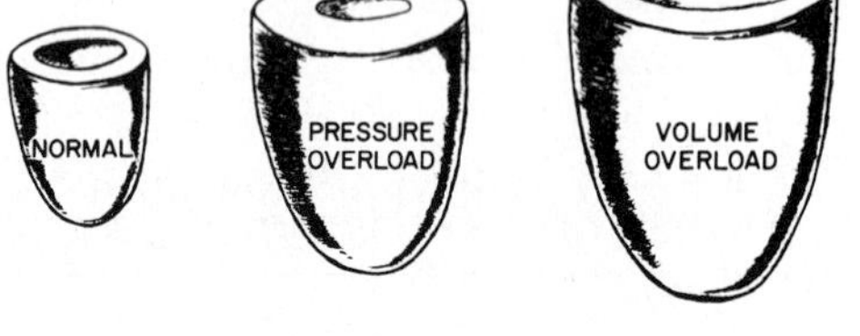

LV PRESSURE (mmHg)	117±7/10±1	226±6*/23±3*	138±7/23±2*
LVMI (gm/m²)	71±8	206±17*	196±17*
LV WALL THICKNESS (mm)	8.2±.6	15.2±.9*	10.6±.5*
h/R	.34±.03	.56±.05*	.33±.02
σ_m (10³ dynes/cm²)			
PEAK SYSTOLIC	151±4	161±24	175±7
END DIASTOLIC	17±2	23±3	41±3*

*p<.01

FIGURE 14–8. Mean values for left ventricular (LV) pressure, mass index (LVMI), left ventricular wall thickness, the ratio of wall thickness to radius (h/R), and peak systolic and end-diastolic meridional wall stress in patients with normal (6 subjects), pressure-overloaded (6 subjects), and volume-overloaded (18 subjects) ventricles. Although mass is increased similarly in both pressure- and volume-overloaded groups, the increase is accomplished primarily by wall thickening in the pressure-overloaded group. The h/R ratio is normal in volume-overload hypertrophy, indicating a "magnification" type of growth. In pressure overload, concentric hypertrophy is quantified by the increase in h/R. Patients were compensated with respect to heart failure, and peak systolic tension (σ_m) was not statistically different from normal. However, end-diastolic stress was consistently elevated in the volume-overloaded group. See text for details. (From Grossman, W., et al.: Wall stress and patterns of hypertrophy in the human left ventricle. J. Clin. Invest. *56*:56, 1975.)

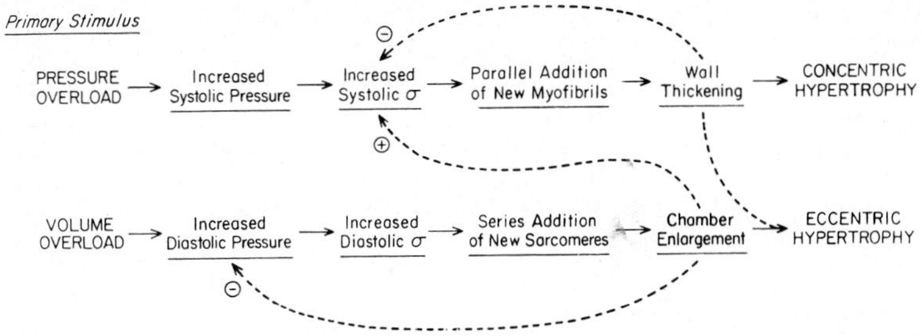

FIGURE 14–9. Hypothesis relating wall stress and patterns of hypertrophy. (From Grossman, W., et al.: Wall stress and patterns of hypertrophy in the human left ventricle. J. Clin. Invest. *56*:56, 1975.)

Left ventricular systolic stress, end-diastolic pressure, and mass were increased approximately equally in both the pressure- and the volume-overloaded groups. There was a substantial increase in wall thickness in the pressure-overloaded ventricles, but only a mild increase in wall thickness in the volume-overloaded ventricles (Fig. 14–8). The latter was just sufficient to counterbalance the increased radius, so that the ratio of wall thickness (h) to radius (R) remained normal for the patients with volume-overloaded hypertrophy, while it was substantially increased in patients with pressure-overloaded hypertrophy, in whom there was disproportionate thickening of the ventricular wall (Fig. 14–8).

These observations are in concert with those of other investigators who have indicated that myocardial hypertrophy develops in a manner that maintains systolic stress within normal limits.[49–52] When the primary stimulus to hypertrophy is pressure overload, the resultant acute increase in systolic wall stress leads to parallel replication of myofibrils, wall thickening of individual myocytes[38] and of the ventricular wall, and concentric hypertrophy (Fig. 14–9). The wall thickening is just sufficient to maintain a normal level of systolic stress. The importance of preventing the development of excessive levels of ventricular wall stress is illustrated in Figure 14–10, obtained from a series of patients with hypertension. As might be anticipated from the inverse relationship between afterload and shortening, as ventricular wall stress increased to excessive levels, both the extent and shortening of velocity declined. When the primary stimulus is ventricular volume overload, increased diastolic wall stress leads to replication of sarcomeres in series, elongation of myocytes, and ventricular dilatation. This, in turn, results in a modest increase in systolic stress (by the Laplace relationship), which then causes wall thickening which again tends to maintain a normal level of systolic stress. Thus, in compensated subjects, both volume and pressure overload alter ventricular geometry and wall thickness, so that systolic stress is not changed greatly.

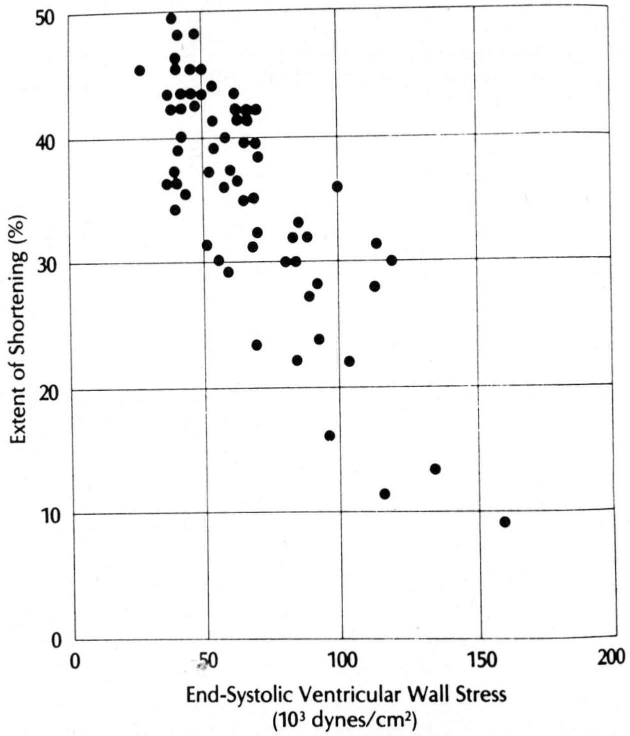

FIGURE 14–10. In a study of hypertensive patients, calculated end-systolic ventricular wall stress (indicative of afterload during ventricular ejection) correlated closely with ventricular performance. A consistent relationship occurred with extent of circumference shortening in the left ventricular wall. A similar relationship was observed between end-systolic ventricular wall stress and the velocity of shortening. (From Tarazi, R. C.: The progression from hypertrophy to heart failure. Hosp. Pract. *18*:104, 1983.)

An inverse correlation between circumferential wall stress and both ejection fraction and velocity of fiber shortening has been described in patients with aortic stenosis and with hypertension, with relationships between stress and shortening indistinguishable from those of normal subjects. This suggests that intrinsic myocardial function is normal in most patients with pressure-overloaded hypertrophy and with depressed ejection fractions and velocity of fiber shortening. Such impairment of ventricular emptying and shortening occurred only when wall thickening (as reflected in the ratio h/R) was not appropriately elevated (Fig. 14–11).[51] These observations suggest that left ventricular wall thickness is a critical determinant of ventricular performance in patients with pressure-overloaded hypertrophy due to aortic stenosis or hypertension. Poor cardiac performance in such patients is not necessarily caused by an intrinsic depression of myocardial contractility, but rather it could be secondary to inadequate hypertrophy leading to increased wall stress (afterload), which in turn may be responsible for inadequate muscle shortening. It is likely that the depression of contractility which occurs in the "exhaustion" phase of ventricular hypertrophy and myocardial ischemia also contributes to the depression of cardiac performance; such depression in intrinsic contractility has been documented in some patients with aortic stenosis and heart failure.[52, 52a]

The experimental studies of Sasayama and associates are in accord with this hypothesis.[53] They found that when the aorta in conscious dogs was suddenly constricted, left ventricular systolic pressure rose and the left ventricular wall became thinned: This was associated with a large increase in wall stress and as a consequence a reduction in the extent and velocity of shortening. During the next few weeks the left ventricle became hypertrophied; therefore, wall stress declined toward normal, although systolic pressure remained elevated, and shortening also rose to normal levels. When the constriction was suddenly released, wall

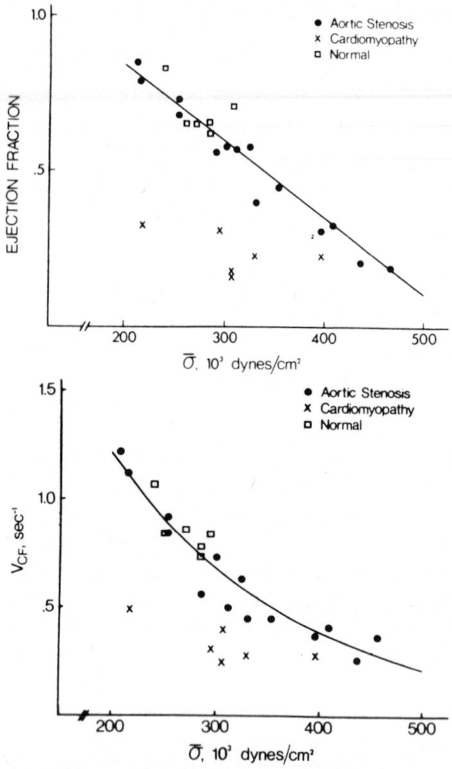

FIGURE 14–11. Relationship between wall stress and muscle fiber shortening characteristics. *A*, Ejection fraction. The line represents the best curve derived from linear regression analysis of the data for patients with aortic stenosis. In these patients, normal values for ejection fraction are associated with normal levels of wall stress, whereas decreasing values for ejection fraction are associated with increasing levels of wall stress. Values for normal controls fall on or near the regression line for the aortic stenosis group. Patients with cardiomyopathy, however, have depressed ejection fractions, regardless of the level of stress. *B*, Mean midwall velocity of circumferential fiber shortening (V_{CF}). Values for patients with aortic stenosis are well approximated as an exponential function of wall stress. Normal patients, again, exhibit a relationship similar to those with aortic stenosis. Patients with cardiomyopathy show depressed values for V_{CF} for any corresponding wall stress. $\bar{\sigma}$ = Mean midwall circumferential stress. (From Gunther, S., and Grossman, W.: Determinants of ventricular function in pressure overload hypertrophy in man. Circulation *59*:679, 1979, by permission of the American Heart Association, Inc.)

stress declined and shortening increased. Similar observations have been made in the spontaneously hypertensive rat (SHR).[30] In the young (6 months) SHR peak tension is elevated. However, it declines progressively with age, to fall to subnormal levels at 24 months, at which time maximum cardiac output is depressed, even though left ventricular mass is increased.

VENTRICULAR RELAXATION AND DIASTOLIC PROPERTIES OF THE VENTRICLE (See also p. 402)

While the development of hypertrophy constitutes a principal compensatory mechanism to an increased load, hypertrophy may have the adverse effect of slowing relaxation and increasing the stiffness (or reducing the compliance) of the ventricle.[53a] While these two aspects of cardiac function, i.e., relaxation and diastolic stiffness, are often considered together, they actually describe different properties of the heart. Relaxation is a dynamic process which begins at the termination of contraction and takes place during isovolumetric relaxation and the rapid filling phase. Diastolic stiffness is measured at end diastole, usually long after filling has terminated. The diastolic stiffness of the ventricle is defined by its curvilinear pressure-volume relation (Fig. 13–24, p. 402). The slope of a tangent (dP/dv) to this curvilinear relation defines the *chamber stiffness* at any level of filling pressure. An increase in chamber stiffness may occur (1) secondary to a rise in filling pressure,[54] i.e., by moving up on the pressure-volume curve; (2) by a shift to a steeper pressure-volume curve at the same ventricular end-diastolic pressure; or (3) through a combination of these two mechanisms. The second of these mechanisms, an alteration of ventricular (chamber) stiffness, in turn can result from (1) an increase in *intrinsic* myocardial stiffness (the stiffness of a unit of cardiac wall regardless of the total mass or thickness of the myocardium), as might occur with amyloid infiltration, fibrosis, or myocardial ischemia; (2) an increase in ventricular mass and wall thickness without any alteration in intrinsic myocardial stiffness; or (3) a combination of these two mechanisms.

An acute increase in ventricular afterload has been shown to delay relaxation[55]; therefore, it is possible that with pressure overload inadequate hypertrophy could augment afterload, thereby slowing ventricular relaxation. Similarly, delayed inactivation of contraction (cross-bridge cycling) can also slow relaxation. The rate of inactivation depends on the uptake of myoplasmic calcium by the sarcoplasmic reticulum, an energy-dependent process that may be slowed by a reduction of intracellular ATP. Morgan et al. have observed that myocardium isolated from patients with hypertrophic cardiomyopathy[56] and from ferrets with pressure-overloaded hypertrophy[57] exhibits a prolonged calcium transient (i.e., elevated myoplasmic calcium concentration), associated with a prolonged tension decay, findings consistent with a delayed uptake of Ca^{++} by the sarcoplasmic reticulum. The presence of pressure-overloaded hypertrophy also enhances the susceptibility to the development of impaired relaxation during hypoxia.[58]

Since ventricular volume and chamber stiffness are interdependent, disease states that modify ventricular size will alter chamber stiffness as a consequence of simple changes of ventricular volume in the absence of a change in myocardial stiffness. Thus, in acute volume overload, as might occur in acute aortic or mitral regurgitation or in acute left ventricular failure due to myocarditis, the left ventricle appears to move up to the steep portion of its pressure-volume curve and the end-diastolic pressure can rise sharply.

CHRONIC CHANGES IN VENTRICULAR DIASTOLIC PRESSURE-VOLUME RELATIONS. In contrast to the relative constancy of the passive end-diastolic pressure-volume relation, i.e., stiffness or compliance, of the left ventricle during acute interventions, prominent changes in this relation frequently occur with chronic heart disease, thus making the ventricular end-diastolic pressure an unreliable guide to end-diastolic volume.[59] Changes in compliance and substantial shifts in the diastolic pressure-volume curve of the left ventricle can be demonstrated experimentally during sustained volume overloading. Dogs with a chronic arteriovenous fistula demonstrate a progressive increase in left ventricular end-diastolic volume, without further elevation of the left ventricular end-diastolic pressure beyond that observed during the early, acute phase of the volume overloading. A rightward displacement (along the volume axis) of the entire diastolic pressure-dimension relationship occurs, and the slope of this curve is steeper, indicating increased chamber stiffness (Fig. 14–5).[37] Some patients with severe overloading due to chronic aortic regurgitation

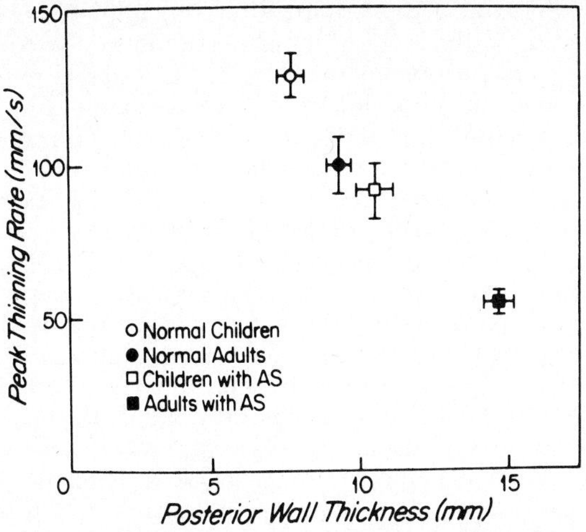

FIGURE 14–12. Relation between left ventricular end-diastolic posterior wall thickness and peak left ventricular early diastolic wall thinning rate for the four groups of subjects. Means and standard errors of the mean are shown. AS = aortic stenosis. (From Fifer, M. A., Borow, D. M., Colan, S. D., and Lorell, B. H.: Early diastolic left ventricular function in children and adults with aortic stenosis. Reprinted by permission of The American College of Cardiology. J. Am. Coll. Cardiol. 5:1151, 1985.)

demonstrate similar shifts of the left ventricular diastolic pressure-circumference relation.

An increase in intrinsic myocardial (as opposed to chamber) stiffness has been described in the ventricular myocardium of dogs subjected to pulmonary artery constriction.[60] When spontaneously hypertensive rats exhibit a depression of ventricular contractility, they also evidence an increase of myocardial stiffness.[61] An increase in myocardial stiffness that may be reversed following surgical treatment has also been reported in patients with aortic stenosis.[50] Thus, it has been postulated that in aortic stenosis, the development of concentric hypertrophy mitigates the increased systolic tension that would otherwise be required to eject blood across the narrowed orifice. There is an inverse relationship between the thickness of the posterior wall and its peak thinning rate during early diastole[62] (Fig. 14–12). An elevation of diastolic ventricular pressure is required to fill the hypertrophied ventricle. However, some patients have not only increased chamber stiffness but increased muscle stiffness as well, and in them the rise in left ventricular diastolic pressure is particularly striking.[50] In patients with hypertension there is a slowing of ventricular filling which has been demonstrated by radionuclide angiography (Fig. 14–13)[63] and echocardiography,[64] even at a time when systolic function is normal.[64a] However, a reduced rate of relaxation is not an inevitable accompaniment of ventricular hypertrophy, since it is not observed in athletes who have an increase in myocardial mass.[65]

The markedly dilated left ventricles of patients with chronic volume overload or with congestive (dilated) cardiomyopathy may be associated with little elevation of left ventricular end-diastolic pressure, indicating a shift of the pressure-volume curve to the right, i.e., along the volume axis (Fig. 14–5).[66] In contrast, concentric left ventricular hypertrophy, as occurs in aortic stenosis, hypertension, and hypertrophic cardiomyopathy, frequently changes the shape and position of the normal pressure-volume relation, so that at any diastolic volume, ventricular diastolic pressure is abnormally elevated, representing a shift to the left along the volume axis. Myocardial stiffness may or may not be altered in the presence of myocardial hypertrophy secondary to pressure overload.[67] However, the speed of ventricular relaxation is impaired in patients with marked left ventricular hypertrophy, regardless of whether it is due to pressure (aortic stenosis) or volume (aortic regurgitation) overload.[68]

ISCHEMIC HEART DISEASE. Marked changes can occur in the diastolic properties of the left ventricle in ischemic heart disease. First, as already pointed out, ventricular relaxation may be slowed and myocardial wall stiffness increased in the presence of acute, reversible myocardial ischemia.[69, 70] Myocardial infarction causes complex changes in ventricular pressure-volume relations,[71] the results depending on (1) whether the infarcted tissue or the entire ventricle is studied, (2) the size of the infarct, and (3) the time following infarction at which the study is carried out. In experimental infarction, the infarcted muscle initially exhibits *increased* stiffness,[72] perhaps related to the stress placed on the noncontracting tissue by the neighboring normal muscle.[73] Edema and the fibrocellular infiltration can contribute to further late stiffening of the necrotic tissue.[74] In a rat model of well-healed infarction, the left ventricular diastolic volume is increased at any diastolic pressure, the extent of displacement of the pressure-volume curve being a function of infarct size.[75] In addition, the diastolic pressure-volume relationship of the entire ventricle is shifted so that at low distending pressures, volume is increased—i.e., the chamber displays decreased stiffness—whereas at higher pressures the slope of the pressure-volume curve is normal.

CLINICAL IMPLICATIONS. Changes in the diastolic properties of the ventricular chambers are of clinical as well as

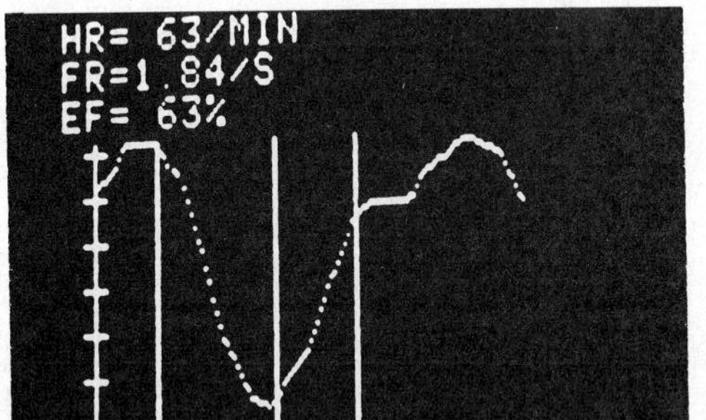

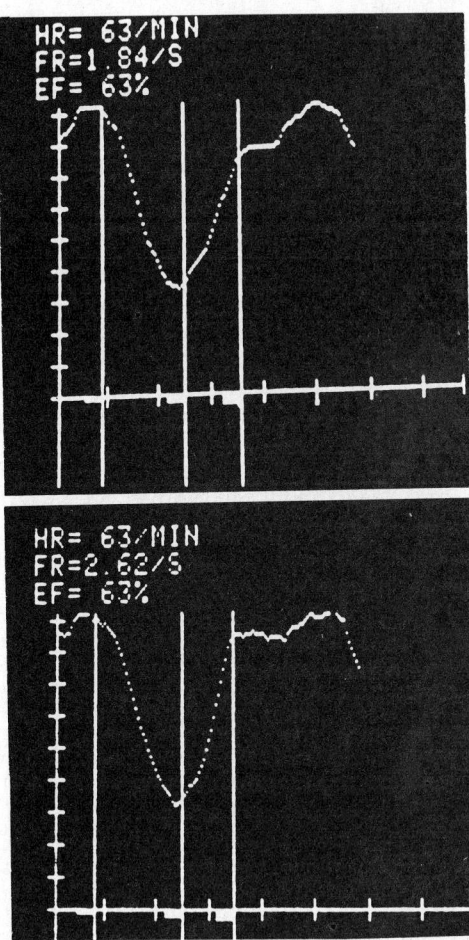

FIGURE 14–13. Radionuclide left ventricular time-activity curves: Patients with mild hypertension (*top*) had a reduced ventricular volume by the end of the rapid filling phase, as compared with normal (*bottom*). This resulted in a low average filling rate in the patient with hypertension. Heart rate and ejection fraction were similar in both. There is also a greater contribution of atrial systole to ventricular filling in hypertension. (From Smith, V. E., and Katz, A. M.: Relaxation abnormalities. Part II: Clinical aspects. Hosp. Pract. 19:166, 1984.)

theoretical importance. Thus, impairment of cardiac relaxation and leftward displacement of the ventricular diastolic pressure-volume curve can interfere with ventricular filling; this situation constitutes a major hemodynamic abnormality in hypertrophic cardiomyopathy as well as other conditions characterized by concentric ventricular hypertrophy such as aortic stenosis and hypertension and by reversible myocardial ischemia. The subendocardial ischemia that is characteristic of severe concentric hypertrophy (even in the presence of a normal coronary circulation) intensifies the failure of relaxation, and when coronary artery obstruction accompanies severe hypertrophy this abnormality may be even more severe.[58] At any given diastolic volume, ventricular end-diastolic pressure and pulmonary venous pressures rise. Tachycardia, by reducing the duration of diastole and, under some circumstances causing ischemia, intensifies this abnormality, whereas bradycardia reduces it. When the pressure-volume curve is shifted by ischemia, the treatment of the ischemia (with a beta-adrenoceptor blocker or calcium antagonist[75a]) improves diastolic relaxation and lowers ventricular diastolic (and pulmonary venous) pressure.

Whereas a defect in ventricular emptying (systolic dysfunction) is the most common form of heart failure, there is increasing evidence that in the presence of ventricular hypertrophy diastolic dysfunction may play a dominant role.[76] In this connection, it is interesting to note that Topol et al. have described a group of elderly patients with hypertension and clinical evidence of severe heart failure with excessive left ventricular emptying and marked prolongation of early diastolic filling.[77] Sometimes isolated diastolic dysfunction can be severe enough to be responsible for severe, even terminal heart failure.[78]

The contribution of atrial contraction to ventricular filling is particularly important in conditions in which ventricular stiffness is increased. Thus, loss of a properly synchronized, powerful atrial contraction in patients with leftward displacement of the ventricular pressure-volume curve (higher pressure at any volume), as occurs in atrial fibrillation or atrioventricular dissociation, raises atrial pressure or lowers cardiac output or both. Pericardial tamponade and constrictive pericarditis also change the apparent diastolic properties of the heart (p. 1494). Early filling is unimpaired in constrictive pericarditis because the myocardium is normal. However, filling is abruptly halted in mid-diastole by the constricted pericardium, which imposes its mechanical properties on those of the ventricle in the latter half of diastole.

The fact that the normal left ventricle operates just below the bend of the pressure-volume curve explains why an acute volume overload or impairment of contractility will result in a marked rise in left ventricular diastolic pressure, which can lead to pulmonary edema as the ventricle moves up to the steep portion of its pressure-volume curve. The rightward displacement of the curve—i.e., an increase in volume at any level of pressure—as occurs with chronic volume overload or cardiomyopathy, is a helpful change, since it lowers the pressure necessary to provide the high preload required by the diseased left ventricle.

MECHANISMS RESPONSIBLE FOR DEPRESSED CONTRACTILITY

Considerable effort has been and is being directed toward elucidating the fundamental mechanism responsible for the contractile abnormality ultimately expressed in a reduction in the work of the myocardium in the common forms of low-output heart failure. The available evidence for the mechanism of myocardial failure analyzed in terms of energy supply, production, storage, and utilization, as well as the structure and function of the contractile proteins, is conflicting. Although a number of metabolic alterations have been identified in the failing, hemodynamically overloaded heart, it is not clear which is the *primary* defect responsible for heart failure and which are *secondary* compensatory mechanisms that aid these hearts in coping with the overload. Therefore, although a single unifying biochemical defect responsible for heart failure has not been identified, a number of possible abnormalities have been excluded, and there is increasing evidence for several possible defects that might be responsible. Some of the confusion in this field results undoubtedly from the various models of heart failure employed, from species differences, from variations in the nature of the inciting stimulus, from the rate and severity of its application, and from the time interval following the inciting stimulus at which the study is conducted.

MYOCARDIAL ENERGY PRODUCTION

In early studies, measurements of coronary blood flow utilizing coronary sinus catheterization, both in humans and in dogs with low-output heart failure, showed that the coronary blood flow per gram of myocardium does not differ significantly from normal.[79] However, other observations on the relation between left ventricular performance and myocardial oxygen consumption have shown that when contractility becomes acutely depressed, myocardial oxygen consumption also declines.[80] Patients with chronic impairment of left ventricular performance and reduction of the velocity of myocardial fiber shortening also exhibit reduction of coronary blood flow and myocardial oxygen consumption per unit of muscle.[81] Marked reductions in oxygen consumption have been described in the Syrian hamster with hereditary cardiomyopathy.[82] Papillary muscles removed from cats with pressure overload–induced right ventricular hypertrophy exhibit a depression of both contractility and oxygen consumption per unit of tension development.[16] Thus, heart failure can certainly occur in the presence of both adequate myocardial perfusion and oxygen availability. In several preparations, failing heart muscle appears to require less oxygen than does normal muscle.

Mitochondrial Function

Considerable dispute has centered on the question of whether or not mitochondrial oxidative phosphorylation, i.e., energy production, is abnormal in heart failure. Some investigators have shown that experimentally produced heart failure is characterized by a defect in mitochondrial energy production.[82] The mitochondrial respiratory control index, i.e., the ratio of active phosphorylating respiration by mitochondria (the rate of oxygen uptake), in the presence of added ADP to the rate of oxygen uptake after phosphorylation of all ADP (normally greater than 4:1) and the number of atoms of inorganic phosphate esterified with ADP to form ATP per atom of oxygen consumed (normally 3:1) have been reported to be markedly abnormal in mitochondria obtained from hearts with experimentally produced failure. Similarly, mitochondria isolated from the hearts of hamsters with hereditary cardiomyopathy[83] and the cardiomyopathy produced by potassium depletion[84] exhibit depression of respiratory activity. Homogenates prepared from hamster hearts with hereditary cardiomyopathy exhibit severe depression of the ability to oxidize fatty acids and acetate.[85] Mitochondria obtained from failing *human* cardiac muscle have also shown reduced oxygen consumption during active phosphorylation and reduced rates of NADH-linked respiratory activity.[82] In contrast to these observations, other data indicate that electron transport and the tightness of respiratory control are normal in mitochondria obtained from failing human hearts[86] and cat hearts with experimental heart failure produced by pressure overload.[87]

MITOCHONDRIAL FUNCTION IN HYPERTROPHY. Mitochondria obtained from hypertrophied, nonfailing rabbit hearts have shown significantly *increased* respiratory activity compared with those of normal hearts, without a change in the ADP/O ratio, i.e., in the rate of energy production to oxygen consumption, or in the respiratory control index, permitting an *increase* in the capacity for synthesizing ATP; in contrast, mitochondria obtained from rabbit hearts with congestive heart failure have shown respiratory rates near or below normal, a decreased respiratory control index, and some lowering of the ADP/O ratio.[88] In the phase of compensatory hypertrophy the ability of mitochondria to generate ATP is increased, due at least in part to the increased mitochondrial mass. However, in the late phase of hypertrophy there is a reduction in the quantity of mitochondria as well as in the capacity of individual mitochondria to generate ATP. According to this concept, a primary cause of contractile failure of the hypertrophic heart might be an inability of the energy-producing system, that is, the mitochondria, to keep pace with the needs of the contractile apparatus.

MITOCHONDRIAL FUNCTION IN HEART FAILURE. Failing muscles removed from cats subjected to an acute pressure overload exhibit decreased efficiency—increased oxygen uptake for any level of tension development. The mitochondria from these papillary muscles exhibit an increase in the rate of oxygen consumption in state 4—basal (so-called nonphosphorylating)—respiration.[89, 90] Ruthenium red, a compound that blocks the mitochondrial uptake of Ca^{++}, reduces the rate of state 4 respiration to normal in these mitochondria. This suggests that nonphosphorylating mitochondrial respiration, linked to Ca^{++} transport and perhaps due to increased cycling of Ca^{++} across the mitochondrial membranes, is responsible for the abnormal myocardial oxygen consumption and the reduced external efficiency that characterizes hypertrophy induced by the acute imposition of a pressure load. Following unbanding of the pulmonary artery, myocardial hypertrophy, the accompanying depression of contractility, elevation of oxygen consumption, and the abnormality of state 4 mitochondrial respiration all return to normal.[34] In addition, no abnormality of mitochondrial function (or, as already noted, of contractility) has been observed in hypertrophy produced by moderately severe volume overload.[22]

The explanation for the conflicting data concerning mitochondrial respiration in experimental heart failure, summarized above, is not clear. It may be related to differences in species or in the nature, severity, and rate of application of the inciting stimulus. However, since, in some studies, oxidative phosphorylation appears to be sustained until very late in the course of heart failure, it is unlikely that the observed changes in mitochondrial function are causally related to the development of heart failure. However, they may well be important in *perpetuating* chronic heart failure.

MYOCARDIAL ENERGY SUPPLIES

As is the case for mitochondrial function, the data concerning myocardial energy supplies in heart failure are conflicting. In the cardiomyopathic Syrian hamster, there is a decrease in high-energy phosphates, and a depression in the free energy of ATP hydrolysis and augmented levels of lactate and inorganic phosphate.[82] Whether these changes are *causally* related to an impairment of contractility is not clear.

In order to determine whether energy supplies are adequate in cardiac hypertrophy and failure, the contents of high-energy phosphate were compared in the papillary muscles of normal cats, cats with hypertrophy without failure, and cats with overt right ventricular failure induced by pulmonary artery constriction. Both the ATP and the creatine phosphate (CP) concentrations were normal in the papillary muscles removed from failing hearts and from nonfailing, hypertrophied hearts which were studied in vitro.[91] Because, as already pointed out (Figs. 14–2 and 14–3), the mechanical performance of these isolated muscles was impaired, *their depression of contractility could not be attributed to a reduction of total myocardial high-energy stores*.[91, 92] In addition, there appear to be no reductions of ATP and CP concentrations in papillary muscles removed from failing human hearts.[86] Thus, it would appear that, just as is the case for abnormalities of mitochondrial function, defects in energy production and the total reserve of high-energy phosphate compounds are not *primarily* responsible for the reduced contractility of the hypertrophied or failing heart. However, it is possible that reduction of ATP in one compartment of the cell which is required for ionic movement or for another vital function does play a key role in the depression of contractility characteristic of heart failure.

One form of heart failure *primarily* related to a reduction of myocardial energy stores is that due to phosphate deficiency. Chronic hypophosphatemia induced by dietary means is associated with reversible depression of myocardial performance in isolated muscle as well as in the intact heart of animals and humans, presumably as a consequence of reduced ATP stores.[93]

MYOCARDIAL ENERGY UTILIZATION

External efficiency, i.e., the ratio of work performed to oxygen utilized, is usually depressed in chronic myocardial failure, probably as a consequence of an abnormality in the conversion of metabolic energy to contractile work. Other possibilities, however, such as abnormalities of cellular alignment, including slippage between adjacent myocytes with ineffective coordination of contraction, must also be considered.

Insofar as the *quantity* of the contractile apparatus is concerned, in a model of stable pressure-induced hypertrophy, as already noted, the fraction of cell volume composed of myofibrils is increased.[35, 94] Patients having aortic stenosis *without* heart failure exhibit a normal fraction of myofibrils per cell, whereas those with left ventricular failure show a significant reduction in cell volume occupied by myofibrils, suggesting that this decrease in the quantity of the contractile machinery may play a role in the development of cardiac decompensation.[95]

Alterations of Myosin ATPase

There is considerable evidence implicating alterations of contractile proteins in heart failure. First, the finding that the reduced velocity of contraction of the hypertrophied myocardium occurs in chemically skinned ventricular fiber suggests that this change reflects intrinsic alterations in the contractile apparatus. Early studies showed that the activity of myofibrillar ATPase was reduced in the hearts of patients who died of heart failure[96, 97] and in dogs with naturally occurring heart failure.[98] Furthermore, reductions in the activities of myofibrillar ATPase, actomyosin ATPase, and myosin ATPase occur in heart failure induced in cats by pulmonary artery constriction,[99] in guinea pigs with constriction of the ascending aorta,[100] in dogs with constriction of the pulmonary artery or aorta,[101] and in rats with renovascular hypertension[102] (Fig. 14–14). These depressions of enzymatic activity could occur if an altered low molecular weight subunit of the myosin molecule, i.e., the portion of the molecule responsible for the ATPase activity, were produced in the overloaded heart and if it

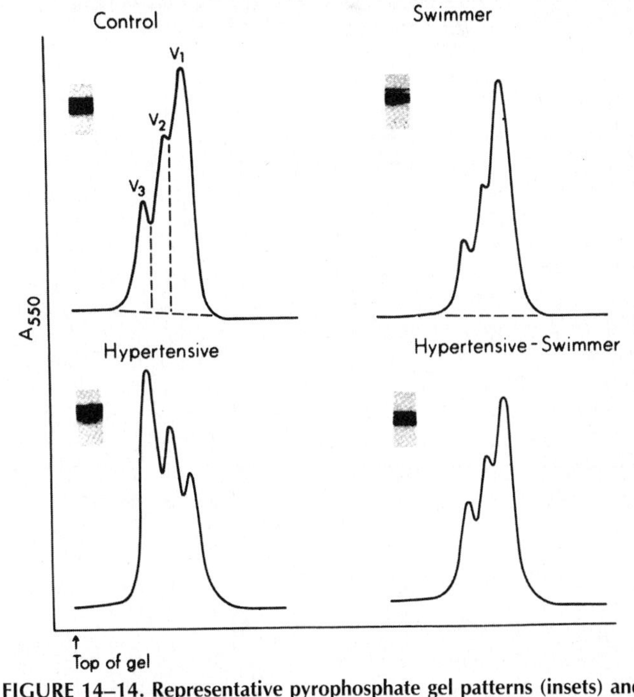

FIGURE 14–14. Representative pyrophosphate gel patterns (insets) and representative densitometric scans of isoenzyme gels for four groups of rats. Hypertension was produced by renal vascular stenosis. (From Sheuer, J., Malhotra, A., Hirsch, C., Capasso, J., and Schaible, T. F.: Physiologic cardiac hypertrophy corrects contractile protein abnormalities associated with pathologic hypertrophy in rats. J. Clin. Invest. *70*:1303, 1982.)

reduced contractility by lowering the rate of interaction between actin and myosin filaments.

It has been shown that the heavy chains of cardiac myosin are composed of several polymorphic forms, termed *isozymes* (p. 387).[103, 104] Thus adaptation of cardiac performance appears to be mediated by a change in myosin. Thyroxin administration,[105] exercise,[102] and mild pressure overload[106] increase the work of the heart and produce a shift in synthesis toward a myosin with increased ATPase activity,[103] that is, myosin V_1 with myosin heavy-chain isozyme (HC)α. However, an increase in cardiac work produced by pressure overload induces the preferential synthesis of cardiac myosin isozyme, i.e., myosin V_3 with myosin (HC)β, which has reduced ATPase activity.[107, 108] However, hypertrophy in the rat produced by swimming caused an increase in the percentage of V_1.[102]

In the human heart, a shift to the V_3 isozyme has been observed in hypertrophied left atria,[109, 110] but the situation in the ventricle is less clear. Increases in myosin *light-chain* isoforms have been observed in hearts subjected to increased mechanical stress.[111]

The synthesis of a myosin with abnormally low intrinsic ATPase activity could explain many of the functional changes in failing heart muscle, such as depression of the force-velocity curve (Fig. 14–2). However, it has been proposed that such a biochemical abnormality might actually be beneficial in heart failure. It would be expected to *increase* the quantity of mechanical energy derived from each mole of ATP utilized, i.e., the "internal efficiency" of cardiac muscle, albeit at the expense of a slowing of the maximum rate at which blood is ejected.[92] This suggestion is compatible with the finding of reduced oxygen consumption per unit of tension development of papillary muscles obtained from cats with pressure overload.[16]

EXCITATION-CONTRACTION COUPLING AND THE ROLE OF CALCIUM

Given the critical role played by Ca^{++} in the contractile process (pp. 389 to 393), it is not surprising that considerable attention has been devoted to examining the role of this ion and of excitation-coupling in the etiology of heart failure. Hypocalcemia secondary to hypoparathyroidism can cause heart failure which is responsive to the infusion of Ca^{++}.[112, 113] Elevation of serum ionized [Ca^{++}] has been shown to augment contractility in patients with renal failure receiving dialysis[114] as well as in patients with severe heart failure secondary to cardiomyopathy who have down-regulation of beta receptors (p. 441) and whose condition is not responsive to sympathomimetic amines.[115]

Studies of a number of in vitro systems indicate that the delivery of Ca^{++} for activation of the contractile process is impaired in heart failure.[116] A variety of cellular structures and membranes, including the sarcolemma, the sarcoplasmic reticulum, and the mitochondria, affect the myoplasmic ionic calcium concentration [Ca^{++}] (Fig. 13–11, p. 392). It has been proposed that damage of these structures or changes in the intracellular concentrations of other cations, adenonucleotides, or free fatty acids may interfere with mechanisms regulating myoplasmic [Ca^{++}] and thereby participate in the production of heart failure.

ABNORMALITIES OF UPTAKE OF Ca^{++} BY SARCOPLASMIC RETICULUM. The uptake of Ca^{++} by the sarcoplasmic reticulum (SR) depends on a Ca^{++}-activated ATPase. Depressed activity of this enzyme, leading to defects in Ca^{++} accumulation by the SR, could play a role in the development of myocardial failure, in that a reduction in Ca^{++} pumping could be responsible for a reduction of Ca^{++} bound to the SR, and this in turn could make less Ca^{++} available for "regenerative release" (p. 389) for the contractile process (Fig. 14–15).

The aforementioned reduction in contractility of papillary muscle obtained from cats with constriction of the pulmonary artery (Figs. 14–1 and 14–2) is accompanied by reduction in the muscle's resting membrane potential, maximum rate of rise, and overshoot, as well as in the duration of the action potential.[117] Prolongation of the action potential has also been observed in myocytes obtained from rats with renovascular hypertension.[19] Although the precise mechanism responsible for these changes in electrical properties is unknown, it may be related to alterations in cellular concentrations of Na^+ and K^+ and thereby affect the entry of Ca^{++} into the myocardium. There is controversy about the response of failing heart muscle to increases in extracellular [Ca^{++}]. Although the contractility of muscle obtained from the failing hearts of cats with pressure overload and of patients with end-stage cardiomyopathy is markedly reduced in a medium containing a normal amount of Ca^{++}, in a medium containing a high [Ca^{++}], the contractility of failing muscles and normal muscles becomes augmented to similar levels.[118] This suggests that the contractile apparatus is not always abnormal in failing heart muscle when it is fully activated and that there may be inadequate activation by Ca^{++}.[115] On the other hand, the contractile response of cardiac muscle from ferrets with pressure-load hypertrophy could not be restored by raising extracellular [Ca^{++}]. Studies with the bioluminescent protein aqueorin indicated that the reduction in peak tension developed by the hypertrophied muscles was *not* due to decreased activator Ca^{++}.[57] These muscles demonstrated a marked prolongation of the Ca^{++} transient, i.e., prolongation of elevation of myoplasmic [Ca^{++}]. This was associated with increased duration of isometric contraction, a finding consistent with a reduced rate of sequestration (and perhaps release) of intracellular stores of Ca^{++}. These findings are compatible with the earlier observation that the rate of Ca^{++} uptake by the SR obtained from failing heart muscle in humans,[119] rabbits,[120] and hamsters[121] is slowed.

An abnormality in the handling of Ca^{++} by the SR in heart failure is also supported by the finding that the ATPase isolated from the SR obtained from the ventricles of dogs with heart failure is depressed.[122] Also, in failing calf hearts the rate of Ca^{++} uptake by the SR and the activity of microsomal Ca^{++}-activated ATPase obtained are reduced to about 50 per cent of normal.[123]

Experimental heart failure in the rabbit produced by aortic regurgitation appears to be associated with a significant alteration in the intracellular distribution of Ca^{++}. Although total intracellular [Ca^{++}] is normal, mitochondrial [Ca^{++}] is increased.[124] The rate and binding of Ca^{++} to the SR are reduced (Fig. 14–15), and it is possible that if the SR can no longer maintain the myoplasmic [Ca^{++}] low enough to initiate muscle relaxation, the mitochondria might become an important storage site as a source of activator Ca^{++} for muscle contraction.[125] Thus, although the total *quantity* of Ca^{++} available to the myocardial cell may not necessarily be diminished in heart failure, *distribution* of this cation might well be altered. With greater quantities of Ca^{++} accumulated in the mitochondria, contractility might then be reduced by limiting the amount of Ca^{++} available to activate the myofilaments; moreover, if enough Ca^{++} enters the mitochondria, their function may become impaired, i.e., uncoupling of oxidative phosphorylation can occur. Interestingly, the uptake of Ca^{++} by the

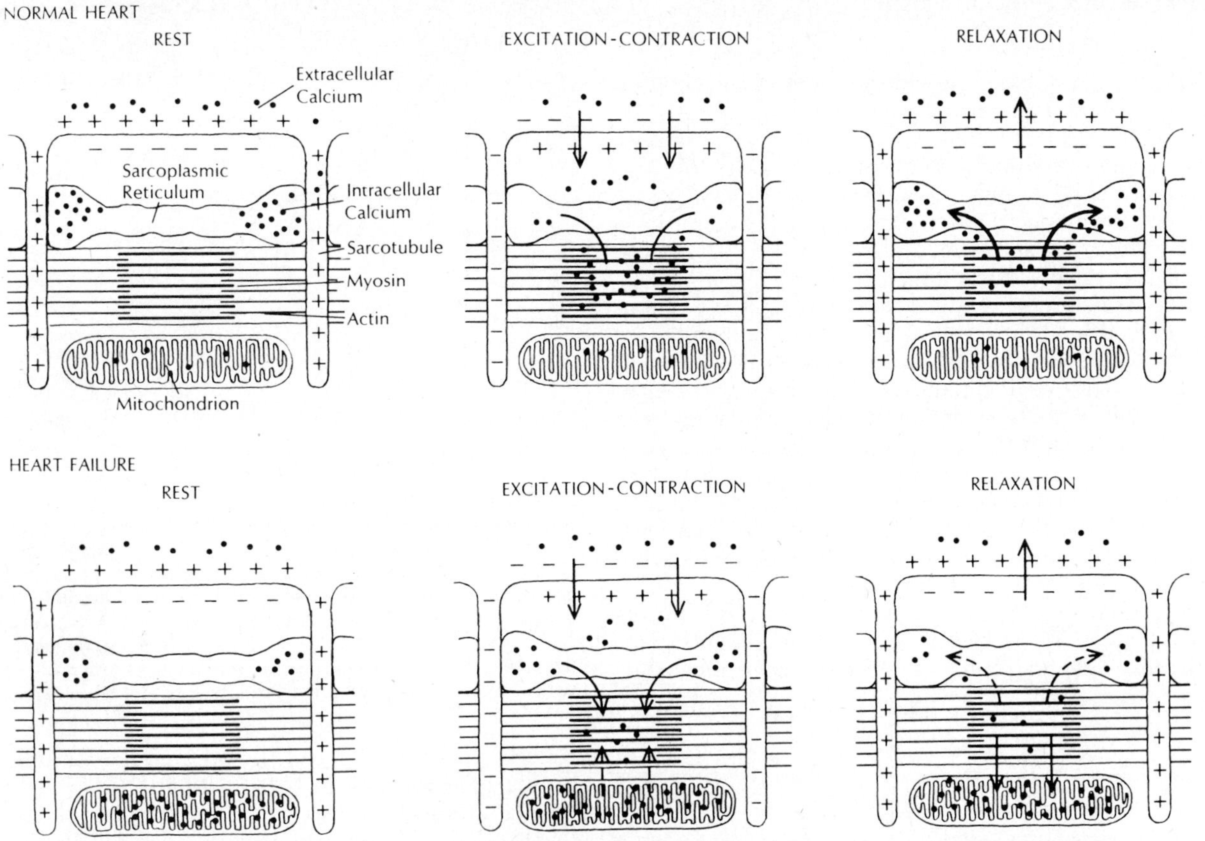

FIGURE 14–15. Hypothetical abnormality in excitation-contraction in heart failure. In the *normal heart* at rest, extracellular calcium is concentrated in the region of the sarcolemmal membrane and its invaginations (sarcotubular system); intracellular calcium sequestered chiefly in the sarcoplasmic reticulum is awaiting delivery to the contractile apparatus. With excitation of the cell membrane and depolarization, there is rapid entry of extracellular calcium; spread of electrical activity via the sarcotubules causes release of intracellular calcium and activation of contraction. For muscle to relax, intracellular calcium must be recaptured by the sarcoplasmic reticulum; efflux of calcium across the cell membrane probably also occurs. In contrast, according to the sequence of events postulated to occur in *heart failure*, ineffective calcium pumping by the sarcoplasmic reticulum may alter the normal relaxation process, rendering the mitochondria the dominant calcium uptake mechanism and a source of activator calcium for contraction. If so, in resting muscle, relatively little calcium would be available for release from the sarcoplasmic reticulum to activate contraction. Although the mitochondria may contain an ample amount, it is likely to be released slowly; thus, with depolarization, a diminished amount of calcium might be supplied to the contractile proteins. Whether the depressed myocardial contractility characteristic of heart failure develops on this basis remains to be determined. (From Chidsey, C. A.: Calcium metabolism in the normal and failing heart. *In* Braunwald, E. [ed.]: The Myocardium: Failure and Infarction. New York, HP Publishing Co., 1974, p. 37.)

SR is significantly reduced in rabbits with aortic regurgitation which were sacrificed *before* the objective signs of heart failure had developed. This finding, very early in the course of failure, suggests that this reduction of Ca^{++} uptake is responsible for, rather than a consequence of, impaired contractility.[126]

The hamster with hereditary cardiomyopathy offers the opportunity for study of the function of the SR in a naturally occurring form of myocardial failure. The Ca^{++} content bound to the sarcolemma is reduced,[123] and there is a depression of the rate of Ca^{++} binding by the SR. This depression becomes more severe as heart failure progresses. Abnormalities of phospholipid and cholesterol composition of the SR, which have been described in the cardiomyopathic hamster,[129] might explain these changes. In addition, both the rate and the extent of energy-linked Ca^{++} binding by mitochondria have been reported to be greatly reduced in these failing hearts.[128]

Abnormalities in the accumulation of Ca^{++} by the SR have been demonstrated in other forms of heart failure as well, including round heart disease, a naturally occurring model of congestive cardiomyopathy in turkeys,[130] spontaneously failing dog heart-lung preparation,[131] failing ischemic heart muscle,[132] the substrate-depleted failing rat heart, and the heart with isoproterenol-induced necrosis,[133] as well as the heart in which hypertrophy and failure are caused by bacterial infection. In the depressed contractile state characteristic of chronic K^+ deficiency, Ca^{++} uptake by SR is reduced, whereas mitochondrial Ca^{++} binding is increased.[134] Cardiac muscle removed from patients with severe heart failure who were recipients of cardiac transplants has yielded SR with slower rates of Ca^{++} accumulation and reduced release compared with normal animal heart preparations.[119, 135] Thus, although disturbances of Ca^{++} transport frequently accompany and may be causally related to heart failure, the nature of the abnormality of Ca^{++} transport appears to vary in different types of heart failure.[126, 136, 137]

ALTERATIONS IN THE FUNCTION OF THE ADRENERGIC NERVOUS SYSTEM

In view of the well-established role of the adrenergic nervous system in the normal regulation of cardiac performance (p. 414), considerable attention has been directed to the activity of this system in patients with heart failure. Measurements of the concentration of norepinephrine (NE) in arterial blood provide an index of the activity of this system at rest and during exercise. At rest, in patients with heart failure the circulating NE concentration is much higher, generally two to three times the level in normal subjects,[138–143] and is accompanied by elevation of circulating dopamine[143] and sometimes by epinephrine, reflecting increased adrenomedullary activity.[139] The elevation of NE results from both increased release of NE from adrenergic nerve endings and its "spillover" into plasma as well as reduced clearance of NE from plasma (Fig. 14–16). Tracer studies have revealed that release of NE from the heart itself is reduced,[144] presumably because of cardiac NE depletion; therefore, the circulating NE appears to be mainly derived from noncardiac sources. Measurements of 24-hour urinary NE excretion have also revealed marked elevations in patients with heart failure.[145] This confirms that the activity of the adrenergic nervous system (and presumably secretion of catecholamines by the adrenal medulla) is augmented at rest.

During comparable levels of moderate exercise, much greater elevations in circulating NE occur in patients with heart failure than in normal subjects. Presumably, this

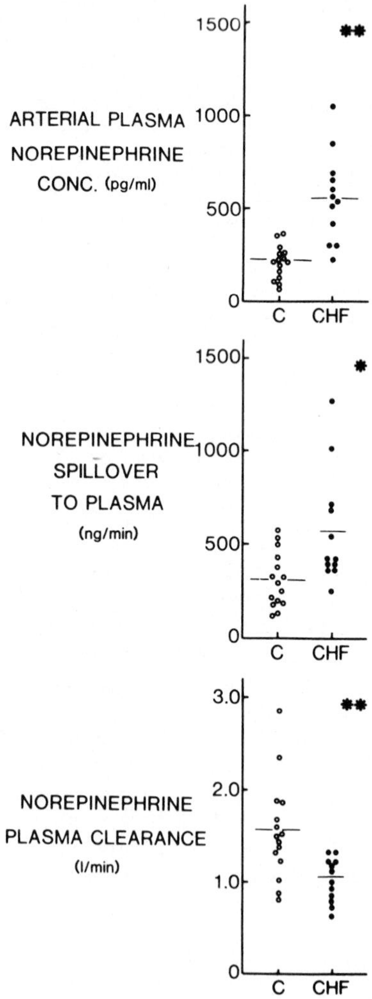

FIGURE 14–16. Plasma norepinephrine (NE) concentration and its determinants in control subjects (C) and in patients with congestive heart failure (CHF). The elevated NE level is related to both increased spillover into the plasma and reduced clearance. *p<.02; **p<.002. (From Hasking, G. J., Esler, M. D., Jennings, G. L., Burton, D., and Korner, P. I.: Norepinephrine spillover to plasma in patients with congestive heart failure: Evidence of increased overall and cardiorenal sympathetic nervous activity. Circulation *73*:618, 1986, by permission of the American Heart Association, Inc.)

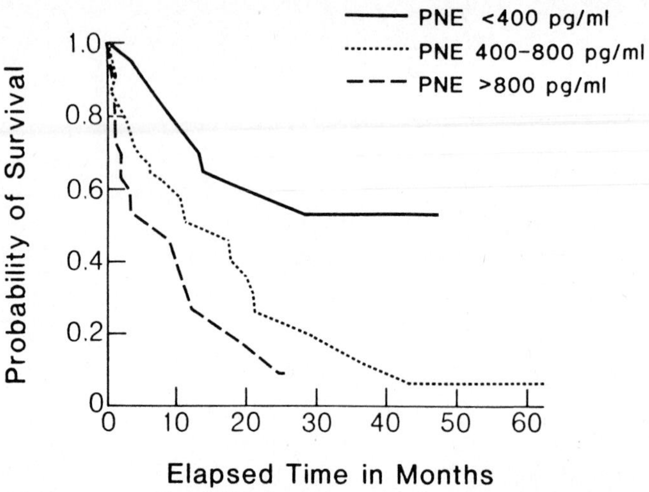

FIGURE 14–17. Life-table analysis of survival, according to tercile based on level of plasma norepinephrine (PNE). Group 1 (<400 pg/ml) contained 27 patients, group 2 (400 to 800 pg/ml) 49 patients, and group 3 (>800 pg/ml) 30 patients. The probability of survival in each group was significantly different from the probabilities in the other two groups. (Reproduced with permission from Cohn, J. N., Levine, T. B., Olivari, M. T., Garberg, V., Lura, D., Francis, G. S., Simon, A. B., and Rector T.: Plasma norepinephrine as a guide to prognosis in patients with chronic congestive heart failure. N. Engl. J. Med. *311*:822, 1984.)

reflects greater activity of the adrenergic nervous system during mild exercise in these patients.[138, 146–148] However, during maximal exercise normal subjects exhibit higher levels of NE than do patients with heart failure, indicating a *relative* attenuation of adrenergic drive during exercise in the latter.[141]

The elevation of plasma NE concentration that occurs in patients with heart failure correlates directly with the degree of left ventricular dysfunction,[149] as reflected in the height of the pulmonary capillary wedge pressure, and inversely with cardiac index and left ventricular ejection time.[150–152] The plasma NE concentration is also directly related to cardiac mortality[142] (Fig. 14–17).

There is evidence that in patients with heart failure beta-adrenoceptors on circulating lymphocytes[153] and $alpha_2$ adrenoceptors on platelets[154] are "down-regulated," presumably as a consequence of prolonged elevation of circulating NE. Most important is the finding that ventricles obtained from patients with heart failure demonstrated a marked reduction of beta-adrenoceptor density, of isoproterenol-mediated adenylate cyclase stimulation, and myocardial contractility[155] (Fig. 14–18). This finding is consistent with an elevation of NE concentration in the immediate vicinity of the cardiac beta-adrenoceptors[155a] and deprives the failing heart of an important compensatory mechanism. In addition, deficient production of cyclic AMP may be an important cause of contractile failure in patients with end-stage heart failure.[155b]

"Down-regulation" of beta-adrenoceptors has also been observed in the hypertrophied left ventricle of renal hypertensive rats. Interestingly, when nephrectomy caused regression of ventricular hypertrophy, both receptor density and responsiveness to isoproterenol were restored.[155c] Ventricular hypertrophy also causes a reduction of the inotropic response to an $alpha_1$-adrenoceptor agonist, phenylephrine, and a reduction of $alpha_1$-adrenergic cardiac receptors.[156]

Further abnormality of adrenergic nervous activity is reflected in the very low concentration of NE in atrial tissue[145] removed at operation from patients with heart failure. In some patients with heart failure, extremely low values were found, with NE concentrations less than 10

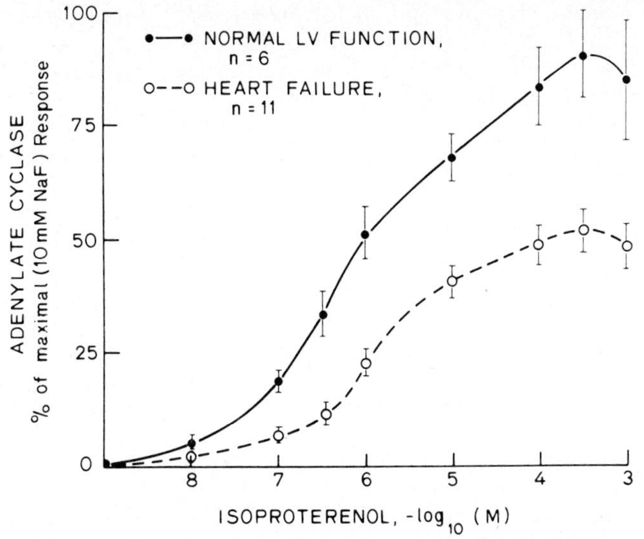

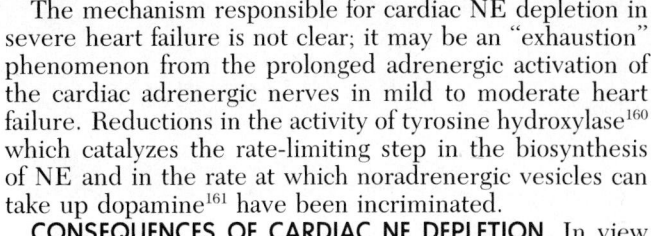

FIGURE 14–18. l-Isoproterenol-stimulated adenylate cyclase activity in human left ventricles in normal human hearts (solid circles) and failing human hearts (open circles), expressed as a percentage of the response to 10 mM sodium fluoride (NaF) stimulation (mean ± SEM). (Reproduced with permission from Bristow, M. R., Ginsburg, R., Minobe, W., et al.: Decreased catecholamine sensitivity and beta-adrenergic receptor density in failing human hearts. N. Engl. J. Med. *307*:205, 1982.)

per cent of normal. NE concentrations were also markedly depressed in papillary muscles removed from the left ventricles of patients undergoing mitral valve replacement for mitral regurgitation and who had been in severe left ventricular failure,[21] and in dogs with right ventricular failure produced by the creation of pulmonary stenosis and tricuspid regurgitation[157] (Fig. 14–19). In NE-depleted failing hearts, fluorescence is absent in the terminal varicosities of sympathetic fibers in close association with cardiac muscle cells.

Following relief from pulmonary artery constriction, many indices of contractile function of the hypertrophied or failing cat right ventricle returned to normal, but NE depletion persisted.[158] It should be noted that local NE stores do *not* play any role in the *intrinsic* contractile state of cardiac muscle. Thus, no differences in contractility were found in papillary muscles removed from normal cats and from cats with NE depletion produced by chronic cardiac denervation or reserpine pretreatment.[159] Length-tension curves, force-velocity relations, and the augmentation of isometric tension achieved by postextrasystolic potentiation and by increasing the frequency of contraction were not altered from the normal state in NE-depleted muscles.

The mechanism responsible for cardiac NE depletion in severe heart failure is not clear; it may be an "exhaustion" phenomenon from the prolonged adrenergic activation of the cardiac adrenergic nerves in mild to moderate heart failure. Reductions in the activity of tyrosine hydroxylase[160] which catalyzes the rate-limiting step in the biosynthesis of NE and in the rate at which noradrenergic vesicles can take up dopamine[161] have been incriminated.

CONSEQUENCES OF CARDIAC NE DEPLETION. In view of the strongly positive inotropic effect exerted by the NE released from its nerves, the adrenergic nervous system may be considered to provide important potential support to the failing myocardium. However, with supramaximal stimulation of the cardiac sympathetic nerves, the increments in heart rate and contractile force that occur in animals with heart failure and cardiac NE depletion are abolished or are much smaller than those in normal dogs[162] (Fig. 14–20). Thus, it is likely that when depletion of cardiac NE stores occurs in heart failure, the quantity of NE released by the sympathetic nerve endings in the heart is deficient in relation to the impulse traffic along these nerves. Furthermore, the reduction in beta-adrenoceptor density in failing heart muscle[155] further limits the response. Therefore, while cardiac stores of NE are not fundamental to maintenance of the *intrinsic* contractile state of the myocardium, diminished release of the neurotransmitter and of beta-adrenoceptor density in heart failure may be responsible for loss of the much-needed adrenergic support of the failing heart and in this manner could intensify the severity of the congestive heart failure state.

ADRENERGIC SUPPORT OF THE FAILING HEART. The importance of the adrenergic nervous system in maintaining ventricular contractility when myocardial function is depressed in congestive heart failure is shown by the effects of adrenergic blockade. Pharmacological blockade of the sympathetic nervous system may cause sodium and water retention as well as intensification of heart failure.[163, 164] Therefore, caution must be exercised in using adrenoceptor blocking agents in the treatment of patients with limited cardiac reserve. Indeed, severe heart failure and occasionally even life-threatening pulmonary edema may be precipitated by the administration of a beta-adrenoceptor blocker in heart failure, attesting to the importance of the adrenergic drive to the heart in these patients. Additional evidence indicating that the NE-depleted failing heart is supported by circulating catecholamines comes from experiments on calves with experimentally produced heart failure and cardiac NE depletion in which beta-adrenoceptor blockade intensifies heart failure, presumably

FIGURE 14–19. Effects of heart failure on cardiac stores of norepinephrine (NE). *A,* Concentration of NE in biopsy specimens of the atrial appendage taken during cardiac operations from 34 patients without heart failure (Classes I and II) and 49 patients with heart failure (Classes III and IV). Average values ± SEM are included. *B,* Total ventricular NE content in normal dogs and in dogs with pulmonary stenosis, tricuspid regurgitation, and congestive heart failure (CHF). Average values ± SEM are given. RV = right ventricle; LV = left ventricle. (From Braunwald, E., Ross, J., Jr., and Sonnenblick, E. H.: Mechanisms of Contraction of the Normal and Failing Heart. 2nd ed. Boston, Little, Brown and Co., 1976.)

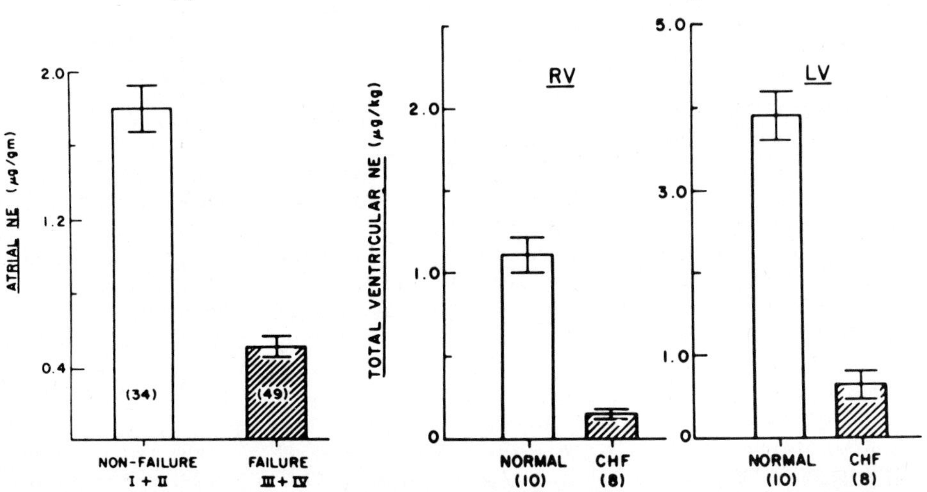

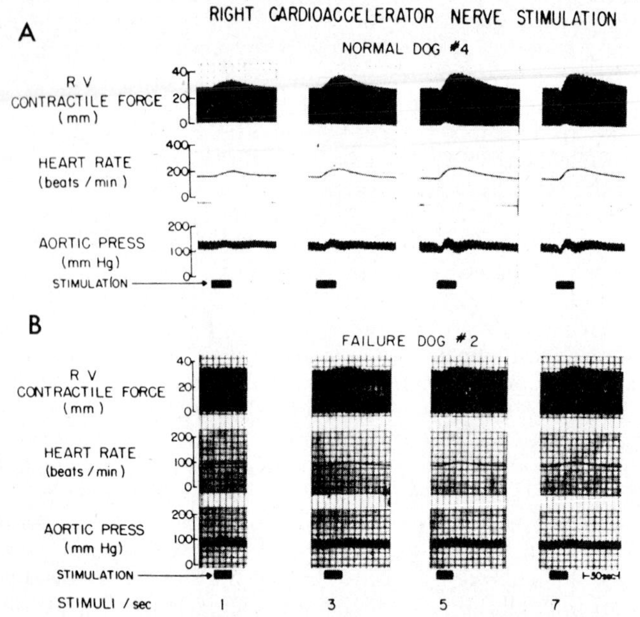

FIGURE 14–20. Records showing the effect of right cardioaccelerator stimulation in a normal dog (*A*) and in a dog with congestive heart failure (*B*). (From Covell, J. W., Chidsey, C. A., and Braunwald, E.: Reduction of the cardiac response to postganglionic sympathetic nerve stimulation in experimental heart failure. Circ. Res. *19*:51, 1966, by permission of the American Heart Association, Inc.)

by blocking the inotropic action of circulating epinephrine.[165] Thus, the increased adrenergic drive presumably serves as a valuable compensatory mechanism in heart failure, stimulating cardiac contractility, redistributing blood flow from nonvital beds, and maintaining arterial pressure in the face of a limited cardiac output. However, it is possible that it becomes deleterious in the late stages of severe failure, by increasing afterload and perhaps exerting a toxic effect on the failing myocardium[155a] and precipitating cardiac arrhythmias. Thus, it has been postulated that in heart failure there actually may be a positive feedback loop causing a vicious circle. According to this theory, heart failure activates the sympathetic nervous system (as well as the renin-angiotensin system and the release of vasopressin); this causes increases in preload and afterload that intensify heart failure.[166] Administration of drugs such as the $alpha_2$ agonist guanabenz (which reduces sympathetic nerve impulse traffic[167]) and bromocriptine (a presynaptic dopamine-2 agonist[168]), reduces plasma NE, indicating that there is a potent presynaptic control mechanism in the heightened sympathetic nervous activity of heart failure.[166] It has been suggested that treatment with such agents might actually be useful in interrupting the vicious circle referred to above.[166]

ABNORMALITIES OF ADRENERGIC CONTROL IN HEART FAILURE. The possibility of defective adrenergic control of heart rate in patients with heart failure has been studied by observing the reflex chronotropic responses to upright tilt and to nitroglycerin-induced hypotension.[169] An attenuation of the normal increase in heart rate in patients with heart failure both before and after administration of atropine confirmed that a defect exists in the adrenergic component of baroreceptor-mediated control of heart rate in patients with cardiac dysfunction; the severity of this defect was, in general, proportional to the impairment of cardiac reserve. In addition, during upright tilt there is a blunted response of the normal rise of plasma NE, of forearm vascular resistance, and of hepatic vascular resistance in patients with heart failure.[170, 171] Some patients with heart failure exhibit a major reduction in arterial pressure during tilting, analogous to what is observed in idiopathic orthostatic hypotension[172] (p. 886). In such patients, not surprisingly, exercise capacity in the upright position is markedly reduced.[173] Further evidence for impairment of baroreflex control of the systemic circulation comes from investigations in which lower body negative pressure failed to cause normal reflex augmentation of forearm vascular resistance.[174]

In dogs with experimental heart failure carotid occlusion elicits a blunted reflex response of heart rate, arterial pressure, and vascular resistance.[175, 176] A reduction in responsiveness of the beta receptors could be excluded as a cause of impaired adrenergic influence, because in many patients there is a normal chronotropic response to isoproterenol,[169] indicating that the adrenergically mediated heart rate response results either from NE depletion or a reduction of adrenergic nerve impulse traffic to the heart. In addition, the heart rate during maximal exercise is reduced in patients with cardiac dysfunction,[169] suggesting that the ability of the adrenergic nervous system to speed the heart rate is impaired in these subjects.

An inappropriately depressed increase in heart rate in humans[177] and in dogs[176] with heart failure was also observed when arterial pressure was reduced through administration of vasodilators. While the changes in mean arterial pressure observed in response to the vasodilators were similar in patients with heart failure and in control subjects, the changes in heart rate after vasodilators correlated significantly with the changes in concentration of circulating NE and with the sum of circulating NE and epinephrine. In normal individuals, both heart rate and catecholamine concentrations rose, whereas in patients with heart failure, in whom resting catecholamine levels were increased, cardiac acceleration was blunted, and catecholamine concentration failed to rise further.[177, 178]

ADRENERGIC NERVOUS FUNCTIONS IN THE PERIPHERAL CIRCULATION. Substantial changes also occur in the function of the adrenergic nerves that innervate peripheral blood vessels in heart failure. Thus, while adrenergically mediated vasoconstriction normally occurs in the vessels supplying the splanchnic viscera and kidneys during exercise, neurogenic vasoconstriction is even more important and much more marked when augmentation of cardiac output is seriously limited, as occurs in heart failure. Thus, it has been shown in dogs with heart failure produced experimentally by inducing tricuspid regurgitation and constriction of the pulmonary artery that exercise induces a much more marked reduction in mesenteric blood flow and elevation of mesenteric vascular resistance than in normal dogs.[9] Similar changes during exercise were observed in other major visceral vascular beds, such as the renal bed. Evidence that this intense vasoconstriction during exercise is mediated by the adrenergic nervous system is provided by observations on dogs with experimentally produced heart failure in which one kidney was denervated. Blood flow through the normal kidney declined precipitously during exercise, and calculated renal vascular resistance increased markedly. In contrast, little change in renal blood flow and calculated renal vascular resistance occurred in the denervated kidney[9] (Fig. 14–21). This intensive visceral vasoconstriction during exercise diverts cardiac output to exercising muscle.

PARASYMPATHETIC FUNCTION IN HEART FAILURE

Cardiac enlargement, with or without heart failure, is associated with marked disturbances of parasympathetic as

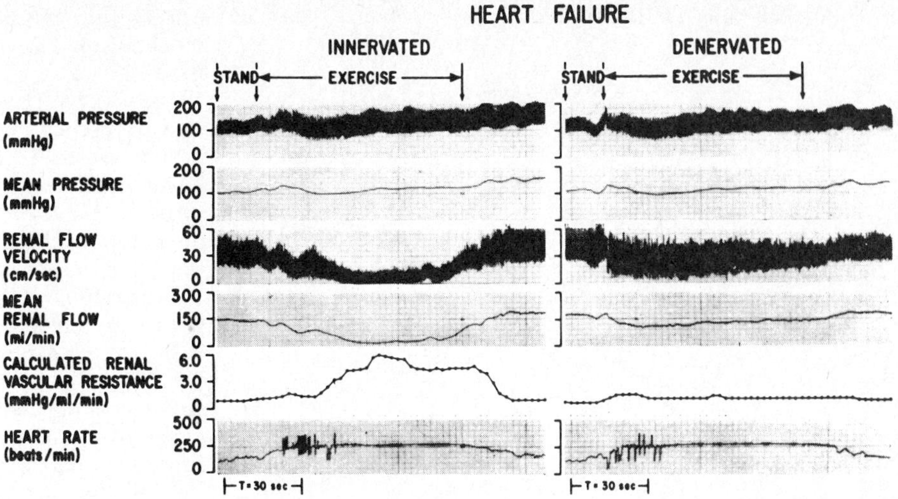

FIGURE 14–21. Tracings comparing the alterations in renal hemodynamics during exercise in the innervated kidney and contralateral denervated kidney in a dog with experimental heart failure. (From Higgins, C. B., et al.: Alterations in regional hemodynamics in experimental heart failure in conscious dogs. Trans. Assoc. Am. Physicians *85*:267, 1972.)

well as sympathetic function.[178, 178a, 179] The parasympathetic restraint on sinoatrial node automaticity is markedly reduced in patients with heart disease who also exhibit less heart rate slowing for any given elevation of systemic arterial pressure than do normal subjects. The sensitivity of the baroreceptor reflex to increase in pressure has also been shown to be significantly reduced in dogs with heart failure.[175] Cardiomyopathic hamster hearts display a reduction in the activity of choline acetyltransferase, an enzyme that provides an estimate of the density of parasympathetic innervation.[179, 180]

Although the mechanism responsible for the demonstrated impairment of parasympathetic function in heart failure is not clear,[181] this disturbance may be of considerable functional importance, since the ability to alter heart rate constitutes an extremely important mechanism for the adjustment of cardiac output; indeed, in normal subjects alterations in heart rate account in large measure for changes in cardiac output. In patients with heart failure, exercise does not elevate stroke volume normally, and when this limitation of stroke volume is combined with defective control of heart rate as a consequence of abnormalities of both the sympathetic and the parasympathetic limbs of the autonomic nervous system, this inability to raise cardiac output appropriately is readily appreciated.

ABNORMALITIES IN AFFERENT IMPULSES

Heart failure also interferes with the afferent limbs of cardiovascular reflexes. According to the schema proposed by Gauer and Henry,[182] under normal circumstances, elevated left atrial pressure increases left atrial stretch and stimulates left atrial stretch receptors.[183] The increased activity of both myelinated and nonmyelinated (C-fiber) afferents[184] normally inhibits the release of ADH, thereby increasing water excretion, which in turn reduces plasma volume, and left atrial pressure returns to normal. In addition, enhanced left atrial stretch receptor activity depresses renal efferent sympathetic nerve activity and increases renal blood flow and glomerular filtration rate, thereby enhancing the ability of the kidney to reduce plasma volume. Indeed, in patients with myocardial infarction and acute heart failure, urine flow and glomerular filtration rate (and sometimes even sodium excretion) are increased despite the decline in arterial pressure. Presumably, activation of atrial or ventricular receptors from a rise in left atrial pressure or bulging left ventricle is responsible.[185] Zucker et al.[186] observed that the decreased sensitivity of left atrial stretch receptors in dogs with heart failure is the result of cardiac dilatation and alterations in atrial compliance and is reversible following reversal of heart failure.[187] This resetting of atrial receptors may be responsible for the inappropriately high plasma ADH levels in heart failure[188] (see below) and may contribute to the renal vasoconstriction, peripheral edema, ascites, and hyponatremia often seen in patients with chronic heart failure (Chap. 59). With chronic heart failure and its attendant cardiac distention and decreased sensitivity of cardiac receptors, the reflex inhibition of adrenergic activity disappears, and the adrenergic drive to the heart, the peripheral vascular bed, and the adrenal medulla is enhanced, resulting in the sodium retention, tachycardia, and the vasoconstricted state characteristic of heart failure (p. 442).

ATRIAL NATRIURETIC FACTOR

Atrial distention also releases atrial natriuretic factor. This is discussed on page 1831.

THE RENIN-ANGIOTENSIN SYSTEM

In low-output states there is activation of the renin-angiotensin-aldosterone axis (as there is of the adrenergic system). Activation of this axis works in concert with the adrenergic system to maintain arterial pressure. Indeed, stimulation of beta$_1$-adrenoceptors in the juxtaglomerular apparatus is probably the principal mechanism responsible for activation of the renin-angiotensin-aldosterone axis in acute heart failure (Fig. 27–16, p. 835). However, in patients with severe chronic heart failure, especially following salt restriction and diuretic treatment, reduction of the sodium presented to the macula densa also contributes to the release of renin. Elevated plasma renin activity is a common, although not universal, finding in heart failure[151, 152, 189, 190]; plasma renin activity often varies inversely with serum potassium.[191] Angiotensin II is a potent vasoconstrictor and contributes, along with increased adrenergic activity, to the excessive elevation of systemic vascular resistance and possibly to the vicious circle referred to above[166] in patients with heart failure. Aldosterone, in turn, has potent sodium-retaining properties. Therefore, it is not surprising that interruption of the renin-angiotensin-aldosterone axis by means of an angiotensin conversion inhibitor reduces systemic vascular resistance, diminishes afterload, and thereby elevates cardiac output in heart failure. In addition, converting enzyme inhibition often acts as a diuretic, presumably by lowering angiotensin II-stimulated production of aldosterone.

ARGININE VASOPRESSIN (AVP)

There is now substantial evidence that circulating AVP is elevated to approximately twice normal levels in many

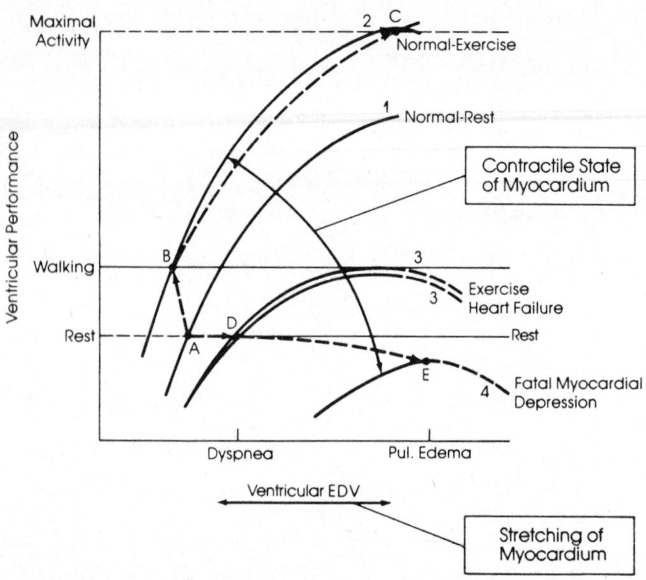

FIGURE 14–22. Diagram showing the interrelationship of influences on ventricular end-diastolic volume (EDV) through stretching of the myocardium and the contractile state of the myocardium. Levels of ventricular EDV associated with filling pressures that result in dyspnea and pulmonary edema are shown on the abscissa. Levels of ventricular performance required during rest, walking, and maximal activity are designated on the ordinate. The dotted lines are the descending limbs of the ventricular performance curves, which are rarely seen during life but which show what the level of ventricular performance would be if end-diastolic volume could be elevated to very high levels. (Modified from Braunwald, E., Ross, J., Jr., and Sonnenblick, E. H.: Mechanisms of Contraction of the Normal and Failing Heart. Boston, Little, Brown and Co., 1968.)

patients with heart failure,[192, 193] even after correction for plasma osmolality. Perhaps the decreased sensitivity of atrial stretch receptors, which normally inhibit AVP release in heart failure and which are discussed above, contributes to the elevation of circulating AVP.[194–196] AVP is a potent vasoconstrictor, and the elevated levels may cause systemic vasoconstriction.

Administration of an AVP antagonist has been shown to reduce systemic vascular resistance and to increase cardiac output in patients with heart failure and elevated AVP. These responses are similar to those evoked by a converting enzyme inhibitor in patients with elevated plasma renin activity and an antiadrenergic agent in patients with elevated circulating NE.[191]

Control of circulating AVP concentration is abnormal in heart failure; patients with heart failure fail to show the normal reduction of AVP with a reduction of osmolality.[197] This may contribute to the inadequate ability to excrete free water, and hence the hypoosmolarity in some patients with heart failure.[192] In addition, patients with heart failure exhibit failure of normal suppression of AVP following administration of ethanol[198] and failure of the normal augmentation of circulating AVP in response to orthostatic stress.[193]

CONCLUSIONS

It may be useful to consider normal and impaired myocardial function, whatever the etiology and pathogenesis, within the framework of the familiar Frank-Starling mechanism. The normal relation between ventricular end-diastolic volume and performance is shown in Figure 14–22, curve 1. Normally, assumption of the upright posture reduces venous return; as a consequence, at any particular level of exercise, cardiac output tends to be lower in the upright than in the recumbent position. On the other hand, the hyperventilation of exercise, the pumping action of the exercising muscles, and the venoconstriction that occur all tend to augment ventricular filling. Simultaneously, the increase in sympathetic nerve impulses to the myocardium and in the concentration of circulating catecholamines and the tachycardia that occur during exercise all augment the myocardial contractility and the stroke volume, with either no change or even a reduction in end-diastolic pressure and volume. This state is represented by a shift from point A to point B in Figure 14–22. Vasodilation occurs in the exercising muscles, reducing peripheral vascular resistance and aortic impedance. This ultimately allows achievement of a greatly elevated cardiac output during exercise at an arterial pressure only slightly greater than that in the resting state. During intense exercise, cardiac output can rise to a maximal level if use is made of the Frank-Starling mechanism, as reflected in increases in the left ventricular end-diastolic volume and pressure (Fig. 14–22, point C).

In heart failure, the fundamental abnormality resides in depressions of the myocardial force-velocity relation and of the length–active tension curve, reflecting reductions in the myocardial contractile state. In many cases, such as those represented by Figure 14–22, curve 3, cardiac output and external ventricular performance at rest are within normal limits, but are maintained at these levels only because the end-diastolic fiber length and the ventricular end-diastolic volume are above normal, i.e., through the operation of the Frank-Starling mechanism. The elevations of left ventricular end-diastolic volume and pressure are associated with greater than normal levels of the pulmonary capillary pressure, contributing to the dyspnea experienced by patients with heart failure (Fig. 14–22, point D).

Since heart failure is frequently accompanied by reductions in (1) cardiac NE stores, (2) myocardial beta-adrenoceptor density, (3) catecholamine sensitivity, and (4) inotropic response to impulses in the cardiac adrenergic nerves, ventricular performance curves cannot be elevated to normal levels by the adrenergic nervous system, and the normal improvement of contractility that takes place during exercise is attenuated or even prevented (Fig. 14–22, curves 3 and 3′). The factors that tend to augment ventricular filling during exercise in the normal subject push the failing myocardium even farther along its flattened length–active tension curve, and although left ventricular performance may be improved slightly, this occurs only as a consequence of an inordinate elevation of ventricular end-diastolic volume and pressure and therefore of pulmonary capillary pressure. The elevation of the latter intensifies dyspnea and therefore plays an important role in limiting the intensity of exercise that the patient can perform. According to this concept, left ventricular failure becomes fatal when the myocardial length–active tension curve becomes depressed (Fig. 14–22, curve 4) to the point at which either cardiac performance fails to satisfy the requirements of the peripheral tissues even at rest or the left ventricular end-diastolic and pulmonary capillary pressures are elevated to levels that result in pulmonary edema, or both (Fig. 14–22, point E).

REFERENCES

COMPENSATORY MECHANISMS

1. Braunwald, E., Mock, M. B., and Watson, J. (eds.): Congestive Heart Failure: Current Research and Clinical Applications. New York, Grune and Stratton, 1982, 384 pp.
2. Eichna, L. S.: Circulatory congestion and heart failure. Circulation *22*:864, 1960.
3. Braunwald, E.: The Myocardium: Failure and Infarction. New York, H. P. Publishing Co., 1974, 409 pp.
4. Guyton, A. C.: The relationship of cardiac output and arterial pressure control. Circulation *64*:1079, 1981.
5. Katz, A. M.: The descending limb of the Starling curve and the failing heart (Editorial). Circulation *32*:871, 1965.
6. Ross, J., Jr., and Braunwald, E.: Studies on Starling's law of the heart. IX. The effects of impeding venous return on performance of the normal and failing human left ventricle. Circulation *30*:719, 1964.
7. Braunwald, E., Ross, J., Jr., and Sonnenblick, E. H.: Mechanisms of Contraction of the Normal and Failing Heart. 2nd ed. Boston, Little, Brown and Co., 1976, 417 pp.
8. Vanhoutte, P. M.: Adjustments in the peripheral circulation in chronic heart failure. Eur. Heart J. *4*(Suppl. A):67, 1983.
9. Higgins, C. B., Vatner, S. F., Millard, R. W., Franklin. D., and Braunwald, E.: Alterations in regional hemodynamics in experimental heart failure in conscious dogs. Trans. Assoc. Am. Physicians *85*:267, 1972.
10. Zelis, R. D., Mason, D. T., and Braunwald, E.: A comparison of the effects of vasodilator stimuli on peripheral resistance vessels in normal subjects and in patients with congestive heart failure. J. Clin. Invest. *47*:960, 1968.
11. Zelis, R. G., Mason, D. T., and Braunwald, E.: Partition of blood flow to the cutaneous and muscular beds of the forearm at rest and during leg exercise in normal subjects and in patients with heart failure. Circ. Res. *24*:799, 1969.
12. Zelis, R., and Flaim, S. F.: Peripheral vascular mechanisms mediating vasoconstriction. *In* Braunwald, E., Mock, M. B., and Watson, J. (eds.): Congestive Heart Failure: Current Research and Clinical Applications. New York, Grune and Stratton, 1982, p. 115.
13. Woodson, R. D., Torrance, J. D., Shappell, S. D., and Lenfant, C.: The effect of cardiac disease on hemoglobin-oxygen binding. J. Clin. Invest. *49*:1349, 1970.

CONTRACTILITY OF HYPERTROPHIED AND FAILING MYOCARDIUM

14. Krayenbuehl, H. P., Hess, O. M., Schneider, J., and Turina, M.: Physiologic or pathologic hypertrophy. Eur. Heart J. *4*(Suppl. A):29, 1983.
15. Spann, J. F., Jr., Buccino, R. A., Sonnenblick, E. H., and Braunwald, E.: Contractile state of cardiac muscle obtained from cats with experimentally produced ventricular hypertrophy and heart failure. Circ. Res. *21*:341, 1967.
16. Cooper, G., IV, Tomanek, R. J., Ehrhardt, J. D., and Marcus, M. L.: Chronic progressive pressure overload of the cat right ventricle. Circ. Res. *48*:488, 1981.
17. Cameron, J. S., Myerburg, R. H., Wong, S. S., Gaide, M. S., Epstein, K., Alvarez, T. R., Gelband, H., Guse, P. A., and Bassett, A. L.: Electrophysiologic consequences of chronic experimentally induced left ventricular pressure overload. J. Am. Coll. Cardiol. 2:481, 1983.
18. Hoffman, H., and Covell, J. W.: Relationship between ejection phase indices of performance and myocardial functions during the development of pressure overload hypertrophy. Am. Heart J. *107*:738, 1984.
19. Capasso, J. M., Aronson, R. S., and Sonnenblick, E. H.: Reversible alterations in excitation-contraction coupling during myocardial hypertrophy in rat papillary muscle. Circ. Res. *51*:189, 1982.
20. Forman, R., Parmley, W. W., and Sonnenblick, E. H.: Myocardial contractility in relation to hypertrophy and failure in myopathic Syrian hamsters. J. Mol. Cell. Cardiol. *4*:203, 1972.
21. Chidsey, C. A., Sonnenblick, E. H., Morrow, A. G., and Braunwald, E.: Norepinephrine stores and contractile force of papillary muscle from the failing human heart. Circulation *33*:43, 1966.
22. Cooper, G., IV, Puga, F., Zujko, K. J., Harrison, C. E., and Coleman, H. N.: Normal myocardial function and energetics in volume-overload hypertrophy in the cat. Circ. Res. *32*:140, 1973.
23. Williams, J. F., Jr., and Potter, R. D.: Normal contractile state of hypertrophied myocardium following pulmonary artery constriction in the cat. J. Clin. Invest. *54*:1266, 1974.
24. Williams, J. F., Matthew, B., Hern, D. L., Potter, R. D., and Deiss, W. P.: Myocardial hydroxyproline and mechanical response to prolonged pressure loading followed by unloading in the cat. J. Clin. Invest. *72*:1910, 1983.
25. Meerson, F. Z.: The myocardium in hyperfunction, hypertrophy, and heart failure. Circ. Res. *25*(Suppl. 2):1, 1969.
26. Ross, J., Jr., Sonnenblick, E. H., Taylor, R. R., and Covell, J. W.: Diastolic geometry and sarcomere length in the chronically dilated canine left ventricle. Circ. Res. *28*:49, 1971.
27. Alyono, D., Ring, W. S., Anderson, M. R., and Anderson, R. W.: Left ventricular adaptation to volume overload from large aortocaval fistula. Surgery *96*:360, 1984.
28. Spann, J. F., Jr., Covell, J. W., Eckberg, D. L., Sonnenblick, E. H., Ross, J., Jr., and Braunwald, E.: Contractile performance of the hypertrophied and chronically failing cat ventricle. Am. J. Physiol. *223*:1150, 1972.
29. Pfeffer, J. M., Pfeffer, M. A., Mirsky, E., and Braunwald, E.: Regression of left ventricular hypertrophy and prevention of left ventricular dysfunction by captopril in the spontaneously hypertensive rat. Proc. Natl. Acad. Sci. *79*:3310, 1982.
30. Pfeffer, J. M., Pfeffer, M. A., Fletcher, P., Fishbein, M. C., and Braunwald, E.: Favorable effects of therapy on cardiac performance in spontaneously hypertensive rats. Am. J. Physiol. *242*:H776, 1982.
30a. Scheuer, J., and Buttrick, P.: The cardiac hypertrophic responses to pathologic and physiologic loads. Circulation *75*(Suppl. I):63, 1987.
31. Mirsky, I., Pfeffer, J. M., Pfeffer, M. A., and Braunwald, E.: The contractile state as the major determinant in the evolution of left ventricular dysfunction in the spontaneously hypertensive rat. Circ. Res. *53*:767, 1983.
32. Pinsky, W. W., Lewis, R. M., Hartley, C. J., and Entman, M. L.: Permanent changes of ventricular contractility and compliance in chronic volume overload. Am. J. Physiol. *237*:H575, 1979.
32a. Sen, S.: Factors regulating myocardial hypertrophy in hypertension. Circulation *75*(Suppl. I):81, 1987.
33. Penpargkul, S., Schaible, T., Yipintsoi, T., and Scheuer, J.: The effect of diabetes on performance and metabolism of rat hearts. Circ. Res. *47*:911, 1980.
34. Cooper, G., IV, Satava, R. M., Harrison, C. E., and Coleman, H. N.: Normal myocardial function and energetics after reversing pressure-overload hypertrophy. Am. J. Physiol. *226*:1158, 1974.
34a. Cooper, G., and Marino, T. A.: Complete reversibility of cat right ventricular chronic progressive pressure overload. Circ. Res. *54*:323, 1984.
35. Zak, R.: Cardiac hypertrophy: Biochemical and cellular relationships. Hosp. Prac. *18*:85, 1983.
35a. Pritzl, N., and Zak, R.: Molecular biology of myocardial proteins. Circulation *75*(Suppl. I):85, 1987.
36. Tan, E., and Taegtmeyer, H.: Mechanisms of cardiac hypertrophy in systemic hypertension: A critical review. J. Appl. Cardiol. *1*:329, 1986.
37. McCullagh, W. H., Covell, J. W., and Ross, J., Jr.: Left ventricular dilatation and diastolic compliance changes during chronic volume overloading. Circulation *45*:943, 1972.
38. Anversa, P., Ricci, R., and Olivetti, G.: Quantitative structural analysis of the myocardium during physiologic growth and induced cardiac hypertrophy: A review. J. Am. Coll. Cardiol. *7*:1140, 1986.
39. Ross, J., Jr.: Afterload mismatch and preload reserve: A conceptual framework for the analysis of ventricular function. Prog. Cardiovasc. Dis. *18*:255, 1976.
40. Breisch, E. A., White, F. C., and Bloor, C. M.: Myocardial characteristics of pressure overload hypertrophy: A structural and functional study. Lab. Invest. *51*:333, 1984.
41. Ferrans, V. J.: Morphology of the heart in hypertrophy. Hosp. Pract. *18*:67, 1983.
41a. Weber, L. T., Janicki, J. S., Pick, R., Abrams, C., Shroff, S. G., Bashey, R. I., and Chen, R. M.: Collagen in the hypertrophied pressure-overloaded myocardium. Circulation *75*:(Suppl. I):40, 1987.
41b. Huston, T. P., Puffer, J. C., and Rodney, W. M.: The athletic heart syndrome. N. Engl. J. Med. *313*:24, 1985.
41c. Maron, B. J.: Structural features of the athlete heart as defined by echocardiography. J. Am. Coll. Cardiol. *7*:190, 1986.
41d. Unverferth, D. V., Fetters, J. K., Unverferth, B. J., Leier, C. V., Magorien, R. D., Arn, A. R., and Baker, P. B.: Human myocardial histologic characteristics in congestive heart failure. Circulation *2*:1194, 1983.
42. Figulla, H. R., Rahlf, G., Nieger, M., Luig, H., and Kreuzer, H.: Spontaneous hemodynamic improvement or stabilization and associated biopsy findings in patients with congestive cardiomyopathy. Circulation *71*:1095, 1985.
43. Braunwald, E., Welch, G. H., Jr., and Sarnoff, S. J.: Hemodynamic effects of quantitatively varied experimental mitral regurgitation. Circ. Res. *5*:539, 1957.
44. Welch, G. H., Jr., Braunwald, E., and Sarnoff, S. J.: Hemodynamic effects of quantitatively varied experimental aortic regurgitation. Circ. Res. *5*:546, 1957.
45. Urschel, C. W., Covell, J. W., Sonnenblick, E. H., Ross, J., Jr., and Braunwald, E.: Myocardial mechanics in aortic and mitral valvular regurgitation: The concept of instantaneous impedance as a determinant of the performance of the intact heart. J. Clin. Invest. *47*:867, 1968.
46. Mason, D. T.: Regulation of cardiac performance in clinical heart disease: Interactions between contractile state, mechanical abnormalities and ventricular compensatory mechanisms. Am. J. Cardiol. *32*:437, 1973.
47. Urschel, C. W., Covell, J. W., Graham, T. P., Clancy, R. L., Ross, J., Jr., Sonnenblick, E. H., and Braunwald, E.: Effects of acute valvular regurgitation on the oxygen consumption of the canine heart. Circ. Res. *23*:33, 1968.
48. Grossman, W., Jones, D., and McLaurin, L. P.: Wall stress and patterns of hypertrophy in the human left ventricle. J. Clin. Invest. *56*:56, 1975.
49. Sandler, H., and Dodge, H. T.: Left ventricular tension and stress in man. Circ. Res. *13*:91, 1963.
50. Peterson, K. L., Tsuji, J., Johnson, A., DiDonna, J., and LeWinter, M.: Diastolic left ventricular pressure-volume and stress-strain relations in patients with valvular aortic stenosis and left ventricular hypertrophy. Circulation *58*:77, 1978.
51. Gunther, S., and Grossman, W.: Determinants of ventricular function in pressure overload hypertrophy in man. Circulation *59*:679, 1979.
51a. Donner, R., Carabello, B. A., Black, I., and Spann, J. F.: Left ventricular wall stress in compensated aortic stenosis in children. Am. J. Cardiol. *51*:946, 1983.
52. Spann, J. F., Bove, A. A., Natarajan, G., and Kreulen, T.: Ventricular performance, pump function and compensatory mechanisms in patients with aortic stenosis. Circulation *62*:576, 1980.
52a. Al-Nouri, M. B., Ford, L. E., and Wix, H.: Dimensional correlates of left ventricular dilation in the presence of hypertrophy. Chest *83*:43, 1983.
53. Sasayama, S., Ross, J., Jr., Franklin, D., Bloor, C. M., Bishop, S., and Dilley,

R. B.: Adaptations of the left ventricle to chronic pressure overload. Circ. Res. 38:172, 1976.

VENTRICULAR RELAXATION AND DIASTOLIC PROPERTIES OF THE VENTRICLE

53a. Lorell, B. H., and Grossman, W.: Cardiac hypertrophy: The consequence for diastole. J. Am. Coll. Cardiol. (*In press*).
54. Gaasch, W. H., Levine, H. J., Quinones, M. A., and Alexander, J. K.: Left ventricular compliance: Mechanisms and clinical implications. Am. J. Cardiol. 38:645, 1976.
55. Brutsaert, D. L., Rademakers, F. E., and Sys, S. U.: Triple control of relaxation: Implications in cardiac disease. Circulation 69:190, 1984.
56. Morgan, J. P., and Morgan, K. G.: Calcium and cardiovascular function: Intracellular calcium levels during contraction and relaxation of mammalian cardiac and vascular smooth muscle as detected with aequorin. Am. J. Med. 77(Suppl. 5A):33, 1984.
57. Gwathmey, J. K., and Morgan, J. P.: Altered calcium handling in experimental pressure-overload hypertrophy in the ferret. Circ. Res. 57:836, 1985.
58. Lorell, B. H., Wexler, L. F., Momomura, S., Weinberg, E., and Apstein, C. S.: The influence of pressure overload left ventricular hypertrophy on diastolic properties during hypoxia in isovolumetrically contracting rat hearts. Circ. Res. 58:683, 1986.
59. Braunwald, E., and Ross, J., Jr.: The ventricular end-diastolic pressure: Appraisal of its value in the recognition of ventricular failure in man (Editorial). Am. J. Med. 34:147, 1963.
60. Mirsky, I., and Laks, M. M.: Time course of changes in the mechanical properties of the canine right and left ventricles during hypertrophy caused by pressure overload. Circulation 46:530, 1980.
61. Mirsky, I., Pfeffer, J. M., Pfeffer, M. A., and Braunwald, E.: The contractile state as a major determinant in the evolution of left ventricular dysfunction in the spontaneously hypertensive rat. Circ. Res. 53:767, 1983.
62. Fifer, M. A., Borow, K. M., Colan, S. D., and Lorell, B. H.: Early diastolic left ventricular function in children and adults with aortic stenosis. J. Am. Coll. Cardiol. 5:1147, 1985.
63. Smith, V. E., Schulman, P., Karimeddini, M. K., White, W. B., Meeran, M. K., and Katz, A. M.: Rapid ventricular filling in left ventricular hypertrophy: II. Pathologic hypertrophy. J. Am. Coll. Cardiol. 5:869, 1985.
64. Papademetriou, V., Gottdiener, J. S., Fletcher, R. D., and Freis, E. D.: Echocardiographic assessment by computer-assisted analysis of diastolic left ventricular function and hypertrophy in borderline or mild systemic hypertension. Am. J. Cardiol. 56:546, 1985.
64a. Fouad, F. M.: Left ventricular diastolic function in hypertensive patients. Circulation 75(Suppl. I):48, 1987.
65. Granger, C. B., Karimeddini, M. K., Smith, V. E., Shapiro, H. R., Katz, A. M., and Riba, A. L.: Rapid ventricular filling in left ventricular hypertrophy. I. Physiologic hypertrophy. Am. J. Cardiol. 5:862, 1985.
66. Lewis, B. S., and Gotsman, M. S.: Current concepts of left ventricular relaxation and compliance. Am. Heart J. 99:101, 1980.
67. Williams, J. F., Jr., Potter, R. D., Hern, D. L., Matthew, B., and Deiss, W. P., Jr.: Hydroxyproline and passive stiffness of pressure-induced hypertrophied kitten myocardium. J. Clin. Invest. 69:309, 1982.
68. Eichhorn, P., Grimm, J., Koch, R., Hess, O., Carroll, J., and Krayenbuehl, H. P.: Left ventricular relaxation in patients with left ventricular hypertrophy secondary to aortic valve disease. Circulation 65:1395, 1982.
69. Serizawa, T., Carabello, B. A., and Grossman, W.: Effect of pacing-induced ischemia on left ventricular diastolic pressure–volume relations in dogs with coronary stenosis. Circ. Res. 46:430, 1980.
70. Hess, O. M., Osakada, G., Lavelle, J. F., Gallagher, K. P., Kemper, W. S., and Ross, J., Jr.: Diastolic myocardial wall stiffness and ventricular relaxation during partial and complete coronary occlusions in the conscious dog. Circ. Res. 52:387, 1983.
71. Forrester, J., Diamond, G., Parmley, W. W., and Swan, H. J. C.: Early increase in left ventricular compliance following myocardial infarction. J. Clin. Invest. 51:598, 1972.
72. Pirzada, F. A., Ekong, E. A., Vokonas, P. S., Apstein, C. S., and Hood, W. B., Jr.: Experimental myocardial infarction. XIII. Sequential changes in left ventricular pressure-length relations in the acute phase. Circulation 53:970, 1976.
73. Swan, H. J. C., Forrester, J. S., Diamond, G., Chatterjee, K., and Parmley, W. W.: Hemodynamic spectrum of myocardial infarction and cardiogenic shock. Circulation 40:1097, 1972.
74. Diamond, G., and Forrester, J. S.: Effect of coronary artery disease and acute myocardial infarction on left ventricular compliance in man. Circulation 45:11, 1972.
75. Fletcher, P. J., Pfeffer, J. M., Pfeffer, M. A., and Braunwald, E.: Left ventricular diastolic pressure-volume relations in rats with healed myocardial infarction. Effects on systolic function. Circ. Res. 49:618, 1981.
75a. Lorell, B. M., Turi, Z., and Grossman, W.: Modification of left ventricular response to pacing tachycardia by nifedipine in patients with coronary artery disease. Am. J. Med. 71:667, 1981.
76. Entman, M. L., VanWinkle, W. B., Tate, C. A., and McMillin-Wood, J. B.: Pitfalls in biochemical studies of hypertrophied and failing myocardium. *In* Braunwald, E., Mock, M. B., and Watson, J. (eds.): Congestive Heart Failure: Current Research and Clinical Applications. New York, Grune and Stratton, 1982, p. 51.
76a. Dougherty, A. H., Naccarelli, G. V., Gray, E. L., Hicks, C. H., and Goldstein, R. A.: Congestive heart failure with normal systolic function. Am. J. Cardiol. 54:778, 1984.
77. Topol, E. J., Traill, T. A., and Fortuin, N. J.: Hypertensive hypertrophic cardiomyopathy of the elderly. N. Engl. J. Med. 312:277, 1985.
78. Warren, S. E., Cohn, L. H., Schoen, F. J., Mudge, G. H., Jr., and Lorell, B. H.: Advanced diastolic heart failure in familial hypertrophic cardiomyopathy managed with cardiac transplantation. Submitted.

MECHANISMS RESPONSIBLE FOR DEPRESSED CONTRACTILITY

79. Bing, R. L.: The biochemical basis of myocardial failure. Hosp. Pract. 18:93, 1983.
80. Graham, T. P., Jr., Ross, J., Jr., and Covell, J. W.: Myocardial oxygen consumption in acute experimental cardiac depression. Circ. Res. 21:123, 1967.
81. Henry, P. D., Eckberg, D., Gault, J. H., and Ross, J., Jr.: Depressed inotropic state and reduced myocardial oxygen consumption in the human heart. Am. J. Cardiol. 31:300, 1973.
82. Sievers, R., Parmley, W. W., James, T., and Coffelt-Wilman, J.: Energy levels at systole vs. diastole in normal hamster hearts vs. myopathic hamster hearts. Circ. Res. 53:759, 1983.
83. Schwartz, A., Lindenmayer, G. E., and Harigaya, S.: Respiratory control and calcium transport in heart mitochondria from the cardiomyopathic Syrian hamster. Trans. N.Y. Acad. Sci. 30(Suppl. II):951, 1968.
84. Harrison, C. E., Jr., Cooper, G., IV, Zujko, K. J., and Coleman, H. N., III: Myocardial and mitochondrial function in potassium depletion cardiomyopathy. J. Mol. Cell. Cardiol. 4:633, 1972.
85. Kako, K. J., Thornton, M. J., and Hegtveit, H. A.: Depressed fatty acid and acetate oxidation and other metabolic defects in homogenates from hearts of hamsters with hereditary cardiomyopathy. Circ. Res. 34:570, 1974.
86. Chidsey, C. A., Weinbach, E. C., Pool, P. E., and Morrow, A. G.: Biochemical studies of energy production in the failing human heart. J. Clin. Invest. 45:40, 1966.
87. Sobel, B. E., Spann, J. F., Jr., Pool, P. E., Sonnenblick, E. H., and Braunwald, E.: Normal oxidative phosphorylation in mitochondria from the failing heart. Circ. Res. 21:355, 1967.
88. Sordahl, L. A., Wood, W. G., and Lazarus, M.: Alterations in heart mitochondria during hypertrophy and progressive failure: Increases and decreases in function and structure. Circ. Res. 42(Suppl. 2):51, 1970.
89. Sordahl, L. A.: Some biochemical lesions in myocardial disease. Tex. Rep. Biol. Med. 38:121, 1979.
90. Cooper, G., IV, Satava, R. M., Harrison, C. E., and Coleman, H. N.: Mechanisms for the abnormal energetics of pressure-induced hypertrophy of cat myocardium. Circ. Res. 33:213, 1973.
91. Pool, P. E., Spann, J. F., Jr., Buccino, R. A., Sonnenblick, E. J., and Braunwald, E.: Myocardial high energy phosphate stores in cardiac hypertrophy and heart failure. Circ. Res. 21:365, 1967.
92. Katz, A. M.: Biochemical "defect" in the hypertrophied and failing heart. Circulation 47:1076, 1973.
93. Capasso, J. M., Aronson, R. S., Strobeck, J. E., and Sonnenblick, E. H.: Effects of experimental phosphate deficiency on action potential characteristics and contractile performance of rat myocardium. Cardiovasc. Res. 16:71, 1982.
94. Page, E., and McCallister, L. P.: Quantitative electron microscopic description of heart muscle cells. Application to normal, hypertrophied and thyroxin-stimulated hearts. Am. J. Cardiol. 31:172, 1973.
95. Schwarz, F., Schaper, J., Kittstein, D., Flameng, W., Walter, P., and Schaper, W.: Reduced volume fraction of myofibrils in myocardium of patients with decompensated pressure overload. Circulation 63:1299, 1981.
96. Alpert, N. R., and Gordon, M. S.: Myofibrillar adenosine triphosphate activity in congestive failure. Am. J. Physiol. 202:940, 1962.
97. Gordon, M. S., and Brown, A. L.: Myofibrillar adenosine triphosphate activity of human heart tissue and congestive failure: Effects of ouabain and calcium. Circ. Res. 19:534, 1966.
98. Luchi, R. J., Dritcher, E. M., and Thyrum, P. T.: Reduced cardiac myosin adenosine triphosphate activity in dogs with spontaneously occurring heart failure. Circ. Res. 24:513, 1969.
99. Chandler, B. M., Sonnenblick, E. H., Spann, J. R., Jr., and Pool, P. E.: Association of depressed myofibrillar adenosine triphosphatase and reduced contractility in experimental heart failure. Circ. Res. 21:717, 1967.
100. Draper, M., Taylor, N., and Alpert, N. R.: Alteration in contractile protein in hypertrophied guinea pig hearts. *In* Alpert, N. (ed.): Cardiac Hypertrophy. New York, Academic Press, 1971, pp. 315–331.
101. Wikman-Coffelt, J., Kamiyama, T., Salel, A. F., and Mason, D. T.: Differential responses of canine myosin ATPase activity and tissue gases in the pressure-overloaded ventricle dependent upon degree of obstruction—mild versus severe pulmonic and aortic stenosis. *In* Kobayashi, T., Yoshio, I., and Rona, G. (eds.): Recent Advances in Studies on Cardiac Structure and Metabolism. Vol. 12. Cardiac Adaption. Baltimore, University Park Press, 1978, pp. 367–372.
102. Scheuer, J., Malhotra, A., Hirsch, C., Capasso, J., and Schaible, T. F.: Physiologic cardiac hypertrophy corrects contractile protein abnormalities associated with pathologic hypertrophy in rats. J. Clin. Invest. 70:1300, 1983.
103. Wikman-Coffelt, J., Parmley, W. W., and Mason, D. T.: Relation of myosin isozymes to the heart as a pump. Am. Heart J. 103:934, 1982.
104. Gorza, L., Pauletto, P., Pessina, A. C., Sartore, S., and Schiaffino, S.: Isomyosin distribution in normal and pressure-overloaded rat ventricular myocardium. An immunohistochemical study. Circ. Res. 49:1003, 1981.
105. Flink, I. L., Rader, J. H., and Morkin, E.: Thyroid hormone stimulates synthesis of cardiac myosin isozymes. J. Biol. Chem. 254:3105, 1979.

106. Wikman-Coffelt, J., Fenner, C., Walsh, R., Salel, A., Kamiyama, T., and Mason, D. T.: Comparison of mild vs. severe pressure overload on the enzymatic activity of myosin in the canine ventricles. Biochem. Med. *14*:139, 1975.
107. Lompre, A.-M., Schwartz, K., d'Albis, A., Lacombe, G., Van Thiem, N., and Swynghedauw, B.: Myosin isoenzyme redistribution in chronic heart overload. Nature 282:105, 1979.
108. Wikman-Coffelt, J., Parmley, W. W., and Mason, D. T.: The cardiac hypertrophy process. Analyses of factors determining pathological vs. physiological development. Circ. Res. *45*:697, 1979.
109. Gorza, L., Mercadier, J. J., Schwartz, K., Thornell, L. E., Sartore, S., and Schiaffino, S.: Myosin types in the human heart: An immunofluorescence study of normal and hypertrophied atrial and ventricular myocardium. Circ. Res. *54*:694, 1984.
110. Bouvagnet, P., Leger, J., Dechesne, C. A., Dureau, G., Anoal, M., and Leger, J. J.: Local changes in myosin types in diseased human atrial myocardium: A quantitative immunofluorescence study. Circulation 72:272, 1985.
111. Hirzel, H. O., Tuchschmid, C. R., Schneider, J., Krayenbuehl, H. P., and Schaub, M.: Relationship between myosin isoenzyme composition, hemodynamics and myocardial structure in various forms of human cardiac hypertrophy. Circ. Res. *57*:729, 1985.
112. Connor, T. B., Rosen, B. L., Blaustein, M. P., Applefeld, M. M., and Doyle, L. A.: Hypocalcemia precipitating congestive heart failure. N. Engl. J. Med. *307*:869, 1982.
113. Levine, S. N., and Rheams, C. N.: Hypocalcemic heart failure. Am. J. Med. *78*:1033, 1985.
114. Henrich, W. L., Hunt, J. M., and Nixon, J. V.: Increased ionized calcium and left ventricular contractility during hemodialysis. N. Engl. J. Med. *310*:19, 1984.
115. Ginsburg, R., Esserman, L. J., and Bristow, M. R.: Myocardial performance and extracellular ionized calcium in a severely failing human heart. Ann. Intern. Med. 98:603, 1983.
116. Fleckenstein, A.: Calcium Antagonism in Heart and Smooth Muscle. New York, John Wiley and Sons, 1983.
117. Gelband, H., and Bassett, A. L.: Depressed transmembrane potentials during experimentally induced ventricular failure in cats. Circ. Res. *32*:625, 1973.
118. Kaufmann, R. L., Hamburger, H., and Wirth, H.: Disorder in excitation-contraction coupling of cardiac muscle from cats with experimentally produced right ventricular hypertrophy. Circ. Res. *28*:346, 1971.
119. Harigaya, S., and Schwartz, A.: Rate of calcium binding and uptake in normal animal and failing human cardiac muscle. Circ. Res. *25*:781, 1969.
120. Sordahl, L. A., Wood, W. G., and Schwartz, A.: Production of cardiac hypertrophy and failure in rabbits with ameroid clips. J. Mol. Cell. Cardiol. *1*:341, 1970.
121. McCollum, W. B., Crow, C., Harigaya, S., Bajusz, E., and Schwartz, A.: Calcium binding by cardiac relaxing system isolated from myopathic Syrian hamsters. J. Mol. Cell. Cardiol. *1*:445, 1970.
122. Mead, R. J., Peterson, M. B., and Welty, J. D.: Sarcolemmal and sarcoplasmic reticular ATPase activities in the failing canine heart. Circ. Res. *29*:14, 1971.
123. Suko, J., Vogel, J. H. K., and Chidsey, C. A.: Intracellular calcium and myocardial contractility. III. Reduced calcium uptake and ATPase of the sarcoplasmic reticular fraction prepared from chronically failing calf hearts. Circ. Res. *27*:235, 1970.
124. Ito, Y., and Chidsey, C. A.: Intracellular calcium and myocardial contractility. IV. Distribution of calcium in the failing heart. J. Mol. Cell. Cardiol. *4*:507, 1972.
125. Sordahl, L. A., McCollum, W. B., Wood, W. G., and Schwartz, A.: Mitochondria and sarcoplasmic reticulum function in cardiac hypertrophy and failure. Am. J. Physiol. *224*:497, 1973.
126. Ito, Y., Suko, J., and Chidsey, C. A.: Intracellular calcium and myocardial contractility. V. Calcium uptake of sarcoplasmic reticulum fractions in hypertrophied and failing rabbit hearts. J. Mol. Cell. Cardiol. *6*:237, 1974.
127. Ma, T. S., and Bailey, L. E.: Excitation-contraction coupling in normal and myopathic hamster hearts. II: Changes in contractility and Ca pools associated with development of the cardiomyopathy. Cardiovasc. Res. *13*:499, 1979.
128. Sulakhe, P. V., and Dhalla, N. S.: Excitation-contraction coupling in heart. VII. Calcium accumulation in subcellular particles in congestive heart failure. J. Clin. Invest. *50*:1019, 1971.
129. Owens, K., Ruth, R. C., Weglicki, W. B., Stam, A. C., and Sonnenblick, E. H.: Fragmented sarcoplasmic reticulum of the cardiomyopathic Syrian hamster: Lipid composition, Ca^{++} transport, and Ca^{++}-stimulated ATPase. *In* Dhalla, N. S. (ed.): Myocardial Biology: Recent Advances in Studies on Cardiac Structure and Metabolism. Baltimore, University Park Press, 1974, pp. 541–550.
130. Staley, N. A., Noren, G. R., and Einzig, S.: Early alterations in the function of sarcoplasmic reticulum in a naturally occurring model of congestive cardiomyopathy. Cardiovasc. Res. *15*:276, 1981.
131. Gertz, E. W., Hess, M. L., Lain, R. F., and Briggs, F. N.: Activity of the vesicular calcium pump in the spontaneously failing heart-lung preparation. Circ. Res. *20*:477, 1967.
132. Lee, K. S., Ladinsky, H., and Stuckey, J. H.: Decreased Ca^{2+} uptake by sarcoplasmic reticulum after coronary artery occlusion for 60 and 90 minutes. Circ. Res. *20*:439, 1967.
133. Varley, K. G., and Dhalla, N. S.: Excitation-contraction coupling in heart: XII. Subcellular calcium transport in isoproterenol-induced myocardial necrosis. Exp. Mol. Pathol. *19*:94, 1973.
134. Kim, N. D., and Harrison, C. E.: $^{45}Ca^{2+}$ accumulation by mitochondria and sarcoplasmic reticulum in chronic potassium depletion cardiomyopathy. *In* Dhalla, N. S., and Rona, G. (eds.): Myocardial Biology. Vol. 4. Baltimore, University Park Press, 1972, pp. 551–562.
135. Lindenmayer, G. E., Sordahl, L. A., Harigaya, S., Allen, J. C., Besch, H. R., Jr., and Schwartz, A.: Some biochemical studies on subcellular systems isolated from fresh recipient human cardiac tissue obtained during transplantation. Am. J. Cardiol. 27:277, 1971.
136. Khatter, J. C., and Prasad, K.: Myocardial sarcolemmal ATPase in dogs with induced mitral insufficiency. Cardiovasc. Res. *10*:637, 1976.
137. Prasad, K., Khatter, J. C., and Bharadwaj, B.: Intra- and extracellular electrolytes and sarcolemmal ATPase in the failing heart due to pressure overload in dogs. Cardiovasc. Res. *13*:95, 1979.

ALTERATIONS IN THE FUNCTION OF THE AUTONOMIC NERVOUS SYSTEM

138. Chidsey, C. A., Harrison, D. C., and Braunwald, E.: Augmentation of plasma norepinephrine response to exercise in patients with congestive heart failure. N. Engl. J. Med. *267*:650, 1962.
139. Hasking, G. J., Esler, M. D., Jennings, G. L., Burton, D., and Korner, P. I.: Norepinephrine spillover to plasma in patients with congestive heart failure: Evidence of increased overall and cardiorenal sympathetic nervous activity. Circulation *73*:615, 1986.
140. Minami, M., Yasuda, H., Yamazaki, N., Kojima, S., Nishijima, H., Matsumura, N., Togashi, H., Koike, Y., and Saito, H.: Plasma norepinephrine concentration and plasma dopamine-beta-hydroxylase activity in patients with congestive heart failure. Circulation *67*:1324, 1983.
141. Francis, G. S., Goldsmith, S. R., Ziesche, S., Nakajima, H., and Cohn, J. N.: Relative attenuation of sympathetic drive during exercise in patients with congestive heart failure. J. Am. Coll. Cardiol. *5*:832, 1985.
142. Cohn, J. N., Levine, T. B., Olivari, M. T., Garberg, V., Lura, D., Francis, G. S., Simon, A. B., and Rector, T.: Plasma norepinephrine as a guide to prognosis in patients with chronic congestive heart failure. N. Engl. J. Med. *311*:819, 1984.
143. Viquerat, C. E., Daly, P., Swedberg, K., Evers, C., Curran, D., Parmley, W. W., and Chatterjee, K.: Endogenous catecholamine levels in chronic heart failure: Relation to the severity of hemodynamic abnormalities. Am. J. Med. *78*:455, 1985.
144. Rose, C. P., Burgess, J. H., and Cousineau, D.: Tracer norepinephrine kinetics in coronary circulation of patients with heart failure secondary to chronic pressure and volume overload. J. Clin. Invest. *76*:1740, 1985.
145. Chidsey, C. A., Braunwald, E., and Morrow, A. G.: Catecholamine excretion and cardiac stores of norepinephrine in congestive heart failure. Am. J. Med. *39*:442, 1965.
146. Goldstein, D. S.: Plasma norepinephrine as an indicator of sympathetic neural activity in clinical cardiology. Am. J. Cardiol. *48*:1147, 1981.
147. Maurer, W., Ablasser, A., Tschada, R., Hausen, M., Saggau, W., and Kubler, W.: Myocardial catecholamine metabolism in patients with chronic aortic regurgitation. Circulation *66*(Suppl. 1):139, 1982.
148. Malliani, A., and Pagani, M.: The role of the sympathetic nervous system in congestive heart failure. Eur. Heart J. *4*(Suppl. A):49, 1983.
149. Thomas, J. A., and Marks, B. H.: Plasma norepinephrine in congestive heart failure. Am. J. Cardiol. *41*:233, 1978.
150. Cody, R. J., Franklin, K. W., Kluger, J., and Laragh, J. H.: Sympathetic responsiveness and plasma norepinephrine during therapy of chronic congestive heart failure with captopril. Am. J. Med. 72:791, 1982.
151. Levine, T. B., Francis, G. S., Goldsmith, S. R., Simon, A. B., and Cohn, J. N.: Activity of the sympathetic nervous system and renin-angiotensin system assessed by plasma hormone levels and their relation to hemodynamic abnormalities in congestive heart failure. Am. J. Cardiol. *49*:1659, 1982.
152. Kluger, J., Cody, R. J., and Laragh, J. H.: The contributions of sympathetic tone and the renin-angiotensin system to severe chronic congestive heart failure: Response to specific inhibitors (prazosin and captopril). Am. J. Cardiol. *49*:1667, 1982.
153. Colucci, W. S., Alexander, R. W., Williams, G. H., Rude, R. E., Holman, B. L., Konstam, M. A., Wynne, J., Mudge, G. H., Jr., and Braunwald, E.: Decreased lymphocyte beta-adrenergic-receptor density in patients with heart failure and tolerance to the beta-adrenergic agonist pirbuterol. N. Engl. J. Med. *305*:185, 1981.
154. Weiss, R. J., Tobes, M., Wertz, C. E., and Smith, C. B.: Platelet $alpha_2$ adrenoreceptors in chronic congestive heart failure. Am. J. Cardiol. *52*:101, 1983.
155. Bristow, M. R., Ginsburg, R., Minobe, W., Cubicciotti, R. S., Sageman, W. S., Lurie, K., Billingham, M. E., Harrison, D. C., and Stinson, E. B.: Decreased catecholamine sensitivity and beta-adrenergic-receptor density in failing human hearts. N. Engl. J. Med. *307*:205, 1982.
155a. Bristow, M. R.: The adrenergic nervous system in heart failure. N. Engl. J. Med. *311*:850, 1984.
155b. Feldman, M. D., Copelas, L., Gwathmey, J. K., Phillips, P., Warren, S. E., Schoen, F. J., Grossman, W., and Morgan, J. P.: Deficient production of cyclic AMP: Pharmacologic evidence of an important cause of contractile dysfunction in patients with end-stage heart failure. Circulation *75*:331, 1987.
155c. Ayobe, M. H., and Tarazi, R. C.: Reversal of changes in myocardial beta-receptors and inotropic responsiveness with regression of cardiac hypertrophy in renal hypertensive rats (RHR). Circ. Res. *54*:125, 1984.
156. Fouad, F. M., Shimamatsu, K., Hanna, M. M., Khairallah, P. A., and Tarazi, R. C.: Impaired inotropic responses to alpha-adrenergic stimulation in experimental left ventricular hypertrophy. Circulation *71*:1023, 1985.
157. Chidsey, C. A., Kaiser, G. A., Sonnenblick, E. H., Spann, J. F., Jr., and Braunwald, E.: Cardiac norepinephrine stores in experimental heart failure in dogs. J. Clin. Invest. *43*:2386, 1964.
158. Coulson, R. L., Yazdanfar, S., Rubio, E., Bove, A. A., Lemole, G. M., and

Spann, J. F.: Recuperative potential of cardiac muscle following relief of pressure overload hypertrophy and right ventricular failure in the cat. Circ. Res. *40*:41, 1977.

159. Spann, J. F., Jr., Sonnenblick, E. H., Cooper, T., Chidsey, C. A., Willman, V. L., and Braunwald, E.: Cardiac norepinephrine stores and the contractile state of heart muscle. Circ. Res. *19*:317, 1966.
160. Pool, P. E., Covell, J. W., Levitt, M., Gibb, J., and Braunwald, E.: Reduction of cardiac tyrosine hydroxylase activity in experimental congestive heart failure. Its role in depletion of cardiac norepinephrine stores. Circ. Res. *20*:349, 1967.
161. Sole, M. J.: Alterations in sympathetic and parasympathetic neurotransmitter activity. *In* Braunwald, E., Mock, M. B., and Watson, J. (eds.): Congestive Heart Failure: Current Research and Clinical Applications. New York, Grune and Stratton, 1982, p. 101.
162. Covell, J. W., Chidsey, C. A., and Braunwald, E.: Reduction of the cardiac response to postganglionic sympathetic nerve stimulation in experimental heart failure. Circ. Res. *19*:51, 1966.
163. Gaffney, T. E., and Braunwald, E.: Importance of the adrenergic nervous system in the support of circulatory function in patients with congestive heart failure. Am. J. Med. *34*:320, 1963.
164. Epstein, S. E., and Braunwald, E.: The effect of beta-adrenergic blockade on patterns of urinary sodium excretion: Studies in normal subjects and in patients with heart disease. Ann. Intern. Med. *75*:20, 1966.
165. Vogel, J. H. K., and Chidsey, C. A.: Cardiac adrenergic activity in experimental heart failure assessed with beta-receptor blockade. Am. J. Cardiol. *24*:198, 1969.
166. Francis, G. S., Goldsmith, S. R., Levine, T. B., Olivary, M. T., and Cohn, J. T.: The neurohumoral axis in congestive heart failure. Ann. Intern. Med. *101*:370, 1984.
167. Van Zweeten, P. A., and Timmermans, P. B.: Cardiovascular alpha-2 receptors. J. Mol. Cell. Cardiol. *15*:717, 1983.
168. Francis, G. S., Parks, R., and Cohn, J. N.: The effects of bromocriptine in patients with congestive heart failure. Am. Heart J. *106*:100, 1983.
169. Goldstein, R. E., Beiser, G. D., Stampfer, M., and Epstein, S. E.: Impairment of autonomically mediated heart rate control in patients with cardiac dysfunction. Circ. Res. *36*:571, 1975.
170. Levine, T. B., Francis, G. S., Goldsmith, S. R., and Cohn, J. N.: The neurohumoral and hemodynamic response to orthostatic tilt in patients with congestive heart failure. Circulation *67*:1070, 1983.
171. Goldsmith, S. R., Francis, G. S., Levine, T. B., and Cohn, J. N.: Regional blood flow response to orthostasis in patients with congestive heart failure. J. Am. Coll. Cardiol. *1*:1391, 1983.
172. Kubo, S. H., and Cody, R. J.: Circulatory autoregulation in chronic congestive heart failure: Responses to head-up tilt in 41 patients. Am. J. Cardiol. *52*:512, 1983.
173. Stone, G. W., Kubo, S. H., and Cody, R. J.: Adverse influence of baroreceptor dysfunction on upright exercise in congestive heart failure. Am. J. Med. *80*:799, 1986.
174. Ferguson, D. W., Abboud, F. M., and Mark, A. L.: Selective impairment of baroreflex-mediated vasoconstrictor responses in patients with ventricular dysfunction. Circulation *69*:451, 1984.
175. Higgins, C. B., Vatner, S. F., Eckberg, D. L., and Braunwald, E.: Alterations in the baroreceptor reflex in conscious dogs with heart failure. J. Clin. Invest. *51*:715, 1972.
176. White, C. W.: Reversibility of abnormal arterial baroreflex control of heart rate in heart failure. Am. J. Physiol. *241*(Heart Circ. Physiol. 10):H778, 1981.
177. Cohn, J. N., Taylor, N., Vrobel, T., and Moskowitz, R.: Contrasting effect of vasodilators on heart rate and plasma catecholamines in patients with hypertension and heart failure. Clin. Res. *26*(Abstr.):547A, 1978.
178. Levine, T. B., Olivari, T., and Cohn, J. N.: Dissociation of the responses of the renin-angiotensin system and sympathetic nervous system to a vasodilator stimulus in congestive heart failure. Int. J. Cardiol. *12*:165, 1986.
178a. Eckberg, D. L., Drabinsky, M., and Braunwald, E.: Defective cardiac parasympathetic control in patients with heart disease. N. Engl. J. Med. 285:877, 1971.
179. Roskoski, R., Jr., Schmid, P. G., Mayer, H. E., and Abboud, F. M.: In vitro acetylcholine biosynthesis in normal and failing guinea pig hearts. Circ. Res. *36*:547, 1975.
180. Schmid, P. G., Lund, D. D., and Roskoski, R., Jr.: Efferent autonomic dysfunction in heart failure. *In* Abboud, F. M., Fozzard, H. A., Gilmore, J. P., and Reis, D. J. (eds.): Disturbances in Neurogenic Control of the Circulation. Bethesda, Md., American Physiological Society, 1981, p. 138.
181. Amorim, D. S., Heer, K., Jenner, D., Richardson, P., Dargie, H. J., Brown, M., Olsen, E. G. J., and Goodwin, J. F.: Is there autonomic impairment in congestive (dilated) cardiomyopathy? Lancet *1*:525, 1981.
182. Gauer, O. H., and Henry, J. P.: Neurohumoral control of plasma volume. *In* Guyton, A. C., and Cowley, A. W. (eds.): International Review of Physiology. Cardiovascular Physiology II. Baltimore, University Park Press, 1976, pp. 145–190.
183. Nonidez, J. F.: Identification of the receptor areas in the venae cavae and pulmonary veins which initiate reflex cardiac acceleration (Bainbridge's reflex). Am. J. Anat. *61*:203, 1937.
184. Thoren, P., and Ricksten, S.-E.: Cardiac C-fiber endings in cardiovascular control under normal and pathophysiological conditions. *In* Abboud, F. M., Fozzard, H. A., Gilmore, J. P., and Reis, D. J. (eds.): Disturbances in Neurogenic Control of the Circulation. Bethesda, Md., American Physiological Society, 1981, p. 17.
185. Abboud, F. M., Thames, M. C., and Mark, A. L.: Role of cardiac afferent nerves in regulation of circulation during coronary occlusion and heart failure. *In* Abboud, F. M., Fozzard, H. A., Gilmore, J. P., and Reis, D. J. (eds.): Disturbances in Neurogenic Control of the Circulation. Bethesda, Md., American Physiological Society, 1981, p. 65.
186. Zucker, I. H., Earle, A. M., and Gilmore, J. P.: The mechanism of adaptation of left atrial stretch receptors in dogs with chronic congestive heart failure. J. Clin. Invest. *60*:323, 1977.
187. Zucker, I. H., Earle, A. M., and Gilmore, J. P.: Changes in the sensitivity of left atrial receptors following reversal of heart failure. Am. J. Physiol. *237*:H555, 1979.
188. Riegger, G. A. J., Leibau, G., and Kocksiek, K.: Antidiuretic hormone in congestive heart failure. Am. J. Med. *72*:49, 1982.
189. Pedersen, E. B., Danielson, H., Jensen, T., Madsen, M., Sorensen, S. S., and Thomsen, O. O.: Angiotensin II, aldosterone and arginine vasopressin in plasma in congestive heart failure. Eur. J. Clin. Invest. *16*:56, 1986.
190. Mettauer, B., Rouleau, J.-L., Bichet, D., Juneau, D., Kortas, C., Barjon, J.-N., and de Champlain, J.: Sodium and water excretion abnormalities in congestive heart failure: Determinant factors and clinical implications. Ann. Intern. Med. *105*:161, 1986.
191. Creager, M. A., Faxon, D. P., Cutler, S. S., Kohlmann, O., Ryan, T. J., and Gavras, H.: Contribution of vasopressin to vasoconstriction in patients with congestive heart failure: Comparison with the renin-angiotensin system and the sympathetic nervous system. J. Am. Coll. Cardiol. *7*:758, 1986.
192. Goldsmith, S. R., Francis, G. S., and Cowley, A. W.: Arginine vasopressin and the renal response to water loading in congestive heart failure. Am. J. Cardiol. *58*:295, 1986.
193. Goldsmith, S. R., Francis, G. S., Levine, T. B., Cowley, A. W., and Cohn, J. N.: Impaired response of plasma vasopressin to orthostatic stress in patients with congestive heart failure. J. Am. Coll. Cardiol. *2*:1080, 1983.
194. Belleau, L., Mion, H., Simard, S., Granger, P., Bertranou, E., Nowacynski, W., Boucher, R., and Genest, J.: Studies on the mechanism of experimental congestive heart failure in dogs. Can. J. Physiol. Pharmacol. *48*:450, 1970.
195. Zehr, J. E., Hawe, A., Tsakiris, A. G., Rastelli, G. C., McGoon, D. C., and Segar, W. E.: ADH levels following nonhypotensive hemorrhage in dogs with chronic mitral stenosis. Am. J. Physiol. *221*:312, 1971.
196. Greenberg, T. T., Richmond, W. H., Stocking, R. A., Gupta, P. D., Meehan, J. P., and Henry, J. P.: Impaired atrial receptor responses in dogs with heart failure due to tricuspid insufficiency and pulmonary artery stenosis. Circ. Res. *32*:424, 1973.
197. Pruszczynski, W., Vahanian, A., Ardaillou, R., and Acar, J.: Role of antidiuretic hormone in impaired water excretion of patients with congestive heart failure. J. Clin. Endocrinol. Metab. *58*:599, 1984.
198. Goldsmith, S. R., and Dodge, D.: Response of plasma vasopressin to ethanol in congestive heart failure. Am. J. Cardiol. *55*:1354, 1985.

15 ASSESSMENT OF CARDIAC FUNCTION

by EUGENE BRAUNWALD, M.D.

THEORETICAL CONSIDERATIONS

Assessment of ventricular performance and function and myocardial contractility is a critically important task in the evaluation of many patients with known or suspected heart disease. *Ventricular performance* is related to the simple pumping function of the ventricle, as reflected in the cardiac output or cardiac work, and expressed per stroke or per minute. *Ventricular function* relates these parameters of ventricular performance to end-diastolic volume, dimension, or pressure. *Myocardial contractility*, also called the contractile or inotropic state, refers to a fundamental property of cardiac muscle which reflects the level of activation of cross-bridge formation.

LIMITATIONS OF CARDIAC OUTPUT IN ASSESSING CARDIAC FUNCTION. Since the heart's prime function is to deliver sufficient oxygenated blood to meet the metabolic requirements of the tissues, it is understandable that measurement of cardiac output and ventricular filling pressure has become a time-honored method of assessing cardiac performance and function and that therapeutic interventions in patients with heart disease frequently are evaluated in terms of their effects on these parameters. Determination of cardiac output does indeed provide a useful measure of the pumping ability of the heart. However, cardiac output critically depends on preload and afterload,* in addition to myocardial contractility. As a consequence, measurement of cardiac output alone provides a limited assessment of ventricular function or of myocardial contractility.[1]

At any level of contractility, the extent of myocardial fiber shortening, and therefore the stroke volume, varies directly with the preload and inversely with the afterload.[2] In the intact organism afterload is closely related to *aortic impedance*, which is defined as the sum of the external factors that oppose ventricular ejection. Aortic impedance is the ratio of pressure to flow in the aorta and is determined by the physical properties of blood and the vascular wall; it includes the viscosity and density of blood, the diameter of the aorta and the viscoelasticity of the aortic wall, and the reflected pressure and flow waves generated in the distal part of the arterial tree. Aortic impedance is generally expressed as the sum of a series of sinusoidal functions of pressure and flow waves ("harmonics") superimposed on the mean pressure and flow.[3] When aortic impedance is progressively raised, an increasing proportion of the muscle's contractile activity is expressed in the generation of tension and a correspondingly smaller fraction in myocardial fiber shortening (Fig. 13–15*C*, p. 395). For example, if ventricular end-diastolic volume (preload) is held constant, when left ventricular afterload (aortic impedance) is raised progressively, stroke volume declines until a level of impedance is reached at which the maximum force-generating capacity of the myocardium is exceeded and ventricular ejection ceases, i.e., the contraction becomes isovolumetric.

Conversely, when at a constant preload the aortic impedance falls, i.e., when afterload is reduced, stroke volume rises. From these considerations, it is clear that when afterload changes, reciprocal changes take place in cardiac output (and related measures, such as stroke volume, ventricular fiber shortening, and its velocity) and that these changes do not reflect changes in myocardial contractility (Fig. 13–34, p. 412). For example, an increase in cardiac output in a patient with heart failure following relief of severe aortic stenosis or the successful treatment of hypertension may be due to a reduction in afterload, an improvement in contractility, or both. Similarly, the elevated cardiac output associated with severe anemia (low blood viscosity), fever (arteriolar dilatation), or patent ductus arteriosus (arteriovenous fistula) may be explained in part or entirely by a reduction in aortic impedance, which reduces afterload (Fig. 25–1, p. 779); an augmentation of contractility need not be invoked.

The effects of simple alterations of preload on cardiac output have been studied by many investigators. Thus, the depression of cardiac output that occurs with hypovolemia (e.g., hemorrhagic shock), displacement of blood from the thorax (e.g., positive-pressure ventilation), or cardiac compression (e.g., pericardial tamponade) may be explained solely on the basis of a reduction of preload. The

*Heart rate, the fourth determinant of cardiac performance (p. 413), is so easily measurable that it will not be considered further, although it is recognized that changes in heart rate per se affect myocardial contractility.

elevation of cardiac output that occurs in patients with hypervolemia, including patients with polycythemia vera and acute glomerulonephritis, does *not* reflect an augmentation of contractility, but rather a higher preload resulting from the hypervolemia.

THE RELATION BETWEEN CARDIAC OUTPUT AND CONTRACTILITY. When myocardial contractility is normal, cardiac output depends less on myocardial contractility than on peripheral factors and their influence on ventricular preload and afterload. For example, both digitalis glycosides and paired electrical stimulation exert powerful inotropic influences yet do not raise cardiac output in normal human subjects or experimental animals. By contrast, in the presence of myocardial failure, these stimuli do elevate cardiac output significantly.[4]

The relationship between a chain and its several links may be a useful, although obviously oversimplified, analogy for explaining the relation between cardiac output and myocardial contractility. The total weight that the chain can support (analogous to the total cardiac output) will increase only if its weakest link is strengthened. Thus, in a patient with heart failure, stimulation of contractility, which may be thought of as strengthening the weakest link in the chain of factors controlling this patient's cardiac output, will elevate cardiac output. On the other hand, when contractility is normal and is not the limiting factor, it is not surprising that stimulation of myocardial contractility will not elevate cardiac output. When reduced preload is the limiting factor, as in hypovolemia, restoration of blood volume will restore cardiac output; when increased afterload is limiting, as in critical aortic stenosis, relief of the obstruction will elevate cardiac output.

From the foregoing discussion and Figure 13–34 (p. 412), it is evident that cardiac output can be lowered by a reduction of contractility and preload and by an elevation of afterload—operating singly or in combination. It is not possible to deduce from the finding of a reduced cardiac output that contractility is depressed. Conversely, cardiac output may be within normal limits when depression of contractility is accompanied by an optimal preload and/or a reduced afterload. (Indeed, such manipulation of loading is an important goal in the management of heart failure [Chap. 17]). Therefore, while assessment of cardiac function should include measurement of cardiac output it must not be limited to this. Rather, it should also provide an analysis both of the heart's loading conditions and of contractility.

THE NEED FOR ASSESSING MYOCARDIAL CONTRACTILITY. It is often helpful to assess the level of myocardial contractility in the basal state and to determine how it is influenced by therapeutic interventions, such as a drug or an operation. In isolated cardiac muscle or in the isolated heart, loading can be readily controlled and the effects of the intervention on the extent and velocity of muscle shortening can be determined. However, it is more difficult to make analogous measurements in patients in whom preload, afterload, or both may be abnormal and cannot be controlled readily or held constant. For example, it is often desirable to ascertain in a patient with valvular heart disease, ventricular hypertrophy, and symptoms of heart failure whether it is the abnormality in loading produced by the valvular lesion or a depression of myocardial contractility (or a combination) that is responsible for the clinical manifestations. Similarly, many drugs that may affect myocardial contractility may also act on the arterial and/or venous beds and therefore may change cardiac loading. These considerations have led to the search for methods of evaluating cardiac function that go beyond simple analysis of the pumping function of the ventricle and that are directed toward quantification of contractility. Although a number of indices of contractility have been proposed and investigated empirically, conclusions drawn about them have involved an element of circular reasoning. Unfortunately, there is no ***absolute*** hemodynamic or mechanical measure of this property of the myocardium, i.e., there is no "gold standard" with which these indices can be compared.

THE FRANK-STARLING MECHANISM AND THE VENTRICULAR FUNCTION CURVE

The earliest efforts to separate loading conditions from contractility in assessing ventricular performance utilized the Frank-Starling relation, i.e., the relation between ventricular filling pressure (or end-diastolic volume) and ventricular mechanical activity, as expressed in the pressure generated, the volume output, or the product of these two variables—that is, stroke work. It was shown early in this century in the heart-lung preparation that stroke volume is a function of both diastolic fiber length (i.e., of preload) and contractility. The failing heart was found to deliver a smaller than normal stroke volume from a normal or elevated end-diastolic volume.[5] Later, Sarnoff and his collaborators examined ventricular stroke work over a range of mean atrial or ventricular end-diastolic pressures and termed the resulting relation "the ventricular function curve."[6] A family of such curves reflects a spectrum of contractile states, and the position of a given curve provides a description of ventricular contractility. Movement along

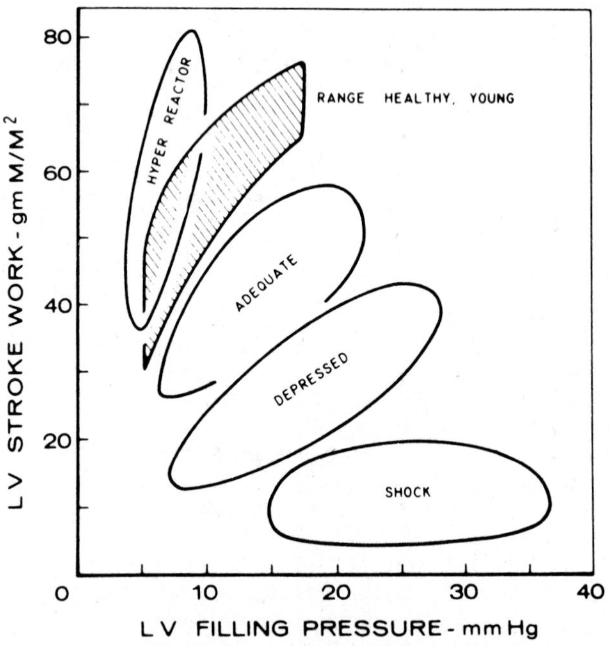

FIGURE 15–1. Hemodynamic consequences of myocardial infarction expressed as varying levels of left ventricular function. The cross-hatched area represents the range of left ventricular (LV) function in healthy, young individuals. Following acute myocardial infarction, there is wide variability in the hemodynamic response. Some patients with small infarcts and increased sympathetic tone may be in the normal or supernormal range. As the size of the infarct increases, however, function is progressively shifted down and to the right, so that all patients with cardiogenic shock fall in the lower right-hand group. (From Parmley, W. W.: Hemodynamic monitoring in acute ischemic disease. *In* Fishman, A. P. [ed.]: Heart Failure. New York, McGraw-Hill Book Co., 1978, p. 114.)

a single curve (Fig. 13–31, p. 409) represents the operation of the Frank-Starling principle, which indicates that stroke work or volume varies with changes in preload. By contrast, upward or downward displacement of the curve represents a positive or negative inotropic effect, i.e., an augmentation or depression of contractility, respectively (Fig. 15–1).

In experimental animal preparations in which left ventricular outflow resistance can be varied, ventricular function curves are often recorded at a constant mean arterial pressure, since the level of stroke work is pressure-dependent, just as the work of isolated muscle is afterload-dependent (Fig. 13–15*C*, p. 395). Thus, at any level of contractility and preload, stroke work is influenced also by the afterload, being low when outflow pressure is low, increasing to a maximal level as pressure is raised, and declining to zero when the afterload is so high as to prevent ventricular ejection (i.e., when ventricular contraction becomes isovolumetric).[7] It should be recognized that even when arterial pressure is held constant, the standard ventricular function curve (Fig. 13–31, p. 409) represents a complex interaction of preload and afterload. This is because as preload is augmented and heart size increases, according to Laplace's law (p. 405), afterload rises at a constant aortic pressure.

ASSESSMENT OF CARDIAC PERFORMANCE BASED ON PRESSURES, FLOWS, VOLUMES, AND DIMENSIONS

Despite the theoretical limitations discussed above, the simplest, most straightforward approaches for assessing cardiac function are still based on measurements of intravascular and intracardiac pressure, stroke volume (or cardiac output), and ventricular volume and/or dimensions.

CARDIAC OUTPUT. Basal State. The normal range for the cardiac index, i.e., the cardiac output corrected for body size, in the basal (resting) state and the supine position is wide—between 2.5 and 4.2 liters/min/m^2—making this variable relatively insensitive in the assessment of cardiac function. Cardiac output can decline by almost 40 per cent as a consequence of myocardial failure and still remain within normal limits. Therefore, when the cardiac output falls below normal, it usually represents a marked disturbance in *circulatory* (although not necessarily *cardiac*) performance. Such a degree of impairment is often readily detectable clinically. (Hypovolemia secondary to hemorrhage or dehydration is the most common noncardiac circulatory cause of a depressed cardiac output.) The aforementioned limitations notwithstanding, measurement of cardiac output in the basal state is valuable because it provides an assessment of the most critical circulatory function, i.e., the delivery of blood to the metabolizing tissues.

Exercise. A measurement that detects milder degrees of cardiac impairment with greater sensitivity than does the cardiac output in the basal state is the level of cardiac output in response to the stress of exercise. Most commonly, the effect of exercise on cardiac output is determined in the cardiac catheterization laboratory as the patient pedals a stationary bicycle in the supine position, and both oxygen consumption and cardiac output are measured at rest and during exercise (p. 258). It can also be determined during treadmill exercise testing (see Fig. 15–21). The increase in cardiac output is a function not only of the heart's pumping capacity but also of the severity of exercise, which can be expressed by the patient's total oxygen consumption. Normally, the increase in cardiac output exceeds 6 milliliters per minute for each milliliter increase in oxygen consumption per minute.

INTRACARDIAC PRESSURES. The assessment of cardiac performance can be greatly increased by adding a measurement of ventricular filling pressure* to that of cardiac (or stroke) output. In the basal state, when the ventricular end-diastolic volume is abnormally elevated *and* cardiac performance (expressed as cardiac [or stroke] index or work) is depressed, myocardial contractility is impaired. However, an elevation of ventricular filling *pressure* does not necessarily indicate an elevation of end-diastolic volume, since cardiac compliance may be reduced (Fig. 13–24, p. 402). Such a reduction of compliance may be caused by pericardial disease, restrictive endocardial or myocardial disease, cardiac hypertrophy, or myocardial ischemia; it can be responsible for an elevation of the ventricular filling pressure while end-diastolic volume remains normal. Therefore, an abnormally elevated left ventricular filling pressure in the presence of a normal cardiac index or stoke work does not necessarily signify an impairment of contractility. Conversely, chronic volume overload may displace the ventricular diastolic pressure-volume curve so that volume is elevated at a normal end-diastolic pressure (Fig. 14–5, p. 430). Thus, changes in the ventricle's diastolic pressure-volume relations can complicate interpretation of ventricular filling pressure and thereby the assessment of cardiac function on the basis of the relationship between filling pressure and cardiac output or work.

Despite these problems, the combination of ventricular end-diastolic pressure and cardiac output or work is often helpful in assessing ventricular function (Fig. 15–1). For example, the combination of a normal cardiac index (>2.5 liters/min/m^2) and ventricular filling pressure (<12 mm Hg) is a far more accurate indicator of normal contractility than is either measurement alone. An obvious limitation of this combination of measurements emerges when cardiac output (or work) is depressed while left ventricular filling pressure is within the normal range (6 to 12 mm Hg). Such findings could reflect either a depression of contractility or a reduction of preload in the presence of normal contractility.

One approach to overcoming these problems is to measure cardiac performance (cardiac or stroke index or work) both in the basal state and after preload has been raised by an increase in intravascular volume. Normally, an elevation of preload is accompanied by an increase in cardiac output or cardiac work, i.e., the product of cardiac output and the difference between arterial and atrial pressures. In addition, the effects of an intervention on the slope of the relation between filling pressure and cardiac work can be evaluated. For example, as shown in Figure 15–2, in a patient recovering from myocardial infarction, cessation of the infusion of glucose-insulin-potassium depressed the slope of the line relating an index of ventricular filling pressure to the stroke work index.[8] This approach to the assessment of ventricular function is commonly

---

*Ventricular filling pressure refers to ventricular end-diastolic pressure, or an index thereof. In the absence of disease of the atrioventricular valve this is reflected in the mean atrial or, preferably, the atrial pressure or onset of ventricular contraction, often termed the *z* point. In the case of the left ventricle, the mean pulmonary capillary wedge pressure or, in the case of the right ventricle, the central venous pressure provides a reasonably accurate approximation of ventricular end-diastolic pressure. However, when there is a tall *a* wave, the end-diastolic ventricular pressure exceeds the mean atrial pressure, or when there is a tall *v* wave, the mean atrial pressure exceeds the end-diastolic ventricular pressure. When pulmonary vascular resistance is normal, the pulmonary artery diastolic pressure is similar to the pulmonary capillary wedge pressure.

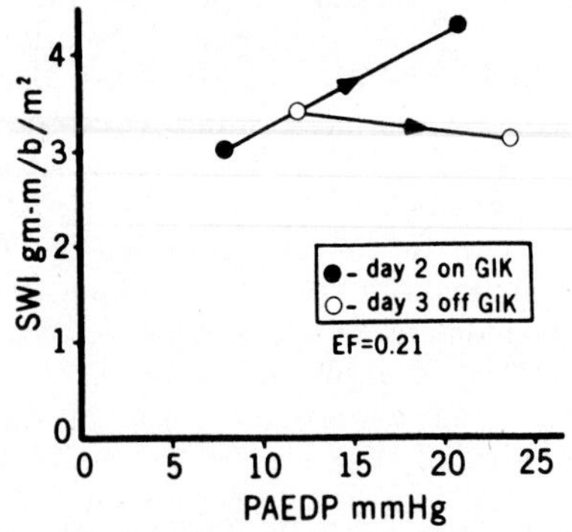

FIGURE 15–2. The hemodynamic effect of glucose-insulin-potassium (GIK) solution on left ventricular (LV) function is illustrated by the slope of the ventricular function curve in a patient with acute myocardial infarction. After the patient had been on the GIK solution for 2 days, the slope of the function curve was steeper than on day 3, 24 hours after the GIK solution had been discontinued. These changes indicate the positive inotropic effect of the metabolic solution on the viable and/or marginally ischemic myocardium surrounding the infarction site. Ventricular function is expressed as the relation between pulmonary artery end-diastolic pressure (PAEDP), reflecting left ventricular filling pressure and left ventricular stroke work index (SWI). (From Rackley, C. E., Russell, R. O., Jr., Rogers, W. J., et al.: Clinical experience with glucose-insulin-potassium therapy in acute myocardial infarction. Am. Heart J. *102*:1038, 1981.)

employed in the intensive care unit. In patients who have low cardiac output and/or hypotension, determining the response of the cardiac output, arterial pressure, and pulmonary capillary wedge pressure to a rapid expansion of blood volume will indicate rapidly whether the depression of ventricular performance is due to hypovolemia or left ventricular failure.

MEASUREMENTS OF VENTRICULAR VOLUME

From the foregoing consideration of the importance of changes in ventricular compliance, it is clear that measurement of ventricular end-diastolic *volume* is superior to that of *filling pressure* in the assessment of left ventricular preload. Angiographic techniques, described below, provide the most widely accepted means for measuring ventricular cavity volumes as well as wall thickness. They allow calculation of the extent and velocity of wall shortening and of regional abnormalities of wall motion. When they are combined with measurements of pressure, both ventricular compliance and afterload (i.e., the forces acting within the wall that oppose shortening) can be determined. Such calculations permit left ventricular performance to be analyzed in terms used for describing isolated heart muscle (Chap. 13). When the results are expressed in units corrected for muscle length or circumferences of the ventricle, comparisons can be made between individuals with widely differing heart sizes. Although noninvasive techniques can also be used in the assessment of ventricular volume or dimensions, their application to the assessment of cardiac function is based on the earlier work using contrast angiography.

Quantitative Angiocardiography

Despite the convenience of noninvasive techniques for measuring ventricular volume and/or dimensions, radiocontrast angiography remains the benchmark for these measurements. Angiography can be carried out utilizing either large cut films or cineangiograms (single-plane or biplane).[9] Cineangiography, which is emerging as the method of choice, provides a larger number of sequential observations per unit of time (30 to 60 frames per second), whereas the large cut films produce sharper margins of the opacified chambers with improved edge detection but are exposed less frequently (6 to 12 per second). Although contrast material can be injected into the pulmonary artery and left atrium, the left ventricle is outlined more clearly by means of direct injection into its cavity. Therefore, this latter mode is used in most patients, except in those with severe aortic regurgitation in whom the contrast material may be injected into the aorta, with the resultant reflux outlining the left ventricular cavity. Digital subtraction angiography (p. 357) utilizing injections into a peripheral vein, pulmonary artery, or left ventricle may also be employed.[10, 11]

Unless the effects of premature contractions and of the resultant postextrasystolic potentiation are to be examined specifically,[12] ventricular irritability should be avoided during injection of the contrast material. The operator should be sure that the tip of the catheter is not in contact with the myocardium and that a multiholed catheter is used to diminish the impact of the jet of contrast agent striking the endocardium. If premature contractions are induced, the results are subject to serious misinterpretation, since the premature contraction itself and the first and second postpremature beats may result in marked changes in cardiac function. The premature ventricular contraction may also induce mitral and/or tricuspid regurgitation. However, since the contrast material is usually injected within 2 or 3 seconds and filming is carried out for 5 to 8 seconds, one or two cardiac cycles are usually available for analysis even if a single premature contraction occurs at the beginning of the injection. Multiple premature contractions during filming make the angiogram virtually useless in assessing ventricular performance.

Injection of the contrast agent does not begin to produce hemodynamic changes (except for premature beats) until approximately the sixth beat after injection.[13] The hyperosmolarity produced by the contrast agent increases the blood volume, which begins to raise preload and heart rate within 30 seconds of the injection, an effect that may persist for as long as 2 hours. Regular contrast agents also depress contractility directly; newer nonionic agents are useful in minimizing these adverse effects. Digital subtraction techniques are also useful since they allow the injection of much smaller quantities of contrast agent and still provide excellent resolution[10, 11] (Chap. 12).

When multiple observations made under comparable conditions are desired, it is essential to monitor hemodynamics to insure that they have returned to control levels before the angiogram is repeated. Ordinarily, the exposure of each pair of angiographic films or cineangiographic frames is recorded and related to a simultaneously recorded electrocardiogram and intracardiac pressure pulse.

In calculating ventricular volumes or dimensions from angiograms, it is essential to take into account and apply appropriate correction factors for magnification as well as for distortion resulting from nonparallel x-ray beams.[14, 15] In order to apply these correction factors, care must be exercised to determine with accuracy the tube-to-patient and tube-to-film distances. With cine technique, correction is best accomplished by filming a calibrated grid at the position of the ventricle.[16]

Noninvasive Methods

Cardiac catheterization and quantitative selective angiography are the standard tools for evaluating the function and contractility of the heart, but these invasive procedures are not free of risk or discomfort, and they are generally not suitable for repeated application at intervals in the same patient. Therefore, a continuing search has been made for reliable noninvasive methods of assessing cardiac performance.[17] Such methods are needed particularly in detecting serial changes in cardiac function and in evaluating both acute and chronic effects of interventions such as drug therapy and cardiac operations. Discussed elsewhere in this book are the five principal noninvasive methods for assessing cardiac performance: systolic time intervals[18] (p. 53), M-mode and two-dimensional echocardiography[19–22] (p. 96), radionuclide angiography[23, 24] (p. 314), gated computerized tomography (CT scanning)[25, 26] (p. 361), and gated magnetic resonance imaging (MRI) (p. 376). All but the first of these are alternatives to contrast angiography for measurement of ventricular volumes and/or dimensions and therefore permit the noninvasive estimation of ejection phase indices (see below). Other than in patients with obstruction to left ventricular outflow, wall stress (afterload) can be estimated from a combination of systemic arterial pressure, ventricular radius, and wall thickness. All four noninvasive imaging methods allow estimation of ventricular systolic and diastolic volumes and ejection fraction (EF).

Mean velocity of circumferential fiber shortening (V_{cf}) can be determined simply from measurements of end-diastolic and end-systolic dimensions by echocardiography, CT scanning, or MRI. Since the ventricle is approximately circular at its minor axis, the circumference is equal to diameter (D) • π. Mean V_{cf} (in circumference/sec) is therefore the difference between end-diastolic and end-systolic circumference (in cm) divided by the product of the duration of ejection (in sec) and the end-diastolic circumference. Values of V_{cf} obtained by echocardiography compare closely with those determined from cineangiograms.

Thus, while the discussion in this chapter refers primarily to measurements made with angiography, they can be modified readily and applied to noninvasively derived images of the ventricles.

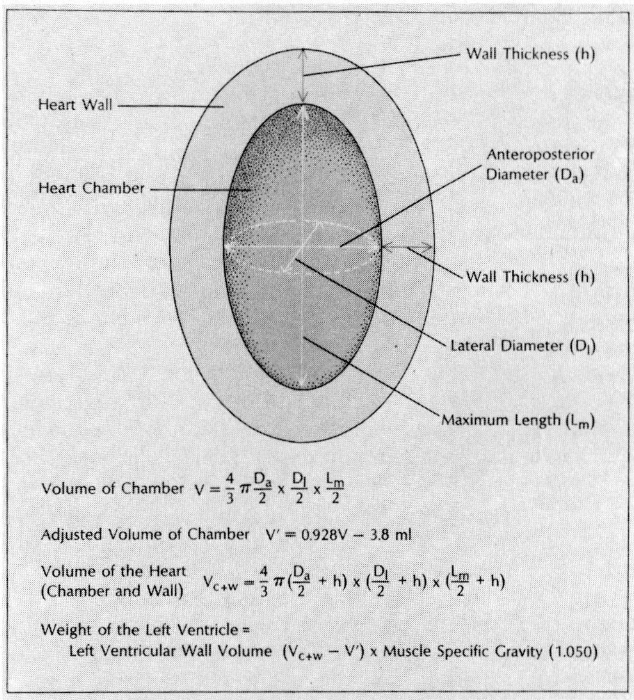

FIGURE 15–3. Diagram illustrating the approach used to calculate left ventricular volume by means of quantitative angiocardiography. Margins of the projected image of the left ventricular chamber are traced, and maximum length is measured in the anteroposterior and lateral views. Minor axes are derived from the planimetered areas of the chamber in both views; all dimensions are corrected to allow for distortion due to nonparallel x-rays. Left ventricular volumes are calculated using the formula for the volume of an ellipsoid, since (with regression-equation adjustment) this has given results that tally closely with directly measured ventricular volume. To determine left ventricular mass, volume of the ventricular chamber is subtracted from volume of chamber plus wall; multiplying wall volume by the specific gravity of cardiac muscle converts volume to heart weight or mass. (From Dodge, H. T.: Hemodynamic aspects of cardiac failure. *In* Braunwald, E. [ed.]: The Myocardium: Failure and Infarction. New York, HP Publishing Co., 1974, p. 70.)

Left Ventricular Volume, Mass, and Force

The area-length method developed by Dodge remains the most useful for calculating left ventricular volume[14] (Fig. 15–3). The longest length (L) of the ventricular chamber, i.e., from the apex to the root of the aortic valve, is measured, and the diameter (D) of the ventricle is calculated from the formula D = 4A/L, where A = area of left ventricular cavity determined by planimetry. Ordinarily this calculation is made for images exposed in both anteroposterior (AP) and lateral projections. The shape of the left ventricle usually resembles a prolate ellipsoid with one major and two minor diameters.[14, 27] With this assumption, left ventricular volume is calculated from the formula

$$V = 4/3\pi\ (L/2) \cdot (D_{AP}/2) \cdot (D_{lat}/2)$$

where V = volume in ml; L = longest length in cm in the AP or lateral projections; and D_{AP} and D_{lat} = the diameters (minor axes) calculated from the AP and lateral projections, respectively. These diameters in turn are calculated from the formula for the area of an ellipse (A) as follows:

$$D = \frac{4A}{\pi L}$$

A, the area of the opacified ventricle, can be conveniently determined by a hand or electronic planimeter and an X-Y plotter. The actual ventricular volume is determined from the calculated volume using a regression formula that takes into account the volume occupied by the papillary muscles and chordae tendineae within the ventricular chamber as well as corrections for distortion of x-ray beams (Fig. 15–3). Studies based on human autopsy specimens as well as on models and casts thereof have proved the accuracy of this approach.[9]

It is customary to obtain biplane angiograms in the 30-degree right anterior oblique (RAO) and 60-degree left anterior oblique (LAO) projections. Ventricular volume is calculated using a formula derived elsewhere[16]

$$V = \frac{8}{3\pi} \cdot \frac{A_{RAO} - A_{LAO}}{L_{min}}$$

where L_{min} is the shorter of L in the RAO or LAO projections.

Biplane angiographic methods are superior to single-plane methods for the calculation of left ventricular volumes. However, in patients without serious regional wall motion disorders, ventricular aneurysm, or distortion of the ventricular cavity, a reasonable estimate of ventricular volume can be obtained by utilizing either the AP or the RAO projection. Assuming that the two diameters of the left ventricle are equal, ventricular volume is calculated from the formula

$$V = L \cdot D^2 \cdot CF^3 \cdot \pi/6$$

where CF represents a one-dimensional correction factor.[9] Standardization of the degee of obliquity—usually 30-degree RAO and 60-degree LAO—is required for application of any particular correction factor in the calculation of ventricular volume. A close correlation has been found between left ventricular volume determined in the RAO projection and true cardiac volume; however, the overestimation of true volume is greater than with the biplane oblique volume method, and appropriate corrections must be made.[16, 29]

The normal left ventricular end-diastolic volume averages 70 ± 20 (SD) ml/m² (Table 15–1).[16, 32] Left ventricular function ordinarily is considered to be depressed when ventricular end-diastolic volume is clearly elevated (i.e., >110 ml/m², or > 2 SD's above the normal average) and *total* stroke volume and/or cardiac index and work are either reduced or within normal limits, while heart rate and arterial pressure are normal.

Left ventricular stroke volume (SV) is calculated as the difference between end-diastolic volume (EDV) and end-systolic volume (ESV). An important validation of the angiographic method for measuring ventricular volume in any laboratory is provided by insuring that SV, calculated by angiocardiography, correlates closely with that determined by an independent measurement utilizing the Fick or indicator dilution method. When the total SV, determined by angiocardiography, and the effective forward SV, determined by the Fick or indicator dilution method, are not equal, as occurs with aortic or mitral valvular regurgitation or with certain cardiac shunts, the difference between the two represents the regurgitant (or shunt) flow per cardiac cycle.

The ejection fraction (EF) represents the ratio between SV and EDV

$$EF = \frac{(EDV - ESV)}{EDV} = SV/EDV$$

In the presence of valvular regurgitation, the total SV ejected by the ventricle, i.e., the sum of forward and regurgitant volumes, is used in this calculation. The regurgitant fraction (RF) represents the ratio of regurgitant flow per stroke to the total left ventricular SV

$$RF = \frac{\text{SV total} - \text{SV forward}}{\text{SV total}}$$

where total SV is determined by angiography and forward SV by the Fick or indicator-dilution method.

Since there are errors in both techniques for measuring SV, these errors may summate in the calculation of the regurgitant volume and the regurgitant fraction. Also, when mitral and aortic regurgitation coexist, the regurgitant fraction reflects the sum of the two regurgitant volumes and does not distinguish between them.

Just as the prolate ellipsoid provides a frame of reference for the shape of the left ventricle, the *right ventricle* is shaped like a pyramid with a triangular base, and the formula for deriving the volume of this geometrical figure should be employed in the calculation of right ventricular volume.[30] The atria resemble ellipsoids, and their volumes can be determined using the area-length method.[31]

Two-dimensional echocardiography can be used readily to calculate left ventricular end-diastolic volume (EDV). In one approach,[20] EDV = $(D_{max} \times L_{max}/4 \times 4.35) - 6.44$, where D_{max} is the longest minor diameter determined from the parasternal long axis and the apical four-chamber and two-chamber views, and L_{max} is the major long axis derived from the apical views. The EDV, ESV, and EF calculated utilizing this method correlated well with those obtained by biplane angiography.

LEFT VENTRICULAR MASS. This value can also be determined by angiocardiography. Wall thickness, h, as visualized and measured along the free lateral wall of the left ventricle just below the equator at end-diastole (best measured on the AP or RAO projections), is added to the major and minor semiaxes to obtain the sum of volumes of the chamber and wall. This volume minus the chamber volume equals the volume of the wall. The product of wall volume and the specific gravity of heart muscle (1.050) equals left ventricular mass.[32] Thus, left ventricular mass (M) in grams can be calculated from the formula

$$M = ([4/3 \cdot \pi \frac{(L + 2h)}{2} \cdot \frac{(D_{AP} + 2h)}{2} \cdot \frac{(D_{lat} + 2h)}{2}] - V) \cdot (1.050)$$

where h = ventricular wall thickness in cm; 1.050 = specific gravity of heart muscle; D_{AP} and D_{lat} are the ventricular diameters in centimeters in the AP and lateral views, respectively; and V = left ventricular volume in milliliters. In addition, the ventricular volume must be corrected for the volume of the papillary muscles and trabeculae. A major assumption made with this method and one that undoubtedly introduces some inaccuracy is that left ventricular wall thickness is uniform around the entire left ventricular cavity. However, this method has been appropriately validated by postmortem studies comparing actual and projected left ventricular weights.[16]

Left ventricular mass can also be determined by two-dimensional echocardiography as the difference between total ventricular volume, estimated from the product of the epicardial left ventricular length and the area of the left ventricle in the short axis and the volume of the left ventricular cavity. This method too has been validated against actual ventricular weights.[21]

Left ventricular wall thickness normally averages 10.9 ± 2.0 mm (SD) and left ventricular mass, 92 ± 16 gm/m² (Table 15–1).[9, 32] Chronic cardiac dilatation secondary to volume overload or primary myocardial disease increases left ventricular mass, as does chronic pressure overload. Characteristically, hypertrophy due to pressure overload is characterized by an increased muscle mass resulting from an augmentation of wall thickness with, at first, little change in ventricular chamber volume (concentric hypertrophy). In contrast, hypertrophy due to volume overload or to primary myocardial disease is characterized by an increased muscle mass resulting from ventricular dilatation, with only a slight increase in wall thickness (eccentric hypertrophy) (Fig. 14–8, p. 432). There is often a correlation between left ventricular stroke work and left ventricular mass in chronic valvular heart disease, but no such relation exists in primary myocardial disease (Table 15–1).

LEFT VENTRICULAR FORCES. In order to assess myocardial function it is necessary to calculate the forces acting on the myocardial fibers within the ventricular wall. This requires knowledge of the dimensions of the left ventricular cavity, wall thickness, and intraventricular pressure.[33] *Tension* (force/cm), which, according to Laplace's law, is a product of the intraventricular pressure and radius (p. 405), may be defined as the force acting on a hypothetical slit in the ventricular wall that would tend to pull its edges apart. *Wall stress*, designated σ, is the force or tension (in dynes) per unit of cross-sectional area of the ventricular wall in cm². Wall stress may be considered to act in three directions—circumferential, meridional, and radial (Fig. 15–4). The most useful calculation is that of *circumferential wall stress*, which is the strongest force generated and supported within the ventricular wall at the equator

TABLE 15–1 LEFT VENTRICULAR VOLUME DATA IN PATIENTS

Group	Number of Patients	End-Diastolic Volume (ml/m²)	Stroke Volume (ml/m²)	Mass (gm/m²)	Ejection Fraction
Normal*	–	70 ± 20.0	45 ± 13.0	92 ± 16.0	0.67 ± 0.08
AS	14	84 ± 22.9	44 ± 10.1	172 ± 32.7	0.56 ± 0.17
AR	22	193 ± 55.4	92 ± 30.9	223 ± 73.0	0.56 ± 0.13
AS and AR	13	138 ± 36.5	75 ± 19.1	231 ± 56.9	0.53 ± 0.10
MS	37	83 ± 21.2	43 ± 11.9	98 ± 24.1	0.57 ± 0.14
MR	29	160 ± 53.1	87 ± 21.3	166 ± 49.9	0.47 ± 0.10
MS and MR	29	106 ± 34.4	58 ± 14.7	119 ± 27.8	0.57 ± 0.12
A and M combined	45	130 ± 55.8	69 ± 25.5	156 ± 55.9	0.55 ± 0.12
Myocardial disease	15	199 ± 75.7	44 ± 14.5	145 ± 27.6	0.25 ± 0.09

*Normal values from Kennedy, J. W., et al.: Quantitative angiocardiography. The normal left ventricle in man. Circulation *34*:272, 1966.
AS = aortic valve stenosis with peak systolic pressure gradient >30 mm Hg.
AR = aortic valve insufficiency with regurgitant flow >30 ml per beat.
MS = mitral valve area <1.5 sq cm.
MR = mitral valve regurgitant flow >20 ml per beat.
A and M combined = combined aortic and mitral valve disease.
Myocardial disease = primary cardiomyopathy or myocardial disease secondary to coronary atherosclerosis.
From Dodge, H. T., and Baxley, W. A.: Left ventricular volume and mass and their significance in heart disease. Am. J. Cardiol. *23*:528, 1969.

$$CWS = \frac{(P \bullet b)}{h}(1 - b^2/2a^2 - h/2b + h^2/8a^2)$$

where CWS = circumferential wall stress in dynes/cm^2 × 10^3; P = left ventricular pressure in dynes/cm^2; a and b are major and minor semiaxes (i.e., half the longest lengths), respectively, in cm, and h = left ventricular wall thickness in cm^2.[34] Also of value clinically is *meridional wall stress* (MWS), which is calculated as[35]

$$MWS = \frac{Pr}{2h\,(1 + h/2r)}$$

where r is the internal radius of the ventricle in cm.

Simultaneous recording of an angiogram (preferably biplane) and intraventricular pressure pulse (recording preferably with a high-fidelity micromanometer to avoid the artifacts inherent in the usual catheter-external manometer systems) allows calculation of *left ventricular tension* and *stress* throughout the cardiac cycle.

A somewhat simpler method of analyzing the instantaneous left ventricular tension throughout the cardiac cycle consists of recording left ventricular pressure simultaneously with left ventricular diameter across the minor axis of the left ventricle by means of an M-mode or two-dimensional echocardiogram. Alternatively, cine CT or MRI can be employed to obtain ventricular volumes and dimensions. This combination of measurements provides the data necessary to calculate ventricular circumferential fiber shortening (at either the endocardium or the midwall) and midwall circumferential stress, using minor modifications of the equations presented above.[36] However, the use of M-mode echocardiography for these calculations is based on the assumption of uniform wall motion. This assumption can be made with reasonable assurance only in conditions that affect left ventricular function relatively uniformly, such as dilated cardiomyopathy or aortic regurgitation, but not in conditions that produce localized or regional dysfunction, such as ischemic heart disease.

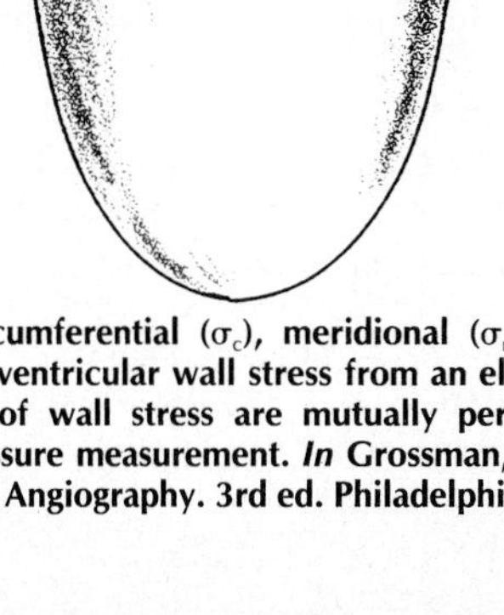

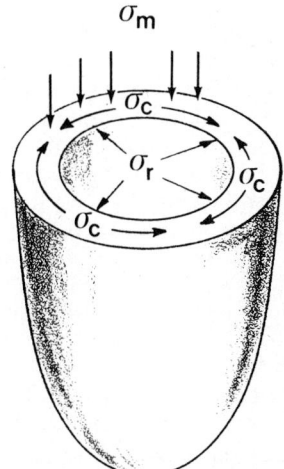

FIGURE 15–4. Circumferential (σ_c), meridional (σ_m), and radial (σ_r) components of left ventricular wall stress from an ellipsoid model. The three components of wall stress are mutually perpendicular. (From Grossman, W.: Pressure measurement. *In* Grossman, W. [ed.]: Cardiac Catheterization and Angiography. 3rd ed. Philadelphia, Lea and Febiger, 1986, p. 293.)

Ventricular *preload* may be expressed as end-diastolic wall stress and *afterload* as peak or mean systolic wall stress. During ejection, as the left ventricular cavity decreases in size and wall thickness increases, systolic wall stress and tension decline rapidly even though pressure is maintained (Fig. 15–5). *Left ventricular power* can be calculated as the product of intracavitary pressure and the rate of change of ventricular volume. Simultaneously recorded ventricular volumes and pressures during diastole allow the calculation of *left ventricular chamber and muscle* compliance[37] (Fig. 13–24, p. 402).

The use of automated methods has simplified greatly the calculations of all of these variables. For example, videodensitometric analysis of digital subtraction angiograms obtained following intravenous injection can provide in a simple manner an accurate measurement of EF.[10]

VENTRICULAR WALL MOTION

Contrast angiography and other imaging techniques also permit study of ventricular wall motion. Marked focal abnormalities of contraction can be appreciated by visual inspection of cineventriculograms; segments of abnormal ventricular contraction can be localized by superimposing end-diastolic and end-systolic outlines of the left ventricular cavity and tracing both the central x-ray beam and the cavity silhouette on paper or by using a computer. *Akinesis* is present when a portion of each of the two silhouettes shares a common line; *dyskinesis* is present when the end-systolic silhouette extends outside the end-diastolic silhouette.[38] The abnormally contracting segments (both akinetic and dyskinetic) may be expressed simply as percentages of the total end-diastolic circumference (Fig. 15–6). *Hypokinesis* (focal decreases in the extent of contraction) as well

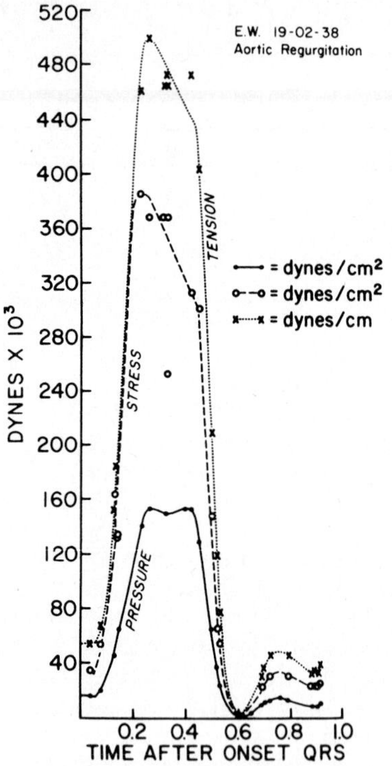

FIGURE 15–5. Sequential changes in left ventricular tension, stress, and pressure are illustrated throughout the cardiac cycle in a patient with aortic regurgitation. Note that tension, but particularly stress, declines during ejection (i.e., while the left ventricular volume decreases), although left ventricular pressure is maintained. (From Rackley, C. E.: Quantitative evaluation of left ventricular function by radiographic techniques. Circulation *54*:862, 1976, by permission of the American Heart Association, Inc.)

as *asynchrony* (abnormalities of timing contraction) are less severe disturbances of contraction. High filming rates, with analysis of wall motion from multiple cine frames, and the use of computer techniques to assist in data reduction and analysis are necessary for the detection of these more subtle abnormalities.[39] By use of such techniques, it is apparent that focal hypokinesis that cannot be detected readily by visual inspection of cineangiograms is a common disturbance, especially in ischemic heart disease, and that abnormalities of timing of segmental wall motion are nearly as common.

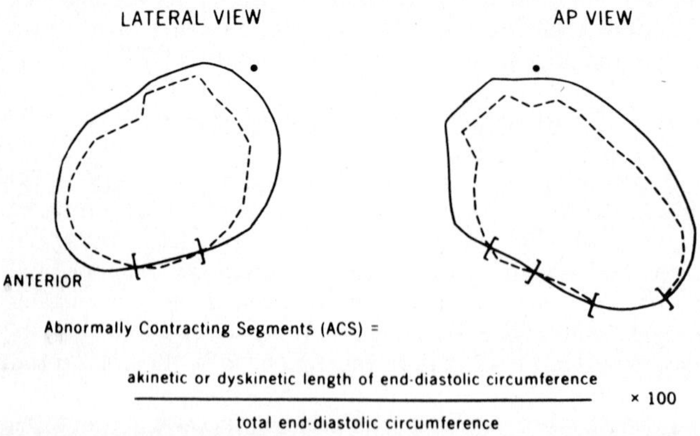

FIGURE 15–6. Systolic (dashed) and diastolic (solid) lateral and anteroposterior (AP) angiocardiograms are superimposed with a central lead marker as a reference point. The abnormally contracting segments are enclosed by brackets on the diastolic silhouette. (From Rackley, C. E.: Quantitative evaluation of left ventricular function by radiographic techniques. Circulation *54*:862, 1976, by permission of the American Heart Association, Inc.)

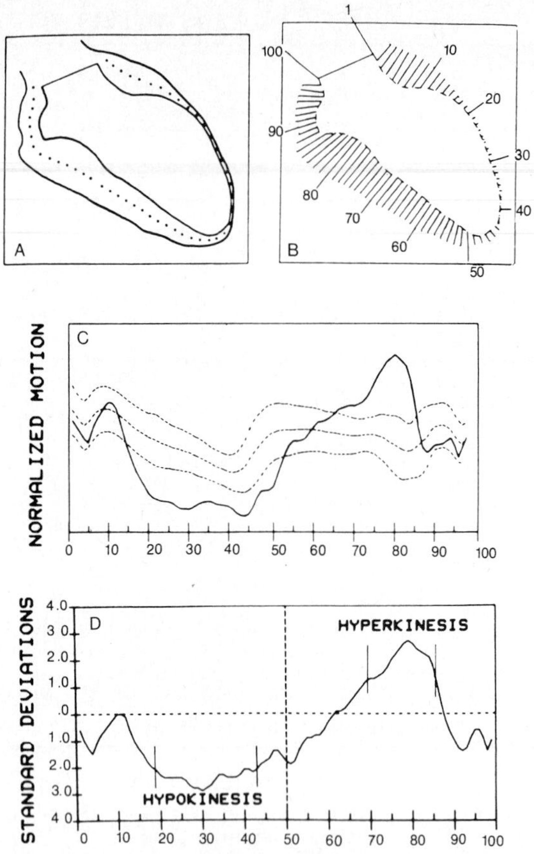

FIGURE 15–7. Centerline method of regional wall motion analysis. *A*, End-diastolic and end-systolic left ventricular endocardial contours and centerline constructed by the computer midway between the two contours. *B*, Motion is measured along 100 chords constructed perpendicular to the centerline. *C*, Motion at each chord is normalized by the end-diastolic perimeter to yield a shortening fraction. Motion along each chord is plotted for each patient (solid line). The mean motion in the normal ventriculogram group (dashed line) and one SD above and below the mean (dotted lines) are shown for comparison. *D*, The wall motion of the patient is plotted in units of SD's from the normal mean (dotted line). The normal group mean is represented by the horizontal zero line. Vertical lines delimit the most hyperkinetic and most hypokinetic parts of the anterior and inferior regions. (From Sheehan, F. H., Mathey, D. G., Schofer, J., Dodge, H. T., and Bolson, E. L.: Factors that determine recovery of left ventricular function after thrombolysis in patients with acute myocardial infarction. Circulation *71*:1122, 1985, by permission of the American Heart Association, Inc.)

Sheehan and Dodge have developed a useful technique in which end-diastolic and end-systolic endocardial contours are traced from a normal nonpostpremature sinus beat[40, 41] (Fig. 15–7*A*). A center line is drawn midway between the end-systolic and end-diastolic silhouettes (Fig. 15–7*A*); 100 chords are then constructed perpendicular to this center line (Fig. 15–7*B*). The length of each chord is determined, and after appropriate corrections for ventricular size, it is then compared with that of a group of normal subjects (Fig. 15–7*C*) and is expressed in units of standard deviation from the mean normal (Fig. 15–7*D*). A similar method developed by Fujita et al. involves the construction of 128 radial grids from the center of the left ventricular cavity and measurement of each grid between end-systole and end-diastole.[42] In many patients with ischemic heart disease, such as the one whose data are shown in Figure 15–7, hyperkinesis of the normal wall can compensate for large areas of hypokinesis or even akinesis and maintain ejection fraction despite substantial focal myocardial damage.

EJECTION FRACTION (EF) AND FRACTIONAL MYOCARDIAL SHORTENING

The ratio of SV to EDV, i.e., the EF, is a global index of the extent of ventricular fiber shortening and is considered, on the basis of a number of empirical studies, to provide a useful measure of left ventricular pump function. Left ventricular EF averages 0.67 ± 0.08 (SD) in normal subjects[16, 32] and ranges from 0.45 to 0.70 in experimental animals; it varies inversely with heart rate, and is influenced by the method used to measure cardiac volume, whether the animal is anesthetized or awake, and whether the chest is open or closed.[43] In normal subjects EF in the two ventricles is approximately equal.[44]

EF is closely related to and can be predicted accurately from the percentage of shortening of the left ventricular minor axis during systole, and this provides the basis for estimating EF by echocardiography.[45, 46] Most commonly, the diameter perpendicular to the midpoint of the long axis is used, and its fractional shortening (FS) is calculated as follows:

$$FS = \frac{\text{(Left ventricular) end-diastolic dimension} - \text{end-systolic dimension}}{\text{end-diastolic dimension}}$$

and is expressed as a percentage.

EF is a relatively insensitive index of ventricular function since focal hypokinesis of impaired myocardium, as occurs in ischemic heart disease, is often compensated for by hyperkinesis of normal myocardium (Fig. 15–7), resulting in a normal global EF. In addition to myocardial contractility, both preload and afterload affect EF, FS, and the mean velocity of circumferential fiber shortening (V_{cf}), i.e., the so-called ejection phase indices of ventricular performance. However, while studies in conscious or lightly sedated baboons[47] and conscious human subjects[48] have shown that moderate changes in preload have relatively little effect on these indices, they are quite sensitive to (and vary inversely with) afterload. Thus, values of EF, FS, and V_{cf}, like values of cardiac output or stroke volume, do not simply reflect levels of contractility. However, as pointed out below, the ejection phase indices are often useful for determining the level of contractility in the basal state in the presence of chronic heart disease, in which the influence of changes in preload and afterload tends to be corrected for by compensatory dilatation and hypertrophy.

VENTRICULAR DIMENSIONS AND THE VELOCITY OF SHORTENING. The extent, mean, and peak velocity of ventricular wall shortening during ejection have been employed to determine the effects of a variety of interventions on contractility using implanted ultrasonic dimension gauges in conscious dogs and primates and by cineradiographic recording of the motion of radiopaque markers sutured to the epicardium at the time of cardiac operations in patients.[49] Angiography and noninvasive imaging techniques, especially two-dimensional echocardiography, can also be used to measure ventricular dimensions, and the extent and velocity of their shortening. However, care must be taken that rotation and motion of the ventricle during systole are taken into consideration (a problem that may be avoided by recording signals from implanted markers). Changes in mean and peak V_{cf} can be used to evaluate acute inotropic interventions provided that afterload remains constant or almost so, or is corrected for. Fortuitously, V_{cf} shows little change during acute elevations in preload because the modest increases in systolic pressure and heart size that take place result in some augmentation of afterload, which offsets the increase of V_{cf} that would have occurred with an increase in preload alone had afterload remained constant.[45, 46, 50] Mean and peak V_{cf} incorporate the important element of the *velocity* of myocardial fiber shortening and appear to be more sensitive measures of contractility than EF and FS, which reflect simply the pumping function of the ventricle.

THE VENTRICULAR PRESSURE-VOLUME LOOP

When ventricular pressure and volume are related to each other over an entire cardiac cycle, a pressure-volume loop can be constructed (Fig. 15–8). The timing of valve opening and closing can be indicated on such a loop; the height and width of the loop are determined by the systolic pressure and stroke volume, respectively.[32, 51] The area subtended by the systolic portion of the curve provides a measure of stroke work performed *by* the left ventricle during systole, whereas the area subtended by the diastolic limb provides a measure of diastolic work performed *on* the left ventricle in distending it during diastole. Net work is the difference between the two. Diastolic work may be thought of as the energy supplied to the ventricle required for "priming the pump." In the absence of valvular regurgitation, diastolic work of the left ventricle is largely generated by the left atrium and right ventricle, and its elevation is the physiological basis for the right ventricular hypertrophy and sometimes failure observed in patients with left ventricular failure and secondary pulmonary hypertension.[32]

The position and slope of the ventricular pressure-volume loop in diastole (Fig. 13–24, p. 402 and Fig. 14–5, p. 430) provide important information concerning the ventricle's diastolic properties.[16] With left ventricular failure and an elevation of left ventricular diastolic pressure, there is an increase in diastolic work relative to systolic work and thus a reduction in net work. Characteristic changes in the left ventricular pressure-volume loops occur in various disease states (Fig. 15–9).

The use of radionuclide ventriculography[23, 24] or an

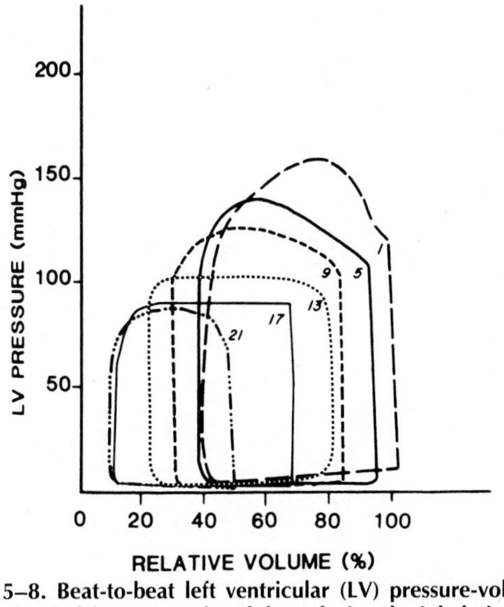

FIGURE 15–8. Beat-to-beat left ventricular (LV) pressure-volume diagrams constructed from every fourth beat during the inhalation of amyl nitrite in a patient in whom relative volume was measured with an impedance catheter. (From McKay, R. G., Spears, J. R., Aroesty, J. M., Baim, D. S., Royal, H. D., Heller, G. V., Lincoln, W., Salo, R. W., Braunwald, E., and Grossman, W.: Instantaneous measurement of left and right ventricular stroke volume and pressure-volume relationships with an impedance catheter. Circulation 69:709, 1984, by permission of the American Heart Association, Inc.)

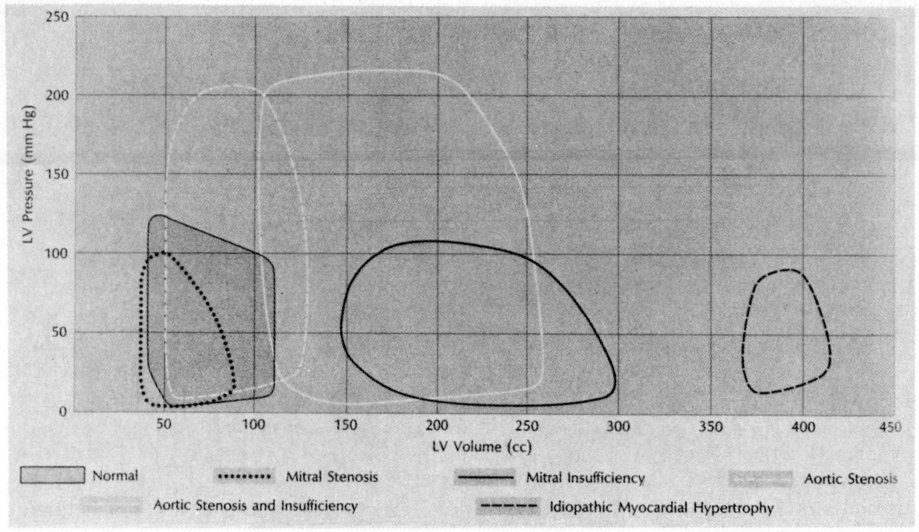

FIGURE 15–9. Left ventricular pressure-volume curves from patients with different varieties of heart disease. The height of each curve is determined by systolic pressure and the width by stroke volume. The two smallest curves—one from a patient with mitral stenosis, the other from a patient with primary cardiomyopathy—indicate similar stroke volumes; however, in the latter, the dilated left ventricle is functioning at an inappropriately large volume, and the ejection fraction is low. The curve in mitral insufficiency demonstrates volume overload by the large excursion along the volume axis and the absence of an isovolumetric contraction period. The shape of the curve in aortic stenosis shows the effect of pressure overload. In aortic stenosis and insufficiency the curve demonstrates the influence of pressure and volume overload, with the large area subtended by the curve. (From Dodge, H. T.: Hemodynamic aspects of cardiac failure. *In* Braunwald, E. [ed.]: The Myocardium: Failure and Infarction. New York, HP Publishing Co., 1974, p. 70.)

impedance catheter[52, 53] (Fig. 15–8) for the continuous or almost continuous measurement of ventricular volume has greatly facilitated the construction of pressure-volume loops and therefore their application in the assessment of left ventricular function.

VENTRICULAR END-SYSTOLIC PRESSURE-VOLUME RELATIONS

The extent of myocardial fiber shortening reflects the interactions among preload, afterload, and contractility. As already noted, as afterload increases, the extent of systolic fiber shortening declines (Figs. 13–15*C*, p. 395; 13–27 and 13–28, p. 406), resulting in progressively greater end-systolic fiber lengths.[54, 55] There is little difference between the end-systolic pressure-volume relation in isovolumetric and ejecting contractions. Indeed, the virtual identity of isometric and isotonic length-tension curves has been demonstrated in isolated cat papillary muscle[56, 57] (Fig. 15–10) and in the intact heart[58–60] and forms the basis for evaluating contractility. Thus, at any level of contractility, end-systolic fiber length is a direct function of and varies inversely with afterload (Fig. 15–11).

Myocardial contractility can be assessed by making use of this fundamental property of heart muscle. This is accomplished in the intact heart by focusing attention on the relation between the end-systolic volume (ESV), i.e., the volume remaining in the ventricle at the end of contraction, and the ventricular pressure at that instant. Since ESV varies inversely and end-systolic pressure directly with contractility, at a given level of contractility there is a unique line relating end-systolic pressure to ESV

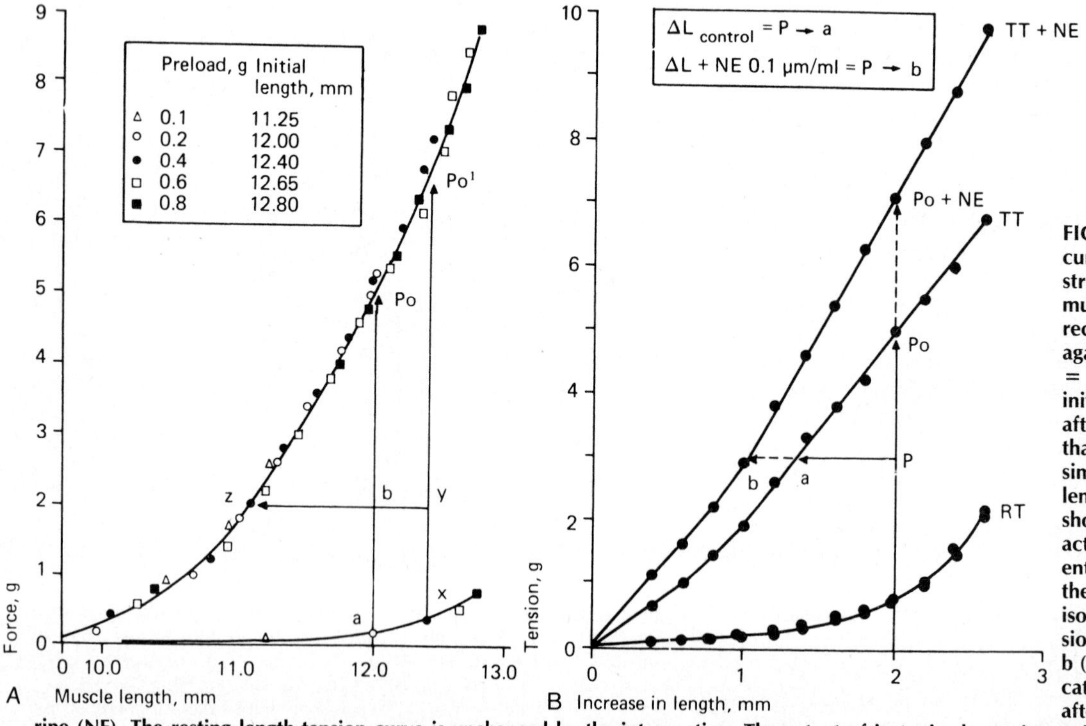

FIGURE 15–10. *A*, Length-tension curve of cat papillary muscle constructed by establishing the initial muscle length with a preload, and recording the extent of shortening against increasing afterloads. Po = total tension developed from initial length, a (*left*), when the afterload was of such magnitude that shortening did not occur; Po′ similar to Po but from initial length, x. Note that the muscle shortens to the same point on the active tension curve (z) independent of its initial length so long as the load is constant. Thus, the isometric and isotonic length-tension curves are virtually identical. b (*right*), Length-tension curves of cat papillary muscle before and after the addition of norepinephrine (NE). The resting length-tension curve is unchanged by the intervention. The extent of isotonic shortening at load P is increased from a to b with addition of NE, while total isometric tension is increased from Po to Po + NE. (From Downing, S. E., and Sonnenblick, E. H.: Cardiac muscle mechanics and ventricular performance: Force and time parameters. Am. J. Physiol. *207*:705, 1964.)

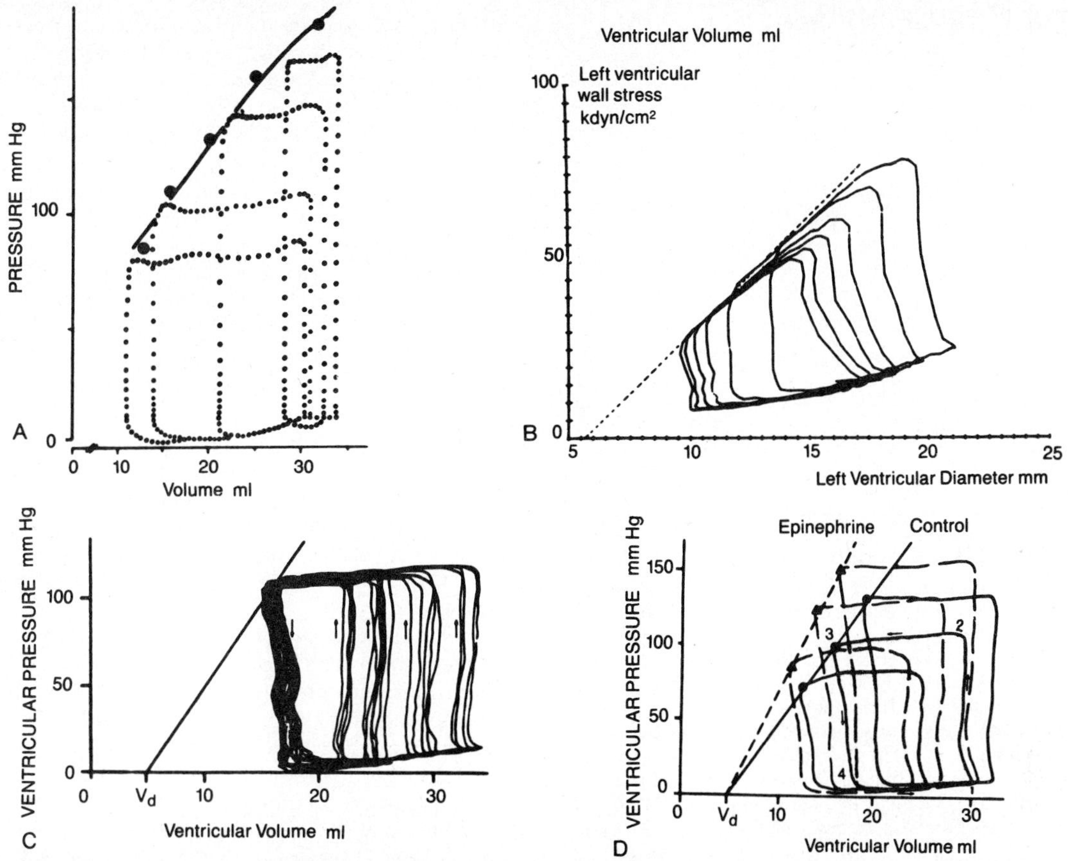

FIGURE 15–11. Pressure-volume (P-V) diagrams in canine ventricles. ***A*****, P-V diagram obtained in an isolated left ventricle that ejected liquid against a hydraulic servo-controlled loading system. The large dots near the solid line represent the peak isovolumetric pressures at various volumes. (From Weber, K. T., et al.: Left ventricular force-length relations of isovolumic and ejection beats. Am. J. Physiol.** ***231*****:337, 1976.)** ***B*****, Beat-to-beat changes in left ventricular stress-diameter loop during a decrease in venous return in an open-chest but otherwise intact dog. The dashed line corresponds to the end-systolic stress end-systolic diameter line. The stress-diameter relations are linear during most of ejection. (From Pouleur, H., Rousseau, M. F., van Eyll, C., van Mechelen, H., Brasseur, L. A., and Charlier, A. A.: Assessment of left ventricular contractility from late systolic stress-volume relations. Circulation** ***65*****:1204, 1982, by permission of the American Heart Association, Inc.)** ***C*****, Observations in the dog in which mean arterial pressure was kept constant while cardiac output was varied extensively in the control contractile state by changes in preload. Note that large changes in preload did not affect the end-systolic pressure-volume relation.** ***D*****, Mean arterial blood pressure was fixed at three different levels while cardiac output was kept constant during both the control (solid loops) and epinephrine infusion 2 μg/kg min^{-1} (broken loops). 1-2 = isovolumetric contraction, 2-3 = ejection, 3-4 = isovolumetric relaxation, 4-1 = filling. The diagonal lines represent the end-systolic pressure-volume relation (E_{es}). Epinephrine increased the slope, signifying an increase in contractility. (*C* and *D* from Suga, H., Sagawa, K., and Shoukas, A. A.: Load independence of the instantaneous pressure-volume ratio of the canine left ventricle and effects of epinephrine and heart rate on the ratio. Circ. Res.** ***32*****:317, 1973, by permission of the American Heart Association, Inc.)**

which is independent of load. The slope of this line defines contractility.

The end-systolic pressure-volume relations can be obtained from the pressure-volume loop, and the relation between these two variables at different levels of aortic pressure can be obtained by varying loading conditions (Fig. 13–28, p. 406). In experimental animals this is usually accomplished by volume expansion and vena caval occlusion. In intact human subjects, loading may be altered by infusion of a noninotropic vasoconstrictor such as phenylephrine and/or a vasodilator such as nitroglycerin (Fig. 15–12).

Figure 15–11*A* shows the pressure-volume diagrams from a canine left ventricle connected to a pump system, which allowed the ventricle to eject the fluid at any desired afterload.[59] The large dots, which represent the peak pressures that this ventricle reached in isovolumetric contractions, lie very close to the solid line, which connects the end-systolic pressure-volume relations of ejection beats. Figure 15–11*B* shows the effects of decreasing venous return; there was a progressive reduction in end-diastolic and end-systolic diameters as well as left ventricular wall stress. However, the stress-diameter relation remained constant.[61, 62] Figure 15–11*C* shows pressure-volume loops from a left ventricle that ejected blood from different end-diastolic volumes but at identical systolic pressures; the end-systolic pressure-volume relations are identical.

The end-systolic pressure-volume relationship for both isovolumetric and ejecting contractions can be expressed as $P_{es} = E_{es} (V_{es} - V_d)$ where P_{es} and V_{es} are the end-systolic pressure and end-systolic volume, respectively. E (not in the equation) is the ratio of ventricular pressure/volume (systolic elastance) at any time during the cardiac cycle; the maximum value for E, i.e., E_{max}, occurs at end-systole. E_{es} is the slope of the line relating E_{max} at various loading conditions (the solid lines in Figures 15–11*A*, *B*, and *D*); V_d is the intercept of this line on the volume (x) axis (Fig. 15–11*C* and *D*). Thus, E_{es} is a numerical expression of myocardial contractility; a higher value, i.e., a steeper slope, indicates a smaller end-systolic volume, i.e., more complete systolic emptying, at any given end-systolic pressure (Fig. 15–11*D*). (There is controversy concerning the interpretation of the intercept on

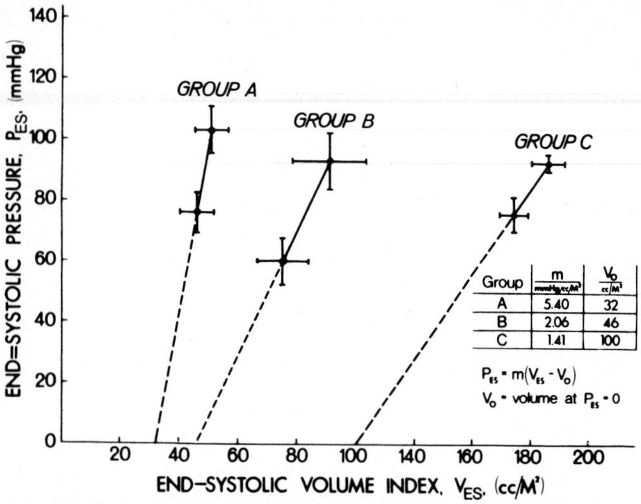

FIGURE 15–12. Average values for left ventricular end-systolic volume and pressure at two levels of systolic load are plotted for subjects with normal contractile function (group A, ejection fraction ≥ 0.60), intermediate function (group B, ejection fraction = 0.41 to 0.59), and poor contractile function (group C, ejection fraction ≤ 0.40). Points represent average values, and brackets indicate standard errors of the means. Volumes are index for body surface area in square meters. (From Grossman, W., Braunwald, E., Mann, T., McLaurin, L. P., and Green, L. H.: Contractile state of the left ventricle in man as evaluated from end-systolic pressure-volume relations. Circulation *56*:845, 1977, by permission of the American Heart Association, Inc.)

the volume axis of the line relating end-systolic pressure to volume.[63]) E_{es} can be measured by rearranging the equation as follows:

$$E_{es} = P_{es}/(V_{es} - V_d)$$

P_{es} and V_{es} can be measured relatively easily in patients; the determination of V_d requires measurement of P_{es} and V_{es} from contractions at a constant contractility but at different afterloads.

Although measurements of P_{es} appear to be useful clinically,[54] pressure is not an accurate estimate of end-systolic afterload. Rather, it is more accurate to use end-systolic wall *stress* rather than pressure[63–67]; stress can be calculated from considerations of intraventricular pressure and from cavity diameter and thickness[65] (p. 455).

There appear to be a number of theoretical advantages to the use of the slope of the end-systolic pressure (stress)-volume (dimension) relation (E_{es}) in assessment of myocardial contractility.[62, 63] First, since afterload is already incorporated into the calculation of E_{es}, any observed changes in this variable assess contractility directly; in contrast, the ejection phase indices provide a complex mixture of contractility and afterload. Second, because E_{es} is independent of preload, difficulties with the ejection phase indices that are affected by end-diastolic volume are obviated.[61]

SIMPLIFICATIONS. This approach can further be simplified by determining V_{es} noninvasively. Radionuclide angiography[23, 24] and an impedance (volume) catheter technique[52, 53] and M-mode or two-dimensional echocardiography[19, 22, 65–68] have been employed. In the absence of obstruction to left ventricular outflow, cuff pressure can be used to estimate ventricular systolic pressure. An indirect carotid pulse can indicate end-systole and with cuff pressure provides a noninvasive assessment of the end-systolic pressure.

This approach can be simplified further by determining the ratio of peak systolic pressure to end-systolic volume, the numerator determined by sphygmomanometry and the denominator by radionuclide ventriculography.[69–71] In normal subjects this ratio rises markedly during exercise but fails to do so in patients with left ventricular dysfunction.[72] An even simpler, albeit less accurate, assessment of contractility may be provided by the end-systolic volume (or end-systolic dimension) at the operating end-systolic pressure, if the latter is normal or almost so. Under these circumstances the end-systolic volume (corrected for body surface area) correlates inversely with contractility.[54, 73] The left ventricular end-systolic pressure-volume relation is of particular value in assessing contractility in patients with mitral regurgitation, in whom this assessment is otherwise particularly difficult[64] (see below).

VENTRICULAR dP/dt

Since *changes* in the maximum rate of rise of ventricular pressure (peak dP/dt) are known to be highly sensitive to acute *changes* in contractility[74, 75] (Fig. 15–13), measure-

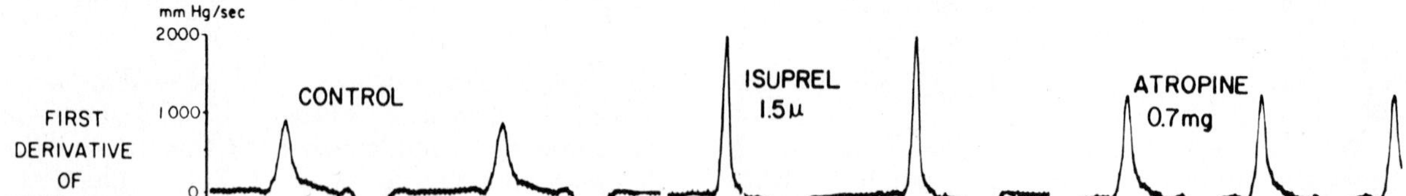

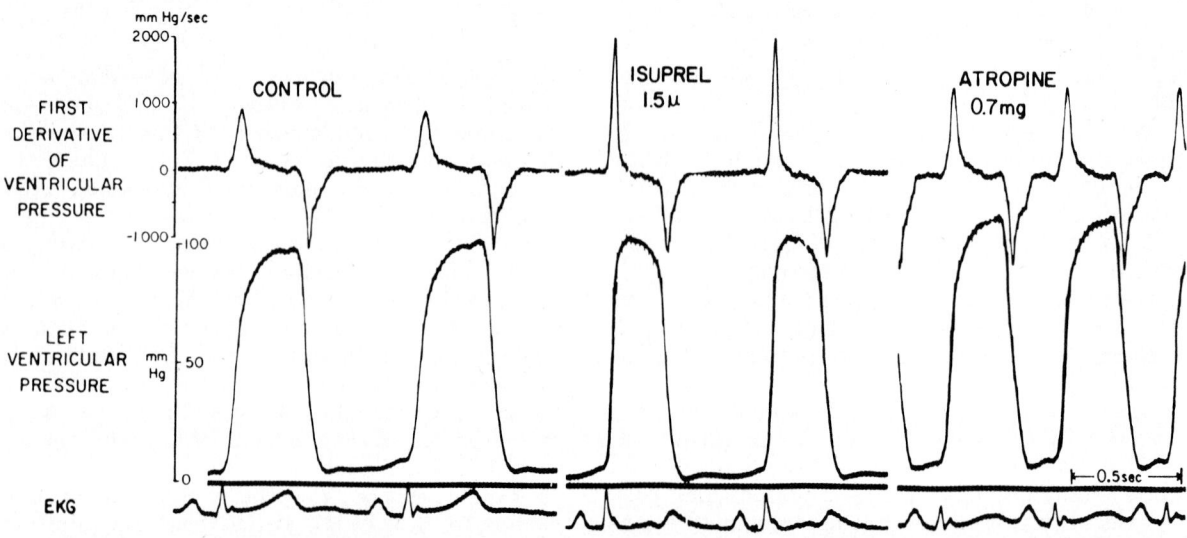

FIGURE 15–13. Serial recordings of left ventricular pressure and of the first derivative of left ventricular pressure (dP/dt) in a 12-year-old girl with mild pulmonic valvular stenosis. The first record (control) is in the basal state, the middle record after the administration of 1.5 µg isoproterenol, and the final record after 0.7 mg atropine. (From Gleason, W. L., and Braunwald, E.: Studies on the first derivative of the ventricular pressure pulse in man. J. Clin. Invest. *41*:80, 1962.)

ment of this variable may be employed along with ventricular end-diastolic volume and filling pressure in the assessment of *directional changes* in contractility with an intervention. Peak dP/dt cannot be measured reliably with the catheter-manometer systems ordinarily used during cardiac catheterization, unless special precautions are taken to prevent artifacts and the frequency response of the system is carefully determined.[76] High-fidelity catheter-tip micromanometers should be employed, but even with these, artifacts due to flicking catheter motion during the cardiac cycle must be assiduously avoided.

Peak dP/dt is largely independent of changes in afterload, provided that it occurs *before* aortic valve opening.[50, 77] Studies carried out in dogs[78] and humans[50] have shown that peak dP/dt is little changed by steady-state alterations in aortic pressure, and although it appears to be much more markedly affected by changes in contractility than by alterations in preload, the influence of the latter cannot be disregarded. Therefore, even when contractility is constant, a major change in preload can cause a modest alteration in dP/dt in the same direction. Another difficulty with peak dP/dt is that it cannot be corrected for changes in muscle mass produced by ventricular hypertrophy. This difficulty can be surmounted, however, by calculating the peak rate of rise of *stress*.[78a] Although the absolute level of peak dP/dt, in general, correlates with the basal level of contractility, it is not as useful for assessing this property of cardiac function as are the ejection phase indices (see below). Instead, it is more useful in assessing *directional* changes in contractility with acute interventions.

ASSESSMENT OF CARDIAC FUNCTION DERIVED FROM CONSIDERATION OF MUSCLE MECHANICS

In the final analysis, and irrespective of theoretical considerations, any index that is proposed for assessing ventricular contractility must be reproducible in the same individual under constant conditions and must be capable of differentiating patients with normal cardiac function from those with reduced cardiac function. The principles of myocardial muscle mechanics, outlined in Chapter 13, provide a framework for analysis for two classes of indices: one group based on events during isovolumetric contraction and a second based on events during ejection.

ISOVOLUMETRIC PHASE INDICES. V_{max}, the maximum velocity of shortening of the unloaded contractile elements (CE), theoretically provides a measure of myocardial contractility which is independent of preload or afterload. Controversy continues to surround calculation of CE V_{max}, in isolated muscle and even more so in the intact heart, in which case the calculation must be based on many assumptions.[79] Despite these difficulties, observations in the intact left ventricle (p. 412) indicate that its V_{max}, determined by extrapolation of the force-velocity relation derived from multiple variably afterloaded beats, is, like the V_{max} of isolated cardiac muscle, not altered significantly by changes of preload within the physiological range but is markedly sensitive to inotropic stimuli.[80]

V_{max} (The Maximum Velocity of Shortening of the Contractile Elements). It is obviously impractical in patients to determine the V_{max} either in variably afterloaded or completely isovolumetric beats. However, a mathematical derivation of CE V_{max} can be obtained in the normally ejecting heart using only the isovolumetric phase of contraction and employing one of the so-called isovolumetric phase indices described below. In one approach that has been applied clinically,[81] V_{CE} is calculated as dP/dt/KP (where K is an assumed stiffness constant for the series elastic element) and is plotted against instantaneous wall stress (calculated from intraventricular pressure, volume, and wall thickness) during the isovolumetric phase of left ventricular systole, and the curve is then extrapolated to zero stress to obtain V_{max}. If it is further assumed that contraction of the myocardium during isovolumetric contraction is truly isometric, then pressure and wall stress are linearly related to one another, and no calculation of wall stress is required to determine V_{max}[82]; calculated V_{CE} is simply plotted against the instantaneous intraventricular pressure and extrapolated to zero pressure. This index of V_{max} is relatively independent of acute changes in preload at low left ventricular end-diastolic pressure[83] but declines at end-diastolic pressures exceeding 10 mm Hg.[84]

Determination of V_{max} in the intact heart, as described above, requires a number of assumptions concerning the characteristics of the SE and PE (parallel elastic elements) and the type of muscle model that exists in the intact heart. Little information is available about how chronic heart disease alters these characteristics.[79] Furthermore, the validity of the assumption that isovolumetric contraction is truly isometric has been questioned.[85]

Some of the difficulties cited above involving the calculation of V_{max} can be partially avoided by the selection of certain points on the curve relating dP/dt/DP, where DP is the developed left ventricular pressure (i.e., left ventricular pressure minus end-diastolic pressure) to the corresponding DP. These measures tend to be relatively independent of changes in afterload, since they are usually computed at a DP of 40 mm Hg, a level of pressure generation which in most clinical circumstances occurs before the opening of the aortic valve.[86] The ratio dP/dt/DP at a DP of 40 mm Hg, although somewhat less sensitive to acute changes in contractility than simple peak dP/dt, is nonetheless useful for assessing *directional* changes in contractility,[50, 86, 87] since it is unaffected by changes in afterload and is relatively insensitive to changes in preload. The peak level of dP/dt/TP (where TP refers to total pressure development), termed "V_{pm}," is also relatively independent of both preload and afterload but is sensitive to changes in the inotropic state.[88] It has been advocated as an index of the contractility in the basal state, as discussed further below.

EJECTION PHASE INDICES. The most commonly used ejection phase indices include ejection fraction (EF), peak and mean fractional shortening (FS) of ventricular myocardium, and peak and mean velocity of circumferential fiber shortening. V_{CF} at peak wall stress has been chosen for many estimates of contractility since at that instant the rate of change in wall force (and therefore the rate of change in the length of SE) is zero, and V_{CF} equals V_{CE}.

The end-systolic pressure (or stress) to end-systolic volume (or dimension) relation described above (Fig. 15–11) and the relation between ejection fraction or the fractional shortening of the left ventricle and left ventricular end-systolic wall stress (see Fig. 15–15) are special cases of ejection phase indices because they are based on the characteristics of the ventricle during ejection. They are, however, superior to the "classical" ejection phase indices in that they correct, at least in part, for variations in loading conditions.

DETERMINATION OF DIRECTIONAL CHANGES IN CONTRACTILITY

As already noted, at constant levels of ventricular filling pressure, end-diastolic volume or dimensions (as evidence of constant ventricular preload) and of aortic or left ventricular systolic pressure (as evidence of constant afterload), a variety of measures of left ventricular performance, such as the ejection phase indices (EF, peak and mean FS, and V_{CF}) as well as stroke volume, stroke work and stroke power, all vary as functions of myocardial contractility. Thus, it may be assumed that an acute enhancement of contractility has occurred if any of these indices of mechanical performance increases while filling pressure or end-diastolic volume remains unchanged or declines and aortic pressure remains unchanged or rises.

Although the absolute levels of ventricular filling pressure do not correlate with end-diastolic volume in chronic heart disease[32, 89] (Fig. 15–9), acute changes in ventricular filling pressure are directionally similar to changes in end-diastolic volume (except in the presence of myocardial ischemia or marked tachycardia [p. 434]). Therefore, when the effect of an intervention is studied, a change in ventricular filling pressure may be related to a change in one of the hemodynamic measures of left ventricular performance enumerated above in order to assess directional changes of contractility.[58, 89] This approach is *not* applicable when preload or afterload or both are altered by the intervention under study so as to cause a change in performance in the same direction as the presumed effect of the alteration in contractility, such as occurs when ventricular filling pressure rises and/or left ventricular systolic pressure declines as one of the aforementioned indices of ventricular performance increases.

ISOVOLUMETRIC PHASE INDICES. In assessing acute

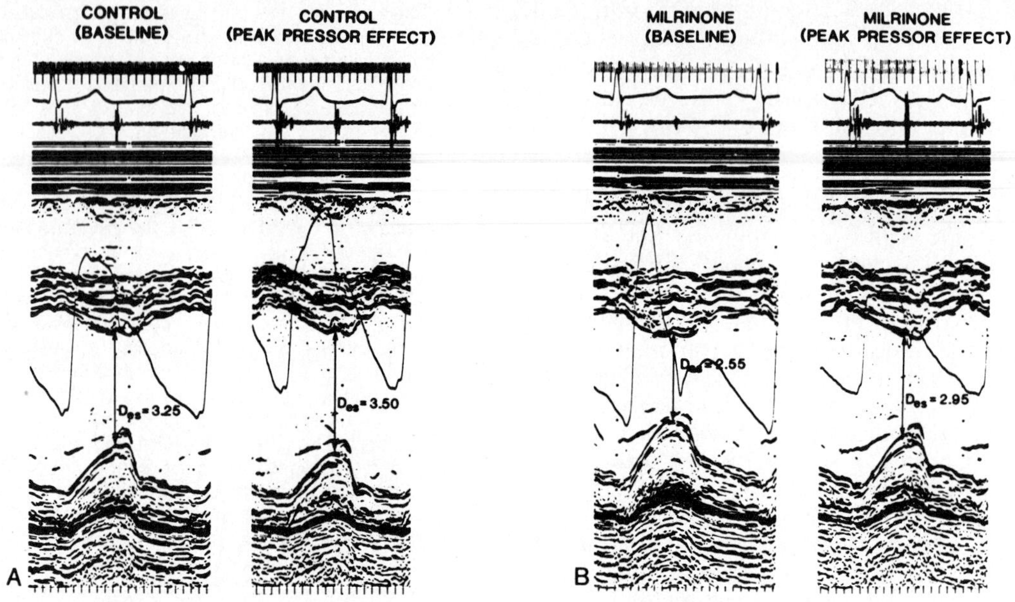

	A Control (Baseline)	A Control (Peak Pressor Effect)	B Milrinone (Baseline)	B Milrinone (Peak Pressor Effect)
HR	72	79	69	77
P_{PS}/P_D	130/73	161/107	104/61	162/101
P_{es}	105	134	67	127
h_{es}	1.75	1.65	1.90	1.80
σ_{es}	43	65	17	44
%ΔD	36.3	34.6	44.0	40.4
V_{cf_c}	0.99	0.92	1.29	1.13
m	116		150	

FIGURE 15–14. *A*, Simultaneous recordings of the left ventricular echocardiogram, phonocardiogram, carotid pulse tracing, and electrocardiogram under control baseline conditions (before methoxamine infusion) and at peak pressor effect. *B*, Recordings from the same subject as in panel A, performed during milrinone administration (before methoxamine infusion) and at peak pressor effect. The carotid pulse dicrotic notch is low and early peaking takes place under baseline conditions, reflecting the significant vasodilator effect of milrinone. The carotid pulse morphology normalized with the afterload challenge. The end-systolic pressure-dimension (P_{es}-D_{es}) slope (m) increased significantly over the control value (from 116 to 150 mm Hg/cm). P_D = aortic diastolic pressure (mm Hg), σ_{es} = end-systolic wall stress (gm/cm²); h_{es} = end-systolic wall thickness (cm), HR = heart rate (beats/min), P_{ps} = peak systolic pressure (mm Hg), Vcf_c = rate-corrected velocity of fiber shortening in circumferences/sec, %Δ = percentage of fractional shortening. (From Borow, K. M., Come, P. C., Neumann, A., Baim, D. S., Braunwald, E., and Grossman, W.: Physiological assessment of the inotropic, vasodilator and afterload reducing effects of milrinone in subjects without cardiac disease. Am. J. Cardiol. *55*:1208, 1985.)

changes in contractility, there does not seem to be an advantage in the use of derived measures such as "V_{max}," which is calculated from the isovolumetric phase pressure tracings, over the more directly obtained peak dP/dt/DP_{40}. Both of these isovolumetric phase indices are highly responsive to changes in the inotropic state and are relatively insensitive to changes in preload and afterload.[90]

EJECTION PHASE INDICES. Changes in the relation between the extent or velocity of myocardial wall shortening and the simultaneous ventricular wall stress (at any given ventricular dimension) reflect acute changes in contractility. For instance, an augmentation of instantaneous velocity of minor axis shortening (V_{CF}) at any given ventricular length and wall stress signifies an improvement of contractility. The relation between end-systolic meridional wall stress and of left ventricular fractional shortening provides a sensitive index by which an inotropic intervention can be assessed[67] (Figs. 15–14 and 15–15). As already noted (p. 459), a change in the slope of E_{es}, the end-systolic pressure (stress) to end-systolic volume (dimension) relation, an ejection phase index, is also an excellent indicator of a change in contractility.

DETERMINATION OF CONTRACTILITY IN THE BASAL STATE (Table 15–2)

ISOVOLUMETRIC PHASE INDICES. These indices[90a]—peak dP/dt, dP/dt/DP_{40}, V_{pm}, and V_{max}—are usually of little value in assessing *basal levels* of contractility and in *com-*

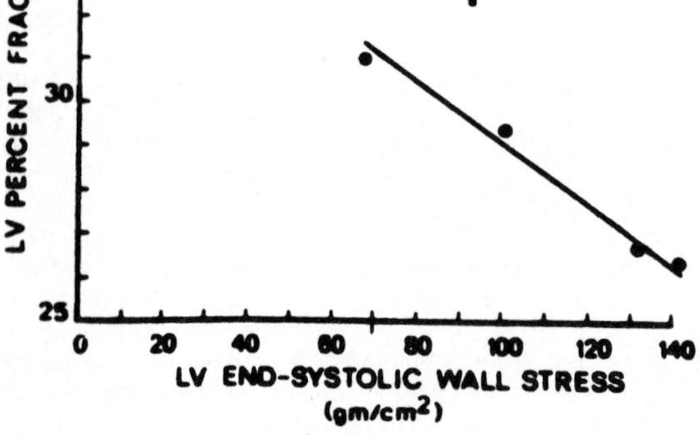

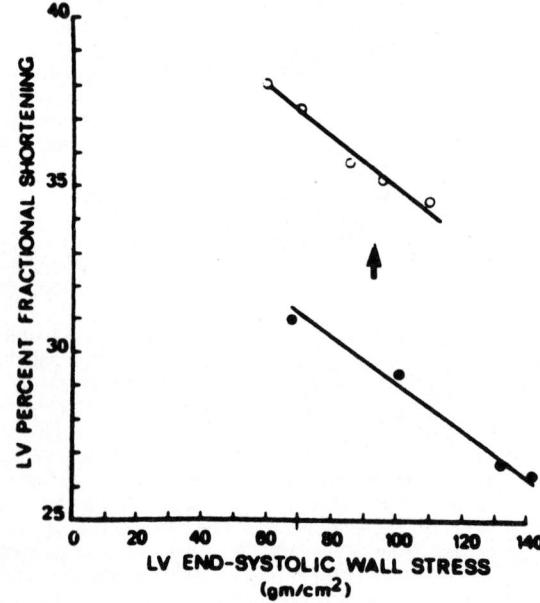

FIGURE 15–15. Comparison of the LV end-systolic wall stress-shortening lines joining points at different afterloads for control (closed circles) and increased (open circles) contractile states produced by dobutamine in a representative subject. With the dobutamine infusion, the percentage of ΔD is higher for any level of end-systolic wall stress. (From Borow, K. M., Green, L. H., Grossman, W., and Braunwald, E.: Left ventricular end-systolic stress-shortening and stress-length relations in humans. Am. J. Cardiol. *50*:1301, 1982.)

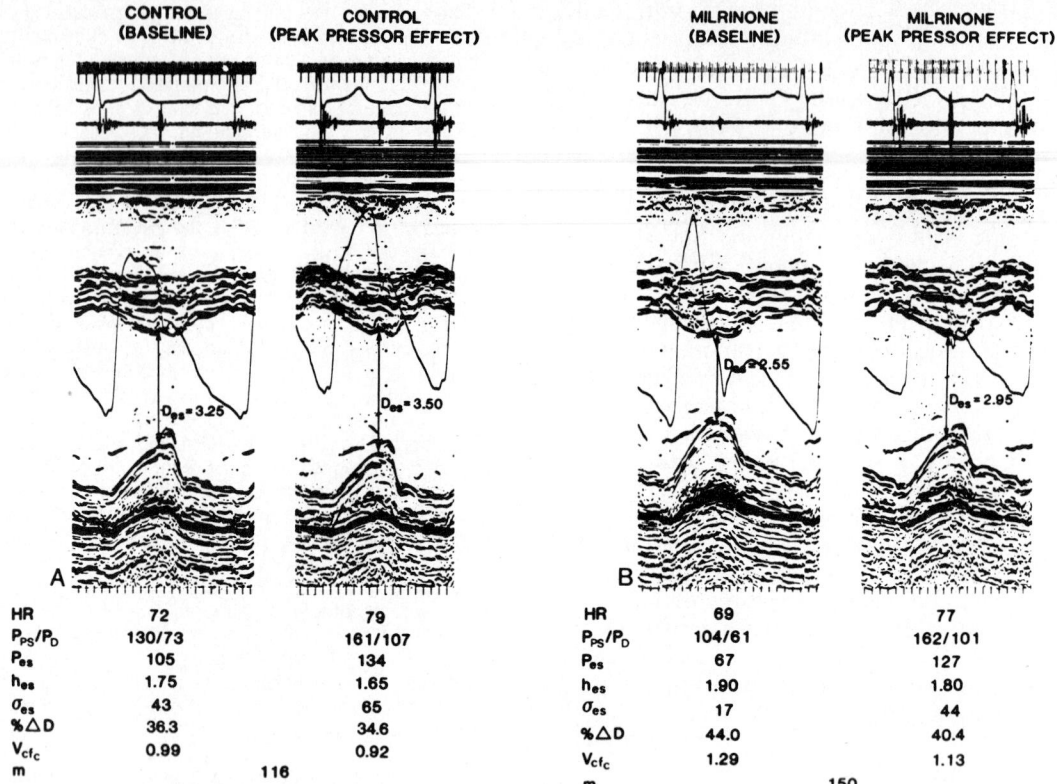

TABLE 15–2 EVALUATION OF LEFT VENTRICULAR SYSTOLIC PERFORMANCE: NORMAL VALUES FOR SOME ISOVOLUMIC AND EJECTION PHASE INDICES

CONTRACTILITY INDICES		NORMAL VALUES (MEAN ± S.D.)
Isovolumic Indices:		
Maximum dP/dt		1610 ± 290 mm Hg/sec
		1670 ± 320 mm Hg/sec
		1661 ± 323 mm Hg/sec
Maximum (dP/dt/P)		44 ± 8.4 sec^{-1}
V_{PM} or peak $\left[\frac{dP/dt}{28P}\right]$		1.47 ± 0.19 ML/sec
dPdt/DP at DP = 40 mm Hg		37.6 ± 12.2 sec^{-1}
Ejection Phase Indices:		
LVSW		81 ± 23 gm-m
LVSWI		53 ± 22 gm-m/M^2
		41 ± 12 gm-m/M^2
EF	angio:	0.72 ± 0.08
MNSER	angio:	3.32 ± 0.84 EDV/sec
	echo:	2.29 ± 0.30 EDV/sec
Mean V_{CF}	angio:	1.83 ± 0.56 ED circ/sec
		1.50 ± 0.27 ED circ/sec
	echo:	1.09 ± 0.12 ED circ/sec

dP/dt = rate of rise of left ventricular (LV) pressure; DP = developed LV pressure; ML = muscle lengths; MNSER = mean normalized systolic ejection rate; ED = end-diastolic; V = volume; circ = circumference; EF = ejection fraction.

Adapted from Grossman, W.: Evaluation of systolic and diastolic function of the myocardium. *In* Grossman, W. (ed.): Cardiac Catheterization and Angiography. 3rd ed. Philadelphia, Lea & Febiger, 1986, p. 308. Original references for each item are given in Grossman, p. 308.

paring contractility among different patients or in any given patient at different times. Empirically, it has been observed that of these several indices, V_{pm}—i.e., the physiological maximum observed velocity of myocardial shortening, calculated as the maximum dP/dt/P—is superior to the others in separating *groups* of patients with normal and depressed contractility. However, even this index is not always reliable in classifying individual patients.[91]

EJECTION PHASE INDICES. In contrast to the limitations of the isovolumetric phase indices, the ejection phase indices (EF, FS, and mean and peak V_{CF},[92] the rate of left ventricular wall thickening during systole[93]) and the closely related mean systolic ejection rate can all be employed in the assessment of basal contractility despite their sensitivity to variations in loading. Acute alterations of afterload cause an inverse change in ejection phase indices at any level of contractility; therefore, these indices should not be employed in the assessment of myocardial contractility in the face of an acute change in afterload. However, these indices are less sensitive to changes in preload. In experimental animals, both FS and V_{CF} remain normal when measured at various time intervals following establishment of a chronic volume overload during the stable, compensatory stage of ventricular hypertrophy.[94] Therefore, chronic dilatation and hypertrophy in the presence of a chronic volume overload do *not* preclude the usefulness of ejection phase indices for assessing the basal level of contractility. An exception occurs in the case of mitral regurgitation when, as noted below, the volume overload (increased preload) is accompanied by a reduction in afterload, thereby resulting in inappropriately elevated levels of ejection phase indices (Fig. 15–16).

Ejection phase indices may also be useful in assessing basal levels of contractility in the chronically pressure-overloaded heart that has adapted to the change in afterload by means of concentric hypertrophy, thereby tending to maintain afterload at a normal level. As left ventricular hypertrophy develops in dogs with chronic experimental aortic constriction, FS as well as mean and peak V_{CF} at first decline but then return to and stabilize at close to normal levels.[95] Indeed, when the obstruction develops slowly and compensatory hypertrophy keeps pace with it, so that wall stress does not rise, the ejection phase indices remain normal[96] until the "exhaustion phase" of ventricular hypertrophy, when contractility deteriorates. The relation between percentage of fractional myocardial shortening, determined noninvasively, and left ventricular end-systolic stress,[67] obtained in the basal state (Fig. 15–17) or during the stress of an increased afterload (Fig. 15–18), provides a useful, practical framework for assessing the basal level of left ventricular contractility.[96a, 96b] This relationship is particularly useful in patients who have reduced ejection phase indices and distinguishes between reduced myocardial shortening due to excessive afterload from that due to depressed myocardial contractility. However, as is the case with other ejection phase indices, this relationship may be altered, albeit modestly, by acute changes in preload.

Only the end-systolic pressure (or stress) to volume (or dimension) relation, i.e., E_{es} (p. 459), is not affected by either preload or afterload. However, the normal range of

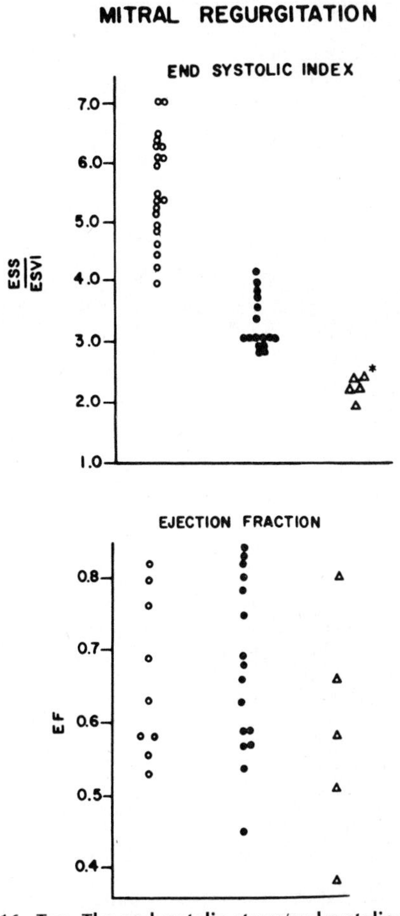

FIGURE 15–16. *Top,* The end-systolic stress/end-systolic volume index ratio for normal subjects (open circles), patients with mitral regurgitation who improved clinically after valve replacement (solid circles), and patients with mitral regurgitation who died or did not improve with surgery (open triangles). The ratio allowed separation of these groups of patients, whereas use of ejection fraction (*bottom*) did not. (From Carabello, B. A., Nolan, S. P., and McGuire, L. D.: Assessment of preoperative left ventricular function in patients with mitral regurgitation: Value of end-systolic wall stress/end-systolic volume ratio. Circulation *64*:1212, 1986, by permission of the American Heart Association, Inc.)

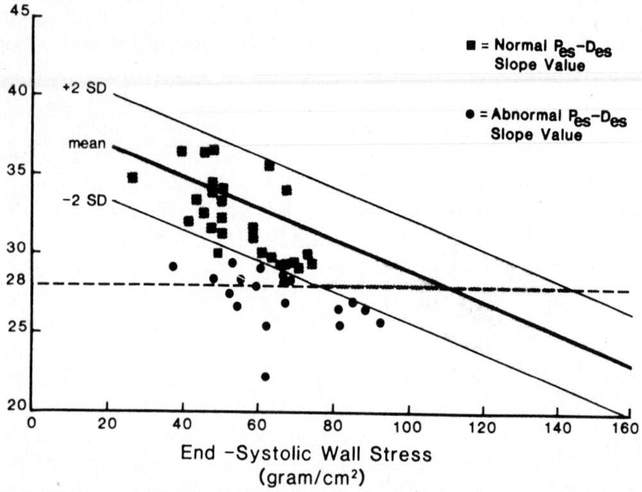

FIGURE 15–17. Plot of the left ventricular end-systolic wall stress (σ_{es}) = per cent fractional shortening (%ΔD) relation under resting conditions for the patient treated with doxorubicin. Previously reported normal values are shown by the solid lines. The normal lower limit for %ΔD is shown by the dashed line. All 10 patients with abnormalities of both resting %ΔD and P_{es}-D_{es} slope value had depressed σ_{es}-%ΔD relations. Ten of 36 patients with normal resting %ΔD had σ_{es}-%ΔD values outside the 95 per cent confidence limits, showing inappropriately low %ΔD for the level of afterload. (From Borow, K. M., et al.: Assessment of left ventricular contractility in patients receiving doxorubicin. Ann. Intern. Med. 99:750, 1983.)

values for this relation, i.e., the slope E_{es}, has not yet been clearly established.

AORTIC REGURGITATION. The usefulness of ejection phase indices in assessing left ventricular contractility has been demonstrated in patients before and after aortic valve replacement for aortic regurgitation. Although in one series[97] all patients studied demonstrated an improved forward cardiac index, increased aortic diastolic pressure, and decreased left ventricular end-diastolic pressure postoperatively, the majority manifested no improvement in the depressed V_{CF}. This indicates that the contractility remained depressed even though correction of the valvular leak improved apparent ventricular performance.

AORTIC STENOSIS AND HYPERTENSION. Under conditions of chronic pressure overload, such as occur in aortic stenosis or hypertension, the ventricle compensates by means of hypertrophy, adding more contractile units in parallel in an attempt to maintain afterload relatively constant (p. 431). If hypertrophy is inadequate or fails to keep pace with an increasingly severe pressure overload, wall stress rises. In keeping with the inverse force-velocity relation of cardiac muscle, there are reciprocal reductions in the various ejection phase indices, which under these circumstances do not signify a depression in contractility. Therefore, for ejection phase indices to provide an index of contractility in the presence of pressure overload, they must be related to wall stress. A true depression of contractility is present when these indices of shortening are low even when the existing level of afterload is taken into account.[98]

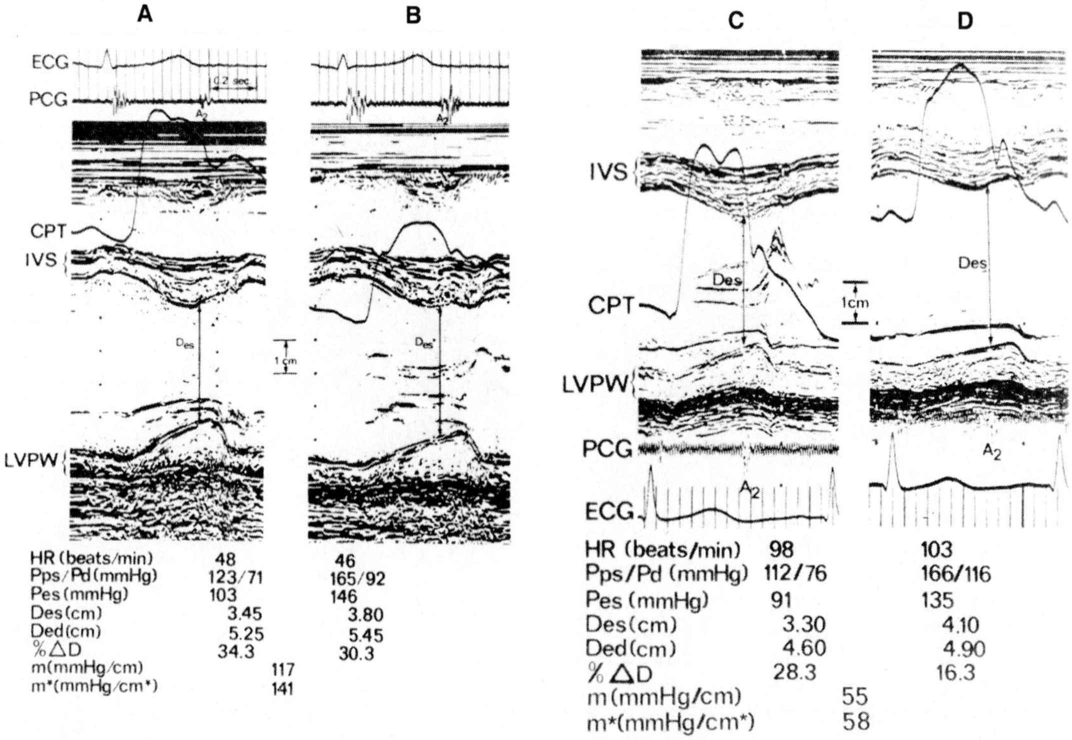

FIGURE 15–18. *Left,* Simultaneous recordings of left ventricular echocardiogram, phonocardiogram (PCG), carotid pulse tracing (CPT), and electrocardiogram (ECG) in a control subject. Recordings were made under baseline conditions (A) and at peak methoxamine effect (B). The 43-mm Hg increase in end-systolic pressure (P_{es}) resulted in a 0.35-cm increase in end-systolic dimension (D_{es}). *Right,* Recordings from a 16-year-old patient with thalassemia major during baseline conditions (C) and at peak methoxamine effect (D). Both the actual and corrected slope values (m and m*) were abnormal despite normal resting fractional shortening (%ΔD). The 44-mm Hg increase in end-systolic pressure (P_{es}) resulted in a 0.80-cm increase in end-systolic dimension (D_{es}). IVS = interventricular septum, LVPW = left ventricular posterior wall, A_2 = aortic component of the second heart sound, HR = heart rate, Pps = peak systolic pressure, Pd = aortic diastolic pressure; %ΔD = per cent fractional shortening, m = slope relating P_{es} to D_{es}, m* = slope corrected for body surface area. (From Borow, K. M., Propper, R., Bierman, F. Z., Grady, S., and Inati, A.: The left ventricular end-systolic pressure-dimension relation in patients with thalassemia major. Circulation 66:982, 1982, by permission of the American Heart Association, Inc.)

MITRAL REGURGITATION. Studies in experimental animals have demonstrated that acute mitral regurgitation is associated with a marked reduction in intramyocardial wall tension (afterload) and as a consequence ventricular emptying and ejection phase indices are enhanced.[99, 100] In patients with severe mitral regurgitation in the clinically compensated state, these ejection phase indices may also be elevated, with ejection fractions sometimes rising to exceed 0.80 (Fig. 15–16). Thus left ventricular fiber shortening and ejection phase indices may be normal[101, 102] in patients with chronic mitral regurgitation and clinical evidence of heart failure. In chronic severe mitral regurgitation, myocardial contractility is affected by two opposing influences: the tendency of a low-impedance leak to increase myocardial shortening and thereby to elevate the ejection phase indices, and of impaired myocardial function secondary to prolonged volume overload to reduce them. The important implication is that when ejection phase indices are in the normal range in patients with severe mitral regurgitation, impaired myocardial function is often present. Moderately reduced values of these indices, such as an EF of 40 to 50 per cent, usually indicate much more severe myocardial impairment than similar values recorded in patients with other forms of heart disease. Thus, many patients with chronic mitral regurgitation, marked left ventricular dilatation, moderate depression of EF, and eccentric cardiac hypertrophy manifest progressive worsening of myocardial shortening and lack of regression of hypertrophy after mitral valve replacement. Presumably, this is a consequence of the sudden increase in left ventricular afterload acting on a severely depressed myocardium when the regurgitant leak is abolished.[102]

CARDIOMYOPATHY. Patients with cardiomyopathy without volume or pressure overload can be distinguished from normal persons by the presence of depressed ejection phase indices.[91] These indices of global left ventricular function, although relatively insensitive to the consequence of focal ischemia, are far more useful than simple measurements of cardiac output, stroke volume, and stroke work in establishing prognosis in patients who have suffered extensive infarcts and/or who have generalized ischemia. Impaired left ventricular function can also be detected in patients with deviated cardiomyopathy by examining the relationship between ventricular dimensional shortening as arterial pressure is altered (Fig. 15–18*B*).

ISCHEMIC HEART DISEASE. The mildest disturbance of ventricular performance in ischemic heart disease consists of focal abnormalities of contraction and relaxation present only when ischemia is induced by a stress such as pacing,[51] but with maintenance of global ventricular function, as reflected in normal end-diastolic, end-systolic, and stroke volumes and EF. As already noted (Fig. 15–7), this discrepancy between regional wall motion and ventricular volumes may result from augmented motion of the normal segment of the ventricle. As ischemia progresses, wall motion abnormalities become present at rest. A slightly more severe disturbance is characterized by a normal EF at rest, which fails to rise during exercise. In this situation exercise induces ischemia of a segment of the ventricle that is of sufficient size that even a compensatory hypercontractile response of the remaining portion is not sufficient to maintain global ventricular function. With more severe ischemia EF declines and filling pressure rises, at first only during stress (atrial pacing or exercise) and then even at rest. The latter usually occurs in patients who have suffered infarcts of substantial size, in whom the elevated filling pressure reflects reduced compliance of the scarred ventricle. With severe ischemic damage the ventricular end-diastolic volume at rest rises; ultimately, cardiac output declines, at first only during exercise and finally at rest.

CONCLUSIONS

The *isovolumetric phase indices* are most useful for measuring acute directional changes in contractility. Left ventricular dP/dt/DP_{40} is relatively simple to obtain and has the advantage over maximum dP/dt in that it is relatively independent of the time and level of arterial pressure at the instant of aortic valve opening; it is insensitive to changes in afterload but increases slightly with large changes in preload. Although V_{max}, calculated using developed pressure, is not preload- or afterload-dependent, its determination is beset by many theoretical and practical problems, and it appears to have little advantage over V_{pm}, i.e., the maximum dP/dt/P, or over dP/dt/DP_{40}.

The *ejection phase indices* (ejection fraction, fractional shortening of the ventricular circumference or a ventricular dimension, and the mean and peak velocities of circumferential fiber shortening) are responsive to acute changes in contractility and are relatively insensitive to acute changes in preload. However, unlike the isovolumetric indices, they are markedly influenced by acute alterations in afterload,[50, 103] so that they cannot be used to assess variations in contractility when acute changes in aortic pressure occur.

When a ventricle is stressed by a hemodynamic overload, at first it utilizes all of its compensatory mechanisms to maintain normal mechanical performance, and the ejection phase indices are maintained within normal limits. However, when the Frank-Starling mechanism, the development of hypertrophy, and endogenous adrenergic stimulation are all maximally utilized, ejection phase indices decline, reflecting a depression of contractility, which may occur despite maintenance of a normal cardiac output at rest.[103] As contractility continues to decline, these indices fall further, ultimately resulting in a reduction in stroke volume, a rise in ventricular filling pressure, and the clinical manifestations of heart failure (Chap. 16).

A number of invasive and noninvasive approaches are useful for separating groups of patients with normal left ventricular function from those with abnormal function. Of the isovolumetric phase indices, V_{pm} and V_{max} based on total pressure appear to be the most reliable, although considerable overlap exists between individuals in normal and abnormal groups. Ejection phase indices are capable of detecting depressed contractility in the basal state in individual patients and are clearly preferable to the isovolumetric phase indices for this purpose. End-systolic pressure-volume, stress-dimension, and stress-shortening relationships provide a useful approach to assessing basal levels of contractility in individual patients (Fig. 15–18) and in groups of patients (Fig. 15–17). Noninvasive techniques may be used for assessing left ventricular ejection phase indices and are particularly useful in serial assessments of cardiac performance in individual patients.

ASSESSMENT OF THE VENTRICULAR RESPONSE TO STRESS

Patients with impaired cardiac function characteristically have few and often no symptoms at rest but become symptomatic during exertion (Chap. 16). Similarly, the various indices of cardiac function discussed above may be normal in the basal state of patients with severe heart disease and are altered relatively late in the course. A number of approaches in which the ventricle is stressed have been used to detect mild to moderate left ventricular

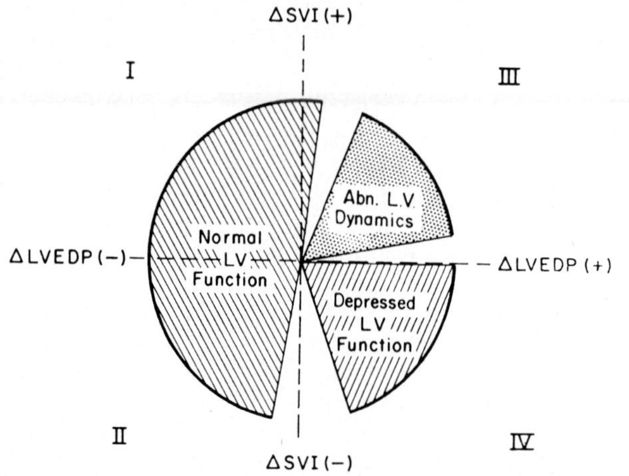

FIGURE 15–19. Patterns of left ventricular response to supine muscular exercise. Normal LV function (quadrants I and II, cross-hatched area) includes a variable change in stroke volume, usually an increase, and a fall or no change in LVEDP. Abnormal left ventricular dynamics (quadrant III, stippled area) is associated with an increase in stroke volume index (SVI) and an increase in LVEDP. Depressed LV function (quadrant IV, cross-hatched area) is characterized by no change or a fall in SVI and an increase in LVEDP. The areas between the shaded sectors include responses that cannot be definitively classified. (From Ross, J., Jr., and Braunwald, E.: Left ventricular performance during muscular exercise in patients with and without cardiac dysfunction. Circulation *34*:597, 1966, by permission of the American Heart Association, Inc.)

dysfunction, when the basal values of left ventricular pump performance are within the normal range. The stresses most commonly employed are isotonic exercise, isometric exercise, pacing, and increased afterload.

DYNAMIC EXERCISE. In the supine posture, the cardiac output normally rises by more than 6 ml/min for each milliliter of increase in oxygen consumption per minute; stroke volume and ejection fraction usually rise, and left ventricular end-diastolic pressure either remains unchanged or decreases or rises slightly. When left ventricular end-diastolic pressure rises by more than 6 mm Hg, to exceed 17 mm Hg, and stroke volume and ejection fraction either remain constant or decline,[104–106] left ventricular function may be considered to be impaired. There are various intermediate degrees of impairment between the normal response and that of the failing left ventricle (Fig. 15–19).

When upright posture is assumed, the pooling of blood below the thorax reduces end-diastolic pressure and volume, both of which may then rise during exercise in normal subjects to the levels achieved in the supine position.[107] Both end-diastolic and end-systolic volumes rise abnormally in patients with impaired left ventricular function.

It is important to recognize that the response to exercise is altered by age and physical training. In normal elderly subjects (>65 years) during upright exercise EF declines rather than increases,[108] as it does in normal young subjects (Chap. 11). It is possible that stiffening of the arterial system with age results in a greater afterload during exercise, thereby reducing the ejection fraction.[109] Although both untrained and trained healthy young subjects develop an increased EF during supine exercise, this tends to be associated with an increase in end-diastolic volume in untrained subjects and a reduction in end-systolic volume in athletes.[110] These variations must be kept in mind in interpreting the results of exercise in patients with suspected heart disease.

ISOMETRIC EXERCISE. This form of exercise—most often sustained handgrip[111]—has the advantage over dynamic exercise in that it requires minimal movement of the patient and therefore allows simultaneous recording of other variables such as the echocardiogram.[112] It is a simple, convenient test of left ventricular function. The centrally mediated increases in heart rate, arterial pressure, and cardiac output appear to be designed to maintain flow in the compressed vascular bed of skeletal muscle.[113] The normal left ventricle responds to the stress of isometric exercise with little change in or a decline in filling pressure and end-diastolic volume, but with an increase in stroke work. In contrast, the ventricle whose function is impaired displays an increase in filling pressure and end-diastolic volume but little change or an actual fall in stroke work.[114, 115]

The response of stroke volume, stroke work, and ventricular end-diastolic pressure before and during an increase in left ventricular afterload induced by the infusion of a pressure agent such as angiotensin is another useful method of evaluating the response of the left ventricle to stress.[116] The normal left ventricle responds to this stress with little change or even a small increase in stroke volume, an increase in stroke work, and a small rise in filling pressure and end-diastolic volume. However, when left ventricular contractility is impaired, filling pressure rises markedly but stroke volume falls, so that stroke work either remains constant or declines.

TACHYCARDIA. With atrial pacing in normal subjects, cardiac output and arterial pressure remain constant and stroke volume varies inversely with heart rate[117]; both end-diastolic and end-systolic volumes decline. In patients with coronary artery disease not severe enough to cause ischemia in the basal state, tachycardia may induce ischemia with impairment of wall motion in the distribution of the involved artery. If a sufficiently large area of the ventricle is involved, the left ventricular end-diastolic pressure will rise as a consequence of the ischemia-induced reduction of ventricular compliance (p. 435).

CONCLUSIONS. The left ventricular responses to the various forms of stress are useful not only in detecting mild impairment of myocardial functional reserve but also in expressing the severity of this impairment quantitatively and in studying the effects of interventions such as drugs and operation on cardiac function. Considerable effort is now under way to apply such stresses in a standardized manner by employing noninvasive techniques to evaluate the effects on ventricular performance.

CARDIOPULMONARY EXERCISE TESTING

Weber and his associates have developed a systemic approach to cardiopulmonary exercise testing which allows the noninvasive assessment of total oxygen and carbon dioxide.[118–121] Progressively increasing isotonic exercise is carried out on a treadmill or bicycle ergometer. End tidal oxygen and carbon dioxide concentrations and ventilation are measured continuously, allowing the monitoring of oxygen uptake ($\dot{V}O_2$) and carbon dioxide production ($\dot{V}CO_2$) on a breath-by-breath basis. This permits determination of (1) the maximal oxygen uptake ($\dot{V}O_{2\,max}$ or aerobic capacity), defined as the value achieved when $\dot{V}O_2$ remains stable despite an increase in the intensity of exercise (Fig. 15–20); and (2) the anaerobic threshold. The latter is reached when oxygen availability to the tissues becomes inadequate. At this point energy is generated inefficiently by anaerobic metabolism, a process producing lactate which is buffered by bicarbonate, leading to the production of carbon dioxide. This can be recognized by a rise in $\dot{V}CO_2$ which

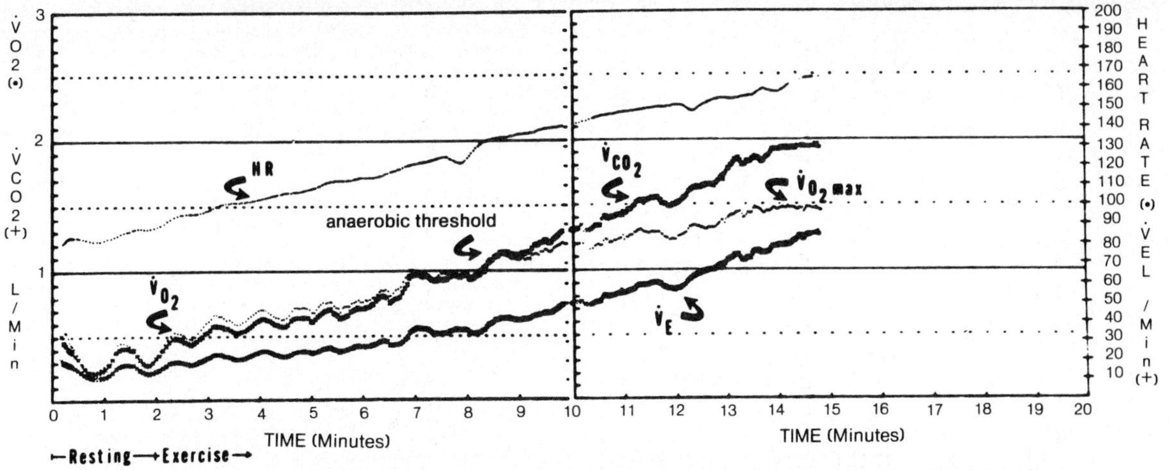

FIGURE 15–20. Breath-by-breath response in oxygen uptake (VO$_2$), carbon dioxide production (VCO$_2$) and minute ventilation ($\dot{V}_E$) to incremental (2-minute stages) treadmill exercise in a 65-year-old man with enlarged heart and mitral valve incompetence. Appearance of anaerobic metabolism is indicated by crossover in $\dot{V}O_2$ and $\dot{V}CO_2$; the corresponding $\dot{V}O_2$ is termed anaerobic threshold. Maximal oxygen uptake ($\dot{V}O_{2max}$) is achieved when $\dot{V}O_2$ fails to increase more than 1 ml/min/kg after an increment in treadmill work. Heart rate (HR) response is also shown. (From Weber, K. T., and Janicki, J. S.: Cardiopulmonary exercise testing for evaluation of chronic cardiac failure. Am. J. Cardiol. *55*:25A, 1985.)

exceeds the rise in $\dot{V}O_2$ and a rise in the respiratory quotient (R), i.e., the ratio $\dot{V}CO_2/\dot{V}O_2$. These two endpoints—the maximal oxygen uptake and the anaerobic threshold—are objective and are not limited by the subjectivity and patient and physician bias of symptom-limited exercise tests. Although both exercise capacity as reflected in treadmill time and heart rate correlate with maximal oxygen uptake, these correlations are not good enough to allow the former to serve as a substitute for the latter. The repeatability of maximal oxygen uptake and the anaerobic threshold, when measured days or weeks apart, is excellent.[120, 120a]

Normal values of maximal oxygen uptake and anaerobic threshold decline with age after 20 years and are higher in men than in women, but in any case exceed 20 and 14 ml/min/kg, respectively. Functional capacity can be categorized into five classes (A to E); impairment in group E is so severe that the patients cannot (or should not) exercise (Table 15–3).

The maximal oxygen uptake is a function of both the maximal cardiac output and the maximal extraction of oxygen by the tissues. The latter does not vary systematically in patients of various classes and generally exceeds 70 per cent at maximal oxygen uptake. Therefore $\dot{V}O_{2\ max}$ reflects the maximum cardiac output, which is a far more sensitive measurement than the resting cardiac output in discriminating among patients in different classes (Fig. 15–21A).

TABLE 15–3 FUNCTIONAL IMPAIRMENT IN AEROBIC CAPACITY AND ANAEROBIC THRESHOLD AS MEASURED DURING INCREMENTAL TREADMILL CPX

Class	Severity	$\dot{V}O_2$Max (ml/min/kg)	Anaerobic Threshold (ml/min/kg)
A	Mild to none	>20	>14
B	Mild to moderate	16 to 20	11 to 14
C	Moderate to severe	10 to 16	8 to 11
D	Severe	6 to 10	5 to 8
E	Very severe	<6	<4

From Weber, K.T., Janicki, J. S., and McElroy, P. A.: Cardiopulmonary exercise (CPX) testing. *In* Weber, K. T., and Janicki, J. S. (eds.): Cardiopulmonary Exercise Testing. Philadelphia, W. B. Saunders Company, 1986, p. 153.

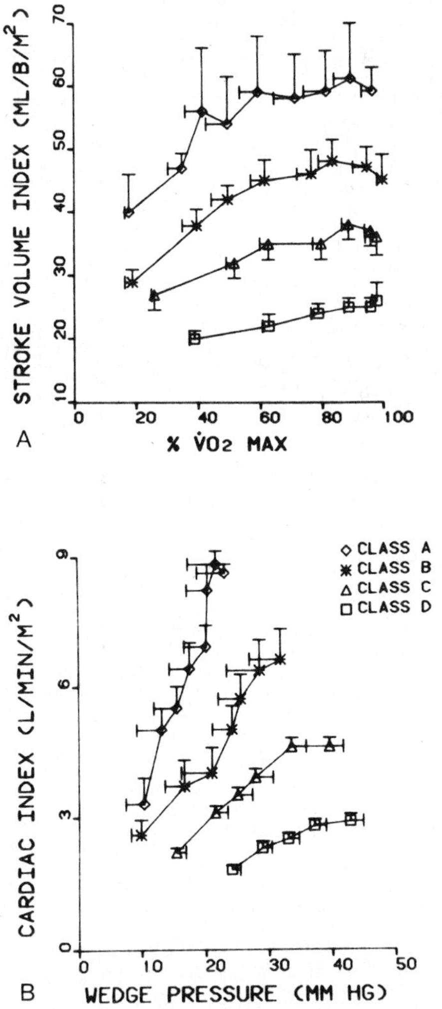

FIGURE 15–21. *A,* The cardiac output during exercise expressed as a percentage of maximal oxygen uptake ($\dot{V}O_{2max}$) for the four functional classes. *B,* Ventricular function curves, obtained during incremental treadmill exercise, while gas exchange was continuously monitored, is shown for the four functional classes of patients with chronic cardiac failure. (From Weber, K. T., and Janicki, J. S.: Cardiopulmonary exercise testing for evaluation of chronic cardiac failure. Am. J. Cardiol. *55*:22A, 1985.)

Further information concerning left ventricular function can be obtained by measuring pulmonary capillary wedge pressure together with arterial pressure, cardiac output, and gas exchange at each stage of exercise. A triple-lumen balloon flotation thermodilution catheter can be utilized conveniently to make these measurements. An inverse relationship between wedge pressure and cardiac output is observed at peak exercise as function deteriorates (Fig. 15–21*B*). The response of systolic arterial pressure to peak exercise is a function of the increment in cardiac output, rising substantially in class A and progressively less in classes B and C and remaining virtually unchanged in class D.

Cardiopulmonary exercise testing is valuable in assessing objectively exercise tolerance and functional capacity, in evaluating the possible causes of exertional dyspnea and fatigue, in determining the severity of disease, in following its progress, and in assessing the response to therapy. Obviously, impairment of pulmonary function can interfere with oxygen uptake during exertion. Therefore, in a patient with a reduced maximal oxygen uptake and clinical manifestations of lung disease, pulmonary function should be evaluated.[122]

REFERENCES

THEORETICAL CONSIDERATIONS

1. Braunwald, E.: On the difference between the heart's output and its contractile state (Editorial). Circulation *43*:171, 1971.
2. Ross, J., Jr.: Cardiac function and myocardial contractility: A perspective. J. Am. Coll. Cardiol. *1*:52, 1983.
3. Nichols, W. W., Conti, C. R., Walker, W. E., and Milnor, W. R.: Input impedance of the systemic circulation in man. Circ. Res. *40*:451, 1977.
4. Frommer, P. L., Robinson, B. F., and Braunwald, E.: Paired electrical stimulation. A comparison of the effects on performance of the failing and nonfailing heart. Am. J. Cardiol. *18*:738, 1966.
5. Starling, E. H.: Linacre Lecture on the Law of the Heart (1915). London, Longmans, 1918.
6. Sarnoff, S. J., and Mitchell, J. H.: Control of function of heart. *In* Hamilton, W. F., and Dow, P. (eds.): Handbook of Physiology. Section 2. Circulation, Vol. 1. Washington, D.C., American Physiological Society, 1962, pp. 489–532.
7. Suga, H., Sagawa, K., and Demer, L.: Determinants of instantaneous pressure in canine left ventricle: Time and volume specification. Circ. Res. *46*:256, 1980.

ASSESSMENT OF CARDIAC PERFORMANCE BASED ON PRESSURES, FLOWS, VOLUMES, AND DIMENSIONS

8. Rackley, C. E., Russell, R. O., Rogers, W. J., Mantle, J. A., McDaniel, H. G., and Papapietro, S. E.: Clinical experience with glucose-insulin-potassium therapy in acute myocardial infarction. Am. Heart J. *102*:1038, 1981.
9. Rackley, C. E.: Quantitative evaluation of left ventricular function by radiographic techniques. Circulation *54*:862, 1976.
10. Tobis, J., Nalcioglu, O., Seibert, A., Johnston, W. D., and Henry, W. L.: Measurement of left ventricular ejection fraction by videodensitometric analysis of digital subtraction angiograms. Am. J. Cardiol. 52:871, 1983.
11. Kronenberg, M. W., Price, R. R., Smith, C. W., Robertson, R. M., Perry, J. M., Pickens, D. R., Domanski, M. J., Partain, C. L., and Friesinger, G. C.: Evaluation of left ventricular performance using digital subtraction angiography. Am. J. Cardiol. *51*:837, 1983.
12. Popio, K. A., Gorlin, R., Bechtel, D., and Levine, J. A.: Postextrasystolic potentiation as a predictor of myocardial viability: Preoperative analyses compared with studies after coronary bypass surgery. Am. J. Cardiol. *39*:944, 1977.
13. Vine, D. L., Hegg, T. D., Dodge, H. T., Stewart, D. K., and Frimer, M.: Immediate effect of contrast medium injection of left ventricular volumes and ejection fraction. Circulation *56*:379, 1977.
14. Dodge, H. T., and Sheehan, F. H.: Quantitative contrast angiography for assessment of ventricular performance in heart disease. J. Am. Coll. Cardiol. *1*:73, 1983.
15. Rackley, C. E., and Hood, W. P., Jr.: Quantitative angiographic evaluation and pathophysiological mechanisms in valvular heart disease. Prog. Cardiovasc. Dis. *15*:427, 1973.
16. Fifer, M. A., and Grossman, W.: Measurement of ventricular volumes, ejection fraction, mass and wall stress. *In* Grossman, W. (ed.): Cardiac Catheterization and Angiography. 3rd ed. Philadelphia, Lea and Febiger, 1986, pp. 282–300.
17. Luisada, A. A., Singhal, A., and Portaluppi, F.: Assessment of left ventricular function by noninvasive methods. Adv. Cardiol. *32*:111, 1985.
18. Boudoulas, H., Geleris, P., Bush, C. A., Lewis, R. P., Fulkerson, P. K., Kolibash, A. J., and Weissler, A. M.: Assessment of ventricular function by combined noninvasive measures: Factors accounting for methodologic disparities. Int. J. Cardiol. *2*:493, 1983.
19. Borow, K. M., Green, L. H., Grossman, W., and Braunwald, E.: Left ventricular end-systolic stress-shortening and stress-length relations in humans: Normal values and sensitivity to inotropic state. Am. J. Cardiol. *50*:1301, 1982.
20. Tortoledo, F. A., Quinones, M. A., Fernandez, G. C., Waggoner, A. D., and Winters, W. L., Jr.: Quantification of left ventricular volumes by two-dimensional echocardiography: A simplied and accurate approach. Circulation *67*:579, 1983.
21. Reichek, N., Helak, J., Plappert, T., St. John Sutton, M., and Weber, K. T.: Anatomic validation of left ventricular mass estimates from clinical two-dimensional echocardiography: Initial results. Circulation *67*:348, 1983.
22. Borow, K. M., Come, P. C., Neumann, A., Baim, D. S., Braunwald, E., and Grossman, W.: Physiological assessment of the inotropic, vasodilator and afterload reducing effects of milrinone in subjects without cardiac disease. Am. J. Cardiol. *55*:1204, 1985.
23. McKay, R. G., Aroesty, J. M., Heller, G. V., Royal, H., Parker, J. A., Silverman, K. J., Kolodny, G. M., and Grossman, W.: Left ventricular pressure-volume diagrams and end-systolic pressure-volume relations in human beings. J. Am. Coll. Cardiol. *3*:301, 1984.
24. Kronenberg, M. W., Parrish, M. D., Jenkins, D. W., Jr, Sandler, M. P., Friesinger, G. C., James, J., and Wolfe, O. H.: Accuracy of radionuclide ventriculography for estimation of left ventricular volume changes and end-systolic pressure volume relations. J. Am. Coll. Cardiol. *6*:1064, 1985.
25. Rich, S., Chomka, E. V., Stagl, R., Shanes, J. G., Kondos, G. T., and Brundage, B. H.: Determination of left ventricular ejection fraction using ultrafast computed tomography. Am. Heart J. *112*:392, 1986.
26. Osbakken, M., and Yuschok, T.: Evaluation of ventricular function with gated cardiac magnetic resonance imaging. Catheter. Cardiovasc. Diag. *12*:156, 1986.
27. Herman, H. J., and Bartle, S. H.: Left ventricular volumes by angiocardiography: Comparison of methods and simplification of techniques. Cardiovasc. Res. *4*:404, 1968.
28. Dodge, H. T., Hay, R. E., and Sandler, H.: An angiocardiographic method for directly determining left ventricular stroke volume in man. Circ. Res. *11*:739, 1962.
29. Wynne, J., Green, L. H., Mann, T., Levin, D., and Grossman, W.: Estimation of left ventricular volumes in man from biplane cineangiograms filmed in oblique projections. Am. J. Cardiol. *41*:726, 1978.
30. Sandler, H., and Dodge, H. T.: Angiographic methods for determination of left ventricular geometry and volume. *In* Mirsky, I., Ghista, D. N., and Sandler, H. (eds.): Cardiac Mechanics: Physiological, Clinical and Mathematical Considerations. New York, John Wiley and Sons, 1974.
31. Graham, T. P., Jr., Atwood, G. F., Faulkner, S. L., and Nelson, J. H.: Right atrial volume measurements from biplane cineangiocardiography. Circulation *49*:709, 1974.
32. Dodge, H. T.: Hemodynamic aspects of cardiac failure. *In* Braunwald, E. (ed.): The Myocardium: Failure and Infarction. New York, H. P. Publishing Co., 1974, pp. 70–79.
33. Yin, F. C. P.: Ventricular wall stress. Circ. Res. *49*:829, 1981.
34. Mirsky, I.: Elastic properties of the myocardium: A quantitative approach with physiological and clinical applications. *In* Berne, R. M. (ed.): Handbook of Physiology. Section 2, The Cardiovascular System. Vol. 1, Heart. Bethesda, Md., American Physiological Society, 1979, p. 501.
35. Grossman, W., Jones, D., and McLaurin, L. P.: Wall stress and patterns of hypertrophy in the human left ventricle. J. Clin. Invest. *56*:56, 1974.
36. Peterson, K. L.: Instantaneous force-velocity-length relations of the left ventricle: Methods, limitations and applications in humans. *In* Fishman, A. P. (ed.): Heart Failure. Washington, D.C., Hemisphere Publishing Co., 1978, pp. 121–132.
37. Smith, M., Russell R. O., Jr., Feild, B. J., and Rackley, C. E.: Left ventricular compliance and abnormally contracting segments in post-myocardial infarction patients. Chest *65*:368, 1974.
38. Herman, M. V., Heinle, R. A., Klein, M. D., and Gorlin, R.: Localized disorders in myocardial contraction: Asynergy and its role in congestive heart failure. N. Engl. J. Med. *277*:222, 1967.
39. Dodge, H. T., Stewart, D. K., and Frimer, M.: Implications of shape, stress and wall dynamics in clinical heart disease. *In* Fishman, A. P. (ed.): Heart Failure. Washington, D.C., Hemisphere Publishing Co., 1978, p. 43.
40. Sheehan, F. H., Dodge, H. T., Mathey, D. G., Brown, B. G., Bolson, E. L., and Mitten, S.: Application of the centerline method: Analysis of change in regional left ventricular wall motion in serial studies. IEEE Comput. Cardiol. 1982, p. 9.
41. Sheehan, F. H., Stewart, D. K., Dodge, H. T., Mitten, S., Bolson, E. L., and Brown, B. G.: Variability in the measurement of regional left ventricular wall motion from contrast angiograms. Circulation *68*:550, 1983.
42. Fujita, M., Sasayama, S., Kawai, C., Eiho, S., and Kuwahara, M.: Automatic processing of cine ventriculograms for analysis of regional myocardial function. Circulation *63*:1065, 1981.
43. Tsakiris, A. G., Donald, D. E., Sturm, R. E., and Wood, E. H.: Volume, ejection fraction, and internal dimensions of left ventricle determined by biplane videometry. Fed. Proc. *28*:1358, 1969.
44. Marving, J., Hoilunk-Carlsen, P. F., Chraemmer-Jorgensen, B., and Gadsboll, N.: Are right and left ventricular ejection fractions equal? Ejection fractions in normal subjects and in patients with first acute myocardial infarction. Circulation 72:502, 1985.
45. Stamm, R. B., Carabello, B. A., Mayers, D. L., and Martin, R. P.: Two-

dimensional echocardiographic measurement of left ventricular ejection fraction: Prospective analysis of what constitutes an adequate determination. Am. Heart J. *104*:136, 1982.
46. Quinones, M. A., Waggoner, A. D., Reduto, L. A., Nelson, J. G., Young, J. B., Winters, W. L., Jr., Ribeiro, L. G., and Miller, R. R.: A new simplified and accurate method for determining ejection fraction with two-dimensional echocardiography. Circulation *64*:744, 1981.
47. Zimpfer, M., and Vatner, S. F.: Effects of acute increases in left ventricular preload on indices of myocardial function in conscious, unrestrained and intact, tranquilized babooons. J. Clin Invest. *67*:430, 1981.
48. Nixon, J. V., Murray, R. G., Leonard, P. D., Mitchell, J. H., and Blomqvist, C. G.: Effect of large variations in preload on left ventricular performance characteristic in normal subjects. Circulation *65*:698, 1982.
49. Braunwald, E., Goldblatt, A., Harrison, D. C., and Mason, D. T.: Studies on cardiac dimensions in intact unanesthetized man. III. Effects of muscular exercise. Circ. Res. *13*:460, 1963.
50. Quinones, M. A., Gaasch, W. H., and Alexander, J. K.: Influence of acute changes in preload, afterload, contractile state and heart rate on ejection and isovolumic indices of myocardial contractility in man. Circulation *53*:293, 1976.

VENTRICULAR END-SYSTOLIC PRESSURE-VOLUME RELATIONS

51. Grossman, W.: Evaluation of systolic and diastolic function of the myocardium. *In* Grossman, W. (ed.): Cardiac Catheterization and Angiography, 3rd ed. Philadelphia, Lea and Febiger, 1986, pp. 301–319.
52. McKay, R. G., Spears, J. R., Aroesty, J. M., Baim, D. S., Royal, H. D., Heller, G. V., Lincoln, W., Salo, R. W., Braunwald, E., and Grossman, W.: Instantaneous measurement of left and right ventricular stroke volume and pressure-volume relationships with an impedance catheter. Circulation *69*:703, 1984.
53. Kass, D. A., Yamazaki, T., Burkhoff, D., Maughan, W. L., and Sagawa, K.: Determination of left ventricular end-systolic pressure-volume relationships by the conductance (volume) catheter technique. Circulation *73*:586, 1986.
54. Grossman, W., Braunwald, E., Mann, T., McLaurin, L. P., and Green, L. H.: Contractile state of the left ventricle in man as evaluated from end-systolic pressure-volume relations. Circulation *56*:845, 1977.
55. Imperial, E. S., Levy, M. N., and Zieske, H., Jr.: Outflow resistance as an independent determinant of cardiac performance. Circ. Res. *9*:148, 1961.
56. Noble, M. I. M.: Problems concerning the application of concepts of muscle mechanics to the determination of contractile state of the heart. Circulation *45*:252, 1972.
57. Downing, S. E., and Sonnenblick, E. H.: Cardiac muscle mechanics and ventricular performance. Force and time parameters. Am. J. Physiol. *207*:705, 1964.
58. Suga, H., Katabatake, A., and Sagawa, K.: End-systolic pressure determines stroke volume from fixed end-diastolic volume in the isolated canine left ventricle under a constant contractile state. Circ. Res. *44*:238, 1979.
59. Weber, K. T., and Janicki, J. S.: Muscle-pump function of the intact heart. *In* Fishman, A. P. (ed.): Heart Failure. Washington, D. C., Hemisphere Publishing Co., 1978, pp. 29–42.
60. Mahler, F., Covell, J. W., and Ross, J., Jr.: Systolic pressure-diameter relations in the normal conscious dog. Cardiovasc. Res. *9*:447, 1975.
61. Pouleur, H., Rousseau, M. F., van Eyll, C., van Mechelen, H., Brasseur, L. A., and Charlier, A. A.: Assessment of left ventricular contractility from late systolic stress-volume relations. Circulation *65*:1204, 1982.
62. Sunagawa, K., Maughan, W. L., and Sagawa, K.: Effect of regional ischemia on the left ventricular end-systolic pressure-volume relationship of isolated canine hearts. Circ. Res. *52*:170, 1983.
63. Carabello, B. A., and Spann, J. F.: The uses and limitations of end-systolic indexes of left ventricular function. Circulation *69*:1058, 1984.
64. Carabello, B. A., Nolan, S. P., and McGuire, L. B.: Assessment of preoperative left ventricular function in patients with mitral regurgitation: Value of the end-systolic wall stress–end-systolic volume ratio. Circulation *64*:1212, 1981.
65. Reichek, N., Wilson, J., Sutton, M. St.J., Plappert, T. A., Goldberg, S., and Hirshfeld, J. W.: Noninvasive determination of left ventricular end-systolic stress: Validation of the method and initial application. Circulation *65*:99, 1982.
66. Sagawa, K.: The end-systolic pressure-volume relation of the ventricle: Definition, modifications and clinical use (Editorial). Circulation *63*:1223, 1981.
67. Borow, K. M., Green, L. H., Grossman, W., and Braunwald, E.: Left ventricular end-systolic stress-shortening and stress-length relations in humans. Am. J. Cardiol. *50*:1301, 1982.
67a. Colan, S. D., Borow, K. M., and Neumann, A.: Left ventricular end-systolic wall stress-velocity of fiber shortening relation: A load independent index of myocardial contractility. J. Am. Coll. Cardiol. *4*:715, 1984.
68. Fifer, M. A., and Braunwald, E.: End-systolic pressure-volume and stress-length relations in the assessment of ventricular function in man. Adv. Cardiol. *32*:36, 1985.
69. Takahashi, M., Sasayama, S., Kawai, C., and Kotoura, H.: Contractile performance of the hypertrophied ventricle in patients with systemic hypertension. Circulation *62*:116, 1980.
70. Watkins, J., Slutsky, R., Tubau, J., and Karliner, J.: Scintigraphic study of relation between left ventricular peak systolic presure and end-systolic volume in patients with coronary artery disease and normal subjects. Br. Heart J. *48*:39, 1982.
71. Iskandrian, A. S., Hakki, A-H., Bemmis, C. E., Kane, S. A., Boston, B., and Amenta, A.: Left ventricular end-systolic pressure-volume relation. A combined radionuclide and hemodynamic study. Am. J. Cardiol. *51*:1057, 1983.
72. Anderson, K., and Vik-Mo, H.: Increased left ventricular emptying at maximal exercise after reduction in afterload. Circulation *69*:492, 1984.
73. Magorien, D. J., Shaffer, P., Bush, C. A., Magorien, R. D., Kolibash, A. J., Leier, C. V., and Bashore, T. M.: Assessment of left ventricular pressure-volume relations using gated radionuclide angiography, echocardiography, and micromanometer pressure recordings. A new method for serial measurements of systolic and diastolic function in man. Circulation *67*:844, 1983.

VENTRICULAR dP/dt

74. Gleason, W. L., and Braunwald, E.: Studies on the first derivative of the ventricular pressure pulse in man. J. Clin. Invest. *41*:80, 1962.
75. Mason, D. T.: Usefulness and limitations of the rate of rise of intraventricular pressure (dP/dt) in the evaluation of myocardial contractility in man. Am. J. Cardiol. *23*:516, 1969.
76. Fry, D. L., Noble, F. W., and Mallos, A. J.: An evaluation of modern pressure recording systems. Circ. Res. *5*:40, 1957.
77. Wallace, A. G., Skinner, N. S., Jr., and Mitchell, J. H.: Hemodynamic determinants of the maximal rate of left ventricular pressure. Am. J. Physiol. *205*:30, 1963.
78. Furnival, C. M., Linden, R. J., and Snow, H. M.: Inotropic changes in the left ventricle: The effect of changes in heart rate, aortic pressure and end-diastolic pressure. J. Physiol. (Lond.) *211*:359, 1970.
78a. Fifer, M. A., Gunther, S., Grossman, W., Mirsky, I. Carabello, B., and Barry, W. H.: Myocardial contractile function in aortic stenosis as determined from the rate of stress development during isovolumic stress. Am. J. Cardiol. *44*:1318, 1979.
79. Ross, J., Jr., and Sobel, B. E.: Regulation of cardiac contraction. Ann. Rev. Physiol. *34*:47, 1972.
80. Burns, J. W., Covell, J. W., and Ross, J., Jr.: Mechanics of isotonic left ventricular contractions. Am. J. Physiol. *224*:725, 1973.
81. Hugenholtz, P. G., Ellison, R. C., Urschel, C. W., Mirsky, I., and Sonnenblick, E. H.: Myocardial force-velocity relationships in clinical heart disease. Circulation *41*:191, 1970.
82. Mirsky, I., and Parmley, W. W.: Force-velocity studies in isolated and intact heart muscle. *In* Mirsky, I., Ghista, D. N., and Sandler, H. (eds.): Cardiac Mechanics: Physiological, Clinical and Mathematical Considerations. New York, John Wiley and Sons, 1974, pp. 87–112.
83. Wolk, M. J., Keefe, J. F., Bing, O. H. L., Finkelstein, L. J., and Levine, H. J.: Estimation of V_{max} in auxotonic systoles from the rate of relative increase of isovolumic pressures: (dP/dt)dP. J. Clin. Invest. *50*:1276, 1971.
84. Grossman, W., Haynes, F., Paraskos, J. A., Saltz, S., Dalen, J. E., and Dexter, L.: Alterations in preload and myocardial mechanics in the dog and in man. Circ. Res. *31*:83, 1972.
85. Van Den Box, G. C., Elzinga, G., Westerhof, N., and Noble, M. I. M.: Problems in the use of indices of myocardial contractility. Cardiovasc. Res. *7*:834, 1973.
86. Mason, D. T., Braunwald, E., Covell, J. W., Sonnenblick, E. H., and Ross, J., Jr.: Assessment of cardiac contractility: The relation between the rate of pressure rise and ventricular pressure during isovolumic systole. Circulation *44*:47, 1971.
87. Davidson, D. M., Covell, J. W., Malloch, C. I., and Ross, J., Jr.: Factors influencing indices of left ventricular contractility in the conscious dog. Cardiovasc. Res. *8*:299, 1974.
88. Mehmel, H., Krayenbuehl, H. P., and Rutishauser, W.: Peak measured velocity of shortening in the canine left ventricle. J. Appl. Physiol. *29*:637, 1970.
89. Braunwald, E., and Ross, J., Jr.: The ventricular end-diastolic pressure. An appraisal of its value in the recognition of ventricular failure in man (Editorial). Am. J. Med. *34*:147, 1963.
90. Mahler, F., Covell, J. W., O'Rourke, R. A., and Ross, J., Jr.: Effects of acute changes in loading and inotropic state on left ventricular performance and contractility measures in the conscious dog. Am. J. Cardiol. *35*:626, 1975.
90a. Lambert, C. R., Jr., Nichols, W. W., and Pepine, C. J.: Indices of ventricular contractile state: Comparative sensitivity and specificity. Am. Heart J. *106*:136, 1983.
91. Peterson, K. L., Sklovan, D., Ludbrook, P., Uther, J. B., and Ross, J., Jr.: Comparison of isovolumic and ejection phase indices of myocardial performance in man. Circulation *49*:1088, 1974.
92. Karliner, J. S., Gault, J. H., Eckberg, D. L., Mullins, C. B., and Ross, J., Jr.: Mean velocity of fiber shortening: A simplified measure of left ventricular myocardial contractility. Circulation *44*:323, 1971.
93. Gould, K. L.: Analysis of wall dynamics and directional components of left ventricular contraction in man. Am. J. Cardiol. *38*:322, 1976.
94. Ross, J., Jr., and McCullagh, W. H.: The nature of enhanced performance of the dilated left ventricle during chronic volume overloading. Circ. Res. *30*:549, 1972.
95. Sasayama, S., Theroux, P., Romero, M., Bishop, S., Bloor, C., Franklin, D., and Ross, J., Jr.: Adaptations of the left ventricle to chronic pressure overload. Am. J. Cardiol. *35*:167, 1975.
96. Carabello, B. A., Mee, R., Collins, J. J., Jr., Kloner, R. A., Levin, D., and Grossman, W.: Contractile function in chronic gradually developing subcoronary aortic stenosis. Am. J. Physiol. *240*:H80, 1981.
96a. Borow, K. M., Propper, R., Bierman, F. Z., Grady, S., and Inati, A.: The left ventricular end-systolic pressure-dimension relation in patients with thalassemia major. Circulation *66*:980, 1982.
96b. Borow, K. M., Henderson, I. C., Neumann, A., Colan, S., Grady, S., Papish, S., and Goorin, A.: Assessment of left ventricular contractility in patients receiving doxorubicin. Ann. Intern. Med. *99*:750, 1983.

97. Gault, J. H., Covell, J. W., Braunwald, E., and Ross, J., Jr.: Left ventricular performance following correction of the free aortic regurgitation. Circulation *42*:773, 1970.
98. Carabello, B. A., Green, L. H., Grossman, W., Cohn, L. H., Koster, J. K., and Collins, J. J., Jr.: Hemodynamic determinants of prognosis of aortic valve replacement in critical aortic stenosis and advanced congestive heart failure. Circulation *62*:42, 1980.
99. Urschel, C. W., Covell, J. W., Sonnenblick, E. H., Ross, J., Jr., and Braunwald, E.: Myocardial mechanics in aortic and mitral valvular regurgitation: The concept of instantaneous impedance as a determinant of the performance of the intact heart. J. Clin. Invest. *47*:867, 1968.
100. Ross, J., Jr.: Left ventricular function and the timing of surgical treatment in valvular heart disease. Ann. Intern. Med. *94*:498, 1981.
101. McDonald, I. G.: Echocardiographic assessment of left ventricular function in mitral valve disease. Circulation *53*:865, 1976.
102. Schuler, G., Peterson, K. L., Johnson, A., Francis, G., Dennosh, G., Utley, J., Daily, P., Ashburn, W., and Ross, J., Jr.: Temporal response of left ventricular performance to mitral valve surgery. Circulation *59*:1218, 1979.

ASSESSMENT OF THE VENTRICULAR RESPONSE TO STRESS

103. Ross, J., Jr.: Afterload mismatch and preload reserve: A conceptual framework for the analysis of ventricular function. Prog. Cardiovasc. Dis. *18*:255, 1976.
104. Ross, J., Jr., Gault, J. H., Mason, D. T., Linhart, J. W., and Braunwald, E.: Left ventricular performance during muscular exercise in patients with and without cardiac dysfunction. Circulation *34*:597, 1966.
105. Gelberg, H. J., Rubin, S. A., Ports, T. A., Brundage, B. H., Parmley, W. W., and Chatterjee, K.: Detection of left ventricular functional reserve by supine exercise hemodynamics in patients with severe, chronic heart failure. Am. J. Cardiol. *44*:1062, 1979.
106. Boucher, C. A., Wilson, R. A., Kanarek, D. J., Hutter, A. M., Jr., Okada, R. D., Libethson, R. R., Strauss, H. W., and Pohost, G. M.: Exercise testing in asymptomatic or minimally symptomatic aortic regurgitation: Relationship of left ventricular ejection fraction to left ventricular filling pressure during exercise. Circulation *67*:1091, 1983.
107. Upton, M. T., Rerych, S. K., Roeback, J. R., Jr., Newman, G. E., Douglas, J. M., Jr., Wallace, A. G., and Jones, R. H.: Effect of brief and prolonged exercise on left ventricular function. Am. J. Cardiol. *45*:1154, 1980.
108. Port, S., Cobb, F. R., Coleman, R. E., and Jones, R. H.: Effect of age on the response of the left ventricular ejection fraction to exercise. N. Engl. J. Med. *303*:1133, 1980.
109. Yin, F. C. P., Weisfeldt, M. L., and Milnor, W. R.: Role of aortic input impedance in the decreased cardiovascular response to exercise with aging in dogs. J. Clin. Invest. *68*:28, 1981.
110. Bar-Shlomo, B.-Z., Druck, M. N., Morch, J. E., Jablonsky, G., Hilton, J. D., Feiglin, D. H. I., and McLaughlin, P. R.: Left ventricular function in trained and untrained healthy subjects. Circulation *65*:484, 1982.
111. Donald, K. W., Lind, A., McNicol, G. W., Humphreys, P. W., Taylor, S. H., and Staunton, H. P.: Cardiovascular responses to sustained (static) contractions. Circ. Res. *21*(Suppl. 1):15, 1967.
112. Corya, B. C., and Rasmussen, S.: Assessing left ventricular function with intervention echocardiography. J. Cardiovasc. Med. *6*:574, 1981.
113. Awan, N., Vismara, L. N., Miller, R. R., DeMaria, A. N., and Mason, D. T.: Effects of isometric exercise and increased arterial impedance on left ventricular function in severe aortic valvular stenosis. Br. Heart J. *39*:651, 1977.
114. Helfant, R. H., deVilla, M., and Meister, S. G.: Effect of sustained isometric handgrip exercise on left ventricular performance. Circulation *44*:982, 1971.
115. Kivowitz, C., Parmley, W. W., Donoso, R., Marcus, H., Ganz, W., and Swan, H. J. C.: Effects of isometric exercise on left cardiac performance: The grip test. Circulation *44*:994, 1971.
116. Ross, J., Jr., and Braunwald, E.: A study of left ventricular function in man by increasing resistance to ventricular ejection with angiotensin. Circulation *29*:739, 1964.
117. Parker, J. D.: Atrial pacing: Pacing ventricular function curves. *In* Grossman, W. (ed.): Cardiac Catheterization and Angiography. 2nd ed. Philadelphia, Lea and Febiger, 1980, pp. 223–231.
118. Weber, K. T., and Janicki, J. S.: Lactate production during maximal and submaximal exercise in patients with chronic heart failure. J. Am. Coll. Cardiol. *6*:717, 1985.
119. Wilson, J. R., Ferraro, N., and Weber, K. T.: Respiratory gas analysis during exercise as a noninvasive measure of lactate concentration in chronic congestive heart failure. Am. J. Cardiol. *51*:1639, 1983.
120. Weber, K. T., and Janicki, J. S.: Cardiopulmonary exercise testing. Philadelphia, W. B. Saunders Company, 1986, 378 pp.
120a. Hansen, J. E., Sue, D. Y., Oren, A., and Wasserman, K.: Relation of oxygen uptake to work rate in normal men and men with circulatory disorders. Am. J. Cardiol. *59*:669, 1987.
121. Matsumura, N., Nishijima, H., Kojima, S., Hashimoto, F., Minami, M., and Yasuda, H.: Determination of anaerobic threshold for assessment of functional state in patients with chronic heart failure. Circulation *68*:360, 1983.
122. Franciosa, J. A., Baker, B. J., and Seth, L.: Pulmonary versus systemic hemodynamics in determining exercise capacity of patients with chronic left ventricular failure. Am. Heart J. *110*:807, 1985.

16 CLINICAL MANIFESTATIONS OF HEART FAILURE

by EUGENE BRAUNWALD, M.D.

> It is impossible thoughtfully to survey, in the light of early experience, the field of medical work covering diseases of the heart without realizing the central problem to be failure of the heart to accomplish its work in lesser or greater degree. . . . The very essence of cardiovascular practice is recognition of early heart failure and discrimination between different grades of failure. . . . When a patient seeks advice and heart disease is suspected, or is known to be present, two questions are of chief importance. Firstly, has the heart the capacity to do the work demanded of it when the body is at rest? Secondly, what is the condition of the heart's reserve? These questions can be correctly answered in almost all cases by simple interrogations and by bedside signs.

In this, the opening paragraph of his classic text *Diseases of the Heart*, published in 1933, Sir Thomas Lewis identified the diagnosis and assessment of heart failure as the cardinal problem in clinical cardiology.[1] Now, more than a half century later, the situation has changed little, in that a principal complication of virtually all forms of heart disease is heart failure, defined as the pathophysiological state in which an abnormality of cardiac function is responsible for the failure of the heart to pump blood at a rate commensurate with the requirements of the metabolizing tissues and/or to be able to do so only from an elevated filling pressure (p. 426). Included in this definition is a wide spectrum of clinicophysiological states, ranging from the rapid impairment of pumping function, occurring when a massive myocardial infarction or tachyarrhythmia or bradyarrhythmia develops suddenly, to the gradual impairment of myocardial function, observed only during stress and occurring in a patient whose heart sustains a pressure or volume overload for a prolonged period.[2]

The clinical manifestations of heart failure vary enormously and depend on a variety of factors, including the age of the patient, the extent and rate at which cardiac performance becomes impaired, the etiology of the heart disease, the precipitating causes of heart failure, and the specific ventricle initially involved in the disease process.[3–5] It must also be emphasized that there is a broad spectrum of severity of impairment of cardiac function, ranging from the mildest, which is manifest clinically only during marked stress, to the most advanced form, in which cardiac pump function is unable to sustain life without external support.

FORMS OF HEART FAILURE

FORWARD VS. BACKWARD HEART FAILURE

The clinical manifestations of heart failure arise as a consequence of inadequate cardiac output and/or damming up of blood behind one or both ventricles. These two principal mechanisms are the basis of the so-called forward and backward pressure theories of heart failure. The *backward failure hypothesis*, first proposed in 1832 by James Hope, indicates that when the ventricle fails to discharge its contents, blood accumulates and pressure rises in the atrium and the venous system emptying into it.[6] There is substantial physiological evidence in favor of this theory. As discussed on page 428, the inability of cardiac muscle to shorten against a load alters the relationship between ventricular end-systolic pressure and volume, so that residual volume rises. The following sequence of adaptations then occurs that at first tends to maintain normal cardiac output: (1) Ventricular end-diastolic volume and pressure increase; (2) the volume and pressure rise in the atrium behind the failing ventricle; (3) the atrium contracts more vigorously (a manifestation of Starling's Law, operating on the atrium)[7]; (4) the pressure in the venous and capillary beds behind (upstream to) the failing ventricle rises; and (5) transudation of fluid from the capillary bed into the interstitial space (pulmonary or systemic) increases. Many of the symptoms characteristic of heart failure can be traced to this sequence of events and the resultant increase in fluid in the interstitial spaces of the lungs, liver, subcutaneous tissues, and serous cavities.

Cardiac output in the basal state is a relatively *insensitive* index of cardiac function (p. 449). In many patients the entire sequence of events outlined above may transpire while cardiac output *at rest* is still within normal limits. Indeed, the backward pressure theory of heart failure reflects one of the principal compensatory mechanisms in heart failure, i.e., the operation of Starling's Law of the Heart,[8] in which distention of the ventricle helps to maintain cardiac output. The failing ventricle operates on an ascending, albeit depressed and flattened, function curve[9] (Fig. 15–1, p. 450), and the augmented ventricular end-diastolic volume and pressure characteristic of heart failure must be regarded as aiding in the maintenance of cardiac output. When this compensatory mechanism is interfered with (e.g., by means of dietary sodium restriction and treatment with diuretics), the patient may be less symptomatic owing to loss of extracellular fluid volume, with its accompanying reduction in congestion of the lungs, liver, and lower extremities, but at the same time cardiac output may decline,[10] and the symptoms secondary to a reduction of cardiac output may actually intensify. Thus, although many of the clinical manifestations of heart failure are secondary to excessive retention of extracellular fluid, the elevation of ventricular preload associated with this excess fluid constitutes an important compensatory mechanism.

"BACKWARD" FAILURE. Hope's backward pressure theory of cardiac failure incorporates the concept that the cardiac chambers may fail independently and that an imbalance in performance of the ventricles may result. If one considers, for simplicity, the development of left ventricular failure consequent to aortic stenosis or of right ventricular failure secondary to pulmonic stenosis, the initial clinical manifestations of each relate primarily to the damming up of blood behind the affected ventricle. An important extension of the backward failure theory is the sequential development of right ventricular failure as a consequence of left ventricular failure. According to this concept, the elevation of left ventricular diastolic, left atrial, and pulmonary venous pressures results in backward transmission of pressure and leads to pulmonary hypertension, which ultimately causes right ventricular failure. Often, pulmonary vasoconstriction plays a part in this form of pulmonary hypertension as well (p. 797).

"FORWARD" FAILURE. Eighty years after publication of Hope's work, Mackenzie proposed the *forward failure hypothesis*, which relates clinical manifestations of heart failure to inadequate delivery of blood into the arterial system.[11] According to this hypothesis, the principal clinical manifestations of heart failure are due to reduced cardiac output, which results in diminished perfusion of vital organs, including the brain, leading to mental confusion; skeletal muscles, leading to weakness; and kidneys, leading to sodium and water retention through a series of complex mechanisms (Chap. 59). This renal effect, in turn, augments extracellular fluid volume and ultimately leads to symptoms of heart failure which are caused by congestion of organs and tissues. The heart then fails "as a whole," since there can be no imbalance between the output of the two ventricles in the steady state.

Although these two seemingly opposing views concerning the pathogenesis of heart failure led to lively controversy during the first half of this century, it no longer seems fruitful to make a rigid distinction between backward and forward heart failure, since *both* mechanisms appear to operate in the majority of patients with *chronic* heart failure. Exceptions may occur, however, and some patients, particularly those with *acute* decompensation, develop relatively pure forms of forward or backward failure. An example of relatively pure forward failure occurs in the patient with acute right ventricular failure secondary to massive pulmonary embolism in whom shock—perhaps even death—owing to inadequate cardiac output may ensue within minutes or hours. Although right ventricular diastolic pressure and volume and right atrial and systemic venous pressure all rise markedly, the patient may succumb before sufficient extracellular fluid has accumulated to produce symptoms of systemic venous congestion. This presentation may be contrasted with that of the patient who develops chronic cor pulmonale as a result of multiple pulmonary emboli with organization and gradually rising pressures in the pulmonary artery, right side of the heart, and systemic venous bed. Cardiac output and perfusion of the renal bed may be normal, at least in the resting state, but abnormal retention of extracellular fluid volume, with congestive hepatomegaly, ankle edema, and ascites, may occur. Such a patient manifests relatively pure backward failure.

Similar considerations apply to disorders affecting the left ventricle. For instance, a massive myocardial infarction may result in either (1) forward failure with a marked reduction of left ventricular output and cardiogenic shock (p. 572) and clinical manifestations secondary to impaired perfusion (hypotension, mental confusion, oliguria, and so on) or (2) backward failure with a transient inequality of output between the two ventricles, resulting in acute pulmonary edema. More commonly, patients with large myocardial infarctions develop a combination of forward and backward failure, with symptoms resulting from both inadequate cardiac output and pulmonary congestion. Early in the course of acute myocardial infarction, patients might succumb to these forms of heart failure long before renal retention of salt and water can occur. However, if the patient survives the acute insult, expansion of the extracellular fluid volume and manifestations resulting therefrom usually occur.

The relative importance of forward and backward failure in the genesis of the clinical manifestations of heart failure also depends on the specific anatomical abnormality. For instance, in conditions in which the filling of the right side of the heart is interfered with, such as tricuspid stenosis or constrictive pericarditis, systemic venous pressure is markedly elevated; one can readily appreciate how this leads to capillary transudation, hepatomegaly, edema, and ascites (i.e., to backward heart failure). Patients with chronic left ventricular failure secondary to coronary artery disease or hypertension may exhibit marked accumulation of sodium and water in the systemic venous bed with no or only minimal elevation of systemic venous pressure. In such patients, accumulation of fluid is largely due to impairment of renal perfusion (i.e., forward heart failure accompanied by excessive renal tubular sodium reabsorption).

There is general agreement that fluid retention in heart failure (Fig. 59–2, p. 1829) is due in part to reduction in glomerular filtration rate and in part to activation of the renin-angiotensin-aldosterone system.[12] Reduced cardiac output is associated with a lowered glomerular filtration rate and an increased elaboration of renin, which, through the activation of angiotensin, results in the release of aldosterone. The combination of impaired hepatic function owing to hepatic venous congestion, and reduced hepatic blood flow interferes with the metabolism of aldosterone,[13] further raising its plasma concentration and augmenting the retention of sodium and water.

As already noted, cardiac output (and glomerular filtration rate) may be normal in many patients with heart failure, particularly when they are at rest. However, during stress, such as physical exercise and fever, the cardiac output fails to rise normally, the glomerular filtration rate declines, and the renal mechanisms for salt and water retention described above come into play. In addition, ventricular filling pressure, and therefore pressures in the atrium and systemic veins behind (upstream to) the ventricle, may be normal at rest, only to rise abnormally during the stress, causing transudation and symptoms of tissue congestion (pulmonary in the case of the left ventricle and systemic in the case of the right) during exercise. For this reason simple rest may induce a diuresis and relieve symptoms in many patients with mild heart failure.

RIGHT-SIDED VS. LEFT-SIDED HEART FAILURE

Implicit in the backward failure theory is the idea that fluid localizes behind the specific cardiac chamber that is *initially* affected. Thus, symptoms secondary to pulmonary congestion initially predominate in patients with left ventricular infarction, hypertension, and aortic and mitral valve disease, i.e., they manifest *left heart failure*. With time, however, fluid accumulation becomes generalized, and ankle edema, congestive hepatomegaly, ascites, and pleural effusion occur (i.e., the patients later exhibit *right heart failure* as well). Less commonly, prolonged right ventricular failure with massive accumulation of extracellular fluid may be associated with dyspnea, particularly when the patient is in the supine position and when large pleural effusions are present.

Although a disturbance of contractile function initially takes place in the ventricle subjected to the abnormal burden, with the passage of time the other ventricle undergoes changes as well. For example, the depletion of norepinephrine that occurs in experimental animals subjected to ventricular pressure overload is not confined to the stressed ventricle, but also involves the opposite ventricle.[14] Similarly, alterations in the activity of actomyosin ATPase have been described in both ventricles of animals in which the hemodynamic burden was placed on only one.[15] These findings are not surprising when one considers that both ventricles share a common wall—the interventricular septum—and that the muscle bundles constituting the ventricles are continuous. In addition, all four cardiac chambers are enclosed within and share space within the pericardial sac. As a consequence, when the cardiac expansion is limited by the pericardium, as occurs in pericardial constriction, with large pericardial effusions, or even with a normal pericardium when the size of one side of the heart suddenly increases (e.g., the left ventricle and atrium in acute severe aortic regurgitation), the opposite chambers are compressed, and the filling pressure of the normal ventricle rises. This condition is called *ventricular interdependence*. Therefore, specific lesions that place an abnormal load on only one ventricle may eventually be responsible for failure of the heart as a whole.

ACUTE VS. CHRONIC HEART FAILURE

As already noted, the clinical manifestations of heart failure depend importantly on the rate at which the syndrome develops and specifically on whether sufficient time has elapsed for compensatory mechanisms to become operative and for fluid to accumulate in the interstitial space. For example, when a previously normal person suddenly develops a serious anatomical or functional abnormality of the heart (such as massive myocardial infarction, heart block with a very slow ventricular rate [<35/min], a tachyarrhythmia with a very rapid rate [>180/min], rupture of a valve secondary to infective endocarditis, or occlusion of a large segment of the pulmonary vascular bed by a pulmonary embolus), either a marked, sudden reduction in cardiac output with symptoms due to inadequate organ perfusion and/or acute congestion of the venous bed behind the affected ventricle will occur. If the same anatomical abnormality develops gradually, or if a patient survives the acute insult, a host of compensatory mechanisms develop, especially cardiac hypertrophy, and these allow the patient to adjust to and tolerate not only the anatomical abnormality, but also a reduction in cardiac output, with less difficulty. Frequently, the important clinical manifestations of chronic heart failure secondary to tissue congestion may be suppressed by dietary sodium restriction and diuretics. Cardiac function may not have been improved, and such patients still are in "heart failure," albeit with fewer clinical manifestations thereof. Under these circumstances, an acute event such as an infection, an arrhythmia, or discontinuation of therapy may precipitate manifestations of acute heart failure.

LOW-OUTPUT VS. HIGH-OUTPUT HEART FAILURE

Low cardiac output at rest, or in milder cases only during exertion and other stresses, characterizes heart failure occurring in most forms of heart disease (i.e., congenital, valvular, rheumatic, hypertensive, coronary, and cardiomyopathic). A variety of high-output states, including thyrotoxicosis, arteriovenous fistulas, beriberi, Paget's disease of bone, anemia, and pregnancy (described in detail in Chap. 25), may lead to heart failure as well. Low-output heart failure is characterized by clinical evidence of impairment of the peripheral circulation, with systemic vasoconstriction and cold, pale, and sometimes cyanotic extremities; in advanced forms of low-output failure, as the stroke volume declines, the pulse pressure narrows. In contrast, in high-output heart failure the extremities are usually warm and flushed, and the pulse pressure is widened or at least normal. The ability of the heart to deliver the quantity of oxygen required by the metabolizing tissues is reflected in the arterial–mixed venous oxygen difference, which is abnormally widened (i.e., >5.0 ml/liter in the resting state) in patients with low-output heart failure but is normal or even reduced in high-output states, owing to elevation of the mixed venous oxygen saturation by the admixture of blood that has been shunted away from metabolizing tissues. However, regardless of the absolute level of the arterial–mixed venous oxygen (high in low-output heart failure and normal or low in high-output heart failure) in the presence of heart failure, this difference still exceeds the level that existed *before* the development of heart failure, and cardiac output, regardless of its absolute level, is lower than it had been before the development of heart failure.

SYSTOLIC VS. DIASTOLIC HEART FAILURE

Implicit in the definition of heart failure (inability to pump an adequate volume of blood and/or to do so only from an abnormally elevated filling pressure) is that heart failure can be caused by an abnormality in systolic contraction, an inability to expel sufficient blood (i.e., *systolic heart failure*), or an abnormality in diastolic filling (i.e., *diastolic heart failure*). The former is the more familiar, classic heart failure in which an impaired inotropic state is responsible for the sequence known as heart failure, described above. Less familiar, but perhaps as important, is diastolic heart failure, in which the ability of the ventricle(s) to accept blood is impaired. This may be due to slowed or incomplete ventricular relaxation which may be transient, as occurs in acute ischemia, or sustained, as noted in concentric myocardial hypertrophy or restrictive cardiomyopathy secondary to infiltrative conditions such as amyloidosis (p. 1431). The principal clinical manifestations of systolic failure result from an inadequate forward cardiac output, while the major consequences of diastolic failure relate to elevation of the ventricular filling pressure and the high venous pressure upstream to the ventricle, causing pulmonic and/or systemic congestion.

There are many examples of pure systolic or diastolic heart failure. Examples of the former are patients with acute massive pulmonary embolism or dilated cardiomyopathy, while examples of the latter are patients with hypertrophic cardiomyopathy or subendocardial fibrosis. However, in many patients systolic and diastolic heart failure coexist. Perhaps the most common form of heart failure, that caused by coronary atherosclerosis, is an example of combined systolic and diastolic failure. Systolic failure is caused by both the chronic loss of contracting myocardium secondary to myocardial necrosis resulting from previous infarction as well as the acute loss of myocardial contractility induced by a transient episode of ischemia. Diastolic failure is due to the ventricle's reduced compliance caused by replacement of normal, distensible myocardium with nondistensible fibrous scar tissue and by the acute reduction of diastolic distensibility of reversibly injured myocardium during a transient episode of ischemia.

HEART FAILURE IN THE NEONATE AND INFANT

Heart failure in the neonate or infant has a different clinical expression from that in the older child or adult[16] (Table 30–3, p. 903). Feeding difficulties, failure to gain weight and grow, tachypnea, and excessive diaphoresis are manifestations of heart failure occurring in the first year of life. Obstruction of the airways because of enlargement of the left atrium and main pulmonary artery may result in either emphysematous expansion of the left lung or, in severer cases, atelectasis. Excessive sweating and repeated pulmonary infections are common features of heart failure in infants. Interstitial pulmonary edema causes a reduction in tidal volume; this in turn causes tachypnea, which contributes to the tachycardia. Respiratory distress is manifested by flaring of the alae nasi, grunting, and retraction of the ribs, features seldom seen in adults. Peripheral perfusion is poor, with cool limbs and delayed capillary filling. Hepatomegaly is a common manifestation of both left and right heart failure in infants, as is a paradoxical pulse secondary to wide variations in ventricular filling as a consequence of marked swings in intrapulmonary pressure. Peripheral edema, ascites, and pulsus alternans occur far less frequently in infants than in older children or adults with heart failure. On the other hand, facial edema, an uncommon finding in adults, is more common than peripheral edema in infants.

Because of the short neck of infants, distention of the jugular veins is difficult to detect. However, prominence of the veins on the back of the hand may be a valuable sign of systemic venous congestion. Although most neonates and infants (as well as adults) with cardiac failure have heart disease that is obvious on clinical examination, sometimes it is difficult to distinguish respiratory distress arising from cardiac disease from that associated with primary pulmonary disorders. Specifically, heart failure may be confused with bronchiolitis, asthma, or pneumonia. The presence of cyanosis and heart murmurs on physical examination and of cardiomegaly and pulmonary congestion on radiological examination are helpful although not decisive signs in the differential diagnosis. The differentiation of primary cardiac and pulmonary disease is discussed in Chap. 61.

CAUSES OF HEART FAILURE

From a clinical viewpoint, it is useful to classify the causes of heart failure into three categories: (1) *underlying causes*, comprising the structural abnormalities—congenital or acquired—that affect the peripheral and coronary vessels, pericardium, myocardium, or cardiac valves and lead to the increased hemodynamic burden or myocardial or coronary insufficiency responsible for heart failure; (2) *fundamental causes*, comprising the biochemical and physiological mechanisms through which either an increased hemodynamic burden or a reduction in oxygen delivery to the myocardium results in impairment of myocardial contraction (Chap. 14); and (3) *precipitating causes*, comprising the specific causes or incidents that precipitate heart failure in approximately 50 per cent of episodes of clinical heart failure.[17]

It is helpful to recognize both the underlying and the precipitating causes of heart failure. Appropriate management of the underlying heart disease (e.g., surgical correction of a congenital heart defect or an acquired valvular abnormality, or pharmacological management of hypertension) may prevent the development or recurrence of heart failure. Similarly, treatment of the precipitating cause will usually rapidly terminate an episode of heart failure and may be life-saving.

Overt heart failure may, of course, also be precipitated if there is progression of the underlying heart disease. A previously stable, compensated patient may develop heart failure that is apparent clinically for the first time when the intrinsic process has advanced to a critical point, such as with progressive obliteration of the pulmonary vascular bed in a patient with cor pulmonale or further narrowing of a stenotic aortic valve. Alternatively, decompensation may occur as a result of failure or exhaustion of the compensatory mechanisms but without any change in the volume load on the heart, or by progressive depression of intrinsic myocardial contractility which occurs with persistent severe pressure or volume overload.

PRECIPITATING CAUSES OF HEART FAILURE

INAPPROPRIATE REDUCTION OF THERAPY. Perhaps the most common cause of decompensation in a previously compensated patient with heart failure is inappropriate reduction in the intensity of treatment—be it dietary sodium restriction, reduced physical activity, a drug regimen, or, most commonly, a combination of these measures. Many patients with serious underlying heart disease, regardless of whether they previously experienced heart failure, may be relatively asymptomatic for as long as they carefully adhere to their treatment regimen. However, without proper instruction, the patient who has become asymptomatic may incorrectly assume that the underlying condition has been cured and may voluntarily diminish the intensity of therapy, precipitating a bout of congestive heart failure. Perhaps the most serious example of this situation is the patient who adjusts his digitalis dosage on the basis of symptoms, discontinuing the drug when there are no symptoms of heart failure but taking three, four, or even more times the maintenance dose when symptoms of heart failure are present. Obviously this practice can lead to wide variations in digitalis levels, exacerbation of heart failure, and digitalis intoxication. Dietary excesses of sodium, incurred particularly on vacations or holidays or during an illness of the spouse responsible for preparing the patient's meals, are related frequent causes of sudden cardiac decompensation. Careful and repeated instruction of the patient is a simple yet effective measure of preventing this common clinical problem.

ARRHYTHMIAS (See also Chap. 22). Cardiac arrhythmias are far more common in patients with underlying structural heart disease than in normal subjects and commonly precipitate or intensify heart failure. The development of arrhythmias may precipitate heart failure through several mechanisms. (1) *Tachyarrhythmias* reduce the time available for ventricular filling. When there is already an impairment of ventricular filling, as in mitral stenosis, or reduced ventricular compliance (diastolic failure, see below), tachycardia will raise atrial pressure and further reduce cardiac output. In addition, tachyarrhythmias increase myocardial oxygen demands and, in a patient with obstructive coronary artery disease, may induce or intensify myocardial ischemia, which, in turn, impairs both cardiac relaxation and systolic function, thereby raising left atrial pressure further and causing symptoms secondary to pulmonary congestion. (2) *Marked bradycardia* in a patient with underlying heart disease usually depresses cardiac output, since stroke volume may already be maximal and cannot rise further to maintain cardiac output. (3) *Dissociation between atrial and ventricular contraction*, which occurs in many arrhythmias, results in loss of the atrial booster pump mechanism, which impairs ventricular filling, lowers cardiac output, and raises atrial pressure.[18] This loss is particularly deleterious in patients with impaired ventricular filling owing to concentric cardiac hypertrophy (e.g., in systemic hypertension, aortic stenosis, and hypertrophic cardiomyopathy). (4) *Abnormal intraventricular conduction*, which occurs in many arrhythmias such as ventricular tachycardia, impairs myocardial performance because of loss of the normal synchronicity of ventricular contraction. In addition to precipitating heart failure, arrhythmias—sometimes fatal—may be *caused* by heart failure.

SYSTEMIC INFECTION. Although patients with congestive heart failure are particularly susceptible to pulmonary infections, presumably because of the diminished ability of congested lungs to expel respiratory secretions, *any* infection may precipitate cardiac failure. The mechanisms include increased total metabolism as a consequence of fever, discomfort, and cough, which increase the hemodynamic burden on the heart; the accompanying sinus tachycardia, secondary to fever and discomfort, plays an additional adverse role.

PULMONARY EMBOLISM. Patients with congestive heart failure, particularly when confined to bed, are at high risk of developing pulmonary emboli, which may increase the hemodynamic burden on the right ventricle by further elevating right ventricular systolic pressure and may cause fever, tachypnea, and tachycardia (Chap. 47), the deleterious effects of which have already been discussed.

PHYSICAL, ENVIRONMENTAL, AND EMOTIONAL EXCESSES. Intense, prolonged exertion or severe fatigue, such as may result from prolonged travel or emotional crises, and a severe climatic change, such as to a hot, humid environment, are relatively common precipitants of cardiac decompensation.

CARDIAC INFECTION AND INFLAMMATION. Myocarditis owing to a recurrence of acute rheumatic fever (Chap. 54) or to infective endocarditis (Chap. 34) or as a consequence of a variety of allergic inflammatory or infectious processes (including viral myocarditis) may impair myocardial function directly and exacerbate existing heart disease. The anemia, fever, and tachycardia that frequently accompany these processes are also deleterious. In patients with infective endocarditis, additional valvular damage may also precipitate cardiac decompensation.

HIGH-OUTPUT STATES. As indicated in Chap. 25, anemia, thyrotoxicosis, or pregnancy and other high-output states by themselves seldom, if ever, produce heart failure; however, the development of these conditions in the presence of underlying heart disease often precipitates heart failure. In these states the requirements of the peripheral tissues for oxygen can be satisfied only by an increase in cardiac output. Although the normal heart is capable of augmenting its output, this may not be true of the diseased heart. Thus acute heart failure may be precipitated in patients with underlying heart disease who develop one of the hyperkinetic circulatory states.

DEVELOPMENT OF AN UNRELATED ILLNESS. Heart failure may be precipitated in patients with compensated heart disease when an unrelated illness develops. For example, the development of intrinsic renal disease may further impair the ability of patients with heart failure to excrete sodium and thus may intensify the accumulation of fluid. Similarly, blood transfusion or the administration of sodium-containing fluid after a noncardiac operation may result in sudden heart failure in patients with underlying heart disease. Prostatic obstruction in the elderly male, parenchymal liver disease, and the administration of corticosteroids or estrogens with sodium-retaining properties may also precipitate heart failure in patients with underlying heart disease.

ADMINISTRATION OF A CARDIAC DEPRESSANT OR SALT-RETAINING DRUG. A variety of drugs depress myocardial function; among these are alcohol, beta-adrenoceptor blocking agents, disopyramide, verapamil, and antineoplastic drugs such as doxorubicin (Adriamycin) and cyclophosphamide. Others, such as estrogens, androgens, glucocorticoids, and nonsteroidal antiinflammatory agents, may cause salt and water retention. Any of these agents, when administered to a patient with heart disease, can precipitate or aggravate heart failure.

DEVELOPMENT OF A SECOND FORM OF HEART DISEASE. Patients with one form of heart disease often remain compensated until they develop a second form of heart disease. For example, a patient with chronic hypertension and left ventricular hypertrophy but without left ventricular failure may be asymptomatic until a myocardial infarction develops (which may be silent) and precipitates heart failure.

It is essential to carefully and systematically search for these precipitating causes in all patients with congestive heart failure, since lack of recognition or treatment or both may be responsible for otherwise refractory heart failure. In most instances these precipitating causes can be treated effectively, after which appropriate measures should be instituted to avoid any recurrence. When a precipitating cause of heart failure can be identified, it generally signifies a better prognosis than when a similar degree of heart failure is due simply to progression of the underlying cardiac disease.

SYMPTOMS OF HEART FAILURE

RESPIRATORY DISTRESS

Breathlessness, a cardinal manifestation of left ventricular failure,[19] may present with progressively increasing severity as (1) exertional dyspnea, (2) orthopnea, (3) paroxysmal nocturnal dyspnea, (4) dyspnea at rest, and (5) acute pulmonary edema.

EXERTIONAL DYSPNEA (See also p. 2). The principal difference between exertional dyspnea in normal subjects and in patients with heart failure is the degree of activity necessary to induce the symptom. Indeed, as heart failure first appears, exertional dyspnea may simply represent an aggravation of the breathlessness that occurs in normal subjects during activity. Because dyspnea occurs on exertion in all individuals, normal and abnormal, an effort should be made to elicit in the history that a *change* in the extent of exertion which causes dyspnea has actually occurred. It is also important to attempt to distinguish dyspnea secondary to poor conditioning from that caused by cardiac (or pulmonary) disease. Patients usually report that a specific task which they were able to carry out without difficulty for many years (e.g., climbing three flights of stairs) evokes more breathlessness than previously or requires them to stop briefly midway or both. As left ventricular failure advances, the intensity of exercise resulting in breathlessness declines progressively. However, there is no close correlation between subjective exercise capacity and objective measures of left ventricular performance at rest in patients with heart failure.[5, 20] It is important to remember that exertional dyspnea can occur only in a patient who exerts himself. This cardinal symptom of left ventricular failure may be absent in patients who are sedentary for a variety of reasons—habit, the presence of a cardiovascular disease (e.g., severe angina or intermittent claudication) or a noncardiovascular disease (e.g., crippling arthritis). Any of these conditions may mask the presence of heart failure.

ORTHOPNEA. This symptom may be defined as dyspnea that develops in the recumbent position and is relieved by elevation of the head with pillows. Again, as in the case of exertional dyspnea, it is a *change* in the number of pillows required that is important, since many normal individuals prefer to sleep with their heads elevated by two or three pillows. In the recumbent position there is reduced pooling of fluid in the lower extremities and abdomen; blood is displaced from the extrathoracic to the thoracic compartment. The failing left ventricle, operating on the flat portion of its depressed Starling curve (Fig. 15–1, p. 450), cannot accept and pump out the extra volume of blood delivered to it by the competent right ventricle, and pulmonary venous and capillary pressures rise further, causing interstitial edema, reduced pulmonary compliance, increased airway resistance, and dyspnea. In contrast to paroxysmal nocturnal dyspnea (see below), orthopnea occurs rapidly, often within a minute or two of assuming recumbency, and develops when the patient is awake. Orthopnea is an important symptom of heart failure but is far from specific; it may occur in any condition in which vital capacity is low; dyspnea is exacerbated when recumbency elevates the diaphragm, reducing vital capacity even further. This problem is frequently associated with marked ascites, whatever its etiology.

The patient with orthopnea generally elevates his head on several pillows to prevent nocturnal breathlessness and the development of paroxysmal nocturnal dyspnea (see below); in fact, the severity of orthopnea is conveniently estimated from the number of pillows required. Patients frequently awaken short of breath if the head has slipped off the pillows, and they then often seek and find relief by sitting in front of an open window. In advanced left ventricular failure, orthopnea may be so severe that the patient cannot lie down and must spend the night in the sitting position. Often such patients are observed sitting at the side of the bed, slumped over a bedside table.

A nonproductive *cough* in patients with heart failure is often a "dyspnea equivalent," whereas a nocturnal cough may be considered an "orthopnea equivalent." Cough may be caused by pulmonary congestion, occurs under the same circumstances as dyspnea (i.e., during exertion or recumbency), and is relieved by treatment of heart failure.

PAROXYSMAL NOCTURNAL DYSPNEA. Attacks of paroxysmal nocturnal dyspnea usually occur at night. The patient awakens, often quite suddenly and with a feeling of extreme suffocation, sits bolt upright, and gasps for breath. Bronchospasm, which may be caused by congestion of the bronchial mucosa and which increases ventilatory difficulty and the work of breathing, is a common complicating factor of paroxysmal nocturnal dyspnea. The commonly associated wheezing is responsible for the alternate name of this condition, *cardiac asthma*. In contrast to orthopnea, which may be relieved immediately by sitting upright at the side of the bed with the legs dependent, attacks of paroxysmal nocturnal dyspnea may require 30 minutes or longer in this position for relief. Episodes of paroxysmal nocturnal dyspnea may be so frightening that the patient may be afraid to go back to sleep, even after the symptoms have abated. The reason for the common occurrence of these episodes at night is not clear, but it seems likely that the combination of (1) reduced adrenergic support of left ventricular function during sleep, (2) sudden elevation of thoracic blood volume and of the diaphragm which occurs immediately on assuming recumbency (as described above for orthopnea), (3) the slow resorption of interstitial fluid from the dependent portion of the body and the resultant expansion of (thoracic) blood volume, and (4) normal nocturnal depression of the respiratory center plays a major role. Attacks of paroxysmal dyspnea seldom occur during the daytime and are provoked by effort or excitement. When accompanied by chest heaviness, these episodes may be "anginal equivalents" and caused by myocardial ischemia.

PULMONARY EDEMA. The severest form of breathlessness, pulmonary edema, is associated with a number of unique pathophysiological and clinical features and is described in Chap. 18.

Mechanisms of Dyspnea

Increased awareness of respiration or difficulty in breathing is associated with pulmonary capillary hypertension caused by an elevation of left atrial or left ventricular filling pressure. Patients with left ventricular failure typically exhibit a restrictive ventilatory defect, characterized by a reduction of vital capacity as a consequence of the replacement of the air in the lungs with blood or interstitial fluid or both. Consequently, the lungs become stiffer, air trapping occurs because of earlier than normal closure of dependent airways,[21] and the work of breathing is increased because higher intrapleural pressures are needed to distend the stiff lungs.[22] Tidal volume is reduced, and respiratory frequency rises in a compensatory fashion. Engorgement of blood vessels may reduce the caliber of the peripheral airways, increasing airway resistance. In addition, there are alterations in the distribution of ventilation and perfusion, resulting in widened alveolar–arterial differences for oxygen, hypoxemia, and an increased ratio of dead space to tidal volume. Thus, dyspnea (during exertion or at rest) and orthopnea are clinical expressions of pulmonary venous and capillary congestion. Paroxysmal noc-

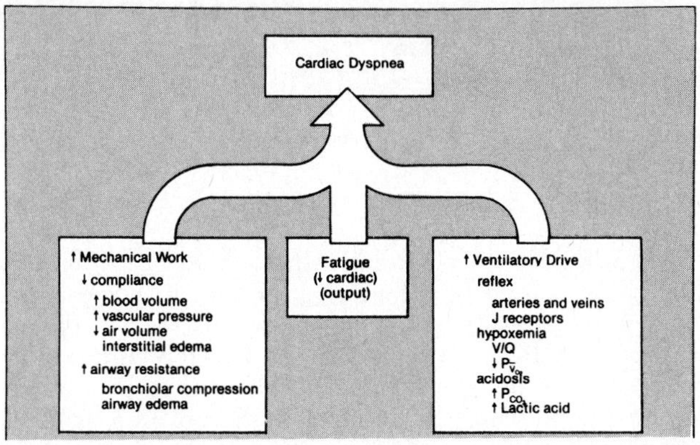

FIGURE 16–1. Factors that induce an increase in mechanical work of ventilation and ventilatory drive in states of pulmonary venous hypertension resulting from increased left heart filling pressure. The simultaneous occurrence of these factors and muscular fatigue converge to produce the sensation of dyspnea. (Reproduced with permission from Turino, G. M.: Origins of cardiac dyspnea. Primary Cardiol. *7*:76, 1981.)

turnal dyspnea reflects the presence of *interstitial* edema, whereas pulmonary edema, in which there is transudation and expectoration of blood-tinged fluid (Chap. 18), is a manifestation of *alveolar* edema.

Whatever abnormalities in mechanics and gas exchange function of the lung that exist at rest are aggravated during exercise (and sometimes during recumbency) when pulmonary venous and capillary pressures rise further. Transudation of fluid from the intravascular to the extravascular space results in greater stiffening of the lungs, an augmentation in the work of breathing, and increased resistance to air flow.[23] There is an increased ventilatory drive, as a consequence of the stimulation of stretch receptors in the pulmonary vessels and interstitium, as well as a result of hypoxemia and metabolic acidosis. The increased work of breathing, combined with a low cardiac output and resulting impaired perfusion of the respiratory muscles, causes fatigue[24] and ultimately the sensation of dyspnea.[25]

The precise mechanism (or mechanisms) responsible for the respiratory distress of heart failure has not been definitively elucidated,[26] but a number of factors may be in operation (Figs. 16–1 and 16–2). It is well known that dyspnea occurs whenever the work of respiration is excessive. Increased force generation is required for the respiratory muscles to move a given volume of air if the compliance of the lungs is reduced or the resistance to air flow is increased; both these changes occur in left heart failure. Although patients are more likely to become dyspneic when the work of respiration is augmented, this increased work does not account for the perceptual difference between a deep breath with a normal mechanical load and a normal-sized breath with an increased mechanical load. The amount of work may be the same with both breaths, but the normal breath with the increased load will be associated with discomfort. A more appealing theory of the mechanism of dyspnea involves the inappropriateness of length to tension in the respiratory muscles. It has been proposed that discomfort arises when there is misalignment of the nerve spindles, which sense tension, in relation to muscle length. This misalignment could lead to the sensation of getting an insufficient breath for the tension generated by the respiratory muscles.[27]

Differentiation Between Cardiac and Pulmonary Dyspnea (See also Chap. 61)

In most patients with dyspnea there is obvious clinical evidence of disease of either the heart or the lungs, but in some the differentiation between cardiac and pulmonary dyspnea may be difficult. The dyspnea of chronic obstructive lung disease tends to develop more gradually than that of heart disease; exceptions, of course, occur in patients with *obstructive lung disease* who experience an episode of infectious bronchitis, pneumonia, or pneumothorax or an exacerbation of asthma. Like patients with cardiac dyspnea, patients with chronic obstructive lung disease may also waken at night with dyspnea, but this is usually associated with sputum production; the dyspnea is relieved after the patient rids himself of secretions by coughing rather than specifically by sitting up.

Acute cardiac asthma (paroxysmal nocturnal dyspnea with prominent wheezing) usually occurs in patients who have obvious clinical evidence of heart disease and may be further differentiated from acute bronchial asthma by diaphoresis, bubblier airway sounds, and the more common occurrence of cyanosis. The difficulty in distinguishing between cardiac and pulmonary dyspnea may be compounded by the coexistence of diseases involving both organ systems. Thus, patients with a history of chronic bronchitis or asthma who develop left ventricular failure tend to develop particularly severe bronchoconstriction

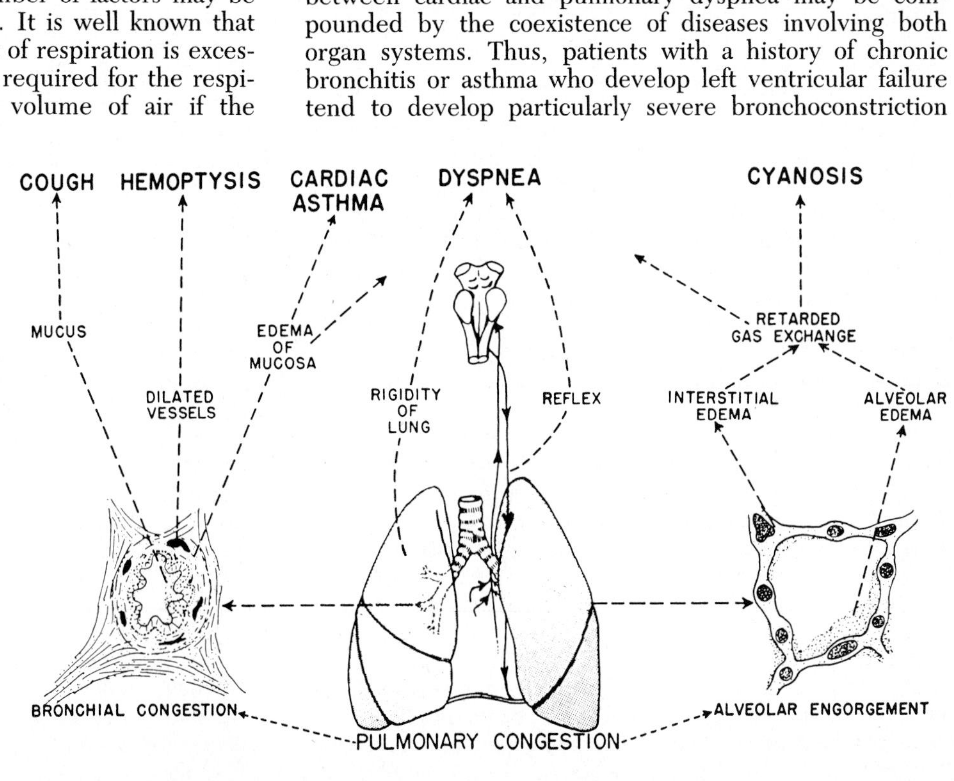

FIGURE 16–2. Etiology of respiratory symptoms from pulmonary congestion. Since most bronchial capillaries drain by way of the pulmonary veins, congestion develops simultaneously in alveolar and bronchial vascular networks. Bronchial congestion tends to stimulate production of mucus, leading to a productive cough. The distended bronchial capillaries may rupture, causing the patient to cough up blood-tinged sputum (hemoptysis). Edema of the bronchial mucosa increases resistance to air flow, producing respiratory distress similar to asthma. Dyspnea results primarily from reflexes initiated by vascular distention but may be supplemented by increased rigidity of the lungs and by impaired gas exchange resulting from interstitial edema and the accumulation of fluid in alveolar sacs. (From Rushmer, R. F.: Cardiac compensation, hypertrophy and myopathy and congestive heart failure. *In* Rushmer, R. F. [ed.]: Cardiovascular Dynamics. Philadelphia, W. B. Saunders Company, 1976, p. 532).

and wheezing in association with bouts of paroxysmal nocturnal dyspnea and pulmonary edema.

PULMONARY FUNCTION TESTING. This testing should be carried out in patients in whom the etiology of dyspnea is unclear despite detailed clinical evaluation. The results may be helpful in determining whether dyspnea is produced by heart disease, lung disease, a combination of the two, or neither. In the latter case, it may be a manifestation of anxiety. In addition to the usual clinical means of assessing patients for heart disease (Chaps. 1 and 2), the arm-to-tongue circulation time may be useful, since in patients with cardiac dyspnea, this value usually exceeds the upper limit of normal (16 seconds) by 4 or more seconds (unless high-output heart failure is present).

The major alterations in pulmonary function tests in congestive heart failure are reductions of vital capacity, total lung capacity, pulmonary diffusion capacity at rest and particularly during exercise, and pulmonary compliance; resistance to air flow is moderately increased. Often there is hyperventilation at rest and during exercise, an increase in dead space, and some abnormalities of ventilation–perfusion relations with slight reductions in arterial PCO_2 and PO_2.

Rarely, it may be difficult to differentiate between cardiac dyspnea, dyspnea based on *malingering*, and dyspnea caused by an *anxiety neurosis*. Careful observation for the appearance of effortless or irregular respiration during exercise testing often helps to identify the patient in whom dyspnea is related to the latter two, noncardiac causes. Patients whose anxiety neurosis focuses on the heart may fear the presence of (nonexistent) heart disease and may exhibit sighing respiration and difficulty in taking a deep breath as well as dyspnea at rest. Their breathing patterns are not rapid and shallow, as in cardiac dyspnea. In some patients a "therapeutic test" is helpful, and amelioration of dyspnea, accompanied by a weight loss exceeding 2 kg induced by administration of a diuretic, supports a cardiac origin for the dyspnea. Conversely, failure of these measures to achieve weight reduction in excess of 2 kg and to diminish dyspnea weighs heavily against a cardiac origin.

Exercise Testing (See also Chap. 8 and p. 466)

Exercise stress testing may be an exceedingly useful adjunct in the *clinical* assessment of patients with suspected or known heart failure.[5, 28] By using a bicycle ergometer or treadmill with a progressively increasing load, the maximum level of exercise which can be achieved can be determined; the latter correlates closely with the total oxygen uptake ($\dot{V}O_2$). Close observation of the patient during an exercise test may disclose obvious difficulty in breathing at a low level of exercise (or the opposite). Thus, this simple test may be considered to be an adjunct of the clinical examination.

A more formal assessment in which $\dot{V}O_2$ is measured at each stage of exercise, or preferably in which $\dot{V}O_2$ and $\dot{V}CO_2$ are measured continuously, allows determination of maximum $\dot{V}O_2$, and the anaerobic threshold (i.e., the point during the exercise test at which the respiratory quotient rises as a consequence of the production of excess lactate)[29] (Fig. 15–20, p. 467). When a progressive exercise test is carried out until (1) $\dot{V}O_2$ fails to rise with further increases in activity; or (2) the patient is limited by severe dyspnea and/or fatigue, $\dot{V}O_2$ less than 25 mg/kg/min represents a reduction of maximum $\dot{V}O_2$. When this reduction is caused by a cardiac abnormality (rather than by pulmonary disease, anemia, peripheral vascular disease or skeletal muscle deformity, marked obesity, severe deconditioning, or malingering), it may be used to classify the severity of heart failure, to follow the progress of the patient and assess the efficacy of therapeutic maneuvers.[29, 30]

OTHER SYMPTOMS

FATIGUE AND WEAKNESS. Although these symptoms, often accompanied by a feeling of heaviness in the limbs, are generally related to poor perfusion of the skeletal muscles in patients with a lowered cardiac output, they are notoriously nonspecific and may be caused by a variety of noncardiopulmonary diseases as well as by neurasthenia; they may also be caused by sodium depletion, hypovolemia, or both, as a consequence of excessive treatment with diuretics and restriction of dietary sodium.

URINARY SYMPTOMS. *Nocturia* occurs relatively early in the course of heart failure. Urine formation is suppressed during the day when the patient is upright and active; this is due, at least in part, to a redistribution of blood flow away from the kidneys during activity[31] (Fig. 14–21, p. 443). When the patient rests in the recumbent position at night, the deficit in cardiac output in relation to oxygen demands is reduced, renal vasoconstriction diminishes, and urine formation increases. Nocturia may be troublesome in that it prevents the patient with heart failure from obtaining much-needed rest. The diurnal pattern of urine flow characteristic of heart failure contrasts sharply with that existing in renal failure, in which urine formation occurs at a reasonably constant rate, both day and night. *Oliguria* is a sign of late cardiac failure and is related to the suppression of urine formation as a consequence of severely reduced cardiac output.

CEREBRAL SYMPTOMS. Confusion, impairment of memory, anxiety, headache, insomnia, bad dreams or nightmares, and, rarely, psychosis with disorientation, delirium, and even hallucinations may occur in elderly patients with advanced heart failure, particularly in those with accompanying cerebral arteriosclerosis.

SYMPTOMS OF PREDOMINANT RIGHT HEART FAILURE. Breathlessness, the cardinal manifestation of left ventricular failure, is uncommon in isolated right ventricular failure because pulmonary congestion is usually absent. Indeed, when a patient with mitral stenosis or left ventricular failure develops right ventricular failure, the severer forms of dyspnea (i.e., paroxysmal nocturnal dyspnea and episodic pulmonary edema) tend to diminish in frequency and intensity because the inability of the right ventricle to augment its output prevents the temporary imbalance between blood flow into and out of the pulmonary vascular bed. On the other hand, when cardiac output becomes markedly reduced in patients with terminal right heart failure, as may occur in isolated right ventricular infarction and in the terminal phases of primary pulmonary hypertension and of pulmonary thromboembolic disease, severe dyspnea (air hunger) may occur, presumably as a consequence of the reduced cardiac output, poor perfusion of respiratory muscle, hypoxemia, and metabolic acidosis. In addition, dyspnea may be a prominent symptom in some patients with right ventricular failure and anasarca, hydrothorax, and ascites as a consequence of lung compression; such patients may even have orthopnea.

As in patients with predominant left ventricular failure, fatigue, a sense of heaviness of the limbs, and anorexia may be troubling symptoms in patients with predominant right heart failure. In patients with severe obstruction of right ventricular outflow of any cause and right ventricular failure, right ventricular stroke volume cannot be augmented, and dizziness and syncope may occur on exertion, just as in patients with aortic stenosis.

Congestive hepatomegaly may produce discomfort in the right upper quadrant or epigastrium, generally described as a dull ache or heaviness. This discomfort, which is caused by stretching of the hepatic capsule, may be severe when the liver enlarges rapidly, as in acute right heart failure. In contrast, chronic, slowly developing hepatic enlargement is generally painless. Other gastrointestinal symptoms, including anorexia, nausea, bloating, a sense of fullness after meals, and constipation, occur owing to congestion of the liver and gastrointestinal tract. In severe, preterminal heart failure, inadequate bowel perfusion can cause abdominal pain, distention, and bloody stools. Nausea, anorexia, and emesis may also be due to cardiac drugs, particularly digitalis (p. 489) and quinidine (p. 628).

Functional Classification

A classification of patients with heart disease based on the relation between symptoms and the amount of effort required to provoke them has been developed by the New York Heart Association.[32] Although there are obvious limitations to assigning numerical values to subjective findings, this classification is nonetheless useful in comparing groups of patients as well as the same patient at different times.

Class I—*No limitation:* Ordinary physical activity does not cause undue fatigue, dyspnea, or palpitation.

Class II—*Slight limitation of physical activity:* Such patients are comfortable at rest. Ordinary physical activity results in fatigue, palpitation, dyspnea, or angina.

Class III—*Marked limitation of physical activity:* Although patients are comfortable at rest, less than ordinary activity will lead to symptoms.

Class IV—*Inability to carry on any physical activity without discomfort:* Symptoms of congestive failure are present even at rest. With any physical activity, increased discomfort is experienced. As discussed on page 11, the accuracy and reproducibility of this classification are limited. To overcome these limitations, Goldman et al. have developed a useful classification based on the estimated metabolic cost of various activities (Table 1–2, p. 4).[33]

PHYSICAL FINDINGS

GENERAL APPEARANCE. Patients with mild or moderate heart failure appear to be in no distress after a few minutes of rest. However, they may be obviously dyspneic during and immediately after activity, such as walking to the physician's office or even after undressing. Patients with left ventricular failure may become uncomfortable if asked to lie flat for more than a few minutes.[34] Those with severe heart failure appear anxious and may exhibit signs of air hunger. Patients with heart failure of recent onset appear acutely ill but are usually well nourished, whereas those with chronic cardiac failure often appear malnourished and sometimes even cachectic. Chronic, marked elevation of systemic venous pressure may produce exophthalmos and severe tricuspid regurgitation and may lead to visible systolic pulsation of the eyes.[35] Cyanosis, icterus, and a malar flush may be evident in patients with severe heart failure.

In mild or moderately severe heart failure, stroke volume is normal at rest; in severe heart failure, it is reduced and this is reflected in a diminished pulse pressure and dusky discoloration of the skin. With very severe failure, particularly if cardiac output has declined acutely, systolic arterial pressure may be reduced. The pulse may be rapid, weak, and thready.

EVIDENCE OF INCREASED ADRENERGIC ACTIVITY. Increased activity of the adrenergic nervous system is a principal compensatory mechanism for support of the circulation in the presence of reduced cardiac output (p. 439). It is responsible for a number of physical signs, including peripheral vasoconstriction, which is manifested as pallor and coldness of the extremities and cyanosis of the digits. There may be diaphoresis with tachycardia, loss of normal sinus arrhythmia, and obvious distention of the peripheral veins secondary to venoconstriction. Diastolic arterial pressure may even be slightly elevated.

PULMONARY RALES. Moist rales result from the transudation of fluid into the alveoli, which then moves into the airways. Rales are heard over the lung bases and are often accompanied by some dullness to percussion. They are characteristic of congestive heart failure of at least moderate severity. (In acute pulmonary edema, coarse, bubbling rales and wheezes are heard over both lung fields and are accompanied by the expectoration of frothy, blood-tinged sputum [p. 554].) With congestion of the bronchial mucosa, excessive bronchial secretions or bronchospasm or both may give rise to rhonchi and wheezes. Rales are usually heard at both lung bases, but if unilateral, they occur more commonly on the right side. When rales are audible *only* over the left lung in a patient with heart failure, they may signify the presence of pulmonary embolism to that lung.

SYSTEMIC VENOUS HYPERTENSION (See also p. 19). This can be detected more readily by inspection of the jugular veins, which provides a useful index of right atrial pressure. The upper limit of normal of the jugular venous pressure is approximately 4 cm above the sternal angle. The patient should be examined at a 45-degree angle. When tricuspid regurgitation is present, the v wave and y descent are most prominent; however, with impedance to right ventricular filling (tricuspid stenosis) or right ventricular emptying (pulmonary hypertension, pulmonic stenosis), the a wave is most prominent. The jugular venous pressure normally declines on exertion, but in patients with heart failure (and in those with constrictive pericarditis, p. 1501) it rises, a finding known as *Kussmaul's sign.* Rarely, venous pressure may be so high that the peripheral veins on the dorsum of the hands or in the temporal region are dilated.

ABDOMINOJUGULAR REFLUX. In patients with mild right heart failure, the jugular venous pressure may be normal at rest but rises to abnormal levels with compression of the abdomen, a sign known as the *abdominojugular reflux.* In order to elicit this sign, the periumbilical region should be compressed firmly, gradually, and continuously for 1 minute while the veins of the neck are observed. The patient should be advised to avoid straining, holding the breath, or carrying out a Valsalva maneuver. A positive test (i.e., expansion of the jugular veins during and immediately after compression) usually reflects the combination of a congested abdomen (particularly liver) and inability of the right side of the heart to accept or eject the transiently increased venous return. Thus, a positive abdominojugular reflux is helpful in differentiating hepatic enlargement caused by heart failure from that caused by other conditions.

CONGESTIVE HEPATOMEGALY. The liver often enlarges *before* overt edema develops, and it may remain so even after other symptoms of right-sided heart failure have disappeared. Inspection of the abdomen may reveal epigastric fullness and, on percussion, dullness in the right upper quadrant. If hepatomegaly has occurred rapidly and relatively recently, the liver is usually tender, owing to stretching of its capsule. In longstanding heart failure this tenderness disappears, even though the liver remains enlarged.

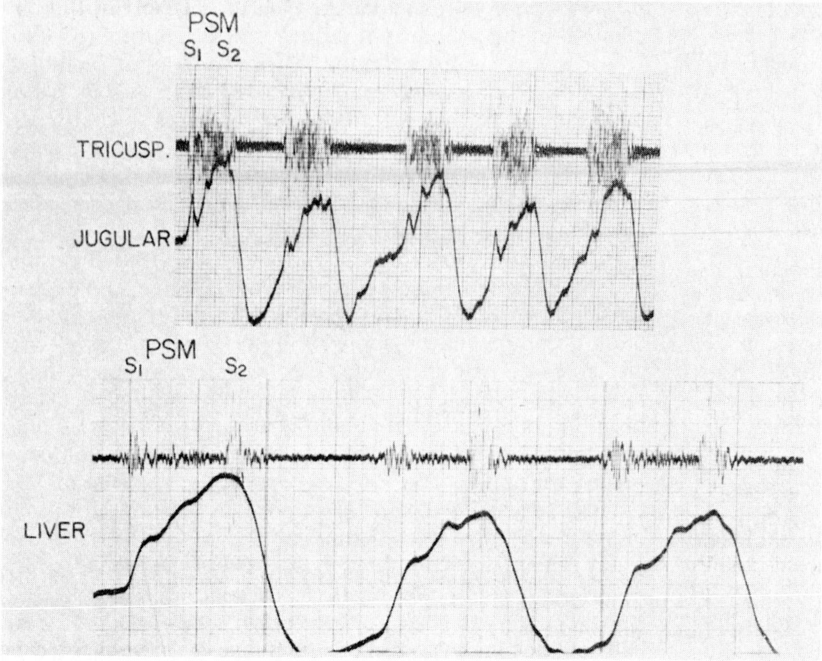

FIGURE 16–3. Jugular venous and hepatic pulse tracings and phonocardiogram from a 42-year-old woman with mitral stenosis and marked tricuspid regurgitation. A pansystolic murmur (PSM) was heard in the tricuspid area. Atrial fibrillation was present. The phonocardiogram shows the pansystolic murmur in the tricuspid region. Graphs of the jugular vein and liver show "ventricularization" of the systolic pulse wave. The rise of the regurgitant venous and liver pulses is synchronous with the first sound. Paper speed at the top tracing is 25 mm/sec, in the bottom tracing 75 mm/sec. (From Dressler, W.: Pulsations of the cervical veins and liver. *In* Dressler, W. [ed.]: Clinical Aids in Cardiac Diagnosis. New York, Grune and Stratton, 1970, p. 190, by permission of Grune and Stratton.)

In patients with tricuspid regurgitation, the prominent right atrial *v* wave may be transmitted to the liver, which pulsates during systole (Fig. 16–3). A prominent presystolic pulsation in the liver owing to an enlarged right atrial *a* wave can occur in tricuspid stenosis, constrictive pericarditis, restrictive cardiomyopathy involving the right ventricle, pulmonary hypertension, and pulmonic stenosis.

EDEMA. Although a cardinal manifestation of congestive heart failure, edema does not correlate well with the level of systemic venous pressure. In patients with chronic left ventricular failure and a low cardiac output, extracellular fluid volume may be sufficiently expanded to cause edema in the presence of normal or only minimal elevations of systemic venous pressure. A substantial gain of extracellular fluid volume, a minimum of 5 liters in adults, must usually take place before peripheral edema is manifested. Therefore, edema may develop over a number of days and may not be present initially in patients with acute heart failure and marked systemic venous hypertension.

Edema is usually symmetrical and generally occurs first in the dependent portions of the body, where the systemic venous pressure rises to its highest levels. Accordingly, cardiac edema in ambulatory patients is usually first noted in the feet or ankles at the end of the day and generally resolves after a night's rest. In bedridden patients it is most commonly found over the sacrum. Facial edema seldom appears in adults with heart failure but, as mentioned earlier, may occur in infants and young children. Late in the course of heart failure, edema may become massive and generalized (anasarca); it can involve the upper extremities, the thoracic and abdominal walls, and particularly the genital area. Rarely, when edema is severe and develops suddenly, it may cause rupture of the skin and extravasation of fluid. Long-standing edema results in pigmentation, reddening, and induration of the skin of the lower extremities, usually the dorsum of the feet and the pretibial areas. In patients with hemiplegia, edema is usually more marked on the paralyzed side. Unilateral edema of the lower extremity may be secondary to unilateral venous obstruction or a cerebrovascular accident.

HYDROTHORAX. Because the pleural veins drain into both the systemic and the pulmonary venous beds, hydrothorax is observed most commonly in patients with hypertension involving both venous systems, but it may also occur when there is marked elevation of pressure in either venous bed. An increase in capillary permeability probably also plays a role in the pathogenesis of cardiac hydrothorax, since the protein content of the pleural fluid may be significantly greater (2 to 3 gm/dl) than that found in edema fluid (0.5 gm/dl). Hydrothorax is usually bilateral, but when unilateral it is usually confined to the right side of the chest and is caused most commonly by severe systemic venous hypertension, as occurs in tricuspid stenosis or constrictive pericarditis. If pleural effusion is limited to the left side, it should suggest pulmonary embolism, a common complication of heart failure. When hydrothorax develops, dyspnea usually intensifies, owing to a further reduction in vital capacity. Although the excess fluid in hydrothorax is usually resorbed as heart failure improves, sometimes interlobar effusions persist.

ASCITES. This finding occurs in patients with increased pressure in the hepatic veins and in the veins draining the peritoneum. Ascites usually reflects longstanding systemic venous hypertension, and in patients with organic tricuspid valve disease and chronic constrictive pericarditis, it may be more prominent than subcutaneous edema. As in the case of hydrothorax, there is increased capillary permeability because the protein content is similar to that of hepatic lymph (i.e., four to six times that of edema fluid). Protein-losing enteropathy may occur in patients with visceral congestion,[36] and the resultant reduced plasma oncotic pressure may lower the threshold for the development of ascites.

Cardiac Findings

The presence of cardiac disease is usually readily evident on clinical examination of patients with congestive heart failure.

CARDIOMEGALY. This finding is nonspecific and occurs in the majority of patients with chronic heart failure. Notable exceptions are heart failure owing to chronic constrictive pericarditis, restrictive cardiomyopathy, and a variety of acute insults such as acute myocardial infarction, the sudden development of tachyarrhythmias or bradyarrhythmias, or rupture of a valve or chordae tendineae; in such circumstances heart failure may develop before the heart has had a chance to enlarge.

GALLOP SOUNDS. Protodiastolic sounds, generally emanating from the left ventricle (but occasionally from the right) and occurring 0.13 to 0.16 second after the second heart sound, are common findings in healthy children and young adults. Such physiological sounds are seldom audible in healthy persons after the age of 40 years but occur in patients of all ages with heart failure and are referred to as protodiastolic, or S_3, gallops. In older adults they generally signify the presence of heart failure (p. 31). Protodiastolic gallops are caused by the sharp deceleration of ventricular inflow that occurs immediately after the early filling phase, perhaps accompanied by simultaneous closure of the atrioventricular valve; a reduction in ventricular distensibility, i.e., the ventricle operating on the steep portion of its diastolic pressure-volume curve (Fig. 13–24, p. 402), may contribute to their genesis. In patients with mitral or tricuspid regurgitation or left-to-right shunts, torrential flow into the ventricle in early diastole contributes to the generation of an S_3 (p. 50), but under these conditions this sound is not to be interpreted as signifying the presence of heart failure. In heart failure the atrioventricular pressure gradient during early filling may be high as a consequence of elevated atrial pressure, and the distensibility of the ventricle may be altered, resulting in a protodiastolic gallop. Thus, a protodiastolic gallop sound is an excellent sign of heart failure when other causes, such as a physiological S_3 occurring in a healthy child or young adult, constrictive pericarditis, mitral and tricuspid regurgitation, or a left-to-right shunt, can be excluded.

Left ventricular gallop sounds are best heard at the apex with the patient in the left lateral recumbent position and are frequently palpable, whereas right ventricular gallop sounds are best heard at the left sternal edge in the fourth or fifth interspace with the patient supine. Protodiastolic gallop sounds originating from the left ventricle tend to be louder *after* inspiration, whereas those originating from the right ventricle are best heard *during* inspiration. Gallop sounds are more readily audible in the presence of a rapid heart rate and sometimes may be elicited by a brief bout of exercise.

PULSUS ALTERNANS (See also p. 23). This condition is characterized by a regular rhythm with alternation of strong and weak contractions. It should be distinguished from the alternation of strong and weak beats that occurs in pulsus bigeminus, in which the weak beat follows the strong beat by a shorter time interval than the strong beat follows the weak, whereas in pulsus alternans they are equally spaced or the weak beat is slightly closer to the succeeding than to the preceding beat. Severe pulsus alternans may be detected either by palpation of the peripheral pulses (the femoral more readily than the brachial, radial, or carotid) or by sphygmomanometry. As the cuff is slowly deflated, only alternate beats are audible for a variable number of millimeters of mercury below the systolic level, depending on the severity of the alternans, and then all beats are heard. Occasionally the weak beat is so small that the aortic valve is not opened, and this results in an apparent halving of the pulse rate, a condition referred to as *total alternans*. Pulsus alternans may be accompanied by alternation in the intensity of the heart sounds and of existing heart murmurs. With total alternans there is a first heart sound for each contraction, but the second heart sound may be absent, with the weak contractions owing to failure of the semilunar valves to open.

Pulsus alternans occurs most commonly in heart failure secondary to increased resistance to left ventricular ejection, as occurs in systemic hypertension and aortic stenosis, as well as in coronary atherosclerosis and dilated cardiomyopathy. It is usually associated with a ventricular protodiastolic gallop sound (S_3), signifies advanced myocardial disease, and often disappears with treatment of heart failure. In patients with heart failure, pulsus alternans can often be elicited by reduction in systemic venous return, as occurs with assumption of the erect posture or application of venous tourniquets, and it is reduced by an increase in venous return, as in recumbency or with exercise. In patients with heart disease, it tends to be present during tachycardia and is often initiated by a premature beat.

Pulsus alternans is attributed to an alternation in the stroke volume ejected by the left ventricle[37] and, ultimately, to a deletion in the number of contracting cells in every other cycle owing to incomplete recovery. Alternans is almost always concordant in the two sides of the circulation, i.e., the strong and weak beats occur simultaneously in the two ventricles. Rarely, pulsus alternans is accompanied by *electrical alternans*; however, the latter condition is usually not due to mechanical alternans, but to alternating position of the heart within the fluid-filled pericardial sac (Fig. 5–103, p. 128).

ACCENTUATION OF P_2. With the development of left ventricular failure, pulmonary artery pressure rises, and P_2 becomes accentuated—often louder than A_2—and more widely transmitted. As left ventricular failure improves, P_2 becomes softer.

Systolic murmurs are common in heart failure owing to the relative mitral or tricuspid regurgitation that may occur secondary to ventricular dilatation. Often these murmurs diminish or disappear when compensation is restored.

FEVER. A low-grade temperature (<38°C), which results from cutaneous vasoconstriction and therefore impairment of heat loss, may occur in severe heart failure; fever usually subsides when compensation is restored. Greater elevations of temperature usually signify the presence of an infection, pulmonary infarction, or infective endocarditis.

CARDIAC CACHEXIA. Longstanding, severe congestive heart failure, particularly of the right ventricle, may lead to anorexia, owing to hepatic and intestinal congestion and sometimes to digitalis intoxication. Occasionally there is impaired intestinal absorption of fat[38] and rarely protein-losing enteropathy.[36] Patients with heart failure may also exhibit increased total metabolism, secondary to (1) an augmentation of myocardial oxygen consumption, as occurs in patients with aortic stenosis and hypertension; (2) excessive work of breathing; and (3) low-grade fever. The combination of a reduced caloric intake and increased caloric expenditure may lead to a marked reduction of tissue mass and, in severe cases, to cardiac cachexia.[39] In some patients the cachexia may be severe enough to suggest the presence of disseminated malignant disease. In others, the loss of lean body mass may be masked by the accumulation of edema.

CHEYNE-STOKES RESPIRATION. This condition, also known as periodic or cyclic respiration, is characterized by the combination of depression in the sensitivity of the respiratory center to carbon dioxide and left ventricular failure.[40] During the apneic phase, arterial P_{O_2} falls and P_{CO_2} rises; this combination excites the depressed respiratory center, resulting in hyperventilation and, subsequently, hypocapnia, followed by another period of apnea. The principal cause of Cheyne-Stokes respiration is a cerebral lesion such as cerebral arteriosclerosis, stroke, or head injury. These causes are often exaggerated by sleep, barbiturates, and narcotics, all of which further depress the sensitivity of the respiratory center. Left ventricular failure, which prolongs the circulation time from the lung to the brain, results in a sluggish response of the system and is responsible for the oscillations between apnea and hyperpnea and prevents return to a steady state of ventilation and blood gases. Occasionally the patient with heart failure awakens at night with dyspnea precipitated by periodic (Cheyne-Stokes) respiration; this form of nocturnal dyspnea is not considered as ominous as classic paroxysmal nocturnal dyspnea.[41] Usually patients are not aware of Cheyne-Stokes respiration. However, it can be readily observed in a sleeping patient, or a history can be elicited from the patient's bed partner.

PATHOLOGICAL FINDINGS

LUNGS. In patients who have died of left ventricular failure the lungs are enlarged, firm, and dark and may be filled with bloody fluid. When pulmonary congestion has been longstanding, they are brown with deposition of hemosiderin and usually do not seep edema fluid. On microscopic examination, the capillaries are engorged and there is thickening of the alveolar septa as well as extravasation of large mononuclear cells containing red blood cells or hemosiderin granules or both.[42] Often the pulmonary vessels show medial hypertrophy and intimal hyperplasia (p. 800).

LIVER. In acute right heart failure, the liver is enlarged, firm, and filled with fluid. On microscopic examination, the central hepatic veins and sinusoids are dilated.[43, 44] With longstanding right heart failure, the liver returns to normal size, subsequently atrophies, and becomes "nutmeg" in appearance as a consequence of the dark red areas of central venous congestion and the lighter, fatty area in the periphery of the lobule. Cardiac cirrhosis is characterized by central lobular necrosis and atrophy as well as extensive fibrous retraction; sometimes there is sclerosis of the hepatic veins. Because cardiac cirrhosis develops as a function of the level of hepatic venous pressure and the duration of its elevation, it is not surprising that it occurs most commonly in patients with chronic constrictive pericarditis and organic tricuspid valve disease and in children after a Fontan procedure for tricuspid atresia,[45] who often have prolonged elevation of systemic venous pressure. In patients with left ventricular failure, central hepatic necrosis without evidence of passive congestion may be present.[46, 47, 48] Liver biopsies in patients with acute heart failure exhibiting fulminant hepatic failure showed replacement of hepatocytes by red blood cells. Presumably, the hypoxia caused by hypoperfusion produces hepatocyte necrosis[49, 50]; erythrocytes may then enter the space of Disse between damaged endothelial cells. These changes resulting from acute heart failure may be transient if there is hemodynamic recovery.

OTHER VISCERA. Patients with chronic hepatic venous hypertension develop portal hypertension that results in congestive splenomegaly. On microscopic examination, the spleen reveals dilatation of the sinusoids and fibrosis, and there is chronic passive congestion of the pancreas and of the veins and capillaries of the gastrointestinal tract. Rarely, intense mesenteric vasoconstriction without thrombotic or embolic occlusion of a mesenteric artery may lead to a hemorrhagic, nonbacterial enterocolitis,[51] with hemorrhagic necrosis.

Chronic venous congestion also occurs in the kidney and brain, with dilatation and engorgement of the capillaries. Small infarcts are frequently observed in the spleen and kidneys of patients with longstanding atrial fibrillation.

LABORATORY FINDINGS

Proteinuria and a high urine specific gravity are common findings in heart failure. Blood urea nitrogen and creatinine levels are often moderately elevated secondary to reductions in renal blood flow and glomerular filtration rate[12] (prerenal azotemia). The erythrocyte sedimentation rate is usually quite low secondary to impaired fibrinogen synthesis and resultant decreased fibrinogen concentrations.

SERUM ELECTROLYTES. Serum electrolyte values are generally normal in patients with heart failure before treatment. However, in severe heart failure, prolonged, rigid sodium restriction, coupled with intensive diuretic therapy as well as the inability to excrete water, may lead to hyponatremia (p. 1830). The hyponatremia is dilutional and occurs despite an expansion of extracellular fluid volume and a normal increased level of total body sodium. It may be accompanied by, and presumably is caused in part by, elevated concentrations of circulating vasopressin.[52] Serum potassium levels are usually normal, although the prolonged administration of kaliuretic diuretics, such as the thiazides or loop diuretics, may result in hypokalemia (p. 514). Hyperkalemia may occur in patients with severe heart failure who show marked reductions in glomerular filtration rate and inadequate delivery of sodium to the distal tubular sodium–potassium exchange sites, particularly if such patients are also receiving potassium-retaining diuretics (p. 1834).

Congestive hepatomegaly and cardiac cirrhosis are often associated with impaired hepatic function, characterized by abnormal values of serum glutamic oxaloacetic transaminase (SGOT) and other liver enzymes.[53, 54] Hyperbilirubinemia, secondary to an increase in both the directly and the indirectly reacting bilirubins, is common, and in severe cases of acute (right or left) ventricular failure, frank jaundice may occur. *Acute* hepatic venous congestion can result in severe jaundice with a bilirubin level as high as 15 to 20 mg/dl, elevation of SGOT to more than 10 times the upper limit of normal, and elevation of the serum alkaline phosphatase level, as well as prolongation of the prothrombin time. Both the clinical and the laboratory pictures may resemble viral hepatitis, but the impairment of hepatic function is rapidly ameliorated by successful treatment of heart failure. In patients with longstanding cardiac cirrhosis, albumin synthesis may be impaired, with resultant hypoalbuminemia, intensifying the accumulation of fluid. Hepatic hypoglycemia, fulminant hepatic failure, and hepatic coma are uncommon, late, and sometimes terminal complications of cardiac cirrhosis.[55, 56]

Venous pressure can be conveniently measured with a spinal fluid manometer while the patient is in the recumbent position and the arm is abducted from the thorax. The baseline for the measurement should be 5 cm below the sternal angle (i.e., the estimated position of the right atrium). The venous pressure is often elevated (i.e., >12 cm H_2O) at rest, but in mild or borderline cases it may be normal at rest but rises with hepatic compression or during exercise.

Circulation time can be measured by rapid intravenous injection of 3 to 5 ml of 20 per cent dehydrocholic acid (Decholin), with a bitter taste designating the endpoint. The normal range in adults is 9 to 16 seconds. Circulation time varies directly with the volume of blood in which the indicator is diluted and inversely with the velocity of blood flow. Therefore, pulmonary and/or systemic venous congestion, as well as reduced cardiac output, causes prolongation. Because of the high velocity of blood flow, circulation time tends to be normal or even shortened in patients with high-output heart failure. Although circulation time is not a particularly sensitive test for heart failure, it may be useful in differentiating between pulmonary and cardiac dyspnea and between low- and high-output cardiac failure (Chap. 25).

THE VALSALVA MANEUVER. This maneuver—forced expiration against a closed glottis—is helpful in the diagnosis of heart failure.[57] The standard test consists of asking the patient to blow against an aneroid manometer and maintain a pressure of 40 mm Hg for 30 seconds. During the Valsalva maneuver, intrathoracic pressure rises, venous return to the heart diminishes, stroke volume falls, and venous pressure rises. Arterial pressure tracings normally show four distinct phases (Fig. 16–4*A*): (1) an initial rise in arterial pressure, which represents transmission to the periphery of the increased intrathoracic pressure; (2) with continuation of the strain and the accompanying reduction

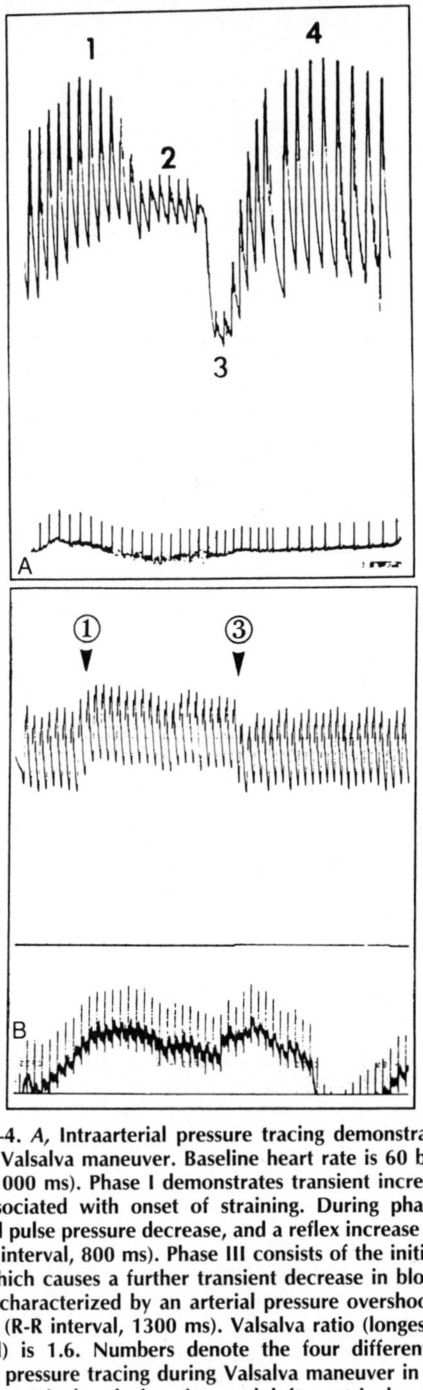

FIGURE 16–4. *A,* Intraarterial pressure tracing demonstrating normal response to Valsalva maneuver. Baseline heart rate is 60 beats/min (R-R interval, 1000 ms). Phase I demonstrates transient increase in blood pressure associated with onset of straining. During phase II, blood pressure and pulse pressure decrease, and a reflex increase in heart rate occurs (R-R interval, 800 ms). Phase III consists of the initial release of straining, which causes a further transient decrease in blood pressure. Phase IV is characterized by an arterial pressure overshoot and reflex bradycardia (R-R interval, 1300 ms). Valsalva ratio (longest to shortest R-R interval) is 1.6. Numbers denote the four different phases. *B,* Intraarterial pressure tracing during Valsalva maneuver in patient with severe left ventricular dysfunction and left ventricular end-diastolic pressure of 35 mm Hg demonstrates square-wave response (absence of decreased pulse pressure and stroke volume normally seen in phase II) and loss of arterial pressure overshoot in phase IV. R-R intervals do not change during the four phases, and the Valsalva ratio is 1.0. Encircled numbers denote onset of first and third phases. (From Nishimura, R. A., and Tajik, A. J.: The Valsalva maneuver and response revisited. Mayo Clin. Proc. *61*:211, 1986.)

of venous return, reductions in systolic, diastolic, and pulse pressures accompanied by a reflex increase in heart rate; (3) on release of the strain, a sudden drop of arterial pressure equivalent to the fall in intrathoracic pressure; and (4) an overshoot of arterial pressure to above control levels, with a wide pulse pressure and bradycardia due to the combination of the inrush into the heart of blood that had been dammed up in the venous bed and reflex vasoconstriction and tachycardia secondary to the low perfusion pressure of the carotid and baroreceptors during phase 3.

In heart failure[57] (Fig. 16–4*B*), phases 1 and 3 are normal; that is, there is normal transmission of the elevated intrathoracic pressure into the arterial tree during phase 1 and sudden loss of this with the release of the strain during phase 3. However, because the heart operates on the flat portion of its Starling curve (Fig. 14–3, p. 429), the impedance of venous return during phase 2 does not affect stroke volume. Therefore, the baroreceptor reflex is not activated, and there is no overshoot on release of the strain. This results in a "square-wave" appearance of the tracing. Although the Valsalva maneuver can be recorded most accurately through an indwelling needle, careful palpation of the pulse in normal individuals allows detection of phases 2 and 4 and their absence, in particular, slowing of the pulse in phase 4 in heart failure.[58]

THE CHEST ROENTGENOGRAM

(See also Chap. 6)

Two principal features of the chest roentgenogram are useful in the patient with congestive heart failure.

The *size and shape of the cardiac silhouette* provide important information concerning the precise nature of the underlying heart disease. Both the cardiothoracic ratio (Fig. 6–16, p. 150) and the heart volume determined on the plain film (Fig. 6–17, p. 151) are relatively specific but insensitive indicators of increased left ventricular end-diastolic volume.

In the presence of normal pulmonary capillary and venous pressure in the erect position, the lung bases are better perfused than the apices, and the vessels supplying the lower lobes are significantly larger than are those supplying the upper lobes. With elevation of left atrial, pulmonary venous, and capillary pressures, interstitial and perivascular edema develops and is most prominent at the lung bases because hydrostatic pressure is greater there.[54] When pulmonary capillary pressure is slightly elevated, i.e., approximately 13 to 17 mm Hg,[59, 60] the resultant compression of pulmonary vessels in the lower lobes causes equalization in size of the vessels to the apices and bases. With greater pressure elevation (approximately 18 to 23 mm Hg), actual pulmonary vascular redistribution occurs (i.e., further constriction of vessels leading to the lower lobes and dilatation of vessels leading to the upper lobes). When pulmonary capillary pressures exceed approximately 20 to 25 mm Hg, interstitial pulmonary edema occurs (Fig. 6–38, p. 163; Fig. 6–39, p. 164, and Fig. 6–40, p. 164). This may be of several varieties: (1) *septal,* producing Kerley's lines (i.e., sharp, linear densities of interlobular interstitial edema); (2) *perivascular,* producing loss of sharpness of the central and peripheral vessels; and (3) *subpleural,* producing spindle-shaped accumulations of fluid between the lung and adjacent pleural surface. When pulmonary capillary pressure exceeds 25 mm Hg, alveolar edema, with a cloudlike appearance and concentration of the fluid around the hili in a "butterfly pattern" (Fig. 6–42, p. 151), and large pleural effusions may occur.[60] With elevation of systemic venous pressure, the azygos vein and superior vena cava may enlarge.[61]

PROGNOSIS

The prognosis of patients with overt heart failure (New York Heart Association Classes III and IV) is poor[61a]; in seven separate studies involving a total of almost 900 patients, the overall 1-year mortality ranged from 34 to 58 per cent.[62] In these seven studies the percentage of total deaths that were sudden ranged from 33 to 47 per cent; 24-hour ambulatory electrocardiographic monitoring has shown that approximately three-fourths of patients with heart failure have frequent or complex ventricular ectopy and one-half have nonsustained ventricular tachycardia.[63]

REFERENCES

1. Lewis, T.: Diseases of the Heart. New York, The Macmillan Co., 1933, p. 1.
2. Braunwald, E., Mock, M. B., and Watson, J. (eds.): Congestive Heart Failure. Current Research and Clinical Applications. Orlando, Fla., Grune and Stratton, 1982.
3. O'Brien, C. P.: Approaches to heart failure. *In* Brandenburg, R. O. (ed.): Office cardiology. Cardiovasc. Clin. *10*:33, 1980.
4. Selzer, A.: Principles and Practice of Clinical Cardiology. 2nd ed. Philadelphia, W. B. Saunders Company, 1983, pp. 172–181.
5. Cohn, J. N. (ed.): Drug Treatment of Heart Failure. New York, Yorke Medical Books, 1983.

FORMS OF HEART FAILURE

6. Hope, J. A.: Treatise on the Diseases of the Heart and Great Vessels. London, Williams-Kidd, 1832.
7. Williams, J. F., Jr., Sonnenblick, E. H., and Braunwald, E.: Determinants of atrial contractile force in intact heart. Am. J. Physiol. *209*:1061, 1965.
8. Starling, E. H.: Linacre Lecture on the Law of the Heart (1915). London, Longmans, 1918.
9. Ross, J., Jr., and Braunwald, E.: Studies on Starling's law of the heart. IX. The effects of impeding venous return on performance of the normal and failing human left ventricle. Circulation *30*:719, 1964.
10. Stampfer, M., Epstein, S. E., Beiser, G. D., and Braunwald, E.: Hemodynamic effects of diuresis at rest and during intense upright exercise in patients with impaired cardiac function. Circulation *37*:900, 1968.
11. Mackenzie, J.: Disease of the Heart. 3rd ed. London, Oxford University Press, 1913.
12. Hricik, D. E., and Kassirer, J. P.: How to interpret azotemia in cardiac failure. J. Cardiovasc. Med. *8*:397, 1983.
13. Tan, S. Y., and Mulrow, P. J.: Aldosterone in hypertension and edema. *In* Bondy, P. K., and Rosenberg, L. E. (eds.): Metabolic Control and Disease. 8th ed. Philadelphia, W. B. Saunders Company, 1980, p. 1516.
14. Chidsey, C. A., Kaiser, G. A., Sonnenblick, E. H., Spann, J. F., and Braunwald, E.: Cardiac norepinephrine stores in experimental heart failure in the dog. J. Clin. Invest. *43*:2386, 1964.
15. Chandler, B. M., Sonnenblick, E. H., Spann, J. F., and Pool, P. E.: Association of depressed myofibrillar adenosinetriphosphate and reduced contractility in experimental heart failure. Circ. Res. *21*:717, 1967.
16. Artman, M., and Graham, T. P., Jr.: Congestive heart failure in infancy: Recognition and management. Am. Heart J. *103*:1040, 1982.

CAUSES OF HEART FAILURE

17. Sodeman, W. A., and Burch, G. E.: The precipitating causes of congestive heart failure. Am. Heart J. *15*:22, 1938.
18. Braunwald, E., and Frahm, C. J.: Studies on Starling's law of the heart. IV. Observations on the hemodynamic functions of the left atrium in man. Circulation *24*:633, 1961.
19. Srebro, J., and Karliner, J. S.: Congestive heart failure. Curr. Probl. Cardiol. *23*:1, 1986.
20. Franciosa, J. A., Park, M., and Levine, T. B.: Lack of correlation between exercise capacity and indexes of resting left ventricular performance in heart failure. Am. J. Cardiol. *47*:33, 1981.

SYMPTOMS OF HEART FAILURE

21. Collins, J. V., Clark, T. J. H., and Brown, D. J.: Airway function in healthy subjects and in patients with left heart disease. Clin. Sci. Molec. Med. *49*:217, 1975.
22. Marshall, R., McIroy, M. B., and Christie, R. V.: The work of breathing in mitral stenosis. Clin. Sci. *17*:667, 1958.
23. Fishman, A. P. (ed.): Pulmonary Diseases and Disorders. New York, McGraw-Hill Book Co., 1980, pp. 44–67.
24. Macklem, P. T.: Respiratory muscles: The vital pump. Chest *78*:753, 1980.
25. Turino, G. M.: Origins of cardiac dyspnea. Primary Cardiol. *7*:76, 1981.
26. Fishman, A. P., and Ledlie, J. F.: Dyspnea. Bull. Eur. Physiopathol. Resp. *15*:789, 1979.
27. Campbell, E. J. M., Agostoni, E., and Newsom Davis, J.: The Respiratory Muscles: Mechanisms and Neural Control. 2nd ed. Philadelphia, W. B. Saunders Company, 1970.
28. Franciosa, J. A.: Exercise testing in chronic congestive heart failure. Am. J. Cardiol. *53*:1447, 1984.
29. Weber, K. T., and Janicki, J. S.: Cardiopulmonary Exercise Testing. Philadelphia, W. B. Saunders Company, 1986.
30. Wasserman, D.: Dyspnea on exertion: Is it the heart or the lungs? J.A.M.A. *248*:2042, 1982.
31. Higgins, C. B., Vatner, S. F., Franklin, D., and Braunwald, E.: Effects of experimentally produced heart failure on the peripheral vascular response to severe exercise in conscious dogs. Circ. Res. *31*:186, 1972.
32. Criteria Committee, New York Heart Association, Inc.: Diseases of the Heart and Blood Vessels. Nomenclature and Criteria for Diagnosis. 6th ed. Boston, Little, Brown and Co., 1964, p. 114.
33. Goldman, L., Hashimoto, B., Cook, E. F., and Loscalzo, A.: Comparative reproducibility and validity of symptoms for assessing cardiovascular functional class. Advantages of a new specific activity scale. Circulation *64*:1227, 1981.
34. Constant, J.: Bedside Cardiology. Boston, Little, Brown and Co., 1985.
35. Earnest, D. L., and Hurst, J. W.: Exophthalmos, stare and increase in intraocular pressure and systolic propulsion of the eyeballs due to congestive heart failure. Am. J. Cardiol. *26*:351, 1970.
36. Strober, W., Cohen, L. S., Waldmann, T. A., and Braunwald, E.: Tricuspid regurgitation: A newly recognized cause of protein-losing enteropathy, lymphocytopenia and immunologic deficiency. Am. J. Med. *44*:842, 1968.
37. Gleason, W. L., and Braunwald, E.: Studies on Starling's law of the heart. VI. Relationships between left ventricular end-diastolic volume and stroke volume in man with observations on the mechanism of pulsus alternans. Circulation *25*: 841, 1962.
38. Berkowitz, D., Croll, M. N., and Likoff, W.: Malabsorption as a complication of congestive heart failure. Am. J. Cardiol. *11*:43, 1963.
39. Pittman, J. G., and Cohen, P.: The pathogenesis of cardiac cachexia. N. Engl. J. Med. *27*:403, 1964.
40. Lange, R. L., and Hecht, H. H.: The mechanism of Cheyne-Stokes respiration. J. Clin. Invest. *41*:42, 1962.
41. Rees, P. J., and Clark, T. J. H.: Paroxysmal nocturnal dyspnoea and periodic respiration. Lancet *2*:1315, 1979.
42. Friedman-Mor, Z., Chalon, J., Turndorf, H., and Orkin, L. R.: Cardiac index and incidence of heart failure cells. Arch. Pathol. Lab. Med. *102*:418, 1978.
43. Wolke, A. M., Brooks, K. M., and Schaffner, F.: The liver in congestive heart failure. Primary Cardiol. *8*:130, 1982.
44. Blasco, V. V.: Features of hepatic involvement in congestive heart failure. Cardiovasc. Rev. Rep. *4*:963, 1983.
45. Lemmer, J. H., Coran, A. G., Behrendt, D. M., Heidelberger, K. P., and Stern, A. M.: Liver fibrosis (cardiac cirrhosis) five years after modified Fontan operation for tricuspid atresia. J. Thorac. Cardiovasc. Surg. *86*:757, 1983.
46. Cohen, J. A., and Kaplan, M. M.: Left-sided heart failure presenting as hepatitis. Gastroenterology *74*:583, 1978.
47. Mace, S., Borkat, G., and Liebman, J.: Hepatic dysfunction and cardiovascular abnormalities: Occurrence in infants, children and young adults. Am. J. Dis. Child. *139*:60, 1985.
48. Kanel, G. C., Ucci, A. A., Kaplan, M. M., and Wolfe, H. J.: A distinctive perivenular hepatic lesion associated with heart failure. Am. J. Clin. Pathol. *73*: 235, 1980.
49. Nouel, O., Henrion, J., Bernuau, J., DeGott, C., Rueff, B., and Benhamou, J.-P.: Fulminant hepatic failure due to transient circulatory failure in patients with chronic heart disease. Dig. Dis. Sci. *25*:49, 1980.
50. Jenkins, J. G., Lynn, A. M., Wood, A. E., Trusler, G. A., and Barker, G. A.: Acute hepatic failure following cardiac operation in children. J. Thorac. Cardiovasc. Surg. *84*:865, 1982.
51. Wilson, R., and Qualheim, R. E.: A form of acute hemorrhagic enterocolitis afflicting chronically ill individuals. Gastroenterology *27*:431, 1954.
52. Szatalowicz, V. L., Arnold, P. E., Chaimovitz, C., Bichet, D., Beri, T., and Schrier, R. W.: Radioimmunoassay of plasma arginine vasopressin in hyponatremic patients with congestive heart failure. N. Engl. J. Med. *305*:263, 1981.
53. West, M., Pilz, C. G., and Zimmerman, H. J.: Serum enzymes in disease. III. Significance of abnormal serum enzyme levels in cardiac failure. Am. J. Med. Sci. *241*:350, 1960.
54. Kaplan, M. M.: Liver dysfunction secondary to congestive heart failure. Practical Cardiol. *6*:39, 1980.
55. Kaymakcalan, H., Dourdourekas, D., Szanto, P. B., and Steigmann, F.: Congestive heart failure as cause of fulminant hepatic failure. Am. J. Med. *65*:384, 1978.
56. Kisloff, B., and Schaffer, G.: Fulminant hepatic failure secondary to congestive heart failure. Am. J. Dig. Dis. *21*:895, 1976.
57. Gorlin, R., Knowles, J. H., and Storey, C. F.: The Valsalva maneuver as a test of cardiac function. Pathologic physiology and clinical significance. Am. J. Med. *22*:197, 1957.
58. Elisberg, E. I.: Heart rate response to the Valsalva maneuver as a test of circulatory integrity. J.A.M.A. *186*:200, 1963.
59. Baumstark, A., Swensson, R. G., Hessel, S. J., Levin, D. C., Grossman, W., Mann, J. T., and Abrams, H. L.: Evaluating the radiographic assessment of pulmonary venous hypertension in chronic heart disease. AJR *142*:877, 1984.
60. Spindola-Franco, H.: Plain film diagnosis of congestive heart failure. J. Med. Soc. N. J. *75*:783, 1978.
61. Daves, M. L.: Cardiac Roentgenology. Chicago, Year Book Medical Publishers, 1981, pp. 78–86.
61a. Likoff, M. J., Chandler, S. L., and Kay, H. R.: Clinical determinants of mortality in chronic congestive heart failure secondary to idiopathic dilated or to ischemic cardiomyopathy. Am. J. Cardiol. *59*:634, 1987.
62. Packer, M.: Sudden unexpected death in patients with congestive heart failure: A second frontier. Circulation *72*:681, 1985.
63. Chakko, C. S., and Gheorghiade, M.: Ventricular arrhythmias in severe heart failure: Incidence, significance and effectiveness of antiarrhythmic therapy. Am. Heart J. *109*:497, 1985.

17 THE MANAGEMENT OF HEART FAILURE

by THOMAS W. SMITH, M.D.,
EUGENE BRAUNWALD, M.D., and
RALPH A. KELLY, M.D.

INTRODUCTION

Three general approaches are employed in the treatment of heart failure:

1. *Removal of the Underlying Cause.* This—the most desirable approach—involves surgical correction of structural abnormalities responsible for heart failure, such as congenital malformations and acquired valvular lesions, or medical treatment of conditions such as infective endocarditis or hypertension. When symptoms of dyspnea on exertion or orthopnea are due to ischemia-induced impairment of ventricular diastolic relaxation rather than to diminished systolic contraction, specific measures to reduce myocardial ischemia are in order (see Chap. 39).

2. *Removal of the Precipitating Cause.* The recognition, prompt treatment, and, whenever possible, prevention of the specific causes or incidents that produce or exacerbate heart failure, such as infections, arrhythmias, and pulmonary emboli (Chap. 47), are critical to successful management of heart failure.

3. *Control of the Congestive Heart Failure State.* This approach, the subject of this chapter, may be divided into three categories (Table 17–1):

a. *Improvement of the heart's pumping performance,* which consists of efforts to restore the contractility of the failing heart toward normal.

TABLE 17–1 CONTROL OF CONGESTIVE HEART FAILURE

1. *Improvement of Pumping Performance*
   (A) Digitalis glycoside
   (B) Sympathomimetic agents
   (C) Other positive inotropic agents
   (D) Pacemaker
2. *Reduction of Workload*
   (A) Physical and emotional rest
   (B) Treatment of obesity
   (C) Vasodilator therapy
   (D) Assisted circulation
3. *Control of Excessive Salt and Water Retention*
   (A) Low-sodium diet
   (B) Diuretics
   (C) Mechanical removal of fluid
      (1) Thoracentesis
      (2) Paracentesis
      (3) Dialysis
      (4) Phlebotomy

TABLE 17–2 OUTLINE OF TREATMENT OF CHRONIC CONGESTIVE HEART FAILURE*

1. *Restriction of Physical Activity*
   (A) Discontinue exhausting sports and heavy labor
   (B) Discontinue full-time work or equivalent activity, introduce rest periods during the day
   (C) Confine to house
   (D) Confine to bed, chair
2. *Restriction of Sodium Intake*
   (A) Eliminate saltshaker at table (Na = 1.6 to 2.8 gm)
   (B) Eliminate salt in cooking and at table (Na = 1.2 to 1.8 gm)
   (C) Institute A and B above plus low-sodium diet (Na = 0.2 to 1.0 gm)
3. *Digitalis Glycoside*
   (A) Usual maintenance dose
   (B) Maximum tolerable dose
4. *Diuretics*
   (A) Moderate diuretics (thiazide†)
   (B) Loop diuretic (ethacrynic acid, furosemide or bumetanide)
   (C) Loop diuretic plus distal tubular (potassium-sparing) diuretic
   (D) Loop diuretic plus thiazide and distal tubular diuretic
5. *Vasodilators*
   (A) Captopril, enalapril, or combination of hydralazine plus isosorbide dinitrate
   (B) Intensification of oral vasodilator regimen
   (C) Intravenous nitroprusside
6. *Other Inotropic Agents* (dopamine, dobutamine, amrinone)
7. *Special Measures*
   (A) Consider cardiac transplantation
   (B) Dialysis
   (C) Assisted circulation (intraaortic balloon, left ventricular assist device, artificial heart)

*Numbers and letters correspond to Figure 17–1.
†Thiazide or a diuretic of approximately equal potency, such as metolazone.

b. *Reduction of the heart's workload,* which involves reduction of the demands placed on the heart to generate pressure and/or to pump blood.

c. *Control of excessive salt and water retention,* i.e., control of the expansion of extracellular fluid volume, which is the principal cause of many manifestations of heart failure, such as dyspnea and edema.

In each of these last three categories, a number of therapeutic measures are available. As outlined in Table 17–2, numbers 3 (digitalis) and 6 (other inotropic agents) contribute to the direct improvement of the heart's pumping performance; numbers 1 (restriction of physical activity) and 5 (vasodilators) involve reducing the heart's workload; while numbers 2 (restriction of sodium intake), 4 (diuretics), and some aspects of 7 (special measures) involve control of excessive salt and water retention.

THERAPEUTIC STRATEGY IN THE TREATMENT OF HEART FAILURE

CHRONIC HEART FAILURE. A condition as variable as congestive heart failure cannot be treated according to a simple formula. Intelligent management depends on an appreciation of the nature of the underlying condition and the rapidity of its progression; the presence of associated illnesses; the patient's age, occupation, personality, life style, family setting, and ability and motivation to cooperate with treatment; and, importantly, the response to therapeutic measures.[1] With the recognition that wide differences exist among individual patients, Figure 17–1 is presented as a general guide to the therapy of adult patients with chronic congestive heart failure in whom the underlying disease is not amenable to further treatment and in whom precipitating causes have been eliminated to the maximum extent possible. The course of heart failure is rarely smoothly progressive; rather, it is usually punctuated by a series of abrupt downward steps due to acute decompensation, generally as a consequence of one of the precipitating causes of heart failure described on page 474. When

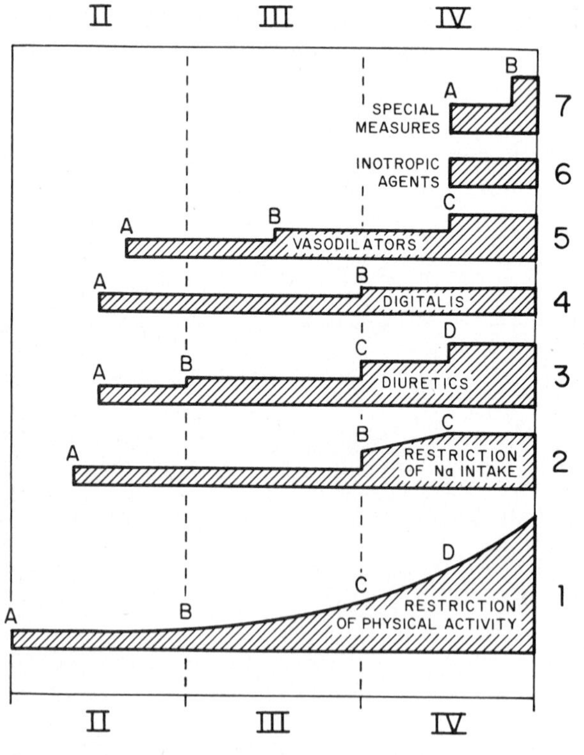

FIGURE 17–1. Strategy of treatment of chronic congestive heart failure in the adult. Various modes of therapy and the intensity of their application at various stages of the patient's course are plotted. For further explanation, see Table 17–2.

the precipitating cause has been removed and treatment has been intensified, the patient's previous condition is often restored. In other patients there are long periods—many months or even years—when the course is stable without any discernible deterioration.

Ordinarily, treatment of heart failure is not begun until the first symptoms of diminished cardiac reserve occur, i.e., until the patient enters functional Class II. The general strategy is to utilize relatively simple means and to utilize progressively stricter and more aggressive measures if clinical manifestations of heart failure persist or recur. As has been pointed out elsewhere (p. 476), the earliest symptoms of heart failure usually appear during heavy exertion. When it has become clear that these symptoms are indeed related to impaired cardiovascular reserve, two forms of treatment are begun simultaneously: discontinuation of intense physical exertion, i.e., heavy labor and competitive or exhausting sports (1A*). Obese patients should be encouraged to lose weight, and systemic hypertension, if present, must be treated vigorously. Many patients initially respond to these relatively simple measures, but if symptoms secondary to extracellular fluid accumulation again appear, dietary sodium intake should be restricted. This may consist merely of eliminating the saltshaker at the table (2A*). If heart failure recurs, persists, or advances despite these measures, an oral diuretic such as a thiazide or an agent of similar potency (3A*) and digitalis (4A*) constitute the next steps. At the same time, consideration should be given to the use of vasodilator therapy (5A*) in selected patients, e.g., those with elevated systemic vascular resistance despite appropriate antihypertensive measures and those with mitral regurgitation.

When, despite the measures outlined above, a patient is symptomatic upon ordinary exertion such as work that does not involve physical labor, shopping, or cleaning the home, i.e., when deterioration into functional Class III (p. 11) has occurred, certain of the measures already taken should be intensified. Full-time work or its equivalent is reduced, the patient is advised to take one or two rest periods during the day (1B*), and a more powerful diuretic—furosemide, bumetanide, or ethacrynic acid—is substituted for the thiazide (3B*). When a patient becomes a "late Class III" and is increasingly symptomatic upon ordinary activity, vasodilators should be given to the maximal extent tolerated (5B*).

In patients who are symptomatic at rest or with minimal activity, i.e., functional Class IV, confinement to the home is necessary (1C*), and the dose of the cardiac glycoside is cautiously raised to achieve the maximum level consistent with an adequate margin of safety (4B*). All salt is elimi-

*These number and letter designations refer to both Figure 17–1 and Table 17–2.

nated at the table and in cooking (2B*), and a potassium-sparing diuretic that acts on the distal tubule, such as spironolactone, triamterene, or amiloride, is added to the "loop" diuretic (3C*). If further deterioration occurs, hospitalization is usually required. At this time, cardiac transplantation (7A*) should be given due consideration in patients who meet relevant clinical criteria (p. 530). Other inotropic agents such as a sympathomimetic amine (6*) are administered, physical activity is drastically curtailed (1D*), a low-sodium (200 mg) diet is instituted (2C*), the number and/or dose of diuretics is increased (3D*), intravenous vasodilators may be administered (5C*), and the application of special measures (7B*) such as the physical removal of fluid (thoracentesis, paracentesis, or dialysis) or, under special circumstances, the application of assisted circulation may be considered.

To reemphasize the importance of individualizing the treatment of heart failure, a few explanations of this therapeutic strategy are in order.

1. In some patients it may be desirable to commence therapy by improving cardiac contractility with a cardiac glycoside and to reduce or eliminate those activities that usually precipitate symptoms of cardiac failure (i.e., to diminish the discrepancy between the heart's ability to pump blood and the requirements of the metabolizing tissues [Fig. 17–2]), as opposed to commencing therapy with diuretics, which treat a complication of heart failure (i.e., the abnormal retention of sodium and water). Nevertheless, certain subsets of patients, such as those with mild symptoms and signs of failure whose physical activity is limited by age or other infirmity, may be treated initially with thiazide diuretics with a more favorable risk-to-benefit ratio. Also, certain patients with an unusual propensity to develop overt digitalis toxicity may be more appropriately treated initially with a diuretic.

2. There is continuing debate about when in the course of heart failure vasodilator treatment should be initiated. The tendency, bolstered by the initial results available from the VHEFT study,[2] has become to introduce vasodilators earlier in the management of heart failure. It has been proposed that the treatment of heart failure can begin with these drugs rather than with digitalis or diuretics. However, while the efficacy of this mode of therapy in selected patients is unquestioned, many patients do not derive long-term benefit (or cannot tolerate side effects) from the chronic oral use of vasodilators (p. 516). Furthermore, in the absence of pulmonary congestion, vasodilators produce little if any rise in cardiac output and may cause a dangerous fall in arterial pressure. Accordingly, it is recommended that vasodilator therapy be begun when the patient has become symptomatic upon mild activity despite optimal use of digitalis and thiazide or comparable diuretics. However, we believe it appropriate to use these agents *before* rigid dietary sodium restriction, multiple diuretics, or intravenous inotropic agents are employed.

3. Restriction of physical activity is carried out in a manner so as to disturb the patient's life style as little as possible (p. 488). Care should be taken to avoid restriction of physical activity to such a severe extent that skeletal muscle deconditioning, rather than cardiac status per se, becomes the factor limiting exercise tolerance.

4. Similarly, restriction of sodium intake need be only mild initially and consist of eliminating the saltshaker at the table, unless heart failure is severe. The availability of potent diuretics allows the patient to eat a nutritious and palatable diet for the major portion of the course of the disease.

*These number and letter designations refer to both Figure 17–1 and Table 17–2.

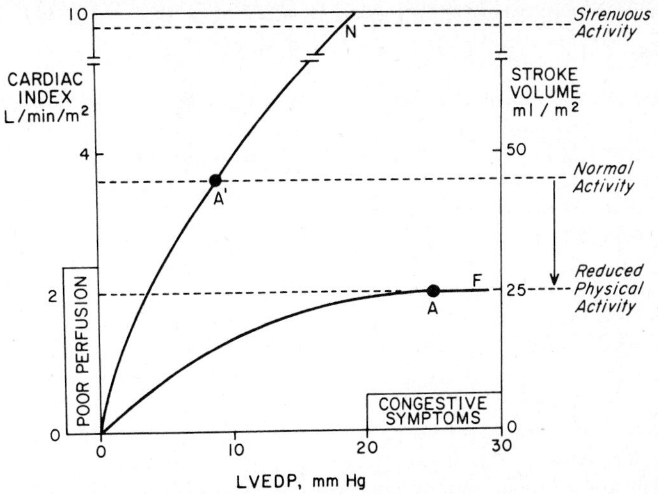

FIGURE 17–2. Diagram demonstrating the relationship between left ventricular end-diastolic pressure (LVEDP) and cardiac index (left ordinate) or stroke volume (right ordinate) in a normal (N) and a failing (F) heart. The upper limit of normal LVEDP (12 mm Hg) and lower limit of normal of CI (2.5 liters/min/m²) are shown, as are the values associated with congestive symptoms (LVEDP > 20 mm Hg) and with impaired perfusion (< 2.2 liters/min/m²). A and A' represent the operating points at rest of a hypothetical patient with heart failure and of a normal person, respectively. Reduction of physical activity allows the failing heart to meet the demands of the metabolizing tissues. A positive inotropic agent displaces the curve from F toward N.

Since there are many exceptions to this general therapeutic strategy, a few examples demonstrate how it may be modified in specific circumstances:

1. If a patient's livelihood is dependent on physical labor and transfer to a more sedentary occupation cannot be readily accomplished, moderate restriction of sodium intake and diuretics can be begun along with digitalis, and marked restriction of physical activity can be deferred, often for a number of years. Also, in a patient with atrial fibrillation and limitation of functional activity, the administration of digitalis (with or without ancillary use of verapamil or a beta-adrenoceptor blocking agent), by controlling ventricular rate, may restore the patient to near-normal cardiac reserve, and restriction of physical activity can be avoided.

2. Occasional patients with left ventricular failure exhibit symptoms of paroxysmal nocturnal dyspnea that are particularly troublesome, yet they are able to engage in almost-normal physical activity during the day. In such patients the paroxysmal nocturnal dyspnea can often be prevented by the administration in the evening of a long-acting venodilator such as nitroglycerin ointment or other transdermal preparation, or by the intensification of diuretic therapy, and they can be maintained in functional Class II.

3. Some patients have difficulty tolerating vasodilators. They become severely hypotensive, develop an adverse reaction to one of the drugs after prolonged use (e.g., the lupus-like syndrome due to hydralazine), or are unwilling (or unable) to take multiple medications several times a day. Such patients may fare better with a change in the vasodilator regimen (e.g., a converting enzyme inhibitor in place of hydralazine plus nitrates), or with more rigid restriction of dietary sodium at an early stage of the disease, and the vasodilator can be held in reserve until later.

4. Occasional patients are particularly prone to accumulate fluid in serous cavities, in which case thoracentesis and/or paracentesis may rapidly relieve dyspnea and need not be reserved until a more advanced phase of the illness.

ACUTE HEART FAILURE (See also p. 553). Treatment of

patients with acute congestive cardiac failure usually involves a choice among diuretics, vasodilators, and inotropic agents. In selecting from these three modes of therapy it is well to ascertain by clinical or laboratory means whether cardiac output and arterial pressure are normal or depressed and whether or not myocardial ischemia is present. It must be appreciated that although *diuretics* diminish filling pressure and symptoms of pulmonary congestion, they do not usually increase cardiac output or relieve hypoperfusion; indeed, they may have precisely the opposite effect (see Fig. 17–12). *Inotropic agents* increase cardiac output but differ widely in their effects on blood pressure. Selection of the specific agent(s) should be influenced by the effect on vascular resistance that is desired. By virtue of increasing myocardial oxygen demands, inotropic agents potentially aggravate myocardial ischemia. In the presence of ischemia, therefore, afterload-reducing agents that increase cardiac output without this potential adverse effect of inotropic agents may be desirable. However, *vasodilators* may lower arterial pressure, which can interfere with perfusion of the coronary bed, thereby potentially intensifying ischemia. They must be used with great caution in patients with ischemic heart disease and borderline arterial pressure (systolic 95–110 mm Hg) and should be avoided in patients who are frankly hypotensive (<95 mm Hg).

An effective therapeutic strategy for most patients with acute heart failure can be developed when these principles are kept in mind. Thus, congestion without hypoperfusion should be treated with diuretics. If blood pressure is elevated or normal, vasodilators are indicated if heart failure is severe. The combination of congestion and hypoperfusion should be treated with a vasodilator and diuretic as long as adequate arterial pressure is maintained, and with positive inotropic agents when blood pressure is depressed.

In transient acute heart failure (e.g., that following acute cardiopulmonary bypass), the most effective therapy may consist of a short period of additional inotropic support with infusion of a sympathomimetic agent, or of reduction of the cardiac workload by applying intraaortic balloon counterpulsation.

GENERAL MEASURES

REST. Reduced physical activity is critical in the care of patients with heart failure throughout their entire course (Fig. 17–1). The intensity of the restriction should depend, of course, on the severity of the heart failure. Until relatively recently it was common practice to reduce markedly the physical activity of patients with enlarged hearts in functional Class II; as a consequence, these patients led unnecessarily restricted lives for many years. Now, the usual recommendation is to tailor the degree of physical activity depending on the symptoms in patients with impaired cardiac reserve. For example, in a patient with heart disease, if dyspnea occurs only while the patient is loading heavy cartons into a truck or climbing four flights of stairs, he or she should be advised to make every effort to discontinue these particular activities. If it is essential for them to be continued, they should be carried out more slowly and should be interrupted by rest periods. Competitive or exhausting sports should be discontinued. Often relatively minor adjustments in activity will allow a patient with mild heart failure to remain gainfully employed or a homemaker to continue routine tasks. Insofar as recreation is concerned, again, minor adjustments, such as the use of a golf cart, may allow the patient many hours of pleasurable activity. As is the case in patients with angina pectoris, regular physical activity to a level that does not regularly produce symptoms is desirable in patients with congestive heart failure.

In patients with more severe heart failure, i.e., those in functional Class III, the problem of continued employment becomes more difficult. Such patients are usually unable, and should not be encouraged, to work full-time, even at a relatively sedentary job. This should not mean, however, that complete cessation of employment is necessary or desirable. Often an adjustment of the work schedule is feasible, e.g., a reduction of the working day from 8 to 5 hours, with two mandatory one-hour rest periods, or a 4-day work week, with a day in the middle of the week during which the patient remains at home to rest. Evening activities should be curtailed. Even some patients who are in functional Class IV and are confined to the home are able to lead more satisfying and productive lives by working for 2 or 3 hours a day at a desk.

In contrast to the situation in chronic heart failure, in which the patient is urged to remain active short of becoming symptomatic, physical activity should be rigidly restricted in the presence of acute cardiac decompensation. Under these circumstances it is almost always desirable to hospitalize the patient, since this will facilitate work-up and the search for a precipitating cause and will allow adjustment of medication and institution of additional therapeutic measures while the patient is under observation. Hospitalization also usually allows more rigid restriction of sodium intake than is possible at home and permits more rigorous control of the restriction of physical activity. Although physical rest plays an important role in the treatment of heart failure, complete physical rest does not mean complete bed rest. Indeed, patients are usually more comfortable and the venous return (and therefore the cardiac preload) is lower when the patient is sitting rather than supine. Also, patients should not be forced to use the bedpan, and trips to the bathroom can usually be allowed. On the other hand, too much relaxation of the rules restricting physical activity can obviate the value of physical rest. For examples, frequent walks to another room on the hospital floor to visit with family or friends, watch television, eat, or use the telephone may nullify the potential benefit of rest in the hospital.

The hazards of phlebothrombosis and pulmonary embolization should be recognized, and deep-breathing exercises, leg exercises, and elastic stockings are advisable. The use of anticoagulants (minidose heparin, p. 1773) should be considered in patients with heart failure with or without a previous history of thromboembolic disease. Patients with marked impairment of ventricular function (e.g., ejection fraction <20 per cent) are at particularly high risk for both systemic and pulmonary emboli, and chronic anticoagulation with coumarin-type drugs should be considered for outpatient use if contraindications do not exist.

Emotional and mental rest are as important as physical rest. Hospitalization is often beneficial because it removes the patient from a situation that is anxiety-provoking. Since emotional stress can retard convalescence from an episode of acute congestive heart failure, visitors and incoming telephone calls should be limited. The physician should serve as a thoughtful, sympathetic listener with whom the patient can discuss a variety of problems. In particular, the patient must be given a realistic appraisal of the prognosis, and it must be emphasized that if a precipitating cause of heart failure can be identified, acute cardiac decompensation does not signify a hopeless outlook. It is important that the patient sleep well each night, and the use of flurazepam (15 to 30 mg) or triazolam (0.125 to 0.25 mg), as a hypnotic may be advisable. Diazepam, 2 to 5 mg twice a day, may be helpful as well in patients with marked anxiety.

There is no formula for deciding on the duration of rigid restriction of physical activity for patients who are being treated for *acute* cardiac decompensation. It should depend principally on the patient's response to the overall treatment program. As a general rule, it is advisable to maintain the patient at rest as long as edema or moist pulmonary rales persist. Although the restriction of physical activity can be relaxed as these and other clinical manifestations of heart failure abate, it should continue in a modified form for 2 to 4 weeks, depending on the course of the patient's convalescence.

DIET. Before effective oral diuretics were available, diet played a more important role in the control of salt and water retention than it does today. It is now possible to recommend only modest restriction of sodium intake in most patients with heart failure, with intensification of the diuretic regimen to prevent accumulation of extracellular fluid. Nonetheless, restriction of sodium intake remains one of the cornerstones of the treatment of congestive heart failure. The normal daily sodium content of the unrestricted American diet ranges from 3.0 to 6.0 gm; simple elimination of the saltshaker at the table and a few common foods such as pretzels, popcorn, salted nuts, potato chips, candy bars, smoked and salt-cured meats (including ham, bacon, and sausage), delicatessen meats, herring, and condiments such as olives and pickles will reduce this to approximately half (1.5 to 3.0 gm). Potassium chloride (salt substitute) may be used in place of ordinary table salt. There is no need to eliminate the salt in cooking and to make the diet unpalatable unless fluid retention occurs despite intensive use of diuretics. Indeed, the monotony and unpalatability of a low-sodium diet has caused unnecessary hardship to patients and their families and has often interfered with adequate nutrition.

Reduction of sodium intake to between 1.2 and 1.5 gm/day can be achieved by simply eliminating all salt from cooking and from the table. If it is necessary to reduce the sodium intake to 0.2 gm daily in patients with Class IV congestive heart failure, many common foods must be eliminated. Spices and herbs can be used to flavor the food in place of sodium chloride, and as wide a variety of foods as possible should be employed to diminish the monotony. A variety of books and pamphlets are available to aid in the preparation of salt-poor diets. It must be recognized that while the elimination of dietary salt may be necessary in patients with severe heart failure, this can result in a marked reduction of caloric intake, leading to malnutrition and even cardiac cachexia (p. 481).

Opinion concerning *water intake* in heart failure has varied widely in the past. At one time rigid restriction of water intake was advised; then it became clear that the total extracellular fluid volume was primarily dependent on the body sodium content. For some years it was thought that excessive water intake (exceeding 3 liters/day) would increase the elimination of salt, i.e., it would "flush out" sodium. There is no evidence in favor of this concept, and therefore it is advisable simply to leave the water intake to the patient's own desire. However, in far-advanced congestive heart failure, the concentration of circulating antidiuretic hormone may be elevated (p. 444) and the ability to excrete a free-water load may be impaired, with resulting dilutional hyponatremia (p. 1830). Only under these circumstances is it desirable to restrict water intake so that the serum sodium concentration does not fall below approximately 130 mEq/liter. Modest reductions of serum sodium (i.e., to 130 to 140 mEq/liter) do not usually require specific therapy.

OXYGEN. The use of oxygen in patients with pulmonary edema and with acute myocardial infarction is discussed elsewhere (p. 555). Oxygen inhalation, most conveniently by means of nasal prongs at 4 to 6 liters/min, should be employed in patients with other forms of congestive heart failure if the arterial oxygen saturation falls below 90 per cent. Oxygen therapy is useful in patients with heart failure precipitated by pulmonary infection or pulmonary infarction. The pulmonary vasorelaxant effect observed when hypoxemia is corrected is particularly valuable in reducing right ventricular afterload in the presence of right-sided failure.

PHYSICAL REMOVAL OF FLUID. Ordinarily, mechanical removal of fluid from the pleural and abdominal cavities is unnecessary in patients with congestive heart failure, because these collections are generally easily mobilized and eliminated with effective diuresis. Occasionally, patients with advanced congestive heart failure who have become resistant to diuretic therapy may regain their sensitivity following mechanical removal of fluid. In some patients with acute respiratory distress in whom the lungs are compressed by large pleural effusion(s) and/or by diaphragms elevated by ascites, mechanical removal of the effusions can bring rapid relief of dyspnea. Mechanical removal of fluid may be associated with a risk, albeit a small one in experienced hands, of pneumothorax or infection. Drainage of ascitic fluid should be carried out slowly, i.e., not more than 200 ml/hr, and the total quantity of pleural fluid removed on a single occasion should not usually exceed 1500 ml; otherwise, fluid may move rapidly from the circulation into the abdominal or pleural cavity, and cause cardiovascular collapse.

Removal of excess fluid by *peritoneal dialysis* or, preferably, *hemodialysis with ultrafiltration*[3, 4] has been employed successfully in patients with congestive heart failure resistant to diuretic therapy.

Severe constipation and consequent straining at stool should be avoided in patients with heart failure. Dioctyl sodium sulfosuccinate, 50 to 200 mg daily, is useful as a stool softener. In addition, a mild laxative may be necessary in patients whose physical activity has been restricted.

DIGITALIS GLYCOSIDES

For more than 200 years, digitalis glycosides have occupied a prominent place in the management of congestive heart failure and certain arrhythmias. Withering recognized in 1785 that optimal use of digitalis requires considerable knowledge and skill on the part of the physician because of the unusually narrow therapeutic:toxic dose ratio of this group of drugs.[5] A sound understanding of the actions and pharmacokinetics of these drugs is essential to minimize the ever-present risk of toxicity and to provide maximum benefit to the patient.

In the discussion that follows, the term *digitalis* is used to refer to any of the steroid or steroid glycoside compounds that exert typical positive inotropic and electrophysiological effects on the heart. Although there are important differences in pharmacokinetics among the more than 300 known compounds with these properties, their pharmacological actions are fundamentally similar, and detailed consideration will therefore be limited to those agents that are in common clinical use.

SOURCES. The majority of digitalis drugs in routine

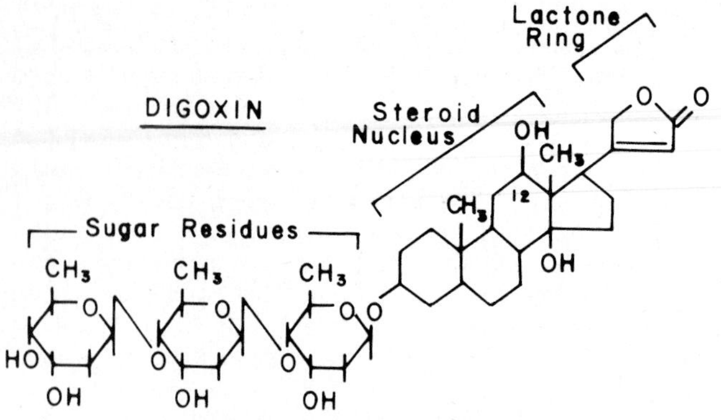

FIGURE 17–3. Structure of digoxin.

clinical use today are steroid glycosides derived from the leaves of the common flowering plant known as foxglove, or *Digitalis purpurea* (digitoxin, gitalin, digitalis leaf), or from the leaves of *D. lanata* (digoxin, lanatoside C, deslanoside). Ouabain, an exception, is obtained from seeds of *Strophanthus gratus*.

STRUCTURE. The steroid nucleus common to all cardiac glycosides contains an α, β-unsaturated lactone ring attached at the C-17 position. Without attached sugars, the steroid and unsaturated lactone part of the molecule is called the *genin* or *aglycone*. Although possessing characteristic digitalis-like pharmacological properties, genins are usually less potent and have more transient actions than do the parent glycosides. Figure 17–3 shows the structure of digoxin; digitoxin differs from digoxin only in the absence of the hydroxyl group at C-12. It is apparent from structure-activity comparisons that considerable variation in the steroid nucleus as well as sugar substituents attached at the C-3 position occurs among the cardioactive glycosides. Potent cardioactivity does, however, require the unsaturated lactone ring, the C-14 β-hydroxyl group, and *cis* fusion of the C and D rings.[6,7] Research continues in pursuit of the goal of improved cardiac glycoside molecules with reduced adverse side effects and enhanced selectivity of action.[8]

MECHANISMS OF CARDIAC GLYCOSIDE ACTION

INOTROPY. The entire spectrum of myocardial cellular activity has been studied in search of the cellular or molecular mechanism underlying the positive inotropic action of digitalis.[9–11] While controversy persists regarding the basic mechanism of digitalis-induced inotropy, it is apparent that cardiac glycosides increase the force and velocity of contraction of the normal as well as the failing heart.

Any comprehensive model of cardiac glycoside–induced inotropy must take into account several fundamental observations, including the following:[12, 13] digitalis glycosides exert a positive inotropic effect on cardiac muscle but not on skeletal muscle; the extent of the positive inotropic response is dependent on contraction frequency, declining on either side of an optimum value; and the magnitude and rate of onset of positive inotropy are dependent on the concentration of a number of ions, including potassium, sodium, calcium, and magnesium. There is not a close correlation between cardiac catecholamine content and the response to cardiac glycosides. Furthermore, marked positive inotropic effects persist in the presence of full beta-adrenoceptor blocking doses of drugs such as propranolol. Therefore, the major inotropic effects of cardiac glycosides are not mediated by catecholamine release or increased sensitivity to catecholamines. Adenylate cyclase activity, although thought to participate in the mediation of positive inotropic effects of beta-adrenoceptor agonists and glucagon, does not appear to be influenced by digitalis glycosides.

Actin, myosin, and the troponin-tropomyosin regulatory system have all been postulated as possible sites of cardiac glycoside action, but convincing evidence is lacking for a primary interaction between these proteins and digitalis glycosides at relevant concentrations.[14] Also, there is no evidence that digitalis has a direct effect on intermediary metabolism or on myocardial energetics, although cardiac glycosides share with other positive inotropic agents the tendency to increase myocardial oxygen consumption. In the failing heart, digitalis may actually reduce myocardial oxygen consumption by decreasing heart size and hence wall tension through the Laplace relation.[15]

CARDIAC GLYCOSIDES, CALCIUM, AND EXCITATION-CONTRACTION COUPLING. Central to the problem of elucidating the mechanism by which digitalis exerts its positive inotropic effect is the still incomplete understanding of myocardial excitation-contraction coupling. As discussed on page 392, the slow inward current that occurs during the plateau phase of the myocardial action potential has been well documented to be carried, in large part, by Ca^{++}; this influx of Ca^{++} appears to be related to excitation-contraction coupling. An increase in the magnitude of slow inward current in cardiac Purkinje and myocardial fibers exposed to cardiotonic steroids has been reported and may be related, at least in part, to inhibition of the Na pump, as discussed below.[16, 17] In any case, the absence of definable primary changes in other cellular functions has led most investigators to conclude that cardiac glycosides, by some mechanism, increase the availability of Ca^{++} to the contractile element at the time of excitation-contraction coupling. In principle, this could be brought about by an increase in the steady-state contractile Ca^{++} pool as a result of increased influx or decreased efflux of Ca^{++}. Alternatively, the mechanism could involve increased influx of Ca^{++} during the action potential, with enhanced excitation-contraction coupling, balanced by increased efflux with no increase in net steady-state myocardial Ca^{++}. The inotropic response requires an intact sarcolemma, since inotropic effects of digitalis are absent in mechanically skinned myocardial fibers[18] despite intact sarcoplasmic reticulum and contractile element structures. The complexity of myocardial Ca^{++} compartmentalization precludes any simple experimental approach to these problems, but cardiac glycoside–induced increases in a rapidly exchangeable Ca^{++} pool that appear to be linked to the contractile state of the cell have been reported.[19–21] Direct evidence for an increase in the intracellular Ca^{++} transient following exposure to digitalis is now available from studies using the photoactive calcium-sensitive protein aequorin (Fig. 13–7, p. 389).[22] Figure 17–4 shows, from the work of Wier and Hess,[23] aequorin signals together with action potential and tension recordings illustrating control, therapeutic, and early toxic responses. In these studies using a canine Purkinje fiber, a 25-minute exposure to 10^{-7} M ouabain (*B*) results in little if any change in the action potential, but systolic aequorin luminescence (reflecting the Ca^{++} transient) and tension are markedly increased. In *C*, an afterdepolarization and aftercontraction occur simultaneously with spontaneous Ca^{++} release from an overloaded sarcoplasmic reticulum.

INHIBITION OF Na^+, K^+-ATPase BY CARDIAC GLYCOSIDES. The noteworthy lack of well-defined effects of

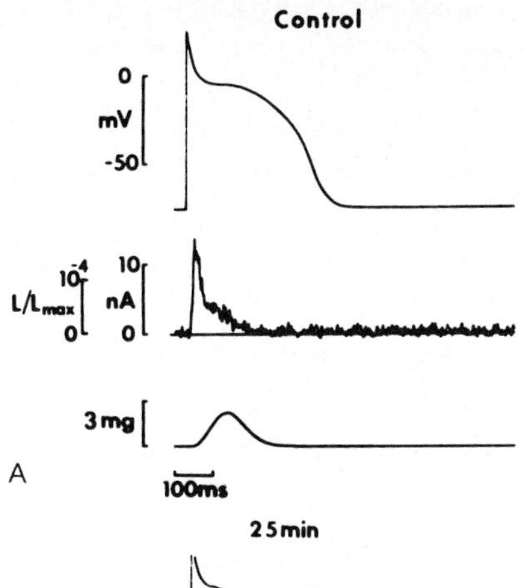

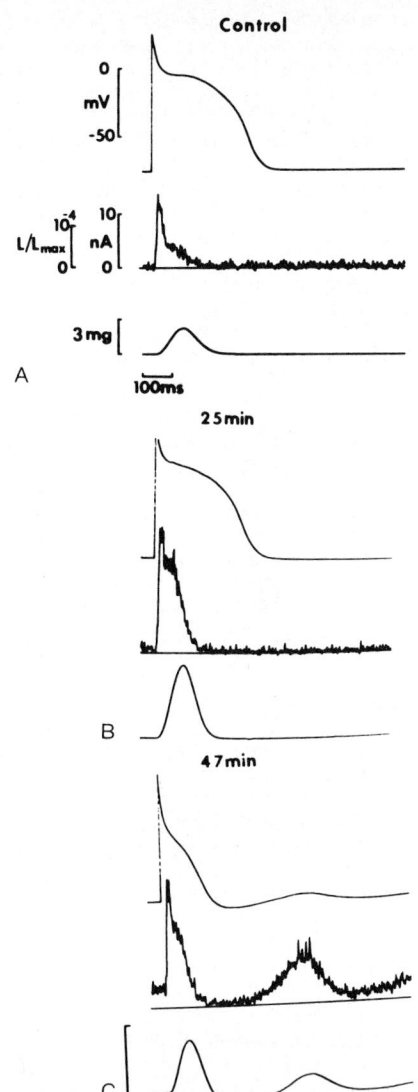

FIGURE 17–4. Calcium transients measured with aequorin during exposure to digitalis. Simultaneous signal-averaged recordings of membrane potential, aequorin luminescence, and tension in a canine cardiac Purkinje fiber before (*A*) and during (*B*, 25 min; *C*, 47 min) exposure to 100^{-7}M ouabain. (From Wier, W. G., and Hess, P.: Excitation-contraction coupling in cardiac Purkinje fibers. Effects of cardiotonic steroids on the intracellular [Ca^{++}] transient, membrane potential, and contraction. J. Gen. Physiol. *83*:395, 1984.)

digitalis on other cellular functions has led to continuing investigative interest in the uniquely specific ability of cardioactive steroids to inhibit the active transmembrane transport of the monovalent cations Na^+ and K^+. All cardioactive steroids share the property of being potent and highly specific inhibitors of the intrinsic membrane monovalent cation active transport protein Na^+, Na^+-ATPase, the enzymatic equivalent of the "sodium pump." This Mg^{++}- and ATP-dependent, Na^+- and K^+-activated transport enzyme complex consists of two polypeptide subunits, termed α (about 100 kd) and β (a sialoglycoprotein with a mass of approximately 50 kd), that occur in 1:1 stoichiometry. The complete primary structure of both α and β subunits has now been deduced from the base sequence of cDNA clones.[24, 25] Na^+, K^+-ATPase sites in the sarcolemma tend to increase in response to interventions that increase intracellular Na^+, including the presence of low extracellular K^+ or cardiac glycosides,[26] thus tending to restore normal intracellular [Na^+]. A 12-kd proteolipid component tends to copurify but has not been proved to be essential to the activity of the enzyme complex.[27] One cardiac glycoside binding site is present per alpha chain. Optimal binding requires Na^+, Mg^{++}, and ATP and is inhibited by extracellular K^+. Cardiac glycoside binding results in complete inhibition of enzymatic and transport functions of each Na^+, K^+-ATPase site occupied. Na^+, K^+-ATPase is generally agreed to be the receptor for the biological actions of digitalis glycosides.

Circumstantial evidence implicating Na^+, K^+-ATPase as a receptor for the inotropic action of cardiac glycosides includes the following observations (see ref. 12 for additional information).

1. Na^+, K^+-ATPase is inhibited by cardioactive but not by inactive digitalis analogs, and a close relationship exists between potency of Na^+, K^+-ATPase inhibition and cardiac activity.[28]
2. Species cardiac sensitivity to digitalis glycosides is directly correlated with the ability of glycosides to inhibit myocardial Na^+, K^+-ATPase from that species. In the rat, for example, which is notably resistant to the cardiac effects of digitalis, myocardial Na^+, K^+-ATPase is about 100 times less sensitive to cardiac glycosides than is enzyme derived from sensitive species.[29]
3. The time course of Na^+, K^+-ATPase inhibition closely parallels that of the inotropic effect in the hearts of several species, in terms of both onset and offset of effects.[21, 30]
4. The positive inotropic effects of cardiac glycosides are enhanced under conditions that increase intracellular Na^+ concentration, such as paired stimulation or the presence of drugs that increase Na^+ influx. Conversely, digitalis-induced inotropy is delayed under conditions that decrease intracellular Na^+ concentration such as a low [Na^+] in the extracellular milieu or the presence of tetrodotoxin.
5. A number of interventions such as lowering temperature, raising extracellular [K^+], and lowering pH all have a parallel tendency to reduce both the inotropic effect on isolated heart muscle and the inhibitory effect of cardiac glycosides on Na^+, K^+-ATPase.
6. Another intervention that inhibits the activity of Na^+, K^+-ATPase, reduction of extracellular [K^+], exerts similar positive inotropic effects, a similar degree of Na^+, K^+-ATPase inhibition, and similar enhancement of intracellular [Na^+].[31, 32]
7. Doses of cardiac glycosides producing a positive inotropic effect in the intact dog have been shown to inhibit Na^+, K^+-ATPase activity in myocardial enzyme preparations from the heart of the same animal.[33] Studies employing myocardial biopsies in dogs have demonstrated that sustained subtoxic plasma and myocardial cardiac glycoside levels sufficient to produce a positive inotropic effect result in appreciable inhibition of myocardial monovalent cation transport capacity.[34, 35]
8. Elevated extracellular [K^+] has been shown to slow the uptake of cardiac glycosides by myocardial tissue, to slow the onset of inotropic effect, and to slow the rate of binding of cardiac glycosides to myocardial Na^+, K^+-ATPase. The ability of potassium to suppress clinical digitalis toxicity adds further substance to this line of reasoning.
9. At least one group of compounds, the erythrophleum alkaloids, differs chemically from the cardiac glycosides yet shares both the positive inotropic effect and the ability specifically to inhibit Na^+, K^+-ATPase.
10. Inhibitors of Na^+, K^+-ATPase such as N-ethylmaleimide and *p*-chloromercuribenzoate have been shown to produce positive inotropic effects, and these effects are accompanied by inhibition of the Na^+ pump.[36] Furthermore, monovalent cations such as Rb^+ and Tl^+ that are capable of inhibiting Na^+, K^+-ATPase in the presence of Na^+ and K^+ produce sustained positive inotropic effects in isolated heart preparations; concentrations of Tl^+ and digitalis that are equieffective in inhibiting the activity of the Na^+ pump produce similar increases in myocardial contractility.

MONOVALENT CATION TRANSPORT INHIBITION AND INOTROPY

A highly specific interaction between cardiac glycosides and Na^+, K^+-ATPase having been defined, the relationship between this interaction and the well-known effects of digitalis on the intact heart remains to be explained. As early as 1931, Calhoun and Harrison observed a decrease in myocardial [K^+] after toxic doses of cardiac glycosides.[37] Many subsequent studies have documented decreases in intracellular [K^+] and, in many cases, increases in intracellular [Na^+] in response to large toxic doses of cardiac glycosides, while results with smaller subtoxic but still inotropic doses have often been more equivocal.

Studies with isotopic uptake and washout techniques have provided evidence that positive inotropic responses are accompanied by a net loss of K^+ and a net uptake of Na^+, accompanied by a net uptake of cellular Ca^{++}.[20] The appearance of toxic manifestations, such as ectopic

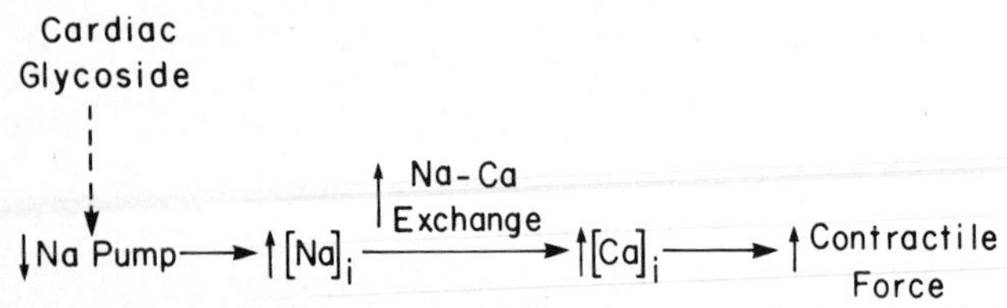

FIGURE 17–5. Schematic representation of the mechanism of inotropic action of cardiac glycosides. Binding of digitalis to NaK-ATPase inhibits this enzyme and hence the active outward transport of Na^+ across the myocardial cell membrane. Na^+ pump inhibition thus leads to increased intracellular Na^+ ($[Na]_i$) content and activity, which in turn enhances Na-Ca exchange with consequent increase in Ca influx, decrease of Ca efflux, or both. The resulting increase in intracellular Ca ($[Ca]_i$) is presumed to mediate the observed increase in myocardial contractile force.

beats and contracture, was accompanied by further changes of still greater magnitude. Positive inotropic responses were not observed without evidence of some degree of inhibition of Na^+ transport. Compelling direct evidence supporting cardiac glycoside–induced increases in intracellular $[Na^+]$ is now available from impalement of cardiac cells with Na^+-sensitive microelectrodes.[38–42] The relation of $[Na]_i$ to tension development is direct and remarkably steep,[41] helping to explain why increases in $[Na]_i$ were difficult to demonstrate at subtoxic cardiac glycoside doses using older and less sensitive methods.

Data from these and other experiments support the view that inhibition of active cellular Na^+ transport may result in augmentation of myocyte Ca^{++} content, which in turn produces a positive inotropic response analogous to that which follows an increase in contraction frequency in the "treppe" or Bowditch staircase phenomenon.[43] The mechanism of this effect appears to involve enhanced exchange of intracellular Na^+ for extracellular Ca^{++} such as has been observed in the squid giant axon[44] as well as mammalian myocardium.[45] This proposed sequence is shown in schematic form in Figure 17–5. Such a mechanism would be consistent with the known dependence of cardiac glycoside–induced inotropy on both the number and the rate of contractions following exposure to the drug. The transmembrane Na^+ influx occurring with each action potential, in the presence of diminished outward Na^+ pumping, would lead to the increased intracellular Na^+ concentration proposed to promote transmembrane exchange of Na^+ and Ca^{++}. At rapid heart rates, Na^+ influx may be of sufficient magnitude to provide the maximum utilizable intracellular Na^+, thus perhaps explaining the diminished effects of cardiac glycosides at these high frequencies.

Studies with spontaneously contracting cultured chick embryo ventricular cells have demonstrated direct correlations between ouabain-induced enhancement of the contractile state and inhibition of monovalent cation active transport as well as increased cell content of both Na^+ and Ca^{++}.[21] These data support the hypothesis that inhibition of the Na^+ pump by cardiac glycosides is causally related to the development of positive inotropy and are consistent with modulation of Ca^{++} content by Na^+ via the Na^+-Ca^{++} exchange carrier mechanism. Further support is provided by studies showing that another intervention, decreasing extracellular $[K^+]$, produces equivalent positive inotropic effects together with similar Na^+ and K^+ transport inhibition, similar increases in intracellular $[Na^+]$, and similar enhancement of Na^+-Ca^{++} exchange compared with cardiac glycosides.[31]

ENHANCED CALCIUM CURRENT. Another way in which digitalis could produce an increase in intracellular $[Ca^{++}]$ is by increasing Ca influx through sarcolemmal Ca channels. Although an increase in the related Ca current was not found in many early studies, reexamination of the question by Weingart et al.[16] yielded evidence that increased Ca current accompanies digitalis inotropy in Purkinje fibers. Marban and Tsien[17] extended this observation to cells of the mammalian ventricle. Figure 17–4 shows membrane potential, current, and tension during depolarizing voltage-clamp pulses in ferret papillary muscle before and during exposure to ouabain. The increase in inward current associated with the increase in force indicates an increase in I_{Ca}. This interpretation was confirmed in Purkinje fibers. Marban and Tsien also proposed a mechanism for the increase in I_{Ca}: a small increase in intracellular free $[Ca^{++}]$ (by Na-pump inhibition or any other mechanism) acts as a positive-feedback signal to increase I_{Ca}. Lederer and Eisner proposed a similar mechanism to explain the changes in membrane current that they observed during Na^+, K^+-ATPase inhibition by extracellular K^+ withdrawal.[46]

The relative contribution of increased I_{Ca} to the inotropic effect of digitalis is still undetermined. It could be important in amplifying small changes in diastolic $[Ca^{++}]_i$ to larger changes in systolic $[Ca^{++}]_i$. Nevertheless, a positive inotropic effect seems to occur without an increase in I_{Ca} in frog ventricle,[47] in mammalian heart when strontium replaces Ca as the cation activating tension,[17] and with high concentrations of digitalis.[16] $[Ca^{++}]_i$ also has negative-feedback effects on I_{Ca}: Ca-channel inactivation is partly Ca-dependent,[48] so that increased $[Ca^{++}]_i$ may actually lead to a net decrease in I_{Ca} at the high $[Ca^{++}]_i$ associated with toxic effects of digitalis.

Despite the weight of evidence implicating Na^+,K^+-ATPase as a receptor for the inotropic effects of digitalis, findings from some laboratories raise questions regarding the concept that positive inotropy results from inhibition of this enzyme system. Further detailed discussions of the vast experimental literature on mechanisms of cardiac glycoside action are found in several reviews.[9, 10, 12, 13, 36, 43, 49, 50]

MYOCARDIAL UPTAKE AND SUBCELLULAR LOCALIZATION

Availability of radioactively labeled cardiac glycosides has allowed detailed studies of uptake by intact heart muscle and of subcellular localization. A general conclusion that can be drawn is that more polar glycosides, such as ouabain, principally undergo specific binding to membrane receptor sites that have many of the properties of Na^+, K^+-ATPase.[9] Less polar glycosides are bound nonspecifically to lipid membrane sites, and there is a high degree of nonspecific binding of nonpolar glycosides such as digitoxin. Digoxin is intermediate both in polarity and in specificity of binding.

The degree of specific binding to myocardial cell membrane components is dependent on specific binding site content, and on extracellular Na^+ and K^+ concentrations, with low K^+ and high Na^+ promoting binding.[9–11] Therefore, it is not surprising that electrolyte disturbances may exert clinically important effects on the myocardial uptake and hence actions of cardiac glycosides. Goldman et al. showed that hyperkalemia inhibited the positive inotropic effect of digoxin in addition to diminishing digoxin binding by the intact canine heart.[53]

Cardiac glycosides can inhibit monovalent cation transport only when present at the outer cell surface.[54] The myocardial receptor is also likely to be accessible only at the outer cell surface, although studies with ouabain and digoxin covalently coupled to macromolecular carrier molecules such as albumin, which are too large to enter intact cells, have not provided conclusive proof of this hypothesis.[56]

ELECTROPHYSIOLOGICAL EFFECTS

(See also p. 217)

Major electrophysiological effects of digitalis on the heart are summarized in Table 17–3. The 80- to 90-mV transmembrane resting potential of cardiac cells (see Fig. 20–6, p. 586) is maintained by Na^+ and K^+ gradients (particularly the latter), which in turn are dependent upon the integrity of the active Na^+-K^+ pump mechanism discussed above. It is therefore not surprising that agents such as cardiac glycosides that inhibit the pump mechanism have profound effects on the electrophysiology of the intact heart as well as on isolated muscle preparations. There is general agreement that inhibition of Na^+,K^+-ATPase underlies direct toxic effects on cardiac rhythm, and thus represents an extension of the therapeutic (inotropic) effect. Cells in various parts of the heart show differing sensitivities to digitalis (Table 17–3), and both direct and neurally mediated effects must be dissected before conclusions can be drawn about the mechanisms involved.[50, 57]

Although usually absent or clinically inapparent at conventional doses, glycoside-induced depression of intraatrial conduction, manifested by increases in P-A interval and atrial effective and functional refractory periods, has been documented.[58] The relative importance of direct and autonomically mediated effects of digoxin has been assessed in man by studying patients undergoing cardiac transplantation.[59, 60] Evaluation of sinus node function showed no change in sinus cycle length after administration of digoxin to patients with hearts denervated by transplantation. Sinoatrial conduction time was unchanged by digoxin in

TABLE 17–3 SOME MAJOR EFFECTS OF DIGITALIS ON THE ELECTROPHYSIOLOGICAL PROPERTIES OF THE HEART

Property	Effect
Pacemaker Automaticity	
SA node	→ ↓ (↑ after atropine or toxic doses)
Purkinje fibers	↑
Excitability	
Atrium	→ *
Ventricle	Variable*
Purkinje fibers	↑ *
Membrane Responsiveness	
Atrium	Variable* (↓ after atropine)
Ventricle	↓ (toxic doses)
Purkinje fibers	↓ (toxic doses)
Conduction Velocity	
Atrium, ventricle	↑ (slight)*
AV node	↓
Purkinje fibers	↓
Effective Refractory Period	
Atrium	↓ (↑ after atropine)
Ventricle	↓
AV node	↑
Purkinje fibers	↑ *

Key: The arrows indicate the direction, not the magnitude, of the changes indicated: ↑ = increased; ↓ = decreased; → = no significant change.

*Decreased with high toxic doses of digitalis.

From Moe, G. K., and Farah, A. E.: Digitalis and allied cardiac glycosides. *In* Goodman, L. S., and Gilman, A. (eds.): The Pharmacological Basis of Therapeutics. 5th ed. New York, Macmillan, 1975, p. 661.

the majority of patients, while first-degree sinoatrial node exit block occurred in one patient and 2:1 sinoatrial node exit block developed in a second.[59] Digoxin did not produce significant changes in atrial effective or functional refractory periods nor in atrioventricular nodal effective or functional refractory periods in denervated patients.[60] These findings underscore the importance of the autonomic nervous system in the modulation of automaticity and conduction by digitalis.

In studies on the cellular electrophysiological effects of digitalis on human atrial fibers obtained at operation, ouabain initially induced increases in maximum diastolic potential, action-potential amplitude, and upstroke velocity of phase 0 depolarization and decreases in duration and automaticity of the action potential.[61] These effects were identical to those produced by acetylcholine and were blocked by atropine. After more prolonged ouabain exposure, opposite responses emerged, and delayed afterdepolarizations and tachyarrhythmias occurred. Thus, the acetylcholine-like effects of digitalis decreased automaticity and increased maximum diastolic potential, while direct effects decreased maximum diastolic potential, increased automaticity, and induced tachyarrhythmias in isolated human atrial fibers.[61]

Most of the antiarrhythmic effects of digitalis are the result of its action on the atria and atrioventricular junction. Within the specialized conduction tissues of the heart the refractory period is increased by digitalis, and conduction velocity is diminished, tending to slow the ventricular response to atrial fibrillation and atrial flutter or to prolong the P-R interval in the presence of normal sinus rhythm. In atrial and ventricular myocardium, the refractory period tends to be shortened, and the more rapid recovery time is reflected in a shortening of the Q-T interval. Effects of digitalis on AV conduction occur predominantly at the level of the AV node rather than more distally in the His-Purkinje system.[62]

Detailed in vitro studies of the effects of digitalis glycosides on cardiac transmembrane action potentials have been carried out for the most part in the mammalian ventricular Purkinje fiber, and the effects observed are generally assumed to be relevant to electrophysiological changes occurring in other cardiac cells. At low concentrations, the resting potential, action potential amplitude, and time course of depolarization and repolarization remain unchanged at a time when inotropic effects are first apparent. At higher concentrations of cardiac glycosides and particularly at more rapid rates of stimulation, there is progressive loss of resting potential. Changes occur in the time course of depolarization and repolarization, including decreased slope of the upstroke of the action potential, shortening of the plateau phase, and increased rate of spontaneous diastolic depolarization. The sensitivity of canine Purkinje fibers to ouabain increases with age,[63] consistent with the clinical observation that younger patients tend to require (and to tolerate) greater cardiac glycoside doses on the basis of dosage per unit of body weight or per square meter of body surface area.[64, 65]

Further details concerning the electrophysiological effects of cardiac glycosides may be found in the discussions of Friedman,[62] Hoffman and Bigger,[7] Weingart,[66] and Rosen.[57]

NEURALLY MEDIATED EFFECTS

Substantial progress has been made in recent years in the delineation of neurally mediated effects of cardiac glycosides.[50, 67] Direct nerve recordings have shown that cardiac glycosides can influence preganglionic cardiac sympathetic nerve activity in anesthetized cats.[67] In the toxic range, sympathetic nerve activity was substantially augmented by digitalis, and high-intensity bursting was temporally correlated with ventricular tachyarrhythmias, including fatal ventricular fibrillation. Spinal-cord section at the C1 level prevented these effects and resulted in an increase in the dose of ouabain required to produce ventricular arrhythmias.[68, 69] Propranolol administration reduced ouabain-induced neural hyperactivity and usually converted ventricular arrhythmias to normal sinus rhythm. These studies support the concept that neural activation by cardiac glycosides may play an important part in the development of cardiac rhythm disturbances.

Studies in a cat experimental model indicate that an important locus of neural augmentation of digitalis-induced arrhythmias lies within an area of the medulla 2 mm above to 2 mm below the obex.[68] Taken together with observations of the effects of highly polar glycoside derivatives that do not appear to cross the normal blood-brain barrier,[70] these findings implicate the area postrema as a likely site of digitalis-induced neural activation. Neurally mediated effects of cardiac glycosides are discussed in greater detail elsewhere,[50] and interactions with the autonomic nervous system are usefully reviewed by Rosen[51] and by Watanabe.[52]

HEMODYNAMIC EFFECTS

MYOCARDIAL CONTRACTILITY. For many decades after the introduction of digitalis into clinical use, clinicians overlooked what is now considered to be one of its major actions: augmentation of the force of myocardial contraction. The drug was not recommended for the treatment of heart failure with normal rhythm but was instead reserved for patients with rapid heart rates. Early in the twentieth century, a series of clinical observations led to recognition that the beneficial effects of digitalis in congestive heart failure were not solely dependent on cardiac rate but were mediated through a positive inotropic effect on the myocardium.[71]

Improved techniques of pharmacological investigation allowed documentation of the positive inotropic actions of digitalis. Wiggers and Stimson showed that digitalis increases the rate of rise in intraventricular pressure during isovolumetric systole when heart rate and aortic pressure are kept constant.[72] The experiments of Cattell and Gold in 1938 showed directly that ouabain increased the force of contraction in isolated, electrically driven cat papillary muscles.[73] The inotropic action of digitalis is manifest in normal as well as in failing heart muscle.[74, 75]

The effect of digitalis on the intact heart is reflected in the ventricular function curve (Fig. 17–2), in which glycoside administration causes the curve to shift upward and to the left, so that at any given ventricular filling pressure more stroke work is generated in the presence of digitalis than in control circumstances. Experimental studies of the velocity of contraction at varying loads demonstrate a shift in the force-velocity relation such that the velocity of muscle shortening is greater at any given load imposed. Effects on the force-velocity relation of heart muscle are similar to those resulting from the action of catecholamines but are independent of cardiac norepinephrine stores, since similar responses occur in reserpine-treated or chronically denervated hearts or after beta-adrenoceptor blockade. The *absolute* increase in tension development induced by digitalis is at least as great in the normal as in the failing myocardium. However, since the failing myocardium has a lower peak tension, the *relative* augmentation of tension may be greater.

Administration of cardiac glycosides results in no change or a slight decline in cardiac output in normal subjects.[76, 77] This is not surprising, since cardiac output is determined not only by contractile state but also by preload, afterload, and heart rate (Fig. 13–34, p. 412). It is now clear that digitalis augments the contractile state of the nonfailing myocardium in the intact human heart, but adjustments in other determinants of cardiac output prevent an appreciable increase in cardiac output.[78]

The effects of digitalis on cardiac function of patients in normal sinus rhythm have undergone considerable study recently, prompted in part by several publications questioning the value of cardiac glycosides in this setting.[79] Studies using both noninvasive and invasive techniques have now documented sustained improvement in cardiac performance of patients with chronic congestive heart failure.[79, 80] The clinical response, however, is critically dependent on patient selection and on the nature and extent of ventricular dysfunction. Arnold and colleagues documented favorable hemodynamic effects of digoxin in a series of patients with functional class III or IV heart failure.[81] Lee et al., using a double-blind placebo-controlled trial design, reported clinical improvement in 14 of 25 patients during outpatient digoxin administration. If one excludes patients with normal left ventricular ejection fractions and those with low steady-state serum digoxin concentrations of 0.5 ng/ml or less from the group reported by Lee et al., then 14 of the 16 patients (all of whom had depressed left ventricular ejection fractions and an audible S_3 gallop) who might have been expected to respond favorably showed objective improvement on digoxin.[82] Griffiths et al. also reported a sustained positive inotropic of digoxin as judged by noninvasive measurements of cardiac function.[83] Murray and colleagues likewise found that both intravenous ouabain and maintenance oral digoxin exerted a modest positive inotropic effect in patients with cardiac failure in sinus rhythm, but hemodynamic benefit was significant only during exertion in this group of 10 patients.[84] However, a group of 30 patients, most of whom were elderly and had ischemic heart disease, studied with a placebo-controlled trial design by Fleg et al., showed no detectable deterioration during the period of digoxin withdrawal.[85] These authors concluded that long-term digoxin therapy has only a minor effect on cardiac performance that is without apparent clinical importance in a "representative" population of ambulatory patients, a little over half of whom were in functional class II; only one subject in this series had an S_3 gallop. Another study showed no objective evidence of clinical deterioration after digoxin withdrawal in a series of 24 patients with coronary artery disease and heart failure who were maintained on diuretic and/or vasodilator therapy.[86] Among infants with a congested circulatory state, 12 of 21 were judged to have benefited clinically from digoxin administration.[87] These studies emphasize the importance of patient selection in predicting clinical responses to cardiac glycosides of patients with normal sinus rhythm, as well as the need for careful observation of patients after institution of such therapy.

DIGITALIS IN HEART FAILURE. The foregoing observations provide a basis for understanding the mechanisms whereby digitalis ameliorates the signs and symptoms of congestive heart failure. As various pathological processes (such as ischemia, volume or pressure loading, or intrinsic cardiac muscle defects) decrease contractility, compensatory reserve mechanisms are brought into play. Elevations in end-diastolic pressure and volume result in increased contractile force through the Frank-Starling mechanism, increased sympathetic tone tends to increase the contractile state, and ventricular hypertrophy may provide more contractile elements. However, each of these three compensatory mechanisms has a price: pulmonary or peripheral edema occurs when end-diastolic ventricular pressures rise excessively; tachycardia may be an undesirable effect of excess sympathetic tone; and increased myocardial oxygen consumption results with all three compensatory mechanisms. If cardiac disease progresses and contractility continues to diminish, the consequences of one of these compensatory mechanisms will become dominant (e.g., pulmonary edema) or the compensatory mechanisms will become insufficient to maintain cardiac output.

Under these circumstances, administration of cardiac glycosides will improve the depressed contractile state, decreasing encroachment on compensatory mechanisms and improving cardiac reserve. The ventricular function curve is shifted upward (Fig. 17–2), so that for any given ventricular end-diastolic pressure, cardiac output is greater. The clinical consequence is a reduction in end-diastolic pressure (and hence diminished pulmonary and systemic venous pressure) and increased cardiac output.[81] As would be expected, the favorable hemodynamic effects of digoxin are additive to those of the vasodilator captopril[88] and also are additive with the favorable effects of the beta-adrenoceptor agonist prenalterol.[89]

Of major clinical importance is the selection of appropriate endpoints or therapeutic goals in the use of digitalis. Although experimental studies have indicated that the positive inotropic action of cardiac glycosides increases progressively until toxic arrhythmias appear,[90] the limited clinical evidence available suggests that little if any further benefit is to be expected by increasing digoxin doses to levels resulting in serum concentrations in excess of about 1.5 to 2.0 ng/ml in patients with congestive heart failure and normal sinus rhythm.[79] Nevertheless, digitalization is not an all-or-none state and the degree of positive inotropic action of the drug increases in a graded manner with increasing dose, at least to the point where steady-state serum digoxin levels are in the range usually considered to be therapeutic. The clinician's task is to determine the appropriate dose consistent with an adequate margin of safety.

DIGITALIS AND THE NONFAILING HEART. Although general agreement exists regarding the beneficial effect of digitalis glycosides in the treatment of the failing heart, considerably less evidence is available to support their usefulness in the absence of overt heart failure. Digitalis is often administered to patients with mitral stenosis regardless of the type of rhythm. It is clearly beneficial in slowing the ventricular response to atrial fibrillation, thereby allowing more complete diastolic filling of the left ventricle. In the presence of right ventricular failure, benefit results from increased contractility and reduced end-diastolic pressure. However, in patients with mitral stenosis and normal sinus rhythm who were studied during maximal exercise, ouabain produced no significant change in heart rate and had no beneficial effect on cardiac output, oxygen consumption, or severity of pulmonary hypertension.[91]

The therapeutic value of digitalis in the hypertrophied or dilated nonfailing heart remains unclear. With the development of hypertrophy, and before the onset of overt failure, the work capacity of the myocardium at any given left ventricular end-diastolic pressure tends to be decreased, and digitalis exerts a positive inotropic action, augments the capacity for performance of cardiac work, and reduces end-systolic volume and end-diastolic pressure.[78] If cardiac output has not been reduced, it does not increase as a result of digitalis administration, but the same stroke work and cardiac output can be delivered from a lower ventricular filling pressure. Thus, digitalis should provide a greater inotropic reserve. However, there is little objective evidence that these considerations can be translated directly into clinical practice. The therapeutic value of digitalis in patients without heart failure (either in altering their prognosis or in retarding the progress of hypertrophy or dilatation) has not been determined in long-term studies. Nevertheless, in the early stages of heart failure, cardiac output may be impaired only on exertion, with a normal output at rest. The clinical diagnosis of this intermediate state between compensation and frank failure is often difficult to make. It is likely that digitalis would improve exercise performance of such patients by increasing cardiac output during exercise and by preventing an undue rise in end-diastolic pressure.

EXTRACARDIAC HEMODYNAMIC EFFECTS. Whereas the direct cardiac effects of digitalis are of primary importance to an understanding of the hemodynamic effects of the drug, it is clear that extracardiac effects are also involved. Digitalis glycosides constrict isolated arterial and venous segments, and arteriolar and venous constriction has been demonstrated in intact laboratory animals.[92, 93] Elevation of total systemic arteriolar resistance has been demonstrated in normal human subjects.[94] These effects appear to be mediated both by the local action of digitalis on vascular smooth muscle and indirectly through the sympathetic nervous system.[95] The latter effect appears to be the predominant mechanism whereby the drug increases the vascular resistance of skeletal muscle. Cross-circulation experiments have shown that the central nervous system may mediate a substantial portion of the vasoconstrictor effect of digoxin.[96] Neurogenic coronary vasoconstrictor effects of digoxin and acetylstrophanthidin have also been documented in a canine model of acute global myocardial ischemia.[97] These effects could be blocked with phenoxybenzamine and hence appear to be mediated by a digitalis-evoked increase in sympathetically mediated vasoconstriction.[97]

Peripheral vasoconstrictor effects of ouabain have also been documented clinically,[98] including observations in patients with cardiogenic shock[99] in whom the vasoconstrictor effect preceded the positive inotropic effect. In some cases this effect was associated with increased left ventricular end-diastolic pressures. These observations indicate the need for caution when digitalis glycosides are administered acutely, particularly in situations in which transient increases in peripheral resistance would be deleterious. There is also evidence that increased mesenteric vascular resistance can compromise splanchnic blood flow, possibly subjecting the patient with marginal perfusion to increased risk of ischemic bowel necrosis.[100]

In clinical circumstances in which the intravenous use of digitalis is required, gradual administration of glycosides over several minutes is preferred to a rapid bolus injection. This preference has been confirmed in a clinically relevant study of the effects of ouabain on coronary and systemic vascular resistance and myocardial oxygen consumption in patients undergoing cardiac catheterization.[101] Ten-second and 2-minute intravenous infusions of ouabain produced increases in mean arterial pressure and systemic vascular resistance, while a 15-minute infusion of the same dose produced no significant change in either variable. Coronary vascular resistance increased after the 10-second infusion but did not change after the 15-minute infusion. The 10-second infusion was also associated with transient deterioration of myocardial lactate metabolism. These findings demonstrate that rapid intravenous infusion of a cardiac glycoside produces systemic and coronary arteriolar constriction that may lead to clinical deterioration. These effects can and should be avoided with slower administration of the drug.

Digitalis produces generalized venoconstriction in the normal dog. This action is particularly marked in the hepatic veins and leads to pooling of blood in the portal venous system and consequently diminished venous return. Effects are probably less striking in man. Extracardiac and coronary vascular effects of digitalis are considered in further detail in the reviews by Longhurst and Ross[102] and by Blatt et al.[95]

In congestive heart failure, sympathetic augmentation of contractility is important in maintaining cardiac output, as discussed in Chapter 14. This increase in sympathetic nervous activity, producing systemic arteriolar and venous constriction, may serve to maintain blood pressure in the face of diminished cardiac output and to redistribute this reduced output among various regional circulations.[103] When digitalis is given to patients with heart failure, generalized vasodilation typically occurs instead of the vasoconstriction observed in normal persons[104]—an effect presumably related to increased cardiac output mediated by the positive inotropic action of the drug and resulting in reflex withdrawal of sympathetic vasoconstriction. This withdrawal may account for the observation that venous pressure is often lowered before diuresis occurs after the administration of digitalis.[104] Digoxin has been shown to suppress plasma renin activity and also to reduce plasma aldosterone activity in patients with chronic congestive heart failure,[104] a finding that may provide a further explanation for this early reduction in venous pressure. However, such decreases in systemic vascular resistance are not invariably observed when digoxin is given to patients with congestive heart failure,[105] and baseline fluid and hormonal status undoubtedly condition the response observed.

Diuresis is a characteristic and important manifestation of digitalis action in edematous patients with congestive heart failure. Digitalis has been shown to inhibit tubular reabsorption of sodium.[106] Direct infusion of ouabain into the renal artery produces substantial inhibition of renal Na^+,K^+-ATPase and impairment of both concentrating and diluting ability.[107] However, relatively large doses are needed to demonstrate these effects, and it is unlikely that any direct renal action of digitalis plays an important part in the diuresis that occurs in the treatment of congestive heart failure. Rather, it is through an improvement of cardiac output and therefore in renal hemodynamics that glycosides induce diuresis.

Finally, a major hemodynamic effect of digitalis in enhancing cardiac performance lies in its ability to slow the ventricular response to supraventricular tachyarrhythmias, particularly in conditions such as mitral stenosis. Slowing of sinus tachycardia in patients with congestive heart failure is often pronounced, through withdrawal of enhanced sympathetic tone, when the failure state is ameliorated by virtue of increased cardiac contractility and output. In usual doses, digitalis has no pronounced direct effect on sinoatrial pacemaker automaticity.

PHARMACOKINETICS AND BIOAVAILABILITY

Many important aspects of pharmacokinetic patterns of commonly used cardiac glycosides were outlined as a result of the studies of Gold and Modell and their coworkers in the 1940's.[108, 109] More recent contributions to the current understanding of digitalis pharmacokinetics have been reviewed recently.[110] Table 17–4 summarizes data related to absorption, onset of action, and excretion times and patterns for cardiac glycosides commonly used in the United States. It is important to recognize that the values cited are averages and that substantial individual variation is to be expected. Extensive discussions of the pharmacokinetics of cardiac glycosides are also available in the volume edited by Greeff.[111]

DIGOXIN. This glycoside has become the digitalis prep-

TABLE 17–4 CARDIAC GLYCOSIDE PREPARATIONS

Agent	Gastrointestinal Absorption	Onset of Action* (min)	Peak Effect (hr)	Average Half-Life**	Principal Metabolic Route (Excretory Pathway)	Average Digitalizing Dose: Oral†	Average Digitalizing Dose: Intravenous†	Usual Daily Oral Maintenance Dose§‡
Ouabain	Unreliable	5 to 10	½ to 2	21 hours	Renal; some gastrointestinal excretion	—	0.03 to 0.50 mg	—
Deslanoside	Unreliable	10 to 30	1 to 2	33 hours	Renal	—	0.80 mg	—
Digoxin	55 to 75%¶ 90 to 100%#	15 to 30	1½ to 5	36 to 48 hours	Renal; some gastrointestinal excretion	1.25 to 1.50 mg#	0.75 to 1.00 mg#	0.25 to 0.50 mg
Digitoxin	90 to 100%	25 to 120	4 to 12	4 to 6 days	Hepatic‖; renal excretion of metabolites	0.70 to 1.20 mg	1.00 mg	0.10 mg
Digitalis leaf	About 40%	—	—	4 to 6 days	Similar to digitoxin	0.08 to 1.20 g	—	0.10 g

*For intravenous dose.
**For normal subjects (prolonged by renal impairment with digoxin, ouabain, and deslanoside and probably by severe hepatic disease with digitoxin and digitalis leaf).
†Divided doses over 12 to 24 hours at intervals of 6 to 8 hours.
‡Given in increments for initial subcomplete digitalization, to be supplemented by further small increments as necessary.
§Average for adult patients without renal or hepatic impairment; varies widely among individual patients and requires close medical supervision.
¶For tablet form of administration (may be less in malabsorption syndromes and in formulations with poor bioavailability).
‖Enterohepatic cycle exists.
#Ninety to 100 per cent gastrointestinal absorption has been reported for the new encapsulated gel formulation Lanoxicaps®, available in capsules containing 0.05, 0.10, and 0.20 mg. When this product is used, the average digitalizing dose should be lowered about 20 per cent.
Modified from Smith, T. W.: Drug therapy: Digitalis glycosides. N. Engl. J. Med. 288:719, 1973.

aration predominantly used in hospitalized patients and to only a slightly lesser extent in outpatients, principally because of the flexibility in its route of administration and its intermediate duration of action. Digoxin is excreted exponentially, with a half-life of about 36 to 48 hours in subjects with normal renal function, resulting in the loss of about one-third of body stores daily.[112] Although the drug is excreted for the most part in unchanged form, some patients excrete appreciable quantities of the relatively inactive metabolite dihydrodigoxin, which arises through bacterial biotransformation in the gut lumen.[113, 114] Renal excretion of digoxin is proportional to glomerular filtration rate (and hence to creatinine clearance) and is largely independent of rate of urine flow in patients with reasonably intact renal function.[110] In patients with prerenal azotemia, digoxin clearance was reported to correlate more closely with urea clearance than with creatinine clearance, suggesting that digoxin may undergo some degree of tubular reabsorption under these circumstances.[115] This point remains unsettled, however, and evidence for secretion of digoxin at the tubular level in humans has also been reported and appears to be more pronounced before puberty.[116] With daily maintenance therapy, a steady state is reached when daily losses are matched by daily intake. For patients not previously given digitalis, institution of daily maintenance therapy without a loading dose results in development of steady-state plateau concentrations after four to five half-lives, or about 7 days, in subjects with normal renal function.[117] If the half-life of the drug is prolonged, the length of time before a steady state is reached on a daily maintenance dose is prolonged accordingly. Because of the high degree of tissue binding of digoxin, the drug is not effectively removed from the body by dialysis.[118] Similarly, it has been shown that cardiopulmonary bypass[119] and exchange transfusion[120] remove only minor amounts of digoxin from the body. Serum digoxin levels and pharmacokinetics are essentially the same before and after the loss of large amounts of adipose tissue in massively obese subjects,[121] suggesting that lean body mass should be used when dosage is being calculated. Acute vasodilator therapy with nitroprusside or hydralazine tends to increase renal digoxin clearance without changing glomerular filtration rate, and may necessitate adjustment of maintenance digoxin dosage.[122]

Infants and children absorb and excrete digoxin in much the same way as adults do,[64] although recent evidence suggests that secretion at the renal tubular level may be quantitatively more important in prepubertal subjects.[116] Digoxin doses in neonates and infants are substantially larger than those in adults when calculated on the basis of milligrams per kilogram of body weight or per square meter of body surface area.[65] These higher doses result in relatively higher serum digoxin concentrations, which are generally well tolerated. Fetal umbilical-cord venous blood digoxin concentrations at term have been found to be similar to those in the venous blood of the mother maintained on digoxin, documenting transplacental passage of the drug.[64]

An important interaction between digoxin and quinidine has been described that leads to an approximately twofold increase in serum digoxin concentration when conventional quinidine doses are added to a standard maintenance digoxin regimen.[123] This increase is associated in some instances with the development of digoxin-toxic rhythm disturbances. A decrease in digoxin dosage, in addition to frequent assessment of serum digoxin concentration and clinical status, is advisable when quinidine is given concurrently. Interactions of digoxin with quinidine, verapamil, and amiodarone (among other drugs) are discussed on page 500.

DIGITOXIN. This glycoside is the least polar and most slowly excreted of the cardiac glycosides in common use. Since it constitutes the principal active agent in digitalis leaf, the two preparations can be considered together. Gastrointestinal absorption of digitoxin is a passive process and is thought to be essentially complete, although patients with malabsorption syndromes or other gastrointestinal diseases have not been studied extensively.

Digitoxin binds avidly to human serum albumin, and about 97 per cent of the serum or plasma content of the drug is bound to albumin at clinically relevant concentrations.[124] It therefore differs considerably in this respect from digoxin, which is only about 23 per cent bound to plasma proteins.[124] Renal clearance of the native compound is relatively minor compared with digoxin,[125] and extensive metabolism of digitoxin occurs, presumably in the liver. An enterohepatic cycle exists for digitoxin and can be interrupted by resins, such as cholestyramine, which bind digitoxin in the gut lumen.[126] A modest acceleration of the excretion of digitoxin has been documented in human subjects given cholestyramine,[126] but the clinical efficacy of this approach in patients with digitoxin intoxication remains to be proved. Digoxin is not ordinarily a quantitatively important metabolic product of digitoxin in man. It is of interest that drugs known to increase the activity of hepatic microsomal enzyme systems, such as phenobarbital and phenylbutazone, can accelerate the metabolism of digitoxin in some patients. Although digitoxin can be displaced from its serum albumin binding sites by high concentrations of other drugs, including phenylbutazone, warfarin, tolbutamide, sulfadimethoxine, and clofibrate, these effects are probably not of consequence at the plasma concentrations encountered in clinical use.[127]

Half-times of digitoxin in plasma appear to vary relatively little from patient to patient, with most studies reporting mean values in the range of 4 to 6 days irrespective of renal function, although estimates of as long as 8 days have been reported.[128] Administration of daily maintenance doses of digitoxin without a loading dose will result in gradual digitalization, with the 4- to 6-day half-life of the drug resulting in establishment of the final steady-state plateau after 3 to 4 weeks.

DESLANOSIDE (CEDILANID-D). This agent is structurally identical to digoxin except for the presence of an additional terminal glucose residue. This alteration results in poor gastrointestinal absorption, and thus the drug is recommended only for parenteral use. Its half-life is essentially identical to that of digoxin. Although its onset of action is somewhat more rapid, it probably enjoys no substantial advantages over parenteral use of digoxin unless rapidity of effect is an overriding consideration; however, if this is the case, ouabain may be preferable.

OUABAIN AND ACETYLSTROPHANTHIDIN. *Ouabain* is the most polar and rapidly acting of the cardiac glycosides currently available for routine clinical use. Like the other cardiac glycosides, its excretion from the body follows first-order pharmacokinetics, with a fixed proportion of the residual drug in the body being excreted each day. For ouabain, the plasma half-life in normal subjects is about 21 hours—similar to the half-life of positive inotropic effect and of ventricular rate slowing in patients with atrial fibrillation.[129] The quantity of ouabain in the body, and also the risk of toxicity, in a patient placed on a regular maintenance dosage schedule without a loading dose will continue to rise for four to five half-lives (4 to 5 days) until a plateau is reached. Impairment of renal function will prolong the half-life of ouabain and also the period during which accumulation will continue.

Although ouabain is predominantly excreted unchanged via the renal route, its gastrointestinal excretion is substantial after intravenous administration in both dog and man.[130] The drug appears to enter the gastrointestinal tract by pathways other than the biliary tract. In normal human subjects, urinary excretion accounted for an average of only 47 per cent of the intravenous dose. Ouabain is poorly absorbed from the gastrointestinal tract and is not available for oral use.

Acetylstrophanthidin, a rapidly acting synthetic C-3 acetyl ester of the aglycone strophanthidin, has been used in both experimental and clinical investigations but is available for clinical use only on an investigative basis. In human subjects, the principal exponential decline of plasma acetylstrophanthidin commences 10 to 30 minutes after intravenous infusion, and the mean half-life in plasma is 2.3 hours, in keeping with the known short duration of clinical effect. Urinary excretion averages only 22 per cent of the intravenous dose.[131]

Detailed reviews of cardiac glycoside pharmacokinetics and metabolism are available.[110, 111]

BIOAVAILABILITY

Three decades ago, Gold and his colleagues evaluated the relative efficacy of cardiac glycosides given by oral and parenteral routes. The ventricular rate of patients in atrial fibrillation was used as a quantitative indicator of digitalis effect.[107] Oral digoxin was found to be about two-thirds as effective in slowing the ventricular rate as an equivalent intravenous dose,[109] whereas digitoxin was almost equally effective when given by either route.[108] Thus, the bioavailability of digoxin as determined by this clinical bioassay was about 67 per cent, whereas that of digitoxin was nearly 100 per cent.

Subsequent studies have documented incomplete absorption of digoxin from the gastrointestinal tract.[132] Individual patient variation, circumstances of drug administration, and characteristics of the pharmaceutical preparation ingested are all known to affect digoxin bioavailability.[133] Patients with malabsorption syndromes may absorb digoxin poorly and erratically.[134] However, patients with maldigestion due to pancreatic insufficiency, despite comparable degrees of steatorrhea, appear to absorb the drug more normally. Administration of digoxin after meals is likely to decrease peak serum levels achieved, but total absorption is not affected to any noteworthy degree. Absorption of digoxin tends to be enhanced by drugs that decrease gastrointestinal motility and to be reduced by drugs that increase motility, particularly if the preparations have limited bioavailability. In addition, nonabsorbed substances, such as cholestyramine, colestipol, kaolin and pectin (Kaopectate), and nonabsorbable antacids, when taken concurrently can interfere with gastrointestinal absorption of digoxin; neomycin has also been shown to interfere with digoxin absorption. Because of previously documented variations in the bioavailability of commercially available digoxin preparations,[135] bioavailability specifications provided by the FDA and USP are currently in effect.[135, 136]

Biological availability uniformly approaching 100 per cent probably cannot be achieved with any oral digoxin preparation, but an encapsulated gel preparation is reported to have 90 to 100 per cent bioavailability. After intravenous administration of digoxin, 6-day urinary recovery by radioimmunoassay averaged 76 per cent of the administered dose. Intramuscular digoxin caused severe pain at the injection site, and bioavailability was only 83 per cent that of intravenous digoxin. Digoxin elixir was significantly more bioavailable (65 per cent of intravenous) than the tablet form studied (55 per cent of intravenous).[133]

Since the studies of Gold et al., oral absorption of digitoxin has generally been considered to be virtually 100 per cent, and no recent studies have cast doubt on that estimate. As with digoxin, binding to nonabsorbable substances such as cholestyramine can interfere with initial absorption.[136] Patients receiving such anion-exchange resins in addition to a cardiac glycoside should be instructed to ingest the cardiac glycoside two hours before the resin to minimize this effect.

CLINICAL USE OF DIGITALIS

A sound working knowledge of the pharmacokinetics of the commonly used cardiac glycosides is essential to the optimal use of these drugs. Computer programs and nomograms[137, 138] can provide initial approximations of optimal dose, but further dosage adjustments based on close clinical observation of the patient are often required. In many cases the variability in serum digoxin concentrations among different patients remains unexplained even after adjustments for dose, body size, and renal function have been made and measurement of digoxin concentrations and their use for feedback dosage adjustments have been suggested.[139]

The clinical use of cardiac glycosides is complicated by the absence of a readily measurable therapeutic objective (except in certain atrial arrhythmias), the lack of reliable means to predict individual cardiac responses, and the difficulty in defining proximity to toxicity.[140]

CONGESTIVE HEART FAILURE. Cardiac glycosides are of potential value in most patients with symptoms and signs of *congestive heart failure* due to ischemic, valvular, hypertensive, or congenital heart disease, dilated cardiomyopathies, and cor pulmonale. Improvement of depressed myocardial contractility increases cardiac output, promotes diuresis, and reduces the filling pressure of the failing ventricle(s), with consequent reduction of pulmonary vascular congestion and central venous pressure.

As previously noted, digitalis is of no demonstrable benefit in isolated *mitral stenosis* with normal sinus rhythm unless right ventricular failure has supervened. Similarly, little benefit may result in patients with *pericardial tamponade* or *constrictive pericarditis* except when there is invasion of the myocardium in the latter. Hypertrophic obstructive cardiomyopathy represents another process in which digitalis is often of little value and may actually be deleterious because it can increase left ventricular outflow obstruction by augmenting the contractility of the hypertrophic outflow-tract segment. It is our impression that patients with left ventricular hypertrophy and well-preserved left ventricular ejection fractions, even in the presence of symptoms related to elevated filling pressures, benefit little from digitalis. In the later stages of hypertrophic cardiomyopathy, in which ventricular dilation and congestive problems may predominate over obstructive ones, cardiac glycosides may be beneficial. Patients who develop congestive heart failure in response to a specific precipitating stress (p. 474) may benefit from temporary use of digitalis but will not necessarily require long-term maintenance digitalization. The risk-to-benefit ratio must be reassessed with any change in clinical status and will often be found to favor discontinuation of digitalis when an acute stress such as infection, anemia, or thyrotoxicosis is no longer present.

Digitalis glycosides may improve symptoms of angina pectoris when it coexists with cardiomegaly and congestive heart failure. As discussed subsequently, however, an increase in angina may occur unless the tendency toward increased oxygen consumption is offset by decreased ventricular size and wall tension.

Prophylactic digitalization of the patient with diminished cardiac reserve about to undergo a major stress such as surgery remains controversial (p. 1699). In the absence of obvious cardiomegaly or other evidence of overt congestive heart failure, most clinicians prefer to withhold digitalis until a specific indication arises. Prophylactic digitalization has been recommended for patients undergoing aortocoronary bypass surgery on the basis of a significant reduction in supraventricular arrhythmias.[141] Evidence of a difference in ultimate outcome between digitalized and nondigitalized patients was not documented, however, and another study of 140 consecutive patients undergoing myocardial revascularization showed a *higher* incidence of supraventricular tachyarrhythmias in patients receiving prophylactic digitalis.[142]

The availability of reliable pervenous catheter endocardial pacing techniques has helped to resolve the problem of digitalis use in patients with marginal atrioventricular conduction or established atrioventricular block. One can now carry out pacemaker implantation at minimal risk even in severely ill patients and then give digitalis without fear of aggravating conduction problems.

Clinical use of cardiac glycosides in congestive heart failure has been considered in further detail by Marsh and Smith.[143]

ARRHYTHMIAS (See also Chap. 23 and reference 144). Digitalis is of potential use in the management of four types of supraventricular tachyarrhythmias.

1. *Paroxysmal supraventricular tachycardia* (p. 680), whether of atrial or atrioventricular junctional origin, usually responds to digitalization when simpler measures such as carotid sinus pressure alone have failed. Many clinicians now prefer to use verapamil as the drug of first choice in this clinical setting (p. 682). When digitalis is used, carotid sinus pressure should be repeated during the course of digitalization, since the combination of partial digitalization and carotid sinus pressure will often succeed when neither measure alone suffices. Maintenance digitalization usually abolishes or reduces the frequency of recurrent attacks. Use of digitalis in the setting of paroxysmal supraventricular tachycardia demands that digitalis intoxication be excluded as a cause of the arrhythmia.

2. *Atrial fibrillation* with a rapid ventricular response is one of the most common indications for the use of digitalis. Both vagal and direct mechanisms result in increased blockade of impulses arriving at the atrioventricular junction, with slowing of the ventricular rate. Conversion to normal sinus rhythm may occur in the course of digitalization. There is a growing consensus that digitalis often is insufficiently effective in controlling the ventricular rate in atrial fibrillation when used alone.[145,146] Addition of beta-adrenoceptor blocking agents or verapamil[147] may be useful in circumstances in which the ventricular rate is difficult to control without the emergence of toxic symptoms (e.g., untreated thyrotoxicosis) and congestive heart failure is absent or minimal.

3. *Atrial flutter,* usually accompanied by 2:1 atrioventricular block in untreated cases, can often be managed with digitalis in doses sufficient to produce a degree of atrioventricular blockade that results in a ventricular rate in the range of 70 to 100/min. This effect may require doses considerably in excess of the usual range. As in atrial fibrillation, when the arrhythmia is poorly tolerated by the patient, it is often advisable to attempt direct-current cardioversion before administration of doses of digitalis that would render the procedure hazardous.

4. *Wolff-Parkinson-White syndrome* tachyarrhythmias (p. 686) may be terminated or prevented by digitalis in cases in which preferential effects on conduction or refractoriness in the normal or anomalous conduction pathways result in interruption of the reentrant circus movement. Other antiarrhythmic drugs may be more effective in other cases. Digitalis exerts a variety of electrophysiological effects in patients with Wolff-Parkinson-White syndrome, the sum of which renders these drugs potentially hazardous in patients with a history of atrial fibrillation or flutter. Sellers et al. concluded on the basis of detailed electrophysiological studies of responses to digoxin in 21 patients that no a priori prediction about the effect of digitalis on the antegrade conduction of accessory pathways can be made, suggesting that formal electrophysiological studies are indicated in many of these patients to predict their response to maintenance digoxin therapy.[148] Potential hazards of digitalis use in patients with the syndrome and episodes of atrial fibrillation are discussed further on page 691. While digoxin has been shown to reduce ventricular ectopic beats in some studies,[148a] there is no evidence that digoxin is useful generally in the management of high-grade ventricular arrhythmias.

DOSAGE SCHEDULES

Specific recommendations for digoxin dosage have been developed on the basis of the pharmacokinetic principles previously discussed. Usually there is no reason to use a loading dose far in excess of what the steady-state body content will be with the usual maintenance dose. Patients with entirely normal renal function who excrete 37 per cent of the digoxin in their bodies each day will, on a maintenance dose of 0.25 or 0.50 mg/day, have a steady-state total body content of about 0.67 or 1.35 mg, respectively. If a reasonable estimation of 75 per cent absorption of the tablet form of digoxin is made, estimates for the oral loading dose are about 0.9 and 1.8 mg, respectively, corresponding to maintenance doses of 0.25 and 0.50 mg/day. This amount can be given over a period of a day or so in several increments, or the same level of digitalization can be achieved over a period of about a week in a patient with normal renal function by administration of the daily maintenance dose without any loading dose. The latter procedure is often preferable in outpatient practice. It must be remembered, however, that severe renal impairment will prolong the half-life of digoxin to a maximum of about 4.4 days and hence extend the period required to reach a steady-state plateau to a maximum of about 3 weeks. Lean body mass should be considered in selection of both loading and maintenance digoxin doses. In adult patients with cardiac disease, initial intravenous loading doses of about 0.50 to 0.75 mg/45 kg (100 lb) of body weight, given in increments, are unlikely to cause toxicity and can be supplemented by further increments if indicated by the clinical course.

The maintenance digoxin dose required to replace daily losses will vary from about 37 per cent of the total body content in patients with normal renal function to nonrenal losses averaging about 14 per cent in patients who are essentially anephric. Between the extremes of normal renal function and no renal function, digoxin excretion is linearly related to glomerular filtration rate or creatinine clearance (C_{Cr}). A reasonable approximation of daily percentage of loss of digoxin is as follows[149]:

$$14 + \frac{C_{Cr} \text{ in ml/min}}{5}$$

Since accurate creatinine clearance values will often not be immediately available, one can use the following estimate based on a stable serum creatinine in mg/100 ml, abbreviated as c:

$$C_{Cr} \text{ (men)} = \frac{100}{c} - 12$$

and

$$C_{Cr} \text{ (women)} = \frac{80}{c} - 7$$

These expressions can be combined so that

$$\% \text{ daily loss (men)} = 11.6 + \frac{20}{c}$$

and

$$\% \text{ daily loss (women)} = 12.6 + \frac{16}{c}$$

The daily maintenance digoxin dose is intended to replace daily losses after an appropriate loading dose, so that the above value for daily percentage of loss multiplied by the loading dose that produced a satisfactory therapeutic response gives a reasonable initial approximation of the proper daily maintenance dose. Jelliffe and Brooker have developed a useful nomogram for digoxin therapy that takes into account body weight and renal function and provides guidelines for determining both loading and maintenance doses.[138]

The recommended oral loading dose of digoxin, based on *lean body weight* and administered in the form of digoxin elixir, is 25 to 35 μg/kg for full-term infants; 35 to 60 μg/kg for infants from 1 to 24 months; 30 to 40 μg/kg for ages 2 to 5 years; 20 to 35 μg/kg for 5 to 10 years; and 10 to 15 μg/kg for children over 10 years. For premature infants a loading dose of 20 to 30 μg/kg is recommended. Daily maintenance doses *for patients with normal renal function* are estimated as 20 to 30 per cent of the oral loading dose for premature infants and as 25 to 35 per cent of the oral loading dose for full-term infants through children 10 years of age and older. Parenteral (intravenous) loading and maintenance dose recommendations are approximately 75 per cent of the oral dosages.[149] Hougen has recently reviewed in detail digoxin use in the young.[65]

For digitoxin, half-lives usually range within 20 per cent of a mean value of 4.8 days, and relatively little variation in the body pool would be expected among individual patients receiving a given maintenance dose of the drug. The average steady-state digitoxin pool in a patient receiving 0.1 mg/day is about 0.8 mg, and as with digoxin, there is usually no reason to give a loading dose substantially in excess of the expected steady-state body pool achieved with usual maintenance doses. A loading dose of about 0.010 to 0.012 mg/kg allows compensation for variations in body size. Gradual digitalization without a loading dose is feasible with digitoxin, but because four to five half-lives are required to reach the steady-state plateau, this will take 3 to 4 weeks.

Estimates of loading and maintenance doses based on the above considerations are average values intended only as initial approximations and in no way diminish the need for further adjustments based on frequent and careful observation of the patient.

THERAPEUTIC ENDPOINTS

In addressing the problem of defining the elusive state of optimal digitalization, one might begin by stating that it is not necessarily the largest dose that can be tolerated without emergence of overt toxicity. The ratio of toxicity to therapy for cardiac glycosides is small at best, and the availability of other measures of treating heart failure, particularly potent oral diuretics and vasodilators, usually obviates balancing therapy at the edge of toxicity. Electrocardiographic ST-segment and T-wave changes of "digitalis effect" are, unfortunately, limited indicators of the state of digitalization. The perils of depending on slowing of sinus tachycardia to gauge the adequacy of digitalis dosage are well known.

In patients with atrial flutter or fibrillation, control of the ventricular response provides a relatively straightforward endpoint. Failure of atropine or exercise to increase the ventricular response has been used as an additional indicator of "full digitalization" in such patients, but overly vigorous pursuit of this goal may result in unduly slow resting heart rates or other evidence of impending or overt toxicity.

When congestive heart failure is the indication for use of digitalis, it is helpful to remember that positive inotropy is a graded response that is appreciable at doses well short of "maximally tolerated doses." As already stated, available data suggest that further inotropic benefit may not occur clinically beyond serum digoxin levels in the 1.0 to 2.0 ng/ml range. Carotid sinus massage can provide useful bedside clues to impending digitalis excess. Rhythm disorders such as second-degree atrioventricular block, accelerated atrioventricular junctional rhythm, and ventricular premature beats or bigeminy may emerge in response to carotid sinus stimulation before they occur spontaneously.[150]

INDIVIDUAL SENSITIVITY TO DIGITALIS. It is considerably easier to calculate theoretical body pools of cardiac glycosides than to decide, at the bedside, when optimal digitalization has been achieved in an individual patient. A number of factors influencing individual sensitivity to cardiac glycosides are listed in Table 17–5. Changes in absorption or bioavailability increase the probability of

TABLE 17–5 FACTORS INFLUENCING INDIVIDUAL SENSITIVITY TO DIGITALIS

Type and severity of underlying cardiac disease
Serum electrolyte derangements
Hypokalemia or hyperkalemia
Hypomagnesemia
Hypercalcemia
Hyponatremia
Acid-base imbalance
Concomitant drug administration
Anesthetics
Catecholamines and sympathomimetics
Antiarrhythmic agents
Thyroid status
Renal function
Autonomic nervous system tone
Respiratory disease

suboptimal digitalization because of fluctuations that can occur on a supposedly fixed dosage regimen. Such changes are reflected by changes in serum glycoside concentrations, however, and do not represent an actual change in sensitivity to the drug's effects. Quite distinct from the clinical problem of variable bioavailability is the enhanced sensitivity to lower serum concentrations of cardiac glycosides noted in up to 10 to 15 per cent of patients.

ELECTROLYTE AND ACID-BASE DISTURBANCES. Disturbances of potassium homeostasis clearly influence the action of digitalis.[50] Myocardial concentrations of digoxin tend to decrease with increasing serum potassium concentration. Furthermore, hypokalemia has a primary arrhythmogenic effect, both decreasing the effective refractory period of Purkinje cells and shortening the coupling interval for ventricular premature beats.[151] Depression of atrioventricular nodal conduction can occur with both digitalis excess and either very low or extremely high levels of serum K^+.[62] Diuretic therapy, insulin administration or carbohydrate loading, renal disease, and acid-base disturbances must all be borne in mind as potential causes of clinically significant alterations in potassium homeostasis, which can, in turn, affect importantly the response to cardiac glycosides.

Disturbances in serum levels of other electrolytes may also influence myocardial sensitivity to digitalis, although less profoundly than K^+ concentration. Administration of Mg^{++} salts suppresses digitalis-induced arrhythmias and hypomagnesemia appears to predispose to digitalis toxicity.[152] There is some evidence that the digitalis-induced K^+ efflux from the myocardium is reduced by Mg^{++} salts.[153] Magnesium depletion may become clinically important with the chronic administration of diuretic agents[154] and with gastrointestinal disease, diabetes mellitus, or poor nutritional states. Moreover, in patients with congestive heart failure, significant depletion of total body Mg^{++} stores may occur owing to prolonged secondary aldosteronism. The clinical importance of Mg^{++} depletion in digitalis therapy remains unresolved,[155, 156] but appears to be a frequent occurrence.[157]

Elevated serum Ca^{++} levels increase ventricular automaticity, and this effect is at least additive to and perhaps synergistic with the effects of digitalis. In one early study, ventricular ectopic activity occurred at lower doses of ouabain in hypercalcemic patients.[158] Furthermore, patients with digitalis intoxication have been reported to respond successfully to calcium-chelating agents.[159] The clinician should be alert for the possibility of enhanced digitalis sensitivity when treating hypercalcemic patients or when administering calcium parenterally to digitalized patients.

The interactions of digitalis with acid-base disturbances are complex. Perturbations in potassium homeostasis that follow shifts in hydrogen ion concentration obviously will affect myocardial binding of cardiac glycosides and the development of digitalis-related arrhythmias, as will primary changes in serum K^+ concentration. Similarly, acid-base status will influence the serum levels of ionized Ca^{++}, with attendant effects on automaticity. Whether alkalosis itself, independent of these changes, increases sensitivity to digitalis is controversial. Acidosis independent of changes in $[K^+]$ does not appear to enhance sensitivity to the arrhythmogenic effects of digitalis[160] and may even render the myocardium more resistant to digitalis intoxication.[161]

DRUG INTERACTIONS. Concomitant drug administration may interact with the effects of digitalis through several mechanisms. Clinically important interactions are summarized in Table 17–6 from the valuable review of Marcus.[162] As noted above, certain drugs such as cholestyramine and neomycin may decrease oral absorption of digoxin, thereby altering the serum and myocardial levels ultimately achieved. In addition, nonabsorbable antacids and Kaopectate may have a similar effect in some patients.

Drugs that affect metabolism or excretion of various digitalis preparations will influence toxicity through variations in the levels of serum and myocardial digitalis achieved rather than through altered sensitivity to the action of the glycosides themselves. Quinidine reduces both the renal and nonrenal elimination of digoxin and also appears to decrease the apparent volume of distribution of this glycoside.[163] The net result is an increase in serum digoxin concentration that averages twofold in patients in whom conventional doses of quinidine are added to a maintenance digoxin regimen; unfortunately, individual responses to quinidine may vary substantially and close surveillance of clinical status (and, if possible, serum digoxin concentration) is needed to reduce the risk of precipitating overt digoxin toxicity. Preliminary studies of a possible interaction between digitoxin and quinidine have yielded conflicting results, and this issue remains unsettled. Procainamide and disopyramide do not appear to alter serum digoxin levels, but verapamil does increase serum digoxin concentration by decreasing volume of distribution and clearance of digoxin.[163] One report indicates that verapamil causes a mean 35 per cent rise in steady-state serum digitoxin levels.[164] Tiapamil can also increase serum digoxin levels,[165] and both short- and long-term amiodarone administration has been found to increase steady-state serum digoxin concentration.[166, 167] Nifedipine appears to produce no clinically significant change in digoxin disposition. Other newly introduced drugs will require close surveillance for interactions with cardiac glycosides.

Diuretic agents potentially enhance the occurrence of digitalis toxicity both by decreasing glomerular filtration rate and through a variety of electrolyte disturbances, including hypokalemia, hypomagnesemia, and (for thiazide diuretics) hypercalcemia. By counteracting the cardiac toxic manifestations of digitalis excess, concurrent administration of some antiarrhythmic agents may create the impression of a relative resistance to digitalis toxicity.

Several anesthetic agents are arrhythmogenic, and experimental studies suggest that this effect may be synergistic with digitalis enhancement of ventricular automaticity in the case of cyclopropane and succinylcholine. The profound systemic effects of general anesthesia introduce many variables that could affect digitalis sensitivity, thus

TABLE 17–6 PHARMACOKINETIC DRUG INTERACTIONS WITH DIGOXIN

Drug	Mechanism of Interaction: Effect on Digoxin	Mean Magnitude of Interaction*	Type of Study: Single-Dose Digoxin	Type of Study: Steady State	Suggested Intervention
Cholestyramine	Absorption of digoxin	↓ 25%		X	1) Give digoxin 8 hours before cholestyramine 2) Use solution or capsule form of digoxin
Antacids	Unclear	↓ 25%	X		Temporal separation of time of administration
Kaolin-pectate	Adsorption of digoxin	?	X		1) Give digoxin 2 hours before kaolin-pectate 2) ? Use solution or capsule form of digoxin
Bran	Adsorption of digoxin	↓ 20%	X		Temporal separation of time of administration
Neomycin	Unknown	↓ 28%	X		Increase dose of digoxin
Sulfasalazine		↓ 18%	X		
PAS		↓ 22%	X		
Erythromycin; Tetracycline (in <10% of subjects)	↑ Bioavailability by ↓ intestinal metabolism of digoxin by certain gut flora	↑ 43 to 116%		X	1) Measure serum digoxin concentration 2) Decrease digoxin dose 3) Use solution or capsule form of digoxin
Quinidine	? ↓ Bioavailability, ↓ volume of distribution, ↓ renal and nonrenal clearance	↑ 100%	X	X	1) Decrease dose by 50% 2) Measure serum digoxin concentration
Amiodarone	↓ Renal and nonrenal clearance	↑ 70 to 100%		X	Same as for quinidine
Verapamil	↓ Renal and nonrenal clearance	↑ 70 to 100%		X	Same as for quinidine
Diltiazem	? ↓ Renal clearance	Zero to ↑ 22%†		X	None
Nicardipine	Unknown	↑ 15%		X	None
Tiapamil	Unknown	↑ 60%		X	Same as for quinidine
Spironolactone	↓ Renal and nonrenal clearance	↑ 30%	X		Measure serum digoxin concentration
Triamterene	↓ Nonrenal clearance	↑ 20%	X		Measure serum digoxin concentration
Indomethacin (preterm infants)	? ↓ Renal clearance	↑ 50%		X	Decrease dose by 25%

*Alteration in bioavailability or serum concentration. For single dose studies, the magnitude of the anticipated change in serum digoxin concentration was estimated from pharmacokinetic data, particularly the change in total body clearance. ↑ = increased; ↓ = decreased; ? = questionable.

†Also see study of Elkayam, et al. 163a.

Adapted, with minor modification, from Marcus, F. I.: Pharmacokinetic interactions between digoxin and other drugs. J. Am. Coll. Cardiol., 5:82A–90A, 1985, where relevant references are found.

greatly complicating the detailed assessment of individual anesthetic agents. The interrelationships between catecholamines and sympathomimetic drugs and cardiac glycosides are intriguing but incompletely characterized. Experimental studies demonstrate that catecholamine-induced increases in ventricular automaticity can add to the arrhythmogenic effects of digitalis; however, detailed clinical correlation has not been forthcoming. It is reasonable for the clinician to assume that sympathomimetic agents increase the likelihood of enhanced automaticity of ectopic pacemakers in patients receiving digitalis.

Drug interactions with digitalis glycosides are considered in further detail elsewhere.[162, 163]

TYPE AND SEVERITY OF UNDERLYING HEART DISEASE

The effects of digitalis on the heart are modified by the type and severity of the underlying heart disease. This is dramatically demonstrated in otherwise healthy subjects who ingest massive doses of digitalis. Toxicity in such situations is frequently manifested by progressively diminished atrioventricular conduction or by sinoatrial exit block, rather than by enhanced automaticity and ventricular ectopic activity as seen in patients with underlying heart disease.[168, 169] In many patients with ischemic, myocardial, or valvular heart disease the effects of digitalis are superimposed on an electrophysiologically unstable condition with preexisting abnormalities of impulse formation and conduction. The more severe and advanced the heart disease, the more likely the occurrence of focal ischemia, myocardial fibrosis, and ventricular dilatation with stretching of Purkinje fibers and resultant tendency toward increased automaticity. The clinical observation that digitalis toxicity is particularly common in patients with amyloidosis involving the heart may be accounted for, at least in part, by digoxin binding by amyloid fibrils.[170]

DIGITALIS AND ISCHEMIC HEART DISEASE. The use of digitalis in patients with ischemic heart disease deserves special attention. In experiments employing an isolated canine cardiac preparation, it was shown that acetylstrophanthidin administration increased myocardial oxygen consumption in the normal heart, whereas consumption was decreased in the failing heart.[171] The increase in oxygen consumption in the normal heart can be explained by the increased velocity of contraction and increased wall tension. In the failing heart, decreased oxygen consumption can be explained by a decrease in left ventricular end-diastolic pressure, resulting in a reduction in end-diastolic volume and consequently, on the basis of the Laplace relation, a decline in intramyocardial tension.

Changes in oxygen consumption are always the net result of two opposing effects of digitalis: a potential reduction in wall tension and an increase in contractility. Thus, in the failing heart the net result depends on the balance of these effects, and either a diminution of oxygen consumption or no change may be observed. In the nonfailing heart, oxygen consumption increases with digitalis administration.[172] These considerations are of clinical importance when a decision must be made about whether to use digitalis in patients with coronary disease. Angina pectoris has been observed to improve after digitalization in patients with heart failure but occasionally to worsen in those who are well compensated. An objective study of the effect of ouabain on the response of the left ventricle in patients with angina pectoris showed that the depressed myocardial performance noted on exercise was improved by digitalization in the majority of patients studied.[173] Despite these beneficial effects on left ventricular performance, however, there was no consistent alteration in exercise tolerance or the pressure-rate product at which angina occurred. Other studies have demonstrated an increased cardiac output on exercise after digitalization, suggesting that the reduction in myocardial oxygen consumption that followed digitalis-induced improvement in left ventricular function probably masked any increase caused by its positive inotropic action.[174] No deterioration of myocardial metabolism with acute ouabain administration was found in patients with chronic coronary artery disease either at rest[175] or with pacing-induced myocardial ischemia.[176] Improved myocardial perfusion judged by means of thallium-201 scans was found in response to maintenance doses of digoxin in patients with coronary artery disease and left ventricular dysfunction.[177] The combination of propranolol and digoxin in patients with angina pectoris appears to be advantageous in the subgroup with angina pectoris and abnormal ventricular function or large hearts.[178]

There are still many unanswered questions concerning the role of digitalis therapy after acute myocardial infarction (Chap. 38). There is little to be gained from administration of the drug to patients who have uncomplicated infarction without cardiomegaly. There is limited clinical documentation of its value in cardiogenic shock, a syndrome in which no pharmacological agent has been demonstrated to be highly effective. Indeed, rapid digitalization may occasionally be harmful, owing to the vasoconstrictor properties of the drug. Small increases in cardiac index and stroke work as well as a reduction in left ventricular end-diastolic pressure have been observed after digitalization in patients with left ventricular failure following myocardial infarction.[179] Although ouabain did not alter cardiac output in another series of patients with acute myocardial infarction,[180] it caused significant improvement in other indices of left ventricular performance, such as end-diastolic pressure and stroke work. Similar benefits were noted in patients convalescing from myocardial infarction.[181]

The issue of increased susceptibility to the toxic effects of digitalis in recent or acute myocardial infarction remains controversial. In animal models, the dose of digitalis required to reach a toxic endpoint clearly is reduced after experimentally induced myocardial infarction.[182] However, in a study of patients with acute myocardial infarction, 89 per cent tolerated a full dose of acetylstrophanthidin, suggesting no significant enhancement of sensitivity to the drug.[140] In patients with acute myocardial infarction treated with intravenous digoxin using a double-blind randomized protocol, no difference in incidence of rhythm disturbances was found between digoxin-treated and control patients.[183] There appears to be no convincing evidence for an increased incidence of arrhythmias complicating digitalization in patients with acute infarction when serum levels do not exceed the conventional therapeutic range.[184]

The clearest indication for digitalis after acute myocardial infarction is in the treatment of atrial fibrillation with a rapid ventricular rate. Electrical cardioversion may be preferred in the treatment of other supraventricular tachyarrhythmias.[185]

Evidence based on a retrospective analysis by Moss et al.[186] suggests that mortality within the first 4 months after myocardial infarction may be increased in a high-risk subset of patients with congestive heart failure and ventricular arrhythmias. Bigger and colleagues also interpreted the results of an observational study of 504 post-myocardial infarction patients as suggesting that digitalis may have adverse effects on survival during follow-up.[187] However, four other studies demonstrated the expected increased mortality after myocardial infarction among patients treated with digoxin for chronic heart failure and/or supraventricular arrhythmias. It was concluded that the excess mortality could be accounted for by baseline prognostic variables without invoking any statistically significant independent effect of digoxin. This latter conclusion was reached by Ryan et al. from the CASS data base,[188] by Madsen et al. from an analysis of 1599 patients studied after infarction,[189] by Byington et al. from the BHAT data base,[190] and by Muller et al. based on clinical experience with patients enrolled in the MILIS study.[191] We believe that the available data do not support the assertion that digoxin therapy is excessively hazardous after infarction, but the existence of an undetected harmful effect can be excluded only with a randomized study. At present, we recommend a three-part approach: (1) careful consideration of whether any treatment of ventricular dysfunction is needed, (2) consideration of alternatives to digoxin therapy, and (3) restriction of digoxin use to the subgroup of patients with chronic congestive heart failure and a dilated left ventricle previously shown to benefit clinically.

In *summary*, current evidence indicates that digitalis has no well-defined role in the management of acute myocardial infarction without congestive heart failure or supraventricular tachyarrhythmias. Judicious patient selection, management of drug doses, and careful monitoring will minimize the potentially deleterious effects of digitalis in acute myocardial infarction.

ADVANCED AGE. Advanced age per se has been considered by some to be a risk factor in the development of digitalis toxicity because of an enhanced sensitivity to the drug.[192] However, diminished glomerular filtration rate with age will alone lead to prolonged half-life of digoxin and thus to increased serum levels and an increased probability of toxicity on a given dosage regimen. Advanced age is frequently associated with other factors that increase the likelihood of digitalis intoxication, including more severe heart disease; impairment of pulmonary, renal, and neurological function; and an increased number of concurrent medications.

RENAL FAILURE (See also p. 1843). Renal failure, particularly in patients requiring hemodialysis, is a disease state in which factors influencing digitalis absorption and elimination and rapid shifts of electrolytes profoundly affect the response to digitalis. The marked diminution of glomerular filtration rate with renal failure prolongs the half-life of digoxin and thus increases serum digoxin levels. Toxicity from this predictable response can be avoided by careful and frequent adjustments of dosage to correlate with the level of renal function present. Less predictably, dialysis can cause at least a transient decrease in serum potassium that will increase the tendency toward digitalis-induced arrhythmias. Depending on the magnesium content of the dialysate and the use of magnesium-containing antacids by the patient, there may be significant aberrations of serum magnesium levels in patients on dialysis.[156] Some evidence suggests that increased serum levels of digoxin may reflect a decreased volume of distribution in renal failure.[193] The clinician is well advised to use the minimum drug dosage that produces the desired clinical effect in this condition noted for its extreme fluctuations in fluid and electrolyte balance.

THYROID DISEASE. It is well known that thyroid disease alters digitalis pharmacokinetics. In hypothyroid patients the serum digoxin half-life is consistently prolonged, while in those with hyperthyroidism serum digoxin levels tend to be decreased.[194] Since some studies have not documented significant changes in metabolism or serum half-life of digoxin in hyperthyroid patients, it has been suggested that an increased distribution space for digoxin may exist. This hypothesis is of interest in light of experimental findings indicating higher levels of Na^+, K^+-ATPase activity in the myocardium[195] and other tissues of hyperthyroid animals.[196] We have documented increased tolerance to cardiac glycosides in heart cells grown in culture in the presence of high thyroid hormone concentrations, associated with an increased number of Na^+, K^+-ATPase sites and enhanced monovalent cation transport capacity.[197] In any event, the apparent resistance or sensitivity to digitalis in thyroid disease probably depends on changes in target organ responsiveness as well as in the pharmacokinetics of digoxin. Changes in the response of the heart to a given serum level of drug (for example, the difficulty in controlling the ventricular response in patients with thyrotoxicosis and atrial fibrillation) have not been well defined in the clinical setting. As discussed previously, autonomic neural influences on the effect of digitalis on the heart have long been appreciated. Such changes in autonomic tone may contribute to the apparent resistance to digitalis effect seen in thyrotoxicosis.

PULMONARY DISEASE. There has been considerable interest in the use of digitalis in patients with pulmonary disease.[198] A number of authors have noted that ventricular ectopic activity consistent with digitalis toxicity frequently occurs in patients with respiratory disease who are receiving digitalis.[199] Such reports are difficult to interpret, however, because respiratory failure and hypoxemia frequently provoke arrhythmias indistinguishable from those associated with digitalis excess.[200] A population of 931 patients admitted consecutively to a medical service and studied prospectively demonstrated an increased incidence of rhythm disturbances consistent with digitalis toxicity among patients with acute or chronic lung disease.[201] Excessive sensitivity to digitalis in patients with pulmonary disease generally correlates with overt cor pulmonale, hypercapnia, and hypoxemia. These findings are corroborated by the relatively frequent discordance between serum digoxin levels and tolerance to acetylstrophanthidin in patients with pulmonary disease.

The degree of hypoxemia may, however, be an index of the severity of the respiratory failure and its associated physiological derangements rather than a factor that by itself is causally related to digitalis sensitivity. Although not adequately subdivided into acute or chronic respiratory illnesses, the available epidemiological data suggest that patients with stable chronic lung disease are at increased risk of developing digitalis intoxication. Particularly as a result of diuretic therapy, these patients are subject to derangements in potassium homeostasis and the development of metabolic alkalosis—both predisposing to digitalis toxicity. What role exogenous catecholamines and the sympathomimetic agents commonly used in the therapy of chronic airway disease may have in the development of digitalis-related arrhythmias is not known. No published studies have shown convincing enhancement of ventricular ectopic activity in patients receiving catecholamines by inhalation in either the presence or the absence of digitalis.

From the data available, then, it is reasonable for the clinician to assume that patients with a variety of pulmonary diseases may be sensitive to the arrhythmogenic effects of digitalis at relatively low serum concentrations.

Further discussion of factors affecting individual tolerance to digitalis may be found in the review by Surawicz.[202]

SERUM OR PLASMA CONCENTRATIONS OF DIGITALIS GLYCOSIDES

It has long been apparent clinically that alterations in cardiac rhythm as well as extracardiac manifestations of digitalis action, such as gastrointestinal and central nervous system symptoms, are dose-related.[203] It has now been demonstrated convincingly in a number of studies that plasma digitalis concentrations are also correlated with the amount of drug administered. One would therefore expect that a correlation would exist between plasma digitalis concentration and the symptoms and signs of toxicity. In both animal and human studies, after attainment of equilibrium, a relatively constant ratio of plasma to myocardial digoxin concentration has been observed,[204, 205] although not all the digoxin present in myocardium is bound to specific receptors relevant to the pharmacological action of the drug. As discussed earlier, the available evidence that digitalis glycosides act on Na^+, K^+-ATPase sites at the cell surface suggests that digitalis concentration at these receptor sites would be influenced readily by the concentration in plasma. Animal experiments have confirmed the expected relation between plasma digoxin concentrations and electrophysiological effects on the heart.[206]

The availability of methods for measuring serum or plasma digitalis concentrations* in the clinical laboratory has led to extensive studies concerning the relation between serum levels and manifestations of toxicity in man.[60] Methods practically applicable to evaluation of patient serum samples are based on physicochemical separation, inhibition of Na^+, K^+-ATPase or its transmembrane cation transport function, or competitive protein binding employing either a specific antibody or a preparation containing Na^+, K^+-ATPase. Available methods are discussed in detail elsewhere.[207]

RADIOIMMUNOASSAY. Most published clinical studies have employed specific antibody as the binding protein in a competitive binding assay. This procedure is readily adaptable to the clinical laboratory. Small volumes of serum or plasma may be used directly, without prior extraction, necessitating a minimal number of manipulations. Appropriately selected antisera have exceptionally high degrees of affinity and specificity for the cardiac glycoside of interest, allowing the measurement of subnanogram amounts. However, as with other radioimmunoassays, these are subject to certain pitfalls that may cause erroneous results if careful attention is not paid to selection of antisera, assurance of purity of standards and tracers, and appropriate counting techniques.

Further details of available techniques for measurement of circulating cardiac glycoside concentrations are provided

*Serum and plasma digoxin, digitoxin, and ouabain concentrations are equivalent and will hereafter be referred to as serum concentrations.

in reviews of this subject. With the proliferation of commercial kits for measuring cardiac glycoside concentrations, it is particularly important for the clinician and clinical investigator to be certain that the values reported by the laboratory are accurate. Moreover, uncertainty can be introduced if sufficient time has not elapsed since the last previous dose to allow full equilibration of the drug between intravascular and peripheral compartments. In practice, a safe time for sampling of serum or plasma is 6 hours or more after the last dose of the cardiac glycoside.

CLINICAL CORRELATIONS. Although several techniques have been used to measure the concentrations of digoxin and digitoxin, there is substantial agreement regarding these values in patients receiving usual maintenance doses of these drugs. Mean serum or plasma digoxin concentrations in groups of patients without evidence of toxicity average about 1.4 ng/ml. As would be expected, increasing digoxin doses or decreasing renal function is correlated with higher mean serum levels. Mean serum digoxin concentrations tend to be two to three times higher in patients with clinical evidence of digoxin toxicity, and the difference in mean levels is statistically significant in the vast majority of studies.[208] It must be emphasized that overlap of levels between groups with and without evidence of toxicity has been observed in most series and tends to be more pronounced in prospective, blind studies than in retrospective studies.[191] Despite this overlap, use of serum digoxin concentration measurements to guide therapy has been associated with a reduction in the incidence of digitalis toxicity.[209]

Analogous data correlating serum digitoxin concentrations with clinical state[50] indicate that although levels average about 10 times higher than those of digoxin because of digitoxin binding to serum proteins, patients with clinical evidence of toxicity again have mean levels about two times higher than those without evidence of a toxic response. As in the case of digoxin, substantial overlap in levels occurs among groups of patients with and without evidence of toxicity despite the statistically significant differences in mean serum concentrations.

Although cardiac digitalis toxicity is accompanied by relatively well-defined relations between rhythm disturbance and serum glycoside concentration, it is more difficult to correlate therapeutic effects with serum levels in humans. A general correlation (albeit not overly close) has been reported between plasma digoxin levels and slowing of previously rapid ventricular rates in patients with atrial fibrillation.[210] Another measure of the degree of digitalization is the cumulative dose of acetylstrophanthidin required to reach a toxic endpoint.[211] Substantial variation in acetylstrophanthidin sensitivity was demonstrated among individual patients at any given serum digoxin level, indicating a continuing need to correlate serum digoxin concentration with other, independent methods of assessing myocardial sensitivity to cardiac glycosides.

The multifactorial determinants of digitalis intoxication and the overlap in serum digitalis concentrations between toxic and nontoxic states preclude the use of these levels as a sole guide to digitalis dosage. A Bayesian approach (p. 235) to the use of serum digoxin levels in clinical decision-making is logical and theoretically attractive.[212] Serum levels considered within a particular clinical context together with other available information can be a valuable aid to therapeutic decision-making. Suspected manifestations of digitalis intoxication in the absence of an adequate history, fluctuating renal function, presence of overt or suspected malabsorption, and use of preparations of uncertain bioavailability are among the circumstances in which knowledge of the serum level is most helpful. More generally, it is our opinion that measurement of serum cardiac glycoside concentrations is indicated whenever an unanticipated response to these drugs (either suspected toxicity or absence of an expected therapeutic effect) is encountered.

DIGITALIS TOXICITY

Toxic manifestations of digitalis persist as one of the most prevalent adverse drug reactions encountered in clinical practice.[50, 201] The true incidence is difficult to determine accurately but at present is probably in the range of 5 to 15 per cent in hospitalized patients receiving these drugs. The variability in available estimates relates to differing definitions of digitalis intoxication, the retrospective nature of many studies, and differences in the groups under study. In a prospective investigation of 931 consecutive admissions to a single medical facility, 23 per cent of the digitalized patients fulfilled criteria for definite digitalis toxicity and another 6 per cent were judged to be possibly toxic.[201] Other prospective studies have reported a comparable incidence of toxicity.[50] There is evidence that increased understanding of pharmacokinetics and the use of serum level data to guide therapy have reduced this alarming incidence,[209] but constant vigilance on the part of the physician is required.

MECHANISMS OF DIGITALIS INTOXICATION

(See also p. 217)

The major manifestations of digitalis intoxication include gastrointestinal and central nervous system symptoms and disturbances of cardiac rhythm. Anorexia, nausea, and vomiting are mediated by chemoreceptors located in the area postrema of the medulla rather than by a direct irritant effect of the drug on the gastrointestinal tract.[213] The precise mechanism underlying this and other central nervous system effects remains unclear, but studies have demonstrated the presence of digoxin in the cerebrospinal fluid of patients treated with this drug.[214] Therefore, the drug clearly penetrates the blood-brain barrier in appreciable amounts and may, in addition, exert effects in regions that lack a normal blood-brain barrier, such as the area postrema of the medulla.[68, 215]

The genesis of cardiac arrhythmias depends, at least in part, on the effect of the drug on the electrical activity of cardiac cells. Digitalis-induced disturbances of impulse formation and conduction are conventionally explained in terms of alterations in refractory period, impulse transmission, and automaticity of cardiac tissues, although alterations in sympathetic activity and changes in vagal tone may also be of considerable importance in some situations, as discussed previously. Interesting data have been obtained from experiments in which isolated canine Purkinje fibers were perfused with the blood of intact donor dogs and ouabain-induced changes in the donor dog's electrocardiogram were correlated with changes in the Purkinje fiber transmembrane potential[216, 217] (Fig. 17–6). At the time of onset of early ouabain toxicity in the donor dog, defined as junctional or ventricular premature contractions or junctional tachycardia, Purkinje fiber recordings showed decreases in action-potential amplitude, resting membrane potential, maximum velocity of the upstroke of the action potential, action-potential duration, and plateau phase. Slowing of conduction was also apparent, often varying in extent from cycle to cycle. With further progression of toxicity to ventricular tachycardia in the donor dog, changes in transmembrane potential became still more marked, as shown in Figure 17–6.

In additional experiments, increased automaticity was found to occur at the time of early toxicity at plasma potassium concentrations below 4 mEq/liter. Increased automaticity was more frequent when Purkinje fibers had been stretched and in the presence of hypokalemia, which correlates well with clinical observations of increased frequency of digitalis toxicity in the dilated failing heart as well as in the presence of hypokalemia. Additional evidence bearing on the particular sensitivity of Purkinje fibers to the toxic electrophysiological effects of digitalis comes from studies showing greater effects of acute and chronic digoxin administration on monovalent cation transport in Purkinje fibers compared with adjacent working myocardium.[35]

Regarding the cellular mechanism of digitalis toxicity, until relatively recently most investigators favored a sequence in which digitalis-induced inhibition of Na^+ and K^+ transport caused increased intracellular $[Na^+]$, decreased intracellular $[K^+]$, and gradual depolarization.

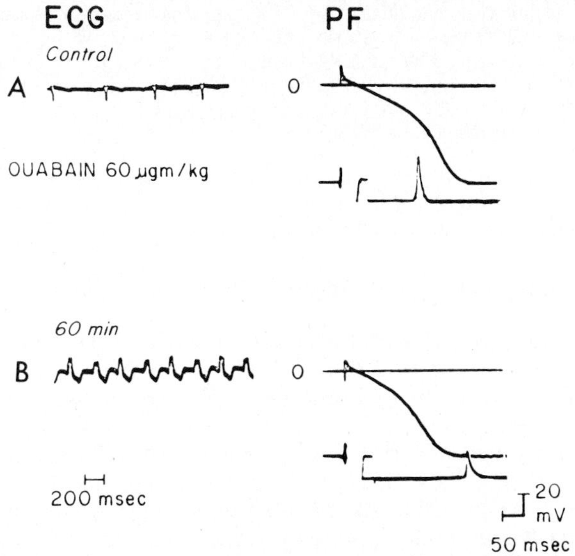

FIGURE 17–6. Effects of ouabain on the electrocardiogram (ECG) of an intact donor dog and on the Purkinje fiber (PF) action potential of an isolated preparation perfused with blood from the donor dog. Sinus rhythm (panel A) is succeeded by ventricular tachycardia (panel B) 60 minutes after administration of a toxic dose of ouabain. At the onset of ventricular tachycardia, the Purkinje fiber action potential shows significant loss of amplitude, duration, and maximum velocity of the phase 0 upstroke. The lower trace in each PF panel shows the first derivative of voltage with respect to time during phase 0. (From Rosen, M. R., et al.: Correlation between effects of ouabain on the canine electrocardiogram and transmembrane potentials of isolated Purkinje fibers. Circulation *47*:65, 1973, by permission of the American Heart Association, Inc.)

This in turn led to increased automaticity, conduction disturbances, and finally inexcitability. Subsequent experimental evidence suggests that cardiac glycosides promote a hitherto unrecognized mechanism of spontaneous activity in specialized cardiac conducting tissue. The underlying cellular event is a depolarizing afterpotential that has been variously called "enhanced diastolic depolarization,"[218] "low-amplitude potential,"[219] "transient depolarization,"[220] or "oscillatory afterpotentials," shown in Figure 17–7. In panel A, a transient depolarization follows a train of six action potentials. It falls short of threshold in this instance but can influence conduction of subsequent impulses.[221] With increased driving frequency, as shown in panel B, the transient depolarization reaches threshold, and excitation occurs. The counterpart of this event in the intact heart would be a ventricular premature beat. Panels C and D show multiple repetitive responses to further increases in driving frequency, which may be analogous to the beat dependence of digitalis-induced ectopic activity in intact hearts of experimental animals.[222] The recent review of Rosen provides additional useful discussion and references.[57]

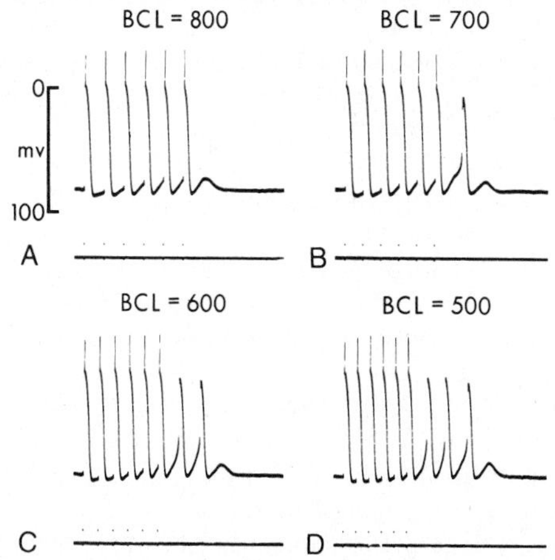

FIGURE 17–7. Sequential development (*A* and *D*) of a train of spontaneous beats due to transient depolarizations (also called oscillatory afterpotentials) in a canine Purkinje fiber exposed to acetylstrophanthidin and then driven at varying basic cycle lengths (BCL), indicated in milliseconds at the top of each panel. (From Ferrier, G. R., et al.: A cellular mechanism for the generation of ventricular arrhythmias by acetylstrophanthidin. Circ. Res. *32*:600, 1973, by permission of the American Heart Association, Inc.)

The cellular mechanism underlying the transient depolarization phenomenon has been studied using voltage-clamp techniques[223] and more recently by the addition of the calcium-sensitive photoluminescent protein aequorin (see Fig. 17–4). A transient inward current closely related to transient depolarizations was observed in response to cardiotonic steroids and was temporally coincident with phasic increases in tension ("aftercontraction").[22, 224] Further evidence supports the view that elevated levels of free intracellular calcium are a crucial factor,[22, 224, 225] just as has been discussed earlier with respect to the mechanism of positive inotropic action of digitalis. The mechanism involved in the generation of digitalis-induced transient depolarizations clearly differs both from that underlying normal phase 4 spontaneous depolarization and from the slow inward current.[226]

Potential or overt toxic effects of digitalis on electrophysiology of the intact heart will now be briefly summarized; additional references may be found in a recent review.[50]

SINUS NODE AND ATRIUM. Digitalis-induced slowing of the sinus rate in patients without congestive heart failure is usually minor in degree and is largely mediated by vagal effects on the sinoatrial node. Patients with transplanted, denervated hearts do not respond to conventional doses of digoxin with any change in sinus rate.[59] As far as direct effects of digitalis are concerned, the atrium seems more sensitive than the sinus node. Experimentally, at higher doses, there is a depression in sinus node automaticity. A combination of vagal and direct effects on the sinus node probably contributes to sinus bradycardia as well as to occasional cases of sinoatrial arrest or exit block seen in digitalis intoxication. This bradycardia predisposes to the emergence of junctional ventricular escape rhythms.

Digitalis, even in therapeutic doses, can impair sinoatrial conduction. Although usually well tolerated in patients with sick sinus syndrome, occasionally sinus node dysfunction is precipitated by digoxin, even in doses not usually associated with toxicity. Digitalis shortens the refractory period of the atrial myocardium in experimental studies, but has relatively minor and variable effects in the human heart.[62]

ATRIOVENTRICULAR NODE. The effective refractory period of the atrioventricular node is prolonged by digitalis. As with the sinus node, this longer period is in part related to increased vagal activity and in part to direct action on nodal fibers, although the vagal effect appears to predominate in subjects without intrinsic diseases of the cardiac conduction system.[168]

The therapeutic effect of digitalis in slowing ventricular response in atrial flutter or fibrillation depends in part on the entry of concealed atrial impulses into the atrioventricular node, with failure to reach the His-Purkinje system by virtue of decremental conduction within the node (p. 600). When atrioventricular block of second or third degree occurs as a result of digitalis intoxication, however, the principal mechanism is failure of propagation within the atrioventricular node.

HIS-PURKINJE SYSTEM. Digitalis-induced increases in the automaticity of the His-Purkinje system may come about because of enhanced spontaneous diastolic (phase 4) depolarization or the more recently described transient depolarization mechanism discussed above and elsewhere.[220] The appearance of new pacemakers is manifest clinically by premature junctional or ventricular beats or by accelerated junctional or ventricular rhythms. The nonuniform effect of digitalis on ventricular and Purkinje fibers and simultaneous enhancement of automaticity, depression of conduction velocity, and local block may also predispose to arrhythmias based on reentry mechanisms that may progress to ventricular tachycardia and fibrillation.

CLINICAL MANIFESTATIONS

GASTROINTESTINAL SYMPTOMS. Anorexia is often an early manifestation of digitalis intoxication.[201] Nausea and vomiting follow as clear consequences of digitalis overdose and result from central nervous system mechanisms.[213] It may be difficult, in clinical situations, to attribute these symptoms to digitalis, since they may also be caused by cardiac failure or by associated illnesses.

NEUROLOGICAL SYMPTOMS. These include headache, fatigue, malaise, neuralgic pain, disorientation, confusion, delirium, and seizures. Visual symptoms are not infrequent and include scotomas, flickering, halos, and changes in color perception.[227, 228] As with gastrointestinal symptoms, it is often difficult to determine whether neurological symptoms are a consequence of digitalis excess, associated fluid and electrolyte disturbances, or associated illnesses.

CARDIAC TOXICITY (See also pp. 217 to 219). Cardiac toxicity manifested by arrhythmias can take the form of essentially every known rhythm disturbance.[50] Common arrhythmias include atrioventricular junctional escape rhythms, ventricular bigeminy or trigeminy, nonparoxysmal atrioventricular junctional tachycardia, unifocal or multifocal ectopic ventricular beats, and ventricular tachycardia. Atrioventricular junctional exit block, paroxysmal atrial tachycardia with atrioventricular block, sinus arrest, and Mobitz type I (Wenckebach) second-degree atrioventricular block also occur. This list should not be considered exhaustive. There are no unequivocal electrocardiographic features that distinguish digitalis-toxic rhythm disturbances from rhythms due to intrinsic cardiac disease, although rhythms combining features of increased automaticity of ectopic pacemakers with impaired conduction, such as paroxysmal atrial tachycardia with atrioventricular dissociation and an accelerated atrioventricular junctional pacemaker, strongly suggest digitalis toxicity. However, even rhythms such as atrial tachycardia with AV block, considered typical of digitalis toxicity, are frequently due to underlying heart disease rather than to digitalis excess.[229] The difficulty in determining whether or not ventricular ectopic activity is due to digitalis excess is exemplified by a study in which 142 patients with this rhythm disturbance, most of whom were on maintenance digoxin doses, were given incremental doses of the rapidly acting agent acetylstrophanthidin to determine their response.[230] Frequency of ventricular premature beats decreased in 46 per cent of patients, remained unchanged in 26 per cent, and increased in 28 per cent in response to the additional doses of digitalis. The cause of an arrhythmia may at times be clarified (but not defined with complete certainty) by demonstration of a reversion to normal rhythm when the drug is withheld. Clinical and electrocardiographic findings associated with digitalis toxicity have been reviewed extensively.[231–233]

OTHER MANIFESTATIONS. Allergic skin lesions are rare but have been reported.[234] Gynecomastia is occasionally induced in men,[235] and sexual dysfunction has been reported.[236]

MASSIVE CARDIAC GLYCOSIDE OVERDOSE

Digitalis overdose, either suicidal or accidental, is occasionally encountered as a life-threatening problem.[168, 169, 237] Patients without underlying heart disease tend to tolerate large doses, with serum digoxin concentrations ranging as high as 10 to 15 ng/ml.

The principal manifestations in patients without intrinsic heart disease are most often sinus bradycardia; atrioventricular block of first, second, or third degree; or sinoatrial exit block. Atropine alone is often successful in reversing these manifestations but is not invariably effective.[50] Ventricular pacing with a pervenous endocardial catheter electrode is usually successful, although ventricular standstill unresponsive to pacing has been reported.[168]

The condition in patients with preexisting heart disease tends to be more difficult to manage, in that ectopic ventricular arrhythmias are frequently the initial manifestation of digitalis intoxication. Phenytoin, lidocaine, procainamide, and potassium have been used in treatment.[238] Direct-current cardioversion may also be required for refractory, life-threatening supraventricular or ventricular tachycardia or for ventricular fibrillation, despite the known hazards of this therapeutic modality in patients with digitalis toxicity. Not infrequently, the ventricular arrhythmias in this group lead to a fatal outcome despite the most vigorous therapeutic efforts.

Refractory hyperkalemia can occur at extremely high digoxin doses and serum concentrations.[191, 238, 238a] Greater elevations of serum K^+ concentration were associated with worsening prognosis in a large series of patients after massive doses, usually of digitoxin.[239] Elevation of serum potassium is a consequence of inhibition of Na^+, K^+-ATPase throughout the body, with consequent impairment of monovalent cation transport across cell membranes.

The half-time for digoxin clearance from plasma is shortened when levels are very high.[168, 240] This effect may be related to an altered ratio between plasma and tissue concentrations, allowing a relatively large quantity of the drug to be presented to the kidney for excretion.

TREATMENT OF DIGITALIS INTOXICATION

The key to successful treatment is early recognition that an arrhythmia is related to digitalis intoxication.[238] The more common manifestations—including occasional ectopic beats, marked first-degree atrioventricular block, or atrial fibrillation with a slow ventricular response—require only temporary withdrawal of the drug, electrocardiographic monitoring (if indicated) until the arrhythmia has disappeared, and subsequent adjustment of the dosage schedule to prevent recurrence. Rhythm disturbances that impair cardiac output because of too rapid or too slow ventricular rates, or those that portend ventricular fibrillation, require more active intervention. Ventricular tachycardia due to digitalis intoxication demands immediate vigorous treatment. Sinus bradycardia, sinoatrial arrest, and atrioventricular block of second or third degree are sometimes treated effectively with atropine, as previously indicated. Occasionally, electrical pacing will be required. It has been recommended that nonparoxysmal atrioventricular junctional rhythms with rates greater than 90 or with exit block be treated actively.[241] Atrioventricular junctional escape rhythms may simply be monitored if the rate is satisfactory.

PHENYTOIN AND LIDOCAINE (See also pp. 632 and 625). Phenytoin and lidocaine are useful drugs in the treatment of ectopic arrhythmias due to digitalis toxicity.[238] They have little adverse effect on sinoatrial rate, atrial conduction, atrioventricular conduction, or conduction in the His-Purkinje system. Indeed, phenytoin may improve sinoatrial block and atrioventricular conduction under some circumstances. A recommended regimen for phenytoin is 100 mg administered by slow intravenous infusion every 5 minutes until onset of toxicity or control of the arrhythmia, followed by an oral maintenance dose of 400 to 600 mg/day if control of the arrhythmia is achieved. Lidocaine is given intravenously in 100-mg bolus doses every 3 to 5 minutes, followed by the continuous infusion of 15 to 50 μg/kg of body weight/min as required to maintain control of the rhythm disturbances.

POTASSIUM. Therapy with potassium is recommended for ectopic tachyarrhythmias when hypokalemia is present but must be used with caution in other circumstances because of the risks associated with hyperkalemia.[238] Particular care is necessary when conduction disturbances are present, since elevations of plasma potassium concentration may impair atrioventricular conduction.

PROPRANOLOL. Propranolol has been useful in the treatment of some digitalis-toxic arrhythmias. Because of its antiadrenergic effects, it causes a decrease in automaticity, whereas by virtue of its direct myocardial effects, it shortens the refractory period of atrial muscle, ventricular muscle, and Purkinje fibers. It also slows the rate of depolarization and slows conduction velocity. Potential undesirable effects include depression of atrioventricular conduction and of sinoatrial and atrioventricular junctional pacemakers, with asystole or marked bradycardia, and depression of myocardial contractility with hemodynamic deterioration.

QUINIDINE AND PROCAINAMIDE (See also pp. 628 and 630). Quinidine and procainamide carry a risk of cardiac toxicity, such as depression of the sinoatrial node and of atrioventricular and His-Purkinje conduction, as well as the potential for eliciting ventricular arrhythmias. They are also capable of depressing myocardial contractility. Quinidine may actually intensify digitalis intoxication by raising the serum digoxin level, as discussed on page 630. Other agents are usually preferable for use in digitalis intoxication.

DIRECT-CURRENT COUNTERSHOCK (See also p. 642). Whereas countershock is generally inadvisable in the presence of digitalis intoxication because of the severe arrhythmias that may ensue, it must occasionally be used when all other methods have failed in the face of a life-threatening rhythm disturbance. The risk is decreased when lower energy levels are employed.[238] In contrast to the increased risk reported in the presence of overt digitalis toxicity, cardioversion appears to be a benign procedure in patients without digitalis-induced rhythm disturbances.[242]

STEROID-BINDING RESINS. As previously noted (p. 496), digitoxin undergoes some enterohepatic circulation, and agents that bind the drug within the gastrointestinal lumen should shorten its half-life. Cholestyramine induced a reduction in serum half-life of chloroform-extractable activity from 6.0 to 4.5 days after tritiated digitoxin administration in humans,[136] and colestipol appears to have a similar effect.[243] These effects may provide a means of reducing the duration of digitoxin toxicity but are probably not of sufficient magnitude or rapidity to be of great importance in the management of severe, life-threatening toxicity. Although digoxin has only a minimal enterohepatic circulation, cholestyramine tends to interfere with its initial absorption from the gastrointestinal tract.[244]

REVERSAL OF TOXICITY BY SPECIFIC ANTIBODY. The use of cardiac glycoside–specific antibodies and their Fab fragments for treatment of advanced digitalis intoxication has been studied in considerable detail.[245–248] A possible mechanism for the reversal of both inotropic and arrhythmogenic effects of cardiac glycosides was suggested in experiments demonstrating that high-affinity cardiac glycoside–specific antibodies are able to reverse established glycoside-induced inhibition of myocardial Na^+, K^+-ATPase[249] and monovalent cation active transport.[250]

Fab fragments provide advantages over purified intact antibodies as potential therapeutic agents. Each intact IgG antibody molecule of molecular weight 150,000 is cleaved by the proteolytic enzyme papain into an Fc fragment and two Fab fragments, each of which contains a specific binding site and has a molecular weight of 50,000. This smaller molecular species has a greater rate and volume of distribution after intravenous infusion and reverses experimentally induced digoxin-toxic arrhythmias more rapidly than does intact antibody.[248] The smaller size of the Fab molecule also allows it to pass through the mammalian glomerulus, unlike intact IgG. Fab fragments are excreted to an appreciable extent in the urine, but intact IgG is not.[251] Whereas injection of intact antibody markedly prolongs the plasma half-life of digoxin (although it is largely antibody-bound), digoxin bound to Fab fragments is excreted much more rapidly.[252] Rapid reversal of otherwise lethal experimentally induced digitoxin toxicity with specific antibodies and Fab fragments has been demonstrated[253] together with substantial acceleration by Fab of the renal excretion of digitoxin. This rapid renal excretion of Fab fragments may be of importance in reducing the immunogenicity of the foreign protein.[251]

More than 400 patients with potentially life-threatening digoxin or digitoxin toxicity have been treated with purified digoxin-specific Fab fragments, the first 63 of whom have been reported in detail.[254] All these patients had advanced cardiac rhythm disturbances and in 29 cases hyperkalemia was present as well, owing, in the majority, to ingestion of very large digitalis doses accidentally or with suicidal intent. All but three patients treated had an initial favorable response to intravenously administered Fab, and the diagnosis of digitalis toxicity was uncertain in each of these three. Four patients eventually died as a result of cerebral or myocardial damage from prolonged low output states prior to Fab administration; available Fab supplies were insufficient to provide adequate treatment in a fifth case. In the remaining patients, cardiac arrhythmias and hyperkalemia were reversed rapidly with full recovery.[254] This therapeutic modality has been released by the U.S. Food and Drug Administration and is commercially available.

DIURETICS

Of the pharmacological modalities available for the treatment of congestive heart failure, diuretics remain the cornerstone. The introduction of the "high ceiling" or "loop" diuretics in the 1960's revolutionized the care of patients with congestive heart failure and substantially reduced the morbidity of this disease. The high efficacy and relatively low and predictable toxicity of these drugs have made them among the most commonly prescribed medicines. Indeed, bed rest, combined with modest salt restriction and a diuretic alone, has been shown to result in a clinically important degree of weight loss,[255] a decline in ventricular filling pressures, and an increase in the cardiac index[256] in patients with advanced congestive failure. In addition, other agents, such as certain vasodilators, may be ineffective or deleterious if not administered appropriately with a diuretic.

The importance of diuretics in the treatment of the syndrome of congestive heart failure relates to the central role of the kidney as the target organ of many of the neurohumoral and hemodynamic changes that occur in response to a failing myocardium, discussed on pages 1828 to 1831. Reduced tissue perfusion leads to activation of the renin-angiotensin system within the kidney, which decreases renal blood flow and increases the glomerular filtration fraction, leading to enhanced resorption of solute and water by the proximal tubules (Fig. 17–8). Elevated plasma angiotensin II contributes to a rise in systemic vascular resistance and also causes release from the adrenal gland of the potent mineralocorticoid aldosterone. Enhanced renal sympathetic nerve activity also reduces renal blood flow, releases renin from macula densa cells, and directly augments sodium resorption along the nephron. Renal blood flow is directed away from superficial cortical nephrons to the more efficient solute-resorbing juxtamedullary nephrons that rely upon the high capacity of the ion transport carriers in their long loops of Henle and the countercurrent mechanism of the medulla to allow the formation of very concentrated urine. Finally, plasma antidiuretic hormone (ADH) levels are also elevated in many patients with congestive heart failure, which causes further reductions in free water clearance by the kidney. This, coupled with the increased thirst of many patients with advanced heart failure perhaps caused by their high angiotensin II levels, often leads to a hypotonic edematous state.[257] As with any other complex biological system, countervailing humoral responses also occur, including increased prostaglandin E_2 and prostacyclin levels within the kidney (tubuloglomerular feedback), and perhaps the release of humoral natriuretic factors.[258] Elevated levels of atrial natriuretic peptide (human ANP) have been described in these patients.[259] This suggests that although the failing heart is capable of producing ANP, the kidney appears to resist the natriuretic effect of the peptide.

The net effect of all the neuronal, hormonal, and hemodynamic influences on the kidney induced by the failing myocardium is retention of solute and water and expansion of extracellular volume. This may serve to sustain cardiac output and, therefore, tissue perfusion in the short run by allowing the ventricle to function further along its function curve. However, increasing cardiac filling pressures may lead to progressive cardiac dilation, worsening congestive symptoms, and a decline in cardiac output that may elicit even more avid salt and water retention by the kidneys. Therefore, although diuretics may not influence the natural history of the primary disease process responsible for myocardial dysfunction, they can dramatically improve symptoms of congestive failure by acting directly on solute and water resorption by the nephron, and may slow the progression of cardiac chamber dilation by reducing ventricular filling pressure (preload).

A diuretic is any drug that increases urine flow. Water or common beverages such as those containing caffeine or ethanol will increase urine flow rate but are useless as agents that promote the loss of solute from the body. Therefore, the term "diuretic" commonly is used to refer to agents that enhance the delivery of NaCl and the other principal small ions that form the extracellular milieu, along with water, into the urine. Certain agents indirectly increase urine production by enhancing renal blood flow and the rate of glomerular filtration, thereby promoting a fall in the filtration fraction and diminished water and solute resorption by the proximal tubule. In patients with decompensated congestive heart failure, digitalis, by improving cardiac output, may enhance renal blood flow. Similarly, dopamine, in doses ranging from 1 to 5 μg/kg/min, induces renal vasodilatation by stimulation of vascular dopaminergic receptors (p. 524). Aside from effects on renal perfusion, the improved cardiac output will lead to reduced renal sympathetic tone and angiotensin II production by the kidney.

Most diuretics, however, act directly on the kidney to inhibit solute and water reabsorption. There are a number of classification schemes for diuretics, based upon their mechanism of action, their anatomical locus of action in the nephron, and the form of diuresis they elicit. Most diuretics can be classified according to whether they induce a "solute" or "water" diuresis. Of the latter, only two agents are of clinical relevance, demeclocycline and lithium, each of which, by differing mechanisms, inhibits the action of ADH on the collecting duct, increasing free water clearance. Drugs that cause a "solute" diuresis are subdivided into two types: those that inhibit active transport of ions across tubular epithelia (the majority of potent, clinically useful diuretics) and those that are nonresorbable solutes that osmotically retain water and other solutes within the tubular lumen. Much information is available regarding sites and cellular mechanisms of action of most diuretic agents. This is discussed below in the context of a description of those segments of the nephron most directly affected by each drug[260, 261] (Figs. 17–8 to 17–11). It should be kept in mind that these drugs may, directly or indirectly, affect solute resorption elsewhere in the nephron, and that many of these drugs have extrarenal effects as well that may be important in determining the overall hemodynamic response.

SITES AND MECHANISM OF ACTION OF DIURETIC AGENTS

(Figs. 17–8 and 17–9, and Table 17–7)

THE PROXIMAL TUBULE. Fluid resorption across the proximal tubule is isosmotic and accounts for approximately two-thirds of the resorption of filtered Na^+ and H_2O. The active resorption of sodium bicarbonate by carbonic anhydrase activity raises the intraluminal chloride concentration, allowing for further isosmotic resorption of NaCl along the proximal tubule. Although active transport processes are important in solute resorption by this segment of the nephron, the most significant influences on the absolute quantity of solute and water resorbed in the proximal tubule are the volume of glomerular filtrate (a function of glomerular capillary permeability and filtration pressure), and the net effect of the Starling forces that govern solute and water movement across and between tubular epithelial cells into peritubular capillaries. A variety of neuronal, hormonal, and hemodynamic factors, both extrinsic and intrinsic to the kidney, may affect greatly the volume and content of urine by altering the rate of formation of glomerular filtrate for given renal blood flow ("filtration fraction"). The balance of Starling forces between the proximal tubule and postglomerular peritubular capillaries is thereby altered.[262]

Agents that alter the intrarenal regulation of formation of glomerular filtrate, such as angiotensin-converting enzyme inhibitors, may enhance the delivery of solute and water to more distal segments of the nephron that are sensitive to diuretics that inhibit ion transport. Predictably, other drugs, such as nonsteroidal antiinflammatory drugs, may diminish glomerular filtrate formation, thus reducing the flow of urine to distal diuretic-sensitive portions of the nephron. Clearly, a reduction in systemic blood pressure, or in renal artery pressure distal to a stenotic lesion, below that necessary for formation of glomerular filtrate will render the kidney refractory to any diuretic. The pars recta section of the proximal tubule does resorb some of the glomerular filtrate, and is important to the understanding of diuretic pharmacology because the organic anion secretory transport system exists here. Many diuretics that are not freely filtered at the glomerulus are actively secreted by the tubular cells of the pars recta. Drugs that competitively inhibit the secretion of diuretics, such as probenecid, will delay and/or diminish the desired diuretic effect.[263] In patients with chronic renal failure, in whom the absolute number of transporters may be diminished significantly due to nephron loss, high concentrations of endogenous organic acids may compete with diuretics for secretion into the tubular lumen of the pars recta of the remaining functioning nephrons. This is clearly one cause of "diuretic resistance" in these patients.

THE LOOP OF HENLE. About one-third of the glomerular filtrate arrives at the descending limb of Henle's loop; no active transport of solute occurs here, although the tubular epithelium is highly permeable to water, which leaves the nephron for the increasingly hyperosmotic medullary interstitium. The generation of the hyperosmolar milieu is accomplished as the glomerular filtrate rounds the bend into the thin ascending limb. Most of the solute transport responsible for maintaining the hypertonicity of the medullary interstitium occurs in the water-impermeable thick ascending limb of Henle's loop. Here, a sodium-potassium cotransport system in the luminal membrane is coupled to the uptake of two chloride ions, an electroneutral process. This process is dependent upon the electrochemical gradient for Na^+ and the energy is derived from ATP by Na^+, K^+-ATPase on the basolateral cell membrane.[264] This Na/K/2Cl cotransport system serves mainly to resorb NaCl from the tubular lumen, as most of the resorbed K^+ is recycled back to the lumen due to the high K^+ conductivity of the luminal membrane. This recycled K^+ is responsible for the lumen positive potential in this nephron segment. Substantial amounts of Ca^{++} and Mg^{++} are also resorbed in this segment, largely due to passive transport through the "leaky" epithelial tight junctions. This cation flux mechanism is due to the negative transepithelial electrical potential. The Na/K/2Cl cotransport system is the receptor for the loop diuretics (furosemide,

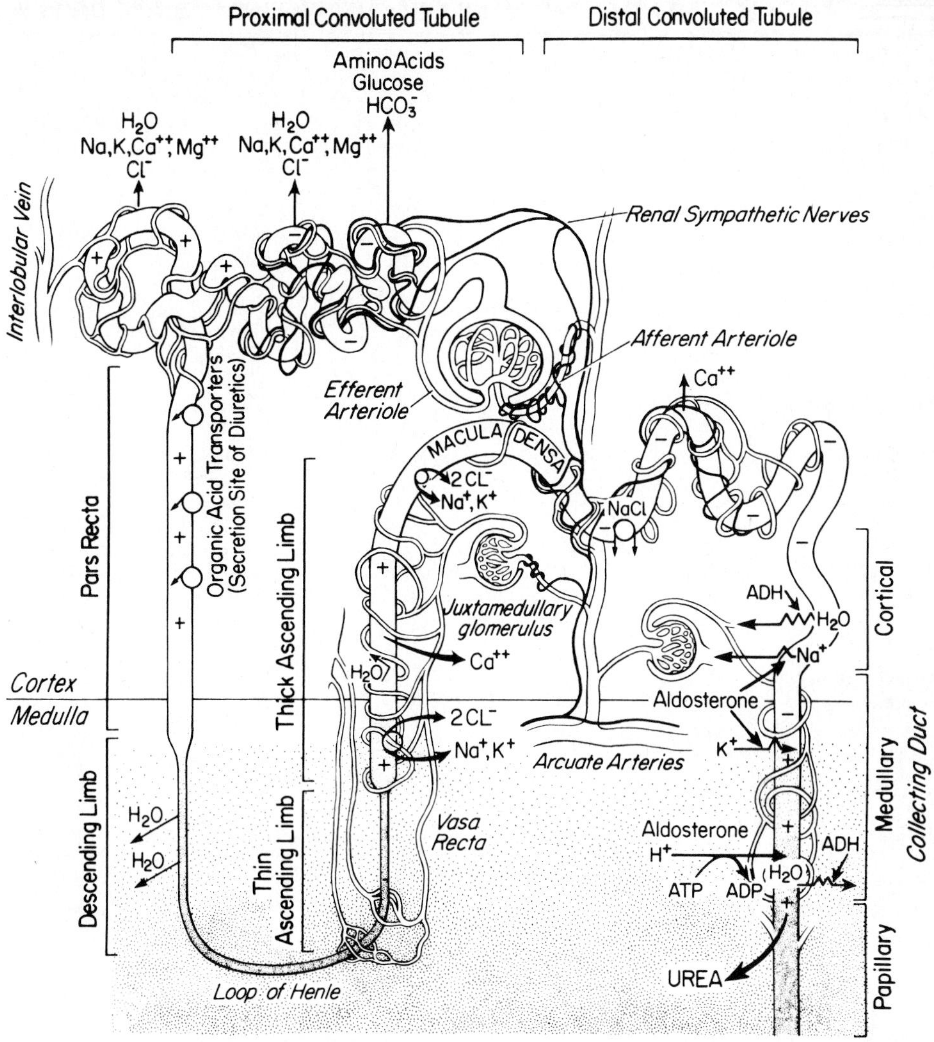

FIGURE 17–8. Transport functions of the anatomical segments of the mammalian nephron.

bumetanide, piretanide, ethacrynic acid) and is illustrated in Figure 17–10. Solute resorption in this segment is under direct hormonal control in some species. ADH stimulates solute uptake in rodents, an effect that would enhance resorption of water by ADH-sensitive cells in the collecting duct; such an effect of ADH on the thick ascending limb in man has not been demonstrated. Prostaglandins (PGE_2) can be shown in animals to inhibit Na/K/2Cl transport in this segment, and perhaps do so in humans as well, as cyclo-oxygenase inhibitors clearly reduce the effectiveness of loop diuretics in some patients.

ACTION OF LOOP DIURETICS. Inhibition of cation transport by loop diuretics has two effects. First, it prevents the normal generation of the hypertonic medullary interstitium thus reducing the osmotic gradient for free water reabsorption by ADH-sensitive epithelium in the collecting duct. Second, it causes delivery of large amounts of solute and water to the distal nephron, thus overwhelming distal Na^+ and Cl^- resorption sites and dramatically affecting K^+ secretion and urinary acidification. However the efficacy of loop diuretics is predicated upon the delivery of a threshold amount of NaCl, at an adequate flow rate, to this nephron segment. This precondition may not be present in severe prerenal azotemia due to factors controlling the formation of glomerular filtrate and proximal tubular resorption, as noted above.

THE DISTAL TUBULE. The thick ascending limb approaches its own glomerulus as it reenters the cortex and passes between the afferent and efferent arterioles to form the juxtaglomerular apparatus (JGA), the tubular contribution to which is termed the macula densa. Loop diuretics may directly stimulate the release of renin by the JGA, an action that may contribute to the extrarenal vascular effects of these drugs. The distal convoluted tubule begins beyond the macula densa. Na^+ and Cl^- as well as other ions (e.g., Ca^{++}) are resorbed in this segment, which is largely ADH-insensitive and impermeant to water. The benzothiadiazides and related drugs inhibit NaCl uptake in this segment, although the mechanism is unknown; they may enhance Ca^{++} resorption by epithelial cells in this segment. NaCl resorption by this distal water-impermeant portion of the nephron allows the formation of a dilute urine, hence the term "cortical diluting segment." Thiazide-induced inhibition of NaCl resorption in this segment therefore may lead to hyponatremia, particularly when accompanied by elevated ADH levels and increased thirst.

THE COLLECTING DUCT. This structure is divided into three segments: the cortical, medullary, and papillary collecting ducts. The cortical collecting duct actively resorbs sodium NaCl via an aldosterone-sensitive mechanism. The primary effect is to increase the permeability of the apical membrane to sodium; the increased sodium entry into the cell is then pumped out by the Na^+, K^+-ATPase on the basolateral membrane. Aldosterone binds to a specific soluble cytoplasmic receptor protein leading to the sequence of events, including synthesis of specific proteins, that leads to the modulation of cation transport in the luminal membrane. The synthesis of new Na^+, K^+-ATPase units is probably secondary to the increase in intracellular sodium concentration. The increasing resorption of Na^+ from the tubule leads to a lumen negative potential difference that favors the secretion of K^+ and H^+ ions. Thus, reduction of Na^+ delivery to the cortical collecting duct reduces the Na^+-linked secretion of K^+ down its electrochemical gradient into the tubular lumen. Conversely, increased Na^+ concentrations and high flow rates in the cortical collecting duct, as after loop or thiazide diuretic administration, leads to enhanced passive K^+ secretion, but only if Na^+ is being absorbed by epithelial cells in this segment. Blockade of apical membrane Na^+ conductance by amiloride reduces the lumen negative potential to zero and greatly reduces the electrochemical driving force for K^+ (and H^+) secretion.

Antialdosterone drugs, such as spironolactone and canrenone, competitively inhibit aldosterone's binding to its receptor and thereby limit Na^+ permeability by the apical membrane and reduce the negative lumen potential. It follows that reduced Na^+ entry into cortical collecting duct epithelial cells will reduce the active flux of Na^+ out of the cell into the blood via the Na^+, K^+-ATPase, which, in turn, will necessarily reduce the amount of K^+ available for secretion into the tubular lumen.

THE MEDULLARY COLLECTING DUCT. This portion of the duct is not a major site of action of any diuretic. It is important for the active secretion of H^+ ion via a H^+-ATPase, a Na^+-independent process. This proton pump is aldosterone-sensitive and can be inhibited by aldosterone antagonists. The entire collecting duct is permeable to water in the

TABLE 17–7 DIURETICS: ACTION, DOSAGE, AND DRUG INTERACTIONS

Diuretic	Brand Name	Principal Site and Mechanism of Action	Effects on Urinary Electrolytes	Effects on Blood Electrolytes and Acid-Base Balance	Extrarenal Effects	Usual Dosage*	Drug Interactions
Thiazides & Related Compounds							
Chlorothiazide	Diuril	*Distal Tubule:*	↑ Na^+	↓ NA^+ particularly in elderly patients	↑ Glucose	500–1000 mg IV or p.o.	Efficacy reduced by prostaglandin inhibitors
Hydrochlorothiazide	Hydrodiuril	Enhance NaCl reabsorption	↑ Cl^- ↑ K^+	↓ Cl ↑ HCO_3-	↑ LDL/ triglycerides	25–100 mg/d	Reduces renal clearance of lithium
Trichlormethiazide	Methahydrin	and ↓ CA^{++} excretion	↑ H^+	mild metabolic alkalosis	(may be dose related)	2–8 mg/d	
Chlorthalidone	Hygroton					25–100 mg/d	
Metolazone	Zaroxolyn		↑ Mg^{++} ↓ Ca^{++}	↑ Uric acid ↑ Ca^{++}		5–10 mg/d	Additive effect on NaCl and K^+ excretion with loop diuretics
Indapamide	Lozol	Smooth muscle vasodilator			Extrarenal effects less marked with indapamide	2.5–5 mg/d	
Acetazolamide	Diamox	*Proximal Tubule:* Carbonic anhydrase inhibitor	↑ Na^+, ↑ K^+ ↑ HCO_3^-	Metabolic acidosis	↑ Ventilatory drive ↓ Intraocular pressure	250–500 mg/d	May be useful in alkalemia due to other diuretics
Osmotic Diuretics							
Mannitol	Osmitrol	Proximal Tubule (Primarily)	↑ Na^+, ↑ Cl	↑ Extracellular volume transiently	↓ Intracranial pressure	50–200 gm/d IV	May enhance loop diuretic effectiveness by maintaining GFR
Glycerol	Glyrol		↑ H_2O		↓ Intraocular pressure	1–1.5 gm/kg p.o.	
Loop Diuretics							
Furosemide	Lasix	*Thick ascending limb of loop*	↑ ↑ Na	Hypochloremic alkalosis (↑ HCO_3)	*Acute:* ↑ Venous capacitance	20–1000 mg/d p.o./IV	Tubular secretion delayed by competing organic acids (renal failure) and some drugs
Bumetanide	Bumex	*of Henle:* inhibition of Na/K/Cl	↑ ↑ Cl ↑ K^+ ↑ H^+	↓ K^+, ↓ Na^+, ↓ Cl	↑ Systemic vascular resistance	0.5–20.0 mg/d	
Piretanide		cotransport	↑ Mg^{++}, ↑ Ca^{++}	↑ Uric acid (less than thiazide)	*Chronic:* ↓ Cardiac preload	6–20 mg/d	Effectiveness reduced by prostaglandin inhibitors
Ethacrynic Acid	Edecrin						Additive ototoxicity with aminoglycosides
Indacrinone				Uricosuric potency depends upon ratio of ± enantiomers in final drug	Ototoxicity	50–150 mg/d	Excessive hypotension may occur in patients treated chronically with diuretics and begun on ACE inhibitors
Potassium-Sparing Diuretics							
Spironolactone	Aldactone	*Collecting Duct:* Aldosterone antagonists	↓ K^+ ↑ Na^+ ↑ Cl^-	↑ K, particularly in patients with ↓ GFR; metabolic acidosis	Gynecomastia	25–100 mg/d	Useful adjunct to therapy with K^+ wasting diuretics; triamterene with indomethacin may cause abrupt ↓ GFR
Triamterene	Dyrenium		↑ HCO_3^-			100–300 mg/d	
Amiloride	Midamor	Inhibit apical membrane Na^+ conductance				5–10 mg/d	

*Route of administration is p.o. except as noted.

presence of ADH; the final osmolality of the urine will depend upon the concentration of solute remaining in the collecting duct, the osmolality of the medullary interstitium and the responsiveness of the tubular epithelium to ADH. Drugs such as demeclocycline and lithium may directly antagonize the effects of ADH, leading to diabetes insipidus.

BLOOD SUPPLY TO NEPHRON. As illustrated in Figure 17–8, the blood supply to each nephron is derived from several sources. The *afferent arteriole* that enters the vascular pole of the glomerulus is a branch of an interlobular artery[265] and is richly innervated with sympathetic nerve endings, particularly as it enters the glomerulus at its vascular pole within the juxtaglomerular apparatus. In the case of a superficial cortical nephron, as illustrated here, the efferent arteriole from the glomerulus perfuses segments of proximal and distal convoluted tubules. Tubular segments lying deeper in the cortex and medulla are perfused by efferent arterioles from juxtamedullary nephrons, and include the long, unbranched peritubular vasa recta.

INNERVATION OF RENAL VESSELS. Postganglionic sympathetic nerves extend from the celiac and aortorenal ganglia along the renal nerves into the hilus of the kidney and then traverse, and innervate, successive branches of the renal arteries, with a concentration of sympathetic fibers surrounding the afferent arteriole and the juxtaglomerular apparatus. Direct sympathetic innervation of proximal and distal tubular epithelia has been described; increased sympathetic discharge to the kidney results in increased net NaCl resorption even in the absence of changes in glomerular hemodynamics.[266] Elevated efferent sympathetic activity, as in decompensated congestive heart failure, thus would be expected to result in avid retention of solute due to reduced renal perfusion, increased renin release, and enhanced tubular resorption of solute.

Dopamine is a potent renal vasodilator and may directly affect tubular epithelia to reduce NaCl resorption, thus acting as a natriuretic agent. Although dopaminergic innervation to the kidney has been described,

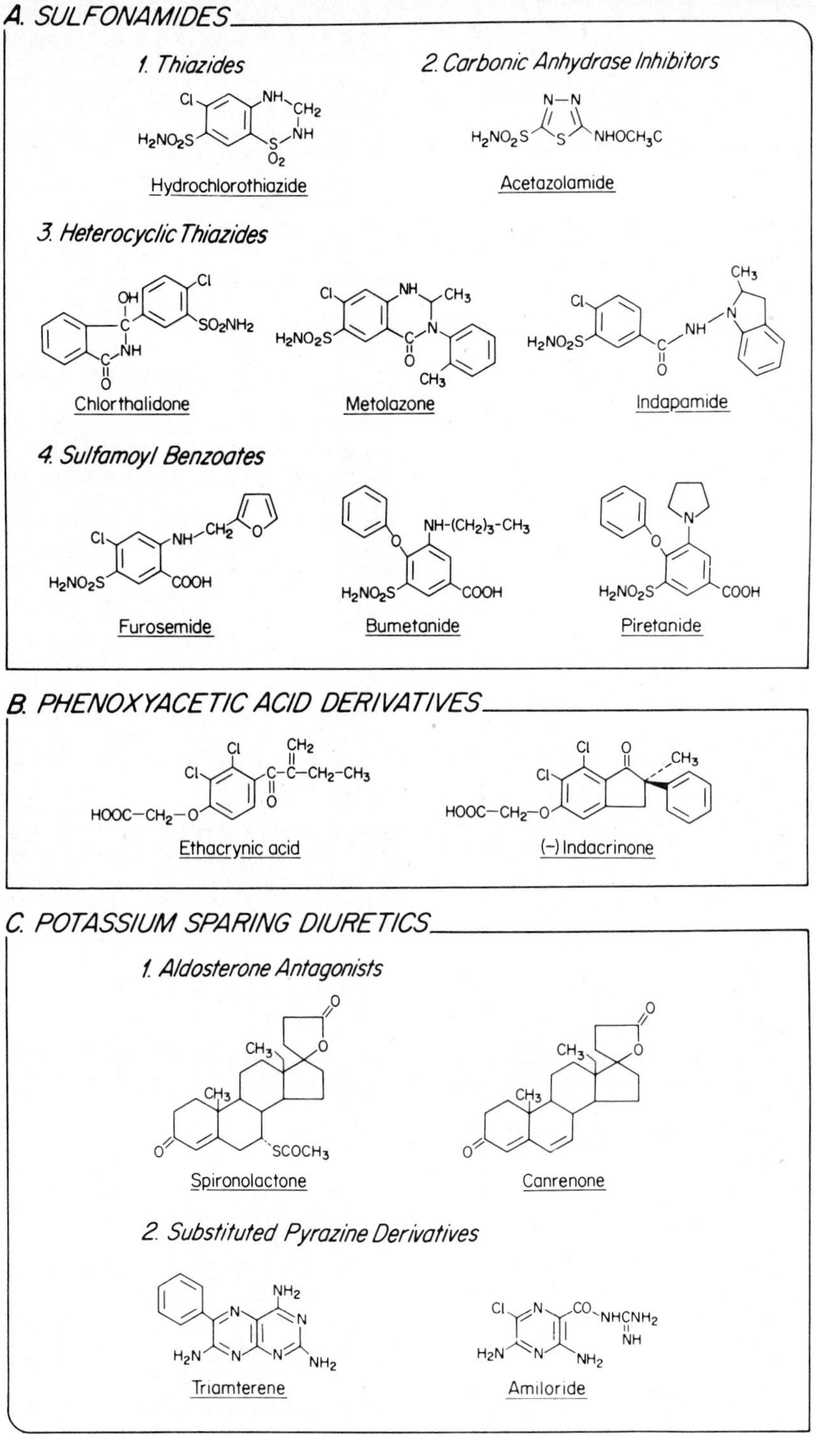

FIGURE 17–9. Chemical structure of diuretics.

most renal dopamine is produced locally by the action of dopa decarboxylase in tubular epithelial cells. Exogenously administered dopamine, particularly when infused at rates of 5 μg/kg/min or less, may be a useful adjunct to diuretic therapy in selected patients with advanced CHF (p. 524).

PHARMACOLOGY OF DIURETICS

The pharmacology of diuretic agents that is relevant to cardiovascular medicine is discussed below. For a more extensive review of the pharmacology of these drugs, the reader is referred to several recent reviews.[267–271]

CARBONIC ANHYDRASE INHIBITORS

Although all the sulfonamide diuretics, including furosemide and the thiazides, are weak carbonic anhydrase inhibitors, only acetazolamide is used clinically for this purpose. Acute administration of acetazolamide results in bicarbonaturia until the plasma bicarbonate falls to the point at which renal tubular bicarbonate resorption (both proximal and distal) exceeds the filtered load of bicarbonate at the glomerulus[272] (Figs. 17–9 and 17–10). This renal loss of bicarbonate can be used to alkalinize the urine transiently to enhance dissolution of uric acid crystals or the clearance of certain drugs. Maintenance of urinary alkalinization with these drugs requires a chronic bicarbonate infusion; otherwise, a mild hyperchloremic (non-anion gap) metabolic acidosis develops, accom-

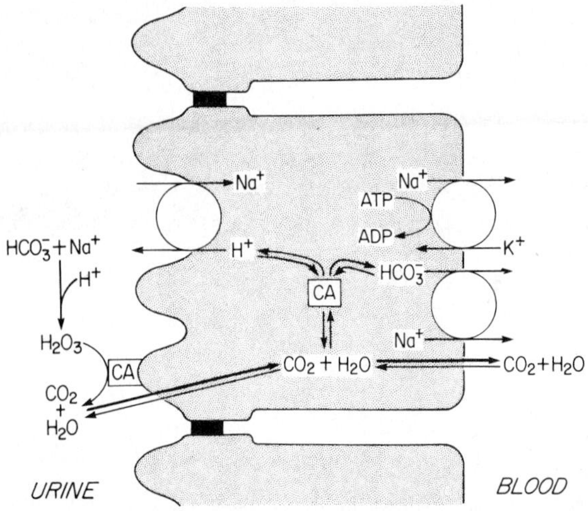

FIGURE 17–10. A proximal tubular cell, the primary site of action of carbonic anhydrase inhibitors. Inhibition of carbonic anhydrase (CA) will lead to a decrease in bicarbonate and Na^+ resorption, eventually producing hyperchloremic metabolic acidosis. Osmotic diuretics also reduce proximal tubular sodium resorption; the reduction in water flow through the epithelium dilutes luminal solute and favors back-leak of Na^+ into the tubular lumen. Although amiloride is an inhibitor of the Na^+/H^+ exchanger (illustrated here in the proximal tubule), as well as in the collecting duct, it has little diuretic effect proximally. This may be the result of reduced diuretic availability at this site, the compensatory reserve of other distal sodium resorptive mechanisms, and the high concentrations of amiloride necessary for inhibition of Na^+/H^+ exchange.

panied by a small volume contraction of extracellular volume and hypokalemia.

Metabolic acidosis may be of use in edematous patients with hypochloremic metabolic alkalosis due to chronic use of loop diuretics, particularly if the acid-base status of these patients is complicated by hypercarbia (either "primary" as in severe chronic obstructive pulmonary disease with cor pulmonale, or a "compensatory" respiratory acidosis due to the diuretic-induced alkalosis, or both).[273, 274] In these patients, a fall in the renal threshold for bicarbonate resorption may stimulate ventilatory drive. However, acetazolamide should be considered only if a patient is not intravascularly volume-depleted and cannot tolerate infusions of NaCl or KCl. Careful monitoring of arterial pH and pCO_2 is necessary to insure that an increased minute ventilation does occur; otherwise, a metabolic acidosis will be added to an already complex acid-base disturbance. Renal potassium losses can be rapid and substantial and may be partially masked by intracellular K^+ shifts induced by mild acidemia.

Another indication of use is in the prevention of acute mountain sickness, including noncardiogenic pulmonary edema and cerebral edema.[275] The acute metabolic acidosis induced by the bicarbonaturia presumably stimulates the respiratory drive and prevents hypoxemia. Acetazolamide also improved exercise performance and decreased loss of muscle mass in individuals acclimatized to high altitude when compared with placebo.[276]

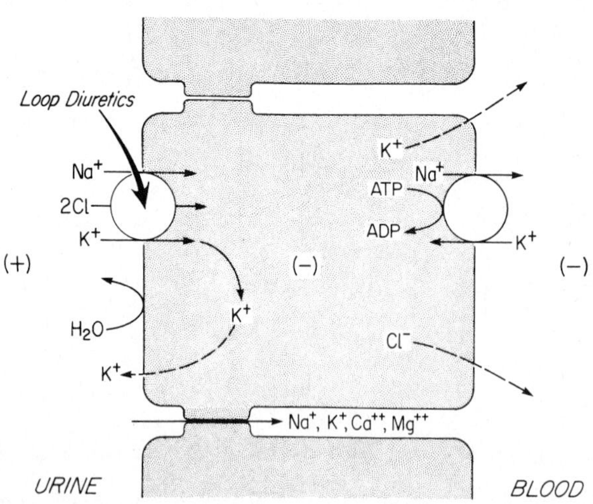

FIGURE 17–11. A medullary thick ascending limb (TAL) cell. The loop diuretics, furosemide, bumetanide, and piretanide, are all known to inhibit the Na/K/2Cl cotransporter in this epithelium. Ethacrynic acid and indacrinone are less specific inhibitors of the cotransporter, but their principal pharmacological action is presumed to be through this mechanism. The loop diuretics also decrease the absorption of Ca^{++} and Mg^{++} by TAL cells, absorption that is indirectly linked to NaCl uptake. Inhibition of NaCl transport in this segment secondarily impairs urinary concentrating ability by preventing the formation of a hypertonic medullary interstitium.

OSMOTIC DIURETICS

Any agent may act as an "osmotic diuretic" if it is freely filtered by the glomerulus, is neither resorbed nor metabolized in the renal tubule, and is relatively inactive pharmacologically so as to allow the intravenous administration of sufficiently large quantities of the drug to affect both plasma and urine osmolality. By these criteria, endogenous products of metabolism such as glucose and urea may act as osmotic diuretics, but only if the tubular capacity for resorption of these solutes is exceeded. Radiographic contrast dyes are also filtered by the glomerulus and are not resorbed by renal tubules; therefore, they act as osmotic diuretics, increasing urinary losses of salt and water. The diuresis induced by these agents is short-lived but may be intense, particularly in the setting of underlying renal disease when the contrast agent must be cleared by a reduced number of functioning nephrons.

An important characteristic of osmotic diuretics is their ability to maintain urine flow even at very low glomerular filtration rates, as occurs in hypotension or dehydration. As long as perfusion pressure in the glomerular capillaries is sufficient to sustain filtration, and the tubular epithelium remains relatively impermeable, mannitol infusions will maintain a flow of salt and water to the distal nephron.[277, 278] This effect of mannitol, glycerol, and related agents is superior to that of resorbable solutes such as NaCl that are avidly absorbed by the proximal tubule in these clinical settings. Mannitol, as an inert extracellular osmotic agent, will increase the extracellular fluid volume; consequently, the drug is contraindicated in patients with decompensated congestive heart failure.

LOOP DIURETICS

The loop diuretics are among the most potent diuretic agents known, capable of inducing a natriuresis of up to 20 per cent of the filtered load of sodium for a short period. Ethacrynic acid, a phenoxyacetic acid derivative, was the first loop diuretic to become available. Following shortly was the sulfonamide derivative of anthranilic acid, furosemide. More potent congeners of furosemide include bumetanide and piretanide. Although the precise site of action of ethacrynic acid in the ascending limb of Henle's loop is not yet known, it is presumed to be similar to that of furosemide and its congeners: the Na/K/2Cl transport system, an apical transmembrane protein responsible for the majority of solute resorption in the thick ascending limb (Fig. 17–11). These drugs maintain solute loss even in the presence of a declining glomerular filtration rate (GFR) and reduced renal perfusion.[279] Unlike thiazides and other diuretics, the loop-active agents do not induce a compensatory decline in GFR via tubuloglomerular feedback mechanisms, perhaps because the drugs themselves inhibit the flow of NaCl into macula densa cells.[280] Each of these drugs is secreted into the tubular lumen by the organic acid secretory pathway. Their pharmacological effect may therefore be delayed or diminished by exogenous (e.g., probenecid, indomethacin) or endogenous (metabolic byproducts in uremia) competitive inhibitors of the transporter.

ABSORPTION. The absorption of orally administered furosemide is highly variable even among normal subjects; the drug has an average bioavailability of 60 per cent,[281] that is markedly diminished when it is given with meals.[282,

[283] Both bumetanide and furosemide, when administered orally, have reduced natriuretic effects in patients with congestive heart failure, in part due to delayed intestinal absorption and delivery of the drug to its tubular site of action,[284] although absolute bioavailability (absorption) is little affected. This increased lag time from administration of the drug to its natriuretic effect, which is exacerbated by decompensated congestive heart failure,[285] not only delays the onset of the natriuresis but may prevent a sufficient amount of drug from arriving at its receptor in the loop of Henle to produce a clinically relevant natriuretic effect.

DOSE-RESPONSE RELATIONS. Even when furosemide is administered intravenously, the dose-response relationship between its urinary levels and sodium excretion rates is shifted to the right, a reflection of enhanced proximal and distal solute resorption in the kidney. To a certain extent, these problems can be overcome simply by giving more drug or by adding a diuretic active at another nephron site (see below). Extremely high-dose furosemide regimens (0.5 to 1 gm/day) have also been advocated for patients with severe refractory cardiac failure but conserved renal function, in order to avoid some of the potential toxicity of a second drug.[286] Although loop diuretics given chronically may induce a hypochloremic metabolic alkalosis, resistance to these agents is not normally affected by arterial pH,[287] although advanced respiratory acidosis combined with hypoxemia may substantially reduce urinary clearance of the drugs,[288] thereby limiting their natriuretic effect.

INTERACTION WITH ANTIINFLAMMATORY DRUGS. The nonsteroidal antiinflammatory drugs (NSAID's), including aspirin, blunt the natriuretic response to all the loop diuretics. Given alone, NSAID's may reduce glomerular filtration and cause sodium retention, particularly in patients with diminished renal perfusion, as in congestive heart failure.[289] The predominant effect of these agents in limiting the response to loop diuretics is to prevent the prostaglandin-induced rise in renal blood flow that accompanies and sustains the natriuretic response to loop diuretics.[290, 291] Prostaglandin synthesis inhibitors also increase chloride uptake by the thick ascending limb of Henle's loop in the mammalian nephron, probably by reducing the effect of chloruretic prostanoids.[292] Clinically, not all the NSAID's are of equivalent potency in inducing this interaction; indomethacin competitively inhibits furosemide excretion into the proximal tubule in addition to inhibiting renal cyclooxygenase,[293] and sulindac, a "prodrug" that is not excreted into the renal tubule in its active form, has much less effect on acute diuretic-induced natriuresis or chronic diuretic antihypertensive effects.[294–296] Low-dose aspirin, in the dosage range that inhibits platelet production of thromboxane A_2 (<1.0 mg/kg/day), has no effect on enhanced urinary prostaglandin production or the natriuresis induced by furosemide.[297]

EFFECTS ON SYSTEMIC HEMODYNAMICS. All loop diuretics cause changes in systemic hemodynamics that are initially unrelated to the degree and extent of the natriuresis they induce. Acute administration of furosemide, the best studied of these agents, results in a rapid increase in venous capacitance and a decline in cardiac filling pressures.[298] This effect is coincident with a rise in plasma renin activity, is blunted by prostaglandin synthesis inhibitors and a high dietary salt intake, and is abolished in anephric subjects.[299] Acute furosemide administration also can result in a rise in systemic vascular resistance, both in normal volunteers and in patients with compensated congestive heart failure, an effect that is blocked by drugs that inhibit renin release (e.g., propranolol) or angiotensin II formation (e.g., captopril).[300, 301] Indeed, this rise in left ventricular afterload can induce worsening congestive symptoms in patients with compensated but borderline systolic function.[301] All these hemodynamic effects are presumed to be due to the rapid release of renin by the juxtaglomerular apparatus following an intravenous dose of furosemide. This results in arteriolar vasoconstriction due to increases in angiotensin II levels and an increase in venous capacitance due to angiotensin II mediated vasodilatory prostaglandin release.[299] In patients with decompensated congestive heart failure or frank pulmonary edema, in whom systemic vascular resistance is already high, the venodilator effects of furosemide predominate and may be prolonged (hours).[302] Unlike the natriuretic effect of furosemide, which increases almost linearly with dose above a threshold, there is little further increase in systemic vascular resistance or venous capacitance above a 20-mg intravenous dose.[303] Dosages of bumetanide that result in an equivalent natriuretic effect to furosemide appear to have diminished vascular effects, both arteriolar and venous, at least in salt-depleted normal subjects.[304]

Furosemide may also have direct effects on arterial oxygen saturation in models of acute pulmonary edema characterized by increased capillary permeability. This effect is apparently due to a redistribution of pulmonary blood flow away from "flooded" alveoli and provides a rationale for use of furosemide in noncardiogenic pulmonary edema, although its clinical use remains controversial for this indication.[305–307]

Another hemodynamic effect of furosemide has been identified in neonates. By increasing renal production of prostaglandin E_2, furosemide promotes shunting through a patent ductus arteriosus in premature infants, thus complicating the respiratory distress syndrome often seen in these infants.[308]

NEUROTOXIC EFFECTS. Although the loop diuretics are potent inhibitors of Na/K/2Cl cotransport, inhibition of this transporter, which exists in most cells, is clinically unimportant in nonrenal cells except in the cochlea. All the loop diuretics possess some toxicity for the eighth nerve, with ethacrynic acid being the most ototoxic. Sensorineuronal hearing loss usually occurs at doses greater than 1 gm/day; transient hearing loss may be common in patients receiving bolus injections of furosemide due to a reversible decrease in endocochlear potential and the eighth nerve action potential.[309] Loop diuretic ototoxicity is synergistic with that of aminoglycoside antibiotics. Electrophysiological effects of furosemide on the heart have also been described.[310] Furosemide, 20 mg intravenously, caused a significant prolongation of A-H intervals at a variety of atrial pacing rates, with no effect on the H-V interval; the sinus node recovery time and atrial refractory period also increased. Sinus exit block or increased AV block due to loop diuretics must be rare but should be considered in patients with underlying conduction system disease receiving large bolus doses of these drugs.

EFFICACY. All the loop diuretics are roughly equivalent in terms of their efficacy. There is little justification for the use of ethacrynic acid because of its increased ototoxicity except in patients with a drug allergy or interstitial nephritis due to sulfonamides. Bumetanide and piretanide both have higher bioavailability and greater potency (40:1 and 6:1, respectively) than furosemide, and may each be slightly less ototoxic. Other differences among these drugs are small and probably clinically insignificant.[311–313]

THIAZIDE DIURETICS

The thiazide diuretics include a number of agents that are chemically and pharmacologically similar, the prototype of which is chlorothiazide. Chlorthalidone and metolazone are heterocyclic variants of the basic benzothiadiazine nucleus. All these drugs inhibit NaCl resorption in the distal tubule, an effect that is independent of the weak carbonic anhydrase inhibitory activity most of these drugs possess. Although these sulfonamide derivatives are the oldest orally effective diuretics in common use, their fundamental cellular mechanism of action remains unclear. By inhibiting NaCl transport in the distal tubule, they prevent dilution of the tubular fluid and augment the delivery of solute and water to the H^+ and K^+ secreting sites in the collecting duct. The thiazides also promote Ca^{++} resorption, probably by directly enhancing Ca^{++} entry into distal tubular epithelial cells, and by inducing mild volume depletion, thus enhancing Ca^{++} resorption at several sites in the nephron. These effects appear to be largely independent of PTH or 1,25-dihydroxy vitamin D_3.[314, 315]

The thiazides are useful in the management of mild to moderate hypertension (p. 869) and as single agents in the initial management of early congestive heart failure. However, their utility is limited by avidity of solute resorption by more proximal nephron segments. They are largely ineffective when the GFR is less than 30 ml/min. They may be useful for refractory edema in combination with loop diuretics, as discussed below. Metolazone may cause a smaller reduction in GFR than other drugs of this class, but it is unclear whether this is a clinically important distinction.[316]

Indapamide is structurally related to the thiazides, and has both a vasodilatory and diuretic effect, making it particularly useful in the treatment of hypertension. With it, the toxicity of electrolyte depletion seen with equipotent antihypertensive doses of the older thiazides is minimized potentially. Although the combination of vasoactive and diuretic properties would appear to be of particular value in congestive heart failure, indapamide appears to offer little advantage over thiazide diuretics unless patients receiving it are also hypertensive or have mild renal insufficiency.[317, 318]

POTASSIUM-SPARING DIURETICS

Two classes of agents fall into this group of diuretic drugs: (1) the aldosterone antagonists, and (2) the direct inhibitors of collecting duct sodium conductance, amiloride and triamterene (Fig. 17–12). The aldosterone antagonist in common use is spironolactone, although the spironolactone congener potassium canrenoate and their common pharmacologically active metabolic byproduct canrenone are also available commercially. The aldosterone antagonists competitively bind to a cytoplasmic receptor protein in aldosterone-responsive cells, leading to enhanced transcription of mRNA and production of new cation transporting proteins.[319] As single-diuretic therapy, their efficacy is likely to be enhanced in conditions characterized by high aldosterone levels, such as ascites due to cirrhosis. They are relatively ineffective in the therapy of heart failure unless combined with a second diuretic. Amiloride and triamterene are structurally related agents that inhibit Na^+ uptake into collecting duct epithelia by reducing Na^+ conductance of the apical membrane.[320] Amiloride has been the better studied of the two agents, although it is presumed that triamterene works via a similar mechanism.

A major effect of these drugs is to diminish renal K^+ secretion, which may lead to clinically important hyperkalemia, particularly in patients with renal insufficiency.[321] These drugs also cause a mild metabolic acidosis due to reduced H^+ secretion into the urine by collecting duct epithelial cells. In patients with chronic obstructive pulmonary disease, potassium-sparing diuretics, alone or in combination with other diuretics, may be preferred to diuretics that enhance renal H^+ wasting and secondarily diminish ventilatory drive.[323]

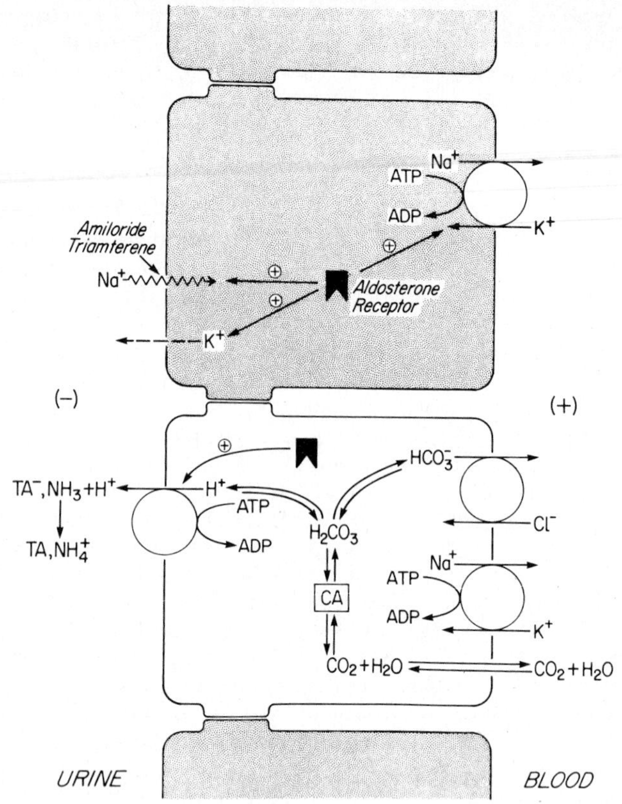

FIGURE 17–12. Diuretics act in the cortical collecting duct primarily on the principal cells. Aldosterone enhances apical membrane permeability by increasing conductance of sodium through the tubular membrane; aldosterone also increases H^+ secretion in intercalated cells by enhancing proton pump activity. Amiloride, and probably triamterene, inhibit the luminal Na^+ conductance channels. Any reduction in Na^+ transport will reduce the luminal potential difference and diminish K^+ secretion; the negative lumen potential difference also enhances proton secretion. Protons secreted into the tubular lumen titrate poorly resorbable anions (titratable acid, TA) and convert ammonia (NH_3) to ammonium (NH_4^+). Inhibition of carbonic anhydrase by acetazolamide is pharmacologically unimportant in the collecting duct.

COMBINED DIURETIC REGIMENS

LOOP DIURETICS COMBINED WITH THIAZIDES. In patients with edema refractory to high doses of loop diuretics or with side effects (generally ototoxicity) from these agents, combinations of diuretics may result in clinically desirable diuresis at lower doses of both drugs. Indeed, the combination of a loop diuretic with a thiazide often results in a synergistic effect on solute and water excretion.[322] This may be due in part to an "unmasking" of the proximal tubular effects of thiazides due to inhibition of NaCl resorption in the loop of Henle, although additive effects in the distal tubule are also important.[324] Treatment of refractory edema due to cardiac failure is also enhanced in children with a combination of a thiazide and loop diuretic.[325] Severe hypoalbuminemia or chronic renal insufficiency (creatinine clearance <25 ml/min/1.73 M^2) diminished the natriuretic response to this combination.[325–326]

Although this combination of diuretics may be very efficacious in selected patients with refractory edema formation, profound intravascular volume depletion and electrolyte disturbances may complicate its use. K^+ wasting is severe and potentially life-threatening unless serum K^+ is carefully monitored. Advanced prerenal azotemia may occur, leading to irreversible renal insufficiency in some patients.[326] A rapid reduction in GFR will directly affect the clearance of many drugs, and hypokalemia enhances the toxicity of cardiac glycosides. Consequently, this combination of diuretics should be initiated only with careful observation, preferably in a hospital setting. Subsequent outpatient therapy should be regulated carefully by monitoring of daily weights and appropriate checks of serum electrolytes and digoxin levels.

LOOP AND THIAZIDE DIURETICS IN COMBINATION WITH POTASSIUM-SPARING AGENTS. A potassium-sparing diuretic combined with a more proximally acting diuretic is the most commonly prescribed diuretic combination. The rationale for limiting potassium losses with routine diuretic administration is discussed in more detail below. All the potassium-sparing diuretics limit K^+ and H^+ loss induced by diuretics acting more proximally. However, some combinations of these drugs may lead to a less than additive effect on NaCl excretion.[327] Triamterene, but not amiloride or spironolactone, inhibits the tubular secretion of furosemide, thus delaying and possibly limiting its pharmacological effect.[328] In addition, loop diuretics tend to attenuate the inhibitory effect of amiloride or triamterene on collecting duct Na^+ conductance due to the high luminal sodium concentration present in the collecting duct during a furosemide natriuresis.[327] Nevertheless, these combinations of agents are useful in some patients with congestive failure, provided that a careful watch is kept for the development of hyperkalemia and metabolic acidosis, particularly in patients with renal insufficiency.[328, 329]

COMPLICATIONS OF DIURETIC THERAPY

DISTURBANCES OF POTASSIUM HOMEOSTASIS. All the diuretics discussed in this chapter affect renal potassium handling.[330] In patients with congestive heart failure, both hypokalemia due to potassium-wasting diuretics and hyperkalemia due to potassium supplements or potassium-sparing diuretics may contribute to morbidity and mortality. Renal potassium losses due to diuretic use can be exacerbated by hyperaldosteronism and persistent chloride depletion with the development of a metabolic alkalosis. Dietary salt intake may also contribute to the extent of renal potassium wasting with diuretics: very high salt diets increase delivery of NaCl to distal tubular K^+ secretory sites, while very low salt diets may stimulate aldosterone-induced K^+ secretion[331, 332] (Fig. 17–11). Extrarenal regulators of the serum potassium concentration may also serve to exacerbate renal losses of K^+, such as the release of epinephrine in response to stress, myocardial ischemia, or pulmonary edema,[333] or the administration of insulin, whether or not concurrent glucose is given.[334]

The controversy over whether diuretic-induced hypokalemia justifies therapy with oral potassium or potassium-sparing diuretics has been summarized in several recent reviews[335–338] and is discussed in Chapter 28. Patients with congestive heart failure, a majority of whom have underlying ischemic heart disease, are a population at risk for malignant ventricular arrhythmias.[339–341] Many of these patients are on maintenance cardiac glycosides. It is prudent in this population to administer potassium supplements or a potassium-sparing diuretic, or to any patient with a serum potassium below 3.5 mEq/liters. In patients with severe hepatic dysfunction due to advanced right heart failure or to other causes, K^+ supplements should be administered to reduce hepatic (and renal) ammonia production. Hypokalemia may also exacerbate glucose intolerance in certain patients. There is little justification for treating all patients with congestive heart failure on diuretic therapy with costly potassium supplements, and there is a small, but definite, risk of inducing hyperkalemia with its attendant cardiovascular morbidity, particularly in patients with reduced renal function (which includes a majority of geriatric patients). It should also be noted that concomitant administration with diuretics of prostaglandin synthetase inhibitors, beta-blockers, and angiotensin-converting enzyme inhibitors may result in a rise in serum potassium levels.[333, 342]

HYPONATREMIA. This is a common complication of diuretic therapy, particularly in patients with congestive heart failure. The origin of hyponatremia in these patients is multifactorial and includes diuretic-induced defects in renal diluting ability, inappropriately high vasopressin levels due to a reduced cardiac output and high angiotensin II levels, and excessive thirst. Hyponatremic patients tend to have high plasma renin activity and norepinephrine and epinephrine levels and reduced renal plasma flows compared with nonhyponatremic ($\geq$135 mEq/liter) subjects.[343–345] Indeed, hyponatremia per se is a powerful predictor of cardiovascular mortality, as one would expect if it were the result of increasing and relatively ineffective diuretic therapy and heightened stimulation of neurohumoral compensatory systems due to worsening myocardial failure.[346] Mild hyponatremia will generally respond to fluid restriction below urinary and insensible losses, usually less than 1000 ml/day, coupled with a moderate (not severe) salt restriction. More severe hyponatremia ($<$120 mEq/liter) should be treated more rapidly but cautiously, with a combination of loop diuretics and administration of 0.9 per cent NaCl (or, rarely, 3 per cent NaCl) administered intravenously.[347] This therapy may require concomitant monitoring of cardiac filling pressures. Combined therapy with angiotensin-converting enzyme inhibitors, but not other vasodilators, with a loop diuretic often results in improved control of hyponatremia in these patients.[346, 348, 349]

HYPOMAGNESEMIA. Unlike urinary excretion of calcium, which is enhanced only by loop diuretics in volume-replete subjects, urinary magnesium wasting occurs with both loop and thiazide (but not potassium-sparing) diuretics. Total body magnesium stores, which may not be reflected accurately by the serum magnesium level, are invariably depleted in chronic diuretic therapy. Although a role for hypomagnesemia in the generation of cardiac arrhythmias has been hypothesized, the clinical manifestations of lowered total body magnesium stores remain poorly defined.[350–352] Deficiencies in this intracellular divalent cation may play a critical role in cardiac arrhythmias and vascular spasm. Nevertheless, given our present state of knowledge, no justification exists for magnesium supplementation in diuretic-treated patients in the absence of documented magnesium depletion.

HYPERURICEMIA. This is a common complication of chronic diuretic therapy with all loop and thiazide diuretics except indacrinone. Competition by diuretics for the proximal tubular organic acid secretory pathway and enhanced proximal and distal tubular resorption of uric acid by diuretics causes the hyperuricemia. Although sustained plasma urate levels of up to 13 mg/100 ml may sometimes occur, attacks of gout or uric acid nephropathy are rarely a problem clinically; however, if higher levels of hyperuricemia occur, allopurinol may be given.[352a, 353] Indacrinone is an orally active loop diuretic that may become the only commercially available uricosuric diuretic. It structurally resembles both ethacrynic acid and ticrynafen; the latter was marketed in the United States only briefly because of its hepatotoxicity.

CARBOHYDRATE INTOLERANCE AND HYPERLIPIDEMIA. Carbohydrate intolerance is commonly seen in patients receiving thiazide diuretics. Hypokalemia may be partly responsible for this effect, but the principal mechanism is probably a blunted insulin response to increases in plasma glucose, although peripheral insulin resistance has not been ruled out.[354] This is supported by the description of normal hemoglobin A_{1C} levels in patients treated with furosemide, as opposed to elevated levels in those treated with hydrochlorothiazide.[355] Ketoacidosis is rare, although hyperosmolar nonketotic coma may develop in volume-depleted patients with adult-onset Type II diabetes.

The impact of thiazide diuretics on serum lipid levels remains controversial. LDL levels have been shown to be elevated in patients on thiazides (but not loop diuretics[355]), including an increase in the ratio of LDL to HDL.[356] Serum triglyceride levels are also significantly higher in patients receiving thiazide diuretics.[357, 358] Although in studies aerobic exercise and diet lowered both serum triglycerides and the LDL/HDL ratio, independent effects of diuretics appeared to persist.[357, 358] Unlike in hypertension, for which alternative therapies exist, diuretics remain first-line agents in the treatment of congestive cardiac failure. Therefore, plasma glucose levels and serum lipids should be monitored periodically in patients receiving thiazide diuretics. These effects may be dose-related; therefore, the lowest effective dose of the appropriate thiazide should be prescribed. Glucose intolerance and lipoprotein abnormalities have been reported to be less marked with the heterocyclic thiazide derivative indapamide.[359, 360]

ACID-BASE DISTURBANCES. These may be seen with any diuretic, and are discussed above, with the description of individual diuretics. Metabolic acidosis is an unusual complication of therapy with potassium-sparing diuretics but is a consistent outcome of acetazolamide administration. Thiazide diuretics may cause a mild "contraction" alkalosis, while loop diuretics typically induce a more severe hypochloremic alkalosis, particularly in salt-restricted, potassium-depleted patients. Because these agents are commonly utilized in patients with multiple metabolic and respiratory acid-base problems, a mixed acid-base disorder tends to be the rule, and the contribution of diuretics to the clinical problem requires careful analysis.

DIURETIC USE IN CONGESTIVE HEART FAILURE

The principal justification for using a diuretic in therapy is the reduction of cardiac filling pressures, thereby diminishing congestive symptoms. For the loop diuretics, which are most commonly used for this indication, this results from both a decrease in extracellular volume caused by the diuretic-induced natriuresis and an increase in venous capacitance. Intravascular volume (blood volume) may change little immediately after intravenous furosemide administration to patients in pulmonary edema, even if a substantial natriuresis occurs, due to alterations in Starling forces across capillary endothelia that result in shifts of solute and fluid into the vascular space.[361] The fall in cardiac preload with intravenous loop diuretics usually leads to a rapid improvement in pulmonary congestive symptoms. Chronic diuretic administration, in conjunction with a low salt diet, will result in substantial losses of edema fluid with little change in the cardiac index.[362] Excessive diuretic use may lead to hyponatremia, metabolic alkalosis, prerenal azotemia, and orthostatic hypotension, even in patients who remain edematous, if insufficient time is allowed for redistribution of edema fluid into the intravascular space.

Although diuretics are relatively safe drugs with predictable and often easily manageable toxicity, certain cardiac patients may suffer increased morbidity when given a diuretic. Patients with congestive heart failure will benefit from the hemodynamic and natriuretic effects of diuretics if the reduction in cardiac filling pressures does not result in a clinically significant fall in cardiac output. This is the case when, before diuretic administration, the patient's cardiac function is situated on a relatively flat portion of the ventricular function curve and not on its ascending limb. Patients with chronic heart failure characterized by poor ventricular compliance, such as hypertrophic subaortic stenosis, concentric left ventricular hypertrophy due to aortic stenosis, and long-standing hypertension, or by constrictive pericardial or myocardial disease, may experience a sharp fall in cardiac output as filling pressures are reduced. In these patients, diuretics should be given cautiously, with careful monitoring of blood pressure, heart rate, and urine output, and, if necessary, direct measurement of hemodynamics. As discussed previously, some patients with chronic congestive failure and relatively normal ventricular compliance—particularly those not acutely ill—may experience transient worsening of their congestive symptoms after being given an intravenous loop diuretic due to the rapid release of renin by the kidney and subsequent increase in systemic vascular resistance.[307]

Most patients with acute congestive heart failure can be treated safely with diuretics without a clinically significant fall in cardiac output, in part because these patients are likely to be operating on a relatively flat portion of their ventricular function curves, and in part because relief of pulmonary edema and improved tissue oxygenation results in a reduction in sympathetic vasomotor tone and a fall in afterload that offsets the fall in preload. However, there is no justification for *routinely* treating patients with acute myocardial infarction with a diuretic, in part because the magnitude of the fall in pulmonary capillary wedge pressures is unpredictable, and because their reduced ventricular compliance may require higher filling pressures to sustain cardiac output.[363, 364] Diuretics are, of course, useful in the treatment of heart failure in patients with myocardial infarction.

VASODILATORS

GENERAL CONSIDERATIONS

Cardiac performance can be affected profoundly by alterations in the resistance and capacitance of the peripheral vascular bed. Thus, it has been appreciated for many years that both in animals with experimentally induced mitral regurgitation[365, 366] and in patients with this valvular lesion[367] the volume of regurgitant flow varies directly, and the forward stroke volume varies inversely, with afterload. It is also well known that the response of the left ventricle to an augmentation of afterload is a direct function of myocardial contractility. When contractility is normal, elevating afterload leads to an increase in stroke work, with little elevation of ventricular end-diastolic volume or pressure, and little decline in stroke volume. In patients with left ventricular dysfunction, as afterload is increased further, stroke work fails to rise or even declines and left ventricular end-diastolic pressure and volume rise even further.

In patients with congestive heart failure the arterial and venous beds are often inappropriately constricted.[368] The vasoconstriction is related to the same phenomenon observed in other conditions, such as hypovolemic shock, in which there is a reduction of cardiac output; the survival value of this fundamental response is to maintain perfusion of vital organs, such as the brain and the heart, at the expense of less immediately essential vascular beds, such as the skin, gut, and kidney. While this maintenance of perfusion pressure may be a desirable evolutionary development insofar as hypovolemic shock is concerned, it is of

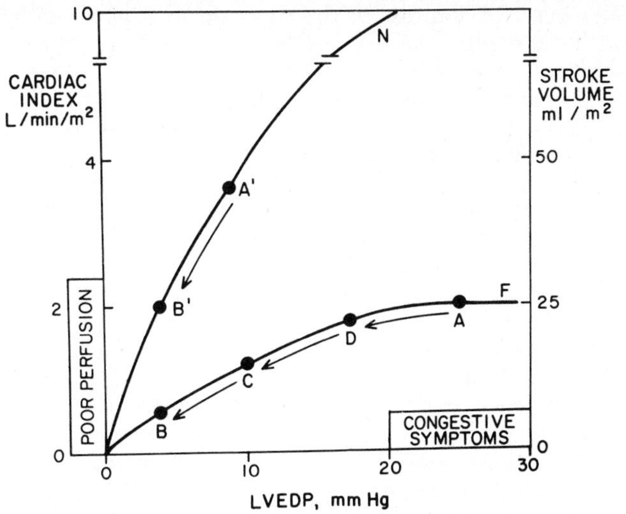

FIGURE 17–13. Effect of venodilator or diuretic therapy in a normal (N) subject (A′ → B′) and in patients with heart failure (F) and markedly elevated left ventricular filling pressure (A → D), moderately elevated filling pressure (D → C), and normal filling pressure (C → B). In all instances venodilators or diuretic therapy results in a decline in filling pressure; except in the patient with marked elevation of filling pressure, cardiac output declines.

little value and actually may be deleterious in patients with heart failure. (Presumably there is little evolutionary advantage to the survival of individuals with heart failure.) At least five mechanisms appear to be involved in the inappropriate vasoconstriction in heart failure (pp. 439 to 444): (1) increased adrenergically mediated vasoconstrictor tone; (2) elevated concentrations of circulating catecholamines; (3) elaboration of renin, with resultant increases in the potent vasoconstrictor angiotensin II; (4) elevated levels of circulating arginine vasopressin; (5) increased thickness of arteriolar walls, presumably related to extracellular fluid accumulation in the blood vessels themselves.[369]

Venoconstriction tends to displace blood into the thorax, causing pulmonary congestion while arteriolar constriction increases the impedance to left ventricular emptying. The combination of ventricular dilatation induced by the cardiac lesion (augmented by the blood volume redistribution resulting from venoconstriction) and elevated vascular resistance operating through Laplace's law (p. 405) increases the afterload on the failing myocardium, which is operating on the flat portion of its function curve (Fig. 17–13). Under these circumstances further elevation of preload increases pulmonary congestion but will not raise cardiac output. Instead, the augmented afterload reduces myocardial fiber shortening that reduces cardiac output further, leading to a vicious circle (Fig. 17–14).

Intra-arterial counterpulsation, a mechanical technique that reduces left ventricular afterload (p. 573), appears to have been the first deliberate clinical use of afterload reduction in the treatment of left ventricular failure,[370] although effective treatment of hypertension with antihypertensive drugs undoubtedly had also achieved this goal. Majid et al. took an important step forward when they infused the alpha-adrenoceptor blocking agent phentolamine into normotensive patients with persistent left ventricular dysfunction after myocardial infarction and demonstrated that the induced fall in systemic vascular resistance was accompanied by considerable elevation of cardiac output and reduction in pulmonary artery pressure.[371] Since that report, vasodilators have achieved wide use in the treatment of heart failure.[372–378a]

With few exceptions, vasodilators do not exert a direct effect on myocardium, but their ability to relax vascular smooth muscle, directly or indirectly, can result in marked improvement in both the clinical and hemodynamic state of the patient. By dilating arterioles and/or veins, these agents have the capacity to alter profoundly the loading conditions on the heart and thereby to modify cardiac performance. Arteriolar dilatation results in a reduction in afterload and may augment cardiac output, while venodilatation may produce a reduction in preload, may lower ventricular filling pressure, and may reduce symptoms of pulmonary congestion.

Venodilators tend to reduce to normal the elevated intrathoracic blood volume characteristic of heart failure. Since the capacity of the venous bed (also referred to as the capacitance bed) is large, a relatively small reduction in venous tone can result in the pooling of substantial quantities of blood into this bed and its redistribution from the pulmonary to the systemic circuit.[378] The acute hemodynamic effects of a pure systemic venodilator resemble those of a diuretic (Fig. 17–13) and cause the left ventricular function curve to shift to the left. In a normal subject this reduction in preload can result in an undesirable decline of cardiac output (A′→B′) and can cause postural hypotension, often observed in patients without heart failure who take large doses of nitrates. In contrast, patients with heart failure and elevated filling pressure generally tolerate even large doses of nitrates quite well. In patients with heart failure but normal filling pressure, perhaps from previous diuresis, venodilatation may also result in a decline in cardiac output (C→B). Only in the patient with heart failure and an elevated filling pressure can venodilation reduce filling pressure and thereby relieve symptoms of pulmonary congestion without depressing cardiac output (A→D). Intermediate responses are observed in patients with moderate elevation of filling pressures (D→C).

CHOICE OF VASODILATOR. From a theoretical point of view, the administration of a vasodilator whose principal action is on the venous system is: (1) *desirable* in patients whose principal clinical manifestation of heart failure is pulmonary congestion secondary to elevated left ventricular filling pressure, (2) *undesirable* in patients in whom the preload or filling pressure has already been restored to normal by means of diuretic therapy and/or dietary sodium restriction, and (3) *useful* in combination with arteriolar dilators in patients whose clinical manifestations of failure are related to both reduction of perfusion and pulmonary congestion.[379]

Arteriolar dilators act as *afterload-reducing agents.* As shown in Figure 17–15, as well as in Figures 13–15C

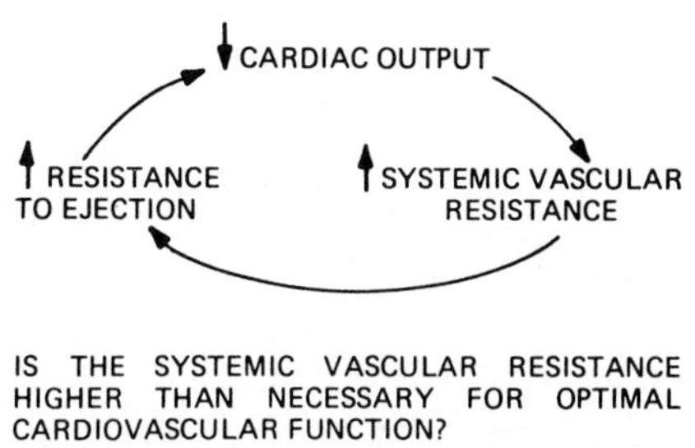

FIGURE 17–14. Potential vicious circle of chronic heart failure. With the onset of heart failure, cardiac output decreases. As a compensatory mechanism to maintain arterial blood pressure, systemic vascular resistance increases. This further increases the resistance or impedance to ejection of the left ventricle, which will result in a further reduction in cardiac output. The patient will spiral down this cycle until a new steady-state relation is reached in which cardiac output may be lower and systemic vascular resistance higher than is really optimal for the patient. (From Parmley, W. W., and Chatterjee, K.: Vasodilator therapy. Curr. Probl. Cardiol. Vol. 2, No. 12, 1978, p. 15.)

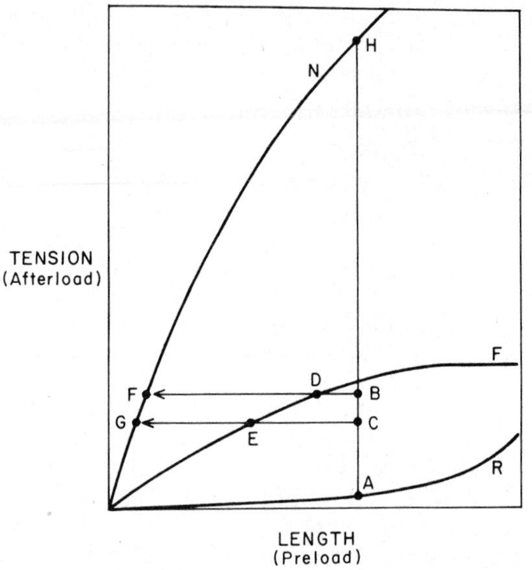

FIGURE 17–15. Length-tension relations in normal (N) and failing (F) heart muscle. R = length–resting tension curve for both normal and failing heart muscle. The effects of reducing afterloads from B to C on shortening are contrasted. In the normal muscle, shortening increases only slightly (from B → F to C → G). In failing muscle, there is substantial enhancement of shortening (B → D to C → E). H represents isometric tension development by normal muscle.

(p. 395) and 13–16 (p. 396), at any level of preload and myocardial contractility, the extent of myocardial fiber shortening (and therefore stroke volume) is inversely related to the afterload. Afterload is related to the instantaneous stress in the muscle fibers of the ventricle (p. 410), which is also closely related to the aortic impedance, i.e., the instantaneous relationship between pressure and flow in the aorta during ejection, and, in turn, to systemic vascular resistance. Just as the hemodynamic and clinical effects of venodilatation and the resultant reduction of ventricular preload depend on the filling pressure so do the effects of afterload depend on myocardial contractility. Figure 17–15 displays, in schematic form, the acute effects of afterload reduction on ventricular fiber shortening in normal and failing hearts. In the normal heart a reduction of afterload (B→C) results in only a minor augmentation of myocardial fiber shortening (B→F to C→G). In contrast, an identical reduction in afterload in the failing heart causes a substantial augmentation of myocardial fiber shortening (B→D to C→E). In the intact heart, as schematized in Figure 17–16, the reduction of stroke volume caused by an increased afterload is substantially greater in the presence of myocardial dysfunction than in the normal heart. A corollary is that any given reduction of afterload will cause a much greater increase in stroke volume in the failing than in the normal heart.

In patients with heart failure the reduction in systemic vascular resistance induced by vasodilators is usually offset by an increase in cardiac output, and arterial pressure may decline only slightly or not at all. In normal subjects the reduction of systemic vascular resistance induced by arteriolar vasodilators is associated with no or only small increases in cardiac output (Fig. 17–17) (A′→H′), and their administration to normotensive subjects without heart failure may cause postural hypotension accompanied by reflex tachycardia. In patients with depressed contractility without elevation of filling pressure, arteriolar dilatation may produce a small augmentation of cardiac output (C→H″). However, in contrast to the situation existing in patients with markedly elevated preload, arterial pressure may decline.

Many vasodilators act on both the arterial and the venous beds (so-called balanced vasodilators), and their actions are intermediate between those of pure venous and pure arterial dilators and resemble those of a combination (Fig. 17–17). In normal subjects (A′→P′), and in patients with heart disease but without elevated ventricular filling pressure (C→P″), balanced dilators usually cause reductions in filling pressure, arterial pressure, and cardiac output. Patients with heart failure and pulmonary congestion who are given balanced vasodilators display favorable effects (A→P), with augmentation of cardiac output and reduction of pulmonary capillary pressure but little decline in arterial pressure or elevation of heart rate.

From these considerations, it is apparent that patients with depressed myocardial contractility and an elevation of filling pressure are likely to benefit significantly from vasodilator therapy. Arterial dilators cause an increase in cardiac output, while venodilators reduce pulmonary congestion and balanced dilators cause a combination of these effects. Patients with heart disease without elevated vascular resistance, depressed cardiac output, and elevated filling pressures are unlikely to benefit immediately from the use of vasodilators.

Although the classification of vasodilators as arterial, venous, or balanced has proved to be useful in understanding their action and in the rational selection of a particular agent for a specific patient, the intimate interactions between cardiac preload and afterload that exist in the intact circulation must be considered. Since afterload is a function of intraventricular pressure and ventricular volume, a venodilator will, by reducing ventricular volume, also lower afterload. Conversely, an arterial dilator, by enhancing stroke volume and ventricular emptying, will reduce

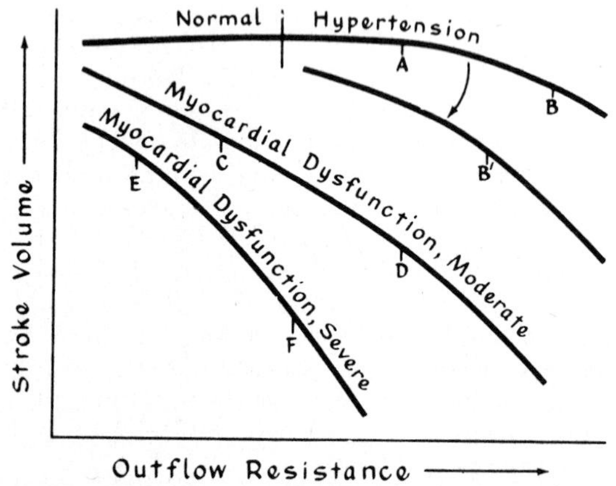

FIGURE 17–16. Relation of left ventricular stroke volume to systemic outflow resistance in normal and diseased hearts. A family of curves may be described, depending on the severity of the myocardial disease. If cardiac function is normal, a rise in resistance results in hypertension, since cardiac output remains fairly constant. Heart failure in a hypertensive patient could be shown by a move to either point B, a high resistance with normal function, or point B′, which represents a shift to a slightly depressed ventricular function curve. When myocardial dysfunction is more severe, as shown by the lower two curves, blood pressure is no longer directly determined by resistance, since stroke volume and resistance are inversely related. Consequently, arterial pressure may be similar at points E and F despite marked differences in cardiac output and resistance. It is also apparent that a reduction in outflow resistance will not affect significantly the stroke volume of the normal ventricle. However, it can produce a marked increase in the stroke volume of the failing ventricle (F → E). (Reproduced with permission from Cohn, J. N., and Franciosa, J. A.: Vasodilator therapy of cardiac failure. N. Engl. J. Med. *297*:27, 1977.)

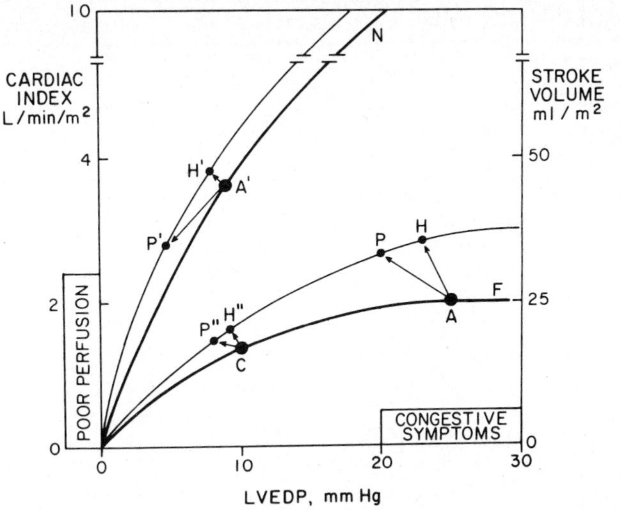

FIGURE 17–17. Effects of various vasodilators on the relationship between left ventricular end-diastolic pressure (LVEDP) and cardiac index or stroke volume in normal (N) and failing (F) hearts. H represents hydralazine or any other pure arterial dilator. It produces only a minimal increase in cardiac index in the normal subject (A′ → H′) or in the patient with heart failure with normal LVEDP (C → H″). In contrast, it elevates output in the patient with heart failure and elevated LVEDP (A → H). P represents a balanced vasodilator, such as sodium nitroprusside or prazosin. It reduces filling pressure in all patients, elevates cardiac output in patients with heart failure and elevated LVEDP (A → P), lowers cardiac output in normal subjects (A′ → P′), and has little effect on cardiac output in heart failure patients with normal filling pressures (C → P″).

ventricular volume (preload). This reduction in ventricular size combines with lowering arterial pressures to cause a proportionately greater reduction of systolic wall tension (afterload) than of arterial pressure.

Because wall tension is a principal determinant of myocardial oxygen consumption ($M\dot{V}O_2$) and because both arteriolar and venodilators reduce wall tension in patients with heart failure, vasodilators reduce $M\dot{V}O_2$ while increasing cardiac output. These actions of vasodilators compare favorably with those of positive inotropic agents or beta-adrenoceptor blocking agents. The former (like vasodilators) augment cardiac output but either increase $M\dot{V}O_2$ or maintain it at a constant level; the latter (like vasodilators) reduce $M\dot{V}O_2$ but depress cardiac performance.

MONITORING. The monitoring of vasodilators when they are used in the treatment of acute myocardial infarction is discussed on page 1247. It is important to bear in mind that, when these drugs are given to patients with critical coronary artery obstructions, particularly with acute ischemia reductions in coronary perfusion pressure in the face of critical coronary obstruction can impair further blood flow through narrowed coronary arteries, and through collateral vessels, and thereby this therapy can intensify ischemia. Therefore, vasodilator therapy must be employed cautiously in patients with coronary artery disease, particularly in those with acute myocardial infarction or other acute ischemic syndromes. Arterial pressure should be monitored carefully during acute vasodilator therapy, particularly in patients with known or suspected coronary artery disease. In view of the importance of ventricular filling pressure as a determinant of the response to vasodilators (Figs. 17–13 and 17–17), the monitoring of pulmonary capillary wedge or pulmonary artery pressure by means of a Swan-Ganz catheter is extremely helpful in regulating the dosage of vasodilators during intravenous therapy. Because in addition to the reduction in pulmonary wedge pressure, the elevation of cardiac output is an important endpoint, it is desirable to make serial measurements of cardiac output in acutely ill patients receiving intravenous vasodilators.

In patients without ischemic heart disease, monitoring of intraarterial pressure during intravenous vasodilator therapy is desirable but is not essential as long as indirect pressure is measured at frequent intervals. Invasive monitoring is obviously not practical or necessary in patients treated for prolonged periods with agents administered orally, sublingually, or transdermally. However, it is desirable to make frequent measurements of arterial pressure in the supine and upright positions when therapy is initiated or the dosage is being adjusted.

VASODILATOR AGENTS (Table 17–8)

SODIUM NITROPRUSSIDE. Probably the most widely used vasodilator in the treatment of *acute* congestive heart failure, sodium nitroprusside is extremely short-acting and must be given intravenously. It acts directly to relax vascular smooth muscle in both arterioles and veins. Sodium nitroprusside had been employed successfully for many years to treat hypertensive crisis (p. 880) and subsequently was introduced for the treatment of congestive heart failure.[380, 381] Since sodium nitroprusside is a balanced dilator, its hemodynamic action in the presence of severe impairment of left ventricular failure is both to increase cardiac output and diminish pulmonary congestion (Fig. 17–17). It is particularly useful in patients with severe hypertension associated with left ventricular failure, severe heart failure associated with mitral and/or aortic regurgitation, acute myocardial infarction, acute heart failure following cardiac surgery, and in patients with acute intensification of chronic heart failure. It should not be administered to patients with hypotension. The initial infusion rate in adults is usually 10 μg/min and may be increased by increments of 5 to 10 μg/min every 5 minutes until the desired effect is achieved or until hypotension or other side effects limit further dose increments; the maximum dose in adults is 300 μg/min.

The most important adverse effect of sodium nitroprusside is hypotension, an extension of its therapeutic action, which is typically reversed within 10 minutes after discontinuation of the drug. If this waiting period poses a danger, hypotension can be treated more rapidly by infusion of a vasoconstrictor such as phenylephrine or norepinephrine. Nitroprusside releases hydrocyanic acid, which could lead to cyanide poisoning.[382] However, this is an extremely uncommon complication, since hydrocyanic acid is converted to thiocyanate in the presence of thiosulfate. Thiocyanate is excreted by the kidney, and in the presence of renal insufficiency the infusion of large doses of nitroprusside for prolonged periods may lead to thiocyanate toxicity, which is characterized by convulsions, psychosis, abdominal pain, hypothyroidism, muscle twitching, and dizziness. Therefore, when patients receive nitroprusside for more than a few days, serum levels of thiocyanate should be measured and not allowed to exceed 6 mg/100 ml. Methemoglobinemia and vitamin B_{12} deficiency are two other rare complications of nitroprusside therapy. In patients with chronic pulmonary disease, nitroprusside can cause hypoxia due to pulmonary vascular dilatation and perfusion of poorly ventilated alveoli.

As described below (p. 529), for enhanced effect, nitroprusside may be infused in combination with positive inotropic agents such as dobutamine.

PHENTOLAMINE. This agent was the first vasodilator used to increase cardiac output in patients with heart failure.[371] Phentolamine is a complex drug. It is an $alpha_1$ (postsynaptic) and $alpha_2$ (presynaptic) adrenoceptor

TABLE 17–8 MAJOR VASODILATOR DRUGS*

Drug	Mechanism of Action	Venous Dilating Effect (Preload Reduction)	Arteriolar Dilating Effect (Afterload Reduction)	Usual Dosage	Comments
Nitroglycerin	Direct	+ + +	+	25–500 μg/min IV 5–60 mg transdermal	Tolerance may be a problem with sustained continuous use.
Isosorbide dinitrate	Direct	+ + +	+	5–20 mg q 2 hr sl 10–60 mg q 4 hr p.o.	Improved survival shown in chronic CHF when used with hydralazine.
Nitroprusside	Direct	+ + +	+ + +	5–150 μg/min IV	Used IV only. Drug is light-sensitive.
Hydralazine	Direct	–	+ + +	10–100 mg q 6 hr p.o.	Sustained benefit in heart failure not shown when used as sole vasodilator.
Prostacyclin	Direct	+ + +	+ + +	5–15 ng/kg/min IV	Investigational use only.
Phenoxybenzamine	Alpha-adrenoceptor blockade (nonselective)	+ +	+ +	10–20 mg q 8 hr p.o.	Limited current use.
Phentolamine	Alpha-adrenoceptor blockade (nonselective)	+ +	+ +	50 mg q 4–6 hr p.o.	Limited current use.
Prazosin	Alpha-adrenoceptor blockade (α selective)	+ + +	+ +	1–5 mg q 6 hr p.o.	Extra caution required with initial doses.
Trimazosin	Alpha-adrenoceptor blockade plus undetermined mechanism	+ + +	+ +	50–450 mg b.i.d. p.o.	Investigational use only.
Captopril	Angiotensin-converting enzyme inhibitor	+ +	+ +	6.25–25.0 mg q 6–8 hr p.o.	Approved by FDA for use in chronic CHF. Acute renal failure can occur with initial doses; initiate use with extra caution.
Enalapril	Angiotensin converting enzyme inhibitor	+ +	+ +	2.5 mg q.i.d. to 15 mg b.i.d.	Approved by FDA for treatment of hypertension.
Nifedipine	Calcium channel blockade	+	+ +	10–40 mg q 6 hr p.o. 10–40 mg q 6 hr sl	Negative inotropic effect may be unmasked in severe CHF.

*All of these agents may cause severe hypotension, and special caution is required with initial use, particularly in patients with severe CHF.

blocker of both arterioles and veins, but predominantly of the former[383]; it releases cardiac norepinephrine stores and thereby exerts transient positive chronotropic and inotropic effects. (The positive chronotropic effect is usually undesirable in patients with heart failure.) Like nitroprusside, phentolamine has a short duration of action when used intravenously, and excessive hypotension is its major adverse effect. The initial dose in adult patients is 0.1 mg/min, and it may be increased in steps of 0.1 mg/min every 5 minutes to a maximum of 2.0 mg/min. It has been reported to be effective in the treatment of low-output chronic heart failure[384] and pulmonary edema.[385] In addition to gastrointestinal symptoms of nausea, vomiting, and abdominal pain, the aforementioned tachycardia and the high cost of the drug make phentolamine less desirable than nitroprusside in the treatment of acute heart failure. It is now rarely used in the treatment of heart failure.

NITRATES (See also p. 1327). Nitroglycerin and the closely related long-acting nitrates such as isosorbide dinitrate and pentaerythritol tetranitrate are vasodilators that act on vascular smooth muscle, principally on the venous bed, the pulmonary arterial bed, and to a lesser extent on the systemic arteriolar bed. These drugs are available in a variety of formulations[374, 386, 387] and can be administered by various routes (Table 39–1, p. 1329), making them useful in a number of situations. In normal individuals and in patients with heart failure but without elevated filling pressure, the prominent venodilator action results in reduction of cardiac output (Fig. 17–13) and often postural hypotension. This hypotensive response, which had been observed many years ago in some patients with acute myocardial infarction without heart failure, was responsible for cessation of nitroglycerin use in this condition. However, in patients with heart failure and elevated pulmonary capillary pressure, even when secondary to myocardial infarction, nitroglycerin reduces ventricular filling pressure and relieves congestive symptoms. The pulmonary vasodilating and slight systemic arteriolar dilating effects of the drug are sufficient to cause a modest increase in cardiac output as well,[388] if ventricular filling pressures are maintained in an adequate range.

Nitroglycerin. When administered sublingually, nitroglycerin is useful in the treatment of acute congestive heart failure in the absence of hypotension. It is usually administered in a dose of 0.3 to 1.2 mg; the effect usually begins within 2 minutes, becomes maximal in 8 minutes and persists for 15 to 30 minutes. In patients in whom left ventricular filling pressure is elevated to 20 mm Hg, it usually declines to approximately 10 mm Hg in 5 to 10 minutes following nitroglycerin use.[389] Although the slight reduction of arterial pressure may be accompanied by a mild acceleration of heart rate, MVO_2 declines, and this is a major mechanism for the antianginal effect of the drug (p. 1328). Since the absorption of sublingual nitroglycerin may be erratic, continuous *intravenous infusion* has been utilized to produce a sustained, controllable effect in patients with acute heart failure and pulmonary congestion in whom predominant venodilation is desired. The initial dose is 10 μg/min and may be increased by increments of 10 μg/min every 5 minutes to a maximal dose of 100 μg/min.

For prolonged duration of action, *topical nitroglycerin* may be used; effects of the ointment last at least 3 hours. Depending on the dose desired, a 0.5 to 4.0 inch strip is applied to the skin, usually on the chest. Although topical administration does not make nitroglycerin ointment convenient for ambulatory patients, an advantage of this formulation is that it can be removed readily in case of adverse effects. It can be applied conveniently before retiring and is useful to combat attacks of paroxysmal nocturnal dyspnea. Any of several available transdermal administration systems (nitroglycerin patches or discs) provide a steady rate of absorption and stable venous plasma level for 24 hours. It is more convenient than the ointment for ambulatory patients and allows showering.

Isosorbide Dinitrate. This long-acting nitrate is available in sublingual and oral formulations. The sublingual dose is 2.5 to 10 mg every 2 hours, and the oral dose is 20 to 60 mg every 4 hours. In addition, other long-acting nitrates such as oral pentaerythritol tetranitrate (10 to 40 mg four times a day) or oral controlled-release nitroglycerin preparations (one 6.5 mg capsule every 4 hours) have been employed to achieve a prolonged nitrate effect and have been found useful in the treatment of chronic heart failure.[390, 391] The side effects of all nitrates include headache and postural hypotension, but these symptoms are more prominent in patients with mild than with severe heart failure and can be controlled by decreasing the dose. Methemoglobinemia, an extremely rare complication, may occur with long-term use of large doses.

A major problem with all sustained-use nitrate preparations is the development of partial tolerance.[392] With transdermal patches, relatively high doses (60 mg/24 hr) are necessary for effectiveness and even these are associated with a diminished action after 18 hours. It may be desirable to allow the patient several hours each day when he is not exposed to nitrates, since recovery from tolerance occurs rapidly.

There is some evidence from controlled trials that chronic administration of long-acting nitrates reduces symptoms of heart failure and increases exercise tolerance.[387] When used in combination with hydralazine, chronic administration of isosorbide dinitrate, 40 mg four times daily, was found in the VHEFT trial to prolong survival in patients with heart failure[374] (Fig. 17–18).

HYDRALAZINE (See p. 876). This orally effective vasodilator acts directly on arteriolar smooth muscle.[392a] Hydralazine's predominant action on the arterial bed results

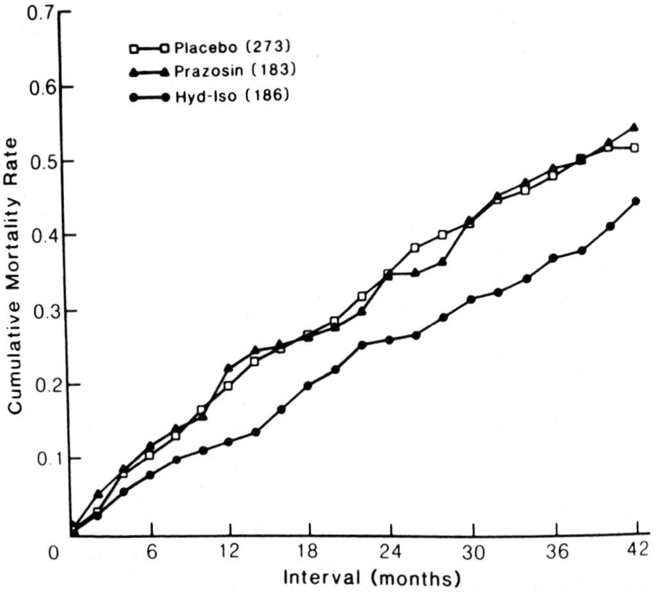

FIGURE 17–18. Cumulative mortality from the time of randomization in three groups of patients with heart failure in the VHEFT trial. Mortality in placebo and prazosin treated patients was identical; mortality was reduced in patients treated with hydralazine and isosorbide dinitrate. (Reproduced with permission from Cohn, J. N., Archibald, D. G., Ziesche, S., et al: Effect of vasodilator therapy on mortality in chronic congestive heart failure: Results of a Veterans Administration Cooperative Study. N. Engl. J. Med. *374*:1550, 1986.)

in an increase in cardiac output with relatively minor reductions in ventricular filling and arterial pressures and increases in heart rate in patients with heart failure.[393] The usual dose ranges from 25 to 100 mg three to four times daily, and its effects commence within 30 minutes and persist for about 6 hours.

The degree of left ventricular enlargement[394] and the level of peripheral vascular resistance appear to be important determinants of the response to hydralazine in patients with chronic heart failure. Patients with marked cardiomegaly and markedly elevated systemic vascular resistance exhibit the most salutary responses. Side effects include vascular headaches, flushing, nausea, and vomiting, which often disappear with continued therapy. Drug fever and skin rash are seen occasionally; fluid retention and increased edema occur commonly when this drug, as well as other vasodilators, is administered over the long term. The latter complication usually responds readily to an increase in the dose of diuretics. In addition to fluid retention, tolerance to the favorable hemodynamic effects of hydralazine develops in a minority of patients, apparently due to an altered responsiveness to the drug of vascular smooth muscle.[395] A more serious adverse effect, a lupus-like syndrome, is seen in approximately 15 per cent of patients receiving 400 mg of hydralazine daily, and an even higher percentage of patients develops circulating antinuclear antibodies. Although this syndrome is not usually observed in patients who receive less than 200 mg of the drug daily, the average dose required for effective afterload reduction is about 75 mg four times a day, making this complication significant in patients receiving hydralazine. Hydralazine is metabolized principally by acetylation, and patients in whom this process is slow are more likely to develop both the lupus-like syndrome and a peripheral neuropathy due to pyridoxine deficiency. Fortunately, the lupus-like syndrome subsides when hydralazine is discontinued. The peripheral neuropathy can be treated or prevented by pyridoxine administration.

The ultimate role of hydralazine in the management of chronic congestive heart failure remains controversial. Some studies have yielded favorable long-term results with improved exercise capacity and reduced cardiac size on x-ray,[396] especially when hydralazine is used in combination with nitrates.[397] Other trials have not demonstrated a difference between hydralazine and placebo in long-term treatment of chronic heart failure.[398] As mentioned above, in the VHEFT study, a multicenter, randomized double-blind trial, 300 mg hydralazine daily combined with isosorbide dinitrate resulted in improved survival (compared to placebo or prazosin) (Fig. 17–18).[374] This represents the first trial of vasodilators demonstrating a beneficial effect on survival.

Endralazine. This experimental drug, which is structurally related to hydralazine, may have the distinct advantage of not causing the lupus-like syndrome.[399]

PRAZOSIN (See p. 873). This antihypertensive drug, a quinazoline derivative, is a potent alpha-adrenoceptor blocking agent, the action of which is limited to the vascular adrenergic (alpha$_1$) receptors with little effect on presynaptic (alpha$_2$) receptors (Fig. 28–7, p. 872).[400] As a consequence, neuronally released norepinephrine is available to act on the alpha$_2$ receptors, inhibiting its own release and preventing the development of reflex tachycardia. Prazosin differs from phentolamine and phenoxybenzamine, which block both presynaptic (alpha$_2$) and postsynaptic (alpha$_1$) receptors. In addition, prazosin exerts direct relaxing effects on vascular smooth muscle, but this mechanism is probably not important at clinically relevant serum or tissue levels of the drug.

Prazosin is an orally effective, balanced vasodilator, equally effective on arterioles and veins, and its circulatory effects resemble those of intravenous nitroprusside.[401] Oral doses show maximum effectiveness in 45 minutes and persist for 6 hours. Tolerance to the drug has been reported,[402] and in a long-term comparison of prazosin and captopril the latter was found to be superior in terms of clinical benefit and long-term hemodynamic improvement.[402] As noted above, in the VHEFT study prazosin did not improve long-term patient survival in comparison with placebo[374] (Fig. 17–18).

While the vascular headaches, flushing, and lupus-like syndrome that occur with the use of hydralazine are not observed with prazosin, polyarthralgias, transient headache, mild nausea, urinary incontinence, rash, mental depression, dry mouth, and fluid retention have been reported.[404] An important problem with the use of the drug, although uncommon in patients with congestive heart failure, is the so-called "first-dose phenomenon," in which transient faintness, dizziness, palpitation, and, uncommonly, syncope occur after the initial dose, owing to postural hypotension. This dose is therefore quite low, 1 mg, and may be adjusted upward during the first few days of administration, but the total dosage should not exceed 10 mg three times a day. Despite the favorable acute hemodynamic effects exerted by prazosin in heart failure, and its value as an antihypertensive (p. 873), the side effects, frequent development of tolerance, and the unimpressive long-term effects do not argue for its use in the chronic treatment of heart failure.

ANGIOTENSIN-CONVERTING ENZYME (ACE) INHIBITORS (p. 877). The renin-angiotensin-aldosterone axis is activated in many patients with congestive heart failure (p. 443) and circulating levels of all three substances are often elevated.[405] This has led to the use of captopril[375, 376, 378, 403, 406-408] and enalapril,[377, 409-413] orally active drugs that block the enzymatic conversion of angiotensin I to angiotensin II, in the management of heart failure.

ACE inhibitors depress circulatory levels of angiotensin I and markedly elevate plasma renin activity. Also, by interfering with the breakdown of bradykinin, ACE inhibition increases the circulating level of this vasodilator; this action, as well as possible increases in circulating prostaglandins, may play a role in the vasodilator action of these drugs.[414] In addition, ACE inhibitors decrease circulating catecholamine concentrations. ACE inhibitors are balanced vasodilators with actions on both the arteriolar and venous beds, and in sufficient doses cause marked reductions in systemic vascular resistance and arterial pressure. ACE inhibition is particularly marked in arterioles that are highly sensitive to angiotensin II, such as those in the renal arterial bed.

In patients with heart failure, left and right ventricular filling pressures decline and cardiac output rises, but there is usually little or no change in heart rate[415] and arterial pressure. With captopril the action commences one-half hour after ingestion, is maximal at 1 to 1½ hours, and persists for 6 to 8 hours. Maximal effects are observed with 25 to 50 mg t.i.d. Enalapril[411] resembles captopril except that it has a slower onset and a longer duration (12 to 24 hours) of action. The "pro-drug" enalapril is deesterified in the liver to the active form, enalaprilat. The initial dose, which rarely causes hypotension and renal failure, is 2.5 mg, and the maintenance dose ranges from 10 mg q.i.d. to 15 mg b.i.d.

Captopril and enalapril have been reported to improve hemodynamics in patients with congestive heart failure that is poorly controlled by digitalis and diuretics,[416-418] to restore responsiveness to diuretics, and to restore serum sodium levels in azotemic hyponatremic patients with heart failure.[419]

As is the case with hypertension, ACE inhibitors appear to be effective in heart failure, regardless of the level of plasma renin[420]; they have been shown to be effective clinically even in patients with low plasma renin activity.[407] The overall clinical response to ACE inhibition appears to be less impressive in patients with renal failure.[421, 422] ACE inhibition augments skeletal muscle flow in normal subjects; it reduces renal vascular resistance and elevates renal blood flow in patients with heart failure.[423] By reducing arterial pressure without causing reflex tachycardia, captopril lowers myocardial oxygen demands and thereby may exert an antianginal effect.[427]

The clinical benefits of ACE inhibitors in heart failure are impressive. These drugs enhance the sense of well-being in the majority of patients. In double-blind, placebo-controlled trials, ACE inhibition exerts a number of salutary effects, including symptomatic improvement,[376] less frequent clinical deterioration during follow-up[375, 410] sustained improvement of exercise tolerance[375-377, 412] (Fig. 17–19), and hemodynamic improvement and reduction in cardiac dimensions.[377] ACE inhibition is effective in patients with mild[409] as well as with severe heart failure.

In a randomized trial carried out on 253 patients with severe heart failure, the so-called CONSENSUS trial,[425] the 6 month survival of patients who received enalapril, digitalis, and diuretics was 74 per cent, significantly greater than that of patients on diuretics and digitalis alone (56 per cent). This study, together with VHEFT,[374] indicates that survival of patients with heart failure can be improved with vasodilator therapy.

ACE inhibitors should not be administered with potassium-sparing diuretics (except in the presence of hypokalemia), and excessive hypotension is the major hazard. The drugs are contraindicated in intrinsic renal disease with renal failure, bilateral renal artery stenosis, and systemic hypotension. The lack of arterial unsaturation, regularly observed with the use of other vasodilators, suggests that ACE inhibitors do not produce significant pulmonary arteriovenous shunting.

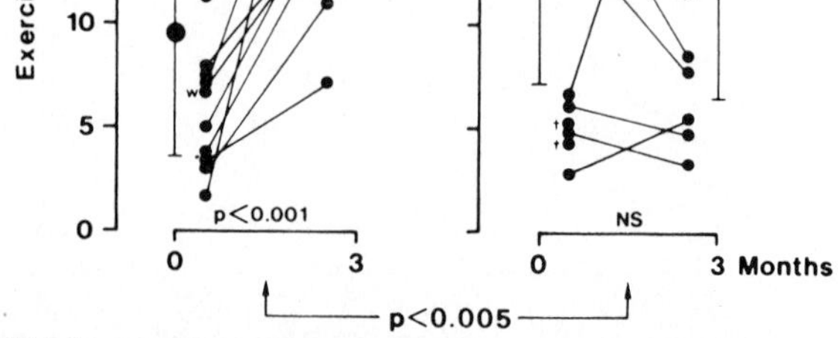

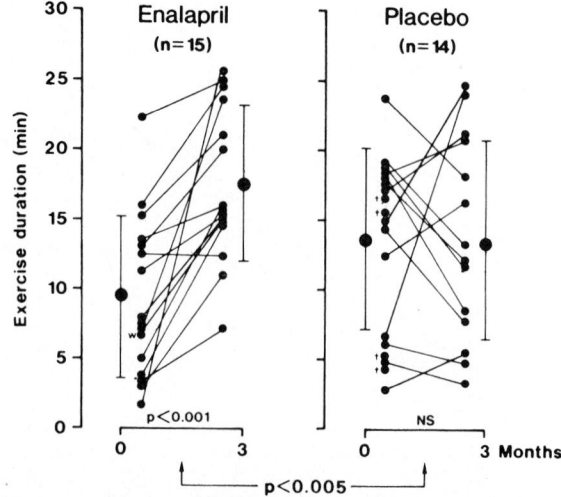

FIGURE 17–19. Effects of 3 months of enalapril and placebo treatment on exercise duration in patients with heart failure. The groups were significantly different at baseline, but the change within the enalapril group from baseline to 3 months was significant (p<0.001). This change was quite dissimilar in the two groups. W = withdrawn; + = died. (From Sharpe, D. N., Murphy, J., Coxon, R., and Hannan, S. F.: Enalapril in patients with chronic heart failure: A placebo-controlled, randomized, double-blind study. Circulation *70*:271, 1984, by permission of the American Heart Association, Inc.)

CLINICAL APPLICATIONS OF VASODILATOR THERAPY

The use of vasodilators in two specific situations, acute pulmonary edema and acute myocardial infarction, is discussed elsewhere (p. 555).

LEFT VENTRICULAR FAILURE. Vasodilator therapy has proved to be very effective in patients with acute left ventricular decompensation. The intravenous infusion of sodium nitroprusside is generally associated with clinical improvement, clearing of pulmonary rales, elevation of cardiac output, improvement of peripheral perfusion, and augmented responsiveness to diuretics. When left ventricular filling pressure has declined to approximately 15 mm Hg and cardiac output has risen to above 2.1 liters/min/m^2, an attempt should be made to wean the patient from the intravenous vasodilator and to convert to one of the oral (or transdermal) medications. Although the infusion of sodium nitroprusside usually can be discontinued after 48 to 72 hours, it may be necessary to continue it for as long as 7 to 10 days in patients with severe heart failure. The major problem with sodium nitroprusside infusion is hypotension. If, in a previously normotensive patient, systolic arterial pressure falls to below 90 mm Hg or decreases by more than 30 mm Hg from the control level, the drug should be discontinued or the dosage reduced. In patients who become hypotensive but require vasodilator therapy to improve perfusion, a combination of nitroprusside and an inotropic agent (dopamine or dobutamine) should be considered (p. 529). Particular care must be taken to avoid hypotension (and therefore hypoperfusion of myocardium in the distribution of stenotic coronary vessels) in patients with known or suspected coronary artery disease.

Transient myocardial depression during the perioperative period in patients who have undergone cardiac surgery may be associated with an elevated systemic vascular resistance, and in such cases sodium nitroprusside may be useful. In patients with perioperative depression of cardiac function and hypotension, a sympathomimetic agent and/or intraaortic balloon counterpulsation usually is used in combination with the vasodilator.

Infusion of sodium nitroprusside for several days may also be effective in *chronic heart failure* that has become refractory to therapy with digitalis and diuretics,[426] although most such patients can be managed with one of the orally active vasodilators. Patients with borderline elevations of left ventricular filling pressure (12 to 15 mm Hg) derive little benefit from nitroprusside, because the venodilator action results in further reduction of filling pressure with little change, or even a decline, in cardiac output. When filling pressure has been reduced to normal by nitroprusside and the principal hemodynamic abnormality is low cardiac output, cautious expansion of blood volume with dextran and the simultaneous administration of nitroprusside can result in striking elevation in cardiac output.[392] Rebound increases in systemic vascular resistance above baseline, with consequent reduction in cardiac output, have been reported immediately after withdrawal of nitroprusside and are most pronounced in patients who developed tachycardia during infusion of the drug.[427] This phenomenon is presumably due to unopposed vasoconstrictor influences and can be managed by the gradual tapering of nitroprusside and the substitution of an orally effective vasodilator.

MECHANICAL LESIONS. In patients with mitral regurgitation or ventricular septal defect,[428] the abnormal regurgitant or shunt flow is a direct function of the systemic vascular resistance; reduction of the latter augments systemic output and diminishes the load on the left ventricle by reducing the abnormal flow. Ordinarily when these lesions are severe enough to cause heart failure, they should be treated surgically, but when they occur in the course of acute myocardial infarction, it may be best to defer operation for several weeks if the patient's condition is stable. Treatment with vasodilators, at first with sodium nitroprusside and then sustained with orally active drugs, may aid in stabilizing the patient's condition during this interval.[429]

Increased systemic vascular resistance also augments the regurgitant volume in patients with aortic regurgitation, and vasodilator therapy reduces the regurgitation and increases the forward stroke volume and cardiac output.[430] However, caution must be exercised in the treatment of aortic regurgitation with vasodilators, since these drugs may lower further the already depressed aortic diastolic pressure and interfere with coronary filling. Vasodilator therapy is of little benefit and generally should not be used in patients with obstructive valvular lesions.

Although systemic vasodilators often have relatively little effect on the pulmonary vascular bed, oral hydralazine has been reported to exert favorable hemodynamic effects in some patients with cor pulmonale.[431] Prazosin can improve right ventricular function by lowering left ventricular diastolic pressure and, secondarily, pulmonary artery and right ventricular systolic pressure in patients with severe congestive heart failure.[432] Oxygen may also be considered to be a right ventricular afterload reducing agent, since high concentrations may be used to counteract the pulmonary vasoconstrictor effect of hypoxia.

LONG-TERM THERAPY WITH VASODILATORS

There is general agreement that patients with chronic left ventricular failure that does not respond adequately to measures such as modest restriction of sodium intake, diuretics and digitalis, and who have no contraindications (hypotension, renal failure), should receive chronic therapy with an orally active vasodilator. Although clear-cut evidence of improvement in survival as a result of such therapy has been demonstrated only with the combination of hydralazine and isosorbide dinitrate[374] (Fig. 17–18), and with enalapril[425a] the available clinical and hemodynamic data with the use of ACE inhibitors are quite impressive. These drugs usually are well tolerated and increasingly are the agents of choice when chronic vasodilator therapy is indicated. There is interest in commencing treatment with these agents earlier than heretofore, i.e., before the patient has become unresponsive to the combination of diuretics and glycosides. Indeed, there is some rationale, based on animal investigations,[432a] for reducing intraventricular wall tension in patients who have cardiac dilation and/or a reduced ejection fraction without overt heart failure, in an effort to delay the deterioration of cardiac function and the development of heart failure. The use of vasodilators prophylactically in this manner is currently under active investigation.

NONGLYCOSIDE INOTROPIC AGENTS

SYMPATHOMIMETIC AMINES

Catecholamines and other sympathomimetic amines exert potent inotropic effects by interacting with myocardial ($beta_1$) adrenoceptors. For many years attempts were made to utilize these properties in the treatment of heart failure. However, these efforts were largely unsuccessful because of the potent positive chronotropic, vasoconstrictor, or vasodilator actions of these agents (Tables 17–9 and 17–10), the development of tolerance and "down-regulation" of $beta_1$ receptors with prolonged administration, and the lack of sensitivity of failing myocardium to beta agonists (Fig. 14–18, p. 441). Isoproterenol, and to a lesser extent epinephrine, cause tachycardia and hypotension by stimulating $beta_1$-adrenoceptors in the sinoatrial node and $beta_2$ receptors in the systemic vascular bed. Norepinephrine, on the other hand, a powerful stimulant not only of $beta_1$- but also of $alpha_1$-adrenoceptors, causes vasoconstriction and hypertension. Two sympathomimetic agents, dopamine and dobutamine, cause less tachycardia and fewer systemic vascular effects. They are employed frequently and are useful for short periods in the treatment of severe heart failure.

DOPAMINE

This endogenous catecholamine, the immediate biosynthetic precursor of norepinephrine, stimulates myocardial contractility by acting directly on $beta_1$-adrenoceptors in the myocardium and indirectly by releasing norepinephrine from sympathetic nerve terminals, which in turn also stimulates $beta_1$ receptors[433] (Tables 17–9 and 17–10). The cardiac effects of dopamine are antagonized by beta-adrenoceptor blockers. Dopamine-induced vasodilation is not blocked by propranolol and therefore is not related to activation of $beta_2$ receptors; also, it is not due to release of acetylcholine,[434] histamine,[433] or prostaglandins.[435] However, dopaminergic vasodilation is antagonized by phenothiazines, such as chlorpromazine, and butyrophenone compounds, such as haloperidol.[436] It is now clear that the vasodilation mediated by dopamine is secondary to activation of specific dopaminergic receptors, which exist in a variety of tissues including blood vessels as well as the central and peripheral nervous systems (Fig. 17–20).[437] Activation of so-called $dopamine_1$ receptors causes vasodilation in the coronary, renal, mesenteric, and cerebral vascular beds; these actions result from stimulation of adenylate cyclase and elevation of intracellular cyclic AMP. The activation of $dopamine_2$ receptors is also responsible for vasodilation but does so by inhibiting transmission in sympathetic nerve endings, presumably by *inhibiting* adenylate cyclase.[437] Dopamine-induced diuresis is a prominent and clinically important action in patients with heart failure (Fig. 17–21)[438] and is secondary to a combination of inotropic and, at lower doses, selective renal vasodilator effects.[443, 447] Studies in both dogs[439] and humans[440] have demonstrated that dopamine preferentially dilates vessels in the renal cortex.

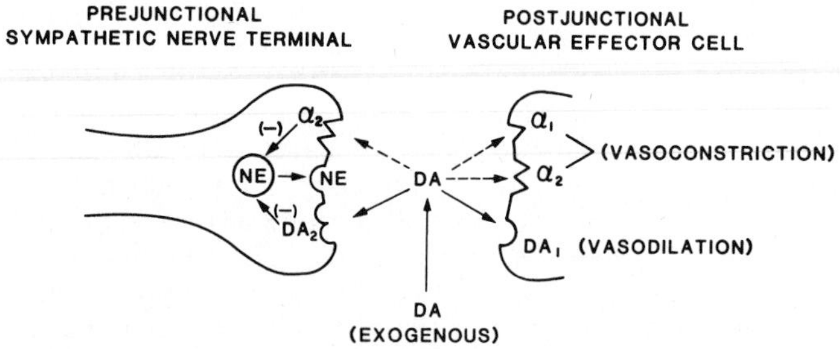

FIGURE 17–20. Location of dopamine-1 (DA_1) receptors, $alpha_1$- and $alpha_2$-adrenoceptors on postganglionic vascular effector cells, and DA_2 receptors and $alpha_2$-adrenoceptors on the prejunctional sympathetic nerve terminal. When dopamine is administered, activation of DA_1 receptors causes vasodilation and activation of DA_2 receptors causes inhibition (−) of norepinephrine (NE) release from storage granules. A larger dose of dopamine activates $alpha_1$- and $alpha_2$-adrenoceptors on the postjunctional effector cells to cause vasoconstriction and on $alpha_2$-adrenoceptors on the prejunctional sympathetic terminal to inhibit release of norepinephrine. Norepinephrine released from the prejunctional sympathetic terminal also acts on the two types of adrenoceptors. (From Goldberg, L. I., and Rajfer, S. I.: Dopamine receptors: Applications in clinical cardiology. Circulation *72*:245, 1985, by permission of the American Heart Association, Inc.)

When larger doses of dopamine are administered, the dilatation is reversed, and dopamine causes constriction of arteries and veins in all vascular beds.[433] Although the vasoconstriction has been attributed to action of the drug on alpha-adrenoceptors, the doses of the alpha receptor blockers phentolamine and phenoxybenzamine required to prevent the dopamine-induced vasoconstriction are higher than those required to antagonize the vasoconstriction caused by other alpha-adrenoceptor agonists. Dopamine-induced contractions of isolated canine vessels can be attenuated by concentrations of the serotonin-blocking agent cyproheptadine that do not antagonize the actions of norepinephrine. These findings suggest that the vasoconstrictor action of larger doses of dopamine results from contraction of vascular smooth muscle, caused in part by action on serotonin-sensitive receptors as well as on $alpha_1$-adrenoceptors.[441]

Thus, effects of dopamine on vascular resistance and arterial pressure are dose-dependent. With infusion rates below 2 μg/kg/min the major action of the drug is to reduce resistance in the renal, mesenteric, and coronary vascular

TABLE 17–9 SOME RECEPTOR ACTIONS OF CATECHOLAMINES

Adrenoceptor	Site	Action
$Beta_1$	Myocardium	Increase atrial and ventricular contractility
	Sinoatrial node	Increase heart rate
	Atrioventricular conduction system	Enhance atrioventricular conduction
$Beta_2$	Arterioles	Vasodilation
	Lungs	Bronchodilation
Alpha	Peripheral arterioles	Vasoconstriction

TABLE 17–10 ADRENERGIC RECEPTOR ACTIVITY OF SYMPATHOMIMETIC AMINES

	Alpha Peripheral	$Beta_1$ Cardiac	$Beta_2$ Peripheral
Norepinephrine	++++	++++	0
Epinephrine	++++	++++	++
Dopamine*	++++	++++	++
Isoproterenol	0	++++	++++
Dobutamine	+	++++	+
Methoxamine	++++	0	0

*Causes renal and mesenteric dilatation by stimulating dopaminergic receptors.
Tables 9 and 10 from Sonnenblick, E. H., et al: Dobutamine: A new synthetic cardioactive sympathetic amine. N. Engl. J. Med. *300*:18, 1979.

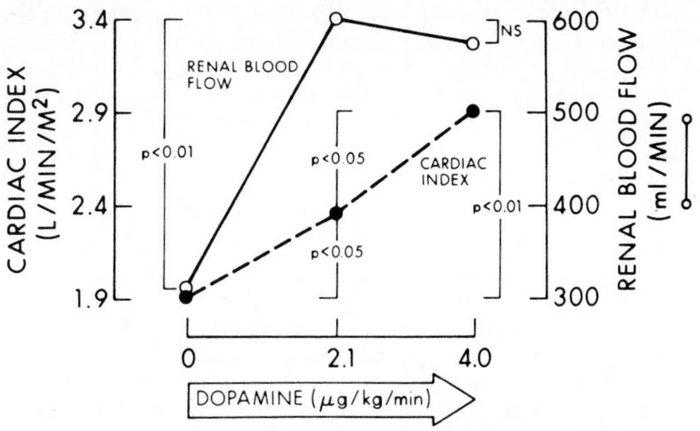

FIGURE 17–21. Changes in cardiac index and renal blood flow in response to ascending doses of dopamine. (From Maskin, C. S., Ocken, S., Chadwick, B., and LeJemtel, T. H.: Comparative systemic and renal effects of dopamine and angiotensin-converting enzyme inhibition with enalaprilat in patients with heart failure. Circulation *72*:846, 1985, by permission of the American Heart Association, Inc.)

beds. Doses of 2 to 5 μg/kg/min exert a positive inotropic effect; cardiac contractility and cardiac output increase, with little change in heart rate and either a reduction or no change in total peripheral resistance.[442] With higher infusion rates (5 to 10 μg/kg/min), arterial pressure, peripheral resistance, and heart rate increase[443] and renal blood flow may decline.

Like other sympathomimetic amines that increase cardiac contractility, dopamine increases coronary blood flow[433] secondary to the increase in myocardial oxygen consumption that results from increased cardiac work.[444] Direct coronary vasodilatation mediated through action on dopaminergic receptors in the coronary arteries is a secondary mechanism involved in the increase in coronary flow.[445] However, as is the case in other vascular beds, large doses of dopamine may increase coronary artery resistance by direct action on alpha$_1$-adrenergic (and perhaps serotonergic) receptors.[433] Ultimately, the effects of dopamine in patients with myocardial ischemia, like those of other catecholamines, depend on the balance between myocardial oxygen utilization and coronary blood flow, which in turn are affected by the sum total of its several actions. Augmented heart rate, contractility, and arterial pressure—all resulting from high doses—increase oxygen utilization, whereas reduced peripheral resistance and heart size lower oxygen utilization. In addition, low doses of dopamine reduce coronary vascular resistance, while high doses increase it.

In early investigations, Goldberg et al. found that in patients with heart failure dopamine increased sodium excretion and cardiac output[446]; infusion rates of 2.1 to 5.8 μg/kg/min increased cardiac index (+26 per cent) without causing significant changes in heart rate or total body oxygen consumption. Peripheral resistance was reduced, and pulmonary vascular resistance, when elevated, also fell. Left ventricular dP/dt increased by 58 per cent, glomerular filtration rate by 38 per cent, renal plasma flow by 79 per cent, and sodium excretion by an average of 48 per cent. Thus, in patients with congestive heart failure, dopamine exerts important beneficial hemodynamic and renal effects.[447] However, care must be taken to adjust the infusion rate carefully to prevent excessive positive inotropic effect, tachycardia, and increased peripheral resistance.

In normotensive patients with refractory heart failure, infusions are begun at low rates (0.5 to 1.0 μg/kg/min) and are gradually increased until urine flow is augmented or until increments in diastolic pressure and heart rate are observed. The infusion rate should then be decreased and if possible discontinued. In patients with cardiogenic shock, both the vasoconstrictor and the more intense inotropic effects of higher doses may be desirable (p. 573). When large doses of dopamine are required for its positive inotropic action, it may be infused together with nitroprusside[448] or nitroglycerin to counteract the vasoconstrictor action.

USE DURING AND FOLLOWING CARDIAC SURGERY. Dopamine is widely used for the treatment of acute heart failure following cardiopulmonary bypass.[449, 450] In a comparison of the effects of three catecholamines in 22 patients with low cardiac output states following surgery, dopamine increased cardiac index by 1.1 liters/min/m^2, mean arterial pressure by 7 mm Hg, heart rate by 19 beats/min, and urine flow by 75 ml/hr. In contrast, norepinephrine increased cardiac index by much less (only 0.2 liter/min/m^2) and mean arterial pressure by much more (23 mm Hg), while heart rate rose by 9 beats/min and urine flow *decreased* by 8 ml/hr. The action of isoproterenol was similar to that of dopamine by increasing cardiac index by 0.95 liter/min/m^2, but the former caused a more severe tachycardia, increasing heart rate by 28 beats/min. Urine flow increased by 28 ml/hr, while mean arterial pressure decreased by 7 mm Hg. These observations demonstrate the superiority of dopamine over isoproterenol and norepinephrine in this clinical setting.[451] The use of dopamine (or dobutamine, see below), sometimes combined with intraaortic balloon counterpulsation, permits the discontinuation of cardiopulmonary bypass in some patients with severe depression of cardiac function who cannot otherwise be weaned from the heart-lung machine.[452] Here also dopamine appears to be superior to isoproterenol.

The low cardiac output state in the early postoperative period may be due to severe depression of myocardial contractility resulting in a hemodynamic picture of cardiogenic shock. If the operation has successfully corrected the underlying mechanical defect, the depression of contractility is often reversible. Support with a sympathomimetic agent (dopamine or dobutamine) or with amrinone (p. 527) together with intraaortic balloon counterpulsation is often successful in tiding the patient over until myocardial function recovers.

DOBUTAMINE

Dobutamine is a synthetic cardioactive sympathomimetic amine that stimulates beta$_1$-, beta$_2$-, and alpha-adrenoceptors.[453-455] Radioligand binding studies suggest that beta$_1$ activity predominates over beta$_2$, and that alpha$_1$ predominates over alpha$_2$ activity of this drug.[456] Dobutamine is a racemic mixture; the l isomer is predominantly a potent alpha$_1$ agonist while the d isomer is a potent stimulant of beta$_1$ and beta$_2$ receptors. Myocardial contractility is augmented by the stimulation of alpha and beta$_1$ receptors, while stimulation of each of these receptors counteracts the other so that there is little net action on the systemic vascular bed. Dobutamine does not activate dopaminergic receptors and does not release norepinephrine from adrenergic nerve endings. At equivalent cardiac contractile force responses, dobutamine exerts a much weaker beta$_2$-adrenergic action than does isoproterenol and a much weaker alpha-adrenergic action than does either norepinephrine or dopamine. When given to patients with heart failure, dobutamine results in a reduction in systemic vascular resistance as cardiac output rises, so that arterial pressure remains relatively constant.[457, 458]

In contrast to dopamine, dobutamine is not a renal vasodilator; it does cause a redistribution of cardiac output in favor of the coronary and skeletal muscle beds over the mesenteric and renal vascular beds.[459, 460] A low-dose infusion of dopamine may be added to dobutamine in order to obtain a renal vasodilator effect from the former and a positive inotropic effect from the latter. Gillespie and colleagues administered dobutamine to patients with acute myocardial infarction and found that the drug improved hemodynamics without provoking undesirable side effects and without increasing the extent of myocardial injury.[461] Improvement in cardiac index (mean increase 54 per cent) and stroke work index (mean increase 65 per cent) has been reported in response to dobutamine infusion in patients with chronic heart failure associated with ischemic heart disease, with infrequent precipitation of overt myocardial ischemia.[462] Patients with dilated cardiomyopathy treated continuously for 2 or 3 days or on a weekly basis with intravenous dobutamine have been reported to exhibit favorable hemodynamic effects which were sustained for weeks to a few months.[463–466] Portable infusion devices have been used to administer intravenous dobutamine to ambulatory patients with severe heart failure awaiting cardiac transplantation.[467] However, this long-term treatment has been ineffective; indeed, evidence suggests that it may have increased mortality. Dobutamine, like dopamine, is also useful in the treatment of low cardiac output states following cardiac surgery.[449, 450]

The usual dosage ranges from 2.5 to 10 μg/kg/min, although occasionally doses as low as 0.5 or as high as 40 μg/kg/min have been used. It is important to be sure by clinical examination or invasive monitoring that hypovolemia is not present.

ADVERSE EFFECTS OF DOPAMINE AND DOBUTAMINE. The development of sinus tachycardia and other cardiac arrhythmias constitute the most serious adverse effects of dopamine and dobutamine. The electrophysiological properties of these drugs resemble those of other sympathomimetic amines[433, 468, 469] and consist of accelerating the spontaneous depolarization of sinoatrial cells (thereby increasing heart rate), accelerating diastolic depolarization and facilitating activation of latent pacemaker cells (thereby causing tachyarrhythmias), shortening the refractory period of atrial and ventricular muscle, and speeding atrioventricular conduction. Ventricular arrhythmias have been observed with the use of both drugs.[433, 470] In patients with coronary artery disease, both dobutamine and dopamine may precipitate angina pectoris.[433, 470, 471]

In patients with preexisting vascular disease, the vasoconstriction induced by high doses of dopamine may cause gangrene of the digits.[472] Tissue necrosis similar to that produced by norepinephrine can also occur if an infusion of dopamine extravasates into tissue; this can be prevented by infiltrating the area promptly with 5 to 10 mg of phentolamine diluted in saline. Dopamine differs from the other catecholamines in that it causes nausea and vomiting in some patients, a central nervous system effect more commonly observed with high dosage.[433, 440] Since the cardiovascular effects of dopamine (in contrast to dobutamine) are potentiated by previous therapy with monoamine oxidase inhibitors, the dosage of dopamine in such patients should be reduced to approximately 10 per cent of the usual.[433]

COMPARISONS AMONG DOPAMINE, DOBUTAMINE, AND NITROPRUSSIDE. There has been considerable interest in comparing the effects of these drugs in patients with severe congestive heart failure.[473-475] In one study, dobutamine raised cardiac index while lowering left ventricular end-diastolic pressure and leaving mean aortic pressure unchanged. Dopamine also improved cardiac index but at the expense of a greater increase in heart rate than occurred with dobutamine. Dopamine increased mean aortic pressure but was ineffective in lowering left ventricular end-diastolic pressure. Both dopamine and dobutamine increase myocardial contractility and thereby augment myocardial oxygen consumption. Because dobutamine has little effect on two other major determinants of myocardial oxygen consumption, heart rate and aortic pressure, and reduces a third, ventricular filling pressure (a determinant of ventricular size), it may be superior to dopamine in patients with low-output syndrome associated with ischemic heart disease.[473] Dobutamine effected a more favorable balance between myocardial oxygen supply and demand in patients with severe myocardial depression following cardiac surgery.[449, 450]

In a study comparing the acute hemodynamic effects of dobutamine and dopamine in patients with chronic low-output cardiac failure, it was observed that at dosages adjusted to achieve similar increments in cardiac output, dobutamine reduced left ventricular filling pressure from an average of 25 to 17 mm Hg, while dopamine increased it to 30 mm Hg.[474] This response to dopamine was probably the result of its vasoconstrictor actions and illustrates the potential advantages of using a more cardioselective agent such as dobutamine when the desired goal of therapy is to improve ventricular function by direct inotropic stimulation.

In a comparison between these two sympathomimetic amines in patients with severe heart failure, dobutamine in doses up to 10 μg/kg/min progressively increased cardiac output while decreasing systemic and pulmonary vascular resistance and filling pressure, without a significant effect on heart rate and ventricular irritability. In contrast, dopamine at doses above 4 μg/kg/min increased not only cardiac output but also left ventricular filling pressure and ventricular ectopic activity; at doses greater than 6 μg/kg/min, dopamine also increased heart rate and systemic and pulmonary vascular resistance.[475] The heart rate–systolic blood pressure product, an index related to myocardial oxygen demands, increases with both agents but more so with dopamine than with dobutamine. Furthermore, at any increase in the heart rate–systolic pressure product, the increase in cardiac output with dobutamine is greater than with dopamine.

Thus, in *normotensive* patients with advanced heart failure, large doses of dopamine cause vasoconstriction and raise left ventricular filling pressure. However, filling pressures decline with dobutamine, or with a combination of dopamine or dobutamine and a vasodilator. The inotropic effects of dopamine are in part mediated by release of endogenous norepinephrine, which may be reduced in the hearts of patients with chronic heart failure (p. 440), therefore, low doses of this drug may be insufficient to achieve the desired inotropic effect of an increase in cardiac output, while larger doses may produce unwanted vasoconstriction.

Although dopamine can improve renal and mesenteric perfusion by selective dopaminergic vasodilation (and this unique property of dopamine is not shared by dobutamine), this beneficial effect on regional perfusion is often reversed when dopamine is given in the large doses sometimes required to achieve a sufficient inotropic effect. It is possible, however, to use dopamine in low doses (1.2 to 2.5 μg/kg/min) to provide selective vasodilation of mesenteric and renal vascular beds and combine it with dobutamine, or with a vasodilator, to achieve optimal hemodynamic improvement (p. 529). In conclusion, both drugs are useful in the treatment of refractory heart failure; overall dobutamine is preferred to dopamine, especially in patients with sinus tachycardia who are not hypotensive. However, in patients with heart failure and hypotension, dopamine, with its greater vasoconstrictor properties, may be the sympathomimetic of choice.

In a comparison between sodium nitroprusside and dobutamine, it was found that both drugs reduced systemic vascular resistance.[476] The reduction produced by dobutamine results primarily from withdrawal of compensatory vasoconstriction as a consequence of elevation of cardiac output. On the other hand, sodium nitroprusside infusion reduces systemic vascular resistance more than does dobutamine, suggesting that dobutamine might be preferable to nitroprusside for augmenting cardiac output in patients with borderline hypotension. When the major objective is to lower elevated filling pressure, especially in hypertensive patients, nitroprusside is superior to dobutamine.

ORALLY ACTIVE SYMPATHOMIMETIC AMINES

Several orally active beta-adrenoceptor agonists have undergone clinical study recently, although none has, at the time of this writing, been approved for clinical use in the United States.

LEVODOPA AND DOPAMINE ANALOGUES. Levodopa is the biosynthetic precursor of dopamine; when administered orally with pyridoxine it is decarboxylated to dopamine[477] and exerts a similar salutary hemodynamic effect in heart failure.[478] A central action may be responsible for the nausea and vomiting that are prominent side effects. *Ibopamine*, also orally active, is converted to N-methyl dopamine, and has hemodynamic actions that resemble those of dopamine.[479, 480] Propylbutyldopamine[481] and dopexamine[482] are orally active dopamine analogues that stimulate dopaminergic and beta-adrenergic receptors. While all of these orally active precursors or analogues of dopamine exert favorable hemodynamic effects in patients with heart failure, it is not clear that these effects are sustained with prolonged administration.

Pirbuterol has been found to exert favorable hemodynamic effects in patients with refractory congestive heart failure. These effects may derive from both positive inotropic and vasodilator actions as a consequence of stimulating the $beta_1$- and $beta_2$-adrenoceptors.[483] Cardiac output rises and ventricular filling pressures decline in patients with chronic severe congestive heart failure,[484] responses that resemble those observed with intravenous dobutamine.[485, 486] No provocation of myocardial ischemia was noted in six patients with coronary artery disease and chronic congestive heart failure whose conditions were refractory to digitalis and diuretics.[487] Of concern, however, is the finding that tolerance to the favorable hemodynamic effects of pirbuterol developed over a one-month period of administration. This was accompanied by decreased numbers of beta-adrenoceptors on the lymphocytes of these patients, suggesting a possible mechanism for reduced responsiveness after long-term therapy with pirbuterol, or for that matter with any beta-adrenoceptor agonist administered continuously for long periods.[488]

Prenalterol is an orally active $beta_1$ selective adrenoceptor agonist with positive inotropic effects that has undergone recent clinical testing. At appropriate doses, positive inotropic effects have been observed with little increase in heart rate[489, 490]; however, increased ventricular ectopic activity has also been observed in some patients.

Other beta-adrenoceptor agonists originally introduced as bronchodilators, including *terbutaline* and *salbutamol*,[491] have also been found to exert favorable hemodynamic effects consequent to vasodilator and/or positive inotropic activities.

PHOSPHODIESTERASE INHIBITORS

The action of this group of agents, which exerts both positive inotropic and vasodilator effects, is through the

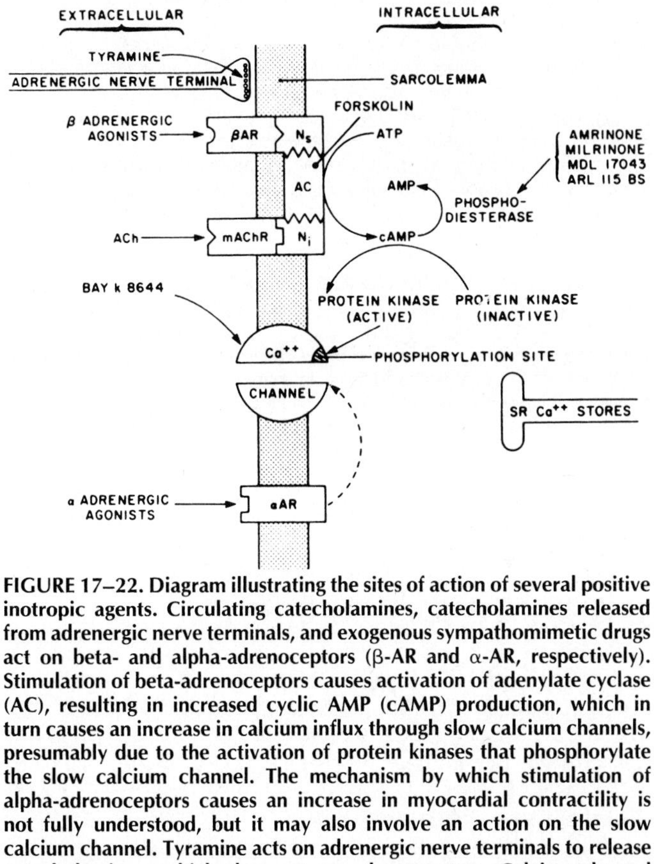

FIGURE 17–22. Diagram illustrating the sites of action of several positive inotropic agents. Circulating catecholamines, catecholamines released from adrenergic nerve terminals, and exogenous sympathomimetic drugs act on beta- and alpha-adrenoceptors (β-AR and α-AR, respectively). Stimulation of beta-adrenoceptors causes activation of adenylate cyclase (AC), resulting in increased cyclic AMP (cAMP) production, which in turn causes an increase in calcium influx through slow calcium channels, presumably due to the activation of protein kinases that phosphorylate the slow calcium channel. The mechanism by which stimulation of alpha-adrenoceptors causes an increase in myocardial contractility is not fully understood, but it may also involve an action on the slow calcium channel. Tyramine acts on adrenergic nerve terminals to release catecholamines, which then act on adrenoceptors. Calcium-channel agonists (e.g., the drug Bay K 8644) act directly on the calcium channel to increase calcium influx. Intracellular cAMP is degraded by phosphodiesterases; therefore, inhibition of cardiac phosphodiesterase results in an increase in intracellular cAMP levels. Several of the newer positive inotropic agents appear to act largely by this mechanism. cAMP can also be increased independently of beta-adrenoceptors by direct stimulation of adenylate cyclase with forskolin. N_s = guanine nucleotide stimulatory subunit, ACh = acetylcholine, mAChR = muscarinic ACh receptor, N_i = guanine nucleotide inhibitory subunit, and SR = sarcoplasmic reticulum. Schema prepared by Dr. T. Smith. (Reproduced with permission from Colucci, W. S., Wright, R. F., and Braunwald, E.: New positive inotropic agents in the treatment of congestive heart failure. N. Engl. J. Med. *314*:292, 1986.)

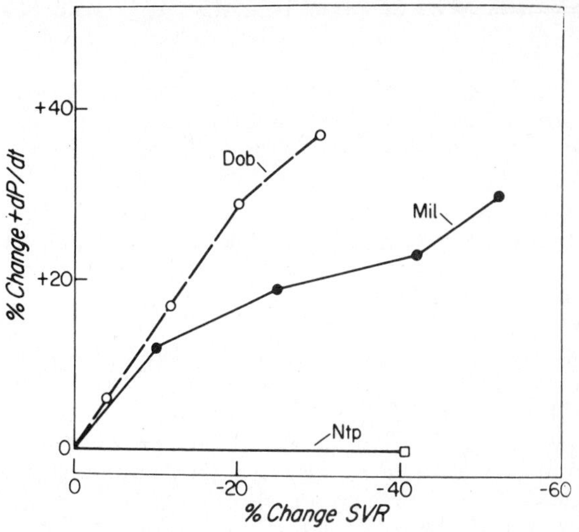

FIGURE 17–23. The relative effects of dobutamine (Dob), nitroprusside (Ntp) and milrinone (Mil) on systemic vascular resistance (SVR) and the peak positive rate of left ventricular pressure development (+dP/dt) in patients with severe congestive heart failure. Nitroprusside, a pure vasodilator agent, causes only a decrease in systemic vascular resistance, without evidence of a positive inotropic action. Dobutamine, a pure positive inotropic agent, causes a marked increase in +dP/dt, a measure of the myocardial inotropic state. In addition, there is a decrease in the systemic vascular resistance with dobutamine, which is most likely caused by reflex withdrawal of sympathetic tone. The new positive inotropic agent milrinone has an effect that is intermediate between those of nitroprusside and dobutamine, causing both a substantial increase in +dP/dt and a substantial reduction in systemic vascular resistance. Milrinone and several of the other new positive inotropic agents appear to exert both positive inotropic and direct vasodilator actions in patients with congestive heart failure, and both actions probably contribute markedly to the net hemodynamic response to the drug. (From Colucci, W. S., Wright, R. F., Jaski, B. E., Fifer, M. A., Braunwald, E.: Milrinone and dobutamine in severe heart failure: Differing hemodynamic effects and individual patient responsiveness. Circulation *73*(Suppl. 3):178, 1986, by permission of the American Heart Association, Inc.)

inhibition of phosphodiesterase F-III.[492] This membrane-bound enzyme is responsible for the breakdown of cyclic AMP, and its inhibition raises intracellular cyclic AMP concentrations. The latter action appears to be responsible for both the positive inotropic and vasodilator effects of these agents (Fig. 17–22). This mechanism is supported by the observation that the muscarinic agonist carbachol, which inhibits adenylate cyclase, interferes with the positive inotropic action of these agents.[493] As is the case for other positive inotropic agents, an increased calcium flux into myocardial cells appears to be the ultimate mechanism of action. It has been demonstrated that these drugs do not inhibit Na^+, K^+-ATPase, nor do they act on adrenergic or histaminergic receptors.

AMRINONE. This bipyridine is the only agent in this class that has been approved for clinical use (by intravenous administration).[494-498] Its administration to patients with heart failure causes dose-dependent increases in cardiac output and reductions in right- and left-sided filling pressures and systemic vascular resistance. Studies in isolated hearts and vascular beds have shown that amrinone exerts both a direct positive inotropic and direct systemic vasodilator action; it causes reductions in pulmonary vascular and coronary vascular resistances. Amrinone's (and milrinone's) hemodynamic effects can be likened to those of a combination of dobutamine, a positive inotropic agent with little direct vascular action, and nitroprusside, a balanced arterial and venous dilator (Fig. 17–23). The drug's effects are additive to those of the digitalis glycosides and are synergistic with direct-acting sympathomimetics. The development of tolerance has not been a problem as it has with the latter agents. The vasodilator action tends to offset the effects of the positive inotropic action, resulting in little change in myocardial oxygen consumption.[499] Therefore, amrinone tends not to intensify ischemia in patients with coronary artery disease. There is facilitation of atrioventricular conduction, causing an acceleration of ventricular rate in patients with atrial fibrillation, but it is usually not otherwise arrhythmogenic.[500]

Amrinone, administered intravenously, is useful in the treatment of heart failure that is refractory to the combination of digitalis glycosides, diuretics, and vasodilators.[501-504] After an initial bolus of 0.75 mg/kg, it is infused intravenously at a dose of 5 to 10 μg/kg/min. Amrinone's vasodilator effects may cause hypotension in patients who are hypovolemic or who are already taking large dosages of other vasodilators. It is useful when infused for several hours to several days in patients with severe heart failure in whom a reversible component is present. It is particularly helpful in patients with postcardiac surgical myocardial depression,[504] in patients with acute exacerbation of chronic heart failure, and in some patients with myocardial infarction and left ventricular failure.[503] While the mechanism of action of amrinone is quite different, its hemodynamic effects resemble those of dobutamine. However, several differences may confer some advantages on amrinone. First, it possesses a direct vasodilator action, which is useful in patients with heart failure who are not hypotensive. The effects of a combination of dobutamine and nitroprusside resemble those produced by amrinone. Second, in contrast to dobutamine, amrinone does not appear to cause tolerance with prolonged infusion and perhaps has less tendency to cause ischemia and ventricular tachyarrhythmias. Since amrinone is available only for intravenous use, it is not recommended for long-term management of heart failure, although it has been administered continuously for as long as 10 days.

Amrinone is well absorbed from the gastrointestinal tract, and the hemodynamic effects produced after oral administration resemble those following intravenous infusion.[505] However, it is not suitable for long-term oral administration because of the high incidence of adverse side effects (gastrointestinal intolerance, fever, abnormalities in hepatic function, and reversible thrombocytopenia). While oral (and intravenous) amrinone initially improves exercise tolerance, there is controversy whether it delays or hastens deterioration of cardiac performance, even among patients who tolerate long-term oral administration.[506] There is concern that prolonged inotropic stimulation of failing hearts may actually hasten deterioration of the underlying myocardial disease ("whipping a tired horse").[507, 508]

The following phosphodiesterase inhibitors are currently in investigational use.

MILRINONE. This congener of amrinone is 15 to 20 times as potent on a per milligram basis and except for a somewhat shorter duration of action has essentially identical pharmacological and hemodynamic effects when administered intravenously.[509-518] In contrast to amrinone, it is well tolerated when administered orally and initially exerts profound salutary effects in patients with refractory heart failure who initially exhibit striking clinical improvement with augmentation of maximum oxygen uptake, anaerobic threshold, and exercise capacity,[519] which are sometimes sustained.[520] However, it is not clear whether its chronic administration exerts a beneficial or detrimental effect on patient survival. The available data suggest that it does not alter the overall natural history when it is administered to patients with advanced heart failure.[521] Milrinone and the other new phosphodiesterase inhibitors have been administered primarily to patients with advanced heart failure. It is important to determine whether they are useful in patients with less severe failure and whether certain subgroups who are likely to benefit from these drugs can be identified.

ENOXIMONE AND PIROXIMONE. These two related agents[522-526] are imidazolones, dissimilar chemically from the bipyridines (amrinone and milrinone) but with quite similar biochemical actions (they are inhibitors of phosphodiesterase F-III) and pharmacological actions (positive inotropic and vasodilator effects). They also initially cause improvement in the clinical manifestations of heart failure, but there is no evidence for any long-term beneficial effects.[526]

OTHER PHOSPHODIESTERASE INHIBITORS. A variety of other compounds, including sulmazole[527] (a phenyl imidazopyridine), RO-13-6438,[528] an imidazoquinazoline derivative, and UD-CG 212,[529] a benzimidazole-pyridazinone, are all orally active, potent phosphodiesterase inhibitors that exert both positive inotropic and vasodilator actions similar to those of the bipyridines. Clinical trials are needed to determine the long-term safety and efficacy of these positive inotropic agents.

REFRACTORY AND INTRACTABLE HEART FAILURE

Heart failure is considered to be *refractory* when it persists or the patient's condition deteriorates despite intensive therapy. It is considered to be *intractable* when it is resistant to all regular therapeutic measures. The first step in dealing with a patient supposedly in refractory failure is to "step back and take a fresh look" and determine whether or not the patient is truly in refractory heart failure. There are, of course, other conditions that could be responsible for clinical deterioration. Has excessive diuresis occurred, and are lethargy and weakness due to a low cardiac output state secondary to an inadequate preload? Could digitalis intoxication be present? Digitalis toxicity can occur despite a serum glycoside level in the usual therapeutic range and can cause fatigue, lethargy, and anorexia that may mimic refractory heart failure. Are the symptoms due to electrolyte imbalance, such as hypokalemic alkalosis or hyponatremia, which have developed as a consequence of excessive diuresis and restriction of sodium intake? Could the patient with established heart disease be suffering from an unrelated illness, such as an occult neoplasm, viral hepatitis, or hepatic cirrhosis?

Once it has been established that the patient is truly in refractory heart failure, one must next consider whether some precipitating event has occurred. A number of possibilities should be considered:

1. Could the patient be "cheating" on the restricted sodium diet?

2. Is the patient not complying with the medication schedule prescribed despite protestations to the contrary? A "pill count" is often helpful in determining compliance.

3. Has the patient been receiving optimal doses of cardiac glycosides? A glycoside level in the usual therapeutic range does not necessarily mean that the patient has been receiving an optimal dose. A greater inotropic effect may sometimes be provided by the addition of a very small dose of digitalis (0.125 mg digoxin daily or every other day) above the maintenance dose without precipitating signs or symptoms of toxicity.

4. Could the patient be suffering from unrecognized pulmonary embolism (Chap. 48)? This condition occurs frequently in heart failure, is often silent, and may be manifested only by slight tachycardia, anxiety, tachypnea, and intensification of heart failure. Densities on the chest roentgenogram may make it difficult or impossible to interpret lung scans, and a pulmonary angiogram may be required to establish the diagnosis. Although this procedure is not without risk, a positive result may lead to treatment with anticoagulants and/or vena caval interruption that could prevent further emboli and prove to be life-saving.

5. Could pulmonary infection be present? Pneumonitis, a frequent complication of left ventricular failure, may be difficult to recognize in patients with chronic congestive heart failure who often have a chronic low-grade fever as well as increased interstitial markings on chest roentgenogram and pulmonary rales on clinical examination. Is the suspicion of pulmonary infection high enough to warrant sputum culture and consideration of a course of antibiotics?

6. Could hyperthyroidism or infective endocarditis be present? Thyrotoxicosis (often apathetic in the elderly) and infective endocarditis may not present with typical clinical manifestations in the presence of heart failure, but they can lead to refractory heart failure. Should tests, including an assessment of thyroid function and multiple blood cultures, be obtained?

7. Could alcohol, a potent myocardial depressant, be playing a role? In addition to producing cardiomyopathy (p. 1417), alcohol can contribute to heart failure even when it is not the primary cause but its use is superimposed on some other form of heart disease.

8. Does the patient have inappropriate bradycardia due to sinus node dysfunction or atrioventricular block that could be corrected by means of a pacemaker?

9. Is the patient receiving any medications with salt-retaining effects, such as corticosteroids, estrogens, or nonsteroidal antiinflammatory drugs, or drugs with negative inotropic actions, such as disopyramide, beta-adrenoceptor blocking agents, or verapamil?

10. Could vasodilator therapy be responsible for an increased tendency to salt and water retention?

11. Can any aspect of therapy be intensified without producing untoward effects?

After any issues raised by these questions have been dealt with and refractory heart failure persists, both the nature and hemodynamic consequences of the underlying illness should be reassessed, and surgical treatment should be considered or reconsidered; often cardiac catheterization and angiography should be carried out or repeated at this time. For example, resection of a large ventricular aneurysm might have been deferred as long as the patient responded to medical treatment for heart failure because of the surgical risk, but reconsideration might be in order when the response to medical therapy wanes. Similar considerations may apply to patients with known multivessel coronary artery disease or advanced valvular heart disease and poor left ventricular function. Elderly patients who might not have been considered to be suitable for surgical treatment when symptoms of heart failure were controlled might become surgical candidates, albeit at a significantly heightened risk. Other forms of heart disease that may lead to refractory heart failure and that may be amenable to surgical treatment, but which are not readily recognized on clinical examination, include cardiac tumors (Chap. 43), endomyocardial fibrosis (p. 1437), and constrictive pericarditis without calcification (Chap. 44). Such

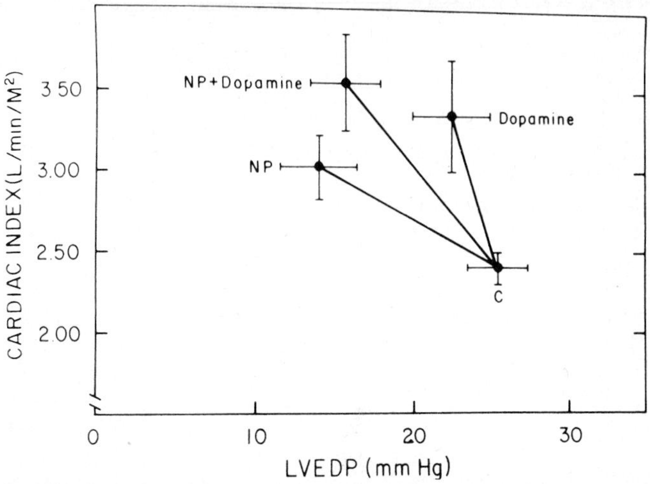

FIGURE 17–24. Effect of nitroprusside (NP), dopamine, and the combination of NP and dopamine on left ventricular end-diastolic pressure and cardiac index. Data are from 9 patients with chronic congestive heart failure (Class III) despite use of digitalis and diuretics; digitalis was discontinued 72 hours before this study. (From Miller, R. R., et al.: Combined dopamine and nitroprusside therapy in congestive heart failure. Circulation *55*:881, 1977, by permission of the American Heart Association, Inc.)

conditions should be considered and, if possible, excluded.

If every aspect of the diagnosis including the underlying and precipitating causes of heart failure is carefully assessed, if every aspect of therapy is meticulously reconsidered, if the patient has been placed at bed rest and has received optimal doses of cardiac glycosides, diuretics, and oral vasodilators, if any electrolyte imbalance has been corrected and large volumes of fluid in the serous cavities not mobilized by diuretics have been removed mechanically, then the patient should receive a course of intravenous therapy with a vasodilator, an inotropic agent (amrinone or dobutamine), or a combination of an inotropic agent and vasodilator for 2 to 3 days. Combinations of nitroprusside or nitroglycerin[530] with dobutamine or dopamine may be effective (Fig. 17–24). Such combined administration of a sympathomimetic amine and vasodilator may be of benefit in patients with severe heart failure in whom the use of one of these agents alone is insufficient. Thus, in one series of patients with severe chronic congestive heart failure, nitroprusside alone reduced left ventricular end-diastolic pressure from 25 to 14 mm Hg and increased cardiac index from 2.4 to 3.0 liters/min/m^2 but did not reduce end-diastolic pressure. Simultaneous infusion of the two agents resulted in favorable alterations in both hemodynamic variables: left ventricular end-diastolic pressure declined to 16 mm Hg and cardiac index rose to 3.5 liters/min/m^2.[448]

Such treatment ordinarily can be carried out only in the hospital, with careful monitoring of filling pressure, cardiac output, and arterial pressure. If it is successful and the patient can be weaned from the intravenous therapy, larger doses of oral vasodilators and experimental drugs such as oral sympathomimetics, milrinone, or one of the other new orally active phosphodiesterase inhibitors may provide benefit.

Heart failure can properly be termed intractable if it persists despite the judicious application of all of the aforementioned measures. Then the possibility of cardiac transplantation and assisted circulation may be considered in selected instances.

CARDIAC TRANSPLANTATION

This procedure was first performed in humans in 1967.[531, 532] Despite its technical feasibility, initially the high mortality rates resulting from graft rejection led to its abandonment in most institutions. However, in the past few years, there has been a rekindling of interest in cardiac transplantation. At the time of this writing, a total of 74 active cardiac transplantation programs exist in the United States. During 1986, 1050 cardiac transplants were carried out. As of June 1, 1987, a total of 448 patients have undergone cardiac transplantation at Stanford University Medical Center. There are a total of 256 1-year survivors, and 206 patients are currently surviving. The longest survivor at 17½ years post cardiac transplantation is doing well without evidence of cardiac dysfunction or accelerated coronary artery disease. The youngest patient to undergo transplant in the Stanford program was 5 months old at the time of transplant and is currently doing well 11 months after transplant. As of January 1, 1987, the 1-year survival is 80 per cent and 3 years, 70 per cent. Five-year survival is 55 per cent for patients who have had transplantation since December 1980, when cyclosporine immunosuppression was introduced.[533] These results are comparable to those obtained with cadaver kidney transplant programs. Recent improved results reflect the potency and effectiveness of the immunosuppressive agent cyclosporine.[534]

Potential recipients of cardiac transplants must have end-stage heart disease with severe heart failure and a life expectancy of less than one year.[534a] Candidates should be stable psychologically and should have a history of compliance with medical therapy. Since younger patients have better survival rates, 50 to 55 years is the usual upper age limit of potential recipients. Contraindications to cardiac transplantation include pulmonary hypertension, parenchymal pulmonary disease, recent pulmonary infarction, donor-specific cytotoxic antibodies, active infection, diabetes mellitus requiring insulin, a history of coexisting liver or renal disease, active duodenal ulcer, drug addiction, psychosis, continued excessive alcohol consumption, clinically significant cerebral or peripheral vascular disease, and other diseases (such as malignant disease) that are considered likely to limit survival or rehabilitation. The ideal recipient is a young person who is dying of end-stage cardiac disease and who is otherwise well, emotionally stable, and willing to risk a complex procedure and course for the chance of functional improvement. Over half the recipients have had coronary artery disease while most of the remainder have had idiopathic, viral, or rheumatic cardiomyopathies.[535] Combined transplantation of the heart and lungs has been employed successfully in the treatment of severe, irreversible pulmonary hypertension.[536]

The majority of heart donors have sustained irreversible cerebral damage due to trauma or intracranial hemorrhage. Donor supply remains limited,[536a] and approximately one-third of recipients awaiting transplant die before a suitable donor heart becomes available. The number of suitable donor hearts is unlikely to exceed 2,000 per year and there may be more than 15,000 suitable candidates per year. The success of using hearts removed from donors and transported under conditions of hypothermic ischemia for up to 3 hours[537] and the use of hypothermic perfusion with an oxygenated hyperosmolar solution[538] is broadening the sources of donor supply. Public educational programs are likely to add to the donor pool, while legislation to reduce traumatic death (e.g., seat belt and helmet laws) will reduce it. Other than choosing a heart from a donor less than 35 years of age, of appropriate weight, ABO type, and absence of a positive lymphocyte cross-match, no prospective histocompatibility typing has been used for cardiac transplantation. The results of HLA typing have been disappointing in predicting long-term survival.

In carrying out orthotopic heart transplantation, after the recipient undergoes cardiopulmonary bypass, the heart is removed, leaving the posterior walls of the atria with their venous connections in place.[532] The donor atria are sutured to the corresponding structures of the in situ residual atria of the recipient, and the great vessels are anastomosed last. Alternatively, in *heterotopic* heart transplantation, the recipient's heart is left in situ and the donor heart is placed in parallel, with anastomoses between the two right atria, pulmonary arteries, left atria, and aortae. The stated advantage of the latter technique is that should the donor heart fail, most commonly as a consequence of acute rejection, chances for the patient's survival are improved by the patient's own heart; retransplantation may be possible if the donor heart becomes nonfunctional.[539] Immunosuppression has been accomplished with the combination of cyclosporine, azathioprine, prednisone, and antithymocyte globulin.[539a] The regimen utilized at Stanford University Hospital is shown in Table 17–11. It attempts to balance inadequate immunosuppression with the accompanying hazards of rejection on the one hand with the risks of infection and the development of nephrotoxicity as a consequence of vigorous immunosuppression with cyclosporine on the other.

In the absence of rejection, the transplanted heart, which is denervated and lacks autonomic neural control, exhibits normal contractility and contractile reserve.[515] It has the capacity to maintain a normal resting cardiac output; during exercise, stroke volume rises first, after which increased levels of circulating catecholamines cause tachycardia. As a consequence of this near-normal circulatory response, the transplanted heart permits excellent functional and social and vocational rehabilitation in 90 per cent of long-term survivors.[541]

Acute rejection is monitored by right ventricular endomyocardial biopsy[542, 542a] (p. 262), carried out routinely at weekly intervals for the first 3 weeks postoperatively, biweekly for the next month, and in patients who are clinically stable at 6-month intervals thereafter. Between biopsies a fall in electrocardiographic QRS voltage (reflecting myocardial edema), atrial arrhythmia, and a S_3 gallop are clinical signs of rejection and their appearance should lead to endocardial biopsy. Magnetic resonance imaging may also reveal the presence of edema during rejection.[543] Treatment of acute rejection consists of 1 gm methylpred-

TABLE 17–11 IMMUNOSUPPRESSIVE PROTOCOL UTILIZED AT STANFORD UNIVERSITY HOSPITAL

PREOPERATIVE INDUCTION:	
Cyclosporine-A	10–16 mg/kg
	4 mg/kg IV
POSTOPERATIVE MAINTENANCE:	
Cyclosporine	Dose to target serum level of 200–300 ng/ml during *first postop month* and 50–150 ng/ml *thereafter*
Prednisone	0.2 mg/kg/day; minimal tapering schedule to tolerance beginning late postop.
Azathioprine	1.5–2.0 mg/kg/day; adjust to WBC tolerance
Equine ATG (ATGAM)	10 mg/kg/day for seven days

From Oyer, P. E.: Transplantation and Immunology Letter, Vol. 3, No. 3, p. 3, 1986.

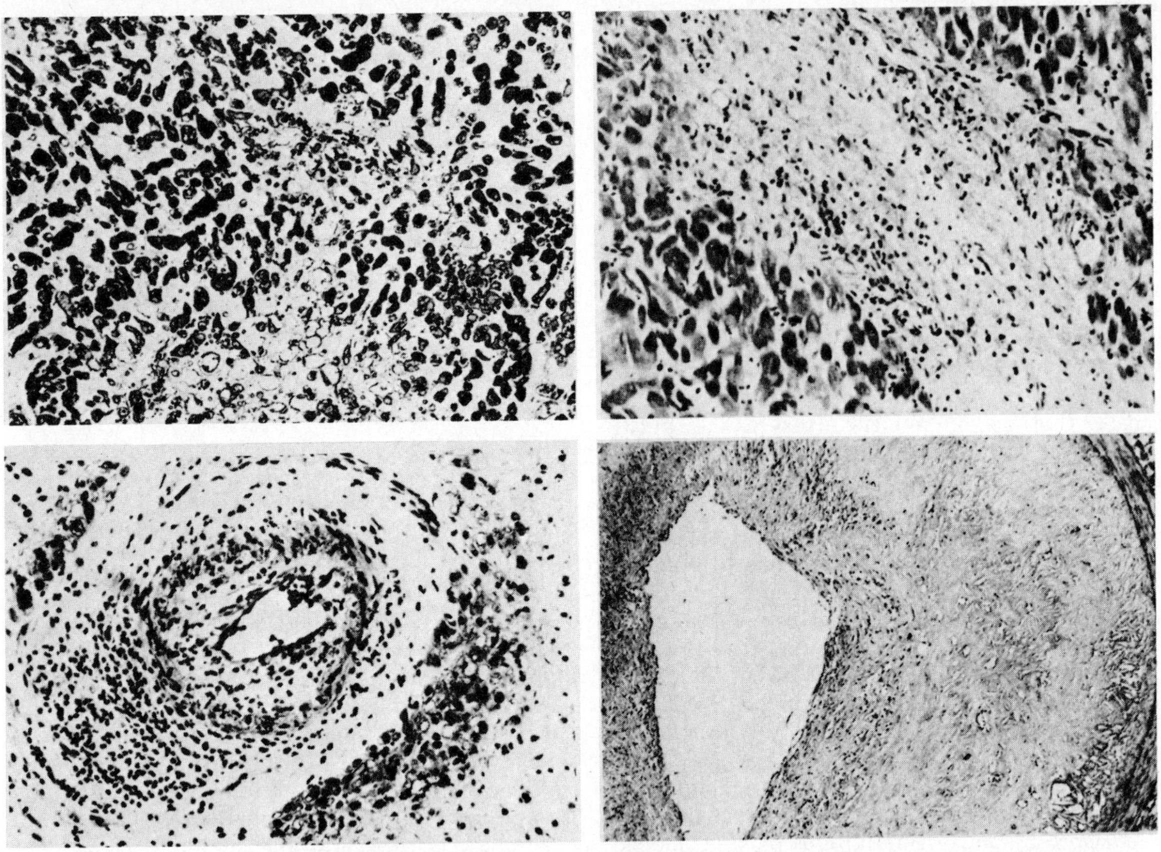

FIGURE 17–25. Histological findings in rejection of cardiac transplant. *Top left,* Myocytolysis of acute rejection. Graft survival was 1.6 years (hematoxylin-eosin, × 175). *Top right,* Stromal collapse fibrosis with focal scarring following earlier myocytolysis. Lymphoid and plasma cell infiltrate illustrate persistent cellular rejection. Patient survival was 1.6 years (hematoxylin-eosin, × 175). *Bottom left,* Intense lymphoid infiltrate of small coronary artery wall, perivascular connective tissue, and adjacent myocardium, indicating persistent acute rejection. Intimal thickening and lumen narrowing indicate development of early chronic vascular rejection. Graft survival was 1.2 years. Donor was 35 years old (hematoxylin-eosin, × 175). *Bottom right,* Advanced chronic vascular rejection of large coronary artery radicle. Medial fibrous replacement and fragmentation of elastic intima are present. Intima shows striking fibrous intimal thickening with substantial lumen encroachment. Lipid deposits as illustrated by cholesterol clefts are present in depths of thickened intima. Lesion resembles advanced atherosclerosis. Patient survival was 4.2 years. Donor was 35 years old (hematoxylin-eosin, × 70). (From Uys, C. J., and Rose, A. G.: Pathologic findings in long-term cardiac transplants. Arch. Pathol. Lab. Med. *108*:112, 1984.)

nisolone intravenously per day for 3 days followed by repeat cardiac biopsies (Fig. 17–25).

Infections complicating intense immunosuppression are still a major hazard to survival, and continued medical surveillance is required at 2- to 4-week intervals to look for infection and rejection. In the late postoperative course the threat of rejection continues, but its likelihood diminishes considerably. However, accelerated coronary atherosclerosis, presumably due to rejection-induced injury to the coronary arterial intima, develops in the transplanted heart of some patients[544, 545] (Fig. 17–25*D*). Hypercholesterolemia is an added risk factor and should be treated vigorously with diet and drugs (Chap. 36). As in renal transplantation involving chronic immunosuppression, malignant neoplasms, usually of the lymphoreticular type, have been observed in a few recipients.

Patients who survive for 3 months have a better than 80 per cent 2-year survival rate. Patients younger than 40 years and those who have had previous cardiac surgery associated with blood transfusions exhibit even better survival. Subsequent attrition is approximately 5 per cent per year and reflects the continuing hazards threatening immunosuppressed patients.[533] Despite the aforementioned advances in heart procurement and preservation, it is likely that the supply of donor hearts will continue to be a limiting factor in the number of cardiac transplants performed. Initial experience with xeno-transplantation suggests that this approach will not provide a solution to the problem in the near future.[546] The enormous costs of cardiac transplantation in an era of cost consciousness and control must also be considered.[546a]

MECHANICAL CIRCULATORY SUPPORT

INTRAAORTIC BALLOON COUNTERPULSATION (See p. 573). The phased inflation during diastole of a balloon inserted into the descending aorta through the femoral artery generally increases cardiac output by 10 to 20 per cent and elevates arterial diastolic pressure while reducing arterial systolic pressure.[547, 548] A major application of this technique has been in the treatment of patients with acute left ventricular failure secondary to acute myocardial infarction (cardiogenic shock), but it has also been utilized to support the circulation in patients with acute ischemic syndromes who are undergoing cardiac catheterization, angiocardiography, and coronary arteriography.[549] Of increasing importance is the use of intraaortic balloon counterpulsation during the perioperative period in patients undergoing cardiac surgery and developing acute heart failure. In most cases this method of therapy is applied for

24 to 48 hours, often together with the combination of a positive inotropic agent, such as dopamine or dobutamine, and a vasodilator, usually nitroprusside, after which an attempt is made to wean the patient from this support. In some instances, counterpulsation has been continued for as long as 2 weeks.

The device can be inserted percutaneously. The principal advantage of the intraaortic balloon technique is its relative simplicity and low risk. The major disadvantage is that it offers only modest circulatory support (elevation of cardiac index up to 0.8 liter/min/m^2) and cannot sustain life in extremely severe heart failure or in the presence of chaotic cardiac rhythms. Pulmonary artery counterpulsation can be used to support the right ventricle.[548] The major risks of intraaortic balloon counterpulsation are (1) laceration or other damage to the arterial bed, (2) ischemia of the lower extremity distal to the femoral arterial insertion site (particularly common in smaller elderly women), and (3) infection originating at the site of insertion in the groin and subsequent bacteremia in patients who require prolonged assistance.

TEMPORARY LEFT VENTRICULAR ASSISTANCE. More drastic means of circulatory support must be considered for patients who cannot be sustained by pharmacological therapy and intraaortic balloon assistance. For patients in whom recovery of left ventricular function is anticipated and removal of the pump is expected (perhaps at the time of cardiac transplantation), several groups have developed left ventricular assist devices consisting of a pump with afferent and efferent conduits attached to the left ventricular apex and ascending thoracic aorta, respectively.[549–551]

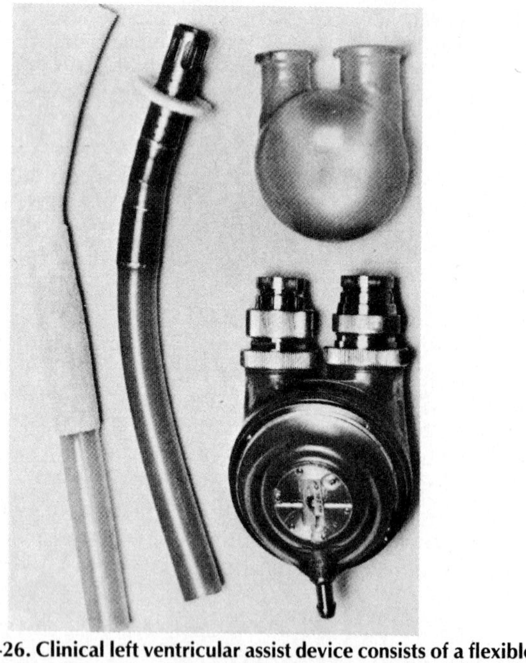

FIGURE 17–26. Clinical left ventricular assist device consists of a flexible polyurethane blood sac (*top right*) and diaphragm within a rigid polysulfone case (*bottom right*). The lighthouse tip cannula is coated with segmented polyurethane (*center*). It is inserted into the left ventricular apex and secured in place with pledget-supported sutures through the felt skirt. Blood return is achieved through the composite segmented polyurethane-woven Dacron prosthesis anastomosed to the ascending aorta (*left*). (Reproduced with permission from Pennock, J. L., Pierce, W. S., Campbell, D. B., Pae, W. E., Jr., Davis, D., Hensley, F. A., Richenbacher, W. E., and Waldhausen, J.: Mechanical support of the circulation followed by cardiac transplantation. J. Thorac. Cardiovasc. Surg. *92*:994, 1986.)

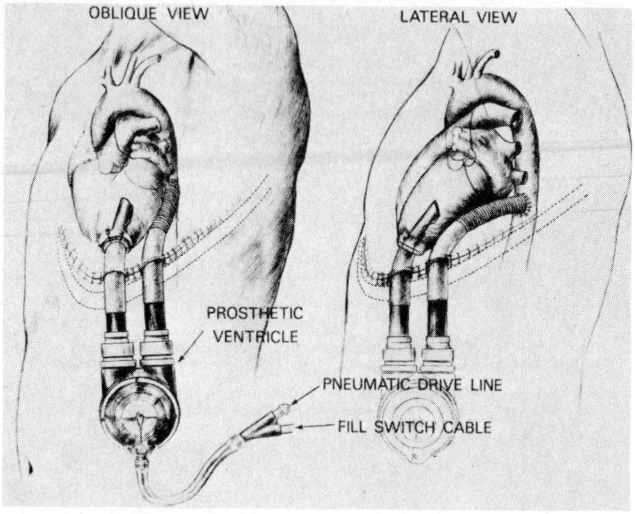

FIGURE 17–27. Prosthetic ventricle connected from the left ventricular apex and returning blood flow to the descending aorta. (Reproduced with permission from Hill, J. D., Farrar, D. J., Hershon, J. J., Compton, P. G., Avery, G. J., Levin, B. S., and Brent, B. N.: Use of a prosthetic ventricle as a bridge to cardiac transplantation for postinfarction cardiogenic shock. N. Engl. J. Med. *314*:626, 1986.)

The ventricular assist device developed and used clinically at Pennsylvania State University consists of a flexible polyurethane blood sac and diaphragm placed within a rigid case (Fig. 17–26). Björk-Shiley valves (p. 1078) are used to provide unidirectional flow. Blood flows through a cannula inserted into the left ventricular apex and is returned by the device into the ascending aorta through a Dacron graft. The device is positioned externally (Fig. 17–27) and is powered by an external unit that delivers pulses of compressed carbon dioxide between the case and the diaphragm. Another device* is titanium-cased,[550] uses porcine heterograft (or Björk-Shiley) valves, and is powered by an air-driven console. It is placed either externally on the patient's chest (for short-term use) or in the abdomen (for long-term use).[552]

Clinical trials with temporary left ventricular assist devices are currently under way in patients who have had corrective cardiac surgery and in whom (1) pump oxygenator dependence develops in spite of intensive treatment with conventional measures, including intraaortic balloon counterpulsation, and/or (2) refractory cardiogenic shock occurs within 72 hours of operation. In addition, they are being tested in patients with terminal heart failure secondary to acute (presumably viral) myocarditis and in patients with acute myocardial infarction and refractory cardiogenic shock. Rose et al. have reported clinical experiences in 16 patients with perioperative myocardial infarction and shock who could not be weaned from cardiopulmonary bypass despite use of inotropic agents and the intraaortic balloon pump and were treated with partial left heart (left atrium-aorta) bypass; eight patients survived.[553] Increasingly, these devices are used as "bridges" in patients who are terminally ill and are candidates for cardiac transplantation awaiting a donor heart.[554, 555]

When the left ventricular assist device is first applied to the patient, it handles almost the total left heart output, while the patient's left ventricle performs little work. If, as a result of this "rest" period for 48 to 72 hours, the myocardium recovers, the left ventricle may be allowed to resume pumping a gradually increasing portion of systemic blood flow. Temporary reductions in the output of the device are made, and if adequate cardiac output and

*Thermedics Corp., Woburn, Massachusetts.

arterial pressures are maintained without a marked increase in left atrial pressure, withdrawal of mechanical support can be planned. A major disadvantage of all left ventricular assist devices is that they require reasonable function of the right ventricle. Severe right-heart failure leads to inadequate filling of the left heart, and the low preload precludes adequate inflow into the left ventricular assist device. Inotropic support of the right heart with catecholamines is therefore frequently necessary. Norman and colleagues have developed an intracorporeal (abdominal) left ventricular assist device that is undergoing clinical testing.[552]

There is increasing evidence that approximately 20 per cent of patients whose hearts cannot sustain life despite pharmacological therapy and intraaortic balloon counterpulsation can be maintained alive, can survive discontinuation of left ventricular assistance, and sometimes can leave the hospital. Obviously, long-term survival from this temporary period of support can be attained only if the cardiac insult is reversible, which occurs most frequently in postcardiotomy cardiac failure.

PERMANENT LEFT VENTRICULAR ASSISTANCE. Patients whose left ventricles have sustained permanent damage and in whom recovery of function sufficient to support the circulation is not anticipated are potential candidates for permanent left ventricular assistance. These include patients with end-stage left ventricular disease resulting from ischemic or other cardiomyopathies, patients with left ventricular infarction and shock, and postoperative patients with intractable left ventricular failure who are dependent on and cannot be weaned from temporary left ventricular assistance. These permanent devices, currently undergoing refinement and chronic testing in animals, are similar to those described above for temporary left ventricular assistance, except that the pump that fills from the left atrium or left ventricle and ejects blood into the aorta is implanted into the thorax or abdominal cavity. The energy source for these pumps is external and either an air tube or a wire passes through the skin. The native heart remains in situ, and survival requires continued function of the right ventricle. Such devices have functioned in calves for several months and over a month in humans.[556]

THE TOTAL ARTIFICIAL HEART. Also known as the biventricular replacement device, the total artificial heart involves the use of two mechanical pumps that replace the natural ventricles and support both the systemic and pulmonary circulations (Fig. 17–28). With such a device the natural heart is excised, the inlet connectors are attached to the atrial remnants and the outlet connectors to the great arteries through Dacron-covered vascular prostheses (Fig. 17–29). The pneumatic power units and control systems are housed externally. The total artificial heart might be used in patients who could not otherwise survive and in whom the natural heart is permanently useless or even a threat to life, such as patients with large left ventricular infarctions and rupture of the left ventricle or with an irreparable ventricular septal defect or patients in whom catastrophic injury to the heart occurs during operation.

Since the first report describing the implantation of an artificial heart in an experimental animal in 1958, progress has been made, albeit gradually, toward the goal of developing a practical, totally implanted device that will support the circulation. A variety of devices are now being tested in experimental animals. A promising artificial heart which was recently developed[547a] consists of an electronic control system and two smooth-surfaced, sac-type pumps made of polyurethane.[557–559] Two pneumatic power units pulse air intermittently to move the diaphragm, thereby moving blood into and out of the blood chamber. The control system has the capability of balancing the output automatically during exercise. Bulky, electrically driven air-powered units positioned alongside the recipient power the artificial ventricles through air tubes. Such devices have assumed the total function of the heart for more than a year in calves, which ate well and gained weight.[559] The Jarvik heart has successfully supported the circulation for more than a year in two patients.[557] However, serious problems have not been solved that involve thrombosis of the prosthesis and hemorrhage as a result of the vigorous anticoagulation required to reduce thrombosis. Current research centers on the development of nonthrombogenic

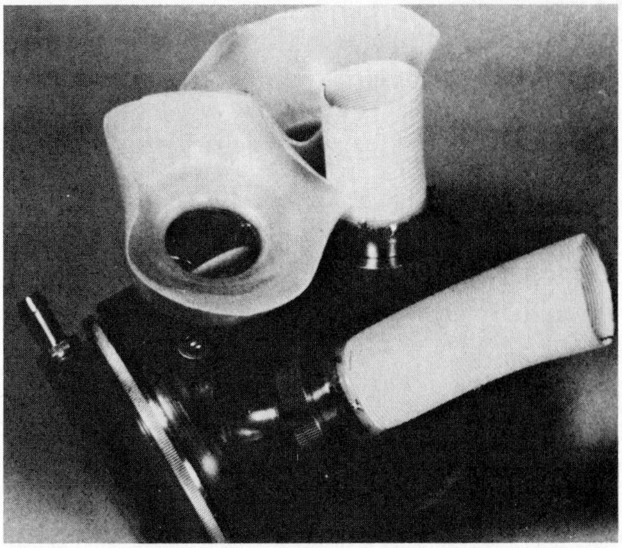

FIGURE 17–28. The air-driven artificial heart designed and constructed by Pierce and associates at the Pennsylvania State University. Each prosthetic ventricle consists of a flexible blood sac housed in a rigid case. Wide atrial connectors are anastomosed to the atrial remnants, while outlet grafts, composed of Dacron, are sutured to the appropriate great vessel. Air pulses are transmitted to the ventricles by way of percutaneous drive lines. (From Richenbacher, W. E., Pennock, J. L., Pae, W. E., Jr., and Pierce, W. S.: Artificial heart implantation for end-stage cardiac disease. J. Cardiac Surg. *1*:3, 1986.)

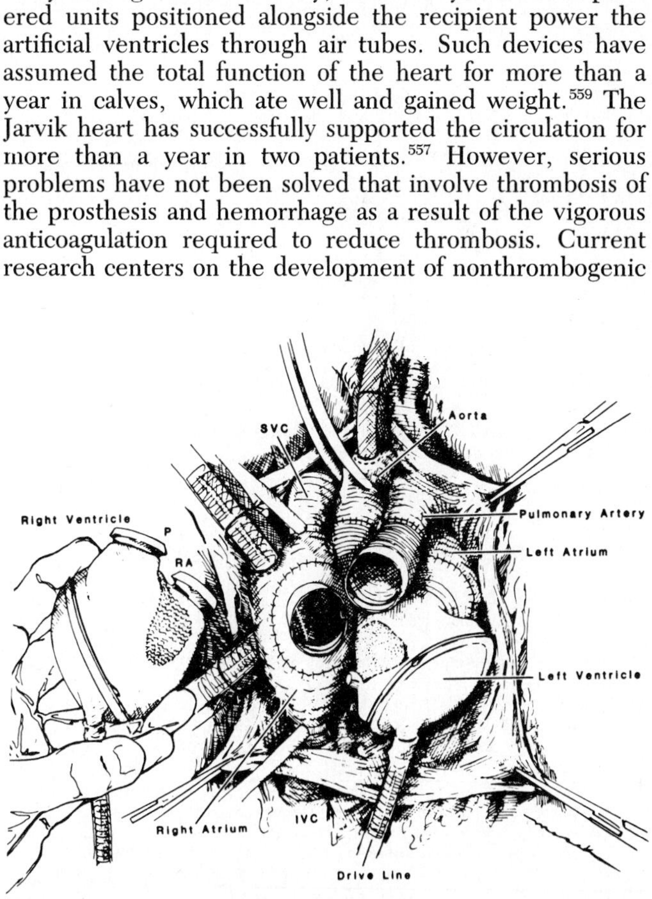

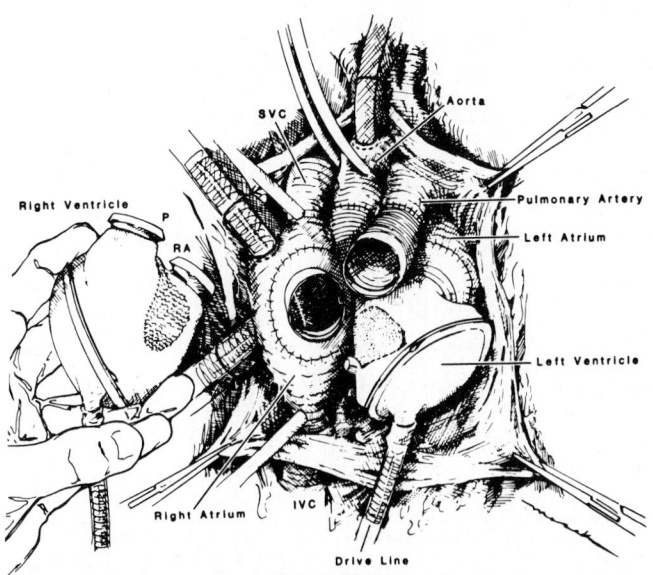

FIGURE 17–29. Diagrammatic representation of the Utah (Jarvik-7) total artificial heart. (Reproduced with permission from DeVries, W. C., Anderson, J. L., Joyce, L. D., Anderson, F. L., Hammond, E. H., Jarvik, R. K., and Kolff, W. J.: Clinical use of the total artificial heart. N. Engl. J. Med. *310*:273, 1984.)

surfaces and of pumps powered by implanted compact electrical motors.

At this time the most important application of the totally implanted heart is as a temporary bridge to transplantation.[558, 563] In a review of the world experience with the clinical use of total artificial hearts in June 1986, it was reported that a total of 27 artificial hearts of eight different types had been implanted into 26 patients.[559] Five patients had implants for permanent support. Four of the five survived more than one month and although two patients survived more than one year, there have been no long-term survivors who had no serious complications. In the other 21 patients, nine had successful transplantation and were living at the time of the survey and two were alive and awaiting transplantation.

The problems inherent in the development of a totally implanted heart capable of permanent support of the circulation, although they have not yet been solved, do not appear to be insurmountable. Problems dealing with ethics and financing of the application of the artificial heart should be addressed simultaneously with the improvement of the device itself.

REFERENCES

1. Opie, L. H.: Principles of therapy for congestive heart failure. Eur. Heart J. *4*(Suppl. A):199, 1983.
2. Cohn, J. N., Archibald, D. G., Phil, M., Ziesche, S., Franciosa, J. A., Harston, W. E., Tristani, F. E., Dunkman, W. B., Jacobs, W., Francis, G. S., Flohr, K. H., Goldman, S., Cobb, F. R., Shah, P. M., Saunders, R., Fletcher, R. D., Loeb, H. S., Hughes, V. C., and Baker, B.: Effect of vasodilator therapy on mortality in chronic congestive heart failure. N. Engl. J. Med. *314*:1547, 1986.
3. Morgan, S. H., Mansell, M. A., and Thompson, F. D.: Fluid removed by haemofiltration in diuretic-resistant cardiac failure. Br. Heart J. *54*:218, 1985.
4. Simpson, I. A., Rae, A. P., Simpson, K., Gribben, J., Allison, M. E. M., and Hutton, I.: Ultrafiltration in the management of refractory congestive heart failure. Br. Heart J. *55*:344, 1986.

DIGITALIS GLYCOSIDES

5. Withering, W.: An account of the foxglove and some of its medical uses, with practical remarks on dropsy, and other diseases. *In* Willis, F. A., and Keys, T. E. (eds.): Classics of Cardiology. New York, Henry Schuman, Inc. 1941, p. 231.
6. Marshall, P. G.: Steroids: Cardiotonic glycosides and aglycons: Toad poisons. *In* Coffey, S. (ed.): Rodd's Chemistry of Carbon Compounds. 2nd ed. Vol. 2D, Steroids. Amsterdam, Elsevier Publishing Co., 1970, p. 360.
7. Hoffman, B. F., and Bigger, J. T., Jr.: Digitalis and allied cardiac glycosides. *In* Gilman, A. G., et al. (eds.): The Pharmacological Basis of Therapeutics. 7th Ed. New York, Macmillan, 1985.
8. Repke, K. R. H.: New developments in cardiac glycoside structure-activity relationships. Trends in Pharmacological Science, July 1985, pp. 275–278.

Mechanisms of Cardiac Glycoside Action

9. Schwartz, A., Lindenmayer, G. E., and Allen, J. C.: The sodium-potassium adenosine triphosphatase: Pharmacological, physiological and biochemical aspects. Pharmacol. Rev. *27*:1, 1975.
10. Akera, T., and Brody, T. M.: The role of Na^+, K^+-ATPase in the inotropic action of digitalis. Pharmacol. Rev. *29*:187, 1977.
11. Kim, D., Barry, W. H., and Smith, T. W.: Kinetics of ouabain binding and changes in cellular sodium content, $^{42}K^+$ transport, and contractile state during ouabain exposure in cultured chick heart cells. J. Pharmacol. Exp. Ther. *231*:326, 1984.
12. Marban, E., and Smith, T.W.: Digitalis. *In* Fozzard, H. M., et al. (eds.): The Heart and Cardiovascular System. New York, Raven Press, 1986.
13. Lee, C. O.: 200 years of digitalis: The emerging central role of the sodium ion in the control of cardiac force. Am. J. Physiol. *249*:C367, 1985.
14. Katz, A. M.: Contractile proteins of the heart. Physiol. Rev. *50*:63, 1970.
15. Coleman, H. N.: Role of acetylstrophanthidin in augmenting myocardial oxygen consumption. Circ. Res. *21*:487, 1967.
16. Weingart, R., Kass, R. S., and Tsien, R. W.: Is digitalis inotropy associated with enhanced slow inward calcium current? Nature *273*:389, 1978.
17. Marban, E., and Tsien, R. W.: Enhancement of cardiac calcium current during digitalis inotropy: Positive feedback regulation by intracellular calcium? J. Physiol. (Lond.) *329*:589, 1982.
18. Fabiato, A., and Fabiato, F.: Activation of skinned cardiac cells. Subcellular effects of cardioactive drugs. Eur. J. Cardiol. *1*:145–155, 1973.
19. Bailey, L. E., and Harvey, S. C.: Effects of ouabain on cardiac ^{45}Ca kinetics measured by indicator dilution. Am. J. Physiol. *16*:123, 1969.
20. Langer, G. A., and Serena, S. D.: Effects of strophanthidin upon contraction and ionic exchange in rabbit ventricular myocardium: Relation to control of active state. J. Molec. Cell. Cardiol. *1*:65, 1970.
21. Biedert, S., Barry, W. H., and Smith, T. W.: Inotropic effects and changes in sodium and calcium contents associated with inhibition of monovalent cation active transport by ouabain in cultured myocardial cells. J. Gen. Physiol. *74*:479, 1979.
22. Morgan, J. P., and Blinks, J. R.: Intracellular Ca^{++} transients in the cat papillary muscle. Can. J. Physiol. Pharmacol. *60*:524, 1982.
23. Weir, W. G., and Hess, P.: Excitation-contraction coupling in cardiac Purkinje fibers. Effects of cardiotonic steroids on the intracellular $[Ca^{2+}]$ transient, membrane potential, and contraction. J. Gen. Physiol. *83*:395, 1984.
24. Kawakami, K., Noguchi, S., Noda, M., Takahashi, H., Ohta, T., Kawamura, M., Nojima, H., Nagano, K., Hirose, T., Inayama, S., Hayashida, H., Miyata, T., and Numa, S.: Primary structure of the α-subunit of Torpedo californica (Na^+ + K^+) ATPase deduced from cDNA sequence. Nature *316*:733, 1985.
25. Shull, G. E., Schwartz, A., and Lingrel, J. B.: Amino-acid sequence of the catalytic subunit of the (Na^+ + K^+) ATPase deduced from a complementary DNA. Nature *316*:691, 1985.
26. Kim, D., Marsh, J. D., Barry, W. H., and Smith, T. W.: Effects of growth in low potassium medium or ouabain on membrane Na^+, K^+-ATPase, cation transport, and contractility in cultured chick heart cells. Circ. Res. *55*:39, 1984.
27. Forbush, B., III, Kaplan, J. H., and Hoffman, J. F.: Characterization of a new photoaffinity derivative of ouabain: Labelling of the large polypeptide and of a proteolipid component of the Na^+, K^+-ATPase. Biochemistry *17*:3667, 1978.
28. Flasch, H., and Heinz, N.: Correlation between inhibition of NaK-membrane-ATPase and positive inotropic activity of cardenolides in isolated papillary muscles of guinea pig. Naunyn Schmiedebergs Arch. Pharmakol. *304*:37, 1978.
29. Allen, J. C., and Schwartz, A.: A possible biochemical explanation for the sensitivity of the rat to cardiac glycosides. J. Pharmacol. Exp. Ther. *168*:42, 1969.
30. Akera, T., Baskin, S. I., Tobin, T., and Brody, T. M.: Ouabain: Temporal relationship between the inotropic effect and the in vitro binding to, and dissociation from, (Na^+, K^+)-activated ATPase. Naunyn Schmiedebergs Arch. Pharmakol. *277*:151, 1973.
31. Barry, W. H., Hasin, Y., and Smith, T. W.: Sodium pump inhibition, enhanced Ca-influx via Na-Ca exchange, and positive inotropic response in cultured heart cells. Circ. Res. *56*:231, 1985.
32. Eisner, D. A., and Lederer, W. J.: The role of the sodium pump in the effects of potassium-depleted solutions on mammalian cardiac muscle. J. Physiol. *294*:279, 1979.
33. Akera, T., Larsen, F. S., and Brody, T. M.: Correlation of cardiac sodium- and potassium-activated adenosine triphosphatase activity with ouabain-induced inotropic stimulation. J. Pharmacol. Exp. Ther. *173*:145, 1970.
34. Hougen, T. J., and Smith, T. W.: Inhibition of myocardial monovalent cation active transport by subtoxic doses of ouabain in the dog. Circ. Res. *42*:856, 1978.
35. Somberg, J. C., Barry, W. H., and Smith, T.W.: Differing sensitivities of Purkinje fibers and myocardium to inhibition of monovalent cation transport by digitalis. J. Clin. Invest. *67*:116, 1981.
36. Akera, T.: Membrane adenosine triphosphatase: A digitalis receptor? Science *198*:569, 1977.
37. Calhoun, J. A., and Harrison, T. R.: Studies in congestive heart failure. IX. The effect of digitalis on the potassium content of the cardiac muscle of dogs. J. Clin. Invest. *10*:139, 1931.
38. Ellis, D.: The effects of external cations and ouabain on the intracellular sodium activity of sheep heart Purkinje fibers. J. Physiol. *273*:211, 1977.
39. Lee, C. O., Kang, D. H., Sokol, J. H., and Lee, K. S.: Relation between intracellular Na ion activity and tension of sheep cardiac Purkinje fibers exposed to dihydro-ouabain. Biophys. J. *29*:315, 1980.
40. Cohen, C. J., Fozzard, H. A., and Sheu, S-S.: Increase in intracellular sodium ion activity during stimulation in mammalian cardiac muscle. Circ. Res. *50*:651, 1982.
41. Eisner, D. A., Lederer, W. J., and Vaughan-Jones, R. D.: The quantitative relationship between twitch tension and intracellular sodium activity in sheep cardiac Purkinje fibres. J. Physiol. *355*:251, 1984.
42. Grupp, I, Im, W. B., Lee, C. O., Lee, S. W., Pecker, M. S., and Schwartz, A.: Relation of sodium pump inhibition to positive inotropy at low concentrations of ouabain in rat heart muscle. J. Physiol. *360*:149, 1985.
43. Langer, G. A.: Relationship between myocardial contractility and the effects of digitalis on ionic exchange. Fed. Proc. *36*:2231, 1977.
44. Baker, P. F., Blaustein, M. P., Hodgkin, A. L., and Steinhardt, R. A.: The influence of calcium on sodium efflux in squid axons. J. Physiol. *200*:431, 1969.
45. Glitsch, H. G., Reuter, H., and Scholz, H.: The effect of the internal sodium concentration on calcium fluxes in isolated guinea pig auricles. J. Physiol. *209*:25, 1970.
46. Lederer, W. J., and Eisner, D. A.: The effects of sodium pump activity on the slow inward current in sheep cardiac Purkinje fibers. Proc. R. Soc. Lond. *B214*:249, 1982.
47. Greenspan, A. M., and Morad, M.: Electromechanical studies on the inotropic effects of acetylstrophanthidin in ventricular muscle. J. Physiol. *253*:357, 1975.
48. Lee, K. S., Marban, E., and Tsien, R. W.: Inactivation of calcium channels in mammalian heart cells. Joint dependence on membrane potential and intracellular calcium. J. Physiol. *364*:395, 1985.

49. Noble, D.: Mechanism of action of therapeutic levels of cardiac glycosides. Cardiovasc. Res. *14*:495, 1980.
50. Smith, T. W., Antman, E. M., Friedman, P. L., Blatt, C. M., and Marsh, J. D.: Digitalis glycosides: Mechanisms and manifestations of toxicity. Progr. Cardiovasc. Dis. *26*:413, 1984; *26*:495, 1984; *27*:21, 1985.
51. Rosen, M. R.: Interactions of digitalis with the autonomic nervous system and their relationship to cardiac arrhythmias. *In* Disturbances in Neurogenic Control of the Circulation. Bethesda, Am. Physiol. Soc., 1981, pp. 251–263.
52. Watanabe, A. M.: Digitalis and the autonomic nervous system. J. Am. Coll. Cardiol. *5*:35A, 1985.
53. Goldman, R. H., Deutscher, R. N., Schweizer, E., and Harrison, D. C.: Effect of a pharmacologic dose of digoxin on inotropy in hyper- and normokalemic dogs. Am. J. Physiol. *223*:1438, 1972.
54. Perrone, J. R., and Blostein, R.: Asymmetric interaction of inside-out and right-side-out erythrocyte membrane vesicles with ouabain. Biochim. Biophys. Acta *291*:680, 1973.
55. Okarma, T. B., Tramell, P., and Kalman, S. M.: The surface interaction between the digoxin and cultured heart cells. J. Pharmacol. Exp. Ther. *183*:559, 1972.
56. Smith, T. W., Wagner, H., Jr., Markis, J. E., and Young, M.: Studies on the localization of the cardiac receptor. J. Clin. Invest. *51*:1777, 1972.
57. Rosen, M. R.: Cellular electrophysiology of digitalis toxicity. J. Am. Coll. Cardiol. *5*:22A, 1985.
58. Dhingra, R. C., Amat-Y-Leon, F., Wyndham, C., Wu, D., Denes, P., and Rosen, K. M.: The electrophysiological effects of ouabain on sinus node and atrium in man. J. Clin. Invest. *56*:555, 1975.
59. Goodman, D. J., Rossen, R. M., Ingham, R., Rider, A. K., and Harrison, D. C.: Sinus node function in the denervated human heart: Effects of digitalis. Br. Heart J. *37*:612, 1975.
60. Goodman, D. J., Rossen, R. M., Cannom, D. S., Rider, A. K., and Harrison, D. C.: Effect of digoxin on atrioventricular conduction: Studies in patients with and without cardiac autonomic innervation. Circulation *51*:251, 1975.
61. Hordof, A. J., Spotnitz, A., Mary-Rabine, L., Edie, R., and Rosen, M. R.: The cellular electrophysiologic effects of digitalis on human atrial fibers. Circulation *56*:223, 1978.
62. Friedman, P. L.: Therapeutic and toxic electrophysiologic effects of cardiac glycosides. *In* Smith, T. W. (ed.): Digitalis Glycosides. Orlando, Grune and Stratton, 1985, pp. 29–44.
63. Rosen, M. R., Hordof, A. J., Hodess, A. B., Verosky, M. and Vulliemoz, Y.: Ouabain-induced changes in electrophysiologic properties of neonatal, young and adult canine cardiac Purkinje fibers. J. Pharmacol. Exp. Ther. *194*:255, 1975.
64. Rogers, M. C., Willerson, J. T., Goldblatt, A., and Smith, T. W.: Serum digoxin concentrations in the human fetus, neonate, and infant. N. Engl. J. Med. *287*:1010, 1972.
65. Hougen, T. J.: Use of digoxin in the young. *In* Smith, T. W. (ed.): Digitalis Glycosides. Orlando, Grune and Stratton, 1985, pp. 169–207.
66. Weingart, R.: Influence of cardiac glycosides on electrophysiologic processes. *In* Greeff, K. (ed.): Cardiac Glycosides. Vol. 56, Part I, Handbook of Experimental Pharmacology. Berlin, Springer-Verlag, 1981.
67. Gillis, R. A., and Quest, J. A.: The role of the nervous system in the cardiovascular effects of digitalis. Pharmacol. Rev. *31*:19–97, 1979.
68. Somberg, J. C., and Smith, T. W.: Localization of the neurally mediated arrhythmogenic properties of digitalis. Science *204*:321, 1979.
69. Somberg, J. C., Risler, T., and Smith, T. W.: Neural factors in digitalis toxicity: Protective effect of C-1 spinal cord transection. Am. J. Physiol. *235*:H531, 1978.
70. Mudge, G. H., Jr., Lloyd, B. L., Greenblatt, D. J., and Smith, T. W.: Inotropic and toxic effects of a polar cardiac glycoside derivative in the dog. Circ. Res. *43*:847, 1978.

Hemodynamic Effects

71. Smith, T. W.: The future of inotropic drugs in clinical practice. Eur. Heart J. *3*:149, 1982.
72. Wiggers, C. J., and Stimson, B.: Studies on cardiodynamic action of drugs. III. The mechanism of cardiac stimulation by digitalis and g-strophanthin. J. Pharmacol. Exp. Ther. *30*:251, 1927.
73. Cattell, M., and Gold, H.: The influence of digitalis glycosides on the force of contraction of mammalian cardiac muscle. J. Pharmacol. Exp. Ther. *62*:116, 1938.
74. Braunwald, E., Bloodwell, R. D., Goldberg, L. I., and Morrow, A. G.: Studies on digitalis. IV. Observations in man on the effects of digitalis preparations on the contractility of the non-failing heart and on total vascular resistance. J. Clin. Invest. *40*:52, 1961.
75. Cotten, M. deV., and Stopp, P. E.: Action of digitalis on the nonfailing heart of the dog. Am. J. Physiol. *192*:114, 1958.
76. Burwell, C. S., Neighbors, DeW., and Regen, E. M.: The effect of digitalis upon the output of the heart in normal man. J. Clin. Invest. *5*:125, 1927.
77. Harvey, R. M., Ferrer, M. I., Cathcart, R. T., and Alexander, J. K.: Some effects of digoxin on the heart and circulation in man: Digoxin in enlarged hearts not in clinical congestive failure. Circulation *4*:366, 1951.
78. Braunwald, E.: Effects of digitalis on the normal and the failing heart. J. Am. Coll. Cardiol. *5*:51A, 1985.
79. Smith, T. W.: Medical treatment of advanced congestive heart failure: Digitalis and diuretics. *In* Braunwald, E., Moch, M. B., and Watson, J. T. (eds.): Congestive Heart Failure. New York, Grune and Stratton, 1982, pp. 261–278.
80. Ware, J. A., Snow, E., Luchi, J. M., and Luchi, R. J.: Effect of digoxin on ejection fraction in elderly patients with congestive heart failure. J. Am. Geriatr. Soc. *32*:631, 1984.
81. Arnold, S. B., Byrd, R. C., Meister, W., Melmon, K., Cheitlin, M. D., Bristow, J. D., Parmley, W. W., and Chatterjee, K.: Long-term digitalis therapy improves left ventricular function in heart failure. N. Engl. J. Med. *303*:1443, 1980.
82. Lee, D. C.-S., Johnson, R. A., Bingham, J. B., Leahy, M., Dinsmore, R. E., Goroll, A. H., Newell, J. B., Strauss, H. W., and Haber, E.: Heart failure in outpatients. A randomized trial of digoxin versus placebo. N. Engl. J. Med. *306*:699, 1982.
83. Griffiths, B. E., Penny, W. J., Lewis, M. J., and Henderson, A. H.: Maintenance of the inotropic effect of digoxin on long-term treatment. Br. Med. J. *284*:1819, 1982.
84. Murray, R. G., Tweddel, A. C., Martin, W., Pearson, D., Hutton, I., and Lawrie, T. D. V.: Evaluation of digitalis in cardiac failure. Br. Med J. *284*:1526, 1982.
85. Fleg, J. L., Gottlieb, S. H., and Lakatta, E. G.: Is digoxin really important in treatment of compensated heart failure? Am. J. Med. *73*:244, 1982.
86. Gheorghiade, M., and Beller, G. A.: Effects of discontinuing maintenance digoxin therapy in patients with ischemic heart disease and congestive heart failure in sinus rhythm. Am. J. Cardiol. *51*:1243, 1983.
87. Berman, W., Yabek, S. M., Dillon, T., Niland, C., Corlew, S., and Christensen, D.: Effects of digoxin in infants with a congested circulatory state due to a ventricular septal defect. N. Engl. J. Med. *308*:363, 1983.
88. Cantelli, I., Vitolo, A., Lombardi, G., Bomba, E., and Bracchetti, D.: Combined hemodynamic effects of digoxin and captopril in patients with congestive heart failure. Curr. Ther. Res. *36*:323, 1984.
89. Boström, P. A., Andersson, J., Johansson, B. W., Lilja, B., Thorell, J., Tidfalt, K., and Westerling, S.: Haemodynamic effects of prenalterol and cardiac glycosides in patients with recent myocardial infarction. Eur. J. Clin. Invest. *14*:175, 1984.
90. Klein, M., Nejad, N. S., Lown, B., Hagemeijer, F., and Barr, I.: Correlation of the electrical and mechanical changes in the dog heart during progressive digitalization. Circ. Res. *29*:635, 1971.
91. Beiser, G. D., Epstein, S. E., Stampfer, M., Robinson, B., and Braunwald, E.: Studies on digitalis. XVII. Effects of ouabain on the hemodynamic response to exercise in patients with mitral stenosis in normal sinus rhythm. N. Engl. J. Med. *278*:131, 1968.
92. Ross, J., Jr., Waldhausen, J. A., and Braunwald, E.: Studies on digitalis. I. Direct effects on peripheral vascular resistance. J. Clin. Invest. *39*:930, 1960.
93. Goldman, M. R., Wold, S. W., Rulten, D. L., and Powell, W. J., Jr.: Effect of ouabain on total vascular capacity in the dog. J. Clin. Invest. *69*:175–184, 1982.
94. Mason, D. T., and Braunwald, E.: Studies on digitalis. X. Effects of ouabain on forearm vascular resistance and venous tone in normal subjects and in patients in heart failure. J. Clin. Invest. *43*:532, 1964.
95. Blatt, C. M., Marsh, J. D., and Smith, T. W.: Extracardiac effects of digitalis. *In* Smith, T. W. (ed.): Digitalis Glycosides. Orlando, Grune and Stratton, 1985. pp. 209–215.
96. Garan, H., Smith, T. W., and Powell, W. J., Jr.: The central nervous system as a site of action for the coronary vasoconstrictor effect of digoxin. J. Clin. Invest. *54*:1365, 1974.
97. Sagar, K. B., Hanson, E. C., and Powell, W. J.: Neurogenic coronary vasoconstrictor effects of digitalis during acute global ischemia in dogs. J. Clin. Invest. *60*:1248, 1977.
98. Kumar, R., Yankopoulos, N. A., and Abelmann, W. H.: Ouabain-induced hypertension in a patient with decompensated hypertensive heart disease. Chest *63*:105, 1973.
99. Cohn, J. N., Tristani, F. E., and Khatri, I. M.: Cardiac and peripheral vascular effects of digitalis in clinical shock. Am. Heart J. *78*:318, 1969.
100. Shanbour, L. L., and Jacobson, E. D.: Digitalis and the mesenteric circulation. Am. J. Dig. Dis. *17*:826, 1972.
101. DeMots, H., Rahimtoola, S. H., McAnulty, J. H., and Porter, G. A.: Effects of ouabain on coronary and systemic vascular resistance and myocardial oxygen consumption in patients without heart failure. Am. J. Cardiol. *41*:88, 1978.
102. Longhurst, J. C., and Ross, J.: Extracardiac and coronary vascular effects of digitalis. J. Am. Coll. Cardiol. *5*:99A, 1985.
103. Zelis, R., and Mason, D. T.: Compensatory mechanisms in congestive heart failure: The role of the peripheral resistance vessels. N. Engl. J. Med. *282*:962, 1970.
104. Covpit, A. B., Schaer, G. L., Scaley, J. E., Laragh, J. H., and Cody, R. J.: Suppression of the renin-angiotensin system by IV digoxin in chronic congestive heart failure. Am. J. Med. *75*:445, 1983.
105. Ribner, H. S., Plucinski, D. A., Hsieh, A. M., Bresnahan, D., Molteni, A., Askenazi, J., and Lesch, M.: Acute effects of digoxin on total systemic vascular resistance in congestive heart failure due to dilated cardiomyopathy: A hemodynamic-hormonal study. Am. J. Cardiol. *56*:896, 1985.
106. Strickler, J. C., and Kessler, R. H.: Direct renal action of some digitalis steroids. J. Clin. Invest. *40*:311, 1961.
107. Torretti, J., Hendler, E., and Weinstein, E.: Functional significance of Na-K-ATPase in the kidney: Effects of ouabain inhibition. Am. J. Physiol. *222*:1398, 1972.

Pharmacokinetics and Bioavailability

108. Gold, H., Cattell, M., Modell, W., Kwit, N. T., Kramer, M. L., and Zahm, W.: Clinical studies on digitoxin (Digitaline Nativelle): With further observations on its use in the single average full dose method of digitalization. J. Pharmacol. Exp. Ther. *82*:187, 1944.
109. Gold, H., Cattell, M., Greiner, T., Hanlon, L. W., Kwit, N. T., Modell, W., Cotlove, E., Benton, J., and Otto, H. L.: Clinical pharmacology of digoxin. J. Pharmacol. Exp. Ther. *109*:45, 1953.

110. Antman, E. M., and Smith, T. W.: Pharmacokinetics of digitalis glycosides. *In* Smith, T. W. (ed.): Digitalis Glycosides. Orlando, Grune and Stratton, 1985, pp. 45–60.
111. Cardiac Glycosides. Part II: Pharmacokinetics and Clinical Pharmacology. *In* Greeff, K. (ed.): Handbook of Experimental Pharmacology, Vol. 56. Berlin, Springer-Verlag, 1981.
112. Smith, T. W.: Drug therapy: Digitalis glycosides. N. Engl. J. Med. *288*:719, 1973.
113. Peters, V., Falk, L. C., and Kalman, S. M.: Digoxin metabolism in patients. Arch. Intern. Med. *138*:1074, 1978.
114. Lindenbaum, J., Rund, D. G., and Butler, V. P., Jr.: Inactivation of digoxin by the gut flora: reversal by antibiotic therapy. N. Engl. J. Med. *305*:789, 1981.
115. Halkin, H., Sheiner, L. B., Peck, C. C., and Melmon, K. L.: Determinants of the renal clearance of digoxin. Clin. Pharmacol. Ther. *385*:394, 1975.
116. Linday, L. A., Drayer, D. E., Khan, M. A. A., Cicalese, C., and Reidenberg, M. M.: Pubertal changes in net renal tubular secretion of digoxin. Clin. Pharmacol. Ther. *35*:438, 1984.
117. Marcus, F. L., Burkhalter, L., Cuccia, C., Pavlovich, J., and Kapadia, G. G.: Administration of tritiated digoxin with and without a loading dose: A metabolic study. Circulation *34*:865, 1966.
118. Ackerman, G. L., Doherty, J. E., and Flanigan, W. J.: Peritoneal dialysis and hemodialysis of tritiated digoxin. Ann. Intern Med. *67*:718, 1967.
119. Coltart, D. J., Chamberlain, D. A., Howard, M. R., Kettlewell, M. G., Mercer, J. L., and Smith, T. W.: The effect of cardiopulmonary bypass on plasma digoxin concentrations. Br. Heart J. *33*:334, 1971.
120. Coltart, D. J., Watson, D., and Howard, M. R.: Effect of exchange transfusions on plasma digoxin levels. Arch. Dis. Child. *47*:814, 1972.
121. Ewy, G. A., Groves, B. M., Ball, M. F., Nimmol, L., Jackson, B., and Marcus, F.: Digoxin-metabolism in obesity. Circulation *44*:810, 1971.
122. Cogan, J. J., Humphreys, M. H., Carlson, C. J., Benowitz, N. L., and Rapaport, E.: Acute vasodilator therapy increases renal clearance of digoxin in patients with congestive heart failure. Circulation *64*:973, 1981.
123. Leahey, E. B., Jr., Reiffel, J. A., Drusin, R. E., Heissenbuttel, R. H., Lovejoy, W. P., and Bigger, J. T., Jr.: Interaction between quinidine and digoxin. J.A.M.A. *240*:533, 1978.
124. Lukas, D. S., and DeMartino, A. G.: Binding of digitoxin and some related cardenolides to human plasma proteins. J. Clin. Invest. *48*:1041, 1969.
125. Storstein, L.: Studies on digitalis. I. Renal excretion of digitoxin and its cardioactive metabolites. Clin. Pharmacol. Ther. *16*:14, 1974.
126. Caldwell, J. H., Bush, C. A., and Greenberger, N. J.: Interruption of the enterohepatic circulation of digitoxin by cholestyramine. II. Effect on metabolic disposition of tritium-labeled digitoxin and cardiac systolic intervals in man. J. Clin. Invest. *50*:2638, 1971.
127. Solomon, H. M., and Abrams, W. B.: Interactions between digitoxin and other drugs in man. Am. Heart J. *83*:277, 1972.
128. Ochs, H. R., Pabst, J., Greenblatt, D. J., and Hartlapp, J.: Digoxin accumulation. Br. J. Clin. Pharmacol. *14*:225, 1982.
129. Selden, R., and Smith, T. W.: Ouabain pharmacokinetics in dog and man: Determination by radioimmunoassay. Circulation *45*:1176, 1972.
130. Selden, R., Margolies, M. N., and Smith, T. W.: Renal and gastrointestinal excretion of ouabain in dog and man. J. Pharmacol. Exp. Ther. *188*:615, 1974.
131. Selden R., Klein, M. D., and Smith, T. W.: Plasma concentration and urinary excretion kinetics of acetylstrophanthidin. Circulation *47*:744, 1973.
132. Beermann, B., Hellstrom, K., and Rosen, A.: The absorption of orally administered (12α-^{3}H) digoxin in man. Clin. Sci. *43*:507, 1972.
133. Greenblatt, D. J., Smith, T. W., and Koch-Weser, J.: Bioavailability of drugs: The digoxin dilemma. Clin. Pharmacokinet. *1*:36–51, 1976.
134. Heizer, W. D., Smith, T. W., and Goldfinger, S. E.: Absorption of digoxin in patients with malabsorption syndromes. N. Engl. J. Med. *285*:257, 1971.
135. Lindenbaum, J., Mellow, M. H., Blackstone, M. O., and Butler, V. P.: Variation in biologic availability of digoxin from four preparations. N. Engl. J. Med. *285*:1344, 1971.
136. Harter, J. G., Skelly, J. P., and Steers, A. W.: Digoxin—The regulatory viewpoint. Circulation *49*:395, 1974.

Clinical Use of Digitalis

137. Jelliffe, R. W., Buell, J., and Kalaba, R.: Reduction of digitalis toxicity by computer-assisted glycoside dosage regimens. Ann. Intern. Med. *77*:891, 1972.
138. Jelliffe, R. W., and Brooker, G.: A nomogram for digoxin therapy. Am. J. Med. *57*:63, 1974.
139. Peck, C. C., Sheiner, L. B., Martin, C. M., Combs, D. L., and Melmon, K. L.: Computer-assisted digoxin therapy. N. Engl. J. Med. *289*:441, 1973.
140. Lown, B., Klein, M. D., Barr, I., Hagemeijer, F., Kosowsky, B. D., and Garrison, H.: Sensitivity to digitalis drugs in acute myocardial infarction. Am. J. Cardiol. *30*:388, 1972.
141. Johnson, L. W., Dickstein, R. A., Freuhan, C. T., Kane, P., Potts, J. L., Smulyan, H., Webb, W. R., and Eich, R. H.: Prophylactic digitalization for coronary artery bypass surgery. Circulation *53*:819, 1976.
142. Tyras, D. H., Stothert, J. C., Jr., Kaiser, G. C., Barner, H. B., Codd, J. E., and Willman, V. L.: Supraventricular tachyarrhythmias after myocardial revascularization: A randomized trial of prophylactic digitalization. J. Thorac. Cardiovasc. Surg. *77*:310, 1979.
143. Marsh, J. D., and Smith, T. W.: Clinical use of cardiac glycosides in congestive heart failure. *In* Smith, T. W. (ed.): Digitalis Glycosides. Orlando, Grune and Stratton, 1985, pp. 83–113.
144. Antman, E. M., and Friedman, P. L.: Use of digitalis glycosides in the management of cardiac arrhythmias. *In* Smith, T. W. (ed.): Digitalis Glycosides. Orlando, Grune and Stratton, 1985, pp. 127–151.
145. Simpson, R. J., Foster, J. R., Woelfel, A. K., and Gettes, L. S.: Management of atrial fibrillation and flutter—A reappraisal of digitalis therapy. Postgrad. Med. *79*:241, 1986.
146. Beasley, R., Smith, D. A., and McHaffie, D. J.: Exercise heart rates at different serum digoxin concentrations in patients with atrial fibrillation. Br. Med. J. *290*:9, 1985.
147. Schwartz, J. B., Keefe, D., Kates, R. E., Kirsten, E., and Harrison, D. C.: Acute and chronic pharmacodynamic interaction of verapamil and digoxin in atrial fibrillation. Circulation *65*:1162, 1982.
148. Sellers, T. D., Bashore, T. M., and Gallagher, J. J.: Digitalis in pre-excitation syndrome—Analysis during atrial fibrillation. Circulation *56*:260, 1977.
148a. Gradman, A. H., Cunningham, M., Harbison, M. A., Berger, H. J., and Zaret, B. L.: Effects of oral digoxin on ventricular ectopy and its relation to left ventricular function. Am. J. Cardiol. *51*:765, 1983.

Dosage Schedules and Therapeutic Endpoints

149. Package Insert—Lanoxin Brand of Digoxin. Burroughs Wellcome Company, March, 1981.
150. Lown, B., and Levine, S. A.: The carotid sinus: Clinical value of its stimulation. Circulation *23*:766, 1961.
151. Fisch, C.: Relation of electrolyte disturbances to cardiac arrhythmias. Circulation *47*:408, 1973.
152. Ghani, M. F., and Smith, J. R.: The effectiveness of magnesium chloride in the treatment of ventricular tachyarrhythmias due to digitalis intoxication. Am. Heart J. *88*:621, 1974.
153. Neff, M. S., Mendelssohn, S., Kim, K. E., Banach, S., Swartz, C., and Seller, R. H.: Magnesium sulfate in digitalis toxicity. Am. J. Cardiol. *29*:377, 1972.
154. Editorial: Calcium, magnesium, and diuretics. Br. Med. J. *1*:170, 1975.
155. Holt, D. W., and Goulding, R.: Magnesium depletion and digoxin toxicity. Br. Med. J. *1*:627, 1975.
156. Beller, G. A., Hood, W. B., Jr., Smith, T. W., Abelmann, W. H., and Wacker, W. E. C.: Correlation of serum magnesium levels and cardiac digitalis intoxication. Am. J. Cardiol. *33*:225, 1974.
157. Whang, R., Qei, T. O., and Watanabe, A.: Frequency of hypomagnesemia in hospitalized patients receiving digitalis. Arch. Int. Med. *145*:655, 1985.
158. Gold, H., and Edwards, D. J.: The effects of ouabain on the heart in the presence of hypercalcemia. Am. Heart J. *3*:45, 1927.
159. Surawicz, B.: Use of the chelating agent, EDTA, in digitalis intoxication and cardiac arrhythmias. Progr. Cardiovasc. Dis. *2*:432, 1959.
160. Williams, J. F., Jr., Boyd, D. C., and Border, J. F.: Effects of acute hypoxia and hypercapnic acidosis on the development of acetylstrophanthidin induced arrhythmias. J. Clin. Invest. *47*:1885, 1968.
161. Tisi, G. M., and Moser, K. M.: Effect of acute changes in pO_2, pCO_2, and pH on digitalis toxicity. Circulation *36*:11, 1967.
162. Marcus, F. I.: Pharmacokinetic interactions between digoxin and other drugs. J. Am. Coll. Cardiol. *5*:82A, 1985.
163. Antman, E. M., and Smith, T. W.: Drug interactions with digitalis glycosides. *In* Smith, T. W. (ed.): Digitalis Glycosides. Orlando, Grune and Stratton, 1985, pp. 65–81.
163a. Elkayam, U., Parikh, K., Torkan, B., Weber, L., Cohen, J. L., and Rahimtoola, S. H.: Effect of diltiazem on renal clearance and serum concentration of digoxin in patients with cardiac disease. Am. J. Cardiol. *55*:1393, 1985.
164. Kuhlmann, J., and Marcin, S.: Effects of verapamil on pharmacokinetics and pharmacodynamics of digitoxin in patients. Am. Heart J. *110*:1245, 1985.
165. Lessem, J., and Bellinetto, A.: Interaction between digoxin and calcium antagonists. Am. J. Cardiol. *49*:1025, 1982.
166. Moysey, J. O., Jaggarao, N. S. V., Grundy, E. N., and Chamberlain, D. A.: Amiodarone increases plasma digoxin concentrations. Br. Med. J. *282*:272, 1981.
167. Nademanee, K., Kannan, R., Hendrickson, J., Burnam, M., Kay, I., and Singh, B.: Amiodarone-digoxin interaction during treatment of resistant cardiac arrhythmias. Am. J. Cardiol. *49*:1026, 1982.
168. Smith, T. W., and Willerson, J. T.: Suicidal and accidental digoxin ingestion: Report of five cases with serum digoxin level correlations. Circulation *44*:29, 1971.
169. Smith, T. W., Butler, V. P., Jr., Haber, E., Fozzard, H., Marcus, F. I., Bremner, W. F., Schulman, I. C., and Phillips, A.: Treatment of life-threatening digitalis intoxication with digoxin-specific Fab fragments: Experience in 26 cases. N. Engl. J. Med. *307*:1357, 1982.
170. Rubinow, A., Skinner, M., and Cohen, A. S.: Digoxin sensitivity in amyloid cardiomyopathy. Circulation *63*:1285, 1981.
171. Covell, J. W., Braunwald, E., Ross, J., Jr., and Sonnenblick, E. H.: Studies on digitalis. XVI. Effects on myocardial oxygen consumption. J. Clin. Invest. *45*:1535, 1966.
172. Sonnenblick, E. H., Ross, J., Jr., and Braunwald, E.: Oxygen consumption of the heart: Newer concepts of its multifactorial determination. Am. J. Cardiol. *22*:328, 1968.
173. Glancy, D. L., Higgs, L. M., O'Brien, K. P., and Epstein, S. E.: Effects of ouabain on the left ventricular response to exercise in patients with angina pectoris. Circulation *43*:45, 1971.
174. Sharma, B., Majid, P. A., Meeran, M. K., Whitaker, W., and Taylor, S. H.: Clinical, electrocardiographic and haemodynamic effects of digitalis (ouabain) in angina pectoris. Br. Heart J. *34*:631, 1972.

175. DeMots, H., Rahimtoola, S. H., Kremkau, E. L., Bennett, W., and Mahler, D.: Effects of ouabain on myocardial oxygen supply and demand in patients with chronic coronary artery disease: A hemodynamic, volumetric, and metabolic study in patients without heart failure. J. Clin. Invest. *58*:312, 1976.
176. Loeb, H. S., Streitmatter, N., Braunstein, D., Jacobs, W. R., Croke, R. P., and Gunnar, R. M.: Lack of ouabain effect on pacing-induced myocardial ischemia in patients with coronary artery disease. Am. J. Cardiol. *43*:995, 1979.
177. Vogel, R., Kirch, D., LeFree, M., Frischknecht, J., and Steele, P.: Effects of digitalis on resting and isometric exercise myocardial perfusion in patients with coronary artery disease and left ventricular dysfunction. Circulation *56*:355, 1977.
178. Crawford, M. H., LeWinter, M. M., O'Rourke, R. A., Karliner, J. S., and Ross, J.: Combined propranolol and digoxin therapy in angina pectoris. Ann. Intern. Med. *83*:449, 1975.
179. Ratshin, R. A., Rackley, C. E., and Russell, R. O., Jr.: Hemodynamic evaluation of left ventricular function in shock complicating myocardial infarction. Circulation *45*:127, 1972.
180. Rahimtoola, S. H., Sinno, M. Z., Chuquimia, R., Loeb, H. S., Rosen, K. M., and Gunnar, R. M.: Effects of ouabain on impaired left ventricular function in acute myocardial infarction. N. Engl. J. Med. *287*:527, 1972.
181. Rahimtoola, S. H., DiGilio, M. M., Sinno, M. Z., Loeb, H. S., Rosen, K. M., and Gunnar, R. M.: Effects of ouabain on impaired left ventricular function during convalescence after acute myocardial infarction. Circulation *44*:866, 1971.
182. Kumar, R., Hood, W. B., Jr., Joison, J., Gilmour, D. P., Norman, J. C., and Abelmann, W. H.: Experimental myocardial infarction. VI. Efficacy and toxicity of digitalis in acute and healing phase in intact conscious dogs. J. Clin. Invest. *49*:358, 1970.
183. Reičansky, I., Conradson, T. B., Holmberg, S., Rydén, L., Waldenström, A., and Wennerblom, B.: The effect of intravenous digoxin on the occurrence of ventricular tachyarrhythmias in acute myocardial infarction in man. Am. Heart J. *91*:705, 1976.
184. Rahimtoola, S. H., and Gunnar, R. M.: Digitalis in acute myocardial infarction: Help or hazard? Ann. Intern. Med. *82*:234, 1975.
185. Selzer, A.: The use of digitalis in acute myocardial infarction. Progr. Cardiovasc. Dis. *10*:518, 1968.
186. Moss, A. J., Davis, H. T., Conard, D. L., DeCamilla, J. J., and Odoroff, C. L.: Digitalis-associated cardiac mortality after myocardial infarction. Circulation *64*:1150, 1981.
187. Bigger, J. T., Fleiss, J. L., Rolnitsky, L. M., Merab, J. P., and Ferrick, K. J.: Effect of digitalis treatment on survival after acute myocardial infarction. Am. J. Cardiol. *55*:623, 1985.
188. Ryan, T. J., Bailey, K. R., McCabe, C. H., Luk, S., Fisher, L. D., Mock, M. B., and Killip, T.: The effects of digitalis on survival in high-risk patients with coronary artery disease. Circulation *67*:735, 1983.
189. Madsen, E. B., Gilpin, E., Henning, H., Ahnve, S., LeWinter, M., Mazur, J., Shabetai, R., Collins, D., and Ross, J.: Prognostic importance of digitalis after acute myocardial infarction. J. Am. Coll. Cardiol. *3*:681, 1984.
190. Byington, R., Goldstein, S., and the BHAT Research Group: Association of digitalis therapy with mortality in survivors of acute myocardial infarction: Observations in the beta-blocker heart attack trial. J. Am. Coll. Cardiol. *6*:976, 1985.
191. Muller, J. E., Turi, Z. G., Stone, P. H., Rude, R. E., Raabe, D. S., Jaffe, A. S., Gold, H. K., Gustafson, N., Poole, W. K., Passamani, E., Smith, T. W., Braunwald, E., and the MILIS Study Group. Digoxin therapy and mortality after myocardial infarction: experience in the MILIS study. N. Engl. J. Med. *314*:265, 1986.
192. Dall, J. L.: Digitalis intoxication in the elderly. Lancet *1*:194, 1965.
193. Szefler, S. J., and Jusko, W. J.: Decreased volume of distribution of digoxin in a patient with renal failure. Res. Commun. Chem. Pathol. Pharmacol. *6*:1095, 1973.
194. Croxson, M. S., and Ibbertson, H. K.: Serum digoxin in patients with thyroid disease. Br. Med. J. *3*:566, 1975.
195. Curfman, G. D., Crowley, T. J., and Smith, T. W.: Thyroid-induced alterations in myocardial sodium- and potassium-activated adenosine triphosphatase, monovalent cation active transport, and cardiac glycoside binding. J. Clin. Invest. *59*:586, 1977.
196. Ismail-Beigi, F., and Edelman, I. S.: The mechanism of the calorigenic action of thyroid hormone: Stimulation of $Na^+ + K^+$-activated adenosine-triphosphatase. J. Gen. Physiol. *57*:710, 1971.
197. Kim, D., and Smith, T. W.: Effects of thyroid hormone on sodium pump sites, sodium content, and contractile responses to cardiac glycosides in cultured chick ventricular cells. J. Clin. Invest. *74*:1481, 1984.
198. Green, L. H., and Smith, T. W.: The use of digitalis in patients with pulmonary disease. Ann. Intern. Med. *87*:459, 1977.
199. Hargreave, F. D.: Digitalis and cor pulmonale. Br. Med. J. *2*:943, 1965.
200. Hudson, L. D., Kurt, T. L., Petty, T. L., and Genton, E.: Arrhythmias associated with acute respiratory failure in patients with chronic airway obstruction. Chest *63*:661, 1973.
201. Beller, G. A., Smith, T. W., Abelmann, W. H., Haber, E., and Hood, W. B., Jr.: Digitalis intoxication: Prospective clinical study with serum level correlations. N. Engl. J. Med. *284*:989, 1971.
202. Surawicz, B.: Factors affecting tolerance to digitalis. J. Am. Coll. Cardiol. *5*:69A, 1985.

Serum or Plasma Concentrations of Digitalis Glycosides

203. Lely, A. H., and van Enter, C. H. J.: Non-cardiac symptoms of digitalis intoxication. Am. Heart J. *83*:149, 1972.
204. Doherty, J. E., and Perkins, W. H.: Tissue concentration and turnover of tritiated digoxin in dogs. Am. J. Cardiol. *17*:47, 1966.
205. Doherty, J. E., Perkins, W. H., and Flanigan, W. J.: The distribution and concentration of tritiated digoxin in human tissues. Ann. Intern. Med. *66*:116, 1967.
206. Barr, I., Smith, T. W., Klein, M. D., Hagemeijer, F., and Lown, B.: Correlation of the electrophysiologic action of digoxin with serum digoxin concentration. J. Pharmacol. Exp. Ther. *180*:710, 1972.
207. Smith, T. W., and Curfman, G. D.: Radioimmunoassay of cardiac glycosides. *In* Strauss, W., and Pitt, B. (eds.): Cardiovascular Nuclear Medicine. 2nd ed. St. Louis, C. V. Mosby Co., 1979, p. 394.
208. Smith, T. W.: Serum and plasma cardiac glycoside concentrations: Clinical use and misuse. *In* Smith, T. W. (ed.): Digitalis Glycosides. Orlando, Grune and Stratton, 1985, pp. 153–167.
209. Duhme, D. W., Greenblatt, D. J., and Koch-Weser, J.: Reduction of digoxin toxicity associated with measurement of serum levels. Ann. Intern. Med. *80*:516, 1974.
210. Chamberlain, D. A., White, R. J., Howard, M. R., and Smith, T. W.: Plasma digoxin concentrations in patients with atrial fibrillation. Br. Med. J. *3*:429, 1970.
211. Klein, M. D., Lown, B., Barr, I., Hagemeijer, F., Garrison, H., and Axelrod, P.: Comparison of serum digoxin level measurement with acetyl strophanthidin tolerance testing. Circulation *49*:1053, 1974.
212. Eraker, S. A., and Sasse, L.: The serum digoxin test and digoxin toxicity: A Bayesian approach to decision-making. Circulation *64*:409, 1981.

Digitalis Toxicity

213. Borison, H. L., and Wang, S. C.: Physiology and pharmacology of vomiting. Pharmacol. Rev. *5*:193, 1953.
214. Gayes, J. M., Greenblatt, D. J., Lloyd, B. L., Harmatz, J. S., and Smith, T. W.: Cerebrospinal fluid digoxin concentrations in humans. J. Clin. Pharmacol. *18*:16, 1978.
215. Somberg, J. C., Kuhlman, J. E., and Smith, T. W.: Localization of the neurally mediated coronary vasoconstrictor properties of digitalis in the cat. Circ. Res. *49*:226, 1981.
216. Rosen, M. R., Gelband, H., and Hoffman, B. F.: Correlation between effects of ouabain on the canine electrocardiogram and transmembrane potentials of isolated Purkinje fibers. Circulation *47*:65, 1973.
217. Rosen, M. R., and Gelband, H.: Effect of ouabain on canine Purkinje fibers in situ or perfused with blood. J. Pharmacol. Exp. Ther. *186*:366, 1973.
218. Davis, L. D.: Effect of changes in cycle length on diastolic depolarization produced by ouabain in canine Purkinje fibers. Circ. Res. *32*:206, 1973.
219. Rosen, M. R., Gelband, H., Merker, C., and Hoffman, B. F.: Mechanisms of digitalis toxicity. Effects of ouabain on phase 4 of canine Purkinje fiber transmembrane potentials. Circulation *47*:681, 1973,
220. Ferrier, G. R.: Digitalis arrhythmias: Role of oscillatory afterpotentials. Prog. Cardiovasc. Dis. *19*:459, 1977.
221. Saunders, J. H., Ferrier, G. R., and Moe, G. K.: Conduction block associated with transient depolarizations induced by acetylstrophanthidin in isolated canine Purkinje fibers. Circ. Res. *32*:610, 1973.
222. Zipes, D. P., Arbel, E., Knope, R. F., and Moe, G. K.: Accelerated cardiac escape rhythms caused by ouabain intoxication. Am. J. Cardiol. *33*:248, 1973.
223. Lederer, W. J., and Tsien, R. W.: Transient inward current underlying arrhythmogenic effects of cardiotonic steroids in Purkinje fibers. J. Physiol. *263*:73, 1976.
224. Kass, R. S., Lederer, W. J., Tsien, R. W., and Weingart R.: Role of calcium ions in transient inward currents and aftercontractions induced by strophanthidin in cardiac Purkinje fibers. J. Physiol *281*:187, 1978.
225. Tsien, R. W., Weingart, R., Lederer, W. J., and Kass, R. S.: On the inotropic and arrhythmogenic effects of digitalis. *In* Riecker, G., Weber, A., and Goodwin, J. (eds.): Myocardial Failure. New York, Springer-Verlag, 1977, p. 331.
226. Kass, R. S., Tsien, R. W., and Weingart, R.: Ionic basis of transient inward current induced by strophanthidin in cardiac Purkinje fibers. J. Physiol. *281*:209, 1978.
227. Lely, A., and van Enter, C.: Large-scale digitoxin intoxication. Br. Med. J. *3*:737, 1970.
228. Blatt, C. M., Marsh, J. D., and Smith, T. W.: The role of neural factors in digitalis intoxication. *In* Smith, T. W. (ed.): Digitalis Glycosides. Orlando, Grune and Stratton, 1985, pp. 227–293.
229. Storstein, O., and Rasmussen, K.: Digitalis and atrial tachycardia with block. Br. Heart J. *36*:171, 1974.
230. Lown, B., Graboys, T. B., Podrid, P. J., Cohen, B. H., Stockman, M. B., and Gaughan, C. E.: Effect of a digitalis drug on ventricular premature beats. N. Engl. J. Med. *296*:301, 1977.
231. Fisch, C., and Knoebel, S. B.: Digitalis cardiotoxicity. J. Am. Coll. Cardiol. *5*:91A, 1985.
232. Wellens, H. J. J.: The electrocardiogram in digitalis intoxication. *In* Yu, P. N., and Goodwin, J. F. (eds.): Progress in Cardiology. Vol. 5. Philadelphia, Lea and Febiger, 1976, p. 271.
233. Friedman, P. L., Antman, E. M.: Electrocardiographic manifestations of digitalis toxicity. *In* Smith, T. W. (Ed.): Digitalis Glycosides. Orlando, Florida, Grune & Stratton, 1985, pp. 241–275.
234. Brauner, G. J., and Greene, M. H.: Digitalis allergy: Digoxin-induced vasculitis. Cutis *10*:441, 1972.
235. LeWinn, E. B.: Gynecomastia during digitalis therapy: Report of eight additional cases with liver-function studies. N. Engl. J. Med. *248*:316, 1953.
236. Neri, A., Aygen, M., Zuckerman, A., and Bahary, C.: Subject of assessment of sexual dysfunction of patients on long-term administration of digoxin. Arch. Sexual Behav. *9*:343, 1980.

237. Bismuth, C., Motte, G., Conso, F., Chauvin, M., and Gaultier, M.: Acute digitoxin intoxication treated by intracardiac pacemaker: Experience in sixty-eight patients. Clin. Toxicol. *10*:443, 1977.
238. Citrin, D., Stevenson, I. H., and O'Malley, K.: Massive digoxin overdose: Observations on hyperkalaemia and plasma digoxin levels. Scott. Med. J. *17*:275, 1972.
238a. Friedman, P. L., Antman, E. M., Smith, T. W.: Clinical management of digitalis toxicity. *In* Smith, T. W. (Ed): Digitalis Glycosides. Orlando, Florida, Grune & Stratton, 1985, pp. 295–309.
239. Gaultier, M., Fournier, E., Efthymiou, M. L., Frejaville, J. P., Jouannot, P., and Dentan, M.: Intoxication digitalique aiguë (70 observations). Bull. Soc. Med. Hop. Paris *119*:247, 1968.
240. Hobson, J. D., and Zettner, A.: Digoxin serum half-life following suicidal digoxin poisoning. J.A.M.A. *223*:147, 1973.
241. Bigger, J. T., Jr., and Strauss, H. C.: Digitalis toxicity: Drug interactions promoting toxicity and the management of toxicity. Semin. Drug Treat. *2*:147, 1972.
242. Ditchey, R. V., and Karliner, J. S.: Safety of electrical cardioversion in patients without digitalis toxicity. Ann. Intern. Med. *95*:676, 1981.
243. Bazzano, G., and Bazzano, G. S.: Digitalis intoxication: Treatment with a new steroid-binding resin. J.A.M.A. *220*:828, 1972.
244. Goldfinger, S. E., Heizer, W. D., and Smith, T. W.: Absorption of digoxin in patients with malabsorption syndrome. *In* Storstein, O. (ed.): International Symposium on Digitalis. Oslo, Gyldendal Norsk Forlag, 1973, p. 224.
245. Smith, T. W.: Digitalis toxicity: Clinical management of advanced life-threatening toxicity resistance to conventional therapy. *In* Smith, T. W. (Ed): Digitalis Glycosides. Orlando, Florida, Grune & Stratton, 1985, pp. 311–321.
246. Smith, T. W., Butler, V. P., Jr., and Haber, E.: Cardiac glycoside-specific antibodies in the treatment of digitalis intoxication. *In* Haber, E., and Krause, R. M. (eds.): Antibodies in Human Diagnosis and Therapy. New York, Raven Press, 1977.
247. Butler, V. P., Jr., Smith, T. W., Schmidt, D. H., and Haber, E.: Immunological reversal of the effects of digoxin. Fed. Proc. *36*:2235, 1977.
248. Lloyd, B. L., and Smith, T. W.: Contrasting rates of reversal of digoxin toxicity by digoxin-specific IgG and Fab fragments. Circulation *58*:280, 1978.
249. Smith, T. W.: Ouabain-specific antibodies: Immunochemical properties and reversal of Na^+, K^+-activated adenosine triphosphatase inhibition. J. Clin. Invest. *51*:1583, 1972.
250. Hougen, T. J., Lloyd, B. L., and Smith, T. W.: Effects of inotropic and arrhythmogenic digoxin doses and of digoxin-specific antibody on myocardial monovalent cation transport in the dog. Circ. Res. *44*:23, 1979.
251. Smith, T. W., Lloyd, B. L., Spicer, N., and Haber, E.: Immunogenicity and kinetics of distribution and elimination of sheep digoxin-specific IgG and Fab fragments in the rabbit and baboon. Clin. Exp. Immunol. *36*:384, 1979.
252. Butler, V. P., Jr., Schmidt, D. H., Smith, T. W., Haber, E., Raynor, B. D., and McMartini, P.: Effects of sheep digoxin-specific antibodies and their Fab fragments on digoxin pharmacokinetics in dogs. J. Clin. Invest. *59*:345, 1977.
253. Ochs, H. R., and Smith, T. W.: Reversal of advanced digitoxin toxicity and modification of pharmacokinetics by specific antibodies and Fab fragments. J. Clin. Invest. *60*:1303, 1977.
254. Wenger, T. L., Butler, V. P., Haber, E., and Smith, T. W.: Treatment of 63 severely digitalis-toxic patients with digoxin-specific antibody fragments. J. Am. Coll. Cardiol. *5*:118A, 1985.

DIURETICS

255. Abildgaard, U., Aldershville, J., Ring-Larsen, H., Falk, J., Christensen, N. J., Giese, J., Hammer, M., and Henriksen, J.H.: Bed rest and increased diuretic treatment in chronic congestive heart failure. Eur. Heart J. *6*:1040, 1985.
256. Nishijima, H., Yasuda, H., Ito, K., Murakami, R., Hayashi, K., Yamazaki, M., and Hatori, T.: Acute and chronic hemodynamic effects of the basic therapeutic regimen for congestive heart failure; Diuretics, low-salt diets, and bed rest. Jpn. Heart J. *25*:(4):571, 1984.
257. Cody, R. J., Covit, A. B., Schaer, G. L., Laragh, J. H., Sealey, J. E., and Fedlshuk, J.: Sodium and water balance in chronic congestive heart failure. J. Clin. Invest. *77*:1441, 1986.
258. Atlas, S. A., and Laragh, J. H.: Atrial natriuretic peptide: A new factor in hormonal control of blood pressure and electrolyte homeostasis. Am. Rev. Med. *37*:397, 1986.
259. Barnett, J. C., Kao, P. C., Hu, D. C., Heser, D. W., Heublein, D., Granger, J. P., Opgenorth, T. J., and Reeder, G. S.: Atrial natriuretic peptide elevation in congestive heart failure in the human. Science *231*:1145, 1986.
260. Lant, A.: Diuretics: Clinical pharmacology and therapeutic use. Drugs, Part I *29*:57; Part II 29:162, 1985.
261. Puschett, J. B.: Clinical pharmacologic implications in diuretic selection. Am. J. Cardiol. *57*:6A, 1986.

Sites and Mechanism of Action

262. Burg, M.: Renal handling of sodium, chloride, water, amino acids, and glucose. *In* Brenner, B. M., Rector, F. C. (eds.); The Kidney. Philadelphia, W. B. Saunders Company, 1986, pp. 145–175.
263. Brater, D. C.: Pharmacodynamic considerations in the use of diuretics. Ann. Rev. Pharmacol. Toxicol. *23*:45, 1983.
264. Greger, R.: Ion transport mechanisms in the thick ascending limb of Henle's loop of mammalian nephron. Physiol. Rev. *65*:760, 1985.
265. Brenner, B. M., Zatz, R., and Ichikawa, I.: The renal circulations. *In* Brenner, B. M., and Rector, F. C. (eds.): The Kidney. Philadelphia, W. B. Saunders Company, 1986, pp. 93–123.
266. Gottschalk, C. W., Moss, N. G., and Colindres, R. E.: Neuronal control of renal function in health and disease. *In* Seldin, D. W., and Giebisch, G. (eds.): The Kidney: Physiology and Pathophysiology. New York, Raven Press, 1986, pp. 581–611.

Pharmacology

267. Kokko, J. P.: Site and mechanism of action of diuretics. Am. J. Med. *77*:11, 1984.
268. Suki, W. N., Steinbaugh, B. J., Frommer, J. P., and Eknoyan, G.: Physiology of diuretic action. *In* Seldin, D. W., and Giebisch, G. (eds.) The Kidney: Physiology and Pathophysiology. New York, Raven Press, 1985, pp. 2127–2162.
269. Berger, B. E., and Warnock, D. G.: Clinical uses and mechanisms of action of diuretic agents. *In* Brenner, B. M., and Rector, F. C. (eds.): The Kidney. Philadelphia, W. B. Saunders Company, 1986, pp. 433–455.
270. Mudge, G. H., and Wainer, I. M.: Drugs affecting renal function and electrolyte metabolism. *In* Gilman, A. F., et al. (eds.) The Pharmacologic Basis of Therapeutics. 7th ed. New York, Macmillan, 1985, pp. 879–907.
271. Eknoyan, G., and Martinez-Maldonado, M. (eds.): The Physiologic Basis of Diuretic Therapy in Clinical Medicine. Orlando, Grune and Stratton, 1986.
272. Lucci, M. S., Tinker, J. P., Weiner, I. M., and DuBose, T. P.: Function of proximal tubular carbonic anhydrase defined by selective inhibition. Am. J. Physiol. *245*:F443, 1983.
273. Miller, P. D., and Berns, A. S.: Acute metabolic acidosis perpetuating hypercarbia: A role for acetazolamide in chronic obstructive pulmonary disease. J.A.M.A. *248*:2400, 1977.
274. Bear, R., Goldstein, M., Phillipson, E., Ho, M., Hammeke, M., Feldman, R., Handelsman, S., and Halperin, M.: Effect of metabolic alkalosis on respiratory function in patients with chronic obstructive lung disease. Can. Med. Assoc. J. *117*:900, 1977.
275. Greene, M. K., Kerr, A. M., McIntosh, I. B., and Prescott, R. J.: Acetazolamide in prevention of acute mountain sickness: A double-blind controlled crossover study. Br. Med. J. *283*:811, 1981.
276. Brodwell, A. R., Coote, J. H., Milles, J. F., Dykes, P. W., Forster, P. G. E., Chesner, I., and Richardson, N. V.: Effect of acetazolamide on exercise tolerance and muscle mass at high altitude. Lancet *1*:1001, 1986.
277. Levinsky, N. G., Bernard, D. B., and Johnston, P. A.: Mannitol and loop diuretics in acute renal failure. *In* Brenner, B. M., and Lazarus, J. M. (eds.): Acute Renal Failure. Philadelphia, W. B. Saunders Company, 1983, pp. 712–722.
278. Narins, R. G., and Chusid, P.: Diuretic use in critical care. Am J. Cardiol. *57*:26A, 1986.
279. Feig, P. U.: Cellular mechanism of action of loop diuretics: Implications for drug effectiveness and adverse effects. Am. J. Cardiol. *57*:14A, 1986.
280. Wright, F. S., and Schnermann, J.: Interference with feedback control of glomerular filtration rate by furosemide, triflocin, and cyanide. J. Clin. Invest. *53*:1695, 1974.
281. Grahnen, A., Hammarlund, M., and Lundquist, T.: Implications of intraindividual variability in bioavailability studies of furosemide. Eur. J. Clin. Pharmacol. *27*:595, 1984.
282. Beermann, B., and Midskov, C.: Reduced bioavailability and effect of furosemide given with food. Eur. J. Clin. Pharmacol. *29*:725, 1986.
283. Ogata, H., Kawatsu, Y., Maruyama, Y., Machida, K., and Haga, T.: Bioavailability and diuretic effect of furosemide during long-term treatment of chronic respiratory failure. Eur. J. Clin. Pharmacol. *28*:53, 1985.
284. Brater, D. C., Day, B., Burdette, A., and Anderson, S.: Bumetanide and furosemide in heart failure. Kidney Int. *26*:183, 1984.
285. Vasko, M. R., Brown-Cartwright, D., Knochel, J. P., Nixon, J. V., and Brater, D. C.: Furosemide absorption altered in decompensated congestive heart failure. Ann. Intern. Med. *102*:314, 1985.
286. Kuchar, D. L., and O'Rourke, M. F.: High-dose furosemide in refractory cardiac failure. Eur. Heart J. *6*:954, 1985.
287. Colice, G. L., and Ramirez, G.: The effect of furosemide during normoxemia and hypoxemia. Am. Rev. Respir. Dis. *133*:279, 1986.
288. Babini, R., and du Souich, P.: Furosemide pharmacodynamics: Effects of respiratory and acid base disturbances. J. Pharmacol. Exp. Ther. *237*:623, 1986.
289. Blackshear, J. L. et al: Identification of risk for renal insufficiency from nonsteroidal anti-inflammatory drugs. Arch. Intern. Med. *143*:1130, 1983.
290. Nies, A. S., Gal, S., Fadul, S., and Gerker, J. G.: Indomethacin-furosemide interaction: The importance of renal blood flow. J. Pharmacol. Exp. Ther. *226*:27, 1983.
291. Webster, J.: Interactions of NSAIDs with diuretics and β-blockers. Mechanisms and clinical implications. Drugs *30*:32, 1985.
292. Kirchner, K. A.: Prostaglandin inhibitors after loop segment chloride uptake during furosemide diuresis. Am. J. Physiol. *248*:F698, 1985.
293. Chennavasin, P., Seiwell, R., and Brater, D. C.: Pharmacokinetic-dynamic analysis of the indomethacin-furosemide interaction in man. J. Pharmacol. Exp. Ther. *215*:77, 1980.
294. Koopmans, P. P., Thien, T. H., Thomas, C. M. G., Vandenberg, R. J., and Gribrane, W. J.: The effects of sulindac and indomethacin on antihypertensive and diuretic action of hydrochlorothiazide in patients with mild to moderate essential hypertension. Br. J. Clin. Pharmacol. *21*:417, 1986.

295. Eriksson, L. O., Beermann, B., and Kallner, M.: Aspects of the effects of NSAIDs on renal function in congestive heart failure. Agents Actions (Suppl) *17*:99, 1985.
296. Wong, D. G., Lamki, L., Spencer, J. P., Freeman, P., and McDonald, J. W. D.: Effect of non-steroidal antiinflammatory drugs on control of hypertension by beta-blockers and diuretics. Lancet *1*:997, 1986.
297. Wilson, T. W., McCauley, F. A., and Wells, H. D.: Effects of low-dose aspirin on responses to furosemide. J. Clin. Pharmacol. *26*:100, 1986.
298. Dikshit, K., Vyden, J. K., Forrester, J. S., Chatterjee, K., Prakosh, R., and Swan, H. J. C.: Renal and extrarenal hemodynamic effects of furosemide in congestive heart failure after acute myocardial infarction. N. Engl. J. Med. *288*:1087, 1973.
299. Gerber, J. G.: Role of prostaglandins in the hemodynamic and tubular effects of furosemide. Fed. Proc. *42*:1707, 1983.
300. Kelly, R. A., Wilcox, C. S., Meyer, T. W., Souney, P. F., Rayment, C., Friedman, P. A., Swartz, S. L., and Mitch, W. E.: The response of the kidney to furosemide II; Effect of captopril on sodium balance. Kidney Int. *24*:233, 1983.
301. Francis, G. S., Siegel, R. M., Goldsmith, S. R., Olivari, M. T., Levine, B., and Cohn, J. N.: Acute vasoconstrictor response to intravenous furosemide in patients with chronic congestive failure. Ann. Intern. Med. *103*:1, 1985.
302. Brater, D. C., Chennavasin, P., and Dehmer, G. J.: Prolonged hemodynamic effect of furosemide in congestive heart failure. Am. Heart J. *108*:1031, 1984.
303. Johnston, G. D., Nicholls, D. P., and Leahey, W. J.: The dose response characteristics of the acute non-diuretic peripheral vascular effects of furosemide in normal subjects. Br. J. Clin. Pharmacol. *18*:75, 1984.
304. Johnston, G. D., Nicholls, D. P., Kondowe, G. B., and Finch, M. B.: Comparison of the acute vascular effects of furosemide and bumetanide. Br. J. Clin. Pharmacol. *21*:359, 1986.
305. Ali, J., Chernicki, W., and Wood, L. D. H.: Effect of furosemide in canine low-pressure pulmonary edema. J. Clin. Invest. *64*:1494, 1979.
306. Ali, J., and Wood, L. D. H.: Pulmonary vascular effects of furosemide on gas exchange in pulmonary edema. Am. J. Physiol. *57*:160, 1984.
307. Lydon, J. C., Ebert, J. P., Grimes, B., and Niemann, K. M.: Furosemide may be detrimental in the treatment of pulmonary edema. Anesthesiology *64*:298, 1986.
308. Green, T. P., Thompson, T. R., Johnson, D. E., and Lock, J. E.: Furosemide promotes patent ductus arteriosus in preparative infants with the respiratory distress syndrome. N. Engl. J. Med. *308*:743, 1983.
309. Rybak, L.: Furosemide ototoxicity: Clinical and experimental aspects. Laryngoscope *95* (Suppl. 38):1, 1985.
310. Gould, L., Chokski, A. B., Patel, S., and Gomes, G. I.: Electro-physiologic properties of furosemide in man. Angiology *34*:53, 1983.
311. Marsh, J. D., and Smith, T. W.: Piretanide: A loop-active diuretic. Pharmacology, therapeutic efficacy, and adverse effects. Pharmacotherapy *4*:170, 1984.
312. Ward, A., and Heel, R. C.: Bumetanide: A review of its pharmacodynamic and pharmacokinetic properties and therapeutic use. Drugs *28*:426, 1984.
313. Brater, D. C.: Disposition and response to bumetanide and furosemide. Am. J. Cardiol. *57*:20A, 1986.
314. Stier, C. T., and Itskovitz, H. D.: Renal calcium metabolism and diuretics. Ann. Rev. Pharmacol. Toxicol. *26*:101, 1986.
315. Sutton, R. A. L.: Diuretics and calcium metabolism. Am. J. Kidney Dis. *5*:4, 1985.
316. Croswell, P. W., Ezzat, E., Kopstein, J., Varghese, Z., and Moorhead, J. F.: Use of metolazone, a new diuretic in patients with renal disease. Nephron *12*:63, 1973.
317. Slotkoss, L.: Clinical efficacy and safety of indapamide in the treatment of edema. Am. Heart J. *106*:233, 1983.
318. Thomas, J. R.: A review of 10 years of experience with indapamide as an antihypertensive agent. Hypertension 7 (Suppl. II):152–156, 1985.
319. Corvol, P., Claire, M., Oblin, M. E., Geening, K., and Rossier, B.: Mechanisms of the antimineralocorticoid effects of spironolactone. Kidney Int. *242*:C131, 1982.
320. Sariban-Sohraby, S., and Benos, D. G.: The amiloride-sensitive sodium channel. Am. J. Physiol. *250*:C175, 1986.
321. Favre, L., Glasson, P., and Vallotton, M. B.: Reversible acute renal failure from combined triamterene and indomethacin. Ann. Intern. Med. *96*:317, 1982.
322. Oster, J. R., Epstein, M., and Smaller, S.: Combined therapy with thiazide-type and loop diuretic agents for resistant sodium retention. Ann. Intern. Med. *99*:104, 1983.
323. Hill, N. S.: Fluid and electrolyte considerations in diuretic therapy for hypertensive patients with chronic obstructive pulmonary disease. Arch. Intern. Med. *146*:129, 1986.
324. Marone, C., Muggli, F., Lahn, W., and Frey, F. J.: Pharmacokinetic and pharmacodynamic interaction between furosemide and metolazone in man. Eur. J. Clin. Invest. *15*:253, 1985.
325. Arnold, W. C.: Efficacy of metolazone and furosemide in children with furosemide-resistant edema. Pediatrics *74*:872, 1984.
326. Wollam, G. L., Tarazi, R. C., Bravo, E. L., and Dustan, H. P.: Diuretic potency of combined hydrochlorothiazide and furosemide therapy in patients with azotemia. Am. J. Med. *72*:929, 1982.
327. Hropot, M., Fowler, N., Karlmark, B., and Giebisch, G.: Tubular action of diuretics: distal effects on electrolyte transport and acidification. Kidney Int. *28*:477, 1985.
328. Funke Kupper, A. J., Fintelman, H., Hurge, M. C., Koolen, J. J., Lien, K. L., and Lustermans, F. A.: Crossover comparison of the fixed combination of furosemide and triamterene and the free combination of furosemide and triamterene in the maintenance treatment of congestive heart failure. Eur. J. Clin. Pharmacol. *30*:341, 1986.
329. Ridgeway, N. A., Ginn, D. R., and Alley, K.: Outpatient conversion of treatment to potassium sparing diuretics. Am. J. Med. *80*:785, 1986.

Complications of Diuretic Therapy

330. Velazquez, H., and Wright, F. S.: Control by drugs of renal potassium handling. Ann. Rev. Pharmacol. Toxicol. *26*:293, 1986.
331. Ram, C. V. S., Garrett, B. N., and Kaplan, N. M.: Moderate sodium restriction and various diuretics in the treatment of hypertension. Arch. Intern. Med. *141*:1015, 1981.
332. Wilcox, C. S., Mitch, W. E., Kelly, R. A., Friedman, P. A., Souney, P. F., Rayment, C. A., Meyer, T. W., and Skorecki, K. L.: Factors affecting potassium balance during furosemide administration. Clin. Sci. *67*:195, 1984.
333. Epstein, F. H., and Rosa, R. M.: Adrenergic control of serum potassium. N. Engl. J. Med. *309*:1450, 1983.
334. Thier, S. O.: Potassium physiology. Am. J. Med. *80* (Suppl. 4A):3, 1986.
335. Tannen, R. L.: Diuretic-induced hypokalemia. Kidney Int. *28*:988, 1985.
336. Hollenberg, N. K.: Potassium, magnesium, and cardiovascular morbidity. Am. J. Med. *80* (4A):1, 1986.
337. Papademetriou, V.: Diuretics, hypokalemia, and cardiac arrhythmias: A critical analysis. Am. Heart J. *111*:1217, 1986.
338. Atwood, J. E., and Gardin, J. M.: Diuretics, hypokalemia, and ventricular ectopy. Arch. Intern. Med. *145*:1185, 1985.
339. Parker, M.: Sudden unexpected death in patients with congestive heart failure: A second frontier. Circulation *72*:681, 1985.
340. Chakko, C. S., and Gheorghide, M.: Ventricular arrhythmias in severe heart failure: Incidence, significance and effectiveness of antiarrhythmic therapy. Am. Heart J. *109*:497, 1985.
341. Papademetriou, V., Price, M., Notorgiacomo, A., Gottdiener, J., Fletcher, R. D., and Freis, E. D.: Effect of diuretic therapy on ventricular arrhythmias in hypertensive patients with or without left ventricular hypertrophy. Am. Heart J. *110*:595, 1986.
342. Cleland, J. G. F., Dargie, H. O., East, B. W., Robertson, I., Hodsman, G. P., Ball, S. G., Gillen, G., Robertson, J. I. S., and Morton, J. J.: Total body and serum electrolyte composition in heart failure: The effect of captopril. Eur. Heart J. *6*:681, 1985.
343. Lilly, L. S., Dzau, V. J., Williams, G. H., Rydstedt, L., and Hollenberg, N. K.: Hyponatremia in congestive heart failure: Implication for neurohumoral activation and response to orthostasis. J. Clin. Endocrinol. Metab. *59*:924 1984.
344. Schaer, G. L., Covit, A. B., Laragh, J. H., and Cody, R. J.: Association of hyponatremia with increased renin activity in chronic congestive heart failure. Impact of diuretic therapy. Am. J. Cardiol. *51*:1635, 1983.
345. Hamilton, R. W., and Buckalew, V. M.: Sodium, water and congestive failure. Ann. Intern. Med. *100*:902, 1984.
346. Lee, W. H., and Packer, M.: Prognostic importance of serum sodium concentration and its modification by converting enzyme inhibition in patients with severe chronic heart failure. Circulation *73*:257, 1986.
347. Narins, R. G.: Therapy of hyponatremia. Does haste make waste? N. Engl. J. Med. *314*:1573, 1986.
348. Packer, M., Medina, N., and Yashak, M.: Correction of dilutional hyponatremia in severe chronic heart failure by converting enzyme inhibition. Ann. Intern. Med. *100*:782, 1984.
349. Dzau, V. J., and Hollenberg, N. K.: Renal response to captopril in severe heart failure: Role of furosemide in natriuresis and reversal of hyponatremia. Ann. Intern. Med. *100*:777, 1984.
350. Altura, B. M., and Altura, B. T.: Magnesium, electrolyte transport, and coronary vascular tone. Drugs *28* (Suppl. 1):120, 1984.
351. Ryan, M. P., Devane, J., Ryan, M. F., and Conihan, T. B.: Effects of diuretics on the renal handling of magnesium. Drugs *28* (Suppl. 1):167, 1984.
352. Reyes, A. J., and Leary, W. P.: Cardiovascular toxicity of diuretics related to magnesium depletion. Hum. Toxicol. *3*:351, 1984.
352a. Fessel, W. J.: Renal outcomes of gout and hyperuricemia. Am. J. Med. *67*:74, 1979.
353. Johnson, M. W., and Mitch, W. E.: The risks of asymptomatic hyperuricemia and the use of uricosuric diuretics. Drugs *21*:220, 1981.
354. Struthers, A. D., Murphy, M. B., and Dolley, C. T.: Glucose tolerance during antihypertensive therapy in patients with diabetes mellitus. Hypertension 7 (Suppl. II):II-95–II-109, 1985.
355. Bloomgarden, Z. T., Ginsberg-Fellner, F., Rayfield, E. J., Boohman, J., and Brown, W. V.: Elevated hemoglobin A_{1C} and low-density cholesterol levels in thiazide-treated diabetes. Am. J. Med. *77*:823, 1984.
356. Percy-Stable, E., and Caralis, P. V.: Thiazide-induced disturbances in carbohydrate, lipid, and potassium metabolism. Am. Heart J. *106*:245, 1983.
357. Hietanen, E., Hamalainen, H., Maki, J., Seppanen, A., Kallio, V., and Marniemi, J.: Beta blockers, diuretics and physical fitness as determinants of serum lipids in myocardial infarction patients. Scand. J. Clin. Lab. Invest. *46*:97, 1986.
358. Kahns, S. J., Weinstein, C., Dooures, J., Alexander, J., and Weinstein, D.: Effect of exercise training and diet modification on serum lipids and lipoproteins in coronary artery disease patients treated with thiazides. Clin. Cardiol. *8*:636, 1985.
359. Gerber, A., Weidmann, P., Bianchetti, M. G., Ferrier, C., Laederach, K., Mordasini, R., Riesen, W., and Bachmonn, C.: Serum lipoproteins during treatment with the antihypertensive agent, indapamide. Hypertension 7(Suppl. II):II-164–II-169, 1985.
360. Raggi, U., Palumbo, P., Moro, B., Bevilaegero, M., and Norbiato, G.: Indapamide in the treatment of hypertension in non-insulin dependent diabetes. Hypertension 7(Suppl. II):II-157–II-160, 1985.

Diuretic Use in Congestive Heart Failure

361. Schuster, C. J., Weil, M. H., Besso, J., Carpio, M., and Henning, R. J.: Blood volume following diuresis induced by furosemide. Am. J. Med. *76*:585, 1984.
362. Wilson, J. R., Reichek, N., Dunkman, W. B., and Goldberg, S.: Effect of diuresis on the performance of the failing left ventricular in man. Am. J. Med. *70*:234, 1981.
363. Larsen, F. F.: Prophylactic furosemide treatment in acute myocardial infarction. Acta Med. Scand. *218*:63, 1985.
364. Kiely, J., Kelly, D. T., Taylor, D. R., and Pitt, B.: The role of furosemide in the treatment of left ventricular dysfunction associated with acute myocardial infarction. Circulation *48*:581, 1973.

VASODILATORS

365. Wiggers, C. J., and Feely, H.: The cardiodynamics of mitral insufficiency. Heart *9*:141, 1921–22.
366. Braunwald, E., Welch, G. H., Jr., and Sarnoff, S. J.: Hemodynamic effects of quantitatively varied experimental mitral regurgitation. Circ. Res. *5*:539, 1957.
367. Braunwald, E., Welch, G. H., Jr., and Morrow, A. G.: The effects of acutely increased systemic resistance on the left atrial pressure pulse: A method for the clinical detection of mitral insufficiency. J. Clin. Invest. *37*:35, 1958.
368. Zelis, R., and Flaim, S. F.: Alterations in vasomotor tone in congestive heart failure. Prog. Cardiovasc. Dis. *24*:437, 1982.
369. Zelis, R., Mason, D. T., and Braunwald, E.: A comparison of the effects of vasodilator stimuli on peripheral resistance vessels in normal subjects and in patients with congestive heart failure. J. Clin. Invest. *47*:960, 1968.
370. Clauss, R. H., Birtwell, W. C., Albertel, G. A., Lunzer, S., Taylor, W. J., Fosberg, A. M., and Harkin, D. E.: Assisted circulation. I. The arterial counterpulsator. J. Thorac. Cardiovasc. Surg. *41*:447, 1961.
371. Majid, P. A., Sharma, B., and Taylor, S. H.: Phentolamine for vasodilator treatment of severe heart failure. Lancet *2*:719, 1971.
372. Cohn, J. N.: Vasodilators: Rationale, application, and future prospects. *In* Braunwald, E., Mock, M. B., and Watson, J. (eds.): Congestive Heart Failure: Current Research and Clinical Applications. New York. Grune and Stratton, 1982, p. 279.
373. Srebro, J., and Karliner, J. S.: Congestive Heart Failure. Current Problems in Cardiology 22:303, 1986.
374. Cohn, J. N., Archibald, D. G., Ziesche, S., Franciosa, J. A., Harston, W. E., Tristani, F. E., Dunkman, W. B., Jacobs, W., Francis, G. S., Flohr, K. H., Goldman, S., Cobb, F. R., Shah, P. M., Saunders, R., Fletcher, R. D., Loeb, H. S., Hughes, V. C., and Baker, B.: Effect of vasodilator therapy on mortality in chronic congestive heart failure: Results of a Veterans Administration Cooperative Study. N. Engl. J. Med. *314*:1547, 1986.
375. The Captopril Multicenter Research Group: A cooperative multicenter study of captopril in congestive heart failure: Hemodynamic effects and long-term response. Am. Heart J. *110*:439, 1985.
376. Cleland, J. G., Dargie, H. J., Hodsman, G. P., Ball, S. G., Robertson, J. I., Morton, J. J., East, B. W., Robertson, I., Murray, G. D., and Gillen, G.: Captopril in heart failure. A double-blind controlled trial. Br. Heart. J. 52:530, 1984.
377. Sharpe, D. N., Murphy, J., Coxon, R., and Hannon, S. F.: Enalapril in patients with chronic heart failure: A placebo-controlled, randomized, double-blind study. Circulation *70*:271, 1984.
378. The Captopril Multicenter Research Group: A placebo-controlled trial of captopril in refractory chronic congestive heart failure. J. Am. Coll. Cardiol. 2:755, 1983.
378a. Braunwald, E., Ross, J., Jr., Kahler, R. L., Gaffney, T. E., Goldblatt, A., and Mason, D. T.: Reflex control of the systemic venous bed: Effects on venous tone of vasoactive drugs and of baroreceptor and chemoreceptor stimulation. Circ. Res. *12*:539, 1963.
379. Miller, R. M., Fennell, W. H., Young, J. B., Palomo, A. R., and Quinones, M. A.: Differential systemic arterial and venous actions and consequent cardiac effects of vasodilator drugs. Prog. Cardiovasc. Dis. *24*:353, 1982.
380. Franciosa, J. A., Guiha, N. M., Limas, C. J., Rodriguera, E., and Cohn, J. N.: Improved left ventricular function during nitroprusside infusion in acute myocardial infarction. Lancet *1*:650, 1972.
381. Pouleur, H., Covell, J. W., and Ross, J., Jr.: Effects of nitroprusside on venous return and central blood volume in the absence and presence of acute heart failure. Circulation *61*:328, 1980.
382. Davies, D. W., Kadar, D., Steward, D. J., and Munro, I. R.: A sudden death associated with the use of sodium nitroprusside for induction of hypotension during anesthesia. Can. Anaesth. Soc. J. *22*:547, 1975.
383. Miller, R. R., Vismara, L. A., Williams, D. O., Amsterdam, E. A., and Mason, D. T.: Pharmacological mechanisms for left ventricular unloading in clinical congestive heart failure. Differential effects of nitroprusside, phentolamine, and nitroglycerin on cardiac function and peripheral circulation. Circ. Res. *39*:127, 1976.
384. Stern, M. A., Gohlke, H. K., Loeb, H. S., Croke, R. P., and Gunnar, R. M.: Hemodynamic effects of intravenous phentolamine in low output cardiac failure. Dose-response relationships. Circulation *58*:157, 1978.
385. Henning, R. J., Shubin, H., and Weil, M. H.: Afterload reduction with phentolamine in patients with acute pulmonary edema. Am. J. Med. *63*:568, 1977.
386. Jordan, R. A., Seth, L., Casebolt, P., Hayes, M. J., Wilen, M. M., and Franciosa, J.: Rapidly developing tolerance to transdermal nitroglycerin in congestive heart failure. Ann. Intern. Med. *104*:295, 1986.
387. Cohn, J. N.: Nitrates for congestive heart failure. Am. J. Cardiol. *56*:19A, 1985.
388. Packer, M.: Mechanisms of nitrate action in patients with severe left ventricular failure: Conceptual problems with the theory of venosequestration. Am. Heart J. *110*:259, 1985.
389. Williams, D. O., Amsterdam, E. A., and Mason, D. T.: Hemodynamic effects of nitroglycerin in acute myocardial infarction. Decrease in ventricular preload at the expense of cardiac output. Circulation. *51*:421, 1975.
390. Franciosa, J. A., and Cohn, J. N.: Sustained hemodynamic effects without tolerance during long-term isosorbide dinitrate treatment of chronic left ventricular failure. Am. J. Cardiol. *45*:648, 1980.
391. Leier, C. V., Huss, P., Magorien, R. D., and Unverferth, D. V.: Improved exercise capacity and differing arterial and venous tolerance during chronic isosorbide dinitrate therapy for congestive heart failure. Circulation *67*:817, 1983.
392. Jordon, R. A., Seith, L., Henry, D. A., Wilen, M. M., and Franciosa, J. A.: Dose requirements and hemodynamic effects of transdermal nitroglycerin compared with placebo with congestive heart failure. Circulation *71*:980, 1985.
392a. Pierpont, G. L., Brown, D. C., Franciosa, J. A., and Cohn, J. N.: Effect of hydralazine on renal failure in patients with congestive heart failure. Circulation *61*:323, 1980.
393. Packer, M., Meller, J., Medina, N., Gorlin, R., and Herman, M. V.: Dose requirements of hydralazine in patients with severe chronic congestive heart failure. Am. J. Cardiol. *45*:655, 1980.
394. Packer, M., Meller, J., Medina., N., Gorlin, R., and Herman, M. V.: Importance of left ventricular chamber size in determining the response to hydralazine in severe chronic heart failure. N. Engl. J. Med. *303*:250, 1980.
395. Packer, M., Meller, J., Medina, N., Yushak, M., and Gorlin, R.: Hemodynamic characterization of tolerance to long-term hydralazine therapy in severe chronic heart failure. N. Engl. J. Med. *306*:57, 1982.
396. Conradson, T. B., Ryden, L., Ahlmark, G., Saetre, H., Persson, S., Nyquist, O., and Wernersson, B.: Clinical efficacy of hydralazine in chronic heart failure: One-year double-blind placebo-controlled study. Am. Heart J. *108*:1001, 1984.
397. Massie, B., Ports, T., Chatterjee, K., Parmley, W., Ostland, J., O'Young, J., and Haughom, F.: Long-term vasodilator therapy for heart failure: Clinical response and its relationship to hemodynamic measurements. Circulation *63*:269, 1981.
398. Franciosa, J. A., Weber, K. T., Levine, T. B., Kinasewitz, G. T., Janicki, J. S., West, J., Henis, M. M., and Cohn, J. N.: Hydralazine in the long-term treatment of chronic heart failure: Lack of difference from placebo. Am. Heart J. *104*:587, 1982.
399. Quyyumi, A. A., Wagstaff, D., and Evans, T. R.: Acute hemodynamic effects of endralazine: A new vasodilator for chronic refractory congestive heart failure. Am. J. Cardiol. *51*:1353, 1983.
400. Colucci, W. S.: Alpha-adrenergic receptor blockade with prazosin: Consideration of hypertension, heart failure, and potential new applications. Ann. Intern. Med. 97:67, 1982.
401. Awan, N. A., Miller, R. R., and Mason, D. T.: Comparison of effects of nitroprusside and prazosin on left ventricular function and the peripheral circulation in chronic refractory congestive heart failure. Circulation *57*:152, 1978.
402. Packer, M., Meller, J., Gorlin, R., and Herman, H. V.: Hemodynamic and clinical tachyphylaxis to prazosin-mediated afterload reduction in severe congestive heart failure. Circulation *59*:531, 1979.
403. Packer, M., Medina, N., and Yushak, M.: Comparative hemodynamic and clinical effects of long-term treatment with prazosin and captopril for severe chronic congestive heart failure secondary to coronary artery disease or idiopathic dilated cardiomyopathy. Am. J. Cardiol. *57*:1323, 1986.
404. Awan, N. A., Miller, R. R., Miller, M. P., Specht, K., Vera, Z., and Mason, D. T.: Clinical pharmacology and therapeutic application of prazosin in acute and chronic refractory congestive heart failure. Balanced systemic venous and arterial dilation improving pulmonary congestion and cardiac output. Am. J. Med. *65*:146, 1978.
405. Dzau, V. J., Colucci, W. S., Hollenberg, N. K., and Williams, G. H.: Relation of the renin-angiotensin-aldosterone system to clinical state in congestive heart failure. Circulation *63*:645, 1981.
406. Massie, B. M., Kramer, B. L., and Topic, N.: Long-term captopril therapy for chronic congestive heart failure. Am. J. Cardiol. *53*:1316, 1984.
407. Packer, M., Medina, N., and Yushak, M.: Efficacy of captopril in low-renin congestive heart failure: Importance of sustained reactive hyperreninemia in distinguishing responders from nonresponders. Am. J. Cardiol. *54*:771, 1984.
408. Cleland, J. G. F., Dargie, H. J., Hodsman, G. P., Ball, S. G., Robertson, J. I. S., Morton, J. J., East, B. W., Robertson, I., Murray, G. D., and Gillen, G.: Captopril in heart failure: A double-blind controlled trial. Br. Heart J. *52*:530, 1984.
409. Kromer, E. P., Riegger, G. A. J., Liebau, G., Kochsiek, K.: Effectiveness of converting enzyme inhibition (enalapril) for mild congestive heart failure. Am. J. Cardiol. *57*:459, 1986.
410. McGrath, B. P., Arnold, L., Matthews, P. G., Jackson, B., Jennings, G., Kiat, H., and Johnston, C. I.: Controlled trial of enalapril in congestive cardiac failure. Br. Heart J. *54*:405, 1985.
411. Riley, L. J., Jr., Vlasses, P. H., and Ferguson, R. K.: Clinical pharmacology and therapeutic applications of the new oral converting enzyme inhibitor, enalapril. Am. Heart J. *190*:1085, 1985.
412. Creager, M. A., Massie, B. M., Faxon, D. P., Friedman, S. D., Kramer, B. L., Weiner, D. A., Ryan, T. J., Topic, N., and Melidossian, C. D.: Acute and long-term effects of enalapril on the cardiovascular response to exercise

and exercise tolerance in patients with congestive heart failure. J. Am. Coll. Cardiol. *6*:163, 1985.

413. McGrath, B. P., Arnold, L., Matthews, P. G., Jackson, B., Jennings, G., Kiat, H., and Johnston, C. I.: Controlled trial of enalapril in congestive cardiac failure. Br. Heart J. *54*:405, 1985.
414. Lijnen, P., Fagard, R., Staessen, J., VerSchueren, L. J., and Amery, A.: Role of various vasodepressor systems in the acute hypotensive effect of captopril in man. Eur. J. Clin. Pharmacol. *20*:1, 1981.
415. Creager, M. A., Halperin, J. L., Bernard, D. B., Faxon, D. P., Melidossian, C. D., Gavras, H., and Ryan, T. J.: Acute regional circulatory and renal hemodynamic effects of converting enzyme inhibition in patients with congestive heart failure. Circulation *64*:483, 1981.
416. Kramer, B. L., Massie, B. M., and Topic, N.: Controlled trial of captopril in chronic heart failure: A rest and exercise hemodynamic study. Circulation *67*:807, 1983.
417. Awan, N. A., Amsterdam, E. A., Hermanovich, J., Bommer, W. J., Needham, K. E., and Mason, D. T.: Long-term hemodynamic and clinical efficacy of captopril therapy in ambulatory management of severe chronic congestive heart failure. Am. Heart J. *103*:474, 1982.
418. DiCarlo, L., Chatterjee, K., Parmley, W. W., Swedberg, K., Atherton, B., Curran, D., and Cucci, M.: Enalapril: A new angiotensin-converting enzyme inhibitor in chronic heart failure. Acute and chronic hemodynamic evaluations. J. Am. Coll. Cardiol. *2*:865, 1983.
419. Packer, M., Medina, N., and Yushak, M.: Correction of dilutional hyponatremia in severe chronic heart failure by converting-enzyme inhibition. Ann. Intern. Med. *100*:782, 1984.
420. Packer, M., Medina, N., Yushak, M., and Lee, W. H.: Usefulness of plasma renin activity in predicting hemodynamic and clinical responses and survival during long-term converting enzyme inhibition in severe chronic heart failure. Experience in 100 consecutive patients. Br. Heart J. *54*:298, 1985.
421. Lee, W. H., and Packer, M.: Prognostic importance of serum sodium concentration and its modification by converting-enzyme inhibition in patients with severe chronic heart failure. Circulation *73*:257, 1986.
422. Packer, M., Lee, W. H., Medina, N., and Yushak, M.: Influence of renal function on the hemodynamic and clinical responses to long-term captopril therapy in severe chronic heart failure. Ann. Intern. Med. *104*:147, 1986.
423. Faxon, D. P., Creager, M. A., Halperin, J. L., Bernard, D. B., and Ryan, T. J.: Redistribution of regional blood flow following angiotensin-converting enzyme inhibition: Comparison of normal subjects and patients with heart failure. Am. J. Med. *76*:104, 1984.
424. Daly, P., Mettauer, B., Rouleau, J-L, Cousineau, D., and Burgess, J. H.: Lack of reflex increase in myocardial sympathetic tone after captopril: Potential antianginal effect. Circulation *71*:317, 1985.
425. The Consensus Trial Group: Effects of enalapril on mortality in severe congestive heart failure: Results of the Cooperative North Scandinavian Enalapril Survival Study. N. Engl. J. Med. *316*:1429, 1987.

Clinical Applications of Vasodilator Therapy

426. Franciosa, J. A.: Effectiveness of long-term vasodilator administration in the treatment of chronic left ventricular failure. Prog. Cardiovasc. Dis. *24*:319, 1982.
427. Packer, M., and LeJemtel, T. H.: Physiologic and pharmacologic determinants of vasodilator response: A conceptual framework for rational drug therapy for chronic heart failure. Prog. Cardiovasc. Dis. *24*:275, 1982.
428. DiSegni, E., Kaplinsky, E., Klein, H. O., and Levy, M.: Treatment of ruptured interventricular septum with afterload reduction. Arch. Intern. Med. *138*:1427, 1978.
429. Greenberg, B. H., Massie, B. M., Brundage, B. H., Botvinick, E. H., Parmley, W. W., and Chatterjee, K.: Beneficial effects of hydralazine in severe mitral regurgitation. Circulation *58*:273, 1978.
430. Fioretti, P., Benussi, B., Scardi, S., Klugmann, S., Brower, R. W., and Camerini, F.: Afterload reduction with nifedipine in aortic insufficiency. Am. J. Cardiol. *49*:1728, 1982.
431. Rubin, L. J., and Peter, R. H.: Hemodynamics at rest and during exercise after oral hydralazine in patients with cor pulmonale. Am. J. Cardiol. *47*:116, 1981.
432. Colucci, W. S., Holman, L., Wynne, J., Carabello, B., Malacoff, R., Grossman, W., and Braunwald, E.: Improved right ventricular function and reduced pulmonary vascular resistance during prazosin therapy of congestive heart failure. Am. J. Med. *71*:75, 1981.
432a. Pfeffer, J. M., Pfeffer, M. A., and Braunwald, E.: Hemodynamic benefits and prolonged survival with long-term captopril therapy in rats with myocardial infarction and heart failure. Circulation 75:I-149, 1987.

NONGLYCOSIDE INOTROPIC AGENTS
Sympathomimetic Amines

433. Goldberg, L. I.: Cardiovascular and renal actions of dopamine: Potential clinical applications. Pharmacol. Rev *24*:1, 1972.
434. Toda, N., Hojo, M., Sakae, K., and Usui, H.: Comparison of the relaxing effect of dopamine with that of adenosine, isoproterenol and acetylcholine in isolated canine coronary arteries. Blood Vessels *12*:290, 1975.
435. Dressler, W. E., Rossi, G. V., and Orzechowski, R. F.: Evidence that renal vasodilation by dopamine in dogs does not involve release of prostaglandin. J. Pharm. Pharmacol. *27*:203, 1975.
436. Yeh, B. K., McNay, J. L., and Goldberg, L. I.: Attenuation of dopamine renal and mesenteric vasodilation by haloperidol: Evidence for a specific receptor. J. Pharmacol. Exp. Ther. *168*:303, 1969.
437. Goldberg, L. I., and Rajfer, S. I.: Dopamine receptors: Applications in clinical cardiology. Circulation 72:245, 1985.
438. Maskin, C. S., Ocken, S., Chadwick, B., and LeJemtel, T. H.: Comparative systemic and renal effects of dopamine and angiotensin-converting enzyme inhibition with enalaprilat in patients with heart failure. Circulation, *72*:846, 1985.
439. Hardaker, W. T., Jr., and Wechsler, A. S.: Redistribution of renal intracortical blood flow during dopamine infusion in dogs. Circ. Res. *33*:437, 1973.
440. Hollenberg, N. K., Adams, D. F., Mendell, P., Abrams, H. L., and Merrill, J. P.: Renal vascular responses to dopamine. Haemodynamics and angiographic observations in normal man. Clin. Sci. Molec. Med. *45*:733, 1973.
441. Gilbert, J. C., and Goldberg, L. I.: Characterization by cyproheptadine of the dopamine-induced contraction in canine isolated arteries. J. Pharmacol. Exp. Ther. *193*:435, 1975.
442. Goldberg, L. I.: Dopamine: Clinical uses of an endogenous catecholamine. N. Engl. J. Med. *291*:707, 1974.
443. Allwood, M. J., and Ginsburg, J.: Peripheral vascular and other effects of dopamine infusion in man. Clin. Sci. *27*:271, 1964.
444. Brooks, H. L., Stein, P. D., Matson, J. L., and Hyland, J. W.: Dopamine-induced alterations in coronary hemodynamics in dogs. Circ. Res. *24*:699, 1969.
445. Toda, N., and Goldberg, L. I.: Effects of dopamine on isolated canine coronary arteries. Cardiovasc. Res. *9*:384, 1975.
446. Goldberg, L. I., McDonald, R. H., Jr., and Zimmerman, A. M.: Sodium diuresis produced by dopamine in patients with congestive heart failure. N. Engl. J. Med. *269*:1060, 1963.
447. Rosenblum, R., Tai, A. R., and Lawson, D.: Dopamine in man: Cardiorenal hemodynamics in normotensive patients with heart disease. J. Pharmacol. Exp. Ther. *183*:256, 1972.
448. Miller, R. R., Awan, N. A., Joye, J. A., Maxwell, K. S., DeMaria, A. N., Amsterdam, E. A., and Mason, D. T.: Combined dopamine and nitroprusside therapy in congestive heart failure. Circulation *55*:881, 1977.
449. van Trigt, P., Spray, T. L., Pasque, M. K., Peyteon, R. B., Pellom, G. L., and Wechsler, A. S.: The comparative effects of dopamine and dobutamine on ventricular mechanics after coronary artery bypass grafting: A pressure-dimension analysis. Circulation *70* (Suppl. I):I-112, 1984.
450. Fowler, M. B., Alderman, E. L., Oesterle, S. N., Derby, G., Daughters, G. T., Stinson, E. B., Ingels, N. B., Mitchell, R. S., Miller, D. C.: Dobutamine and dopamine after cardiac surgery: Greater augmentation of myocardial blood flow with dobutamine. Circulation *70* (Suppl. I):I-103, 1984.
451. Marino, R. J., Romagnoli, A., and Keats, A. S.: Selective venoconstriction by dopamine in comparison with isoproterenol and phenylephrine. Anesthesiology *43*:570, 1975.
452. Sturm, J. T., Guhrman, T. M., Sterling, R., Turner, S. A., Igo, S. R., and Norman, J. C.: Combined use of dopamine and nitroprusside therapy in conjunction with intra-aortic balloon pumping for the treatment of post-cardiotomy low-output syndrome. J. Thorac. Cardiovasc. Surg. *82*:13–17, 1981.
453. Vatner, S. F., McRitchie, R. J., and Braunwald, E.: Effects of dobutamine on left ventricular performance, coronary dynamics, and distribution of cardiac output in conscious dogs. J. Clin. Invest. *53*:1265, 1974.
454. Tuttle, R. R., and Mills, J.: Dopamine: development of a new catecholamine to selectively increase cardiac contractility. Circ. Res. *36*:185, 1975.
455. Sonnenblick, E. H., Frishman, W. H., and LeJemtel, T. H.: Dobutamine: A new synthetic cardioactive sympathetic amine. N. Engl. J. Med. *300*:17, 1979.
456. Williams, R. S., and Bishop, T.: Selectivity of dobutamine for adrenergic receptor subtypes. *In vitro* analysis by radioligand binding. J. Clin. Invest. *67*:1703, 1981.
457. Kenakin, T. P.: An in vitro quantitative analysis of the alpha adrenoceptor partial agonist activity of dobutamine and its relevance to inotropic selectivity. J. Pharmacol. Exp. Ther. *9*:216, 1981.
458. Ruffolo, R. R., Jr., Sporadlin, T. A., Pollock, G. D., Waddell, J. E., and Murphy, R. T.: Alpha- and beta-adrenergic effects of the stereoisomers of dobutamine. J. Pharmacol. Exp. Ther. *219*:447, 1981.
459. Robie, N. W., and Goldberg, L. I.: Comparative systemic and regional hemodynamic effects of dopamine and dobutamine. Am. Heart J. *90*:340, 1975.
460. Magorien, R. D., Unverferth, D. V., Brown, G. P., and Leier, C. V.: Dobutamine and hydralazine: Comparative influences of positive inotropy and vasodilation on coronary blood flow and myocardial energetics in non-ischemic congestive heart failure. J. Am. Coll. Cardiol. *1*:499, 1983.
461. Gillespie, J. A., Ambros, H. D., Sobel, B. E., and Roberts, R.: Effects of dobutamine in patients with acute myocardial infarction. Am. J. Cardiol. *39*:588, 1977.
462. Bendersky, R., Chatterjee, K., Parmley, W. W., Brundage, B. H., and Ports, T. A.: Dobutamine in chronic ischemic heart failure. Alterations in left ventricular function and coronary hemodynamics. Am. J. Cardiol. *48*:554, 1981.
463. Unverferth, D. V., Magorien, R. D., Lewis, R. P., and Leier, C. V.: Long-term benefit of dobutamine in patients with congestive cardiomyopathy. Am. Heart J. *100*:622, 1980.
464. Applefeld, M. M., Newman, K. A., Grove, W. R., Stutton, F. J., Roffman, D. S., Reed, W. P., and Linberg, S.: Intermittent, continuous outpatient dobutamine infusion in the management of congestive heart failure. Am. J. Cardiol. *51*:455, 1983.
465. Krell, M. J., Kline, E. M., Bates, E. R., Hodgson, J. M., Dilworth, L. R., Laufer, N., Vogel, R. A., and Pitt, B.: Intermittent, ambulatory dobutamine infusions in patients with severe congestive heart failure. *112*:787, 1986.
466. Leier, C. V., Magorien, R. D., Altschuld, R., Kolibash, A. J., and Lewis, R. P.: The hemodynamic and metabolic advantages gained by a three-day infusion of dobutamine in patients with congestive cardiomyopathy. Am. Heart J. *106*:29, 1983.
467. Hodgson, J. M., Aja, M., and Sorkin, R. P.: Intermittent ambulatory dobu-

tamine infusions for patients awaiting cardiac transplantation. Am. J. Cardiol. 53:375, 1984.

468. Aronson, R. S., and Gelles, J. M.: Electrophysiologic effects of dopamine on sheep cardiac Purkinje fibers. J. Pharmacol. Exp. Ther. 188:596, 1974.
469. Loeb, H. S., Sinno, M. Z., Saudye, A., Towne, W. D., and Gunnar, R. M.: Electrophysiologic properties of dobutamine. Circ. Shock 1:217, 1974.
470. Loeb, H. S., Khan, M., Klodnycky, M. L., Sinno, M. Z., Towne, W. D., and Gunner, R. M.: Haemodynamic effects of dobutamine in man. Circ. Shock 2:29, 1975.
471. Pozen, R. G., DiBianco, R., Katz, R. J., Bortz, R., Myerburg, R. J., and Fletcher, R. D.: Myocardial metabolic and hemodynamic effects of dobutamine in heart failure complicating coronary artery disease. Circulation 63:1279, 1981.
472. Greene, S. I., and Smith, J. W.: Dopamine gangrene. N. Engl. J. Med. 294:114, 1976.
473. Stoner, J. D., Bolen, J. L., and Harrison, D. C.: Comparison of dobutamine and dopamine in treatment of severe heart failure. Br. Heart J. 39:536, 1977.
474. Loeb, H. S., Bredakis, J., and Gunnar, R. M.: Superiority of dobutamine over dopamine for augmentation of cardiac output in patients with chronic low output cardiac failure. Circulation 55:375, 1977.
475. Leier, C. V., Heban, P. T., Huss, P., Bush, C. A., and Lewis, R. P.: Comparative systemic and regional hemodynamic effects of dopamine and dobutamine in patients with cardiomyopathic heart failure. Circulation 58:466, 1978.
476. Berkowitz, C., McKeever, L., Croke, R. P., Jacobs, W. R., Loeb, H. S., and Gunnar, R. M.: Comparative responses to dobutamine and nitroprusside in patients with chronic low output cardiac failure. Circulation 56:918, 1977.
477. Goldberg, L. I., and Rajfer, S. I.: Dopamine receptors: Applications in clinical cardiology. Circulation 72:245, 1985.
478. Rajfer, S. I., Anton, A. H., Rossen, J. D., and Goldberg, L. I.: Beneficial hemodynamic effects of oral levodopa in heart failure: Relation to the generation of dopamine. N. Engl. J. Med. 310:1357, 1984.
479. Dei Cas, L., Manca, C., Bernardini, B., Vasini, G., and Visioli, O.: Noninvasive evaluation of the effects of oral ibopamine (SB 7505) on cardiac and renal function in patients with congestive heart failure. J. Cardiovasc. Pharmacol. 4:436, 1982.
480. Dei Cas, L., Bolognesi, R., Cucchini, F., Fappani, A., Riva, S., and Visioli, O.: Hemodynamic effects of ibopamine in patients with idiopathic congestive cardiomyopathy. J. Cardiovasc. Pharmacol. 5:249, 1983.
481. Fennell, W. H., Taylor, A. A., Young, J. B., et al.: Propylbutyldopamine: hemodynamic effects in conscious dogs, normal human volunteers and patients with heart failure. Circulation 67:829, 1983.
482. Brown, R. A., Farmer, J. B., Hall, J. C., Humphries, R. G., O'Connor, S. E., and Smith G. W.: The effects of dopexamine on the cardiovascular system of the dog. Br. J. Pharmacol. 85:609, 1985.
483. Sharma, B., Hoback, J., Francis, G. S., Hodges, M., Asinger, R. W., Cohn, J. N., and Taylor C. R.: Pirbuterol: A new oral sympathomimetic amine for the treatment of congestive heart failure. Am. Heart J. 102:533, 1981.
484. Awan, N. A., Evenson, M. K., Needham, K. E., Evans, T. O., Hermanovich, J., Taylor, C. R., Amsterdam, E., and Mason, D. T.: Hemodynamic effects of oral pirbuterol in chronic severe congestive heart failure. Circulation 63:96, 1981.
485. Awan, N. A., Needham, K. E., Evenson, M. K., and Mason, D. T.: Comparison of hemodynamic actions of pirbuterol and dobutamine on cardiac function in severe congestive heart failure. Am. J. Cardiol. 47:665, 1981.
486. Dawson, J. R., Canepa-Anson, R., Kuan, P., Whitaker, N. H. G., Carnie, J., Warnes, C., Ruben, S. R., Poole-Wilson, P. A., and Sutton, G. C.: Treatment of chronic heart failure and pirbuterol: Acute haemodynamic responses. Br. Med. J. 282:1423, 1981.
487. Rude, R. E., Turi, Z., Brown, E. J., Lorell, B. H., Colucci, W. S., Mudge, G. H., Jr., Taylor, C. R., and Grossman, W.: Acute effects of oral pirbuterol on myocardial oxygen metabolism and systemic hemodynamics in chronic congestive heart failure. Circulation 64:139, 1981.
488. Colucci, W. S., Alexander, R. W., Williams, G. H., Rude, R. E., Holman, B. L., Konstam, M. A., Wynne, J., Mudge, G. H., Jr., and Braunwald, E.: Decreased lymphocyte beta-adrenergic-receptor density in patients with heart failure and tolerance to the beta-adrenergic agonist pirbuterol. N. Engl. J. Med. 305:185, 1981.
489. Wahr, D. W., Swedberg, K., Rabbino, M., Hoyle, M. J., Curran, D., Parmley, W. W., and Chatterjee, K.: Intravenous and oral prenalterol in congestive heart failure: Effects on systemic and coronary hemodynamics and myocardial catecholamine balance. Am. J. Med. 76:999, 1984.
490. Tweddel, A. C., Murray, R. G., Pearson, D., Martin, W., and Hutton, I.: Cardiovascular effects of prenalterol on rest and exercise haemodynamics in patients with chronic congestive heart failure. Br. Heart J. 47:375, 1982.
491. Sharma, B., and Goodwin, J. F.: Beneficial effects of salbutamol on cardiac function in severe congestive cardiomyopathy: Effect on systolic and diastolic function of the left ventricle. Circulation 58:449, 1978.

Phosphodiesterase Inhibitors

492. Colucci, W. S., Wright, R. F., and Braunwald, E.: New positive inotropic agents in the treatment of congestive heart failure. Mechanisms of action and recent clinical developments. N. Engl. J. Med. 314:349, 1986.
493. Endoh, M., Yamashita, S., and Taira, N.: Positive inotropic effect of amrinone in relation to cyclic nucleotide metabolism in the canine ventricular muscle. J. Pharmacol. Exp. Ther. 22:775, 1982.
494. Braunwald, E.: Introduction—A Symposium on Amrinone, Am. J. Cardiol. 56: (No. 3):1B-2B, 1985.
495. Alousi, A. A., Farah, A. E., Lesher, G. Y., and Opalka, C. J., Jr.: Cardiotonic activity of amrinone. Circ. Res. 45:666, 1979.
496. Endoh, M., Yamashita, S., and Taira, N.: Positive inotropic effect of amrinone in relation to cyclic nucleotide metabolism in the canine ventricular muscle. J. Pharmacol. Exp. Ther. 22:775, 1982.
497. Honerjäger, P., Schäfer-Koeting, M., and Reiter, M.: Involvement of cyclic AMP in the direct inotropic action of amrinone: Biochemical and functional evidence. Naunyn Schmiedebergs Arch. Pharmacol. 318:112, 1981.
498. Benotti, J. R., Grossman, W., Braunwald, E., Davolos, D. D., and Alousi, A. A.: Hemodynamic assessment of amrinone: A new inotropic agent. N. Engl. J. Med. 299:1373, 1978.
499. Benotti, J. R., Grossman, W., Braunwald, E., and Carabello, B. A.: Effects of amrinone on myocardial energy metabolism and hemodynamics in patients with severe congestive heart failure due to coronary artery disease. Circulation 62:28, 1980.
500. Naccarelli, G. V., Gray, E. L., Dougherty, A. H., Hanna, J. E., and Goldstein, R. A.: Amrinone: Acute electrophysiologic and hemodynamic effects in patients with congestive heart failure. Am. J. Cardiol. 54:600, 1984.
501. Hartman, A., and Saeed, M.: Phosphodiesterase inhibition in positive inotropic therapy of congestive heart failure. J. Appl. Cardiol. 1:361, 1986.
502. Mancini, D., LeJemtel, T., and Sonnenblick, E.: Intravenous use of amrinone for the treatment of the failing heart. Am. J. Cardiol. 56:8B, 1985.
503. Taylor, S. H., Verma, S. P., Hussain, M., Reynolds, G., Jackson, N. C., Hafizullah, M., Richmond, A., and Silke, B.: Intravenous amrinone in left ventricular failure complicated by acute myocardial infarction. Am. J. Cardiol. 56:29B, 1985.
504. Goenen, M., Pedemonte, O., Baele, P., and Col, J.: Amrinone in the management of low cardiac output after open heart surgery. Am. J. Cardiol. 56:33B, 1985.
505. Wynne, J., Malacoff, R. F., Benotti, J. R., Curfman, G. C., Grossman, W., Holman, B. L., Smith, T. W., and Braunwald, E.: Oral amrinone in refractory congestive heart failure. Am. J. Cardiol. 45:1245, 1980.
506. Massie, B., Bourassa, M., DiBianco, R., Hess, M., Konstam, M., Likoff, M., and Packer, M.: Long-term oral administration of amrinone for congestive heart failure: Lack of efficacy in a multicenter controlled trial. Circulation 71:963, 1985.
507. Katz, A. M.: Potential deleterious effects of inotropic agents in the therapy of chronic heart failure. Circulation 73(Suppl. III):184, 1986.
508. LeJemtel, T. H., Sonnenblick, E. H.: Should the failing heart be stimulated? (editorial) N. Engl. J. Med. 310:1384, 1984.
509. Kloner, R. A., Ellis, S. G., Lange, R., and Braunwald, E.: Studies of experimental coronary artery reperfusion. Effects on infarct size, myocardial function, biochemistry, ultrastructure and microvascular damage. Circulation 68(Suppl. II):8, 1983.
510. Monrad, E. S., Baim, D. S., Smith, H. S., Lanoue, A., Braunwald, E., and Grossman, W.: Effects of milrinone on coronary hemodynamics and myocardial energetics in patients with congestive heart failure. Circulation 71:972, 1985.
511. Jaski, B. E., Fifer, M. A., Wright, R. F., Braunwald, E., and Colucci, W. S.: Positive inotropic and vasodilator actions of milrinone in patients with severe congestive heart failure: Dose-response relationships and comparison to nitroprusside. J. Clin. Invest. 75:643, 1985.
512. Timmis, A. D., Smyth, P., Monaghan, M., Walker, L., Daly, K., McLeod, A. A., and Jewitt, D. E.: Milrinone in heart failure: Acute effects on left ventricular systolic function and myocardial metabolism. Br. Heart J. 54:36, 1985.
513. Grose, R., Strain, J., Greenberg, M., and LeJemtel, T. H.: Systemic and coronary effects of intravenous milrinone and dobutamine in congestive heart failure. J. Am. Coll. Cardiol. 7:1107, 1986.
514. Goldstein, R. A., Geraci, S. A., Gray, E. L., Rinkenberger, R. L., Dougherty, H., and Naccarelli, G. V.: Electrophysiologic effects of milrinone in patients with congestive heart failure. Am. J. Cardiol. 57:624, 1986.
515. Cody, R. J., Kubo, S. H., Covit, A. B., Muller, F. B., Rutman, H., Leonard, D., Laragh, J. H., Feldschuh, J., and Preibisz, J.: Regional blood flow and neurohumoral responses to milrinone in congestive heart failure. Clin. Pharmacol. Ther. 39:128, 1986.
516. Sonnenblick, E. H., Grose, R., Strain, J., Zelcer, A. A., and LeJemtel, T. H.: Effects of milrinone on left ventricular performance and myocardial contractility in patients with severe heart failure. Circulation 73(Suppl. III):162, 1986.
517. Ludmer, P. L., Wright, R. F., Arnold, J. M., Ganz, P., Braunwald, E., and Colucci, W. S.: Separation of the direct myocardial and vasodilator actions of milrinone administered by an intracoronary infusion technique. Circulation 73:130, 1986.
518. Braunwald, E. (ed.): Newer positive inotropic agents. Circulation 73(Suppl. III):237, 1986.
519. White, H. D., Ribeiro, J. P., Hartley, L. H., and Colucci, W. S.: Immediate effects of milrinone on metabolic and sympathetic responses to exercise in severe congestive heart failure. Am. J. Cardiol. 56:93, 1985.
520. LeJemtel, T. H., Gumbardo, D., Chadwick, B., Rutman, H. I., and Sonnenblick, E. H.: Milrinone for long-term therapy of severe heart failure: Clinical experience with special reference to maximal exercise tolerance. Circulation 73(Suppl. III):213, 1986.
521. Baim, D. S., Colucci, W. S., Monrad, E. S., Smith, H. S., Wright, R. F., Lanoue, A., Gauthier, D. F., Ransil, B. J., Grossman, W., and Braunwald, E.: Survival of patients with severe congestive heart failure treated with oral milrinone. J. Am. Coll. Cardiol. 7:661, 1986.
522. Likoff, M. J., Ulrich, S., Hakki, A.-H., and Iskandrian, A. S.: Comparison of acute hemodynamic response to dobutamine and intravenous MDL 17,043 (Enoximone) in severe congestive heart failure secondary to ischemic cardiomyopathy or idiopathic dilated cardiomyopathy. Am. J. Cardiol. 57:1328, 1986.

523. Uretsky, B. F., Valdes, A. M., and Reddy, P. S.: Positive inotropic therapy for short-term support and long-term management of patients with congestive heart failure: Hemodynamic effects and clinical efficacy of MDL 17,043. Circulation *73*(Suppl. III):219, 1986.
524. Shah, P. K., Amin, D. K., Hulse, S., Shellock, F., and Swan, H. J.: Inotropic therapy for refractory congestive heart failure with oral fenoximone (MDL 17,043): Poor long-term results despite early hemodynamic and clinical improvement. Circulation *71*:326, 1985.
525. Martin, J. L., Likoff, M. J., Janicki, J. S., Laskey, W. K., Hirshfeld, J. W., and Weber, K. T.: Myocardial energetics and clinical response to the cardiotonic agent MDL 17043 in advanced heart failure. J. Am. Coll. Cardiol. *4*:875, 1984.
526. Petein, M., Levine, T. B., and Cohn, J. N.: Persistent hemodynamic effects without long-term clinical benefits in response to oral piroximone (MDL 19,205) in patients with congestive heart failure. Circulation *73*(Suppl. III):230, 1986.
527. Renard, M., Jacobs, P., Dechamps, P., Dresse, A., and Bernard, R.: Hemodynamic and clinical response to three-day infusion of sulmazol (AR-L 115 BS) in severe congestive heart failure. Chest *84*:408, 1983.
528. Daly, P. A., Chatterjee, K., Viquerat, C. E., Parmley, W. W., Curran, D., Scheinbaum, M., and Anderson, S.: RO13–6438, a new inotropic-vasodilator: Systemic and coronary hemodynamic effects in congestive heart failure. Am. J. Cardiol. *55*:1539, 1985.
529. Meyer, W.: Effect of a new benzimidazole derivative (UD–CG 212) on force of contraction and phosphodiesterase activity in guinea pig hearts (abstract). Naunyn Schmiedebergs Arch. Pharmacol. *325*(Suppl.):R46, 1984.
530. Gagnon, R. M., Fortin, L., Boucher, R., Gilbert, S., Morrisette, M., Present, S., Lemire, J., and David, A.: Combined hemodynamic effects of dobutamine and IV nitroglycerin in congestive heart failure. Chest *78*:694, 1980.

CARDIAC TRANSPLANTATION

531. Barnard, C. N.: The operation. S. Afr. Med. J. *41*:1271, 1967.
532. Stinson, E. B., Dong, E., Jr., Iben, A. R., and Shumway, N., E.: Cardiac transplantation in man. III. Surgical aspects. Am. J. Surg. *118*:182, 1969.
533. Schroeder, J.: Personal communication, 1987.
534. Emery, R. W., Cork, R., Christensen, R., Levinson, M. M., Icenogle, T. B., Riley, J., Ott, R. A., and Copeland, J. G.: Cardiac transplant patient at one year. Cyclosporine vs. conventional immunosuppression. Chest *90*:29, 1986.
534a. Copeland, J. G., Emery, R. W., Levinson, M. M., Icenogle, T. B., Carrier, M., Ott, R. A., Copeland, J. A., McAleer-Rhenman, M. J., and Nicholson, S. M.: Selection of patients for cardiac transplantation. Circulation *75*:2, 1987.
535. Lanza, R. P., Cooper, D. K. C., Boyd, S. T., and Barnard, C. N.: Comparison of patients with ischemic, myopathic, and rheumatic heart diseases as cardiac transplant recipients. Am. Heart J. *107*:8, 1984.
536. Jamieson, S. W., Baldwin, J., Stinson, E. B., Reitz, B. A., Oyer, P. E., Hunt, S., Billingham, M., Theodore, J., Modry, D., Bieber, C. P., and Shumway, N. E.: Clinical heart-lung transplantation. Transplantation *37*:81, 1984.
536a. Evans, R. W.: The economics of heart transplantation. Circulation *75*:63, 1987.
537. Billingham, M. E., Baumgartner, W. A., Watson, D. C., Reitz, B. A., Masek, M. A., Raney, A. A., Oyer, P. E., Stinson, E. B., and Shumway, N. E.: Distant heart procurement for human transplantation. Circulation *62*(Suppl. I):11, 1980.
538. Wicomb, W. N., Cooper, D. K. C., Novitzky, D., and Barnard, C. N.: Cardiac transplantation following storage of the donor heart by a portable hypothermic perfusion system. Ann. Thorac. Surg. *37*:243, 1984.
539. Losman, J. G., Levine, H., Campbell, C. D., Replogie, R. L., Hassoulas, J., Novitsky, D., Cooper, D. K., and Barnard, C. N.: Changes in indications for heart transplantation. An additional argument for the preservation of the recipient's own heart. J. Thorac. Cardiovasc. Surg. *85*:716, 1982.
539a. Kahan, B. D.: Immunosuppressive therapy with cyclosporine for cardiac transplantation. Circulation *75*:40, 1987.
540. Borow, K. M., Neumann, A., Arensman, F. W., and Yacoub, M. H.: Left ventricular contractility and contractile reserve in humans after cardiac transplantation. Circulation *71*:866, 1985.
541. Samuelsson, R. G., Hunt, S. A., and Schroeder, J. S.: Functional and social rehabilitation of heart transplant recipients under age thirty. Scand. J. Thorac. Cardiovasc. Surg. *18*:97, 1984.
542. Caves, P. K., Stinson, E. B., Billingham, M. E., and Shumway, N. E.: Serial transvenous biopsy of the transplanted human heart: Improved management of acute rejection episodes. Lancet *1*:821, 1974.
542a. Uys, C. J., and Rose, A. G.: Pathologic findings in long-term cardiac transplants. Arch. Pathol. Lab. Med. *108*:112, 1984.
543. Aherne, T., Tscholakoff, D., Finkbeiner, W., Sechtem, U., Derugin, N., Yee, E., and Higgins, C. B.: Magnetic resonance imaging of cardiac transplants: the evaluation of rejection of cardiac allografts with and without immunosuppression. Circulation *74*:145, 1986.
544. Nitkin, R. S., Hunt, S. A., and Schroeder, J. S.: Accelerated atherosclerosis in a cardiac transplant patient. J. Am. Coll. Cardiol. *6*:243, 1985.
545. Hess, M. L., Hastillo, A., Mohanakumar, T., Cowley, M. J., Vetrovac, G., Szentpetery, S., Wolfgang, T. C., and Lower, R. R.: Accelerated atherosclerosis in cardiac transplantation: Role of cytotoxic B-cell antibodies and hyperlipidemia. Circulation *68*(Suppl. II):94, 1983.
546. Bailey, L. L., Nehlsen-Cannarella, S. L., Concepcion, W., and Jolley, W. B.: Baboon-to-human cardiac xenotransplantation in a neonate. J.A.M.A. *254*:3321, 1985.
546a. Robertson, J. A.: Supply and distribution of hearts for transplantation: Legal, ethical, and policy issues. Circulation *75*:77, 1987.

MECHANICAL CIRCULATORY SUPPORT

547. Sanfelippo, P. M., Baker, N. H., Ewy, H. G., Moore, P. J., Thomas, J. W., Brahos, G. J., and McVicker, R. F.: Experience with intraaortic balloon counterpulsation. Ann. Thorac. Surg. *41*:36, 1986.
548. Bregman, D.: Assessment of intra-aortic balloon counterpulsation in cardiogenic shock. Crit. Care Med. *3*:90, 1975.
548a. Moran, J. M., Opravil, M., Gorman, A. J., Rastegar, H., Meyers, S. N., and Michaelis, L. L.: Pulmonary artery balloon counterpulsation for right ventricular failure. II. Clinical experience. Ann. Thorac. Surg. *38*:254, 1984.
549. Leinbach, R. C., Dinsmore, R. E., Mundth, E. D., Buckley, M. J., Dunkman, W. B., Austen, W. G., and Sanders, C. A.: Selective coronary and left ventricular cineangiography during intraaortic balloon pumping for cardiogenic shock. Circulation *45*:845, 1972.
549a. Pennock, J. L., Pierce, W. S., Campbell, D. B., Pae, W. E., Jr., Davis, D., Hensley, F. A., Richenbacher, W. E., and Waldhausen, J. A.: Mechanical support of the circulation followed by cardiac transplantation. J. Thorac. Cardiovasc. Surg. *92*:994, 1986.
550. Schoen, F. J., Palmer, D. C., Bernhard, W. F., Pennington, D. G., Haudenschild, C. C., Ratliff, N. B., Berger, R. L., Golding, L. R., and Watson, J. T.: Clinical temporary ventricular assist. Pathologic findings and their implications in a multi-institutional study of 41 patients. J. Thorac. Cardiovasc. Surg. *92*:1071, 1986.
551. Pierce, W. S.: Artificial hearts and blood pumps in the treatment of profound heart failure. Circulation *68*:883, 1983.
552. Norman, J. C., Duncan, J. M., Frazier, O. H., Hallman, G. L., Ott, D. A., Ruel, G. J., and Cooley, D. A.: Intracorporeal (abdominal) left ventricular assist devices or partial artificial hearts. Arch. Surg. *116*:1441, 1981.
553. Rose, D. M., Culvin, S. B., Culliford, A. T., Cunningham, J. N., Adams, P. X., Glassman, E., Isom, O. W., and Spencer, F. C.: Long-term survival with partial left heart bypass following perioperative myocardial infarction and shock. J. Thorac. Cardiovasc. Surg. *83*:483, 1982.
554. Magovern, J. A., Pennock, J. L., Campbell, D. B., Pae, W. E., Jr., Pierce, W. S., and Waldhausen, J. A.: Bridge to heart transplantation: The Penn State Experience. J. Heart Transplant. *5*:196, 1986.
555. Hill, J. D., Farrar, D. J., Hershon, J. J., Compton, P. G., Avery, G. J., II, Levin, B. S., and Brent, B. N.: Use of a prosthetic ventricle as a bridge to cardiac transplantation for postinfarction cardiogenic shock. N. Engl. J. Med. *314*:626, 1986.
556. Pierce, W. S.: The use of mechanical circulatory support in advanced congestive heart failure. *In* Braunwald, E., Mock, M. B., and Watson, J. (eds.): Congestive Heart Failure. New York, Grune and Stratton, 1982, pp. 329–340.
557. DeVries, W. C., Anderson, J. L., Joyce, L. D., Anderson, F. L., Hammond, E. H., Jarvik, R. K., and Kolff, W. J.: Clinical use of the total artificial heart. N. Engl. J. Med. *310*:273, 1984.
558. Richenbacher, W. E., Pennock, J. L., Pae, W. E., Jr., and Pierce, W S.: Artificial heart implantation for end-stage cardiac disease. J. Cardiac Surg. *1*:3, 1986.
559. Joyce, L. D., Johnson, K. E., Pierce, W. S., DeVries, W. C., Sembe, B. K. H., Copeland, J. G., Griffith, B. P., Cooley, D. A., Frazier, O. H., Cabrol, C., Keon, W. J., Unger, F., Bucherl, E. S., and Wolner, E.: Summary of the world experience with clinical use of total artificial hearts as heart support devices. J. Heart Transplant. *5*:229, 1986.
560. Joyce, L. D., Pritzker, M. R., Kiser, J. C., Nicoloff, D. M., Kersten, T. E., Von Rueden, T. J., Eales, F., Johnson, K. E., Jorgensen, C. R., Gobel, F. L., and Van Tassel, R. A.: Use of the mini Jarvik-7 total artificial heart as a bridge to transplantation. J. Heart Transplant. *5*:203, 1986.
561. Griffith, B. P., Kormos, R. L., Wei, L. M., Borovetz, H. S., Trento, A., and Hardesty, R. L.: Use of the total artificial heart as an interim device. Initial experience in Pittsburgh with four patients. J. Heart Transplant. *5*:210, 1986.
562. Levinson, M. M., Smith, R. G., Cork, R., Gallo, J., Icenogle, T., Emery, R., Ott, R., and Copeland, J. G.: Three recent cases of the total artificial heart before transplantation. J. Heart Transplant. *5*:215, 1986.
563. Griffith, B. P., Hardesty, R. L., Kormos, R. L., Trento, A., Borovetz, H. S., Thompson, M. E., and Bahnson, H. T.: Temporary use of the Jarvik-7 total artificial heart before transplantation. N. Engl. J. Med. *316*:130, 1987.

18 PULMONARY EDEMA: Cardiogenic and Noncardiogenic

by ROLAND H. INGRAM, Jr., M.D., and EUGENE BRAUNWALD, M.D.

THE ALVEOLAR-CAPILLARY MEMBRANE AND PULMONARY EDEMA

Pulmonary edema develops when the movement of liquid from the blood to the interstitial space and in some instances to the alveoli exceeds the return of liquid to the blood and its drainage through the lymphatics.[1] Integral to an understanding of the pathogenesis of pulmonary edema is a comprehension of the structure of the alveolar-capillary membrane.

STRUCTURE OF THE ALVEOLAR-CAPILLARY MEMBRANE

The barrier between pulmonary capillaries and alveolar gas consists of a series of three anatomical layers with distinct structural characteristics (Figs. 18–1 and 18–2).

(1) The cytoplasmic projections of the *capillary endothelial cells* join by abutment or interdigitation or overlap to form a continuous cytoplasmic tube. At the overlapping junctions of these cytoplasmic projections are clefts of varying sizes, averaging approximately 4 nm in width, which provide communication between pulmonary capillaries and the interstitial space. Because these clefts can be widened with relatively small increases in vascular pressure, they are referred to as "loose" junctions. Although thin cytoplasmic projections result in maximal area for gas exchange with minimal tissue mass, these tenuous projections and junctions may be unusually vulnerable to disruption.[2] One side of the pulmonary capillary generally abuts the interalveolar septum (Fig. 18–2); with elevation of pressure, the pulmonary capillary endothelial cells may swell.[1]

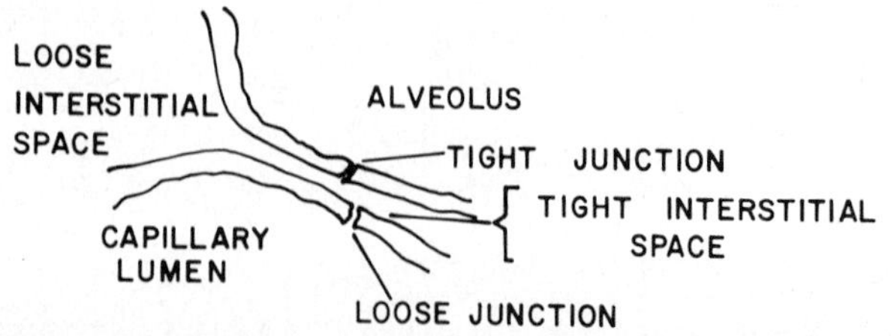

FIGURE 18–1. Schematic representation of the ultrastructure of the alveolar-capillary membrane. (Labeling corresponds to the discussion in the text.)

(2) The *interstitial space* varies in thickness and may contain connective tissue fibrils, fibroblasts, and macrophages between the capillary endothelium and the alveolar epithelium. There are no lymphatics in the alveolar-capillary interstitium.[3] This interstitial space of the alveolar-capillary septum is continuous with the wider and more compliant space surrounding terminal bronchioles, small arteries, and veins, and it is in this latter portion of the interstitial space that lymphatic channels first appear.[3] The lymphatics serve to remove solutes, colloids, and liquid derived from the blood vessels. Because of the increased compliance of the nonalveolar interstitial space and the peribronchial and perivascular interstitial space, liquid is more apt to increase here once the pumping capacity of the lymphatic channels is exceeded. As a consequence, small airways and blood vessels may become compressed.

(3) The *lining of the alveolar wall*, which is continuous with the bronchial epithelium, is composed predominantly of large squamous cells (Type I) with thin cytoplasmic projections. Many fewer granular pneumocytes (Type II) join with the Type I cells to form the alveolar epithelium. Similar to the junctions of capillary endothelium, the projections of the alveolar cells abut and overlap. In contrast to the endothelial junctions, which allow for variable continuity between blood vessels and interstitial space, the alveolar epithelial clefts are obliterated by complete fusion of the membranes of the adjacent cells.

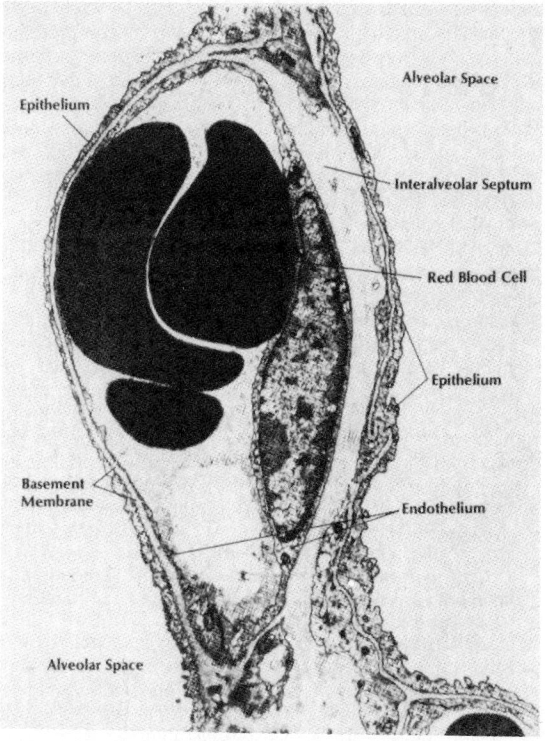

FIGURE 18–2. Electrophotomicrograph showing alveolar-capillary function. Capillaries in alveolar wall are arranged to create a "thin" portion of the alveolar-capillary barrier on one side (*left*); alveolar epithelium, basement membrane, and endothelium are attenuated in this region and air-to-blood gas diffusion distance is less than 1 μm. The "thick" side of the capillary in the alveolar wall (*right*) faces the interalveolar septum and contains abundant interstitial connective tissue fibrils, ground substance, and cells. (From Murray, J. F.: The lungs and heart failure. Hosp. Pract. *20*:63, 1985.)

Because the alveolar intercellular unions require much greater distending forces for their disruption than do the capillary endothelial connections, the former are referred to as "tight" junctions. The *tightness* of these junctions helps to forestall alveolar flooding, which represents the third and final stage of pulmonary edema. Although its principal function is to maintain alveolar stability, surfactant, the hydrophobic lipoprotein that lines the alveoli, may represent an additional mechanism for maintaining a dry alveolus.

CAPILLARY-INTERSTITIAL LIQUID EXCHANGE IN THE LUNG (THE STARLING RELATIONSHIP). As in other tissues, there is normally a continuous exchange of liquid, colloid, and solutes between the vascular bed and interstitium.[4,5] A pathological state exists only when there is an increase in the net flux of liquids, colloids, and solutes from the vasculature into the interstitial space (Fig. 18–3). Experimental studies have confirmed that the basic principles outlined in the classic Starling equation apply to the lung as well as to the systemic circulation. The equation describes the net flux of liquid between capillaries and interstitium in terms of hydraulic conductance (K_f), which is a function of area and conductivity per unit area, and the balance of the total forces tending to move liquid out of the capillary into the interstitial space and those that act to move liquid into the capillary from the interstitial space. Liquid accumulation in the lung is determined by the net flux between the vascular and interstitial spaces (which is in turn determined by the algebraic sum of vascular and interstitial hydrostatic and colloid osmotic pressures) and the rate of lymphatic drainage. That is to say, there will be an undetectable net accumulation of liquid in the lung with time if the rate of transudation of liquid from the blood vessels to the interstitial space is equal to the rate of removal of liquid from the interstitial space by way of the lymphatics ($\dot{Q}_{lymph}$). The rate of transudation from blood vessels can be expressed either as the balance of those forces acting to move liquid out of and those acting to move liquid into the vessels (Eq. 1) or as the balance of hydrostatic and colloid osmotic forces (Eq. 2):

$$\dot{Q}_{(iv\text{-}int)} \propto K_f[\underbrace{(P_{iv} + \Pi_{int})}_{\text{Outward force}} - \underbrace{(P_{int} + \Pi_{iv})}_{\text{Inward force}}] \qquad (1)$$

$$\dot{Q}_{(iv\text{-}int)} = K_f[\underbrace{P_{iv} - P_{int})}_{\text{Hydrostatic force}} - \underbrace{\sigma_f(\Pi_{iv} - \Pi_{int})}_{\text{Colloid osmotic force}}] \qquad (2)$$

where $\dot{Q}$ = net rate of transudation (flow of liquid from blood vessels to interstitial space
P_{int} = interstitial hydrostatic pressures
P_{iv} = intravascular hydrostatic pressures
Π_{int} = interstitial colloid osmotic pressure
Π_{iv} = intravascular colloid osmotic pressure
σ_f = reflection coefficient for proteins
K_f = hydraulic conductance. Thus, the Starling relationship is analogous to Ohm's law, because transvascular flow equals conductance times driving pressure.

Although the traditional Starling relationship has in the past been considered to apply to the transfer of liquid between pulmonary vasculature and alveolar space, it is clear from both the structural and the functional standpoints outlined above that this relationship applies mainly to the transfer between blood vessels and interstitial space. Although the equations are straightforward and set the stage for designating cardiogenic versus noncardiogenic pulmonary edema, there are many specific points to be made with regard to quantitative assessments.

VARIABLES AMENABLE TO MEASUREMENT. An estimate of pulmonary capillary pressure (P_{iv}) can be obtained from capillary wedge or left atrial pressure measurements. Also, plasma colloid osmotic pressure (Π_{iv}) can be determined by means of an osmometer. However, accurate measurements of interstitial fluid colloid osmotic pressures (Π_{int}) and interstitial hydrostatic pressures (P_{int}) continue to be elusive. With regard to Π_{int}, it has been frequently assumed in experimental studies that values obtained for lymph or for the free space of implanted capsules are representative of interstitial fluid. However, Staub has pointed out that such assumptions are ill-founded, since interstitial liquid is not homogeneous, and lymph from the lung collected experimentally may be contaminated with lymph from other tissues. Interstitial hydrostatic pressure is equally elusive, but the assumption is often made that pleural pressures or hydrostatic pressures in implanted capsules are closely related to interstitial pressure.[3] Direct measurements using micropipettes inserted into the perivascular interstitium of hilar vessels of dog lungs indicate, indeed, that P_{int} is more negative than pleural pressure and that the difference increases at higher lung volumes.[6] However, the difference is small, and pleural pressure is probably sufficiently close to interstitial hydrostatic pressure to be useful as a clinical index. It has been suggested that the mean negative intrapleural pressures seen in asthma may promote the formation and accumulation of interstitial liquid.[7]

It is worthwhile to note that the reflection coefficient (σ_f in Equation 2 above) is often considered to be 1.0 in experimental studies, i.e., the capillary membrane does not allow colloids to pass. In fact, as can be anticipated from the existence of the clefts between cells (loose

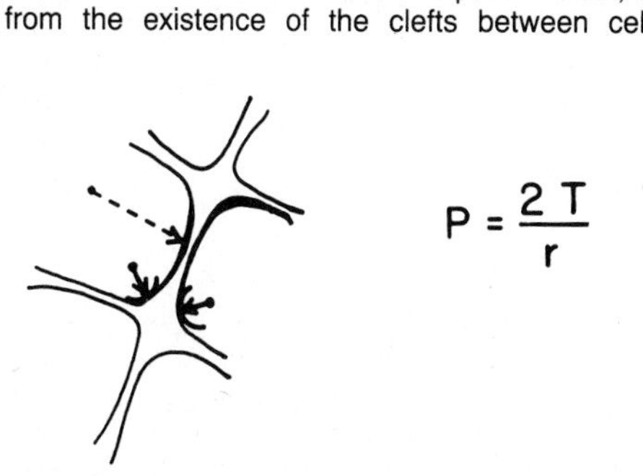

FIGURE 18–3. Schematic representation of the junction of several alveoli. The radii of curvature of a single alveolus vary considerably. The portion of the alveolar wall at which the radius of curvature is small (solid arrows) will tend toward greater local recoil pressures according to the Laplace relationship (P = 2T/r, where P = transmural pressure, T = surface tension, and r = the local radius of curvature). Since pressure in communicating alveoli is the same relative to atmospheric pressure, differences in transmural pressure result in different local interstitial pressures. It is in that portion of the interstitial space beneath smaller radii that liquid would first accumulate under conditions of increased transduction. These portions of the wall with greater radii of curvature (dashed arrow) would have smaller transmural pressures and hence would accumulate less liquid.

junctions) described above and possibly through pinocytotic vesicles in the capillary endothelial projections, macromolecules can and do pass into the interstitial space. This is reflected by the fact that the mean lymph to plasma protein ratio is 0.75 in experimental animals. The larger the molecule, the higher the reflection coefficient and the smaller the lymph to plasma ratio.[8] Hence the lymphatic proteins are predominantly of the smaller variety. Any disruption of the endothelial barrier produced either by increasing P_{iv} or by direct toxins will result in greater passage of macromolecules into the interstitium, which in turn increases Π_{int} and results in the passage of greater quantities of liquid.

ROLE OF LYMPHATICS IN THE LUNGS. As stated above, the lymphatics play a key role in removing liquid from the interstitial space, and unless the pumping capacity of the lymphatic channels is exceeded, edema will occur.

$$\dot{Q}_{(iv\text{-}int)} - \dot{Q}_{lymph} = \text{Rate of accumulation} \quad (3)$$

where $\dot{Q}$ = flow, iv = intravascular, and int = interstitial.

Although there is no direct way to measure lymph flow in humans, on the basis of extrapolation from animal data, Staub has estimated that an average 70-kg person at rest has a $\dot{Q}_{lymph}$ of approximately 20 ml per hour.[9] Experimentally, lymph flow rates of up to 10 times control values have been reported. Thus, it is possible that lymphatic pumping capacity can be as much as 200 ml per hour in an average-sized adult. It is probable that there would be some measurable accumulation of liquid in the lung before this capacity were reached, but it should be clear that there is an enormous lymphatic reserve. Given the capacity of lymphatic pumping, it can readily be comprehended that complete interruption of lymph flow, as with experiments on isolated lungs or in animals that have had surgical excision and reimplantation of the lung,[10] would result in much more rapid accumulation of interstitial liquid at any given rate of transudation from vessels.

Studies in the dog have shown that with chronic elevations of left atrial pressure, the pulmonary lymphatic system hypertrophies and is able to transport greater quantities of capillary filtrate during acute edematogenic incidents, thus prolonging survival.[11] On the basis of these experimental findings it is tempting to speculate that chronic increases in left atrial pressure in human disease might result in the same adaptive changes in the lymphatics that protect the lungs from edema during acute insults. A sudden marked increase in pulmonary capillary pressure can be rapidly fatal in a patient or animal not preconditioned by growth of the lymphatic drainage system. The same hemodynamic abnormality may be well tolerated in the presence of well-developed lymphatics. Also, since pulmonary lymph drains into the thoracic duct and from these into the systemic venous bed, when systemic venous pressure is elevated, lymph flow is impeded and the formation of pulmonary edema at any given level of pulmonary microvascular pressure is enhanced.[12]

Since the lymphatic channels are so important in determining the net accumulation of interstitial liquid in the lung, it is worthwhile to consider how liquids and colloids get into these channels and the manner by which they are then transferred to the systemic circulation. Normally, filtered liquid does not accumulate in the less compliant interstitial space of the alveolar-capillary septum but moves into the more compliant interstitial space that surrounds the bronchioles, venules, and arterioles. As noted earlier, it is in this latter interstitial space that the lymphatic channels are found.

MOVEMENT OF LIQUIDS AND COLLOIDS FROM THE TIGHT INTERSTITIUM OF THE ALVEOLAR-CAPILLARY SEPTUM TO THE MORE COMPLIANT INTERSTITIAL SPACE. It has been suggested that the forces resulting from the geometrical configuration of adjacent alveoli serve as a means of collecting liquid.[13] Figure 18–3 shows this configuration schematically. Through the Laplace relationship, the smaller radius of curvature at the corners results in greater local recoil pressures (hence more negative interstitial pressures) than occur at portions with greater radii of curvature. The resulting hydrostatic gradient would result in transfer of liquid to those junctions with smaller radii of curvature.[3] Indeed, after subpleural injections of dye-containing saline into cat lung, rapid accumulation of dye at such corners has been demonstrated. Within several minutes, the dye appears in the loose connective tissue spaces where the lymph capillaries are located.[3] Thus, there is a relatively direct pathway from the alveolar-capillary septum to the site of lymphatic channels. How liquids and colloids get into the lymphatic channels is not known. Increased permeability of the lymphatic walls with passive movement according to hydrostatic pressure gradients has been suggested,[14] yet with no experimental support. It has also been suggested that the pinocytotic vesicles within the lymphatic capillary endothelium serve to transfer liquid and protein into these channels; however, two studies have failed to demonstrate active transport.[15, 16] Some structural data have supported the proposition that the fine fibrillar attachments of connective tissue to the edges of the cytoplasmic projections at points of juncture serve as one-way valve mechanisms.[17] These fibrils are thought to expand the lymph-capillary lumen and open junctions during tissue swelling, thus opening the drainage pathway when tissue pressure rises. Conversely, as lymph pressure rises, the junctions close.

MOVEMENT THROUGH THE LYMPHATICS. Once inside the lymphatic channels, liquids and colloids are driven to major channels and ultimately to the systemic venous circulation. It had long been thought that only extrinsic forces were responsible for the propulsion of lymph through these valved channels, i.e., respiratory movements and vascular pulsations were thought to massage the lymphatics and result in unidirectional movement due to the valves in the lymphatic capillaries. Although there is no doubt that extrinsic forces influence the rate of lymph movement, it is now well established in experimental animals that lymphatic capillaries are actively contractile.[18] Factors that control or regulate contraction of lymphatic capillaries and any change in their contractile properties under conditions of increased liquid and colloid filtration remain to be elucidated.

QUANTITATION OF PULMONARY EDEMA

DIRECT MEASURES. Constant weighing of an isolated perfused lung has often been used as an index of edema based simply upon weight gain. However, as pointed out above, an isolated lung has no active lymphatic pump; hence the findings in this preparation do not take into account the important role that lymphatics play in vivo. The most commonly used and still standard quantitative assessment of pulmonary edema in experimental studies is the ratio of wet-to-dry lung weight. All the blood possible is drained from the vessels, and the lung is weighed, desiccated, and weighed again. This technique invariably includes the effects of a variable amount of retained blood and clearly measures the end result of a prolonged experiment rather than giving insights into the rate of change in response to a perturbation across the alveolar-capillary membrane.[19]

INDIRECT MEASURES. Attempts have been made to gain quantitative information concerning the rate of change in lung water both during experimental interventions in animals and for assessment of disease and effects of treatment in human beings. These include the measurement of transthoracic electrical impedance, emission or absorption of radiation, magnetic resonance imaging, and simultaneous indicator-dilution curves. The potential advantage of these less invasive measures lies in the fact that multiple determinations can be made for rapid assessment of changes in response to interventions.

Methods Employing Detection of Radiation. These assess either the appearance or the disappearance of radioactive substances introduced through the airways or blood vessels (emission) or the changes in absorption of roentgen rays or gamma irradiation across the chest from external sources (absorption). Emission techniques, although not completely tested, do not show great promise for clinical use. In contrast, quantitation of roentgen ray transmission using a filtered, monochromatic roentgen source and a photomultiplier detector offers some promise,[20] as does computerized axial tomography. The latter has been combined with radionuclide emission to quantitate edema in an experimental setting.[21] Intravascular marker (^{14}CO) signals were subtracted from those of a marker contained in both intra- and extravascular spaces ($C^{15}O_2$) to give extravascular lung water. Although interesting and possibly sensitive, the application of this technique requires expensive and rarely available equipment, including a cyclotron for generation of short-lived isotopes and a positron camera. To date, methods involving the use of radiation or radioisotopes have not been systematically applied to the clinical study of pulmonary edema.

Magnetic Resonance Imaging (See also p. 368). This procedure offers some promise as a quantitative technique to separate vascular engorgement from interstitial and alveolar liquid accumulation. This is based upon the effect of oxygen tension on spin-lattice relaxation rate of blood in vivo,[22, 23] so that blood vessels should be identifiable through changing the fraction of inspired oxygen. However, as of this writing, this cumbersome and expensive technology has not been used to quantitate pulmonary edema in either experimental or clinical settings.

Simultaneous Indicator-Dilution Curves. When derived from measurements of a detectable tracer substance that remains in the vasculature and one that quickly diffuses into the interstitial space, double indicator-dilution curves offer the advantages of safety, theoretical soundness, and a numerical value.[24, 25] Theoretically, the tracer for water must equilibrate with tissue water during a single-transit interval.

However, this condition is rarely met, since, in human lungs, only about half the interstitial lung water is measured by this technique.[3] Thus, although the double indicator-dilution method is simple, safe, and rapid, it is relatively insensitive and therefore does not serve a useful function in detecting the interstitial phase of acute pulmonary edema. Certainly, with the alveolar flooding in Stage 3 of pulmonary edema (Fig. 18–4), more water is in contact with the microvasculature than at any other stage, so that, as would be expected, the technique shows quite high values at a time when both the clinical and the routine radiographic methods of diagnosis probably suffice.

To sum up, attempts to quantitate pulmonary edema in its various stages of development are not yet sufficiently successful in terms of accuracy, sensitivity, and reproducibility to be clinically applicable.

SEQUENCE OF LIQUID ACCUMULATION DURING PULMONARY EDEMA

Whether initiated by an imbalance of Starling forces or by primary damage to the various components of the alveolar-capillary membranes, the sequence of liquid exchange and accumulation in the lungs is the same and can be represented as three separate stages, the last of which has two substages that occur closely in time.[26, 27] These three stages of liquid accumulation in the lungs are shown schematically in Figure 18–4. As just discussed, the top portion demonstrates that normally there is continuous movement of liquid and colloid from the vessels to the interstitial space and that lymphatic channels constantly pump this liquid and colloid into the systemic venous system to maintain a constant interstitial volume.

In *Stage 1*, there is an increase in mass transfer of liquid and colloid from blood capillaries through the interstitium. The pulmonary capillary endothelial junctions may have been widened by an increase in filtrative forces or by toxic damage. Despite the increased filtration, there is no measurable increase in interstitial volume because there is an equal increase in lymphatic outflow. The stimulus or mechanism for increased lymph flow is not clear, yet it is possible that small increases in interstitial volume that defy detection by present techniques stimulate stretch receptors, resulting in tachypnea and, in turn, extrinsically augmenting lymphatic pumping.[2] Furthermore, it is possible that the same stimulus somehow augments the intrinsic lymphatic pumping capacity.

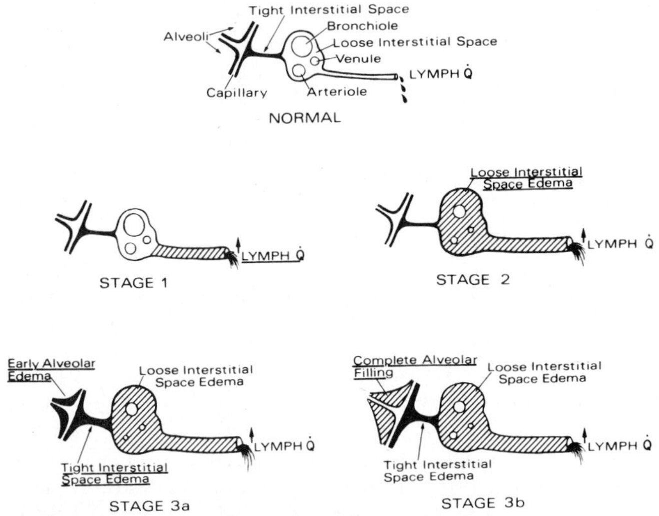

FIGURE 18–4. Schematic representation of alveolar-capillary membrane, loose interstitial space, and lymphatic system at the several stages of pulmonary edema—from the normal situation to fully developed alveolar edema, the new feature at each stage being underlined. (Drawn from Staub, N. C., et al.: Pulmonary edema in dogs, especially the sequence of fluid accumulation in lungs. J. Appl. Physiol. *22*:227, 1967.)

When the filtered load from the pulmonary capillaries is sufficiently large, the pumping capacity of the lymphatics is approached or exceeded, and liquid and colloid then begin to accumulate in the more compliant interstitial compartment surrounding bronchioles, arterioles, and venules. This is designated *Stage 2*.

With further increments in filtered load, the volume limits of the loose interstitial spaces are exceeded, causing distention of the less compliant interstitial space of the alveolar-capillary septum. Pressures sufficient to disrupt the tight junctions of the alveolar membranes ensue, and alveolar edema results. In early alveolar edema (*Stage 3a*), liquid accumulates at the corners of alveolar-capillary membranes where the radii of curvature are the smallest. Alveolar flooding (*Stage 3b*) occurs when alveoli reach a critical configuration at which inflation pressures can no longer maintain the existing configuration, and the alveolar gas volume rapidly decreases, being replaced by liquid and macromolecules. At this final stage of alveolar flooding, disruption of all components of the alveolar-capillary membrane occurs, irrespective of the initiating events.

GRAVITY-DEPENDENT DISTRIBUTION OF PULMONARY EDEMA AND PULMONARY BLOOD FLOW

The foregoing discussion dealt with the forces across the alveolar-capillary membranes as if they were homogeneously distributed throughout the lung. However, it is well known that neither lung tissue forces nor intravascular pressures are homogeneous and that major interregional nonhomogeneities exist owing to the differential effects of gravity on blood, gas-containing lung tissue, and air. Since blood is more dense (i.e., heavier) than gas-containing lung, the effects of gravity are much greater on the distribution of blood flow than on the distribution of tissue forces in the lung. From apex to base, the effective perfusion pressure of the pulmonary circulation (P_{pa}) increases by approximately 1.00 cm H_2O/cm vertical distance, whereas pleural pressures (P_{pl}) increase by only 0.25 cm H_2O/cm vertical distance.[28] Pulmonary capillaries (or alveolar vessels) are exposed to alveolar pressure (P_{alv}), which does not vary from apex to base. In contrast, pulmonary arteries, arterioles, veins, and venules (extraalveolar vessels) are exposed to pleural pressure, which does vary from apex to base. The consequences of these differences in forces on ventilation-perfusion relationships have been well described.[29]

ZONE 1. As shown in Figure 18–5, in Zone 1, pulmonary arterial pressure is less than alveolar pressure; thus there is no flow. Indeed, rapid-freezing techniques in animals have confirmed that apical capillaries are bloodless.[30] On the other hand, gamma-emitting isotope studies in normal humans indicate that, although blood flow is strikingly diminished at the apex, no *true* Zone 1 (with total absence of flow) exists.[31]

ZONE 2. In this zone, arterial pressure exceeds alveolar pressure, which in turn exceeds venous pressure. Here, each vessel is similar to a collapsible tube in a pressure chamber. An analogy has been drawn between these vessels and a Starling resistor, which has the following interesting property: When chamber pressure (analogous to alveolar pressure) exceeds the downstream pressure (analogous to venous pressure), the pressure drop for flow is not equal to the difference between upstream (arterial) and downstream (venous) pressures but rather to the difference between upstream (arterial) and chamber (alveolar) pressures. It is in this zone that large increases in flow

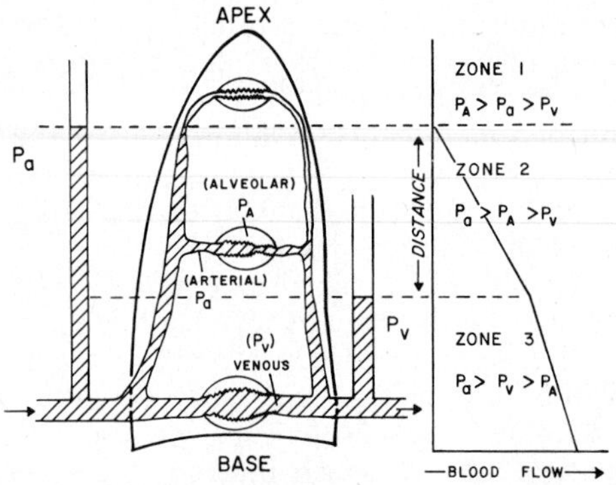

FIGURE 18–5. Schematic representation of the gravity-dependent, apex-to-base distribution of pulmonary blood flow in an upright lung according to West.[29] Pulmonary artery pressure (P_a) and pulmonary venous pressure (P_v) increase on a hydrostatic basis as the base is approached. Alveolar pressure (P_A) is constant with vertical distance. (The three zones are described at length in the text.)

occur per unit of distance of descent down the lung. These are due to large increases in perfusing pressures with no change in alveolar pressures.

ZONE 3. In this zone, venous pressure exceeds alveolar pressure, resulting in distention of collapsible capillaries. Mean intravascular pressures are greatest in this zone; hence, with elevations of venous pressure or with disruption of alveolar-capillary membranes, edema formation is both more rapid and greatest here. It is only in this zone that the usual calculation of pulmonary vascular resistance is valid, and it is the only zone in which a valid pulmonary capillary wedge pressure measurement can be obtained. Increases in blood flow with increasing distance from the apex are more gradual in this zone because increases in pulmonary arterial pressures are offset by identical increases in venous pressures. The basis for the increase in flow with distance is the greater mean distending intravascular pressure with greater distention of the vessels as the base is approached.

VASCULAR REDISTRIBUTION. Thus, in normal, erect humans, perfusion is greater in the basilar lung regions than in the more apical ones. Deviation from this gravity-dependent pattern has been called vascular redistribution. There are several ways to view the phenomenon of redistribution. Any encroachment of Zone 1 upon Zone 2 secondary to increased pulmonary venous pressure is, in a sense, redistribution, since regional blood flow is distributed differently after such a change. In like manner, greater relative perfusion of Zone 2 with increases in pulmonary artery pressure distributes more blood to the apex. However, true redistribution is generally considered to be a relative reduction in perfusion of the bases with a relative increase in apical perfusion. This phenomenon is most likely due to compression of the lumina of basilar vessels secondary to the greater and more rapid formation of edema at the lung bases and the tendency for extravascular liquid formed elsewhere to gravitate toward the bases.[3] In addition, pulmonary arteriolar constriction secondary to alveolar hypoxia, which may also contribute to this redistribution, is more prominent at the lung bases.[32] Several experimental studies either imply[33] or demonstrate[34] that vascular redistribution occurs only *after* the acute onset of alveolar edema. If this were the case in human disease, as it seems likely to be, redistribution should be no more subtle a finding than auscultatory abnormalities.

The situation with *chronic* elevations of left atrial pressure, as in mitral stenosis or chronic congestive heart failure, should be contrasted with that of *acute* pulmonary edema. Clinical experience with such chronic conditions suggests that redistribution of flow does occur with minimal or no evidence of interstitial edema and in the absence of alveolar edema. Because of the pathological changes found in such lungs at postmortem examination,[35] i.e., interstitial fibrosis of basilar lung regions and narrowing of basilar arteries and arterioles by lesions that often occur with pulmonary hypertension (p. 796), it is more likely that redistribution is secondary to such changes.

CLASSIFICATION OF PULMONARY EDEMA

The two most common forms of pulmonary edema are those initiated by an imbalance of Starling forces and those initiated by disruption of one or more components of the alveolar-capillary membrane (Table 18–1).[36–38] Less often, lymphatic insufficiency can be involved as a predisposing, if not initiating, factor in the genesis of edema. Although the initiating or primary mechanism may be clearly identifiable, multiple factors come into play during the development of edema, and irrespective of the initiating event, the stage of alveolar flooding is characterized most often by disruption of the alveolar-capillary membrane.

IMBALANCE OF STARLING FORCES

Increased pulmonary capillary pressure is a straightforward initiating event, whether due to mitral stenosis, left ventricular failure, or pulmonary venoocclusive disease. It has been found in experimental animals that pulmonary edema will occur only when the pulmonary capillary pressure rises to values exceeding the plasma colloid osmotic pressure, which is approximately 28 mm Hg in the human. Since the normal pulmonary pressure is about 8 mm Hg, there is a margin of safety of approximately 20 mm Hg in the development of pulmonary edema.[5] Although pulmonary capillary wedge pressures must be abnormally high to increase the flow of interstitial liquid, at a time when edema is clearly present, these pressures may not correlate with the severity of pulmonary edema.[39] In fact, pulmonary capillary wedge pressures may have returned to normal at a time when there is still considerable pulmonary edema, since the rate of removal of both interstitial and alveolar edema appears to be relatively slow. Other factors obscure the relationship between the severity of edema and measured pulmonary capillary pressures in addition to slower rates of removal after edema has collected. The rate of increase in lung liquid at any given elevation of capillary pressure is related to the functional capacity of lymphatics,[40] which may vary from patient to patient, and to variations in interstitial oncotic and hydrostatic pressures.

The question of increased capillary pressures secondary to increased pulmonary artery pressure due to overperfusion is difficult to place in a clinical context.[41] Indeed, experimental resection of well over half the pulmonary capillary bed has been required to produce pulmonary edema.[42] The most relevant clinical observation has been the description of pulmonary edema in one lung or lobe following the creation of an end-to-end shunt from a systemic artery to a single pulmonary artery for the treatment of cyanotic congenital heart disease.[43] The question might be raised of why pulmonary edema does not occur with severe pulmonary hypertension (e.g., primary pulmonary hypertension). The obvious answer is that the

TABLE 18–1 CLASSIFICATION OF PULMONARY EDEMA BASED UPON INITIATING MECHANISM

I. Imbalance of Starling Forces
 A. Increased pulmonary capillary pressure
  1. Increased pulmonary venous pressure without left ventricular failure (e.g., mitral stenosis)
  2. Increased pulmonary venous pressure secondary to left ventricular failure
  3. Increased pulmonary capillary pressure secondary to increased pulmonary arterial pressure (so-called overperfusion pulmonary edema)*
 B. Decreased plasma oncotic pressure
  1. Hypoalbuminemia secondary to renal, hepatic, protein-losing enteropathic, or dermatological disease or nutritional causes**
 C. Increased negativity of interstitial pressure
  1. Rapid removal of pneumothorax with large applied negative pressures (unilateral)
  2. Large negative pleural pressures due to acute airway obstruction along with increased end-expiratory volumes (asthma)*
 D. Increased interstitial oncotic pressure
  1. No known clinical or experimental example

II. Altered Alveolar-Capillary Membrane Permeability (Adult Respiratory Distress Syndrome)
 A. Infectious pneumonia—bacterial, viral, parasitic
 B. Inhaled toxins (e.g., phosgene, ozone, chlorine, Teflon fumes, nitrogen dioxide, smoke)
 C. Circulating foreign substances (e.g., snake venom, bacterial endotoxins, alloxan†, alpha-naphthyl thiourea†)
 D. Aspiration of acidic gastric contents
 E. Acute radiation pneumonitis
 F. Endogenous vasoactive substances (e.g., histamine, kinins*)
 G. Disseminated intravascular coagulation
 H. Immunological—hypersensitivity pneumonitis, drugs (nitrofurantoin), leukoagglutinins
 I. Shock lung in association with nonthoracic trauma
 J. Acute hemorrhagic pancreatitis

III. Lymphatic Insufficiency
 A. Post lung transplant
 B. Lymphangitic carcinomatosis
 C. Fibrosing lymphangitis (e.g., silicosis)

IV. Unknown or Incompletely Understood
 A. High-altitude pulmonary edema
 B. Neurogenic pulmonary edema
 C. Narcotic overdose
 D. Pulmonary embolism
 E. Eclampsia
 F. Post cardioversion
 G. Post anesthesia
 H. Post cardiopulmonary bypass

*Not certain to exist as a clinical entity.
**Not certain that this, as a single factor, leads to clinical pulmonary edema.
†Predominantly an experimental technique.

arteriolar bed is severely narrowed in the latter instance, and thus capillaries are not exposed to the increased pressure, whereas in the former instance, the arteriolar bed is not narrowed, and increased pressures are found in the pulmonary capillaries.

HYPOALBUMINEMIA. This is well known to produce dependent systemic edema without elevations of systemic venous pressures. In contrast, pulmonary edema does *not* develop with hypoalbuminemia alone. Hypoalbuminemia may alter the fluid conductivity of the interstitial gel so that liquid moves more easily between capillaries and lymphatics to add to the lymphatic safety factor.[44] Thus, there must be, in addition to hypoalbuminemia, some elevations of pulmonary capillary pressure, albeit only small increases are necessary before pulmonary edema ensues. Indeed, in such patients, only moderate fluid overload can precipitate overt pulmonary edema in the absence of left ventricular failure.

INCREASED NEGATIVITY OF INTERSTITIAL PRESSURE. When this is due to rapid removal of pleural air for relief of a relatively complete pneumothorax it may be associated with pulmonary edema. Usually, the pneumothorax has been present for several hours to days, allowing time for alterations in surfactant, so that large negative pressures are necessary to open collapsed alveoli.[45] In this instance the edema is unilateral and is most often only a radiographic finding with few clinical findings.

Large negative pleural pressures thought to approximate interstitial pressures have been shown experimentally to increase the rate of edema formation in sheep.[46] It has been shown that the degree of negativity of the mean intrapleural pressure in asthma correlates with the severity of an attack and speculated that there might be associated pulmonary edema, although it is radiographically inapparent owing to the hyperinflation of the lung in this condition.[7] This interesting hypothesis should be tested, since asthma is a common condition that is often treated with large volumes of intravenous fluids. Animal experiments involving inspiratory loading and increased lung volume as a means of increasing pleural pressure swings have demonstrated increases in left atrial transmural pressures along with diminution in left ventricular end-diastolic dimensions and decreases in cardiac output.[47–49] Thus, it is possible that diminution of left ventricular diastolic filling and an elevation of left atrial pressures accompany such large negative intrapleural pressures.

INCREASED INTERSTITIAL ONCOTIC PRESSURE. There is no known clinical or experimental example of pulmonary edema initiated by this mechanism. However, after the appearance of increased concentrations of macromolecules in the liquid of the interstitium or in alveoli, extravascular oncotic forces undoubtedly serve to intensify and perpetuate the process of edema formation.

PRIMARY ALVEOLAR-CAPILLARY MEMBRANE DAMAGE

Many diverse medical and surgical conditions are associated with pulmonary edema that appears to be due not to primary alteration in Starling forces but rather to damage of the alveolar-capillary membrane (Table 18–1). These conditions include acute pulmonary infections and pulmonary effects of gram-negative septicemia and nonthoracic trauma as well as any condition associated with disseminated intravascular coagulation.[36, 37, 50–52] Despite the diversity of underlying causes, once diffuse alveolar-capillary injury has occurred, the pathophysiological and clinical sequence of events is quite similar in most patients. Because of the resemblance of the clinical picture to that seen with respiratory distress of the neonate, these conditions have been referred to as the *adult respiratory distress syndrome* (ARDS).[53] This similarity includes the superimposition of secondary factors, either occurring spontaneously or induced by therapeutic interventions, that serve to perpetuate or worsen the clinical course. An example of a spontaneously occurring secondary factor is the appearance of left ventricular failure with elevation of pulmonary capillary pressure during the course of the illness; a frequent consequence of therapeutic intervention is liquid overload of the patient due to the administration of excessive volumes of intravenous liquids.

Direct evidence for increased capillary permeability has come mainly from experimental studies in which pulmonary edema has been produced by endotoxin infusion[54]; hemorrhagic shock[55]; infusion of oleic acid[56, 57]; ethchlorvynol, alloxan, thiourea, phorbol myristate acetate, complement fragments, and cobra venom factor[57–62]; and inhalation of high concentrations of oxygen[63] or toxic gases, such as phosgene,[64] ozone,[65] and nitrogen dioxide.[66] Reliable clinical data are far more difficult to obtain, since (1) macromolecules in alveolar liquid may be diluted by tracheobronchial secretion, resulting in an underestimation of the extent of the alveolar-capillary leak, and (2) such macromolecules, secondary to previously elevated capillary pressures, can be present at a time when intravascular pressures have returned to normal levels, hence leading to the erroneous conclusion that alveolar-capillary membrane damage was the primary event. Nonetheless, clinical studies of ARDS with normal pulmonary capillary wedge pressures have been reported and have shown either an elevation of protein in the liquid aspirated from the tra-

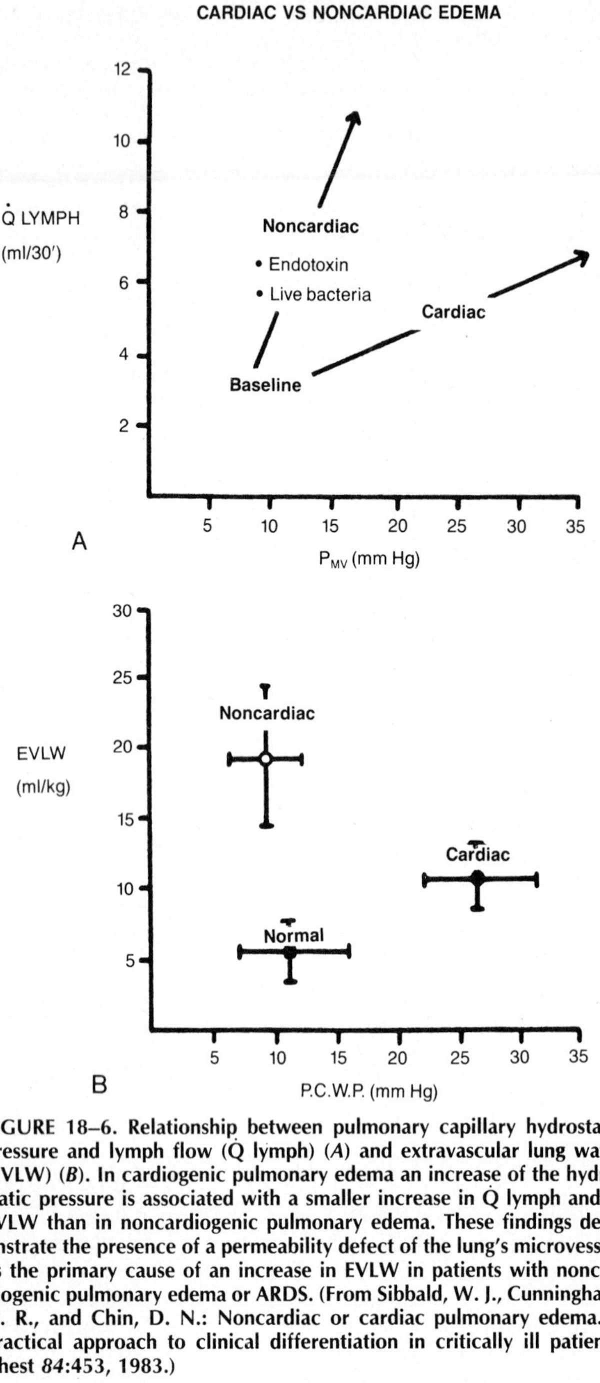

FIGURE 18–6. Relationship between pulmonary capillary hydrostatic pressure and lymph flow (Q̇ lymph) (*A*) and extravascular lung water (EVLW) (*B*). In cardiogenic pulmonary edema an increase of the hydrostatic pressure is associated with a smaller increase in Q̇ lymph and in EVLW than in noncardiogenic pulmonary edema. These findings demonstrate the presence of a permeability defect of the lung's microvessels as the primary cause of an increase in EVLW in patients with noncardiogenic pulmonary edema or ARDS. (From Sibbald, W. J., Cunningham, D. R., and Chin, D. N.: Noncardiac or cardiac pulmonary edema. A practical approach to clinical differentiation in critically ill patients. Chest *84*:453, 1983.)

cheobronchial tree[67–69] or appearance in this liquid of foreign macromolecules injected intravenously.[70] Thus, it is probable, though not yet proved, that increased permeability of the alveolar-capillary membrane is an initiating event in most of the cases designated as ARDS. There is some experimental evidence that electrical charge of the involved membranes (the pulmonary capillary endothelium and alveolar basement membrane are negatively charged while capillary basement membrane is positively charged) as of macromolecules can affect the movement of the latter into the alveolar space.[71] The relationship between pulmonary capillary pressures and lymph flow (Fig. 18–6*A*) and extracellular lung water (Fig. 18–6*B*) differs in cardiogenic pulmonary edema from that edema caused primarily by alveolar capillary damage. In the former, both lymph flow and lung water increase modestly, as a consequence of a large increase in microvascular hydrostatic pressure; in the latter, lymph flow and lung water increase markedly in the absence of or with only a slight rise in hydrostatic pressure.

There are many similarities between ARDS from diverse etiologies and the respiratory distress syndrome seen in infants, which is due only to immaturity of the surfactant system. Although surfactant deficiency cannot be assigned a *primary* role in the pathogenesis of ARDS, there are many data to support the idea that changes in the properties of surfactant are added to the initial impairment and serve to perpetuate pulmonary dysfunction. Impairment of surfactant has been shown to occur with cardiogenic pulmonary edema,[72] exposure to various plasma constituents,[73] and high concentrations of oxygen[74] and in association with systemic hypotension.[75] Closely related to the pulmonary edema in the ARDS is that which is commonly associated with all forms of shock—the so-called "shock lung." The theories of pathogenesis of shock lung are shown in Table 18–2. (For further discussion of ARDS and shock lung, see p. 567.)

ROLE OF POLYMORPHONUCLEAR LEUKOCYTES. Experimental data strongly imply a major role for interaction of polymorphonuclear leukocytes in the blood and circulating or cellular chemotactic macromolecules for the initiation, perpetuation, or amplification of lung injury leading to most forms of ARDS. The precise sequence of events is not truly settled but comprises some combination of items II, III, IVA, and B in Table 18–2. Figure 18–7 gives the elements of the potential role of leukocytes and chemotactic agents.[76] Chemotaxins in the circulating blood (e.g., the fifth component of complement, C5a) or from alveolar macrophages can recruit polymorphonuclear leukocytes, cause them to adhere to the pulmonary capillary endothelium, and activate them to produce several toxic substances that alter alveolar-capillary membrane permeability or cause circulatory changes or both. Because of the location of the polymorphonuclear leukocytes, their peripheral depletion and pulmonary vascular sequestration in many forms of acute lung injury, and their ability, when activated, to produce arachidonic acid metabolites (by both cyclo- and lipo-oxygenase pathways), oxygen radicals, proteases, and other mediators that alter permeability and influence vasomotoricity, the hypothesis is an appealing, though not unchallenged,[77] one. Experimental challenge, mainly in sheep, has been based upon leukocyte depletion studies which have shown for some agents (e.g., phorbol myristate acetate)[78] that leukocytes play a minimal role. However, leukocyte depletion is never complete, and extremely toxic drugs, which may alter a series of responses, are used to produce the leukopenic state. Hence at this stage of knowledge it is believed that the balance is strongly in favor of a role for the polymorphonuclear leukocyte in clinically important forms of ARDS.

Since chemotaxins can arrive from distal sources in the body to inflict injury or can be derived from the alveolar macrophages of the alveolar

TABLE 18–2 THEORIES OF PATHOGENESIS OF SHOCK LUNG

I. Hemodynamic
  A. Backward theory—pulmonary venular constriction (? centrally mediated; ? cerebral hypoxia)
  B. Forward theory—pulmonary hypertension. See IV, Microemboli (below)
II. Circulating humoral agent(s)
  A. Soluble factor(s) released from extrapulmonary cells injures vascular endothelium
III. Cellular agent(s)
  A. Locally released in lung injures vascular endothelium
IV. Microemboli—altered permeability arises from diffuse microembolization of lung
  A. Subtheories: why emboli form
    1. Exogenous from transfusions
    2. Increased rate of formation (platelet, leukocyte, or erythrocyte aggregates)
    3. Decreased breakdown (altered fibrinolysis)
    4. Decreased removal by reticuloendothelial system (liver)
      a. Humoral—deficient opsonin
      b. Decreased hepatic phagocytosis
  B. Mechanism of injury
    1. Hemodynamic (forward theory—severe, unevenly distributed pulmonary arterial hypertension transmitted to pulmonary capillaries, leading to shear stress and mechanical injury)
    2. Chemical (endothelium is injured by clot products: platelet, leukocyte, or erythrocyte aggregates)

From Robin, E. D.: Permeability pulmonary edema. *In* Fishman, A. P., and Renkin, E. M. (eds.): Pulmonary Edema. Bethesda, American Physiological Society, 1979, p. 217.

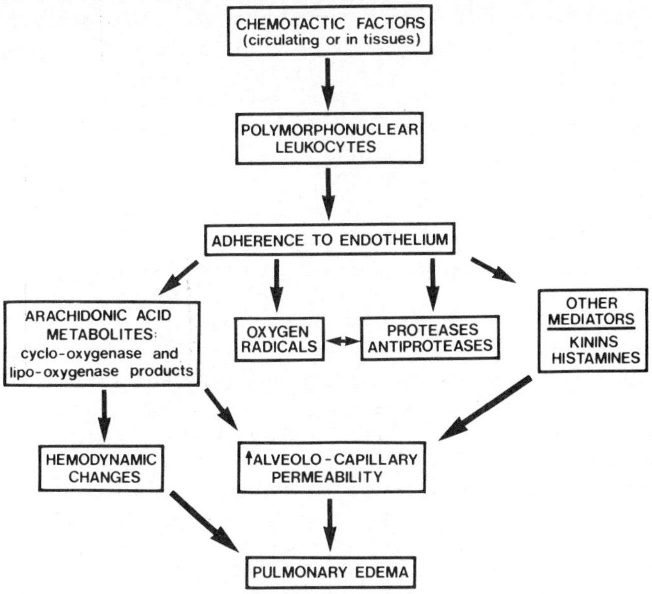

FIGURE 18–7. Flow chart showing the proposed mechanisms for chemotaxin and leukocyte interactions to produce alveolar-capillary membrane damage and pulmonary edema. (Adapted from Repine, J. E., Bowman, C. M., and Tate, R. M.: Neutrophils and lung edema. Chest *81*(Suppl.):5, 1982.)

side, systemic events such as gram-negative septicemia, distal events such as pancreatitis, and local pulmonary events such as inhalational injury can all be accommodated by this hypothesis.[79, 80] Moreover, since the leukocyte aggregates often include platelets, the thrombocytopenic and consumptive coagulopathic states often accompanying ARDS can be explained. Clinical studies appear to support this hypothesis.[79] Bronchoalveolar lavage liquid from patients with ARDS has shown a predominance of neutrophils, leukocytic elastase, and partially inactivated alpha$_1$ antitrypsin.[81–83] Further, there is a strong correlation between neutrophil-aggregating activity in the plasma and the subsequent development of ARDS in clinical conditions that are often associated with this syndrome.[84] In addition, the numbers of neutrophils obtained by bronchoalveolar lavage correlate strongly with abnormalities in gas exchange and indices of permeability.[83] To date, no observations are available to negate this hypothesis, yet the many potential and complex interactions await elucidation before preventive or therapeutic measures can be devised and translated into clinical practice for the avoidance or arrest of lung injury.

LYMPHATIC DYSFUNCTION

Abnormalities in pulmonary lymphatics can produce abnormalities of liquid transport in the lung. However, the question remains whether such alterations alone ever account for pulmonary edema. Experimental studies have been in direct conflict on this point.[85] From the clinical standpoint, however, there are clear examples to suggest the importance of pulmonary lymphatics. In silicosis, with the invariably associated obliterative lymphangitis, only moderate elevations of left atrial pressures result in impressive pulmonary edema.[40] Similar observations have been made following lung transplantation with complete disruption of lymphatics[10] and in association with obstruction of lymphatics due to lymphangitic carcinomatosis.[86]

There are experimental studies showing that lymphatic dysfunction can be present *without structural abnormalities*. For example, Hall and colleagues have shown that the normal rhythmic contractions of pulmonary lymphatic vessels in sheep disappear when the animals are anesthetized.[87] Cessation of lymphatic pumping would be expected to result in a net gain of interstitial liquid, and this may leave a clinical counterpart of pulmonary edema following anesthesia or sedative drug overdose. Impairment of lymphatic flow with a net gain of lung liquid content has also been shown to occur in sheep given continuous positive airway pressure.[88] The clinical occurrence or importance of this finding has yet to be established, but the question is a significant one, since both continuous positive airway pressure and positive end-expiratory pressure with mechanical ventilation are often used to improve gas exchange in patients with pulmonary edema.

PULMONARY EDEMA OF UNKNOWN PATHOGENESIS

HIGH-ALTITUDE PULMONARY EDEMA (HAPE). Victims of this disorder are usually persons mostly in their teens or early twenties who have quickly ascended to altitudes in excess of 2700 meters and who then engage in strenuous physical exercise at that altitude before they have become acclimatized.[67, 89–91] At one time this syndrome was considered to be rare; however, recent estimates place the incidence at 6.4 clinically apparent cases per 100 exposures to high altitude in persons less than 21 years of age and 0.4 case per 100 exposures in those older than 21 years.[92] Gradual ascent, allowing time for acclimatization, and limiting physical exertion upon more rapid ascent are thought to be preventive. Usually within one day of ascent, affected patients complain of cough, dyspnea, and, in some cases, chest pain in association with tachycardia, bilateral rales, and cyanosis accompanied by radiographic evidence of discrete patches of pulmonary infiltrate (Fig. 18–8).

Reversal of this syndrome is both rapid (less than 48 hours) and certain either by returning the patient to a lower altitude and/or by administering a high inspiratory concentration of oxygen. Sleeping below 8000 ft, gradual acclimatization, and avoidance of heavy exertion for the first 2 or 3 days at high altitude appear to be preventive. Although formerly thought to occur only in persons from low altitudes who ascend quickly for mountaineering or skiing, it has now been documented to occur among natives of high-altitude regions upon their return from altitudes below 2200 meters.[93]

Although no single mechanism satisfactorily explains the pathogenesis of HAPE, several possible mechanisms have been proposed. Although most patients have shown pulmonary arterial hypertension, the pulmonary capillary wedge pressures have been near normal,[94] a finding which has led to the suggestion that direct disruption of the walls of small arteries proximal to the hypoxically constructed arterioles in patients with hyperresponsive pulmonary vessels with resultant leakage of liquid may be responsible.[95] No hemodynamic data have been obtained during the development of, nor at the peak of, pulmonary edema, so that transitory elevations of pulmonary capillary pressures

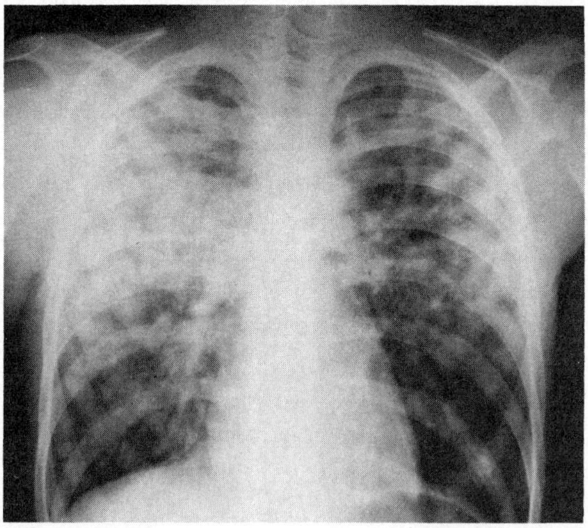

FIGURE 18–8. Chest x-ray of a 10-year-old boy in whom pulmonary edema developed on his return to his home at an elevation of 3100 meters after a visit to low altitude. Note patchy infiltrates scattered throughout both lung fields. Normal heart size indicates absence of left heart failure. (From Grover, R. F., et al.: High-altitude pulmonary edema. *In* Fishman, A. P., and Renkin, E. M. [eds.]: Pulmonary Edema. Bethesda, American Physiological Society, 1979, p. 229.)

could have been present and could have returned to normal at the time of measurement. However, in view of the existing data showing normal pulmonary capillary wedge pressures, other mechanisms have been proposed. The direct effect of alveolar hypoxia on increasing alveolar-capillary membrane permeability was initially considered, yet more recent studies do not support that idea.[96] Transient intravascular coagulation secondary to hypoxic sequestration of platelets in the pulmonary circulation has also been implicated[97]; however, it is possible that the intravascular coagulation is secondary to alveolar-capillary membrane disruption rather than a cause. At this point, it is fair to state that the pathogenesis is unknown,[98] but the response to simple treatment is dramatic.

NEUROGENIC PULMONARY EDEMA. Central nervous system disorders ranging from head trauma to grand mal seizures can be associated with acute pulmonary edema (without detectable left ventricular disease).[99] An early experimental model for this syndrome, consisting of fibrin injections into the fourth ventricle of dogs,[100] has been used to show that sympathectomy completely prevented the accumulation of lung liquid.[101] Indeed, observation that a variety of sympatholytic drugs serve to prevent neurogenic pulmonary edema makes it likely that the sympathetic nervous system plays a key role. Although not completely supported by direct measurements, the current idea is that sympathetic overactivity produces shifts of blood volume from the systemic to the pulmonary circulation, with secondary elevations of left atrial and pulmonary capillary pressures.[102] Thus, it would appear that an imbalance of Starling forces is the basis for this form of pulmonary edema, although capillary pressure quickly returns to normal after the acute and transitory sympathetic discharge. An unusually timely set of observations made on a patient with a pulmonary arterial catheter who experienced a grand mal seizure lent support to this idea. Wray and Nicotra observed transitory and severe elevations of pulmonary capillary wedge pressure in this patient during and immediately following the seizure.[103] Pulmonary edema diagnosed by both radiographic and clinical criteria was clearly present after wedge pressures had returned to normal levels. It should be emphasized that although sympatholytics prevent neurogenic pulmonary edema, they appear to have no place in the *treatment* of this syndrome, since it appears that pulmonary capillary pressures have returned to near normal by the time the syndrome is diagnosed.

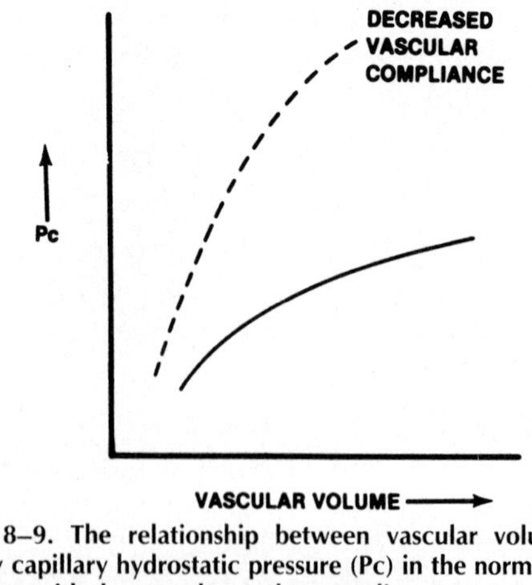

FIGURE 18–9. The relationship between vascular volume and the pulmonary capillary hydrostatic pressure (Pc) in the normal lung (——) and the lung with decreased vascular compliance (- - - - -). For a given increase in blood volume, the increase in Pc is greater in the lung with reduced vascular compliance. (From Malil, A. B.: Mechanisms of neurogenic pulmonary edema. Circ. Res. *57*:10, 1985, by permission of the American Heart Association, Inc.)

The idea of a transitory sympathetic neural discharge of sufficient magnitude to account for high-pressure pulmonary edema as the basis for the neurogenic variety has not gone without challenge. It has been shown that modest increases in pulmonary endothelial permeability can be produced by stellate ganglion stimulation in dogs without elevation of pressures.[104] Also, neurally mediated elevations in permeability during status epilepticus in anesthetized and paralyzed sheep, also without elevations of pulmonary capillary pressures,[105] have been demonstrated. Both of these observations, although demonstrating only a modest effect, suggest that neural mechanisms can alter membrane permeability. However, whether these changes are of sufficient magnitude to produce pulmonary edema is open to question. Recently Malik[106] reviewed the combined experimental and clinical data and concluded that a combination of hemodynamic and permeability changes probably contributes to the genesis of pulmonary edema of neurogenic origin. While both factors undoubtedly contribute, it is believed that the major alteration is due to hemodynamics. One way that sympathetic stimulation can magnify the hydrostatic gradient is illustrated in Figure 18–9.

NARCOTIC OVERDOSE PULMONARY EDEMA. Acute pulmonary edema is a well-recognized sequence of heroin overdose.[107] Because of the illicit traffic in this drug given by the intravenous route, the syndrome was initially thought to be due to injected impurities rather than to the heroin itself. However, since oral methadone and dextropropoxyphene can also be associated with pulmonary edema,[108, 109] the syndrome cannot be attributed entirely to injected impurities.

The well-known respiratory depressant effects of opiates lead to severe hypoxemia and hypercapnia with respiratory acidosis, which may account for the cerebral edema seen in many of these patients.[110] Cerebral edema, along with opiate-induced hypothalamic dysfunction,[111] raises the possibility of a neurogenic mechanism. Transient impairment of lymphatic pumping capacity may be a contributory factor.[87] The fact that edema fluid contains protein concentrations nearly identical to those found in plasma[112] and that pulmonary capillary wedge pressures, when measured, are normal[113] argues for an alveolar-capillary membrane leak as the initiating cause. In animal experiments, histamine has been shown to be released in the lung after both heroin and morphine administration.[114] Thus, it is possible that the well-known effects of histamine on increasing vascular permeability might play a role in this syndrome. However, there is not sufficient experimental or clinical evidence in support of such a role. As with several other pulmonary edema syndromes of uncertain etiology that develop quickly, the possibility must be considered that transitory pulmonary capillary pressure elevations account for the edema and that the reported normal measurements were made during the phase of resolution.

PULMONARY EMBOLISM. Acute pulmonary edema in association with either a massive embolus or multiple smaller emboli has been well described and most often attributed to concomitant left ventricular dysfunction due to a combination of hypoxemia and encroachment of the interventricular septum on the left ventricular cavity. Although this sequence is quite likely to be applicable in the case of massive embolism, whether it applies equally well to instances of multiple small emboli or microemboli is open to question. There are data to suggest, in the latter instance, that an increase in permeability of the alveolar-capillary membrane occurs.[51] It has been suggested that both clotting factors and formed elements in the pathogenesis of a pulmonary capillary leak due to microembolism.[115] Thrombin generated by the clotting process and in association with the embolus causes aggregation of platelets, complement activation, and leukostasis. It is proposed that

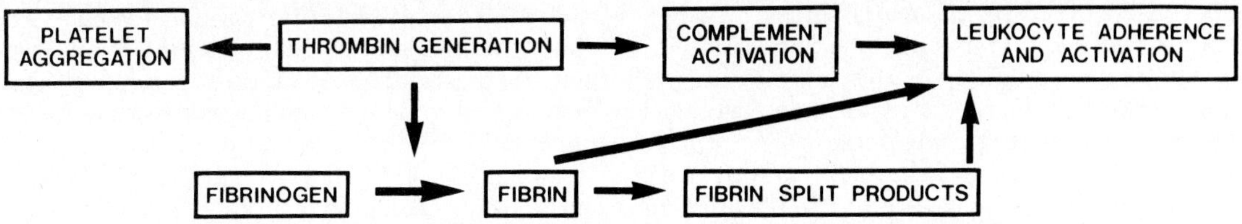

FIGURE 18–10. Flow chart showing the proposed mechanism for microembolic generation of increased permeability through the route shown in Figure 18–7. (Adapted from Malik, A. B.: Pulmonary microembolism. Physiol. Rev. *63*:1114, 1983.)

the sequence then follows that outlined in Figure 18–10. Experimental support for this notion comes from the blunting of the capillary leak process following defibrinogenation[116] or leukocyte depletion.[117]

ECLAMPSIA. Acute pulmonary edema frequently complicates eclampsia.[118] Multiple factors such as cerebral dysfunction with massive sympathetic discharge, left ventricular dysfunction secondary to acute systemic hypertension, hypervolemia, hypoalbuminemia (secondary to renal losses), and disseminated intravascular coagulation probably play a role in the pathogenesis.

POST CARDIOVERSION. Although pulmonary edema has been documented to occur following cardioversion,[119] the mechanism is poorly understood. Ineffective left atrial function immediately following cardioversion has been suggested as a contributing factor, yet left ventricular dysfunction and neurogenic mechanisms are also possible.

POST ANESTHESIA. In previously healthy subjects, pulmonary edema has been found in the early postanesthesia period without a clear relationship to fluid overload or any subsequent evidence of left ventricular disease.[120] The basis for this disorder is unknown, but it is tempting to invoke some role for temporary lymphatic dysfunction under anesthesia, as previously shown in sheep.[87]

POST CARDIOPULMONARY BYPASS. Although all patients who undergo cardiopulmonary bypass obviously have significant heart disease, the development of edema has been associated with normal left atrial pressures.[120–122] Alterations of surfactant due to prolonged collapse of the lung during the procedure, with subsequent need to apply high negative intrapleural pressures for reexpansion, and release of toxic substances have been suggested as mechanisms. Some data suggest that anaphylactic reactions to fresh frozen plasma may account for some episodes.[121] The matter is far from settled, but the syndrome is fortunately rare.

DIFFERENTIAL DIAGNOSIS

The differentiation between the two principal forms of pulmonary edema, i.e., cardiogenic (hemodynamic) and noncardiogenic (caused by alterations in the pulmonary capillary membrane) can usually be made readily by history, physical examination, and laboratory examination (Table 18–3).

TABLE 18–3 INITIAL DIFFERENTIATION OF CARDIOGENIC FROM NONCARDIOGENIC PULMONARY EDEMA

Cardiac Pulmonary Edema	Noncardiac Pulmonary Edema
History	
Acute cardiac event	Acute cardiac event is uncommon in immediate history (but possible!)
	Underlying disease? (Table 18–1)
Clinical Examination	
Low flow state = cool periphery	Usually high flow state = warm periphery
S_3 gallop/cardiomegaly	Bounding pulses
Jugular venous distention	No gallop
Crackles (wet)	No jugular venous distention
	Crackles (dry)
	Evidence of underlying disease (e.g., peritonitis)
Laboratory Tests	
ECG, ischemia/infarct?	ECG, usually normal
CXR, perihilar distribution	CXR, peripheral distribution
Cardiac enzymes may be ↑	Cardiac enzymes usually normal
PCWP > 18 mm Hg	PCWP < 18 mm Hg
Intrapulmonary shunting: small ↑	Intrapulmonary shunting: large ↑
Edema fluid/serum protein < .5	Edema fluid/serum protein > .7

From Sibbald, W. J., Cunningham, D. R., and Chin, D. N.: Noncardiac or cardiac pulmonary edema? A practical approach to clinical differentiation in critically ill patients. Chest *84*:460, 1983.

CARDIOGENIC PULMONARY EDEMA

CLINICAL MANIFESTATIONS. It would be satisfying to relate signs, symptoms, radiographic changes, and measurable dysfunction to all three stages of pulmonary edema. Unfortunately, there is currently no reliable way to detect pulmonary edema clinically or to quantitate it in its earliest stage—i.e., increased lymph flow without net gain of interstitial liquid. If the process is initiated by an increase in left atrial or pulmonary venous pressures, prominent pulmonary veins with secondary prominence of pulmonary arteries would be an expected radiographic finding. Although earlier studies were able to relate vascular dimensions to intravascular pressures, those measurements were made only under conditions of *chronic* pressure elevations[123]; therefore, the findings might not apply to acute changes. Nonetheless, it is likely, given the pressure-diameter characteristics of both pulmonary veins and pulmonary arteries, that acute changes could be easily detectable radiographically, especially if serial films were available. Concerning measurable dysfunction, Hogg and coworkers have demonstrated in animal studies an increase in resistance of peripheral airways during pulmonary venous hypertension and have shown that this finding could be attributed to competition for space between vessels and airways within the bronchovascular sheaths, with consequent compression of small airways.[124] The same phenomenon may occur in human disease in which there is increased pulmonary blood volume.[125] Compromise of the lumina of small airways, predominantly in the more dependent portions of the lung, would be expected to increase both the alveolar-to-arterial difference for oxygen and the wasted ventilation ratio (Chap. 61).

Stage 1. The distention and recruitment of small pulmonary vessels in Stage 1 edema may actually improve gas exchange in the lung and augment slightly the diffusion capacity for carbon monoxide by causing a more uniform distribution of blood in the lungs.[126] Since such mild changes in other settings rarely lead to symptoms, it is doubtful that any symptoms, except for exertional dyspnea, would accompany these abnormalities in Stage 1 edema. In like manner, physical findings in the lungs would be scarce except for mild inspiratory rales due to opening of closed airways.

Stage 2. In this stage interstitial edema presents similar problems, in that correlative studies are scarce or nonexistent. Radiographic changes have been attributed to the increase in liquid in the loose interstitial space contiguous with the perivascular tissue of larger vessels and containing venules and arterioles. These changes (Figs. 6–38 to 6–41, pp. 163–165) are a loss of the normally sharp radiographic definition of pulmonary vascular markings, haziness and loss of demarcation of hilar shadows, and thickening of interlobular septa (Kerley B lines). Competition for space between vessels, airways, and increased liquid within the loose interstitial space produces greater compromise of small airway lumina, particularly in the dependent portions of the lungs, than does Stage 1 edema. There may also be reflex bronchoconstriction.[126] A mismatch exists between ventilation and perfusion that results in hypoxemia and more wasted ventilation. Indeed, in the setting of acute myocardial infarction, the degree of hypoxemia correlates with the degree of elevation of the pulmonary capillary wedge pressure.[127] *Tachypnea* is a frequent finding with interstitial edema and has been attributed to stimulation by the edema of interstitial J-type receptors or to stretch receptors in the interstitium rather than to hypoxemia, which is rarely of sufficient magnitude to stimulate breathing.[2] Although the tachypnea itself is a sign of dysfunction, it augments the pumping action of lymphatic vessels and may serve to minimize or delay the increase in interstitial liquid. There are few changes in the standard spirometric indices.

Stage 3. With the onset of alveolar flooding, or Stage 3 edema, gas exchange is extremely abnormal, with severe hypoxemia and hypocapnia. Alveolar flooding can proceed to such a degree that many large airways are filled with blood-tinged foam that can be expectorated. Vital capacity and other lung volumes are, of course, markedly reduced. A right-to-left intrapulmonary shunt develops as a consequence of perfusion of the flooded alveoli. Although hypocapnia is the rule, it has been well documented that hypercapnia with acute respiratory acidemia can occur in more severe cases.[128] It is in such instances that morphine, with its well-known respiratory depressant effects, should be used with caution.

As indicated above, pulmonary edema developing during acute myocardial infarction most often is thought to be due to pulmonary capillary hypertension, yet experimental data in dogs with acute ligation of coronary arteries indicate another possible contributory mechanism. Edema developing after coronary artery ligation occurred when pulmonary capillary pressures were normal and the increases in lung water were blocked when animals were pretreated with indomethacin.[129] This finding suggests that inhibition of cyclooxygenase or cyclic nucleotide phosphodiesterase reduced pulmonary edema secondary to increased permeability of the alveolar-capillary membrane. Whether and to what extent these findings will apply to the human illness must await further study. Occasionally, patients with acute myocardial infarction and pulmonary edema present with normal pulmonary capillary wedge pressures.[130] It is possible that delay in radiographing clearance after a fall in pulmonary venous pressure is responsible, but it is also possible that in some patients an increase in permeability of the alveolar-capillary membrane secondary to low cardiac output, i.e., a form of "cardiogenic shock" lung, causes the pulmonary edema.

DIAGNOSIS. Acute cardiogenic pulmonary edema is the most dramatic symptom of left heart failure. Impaired left ventricular systolic and/or diastolic function, mitral stenosis, or whatever cause of elevated left atrial and pulmonary capillary pressures leading to cardiogenic pulmonary edema interferes with oxygen transfer in the lungs and, in turn, depresses arterial oxygen tension. At the same time the sensation of suffocation and oppression in the chest intensifies the patient's fright, elevates heart rate and blood pressure, and further restricts ventricular filling. The increased discomfort and work of breathing place an additional load on the heart, and cardiac function becomes further depressed by the hypoxia. If this vicious circle is not interrupted, it may rapidly lead to death.

Acute cardiogenic pulmonary edema differs from orthopnea and paroxysmal nocturnal dyspnea in the more rapid development of extreme pulmonary capillary hypertension. Acute pulmonary edema is a terrifying experience for both patient and bystander; usually extreme breathlessness develops suddenly, and the patient becomes extremely anxious, coughs, and expectorates pink, frothy liquid, causing him to feel as if he is literally drowning. The patient sits bolt upright, or may stand, exhibits air hunger, and may thrash about. The respiratory rate is elevated, the alae nasi are dilated, and there is inspiratory retraction of the intercostal spaces and supraclavicular fossae that reflects the large negative intrapleural pressures required for inspiration. The patient often grasps the sides of the bed in order to allow use of the accessory muscles of respiration. Respiration is noisy, with loud inspiratory and expiratory gurgling sounds that are often easily audible across the room. Sweating is profuse, and the skin is usually cold, ashen, and cyanotic, reflecting low cardiac output and increased sympathetic drive.

On auscultation the lungs are noisy, with rhonchi, wheezes, and moist and fine crepitant rales that appear at first over the lung bases but then extend upward to the apices as the condition worsens. Cardiac auscultation may be difficult because of the respiratory sounds, but a third heart sound and an accentuated pulmonic component of the second heart sound are frequently present.

The patient may suffer from intense precordial pain if the pulmonary edema is secondary to acute myocardial infarction. Unless cardiogenic shock is present, arterial pressure is usually elevated above the patient's normal level as a result of excitement and sympathetic vasoconstriction. Because of the presence of systemic hypertension, it may be inappropriately suspected that the pulmonary edema is due to hypertensive heart disease. However, it should be noted that this condition is now quite rare, and if arterial pressure is elevated, examination of the fundi will usually indicate whether or not hypertensive heart disease is actually present. Obviously, if the attack is not terminated, arterial pressure declines preterminally.

Differentiation from Bronchial Asthma. It may be difficult to differentiate severe bronchial asthma from acute pulmonary edema, since both conditions may be associated with extreme dyspnea, pulsus paradoxicus, demands for an upright posture, and diffuse wheezes that interfere with cardiac auscultation. In bronchial asthma, there is most often a history of previous similar episodes, and the patient is frequently aware of the diagnosis. During the acute attack, the asthmatic patient does not usually sweat profusely, and arterial hypoxemia, although present, is not usually of sufficient magnitude to produce cyanosis. In addition, the chest is hyperexpanded and hyperresonant, and use of accessory muscles is prominent. The wheezes are more high-pitched and musical than in pulmonary edema, and other adventitious sounds such as rhonchi and rales are less prominent in asthma. The patient with acute pulmonary edema most often perspires profusely and is frequently cyanotic owing to desaturation of arterial blood *and* decreased cutaneous blood flow. The chest is often dull to percussion, there is no hyperexpansion, accessory muscle use is less prominent than in asthma, and moist, bubbly rales and rhonchi are heard in addition to wheezes. The radiological changes in pulmonary edema are discussed on page 163 and illustrated in Figures 6–38 through 6–42, pages 163 to 165. As the patient recovers, the radiological appearance of pulmonary edema usually resolves more slowly than the elevated pulmonary capillary wedge pressure.

Pulmonary Artery Wedge Pressure Measurements. Measurement of pulmonary artery wedge pressure by means of a Swan-Ganz catheter may be critical to the differentiation between pulmonary edema secondary to an imbalance of Starling forces, i.e., cardiogenic pulmonary edema, and that secondary to alterations of the alveolar-capillary membrane. Specifically, a pulmonary capillary wedge or pulmonary artery diastolic pressure exceeding 25 mm Hg in a patient without previous pulmonary capillary pressure elevation (or exceeding 30 mm Hg in a patient with chronic pulmonary capillary pressure elevation) and with the clinical features of pulmonary edema strongly suggests that the edema is cardiogenic in origin.

Following effective treatment of the pulmonary edema, patients are often rapidly restored to the condition that existed before the attack, although they usually feel exhausted; between attacks of pulmonary edema there may be few symptoms or signs of heart failure.

TREATMENT

In the treatment of acute pulmonary edema, a physician cannot usually work alone, since multiple simultaneous maneuvers are required. Therefore, if logistics and time permit, the patient should be transferred to an intensive care unit, and cardiac rhythm should be monitored.[131] However, it is important to emphasize that transfer of the patient and institution of monitoring *must not delay initial therapy*, which must often be begun in the home or ambulance. While initial treatment is under way, it is frequently advisable to place an arterial catheter to record intraarterial pressure and obtain frequent samples for arterial blood gas measurements. If possible, a Swan-Ganz catheter should be inserted, so that pulmonary arterial diastolic and capillary wedge pressures can be measured and monitored.

The strategy of treatment of cardiogenic pulmonary edema is threefold: (1) a series of nonspecific measures is applied; (2) the precipitating factor is identified, if possible, and treated; and (3) attention is directed to the underlying condition, which is then corrected, if possible.

Nonspecific Measures

1. *Inhalation of oxygen-enriched inspired gas*, often with the aid of mechanical ventilation, is useful, as discussed below (p. 557).

2. The patient should be placed in the *sitting position*. Usually this is not necessary, because patients recognize that distress is increased when they lie down and that they are more comfortable sitting up. However, it is often helpful to seat the patient at the side of the bed or in a chair in order to lower the feet and thereby further diminish venous return.

3. *Morphine sulfate* remains an extremely valuable drug in the treatment of cardiogenic pulmonary edema. By its narcotic action it diminishes the patient's distress, reduces the work of breathing, and, perhaps most importantly, diminishes the central sympathetic outflow which causes venous and arteriolar constriction. Thus, even though morphine does not relax vascular smooth muscle directly, in the setting of acute pulmonary edema it results in arteriolar and especially in venous dilation.[132]

Three to 5 mg of morphine sulfate may be injected intravenously over a 3-minute period, while the patient is observed for both its beneficial action (i.e., relief of pulmonary edema) and its principal adverse effect (i.e., respiratory depression). This dose may usually be repeated two or three times at 15-minute intervals, if necessary. When the situation is somewhat less urgent, 8 to 15 mg of morphine sulfate may be injected subcutaneously or intramuscularly, and this dose can be repeated every 3 to 4 hours. Morphine antagonists should be readily available whenever morphine is administered. Morphine should be avoided if acute pulmonary edema is associated with intracranial bleeding, disturbed consciousness, bronchial asthma, chronic pulmonary disease, or reduced ventilation, as reflected in an elevated arterial P_{CO_2}.

4. *Furosemide* or *ethacrynic acid*, 40 to 60 mg injected intravenously over a 2-minute period, is another mainstay of therapy. With furosemide, diuresis commences within 5 minutes, reaches a peak effect at approximately 30 minutes, and lasts for approximately 2 hours.[133, 134] However, pulmonary edema is relieved even before diuresis has occurred, suggesting that the initial effect of furosemide is not on the kidney but on venodilation.[135] In addition, there is evidence that furosemide reduces afterload and may act in part to relieve pulmonary edema by improving left ventricular emptying (p. 513).[136]

5. *Reduction of preload* can be accomplished by applying rotating tourniquets of wide, soft rubber tubing or blood pressure cuffs to the extremities. These should be placed several inches below the groin and shoulders, and the cuffs should be inflated to approximately 10 mm Hg below diastolic pressure, thus permitting arterial inflow to the limbs but restricting venous outflow. Only three of the four extremities should be compressed at one time, and every 15 to 20 minutes one of the tourniquets should be released and rotated to the free extremity. Rotating tourniquets are used less frequently than previously because of the effectiveness of the intravenously administered diuretics, described above.

6. Since acute cardiogenic pulmonary edema, even in patients without hypertensive heart disease, is frequently associated with elevation of arterial and left ventricular end-diastolic pressures, cardiac output is depressed and systemic vascular resistance is elevated. Diuretic therapy, although of considerable value in reducing pulmonary capillary pressure, often does little to elevate cardiac output. *Vasodilators* promptly reduce systemic and pulmonary vascular pressures and relieve symptoms of acute pulmonary edema. A most appropriate vasodilator is *nitroprusside* (p. 519), which has a dual action: (1) it lowers systemic vascular resistance (afterload), thereby elevating cardiac output; and (2) it produces venodilatation (preload), thereby reducing pulmonary capillary pressure. A useful regimen is as follows: An initial dose of 40 to 80 μg/min can be employed, with the dose increased by increments of 5 μg/min every 5 minutes until pulmonary edema is relieved or until systemic arterial systolic pressure falls below approximately 100 mm Hg. If possible, arterial pressure should be recorded directly by means of an indwelling cannula during administration of this agent.

Nitroglycerin, 0.3 to 0.6 mg sublingually, also reduces ventricular preload by inducing venous dilation. The difficulty with this drug is that buccal absorption may be erratic; some patients develop marked reductions in arterial pressure. The hypotensive effect may be beneficial in patients with acute cardiogenic pulmonary edema and hypertension. However, it may be hazardous in patients with pulmonary edema secondary to acute myocardial infarction in whom arterial pressure is normal or reduced. Arterial pressure usually declines little in patients with hypervolemia and systemic edema.

7. The combination of morphine, rotating tourniquets, a diuretic, and sublingual nitroglycerin generally diminishes preload sufficiently to obviate *phlebotomy*. Although the removal of approximately 500 ml of blood certainly diminishes preload, it is a time-consuming and often cumbersome procedure for an acutely ill patient, and it is therefore rarely, if ever, necessary to employ this technique.

8. In a patient known not to be receiving *digitalis*, a rapidly acting cardiac glycoside given intravenously may be helpful, depending on the etiology of the pulmonary edema. It is most useful in patients in whom pulmonary edema is secondary to severe mitral stenosis, in whom atrial fibrillation or other supraventricular tachycardias and an excessive ventricular rate have developed, and in whom the abbreviated diastolic filling period has caused increased left atrial pressure (Chap. 33). The slowing of ventricular rate accomplished by the glycoside, either by conversion of the arrhythmia to sinus rhythm or by increasing the effective refractory period of the atrioventricular conduction system, can exert a rapid and salutary effect. Specific glycosides and dosages are discussed in Chapter 17. Digitalis is also useful in patients in sinus rhythm, who are known not to be taking glycosides and who have impaired systolic function of the left ventricle, such as those with acute pulmonary edema secondary to severe aortic valve disease and hypertension.

The problem is much more difficult in patients with acute pulmonary edema with sinus rhythm who have been taking an unknown dose of digitalis. Time usually does not allow one to wait for a serum glycoside level, and one must decide whether the pulmonary edema has been precipitated by digitalis intoxication or whether the patient requires more drug on the basis of clinical examination and the electrocardiogram (p. 504). A history of previous digitalis intoxication and/or nausea, vomiting, paroxysmal atrial tachycardia with atrioventricular block, nonparoxysmal atrioventricular junctional tachycardia, frequent ventricular premature contractions, ventricular tachycardia, and hypokalemia all imply digitalis intoxication. If these signs are absent, it is well to remember that when patients on a maintenance dose of a cardiac glycoside suddenly develop atrial fibrillation or other supraventricular tachycardia, the ventricular rate may be almost as rapid as if they had not been receiving the glycoside previously, and almost full doses may be required to slow the ventricular rate.

9. *Aminophylline* (theophylline ethylenediamine) is particularly useful when bronchospasm complicates pulmonary edema or in the occasional patient in whom it is not clear whether the attack of breathlessness is due to bronchial or cardiac asthma. Aminophylline is useful because it exerts a direct myocardial stimulating effect, analogous to that of caffeine. The reduction of ventricular filling pressure induced by aminophylline is caused not only by its positive inotropic effect but by mild venodilatation as well. In addition, it is a central nervous system stimulant, although less so than caffeine, and it exerts mild diuretic and bronchodilator effects.

The usual dose is 5 mg/kg intravenously in 10 minutes, followed by a constant infusion of 0.5 mg/kg/hr. This dose should be decreased in older persons and in those with hepatic or renal dysfunction.[137] After 12 hours the dose should be reduced to 0.1 mg/kg/hr. Optimal blood levels range from 10 to 20 mg/liter. Measurements of blood levels are important in the clinical use of this drug, since there are surprisingly wide individual variations in the kinetics of aminophylline degradation and since symptoms of nausea and vomiting are frequently due to other drugs used in the treatment of pulmonary edema rather than to aminophylline. Other side effects include headache, flushing, palpitations, precordial pain, hypotension, and, rarely, convulsions. The more serious side effects are sudden death from ventricular arrhythmias and hypotension due to vasodilation. Arterial unsaturation may occur owing to pulmonary vasodilatation and perfusion of poorly ventilated alveoli in patients with pulmonary edema.[138]

IDENTIFICATION AND TREATMENT OF PRECIPITATING FACTORS. In most patients with pulmonary edema, it is possible to identify one or more precipitating factors, similar to those that exacerbate congestive heart failure (p. 474). Most frequently, pulmonary edema is brought on by acute myocardial ischemia or infarction,[139] the development of a tachyarrhythmia, fluid overloading, an infection in a patient with established underlying heart disease, pulmonary embolism (Chap. 47), thyrotoxicosis (Chaps. 25 and 58), or severe anemia (Chaps. 25 and 55).

In addition to applying the nonspecific measures for the treatment of pulmonary edema outlined above, additional attention must be directed to identifying and treating the precipitating factors (e.g., lowering body temperature in a patient with a high fever or treating thyroid storm or severe anemia). If acute pulmonary edema has been precipitated by a *tachyarrhythmia* that does not respond to appropriate medical therapy and does not appear to be secondary to digitalis intoxication, it may be necessary to institute cardioversion with direct-current countershock (p. 642). On the other hand, if acute pulmonary edema occurs in a patient with a *bradyarrhythmia* that does not respond to appropriate medical therapy, a temporary pacemaker should be inserted and the heart rate restored to normal (Chap. 23).

If acute pulmonary edema is precipitated or aggravated by a *hypertensive crisis*, treatment of the pulmonary edema clearly requires a rapidly acting hypotensive drug such as sodium nitroprusside (as discussed above). Alternatively, diazoxide, 300 mg as an intravenous bolus, or other vasodilators (Table 28–9, p. 880) may be employed.

RECOGNITION AND TREATMENT OF THE UNDERLYING CONDITION. After emergency therapeutic measures have been instituted, an attempt must be made rapidly to establish the diagnosis of the underlying cardiac disorder responsible for the pulmonary edema, when this is not already clear. Obviously, the history, physical examination, chest x-ray, and electrocardiogram are of great value. The echocardiogram may be helpful in the diagnosis of mitral valve disease, particularly silent mitral stenosis, as well as in the recognition of left atrial myxoma, which may be responsible for acute pulmonary edema (Chap. 43). The diagnosis of congestive cardiomyopathy and of hypertrophic obstructive cardiomyopathy, both of which may be responsible for pulmonary edema, can also be strongly suggested by the echocardiogram. Although the echocardiogram may be enormously helpful in establishing an anatomical diagnosis, it must be recognized that the *quality* of echocardiographic tracings may be poor in patients who are acutely ill.

Catheterization of the right side of the heart and pulmonary artery with a Swan-Ganz catheter is useful not only in the diagnosis of pulmonary edema, as indicated above, but also in aiding in the recognition of underlying cardiac disorders such as ventricular septal defect and mitral regurgitation, which may be responsible for pulmonary edema in patients with acute myocardial infarction. In addition, blood cultures for infective bacterial endocarditis and emergency creatine kinase isoenzyme (CK-MB) determinations for the diagnosis of acute myocardial infarction are critical tests in a patient in whom the cause of the pulmonary edema is obscure. Radioisotope angiography (Chap. 11) may be helpful in revealing the status of left ventricular function.

Rarely, *surgical treatment* is necessary to relieve pulmonary edema in patients with acute infective endocarditis (Chap. 34), prosthetic valve dysfunction (Chap. 33), prolapsing atrial myxoma (Chap. 43), end-stage critically severe aortic or mitral stenosis, ventricular septal defect, or mitral regurgitation complicating acute myocardial infarction (Chap. 39). Whenever possible, the patient's condition should first be stabilized, so that operation is not carried out on an emergency basis. Occasionally, however, when pulmonary edema persists despite optimal application of the nonspecific measures and removal of the precipitating factors, preoperative stabilization is not possible, and emergency surgery must be employed as a life-saving maneuver. Balloon valvuloplasty (p. 1390) may be employed in patients with aortic and/or mitral stenosis who are poor surgical candidates.

LONG-TERM MANAGEMENT. The initial management of pulmonary edema, outlined above, blends in with the long-term management of heart failure described in Chapter 17. If the nature of the patient's underlying heart disease is known, it is necessary to assess its severity, attempt to ascertain the precipitating cause of the pulmonary edema, and develop a therapeutic strategy to prevent its recurrence. In many instances this consists merely of instructing the patient to remain on a salt-poor diet and to continue administration of a cardiac glycoside, a diuretic, and a vasodilator. In other instances, the development of pulmonary edema in a patient with chronic heart disease signals a process of such severity that, following recovery from the acute decompensation, it may be advisable to assess carefully the patient's hemodynamic status and consider or reconsider surgical treatment. If the patient is seen for the first time during an acute episode of pulmonary edema, and the nature of the underlying heart disease is not clear, a detailed cardiac work-up should be undertaken soon after recovery in order to elucidate the nature and severity of the underlying disorder with a view to identification of a lesion which can be corrected surgically.

PULMONARY EDEMA SECONDARY TO ALTERATIONS OF THE ALVEOLAR-CAPILLARY MEMBRANE

CLINICAL MANIFESTATIONS. Since the sequence of liquid accumulation is similar whether primary membrane damage or alteration of Starling forces is responsible, both radiographic and clinical signs described above for patients with cardiogenic pulmonary edema also apply in patients with pulmonary edema due to primary alterations of the alveolar-capillary membrane.[140] At the time of initial injury and for several hours thereafter, the patient may be free of respiratory symptoms or signs. The earliest sign is an increase in respiratory frequency followed shortly by dyspnea. Arterial blood gas measurement in the earlier period will disclose a depressed Po_2 despite a decreased Pco_2, so that the alveolar-to-arterial difference for oxygen is increased. At this point, oxygen given by mask or nasal prongs results in a significant increase in the arterial Po_2. Physical examination may be unremarkable, although a few fine inspiratory rales may be audible. With progression, the patient becomes cyanotic and increasingly dyspneic and tachypneic. Rales are more prominent and easily heard throughout both lung fields along with regions of tubular breath sounds. At this stage, hypoxemia cannot be corrected by the simple administration of oxygen, and mechanical ventilatory assistance or control must be initiated in order to provide adequate oxygenation of arterial blood. Should this more aggressive therapy be delayed, the combination of increasing tachypnea and smaller tidal volumes results in a rising Pco_2 and further fall in Po_2 to near fatal levels.

TREATMENT

Whatever the underlying cause of pulmonary edema, analysis of arterial blood to assess the type and degree of gas exchange abnormality is necessary, followed by institution of appropriate inhalation therapeutic measures. When there is hypoxemia ($Pao_2 < 60$ mm Hg) without hypercapnia, oxygen enrichment of the inspired gas may suffice and can be given by nasal prongs, Venturi masks, or reservoir bag masks, depending upon the degree of oxygen enrichment required to elevate the Pao_2 sufficiently. If arterial oxygen tensions cannot be maintained at or near 60 mm Hg despite inhalation of 100 per cent O_2 at 20 liters per minute, or if there is progressive hypercapnia, intubation and institution of mechanical ventilation are usually necessary.

MECHANICAL VENTILATION. In the instance of progressive hypoxemia without hypercapnia, the role of mechanical ventilation is not to increase alveolar ventilation but to increase mean lung volume during the respiratory cycle, which in turn opens more alveoli for gas exchange. If hypoxemia is not corrected by mechanical ventilation or if toxic doses of oxygen are necessary for prolonged periods, further improvements in arterial oxygenation at the same inspired oxygen concentration or equivalent levels of arterial oxygenation at lower concentrations of oxygen can be achieved by increasing end-expiratory lung volumes by the addition of positive end-expiratory pressure (PEEP).[141] Early use of PEEP to avoid or delay the onset of more severe respiratory failure has not been found to be effective.[142] Since maintenance of oxygenation is absolutely necessary for survival, reports that mechanical ventilation with positive end-expiratory pressure actually increases the liquid content of the lung[88] may unsettle physicians who must utilize these techniques but will make them aware that this form of treatment should be discontinued as soon as possible.

Two complications of mechanical ventilation with positive end-expiratory pressure deserve special mention. The first is that high intrathoracic pressures and increasing lung volumes serve to impede venous return and increase the afterload to the right ventricle, with attendant decreases in cardiac output.[47] In the case of cardiogenic pulmonary edema, the impedance of venous return may provide some benefit with decreases in central pressures but no decline in cardiac output. However, in other forms of pulmonary edema, a fall in cardiac output may be detrimental to the oxygen transport system. A fall in blood pressure or urine output or both may indicate that a severe diminution in cardiac output has occurred unless cardiac output is monitored during this form of therapy. The predominant basis for the decrease in cardiac output is increased intrathoracic pressure, which directly impedes venous return.[47, 48] An additional contribution may come from greater pulmonary vascular resistance due to increased lung volume.[47] The result of increased right ventricular afterload is a displacement of the interventricular septum, which impedes left ventricular diastolic filling.[49, 143–145] It is also likely that direct compression of the left ventricle by the inflated lung also restricts diastolic filling.[146, 147] The second complication of mechanical ventilation is barotrauma (pneumomediastinum, pneumothorax, and subcutaneous emphysema). Pneumothorax may require appropriate decompressive therapy by means of a chest tube.[148]

OTHER MEASURES. When it is not possible to maintain oxygenation utilizing the above techniques, *extracorporeal membrane oxygenators* have been tried with the hope that life could be maintained during critical periods while reparative processes in the heart or lung or both are taking

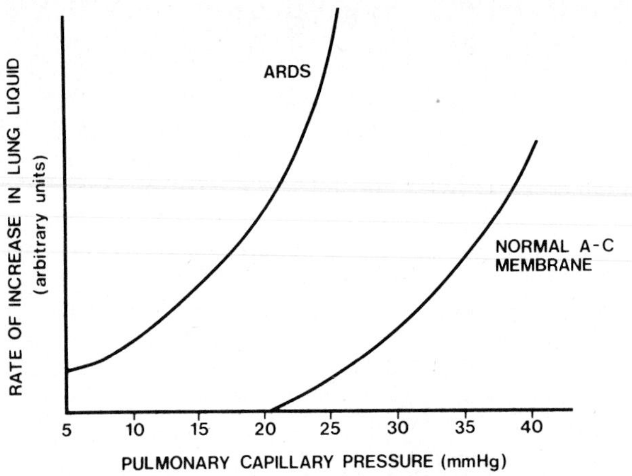

FIGURE 18–11. Schematic representation of the deleterious effects of acceptably normal capillary pressures in combination with pulmonary capillary leak. (Based upon the data of Prewitt, R. M., McCarthy, J., and Wood, L. D. H.: Treatment of acute low pressure pulmonary edema in dogs: Relative effects of hydrostatic and oncotic pressure, nitroprusside, and positive end-expiratory pressure. J. Clin. Invest. *67*:409, 1981.)

place. However, a National Heart, Lung, and Blood Institute trial designed to evaluate this heroic and costly form of life support has shown that it does not improve the clinical outcome.

When hypercapnia with respiratory acidosis is present, mechanical ventilatory support may be necessary for improving alveolar ventilation in addition to improving oxygenation. If hypercapnia has resulted from excessively vigorous use of morphine, *morphine antagonists* (naloxone) might avert the need for mechanical ventilation.

In any situation in which cardiac output is diminished and arterial oxygenation is impaired, there may be insufficient oxygen delivered for aerobic metabolic demands; hence anaerobic metabolism with excessive production of lactic acid results in metabolic acidemia. Clearly, the primary aim is to improve both cardiac output and arterial oxygenation; however, *sodium bicarbonate* may be given intravenously as a temporary measure while more basic therapeutic measures are undertaken. Occasionally, when large quantities of sodium bicarbonate are required, there is a danger of sodium overload.

An obvious and not often emphasized principle is to *maintain pulmonary capillary pressures at the lowest possible levels* (i.e., compatible with maintaining cardiac and urinary outputs and blood pressure) when there is increased permeability. Prewitt et al. have shown, using a dog model of oleic acid–induced pulmonary edema, that the rate of formation of pulmonary edema is cut to less than half when pulmonary capillary wedge pressures are decreased from 12 to 6 mm Hg.[149] The principle is schematized in Figure 18–11.

THE CASE AGAINST INTRAVENOUS COLLOIDS. Since both increases in pulmonary capillary pressure and primary alveolar-capillary damage result in interstitial edema and alveolar flooding with liquid containing erythrocytes and macromolecules, indicating severe membrane disruption, it is difficult to evolve a rationale for the use of intravenous colloids such as albumin or high molecular weight dextrans. In fact, high molecular weight compounds administered intravenously have been shown to appear rapidly in alveolar liquid.[70] Furthermore, there is experimental evidence that the administration of colloid to dogs with experimental lung injury actually *slows* the resolution of ultrastructural changes in the interstitium.[150] Since there is no firm clinical evidence that treatment with protein-containing solutions results in more rapid recovery from acute pulmonary edema,[148] and since there are strong intuitive reasons and some experimental data to suggest detrimental results, the use of albumin and other colloids should generally be avoided. There are, however, two situations in which albumin can be reasonably considered. First, if hypoalbuminemia is present, administration of albumin in addition to interventions designed to lower pulmonary capillary pressures is rational. Second, the suggestion has been made that albumin might hasten the rate of resolution of pulmonary edema once alveolar-capillary membrane integrity has been reestablished.[151]

Measures aimed at combating increased capillary permeability in ARDS are nonspecific and have not been shown to alter the time course or outcome of the illness. A possible exception is the use of specific antibiotic therapy directed against a causative or complicating bacterial infection. Adrenal glucocorticosteroid therapy leads the list of nonspecific measures that have yet to be proved beneficial in properly designed prospective studies.[152] In cases of pulmonary edema related to or complicated by disseminated intravascular coagulation, low-molecular weight dextran and heparin have been used without any clear evidence of an effect on the severity of the lung lesion.

Based upon alterations of multiple models of lung injury, agents will undoubtedly be tried that reduce chemotaxis, adherence, and activation of polymorphonuclear leukocytes (e.g., prostaglandins of the E series), that inhibit the formation of cell membrane–derived arachidonic acid metabolites (e.g., cyclo-oxygenase, lipoxygenase, and thromboxane synthase inhibitors), that competitively inhibit the various products (e.g., leukotriene D_4, E_4 antagonists), and that scavenge toxic metabolites of oxygen (e.g., glutathione, catalase). The rationale for and effectiveness of each are well documented in various experimental systems. However, the ultimate safety of such agents and their efficacy against the onset or continuation of membrane leaks in the clinical setting must await prospective trials.

REFERENCES

THE ALVEOLAR-CAPILLARY MEMBRANE AND PULMONARY EDEMA

1. Harris, P., and Heath, D.: Pulmonary edema. *In* The Human Pulmonary Circulation, 3rd ed. New York, Churchill Livingstone, 1986, pp. 373–383.
2. Szidon, J. P., Pietra, G. G., and Fishman, A. P.: The alveolar-capillary membrane and pulmonary edema. N. Engl. J. Med. *286*:1200, 1972.
3. Staub, N. C.: Pulmonary edema. Physiol. Rev. *54*:678, 1974.
4. Guyton, A. C., Parker, J. C., Taylor, A. E., Jackson, T. E., and Moffatt, D. S.: Forces governing water movement in the lung. *In* Fishman, A. P., and Renkin, E. M. (eds.): Pulmonary Edema. Bethesda, American Physiological Society, 1979, p. 70.
5. Guyton, A. C.: Textbook of Medical Physiology, 7th ed. Philadelphia, W. B. Saunders Company, 1986, p. 372.
6. Lai-Fook, S. J.: Perivascular interstitial fluid pressure measured by micropipettes in isolated dog lung. J. Appl. Physiol. *52*:9, 1982.
7. Stalcup, S. A., and Mellins, R. B.: Mechanical forces producing pulmonary edema in acute asthma. N. Engl. J. Med. *297*:592, 1977.
8. Parker, J. C., Parker, R. E., Granger, D. N., and Taylor, A. E.: Vascular permeability and transvascular fluid and protein transport in the dog lung. Circ. Res. *48*:549, 1981.
9. Staub, N. C.: Pulmonary edema due to increased microvascular permeability to fluid and protein. Circ. Res. *43*:143, 1978.
10. Ersalan, S., Turner, M. D., and Hardy, J. D.: Lymphatic regeneration following lung reimplantation in dogs. Surgery *56*:970, 1964.
11. Sampson, J. J., Leeds, S. E., Uhley, H. N., and Friedman, M.: The lymphatic system and pulmonary disease. *In* Mayerson, H. S. (ed.): Lymph and the Lymphatic System. Springfield, Ill., Charles C Thomas, 1968, p. 200.
12. Laine, G. A., Allen, S. J., Katz, J., Gabel, J. C., and Drake, R. E.: Effect of systemic venous pressure elevation on lymph flow and lung edema formation. J. Appl. Physiol. *61*:1634, 1986.
13. Bruderman, I., Somers, K., Hamilton, W. K., Tooley, W. H., and Butler, J.: Effect of surface tension on circulation in the excised lungs of dogs. J. Appl. Physiol. *19*:707, 1964.
14. Yoffey, J. M., and Courtice, F. C.: Lymphatics, Lymph and the Lymphomyeloid Complex. London, Academic Press, 1970.

15. Rusznyak, J., Földi, M., and Szabo, G.: Lymphatics and Lymph Circulation: Physiology and Pathology. 2nd ed. Oxford, Pergamon Press, 1967.
16. Hammersen, F.: Ultrastructure and functions of capillaries and lymphatics. Arch. Physiol. *336* (Suppl.):S43, 1972.
17. Casley-Smith, J. R.: The role of the endothelial intercellular junctions in the functioning of the initial lymphatics. Angiologica *9*:106, 1972.
18. Hall, J. G., Morris, B., and Wooley, G.: Intrinsic rhythmic propulsion of lymph in the unanesthetized sheep. J. Physiol. *180*:336, 1965.
19. Lambert, R. K., and Gremels, H.: On the factors concerned in the production of pulmonary edema. J. Physiol. (London) *61*:98, 1926.
20. Vanselow, K., and Heuck, F.: Theoretische Untersuchungen über eine Messmethode zur quantitativen Bestimmung des Wasser-Luft-Verhältnisses des Lungengewebes. Fortschr. Röntgenstr. *100*:441, 1964.
21. Ahluwalia, B. D., Brownell, G. L., Hales, C. A., and Kazemi, H.: An index of pulmonary edema measured with emission computed tomography. J. Comput. Assist. Tomogr. *5*:690, 1981.
22. Tripathi, A., Bydder, G. M., Hughes, J. M. B., Pennock, J. M., Goatcher, A., Orr, J. S., Steiner, R. E., and Greenspan, R. H.: Effect of oxygen tension on NMR spin-lattice relaxation rate of blood in vivo. Invest. Radiol. *19*:174, 1984.
23. Schmidt, H. C., Tsay, D. G., and Higgins, C. B.: Pulmonary edema: An MR study of permeability and hydrostatic types in animals. Radiology *158*:297, 1986.
24. Chinard, F. P.: Estimation of extravascular lung water by indicator-dilution techniques. Circ. Res. *37*:137, 1975.
25. Sibbald, W. J., Warshawski, F. J., Short, A. K., Harris, J., Lefcoe, M. S., and Holliday, R. L.: Clinical studies of measuring extravascular lung water by the thermal dye technique in critically ill patients. Chest *83*:725, 1983.
26. Fishman, A. P.: Pulmonary edema. *In* Fishman, A. P. (ed.): Pulmonary Diseases and Disorders. New York, McGraw-Hill Book Co., 1980, p. 733.
27. Staub, N. C., Nagano, H., and Pearce, M. L.: Pulmonary edema in dogs, especially the sequence of fluid accumulation in lungs. J. Appl. Physiol. *22*:227, 1967.
28. Agostoni, E.: Mechanics of the pleural space. Physiol. Rev. *52*:57, 1972.
29. West, J. B.: Ventilation Blood Flow and Gas Exchange. Oxford, Blackwell Scientific Publications, 1970.
30. Glazier, J. B., Hughes, J. M. B., Maloney, J. E., and West, J. B.: Measurements of capillary dimensions and blood volume in rapidly frozen lung. J. Appl. Physiol. *26*:65, 1969.
31. Dollery, C. T., Heimberg, P., and Hugh-Jones, P.: Relationships between blood flow and clearance rate of radioactive carbon dioxide and oxygen in normal and oedematous lungs. J. Physiol. (London) *162*:93, 1962.
32. Dawson, A.: Regional pulmonary blood flow in sitting and supine man during and after acute hypoxia. J. Clin. Invest. *48*:301, 1969.
33. Ritchie, B. C., Schauberger, G., and Staub, N. C.: Inadequacy of perivascular edema hypothesis to account for distribution of pulmonary blood flow in lung edema. Circ. Res. *24*:807, 1969.
34. Muir, A. L., Hogg, J. C., Naimark, A., Hall, D. L., and Chernecki, W.: Effect of alveolar liquid on distribution of blood flow in dog lungs. J. Appl. Physiol. *39*:885, 1975.

CLASSIFICATION OF PULMONARY EDEMA

35. Parker, F., Jr., and Weiss, S.: The nature and significance of the structural changes in the lungs in mitral stenosis. Am. J. Pathol. *12*:573, 1936.
36. Bernard, G. R., and Brigham, K. L.: Pulmonary edema. Pathophysiologic mechanisms and new approaches to therapy. Chest *89*:594, 1986.
37. Snapper, J. R., and Brigham, K. L.: Pulmonary edema. Hosp. Pract. *21*:87, 1986.
38. Sprung, C. L., Rackow, E. C., Fein, I. A., Jacob, A. I., and Isikoff, S. K.: The spectrum of pulmonary edema: Differentiation of cardiogenic, intermediate, and noncardiogenic forms of pulmonary edema. Ann. Rev. Respir. Dis. *124*:718, 1981.
39. Minnear, F. L., Barie, P. S., and Malik, A. B.: Effects of large, transient increases in pulmonary vascular pressures on lung fluid balance. J. Appl. Physiol. *55*:983, 1983.
40. Cross, C. E., Shaver, J. A., Wilson, R. J., and Robin, E. D.: Mitral stenosis and pulmonary fibrosis: Special reference to pulmonary edema and lung lymphatic function. Arch. Intern. Med. *125*:248, 1970.
41. Landolt, C. C., Matthay, M. A., Albertine, K. H., Roos, P. J., Wiener-Kronish, J. P., and Staub, N. C.: Overperfusion, hypoxia, and increased pressure cause only hydrostatic pulmonary edema in anesthetized sheep. Circ. Res. *52*:335, 1983.
42. Hultgren, H. N., and Grover, R. F.: Circulatory adaptation to high altitude. Annu. Rev. Med. *19*:119, 1968.
43. Albers, W. H., and Nadas, A. S.: Unilateral chronic pulmonary edema and pleural effusion after systemic-pulmonary arterial shunts for cyanotic congenital heart disease. Am. J. Cardiol. *19*:861, 1967.
44. Kramer, G. C., Harms, B.A., Gunther, R. A., Renkin, E. M., and Demling, R. H.: The effects of hypoproteinemia on blood-to-lymph fluid transport in sheep lung. Circ. Res. *49*:1173, 1981.
45. Trapnell, D. H., and Thurston, J. G. B.: Unilateral pulmonary oedema after pleural aspiration. Lancet *1*:1367, 1970.
46. Loyd, J. E., Nolop, K. B., Parker, R. E., Roselli, R. J., and Brigham, K. L.: Effects of inspiratory resistance loading on lung fluid balance in awake sheep. J. Appl. Physiol. *60*:198, 1986.
47. Scharf, S. M., Caldini P., and Ingram, R. H., Jr.: Cardiovascular effects of increasing airway pressure. Am. J. Physiol. *1*:35, 1977.
48. Scharf, S. M., Brown, R., Saunders, N. A., Green, L. H., and Ingram, R. H., Jr.: Changes in left ventricular size and configuration with positive end-expiratory pressure. Circ. Res. *44*:672, 1979.
49. Scharf, S. M., and Brown, R.: Influence of the right ventricle on canine left ventricular function with PEEP. J. Appl. Physiol. *52*:254, 1982.
50. Malik, A. B., and Staub, N. C. (eds.): Mechanisms of Lung Microvascular Injury. New York, New York Academy of Sciences, 1982.
51. Staub, N. C.: Pulmonary edema due to increased microvascular permeability. Ann. Rev. Med. *32*:291, 1981.
52. Carlson, R. W., Schaeffer, R. C., Jr., Puri, V. K., Brennan, A. P., and Weil, M. H.: Hypovolemia and permeability pulmonary edema associated with anaphylaxis. Crit. Care Med. *9*:883, 1981.
53. Ashbaugh, D. G., Bigelow, D. B., Petty, T. L., and Levine, B. E.: Acute respiratory distress in adults. Lancet *2*:319, 1967.
54. Snell, J. D., Jr., and Ramsey, L. H.: Pulmonary edema as a result of endotoxemia. Am. J. Physiol. *217*:170, 1969.
55. Ratliff, N. B., Wilson, J. W., Horckel, D. B., and Martin, A. M., Jr.: The lung in hemorrhagic shock. II. Observations on alveolar and vascular ultrastructure. Am. J. Pathol. *58*:353, 1970.
56. Henning, R. J., Heyman, V., Alcover, I., and Romeo, S.: Cardiopulmonary effects of oleic acid-induced pulmonary edema and mechanical ventilation. Anesth. Analg. *65*:925, 1986.
57. Glauser, F. L., Fairman, R. P., Miller, J. E., and Falls, R. K.: Indomethacin blunts ethchloryne induced pulmonary hypertension but not pulmonary edema. J. Appl. Physiol. *53*:563, 1982.
58. Havill, A. M., Gee, M. H., Washburne, J. D., Premkumar, A., Ottaviano, R., and Flynn, J. T.: Alpha naphthyl thiourea produces dose dependent lung vascular injury in sheep. Am. J. Physiol. *243*:505, 1982.
59. Weinberg, P. F., Mathey, M. A., Webster, R. O., Roskos, K. V., Goldstein, R. M., and Murray, J. F.: Biologically active products of complement in acute lung injury in patients with sepsis syndrome. Am. Rev. Resp. Dis. *130*:791, 1984.
60. Rinaldo, J. E., Dauber, G. H., Christman, J., and Rogers, R. M.: Neutrophil alveolitis endotoxemia. Am. Rev. Respir. Dis. *130*:1065, 1984.
61. Biermann, G. J., Dockey, B. F., and Thrall, R. S.: Polymorphonuclear leukocyte participation in acute oleic acid induced lung injury. Am. Rev. Respir. Dis. *128*:845, 1983.
62. Taylor, R. G., McCall, C. E., Thrall, R. S., Woodruff, R. D., and O'Flaherty, J. T.: Histological features of PMA-induced lung injury. Lab. Invest. *52*:61, 1985.
63. Kapanci, Y., Weibel, E. R., Kaplan, H. P., and Robinson, P. V. M.: Pathogenesis and reversibility of the pulmonary lesions of oxygen toxicity in monkey. II. Ultrastructural and morphometric studies. Lab. Invest. *20*:101, 1969.
64. Cameron, G. R., and Courtice, F. C.: The production and removal of oedema fluid in the lungs after exposure to carbonyl chloride (phosgene). J. Physiol. (London) *105*:175, 1946.
65. Bils, R. F.: Ultrastructural alterations of alveolar tissue of mice. III. Ozone. Arch. Environ. Health *20*:468, 1970.
66. Sherwin, R. P., and Richters, V.: Lung capillary permeability: nitrogen dioxide exposure and leakage of tritiated serum. Arch. Intern. Med. *128*:61, 1971.
67. Schoene, R. B., Hackett, P. H., Henderson, W. R., Sage, E. H., Chow, M., Roach, R. C., Mills, W. J., Jr., and Martin, T. R.: High-altitude pulmonary edema. Characteristics of lung lavage fluid. J.A.M.A. *256*:63, 1986.
68. Gelb, A. F., and Klein, E.: Hemodynamic and alveolar protein studies in non-cardiac pulmonary edema. Am. Rev. Respir. Dis. *114*:831, 1976.
69. Sprung, C. L., Rackow, E. C., Fein, I. A., Jacob, A. I., and Isikoff, S. K.: The spectrum of pulmonary edema: differentiation of cardiogenic, intermediate, and noncardiogenic forms of pulmonary edema. Am. Rev. Respir. Dis. *124*:718, 1981.
70. Robin, E. D., Carey, L. C., Grenvik, A., Glauser, F., and Gaudio, R.: Capillary leak syndrome with pulmonary edema. Arch. Intern. Med. *130*:66, 1972.
71. Brady, J. S., Vaccara, C. A., Hill, N. S., and Rounds, S.: Binding of charged ferritin to alveolar wall components and charge selectivity of macromolecular transport in permeability pulmonary edema in rats. Circ. Res. *55*:155, 1984.
72. Pattle, R. E.: Properties, function, and origin of the alveolar lining layer. Nature (London) *175*:1125, 1955.
73. Said, S. I., Avery, M. E., Davis, R. K., Banjaree, C. M., and El-Gohar, M.: Pulmonary surface activity in induced pulmonary edema. J. Clin. Invest. *44*:458, 1965.
74. Miller, W. W., Waldhausen, J. A., and Rashkind, W. J.: Comparison of oxygen poisoning of the lung in cyanotic and acyanotic dogs. N. Engl. J. Med. *282*:943, 1970.
75. Henry, J. N.: The effect of shock on pulmonary alveolar surfactant. Its role in refractory respiratory insufficiency of the critically ill or severely injured patient. J. Trauma *8*:756, 1968.
76. Repine, J. E., Bowman, C. M., and Tate, R. M.: Neutrophils and lung edema. Chest *81*(Suppl.):5, 1982.
77. Glauser, F. L., and Fairman, R. P.: The uncertain role of the neutrophil in increased permeability pulmonary edema. Chest *88*:601, 1985.
78. Dyer, E. L., and Snapper, J. R.: Role of circulating granulocytes in sheep lung injury produced by phorbol myristate acetate. J. Appl. Physiol. *60*:576, 1986.
79. Rinaldo, J. E., and Rogers, R. M.: Adult respiratory-distress syndrome: Changing concepts of lung injury and repair. N. Engl. J. Med. *306*:900, 1982.
80. Brigham, K. L., Loyd, J. E., Newman, J. H., Snapper, J. R., Ogletree, M. L., and English, D. K.: Granulocytes in acute lung vascular injury in unanesthetized sheep. Chest *81*(Suppl.):5, 1982.
81. Lee, C. T., Fein, A. M., Lippman, M., Holtzman, H., Kimbel, P., and Weinbaum, G.: Elastolytic activity in pulmonary lavage fluid from patients with adult respiratory distress syndrome. N. Engl. J. Med. *304*:192, 1981.
82. Cohen, A. B., and Cochrane, C. G.: Studies on the pathogenesis of the adult respiratory distress syndrome. J. Clin. Invest. *69*:543, 1982.

83. Welland, J. E., David, W. B., Holter, J. F., Mohammed, J. R., Dorinsky, P. M., and Gadek, J. E.: Lung neutrophils in ARDS: Clinical and pathological significance. Am. Rev. Respir. Dis. *133*:218, 1986.
84. Hammerschmidt, D. E., Weaver, L. J., Hudson, L. D., Craddock, P. R., and Jacob, H. S.: Association of complement activation and elevated plasma-C5a with adult respiratory distress syndrome: Pathophysiological relevance and possible prognostic value. Lancet *1*:947, 1980.
85. Magno, M., and Szidon, J. P.: Hemodynamic pulmonary edema in dogs with acute and chronic lymphatic ligation. Am. J. Physiol. *231*:1777, 1976.
86. Trapnell, D. H.: Radiological appearances of lymphangitis carcinomatosa of the lung. Thorax *19*:251, 1964.
87. Hall, J. G., Morris, B., and Wooley, G.: Intrinsic rhythmic propulsion of lymph in the unanesthetized sheep. J. Physiol. (London) *180*:336, 1965.
88. Permutt, S.: Mechanical influences on water accumulation in the lungs. *In* Fishman, A. P., and Renkin, E. M. (eds.): Pulmonary Edema. Bethesda, American Physiological Society, 1979, p. 175.
89. Naeije, R., Melot, C., and Lejeune, P.: Hypoxic pulmonary vasoconstriction and high altitude pulmonary edema. Am. Rev. Respir. Dis. *134*:332, 1986.
90. Sophocles, A. M., Jr.: High-altitude pulmonary edema in Vail, Colorado, 1975–1982. West. J. Med. *144*:569, 1986.
91. Lockhart, A., and Saiag, B.: Altitude and the human pulmonary circulation. Clin. Sci. *60*:599, 1981.
92. Hultgren, H. N.: High altitude pulmonary edema. Adv. Cardiol. *5*:24, 1970.
93. Harris, P., and Heath, D.: The pulmonary circulation at high altitude. *In* The Human Pulmonary Circulation. 3rd ed. New York, Churchill Livingstone, 1986, pp. 499–503.
94. Hultgren, H. N., Lopez, C. E., Lundberg, E., and Miller, H.: Physiologic studies of pulmonary edema at high altitude. Circulation *29*:393, 1964.
95. Whayne, T. F., Jr., and Severinghaus, J. W.: Experimental hypoxic pulmonary edema in the rat. J. Appl. Physiol. *25*:279, 1968.
96. Goodale, R. L., Goetzman, B., and Visscher, M. B.: Hypoxia and iodoacetic acid and alveolo-capillary membrane permeability to albumin. Am. J. Physiol. *219*:1226, 1970.
97. Gray, G. W., Bryan, A. C., Freedman, M. H., Houston, C. S., Lewis, W. F., McFadden, D. M., and Newell, G.: Effect of altitude exposure on platelets. J. Appl. Physiol. *39*:648, 1975.
98. Grover, R. F., Hyers, R. M., McCurty, I. F., and Reeves, J. T.: High-altitude pulmonary edema. *In* Fishman, A. P., and Renkin, E. M. (eds.): Pulmonary Edema. Bethesda, American Physiological Society, 1979, p. 229.
99. Yabumoto, M., Kuriyama, T., Iwamoto, M., and Kinoshita, T.: Neurogenic pulmonary edema associated with ruptured intracranial aneurysm: Case report. Neurosurgery *19*:300, 1986.
100. Cameron, G. R., and De, S. N.: Experimental pulmonary oedema of nervous origin. J. Pathol. Bacteriol. *61*:375, 1949.
101. Sarnoff, S. J., and Sarnoff, L. C.: Neurohemodynamics of pulmonary edema. II. The role of sympathetic pathways in the elevation of pulmonary and systemic vascular pressures following the intracisternal injection of fibrin. Circulation *6*:51, 1952.
102. Theodore, J., and Robin, E. D.: Speculations on neurogenic pulmonary edema (NPE). Am. Rev. Respir. Dis. *113*:405, 1976.
103. Wray, N. P., and Nicotra, M. B.: Pathogenesis of neurogenic pulmonary edema. Am. Rev. Respir. Dis. *118*:783, 1978.
104. Hakim, T. S., van der Zee, H., and Malik, A. B.: Effects of sympathetic nerve stimulation on lung fluid and protein exchange. J. Appl. Physiol. *47*:1025, 1979.
105. Simon, R. P., Bayne, L. L., Tranbaugh, R. F., and Lewis, F. R.: Elevated pulmonary lymph flow and protein content during status epilepticus in sheep. J. Appl. Physiol. *52*:91, 1982.
106. Malik, A. B.: Mechanisms of neurogenic pulmonary edema. Circ. Res. *57*:1, 1985.
107. Steinberg, A. D., and Karliner, J. S.: The clinical spectrum of heroin pulmonary edema. Arch. Intern. Med. *122*:122, 1968.
108. Fraser, D. W.: Methadone overdose: Illicit use of pharmaceutically prepared narcotics. J.A.M.A. *217*:1387, 1971.
109. Bogartz, L. J., and Miller, W. C.: Pulmonary edema associated with propoxyphene intoxication. J.A.M.A. *215*:259, 1971.
110. Richter, R. W., Baden, M. N., and Pearson, J.: Cerebral edema seen in many "sudden death" heroin victims. J.A.M.A. *212*:967, 1970.
111. Jaffe, J. H.: Narcotic analgesics. *In* Goodman, L. S., and Gilman, A. (eds.): The Pharmacological Basis of Therapeutics. 4th ed. New York, Macmillan, 1970, p. 237.
112. Katz, S., Aberman, A., Frand, U. I., Stein, I. M., and Fulop, M.: Heroin pulmonary edema: Evidence for increased pulmonary capillary permeability. Am. Rev. Respir. Dis. *106*:472, 1972.
113. Gopinathan, K., Saroja, D., Spears, J. R., Gelb, A., and Emmanuel, G. E.: Hemodynamic studies in heroin induced acute pulmonary edema. Circulation *42* (Suppl. 3):44, 1970.
114. Brashear, R. E., Kelly, M. T., and White, A. C.: Elevated plasma histamine after heroin and morphine. J. Lab. Clin. Med. *83*:451, 1974.
115. Malik, A. B., Tahamont, M. V., Minnear, F. L., Johnson, A., and Kaplan, J. E.: Lung fluid and protein exchange after pulmonary vascular thrombosis. Chest *81*:5, 1982.
116. Johnson, A., and Malik, A. B.: Effect of defibrinogenation on lung water accumulation after pulmonary microembolism in dogs. J. Appl. Physiol. *49*:841, 1980.
117. Flick, M. R., Perel, A., and Staub, N. C.: Leukocytes are required for increased lung microvascular permeability after microembolization in sheep. Circ. Res. *48*:344, 1981.
118. Rovinsky, J. J., and Guttmacher, A. F.: Medical, Surgical, and Gynecologic Complications of Pregnancy. 2nd ed. Baltimore, Williams and Wilkins Co., 1965.
119. Goldbaum, T. S., Bacos, J. M., and Lindsay, J., Jr.: Pulmonary edema following conversion of tachyarrhythmia. Chest *89*:465, 1986.
120. Cooperman, L. H., and Price, H. L.: Pulmonary edema in the operative and postoperative period: A review of 40 cases. Ann. Surg. *172*:883, 1970.
121. Hashim, S. E., Kay, H. R., Hammond, G. L., Kopf, G. S., and Geha, A. S.: Noncardiac pulmonary edema after cardiopulmonary bypass. Am. J. Surg. *147*:560, 1984.
122. Culliford, A. T., Thomas, S., and Spencer, F. C.: Fulminating noncardiogenic pulmonary edema: A newly recognized hazard during cardiac operations. J. Thorac. Cardiovasc. Surg. *80*:868, 1980.
123. Teichmann, V., Jezek, V., and Herles, F.: Relevance of width of right descending branch of pulmonary artery as a radiological sign of pulmonary hypertension. Thorax *25*:91, 1970.
124. Hogg, J. C., Agarawal, J. B., Gardiner, A. J. S., Palmer, W. H., and Macklem, P. T.: Distribution of airway resistance with developing pulmonary edema in dogs. J. Appl. Physiol. *32*:20, 1972.
125. DeTroyer, A., Yernault, J., and Englert, M.: Mechanics of breathing in patients with atrial septal defect. Am. Rev. Respir. Dis. *115*:413, 1977.
126. Murray, J. F.: The lungs and heart failure. Hosp. Prac. *20*:55, 1985.
127. Fillmore, S. J., Giumaraes, A. C., Scheidt, S. S., and Killip, T.: Blood gas changes and pulmonary hemodynamics following acute myocardial infarction. Circulation *45*:583, 1972.
128. Aberman, A., and Fulop, M.: The metabolic and respiratory acidosis of acute pulmonary edema. Ann. Intern. Med. *76*:173, 1972.
129. Richeson, J. F., Paulshock, C., and Yu, P. N.: Non-hydrostatic pulmonary edema after coronary artery ligation in dogs. Circ. Res. *50*:301, 1982.
130. Timmis, A. D., Fowler, M. B., Burwood, R. J., Gishen, P., Vincent, R., and Chamberlain, D. A.: Pulmonary oedema without critical increase in left atrial pressure in acute myocardial infarction. Br. Med. J. *283*:636, 1981.
131. Donat, W. E., and Weiner, B. H.: Syndromes of left ventricular failure. *In* Rippe, J. M., Irwin, R. S., and Alpert, J. S. (eds.): Intensive Care of Medicine. Boston, Little, Brown and Co., 1985, pp. 322–336.
132. Vismara, L. A., Leaman, D. M., and Zelis, R.: The effects of morphine on venous tone in patients with acute pulmonary edema. Circulation *54*:335, 1976.
133. Iff, H. W., and Flenley, D. C.: Blood-gas exchange after furosemide in acute pulmonary edema. Lancet *1*:616, 1971.
134. Scheinman, M., Brown, M., and Rapaport, E.: Hemodynamic effects of ethacrynic acid in patients with refractory acute left ventricular failure. Am. J. Med. *50*:291, 1971.
135. Dikshit, K., Vyden, J. K., Forrester, J. S., Chatterjee, K., Prakash, R., and Swan, H. J. C.: Renal and extrarenal hemodynamic effects of furosemide in congestive heart failure after acute myocardial infarction. N. Engl. J. Med. *288*:1087, 1973.
136. Wilson, J. R., Reichek, N., Dunkman, W. B., and Goldberg, S.: Effect of diuresis on the performance of the failing left ventricle in man. Am. J. Med. *70*:234, 1981.
137. Mitenko, P. A., and Ogilvie, R. I.: Rational intravenous doses of theophylline. N. Engl. J. Med. *289*:600, 1973.
138. Tai, E., and Read, J.: Response of blood gas tensions to aminophylline and isoprenaline in patients with asthma. Thorax *22*:543, 1967.
139. Goldberger, J. J., Peled, H. B., Stroh, J. A., Cohen, M. N., and Frishman, W. H.: Prognostic factors in acute pulmonary edema. Arch. Intern. Med. *146*:489, 1986.
140. Hildner, F. J.: Pulmonary edema associated with low left ventricular filling pressures. Am. J. Cardiol. *44*:1410, 1979.
141. Rizk, N. W., and Murray, J. F.: PEEP and pulmonary edema. Am. J. Med. *72*:381, 1982.
142. Pepe, P. E., Hudson, L. D., and Carrico, C. J.: Early application of PEEP in patients at risk for the adult respiratory distress syndrome. N. Engl. J. Med. *311*:281, 1984.
143. Cassidy, S. S., and Mitchell, J. H.: Effects of positive pressure breathing on right and left ventricular preload and afterload. Fed. Proc. *40*:2178, 1981.
144. Jardin, F., Farcot, J.-C., Boisante, L., Curien, N., Margairaz, A., and Bourdarias, J.-P.: Influence of positive end-expiratory pressure on left ventricular performance. N. Engl. J. Med. *304*:387, 1981.
145. Lorell, B. H., Palacios, I., Daggett, W. M., Jacobs, M. L., Fowler, B. N., and Newell, J. B.: Right ventricular distension and left ventricular compliance. Am. J. Physiol. *240*:H87, 1981.
146. Wead, W. B., and Norton, J. F.: Effects of intrapleural pressure changes on canine left ventricular function. J. Appl. Physiol. *50*:1027, 1981.
147. Fewell, J. E., Abendschein, D. R., Carlson, C. J., Rapaport, E., and Murray, J. F.: Continuous positive-pressure ventilation does not alter ventricular pressure-volume relationship. Am. J. Physiol. *240*:H821, 1981.
148. Pontoppidan, H., Wilson, R. S., Rie, M. A., and Schneider, R. C.: Respiratory intensive care. Anesthesiology *47*:96, 1977.
149. Prewitt, R. M., McCarthy, J., and Wood, L. D. H.: Treatment of acute low pressure pulmonary edema in dogs: Relative effects of hydrostatic and oncotic pressure, nitroprusside, and positive end-expiratory pressure. J. Clin. Invest. *67*:409, 1981.
150. Lowe, R. J., and Moss, G. S.: Pulmonary failure after trauma. Surg. Annu. *8*:63, 1976.
151. Tullis, J. L.: Albumin. I. Background and use. J.A.M.A. *237*:355 and 460, 1977.
152. Andreadis, N., and Petty, T. L.: Adult respiratory distress syndrome: Problems and prognosis. Am. Rev. Respir. Dis. *132*:1344, 1985.

19 ACUTE CIRCULATORY FAILURE (SHOCK)

by MAX HARRY WEIL, M.D., Ph.D.,
MARTIN von PLANTA, M.D., and
ERIC C. RACKOW, M.D.

PATHOPHYSIOLOGY

DEFINITIONS

Acute circulatory failure, for purposes of this chapter, encompasses the syndromes associated with an acute reduction in effective blood flow with failure to maintain the transport and delivery of essential substrates to sustain the function of vital organ systems.[1, 2] The fully developed syndrome is clinically recognized as circulatory shock. There is usually little controversy regarding the serious clinical status of the patient who presents with prostration, hypotension, pallor, coldness and moistness of the skin, collapse of superficial veins, suppression of the formation of urine, and mental obtundation. The term "shock" of itself is descriptive of these signs and spotlights the dire threat of a critical reduction in systemic blood flow.

A WORKING MODEL OF THE CIRCULATION

For purposes of defining primary hemodynamic mechanisms of circulatory shock and implications for its management, conceptualization of a simple working model of the circulatory system is likely to be helpful (Fig. 19–1). Eight primary components of the circulatory system may be identified. The first component is the *intravascular volume*, which moderates the venous return or preload. The second, the *heart*, serves as the pump and provides contractile power for circulation. Contractility, rate (and rhythm), and loading conditions determine cardiac output (p. 404). Third is the *resistance circuit*, which includes the arteries and arterioles. It is the mainstream by which blood is carried from the heart to the capillary beds; changes in arteriolar resistance moderate the afterload on the heart. The fourth component is the *capillary exchange bed*, a largely passive circuit which provides for exchange of fluid and metabolites between the intravascular and extravascular compartments. The fifth is the *venous resistance bed*, which includes the postcapillary venules and probably the small veins. Blood flow through the capillary bed and both fluid and substrate filtration between the intravascular and interstitial fluid compartments are largely regulated by humoral and neurogenic controls on precapillary arterioles and postcapillary venules.[3–6] The sixth component is represented by *metarterioles* that bridge the arterial resistance and postcapillary venous vessels. Blood may be shunted through these vessels from the resistance to the capacitance circuits.[7, 8] It thereby bypasses the capillary exchange vessels. The seventh extends from the medium-sized veins to the large veins including the cavae. This venous capacitance bed acts as the primary storage reservoir for the intravascular compartment. Approximately 70 to 80 per cent of the total blood volume is contained within the venous capacitance bed.[9, 10] Changes in venous compliance moderate venous capacitance. This,

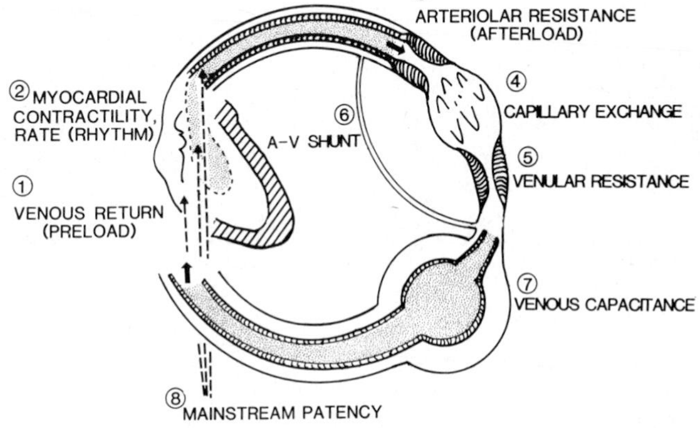

FIGURE 19–1. Functional components of the circulatory system of import in the regulation of systemic perfusion.

in turn, regulates the "effective circulating volume" and therefore the venous return of blood to the heart. Accordingly, it is the major determinant of preload. The eighth component represents obstruction in the mainstream of blood flow. Such obstruction may be due to vena caval or pericardial compression, intracardiac or pulmonary obstruction, or dissection or compression of the aorta.

The eight discrete *hemodynamic defects* which may account for perfusion failure are listed in Table 19–1. These include (1) critical reductions in the volume of fluid contained within the vascular compartment because of loss of red cells, plasma water, plasma protein, and/or electrolytes; (2) pump failure and, more specifically, failure of the contractile capacity of the heart and/or defects in rate or rhythm of the heart so that it no longer serves as an effective pump; (3) excessive resistance in the arterial circuit such that impedance to left ventricular outflow is increased and capillary blood flow may be reduced by arteriolar constriction; (4) impaired delivery and removal of vital substrates in the capillary exchange vessels; (5) excessive resistance in the postcapillary venous bed by which capillary hydrostatic pressure may be increased; (6) shunting of blood through arteriovenous communications or through capillary vessels that no longer function as effective exchange vessels; (7) pooling of blood in an expanded venous capacitance bed such that venous return and therefore preload are decreased; and (8) obstruction to the mainstream of blood flow through the central circuit. One or more of these hemodynamic mechanisms account for the clinical signs of circulatory shock.

HEMODYNAMIC PARAMETERS

The parameters which indicate the hemodynamic status of the patient during circulatory shock include heart rate, rhythm, and cardiac output. Central venous and right atrial pressure reflect the right ventricular filling pressure; and pulmonary artery occlusion or left atrial pressure is a measure of left ventricular filling pressure. The ratio of arterial (and pulmonary artery) pressure to cardiac output reflects systemic (and pulmonary) vascular resistance. When changes in venous pressure are related to changes in intravascular volume during fluid infusion, they reflect both venous capacitance and ventricular function. The ventricular systolic and diastolic volumes, and consequently ventricular ejection fractions, together with corresponding pressures reflect cardiac performance.[11–14]

TRANSPORT OF SUBSTRATES. Oxygen is the most critical substrate.[15–17] Mitochondrial function is obligatorily aerobic and the regeneration of high-energy phosphates cannot be sustained, except for brief periods, by anaerobic pathways. This emergency pathway yields lactic acid as an end product. Accordingly, critical reduction in tissue perfusion, and the consequent reduction in oxygen delivery, is accompanied by production of lactate, which is rapidly distributed throughout body water.

TABLE 19–1 HEMODYNAMIC MECHANISMS OF SHOCK

1. Reduction in intravascular volume
2. Heart (pump) failure
3. Increased arterial resistance
4. Impaired capillary exchange
5. Excessive resistance in postcapillary venules and small veins
6. Arteriovenous shunting
7. Pooling in the venous capacitance circuit
8. Obstruction to mainstream

ARTERIAL PRESSURE

Before the 1960's, before invasive hemodynamic measurements were adapted for bedside use, the indirect (cuff) measurement of blood pressure was accepted as the primary objective measurement of the presence and severity of clinical shock states. After measurements of blood flow and particularly cardiac output became available to the clinician, the blood pressure measurement was no longer the sole, or even the predominant, indicator of perfusion failure.[18–20] Substantial reductions in arterial pressure to levels of less than 90 mm Hg were recognized, in some circumstances, as relatively benign reductions in arterial resistance without impairment in perfusion.[21] In addition, the indirect measurement of blood pressure lacked precision in patients with low-flow states.[22] With the possible exception of patients with hyperdynamic septic shock, circulatory shock is characterized by marked increases in both neurogenic and humoral adrenergic vasoconstriction. Such increases in vascular resistance to blood flow in muscular arteries of the extremities reduce the accuracy of both auscultatory and palpable blood pressure.

The pulsatile ejection of left ventricular stroke volume is the hemodynamic event which normally produces the Korotkoff sounds in the brachial artery. When stroke volume is reduced and arterial resistance in the brachial artery increases, the Korotkoff sounds are critically decreased.[22] As a rule, arterial pressure is considerably

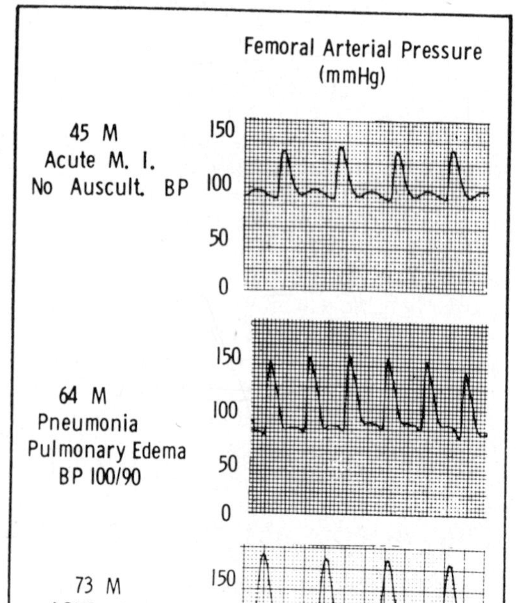

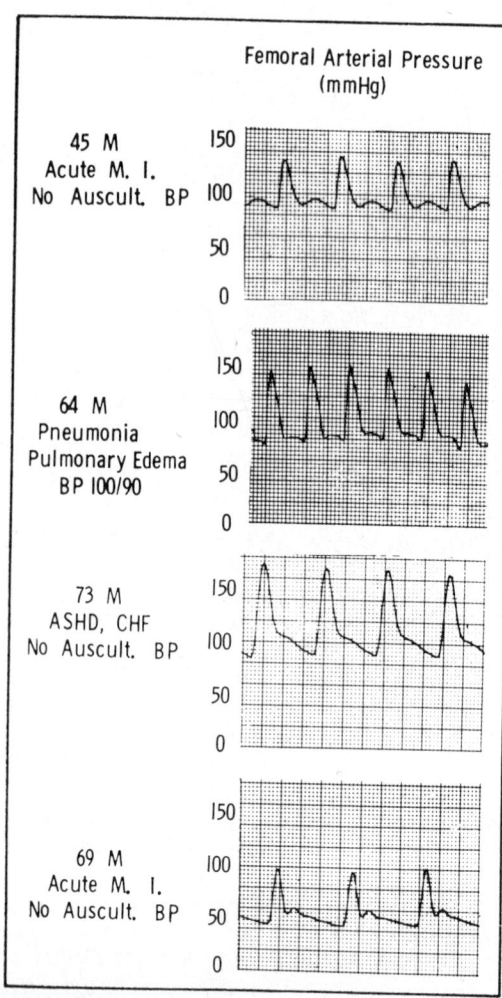

FIGURE 19–2. Differences between auscultatory and intraaortic measurements of blood pressure during circulatory shock. (From Cohn, J. N.: Blood pressure measurement in shock: Mechanism of inaccuracy in auscultatory and palpatory methods. J.A.M.A. *199*:118, 1967. Copyright 1967, American Medical Association.)

greater than would be indicated by the cuff pressure under conditions of decreased blood flow and increased arterial resistance (Fig. 19–2). This applies to measurements obtained by auscultation or palpation. Even with Doppler techniques of indirect measurement, a substantial discrepancy between intraarterial and cuff blood pressure should be anticipated.[23] For these reasons, intraarterial rather than cuff blood pressure is now routinely monitored in patients with circulatory shock. Substantial gradients of pressure may be observed during the low perfusion state between the aorta and distal arteries of extremities. For instance, systolic pressure gradients in excess of 40 mm Hg have been documented between the aorta and a radial artery. Even the more precise measurement of intraarterial pressure is viewed as an indication of arterial side wall pressure at the site of measurement and interpreted in close relationship to concurrent clinical signs and measurements of perfusion.

BLOOD FLOW AND PERFUSION

Among quantitative measurements of flow, the principal measurement is cardiac output.[24] Peripheral perfusion may be estimated by measurements of skin temperature, especially the temperature of the great toe,[25] and by transcutaneous and conjunctival oxygen tension.[26] Blood lactate provides a practical measure of the metabolic severity of the perfusion deficit, and the blood level of lactate now constitutes the single best measurement of systemic perfusion deficits[27] (p. 565).

CLINICOPATHOPHYSIOLOGICAL CORRELATIONS

The clinical signs of shock reflect decreases in blood flow. A decrease in mental alertness is related to decrease in the cerebral blood flow. Cold, pale, and clammy skin together with cyanotic distal extremities, the earlobes, and the tip of the nose reflect a combination of reduced skin blood flow and excessive adrenergic activity. An important exception is "*warm shock*" of the hyperdynamic septic state, which is characterized by a marked reduction in peripheral arterial resistance.[28] However, it shares with other types of shock a reduction in cerebral, renal, and coronary blood flow with altered mental alertness, reduced urine flow, and electrocardiographic abnormalities. Electrocardiographic signs of myocardial ischemia are not of themselves indicative of the primary cardiac cause of shock, particularly in elderly patients with noncritical coronary artery disease. Both ST and T-wave changes stem from a reduction in regional blood flow like that of reduced cerebral and renal blood flow and impaired skin perfusion.[29, 30]

To the extent that circulatory shock, regardless of cause, represents a generalized defect of perfusion, the pathophysiological processes that stem therefrom may be discussed as a group. Excepted are the more transient low-flow (hypotensive) states which account for syncopal episodes; these are addressed separately (Chap. 29).

In translating concepts of circulatory shock derived from the animal laboratory, the clinician must do so with an awareness of the large number of variables which moderate the shock insult. For instance, observations made on the low-flow state which stems from hypovolemia cannot be directly translated to the low-flow state which stems from cardiac failure, bacterial infection, or mechanical obstruction to blood flow. Even within the gamut of septic shock states, there are substantial differences in the pathophysiology and clinical manifestations of shock states produced by various gram-positive and gram-negative organisms. Moreover, even a single bacterial species may provoke different pathophysiological effects dependent on whether shock is produced by spontaneous infection, the infusion of live bacteria into the bloodstream, or the injection of bacterial toxins. For instance, the high-output state characteristic of septic shock cannot be readily duplicated by the injection of gram-negative endotoxin.

There are also substantial differences between animal species. The major target organ of endotoxin in the dog is the gastrointestinal tract, and particularly the liver, whereas it is the lung in the cat. Neither the gastrointestinal tract nor the lung is a major shock organ in the primate.

Age and even sex differences are of significance.[28, 31] Circulatory shock in the newborn is frequently associated with bacteremia caused by gram-negative bacilli. This susceptibility continues until the age of approximately 3 months. However, the incidence of shock caused by gram-negative bacteremia is relatively low until ages 35 to 40. The endocrine, immunological, and neurological status of the patient is also of importance. During pregnancy or in the immunosuppressed patient, this age-related protection is lost.[32] Neural blockade, anesthesia, and alpha-adrenoceptor blockade decrease the severity and improve the prognosis of experimental shock states.[33]

HEMODYNAMIC ALTERATIONS

When the cardiac output declines, there is a redistribution of blood flow. Coronary and cerebral blood flow are protected. However, alpha-adrenergic arterial constriction accounts for a reduction in cutaneous, voluntary muscle, splanchnic, and renal blood flows.[5, 34] Decreases in the perfusion of the kidney and the gut account for ischemic injury to these organs. In patients with septic shock, pulmonary arteriovenous shunts appear.[35] When cardiac output is increased by augmenting preload or by the administration of inotropic or vasodilator drugs, such shunts owing to mismatching of ventilation and pulmonary blood flow are further augmented.[36] Increases in sympathetic autonomic function account for arterial vasoconstriction. Arterial constriction is accompanied by alpha-adrenergically induced post-capillary venular constriction. The net effect is an increase in capillary hydrostatic pressure which explains an egress of plasma water during low-flow, high-resistance states (Fig. 19–3). This explains the decrease in intravascular volume and hemoconcentration which follows shock, regardless of cause. Such volume depletion is also observed after the administration of exogenous alpha-adrenergic agonists and, in the clinical setting, in patients with catecholamine excess owing to pheo-

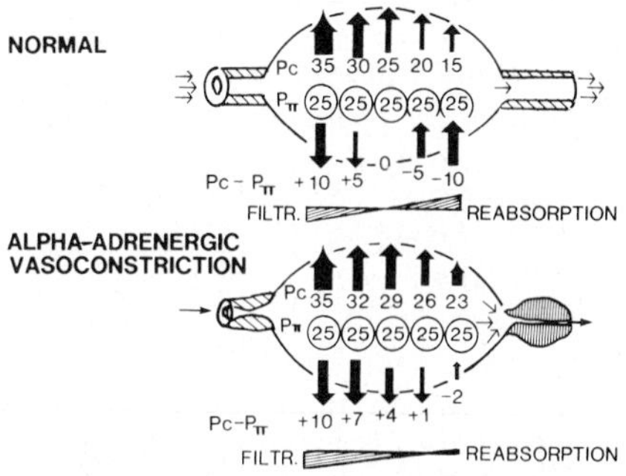

FIGURE 19–3. Depletion in plasma water during the course of circulatory shock is related to increases in capillary hydrostatic pressure. These are attributed to alpha-adrenergically primed increases in venular resistance which override effects of arteriolar vasoconstriction.

chromocytomas.[37] Alpha-adrenoceptor agents such as phentolamine reverse the process and increase intravascular volume.[38]

Intravascular volume is also moderated by neuroendocrine responses involving ventricular afferent nerves and stretch receptors in the atria and cava, in part acting through the Bainbridge reflex.[39] Reductions in renal blood flow prompt increases in intravascular volume by the secretion of renin and in turn angiotensin and aldosterone. Water may also be retained because of increased secretion of antidiuretic hormone (ADH).[40] In addition to the effects of epinephrine, norepinephrine, and angiotensin, there is increased secretion of vasopressin.[40, 41] Prostaglandins have also been implicated.[42] No significant role for atrial natriuretic factor (p. 1831) is currently recognized.[43]

MYOCARDIAL FUNCTION

Decreases in coronary perfusion are minimized by increases in diastolic aortic pressure owing to peripheral vasoconstriction. The distribution of myocardial blood flow is altered. Intramural coronary arteries penetrate perpendicularly from the epicardium to the ventricular wall. When coronary pressure and flow are reduced, there is a substantial decrease in blood flow to the endocardium.[44] This may account for myocyte necrosis and hemorrhage in the subendocardium, which frequently occur during shock states regardless of cause.[45] Such hemorrhages appear in the absence of coronary artery disease in both laboratory animals and humans. They are also observed after excessive endogenous catecholamine stimulation or exogenous administration of alpha-adrenergic vasopressor agents.[46–48] Experimentally, such lesions may also be prevented by adrenoceptor blockade.[49]

So-called irreversibility of both hemorrhagic and septic shock has been attributed to a large number of metabolic and circulatory mechanisms, but especially to a cardiac mechanism.[50, 51] The evidence implicating myocardial depression during shock states is rather secure. Gram-negative endotoxins reduce left ventricular performance.[52] However, the assumption that this is entirely explained by decreases in coronary perfusion pressure and coronary blood flow has not been sustained. Myocardial oxygen availability is sharply reduced only as a late event.[53]

Reductions in left ventricular ejection fraction and ventricular dilation occur in the absence of reductions in coronary perfusion pressure or coronary flow.[14, 54] The extent to which one or more humoral factors account for such decreases in myocardial function is unsettled.[55–57] The myocardial depressant factor described by Lefer[55] is believed to be a small peptide produced by lysosomal hydrolases in ischemic pancreas. Goldfarb[56] implicated L-leucine as a cardiodepressant during shock. A high-molecular-weight cardiodepressive has also been described.[57] Its effects are reversed by intravenous infusion of a glucose-insulin-potassium mixture.[57] Perhaps most persuasive have been the recent investigations by Parrillo and his associates,[58] who identified a myocardial depressant substance in the serum of patients with septic shock. Decreases in ejection fraction of patients with systemic sepsis were correlated with reductions in the in vitro contractility of beating rat myocardial cells when exposed to the serum of the same patients. Meningococcal bacteremia is associated with reversible myocardial depression, including reductions in cardiac output and increases in left ventricular filling pressure.[59] During experimental hemorrhagic shock in dogs, perfusion of the anterior and posterior papillary muscles is impaired.[60] Histologically, myocyte injury with "zonal lesions," including fragmentation of Z bands, distortion of microfilaments, and displacement of mitochondria away from the intercalated discs, is observed after hemorrhagic shock.[61]

Impaired ventricular function during shock is associated with substantial decreases in left ventricular compliance, together with decreases in end-diastolic volume.[62, 63] This may be due to myocardial fluid retention with swelling of myocytes.[64] Glucose-insulin-potassium dilution may also minimize such cell swelling and improve compliance after endotoxin shock.[65]

Aerobic myocardial metabolism is required for efficient generation of energy to maintain contraction of myofibrillar proteins.[66] Anaerobic metabolism yields lactic acid with reduced adenosine triphosphate (ATP) production. Without regeneration of high-energy phosphate, ion pump function and myocardial contractility are impaired. The inorganic phosphate concentration of myocardium increases. There is impaired cation transport, with an efflux of potassium and an influx of sodium. Consequently, myocytes swell and the compliance of the myocardium is decreased.[67] Although oxygen supply to the myocardium is decreased, the oxygen requirements of the myocardium are augmented because of increased adrenergic activity and increases in afterload because of arterial constriction.[68] As myocardial ischemia and cell swelling progress, maldistribution of blood flow is intensified. As the heart becomes less compliant, myocardial contractility becomes less efficient and the imbalance between myocardial oxygen requirements and oxygen delivery increases.

Reflex increases in heart rate and the onset of cardiac arrhythmias may of themselves curtail cardiac output. The problem may be further complicated in patients with preexisting heart disease and especially in patients who are treated with digitalis glycosides. During shock there is decreased myocardial clearance of the glycoside, and hence substantially greater risk of digitalis toxicity and, therefore, ectopic dysrhythmia.[69]

OXYGEN CONSUMPTION AND ANAEROBIC METABOLISM

Fundamental to the understanding of metabolic defects during the low perfusion state is the critical reduction in cardiac output and the reduced delivery of oxygen stemming therefrom. A decline in oxygen consumption is an almost inevitable feature of fatal progression of shock states.[17] This also applies to high or normal cardiac output states during septic shock in which disproportionate increases in oxygen consumption accompany the low-resistance, hyperdynamic state.[70] More precisely, however, the fundamental defect stems from failure to maintain oxygen delivery in amounts which fulfill the oxygen requirements of the organism.

The metabolic requirements for oxygen are contingent on the metabolic state of the patient, which reflects the underlying illness, the presence or absence of fever, effects of both endogenous and exogenous hormones (especially beta-adrenergic agonists and thyroid hormones), and the physical activity status of the patient. Accordingly, the oxygen consumption during shock is highly variable and not of itself a clinically useful measurement for diagnosis or prognosis.[17, 71] A substantial reduction in oxygen consumption during the more advanced stages of perfusion failure is almost always preceded by a major deterioration of hemodynamic status.[17] This does not detract from the fact that a marked decline in oxygen consumption often

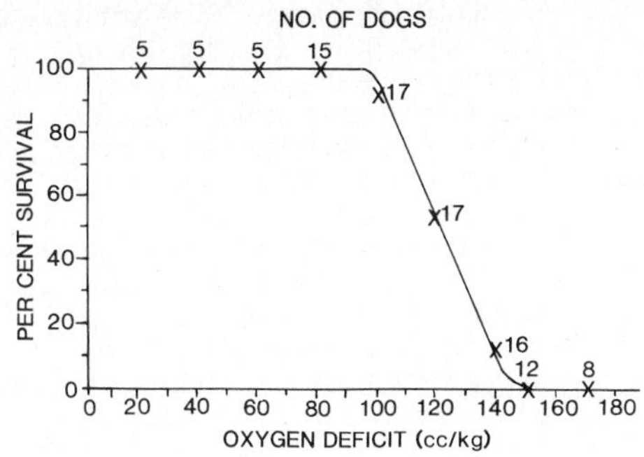

FIGURE 19–4. The relationship between oxygen deficit and survival during experimental shock produced by hemorrhage. (From Crowell, J. W., and Smith, E. E.: Oxygen deficit and irreversible hemorrhagic shock. Am. J. Physiol. *206*:313, 1964.)

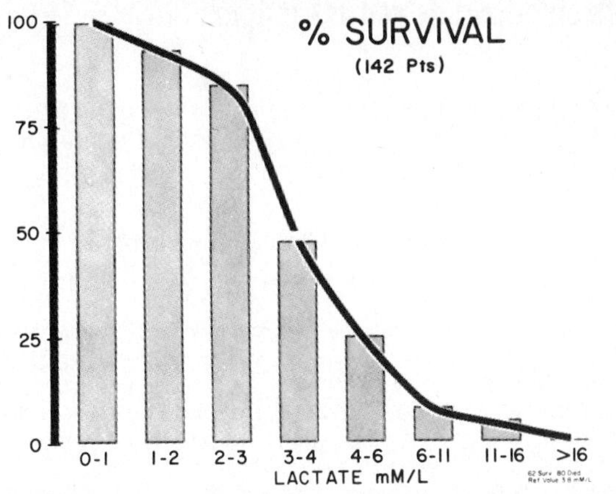

FIGURE 19–6. Relationship between concentrations of arterial blood lactate and survival in clinical shock states. (From Weil, M. H., and Shubin, H.: Metabolic consequences of cardiogenic shock. *In* Meltzer, L. E., and Dunning, A. J. (eds.): Textbook of Coronary Care. Amsterdam, Excerpta Medica 1972, p. 634).

ushers in the terminal cause of perfusion failure. Experimentally, there is a close relationship between the cumulative oxygen deficit during hemorrhagic shock, and survival. When oxygen deficit increases from 100 to 150 ml/kg during hemorrhage in dogs, survival declines from 100 to 0 per cent[15] (Fig. 19–4).

When oxygen delivery is critically reduced, the regeneration of high-energy phosphate compounds is impaired. For oxidation of pyruvate derived from carbohydrates, amino acids, and fatty acids, the final common pathway of aerobic energy production by mitochondria is aerobic oxidation by way of the citric acid (Krebs) cycle (Fig. 19–5). Electron transfer occurs through pyridine nucleotides and flavoproteins. Final electron transfer is to oxygen, which is then converted to water. This produces ATP, which is the energy source for the cell. During shock, however, oxidation through the citric acid cycle is inhibited because of the lack of an external electron acceptor (i.e., oxygen). Therefore, ATP is produced only by anaerobic glycolysis in cytoplasm, which cannot proceed beyond the metabolism of pyruvate to lactate. The pyruvate-to-lactate shunt is then activated as an emergency pathway of anaerobic metabolism. Anaerobic metabolism of 1 mole of glucose provides less than 10 per cent of the amount of ATP which would be generated by aerobic metabolism of the same quantity of glucose.

ELEVATIONS OF BLOOD LACTATE. The quantitative increases in blood lactate of the intact organism are in turn related to the oxygen deficit.[27] When lactic acid concentration increases from 2 to 8 mM/liter in human patients during circulatory shock, survival progressively decreases from approximately 90 to 10 per cent (Fig. 19–6). The lactate concentration, measured in either arterial or mixed venous blood, therefore quantitates the cumulative oxygen

CELLULAR METABOLISM

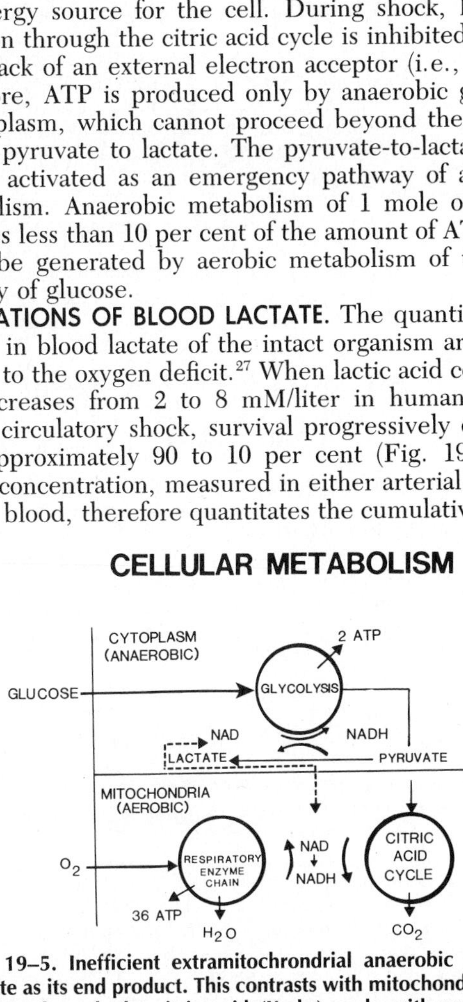

FIGURE 19–5. Inefficient extramitochrondrial anaerobic metabolism has lactate as its end product. This contrasts with mitochondrial aerobic metabolism through the citric acid (Krebs) cycle with production of carbon dioxide and water.

deficit and serves as a close correlate of survival. This is of great practical moment in the clinical setting, since the measurement of blood lactate, which can now be performed with technical ease and rapidity as part of blood gases by an electrode technique,[72] serves as an objective measure of both the presence and the severity of the shock state.[27, 73, 74] The clinical diagnosis of perfusion failure (shock) is confirmed only if the blood lactate exceeds 1.5 mM/liter. Reversal of the perfusion deficit is accompanied by a reduction in arterial blood lactate, and the effectiveness of therapy may therefore be gauged by repetitive measurement of blood lactic acid concentration. Transient increases in blood lactate occur during hyperventilation, physical exertion, shivering, and convulsive seizures.[75, 76] Accordingly, the activity status of the patient at the time of measurement should be taken into account in the interpretation of the lactate measurement.

When lactate is generated during exertion under physiological conditions, it is cleared over an interval of minutes by liver, skeletal muscle, and myocardium when physical exertion ceases. However, lactate is cleared much more slowly (over periods of hours) during recovery from circulatory shock. After cardiac arrest and resuscitation, substantial but transient increases in blood lactate are observed more like those which occur during physical exertion.[77]

Exercise physiologists have traditionally measured both lactate and pyruvate and computed the lactate:pyruvate ratio (L/P) as a correlate of oxygen deficit. Huckabee[78, 79] proposed the concept of excess lactate (XL) as a preferred quantitator of the severity of the perfusion defect. Both L/P and XL are based on the assumption that increases in "metabolic" lactate are accompanied by corresponding increases in pyruvate in the absence of anaerobic metabolism. Such may occur during infusions of glucose, bicarbonate, and pyruvate. However, both experimental and clinical investigations fail to confirm that, in the setting of circulatory shock, either the diagnostic or the prognostic value of the lactate measurement is enhanced by the concurrent measurement of pyruvate.[27, 80]

Increases in blood lactate are also observed after majoı vascular obstruction and especially after aortic occlusion in which there is so-called *regional shock*.[81] It is assumed that restoration of blood flow is accompanied by a "washout" of lactate, with transient elevations in systemic lactate during restoration of more normal perfusion. However, this has not been objectively documented.[82] There is rapid diffusion of lactate throughout the central circulation. Even in the setting of "regional shock" owing to aortic obstruction, the lactate concentrations measured in carotid artery blood are essentially the same as those of blood simultaneously sampled from a femoral vein.

METABOLIC AND ENDOCRINE ABNORMALITIES

Other abnormalities of carbohydrate and lipid metabolism accompany circulatory shock. Hyperglycemia during the initial stages of shock is attributed to increased secretion of catecholamines, glucagon, and glucocorticoids.[83, 84] When glycogen stores are depleted, in the more advanced stages of perfusion failure, hypoglycemia is more likely.[83] Increased lipolysis is also attributed to excessive catecholamine secretion together with reduced lipoprotein lipase activity. This accounts for hypertriglyceridemia.[85] The concentration of free fatty acids is inversely related to increases in blood lactate, presumably because of reduced perfusion of adipose tissue.[86, 87]

A large number of humoral substances have been identified, both experimentally and clinically, during the low-flow states. Among hormones, increases in epinephrine, norepinephrine, renin-angiotensin-aldosterone, glucocorticoids, and vasopressin levels have already been cited. The actions of these hormones account for vasoconstriction, inotropic and chronotropic effects on the myocardium, expansion and contraction of intravascular volume, and altered glucose, fat, and protein metabolism.

OTHER MEDIATORS IN SHOCK

Increased release of *histamine* in part related to a reduction in histaminase has been identified in shock states and particularly during the course of sepsis and anaphylaxis.[88, 89] *Kinins* are released by the action of a group of enzymes termed kallikreins acting on kininogen, a plasma globulin.[90] The predominant vasoactive peptide is bradykinin, which mediates vasodilation and increases vascular permeability. It also accounts for margination of leukocytes at local sites of inflammation, where kinins are released from granulocytes.[91] Serotonin is a potentially potent vasoconstrictor found in large concentrations in circulating platelets. Rapid destruction of platelets, especially in the settings of septic (endotoxin) shock and anaphylactic shock, is accompanied by *serotonin* release.[92] Serotonin increases pulmonary vascular resistance and therefore has been implicated in the development of pulmonary hypertension after sepsis and trauma.[93] It has also been implicated in the development of adult respiratory distress syndrome (ARDS).[94]

The products of the *arachidonic acid* cascade have been implicated in cellular injury of a variety of causes. The concentrations of various prostanoids in blood are increased in shock, but the precise role of prostanoids in the pathophysiology of shock is as yet unclear. The vasoconstrictor actions of thromboxane are prevented after injection of endotoxin when rats are pretreated with a thromboxane synthetase inhibitor such as imidazole.[95, 96] The vasodilator effects of prostaglandins, and more specifically prostaglandin E_2 (PGE_2) and prostacyclin (PGI_2), may, at least in part, account for the typical hyperdynamic abnormalities characteristic of septic shock.[96, 97] The hyperdynamic state is reversed by the administration of indomethacin and ibuprofen, which inhibit prostglandin synthesis.[98]

Increases in *endorphins*, endogenous opiates liberated from the pituitary gland, have been implicated in the progression of septic shock.[40, 99] These peptides are regarded as mediators of hypotension during sepsis and hemorrhage. Naloxone, an antagonist to endogenous opiates, has reversed endotoxin-mediated hypotension and increased survival. However, it has not as yet proved to have long-term survival benefits in patients.[100, 101]

The primary toxic component of gram-negative lipopolysaccharides is *lipid-A*.[102] When endotoxin is administered to laboratory animals, diffuse endothelial cell damage occurs. There is abrupt onset of thrombocytopenia and granulocytopenia.[103] A variety of *lysosomal enzymes* and especially proteases, serotonin, epinephrine, and thromboxanes are released. Antiproteases are disabled and there is lipid peroxidation of cell membranes. Among cytotoxic products, *free oxygen radicals* are liberated. There is lipid peroxidation of cell membranes and fragmentation of the interstitial hyaluronic acid lattices. Consequently, both proteases and free oxygen radicals cause diffuse tissue injury.[104–107]

The *complement system* is activated directly by endotoxin, chiefly through the intrinsic coagulation cascade. This accounts for intravascular coagulation with consumption of clotting factors, fibrinolysis with generation of fibrin monomers and fibrin split products.[108] Together with progressive thrombocytopenia and fibrinogen depletion, this characterizes the clinical syndrome of disseminated intravascular coagulation.

These injuries are additive to those of tissue hypoxia and impaired mitochondrial capability for oxidative phosphorylation. The therapeutic administration of an exogenous high-energy phosphate source, ATP magnesium chloride ($MgCl_2$), has been proposed as an adjunct for treatment of shock with the anticipation that it would restore more normal membrane permeability, decrease cellular edema, reduce enzyme leakage, and thereby improve cell function.[109] However, confirmation of its efficacy and safety for clinical management is still required.

IMMUNOLOGICAL MECHANISMS

Altered immunological function is in evidence during circulatory shock. It is the primary cause of anaphylaxis, which is mediated by antigen-antibody reactions with IgE antibody. This antibody, also known as reagin, acts directly on tissue-bound mast cells and circulating basophils to release primary mediators, including histamine, slow-reacting substances of anaphylaxis, eosinophil chemotactic factor of anaphylaxis, and a platelet-activating factor.[110–112] The activation of complement by classic and alternative pathways generates the kinins from platelets, eosinophils, and neutrophils. The kinins increase capillary permeability and stimulate mast cells and basophils to increase their release of primary mediators. Complement fractions also act as opsonins, which facilitate phagocytosis.[113] These cascading reactions trigger the release of Hageman factor (factor XII), and therefore the intrinsic coagulation cascade. The end result is bronchoconstriction, increased capillary permeability with pulmonary and systemic edema, increased leukocyte aggregation, release of lysosomal enzymes, intravascular coagulation, thrombocytopenia, and progressive hypovolemia with perfusion failure. These pathophysiological processes are of major importance in anaphylactic shock (p. 574).

Although the side effects of complement activation are detrimental, the more fundamental biological role of complement may be beneficial for enhancing phagocytosis and curtailing infection. However, the reticuloendothelial system (RES), and therefore the capability for clearing circulating microorganisms from the bloodstream, is impaired during shock states.[114] The principal components of the RES, which is made up of tissue-based phagocytes, include macrophages in the lung, spleen, lymph nodes, and Kupffer cells of the liver.[115, 116] RES function is impaired during both hypovolemic and endotoxin shock. Both histamine and serotonin reduce the capability of the RES to clear particulate matter, and a dialyzable RES-depressant substance has been described.[117] In the clinical setting in which the RES is impaired, as it is in debilitated patients after cytotoxic or radiation therapy, in patients with neoplastic diseases, or in patients with hepatic cirrhosis, the mortality of shock, and particularly septic shock, is increased.

SECONDARY EFFECTS OF SHOCK

THE HEART

Except in instances of cardiogenic shock when primary abnormalities in cardiac function are responsible, the heart, like the brain, is remarkably accommodating to decreases in systemic blood flow during the early stages of shock.[118] In the late stages of shock, the decreases in left ventricular compliance which are associated with cellular injury and particularly cell swelling may be important. However, these are not likely to be the major causes for fatal progression of shock. The same applies to the as-yet-not-fully-elucidated role of several myocardial depressant substances.

THE KIDNEYS (See also Ch. 59)

Renal failure is a major complication of circulatory shock. It typically appears within an interval of 36 to 72 hours after the onset of acute circulatory failure and in close association with other manifestations of tissue catabolism.

PATHOPHYSIOLOGY. During low-perfusion states, and most especially during hypovolemic shock, renal blood flow may be reduced to as low as 10 per cent of normal. There is redistribution of renal blood flow with diminished cortical blood flow. Such redistribution of renal blood flow is in part attributed to endogenous alpha-adrenergic action and accentuated by renal sympathetic nerve activity. It is accentuated by the vasoconstrictor actions of exogenous alpha-adrenergic agonists and probably by angiotensin II, especially when cardiac output and arterial perfusion pressures are critically reduced. Renal tubular injury progresses to cell necrosis with tubular obstruction. Proteinaceous and cellular debris accumulate within the tubular lumens. There is back diffusion and ultimately leakage of the glomerular filtrate, which, together with peritubular interstitial edema, may cause tubular collapse.[119, 120] Contrary to earlier reports, there is rather good correlation between histological changes in the kidney and renal function.[121]

Under conditions of extremely low flow, there may be critical limitations in renal tissue oxygen tension, especially in the medullary thick ascending limb of the nephron.[122–125] During the low-flow state there is initial increase in sodium and free water reabsorption, in part caused by increases in the secretion of aldosterone and ADH, which may enhance back diffusion. Nevertheless, the mineralocorticoids and ADH subsequently fail to maintain sodium reabsorption. Both sodium and urea concentration in the medulla are reduced so that the hypertonic gradient for reabsorption of water by the countercurrent mechanism is disabled. The capability of renal solute concentration is therefore rapidly lost.[126]

CLINICAL FEATURES. In acute renal failure these include proteinuria, hematuria, isosthenuria, and iso-osmolality with plasma. Progressive increases in serum urea nitrogen, creatinine, potassium, phosphate, and sulfate are frequently observed, together with decreases in serum sodium, calcium, and bicarbonate. Initial reduction in urine output to volumes of less than 400 ml per day ushers in the oliguric phase. The urine typically contains protein, red cells, epithelial cells, and characteristic brown granular casts of renal failure. *Hypertension* frequently develops during the recovery stage of acute renal failure. It is important to adjust potassium intake to avoid hyperkalemia and consequent cardiac arrhythmias and neuromuscular depression. In the absence of dialysis, the onset of the diuretic phase between 6 days and 2 weeks after the clinical shock state signals recovery, but renal concentration capability returns much more slowly.[127]

The typical laboratory findings of acute renal failure include urine osmolality of less than 350 mOsm, urine:plasma urea ratio of less than 10, urine:plasma creatinine ratio of less than 20, and urinary sodium concentration of greater han 40 mEq/liter. Renal failure indices based on measurements of urine flow and either or both renal clearance of creatinine and sodium may increase precision for purposes of monitoring and prognosis.[128] When renal failure occurs as part of multisystemic failure, the prognosis diminishes contingent on the number of major organ systems that fail.[129] However, when renal failure occurs after reversal of shock, it does not of itself prognosticate an unfavorable outcome. With the availability of intermittent dialysis or hemofiltration, recovery of essentially normal renal function is the rule.[130]

MANAGEMENT. This is directed to the treatment of the shock state, control of infection, appropriate nutrition, careful control of fluid intake, and appropriate electrolyte replacement. Hemodialysis, peritoneal dialysis, and hemofiltration are liberally used for the control of uremia and for fluid and electrolyte management. The routine use of diuretic agents for reversal of oliguria is not advised, not only because it is unlikely to be effective but also because it invalidates both diagnostic and prognostic measurement of renal function and particularly the tests of urea, creatinine, sodium, and osmolal clearance.

THE LUNGS (See also p. 557)

Early changes of pulmonary function include increments in ventilation so that the ventilation-perfusion ratio is markedly increased, with augmented physiological dead space and alveolocapillary gradients for oxygen. Pulmonary vascular resistance is usually only mildly elevated except for disproportionate increases in patients with arterial hypoxemia.

Progressive pulmonary injury, associated with circulatory shock, termed the adult respiratory distress syndrome (ARDS), represents impairment of alveolocapillary membrane integrity.[131] This is attributed to injury of alveolocapillary endothelium. Injury to Type 2 pneumocytes contributes to permeability defects and accounts for reduced synthesis of surfactin. There is sequestration of platelets and neutrophils in the pulmonary capillaries with liberation of proteases. Macrophage-mediated neutrophil sequestration is associated with complement activation and generation of lipid peroxidases from oxygen free radicals. The RES response is blunted and immunological resistance to infection is decreased.[132] An increase in T lymphocyte killer cells has been identified with decreases in fibronectin and immunoglobulin (IgG).[133] Perivascular leakage, potentiated by histamine and bradykinin, augments the increases in extravascular lung water produced by increased capillary permeability. In advanced stages of pulmonary failure, there is more extensive loss of capillary endothelial integrity with perivascular interstitial and intraalveolar hemorrhage.

Pulmonary failure is much more often observed in the setting of hypovolemic and septic shock, and after pulmonary embolization; it is relatively uncommon in patients with cardiogenic shock. There is some hope that prostaglandin E_1 may curtail pulmonary injury.[134, 135] However, objective clinical studies have given contradictory results after high-dose glucocorticoid therapy.[131, 136]

THERAPY. This is largely supportive. Positive end-expiratory pressure (PEEP) improves oxygenation such that FIO_2 of more than 0.6 may be avoided. Prolonged administration of higher concentrations of inspired oxygen may be an iatrogenic cause of pulmonary damage owing to oxygen toxicity.[137] When continuous positive airway pressure (CPAP) or PEEP is used at levels of 5 to 10 cm H_2O, it does not usually impede venous return (i.e., preload). When CPAP or PEEP of larger magnitudes is used, especially in patients with hypovolemia, venous return is impeded such that cardiac output is further reduced.[138, 139] A careful balance between volume expansion and positive airway pressure is therefore required (see p. 558). Positive airway pressure usually reduces the magnitude of pulmonary arteriovenous shunts, most likely by preventing collapse of alveoli, but increases the risk of barotrauma and especially pneumothorax, pneumomediastinum, and subcutaneous emphysema.

THE SKELETAL MUSCLE

With decreases in cell muscle blood flow, the resting transmembrane potential declines and there is impaired membrane transport. Respiratory muscle function, and particularly that of the diaphragm, may be compromised, accounting for decreased efficiency and increased oxygen requirements of breathing.[140, 141] This in part accounts for respiratory muscle fatigue. When metabolic demands are increased and oxygen delivery is severely curtailed, the increased work requirements of breathing may exceed the patient's capability, leading to alveolar hypoventilation with hypercarbia and hypoxemia.[142] The clinician may then have little option other than to intubate the trachea and mechanically assist or control ventilation.

THE LIVER

Isolated zones of centrilobular necrosis are observed in laboratory animals and in humans, but massive hepatic necrosis is uncommon except when circulatory shock occurs in patients with underlying hepatocellular disease. Nonspecific increases in aspartate aminotransferase (SGOT, AST), alanine aminotransferase (SGPT, ALT), and lactic dehydrogenase (LDH) appear early in patients with circulatory shock of diverse causes.[143] Cytoplasmic lysosomal enzymes increase and RES function decreases, accounting for decreases in circulating opsonins and $alpha_2$ glycoproteins.[114, 116] The decreased efficiency of protein and carbohydrate metabolism disables the detoxification function of the liver.[144] This may account for impaired coagulation because of inadequate regeneration of essential clotting factors. Nevertheless, liver failure is a late complication of shock, even though subtle changes in liver architecture are seen early on electron microscopy.[145] Increases in serum bilirubin, in part caused by intravascular hemolysis, are more often observed in patients with septic shock.

THE STOMACH AND INTESTINE

Mucosal congestion and bleeding of the stomach and intestines may account for hypermotility and hypomotility.[41] Submucosal hemorrhage, particularly in the colon, with progressive hemorrhagic necrosis and ulceration is commonly observed on autopsy after hemorrhagic and endotoxic shock, especially in dogs. Similar lesions have been observed in humans.[146] The barrier function of the gut may be decreased so that gram-negative bacilli or their endotoxins may enter the circulation.[147] There is sequestration of blood in the portal venous system. Splanchnic ischemia is attributed to alpha-adrenergically induced vasoconstriction with disproportionate reduction in mucosal blood flow. Elderly patients are likely to exhibit a higher incidence of intestinal ischemia because of preceding atherosclerotic disease of the splanchnic arteries. Nevertheless, transmural infarction complicated by perforation is an uncommon complication. However, mucosal necrosis may cause pseudomembraneous enterocolitis during recovery.

The intestinal tract, like many other systems or organs, has been cited as responsible for irreversibility of shock.[148] However, such hypotheses of "irreversibility" have not proved to be clinically applicable and do not currently call for specific prophylactic or therapeutic interventions.

THE PANCREAS

Blood flow to the pancreas is markedly reduced during shock,[149] and this may account for pancreatic sources of proteases, especially the cathepsins.[150] Experimentally, the pancreas has also been viewed as the source of the myocardial depressant factor, which decreases contractility of an isolated papillary muscle preparation.[151, 152] Subcellular alterations in the pancreas, including dilated endoplasmic reticulum and swollen mitochrondria, are reversible.[153] Local areas of necrosis have been observed in the pancreas. Although this organ is also cited as a primary shock organ which determines reversibility,[154] an important limiting role for the pancreas, or of toxic substances produced by it during clinical shock states, has not been established.

THE BLOOD

With slowing of blood flow, there is intravascular aggregation and clumping of red cells, leukocytes, and platelets, called "sludging." Although this process of itself may increase vascular resistance, it is usually reversible. However, a serious complication of shock is *disseminated intravascular coagulation* (DIC). It results from intravascular activation of the coagulation process by infection, by the abnormal production or liberation of coagulant tissue factors such as endotoxin, amniotic fluid, snake bites, or crush injury, or by generation of procoagulants in the blood as may be the case during hemolytic transfusion reactions.[155, 156] *Purpura fulminans* is an uncommon and extreme complication of DIC and may cause extensive tissue necrosis with gangrene of extremities.[157] Microthrombi are formed within small blood vessels by fibrin deposition, and this triggers fibrinolysis. High levels of fibrin split products have of themselves antihemostatic properties, and they act as circulating anticoagulants and impair platelet function with enhancement of bleeding. The microthrombi and the intravascular fibrin strands associated with them obstruct blood flow so as to produce microangiopathic hemolysis caused by sheer damage to red cells. Both injured endothelium and microthrombi activate fibrinolysis. The fibrinogen concentration of plasma is reduced. There is diffuse tissue injury because of small vessel obstruction by thrombosis, embolization, and bleeding into tissues.[108] The contact of blood with subendothelial components such as collagen may activate factor XII, the Hageman factor, and trigger coagulation through the intrinsic pathway. Plasma levels of the various plasma serum protease inhibitors, such as antithrombin III, alpha$_2$ macroglobulin, and alpha$_2$ antiplasma, are decreased.

Typical laboratory findings include thrombocytopenia, prolongation of prothrombin time and partial thromboplastin time, decreased factors V and VIII and fibrinogen concentrations, and increased concentration of fibrin monomers and fibrin split products.

Therapy is directed first at the control of the underlying cause of the shock state, particularly sepsis. If bleeding and thrombosis are mild, no specific therapy is advised. If bleeding is serious, replacement of clotting factors with fresh frozen plasma, cryoprecipitate, and platelet transfusions may be required in conjunction with heparin. If the primary defect is thrombosis in contrast to bleeding, the administration of a therapeutic anticoagulant loading dose of heparin followed by continuous infusion is advocated to interrupt the cycle of coagulation and fibrinolysis.[158] Replacement of fibrinogen and antithrombin III by the administration of fresh frozen plasma may also be indicated when the fibrinogen level is decreased to less than 150 mg/dl. Fresh frozen plasma replaces depleted clotting factors and serum protease inhibitors. Cryoprecipitate contains a high concentration of fibrinogen and may be used when fibrinogen levels decrease to less than 100 mg/dl.

The role of altered oxyhemoglobin dissociation is unclear. During shock states the affinity of hemoglobin for oxygen is decreased such that the P_{50} (the oxygen tension at which 50 per cent of hemoglobin is saturated with oxygen) is increased[159, 160] (see Figure 55–1, p. 1735). This facilitates the unloading of oxygen at tissue levels. However, when the blood pH is decreased with metabolic acidosis, the erythrocyte 2,3-diphosphoglycerate (2,3-DPG) declines, which decreases P_{50}. At the present time there are no indications for routine measurement or treatment of abnormalities of either P_{50} or 2,3-DPG.[161]

THE BRAIN

The cerebral circulation is remarkably well protected in shock.[162] Except when there is intrinsic cerebrovascular disease, there is preferential flow to the cerebral circuit in a manner analogous to that which occurs during cardiac arrest. Autoregulation maintains constancy of cerebral blood flow.[163] During hypotension there is a reduction in cerebrovascular resistance associated with cerebral vasodilation. Symptoms of ischemia emerge only when cerebral blood flow decreases to less than 50 per cent of normal values, and this is not likely until mean arterial pressure decreases to less than 50 mm Hg.[164]

The arterial carbon dioxide tension exerts a profound effect on cerebral blood flow.[165] Cerebral blood flow is reduced when Pa_{CO_2} declines because of cerebral vasoconstriction and increases when arterial P_{CO_2} increases because of cerebral arterial vasodilation. The response is highly sensitive; for each 1 mm Hg change, cerebral blood flow normally changes by approximately 4 per cent. Alterations in arterial oxygen tension also affect cerebral blood flow. When arterial P_{O_2} declines, there is progressive cerebral vasodilation. Cerebral blood flow may increase fivefold when arterial P_{O_2} falls below 50 mm Hg.

CLINICAL SHOCK STATES

CLASSIFICATION

Earlier classifications of circulatory shock related etiology and hemodynamic mechanisms.[1] A widely used classification included hypovolemic, cardiogenic, hypersensitivity (anaphylactic), bacteremic, neurogenic, obstructive, and endocrine types of shock.[1] Subsequent investigations, however, indicated that anaphylactic shock is predominantly hypovolemic shock and that shock associated with major neurological defects, such as transection of the spinal cord, in fact represented increases in venous capacitance. Endocrine types of shock such as those which occur in the course of pheochromocytoma were demonstrated to be caused by hypovolemia.[37] Consequently, a classification[166] based on four discrete hemodynamic defects was evolved. These defects are shown in Figure 19–7.

The most common cause of reduced systemic blood flow is *hypovolemia*, which results from a reduction of volume within the intravascular compartment. *Cardiogenic shock* represents failure of the cardiac pump to maintain systemic blood flow in amounts that will fulfill metabolic requirements. *Obstruction* may occur in the great veins, including the vena cava, by compression caused by the gravid uterus (the supine hypotensive syndrome [p. 1850]); in the heart itself owing to pericardial tamponade (p. 1492), ball valve thrombi, or pulmonary embolism (Chap. 47); or in the aorta owing to dissection and may physically impede the main stream of blood flow (Chap. 46). This represents obstructive shock. The important new category is that of distributive shock, which represents major alterations in the distribution of blood flow without critical decreases in intravascular volume, cardiac function, or obstruction of

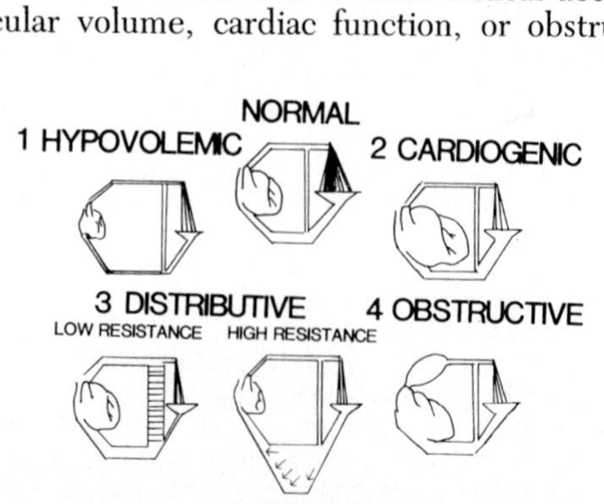

FIGURE 19–7. Hemodynamic classification of circulatory shock states. The common denominator is a critical reduction in blood flow.

TABLE 19–2 CLASSIFICATION OF SHOCK STATES

TYPE OF SHOCK	PRIMARY MECHANISM	CLINICAL CAUSES
Hypovolemic	Volume loss	Exogenous Blood loss due to hemorrhage Plasma loss due to burn, inflammation Fluid and electrolyte loss due to vomiting, diarrhea, dehydration, osmolal diuresis (diabetes) Endogenous Extravasation due to inflammation, trauma, tourniquet, anaphylaxis, snake venom, and adrenergic stimulation (pheochromocytoma)
Cardiogenic	Pump failure	Myocardial infarction Other causes Cardiac arrhythmias Intracardiac obstruction, including valvular stenosis Heart failure
Distributive (vasomotor dysfunction)		
(1) High or normal resistance	Expanded venous capacitance (pooling)	Hypodynamic septic shock due to gram-negative enteric bacillemia Autonomic blockade, spinal shock Tranquilizer, sedative, narcotic overdose
(2) Low resistance	Arteriovenous shunting	Pneumonia, peritonitis, abscess, reactive hyperemia
Obstructive	Extracardiac obstruction of main channel of blood flow	Vena caval obstruction (supine hypotensive syndrome) Pericarditis (tamponade) Pulmonary embolism Dissecting aneurysm or compression of aorta

blood flow. Abnormalities in distribution may be due to either low arterial resistance in association with inflammatory vasodilation or arteriovenous shunting as in hyperdynamic states of septic shock. In the more advanced stages of gram-negative sepsis with shock, there is an increase in arterial resistance and a concomitant increase in venous capacitance with deceased venous return. This also applies to shock states which are associated with altered neural control, including barbiturate intoxication, ganglionic blockade, or spinal shock resulting from transection of the spinal cord. In Table 19–2 the hemodynamic classification is related to commonly encountered clinical circulatory shock states.

In the instance of low-resistance distributive shock, the cardiac output may be normal or increased, but blood pressure is low. Accordingly, the shock state represents a failure to maintain capillary perfusion, which, in the instance of low-resistance distributive states, is largely independent of cardiac output. The common denominator is *failure of tissue perfusion* so that oxygen delivery is not sufficient to sustain normal aerobic metabolism. Consequently, it is lactic acidosis, as the metabolic consequence of anaerobic metabolism, which is the sine qua non of the low-perfusion state, regardless of cause.

GENERAL PRINCIPLES OF DIAGNOSIS AND MANAGEMENT: THE VIP'S

For the patient who presents with clinical signs of shock, a useful guide to initial evaluation and management is provided by the acronym VIP.[167] "V" refers to ventilation to insure adequate pulmonary exchange of oxygen and carbon dioxide. "I" refers to infusion and, in turn, the adequacy of intravascular volume. "P" refers to pump function, and therefore cardiac competence. These priorities apply to the initial management of patients with circulatory shock, regardless of cause.

VENTILATION

In addition to overt physical signs which indicate inadequate chest movement or respiratory distress, analysis of arterial blood gases provides quantitative measurement of the adequacy of both ventilation and acid-base status. When hypoxemia appears in the absence of hypercarbia and respiratory acidosis, the initial intervention is that of increasing inspired concentrations of oxygen. Oxygen therapy by mask or nasal catheter may suffice. If alveolar ventilation is impaired, arterial blood gas measurements will demonstrate respiratory acidosis with substantial increases in arterial carbon dioxide tension.

Either failure to reverse hypoxemia (Pa_{O_2} <60 mm Hg) by increasing the concentration of oxygen in inspired gas to 60 per cent or progressive respiratory acidosis (Pa_{CO_2} >60 mm Hg) would ordinarily require endotracheal intubation and mechanical ventilation with a volume-controlled respirator. It is especially in patients with reduced pulmonary compliance caused by pulmonary edema or pneumonia that positive pressure ventilation is likely to overcome life-threatening hypoxemia. Intubation of the airway facilitates suctioning, and therefore control of secretions. Mechanical ventilation is also likely to decrease the oxygen cost owing to the work of breathing.[140, 168] When pulmonary compliance is decreased in the absence of hypoxemia and hypercarbia, the increased oxygen requirement for breathing nevertheless augments the oxygen deficit, and therefore the severity of the shock state. Ventilation may be either assisted or intermittent so that it is coordinated with the voluntary ventilatory drive of the patient. Fully controlled ventilation in patients who "fight" the ventilator is facilitated by the administration of tranquilizer-sedatives (e.g., diazepam) in intravenous doses of 5 to 20 mg at intervals of 1 to 3 hours or by narcotic drugs. In extreme cases, when mechanical ventilation is opposed by spontaneous ventilation of the patient, neuromuscular blockade with an agent such as pancuronium in initial doses of 0.1

mg/kg and subsequently 0.01 to 0.02 mg/kg, which are repeated at intervals of 20 to 60 minutes as required in addition to the tranquilizer-sedative or narcotic. The frequency and minute volume of mechanical ventilation are adjusted to maintain physiological levels of arterial blood gases.

With decreases in pulmonary compliance, increasingly larger airway pressures are required to maintain adequate minute volumes. When patients develop ARDS (shock lung), PEEP or CPAP with or without mechanical ventilation improves the patency of small airways, recruits alveoli, and decreases pulmonary arterial venous shunting.[169] Because increases in airway pressure produced by mechanical ventilation, PEEP, and CPAP are accompanied by corresponding increases in intrathoracic pressure, these mechanical interventions impede venous return, and therefore preload and cardiac output (p. 410). Accordingly, the clinician is required to balance the effects of positive airway pressures on cardiac output and, more specifically, oxygen delivery.[139] The computation of oxygen transport, represented by the product of cardiac output and arterial oxygen content, is useful for this purpose. Decreases in venous return, and therefore cardiac output, which stem from increases in intrathoracic pressure are usually overcome by expansion of the intravascular volume by judicious fluid challenge.

INFUSION

It is not only that hypovolemia is the most common cause of shock, but progression of shock states, regardless of cause, is likely to be accompanied by reductions in intravascular volume owing to increased hydrostatic pressure and increased permeability of capillary exchange vessels. Volume expansion is therefore routinely required to increase oxygen delivery, not only during hypovolemic shock but in all shock states, including cardiogenic and distributive (septic) shock states.[16]

In the absence of impaired left heart function, the central venous pressure may serve as an appropriate monitor for volume infusion.[170] The changes in central venous pressure parallel those of the pulmonary artery occlusive (wedge) pressure, the pulmonary artery diastolic pressure, and the left ventricular end-diastolic pressure in the normal heart (Fig. 19–8). However, this clearly does not apply in patients with impaired left ventricular function, especially after acute myocardial infarction, in whom changes in left ventricular filling pressure are not reflected in the central venous pressure (Fig. 19–9).[171] Nevertheless, it is important to monitor right-sided filling pressure routinely in addition to left-sided pressures, which is easily accomplished through the right atrial port of the conventional flow-directed, balloon-tipped (Swan-Ganz) catheter. Increases in right-sided filling pressures are of import in the diagnosis and management of right ventricular failure from a diversity of causes in the setting of circulatory shock, including right ventricular infarction with cardiogenic shock, right and left ventricular failure in the late stages of distributive shock resulting from sepsis, or with pulmonary embolism, primary pulmonary hypertension, and ARDS.

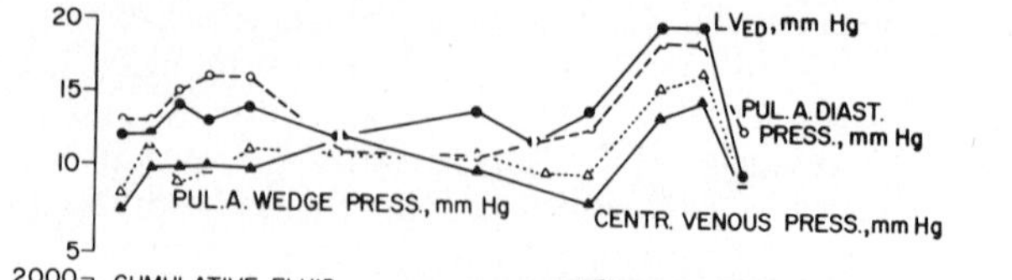

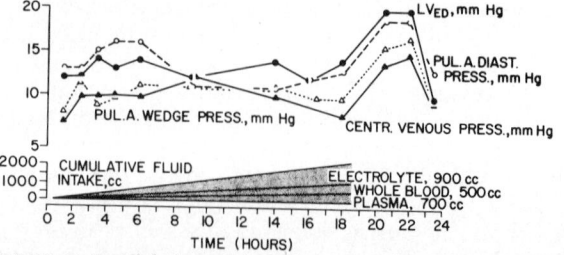

FIGURE 19–8. Parallel changes in right ventricular and left ventricular filling pressures during fluid challenge in the absence of myocardial impairment in a 67-year-old woman who had hypovolemia following total hip replacement.

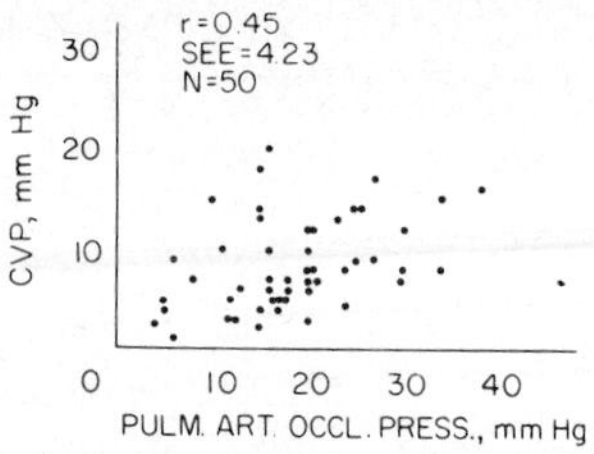

FIGURE 19–9. The relationship between central venous pressure (CVP) and pulmonary artery occlusive pressure in patients after acute myocardial infarction. (Redrawn from Forrester, J. S., et al.: Filling pressures in the right and left sides of the heart in acute myocardial infarction. N. Engl. J. Med. *285*:190, 1971.)

The pulmonary diastolic pressure is typically between 1 and 5 mm Hg less than the pulmonary artery occlusive pressure, except in patients who have increased pulmonary vascular resistance and when pulmonary systolic pressures exceed 45 mm Hg.[172] Because changes in pulmonary artery diastolic pressure usually reflect those of the left-sided filling pressure, they provide a useful check on the validity of the pulmonary artery occlusive pressure. Monitoring of the pulmonary diastolic pressure makes it possible to avoid repetitive inflation of the distal balloon for measurement of pulmonary artery occlusive pressure during fluid challenge. Minute-to-minute monitoring of pulmonary diastolic pressure allows for only intermittent measurement of occlusive (wedge) pressure, and thereby decreases the risk of iatrogenic complications, especially pulmonary infarction by prolonged balloon occlusion of a distal pulmonary artery. When it is technically impossible to advance the balloon into the occluded position, or with malfunction of the balloon, monitoring of diastolic pressure may provide a relatively useful alternative.

STANDARDIZED FLUID CHALLENGE. A constant volume of fluid is infused intravenously over a defined interval.[170] More specifically, aliquots of 200, 100, or 50 ml of fluid (depending on the judgment of the clinician based on the initial pulmonary occlusive pressure) are infused through a site other than that of the monitoring catheter over an interval of 10 minutes. The pulmonary artery occlusive (wedge) pressure or the pulmonary artery diastolic pressure is monitored. If, during the infusion, the pressure increases by no more than 3 mm Hg, there is little risk of fluid overload to the point of heart failure and infusion at the same rate may be continued. The total volume of fluid infused when fluid challenge rules are not violated is guided by clinical, hemodynamic, and metabolic measurements which indicate reversal of the shock state. However, if the pressure increases by more than 3 but less than 7 mm Hg, the fluid challenge should be stopped at the end of 10 minutes and continued only if the pressure recedes to 3 mm Hg or less after an additional 10-minute interval. In instances in which the pressure increases by 7 mm Hg or more during the 10-minute challenge, it suggests serious left ventricular systolic and/or diastolic dysfunction, and the fluid challenge should be stopped, pending pharmacological or mechanical interventions for improving cardiac function (Fig. 19–10). (This has been termed the "7–3" rule.) The corresponding values for fluid challenge when only central venous pressure is monitored are 5 and 2 mm Hg, respectively.

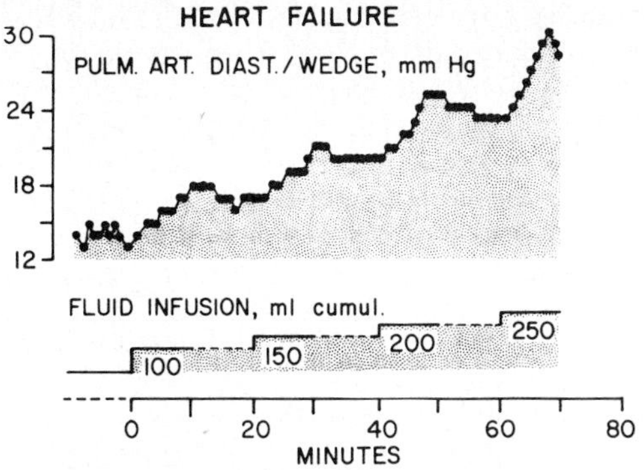

FIGURE 19–10. Standardized fluid challenge, initially with 100-ml and subsequently with 50-ml aliquots of fluid in a patient with hypovolemic hypotension complicating congestive heart failure. The darkened lines indicate a 10-minute wait. The steep rise in pressure between 60 and 68 minutes which exceeded 7 mm signaled the obligatory end of the fluid challenge.

The optimal filling pressure is increased when ventricular compliance is reduced. This applies particularly to patients with ventricular hypertrophy or after myocardial infarction in whom optimal left ventricular filling pressure approximates 18 mm Hg.[173, 174] However, *relative* changes in filling pressures by the standardized fluid challenge technique have greater reliability and safety because of the difficulty of precise measurement of absolute levels of left ventricular filling pressure.

The choice of fluid is contingent on the cause of fluid loss complemented by simple measurements, including hemoglobin and hematocrit, albumin or colloid osmotic pressure, and plasma or serum sodium or osmolality. The rationale for the choice of fluid is summarized in Table 19–3. Either crystalloid or colloid fluids effectively reverse the hypovolemic state. Because sodium-containing fluids are distributed through both the intravascular and interstitial compartments, the total volume of isotonic sodium chloride required for expansion of the intravascular compartment compared with colloid is threefold to fourfold greater.[175] Although the excess of crystalloid fluid may produce edema, it is not usually hazardous. In patients with limited cardiac competence, however, iso-oncotic colloids increase precision of fluid titration against filling pressures. When the plasma concentration of albumin is reduced and left ventricular filling pressures are increased, the colloid-hydrostatic gradient is reduced so that the risk of pulmonary edema is increased.[176] Hypertonic sodium chloride solutions which greatly expand extracellular volume but reduce intracellular volume have, in animal experiments, improved survival under select conditions of hypovolemic shock, including shock after burn injuries.[177–179] Hyperoncotic colloid, especially 25 per cent human serum albumin, selectively increases intravascular volume for up to 16 hours and simultaneously decreases both interstitial and intracellular volumes. It has been advised for management of hypermetabolic or nutritionally deprived patients in whom the plasma protein concentration is critically reduced.[180] The initial effects of fluid infusion on the three major fluid compartments are summarized in Table 19–4.

TABLE 19–3 FLUID CHALLENGE: CHOICE OF FLUID

Clinical	Fluid	Hgb Hct	Alb COP	Osm Na^+
Blood loss	RBC + NACl	↓	–	–
	RBC + colloid	↓	↓	–
Inflammatory plasma loss	Albumin	↑	↓	—
	Hydroxyethyl starch			
Dehydration				
GI	Electrolytes (NaCl)	↑	↑	–
Inanition	Crystalloid (G/W)	↑	↑	↑

TABLE 19–4 INITIAL EFFECTS OF FLUID INFUSION

Fluid Compartment	5% Gluc.	Iso-tonic NaCl	Hyper-tonic NaCl	Iso-oncotic (5%)	Hyper-oncotic (25%)
Intravascular	↑	↑	↑	↑	↑
Interstitial	↑	↑	↑	—	↓
Intracellular	↑	—	↓	—	↓

PNEUMATIC ANTISHOCK GARMENTS. These have been used as an alternative to volume expansion, especially for patients in hypovolemic shock after traumatic injuries. Such garments may augment venous return, and thereby cardiac output, but they may also impede venous return and produce injury to soft tissues by compression.[181] Their primary benefit is to tamponade venous bleeding and splint injured extremities. Experimentally, such pneumatic garments may transiently increase coronary and cerebral perfusion, but there is no proof of ultimate benefit.[182, 183]

PUMPING

After ventilation and intravascular volume are optimized, the next priority is that of maintaining adequate pump function for effective circulation. The routinely monitored electrocardiogram provides an indication of rhythm. Primary hemodynamic measurements, in addition to ventricular filling pressures, include cardiac output, arterial pressure, and heart rate. From these measurements the relationship between average stroke volume and work, and arterial resistance may be computed to facilitate decision making for inotropic, vasodilator, and mechanical support (Fig. 19–11). The difference between the diastolic arterial pressure, preferably measured at a site close to the aorta, and the right atrial diastolic pressure is an indication of coronary perfusion pressure.

These hemodynamic measurements help to distinguish between the four major categories of shock. The characteristic hemodynamic changes in hypovolemic, distributive, and obstructive shock are shown in Table 19–5. The decision-making which follows the initial interventions is largely based on this differential diagnosis and guided by continued monitoring of these hemodynamic variables.

Among inotropic agents, beta-adrenoceptor agonists have the disadvantage of disproportionately increasing myocardial oxygen requirements.[184, 185] Digitalis glycosides (p. 489) are not generally viewed as beneficial in the setting of shock, and the risk of digitalis toxicity increases.[69] One report, however, suggests potential benefit in the setting of septic shock.[186]

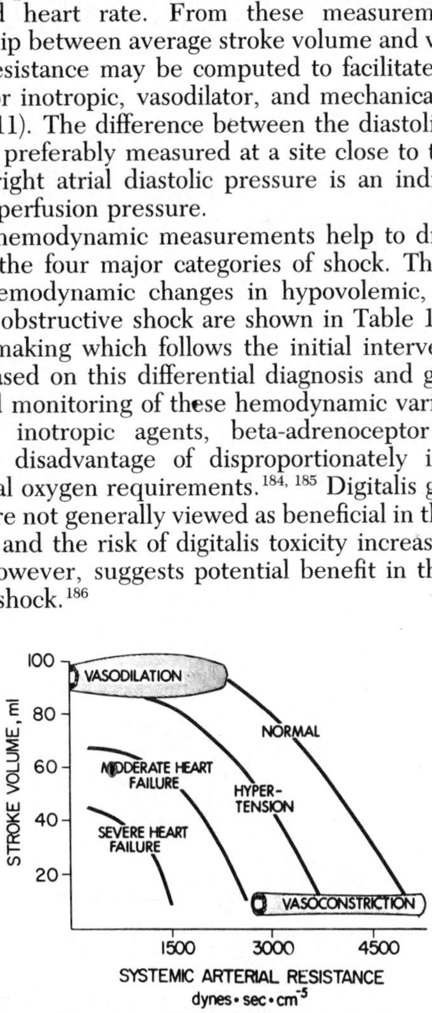

FIGURE 19–11. The reciprocal relationships between systemic arterial resistance and cardiac output (stroke volume).

TABLE 19–5 HEMODYNAMIC DIAGNOSIS OF CIRCULATORY SHOCK*

	Cardiac Output	Intracardiac Pressures			
		RA	RV_S	$PA_{S/D}$	PA_O
Hypovolemic	↓	↓	↓	↓	↓
Distributive (bacterial)	↓↑	—	—	—	—(↑)
Obstructive (pulmonary embolism)	↓	↑	↑	↑	—

*For cardiogenic shock, see Table 19–6.

With greater understanding of the fact that increases in arterial resistance induced by vasopressor agents increase the workload on the heart and do not necessarily improve perfusion, their routine use for treatment of shock states is controversial.[24, 187, 188] To the contrary, there is increasing interest in the use of drugs which decrease arterial resistance. Among vasodilator drugs, both phentolamine and nitroprusside have been used.[38, 188–190] Decreases in arterial resistance are typically followed by increases in cardiac output and tissue perfusion (Fig. 19–11). A disproportionately greater increase in cardiac output with more moderate decline in arterial resistance accounts for the fact that arterial pressure may be increased rather than decreased after the administration of vasodilators. However, the administration of vasodilators must be moderated by the arterial perfusion pressure. In instances where the systolic arterial pressure is less than 80 mm Hg and the mean arterial pressure is less than 55 mm Hg, further reductions in arterial perfusion pressure, and particularly coronary perfusion pressure, may threaten hemodynamic stability.

Dobutamine (p. 525) is currently the preferred adrenergic inotropic agent. Unlike isoproterenol, it has only minor chronotropic actions and more moderate vasodilator effects.[191] When conventional adrenergic amines with combined alpha- and beta-agonist actions (levarterenol, epinephrine, metaraminol, and dopamine) are used in higher doses which exert primarily alpha-adrenoceptor effects, or when a relatively pure alpha-agonist (phenylephrine or methoxamine) is used for predominant alpha-adrenoceptor effects, the routine measurement of intraarterial pressure is advised. The use of such agents is best limited to circulatory shock states in which decreases in perfusion pressure threaten immediate survival because of (1) compromised coronary blood flow manifested by ectopic ventricular arrhythmias; (2) impaired cerebral survival when intracranial pressure is increased and the cerebral-perfusion pressures are therefore critically reduced; and (3) when renal clearances of water and metabolites must be maintained, as in patients with acute pulmonary edema, hypercalcemia, drug overdose, or cerebral edema.

There is currently no established indication for the use of mechanical cardiac assist techniques in the setting of circulatory shock, except in patients with cardiogenic shock.

CARDIOGENIC SHOCK

ACUTE MYOCARDIAL INFARCTION

(See also p. 1222)

PATHOPHYSIOLOGY. The predominant cause of cardiogenic shock is acute myocardial infarction. Both the onset and the severity are closely related to the quantitative loss in functional myocardium.[192, 193] This may be due to recent myocardial infarction superimposed on old infarction. Because ischemic injury and necrosis are progressive over time, there is typically progressive hemodynamic deterioration so that the hemodynamic deficits which account for cardiogenic shock evolve over periods of hours and occasionally days after onset of symptoms of myocardial infarction. Progressive injury and expanding necrosis are associated with high serum levels of the MB fraction of creatine phosphokinase.

Because the left anterior descending coronary artery ordinarily supplies the largest mass of myocardium, cardiogenic shock occurs predominantly in the setting of anterior and anteroseptal myocardial infarction with recent or old infarction of the apex. This typically follows proximal obstruction of the left anterior descending coronary artery. However, a majority of patients in cardiogenic shock secondary to myocardial infarction present with three-vessel coronary artery disease and with acute infarction of more than 40 per cent of the left ventricular myocardium.[194, 195] In a minority of instances, cardiogenic shock may occur in patients with inferior myocardial infarction after infarction of the right ventricle. Approximately 25 per cent of patients who sustain inferior myocardial infarction also have associated right ventricular infarction. However, isolated infarction of the right ventricle is uncommon.[196]

Specific hemodynamic complications, in addition to loss of viable myocardium, may trigger the onset of shock. These include major cardiac arrhythmias with excessively rapid or slow heart rates and loss of atrial transfer function with atrial arrhythmias, atrioventricular block, perforation of the interventricular septum, papillary muscle dysfunction or rupture, myocardial rupture with consequent pericardial tamponade, and pulmonary embolism. Congestive heart failure may progress to cardiogenic shock.

HEMODYNAMIC FEATURES. Routine bedside hemodynamic measurements in cardiogenic shock demonstrates increases in left ventricular filling pressure, as reflected in pulmonary artery occlusive pressure, to levels greater than 18 mm Hg in combination with a decline in the cardiac index to less than 2.2 liters/min/M^2. Except in the setting of right ventricular infarction, pulmonary embolism, cardiac tamponade, or pulmonary hypertension induced by hypoxemia or preexisting pulmonary heart disease, the right-sided filling pressures are normal or only slightly increased.

DIFFERENTIAL DIAGNOSIS. Hemodynamic diagnosis of complications of acute myocardial infarction which may usher in or increase the severity of cardiogenic shock is also facilitated by measurements obtained with the flow-directed, balloon-tipped thermodilution catheter (Table 19–6). Papillary muscle dysfunction is characterized by prominent *v* waves with characteristic morphology in pressure waveforms obtained from the pulmonary artery occlusive and pulmonary artery pressure measurements per-

TABLE 19–6 CARDIAC CAUSES OF SHOCK BY HEMODYNAMIC DIAGNOSIS

	Flow	Intracardiac Pressures				Saturation
Mechanism	CO	RA	$RV_{S/D}$	$PA_{S/D}$	PA_O	SaO_2
LV failure	↓	—↑	—↑	↑	↑↑	—
Mitral regurgitation	↓	—↑	—↑	↑ ("V wave")		—
VSD	±	—↑	↑	↑	—↑	↑ (RV, PA)
Pulmonary hypertension pulmonary embolism	↓	↑	↑	↑	—	—
RV (Infarction)	↓	↑	↑	↓↑	↓↑	—
Tamponade	↓	↑	↑	↑	↑	—

formed. Septal perforation is characterized by arterialization of blood sampled from the right ventricle and pulmonary artery. Pulmonary hypertension and pulmonary embolism are characterized by disproportionate increases in right-sided pressures, including the pulmonary artery pressure. With right ventricular infarction in the setting of inferior myocardial infarction, there is selective increase in right ventricular filling pressure and typically lower pulmonary artery occlusive pressure. For the diagnosis of pericardial tamponade, the right atrial pressure pulse demonstrates a characteristic steep *y* descent, with equilibration of mean right atrial, pulmonary artery diastolic, and pulmonary artery occlusive pressures (p. 1493). These hemodynamic abnormalities complement characteristic physical signs, together with electrocardiographic, radiographic, and echocardiographic findings.

PROGNOSIS. Of the correlates of survival, measurements of blood flow and perfusion have been substantially better than those of arterial pressure. Arterial blood lactate, cardiac output or stroke work, and arterial pressure are prognostic of outcome, in that order.[73] There is substantial variability in the reported acute mortality in cardiogenic shock because of differences in definition of this condition. When lactate is increased to levels exceeding 4 mM/liter, cardiac index is reduced to less than 2.2 liters/min/M^2, arterial resistance is increased to more than 2,000 dyne/sec/cm^{-5}, left ventricular filling pressure exceeds 18 mm Hg, mean arterial pressure is less than 60 mm Hg, and there is no prompt reversal after fluid challenge, mortality approaches 100 per cent. With less rigorous criteria, mortality is generally stated to be between 85 and 95 per cent with medical management, and there has been little improvement over the past 30 years.[193, 196a]

MANAGEMENT. Routine measures include the amelioration of pain by the intravenous administration of morphine in titrated doses of 2 to 5 mg at intervals of 30 minutes to 1 hour. Morphine may increase venous capacitance, and therefore decrease preload and ventricular filling pressures, but this is readily reversed with fluid challenge. Morphine may also provoke increased vagal activity, which may be controlled by the intravenous injection of 0.5 to 1.0 mg of atropine sulfate. Anxiety may be relieved by slow intravenous bolus injection of diazepam in doses of 3 to 5 mg repeated as frequently as necessary, usually at intervals of 30 to 60 minutes.

Optimization of preload by fluid challenge provides the single best option for improving left ventricular performance (Table 19–3). If pulmonary artery occlusion pressure is less than 18 mm Hg, 50-ml fluid challenges by standard protocol with either physiological salt solution or 6 per cent hydroxyethyl starch should be undertaken.[196b] If the safe limits of fluid challenge have been exceeded, and provided that mean arterial pressure is not reduced to less than 50 mm Hg, vasodilator therapy with sodium nitroprusside in amounts of 15 to 400 μg/min by continuous intravenous infusion is titrated to maintain constancy of arterial perfusion pressure.

INOTROPIC AGENTS. These drugs, including digitalis glycosides, dopamine, dobutamine, and amrinone, may be tried in unresponsive patients in whom fluid challenge and afterload reduction are of no avail. However, *digitalis glycosides* (p. 489) are not generally effective and increase the risk of dysrhythmias. Nevertheless, digitalis may be used judiciously for the treatment of atrial fibrillation with rapid ventricular rates. *Dopamine*, (p. 524) when used in doses which exceed 6 μg/kg/min, has a predominant alpha-adrenoceptor effect, and therefore increases afterload, but may be used for transient vasopressor support when marked reduction in arterial pressure with ventricular ectopy threatens immediate survival. However, this agent should be used only for brief periods with the understanding that increases in cardiac output and coronary blood flow are likely to be transient and at the risk of increased ischemic injury and depletion of plasma volume.[196c, 197] *Dobutamine* (p. 525) is an effective inotropic agent with predominant beta-adrenoceptor inotropic effect but potentially at the cost of increased myocardial oxygen requirements, and therefore the risk of extending the infarction. The benefits of nonadrenergic inotropic agents like amrinone are not well defined. Except for the temporary management of bradycardia resulting from heart block, *isoproterenol* is contraindicated because its conjoint chronotropic and inotropic effects extract disproportionately large myocardial oxygen requirements which are likely to increase myocardial ischemic injury.[185]

Improved outcome after reperfusion, whether induced by pharmacological thrombosis and/or percutaneous transluminal coronary angioplasty, has not been well documented.[198]

INTRAAORTIC BALLOON COUNTERPULSATION. There is increasing enthusiasm for mechanical support of the failing pump. The largest experience has been gained with intraaortic counterpulsation. Although the technique which was first described in the early 1960's was slow to gain acceptance, there is little doubt that it provides an effective option for *temporary* hemodynamic stabilization. With the development of percutaneous techniques for balloon insertion through the femoral artery, mechanical support need not be delayed when pharmacological interventions have failed. The outcome is generally more favorable if counterpulsation is initiated early.[199–201]

Technique. The balloon is advanced into the thoracic aorta just distal to the left subclavian artery with the aid of an image intensifier. The controller is so adjusted that the balloon is immediately inflated after closure of the aortic valve so that diastolic aortic runoff is decreased and diastolic aortic pressure is augmented. This increases coronary perfusion. Deflation is initiated just before the onset of systole so that there is systolic unloading with decreased aortic impedance to left ventricular ejection. The mechanically induced increases in diastolic aortic pressure are counterbalanced by decreases in aortic systolic pressure so that there is relatively little change in mean aortic pressure. Left ventricular pressure is decreased by approximately 20 per cent and cardiac output is typically increased by 40 per cent (Table 19–7). Decreases in coronary venous and systemic lactate concentrations, together with improvements in systemic perfusion with increases in urine output, are typically observed.[202]

However, the benefits of balloon counterpulsation are primarily those of gaining time for more definitive interventions. This technique stabilizes the patients, who may then be taken to the invasive laboratory on an urgent basis for diagnosis with view to surgical or other mechanical intervention. Contingent on the angiographic findings, early revascularization, resection of ventricular aneurysm, repair of ruptured ventricular septum, and mitral valve replacement for control of valvular insufficiency stemming

TABLE 19–7 EFFECTS OF INTRAAORTIC BALLOON PUMPING (IABP) IN 35 PATIENTS WITH CARDIOGENIC SHOCK

	BEFORE	IABP	CHANGE (%)
Pulmonary artery occlusive pressure mm Hg	24	19	−21
Aortic systolic/diastolic mm Hg	78/55	68/95	−13/+73
Cardiac index l/min/M^2	1.7	2.4	+41

Adapted from Resnekov, L.: Cardiogenic shock. Chest 83:893, 1983.

from rupture or dysfunction of papillary muscle may then be undertaken. If the patient is stabilized by balloon counterpulsation, both the timing and the preparations for surgical intervention may be optimized with a generally more favorable outcome.[200, 201] However, if surgical intervention is indicated and hemodynamic stability cannot be maintained, surgical operation should not be deferred.

In patients in whom there has been an orderly sequence of intraaortic balloon pumping, invasive diagnosis, and appropriate surgical intervention, the outcome may be more favorable and immediate survival of between 30 and 75 per cent of patients has been reported.[201, 202] However, the benefits of balloon pumping are not without cost. One or more complications of balloon counterpulsation have been reported in 36 per cent of patients, especially during *insertion* of the aortic balloon.[203] Complications, occasionally fatal, are due to perforation of the aorta, aortic dissection, ischemic injury to the lower extremities caused by critical reduction in femoral blood flow, embolism, thrombocytopenia, and hemolysis.[204] A minority of complications are due to mechanical failure of the counterpulsation system or rupture of the intraaortic balloon. However, infection at the site of balloon insertion constitutes a significant problem.[204] Increased incidence of left ventricular rupture has been reported in patients maintained on aortic counterpulsation. However, this may be due to more protracted survival of patients with extensive infarction attributable to counterpulsation rather than an adverse effect of counterpulsation itself.[202]

Contraindications. These include aortic regurgitation, aortic aneurysm, and major rhythm defects which preclude synchronization of the patient's rhythm with inflation and deflation of the balloon. Inotropic therapy, and particularly dobutamine, may be used in conjunction with counterpulsation to augment cardiac output with lesser risk of extending myocardial infarction.[205]

For management of cardiogenic shock associated with *right ventricular infarction*, fluid challenge without other intervention has high likelihood of reversing the clinical signs of shock. When right ventricular infarction is unresponsive to fluids, intraaortic balloon counterpulsation is an appropriate option, followed by invasive diagnosis and surgical intervention, which may include tricuspid valve replacement.

An alternative cardiac assist technique is ventricular assist pumping (left atrial or left ventricular bypass; p. 532), but this has not yet come into routine use.[206, 207]

NONISCHEMIC CAUSES OF CARDIOGENIC SHOCK

Causes of cardiogenic shock, other than myocardial infarction, include extremes of tachycardia, in which there is inadequate diastolic filling time; extremes of bradycardia, with inadequate cardiac output; and ventricular ectopic rhythms, with disorganized or asynchronous myocardial contraction for which pharmacological, electrical, and surgical interventions are indicated.

Intracardiac obstruction may be due to valvular obstruction, with marked reductions in cardiac output of either congenital or acquired cause. Newly developed techniques of balloon valvuloplasty (p. 1390) may be useful for emergency intervention.[208–211] Intracardiac obstruction caused by ball valve thrombus or atrial myxoma may now be diagnosed at the bedside with conventional echocardiographic techniques; urgent surgery may be lifesaving. Previously undetected hypertrophic obstructive cardiomyopathies may present wih cardiogenic shock, especially when provoked by the administration of beta-adrenoceptor agents, inotropic drugs, or vasodilator agents. Beta-adrenoceptor blockade and calcium channel blocking agents may be lifesaving. Acute pump failure may also threaten immediate survival after open heart surgery as a complication of prolonged cardiopulmonary bypass or impairment of contractility owing to incision or resection of myocardium. Temporary inotropic support with beta-adrenoceptors such as dobutamine, epinephrine, dopamine, and isoproterenol is appropriate for improving contractility, especially when coronary blood flow is not compromised.

HYPOVOLEMIC SHOCK

ETIOLOGY. Intravascular volume is depleted by overt or occult extravasation of blood, by increases in capillary permeability after traumatic injuries, by infection, or by hypersensitivity reactions with extravasation of plasma and hemoconcentration. Low-perfusion states may also be due to marked increases in capillary hydrostatic pressure with extravasation of plasma water, and therefore hemoconcentration. Water and electrolyte losses from the gastointestinal tract, the skin, the airways, and the kidneys account for hypovolemia with hemoconcentration. Hemoconcentration is characterized by increases in hemoglobin and hematocrit and in the concentration of plasma proteins, and therefore oncotic pressure. These parameters should be measured at intervals to follow the response to therapy.

COMPENSATORY VOLUME SHIFTS. When intravascular volume is depleted in the absence of protein depletion or marked increases in capillary permeability, lowering of capillary hydrostatic pressure increases the effective capillary oncotic pressures. Consequently, fluid diffuses into the vascular compartment from the interstitial and intracellular compartments. This compensatory restoration of intravascular volume is known as "transcapillary refill" and accounts for the usual reductions in hematocrit and hemoglobin, together with transient reductions in plasma oncotic pressure. However, when intravascular volume is depleted by the selective loss of plasma water with or without protein, the vascular volume deficit is initially accompanied by hemoconcentration. Such hemoconcentration is observed after protracted vomiting and diarrhea, renal losses of water in association with osmolar diuresis owing to hyperosmolar states and especially diabetes mellitus, endocrine abnormalities including diabetes insipidus, adrenocortical insufficiency, pheochromocytoma, and primary renal diseases with impaired salt and water conservation.

ANAPHYLAXIS. Signifiant quantities of plasma water may also be lost during acute hypersensitivity reactions, especially anaphylaxis. Giant urticaria and angioneurotic edema represent localized extravasations of plasma water and protein. The shock state which accompanies systemic anaphylaxis may occur with or without respiratory distress. Respiratory distress is due to mucosal edema of the airway with the clinical manifestation of stridor and/or by bronchiolar constriction with clinical manifestations of acute asthma. Perfusion failure is usually of later onset than the respiratory distress, which typically occurs within 3 minutes. The onset of shock is associated with a marked decrease in cardiac output and arterial pressure.[212] This is now known to be due to a loss of plasma volume with a concurrent increase in the hematocrit and hemoglobin. The features of perfusion failure are usually characteristic of hypovolemic shock with a reduction in right heart filling pressure, marked increases in arterial resistance, decreased peripheral blood flow, anuria, and lactic acidosis. Shock is promptly reversed by the administration of large volumes of fluid, although there may be evidence of bleeding owing to disseminated intravascular coagulation. The immediate administration of epinephrine in amounts of 0.5 mg (5 ml of 1/10,000 concentration) intravenously or 1.0 mg (10 ml) into the trachea, if an intravenous route is not immediately available, remains the therapy of choice for reversal of the respiratory defect. It is possible that epinephrine also ameliorates the circulatory defect of anaphylaxis.

CLINICAL FEATURES. Except for the history and for external signs of bleeding or other fluid loss, the physical findings in patients with hypovolemic shock are not specific. Pallor and postural hypotension may be useful, but sinus tachycardia is not of itself a reliable sign of volume depletion. Reduction in arterial blood pressure is a relatively late manifestation of hypovolemia. With progressive reduction in blood volume by bleeding to aproximately 50 per cent of normal, there is a progressive decline in cardiac

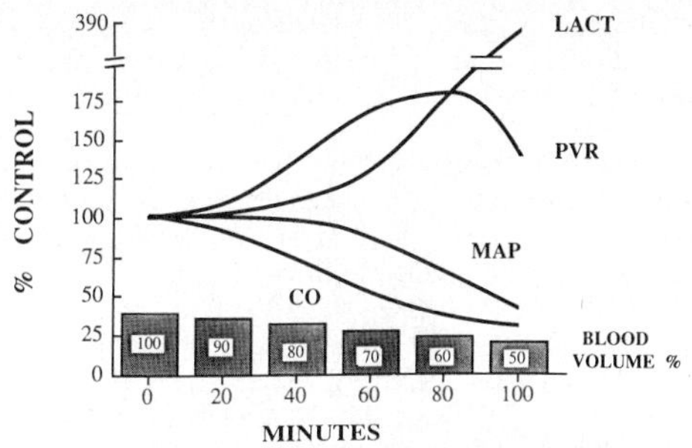

FIGURE 19–12. Relationship between percentage of changes in cardiac output, mean arterial pressure, computed peripheral (arterial) resistance, and lactate concentrations during graded hemorrhage in dogs. (From the data of Nelimarkka, et al.: Effect of graded hemorrhage on renal cortical perfusion in dogs. Am. J. Surg. *141*:235, 1981.)

output to less than 50 per cent of control (Fig. 19–12).[213] Mean arterial pressure is maintained by compensatory increases in peripheral vascular resistance. Significant increases in arterial blood lactate appear only after blood volume is rapidly depleted to 60 per cent of normal. Consequently, decreases in cardiac output are compensated for by arterial vasoconstriction. Lactic acidosis usually occurs only after more than 20 per cent of the blood volume has been depleted and cardiac output is reduced by approximately 50 per cent. Transcapillary refill mitigates decreases in intravascular volume, but this compensatory process occurs over hours and is of little event during rapid blood loss.

Bedside hemodynamic measurements disclose decreases in both right and left ventricular filling pressures, the pulmonary artery pressures, and cardiac output (Table 19–5).

MANAGEMENT. Rapid repletion of intravascular volume by fluid challenge is likely to be curative. General guidelines for the selection of appropriate fluids has already been discussed (p. 571). For practical purposes, red cell mass is most efficiently repleted with type-specific, washed red blood cells. Five per cent human serum albumin is the colloid of choice, but its use is restricted by high cost and limited availability. A 6 per cent solution of hydroxyethyl starch[214, 215] is a satisfactory alternative and generally is preferred over Dextran 70, which has somewhat less favorable effects on blood coagulation and may interfere with cross matching of blood because of red cell agglutination. If blood loss is associated with a coagulation defect, a specific diagnosis of the defect guides component therapy with platelet concentrates, fresh frozen plasma, and cryoprecipitate. Under most conditions, initial volume repletion is carried out with crystalloid solutions and, more specifically, physiological salt or lactated Ringer's solution. However, for treatment of hypovolemic shock, especially in the setting of massive body burns, hypertonic saline solutions containing up to 7.5 per cent sodium chloride have been used and well tolerated.[179, 216]

Citrate is used as an anticoagulant for liquid storage of red blood cells. Infusion of citrate may induce hypocalcemia after the administration of multiple units of citrate-phosphate-dextrose, but this is an unusual complication. It may be recognized by prolongation of the electrocardiographic Q-T interval and confirmed by measurement of plasma-ionized calcium.

There is controversy regarding the benefits of glucocorticoids administered in pharmacological doses for ancillary treatment of hypovolemic shock. Except in the setting of iatrogenic adrenal insufficiency and, rarely, when addisonian crises masquerade as hypovolemic shock after trauma or surgical operation, there is no specific indication for the administration of glucocorticoids.[217]

DISTRIBUTIVE SHOCK

ETIOLOGY. This form of shock is due to alterations in the distribution of blood flow such that tissue perfusion is compromised in the setting of infection or altered neurological function, or due to the effects of drugs and other substances which alter vascular reactivity. The predominant cause of distributive types of shock, however, is bacterial sepsis and particularly infections caused by gram-negative enteric bacilli.[218] The second most common cause is altered arterial resistance and venous capacitance produced by overdoses of barbiturate, narcotic, sedative-tranquilizer, and some anesthetic agents. Neurogenic causes include transection of the spinal cord and ganglionic blockade.

A diversity of microorganisms and toxic substances derived from them have been implicated as causative agents of septic shock, and the hemodynamic, metabolic, and immunological disturbances which accompany the septic shock state are complex. Accordingly, the pathophysiological mechanisms and clinical features are variable, depending on the causative organism, the host, and the magnitude and site of the primary infectious process. This contrasts with either neurological injury or drug-induced alterations of vasomotor function in which the predominant defect is decreased arterial resistance or, more frequently, expanded venous capacitance. Such defects of vasomotion are fully reversed with a high level of predictability by conventional fluid challenge to expand intra-vascular volume.

Gram-Negative Sepsis

The most frequent cause of septic shock is bacteremia caused by gram-negative enteric bacilli, and these constitute approximately two-thirds of clinical cases of septic shock.[219] Between one-fourth and one-half of patients with such bacteremia develop shock.[220] These organisms are largely hospital acquired and often gain entrance into the bloodstream at sites of instrumentation or injury. Accordingly, a majority of instances are related to invasive procedures. In the case of arterial catheters, for instance, there is a progressive increase in the incidence of subcutaneous infection at the site of catheterization so that pathogenic bacteria are recovered from one-third of the patients by the fifth day, approximately one-third of whom develop bacteremias.[221] The morbidity and mortality stemming from protracted vascular catheterizations are therefore substantial.

The incidence of bacteremia and shock is greatly increased when immunological competence is compromised by neoplastic disease, malnutrition, cytotoxic agents, or radiation therapy. Bacteremia caused by gram-negative bacilli has substantially increased in incidence over the past 30 years partly because of more extensive surgical procedures, the much greater use of invasive diagnostic and therapeutic interventions, and the proliferation of gram-negative enteric organisms which are resistant to commonly used antimicrobial drugs in the hospital setting. Most gram-negative infections that occur in the urinary tract are caused by *Escherichia coli*, and bacteremia follows invasion of the urinary tract by catheterization, cystoscopy, or urological surgery. Invasion of the airway by endotracheal tubes or tracheostomy, or seeding of the airway with organisms from contaminated mechanical ventilators and aerosols, accounts for respiratory infections by gram-negative enteric bacilli, especially the *Pseudomonas* and *Klebsiella* species. Surgical manipulation in the gastrointestinal and genitourinary tracts provokes bacteremia resulting from bacteroides. Contaminations at the site of skin penetration of intravenous infusion of contaminated solutions, including blood and drugs, and decubitus ulcers occur in the hospital setting.[222] In the community setting such contamination is found in intravenous drug abusers and in patients with chronic indwelling catheters. The primary site of infection may be a surgical skin wound or the vagina or uterus after delivery or abortion. Specific species of opportunistic bacteria are predominant causes in given hospital locales, but these change from time to time, in part related to the local preferences for antimicrobial agents.

DIAGNOSIS OF GRAM-NEGATIVE SEPSIS. A characteristic sequence of clinical events follows bloodstream invasion by gram-negative bacilli. The onset is usually heralded by a teeth-chattering chill, followed by an increase in body temperature to levels of as high as 41°C (106°F). This typically occurs between 2 and 24 hours after a surgical procedure or mechanical invasion of an infected site. Hyperventilation and therefore respiratory alkalosis occur in the early stages of shock followed by metabolic (lactic) acidosis. Because the skin is warm and dry during the early hyperdynamic stage of septic shock, the physician may not suspect that the blood pressure is falling. An early clue to shock is a relatively abrupt alteration in mental status often with inappropriate behavior, presumably caused by reduction in cerebral blood flow. The cause becomes apparent as soon as the blood pressure is measured. An average fall in arterial pressure from 138/70 to 70/36 mm Hg was observed in one series.[223] When the hemodynamic defect becomes more profound over the subsequent 12 to 24 hours, the skin may become pale, cool, and moist. Approximately one-half of the patients present with gastrointestinal signs, including hyperperistalsis, followed by vomiting and diarrhea, often with green and sometimes bloody stools which have a characteristic "laundry room" odor.

LABORATORY FINDINGS. At the time of onset of hypotension, these include abrupt reduction in the white blood cell count to levels as low as 1,000/mm^3, primarily caused by reduction in the number of polymorphonuclear cells. This is followed within 4 hours by an overall increase in white cells, typically to levels exceeding 20,000 mm^3, with a marked increase in the number of polymorphonuclear cells and immature forms. Increases in serum enzymes, including AST (SGOT), ALT (SGPT), and LDH, reflect nonspecific cellular injury associated with perfusion failure.[143] An increase in blood sugar is most likely caused by increased secretion of catecholamines from the adrenal medulla. Urine flow is decreased, together with decreased renal clearance of amylase such that serum amylase may be increased in the absence of pancreatic injury. The electrocardiographic findings should be interpreted with caution, since T-wave and ST-segment abnormalities are not unusual in older patients after the onset of shock.[28] In the absence of antibiotic therapy, gram-negative enteric organisms are recovered from the bloodstream with three cultures of more than 10 ml of blood in approximately 99 per cent of patients.[223]

HEMODYNAMIC MEASUREMENTS. Bedside hemodynamic measurements usually demonstrate normal or increased cardiac output with decreased arterial resistance in the absence of increases in either right or left ventricular filling pressure. In the setting of fever, hypotension with normal or increased cardiac output, together with lactic acidosis, distinguishes this type of shock from low-output states associated with hypovolemia, cardiogenic causes, and vascular obstruction. Fatal progression of shock is associated with decreases in cardiac output and decreases in both right and left ventricular stroke work.[51] Decreases in cardiac output in the later stages of shock are highly correlated with mortality.[224] Such decreases in cardiac output are, in turn, associated with rather striking impairment in both left and right ventricular function. In Figure 19–13 fatal progression of sepsis is associated with marked decreases in the left ventricular stroke work and increases in pulmonary artery occlusive pressure. Comparable changes were observed in right ventricular function.[51]

Reductions in intravascular volume occur during progression of the shock state. As the total blood volume decreases, mortality strikingly increases.[19] Accordingly, this type of septic shock is characterized by vasodilation with decreased peripheral arterial resistance during the hyperdynamic stage of shock and vasoconstriction, with more typical physical signs of circulatory shock during the late hypodynamic state. However, some patients succumb in the hyperdynamic stage of shock.[20]

The reason for the hyperdynamic state is not fully understood. Experimentally, the injection of live organisms produces vasodilation, and lipopolysaccharides (endotoxins) derived from these organisms produce vasoconstriction. As in shock states resulting from other causes, there is progressive lactic acidosis even though total oxygen consumption remains at near normal levels.[17] However, it is not known whether this represents an inadequate capability to augment oxygen delivery when oxygen requirements are increased, whether there is a reduced capability for oxygen utilization at the exchange site, or whether

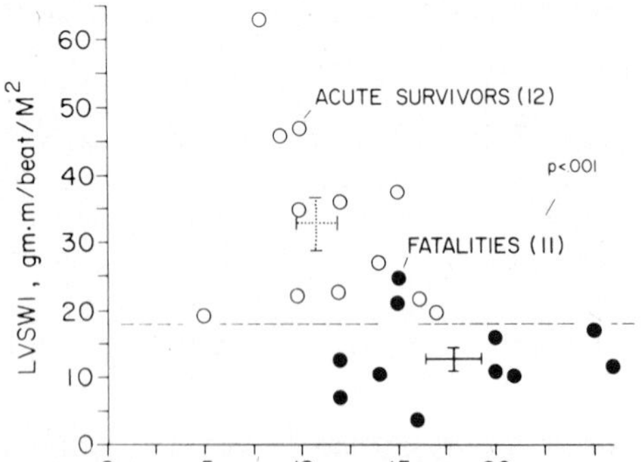

FIGURE 19–13. Stroke work index vs. left ventricular filling pressure at 24 hours in patients with purulent peritonitis. (From Vincent, J.-L., et al.: Circulatory shock associated with purulent peritonitis. Am. J. Surg. *142*:262, 1981.)

there is anatomical bypass of the capillary exchange vessels by arteriovenous shunts. Because the mixed venous oxygen content during the hyperdynamic septic state is maintained at relatively high levels, the concept of arteriovenous shunting with "wasted flow" predominates. Yet measurements of capillary blood flow through muscle during the hyperdynamic shock state have failed to demonstrate reductions in capillary flow in suport of this hypothesis.[225] However, there is evidence of splanchnic and renal shunting during shock produced by endotoxin.[10]

MANAGEMENT. As in other shock states, therapy is primarily directed to management of the underlying cause, in this instance, the control of infection. There is a close relationship between the concentration of bacteria in the bloodstream and the outcome.[226] Both the fatality of bacteremia and the incidence of shock is reduced by one-half if appropriate antibiotic therapy is instituted promptly.[220] When the source of infection is due to continuous seeding of organisms from an open viscus, an abscess, or necrotic tissue, antibiotic therapy is not likely to suffice. Prompt surgical drainage or control with excision of nonviable tissue is lifesaving. Supportive therapy, as in other shock states, includes attention to ventilation and blood gas exchange and adequacy of intravascular volume. Although vasopressor agents continue to be widely used, their efficacy is unproved and they may accentuate the shock state by their vasoconstrictor action. Consequently, they may further compromise tissue perfusion, reduce intravascular volume, and increase the workload on the heart when left ventricular function is already compromised. To the contrary, there is more persuasive evidence favoring the use of vasodilator agents and particularly alpha-adrenoceptor drugs.[187, 227]

Glucocorticoids in high doses increase cardiac output and decrease arterial resistance in both normal subjects and in patients.[228] In laboratory animals they uniformly protect against the fatal effects of endotoxins and, when used in conjunction with antibiotic therapy, improve outcome when bacteremia is experimentally produced by liver gram-negative organisms.[229] Nevertheless, a prospective study suggests that glucocorticoid therapy may only prolong initial survival without benefit of improved hospital survival.[230] Two recently completed but not yet published multicenter randomized trials of methylprednisolone therapy in septic shock have not confirmed statistical benefit from this therapy.

Passive immunotherapy may be more promising. Human antiserum to the lipopolysaccharide core of endotoxin from heat-killed *E. coli* have decreased mortality caused by bacteremia and shock.[231] With securer understanding that the predominant lethal substance of the bacterial cell wall is lipid-A, immunotherapy may have special promise, but this is without immediate applicability.

Disseminated intravascular coagulation (DIC) is a major complication of gram-negative sepsis. While thrombocytopenia occurs in a majority of patients, gross bleeding is observed in only about 3 per cent of patients.[220] Except in patients with uncontrolled bleeding caused by DIC who fail to respond to replacement of clotting factors, or in rare instances of ischemic necrosis caused by thrombosis with purpura, anticoagulation with heparin is not likely to be redeeming.

PROGNOSIS. The mortality of shock complicating gram-negative sepsis ranges from 25 to 90 per cent.[28, 219, 232] This large range reflects not only the age of the patients, but also, more important, the severity of the underlying diseases. This was documented by Kreger and his colleagues,[220] who observed increasing mortality of gram-negative bacteria in close relationship to the estimated severity of the underlying diseases.

Septic Shock Caused by Other Organisms

Approximately one-third of the patients in whom shock is of infectious cause, the causative organisms are gram-positive cocci, meningococci, clostridia, or fungi. Primary treatment in such cases is also directed to control of the infection. In contrast to gram-negative sepsis, shock more often occurs as a final event, except for toxic shock.

Toxic Shock

The syndrome now termed "toxic shock" may be indistinguishable from shock associated with gram-negative sepsis except for a characteristic rash. It was initially described as a febrile illness in children with an exanthematous rash complicated by hypotension. The rash was typically diffuse and macular with blanching on pressure. The syndrome was further characterized by marked neutrophilia, mucosal hyperemia, and nonpurulent conjunctivitis. Multisystem dysfunction with early renal and hepatic impairment was observed.[233] An adult form of toxic shock was identified in 1980 in menstruating women averaging 25 years in age and related to the use of vaginal tampons. Since then between 10 and 20 per cent of instances of toxic shock have been identified in nonmenstruating women and in men.[234] The causative organism is *Staphylococcus aureus*, and toxic shock is believed to be due to a pyrogenic exotoxin produced by some strains of this bacterial species.[235]

The staphylococcal infection occurs typically in a closed space, such as in the vagina and uterus or in the nares, in a surgical wound, or in a joint after arthroscopy.[236–238] Progression is characterized by multiorgan failure with high concentrations of creatine phosphokinase. Because the organism may not be recovered in smear and culture, differential diagnosis includes serological tests for streptococci, Rocky Mountain spotted fever, leptospirosis, and measles. Toxic shock, like gram-negative sepsis, is often complicated by thrombocytopenia and sometimes by DIC.

The most immediate intervention is removal of packing in closed spaces, such as in the nose and in the vagina, and vigorous therapy with antistaphylococcal antimicrobials. Within 1 to 2 weeks after recovery, there is typically desquamation of skin.

Obstructive Shock

The primary causes of obstructive shock have already been reviewed (p. 568). The management of obstructive shock states is singularly directed to rapid reestablishment of patency of the mainstream of blood flow. Thrombolysis with streptokinase, urokinase, or tissue plasminogen activator, or transvenous removal of emboli after major pulmonary artery obstruction may be attempted. Pericardial temponade may be relieved by conventional pericardiocentesis. For practical purposes, however, the successful management of obstructive shock states requires early diagnosis and intervention, often surgical, for prompt restoration of blood flow.

REFERENCES

PATHOPHYSIOLOGY

1. Weil, M. H.: Bacterial shock. *In* Weil, M. H., and Shubin, H. (eds.): Diagnosis and Treatment of Shock. Baltimore, Williams and Wilkins Co., 1967, p. 10.
2. Weil, M. H.: Current understanding of mechanisms and treatment of circulatory shock caused by bacterial infections. Ann. Clin. Res. 9:181, 1977.
3. Zweifach, B. W.: Quantitative studies of microcirculatory structure and function. I. Analysis of pressure distribution in the terminal vascular bed in cat mesentery. Circ. Res. *34*:843, 1974.
4. Zweifach, B. W.: Quantitative studies of microcirculatory structure and function. II. Direct measurement of capillary pressure in splanchnic mesenteric vessels. Circ. Res. *34*:848, 1974.
5. Abboud, F. M., Heistad, D. D., Mark, A. L., and Schmid, P. G.: Reflex control of the peripheral circulation. Prog. Cardiovasc. Dis. *18*:371, 1976.
6. Bond, R. F., and Johnson, G. S.: Vascular adrenergic interactions during hemorrhagic shock. Fed. Proc. *44*:281, 1985.
7. Hinshaw, L. B., and Owen, S. E.: Correlation of pooling and resistance changes in the canine forelimb in septic shock. J. Appl. Physiol. *30*:331, 1971.
8. Archie, J. P., Jr.: Anatomic arterial-venous shunting in endotoxic and septic shock in dogs. Ann. Surg. *186*:171, 1972.
9. Wiedeman, M. P.: Dimensions of blood vessels from distributing artery to collecting vein. Circ. Res. *12*:375, 1963.
10. Kerr, A. R., and Kirklin, J. W.: Changes in canine venous volume and pressure during hemorrhage. Surgery 68:3, 1970.
11. Scheidt, S., Arscheim, R., and Killip, T., III: Shock after acute myocardial infarction. Am. J. Cardiol. *26*:556, 1970.
12. Diamond, G., and Forrest, J. S.: Effect of coronary artery disease and acute myocardial infarction on left ventricular compliance in man. Circulation *45*:11, 1972.
13. Parker, M. M., and Parillo, J. E.: Septic shock. Hemodynamics and pathogenesis. J.A.M.A. *250*:3324, 1983.
14. Ellrodt, A. G., Riedinger, M. S., Kimchi, A., Berman, D. S., Maddahi, J., Swan, H. J. C., and Murata, G. H.: Left ventricular performance in septic shock: Reversible segmental and global abnormalities. Am. Heart J. *110*:402, 1985.
15. Crowell, J. W., and Smith, E. E.: Oxygen deficit and irreversible hemorrhagic shock. Am. J. Physiol. *206*:313, 1964.
16. Kaufman, B. S., Rackow, E. C., and Falk, J. L.: The relationship between oxygen delivery and consumption during fluid resuscitation of hypovolemic and septic shock. Chest *85*:336, 1984.
17. Houtchens, B. A., and Westenskow, D. R.: Review article. Oxygen consumption in septic shock: Collective review. Circ. Shock *13*:361, 1984.
18. Weil, M. H.: Measurement of cardiac output. Crit. Care Med. 5:117, 1977.
19. Weil, M. H., and Nishijima, H.: Cardiac output in bacterial shock. Am. J. Med. *64*:920, 1978.
20. Groeneveld, A. B. J., Bronsveld, W., and Thijs, L. G.: Hemodynamic determinants of mortality in human septic shock. Surgery *99*:140, 1984.
21. Hinshaw, L. B., Gilbert, R. P., Kuida, H., and Visscher, M. B.: Peripheral resistance changes and blood pooling after endotoxin in eviscerated dogs. Am. J. Physiol. *195*:631, 1958.
22. Cohn, J. N.: Blood pressure measurement in shock: Mechanism of inaccuracy in auscultatory and palpatory methods. J.A.M.A. *199*:118, 1967.
23. Kazamias, T. M., Gander, M. P., Franklin, D. L., and Ross, J., Jr.: Blood pressure measurement with doppler ultrasonic flow meter. J. Appl. Physiol. *30*:585, 1971.
24. Weil, M. H., Shubin, H., and Carlson, R. W.: Treatment of circulatory shock: Use of sympathomimetic and related vasoactive agents. J.A.M.A. *231*:1280, 1975.
25. Henning, R. J., Wiener, F., Valdes, S., and Weil, M. H.: Measurement of toe temperature for assessing the severity of acute circulatory failure. Surg. Gynecol. Obstet. *149*:1, 1979.
26. Shoemaker, W. C., Fink, S., Ray, C. W., and McCartney S.: Effect of hemorrhagic shock on conjunctival and transcutaneous oxygen tensions in relation to hemodynamic and oxygen transport changes. Crit. Care Med. *12*:949, 1984.
27. Weil, M. H., and Afifi, A. A.: Experimental and clinical studies on lactate and pyruvate as indicators of the severity of acute circulatory failure (shock). Circulation *41*:989, 1970.
28. Weil, M. H., Shubin, H., and Biddle, M.: Shock caused by gram-negative microorganisms. Analysis of 169 cases. Ann. Int. Med. *60*:384, 1964.
29. Terradellas, J. B., Bellot, J. F., Saris, A. B., Gil, C. L., Torrallardona, A. T., and Garriga, J. R.: Acute and transient ST segment elevation during bacterial shock in seven patients without apparent heart disease. Chest *81*:444, 1982.
30. Thomas, F., Smith, J. L., Orme, J. F., Jr., Clemmer, T. P., Hagan, A. D., Elliott, C. G., and Vincent, G. M.: Reversible segmental myocardial dysfunction in septic shock. Crit. Care Med. *14*:587, 1986.
31. McArdle, C. S., MacDonald, J. A. E., and Ledingham, I. M.: A three-year retrospective analysis of septic shock in a general hospital. Scott. Med. J. *20*:79, 1975.
32. Ollodart, R., and Mansberger, A. R.: The effect of hypovolemic shock on bacterial defense. Am. J. Surg. *110*:302, 1965.
33. Chien, S.: Role of the sympathetic nervous system in hemorrhage. Physiol. Rev. *47*:214, 1967.
34. Rutherford, R. B., Balis, J. V., Trow, R. S., and Graves, G. M.: Comparison of hemodynamic and regional blood flow changes at equivalent stages of endotoxin and hemorrhagic shock. J. Trauma *16*:886, 1976.
35. DelGuercio, L. R., Cohn, S. D., Feins, N. R., Greenspan, M., and Kornitzer, G.: Pulmonary and systemic arteriovenous shunting in clinical septic shock. *In* Third International Conference on Hyperbaric Medicine. Washington, D.C., National Academy of Sciences, 1966, p. 337.
36. Jardin, F., Eveleigh, M. C., Gurdjian, F., Delille, F., and Margairaz, A.: Venous admixture in human septic shock. Comparative effects of blood volume expansion, dopamine infusion and isoproterenol infusion on mismatching of ventilation and pulmonary blood flow in peritonitis. Circulation *60*:155, 1979.
37. Brunjes, S., Johns, V. J., Jr., and Crane, M. G.: Pheochromocytoma: Postoperative shock and blood volume. N. Engl. J. Med. *262*:393, 1960.
38. Henning, R. J., Shubin, H., and Weil, M. H.: Afterload reduction with phentolamine in patients with acute pulmonary edema. Am. J. Med. *63*:568, 1977.
39. Zucker, I. H., Earle, A. M., and Gilmore, J. P.: The mechanism of adaptation of left atrial stretch receptors in dogs with chronic congestive heart failure. J. Clin. Invest. *60*:323, 1977.
40. Feuerstein, G., Johnson, A. K., Zerbe, R. L., Davis-Kramer, R., and Faden, A. I.: Anteroventral hypothalamus and hemorrhagic shock: Cardiovascular and neuroendocrine responses. Am. J. Physiol. *246*:551, 1984.
41. Errington, M. L., and Rocha e Silva, M., Jr.: On the role of vasopressin and angiotensin in the development of irreversible hemorrhagic shock. J. Physiol. *24*:119, 1974.
42. Henrich, W. L., Berl, T., McDonald, K. M., Anderson, R. J., and Schrier, R. W.: Angiotensin II, renal nerves, and prostaglandins in renal hemodynamics during hemorrhage. Am. J. Physiol. *235*:F46, 1978.
43. Scriven, T. A., and Burnett, J. C.: The natriuretic response to atrial natriuretic peptide is attenuated in acute low output failure. Clin. Res. *33*:498, 1985.
44. Carlson, E. L., Selinger, S. L., Utley, J., and Hoffman, J. I. E.: Intramyocardial distribution of blood flow in hemorrhagic shock in anesthetized dogs. Am. J. Physiol. *230*:41, 1976.
45. Hackel, D. B., Ratliff, N. B., and Mikat, E.: The heart in shock. Circ. Res. *35*:805, 1974.
46. Schenk, E. A., and Moss, A. J.: Cardiovascular effects of sustained norepinephrine infusions. II. Morphology. Circ. Res. *18*:605, 1966.
47. Klouda, M. A., and Brynjolfsson, G.: Cardiotoxic effects of electrical stimulation of the stellate ganglia. Ann. N.Y. Acad. Sci. *156*:271, 1969.
48. Greenhout, J. H., and Reichenbach, D. D.: Cardiac injury and subarachnoid hemorrhage. J. Neurosurg. *30*:521, 1969.
49. Nickerson, M., and Gourzis, J. T.: Blockade of sympathetic vasoconstriction in the treatment of shock. J. Trauma 2:399, 1962.
50. Crowell, J. W., and Guyton, A. C.: Further evidence favoring a cardiac mechanism in irreversible hemorrhagic shock. Am. J. Physiol. *203*:248, 1962.
51. Vincent, J.-L., Weil, M. H., Puri, V., and Carlson, R. W.: Circulatory shock associated with purulent peritonitis. Am. J. Surg. *142*:262, 1981.
52. Guntheroth, W., Warren, G., Jacky, J. P., Kawabori, I., Stevenson, J. G., and Moreno, A. H.: Left ventricular performance in endotoxin shock in dogs. Am. J. Physiol. *242*:H172, 1982.
53. Lee, J. C., and Downing, S. E.: Myocardial oxygen availability and cardiac failure in hemorrhagic shock. Am. Heart J. 92:201, 1976.
54. Cunnion, R. E., Schaer, G. L., Parker, M. M., Natanson, C., and Parrillo, J. E.: The coronary circulation in human septic shock. Circulation *73*:637, 1986.
55. Lefer, A. M.: Blood-borne humoral factors in the pathophysiology of circulatory shock. Circ. Res. *32*:129, 1973.
56. Goldfarb, R. D.: Characteristics of shock-induced circulating cardiodepressant substances: A brief review. Circ. Shock (Suppl.) *1*:23, 1979.

57. McConn, R., Greineder, J. K., Wasserman, F., and Clowes, G. H. A., Jr.: Is there a humoral factor that depresses ventricular function in sepsis? Circ. Shock (Suppl.) *1*:9, 1979.
58. Parrillo, J. E., Burch, C., Shelhamer, J. H., Parker, M. M., Natanson, C., and Schuette, W.: A circulating myocardial depressant substance in humans with septic shock. J. Clin. Invest. *76*:1539, 1976.
59. Monsalve, F., Rucabado, L., Salvador, A., Bonastre, J., Cunat, J., and Ruano, M.: Myocardial depression in septic shock caused by meningococcal infection. Crit. Care Med. *12*:1021, 1984.
60. Jones, C. E., Smith, E. E., DuPont, E., and Williams R. D.: Demonstration of nonperfused myocardium in late hemorrhagic shock. Circ. Shock *5*:97, 1978.
61. Geft, I. L., Fishbein, M. C., Ninomiya, K., Hashida, J., Chaux, E., Yano, J., Y-Rit, J., Genov, T., Shell, W., and Ganz, W.: Intermittent brief periods of ischemia have a cumulative effect and may cause myocardial necrosis. Circulation *66*:1150, 1982.
62. Alyono, D., Ring, W. S., Chao, R. Y. N., Alyono, M. M., Crumbley, A. J., Larson, V. E., and Anderson, R. W.: Characteristics of ventricular function in severe hemorrhagic shock. Surgery *94*:250, 1983.
63. Horton, J. W., Coln, D., and Mitchell, J. H.: Left ventricular volumes and contractility during hemorrhagic hypotension: Dimensional analysis and biplane cinefluorography. Circ. Shock *11*:73, 1983.
64. Willerson, J. T., Scales, F., Mukherjee, A., Platt, M., Templeton, G. H., Fink, G. S., and Buja, L. M.: Abnormal myocardial fluid retention as an early manifestation of ischemic injury. Am. J. Pathol. *87*:159, 1977.
65. Bronsveld, W., van Lambalgen, A. A., van den Bos, G. C., Thijs, L. G., and Koopman, P. A. R.: Effects of glucose-insulin-potassium (GIK) on myocardial blood flow and metabolism in canine endotoxin shock. Circ. Shock *13*:325, 1984.
66. Braunwald, E., and Kloner, R. A.: The stunned myocardium: Prolonged, postischemic ventricular dysfunction. Circulation *66*:1146, 1982.
67. Jennings, R. B.: Early phase of myocardial ischemic injury and infarction. Am. J. Cardiol. *24*:753, 1969.
68. Udhoji, V. N., and Weil, M. H.: Circulatory effects of angiotensin, levarterenol and metaraminol in the treatment of shock. N. Engl. J. Med. *270*:501, 1964.
69. Lloyd, B. L., and Taylor, R. R.: Augmentation of myocardial digoxin concentration in hemorrhagic shock. Circulation *51*:718, 1975.
70. Cohn, J. D., Greenspan, M., Goldstein, C. R., Gudwin, A. L., Siegel, J. H., and Del Guercio, L. R. M.: Arteriovenous shunting in high cardiac output shock syndromes. Surg. Gynecol. Obstet. *127*:282, 1968.
71. Hillir, C., Bone, R., Wilson, F.: Comparison of tissue and mixed venous oxygen tension in endotoxic shock. Am. Rev. Resp. Dis. *119a*:127, 1979.
72. Weil, M. H., Leavy, J. A., Rackow, E. C., Halfman, C. J., and Bruno, S. J.: Validation of a semi-automated technique for measurement of whole blood lactate. Clin. Chem. *32*:2175, 1986.
73. Afifi, A. A., Chang, P. C., Liu, V. Y., da Luz, P. L., Weil, M. H., and Shubin, H.: Prognostic indexes in acute myocardial infarction complicated by shock. Am. J. Cardiol. *33*:826, 1974.
74. Weisel, R. D., Vito, L., Dennis, R. C., Valeri, C. R., and Hechtman, H. B.: Myocardial depression during sepsis. Am. J. Surg. *133*:512, 1977.
75. Oliva, P. B.: Lactic acidosis. Am. J. Med. *48*:209, 1970.
76. Orringer, C. E., Eustace, J. C., Wunsch, C. D., and Gardner, L. B.: Natural history of lactic acidosis after grand-mal seizure. A model for the study of an anion-gap acidosis not associated with hyperkalemia. N. Engl. J. Med. 297:796, 1977.
77. Weil, M. H., Ruiz, C. E., Michaels, S., Rackow, E. C.: Acid-base determinants of survival after cardiopulmonary resuscitation. Crit. Care Med. *13*:888, 1985.
78. Huckabee, W. E.: Relationships of pyruvate and lactate during anaerobic metabolism. II. Exercise and formation of O_2-debt. J. Clin. Invest. *37*:255, 1958.
79. Huckabee, W. E.: Relationship of pyruvate and lactate during anaerobic metabolism. V. Coronary adequacy. Am. J. Physiol. *200*:1169, 1961.
80. Blair, E., Cowley, R. A., and Tait, M. K.: Refractory septic shock in man. Role of lactate and pyruvate metabolism and acid-base balance in prognosis. Am. Surg. *31*:537, 1965.
81. Puri, V. K., Schaeffer, R. C., Carlson, R. W., and Weil, M. H.: Experimental aortic occlusion: A model for the study of regional shock with specific reference to blood lactate. Circ. Shock *7*:447, 1980.
82. Leavy, J. A., Weil, M. H., and Rackow, E. C.: Failure to confirm "lactate washout" after circulatory arrest. Fed. Proc. *44*:1130, 1985.
83. Naylor, J. M., and Kronfeld, D. S.: In vivo studies of hypoglycemia and lactic acidosis in endotoxic shock. Am. J. Physiol. *248*:E309, 1985.
84. Togari, H., Sugiyama, S., Ogino, T., Suzuki, S., Ito, T., Ichiki, T., Kamiya, K., Watanabe, I., Ogawa, Y., Wada, Y., and Takaoka, T.: Interactions of endotoxin with cortisol and acute phase proteins in septic shock neonates. Acta Paediatr. Scand. *75*:69, 1986.
85. Bagby, G. J., and Spitzer, J. A.: Decreased rat heart and skeletal muscle lipoprotein lipase activity following endotoxin administration. Circ. Shock *6*:170, 1979.
86. Kashyap, M. L., Tay, J. S. L., Sothy, S. P., and Morrison, J. A.: Role of adipose tissue in free fatty acid metabolism in hemorrhagic hypotension and shock. Metabolism *24*:855, 1975.
87. Daniel, A. M., Pierce, C. H., Shizgal, H. M., and MacLean, L. D.: Protein and fat utilization in shock. Surgery *84*:588, 1978.
88. Hinshaw, L. B., Jordan, M. M., and Vick, J. A.: Histamine release and endotoxin shock in the primate. J. Clin. Invest. *40*:1631, 1961.
89. David, R. B., Bailey, W. L., and Hanson, N. P.: Modification of serotonin and histamine release after *E. coli* endotoxin administration. Am. J. Physiol. *205*:560, 1963.
90. Miller, R. L., Reichgott, M. J., and Melmon, K. L.: Biochemical mechanisms of generation of bradykinin by endotoxin. J. Infect. Dis. *128*:S144, 1973.
91. Hallett, J. W., Jr., Sneiderman, C. A., and Wilson, J. W.: Pulmonary effects of arterial infusion of filtered blood in experimental hemorrhagic shock. Surg. Gynecol. Obstet. *138*:517, 1974.
92. Davis, R. B., Meeker, W. R., and Bailey, W. L.: Serotonin release by bacterial endotoxin. Proc. Soc. Exp. Biol. Med. *108*:774, 1961.
93. Glazier, J. C., and Murray, J. F.: Sites of pulmonary vasomotor reactivity in the dog during alveolar hypoxia and serotonin and histamine infusion. J. Clin. Invest. *50*:2550, 1971.
94. Brigham, K. L., and Owen, P. J.: Mechanism of the serotonin effect on lung transvascular fluid and protein movement in awake sheep. Circ. Res. *36*:761, 1975.
95. Cook, J. A., Wise, W. C., and Halushka, P. V.: Elevated thromboxane levels in the rat during endotoxic shock. Protective effects of imidazole 13-azaprostanoic acid, or essential fatty acid deficiency. J. Clin. Invest. *65*:227, 1980.
96. Wise, W. C., Cook, J. A., Halushka, P. V., and Knapp, D. R.: Protective effects of thromboxane synthetase inhibitors in rats in endotoxin shock. Circ. Res. *46*:854, 1980.
97. Carmona, R. H., Tsao, T. C., and Trunkey, D. D.: The role of prostacyclin and thromboxane in sepsis and septic shock. Arch. Surg. *119*:189, 1984.
98. Fink, M. P., MacVittie, T. J., and Casey, L. C.: Inhibition of prostaglandin synthesis restores normal hemodynamics in canine hyperdynamic sepsis. Ann. Surg. *200*:619, 1984.
99. Bernton, E. W., Long, J. B., and Holaday, J. W.: Opioids and neuropeptides: Mechanisms in circulatory shock. Fed. Proc. *44*:290, 1985.
100. Curtis, M. T., and Lefer, A. M.: Protective actions of naloxone in hemorrhagic shock. Am. J. Physiol. *239*:H416, 1980.
101. Rock, P., Silverman, H., Plump, D., Kecala, Z., Smith, P., Michael, J. R., and Summer, W.: Efficacy and safety of naloxone in septic shock. Crit. Care Med. *13*:28, 1985.
102. Kalter, E. S., Jaspers, F. C., van Dijk, W. C., Nijkamp, E. P., de Jong, W., and Verhoef, J.: Induction of the early hypotensive phase by *Escherichia coli*: Role of bacterial surface structures and inflammatory mediators. J. Infect. Dis. *152*:493, 1985.
103. Krausz, M. M., Utsunomiya, T., Feuerstein, G., Wolfe, J. H. N., Shepro, N., and Hechtman, H. B.: Prostacyclin reversal of lethal endotoxemia in dogs. J. Clin. Invest. *67*:1118, 1981.
104. Sacks, T., Moldow, C. F., Craddock, P. R., Bowers, T. K., and Jacob, H. S.: Oxygen radicals mediate endothelial cell damage by complement-stimulated granulocytes. J. Clin. Invest. *61*:1161, 1978.
105. Weissman, G., Smolen, J. E., and Korchak, H. M.: Release of inflammatory mediators from stimulated neutrophils. N. Engl. J. Med. *303*:27, 1980.
106. Casey, L. C., Fletcher, J. R., Zmudka, M. I., and Ramwell, P. W.: The role of thromboxane in primate endotoxin shock. J. Surg. Res. *39*:140, 1985.
107. Zimmerman, J. J., Shelhamer, J. H., and Parrillo, J. E.: Quantitative analysis of polymorphonuclear leukocyte superoxide anion generation in critically ill children. Crit. Care Med. *13*:143, 1985.
108. Siegal, T., Seligsohn, U., Aghai, E., and Modan, M.: Clinical and laboratory aspects of disseminated intravascular coagulation (DIC): A study of 118 cases. Thromb. Haemost. *39*:122, 1978.
109. Chaudry, I. H.: Cellular mechanisms in shock and ischemia and their correction. Am. J. Physiol. *245*:R117, 1983.
110. Demopoulos, C. A., Pinckard, R. N., and Hanahan, D. J.: Platelet-activating factor. Evidence for 1-0-alkyl-2-acetyl-sn-glyceryl-3-phosphorylcholine as the active component (a new class of lipid chemical mediators). J. Biol. Chem. *254*:9355, 1979.
111. Cusack, N. J.: Platelet-activating factor. Nature *285*:193, 1980.
112. Creticos, P. S., Peters, S. P., Adkinson, F., Jr., Naclerio, R. M., Hayes, E. C., Norman, P. S., and Lichtenstein, L. M.: Peptide leukotriene release after antigen challenge in patients sensitive to ragweed. N. Engl. J. Med. *310*:1626, 1984.
113. McCafferty, M. H., and Saba, T. M.: Influence of septic peritonitis on circulating fibronectin, immunoglobulin, and complement: Relationship to reticuloendothelial phagocytic function. Adv. Shock Res. *9*:241, 1983.
114. Loegerling, D. J.: Humoral factor depletion and reticuloendothelial depression during hemorrhagic shock. Am. J. Physiol. *232*:H283, 1977.
115. Carlson, R. P., and Lefer, A. M.: Hepatic cell integrity in hypodynamic states. Am. J. Physiol. *231*:1408, 1976.
116. Loegering, D. J., and Saba, T. M.: Hepatic Kupffer cell dysfunction during hemorrhagic shock. Circ. Shock *3*:107, 1976.
117. Blattberg, B., and Levy, M. N.: Vasoactive substances and reticuloendothelial function. Am. J. Physiol. *210*:569, 1966.

SECONDARY EFFECTS OF SHOCK

118. Mosher, P., Ross, J., Jr., McFate, P. A., and Shaw, R. F.: Control of coronary blood flow by an autoregulatory mechanism. Circ. Res. *14*:250, 1964.
119. Donohoe, J. F., Venkatachalam, M. A., Bernard, D. B., and Levinsky, N. G.: Tubular leakage and obstruction after renal ischemia: Structural-functional correlations. Kidney Int. *13*:208, 1978.
120. Venkatachalam, M. A., Bernard, D. B., Donohoe, J. F., and Levinsky, N. G.: Ischemic damage and repair in the rat proximal tubule: Differences among the S_1, S_2, and S_3 segments. Kidney Int. *14*:31, 1978.
121. Solez, K.: Pathogenesis of acute renal failure. Int. Rev. Exp. Pathol. *24*:277, 1983.

122. Mason, J., Welsch, J., and Takabatake, T.: Disparity between surface and deep nephron function early after renal ischemia. Kidney Int. *24*:27, 1985.
123. Brezis, M., Rosen, S., Silva, P., and Epstein, F. H.: Selective vulnerability of the medullary thick ascending limb to anoxia in the isolated perfused rat kidney. J. Clin. Invest. *73*:182, 1984.
124. Brezis, M., Rosen, S., Silva, P., and Epstein, F. H.: Renal ischemia: A new perspective. Kidney Int. *26*:375, 1984.
125. Brezis, M., Rosen, S., Spokes, K., Silva, P., and Epstein, F. H.: Transport-dependent anoxic cell injury in the isolated perfused rat kidney. Am. J. Pathol. *116*:327, 1984.
126. Brown, R., Babcock, R., Talbert, J., Gruenberg, J., Czurak, C., and Campbell, M.: Renal function in critically ill postoperative patients: Sequential assessment of creatinine osmolar and free water clearance. Crit. Care Med. *8*:68, 1980.
127. Lucas, C. E., Harrigan, C., Denis, R., and Ledgerwood, A. M.: Impaired renal concentrating ability during resuscitation from shock. Arch. Surg. *118*:642, 1983.
128. Miller, T. R., Anderson, R. J., Stuart, L. L., Henrich, W. L., Berns, A. S., Gabow, P. A., and Schrier, R. W.: Urinary diagnostic indices in acute renal failure. A prospective study. Ann. Intern. Med. *89*:47, 1978.
129. Knaus, W. A., Draper, E., Wagner, D. P., and Zimmerman, J. E.: Prognosis in acute organ-system failure. Ann. Surg. *202*:685, 1985.
130. Finn, W. F.: Recovery from renal failure. *In* Brenner, B. M., and Lazarus, J. M. (eds.): Acute Renal Failure. Philadelphia, W. B. Saunders Company, 1983, p. 753.
131. Rinaldo, J. E., and Rogers, R. M.: Adult respiratory-distress syndrome. Changing concepts of lung injury and repair. N. Engl. J. Med. *306*:900, 1982.
132. Dillon, B. C., and Saba, T. M.: Fibronectin deficiency and intestinal transvascular fluid balance during bacteremia. Am. J. Physiol. *242*:H557, 1982.
133. Saba, T. M., and Jaffe, E.: Plasma fibronectin (opsonic glycoprotein): Its synthesis by vascular endothelial cells and role in cardiopulmonary integrity after trauma as related to reticuloendothelial function. Am. J. Med. *68*:577, 1980.
134. Appel, P. L., and Shoemaker, W. C.: Hemodynamic and oxygen transport effects of prostaglandin E_1 in patients with adult respiratory distress syndrome. Crit. Care Med. *12*:528, 1984.
135. Holcroft, J. W., Vassar, M. J., and Weber, C. J.: Prostaglandin E_1 and survival in patients with the adult respiratory distress syndrome. Ann. Surg. *203*:371, 1986.
136. Nicholson, D. P.: Corticosteroids in the treatment of septic shock and the adult respiratory distress syndrome. Med. Clin. North Am. *67*:717, 1983.
137. Hackney, J. D., Evans, M. J., Spier, C. E., Anzar, U. T., and Clark, K. W.: Effect of high concentrations of oxygen on reparative regeneration of damaged alveolar epithelium in mice. Exp. Mol. Pathol. *34*:338, 1981.
138. Lutch, J. S., and Murray, J. F.: Continuous positive-pressure ventilation: Effects on systemic oxygen transport and tissue oxygenation. Ann. Intern. Med. *76*:193, 1972.
139. Suter, P. M., Fairley, H. B., and Isenberg, M. D.: Optimum end-expiratory airway pressure in patients with acute pulmonary failure. N. Engl. J. Med. *292*:284, 1975.
140. Aubier, M., Trippenbach, T., and Roussos, C.: Respiratory muscle fatigue during cardiogenic shock. J. Appl. Physiol. *51*:449, 1981.
141. Johnson, G., III, Henderson, D., and Bond, R. F.: Morphological differences in cutaneous and skeletal muscle vasculature during compensatory and decompensatory hemorrhagic hypotension. Circ. Shock *15*:111, 1985.
142. Henning, R. J., Shubin, H., and Weil, M. H.: The measurement of the work of breathing for the clinical assessment of ventilator dependence. Crit. Care Med. *5*:264, 1977.
143. Shubin, H., and Weil, M. H.: Acute elevation of serum transaminase and lactic dehydrogenase during circulatory shock. Am. J. Cardiol. *11*:327, 1963.
144. Bor, N. M., Alvur, M., Ercan, M. T., and Bekdik, C. F.: Liver blood flow rate and glucose metabolism in hemorrhagic hypotension and shock. J. Trauma *22*:753, 1982.
145. Cowley, R. A., Mergner, W. J., Fisher, R. S., Jones, R. T., and Trump, B. F.: The subcellular pathology of shock in trauma patients: Studies using the immediate autopsy. Am. Surg. *45*:255, 1979.
146. Bhagwat, A. G., and Hawk, W. A.: Terminal hemorrhagic necrotizing enteropathy (THNE). Am. J. Gastroenterol. 45:163, 1966.
147. Cuevas, P., and Fine, J.: Demonstration of a lethal endotoxemia in experimental occlusion of the superior mesenteric artery. Surg. Gynecol. Obstet. 133:81, 1971.
148. Lillehei, R. C., and MacLean, L. D.: The intestinal factor in irreversible endotoxin shock. Ann. Surg. *148*:513, 1958.
149. Spath, J. A., Jr., Gorczynski, R. J., and Lefer, A. M.: Pancreatic perfusion in the pathophysiology of hemorrhagic shock. Am. J. Physiol. *226*:443, 1974.
150. Hock, C. E., Su, J., and Lefer, A. M.: Role of AVP in maintenance of circulatory homeostasis during hemorragic shock. Am. J. Physiol. *246*:H174, 1984.
151. Lefer, A. M.: Vascular mediators in ischemia and shock. *In* Cowley, R. A., and Trump, B. F. (eds.): Pathophysiology of Shock, Anoxia, and Ischemia. Baltimore, Williams and Wilkins Co., 1982, p. 165.
152. Lefer, A. M.: Pharmacologic and surgical modulation of myocardial depressant factor formation and action during shock. Prog. Clin. Biol. Res. *111*:111, 1983.
153. Jones, R. T., and Linhardt, G. E.: Pathology and pathophysiology of the exocrine pancreas in shock. *In* Cowley, R. A., and Trump, B. F. (eds.): Pathophysiology of Shock, Anoxia, and Ischemia. Baltimore, Williams and Wilkins Co., 1982, p. 309.
154. Herlihy, B. L., and Lefer, A. M.: Alterations in pancreatic acinar cell organelles during circulatory shock. Circ. Shock 2:143, 1975.
155. McManus, W. F., Eurenius, K., and Pruitt, B. A.: Disseminated intravascular coagulation in burned patients. J. Trauma *13*:416, 1973.
156. Hasiba, U., Rosenbach, L. M., Rockwell, D., and Lewis, J. H.: DIC-like syndrome after envenomation by the snake, *Crotalus horridus horridus*. N. Engl. J. Med. *292*:505, 1975.
157. Spicer, T. E., and Rau, J. M.: Purpura fulminans. Am. J. Med. *61*:566, 1976.
158. Feinstein, D. I.: Diagnosis and management of disseminated intravascular coagulation: The role of heparin therapy. Blood *60*:284, 1982.
159. Agostoni, A., Lotto, A., Stabilin, R., Bernascon, C., Gerli, G., Gattinoni, L., Iapickino, G., and Salvade, P.: Hemoglobin oxygen affinity in patients with low-output heart failure and cardiogenic shock after acute myocardial infarction. Eur. J. Cardiol. *3*:53, 1975.
160. da Luz, P. L., Cavanilles, J. M., Michaels, S., Weil, M. H., and Shubin, H.: Oxygen delivery, anoxic metabolism and hemoglobin-oxygen affinity (P_{50}) in patients with acute myocardial infarction and shock. Am. J. Cardiol. *36*:148, 1975.
161. Kalter, E. S., Henning, R. J., Thijs, L., Vincent, J. L., Becker, H., Carlson, R. W., and Weil, M. H.: Effects of methylprednisolone on P_{50}, 2,3-diphosphoglycerate and arteriovenous oxygen difference in acute myocardial infarction. Circulation *62*:970, 1980.
162. Tindall, G. T., Greenfield, J. C., Jr., Dillon, M. L., and Odom, G. L.: Effect of hemorrhage on blood flow in the carotid arteries. Studies in ten rhesus monkeys. J. Neurosurg. *21*:763, 1964.
163. Johansson, B., Strandgaard, S., and Lassen, N. A.: On the pathogenesis of hypertensive encephalopathy. The hypertensive "breakthrough" of autoregulation of cerebral blood flow with forced vasodilatation, flow increase, and blood-brain-barrier damage. Circ. Res. *35*:167, 1974.
164. Harper, A. M.: Autoregulation of cerebral blood flow: Influence of the arterial blood pressure on the blood flow through the cerebral cortex. J. Neurol. Neurosurg. Psychiatry *29*:398, 1966.
165. Lambertson, C. J., Semple, S. J. G., Smyth, M. G., and Gelfand, R.: $H+$ and pCO_2 as chemical factors in respiratory and cerebral circulatory control. J. Appl. Physiol. *16*:473, 1967.

CLINICAL SHOCK STATES

166. Hinshaw, L. B., and Cox, B. G.: The fundamental mechanisms of shock. New York, Plenum Press, 1972, p. 13.
167. Weil, M. H., and Shubin, H.: The "VIP" approach to the bedside management of shock. J.A.M.A. *207*:337, 1969.
168. Viires, N., Sillye, G., Auber, M., Rassidakis, A., and Roussos, C.: Regional blood flow distribution in dog during induced hypotension and low cardiac output: Spontaneous breathing versus artificial ventilation. J. Clin. Invest. *72*:935, 1983.
169. Kumar, A., Falke, K. J., Geffin, B., Aldredge, C. F., Laver, M. B., Lowenstein, E., and Pontoppidan, H.: Continuous positive-pressure ventilation in acute respiratory failure. N. Engl. J. Med. *283*:1430, 1970.
170. Weil, M. H., and Henning, R. J.: New concepts in the diagnosis and fluid treatment of circulatory shock. Anesth. Analg. *58*:124, 1979.
171. Forrester, J. S., Diamond, G., McHugh, T. J., and Swan, H. J. C.: Filling pressures in the right and left sides of the heart in acute myocardial infarction. N. Engl. J. Med. 285:190, 1971.
172. Hanashiro, P. K., and Weil, M. H.: Reliability of central venous pressure as a measure of changes in left sided intracardiac pressures. Chest *62*:479, 1972.
173. Forrester, J. S., Diamond, G., Chatterjee, K., and Swan, H. J. C.: Medical therapy of acute myocardial infarction by application of hemodynamic subsets (first of two parts). N. Engl. J. Med. *295*:1356, 1976.
174. Forrester, J. S., Diamond, G., Chatterjee, K., and Swan, H. J. C.: Medical therapy of acute myocardial infarction by application of hemodynamic subsets (second of two parts). N. Engl. J. Med. 295:1404, 1976.
175. Lamke, L. O., and Liljedahl, S. O.: Plasma volume changes after infusion of various plasma expanders. Resuscitation *5*:93, 1976.
176. Weil, M. H.: Pulmonary edema. *In* Parmley, W., and Chatterjee, K. (eds.): Cardiology. Philadelphia, J. B. Lippincott (*in press*).
177. Monafo, W. M., Chuntrasakul, C., and Ayvazian, V. H.: Hypertonic sodium solutions in the treatment of burn shock. Am. J. Surg. *126*:778, 1973.
178. Moylan, J. A., Jr., Reckler, J. M., and Mason, A. D., Jr.: Resuscitation with hypertonic lactate saline in thermal injury. Am. J. Surg. *125*:580, 1973.
179. Nakayama, S., Sibley, L., Gunther, R. A., Holcroft, J. W., and Kramer, G. C.: Small-volume resuscitation with hypertonic saline (2,400 mOsm/liter) during hemorrhagic shock. Circ. Shock *13*:149, 1984.
180. Shoemaker, W. C.: Evaluation of colloids, crystalloids, whole blood and red cell therapy in the critically ill patients. Clin. Lab. Med. 2:35, 1982.
181. Holcroft, J. W., Link, D. P., Lantz, B. M. T., Green, J. F., and Weber, C. J.: Venous return and the pneumatic antishock garment in hypovolemic baboons. J. Trauma *24*:928, 1984.
182. Mackersie, R. C., Christensen, J. M., and Lewis, F. R.: The prehospital use of external counterpressure: Does MAST make a difference? J. Trauma *24*:882, 1984.
183. Mattox, K. L., Bickell, W. H., Pepe, P. E., and Mangelsdorff, A. D.: Prospective randomized evaluation of antishock MAST in post-traumatic hypotension. J. Trauma *26*:779, 1986.
184. Weil, M. H., and Shubin, H.: Isoproterenol for the treatment of circulatory shock. Ann. Intern. Med. *70*:638, 1969.
185. Mueller, H., Ayres, S. M., Gregory, J. J., Giannelli, S., and Grace, W. J.: Hemodynamics, coronary blood flow, and myocardial metabolism in coronary shock; response to L-norepinephrine and isoproterenol. J. Clin. Invest. *49*:1885, 1970.
186. Karras, G. E., Rackow, E. C., Astiz, M. E., and Weil, M. H.: Inotropic response to dopamine versus digoxin during sepsis. Clin. Res. *34*:896A, 1986.
187. Nicolas, F., Villers, D., and Blanloeil, Y.: Hemodynamic pattern in anaphylactic shock with cardiac arrest. Crit. Care Med. *12*:144, 1984.

188. Ruiz, C. E., Weil, M. H., and Carlson, R. W.: Treatment of circulatory shock with dopamine. J.A.M.A. *242*:165, 1979.
189. Da Luz, P. L., Shubin, H., and Weil, M. H.: Effectiveness of phentolamine for reversal of circulatory failure (shock). Crit. Care Med. *1*:135, 1973.
190. Guiha, N. H., Cohen, J. N., Mikulic, E., Franciosa, J. A., and Limas, C. J.: Treatment of refractory heart failure with infusion of nitroprusside. N. Engl. J. Med. *291*:587, 1974.

CARDIOGENIC SHOCK

191. Sonnenblick, E. H., Frishman, W. H., and LeJemtel, T. H.: Dobutamine: A new synthetic cardioactive sympathetic amine. N. Engl. J. Med. *300*:17, 1979.
192. Page, D. L., Caulfield, J. B., Kastor, J. A., DeSanctis, R. W., and Sanders, C. A.: Myocardial changes associated with cardiogenic shock. N. Engl. J. Med. *285*:133, 1971.
193. Resnekov, L.: Cardiogenic shock. Chest *83*:893, 1983.
194. Harnarayan, C., Bennett, M. A., Pentecost, B. L., and Brewer, D. B.: Quantitative study of infarcted myocardium in cardiogenic shock. Br. Heart J. *32*:728, 1970.
195. Wackers, F. J., Lie, K. I., Becker, A. E., Durrer, D., and Wellens, H. J.: Coronary artery disease in patients dying from cardiogenic shock or congestive heart failure in the setting of acute myocardial infarction. Br. Heart J. *38*:906, 1976.
196. Roberts, N., Harrison, D. G., Reimer, K. A., Crain, B. S., and Wagner, G. S.: Right ventricular infarction with shock but without significant left ventricular infarction: A new clinical syndrome. Am. Heart J. *110*:1047, 1985.
196a. Gunnar, R. M., Cruz, A., Boswell, J., Co, B. S., Pietras, R. J., and Tobin, J. R., Jr.: Myocardial infarction with shock. Hemodynamic studies and results of therapy. Circulation *33*:753, 1966.
196b. Da Luz, P., Weil, M. H., Liu, V. Y., and Shubin, H.: Plasma volume prior to and following volume loading during shock complicating acute myocardial infarction. Circulation *49*:98, 1974.
196c. Puri, P. S., and Bing, R. J.: Effects of drugs on myocardial contractility in the intact dog and in experimental myocardial infarction. Basis for their use in cardiogenic shock. Am. J. Cardiol. *21*:886, 1968.
197. Perlroth, M. G., and Harrison, D. C.: Cardiogenic shock: A review. Clin. Pharmacol. Ther. *10*:449, 1969.
198. Lew, A. S., Weiss, A. T., Shah, P. K., Fishbein, M. C., Berman, D. S., and Maddahi, J.: Extensive myocardial salvage and reversal of cardiogenic shock after reperfusion of the left main coronary artery by intravenous streptokinase. Am. J. Cardiol. *54*:450, 1984.
199. Dunkman, W. B., Leinbach, R. C., Buckley, M. J., Mundth, E. D., and Kantrowitz, A. R., Austen, W. G., and Sanders, C. A.: Clinical and hemodynamic results of intraaortic balloon pumping and surgery for cardiogenic shock. Circulation *46*:465, 1972.
200. Bardet, J., Masquet, C., Kahn, J., Gourgon, R., Bourdarias, J., Mathivat, A., and Bouvrain, Y.: Clinical and hemodynamic results of intra-aortic balloon counterpulsation and surgery for cardiogenic shock. Am. Heart J. *93*:280, 1977.
201. DeWood, M. A., Notske, R. N., Hensley, G. R., Shields, J. P., O'Grady, W. P., Spores, J., Goldman, M., and Ganji, J. H.: Intra-aortic balloon counterpulsation with and without reperfusion for myocardial infarction shock. Circulation *61*:1105, 1980.
202. Scheidt, S., Wilner, G., Mueller, H., Summers, D., Lesch, M., Wolff, G., Krakauer, J., Rubenfire, M., Fleming, P., Noon, G., Oldham, N., Killip, T., and Kantrowitz, A.: Intra-aortic balloon counterpulsation in cardiogenic shock. N. Engl. J. Med. *288*:979, 1973.
203. Isner, J. M., Cohen, S. R., Virmani, R., Lawrinson, W., and Roberts, W. C.: Complications of the intraaortic balloon counterpulsation device: Clinical and morphologic observations in 45 necropsy patients. Am. J. Cardiol. *45*:260, 1980.
204. McCabe, J. C., Abel, R. M., Subramanian, V. A., and Gay, W. A., Jr.: Complications of intra-aortic balloon insertion and counterpulsation. Circulation *57*:769, 1978.
205. Iqbal, M. Z., and Liebson, P. R.: Counterpulsation and dobutamine. Their use in treatment of cardiogenic shock due to right ventricular infarct. Arch. Intern. Med. *141*:247, 1981.
206. Bernhard, W. F., Poirer, B. S., La-Farge, G., and Carr, J.: A new method for temporary left ventricular bypass. J. Thorac. Cardiovasc. Surg. *70*:880, 1975.
207. Pierce, W. S., Parr, G. V. S., Myers, J. L., Pae, W. E., Jr., Bull, A. P., and Waldhausen, J. A.: Ventricular-assist pumping in patients with cardiogenic shock after cardiac operations. N. Engl. J. Med. *305*:1606, 1981.
208. Inoue, K., Owaki, T., Nakamura, T., Kitamura, F., and Miyamoto, N.: Clinical application of transvenous mitral commissurotomy by a new balloon catheter. J. Thorac. Cardiovasc. Surg. *87*:394, 1984.
209. McKay, R. G., Safian, R. D., Lock, J. E., Mandell, V. S., Thurer, R. L., Schnitt, S. J., and Grossman, W.: Balloon dilatation of calcific aortic stenosis in elderly patients: Postmortem, intraoperative, and percutaneous valvuloplasty studies. Circulation *74*:119, 1986.
210. McKay, R. G., Lock, J. E., Keane, J. F., Safian, R. D., Aroesty, J. M., and Grossman, W.: Percutaneous mitral valvuloplasty in an adult patient with calcific rheumatic mitral stenosis. J. Am. Coll. Cardiol. *7*:1410, 1986.
211. Palacios, I. F., Lock, J. E., Keane, J. F., and Block, P. C.: Percutaneous transvenous balloon valvotomy in a patient with severe calcific mitral stenosis. J. Am. Coll. Cardiol. *7*:1416, 1986.
212. Hanashiro, P. K., and Weil, M. H.: Anaphylactic shock in man: Report of two cases with detailed hemodynamic and metabolic studies. Arch. Intern. Med. *119*:129, 1967.
213. Nelimarkka, O., Halkola, L., and Ninikoski, J.: Effect of graded hemorrhage on renal cortical perfusion in dogs. Am. J. Surg. *141*:235, 1981.
214. Rackow, E. C., Falk, J. L., Fein, A., Siegel, J. S., Packman, M. I., Haupt, M. T., Kaufman, B. S., and Putnam, D.: Fluid resuscitation in circulatory shock: A comparison of the cardiorespiratory effects of albumin, hetastarch, and saline solutions in patients with hypovolemic and septic shock. Crit. Care Med. *11*:839, 1983.
215. Shatney, C. H., Deepika, K., Militello, P. R., Majerus, T. C., and Dawson, R. B.: Efficacy of hetastarch in the resuscitation of patients with multisystem trauma and shock. Arch. Surg. *118*:804, 1983.
216. Maningas, P. A., and Bellamy, R. F.: Hypertonic sodium chloride solutions for the prehospital management of traumatic hemorrhagic shock: A possible improvement in the standard of care? Ann. Emergency Med. *15*:1411, 1986.
217. Shubin, H., and Weil, M. H.: Failure of corticosteroid to potentiate sympathomimetic pressor response during shock. J.A.M.A. *197*:808, 1966.
218. Shubin, H., and Weil, M. H.: Bacterial shock. J.A.M.A. *235*:421, 1976.
219. Hruska, J. F., and Hornick, R. B.: Treatment of infection in septic shock. *In* Cowley, R. A., and Trump, B. F. (eds.): Pathophyiology of Shock, Anoxia, and Ischemia. Baltimore, Williams and Wilkins Co., 1982, p. 482.
220. Kreger, B. E., Craven, D. E., and McCabe, W. R.: Gram-negative bacteremia. IV. Re-evaluation of clinical features and treatment in 612 patients. Am. J. Med. *68*:344, 1980.
221. Band, J. D., and Maki, D. G.: Infections caused by arterial catheters used for hemodynamic monitoring. Am. J. Med. *67*:735, 1979.
222. Goldmann, D. A., Maki, M. G., Rhame, F. S., Kaiser, A. B., Tenney, J. H., and Bennett, J. V.: Guidelines for infection control in intravenous therapy. Ann. Intern. Med. *79*:848, 1973.
223. Washington, J. A., II, and Ilstrup, D. M.: Blood cultures: Issues and controversies. Rev. Infect. Dis. *8*:792, 1986.
224. Nishijima, H., Weil, M. H., Shubin, H., and Cavanilles, J.: Hemodynamic and metabolic studies on shock associated with gram-negative bacteremia. Medicine *52*:287, 1973.
225. Finley, R. J., Duff, J. H., Holliday, R. L,, Jones, D., and Marchuk, J. B.: Capillary muscle blood flow in human sepsis. Surgery *78*:87, 1975.
226. Kreger, B. E., Craven, D. E., Carling, P. C., and McCabe, W. R.: Gram-negative bacteremia. III. Reassessment of etiology, epidemiology and ecology in 612 patients. Am. J. Med. *68*:332, 1980.
227. Weil, M. H., and Allen, K. S.: Comparison of sympathetic blocking drugs in prevention of lethal effects of endotoxin. Proc. Soc. Exp. Biol. Med. *115*:627, 1964.
228. Sambhi, M. P., Weil, M. H., and Udhoji, V. N.: Acute pharmacodynamic effects of glucocorticoids: Cardiac output and related hemodynamic changes in normal subjects and patients in shock. Circulation *31*:523, 1965.
229. Hinshaw, L. B., Solomon, L. A., Holmes, D. D., and Greenfield, J. L.: Comparison of canine responses to *Escherichia coli* organisms and endotoxin. Surg. Gynecol. Obstet. *127*:981, 1968.
230. Sprung, C. L., Caralis, P. V., Marcial, E. H., Pierce, M., Gelbard, M. A., Long, W. M., Duncan, R. C., Tendler, M. D., and Karpf, M.: The effects of high-dose corticosteroids in patients with septic shock. N. Engl. J. Med. *311*:1137, 1984.
231. Ziegler, E. J., McCutchan, J. A., Fierer, J., Glauser, M. P., Sadoff, J. C., Douglas, H., and Braude, A. I.: Treatment of gram-negative bacteremia and shock with human antiserum to a mutant *Escherichia coli*. N. Engl. J. Med. *307*:1225, 1982.
232. Ledingham, I., McA., McArdle, C. S., and Macdonald, R. C.: Septic shock. *In* Ledingham, I., McA. (eds.): Recent Advances in Intensive Therapy. New York, Churchill Livingstone, 1977, p. 161.
233. Todd, J. K., Ressman, M., Caston, S. A., Todd, B. H., and Wiesenthal, A. M.: Corticosteroid therapy for patients with toxic shock syndrome. J.A.M.A. *252*:3399, 1984.
234. Todd, J.: Toxic shock syndrome. Disease-a-Month. *32*(2):82, 1986.
235. Hayes, P. S., Graves, L. M., Feeley, J. C., Hancock, G. A., Cohen, M. L., Reingold, A. L., Broome, C. V., and Hightower, A. W.: Production of toxic-shock-associated protein(s) in *Staphylococcus aureus* strains isolated from 1956 through 1982. J. Clin. Microbiol. *20*:43, 1984.
236. Hull, H. F., Mann, J. M., Sands, C. J., Gregg, S. H., and Kaufman, P. W.: Toxic shock syndrome related to nasal packing. Arch. Otolaryngol. *109*:624, 1983.
237. Toback, J., and Fayerman, J. W.: Toxic shock syndrome following septorhinoplasty. Arch. Otolaryngol. *109*:627, 1983.
238. Farber, B. F., Broome, C. V., and Hopkins, C. C.: Fulminant hospital-acquired toxic shock syndrome. Am. J. Med. *77*:331, 1984.

20 GENESIS OF CARDIAC ARRHYTHMIAS: Electrophysiological Considerations

by DOUGLAS P. ZIPES, M.D.

ANATOMY OF THE CARDIAC CONDUCTION SYSTEM

SINUS NODE

In man, the sinus node is a spindle-shaped structure composed of a fibrous tissue matrix with closely packed cells. It is 10 to 20 mm long, 2 to 3 mm wide, and thick, tending to narrow caudally toward the inferior vena cava. It lies less than 1 mm from the epicardial surface, laterally in the right atrial sulcus terminalis, at the junction of the superior vena cava and right atrium[1,2] (Fig. 20–1). The artery supplying the sinus node branches from the right (55 to 60 per cent of the time) or the left circumflex (40 to 45 per cent) coronary artery,[1] approaching the node from a clockwise or counterclockwise direction around the superior vena caval–right atrial junction.[2]

CELLULAR STRUCTURE. Cell types in the sinus node include nodal cells, transitional cells, and atrial muscle cells. *Nodal cells*, also called P cells, thought to be the source of normal impulse formation in the sinus node, are small (5 to 10 μm), ovoid, primitive-appearing cells with cytoplasm that contains relatively few organelles and myofibrils. The few mitochondria are distributed randomly and are variable in size and shape.[1] No transverse tubular system exists. Nodal cells stain poorly, have a pale appearance on light and electron microscopy, and are grouped in elongated clusters located centrally in the sinus node.[1] Contact between nodal cells appears to occur via nexus connections.

Transitional Cells. Also known as T cells, these are elongated cells intermediate in size and complexity between nodal cells and atrial muscle cells. These plentiful cells have large numbers of myofibrils and are heterogeneous, with some T cells more organized and complex than others. T cells near nodal cells have simple intercellular connections, while more fully developed intercalated discs exist between T cells and atrial myocardium. Since nodal cells make contact only with each other or T cells, the latter may provide the only functional pathway for distribution of the sinus impulse formed in the nodal cells to the rest of the atrial myocardium.[1] T cells constitute a spectrum of morphologies ranging from "typical" nodal cells on the one hand and "typical" working atrial myocardium on the other.

The third cell type present in the sinus node is the working *atrial myocardial cell*. These cells extend as peninsulas into the nodal boundaries, with overlapping zones of sinus and atrial cells most prominent on the nodal surface that abuts the crista terminalis.[2]

Some investigators have described large, *clear cells* that are Purkinje-like anatomically and are numerous at the margins of the sinus node.[1] The nature, and even presence, of these cells is unsettled.

Very probably there is no single cell in the sinus node that serves as *the* pacemaker. Rather, sinus nodal cells function as electrically coupled oscillators, discharging synchronously because of mutual entrainment. Thus, faster discharging cells are slowed by cells firing more slowly, while they themselves are sped so that a "democratically derived" discharge rate occurs.[3,4] In the dog, sinus rhythm results from impulse origin at widely separated sites, creating two or three individual wavefronts that merge to form a single widely disseminated wavefront.[5]

INNERVATION. The sinus node is richly innervated with postganglionic adrenergic and cholinergic nerve terminals. Vagal nerves in the dog enter the sinus node region over the superior vena caval–right atrial junction and the azygous and pulmonary veins.[6] The concentration of norepinephrine is two to four times higher in atrial than in ventricular tissue in canine and guinea pig hearts. Although the sinus nodal region contains amounts of norepinephrine equivalent to those in other parts of the right atrium,[7] acetylcholine, acetylcholinesterase, and choline acetyltransferase (the enzyme necessary for the synthesis of acetylcholine) have all been found in greatest concentration in the sinus node, with the next highest concentration in the right and then the left atrium. The concentration of acetylcholine in the ventricles is only 20 to 50 per cent of that in the atria.[7]

Vagal stimulation, by releasing acetylcholine, slows sinus nodal discharge rate and prolongs intranodal conduction time, at times to the point of sinus nodal exit block (p. 583).[8] Adrenergic stimulation speeds sinus discharge rate. The phase (timing) in the cardiac cycle at which vagal discharge occurs[8] and the background sympathetic tone[9] importantly influence vagal effects on sinus rate and conduction (see below). Acetylcholine increases and norepinephrine decreases refractoriness in the center of the sinus node.[10] Negative chronotropic effects of acetylcholine are due to increased potassium conductance and hyperpolarization of the membrane potential. After cessation of vagal stimulation, sinus nodal automaticity may accelerate transiently (postvagal tachycardia).[11]

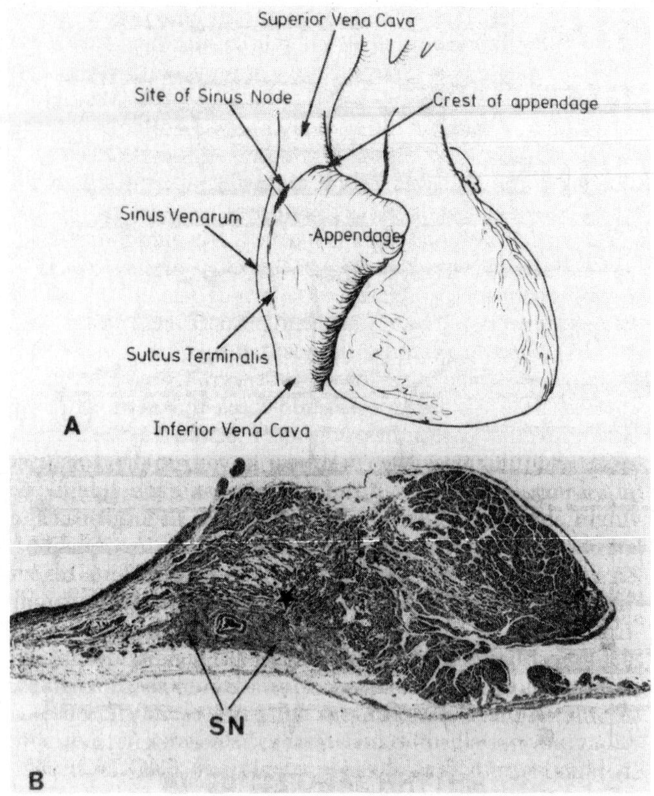

FIGURE 20–1. The human sinus node. *A,* Drawing showing location of the sinus node. *B,* Histological section taken perpendicular to the long axis of the sinus node (thin line in *A*). The sinus node (sn) rests on atrial myocardium of the crista terminalis. The star indicates a portion of nodal tissue blending with the crista terminalis. A layer of adipose tissue covers the epicardial margin of the sinus node (lower portion of the figure). (Masson's trichrome stain [× 6]). (From Becker, A. E., et al.: Functional anatomy of the cardiac conduction system. *In* Harrison, D. C. [ed.]: Cardiac Arrhythmias: A Decade of Progress. Boston, G. K. Hall, 1981.)

INTERNODAL AND INTERATRIAL CONDUCTION

Whether impulses travel from the sinus to the AV node over preferentially conducting pathways—and if they do, over what kind of pathways—is still unsettled. Anatomical evidence has been interpreted to indicate the presence of three pathways. The *anterior internodal pathway* begins at the anterior margin of the sinus node and curves anteriorly around the superior vena cava to enter the anterior interatrial band, called *Bachmann's bundle.* Near the anterior margin of the interatrial septum, the fibers divide, with Bachmann's bundle continuing to the left atrium and the anterior internodal pathway diving inferiorly behind the aorta within the interatrial septum to enter the superior margin of the AV node. The *middle internodal tract* begins at the superior and posterior margins of the sinus node and travels behind the superior vena cava to the crest of the interatrial septum where a few strands continue to the left atrium, but the bulk of the fibers descends in the interatrial septum to the superior margin of the AV node. The *posterior internodal tract* starts at the posterior margin of the sinus node and travels posteriorly around the superior vena cava and along the crista terminalis to the eustachian ridge and then into the interatrial septum above the coronary sinus, joining the posterior portion of the AV node. The anterior and posterior tracts appear to be most constant. Some fibers from all three tracts bypass the crest of the AV node and enter its more distal segment.[1] These groups of internodal tissue are best referred to as internodal atrial myocardium, not tracts, because they do not appear to be histologically discrete specialized tracts, only plain atrial myocardium.[2]

The basis for specialized tracts stems from finding cell types in the atrium that differ electrophysiologically[12] and anatomically,[13] but it is not clear that these different cells are responsible for more rapid conduction velocity. Also, differential sensitivity of atrial fibers to potassium, giving rise to an apparent sinoventricular rhythm (i.e., impulse propagation from the sinus node to the ventricle without activating atrial myocardium), and activation changes following localized surgical lesions designed to interrupt discrete pathways[14] provide further functional data to support the presence of specialized tracts. However, conclusions from these studies have been challenged, and it appears more likely that the entire atrial septum conducts impulses from the sinus to the AV node and that no functional evidence exists for narrow, specialized internodal tracts of fixed location. The issue is not entirely settled, but the *weight of evidence does not support the presence of specialized internodal tracts resembling the bundle branches, i.e., discrete histologically identifiable tracts of tissue.* However, preferential internodal conduction, i.e., more rapid conduction velocity between the nodes in some parts of the atrium compared to other parts, probably does exist and may be due to fiber orientation, size, geometry, or other factors rather than to specialized tracts located between the nodes.[15]

INTERATRIAL CONDUCTION. *Bachmann's bundle*, a large muscle bundle beginning along the anterior internodal pathway and traveling posteriorly around the aorta to the left atrium, appears to conduct the cardiac impulse preferentially from right to left atrium. The middle and posterior internodal tracts may also extend fibers to the left atrium, but little is known about their anatomical or functional importance.[1]

THE ATRIOVENTRICULAR JUNCTIONAL AREA AND INTRAVENTRICULAR CONDUCTION SYSTEM

The normal AV junctional area (Fig. 20–2) can be divided into distinct regions: transitional cell zone, also called nodal approaches; compact portion, or the AV node itself; and the penetrating part of the AV bundle (His bundle), which continues as a nonbranching portion. Some investigators consider the branching portion of the AV bundle (i.e., the bundle

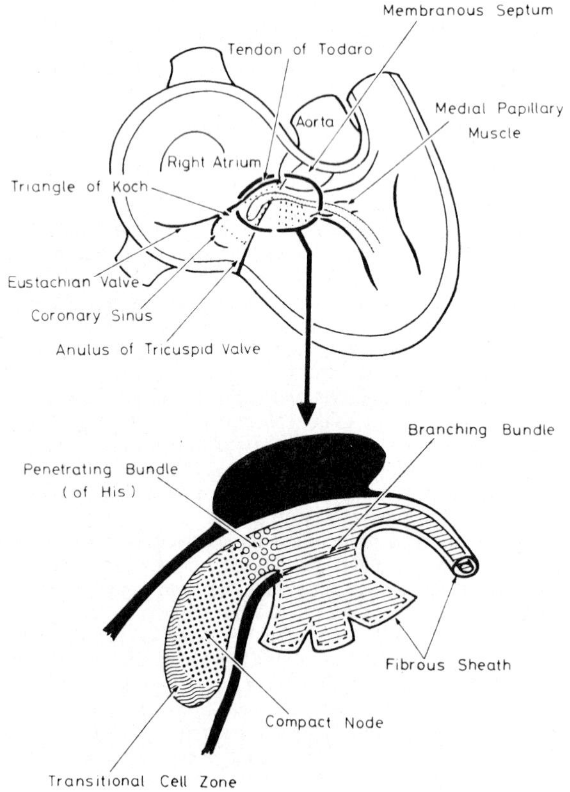

FIGURE 20–2. Schematic display of the atrioventricular junctional area. The area bounded by the dark circle in the top panel has been enlarged in the bottom panel, in which the central fibrous body (dark cap) overlies the AV node–His bundle. (See text for explanation.) (From Becker, A. E., et al.: Functional anatomy of the cardiac conduction system. *In* Harrison, D. C. [ed.]: Cardiac Arrhythmias: A Decade of Progress. Boston, G. K. Hall, 1981.)

branches) to be part of the AV junctional area anatomically, while others, relying more on electrophysiological function, separate the branching from the nonbranching portion.

TRANSITIONAL CELL ZONE. In the rabbit AV node, the transitional cells or nodal approaches are located in posterior, superficial, and deep groups of cells. They differ histologically from atrial myocardium and connect the latter with the compact portion of the AV node. Some fibers may pass from the posterior internodal tract to the distal portion of the AV node or His bundle and provide the anatomical substrate for conduction to bypass AV nodal slowing. However, the importance of this structure is unclear[16] (see p. 684).

THE AV NODE. The compact portion of the AV node is a superficial structure, lying just beneath the right atrial endocardium, anterior to the ostium of the coronary sinus, and directly above the insertion of the septal leaflet of the tricuspid valve. It is at the apex of a triangle formed by the tricuspid annulus and the tendon of Todaro, which originates in the central fibrous body, and passes posteriorly through the atrial septum to continue with the eustachian valve (Fig. 20–2). The compact portion of the AV node is divided from and becomes the penetrating portion of the His bundle at the point where it enters the central fibrous body. In 85 to 90 per cent of human hearts, the arterial supply to the AV node is a branch from the right coronary artery that originates at the posterior intersection of the AV and interventricular grooves (crux). A branch of the circumflex coronary artery provides the AV nodal artery in the remaining hearts.[1]

THE BUNDLE OF HIS, OR PENETRATING PORTION OF THE AV BUNDLE. This connects with the distal part of the compact AV node and perforates the central fibrous body, continuing through the annulus fibrosis, where it is called the nonbranching portion as it penetrates the membranous septum. Proximal cells of the penetrating portion are heterogeneous, resembling those of the compact AV node, while distal cells are similar to cells in the proximal bundle branches. Connective tissue of the central fibrous body and membranous septum encloses the penetrating portion of the AV bundle, which may send out extensions into the central fibrous body. However, large well-formed fasciculoventricular connections between the penetrating portion of the AV bundle and the ventricular septal crest are rarely found in adult hearts. Branches from the anterior and posterior descending coronary arteries supply the upper muscular interventricular septum with blood, making the conduction system at this site more impervious to ischemic damage unless the damage is extensive.[1]

THE BUNDLE BRANCHES, OR BRANCHING PORTION OF THE AV BUNDLE. These structures begin at the superior margin of the muscular interventricular septum, immediately beneath the membranous septum, with the cells of the left bundle branch cascading downward as a continuous sheet onto the septum beneath the noncoronary aortic cusp (Fig. 20–2). The AV bundle then may give off other left bundle branches, sometimes constituting a true bifascicular system with an anterosuperior branch, in other hearts giving rise to a group of central fibers, and in still others appearing more as a network without a clear division into a fascicular system. The right bundle branch continues intramyocardially as an unbranched extension of the AV bundle down the right side of the interventricular septum to the apex of the right ventricle and base of the anterior papillary muscle. In some human hearts, the His bundle traverses the right interventricular crest, giving rise to a right-sided narrow stem origin of the left bundle branch. Clearly the anatomy of the left bundle branch system may be variable and may not conform to a constant bifascicular division represented as anterosuperior (thin) and posteroinferior (broad) fascicles. However, despite these anatomical variabilities, the concept of a trifascicular system remains useful[17] to both the electrocardiographer and the clinician.

TERMINAL PURKINJE FIBERS. These fibers connect with the ends of the bundle branches to form interweaving networks on the endocardial surface of both ventricles that transmit the cardiac impulse almost simultaneously to the entire right and left ventricular endocardium. Purkinje fibers tend to be less concentrated at the base of the ventricle and at the papillary muscle tips. They penetrate the myocardium for varying distances depending on the animal species; in man, they apparently penetrate only the inner third of the endocardium, while in the pig they almost reach the epicardium. Such variations could influence changes produced by myocardial ischemia, for example, since Purkinje fibers appear more resistant to ischemia than are ordinary myocardial fibers.

CELLULAR COMPOSITION OF THE AV JUNCTIONAL AREA. Transitional cells in the rabbit are elongated, smaller than atrial cells, stain more palely, and are separated by numerous strands of connective tissue. They merge at the entrance of the compact portion of the AV node, which in the rabbit is surrounded by a fibrous collar that is a posterior extension of the central fibrous body. Tightly packed midnodal

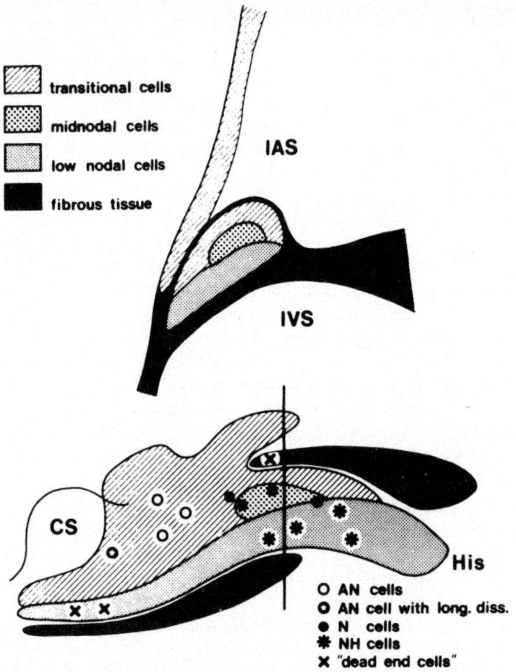

FIGURE 20–3. Diagram showing distribution of morphologically different cell types in AV node. *Upper panel,* Transverse section showing trilaminar appearance of the interior part of the node. The level of sectioning is indicated by the vertical dark line in the lower panel. *Lower panel,* Diagram of the AV node indicating the different sites identified histologically after recording typical action potentials. (From Janse, M. J., et al.: Electrophysiology and structure of the atrioventricular node of the isolated rabbit heart. *In* Wellens, J. H. H., et al. [eds.]: The Conduction System of the Heart. Philadelphia, Lea and Febiger, 1976, p. 296.)

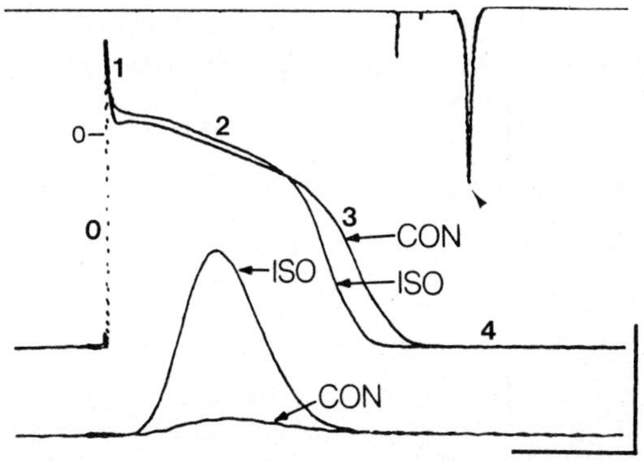

FIGURE 20–4. Recordings of canine Purkinje fiber action potential and developed tension before and during isoproterenol administration. Tracings from above downward show upstroke velocity of phase 0 ($\dot{V}$max, arrowhead), action potential configuration of Purkinje fiber, and developed tension in the Purkinje fiber bundle during control (CON) and after exposure to isoproterenol (ISO, 0.1 ml/10^{-5} M, added directly to the tissue bath). The five phases of the action potential are indicated by the large numerals. The short horizontal line to the left with a zero near the peak of the action potential indicates the zero voltage potential. Vertical calibration: 400 V/sec for $\dot{V}$max/sec, 50 mV for action potential amplitude, and 400 mg for the developed tension, respectively. Horizontal calibration: 4 msec for the upper record and 100 msec for the middle and lower records. (V = volts; mV = millivolts; msec = milliseconds.) Isoproterenol increased plateau height of the action potential and developed tension and decreased action potential duration during the terminal phase of repolarization, without significantly affecting resting membrane potential or phase 0. (From Gilmour, R. F., Jr., and Zipes, D. P.: Basic electrophysiology of the slow inward current. *In* Antman, E., and Stone, P. [eds.]: Calcium Blocking Agents in the Treatment of Cardiovascular Disorders. Mt. Kisco, N.Y., Futura Publishing Co. Inc., 1983, pp. 1–37.)

cells in the compact portion of the AV node are small and spherical, are not separated by muscle or connective tissue, and have very few nexuses. They interweave in interconnecting whorls of fasciculi. A group of lower nodal cells underlies the midnodal grouping and is continuous with the His bundle. The AV node is divided, based on electrophysiological characteristics, into AN, N, and NH regions[18] (Fig. 20–3). In the rabbit, the AN region corresponds to the transitional cell groups of the posterior portion of the node, the NH region to the anterior portion of the bundle of lower nodal cells, and the N region to the small enclosed node where transitional cells merge with midnodal cells. *Dead-end pathways*—groups of cells that form an apparent electrophysiological cul-de-sac that does not contribute to overall conduction in the node—are also found at several sites.[19] Cells in the penetrating bundle remain similar to compact AV nodal cells. In the dog, P cells, similar to those found in the sinus node, and several types of transitional cells have been noted and related to the automaticity and conduction properties of the AV node.[20] Cellular morphology alone does not determine the functional characteristics of these cells, which are influenced by the overall nodal architecture as well as by the nature and direction of the excitatory wavefront.

Purkinje cells are found in the His bundle and bundle branches and cover much of the endocardium of both ventricles. In the His bundle and bundle branches, Purkinje cells align to form multicellular bundles in longitudinal strands separated by collagen. They are large, clear cells (10 to 30 μm in diameter, 20 to 50 μm long) with loosely arrayed mitochondria distributed between few linearly aligned myofibrils that have few myofilaments. Round nuclei occupy the center of the cell. Although conduction of the cardiac impulse appears to be their major function, it is quite clear that free-running Purkinje fibers, sometimes called false tendons, which are composed of many Purkinje cells in a series, are capable of contraction (Fig. 20–4). While also exhibiting side-to-side connections, the major intercellular connection of Purkinje fibers is end-to-end through well-developed intercalated discs[1] (see p. 585) that may facilitate rapid longitudinal conduction.

INNERVATION OF AV NODE AND HIS BUNDLE

The AV node and His bundle region are innervated by a rich supply of cholinergic and adrenergic fibers with a density exceeding that found in the ventricular myocardium. Somatostatin is a neuroregulatory peptide abundant in the atria and AV node that may be important electrophysiologically.[21] Ganglia, nerve fibers, and nerve nets lie close to the AV node. Parasympathetic nerves to the AV node region enter the canine heart at the junction of the inferior vena cava and the inferior left atrium, adjacent to the coronary sinus entrance.[6] Nerves in direct contact with AV nodal fibers have been noted, along with agranular and granular vesicular processes, presumably representing cholinergic and adrenergic processes.

In general, autonomic neural input to the heart exhibits some degree of "sidedness," with the right sympathetic and vagal nerves affecting the sinus node more than the AV node and the left sympathetic and vagal nerves affecting the AV node more than the sinus node. The distribution of the neural input to the sinus and AV nodes is complex because of substantial overlapping innervation. Despite the overlap, specific branches of the vagal and sympathetic nerves can be shown to innervate certain regions preferentially, and sympathetic or vagal nerves to the sinus node can be interrupted discretely without affecting AV nodal innervation. Similarly, vagal or sympathetic neural input to the AV node can be interrupted without affecting sinus innervation.[6] Stimulation of the right stellate ganglion produces sinus tachycardia with less effect on AV nodal conduction, while stimulation of the left stellate ganglion generally produces a shift in the sinus pacemaker to an ectopic site and consistently shortens AV nodal conduction time and refractoriness, but inconsistently speeds the sinus nodal discharge rate. Stimulation of the right cervical vagus nerve primarily slows the sinus nodal discharge rate, while stimulation of the left vagus primarily prolongs AV nodal conduction time and refractoriness when "sidedness" is present. Neither sympathetic nor vagal stimulation affects normal conduction in the His bundle.

Most efferent sympathetic impulses reach the canine ventricles over the ansae subclaviae, branches from the stellate ganglia. Sympathetic impulses then synapse primarily in the caudal cervical ganglia and form individual cardiac nerves that innervate relatively localized parts of the ventricles. On the right side, the major route to the heart is the recurrent cardiac nerve, and on the left, the ventrolateral cardiac nerve. In general, the right sympathetic chain shortens refractoriness primarily of the anterior portion of the ventricles while the left affects primarily the posterior surface of the ventricles, although overlapping areas of distribution occur.

The intraventricular route of sympathetic nerves generally follows coronary arteries. Functional data suggest that afferent and efferent sympathetic nerves travel in the superficial layers of the epicardium and dive to innervate the endocardium, while vagal fibers travel intramurally or subendocardially, rising to the epicardium at the AV groove.[22–24]

EFFECTS OF VAGAL STIMULATION. The vagus modulates cardiac sympathetic activity at prejunctional and postjunctional sites[25, 26] by regulating the amount of norepinephrine released[7] and possibly by inhibiting cyclic AMP-induced phosphorylation of cardiac proteins such as phospholamban. The latter inhibition occurs at more than one level in the series of reactions comprising the adenylate cyclase, cyclic AMP-dependent, protein kinase system.[27]

Tonic vagal stimulation produces a greater absolute reduction in sinus rate in the presence of tonic background sympathetic stimulation, a sympathetic-parasympathetic interaction termed accentuated antagonism.[7] In contrast, changes in AV conduction during concomitant sympathetic and vagal stimulation are essentially the "algebraic sum" of the individual AV conduction responses to tonic vagal and sympathetic stimulation alone.[7] Cardiac responses to brief vagal bursts begin after a short latency and dissipate quickly; in contrast, cardiac responses to sympathetic stimulation commence and dissipate slowly. The rapid onset and offset of responses to vagal stimulation allow for dynamic vagal modulation of heart rate and AV conduction (phase-dependent), whereas the slow temporal response to sympathetic stimulation precludes any beat-to-beat regulation by sympathetic activity (phase-independent).[9] Periodic vagal bursting (as may occur each time a systolic pressure wave arrives at the baroreceptor regions in the aortic and carotid sinuses) induces phasic changes in sinus cycle length and can entrain the sinus node to discharge faster or slower at periods that are identical to those of the vagal burst.[8, 28] In a similar phasic manner, vagal bursts prolong AV nodal conduction time and are influenced by background levels of sympathetic tone.[9] Because the peak vagal effects on sinus rate and AV nodal conduction occur at different times in the cardiac cycle, a brief vagal burst can slow the sinus rate without affecting AV nodal conduction or can prolong AV nodal conduction time and not slow the sinus rate.[9] Shifts in pacemaker location can occur.[29]

EFFECTS OF SYMPATHETIC STIMULATION WITH VAGAL STIMULATION. Stimulation of sympathetic ganglia shortens the refractory period equally in the epicardium and underlying endocardium of the left ventricular free wall,[29a] although dispersion of recovery properties occurs, i.e., different degrees of shortening of refractoriness occur when measured at different epicardial sites. Nonuniform distribution of norepinephrine may, in part, contribute to some of the nonuniform electrophysiological effects following sympathetic neural stimulation, since the ventricular content of norepinephrine, for example, is greater at the base than at the apex of the heart,[30] with greater distribution to muscle than to Purkinje fibers. Afferent vagal activity appears to be greater in the posterior ventricular myocardium.[31] This may account for the vagomimetic effects of inferior myocardial infarction.

EFFECTS OF AUTONOMIC NERVES. The vagi exert minimal but measurable effects on ventricular tissue, decreasing the strength of myocardial contraction and prolonging refractoriness.[38] Surprisingly, acetylcholine causes a positive inotropic effect in canine Purkinje fibers.[32] It is still not clear whether some or all of the vagal effects on the ventricle are direct or indirect, by modulating sympathetic influences.

Alterations in vagal and sympathetic innervation may influence the development of arrhythmias. Damage to nerves extrinsic to the heart, such as the stellate ganglia, as well as to intrinsic cardiac nerves from diseases that may affect nerves primarily, e.g., viral infections, or secondarily, from diseases that cause cardiac damage, may produce cardioneuropathy.[33, 34] Such neural changes may create electrical instability via a variety of electrophysiological mechanisms. For example, myocardial infarction can interrupt afferent and efferent neural transmission[35] and create areas of sympathetic supersensitivity[36] that may be conducive to the development of arrhythmias.[37]

BASIC ELECTROPHYSIOLOGICAL PRINCIPLES

CELL MEMBRANE (SARCOLEMMA)

The cell membrane constitutes a bilayer boundary of phospholipid molecules (Fig. 20–5). The tail end of the phospholipid molecules is nonpolar and hydrophobic, pointing toward the center of the membrane, while the head end is polar and hydrophilic, pointing toward the outer and inner layers of the membrane, in contact with the aqueous extracellular and intracellular environment. The sarcolemma, particularly the hydrophobic core, provides a high-resistance, insulated wrapping around the cell that exhibits selective permeability to ions—a property responsible for creating an electrical potential across the cell membrane. Ions are positively (cations) or negatively (anions) charged atoms such as Na, K, Ca, or Cl and other molecules whose movement inside the cell or across the cell membrane constitutes a flow of current that generates signals in excitable membranes. At rest, the resistance to ion flow is greater across the cell membrane than in the cytoplasm of the cell interior. The cell membrane has openings called channels that serve as conduits through which ions move. The different protein or phospholipoprotein channels are selective, favoring passage of one ion over another. In contrast to the membrane lipids that act primarily as inert barriers, membrane proteins appear to be responsible for most of the known biological activities of membranes.[39] Gates, influenced by the electric field and by time, control ion movement through the channels and, when opened or closed, permit or prevent ion travel.

In addition to the channels, other protein complexes serve as a major supplementary transport system through the cell membrane and provide for neutral exchange of some ions and small organic molecules along their concentration gradients (passive ion transport) and for transporting ions against their electrochemical energy gradients (active ion transport). Some protein complexes penetrate only the outer cell membrane and may serve as receptor sites for neurotransmitters and hormones, while others, such as the adenylate cyclase system, protrude through the inner cell membrane and may be involved in various enzymatic activities. Protein molecules protruding through the entire cell membrane, such as the Na-K pump, may help regulate the ionic fluxes that determine the electrical status of the resting and excited membrane.[39] The Na-K pump requires adenosine triphosphate (ATP) to extrude intracellular NA

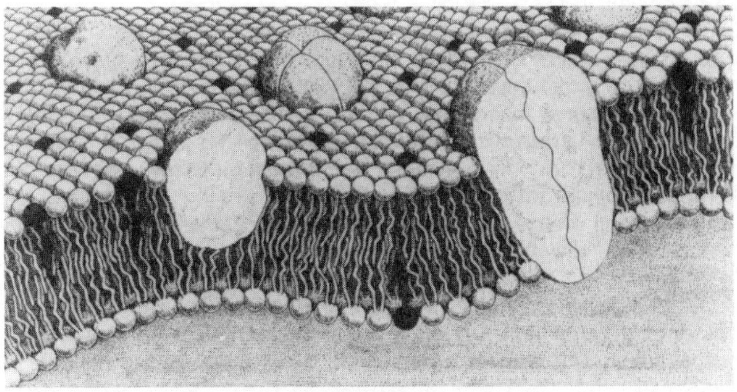

FIGURE 20–5. Membrane model showing proteins embedded in the phospholipid bilayer. Proteins that span the entire bilayer can serve as ion channels by providing a hydrophilic environment through which the ions can traverse the hydrophilic phospholipid bilayer. (From Singer, S. J.: Architecture and topography of biologic membranes. *In* Weissman, G., and Clairborne, R. [eds.]: Cell Membranes, Biochemistry, Cell Biology, and Pathology. New York, HP Publishing Co., 1975, pp. 35–44.)

TABLE 20–1 INTRACELLULAR AND EXTRACELLULAR ION CONCENTRATIONS IN CARDIAC MUSCLE

Ion	Extracellular Concentration	Intracellular Concentration	Ratio of Extracellular to Intracellular Concentration	E_i
Na	145 mM	15 mM	9.7	+60 mV
K	4 mM	150 mM	0.027	−94 mV
Cl	120 mM	5 mM	24	−83 mV
Ca	2 mM	10^{-7} M	2×10^4	+129 mV

E_i = equilibrium potential for a particular ion.

Although intracellular Ca content is about 2 mM/kg, most of this is bound or sequestered in intracellular organelles (mitochondria and sarcoplasmic reticulum). For the same reason, the actual free Na concentration may be less. Intracellular Cl concentration depends on the average membrane potential, if Cl is passively distributed, and therefore on heart rate.

From Sperelakis, N.: Origin of the cardiac resting potential. *In* Berne, R. M., et al. (eds.): Handbook of Physiology, The Cardiovascular System, Bethesda, Md., American Physiological Society, 1979, p. 190.

against its concentration and electrical gradients and to move K intracellularly, against its concentration gradient, resulting in high concentrations of K inside and of Na outside the cell (Table 20–1). Membrane proteins are considered to be "floating," moving from one area of the membrane to another.

INTERCALATED DISCS. The cell membranes of some types of adjacent cells form close margins called *intercalated discs* (p. 385). Three types of specialized junctions make up each intercalated disc. The macula adherens or desmosome and fascia adherens form the areas of strong adhesions between cells and may provide a linkage for the transfer of mechanical energy from one cell to the next. The *nexus*, also called tight or gap junction, is a region in the intercalated disc where cells are in functional contact with each other. Membranes at these junctions are separated by only about 10 to 20 Å and are connected by a series of hexagonally packed subunit bridges. Nexuses probably provide low-resistance electrical coupling between adjacent cells[40–43] at their longitudinal ends, reducing cell-to-cell resistance. Nexuses also occur along the sides of cells, connecting lateral surfaces. The nexuses may form water-filled channels complexed with protein units that allow movement of ions and perhaps of small molecules between cells. The size of the channels is variable. They link interiors of adjacent cells and are stable in their open state, closing when intracellular calcium rises.[39] The nexuses permit a multicellular structure like the heart to function electrically like an orderly, synchronized, interconnected unit. Nexuses may also provide "biochemical coupling" that might permit cell-to-cell movement of ATP or other high-energy phosphates and can change their electrical resistance, possibly controlled in part by calcium. When intracellular calcium rises, as in myocardial infarction, the nexus may close to help "seal off" the effects of injured from noninjured cells. Acidosis increases and alkalosis decreases gap junctional resistance. Increased gap junctional resistance tends to slow the rate of action potential propagation, a condition that could lead to conduction delay or block.

In ventricular muscle cells, but apparently not in atrial or His-Purkinje cells, the cell membrane invaginates to form a transverse tubular system that introduces the cell membrane and extracellular space deep into the cells. Because of reduced diffusion in that space, ions, metabolites, or other constituents may be present in greater or lower concentrations than are found intracellularly or extracellularly. Such surface scalloping can greatly increase the surface area of the ventricular cell.

PHASES OF THE CARDIAC ACTION POTENTIAL

The cardiac transmembrane potential consists of five phases: phase 0—the upstroke or rapid depolarization; phase 1—early rapid repolarization; phase 2—plateau; phase 3—final rapid repolarization; phase 4—resting membrane potential and diastolic depolarization (Fig. 20–4). These phases are the result of ion fluxes that are passive: Ions move down electrochemical gradients established by active ion pumps and exchange mechanisms. Each ion moves primarily through its own ion-specific channel.[39] Impulses spread from one cell to the next without requiring neural input. The transplanted heart dramatically demonstrates this fact. The following discussion will explain the electrogenesis of each of these phases. For an in-depth discussion, the reader is referred to other reference sources.[44–46]

PHASE 4—THE RESTING MEMBRANE POTENTIAL

Intracellular electrical activity can be recorded by inserting a glass microelectrode with a tip diameter less than 0.5 μm into a single cell. The electrode produces minimal damage, its entry point apparently being sealed by the cell. The transmembrane potential is recorded using this electrode in reference to an extracellular ground electrode placed in the tissue bath near the cell membrane and represents the potential difference between intracellular and extracellular voltages (Fig. 20–6 *Left*). A variety of other techniques, including voltage and patch clamp procedures, can be used to study the passage of individual ionic species across specific channels in the cell membrane[44, 45] (Fig. 20–6 *Right*).

Intracellular potential during electrical quiescence in diastole is −50 to −95 mV, depending on the cell type (Table 20–2). This means that the inside of the cell is 50 to 95 mV negative relative to the outside of the cell owing to the distribution of ions such as K, Na, Cl, and Ca across the cell membrane.

K is the major ion determining the resting potential. During diastole the cell membrane is quite permeable to K and relatively impermeable to Na. Because of the Na-K pump, which pumps Na out of the cell against its electrochemical gradient and simultaneously pumps K into the cell against its chemical gradient, intracellular K concentration remains high and intracellular Na concentration remains low. This pump, fueled by an Na^+,K^+-ATPase enzyme that hydrolyzes ATP for energy, is bound to the membrane. It requires both Na and K to function and can transport three Na ions outward for two K ions inward. Therefore the pump can be electrogenic, generating a net outward movement of positive charges. The rate of Na-K pumping to maintain the same ionic gradients must in-

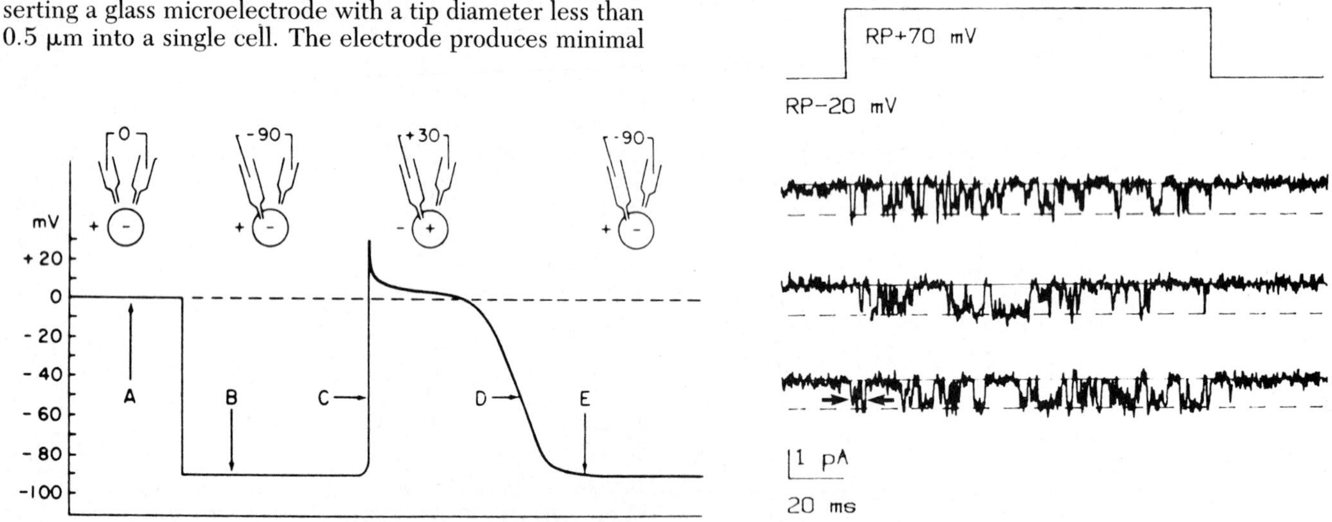

FIGURE 20–6. ***Left,*** **A demonstration of action potentials recorded during impalement of a cardiac cell. The upper row of diagrams shows a cell (circle), two microelectrodes, and stages during impalement of the cell and its activation and recovery. *A,* Both microelectrodes are extracellular, and no difference in potential exists between them (0 potential). The environment inside the cell is negative and the outside is positive, since the cell is polarized. *B,* One microelectrode has pierced the cell membrane to record the intracellular resting membrane potential, which is −90 mV with respect to the outside of the cell. *C,* The cell has depolarized and the upstroke of the action potential is recorded. At its peak voltage, the inside of the cell is about +30 mV with respect to the outside of the cell. *D,* Phase of repolarization, returning the membrane to its former resting potential (*E*). (From Cranefield, P. F.: The Conduction of the Cardiac Impulse. Mt. Kisco, N.Y., Futura Publishing Co. Inc., 1975.)**

Right, **Calcium channel recording. A portion or patch of the sarcolemmal membrane from a single guinea pig ventricular muscle cell is sucked up into a micropipette to record the opening and closing of single calcium channels. The pipette is filled with 110 mM Ba^{+2}. The Ba^{+2} crosses the membrane through the calcium channel when it opens and generates a current, recorded as the large downward pulses that reach the interrupted line (first in the bottom tracing). The solid line indicates average baseline current while the interrupted line (about 1 pA) indicates average single channel current. The channel stays open for brief but varied durations and then closes (upward deflection back to solid line, second). Three sequentially obtained current records are shown. Resting membrane potential (RP) was near −60 mV by addition of 10 mM [K]o. The RP was then reduced by 20 mV (RP −20 mV) and virtually no Ca channel openings occurred. When RP was made 70 mV more positive (RP + 70 mV) Ca channel activity was generated. (Square wave-shaped tracing at very top indicates RP changes). Thus, this figure illustrates opening and closing of single calcium channels when the RP is reduced to the range at which the slow inward current functions. (From Tsien, R.: Excitable tissues: The heart. *In* Andreoli, T.E., et al. [eds.]: *Physiology of Membrane Disorders.* New York, Plenum, 1986, p. 478.)**

TABLE 20–2 PROPERTIES OF TRANSMEMBRANE POTENTIALS IN MAMMALIAN HEARTS

	Sinus Nodal Cell	Atrial Muscle Cell	AV Nodal Cell	Purkinje Fiber	Ventricular Muscle Cell
Resting potential (mV)	−50 to −60	−80 to −90	−60 to −70	−90 to −95	−80 to −90
Action potential					
Amplitude (mV)	60 to 70	110 to 120	70 to 80	120	110 to 120
Overshoot (mV)	0 to 10	30	5 to 15	30	30
Duration (msec)	100 to 300	100 to 300	100 to 300	300 to 500	200 to 300
$\dot{V}$max (V/S)	1 to 10	100 to 200	5 to 15	500 to 700	100 to 200
Propagation velocity (M/sec)	<0.05	0.3 to 0.4	0.1	2 to 3	0.3 to 0.4
Fiber diameter (μm)	5 to 10	10 to 15	5 to 10	100	10 to 16

Modified from Sperelakis, N.: Origin of the cardiac resting potential. *In* Berne, R. M., Sperelakis, N., and Geiger, S. R. (eds.): Handbook of Physiology, The Cardiovascular System, Bethesda, Md., American Physiological Society, 1979, p. 190.

crease as heart rate increases, since the cell gains a slight amount of Na and loses a slight amount of K with each depolarization. Heart rate becomes important when we consider the electrophysiological basis of some types of digitalis-induced cardiac arrhythmias, because cardiac glycosides block this pump.

THE NERNST EQUATION. Little Na, despite its concentration gradient, can diffuse into the cell, owing to the relative impermeability to Na of the polarized cell membrane. However, K can diffuse freely out of the cell down its concentration gradient, and does so, removing with it a positive charge and leaving the inside of the cell more negative. Negative intracellular charges, presumably due to large polyvalent ions such as proteins, do not cross the membrane and help maintain intracellular negativity. K continues to leave the cell until the forces driving it down its concentration gradient are balanced by the negative intracellular electrical charges that attract K back into the cell. The transmembrane voltage at which the electrical gradient is equal and opposite to the concentration gradient, so that the algebraic sum of these two passive forces equals zero, is the K electrochemical equilibrium potential E_k, and is described by the Nernst equation

$$E_k = \frac{RT}{F} \ln \frac{[K]_o}{[K]_i} \qquad (1)$$

where R is the gas constant, T is the absolute temperature, F is the Faraday number, ln is the logarithm to the base E, $[K]_o$ is the extracellular K concentration and $[K]_i$ the intracellular K concentration.

Solving this equation predicts a transmembrane voltage of about −96 mV in cardiac muscle, which is very near the observed voltages. However, certain factors make the equation an approximation. Because the $[K]_o/[K]_i$ ratio primarily determines transmembrane voltage, the cell membrane is said to behave as a K electrode during diastole, and more closely follows the values predicted by the Nernst equation at $[K]_o$ greater than 10 mM. When $[K]_o$ is reduced, membrane permeability to K also decreases, the small inward movement of Na, negligible at high $[K]_o$, becomes more important, and the actual resting membrane voltage becomes less than that predicted by the Nernst equation for a K electrode. The difference between predicted and observed voltages increases as $[K]_o$ is reduced further. The contribution of the minimal inward movement of Na to the resting membrane potential can be incorporated into an equation called the Goldman constant-field equation and is a slight modification of the Nernst equation. If one assumes that the membrane is permeable to only Na and K, the resting membrane potential (V_r) would be

$$V_r = \frac{RT}{F} \ln \frac{[K]_o + P_{Na}/P_K\,[Na]_o}{[K]_i + P_{Na}/P_K\,[Na]_i} \qquad (2)$$

where P_{Na}/P_K is the ratio of the sodium to the potassium permeability coefficient of the cell membrane, $[Na]_o$ is the extracellular sodium concentration, and $[Na]_i$ is the intracellular sodium concentration. The equation can be modified further to include the minimal contributions of other ions.[47]

Calcium contributes little to the resting membrane potential, although changes in Ca concentration can affect the permeability of the cell membrane to other ions. An increase in $[Ca]_i$ increases potassium conductance. Ca is handled by several mechanisms, including uptake by the sarcoplasmic reticulum. Also, there appears to be a passive transarcolemmal Ca-Na exchange reaction. This exchange depends in part on maintenance of the Na concentration gradient by the Na-K pump (Fig. 13–3, p. 386). Under normal conditions, one internal Ca ion is probably exchanged for two or three external Na ions. Under some pathological conditions or drug actions when $[Na]_i$ is abnormally high, external Ca may be exchanged for internal Na. Cells that gain Na, in general, gain Ca—a reaction important to the genesis of some digitalis-induced arrhythmias. The role of calcium is further considered on page 389.

PHASE 0—UPSTROKE OR RAPID DEPOLARIZATION

A stimulus delivered to excitable tissue evokes an action potential characterized by a sudden voltage change due to transient depolarization followed by repolarization. The action potential is conducted throughout the heart and is responsible for initiating each "heart beat." Electrical changes of the action potential follow a relatively fixed time and voltage relationship that differs according to specific cell types (Fig. 20–7). In nerve, the entire process takes several milliseconds, while action potentials in cardiac fibers last several hundred milliseconds. Normally the action potential is independent of the size of the depolarizing stimulus, if the latter exceeds a certain threshold potential. Small subthreshold depolarizing stimuli depolarize the membrane proportional to the strength of the stimulus. However, once the stimulus is sufficiently intense to reduce membrane potential to a threshold value in the range of −70 to −65 mV for normal Purkinje fibers, more intense stimuli do not produce larger action potential responses, and an "all-or-none" response results. In contrast, hyperpolarizing pulses, i.e., stimuli that render the membrane potential more negative, elicit a response proportional to the strength of the stimulus.

MECHANISM OF PHASE 0. The upstroke of the cardiac action potential in atrial and ventricular muscle and His-Purkinje fibers is due to a sudden increase in membrane conductance to Na (Fig. 20–8). An externally applied stimulus, or a spontaneously generated local membrane circuit current in advance of a propagating action potential, depolarizes a sufficiently large area of membrane at a sufficiently rapid rate to open the Na channels and depolarize the membrane further. When the membrane voltage reaches threshold, Na rushes through ion-specific channels into the cell, down its electrochemical gradient—i.e., Na is "drawn" into the cell by the low $[Na]_i$ and the negatively charged intracellular environment. The excited membrane no longer behaves like a K electrode, i.e., exclusively permeable to K, but more closely approximates an Na electrode, and the membrane moves toward the Na equilibrium potential.

The rate at which depolarization occurs during phase 0, i.e., the maximum rate of change of voltage over time, is indicated by the expression dV/dt_{max} or $\dot{V}_{max}$ (Table 20–2), which is a reasonable approximation of the rate and magnitude of Na entry into the cell and a determinant of conduction velocity for the propagated action potential The transient increase in sodium conductance lasts 1 to 2 msec. The action potential, or more properly the Na current, is said to be regenerative; that is, intracellular movement of a little Na depolarizes the membrane more, which increases conductance to Na more, which allows more Na to enter, and so on. As this is occurring, however, $[Na]_i$ and positive intracellular charges increase and reduce the driving force

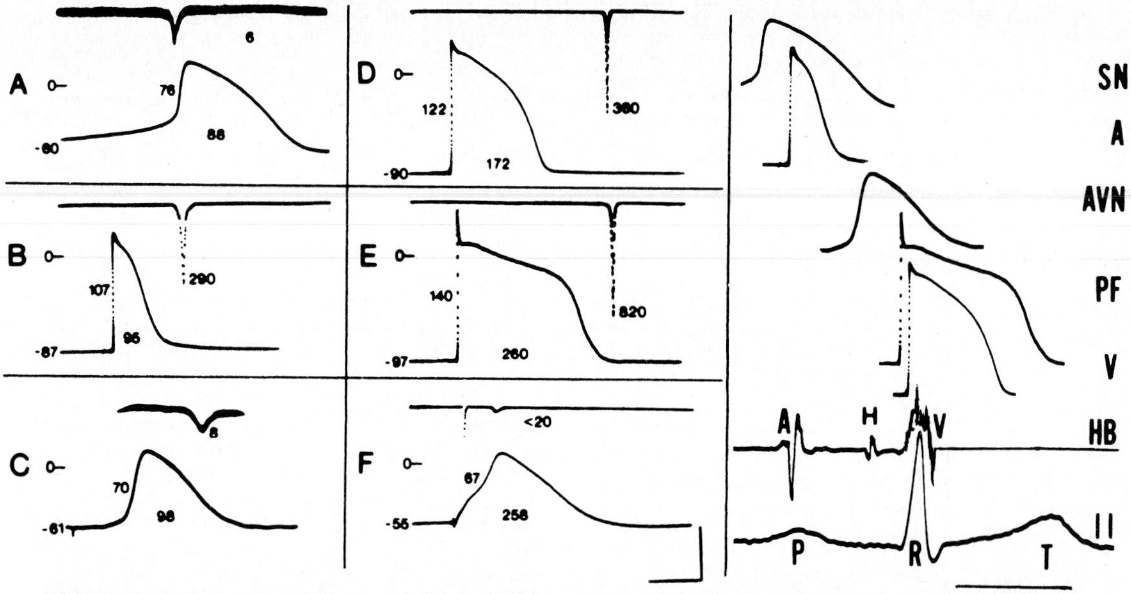

FIGURE 20–7. Action potentials recorded from different tissues in the heart (*left*), remounted along with a His bundle recording and scalar ECG from a patient (*right*) to illustrate the timing during a single cardiac cycle. In panels *A* to *F*, the top tracing is dV/dt of phase 0 and the second tracing is the action potential. For each panel, the numbers (from left to right) indicate maximum diastolic potential (mV), action potential amplitude (mV), action potential duration at 90 per cent of repolarization (msec), and V̇max of phase 0 (V/sec). Zero potential is indicated by the short horizontal line next to the zero on the upper left of each action potential. *A*, Rabbit sinoatrial node; *B*, canine atrial muscle; *C*, rabbit atrioventricular node; *D*, canine ventricular muscle; *E*, canine Purkinje fiber; *F*, diseased human ventricle. Note that the action potentials recorded in *A, C,* and *F* have reduced resting membrane potentials, amplitudes and V̇max compared to the other action potentials. In the right panel, SN = sinus nodal potential; A = atrial muscle potential; AVN = atrioventricular nodal potential; PF = Purkinje fiber potential; V = ventricular muscle potential; HB = His bundle recording; II = lead II. Horizontal calibration on the left: 50 msec for *A* and *C*, 100 msec for *B, D, E,* and *F*; 200 msec on the right. Vertical calibration on the left: 50 mV. Horizontal calibration on the right: 200 msec. (Modified from Gilmour, R. F., Jr., and Zipes, D. P.: Basic electrophysiology of the slow inward current. *In* Antman, E., and Stone, P. H. [eds.]: Calcium Blocking Agents in the Treatment of Cardiovascular Disorders. Mt. Kisco, N.Y., Futura Publishing Co. Inc., 1983, pp. 1–37).

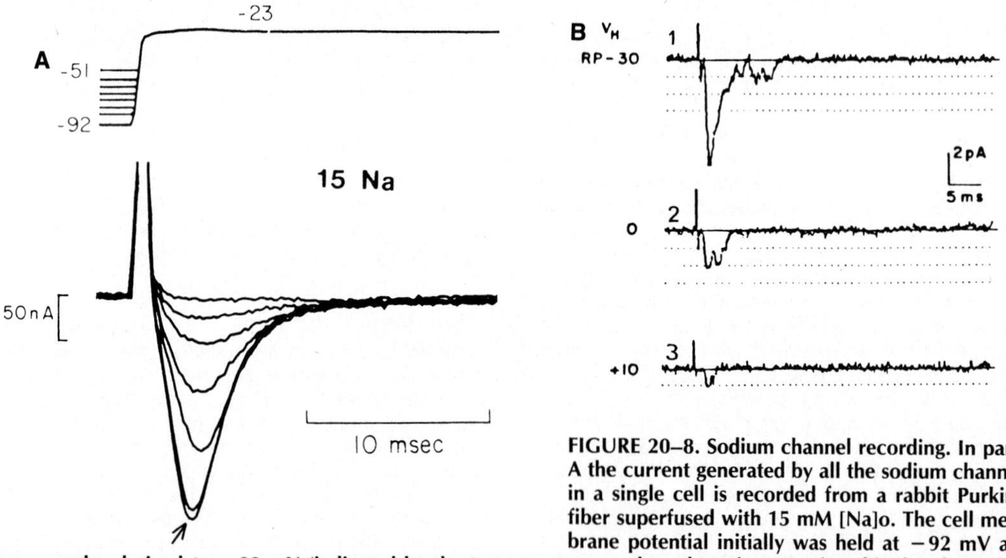

FIGURE 20–8. Sodium channel recording. In panel A the current generated by all the sodium channels in a single cell is recorded from a rabbit Purkinje fiber superfused with 15 mM [Na]o. The cell membrane potential initially was held at −92 mV and then was depolarized to −23 mV (indicated by the top square wave-shaped tracing). During this depolarization, I_{Na} was generated, recorded as the large negative deflection (arrow). The membrane potential was then reduced in steps to −51 mV. At each step the cell was depolarized to −23 mV. The I_{Na} produced was recorded in superimposed sweeps.

Panel A illustrates that depolarization (to −23 mV) of the cell, starting from progressively less negative membrane potentials (−92 to −51 mV) generated less I_{Na} because the sodium channels became inactivated at reduced membrane potentials.

Shown in panel B is the sodium current generated in single channels of a cell, rather than all the channels together, as in panel A. The patch recording of single channels is as described in Figure 20–6. The membrane potential just prior to depolarization (holding potential, V_H) was made progressively more positive in relation to the resting potential (1 = −30 mV; 2 = 0 mV; 3 = +10 mV). The I_{Na} generated in single channels was recorded when the cell was depolarized to a value 40 mV above the resting membrane potential. Solid and interrupted lines indicate average baseline and single channel current levels, respectively. As the holding potential was made less negative, the number of sodium channels that opened in response to the test depolarization decreased (from 6 to 2 to 1). This panel illustrates for single channels the same finding as in panel A for the global I_{Na}. (From Tsien, R.: Excitable tissues: The heart. *In* Andreoli, T. E., et al.: Physiology of Membrane Disorders. New York, Plenum, 1986, p. 475.)

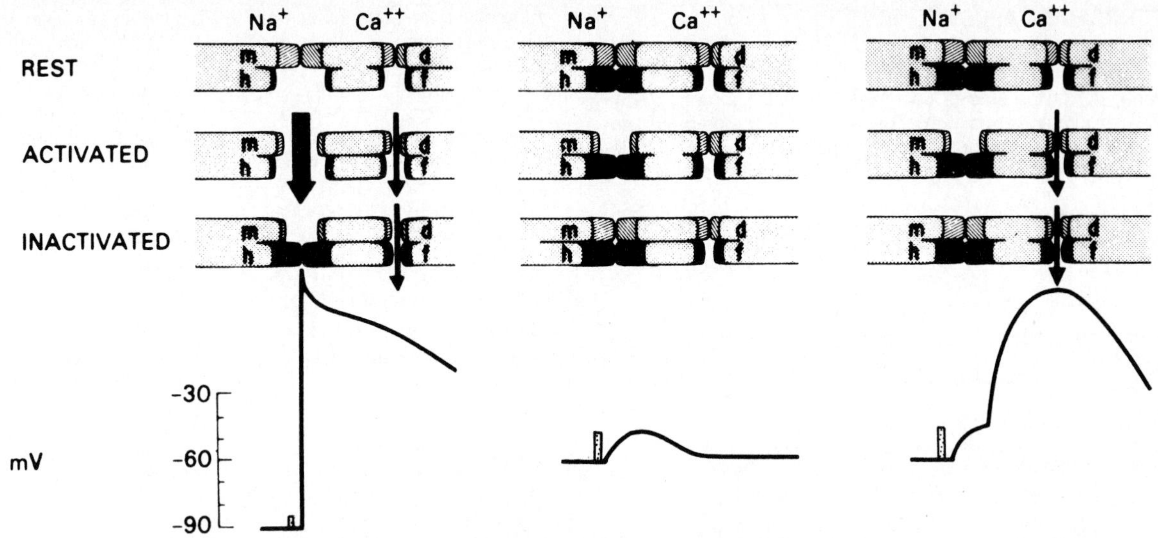

FIGURE 20–9. Schematic representation of membrane channels for rapid and slow inward currents at resting membrane potential (*top row*), during the activated state (*middle row*), and during the inactivated state (*bottom row*). Vertically separated panels depict fibers with a normal resting potential of −90 mV (*left*), with resting membrane potential reduced to less than −60 mV (*middle*), and after stimulation of the cell with catecholamines (*right*). The activation (m) and inactivation (h) gates of the fast channel and the activation (d) and inactivation (f) gates of the slow channel are depicted.

During the resting state (*left panel*), the activation gates of both channels are closed while the inactivation gates are open. When the cell is stimulated, the m gates of the fast channel open, and for a brief period of time, the open m gates and h gates allow inward sodium current to flow, depolarize the cell, and produce its upstroke. The action potential is depicted below. The h gates then close the channel and inactivate sodium conductance. When the upstroke of the action potential exceeds the threshold for activation of the slow inward current, the d gates open, allowing ingress of the slow inward current that contributes to the plateau phase of the action potential. The f gates of the slow channel close more slowly than the h gates. Although the slow inward channel remains open longer than does the fast channel, less total current flows.

When the resting membrane potential is reduced below −60 mV by increasing $[K]_o$ from 4.0 to 14.0 mm (*middle panel*), the cell depolarizes to −60 mV and the fast channel becomes inactivated because the h gates remain closed. Even though the m gate may open during activation, the amount of sodium current is too small to elicit an action potential. The inactivation gates of the slow channel (f gates) are only partially closed, and when the cell is excited after addition of catecholamine (*right panel*), the d gates open and permit flow of a slow inward current that causes a slow-response action potential. This action potential resembles those in panels *A, C,* and *F* of Figure 19–7. (From Wit, A. L., and Bigger, J. T., Jr.: Possible electrophysiological mechanisms for lethal arrhythmias accompanying myocardial ischemia and infarction. Circulation *52*(Suppl. 3):96, 1975, by permission of the American Heart Association, Inc.)

for Na. When the equilibrium potential for Na (E_{Na}) is reached, Na no longer enters the cell, i.e., when the driving force acting on the ion is zero, no current will flow. In addition, Na conductance is time dependent so that when the membrane spends some time at voltages less negative than the resting potential, Na conductance decreases. Therefore an intervention that reduces membrane potential for a time—but not to threshold—partially inactivates Na channels, so that if threshold is now achieved, the magnitude and rate of Na influx are reduced.

At this point, several concepts need to be expanded. Ohm's law states that voltage equals current times resistance. The term conductance (g) is the inverse or reciprocal of resistance and is related to the ease with which ions can cross the cell membrane when driven by a potential difference across the membrane. As resistance of the membrane to passage of an ion increases, conductance decreases. Membrane permeability or conductance of the Na channel during phase 0 is regulated hypothetically by two types of gates, the "m" gate and the "h" gate, which modulate Na ion passage through the channel (Fig. 20–9).

THE GATED SYSTEM—A HYPOTHETICAL MODEL. In this hypothetical model, three m (activation) gates and one h (inactivation) gate can be considered to be lined up in series in the membrane Na channel (Fig. 20–9), with the m gate on the extracellular side and the h gate on the intracellular side of the membrane. When the membrane is in a resting polarized state, the m gates are almost completely closed, the h gate is open, and no Na can cross the membrane. Although depolarization of the membrane opens the m gates and closes the h gate, the m gates open faster than the h gate closes, i.e., activation of the channel proceeds faster than inactivation can occur, and Na flows through the Na channel for about 1 msec while both gates are open simultaneously. When the membrane repolarizes to fairly high negative values, i.e., membrane potential becomes more negative than about −60 mV, the m gates shut rapidly, the h gate opens more slowly (reactivation or recovery from inactivation), and the membrane is once again capable of depolarization. Until that time, the cell is absolutely refractory, i.e., no stimulus, regardless of intensity, can activate the cell. If the membrane is activated a second time before reaching a large negative value, all the h gates have not yet reopened so that the maximum number of Na channels that can open is reduced. The resulting action potential will have reduced $\dot{V}_{max}$, amplitude, duration, and conduction velocity. The state of the gates at any time depends on the membrane potential and the length of time the potential has been maintained.

Recent evidence suggests that the three distinct states in this Hodgkin-Huxley model—closed resting, open activated, and closed inactivated—may not be applicable to mammalian cells. When single Na channel currents are studied, Na channels are noted to open only once and rapidly move from the open to the inactivated state.[48, 49] Thus, true inactivation may be faster than the model predicts. Calcium channels have three modes of gating behavior: brief openings, no openings because of channel unavailability, and long-lasting openings with rare, very brief closings[50] (Fig. 20–6, *right*).

However, using this model, the amount of current (I) generated by a specific ion (I_i) equals the membrane conductance for the ion (g_i) multiplied by the driving force for that ion. The driving force is the difference between the actual membrane voltage (V_m) and the equilibrium potential for that ion (E_i). Thus

$$I_i = g_i\,(V_m - E_i)$$

Conductance can be determined by rearranging the equation:

$$g_i = \frac{I_i}{(V_m - E_i)}$$

The equations indicate that the current flow is voltage dependent, i.e., as the voltage of the membrane (V_m) changes relative to the equilibrium potential (E_i), the electrical driving force for an ion ($V_m - E_i$) changes and so does the current. The relationship between membrane voltage, V_m, at the time of depolarization, and I_{Na}, measured in terms of $\dot{V}_{max}$ (maximum rate of rise of phase 0), is indicated by the so-called membrane responsiveness curve. Depolarization results in decreased I_{Na} and $\dot{V}_{max}$ when it occurs at reduced membrane potentials (Fig. 20–8).

Membrane voltage may also regulate current flow by altering the status of the channel gates, thereby altering conductance. For the Na channel,

$$gi_{Na} = \bar{g}_{Na}\, m^3 h$$

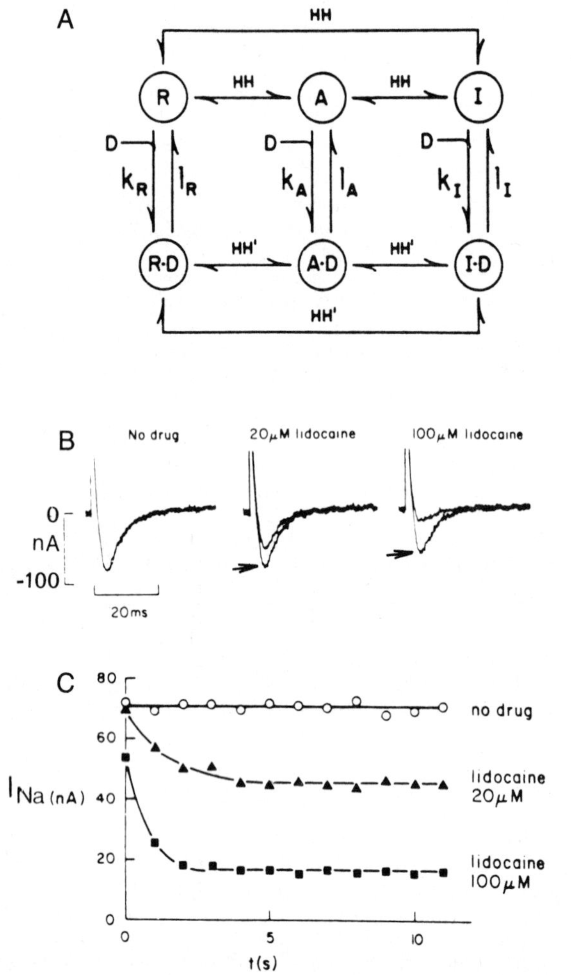

FIGURE 20–10. Interaction between sodium channels and lidocaine. *A*, Schematic of the modulated receptor hypothesis is presented. Sodium channel gating is represented by transitions between a resting state (R), an open state (A), and an inactivated state (I). The rate constants for binding and unbinding of drug to the channel (k's, l's) depend on the gating state. The presence of bound drug alters the gating transitions from their normal kinetics (HH for Hodgkin-Huxley) to modified kinetics (HH'). Application of this hypothesis explains why some drugs affect cardiac electrophysiologic properties according to different channel states, e.g., depolarized or repolarized conditions. *B*, An example of use dependent block of I_{Na} by lidocaine is demonstrated. I_{Na} was measured (nA) during trains of 500 msec pulses when the cell was depolarized from a holding potential of −105 mV to −35 mV at 1Hz following a period of rest. The traces show membrane currents associated with the 1st and 12th pulses superimposed, and the graph (C) plots measured I_{Na} amplitudes for each of the 12 pulses. Lidocaine exerted relatively little effect on the first inward current signal following the rest period (arrows B), but it substantially reduced peak I_{Na} following repetitive depolarizations. Lidocaine exerted a greater effect at the higher concentration. This figure illustrates that lidocaine blocks the sodium channel and reduces I_{Na} to a greater degree after repeated depolarizations of the cell compared with the first depolarization when the cell has been resting (use-dependence). (From Bean, B. P., Cohen, C. J., and Tsien, R. W.: Lidocaine block of cardiac sodium channels. J. Gen. Physiol. *87*:613, 1983.)

where gi_{Na} is the conductance of the Na channel at a given voltage, $\bar{g}_{Na}$ is the maximum possible conductance of the channel, m^3 represents the status of the activation gate (m = 1, the gate is open; m = 0, the gate is closed) and h represents the status of the inactivation gate (h = 1, gate open; h = 0, gate closed). Since the opening and closing of the gates are voltage and time dependent, the conductance of the channel (g) will be some fraction of the maximum possible conductance ($\bar{g}_{Na}$), depending on membrane voltage and the period during which the membrane has been at that voltage. The state of the channel influences the effects of drugs (Fig. 20–10, see also Chap. 21).

UPSTROKE OF THE ACTION POTENTIAL. In normal atrial and ventricular muscle and in the fibers in the His-Purkinje system, action potentials have very rapid upstrokes with a large $\dot{V}_{max}$ and are called fast responses. Action potentials in the normal sinus and atrioventricular (AV) nodes have very slow upstrokes with a reduced $\dot{V}_{max}$ and are called slow responses (Fig. 20–7). Upstrokes of "slow responses" are mediated by a slow inward, predominantly Ca current rather than the fast inward Na current.[51–53] These potentials received the name *slow response* because the time required for activation and inactivation of the slow inward current (I_{si}) is approximately an order of magnitude slower than that for the fast inward Na current (I_{Na}).[44] Recovery from inactivation also takes longer. Calcium entry and $[Ca]_i$ help promote inactivation. Thus the slow channel opens (activation gates "d") and closes (inactivation gates "f") more slowly than the fast channel, remains open for a longer time, and requires more time following a stimulus to be reactivated (Fig. 20–9). In fact, recovery of excitability outlasts full restoration of maximum diastolic potential. This means that even though the membrane potential has returned to normal, the cell has not recovered excitability completely because the latter depends on elapse of a certain amount of time (i.e., is time dependent) and not just on recovery of a particular membrane potential (i.e., voltage dependence).

Calcium channels are much more selective for Ca than sodium channels are for Na. Selectivity results from the presence of binding sites for which the permeant ions must compete, and under physiological conditions, more than 90 per cent of the inward current through the calcium channel is carried by Ca ions. Other divalent cations such as barium and strontium may also carry I_{si}. The magnitude of I_{si} is determined by the probability of calcium channel opening (P), the current through an open channel (i) and the number of channels (N): $I_{si} = N{\cdot}P{\cdot}i$. There are estimated to be 1 to 10 functional Ca channels/μM^2 surface area. At 3mM$[Ca]_o$ and a membrane potential of 0mV, i approximates 0.05 pA.[44]

The threshold for activation of I_{si}, i.e., the voltage the cell must reach to "turn on" the slow inward current, is about −30 to −40 mV. In fast-response type fibers, I_{si} is normally activated during phase 0 by the regenerative depolarization caused by the fast sodium current. Current flows through both fast and slow channels during the latter part of the action potential upstroke. However, I_{si} is much smaller than the peak Na current and therefore contributes little to the action potential until the fast Na current is inactivated, after completion of phase 0. Thus, I_{si} affects mainly the plateau of action potentials recorded in atrial and ventricular muscle and His-Purkinje fibers. When the fast Na current inactivates rapidly, such as in frog ventricle, I_{si} may contribute noticeably to the peak of phase 0. In addition, I_{si} can be activated and may play a prominent role in partially depolarized cells in which the fast Na channels have been inactivated, if conditions are appropriate for slow-channel activation.

Other significant differences exist between the fast and slow channels (Table 20–3). The following features are of some clinical relevance (Table 20–4). Drugs that elevate

TABLE 20–3 CHARACTERISTICS OF FAST AND SLOW INWARD CURRENTS IN CARDIAC TISSUE

	FAST	SLOW
Primary charge carrier	Na	Ca (Na)
Activation threshold	−70 to −55 mV	−55 to −30 mV
Magnitude	1 to 30 μA	0.1 to 3.0 μA
Time constant of		
Activation	< 1 msec	10 to 20 msec
Inactivation	< 1 msec	50 to 500 msec
Inhibitors	Tetrodotoxin, local anesthetics, sustained depolarization at < −40 mV	Verapamil, D-600, nifedipine, diltiazem, Mn, Co, Ni, La
Resting membrane potential	−80 to −95 mV	−40 to −70 mV
Conduction velocity	0.3 to 3.0 M/sec	0.01 to 0.10 M/sec
Rate of rise ($\dot{V}_{max}$) of action potential upstroke	200 to 1000 V/sec	1 to 10 V/sec
Action potential amplitude	100 to 130 mV	35 to 75 mV
Response to stimulus	All-or-none	Affected by characteristics of stimulus
Recovery of excitability	Prompt, ends with repolarization	Delayed, outlasts full repolarization
Safety factor for conduction	High	Low
Major current of action potential upstroke in the following:		
SA node	−	+
Atrial myocardium	+	−
AV node (N region)	−	+
His-Purkinje system	+	−
Ventricular myocardium	+	−
Neurotransmitter influence		
Beta-adrenergic	−	↑ ↑
Alpha-adrenergic	−	↑ (?)
Muscarinic cholinergic	−	↓ in atrium ↓ (?) in ventricle

cyclic AMP levels such as beta-adrenergic agonists, phosphodiesterase inhibitors such as theophylline and the lipid-soluble derivative of cyclic AMP, dibutyryl cyclic AMP, increase I_{si}. It has been proposed[54] that the beta-adrenergic agonist, binding to specific sarcolemmal receptors, facilitates the dissociation of two subunits of a regulatory protein, one of which activates adenylate cyclase and thus increases intracellular levels of cyclic AMP. The latter binds to a regulatory subunit of a cyclic AMP–dependent protein kinase that promotes phosphorylation of specific membrane proteins controlling the permeability of the slow channel. This putative conformational change in the channel increases the magnitude of the current or the conductance to the ion, presumably by increasing the amount of time the individual channels are open, without increasing the total number of calcium channels. The probability of channel opening increases. Acetylcholine reduces I_{si} in a variety of preparations, although the mechanism(s) by which this occurs may vary. Possibilities include a direct effect on I_{si} conductance, an increase in outward K currents with hyperpolarization, and an antisympathetic effect.[55–57]

Fast and slow channels can be differentiated on the basis of their pharmacological sensitivity. Drugs that block the slow channel with a *fair* degree of specificity (p. 635) include verapamil, nifedipine, diltiazem, D-600 (a methoxy derivative of verapamil), and compounds like manganese, lanthanum, nickel, and cobalt. D-600 reduces I_{si} by reducing open-channel probability, as does nifedipine. Other drugs of the same dihydropyridine family as nifedipine can enhance I_{si} by stabilizing the channel in the open mode. Antiarrhythmic agents such as lidocaine, quinidine, procainamide, and disopyramide (see Chap. 21) affect the fast channel and not the slow channel. The puffer fish poison, tetrodotoxin (TTX), which is too toxic to be used clinically, blocks the fast channel with considerable specificity.

While fast-response action potentials are characteristic of atrial and ventricular muscle and His-Purkinje tissue, slow-response type action potentials are found in the normal sinus and AV nodes and many kinds of diseased tissue (Table 20–4). Normal action potentials recorded from the sinus node and the N region of the AV node have a reduced resting membrane potential, action potential amplitude, overshoot, upstroke, and conduction velocity com-

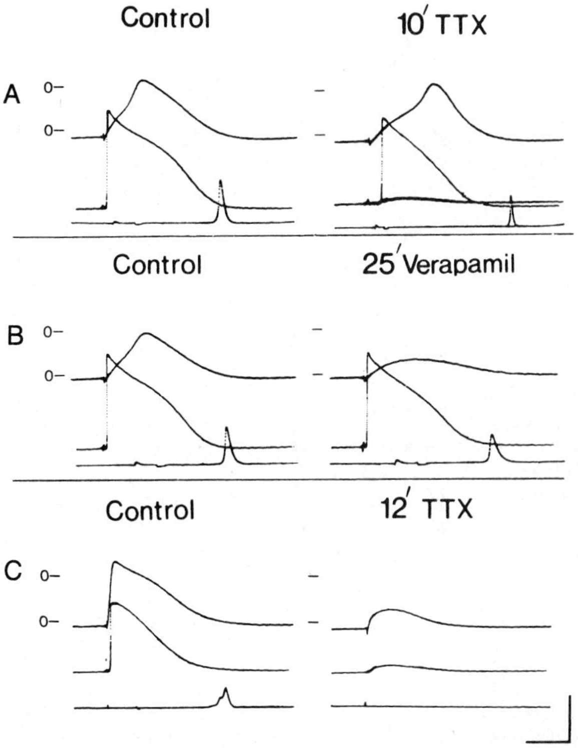

FIGURE 20–11. Effects of tetrodotoxin (TTX) and verapamil on action potentials in diseased human ventricle, removed from a patient at the time of endocardial resection for recurrent ventricular tachycardia. *A*, Action potentials and upstroke velocity recordings from an abnormal cell (upper action potential recording) and a relatively normal cell (lower action potential recording) before (*left*) and after (*right*) exposure to TTX for 10 minutes. $\dot{V}$max for the lower cell is shown in the bottom tracing. TTX produced activation delay and intermittent conduction block in the normal cell but had little effect on the action potential of the abnormal cell (right panel). Two consecutive cycles are superimposed in the right panel. *B*, After washout of TTX, the same two cells were exposed to verapamil for 25 minutes. Verapamil reduced both the action potential and the amplitude of the abnormal cell without affecting its resting membrane potential and slightly reduced both the action potential amplitude and $\dot{V}$max in the normal cell (right panel). *C*, Effects of TTX on a different specimen of myocardium from the same patient. Control recordings are shown on the left. In these cells, TTX markedly reduced action potential amplitude and Vmax (right panel) while verapamil only slightly reduced action potential amplitude (not shown). (From Gilmour, R. F., Jr., et al.: Cellular electrophysiological abnormalities of diseased human ventricular myocardium. Am. J. Cardiol. 51:137, 1983.)

TABLE 20–4 IONIC CURRENTS

TISSUE TYPE	I_{Na}	I_{si}	I_{k1}	$I_K(I_x)$	I_{to}	$I_f(I_h)$	I_{TI}
Atrial and ventricular myocardium	Responsible for action potential upstroke	Responsible for action potential plateau, excitation contraction coupling, activation in depolarized cells exhibiting the slow response; inactivates to terminate plateau; increased by beta stimulation, inhibited by ACh	Responsible for resting potential; repolarizing current in last phase of action potential. Exhibits inward rectification. Time independent, voltage dependent	Responsible for duration of plateau; time-dependent rate-limiting effect; increased by beta stimulation	Responsible for early, transient repolarization preceding plateau; two separate components	Not prominent but may be present	Responsible for delayed afterdepolarization; carried by influx of Na due to increase in [Ca]; easily produced with digitalis
His Purkinje tissue	As in myocardium	As in myocardium; can be responsible for automaticity in all cells that are sufficiently depolarized	As in myocardium	As in myocardium	Prominent; causes phase I; modulates action potential duration in Purkinje fibers	Responsible for automaticity; prominent; increased by beta stimulation	Prominent
SA node and AV node	If present, largely inactivated at reduced membrane potentials	Responsible for action potential upstroke in normal SA and AV nodes. Probably contributes to automaticity	Not prominent	Decay important for normal automaticity	Present	May contribute to automaticity	Present

Abbreviations
I_{Na}, sodium current; I_{si}, slow inward current; I_{kI}, time independent inwardly rectifying potassium current; I_K, delayed rectifier, time dependent potassium current; I_{to}, transient outward current; I_f (also called I_h), pacemaker current; I_{TI}, Ca^{+2}, calcium activated transient inward current.

pared to action potentials in muscle or Purkinje fibers (Fig. 20–7).

Slow-channel blockers, but not TTX, suppress sinus and AV nodal action potentials. The prolonged time for reactivation of the I_{si} probably accounts for the fact that these cells remain refractory longer than the time it takes for full voltage repolarization to occur. Thus, premature stimulation immediately after the membrane potential reaches full repolarization leads to action potentials with reduced amplitudes and upstroke velocities. Therefore, slow conduction and prolonged refractoriness are characteristic features of nodal cells. These cells also have a reduced "safety factor for conduction," which means that the stimulating efficacy of the propagating impulse is low and conduction block easily occurs. Membranes of nodal cells probably do have Na channels that are inactivated by the relatively depolarized range of potentials over which activity takes place. Hyperpolarization exposes a fast TTX-sensitive sodium current in nodal cells.

These and many other observations support the conclusion that, in the *normal* heart, the I_{si} mediates not only the plateau but also the upstroke of the action potential in the sinus and AV nodes. A small fast component, enhanced by hyperpolarization, may contribute to the slow-response upstroke of sinus nodal potentials. However, the slow diastolic depolarization preceding the upstroke of sinus action potentials probably largely inactivates this fast-current component at the usual thresholds.

A variety of manipulations, including those that block or inactivate the fast inward current (such as administration of TTX or depolarization of the cell membrane with K), those that increase the slow current (such as administration of Ca or catecholamines), or those that decrease the outward potassium currents (such as barium), can transform a fast-channel–dependent fiber (e.g., a Purkinje fiber) to a slow-channel–dependent fiber. Whether these artificial in vitro alterations have clinical relevance is not known, but it is possible that myocardial ischemia or infarction, for example, can produce this transformation[51] (Fig. 20–7*F*). Current data suggest that the electrophysiological changes accompanying *acute* myocardial ischemia represent a depressed form of a fast response rather than a slow response.[58] However, probable slow-response activity has been shown in myocardium resected from patients undergoing surgery for recurrent ventricular tachyarrhythmias[59–61] (Fig. 20–11). Whether these responses play a role in the genesis of ventricular arrhythmias in these patients has not been established.

PHASE 1—EARLY RAPID REPOLARIZATION

Following phase 0, the membrane repolarizes rapidly and transiently to near 0 mV, partly owing to inactivation of I_{Na} or activation of a transient outward current carried mostly by K ions and also possibly related to Cl moving intracellularly through a Cl channel. Cl distributes itself passively according to the membrane potential. Therefore, $[Cl]_i$ is low when the membrane is polarized because of the intracellular negative environment. However, the Cl channel may open upon depolarization and permit Cl to enter the cell down its concentration gradient.[62–64] The increase in intracellular negative ions reduces the positive membrane voltage, and the membrane potential returns to near 0 mV, from which the plateau, or phase 2, arises. Sometimes a slight transient depolarization follows phase 1 repolarization. Phase 1 is well defined and separated from phase 2 in Purkinje fibers and some muscle fibers.

PHASE 2—PLATEAU

During the plateau phase, which may last several hundred milliseconds, membrane conductance to all ions falls to rather low values. Potassium conductance (g_K) falls almost immediately upon depolarization, in spite of the large electrochemical gradient for K, owing to "inward-going rectification" (sometimes called "anomalous rectification," since it is opposite to that observed in the squid giant axon). This ponderous term simply means that when the membrane depolarizes it passes inward current more easily than it passes outward current, or, in this instance, K can enter the cell more easily than it can exit, and therefore, in spite of at least three important outward K currents and a large electrochemical gradient, g_K is low and few K ions leave the cell. Sodium conductance (g_{Na}) is low because of inactivation of sodium channels. Minor contributions to repolarization include a small inward Cl flux and electrogenic Na-K exchange, pumping out 3 Na ions in exchange for 2 K ions. The Na-K exchange does not turn on and off with each single action potential but restores the ionic gradient over a cumulative time period. The slow inward current, active during the plateau, supplies a small (compared to the Na or fast current) inward current and balances these outward currents, and membrane voltage remains near zero for more than 100 msec. A recently studied inward Na current, blocked by tetrodotoxin, also contributes to the plateau.[65]

PHASE 3—FINAL RAPID REPOLARIZATION

In this portion of the action potential, repolarization proceeds rapidly, owing at least in part to two currents: time-dependent inactivation of the slow inward current, so that intracellular movement of positive charges decreases, and activation of an outward K current (reversal of "inward-going rectification"), so that extracellular movement of positive charges increases. The outward K current is called I_x (or I_K). The net membrane current becomes more outward, and the membrane potential shifts in a negative direction. As repolarization continues, g_K increases, and these repolarization changes self-perpetuate in a regenerative manner.

PHASE 4—RESTING MEMBRANE POTENTIAL AND DIASTOLIC DEPOLARIZATION

Under normal conditions, the membrane potential of atrial and ventricular muscle cells remains steady throughout diastole. Factors responsible for this resting membrane potential were described earlier. In other fibers found in certain parts of the atria, in the muscle of the mitral and tricuspid valves, in His-Purkinje fibers, and in the sinus node and distal portion of the AV node, the resting membrane potential does not remain constant in diastole but gradually depolarizes (Fig. 20–7A). If a propagating impulse does not depolarize the cell—or more likely, a group of cells—it may reach threshold by itself and produce a spontaneous action potential. The property possessed by spontaneously discharging cells is called phase 4 diastolic depolarization; when it leads to initiation of action potentials, automaticity results. The discharge rate of the sinus node normally exceeds the discharge rate of other potentially automatic pacemaker sites and thus maintains dominance of the cardiac rhythm. Normal or abnormal automaticity at other sites may discharge at rates faster than the sinus nodal discharge rate and may usurp control of the cardiac rhythm for one cycle or many. This will be discussed subsequently.

NORMAL AUTOMATICITY

The ionic basis of automaticity must be explained by a net gain in intracellular positive charges during diastole. Until recently it was thought that in cardiac Purkinje fibers a decrease in an outward K current (I_{K2}) occurred during a relatively constant background inward current and caused pacemaker activity. It is now clear that all cardiac pacemaker cells exhibit a voltage-dependent channel that is activated by potentials negative to −50 to −60 mV. At this potential an inward current becomes activated and is carried by a channel relatively nonselective for monovalent cations. Hyperpolarization increases its rate of activation and, at −70 mV, the time constant ranges from 2 to 4 sec. This pacemaker current (I_h or I_f) probably underlies the slow diastolic depolarization that occurs between −90 and −60 mV in Purkinje fibers.[66] Although either K or Na can serve as ion transporters, I_f carries largely Na at the more negative intracellular voltages. Extracellular K ions activate I_f, but $[Na]_o$ does not influence its conductance.[67] Cesium fairly specifically blocks I_f. Reduction in K conductance by barium or amantidine seemingly can unmask I_f in ventricular muscle to produce automaticity at relatively normal membrane potentials (Fig. 20–12).[68]

AUTOMATICITY IN SINUS NODAL CELLS. This is primarily dependent on I_k and I_{si},[69] and not I_f because at the reduced membrane potentials of sinus nodal cells, I_f contributes only about 20 per cent of the pacemaker current. Conversely, I_k in normally polarized Purkinje fibers adds little to the pacemaker current. The decay of I_k, together with the presence of an unidentified background inward current, and I_{si} are the essential processes governing the rate of pacemaker depolarization in sinus and AV nodal cells[70] and in Purkinje fibers whose membrane potential has been depolarized to voltages largely positive to the activation range of I_f. I_{K1} is negligible in sinus nodal cells, which therefore are quite resistant to changes in $[K]_o$. Sinus nodal cells do possess the I_f current if they are hyperpolarized in the range of −50 to −100 mV. Both Na and K carry the current I_f, which is strongly depressed by cesium.[71] The exact location of pacemaking cells within the AV nodal region still has not been demonstrated conclusively, and it is likely that several potential pacemaker sites exist. Also, whether AV nodal cells themselves possess the property of automaticity has not been completely resolved. Automaticity in canine AV nodal cells has been noted, and more recent evidence from studies of rabbit AV nodal cells suggests that they, too, exhibit automaticity.[72]

Sinus nodal discharge rate maintains dominance over latent pacemaker sites because it depolarizes more rapidly and because of the mechanism called *overdrive suppression*, a phenomenon characterized by prolonged suppression of normal pacemakers (Fig. 20–12 and Fig. 22–46, p. 706) in proportion to the duration and rate of stimulation by a more rapidly discharging pacemaker. The mechanism may relate to active Na extrusion during the more rapid rate that maintains diastolic

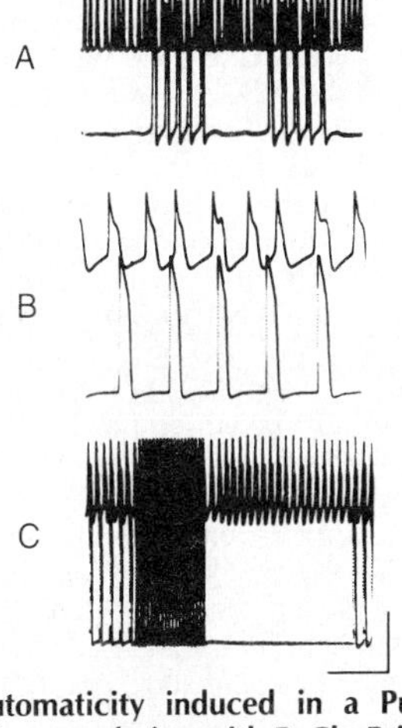

FIGURE 20–12. Automaticity induced in a Purkinje fiber-papillary muscle preparation by superfusion with $BaCl_2$. Prior to superfusion with $BaCl_2$, the preparation had been superfused with 8.0 mM $CaCl_2$ Tyrode solution to produce irreversible unidirectional block from the Purkinje fiber to papillary muscle. The preparation subsequently was superfused with 2.0 mM $CaCl_2$ Tyrode solution containing 0.25 mM $BaCl_2$. *A*, $BaCl_2$-induced depolarization and sustained automaticity in the Purkinje fiber (upper recording) and intermittent spontaneous activity in the papillary muscle (lower recording) that was not accompanied by a significant loss of maximum diastolic membrane potential. This figure shows that, under certain circumstances, muscle can exhibit diastolic depolarization, even at fairly normal resting membrane potentials. *B*, Purkinje fiber automaticity did not propagate to papillary muscle, but spontaneous papillary muscle action potentials propagated to the Purkinje fiber. (Purkinje fiber action potentials 3 and 6 occur early due to capture from muscle propagation when they occurred outside the Purkinje fiber refractory period. Thus, this preparation exhibits unidirectional block.) *C*, Following simultaneous overdrive pacing of Purkinje fiber and papillary muscle, automaticity was suppressed only in papillary muscle possibly because it was not depolarized as was the Purkinje fiber. Vertical calibration 50 mV. Horizontal calibration 10 seconds for panels A and C and 2 seconds for panel B. (From Gilmour, R. F., Jr., Evans, J. J., and Zipes, D. P.: Preferential interruption of impulse transmission across Purkinje-muscle junctions by interventions that depress conduction. *In* Zipes, D. P., and Jalife, J. [eds.]: Cardiac Electrophysiology and Arrhythmias. Orlando, Grune and Stratton, 1985, p. 292.)

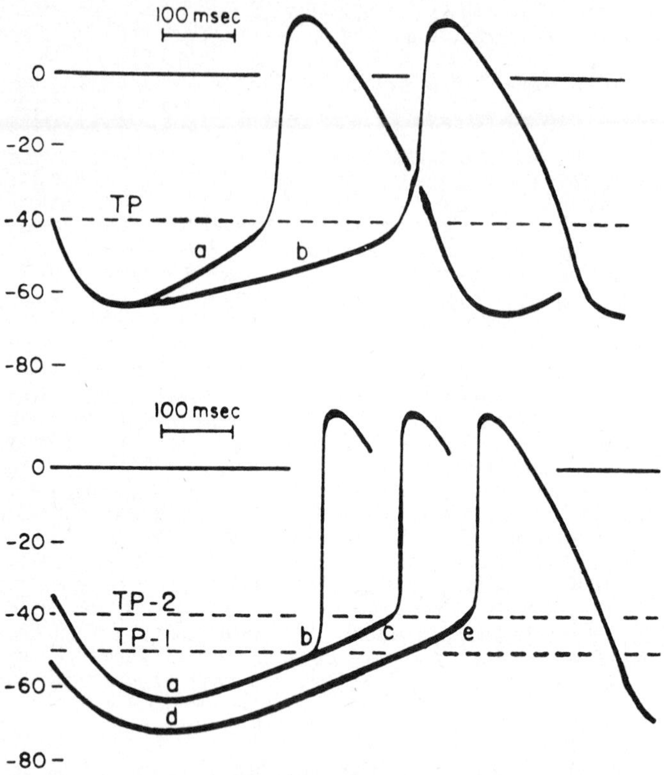

FIGURE 20–13. Significant mechanisms responsible for changes in discharge frequency of a pacemaker cell. *Top*, A decrease in the slope of phase 4 diastolic depolarization (from a to b) decreases the rate by increasing the time required for the transmembrane potential to reach the threshold potential (TP). *Bottom*, A change in the level of threshold potential from TP-1 to TP-2 increases the cycle length from a-b to a-c, and an increase in resting potential from a to d slows the discharge rate from a-c to d-e. (From Hoffman, B. F., and Cranefield, P. F.: Electrophysiology of the Heart. New York, McGraw-Hill Book Co., 1960.)

depolarization of latent pacemakers at a level more negative than the threshold potential for automatic discharge.

The rate of sinus nodal discharge can be varied by several mechanisms in response to autonomic or other influences. The pacemaker locus can shift within or outside[29] the sinus node to cells discharging faster or more slowly than the present rhythm. If the pacemaker site remains the same, alterations in the slope of diastolic depolarization, maximum diastolic potential, or threshold potential can speed or slow the discharge rate (Fig. 20–13). For example, if the slope of diastolic depolarization steepens and if the resting membrane potential becomes less negative or the threshold potential more negative (within limits), discharge rate increases. Opposite changes slow the discharge rate.

PASSIVE MEMBRANE ELECTRICAL PROPERTIES

We have just discussed many of the features of active membrane properties. In addition, it is important to be aware of some features of the passive membrane properties, such as membrane resistance, capacitance, and cable properties. The important difference between the active and passive states is that the active system responds out of proportion to the applied stimulus and thereby adds energy to the electrical system; the passive system responds proportionately to the size of the stimulus and does not add energy.

Although the cardiac cell membrane is resistant to current flow, it also has capacitative properties, which means it behaves like a battery and can store charges of opposite sign on its two sides: an excess of negative charges inside the membrane balanced by equivalent positive charges outside the membrane. These resistive and capacitative charges cause the membrane to take a certain amount of time to respond to an applied stimulus, rather than responding instantly, because the charges across the capacitative membrane must be altered first. A subthreshold rectangular-shaped current pulse applied to the membrane produces a slowly rising and decaying membrane-voltage change rather than a rectangular voltage change. A value called the time constant of the membrane reflects this property and is the time taken by the membrane voltage to reach 63 per cent of its final value after application of a steady current.

When aligned end to end, cardiac cells, particularly the His-Purkinje system, behave like a long cable in which current flows more easily inside the cell and to the adjacent cell across the intercalated disc than it does across the cell membrane to the outside. When current is injected at a point, most of it flows along the cell, but some leaks out. Because of this loss of current, the voltage change of a cell at a site distant from the point of applied current is less than the change in membrane voltage where the stimulus was given. A measure of this property of a cable is called the space or length constant (λ); it is the distance along the cable from the point of stimulation that the voltage at steady state is 1/e (37 per cent) of its value at the point of introduction. Restated, λ describes how far current flows before leaking passively across the surface membrane to a value about one-third its initial value. This distance is normally about 2 mm for Purkinje fibers, 0.5 mm for the sinus node, and 0.8 mm for ventricular muscle fibers. λ is about 10 times the length of an individual cell.[44] As an example, if e is about 2.7 and a hyperpolarizing current pulse in a Purkinje fiber produces a membrane-voltage change of 15 mV at the site of current injection, the membrane potential change one space constant (2 mm) away would be 15/2.7 = 5.5 mV.

Since the current loop in any circuit must be closed, current must flow back to its point of origin. Local circuit currents pass across nexuses between cells and exit across the sarcolemmal membrane to close the loop and complete the circuit. Inward excitation currents in one area (carried by Na in most regions) flow intracellularly along the length of the tissue (carried mostly by K), escape across the membrane, and flow extracellularly in a longitudinal direction.[44] The outside local circuit current is the current recorded in an electrocardiogram. Through these local circuit currents the transmembrane potential of each cell influences the transmembrane potential of its neighbor because of the passive flow of current from one segment of the fiber to another across the low-resistance intercellular junctions. A cell hyperpolarized compared to its neighbor depolarizes slightly while the neighboring cell hyperpolarizes slightly. Conversely, a depolarized cell adjacent to a polarized cell polarizes slightly while the neighbor depolarizes slightly. This "electrotonic" influence of neighboring cells on each other is determined chiefly by the length constant of the fiber and is due to the passive spread of current.

As discussed earlier, the speed of conduction depends on active membrane properties such as the magnitude of the Na current, a measure of which is $\dot{V}_{max}$. Passive membrane properties also contribute to conduction velocity and include excitability threshold, which influences the capability of cells adjacent to the one that has been discharged to reach threshold; the intracellular resistance of the cell, which is determined by the free ions in the cytoplasm, the resistance of the gap junction, and the cross-sectional area of the cell. Direction of propagation is critically important.[15] Longitudinal conduction velocity is about three times greater than transverse conduction velocity, at least in part because of a much more tortuous transverse path and fewer nexuses per unit distance with transverse conduction.[44]

LOSS OF MEMBRANE POTENTIAL

Most acquired abnormalities of cardiac muscle or specialized fibers that result in arrhythmias produce a loss of membrane potential, i.e., maximum diastolic potential becomes less negative. This change should be viewed as a symptom of an underlying abnormality, analogous to fever or jaundice, rather than a diagnostic category in and of itself, because both the ionic changes resulting in cellular depolarization and the more fundamental biochemical or metabolic abnormalities responsible for the ionic alterations are probably multicausal. Cellular depolarization can result from elevated $[K]_o$ or decreased $[K]_i$, an increase in membrane permeability to Na (P_{Na} increases), or a decrease in membrane permeability to K (P_K decreases). Reference to Equation 2 (p. 587) illustrates that these changes alone or in combination make V_r less negative. Normal cells perfused by an abnormal milieu (e.g., hyperkalemia), abnormal cells with probable membrane changes perfused by a normal milieu (e.g., healed myocardial infarction), or abnormal cells perfused by an abnormal milieu (e.g., acute myocardial ischemia and infarction) may exist alone or in combination to reduce resting membrane voltage. Each of these changes can have one or more biochemical or metabolic causes. For example, acute myocardial ischemia[73] results in decreased $[K]_i$ and increased $[K]_o$[74] possibly because of reduced Na-K exchange pump activity caused by a fall in available ATP as well as release of substances such as lysophosphatidylcholine.[75] Also, $[Ca]_i$ may accumulate and further reduce V_r.[76] Oxygen-free radicals may be important in ischemic-related myocardial injury.[77, 78] Knowledge of these changes may provide insight into therapy that actually reverses basic defects and restores membrane potential or other abnormalities to normal.[79]

EFFECTS OF REDUCED RESTING POTENTIAL. The reduced resting membrane potential alters depolarization and repolarization phases of the cardiac action potential. For example, partial membrane depolarization prevents complete recovery from inactivation (h gate) of the rapid Na channel. This reduces the number of available Na channels for depolarization and decreases the magnitude of the rapid Na current during phase 0. The subsequent reduction in $\dot{V}_{max}$ and action potential amplitude prolongs conduction time of the propagated impulse, at times to the point of block. Action potentials with upstrokes dependent on the rapid Na current flowing through partially inactivated Na channels are called *depressed fast responses* (Fig. 20–11*C*). Their contours often resemble, and may be difficult to distinguish from, slow responses, in which upstrokes are due to I_{si} (Fig. 20–7*F*). Membrane depolarization to levels of −60 to −70 mV may inactivate half the Na channels, while depolarization to −50 mV or less may inactivate all the Na channels. At membrane potentials positive to −50 mV, I_{si} can be activated to generate phase 0[51, 52, 55] if conditions are appropriate. These action potential changes are likely to be heterogeneous with unequal degrees of Na inactivation that create areas with minimally reduced velocity, more severely depressed zones, and areas of complete block. These uneven changes are propitious for the development of arrhythmias (Figs. 20–14 and 20–15).

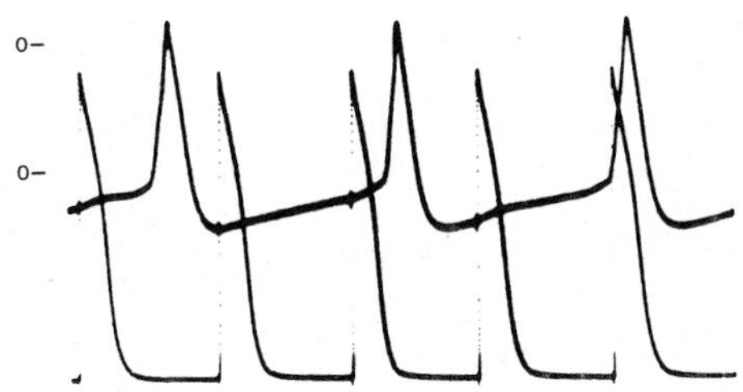

FIGURE 20–14. Bidirectional block and automaticity at reduced membrane potentials in diseased human ventricular myocardium. The upper recording was obtained from an area near the infarcted segment of endocardium resected from a patient with recurrent ventricular tachycardia. The lower recording was obtained from more normal-appearing myocardium in another area of the same resected specimen. Maximum diastolic potentials in the upper and lower recordings were −67 mV and −84 mV, respectively. The abnormal area exhibited spontaneous automatic activity, whereas the normal area was quiescent (not shown). Pacing the normal area at a cycle length of 1000 msec produced action potentials that did not propagate to the abnormal zone, nor did spontaneous action potentials in the abnormal zone propagate to the normal zone. Thus, in a small piece of human ventricle, automaticity could be recorded in cells that probably were depolarized ventricular muscle, and bidirectional block existed between this abnormal and an adjacent normal area. Such heterogeneity is probably the basis for some types of arrhythmias. Vertical calibration, 50 mV, horizontal calibration, 2 seconds. (From Gilmour, R. F., Jr., and Zipes, D. P.: Abnormal automaticity and interrelated phenomena. *In* Fozzard, H. M., et al. [eds.]: The Heart and Cardiovascular System. New York, Raven Press, 1986.)

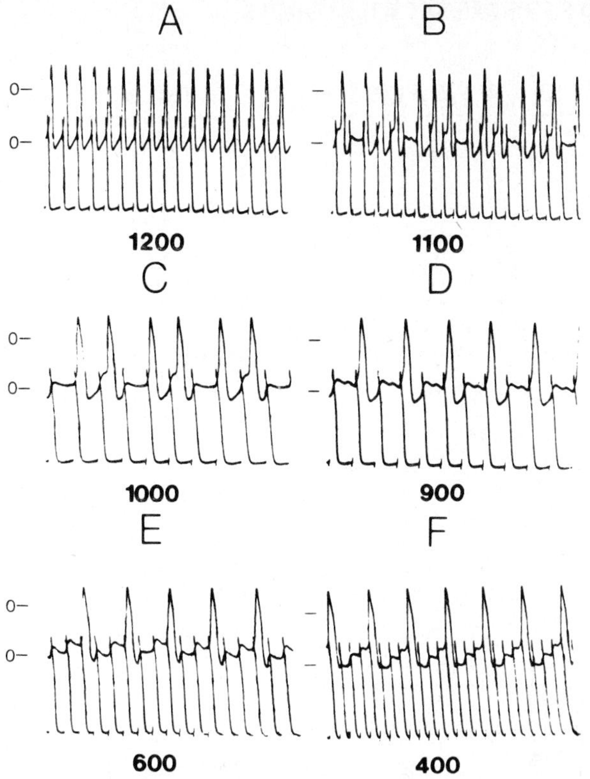

FIGURE 20–15. Rate-dependent conduction from the normal zone into the abnormal zone. When the pacing cycle length in the normal zone was shortened from 1200 to 400 msec (panels A to F), increasing degrees of entrance block into the abnormal area occurred, progressing from 1:1 conduction at a cycle length of 1200 msec, to 4:3 conduction at 1100 msec, 3:2 conduction at 1000 msec, 2:1 conduction at 900 msec, 3:1 conduction at 600 msec, and 4:1 conduction at 400 msec. Pacing the abnormal zone (not shown) resulted in block to the normal zone (unidirectional propagation). Vertical calibration: 50 mV. Horizontal calibration: 4 sec in *A* and *B* and 2 sec in *C* to *F*. (From Gilmour, R. F., Jr., et al.: Cellular electrophysiologic abnormalities of diseased human ventricular myocardium. Am. J. Cardiol. *51*:137, 1983.)

In these cells with reduced membrane potential, refractoriness may outlast voltage recovery of the action potential, i.e., the cell may still be refractory or partially refractory after the resting membrane potential returns to its most negative value. Further, if block of the cardiac impulse occurs in a fairly localized area without significant slowing of conduction proximal to the site of block, cells in this proximal zone exhibit short action potentials and refractory periods because unexcited cells distal to the block (still in a polarized state) electrotonically speed recovery in cells proximal to the site of block. If conduction slows gradually proximal to the site of block, the duration of these action potentials and their refractory periods may be prolonged. Some cells may exhibit abnormal electrophysiological properties even though they have a relatively normal resting membrane potential.[61]

MECHANISMS OF ARRHYTHMOGENESIS

(Table 20–5)

Cardiac arrhythmias are generally divided into categories of disorders of impulse formation, disorders of impulse conduction, or combinations of both.[47, 80–85] It is important to realize, however, that our present diagnostic tools do not permit unequivocal determination of the electrophysiological mechanisms responsible for most clinically occurring arrhythmias or their ionic bases. It is very difficult to separate reentry from automaticity clinically. At best, one can postulate only that a particular arrhythmia is "most consistent with" or "best explained by" one or the other electrophysiological mechanism. Some tachyarrhythmias may be started by one mechanism and perpetuated by another. For example, premature ventricular depolarization due to abnormal automaticity may precipitate a ventricular tachycardia sustained by reentry. Conceivably, an antiarrhythmic drug could affect the abnormal automaticity and not the reentry, or vice versa. Given these comments, mechanisms demonstrated to cause electrical activity in a variety of myocardial preparations will be considered and, when possible, related to clinical situations.

TABLE 20–5 MECHANISMS OF ARRHYTHMOGENESIS

I. Disorders of Impulse Formation
  A. Automaticity
    1. Normal automaticity
      a. Experimental examples–Normal in vivo or in vitro sinus node, Purkinje fibers, others
      b. Clinical examples–Sinus tachycardia or bradycardia inappropriate for the clinical situation, possibly ventricular parasystole
    2. Abnormal automaticity
      a. Experimental example—Depolarization-induced automaticity in Purkinje fibers or ventricular muscle
      b. Clinical example–Possibly accelerated ventricular rhythms after myocardial infarction
  B. Triggered Activity
    1. Early afterdepolarizations (EAD's)
      a. Experimental examples–EAD's produced by barium, hypoxia, high concentrations of catecholamines, drugs such as sotalol, *N*-acetylprocainamide, cesium
      b. Clinical examples–Possibly acquired long Q-T syndrome and associated ventricular arrhythmias
    2. Delayed afterdepolarizations (DAD's)
      a. Experimental example–DAD's produced in Purkinje fibers by digitalis
      b. Clinical example–Possibly some digitalis-induced arrhythmias
II. Disorders of Impulse Conduction
  A. Block
    1. Bidirectional or unidirectional without reentry
      a. Experimental example–SA, AV, bundle branch, Purkinje-muscle, others
      b. Clinical example–SA, AV, bundle branch, others
    2. Unidirectional block with reentry
      a. Experimental examples–AV node, Purkinje-muscle junction, infarcted myocardium, others
      b. Clinical examples–Reciprocating tachycardia in WPW syndrome, AV nodal reentry, VT due to bundle branch reentry, others
    3. Reflection
      a. Experimental example—Purkinje fiber with area of inexcitability
      b. Clinical example–Unknown
III. Combined Disorders
  A. Interactions between automatic foci
    1. Experimental examples—Depolarizing or hyperpolarizing subthreshold stimuli speed or slow automatic discharge rate
    2. Clinical examples–Modulated parasystole
  B. Interactions between automaticity and conduction
    1. Experimental examples–Deceleration-dependent block, overdrive suppression of conduction, entrance and exit block
    2. Clinical examples–Similar to experimental

DISORDERS OF IMPULSE FORMATION

This category is defined as inappropriate discharge rate of the normal pacemaker, the sinus node (e.g., sinus rates too fast or too slow for the physiological needs of the patient), or discharge from an ectopic pacemaker that controls the atrial or ventricular rhythm for one complex or more. Pacemaker discharge from ectopic sites, often called latent or subsidiary pacemakers, can occur in fibers located in several parts of the atria, the coronary sinus, atrioventricular valves, portions of the AV junction, and the His-Purkinje system. Ordinarily kept from reaching the level of threshold potential because of overdrive suppression by the more rapidly firing sinus node,[85] ectopic pacemaker activity at one of these latent sites can become manifest when sinus nodal discharge rate slows or block occurs at some level between the sinus node and the ectopic pacemaker site, permitting *escape* of the latent pacemaker at the latter's normal discharge rate. A clinical example would be sinus bradycardia to a rate of 45 beats/min that permits an AV junctional escape complex to occur at a rate of 50 beats/min.

Alternatively, the discharge rate of the latent pacemaker can speed up inappropriately and usurp control of the cardiac rhythm from the sinus node that has been discharging at a normal rate. A clinical example would be interruption of normal sinus rhythm by a premature ventricular complex or a burst of ventricular tachycardia. It is important to remember that such disorders of impulse formation can be due to a speeding or slowing of a *normal* pacemaker mechanism (e.g., phase 4 diastolic depolarization that is ionically normal for the sinus node or for an ectopic site such as a Purkinje fiber but occurs inappropriately fast or slow) or due to an ionically *abnormal* pacemaker mechanism. The patient with persistent sinus tachycardia at rest or sinus bradycardia during exertion exhibits inappropriate sinus nodal discharge rates, but the ionic mechanisms responsible for sinus nodal discharge may still be normal although the kinetics or magnitude of the currents may be altered. Conversely, when a patient experiences ventricular tachycardia during an acute myocardial infarction, ionic mechanisms ordinarily not involved in formation of spontaneous impulses for this fiber type may be operative to generate this tachycardia. For example, although pacemaker activity generally is not found in ordinary working myocardium, the effects of myocardial infarction perhaps can depolarize these cells to membrane potentials at which inactivation of I_K and activation of I_{si} cause automatic discharge. Experimental evidence suggests, however, that *acute* myocardial ischemia does not enhance, or may actually suppress, automaticity.[58] Enhanced automaticity has been found in depolarized Purkinje fibers surviving myocardial infarction. Areas of conduction block that may produce entrance block to the automatic focus may protect it from the effects of overdrive suppression and favor the development of automatic discharge (Fig. 20–14). Based on the rate response to catecholamine administration of isolated fibers exhibiting normal phase 4 diastolic depolarization and on in vivo studies during stellate ganglion stimulation, it is likely that rates much in excess of 200 beats/min are not due to enhanced normal automaticity.[51]

ABNORMAL AUTOMATICITY. Mechanisms responsible for *normal* automaticity were described earlier (p. 593). *Abnormal* automaticity may arise from cells that have reduced maximum diastolic potentials, often at membrane potentials positive to -50 mV, when I_K and I_{si} may be operative. Automaticity at membrane potentials more negative than -70 mV may be due to I_f. When the membrane potential is between -50 and -70 mV the cell may be quiescent.[86] Electrotonic effects from surrounding normally polarized or more depolarized myocardium will influence the development of automaticity. Abnormal automaticity has been found in Purkinje fibers removed from dogs subjected to myocardial infarction, in rat myocardium damaged by epinephrine (Fig. 20–16), in human atrial samples, and in ventricular myocardial specimens from patients undergoing aneurysmectomy and endocardial resection for recurrent ventricular tachyarrhythmias. Abnormal automaticity can be produced in normal muscle or Purkinje fibers by appropriate interventions such as current passage that reduces diastolic potential[68] (Fig. 20–17). Automatic discharge rate speeds up with progressive depolarization, while hyperpolarizing pulses slow the spontaneous firing. Other interventions, such as barium administration, produce automaticity during which action potentials are similar to those produced by current passage. Both may be due to I_K and I_{si}. It is possible that partial depolarization and failure to reach normal maximal diastolic

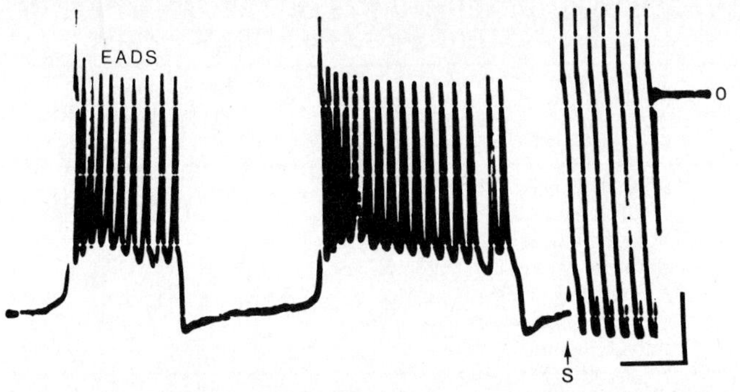

FIGURE 20–16. Early afterdepolarizations (EAD's). Early afterdepolarizations occur spontaneously in an isolated canine cardiac Purkinje fiber when exposed to reduced extracellular potassium concentration. Note spontaneous phase four diastolic depolarization is present. In the initial two action potentials, a series of spontaneous depolarizations (EAD's) result before the membrane returns to its maximum diastolic potential. Following the second series of EAD's, pacing is begun (S) and normal action potentials follow. Horizontal calibration bar = 5 seconds, vertical bar = 25 mV. (From Kovacs, R. J., Bailey, J. C., and Zipes, D. P.: Mechanisms of cardiac arrhythmias. *In* Parmley, W. W., et al. [eds.]: Cardiology. Philadelphia, J.B. Lippincott Co., in press.)

potential can induce automatic discharge in most if not all cardiac fibers. Although this type of spontaneous automatic activity has been found in human atrial and ventricular[59–61] fibers, its relation to the genesis of clinical arrhythmias has not been established. Rhythms due to automaticity may be slow atrial, junctional and ventricular escape rhythms, certain types of atrial tachycardias (such as those produced by digitalis[87]), accelerated junctional (nonparoxysmal junctional tachycardia), and idioventricular rhythms and parasystole (see Chap. 22).

TRIGGERED ACTIVITY

The demonstration of triggered activity requires a more precise consideration of the term "automaticity." Triggered activity is pacemaker activity that results *consequent to* a preceding impulse or series of impulses, without which electrical quiescence occurs (Fig. 20–18). Technically, that is not an automatic self-generating mechanism. *Automaticity* is the property of a fiber to initiate an impulse *spontaneously*, without need for prior stimulation, so that electrical quiescence does not occur. *Triggered activity* is initiated by afterdepolarizations. These depolarizations may occur before or after full repolarization of the fiber (Figs. 20–16 and 20–18) and are best termed *early afterdepolarizations* (EAD's) when they arise from a low level of membrane potential during phases 2 and 3 of the cardiac action potential, and *late* or *delayed afterdepolarizations* (DAD's) when they occur after completion of repolarization (phase 4) generally at a more negative membrane potential (Table 20–6). All afterdepolarizations may not reach threshold potential and may trigger another afterdepolarization and thus self-perpetuate.

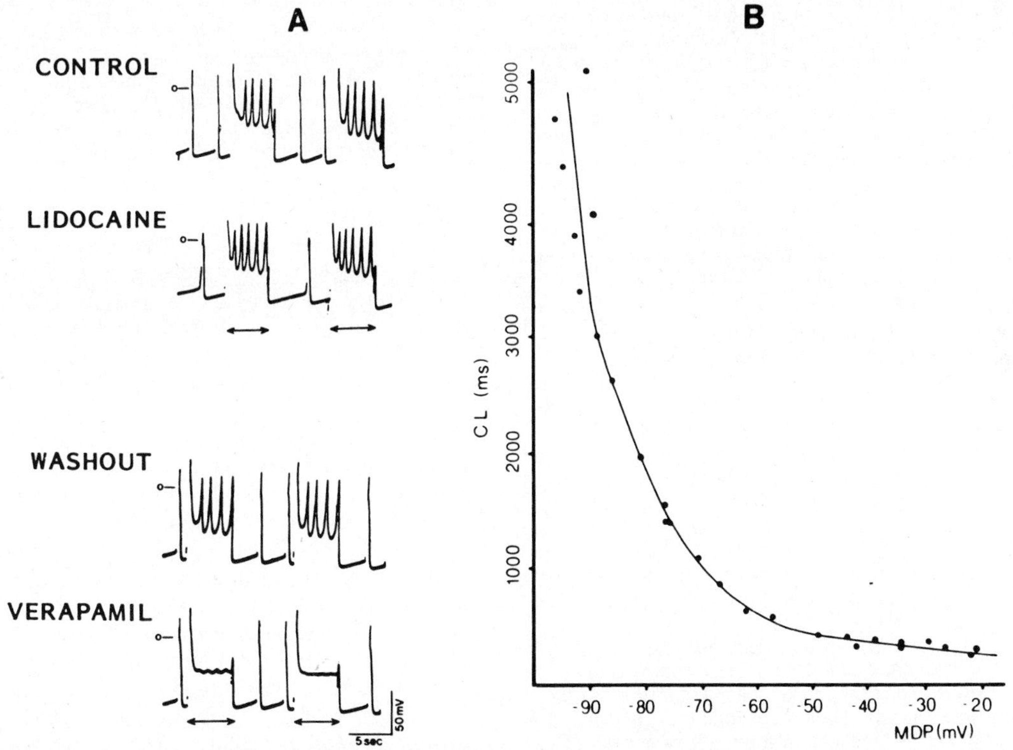

FIGURE 20–17. Automaticity at two levels of membrane potential in canine Purkinje fiber. *A*, Depolarizing current pulses were delivered (across a single sucrose gap) at various times, as indicated by the intervals between arrowheads. Depolarization reduced membrane potential from −85 to −50 mV and initiated more rapid automaticity. While the fiber was at the more negative resting potential it also spontaneously discharged. Lidocaine (3 mg/L) and verapamil (3 × 10^{-6} M) exerted differential effects on automaticity initiated at high and low levels of transmembrane potential. Lidocaine slowed the spontaneous discharge rate and reduced the amplitude of action potentials arising from the high (more negative) levels of membrane potential but did not alter action potentials or spontaneous rate at the low (less negative) level of membrane potential. Verapamil suppressed automaticity at the low (less negative) level of membrane potential without altering the spontaneous discharge rate at the high level of membrane potential. *B*, Relationship between the maximum diastolic membrane potential (abscissa) and the cycle length of spontaneous discharges (ordinate) in a canine Purkinje fiber similar to that shown in panel A. Spontaneous cycle length shortened as the membrane potential was reduced from −90 to −60 mV, with less shortening of the cycle length as the membrane potential was reduced further to −20 mV. (From Elharrar, V., and Zipes, D. P.: Voltage modulation of automaticity in cardiac Purkinje fibers. *In* Zipes, D. P., et al. [eds.]: The Slow Inward Current and Cardiac Arrhythmias. The Hague, Martinus Nijhoff, 1980, p. 357.)

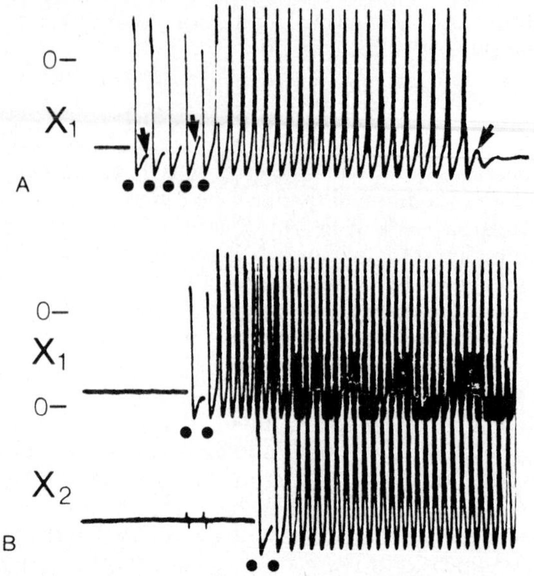

FIGURE 20–18. Triggered sustained rhythmic activity and delayed afterdepolarizations in diseased human ventricle. ***A,*** **Spontaneous activity triggered by a series of driven action potentials (indicated by the dots) at a recording site X1. Note the gradual increase in the size of the delayed afterdepolarizations (arrows) until the afterdepolarization reaches threshold and maintains sustained rhythmic activity after cessation of pacing. The sustained rhythmic activity finally terminates when the last afterdepolarization fails to reach threshold (arrow).** ***B,*** **Initiation of triggered activity by intracellular current injection (indicated by dots beneath the respective action potential recordings) at sites X1 and X2, which lie along the same trabeculum. Although sites X1 and X2 were only about 4 mm apart, triggered sustained rhythmic activity from one site did not propagate to the other site, indicating complete dissociation between these two sites. For current pulses, cycle length = 2000 msec; pulse duration = 10 msec; pulse intensity = 200 na. Vertical calibration: 50 mV. Horizontal calibration: 10 sec. (From Gilmour, R. F., Jr., et al.: Cellular electrophysiological abnormalities of diseased human ventricular myocardium. Am. J. Cardiol. *51*:137, 1983.)**

An increase in background inward current (hypoxia, injury, aconitine) or a decrease in repolarizing outward current (abrupt decrease in $[K]_o$ cooling) may cause EAD's.[80] Also, EAD's may be precipitated by high concentrations of catecholamines and by some antiarrhythmic drugs like sotalol and N-acetylprocainamide and may also be found in myocardium damaged by catecholamines[68] or in myocardium removed from patients who have ventricular arrhythmias.[60, 61] Cesium results in EAD's[88] that have been implicated in the genesis of some ventricular tachyarrhythmias,[89] possibly associated with the long Q-T syndrome and torsades de pointes (p. 698).[90, 91] It is not clear whether all of the oscillations at the reduced membrane potential are EAD's or whether only the first is, and subsequent activity is simply a form of abnormal automaticity at a reduced membrane potential.

DAD's and triggered activity have been demonstrated in Purkinje fibers, specialized atrial fibers and ventricular muscle fibers exposed to digitalis preparations and in normal Purkinje fibers exposed to Na-free superfusates. When fibers in the rabbit, canine, simian, and human mitral valves and in the canine tricuspid valve and coronary sinus are superfused with norepinephrine, they exhibit the capacity for sustained triggered rhythmic activity. In general, the fibers exhibit delayed after-hyperpolarizations (i.e., membrane potential following depolarization transiently becomes more negative than the resting potential), followed by DAD's capable of reaching threshold and triggering sustained rhythmic activity. Triggered activity not requiring norepinephrine for initiation has been recorded in the rabbit atrial pectinate muscle. Triggered activity due to DAD's has also been noted in diseased human atrial and ventricular[60, 61] fibers studied in vitro. In vivo, atrial and ventricular arrhythmias apparently due to triggered activity have been reported in the dog and possibly in humans. However, as indicated earlier, it is very difficult to be certain that a particular mechanism is operative in vivo, given our present state of knowledge. It is tempting to ascribe certain clinical arrhythmias to DAD's, such as some arrhythmias precipitated by digitalis,[92] but this remains speculative.[93]

TABLE 20–6 DETERMINANTS OF THE AMPLITUDE OF AFTERDEPOLARIZATIONS

Intervention	Effect on Amplitude of EAD's	Effect on Amplitude of DAD's
Long cycles (Basic and Premature)	↑	↓
Long action potential duration	↑	↑
Reduced membrane potential	↑	↓
Na channel blockers	No effect	↓
Ca channel blockers	↓	↓
Catecholamines	↑	↑

↑ Increase amplitude
↓ Decrease amplitude
EAD's = Early afterdepolarizations
DAD's = Delayed afterdepolarizations

IONIC BASIS OF DELAYED AFTERDEPOLARIZATIONS. DAD's appear to be caused by a transient inward current (I_{TI}) that is small or absent under normal physiological conditions. When intracellular calcium overload occurs, as during extensive sympathetic stimulation, high $[Ca]_o$, or after large doses of digitalis, oscillatory release of Ca from the sarcoplasmic reticulum activates a nonselective cation channel (or an electrogenic Na-Ca exchange). This results in a transient inward current, carried primarily by Na, that generates the DAD. Drugs that block the diastolic Ca transient, by reducing Ca overload (e.g., Ca channel blockers, beta receptor blockers) or by inhibiting Ca release from the sarcoplasmic reticulum (caffeine, ryanodine), inhibit the DAD. Drugs that reduce the Na current also reduce $[Na]_i$ (tetrodotoxin, lidocaine, phenytoin), relieve the Ca overload, and also can abolish DAD's.[44, 94]

DAD's due to *digitalis toxicity* (p. 504) behave differently from DAD's due to catecholamines. Catecholamine-induced triggering often slows slightly after initiation, then regularizes but slows still further prior to termination, without a progressive increase in maximum diastolic potential. A subthreshold DAD often follows termination of triggered activity. Spontaneous termination may be due, in part, to an increase in the rate of electrogenic sodium extrusion. Termination of digitalis-induced triggering is often characterized by speeding of the rate, decrease in action potential amplitude, and decrease in membrane potential, possibly due to $[Na]_i$ or $[Ca]_i$ accumulation.[80, 83]

The amplitude of the DAD determines whether it is capable of bringing the membrane to threshold and producing a propagated response (Table 20–6). The cycle length of triggered activity due to DAD's often is in the range of 500 to 1000 msec and is related to the cycle lengths of the initiating stimuli.

Short coupling intervals or pacing at rates more rapid than the triggered activity rate (overdrive pacing) increases the amplitude and shortens the cycle length of the delayed afterdepolarization following cessation of pacing (overdrive acceleration) rather than suppressing and delaying the escape rate of the afterdepolarization, as in normal automatic mechanisms (Fig. 20–12) (Table 20–7). Premature stimulation exerts a simlar effect; the shorter the premature interval, the larger the amplitude and shorter the escape interval of the triggered event. The mechanisms responsible for overdrive acceleration are not clear, but may relate to steepening of the slope of diastolic depolarization and the influence of Na/K electrogenic pumping. The clinical implication might be that tachyarrhythmias due to DAD-triggered activity may not be suppressed easily or, indeed, may be precipitated by rapid rates, either spon-

TABLE 20–7 EFFECTS OF ELECTRICAL STIMULATION ON AUTOMATICITY AND TRIGGERED ACTIVITY

	Normal Automaticity	EAD's	DAD's
Suppressed by overdrive pacing	Yes	Not usually	Not usually
Terminated by premature stimulation	Not usually	Not usually	Usually

EAD's = early afterdepolarizations; DAD's = delayed afterdepolarizations taneous (such as a sinus tachycardia) or pacing induced. Finally, because a single premature stimulus can both initiate and terminate triggered activity, differentiation from reentry (see below) becomes quite difficult.

PARASYSTOLE

Classically, parasystole has been likened to the function of a fixed-rate asynchronously discharging pacemaker: Its timing is not altered by the dominant rhythm, it produces depolarization when the myocardium is excitable, and the intervals between discharges are multiples of a basic interval. Complete *entrance block*, constant or intermittent, insulates and protects the parasystolic focus from surrounding electrical events and accounts for such behavior. Occasionally the focus may exhibit *exit block*, during which it may fail to depolarize excitable myocardium.[95] Data from recent experiments indicate that, in fact, the dominant cardiac rhythm may modulate parasystolic discharge to speed up or slow down its rate.[96, 97] Experimental simulations of parasystole (using a sucrose gap technique, in which a segment of block is created in a fiber by superfusing it with a solution that prevents active impulse propagation across a localized area) demonstrate that the discharge rate of an isolated, "protected" focus can be modulated by electrotonic interactions with the dominant rhythm across an area of depressed excitability. Brief subthreshold depolarizations induced during the first half of the cardiac cycle of a spontaneously discharging pacemaker will delay the subsequent discharge, while similar depolarizations induced in the second half of the cardiac cycle will accelerate it (Figs. 20–19 and 20–20). The ionic basis for these rate changes is not totally established, but it is probable that early depolarizing stimuli reactivate outward potassium currents and retard depolarization while late stimuli contribute depolarizing current that enables the cell to reach threshold more quickly. Early hyperpolarizing subthreshold stimuli accelerate, while late hyperpolarizing stimuli retard discharge. Complex interactions of complete silence, concealed or manifest bigeminy, trigeminy, quadrigeminy, and periods of more complex group beating may occur owing to the entraining effects of the dominant rhythm on the ectopic focus. Similar examples have been noted in human ventricular tissue and interactions may be predicted according to the general rules of biological oscillators (Fig. 20–20).[61] There appear to be clinical examples[98] to support these experimental observations (see p. 708).

DISORDERS OF IMPULSE CONDUCTION

Conduction delay and block can result in bradyarrhythmias or tachyarrhythmias, the former when the propagating impulse blocks and is followed by asystole or a slow escape rhythm, and the latter when the delay and block produce reentrant excitation (see below). Various factors, involving both active and passive membrane properties, determine the conduction velocity of an impulse and whether or not conduction is successful. Among these factors are the

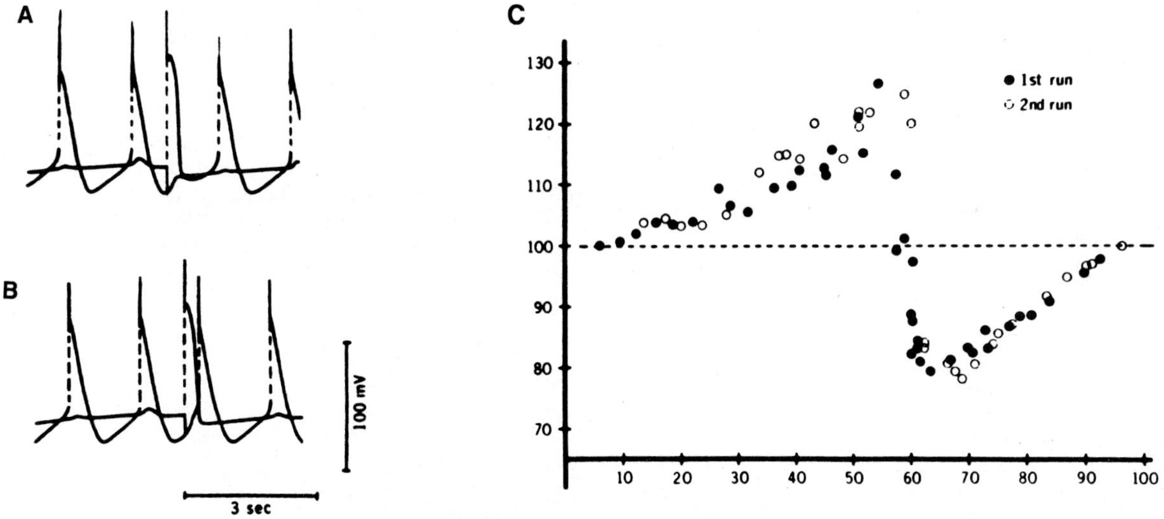

FIGURE 20–19. Phase-dependent acceleration and delay of Purkinje fiber automaticity induced by subthreshold depolarizations. The Purkinje fiber was mounted in a three chamber bath. The left segment was superfused with Tyrode solution containing 2 mM K and 0.1 μg/ml epinephrine to produce automaticity. The middle segment was superfused with isotonic sucrose solution to create an area of inexcitable cells, and the right segment was superfused with normal Tyrode solution. Stimulation of the right segment of the fiber produced action potentials that propagated to the border with the middle segment, at which point active propagation ceased because of the inexcitable gap. However, the middle segment acted as a conduit for passive flow of current from right to left segments. Thus, action potentials in the right segment generated an electrotonic potential that produced subthreshold depolarizations in the left segment. *A*, Action potentials were recorded from the right (upper recording) and left (lower recording) segments of the fiber. The control spontaneous cycle length of the left segment was 1500 msec. Stimulation of the right segment of the fiber 800 msec after the left segment had discharged spontaneously produced a subthreshold depolarization in the left segment and prolonged the cycle length of the next spontaneous discharge to 1850 msec (a 23 per cent increase). *B*, Stimulation of the right segment 1000 msec after the left had discharged spontaneously shortened the spontaneous cycle length to 1230 msec (an 18 per cent decrease). *C*, Complete phase response curves for the experiment shown in *A* and *B*. Two different runs are shown. Ordinate: percentage increase or decrease in the spontaneous cycle length of the left segment (control cycle length = 100 per cent). Abscissa: percentage of the control left segment spontaneous cycle length at which the cycle length was stimulated. The spontaneous cycle length was maximally prolonged (by 26 per cent) or shortened (by 20 per cent) by subthreshold depolarizations that entered the left segment after approximately 50 and 60 per cent of cycle had elapsed, respectively. (From Jalife, J., and Moe, G. K.: Effect of electrotonic potentials on pacemaker activity of canine Purkinje fibers and relation to parasystole. Circ. Res. *39*:801, 1976, by permission of the American Heart Association, Inc.)

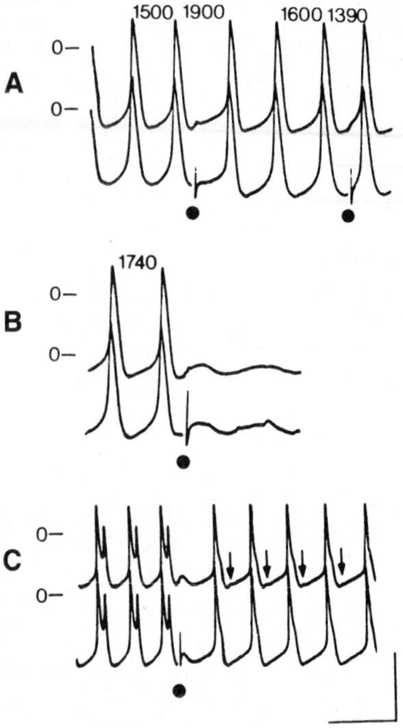

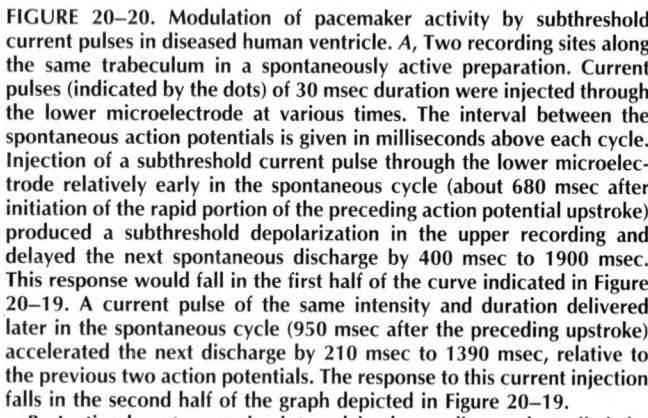

FIGURE 20–20. Modulation of pacemaker activity by subthreshold current pulses in diseased human ventricle. *A,* Two recording sites along the same trabeculum in a spontaneously active preparation. Current pulses (indicated by the dots) of 30 msec duration were injected through the lower microelectrode at various times. The interval between the spontaneous action potentials is given in milliseconds above each cycle. Injection of a subthreshold current pulse through the lower microelectrode relatively early in the spontaneous cycle (about 680 msec after initiation of the rapid portion of the preceding action potential upstroke) produced a subthreshold depolarization in the upper recording and delayed the next spontaneous discharge by 400 msec to 1900 msec. This response would fall in the first half of the curve indicated in Figure 20–19. A current pulse of the same intensity and duration delivered later in the spontaneous cycle (950 msec after the preceding upstroke) accelerated the next discharge by 210 msec to 1390 msec, relative to the previous two action potentials. The response to this current injection falls in the second half of the graph depicted in Figure 20–19.

B, A stimulus at a precise interval in the cardiac cycle (called the singular point [in this example, 930 msec after the preceding action potential upstroke]) abolished pacemaker activity.

C, A single subthreshold pulse (dot) can also alter the contour of the subsequent spontaneous action potentials and convert biphasic action potentials to action potentials with a single active component followed by delayed afterdepolarizations (arrows). Vertical calibration: 50 mV. Horizontal calibration: 2 sec in *A* and *B* and 4 sec in *C*. (From Gilmour, R. F., Jr., et al.: Cellular electrophysiological abnormalities of diseased human ventricular myocardium. Am. J. Cardiol. *51*:137, 1983.)

stimulating efficacy of the propagating impulse, which is related to the amplitude and rate of rise of phase 0, and the excitability of the tissue into which the impulse conducts.

INFLUENCE OF AUTOMATICITY ON CONDUCTION. Diastolic depolarization has been suggested as a cause of conduction block at slow rates.[99] Yet excitability increases as the membrane depolarizes until about −70 mV, despite a reduction in action potential amplitude and $\dot{V}_{max}$. Evidently inactivation of fast sodium channels is offset by other factors such as reduction in the difference between membrane potential and threshold potential. Recently it has been shown that action potential amplitude and excitability are reduced at long diastolic intervals in continuously depolarized Purkinje fibers[100, 101] and atrial muscle,[102] and may explain deceleration-dependent block (Fig. 20–21). Rapid pacing can produce overdrive suppression of conduction, with a mechanism related to the biphasic changes in action potential amplitude and excitability noted above (Fig. 20–22). Action potential amplitude and excitability in the depressed segment are reduced further by rapid pacing,[101, 103] and conduction block follows (Fig. 20–22). These observations may explain a variety of electrocardiographic phenomena, including deceleration-dependent block or aberrancy,[68] explained previously by the effects of diastolic depolarization.[99]

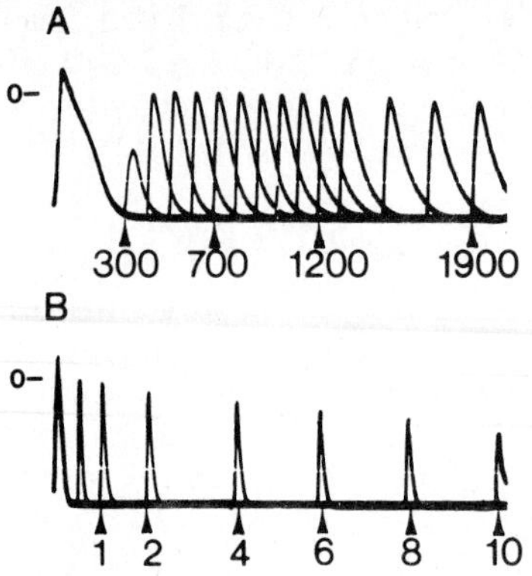

FIGURE 20–21. Biphasic time-dependent changes of action potential amplitude in the middle segment of a Purkinje fiber mounted in a three-chamber bath. The left, middle, and right segments of the fiber were superfused with normal Tyrode solution, Tyrode solution containing 16 mM KCl at a pH 6.7 and a P_{O_2} less than 40 mmHg, and Tyrode solution containing 6 mM KCl, respectively. *A,* Following the last stimulus of a train of 20 stimuli delivered to the left segment of the fiber (basic cycle length, 500 msec), single stimuli were delivered to the right segment at coupling intervals that varied from 300 to 1900 msec. The middle segment action potential elicited by the last stimulus of the train is shown to the left, and the action potentials elicited by stimulation of the right segment at various coupling intervals are superimposed to the right. Action potential amplitude was low at short coupling intervals (300 msec) and increased to a maximum at intermediate coupling intervals (700 msec). At coupling intervals exceeding 1200 msec, action potential amplitude began to decline. *B,* Same format as *A,* except that the time scale has been expanded to show the decline of action potential amplitude as coupling intervals were prolonged from 1 to 10 seconds. Vertical calibration, 50 mV, horizontal calibration, 400 msec for panel A and 2 seconds for panel B. (From Gilmour, R. F., Jr., and Zipes, D. P.: Abnormal automaticity and related phenomena. *In* Fozzard, H. M., et al. (eds.): The Heart and Cardiovascular System. New York, Raven Press, 1986.)

DECREMENTAL CONDUCTION. This term is used commonly in the clinical literature but often is misapplied to describe any Wenckebach-like conduction block, i.e., responses similar to block in the AV node during which progressive conduction delay precedes the nonconducted impulse (p. 704). Correctly used, decremental conduction refers to the situation in which the properties of the fiber change along its length so that the action potential loses its efficacy as a stimulus to excite the fiber ahead of it.[18, 47] Thus the stimulating efficacy of the propagating action potential diminishes progressively, possibly as a result of its decreasing amplitude and $\dot{V}_{max}$. Whether or not decremental conduction, as defined above, accounts for Wenckebach AV block is not yet resolved.

REENTRY

Electrical activity during each normal cardiac cycle begins in the sinus node and continues until the entire heart has been activated. Each cell, interconnected electrically, becomes activated in turn and the cardiac impulse dies out when all fibers have been discharged and are completely refractory. During this absolute refractory period, the cardiac impulse has "no place to go" and must be extinguished. If, however, a group of fibers not activated

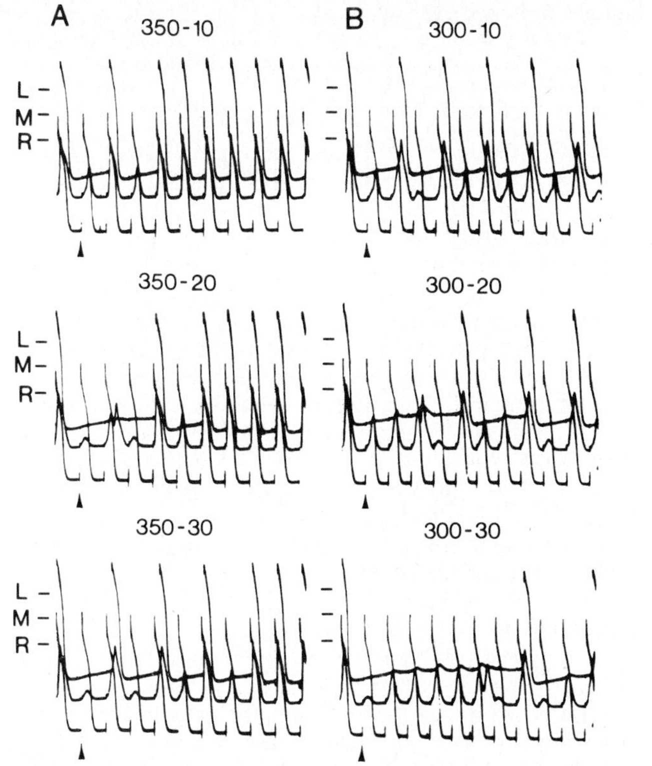

FIGURE 20–22. Overdrive suppression of conduction in a canine Purkinje fiber mounted in a three-chamber bath. The preparation was similar to that described in Figure 20–21. The upper, middle, and lower recordings in each set of recordings were obtained from the left (L), middle (M), and right (R) segments of the fiber, respectively. The horizontal lines to the left of each recording represent zero potential. *A,* Following delivery of a train of 10, 20, or 30 stimuli at a cycle length of 350 msec to the left segment of the fiber (upper, middle, and lower sets of recordings, respectively) the right segment was paced at a cycle length (450 msec) that had produced 1:1 right to left conduction prior to overdrive pacing. Action potentials produced by the last stimulus of the train are shown to the left, and the beginning of right segment pacing is indicated by the arrowheads. As the number of overdrive pacing stimuli was increased from 10 to 30, the time to the first conducted action potential and the time to restoration of 1:1 right to left conduction increased. *B,* Same experiment and stimulation protocol as in *A,* except that the cycle length of overdrive pacing was reduced to 300 msec. Shortening the cycle length of overdrive pacing further increased the time to the first conducted potential and the time for restoration of 1:1 conduction. Vertical calibration, 50 mV. Horizontal calibration, 1 second. (From Gilmour R. F., Jr., and Zipes, D. P.: Abnormal automaticity and related phenomena. *In:* Fozzard, H. M., et al. (eds.): The Heart and Cardiovascular System. New York, Raven Press, 1986.)

because of unidirectional block during the initial wave of depolarization recovers excitability in time to be discharged before the impulse dies out, they may serve as a link to reexcite areas that were just discharged and have now recovered from the initial depolarization. Such a process is given various names, all meaning approximately the same thing: reentry, reentrant excitation, circus movement, reciprocal or echo beat, or reciprocating tachycardia.

Mines[104, 105] noted that, to prove reentry, three features had to be established: (1) an area of unidirectional block, (2) recirculation of the impulse to its point of origin, and (3) elimination of the arrhythmia by cutting the pathway. The development of unidirectional block is due to the presence of tissues, either contiguous, such as adjacent AV nodal cells or Purkinje fibers, or anatomically separated, such as the AV node and an accessory pathway (see p. 687), with disparate electrophysiological properties. Because the two (or more) pathways have different properties—e.g., a refractory period longer in one pathway than the other, decreased excitability in one pathway, ineffectiveness of the wavefront to activate all fibers, or other reasons—the impulse (1) blocks in one pathway (site x in Fig. 20–23A; site A in Fig. 20–23*B*) and (2) propagates slowly in the adjacent pathway (arrow from x to y in Fig. 20–23*A*; serpentine arrow, D to C, Fig. 20–23*B*). If conduction in this alternative route is sufficiently depressed, the slowly propagating impulse excites tissue beyond the blocked pathway (y to 5 in Fig. 20–23*A* and horizontal lined area in Fig. 20–23*B*) and returns in a reversed direction along the pathway initially blocked (y to x in Fig. 20–23*A*; B to A in Fig. 20–23*B*) to (3) reexcite tissue proximal to the site of block (x to 1 in Fig. 20–23*A*: A to D in Fig. 20–23*B*). For reentry of this type to occur, the time for conduction within the depressed but unblocked area and for excitation of the distal segments must exceed the refractory period of the initially blocked pathway (x in Fig. 20–23*A*; A in Fig. 20–23*B*) and the tissue proximal to the site of block (A in Fig. 20–23*A*; D in Fig. 20–23*B*). Stated another way, continuous reentry requires the anatomical length of the circuit traveled to equal or exceed the reentrant wavelength. The latter is equal to mean conduction velocity of the impulse multiplied by the longest refractory period of the elements in the circuit. Conditions that depress conduction velocity or abbreviate the refractory period will promote the development of reentry in this model, while prolonging refractoriness and speeding

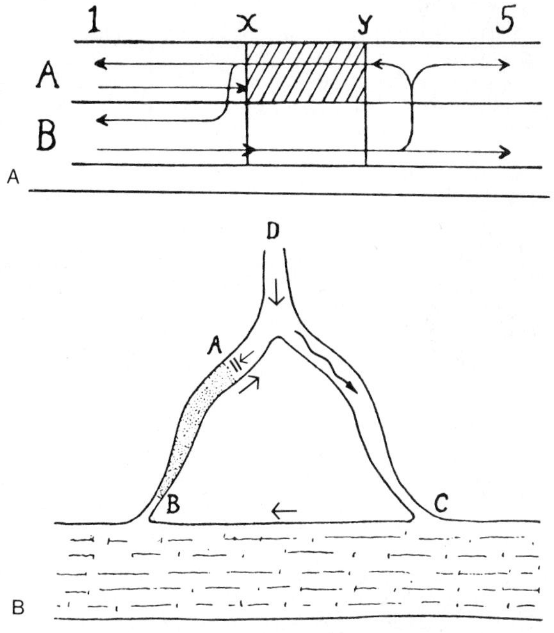

FIGURE 20–23. Diagrams of reentry published by Schmitt and Erlanger in 1928.

A, Reentry is depicted as occurring in contiguous pathways, based on observations that these pathways can undergo functional longitudinal dissociation. Initial propagation begins at site 1 but is able to reach site 5 only in pathway B (lower arrow). Pathway A exhibits unidirectional block (from left to right) at site x in the cross-hatched area. The impulse can then reenter pathway A from pathway B and travel from y to x, reexciting tissue proximal to the site of block. Such concepts of reentry can be applied to any site in the heart.

B, A Purkinje fiber (D) divides into two pathways (B and C), both of which join ventricular muscle (stippled area). It is assumed that the original impulse travels down D, blocks in its anterograde direction at site A (arrow followed by double bar), but continues slowly down C (serpentine arrow) to excite ventricular muscle. The impulse then reenters the Purkinje twig at B and retrogradely excites A and D. If the impulse continues to propagate through D to the ventricular myocardium and elicits ventricular depolarization, a reentrant ventricular extrasystole results. Continued reentry of this type would produce ventricular tachycardia.

conduction velocity will hinder its development. For example, if conduction velocity (0.30 M/sec) and refractoriness (350 M/sec) for ventricular muscle were normal, a pathway of 105 mm (0.30 M/sec × 0.35 sec) would be necessary for reentry to occur. However, under certain conditions, conduction velocity in ventricular muscle and Purkinje fibers can be very slow (0.03 M/sec), and if refractoriness is not greatly prolonged (600 msec), a pathway of only 18 mm (0.03 M/sec × 0.60 sec) may be necessary.

THE LEADING CIRCLE HYPOTHESIS. Reentry over pathways with anatomical boundaries (above) differs from reentry with functional boundaries, explained by the *leading circle hypothesis*.[106] The former frequently exhibits an excitable gap, i.e., a time interval between the end of refractoriness from one cycle and beginning of depolarization in the next, when tissue in the circuit is excitable. According to the leading circle hypothesis, the reentrant circuit propagates around a functionally refractory core and follows a course along fibers that have a shorter refractory period, blocking in one direction in fibers with a longer refractory period. The pathway is determined by the smallest circuit in which the leading wavefront is just able to excite tissue ahead that is still relatively refractory. Shorter wavelengths may predispose to fibrillation.[107] No excitable gap exists, and the duration of the refractory period of the tissue in the circuit primarily determines the cycle length of the tachycardia. In reentry with an excitable gap and anatomical circuits, changes in conduction velocity, rather than changes in refractoriness (as long as the duration of refractoriness does not exceed the duration of the excitable gap), primarily determine cycle length of the tachycardia.

Theoretically, drugs that prolong refractoriness and do not delay conduction would slow tachycardia due to the leading circle mechanism and not affect tachycardia with an excitable gap until the prolongation of refractoriness exceeded the duration of the excitable gap. Drugs that primarily slow conduction would have major effects on tachycardia with an excitable gap and not on tachycardias due to the leading circle concept. Mixed circuits with both anatomical and functional pathways obfuscate these differences, and circuits due to the leading circle phenomenon also may have an excitable gap.

REFLECTION.[51, 108, 109] This can be considered a special subclass of reentry. As in reentry, an area of conduction delay is required, and the total time for the impulse to leave and return to its site of origin must exceed the refractory period of the proximal segment. Reflection differs from reentry in that the impulse does not require a circuit, as diagrammed in Figure 20–23*A* and *B*, but appears to travel along the *same* pathway in both directions. The impulse travels in one direction and meets an area of impaired conduction where active transmission pauses (Fig. 20–24 segment 4). Electrotonically, the impulse spans the zone of impairment, activates the distal segment, and returns electrotonically across the zone of impaired conduction to reexcite the proximal segment. A single reflection could cause a coupled premature complex, while continued reflection back and forth across an inexcitable zone could cause a tachycardia. Data[108] suggest that reflection and parasystole (or reentry) are part of a continuous spectrum, without a critical boundary to separate them.

Reentry is probably the cause of many tachyarrhythmias, including various kinds of supraventricular and ventricular tachycardias, flutter, and fibrillation. It is important to remember, however, that, circa 1900, investigators were able to demonstrate reentry by using simple preparations. In more complex preparations, such as large pieces of tissue in vitro or the intact heart, it becomes much more difficult to prove that reentry exists. It is very hard

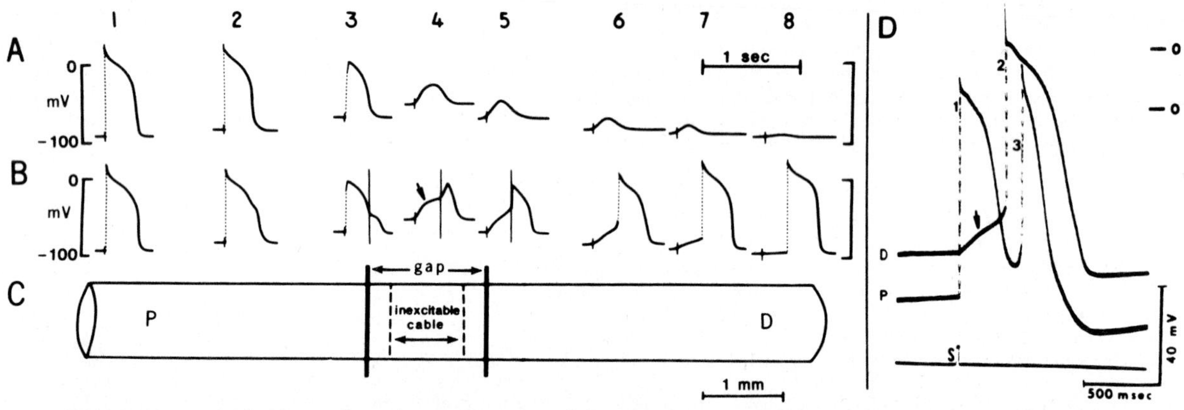

FIGURE 20–24. Reflection. Schematic representation of electrotonic transmission across an area of inexcitability in a Purkinje fiber. The central compartment (gap) of the tissue bath contains a solution that prevents active conduction in the central segment (inexcitable cable) of the Purkinje fiber. Action potentials from various locations along the Purkinje fiber are presented in panel A when transmission across the inexcitable area is unsuccessful and in panel B when transmission is successful. In panel A, the regenerative impulse encountering the region of block decays along the length of the blocked segment. In panel B, the slowly rising electrotonic potential (arrow) resulting from the activity in the proximal tissue brings the distal segment to threshold and thus restores, after a delay, active propagation via electrotonic transmission. The amplitude of the electrotonic potential emerging from the distal end of the inexcitable cable must be sufficiently large to bring that membrane to the threshold if transmission is to succeed.

When the delay in transmission across the gap is sufficiently long, electrotonic transmission in the reverse direction over the same blocked segment can reexcite the proximal segment and generate a repetitive response, which, under these experimental conditions, is termed *reflection*. This is illustrated in panel D. The two traces were recorded from the two active segments on the proximal (P) and distal (D) sides of the inexcitable gap. The bottom trace is the stimulus marker (S). Stimulation of the proximal segment (1) was transmitted to the distal segment (2) following a slowly developing electrotonic depolarization (arrow) that reached the threshold of the tissue beyond the inexcitable gap after the delay of 300 msec. Electrotonic transmission in the reverse direction induced a closely coupled (404 msec), reflected response (3) in the proximal segment after expiration of its refractory period. Thus, to-and-fro electrotonic transmission across an inexcitable segment of tissue occurs over the *same pathway* and must be differentiated conceptually from a micro-reentrant circuit that uses *different pathways* in each direction. (From Antzelevitch, C., and Moe, G. K.: Electrotonically mediated delayed conduction and reentry in relation to "slow responses" in mammalian ventricular conducting tissue. Circ. Res. *49*:1129, 1981, by permission of the American Heart Association, Inc.)

technically to record from sufficient sites to meet Mines' criteria. Initiation or termination of tachycardia by pacing stimuli, the demonstration of electrical activity bridging diastole, fixed coupling, and a variety of other clinically used techniques, while consistent with reentry, do not constitute proof of its existence.

ATRIAL FLUTTER. Reentry is the most likely cause of atrial flutter,[110–112] with the wavefront traveling a pathway established by atrial anatomy, distribution of refractoriness,[113] and conduction delay.[114, 115] Entrainment of atrial flutter, i.e., an increase to the pacing rate of all tissue responsible for sustaining the tachycardia, with resumption of the intrinsic rate of the tachycardia upon either abrupt cessation of pacing or slowing of the pacing rate below the intrinsic rate of the tachycardia, strongly supports a reentrant mechanism with an excitable gap.[116, 117] Constant fusion beats (except for the last captured beat after cessation of pacing, which is entrained but is not a fusion beat), different degrees of fusion at different paced rates, and interruption of tachycardia during rapid pacing with localized conduction block are other features of entrainment and are influenced by the pacing site.[117].

ATRIAL AND VENTRICULAR FIBRILLATION. A critical mass of myocardium, either atrial or ventricular, is required to maintain fibrillation.[118] For example, ventricular myocardium cut into small pieces ceases fibrillating when the pieces reach a critically small size.

Ventricles of small animals stop fibrillating spontaneously, while that rarely if ever occurs in the canine or human heart. In the canine ventricle, the left ventricular free wall and septum appear to be required as a critical mass to maintain fibrillation, since, if they are depolarized, the right ventricle stops fibrillating spontaneously. Fibrillation in the atrial appendage stops when it is clamped off from the rest of the atria in which fibrillation is induced by rapid atrial pacing and vagal stimulation. Atrial fibrillation is much less stable than ventricular fibrillation. All these observations support Moe's hypothesis that multiple wavelets of reentry, influenced by the mass of the tissue, refractory periods, and conduction velocity, maintain fibrillation. These factors influence the number of wavelets present, which determines the likelihood of the fibrillation to continue. Recently, elegant atrial mapping studies have demonstrated that intraatrial reentry of the leading circle type (p. 602) forms the basis of the reentry in atrial fibrillation. The reentry is random, with a single wavelet seldom lasting longer than a few hundred milliseconds.[119] These findings do not exclude the possibility that concomitantly discharging automatic foci contribute to the maintenance of fibrillation in some patients.[120]

SINUS REENTRY. Reentry in parts of the atrium has been reported to occur in several experimental models as well as in humans. The sinus node shares with the AV node electrophysiological features such as the potential for *dissociation of conduction*, i.e., an impulse can conduct in some nodal fibers but not in others. For example, premature stimulation can produce slow propagation in the sinus node, block in some areas, and the development of repetitive responses most likely due to reentry. The reentrant circuit may be located entirely within the sinus node; the atrium is not an essential link.[121] Supraventricular tachycardias interpreted to be due to sustained reentry in the sinus node do occur and can cause symptoms.[122, 123]

ATRIAL REENTRY. Reentry within the atrium, unrelated to the sinus node, has been shown experimentally to occur in the rabbit,[106, 124] and dog atrium,[125] with or without an anatomical obstacle, and may be a cause of supraventricular tachycardia in man. Examples of supraventricular tachycardia purported to be due to atrial reentry appear to be less frequently reported than other types of supraventricular tachycardia[126] which suggests that this is not a commonly recognized cause of supraventricular tachycardia in man.[123] Distinguishing atrial tachycardia due to automaticity from atrial tachycardia sustained by reentry over very small areas, i.e., microreentry of the leading circle type,[106, 124] is very difficult, and therefore conclusions regarding clinical electrophysiological mechanisms of this supraventricular tachycardia based on currently available information must be accepted cautiously.

AV NODAL REENTRY (AVNR). It has been known for 80 years that stimulation of the ventricle could propagate to the atrium and then back to the ventricles to produce a ventricular echo, sometimes being sustained to cause a reciprocating rhythm. Longitudinal dissociation into two or more pathways within the AV node, where reentry most likely occurs, remains a plausible mechanism. Microelectrode studies on isolated rabbit AV nodal preparations reveal that cells in the upper portion of the AV node can be dissociated during propagation of premature stimuli, so that one group of cells, called alpha, can discharge in response to a premature stimulus at a time when another group of cells, called beta, fails to discharge.[127] The impulse can then propagate to the mid and lower portions of the AV node and turn around (without needing to activate the His bundle) to reexcite the beta group of cells and produce an atrial echo (Fig. 20–25).

Episodes of sustained AV nodal tachycardia can be initiated in isolated rabbit preparations. These studies provide very convincing animal experimental evidence supporting the presence of AV nodal reentry.

The observations in dogs and humans (Fig. 20–26), that an impulse traveling from ventricle to atrium, if timed properly, need not prevent another impulse traveling simultaneously from atrium to ventricle from reaching the His bundle, provides one of the most definitive pieces of evidence to support the presence of dual AV nodal pathways. For this event to occur, the impulses traveling in opposite directions must be conducting in different AV nodal pathways. A second convincing fact is the finding of two ventricular responses to a single atrial depolarization due to simultaneous transmission over both the slow and fast AV nodal pathways.

Because it is not possible at present using extracellular catheter electrodes to record directly from the AV node in situ, it has not been possible to demonstrate in man that reentry unquestionably is the mechanism of AVNR and that it is confined to the AV node. Indirect evidence mentioned above plus the observations that the onset of AVNR depends on a critical increase in the A-H interval and that retrograde atrial activation is normal, is consistent with dual AV nodal pathways that have different electrophysiological properties.

The premature atrial response can block anterogradely in one AV nodal pathway that conducts more rapidly (fast pathway, or beta pathway in Figure 20–25), but has a longer refractory period than a second pathway (slow pathway, or alpha pathway in Figure 20–25). The premature atrial response travels to the ventricle over the slow (alpha) pathway and back to the atrium over the fast (beta) pathway. Less commonly, the slow pathway has a long refractory period and the premature atrial response can block anterogradely in the slow pathway and travel in the fast pathway, using the slow pathway retrogradely; this is called the uncommon form of AVNR. Conceivably, some patients may have three or more pathways.[128]

In patients who have dual AV nodal physiology, both pathways exhibit electrophysiological responses in the anterograde direction characteristic of AV nodal fibers. However, the electrophysiological features of the pathway conducting retrogradely during the tachycardia differ greatly from those of either anterogradely conducting pathways, in response not only to atrial or ventricular pacing but also to various drugs. For example, drugs such as procainamide prolong conduction time in the retrogradely conducting, but not in either anterogradely conducting, pathway.[129] Also, pacing at short cycle lengths prolongs anterograde, but not retrograde, AV nodal conduction time. Yet, verapamil prolongs retrograde AV nodal conduction time, consistent with an effect on nodal fibers.[130]

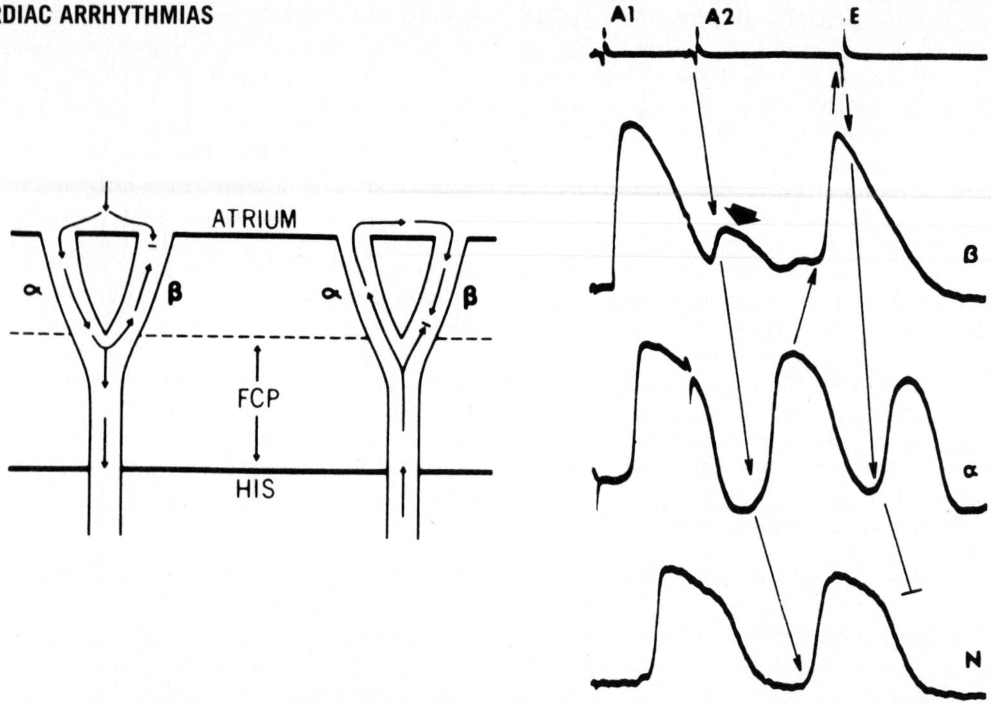

FIGURE 20–25. Atrial echoes. *Left,* Schematic representation of intranodal dissociation responsible for an atrial echo. A premature atrial response fails to penetrate the beta pathway, which exhibits unidirectional block, but propagates anterogradely through the alpha pathway. Once the final common pathway (FCP) is engaged, the impulse may return to the atrium via the now recovered beta pathway to produce an atrial echo. The neighboring diagram illustrates the pattern of propagation during generation of a ventricular echo. A premature response in the His bundle traverses the final common pathway, encounters a refractory beta pathway (unidirectional block), reaches the atrium over the alpha pathway, and returns through a now recovered beta pathway to produce a ventricular echo. Such events can explain the findings in Figure 20–22.

Right, Actual recordings from the atrium (top tracing), cells impaled in the beta region (second tracing), alpha region (third tracing), and N portion of the AV node (bottom tracing) in an isolated rabbit preparation. The basic response to A_1 activated both alpha and beta pathways and the N cell (first tier of action potentials). The premature atrial response, A_2, caused only a local response in the beta cell (heavy arrow), was delayed in transmission to the alpha cell, and was further delayed in propagation to the N cell. Following the alpha response, a retrograde spontaneous response occurred in the beta cell and propagated to the atrium (E). This atrial response represents an atrial echo. The echo returned to stimulate the alpha cell but was not propagated to the N cell. (From Mendez, C., and Moe, G. K.: Demonstrations of a dual AV nodal conduction system in the isolated rabbit heart. Circ. Res. *19*:378, 1966, by permission of the American Heart Association, Inc.)

Thus, it is not clear whether the retrogradely conducting pathway is extranodal, composed of non-nodal tissue, is intranodal but insulated from the rest of the AV node, or includes only a small amount of AV nodal tissue, and whether the retrogradely conducting pathway is distinct from the fast and slow anterogradely conducting pathways. The geometry and direction of conduction,[131] effects of summation,[132] autonomic tone,[133] as well as the electrophysiological characteristics of the fibers, all may influence conduction and the response to drugs. It is likely that the anatomical as well as the electrophysiological features of AV nodal pathways may not be the same in all patients who have AV nodal reentrant supraventricular tachycardia.[134]

While it is clear that activation of the ventricle is not necessary for AVNR (Fig. 20–27) and activation of the His bundle is also probably not required in some patients, the necessary role of atrial participation in the reentrant circuit is still debated. Mendez et al.[127] demonstrated the need for the atrium in generating ventricular echoes caused by AV nodal reentrant activity in dogs, and such a circuit is implicit in their diagram in Figure 20–25. Studies in animals[135] and patients[136] have challenged the interpretations of Mendez et al. and have suggested that ventricular echoes due to AV nodal reentry can occur *without* activation of the atrium. Figure 20–28 is an example of apparent dissociation of the atrium with uninterrupted continuation of the supraventricular tachycardia, leading to the conclusion that the atrium may *not* be a necessary part of the reentrant circuit in humans. However, since rhythms in the atria may become dissimilar—that is, electrical activity in one part of the atrium may differ from that in another—a portion of the atrium may control, or participate in, the cardiac rhythm without recognition of this fact from observation of a scalar ECG or, indeed, from recordings within the right atrium or coronary sinus.[137] Therefore, data refuting the role of the atrium as a necessary link in the reentrant pathway must be obtained from studies in which both atria are carefully mapped for the presence of localized atrial activity, particularly near the upper AV node. Elimination of AVNR with an atriotomy in 1 patient[138] and by disconnecting the perinodal atrium in 10 patients[139] supports the conclusion that the atrium is a necessary participant in the AVNR circuit.

PREEXCITATION SYNDROME (See also p. 685). The accumulated anatomical and electrophysiological data support a reentrant mechanism to explain tachycardias related to an accessory pathway more than they support that mechanism for any other kind of tachycardia.[140–144] In fact, the bundle described by Kent[145, 146] was used to explain a reentrant mechanism for paroxysmal tachycardia even before the preexcitation syndrome was ever described in man.

In most patients who have reciprocating tachycardia

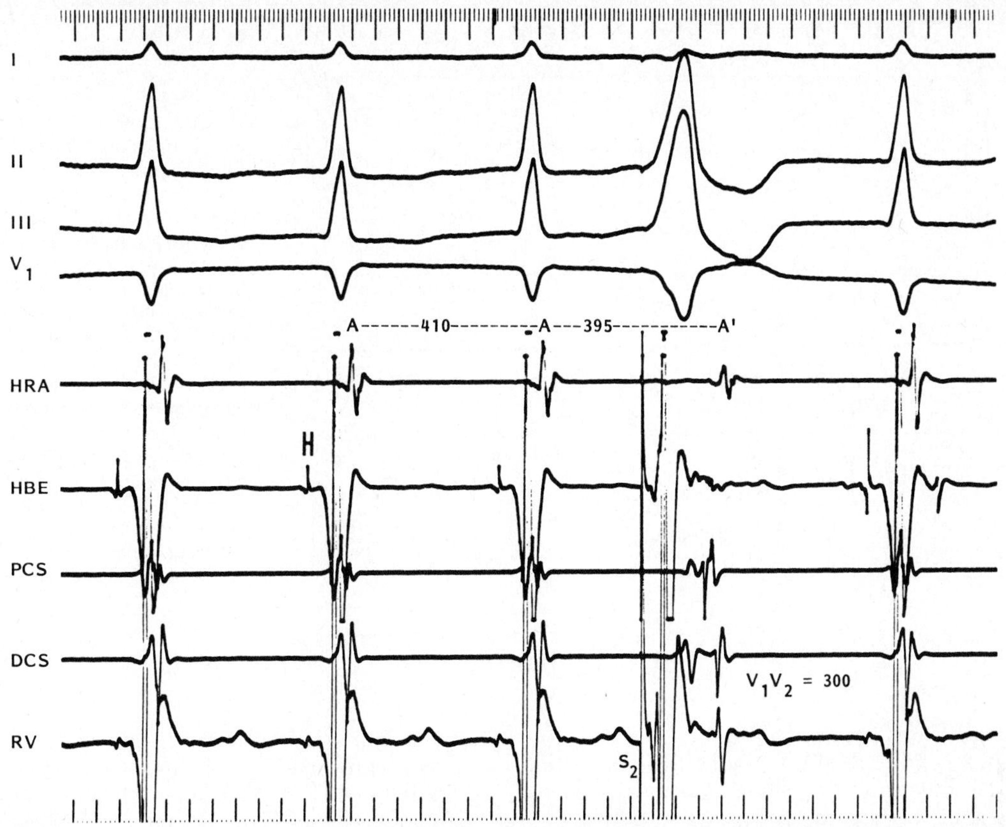

FIGURE 20–26. Atrial preexcitation during AV nodal reentry. AV nodal reentrant tachycardia is present with a cycle length of 410 msec. A premature ventricular complex (S2) from the right ventricular outflow tract with a coupling interval of 300 msec is introduced during the tachycardia before His is activated and penetrates the AV node retrogradely to shorten the AA interval to 395 msec. Shorter V1V2 intervals decreased the AA interval to 355 msec. Dual AV nodal pathways best explain how two impulses can travel in opposite directions in the AV node, i.e., the impulse from the tachycardia traveling anterogradely and the impulse from premature ventricular stimulation traveling retrogradely and not collide. Surface leads I, II, III, and V1 are displayed along with high right atrial (HRA), His bundle (HBE), proximal coronary sinus (PCS), distal coronary sinus (DCS), and right ventricular (RV) electrograms. Numbers indicated in msec. Premature ventricular stimulus indicated by S2. His bundle activation indicated by H and atrial activation indicated by A. Large time 50 msec, small time 10 msec. (From Miles, W. M., Yee, R., Klein, G., Zipes, D. P., and Prystowsky, E. N.: The preexcitation index: An aid in determining the mechanism of supraventricular tachycardia and localizing accessory pathways. Circulation *74*:493, 1986, by permission of the American Heart Association, Inc.)

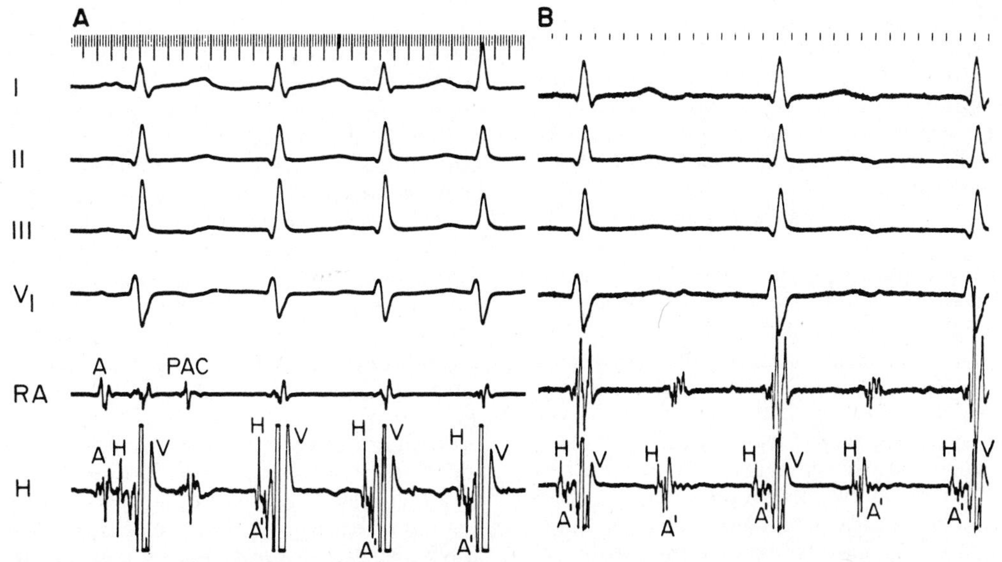

FIGURE 20–27. 2:1 His Purkinje block during AV nodal reentry. In panel A, a spontaneous premature atrial complex (PAC) is followed by PR (AH) prolongation and the initiation of AV nodal reentry. Retrograde atrial activation (A′) occurs simultaneously with the onset of the QRS complex. In panel B, 2:1 block distal to the His bundle recording site is present, with continuation of the AV nodal reentry, indicating that activation of the ventricle is not required for perpetuation of the tachycardia. Such an event could not occur during reciprocating tachycardia utilizing an accessory atrioventricular connection in the Wolff-Parkinson-White syndrome. Conventions as in Figure 20–26. (Patient studied by E. N. Prystowsky, M.D., and W. M. Miles, M.D.)

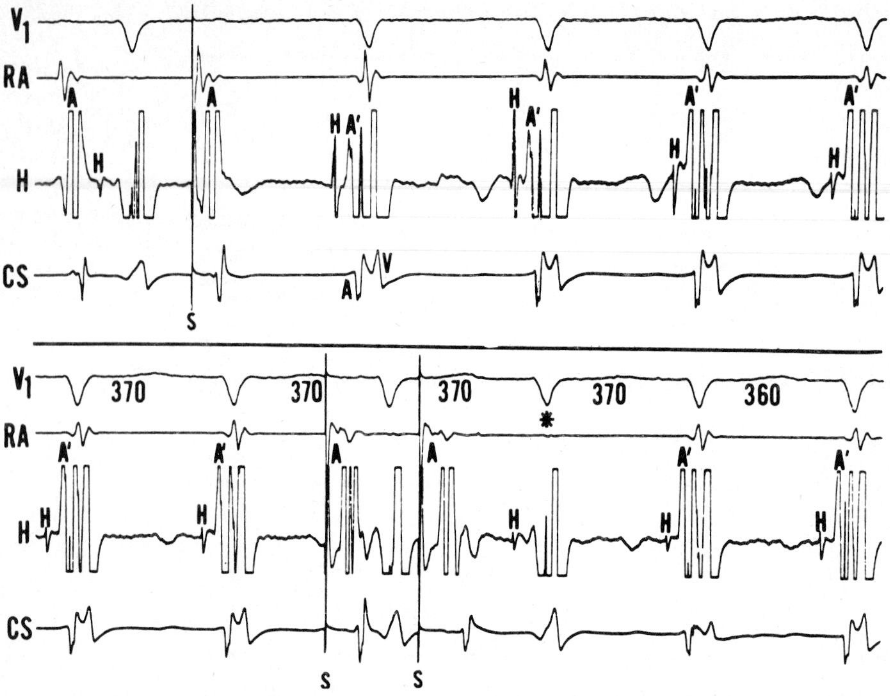

FIGURE 20–28. Dissociation of atria from ventricles without interrupting AV nodal reentrant supraventricular tachycardia. During sinus rhythm, a single premature atrial complex (S, *top panel*) was conducted with AV nodal delay (prolonged A-H interval) and initiated an AV nodal reentrant supraventricular tachycardia. Note that retrograde atrial activation (A′) occurred prior to onset of the QRS complex. Two premature atrial stimuli (S-S, *bottom panel*) captured the atria on both occasions without altering the regular cycle length of the AV nodal reentrant supraventricular tachycardia. Note that the QRS complex marked by an asterisk has no accompanying atrial complex, suggesting that atrial participation in the reentrant circuit was not required. V_1 = scalar lead; RA = right atrial electrogram; H = His bundle electrogram; CS = coronary sinus electrogram.

associated with the Wolff-Parkinson-White syndrome, the accessory pathway conducts more rapidly than does the normal AV node but takes a longer time to recover excitability, i.e., the anterograde refractory period of the accessory pathway exceeds that of the AV node.[141] Consequently, a premature atrial complex that occurs sufficiently early blocks anterogradely in the accessory pathway and continues to the ventricle over the normal AV node and His bundle. After the ventricles have been excited, the impulse is able to enter the accessory pathway retrogradely and return to the atrium. A continuous conduction loop of this kind establishes the circuit for the tachycardia. Although exceptions occur, the usual activation wave during such a reciprocating tachycardia in a patient with an accessory pathway occurs in this fashion: anterogradely over the normal AV node–His-Purkinje system and retrogradely over the accessory pathway, resulting in a normal QRS complex (Fig. 20–29). Because the circuit requires both atria and ventricles, the term *supraventricular tachycardia* is not precisely correct and the tachycardia is more accurately called atrioventricular reciprocating tachycardia (AVRT). In some patients, the accessory pathway may be capable only of retrograde conduction, but the circuit and mechanism of tachycardia remain the same. Less commonly, the accessory pathway may conduct only anterogradely.[142, 147]

In addition to the response of the reciprocating tachycardia to premature stimulation, one of the strongest lines of evidence supporting a reentrant mechanism is that interruption of the reentrant loop at widely separated points (i.e., by surgically cutting the normal AV node–His bundle pathway *or* the accessory pathway) eliminates the ability to develop supraventricular tachycardia.

Other pathways, such as those having an unusual accessory pathway with AV nodal–like electrophysiological properties,[148] nodofascicular or nodoventricular fibers,[149, 150] may constitute the circuit for reciprocating tachycardias in patients who have some form of the Wolff-Parkinson-White syndrome.[150] Tachycardia in patients with nodoventricular fibers may be due to reentry using these fibers as the anterograde pathway and the His-Purkinje fibers and a portion of the AV node retrogradely. No direct relationship may exist between fasciculoventricular fibers and tachycardia, so-called *antidromic tachycardia*. Conduction proceeds anterogradely over the accessory pathway and retrogradely over the AV node–His bundle. Two accessory pathways may form the circuit.[151, 152] In the Lown-Ganong-Levine syndrome (short P-R interval and normal QRS complex),[153, 154] conduction over a James fiber that connects atrium to the distal portion of the AV node and His bundle has been proposed, although the presence of this entity as a distinct syndrome is unsettled[16] (p. 687).

VENTRICULAR REENTRY (see also p. 694). Reentry in the ventricle as a cause of sustained ventricular arrhythmias was suggested by the work of Mines[104, 105] and, later, Schmitt and Erlanger.[155] Their diagram (Fig. 20–23*A* and *B*) has been reproduced many times. While bundle branch reentry has been demonstrated to occur in dogs (Fig. 20–30) and man, it does not appear to be a common cause of sustained ventricular tachycardia. More likely reentry in ventricular muscle,[156–158] with or without contribution from specialized tissue,[159] is responsible for many or most ventricular tachycardias, particularly in patients with ischemic heart disease. Although reentry in ventricular muscle is difficult to move by Mines' criteria because the large muscle mass makes complete mapping of the reentrant loop and interruption of the pathway difficult, studies by several investigators, utilizing a dog model subjected to coronary occlusion, have provided compelling evidence to support reentry.

Complete coronary occlusion in the dog results in a surviving epicardial layer of tissue—almost two-dimensional—in which electrical activity can be mapped accurately during normal sinus rhythm and during ventricular tachycardia induced by premature ventricular stimulation. Both figure-of-eight (Fig. 20–31)[156, 160] and single circle[157] reentrant loops have been described, circulating around an area of functional block in a manner consistent with the leading circle hypothesis.[106] Cooling epicardial regions involved in the reentrant circuit can terminate the ventricular tachycardia, providing further evidence to support a reentrant circuit.[161, 162] The location of the infarction and structure of surviving myocardium importantly influence the development of reentry as well as the location of the circuit.[163, 164] When intramural myocardium survives, it may form part of the reentrant loop.[165] Structural discon-

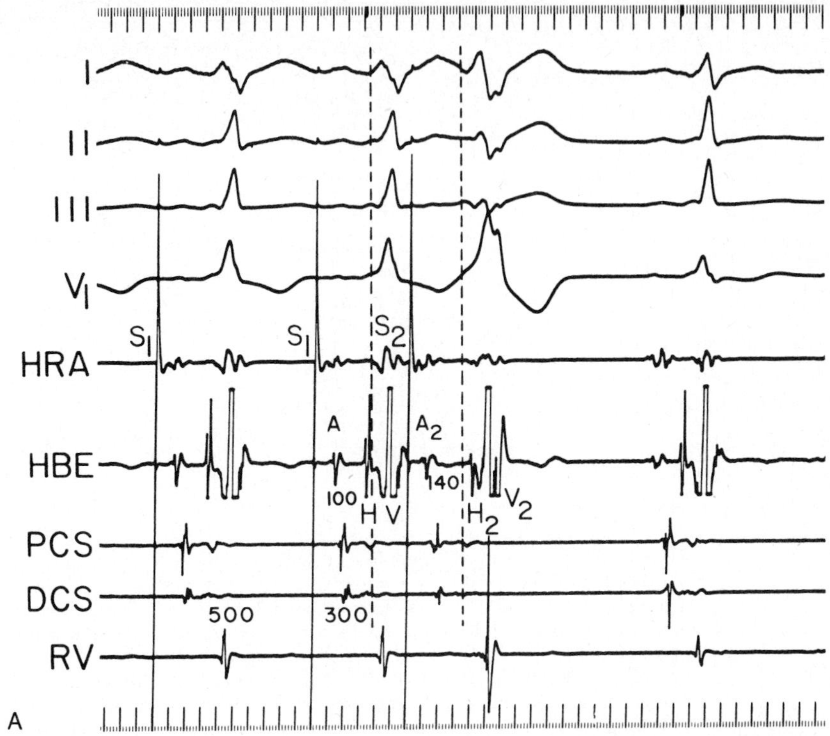

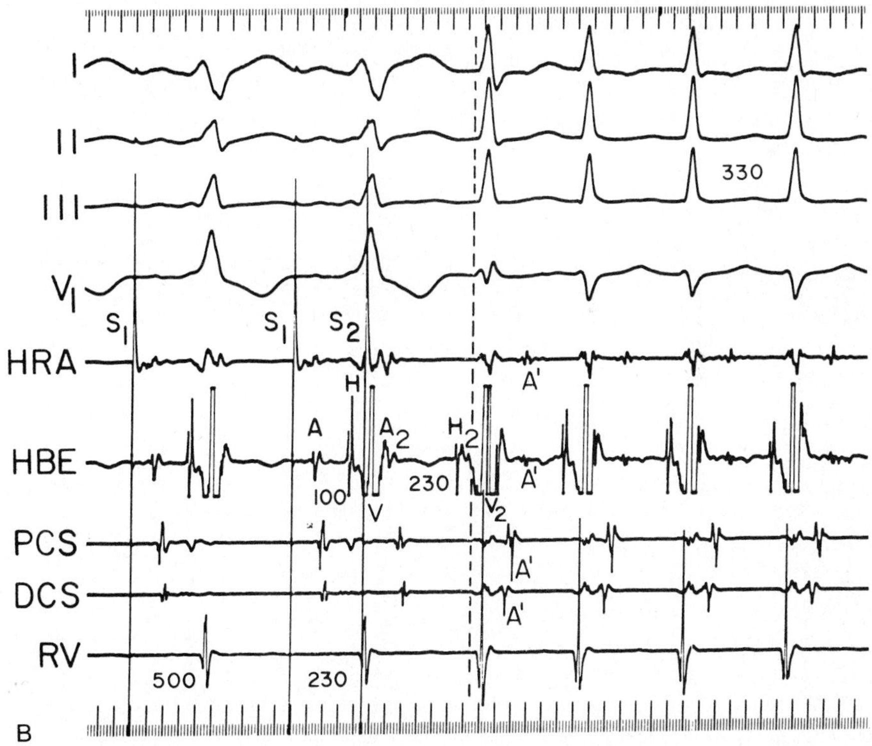

FIGURE 20–29. *A,* Wolff-Parkinson-White syndrome. Following high right atrial pacing at a cycle length of 500 msec (S1–S1), premature stimulation at a coupling interval of 300 msec (S1–S2) produces physiological delay in AV nodal conduction resulting in an increase in the AH interval from 100 to 140 msec but no delay in the AV interval. Consequently, activation of the His bundle occurs following activation of the QRS complex (second interrupted line) and the QRS complex becomes more anomalous in appearance due to increased ventricular activation over the accessory pathway. I, II, III, and V1 are scalar leads. HRA, high right atrium; HBE, His bundle electrogram; PCS, proximal coronary sinus electrogram; DCS, distal coronary sinus electrogram; RV, right ventricular electrogram. Time lines 50 and 10 msec intervals. S1, stimulus of the drive train; S2, premature stimulus. A, H, V, atrial His bundle, and ventricular activation during the drive train. A2, H2, V2, atrial His bundle, and ventricular activation during the premature stimulus.

B, Induction of reciprocating atrioventricular tachycardia. Premature stimulation at a coupling interval of 230 msec prolongs the AH interval to 230 msec and results in anterograde block in the accessory pathway and normalization of the QRS complex (slight functional aberrancy in the nature of incomplete right bundle branch block occurs). Note that H2 precedes the onset of the QRS complex (interrupted line). Following V2, the atria are excited retrogradely (A′) beginning in the distal coronary sinus, then followed by atrial activation in leads recording from the proximal coronary sinus, His bundle, and high right atrium. A supraventricular tachycardia is initiated at a cycle length of 330 msec. Conventions as in panel A. (From Zipes, D. P., Mahomed, Y., King, R. D., Heger, J. J., Miles, W. M., Brown, J., Adams, D. E., and Prystowsky, E. N.: Wolff-Parkinson-White syndrome: Cryosurgical treatment. Indiana Med. *89*:432, 1986.)

tinuities that separate muscle bundles, owing to naturally occurring myocardial fiber orientation and anisotropic conduction,[15] as well as collagen matrices, formed from the fibrosis after a myocardial infarction,[163, 166] establish the basis for slowed conduction, fragmented electrograms,[167] and continuous electrical activity[168] that can lead to reentry.[163] The presence of continuous electrical activity is not proof of reentry.[167, 167a] After the infarction, action potential recordings from surviving cells return to normal, suggesting that depressed activity in these cells does not account for the slowed conduction. During acute ischemia, however, a variety of factors, including elevated $[K]_o$ and reduced pH, combine to create depressed action potentials in ischemic cells that certainly retards conduction and can lead to reentry.[169]

Ventricular myocardium resected from humans with recurrent ventricular tachycardia demonstrates abnormal action potentials, suggesting that causes of depressed conduction in humans may be multifactorial (Figs. 20–14, 20–15, and 20–18). In addition, since endocardial resection often eliminates ventricular tachycardia in patients with coronary artery disease, it is likely that the origin of the tachycardia, part of its reentrant loop, or a necessary pathway for its exit to the rest of the ventricle resides in the endocardium. However, although human ventricles cannot be mapped as completely as the animal models,[170, 171]

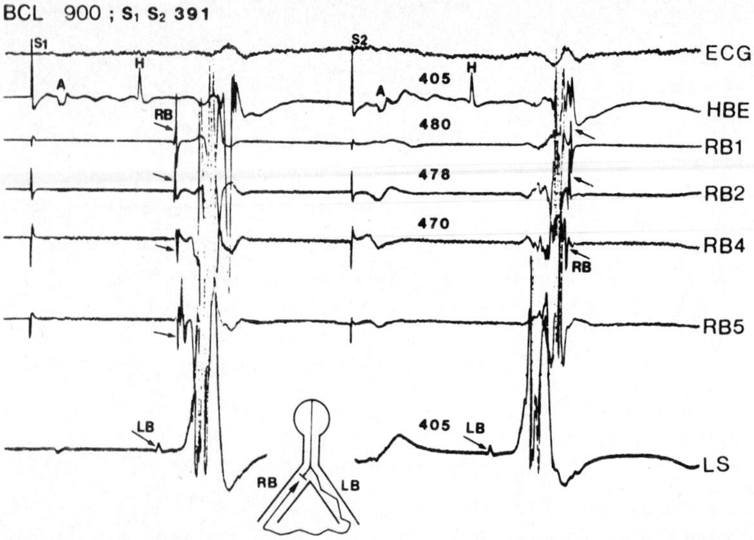

FIGURE 20–30. Reentry in the bundle branches of the dog heart. Recordings have been made with an electrode in the His bundle area (HBE), a multipolar plaque electrode sewn on the right bundle branch portraying activation from base to apex direction in electrograms RB_1 to RB_5 and from the left bundle branch (LB) in the left septal lead (LS). During the last basic cycle, S_1 applied to the atrium causes conduction to proceed from the His bundle through the left and right bundle branches to the ventricle. Note orderly progression of conduction from RB_1 to RB_5. At a premature right atrial interval of 391 msec, conduction is blocked distal to His, travels to the ventricle over the left bundle branch without any delay between left bundle branch deflections, and then activates the right bundle branch retrogradely from RB_4 to RB_2 to RB_1. Retrograde right bundle branch deflection in RB_5 cannot be seen. *Insert* shows activation sequence in bundle branches following S_2. (From Glassman, R. D., and Zipes, D. P.: Site of anterograde and retrograde functional right bundle branch block in the intact canine heart. Circulation *64*:1277, 1981, by permission of the American Heart Association, Inc.)

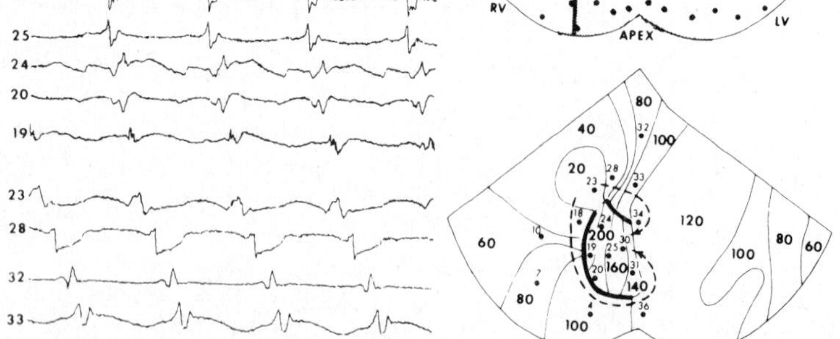

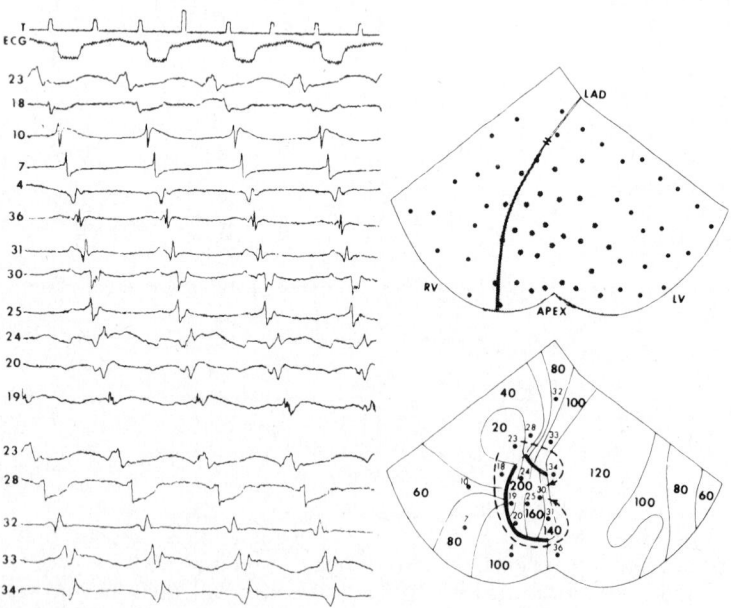

FIGURE 20–31. Isochronal map of epicardial activation during a monomorphic reentrant ventricular tachycardia. Recordings were obtained from a dog with a four day old infarction. The double bar represents the site of the left anterior descending coronary artery (LAD) ligation. The shaded area represents the visible epicardial border of the infarction. The solid circles indicate the position of the epicardial electrodes. The reentrant circuit has a figure-of-eight activation pattern. The left panel shows selected simultaneous electrograms recorded along the two arcs of functional conduction block and the common reentrant wave front, and depicts the presence of diastolic bridging between the reentrant beats. In the right lower panel the solid lines indicate the sites of functional block. The interrupted lines with the arrows indicate the figure-of-eight propagation pattern around the sites of block. RV = right ventricle; LV = left ventricle. (From El-Sherif, N.: The figure 8 model of reentrant excitation in the canine post infarction heart. *In* Zipes, D. P., and Jalife, J. [eds.]: Cardiac Electrophysiology and Arrhythmias. Orlando, Grune and Stratton, 1985, p. 367.)

anatomical similarities of the subendocardial region in these patients who have ischemic heart disease to those found in the epicardium of the animal models, as well as electrophysiological similarities of the ventricular tachycardias, suggest that data relevant to mechanisms responsible for the animal arrhythmias may be applicable to humans. In addition, response to electrical stimulation, including features such as initiation and termination of tachycardia, resetting,[157a] and entrainment, are all consistent with reentry.[158] Thus, even though more evidence meeting Mines' postulates is required to exclude completely other mechanisms responsible for ventricular tachycardia, current information suggests that a great many ventricular tachycardias occurring in man are due to reentrant excitation.

APPROACH TO THE DIAGNOSIS OF CARDIAC ARRHYTHMIAS

It is important to remember that the physician evaluates a *patient* who has a rhythm disturbance and does not evaluate a rhythm disturbance in isolation. Some rhythm disturbances are hazardous to the patient regardless of the clinical setting, while others are hazardous *because* of the clinical setting. Evaluation of the patient should usually progress from the simplest to the most complex test, from the least invasive and safest to the most invasive and risky, and from the least expensive out-of-hospital evaluations to those that require hospitalization and sophisticated, costly procedures. Occasionally, depending on the clinical circumstances, the physician may wish to proceed directly to a high-risk, expensive procedure, such as an electrophysiological study, prior to obtaining a 24-hour electrocardiographic (ECG) recording.

Patients with cardiac rhythm disturbances may present with a variety of complaints, but commonly symptoms such as palpitations, syncope, presyncope, or congestive heart failure cause them to seek a physician's help. Their awareness of regular or irregular cardiac rhythm varies greatly. Some patients perceive slight variations in their heart rhythm with uncommon accuracy, while others are oblivious even to sustained episodes of ventricular tachycardia; still others complain of palpitations when they actually have regular sinus rhythm. The following tests can be used to evaluate patients who have cardiac arrhythmias.

EXERCISE TESTING

(See also Chap. 8)

About one-third of normal subjects develop ventricular ectopy in response to exercise testing. Ectopy is more likely to occur at faster heart rates, usually in the form of occasional, premature ventricular complexes (PVC's) of constant morphology, or even pairs of PVC's, and is often not reproducible from one stress test to the next. Three to six beats of nonsustained ventricular tachycardia can occur in normal patients, especially the elderly, and its occurrence does not establish the existence of ischemic or other forms of heart disease or predict increased cardiovascular morbidity or mortality.[172] Supraventricular premature complexes are often more common during exercise than at rest and increase in frequency with age; their occurrence does not suggest the presence of structural heart disease.

Approximately 50 per cent of patients who have coronary artery disease develop PVC's in response to exercise testing. Ventricular ectopy appears in these patients at lower heart rates (less than 130 beats/min) than in the normal population and often occurs in the early recovery period as well. Exercise-provoked ventricular arrhythmias have been reported to be[173] and not to be[174, 175] associated with a higher cardiovascular risk in patients with coronary artery disease.

Patients who have symptoms consistent with an arrhythmia induced by exercise (e.g., syncope, sustained palpitation) should be considered for stress testing. Stress testing may be indicated[176] to uncover more complex grades of ventricular arrhythmia, to determine the relationship of the arrhythmia to activity, to aid in choosing antiarrhythmic therapy, and possibly provide some insight into the mechanism of the tachycardia.[177] The test can be performed safely; in one study,[178] maximal exercise testing of patients who experienced serious ventricular arrhythmias was associated with a 2.3 per cent incidence of sustained arrhythmias requiring prompt intervention. Stress testing appears to be more sensitive than a standard 12-lead resting ECG to detect ventricular ectopy. However, prolonged ambulatory recording is more sensitive than exercise testing in detecting ventricular ectopy.[179] Since either technique may uncover serious arrhythmias that the other technique misses, both examinations may be indicated for selected patients.[180]

LONG-TERM ELECTROCARDIOGRAPHIC RECORDING

Prolonged ECG recording in a patient engaged in normal daily activity is the most useful noninvasive method to document and quantitate frequency and complexity of arrhythmia, correlate arrhythmia with the patient's symptoms, and evaluate the effect of antiarrhythmic therapy on arrhythmia.[179–186] In addition, some recorders can document alterations in QRS, ST, and T contours (Fig. 20–32).

Several modes of recordings are available: (1) A recording may be continuous. In this case every beat is recorded and is available for analysis. (2) A recording may be patient activated. This is useful if the patient is able to perceive symptoms of the arrhythmia and activate the recorder. (3) A recording may be arrhythmia (event) activated. This is an effective mode, but is dependent on the accuracy and reliability of the device's arrhythmia-detection algorithm.

Transmitters that send an electrocardiographic signal transtelephonically to a receiver unit may be used to transmit on-line or stored electrocardiographic information.[181, 187–189] Such an instrument converts the patient's electrocardiogram to an audiotone, which, when transmitted to a recorder-receiver, is converted back to an electrocardiographic signal for interpretation. This device may be indicated when the rhythm disturbance is sufficiently infrequent and short lasting that continuous ECG recording is impractical. The arrhythmia must be of sufficient duration to permit real-time actual transmission or for storage and later transmission. It must not be associated with syncope or other symptoms that prevent the patient from transmitting or recording, or the patient must have another

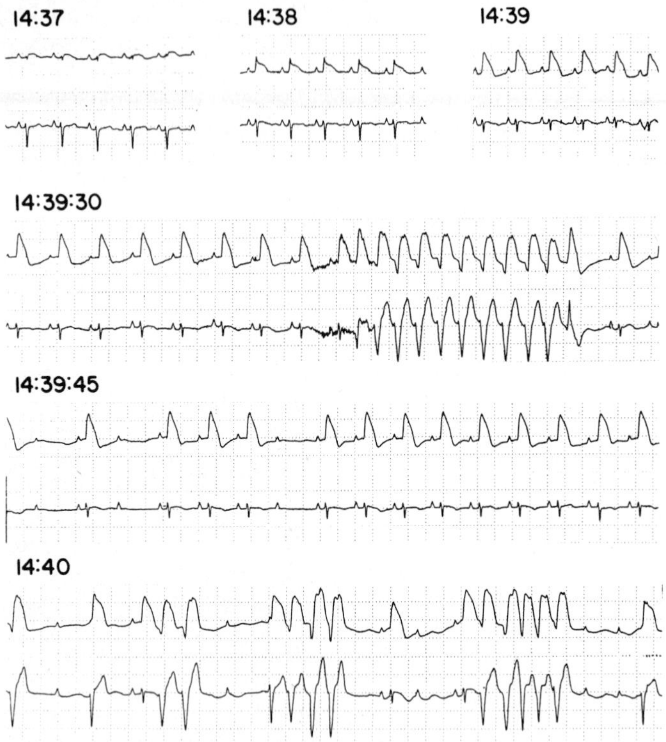

FIGURE 20–32. Long-term ECG recording in a patient with atypical angina. The top channel reflects an inferior lead while the bottom channel records an anterior lead. Note progressive ST segment elevation in the inferior lead, eventually resembling a monophasic action potential. Bursts of nonsustained ventricular tachycardia result. Then, sinus slowing and Wenckebach AV block occur from a vasodepressor reflex response elicited by ischemia of the inferior myocardial wall, or possibly caused by ischemia of the sinus and AV nodes. In the bottom tracing, both AV block and ventricular arrhythmias are apparent. Numbers indicate time, e.g., 2:37 PM. (Tracing of a patient of D. A. Chilson, M.D.)

individual available to record the event. A disadvantage to this approach is that it relies on the patient's perception of a cardiac rhythm disturbance, and many patients may be unaware of significant or serious bradyarrhythmias and tachyarrhythmias. In addition, the technique requires access to a receiver and some sort of receiving mechanism, preferably available 24 hours a day. Recording normal sinus rhythm during the patient's typical symptomatic episode effectively excludes cardiac arrhythmia as a cause.

Home monitoring systems, presently not widely available, operate in a fashion similar to telemetry monitoring in hospital, but transmit ECG data over telephone lines. Effective use of this system may shorten hospital stay and provide safer home care for many patients with cardiac arrhythmias.

HOLTER MONITORING. Continuous ECG recorders represent the traditional Holter monitor and typically record on tape two ECG channels for 24 hours. Interpretative accuracy of long-term tape recordings varies with the system used. When technicians interpret the tape without semiautomated computer systems, an excellent qualitative analysis may be provided, i.e., detection of PVC's, ventricular tachycardia, asystolic intervals, and so forth, but not a quantitative account of the actual number of each event. With semiautomated interpreting systems, the error rate is 5 to 10 per cent of ectopic complexes. Recently developed fully automated computers reportedly miscount or misinterpret less than 3 per cent of ectopic complexes. The clinical utility of such accuracy is questionable, since it is not clear that it really matters whether a patient demonstrates 97 or 100 PVC's over a 24-hour period. All systems can potentially record more information than the physician knows how to assimilate. So long as the system detects ectopy, ventricular tachycardia, or asystolic intervals and semiquantitates those abnormalities, the physician probably receives all the clinical information that is needed. Though some physicians and regulatory agencies request information on the actual number of PVC's, until it is clearly demonstrated that reducing the number of PVC's improves prognosis, the necessity for such PVC quantitation is uncertain.

Significant rhythm disturbances are fairly uncommon in healthy young persons. However, sinus bradycardia with heart rates of 35 to 40 beats/min, sinus arrhythmia with pauses of even 2 secs, sinoatrial exit block, Wenckebach second-degree AV block (often during sleep), a wandering atrial pacemaker, junctional escape complexes, and premature atrial complexes (PAC's) and PVC's are not necessarily abnormal.[186, 190–196] Frequent and complex atrial and ventricular rhythm disturbances are rarely recorded, however, and type II second-degree AV conduction disturbances are not recorded in normal patients. Elderly patients may have a greater prevalence of arrhythmias,[197] some of which may be responsible for neurological symptoms.[198, 199] The long-term prognosis in asymptomatic healthy subjects with frequent and complex PVC's resembles that of the healthy U.S. population without an increased risk of death.[200]

A majority of patients who have ischemic heart disease, particularly those recovering from acute infarction, exhibit PVC's when monitored for periods of 6 to 24 hours (p. 669). The frequency of PVC's progressively increases over the first several weeks, decreasing at about 6 months after infarction. Although the presence of simple PVC's in some but not all studies appears to be of little therapeutic or prognostic significance, PVC's that are frequent, multiform, closely coupled (R-on-T phenomenon), paired, bigeminal, and episodes of ventricular tachycardia have been reported to be associated with increased mortality in patients with ischemic heart disease. There is no universal agreement as to the significance of each of these characteristics, but it is generally conceded that increased frequency and more complex forms of ventricular ectopy imply an increased risk of sudden cardiac death.[201–207] Whether the ventricular ectopy is related causally to the subsequent sudden death or is only a marker identifying the patient at increased risk is unknown, but it is thought to be an independent risk factor.[208, 209] An increase in the frequency of PVC's and ventricular tachycardia has been reported to precede the onset of ventricular fibrillation.[210–212] Serious ventricular ectopy correlates closely with the degree of impaired left ventricular function and persistent ST-segment elevation and with the extent of obstructive coronary vascular disease.

Long-term ECG recording has also exposed potentially serious arrhythmias and complex ventricular ectopy in patients with hypertrophic cardiomyopathy[213, 214] (p. 1418), mitral valve prolapse[215] (p. 1045), in patients who have otherwise unexplained syncope (Chap. 29) or transient vague cerebrovascular symptoms,[198, 199] in patients with conduction disturbances, sinus node dysfunction, the bradycardia-tachycardia syndrome, the Wolff-Parkinson-White syndrome, or pacemaker malfunction (p. 734).

In patients with ventricular arrhythmias, programmed stimulation studies commonly provoke ventricular arrhythmias not found on the long-term ECG recording, but it has not yet been clearly established which technique is more useful for predicting therapeutic response to pharmacological therapy.[216–219]

In normal subjects and in patients with serious rhythm disturbances, the cardiac rhythm may vary markedly from one recording period to the next.[220] To prove the efficacy of antiarrhythmic therapy, it is essential to demonstrate that the frequency of the abnormal rhythm disturbance is reduced more by the agent than by chance alone. Spontaneous reductions in the frequency of PVC's of up to 90 per cent have been demonstrated to occur between two recording periods. Therefore, an antiarrhythmic agent must reduce the frequency of premature ventricular complexes by about 75 to 85 per cent, and the frequency of complex ventricular complexes 70 per cent, from one 24-hour recording period to another to be considered effective.[221]

INVASIVE ELECTROPHYSIOLOGICAL STUDIES

An invasive electrophysiological procedure involves introducing multipolar catheter electrodes into the venous and/or arterial system, positioning the electrodes at various intracardiac sites to record electrical activity from portions of the atria or ventricles, from the region of the His bundle, bundle branches, accessory pathways, and stimulating the atria or ventricles electrically.[222–227] Such studies are performed *diagnostically* to provide information on the type of rhythm disturbance and insight into its electrophysiological mechanism; *therapeutically* to terminate a tachycardia by electrical stimulation, to evaluate effects of therapy by determining whether a particular intervention prevents electrical induction of a tachycardia or whether an electrical device properly senses and terminates an induced tachyarrhythmia, and to ablate (fulgurate) myocardium involved in the tachycardia. Finally, these tests have been used *prognostically* to identify patients at risk for sudden cardiac death. The study may be helpful in patients who have AV block, intraventricular conduction disturbance, sinus node dysfunction, tachycardia, and unexplained syncope or palpitations.

False-negative responses—not finding a particular electrical abnormality known to be present—as well as false-positive ones—induction of a nonclinical arrhythmia—may complicate interpretation of the results, as may lack of reproducibility.[228–230] Altered autonomic tone in a supine patient undergoing study, hemodynamic or ischemic influences, changing anatomy after the study, and the fact that the test employs an artificial "trigger" (electrical stimulation) to induce the arrhythmia are several of many factors that may explain the disparity between test results and spontaneous clinical occurrences. Overall, these studies are quite safe[231] when performed by skilled physicians.[232]

AV BLOCK (See also pp. 674, and 702 to 707). In patients with AV block, the site of block usually dictates the clinical course of the patient and whether or not a pacemaker is needed. Generally the site of AV block can be determined from an analysis of the scalar ECG. When the site of block cannot be determined from such an analysis, and when knowing the site of block is imperative for patient management, an invasive electrophysiological study is indicated. Candidates include patients who have Wenckebach (type I) second-degree AV block and bundle branch block, fixed 2:1 AV block when associated with bundle branch block; possible intra-His AV block (apparent type II AV block with a normal QRS complex); and syncope and AV block. Patients with block in the His-Purkinje system more commonly become symptomatic because of periods of bradycardia or asystole and require pacemaker implantation than do patients who have AV nodal block.[233–235] Wenckebach (type I) AV block in older patients may have clinical implications similar to type II AV block.[236] The mechanism responsible for the block, such as concealed His extrasystoles (Fig. 20–33), can sometimes be determined from such a study and can also influence the therapeutic course.

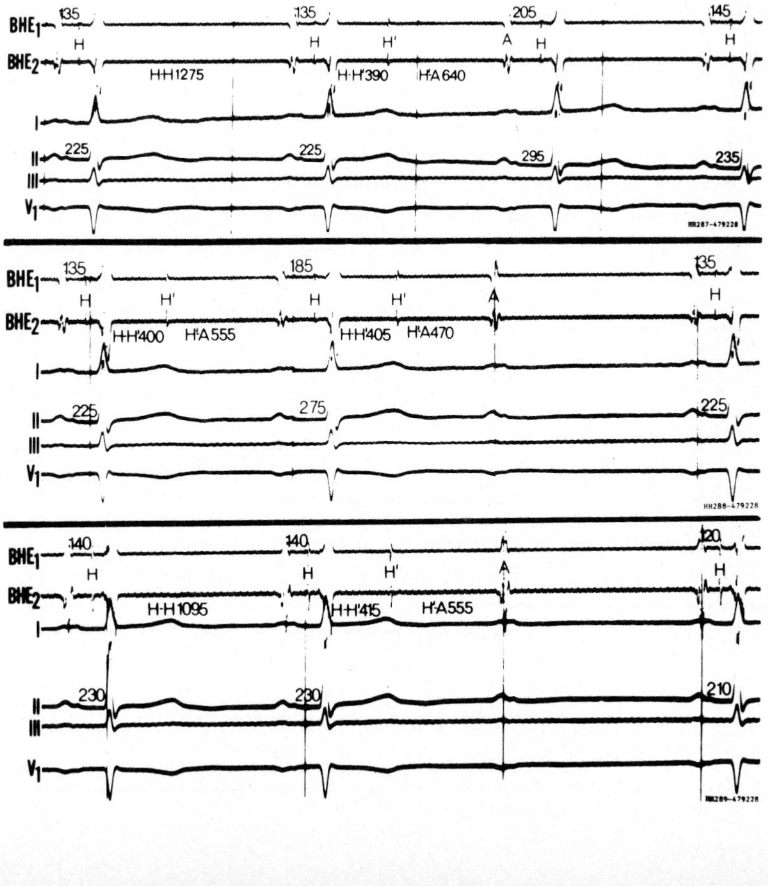

FIGURE 20–33. Concealed discharge from the bundle of His mimicking first-degree (top), type I (middle), and type II (bottom) second-degree AV block. Numbers are in milliseconds. Time lines are one second. (Magnification differs in the three panels.) Numbers in the bipolar His electrogram (BHE_1) indicate A-H intervals; the H-V interval is constant. Numbers in lead II indicate the P-R interval. H-H = interval between His responses in normal conducted cycles. H-H' = interval between the last normal His discharge and the premature His discharge. H'-A = interval between the premature His depolarization and the next normal sinus-initiated atrial discharge. H' invaded the AV node and lengthened the A-H interval or produced AV nodal block of the next atrial depolarization. (From Bonner, A. J., and Zipes, D. P.: Lidocaine and His bundle extrasystoles. His bundle discharge conducted normally, conducted with functional right or left bundle branch block or blocked entirely (concealed). Arch. Intern Med. *136*:700, 1976.)

INTRAVENTRICULAR CONDUCTION DISTURBANCE. For patients with an intraventricular conduction disturbance, an electrophysiological study provides information on the duration of the H-V interval, which can be prolonged with a normal P-R interval or normal with a prolonged P-R interval (see Figure 22–49, p. 709). A prolonged H-V interval (>55 msec) is associated with a greater likelihood of developing trifascicular block (but the rate of progression is slow), having organic disease, and higher mortality.[237] Some data suggest that finding very long H-V intervals (>80 to 90 msec) identifies patients at significant risk of developing AV block. During the study, atrial pacing is used to uncover abnormal His-Purkinje conduction.[238] Drug infusion, such as with procainamide or ajmaline, sometimes exposes abnormal His-Purkinje conduction. Ajmaline may cause arrhythmias and should be used cautiously.[239]

An electrophysiological study is indicated only if the patient has symptoms that appear to be related to a bradyarrhythmia (syncope or presyncope) and when no other cause for syncope is found. For many of these patients, ventricular *tachyarrhythmias* rather than AV block may be the cause of their symptoms.[237]

SINUS NODAL DYSFUNCTION. The demonstration of slow sinus rates, sinus exit block, or sinus pauses temporally related to symptoms suggests a causal relationship and usually obviates further diagnostic studies. Carotid sinus pressure that results in complete cardiac asystole or AV block with the patient's usual symptoms exposes the presence of a hypersensitive carotid sinus reflex[240] (p. 666). Carotid sinus massage must be done cautiously.[241] Neurohumoral agents[242, 243] or stress testing may be employed to evaluate effects of autonomic tone on sinus nodal function. Invasive electrophysiological studies include assessment of sinus node automaticity and sinoatrial conduction time. Electrophysiological studies should be considered in patients who have symptoms attributable to bradycardia or asystole, such as presyncope or syncope, and for whom noninvasive approaches have provided no explanation for the symptoms.

Overdrive Suppression. This technique may be a useful and sensitive test to evaluate sinus node function.[244] The interval between the last paced high right atrial response and the first spontaneous (sinus) high right atrial response after termination of pacing is measured to determine the *sinus node recovery time* (SNRT), by subtracting the spontaneous sinus node cycle length (prior to pacing) from the sinus recovery time (Fig. 20–34). Normal values are generally less than 525 msec. Prolonged SNRT has been found in patients suspected of having sinus node dysfunction. Direct recordings of sinus node electrogram have documented that SNRT is influenced by prolongation of sinoatrial conduction time, as well as by changes in sinus nodal automaticity, especially in the first beat after cessation of pacing.[245] After cessation of pacing, the first return sinus cycle may be normal and may be followed by secondary pauses (Fig. 20–34). Secondary pauses appear to be more common in patients whose sinus node dysfunction is caused by sinoatrial exit block. Sinoatrial exit block may cause some sinus pauses.[246] It is important to evaluate AV nodal and His-Purkinje function in patients with sinus node dysfunction, since many also exhibit impaired AV conduction.

Sinoatrial Conduction Time (SACT). This time can be estimated, based on the assumptions that (1) conduction times into and out of the sinus node are equal, (2) no depression of sinus node automaticity occurs, and (3) the pacemaker site does not shift following premature stimulation. Since these assumptions cannot be applied to all patients, indirectly determining sinus node conduction time is less useful than determining corrected sinus node recovery time when sinus node function in human beings is evaluated.[247] The sensitivity of the SACT and SNRT tests is only about 50 per cent for each test alone and about 70

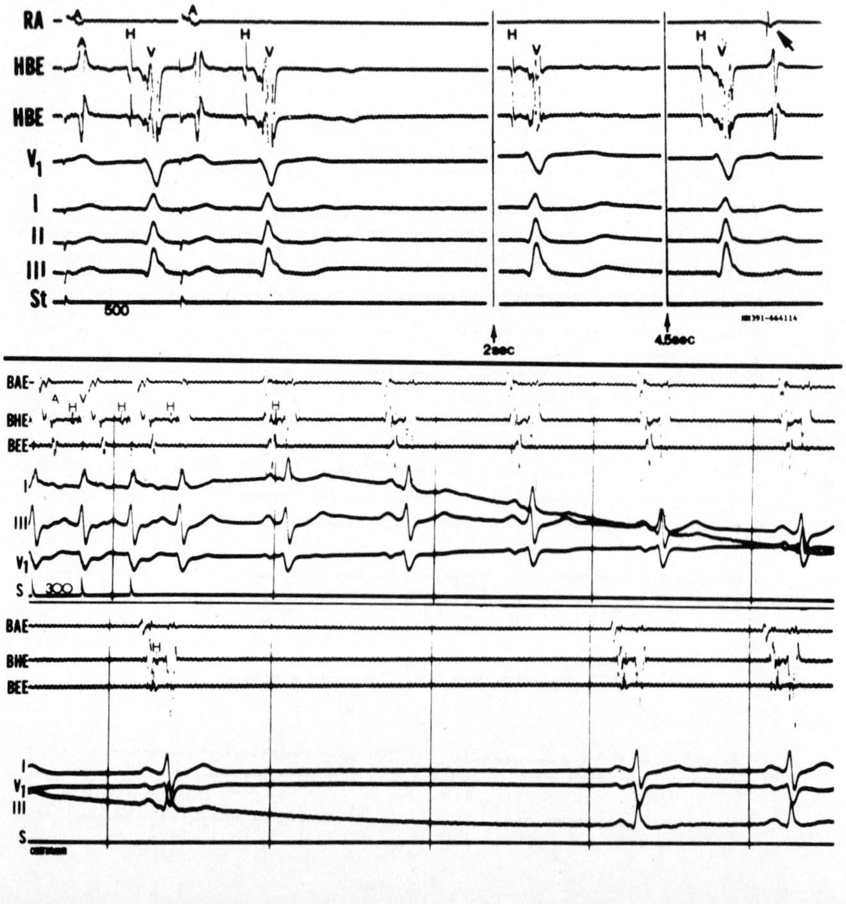

FIGURE 20–34. Abnormal response of sinus node to overdrive pacing. *Top,* After 30 sec of right atrial pacing at a cycle length of 500 msec, sinus nodal discharge (arrow) is suppressed for more than 8 sec. (Sections of 2 sec and 4.5 sec removed for mounting.) *Bottom,* Right atrial pacing at a cycle length of 300 msec was followed by initial P waves occurring at an appropriate rate. The rate then slowed progressively, with P-P prolongation reaching 3 seconds and reproducing the patient's symptoms. Continuous recording; time lines = 1 sec. RA and BAE = bipolar right atrial electrogram; HBE and BHE = bipolar His electrogram; BEE = bipolar esophageal electrogram; I, II, III, and V = scalar leads; St and S = stimulus. (Modified from Zipes, D. P., and Noble, R. J.: Assessment of electrical abnormalities. *In* Hurst, J. W. [ed.]: The Heart. 5th ed. New York, McGraw-Hill Book Co., 1982, pp. 333–357.)

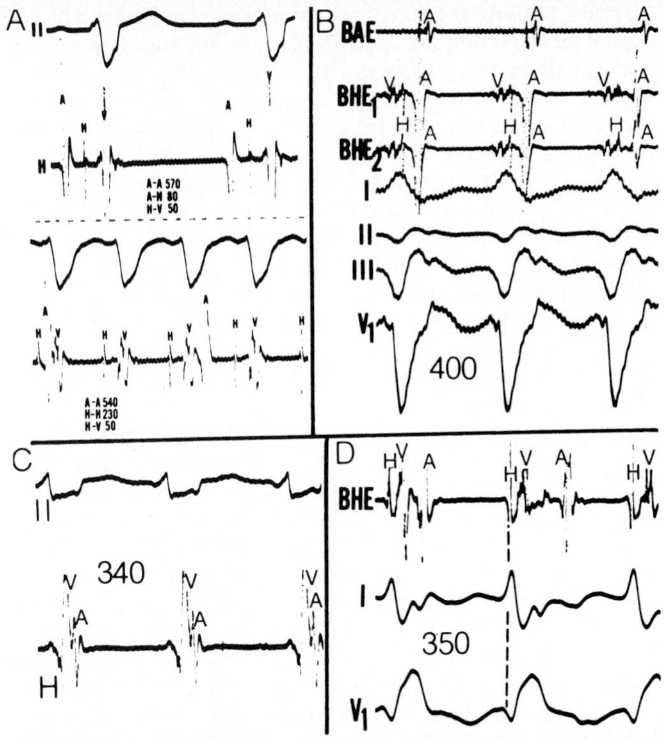

FIGURE 20–35. His bundle recording in four different patients with tachycardias. *A,* The top portion of the tracing shows His bundle recording during sinus rhythm. The H-V interval is 50 msec. The bottom portion shows His bundle recording during tachycardia. Since the QRS complex and H-V interval are the same as those recorded during sinus rhythm, this is a supraventricular tachycardia. Of note is the fact that the atria discharged at a rate that was different from (not a multiple of) the ventricular rate. Thus, AV dissociation is present during this supraventricular tachycardia. *B,* His bundle activity occurred after the onset of the QRS complex, during ventricular septal depolarization, which confirmed the diagnosis of ventricular tachycardia. (WPW had been excluded.) The R-P interval remained constant, and the atria were captured retrogradely from the ventricles. Thus, AV dissociation is not present during this ventricular tachycardia. *C,* His bundle activity was not recorded despite careful exploration of the His bundle area with the catheter electrode tip. This most likely represents ventricular tachycardia with 1:1 retrograde atrial capture, but the diagnosis cannot be as clear as in panels *B* and *D,* His bundle activity preceded the onset of ventricular septal depolarization (interrupted line) but followed the onset of the QRS complex. Thus, this must be ventricular tachycardia. Retrograde (VA) Wenckebach conduction (not shown in its entirety) was also present. (From Zipes, D. P., et al.: Clinical electrophysiology and electrocardiography. *In* Willerson, J. T., and Sanders, C. A. [eds.]: The Science and Practice of Clinical Medicine. Clinical Cardiology. New York, Grune and Stratton, 1977, pp. 235–248.)

per cent when combined. The specificity, when combined, is about 88 per cent, with a low predictive value.[224]

TACHYCARDIA. In patients with tachycardias, an electrophysiological study may be used to diagnose the arrhythmia, determine therapy, deliver therapy, determine anatomical site(s) involved in the tachycardia, identify patients at high risk for developing serious arrhythmias, and gain insights into mechanisms responsible for the arrhythmia. For example, results of the study can differentiate aberrant supraventricular conduction from ventricular tachyarrhythmias (p. 694). Since all the electrocardiographic manifestations of ventricular tachycardia can be mimicked, under certain circumstances, by aberrantly conducted supraventricular tachycardia, exceptions exist to the criteria that help to differentiate supraventricular tachyarrhythmias with abnormal QRS complexes from ventricular tachyarrhythmias.[248] A *supraventricular tachycardia* is recognized electrophysiologically by the presence of an H-V interval equaling or exceeding that recorded during normal sinus rhythm (Fig. 20–35). In contrast, during *ventricular tachycardia,* the H-V interval is shorter than normal or, more commonly, cannot be recorded clearly. Only two situations exist when a consistently short H-V interval occurs: during retrograde activation of the His bundle from a complex originating in the ventricle or during conduction over an accessory pathway (preexcitation syndrome).[249] Atrial pacing at rates exceeding the tachycardia rate can demonstrate ventricular origin of the wide QRS tachycardia by producing fusion and capture beats and normalization of the H-V interval (Fig. 20–36). Atropine administration to improve AV nodal conduction may facilitate ventricular capture by the atria.

Initiation and termination with programmed electrical stimulation of supraventricular or ventricular tachycardia to test the potential efficacy of pharmacological, pacemaker, or surgical therapy represent a second important application of electrophysiological studies in patients with tachycardia.[224, 250] Determination of drug efficacy based on results from long-term ECG recordings may be insufficient to predict a patient's therapeutic response, particularly in the patient with a low frequency of spontaneous ventricular arrhythmias. A drug that prevents electrical induction of a sustained monomorphic tachycardia that was induced during the pre-drug control state has a high probability of achieving long-term successful suppression of spontaneous episodes. A drug that fails to prevent electrical induction may still prevent spontaneous clinical episodes, but in a lesser percentage of patients.[224, 250] The patient's hemody-

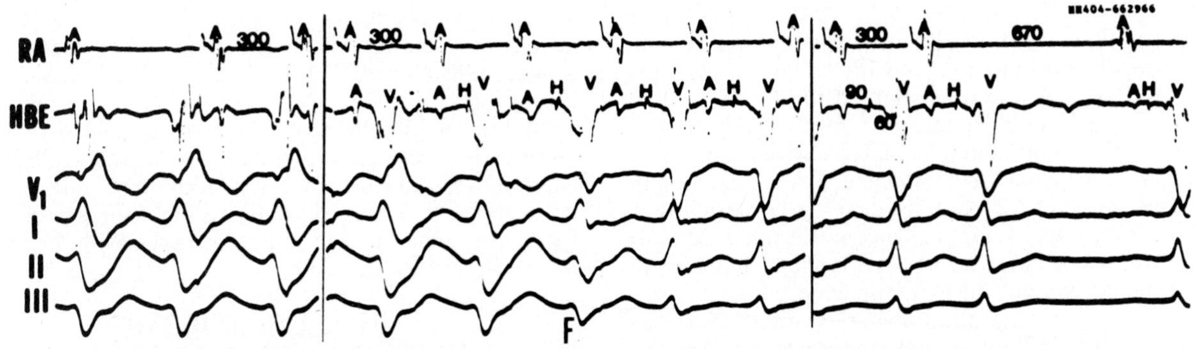

FIGURE 20–36. Termination of ventricular tachycardia by rapid atrial pacing. Ventricular tachycardia (*left panel*) with AV dissociation became captured by rapid atrial pacing (200 bpm) (*middle panel*) and was terminated after cessation of atrial pacing (*right panel*). Note fusion beat (F) in the midportion of panel 2 and normalization of the H-V interval. (From Foster, P. R., and Zipes, D. P.: Pacing and cardiac arrhythmias. *In* Mandel, W. J. [ed.]: Cardiac Arrhythmias. Their Mechanisms, Diagnosis and Management. Philadelphia, J. B. Lippincott Co., 1980, pp. 605–624.)

namic response to the tachycardia can be assessed. Often, drugs slow the rate of a tachycardia, even though they fail to prevent its induction, and the patient may have a better hemodynamic response to the tachycardia. Electrical therapy also can be delivered via the catheter electrode (pacing, cardioversion, defibrillation, ablation; see p. 642).

Finding the site of origin and/or the pathways involved in maintenance of some tachycardias, localized by endocardial mapping, in patients with the Wolff-Parkinson-White syndrome or its variants[251, 252] and in selected patients with ventricular tachycardia[170] is a prerequisite for almost any type of arrhythmic surgery (p. 645).

Electrophysiological testing may help identify patients with the *Wolff-Parkinson-White* syndrome[252, 253] or with coronary artery disease[254–255a] who are at risk for the subsequent development of serious supraventricular or ventricular tachycardias or sudden cardiac death. Complete agreement does not exist regarding use of electrophysiological testing in this area.

Finally, an electrophysiological study may provide some insight into possible electrophysiological mechanisms responsible for the tachycardia.[256] Conduction and refractoriness of various cardiac tissues involved in the tachycardia can be assessed. Although it is difficult in most instances to differentiate reentry from automaticity reliably (p. 595), evidence in favor of one or the other mechanism may be obtained.

INDICATIONS. An electrophysiological study should be considered (1) in patients who have symptomatic, recurrent, or drug-resistant supraventricular or ventricular tachyarrhythmias, particularly when the tachycardia produces hemodynamically significant consequences; (2) in patients with tachyarrhythmias occurring too infrequently to permit adequate diagnostic or therapeutic assessment; or (3) to differentiate supraventricular tachycardia and aberrant conduction from ventricular tachycardia; (4) whenever nonpharmacological therapy such as the use of electrical devices, catheter ablation, or surgery is contemplated.[224, 225]

Patients with Unexplained Syncope or Palpitations (see p. 887). The three common arrhythmic causes of syncope include sinus node dysfunction, tachyarrhythmias, and AV block. Of the three, tachyarrhythmias are probably most reliably initiated in the electrophysiology laboratory, followed by sinus node abnormalities and then His-Purkinje block.

The cause of syncope goes undetected in 13 to 47 per cent of patients, depending in part on the extent of the evaluation.[257–259] A careful, accurately performed history and physical examination are the most important tests performed.[260] The 1-year mortality is about 6 per cent in patients with unknown cause, 1 to 12 per cent in patients with noncardiovascular causes, but 19 to 30 per cent in patients with cardiovascular causes.[257, 258, 261] The incidence of sudden death is also higher in patients with a cardiovascular cause of syncope. A very small percentage (2 per cent in one series)[261] of patients develop an arrhythmia coincident with syncope or presyncope during a 24-hour ECG recording, while a large percentage (15 per cent) have symptoms without an arrhythmia, excluding an arrhythmic cause.[261] Diagnostic difficulties arise in patients in whom bradyarrhythmias or tachyarrhythmias are recorded without associated symptoms. Often a probable diagnosis must be inferred from the ECG findings.[257, 258, 261]

In an analogous fashion, the electrophysiological study may fail to explain the patient's symptoms if the arrhythmia cannot be induced or if an abnormal rhythm is induced and the patient remains asymptomatic. However, induction of an arrhythmia that replicates the patient's symptoms may explain the cause of the palpitations or syncope. Patients considered for a study are those whose recurrent syncopal spells remain undiagnosed despite complete general and neurological evaluation, repeated 24-hour ECG recordings, stress testing, and other noninvasive cardiac tests. The presence of palpitations alone is *not* an indication for an electrophysiological study. However, an electrophysiological study may be useful if the patient complains of symptoms such as angina, shortness of breath, or lightheadedness during the palpitations; if there is evidence that the palpitations may represent a significant rhythm disturbance, and if noninvasive studies fail to reveal a cause of the palpitations.[224, 225, 262, 263]

Electrophysiological testing has been reported to uncover the cause of syncope in 12[264] to 68 per cent[265] of patients, the lower percentage in patients with no recognizable structural heart disease. Therapy of a putative cause found during electrophysiological testing prevents recurrence of syncope in about 80 per cent of patients.[265] Thus, depending on the population studied, the sensitivity of the electrophysiological test may be very low, but may be increased at the expense of specificity. For example, more aggressive pacing techniques (e.g., using three or four premature stimuli), administration of drugs (e.g., isoproterenol), or left ventricular pacing may increase the success rate of ventricular tachycardia induction, but by precipitating nonclinical ventricular tachyarrhythmias such as nonsustained polymorphic or monomorphic ventricular tachycardia or ventricular fibrillation.[266–269] Similarly, aggressive techniques during atrial pacing may induce nonspecific episodes of atrial flutter or atrial fibrillation. A diagnostic dilemma arises when the patient's clinical, symptom-producing arrhythmia is one of these nonspecific arrhythmias that can be produced in the normal patient who has no arrhythmia. Induction of *sustained* supraventricular (e.g., AV nodal reentry, AV reciprocating tachycardia) or monomorphic ventricular tachycardia in patients who are not subject to the spontaneous development of the tachycardia appears to be uncommon and provides important information that the induced tachyarrhythmia may be clinically significant and responsible for the patient's symptoms. Generally, other abnormalities such as prolonged pauses following overdrive atrial pacing or type II AV block are not induced in patients who do not or may not experience these abnormalities spontaneously. Induction of these arrhythmias has a high degree of specificity.

COMPLICATIONS OF ELECTROPHYSIOLOGICAL STUDIES. The risks of these studies are small.[270] Five deaths have been noted in 4015 patients (0.12 per cent) undergoing 8545 studies (0.06 per cent) in six major institutions; 19 patients had cardiac perforation, 4 had major hemorrhage, 8 had arterial injury, and 20 had major venous thromboses.[231]

Since precipitation of AV block or a tachyarrhythmia is often a desirable goal of the study, symptoms from such rhythm disturbances may result, sometimes requiring electrical shock to restore rhythm. Adding therapeutic maneuvers, e.g., ablation, to the procedure will increase the incidence of complication.

OTHER DIAGNOSTIC ELECTROCARDIOGRAPHIC TECHNIQUES

ESOPHAGEAL ELECTROCARDIOGRAPHY. Esophageal electrocardiography is a useful noninvasive technique to diagnose arrhythmias.[271] The esophagus is adjacent to the posterior atria, and an electrode inserted into the esophagus can record atrial potentials. Bipolar recording is superior to unipolar recording.[272] In addition, atrial and occasionally ventricular pacing can be performed via a catheter electrode inserted into the esophagus, and initiation and termination of tachycardias can be accomplished.[273, 274] Optimal electrode position for pacing correlates with patient height and is within about 1 cm of the site at which the maximum amplitude of the atrial electrogram is recorded. No serious immediate complications of transesophageal pacing have been reported.[273] A capsule electrode that is easily swallowed has been used to record continuous atrial electrograms from the esophagus.[271]

The esophageal atrial electrogram is useful for differentiating supraventricular tachycardia with aberrancy from ventricular tachycardia. During a wide QRS tachycardia when the ventricular rate exceeds the atrial rate, AV dissociation is often present, and the most likely diagnosis is ventricular tachycardia (see p. 694). If each ventricular depolarization is coupled to an atrial depolarization, either supraventricular tachycardia or ventricular tachycardia with 1:1 ventriculoatrial conduction may be present. Uncommonly, junctional tachycardia with aberrancy may mimic ventricular tachycardia, and His bundle recordings are needed for a definitive diagnosis. When the same number of atrial and ventricular depolarizations occurs, the autonomic nervous system may be manipulated to evoke AV nodal block or to slow the supraventricular rate to differentiate ventricular tachycardia from supraventricular tachycardia.

Esophageal atrial electrograms are also helpful to define the mechanism of supraventricular tachycardias. For example, a narrow QRS tachycardia with a ventricular rate of 150 beats/min may be due to atrial flutter with a 2:1 ventricular response, confirmed by finding an atrial rate of 300 beats/min. If atrial and ventricular depolarization occur simultaneously during paroxysmal supraventricular tachycardia, reentry utilizing an accessory AV pathway (Wolff-Parkinson-White) can be excluded, and AV nodal reentry is the most likely mechanism for the tachycardia (p. 680).

BODY SURFACE MAPPING. Isopotential body surface maps are used to provide a complete picture of the effects of the currents from the heart on the body surface. The potential distributions are represented by contour lines of equal potential, and each distribution is displayed instant by instant throughout activation or recovery, or both.

Body surface maps have been used for preliminary clinical application in the following areas: localizing and sizing myocardial infarction,[275] detecting areas of ischemia (especially those apparent only with exercise), localizing ectopic foci[276] or accessory pathways,[277] differentiating aberrant supraventricular conduction from ventricular origin, recognizing the patient prone to developing arrhythmias, and possibly understanding the mechanisms involved.[278, 279] Although these procedures are of interest, their clinical utility has not yet been established.[224]

DIRECT CARDIAC MAPPING: RECORDING POTENTIALS DIRECTLY FROM THE HEART. Cardiac mapping is a method whereby potentials recorded directly from the heart are spatially depicted as a function of time in an integrated manner. The location of recording electrodes (epicardial, intramural, or endocardial) and the recording mode used (unipolar versus bipolar) as well as the method of display (isopotential versus isochrone maps) depend upon the problem under consideration.

Direct cardiac mapping via catheter electrodes or at the time of cardiac surgery can be used to localize accessory pathways associated with the Wolff-Parkinson-White syndrome, to delineate the anatomical course of the His bundle during open-heart surgery to avoid injury during procedures to correct congenital heart defects, and to identify the site of rhythm disturbances in patients with supraventricular and ventricular tachyarrhythmias for electrical or surgical ablation, isolation, or resection (p. 645).[225] These approaches are discussed in greater detail under the individual arrhythmias in Chap. 22.

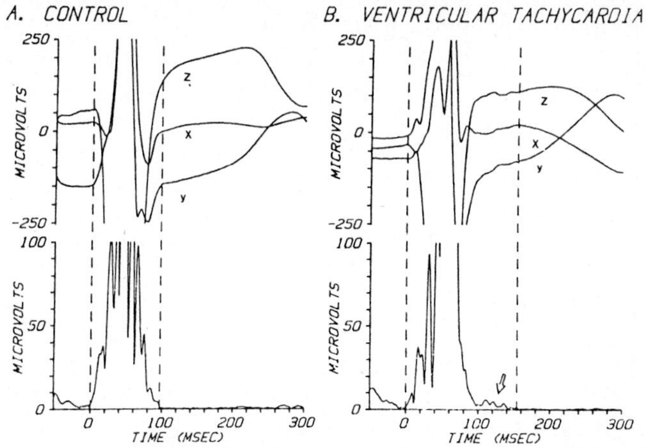

FIGURE 20–37. Signal averaged ECG's from two patients with anterior myocardial infarctions. Unfiltered bipolar leads are shown at high gain (*top*). The filtered QRS complex (*bottom*) is the vector magnitude of the three leads after high pass filtering (more than 25 Hz). Control patient (A) had no complex ventricular ectopy on prolonged ECG recordings. The patient with ventricular tachycardia (B) had sustained, inducible ventricular tachycardia, and the recording demonstrates a late potential (arrow) at the end of the filtered QRS complex. The voltage in the last 40 msec was 52 μV for the control patient and 4 μV for the patient with ventricular tachycardia. (From Simson, M. B.: Signal averaging. Circulation April supplement 1987, by permission of the American Heart Association, Inc.)

SIGNAL-AVERAGING TECHNIQUES. Signal averaging is a method that improves signal-to-noise ratio when signals are recurrent and the noise is random, i.e., not synchronous with the signal. In conjunction with other methods of noise reduction, signal averaging can detect cardiac signals of a few microvolts, reducing noise amplitude, typically 5 to 20 μV to less than 1 μV. With this method, potentials generated by the sinus and AV nodes,[280] His bundle, and bundle branches are detectable at the body surface.[281–283] Fourier transformation has been applied to extract diagnostic high-frequency content.[284]

Signal averaging has been applied clinically most often to detect late ventricular potentials of 1 to 25 μV at the end of the QRS complex, probably corresponding to delayed and fragmented conduction in the ventricle[285] (Fig. 20–37). These late potentials have been recorded in 73 to 92 per cent of patients with sustained and inducible ventricular tachycardia after myocardial infarction, in only 0 to 6 per cent of normal volunteers, and in 7 to 15 per cent of patients after myocardial infarction who do not have ventricular tachycardia.[282] They have also been recorded in patients with ventricular tachycardia not related to ischemia.[286] Successful surgical control of the ventricular tachycardia can eliminate late potentials.[287] Antiarrhythmic drug therapy, on the other hand, decreases the amplitude of the late potentials without abolishing them. Late potentials after myocardial infarction may identify patients prone to develop ventricular tachycardia,[288, 289] and thus, combined with other data such as ejection fraction, spontaneous ventricular ectopy on a 24-hour ECG recording, response to stress testing, and so forth, may be used to identify patients at risk for sudden cardiac death (Chap. 24).

Acknowledgment

The author thanks Robert F. Gilmour, Jr., Ph.D., and William M. Miles, M.D., for critical review of this chapter.

REFERENCES

ANATOMY OF THE CARDIAC CONDUCTION SYSTEM

1. James, T. N.: Anatomy of the conduction system of the heart. *In* Hurst, J. W. (ed): The Heart. 6th ed. New York, McGraw-Hill Book Co., 1982.
2. Anderson, R. H., and Becker, A. E.: Gross anatomy and microscopy of the conducting system. *In* Mandel, W. J. (ed.): Cardiac Arrhythmias, Their Mechanisms, Diagnosis and Management. Philadelphia, J. B. Lippincott Co., 1980.
3. Jalife, J.: Mutual entrainment and electrical coupling as mechanisms for synchronous firing of rabbit sino-atrial pace-maker cells. J. Physiol. *356*:221, 1984.
4. Michaels, D. C., Matyas, E. P., and Jalife, J.: Dynamic interactions and mutual synchronization of sinoatrial node pacemaker cells. A mathematical model. Circ. Res. *58*:706, 1986.
5. Boineau, J. P., Miller, C. B., Schuessler, R. B., Roeske, W. R., Autry, L. J., Wylds, A. C., and Hill, D. A.: Activation sequence and potential distribution maps demonstrating multi-centric atrial impulse origin in dogs. Circ. Res. *54*:332, 1984.
6. Randall, W. C., and Ardell, J. L.: Selective parasympathectomy of autonomic and conductile tissues of the canine heart. Am. J. Physiol. *248*(Heart Circ. Physiol. 17):H61, 1985.
7. Levy, M. N., and Martin, P. J.: Neural control of heart rate and atrioventricular conduction. *In* Abboud, F. M., et al. (eds.): Disturbances in Neurogenic Control of the Circulation. Clinical Physiology Series. Bethesda, Md., American Physiological Society, 1981, p. 205.
8. Slenter, V. A. J., Salata, J. J., Jalife, J.: Vagal control of pacemaker periodicity and intranodal conduction in the rabbit sinoatrial node. Circ. Res. *54*:436, 1984.
9. Salata, J. J., Gill, R. M., Gilmour, R. F., Jr., and Zipes, D. P.: Effects of sympathetic tone on vagally-induced phasic changes in heart rate and A-V nodal conduction in the anesthetized dog. Circ. Res. *58*:584, 1986.
10. Bonke, F. I. M., Allessie, M. A., Kirchhof, C. J. H. J., and Roos, A. G. J. M.: Investigation of the conduction properties of the sinus node. *In* Zipes, D. P., and Jalife, J. (eds.): Cardiac Electrophysiology and Arrhythmias. Orlando, Grune and Stratton, 1985, p. 73.
11. Prystowsky, E. N., and Zipes, D. P.: Observations on postvagal tachycardia in humans. *In* Zipes, D. P., and Jalife, J. (eds.): Cardiac Electrophysiology and Arrhythmias. Orlando, Grune and Stratton, 1985, p. 177.
12. Hogan, P. M., and Davis, L. D.: Electrophysiological characteristics of canine atrial plateau fibers. Circ. Res. *28*:62, 1971.
13. Sherf, L., and James, T. N.: Fine structure of cells and their histologic organization within internodal pathways of the heart: Clinical and electrocardiographic implications. Am. J. Cardiol. *44*:345, 1979.
14. Waldo, A. L., Bush, H. L., Jr., Gelband, H., Zorn, G. L., Vitikainen, K. J., and Hoffman, B. F.: Effects on the canine P wave of discrete lesions in the specialized atrial tracts. Circ. Res. *29*:452, 1971.
15. Spach, M. S., and Dolber, P. C.: Relating extracellular potentials and their derivatives to anisotropic propagation at a microscopic level in human cardiac muscle. Cir. Res. *58*:356, 1986.
16. Jackman, W. M., Prystowsky, E. N., Naccarelli, G. B., Heger, J. J., and Zipes, D. P.: Enhanced AV nodal conduction: Prevalence and anatomic substrate. Circulation *67*:441, 1983.
17. Rosenbaum, M. B., Elizari, M. V., and Lazzari, J. O.: The Hemiblocks. Oldsmar, Fla., Tampa Tracings, 1970.
18. Paes de Carvalho, A., and de Almeida, D. F.: Spread of activity through the atrioventricular node. Circ. Res. *8*:801, 1960.
19. Anderson, R. H., Janse, M. J., van Capelle, F. J. L., Billette, J., Becker, A. E., and Durrer, D.: A combined morphological and electrophysiological study of the atrioventricular node of the rabbit heart. Circ. Res. *35*:909, 1974.
20. Sherf, L., James, T. N., and Woods, W. T.: Function of the atrioventricular node considered on the basis of observed histology and fine structure. J. Am. Coll. Cardiol. *5*:770, 1985.
21. Webb, S. C., Krikler, D. M., Hendry, W. G., Adrian, T. E., and Bloom, S. R.: Electrophysiological actions of somatostatin on the atrioventricular junction in sinus rhythm and reentry tachycardia. Br. Heart J. *56*:236, 1986.
22. Martins, J. B., and Zipes, D. P.: Epicardial phenol interrupts refractory period responses to sympathetic but not vagal stimulation in canine left ventricular epicardium and endocardium. Circ. Res. *47*:33, 1980.
23. Barber, M. J., Mueller, T. M., Davies, B. G., and Zipes, D. P.: Phenol topically applied to canine left ventricular epicardium interrupts sympathetic but not vagal afferents. Circ. Res. *55*:532, 1984.
24. Takahashi, N., Barber, M. J., and Zipes, D. P.: Efferent vagal innervation of the canine ventricle. Am. J. Physiol. *248*(Heart Circ. Physiol. 17):H89, 1985.
25. Takahashi, N., and Zipes, D. P.: Vagal modulation of adrenergic effects on canine sinus and atrioventricular nodes. Am. J. Physiol. *244*(Heart Circ. Physiol. 13):H775, 1983.
26. Gilmour, R. F., Jr., and Zipes, D. P.: Evidence for prejunctional and postjunctional antagonism of the sympathetic neuroeffector junction by acetylcholine in canine cardiac Purkinje fibers. J. Am. Coll. Cardiol. *3*:760, 1984.
27. Lindemann, J. P., and Watanabe, A.: Muscarinic cholinergic inhibition of phospholamban phosphorylation and calcium transport in guinea pig ventricles. J. Biol. Chem. *260*:13122, 1985.
28. Jalife, J., Slenter, V. A. J., Salata, J. J., and Michaels, D. C.: Dynamic vagal control of pacemaker activity in the mammalian sinoatrial node. Circ. Res. *52*:642, 1983.
29. Schuessler, R. B., Boineau, J. B., Wylds, A. C., Hill, D. A., Miller, C. B., and Roeske, W. R.: Effect of canine cardiac nerves on heart rate, rhythm and pacemaker location. Am. J. Physiol. *250*(Heart Circ. Physiol. 19) (*in press*).
29a. Martins, J. B., and Zipes, D. F.: Effects of sympathetic and vagal nerves on recovery properties of the endocardium and epicardium of the canine left ventricle. Circ. Res. *46*:100, 1980.
30. Pierpont, G. L., DeMaster, E. G., and Cohn, J. N.: Regional differences in adrenergic function within the left ventricle. Am. J. Physiol. *246*(Heart Circ. Physiol. 15):H824, 1984.
31. Inoue, H., Gill, R. M., and Zipes, D. P.: Increased afferent vagal responses produced by nicotine on the canine posterior left ventricular epicardium, abstracted. Clin. Res. *33*:867A, 1985.
32. Gilmour, R. F., Jr., and Zipes, D. P.: Positive inotropic effect of acetylcholine in canine Purkinje fibers. Am. J. Physiol. *249*(Heart Circ. Physiol. 18):H735, 1985.
33. Rossi, L.: Cardioneuropathy and extracardiac neural disease. J. Am. Coll. Cardiol. *5*:66B, 1985.
34. James, T. N.: Primary and secondary cardioneuropathies and their functional significance. J. Am. Coll. Cardiol. *2*:983, 1983.
35. Barber, M. J., Mueller, T. M., Davies, B. G., Gill, R. M., and Zipes, D. P.: Interruption of sympathetic and vagal mediated afferent responses by transmural myocardial infarction. Circulation *72*:623, 1985.
36. Kammerling, J. M., Barber, M. J., Henry, D. P., and Zipes, D. P.: Transmural myocardial infarction produces denervation supersensitivity in noninfarcted areas apical to the infarct, abstracted. Circulation *70*(Suppl 2):125, 1984.
37. Inoue, H., Davies, B., and Zipes, D. P.: Denervation supersensitivity is arrhythmogenic. Circulation *72*(Suppl 3):243, 1985.
38. Prystowsky, E. N., Jackman, W. M., Rinkenberger, R. L., Heger, J. J., and Zipes, D. P.: Effect of autonomic blockade on ventricular refractoriness and atrioventricular conduction in humans: Evidence supporting a direct cholinergic action on ventricular muscle refractoriness. Circ. Res. *49*:511, 1981.

BASIC ELECTROPHYSIOLOGICAL PRINCIPLES

39. Katz, A. M., Messineo, F. C., and Herbette, L.: Ion channels in membranes. Circulation *65*(Suppl 1):2, 1982.
40. McNutt, N. S.: Ultrastructure of intercellular junctions in adult and developing cardiac muscle. Am. J. Cardiol. *25*:169, 1970.
41. Mazet, F., Wittenberg, B. A., and Spray, D. C.: Fate of intercellular junctions in isolated adult rat cardiac cells. Circ. Res. *56*:195, 1985.
42. DeMello, W.: Intercellular communication in cardiac muscle: Physiological and pathological implications. *In* Zipes, D. P., and Jalife, J. (eds.): Cardiac electrophysiology and arrhythmias. Orlando, Grune and Stratton, 1985, p. 65.
43. Spray, D. C., and Bennett, M. V. L.: Physiology and pharmacology of gap junctions. Ann. Rev. Physiol. *47*:281, 1985.
44. Tsien, R. W., and Hess, P.: Excitable tissues. The Heart. *In* Andreoli, T. E., et al. (eds.): Physiology of Membrane Disorders. New York, Plenum Publishing Co., 1986.
45. Fozzard, H. M., Haber, E., Jennings, R. B., Katz, A. M., Morgan, H. E. (eds.): The Heart and Cardiovascular System. New York, Raven Press, 1986.
46. Coraboeuf, E.: Ionic basis of electrical activity in cardiac tissues. *In* Levy, M. N., and Vassalle, M. (eds.): Excitation and Neural Control of the Heart. Bethesda, Md., American Physiological Society, 1982, p. 1.
47. Hoffman, B. F., and Cranefield, P. F.: Electrophysiology of the Heart. New York, McGraw-Hill Book Co., 1960.
48. Aldrich, R. W., Corey, D. P., and Stevens, C. F.: A reinterpretation of mammalian sodium channel gating based on single channel recording. Nature *306*:436, 1983.
49. Reuter, H., Cachelin, A. B., dePeyer, J. E., and Kokubun, S.: Whole cell Na^+ current and single Na^+–channel measurements in cultured cardiac cells. *In* Zipes, D. P., and Jalife, J. (eds.): Cardiac Electrophysiology and Arrhythmias. Orlando, Grune and Stratton, 1985, p. 13.
50. Hess, P., Lansman, J. B., and Tsien, R. W.: Different modes of Ca channel gating behavior favoured by dihydropyridine Ca agonists and antagonists. Nature *311*:538, 1984.
51. Cranefield, P. F.: The Conduction of the Cardiac Impulse. Mt. Kisco, N.Y., Futura Publ. Co., 1975.
52. Zipes, D. P., Bailey, J. C., and Elharrar, V.: The Slow Inward Current and Cardiac Arrhythmias. The Hague, Martinus Nijhoff, 1980.
53. Trautwein, W., and Pelzer, D.: Gating of single calcium channels in the membrane of enzymatically isolated ventricular myocytes from adult mammalian hearts. *In* Zipes, D. P., and Jalife, J. (eds.): Cardiac Electrophysiology and Arrhythmias. Orlando, Grune and Stratton, 1985, p. 31.
54. Watanabe, A.: Recent advances in the knowledge about beta adrenergic receptors: Application to clinical cardiology. J. Am. Coll. Cardiol. *1*:82, 1983.
55. Gilmour, R. F., Jr., and Zipes, D. P.: Basic electrophysiology of the slow inward current. *In* Antman, E., and Stone, P. H.: Calcium Blocking Agents in the Treatment of Cardiovascular Disorders. Futura Publ. Co., Mt. Kisco, N.Y., 1983, pp. 1–37.
56. Reuter, H.: Calcium channel modulation by neurotransmitters, enzymes and drugs. Nature *301*:569, 1983.
57. Sperelakis, N.: Phosphorylation hypothesis of the myocardial slow channels and control of Ca^{2+} influx. *In* Zipes, D. P., and Jalife, J. (eds.): Cardiac Electrophysiology and Arrhythmias. Orlando, Grune and Stratton, 1985, p. 123.
58. Gilmour, R. F., Jr., and Zipes, D. P.: Electrophysiological response of vascularized hamster cardiac transplants to ischemia. Circ. Res. *50*:599, 1982.
59. Spear, J. F., Horowitz, L. N., and Moore, E. N.: The slow response in human ventricle. Zipes, D. P., et al. (eds.): The Slow Inward Current and Cardiac Arrhythmias. The Hague, Martinus Nijhoff, 1980, p. 309.
60. Singer, D. H., Baumgarten, C. M., and Ten Eick, R. E.: Cellular electro-

physiology of ventricular and other dysrhythmias: Studies on diseased and ischemic heart. Progr. Cardiovasc. Dis. *24*:97, 1981.

61. Gilmour, R. F., Jr., Heger, J. J., Prystowsky, E. N., and Zipes, D. P.: Cellular electrophysiological abnormalities of diseased human ventricular myocardium. Am. J. Cardiol. *51*:137, 1983.
62. Noble, D.: Ionic bases of rhythmic activity in the heart. *In* Zipes, D. P., and Jalife, J. (eds.): Cardiac Electrophysiology and Arrhythmias. Orlando, Grune and Stratton, 1985, p. 3.
63. Sperelakis, N.: Origin of the cardiac resting potential. *In* Berne, R. M., et al. (eds.): Handbook of Physiology, The Cardiovascular System. Bethesda, Md., American Physiological Society, 1979, p. 187.
64. Carmeliet, E., and Vereecke, J.: Electrogenesis of the action potential and automaticity. *In* Berne, R. M., et al. (eds.): Handbook of Physiology. Bethesda, Md., American Physiological Society, 1979, p. 269.
65. Coraboeuf, E., Deroubaix, E., and Coulombe, A.: Effect of tetrodotoxin on action potentials of the conducting system in the dog. Am. J. Physiol. *236*:H561, 1979.
66. DiFrancesco, D.: The cardiac hyperpolarizing-activated current, i_f. Origins and development. Prog. Biophys. Mol. Biol. *46*:163, 1985.
67. Callewaert, G., Carmeliet, E., and Vereecke, J.: Single cardiac Purkinje cells: General electrophysiology and voltage-clamp analysis of the pacemaker current. J. Physiol. *349*:643, 1984.
68. Gilmour, R. F., Jr., and Zipes, D. P.: Abnormal automaticity and related phenomena. *In* Fozzard, H. M., et al. (eds.): The Heart and Cardiovascular System. New York, Raven Press, 1986, pp. 1239–1258.
69. Kreitner, D.: Electrophysiological study of the two main pacemaker mechanisms in the rabbit sinus node. Cardiovasc. Res. *19*:304, 1985.
70. Brown, H. F.: Electrophysiology of the sinoatrial node. Physiol. Rev. *62*:505, 1982.
71. DiFrancesco, D., Ferroni, A., Mazzanti, M., and Tromba, C.: Properties of the hyperpolarizing-activated current (i_f) in cells isolated from the rabbit sinoatrial node. J. Physiol. (*in press*).
72. Wit, A. L., and Cranefield, P. F.: Mechanisms of impulse initiation in the atrioventricular junction and the effects of acetylstrophanthidin. Am. J. Cardiol. *49*:921, 1982.
73. Carmeliet, E.: Myocardial ischemia: Reversible and irreversible changes. Circulation *70*:149, 1984.
74. Hill, J. L., and Gettes, L. S.: Effect of acute coronary artery occlusion on local myocardial extracellular K^+ activity in swine. Circulation *61*:768, 1980.
75. Sawicki, G. J., and Arnsdorf, M. F.: Electrophysiologic actions and interactions between lysophosphatidylcholine and lidocaine in the nonsteady state: The match between multiphasic arrhythmogenic mechanisms and multiple drug effects in cardiac Purkinje fibers. J. Pharmacol. Exp. Ther. *235*:829, 1985.
76. Clusin, W. T., Buchbinder, M., Ellis, A. K., Kernoff, R. S., Giacomini, J. C., and Harrison, D. C.: Reduction of ischemic depolarization by the calcium channel blocker diltiazem. Circ. Res. *54*:10, 1984.
77. Woodward, B., and Zakaria, M. N.: Effect of some free radical scavengers on reperfusion induced arrhythmias in the isolated rat heart. J. Mol. Cell. Cardiol. *17*:485, 1985.
78. Werns, S. W., Shea, M. J., and Lucchesi, B. R.: Free radicals and myocardial injury: Pharmacologic implications. Circulation *74*:1, 1986.
79. Zipes, D. P.: A consideration of antiarrhythmic therapy. Circulation *72*:949, 1985.

MECHANISMS OF ARRHYTHMOGENESIS

80. Frame, L. H., and Hoffman, B. F.: Mechanisms of tachycardia. *In* Surawicz, B., et al. (eds.): Tachycardias. Boston, Martinus Nijhoff, 1984, p. 7.
81. Lazzara, R., and Scherlag, B. J.: Electrophysiologic basis for arrhythmias in ischemic heart disease. Am. J. Cardiol. *53*:1B, 1984.
82. Zipes, D. P., and Jalife, J. (eds.): Cardiac Electrophysiology and Arrhythmias. Orlando, Grune and Stratton, 1985.
83. Wit, A. L.: Cellular electrophysiologic mechanisms of cardiac arrhythmias. Ann. N.Y. Acad. Sci. *432*:1, 1984.
84. Rozanski, G. J., Lipsius, S. L., and Randall, W. C.: Functional characteristics of sinoatrial and subsidiary pacemaker activity in the canine right atrium. Circulation *6*:1378, 1983.
85. Gilmour, R. F., Jr., and Zipes, D. P.: Pathophysiology of cardiac arrhythmias. *In* Andreoli, T. E., et al. (eds.): Physiology of Membrane Disorders. New York, Plenum Publishing Co., 1986, p. 841.
86. Noble, D.: The surprising heart: A review of recent progress in cardiac electrophysiology. J. Physiol. (Lond) *353*:1, 1984.
87. Ferrier, G. R.: Digitalis arrhythmias: Role of oscillatory afterpotentials. Progr. Cardiovasc. Dis. *19*:459, 1977.
88. Damiano, B. P., and Rosen, M. R.: Effects of pacing on triggered activity induced by early afterdepolarizations. Circulation *69*:1013, 1984.
89. Levine, J. H., Spear, J. F., Guarnieri, T., Weisfeldt, M. L., deLangen, C. D. J., Becker, L. C., and Moore, E. N.: Cesium chloride–induced long QT syndrome: Demonstration of afterdepolarizations and triggered activity in vivo. Circulation *72*:1092, 1985.
90. Brachmann, J., Scherlag, B. J., Rosenstraukh, L. V., and Lazzara, R.: Bradycardia-dependent triggered activity: Relevance to drug-induced multiform ventricular tachycardia. Circulation *68*:846, 1983.
91. Moss, A. J., Schwartz, P. J., Crampton, R. S., Locati, E., and Carleen, E.: The long QT syndrome: A prospective international study. Circulation *71*:17, 1985.
92. Rosen, M. R.: Cellular electrophysiology of digitalis toxicity. J. Am. Coll. Cardiol. *5*(Suppl. A):22A, 1985.
93. Fisch, C., and Knoebel, S. B.: Accelerated junctional escape: A clinical manifestation of "triggered" automaticity. *In* Zipes, D. P., and Jalife, J. (eds.): Cardiac Electrophysiology and Arrhythmias. New York, Grune and Stratton, 1985, p. 467.
94. Rosen, M. R., and Danilo, P.: Effects of tetrodotoxin, lidocaine, verapamil and AHR-2666 on ouabain-induced delayed afterdepolarizations in canine Purkinje fibers. Circ. Res. *46*:117, 1980.
95. Nau, G. J., Aldariz, A. E., Aconzo, R. S., Chiale, P. A., Elizari, M. V., and Rosenbaum, M. B.: Concealed ventricular parasystole uncovered in the form of ventricular escapes of variable coupling. Circulation *64*:199, 1981.
96. Jalife, J., Antzelevitch, C., and Moe, G. K.: Models of parasystole and reflection. *In* Rosenbaum, M. B. (ed.): Cardiac Arrhythmias. The Hague, Martinus Nijhoff, 1982.
97. Antzelevitch, C., Moe, G. K., and Jalife, J.: Electrotonic modulation of pacemaker activity. Further biological and mathematical observations in the behavior of modulated parasystole. Circulation *66*:1225, 1982.
98. Nau, G. T., Aldariz, A. E., Aconzo, R. S., Halpern, S., Davidenko, J. M., Elizari, M. V., and Rosenbaum, M. B.: Modulation of parasystolic activity by non-parasystolic beats. Circulation *66*:462, 1982.
99. Singer, D. H., Lazzara, R., and Hoffman, B. F.: Interrelationships between automaticity and conduction in Purkinje fibers. Circ. Res. *21*:537, 1967.
100. Jalife, J., Antzelevitch, C., LaManna, V., and Moe, G. K.: Rate-dependent changes in excitability of depressed cardiac Purkinje fibers as a mechanism of intermittent bundle branch block. Circ. Res. *67*:912, 1983.
101. Gilmour, R. F., Jr., Salata, J. J., and Zipes, D. P.: Rate related suppression and facilitation of conduction in isolated canine cardiac Purkinje fibers. Circ. Res. *57*:35, 1985.
102. Matsuda, M. D., and Paes de Carvalho, A.: Rate and rhythm dependency of propagation from normal myocardium to a Ba^{++}, K^+–induced slow response zone in rabbit left atrium. Circ. Res. *50*:419, 1982.
103. Takahashi, N., Gilmour, R. F., Jr., and Zipes, D. P.: Overdrive suppression of conduction in the canine His-Purkinje system following anterior septal artery occlusion. Circulation *70*:495, 1984.
104. Mines, G. R.: On dynamic equilibrium in the heart. J. Physiol. (Lond) *46*:349, 1913.
105. Mines, G. R.: On circulating excitations in heart muscles and their possible relation to tachycardia and fibrillation. Trans. R. Soc. Can. (Sec. IV) *8*:43, 1914.
106. Allessie, M. A., Bonke, F. I. M., and Schopman, F. J. G.: Circus movement in rabbit atrial muscle as a mechanism of tachycardia: III. The "leading circle" concept: A new model of circus movement in cardiac tissue without the involvement of an anatomical obstacle. Circ. Res. *41*:9, 1977.
107. Smeets, J. L. R. M., Allessie, M. A., Lammers, W. J. E. P., Bonke, F. I. M., and Hollen, J.: The wavelength of the cardiac impulse and reentrant arrhythmias in isolated rabbit atrium. Circ. Res. *58*:96, 1986.
108. Antzelevitch, C., Jalife, J., and Moe, G. K.: Frequency-dependent alterations of conduction in Purkinje fibers. A model of phase 4 facilitation and block. *In* Rosenbaum, M. B. (ed.): Cardiac Arrhythmias. The Hague, Martinus Nijhoff, 1982.
109. Antzelevitch, C., Jalife, J., and Moe, G. K.: Characteristics of reflection as a mechanism of reentrant arrhythmias and its relationship to parasystole. Circulation *61*:182, 1980.
110. Allessie, M. A., Lammers, W. J. E. P., Bonke, F. I. M., and Hollen, J.: Intra-atrial reentry as a mechanism for atrial flutter induced by acetylcholine and rapid pacing in the dog. Circulation *70*:123, 1984.
111. Inoue, H., Matsuo, H., Takayanagi, K., and Murao, S.: Clinical and experimental studies of the effects of atrial extrastimulation and rapid pacing on atrial flutter cycle. Am. J. Cardiol. *48*:623, 1981.
112. Disertori, M., Inama, G., Vergara, G., Guarnerio, M., Favero, A. D., and Furlanello, F.: Evidence of a reentry circuit in the common type of atrial flutter in man. Circulation *67*:434, 1983.
113. Boineau, J. P.: Atrial flutter: A synthesis of concepts. Circulation *72*:249, 1985.
114. Dobmeyer, D. J., Stine, R. A., Leier, C. V., and Schaal, S. F.: Electrophysiologic mechanisms of provoked atrial flutter in mitral valve prolapse syndrome. Am. J. Cardiol. *56*:602, 1985.
115. Frame, L. H., Page, R. L., and Hoffman, B. F.: Atrial reentry around an anatomic barrier with a partially refractory excitable gap. A canine model of atrial flutter. Circ. Res. *58*:495, 1986.
116. Waldo, A. L., Plumb, V. J., and Henthorn, R. W.: Observations on the mechanism of atrial flutter. *In* Surawicz, B., et al. (eds.): Tachycardias. Boston, Martinus Nijhoff, 1984, p. 213.
117. Okumura, K., Henthorn, R. W., Epstein, A. E., Plumb, V. J., and Waldo, A. L.: Further observations on transient entrainment: Importance of pacing site and properties of the components of the reentrant circuit. Circulation *72*:1293, 1985.
118. Gettes, L. S.: Ventricular fibrillation. *In* Surawicz, B., et al. (eds.): Tachycardias. Boston, Martinus Nijhoff, 1984, p. 37.
119. Allessie, M. A., Lammers, W. J. E. P., Bonke, F. I. M., and Hollen, J.: Experimental evaluation of Moe's multiple wavelet hypothesis of atrial fibrillation. *In* Zipes, D. P., and Jalife, J. (eds.): Cardiac Electrophysiology and Arrhythmias. Orlando, Grune and Stratton, 1985, p. 265.
120. Coumel, P.: Atrial fibrillation. *In* Surawicz, B., et al.: Tachycardias. Boston, Martinus Nijhoff, 1984, p. 231.
121. Allessie, M. A., and Bonke, F. I. M.: Direct demonstration of sinus nodal reentry in the rabbit heart. Circ. Res. *44*:557, 1979.
122. Gomes, J. A., Hariman, R. J., Kang, P. S., and Chowdry, I. H.: Sustained symptomatic sinus node reentrant tachycardia: Incidence, clinical significance, electrophysiologic observations and the effects of antiarrhythmic agents. J. Am. Coll. Cardiol. 5:45, 1985.
123. Akhtar, M.: Supraventricular tachycardia. Electrophysiologic mechanisms, diagnosis and pharmacologic therapy. *In* Josephson, M. E., and Wellens, H.

J. J. (eds): Tachycardias: Mechanisms, Diagnosis, and Treatment. Philadelphia, Lea and Febiger, 1984, p. 137.
124. Allessie, M. A., Bonke, F. I. M., and Schopman, F. J. G.: Circus movement in rabbit atrial muscle as a mechanism of tachycardia: II. The role of nonuniform excitability in the occurrence of unidirectional block, as studied with multiple microelectrodes. Circ. Res. 39:168, 1976.
125. Boineau, J. P., Schuessler, R. B., Mooney, C. R., Miller, C. B., Wylds, A. C., Hudson, R. D., Borremans, J. M., and Brockus, C. W.: Natural and evoked atrial flutter due to circus movement in dogs. Am. J. Cardiol. *45*:1167, 1980.
126. Coumel, P., Flammang, D., Attuel, P., and Leckercq, J. F.: Sustained intra-atrial reentrant tachycardia. Electrophysiologic study of 20 cases. Clin. Cardiol. 2:176, 1979.
127. Mendez, C., Han, J., Garcia de Jalon, P. D., and Moe, G. K.: Some characteristics of ventricular echoes. Circ. Res. *16*:562, 1965.
128. Wu, D.: Dual atrioventricular nodal pathways: A reappraisal. PACE 5:72, 1982.
129. Shenasa, M., Gilbert, C. J., Schmidt, D. H., and Akhtar, M.: Procainamide and retrograde atrioventricular nodal conduction in man. Circulation *65*:355, 1982.
130. Reddy, C. P., and McAllister, R. G., Jr.: Effect of verapamil on retrograde conduction in atrioventricular nodal reentrant tachycardia. Am. J. Cardiol. *54*:535, 1984.
131. Janse, M. J.: Influence of the direction of the atrial wavefront on AV nodal transmission in isolated hearts and rabbits. Circ. Res. *25*:439, 1969.
132. Zipes, D. P., Mendez, C., and Moe, G. K.: Evidence for summation and voltage dependency in rabbit atrioventricular nodal fibers. Circ. Res. *32*:170, 1973.
133. Rahilly, G. T., Zipes, D. P., Naccarelli, G. V., Jackman, W. M., Heger, J. J., and Prystowsky, E. N.: Autonomic blockade in patients with normal and abnormal atrioventricular nodal function. Am. J. Cardiol. *49*:898, 1982.
134. Wah, J. Y. L., Friday, K., Sakurai, M., Lazzara, R., and Jackman, W.: Is the His bundle part of the AV nodal reentry circuit? Circulation 72(Suppl 3):271, 1985.
135. Mignone, R. J., and Wallace, A. G.: Ventricular echoes: Evidence for dissociation of conduction and reentry within the AV node. Circ. Res. *19*:638, 1966.
136. Kerr, C. R., Benson, D. W., and Gallagher, J. J.: Role of specialized conducting fibers in the genesis of "AV nodal" reentry tachycardia. PACE 6:171, 1983.
137. Zipes, D. P., Gaum, W. E., Genetos, B. C., Glassman, R. D., Noble, R. J., and Fisch, C.: Atrial tachycardia without P waves masquerading as an AV junctional tachycardia. Circulation *55*:253, 1977.
138. Marquez-Montes, J., Rufilanchas, J. J., Esteve, J. J., Alvarez, L., Benezet, J., Burgos, R., and Figuera, D.: Paroxysmal nodal reentrant tachycardia. Surgical cure with preservation of atrioventricular conduction. Chest *83*:690, 1983.
139. Ross, D. L., Johnson, D. C., Denniss, A. R., Cooper, M. J., Richards, D. A., and Uther, J. B.: Curative surgery for atrioventricular junctional ("AV nodal") reentrant tachycardia. J. Am. Coll. Cardiol. *6*:1383, 1985.
140. Wolff, L., Parkinson, J., and White, P. D.: Bundle branch block with short P-R interval in healthy young people prone to paroxysmal tachycardia. Am. Heart J. 5:685, 1950.
141. Durrer, D., Schoo, L., Schulienburg, R. M., and Wellens, H. J. J.: The role of premature beats in the initiation and the termination of supraventricular tachycardia in the Wolff-Parkinson-White syndrome. Circulation *36*:644, 1967.
142. Zipes, D. P., DeJoseph, R. L., and Rothbaum, D. A.: Unusual properties of accessory pathways. Circulation *49*:1200, 1974.
143. Gallagher, J. J., Pritchett, E. L. C., Sealy, W. C., Casell, J., and Wallace, A. G.: The pre-excitation syndromes. Progr. Cardiovasc. Dis. *20*:285, 1978.
144. Prystowsky, E. N., Miles, W. M., Heger, J. J., and Zipes, D. P.: Preexcitation syndromes: Mechanisms and management. Med. Clin. North Am. *68*:831, 1984.
145. Kent, A. F. S.: Researches on the structure and function of the mammalian heart. J. Physiol. *14*:233, 1893.
146. Kent, A. F. S.: Observations on the auriculo-ventricular junction of the mammalian heart. Q. J. Exp. Physiol. 7:193, 1913.
147. Hammill, S. C., Pritchett, E. L. C., Klein, G. J., Smith, W. M., and Gallagher, J. J.: Accessory atrioventricular pathways that conduct only in the antegrade direction. Circulation *62*:1335, 1980.
148. Critelli, G., Gallagher, J. J., Thiene, G., Perticone, F., Coltorti, F., and Rossi, L.: Electrophysiologic and histopathologic correlations in a case of permanent form of reciprocating tachycardia. Eur. Heart J. *6*:130, 1985.
149. Gureiner, R., Ng, C. K., Hammer, I., and Becker, A. E.: Tachycardia caused by an accessory nodoventricular tract: A clinico-pathologic correlation. Eur. Heart J. 5:233, 1984.
150. Gallagher, J. J., Smith, W. M., Kasell, J. H., Benson, D. W., Jr., Sterba, R., and Grant, A. O.: Role of Mahaim fibers in cardiac arrhythmias in man. Circulation *64*:176, 1981.
151. Gallagher, J. J.: Variants of preexcitation: Update 1984. *In* Zipes, D. P., and Jalife, J. (eds.): Cardiac Electrophysiology and Arrhythmias. Orlando, Grune and Stratton, 1985, p. 419.
152. Murabit, I., Sosa, E., Pileggi, F., and Denes, P.: Multiple reentry tachycardia in patients with ventricular preexcitation: Report of three patients. Am. Heart J. *111*:69, 1986.
153. Ward, D. E., Bexton, R., and Camm, A. J.: Characteristics of atrio-His conduction in the short PR interval, normal QRS complex syndrome. Evidence for enhanced slow pathway conduction. Eur. Heart J. *4*:882, 1983.
154. Lown, B., Ganong, W. F., and Levine, S. A.: The syndrome of short PR interval, normal QRS complex and paroxysmal rapid heart action. Circulation 5:693, 1952.
155. Schmitt, F. O., and Erlanger, J.: Directional differences in the conduction of the impulse through heart muscle and their possible relation to extrasystolic and fibrillatory contractions. Am. J. Physiol. *87*:326, 1929.
156. Mehra, R., Zeiler, R. H., Gough, W. B., and El Sherif, N.: Reentrant ventricular arrhythmias in the late myocardial infarction period: IX. Electrophysiologic anatomic correlation of reentrant circuits. Circulation *67*:11, 1983.
157. Wit, A. L., Allessie, M. A., Bonke, F. I. M., Lammers, W., Smeets, J., and Fenoglio, J. J., Jr.: Electrophysiologic mapping to determine the mechanism of experimental ventricular tachycardia initiated by premature impulses. Am. J. Cardiol. *49*:166, 1982.
157a. Almendral, J. M., Stamato, N. J., Rosenthal, M. E., Marchlinski, F. E., Miller, J. M., and Josephson, M. E.: Resetting response patterns during sustained ventricular tachycardia: Relationship to the excitable gap. Circulation *74*:722, 1986.
158. Josephson, M. E., Almendral, J. M., Buxton, A. E., and Marchlinski, F. E.: Mechanisms of ventricular tachycardia. Circulation (*in press*).
159. Cardinal, R., Savard, P., Carson, D. L., Perry, J. B., and Page, P.: Mapping of ventricular tachycardia induced by programmed stimulation in canine preparations of myocardial infarction. Circulation *70*:136, 1984.
160. El Sherif, N.: The figure 8 model of reentrant excitation in the canine post infarction heart. *In* Zipes, D. P., and Jalife, J. (eds.): Cardiac Electrophysiology and Arrhythmias. Orlando, Grune and Stratton, 1985, p. 363.
161. Gessman, L. J., Agarwal, J. B., Endo, T., and Helfant, R. H.: Localization and mechanism of ventricular tachycardia by ice mapping 1 week after the onset of myocardial infarction in dogs. Circulation *68*:657, 1983.
162. El Sherif, N., Mehra, R., Gough, W. B., and Zeiler, R. H.: Reentrant ventricular arrhythmias in the late myocardial infarction period: Interruption of reentrant circuits by cryothermal techniques. Circulation *68*:644, 1983.
163. Gardner, P. I., Ursell, P. C., Pham, T. D., Fenoglio, J. J., and Wit, A. L.: Experimental chronic ventricular tachycardia: Anatomic and electrophysiologic substrates. *In* Josephson, M. E., and Wellens, H. J. J. (eds.): Tachycardias: Mechanisms, Diagnosis, and Treatment. Philadelphia, Lea and Febiger, 1984, p. 29.
164. Scherlag, B. J., Brachmann, J., Kabell, G., Harrison, L., Guse, P., and Lazzara, R.: Sustained ventricular tachycardia: Common functional properties of different anatomic substrates. *In* Zipes, D. P., and Jalife, J. (eds.): Cardiac Electrophysiology and Arrhythmias. Orlando, Grune and Stratton, 1985, p. 379.
165. Kramer, J. B., Saffitz, J. E., Witkowski, F. X., and Corr, P. B.: Intramural reentry as a mechanism of ventricular tachycardia during evolving canine myocardial infarction. Circ. Res. *56*:736, 1985.
166. Richards, D. A., Blake, G. J., Spear, J. F., and Moore, E. N.: Electrophysiologic substrate for ventricular tachycardia: Correlation of properties in vivo and in vitro. Circulation *69*:369, 1984.
167. Josephson, M. E., and Wit, A. L.: Fractionated electrical activity and continuous electrical activity: Fact or artifact? Circulation *70*:529, 1984.
167a. Berrgada, P., Abdollah, H., and Wellens, H. J. J.: Continuous electrical activity during sustained monomorphic ventricular tachycardia. Am. J. Cardiol. *55*:402, 1985.
168. Garan, H., and Ruskin, J. N.: Localized reentry. Mechanism of induced sustained ventricular tachycardia in canine model of recent myocardial infarction. J. Clin. Invest. *74*:377, 1984.
169. Fleet, W. F., Johnson, T. A., Graebner, C. A., Engle, C. L., and Gettes, L. S.: Effects of verapamil on ischemia-induced changes in extracellular K^+, pH and local activation in the pig. Circulation *73*:837, 1986.
170. Miller, J. M., Harken, A. H., Hargrove, W. C., and Josephson, M. E.: Pattern of endocardial activation during sustained ventricular tachycardia. J. Am. Coll. Cardiol. *6*:1280, 1985.
171. Mason, J. W., Stinson, E. B., Oyer, P. E., Winkle, R. A., Hunt, S., Anderson, K. P., and Derby, G. C.: Mechanisms of ventricular tachycardia in humans determined by intraoperative recording of the electrical activation sequence. Int. J. Cardiol. *8*:163, 1985.

APPROACH TO THE DIAGNOSIS OF CARDIAC ARRHYTHMIAS

172. Fleg, J. L., and Lakatta, E. G.: Prevalence and prognosis of exercise-induced nonsustained ventricular tachycardia in apparently healthy volunteers. Am. J. Cardiol. *54*:762, 1984.
173. Califf, R. M., McKinnis, R. A., McNeer, J. F., Harrell, F. E., Jr., Lee, K. L., Pryor, D. B., Waugh, R. A., Harris, P. J., Rosati, R. A., and Wagner, G. S.: Prognostic value of ventricular arrhythmias associated with treadmill exercise testing in patients studied with cardiac catheterization for suspected ischemic heart disease. J. Am. Coll. Cardiol. *2*:1060, 1983.
174. Weiner, D. A., Levine, S. R., Klein, M. D., and Ryan, T. J.: Ventricular arrhythmias during exercise testing: Mechanism, response to coronary bypass surgery and prognostic significance. Am. J. Cardiol. *53*:1553, 1984.
175. Sami, M., Chaitman, B., Fisher, L., Holmes, D., Fray, D., and Alderman, E.: Significance of exercise-induced ventricular arrhythmia in stable coronary artery disease: A coronary artery surgery study project. Am. J. Cardiol. *54*:1182, 1984.
176. Podrid, P. J., and Graboys, T. B.: Exercise stress testing in the management of cardiac rhythm disorders. Med. Clin. North Am. *68*:1139, 1984.
177. Woelfel, A., Foster, J. R., McAllister, R. G., Jr., Simson, R. T., Jr., and Gettes, L. S.: Efficacy of verapamil in exercise-induced ventricular tachycardia. Am. J. Cardiol. *56*:292, 1985.

178. Young, D. Z., Lampert, S., Graboys, T. B., and Lown, B.: Safety of maximal exercise testing in patients at high risk for ventricular arrhythmia. Circulation *70*:184, 1984.
179. Kennedy, H. L.: Comparison of ambulatory electrocardiography and exercise testing. Am. J. Cardiol. *47*:1359, 1981.
180. Rauscha, F., Glogar, D., Weber, H., Niederberger, M., and Kaindl, F.: Diagnostic value of exercise testing versus long-term ECG in evaluation of arrhythmias in old age. Eur. Heart J. *5*(Suppl E):79, 1984.
181. Winkle, R. A.: Long-term ECG and event recorders for the diagnosis and treatment of cardiac arrhythmias. Circulation (*in press*).
182. Holter, N. J.: New method for heart studies: Continuous electrocardiography of active subjects over long periods is now practical. Science *134*:1214, 1961.
183. Kennedy, H. L.: Ambulatory Electrocardiography and Holter Recording Technology. Philadelphia, Lea and Febiger, 1981.
184. Wenger, N. K., Mock, M. B., and Ringquist, I.: Ambulatory Electrocardiographic Recording. Chicago, Year Book Medical Publishers, 1981.
185. Winkle, R. A.: Recent status of ambulatory electrocardiography. Am. Heart J. *102*:757, 1981.
186. Smith, M. S., and Pritchett, E. L. C.: Electrocardiographic monitoring in ambulatory patients with cardiac arrhythmias. Cardiol. Clin. *1*:293, 1983.
187. Morganroth, J.: Ambulatory Holter electrocardiography: Choice of technologies and clinical uses. Ann. Intern. Med. *102*:73, 1985.
188. Fyfe, D. A., Holmes, D. R., Jr., Neubauer, S. A., and Feldt, R. H.: Transtelephonic monitoring in pediatric patients with clinically suspected arrhythmias. Clin. Pediatr. (Phila.) *23*:139, 1984.
189. Pritchett, E. L., Hammill, S. C., Reith, M. J., Lee, K. L., McCarthy, E. A., Zimmerman, J. M., and Schand, D. G.: Life-table methods for evaluating antiarrhythmic drug efficacy in patients with paroxysmal atrial tachycardia. Am. J. Cardiol. *52*:1007, 1983.
190. Barrett, P. A., Peter, C. T., Swan, H. J., Singh, B. N., and Mandel, W. J.: The frequency and prognostic significance of electrocardiographic abnormalities in clinically normal individuals. Progr. Cardiovasc. Dis. *23*:299, 1981.
191. Sobotka, P. A., Mayer, J. H., Bauernfeind, R. A., Kanakis, C., Jr., and Rosen, K. M.: Arrhythmias documented by 24 hour continuous ambulatory electrocardiographic monitoring in young women without apparent heart disease. Am. Heart J. *101*:753, 1981.
192. Scott, O., Williams, G. J., and Fiddler, G. I.: Results of 24 hour ambulatory monitoring of electrocardiogram in 131 healthy boys aged 10 to 13 years. Br. Heart J. *44*:304, 1980.
193. Olec, M. D., Smith, N., McNeill, G. P., and Wright, D. S.: Dysrhythmias in apparently healthy subjects. Age-Aging *8*:173, 1979.
194. Romhilt, D. W., Chaffin, C., Choi, S. C., and Irby, E. C.: Arrhythmias on ambulatory monitoring in women without apparent heart disease. Am. J. Cardiol. *54*:582, 1984.
195. Roifman, C., Dembo, L., Grenadier, E., Margolis, T., Palant, A., and Iancu, T. C.: Sinus node dysfunction in a healthy pediatric population. Isr. J. Med. Sci. *20*:497, 1984.
196. Pilcher, G. F., Cook, A. J., Johnston, B. L., and Fletcher, G. F.: Twenty-four-hour continuous electrocardiography during exercise and free activity in 80 apparently healthy runners. Am. J. Cardiol. *52*:859, 1983.
197. Kantelip, J. P., Sage, E., and Duchene-Marullaz, P.: Findings on ambulatory electrocardiographic monitoring in subjects older than 80 years. Am. J. Cardiol. *57*:398, 1986.
198. Abdon, N. J.: Frequency and distribution of long-term ECG recorded cardiac arrhythmias in an elderly population. With special reference to neurological symptoms. Acta Med. Scand. *290*:175, 1981.
199. Mikolich, J. R., Jacobs, W. C., and Fletcher, G. F.: Cardiac arrhythmias in patients with acute cerebrovascular accidents. JAMA *246*:1314, 1981.
200. Kennedy, H. L., Whitlock, J. A., Sprague, M. K., Kennedy, L. J., Buckingham, T. A., and Goldberg, R. J.: Long-term followup of asymptomatic healthy subjects with frequent and complex ventricular ectopy, N. Engl. J. Med. *312*:193, 1985.
201. Bigger, J. T., Jr., Weld, F. M., and Rolnitzky, L. M.: Prevalence characteristics and significance of ventricular tachycardia (three or more complexes) detected with ambulatory electrocardiographic recording in the late hospital phase of acute myocardial infarction. Am. J. Cardiol. *48*:815, 1981.
202. Rozanski, J. J., Castellanos, A., and Myerburg, R. J.: Ventricular ectopy and sudden death. Cardiovasc. Clin. *11*:127, 1980.
203. Ruberman, W., Weinblatt, E., Frank, C. W., Goldberg, J. D., and Shapiro, S.: Repeated one hour of electrocardiograph monitoring of survivors of myocardial infarction at 6 month intervals: Arrhythmia detection and relation to prognosis. Am. J. Cardiol. *47*:1197, 1981.
204. Ruberman, W., Weinblatt, E., Goldberg, J. D., Frank, C. W., Chaudhary, B. S., and Shapiro, S.: Ventricular premature complexes and sudden death after myocardial infarction. Circulation *64*:297, 1981.
205. Weaver, W. D., Cobb, L. A., and Hallstrom, A. P.: Ambulatory arrhythmias in resuscitated victims of cardiac arrest. Circulation *66*:212, 1982.
206. Nikolic, G., Bishop, R. L., and Singh, J. B.: Sudden death recorded during Holter monitoring. Circulation *66*:218, 1982.
207. Olson, H. G., Lyons, K. P., Troop, P., Butman, S. M., and Piters, K. M.: Prognostic implications of complicated ventricular arrhythmias early after hospital discharge in acute myocardial infarction: A serial ambulatory electrocardiography study. Am. Heart J. *108*:1221, 1984.
208. Bigger, J. T., Jr., Fleiss, J. L., Kleiger, R., Miller, J. P., Rolnitzky, L. M., and the Multicenter Post-Infarction Research Group: The relationships among ventricular arrhythmias, left ventricular dysfunction and mortality in the 2 years after myocardial infarction. Circulation *69*:250, 1984.
209. Maisel, A. S., Scott, N., Gilpin, E., Ahnve, S., LeWinter, M., Henning, H., Collins, D., and Ross, J., Jr.: Complex ventricular arrhythmias in patients with Q wave versus non-Q wave myocardial infarction. Circulation *72*:963, 1985.
210. Pratt, C. M., Francis, M. J., Luck, J. C., Wyndham, C. R., Miller, R. R., and Quinones, M. A.: Analysis of ambulatory electrocardiograms in 15 patients during spontaneous ventricular fibrillation with special reference to preceding arrhythmic events. J. Am. Coll. Cardiol. *2*:789, 1983.
211. Panidis, I. P., and Morganroth, J.: Sudden death in hospitalized patients: Cardiac rhythm disturbances detected by ambulatory electrocardiographic monitoring. J. Am. Coll. Cardiol. *2*:806, 1983.
212. Lewis, B. H., Antman, E. M., and Graboys, T. B.: Detailed analysis of 24-hour ambulatory electrocardiographic recordings during ventricular fibrillation or torsade de pointes. J. Am. Coll. Cardiol. *2*:426, 1983.
213. Maron, B. J., Savage, D. D., Wolfson, J. K., and Epstein, S. E.: Prognostic significance of 24 hour ambulatory electrocardiographic monitoring in patients with hypertrophic cardiomyopathy: A prospective study. Am. J. Cardiol. *48*:252, 1981.
214. McKenna, W. J., Krikler, D. M., and Goodwin, J. F.: Arrhythmias in dilated and hypertrophic cardiomyopathy. Med. Clin. North Am. *68*:983, 1984.
215. Mason, D. T., Lee, G., Chan, M. C., and DeMaria, A. N.: Arrhythmias in patients with mitral valve prolapse: Types, evaluation and therapy. Med. Clin. North Am. *68*:1039, 1984.
216. Kim, S. G., Seiden, S. W., Matos, J. A., Waspe, L. E., and Fisher, J. D.: Discordance between ambulatory monitoring and programmed stimulation assessing efficacy of class IA antiarrhythmic agents in patients with ventricular tachycardia. J. Am. Coll. Cardiol. *6*:539, 1985.
217. Swerdlow, C. D., and Peterson, J.: Prospective comparison of Holter monitoring and electrophysiologic study in patients with coronary artery disease and sustained ventricular tachycardias. Am. J. Cardiol. *56*:577, 1985.
218. Gradman, A. H., Batsford, W. P., Rieur, E. C., Leon, L., and VanZetta, A. M.: Ambulatory electrocardiographic correlates of ventricular inducibility during programmed electrical stimulation. J. Am. Coll. Cardiol. *5*:1087, 1985.
219. Heger, J. J., Prystowsky, E. N., Jackman, W. M., Naccarelli, G. V., and Zipes, D. P.: Comparison between results obtained from electrophysiologic testing, exercise testing and ambulatory ECG recording. *In* Wenger, N. K., et al. (eds.): Ambulatory Electrocardiographic Recording. Chicago, Year Book Medical Publishers, 1981, p. 379.
220. Pratt, C. M., Declos, G., Wierman, A. M., Mahler, S. A., Seals, A. A., Leon, C. A., Young, J. B., Quinones, M. A., and Roberts, R.: The changing baseline of complex ventricular arrhythmias. A new consideration in assessing long-term drug therapy. N. Engl. J. Med. *313*:1444, 1985.
221. Morganroth, J., Michelson, E., Horowitz, L. N., Josephson, M. E., Pearlman, A. S., and Dunkman, W. B.: Limitations of routine long-term ambulatory electrocardiographic monitoring to assess ventricular ectopy frequency. Circulation *58*:408, 1978.
222. Denes, P., and Ezri, M. D.: Clinical electrophysiology . . . a decade of progress. J. Am. Coll. Cardiol. *1*:292, 1983.
223. Scheinman, M., and Morady, F.: Invasive cardiac electrophysiologic testing. Circulation *67*:1169, 1983.
224. Rahimtoola, S. H., Zipes, D. P., Akhtar, M., Burchell, H., Mason, J., Myerburg, R., O'Rourke, R., Ruskin, J., Schlant, R., and Surawicz, B.: Consensus statement of the conference on the state of the art of electrophysiological testing in the diagnosis and treatment of patients with cardiac arrhythmias. Circulation (*in press*).
225. Akhtar, M., Fisher, J. D., Gillette, P. G., Josephson, M. E., Prystowsky, E. N., Ruskin, J. N., Saksena, S., Scheinman, M. M., Waldo, A., and Zipes, D. P.: NASPE Ad Hoc Committee on Guidelines for Cardiac Electrophysiologic Studies. PACE *8*:611, 1985.
226. Waldo, A. L., Akhtar, M., Brugada, P., Henthorn, R. W., Scheinman, M., Ward, D. E., and Wellens, H. J. J.: The minimally appropriate electrophysiologic study for the initial assessment of patients with documented sustained monomorphic ventricular tachycardia. J. Am. Coll. Cardiol. *6*:1174, 1985.
227. Prystowsky, E. N., Miles, W. M., Evans, J. J., Hubbard, J. E., Skale, B. T., Windle, J. R., Heger, J. J., and Zipes, D. P.: Induction of ventricular tachycardia during programmed electrical stimulation: Analysis of pacing methods. Circulation *73*(Suppl 2):32, 1986.
228. McPherson, C. A., Rosenfeld, L. E., and Batsford, W. P.: Day-to-day reproducibility of responses to right ventricular programmed electrical stimulation: Implications for serial drug testing. Am. J. Cardiol. *55*:689, 1985.
229. Kudenchuck, P. J., Kron, J., Walance, C. G., Murphy, E. S., Morris, C. D., Griffith, K. K., and McAnulty, J. H.: Reproducibility of arrhythmia induction with intracardiac electrophysiologic testing: Patients with clinical sustained ventricular tachyarrhythmias. J. Am. Coll. Cardiol. *7*:819, 1986.
230. Schoenfeld, M. H., McGovern, B., Garan, H., and Ruskin, J. N.: Long term reproducibility of responses to programmed cardiac stimulation in spontaneous ventricular tachyarrhythmias. Am. J. Cardiol. *54*:564, 1984.
231. Horowitz, L. N.: Safety of electrophysiologic studies. Circulation *73*(Suppl. II):28, 1986.
232. Gettes, L., Zipes, D. P., Gillette, P. G., Josephson, M. E., Laks, M. M., Mirvis, D. M., Scheinman, M., Sheffield, L. T., and Wu, D.: Personnel and equipment required for electrophysiologic testing. Circulation *69*:1219A, 1984.
233. Langendorf, R., and Pick, A.: Atrioventricular block, type II (Mobitz). Its nature and clinical significance. Circulation *38*:819, 1968.
234. Strasberg, B., Amat-y-Leon, F., Dhingra, R. C., Palileo, E., Swiryn, S., Bauernfeind, R., Wyndham, C., and Rosen, K. M.: Natural history of chronic second degree atrioventricular nodal block. Circulation *63*:1043, 1981.
235. Puech, P., and Wainwright, R. J.: Clinical electrophysiology of atrioventricular block. Cardiol. Clin. *1*:209, 1983.
236. Shaw, D. B., Kekwick, C. A., Veale, D., Gowers, J., and Whistance, T.: Survival in second degree atrioventricular block. Br. Heart J. *53*:587, 1985.

237. Dhingra, R. C., Palileo, E., Strasberg, B., Swiryn, S., Bauernfeind, R. A., Wyndham, C. R., and Rosen, K. M.: Significance of the HV interval in 517 patients with chronic bifascicular block. Circulation *64*:1265, 1981.
238. Gallastegui, J., and Hariman, R. J.: Indications for intracardiac electrophysiologic studies in patients with atrioventricular and intraventricular blocks not associated with myocardial infarction. Circulation (*in press*).
239. Wellens, H. J. J., Bar, F. W., and Vanagt, E. J.: Death after ajmaline administration. Am. J. Cardiol. *45*:905, 1980.
240. Peretz, D. I., and Abdullah, A.: Management of cardioinhibitory hypersensitive carotid sinus syncope with permanent cardiac pacing—a seventeen year prospective study. Can. J. Cardiol. *1*:86, 1985.
241. Beal, M. F., Park, T. S., and Fisher, C. M.: Cerebral atheromatous embolism following carotid sinus pressure. Arch. Neurol. *38*:310, 1981.
242. Kang, P. S., Gomes, J. A., Kelen, G., and El-Sherif, N.: Role of autonomic regulatory mechanism in sinoatrial conduction and sinus nodal automaticity in sick sinus syndrome. Circulation *64*:832, 1981.
243. Desae, J. M., Scheinman, M. M., Strauss, H. C., Massie, B., and O'Young, J.: Electrophysiologic effects of combined autonomic blockade in patients with sinus node disease. Circulation *63*:953, 1981.
244. Strauss, H. C., Bigger, J. T., Sardoff, A. C., and Giardina, E. G.: Electrophysiologic evaluation of sinus node function in patients with sinus node dysfunction. Circulation *53*:763, 1976.
245. Gomes, J. A., Hariman, R. J., and Chowdry, I. A.: New application of direct sinus node recordings in man: Assessment of sinus node recovery time. Circulation *70*:663, 1984.
246. Asseman, P., Berzin, B., Desry, D., Vilarem, D., Durand, P., Delmotte, C., Sarkis, E. H., Lekieffre, J., and Thery, C.: Persistent sinus nodal electrograms during abnormally prolonged postpacing atrial pauses in sick sinus syndrome in humans: Sinoatrial block versus overdrive suppression. Circulation *68*:33, 1983.
247. Kerr, C. R., Grant, A. O., Wenger, T. L., and Strauss, H. C.: Sinus node dysfunction. Cardiol. Clin. *1*:187, 1983.
248. Wellens, H. J. J., Bär, F. W. H. M., and Lie, K. I.: The value of the electrocardiogram in the differential diagnosis of a tachycardia with a widened QRS complex. Am. J. Med. *64*:27, 1978.
249. Miles, W. M., Prystowsky, E. N., Heger, J. J., and Zipes, D. P.: Evaluation of the patient with a wide QRS tachycardia. Med. Clin. North Am. *68*:1015, 1984.
250. Horowitz, L. N.: Intracardiac electrophysiologic studies for drug selection in ventricular tachycardia. Circulation *75*:III–134, 1987.
251. Kramer, J. B., Corr, P. B., Cox, J. L., Witkowski, F. X., and Cain, M. E.: Simultaneous computer mapping to facilitate intraoperative localization of accessory pathways in patients with Wolff-Parkinson-White syndrome. Am. J. Cardiol. *56*:571, 1985.
252. Gallagher, J. J.: Accessory pathway tachycardia: Techniques of electrophysiologic study and mechanisms. Circulation *75*:III–31, 1987.
253. Zipes, D. P., Cobb, L. A., Garson, A., Jr., Gillette, P. C., James, T. N., Lazzara, R., Rink, L., and 16th Bethesda Conference: Cardiovascular abnormalities in the athlete: Recommendations regarding eligibility for competition. Task Force VI: Arrhythmias. J. Am. Col. Cardiol. *6*:1225, 1985.
254. Uther, J. B., Richards, M. D., Denniss, A. R., and Ross, D. L.: The prognostic significance of programmed ventricular stimulation after myocardial infarction: A review. Circulation *75*:III–161, 1987.
255. Bhandari, A., and Rahimtoola, S. H.: Indications for intracardiac electrophysiological testing in survivors of acute myocardial infarction. Circulation *75*:III–166, 1987.
255a. Denniss, A. R., Richards, D. A., Cody, D. V., Russell, P. A., Young, A. A., Cooper, M. J., Ross, D. L., and Uther, J. B.: Prognostic significance of ventricular tachycardia and fibrillation induced at programmed stimulation and delayed potentials detected on the signal averaged ECGs of survivors of acute myocardial infarction. Circulation *74*:731, 1986.
256. Lerman, B., Belardinelli, L., West, G., Berne, R., and DiMarco, J.: Adenosine sensitive ventricular tachycardia. Circulation *74*:270, 1986.
257. Kapoor, W. N., Karpf, M., Wieland, S., Peterson, J. R., and Levey, G. S.: A prospective evaluation and followup of patients with syncope. N. Engl. J. Med. *309*:197, 1983.
258. Eagle, K. A., Black, H. R., Cook, E. F., and Goldman, L.: Evaluation of prognostic classifications for patients with syncope. Am. J. Med. *79*:455, 1985.
259. Day, S. C., Cook, E. F., Funkenstein, H., and Goldman, L.: Evaluation and outcome of emergency room patients with transient loss of consciousness. Am. J. Med. *73*:15, 1982.
260. Lipsitz, L. A.: Syncope in the elderly. Ann. Intern. Med. *99*:92, 1983.
261. Gibson, T. C., and Heitzman, M. R.: Diagnostic efficacy of 24-hour electrocardiographic monitoring for syncope. Am. J. Cardiol. *53*:1013, 1984.
262. Reid, P. R.: Indications for intracardiac electrophysiological studies: Unexplained palpitations. Circulation (*in press*).
263. Schlant, R. C.: Indications for intracardiac electrophysiological studies: Unexplained palpitations. Circulation (*in press*).
264. Gulamhusein, S., Naccarelli, G. V., Ko, P. T., Prystowsky, E. N., Zipes, D. P., Barnett, H. J. M., Heger, J. J., and Klein, G. J.: Value and limitations of the clinical electrophysiologic study in the assessment of patients with unexplained syncope. Am. J. Med. *73*:700, 1982.
265. DiMarco, J. P., Garan, H., and Ruskin, J. N.: Approach to the patient with recurrent syncope of unknown cause. Mod. Concepts Cardiovasc. Dis. *52*:11, 1983.
266. Brugada, P., Abdollah, H., Heddle, B., and Wellens, H. J. J.: Results of ventricular stimulation protocol using a maximum of 4 premature stimuli in patients without documented or suspected ventricular arrhythmias. Am. J. Cardiol. *52*:1214, 1983.
267. Brugada, P., Green, M., Abdollah, H., and Wellens, H. J. J.: Significance of ventricular arrhythmias initiated by programmed ventricular stimulation: The importance of the type of ventricular arrhythmia induced and the number of premature stimuli required. Circulation *69*:87, 1984.
268. Bigger, J. T., Jr., Reiffel, J. A., Livelli, F. D., Jr., and Wang, P. J.: Sensitivity, specificity and reproducibility of programmed ventricular stimulation. Circulation *73*(Suppl 2):73, 1986.
269. Wellens, H. J. J., Brugada, P., and Stevenson, W. G.: Programmed electrical stimulation of the heart in patients with life-threatening ventricular arrhythmias: What is the significance of induced arrhythmias and what is the correct stimulation protocol? Circulation *72*:1, 1985.
270. DiMarco, J. P., Garan, H., and Ruskin, J. N.: Morbidity associated with electrophysiologic procedures. Am. J. Cardiol. *49*:959, 1982.
271. Jenkins, J. M., Wu, D., and Arzbacher, R. C.: Computer diagnosis of supraventricular and ventricular arrhythmias. A new esophageal technique. Circulation *60*:977, 1979.
272. Hammill, S. C., and Pritchett, E. L.: Simplified esophageal electrocardiography using bipolar recording leads. Ann. Intern. Med. *95*:14, 1981.
273. Benson, D. W., Jr.: Transesophageal electrocardiography and cardiac pacing: State of the art. Circulation *75*:III–86, 1987.
274. Gallagher, J. J., Smith, W. M., Kerr, C. R., Kasell, J., Cook, L., Reiter, M., Sterba, R., and Harte, M.: Esophageal pacing: A diagnostic and therapeutic tool. Circulation *65*:336, 1982.
275. Mirvis, V. M.: Body surface distributions of repolarization potentials after acute myocardial infarction: II. Relationship between isopotential mapping and ST segment potential summation methods. Circulation *63*:623, 1981.
276. Eifler, W. J., Macchi, E., Ritsema van Eck, H. J., Horacek, B. M., and Rautaharju, P. M.: Mechanism of generation of body surface electrocardiographic P waves in normal middle and lower sinus rhythms. Circ. Res. *48*:168, 1981.
277. Benson, D. W., Jr., Sterba, R., Gallagher, J. J., Walston, A., and Spach, M. S.: Localization of the site of preexcitation with body surface maps in patients with Wolff-Parkinson-White syndrome. Circulation *65*:1259, 1982.
278. Abildskov, J. A., and Green, L. S.: The recognition of arrhythmia vulnerability by body surface electrocardiographic mapping. Circulation (*in press*).
279. Spach, M. S., and Barr, R.: Discussant paper of the recognition of arrhythmia vulnerability by body surface electrocardiographic mapping. Circulation *75*:III–84, 1987.
280. Hombach, V., Braun, V., Hopp, H. W., Gil-Sanchez, D., Scholl, H., Behrenbeck, D. W., Pauchert, M., and Hilger, H. H.: The applicability of the signal-averaging technique in clinical cardiology. Clin. Cardiol. *5*:107, 1982.
281. Flowers, N. C., Shvartsman, V., Kennelly, B. M., Sohi, G. S., and Horan, L. G.: Surface recording of His-Purkinje activity on an every-beat basis without digital averaging. Circulation *63*:948, 1981.
282. Simson, M. B.: Signal averaging. Circulation *75*:III–69, 1987.
283. Flowers, N. C.: Procedure for arrhythmia detection and diagnosis. Signal averaging. Circulation *75*:III–74, 1987.
284. Cain, M. E., Ambos, H. D., Markham, J., Fischer, A. E., and Sobel, B. E.: Quantification of differences in frequency content of signal-averaged electrocardiograms in patients with compared to those without sustained ventricular tachycardia. Am. J. Cardiol. *55*:1500, 1985.
285. Simson, M. B., and Untereker, W. J., Spielman, S. R., Horowitz, L. N., Marcus, N. H., Falcone, R. A., Harken, A. H., and Josephson, M. E.: Relation between late potentials on the body surface and directly recorded fragmented electrograms in patients with ventricular tachycardia. Am. J. Cardiol. *51*:105, 1983.
286. Poll, D. S., Marchlinski, F. E., Falcone, R. A., Josephson, M. E., and Simson, M. B.: Abnormal signal-averaged electrocardiograms in patients with nonischemic congestive cardiomyopathy: Relationship to sustained ventricular tachyarrhythmias. Circulation *72*:1308, 1985.
287. Marcus, N. H., Falcone, R. A., Harken, A. H., Josephson, M. E., and Simson, M. B.: Body surface late potentials: Effects of endocardial resection in patients with ventricular tachycardia. Circulation *70*:632, 1984.
288. Breithardt, G., Schwarzmaier, J., Borggrefe, M., Haerten, K., and Seipel, L.: Prognostic significance of late ventricular potentials after acute myocardial infarction. Eur. Heart J. *4*:487, 1983.
289. Gomes, J. A., Mehra, R., Barreca, P., El Sherif, N., Hariman, R., and Holtzman, R.: Quantitative analysis of the high frequency components of the signal-averaged QRS complex in patients with acute myocardial infarction: A prospective study. Circulation *72*:105, 1985.

21 MANAGEMENT OF CARDIAC ARRHYTHMIAS: Pharmacological, Electrical, and Surgical Techniques

by DOUGLAS P. ZIPES, M.D.

PHARMACOLOGICAL THERAPY

PRINCIPLES OF CLINICAL PHARMACOKINETICS

Pharmacological treatment of a patient with a cardiac arrhythmia has as its primary objectives to reach an effective and well-tolerated serum drug concentration as rapidly as possible and to maintain this concentration for as long as required without producing adverse effects. In many but not all situations and not with all drugs,[1] serum concentration after equilibration strongly correlates with the antiarrhythmic as well as adverse effects of the drug. Therapeutic serum concentrations for the most important available antiarrhythmic agents are listed in Table 21–1 and are based on concentrations of drugs that exert therapeutic effects without adverse effects in a majority of patients. However, the therapeutic concentration for any individual patient is the amount of drug required *for that patient* to suppress or terminate the cardiac arrhythmia without producing adverse effects. For a specific patient, one must consider the response both of the patient and of the arrhythmia to the drug, and the actual serum concentration of the drug is often of secondary importance. In some patients measured serum concentrations can be useful to establish concentrations needed for prophylaxis, to judge the sensitivity or resistance of the arrhythmia to the drug, and to evaluate symptoms that suggest drug toxicity. Serum concentrations can also be used to determine the effects of changing physiological states on drug concentrations, establish drug compliance or abuse, search for drug interactions, and establish the importance of physiologically active metabolites of the parent compound.[2] Active metabolites may be suspected when the clinical effect of the drug outlasts the therapeutic serum concentration of the drug or when results immediately following intravenous drug administration differ from those after oral administration of the drug.[3]

Normally, because antiarrhythmic agents have a narrow toxic-therapeutic relationship, important complications of therapy may result from amounts of drug that only slightly exceed the amount necessary to produce beneficial effects; lesser concentrations are often subtherapeutic. It is obvious that careful dosing with these agents is essential to maintain adequate but nontoxic amounts of drug in the body, a task facilitated by understanding drug pharmacokinetics, which consists of a quantitative assessment of drug absorption, distribution, metabolism, and excretion. Alterations in the rate of any of these processes may account for significant intra- and interpatient variations in serum concentrations.[3–5] In addition, changes in the functional status of any of the organs involved, primarily the liver and kidneys, may significantly alter dose requirements in a given patient.

ABSORPTION. Drug absorption from the intestinal tract occurs for most drugs with a half-time of absorption in the range of 20 to 30 minutes. Completeness of absorption may vary between 50 and over 90 per cent, depending on the drug, with most absorption occurring in the small intestine. Different preparations of the same drug, e.g., digoxin or phenytoin, may undergo different rates of absorption in the same patient because the tablet preparations have different dissolution rates. Thus, two brands of drug may not result in the same serum concentration.[4] By altering the properties of the tablet, a slow release form of a drug ordinarily rapidly absorbed and metabolized, such as procainamide, can be developed. Large amounts of some orally administered drugs, such as propranolol or verapamil, are transformed to inactive metabolites in the liver before they reach the systemic circulation—the so-called first-pass hepatic effect. For such an agent, much more drug must be administered orally than intravenously to achieve the same physiological effect.

Disease states and other factors can alter the rate and completeness of drug absorption. For example, heart failure can cause mucosal edema of the gut and impair the absorption of orally administered drugs, as can decreased intestinal blood flow. Malabsorption syndromes, concomitant use of other drugs, or changes in gut motility or flora caused by diarrheal states, antibiotics, or the use of cathartics may alter absorption. Since most antiarrhythmic agents are basic compounds, they are ionized and poorly absorbed at normal gastric pH, and some drugs may decompose at gastric pH. Conditions that delay gastric emptying increase the absorption lag phase between ingestion of these drugs and their arrival in the small intestine, where most absorption takes place, and therefore may decrease absorption. In patients with severe hypotension, shock, or cardiac arrest, impaired tissue perfusion prevents reliable absorption of intramuscularly administered agents; these patients should receive all medications by the intravenous (IV) route.

BIOAVAILABILITY. The rate of drug absorption, determined by the

TABLE 21–1 DOSAGE AND THERAPEUTIC SERUM CONCENTRATIONS

Usual Dose Ranges

	Intravenous (mg)		Oral (mg)	
Drug	Loading	Maintenance	Loading	Maintenance
Lidocaine	1 to 3 mg/kg at 20 to 50 mg/min	1 to 4 mg/min	N/A	N/A
Quinidine	6 to 10 mg/kg at 0.3 to 0.5 mg/kg/min		600 to 1000	300 to 600 q6h
Procainamide	6 to 13 mg/kg at 0.2 to 0.5 mg/kg/min	2 to 6 mg/min	50 to 1000	350 to 1000 q3–6h
Disopyramide	1 to 2 mg/kg over 15 min* 1 to 2 mg/kg over 45 min	1 mg/kg/hr*		100 to 400 q6–8h
Phenytoin	100 mg q5min for ≤ 1000 mg		1000	100 to 400 q12–24h
Propranolol	0.25 to 0.5 mg, q5min for ≤0.15 to 0.20 mg/kg			10 to 200 q6–8h
Bretylium	5 to 10 mg/kg at 1 to 2 mg/kg/min	½ to 2 mg/min	N/A	4 mg/kg/day*
Verapamil	10 mg over 1 to 2 min	0.005 mg/kg/min		80 to 120 q6–8h
Amiodarone**	5 to 10 mg/kg over 20–30 min then 1 gm/24 hr		800 to 1600 QD for 1 to 3 weeks	200 to 400 QD
Mexiletine**	500 mg	0.5 to 1.0 gm/24 hr	400 to 600	150 to 300 q6–8h
Tocainide**	750 mg		400 to 600	400 to 600 q8–12h
Flecainide**	2 mg/kg			100 to 200 q12h
Encainide*	0.6 to 0.9 mg/kg			25 to 75 q6–8h
Ethmozine*			300	100 to 400 q8h
Lorcainide*	1 to 2 mg/kg			100 q8h
Propafenone*	1 to 2 mg/kg		600 to 900	150 to 300 q8–12h

*Investigational.
**Intravenous administration; investigational only.

time required to achieve maximum serum concentration, and the fraction of drug absorbed influence the drug's *bioavailability*, which is a measure of the amount of drug that reaches the systemic circulation intact. Bioavailability of a drug is influenced by factors such as lack of pill dissolution, metabolism by gut mucosa, hepatic metabolism and binding, and absorption. It is a most important property of the drug. Absorption is thus only one component affecting bioavailability. The fraction of an orally administered drug reaching the systemic circulation intact, or *systemic availability*, can be calculated (assuming equal clearances for IV and oral forms of drug) by comparing the area under the plasma concentration curve achieved with oral and intravenous administrations from the following relationship: systemic availability equals the area under the plasma concentration curve following oral administration/the area under the plasma concentration curve following IV administration times 100 (assuming equal IV and oral doses).

DRUG DISTRIBUTION. Most antiarrhythmic drugs in the therapeutic range are eliminated according to *first-order kinetics*, which means that the amount of drug eliminated per unit time is directly proportional to the amount (or concentration) of drug in the body. More drug in the body results in more drug excreted by the kidneys or metabolized by the liver, so that the *fraction* of drug eliminated per unit of time remains constant regardless of the amount of drug in the body. For example, one-half the drug may be eliminated in 6 hours whether the total amount of drug in the body is 4 gm or 10 gm, resulting in elimination of 2 gm in the first example and 5 gm in the second. As a consequence, the elimination half-life, or time required to eliminate half the body load (or to halve the plasma concentration) of such a drug is constant and independent of the total body load. The following discussion will assume first-order kinetics unless otherwise stated. (*Zero-order kinetics* indicates that the reaction occurs at a constant, usually maximal, rate and cannot increase further despite increased drug concentrations. Such nonlinear or saturable kinetics may occur at high concentrations of the drug, which at usual concentrations exhibits first-order kinetics.)

Generally two models, a *one-compartment open model* and a *two-compartment open model*, are used with relative accuracy to describe and predict serum concentrations at a given time for a variety of dose regimens. Even though these models are oversimplified representations of drug disposition, they provide guidelines for choosing loading doses and maintenance dose schedules for a given patient. In the one-compartment open model, drugs are considered to enter and to be eliminated from a single homogeneous unit that represents the entire body. Drugs entering the compartment are considered to be distributed immediately throughout the compartment, making the concentration of the drug equal to the amount of drug in the compartment divided by the volume of the compartment. The latter equals the amount of the drug in the compartment divided by the drug concentration.

In reality, a one-compartment open model is not entirely appropriate because a certain amount of time is needed to distribute the drug throughout the volume of the compartment. However, the one-compartment model predicts plasma concentration as a function of time and dose, if distribution is significantly faster than the rate of administration or of excretion, which is the case for many antiarrhythmic drugs.

If the rate of drug administration is rapid in relation to drug distribution (e.g., intravenous administration), a two-compartment open model more accurately predicts drug concentrations (Fig. 21–1). In this model the drug enters the system by the central compartment and can leave the system only by distribution into a peripheral compartment or elimination from the central compartment. The central compartment, in dynamic equilibrium with the more slowly equilibrating peripheral compartment, is assumed to consist of the blood volume and extracellular fluid of highly perfused tissues such as heart, lungs, kidneys, and liver, while the peripheral compartment, acting as a reservoir, consists of less well perfused tissue such as muscle, skin, and adipose tissue. The first-order rate constants $K_{1\rightarrow 2}$ and $K_{2\rightarrow 1}$ determine the rate of transfer of drug between the central and peripheral compartments or vice versa, with K_e representing the overall elimination rate constant. K_e relates the

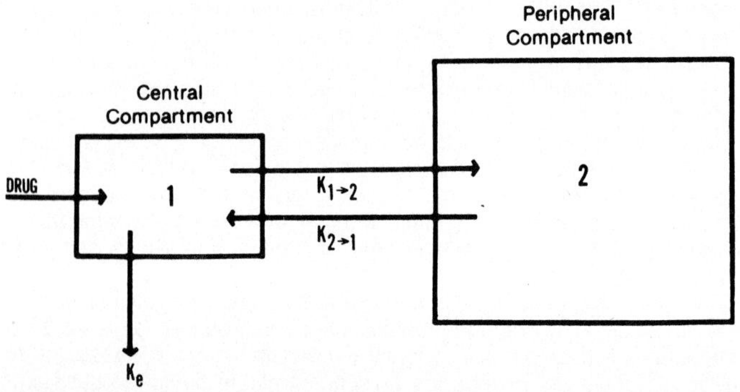

FIGURE 21–1. Two-compartment open model. A smaller central compartment into which drug is administered and from which it is eliminated (K_e) connects in dynamic equilibrium with a larger peripheral compartment.

Time to Peak Plasma Concentration (Oral) (Hr)	Effective Serum or Plasma Concentration (μg/ml)	Elimination Half-life After Oral Dose (hr)	Bioavailability (%)	Major Route of Elimination
N/A	1 to 5	1 to 2	N/A	Liver
1.5 to 3.0	3 to 6	5 to 9	60 to 80	Liver
1	4 to 10	3 to 5	70 to 85	Kidneys
1 to 2	2 to 5	8 to 9	80 to 90	Kidneys
8 to 12	10 to 20	18 to 36	50 to 70	Liver
2 to 4	0.04 to 0.90	3 to 6	20 to 50	Liver
	0.5 to 1.5	8 to 14	25	Kidneys
1 to 2	0.10 to 0.15	3 to 8	10 to 35	Liver
4	1 to 2.5	50 days	35 to 65	Liver
2 to 4	0.75 to 2	10 to 17	90	Liver
0.5 to 2	4 to 10	11	90	Liver
3 to 4	0.2 to 1.0	20	95	Liver
1 to 2	0.5 to 1.0	3 to 4	40	Liver
	0.1			
	0.3 to 1.0	5 to 12	50	Liver
1 to 3	0.2 to 3.0	5 to 8	25 to 75	Liver

Results presented may vary according to doses, disease state, and IV or oral administration.

sum of all methods of irreversible drug elimination from the central compartment to the concentration of drug in that compartment (Fig. 21–1). For antiarrhythmic drugs, the peripheral compartment is generally larger than the central compartment. The concepts of distribution volumes and drug movement are more complex in the two-compartment open model than in the one-compartment open model. The two-compartment model may behave similarly to the one-compartment model when drugs are infused slowly or given orally and K_1 approximates K_2, but pronounced differences exist when injections are given rapidly.

Following administration of drugs for which the kinetics are described by a two-compartment model, the curve of plasma drug concentration demonstrates two distinct phases: an early phase (alpha, or distribution phase), characterized by rapidly falling plasma drug concentrations due to distribution between the central compartment and the peripheral compartment, and a second phase (beta, or elimination phase) of slower decline in plasma drug concentration, representing primarily elimination of drugs from the central compartment (Fig. 21–2). *Alpha*

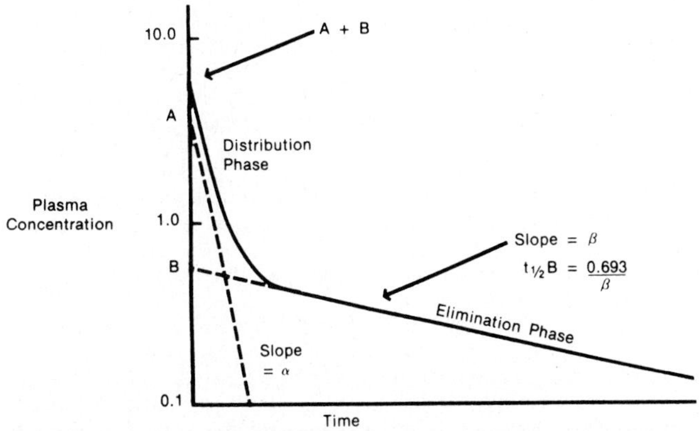

FIGURE 21–2. Schematic diagram of the semilogarithmic plot of drug plasma concentration as a function of time following rapid intravenous injection, according to the principles outlined for a two-compartment open model. (From Gibaldi, M., and Perrier, D.: Drugs and the pharmaceutical sciences. *In* Pharmacokinetics, Vol. 1. New York, Marcel Dekker, 1975.)

is often referred to as the *rate constant for distribution* and *beta* as the *rate constant for elimination*. During the latter beta phase, when the drug is in distribution equilibrium, serum concentrations correlate with the pharmacological effects of the drug. The distribution of quinidine is shown in Figure 21–3.

The extent of extravascular distribution of a drug is obtained by measuring the apparent *volume of distribution*, which is the hypothetical volume into which a dose of drug would have to be diluted to give the observed plasma concentration. It is determined by the dose administered divided by the plasma concentration at time 0. The latter equals the sum of A and B on the logarithmic plasma concentration axis obtained by extrapolating the alpha and beta phases back to 0 time (Fig. 21–2). It is also calculated by dividing the systemic clearance of the drug by beta, the rate constant of elimination.[4] A large volume of distribution indicates a wide distribution and extensive tissue uptake of the drug and often exceeds by several times the actual amount of total body water. The large volume of distribution for most antiarrhythmic agents indicates that they are present in higher concentrations in some tissues than in the plasma. The volume of distribution is dependent on the relative serum and tissue binding characteristics of the drug and may be constricted in some patients, such as those with renal failure, during which a change in serum protein or tissue binding may occur. Quinidine decreases the volume of distribution of digoxin, probably as a result of a decrease in tissue binding of digoxin.

DRUG METABOLISM AND EXCRETION. Approximately 97 per cent of the dose of any drug is removed from the body in a time equal to five half-lives. *Serum elimination half-life* is defined as the time interval for 50 per cent of the drug present in the body at the beginning of the interval to be eliminated. After one half-life, 50 per cent of the drug remains in the body (assuming no further drug is administered), after two half-lives 25 per cent remains, after three half-lives 12.5 per cent remains, and so forth. Half-life is determined from the relationship $t\frac{1}{2} = 0.693/\text{beta}$ for a two-compartment model (Fig. 21–2). Since changes in drug distribution influence elimination half-life, the equation can be rewritten as $t\frac{1}{2} = 0.693 \times$ volume of distribution/total body clearance.

Drug clearance is analogous to renal clearance and is the volume of blood totally cleared of drug in unit time. It is the sum of the clearances for each process by which the drug is eliminated and can be calculated from the relationship: clearance = dose of the drug/area under the plasma concentration time curve (AUC). Expressed differently, clearance equals volume of distribution × beta, or volume of distribution × 0.693/half-life. A larger volume of distribution increases the elimination half-life at a given clearance. The larger volume of

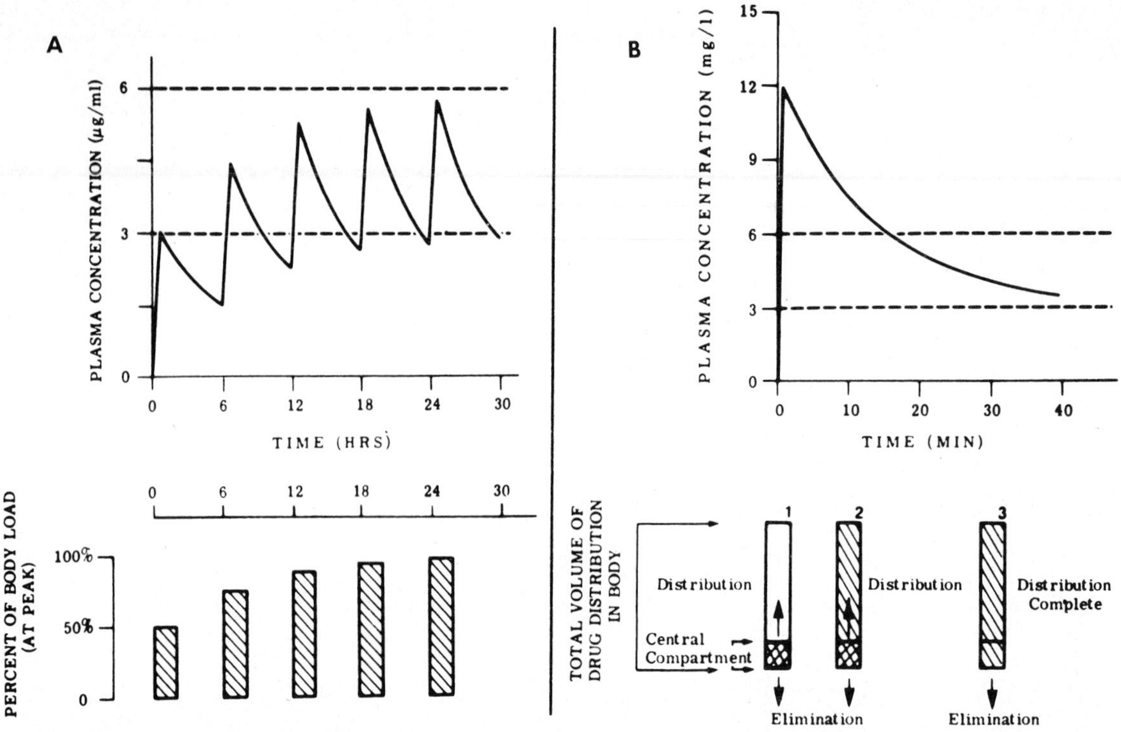

FIGURE 21–3. *A*, Changes in plasma concentration over time after beginning treatment with quinidine. *Top*, Quinidine plasma concentration over time, with the dashed line indicating the therapeutic range. *Bottom*, The hatched bars represent the body load immediately after each dose of quinidine, expressed as a percentage of the load after a dose when a steady state has been achieved. Quinidine is administered every 6 hours (the half-life in this case). Four half-lives, or 24 hours, are required to achieve a body load of quinidine that exceeds 90 per cent of the load at steady state. *B*, *Top*, Plasma concentrations produced by administering a full intravenous loading dose of quinidine as a bolus, with the therapeutic range shown by a dashed line. *Bottom*, The numbered vertical boxes indicate the volume of distribution of quinidine. Just after the drug is given, it is dissolved only in the small central compartment, as in box 1, and very high peak concentrations are achieved (in the toxic range). The drug then distributes throughout the rest of the body. Distribution has a half-life of about 8 minutes and is complete by 30 minutes (box 3). Quinidine concentration is now in the therapeutic range, and further decreases in plasma concentration are due solely to drug elimination. (From Nattel, S., and Zipes, D. P.: Clinical pharmacology of old and new antiarrhythmic drugs. Cardiovasc. Clin. *11*:221, 1980.)

distribution of antiarrhythmic drugs accounts for the relatively long half-life despite their large clearance rates. Quinidine prolongs digitoxin's half-life by decreasing total body clearance.[4] Clearance of drugs with high extraction ratios strongly depends on blood flow to the organ from which they are eliminated, such as propranolol, verapamil, or lidocaine in the liver. For antiarrhythmic drugs that have a high renal extraction ratio, such as procainamide and quinidine, reduction of renal flow decreases their clearance.

Elimination Half-Life. Function of the organ system that eliminates a given drug from the body determines the elimination half-life. Primary routes of elimination are hepatic metabolism and renal clearance. The kidneys may remove unchanged drug or metabolites. For drugs rapidly metabolized in the liver, hepatic blood flow limits the rate of drug elimination. Disorders that reduce liver blood flow (e.g., low cardiac output, hepatic disease with portacaval shunting) markedly slow the elimination of such drugs. Drugs with a short half-life are convenient to use by intravenous infusion but not by chronic oral dosing, since the short half-life requires frequent oral doses to maintain a fairly constant plasma concentration. Generally, maintenance dosing involves giving a certain amount of the drug at a time interval that equals the elimination half-life. However, with drugs that have very long half-lives, such as 12 hours, this may result in excessive peak values shortly after administration and consequent side effects.[3] Maintaining constant plasma concentrations is necessary because of the narrow toxic-therapeutic ratios exhibited by antiarrhythmic agents. Also, some drugs such as encainide (p. 641) have active metabolites with half-lives considerably longer than the parent compound, allowing dosing intervals to be more widely spaced than those predicted by the half-life of the parent drug. Procainamide (p. 630) has an active metabolite, *N*-acetylprocainamide (NAPA) that is eliminated unchanged by the kidneys and may accumulate in high concentrations in patients with renal disease. The rate and extent of metabolism of the same drug may vary greatly from patient to patient owing to a variety of factors, including environment, genetics, age, disease states, and influence of other drugs given concomitantly. A genetically controlled acetyltransferase enzyme system influences the metabolism of some drugs, making about half the American population "rapid" and half "slow acetylators." Rapid acetylators metabolize a greater proportion of a drug dose than do slow acetylators, who may require less drug to achieve any desired serum level or pharmacological effect. Also, rapid acetylators may be more prone to develop reactions from the metabolites of drugs[4] or are less likely to develop side effects from the parent compound for a constant drug dose.

DRUG BINDING. Drugs exist in plasma both in the free form and bound to plasma proteins. Only free drug is capable of distributing into tissues and exerting a pharmacological action. Some drugs, e.g., verapamil and disopyramide, have optical isomers, with different potencies and effects. Virtually all assays for drug concentration in the blood measure *both* free and protein-bound drug. For antiarrhythmic drugs, the fraction of drug that is bound varies greatly among the different agents but is fairly constant for individual drugs over the clinically relevant range of plasma concentrations with the exception of phenytoin, lidocaine, and disopyramide. With these drugs, binding sites become saturated at high concentrations and therefore a doubling of total drug concentration represents more than a doubling of unbound drug. Total serum concentrations of a given drug therefore generally correlate well with its clinical effects, and it has not been necessary to develop assays to measure free drug concentrations for antiarrhythmic agents. Some drugs, such as quinidine, bind to an α_1 glycoprotein that increases in acute disease states, which may decrease the concentration of free drug.

When a constant dose of a drug is administered repeatedly (orally or parenterally) at a constant dosing interval, accumulation occurs until drug concentration approaches a constant steady-state level, at which time the rate of drug administration equals the rate of drug elimination. The time it takes to reach steady state is a function of the half-life of the drug; 94 per cent of steady state is achieved after four half-lives and 99 per cent after seven half-lives. A drug with a long half-life takes longer to reach steady state than does one with a short half-life. The average steady-state concentration of a drug equals the fraction of the dose absorbed (F) $\times$ the maintenance dose ($dose_m$) divided by the total body clearance (Cl_s) $\times$ the dosing interval (τ).

$$\text{Average steady-state concentration} = \frac{F \times dose_m}{Cl_s \times \tau} = \frac{F \times dose_m t_{1/2}}{0.693 \times V_d \tau}$$

If the drug is given intravenously,[4]

$$\text{Steady-state concentration} = \frac{\text{Infusion rate}}{Cl_s} = \frac{\text{Infusion rate } t_{1/2}}{0.693\ V_d}$$

Finally, it is important to stress that drug pharmacokinetics may differ in normal healthy volunteers compared to patients who have a variety of illnesses. Therefore, information derived from patients as well as normal subjects must be considered when one is planning dosing regimens.

GENERAL CONSIDERATIONS REGARDING ANTIARRHYTHMIC DRUGS

The available antiarrhythmic drugs can be divided into those that exert blocking actions predominantly on sodium, potassium, or calcium channels, and those that block beta-adrenoreceptors.[6] Subclassifications[7] are limited because they are based on the electrophysiological effects exerted by an arbitrary concentration of the drug, generally on a normal Purkinje fiber, often not even in an arrhythmic preparation. The effects of these drugs depend on tissue type, species, the degree of acute or chronic damage, heart rate, membrane potential, the ionic composition of the extracellular milieu, and other factors. Many drugs exhibit actions that belong in multiple categories, or operate indirectly, such as by altering hemodynamics, myocardial metabolism, or autonomic neural transmission. Some drugs have active metabolites that exert different effects from the parent compound.[2] Not all drugs in the same class have identical effects, while some drugs in different classes have similar actions. In vitro studies on healthy fibers usually establish the properties of antiarrhythmic agents rather than their antiarrhythmic properties.[6]

Despite these limitations, subclassifications provide a useful communication shorthand.[7–9]

Class I drugs that block the fast sodium channel:

A. Drugs that reduce $\dot{V}_{max}$ and prolong action potential duration: quinidine, procainamide, disopyramide.

B. Drugs that do not reduce $\dot{V}_{max}$ and that shorten action potential duration: tocainide, mexiletine, phenytoin, lidocaine, ethmozine.

C. Drugs that reduce $\dot{V}_{max}$, primarily slow conduction, and may prolong refractoriness minimally: flecainide, encainide, lorcainide, propafenone.

Class II drugs that block beta-adrenoreceptors: propranolol, timolol, metoprolol, and others.

Class III drugs that block potassium channels and prolong repolarization: sotalol, amiodarone, bretylium.

Class IV drugs that block the slow calcium channel: verapamil, diltiazem, nifedipine, bepridil.

A recently proposed model suggests that antiarrhythmic drugs cross the cell membrane and interact with receptors in the membrane channels when the latter are in the rested, activated, or inactivated states and that each of these interactions is characterized by a different association and dissociation rate constant (Fig. 20–10, p. 590). Such interactions are voltage- and time-dependent. Transitions among rested, activated, and inactivated states are governed by standard Hodgkin-Huxley–type equations. When the drug is bound (associated) to a receptor site at or very close to the ionic channel (the drug probably does not actually plug the channel), the latter cannot conduct, even in the activated state.[10, 11]

USE DEPENDENCE. Some drugs exert greater inhibitory effects on the upstroke of the action potential at more rapid rates of stimulation and after longer periods of stimulation, a characteristic called *use dependence*. Use-dependence means that depression of $\dot{V}_{max}$ is greater after the channel has been "used," i.e., after action potential depolarization rather than after a rest period. It is possible that this use-dependence results from preferential interaction of the antiarrhythmic drug with either the open or the inactive channel and little interaction with the resting channels of the unstimulated cell. Agents in class IB exhibit fast kinetics of onset and offset or use-dependent block of the fast channel, that is, they bind and dissociate quickly from the receptors; class IC drugs have slow kinetics, and class IA drugs are intermediate.[8] With increased time spent in diastole (slower rate), a greater proportion of receptors become drug-free and the drug exerts less effect. Cells with reduced membrane potentials recover more slowly than cells with more negative membrane potentials[12] (Fig. 20–10, p. 590).

Given the fact that enhanced automaticity or reentry can cause cardiac arrhythmias, mechanisms by which antiarrhythmic agents suppress arrhythmias can be postulated.[13] Antiarrhythmic agents can slow the spontaneous discharge frequency of an automatic pacemaker by depressing the slope of diastolic depolarization, shifting the threshold voltage toward zero, or hyperpolarizing the resting membrane potential (Fig. 20–13, p. 594). Mechanisms by which different drugs suppress normal or abnormal automaticity may not be the same. In general, however, most antiarrhythmic agents in therapeutic doses depress the automatic firing rate of spontaneously discharging ectopic sites while minimally affecting the discharge rate of the normal sinus node. Slow-channel blockers like verapamil, beta blockers like propranolol, and some antiarrhythmic agents like amiodarone also depress spontaneous discharge of the normal sinus node, while drugs that exert vagolytic effects, such as disopyramide or quinidine, may increase the sinus discharge rate.

As mentioned earlier, reentry depends critically on the timing interrelationships between refractoriness and conduction velocity, the presence of unidirectional block in one of the pathways, and other factors that influence refractoriness and conduction, such as excitability. An antiarrhythmic agent can stop reentry that is already present or prevent it from starting if the drug improves *or* depresses conduction. For example, *improved conduction* can (1) eliminate the unidirectional block so that reentry cannot begin or (2) facilitate conduction in the reentrant loop so that the returning wavefront reenters too quickly, encroaches on fibers still refractory, and becomes extinguished. A drug that *depresses conduction* can transform the unidirectional block to bidirectional block and thus terminate reentry or prevent it from occurring by creating an area of complete block in the reentrant pathway. Conversely, a drug that slows conduction without producing block or lengthening refractoriness significantly may promote reentry. Finally, most antiarrhythmic agents share the ability to prolong refractoriness relative to their effects on action potential duration, i.e., the ratio of effective refractory period to action potential duration exceeds 1.0. If a drug *prolongs refractoriness* of fibers in the reentrant pathway, the pathway may not recover excitability in time to be depolarized by the reentering impulse, and the reentrant propagation ceases.

When one is discussing any of the properties of a drug, it is important that the situation and/or model from which conclusions are drawn be defined with care.[14] Electrophysiological, hemodynamic, autonomic, pharmacokinetic, and adverse effects all may differ in normal subjects compared to patients, in normal tissue compared to abnormal tissue, in muscle compared to specialized fibers, and in different species.

LIDOCAINE

ELECTROPHYSIOLOGICAL ACTIONS (Tables 21–2 and 21–3). Lidocaine does not affect normal sinus nodal automaticity but does depress both normal and abnormal forms of automaticity such as early and late afterdepolarizations[13, 15] in Purkinje fibers in vitro. External environment significantly influences the effects of lidocaine. It exhibits only a modest depressant effect on $\dot{V}_{max}$ and has no effect on maximal diastolic potential of normal muscle and specialized tissue in concentrations of about 1.5 μg/ml. However, faster rates of stimulation, reduced pH,[16] increased extracellular K^+ concentration, and reduced membrane potential—all changes that may result from ischemia—increase the ability of lidocaine to block the fast sodium channels, perhaps in part accounting for its efficacy in patients with acute myocardial infarction (Ch. 38).

Lidocaine may increase refractoriness in partially depolarized fibers. Lidocaine appears to have greatest affinity for open channels but dissociates rapidly from them when membrane potential returns to its maximum diastolic value. Both nonuse-dependent (tonic) and use-dependent block are greater and develop more rapidly in Purkinje fibers from old dogs as compared with young dogs. Fibers from young dogs recover more quickly.[17] Lidocaine reduces intracellular sodium activity and the magnitude of the transient inward current responsible for some forms of afterdepolarizations. Intracellular calcium activity may be reduced because of the sodium-calcium exchange mechanism.[18] Lidocaine may convert areas of unidirectional block into bidirectional block during ischemia and prevent development of ventricular fibrillation by preventing fragmentation of organized large wavefronts into heteroge-

TABLE 21–2 IN VIVO ELECTROPHYSIOLOGICAL CHARACTERISTICS OF ANTIARRHYTHMIC DRUGS

	Electrocardiographic Intervals						Electrophysiological Intervals				
Drug	Sinus Rate	P-R	QRS	Q-T	A-H	H-V	ERP AVN	ERP HPS	ERP A	ERP V	ERP AP
Lidocaine	0	0	0	0	0↓	0↑	0↓	0↑	0	0	0
Quinidine	0↑	↓0↑	↑	↑	↓0↑	0↑	↓0↑	0↑	↑	↑	↑
Procainamide	0	0↑	↑	↑	0↑	0↑	0↑	0↑	↑	↑	↑
Disopyramide	0↑	0	0↑	0↑	0	0↑	0↓	↑	↑	↑	↑
Phenytoin	0	0	0	0↓	0↓	0	0↓	↓	0	0	0
Propranolol	↓	0↑	0	0↓	0	0	↑	0	0	0	0
Bretylium	0↓	0↑	0	0↑			0↑	↑	↑	↑	0
Verapamil	0↓	↑	0	0	↑	0	↑	0	0	0	0
Amiodarone	↓	0↑	↑	↑	↑	↑	↑	↑	↑	↑	↑
Mexiletine	0	0	0	0	0↑	0↑	0↑	0↑	0	0	0
Tocainide	0↓	0	0	0↓	0↑	0	↓	0	0↓	0↓	0
Flecainide	0↓	↑	↑	↑	↑	↑	↑	↑	↑	↑	↑
Encainide	0	↑	↑	↑	↑	↑	↑	↑	↑	↑	↑
Ethmozine	0↓	0↑	0↑	0	↑	↑	0	0	0↑	0↑	↑
Lorcainide		0↑	↑	↑	0	↑	0	0↑	0	0	↑
Propafenone	0↓	↑	↑	0↑	↑	↑	0↑	0	0↑	↑	↑

Results presented may vary according to tissue type, experimental conditions, and drug concentration. ↑ = increase; ↓ = decrease; 0 = no change; 0↑ or 0↓ = slight inconsistent increase or decrease. A = atrium; AVN = AV node; HPS = His-Purkinje system; V = ventricle; AP = accessory pathway (WPW); ERP = effective refractory period—longest S_1-S_2 interval at which S_2 fails to produce a response.

neous wavelets.[19] Lidocaine may be arrhythmogenic if it depresses conduction but not to the point of bidirectional block.[20] For example, it may create an area of unidirectional block and another area of conduction delay and promote reentry.

Lidocaine, except in very high concentrations, does *not* affect slow-channel–dependent action potentials. In fact, its depressant effect on electrical potentials from ischemic myocardium supports the notion that these ischemic potentials are depressed fast responses rather than slow responses.[19, 21] Lidocaine significantly reduces the action potential duration and the effective refractory period of Purkinje fibers and ventricular muscle due to blocking of tetrodotoxin-sensitive sodium channels, and decreasing entry of sodium into the cell.[22] It has little effect on atrial fibers and does not affect conduction in accessory pathways. In some in vitro preparations, lidocaine can improve conduction by hyperpolarizing tissues depolarized as a result of stretch or low external potassium concentration.

In vivo, lidocaine has a minimal effect on automaticity or conduction except in unusual circumstances. Patients with preexisting sinus nodal dysfunction, abnormal His-Purkinje conduction, or junctional or ventricular escape rhythms may develop depressed automaticity or conduction. This drug may shorten His-Purkinje refractoriness in man. Part of its effects may be to inhibit cardiac sympathetic nerve activity.[23, 24]

HEMODYNAMIC EFFECTS. Clinically significant adverse hemodynamic effects are rarely noted at usual drug concentrations unless left ventricular function is severely impaired.

PHARMACOKINETICS (Table 21–1). Lidocaine is used only parenterally because oral administration results in extensive first-pass hepatic metabolism and unpredictable, low plasma levels with excessive metabolites that may produce toxicity. Hepatic metabolism of lidocaine depends greatly on hepatic blood flow, so that clearance of this drug almost equals (and can be approximated by) measurements

TABLE 21–3 IN VITRO ELECTROPHYSIOLOGICAL CHARACTERISTICS

Drug	APA	APD	dV/dt	MDP	ERP	Conduction Velocity	Sinus Nodal Automaticity	PF Nodal Phase 4
Lidocaine	0↓	↓	0↓	0	↓	0↓	0	↓
Quinidine	↓	↑	↓	0	↑	↓	0	↓
Procainamide	↓	↑	↓	0	↑	↓	0	↓
Disopyramide	↓	↑	↓	0	↑	↓	↑0↓	↓
Phenytoin	0	↓	↑0↓	0	↓	0	0	↓
Propranolol	0↓	0↓	0↓	0	↓	0	↓	↓*
Bretylium	0	↑	0	0	↑	0	0↓	0↓*
Verapamil	0	↓	0	0	0	0	↓	↓*
Amiodarone	0	↑	0↓	0	↑	↓	↓	↓
Mexiletine	0	↓	0↓	0	↓	↓	0	↓
Tocainide	0	↓	0↓	0	↓	↓	0	↓
Flecainide	↓	↑	↓	0	↑	↓	0	↓
Encainide	↓	↓	↓	0	↑	↓	0	↓
Ethmozine	↓	↓	↓	0	↓	↓	0	0
Lorcainide	↓	↑	↓	0	↑	↓	0	↓
Propafenone	↓	0↑	↓	0	0↑	↓	↓	↓

*With a background of sympathetic activity.

Key: APA = action potential amplitude; APD = action potential duration; dV/dt = rate of rise of action potential; MDP = maximum diastolic potential; ERP = effective refractory period; PF = Pukinje fibers; ET = excitability threshold; VFT = ventricular fibrillation threshold.

of this flow. Severe hepatic disease or reduced hepatic blood flow, as in heart failure or shock, can markedly decrease the rate of lidocaine metabolism. Prolonged infusion can reduce lidocaine clearance. Its elimination half-life averages about 1 to 2 hours in normal subjects, more than 4 hours in patients after relatively uncomplicated myocardial infarction, more than 10 hours in patients after myocardial infarction complicated by cardiac failure, and even longer in the presence of cardiogenic shock. Maintenance doses should be reduced by one-third to one-half for patients with low cardiac output.

DOSAGE AND ADMINISTRATION (Table 21–1). Although lidocaine may be given intramuscularly,[25] the intravenous route is most commonly used (Fig. 21–4). Intramuscular lidocaine is given in doses of 4 to 5 mg/kg (250 to 350 mg), resulting in effective serum levels at about 15 minutes and lasting for about 90 minutes.[26] Intravenously, lidocaine is given as an initial bolus of 1 to 2 mg/kg body weight at a rate of approximately 20 to 50 mg/min, with a second injection of one-half the initial dose 20 to 40 minutes later. Patients treated with an initial bolus followed by a maintenance infusion may experience transient subtherapeutic plasma concentrations at 30 to 120 minutes after initiation of therapy.[27] A second bolus of about 0.5 mg/kg without increasing the maintenance infusion rate reestablishes therapeutic serum concentrations. If recurrence of arrhythmia appears after a steady state has been achieved (e.g., 6 to 10 hours after starting therapy), a similar bolus should be given and the maintenance infusion rate increased. Increasing the maintenance infusion rate only without an additional bolus results in a very slow increase in plasma lidocaine concentrations, reaching a new plateau in over 6 hours (four elimination half-lives), and is therefore not recommended. Another recommended intravenous dosing is 1.5 mg/kg initially and 0.8 mg/kg at 8-minute intervals for three doses. Doses are reduced by about 50 per cent for patients with heart failure.

If the initial bolus of lidocaine is ineffective, up to two more boluses of 1 mg/kg may be administered at 5-minute intervals. Patients who require more than one bolus to achieve a therapeutic effect have arrhythmias that respond only to higher lidocaine plasma concentrations, and a greater maintenance dose may be necessary to sustain these higher concentrations. Patients requiring only a single initial bolus of lidocaine should probably receive a maintenance infusion of 30 μg/kg/min, while those requiring two or three boluses may need infusions at 40 to 50 μg/kg/min.[27] Loading doses may also be administered by rapid infusion and a constant-rate intravenous infusion may be used to maintain an effective concentration. Maintenance infusion rates in the range of 1 to 4 mg/min produce steady-state plasma levels of 1 to 5 μg/ml in patients with uncomplicated myocardial infarction, but these rates must be reduced during heart failure or shock because of concomitant reduced hepatic blood flow.[1] A loading dose in the range of 75 mg followed by an initial infusion rate of 5.33 mg/min that declines exponentially to 2 mg/min with a half-life of 25 min has been recommended.[27a]

CLINICAL INDICATIONS. Lidocaine demonstrates great efficacy against ventricular arrhythmias of diverse etiology, the ability to achieve effective plasma concentrations rapidly, and a fairly wide toxic-to-therapeutic ratio with a low incidence of hemodynamic complications and other side effects. However, its first-pass hepatic effect precludes oral use, and it is generally ineffective against supraventricular arrhythmias. In patients with the Wolff-Parkinson-White syndrome, when the effective refractory period of the accessory pathway is relatively short, lidocaine generally has no significant effect and may even accelerate the ventricular response during atrial fibrillation.[28]

Lidocaine is used primarily for patients with acute myocardial infarction or recurrent ventricular tachyarrhythmias. In patients resuscitated from out-of-hospital ventricular fibrillation and studied in a randomized, blinded trial,[29] lidocaine was comparable to bretylium in preventing recurrent episodes of ventricular tachyarrhythmia. In patients less than 70 years old who were admitted within six hours of onset of symptoms associated with acute myocardial infarction, lidocaine prophylaxis reduced episodes of ventricular fibrillation compared to results of an untreated control group (p. 1270). However, treated patients had a 15 per cent incidence of lidocaine toxicity, which was greater in older patients, and hospital mortality did not differ between treated and control groups, since

OF ANTIARRHYTHMIC DRUGS

Membrane Responsiveness	ET	VFT	Contractility	Slow Inward Current	Autonomic Nervous System	Local Anesthetic Effect
0 ↓	0 ↑	↑	0	0	0	Yes
↓	↑	↑	0	0	Antivagal alpha blocker	Yes
↓	↑	↑	0	0	Slight antivagal	Yes
↓	↑	↑	↓	0	Central: antivagal, antisympathetic	Yes
0 ↑	0			0	0	No
0 ↑	0	0 ↑	↓	0	Antisympathetic	Yes
0	0	↑	0 ↑	0	Antisympathetic	Yes
0	0	0	↓	Inhibit	? Block alpha receptors	Yes
↓			↓	0 ↓	Antisympathetic	No
↓	↑	↑	↓	0	0	Yes
↓	↑	↑	0	0	0	Yes
↓			↓	0	0	Yes
↓	↑		↓	0	0	Yes
↓	↑	0		0	0	No
↓			↓	0		Yes
↓	↑	↑	↓	May inhibit	Antisympathetic	Yes

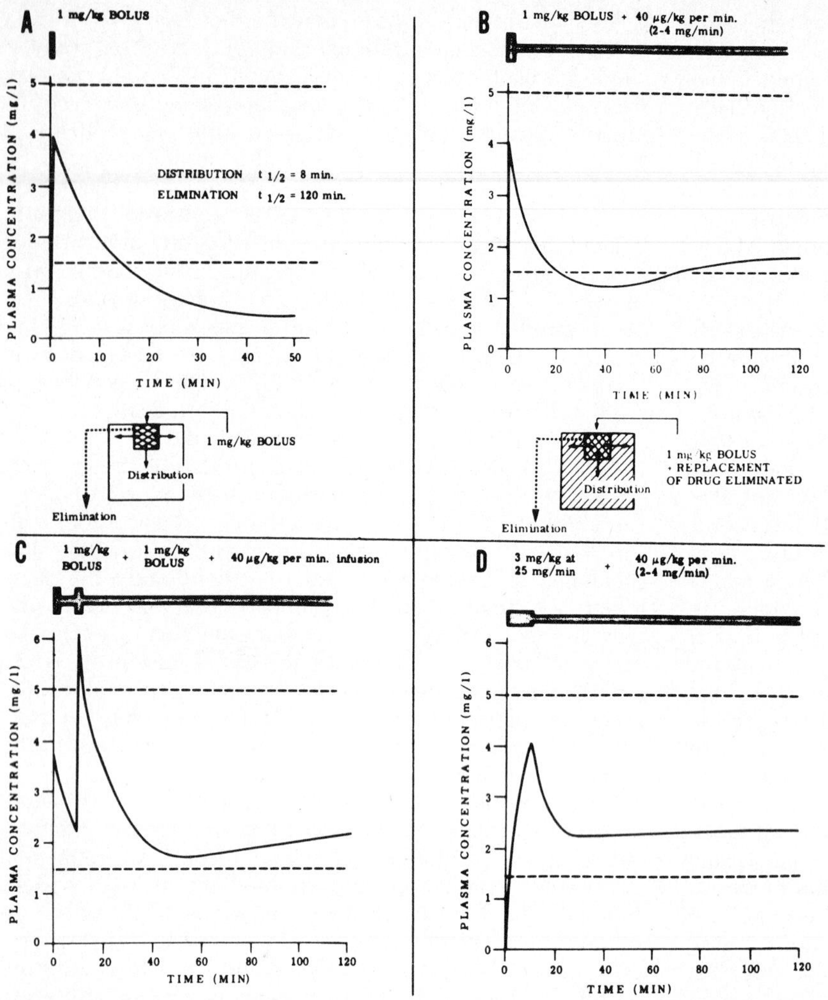

FIGURE 21–4. *A, Top,* Plasma concentrations after a bolus of lidocaine, with the therapeutic range indicated by a dashed line. *Bottom,* The disposition of the drug in the body, with the larger box indicating the total volume of distribution and the smaller box the central compartment. The bolus initially produces therapeutic lidocaine concentrations in the small central compartment. Rapid distribution of the drug to the rest of the body produces subtherapeutic concentrations within 15 minutes. *B,* Lidocaine is administered by an initial bolus as in *A*, with a maintenance infusion begun just after the bolus. The maintenance infusion replaces drug eliminated from the body, but drug is also lost from the central compartment by distribution, which is more rapid than elimination. As a result, plasma concentrations decrease transiently. In this instance, lidocaine concentration is subtherapeutic between 30 and 70 minutes after initiation of therapy. *C,* Subtherapeutic lidocaine concentrations after an initial bolus (as in *B*) can be prevented by giving a second lidocaine bolus 10 minutes after the first. A maintenance infusion should be started after the second bolus rather than after the first, as shown here. This will prevent excessive lidocaine concentrations after the second bolus. *D,* An alternative method to produce therapeutic lidocaine concentrations rapidly. This illustration indicates plasma concentrations after the administration of a loading dose of lidocaine given over 10 minutes. A maintenance infusion is begun after the loading dose has been given. (From Nattel, S., and Zipes, D. P.: Clinical pharmacology of old and new antiarrhythmic drugs. Cardiovasc. Clin. *11*:221, 1980.)

in all instances prompt defibrillation terminated the ventricular fibrillation.[30] Other studies have not shown a protective effect of lidocaine in preventing ventricular arrhythmias due to infarction,[31, 32] and of 15 randomized trials, most showed no apparent benefit.[33] Thus, it has not been unequivocally demonstrated that the benefits of prophylactic lidocaine therapy in hospitalized patients who have acute myocardial infarction outweigh the risks[33, 34] (p. 1270). Because of these conflicting reports, prophylaxis is probably not indicated for all patients, since death from primary ventricular fibrillation occurs uncommonly in a well-staffed coronary care unit and because of the adverse effects accompanying lidocaine administration.

ADVERSE EFFECTS. The most commonly reported adverse effects of lidocaine are dose-related manifestations of central nervous system toxicity: dizziness, paresthesias, confusion, delirium, stupor, coma, and seizures. Occasional sinus node depression and His-Purkinje block have been reported. In patients with atrial tachyarrhythmias, ventricular rate acceleration has been noted.

QUINIDINE

Quinidine and quinine are isomeric alkaloids isolated from the cinchona bark. Although quinidine shares the antimalarial, antipyretic, and vagolytic actions of quinine, the latter lacks the significant electrophysiological and antiarrhythmic effects of quinidine.[35]

ELECTROPHYSIOLOGICAL ACTIONS (Tables 21–2 and 21–3). Quinidine exerts little effect on automaticity of the isolated normal sinus node[1] or on the denervated[36] sinus node in vivo but suppresses automaticity in normal Purkinje fibers, especially in ectopic pacemakers, by decreasing the slope of phase 4 diastolic depolarization and shifting threshold voltage toward zero. It does not affect abnormal automaticity in depolarized Purkinje fibers or delayed afterdepolarizations, and in high doses can cause abnormal automatic discharge in Purkinje fibers. Because of its significant anticholinergic effect[37] and reflex sympathetic stimulation resulting from alpha-adrenergic blockade that causes peripheral vasodilation, quinidine may increase sinus nodal discharge rate and may improve AV nodal conduction in the innervated heart in vivo. Changes in sinus rate and AV nodal conduction were minimal in one recent study.[38] In patients with the sick sinus syndrome, quinidine can depress sinus nodal automaticity. Direct myocardial effects may prolong AV nodal and His-Purkinje conduction times. Quinidine prolongs the duration of action potential of atrial and ventricular muscle and Purkinje fibers slightly (quinine shortens it[35]), while also prolonging the effective refractory period without significantly changing resting membrane potential. Action potential amplitude, overshoot, and V_{max} of phase 0 are reduced, more so during ischemia, hypoxia, and in depolarized fibers, especially at fast rates.[36] Because of its vagolytic actions, produced through muscarinic blockade,[37] quinidine can shorten Purkinje fiber action potential when the latter has been prolonged by vagal inhibition of beta-adrenoreceptor stimulation.[39] The open channel has a high affinity for quinidine, resulting in block of a fraction of sodium channels with each action potential upstroke. For the duration of the plateau of the action potential (inactivated state) or in depolarized fibers, the rate of unblocking is slow, proceeding much faster in polarized fibers. Therefore, faster rates result in more block of sodium channels and less unblocking because of a lesser percentage of time spent in a polarized state (use-dependence).[40]

HEMODYNAMIC EFFECTS. Quinidine decreases peripheral vascular resistance and may cause significant hypotension because of its alpha-adrenoreceptor blocking effects. Concomitant administration of vasodilators may exaggerate the potential for hypotension. In some patients, quinidine can increase cardiac output, possibly by reducing afterload and preload. No significant direct myocardial depressant action occurs unless large doses are given rapidly, intravenously. Most of the adverse effects of intravenous quinidine are probably the result of excessive vasodilation.

PHARMACOKINETICS (Table 21–1). Although orally administered quinidine sulfate and quinidine gluconate exhibit similar degrees of systemic availability, plasma quinidine concentrations peak at about 90 minutes after oral administration of quinidine sulfate and at 3 to 4 hours after oral administration of quinidine gluconate. Intramuscular quinidine produces a higher and an earlier peak plasma concentration but results in incomplete absorption and tissue necrosis. Quinidine may be given intravenously if it is infused slowly. Approximately 80 per cent of plasma quinidine is protein-bound. Both the liver and the kidneys remove quinidine, hepatic metabolism being more important. Approximately 20 per cent is excreted unchanged in the urine. Because congestive heart failure, hepatic disease, or poor renal function may reduce quinidine elimination and increase plasma concentration, dosage probably should be reduced and the drug given cautiously to patients with these disorders while serum quinidine concentration is monitored. Elimination half-life is 5 to 8 hours after oral administration.

DOSAGE AND ADMINISTRATION (Table 21–1). The usual oral dose of quinidine sulfate for an adult is 300 to 600 mg four times daily, which results in a steady state level within about 24 hours. A loading dose of 600 to 1000 mg produces an earlier effective concentration. Similar doses of quinidine gluconate are used intramuscularly, while the intravenous dose of quinidine gluconate is about 10 mg/kg given at a rate of about 0.5 mg/kg/min as blood pressure and ECG parameters are checked frequently.[41,42] Oral doses of the gluconate are about 30 per cent greater than those of sulfate. Anticonvulsant drugs may shorten quinidine's half-life and reduce quinidine serum concentration for a given dose. A new once-a-day quinidine preparation has been tested.[43]

CLINICAL INDICATIONS. Quinidine is a versatile antiarrhythmic agent, useful for treating premature supraventricular and ventricular complexes and sustained tachyarrhythmias. It may prevent spontaneous recurrences of AV nodal reentrant tachycardia and inhibit tachycardia induced by programmed electrical stimulation by prolonging atrial and ventricular refractoriness and depressing conduction in the retrograde fast pathway.[44] In patients with the Wolff-Parkinson-White syndrome, quinidine prolongs the effective refractory period of the accessory pathway and, by so doing, may prevent reciprocating tachycardias and slow the ventricular response from conduction over the accessory pathway during atrial flutter or atrial fibrillation. Quinidine and other antiarrhythmic agents may also prevent recurrences of tachycardia by suppressing the "trigger," i.e., the premature atrial or ventricular complex that initiates a sustained tachycardia.

Quinidine successfully terminates atrial flutter or atrial fibrillation in about 10 to 20 per cent of patients, with higher success rates if the arrhythmia is of more recent onset and if the atria are not enlarged. Incremental dosing with quinidine at 2-hour intervals is no longer indicated to terminate atrial flutter or fibrillation. Prior to administering quinidine to these patients, the ventricular response should be slowed sufficiently with digitalis, propranolol, or verapamil, since quinidine-induced slowing of the atrial flutter rate—e.g., from 300 to the range of 200 beats/min—plus its vagolytic effect on AV nodal conduction may convert a 2:1 atrioventricular response (two atrial impulses for each QRS complex) to a 1:1 atrioventricular response, with an *increase* in the ventricular rate. Prior to elective cardioversion of patients with atrial fibrillation, quinidine should probably be given for one to two days, since this regimen restores sinus rhythm in some patients, thus obviating the need for DC cardioversion, and helps maintain sinus rhythm once it is achieved.[45] In most patients, quinidine should probably be administered as long as sinus rhythm continues.

Quinidine has prevented sudden death in patients resuscitated because of out-of-hospital cardiac arrest.[46] Efficacy may be judged during electrophysiological testing.[47] Quinidine may be combined with other antiarrhythmic agents for increased efficacy.[48] Because it crosses the placenta, quinidine can be used to treat arrhythmias in the fetus.[49]

ADVERSE EFFECTS. The most common adverse effects of chronic oral quinidine therapy are gastrointestinal, including nausea, vomiting, diarrhea, abdominal pain, and anorexia. Central nervous system toxicity includes tinnitus, hearing loss, visual disturbances, confusion, delirium, and pychosis. *Cinchonism* is the term usually applied to these side effects. Allergic reactions may be manifest as rash, fever, immune-mediated thrombocytopenia, hemolytic anemia, and rarely anaphylaxis. Thrombocytopenia is due to the presence of antibodies to quinidine-platelet complexes, causing platelets to agglutinate and lyse. In patients receiving oral anticoagulants, quinidine may cause bleeding. Side effects may preclude long-term administration of quinidine in 30 to 40 per cent of patients.

A prominent electrocardiographic feature of quinidine toxicity is slowing of cardiac conduction, sometimes to the point of block. This may become manifest as prolongation of the QRS duration and Q-T interval or SA or AV nodal conduction disturbances. Quinidine-induced cardiac toxicity may be treated with molar sodium lactate.

Quinidine may produce syncope in 0.5 to 2.0 per cent of patients, most often the result of a self-terminating episode of a polymorphic ventricular tachyarrhythmia,[50,51] commonly of a specific variety called *torsades de pointes*[52,53] (see pp. 698 and 699). The mechanism of torsades de pointes is not clear, but the development of early afterdepolarizations[54] and dispersion of refractoriness[55] have been suggested as causes. Quinidine prolongs the Q-T interval in most patients, whether or not ventricular arrhythmias occur, but significant Q-T prolongation (Q-T interval of 500 to 600 msec) is a general characteristic of quinidine syncope. Many of these patients were also receiving digitalis. Apparently syncope is not related to plasma concentrations of quinidine or duration of therapy.[50] Hypokalemia often is a prominent feature. The incidence of torsades de pointes may be less in patients without sustained ventricular tachycardia or ventricular fibrillation.[56] Therapy for quinidine syncope requires immediate discontinuation of the drug and avoidance of other drugs that have similar pharmacological effects, such as disopyramide. Despite the observations regarding use-dependence, atrial or ventricular pacing may be used to suppress the ventricular tachyarrhythmia and may act by shortening refractoriness at faster rates. For some patients, drugs that do not prolong the Q-T interval, such as lidocaine or phenytoin, may be tried. When pacing is not available, isoproterenol may be given *with caution*. Magnesium given intravenously has been successful in suppressing quinidine-induced torsades de pointes.[57]

Drugs that induce hepatic enzyme production, such as phenobarbital and phenytoin, may shorten the duration of quinidine's action by increasing its rate of elimination. Quinidine may elevate serum digoxin[58] and digitoxin[4] concentrations by decreasing total body clearance of digitoxin and by decreasing the clearance, volume of distribution, and affinity of tissue receptors for digoxin[59] (see p. 500).

PROCAINAMIDE

ELECTROPHYSIOLOGICAL ACTIONS (Tables 21–2 and 21–3). The cardiac actions of procainamide on automaticity, conduction, excitability, and membrane responsiveness resemble those of quinidine and result in depression of excitability in atrium and ventricle, slowing of conduction, and prolongation of the effective refractory period. Like quinidine, procainamide usually prolongs the effective refractory period (ERP) more than it prolongs the action potential duration (APD). When the ERP duration/APD exceeds 1.0, the earliest premature impulse that can be initiated during repolarization arises when the cell has returned to its most negative potential. Premature responses induced at this potential are more likely to have greater $\dot{V}_{max}$ and amplitude, presumably establishing better conduction (see p. 594). Thus the antiarrhythmic agent prevents early responses, arising from less negative resting potentials, that might conduct slowly or block, thereby potentiating the development of arrhythmias. A drug that decreases the ratio of ERP duration/APD may allow earlier premature responses to occur at a time when the membrane potential is more positive. Compared to disopyramide and quinidine, procainamide exerts the least anticholinergic effects[37] but does produce more local anesthetic effects than quinidine. It does not affect normal sinus nodal automaticity.

In vitro studies on cat myocardium subjected to acute and chronic myocardial infarction reveal that procainamide decreases differences in refractoriness between tissue types by prolonging action potential duration and refractoriness most markedly in acutely ischemic cells with the shortest action potential duration and refractoriness and least in chronically injured cells with the longest action potential duration and refractoriness; the drug produced intermediate changes in normal cells.[60]

The electrophysiological effects of *N*-acetylprocainamide (NAPA), procainamide's major metabolite, differ from those of the parent compound.[61] NAPA (10 to 40 mg/liter) does not suppress the rate of phase 4 diastolic depolarization of Purkinje fibers and does not alter resting membrane potential, action potential amplitude, or $\dot{V}_{max}$ of phase 0 of the action potential of Purkinje fibers or ventricular muscle. However, NAPA prolongs the action potential duration of ventricular muscle and Purkinje fibers in a dose-dependent manner. Toxic doses produce early afterdepolarizations and triggered activity. NAPA given to dogs (50 to 100 mg/kg intravenously) produces single instances as well as salvos of ventricular extrasystoles that at times degenerate to ventricular fibrillation. Doses up to 100 mg/kg intravenously exert slight antiarrhythmic effects in dogs subjected to myocardial infarction 24 hours previously.[62] Procainamide appears to exert greater electrophysiological effects than NAPA.[63, 64]

HEMODYNAMIC EFFECTS. Procainamide may depress myocardial contractility in high doses. It does not produce alpha blockade but may result in peripheral vasodilation via a mild ganglionic blocking action that impairs cardiovascular reflexes.

PHARMACOKINETICS (Table 21–1). Oral administration produces peak plasma concentrations in about one hour. Absorption may be reduced in the first week after myocardial infarction. Approximately 80 per cent of oral procainamide is bioavailable, with 20 per cent bound to serum proteins. The overall elimination half-life for procainamide is 3 to 5 hours, with 50 to 60 per cent of the drug eliminated by the kidney and 10 to 30 per cent eliminated by hepatic metabolism.[4] A prolonged-release form of procainamide given every 6 hours provides steady-state plasma levels of the drug equivalent to an equal total daily dose of short-acting procainamide given every 3 hours.

The drug is acetylated to NAPA, which is excreted almost exclusively by the kidneys. As renal function decreases and in patients with heart failure, procainamide levels—and particularly NAPA levels—increase and, because of the risk of serious cardiotoxicity, need to be carefully monitored in such situations. NAPA has an elimination half-life of 7 to 8 hours but exceeds 10 hours if high doses are used. Small amounts of procainamide are present in patients receiving NAPA because of deacetylation.

DOSAGE AND ADMINISTRATION (Table 21–1). Procainamide may be given by the oral, intravenous, or intramuscular route to achieve serum concentrations that produce an antiarrhythmic effect in the range of 44 to 10 μg/ml. Occasionally plasma concentrations exceeding 10 μg/ml have been required,[65] but the probability of adverse effects generally preclude long-term administration at these higher plasma concentrations.[66] Several intravenous regimens have been used to administer procainamide. Twenty-five to 50 mg can be given over a one-minute period and then repeated every 5 minutes until the arrhythmia is controlled, hypotension results, or the QRS complex is prolonged more than 50 per cent. Rather large doses of 6 to 13 mg/kg at a maximum infusion rate of 0.5 mg/kg/min have been used. Another method employs 50 mg/min with the same endpoints. A constant-rate intravenous infusion of procainamide can be given at a dose of 2 to 6 mg/min. The upper limits regarding total dose are flexible and range between 1000 and 2000 mg, depending upon the patient's response.

Oral administration of procainamide requires a 3- or 4-hour dosing interval at a total daily dose of 2 to 6 gm, with a steady state reached within one day. When a loading dose is used, it should be twice the maintenance dose. Frequent dosing is required because of the short elimination half-life in normal subjects. For the prolonged-release form of procainamide, dosing is at 6-hour intervals.[67] A longer half-life may be seen in some cardiac patients, allowing longer intervals between drug administration, but this needs to be documented for the individual patient. Procainamide is well absorbed after intramuscular injection, with virtually 100 per cent of the dose bioavailable. The plasma concentration of procainamide required to suppress premature ventricular complexes (PVC's) may be higher or lower, depending on the patient, than the plasma concentration required to prevent sustained ventricular tachycardia.[68]

CLINICAL INDICATIONS. Procainamide is used to treat both supraventricular and ventricular arrhythmias and has a spectrum of application comparable to that of quinidine. Although both drugs have similar electrophysiological actions, either drug may effectively suppress a supraventricular or ventricular arrhythmia that is refractory to the other drug.

Procainamide may be used to convert atrial fibrillation of recent onset to sinus rhythm.[69] As with quinidine, prior treatment with digitalis, propranolol, or verapamil is recommended to prevent acceleration of the ventricular response following procainamide therapy. In patients with paroxysmal supraventricular tachycardia, procainamide may inhibit the induction of sustained AV nodal reentrant tachycardia as a result of selective depression of retrograde AV nodal conduction in the fast pathway. Procainamide may block conduction in the accessory pathway of patients with the Wolff-Parkinson-White syndrome and has been used intravenously to identify those patients who have a short anterograde effective refractory period of the accessory pathway[70] (p. 685).

Procainamide has been only partially effective in preventing the induction of ventricular tachycardia by programmed stimulation during electrophysiological studies in patients with a history of ventricular tachycardia or ventricular fibrillation. The electrophysiological response to procainamide given intravenously predicts the response to the drug given orally.[71] High doses, 500 to 1000 mg orally every 4 hours, resulting in a plasma concentration exceeding 10.0 μg/ml may be necessary to suppress ventricular tachycardia in some patients. Procainamide also has been given successfully as a single oral dose to terminate nonlife-threatening tachycardias.[72] Most consistently, procainamide slows the rate of the induced ventricular tachycardia. It has been suggested that the response to programmed electrical stimulation of patients receiving procainamide could predict their response to other conventional agents,[73] but this suggestion is not universally accepted.[74] Similarly, the antiarrhythmic response to procainamide does not predict the response to NAPA.

ADVERSE EFFECTS. Multiple adverse noncardiac effects have been reported with procainamide administration and include skin rashes, myalgias, digital vasculitis, and Raynaud's phenomenon. Gastrointestinal side effects are less frequent than with quinidine, and adverse central nervous system side effects are less frequent than with lidocaine. Procainamide may cause giddiness, psychosis, hallucinations, and depression. Toxic concentrations of procainamide can diminish myocardial performance and promote hypotension. A variety of conduction disturbances or ventricular tachyarrhythmias may occur similar to those produced by quinidine, including prolonged Q-T syndrome and polymorphous ventricular tachycardia.[75] NAPA can also induce Q-T prolongation and a polymorphous ventricular tachycardia. Ventricular tachyarrhythmias do not appear to occur as frequently following procainamide therapy as they do following treatment with quinidine. In the absence of sinus node disease, procainamide does not adversely affect sinus node function. In patients with sinus dysfunction, procainamide tends to prolong corrected sinus node recovery time and may worsen symptoms in some patients who have the bradycardia-tachycardia syndrome.[76] Fever and agranulocytosis may be due to hypersensitivity reactions, and white blood cell and differential blood counts should be performed at regular intervals. Procainamide does not increase the serum digoxin concentration.

Arthralgia, fever, pleuropericarditis, hepatomegaly, and hemorrhagic pericardial effusion with tamponade have been described in a systemic lupus erythematosus (SLE)-like syndrome (Table 21–4). The syndrome may occur more frequently and earlier in patients who are "slow acetylators" of procainamide, although this is not entirely clear. The aromatic amino group on procainamide appears important for induction of SLE syndrome, since acetylating this amino group to form NAPA appears to block the SLE-inducing effect.[77] Sixty to 70 per cent of patients who receive procainamide on a chronic basis develop antinuclear antibodies, with clinical symptoms in 20 to 30 per cent, but this is reversible when procainamide is stopped. When symptoms occur, SLE cell preparations are often positive. Positive serological tests are not necessarily a reason to discontinue drug therapy, but the development of symptoms or a positive anti-DNA antibody is, except for patients whose life-threatening arrhythmia is controlled only by procainamide. Steroid administration in those patients may eliminate the symptoms.

TABLE 21–4 COMPARISON OF NATURALLY OCCURRING AND PROCAINAMIDE-INDUCED SYSTEMIC LUPUS ERYTHEMATOSUS

	Naturally Occurring	Procainamide Induced
Brain and kidney involvement	Yes	No
Hematologic complications	Yes	Uncommon
False positive test for syphilis	Yes	No
Antibodies vs. single-stranded DNA	No	Yes
Antibodies vs. double-stranded DNA	Yes	No
Antibodies vs. histones	1/3 of pts.	Almost 100% of pts.

DISOPYRAMIDE

Disopyramide has been approved in the United States for oral but not intravenous administration to treat patients with ventricular arrhythmias.

ELECTROPHYSIOLOGICAL ACTIONS (Tables 21–2 and 21–3). Although structurally different from quinidine and procainamide, disopyramide produces similar electrophysiological effects in vitro. It decreases the slope of phase 4 diastolic depolarization in Purkinje fibers, produces a rate-dependent depression of $\dot{V}_{max}$ of phase 0, prolongs the effective refractory period more than it prolongs the action potential duration, lengthens conduction time in normal and depolarized Purkinje fibers, and does not affect slow response action potentials,[78] except possibly at very high concentrations. Disopyramide, like procainamide,[60] reduces the differences in action potential duration between normal and infarcted tissue by lengthening the action potential of normal cells more than it lengthens the action potential of cells from infarcted regions of the heart.[79]

Stereochemical properties influence the effects of disopyramide. Racemic (clinically used) and (+) disopyramide prolong canine Purkinje fiber action potential, while (−) disopyramide shortens it. The (+) isomer exerts approximately three times more vagolytic effects than does the (−) isomer.[37] Disopyramide can speed the sinus nodal discharge rate and shorten AV nodal conduction time and refractoriness when the nodes are restrained by cholinergic influences. Atropine tends to nullify or even reverse this effect. Disopyramide also can slow the sinus nodal discharge rate by a direct action when given in high concentration[80] and can significantly depress sinus nodal activity in patients with sinus node dysfunction. Disopyramide exerts greater anticholinergic effects than quinidine and does not appear to affect alpha- or beta-adrenoreceptors.

Atrial and ventricular refractory periods increase, as do conduction time and refractoriness of the accessory pathway in patients with the Wolff-Parkinson-White syndrome.[81] Disopyramide's effect on AV nodal conduction and refractoriness in vivo is not consistent. Disopyramide prolongs His-Purkinje conduction time, but infra-His block results infrequently.[82, 83] Disopyramide may be administered safely to patients who have first degree or Type I second degree AV block and narrow QRS complexes.[84]

HEMODYNAMIC EFFECTS. Disopyramide administered intravenously reduces systemic blood pressure, cardiac and stroke index, and increases right atrial pressures and total peripheral resistance.[85] Profound hemodynamic deterioration can occur, and patients who have abnormal ventricular function tolerate the negative inotropic effects of disopyramide quite poorly. In these patients the drug should be used with extreme caution or not at all.[86]

PHARMACOKINETICS (Table 21–1). Disopyramide is 80 to 90 per cent absorbed, with a mean elimination half-life of 8 to 9 hours in healthy volunteers but almost 10 hours in patients with heart failure and sometimes longer in some patients with ventricular arrhythmias. Total body clearance and volume of distribution decrease in patients, and mean serum concentration is higher than reported in normal subjects.[87] Renal insufficiency prolongs the elimination time. Thus, in patients who have renal, hepatic, or cardiac insufficiency, loading and maintenance doses need to be reduced. Peak blood levels after oral administration result in 1 to 2 hours, and bioavailability exceeds 80 per cent. The fraction of disopyramide bound to serum protein varies inversely with the total plasma concentration of the drug but may be more stable (30 to 40 per cent) at clinically relevant concentrations of 3 μg/ml. About half an oral dose is recovered unchanged in the urine, with about 30 per cent as the mono N-dealkylated metabolite. The metabolites appear to exert less effect than the parent compound.

DOSAGE AND ADMINISTRATION (Table 21–1). Doses are generally 100 to 200 mg orally every 6 hours with a range of 400 to 1200 mg/day. The intravenous (investigational) dose is 1 to 2 mg/kg as an initial bolus given over 5 to 10 minutes, which may be followed by an infusion of 1 mg/kg/hour.[81]

CLINICAL INDICATIONS. Disopyramide appears comparable to quinidine in reducing the frequency of premature ventricular complexes and initial data suggest that it effectively prevents recurrence of ventricular tachycardia in selected patients.[82] Disopyramide has been combined safely and effectively with mexiletine to treat patients who had recurrent ventricular tachycardia and/or ventricular fibrillation and were evaluated during electrophysiological study.[88]

Disopyramide terminates and prevents recurrent episodes of paroxysmal supraventricular tachycardia due to AV[81] and AV nodal reentry.[89] It prolongs the anterograde and retrograde refractory period of the accessory pathway in patients with the Wolff-Parkinson-White syndrome,[81] helps prevent recurrence of atrial fibrillation after successful cardioversion as effectively as quinidine,[82] and may terminate atrial flutter. In treating patients with atrial fibrillation, and particularly atrial flutter, the ventricular rate must be controlled prior to administering disopyramide, or the atrial rate may decrease sufficiently, aided by the vagolytic effects of disopyramide, to create 1:1 conduction during atrial flutter.[90]

ADVERSE EFFECTS. Three categories of adverse effects are seen following disopyramide administration. The most common adverse effect relates to the drug's potent parasympatholytic properties and includes urinary hesitancy or retention, constipation, blurred vision, closed-angle glaucoma, and dry mouth. Symptoms may be minimized by concomitant administration of pyridostigmine.[91] Second, disopyramide may produce ventricular tachyarrhythmias that are commonly associated with Q-T prolongation and torsades de pointes.[52, 82, 92] Some patients may have "cross sensitivity" to both quinidine and disopyramide and develop torsades de pointes while receiving either drug.[93] When drug-induced torsades de pointes occur, agents that prolong the Q-T interval should be used very cautiously. Finally, disopyramide may reduce contractility of the normal ventricle but the depression of ventricular function is much more pronounced in patients with preexisting ventricular failure.[86] Occasionally, cardiovascular collapse can result.[94]

Disopyramide does not appear to alter digitalis metabolism, but phenytoin may alter the metabolism of disopyramide and decrease its plasma concentration.

PHENYTOIN (DIPHENYLHYDANTOIN)

Phenytoin was employed originally to treat seizure disorders and was noted subsequently to abolish ventricular tachycardia in dogs after coronary artery ligation. Phenytoin's value as an antiarrhythmic agent remains limited.

ELECTROPHYSIOLOGICAL ACTIONS (Tables 21–2 and 21–3). Therapeutic concentrations of phenytoin do not alter the discharge rate of rabbit sinus nodal tissue but may depress normal automaticity in cardiac Purkinje fibers in vitro or spontaneous ventricular rate in vivo. Phenytoin effectively abolishes abnormal automaticity caused by digitalis-induced delayed afterdepolarizations in cardiac Purkinje fibers[95] and suppresses certain digitalis-induced arrhythmias in man. Similar to lidocaine, phenytoin abbreviates Purkinje fiber action potential duration more than it shortens the effective refractory period, thus increasing the ratio of effective refractory period to action potential duration. Phenytoin can cause depolarized cells to repolarize by increasing potassium conductance and, in so doing, may increase the $\dot{V}_{max}$ of phase 0 in Purkinje fibers, particularly when these are depressed by digitalis. The rate of rise of action potentials initiated early in the relative refractory period is increased, as is membrane responsiveness, possibly reducing the chance for impaired conduction and block. Phenytoin may slow conduction at high potassium concentrations but minimally affects sinus discharge rate and AV conduction in man. As with other Class 1B agents, it has little effect on $\dot{V}_{max}$ in normally polarized fibers at slow rates, and shows use-dependence and rapid kinetics for onset and termination of effects.[12, 96]

Some of phenytoin's antiarrhythmic effects may be neurally mediated, since phenytoin may reduce the increase in impulse traffic in cardiac sympathetic nerves caused by ouabain toxicity. Injected into the central nervous system, phenytoin protects against digitalis-induced ventricular arrhythmias.[97] The drug may also modulate vagal efferent activity centrally. It has no peripheral cholinergic or beta-adrenergic blocking actions.

Phenytoin exerts minimal *hemodynamic effects.*

PHARMACOKINETICS (Table 21–1). The pharmacokinetics of phenytoin are less than ideal. Absorption following oral administration is incomplete and delayed and varies with the brand of drug. Plasma concentrations peak 8 to 12 hours after an oral dose. Ninety per cent of the drug is protein-bound. Phenytoin has limited solubility at physiologic pH, and intramuscular administration is associated with pain, muscle necrosis, sterile abscesses, and variable absorption. Therapeutic serum concentrations of phenytoin (10 to 20 μg/ml) are similar for treating both cardiac arrhythmias and epilepsy. Lower concentrations may suppress certain digitalis-induced arrhythmias or other arrhythmias when decreased plasma protein binding occurs (as in uremia), since a larger fraction of drug is free and pharmacologically active.

Over 90 per cent of a dose is hydroxylated in the liver to presumably inactive compounds. Some families have a genetically determined inability to hydroxylate phenytoin, while others have a higher than usual capability for hydroxylation. Elimination half-time is about 24 hours and may be slowed in the presence of liver disease or when phenytoin is administered concomitantly with drugs such as phenylbutazone, dicumarol, isoniazid, chloramphenicol, and phenothiazines that compete with phenytoin for hepatic enzymes. Because of the large number of medications that may increase or decrease phenytoin levels during chronic therapy, phenytoin plasma concentration should be determined frequently when changes are made in other medications. In some patients, maintenance dose regimens of phenytoin are difficult to predict because the enzyme system that metabolizes phenytoin becomes saturated at plasma concentrations within the therapeutic range. The half-life then increases with increasing phenytoin load. Above the saturation point, phenytoin elimination follows zero-order kinetics, so that only a fixed amount of drug is eliminated per unit time. These concentration-dependent kinetics for elimination can cause unexpected toxicity, since disproportionately large changes in plasma concentration may follow dose increases.

DOSAGE AND ADMINISTRATION (Table 21–1). To achieve therapeutic plasma concentration rapidly, 100 mg of phenytoin should be administered intravenously every 5 minutes until the arrhythmia is controlled, adverse side effects result, or about 1 gm has been given. Generally, 700 to 1000 mg will control the arrhythmia. A large central vein should be used to avoid pain and development of phlebitis produced by the severely alkalotic (pH 11.0) vehicle in which phenytoin is dissolved. Orally, phenytoin is given as a loading dose of approximately 1000 mg the first day, 500 mg on the second and third days, and 400 mg daily thereafter. All maintenance doses can be given once or twice daily, depending on the brand, because of the long half-life of elimination.

CLINICAL INDICATIONS. Phenytoin has been used successfully to treat atrial and ventricular arrhythmias caused by digitalis toxicity but is much less effective in treating ventricular arrhythmias in patients with ischemic heart disease[98] or with atrial arrhythmias not due to digitalis toxicity. The drug has been somewhat more successful in treating ventricular arrhythmias associated with general anesthesia and cardiac surgery.

ADVERSE EFFECTS. The most common manifestations of phenytoin toxicity are central nervous system effects of nystagmus, ataxia, drowsiness, stupor, and coma. Progression of such symptoms can be correlated with increases in plasma drug concentration. Neurological signs, such as nystagmus on lateral gaze, develop at plasma drug levels of about 20 μg/ml. Nausea, epigastric pain, and anorexia are also relatively common effects of phenytoin. Long-term administration may result in hyperglycemia, hypocalcemia, skin rashes, megaloblastic anemia, gingival hypertrophy, lymph node hyperplasia (a syndrome resembling malignant lymphoma), peripheral neuropathy, and drug-induced systemic lupus erythematosus.

BETA-ADRENORECEPTOR BLOCKING AGENTS

Although seven beta-adrenoreceptor blocking drugs have been approved for use in the United States (Table 39–2, p. 1331), only propranolol, metoprolol, acebutolol, and timolol have been approved to treat arrhythmias or to prevent sudden death after myocardial infarction. It is generally considered that no beta blocker offers distinct advantages over the others and that, when titrated to the proper dose, all can be used effectively to treat cardiac arrhythmias, hypertension, or other disorders.[99] However, differences in pharmacokinetic or pharmacodynamic properties that confer safety, reduce adverse effects, or affect dosing intervals or drug interactions influence the choice of agent.

Beta receptors can be separated into those that affect predominantly the heart (beta$_1$) or the bronchi and blood vessels (beta$_2$). In low doses, selective beta blockers can block beta$_1$ receptors more than they block beta$_2$ receptors and might be preferable for treating patients with pulmonary or peripheral vascular diseases. In high doses, the selective beta$_1$ blockers also block beta$_2$ receptors.

Some beta blockers exert intrinsic sympathomimetic activity, i.e., they slightly activate the beta receptor. These drugs appear to be as efficacious as beta blockers without intrinsic sympathomimetic actions and may cause less slowing of heart rate at rest and less prolongation of AV nodal conduction time.[99] They have been shown to induce less depression of left ventricular function than beta blockers without intrinsic sympathomimetic activity.[100] Beta blockers with intrinsic sympathomimetic activity have not been shown to reduce mortality in patients after myocardial infarction.

The following discussion will concentrate on the use of propranolol as a prototypical antiarrhythmic agent.

ELECTROPHYSIOLOGICAL ACTIONS. Beta blockers may exert an electrophysiological action by competitively inhibiting catecholamine binding at beta-adrenoreceptor sites, an effect almost entirely due to the (−) levorotatory stereoisomer,[99] or by their quinidine-like or direct membrane-stabilizing action. The latter is a local anesthetic effect that depresses I_{Na} and membrane responsiveness in cardiac Purkinje fibers, occurs at concentrations generally 10 times that necessary to produce beta blockade, and most likely plays an insignificant antiarrhythmic role. At beta-blocking concentrations, propranolol slows spontaneous automaticity in the sinus node or in Purkinje fibers that are being stimulated by adrenergic tone. In the absence of adrenergic tone, only high concentrations of propranolol slow normal automaticity in Purkinje fibers, probably by a direct membrane action. In concentrations that cause beta-receptor blockade but no local anesthetic effects, beta-blocking drugs do not alter the normal resting membrane potential, maximum diastolic potential, amplitude, $\dot{V}_{max}$, repolarization, or refractoriness of atrial, Purkinje, or ventricular muscle cells when these tissues are not being superfused with catecholamines. However, in the presence of isoproterenol, a pure beta-receptor stimulator, beta blockers reverse isoproterenol's accelerating effects on repolarization; in the presence of norepinephrine, beta blockade permits unopposed alpha-adrenoreceptor stimulation to prolong action potential duration in Purkinje fibers. Propranolol (2×10^{-6}M) reduces the amplitude of digitalis-induced delayed afterdepolarizations and suppresses triggered activity in Purkinje fibers.[101]

If values for these action potential parameters were abnormally reduced to start and were increased by catecholamines, such as a slow response generated in a high-potassium, catecholamine environment, beta-receptor blockade might depress conduction by removing the catecholamine stimulatory effect. At higher concentrations exceeding 3 μg/ml, propranolol depresses $\dot{V}_{max}$ action potential amplitude, membrane responsiveness, and conduction in normal atrial, ventricular, and Purkinje fibers without altering resting membrane potential. These effects probably result from depression of sodium conductance. The direct effect of propranolol shortens the action potential duration of Purkinje fibers and, to a lesser extent, of atrial and ventricular muscle fibers. Long-term administration of propranolol may lengthen action potential duration.[102] Similar to the effects of lidocaine, acceleration of repolarization of Purkinje fibers is most marked in areas of the ventricular conduction system in which the action potential duration is greatest. The reduction in refractory period is not as great as the reduction in action potential duration (effective refractory period duration/action potential duration >1.0). At least one beta blocker, sotalol, markedly increases the time course of repolarization in Purkinje fibers and ventricular muscle.

Propranolol slows the sinus discharge rate in humans by 10 to 20 per cent, while severe bradycardia occasionally results if the heart is particularly dependent on sympathetic tone or if sinus node dysfunction is present. The slowing is probably due to beta blockade because D-propranolol does not significantly slow the sinus discharge rate in doses comparable to the racemic mixture. The P-R interval lengthens, as does AV nodal conduction time and refractoriness (if the heart rate is maintained constant), but refractoriness and conduction in the normal His-Purkinje system remain unchanged even after high doses of propranolol. Therefore, therapeutic doses of propranolol in humans do not exert a direct depressant or "quinidine-like" action but influence cardiac electrophysiology via a beta-blocking action. Beta blockers do not affect conduction in ventricular muscle, as evidenced by their lack of effect on the QRS complex, and they insignificantly prolong the right ventricular effective refractory period[103] and uncorrected Q-T interval.[104, 105]

Because beta blockade with beta blockers that do not have direct membrane action prevents many arrhythmias resulting from activation of the autonomic nervous system, it is thought that the beta-blocking action is responsible for their antiarrhythmic effects. However, the possible importance of direct membrane effect of some of these drugs, such as propranolol, oxprenolol, acebutalol, and alprenolol, cannot be discounted totally because beta blockers with direct membrane actions may affect transmembrane potentials of diseased cardiac fibers at much lower concentrations than are needed to affect normal fibers directly. In addition, the role of important metabolites of propranolol and other beta blockers that may exert electrophysiological actions is not clearly established.

HEMODYNAMIC EFFECTS. Beta blockers exert negative inotropic effects and may precipitate or worsen heart failure. By blocking beta receptors, these drugs may cause peripheral vasoconstriction.

PHARMACOKINETICS (Table 21–1). Although various types of beta blockers exert similar pharmacological effects, their pharmacokinetics differ substantially.[99] Propranolol is almost 100 per cent absorbed, but the effects of first-pass hepatic metabolism reduce bioavailability to about 30 per cent and produce significant interpatient variability of plasma concentration for a given dose. Reduction in hepatic blood flow, as in patients with heart failure, decreases the hepatic extraction of propranolol, and in these patients propranolol may further decrease its own elimination rate by reducing cardiac output and hepatic blood flow. Beta blockers eliminated by the kidney tend to have longer half-lives and exhibit less interpatient variability of drug concentration than do those beta blockers metabolized by the liver.

DOSAGE AND ADMINISTRATION (Table 21–1). The appropriate dose of propranolol is best determined by a measure of the patient's physiological response, such as changes in resting heart rate or in the prevention of exercise-induced tachycardia, since wide individual differences exist between the observed physiological effect and plasma concentration. For example, intravenous dosing is best achieved by titrating the dose to a clinical effect, beginning with 0.25 to 0.50 mg, increasing to 1.0 mg if necessary, and administering doses every 5 minutes until either a desired effect or toxicity is produced or a total of 0.15 to 0.20 mg/kg has been given. Orally, propranolol is given in four divided doses, usually ranging from 40 to 160 mg a day to more than 1 gram a day. Generally, if one agent in adequate doses proves to be ineffective, other beta blockers will be ineffective also.

CLINICAL INDICATIONS. As an antiarrhythmic agent, propranolol is used most commonly to treat supraventricular tachyarrhythmias. Its effectiveness and mechanism of action vary depending on the arrhythmia. Propranolol may be employed to decrease the rate of persistent sinus tachycardia that results from excessive sympathetic stimulation. Arrhythmias associated with thyrotoxicosis, pheochromocytoma, and anesthesia with cyclopropane or halothane or arrhythmias largely due to excessive cardiac adrenergic stimulation, such as those initiated by exercise or emotion, often respond to propranolol therapy. Beta-blocking drugs usually do not convert chronic atrial flutter or atrial fibrillation to normal sinus rhythm but may be successful if the arrhythmia is of recent onset. The rate of the atrial flutter generally is not changed, but the ventricular response during atrial flutter and atrial fibrillation decreases because beta blockade prolongs AV nodal conduction time and refractoriness. For reentrant supraventricular tachycardias using the AV node as one of the reentrant pathways, such as AV nodal reentrant tachycardia and reciprocating tachycardias in Wolff-Parkinson-White syndrome, or for sinus reentrant tachycardia, propranolol may terminate the tachycardia and be used prophylactically to prevent a recurrence. Combining propranolol with digitalis, quinidine, or a variety of other agents may be effective when propranolol as a single agent fails.

Several other groups of arrhythmias respond particularly well to beta blockade. These include digitalis-induced arrhythmias such as atrial tachycardia, nonparoxysmal AV junctional tachycardia, premature ventricular complexes, or ventricular tachycardia. Part of the effects of propranolol against arrhythmias induced by digitalis may result from its action on the central nervous system. If a significant degree of AV block is present during a digitalis-induced arrhythmia, lidocaine or phenytoin may be preferable to propranolol. Propranolol may also be useful to treat ventricular arrhythmias associated with the prolonged Q-T interval syndrome[106, 107] and with mitral valve prolapse. For patients with ischemic heart disease, propranolol generally has not prevented episodes of chronic recurrent ventricular tachycardia that occur in the absence of acute ischemia. However, several clinical trials have demonstrated a reduction in the incidence of overall death and sudden cardiac death after myocardial infarction in patients treated chronically with a variety of beta blockers.[108–112] The mechanism of this reduction in mortality is not entirely clear and may relate to reduction in the extent of ischemic damage, autonomic effects,[113] a direct antiarrhythmic effect, or combinations. Decrease in ventricular arrhythmias documented by 24-hour ECG recordings has been noted after propranolol treatment[114] and a reduction in the incidence of ventricular fibrillation after metoprolol administration following acute myocardial infarction.[115] Timolol has been reported to decrease the frequency and severity of supraventricular tachyarrhythmias after coronary artery bypass surgery.[116] Survival benefits seem most striking in the first one to two years after myocardial infarction.[108–111]

ADVERSE EFFECTS. Adverse cardiovascular effects from propranolol include unacceptable hypotension, bradycardia, and congestive heart failure. The bradycardia may be due to sinus bradycardia or AV block. Uncommonly, propranolol may precipitate left ventricular failure in the absence of previous failure. Sudden withdrawal of propranolol in patients with angina pectoris can precipitate worsening of angina, cardiac arrhythmias, and acute myocardial infarction, possibly owing to heightened sensitivity to beta agonists caused by previous beta blockade. Heightened sensitivity may begin several days after cessation of propranolol therapy and may last 5 or 6 days.[117] Other adverse effects of propranolol include worsening of asthma or chronic obstructive pulmonary disease, intermittent claudication, Raynaud's phenomenon, mental depression, increased risk of hypoglycemia among insulin-dependent diabetic patients, easy fatigability, disturbingly vivid dreams or insomnia, and impaired sexual function.

BRETYLIUM TOSYLATE

Bretylium was introduced as an antihypertensive agent in 1959, and its antiarrhythmic potential was recognized several years later.

ELECTROPHYSIOLOGICAL ACTIONS (Tables 21–2 and 21–3). Bretylium is selectively concentrated in sympathetic ganglia and their postganglionic adrenergic nerve terminals. After initially *causing* norepinephrine release, bretylium *prevents* norepinephrine release from sympathetic nerve terminals, without depressing pre- or postganglionic sympathetic nerve conduction, impairing conduction across sympathetic ganglia, depleting the adrenergic neuron of norepinephrine, or decreasing the responsiveness of adrenergic receptors. During chronic bretylium treatment, the beta-adrenergic responses to circulating catecholamines are increased. The initial release of catecholamines results in several transient electrophysiological responses such as an increase in the discharge rates of the isolated perfused sinus node and of in vitro Purkinje fibers, often making quiescent fibers automatic. Bretylium initially increases conduction velocity and excitability and decreases refractoriness in the rabbit atrium, and partially depolarized fibers may hyperpolarize. Pretreatment with reserpine or propranolol prevents these early changes. Initial catecholamine release may aggravate some arrhythmias, such as those caused by digitalis excess or myocardial infarction.[118] Prolonged drug administration lengthens the duration of the action potential and refractoriness of atrial and ventricular muscle and Purkinje fibers. The ratio of effective refractory period to action potential duration does not change, nor do membrane responsiveness and conduction velocity. Bretylium exerts little effect on diastolic excitability but increases ventricular fibrillation thresholds significantly.[119] It is not clear whether the chemical sympathectomy-like state alone, or together with other actions, exerts the antifibrillatory effect.[120–122] Reduced disparity between action potential duration and refractory period in regions of normal and infarcted myocardium may account for some of its antifibrillatory effects. Procainamide[60] and disopyramide[79] exert similar effects. Bretylium also reduces disparity of refractoriness in dogs with quinidine-induced long Q-T interval.[123] Bretylium has no effect on vagal reflexes and does not alter the responsiveness of cholinergic receptors in the heart.

HEMODYNAMIC EFFECTS. Bretylium does not depress myocardial contractility. After an initial increase in blood pressure, the drug may cause significant hypotension by blocking the efferent limb of the baroreceptor reflex. Hypotension results most commonly when patients are sitting or standing but may also occur in the supine position in seriously ill patients. Bretylium reduces the extent of the vasoconstriction and tachycardia reflexes during standing. Orthostatic hypotension may persist for several days after the drug has been discontinued.

PHARMACOKINETICS (Table 21–1). Bretylium is effective orally as well as parenterally, but it is absorbed poorly and erratically from the gastrointestinal tract. Bioavailability may be less than 50 per cent and elimination is almost exclusively by renal excretion without significant metabolism or active metabolites being recognized. Elimination half-life is 5 to 10 hours but with fairly wide variability. Doses should be reduced in patients with renal insufficiency. In survivors of ventricular tachycardia or ventricular fibrillation, bretylium had an elimination half-life of 13.5 hours following single intravenous dosing, which was similar to previous results in normal subjects. Renal clearance accounted for virtually all elimination. Onset of action after intravenous administration occurs within several minutes, but full antiarrhythmic effects may not be seen for 30 minutes to 2 hours.[124]

DOSAGE AND ADMINISTRATION (Table 21–1). Bretylium is approved for parenteral administration only and can be given intravenously in doses of 5 to 10 mg/kg body weight diluted in 50 to 100 ml of 5 per cent dextrose in water and administered slowly over 10 to 20 minutes. This dose can be repeated in 1 to 2 hours if the arrhythmia persists. The total daily dose should probably not exceed 30 mg/kg. A similar initial dose, but undiluted, can be given intramuscularly. The maintenance intravenous dose is 0.5 to 2.0 mg/min. Intramuscular injection during cardiopulmonary resuscitation from cardiac arrest and in shock states should be avoided because of unreliable absorption during reduced tissue perfusion. In this situation, bretylium should be given intravenously.

CLINICAL INDICATIONS. Bretylium is currently recommended for use in patients who are in an intensive care setting and who have life-threatening recurrent ventricular tachyarrhythmias that have not responded to lidocaine, quinidine, procainamide, or disopyramide. Bretylium has been remarkably effective in treating some patients with drug-resistant tachyarrhythmias.[125–128] It exerts no effect on the energy required for defibrillating dogs.[128] It is certainly useful in treating victims of out-of-hospital ventricular fibrillation,[29, 125–128] but whether it is superior to lidocaine has not been clearly established.

ADVERSE EFFECTS. Hypotension, most prominently orthostatic but also supine, appears to be the most significant side effect and can be prevented with tricyclic drugs such as protriptyline. Transient hypertension, increased sinus rate, and worsening of arrhythmias,[124] often those due to digitalis excess, may follow initial drug administration and may be due to initial release of catecholamines. Bretylium should be used cautiously or not at all in patients who have a relatively fixed cardiac output, such as those with severe aortic stenosis. Vasodilators or diuretics may enhance these hypotensive effects. Nausea and vomiting may occur following parenteral administration. Parotid pain primarily during meals commonly occurs after 2 to 4 months of oral therapy and is associated with increased salivation without parotid swelling or inflammation.

VERAPAMIL

Verapamil, a synthetic papaverine derivative, was first introduced in 1962 as a smooth muscle relaxant that produced peripheral and coronary vasodilation in animals and man. Representing a new class of drugs called "calcium antagonists,"[129–133] verapamil is an effective antiarrhythmic agent in selected circumstances. Nifedipine exhibits minimal electrophysiological effects at clinically used doses, and will not be discussed here (see p. 1332). Diltiazem has electrophysiological actions similar to verapamil[134–139] but at the time of this writing is approved for use only in the treatment of angina in the United States.

ELECTROPHYSIOLOGICAL ACTIONS (Tables 21–2 and 21–3). By blocking the slow inward current in all cardiac fibers, verapamil in concentrations comparable to those achieved clinically, reduces the plateau height of the action potential, slightly shortens muscle action potential, and slightly prolongs total Purkinje fiber action potential.[130, 140] It does not affect the action potential amplitude, $\dot{V}_{max}$ of phase 0, or resting membrane voltage in cells that have fast-response characteristics (atrial and ventricular muscle, the His-Purkinje system). However, in fast-channel cells rendered abnormal by disease, these concentrations of verapamil may suppress electrical activity in atrial or ventricular[141, 142] muscle fibers that have reduced resting potentials, suggesting that activity in these cells depends on transmembrane ionic flux through the slow channel. Similarly, verapamil suppresses slow responses elicited by a variety of experimental methods.[129–133] Verapamil also suppresses triggered sustained rhythmic activity and early and late afterdepolarizations (see p. 597). Verapamil and other slow-channel blockers in concentrations that do not affect action potentials of fast-channel dependent cells suppress activity in the normal sinus and AV nodes. Verapamil depresses the slope of diastolic depolarization in sinus nodal cells, $\dot{V}_{max}$ of phase 0, maximum diastolic potential, and action potential amplitude in the sinus and AV nodal cells and prolongs conduction time and the effective and functional refractory periods of the AV node. The blocking effects of verapamil are more apparent at faster rates of stimulation (use-dependency) and in depolarized fibers (voltage-dependency). Verapamil probably slows the activation and delays recovery from inactivation of the slow channel. Unbinding of the drug from its receptor occurs more rapidly if this tissue is hyperpolarized.

Verapamil does exert some local anesthetic activity because the dextrorotatory stereoisomer of the clinically used racemic mixture exerts slight blocking effects on the fast sodium current. The levorotatory stereoisomer blocks the slow inward current carried by calcium, as well as other ions, traveling through the slow channel. Verapamil does not modify calcium uptake, binding, or exchange by cardiac microsomes nor does it affect calcium-activated ATPase. Verapamil does not block beta receptors, but recent data suggest that it may block alpha receptors. Verapamil may also exert other effects that indirectly alter cardiac electrophysiology, such as decreasing platelet adhesiveness or reducing the extent of myocardial ischemia.[143, 144]

In vivo, both in experimental animals and man, verapamil prolongs conduction time through the AV node (the A-H interval) without affecting the P-A, H-V, or QRS intervals and lengthens the functional and effective refractory periods of the AV node. Spontaneous sinus rate may decrease slightly, an event only partially reversed by atropine. More commonly, the sinus rate does not change significantly in vivo because verapamil causes peripheral vasodilation, transient hypotension, and reflex sympathetic stimulation that mitigates any direct slowing effect verapamil may exert on the sinus node. If verapamil is given to a patient who is also receiving a beta blocker, the sinus nodal discharge rate may slow because reflex sympathetic stimulation is blocked. Verapamil does not exert a direct effect on atrial or ventricular refractoriness or on antegrade or retrograde properties of accessory pathways.[145–147] However, reflex sympathetic stimulation may increase the ventricular response over the accessory pathway during atrial fibrillation in patients with the Wolff-Parkinson-White syndrome.[145, 147, 148]

HEMODYNAMIC EFFECTS. Since verapamil interferes with excitation-contraction coupling, it inhibits vascular smooth muscle contraction and causes marked vasodilation in coronary and other peripheral vascular beds. Propranolol does not block the vasodilation produced by verapamil. Reflex sympathetic effects may reduce in vivo the marked negative inotropic action of verapamil on isolated cardiac muscle, but direct myocardial depressant effects of verapamil may predominate when the drug is given in high doses. In patients with well-preserved left ventricular function, combined therapy with propranolol and verapamil appears to be well tolerated,[149] but beta blockade can accentuate the hemodynamic depressant effects produced by oral verapamil.[150] Patients who have reduced left ventricular function may not tolerate the combined blockade of beta receptors and of slow channels and the combined use of verapamil and propranolol in these patients must be undertaken cautiously or not at all. Verapamil decreases myocardial oxygen demand while decreasing coronary vascular resistance and reduces the extent of ischemic damage in experimental preparations. Such changes may be antiarrhythmic.[144, 151] Diltiazem, possibly by preventing calcium overload, also reduces ventricular arrhythmias during coronary occlusion in the dog.[152]

Peak alterations in hemodynamic variables occur 3 to 5 minutes after completion of the verapamil injection, the major effects being dissipated within 10 minutes. Mean arterial pressure decreases and left ventricular end-diastolic pressure increases; systemic resistance decreases and left ventricular dP/dt max decreases. Heart rate, cardiac index, left ventricular minute work, and mean pulmonary artery pressure do not change significantly. Thus, afterload reduction produced by verapamil significantly minimizes its negative inotropic action so that cardiac index may not be reduced. In addition, when verapamil slows the ventricular rate in a patient with a tachycardia, cardiac slowing may also improve hemodynamics. Nevertheless, caution should be exercised when giving verapamil to patients with severe myocardial depression or those receiving beta blockers or disopyramide, because hemodynamic deterioration may progress in some patients.[153]

PHARMACOKINETICS (Table 21–1). Following single oral doses of verapamil, measurable prolongation of AV nodal conduction time occurs in 30 minutes and lasts 4 to 6 hours. After intravenous administration, AV nodal conduction delay occurs within 1 to 2 minutes and A-H interval prolongation is still detectable after 6 hours. Effective plasma concentrations necessary to terminate supraventricular tachycardia are in the range of 125 ng/ml following doses of 0.075 mg/kg to 0.150 mg/kg.[154] After oral administration absorption is almost complete, but an overall bioavailability of 10 to 35 per cent suggests substantial first-pass metabolism in the liver, particularly of the l-isomer. The elimination half-life of verapamil is 2 to 5 hours, with up to 70 per cent of the drug excreted by the kidneys. Norverapamil is a major metabolite that may contribute to verapamil's electrophysiological actions.[155] Serum protein binding is approximately 90 per cent.

DOSAGE AND ADMINISTRATION (Table 21–1). The most commonly used intravenous dose is 10 mg infused over 1 to 2 minutes while cardiac rhythm and blood pressure are monitored. A second injection of equal dose may be given 30 minutes later. The initial effect achieved with the first bolus injection, such as slowing of the ventricular response during atrial fibrillation, may be maintained by a continuous infusion of the drug at a rate of 0.005 mg/kg/min. The oral dose is 80 to 120 mg, given three or four times a day.[145]

CLINICAL INDICATIONS. Intravenous verapamil is the treatment of choice for terminating sustained sinus nodal reentry, AV nodal reentry, or reciprocating tachycardias associated with the Wolff-Parkinson-White syndrome, when one of the reentrant pathways is the AV node, after simple vagal maneuvers have been tried and fail. Verapamil should definitely be tried prior to attempting termination by digitalis administration, pacing, electrical direct-current cardioversion, or acute blood pressure elevation with vasopressors. Verapamil terminates 60 to 80 per cent of episodes of paroxysmal supraventricular tachycardias within several minutes.[145, 154, 156] In patients with AV nodal reentry, the most common mechanism of termination appears to be block in the anterograde or slowly conducting pathway, with block less often in the fast pathway conducting retrogradely.[145, 154] In patients who experience reciprocating tachycardias during the Wolff-Parkinson-White syndrome, block terminating the tachycardia most often occurs in the AV node, not in the accessory pathway.[145] Although intravenous verapamil has been given along with intravenous propranolol[157] this combination should be used only with great caution.

Verapamil decreases the ventricular response over the AV node in the presence of atrial fibrillation or atrial flutter,[158] possibly converting a small number of episodes to sinus rhythm, particularly if the atrial flutter or fibrillation is of recent onset. Some patients who exhibit atrial flutter may develop atrial fibrillation following verapamil administration. Quinidine appears to be more effective than verapamil in establishing and maintaining sinus rhythm in patients with chronic atrial fibrillation.[45] As noted earlier, in patients with atrial fibrillation associated with the Wolff-Parkinson-White syndrome, verapamil may *accelerate* the ventricular response, and therefore the drug is contraindicated in that situation.[145, 147, 148, 159] Less information is available regarding the efficacy of verapamil in treating other types of supraventricular tachycardia. Verapamil occasionally may terminate ectopic atrial tachycardias. Hemodynamic collapse may occur if intravenous verapamil is given to patients with ventricular tachycardia. A general rule of thumb is not to give intravenous verapamil to any patient with wide-QRS tachycardia.

Orally, verapamil may prevent the recurrence of AV nodal reentrant and reciprocating tachycardias associated with the Wolff-Parkinson-White syndrome as well as help maintain a decreased ventricular response during atrial flutter or atrial fibrillation in patients without an accessory pathway.[160] In this regard, the effectiveness of verapamil appears to be enhanced when given concomitantly with digitalis or propranolol.[145] Verapamil generally has not been effective in treating patients who have recurrent ventricular tachyarrhythmias,[161] although it may suppress some forms of ventricular tachycardia.[162] However, data from animal models suggest that verapamil may be useful in reducing or preventing ventricular arrhythmias due to acute myocardial ischemia[151] and conceivably this agent may be useful to help prevent sudden death after acute myocardial infarction.[143]

ADVERSE EFFECTS. Verapamil must be used cautiously in patients with significant hemodynamic impairment or in those receiving beta blockers, as previously noted. Hypotension, bradycardia, AV block, and asystole are more likely to occur when the drug is given to patients who are already receiving beta blocking agents. Hemodynamic collapse has been noted in infants,[163] and verapamil should be used cautiously in patients less than 1 year old. Verapamil should also be used with caution in patients with sinus nodal abnormalities, since marked depression of sinus nodal function or asystole may result in some of these patients. Isoproterenol, calcium, glucagon infusion, or atropine (which may be only partially effective) and temporary pacing may be necessary to counteract some of the adverse effects of verapamil. Isoproterenol may be more effective for treating bradyarrhythmias and calcium for treating hemodynamic dysfunction. Verapamil may cause accelerated junctional discharge.[164] Contraindications to the use of verapamil include the presence of advanced heart failure, second- or third-degree AV block without a pacemaker in place, atrial fibrillation and anterograde conduction over an accessory pathway, significant sinus node dysfunction, most ventricular tachycardias, cardiogenic shock, or other hypotensive states. While the drug probably should not be used in patients with manifest heart failure,[153] if the latter is due to one of the supraventricular tachyarrhythmias noted earlier, verapamil may restore sinus rhythm or significantly decrease the ventricular rate, leading to hemodynamic improvement. Finally, it is important to note that verapamil may decrease the excretion of digoxin by about 30 per cent. Hepatotoxicity may occur on occasion.

AMIODARONE

Amiodarone is a benzofuran derivative that was introduced more than 15 years ago as a smooth muscle relaxant and coronary vasodilator to treat patients with angina. Subsequently, its antiarrhythmic actions were noted.[165–167]

ELECTROPHYSIOLOGICAL ACTIONS. When given orally chronically, amiodarone prolongs action potential duration and refractoriness of all cardiac fibers without affecting resting membrane potential. If drug effects are tested acutely in vitro, amiodarone and its metabolite, desethylamiodarone, prolong the action potential duration of ventricular muscle but shorten the action potential duration of Purkinje fibers.[168] Desethylamiodarone has relatively greater effects on fast-channel tissue in vivo than does amiodarone.[168a] Injected into the sinus and AV nodal arteries, amiodarone reduces sinus and junctional discharge rates and prolongs AV nodal conduction time.[169] It decreases the slope of diastolic depolarization of the sinus node and markedly depresses $\dot{V}_{max}$ in guinea pig papillary muscle in a rate or use-dependent manner. Such depression of $\dot{V}_{max}$ is caused by blocking of inactivated sodium channels, an effect that is accentuated by depolarized, and reduced by hyperpolarized, membrane potentials. Amiodarone also inhibits depolarization-induced automaticity.[170]

In vivo, amiodarone noncompetitively antagonizes alpha and beta receptors and blocks conversion of thyroxine (T_4) to triiodothyronine (T_3). Although slow-channel blocking effects are incompletely established, chronic oral therapy slows spontaneous sinus nodal discharge rate in anesthetized dogs even after pretreatment with propranolol and atropine. With oral administration it prolongs the Q-T interval, at times changing the contour of the T wave and producing U waves, and slows the sinus rate by 20 to 30 per cent. Right atrial monophasic action potentials are prolonged, as is the effective refractory period of all cardiac tissue. His-Purkinje conduction time increases and QRS duration lengthens, especially at fast rates.[171, 172] Amiodarone given intravenously modestly prolongs the refractory period of atrial and ventricular muscle.[171] P-R interval and AV nodal conduction time lengthen.[173–175] The duration of the QRS complex lengthens at increased rates[171] but less than after oral amiodarone. Thus, far less increase in prolongation of conduction time (except for the AV node), duration of repolarization, and refractoriness occurs after intravenous administration, compared with the oral route.[173]

HEMODYNAMIC EFFECTS. Amiodarone is a peripheral and coronary vasodilator. When administered intravenously in doses of 2.5 to 10 mg/kg, amiodarone decreases heart rate, systemic vascular resistance, left ventricular contractile force, and left ventricular dP/dt. Left ventricular output may increase. Oral doses of amiodarone sufficient to control cardiac arrhythmias do not depress left ventricular ejection fraction, even in patients with reduced ejection fractions measured by radionuclide ventriculography. However, because amiodarone does exert antiadrenergic effects and may block I_{si} to some degree, it does exert some negative inotropic action and should be given cautiously, particularly intravenously, to patients with marginal cardiac compensation.[176]

PHARMACOKINETICS. Amiodarone is slowly, variably, and incompletely absorbed, with systemic bioavailability of 35 to 65 per cent. Plasma concentrations peak 3 to 7 hours after a single oral dose. There is minimal first-pass effect, indicating little hepatic extraction. Elimination is by hepatic excretion into bile with some enterohepatic recirculation. Extensive hepatic metabolism occurs with desethylamiodarone as a major metabolite. It exerts electrophysiologic actions similar to amiodarone. The plasma concentration ratio of parent to metabolite is 3:2. Both extensively accumulate in liver, lung, fat, "blue" skin, and other tissues.[177] Myocardium develops a concentration 10 to 50 times that found in the plasma.[165] Plasma clearance of amiodarone is low and renal excretion negligible. Doses need not be reduced in patients with renal disease. Amiodarone and desethylamiodarone are not dialyzable. Volume of distribution is large but variable, averaging 60 liters/kg. Amiodarone is highly protein bound (96 per cent), crosses the placenta (10 to 50 per cent), and is found in breast milk.

The onset of action after intravenous administration generally is within several hours. Following oral administration the onset of action may require 2 to 3 days, often 1 to 3 weeks and, on occasion, even longer. Loading doses reduce this time interval. Plasma concentrations relate well to oral doses during chronic treatment, averaging about 0.5 μg/ml for each 100 mg/day at doses between 100 and 600 mg/day. Elimination half-life is multiphasic with an initial 50 per cent reduction in plasma concentration 3 to 10 days after cessation of drug ingestion (probably representing elimination from well-perfused tissues) followed by a terminal half-life of 26 to 107 days, mean 53 days, with most patients in the 40- to 55-day range. To achieve steady-state without a loading dose takes about 265 days. Interpatient variability of these pharmacokinetic parameters mandates close monitoring of the patient. Therapeutic serum concentrations range from 1 to 2.5 μg/ml. Greater suppression of arrhythmias may occur up to 3.5 μg/ml, but the risk of side effects increases.[178–180]

DOSAGE AND ADMINISTRATION. An optimal dosing schedule for all patients has not been achieved. One recommended approach is to treat with 800 to 1600 mg daily for 1 to 3 weeks, reduced to 800 mg daily for the next 2 to 4 weeks, then 600 mg daily for 4 to 8 weeks, and finally, after 2 to 3 months of treatment, a maintenance dose of 400 mg per day attained after 2 to 3 months of treatment. Maintenance drug can be given once or twice daily, and should be titrated to the lowest effective dose to minimize the occurrence of side effects. Regimens must be individualized for a given patient and clinical situation. Amiodarone may be administered intravenously (not approved for this route of administration by the FDA at the time of this writing) to achieve more rapid loading[171, 173, 176, 181, 182] at initial doses of 5 to 10 mg/kg over 20 to 30 minutes, followed by 1 gm/24 hours for several days. Additional boluses of 1 to 3 mg/kg may be given several hours after the first bolus if necessary. An alternative, well-studied approach[181] is to infuse 2.0 to 2.5 mg/min for 12 hours followed by a maintenance dose of 0.7 mg/min for the next 36 hours. Patients with depressed ejection fractions should receive intravenous amiodarone with great caution. High-dose oral loading (800 to 2000 mg two or three times a day to maintain trough serum concentrations of 2 to 3 μg/ml) may suppress ventricular arrhythmias in 1 to 2 days.[183]

CLINICAL INDICATIONS. Amiodarone has been used to suppress a wide spectrum of supraventricular and ventricular tachyarrhythmias in adults and children,[166, 184–187] including AV nodal and AV entry,[188, 189] atrial flutter and fibrillation,[190, 191] ventricular tachycardia and ventricular fibrillation associated with coronary artery disease, and hypertrophic cardiomyopathy.[192] Success rates vary widely depending on patient population, arrhythmia, underlying heart disease, length of follow-up, definition and determination of success, and other factors. In general, however, amiodarone's efficacy equals or exceeds that of all other antiarrhythmic agents, and may be conservatively in the range of 60 to 80 per cent for most supraventricular tachyarrhythmias (including those associated with the WPW syndrome) and 40 to 60 per cent for ventricular tachyarrhythmias. Most, but not all,[193, 194] studies report success in the higher end of those ranges. Amiodarone has been approved by the FDA to treat patients with recurrent, hemodynamically unstable ventricular tachycardia or ventricular fibrillation, when these arrhythmias have not responded to other available antiarrhythmic drugs or when these other agents were not tolerated. Because of its long half-life and the difficulty involved in starting another antiarrhythmic drug (while not knowing if amiodarone's effects are still present), and its side effects profile, *amiodarone should be among the last antiarrhythmic agents tried.*

Predicting effectiveness of antiarrhythmic drugs is a difficult problem (see p. 625), and controversy exists regarding amiodarone and ventricular tachyarrhythmias. Clinical assessment,[195] suppression of spontaneous ventricular arrhythmias as documented by 24-hour ECG recordings,[196, 197] and response to electrophysiological testing[198, 199] have served as endpoints to judge therapy. In the patient with a history of sustained ventricular tachycardia or fibrillation and minimal spontaneous ventricular arrhythmias in between symptomatic episodes, an invasive electrophysiologic study would be indicated to judge drug efficacy. Whether such studies are necessary for the patient who manifests spontaneous episodes of life-threatening arrhythmia that can be used as an endpoint to determine drug efficacy is more controversial. In the 10 to 40 per cent of patients whose electrically induced clinical ventricular tachyarrhythmias become no longer inducible while they are receiving amiodarone, the chances for a spontaneous recurrence of the arrhythmias are low while the patients are taking amiodarone, probably less than 5 to 10 per cent at 1 year. For those patients whose ventricular tachyarrhythmias are still inducible, the recurrence rate is 40 to 50 per cent at 1 year.[194, 198, 199] However, in this latter group, greater difficulty in inducing the arrhythmias may predict a less likely possibility of a recurrence.[198] Patients' hemodynamic responses to the induced arrhythmia also may predict how they tolerate a spontaneous recurrence.[199] It is important to remember, however, that the supine patient in the electrophysiology laboratory may tolerate the same tachycardia better than when in an erect position.

Because of the serious nature of the arrhythmias being treated, the unusual pharmacokinetics of the drug, and the adverse effects (see below), amiodarone therapy should be started with the patient hospitalized and monitored for generally a week or longer.

ADVERSE EFFECTS. Adverse effects occur in about 75 per cent of patients treated with 400 mg/day and require discontinuation of treatment in 10 to 20 per cent.[200, 201] Most adverse effects are reversible with dose reduction or cessation of treatment. Adverse effects may become more frequent when therapy is continued beyond 6 months but begin to stabilize after a year or so. Of the noncardiac adverse reactions, pulmonary toxicity is the most serious,[202] usually occurring within the first 30 months of treatment, occasionally as early as 2 to 3 weeks. The mechanism is unclear but may relate to a hypersensitivity reaction and/or widespread phospholipidosis.[165] Frequency varies from 5 or 7 per cent to 13 or 15 per cent at 1 year, possibly increasing with continued drug administration. Dyspnea, nonproductive cough, and fever are common symptoms with rales, hypoxia, a positive gallium scan, reduced diffusion capacity, and radiographic evidence of pulmonary infiltrates noted. Amiodarone must be discontinued if such pulmonary inflammatory changes occur. Steroids may be tried but no controlled studies have been done to support their use. A 10 per cent mortality in patients with pulmonary inflammatory changes has been reported, often in patients with unrecognized pulmonary involvement that is allowed to progress. Chest roentgenograms at 3-month intervals for a year and then twice a year have been recommended.

Although asymptomatic elevations of liver enzymes are found in most patients, the drug is not stopped unless values exceed three times normal or double in a patient with initially abnormal values. Cirrhosis occurs uncommonly but may be fatal. Neurological dysfunction, photosensitivity (perhaps minimized by sunscreens), bluish skin discoloration, corneal microdeposits (in almost 100 per cent of adults receiving the drug more than 6 months), gastroenterological disturbances, and hyperthyroidism (1 to 2 per cent) or hypothyroidism (2 to 4 per cent) may occur.[203, 203a] Amiodarone appears to inhibit the peripheral conversion of T_4 to T_3 so that chemical changes result characterized by a slight increase in T_4, reverse T_3, and TSH, and a slight decrease in T_3. Reverse T_3 concentration has been used as an index of drug efficacy.[12] During hypothyroidism, TSH increases greatly while T_3 increases in hyperthyroidism.

Cardiac side effects include symptomatic bradycardias in about 2 per cent, aggravation of ventricular tachyarrhythmias (with occasional development of torsades de pointes) in 2 to 3 per cent, and worsening of congestive heart failure in 2 per cent. Hypotension after open heart surgery has been noted, possibly due to interactions with anesthetics.[204]

Important interactions with other drugs occur and, when given concomitantly with amiodarone, the dose of warfarin, digoxin, and other antiarrhythmic drugs should be reduced by one-third to one-half, and the patient watched closely. Drugs with synergistic actions, such as beta blockers or calcium channel blockers, must be given cautiously.

MEXILETINE

Mexiletine, a local anesthetic with anticonvulsant properties, is approved by the FDA for oral treatment of patients with symptomatic ventricular arrhythmias.

ELECTROPHYSIOLOGICAL ACTIONS. Mexiletine is similar to lidocaine in many of its electrophysiological actions. In vitro, mexiletine shortens the duration of the action potential and refractory period of Purkinje fibers and to a lesser extent of ventricular muscle. It depresses $\dot{V}_{max}$ of phase 0 by blocking the fast sodium channel, especially at faster rates, and depresses automaticity of Purkinje fibers but not of the normal sinus node. Its onset kinetics are rapid.[8] Hypoxia or ischemia may increase its effects on $\dot{V}_{max}$.

Mexiletine may result in severe bradycardia and abnormal sinus nodal recovery time in patients with sinus node disease but not in patients with a normal sinus node. It may depress His-Purkinje conduction but not greatly unless conduction was abnormal initially. Mexiletine does not appear to affect the refractory period of human atrial and ventricular muscle. The duration of the QT interval does not increase. Because of its rate-dependent effects, theoretically mexiletine might be expected to suppress closely coupled rather than late coupled ventricular extrasystoles or faster tachycardias.[205]

HEMODYNAMIC EFFECTS. Mexiletine exerts no major hemodynamic effects. It does not depress myocardial performance when given orally, although intravenous administration may produce hypotension.[206, 207]

PHARMACOKINETICS. Mexiletine has been reported to be rapidly and almost completely absorbed after oral ingestion by volunteers, with peak plasma concentrations attained in 2 to 4 hours.[208] Elimination half-life in healthy subjects is approximately 10 hours and in patients after myocardial infarction, 17 hours. Therapeutic plasma levels of 1 to 2 μg/ml are maintained by oral doses of 200 to 300 mg every 6 to 8 hours. Absorption with less than 10 per cent first-pass hepatic effect occurs in the upper small intestine and is delayed and incomplete in patients who have myocardial infarction and in patients receiving narcotic analgesics, antacids, or atropine-like drugs that retard gastric emptying. Bioavailability of orally administered mexiletine is approximately 90 per cent, and about 70 per cent of the drug is protein-bound. The apparent volume of distribution is large, reflecting extensive tissue uptake. Normally, mexiletine is eliminated metabolically by the liver, with less than 10 per cent excreted unchanged in the urine. Doses probably should be reduced in patients with cirrhosis and those with left ventricular failure. Renal clearance of mexiletine decreases as urinary pH increases. Known metabolites exert no electrophysiological effects.

DOSAGE AND ADMINISTRATION. Recommended starting dose is 200 mg orally every 8 hours when rapid arrhythmia control is not essential. Doses may be increased or decreased by 50 to 100 mg every 2 to 3 days, and are better tolerated when given with food. Total daily dose should not exceed 1200 mg. In some patients, administration every 12 hours may be effective. For rapid loading, 400 mg followed in 8 hours by a 200 mg dose is suggested.

CLINICAL INDICATIONS. Mexiletine is an effective antiarrhythmic agent for treating patients with both acute and chronic ventricular tachyarrhythmias but not with supraventricular tachycardias. Success rates vary from 6 to

60 per cent.[209, 210] Mexiletine combined with other drugs such as procainamide, beta blockers, quinidine, disopyramide, or amiodarone may become a major application of the drug. Most studies show no clear superiority of mexiletine over other class I agents.[209, 211–215] In treating patients with a long Q-T interval, mexiletine probably would be safer than drugs such as quinidine that increase the Q-T interval further.

ADVERSE EFFECTS. Thirty to 40 per cent of patients may require a change in dose or discontinuation of mexiletine therapy as a result of adverse effects, including tremor, dysarthria, dizziness, paresthesia, diplopia, nystagmus, mental confusion, anxiety, nausea, vomiting, and dyspepsia. Cardiovascular side effects are most often seen after intravenous dosing and include hypotension, bradycardia, and exacerbation of arrhythmia.[209, 216] Adverse effects of mexiletine appear to be dose-related, and toxic effects occur at plasma concentrations only slightly higher than therapeutic levels. Therefore, effective use of this antiarrhythmic drug requires careful titration of dose and monitoring of plasma concentration.

TOCAINIDE

Tocainide is a primary amine analog of lidocaine that lacks two ethyl groups; this characteristic protects it from first-pass hepatic elimination and makes it effective orally.[217]

ELECTROPHYSIOLOGICAL AND HEMODYNAMIC ACTIONS. Electrophysiological effects are virtually the same as those exerted by lidocaine and mexiletine. In patients with compensated left ventricular dysfunction, intravenous infusion of tocainide moderately decreases mean arterial pressure and slightly increases pulmonary and systemic vascular resistance and left ventricular end-diastolic pressure without altering heart rate, cardiac index, or left ventricular dP/dt. It has a small negative inotropic effect and increases peripheral vascular resistance slightly. Oral administration in patients after myocardial infarction does not appear to affect hemodynamic compensation adversely.

PHARMACOKINETICS. Bioavailability of tocainide is almost 100 per cent. The drug is rapidly and completely absorbed, yielding peak plasma concentrations 0.5 to 2 hours after oral ingestion. Approximately 40 per cent is excreted unchanged in the urine. It is not extensively bound by plasma proteins and there are no known active metabolites. Mean elimination half-life is 11 hours in normal volunteers, possibly longer in patients. There appears to be no pharmacokinetic interaction with other drugs,[217] but caution must be used when combining drugs because of additive antiarrhythmic effects.

DOSAGE AND ADMINISTRATION. Oral regimens of 400 to 600 mg every 8 hours produce therapeutic plasma concentrations of 4 to 10 μg/ml. Dosing increases should not be made more often than every 3 or 4 days. Twice daily doses can be tried in patients who respond to dosing three times a day. Doses should be reduced in patients with heart failure, liver, or renal disease.

CLINICAL INDICATIONS. Although tocainide effectively reduces the frequency of premature ventricular complexes, it has been less effective in preventing chronic recurrent ventricular tachycardia–ventricular fibrillation in some but not all studies.[218–221] It is slightly less effective than quinidine in suppressing ventricular arrhythmias,[222] and may be effective when mexiletine is not.[223] Response to intravenous lidocaine may help predict an individual's response to oral tocainide. If lidocaine fails to suppress the ventricular arrhythmia, tocainide has only about a 15 per cent chance of being effective. On the other hand, if lidocaine suppresses the ventricular arrhythmia, tocainide has about a 60 per cent possibility of being effective.[220] Tocainide and mexiletine may be acceptable choices for patients with ventricular arrhythmias in whom the Q-T interval is prolonged.

ADVERSE EFFECTS. Adverse effects are dose-related, similar to those produced by lidocaine, and include nausea, vomiting, anorexia, tremulousness, memory impairment, skin rash, sweating, paresthesia, diplopia, dizziness, anxiety, and tinnitus. Dosing with meals may reduce side effects, possibly by reducing peak serum concentrations of the drug. Occasionally, tocainide may produce pulmonary fibrosis or induce or aggravate ventricular arrhythmias.[217, 220, 224] Hematological disorders including agranulocytosis, bone marrow depression, leukopenia, hypoplastic anemia, and thrombocytopenia have been reported with an estimated incidence of 0.18 per cent and may seriously limit the use of tocainide.

FLECAINIDE

Flecainide is approved by the FDA for the treatment of patients with symptomatic ventricular arrhythmias.[225, 225a]

ELECTROPHYSIOLOGICAL ACTIONS. Flecainide exhibits marked use-dependent depressant effects on the rapid sodium channel, decreasing V_{max} with slow onset and offset kinetics.[226] Drug dissociation from the sodium channel is very slow, with time constants of 10 to 30 sec (compared with 4 to 8 sec for quinidine and <1 second for lidocaine). Marked drug effects occur at physiological heart rates. Flecainide shortens the duration of Purkinje fiber action potential but prolongs it in ventricular muscle,[227] actions that, depending on the circumstances, could enhance or reduce electrical heterogeneity and create or suppress arrhythmias. Flecainide profoundly slows conduction in all cardiac fibers, and, in high concentrations, inhibits the slow channel.[227] Clinically, conduction time in the atria, ventricles, AV node, and His-Purkinje system is prolonged. Minimal increases in atrial or ventricular refractoriness, or in the Q-T interval, result. Anterograde and retrograde refractoriness in accessory pathways may increase by 100 msec or more. Normal sinus node function remains unchanged, but abnormal sinus node discharge may be depressed.[228, 229]

HEMODYNAMIC EFFECTS. Flecainide modestly depresses cardiac performance, particularly in patients with compromised myocardial function. Left ventricular ejection fraction decreased by 15 per cent in patients given 1 mg intravenously.[230] Changes may be less after oral dosing, but caution is warranted, particularly in patients with a history of heart failure. It should be used cautiously, if at all, in patients with severely compromised cardiac function.[225]

PHARMACOKINETICS. Flecainide is at least 90 per cent absorbed with peak plasma concentrations in 3 to 4 hours. Elimination half-life in patients with ventricular arrhythmias is 20 hours, 85 per cent of the drug being excreted unchanged or as an inactive metabolite in urine. Two major metabolites exert less effects than the parent drug. Rate of elimination is slower in patients with renal disease and heart failure and doses should be reduced in these situations. Therapeutic plasma concentrations range from 0.2 to 1.0 μg/ml. About 40 per cent of the drug is protein bound. Small increases in serum concentrations of digoxin

(13 per cent) and propranolol (30 per cent) result during co-administration with flecainide.[231] Propranolol may increase flecainide serum concentration and both drugs may produce combined detrimental hemodynamic effects. Five to 7 days of dosing may be required to reach steady-state in some patients.[232]

DOSAGE AND ADMINISTRATION. Starting dose is 100 mg every 12 hours, increased in increments of 50 mg twice daily, no sooner than every 4 days, until efficacy is achieved, an adverse effect is noted, or to a maximum of 400 mg/day.

CLINICAL INDICATIONS. Flecainide is indicated for the treatment of life-threatening ventricular tachyarrhythmias and to suppress episodes of nonsustained ventricular tachycardia or premature ventricular complexes that produce symptoms. Therapy should begin in the hospital while the ECG is being monitored because of the high incidence of proarrhythmia events (see below). Serum concentration should not exceed 1.0 μg/ml. Flecainide is particularly effective, more so than quinidine, in almost totally suppressing premature ventricular complexes and short runs of nonsustained ventricular tachycardia,[233, 234] although the importance of such a response on the subsequent outcome of the patient has not been established. Flecainide prevents electrical induction of ventricular tachyarrhythmias in a small percentage of patients (20 to 30 per cent) and eliminates recurrence of life-threatening ventricular tachyarrhythmias in about 40 per cent.[235] Although not approved for these indications, flecainide may be very useful in patients with AV nodal and AV reentry tachycardias and other supraventricular tachycardias.[236, 237]

ADVERSE EFFECTS. Proarrhythmic effects[217, 237a] are one of the most important adverse effects of flecainide. Its marked slowing of conduction precludes its use in patients with second degree AV block without a pacemaker and warrants cautious administration in patients with intraventricular conduction disorders. Aggravation of existing ventricular arrhythmias or onset of new ventricular arrhythmias may occur in 5 to 25 per cent of patients, the increased percentage in patients with preexisting sustained ventricular tachycardia, cardiac decompensation, and higher doses of the drug. Failure of the flecainide-related arrhythmia to respond to therapy, including electrical cardioversion-defibrillation, may result in a mortality as high as 10 per cent in patients who develop proarrhythmic events. Negative inotropic effects may cause or worsen heart failure. Patients with sinus node dysfunction may experience sinus arrest and those with pacemakers may develop an increase in pacing threshold. Central nervous system complaints, including confusion and irritability, represent the most frequent noncardiac adverse effect.

NEW ANTIARRHYTHMIC DRUGS

ENCAINIDE

Encainide resembles flecainide electrophysiologically. The rate-dependent block of the fast sodium channel has slow onset and offset kinetics and is greater in depolarized fibers. It shortens the action potential duration of Purkinje fibers but exerts little effect on atrial or ventricular muscle. It markedly slows conduction in all cardiac tissue. Encainide does not affect the slow response in vitro. Encainide has several active metabolites,[238] one of which is more potent than the parent compound.[239] Active metabolites may contribute to its antiarrhythmic efficacy,[240] and variation in the conversion of encainide to its active metabolites may be a source of interpatient differences in drug response.[238] In patients, oral encainide prolongs atrial, ventricular, and accessory pathway refractory periods, A-H and H-V intervals, and P-R, QRS, and Q-T intervals.[240] Encainide does not alter myocardial contractility or ejection indices in patients with relatively normal ventricular function; in those with reduced ventricular function, as evidenced by elevated left ventricular and end-diastolic pressures and reduced cardiac output, encainide further decreases cardiac output slightly.

Encainide exhibits a wide range of bioavailability and a relatively short half-life of 3 to 4 hours. However, the existence of one or more active metabolites permits a long interval between dosing during which the concentration of encainide metabolites exceeds that of the parent compound and is probably responsible for the delayed return (13 hours) of arrhythmias following drug withdrawal.[241] The drug is useful in treating some patients who have supraventricular tachycardias associated with AV nodal reentry or Wolff-Parkinson-White syndrome.[240, 242, 243] It is effective in about 25 to 30 per cent of patients with chronic recurrent ventricular tachyarrhythmias refractory to conventional agents, and may be more effective than quinidine.[244, 244a]

Encainide is generally administered orally four times daily in doses of 100 to 300 mg/day. Dose changes should not be made more frequently than every 48 hours. Adverse effects include dizziness, diplopia, vertigo, paresthesia, leg cramps, and a metallic taste in the mouth. Most significant is its potential to cause or exacerbate serious ventricular tachyarrhythmias in approximately 10 per cent of patients treated. Commonly, a polymorphous ventricular tachycardia ensues and may result in hemodynamic collapse. Often, this is not associated with marked Q-T prolongation and may be difficult to terminate electrically.[245, 246]

ETHMOZINE

Ethmozine is a phenothiazine derivative that exerts its major effect on the fast sodium channel. It depresses $\dot{V}_{max}$ of phase 0, action potential amplitude, and action potential duration in canine Purkinje fibers and decreases the force of Purkinje fiber contraction. Ethmozine suppresses abnormal automaticity arising from depolarized fibers and delayed afterdepolarizations.[247] Injected into the sinus or AV nodal arteries of dogs, ethmozine does not alter sinus discharge rate or AV nodal conduction at therapeutic concentrations[248] and produces minimal electrophysiological changes in patients.[249] It is well absorbed and extensively metabolized, but little is known about the potential activity of its metabolites. Ethmozine suppresses supraventricular[249] and ventricular[250, 251] arrhythmias but the data from controlled studies are too preliminary at present to draw meaningful conclusions.[252]

LORCAINIDE

Lorcainide is an acetanilide derivative with local anesthetic effects that decreases $\dot{V}_{max}$ of phase 0 and conduction velocity and slightly prolongs the effective refractory period of Purkinje fibers. It does not affect the slow response and prolongs conduction time in the atria, His-Purkinje system, and ventricles. Elimination half-life ranges in different studies between 5 and 12 hours. Important first-pass hepatic effects that reduce bioavailability occur with single 100 mg doses, but bioavailability increases after higher and multiple doses. Lorcainide appears effective against ventricular arrhythmias.[253, 254] Insomnia is an important side effect that is treated with diazepam and gradually disappears after continued dosing.

PROPAFENONE

Propafenone exerts weak blocking effects on beta receptors and on the slow calcium channel. However, it blocks the fast sodium channel as its major action,[255] in a phasic or rate-dependent fashion, but also at rest. Resting state block is enhanced more than phasic block when the membrane potential becomes depolarized.[256] Its slow dissociation constant, like that of encainide and flecainide, may make it effective against both slow and fast tachycardias. Propafenone has been shown to prolong the duration of rabbit[255] and shorten that of guinea pig[256] action potential. It depresses sinus nodal automaticity. In patients, the A-H, H-V, P-R and QRS intervals increase, as do refractory periods of the atria, ventricles, and accessory pathways.[257, 258] It exerts a minimal negative inotropic effect.

More than 95 per cent absorbed, the drug's maximum plasma concentration results in 2 to 3 hours. Systemic bioavailability of only 12 per cent indicates extensive presystemic clearance. Bioavailability increases as the dose increases and plasma concentration is therefore nonlinear. A threefold increase in dosage (300 to 900 mg/day) results in a ten-fold increase in plasma concentration. Propafenone is highly protein bound with an elimination half-life of 5 to 8 hours. Marked interpatient variability of pharmacokinetics and pharmacodynamics may be due to genetically determined differences in metabolism. One or more active metabolites may exist.[259, 260] Doses are 150 to 300 mg every 8 to 12 hours. Propafenone has been effective in suppressing both ventricular[257, 261] and supraventricular tachyarrhythmias,[262] and those associated with the WPW syndrome.[258, 262] Tachyarrhythmias still induced despite propafenone administration occur at slower rates and are often better tolerated. Adverse effects include arrhythmia aggravation,[257, 263] worsening of congestive heart failure,[261] and neurologic symptoms.[257]

OTHER ANTIARRHYTHMIC AGENTS

Other antiarrhythmic agents, such as bethanidine,[264] meobentine,[265] cibenzoline,[266, 267] sotalol,[268] bepridil,[269, 270] adenosine,[271, 272] esmolol,[273] recainam,[273a] pirmenol,[273b] antidepressant drugs such as imipramine and nortriptyline,[274] and other agents, are currently undergoing evaluation.

ELECTRICAL THERAPY OF CARDIAC ARRHYTHMIAS

DIRECT CURRENT CARDIOVERSION

Electrical cardioversion offers obvious advantages over drug therapy to terminate tachycardia. Under conditions optimal for close supervision and monitoring, a precisely regulated "dose" of electricity can restore sinus rhythm immediately and safely. The distinction between supraventricular and ventricular tachyarrhythmias—crucial to the proper medical management of arrhythmias—becomes less significant, and the time-consuming titration of drugs with potential side effects is abolished.

MECHANISMS. Electrical cardioversion appears to terminate most effectively those tachycardias presumed to be due to reentry, including atrial flutter and atrial fibrillation, AV nodal reentry, reciprocating tachycardias associated with Wolff-Parkinson-White syndrome, most forms of ventricular tachycardia, ventricular flutter, and ventricular fibrillation. The electric shock, by depolarizing all excitable myocardium, interrupts reentrant circuits, discharges foci, and establishes electrical homogeneity that terminates reentry. A shock that does not end the tachycardia may fail to depolarize critical areas involved in the maintenance of the tachycardia. A tachycardia that terminates and then restarts may be reinitiated by factors provoking the tachycardia in the first place. If the precipitating factors are no longer present, interrupting the tachyarrhythmia for only the brief time produced by the shock may prevent its return for long duration even though the anatomical and electrophysiological substrates required for the tachycardia are still present.

Tachycardias thought to be due to disorders of impulse formation (automaticity) include parasystole, some forms of atrial tachycardias with or without AV block, nonparoxysmal AV junctional tachycardia, and accelerated idioventricular rhythms. An attempt to cardiovert these tachycardias electrically in most instances is not indicated. It is possible that the shock can terminate tachycardias due to enhanced automaticity or triggered activity, but this notion is conjectural at present.

TECHNIQUE

After the procedure has been explained to the patient, a careful physical examination, including palpation of all pulses, should be performed prior to elective cardioversion. A 12-lead electrocardiogram is obtained before and after cardioversion as well as a rhythm strip during the electroshock. The patient should be in a fasting state and "metabolically balanced," i.e., blood gases, pH, and electrolytes should be normal with no evidence of drug toxicity. It does not seem necessary to withhold digitalis for several days prior to elective cardioversion in patients without clinical evidence of digitalis toxicity.[275] Maintenance quinidine administration 1 to 2 days before electrical cardioversion of patients with atrial fibrillation may revert 10 to 15 per cent to sinus rhythm and help prevent recurrence of atrial fibrillation once sinus rhythm is restored.

Despite the clinical applications of transthoracic cardioversion and defibrillation for more than 30 years, new explorations into the effects of different waveforms,[276] pathways of delivering the shock,[277] effects of multiple shocks,[278] and autonomic influences[279, 280] (fueled by the desire to achieve the lowest defibrillation thresholds for implantable devices), show promise of reducing the energy required to terminate tachycardias electrically. The use of self-adhesive pads applied in the standard apex-anterior or apex-posterior paddle positions represents an advance. They have similar transthoracic impedances as paddles[281] and are very useful in elective cardioversions or other situations when there is time for their application, such as at the start of an electrophysiological study. Paddles 12 to 13 cm in diameter can be used[282] to deliver maximum current to the heart,[283] but the benefits of these paddles as compared with those of 8 to 9 cm diameter have not been clearly established. Defibrillators with larger energies than those currently commercially available probably are not necessary, even for very large patients, particularly if paddles with large diameters are used. Larger paddles may distribute the intracardiac current over a wider area and may reduce shock-induced myocardial necrosis.

A synchronized shock, i.e., one delivered during the QRS complex, is used for all cardioversions except for very rapid ventricular tachyarrhythmias, such as ventricular flutter or fibrillation. Because myocardial damage increases directly with increases in applied energy, the minimum effective energy should be used. Therefore, shocks are "titrated" when the clinical situation permits. Except for atrial fibrillation, shocks in the range of 25 to 50 joules successfully terminate most supraventricular tachycardias and should be tried initially. If unsuccessful, a second shock of higher energy may be delivered. The starting level to terminate atrial fibrillation should probably be 50 to 100 joules. For patients with stable ventricular tachycardia, starting levels in the range of 25 to 50 joules may be employed.[284] If there is some urgency to terminate the tachyarrhythmia, one can begin with higher energies. To terminate ventricular fibrillation, 200 to 400 joules generally are used, although much lower energies (<100 joules) terminate ventricular fibrillation when the shock is delivered at the *very onset* of the arrhythmia, using adhesive pads in the electrophysiology laboratory, for example.

During elective cardioversion, a short-acting barbiturate, such as methohexital in intravenous doses of 25 to 75 mg, or an amnesic, such as diazepam given in incremental intravenous doses of 2.5 to 5 mg at 30-second intervals, may be used. A physician skilled in airway management should be in attendance (preferably an anesthetist, if possible), an intravenous route should be established, and all equipment necessary for emergency resuscitation should be immediately accessible. Before cardioversion, 100 per cent oxygen may be administered for 5 to 15 minutes and is continued throughout the procedure. Manual ventilation of the patient may be necessary to avoid hypoxia during periods of deepest sleep.

INDICATIONS. Before considering electrical cardioversion, the likelihood of establishing and maintaining sinus rhythm using electrical countershock should be weighed against the risks of other forms of therapy. As a rule, any tachycardia that produces hypotension, congestive heart failure, or angina and does not respond promptly to medical management should be terminated electrically. Very rapid ventricular rates in patients with atrial fibrillation and the Wolff-Parkinson-White syndrome are often best treated by electrical cardioversion. In almost all instances, the patient's hemodynamic status improves after cardioversion. An occasional patient may develop hypotension, reduced cardiac output, or congestive heart failure following the shock, possibly related to complications of the cardioversion, such as embolic events, myocardial depression resulting from the anesthetic agent, hypoxia, lack of restoration of left atrial contraction despite return of electrical atrial systole or postshock arrhythmias.[285, 286] Direct-current countershock of digitalis-induced tachyarrhythmias is contraindicated.

Favorable candidates for electrical cardioversion of atrial fibrillation include those patients who (1) have symptomatic atrial fibrillation of less than 12 months' duration and derive significant hemodynamic benefits from sinus rhythm; (2) have embolic episodes; (3) continue to have atrial fibrillation after the precipitating cause has been removed, e.g., following treatment of thyrotoxicosis, and (4) have a rapid ventricular rate that is difficult to slow.

Unfavorable candidates include patients with (1) digitalis toxicity, (2) no symptoms and a well-controlled ventricular rate without therapy, (3) sinus node dysfunction and various unstable supraventricular tachyarrhythmias or bradyarrhythmias (often the bradycardia-tachycardia syndrome) who finally develop and maintain atrial fibrillation (which in essence represents a "cure" of the sick sinus syndrome), (4) little or no benefit from normal sinus rhythm and who promptly revert to atrial fibrillation after cardioversion despite drug therapy, (5) a large left atrium and long-standing atrial fibrillation, (6) infrequent episodes of atrial fibrillation that revert spontaneously to sinus rhythm, (7) no mechanical atrial systole after the return of electrical atrial systole, (8) atrial fibrillation and advanced heart block, (9) cardiac surgery planned in the near future, and (10) antiarrhythmic drug intolerance. Atrial fibrillation is likely to recur after cardioversion in patients who have significant chronic obstructive lung disease, congestive heart failure, or mitral valve disease, particularly mitral insufficiency.

In patients with atrial flutter, slowing the ventricular rate by administering digitalis or terminating the flutter with quinidine may be difficult, so that electrical cardioversion is often the initial treatment of choice. For the patient with other types of supraventricular tachycardia, electrical cardioversion may be employed when maneuvers to enhance vagal tone or simple medical management (e.g., intravenous verapamil) have failed to terminate the tachycardia and the clinical setting indicates that fairly prompt restoration of sinus rhythm is desirable because of hemodynamic decompensation or electrophysiological consequences of the tachycardia. Similarly for patients with ventricular tachycardia, the hemodynamic and electrophysiological consequences of the arrhythmias determine the need and urgency for direct current-cardioversion (p. 642). Electrical countershock is the initial treatment of choice for ventricular flutter or ventricular fibrillation.

If, after the first shock, reversion to sinus rhythm does not occur, a higher energy level should be tried. When transient ventricular arrhythmias result after an unsuccessful shock,[285, 286] a bolus of lidocaine may be given prior to delivering a shock at the next energy level. If sinus rhythm returns only transiently and is promptly supplanted by the tachycardia, a repeat shock may be tried, depending on the tachyarrhythmia being treated and its consequences. Administration of an antiarrhythmic agent intravenously may be useful prior to delivering the next cardioversion shock. After cardioversion, the patient should be monitored at least until full consciousness has been restored and preferably for several hours thereafter.

RESULTS. Cardioversion restores sinus rhythm in 70 to 95 per cent of patients, depending upon the type of tachyarrhythmia. However, sinus rhythm remains after 12 months in less than one-third to one-half the patients with chronic atrial fibrillation. Thus, maintenance of sinus rhythm once established is the difficult problem, not the immediate termination of the tachycardia, and depends on the particular arrhythmia, the presence of underlying heart disease, and the adequacy of antiarrhythmic drug therapy.

COMPLICATIONS. Arrhythmias induced by the shock generally are caused by inadequate synchronization, with the shock occurring during the ST segment or T wave. Occasionally, a properly synchronized shock may produce ventricular fibrillation (Fig. 21–5).[282] Post-shock arrhythmias usually are transient and do not require therapy. Embolic episodes are reported to occur in 1 to 3 per cent of the patients converted to sinus rhythm. Prior anticoagulation for 1 to 2 weeks should be considered for patients who have no contraindication to such therapy and who are at high risk for emboli, such as those with mitral stenosis and atrial fibrillation of recent onset, a history of recent or recurrent emboli, a prosthetic mitral valve, enlarged hearts (including left atrial enlargement), or congestive heart failure. Anticoagulation with warfarin for several weeks afterward is recommended. However, it must be emphasized that few controlled studies to support this approach have been published.

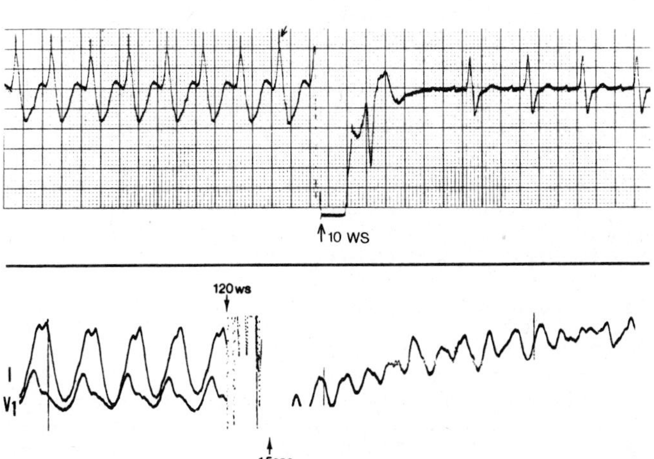

FIGURE 21–5. *Top,* A synchronized shock (note synchronization marks in the apex of the QRS complex [↓]) during ventricular tachycardia is followed by a single repetitive ventricular response and then normal sinus rhythm. *Bottom,* A shock synchronized to the terminal portion of the QRS complex in a patient with atrial fibrillation and conduction to the ventricle over an accessory pathway (WPW syndrome) results in ventricular fibrillation that was promptly terminated by a 400 watt-sec (or joule) shock. Recording was lost for 1.5 sec (↑) owing to baseline drift after the shock.

Although direct-current shock has been demonstrated in animals to cause cardiac injury, studies in man indicate that elevations of myocardial enzymes after cardioversion are not common. ST-segment elevation may occur with elective direct-current cardioversion, although cardiac enzymes and myocardial scintigraphy may be unremarkable.[287]

Cardioversion of ventricular tachycardia can also be achieved by a chest thump. Its mechanism of termination probably relates to a mechanically induced premature atrial or ventricular complex that interrupts a tachycardia. The thump cannot be timed very well and is probably only effective when delivered during a nonrefractory part of the cardiac cycle. Care must therefore be taken, because the thump can alter a ventricular tachycardia[288] and possibly induce ventricular flutter or fibrillation.[289]

IMPLANTABLE ELECTRICAL DEVICES FOR TREATMENT OF CARDIAC ARRHYTHMIAS

Implantable devices[290] that monitor the cardiac rhythm and can deliver competing pacing stimuli[291] and low-[292, 293] and high-energy shocks[294, 295] have been used effectively in selected patients and are discussed fully in Chapter 23.

ELECTRICAL ABLATION THERAPY

The purpose of electrical ablation (fulguration) therapy is to destroy myocardial tissue by delivering a high-energy electrical shock between two electrodes, one of which is located on a catheter that has been placed next to an area of the endocardium integrally related to the arrhythmia.[296, 297] The intracardiac electrode may be the anode, to maximize the effects of the shock, with a large metal plate or conducting adhesive pad on the skin of the thorax serving as the cathode. The shock can also be given over the cathode in the heart or between two electrodes on the same or two separate intracardiac catheters. Energy is delivered from an external cardioverter-defibrillator connected to both electrodes by a switching terminal.

The mechanism by which the shock destroys heart muscle is complex. In vitro studies reveal that the shock produces an incandescent spherical "fireball" approximately 5 to 25 mm in diameter, depending upon the shock size and electrode configuration, centered around the exposed electrode surface of the electrode tips. A shock wave follows collapse of the fireball bubble and creates 2 to 3 atmospheres of pressure 3 cm from the electrode tips.[298] Among the different physical effects of the electrical discharge are electrolysis, heat, mechanical effect, and flow of current.

HIS-BUNDLE ABLATION. For His-bundle ablation, the shock is delivered at a site where the largest His bundle potential amplitude is recorded[296, 297] (Fig. 21–6). His bundle pacing can be used to determine the exact position of the catheter. Atrial fibrillation or atrial flutter with rapid ventricular responses is the most common arrhythmia treated by His bundle ablation. Single shocks of 150 to 400 joules frequently are effective.[299] Screw-in electrodes may reduce the energy needed to destroy the His bundle.[300]

Immediate complications related to the shock include ventricular tachycardia and fibrillation, pericardial tamponade, and transient hypotension. Death may result. Late complications include ventricular tachycardia and ventricular fibrillation, sepsis involving the pacemaker pocket, thrombophlebitis, and hemothorax. Approximately 70 per cent of the treated patients develop chronic complete AV block, 7 per cent have intact AV conduction but do not require drugs for arrhythmia control, and 13 per cent achieve arrhythmia control with drugs. About 10 per cent of patients show no improvement.[299, 301] Recovery of AV conduction has been observed up to a year after a successful attempt at His ablation while AV block can occur several weeks or months after an initially unsuccessful or partially effective attempt.[302, 303] A 2 per cent incidence of late sudden death occurs on long-term follow-up. Thus,

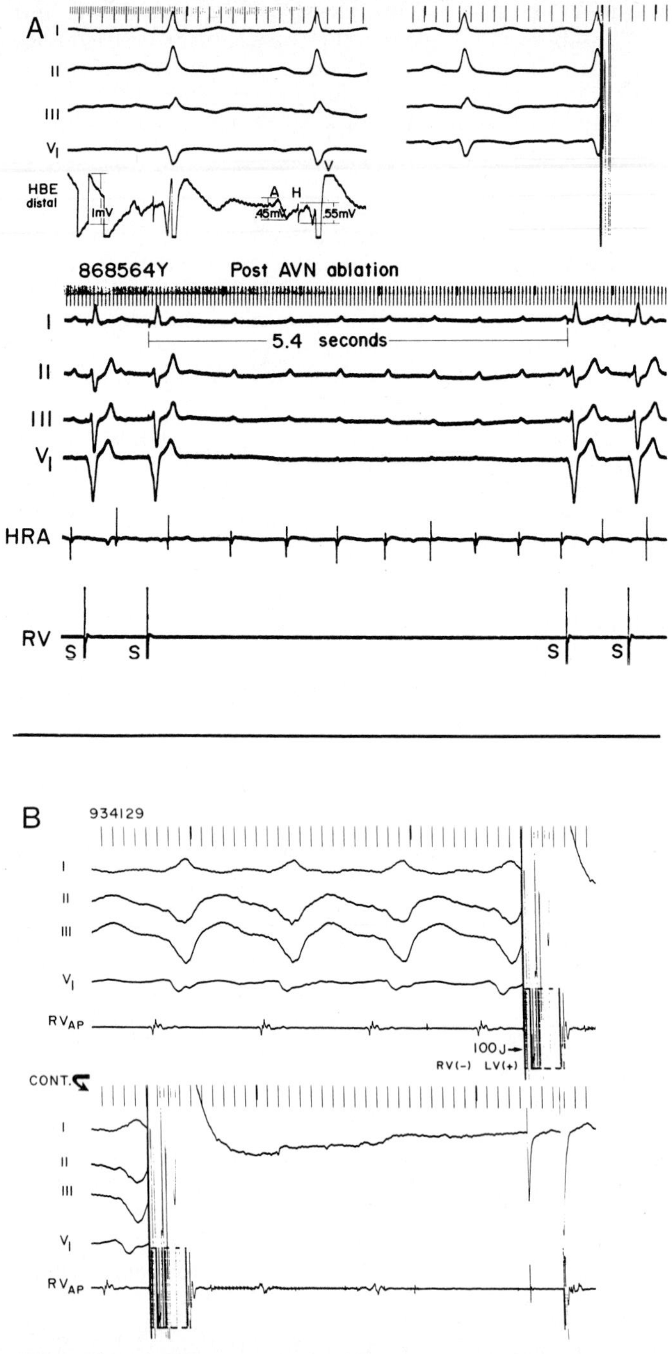

FIGURE 21–6. Electrical catheter ablation of AV conduction and of ventricular tachycardia. Panel A, *top*, illustrates leads I, II, III, and V_1 and a His bundle electrogram during sinus rhythm prior to the delivery of the shock. Amplitude of the atrial and His bundle electrogram is given. At the dark vertical line in the top panel, 200 joules are delivered between the cathodal electrode situated at the His bundle and an anodal patch on the patient's back. In the bottom of panel A, the rhythm immediately following the shock is displayed. The patient is now pacemaker-dependent; turning off the pacemaker for 5.4 seconds illustrates underlying complete AV heart block. HRA, high right atrial electrogram recording; RV, right ventricular electrogram recording; S, stimulus. Panel B illustrates an attempt at ablation of a ventricular tachycardia with the site of origin located near the apical portion of the interventricular septum. The first of several 100-joule shocks was delivered between the anodal electrode placed in the left ventricular apex and the cathodal electrode placed in the right ventricular apex. The delivery of the shock in the top right is reproduced in the bottom left of the panel. The ventricular tachycardia is terminated and the patient's dual chamber pacemaker paces the atrium and then the ventricle after a slight pause. RVap is the right ventricular electrogram recorded at the apex. The electrogram recording at the left ventricular apex occurred 40 msec in advance of the onset of the QRS complex (not shown).

the procedure still must be considered one of last resort because of the possible complications, induction of a pacemaker dependency state, and a small risk of sudden death.[299]

WOLFF-PARKINSON-WHITE SYNDROME. In patients with WPW syndrome an accessory pathway located in a posterior paraseptal position can be ablated by delivering the shock via a quadripolar electrode catheter positioned within the os of the coronary sinus so that the proximal pair of electrodes are just outside the os. The proximal pair of electrodes are made electrically common and connect to the cathodal output of a defibrillator. A patch electrode placed over the midthoracic spine connects to the anodal output of the defibrillator. Cumulative energies of 600 to 900 joules may be used. Long-term success for ablation of posteroseptal accessory pathways in a small number of patients studied appears to be at least 75 per cent. Morbidity rate appears to be low.[304, 305] Ablation of free wall accessory pathways has not been very successful to date, and shocks exceeding 100 to 200 joules may rupture the coronary sinus with exsanguination and pericardial tamponade.[303]

Other tachycardias (including AV nodal reentry,[306] junctional ectopic tachycardia,[307] ectopic atrial tachycardia,[308] permanent form of reciprocating tachycardia,[309, 310] bundle branch reentrant tachycardia,[311] and tachycardias associated with nodofascicular pathways[312, 313]) have been treated successfully with electrical catheter ablation.

VENTRICULAR TACHYCARDIA. For patients with ventricular tachycardia,[314] shocks are synchronized on the QRS complex during the ventricular tachycardia and delivered through the tip electrode of the same catheter that has been used to locate the "origin of the tachycardia" (see below). Arterial blood pressure is monitored throughout the procedure. Clinical success, i.e., no recurrence of ventricular tachycardia after ablation alone or with antiarrhythmic drug therapy, ranges from a low of 10 or 20 per cent to 90 per cent or more.[302] Several ablation attempts are required in some patients and, when ventricular tachycardias with different morphologies are present, multiple sites of ablation are required. Complications are similar to those following His bundle ablation, as well as pump failure or electromechanical dissociation and cerebrovascular accidents.[315]

SEQUELAE OF ELECTRICAL ABLATION. The short- and long-term results of endocardial shocks, in terms of tissue damage and late sequelae, are practically unknown and the procedure needs to be considered experimental. Reported complications are very likely to be underestimated and events such as coronary artery spasm[316] and subsequent damage to coronary arteries may go unnoticed. In dogs, endocardial ablation via a catheter electrode produces significant myocardial injury and sustained ventricular tachycardia and sudden death during the first week after the DC shock.[317] In the initial enthusiasm for this approach, we must not lose sight of these possibilities of significant complications. Further research into electrical and other forms of ablation[318] is clearly indicated.[318a]

SURGICAL THERAPY OF TACHYARRHYTHMIAS

The objectives of a surgical approach to treating a tachycardia are to excise, isolate, or interrupt critical tissue in the heart required for the initiation, maintenance, or propagation of the tachycardia, while preserving or even improving myocardial function.[319, 320] In addition to a direct surgical approach on the arrhythmia, indirect approaches such as aneurysmectomy, coronary artery bypass grafting, and relief of valvular insufficiency or stenosis can be useful in selected patients by improving cardiac hemodynamics and myocardial blood flow. Cardiac sympathectomy alters adrenergic influences on the heart and has been effective in some patients, particularly those who have recurrent ventricular tachycardia with the long Q-T syndrome.[321]

While we understand more about mechanisms responsible for supraventricular tachycardias than we do about mechanisms responsible for ventricular tachycardias, surgical procedures for the former "are complex and are not easily mastered" while "almost any surgical intervention" for ventricular tachycardia will "alter the anatomic-electrophysiologic substrate to alleviate the patient's symptoms or to enhance the effect of subsequent pharmacologic therapy."[320]

SUPRAVENTRICULAR TACHYCARDIAS

Surgical candidates are patients with symptomatic, drug-resistant, recurrent supraventricular tachycardias for whom a surgical procedure exists that offers a high probability of success, minimal morbidity, and for whom alternative therapies are less desirable or have been unsuccessful. Such patients include: (1) those in whom the origin of the tachycardia is confined to a relatively localized area in the atrium, (2) those with the preexcitation syndrome or one of its variants, and (3) those who have uncontrollably rapid ventricular rates during a supraventricular tachycardia and in whom creation of AV block is desirable. However, creation of AV block by electrical ablation using a catheter electrode is preferable to a surgical approach in this last group (p. 643). Selected patients with symptomatic, drug-resistant AV nodal reentrant tachycardia,[322, 323] atrial flutter,[324] and atrial fibrillation[325] may be candidates on occasion.

PREOPERATIVE MAPPING. Preoperatively a cardiac evaluation using noninvasive and invasive means establishes whether concomitant nonarrhythmic cardiac surgery may be necessary. At the electrophysiological study, the tachycardia is initiated, confirmed to be the "clinical tachycardia," and mapped to ascertain areas of the myocardium involved in the arrhythmia. Although more accurate intraoperative mapping refines the preoperative map, the latter is essential because general anesthesia, cooling of the heart when the chest is open, inadvertent trauma to pathways, and other factors may prevent induction of the tachycardia at surgery and preclude the opportunity for intraoperative mapping. (This is particularly true for ventricular tachycardias which, perversely, may not be initiated at surgery.) Also, for types of tachycardia that cannot be induced electrically, the preoperative electrophysiological study can be performed at a time when the tachycardia has begun spontaneously. *Mapping* in the present context is the term applied to the procedure during which the activation sequence—that is, the origin of and the pathways followed by the electrical impulse as it depolarizes the heart—is determined[325a] (Figs. 20–29 and 20–31, p. 607 and p. 608).

WOLFF-PARKINSON-WHITE SYNDROME (p. 202). In patients with the WPW syndrome, the electrophysiological study establishes the presence of preexcitation, number, type, and location of accessory pathways, mechanism of the arrhythmia(s), participation of the accessory pathway in the arrhythmia, functional properties of the normal and accessory pathways, effect of drugs or other interventions, and presence of associated electrophysiological or anatomical anomalies.[326] Catheter electrodes are positioned at various endocardial right atrial sites around the margin of the tricuspid ring, at the His bundle area, and along the length of the coronary sinus to obtain recording of left atrial activity at the region of the AV ring and in the right ventricular apex. The atrial insertion of the accessory pathway is determined by locating the earliest site of atrial activation when the atrium is depolarized over the accessory pathway during ventricular pacing or during reciprocating tachycardia characterized by anterograde conduction over the normal pathway and retrograde conduction over the accessory pathway (Fig. 21–7).

Atrial mapping during tachycardia rather than during ventricular pacing is preferable to be certain that the retrograde atrial activation is due solely to conduction over the accessory pathway and is not a retrograde fusion P wave from simultaneous activation over the accessory pathway and AV node. Verapamil or propranolol can be used to

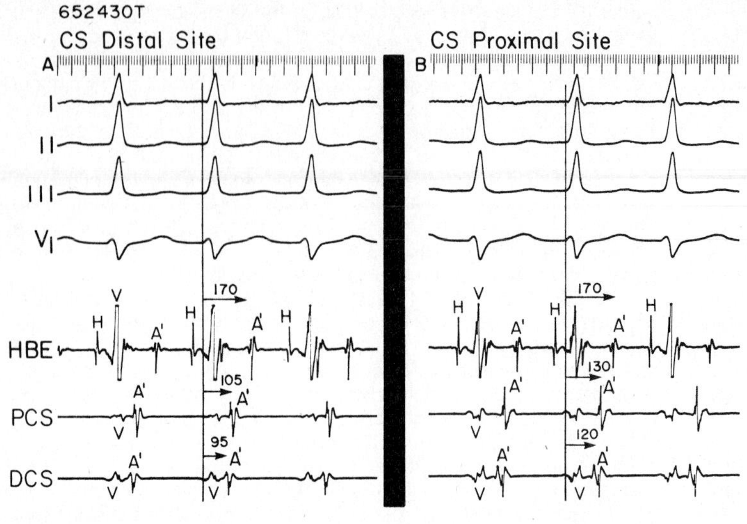

FIGURE 21–7. Atrial map during reciprocating atrioventricular tachycardia. Same patient as in Figure 20–29 (p. 607). In panel A, the catheter is passed far out into the coronary sinus so that its distal pair of electrodes (DCS) lie in close proximity to the lateral border of the heart. In this region the shortest VA conduction time is recorded (95 msec) during tachycardia. The more proximal pair of electrodes (PCS) record a VA time of 105 msec indicating that they are farther away from the site of the pathway. When the catheter is withdrawn to a position closer to the coronary sinus os (panel B) the V-A interval recorded with the distal pair of electrodes increases to 120 msec. This indicates that the catheter tip has been moved farther away from the site of the accessory pathway. I, II, III, V_1 are scalar leads. HBE, PCS, DCS are His bundle electrogram, proximal coronary sinus electrogram, and distal coronary sinus electrogram. Numbers in msec. Large time lines 50 msec, small time lines 10 msec. A, atrial electrogram; H, His bundle electrogram; V, ventricular electrogram. (From Zipes, DP, Mahomed, Y., King, R. D., Heger, J. J., Miles, W. M., Brown, J., Adams, D. E., and Prystowsky, E. N.: Wolff-Parkinson-White syndrome: Cryosurgical treatment. Indiana Med. *79*:432, 1986.)

prolong conduction time selectively over the AV node. About 10 per cent of patients have multiple accessory pathways and the retrograde P wave may be a fusion of activation from two or more accessory pathways.[327] The ventricular insertion can be determined by locating the earliest site of ventricular activation when the ventricle is depolarized over the accessory pathway during stable sinus rhythm, during atrial pacing from a site near the accessory pathway, or during stable reciprocating tachycardia characterized by anterograde conduction over the accessory pathway and retrograde conduction over the normal pathway.[328]

Ventricular mapping with a catheter electrode is very difficult to do and is best done at the time of surgery with epicardial electrodes. Other information such as the vectorial analysis of the delta wave,[326] accessory pathway electrograms,[329, 330] effect of functional bundle branch block on the V-A interval during orthodromic tachycardia,[331] the V-A interval of right ventricular apical extrasystoles,[332] ventricular coupling intervals required to produce atrial preexcitation,[333] phase[334] and echo[335] analysis, and finding the shortest interval between the stimulus applied to various atrial sites and the delta wave of the QRS complex all may be helpful. Mapping is repeated at the time of operation with single or multiple bipolar and/or unipolar electrode probes[319, 326, 336] (Fig. 21–8) to localize more precisely the site of the accessory pathway insertion in the atrium and ventricle. Atrial and ventricular insertions generally are less than 2 cm apart from each other.[319] Usually, complete epicardial maps are not necessary unless a Mahaim connection is present.

SURGICAL TECHNIQUES. Two surgical techniques have evolved, an open heart endocardial[320] and a closed heart epicardial approach.[337] The *open heart procedure* is done after the map is completed, using hypothermic, cardioplegic arrest.[338] An atrial endocardial incision above the annulus is extended to the AV groove fat pad, which is cleaned away; the incision interrupts the pathway. No electrophysiological data can be obtained until after rewarming the heart. If the pathway is not interrupted or a second pathway becomes manifest, the procedure must be repeated.

For the *closed heart approach* using normothermic cardiopulmonary bypass to avoid hypotension when the heart is manipulated or tachycardia occurs, the dissection begins at the atrial epicardium and is extended to the AV groove, which is frozen with the cryoprobe (Fig. 21–9). An atriotomy is required for right anteroseptal pathways but not for those in the posteroseptal or lateral positions. Electrophysiological assessment is continuous and on-line. The successful interruption of the accessory pathway can be pinpointed, damage to the AV node–His bundle (during paraseptal dissections) avoided, multiple pathways discovered, and interruption of tachycardia verified as the dissection is carried out. With both approaches, after the accessory pathway has been interrupted, an attempt is made to reinitiate the tachycardia and another map is obtained to be certain that the operation was successful and that no other accessory pathways exist (Fig. 21–8*C*).

Both procedures have evolved to the point at which, in expert hands, mortality is less than 1 to 2 per cent (depending on associated cardiac abnormalities) and the success rate for interrupting the AV connection and eliminating the tachycardia exceeds 95 per cent.[319, 320, 338–344] Which operation will ultimately become the procedure of choice is still not clear. Another approach for left-sided pathways is to freeze directly through the coronary sinus.[344a] Long-term damage to the coronary artery or sinus is a risk.

Less experience has been acquired with surgical treatment of other supraventricular tachycardias[345] that include basically four types: focal atrial or junctional tachycardia, AV nodal reentry, atrial flutter, and atrial fibrillation. When the atrial tachycardia can be well-mapped and is found to be localized to a portion of the atrium such as in the atrial appendage, focal excision or ablation[342, 346–350] has effectively removed the tachycardia. When precise mapping is impossible, when the tachycardia is located in areas not easily resected or ablated, or when multiple foci are present, an exclusion procedure can be done, based on the principle that a fibrous scar from a surgical incision or cryoinjury that encircles the arrhythmia area effectively isolates it from conducting to the rest of the heart.[347, 351–353] Alteration of AV nodal anatomy by several techniques has been successful in a small number of patients with AV nodal reentry,[320, 322, 323] and interrupting AV nodal–His bundle conduction[297, 354] is useful in selected patients, as noted earlier, but leaves the patient pacemaker-dependent. Very preliminary experience suggests that atrial flutter due to reentry can be eliminated by a strategically placed atrial incision,[324] while atrial fibrillation can be "excluded" by an incision that isolates the sinus and AV nodes.[325]

VENTRICULAR TACHYCARDIA

In contrast to patients with supraventricular arrhythmias, candidates for surgical therapy of ventricular arrhythmias usually have severe left ventricular dysfunction, generally caused by coronary artery disease. The etiology of the underlying heart disease influences the type of surgery performed.[355, 356] Candidates are patients with drug-resistant, symptomatic recurrent ventricular tachyarrhythmias who, ideally, have a localized abnormality, scar, or aneurysm with good left ventricular function. Recently, surgery also has been performed soon after myocardial infarction

FIGURE 21–8. *A*, Panel A is a schematic used as a map to record the site of the accessory pathway. Heart shown from a posterior view can be visualized as being opened anteriorly and spread out, much as if an individual with his back to us unbuttoned a shirt and spread it out so that the right margin of the shirt would be site A and the left margin of the shirt would be site I. Site E represents the right margin of the heart, Q and H the "crux" with the posterior descending coronary artery in that area. Site M represents the left margin of the heart. The contiguous right and left atria are shown. Sites for the location of the left ventricular free wall accessory pathway (LVFWAP), left posterior septal accessory pathway (left PSAP), posterior septal accessory pathway (PSAP), right posterior septal accessory pathway (right PSAP), and right ventricular free wall accessory pathway (RVFWAP) are noted. The AV groove is indicated by the straight line with the letters beneath indicating each recording site. CS indicates the coronary sinus and the dark arrow indicates the mitral valve location. (From Guiraudon, G. M., Klein, G. J., Sharma, A. D., Jones, D. L., and McLellan, D. G.: Surgery for Wolff-Parkinson-White syndrome: Further experience with an epicardial approach. Circulation *74*:525, 1986, by permission of the American Heart Association, Inc.)

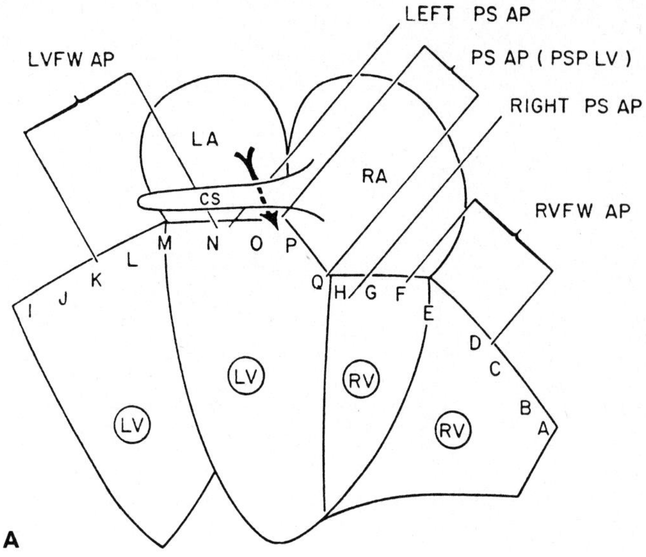

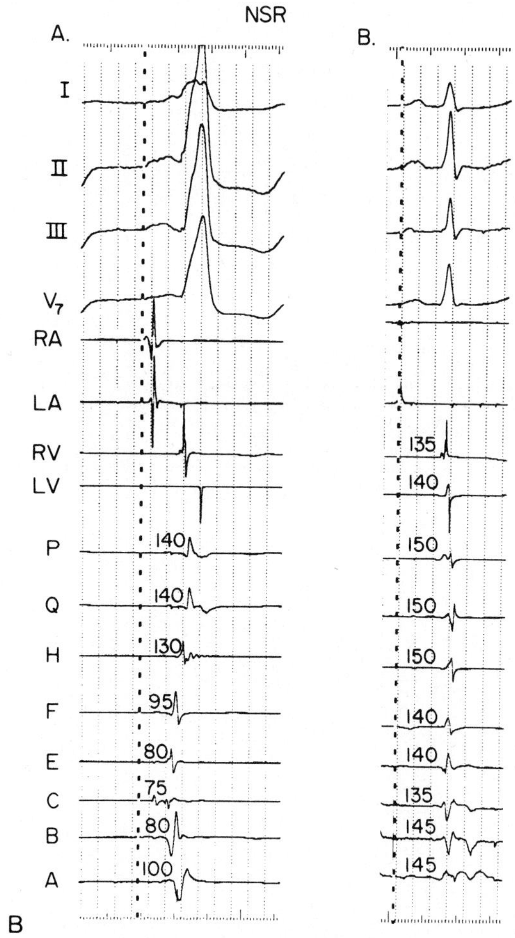

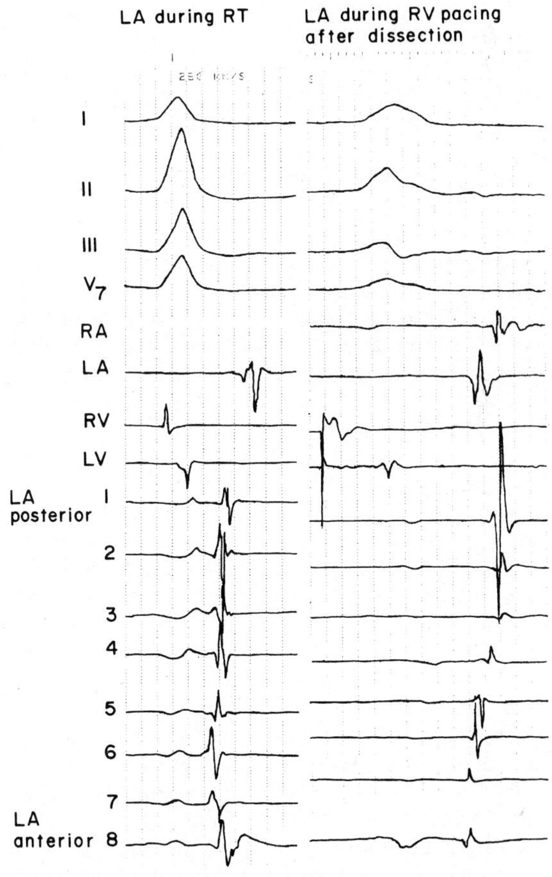

FIGURE 21–8. *B*, Ventricular mapping during sinus rhythm. In panel A, conduction proceeds to the ventricle over the accessory pathway. The QRS complex begins with a delta wave and has a prolonged duration. Note that the shortest A-V interval (75 msec) occurs at site C on the map (Fig. 21–8*A*) indicating a right anterior free wall accessory pathway. When conduction proceeds down the normal pathway (panel B) AV conduction is normal and there is no ventricular preexcitation.

Figure 21–8. *C*, Recorded from another patient, displays the typical "bowing" appearance of an atrial map recorded during reciprocating tachycardia (left panel) and after interruption of the accessory pathway (right panel). Numbers rather than letters are used to indicate the atrial site; 1 corresponds to site Q while 8 corresponds to site K. Activation is recorded early at electrode 6 with a V-A interval of 100 msec, consistent with a left free wall accessory pathway at about site M. After interruption of the accessory pathway, note the prolongation of the V-A interval.

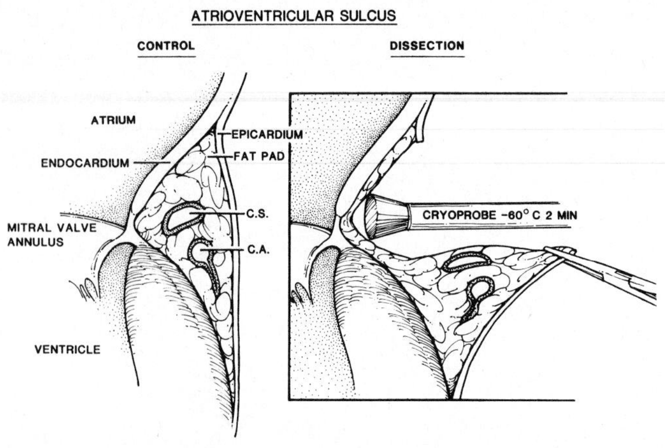

FIGURE 21–9. Schematic illustrating the surgical technique for dissection at the atrioventricular groove and application of the cryoprobe. CS, coronary sinus. CA, coronary artery.

in patients with drug-resistant ventricular tachycardia.[357, 357a] Poorer surgical results are obtained in patients with a history of congestive heart failure and left ventricular dysfunction.[358] Those with no discrete ventricular aneurysm, disparate sites of tachycardia origin, multiple morphologically distinct spontaneous tachycardias, inferior wall origin, and right bundle branch block contour have greater postoperative tachycardia recurrence rates.[359]

ISCHEMIC HEART DISEASE

In almost all patients who have ventricular tachycardia associated with ischemic heart disease, the arrhythmia, regardless of its configuration on the surface ECG, arises in the left ventricle or on the left ventricular side of the interventricular septum.[360] The contour of the ventricular tachycardia may change from a right bundle branch block to a left bundle branch block pattern without a change in the earliest activation site, suggesting that the left ventricular site of origin remains the same, often near the septum, but its exit pathway is altered.[361]

Indirect surgical approaches, including cardiac thoracic sympathectomy, coronary artery bypass grafting (CABG), and ventricular aneurysm or infarct resection with or without CABG, have been successful in about 60 per cent of reported cases.[362] Since most patients have recurrent ventricular tachycardia unrelated to acute ischemia but associated with ischemic heart disease, old myocardial infarction, and scarring, CABG as a primary therapeutic approach is limited to patients who experience ventricular tachycardia during documented exercise-induced ischemia.[363] However, CABG and other procedures are often an adjunct to the direct surgical approach.

SURGICAL TECHNIQUES. Three types of direct surgical procedures have been used: isolation (i.e., encircling endocardial ventriculotomy), resection, and ablation. The *encircling endocardial ventriculotomy* (EEV)[364] involves a transmural ventriculotomy placed perpendicularly or obliquely, relative to the endocardial wall, to isolate areas of endocardial fibrosis that are recognized visually. The incision, sparing the epicardium and overlying coronary vessels, is then repaired. When the septum is involved, the ventriculotomy is approximately 1 cm deep. The rationale for this procedure is to separate arrhythmogenic areas into small islands that become anatomically and electrophysiologically isolated. However, the EEV may reduce cardiac blood flow to the isolated myocardium, adversely affecting myocardial function.[362] A partial EEV has been proposed.[365]

The rationale for the second approach, *endocardial resection*, is based in part on animal data indicating that arrhythmias in dogs subjected to myocardial infarction arise in the subendocardial borders between normal and infarcted tissue.[366] Endocardial resection involves peeling off a layer of endocardium, generally in the rim of an aneurysm, that has been demonstrated by means of mapping procedures to be the site of earliest activation recorded during the ventricular tachycardia (Fig. 21–10). This resection causes less disruption to the left ventricular wall than does the encircling endocardial ventriculotomy.

Tachycardias arising from the papillary muscles cannot be approached in this fashion,[367] and the involved area is *cryoablated*. Cryoablation can also be used to isolate areas of the ventricle that cannot be resected, and can be combined with the above techniques. *Laser approaches* are experimental but appear promising.[368] Combining all approaches as necessary in a given patient to eradicate the

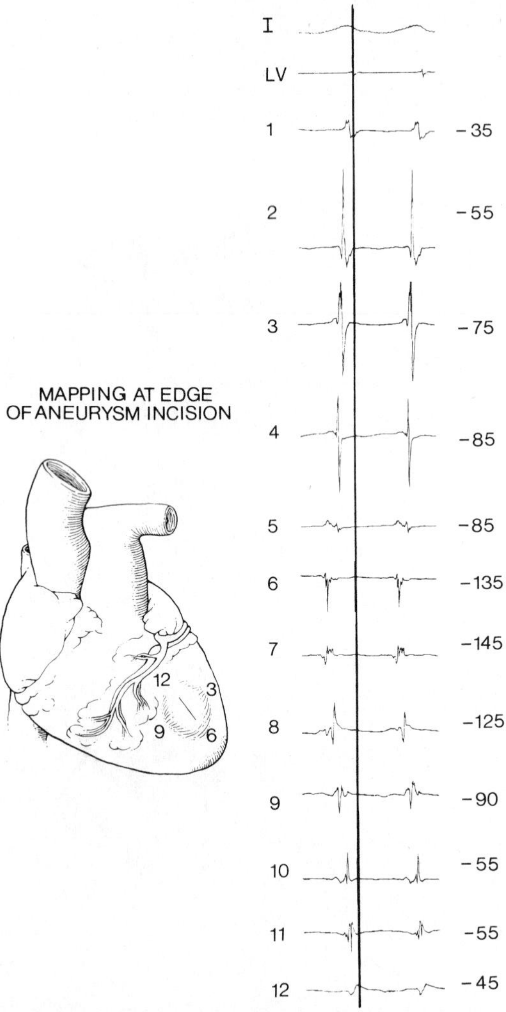

FIGURE 21–10. Activation map during ventricular tachycardia. A left ventricular aneurysm has been opened (straight line between points 12 and 6) and numbered in a clockwise fashion. Left ventricular endocardial recordings (LV) from a handheld exploring electrode are shown. A stationary left ventricular epicardial electrode (LV) has been sewn in place. Ventricular tachycardia was initiated. The left ventricular endocardial recordings at site 7 showed earliest activation during the ventricular tachycardia and occurred 145 msec in advance of the stationary LV electrogram (dark vertical line). Extensive endocardial resection was carried out at site 7 and in the surrounding area, with elimination of ventricular tachycardia. (Tracings have been redrawn for clarity.)

ventricular tachycardia results in elimination or control (with drugs) of the ventricular tachycardia in 80 per cent or more of patients[320] whose conditions could not be controlled by pharmacological therapy.

Preoperative and Intraoperative Electrophysiologic Studies

PREOPERATIVE ELECTROPHYSIOLOGICAL STUDY. This involves induction of the ventricular tachycardia and electrophysiologic mapping to pinpoint the area to be resected. Electrode catheters are positioned generally at the right ventricular apex, in the His bundle area, and often in the coronary sinus to provide reference electrograms and anatomical reference points.[360, 369, 369a] A fourth catheter is moved from site-to-site to record local activation at multiple endocardial sites. Manipulation of this catheter to sample a sufficient number of sites in the left ventricle frequently is very difficult. Fluoroscopy directed in several planes establishes the anatomical position of the catheters. A resolution of 4 to 8 cm^2 of ventricular endocardium is probably achieved,[319] although more accurate anatomical localization of the mapping electrode tip in the ventricle may be possible.[369a] Tachycardias that are too rapid, short in duration, or pleomorphical cannot be mapped accurately unless multiple catheters[370] or a multielectrode array is used.[371–373] Administering a drug such as procainamide may slow the ventricular tachycardia and transform a nonsustained pleomorphic ventricular tachycardia into a sustained ventricular tachycardia of uniform contour that can be mapped.

VENTRICULAR MAPPING. This procedure is also performed at the time of surgery. With the operator using a handheld probe, the ventricular tachycardia must be stable and of uniform configuration, generally for several hundred cycles. Recording from multiple sites simultaneously, coupled with on-line computer techniques that instantaneously provide an activation map cycle-by-cycle, reduces the time necessary to generate an activation sequence map and allows mapping from a single QRS complex. This reduces problems of mapping rapid ventricular tachycardias with changing morphologies and will greatly speed and simplify intraoperative mapping. The sequence of activation during ventricular tachycardia can be plotted and the area of earliest activation determined (Figs. 21–10 and 21–11). Cryothermal mapping and ablation have also been used to confirm the site of origin of a ventricular arrhythmia and then to destroy it. A cryoprobe is cooled to 0°C and its influence on the arrhythmia is noted. If it terminates the tachycardia, the temperature is reduced to −60°C and the area frozen.[374]

Several points are worthy of emphasis. Recording electrical activity in damaged tissue may produce broad low-amplitude electrograms that may originate from the tissue being sampled or from more distant sites; their onset is difficult to measure accurately. Timing of propagation may be distorted because of changing conduction velocities as the wavefront enters specialized conducting tissue, large muscle bundles, or damaged tissue. During ventricular tachycardia, the origin of the arrhythmia is generally ascribed to electrical activity recorded 25 to 50 msec in advance of the QRS complex. However, that is an arbitrary value, and it is quite clear that such activity may be late following the preceding cycle or early in advance of the next cycle (Fig. 21–10). In addition, when such activity is recorded well after termination of the QRS complex, it becomes difficult to determine with certainty whether the deflections represent depolarization or repolarization. Potentials recorded prior to the onset of the surface QRS complex suggest that the origin of the tachycardia is nearby. When the earliest recordable electrical activity occurs after the onset of the QRS complex, the site of origin may be in the interventricular septum.

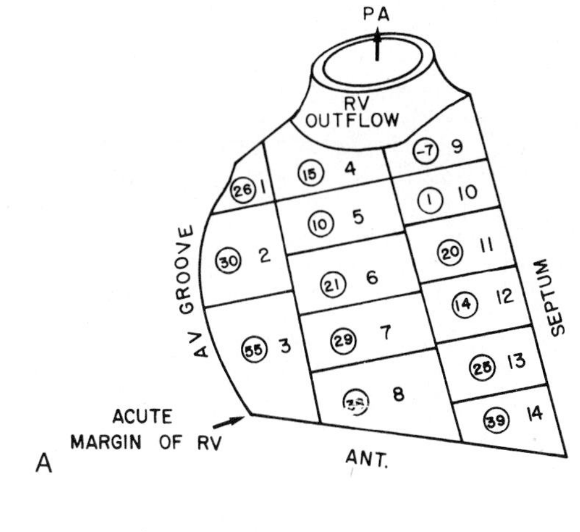

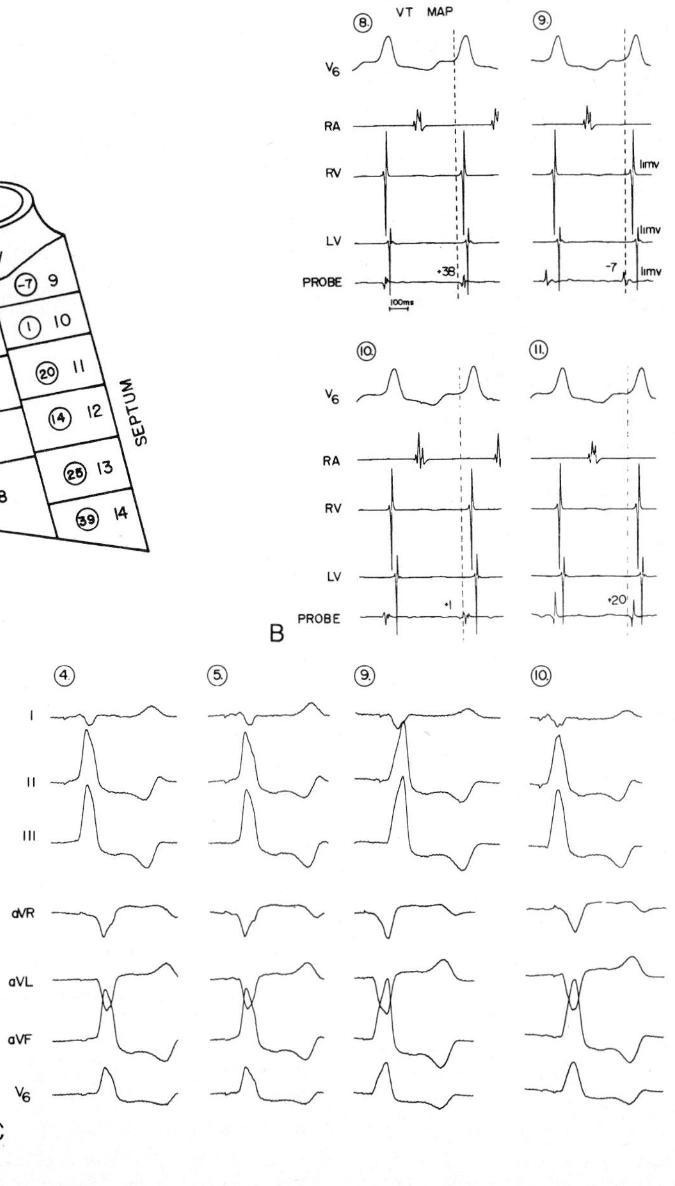

FIGURE 21–11. *A*, Schematic used to display areas of the right ventricle for the map. Circled numbers indicate the activation time (in msec) recorded at that site during the ventricular tachycardia. Earliest epicardial activation recorded only 7 msec in advance of the QRS complex suggests that tachycardia origin may be located in endocardium. *B*, Recordings at 4 sites (denoted in *A*) during the ventricular tachycardia. RA, RV, and LV indicate electrograms from plaques sewn on the right atrium, right ventricle, and left ventricle. Probe indicates the local electrogram recorded with a bipolar electrode at the various sites. Activation times (in msec) in relation to the onset of the QRS complex are indicated. Note that at site 9 the earliest activation was recorded (−7 msec). *C*, Pace mapping. Various QRS contours recorded during electrical stimulation at each of the sites is indicated. Subtle differences exist but the ventricular tachycardia appears to be most closely replicated by stimulation at site 9, where the earliest ventricular activity was recorded during the ventricular tachycardia.

It is important to emphasize that the area of earliest recorded electrical activity during ventricular tachycardia may not actually represent the site or origin of the tachycardia, since the latter may originate several centimeters away, for example in a small scarred area, and be conducted very slowly until it reaches more normally excitable tissue where it generates a recordable extracellular complex. However, this area of early activation is probably closely related to the origin of the tachycardia and, based on our present state of knowledge and results from surgery, warrants surgical intervention at that site. Finding an area of "continuous electrical activity" does not necessarily mean that reentry is present or that this is the origin of the tachycardia, since similar activity can be produced by automatically discharging foci, by recording slowly propagating, overlapping, or fragmented wavefronts from several areas, or by recording repolarization activity. However, it is likely that the origin of the tachycardia is close to the area of continuous electrical activity. Of interest is that the site of epicardial breakthrough may be distant from the earliest area of recordable endocardial activity,[360, 369, 375] further emphasizing the need for endocardial mapping, particularly in patients with coronary artery disease. In some patients, intramural mapping using a plunge needle electrode may be useful.[376]

Mapping during sinus rhythm allows one to detect abnormal areas evidenced by delayed activation, fragmentation, abnormal Q waves, delayed potentials, and potentials with decreased voltage and very slow conduction.[369] This technique may also be useful to demonstrate that areas of early activation during ventricular tachycardia represent late activation during sinus rhythm[362] (Fig. 21–10). While it is argued that mapping during sinus rhythm can be useful to guide the surgical approach,[377] correlation of delayed activity recorded during sinus rhythm with sites of origin recorded during the ventricular tachycardia is imperfect.[378, 379] Sinus rhythm mapping may be helpful if ventricular tachycardia cannot be initiated.

Pacemapping[380, 381] This involves stimulation of various ventricular sites to initiate a QRS contour that duplicates the QRS contour of the ventricular tachycardia, thus establishing the apparent site of origin of the arrhythmia (Fig. 21–11*C*). This technique is limited by several methodological problems and by the possibility that conduction arising from the same site of origin may change and produce a QRS contour with a totally different shape,[361] that stimulating a different site may produce QRS complexes of a similar appearance, and that stimulating closely adjacent sites may produce very different QRS complexes, possibly because of different degrees of penetration of the specialized conduction system.[381] It may be useful, however, when the tachycardia cannot be initiated for mapping.

It is not clear whether mapping improves the surgical success rate in patients with ischemic heart disease,[382–385] as it appears to do in patients with nonischemic heart disease (see below). However, myocardial resection guided by electrophysiological mapping may reduce the amount of tissue removed, thus helping to preserve myocardial contractile function and include in the surgical resection or ablation, areas of normally appearing myocardium that might otherwise have been left undisturbed.

NONISCHEMIC HEART DISEASE

In patients without ischemic heart disease, tachycardias can originate in either the right or the left ventricle, and the type and site or origin of the ventricular tachycardia vary depending on the underlying heart disease (Figs. 21–10 and 21–11). Incessant ventricular tachycardia in children may be due to a cardiac tumor.[386] In patients who have *tetralogy of Fallot*, ventricular tachycardia may arise in the region of the right ventricular infundibulectomy scar.[387] Patients with *arrhythmogenic right ventricular dysplasia*[388] (p. 697) have a right ventricular tachycardia. Some can be treated by a simple ventriculotomy at the apparent site of origin of the ventricular tachycardia or by isolating portions of the right ventricular free wall from the remainder of the heart.[355, 362, 389] Right ventricular disconnection[389] may result in progressive right ventricular dilation.[390] The overall surgical success rate and low mortality for this group of patients are promising but still need improvement.[362, 389, 391] Patients with prolonged Q-T or Q-U syndrome are thought to have arrhythmias due to preponderant left stellate sympathetic tone, and accordingly, left stellate ganglionectomy has been useful in some patients[321, 392] therapeutically. Valve replacement may eliminate the tachycardia in some patients with mitral valve prolapse and associated ventricular tachycardia.[362]

Acknowledgments

The authors thank James J. Heger, M.D., and Robert F. Gilmour, Jr., Ph.D., for critical comments on this chapter.

REFERENCES

PHARMACOLOGICAL THERAPY

1. Heger, J. J., Prystowsky, E. N., and Zipes, D. P.: Clinical choice of antiarrhythmic drugs. *In* Josephson, M. E. (ed.): Ventricular Tachycardia—Mechanisms and Management. Mt. Kisco, N. Y., Futura Publishing Co., 1982.
2. Kates, R. E.: Metabolites of cardiac antiarrhythmic drugs: Their clinical role. Ann. NY Acad. Sci. *432*:75, 1984.
3. Shanks, R. G., and Harrison, D. W.: Pharmacokinetic Principles in Cardiac Arrhythmias: A Decade of Progress. Boston, G. K. Hall, 1981, p. 91.
4. Fenster, P. E.: Clinical pharmacology. Clinical uses of pharmacokinetic principles in prescribing cardiac drugs. Med. Clin. North Am. *68*:1281, 1984.
5. Roden, D. M.: New concepts in antiarrhythmic drug pharmacokinetics. Prog. Cardiol. (*in press*).
6. Zipes, D. P.: A consideration of antiarrhythmic therapy. Circulation 72:949, 1985.
7. Vaughn Williams, E. M.: A classification of antiarrhythmic actions reassessed after a decade of new drugs. J. Clin. Pharmacol. *24*:129, 1984.
8. Campbell, T. J.: Kinetics of onset of rate-dependent effects of class I antiarrhythmic drugs are important in determining their effects on refractoriness in guinea pig ventricle and provide a theoretical basis for their subclassification. Cardiovasc. Res. 17:344, 1983.
9. Harrison, D. C.: Antiarrhythmic drug classification: New science and practice applications. Am. J. Cardiol. *56*:185, 1985.
10. Hondeghem, L. M., and Katzung, B. G.: Antiarrhythmic agents: The modulated receptor mechanism of action of sodium and calcium channel-blocking drugs. Ann. Rev. Pharmacol. Toxicol. *24*:387, 1984.
11. Katzung, B. G.: New concepts of antiarrhythmic drug action. Progr. Cardiol. (*in press*).
12. Singh, B. N.: Effects of antiarrhythmic compounds on the cardiac action potential: Basis for the interpretation of their antiarrhythmic effects. Prog. Cardiol. (*in press*).
13. Binah, O., and Rosen, M. R.: The cellular mechanisms of cardiac antiarrhythmic drug action. Ann. NY Acad. Sci. *432*:31, 1984.
14. Kaplan, H. R.: Advances in antiarrhythmic drug therapy—changing concepts (symposium). Fed. Proc. *45*:2184, 1986.
15. Rosen, M. R., and Danilo, P.: Effects of tetrodotoxin, lidocaine, verapamil, and AHR-2666 on ouabain-induced delayed afterdepolarizations in canine Purkinje fibers. Circ. Res. *46*:117, 1980.
16. Nattel, S., Elharrar, V., Zipes, D. P., and Bailey, J. C.: The pH dependent electrophysiological effects of quinidine and lidocaine on canine cardiac Purkinje fibers. Circ. Res. *48*:55, 1981.
17. Morikawa, Y., and Rosen, M. R.: Developmental changes in the effects of lidocaine on the electrophysiological properties of canine Purkinje fibers. Circ. Res. *55*:633, 1984.
18. Shen, S. S., and Lederer, W. J.: Lidocaine's negative inotropic and antiarrhythmic actions. Dependence on shortening of action potential duration and reduction of intracellular sodium activity. Circ. Res. *57*:578, 1985.
19. Cardinal, R., Janse, M. J., vanEeden, I., Werner, G., d'Alnoncourt, C. N., and Durrer, D.: The effects of lidocaine on intracellular and extracellular potentials, activation, and ventricular arrhythmias during acute regional ischemia in the isolated porcine heart. Circ. Res. *49*:792, 1981.
20. Patterson, E., Gibson, J. K., and Lucchesi, B. R.: Electrophysiologic actions of lidocaine in a canine model of chronic myocardial ischemic damage—arrhythmogenic actions of lidocaine. J. Cardiovasc. Pharmacol. *4*:925, 1982.
21. Gilmour, R. F., Jr., and Zipes, D. P.: Electrophysiological response of vascularized hamster cardiac transplants to ischemia. Circ. Res. *50*:599, 1982.
22. Colatsky, I.: Mechanisms of action of lidocaine and quinidine on action potential duration in rabbit cardiac Purkinje fibers. Circ. Res. *50*:17, 1982.
23. Miller, B. D., Thames, M. D., and Mark, A. L.: Inhibition of cardiac sympathetic nerve activity with intravenous administration of lidocaine. J. Clin. Invest. *71*:1247, 1983.
24. Gilmour, R. F., Jr., Morrical, D. G., Ertel, P. J., Maesaka, J. F., and Zipes, D. P.: Depressant effects of fast channel blockade on the electrical activity of ischemic canine ventricle: Mediation by the sympathetic nervous system. Cardiovasc. Res. *18*:405, 1984.
25. Koster, R. W., and Dunning, A. J.: Intramuscular lidocaine for prevention of lethal arrhythmias in the prehospitalization phase of acute myocardial infarction. N. Engl. J. Med. *313*:1105, 1985.
26. Lie, K. I., Leim, K. L., Louridtz, W. J., Janse, M. J., Willebrands, A. F.,

and Durrer, D.: Efficacy of lidocaine preventing primary ventricular fibrillation within one hour after a 300 mg intramuscular injection. A double-blind randomized study of 300 hospitalized patients with acute myocardial infarction. Am. J. Cardiol. *43*:486, 1978.
27. Nattel, S., and Zipes, D. P.: Clinical pharmacology of old and new antiarrhythmic drugs. Cardiovasc. Res. *11*:221, 1980.
27a. Sefaldt, R. J., Nattel, S., Kreeft, J. H., and Ogilvie, R. I.: Lidocaine therapy with an exponentially declining infusion. Ann. Intern. Med. *101*:632, 1984.
28. Akhtar, M., Gilbert, C. J., and Shenasa, M.: Effect of lidocaine on atrioventricular response via the accessory pathway in patients with Wolff-Parkinson-White syndrome. Circulation *63*:435, 1981.
29. Haynes, R. E., Chinn, T. L., Copass, M. K., and Cobb, L. A.: Comparison of bretylium tosylate and lidocaine in management of out-of-hospital ventricular fibrillation: A randomized clinical trial. Am. J. Cardiol. *48*:353, 1981.
30. Lie, K. I., Wellens, H. J., VanCapelle, F. J., and Durrer, D.: Lidocaine in the prevention of primary ventricular fibrillation. A double-blind randomized study of 212 consecutive patients. N. Engl. J. Med. *291*:132, 1974.
31. Pentecost, B. L., deGiovanni, J. V., Lamb, P., Cadigan, P. J., Evemy, K. L., and Flint, E. J.: Reappraisal of lignocaine therapy in management of myocardial infarction. Br. Heart J. *45*:42, 1981.
32. Dunn, H. M., McComb, J. M., Kinney, C. D., Campbell, N. P., Shanks, R. G., MacKenzie, G., and Adgey, A. A.: Prophylactic lidocaine in the early phase of suspected myocardial infarction. Am. Heart J. *110*:353, 1985.
33. DeSilva, R. A., Hennekens, C. H., Lown, B., and Casscells, W.: Lignocaine prophylaxis in acute myocardial infarction: An evaluation of randomized trials. Lancet *2*:855, 1981.
34. Campbell, R. W. F.: Prophylactic antiarrhythmic therapy in acute myocardial infarction. Am. J. Cardiol. *54*:8E, 1984.
35. Mirro, M. J., Watanabe, A. M., and Bailey, J. C.: Electrophysiologic effects of the optical isomers of disopyramide and quinidine in the dog: Dependence on stereochemistry. Circ. Res. *48*:867, 1981.
36. Mason, J. W., and Hondeghem, L. M.: Quinidine. Ann. NY Acad. Sci. *432*:162, 1984.
37. Mirro, M. J., Manalan, A. S., Bailey, J. C., and Watanabe, A. M.: Anticholinergic effects of disopyramide and quinidine on guinea pig myocardium: Mediation by direct muscarinic receptor blockade. Circ. Res. *47*:855, 1980.
38. Alboni, P., Paparella, N., Pirani, R., Cappato, R., Cucci, A. M., Ruffilli, E., and Tomasi, A. M.: Different electrophysiological modes of action of oral quinidine in man. Eur. Heart J. *6*:946, 1985.
39. Mirro, M. J., Watanabe, A. M., and Bailey, J. C.: Electrophysiological effects of disopyramide and quinidine on guinea pig atria and canine cardiac Purkinje fibers: Dependence on underlying cholinergic tone. Circ. Res. *46*:660, 1980.
40. Weld, F. M., Coromilas, J., Rothman, J. N., and Bigger, J. T., Jr.: Mechanisms of quinidine-induced depression of maximum upstroke velocity in bovine cardiac Purkinje fibers. Circ. Res. *50*:369, 1982.
41. Torres, V., Flowers, D., Miura, D., and Somberg, J.: Intravenous quinidine by intermittent bolus for electrophysiologic studies in patients with ventricular tachycardia. Am. Heart J. *108*:1437, 1984.
42. Swerdlow, C. D., Yu, J. D., Jacobsen, E., Mann, S., Winkle, R. A., Griffin, J. C., Ross, D. L., and Mason, J. W.: Safety and efficacy of intravenous quinidine. Am. J. Med. *75*:36, 1983.
43. Morganroth, J., and Hunter, H.: Comparative efficacy and safety of short-acting and sustained release quinidine in the treatment of patients with ventricular arrhythmias. Am. Heart J. *110*:1176, 1985.
44. Wu, D., Hung, J. S., Kuo, C. T., Hsu, K. S., and Shieh, W. B.: Effects of quinidine on atrioventricular nodal reentrant paroxysmal tachycardia. Circulation *64*:823, 1981.
45. Rasmussen, K., Wang, H., and Fausa, D.: Comparative efficiency of quinidine and verapamil in the maintenance of sinus rhythm after DC conversion of atrial fibrillation. A controlled clinical trial. Acta Med. Scand. *645*(Suppl.):23, 1981.
46. Ruskin, J. N., DiMarco, J. P., and Garan, H.: Out-of-hospital cardiac arrest: Electrophysiologic observations and selection of long-term antiarrhythmic therapy. N. Engl. J. Med. *303*:607, 1980.
47. DiMarco, J. P., Garan, H., and Ruskin, J. N.: Quinidine for ventricular arrhythmias: Value of electrophysiologic testing. Am. J. Cardiol. *51*:90, 1983.
48. Kim, S. G., Seiden, S. W., Matos, J. A., Waspe, L. E., and Fisher, J.: Combination of procainamide and quinidine for better tolerance and additive effects for ventricular arrhythmias. Am. J. Cardiol. *56*:84, 1985.
49. Guntheroth, W. G., Cyr, D. R., Mack, L. A., Benedetti, T., Lenke, R. R., and Petty, C. N.: Hydrops from reciprocating atrioventricular tachycardia in a 27-week fetus requiring quinidine for conversion. Obstet. Gynecol. *66*(Suppl 3):29S, 1985.
50. Selzer, A., and Wray, H. W.: Quinidine syncope: Paroxysmal ventricular fibrillation occurring during treatment of chronic atrial arrhythmias. Circulation *30*:17, 1964.
51. Denes, P., Gabster, A., and Huang, S. K.: Clinical electrocardiographic and followup observations in patients having ventricular fibrillation during Holter monitoring. Role of quinidine therapy. Am. J. Cardiol. *48*:9, 1981.
52. Smith, W. M., and Gallagher, J. J.: "Les torsades de pointes": An unusual ventricular arrhythmia. Ann. Intern. Med. *93*:578, 1980.
53. Roden, D. M., Woosley, R. L., and Primm, K.: Incidence and clinical features of the quinidine-associated long QT syndrome: Implications for patient care. Am. Heart J. *111*:1088, 1986.
54. Roden, D. M., and Hoffman, B. F.: Action potential prolongation and induction of abnormal automaticity by low quinidine concentrations in canine Purkinje fibers: Relationship to potassium and cycle length. Circ. Res. *56*:857, 1985.
55. Inoue, H., Toda, I., Nozaki, A., Matsuo, H., Mashima, S., and Sugimoto, T.: Inhomogeneity of ventricular refractory period in canine heart with quinidine-induced long Q-T interval. Cardiovasc. Res. *19*:623, 1985.
56. Morganroth, J., and Horowitz, L. N.: Incidence of proarrhythmic effects from quinidine in the outpatient treatment of benign or potentially lethal ventricular arrhythmias. Am. J. Cardiol. *56*:585, 1985.
57. Tzivoni, D., Keren, A., Cohen, A. M., Loebel, H., Zahair, I., Chenzbraun, A., and Stern, S.: Magnesium therapy for torsades de pointes. Am. J. Cardiol. *53*:528, 1984.
58. Schenck-Gustafsson, K., Jogestrand, T., Nordlander, R., and Dahlquis, T. R.: Effect of quinidine on digoxin concentration skeletal muscle and serum in patients with atrial fibrillation. Evidence for reduced binding of digoxin in muscle. N. Engl. J. Med. *305*:209, 1981.
59. Ball, W. J., Jr., Tse-Eng, D., Wallick, E. T., Bilezikian, J. P., Schwartz, A., and Butler, V. P., Jr.: Effect of quinidine on the digoxin receptor in vitro. J. Clin. Invest. *68*:1065, 1981.
60. Myerburg, R. J., Bassett, A. L., Epstein, K., Gaide, M. S., Kozlovskis, P., Wong, S. S., Castellanos, A., and Gelband, H.: Electrophysiological effects of procainamide in acute and healed experimental ischemic injury of cat myocardium. Circ. Res. *50*:386, 1982.
61. Giardina, E. G.: Procainamide: Clinical pharmacology and efficacy against ventricular arrhythmias. Ann. NY Acad. Sci. *432*:117, 1984.
62. Dangman, K. H., and Hoffman, B. F.: In vivo and in vitro antiarrhythmic and arrhythmogenic effects of *N*-acetylprocainamide. J. Pharmacol. Exp. Ther. *217*:851, 1981.
63. Roden, D. M., Reele, S. B., Higgins, S. B., Wilkinson, G. R., Smith, R. F., Oates, J. A., and Woosley, R. L.: Antiarrhythmic efficacy, pharmacokinetics and safety of *N*-acetylprocainamide in human subjects: Comparison with procainamide. Am. J. Cardiol. *46*:463, 1980.
64. Wynn, J., Miura, D. S., Torres, V., Flowers, D., Keefe, D., Williams, S., and Somberg, J. C.: Electrophysiologic evaluation of the antiarrhythmic effects of *N*-acetylprocainamide for ventricular tachycardia secondary to coronary artery disease. Am. J. Cardiol. *56*:877, 1985.
65. Greenspan, A. M., Horowitz, L. N., Spielman, S. R., and Josephson, M. E.: Large dose procainamide therapy for ventricular tachycardia. Am. J. Cardiol. *46*:453, 1980.
66. Boccardo, D., Pitchon, R., and Wiener, I.: Adverse reactions and efficacy of high dose procainamide therapy in resistant tachyarrhythmias. Am. Heart J. *102*:797, 1981.
67. Giardina, E. G., Fenster, P., Paul, E., Bigger, J. T., Jr., Mayersohn, M., Perrier, D., and Marcus, F. I.: Efficacy, plasma concentrations and adverse effects of a new sustained release procainamide preparation. Am. J. Cardiol. *46*:855, 1980.
68. Myerburg, R. J., Kessler, K. M., Kiem, I., Pefkaros, K. C., Conde, C. A., Cooper, D., and Castellanos, A.: Relationship between plasma levels of procainamide, suppression of premature ventricular complexes and prevention of recurrent ventricular tachycardia. Circulation *64*:280, 1981.
69. Halpern, S. W., Ellrodt, G., Singh, B. N., and Mandel, W. J.: Efficacy of intravenous procainamide infusion in converting atrial fibrillation to sinus rhythm. Relation to left atrial size. Br. Heart J. *44*:589, 1980.
70. Wellens, H. J. J., Braat, S., Brugada, P., Gorgels, A. P. M., and Bar, F. W.: Use of procainamide in patients with the Wolff-Parkinson-White syndrome to disclose a short refractory period of the accessory pathway. Am. J. Cardiol. *50*:1087, 1982.
71. Marchlinski, F. E., Buxton, A. E., Vassallo, J. A., Waxman, H. L., Cassidy, D. M., Doherty, J. U., and Josephson, M. E.: Comparative electrophysiologic effects of intravenous and oral procainamide in patients with sustained ventricular arrhythmias. J. Am. Coll. Cardiol. *4*:1247, 1984.
72. Benson, D. W., Jr., Dunnigan, A., Green, T. P., Benditt, D. G., and Schneider, S. P.: Periodic procainamide for paroxysmal tachycardia. Circulation *72*:147, 1985.
73. Waxman, H. L., Buxton, A. E., Sadowski, L. M., and Josephson, M. E.: Response to procainamide during electrophysiologic study for sustained ventricular tachycardia predicts response to other drugs. Circulation *67*:30, 1982.
74. Oseran, D. S., Gang, E. S., Rosenthal, M. E., Mandel, W. J., and Peter, T.: Electropharmacologic testing in sustained ventricular tachycardia associated with coronary heart disease: Value of the response to intravenous procainamide in predicting the response to oral quinidine treatment. Am. J. Cardiol. *56*:883, 1985.
75. Strasberg, B., Schlarovsky, S., Erdberg, A., Duffy, C. E., Lan, W., Swiryn, S., Agmon, J., and Rosen, K. M.: Procainamide-induced polymorphous ventricular tachycardia. Am. J. Cardiol. *47*:1309, 1981.
76. Goldberg, D., Reiffel, J. A., Davis, J. C., Gang, E., Livelli, F., and Bigger, J. T., Jr.: Electrophysiologic effects of procainamide on sinus node function in patients with and without sinus node disease. Am. Heart J. *103*:75, 1982.
77. Kluger, J., Drayer, D. E., Reidenberg, M. M., and Lahita, R.: Acetylprocainamide therapy in patients with previous procainamide induced lupus syndrome. Ann. Intern. Med. *95*:18, 1981.
78. Vaughn Williams, E. M.: Disopyramide. Ann. NY Acad. Sci. *432*:189, 1984.
79. Sasyniuk, B. I., and Kus, T.: Cellular electrophysiologic changes induced by disopyramide phosphate in normal and infarcted hearts. J. Int. Med. *4*:20, 1976.
80. Katoh, T., Karagueuzian, H., Jordan, J., and Mandel, W.: The cellular electrophysiologic mechanism of the dual actions of disopyramide on rabbit sinus node function. Circulation *66*:1216, 1982.
81. Kerr, C. R., Prystowsky, E. N., Smith, W. M., Cook, L., and Gallagher, J J.: Electrophysiological effects of disopyramide phosphate in patients with Wolff-Parkinson-White syndrome. Circulation *65*:869, 1982.
82. Morady, F., Scheinman, M. M., and Desai, J.: Disopyramide. Ann. Intern. Med. *96*:337, 1982.

83. Timins, B. I., Gutman, J. A., and Haft, J. I.: Disopyramide-induced heart block. Chest 79:477, 1981.
84. Wilkinson, P. R., Desai, J., Hollister, J., Gonzalez, R., Abbott, J. A., and Scheinman, M. M.: Electrophysiologic effects of disopyramide in patients with atrioventricular nodal dysfunction. Circulation *66*:1211, 1982.
85. Leach, A. J., Brown, J. E., and Armstrong, P. W.: Cardiac depression by intravenous disopyramide in patients with left ventricular dysfunction. Am. J. Med. *68*:839, 1980.
86. Podrid, P. J. Schoeneberger, A., and Lown, B.: Congestive heart failure caused by disopyramide. N. Engl. J. Med. *302*:614, 1980.
87. Landmark, K., Bredesen, J. E., Thaulow, E., Simonsen, S., and Amlie, J. P.: Pharmacokinetics of disopyramide in patients with imminent to moderate cardiac failure. Eur. J. Clin. Pharmacol. *19*:187, 1981.
88. Breithardt, G., Seipel, L., and Abendroth, R. R.: Comparison of the antiarrhythmic efficacy of disopyramide and mexiletine against stimulus induced ventricular tachycardia. J. Cardiovasc. Pharmacol. *3*:1026, 1981.
89. Brugada, P., and Wellens, H. J. J.: Effects of intravenous and oral disopyramide on paroxysmal atrioventricular nodal tachycardia. Am. J. Cardiol. *53*:88, 1984.
90. Robertson, C. E., and Miller, H. C.: Extreme tachycardia complicating the use of disopyramide in atrial flutter. Br. Heart J. *44*:602, 1980.
91. Teichman, S. L., Fisher, J. D., Matos, J. A., and Kim, S. G.: Disopyramide-pyridostigmine: Report of a beneficial drug interaction. J. Cardiovasc. Pharmacol. 7:108, 1985.
92. Tzivoni, D., Keren, A., Stern, S., and Gottlieb, S.: Disopyramide-induced torsades de pointes. Arch. Intern. Med. *141*:946, 1981.
93. Minardo, J. D., Heger, J. J., Zipes, D. P., Miles, W. M., and Prystowsky, E. N.: Drug associated ventricular fibrillation: Analysis of clinical features and QTc prolongation. J. Am. Coll. Cardiol. 7:158A, 1986.
94. Desai, J. M., Scheinman, M. M., Hirschfeld, D., Gonzalez, R., and Peters, R. W.: Cardiovascular collapse associated with disopyramide therapy. Chest 79:545, 1981.
95. Ferrier, G. R.: Digitalis arrhythmias: Role of oscillatory afterpotentials. Progr. Cardiovasc. Dis. *19*:459, 1977.
96. Campbell, T. J.: Resting and rate-dependent depression of maximum rate of depolarization (V_{max}) in guinea pig ventricular action potentials by mexiletine, disopyramide, and encainide. J. Cardiovasc. Pharmacol. *5*:291, 1983.
97. Garan, H., Ruskin, J. N., and Powell, W. J., Jr.: Centrally mediated effect of phenytoin on digoxin-induced ventricular arrhythmias. Am. J. Physiol. *241*:H67, 1981.
98. Peter, T., Ross, D., Duffield, A., Luxton, M., Harper, R., Hunt, D., and Slowman, G.: Effect on survival after myocardial infarction of long-term treatment with phenytoin. Br. Heart J. *40*:1356, 1978.
99. Koch-Weser, J., and Frishman, W. H.: Beta-adrenoreceptor antagonists: New drugs and new indications. N. Engl. J. Med. *305*:500, 1981.
100. Taylor, S. H., Silke, B., and Lee, P. S.: Intravenous beta blockade in coronary heart disease. N. Engl. J. Med. *306*:631, 1982.
101. Hewett, K. W., and Rosen, M. R.: Alpha- and beta-adrenergic interactions with ouabain-induced delayed after depolarizations. J. Pharmacol. Exp. Therapeutics *229*:188, 1984.
102. Raine, A. E. G., and Vaughn Williams, E. M.: Adaptation to prolonged beta-blockade of rabbit atrial, Purkinje and ventricular potentials and papillary muscle contractions. Circ. Res. *48*:804, 1981.
103. Prystowsky, E. N., Jackman, W. M., Rinkenberger, R. L., Heger, J. J., and Zipes, D. P.: Effect of autonomic blockade on ventricular refractoriness and atrioventricular conduction in humans: Evidence supporting a direct cholinergic action on ventricular muscle refractoriness. Circ. Res. *49*:511, 1981.
104. Ahnve, S., and Vallin, H.: Influence of heart rate and inhibition of autonomic tone on the Q-T interval. Circulation *65*:435, 1982.
105. Browne, K. F., Zipes, D. P., Heger, J. J., and Prystowsky, E. N.: The influence of the autonomic nervous system on the Q-T interval. Am. J. Cardiol. *49*:898, 1982.
106. Schwartz, P. J.: Idiopathic long Q-T-syndrome progress and questions. Am. Heart J. *109*:399, 1985.
107. Surawicz, B., and Knoebel, S.: Long Q-T: Good, bad, or indifferent? J. Am. Coll. Cardiol. *4*:498, 1984.
108. Beta Blocker Heart Attack Study Group: The beta blocker heart attack trial. J.A.M.A. *246*:2073, 1981.
109. Hjalmarson, A.: Effect on mortality of metoprolol in acute myocardial infarction. A double-blind randomized trial. Lancet 2:823, 1981.
110. The Norwegian Multicentre Study Group: Timolol-induced reduction in mortality and reinfarction in patients surviving acute myocardial infarction. N. Engl. J. Med. *304*:801, 1981.
111. Gundersen, T., Abrahamsen, A. M., Kjekshus, J., and Ronnevik, P. K. for the Norwegian Multicenter Study Group: Timolol-related reduction in mortality and reinfarction in patients ages 65-75 years surviving acute myocardial infarction. Circulation *66*:1179, 1982.
112. Singh, B. N., and Venkatesh, N.: Prevention of myocardial infarction and of sudden death in survivors of acute myocardial infarction: Role of prophylactic beta-adrenoreceptor blockade. Am. Heart J. *107*:189, 1984.
113. Inoue, H., Davies, B., and Zipes, D. P.: Denervation supersensitivity to norepinephrine is arrhythmogenic. Circulation 72(Suppl 3):243, 1985.
114. Morganroth, J., Lichstein, E., and Byington, R.: Beta-Blocker Heart Attack Trial: Impact of propranolol therapy on ventricular arrhythmias. Prev. Med. *14*:346, 1985.
115. Ryden, L., Ariniego, R., Arnman, K., Herlitz, J., Hjalmarson, A., Holmberg, S., Reyes, C., Sonedgard, P., Svedberg, K., Vedin, A., Waagstein, F., Waldenstrom, A., Wilhelmsson, C., Wedel, H., and Yamamoto, M.: A double-blind trial of metoprolol in acute myocardial infarction. Effects on ventricular arrhythmias. N. Engl. J. Med. *308*:614, 1983.
116. White, H. D., Antman, E. M., Glynn, M. A., Collins, J. J., Cohn, L. H., Shemin, R. J., and Friedman, P. L.: Efficacy and safety of timolol for prevention of supraventricular tachyarrhythmias after coronary artery bypass surgery. Circulation *70*:479, 1984.
117. Nattel, S., Rango, R. E., and Vanloon, G.: Mechanism of propranolol withdrawal phenomenon. Circulation 59:1158, 1979.
118. Duff, H. J., Roden, D. M., Yacobi, A., Robertson, D., Wang, T., Maffucci, R. J., Oates, J. A., and Woosley, R. L.: Bretylium: Relations between plasma concentrations and pharmacologic actions in high-frequency ventricular arrhythmias. Am. J. Cardiol. *55*:395, 1985.
119. Euler, D. E., and Scanlon, P. J.: Mechanisms of the effect of bretylium on the ventricular fibrillation threshold in dogs. Am. J. Cardiol. *55*:1396, 1985.
120. Wenger, T. L., Lederman, S., Starmer, C. F., Brown, T., and Strauss, H. C.: A method for quantitating antifibrillatory effects of drugs after coronary reperfusion in dogs: Improved outcome with bretylium. Circulation *69*:142, 1984.
121. Lucchesi, B. R.: Rationale of therapy in the patient with acute myocardial infarction and life-threatening arrhythmias: A focus on bretylium. Am. J. Cardiol. *54*:14A, 1984.
122. Bacaner, M. B., Clay, J. R., Shrier, A., and Brochu, R. M.: Potassium channel blockade: A mechanism for suppressing ventricular fibrillation. Proc. Natl. Acad. Sci. *83*:2223, 1986.
123. Inoue, H., Toda, I., Nozaki, H., and Sugimoto, T.: Effects of bretylium tosylate on inhomogeneity of refractoriness and ventricular fibrillation threshold in canine hearts with quinidine-induced long Q-T interval. Cardiovasc. Res. *19*:655, 1985.
124. Anderson, J. L., Patterson, E., Wagner, J. G., Johnson, T. A., Lucchesi, B. R., and Pitt, B.: Clinical pharmacokinetics of intravenous and oral bretylium tosylate in survivors of ventricular tachycardia or fibrillation: Clinical application of a new assay for bretylium. J. Cardiovasc. Pharmacol. *3*:485, 1981.
125. Harrison, E. E., and Amey, B. D.: The use of bretylium in prehospital ventricular fibrillation. Am. J. Emerg. Med. *1*:1, 1983.
126. Stang, J. M., Washington, S. E., Barnes, S. A., Dutko, H. J., Cheney, B. D., Easter, C. R., O'Hara, J. T., Kessler, J. H., Schaal, S. F., and Lewis, R. P.: Treatment of prehospital refractory ventricular fibrillation with bretylium tosylate. Ann. Emerg. Med. *13*:234, 1984.
127. Olson, D. W., Thompson, B. M., Darin, J. C., and Milbrath, M. H.: A randomized comparison study of bretylium tosylate and lidocaine in resuscitation of patients from out-of-hospital ventricular fibrillation in a paramedic system. Ann. Emerg. Med. *13*:807, 1984.
128. Kerber, R. E., Pandian, N. G., Jensen, S. R., Constantin, L., Kieso, R. A., Melton, J., and Hunt, M.: Effect of lidocaine and bretylium on energy requirements for transthoracic defibrillation: Experimental studies. J. Am. Coll. Cardiol. 7:397, 1986.
129. Cranefield, P. F.: The Conduction of the Cardiac Impulse. Mt. Kisco, N. Y., Futura Publishing Co., 1975.
130. Zipes, D. P., Bailey, J. C., and Elharrar, V.: The Slow Inward Current and Cardiac Arrhythmias. The Hague, Martinus Nijhoff, 1980.
131. Stone, P. H., and Antman, E. M.: Calcium channel blocking agents in the treatment of cardiovascular disorders. Mt. Kisco, N. Y., Futura Publishing Co., 1983.
132. Sperelakis, N.: Calcium Antagonists. Mechanisms of Action on Cardiac Muscle and Vascular Smooth Muscle. Boston, Martinus Nijhoff, 1984.
133. Fleckenstein, A.: Calcium Antagonism in Heart and Vascular Smooth Muscle. New York, John Wiley and Sons, 1983.
134. Henry, P. D.: Comparative pharmacology of calcium antagonists: Nifedipine, verapamil, and diltiazem. Am. J. Cardiol. *46*:1047, 1980.
135. Lathrop, D. A., Valle-Aguilera, J. R., Millard, R. W., Gaum, W. E., Hannon, D. W., Francis, P. D., Nakaya, H., and Schwartz, A.: Comparative electrophysiologic and coronary hemodynamic effects of diltiazem, nisoldipine and verapamil on myocardial tissue. Am. J. Cardiol. *49*:613, 1982.
136. Roth, A., Harrison, E., Mitani, G., Cohen, J., Rahimtoola, S. H., and Elkayam, U.: Efficacy and safety of medium- and high-dose diltiazem alone and in combination with digoxin for control of heart rate at rest and during exercise in patients with chronic atrial fibrillation. Circulation *73*:316, 1986.
137. Waleffe, A., Hastir, F., and Kulbertus, H. E.: Effects of intravenous diltiazem administration in patients with inducible tachycardia. Eur. Heart J. *6*:882, 1985.
138. Hung, J. S., Yeh, S. J., Lin, F. C., Fu, M., Lee, Y. S., and Wu, D.: Usefulness of intravenous diltiazem in predicting subsequent electrophysiologic and clinical responses to oral diltiazem. Am. J. Cardiol. *54*:1259, 1984.
139. Yeh, S. J., Lin, F. C., Chou, Y. Y., Hung, J. S., and Wu, D.: Termination of paroxysmal supraventricular tachycardia with a single oral dose of diltiazem and propranolol. Circulation *71*:104, 1985.
140. Gilmour, R. F., and Zipes, D. P.: Basic electrophysiology of the slow inward current. *In* Antman, E. M., and Stone, P. H. (eds.): Cardiac Arrhythmias. Mt. Kisco, N. Y., Futura Publishing Co., 1983.
141. Spear, J. F., Horowitz, L. N., and Moore, E. N.: The slow response in human ventricle. *In* Zipes, D. P., Bailey, J. C., and Elharrar, V. (eds.): The Slow Inward Current and Cardiac Arrhythmias. The Hague, Martinus Nijhoff, 1980, p. 309.
142. Gilmour, R. F., Jr., Heger, J. J., Prystowsky, E. N., and Zipes, D. P.: Cellular electrophysiological abnormalities of diseased human ventricular myocardium. Am. J. Cardiol. *51*:137, 1983.
143. Zipes, D. P., and Gilmour, R. F.: Calcium antagonists and their potential

role in the prevention of sudden coronary death. Ann. NY Acad. Sci. *382*:258, 1982.

144. Fleet, W. F., Johnson, T. A., Graebner, C. A., Engle, C. L., and Gettes, L. S.: Effects of verapamil on ischemia-induced changes in extracellular K^+, pH, and local activation in the pig. Circulation *73*:837, 1986.

145. Rinkenberger, R. L., Prystowsky, E. N., Heger, J. J., Troup, P. J., Jackman, W. M., and Zipes, D. P.: Effects of intravenous and chronic oral verapamil administration in patients with supraventricular tachyarrhythmias. Circulation *62*:996, 1980.

146. Matsuyama, E., Konishi, T., Okazaki, H., Matsuda, H., and Kawai, C.: Effects of verapamil on accessory pathway properties and induction of circus movement tachycardia in patients with the Wolff-Parkinson-White syndrome. J. Cardiovasc. Pharmacol. *3*:11, 1981.

147. Harper, R. W., Whitford, E., Middlebrook, K., Federman, J., Anderson, S., and Pitt, A.: Effects of verapamil on the electrophysiologic properties of the accessory pathway in patients with the Wolff-Parkinson-White syndrome. Am. J. Cardiol. *50*:1323, 1982.

148. Gulamhusein, S., Ko, P., Carruthers, S. G., and Klein, G. J.: Acceleration of the ventricular response during atrial fibrillation in the Wolff-Parkinson-White syndrome after verapamil. Circulation *65*:348, 1982.

149. Kieval, J., Kirsten, E. B., Kessler, K. M., Mallon, S. M., and Myerburg, R. J.: The effects of intravenous verapamil on hemodynamic status of patients with coronary artery disease receiving propranolol. Circulation *65*:653, 1982.

150. Packer, M., Mellen, J., Medina, N., Yushak, M., Smith, H., Holt, J., Guerrero, J., Todd, G. D., McAllister, R. G., and Gorlin, R.: Hemodynamic consequences of combined beta-adrenergic and slow calcium channel blockade in man. Circulation *65*:660, 1982.

151. Clusin, W. T., Bristow, M. R., Baim, D. S., Schroeder, J. S., Jaillon, P., Brett, P., and Harrison, D. C.: The effects of diltiazem and reduced serum ionized calcium on ischemic ventricular fibrillation in the dog. Circ. Res. *50*:518, 1982.

152. Clusin, W. T., Buchbinder, M., Ellis, A. K., Kernoff, R. S., Giacomini, J. C., and Harrison, D. C.: Reduction of ischemic depolarization by the calcium channel blocker diltiazem. Circ. Res. *54*:10, 1984.

153. Epstein, M. L., Kiel, E. A., and Victorica, B. E.: Cardiac decompensation following verapamil therapy in infants with supraventricular tachycardia. Pediatrics *75*:737, 1985.

154. Sung, R. J., Elser, B., and McAllister, R. G., Jr.: Intravenous verapamil for termination of reentrant supraventricular tachycardias. Intracardiac studies correlated with plasma verapamil concentrations. Ann. Intern. Med. *93*:682, 1980.

155. Kates, R. E., Keefe, D. L., Schwartz, J., Harapats, S., Kirsten, E. B., and Harrison, D. C.: Verapamil disposition kinetics in chronic atrial fibrillation. Clin. Pharmacol. Ther. *30*:44, 1981.

156. Hamer, A., Peter, T., Platt, M., and Mandel, W. J.: Effects of verapamil on supraventricular tachycardia in patients with overt and concealed Wolff-Parkinson-White syndrome. Am. Heart J. *101*:600, 1981.

157. Yee, R., Gulamhusein, S. S., and Klein, G. J.: Combined verapamil and propranolol for supraventricular tachycardia. Am. J. Cardiol. *53*:757, 1984.

158. Waxman, H. L., Myerburg, R. J., Appel, R., and Sung, R. J.: Verapamil for control of ventricular rate in paroxysmal supraventricular tachycardia and atrial fibrillation or flutter: A double-blind randomized cross-over study. Ann. Intern. Med. *94*:1, 1981.

159. McGovern, B., Garan, H., and Ruskin, J. N.: Precipitation of cardiac arrest by verapamil in patients with Wolff-Parkinson-White syndrome. Ann. Intern Med. *104*:791, 1986.

160. Schwartz, J. B., Keefe, D., Kates, R. E., Kirsten, E., and Harrison, D. C.: Acute and chronic pharmacodynamic interaction of verapamil and digoxin in atrial fibrillation. Circulation *65*:1163, 1982.

161. Wellens, H. J. J., Farre, J., and Bär, F. W.: The role of the slow inward current in the genesis of ventricular tachycardias in man. *In* Zipes, D. P., Bailey, J., and Elharrar, V. (eds.): The Slow Inward Current and Cardiac Arrhythmias. The Hague, Martinus Nijhoff, 1980, p. 507.

162. Sung, R. J., Shapiro, W. A., Shen, E. N., Morady, F., and Davis, J.: Effects of verapamil on ventricular tachycardias possibly caused by reentry, automaticity, and triggered activity. J. Clin. Invest. *72*:350, 1983.

163. Epstein, M., Kiel, E. A., and Victoria, B. E.: Cardiac decompensation following verapamil therapy in infants with supraventricular tachycardia. Pediatrics *75*:737, 1985.

164. Schwartz, J. B., Nielsen, A. P., and Griffin, J. C.: Concentration-dependent enhancement of junctional pacemaker activity by verapamil in man. Circulation *71*:450, 1985.

165. Mason, J. W.: Amiodarone. N. Engl. J. Med. *316*:455, 1987.

166. Zipes, D. P., Prystowsky, E. N., and Heger, J. J.: Amiodarone: Electrophysiologic actions, pharmacokinetics, and clinical effects. J. Am. Coll. Cardiol. *3*:1059, 1984.

167. Haines, D. E., and DiMarco, J. P.: Use of investigational drugs in treating cardiac arrhythmias. Progr. Cardiol. (*in press*).

168. Yabek, S., Kato, R., and Singh, B. N.: Acute electrophysiologic effects of amiodarone and desethylamiodarone in isolated cardiac muscle. J. Cardiovasc. Pharmacol. (*in press*).

168a. Talajic, M., DeRoode, M. R., and Nattel, S.: Comparative electrophysiologic effects of intravenous amiodarone and desethylamiodarone in dogs: Evidence for clinically relevant activity of the metabolite. Circulation *75*:265, 1987.

169. Gloor, H. O., Urthaler, F., and James, T. N.: Acute effects of amiodarone upon the canine sinus node and atrioventricular junctional region. J. Clin. Invest. *71*:1457, 1983.

170. Mason, J. W., Hondeghem, L. M., and Katzung, B. G.: Block of inactivated sodium channels and of depolarization-induced automaticity in guinea pig papillary muscle by amiodarone. Circ. Res. *55*:277, 1984.

171. Morady, F., DiCarlo, L. A., Jr., Krol, R. B., Baerman, J. M., and deBuitleir, M.: Acute and chronic effects of amiodarone on ventricular refractoriness, intraventricular conduction and ventricular tachycardia induction. J. Am. Coll. Cardiol. *7*:148, 1986.

172. Shenasa, M., Denker, S., Mahmud, R., Lehmann, M., Estrada, A., and Akhtar, M.: Effect of amiodarone on conduction and refractoriness of the His Purkinje system in the human heart. J. Am. Coll. Cardiol. *4*:105, 1984.

173. Wellens, H. J. J., Brugada, P., Abdollah, H., and Dassen, W. R.: A comparison of the electrophysiologic effects of intravenous and oral amiodarone in the same patient. Circulation *69*:120, 1984.

174. Heger, J. J., Prystowsky, E. N., Jackman, W. M., Naccarelli, G. V., Warfel, K. A., Rinkenberger, R. L., and Zipes, D. P.: Amiodarone: Clinical efficacy and electrophysiology during long-term therapy for recurrent ventricular tachycardia. N. Engl. J. Med. *305*:539, 1981.

175. Nademanee, K., Hendrickson, J. A., Cannom, D. S., Goldreyer, B. N., and Singh, B. N.: Control of refractory life-threatening ventricular tachyarrhythmias by amiodarone. Am. Heart J. *101*:759, 1981.

176. Kosinski, E. J., Albin, J. B., Young, E., Lewis, S. M., and Leland, O. S., Jr.: Hemodynamic effects of intravenous amiodarone. J. Am. Coll. Cardiol. *4*:565, 1984.

177. Adams, P. C., Holt, D. W., Storey, G. C., Morley, A. R., Callaghan, J., and Campbell, R. W.: Amiodarone and its desethyl metabolite: Tissue distribution and morphologic changes during long-term therapy. Circulation *72*:1064, 1985.

178. Mostow, N. D., Rakita, L., Vrobel, T. R., Noon, D. L., and Blumer, J.: Amiodarone: Correlation of serum concentration with suppression of complex ventricular ectopic activity. Am. J. Cardiol. *54*:569, 1984.

179. Plotmensch, H. H., Belhassen, B., Swanson, B. N., Shoshani, D., Spielman, S. R., Greenspan, A. J., Greenspan, A. M., Vlasses, P. H., and Horowitz, L. N.: Steady-state serum amiodarone concentration: Relationship with antiarrhythmic efficacy and toxicity. Ann. Intern. Med. *101*:462, 1984.

180. Escoubet, B., Caumel, P., Poirier, J. M., Maison-Blanche, P., Jaillon, P., Leclercg, J. F., Manasche, P., Cheymol, G., Piwnica, A., Lagier, G., and Slama, R.: Suppression of arrhythmias within hours after a single oral dose of amiodarone and relation to plasma and myocardial concentrations. Am. J. Cardiol. *55*:696, 1985.

181. Mostow, N. D., Rakita, L., Vrobel, T. R., Noon, D., and Blumer, J.: Amiodarone: Intravenous loading for rapid suppression of complex ventricular arrhythmias. J. Am. Coll. Cardiol. *4*:97, 1984.

182. Kerin, N. Z., Blevins, R. D., Frumin, H., Faitel, K., and Rubenfire, M.: Intravenous and oral loading versus oral loading alone with amiodarone for chronic refractory ventricular arrhythmias. Am. J. Cardiol. *55*:89, 1985.

183. Mostow, N. D., Vrobel, T. R., Noon, D., and Rakita, L.: Rapid suppression of complex ventricular arrhythmias with high dose oral amiodarone. Circulation *73*:1231, 1986.

184. Coumel, P., Lucet, V, and Ngoc, D. D.: The use of amiodarone in children. PACE *6*:930, 1983.

185. Garson, A., Jr., Gillette, P. C., McVey, P., Hesslein, P. S., Porter, C. J., Angell, L. K., Kaldis, L. C., and Hittner, H. M.: Amiodarone treatment of critical arrhythmias in children and young adults. J. Am. Coll. Cardiol. *4*:749, 1984.

186. Haines, D. E., and DiMarco, J. P.: Use of new drugs in treating cardiac arrhythmias. Progr. Cardiol. (*in press*).

187. Haedo, A. H., Chiale, P. A., Bandieri, J. D., Lazzari, J., Elizari, M. V., and Rosenbaum, M. B. Comparative antiarrhythmic efficacy of verapamil, 17-monochloracetyl-ajmaline, mexiletine, and amiodarone in patients with severe chagastic myocarditis: relation with the underlying arrhythmogenic mechanisms. J. Am. Coll. Cardiol. *7*:1114, 1986.

188. Brugada, P., and Wellens, H. J. J.: Effects of oral amiodarone on rate-dependent changes in refractoriness in patients with Wolff-Parkinson-White syndrome. Am. J. Cardiol. *56*:863, 1985.

189. Feld, G. K., Nademanee, K., Weiss, J., Stevenson, W., and Singh, B. N.: Electrophysiologic basis for the suppression by amiodarone of orthodromic supraventricular tachycardias complicating pre-excitation syndromes. J. Am. Coll. Cardiol. *3*:1298, 1984.

190. Horowitz, L. N., Spielman, S. R., Greenspan, A. M., Mintz, G. S., Morganroth, J., Brown, R., Brady, P. M., and Kay, H. R.: Use of amiodarone in the treatment of persistent and paroxysmal atrial fibrillation resistant to quinidine therapy. J. Am. Coll. Cardiol. *6*:1402, 1985.

191. Gold, R. L., Haffajee, C. I., Charos, G., Sloan, K., Baker, S., and Alpert, J. S.: Amiodarone for refractory atrial fibrillation. Am. J. Cardiol. *57*:124, 1986.

192. McKenna, W. J., Harris, L., Rowland, E., Kleinebenne, A., Krikler, D. M., Oakley, C. M., and Goodwin, J. F.: Amiodarone for long-term management of patients with hypertrophic cardiomyopathy. Am. J. Cardiol. *54*:802, 1984.

193. Fogoros, R. N., Anderson, K. P., Winkle, R. A., Swerdlow, C. D., and Mason, J. W.: Amiodarone: Clinical efficacy and toxicity in 96 patients with recurrent drug refractory arrhythmias. Circulation *68*:88, 1983.

194. Winkle, R. A.: Amiodarone and the American way. Editorial. J. Am. Coll. Cardiol. *6*:822, 1985.

195. DiCarlo, L. A., Jr., Morady, F., Sauve, M. J., Malone, P., Davis, J. C., Evans-Bell, T., Winston, S. A., and Scheinman, M. M.: Cardiac arrest and sudden death in patients treated with amiodarone for sustained ventricular tachycardia or ventricular fibrillation: Risk stratification based on clinical variables. Am. J. Cardiol. *55*:372, 1985.

196. Marchlinski, F. E., Buxton, A. E., Flores, B. T., Doherty, J. U., Waxman, H. L., and Josephson, M. E.: Value of Holter monitoring in identifying risk for sustained ventricular arrhythmia recurrence on amiodarone. Am. J. Cardiol. *55*:709, 1985.

197. Veltri, E. P., Reid, P. R., Platia, E. V., and Griffith, L. S.: Amiodarone in the treatment of life threatening tachycardia: Role of Holter monitoring in predicting long term clinical efficacy. J. Am. Coll. Cardiol. *6*:806, 1985.

198. Naccarelli, G. V., Fineberg, N. S., Zipes, D. P., Heger, J. J., Duncan, G., and Prystowsky, E. N.: Amiodarone: Risk factors for recurrence of symptomatic ventricular tachycardia identified at electrophysiologic study. J. Am. Coll. Cardiol. *6*:814, 1985.
199. Horowitz, L. N., Greenspan, A. M., Spielman, S. R., Webb, C. R., Morganroth, J., Rotmensch, H., Sokoloff, N. M., Rae, A. P., Segal, B. L., and Kay, H. R.: Usefulness of electrophysiologic testing in evaluation of amiodarone therapy for sustained ventricular tachyarrhythmias associated with coronary heart disease. Am. J. Cardiol. *55*:367, 1985.
200. Raeder, E. A., Podrid, P. J., and Lown, B.: Side effects and complications of amiodarone therapy. Am. Heart J. *109*:975, 1985.
201. Greene, H. L., Graham, E. L., Werner, J. A., Sears, G. K., Gross, B. W., Gorham, J. P., Kudenchuk, P. J., and Trobaugh, G. B.: Toxic and therapeutic effects of amiodarone in the treatment of cardiac arrhythmias. J. Am. Coll. Cardiol. *2*:1114, 1983.
202. Sobel, S. M., and Rakita, L.: Pneumonitis and pulmonary fibrosis associated with amiodarone treatment: A possible complication of a new antiarrhythmic drug. Circulation *65*:819, 1982.
203. Borowski, G. D., Garofano, C. D., Rose, L. I., Spielman, S. R., Rotmensch, H. R., Greenspan, A. M., and Horowitz, L. N.: Effect of long-term amiodarone therapy on thyroid hormone levels and thyroid function. Am. J. Med. *78*:443, 1985.
203a. Mechlisa, S., Lubin, E., Laor, J., Margaliot, M., and Strasberg, B.: Amiodarone-induced thyroid gland dysfunction. Am. J. Cardiol. *59*:833, 1987.
204. Liberman, B. A., and Teasdale, S. J.: Anesthesia and amiodarone. Can. Anesth. Soc. J. *32*:629, 1985.
205. Schoenfeld, M. H., Whitford, E., McGovern, B., Garan, H., and Ruskin, J. N.: Oral mexiletine in the treatment of refractory ventricular arrhythmias: The role of electrophysiologic techniques. Am. Heart J. *5*:1071, 1984.
206. Sami, M., and Lisbona, R.: Mexiletine: Long-term efficacy and hemodynamic actions in patients with ventricular arrhythmia. Can. J. Cardiol. *1*:251, 1985.
207. Shanks, R. G.: Hemodynamic effects of mexiletine. Am. Heart J. *107*:1065, 1984.
208. Woosley, R. L., Wang, T., Stone, W., Siddoway, L., Thompson, K., Duff, H. J., Cerskus, I., and Roden, D.: Pharmacology, electrophysiology and pharmacokinetics of mexiletine. Am. Heart J. *107*:1058, 1984.
209. Campbell, R. W. F.: Mexiletine. N. Engl. J. Med. *316*:29, 1987.
210. Stein, J., Podrid, P. J., Lampert, S. Hirsowitz, G., and Lown, B.: Long-term mexiletine for ventricular arrhythmia. Am. Heart J. *107*:1091, 1984.
211. Heger, J. J., Nattel, S., Rinkenberger, R. L., and Zipes, D. P.: Mexiletine therapy in 15 patients with a drug-resistant ventricular tachycardia. Am. J. Cardiol. *45*:627, 1980.
212. Podrid, P. J., and Lown, B.: Mexiletine for ventricular arrhythmias. Am. J. Cardiol. *47*:895, 1981.
213. DiMarco, J. P., Garan, H., and Ruskin, J. N.: Mexiletine for refractory ventricular arrhythmias: Results using serial electrophysiologic testing. Am. J. Cardiol. *47*:131, 1981.
214. Waleffe, A., Mary-Rabine, L., Legrand, V., Demoulin, J. C., and Kulbertus, H. E.: Combined mexiletine and amiodarone treatment of refractory recurrent ventricular tachycardia. Am. Heart J. *100*:788, 1980.
215. Nademanee, K., Feld, G., Hendrickson, J., Intarachot, V., Yale, C., Heng, M. K., and Singh, B. N.: Mexiletine: Double-blind comparison with procainamide in PVC suppression and open label sequential comparison with amiodarone in life-threatening ventricular arrhythmias. Am. Heart J. *110*:923, 1985.
216. Cocco, G., Strozzi, C., Chu, D., and Pansini, R.: Torsades de pointes as a manifestation of mexiletine toxicity. Am. Heart J. *100*:878, 1980.
217. Roden, D. M., and Woosley, R. L.: Tocainide. N. Engl. J. Med. *315*:41, 1986.
218. Roden, D. M., Reele, S. B., Higgins, S. B., Carr, R. K., Smith, R. F., Oates, J. A., and Woosley, R. L.: Tocainide therapy for refractory ventricular arrhythmias. Am. Heart J. *100*:15, 1980.
219. Young, M. D., Hadidian, Z., Horn, H. R., Johnson, J. L., and Vassalo, H. G.: Treatment of ventricular arrhythmias with oral tocainide. Am. Heart J. *100*:1041, 1980.
220. Podrid, P. J., and Lown, B.: Tocainide for refractory symptomatic ventricular arrhythmias. Am. J. Cardiol. *49*:1279, 1982.
221. Ryden, L., Arnman, K., Conradson, T. B., Hofvendahl, S., Mortenson, A., and Smedgard, P.: Prophylaxis of ventricular tachyarrhythmias with intravenous and oral tocainide in patients with and recovering from acute myocardial infarction. Am. Heart J. *100*:1006, 1980.
222. Morganroth, J., Oshrain, C., and Steele, P. P.: Comparative efficacy and safety of oral tocainide and quinidine for benign and potentially lethal ventricular arrhythmias. Am. J. Cardiol. *56*:581, 1985.
223. Hession, M., Blum, R., Podrid, P. J., Lampert, S., Stein, J., and Lown, B.: Mexiletine and tocainide: Does response to one predict response to the other? J. Am. Coll. Cadiol. 7:338, 1986.
224. Engler, R. L., and LeWinter, M.: Tocainide-induced ventricular fibrillation. Am. Heart J. *101*:494, 1981.
225. Roden, D. M., and Woosley, R. L.: Flecainide. N. Engl. J. Med. *315*:36, 1986.
225a. Flecainide: A new antiarrhythmic drug. Medical Letter 28:19, 1986.
226. Campbell, T. J., and Vaughn Williams, E. M.: Voltage- and time-dependent depression of maximum rate of depolarization of guinea-pig ventricular action potentials by two new antiarrhythmic drugs, flecainide and lorcainide. Cardiovasc. Res. *17*:251, 1983.
227. Ikeda, N., Singh, B. N., Davis, L. D., and Hauswirth, O.: Effects of flecainide on the electrophysiologic properties of isolated canine and rabbit myocardial fibers. J. Am. Coll. Cardiol. *5*:303, 1985.
228. Hellestrandt, K. J., Bexton, R. S., Nathan, A. W., Spurrell, R. A. J., and Camm, A. J.: Acute, electrophysiological effects of flecainide acetate on cardiac conduction and refractoriness in man. Br. Heart J. *48*:140, 1982.
229. Estes, N. A. M., Garan, H., and Ruskin, J. N.: Electrophysiologic properties of flecainide acetate. Am. J. Cardiol. *53*:26B, 1984.
230. Singh, B. N., Nademanee, K., Josephson, M. A., Ikeda, N., Venkatesh, N., and Kannan, R.: The electrophysiology and pharmacology of verapamil, flecainide, and amiodarone. Correlations with clinical effects and antiarrhythmic actions. Ann. NY Acad. Sci. *432*:210, 1984.
231. Conard, G. J., and Ober, R. E.: Metabolism of flecainide. Am. J. Cardiol. *53*:41B, 1984.
232. Woosley, R. L., Siddoway, L. A., Duff, J. H., and Roden, D. M.: Flecainide dose-response relations in stable ventricular arrhythmias. Am. J. Cardiol. *53*:59B, 1984.
233. The flecainide-quinidine research group. Flecainide versus quinidine for treatment of chronic ventricular arrhythmias. A multicenter clinical trial. Circulation *67*:1117, 1983.
234. Hodges, M., Salerno, D. M., and Granrud, G.: Flecainide versus quinidine: Results of a multicenter trial. Am. J. Cardiol. *53*:66B, 1984.
235. Lal, R., Chapman, P. D., Naccarelli, G. V., Troup, P. J., Rinkenberger, R. L., Dougherty, A. H., and Ruffy, R.: Short- and long-term experience with flecainide acetate in the management of refractory life-threatening ventricular arrhythmias. J. Am. Coll. Cardiol. *6*:772, 1985.
236. Gay, J. J., Grbic, M., Hurni, M., Finci, L ., Maendly, R., Duc, J., and Sigwart, U.: Conversion of supraventricular arrhythmias to sinus rhythm using flecainide. Eur. Heart J. *6*:518, 1985.
237. Camm, A. J., Hellestrand, K. J., Nathan, A. W., and Bexton, R. S.: Clinical usefulness of flecainide acetate in the treatment of paroxysmal supraventricular arrhythmias. Drugs *29*:7, 1985.
237a. Nathan, A. W., Hellestrand, K. J., Bexton, R. S., Banim, S. O., Spurrell, R. A., and Camm, A. J.: Proarrhythmic effects of the new antiarrhythmic agent flecainide acetate. Am. Heart J. *107*:222, 1984.
238. Carey, E. L., Jr., Duff, H. J., Roden, D. M., Primm, R. K., Wilkinson, G. R., Wang, T., Oates, J. A., and Woosley, R. L.: Encainide and its metabolites. Comparative effects in man on ventricular arrhythmias and electrocardiographic intervals. J. Clin. Invest. *73*:539, 1984.
239. Elharrar, V., and Zipes, D. P.: Effects of encainide metabolites (MJI4030 and MJI9444) on canine cardiac Purkinje and ventricular fibers. J. Pharmacol. Exp. Ther. *220*:440, 1982.
240. Jackman, W. M., Zipes, D. P., Naccarelli, G. V., Rinkenberger, R. L., Heger, J. J., and Prystowsky, E. N.: Electrophysiology of oral encainide. Am. J. Cardiol. *49*:1270, 1982.
241. Winkle, R. A., Peters, F., Kates, R. E., Tucker, C., and Harrison, D. C.: Clinical pharmacology and antiarrhythmic efficacy of encainide in patients with chronic ventricular arrhythmias. Circulation *64*:290, 1981.
242. Brugada, P., Abdollah, H., and Wellens, H. J. J.: Suppression of incessant supraventricular tachycardia by intravenous and oral encainide. J. Am. Coll. Cardiol. *4*:1255, 1984.
243. Prystowsky, E. N., Klein, G., Rinkenberger, R. L., Heger, J. J., Nacarelli, G. V., and Zipes, D. P.: Clinical efficacy and electrophysiologic effects of encainide in patients with Wolff-Parkinson-White syndrome. Circulation *69*:278, 1984.
244. Morganroth, J., Somberg, J. C., Pool, P. E., Hsu, P., Lee, I. K., and Durkee, J.: Comparative study of encainide and quinidine in the treatment of ventricular arrhythmias. J. Am. Coll. Cardiol. 7:9, 1986.
244a. Duff, H. J., Roden, D. M., Carey, E. L., Wang, T., Primm, R. K., and Woosley, R. L.: Spectrum of antiarrhythmic response to encainide. Am. J. Cardiol. *56*:887, 1985.
245. Rinkenberger, R. L., Prystowsky, E. N., Jackman, W. M., Heger, J. J., and Zipes, D. P.: Conversion of nonsustained ventricular tachycardia to sustained ventricular tachycardia during drug therapy as determined by serial electrophysiology studies. Am. Heart J. *103*:177, 1982.
246. Winkle, R. A., Mason, J. W., Griffin, J. C., and Ross, D.: Malignant ventricular tachyarrhythmias associated with use of encainide. Am. Heart J. *102*:857, 1981.
247. leMarc, H., Dangman, K. H., Danilo, P., and Rosen, M. R.: An evaluation of automaticity and triggered activity in the canine heart 1 to 4 days after myocardial infarction. Circulation *71*:1224, 1985.
248. Ruffy, R., Rosenshtraukh, L. V., Elharrar, V., and Zipes, D. P.: Electrophysiologic effects of ethmozin on canine myocardium. Cardiovasc. Res. *13*:354, 1979.
249. Chazov, E. I., Shugushev, K. K., and Rosenshtraukh, L.: Ethmozin. I. Effects of intravenous drug administration on paroxysmal supraventricular tachycardia in the ventricular preexcitation syndrome. Am. Heart J. 108:475, 1984.
250. Morganroth J.: Safety and efficacy of twice-daily dosing regimen for moricizine (ethmozine). Am. Heart J. *110*:1188, 1985.
251. Mann, D. E., Luck, J. C., Herre, J. M., Magro, S. A., Yepsen, S. C., Griffith, J. C., Pratt, C. M., and Wyndham, C. R.: Electrophysiologic effects of ethmozine in patients with ventricular tachycardia. Am. Heart J. *107*:674, 1984.
252. Podrid, P. J., Lyakishev, A., Lown, B., and Mazur, N.: Ethmozin: A new antiarrhythmic drug for suppressing ventricular premature complexes. Circulation *61*:450, 1980.
253. Echt, D., Shapiro, M., Trusso, J., Mason, J. W., and Winkle, R. A.: Treatment with oral lorcainide in patients with sustained ventricular tachycardia and fibrillation. Am. Heart J. *109*:28, 1985.
254. Anderson, J. L., Anastasiou-Nana, M., Lutz, J. R., and Writer, S. L.:

Comparison of intravenous lorcainide with lidocaine for acute therapy of complex ventricular arrhythmias: Results of a randomized study with crossover option. J. Am. Coll. Cardiol. 5:333, 1985.
255. Duke, I. S., and Vaughn Williams, E. M.: The multiple modes of action of propafenone. Eur. Heart J. 5:115, 1984.
256. Kohlhardt, M.: Block of sodium channels by antiarrhythmic agents: Analysis of the electrophysiologic effects of propafenone in heart muscle. Am. J. Cardiol. *54*:13D, 1984.
257. Chilson, D. A., Heger, J. J., Zipes, D. P., Browne, K. F., and Prystowsky, E. N.: Electrophysiologic effects and clinical efficacy of oral propafenone therapy in patients with ventricular tachycardia. J. Am. Coll. Cardiol. *5*:1407, 1985.
258. Breithardt, G., Borggrefe, M., Wiebringhaus, E., and Seipel, L.: Effect of propafenone in the Wolff-Parkinson-White syndrome: Electrophysiologic findings and long term followup. Am. J. Cardiol. *54*:29D, 1984.
259. Siddoway, L. A., Roden, D. M., and Woosley, R. L.: Clinical pharmacology of propafenone: Pharmacokinetics, metabolism, and concentration-response relations. Am. J. Cardiol. *54*:9D, 1984.
260. Kates, R. E., Yee, Y. G., and Winkle, R. A.: Metabolite accumulation during chronic propafenone dosing in arrhythmia. Clin. Pharmacol. Ther. *37*:610, 1985.
261. Podrid, P. J., and Lown, B.: Propafenone: A new agent for ventricular arrhythmia. J. Am. Coll. Cardiol. *4*:117, 1984.
262. Manz, M., Steinbeck, G., and Luderitz, B.: Usefulness of programmed stimulation in predicting efficacy of propafenone in long-term antiarrhythmic therapy for paroxysmal supraventricular tachycardia. Am. J. Cardiol. *56*:593, 1985.
263. Stavens, C. S., McGovern, B., Garan, H., and Ruskin, J. N.: Aggravation of electrically provoked ventricular tachycardia during treatment with propafenone. Am. Heart J. *110*:24, 1985.
264. Teichman, S. L., Waspe, L. E., Matos, J. A., Kim, S. G., and Fisher, J. D.: Bethanidine sulfate: Efficacy in prevention of ventricular tachyarrhythmias during programmed stimulation. J. Am. Coll. Cardiol. *6*:510, 1985.
265. Anderson, J. L., Reid, P. R., Platia, E. V., Akhtar, M., Ruskin, J. N., Schaal, S. F., Jeung, P., Long, R. A., and Wenger, T. L.: Meobentine sulfate: Antiarrhythmic and electrophysiologic effects assessed by programmed electrical stimulation and ambulatory monitoring in patients with complex ventricular tachyarrhythmia. Am. Heart J. *110*:774, 1985.
266. Miura, D. S., Keren, G., Torres, V., Butler, B., Aogaichi, K., and Somberg, J. C.: Antiarrhythmic effects of cibenzoline. Am. Heart J. *109*:827, 1985.
267. Browne, K. F., Prystowsky, E. N., Zipes, D. P., Chilson, D. A., and Heger, J. J.: Clinical efficacy and electrophysiologic effects of cibenzoline therapy in patients with ventricular arrhythmias. J. Am. Coll. Cardiol. *3*:857, 1984.
268. Nademanee, K., Feld, G., Hendrickson, J., Singh, P. N., and Singh, B. N.: Electrophysiologic and antiarrhythmic effects of sotolol in patients with life threatening ventricular tachyarrhythmias. Circulation 72:555, 1985.
269. Singh, B. N., Nademanee, K., Feld, G., Piontek, M., and Schwab, M.: Comparative electrophysiologic profiles of calcium antagonists with particular reference to bepridil. Am. J. Cardiol. *55*:14C, 1985.
270. Prystowsky, E. N.: Electrophysiologic and antiarrhythmic properties of bepridil. Am. J. Cardiol. *55*:59C, 1985.
271. DeMarco, J. P., Sellers, T. D., Lerman, B. B., Greenberg, M. L., Berne, R. M., and Belardinelli, L.: Diagnostic and therapeutic use of adenosine in patients with supraventricular tachyarrhythmias. J. Am. Coll. Cardiol. *6*:417, 1985.
272. Wesley, R. C., Jr., and Belardinelli, L.: Role of adenosine on ventricular overdrive suppression in isolated guinea pig hearts and Purkinje fibers. Circ. Res. 57:517, 1985.
273. Morganroth, J., Horowitz, L. N., Anderson, J., and Turlapaty, P.: Comparative efficacy and tolerance of esmolol to propranolol for control of supraventricular tachyarrhythmia. Am. J. Cardiol. *56*:33F, 1985.
273a. Anastasiou-Nana, M. I., Anderson, J. L., Hampton, E. M., Nanas, J. N., and Heath, B. M.: Recainam, a potent new antiarrhythmic agent: Effects on complex ventricular arrhythmias. J. Am. Coll. Cardiol. 8:427, 1986.
273b. Easley, A. R., Mann, D. E., Reiter, M. J., Sakun, V., Sullivan, S. M., Magro, S. A., Luck, J. C., and Wyndham, C. R. C.: Electrophysiologic evaluation of pirmenol for sustained ventricular tachycardia secondary to coronary artery disease. Am. J. Cardiol. *58*:86, 1986.
274. Giardina, E. G., Johnson, L. L., Vita, J., Bigger, J. T., Jr., and Brem, R. F.: Effect of imipramine and nortriptyline on left ventricular function and blood pressure in patients treated for arrhythmias. Am. Heart J. *109*:992, 1985.
275. Mann, D. L., Maisel, A. S., Atwood, J. E., Engler, R. L., and LeWinter, M. M.: Absence of cardioversion-induced ventricular arrhythmias in patients with therapeutic digoxin levels. J. Am. Coll. Cardiol. *5*:882, 1985.
276. Schuder, J. C., McDaniel, W. C., and Stoeckle, H.: Defibrillation of 100 kg calves with asymmetrical bidirectional, rectangular pulses. Cardiovasc. Res. *18*:419, 1984.
277. Kerber, R. E., Klein, S., Kouba, C., and Aronson, A.: Evaluation of a new defibrillation pathway: Tongue-epigastric/tongue-apex route. II. Impedance characteristics in human subjects. J. Am. Coll. Cardiol. *4*:253, 1984.
278. Chang, M. S., Inoue, H., Kallok, M. J., and Zipes, D. P.: Double and triple sequential shocks reduce defibrillation threshold in dogs with and without myocardial infarction. J. Am. Coll. Cardiol. (*in press*).
279. Ruffy, R., Schechtman, K., Monje, E., and Sandza, J.: Adrenergically mediated variations in the energy required to defibrillate the heart: Observations in closed chest, nonanesthetized dogs. Circulation 73:374, 1986.
280. Otto, C. W., Yakaitis, R. W., and Ewy, G. A.: Effect of epinephrine on defibrillation in ischemic ventricular fibrillation. Am. J. Emerg. Med. 3:285, 1985.
281. Kerber, R. E., Martins, J. B., Kelly, K. J., Ferguson, D. W., Kouba, C., Jensen, S. R., Newman, B., Parke, J. D., Kieso, R., and Melton, J.: Self-adhesive preapplied electrode pads for defibrillation and cardioversion. J. Am. Coll. Cardiol. *3*:815, 1984.
282. Kerber, R. E., Jensen, S. R. Grayzel, J., Kennedy, J., and Hoyt, R.: Elective cardioversion: Influence of paddle electrode location and size on success rate and energy requirements. N. Engl. J. Med. *305*:658, 1981.
283. Hoyt, R., Grayzel, J., and Kerber, R. E.: Determinants of intracardiac current in defibrillation. Experimental studies in dogs. Circulation *64*:818, 1981.
284. Geuze, R. H., and deFeijter, P. J.: Evaluation of transthoracic countershock with initial energy levels up to 200 J in a coronary care unit. J. Electrocardiol. *18*:251, 1985.
285. Eysmann, S. B., Marchlinski, F. E., Buxton, A. E., and Josephson, M. E.: Electrocardiographic changes after cardioversion of ventricular arrhythmias. Circulation 73:73, 1986.
286. Waldecker, B., Brugada, P., Zehender, M., Stevenson, W., and Wellens, H. J. J.: Dysrhythmias after direct-current cardioversion. Am. J. Cardiol. *57*:120, 1986.
287. Chun, P. K., Davia, J. E., and Donohue, D. J.: ST segment elevation with elective DC cardioversion. Circulation 63:220, 1981.
288. Sclarovsky, S., Kracoff, O., Arditi, A., Strasberg, B., Zafrir, N., Lewin, R. F., and Agmon, J.: Ventricular tachycardia. "Pleomorphism" induced by chest thump. Chest *81*:97, 1982.
289. Cotoi, S.: Precordial thump and termination of cardiac reentrant tachyarrhythmias. Am. Heart J. *101*:675, 1981.

ELECTRICAL THERAPY OF CARDIAC ARRHYTHMIAS

290. Seger, J. J., and Griffin, J. C.: Electrical treatment of cardiac arrhythmias. Progr. Cardiol. (*in press*).
291. Peters, R. W., Scheinman, M. M., Morady, F., and Jacobson, L.: Long-term management of recurrent paroxysmal tachycardia by cardiac burst pacing. PACE 8:35, 1985.
292. Jackman, W. M., and Zipes, D. P.: Transvenous cardioversion—low energy synchronous cardioversion of ventricular tachycardia using a catheter electrode in a canine model of subacute myocardial infarction. Circulation *66*:187, 1982.
293. Zipes, D. P., Heger, J. J., Miles, W. M., Mahomed, Y., Brown, J. W., Spielman, S. R., and Prystowsky, E. N.: Early experience with the implantable cardioverter. N. Engl. J. Med. *311*:485, 1984.
294. Mirowski, M., Reid, P. R., Mower, M. M., Watkins, L., Gott, V. L., Schauble, J. F., Langer, A., Heilman, M. S., Kolenik, S. A., Fischell, R. E., and Weisfeldt, M. L.: Termination of malignant ventricular arrhythmias with an implantable automatic defibrillator in human beings. N. Engl. J. Med. *303*:322, 1980.
295. Mirowski, M., Reid, P. R., Mower, M. M., Watkins, L., Jr., Platia, E. V., Griffith, L. S., Guarnieri, T., Thomas, A., and Juanteguy, J. M.: Clinical performance of the implantable cardioverter-defibrillator. PACE *7*:1345, 1984.
296. Gonzalez, R., Scheinman, M., Margaretten, W., and Rubinstein, M.: Closed-chest electrode catheter technique for His bundle ablation in dogs. Am. J. Physiol. *10*:H283, 1981.
297. Gallagher, J. J., Svenson, R. H., Kasell, J. H., German, L. D., Bardy, G. H., Broughton, A., and Critelli, G.: Catheter technique for closed-chest ablation of the atrioventricular conduction system: A therapeutic alternative for the treatment of refractory supraventricular tachycardia. N. Engl. J. Med. *306*:194, 1982.
298. Boyd, E. G. C. A., and Holt, P. M.: An investigation into the electrical ablation technique and a method of electrode assessment. PACE *8*:815, 1985.
299. Scheinman, M. M., Evans-Bell, T., and Executive Committee of the Percutaneous Cardiac Mapping and Ablation Registry: Catheter ablation of the atrioventricular junction: A report of the percutaneous mapping and ablation registry. Circulation *70*:1024, 1984.
300. Holt, P. M., Boyde, G., Crick, J. C., and Sowton, E.: Low energies and Helifix electrodes in the successful ablation of atrioventricular conduction. PACE *8*:639, 1985.
301. Nathan, A. W., Bennett, D. H., Ward, D. E., Bexton, R. S., and Camm, A. J.: Catheter ablation of atrioventricular conduction. Lancet *1*(A389):1280, 1984.
302. Fontaine, G., Frank R., Tonet, J. L., Cansell, A., Funck-Brentano, C., Gallais, Y., and Grosgogeat, Y.: Electrode catheter ablation (fulguration) in the treatment of cardiac arrhythmias. Progr. Cardiol. (*in press*).
303. Fisher, J. D., Brodman, R., Waspe, L. E., and Kim, S. G.: Nonsurgical electrical ablation of tachycardias. Circulation (*in press*).
304. Morady, F., Scheinman, M. M., Winston, S. A., DiCarlo, L. A., Jr., Davis, J. C., Griffin, J. C., Ruder, M., Abbott, J. A., and Eldar, M.: Efficacy and safety of transcatheter ablation of posteroseptal accessory pathways. Circulation 72:170, 1985.
305. Ward, D. E., and Camm, A. J.: Treatment of tachycardias associated with the Wolff-Parkinson-White syndrome by transvenous electrical ablation of accessory pathways. Br. Heart J. *53*:64, 1985.
306. McComb, J. M., McGovern, B., Garan, H., and Ruskin, J. N.: Management of patients with refractory supraventricular tachyarrhythmia using low-energy transcatheter shocks. Am. J. Cardiol. (*in press*).
307. Gillette, P. C., Garson, A., Jr., Porter, C. J., Ott, D., McVey, P., Zinner, A., and Blair, H.: Junctional automatic ectopic tachycardia: New proposed treatment by transcatheter His bundle ablation. Am. Heart J. *106*:619, 1983.
308. Gillette, P. C., Wampler, D. G., Garson, A., Jr., Zinner, A., Ott, D., and Cooley, D.: Treatment of atrial automatic tachycardia by ablation procedures. J. Am. Coll. Cardiol. *6*:405, 1985.
309. Gang, E. S., Oseran, D., Rosenthall, M., Mandell, W. J., Deng, Z. W., Meesman, M. N., and Peter, T.: Closed-chest catheter ablation of an accessory pathway in a patient with permanent junctional reciprocating tachycardia. J. Am. Coll. Cardiol. *5*:1167, 1985.

310. Critelli, G., Gallagher, J. J., Perticone, F., Monda, V., Scherillo, M., and Condorelli, M.: Transvenous catheter ablation of the accessory atrioventricular pathway in the permanent form of junctional reciprocating tachycardia. Am. J. Cardiol. *55*:1639, 1985.
311. Touboul, P., Kirkorian, G., Atallah, G., Lavaud, P., Moleur, P., Lamaud, M., and Mathieu, M. P.: Bundle-branch reentrant tachycardia treated by electrical ablation of the right bundle branch. J. Am. Coll. Cardiol. 7:1404, 1986.
312. Bhandari, A., Morady, F., Shen, E. N., Schwartz, A. B., Botvinick, E., and Scheinman, M. M.: Catheter-induced His bundle ablation in a patient with reentrant tachycardia associated with a nodoventricular tract. J. Am. Coll. Cardiol. *4*:611, 1984.
313. Ellenbogen, K. A., O'Callaghan, W. G., Colavita, P. G., Packer, D. L., Gilbert, M. R., and German, L. D.: Catheter atrioventricular junction ablation for recurrent supraventricular tachycardia with nodoventricular fibers. Am. J. Cardiol. *55*:1227, 1985.
314. Hartzler, G. O.: Electrode catheter ablation of refractory focal ventricular tachycardia. J. Am. Coll. Cardiol. *2*:1107, 1983.
315. Evans, G. T., Jr., and Scheinman, M. M.: Executive Committee of the Registry. Catheter ablation of ventricular tachycardia foci; a report of the percutaneous cardiac mapping and ablation registry (abstract). Circulation (*in press*).
316. Hartzler, G. O., Giorgi, L. V., Viehl, A. M., and Hamaker, W. R.: Right coronary spasm complicating electrode catheter ablation of a right lateral accessory pathway. J. Am. Coll. Cardiol. *6*:250, 1985.
317. Lerman, B. B., Weiss, J. L., Bulkley, B. H., Becker, L. C., and Weisfeldt, M. L.: Myocardial injury and induction of arrhythmia by direct current shock delivered via endocardial catheters in dogs. Circulation *69*:1006, 1984.
318. Chilson, D. A., Peigh, P. S., Mahomed Y, Waller, D. F., and Zipes D. P.: Chemical ablation of ventricular tachycardia in the dog. Am. Heart J. *111*:1113, 1986.
318a. Ward, D. E., and Camm, A. J.: The current status of ablation of cardiac conduction tissue and ectopic myocardial foci by transvenous electrical discharges. Clin. Cardiol. 9:237, 1986.

SURGICAL THERAPY OF TACHYARRHYTHMIAS

319. Klein, G. J. Guiraudon, G. M., Sharma, A. D., and Milstein, S: Surgical treatment of tachycardia: Indications and electrophysiological assessment. Circulation (*in press*).
320. Cox, J. L.: The status of surgery for cardiac arrhythmias. Circulation *71*:413, 1985.
321. Moss, A. J., Schwartz, P. J., Crampton, R. S., Locati, E., and Carleen, E.: The long Q-T syndrome: A prospective international study. Circulation *71*:17, 1985.
322. Marquez-Montes, J., Rufilanchas, J. J., Esteve, J. J., Alvarez, L., Benezet, J., Burgos, R., and Figurera, D.: Paraoxysmal nodal reentrant tachycardia. Surgical cure with preservation of atrioventricular conduction. Chest *83*:690, 1983.
323. Ross, D. L., Johnson, D. C., Denniss, A. R., Cooper, M. J., Richards, D. A., and Uther, J. B.: Curative surgery for atrioventricular junctional ("AV nodal") reentrant tachycardia. J. Am. Coll. Cardiol. *6*:1383, 1985.
324. Klein, G. J., Guiraudon, G. M., Sharma, A. D., and Milstein, S.: Demonstration of macro reentry and feasibility of operative therapy in the common type of atrial flutter. Am. J. Cardiol. *57*:587, 1986.
325. Guiraudon, G. M., Campbell, C. S., Jones, D. L., McLellan, D. G., and MacDonald, J. L.: Combined sino-atrial and atrio-ventricular isolation: A surgical alternative to His bundle ablation in patients with atrial fibrillation. Circulation 72 (Suppl 3):220, 1985.
325a. Boineau, J.: Mapping-cardiac activation and repolarization. Circulation *64*:208, 1981.
326. Gallagher, J. J., Cox J. L., German, L. D., and Kasell, J. H.: Nonpharmacologic treatment of supraventricular tachycardia. *In* Josephson, M. E., and Wellens, H. J. J. (eds.): Tachycardias: Mechanisms, Diagnosis, and Treatment. Philadelphia, Lea and Febiger, 1984, p. 271.
327. Sealy, W. C., and Gallagher, J. J.: Surgical problems with multiple accessory pathways of atrioventricular conduction. J. Thorac. Cardiovasc. Surg. *81*:707, 1981.
328. Mitchell, L. B., Mason, W., Scheinman, M. M., Winkle, R. A., and Burchell, H. B.: Recordings of basal ventricular preexcitation from electrode catheters in patients with accessory atrioventricular connections. Circulation *69*:233, 1984.
329. Prystowsky, E. N., Browne, K. F., and Zipes, D. P.: Intracardiac recording by catheter electrode of accessory pathway depolarization. J. Am. Coll. Cardiol. *1*:468, 1983.
330. Jackman, W. M., Friday, K. J., Scherlag, B. J., Dehning, M. M., Schechter, E., Reynolds, D. W., Olson, E. G., Berbari, E. J., Harrison, L. A., and Lazzara, R.: Direct endocardial recording from an accessory atrioventricular pathway; localization of the site of block, effect of antiarrhythmic drugs, and attempt at nonsurgical ablation. Circulation 68:906, 1983.
331. Kerr, C. R., Gallagher, J. J., and German, L. D.: Changes in ventriculoatrial intervals with bundle branch block aberration during reciprocating tachycardia in patients with accessory atrioventricular pathways. Circulation *66*:196, 1982.
332. Weiss, J., Brugada, P., Roy, D., Bar, F. W. H. M., and Wellens, H. J. J.: Localization of the accessory pathway in the Wolff-Parkinson-White syndrome from the ventriculo-atrial conduction time of right ventricular apical extrasytoles. PACE *6*:260, 1983.
333. Miles, W. M., Yee, R., Klein, G., Zipes, D. P., and Prystowsky, E. N.: The preexcitation index: An aid in determining the mechanism of supraventricular tachycardia and localizing accessory pathways. Circulation *74*:493, 1986.
334. Nakajima, K., Bunko, H., Tada, A., Tonami, N., Hisada, K., Misaki, T., and Iwa, T.: Nuclear tomographic phase analysis; localization of accessory conduction pathway in patients with Wolff-Parkinson-White syndrome. Am. Heart J. *109*:809, 1985.
335. Windle, J. R., Armstrong, W. F., Feigenbaum, H., Miles, W. M., and Prystowsky, E. N.: Determination of the earliest site of ventricular activation in Wolff-Parkinson-White syndrome: Application of digital continuous loop two-dimensional echocardiography. J. Am. Coll. Cardiol. 7:1286, 1986.
336. Kramer, J. B., Corr, P. B., Cox, J. L., Witkowski, F. X., and Cain, M. E.: Simultaneous computer mapping to facilitate intraoperative localization of accessory pathways in patients with Wolff-Parkinson-White syndrome. Am. J. Cardiol. *56*:571, 1985.
337. Guiraudon, G. M., Klein, G. J., Sharma, A. D., Jones, D. L., and McLellan, D. G.: Surgery for Wolff-Parkinson-White syndrome: Further experience with an epicardial approach. Circulation *74*:525, 1986.
338. Sealy, W. C.: Role of surgery in the treatment of tachycardias. *In* Surawicz, B., et al (eds.): Tachycardias. Boston, Martinus Nijhoff, 1984, p. 535.
339. Zipes, D. P., Mahomed, Y., King, R. D., Heger, J. J., Miles, W. M., Brown, J. W., Adams, D. E., and Prystowsky, E. N.: Wolff-Parkinson-White syndrome: Cyrosurgical treatment. Indiana Med. *79*:432, 1986.
340. Iwa, T., Mitsui, T., Misaki, T., Mukai, K., Magara, K., and Kamata, E.: Radical surgical cure of Wolff-Parkinson-White syndrome: The Kanazawa experience. J. Thorac. Cardiovasc. Surg. *91*:225, 1986.
341. Bredikis, J., Bukauskas, F., Zebrausas, R., Sakalausas, J., Loschilov, V., Nevsy, V., Bredikis, A., and Liakas, R.: Cyrosurgical ablation of right parietal and septal accessory atrioventricular connections without the use of extracorporeal circulation. A new surgical technique. J. Thorac. Cardiovasc. Surg. *90*:206, 1985.
342. Ott, D. A., Garson A., Cooley, D. A., and McNamara, D. G.: Definitive operation for refractory cardiac tachyarrhythmias in children. J. Thorac. Cardiovasc. Surg. *90*:681, 1985.
343. Cox, J. L., Gallagher, J. J., and Cain, M. E.: Experience with 118 consecutive patients undergoing operation for the Wolff-Parkinson-White syndrome. J. Thorac. Cardiovasc. Surg. *90*:490, 1985.
344. Lawrie, G. M., Wyndham, C. R., Krafchek, J., Luck, J. C., Roberts, R., and DeBakey, M. E.: Progress in the surgical treatment of cardiac arrhythmias. J.A.M.A. *254*:1464, 1985.
344a. Bredikis, J., and Bredikis, A.: Cryosurgical ablation of left parietal wall accessory atrioventricular connections through the coronary sinus without the use of extracorporeal circulation. J. Thorac. Cardiovasc. Surg. *90*:199, 1985.
345. Sealy, W. C., Gallagher, J. J., and Pritchett, E. L.: The surgical approach to supraventricular arrhythmias. Pediatric Cardiovascular Disease. Philadelphia, F. A. Davis, Cardiovascular Clinics *11*:365, 1981.
346. Wyndham, C. R. C., Arnsdorf, M. F., Levitsky, S., Smith, T. C., Dhingra, R. C., Denes, P., and Rosen, K. M.: Successful surgical excision of focal paroxysmal atrial tachycardia. Observations in vivo and vitro. Circulation *62*:1365, 1980.
347. Gillette, P. C., Garson, A., Jr., Hesslein, P. S., Karpawich, P. P., Tierney, R. C., Cooley, D. A., and McNamara, D. G.: Successful surgical treatment of atrial, junctional, and ventricular tachycardia unassociated with accessory connections in infants and children. Am. Heart J. *102*:984, 1981.
348. Iwa, T., Ichihashi, T., Hashizume, Y., Ishida, K., and Okada, R.: Successful surgical treatment of left atrial tachycardia. Am. Heart J. *109*:160, 1985.
349. Josephson, M. E., Spear, J. F., Harken, A. H., Horowitz, L. N., and Dorio, R. J.: Surgical excision of automatic atrial tachycardia: Anatomic and electrophysiologic correlates. Am. Heart J. *103*:1076, 1982.
350. Giorgi, L. V., Hartzler, G. O., and Hamaker, W. R.: Incessant focal atrial tachycardia: A surgically remediable cause of cardiomyopathy. J. Thorac. Cardiovasc. Surg. *87*:466, 1984.
351. Anderson, K. P., Stinson, E. B., and Mason, J. W.: Surgical exclusion of focal paroxysmal atrial tachycardia. Am. J. Cardiol. *49*:869, 1982.
352. Williams, J. M., Ungerleider, R. M., Lofland, G. K., Cox, J. L., and Sabiston, D. C., Jr.: Left atrial isolation. New technique for the treatment of supraventricular arrhythmias. J. Thorac. Cardiovasc. Surg. *80*:373, 1980.
353. Yee, R., Guiraudon, G. M., Gardner, M. J., Gulamhusein, S. S., and Klein, G. J.: Refractory paroxysmal sinus tachycardia: Management by subtotal right atrial exclusion. J. Am. Coll. Cardiol. *3*:400, 1984.
354. Sealy, W. C., Gallagher, J. J., and Kasell, J.: His bundle interruption for control of inappropriate ventricular responses to atrial arrhythmias. Ann. Thorac. Surg. *32*:429, 1981.
355. Fontaine, G., Guiraudon, G., Frank, R., Tereau, Y., Pavie, A., Cabrol, C., Chomette, G., and Grosgogeat, Y.: Surgical management of ventricular tachycardia not related to myocardial ischemia. *In* Josephson, M. E., and Wellens, H. J. J. (eds.): Tachycardias. Mechanisms, Diagnosis, and Treatment. Philadelphia, Lea & Febiger, 1984, p. 451.
356. Harken, A., and Josephson, M. E.: Surgical management of ventricular tachycardia. *In* Josephson, M. E., and Wellens, H. J. J. (eds.): Tachycardias: Mechanisms, Diagnosis, and Treatment. Philadelphia, Lea & Febiger, 1984, p. 475.
357. DiMarco, J. P., Lerman, B. B., Kron, I. L., and Sellers, T. D.: Sustained ventricular tachyarrhythmias within 2 months of acute myocardial infarction: Results of medical and surgical therapy in patients resuscitated from the initial episode. J. Am. Coll. Cardiol. *6*:759, 1985.
357a. Josephson, M. E.: Treatment of ventricular arrhythmias after myocardial infarction. Circulation *74*:653, 1986.

358. Swerdlow, C., Mason, J., Stinson, E., Oyer, P., and Winkle, R.: Results of map-guided surgery in 103 patients with ventricular tachycardia. J. Am. Coll. Cardiol. 5:409, 1985.
359. Miller, J. M., Kienzle, M. G., Harken, A. H., and Josephson, M. E.: Subendocardial resection for ventricular tachycardia: Predictors of surgical success. Circulation *70*:624, 1984.
360. Josephson, M. E., Horowitz, L. N., Spielman, S. R., Waxman, H. L., and Greenspan, A. M.: Role of catheter mapping in the preoperative evaluation of ventricular tachycardia. Am. J. Cardiol. *49*:207, 1982.
361. Josephson, M. E., Horowitz, L. N., Farshidi, A., Spielman, S. R., Michelson, E. L., and Greenspan, A. M.: Recurrent sustained ventricular tachycardia. 4. Pleomorphism. Circulation 59:459, 1979.
362. Boineau, J. P., and Cox, J. L.: Rationale for a direct surgical approach to control ventricular arrhythmias. Relation of specific intraoperative techniques to mechanism and location of arrhythmic circuit. Am. J. Cardiol. *49*:381, 1982.
363. Condini, M. A., Sommerfeldt, L., Eybel, C. E., DeLaria, G. A., and Messer, J. V.: Efficacy of coronary bypass grafting in exercise-induced ventricular tachycardia. J. Thorac. Cardiovasc. Surg. *81*:502, 1981.
364. Guiraudon, G., Fontaine, G., Frank, R., Escande, G., Etievent, P., and Cabrol, C.: Encircling endocardial ventriculotomy: A new surgical treatment for life-threatening ventricular tachycardias resistant to medical treatment following myocardial infarction. Ann. Thorac. Surg. *26*:438, 1978.
365. Ostermeyer, J., Breithardt, G., Borggrefe, M., Godehardt, E., Seipel, L., and Bircks, W.: Surgical treatment of ventricular tachycardias. Complete versus partial encircling endocardial ventriculotomy. J. Thorac. Cardiovasc. Surg. 87:517, 1984.
366. Horowitz, L. N., Spear, J. F., and Moore, E. N.: Subendocardial origin of ventricular arrhythmias in 24 hour old experimental myocardial infarction. Circulation 53:56, 1976.
367. Josephson, M. E., Harken, A. H., and Horowitz, L. N.: Endorcardial excision. A new surgical technique for the treatment of recurrent ventricular tachycardia. Circulation *60*:1430, 1979.
368. Isner, J. M., Michlewitz, H., Clarke, R. H., Estes, N. A., III, Donaldson, R. F., Salem, D. N., Bahn, I, Payne, D. D., and Cleveland, R. J.: Laser photoablation of pathological endocardium: In vitro findings suggesting a new approach to the surgical treatment of refractory arrhythmias and restrictive cardiomyopathy. Ann. Thorac. Surg. *39*:201, 1985.
369. Josephson, M. E., Horowitz, L. N., Farshidi, A., Spear, J. F., Kastor, J. A., and Moore, E. N.: Recurrent sustained ventricular tachycardia. 2. Endocardial mapping. Circulation 57:440, 1978.
369a. Hauer, R. N. W., Heethaar, R. M., deZwart, M. T. W., van Dijk, R. N., Tweel, I. V. D., Borst, C., and de Medina, E. O. R.: Endocardial catheter mapping: Validation of a cineradiographic method for accurate focalization of left ventricular sites. Circulation *74*:862, 1986.
370. Downar, E., Parson, I. D., Yao, L., Cameron, D. C., and Waxman, M. B.: Endocardial catheter mapping of unstable and pleomorphic ventricular tachycardias. Circulation (Abs.) *70*(Suppl 2):1488, 1984.
371. Browne, K. F., Chilson, D. A., Waller, B. F., and Zipes, D. P.: Use of a spatially distributed multielectrode catheter to activation map the left ventricular endocardium simultaneously and destroy selected areas. Circulation 68(Abs.):333, 1983.
372. Chilson, D. A.: Rapid determination of the endocardial electrical activation sequence during ventricular tachycardia using a specially designed multielectrode basket catheter in the dog. J. Am. Coll. Cardiol. *3*(Abs.):511, 1984.
373. Downar, E., Parson, I. D., Mickleborough, L. L., Cameron, D. A., Yao, C. C., and Waxman, B. B.: On-line epicardial mapping of intraoperative ventricular arrhythmias: Initial clinical experience. J. Am. Coll. Cardiol. *4*:703, 1984.
374. Gallagher, J. D., DelRossi, A J., Fernandez, J., Maranhao, V., Strong, M. D., White, M., and Gessman, L. J.: Cyrothermal mapping of recurrent ventricular tachycardia in man. Circulation *71*:732, 1985.
375. Josephson, M. E., Simson, M. B., Harken, A. H., Horowitz, L. N., and Falcone, R. A.: The incidence and clinical significance of epicardial late potentials in patients with recurrent sustained ventricular tachycardia and coronary artery disease. Circulation *66*:1199, 1982.
376. Kramer, J. B., Saffitz, J. E., Witkowski, F. X, and Corr, P. B.: Intramural reentry as a mechanism of ventricular tachycardia during evolving canine myocardial infarction. Circ. Res. *56*:736, 1985.
377. Wiener, I., Mindich, B., and Pitchon, R.: Fragmented endocardial electrical activity in patients with ventricular tachycardia. A new guide to surgical therapy. Am. Heart J. *107*:86, 1984.
378. Cassidy, D. M., Vassallo, J. A., Buxton, A. B., Doherty, J. K., Marchlinski, F. E., and Josephson, M. E.: Catheter mapping during sinus rhythm: Relation to local electrogram duration to ventricular tachycardia cycle length. Am. J. Cardiol. 55:713, 1985.
379. Vassallo, J. A., Cassidy, D., Simson, M. B., Buxton, A. E., Marchlinski, F. E., and Josephson, M. E.: Relation of late potentials to site of origin of ventricular tachycardia associated with coronary heart disease. Am. J. Cardiol. 55:985, 1985.
380. O'Keefe, D. B., Curry, P. V. L., Prior, A. L., Yates, A. K., Deverall, P. B., and Sowton, E.: Surgery for ventricular tachycardia using operative paced mapping. Br. Heart J. *43*:116, 1980.
381. Josephson, M. E., Waxman, H. L., Cain, M. E., Gardner, M. J., and Buxton, A. E.: Ventricular activation during ventricular endocardial pacing. II. Role of pace-mapping to localize origin of ventricular tachycardia. Am. J. Cardiol, *50*:11, 1982.
382. Moran, J. M., Loeb, J. M., and Kehoe, R. F.: Operative therapy for ventricular arrhythmia. Med. Clin. North Am. *68*:1367, 1984.
383. Waldo, A. L., Arciniegas, J. G., and Klein, H.: Surgical treatment of life-threatening ventricular arrhythmias: The role of intraoperative mapping and consideration of the presently available surgical techniques. Progr. Cardiovasc. Dis. 23:247, 1981.
384. Mason, J. W., Stinson, E. B., Winkle, R. A., Oyer, P. E., Griffin, J. C., and Ross, D. L.: Relative efficacy of blind left ventricular aneurysm resection for the treatment of recurrent ventricular tachycardia. Am. J. Cardiol. *49*:241, 1982.
385. Kron, I. L., Lerman, B. B., and DiMarco, J. P.: Extended subendocardial resection. A surgical approach to ventricular tachyarrhythmias that cannot be mapped intraoperatively. J. Thorac. Cardiovasc. Surg. *90*:586, 1985.
386. Garson, A., Jr., Gillette, P. C., Titus, J. L., Hawkins, E., Kearney, D., Ott, D., Cooley, D. A., and McNamara, D. G.: Surgical treatment of ventricular tachycardia in infants. N. Engl. J. Med. *310*:1443, 1984.
387. Garson, A., Jr., Porter, C. B., Gillette, P. C., and McNamara, D. G.: Induction of ventricular tachycardia during electrophysiologic study after repair of tetralogy of Fallot. J. Am. Coll. Cardiol. *1*:1493, 1983.
388. Marcus, F. I., Fontaine, G. H., Guiraudon, G., Frank, R., Laurenceau, J. L., Malergue, C., and Grosgogeat, Y.: Right ventricular dysplasia: A report of 24 adult cases. Circulation *65*:384, 1982.
389. Guiraudon, G. M., Klein, G. J., Gulamhusein, S. S., Painvin, G. A., DelCampo, C., Gonzales, J. C., and Ko, P. T.: Total disconnection of the right ventricular free wall: Surgical treatment of right ventricular tachycardia associated with right ventricular dysplasia. Circulation *67*:463, 1983.
390. Cox, J. L., Bardy, G. H., Damiano, R. J., Jr., German, L. D., Fedor, J. M., Kisslo, J. A., Packer, D. L., and Gallagher, J. J.: Right ventricular isolation procedures for nonischemic ventricular tachycardia. J. Thorac. Cardiovasc. Surg. *90*:212, 1985.
391. Fontaine, G., Guiraudon, G., Frank, R., Fillette, F., Cabrol, C., and Grosgogeat, Y.: Surgical management of ventricular tachycardia unrelated to myocardial ischemia or infarction. Am. J. Cardiol. *49*:397, 1982.
392. Bhandari, A., and Scheinman, M.: The long Q-T syndrome. Mod. Concepts Cardiovasc. Dis. *54*:45, 1985.

22 SPECIFIC ARRHYTHMIAS: Diagnosis and Treatment

by DOUGLAS P. ZIPES, M.D.

DIAGNOSTIC AND THERAPEUTIC CONSIDERATIONS

HISTORY

The initial evaluation of the patient suspected of having a cardiac arrhythmia begins by obtaining a careful history, specifically questioning the patient regarding the presence of palpitations, syncope, spells of lightheadedness, chest pain, or symptoms of congestive heart failure. Palpitations, an awareness of the heartbeat (p. 8), may result from irregularities in cardiac rate or rhythm or a change in contractility of the heart. Some patients may be able to reproduce this sensation by tapping their hand on their chest, knee, or a table top in a fashion similar to the perceived palpitation or recognize a cadence tapped out by a physician. Such a maneuver may help establish the rate and rhythm of the arrhythmia, narrowing it to a particular rate range, a regular or irregular arrhythmia, or one in which a regular rhythm is interrupted by premature beats. The latter often are perceived only upon the contraction that ends a pause following the premature beat, and the patient may feel as if the heart has stopped for a moment. A rapid irregular tapping may suggest the ventricular response to atrial fibrillation while a rapid regular tapping may suggest an atrioventricular (AV) nodal reentrant supraventricular or ventricular tachycardia. Information regarding the nature of onset and termination of the rhythm disturbance is particularly important. Knowing the rate of the arrhythmia is crucial, and a brief demonstration by the physician of how to determine heart rate may yield important dividends. The patient, and sometimes a close relative, should be instructed in how to determine the pulse rate. Answers by the patient to key questions may provide clues to the type of rhythm disturbance, particularly if the physician has some additional information, such as physical findings and a 12-lead electrocardiogram. For example, a young adult with presyncope, normal physical findings, and electrocardiographic changes indicating Wolff-Parkinson-White (WPW) syndrome (p. 685) should be asked whether the palpitations are regular or irregular, how fast they are, and how they start and stop. If the tachycardia is regular, with a rate of approximately 200 beats per minute and of sudden onset and termination, it is likely that the patient is experiencing an AV reciprocating tachycardia (p. 685); on the other hand, if the rhythm is irregular, the patient may have atrial fibrillation, a potentially more serious arrhythmia in the presence of WPW syndrome. In an older patient with presyncope, the physician should suspect ventricular tachycardia (p. 694) if the ventricular rate is fast and AV heart block (p. 702) or sinus nodal disease (p. 667) if the rate is slow. The ventricular rhythm may be regular or irregular. Premature atrial or ventricular beats, perceived as dropped or skipped beats by the patient, are probably the most common cause of palpitations.

The physician should inquire about circumstances that may trigger the tachycardia, such as emotionally upsetting events, ingestion of caffeine-containing beverages,[1] cigarette smoking, exercise, excessive alcohol intake,[2, 3] or fatigue. A careful diet and drug history may be useful, for example, in revealing that the patient develops palpitations only after using a nasal decongestant that contains a sympathomimetic vasoconstrictor. States conducive to the genesis of arrhythmias should be considered, such as thyrotoxicosis, pericarditis, mitral valve prolapse, diuretics with hypokalemia, and so forth.[4, 5, 6,]

PHYSICAL EXAMINATION

In addition to recording cardiac rate and rhythm a number of physical findings may be helpful. For example, changes accompanying AV dissociation (p. 707) include variable peak systolic blood pressure as the atria alter their contribution to ventricular filling, variable intensity of the first heart sound as the P-R interval changes despite a regular ventricular rhythm, intermittent cannon *a* waves in the jugular venous pulse as atrial contraction occurs against closed AV valves, and apparent "intermittent" gallop sounds when atrial systole occurs at various times of the cardiac cycle. The *venous pulse* provides a window through which to judge atrial and ventricular rates and relative timing relationships. It is of interest that Wenckebach first noted the two types of second-degree AV block that bear his name (p. 704) by recording the jugular phlebogram before the electrocardiogram was available.

Examining the *second heart sound* may be helpful (pp. 34 and 46). A paradoxically split second heart sound may occur during a QRS complex with a left bundle branch block contour that results from ventricular tachycardia or supraventricular tachycardia with aberration. A widely split second heart sound that does not become single during expiration may accompany right bundle branch block. Unfortunately, similar physical findings occur with different cardiac arrhythmias. For example, progressive diminution of the intensity of the first heart sound results as the P-R interval lengthens, which may occur during AV dissociation when the atrial rate exceeds the ventricular rate or during Wenckebach second-degree AV block. Similarly, constant cannon *a* waves may occur with 1:1 atrioventricular relationships during ventricular or supraventricular tachycardia. Since AV dissociation may occur (uncommonly) during a supraventricular tachycardia and VA association may occur during a ventricular tachycardia, the clues provided by physical findings may be only suggestive.

CAROTID SINUS MASSAGE. The response to carotid sinus massage provides important diagnostic information by increasing vagal tone and primarily slowing the rate of sinus nodal discharge and prolonging AV nodal conduction time and refractoriness. Sinus tachycardia slows gradually during carotid massage and then returns to the previous rate when massage is discontinued; AV nodal reentry and AV reciprocating tachycardias that involve the AV node in one of its pathways sometimes slow slightly, terminate abruptly, or do not change; and the ventricular response to atrial flutter, atrial fibrillation, and some atrial tachycardias usually decreases (Table 22–1). Rarely, carotid sinus massage terminates a ventricular tachycardia.[7, 8]

To perform carotid massage, the patient is placed in a supine position, with the neck hyperextended and the head turned away from the side being tested, the sternocleidomastoid muscles relaxed or gently pushed out of the way, and the carotid impulse felt at the angle of the jaw. The carotid bifurcation is touched gently initially with the palmar portion of the fingertips to detect patients who have hypersensitive responses. Then, if no change in cardiac rhythm occurs, pressure is applied more firmly for approximately 5 seconds first on one side and then on the other (*never* on both sides simultaneously) with a gentle rotating massaging motion. External pressure stimulates baroreceptors in the carotid sinus to trigger a reflex increase in vagal activity and sympathetic withdrawal. Responses may occur with right-sided massage and not left, or vice versa, so that each side should be tested separately. Generally, the maximal response occurs at the first attempt at massage and lesser responses occur with repeated massages performed at short intervals. Some risk is associated with carotid sinus massage,[9] particularly in older patients. Prior to massage, the carotid artery should be auscultated so that massage is not performed in patients who have carotid bruits indicative of carotid arterial disease.

ELECTROCARDIOGRAPHY

The ECG remains the most important and definitive single noninvasive diagnostic test.[10, 10a] Initially, a 12-lead electrocardiogram is recorded and a long recording employing the lead that shows distinct P waves is obtained for proper analysis. If P waves are not clearly visible, atrial activity can be recorded by placing the right and left arm leads in various chest positions to discern P waves (so-called Lewis leads), using esophageal electrodes or intracavitary right atrial leads (see Fig. 23–11, p. 729).

Each arrhythmia must be approached in a systematic manner to answer the following questions: Are P waves present? What are the atrial and ventricular rates? Are they identical? Are the P-P and R-R intervals regular or irregular? If irregular, is it a consistent, repeating irregularity? Is there a P wave related to each ventricular complex? Does the P wave precede or follow the QRS complex? Is the resultant P-R or R-P interval constant? Are all P waves and QRS complexes identical and normal in contour? To determine the significance of changes in P-wave or QRS contour, or amplitude, one must know the lead being recorded. Are P, P-R, QRS, and Q-T durations normal? Considering the clinical setting, what is the significance of the arrhythmia? Should it be treated and, if so, how? For supraventricular tachycardias with a normal QRS complex, a branching decision tree may be useful (Table 22–2).

THE LADDER DIAGRAM. This is employed to depict depolarization and conduction schematically. Straight or slightly slanting lines drawn on a tiered framework beneath an ECG trace represent electrical events occurring in the various cardiac structures (Fig. 22–1*A* and *B*). Since the ECG and therefore the ladder diagram represent electrical activity against a time base, conduction is indicated by the sloping lines of the ladder diagram in a left to right direction. A less steep line depicts slower conduction. A short bar drawn perpendicular to a sloping line represents blocked conduction (Fig. 22–1*C*). On occasion, activity originating in an ectopic ventricular site may be indicated in another tier drawn beneath the ventricular tier or from the sinus node in a tier drawn above the atrial tier. In general, ectopic atrial, AV junctional, or ventricular activity is diagrammed to begin in the appropriate tier. It is important to remember that sinus nodal discharge and conduction and, under certain circumstances, AV junctional discharge and conduction can only be assumed, since their activity is not recorded on the scalar ECG.

ELECTROPHYSIOLOGICAL STUDY. This may be indicated and is performed by introducing multipolar catheter electrodes into the vascular system and positioning them in various parts of the heart. The catheters are used to record local electrical activity and to stimulate the heart. Multiple leads are recorded simultaneously, usually at a paper speed of 50 to 100 mm/sec. (ECG's generally are recorded at a paper speed of 25 mm/sec.) Because of the rapid recording speed, intervals or complexes of normal duration may appear prolonged. An electrode positioned across the septal leaflet of the tricuspid valve records His bundle activity as well as low right atrial activity and high ventricular septal depolarization. Occasionally, a right bundle branch deflection also may be recorded. Three basic measurements are made using the ECG and the His bundle catheter recording: the P-A, A-H, and H-V intervals (Fig. 22–1*D*). The *P-A interval* is the time between the onset of the P wave in the surface tracing (which generally slightly precedes the onset of the high right atrial recording) and the low right atrial deflection, recorded in the His lead. This interval reflects intraatrial conduction and has not proved to be of much clinical value.

The A-H interval is timed from the onset of the first rapid deflection recorded in the atrial electrogram (A) in the His bundle lead to the beginning of the His (H) deflection. Since the low right atrium and His bundle

TABLE 22–1 ARRHYTHMIA CHARACTERISTICS*

	P Waves			QRS Complexes		
Type of Arrhythmia	Rate	Rhythm	Contour	Rate	Rhythm	Contour
Sinus rhythm	60 to 100	Regular**	Normal	60 to 100	Regular	Normal
Sinus bradycardia	<60	Regular	Normal	<60	Regular	Normal
Sinus tachycardia	100 to 180	Regular	May be peaked	100 to 180	Regular	Normal
AV nodal reentry	150 to 250	Very regular except at onset and termination	Retrograde; difficult to see; lost in QRS complex	150 to 250	Very regular except at onset and termination	Normal
Atrial flutter	250 to 350	Regular	Sawtooth	75 to 175	Generally regular in absence of drugs or disease	Normal
Atrial fibrillation	400 to 600	Grossly irregular	Baseline undulation, no P waves	100 to 160	Grossly irregular	Normal
Atrial tachycardia with block	150 to 250	Regular; may be irregular	Abnormal	75 to 200	Generally regular in absence of drugs or disease	Normal
AV junctional rhythm	40 to 100‡	Regular	Normal	40 to 60	Fairly regular	Normal; may be abnormal but <0.12 second
Reciprocating tachycardias using an accessory (WPW) pathway	150 to 250	Very regular except at onset and termination	Retrograde difficult to see; follow the QRS complex	150 to 250	Very regular except at onset and termination	Normal
Nonparoxysmal AV junctional tachycardia	60 to 100‡	Regular	Normal	70 to 130	Fairly regular	Normal; may be abnormal but <0.12 second
Ventricular tachycardia	60 to 100‡	Regular	Normal	110 to 250	Fairly regular; may be irregular	Abnormal, >0.12 second
Accelerated idioventricular rhythm	60 to 100‡	Regular	Normal	50 to 110	Fairly regular; may be irregular	Abnormal, >0.12 second
Ventricular flutter	60 to 100‡	Regular	Normal; difficult to see	150 to 300	Regular	Sine wave
Ventricular fibrillation	60 to 100‡	Regular	Normal; difficult to see	400 to 600	Grossly irregular	Baseline undulations; no QRS complexes
First-degree AV block	60 to 100¶	Regular	Normal	60 to 100	Regular	Normal
Type I second-degree AV block	60 to 100¶	Regular	Normal	30 to 100	Irregular ‖	Normal
Type II second-degree AV block	60 to 100¶	Regular	Normal	30 to 100	Irregular ‖	Abnormal, >0.12 second
Complete AV block	60 to 100‡	Regular	Normal	<40	Fairly regular	Abnormal, >0.12 second
Right bundle branch block	60 to 100	Regular	Normal	60 to 100	Regular	Abnormal, >0.12 second
Left bundle branch block	60 to 100	Regular	Normal	60 to 100	Regular	Abnormal, >0.12 second

Ventricular Response to Carotid Sinus Massage	Physical Examination: Intensity of S_1	Splitting of S_2	a waves	Treatment
Gradual slowing and return to former rate	Constant	Normal	Normal	None
Gradual slowing and return to former rate	Constant	Normal	Normal	None, unless symptomatic; atropine
Gradual slowing† and return to former rate	Constant	Normal	Normal	None, unless symptomatic; treat underlying disease
Abrupt slowing caused by termination of tachycardia, or no effect	Constant	Normal	Constant cannon *a* waves	Vagal stimulation, verapamil, digitalis, propranolol, DC shock, pacing
Abrupt slowing and return to former rate; flutter remains	Constant; variable if A–V block changing	Normal	Flutter waves	DC shock, digitalis, quinidine, propranolol, verapamil
Slowing; gross irregularity remains	Variable	Normal	No *a* waves	Digitalis, quinidine, DC shock, verapamil
Abrupt slowing and return to former rate; tachycardia remains	Constant; variable if A–V block changing	Normal	More *a* waves than *c–v* waves	Stop digitalis if toxic; digitalis if not toxic; possibly verapamil
None; may be slight slowing	Variable§	Normal	Intermittent cannon waves§	None, unless symptomatic; atropine
Abrupt slowing caused by termination of tachycardia, or no effect	Constant but decreased	Normal	Constant cannon waves	(See AV nodal reentry above)
None, may be slight slowing	Variable§	Normal	Intermittent cannon waves§	None, unless symptomatic; stop digitalis if toxic
None	Variable§	Abnormal	Intermittent cannon waves§	Lidocaine, procainamide, DC shock, quinidine
None	Variable§	Abnormal	Intermittent cannon waves§	None, unless symptomatic; lidocaine, atropine
None	Soft or absent	Soft or absent	Cannon waves	DC shock
None	None	None	Cannon waves	DC shock
Gradual slowing caused by sinus slowing	Constant, diminished	Normal	Normal	None
Slowing caused by sinus slowing and an increase in AV block	Cyclic decrease then increase after pause	Normal	Normal; increasing *a–c* interval; *a* waves without *c* waves	None, unless symptomatic; atropine
Gradual slowing caused by sinus slowing	Constant	Abnormal	Normal; constant *a–c* interval; *a* waves without *c* waves	Pacemaker
None	Variable§	Abnormal	Intermittent cannon waves§	Pacemaker
Gradual slowing and return to former rate	Constant	Wide	Normal	None
Gradual slowing and return to former rate	Constant	Paradoxical	Normal	None

*In an effort to summarize these arrhythmias in a tabular form, generalizations have to be made. For example, response to carotid sinus massage may be slightly different from what is listed. Acute therapy to terminate a tachycardia may be different from chronic therapy to prevent a recurrence. Some of the exceptions are indicated in the footnotes; the reader is referred to the text for a more complete discussion.

**P waves initiated by sinus node discharge may not be precisely regular because of sinus arrhythmia.

†Often, carotid sinus massage fails to slow a sinus tachycardia.

‡Any independent atrial arrhythmia may exist or the atria may be captured retrogradely.

§Constant if atria are captured retrogradely.

¶Atrial rhythm and rate may vary, depending on whether sinus bradycardia or tachycardia, etc., is the atrial mechanism.

‖ Regular or constant if block is unchanging.

Modified with permission from Zipes, D. P.: Arrhythmias. *In* Andreoli, K., Zipes, D. P., Fowkes, V., and Wallace, A. G. (Eds.): Comprehensive Cardiac Care. 6th ed. St. Louis, The C. V. Mosby Co., (*in press*).

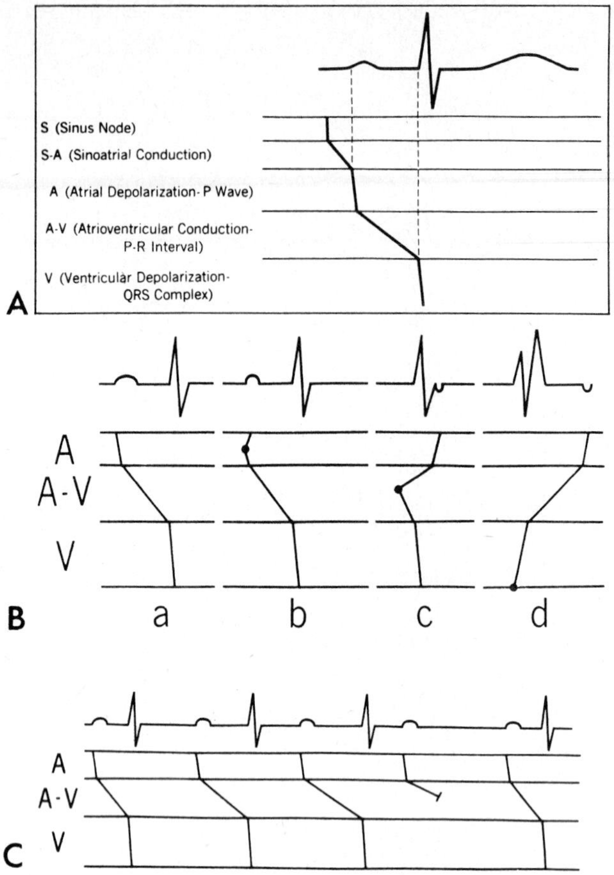

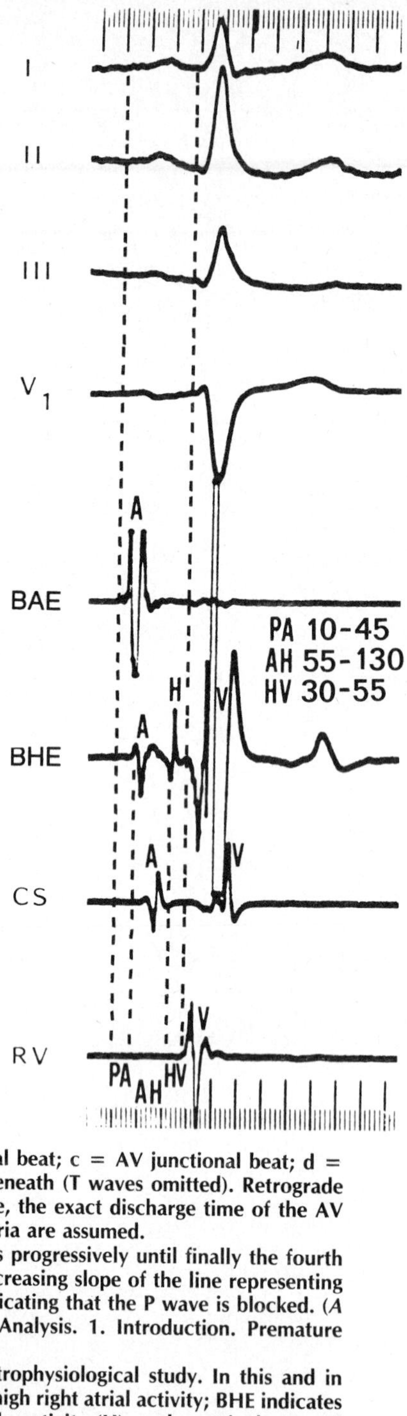

FIGURE 22–1. *A,* Ladder diagram. Straight or slightly sloping lines beginning with the P wave and QRS complex indicate atrial and ventricular depolarization. The time at which the sinus node discharges and the duration of sinoatrial conduction cannot be measured in the surface ECG and are therefore assumed. The sloping line connecting A and V, delimited by the interrupted lines, represents AV conduction.

B, Normal and ectopic beats. a = Normal sinus rhythm; b = ectopic atrial beat; c = AV junctional beat; d = ventricular ectopic beats. All are drawn with appropriate ladder diagrams beneath (T waves omitted). Retrograde atrial conduction is inscribed for the latter two beats. As with the sinus node, the exact discharge time of the AV junctional focus and conduction time from that point to the ventricles and atria are assumed.

C, Second degree Wenckebach type I AV block. The P-R interval lengthens progressively until finally the fourth P wave fails to reach the ventricles. As the P-R interval is prolonged, note decreasing slope of the line representing AV conduction and the small line perpendicular to the fourth sloping line indicating that the P wave is blocked. (*A* to *C* reproduced with permission from Zipes, D. P., and Fisch, C.: ECG Analysis. 1. Introduction. Premature ventricular complexes. Arch. Intern. Med. *128*:140, 1971.)

D, A single cardiac cycle showing the intervals measured during an electrophysiological study. In this and in similar subsequent figures, BAE indicates bipolar atrial electrogram recording high right atrial activity; BHE indicates the bipolar His electrogram recording low right atrial activity (A), His bundle activity (H), and ventricular septal activity (V); CS indicates bipolar electrogram recording of left atrial activity in coronary sinus lead; RV indicates right ventricular electrogram recording right ventricular activity; I = lead I; II = lead II; III = lead III; V_1 = lead V_1; PA = interval representing intraatrial conduction time; AH = interval representing AV nodal conduction time; HV = interval representing His-Purkinje conduction time. All numbers are given in milliseconds. Normal values for P-A, A-H, and H-V intervals are given at the upper right. Paper speed = 100 mm/sec unless otherwise stated. Interrupted lines demarcate the various intervals. Note the normal sequence of atrial activation recorded with this technique: high right atrial activity (BAE) precedes low right atrial activity recorded in the BHE lead, which precedes left atrial activity recorded in the CS lead. Large time lines = 50 msec. Small time lines = 10 msec.

anatomically delimit the boundaries of the AV node, the A-H interval closely approximates AV nodal conduction time. The A-H interval is affected importantly by various interventions: atropine and isoproterenol shorten the A-H interval, while vagal maneuvers, digitalis, propranolol, verapamil, and rapid or premature atrial pacing lengthen it. The normal range for the A-H interval is 55 to 130 msec, depending on heart rate, autonomic tone, and other factors.

The H-V interval is the time from the beginning of the H deflection to the earliest onset of ventricular depolarization recorded in *any* lead. This interval represents conduction from the His bundle through the bundle branch–Purkinje system to the point of ventricular muscle activation and is usually constant—between 30 and 55 msec—regardless of heart rate or autonomic tone.

The ventricular rate and duration of an arrhythmia, its site of origin, and the cardiovascular status of the patient primarily determine the electrophysiological and hemodynamic consequences of a particular rhythm disturbance. Electrophysiological consequences, often influenced by the presence of underlying heart disease such as acute myocardial infarction, include the development of serious arrhythmias as a result of rapid or slow rates, initiation of sustained arrhythmias by premature systoles, or the progression of rhythms like ventricular tachycardia to ventricular fibrillation. Circulatory dynamics may be altered by extremes of heart rate or by loss of the atrial contribution to ventricular filling. Rapid rates greatly shorten the diastolic filling time and, particularly in diseased hearts, the increased heart rate may fail to compensate for the reduced stroke output; as a consequence, arterial pressure, cardiac output, and coronary blood flow decline. Arrhythmias that prevent sequential AV contraction mitigate the hemodynamic benefits of the atrial booster pump, whereas atrial fibrillation causes complete loss of atrial contraction and may reduce cardiac output.[11] Chronic tachycardias can cause cardiac dilation and heart failure.[12, 13]

THERAPY

The therapeutic approach to a patient with a cardiac arrhythmia begins with an accurate electrocardiographic *interpretation* of the arrhythmia and continues with determination of the *cause* of the arrhythmia (if possible), the nature of the underlying *heart disease* (if any), and the *consequences* of the arrhythmias in the individual patient. Thus, one cannot treat arrhythmias as isolated events without having knowledge of the entire clinical situation. Patients who have arrhythmias, *not* arrhythmias themselves, are treated.

When a patient develops a tachyarrhythmia, slowing the ventricular rate is the initial and often most important therapeutic maneuver. Therapy may differ radically for the same arrhythmia in two different patients because the consequences of tachycardia in individual patients differ. For example, a supraventricular tachycardia at a rate of 200 per minute may produce few or no symptoms in a healthy young adult and therefore requires little or no therapy as it is usually self-limited. The same arrhythmia may precipitate pulmonary edema in a patient with mitral stenosis, syncope in a patient with aortic stenosis, shock in a patient with acute myocardial infarction, or hemiparesis in a patient with cerebrovascular disease. In these situations the tachycardia requires prompt electrical conversion.

The *etiology* of the arrhythmia may influence therapy markedly. Electrolyte imbalance (potassium, magnesium, calcium), acidosis or alkalosis, hypoxemia, and many drugs may produce rhythm disturbances (pp. 215 to 216), and their identification and treatment may abolish or prevent these arrhythmias.[6] Because heart failure may cause arrhythmias,[14] treatment of this condition with digitalis, diuretics, or vasodilators may suppress some of the arrhythmias that accompany cardiac decompensation. Similarly arrhythmias secondary to hypotension may respond to leg elevation or vasopressor therapy. Mild sedation or reassurance may be successful in treating some arrhythmias related to emotional stress. Precipitating or contributing disease states such as infection, hypokalemia, anemia, and thyroid disorders should be sought and treated. Since therapy always involves some risk, one must be sure—particularly as the therapeutic regimen escalates—that the risks of *not* treating the arrhythmia continue to outweigh the risks of therapy with potentially hazardous antiarrhythmic measures.

INDIVIDUAL CARDIAC ARRHYTHMIAS

SINUS NODAL DISTURBANCES

NORMAL SINUS RHYTHM

Normal sinus rhythm is arbitrarily limited to impulse formation beginning in the sinus node at frequencies between 60 and 100 beats/min. Infants and children generally have faster heart rates than do adults, both at rest and during exercise. The P wave is upright in leads I, II, and aVf and negative in lead aVr, with a vector in the frontal plane between 0 and +90°. In the horizontal plane, the P vector is directed anteriorly and slightly leftward and therefore may be negative in leads V_1 and V_2 but positive in V_3 to V_6. The P-R interval exceeds 120 msec and may vary slightly with rate. If the pacemaker site shifts, a change in the morphology of the P wave may occur. The rate of sinus rhythm varies significantly and depends on many factors, including age, sex, and physical activity.

The sinus nodal discharge rate responds readily to autonomic stimuli and depends on the effect of the two opposing autonomic influences. Steady vagal stimulation decreases the spontaneous sinus nodal discharge rate and predominates over steady sympathetic stimulation, which increases the spontaneous sinus nodal discharge rate. Single or brief bursts of vagal stimulation may speed, slow, or entrain sinus nodal discharge.[15, 16] A given vagal stimulus produces a greater absolute reduction in heart rate when the basal heart rate has been increased by sympathetic stimulation, a phenomenon known as *accentuated antagonism.*[17]

SINUS TACHYCARDIA

ELECTROCARDIOGRAPHIC RECOGNITION (Fig. 22–2*A*). "Tachycardia" is defined as a rate exceeding 100 beats/min. During sinus tachycardia in the adult, the sinus node exhibits a discharge frequency between 100 and 180 beats/min but may be higher with extreme exertion. The maximum heart rate achieved during strenuous physical activity decreases with age from near 200 beats/min to less than 140 beats/min. Sinus tachycardia generally has a gradual onset and termination. The P-P interval may vary slightly from cycle to cycle. P waves have a normal contour but may develop a larger amplitude and become peaked. They appear before each QRS complex with a stable P-R interval unless concomitant AV block ensues.

Accelerated phase 4 diastolic depolarization of sinus nodal cells generally is responsible for sinus tachycardia. Rate changes may result from a shift in pacemaker cells to a different locus within the sinus node.[18] Carotid sinus massage and Valsalva or other vagal maneuvers gradually slow a sinus tachycardia, which then accelerates to its previous rate upon cessation of enhanced vagal tone. More rapid sinus rates may fail to slow in response to a vagal maneuver.

CLINICAL FEATURES. Sinus tachycardia is common in infancy and early childhood and is the normal reaction to

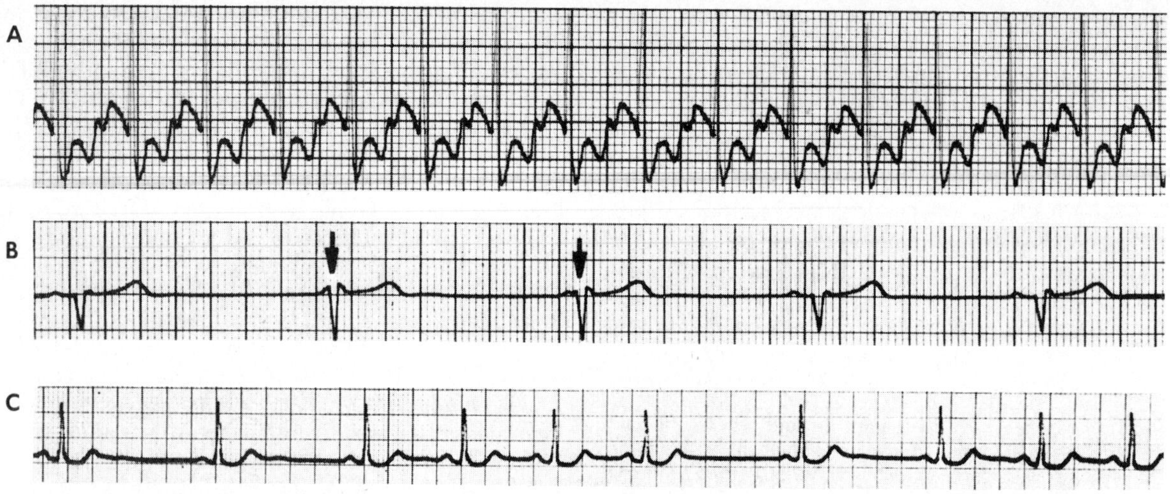

FIGURE 22–2. *A*, Sinus tachycardia (150 beats/min) in a patient during acute myocardial ischemia; note ST-segment depression. *B*, Sinus bradycardia at a rate of 40 to 48 beats/min. The second and third QRS complexes (arrows) represent junctional escape beats. Note P waves at onset of QRS complex. *C*, Nonrespiratory sinus arrhythmia occurring as a consequence of digitalis toxicity. Monitor leads.

a variety of physiological or pathophysiological stresses such as fever, hypotension, thyrotoxicosis, anemia, anxiety, exertion, hypovolemia, pulmonary emboli, myocardial ischemia, congestive heart failure, or shock. Drugs, such as atropine, catecholamines, thyroid, alcohol, nicotine, or caffeine, or inflammation may produce sinus tachycardia. Persistent sinus tachycardia may be a manifestation of heart failure. In patients with mitral stenosis or severe ischemic heart disease,[19] sinus tachycardia may result in a reduced cardiac output or angina, or may precipitate another arrhythmia, in part related to the abbreviated ventricular filling time and compromised coronary blood flow. *Chronic nonparoxysmal sinus tachycardia*[20] has been described in otherwise healthy persons, possibly owing to increased automaticity of the sinus node or an automatic atrial focus located near the sinus node. The abnormality may result from a defect in either sympathetic or vagal nerve control of sinoatrial automaticity, with or without an abnormality of intrinsic heart rate.

Treatment should focus on the *cause* of the sinus tachycardia. Elimination of tobacco, alcohol, coffee, tea, or other stimulants, for example, or the sympathomimetic agents in nose drops may be helpful. Drugs such as propranolol or verapamil may slow the sinus nodal discharge rate. Fluid replacement in a hypovolemic patient or fever reduction in a febrile patient may help slow a sinus tachycardia.

SINUS BRADYCARDIA

ELECTROCARDIOGRAPHIC RECOGNITION (Fig. 22–2*B*). Sinus bradycardia exists in the adult when the sinus node discharges at a rate less than 60 beats/min. P waves have a normal contour and occur before each QRS complex with a constant P-R interval exceeding 120 msec unless concomitant AV block is present. Sinus arrhythmia often coexists.

CLINICAL FEATURES. Sinus bradycardia may result from excessive vagal or decreased sympathetic tone as well as from anatomical changes in the sinus node (see Sick Sinus Syndrome, p. 667). Sinus bradycardia frequently occurs in healthy young adults, particularly well-trained athletes,[21] and decreases in prevalence with advancing age. During sleep the normal heart rate may fall to 35 to 40 beats/min, especially in adolescents and young adults, with marked sinus arrhythmia sometimes producing pauses of 2 seconds or longer[22]; REM sleep has been associated with sinus arrest.[23] Eye surgery,[24] meningitis, intracranial tumors, increased intracranial pressure, cervical and mediastinal tumors, and certain disease states such as myxedema, hypothermia, fibrodegenerative changes, convalescence from some infections, gram-negative sepsis, and mental depression may produce sinus bradycardia. The relationship between obstructive jaundice and sinus bradycardia has been challenged.[25] Sinus bradycardia also occurs during vomiting or vasovagal syncope (p. 889) and may be produced by carotid sinus stimulation or by administration of parasympathomimetic drugs, lithium,[26] amiodarone, beta-adrenoceptor blocking drugs clonidine, or calcium-channel blockers (see Chap. 21). Conjunctival installation of beta blockers may produce sinus or AV nodal abnormalities.[27] In most instances sinus bradycardia is a benign arrhythmia and actually may be beneficial by producing a longer period of diastole and increasing ventricular filling time. Sinus bradycardia occurs in 10 to 15 per cent of patients with acute myocardial infarction and may be even more prevalent when patients are seen in the early hours of infarction. Unless accompanied by hemodynamic decompensation or arrhythmias, sinus bradycardia generally is associated with a more favorable outcome following myocardial infarction than is the presence of sinus tachycardia[19] and occurs more commonly during inferior than anterior myocardial infarction; it has been noted during reperfusion with thrombolytic agents.[28] Bradycardia following resuscitation from cardiac arrest is associated with a poor prognosis.[29]

TREATMENT. Treatment of sinus bradycardia per se is usually not necessary.[30] For example, if the patient with an acute myocardial infarction is asymptomatic, it is probably best not to speed up the sinus rate. If cardiac output is inadequate or if arrhythmias are associated with the slow rate, atropine (0.5 mg IV as an initial dose, repeated if necessary) or, in the absence of myocardial ischemia, isoproterenol (1 to 2 μg/min IV) is usually effective. Lower doses of atropine, particularly when given subcutaneously or intramuscularly, may exert an initial parasympathomimetic effect. Ephedrine, hydralazine,[31] or theophylline[32] may be useful in managing some patients with symptomatic sinus bradycardia.[31] These drugs should be given with caution, so as not to produce too rapid a rate. In some patients who experience congestive heart failure or symptoms of low cardiac output as a result of chronic sinus bradycardia, electrical pacing may be needed. Atrial pacing may be preferable to ventricular pacing in order to preserve sequential atrioventricular contraction and is preferable to drug therapy for long-term management of sinus bradycardia.[33] As a general rule, no available drugs increase the heart rate reliably and safely over long periods without important side effects (see Chap. 23).

SINUS ARRHYTHMIA

Sinus arrhythmia (Fig. 22–2*C*) is characterized by a phasic variation in sinus cycle length during which the maximum sinus cycle length minus minimum sinus cycle length exceeds 120 msec or the maximum sinus cycle length minus minimum sinus cycle length divided by the minimum sinus cycle length exceeds 10 per cent. It is the most frequent form of arrhythmia and is a normal event. P-wave morphology does not vary, and the P-R interval exceeds 120 msec and remains unchanged, since the focus of discharge remains relatively fixed within the sinus node. Occasionally the pacemaker focus may wander within the sinus node, or its exit to the atrium may change, producing P waves of slightly different contour (but not retrograde) and a slightly changing P-R interval that exceeds 120 msec.

Sinus arrhythmia commonly occurs in the young, especially with slower heart rates or following enhanced vagal tone, such as after the administration of digitalis[34, 35] or morphine, and decreases with age or with autonomic dysfunction such as diabetic neuropathy.[35] Sinus arrhythmia appears in two basic forms: In the *respiratory* form, the P-P interval cyclically shortens during inspiration, primarily as a result of reflex inhibition of vagal tone, and slows during expiration; breath-holding eliminates the cycle-length variation. Efferent vagal effects alone have been suggested as responsible for respiratory sinus arrhythmias.[36] *Nonrespiratory* sinus arrhythmia is characterized by a phasic variation in P-P interval unrelated to the respiratory cycle and may be the result of digitalis intoxication.

Symptoms produced by sinus arrhythmia are uncommon, but on occasion, if the pauses between beats are excessively long, palpitations or dizziness may result. Marked sinus arrhythmia can produce a sinus pause sufficiently long to produce syncope if not accompanied by an escape rhythm.

Treatment is usually unnecessary. Increasing the heart rate by exercise or drugs generally abolishes sinus arrhythmia. Symptomatic individuals may experience relief from palpitations with sedatives, tranquilizers, atropine, ephedrine, or isoproterenol administration, as in the treatment of sinus bradycardia.

VENTRICULOPHASIC SINUS ARRHYTHMIA. This arrhythmia occurs when the ventricular rate is slow. The most common example occurs during complete AV block, when P-P cycles that contain a QRS complex are shorter than P-P cycles without a QRS complex. Similar lengthening may be present in the P-P cycle that follows a premature ventricular complex with a compensatory pause. Alterations in the P-P interval are probably due to the influence of the autonomic nervous system responding to changes in ventricular stroke volume.

SINUS PAUSE OR SINUS ARREST

Sinus pause or sinus arrest (Fig. 22–3) is recognized by a pause in the sinus rhythm. The P-P interval delimiting the pause does not equal a multiple of the basic P-P interval. Differentiation of sinus arrest, which is thought to be due to a slowing or cessation of spontaneous sinus

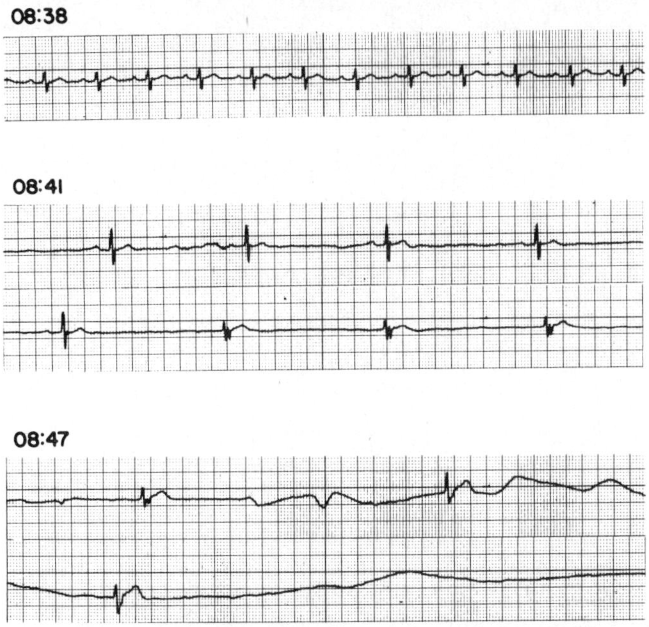

FIGURE 22–3. Sinus arrest. The patient had a long-term ECG recorder connected when he died suddenly due to cardiac standstill. The rhythms demonstrate progressive sinus bradycardia and sinus arrest at 8:41. The rhythm then becomes a ventricular escape rhythm which progressively slows and finally ceases at 08:47. Monitor lead. Double ECG strips are continuous recordings.

nodal automaticity and therefore a disorder of impulse formation (automaticity), from sinoatrial exit block (see below) in patients with sinus arrhythmia may be quite difficult without direct recordings of sinus node discharge.[37, 38]

Failure of sinus nodal discharge results in absence of atrial depolarization and periods of ventricular asystole if escape beats initiated by latent pacemakers do not occur. Involvement of the sinus node by acute myocardial infarction, degenerative fibrotic changes, effects of digitalis toxicity, or excessive vagal tone all may produce sinus arrest. Transient sinus arrest may have no clinical significance by itself if latent pacemakers promptly escape to prevent ventricular asystole or the genesis of other arrhythmias precipitated by the slow rates.

Treatment is as outlined above for sinus bradycardia. In patients who have a chronic form of sinus node disease (p. 667) characterized by marked sinus bradycardia or sinus arrest, permanent pacing is often necessary.

SINOATRIAL (SA) EXIT BLOCK

This arrhythmia is recognized electrocardiographically by a pause due to the absence of the normally expected P wave (Fig. 22–4). The duration of the pause is a multiple of the basic P-P interval. SA exit block is due to a conduction disturbance during which an impulse formed within the sinus node fails to depolarize the atria or does so with delay.[38] An interval without P waves that equals approximately two, three, or four times the normal P-P cycle characterizes type II second degree SA exit block. During type I (Wenckebach) second degree SA exit block, the P-P interval progressively shortens prior to the pause, and the duration of the pause is less than two P-P cycles. (See p. 722 and Fig. 22–42, p. 703), for further discussion of Wenckebach intervals.) First degree SA exit block cannot be recognized electrocardiographically because SA nodal discharge is not recorded. Third degree SA exit block may present as complete absence of P waves and is difficult to diagnose with certainty.

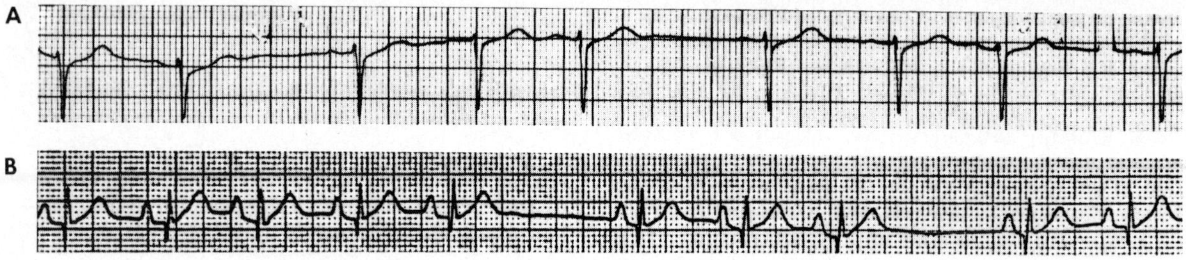

FIGURE 22–4. Sinus nodal exit block. *A,* Type I SA nodal exit block has the following features: the P-P interval shortens from the first to the second cycle in each grouping, followed by a pause. The duration of the pause is less than twice the shortest cycle length, and the cycle after the pause exceeds the cycle before the pause. The P-R interval is normal and constant. Lead V_1. *B,* The P-P interval varies slightly because of sinus arrhythmia. Two pauses in sinus nodal activity occur, equaling twice the basic P-P interval and are consistent with type II 2:1 SA nodal exit block. The P-R interval is normal and constant. Lead III.

Excessive vagal stimulation, acute myocarditis, infarction, or fibrosis involving the atrium as well as drugs such as quinidine, procainamide, or digitalis may produce SA exit block. In contrast to its effects on the AV node, digitalis may produce type II SA exit block. SA exit block is usually transient. It may be of no clinical importance except to prompt a search for the underlying cause. Occasionally, syncope may result if the SA block is prolonged and unaccompanied by an escape rhythm.

Therapy for patients who have symptomatic SA exit block is as outlined for sinus bradycardia.

WANDERING PACEMAKER

This variant of sinus arrhythmia involves the passive transfer of the dominant pacemaker focus from the sinus node to latent pacemakers that have the next highest degree of automaticity located in other atrial sites or in AV junctional tissue. Thus, only one pacemaker at a time controls the rhythm, in sharp contrast to AV dissociation (p. 707). As with other forms of sinus arrhythmia, the change occurs in a gradual fashion over the duration of several beats. The ECG (Fig. 22–5) displays a cyclical increase in R-R interval; a P-R interval that gradually shortens and may become less than 120 msec; and a change in the P-wave contour, which becomes negative in lead I or II (depending on the site of discharge) or is lost within the QRS complex. Generally, these changes occur in reverse as the pacemaker shifts back to the sinus node. Rarely the rate may remain unchanged during these P-wave transitions.

Wandering pacemaker is a normal phenomenon that often occurs in the very young and particularly in athletes, presumably because of augmented vagal tone. Persistence of an AV junctional rhythm for long periods of time, however, may indicate underlying heart disease. *Treatment* is usually not indicated but, if necessary, is the same as that for sinus bradycardia (see above).

HYPERSENSITIVE CAROTID SINUS SYNDROME (See also p. 887)

ELECTROCARDIOGRAPHIC RECOGNITION (Fig. 22–6). This condition is most frequently characterized by ventricular asystole due to cessation of atrial activity from sinus arrest or SA exit block. AV block is observed less frequently, probably in part because the absence of atrial activity due to sinus arrest precludes the manifestations of AV block. However, if an atrial pacemaker maintained an atrial rhythm (Fig. 23–21, p. 738) during the episodes, a higher prevalence of AV block probably would be noted. In symptomatic patients, AV junctional or ventricular escapes generally do not occur or are present at very slow rates, suggesting that heightened vagal tone can suppress subsidiary pacemakers located in the ventricles as well as supraventricular structures.

CLINICAL FEATURES. Two types of hypersensitive carotid sinus responses are noted.[39] *Cardioinhibitory* carotid sinus hypersensitivity is defined as ventricular asystole exceeding 3 seconds during carotid sinus stimulation, although normal limits have not been carefully established. According to one study, asystole exceeding 3 seconds during carotid sinus massage is not common but may occur in asymptomatic subjects,[22] while another suggested it was a cause for pacemaker implantation.[40] *Vasodepressor* carotid sinus hypersensitivity is defined as a decrease in systolic blood pressure of 50 mm Hg or more without associated cardiac slowing, or a decrease in systolic blood pressure exceeding 30 mm Hg when the patient's symptoms are reproduced.[41]

Even if a hyperactive carotid sinus reflex is elicited in patients, particularly in older patients who complain of syncope or presyncope, the hyperactive reflex elicited with carotid sinus massage may not necessarily be responsible for these symptoms.[42] Direct pressure or extension on the carotid sinus from head turning, neck tension, and tight collars may be a source of syncope by reducing blood flow through the vertebral arteries also.

Because intrinsic sinus nodal dysfunction is generally not the major cause for asystole after carotid sinus stimulation in this syndrome,[43] patients with hypersensitive carotid sinus syndrome may be distinguished from those with sick sinus syndrome (p. 667).[41] Hypersensitive carotid sinus reflex is most commonly associated with coronary artery disease.[44] The mechanism responsible for hypersensitive carotid sinus

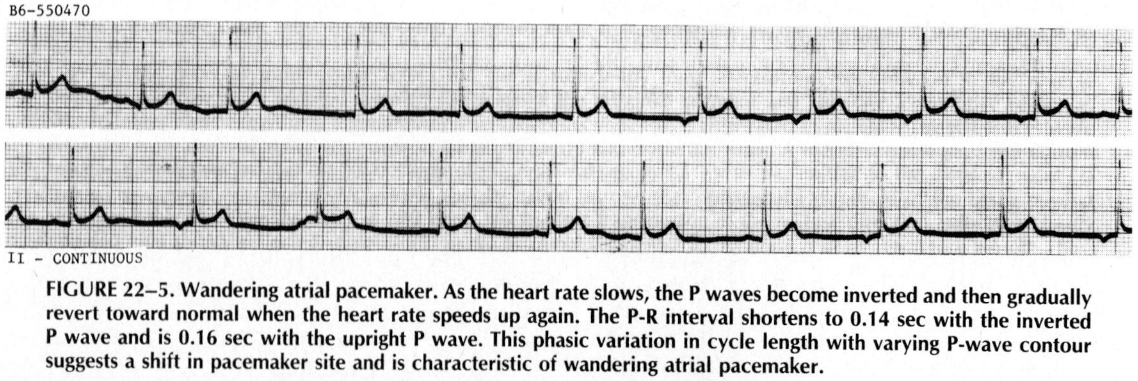

FIGURE 22–5. Wandering atrial pacemaker. As the heart rate slows, the P waves become inverted and then gradually revert toward normal when the heart rate speeds up again. The P-R interval shortens to 0.14 sec with the inverted P wave and is 0.16 sec with the upright P wave. This phasic variation in cycle length with varying P-wave contour suggests a shift in pacemaker site and is characteristic of wandering atrial pacemaker.

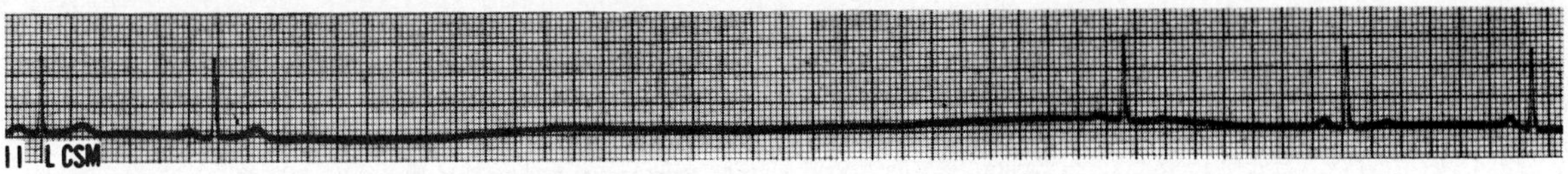

FIGURE 22–6. Hypersensitive carotid sinus syndrome. Gentle left carotid sinus massage (LCSM) produced a prolonged period of asystole. Lead II.

reflex is not known, but possibilities include a high level of resting vagal tone, hyperresponsiveness to acetylcholine, excessive release of acetylcholine, baroreflex hypersensitivity,[45] and inadequate cholinesterase activity to metabolize the acetylcholine released. Carotid sinus receptors, autonomic centers of the brain stem, and the afferent limb of the reflex have all been incriminated.[41]

TREATMENT. Atropine abolishes cardioinhibitory carotid sinus hypersensitivity. However, the majority of symptomatic patients require pacemaker implantation. It must be stressed that because AV block may occur during the periods of hypersensitive carotid reflex, some form of *ventricular* pacing, with or without atrial pacing, is generally required. Atropine does not prevent the decrease in systemic blood pressure in the vasodepressor form of carotid sinus hypersensitivity, which may result from inhibition of sympathetic vasoconstrictor nerves and possibly activation of cholinergic sympathetic vasodilator fibers. Combinations of vasodepressor and cardioinhibitory types may occur, and vasodepression[46, 47] may account for continued syncope after pacemaker implantation in some patients. Patients who have a hyperactive carotid sinus reflex that does not cause symptoms require no treatment.[42] Drugs such as digitalis, alpha-methyldopa, clonidine,[48] and propranolol may enhance the response to carotid sinus massage and be responsible for symptoms in some patients. Severe vasodepressor or mixed vasodepressor and cardioinhibitory responses may require treatment with either radiation therapy or surgical denervation of the carotid sinus.

SICK SINUS SYNDROME

This term[49] is applied to a syndrome encompassing a number of sinus nodal abnormalities that include (1) persistent spontaneous sinus bradycardia not caused by drugs, and inappropriate for the physiological circumstance, (2) apparent sinus arrest or exit block, (3) combinations of SA and AV conduction disturbances, or (4) alternation of paroxysms of rapid regular or irregular atrial tachyarrhythmias and periods of slow atrial and ventricular rates (bradycardia-tachycardia syndrome,[50, 50a] Fig. 22–7). More than one of these conditions can be recorded in the same patient on different occasions, and often their mechanisms can be shown to be causally interrelated and combined with an abnormal state of AV conduction or automaticity.[51]

More than one pathophysiological mechanism can produce the clinical manifestations of sick sinus syndrome. The spontaneous clinical arrhythmia and the response to electrophysiological testing (see Chap. 20) depend on the underlying mechanism of sinus nodal dysfunction. Patients who have sinus node disease may be categorized as having intrinsic sinus node disease unrelated to autonomic abnormalities[52, 53] or combinations of intrinsic and autonomic abnormalities. Symptomatic patients with sinus pauses and/or SA exit block frequently show abnormal responses on electrophysiological testing and can have a relatively high incidence of life-threatening arrhythmias and/or embolic episodes.[51, 54] In children, sinus node dysfunction most commonly occurs in those with congenital or acquired heart disease, particularly following corrective cardiac surgery.[55–57] However, it may occur in the absence of other cardiac abnormalities.[58, 59] Type I, type II, and complete SA exit block apparently can occur in healthy young boys.[60] Also, excessive training apparently can heighten vagal tone and produce syncope related to sinus bradycardia or AV conduction abnormalities in otherwise normal individuals.[21] The course of the disease is frequently intermittent and unpredictable, influenced by the severity of the underlying heart disease.[61, 62]

The anatomical basis of sick sinus syndrome may involve total or subtotal destruction of the sinus node, areas of nodal-atrial discontinuity, inflammatory or degenerative changes of the nerves and ganglia surrounding the node, and pathological changes in the atrial wall. Fibrosis and fatty infiltration occur, and the sclerodegenerative processes generally involve the sinus node and the AV node or the bundle of His and its branches or distal subdivisions.[63, 64]

TREATMENT. For patients with sick sinus syndrome, treatment depends on the basic rhythm problem but generally involves permanent pacemaker implantation when symptoms are manifest (p. 720). Pacing for the bradycardia combined with drug therapy to treat the tachycardia is required in those with the bradycardia-tachycardia syndrome. In these patients, drug therapy without pacing may aggravate the bradycardia. Digitalis should be used cautiously in patients with sick sinus syndrome without a pacemaker.[65] Prolonged sinoatrial conduction time or sinus nodal recovery time at electrophysiological study in the absence of symptoms is not an indication for prophylactic pacing, since therapy is directed toward control of symptoms.

SINUS NODAL REENTRY (See also p. 599)

The rate of sinus nodal reentrant tachycardia varies from 80 to 200 beats/min but is generally slower than the other forms of supraventricular tachycardia, with an average rate of 130 to 140 beats/min (Fig. 22–8). Electrocardiographically, P waves are identical or very similar to the sinus P wave morphologically; the P-R interval is related to the tachycardia rate, but generally the R-P interval is long, with a shorter P-R interval (Fig. 22–9*D*). AV block may occur without affecting the tachycardia, and vagal maneuvers may slow and then abruptly terminate the tachycardia.

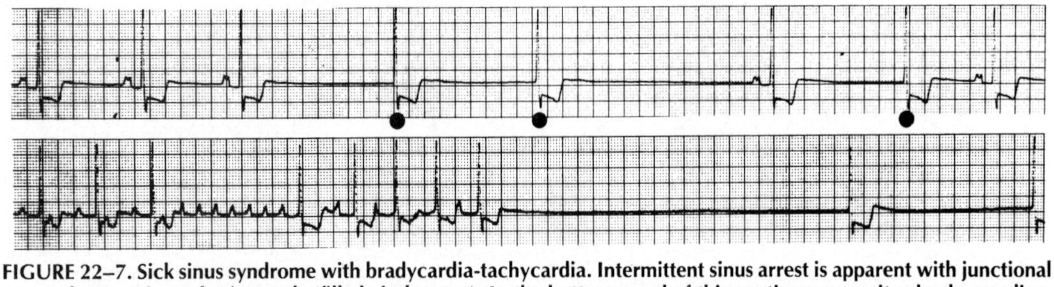

FIGURE 22–7. Sick sinus syndrome with bradycardia-tachycardia. Intermittent sinus arrest is apparent with junctional escape beats at irregular intervals (filled circles, *top*). In the bottom panel of this continuous monitor lead recording, a short episode of atrial flutter is followed by almost 5 sec of asystole before a junctional escape rhythm resumes. The patient became presyncopal at this point.

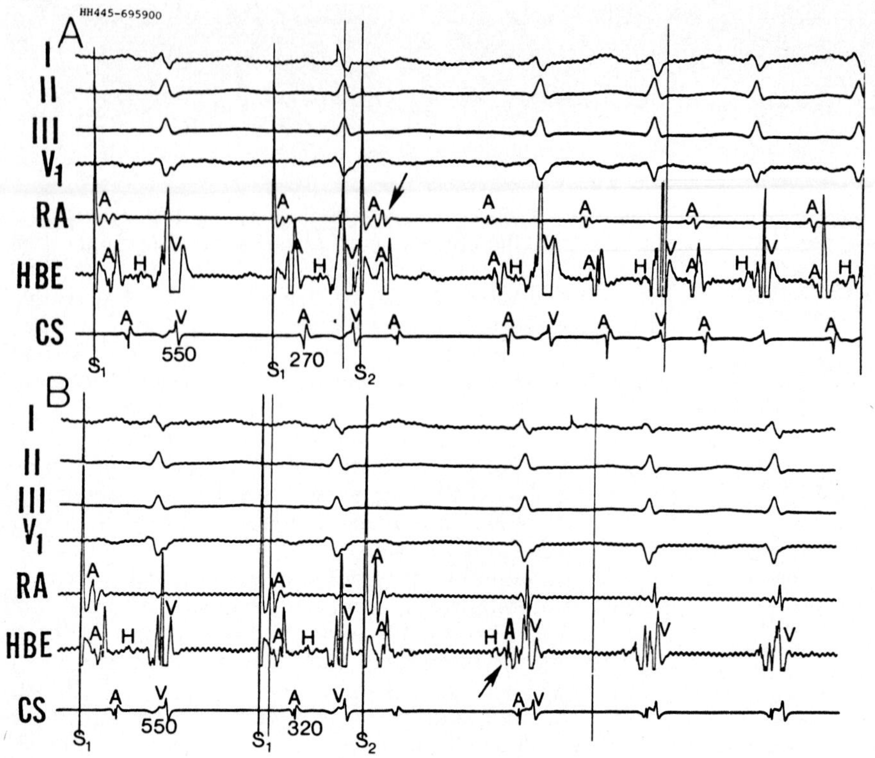

FIGURE 22–8. *A, Sinoatrial nodal reentry.* Premature stimulation of the high right atrium at an S_1-S_2 interval of 270 msec initiates an atrial tachycardia with an activation sequence similar to that occurring during high right atrial pacing. The premature P wave blocks proximal (arrow) to the His bundle but the tachycardia is still initiated. *B, AV nodal reentry.* Premature stimuation of the high right atrium at an S_1-S_2 interval of 320 msec results in a prolonged A-H interval and initiation of *AV nodal reentry.* Retrograde low right atrial activation recorded in the HBE lead occurs before ventricular activation and is followed by left atrial (CS) and high right atrial activation (arrow). This is in sharp contrast to *A,* in which the atrial activation sequence begins in the high right atrium, then the low right atrium (HBE), and then finally the left atrium (CS).

Electrophysiologically, the tachycardia may be initiated and terminated by premature atrial and, uncommonly, premature ventricular stimulation (Fig. 22–8). Initiation of sinus nodal reentry does not depend on a critical degree of intraatrial or AV nodal conduction delay and the atrial activation sequence is the same as during sinus rhythm. AV nodal Wenckebach block during the tachycardia is common.[66, 67] The development of bundle branch block does not affect the cycle length or P-R interval during tachycardia. Prolongation of AV nodal conduction time or development of AV nodal block may occur prior to termination of the tachycardia but does not affect the sinus nodal reentry.

Sinus nodal reentry may account for 5 to 10 per cent of cases of supraventricular tachycardia. It occurs in all age groups without sex predilection. Patients may be slightly older and have a higher incidence of heart disease than do patients with supraventricular tachycardia due to other

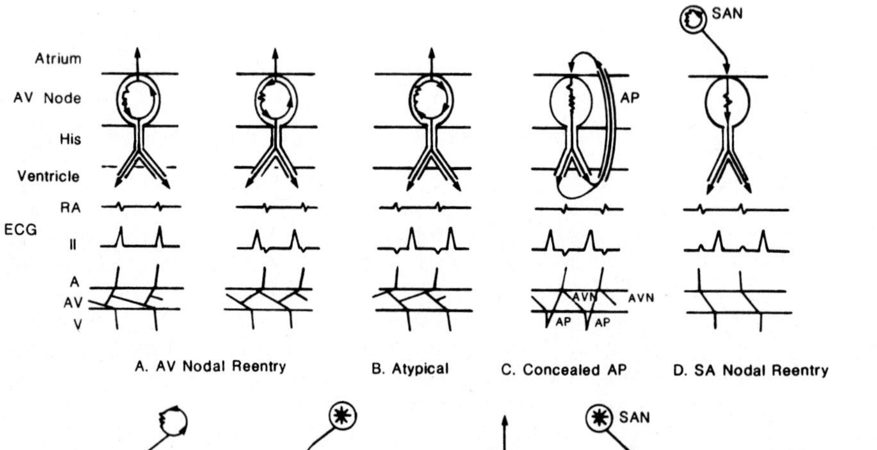

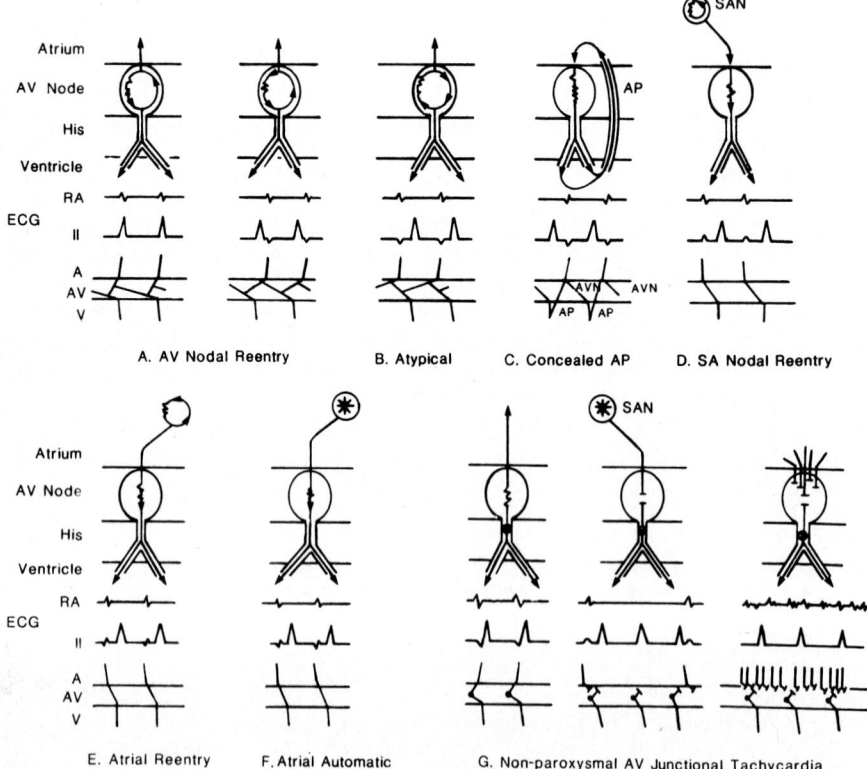

FIGURE 22–9. Diagrammatic representation of various tachycardias. In the top portion of each example, a schematic of the presumed anatomical pathways is drawn; in the bottom half, the ECG presentation and the explanatory ladder diagram are depicted. *A,* AV nodal reentry. In the left example, reentrant excitation is drawn confined to the AV node, with retrograde atrial activity occurring simultaneously with ventricular activity owing to anterograde conduction over the slow AV nodal pathway and retrograde conduction over the fast AV nodal pathway. In the right example, atrial activity occurs slightly later than ventricular activity, owing to retrograde conduction delay. *B,* Atypical AV nodal reentry due to anterograde conduction over a fast AV nodal pathway and retrograde conduction over a slow AV nodal pathway. *C,* Concealed accessory pathway. Reciprocating tachycardia is due to anterograde conduction over the AV node and retrograde conduction over the accessory pathway. Retrograde P waves occur after the QRS complex. *D,* Sinus nodal reentry. The tachycardia is due to reentry within the sinus node, which then conducts to the rest of the heart. *E,* Atrial reentry. Tachycardia is due to reentry within the atrium, which then conducts to the rest of the heart. *F,* Automatic atrial tachycardia. Tachycardia is due to automatic discharge in the atrium, which then conducts to the rest of the heart; it is difficult to distinguish from atrial reentry. *G,* Nonparoxysmal AV junctional tachycardia. Various presentations of this tachycardia are depicted with retrograde atrial capture, AV dissociation with the sinus node in control of the atria, and AV dissociation with atrial fibrillation.

mechanisms. Many may not seek medical attention because the relatively slow rate of the tachycardia does not result in serious symptoms. On the other hand, sinus nodal reentry may be responsible for apparent "anxiety-related sinus tachycardia" in some patients. Drugs such as propranolol, verapamil, and digitalis may be effective in terminating and preventing recurrences of sinus node reentrant tachycardia.

DISTURBANCES OF ATRIAL RHYTHM

PREMATURE ATRIAL COMPLEXES

Premature complexes are one of the most common causes of an irregular pulse. They may originate from any area in the heart—most frequently from the ventricles, less often from the atria and from the AV junctional area, and rarely from the sinus node. Although premature complexes arise in normal hearts, they are more often associated with organic heart disease and increase in frequency with age.

ELECTROCARDIOGRAPHIC RECOGNITION (Fig. 22–10). The electrocardiographic diagnosis of premature atrial complexes is indicated by a premature P wave with a P-R interval exceeding 120 msec (except in WPW syndrome, in which the P-R interval may be less than 120 msec). Although the contour of the premature P wave may resemble the normal sinus P wave, it generally differs. Variations in the basic sinus rate at times may make the diagnosis of prematurity difficult, but differences in the contour of the P waves are usually apparent and indicate a different focus of origin. When a premature atrial complex occurs early in diastole, conduction may not be completely normal. The AV junction may still be refractory from the preceding beat and prevent propagation of the impulse (blocked or nonconducted premature atrial complex, Fig. 22–10*A*) or cause conduction to be slowed (premature atrial complex with a prolonged P-R interval). As a general rule, the R-P interval is inversely related to the P-R interval: thus, a short R-P interval produced by an early premature atrial complex occurring close to the preceding QRS complex is followed by a long P-R interval. When premature atrial complexes occur early in the cardiac cycle, the premature P waves may be difficult to discern because they are superimposed on T waves. Careful examination of tracings from several leads may be necessary before the premature atrial complex can be recognized as a slight deformity of the T wave. Often such premature atrial complexes may block before reaching the ventricle and may be misinterpreted as a sinus pause or sinus exit block (Fig. 22–10*A*).

The length of the pause following any premature complex or series of premature complexes is determined by the interaction of several factors. If the premature atrial complex occurs when the sinus node and perinodal tissue are not refractory, the impulse may conduct into the sinus node, discharge it prematurely, and cause the next sinus cycle to begin from that time. The interval between the two normal P waves flanking a premature atrial complex that has reset the timing of the basic sinus rhythm is less than twice the normal P-P interval and the pause after the premature atrial complex is said to be "noncompensatory." Referring to Figure 22–10*E*, reset (noncompensatory pause) occurs when A_1-A_2 interval + A_2-A_3 interval < two times the A_1-A_1 interval, and A_2-A_3 interval > A_1-A_1 interval. The interval between the premature atrial complex (A_2) and the following sinus-initiated P wave (A_3) exceeds one sinus cycle but is less than "fully compensatory" (see below), because the A_2-A_3 interval is lengthened by the time it takes the ectopic atrial impulse to conduct to the sinus node and depolarize it and then for the sinus impulse to return to the atrium. These factors lengthen the return cycle, i.e., the interval between the premature atrial complex (A_2) and the following sinus-initiated P wave (A_3) (Fig. 22–10*E*). Premature discharge of the sinus node by an early premature atrial complex may temporarily depress sinus nodal automatic activity, causing the sinus node to beat more slowly initially (Fig. 22–10*D*). Often when this happens, the interval between the A_3 and the next sinus initiated P wave exceeds the A_1-A_1 interval.

Less commonly, the premature atrial complex may encounter a refractory sinus node or perinodal tissue, in which case the timing of the basic sinus rhythm is not altered, since the sinus node is not reset by the premature atrial complex and the interval between the two normal, sinus-initiated P waves flanking the premature atrial complex is twice the normal P-P interval. The interval following this premature atrial discharge is said to be a "full compensatory pause," i.e., of sufficient duration so that the P-P interval bounding the premature atrial complex is twice the normal P-P interval. However, sinus arrhythmia may lengthen or shorten this pause. Rarely, an *interpolated premature atrial* complex may occur. In this case, the pause after the premature atrial complex is very short and the interval bounded by the normal sinus-initiated P waves on each side of the premature atrial complex is only slightly longer than or equals one normal P-P cycle length. The interpolated premature atrial complex fails to affect the sinus nodal pacemaker, and the sinus impulse following the premature atrial complex is conducted to the ventricles, often with a slightly lengthened P-R interval. An interpolated premature complex of any type represents the only type of premature systole that does not actually replace the normally conducted beat. Premature atrial complexes may originate in the sinus node and are identified by premature P waves that have a contour identical to the normal sinus P wave.[68] The cycle after the premature sinus complex equals or is slightly shorter than the basic sinus cycle. Premature sinus complexes are not commonly recognized.

On occasion, when the AV node has had sufficient time to repolarize and conduct without delay, the supraventricular QRS complex initiated by the premature atrial complex may be aberrant in configuration because the His-Purkinje system or ventricular muscle has *not* completely repolarized and conducts with functional delay or block (Fig. 22–10*A*). It is important to remember that the refractory period of cardiac fibers is related directly to cycle length. (In the adult, AV nodal effective refractory period prolongs at shorter cycle lengths.) A slow heart rate (long cycle length) produces a longer His-Purkinje refractory period than a faster heart rate. Because of this, a premature atrial complex that follows a long R-R interval (long refractory period) may result in functional bundle branch block (aberrant ventricular conduction, p. 194). Since the right bundle branch at long cycles has a longer refractory period than the left bundle branch, aberration with a right bundle branch block pattern at slow rates occurs more commonly than aberration with a left bundle branch block pattern. At shorter cycles, the refractory period of the left bundle branch exceeds that of the right bundle branch and a left bundle branch block pattern may be more likely to occur.[69]

CLINICAL FEATURES. Premature atrial complexes may occur in a variety of situations, for example, during infection, inflammation, or myocardial ischemia, or they may be provoked by a variety of medications, by tension states, or by tobacco, alcohol, or caffeine. Premature atrial complexes may precipitate or presage the occurrence of sus-

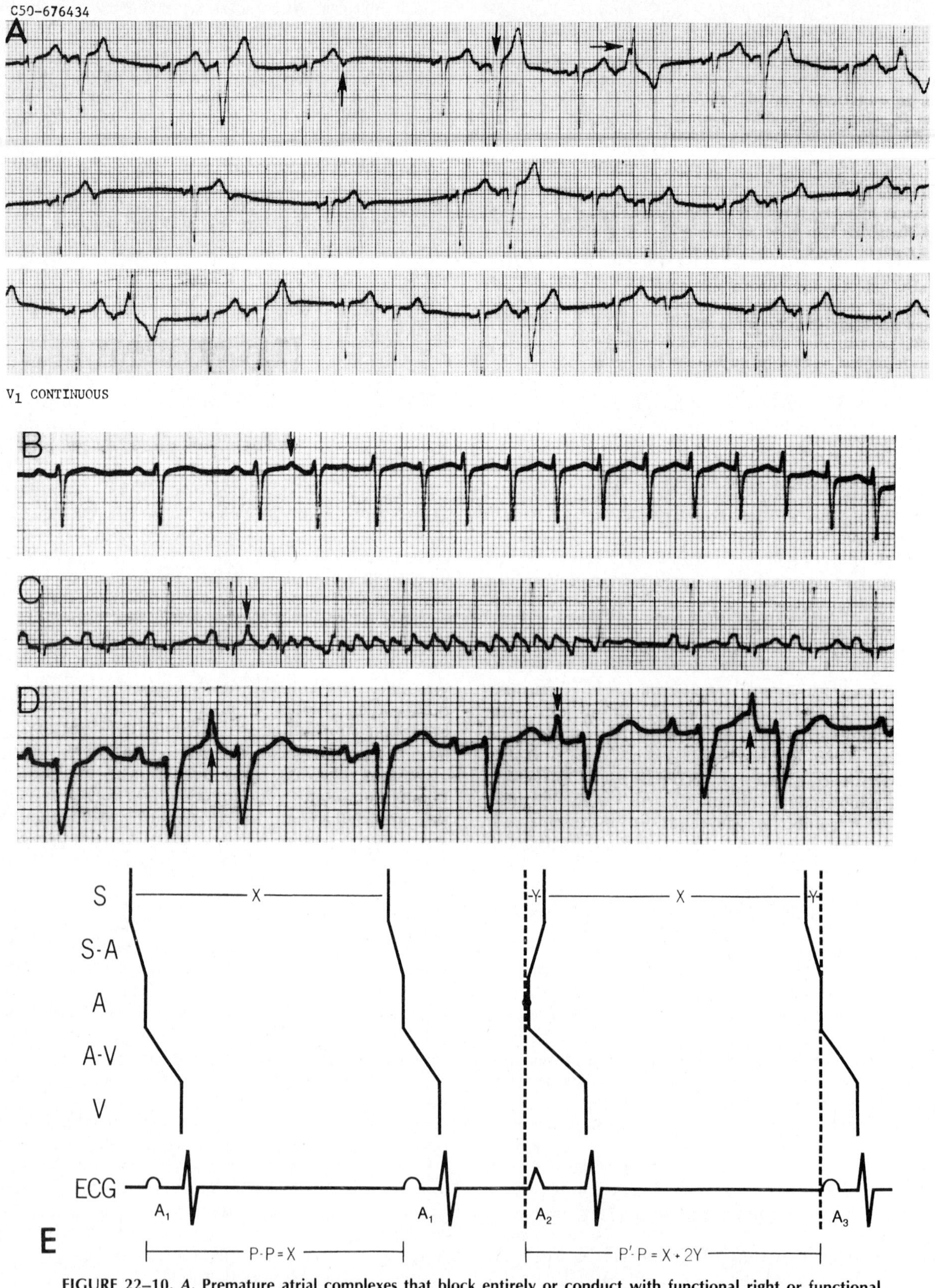

FIGURE 22–10. *A*, Premature atrial complexes that block entirely or conduct with functional right or functional left bundle branch block. Depending on preceding cycle length and coupling interval of the premature atrial complex, the latter blocks entirely in the AV node (↑) or conducts with functional left bundle branch block (↓) or functional right bundle branch block (→).

B, Premature atrial complex (↓) initiates a supraventricular tachycardia probably due to AV nodal reentry.

C and *D*, A premature atrial complex (↓) initiating a short run of atrial flutter (*C*) and a premature atrial complex (↑) depressing the return of the next sinus nodal discharge (*D*). A slightly later premature atrial complex (↓) in D does not depress sinus nodal automaticity. Panels B-D monitor leads.

E, Diagrammatic example of effects of a premature atrial complex. Sinus interval (A_1–A_1) equals X. Third P wave represents premature atrial complex (A_2) that reaches and discharges SA node, causing the next sinus cycle to begin at that time. Therefore, the P′–P (A_2–A_3) equals X + 2Y msec, assuming no depression of SA nodal automaticity. (Modified from Zipes, D. P., and Fisch, C.: Premature atrial contraction. Arch. Intern. Med. *128*:453, 1971.)

tained supraventricular (Fig. 22–10*B* and *C*) and rarely ventricular tachyarrhythmias.[70, 71]

TREATMENT. Premature atrial complexes generally do not require therapy. In symptomatic patients or when the premature atrial complexes precipitate tachycardias, treatment with digitalis, propranolol, or verapamil may be tried. If these drugs are unsuccessful trials with quinidine, procainamide, or disopyramide should be instituted.

ATRIAL FLUTTER (See also p. 603)

ELECTROCARDIOGRAPHIC RECOGNITION (Fig. 22–11). The atrial rate during classical or type I[72] atrial flutter is usually 250 to 350 beats/min, although antiarrhythmic drugs such as quinidine and amiodarone may reduce the rate to the range of 200 beats/min. If this occurs, the ventricles may respond in a 1:1 fashion to the slower atrial rate.[73] Ordinarily the atrial rate is about 300 beats/min, and in untreated patients the ventricular rate is half the atrial rate, i.e., 150 beats/min[74] (Fig. 22–11*A*). A significantly slower ventricular rate (in the absence of drugs) suggests abnormal AV conduction. In children, in patients with the preexcitation syndrome (p. 685), occasionally in patients with hyperthyroidism, and in those whose AV nodes conduct rapidly,[75, 76] atrial flutter may conduct to the ventricle in a 1:1 fashion, producing a ventricular rate of 300 beats/min. The rate in type II flutter is 350 to 450 beats/min.[72]

The ECG reveals identically recurring regular sawtooth flutter waves (Figs. 22–10*C* and 22–11*B*) and evidence of continual electrical activity (lack of an isoelectric interval between flutter waves), often best visualized in leads II, III, aVf, or V_1. The flutter waves are commonly inverted (negative) in these leads and less often are upright (positive). If the AV conduction ratio remains constant, the ventricular rhythm will be regular; if the ratio of conducted beats varies (usually the result of a Wenckebach AV block), the ventricular rhythm will be irregular. Alternation between 2:1 and 4:1 AV conduction often occurs and may be due to two levels of block—2:1 high in the AV node and 3:2 lower down. The irregular ventricular response frequently has the structure that results from Wenckebach periodicity. Recurrent alternation of short and long ventricular intervals may be due to concealed conduction (p. 202). Conduction also may be influenced by various degrees of penetration into the AV junction by the flutter impulses, which then affect conduction of subsequent impulses. The ratio of flutter waves to conducted ventricular complexes most often is an even number (e.g., 2:1, 4:1, and so on).[49] Impure flutter (flutter-fibrillation or "flitter"), occurring at a rate faster than pure flutter, shows variability in the contour and spacing of the flutter waves and in some instances may represent dissimilar atrial rhythms, i.e., fibrillation in one atrium and a slower, more regular rhythm resembling atrial flutter in the opposite atrium.[77, 78] Prolonged atrial conduction time has been found to be a predisposing factor for the development of atrial flutter.[79, 80]

CLINICAL FEATURES. Atrial flutter is less common than is atrial fibrillation. Paroxysmal atrial flutter may occur in

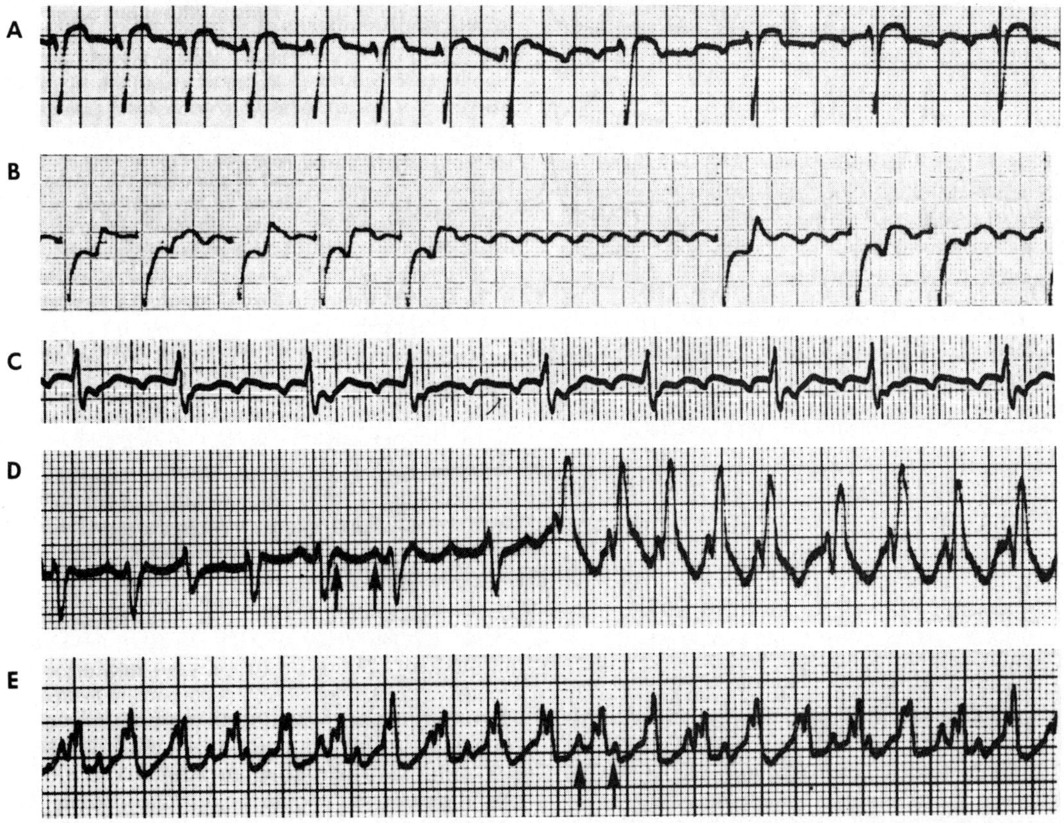

FIGURE 22–11. Various manifestations of atrial flutter. *A*, Atrial flutter at a rate of 300 beats/min conducts to ventricles with 2:1 block. In the midportion of the tracing, carotid sinus massage converts the block to 4:1 and the ventricular rate slows to 75 beats/min. *B*, Carotid sinus massage produces a transient period of AV block clearly revealing the flutter waves. *C*, Quinidine has slowed the atrial flutter rate to approximately 188 beats/min. The block is variable. *D*, Wide QRS complexes with an RSR′ configuration in V_1 begin after a short cycle that follows a long cycle in the midportion of the ECG strip. This represents functional right bundle branch block. Arrows indicate flutter waves. *E*, The QRS complexes are 0.12 sec in duration and have a regular interval at a rate of 200 beats/min. Atrial activity is also regular at a rate of 300 beats/min and independent from the ventricular activity (arrows). Thus, atrial flutter is present with a probable ventricular tachycardia, an example of complete AV dissociation. Monitor leads in *A*, *B*, *C*, and *E*.

patients without organic heart disease, while chronic (persistent) atrial flutter is usually associated with underlying heart disease such as rheumatic or ischemic heart disease or cardiomyopathy. It may occur as a result of atrial dilation from septal defects, pulmonary emboli, mitral or tricuspid valve stenosis or regurgitation, or chronic ventricular failure. Toxic and metabolic conditions that affect the heart, such as thyrotoxicosis, alcoholism, and pericarditis, may cause atrial flutter. Occasionally, it may be congenital[81] or even occur in utero.[82] Atrial flutter tends to be unstable, reverting to sinus rhythm or degenerating into atrial fibrillation. Less commonly, the atria may continue to flutter for months or years. In atrial flutter the atria contract, which may, in part, account for less systemic emboli than during atrial fibrillation. In children, continued episodes of atrial flutter are associated with an increased possibility of sudden death.[83]

Atrial flutter usually responds to carotid sinus massage with a decrease in ventricular rate in stepwise multiples, returning in a reverse manner to the former ventricular rate at the termination of carotid massage (Fig. 22–11*A*). Very rarely sinus rhythm follows carotid sinus massage. Exercise, by enhancing sympathetic or lessening parasympathetic tone, may reduce the AV conduction delay and produce a doubling of the ventricular rate.

Physical examination may reveal rapid flutter waves in the jugular venous pulse. If the relationship of flutter waves to conducted QRS complexes remains constant, the first heart sound will have a constant intensity. Occasionally, sounds caused by atrial contraction may be auscultated.

TREATMENT. Synchronous direct-current (DC) cardioversion (p. 642) is commonly the initial treatment of choice for atrial flutter, since cardioversion promptly and effectively restores sinus rhythm, often requiring relatively low energies (< 50 joules). If the electrical shock results in atrial fibrillation, a second shock at a higher energy level may be used to restore sinus rhythm or, depending on the clinical circumstances, the atrial fibrillation may be left untreated. The latter may revert to atrial flutter or sinus rhythm. If the patient cannot be electrically cardioverted or if electrical cardioversion is contraindicated—for example, after administering large amounts of digitalis—*rapid atrial pacing* can effectively terminate type I atrial flutter in most patients,[84, 85] but not type II,[72] producing sinus rhythm or atrial fibrillation with a slowing of the ventricular rate and concomitant clinical improvement.[86] Termination of atrial flutter by atrial pacing may be associated with entrainment, whereby at critical rates of overdrive atrial pacing the flutter morphology changes but the flutter does not terminate.

Verapamil (p. 636), given as an initial bolus of 5 to 10 mg IV, followed by a constant infusion at a rate of 5 μg/kg/min to slow the ventricular response, may be tried.[87] Verapamil may restore sinus rhythm in patients with atrial flutter of recent onset but less commonly terminates chronic atrial flutter.

If the flutter cannot be electrically cardioverted or terminated by pacing or by verapamil, or if it recurs at frequent intervals, a *short-acting digitalis preparation* (such as digoxin or deslanoside) can be given. The dose of digitalis necessary to slow the ventricular response varies and at times may result in toxic levels because it is often difficult to slow the ventricular rate during atrial flutter. Frequently, atrial fibrillation develops after digitalis administration and may revert to normal sinus rhythm on withdrawal of digitalis; occasionally, normal sinus rhythm may occur without intervening atrial fibrillation. *Propranolol* (p. 634) effectively diminishes the ventricular response to atrial flutter and may be used together with digitalis in patients whose ventricular rate is not decreased after digitalis. Propranolol does not appear to affect the atrial rate during atrial flutter.

If the atrial flutter persists, *quinidine sulfate* (p. 628), 200 to 400 mg orally every 6 hours, can be used to restore sinus rhythm. Large doses of quinidine given every 2 hours to terminate atrial flutter or atrial fibrillation prior to the development of DC cardioversion are no longer warranted. If atrial flutter persists after digitalis and quinidine, administration of disopyramide, procainamide, or amiodarone (Chap. 21) can be tried empirically. If conversion occurs, the patient is given maintenance doses of digitalis and quinidine, disopyramide, or procainamide. Sometimes treatment of the underlying disorder, such as thyrotoxicosis, is necessary to effect conversion to sinus rhythm. In certain instances atrial flutter may continue, and if the ventricular rate can be controlled with digitalis, conversion may not be indicated. Quinidine maintenance therapy should be discontinued if flutter remains.

It is important to reemphasize that quinidine, procainamide, disopyramide and similar drugs should *not* be used unless the ventricular rate during atrial flutter has been *slowed* with digitalis, verapamil, or propranolol. Because of the vagolytic action of quinidine, procainamide, and disopyramide (see Chap. 21) and also their direct effect to slow the atrial rate, AV conduction may be facilitated sufficiently to result in a 1:1 ventricular response to the atrial flutter.[73]

Prevention of recurrent atrial flutter is often difficult to achieve but should be approached as outlined for the prevention of paroxysmal supraventricular tachycardia due to AV nodal reentry (p. 683). If recurrences cannot be prevented, therapy is directed toward controlling the ventricular rate when the flutter does recur, with digitalis alone or combined with propranolol or with oral verapamil.* Surgery and electrical ablation of the His bundle have been successful.

ATRIAL FIBRILLATION (See also p. 603)

ELECTROCARDIOGRAPHIC RECOGNITION (Fig. 22–12). This arrhythmia is characterized by totally disorganized atrial depolarizations without effective atrial contraction. Electrical activity of the atrium may be detected electrocardiographically as small irregular baseline undulations of variable amplitude and morphology, called F waves, at a rate of 350 to 600 beats/min. At times, small, fine, rapid F waves may occur and are detectable only by right atrial leads, intracavitary, or esophageal electrodes. The ventricular response is grossly irregular ("irregularly irregular") and, in the untreated patient with normal AV conduction, is usually between 100 and 160 beats/min. In patients with the WPW syndrome (see p. 202), the ventricular rate during atrial fibrillation at times may exceed 300 beats/min and lead to ventricular fibrillation (Fig. 22–23*B*, p. 686). Atrial fibrillation should be suspected when the ECG shows supraventricular complexes at an irregular rhythm and no obvious P waves. The recognizable F waves probably do not represent total atrial activity but depict only the larger vectors generated by the multiple wavelets of depolarization that occur at any given moment.

---

*At the time of this writing, the use of oral verapamil for this purpose is still investigational, although intravenous verapamil has been approved by the FDA to treat supraventricular tachycardias.

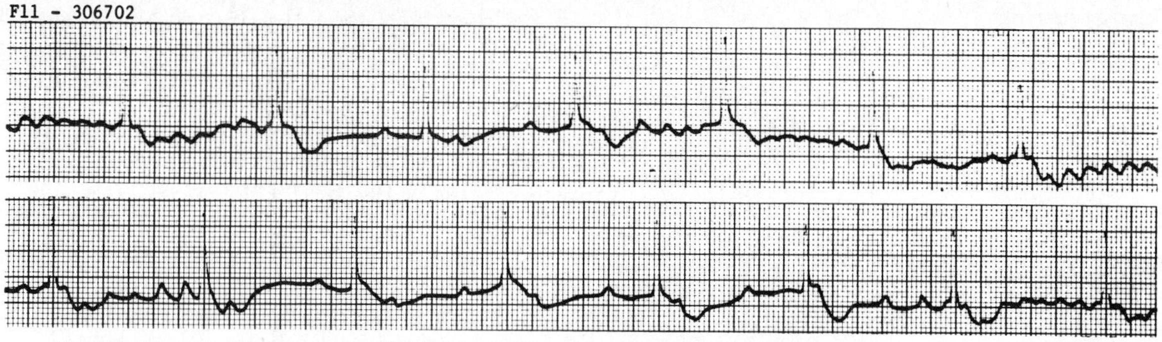

FIGURE 22–12. Intermittent atrial fibrillation and complete AV block. Intermittently through the tracing, discrete P waves are replaced by fibrillatory waves. Despite changing atrial rhythm, ventricular rate and rhythm remain unaltered, indicating complete AV block.

Each recorded F wave is not conducted through the AV junction so that a rapid ventricular response comparable to the atrial rate does not occur. Many atrial impulses are canceled, owing to a collision of wavefronts, or are blocked in the AV junction without reaching the ventricles (i.e., concealed conduction [p. 202]), which accounts for the irregular ventricular rhythm. When the ventricular rate is very rapid or very slow, it may appear to be more regular. Even though the conversion of atrial fibrillation to atrial flutter is accompanied by slowing of the atrial rate, because of less concealed conduction, an increase in the ventricular response may result, since more atrial impulses are transmitted to the ventricle. Also, it is easier to slow the ventricular rate with drugs such as digitalis, propranolol, and verapamil during atrial fibrillation than during atrial flutter because the increased concealed conduction makes it easier to produce AV block.

CLINICAL FEATURES. Atrial fibrillation may be chronic or intermittent; the former is almost always associated with underlying heart disease, while the latter may occur in apparently normal hearts. Underlying heart disease is more frequent in patients with atrial flutter than in those with atrial fibrillation. The arrhythmia commonly results in patients who have rheumatic heart disease, especially with mitral valve involvement, atrial septal defect,[88] cardiomyopathy, pulmonary emboli, coronary heart disease, and after cardiac surgery.[89, 90] Hypertensive cardiovascular disease is the most common antecedent disease, largely because of its frequency in the general population. Pericarditis may be important, although a recent report suggests that pericarditis alone does not cause arrhythmias.[91] Occult or manifest thyrotoxicosis should always be considered in a patient with atrial fibrillation of recent onset.[92] The presence of cardiac failure and rheumatic heart disease are risk factors for the development of atrial fibrillation.

Intermittent episodes of atrial fibrillation may recur in some patients only once or twice and in others more frequently. The duration of a single paroxysm may range from less than 24 hours to several weeks. Atrial fibrillation may become permanent in 25 per cent of these patients observed for more than one year.[93] Mortality is unchanged in patients who have paroxysmal atrial fibrillation with no other identifical cardiovascular impairment. However, paroxysmal atrial fibrillation with associated mitral stenosis or coronary disease incurs a significantly increased mortality. The development of chronic atrial fibrillation is associated with a doubling of overall mortality and of mortality from cardiovascular disease.[94] Mortality is highest in patients with mitral stenosis.[95] Occasionally, patients with longstanding atrial fibrillation may develop spontaneous reversion to sinus rhythm.[96]

Patients with chronic atrial fibrillation are at greatly increased risk of *embolic stroke*, particularly at the onset and termination of the atrial fibrillation. In the absence of rheumatic heart disease, chronic atrial fibrillation is associated with more than a fivefold increase in the incidence of stroke and a seventeenfold increase in patients with rheumatic heart disease. The occurrence of stroke increases directly with the duration of atrial fibrillation.[97–99] Subjects with "lone" atrial fibrillation, i.e., atrial fibrillation in the absence of recognizable structural heart disease, have no increased risk of coronary heart disease and congestive heart failure but have a greater rate of ECG abnormalities and strokes.[100]

Patients who develop atrial fibrillation within one year after acute myocardial infarction are generally older, have a more severe infarction, have higher total mortality, and have a greater frequency of ventricular tachyarrhythmias and right bundle branch block than do patients who do not develop atrial fibrillation.[101] Those who develop atrial fibrillation at the time of their acute myocardial infarction have a higher pulmonary capillary wedge pressure and older age.[102]

The presence of atrial fibrillation appears to be related to the type of underlying heart disease, as well as to left atrial size, which can be determined by cardiac echocardiography but not by the amplitude of the F waves on the ECG. The left atrial diameter measured by echocardiography is smaller in patients with paroxysmal atrial fibrillation that terminates spontaneously compared to that in patients who require DC cardioversion, who have persistent atrial fibrillation,[103] or who have recurrences after electrical reversion.[104] Atrial fibrillation in children is not common and is an indication for a thorough clinical investigation.

The presence or absence of symptoms as a result of atrial fibrillation is determined by multiple factors, the most important of which is cardiac status. The rapid ventricular rate and loss of atrial contraction detrimentally affect cardiac output. Physical findings in patients exhibiting atrial fibrillation include a slight variation in the intensity of the first heart sound, absence of *a* waves in the jugular venous pulse, and an irregularly irregular ventricular rhythm. Often with fast ventricular rates a significant pulse deficit appears, during which the apical rate is faster than the rate palpated at the wrist because each contraction is not sufficiently strong to open the aortic valve or to transmit an arterial pressure wave through the peripheral artery. If the rhythm becomes regular in patients with atrial fibrillation, conversion to one of the following rhythms should be suspected: sinus rhythm, atrial tachycardia, atrial flutter with a constant ratio of conducted beats, or development of junctional or ventricular tachycardia.

TREATMENT. When one is treating the patient with atrial fibrillation for the first time, it is important to search for a precipitating cause, such as thyrotoxicosis, mitral stenosis, pulmonary emboli, or pericarditis, and to treat it appropriately, if found. The patient's clinical status determines initial therapy, the objectives being to slow the ventricular rate and to restore atrial systole. If the sudden onset of atrial fibrillation with a rapid ventricular rate results in acute cardiovascular decompensation, electrical cardioversion is the treatment of choice. In the absence of decompensation, the patient may be treated with digitalis[105] to maintain a resting apical rate of 60 to 80 beats/min that does not exceed 100 beats/min after slight exercise. The speed, route, dosage, and type of digitalis preparation administered are determined by the status of the patient. The combined use of digitalis and a beta or calcium-entry blocker[87] may be useful in slowing the ventricular rate. Quinidine, given with digitalis, is often necessary to convert to sinus rhythm. The use of large doses of quinidine to produce reversion to normal sinus rhythm is no longer indicated. Prior to electrical cardioversion, maintenance doses of quinidine sulfate in the range of 800 to 1600 mg/day should be administered for a few days. During this time normal sinus rhythm will resume in 10 to 15 per cent of patients. DC cardioversion establishes normal sinus rhythm in over 90 per cent of patients, but sinus rhythm remains for 12 months in only 30 to 50 per cent. Patients with atrial fibrillation of less than 12 months' duration have a greater chance of maintaining sinus rhythm after cardioversion. Disopyramide or procainamide[106] may be tried in place of quinidine. Amiodarone is very effective in preventing recurrences of atrial fibrillation but not in terminating the arrhythmia already present.[106a] Rapid atrial pacing will *not* terminate atrial fibrillation.

The role of anticoagulation prior to cardioversion is somewhat controversial because of imperfect studies. Most investigators think that anticoagulation prior to drug or electrical cardioversion is indicated in patients with a high risk of emboli, i.e., those with mitral stenosis, atrial fibrillation of recent onset, recent or recurrent emboli, a prosthetic mitral valve, or cardiomegaly. Some recommend 2 weeks of anticoagulation prior to elective cardioversion of atrial fibrillation present for more than about a week, if no contraindications to anticoagulation exist, and continuing anticoagulation for 2 additional weeks after cardioversion.[107] The incidence of embolization during conversion to normal sinus rhythm is 1 to 2 per cent.

Many elderly patients tolerate atrial fibrillation well without therapy because the ventricular rate is slow as a result of concomitant AV nodal disease. These patients often have associated sick sinus syndrome, and the development of atrial fibrillation represents a cure of sorts. Such patients may demonstrate serious supraventricular and ventricular arrhythmias or asystole after cardioversion, so that the likelihood of establishing and maintaining sinus rhythm should be weighed against the risks of cardioversion or other forms of therapy.

ATRIAL TACHYCARDIAS WITH BLOCK

ELECTROCARDIOGRAPHIC RECOGNITION (Fig. 22–13). In atrial tachycardia, sometimes called atrial tachycardia with block or paroxysmal atrial tachycardia with block (PAT with block), the atrial rate is generally 150 to 200 beats/min. When the tachycardia is due to digitalis excess, the atrial rate may increase gradually as the digitalis is continued (a similar response may occur in nonparoxysmal AV junctional tachycardia) and may be associated with gradual prolongation of the P-R interval. If the atrial rate is not excessive and AV conduction is not significantly depressed by the digitalis, each P wave may conduct to the ventricles. As the atrial rate increases and AV conduction becomes impaired, Wenckebach (Mobitz type I) second degree AV block (p. 703) may ensue, hence the term atrial tachycardia with block. Frequently, other manifestations of digitalis excess, such as premature ventricular complexes, are present. In nearly half the cases of atrial tachycardia with block, the atrial rate is irregular. Characteristic isoelectric intervals between P waves, in contrast to atrial flutter, are usually present in all leads. However, at rapid atrial rates the distinction between atrial tachycardia with block and atrial flutter may be difficult.

The term "paroxysmal" is used to indicate a tachycardia of sudden onset that changes from sinus rhythm to a tachycardia in one beat—for example, a premature atrial complex precipitating a paroxysmal supraventricular tachycardia (Fig. 22–10*B*). In contrast, the term "nonparoxysmal" refers to a tachycardia that has a gradual onset and termination, similar to the warm-up phenomenon characteristic of automaticity (p. 597). Nonparoxysmal AV junctional tachycardia is such a tachycardia. Because the atrial tachycardia described above appears to be a "nonparoxysmal" variety, the term "paroxysmal atrial tachycardia with block" would be inappropriate.

CLINICAL FEATURES. Atrial tachycardia with block occurs most commonly in patients with significant organic heart disease, such as coronary artery disease, with or without myocardial infarction, cor pulmonale, or digitalis intoxication. Digitalis toxicity accounts for 50 to 75 per cent of

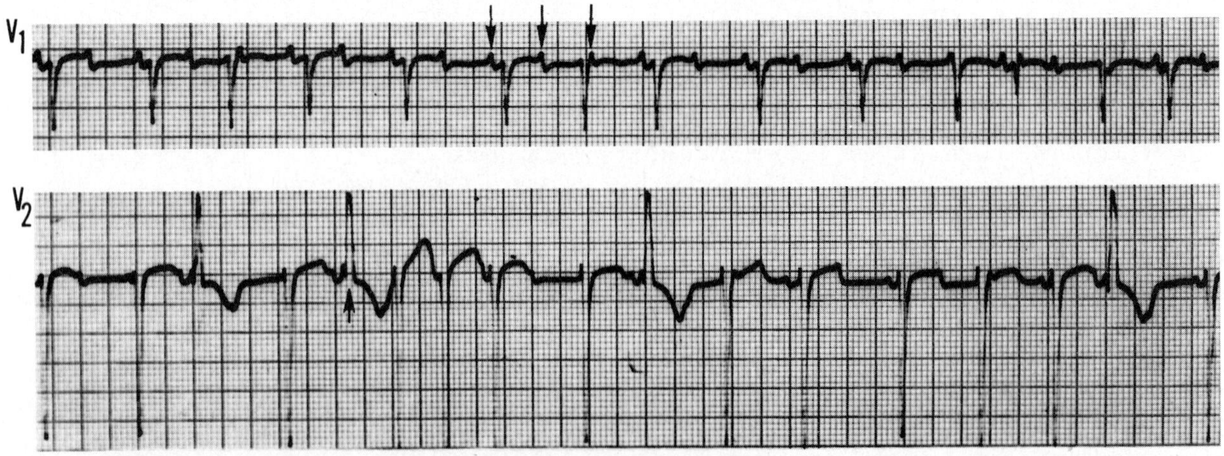

FIGURE 22–13. Atrial tachycardia with varying degrees of AV nodal Wenckebach block. A 3:2 Wenckebach grouping is indicated by the arrows. In V_2, functional right bundle branch block occurs when a short cycle follows a long cycle (arrow).

cases of atrial tachycardia with block. Potassium depletion may precipitate the arrhythmia in patients taking digitalis. The signs, symptoms, and prognosis are usually related to underlying cardiovascular status. Because this arrhythmia occurs primarily in patients suffering from serious heart disease, clinical deterioration may result from the arrhythmia.

Physical findings include a variable rhythm and intensity of the first heart sound, owing to the varying AV block and P-R interval. An excessive number of *a* waves may be seen in the jugular venous pulse. Carotid sinus massage increases the degree of AV block by slowing the ventricular rate in a stepwise fashion, as in atrial flutter. It should be performed cautiously in patients who have digitalis toxicity because serious ventricular arrhythmias may result.

TREATMENT. Atrial tachycardia with block in a patient not receiving digitalis is treated in a manner similar to other atrial tachyarrhythmias. Depending on the clinical situation, digitalis may be administered to slow the ventricular rate and then if atrial tachycardia with block remains, quinidine, disopyramide, or procainamide may be added. If atrial tachycardia with block appears in a patient receiving digitalis, digitalis should initially be assumed to be responsible for the arrhythmia. Therapy includes cessation of digitalis and administration of potassium chloride orally or intravenously if serum [K^+] is not abnormally elevated, or a drug such as lidocaine, propranolol, and phenytoin while cardiac rhythm is monitored. Often, the ventricular response is not excessively fast and simply withholding digitalis is all that is necessary.

AUTOMATIC ATRIAL TACHYCARDIA

Two types of atrial tachycardias have been distinguished electrophysiologically: automatic and reentrant atrial tachycardia. While it is likely that one or both of these atrial tachycardias is responsible for atrial tachycardia with block (described above), the relationship, if any, is not clear at present, and these two tachycardias will be discussed separately.

ELECTROCARDIOGRAPHIC FEATURES (Fig. 22–9*F* and Table 22–2). Automatic atrial tachycardia is characterized electrocardiographically by a supraventricular tachycardia that generally accelerates after its initiation, with heart rates less than 200 beats/min. The P wave contour differs from the sinus P wave, the P-R interval is influenced directly by the tachycardia rate, and AV block may exist without affecting the tachycardia. Vagal maneuvers generally do not terminate the tachycardia, even though they may produce AV nodal block. Thus, pharmacological or physiological maneuvers that selectively result in AV block do not affect the automatic focus nor does the development of bundle branch block alter the P-R or R-P interval unless it is associated with prolongation of the H-V interval.

Electrophysiologically, initiation of tachycardia with premature atrial stimulation is generally not possible but is independent of intraatrial or AV nodal conduction delay when it occurs. The atrial activation sequence usually differs from a sinus-initiated P wave, and the A-H interval is related to the tachycardia rate. The rate may gradually accelerate after initiation. The first P wave of the tachycardia is the same as the subsequent P waves of the tachycardia in contrast to most forms of reentrant supraventricular tachycardias, in which the initial and subsequent P waves differ.[66, 67, 108] Usually the tachycardia cannot be terminated by pacing, although it may exhibit overdrive suppression. The introduction of premature atrial complexes during tachycardia merely resets the timing of the tachycardia. It is very difficult to differentiate this mechanism from micro-reentry, using the leading circle concept (see p. 602).

CLINICAL FEATURES. Many supraventricular tachycardias associated with AV block are probably due to automatic atrial tachycardia, including atrial tachycardia with block due to digitalis intoxication (Fig. 22–13). Automatic atrial tachycardia occurs in all age groups; is thought to be due to enhanced automaticity; and is seen in a setting of myocardial infarction, chronic lung disease (especially with acute infection), acute alcohol ingestion, and a variety of metabolic derangements. Digitalis appears to be a particularly important precipitating agent. Differentiation from other tachycardias such as sinus nodal reentry (if the P waves of the automatic atrial tachycardia resemble the sinus-initiated P waves), atrial reentry (particularly if caused by micro-reentry), and some other mechanisms may be difficult (Table 22–2). In view of the experimental findings of triggered activity from a variety of atrial fibers, including human mitral valve (see p. 597), it is possible that such activity also occurs in man. However, many automatic atrial tachycardias are not suppressed by verapamil.[109]

Therapy is as discussed under atrial tachycardia with block.

ATRIAL TACHYCARDIA DUE TO REENTRY

(See also p. 600)

ELECTROCARDIOGRAPHIC RECOGNITION (Fig. 22–9*E*). This arrhythmia presents electrocardiographically with a P wave that has a contour different from the sinus P wave, a P-R interval influenced directly by the tachycardia rate, and the ability to develop AV block without interrupting the tachycardia (Table 22–2). Electrophysiologically, initiation of the tachycardia occurs with premature stimulation during the atrial relative refractory period, resulting in a critical degree of intraatrial conduction delay, an atrial activation sequence different from that which occurs during sinus rhythm, and an AV nodal conduction time related to the tachycardia rate. Vagal maneuvers generally do not terminate the tachycardia and may produce AV block.[66, 67, 108]

CLINICAL FEATURES. The relative infrequency of published reports suggests that atrial reentry is not a commonly recognized cause of supraventricular tachycardia. The tachycardia rate is about 130 to 150 beats/min, and the tachycardia can be started and stopped by an atrial extrastimulus. Spontaneous termination can be either sudden, with progressive slowing, or alternating long-short cycle lengths.

CHAOTIC ATRIAL TACHYCARDIA

Chaotic (sometimes called multifocal) atrial tachycardia is characterized by atrial rates between 100 and 130 beats/min, with marked variation in P-wave morphology and totally irregular P-P intervals (Fig. 22–14). Generally at least three P-wave contours are noted, with most P waves conducted to the ventricles. This tachycardia occurs commonly in patients with pulmonary disease and in diabetics or older patients and may eventually develop into atrial fibrillation. Digitalis appears to be an unusual cause while theophylline administration has been implicated.[110] Chaotic atrial tachycardia can occur in childhood.[111]

TREATMENT. Therapy is primarily directed toward the underlying disease. Antiarrhythmic agents are often ineffective in slowing either the rate of the atrial tachycardia

TABLE 22–2 ELECTROCARDIOGRAPHIC DIFFERENTIAL DIAGNOSIS OF

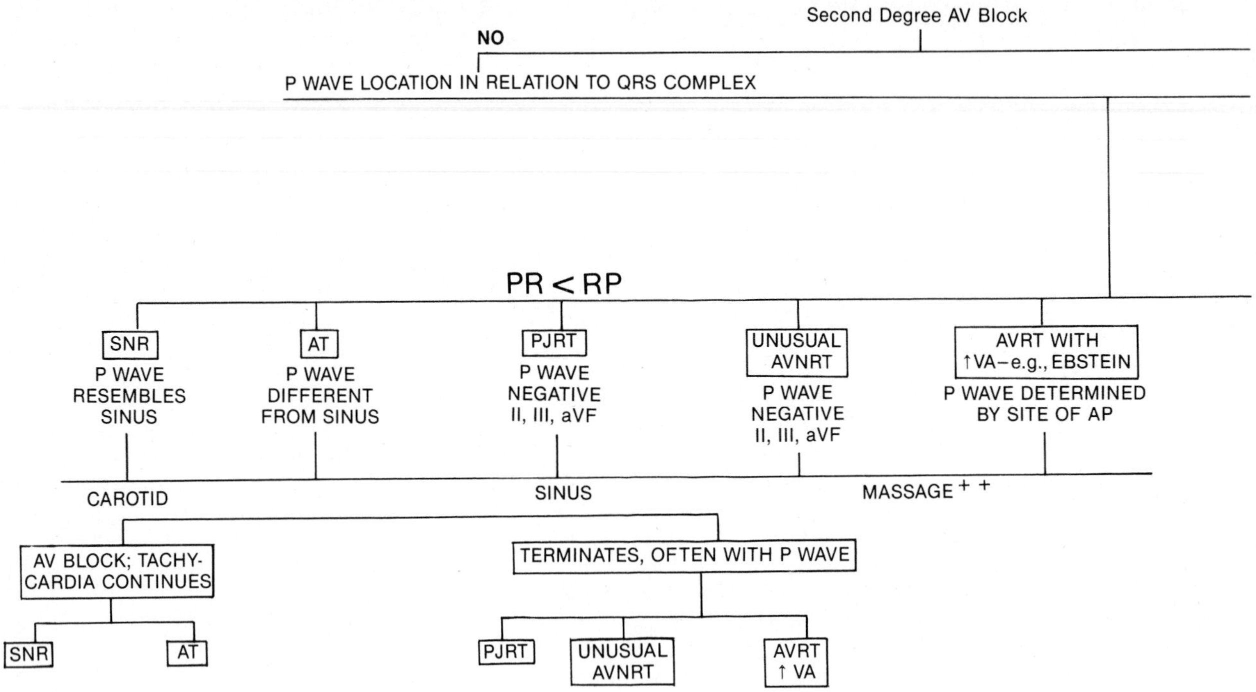

Excludes atrial fibrillation, nonparoxysmal AV junctional tachycardia.
Assumes usual responses/presentations; exceptions occur.
SNR, Sinus node reentry; AT, atrial tachycardia; PJRT, permanent form of AV junctional reciprocating tachycardia; AVNRT, AV nodal reentrant tachycardia; AVRT, AV reciprocating tachycardia; AP, accessory pathway; VA, ventriculoatrial interval; ↑, increase.
*Atrial flutter with 2:1 conduction can mimic PSVT at 150/min if the flutter waves are not recognized.
†Esophageal recording.
‡Tachycardia unaffected by carotid sinus massage provides no useful differential data.

or the ventricular response. Propranolol should be avoided in patients with bronchospastic pulmonary disease. Verapamil[112] may be useful. Potassium and magnesium replacement may suppress the tachycardia.[113]

AV JUNCTIONAL RHYTHM DISTURBANCES

AV JUNCTIONAL ESCAPE BEATS

MECHANISM. Automatic fibers that are prevented from initiating depolarization by a pacemaker such as the sinus node which possesses a more rapid rate of firing are called *latent pacemakers*. Such latent pacemakers are found in some parts of the atrium, in the AV node–His bundle area, in the right and left bundle branches, and in the Purkinje system. Under usual conditions automatic fibers are *not* found in atrial or ventricular myocardium. It is possible that the N region of the AV node may be automatic, at least in some species.[114] A latent pacemaker can become the dominant pacemaker by default or usurpation, that is, by passive or active mechanisms. A decrease in the number of impulses arriving at a latent pacemaker site, the result of slowing of the sinus node or interruption of the propagation of the normal impulse anywhere along its course, allows the latent pacemaker to escape and initiate depolarization passively, by default. An increase in the discharge rate of a latent pacemaker can capture pacemaker control actively, by usurpation. As will be seen, the implication of

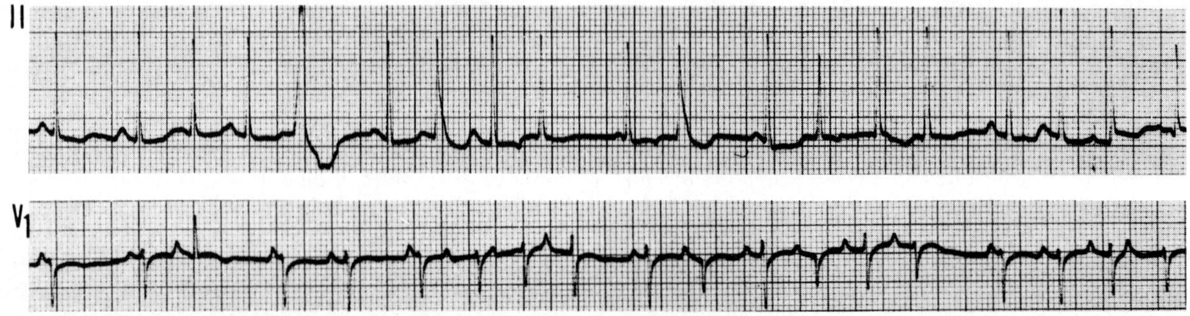

FIGURE 22–14. Chaotic multifocal atrial tachycardia. Premature atrial complexes occur at varying cycle lengths and with differing contours.

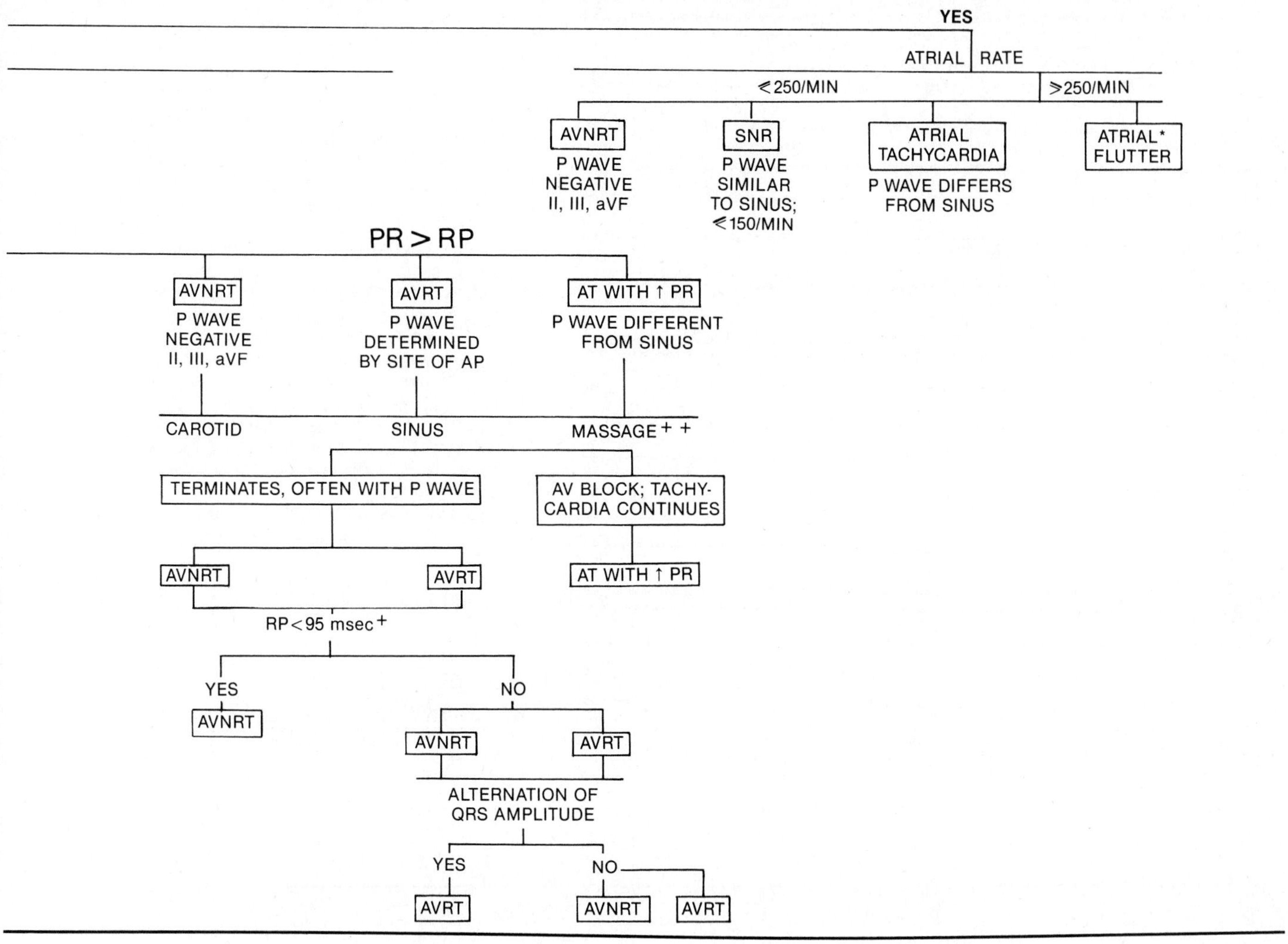

the two different mechanisms of ectopic impulse formation is important therapeutically.

ELECTROCARDIOGRAPHIC RECOGNITION. An AV junctional escape beat occurs when the rate of impulse formation of the primary pacemaker, generally the sinus node, becomes less than that of the AV junctional region, or when impulses from the primary pacemaker do not penetrate to the region of the escape focus and allow the AV junctional focus to reach threshold and discharge. The interval from the last normally conducted beat to the AV junctional escape beat is a measure of the initial discharge rate of the AV junctional focus and generally corresponds to a rate of 35 to 60 beats/min (Fig. 22–2*B*). Although an AV junctional escape rhythm is usually fairly regular, intervals between subsequent escape beats after the initial escape beat may gradually shorten as the rate of discharge of the escape focus increases, the so-called *rhythm of development* or *warm-up phenomenon*.

The electrocardiogram displays pauses longer than the normal P-P interval, interrupted by a QRS complex of supraventricular configuration with absent, retrograde, fusion, or sinus P waves that do not conduct to the ventricle. If P waves precede the QRS, they have a P-R interval generally less than 0.12 sec. The exact site of impulse formation (i.e., AN, N, or NH regions; low atrium; or His bundle) is not known and may differ from patient to patient and be influenced by the cause of the arrhythmia.

Treatment, if any, lies in increasing the discharge rate of the higher pacemakers and improving AV conduction and may require pacing. Frequently, no treatment is necessary.

PREMATURE AV JUNCTIONAL COMPLEXES

Premature AV junctional complexes are characterized by an impulse that arises prematurely in the AV junction (the exact site—i.e., AN, N, or NH regions; low atrium; or His bundle—is not known and may vary from patient to patient) and that attempts conduction in anterograde and retrograde directions. If unimpeded in its course, the impulse discharges the atrium to produce a premature retrograde P wave and a premature QRS complex with a supraventricular contour. The retrograde P wave may occur before, during, or after the QRS complex (Fig. 22–15). Alterations in conduction time may influence the P-R or R-P relationships without a change in the site of origin of the impulse. Premature AV junctional complexes that conduct aberrantly are difficult to distinguish from premature ventricular complexes using the scalar ECG.

Treatment of premature AV junctional complexes is generally not necessary. However, since they may arise distal to the AV node, they may occur early in the cardiac cycle and can initiate a ventricular tachyarrhythmia in some instances. Under these circumstances therapy may be approached as for premature ventricular complexes (see p. 694).

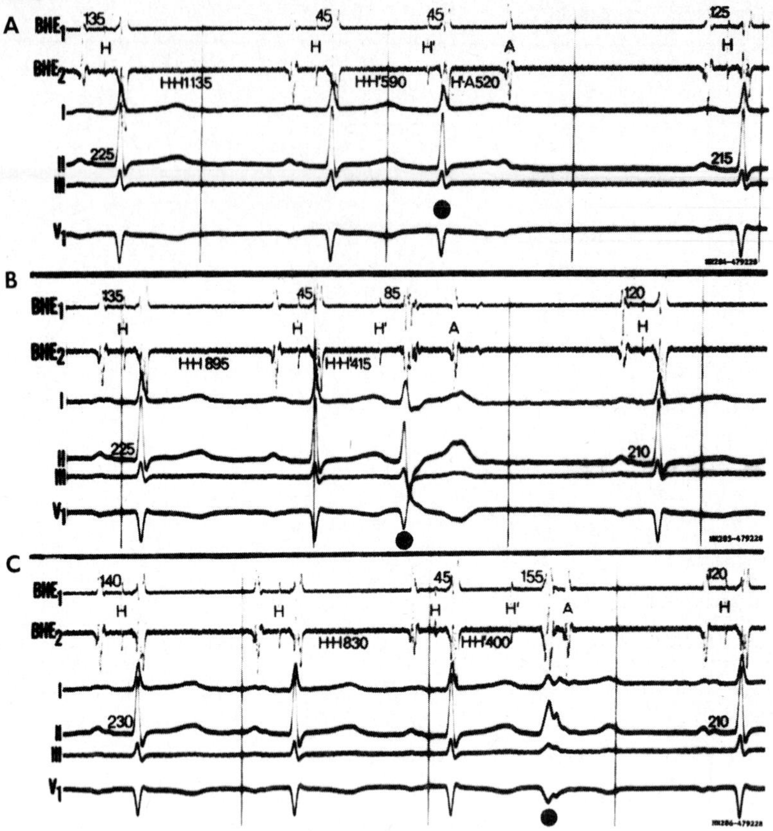

FIGURE 22–15. Premature AV junctional complexes arising in or near the bundle of His (H′) conduct normally (*A*) or with functional right (*B*) and functional left (*C*) bundle branch block. The filled circles indicate the premature junctional complex. Anterograde conduction of the premature junctional (H′) discharges depends on the coupling interval between the last normal His discharge (H) and (H-H′) interval and the spontaneous cycle length (H-H) that preceded H′. When H′ follows a shorter preceding cycle length and occurs at longer coupling intervals, a normal QRS complex results. As the preceding H-H cycle lengthens or as the H-H′ interval shortens, a zone of functional right bundle branch block occurs, followed by a zone of functional left bundle branch block. Not shown are premature His discharges that fail to conduct entirely (Fig. 20–33, p. 611). Numbers in milliseconds. Time lines = 1 sec in each panel. (Magnification is not the same in all three panels.) (From Bonner, A. J., and Zipes, D. P.: Lidocaine and His bundle extrasystoles. His bundle discharge conducted normally, conducted with functional right or left bundle branch block, or blocked entirely [concealed]. Arch. Intern. Med. *136*:700, 1976.)

AV JUNCTIONAL RHYTHM

If the AV junctional escape beats continue for a period of time, the rhythm is called an AV junctional rhythm (Fig. 22–16). Since the inherent rate of the AV junctional tissue is 35 to 60 beats/min, the AV junctional tissue can assume the role of the dominant pacemaker at this rate only by passive default of the sinus pacemaker. The ECG displays a normally conducted QRS complex, which may conduct retrogradely to the atrium or may occur independently of atrial discharge, producing AV dissociation (see p. 707).

An AV junctional escape rhythm may be a normal phenomenon in response to the effects of vagal tone or it may occur during pathological sinus bradycardia or heart block. The escape beat or rhythm serves as a safety mechanism to prevent the occurrence of ventricular asystole. *Physical findings* vary depending on the P-QRS relationship. Large *a* waves in the jugular venous pulse and a loud, soft, or changing intensity of the first heart sound may be present if atrial contraction occurs when the tricuspid valve is shut.

Therapy is discussed under AV junctional escape beats (see above).

NONPAROXYSMAL AV JUNCTIONAL TACHYCARDIA

ELECTROCARDIOGRAPHIC RECOGNITION (Figs. 22–17 and 22–18). To usurp dominant pacemaker status, the AV junctional tissue must exhibit enhanced discharge rate such as during nonparoxysmal AV junctional tachycardia. Nonparoxysmal AV junctional tachycardia is usually of gradual onset and termination, hence the modifier "nonparoxysmal." On occasion, nonparoxysmal AV junctional tachycardia may become manifest abruptly because of slowing of the dominant pacemaker that may then allow sudden capture and control of the rhythm by the AV junctional focus. The rate of discharge is commonly between 70 and 130 beats/min. Accepted terminology confers the label of tachycardia to rates exceeding 100 beats/min. The term nonparoxysmal AV junctional tachycardia, although not entirely correct, has generally been accepted, since rates exceeding 60 beats/min represent in effect a tachycardia for the AV junctional tissue.[115]

Nonparoxysmal AV junctional tachycardia is recognized by a QRS of supraventricular configuration at a fairly regular rate of 70 to 130 beats/min. Enhanced vagal tone may slow while vagolytic agents may speed up the dis-

J5-P539963

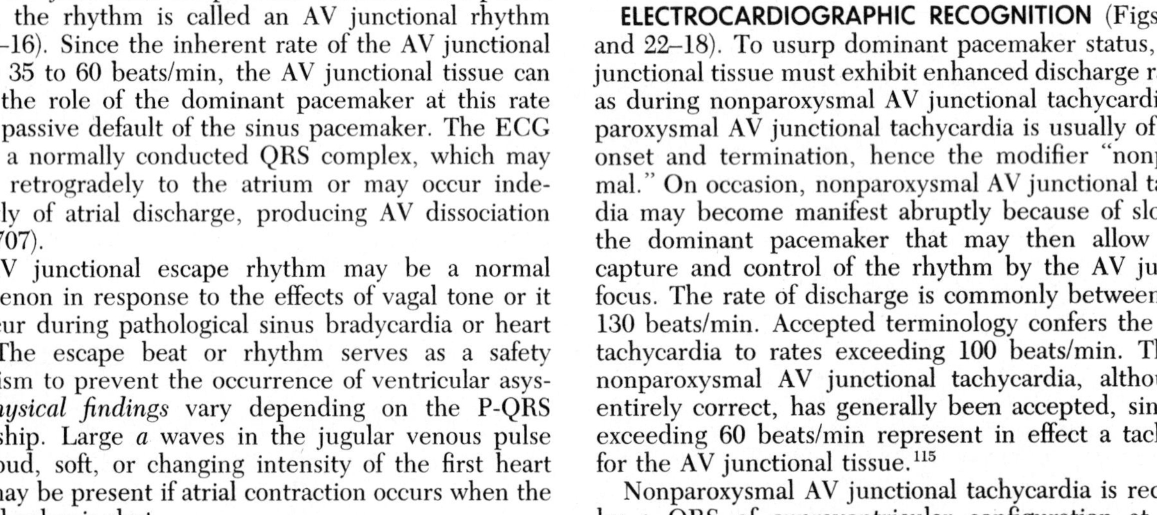

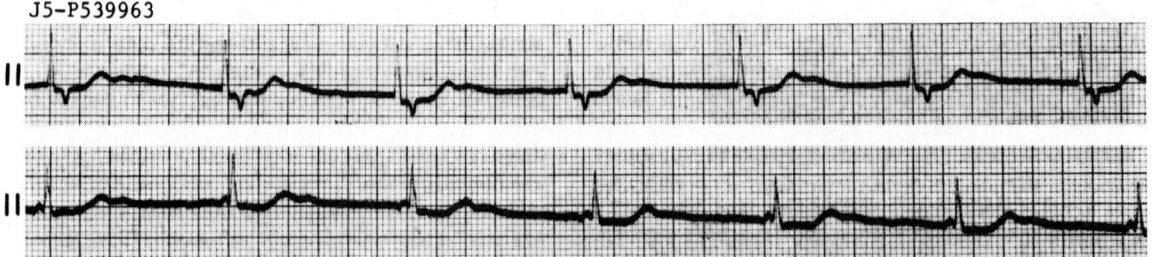

FIGURE 22–16. AV junctional rhythm. *Top*, AV junctional discharge occurs fairly regularly at a rate of approximately 50 beats/min. Retrograde atrial activity follows each junctional discharge. *Bottom*, Recording made on a different day in the same patient; the AV junctional rate is slightly more variable, and retrograde P waves precede the onset of the QRS complex. The positive terminal portion of the P wave gives the appearance of AV dissociation, which was not present.

charge rate. Although retrograde activation of the atria may occur, the atria commonly are controlled by an independent sinus, atrial, or on occasion a second AV junctional focus resulting in AV dissociation (Fig. 22–9*G*). The electrocardiographic diagnosis may be complicated by the presence of entrance and exit blocks at the AV junctional tissue level and incomplete forms of AV dissociation.

The cause of this arrhythmia probably is *accelerated automatic discharge* in or near the His bundle. It is possible that nonparoxysmal AV junctional tachycardia originates in atrial fibers without recognition of the latter's role from analysis of the scalar ECG or on intracardiac electrograms, unless a careful search is made.[116] Wenckebach periods may occur (Fig. 7–48, p. 213), but the presence of exit block has not yet been demonstrated by His bundle recording in humans, and the block may be in the AV node with the origin of the nonparoxysmal AV junctional tachycardia proximal to the site of the His bundle recording.[116, 117] Accelerated junctional escape beats that have shorter escape intervals when following premature atrial complexes has raised the possibility of *overdrive acceleration* (p. 596) in these fibers.[118] In some patients, rapid pacing may suppress junctional automaticity, while in others, acceleration may occur. Lidocaine suppresses automaticity in the first group but not in the second, suggesting normal automaticity as a cause of the rhythm for the first and abnormal automaticity for the second.[119]

CLINICAL FEATURES. Nonparoxysmal AV junctional tachycardia occurs most commonly in patients with underlying heart disease, such as inferior infarction, myocarditis

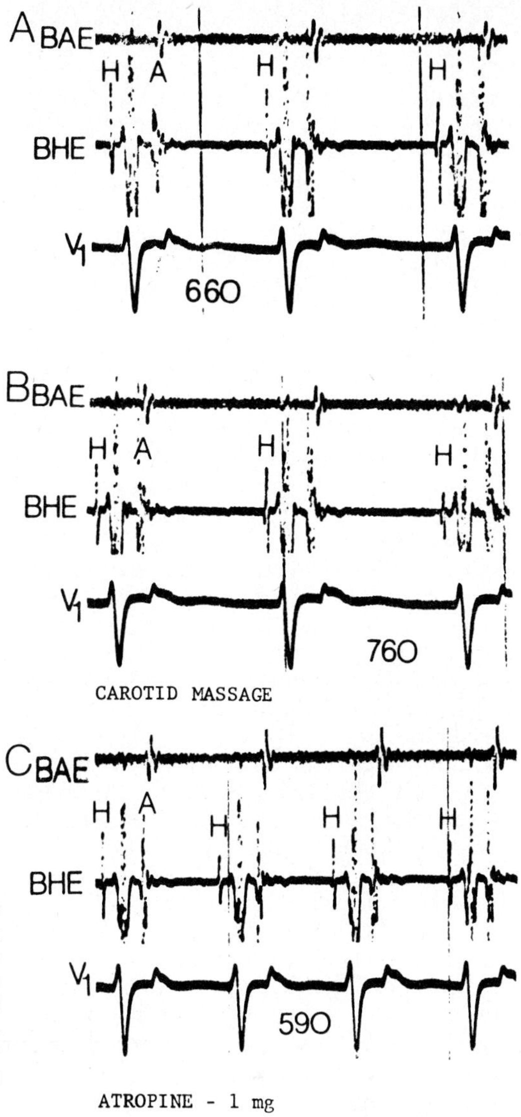

FIGURE 22–17. Nonparoxysmal AV junctional tachycardia. *A*, Control; *B*, response to carotid sinus massage; *C*, response to atropine, 1 mg intravenously. Note that His bundle depolarization is the earliest recordable electrical activity in each cycle. The atria are depolarized retrogradely (low right atrial activity recorded in BHE precedes high right atrial activity recorded in BAE). Note also that carotid sinus massage slows the junctional discharge rate while atropine speeds it up. From these tracings alone one could not distinguish the rhythm from some other types of supraventricular tachycardias. However, onset and termination of this tachycardia was typical of nonparoxysmal AV junctional tachycardia.

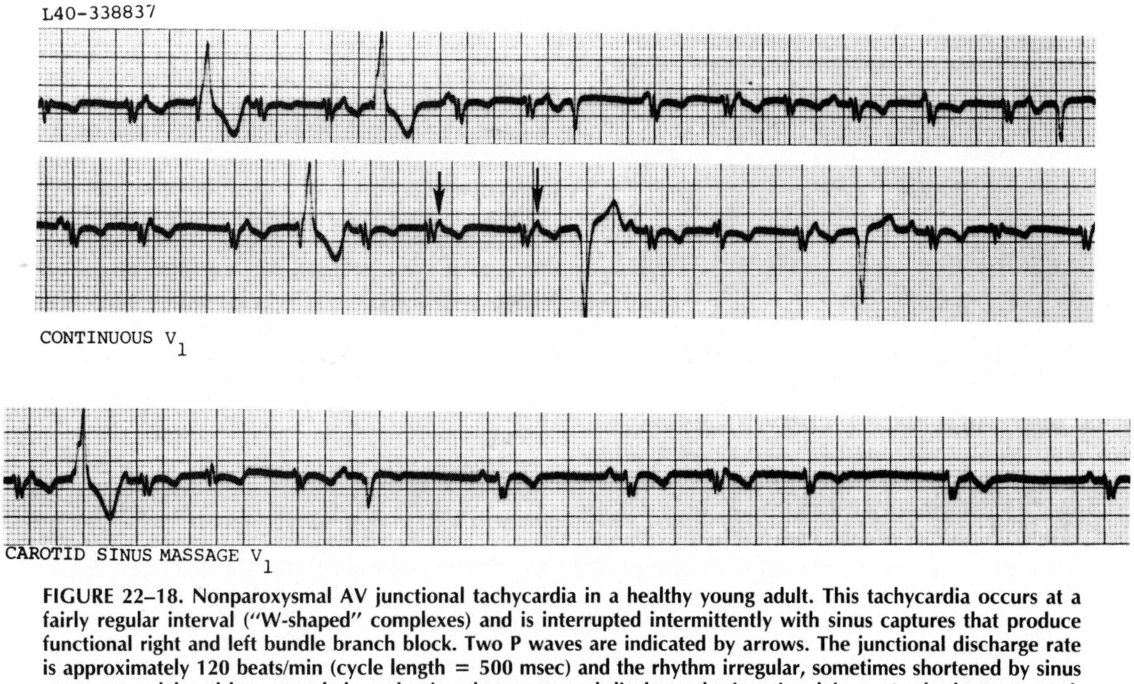

FIGURE 22–18. Nonparoxysmal AV junctional tachycardia in a healthy young adult. This tachycardia occurs at a fairly regular interval ("W-shaped" complexes) and is interrupted intermittently with sinus captures that produce functional right and left bundle branch block. Two P waves are indicated by arrows. The junctional discharge rate is approximately 120 beats/min (cycle length = 500 msec) and the rhythm irregular, sometimes shortened by sinus captures or delayed by concealed conduction that resets and displaces the junctional focus. In the bottom panel, carotid sinus massage slows the junctional as well as the sinus discharge rate.

(often the result of acute rheumatic fever), or after open-heart surgery. Probably the most important cause is excessive digitalis, which may also produce the ECG manifestations of varying degrees of exit block (usually Wenckebach type) from the accelerated AV junctional focus. Nonparoxysmal AV junctional tachycardia can occur in otherwise healthy individuals without symptoms (Fig. 22–18) or can be a serious and difficult to control tachycardia, occasionally chronic and longlasting.[120]

The clinical features vary depending on the rate of the arrhythmia and the underlying etiology and severity of heart disease. As in most arrhythmias, the physical signs are determined by the relationship of the P wave to the QRS complex and the rate of atrial and ventricular discharge. The first heart sound may therefore be constant or varying, and cannon *a* waves may or may not occur in the jugular venous pulse.

The ventricular rhythm may be regular or irregular, often in a constant fashion. It is especially important to recognize slowing and regularization of the ventricular rhythm in a patient with atrial fibrillation as being caused by nonparoxysmal AV junctional tachycardia and as a possible early sign of *digitalis intoxication* (p. 504). Initially, during atrial fibrillation, the regular ventricular rhythm may result from an AV junctional escape rhythm because the depressed AV conduction caused by digitalis blocks the passage of impulses from the fibrillating atria (Fig. 22–9G). As digitalis administration is continued, the ventricular rate may then speed because of increased discharge of the AV junctional pacemaker but may still be regular. Further digitalis administration may produce a rate that is slow and irregular because of varying degrees of AV junctional exit block. The rhythm may be misdiagnosed as resumption of conduction from the fibrillating atria. The rate then may increase further because of development of a ventricular tachycardia.

TREATMENT. This is directed toward the underlying etiological factor and functional support of the cardiovascular system. If the rhythm is regular, the cardiovascular status is compromised, and if the patient is not taking digitalis, digitalis administration should be considered. Cardioversion may be tried if necessary and if digitalis toxicity is excluded; theoretically, however, if the nonparoxysmal AV junctional tachycardia is due to enhanced automaticity, cardioversion may be ineffective. If the patient tolerates the arrhythmia well, careful monitoring and attention to the underlying heart disease is usually all that is required. The arrhythmia usually will abate spontaneously. If digitalis toxicity is the cause, the drug must be stopped and potassium, lidocaine, phenytoin, or propranolol administered.

TACHYCARDIAS INVOLVING THE AV JUNCTION

Much confusion exists regarding the nomenclature of tachycardias characterized by a supraventricular QRS complex, a regular R-R interval, and no evidence of ventricular preexcitation. These tachycardias have often been called paroxysmal atrial tachycardia (PAT) if the P wave occurred in front of the QRS complex or paroxysmal nodal or junctional tachycardia (PJT) if the P wave occurred within or just following the QRS complex and exhibited a retrograde contour. Because it is now apparent that a variety of electrophysiological mechanisms can account for these tachycardias (Fig. 22–9 and Table 22–2), the nonspecific term paroxysmal supraventricular tachycardia (PSVT) has been proposed to encompass the entire group. This term may be inappropriate because tachycardias in patients with accessory pathways (see below) are no more supraventricular than they are ventricular in origin, since they may require participation of both the atria and the ventricles in the reentrant pathway, and they exhibit a QRS complex of normal contour and duration only because anterograde conduction occurs over the normal AV node–His bundle pathways (Fig. 22–9C). If conduction over the reentrant pathway reverses direction and travels in an "antidromic" direction—i.e., to the ventricles over the accessory pathway and to the atria over the AV node–His bundle—the QRS complex exhibits a prolonged duration, although the tachycardia is basically the same. The term *reciprocating tachycardia* has been offered as a substitute for paroxysmal supraventricular tachycardia, but use of such a term presumes the mechanism of the tachycardia to be reentrant (which is probably the case for many supraventricular tachycardias). Reciprocating tachycardia is probably the mechanism of many ventricular tachycardias as well. Thus, no universally acceptable nomenclature exists for these tachycardias. In this chapter, descriptive titles, although cumbersome, will be used for the sake of clarity. In addition, the mechanism of reentry will be assumed operative when the weight of evidence supports its presence even though unequivocal proof is lacking (see p. 599).

ATRIOVENTRICULAR (AV) NODAL REENTRANT TACHYCARDIA

ELECTROCARDIOGRAPHIC RECOGNITION. Reentrant tachycardia in the AV node is characterized by a tachycardia with a QRS complex of supraventricular origin, with sudden onset and termination generally at rates between 150 and 250 beats/min (commonly 180 to 200 beats/min in adults), and with a regular rhythm (Table 22–2). Uncommonly, the rate may be as low as 110 beats/min and occasionally, especially in children, may exceed 250. Unless functional aberrant ventricular conduction or a previous conduction defect exists, the QRS complex is normal in contour and duration. P waves are generally buried in the QRS complex (Table 22–2). AV nodal reentry recorded at the onset begins abruptly, usually following a premature atrial complex that conducts with a prolonged P-R interval (see Figs. 22–9*A* and 22–10*B* and Fig. 20–27, p. 605). The abrupt termination is sometimes followed by a brief period of asystole or bradycardia (Fig. 22–19*A*). The R-R interval may shorten over the course of the first few beats at the onset or lengthen during the last few beats preceding termination of the tachycardia. Variation in cycle length is usually caused by variation in anterograde AV nodal conduction time. Carotid sinus massage may slow the tachycardia slightly prior to its termination or, if termination does not occur, may produce only slight slowing of the tachycardia (see Fig. 22–19*A*).

ELECTROPHYSIOLOGICAL FEATURES. An atrial complex that conducts with a critical prolongation of AV nodal conduction time[66, 121, 122] generally precipitates AV nodal reentry (see Figs. 22–19, 22–20, and 22–21*B*). Premature ventricular stimulation also can induce AV nodal reentry in about one-third of patients.[123] Several AV nodal pathways can be diagrammed to explain this tachycardia. In Figure 20–25 (p. 604), the atria are shown as a necessary link in the reentrant pathway, while in Figure 22–9*A* and *B* (p. 668), the atria are not incorporated in the circuit. In most examples, the retrograde P wave occurs at the onset of the QRS complex, clearly excluding the possibility of an accessory pathway. If an accessory pathway in the ventricle were part of the circuit, the ventricles would have to be activated before the accessory pathway and therefore before the atria were depolarized

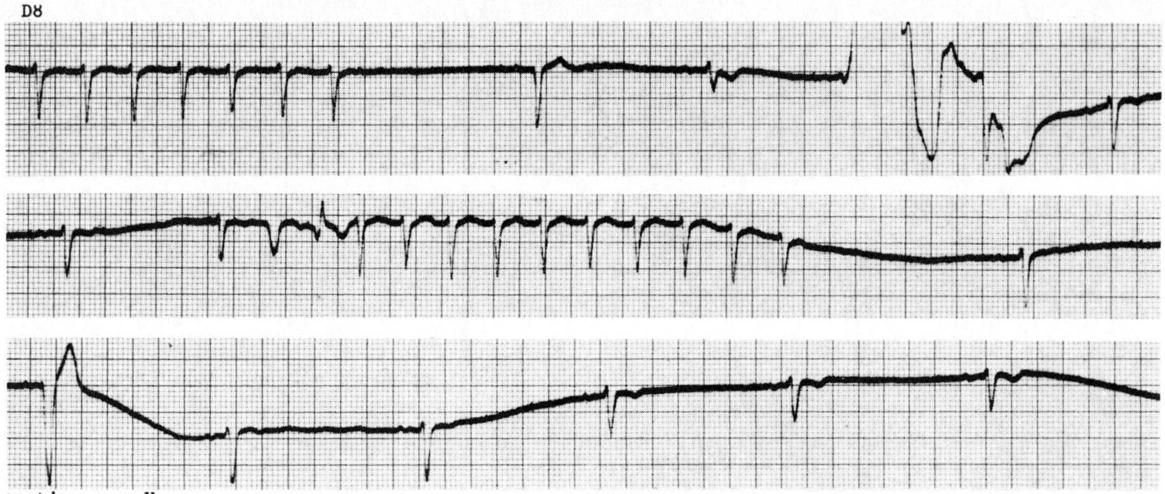

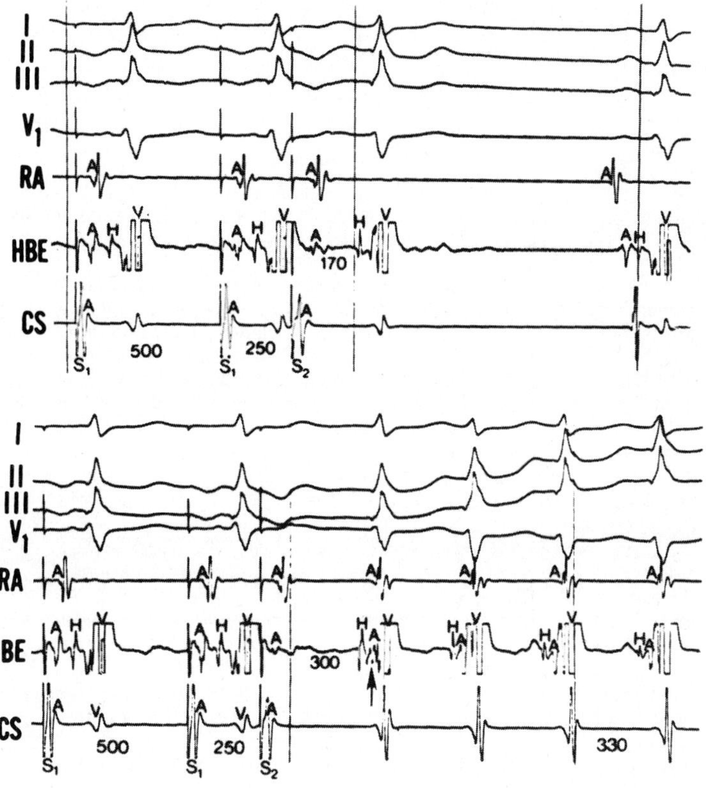

B

FIGURE 22–19. *A,* Sudden termination of paroxysmal supraventricular tachycardia, probably AV nodal reentry. Tachycardia abruptly terminates in the top recording following a short period of carotid sinus massage. Several escape beats occur followed by another short run or paroxysmal supraventricular tachycardia, which again terminates abruptly. A sinus bradycardia ensues and gradually speeds up. Suppression of sinus nodal activity following termination of a tachycardia is common and is a manifestation of overdrive suppression. *B,* Initiation of AV nodal reentrant tachycardia in a patient with dual atrioventricular nodal pathways. Upper and lower panels show the last two paced beats of a train of stimuli delivered to the coronary sinus at a pacing cycle length of 500 msec. The results of premature atrial stimulation at an S_1-S_2 interval of 250 msec on two occasions are shown. In the *upper panel,* S_2 was conducted to the ventricle with an AH interval of 170 msec and then was followed by a sinus beat. In the *lower panel,* S_2 was conducted with an AH interval of 300 msec and initiated AV nodal reentry. Note that the retrograde atrial activity occurs (arrow) prior to the onset of ventricular septal depolarization and is superimposed on the QRS complex. Retrograde atrial activity begins first in the low right atrium (HBE lead) and then progresses to the high right atrium (RA) and coronary sinus (CS) recordings.

(see Preexcitation Syndrome, p. 685). In approximately 30 per cent of instances, atrial activation begins at the end of, or just after, the QRS complex, giving rise to a discrete P wave on the surface ECG (Fig. 22–9*B*), while in the majority of patients P waves are not seen, since they are buried within the inscription of the QRS complex (Fig. 22–9*A*). In the most common variety of AV nodal reentrant tachycardia, the V-A interval (i.e., between onset of QRS and onset of atrial activity) is less than 50 per cent of the R-R interval and the ratio of A-V to V-A interval exceeds 1.0. Most of these patients during tachycardia have a V-A minimum value of ≤61 msec measured to the earliest recorded atrial activity and of ≤95 msec measured to atrial activity recorded in the high right atrial electrogram. These V-A intervals are longer in patients with tachycardia related to accessory pathways as well as in some other forms of AV nodal reentry (Fig. 22–9*B* and Table 22–2).

Slow and Fast Pathways. In the majority of patients, anterograde conduction occurs to the ventricle over the slow (alpha) pathway and retrograde conduction over the fast (beta) pathway (see Fig. 20–25, p. 604, and Fig. 22–9*A* and *B*). An atrial complex blocks in the fast pathway anterogradely, travels to the ventricle over the slow pathway, and returns to the atrium over the previously blocked fast pathway. The proximal and distal final pathways for this circus movement appear to be located within the AV node, so that, as currently conceived, the circus movement is located totally within the AV node (Fig. 22–9*A* and *B*). Exceptions may occur.[124] The reentrant loop is slow AV nodal pathway → final distal common pathway (probably distal AV node) → retrograde fast AV nodal pathway → final proximal common pathway (probably proximal AV node, possibly a portion of low atrium). The cycle length of the tachycardia generally depends on how well the slow pathway conducts, since the fast pathway usually exhibits excellent capability for retrograde conduction and has the shorter refractory period in the retrograde direction. Therefore, conduction time in the anterograde slow pathway is a major determinant of the cycle length of the tachycardia. In one study, patients with shorter A-H intervals appeared more likely to have AV nodal reentrant tachycardia because these patients were more likely to have excellent retrogradely conducting fast pathways.[125]

The Dual Pathway Concept. The evidence supporting the dual pathway concept derives in part from the observation that in these patients, a plot of the A_1-A_2 versus the A_2-H_2 or A_1-A_2 versus the H_1-H_2 intervals shows a discontinuous curve (Fig. 22–20). The explanation is that, at a critical A_1-A_2 interval, the impulse suddenly blocks in the fast pathway and conducts with delay over the slow pathway, with sudden prolongation of the A_2-H_2 (or H_1-H_2) interval. Generally, the A-H interval increases at least 50 msec with only a 10- to 20-msec decrease in the coupling interval of the premature atrial complex. Less commonly, dual pathways may be manifested by different P-R or A-H intervals during sinus rhythm or at identical paced rates or by a sudden jump in the A-H interval during atrial pacing at a constant cycle length. Some patients

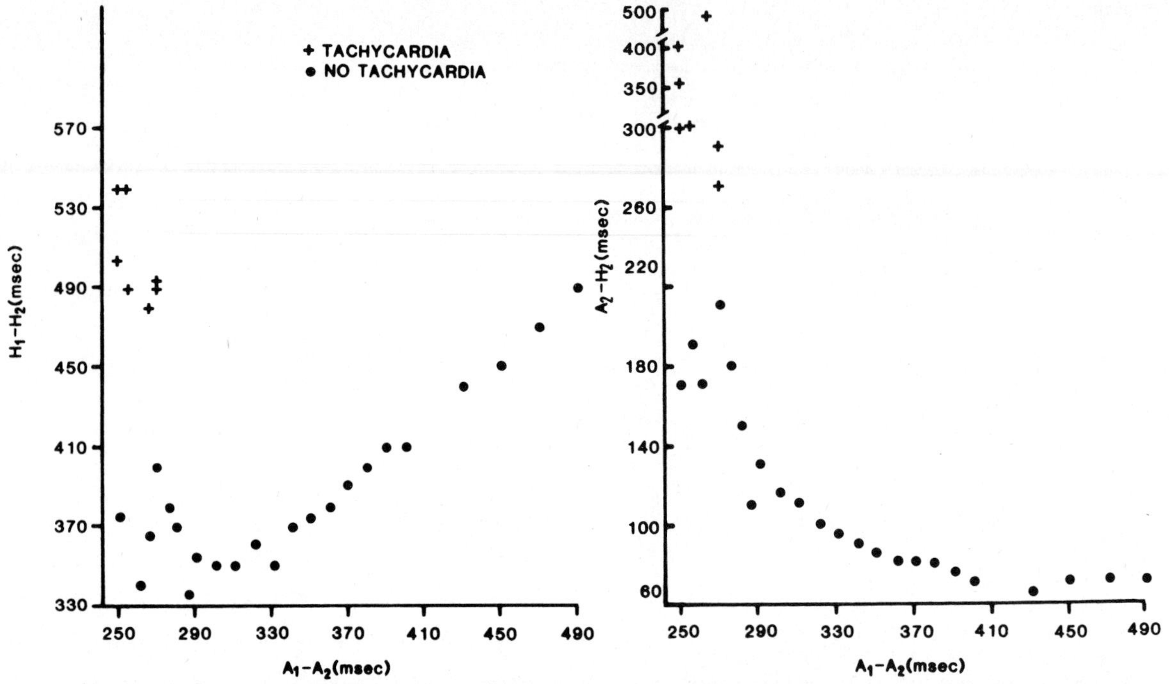

FIGURE 22–20. H_1-H_2 intervals (*left*) and A_2-H_2 intervals (*right*) at various A_1-A_2 intervals. Discontinuous AV nodal curve. At a critical A_1-A_2 interval the H_1-H_2 interval and the A_2-H_2 intervals increase markedly. At the break in the curves, AV nodal reentrant tachycardia is initiated.

with AV nodal reentry may not have discontinuous refractory period curves, and some patients who do not have AV nodal reentry may exhibit discontinuous refractory curves. In the latter patients, dual AV nodal pathways may be a benign finding.[126] Many of these patients exhibit discontinuous curves retrogradely also.[127] Similar mechanisms of tachycardia can occur in children.[128] Triple AV nodal pathways may be demonstrated in occasional patients.[129] Virtually irrefutable proof of dual AV nodal pathways is the simultaneous propagation in opposite directions of two AV nodal wavefronts without collision or the production of two QRS complexes from one P wave or two P waves from one QRS complex.

In less than 5 to 10 per cent of patients with AV nodal reentry, anterograde conduction proceeds over the fast pathway and retrograde conduction over the slow pathway (termed the unusual form of AV nodal reentry), causing atrial activation to begin *after* the QRS complex and producing a long V-A interval and a relatively short A-V interval (generally A-V/V-A < 0.75, Figs. 22–9*B* and 22–21*A*).[130, 131] Finally, it is possible to have tachycardias that use either the anterograde slow or fast pathways and a retrograde concealed accessory pathway (see below).[132]

Certainly the ventricles and apparently the atria are not needed to maintain AV nodal reentry in man, and spontaneous AV block has been noted on occasion, particularly at the onset of the arrhythmia. Such block can take place in the AV node distal to the reentry circuit, between the AV node and bundle of His, within the bundle of His, or distal to it. Rarely the block may be located between the reentry circuit in the AV node and the atrium.[124, 133] Most commonly when block appears, it is below the bundle of His. Termination of the tachycardia generally results from block in the anterogradely conducting slow pathway ("weak link"), so that a retrograde atrial response is not followed by a His or ventricular response.

Retrograde Atrial Activity. The sequence of retrograde atrial activation is normal during AV nodal reentrant supraventricular tachycardia. This means that the earliest site of atrial activation during retrograde conduction over the fast pathway is recorded in the His bundle electrogram followed by electrograms recorded from the os of the coronary sinus and then spreading to depolarize the rest of the right and left atria. During retrograde conduction over the slow pathway in the atypical type of AV nodal reentry, atrial activation recorded in the proximal coronary sinus may precede atrial activation recorded in the low right atrium, suggesting that the slow and fast pathways may enter the atria at slightly different positions.[134] Functional bundle branch block during AV nodal reentrant tachycardia does not modify the tachycardia significantly.

CLINICAL FEATURES. AV nodal reentry commonly occurs in patients who have no organic heart disease. Symptoms frequently accompany the tachycardia and range from feelings of palpitations, nervousness, and anxiety to angina, heart failure, syncope, or shock, depending on the duration and rate of the tachycardia and the presence of organic heart disease. Tachycardia may cause syncope because of the rapid ventricular rate, reduced cardiac output, and cerebral circulation, or because of asystole when the tachycardia terminates, owing to tachycardia-induced depression of sinus node automaticity (Fig. 22–19). The prognosis for patients without heart disease is usually good.

Hemodynamic consequences of supraventricular tachyarrhythmias in patients with normal ventricular function are due primarily to a marked decrease in left ventricular end-diastolic and stroke volumes with an increase in ejection rate and cardiac output without a significant change in ejection fraction as heart rate is increased and the atrial contribution to ventricular filling is lost.[11] Heart disease or tachycardia may reduce the ejection fraction.[135] Initial hypotension during tachycardia evokes a sympathetic response that increases blood pressure and in turn causes a rise in vagal tone that may terminate the tachycardia.[136]

TREATMENT. The Acute Attack. This depends on the underlying heart disease, how well the tachycardia is tolerated, and the natural history of previous attacks in the individual patient. For some patients, rest, reassurance, and sedation may be all that are required to abort an attack. Vagal maneuvers, including carotid sinus massage, Valsalva and Mueller maneuvers, gagging, and exposure of the face to ice water[137] serve as the first line of therapy. These maneuvers may slightly slow the tachycardia rate, which then may speed up to the original rate following cessation of the attempt, or they may terminate the tachycardia. Vagal maneuvers should be tried *again* after each pharmacological approach.

Verapamil[109, 138, 139] (see p. 636), 5 to 10 mg IV, terminates AV nodal reentry successfully in about 2 minutes in over 90 per cent of instances. This drug, or one of the other calcium-entry blockers, such as diltiazem,[140] has become the treatment of choice should simple vagal maneuvers fail. At the time of this writing diltiazem is still an investigational drug for treating arrhythmias.

Cholinergic drugs, particularly *edrophonium chloride* (Tensilon), a short-acting cholinesterase inhibitor, may terminate AV nodal reentry when administered initially at a trial dose of 3 to 5 mg IV and, if unsuccessful, repeated at a dose of 10 mg IV. Its action is rapid in onset and short in duration, with minimal side effects. Edrophonium should be used cautiously or not at all in patients who are hypotensive or who have lung disease, especially a history of asthma. Treating arrhythmias is not an FDA-approved indication for use of edrophonium.

If these initial approaches are unsuccessful, *intravenous digitalis* administration may be attempted using one of the following short-acting digitalis preparations: ouabain, 0.25 to 0.5 mg IV, followed by 0.1 mg every 30 to 60 minutes, if needed, keeping the total dose less than 1.0 mg within a 24-hour period or 0.01 mg/kg as a single dose over 10 to 15 minutes; digoxin, 0.5 to 1.0 mg IV given over 10 to 15 min, followed by 0.25 mg every 2 to 4 hours, with a total dose less than 1.5 mg within any 24-hour period; or deslanoside, 0.8 mg IV, followed by 0.4 mg every 2 to 4 hours, restricting the total dose to less than 2.0 mg within a 24-hour period. *Oral digitalis* administration to terminate an acute attack is generally not indicated. Vagal maneuvers, previously ineffective, may terminate the tachycardia following digitalis administration and therefore should be repeated.

Propranolol given intravenously at a rate of 0.5 to 1.0 mg/min for a total dose of 0.5 to 3.0 mg may be tried if digitalis administration is unsuccessful. Higher doses may be used in some patients (see Chap. 21). Propranolol must be used cautiously, if at all, in patients with heart failure, chronic lung disease, or a history of asthma because its beta-adrenoceptor blocking action depresses myocardial contractility and may produce bronchospasm.

Prior to administering digitalis or propranolol, it is advisable to reassess the clinical status of the patient and consider whether DC cardioversion may be advisable. DC shock, administered to patients who have received excessive amounts of digitalis, may be dangerous and may result in serious post-shock ventricular arrhythmias (p. 643). Particularly if signs or symptoms of cardiac decompensation occur, DC electrical shock should be considered early. DC shock, synchronized to the QRS complex to avoid precipitating ventricular fibrillation, successfully terminates AV nodal reentry with energies in the range of 10 to 50 watt-seconds; higher energies may be required in some instances (pp. 600 and 645).

In the event that digitalis has been given in large doses and DC shock is contraindicated, *atrial or ventricular pacing* may restore sinus rhythm. In some instances, esophageal pacing may be useful (p. 728).

Procainamide, quinidine, or disopyramide may be required to terminate AV nodal reentry in some patients. Unless contraindicated, DC cardioversion generally should be employed prior to using these agents, which are more often administered to prevent recurrences. These three drugs selectively depress conduction in the retrograde fast pathway.[141] Disopyramide may at times depress conduction in the slow pathway anterogradely.[142] Cardiac glycosides and beta and calcium-entry blockers selectively depress anterograde slow pathway conduction but occasionally may depress conduction in the retrograde fast pathway.

Pressor drugs may terminate AV nodal reentry by inducing reflex vagal stimulation mediated by baroreceptors in the carotid sinus and aorta when the systolic blood pressure is acutely elevated to levels of about 180 mm Hg. One of the following drugs, diluted in 5 to 10 ml of 5 per cent dextrose and water, may be given over 1 to 3 minutes: phenylephrine (Neo-Synephrine), 0.5 to 1.0 mg; methoxamine (Vasoxyl), 3 to 5 mg; or metaraminol (Aramine), 0.5 to 2.0 mg. Pressor drugs should be used cautiously or not at all in the elderly and in patients who have organic heart disease, significant hypertension, hyperthyroidism, or acute myocardial infarction. Today, this potentially dangerous and almost always uncomfortable procedure is rarely needed unless the patient is also hypotensive.

Prevention of Recurrences. This is often more difficult than terminating the acute episode. Initially, one must decide whether the frequency and severity of the attacks warrant long-term drug prophylaxis. If the attacks of paroxysmal tachycardia are infrequent, well tolerated, and either terminate spontaneously or are easily terminated by the patient, no prophylactic therapy may be necessary. If the attacks are sufficiently frequent to necessitate therapy, the patient may be treated with drugs empirically or on the basis of serial electrophysiological testing. Because drug responses are variable, serial electrophysiological testing of multiple drugs appears reasonable in some patients with poorly tolerated tachycardias that recur only sporadically (p. 611).[143]

If empirical testing is desirable, the following choices are recommended: Digitalis is generally the initial drug of choice. It has the advantages of being well tolerated and requiring administration only once daily. The clinical situation determines the speed of digitalization. Using digoxin, rapid oral digitalization can be accomplished in 24 to 36 hours with an initial dose of 1.0 to 1.5 mg, followed by 0.25 to 0.5 mg every 6 hours for a total dose of 2.0 to 3.0 mg. A less rapid oral regimen digitalizes in 2 to 3 days with an initial dose of 0.75 to 1.0 mg, followed by 0.25 to 0.50 mg every 12 hours for a total dose of 2.0 to 3.0 mg. Alternatively, digoxin administered as a maintenance dose of 0.125 to 0.500 mg achieves digitalization in about one week. Digitoxin, which has a longer duration of action, may be used instead of digoxin. Oral digitalization with digitoxin may be accomplished in 24 to 36 hours with an initial dose of 0.5 to 0.8 mg, followed by 0.2 mg every 6 to 8 hours until a total dose of 1.2 mg is reached. A slower approach involves administering 0.2 mg three times daily for 2 to 3 days. Complete digitalization can also be accomplished in about one month by simply giving a daily maintenance dose of 0.05 to 0.20 mg.

If digitalis alone is unsuccessful, one can then add verapamil, 80 to 120 mg every 6 or 8 hours, quinidine sulfate, 200 to 400 mg every 6 hours, or propranolol, 10 to 40 mg every 6 hours. Procainamide or disopyramide can be used instead of quinidine. In some patients, concomitant administration of digitalis, propranolol, and quinidine or procainamide or disopyramide may be necessary. Amiodarone alone or combined with digitalis may be effective.

For many patients, pacemaker implantation provides acceptable treatment (p. 728). Competitive atrial pacing promptly terminates AV nodal reentry, restoring sinus rhythm immediately or sometimes after a transient episode of atrial flutter or atrial fibrillation, and avoids the necessity of daily drug administration with potential side effects.

REENTRY OVER A RETROGRADE CONDUCTING (CONCEALED) ACCESSORY PATHWAY

ELECTROCARDIOGRAPHIC RECOGNITION (Fig. 22–22). The presence of an accessory pathway that conducts unidirectionally from the ventricle to the atrium but not in the reverse direction is not apparent by analysis of the scalar ECG during sinus rhythm because the ventricle is not preexcited. Therefore, the ECG manifestations of the

Wolff-Parkinson-White (WPW) syndrome are absent and the accessory pathway is said to be "concealed."[144–147] However, since the mechanism responsible for most tachycardias in patients who have the WPW syndrome is macro-reentry caused by anterograde conduction over the AV node–His bundle pathway and retrograde conduction over an accessory pathway, the latter, even if it only conducts retrogradely, can still participate in the reentrant circuit to cause an *AV reciprocating tachycardia.* Electrocardiographically, a tachycardia due to this mechanism may be *suspected* when the QRS complex is normal and the retrograde P wave occurs *after* completion of the QRS complex, in the ST segment or early T wave (Fig. 22–9C and Table 22–2).[148–151]

MECHANISMS. This relationship between P wave and QRS complex results because the ventricle must be activated before the propagating impulse can enter the accessory pathway and excite the atria retrogradely. Therefore, the retrograde P wave must follow ventricular excitation, in contrast to AV nodal reentry, in which the atria can be excited during ventricular activation (Fig. 22–9*A*). Also, the contour of the retrograde P wave may differ from the usual retrograde P wave, since the atria may be activated eccentrically, i.e., in a manner other than the normal retrograde activation sequence, starting at the low right atrial septum as in AV nodal reentry. This occurs because the concealed accessory pathway in most instances is left-sided, i.e., inserts into the left atrium, making the left atrium the first site of retrograde atrial activation and causing the retrograde P wave to be negative in lead I (Fig. 22–22). Finally, since the tachycardia circuit involves the ventricles, if functional bundle branch block occurs in the same ventricle in which the accessory pathway is located, the cycle length of the tachycardia may become longer. This important change ensues because the bundle branch block lengthens the reentrant circuit (see Preexcitation Syndrome). For example, the normal activation sequence for a reciprocating tachycardia circuit with a left-sided accessory pathway without functional bundle branch block progresses from atrium → AV node–His bundle → right and left ventricles → accessory pathway → atrium. However, during functional left bundle branch block as an example, the tachycardia circuit travels from atrium → AV node–His bundle → right ventricle → septum → left ventricle → accessory pathway → atrium.

The additional time required for the impulse to travel from the right to the left ventricle before reaching the accessory pathway and atrium lengthens the V-A interval, which lengthens the cycle length of the tachycardia by an equal amount, assuming no other changes in conduction times occur within the circuit. Thus, lengthening of the tachycardia cycle length by more than 35 msec during ipsilateral functional bundle branch block is diagnostic of a free wall accessory pathway if the lengthening can be shown to be due to V-A prolongation only and not to prolongation of the H-V interval (which may develop with the appearance of bundle branch block). In an occasional patient, the increase in cycle length due to prolongation of VA conduction may be nullified by a simultaneous decrease in the P-R (A-H) interval.[152]

Septal Accessory Pathway. An exception to these observations occurs in the patient with a septal accessory pathway (see Preexcitation Syndrome, p. 685), in whom retrograde atrial activation is normal and the V-A interval and the cycle length of the tachycardia increases 25 msec or less with the development of ipsilateral functional bundle branch block.[152] Functional bundle branch block in the ventricle contralateral to the accessory pathway does not lengthen the tachycardia cycle if the H-V interval does not lengthen. Functional bundle branch block, particularly functional left bundle branch block, during tachycardia occurs much more commonly in patients who have an accessory pathway than in those with AV nodal reentry, possibly because in the latter, slow pathway anterograde conduction allows for longer recovery time of the His-Purkinje system, while in tachycardias associated with accessory pathways, anterograde conduction over the AV node may be more rapid. Functional left bundle branch block may occur more commonly during rapid tachycardias, perhaps because the refractory period of the right bundle branch appears to be shorter than the left bundle branch at short cycle lengths.[69] Premature right ventricular stimulation that starts an AV reciprocating tachycardia is more likely to induce functional left bundle branch block than is premature atrial stimulation.[153]

Vagal maneuvers, by acting predominantly on the AV node, produce

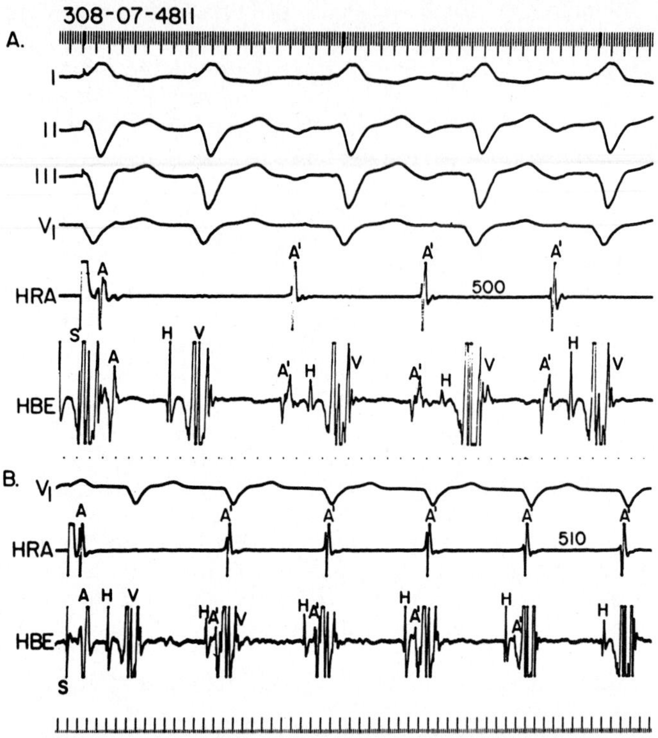

FIGURE 22–21. Unusual and usual forms of AV nodal reentry in the same patient. Panel A, Following the last atrial stimulus (S) of a train of rapid atrial pacing at an increasing rate, a supraventricular tachycardia occurs at a cycle length of 500 msec. The P-R interval is short and the R-P interval is long (see Table 22–2). The retrograde atrial activation sequence is recorded first in the low right atrium (A',HBE lead) and then in the high right atrium (A',HRA). Ventricular stimulation when the His bundle was refractory during the tachycardia did not preexcite the atrium (see Fig. 22–22).

In panel B following the cessation of atrial pacing (S), a supraventricular tachycardia of identical QRS morphology (only V_1 is demonstrated) is initiated at a cycle length of 510 msec. Note, however, that the R-P interval is zero with a long P-R interval. The retrograde atrial activation occurs at the onset of the QRS complex and is recorded first in the low right atrium (A',HBE) and then in the high right atrium (A',HRA).

Thus, panel A most likely represents anterograde conduction down the fast AV nodal pathway and retrograde conduction up the slow AV nodal pathway, while panel B represents anterograde conduction down the slow AV nodal pathway and retrograde conduction up the fast AV nodal pathway (see Chap. 20). Note also that the atrial activation sequence and PR-RP relationships in panel A are similar to that shown in Figure 22–29.

a response similar to AV nodal reentry, and the tachycardia may transiently slow or transiently slow and then terminate. Generally, termination occurs in the anterograde direction, so that the last retrograde P wave fails to conduct to the ventricle.

ELECTROPHYSIOLOGICAL FEATURES. Electrophysiological criteria supporting the diagnosis of tachycardia involving reentry over a concealed accessory pathway include the fact that initiation of tachycardia depends on a critical degree of atrioventricular delay (necessary to allow time for the accessory pathway to recover excitability), but the delay can be in the AV node or His-Purkinje system, i.e., a critical degree of A-H delay is not necessary. Occasionally, a tachycardia may start with little or no measurable lengthening of AV nodal or His-Purkinje conduction time.[154] The AV nodal refractory period curve is smooth, in contrast to the discontinuous curve found in many patients with AV nodal reentry. Dual AV nodal pathways occasionally may be noted as a concomitant but unrelated finding.

Diagnosis of Accessory Pathways. This can be accomplished by demonstrating that during ventricular pacing, premature ventricular stimulation activates the atria prior to retrograde depolarization of the His bundle, indicating that the impulse reached the atria before it depolarized the His bundle and must have traveled a different pathway to do so. Also, if the ventricles can be stimulated prematurely during tachycardia at a time when the His bundle is refractory, and the impulse still conducts to the atrium, this indicates that retrograde propagation traveled to the atrium over a pathway other than the bundle of His[144] (Fig. 22–22*B*). If the premature ventricular complex depolarizes the

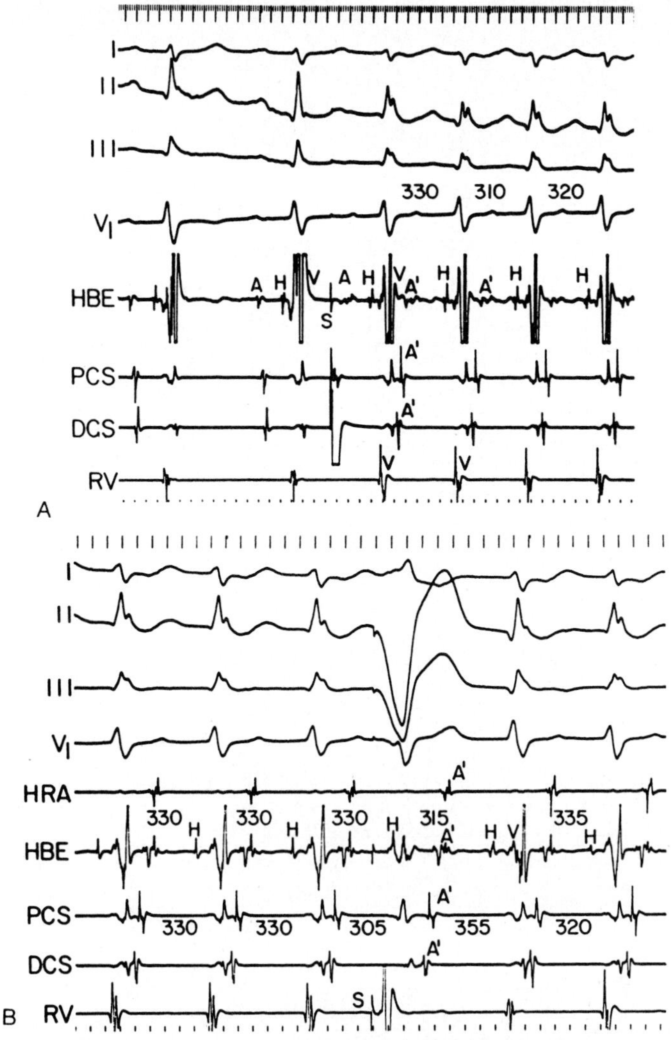

FIGURE 22–22. Atrial preexcitation during atrioventricular reciprocating tachycardia (AVRT) in a patient with a concealed accessory pathway. No evidence of an accessory pathway conduction is present in the two sinus-initiated beats shown in panel A. A premature stimulus in the coronary sinus (S) precipitates a supraventricular tachycardia at a cycle length of approximately 330 msec. The retrograde atrial activation sequence begins first in the distal coronary sinus (A',DCS), followed by activation recorded in the proximal coronary sinus (PCS), low right atrium (HBE), and then high right atrium (not shown). The QRS complex is normal and identical to the sinus-initiated QRS complex. (The terminal portion is slightly deformed by the superimposition of the retrograde atrial recording.) Note that the R-P interval is short and the P-R interval is long (see Table 22–2). The shortest V-A interval exceeds 65 msec, consistent with conduction over a retrogradely conducting atrioventricular pathway.

In panel B, premature ventricular stimulation at a time when the His bundle is still refractory from anterograde activation during tachycardia shortens the A-A interval from 330 to 305 msec without a change in the retrograde atrial activation sequence. (Note that no change occurs in the H-H interval when the right ventricular stimulus, S, is delivered. H-H intervals are in msec in HBE lead.) Thus the ventricular stimulus, despite His bundle refractoriness, still reaches the atrium and produces an identical retrograde atrial activation sequence. The only way this can be explained is via conduction over a retrogradely conducting accessory pathway. Thus the patient has a concealed accessory pathway with the Wolff-Parkinson-White syndrome.

atria at the same coupling interval at which the premature ventricular complex occurred and with the same retrograde atrial activation sequence, one assumes that the stimulation site (i.e., ventricle) is within the reentrant circuit without intervening His-Purkinje or AV nodal tissue that might increase the V-A and therefore A-A intervals. In addition, if a premature ventricular complex delivered at a time when the His bundle is refractory terminates the tachycardia, an accessory pathway is most likely present.[144, 155]

The V-A interval (conduction over the accessory pathway) generally is constant over a wide range of ventricular paced rates and coupling intervals of premature ventricular complexes as well as during the tachycardia in the absence of aberration. Similar short V-A intervals may be observed in patients during AV nodal reentry, but if the VA conduction time or R-P interval is the same during tachycardia *and* ventricular pacing at comparable rates, an accessory pathway is almost certainly present. The V-A interval is usually less than 50 per cent of the R-R interval (Table 22–2). The tachycardia can be easily initiated following premature ventricular stimulation that conducts retrogradely in the accessory pathway but blocks in the AV node or His bundle.[155] Atria and ventricles are required components of the macro-reentrant circuit, and therefore continuation of the tachycardia in the presence of AV or VA block excludes an accessory atrioventricular pathway as part of the reentrant circuit.

CLINICAL FEATURES. The prevalance of concealed accessory pathways is estimated to account for about 30 per cent of patients with apparent supraventricular tachycardia referred for electrophysiological evaluation. The great majority of these accessory pathways are located between left ventricle and left atrium, uncommonly between right ventricle and right atrium. It is important to be aware of the possibility of a concealed accessory pathway being responsible for apparently "routine" supraventricular tachycardia, since therapeutic response at times may not follow the usual guidelines. Antiarrhythmic targeting may need to be directed toward drugs that affect the accessory pathway such as drugs in class 1A and 1C, or amiodarone (Chap. 21). Also, surgical interruption of the accessory pathway may be accomplished (p. 645). The tachycardia rates tend to be somewhat faster than those occurring in AV nodal reentry ($\geq$ 200 beats/min), but a great deal of overlap exists between the two groups. Paroxysmal supraventricular tachycardia may be followed by polyuria after termination. Syncope may occur because the rapid ventricular rate fails to provide adequate cerebral circulation or because the tachyarrhythmia may depress the sinus pacemaker, causing a period of asystole when the tachyarrhythmia terminates. Physical examination reveals an unvarying, regular ventricular rhythm with constant intensity of the first heart sound. The jugular venous pressure may be elevated, but the waveform generally remains constant.

TREATMENT. The therapeutic approach to terminate this form of tachycardia acutely is as outlined for AV nodal reentry (see p. 682). It is necessary to achieve block of a single impulse from atrium to ventricle or ventricle to atrium. Generally, the most successful method is to produce transient AV nodal block, and therefore vagal maneuvers, verapamil, digitalis, and propranolol are acceptable choices. Conventional antiarrhythmic agents that prolong activation time or refractory period in the accessory pathway need to be considered as chronic therapy for prophylactic prevention, similar to that discussed for reciprocating tachycardias associated with the preexcitation syndrome. The presence of atrial fibrillation in *patients with a concealed accessory pathway* should not present a greater therapeutic challenge than it does in patients who do not have such a pathway, because anterograde AV conduction occurs over the AV node. Verapamil and digitalis are not contraindicated. However, it must be remembered that under some circumstances, such as catecholamine stimulation, anterograde conduction in the apparently concealed accessory pathway may occur.[156]

PREEXCITATION SYNDROME

ELECTROCARDIOGRAPHIC RECOGNITION (Fig. 22–23). Preexcitation syndrome[157] occurs when the atrial impulse activates the whole or some part of the ventricle, or the ventricular impulse activates the whole or some part of the atrium, earlier than would be expected if the impulse traveled by way of the normal specific conduction

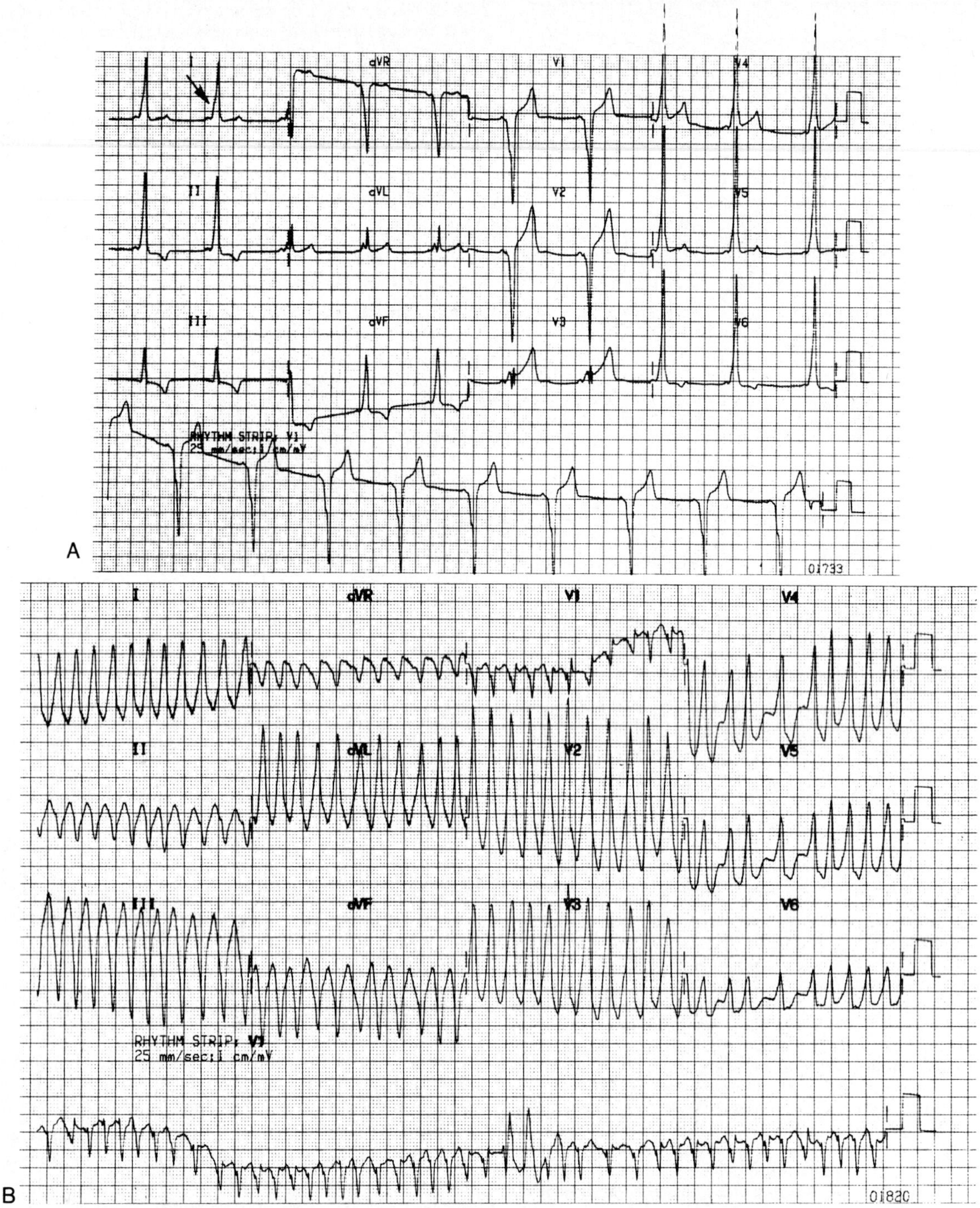

FIGURE 22–23. ***A*, Right anteroseptal accessory pathway. The 12-lead ECG characteristically exhibits a normal to inferior axis. The delta wave is negative in V_1 and V_2, upright in lead I, II, AVL, and AVF, isoelectric in lead III, and negative in AVR. Location verified at surgery. Arrow indicates delta wave (lead I). *B*, Right posteroseptal accessory pathway. Negative delta waves in leads II, III, and AVF, upright in I and AVL, localize this pathway to the posteroseptal region. The negative delta wave in V_1 with sharp transition to an upright delta wave in V_2 pinpoint it to the right posteroseptal area. Atrial fibrillation is present. Location verified at surgery. Arrow indicates delta wave (V_4).**

Illustration continued on the opposite page

system only.[158] In the Wolff-Parkinson-White syndrome,[159] muscular connections composed of working myocardial fibers exist outside the specialized conducting tissue, and connect atrium and ventricle.[160] They are named *accessory atrioventricular pathways* or connections, commonly called *Kent bundles*,[161, 162] and are responsible for the most common variety of preexcitation (incidentally noted in other animals such as monkeys, dogs, and cats).[163, 164] Three basic features typify the ECG abnormalities of patients with the usual form of WPW syndrome caused by an AV connection: (1) P-R interval less than 120 msec during sinus rhythm; (2) QRS complex duration exceeding 120 msec with a slurred, slowly rising onset of the QRS in some leads (delta wave) and usually a normal terminal QRS portion: and (3) secondary ST-T wave changes that are generally directed opposite to the major delta and QRS vectors.[148–150, 165]

The term *Wolff-Parkinson-White* (WPW) *syndrome* is applied when the patient has symptoms, generally due to tachyarrhythmias. The most common tachycardia is characterized by a normal QRS, by ventricular rates of 150 to 250 beats/min (generally faster than AV nodal reentry),

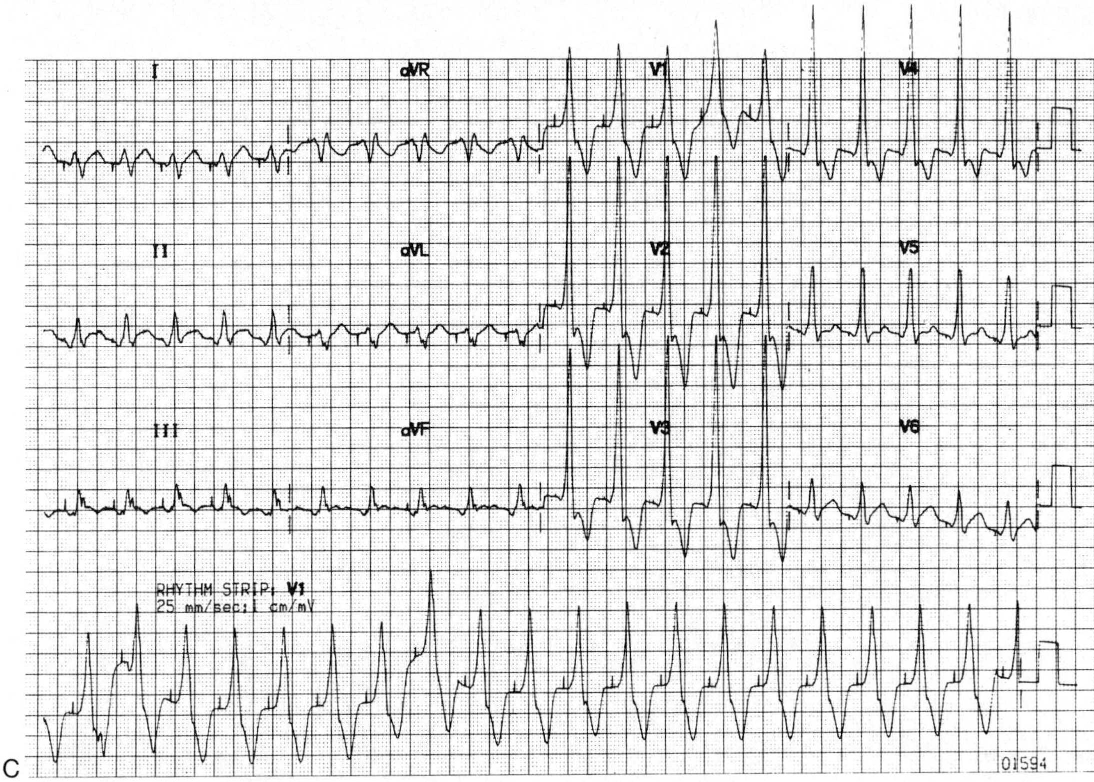

FIGURE 22–23 *Continued.* **C, Left posterolateral accessory pathway. Positive delta wave in the anterior precordial leads and in leads II, III, and AVF, positive or isoelectric in lead I, and AVL and isoelectric or negative in V_5 and V_6 are typical of a left posterolateral accessory pathway. Rapid coronary sinus pacing (450 msec cycle length) was used to enhance preexcitation (negative P wave I, II, III, aVF, V_{3-6}). Location verified at surgery. Arrow indicates delta wave (V_1).**

and by sudden onset and termination, behaving in most respects like the tachycardia described for conduction utilizing a concealed pathway (p. 684). The major difference between the two is the capacity for anterograde conduction over the accessory pathway during atrial flutter or atrial fibrillation (see below).

A variety of other anatomical substrates exist that provide the basis for different ECG manifestations of several variations of the preexcitation syndrome (Fig. 22–24). Fibers from atrium to His bundle bypassing the physiological delay of the AV node are called *atriohisian tracts* (Fig. 22–24*B*) and are associated with a short P-R interval and a normal QRS complex. Although demonstrated anatomically[166] (see below), the electrophysiological significance of these tracts in the genesis of tachycardias with a short P-R interval and a normal QRS complex (Lown-Ganong-Levine, LGL, syndrome) remains to be established. Indeed, evidence does *not* support the presence of a specific LGL syndrome[167] comprising a short P-R interval, normal QRS complex, and tachycardias related to an atriohisian bypass tract. The short P-R intervals reported in many patients probably represent one end of the spectrum of normal AV conduction.[75] Two varieties of Mahaim fibers[168, 169] include those passing from the AV node to the ventricle, called nodoventricular fibers (Fig. 22–24), and those arising in the His bundle or bundle branches and inserting in the ventricular myocardium, called fasciculoventricular fibers (Fig. 22–24). For nodoventricular connections, the P-R interval may be normal or short, and the QRS complex is a fusion beat. Fasciculoventricular connections create a normal P-R interval and a fixed, anomalous QRS complex.[170]

ELECTROPHYSIOLOGICAL FEATURES (Figs. 22–25 to 22–28; see also p. 684). If the Kent bundle accessory pathway is capable of anterograde conduction, two parallel routes of AV conduction are possible, one subject to physiological delay over the AV node and the other passing directly without delay from atrium to ventricle. This produces the typical QRS complex that is a fusion beat due to depolarization of the ventricle in part by the wavefront traveling over the accessory pathway and in part by the wavefront traveling over the normal AV node-His bundle route. The delta wave represents ventricular activation from input over the accessory pathway. The extent of contribution to ventricular depolarization by the wavefront over each route depends upon their relative activation times. If AV nodal conduction delay occurs, for example, because of a rapid atrial pacing rate or premature atrial complex, more of the ventricle becomes activated over the accessory pathway, and the QRS complex becomes more anomalous in contour.

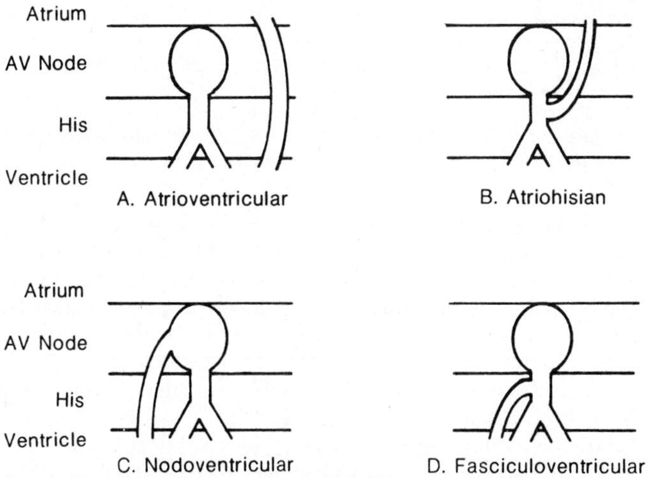

FIGURE 22–24. Schematic representation of accessory pathways.

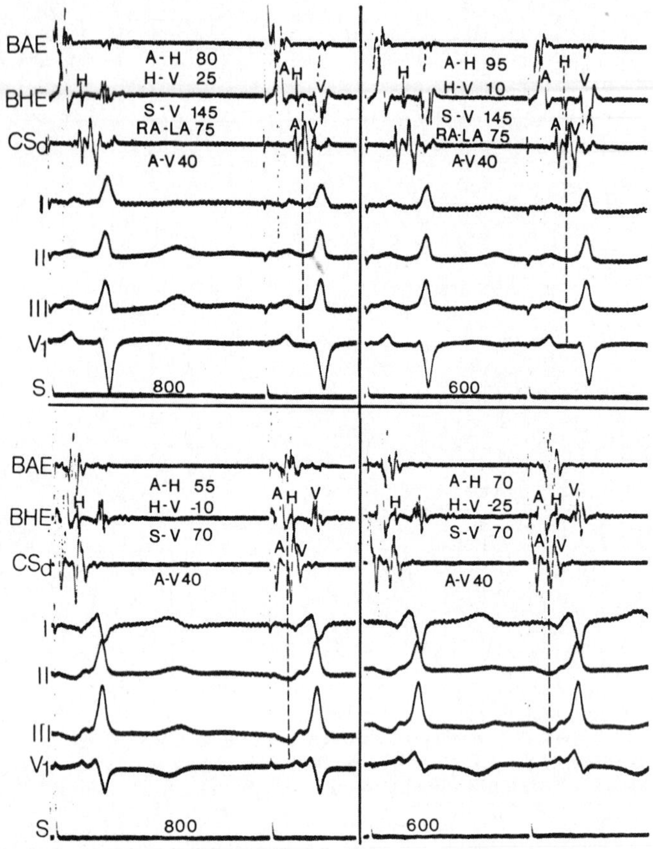

FIGURE 22–25. Influence of pacing site and cycle length on the degree of preexcitation. In this patient with a left anterior accessory pathway, pacing the high right atrium at a cycle length of 800 msec (*top left panel*) produced an A-H interval of 80 msec and an H-V interval of 25 msec. The interval from the stimulus to the onset of ventricular activity (S-V) was 145 msec and the right-to-left atrial activation time was 75 msec. The interrupted line indicates the onset of the delta wave. Little preexcitation is seen in the ECG because the fairly rapid AV conduction time over the normal pathway allows much of the ventricle to be activated normally before the impulse traveling from right to left atrium and then over the accessory pathway can depolarize the ventricles. Shortening the pacing cycle length to 600 msec (*top right panel*) without changing the pacing site lengthened the A-H interval by 15 msec and shortened the H-V interval by 10 msec. The other intervals remained the same and the QRS complex changed very slightly. In the *bottom left panel,* the coronary sinus is paced at a cycle length of 800 msec. Even though the A-H interval shortens to 55 msec because of coronary sinus pacing, the S-V shortens to 70 msec, His bundle activation follows the onset of ventricular depolarization by 10 msec, and the QRS complex becomes more aberrant. By pacing at a site near the atrial insertion of the accessory pathway, conduction rapidly reaches the ventricle over the accessory pathway to activate more of the ventricle than when pacing the right atrium at the same cycle length. In the *bottom right panel,* shortening the pacing cycle length to 600 msec lengthens the A-H interval 15 msec, and His bundle activation begins 25 msec after the onset of QRS complex. The S-V and A-V intervals remain unchanged and the QRS complex becomes even more aberrant.

Total activation of the ventricle over the accessory pathway can occur if the AV nodal delay is sufficiently long. In contrast, if the accessory pathway is relatively far from the sinus node, for example, a left lateral accessory pathway, or if AV nodal conduction time is relatively short, more of the ventricle may be activated by conduction over the normal pathway (Fig. 22–25). The normal fusion beat during sinus rhythm has a short H-V interval, or His bundle activation actually begins after the onset of ventricular depolarization, because part of the atrial impulse bypasses the AV node and activates the ventricle early, at a time when the atrial impulse traveling the normal route just reaches the His bundle. This finding of a short or negative H-V interval occurs *only* during conduction over an accessory pathway or from retrograde His activation during a ventricular tachycardia.

Pacing the atrium at rapid rates, at premature intervals, or from a site close to the atrial insertion of the Kent bundle accentuates the anomalous activation of the ventricles and shortens the H-V interval even more (His activation may become buried in the ventricular electrogram, Fig. 22–25). The position of the accessory pathway can be determined by a careful analysis of the spatial direction of the delta wave in the 12-lead ECG in maximally preexcited beats (Fig. 22–26) as well as by body surface maps. A simple ECG algorithm with 90 per cent accuracy localizes left free wall pathways by a Q wave in the lateral precordial leads, posteroseptal pathways by a Q wave in the inferior leads, anteroseptal pathways by left bundle branch block

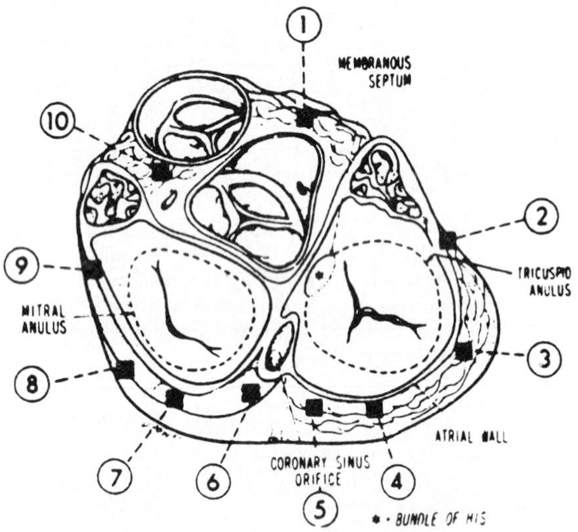

1 RIGHT ANTERIOR PARASEPTAL
2 RIGHT ANTERIOR
3 RIGHT LATERAL
4 RIGHT POSTERIOR
5 RIGHT PARASEPTAL
6 LEFT POSTERIOR PARASEPTAL
7 LEFT POSTERIOR
8 LEFT LATERAL
9 LEFT ANTERIOR
10 LEFT ANTERIOR PARASEPTAL

DELTA WAVE POLARITY

	I	II	III	AVR	AVL	AVF	V1	V2	V3	V4	V5	V6
1	+	+	+(±)	-	±(+)	+	±	±	+(±)	+	+	+
2	+	+	-(±)	-	+(±)	±(-)	±	+(±)	+(±)	+	+	+
3	+	±(-)	-	-	+	-(±)	±	±	±	+	+	+
4	+	-	-	-	+	-	±(+)	±	+	+	+	+
5	+	-	-	-(+)	+	-	±	+	+	+	+	+
6	+	-	-	-	+	-	+	+	+	+	+	+
7	+	-	-	±(+)	+	-	+	+	+	+	+	-(±)
8	-(±)	±	±	±(+)	-(±)	±	+	+	+	+	-(±)	-(±)
9	-(±)	+	+	-	-(±)	+	+	+	+	+	+	+
10	+	+	+(±)	-	±	+	±(+)	+	+	+	+	+

± = Initial 40 msec delta wave isoelectric
+ = Initial 40 msec delta wave positive
- = Initial 40 msec delta wave negative

FIGURE 22–26. In this schematic representation (*top*), sites of the potential position of the accessory pathway are indicated by filled boxes numbered 1 through 10. The delta wave polarity in the 12-lead ECG for each of the 10 sites is depicted in the table at the bottom. (From Gallagher, J. J., et al.: The preexcitation syndromes. Progr. Cardiovasc. Dis. *20*:285, 1978.)

and inferior axis and right free wall pathways by left bundle branch block and left axis deviation.[171] T-wave abnormalities can occur after disappearance of preexcitation with orientation of the T wave according to the site of preexcitation. A variety of electrical (Fig. 22–27), radionuclide, and echocardiographic techniques can be used to localize the insertion site of the accessory pathway.

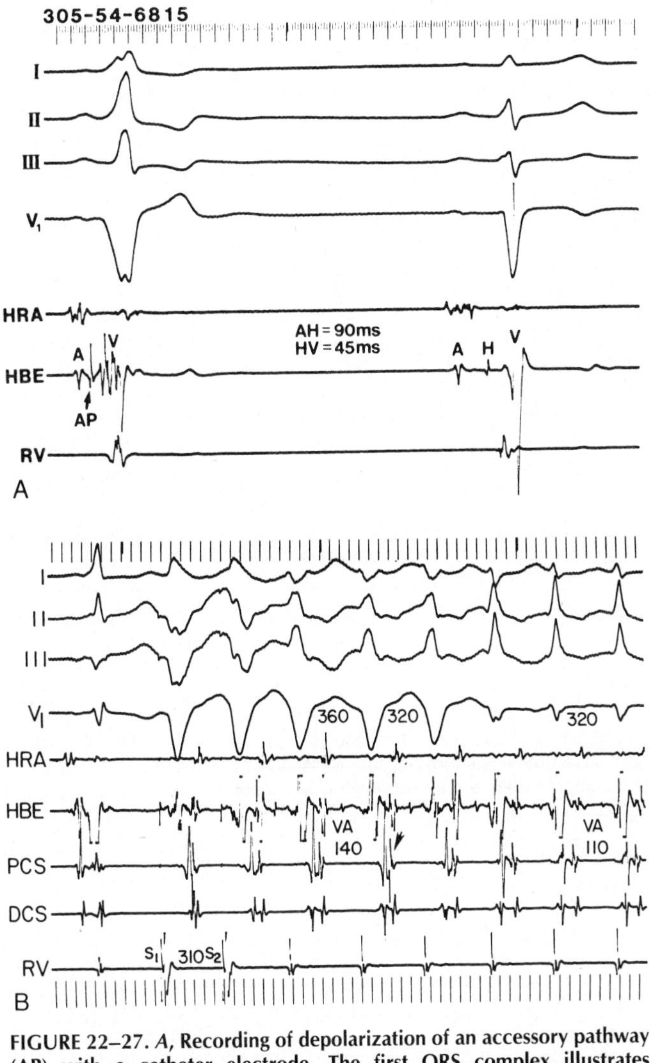

FIGURE 22–27. *A*, Recording of depolarization of an accessory pathway (AP) with a catheter electrode. The first QRS complex illustrates conduction over the accessory pathway (AP). In the scalar ECG a short P-R interval and delta wave (best seen in lead 1 and V_1) are apparent. His bundle activation is buried within the ventricular complex. In the following complex, conduction has blocked over the accessory pathway and a normal QRS complex results. His bundle activation clearly precedes the onset of ventricular depolarization by 45 msec. The A-H interval for this complex is 90 msec. (From Prystowsky, E. N., Browne, K. F., and Zipes, D. P.: Intracardiac recording by catheter electrode of accessory pathway depolarization. J. Am. Col. Cardiol. *1*:468, 1983. *B*, Influence of functional ipsilateral bundle branch block on the V-A interval during an atrioventricular reciprocating tachycardia (AVRT). Partial preexcitation can be noted in the sinus initiated complex (first complex). Two premature ventricular stimuli (S_1, S_2) initiate a sustained supraventricular tachycardia that persists with a left bundle branch block for several complexes, finally reverting to normal. The retrograde atrial activation sequence is recorded first in the proximal coronary sinus lead (arrow, PCS), then in the distal coronary sinus lead (DCS) and low right atrium (HBE) and then high right atrium (HRA). During the functional bundle branch block, the V-A interval in the PCS lead is 140 msec, shortening to 110 msec when the QRS complex reverts to normal. Such behavior is characteristic of a left-sided accessory pathway with prolongation of the reentrant pathway by the functional left bundle branch block.

In patients who have an atriohisian tract, theoretically the QRS complex would remain normal and the short A-H interval fixed or show very little increase during atrial pacing at more rapid rates. The authors have found this response uncommonly. Rapid atrial pacing in patients who have nodoventricular connections shortens the H-V interval and widens the QRS complex but, in contrast to patients who have an atrioventricular connection (Fig. 22–25), the A-V interval also lengthens. In patients who have fasciculoventricular connections, the H-V interval remains short and QRS complex unchanged and anomalous during rapid atrial pacing.

Even though the Kent bundle conducts more rapidly than does the AV node (conduction velocity is faster in the accessory pathway), the Kent bundle usually has a longer refractory period during long cycle lengths (e.g., sinus rhythm)—i.e., it takes longer for the accessory pathway to recover excitability than it does for the AV node. Consequently, a premature atrial complex can occur sufficiently early to block anterogradely in the accessory pathway and conduct to the ventricle only over the normal AV node–His bundle (Fig. 20–28*A,B*). The resultant H-V interval and the QRS complex become normal. Such an event may initiate the most common type of reciprocating tachycardia, which is characterized by anterograde conduction over the normal pathway and retrograde conduction over the accessory pathway (*orthodromic AV reciprocating*)[172] (Fig. 22–28). The accessory pathway, blocking in an anterograde direction, recovers excitability in time to be activated following the QRS complex, in a retrograde direction, completing the reentrant loop. Much less commonly, patients can have tachycardias called *antidromic* tachycardias during which anterograde conduction occurs over the accessory pathway and retrograde conduction over the AV node.[173, 174] The resultant QRS complex is abnormal owing to total ventricular activation over the accessory pathway (Fig. 22–28*C*). In both tachycardias the accessory pathway is an obligatory part of the reentrant circuit.

Ten per cent of patients may have multiple accessory pathways and on occasion tachycardia may be due to a reentrant loop anterogradely over one accessory pathway and retrogradely over the other.[175, 176] Patients who have nodoventricular fibers have tachycardias with a left bundle branch block morphology[177] that may be due to a macroreentrant circuit using the nodoventricular fiber anterogradely and the His-Purkinje system with a portion of the AV node retrogradely[170, 178] (Fig. 22–28*F*). Although this circuit still remains to be established definitively, and it is possible that the nodoventricular pathway is a bystander during an AV nodal reentrant tachycardia without participation in the reentrant circuit,[169] anatomical-electrophysiological correlative evidence supports the presence and functional significance of nodoventricular fibers.[179] No direct relationship between fasciculoventricular fibers and observed arrhythmias has been found.[170]

An incessant form of supraventricular tachycardia has been recognized that generally occurs with a long R-P interval that exceeds the P-R interval (Fig. 22–29 and Table 22–2). A posteroseptal accessory pathway that conducts very slowly, possibly due to a long and tortuous route, appears responsible.[180, 181] Tachycardia is maintained by anterograde AV nodal conduction and retrograde conduction over the accessory pathway[182] (Fig. 22–28*D*). While anterograde conduction over this pathway has been demonstrated, the long anterograde conduction times over the accessory pathway ordinarily may prevent ECG manifestations of accessory pathway conduction during sinus rhythm. The QRS is prolonged during sinus rhythm from conduction over this accessory pathway only when conduction times through the AV node–His bundle exceed those in the accessory pathway.

When retrograde atrial activation during tachycardia occurs over an accessory pathway that connects the left atrium to the left ventricle, the earliest retrograde activity is recorded from a left atrial electrode usually positioned in the coronary sinus (Fig. 22–27*B*). When retrograde atrial activation during tachycardia occurs over an accessory pathway that connects the right ventricle to the right atrium, the earliest retrograde atrial activity generally is recorded from a lateral right atrial electrode. Participation of a septal accessory pathway creates earliest retrograde atrial activation in the low right atrium situated near the septum, anterior or posterior, depending on the insertion site. These mapping techniques with catheter electrodes and at the time of surgery (pp. 615 and 645) provide one of the most accurate assessments of the position of the accessory pathway, which can be anywhere in the AV groove except where the ventricles are contiguous (Fig. 22–26). Recording electrical activity directly from the accessory pathway obviously provides precise localization (Fig. 22–27*A*).

It may be difficult to distinguish AV nodal reentry from participation of a septal accessory connection using the retrograde sequence of atrial activation because activation sequences during both tachycardias are similar. Other approaches to demonstrate retrograde atrial activation over the accessory pathway must be tried and can be accomplished

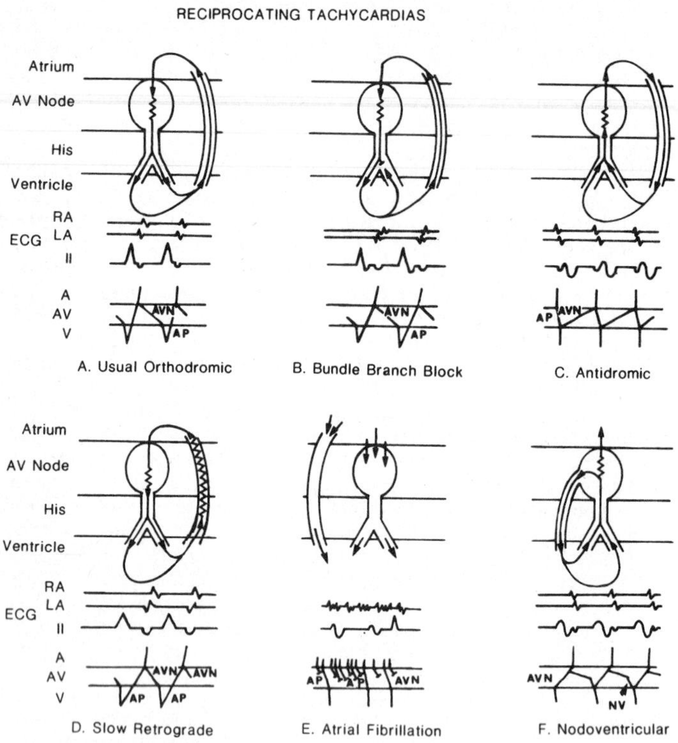

FIGURE 22–28. Schematic diagram of tachycardias associated with accessory pathways. Format as in Figure 22–9. *A*, Orthodromic tachycardia with anterograde conduction over the AV node-His bundle route and retrograde conduction over the accessory pathway (left-sided for this example as depicted by LA activation preceding RA activation). *B*, Orthodromic tachycardia and ipsilateral functional bundle branch block. *C*, Antidromic tachycardia with anterograde conduction over the accessory pathway and retrograde conduction over the AV node-His bundle. *D*, Orthodromic tachycardia with a slowly conducting accessory pathway. *E*, Atrial fibrillation with the accessory pathway as a bystander. *F*, Anterograde conduction over a portion of the AV node and a nodoventricular pathway and retrograde conduction over the AV node.

by inducing premature ventricular complexes during tachycardia to determine whether retrograde atrial preexcitation can occur at a time when the His bundle is refractory (Fig. 22–27*B*). Since ventriculoatrial conduction cannot occur over the normal conduction system because the His bundle is refractory, an accessory pathway must be present for the atria to become preexcited and must be participating in the tachycardia circuit. No patient with a reciprocating tachycardia due to an accessory AV pathway has a V-A interval less than 70 msec measured from the onset of ventricular depolarization to the onset of the earliest atrial activity recorded on an esophageal lead or less than 95 msec when measured to the high right atrium. In contrast, in the majority of patients with reentry in the AV node, intervals from the onset of ventricular activity to the earliest onset of atrial activity recorded in the esophageal lead are less than 70 msec.[150]

OTHER FORMS OF TACHYCARDIA IN PATIENTS WITH WPW SYNDROME. Patients may have other types of tachycardia during which the accessory pathway is a "bystander," i.e., uninvolved in the mechanism responsible for the tachycardia, such as AV nodal reentry or an atrial tachycardia that conducts to the ventricle over the accessory pathway.[144, 182a] In patients with atrial flutter or atrial fibrillation, the accessory pathway is not a requisite part of the mechanism responsible for tachycardia, and the flutter or fibrillation occurs in the atrium unrelated to the accessory pathway (Fig. 22–28*E*). Propagation to the ventricle during atrial flutter or atrial fibrillation therefore can occur over the normal AV node–His bundle or accessory pathway. Patients with WPW syndrome who have atrial fibrillation almost always have inducible reciprocating tachycardias as well, which may develop into the atrial fibrillation (Fig. 22–30). In fact, interruption of the accessory pathway and elimination of AV reciprocating tachycardia prevents recurrence of the atrial fibrillation.[183] Atrial fibrillation presents a potentially serious risk because of the possibility for very rapid conduction over the accessory pathway. At more rapid rates, the refractory period of the accessory pathway may shorten significantly and permit an extremely rapid ventricular response during atrial flutter or atrial fibrillation (Figs. 22–23*B* and 22–30) that may lead to ventricular fibrillation.[164, 184] The rapid ventricular response probably exceeds the ability of the ventricle to follow in an organized fashion, resulting in fragmented disorganized ventricular activation and hypotension, and leads to ventricular fibrillation. Alternatively, supraventricular discharge bypassing AV nodal delay may activate the ventricle during the vulnerable period of the antecedent T wave and precipitate ventricular fibrillation. Patients who have had ventricular fibrillation have ventricular cycle lengths during atrial fibrillation in the range of 200 msec or less.[184]

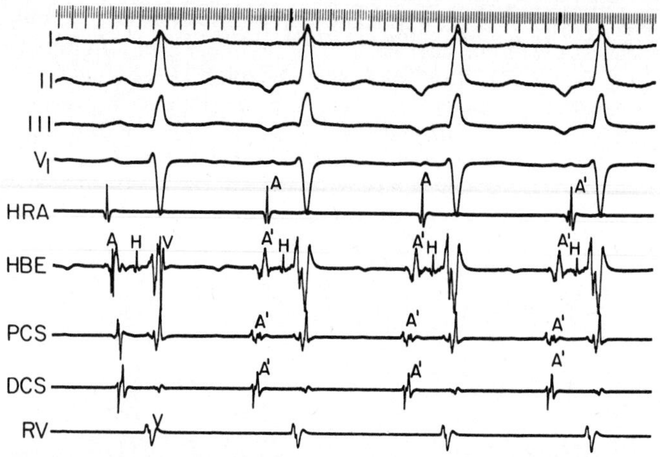

FIGURE 22–29. Permanent form of AV junctional reciprocating tachycardia (PJRT). The first complex is initiated by sinus discharge, while the morphology of the subsequent P waves change. The high right atrium probably is still discharged by the sinus node for the second and third P waves which represent fusion P waves. The fourth P wave represents full activation of the atrium during the tachycardia. The atrial activation sequence during the tachycardia demonstrates initial activation in the proximal coronary sinus (PCS) followed by recording in the distal coronary sinus (DCS), then low right atrium (HBE), and then finally high right atrium (HRA). Premature ventricular stimulation during tachycardia at a time when His bundle was refractory preexcited the atrium retrogradely (during isoproterenol infusion to shorten the refractory period of this slowly conducting accessory pathway), thus proving the existence of an accessory atrioventricular pathway. Note the PR-RP relationship and P wave contour that resemble Figure 22–21*A*. Not shown, during retrograde conduction over the AV node His bundle axis, retrograde atrial activation was recorded first in the HBE lead.

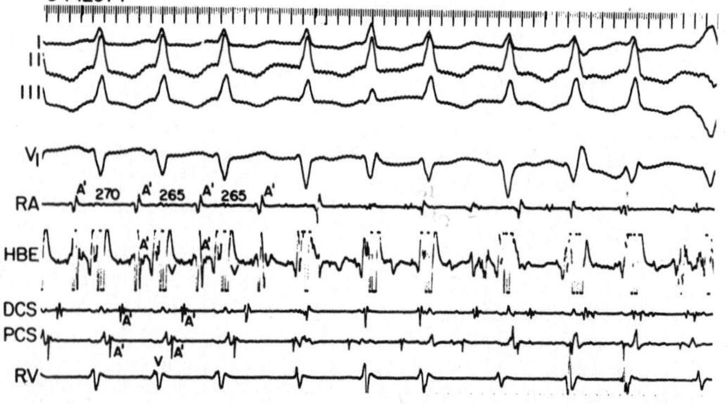

FIGURE 22–30. AV reciprocating tachycardia disorganizing into atrial fibrillation. Same patient as in Figure 22–23*B*. During sustained atrioventricular reciprocating tachycardia at a cycle length of approximately 265 msec, retrograde atrial activation sequence begins first in the right paraseptal region (not shown in this example; location proven at surgery) and was then recorded in the proximal coronary sinus electrogram, followed by atrial activity in the distal coronary sinus, in the low right atrium recorded in the His bundle lead and then in the high right atrium. Spontaneously, the atrial activation sequence becomes irregular (after the last A′) and atrial fibrillation begins. Note that the last QRS complex reflects conduction over the accessory pathway. Such a transformation occurred repeatedly in this patient and was associated with a quickening of the ventricular rate. Atrial fibrillation did not recur following surgical interruption of the accessory pathway.

Finally, it is important to remember that patients with preexcitation syndrome may have other causes of tachycardia such as AV nodal reentry,[144] sometimes with dual AV nodal curves, sinus nodal reentry, or even electrically inducible ventricular tachycardia unrelated to the accessory pathway.[185, 186] Accessory pathways may conduct only anterogradely as well as only retrogradely.[144, 187] If the pathway conducts only anterogradely, it cannot participate in the usual form of reciprocating tachycardia (Fig. 22–28*A*). It can, however, participate in antidromic tachycardia (Fig. 22–28C) as well as conduct to the ventricle during atrial flutter or atrial fibrillation (Fig. 22–28*E*). Some data suggest that the accessory pathway demonstrates automatic activity,[49, 187a] which could conceivably be responsible for some instances of tachycardia.

"Wide QRS tachycardias" in patients with the preexcitation syndrome may be due to multiple mechanisms including sinus or atrial tachycardias, AV nodal reentry, atrial flutter or fibrillation with anterograde conduction over the accessory pathway; orthodromic reciprocating tachycardia with functional or preexisting bundle branch block; antidromic reciprocating tachycardia; reciprocating tachycardia with anterograde conduction over one accessory pathway, and retrograde conduction over a second one; tachycardias using Mahaim fibers; or ventricular tachycardia.

CLINICAL FEATURES. The reported incidence of preexcitation syndrome depends in large measure on the population studied, varying from 0.1 to 3.0 per thousand in apparently healthy subjects, with an average of about 1.5 per thousand. The incidence of the electrocardiographic pattern of Wolff-Parkinson-White conduction in 22,500 healthy aviation personnel was 0.25 per cent with a prevalence of documented tachyarrhythmias of 1.8 per cent. Based on the delta wave vector in the ECG, left-sided pathways are more common than right and are more often associated with paroxysmal tachycardias.[188] WPW is found in all age groups, from the newborn to the elderly, and in identical twins. The prevalence is higher in males and decreases with age, apparently due to loss of preexcitation.[188] The majority of adults with preexcitation syndrome have normal hearts, although a variety of acquired and congenital cardiac defects have been reported, including Ebstein's anomaly,[189] mitral valve prolapse,[190] and cardiomyopathies. Patients with Ebstein's anomaly (p. 951) often have multiple accessory pathways, right-sided either in the posterior septum or posterolateral wall, with preexcitation localized to the atrialized ventricle. They often have reciprocating tachycardia with a long V-A interval and a right bundle branch block morphology.[189]

The frequency of paroxysmal tachycardia apparently increases with age, from 10 per 100 cases of WPW in a 20- to 39-year age group to 36 per 100 in patients more than 60 years old.[188] Approximately 80 per cent of patients with tachycardia have a reciprocating tachycardia, 15 to 30 per cent have atrial fibrillation, and 5 per cent atrial flutter. Ventricular tachycardia occurs uncommonly. The anomalous complexes may mask or mimic myocardial infarction (p. 211), bundle branch block, or ventricular hypertrophy, and the presence of the preexcitation syndrome may call attention to an associated cardiac defect. The prognosis is excellent in patients without tachycardia or an associated cardiac anomaly. In patients with recurrent tachycardia the prognosis is good in most, but sudden death occurs rarely. In one study, it occurred in 1 of 151 patients followed 1 to 11 years.[188]

It is very likely that acquisition of an accessory pathway occurs congenitally, although its manifestations may be detected in later years and appear to be "acquired."[154] Relatives of patients with preexcitation, particularly those with multiple pathways, have an increased prevalence of preexcitation, suggesting a hereditary mode of acquisition.[190a] Some children and adults may lose their tendency to develop tachyarrhythmias as they grow older, possibly owing to fibrotic or other changes at the site of the accessory pathway insertion. Intermittent preexcitation during sinus rhythm[191] and loss of conduction over the accessory pathway after intravenous ajmaline or procainamide and with exercise suggest that the refractory period of the accessory pathway is long and that the patient is not at risk of developing a rapid ventricular rate should atrial flutter or fibrillation develop.[192] Exceptions to these safeguards may occur.[193]

TREATMENT. Patients with ventricular preexcitation may have no or only occasional tachyarrhythmias unassociated with significant symptoms. These patients do not require electrophysiological evaluation or therapy. However, if a patient has frequent episodes of tachyarrhythmias and/or the arrhythmias cause significant symptoms, therapy should be instituted. Those who suffer significant hemodynamic consequences from the tachycardia should be considered for electrophysiological study (p. 611).

Three therapeutic options exist: electrical ablation (p. 644), surgical (p. 645), and pharmacological. Drugs are chosen to prolong conduction time and/or refractoriness in the AV node, the accessory pathway, or both to prevent rapid rates from occurring. If successful, this would prevent maintenance of an AV reciprocating tachycardia or a rapid ventricular response to atrial flutter or atrial fibrillation. Some drugs might suppress premature complexes that precipitate the arrhythmias.

Verapamil, propranolol, and digitalis all prolong conduction time and refractoriness in the AV node. Verapamil[109] and propranolol do not directly affect conduction in the accessory pathway, while digitalis has had variable effects. Because digitalis has been reported to shorten refractoriness in the accessory pathway and speed the ventricular response in some patients with atrial fibrillation, it is advisable *not* to use digitalis as a single drug in patients with the WPW syndrome who have or may develop atrial flutter or atrial fibrillation. Since many patients may develop atrial fibrillation *during* the reciprocating tachycardia (Fig. 22–30), this caveat probably applies to *all* patients who have tachycardia and the WPW syndrome. Rather, drugs that prolong the refractory period in the accessory pathway such as class IA and IC drugs (Chap. 21) should be used. Class IC drugs and amiodarone can affect both the AV node and the accessory pathway. Lidocaine does not prolong refractoriness of the accessory pathway in patients whose effective refractory period $\leq$ 300 msec.[194] Verapamil[109, 195] and lidocaine[194] may increase the ventricular rate during atrial fibrillation in patients with the WPW syndrome. Intravenous verapamil may precipitate *ventricular fibrillation* when given to a patient with WPW syndrome who has a rapid ventricular rate during atrial fibrillation. This does not appear to happen with *oral* verapamil. Isoproterenol may expose WPW syndrome and shorten the refractory period of the accessory pathway.[196]

Termination of the acute episode of reciprocating tachycardia, suspected electrocardiographically by a normal QRS complex, regular R-R intervals, a rate of about 200 beats/min, and a P wave in the ST segment, should be approached as for AV nodal reentry. Following vagal maneuvers, verapamil or a similar calcium-entry blocker or edrophonium should be considered as the initial treatment of choice. For atrial flutter or fibrillation, the latter suspected by an anomalous QRS complex and grossly irregular R-R intervals (Figs. 22–23*B* and 22–30), drugs that prolong refractoriness in the accessory pathway often coupled with drugs that prolong AV nodal refractoriness (e.g., procainamide and propranolol) must be used. In some patients, particularly with a very rapid ventricular response, electrical cardioversion should be the *initial* treatment of choice.

Prevention. For long-term therapy to prevent a recurrence, it is not always possible to predict which drugs may be most effective for an individual patient. Some drugs actually can increase the frequency of episodes of reciprocating tachycardia by prolonging the duration of anterograde and not retrograde refractory periods of the accessory pathway, thereby making it easier for a premature atrial complex to block anterogradely in the accessory pathway and initiate tachycardia. Oral administration of two drugs, such as quinidine and propranolol or procainamide and verapamil, to decrease conduction capabilities in both limbs of the reentrant circuit may be beneficial. Depending on the clinical situation, empirical drug trials or serial electrophysiological drug testing may be employed to determine optimal drug therapy for patients with reciprocating tachycardia. For patients who have atrial fibrillation with a rapid ventricular response, induction of atrial fibrillation while the patient is receiving therapy is essential to be certain that the ventricular rate is controlled.

Electrical or *surgical ablation* of the accessory pathway is advisable for patients with frequent symptomatic arrhythmias that are not fully controlled by drugs or with rapid AV conduction over the accessory pathway during atrial flutter or fibrillation and in whom significant slowing of the ventricular response during tachycardia cannot be obtained by drug therapy. Patients who have accessory pathways with very short refractory periods may be poor candidates for drug therapy, since the refractory periods may be prolonged insignificantly in response to the standard agents.[197] *Pacing therapy* may be useful in this syndrome as in many other supraventricular tachyarrhythmias, with the exception that precipitation of atrial flutter or atrial fibrillation in a patient with an accessory pathway may result in very rapid ventricular rates and clinical deterioration. Interruption of the accessory pathway should be considered before an antitachycardia device is implanted.

In *summary*, electrocardiographic clues are often present that permit differential diagnosis of the various supraventricular tachycardias (Table 22–2). P waves during tachycardia identical to sinus P waves and occurring with a long R-P interval and a short P-R interval are most likely due to sinus nodal reentry. Retrograde (inverted in II, III, and aV_f) P waves generally represent reentry involving the AV junction, either AV nodal reentry or reciprocating tachycardia using a paraseptal accessory pathway. Tachycardia without manifest P waves is probably due to AV nodal reentry (P waves buried in QRS), while a tachycardia with an R-P interval exceeding 60 to 70 msec may be due to an accessory pathway. AV dissociation or AV block during tachycardia excludes the presence of a functioning AV accessory pathway and makes AV nodal reentry less likely. Multiple tachycardias can occur at different times in the same patient.[109]

VENTRICULAR RHYTHM DISTURBANCES

PREMATURE VENTRICULAR COMPLEXES

ELECTROCARDIOGRAPHIC RECOGNITION. A premature ventricular complex is characterized by the premature occurrence of a QRS complex that is bizarre in shape and has a duration usually exceeding the dominant QRS complex, generally greater than 120 msec. The T wave is commonly large and opposite in direction to the major deflection of the QRS. The QRS complex is not preceded by a premature P wave but may be preceded by a sinus P wave occurring at its expected time. The diagnosis of premature ventricular complex can never be made with unequivocal certainty from the scalar electrocardiogram, since a supraventricular beat or rhythm may mimic the manifestations of ventricular arrhythmia (Figs. 22–15 and 22–31). Retrograde transmission to the atria from the premature ventricular complex occurs fairly frequently but is often obscured by the distorted QRS complex and T wave. If the retrograde impulse discharges and resets the sinus node prematurely, it produces a pause that is not fully compensatory. More commonly, the sinus node and atria are not discharged prematurely by the retrograde impulse, since interference of impulses frequently occurs at the AV junction (see p. 707), establishing a collision

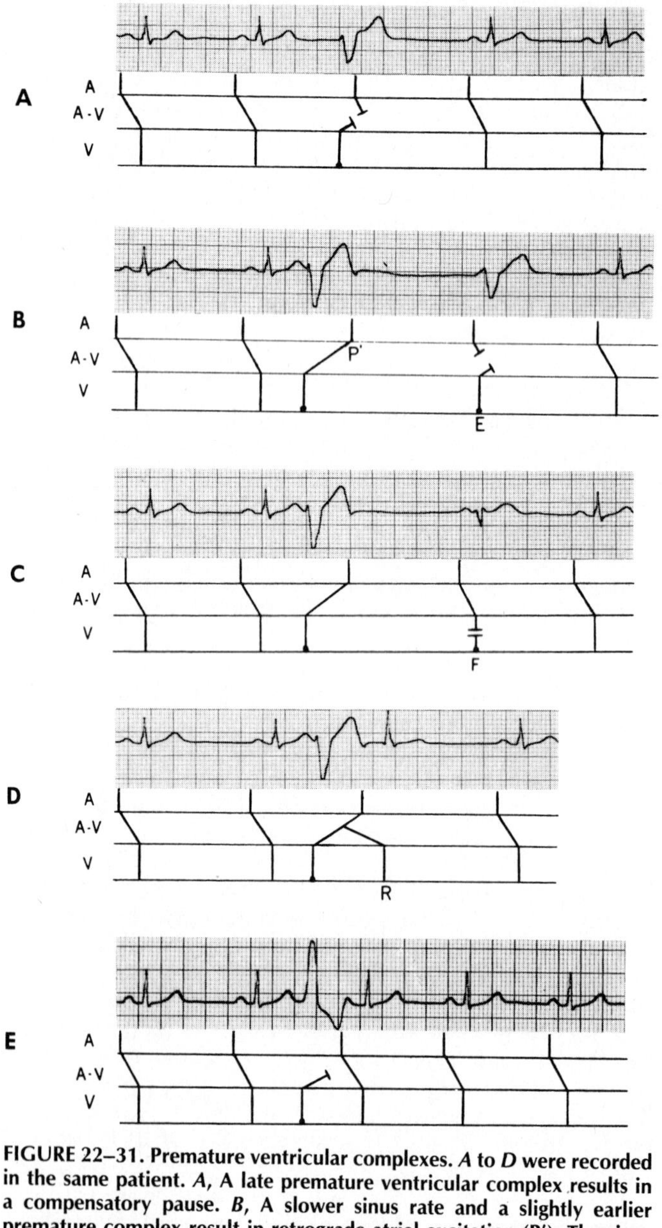

FIGURE 22–31. Premature ventricular complexes. *A* to *D* were recorded in the same patient. *A*, A late premature ventricular complex results in a compensatory pause. *B*, A slower sinus rate and a slightly earlier premature complex result in retrograde atrial excitation (P′). The sinus node is reset, producing a noncompensatory pause. Before the sinus-initiated P wave that follows the retrograde P wave can conduct to the ventricle, a ventricular escape occurs (E). *C*, Events are similar to those in *B* except that a ventricular fusion beat (F) results following the premature ventricular complex owing to a slightly faster sinus rate. *D*, The impulse propagating retrogradely to the atrium reverses its direction after a delay and returns to reexcite the ventricles (R) to produce a ventricular echo. *E*, An interpolated premature ventricular complex is followed by a slightly prolonged P-R interval of the sinus-initiated beat. Lead II.

between the anterograde impulse conducted from the sinus node and the retrograde impulse conducted from the premature ventricular complex. Therefore, a fully compensatory pause usually follows a premature ventricular complex: the R-R interval produced by the two sinus-initiated QRS complexes on either side of the premature complex equals twice the normally conducted R-R interval. The premature ventricular complex may not produce any pause and may therefore be interpolated (Fig. 22–31), or it may produce a postponed compensatory pause when an interpolated premature complex causes P-R prolongation of the first post-extrasystolic beat to such a degree that the P wave of the second post-extrasystolic beat occurs at a very short R-P interval and is therefore blocked.

Interference within the ventricle may result in *ventricular fusion beats* (p. 694), which may be narrower than the dominant beat, as when a right bundle branch block pattern of a premature ventricular complex arising in the left ventricle fuses with the sinus-initiated complex conducting through the AV junction with a left bundle branch block pattern, or when the ventricle with a bundle branch block pattern is paced artificially, producing a narrow ventricular fusion beat between the paced and the sinus-conducted beats. Narrow premature ventricular complexes also have been explained as originating at a point equidistant from each ventricle in the ventricular septum and by arising high in the fascicular system. Whether a compensatory or noncompensatory pause, retrograde atrial excitation, or an interpolated complex, fusion complex, or echo beat occurs (Fig. 22–31), it is merely a function of how the AV junction conducts and the timing of the events taking place.

The term *bigeminy* refers to pairs of complexes and indicates a normal and premature complex; *trigeminy* indicates a premature complex following two normal beats; a premature complex following three normal beats is called *quadrigeminy*, and so on. Two successive premature ventricular complexes are termed a pair or a couplet, while three successive premature ventricular complexes are called a triplet. Arbitrarily, three or more successive premature ventricular complexes are termed ventricular tachycardia. Premature ventricular complexes may have different contours and often are called multifocal (Fig. 22–32). More properly they should be called "multiform," "polymorphic," or "pleomorphic," since it is not known whether multiple foci are discharging or whether conduction of the impulse originating from one site is merely changing.

Premature ventricular complexes may exhibit fixed or variable coupling, i.e., the interval between the normal QRS complex and the premature ventricular complex may be relatively stable or variable. Fixed coupling may be due to reentry, triggered activity (p. 597), or other possible mechanisms. Variable coupling may be due to parasystole (p. 708), to changing conduction in a reentrant circuit, or to changing discharge rates of triggered activity. Usually, it is difficult to determine the precise mechanism responsible for the premature ventricular complex with either constant or variable coupling intervals.

CLINICAL FEATURES. The prevalence of premature complexes increases with age. Their presence may be manifested by symptoms of palpitations or discomfort in the neck or chest because of the greater than normal contractile force of the post-extrasystolic beat or the feeling that the heart has stopped during the long pause after the premature complex. Long runs of frequent premature ventricular complexes in patients with heart disease may produce angina or hypotension. Frequent interpolated premature ventricular complexes actually represent a doubling of the heart rate and may compromise the patient's hemodynamic status. Activity that increases the heart rate may decrease the patient's awareness of the premature systoles or reduce their number. Exercise may increase the number of premature complexes in other patients. Premature systoles may be quite uncomfortable in patients who have aortic regurgitation because of the large stroke volume. Sleep may be associated with a decrease or with an increase in the frequency of ventricular arrhythmias in some patients.[198, 199]

Premature ventricular complexes occur in association with a variety of stimuli and can be produced by direct mechanical, electrical, and chemical stimulation of the myocardium. Often they are noted in patients with left ventricular false tendons,[200] during infection, in ischemic or inflamed myocardium, and during hypoxia,[201] anesthesia, or surgery. They may be provoked by a variety of medications, by electrolyte imbalance, by tension states, and by excessive use of tobacco, caffeine, or alcohol. Both central and peripheral autonomic stimulation have profound effects on heart rate, which may produce or suppress premature complexes.[202]

Physical examination reveals the presence of a premature beat followed by a pause that is longer than normal. A fully compensatory pause may be distinguished from one that is not fully compensatory, since the former does not change the timing of the basic rhythm. The premature beat is often accompanied by a decrease in intensity of the heart sounds, often with just the first heart sound being heard, which may be sharp and snapping, and a decreased or absent peripheral (e.g., radial) pulse. The relationship of atrial to ventricular systole determines the presence of normal *a* waves or giant *a* waves in the jugular venous pulse, and the length of the P-R interval determines the intensity of the first heart sound. The second heart sound may be abnormally split.

The importance of premature ventricular complexes varies depending on the clinical setting. In the absence of underlying heart disease, the presence of premature ventricular complexes usually has no significance regarding longevity or limitation of activity, and antiarrhythmic drugs are not indicated; the patient should be reassured if he or she is symptomatic (see Chap. 20, Exercise Testing and Long-Term ECG Recording). An exception may be middle-aged men, because premature ventricular systoles and

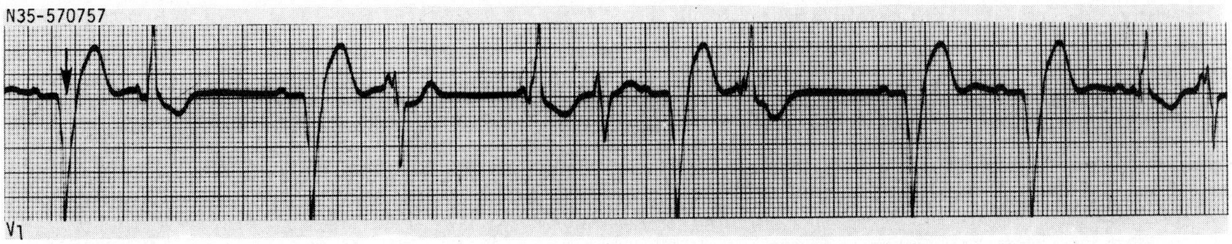

FIGURE 22–32. Multiform premature ventricular complexes. The normally conducted QRS complexes exhibit a left bundle branch block contour (arrow) and are followed by premature ventricular complexes with three different morphologies.

complex ventricular arrhythmias occurring in apparently healthy middle-aged men are associated with the presence of coronary heart disease and with a greater risk of subsequent death from coronary heart disease. However, it has not been demonstrated that premature ventricular systoles or complex ventricular arrhythmias play a *precipitating* role in the genesis of sudden death in these patients, and the arrhythmias may simply be a marker of heart disease. It has not been shown convincingly that antiarrhythmic therapy given to suppress the premature ventricular systoles or complex ventricular arrhythmias reduces the incidence of sudden death in such apparently healthy men. A strong association exists between myocardial infarction size and left ventricular function and frequency of premature ventricular complexes.[203, 204]

In patients suffering from acute myocardial infarction, so-called "warning arrhythmias," such as premature ventricular complexes occurring close to the preceding T wave, greater than five or six per minute, bigeminal, multiform, or occurring in salvoes of two, three, or more, do not occur in about half the patients who develop ventricular fibrillation and about half of those patients who do have "warning arrhythmias" do not develop ventricular fibrillation. Electrophysiological testing may be useful to identify patients at increased risk of developing ventricular tachycardia or sudden cardiac death after myocardial infarction,[205] although such studies presently are controversial.[206] They may be useful in patients with high-grade premature ventricular complexes to identify a high-risk group.[207]

TREATMENT. Extremes of heart rate, both fast and slow, may provoke the development of premature ventricular complexes. Premature ventricular complexes accompanying slow ventricular rates caused by sinus bradycardia or AV block may be abolished by increasing the basic rate with atropine or isoproterenol or by pacing, while slowing the heart rate in some patients with sinus tachycardia may eradicate premature ventricular complexes. In the hospitalized patient, lidocaine given intravenously (p. 625) is generally the initial treatment of choice to suppress premature ventricular complexes. If maximum dosages of lidocaine are unsuccessful, then procainamide intravenously may be tried. Quinidine may be given intravenously slowly and cautiously. The use of disopyramide intravenously is still investigational. Propranolol may be tried if the other drugs have been unsuccessful. For long-term oral maintenance, a variety of class I and III drugs may be useful, as for the prevention of ventricular tachycardia (p. 697). Class IC drugs seem particularly successful in suppressing premature ventricular complexes. Beta blockers have reduced the frequency of ventricular arrhythmias in patients after myocardial infarction.[208]

VENTRICULAR TACHYCARDIA

Ventricular tachycardia (VT) arises in the specialized conduction system distal to the bifurcation of the His bundle, in ventricular muscle, or in combinations of both tissue types. The mechanisms include disorders of impulse formation and conduction (p. 707). The electrocardiographic diagnosis of ventricular tachycardia is suggested by the occurrence of a series of three or more bizarrely shaped premature ventricular complexes whose duration exceeds 120 msec, with the ST-T vector pointing opposite to the major QRS deflection. The R-R interval may be exceedingly regular or may vary. Many patients have VT's with multiple morphologies originating at the same or closely adjacent sites, probably with different exit paths.[209] Others have multiple sites of origin.[210] Atrial activity may be independent of ventricular activity (AV dissociation, p. 707), or the atria may be depolarized by the ventricles retrogradely (VA association). Depending on the particular type of VT, the rate ranges from 70 to 250 beats/min, and the onset may be paroxysmal (sudden) or nonparoxysmal. QRS contours during the VT may be unchanging (uniform, monomorphic), may vary randomly (multiform, polymorphic, or pleomorphic), vary in a more or less repetitive manner (torsades de pointes), vary in alternate complexes (bidirectional ventricular tachycardia), or vary in a stable but changing contour (i.e., right bundle branch contour changing to left bundle branch contour). VT may be sustained, defined arbitrarily as lasting longer than 30 sec or requiring termination because of hemodynamic collapse, or nonsustained (unsustained),[211] when it stops spontaneously in less than 30 sec.[212–214] Patients who present with nonsustained VT and ventricular fibrillation may have electrically inducible arrhythmias easier to suppress with drug treatment than those who present with sustained VT.[215]

Making the electrocardiographic distinction between supraventricular tachycardia with aberration and VT may be extremely difficult at times, since features of both arrhythmias overlap and under certain circumstances a supraventricular tachycardia can mimic all the criteria established for VT. Ventricular complexes with bizarre or prolonged configuration indicate only that conduction through the ventricle is abnormal, and such complexes can occur in supraventricular rhythms due to preexisting bundle branch block, aberrant conduction during incomplete recovery of repolarization, conduction over accessory pathways, and several other conditions. These complexes do not necessarily indicate the origin of impulse formation or the reason for the abnormal conduction. Conversely, ectopic beats originating in the ventricle uncommonly can have a fairly normal duration and shape.

During the course of a tachycardia characterized by widespread, bizarre QRS complexes, the presence of *fusion beats* and *capture beats* provides maximum support for the diagnosis of VT (Table 22–3, p. 702). Fusion beats indicate activation of the ventricle from two different foci, implying that one of the foci had a ventricular origin. Capture of the ventricle by the supraventricular rhythm with a normal configuration of the captured QRS complex at an interval shorter than the tachycardia in question indicates that the impulse has a supraventricular origin (Fig. 22–33). Atrioventricular dissociation (p. 707) has long been considered a hallmark of VT. However, retrograde VA conduction to the atria from ventricular beats occurs in a large percentage of patients, and therefore VT may not exhibit AV dissociation. Atrioventricular dissociation can occur uncommonly during supraventricular tachycardias (see Fig. 20–35A, p. 613). Even if a P wave appears to be related to each QRS complex it is at times difficult to determine whether the P wave is conducted anterogradely to the next QRS complex (i.e., supraventricular tachycardia with aberrancy and a long P-R interval) or retrogradely from the preceding QRS complex (i.e., a VT). As a general rule, however, AV dissociation during a wide QRS tachycardia is strong presumptive evidence that the tachycardia is of ventricular origin.

Because of the overlapping features of ventricular and supraventricular tachycardias, and because differentiating clues may not be present on a given tracing, it appears best to ascribe a certain probability to the diagnosis that may weigh in favor of its ventricular or supraventricular origin. Some electrocardiographic features characterizing supraventricular arrhythmia with aberrancy include (1)

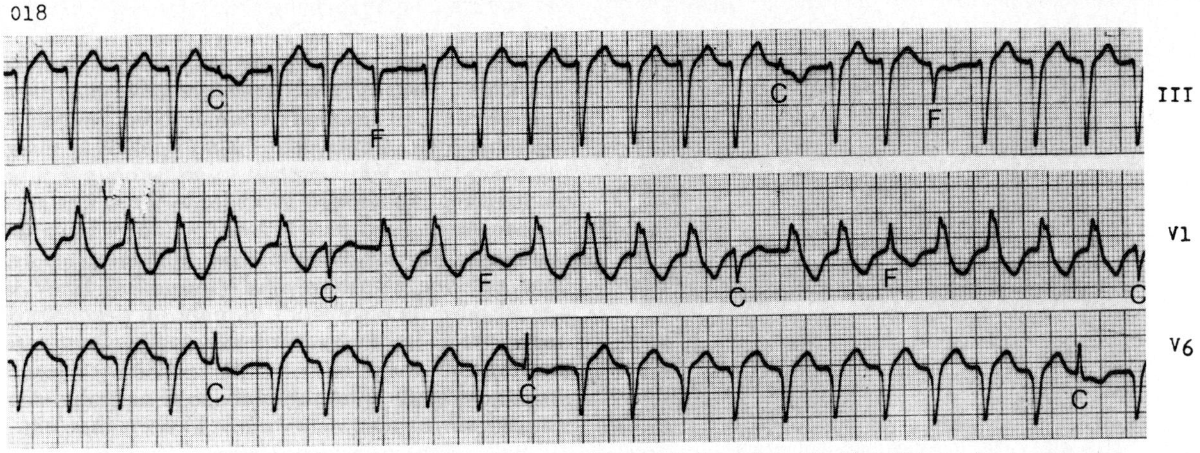

FIGURE 22–33. Fusions and capture beats during a probable ventricular tachycardia. The QRS complex is prolonged, and the R-R interval is regular except for occasional capture beats (C) that have a normal contour and are slightly premature. Complexes intermediate in contour represent fusion beats (F). Thus, even though atrial activity is not clearly apparent, it is likely that AV dissociation is present during a ventricular tachycardia and produces intermittent capture and fusion beats.

consistent onset of the tachycardia with a premature P wave, (2) a very short R-P interval (≤ 0.1 sec) often requiring an esophageal recording to visualize the P waves, (3) a QRS configuration the same as that which occurs from known supraventricular conduction at similar rates, (4) P and QRS rate and rhythm linked to suggest that ventricular activation depends on atrial discharge (e.g., A-V Wenckebach block), and (5) slowing or termination of the tachycardia by vagal maneuvers.

Analysis of specific QRS contours also may be helpful.[216] For example, QRS contours suggesting a VT include left-axis deviation in the frontal plane and a QRS duration exceeding 140 msec with a QRS of normal duration during sinus rhythm. During VT with right bundle branch block appearance, (1) the QRS complex is monophasic or biphasic in V_1 with an initial deflection different from sinus-initiated QRS complex, (2) the amplitude of the R wave in V_1 exceeds the R′, and (3) small R and large S wave or a QS pattern in V_6 may be present. With a VT having a left bundle branch block contour, (1) the axis may be rightward with negative deflections deeper in V_1 than in V_6, (2) a broad prolonged (> 40 msec) R wave in V_1, and (3) a small Q, large R wave or QS pattern in V_6 may exist. A QRS complex that is similar in V_1 through V_6, either all negative or all positive, favors a ventricular origin as does the presence of 2:1 ventriculoatrial block. (An upright QRS complex in V_1 through V_6 also may occur due to conduction over a left-sided accessory pathway.) Supraventricular beats with aberration often have a triphasic pattern in V_1, an initial vector of the abnormal complex similar to that of the normally conducted beats, and a wide QRS complex that terminates a short cycle length which follows a long cycle (long-short cycle sequence). During atrial fibrillation fixed coupling, short coupling intervals, a long pause after the abnormal beat, and runs of bigeminy rather than a consecutive series of abnormal complexes, all favor ventricular origin of the premature complex rather than supraventricular origin with aberration.[217] A grossly irregular, wide QRS tachycardia with ventricular rates faster than 200 beats/min should raise the question of atrial fibrillation with conduction over an accessory pathway (see p. 690 and Figs. 22–23*B* and 22–30).[217–219] In the presence of preexisting bundle branch block, a wide QRS tachycardia with a contour different from that which occurred during sinus rhythm is most likely a VT.[220] Exceptions exist to all the criteria enumerated above, especially in patients who have preexisting conduction disturbances or preexcitation syndrome; when in doubt, one must rely on sound clinical judgment, considering the ECG as only one of several helpful ancillary tests.[216]

ELECTROPHYSIOLOGICAL FEATURES. Electrophysiologically, VT can be distinguished by a short or negative H-V interval (i.e., H begins after the onset of ventricular depolarization) because of retrograde activation from the ventricles (see Fig. 20–35, p. 613, and Fig. 22–34). His bundle deflections dissociated from ventricular activation are diagnostic of VT,[221] with rare exception.[222] His bundle deflections usually are not apparent because they are obscured by simultaneous ventricular septal depolarization or because of inadequate catheter position. The latter must be determined during supraventricular rhythm before the onset or after the termination of the ventricular tachycardia. VT may produce QRS complexes of narrow duration and of short H-V interval, most likely when the site of origin is close to the His bundle in the fascicles.[223]

Successful electrical induction of VT by premature stimulation of the ventricle (Fig. 22–34)[221] depends on the characteristics of the VT and the anatomical substrate. Patients with sustained VT and VT due to coronary artery disease have VT induced more frequently than patients who have nonsustained VT and VT due to noncoronary-related causes.[212] In general, it is more difficult to induce VT with late premature stimuli compared to early premature stimuli, during sinus rhythm compared to ventricular pacing, and with one premature stimulus compared to two or three. The specificity of VT induction using more than two premature ventricular stimuli begins to decrease (while the sensitivity increases), and nonsustained pleomorphic VT or ventricular fibrillation can be induced in patients who have no history of ventricular tachycardia.[224, 225] Occasionally, VT can be initiated only from the left ventricle[221] or from specific sites in the right ventricle.[226] Multiple premature stimuli reduce the need for left ventricular stimulation. Drugs such as isoproterenol, various antiarrhythmic agents, and alcohol can facilitate the induction of ventricular tachycardia..

Termination of VT by pacing depends significantly on the rate of the VT. Slower VT's are more easily terminated and with fewer stimuli than are more rapid VT's. An increasing number of stimuli are required to terminate more rapid VT's, which increases the risks of pacing-induced acceleration of the VT.[227] Following premature

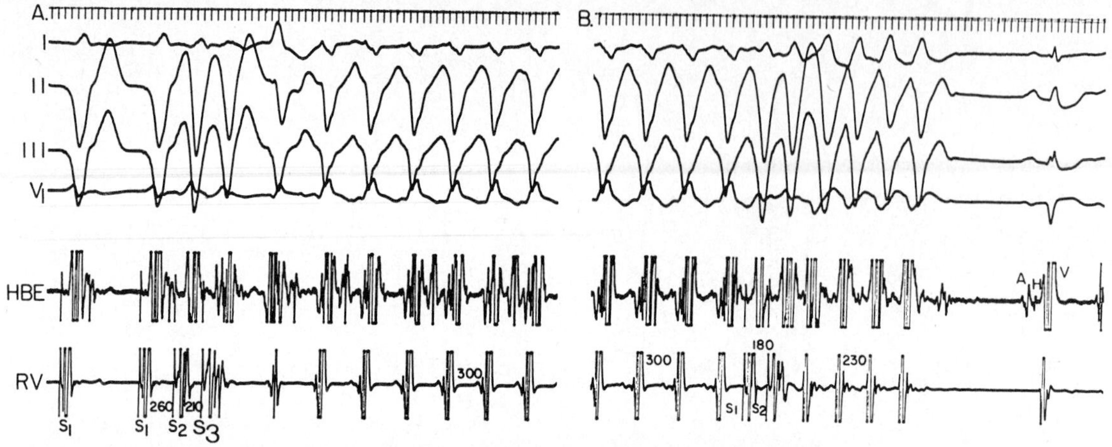

FIGURE 22–34. Initiation and termination of ventricular tachycardia using programmed ventricular stimulation. The last two ventricular-paced beats at a cycle length of 600 msec are shown in panel A. A premature stimulus (S_2) at an S_1-S_2 interval of 260 msec and another premature stimulus (S_3) at a cycle length of 210 msec initiate a sustained monomorphic ventricular tachycardia at a cycle length of 300 msec. Two premature ventricular stimuli (S_1-S_2) in panel B create an unstable ventricular tachycardia which persists for several beats at a shorter cycle length (230 msec) and then terminates, followed by sinus rhythm.

stimulation during VT, a pause may result but the tachycardia continues, suggesting that the origin of the tachycardia is relatively protected.[70, 228] VT can also be induced and terminated during atrial pacing (see Fig. 20–36, p. 613).[70, 71]

With the advent of acceptable surgical techniques to treat some forms of VT (p. 646), it has become important to localize its origin. The 12-lead electrocardiogram may give misleading information regarding the origin of sustained VT[229] and extensive endocardial and epicardial mapping studies are generally necessary (see Chap. 20). *Echocardiography* and *radionuclide phase mapping* of VT may provide additional data on the site of origin of VT[230, 231] (see Chap. 20).

CLINICAL FEATURES. Symptoms occurring during VT depend on the ventricular rate, duration of tachycardia, the presence and extent of the underlying heart disease, and peripheral vascular disease. The location of impulse formation and therefore the way in which the depolarization wave spreads across the myocardium may also be important.[232] Physical findings depend in part on the P to QRS relationship. If atrial activity is dissociated from the ventricular contractions, the findings of AV dissociation (p. 707) will be present. If the atria are captured retrogradely, regularly occurring cannon *a* waves appear when atrial and ventricular contractions occur simultaneously and the signs of AV dissociation are absent.

More than half of the patients treated for symptomatic recurrent VT have ischemic heart disease. The next biggest group has cardiomyopathy (both congestive and hypertrophic), with lesser percentages divided among those with primary electrical disease, mitral valve prolapse, valvular heart disease, and miscellaneous causes. Coronary artery spasm may cause transient myocardial ischemia with severe ventricular arrhythmias (during ischemia and during the apparent reperfusion period) in some patients.[233–237] Complex ventricular arrhythmias may occur *after* coronary artery bypass grafting.[238, 239] In patients resuscitated from sudden cardiac death (Chap. 24) the majority (75 per cent) have severe coronary artery disease and ventricular tachyarrhythmias can be induced by premature ventricular stimulation in approximately 75 per cent.[240, 241] When VT occurs in the ambulatory patient, it is uncommonly induced by R-on-T premature ventricular complexes (see Ventricular Fibrillation).[242] Even short runs of VT consisting of three or four complexes after myocardial infarction portend increased mortality. Left ventricular dysfunction and ventricular arrhythmias are independently related to mortality risk in the 2 years after myocadial infarction.[243] Sustained recurrent VT can also occur in children with or without associated cardiovascular disease.[244, 245] In some patients an acute emotional disturbance may be related temporally to the onset of life-threatening ventricular arrhythmias. While the causal role played by the emotional stress in some patients seems to be established, the mechanism(s) is unclear.[246]

Termination of a tachycardia by triggering vagal reflexes is considered diagnostic of supraventricular tachycardias. However, VT uncommonly can be stopped in a similar manner.[7] Valsalva may terminate VT related to an abrupt reduction in cardiac dimension.[247]

TREATMENT. The most important decision is which patients should be treated. The relative risks of symptoms or sudden death for each type of VT determine the course of therapy. Generally, patients who have sustained VT with or without structural heart disease and those who have nonsustained VT with structural heart disease are treated. Patients who have nonsustained VT without structural heart disease but are symptomatic should be treated while those who are asymptomatic and otherwise healthy may not need therapy and should be followed closely.

VT that does not cause hemodynamic decompensation can be treated medically to achieve acute termination by administering intravenous lidocaine according to the doses indicated on page 627. If lidocaine abolishes the VT, a continuous IV infusion can be given. If maximum doses of lidocaine are unsuccessful, procainamide or bretylium can be administered IV and, if successful, given as an IV infusion. Although quinidine can be used intravenously, great caution is needed because of hypotension. Amiodarone is effective intravenously, although this method of administration has not been approved by the FDA.

If the arrhythmia does not respond to medical therapy, electrical direct current (DC) cardioversion can be employed. VT that precipitates hypotension, shock, angina, or congestive heart failure or symptoms of cerebral hypoperfusion should be treated *promptly* with DC cardioversion (p. 642). Very low energies may terminate VT, beginning with a synchronized shock of 10 to 50 watt-seconds. Digitalis-induced VT is best treated pharmacologically. After reversion of the arrhythmia to a normal rhythm, it is essential to institute measures to prevent a recurrence.

Striking the patient's chest, sometimes called "thumpversion," (p. 761) may terminate VT by mechanically inducing a premature ventricular complex that presumably interrupts the reentrant pathway necessary to support the VT. Stimulation at the time of the vulnerable period during VT may accelerate the VT or possibly provoke ventricular fibrillation.[248, 249]

In patients with recurrent VT, a pacing catheter can be inserted into the right ventricle and single, double, or multiple stimuli can be introduced competitively to terminate the ventricular tachycardia. This procedure incurs the risk of accelerating the VT to ventricular flutter or ventricular fibrillation.[227] A new catheter electrode has been developed recently through which synchronized cardioversion can be performed (see Fig. 23–11, p. 729). Intermittent VT, interrupted by several supravjentricular beats, is generally best treated pharmacologically (see Chap. 21).

A search for reversible conditions contributing to the initiation and maintenance of VT should be made and the conditions corrected if possible. For example, VT related to ischemia,[233, 234] hypotension, or hypokalemia at times may be terminated by antianginal treatment,[250] vasopressors, or potassium, respectively. Correction of heart failure may reduce the frequency of ventricular arrhythmias.[251, 252] Slow ventricular rates that are caused by sinus bradycardia or AV block may permit the occurrence of premature ventricular complexes and ventricular tachyarrhythmias that can be corrected by administering atropine, by temporary isoproterenol administration, or by transvenous pacing (Fig. 23–9, p. 728). Supraventricular tachycardia can initiate VT[253] and should be prevented if possible.

Prevention of Recurrences. This is generally more difficult than is terminating the acute episode. Initial preventive drug therapy for recurrent ventricular arrhythmias in the ambulatory patient should involve one of the class IA drugs quinidine, procainamide, or disopyramide; then the class IC drug, flecainide; and finally the class IB drugs, mexiletine and tocainide. Lastly, amiodarone may be tried. Specific qualities of a drug may influence choices. For example, disopyramide might not be given to a patient with congestive heart failure, while class IB drugs might be chosen early for a patient whose Q-T interval is prolonged. One group of patients may have a unique form of VT that may be due to activity mediated or triggered by cyclic AMP and is suppressed by adenosine, vagal maneuvers, beta-adrenoceptor blockade, and verapamil.[254] Verapamil may be effective in some other types of VT.[255, 256] While propranolol reduces sudden death after myocardial infarction, it does not do so to a greater degree in patients with complex ventricular arrhythmias.[257] This suggests that it may be effective via an antiischemic mechanism.

Combinations of drugs with different mechanisms of action may be successful when single drugs fail and allow one to use low doses of both agents rather than high or toxic doses of one drug. Most of the combinations represent empirical trials, but we generally attempt to combine drugs to which the patient has exhibited a partial therapeutic response.

Different thresholds for arrhythmic suppression may exist. For example, the serum concentration of procainamide necessary to suppress spontaneous VT may be lower than the concentration necessary to achieve a significant suppression of premature ventricular complexes.[258]

A trial of *ventricular* or *atrial pacing*, combined with antiarrhythmic agents if necessary, may be tested; if successful, permanent pacing may be instituted (Chap. 23). Generally, unless the VT is initiated by significant bradycardia, such as ventricular rates less than 40 due to complete AV block, attempts at "overdrive" pacing are ineffective over the long term. Implantable devices that cardiovert and defibrillate, surgery and ablation techniques may be used to treat VT in selected patients (pp. 644 and 646). Evaluating the effectiveness of therapy is often a difficult problem and involves noninvasive and invasive approaches.

Other Clinical States in Which Ventricular Arrhythmias Occur

ARRHYTHMOGENIC RIGHT VENTRICULAR DYSPLASIA. These patients present with ventricular tachycardia that generally has a left bundle branch block contour, often with right-axis deviation, with T waves inverted over the right precordial leads.[259] Supraventricular arrhythmias may also occur.[260] Premature ventricular stimulation can initiate sustained ventricular tachycardia.

Arrhythmogenic right ventricular dysplasia is due to a cardiomyopathy with hypokinetic areas involving the wall of the right ventricle. It may be related to Uhl's anomaly (parchment-thin right ventricular wall) in some patients and can be an important cause of ventricular arrhythmias in children and young adults with an apparently normal heart as well as in older patients.[261] Right heart failure or asymptomatic right ventricular enlargement may be present with normal pulmonary vasculature. Males predominate and all patients show an abnormal right ventricle by echocardiography or right ventricular angiography.[260, 262] ECG during sinus rhythm exhibits complete or incomplete right bundle branch block. Although the conventional pharmacological approaches to therapy may be appropriate, surgical manipulations have been successful in some of these patients.

TETRALOGY OF FALLOT (See also pp. 946 and 988). Chronic serious ventricular arrhythmias may occur in patients some years after repair of *tetralogy of Fallot.*[263] Sustained VT after repair may be caused by reentry at the site of previous operation in the right ventricular outflow tract and may be cured by resection of this area.[264] Conduction delay at multiple right ventricular sites suggests more widespread areas of damage[265] that may include left ventricular dysfunction.[266] Treatment with phenytoin, propranolol, mexiletine, or amiodarone may reduce the likelihood of sudden death in these patients.[267]

CARDIOMYOPATHIES. Both *dilated*[268] and *hypertrophic*[269–272] cardiomyopathies may be associated with VT's and an increased risk of sudden cardiac death. Approximately one-third of patients with hypertrophic cardiomyopathy die suddenly within 10 years of the diagnosis (p. 1430). Amiodarone has been reported to prevent sudden death in these patients.[269] Patients with dilated cardiomyopathy and reduced ejection fraction with ventricular pairs or VT during 24-hour ECG recording are at high risk of dying suddenly.[273] Sustained VT can be induced by programmed stimulation despite drug therapy in these patients.[274]

OTHER CAUSES OF VENTRICULAR TACHYCARDIA. Patients with *mitral valve prolapse* (p. 1045) frequently have ventricular arrhythmias, although a causal relationship is not clearly established. The prognosis for most patients appears good. Although sudden death has been reported, and VT's can be induced by programmed stimulation, their significance is unclear.[275, 276]

Patients may have serious VT's, even ventricular fibrillation, without *recognizable* structural heart disease; they are classified into a group called *primary electrical disease.*[277, 278] Endomyocardial biopsy in some of these patients is abnormal indicating that at least a percentage of those with apparent primary electrical disease do have histological abnormalities of the myocardium.[279, 280] Generally the prognosis for these patients is good,[281] although sudden death may occur.

Some patients may have VT due to a *sensitivity* to the *effects* of *catecholamine stimulation*. Stress or exercise may exacerbate these ventricular arrhythmias, which can be suppressed with beta blocker therapy.[282]

SPECIFIC TYPES OF VENTRICULAR TACHYCARDIA

A variety of fairly specific types of VT have been identified, related either to a constellation of distinctive electrocardiographic and electrophysiological features or to a specific set of clinical events. While our understanding of electrophysiological mechanisms responsible for clinically occurring VT's is still naive, being able to identify different kinds of VT's is the first step toward understanding their mechanisms.

Accelerated Idioventricular Rhythm

ELECTROCARDIOGRAPHIC RECOGNITION. The ventricular rate, commonly between 60 and 110 beats/min, usually hovers within 10 beats of the sinus rate, so that control of the cardiac rhythm may be passed back and forth between these two competing pacemaker sites. Consequently, fusion beats often occur at the onset and termination of the arrhythmia as the pacemakers vie for control of ventricular depolarization (Fig. 22–35). Because of the slow rate, capture beats are common. The onset of this arrhythmia is generally gradual (nonparoxysmal) and occurs when the rate of the ventricular tachycardia exceeds the sinus rate because of sinus slowing or SA or AV block. The ectopic mechanism may also begin after a premature ventricular complex, or the ectopic ventricular focus may simply accelerate sufficiently to overtake the sinus rhythm. The slow rate and nonparoxysmal onset avoid the problems initiated by excitation during the vulnerable period and, consequently, precipitation of more rapid ventricular arrhythmias is rarely seen. Termination of the rhythm generally occurs gradually as the dominant sinus rhythm accelerates or as the ectopic ventricular rhythm decelerates. The ventricular rhythm may be regular or irregular and occasionally may show sudden doubling, suggesting the presence of exit block. Many characteristics incriminate enhanced automaticity as the responsible mechanism.

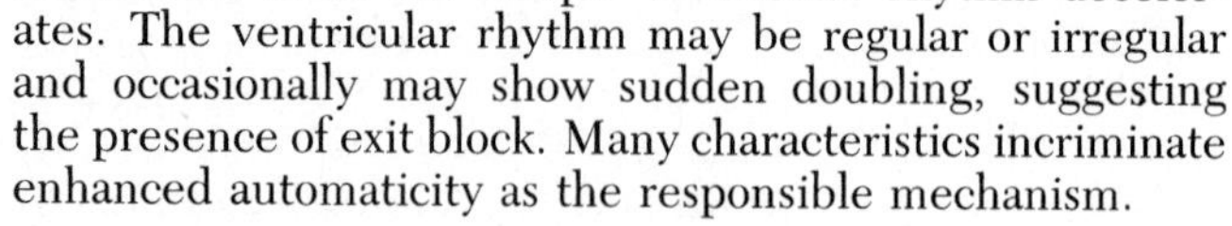

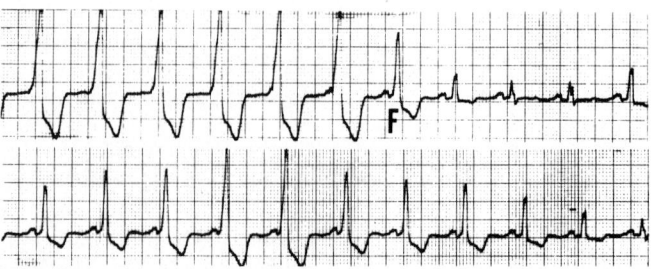

FIGURE 22–35. Accelerated idioventricular rhythm. In this continuous monitor lead recording, an accelerated idioventricular rhythm competes with the sinus rhythm. Wide QRS complexes at a rate of 90 beats/min fuse (F) with the sinus rhythm which takes control briefly, generating the narrow QRS complexes, and then yields once again to the accelerated idioventricular rhythm as the P waves move "in and out" of the QRS complex. This example of isorhythmic AV dissociation may be due to hemodynamic modulation of the sinus rate via the autonomic nervous system.

The arrhythmia occurs as a rule in patients who have heart disease, e.g., those with acute myocardial infarction or with digitalis toxicity. It is transient and intermittent, with episodes lasting a few seconds to a minute, and does not appear to affect seriously the course or prognosis of the patient. It commonly occurs at the moment of reperfusion of a previously occluded coronary artery.[283]

TREATMENT. Suppressive therapy rarely is necessary because the ventricular rate is generally less than 100 beats/min. The following conditions exist during which therapy may be considered: (1) when AV dissociation results in loss of sequential AV contraction and with it the hemodynamic benefits of atrial contribution to ventricular filling; (2) when accelerated idioventricular rhythm occurs together with a more rapid ventricular tachycardia; (3) when accelerated idioventricular rhythm begins with a premature ventricular complex that has a short coupling interval, which causes discharge in the vulnerable period of the preceding T wave; (4) when the ventricular rate is too rapid and produces symptoms; and (5) if ventricular fibrillation develops as a result of the accelerated idioventricular rhythm. This last event appears to be fairly rare. Therapy, when indicated, should be as noted above for VT. Often simply increasing the sinus rate with atropine or atrial pacing suppresses the accelerated idioventricular rhythm.

Torsades De Pointes

ELECTROCARDIOGRAPHIC RECOGNITION. The term "torsades de pointes" refers to a VT characterized by QRS complexes of changing amplitude that appear to twist around the isoelectric line and occur at rates of 200 to 250/min (Fig. 22–36*A*). Originally described in the setting of bradycardia due to complete heart block, torsades de pointes connotes a *syndrome*, not simply an ECG description of the QRS complex of the tachycardia.[284, 285] Prolonged ventricular repolarization with Q-T intervals exceeding 500 msec occurs as part of the syndrome. The U wave may also become prominent, but its role in this syndrome and in the long Q-T syndrome is not clear. Premature ventricular complexes may discharge during the termination of the T wave, precipitating successive bursts of VT during which the peaks of the QRS complexes appear successively on one side and then on the other of the isoelectric baseline, giving the typical twisting appearance with continuous and progressive changes in QRS contour and amplitude. The tachycardia may terminate with progressive prolongation of cycle lengths and larger and more distinctly formed QRS complexes, ending with a return to the basal rhythm, a period of ventricular standstill, or a new attack of torsades de pointes. Ventricular fibrillation may supervene.[285] Long-short cycle sequences commonly precede the onset of torsades de pointes.[286]

ELECTROPHYSIOLOGICAL FEATURES. VT that is similar morphologically to torsades de pointes and occurs in patients without QT prolongation, whether spontaneous or electrically induced, should be classified as polymorphic VT, not as torsades de pointes. The distinction has important therapeutic implications (see below).

Electrophysiological mechanisms responsible for torsades de pointes are not well understood and may be due to intraventricular reentry. However, torsades de pointes is often difficult to initiate by premature stimulation. Reentry appears more probable than the original hypothesis, which suggested the presence of an arrhythmia with two variable opposing foci, although data from one animal study support the latter theory.[287] Afterdepolarizations may be important.[288, 289]

CLINICAL FEATURES. While many predisposing factors

have been cited, the most common are severe bradycardia, potassium depletion, and use of drugs such as quinidine and disopyramide.[290, 291] An imbalance between right and left sympathetic innervations may be important in some patients. When attacks are prolonged, syncope may result.

Management of VT with a polymorphic pattern depends on whether or not it occurs in the setting of a prolonged Q-T interval. For this practical reason and because the mechanism of the tachycardia may differ depending on whether or not a long Q-T interval is present, it is important to restrict the definition of torsades de pointes to the typical morphology in the setting of a long Q-T and/or a polymorphic U wave[285] in the basal complexes. In all patients with torsades de pointes, administration of class IA, possibly class IC, and class III antiarrhythmic agents may increase the abnormal Q-T interval and worsen the arrhythmia. Class IB drugs may be tried. Intravenous magnesium has been successful.[292] Temporary ventricular or atrial pacing suppresses the VT, which often does not recur even after cessation of pacing.[285, 293, 294] Isoproterenol can be tried until pacing is instituted. The cause of the long Q-T should be determined and corrected if possible. When the Q-T interval is normal, polymorphic VT *resembling* torsades de pointes is diagnosed, and standard antiarrhythmic drugs may be given. In borderline cases, the clinical context may help determine whether treatment should be initiated with antiarrhythmic drugs. In doubtful cases when the Q-T interval is at upper limits of normal, treatment with pacing is preferable.

Long Q-T Syndrome

ELECTROCARDIOGRAPHIC RECOGNITION (Fig. 22–36*B*). The upper limit for the duration of the normal Q-T interval *corrected* for heart rate (Q-Tc) is 0.44 sec. However, it is possible that the formulas used to correct for heart rate, derived from normal subjects not receiving drugs, are not applicable to patients with abnormal repolarization syndromes or after drugs such as quinidine are administered or after myocardial infarction.[295] Nevertheless, delayed repolarization has been defined as a Q-Tc exceeding 0.44 sec. Actually, it may be longer, 0.46 for men and 0.47 for women, with a normal range ± 15 per cent of the mean value.[296] The nature of the U-wave abnormality and its relationship to the long Q-T syndrome are not clear. Afterdepolarizations may be important[289, 297, 298] and related to the prolonged notched bifid and sinusoidal T waves.[299] Dispersion of refractoriness has also been suggested as a cause of the long Q-T.[296]

CLINICAL FEATURES. Repolarization abnormalities can be divided into two broad groups: (1) primary or idiopathic, which is a congenital, often familial disorder that is sometimes,[300] but not always,[301, 302] associated with deafness, and (2) an acquired group caused by various drugs such as quinidine,[303] disopyramide,[304] phenothiazines, or tricyclic antidepressants; metabolic abnormalities such as hypokalemia; the results of the liquid protein diet[305] and starvation[306]; central nervous system lesions, autonomic nervous system dysfunction; coronary artery disease with myocardial infarction[307]; cardiac ganglionitis; and mitral valve prolapse. A long Q-T interval may occur during significant bradycardia but this is a normal Q-T interval for the rate. The autonomic dysfunction may result from a preponderance of left sympathetic tone.

Symptomatic patients with long Q-T syndrome develop VT's that in many instances are due to torsades de pointes. Since sudden death may occur in this group of patients, it is obvious that, in some, the ventricular arrhythmia be-

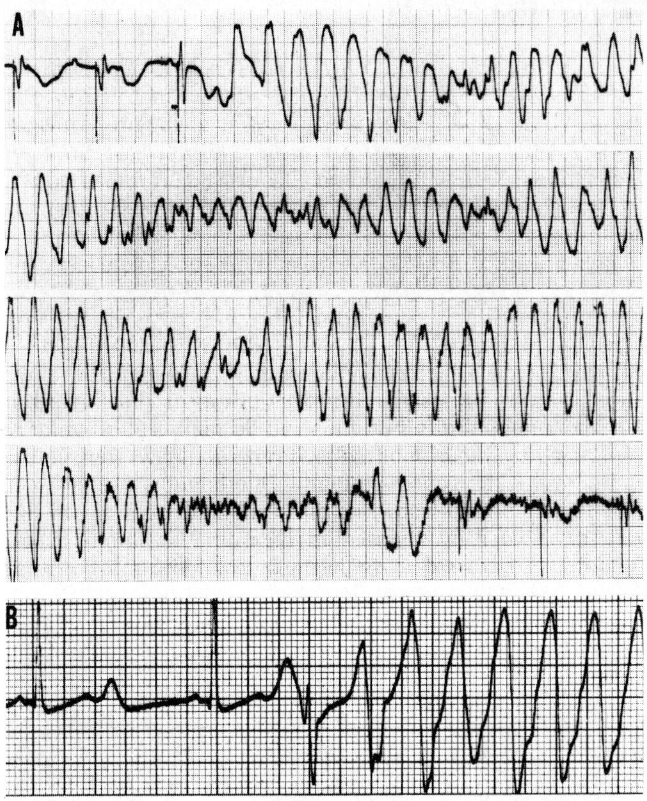

FIGURE 22–36. Torsades de pointes. *A*, Continuous recording monitor lead. A demand ventricular pacemaker (VVI) had been implanted because of type II second degree AV block. After treatment with amiodarone for recurrent ventricular tachycardia, the Q-T interval became prolonged (about 640 msec during paced beats), and the patient developed episodes of torsades de pointes. In this recording, the tachycardia spontaneously terminates and a paced ventricular rhythm is restored. Motion artifact is noted at the end of the recording as the patient lost consciousness. *B*, Tracing from a young boy with a congenital long Q-T syndrome. The Q-TU interval in the sinus beats is at least 600 msec. Note TU wave alternans in the first and second complexes. A late premature complex occurring in the downslope of the TU wave initiates an episode of ventricular tachycardia.

comes sustained and probably results in ventricular fibrillation. Patients with congenital long Q-T syndrome who are at increased risk for sudden death include those who have family members who died suddenly at an early age and those who have experienced syncope. Electrocardiograms should be obtained for all family members when the propositus presents with symptoms. Patients should undergo prolonged ECG recording, with various stresses designed to evoke ventricular arrhythmias, such as auditory stimuli, psychological stress, cold pressor stimulation, and exercise. The Valsalva maneuver may lengthen the Q-T interval and cause T wave alternans and VT in patients who have prolonged Q-T syndromes.[308] Catecholamines may be infused in some patients, but this challenge must be performed cautiously, with resuscitative equipment close at hand. Stellate ganglion stimulation and blockade may be useful to provoke or abolish arrhythmias. Premature ventricular stimulation electrically generally does not induce arrhythmias in this syndrome.[309] Conduction disturbances are common anatomically.[310]

TREATMENT. For patients who have the idiopathic long Q-T syndrome but do not have syncope, complex ventricular arrhythmias, or a family history of sudden cardiac death, no therapy is recommended. In asymptomatic patients with complex ventricular arrhythmias or a family history of premature sudden cardiac death, beta blockers at maximally tolerated doses are recommended. In patients with syncope, beta blockers at maximally tolerated doses, at times combined with phenytoin and phenobarbital, are suggested. For patients who continue to have syncope despite triple drug therapy, left-sided cervicothoracic sympathetic ganglionectomy that interrupts the stellate ganglion and the first three or four thoracic ganglia may be helpful in some[311] but not all[309] patients. Implantation of the automatic cardioverter-defibrillator seems advisable in patients who have syncope despite sympathetic interruption (Chap. 23).

Bidirectional Ventricular Tachycardia

This is an uncommon VT characterized by QRS complexes with a right bundle branch block pattern, alternating polarity in the frontal plane from −60 to −90 degrees to +120 to +130 degrees and a regular rhythm (Fig. 22–37). The ventricular rate is between 140 and 200 beats/min. Although the mechanism and site of origin of this tachycardia has remained somewhat controversial, most evidence supports a ventricular origin.[312]

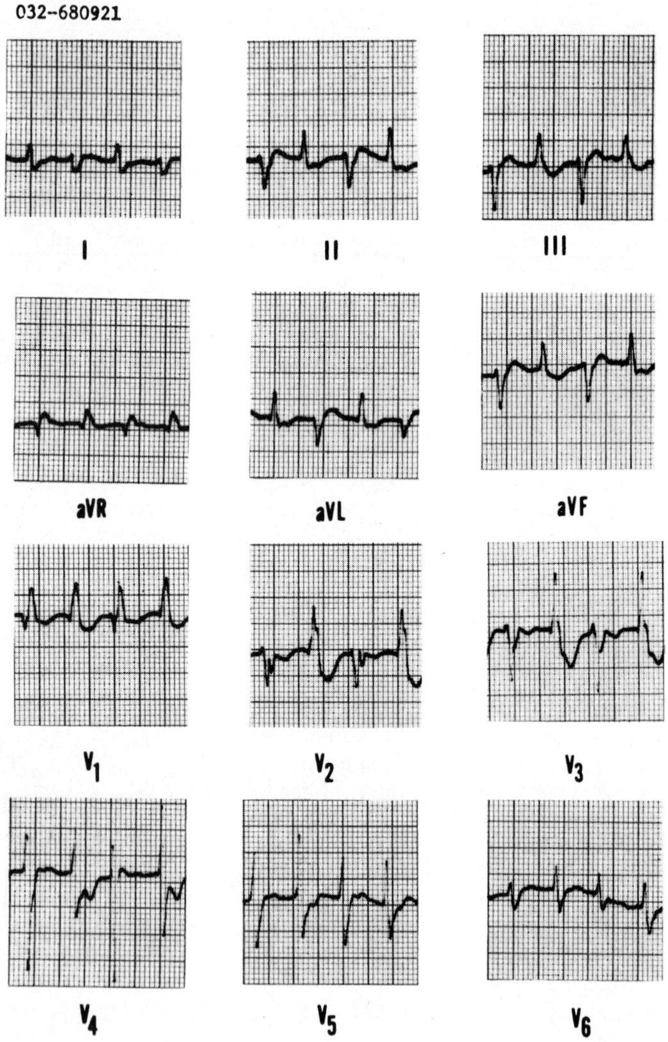

FIGURE 22–37. Bidirectional ventricular tachycardia. The mean frontal plane QRS axis alternates between −60° and +130° in successive beats and all complexes demonstrate a right bundle branch block pattern in V_1. R-R intervals are regular. The tachycardia was shown to be ventricular during an electrophysiological study. (From Morris, S. N., and Zipes, D. P.: His bundle electrocardiography during bidirectional tachycardia. Circulation *48*:32, 1973, by permission of the American Heart Association, Inc.)

Bidirectional VT is usually but not exclusively a manifestation of digitalis excess, typically in older patients and in those with severe myocardial disease. When due to digitalis, the extent of toxicity is often advanced, with a poor prognosis.

Drugs useful to treat digitalis toxicity such as lidocaine, potassium, phenytoin, and propranolol should be considered if excessive digitalis administration is suspected. Otherwise, the usual therapeutic approach to VT (p. 696) is recommended.

Repetitive Monomorphic Ventricular Tachycardia

Repetitive monomorphic VT is defined as three or more consecutive premature ventricular complexes with only brief periods of intervening sinus complexes. Ventricular complexes generally occur in groups of 3 to 15, but occasionally the VT may be almost continuous. Single premature ventricular complexes with the same contour may be present. All ventricular complexes have a uniform QRS morphology. Interectopic, sinus-conducted complexes have a normal QRS without intraventricular conduction delay or pathologic Q waves in patients without structural heart disease (Fig. 22–38). A recent report[313] indicates the presence of repetitive monomorphic VT in patients after myocardial infarction. Cycle lengths of the VT are fairly regular, and the rate ranges between 100 and 150 beats/min, occasionally becoming as rapid as 250 beats/min. Episodes of VT tend to cluster around certain time periods in an individual patient. Late cycle and variably coupled premature ventricular complexes are common. The tachycardia may be difficult to induce with premature electrical stimulation. Isoproterenol may be helpful in some patients.[313] Electrophysiological parameters are normal in patients with structurally normal hearts. Abnormal automaticity may be responsible for the tachycardia,[278, 314] although reentry cannot be excluded.[313]

Repetitive monomorphic VT is often associated with no or minimal structural heart disease and young age. When it occurs in patients who have normal, sinus-conducted QRS complexes and minimal or no structural heart disease, the VT may originate in the right ventricular outflow

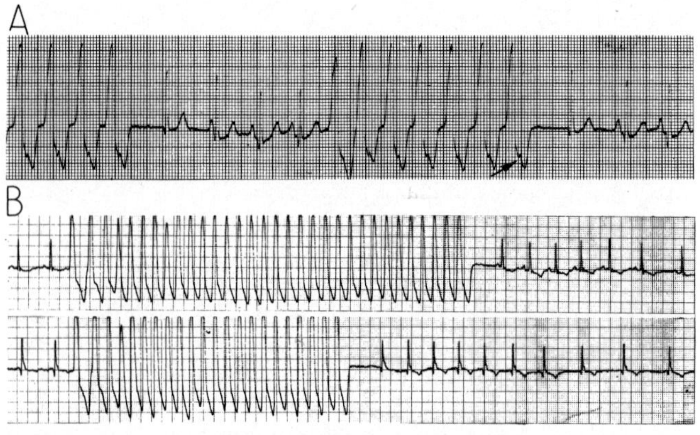

FIGURE 22–38. Repetitive monomorphic ventricular tachycardia. Short episodes of a monomorphic ventricular tachycardia at a rate of 160 beats/min repeatedly interrupt the normal sinus rhythm. Retrograde atrial capture probably occurs (arrow points to the deflection in the ST segment) and the retrograde P wave of the last complex of the repetitive monomorphic ventricular tachycardia conducts over the normal pathway to produce a normal contour QRS complex. Alternatively, these QRS complexes may represent accelerated junctional escape beats. In panel B, short runs of a very rapid (260 beats/min) ventricular tachycardia of uniform contour occur. They probably provoke a compensatory sympathetic response because each is followed by a brief period of sinus tachycardia. The sinus pacemaker appears unstable as changes in P wave morphology result.

tract[313]; it appears to be benign, and the prognosis is favorable.[278] Occurring after myocardial infarction, it appears to originate near the border of the previous infarction.[313] Arrhythmia-related deaths are reported infrequently. The arrhythmia may disappear with time, perhaps accounting for its reduced prevalence in older populations. The exact prevalence of the tachycardia is difficult to assess, since often it produces no symptoms and may be identified only during routine examination.

Therapy, as outlined on p. 696, is reserved for patients who are symptomatic from palpitations or have very rapid rates of the ventricular tachycardia.

Bundle Branch Reentrant Tachycardia

VT due to bundle branch reentry is characterized by a QRS morphology determined by the circuit established over the bundle branches. Retrograde conduction over the left bundle branch system and anterograde conduction over the right bundle branch will create a QRS complex with a left bundle branch block contour. The frontal plane axis may be about +30 degrees. Electrophysiologically, bundle branch reentrant complexes occur only after a critical S_2-H_2 or S_3-H_3 delay. The H-V interval of the bundle branch reentrant complex equals or exceeds the H-V interval of the spontaneous normally conducted QRS complex.[315–317]

Although bundle branch reentry has been clearly demonstrated to occur in animals (Fig. 20–30, p. 608) and probably occurs in humans as well, sustained VT due to bundle branch reentry is a rare event. The long refractory period and rapid conduction velocity of the His-Purkinje system probably prevent sustained circuits of bundle branch reentry from occurring and therefore make it an uncommon mechanism of VT in man.

The therapeutic approach is as for other VT's. Creation of bundle branch block can eliminate the tachycardia.

VENTRICULAR FLUTTER AND VENTRICULAR FIBRILLATION

(See also Chap. 24)

ELECTROCARDIOGRAPHIC RECOGNITION. These arrhythmias represent severe derangements of the heartbeat that usually terminate fatally within 3 to 5 minutes unless corrective measures are undertaken promptly. Ventricular flutter presents as a sine wave in appearance: regular large oscillations occurring at a rate of 150 to 300/min (usually about 200) (Fig. 22–39*A*). The distinction between rapid VT and ventricular flutter may be difficult and is usually of academic interest only. Ventricular fibrillation is recognized by the presence of irregular undulations of varying contour and amplitude (Fig. 22–39*B*). Distinct QRS complexes, ST segments, and T waves are absent. Fine amplitude fibrillatory waves ($<$ 0.2 mV) are present when termination of ventricular fibrillation has been delayed and identifies patients with worse survival rates.[318]

CLINICAL FEATURES. Ventricular fibrillation occurs in a variety of clinical situations, most commonly associated with coronary artery disease and as a terminal event.[319] It may occur during antiarrhythmic drug administration, hypoxia, ischemia, atrial fibrillation and very rapid ventricular rates in the preexcitation syndrome, after electric shock administered during cardioversion or accidentally by improperly grounded equipment, and uncommonly during competitive cardiac pacing at slow rates. Ventricular flutter or ventricular fibrillation results in faintness, followed by loss of consciousness, seizures, and apnea and eventually, if the rhythm continues untreated, death. The blood pressure is unobtainable and heart sounds are usually absent. The atria may continue to beat as an independent rhythm for a time or in response to impulses from the fibrillating ventricles. Eventually, electrical activity of the heart is completely absent.

In patients resuscitated from out-of-hospital cardiac arrest, most have ventricular fibrillation. Bradycardia and asystole may occur in 25 per cent of these patients and is associated with a worse prognosis than is ventricular fibrillation.[320, 321] Some patients with apparent asystole may have ventricular fibrillation with low-amplitude fibrillation waves.[322, 323]

Although 75 per cent of resuscitated patients exhibit significant coronary artery disease, only 20 to 30 per cent develop acute transmural myocardial infarction. Those who do *not* develop a myocardial infarction have a recurrence rate for ventricular fibrillation of approximately 22 per cent in one year and 40 per cent in two years.[324] Patients who have ventricular fibrillation and acute myocardial infarction have a recurrence rate at 1 year of 2 per cent. In one series, R-on-T premature ventricular complexes were the most important initiating factor, with an increase or marked slowing of the sinus rate predisposing to the development of ventricular fibrillation.[325] Predictors of death for resuscitated patients include reduced ejection fraction, abnormal wall motion, history of congestive heart failure, history of myocardial infarction but no acute event, and the presence of ventricular arrhythmias.[326] Sudden death also may occur in a pediatric population.[327]

After the acute phase of myocardial infarction has elapsed, patients who develop ventricular fibrillation in contrast to those who develop VT exhibit no difference in ventricular function or extent of coronary artery disease but show a greater likelihood of having two separate areas of infarction and of developing rapid polymorphic VT or ventricular fibrillation during programmed ventricular stimulation.[328] Patients discharged after an anterior myocardial infarction complicated by ventricular fibrillation appear to represent a subgroup at high risk of sudden death.[329]

TREATMENT (See also pp. 645 and 728). *Immediate* nonsynchronized DC electrical shock using 200 to 400 joules is mandatory treatment for ventricular fibrillation and for ventricular flutter that has caused loss of consciousness. Cardiopulmonary resuscitation is employed only until defibrillation equipment is readied. *Time should not be wasted with cardiopulmonary resuscitation maneuvers if electrical defibrillation can be done promptly.* If the circulation is markedly inadequate despite return to sinus rhythm, closed-chest massage with artificial ventilation as needed should be instituted. The use of anesthesia during electric shock obviously is dictated by the patient's condition and is generally not required. After reversion of the arrhythmia to a normal rhythm, it is essential to monitor the rhythm continuously and to institute measures to prevent a recurrence.

Metabolic acidosis quickly follows cardiovascular collapse. If the arrhythmia is terminated within 30 to 60 seconds, significant acidosis does not occur. The use of sodium bicarbonate to reverse the acidosis may be necessary, but its efficacy is presently being reevaluated (p. 763). Intravenous calcium generally is recommended only for situations characterized by hypocalcemia, hyperkalemia, calcium-channel drug overdose, and possibly electromechanical dissociation.[329a, 329b]

In this short period of time, artificial ventilation by means of a tightly fitting rubber face mask and an Ambu bag is quite satisfactory and eliminates the delay attending intubation by inexperienced personnel. If such a mask and bag are not available, mouth-to-mouth or mouth-to-nose resuscitation is indicated. It is important to reemphasize that there should be *no delay in instituting electrical shock.* If the patient is not monitored and it cannot be established whether asystole or ventricular fibrillation caused the cardiovascular collapse, the electric shock should be administered *without* wasting precious seconds attempting

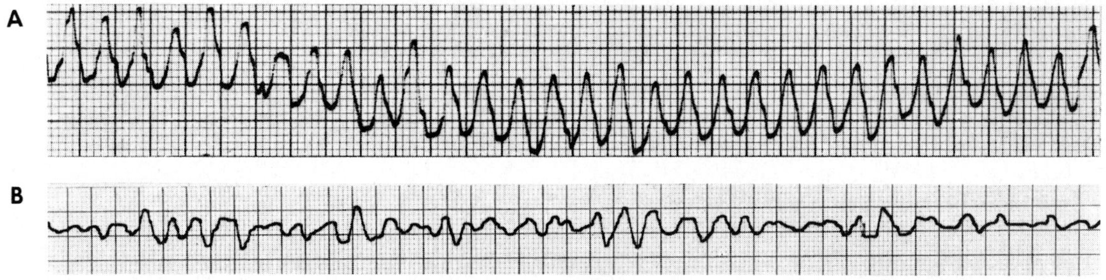

FIGURE 22–39. Ventricular flutter and ventricular fibrillation. ***A,*** **The sine wave appearance of the complexes occurring at a rate of 300 beats/min is characteristic of ventricular flutter.** ***B,*** **The irregular undulating baseline typifies ventricular fibrillation.**

to obtain an electrocardiogram. The DC shock may cause the asystolic heart to begin discharging as well as terminate ventricular fibrillation, if the latter is present.

A search for conditions contributing to the initiation of ventricular flutter or fibrillation should be made and the conditions corrected, if possible. Initial medical approaches to prevent a recurrence of ventricular fibrillation include intravenous administration of licocaine, bretylium, procainamide, quinidine, disopyramide, or amiodarone. (Disopyramide and amiodarone are not approved for IV use by the FDA at the time of this writing.) Beta blockers may reduce the incidence of ventricular fibrillation following acute myocardial infarction.[330] Usually, when ventricular fibrillation occurs, it is irreversible (does not terminate spontaneously) and lethal unless countermeasures are instituted immediately.

HEART BLOCK

Heart block is a disturbance of impulse conduction that may be permanent or transient, owing to anatomical or functional impairment. It must be distinguished from *interference*, a normal phenomenon which is a disturbance of impulse conduction caused by physiological refractoriness due to inexcitability from a preceding impulse. Either interference or block may occur at any site where impulses are conducted, but they are recognized most commonly between the sinus node and atrium (SA block), between the atria and ventricles (AV block), within the atria (intra-atrial block), or within the ventricles (intraventricular block). During AV block, the block may occur in the AV node, His bundle, or bundle branches. In some instances of bundle branch block, for example, the impulse may only be delayed and not completely blocked in the bundle branch, yet the resulting QRS complex may be indistinguishable from a QRS complex generated by complete bundle branch block.

The conduction disturbance is classified by severity in three categories. During *first degree heart block*, conduction time is prolonged but all impulses are conducted. *Second degree heart block* occurs in two forms: Mobitz type I (Wenckebach) and type II. Type I heart block is characterized by a progressive lengthening of the conduction time until an impulse is not conducted. Type II heart block denotes occasional or repetitive sudden block of conduction of an impulse without prior measurable lengthening of conduction time. When no impulses are conducted, *complete or third degree block is present*. The degree of block may depend in part on the direction of impulse propagation. For unknown reasons, normal retrograde conduction can occur in the presence of advanced anterograde AV block.[331] The reverse can also occur.

Certain features of type I second degree block deserve special emphasis because when actual conduction times are not apparent in the electrocardiogram, for example, during SA, junctional, or ventricular exit block (Fig. 22–42), type I conduction disturbance may be difficult to recognize. During typical type I block, the increment in conduction time is greatest in the second beat of the Wenckebach group, and the absolute *increase* in conduction time *decreases* progressively over subsequent beats. These two features serve to establish the characteristics of classic Wenckebach group beating: (1) the interval between successive beats progressively decreases, although the conduction time increases (but by a decreasing function); (2) the duration of the pause produced by the nonconducted impulse is less than twice the interval preceding the blocked impulse (which is usually the shortest interval); and (3) the cycle following the nonconducted beat (beginning the Wenckebach group) is longer than the cycle

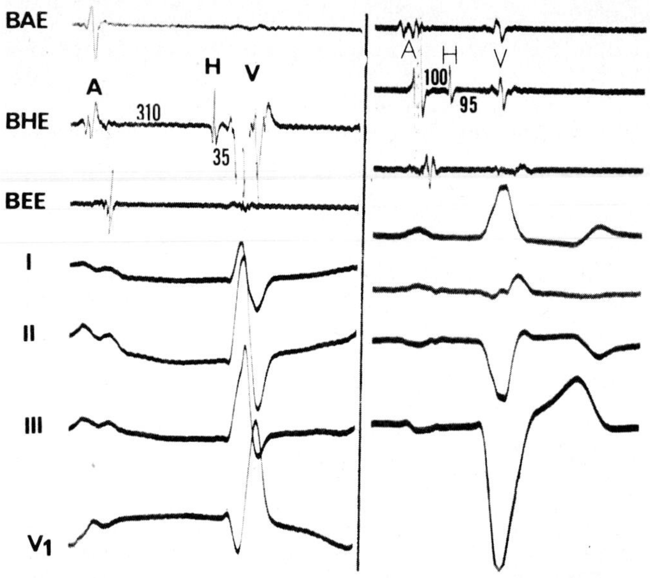

FIGURE 22–40. First degree AV block. One complex during sinus rhythm is shown. The P-R interval in the left panel measured 370 msec (P-A=25 msec; A-H=310 msec; H-V=35 msec) during a right bundle branch block. Conduction delay in the AV node causes the first degree AV block. In the panel on the right, the P-R interval is 230 msec (P-A=35 msec; A-H=100 msec; H-V=95 msec) during a left bundle branch block. The conduction delay in the His-Purkinje system causes the first degree AV block.

preceding the blocked impulse. Although much emphasis has been placed on this characteristic grouping of cycles, primarily to be able to diagnose Wenckebach exit block, this typical grouping occurs in less than 50 per cent of patients who have type I Wenckebach AV nodal block.

Differences in cycle-length patterns may result from changes in pacemaker rate (e.g., sinus arrhythmia), in neurogenic control of conduction, and changes in the increment of conduction delay. For example, if the P-R increment in the last cycle *increases*, the R-R cycle of the last conducted beat may lengthen rather than shorten. In addition, since the last conducted beat is often at a critical state of conduction, it may become blocked, producing a 5:3 or 3:1 conduction ratio instead of a 5:4 or 3:2 ratio. During a 3:2 Wenckebach structure, the duration of the cycle following the nonconducted beat will be the same as the duration of the cycle preceding the nonconducted beat.

ATRIOVENTRICULAR (AV) BLOCK

AV block exists when the atrial impulse is conducted with delay or is not conducted at all to the ventricle at a time when the AV junction is not physiologically refractory.

TABLE 22–3 MAJOR FEATURES IN THE DIFFERENTIAL DIAGNOSIS OF WIDE QRS BEATS OR TACHYCARDIA

Supports SVT	Supports VT
Slowing or termination by ↑ vagal tone	Fusion beats
Onset with premature P wave	Capture beats
RP interval ≤ 100 msec	AV dissociation
P and QRS rate and rhythm linked to suggest ventricular activation depends on atrial discharge, e.g., 2:1 AV block	P and QRS rate and rhythm linked to suggest atrial activation depends on ventricular discharge, e.g., 2:1 VA block
RSR′ V_1	
Long-short cycle sequence	"Compensatory" pause
	Left axis deviation QRS duration > 140 msec specific QRS contours (see text)

SVT = supraventricular tachycardia;
VT = ventricular tachycardia.

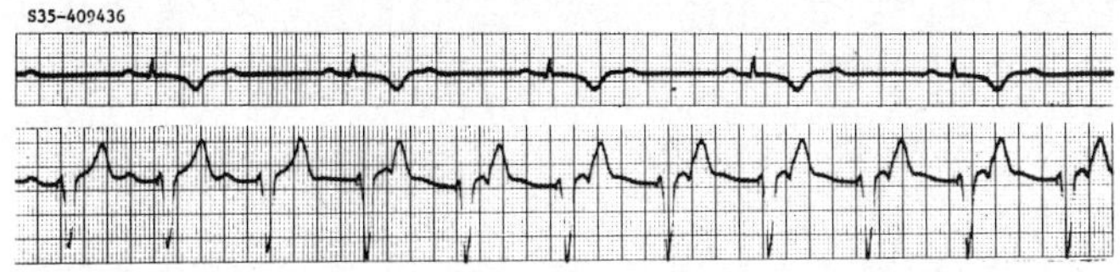

FIGURE 22–41. Unidirectional block. In the top ECG during spontaneous sinus rhythm at a rate of 68 beats/min, 2:1 anterograde AV conduction occurs. In the bottom ECG, during ventricular pacing at a rate of 70 beats/min, 1:1 retrograde conduction is seen.

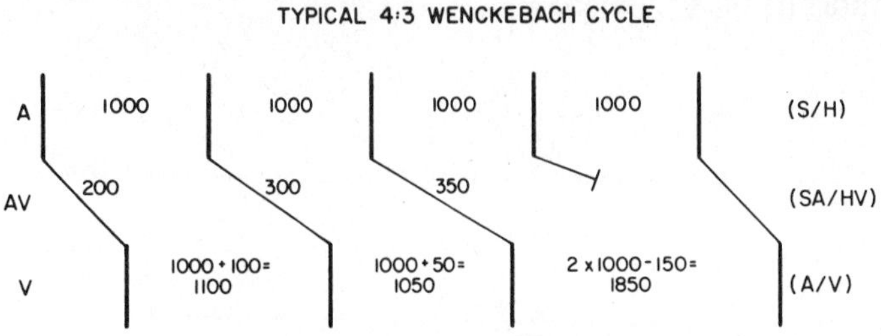

FIGURE 22–42. Typical 4:3 Wenckebach cycle. P waves ("A" tier) occur at a cycle length of 1000 msec. The P-R interval ("A-V" tier) is 200 msec for the first beat and generates a ventricular response ("V" tier). The P-R interval increases by 100 msec in the next complex, resulting in an R-R interval of 1100 msec (1000 + 100). The increment in the P-R interval is only 50 msec for the third cycle, and the P-R interval becomes 350 msec. The R-R interval shortens to 1050 msec (1000 + 50). The next P wave blocks creating an R-R interval that is less than twice the P-P interval by an amount equal to the increments in the P-R interval. Thus, the Wenckebach features explained in the text can be found in this diagram. If the increment in the P-R interval of the last conducted complex *increased* rather than decreased (e.g., 150 msec rather than 50 msec) then the last R-R interval would increase (1150 msec) rather than decrease and thus become an example of atypical Wenckebach (Fig. 22–43).

If this were a Wenckebach exit block from the sinus node to the atrium, the sinus node cycle length (S) would be 1000 msec, the S-A interval would increase from 200 to 300 to 350 msec, culminating in block. These events would be inapparent in the scalar ECG. However, the P-P interval in the ECG would shorten from 1100 to 1050 msec and finally there would be a pause of 1850 msec (A) (Fig. 22–4). If this were a junctional rhythm arising from the His bundle and conducting to the ventricle, the junctional rhythm cycle length would be 1000 msec (H), the H-V interval would progressively lengthen from 200 to 300 to 350 msec, while the R-R interval would decrease from 1100 to 1050 msec and then increase to 1850 msec (V). The only clue to the Wenckebach exit block would be the cycle length changes in the ventricular rhythm.

FIRST DEGREE AV BLOCK. During first degree AV block, every atrial impulse conducts to the ventricles, producing a regular ventricular rate, but the P-R interval exceeds 0.20 sec in the adult. P-R intervals as long as 1.0 sec have been noted and at times may be longer than the P-P interval, a phenomenon known as "skipped" P waves. Clinically important P-R interval prolongation may result from conduction delay in the AV node (A-H interval), in the His-Purkinje system (H-V interval), or at both sites. Equally delayed conduction over both bundle branches uncommonly may produce P-R prolongation without significant QRS complex aberration. Occasionally, intraatrial conduction delay may result in P-R prolongation. If the QRS complex in the scalar ECG is normal in contour and duration, the AV delay almost always resides in the AV node, rarely within the His bundle itself. If the QRS complex shows a bundle branch block pattern, conduction delay may be within the AV node and/or His-Purkinje system (Fig. 22–40). In this latter instance, His bundle electrocardiography is necessary to localize the site of conduction delay. Acceleration of the atrial rate or enhancement of vagal tone by carotid massage may cause first degree AV nodal block to progress to type I second degree AV block. Conversely, type I second degree AV nodal block may revert to first degree block with deceleration of the sinus rate.

SECOND DEGREE AV BLOCK (Figs. 22–41, 22–42, and 22–43). Atrial impulses not conducted to the ventricle at a time when physiological interference is not involved constitutes second degree AV block. The nonconducted P wave may be intermittent or frequent, at regular or irregular intervals, and may be preceded by fixed or lengthening P-R intervals. A distinguishing feature is that conducted P waves relate to the QRS complex with recurring P-R intervals, i.e., the association of P with QRS is not random. Wenckebach and Hay, by analyzing the *a-c* and *v* waves in the jugular venous pulse, described two types of second degree AV block. After the introduction of the electrocardiograph, Mobitz classified them as type I and type II. Electrocardiographically, typical type I second degree AV block is characterized by progressive P-R prolongation culminating in a nonconducted P wave (Figs. 22–42 and 22–43), while in type II second degree AV block, the P-R interval remains constant prior to the blocked P wave (Fig.

FIGURE 22–43. Type I (Wenckebach) atrioventricular nodal block (panel A). During spontaneous sinus rhythm, progressive P-R prolongation occurs, culminating in a nonconducted P wave. From the His bundle recording (HBE), it is apparent that the conduction delay and subsequent block occurs within the AV node. Since the increment in conduction delay does not consistently decrease, the R-R intervals do not reflect the classic Wenckebach structure diagrammed in Figure 22–42. Panel B was recorded 5 min following 0.6 mg IV atropine. Atropine has had its predominant effect on sinus and junctional automaticity at this time, with little improvement in AV conduction. Consequently, more P waves are blocked and AV dissociation, due to a combination of AV block and enhanced junctional discharge rate, is present. At 8 min (not shown) 1:1 atrioventricular conduction occurred, when atropine finally improved AV conduction.

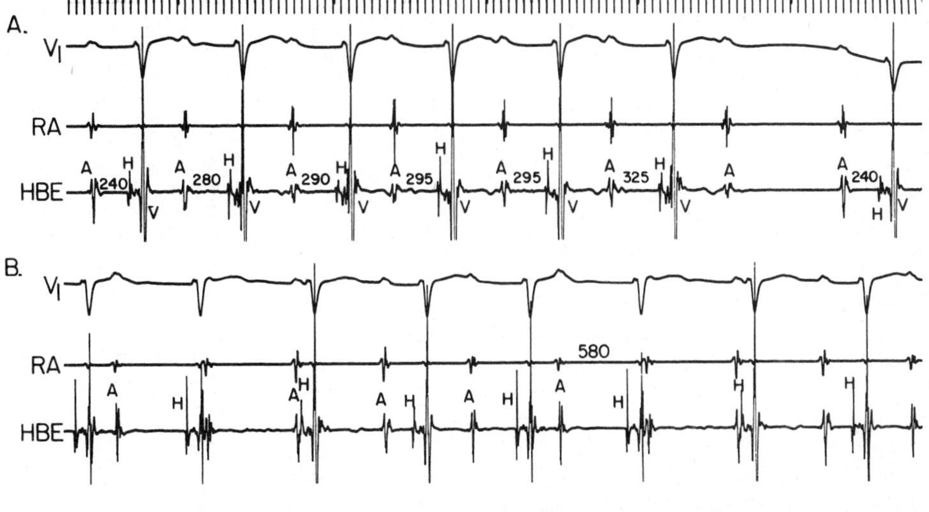

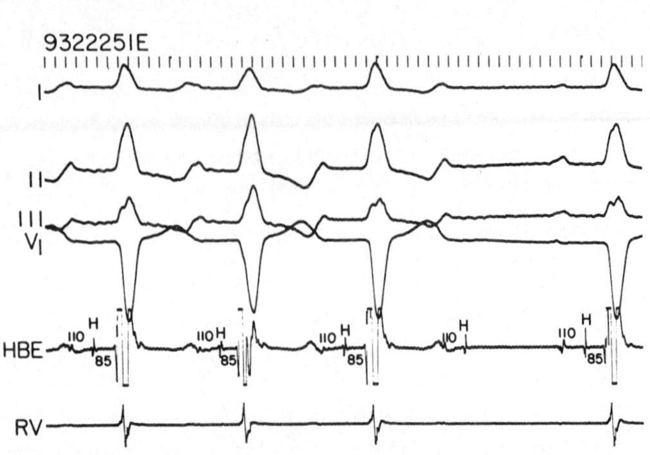

FIGURE 22–44. Sudden development of His-Purkinje block is apparent. The A-H interval and H-V intervals remain constant, as does the P-R interval. Left bundle branch block is present.

22–44). In both instances the AV block is intermittent and generally repetitive and may block several P waves in a row. Often, the eponyms Mobitz type I and Mobitz type II are applied to the two types of block, while the term "Wenckebach block" refers to type I block only.[332, 333]

Although it has been suggested that type I and type II AV block may be different manifestations of the same electrophysiological mechanism, differing only quantitatively in the size of the increments, clinically separating second degree AV block into type I and type II serves a useful function and, in most instances, the differentiation can be made easily and reliably from the surface ECG. Type II AV block often antedates the development of Adams-Stokes syncope and complete AV block, while type I AV block with a normal QRS complex is generally more benign and does not progress to more advanced forms of AV conduction disturbance. In older people, type I AV block with or without bundle branch block has been associated with a clinical picture similar to type II AV block.[334]

In the patient with an acute myocardial infarction, type I AV block usually accompanies inferior infarction (perhaps more often if a right ventricular infarction also occurs),[335] is transient, and does not require temporary pacing, whereas type II AV block results in the setting of an acute anterior myocardial infarction, may require temporary or permanent pacing, and is associated with a high rate of mortality, generally due to pump failure. A high degree of AV block can occur in patients with acute inferior myocardial infarction[336] and is associated with more myocardial damage and a higher mortality rate compared to those without AV block.[336, 337]

While type I conduction disturbance is ubiquitous and may occur in any tissue in the in situ heart, as well as in vitro, the site of block for the usual forms of second degree AV block can be judged with sufficient reliability from the surface ECG to permit clinical decisions without requiring invasive electrophysiological studies in most instances. Type I AV block with a normal QRS complex almost always takes place at the level of the AV node, proximal to the His bundle. An exception is the uncommon patient with type I intrahisian block. Type II AV block, particularly when it occurs in association with a bundle branch block, is localized to the His-Purkinje system. Type I AV block in a patient with a bundle branch block may represent block in the AV node or in the His-Purkinje system. Type II AV block in a patient with a normal QRS complex may be due to intrahisian AV block, but the block is likely to be type I AV nodal block, which exhibits small increments in AV conduction time.

The above generalizations encompass the vast majority of patients who present with second degree AV block. However, certain caveats must be heeded to avoid misdiagnosis because of subtle ECG changes or exceptions:

1. Two:one AV block may be a form of type I or type II AV block (Fig. 22–45). If the QRS complex is normal, the block is more likely to be type I, located in the AV node, and one should search for a transition of the 2:1 block to 3:2 block, during which the P-R interval lengthens in the second cardiac cycle. If a bundle branch block is present, the block may be located either in the AV node or in the His-Purkinje system.
2. AV block may occur simultaneously at two or more levels and may cause difficulty in distinguishing between types I and II.
3. If the atrial rate varies, it may alter conduction times and cause type I AV block to simulate type II or change type II AV block into type I. For example, if the shortest atrial cycle length that just achieved 1:1 AV nodal conduction at a constant P-R interval is decreased by as little as 10 or 20 msec, the P wave of the shortened cycle may block at the level of the AV node without an apparent increase in the antecedent P-R interval. Apparent type II AV block in the His-Purkinje system may be converted to type I in the His-Purkinje system in some patients by increasing the atrial rate.
4. Concealed premature His depolarizations may create electrocardiographic patterns that simulate type I or type II AV block (see Fig. 20–33, p. 611).
5. Abrupt, transient alterations in autonomic tone may cause sudden block of one or more P waves without altering the P-R interval of the conducted P wave before or after block.[338] Thus, apparent type II AV block would be produced at the AV node. Clinically, a burst of vagal tone probably lengthens the P-P interval as well as producing AV block.
6. The response of the AV block to autonomic changes, either spontaneous or induced, to distinguish type I from type II AV block may be misleading. Although vagal stimulation generally increases and vagolytic agents decrease the extent of type I AV block, such conclusions are based on the assumption that the intervention acts primarily on the AV node and fail to consider rate changes. For example, atropine may minimally improve conduction in the AV node and markedly increase the sinus rate, resulting in an increase in AV nodal conduction time and the degree of AV block as a result of the faster atrial rate (Fig. 22–43*B*). Conversely, if an increase in vagal tone minimally prolongs AV conduction time but greatly slows the heart rate, the net effect on type I AV block may be to improve conduction. In general, however, carotid sinus massage improves and atropine worsens AV conduction in patients with His-Purkinje block, while the opposite results are to be expected in patients who have AV nodal block. These two interventions may help differentiate the site of block without invasive study,[339] although recent data suggest that damaged His–Purkinje tissue may be influenced by changes in autonomic tone.[340]
7. During type I AV block with high ratios of conducted beats, the increment in P-R interval may be quite small and simulate type II AV block if only the last few P-R intervals prior to the blocked P wave are measured. By comparing the P-R interval of the first beat in the long Wenckebach cycle with that of the beats immediately preceding the blocked P wave, the increment in AV conduction becomes readily apparent.
8. The classic AV Wenckebach structure depends on a stable atrial rate and a maximal increment in AV conduction time for the second P-R interval of the Wenckebach cycle, with a progressive decrease in subsequent beats. Unstable or unusual alterations in the increment of AV conduction time or in the atrial rate, often seen with long Wenckebach cycles, result in atypical forms of type I AV block in which the last R-R interval may lengthen because the P-R increment *increases*; these are common.
9. Finally, it is important to remember that the P-R interval in the scalar ECG is made up of conduction through the atrium, the AV node, and the His-Purkinje system. An increment in HV conduction, for example, can be masked in the scalar ECG by a reduction in the A-H interval, and the resulting P-R interval will not reflect the entire increment in His-Purkinje conduction time.[332] Very long P-R intervals (> 200 msec) are more likely to result from AV nodal conduction delay (and block), with or without concomitant His-Purkinje conduction delay, although the author recently evaluated a patient with an HV interval of 350 msec.

First degree and type I second degree AV block can occur in normal healthy children,[341] and Wenckebach AV

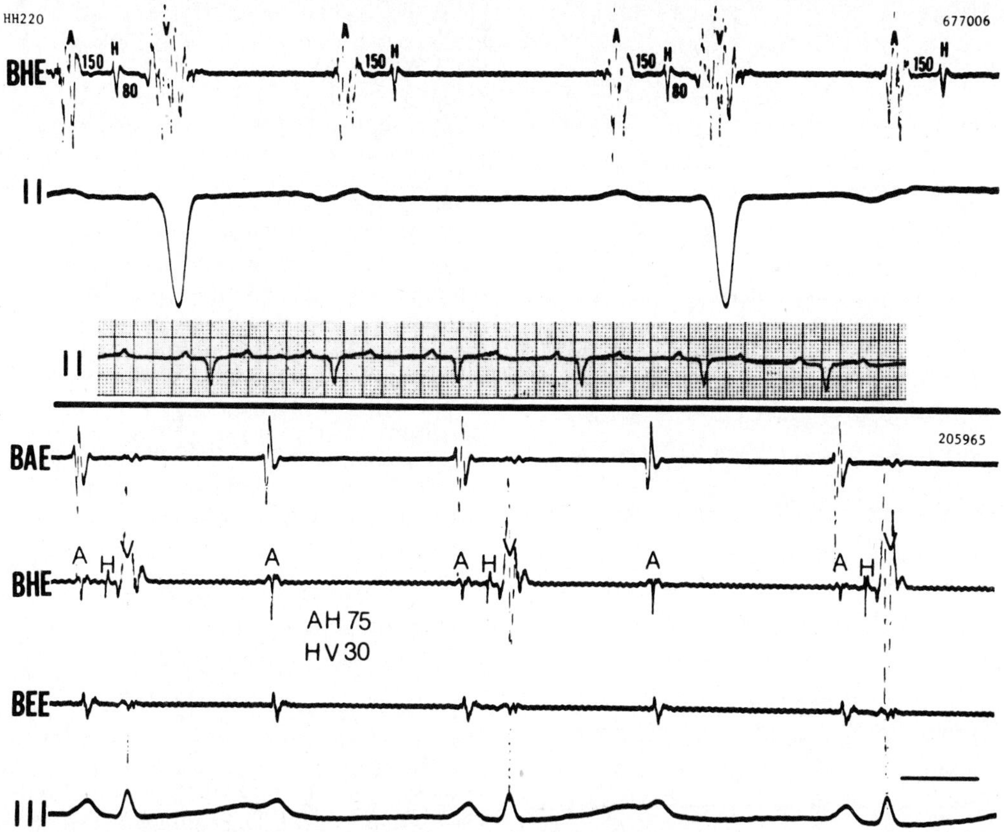

FIGURE 22–45. 2:1 AV block proximal and distal to the His bundle deflection in two different patients. *Top,* 2:1 AV block seen in the scalar ECG occurs distal to the His bundle recording site in a patient with right bundle branch block and left anterior hemiblock. The A-H interval (150 msec) and H-V interval (80 msec) are both prolonged. *Bottom,* 2:1 AV block occurs proximal to the bundle of His in a patient with a normal QRS complex. The A-H interval (75 msec) and the H-V interval (30 msec) remain constant and normal.

block may be a normal phenomenon in well-trained athletes, probably related to an increase in resting vagal tone.[342, 343] Occasionally, progressive worsening of the Wenckebach AV conduction disorder may result so that the athlete becomes symptomatic and has to decondition. In patients who have chronic second degree AV nodal block (proximal to the His bundle) without organic heart disease, the course is relatively benign (except in older age groups[334]), while in those who have organic heart disease the prognosis is poor and related to underlying heart disease.[344]

COMPLETE AV BLOCK

ELECTROCARDIOGRAPHIC RECOGNITION. Complete AV block occurs when no atrial activity conducts to the ventricles and therefore the atria and ventricles are controlled by independent pacemakers. Thus, complete AV block is one type of complete AV dissociation (see p. 707). The atrial pacemaker may be sinus or ectopic (tachycardia, flutter, or fibrillation) or may result from an AV junctional focus occurring above the block with retrograde atrial conduction. The ventricular focus is usually located just below the region of block, which may be above or below the His bundle bifurcation. Sites of ventricular pacemaker activity that are in, or closer to, the His bundle appear to be more stable and may produce a faster escape rate than those located more distally in the ventricular conduction system. The ventricular rate in acquired complete heart block is less than 40 beats/min but may be faster in congenital complete AV block. The ventricular rhythm, usually regular, may vary owing to premature ventricular complexes, a shift in the pacemaker site, an irregularly discharging pacemaker focus, or autonomic influences.

CLINICAL FEATURES. Complete AV block may result from block at the level of the AV node (usually congenital) (Fig. 22–46), within the bundle of His, or distal to it in the Purkinje system (usually acquired) (Fig. 22–47). The first two types of block generally exhibit normal QRS complexes and rates of 40 to 60 beats/min because the escape focus that controls the ventricle arises in or near the His bundle. In complete AV nodal block, the P wave is not followed by a His deflection, but each ventricular complex is preceded by a His deflection (Fig. 22–46). His bundle electrocardiography may be useful to differentiate AV nodal from intrahisian block, since the latter may carry a more serious prognosis than the former. Intrahisian block is recognized infrequently without invasive studies. In patients with AV nodal block atropine usually speeds both the atrial and the ventricular rate. Exercise may reduce the extent of AV nodal block. Acquired complete AV block occurs most commonly distal to the bundle of His owing to trifascicular conduction disturbance. Each P wave is followed by a His deflection, and the ventricular escape complexes are not preceded by a His deflection (Fig. 22–47). The QRS complex is abnormal and the ventricular rate is usually less than 40 beats/min.

Unusual forms such as paroxysmal AV block or AV block following a period of rapid ventricular rate may occur.[345, 346] Paroxysmal AV block in some instances may be due to hyperresponsiveness of the AV node to vagotonic reflexes.[347] Surgery, electrolyte disturbances, endocarditis, tumors, Chagas' disease, rheumatoid nodules, calcific aortic stenosis, myxedema, polymyositis, infiltrative processes

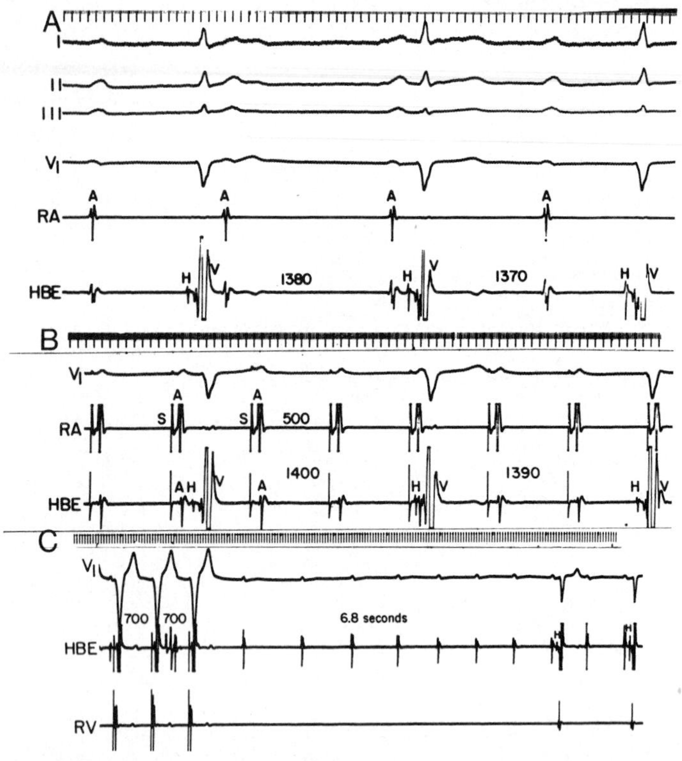

FIGURE 22–46. Congenital third degree AV block. In panel A, complete AV nodal block is apparent. No P wave is followed by a His bundle potential, while each ventricular depolarization is preceded by a His bundle potential. In panel B, atrial pacing (cycle length 500 msec) fails to alter cycle length of the junctional rhythm. Still no P wave is followed by a His bundle potential. In panel C, after 30 seconds of ventricular pacing (cycle length 700 msec), suppression of the junctional focus results for almost 7 sec (overdrive suppression of automaticity; see Chapter 20).

(such as amyloid, sarcoid, or scleroderma), and an almost endless assortment of common and unusual conditions may produce AV block. In the adult, drug toxicity, coronary disease,[348] and degenerative processes appear to be the most common causes of AV heart block. The degenerative process produces partial or complete anatomical or electrical disruption within the AV nodal region, the AV bundle, or both bundle branches.[349]

AV Block in Children. In children, the most common cause of AV block is congenital (Chap. 30). Under such circumstances the AV block may be an isolated finding or associated with other lesions such as atrioventricular discordance.[350] Connective tissue disease[351] (p. 1725) and the presence of anti-Ro negative antibodies[352] in maternal sera of patients with congenital complete AV block raise the possibility that placentally transmitted antibodies play a role in some instances.[353, 353a] Anatomical disruption between the atrial musculature and peripheral parts of the conduction system, and nodoventricular discontinuity are two common histological findings. Children are most often asymptomatic; however, some may develop symptoms that require pacemaker implantation.[354] Mortality from congenital AV block is highest in the neonatal period, is much lower during childhood and adolescence, and increases slowly later in life. Stokes-Adams attacks may occur in patients with congenital heart block at any age. It is difficult to predict the prognosis in the individual patient.[355] A persistent heart rate at rest of 50 beats/min or less correlates with the incidence of syncope, and extreme bradycardia may contribute to the prevalence of Adams-Stokes attacks in children with congenital complete AV block.[356] The site of block may not separate symptomatic children who have congenital or surgically induced complete heart block from those without symptoms. Prolonged recovery times of escape foci following rapid pacing (Fig. 22–46*C*) (see discussion of sinus node recovery time, p. 612) and the occurrence of paroxysmal tachycardias may be predisposing factors to the development of symptoms.[357]

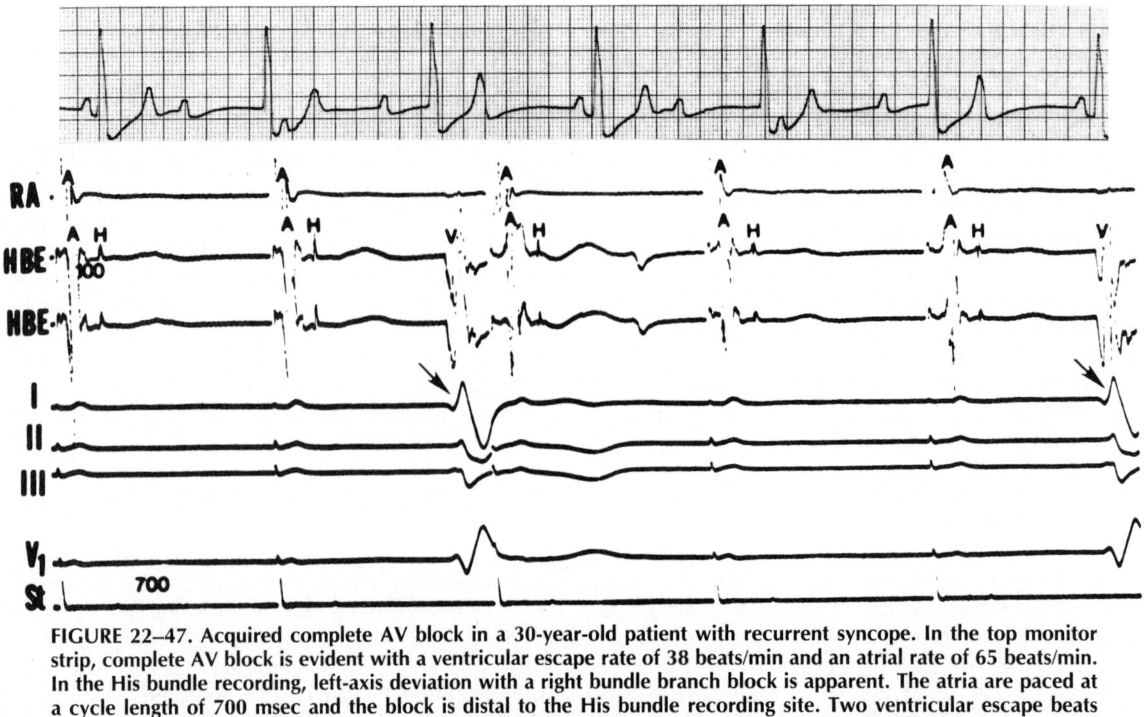

FIGURE 22–47. Acquired complete AV block in a 30-year-old patient with recurrent syncope. In the top monitor strip, complete AV block is evident with a ventricular escape rate of 38 beats/min and an atrial rate of 65 beats/min. In the His bundle recording, left-axis deviation with a right bundle branch block is apparent. The atria are paced at a cycle length of 700 msec and the block is distal to the His bundle recording site. Two ventricular escape beats are seen (*arrows*) at a rate of approximately 30 beats/min and are not preceded by His bundle activation.

CLINICAL FEATURES. Many of the signs of AV block are demonstrated at the bedside. First degree AV block may be recognized by a long *a-c* wave interval in the jugular venous pulse and by diminished intensity of the first heart sound as the P-R interval lengthens. In type I second degree AV block, the heart rate may increase imperceptibly with gradually diminished intensity of the first heart sound, widening the *a-c* interval terminated by a pause, and an *a* wave not followed by a *v* wave. Intermittent ventricular pauses and *a* waves in the neck not followed by *v* waves characterize type II AV block. The first heart sound maintains a constant intensity. In complete AV block, the findings are the same as those in AV dissociation (see below).

Significant clinical manifestations of first and second degree AV block usually consist of palpitations or feelings of the heart "missing a beat." Persistent 2:1 AV block may produce symptoms of chronic bradycardia. Complete AV block may be accompanied by signs and symptoms of reduced cardiac output, syncope or presyncope, angina, or palpitations due to ventricular tachyarrhythmias.

TREATMENT. As discussed in detail in Chapter 23, drugs cannot be relied on to increase the heart rate for more than several hours to several days in patients with symptomatic heart block without producing significant side effects. Therefore, temporary or permanent pacemaker insertion is indicated in patients with symptomatic bradyarrhythmias.[358, 359] For short-term therapy when the block is likely to be evanescent but still requires treatment or until adequate pacing therapy can be established, vagolytic agents such as atropine are useful for patients who have AV nodal disturbances, while catecholamines such as isoproterenol may be used transiently to treat patients who have heart block at any site (see treatment for Sinus Bradycardia, above). Isoproterenol should be used with extreme caution or not at all in patients who have acute myocardial infarction.

ATRIOVENTRICULAR (AV) DISSOCIATION

As the term indicates, dissociated or independent beating of atria and ventricles defines AV dissociation. AV dissociation is never a *primary* disturbance of rhythm but is a "symptom" of an underlying rhythm disturbance produced by one of three causes or a combination of causes (Fig. 22–48), that prevent the normal transmission of impulses from atrium to ventricle, as follows:

1. Slowing of the dominant pacemaker of the heart (usually the sinus node), which allows escape of a subsidiary or latent pacemaker. AV dissociation by *default* of the primary pacemaker to a subsidiary one in this manner is often a normal phenomenon. It may occur during sinus arrhythmia or sinus bradycardia, permitting an independent AV junctional rhythm to arise (Fig. 22–2A, p. 664).

2. Acceleration of a latent pacemaker that *usurps* control of the ventricles. Abnormally enhanced discharge rate of a usually slower subsidiary pacemaker is pathological and commonly occurs during nonparoxysmal AV junctional tachycardia or VT without retrograde atrial capture (see Figs. 22–18 and 22–33).

3. Block, generally at the AV junction, that prevents impulses formed at a normal rate in a dominant pacemaker from reaching the ventricles and allows the ventricles to beat under the control of a subsidiary pacemaker. Junctional or ventricular escape rhythm during AV block, without retrograde atrial capture, are common examples in which block gives rise to AV dissociation. It is important to remember that complete AV block is *not* synonymous with complete AV dissociation: patients who have complete AV block have complete AV dissociation, but patients who have complete AV dissociation may or may not have complete AV block (see Figs. 22–46 and 22–47).

4. A combination of causes may exist, for example, when digitalis excess results in the production of nonparoxysmal AV junctional tachycardia associated with SA or AV block.[115]

With this classification in mind, it is important to emphasize that the term "AV dissociation" is *not* a diagnosis and is analogous to the terms "jaundice" or "fever." One must state that "AV dissociation is present *due to* . . ." and then give the cause. The accelerated rate of a slower, normally subsidiary pacemaker or the slowed rate of a faster, normally dominant pacemaker that prevents conduction due to physiological collision and mutual extinction

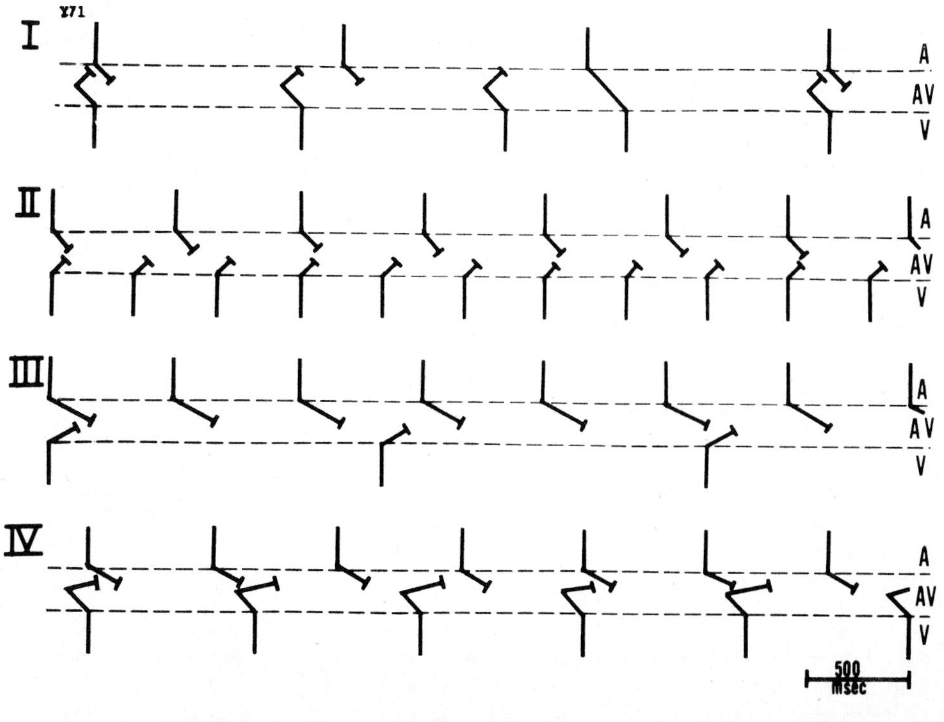

FIGURE 22–48. Diagrammatic illustration of the causes of AV dissociation. A sinus bradycardia that allows the escape of an AV junctional rhythm which does not capture the atria retrogradely illustrates cause I (top panel). Intermittent sinus captures occur (third P wave) to produce incomplete AV dissociation (see Fig. 22–2*B*). For cause II, a ventricular tachycardia without retrograde atrial capture produces complete AV dissociation (see Figs. 22–18 and 22–33). As the third cause, complete AV block with a ventricular escape rhythm is diagrammed (see Fig. 22–47). The combination of causes II and III is shown in panel IV, representing a nonparoxysmal AV junctional tachycardia and some degree of AV block.

of opposing wavefronts (interference), or the manifestations of AV block are the basic disturbances producing AV dissociation. The atria in all these cases beat independently from the ventricles, under control of the sinus node, ectopic atrial, or AV junctional pacemakers, and may exhibit any type of supraventricular rhythms. If a single pacemaker establishes control of both atria and ventricles for one beat (capture) or a series of beats (sinus rhythm, AV junctional rhythm with retrograde atrial capture, VT with retrograde atrial capture, and so forth), AV dissociation is abolished for that period. Conversely, as stated above, whenever the atria and ventricles fail to respond to a single impulse for one beat (premature ventricular complex without retrograde capture of the atrium) or a series of beats (ventricular tachycardia without retrograde atrial capture), AV dissociation exists for that period. The interruption of AV dissociation by one or a series of beats under the control of one pacemaker, either anterogradely or retrogradely, indicates that the AV dissociation is incomplete. Complete or incomplete dissociation may also occur in association with all forms of AV block. Commonly, when AV dissociation occurs as a result of AV block the atrial rate exceeds the ventricular rate. For example, a subsidiary pacemaker with a rate of 40 beats/min may escape in the presence of a 2:1 AV block when the atrial rate is 78. If the AV block is bidirectional, AV dissociation results.

ELECTROCARDIOGRAPHIC AND CLINICAL FEATURES. The electrocardiogram demonstrates the independence of P waves and QRS complexes. The P-wave morphology depends on the rhythm controlling the atria (sinus, atrial tachycardia, junctional, flutter, or fibrillation). During complete AV dissociation both the QRS complex and the P waves appear regularly spaced without a fixed temporal relationship to each other. When the dissociation is incomplete, a QRS complex of supraventricular contour occurs early and is preceded by a P wave at a P-R interval exceeding 0.12 seconds and within a conductable range. This indicates ventricular capture by the supraventricular focus. Similarly, a premature P wave with a retrograde morphology and a conductable R-P interval may indicate retrograde atrial capture by the subsidiary focus.

The physical findings include a variable intensity of the first heart sound as the P-R interval changes, atrial sounds, and *a* waves in the jugular venous pulse lacking a consistent relationship to ventricular contraction. Intermittent large (cannon) *a* waves may be seen in the jugular venous pulse when atrial and ventricular contraction occur simultaneously. The second heart sound may split normally or paradoxically, depending on the manner of ventricular activation. A premature beat representing a ventricular capture may interrupt a regular heart rhythm. When the ventricular rate exceeds the atrial rate, a cyclic increase in intensity of the first heart sound is produced as the P-R interval shortens, climaxed by a very loud sound (bruit de canon). This intense sound is followed by a sudden reduction in intensity of the first heart sound and the appearance of giant *a* waves as the P-R interval shortens and P waves "march through" the cardiac cycle.

TREATMENT. Treatment is directed toward the underlying heart disease and precipitating cause. The individual components *producing the AV dissociation*—not the AV dissociation per se—determine the specific type of antiarrhythmic approaches. Therapy ranges from pacemaker insertion in a patient who has AV dissociation due to complete AV block to lidocaine administration in a patient who has AV dissociation due to a ventricular tachycardia.

OTHER ELECTROPHYSIOLOGICAL ABNORMALITIES LEADING TO CARDIAC ARRHYTHMIAS

SUPERNORMAL CONDUCTION AND EXCITABILITY

SUPERNORMAL CONDUCTION. This is the term applied to situations characterized by conduction that is better than expected but generally not better than normal. The phenomenon almost always occurs when conduction is depressed but can be present in normal cardiac tissues as well.[360] It generally occurs when conduction takes place during the relative refractory period of the preceding complex (Fig. 22–49). The electrophysiological basis may relate, in some examples, to supernormal excitability (see below), but probably to other mechanisms as well.[361, 362] Supernormal conduction commonly has been invoked to explain AV (most probably His-Purkinje rather than AV nodal) conduction that is more rapid than expected or AV conduction that results when AV block is expected. Often the diagnosis is made inappropriately.[362a]

SUPERNORMAL EXCITATION. This phenomenon occurs when a stimulus, normally subthreshold, occurs during the supernormal period of recovery of the preceding complex and produces a propagated response. Stimuli occurring earlier or later fail to produce a propagated response. Demonstrated in vitro in Purkinje fibers but not ventricular muscle, supernormal excitation occurs during phase 3 of the cardiac action potential when the membrane potential, closer to threshold at the end of repolarization, requires less current to produce a propagated response. A similar phenomenon occurs during phase 4 diastolic depolarization or during afterdepolarizations that reduce the membrane potential closer to threshold. The phenomenon is most easily recognized when a nonsensing pacemaker, failing because of battery exhaustion and reduced output, produces a propagated response only when discharge occurs during a specific time period in a cardiac cycle (Fig. 22–50). Similar phenomena probably occur spontaneously with "weak" automatic foci, but the recognition of these events clinically is difficult and often speculative.

CONCEALED CONDUCTION

Concealed conduction[363] describes the phenomenon during which impulses penetrate an area of the conduction tissue, the AV node commonly[364] but other areas as well,[365] without emerging. Since the transmission of the impulse is concealed, that is, electrically silent in the standard electrocardiogram, concealed conduction becomes manifest only by its effects on the conduction and/or formation of subsequent impulses. The most common example follows a premature ventricular complex. Partial retrograde penetration of the AV node by the premature ventricular complex is *deduced* because the following sinus-initiated P wave blocks to produce a compensatory pause (Fig. 22–51) or conducts with a longer P-R interval if the premature ventricular complex is interpolated. The slower ventricular response when the atrial rate increases from atrial flutter to atrial fibrillation is due to a greater number of atrial impulses blocking (conducting into, without emerging) in the AV node and is a manifestation of concealed conduction. Concealed conduction occurs in WPW syndrome[365] and may be manifest by unidirectional block anterogradely or retrogradely in an accessory pathway (p. 689). Concealed junctional extrasystoles (Fig. 20–33) may create electrocardiographic manifestations of apparent heart block. Strict confirmation of concealed conduction should be the demonstration of manifest conduction when possible, such as in the form of conducted junctional extrasystoles (Fig. 22–15, p. 678).

PARASYSTOLE

Parasystole (Fig. 22–52) refers to a cardiac arrhythmia characterized electrocardiographically by: (1) varying coupling interval between the ectopic (parasystolic) complex and the dominant (generally, sinus-initiated) complex; (2) a common minimal time interval between manifest interectopic intervals, with the longer interectopic intervals being multiples of this minimal interval; (3) fusion complexes; and (4) the presence of the parasystolic impulse whenever the cardiac chamber is excitable. Parasystole with exit block is suspected when the parasystolic discharge focus fails to appear even though cardiac tissue is excitable.[366] The analogy commonly invoked to represent parasystole is the behavior of a fixed-rate nonsensing (VOO) pacemaker (Chap. 23). Parasystole can occur in the sinus and AV nodes, atrium and ventricle, and AV

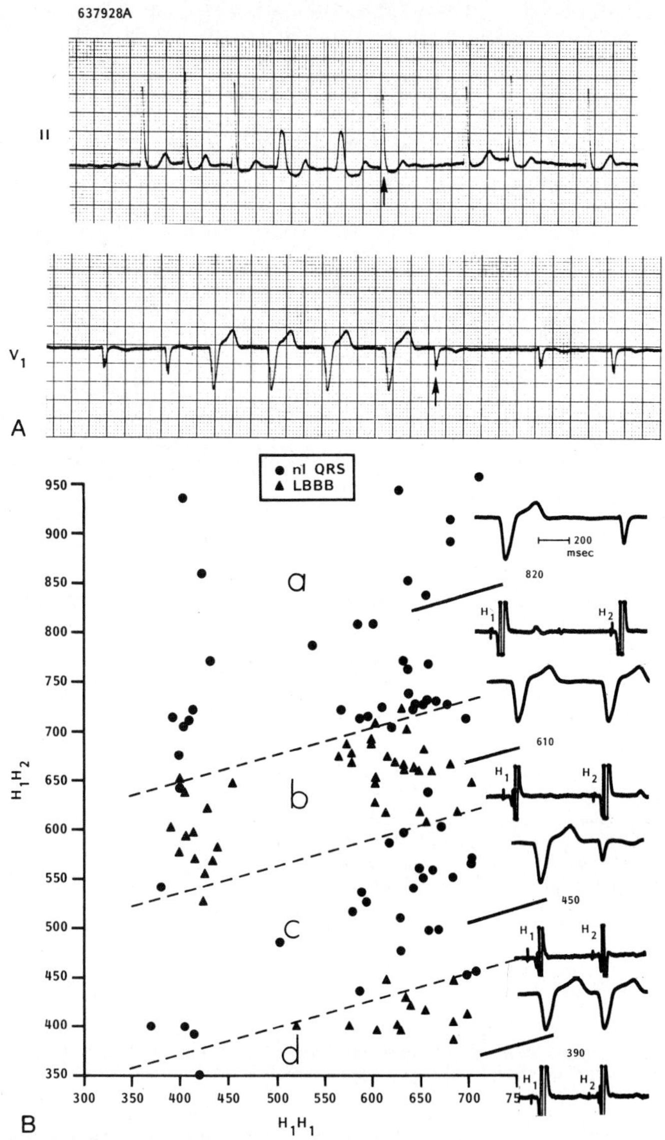

FIGURE 22–49. Supernormal conduction. Panel A illustrates atrial fibrillation with long-short R-R cycle sequences giving rise to QRS complexes conducted with a functional left bundle branch block. In each example, however, a shorter R-R cycle length is terminated by a normal QRS complex (arrow), an example of supernormal conduction.

Panel B shows a graph of the intervals and illustrative recordings during an electrophysiologic study of the patient whose ECG is shown in Panel A. The H-V interval of the complexes conducted with a left bundle branch block morphology is 45 msec, while the H-V interval of those conducted with a normal morphology is 35 msec. The graph indicates the premature interval (H_1-H_2, ordinate) plotted against the preceding cycle length (H_1-H_1, abscissa). All H_1-H_1 intervals were taken from complexes with a left bundle branch block morphology. Normal complexes are represented by filled circles and left bundle branch block contours by filled triangles. Four zones of conduction are identified, and illustrated by the four examples to the right, each connected by a solid line. The longest H_1-H_2 intervals are followed by a normal intraventricular conduction (zone A), while at shorter intervals, left bundle branch block occurs (zone B). When the H_1-H_2 interval shortens further, normal intraventricular conduction returns and the H-V intervals shorten to 35 msec (zone C, supernormal conduction). At the shortest H_1-H_2 interval, left bundle branch block again appears (zone D). (From Miles, W. M., Prystowsky, E. N., Heger, J. J., and Zipes, D. P.: Evaluation of the patient with wide QRS tachycardia. Med. Clin. North Am. *68*:1015, 1984.)

junction. The parasystolic mechanism presumably results from the regular (see below) discharge of an automatic focus that is independent of, and protected from, discharge by the dominant cardiac rhythm. A variety of mechanisms have been postulated to explain the apparent protection enjoyed by the parasystolic rhythm.

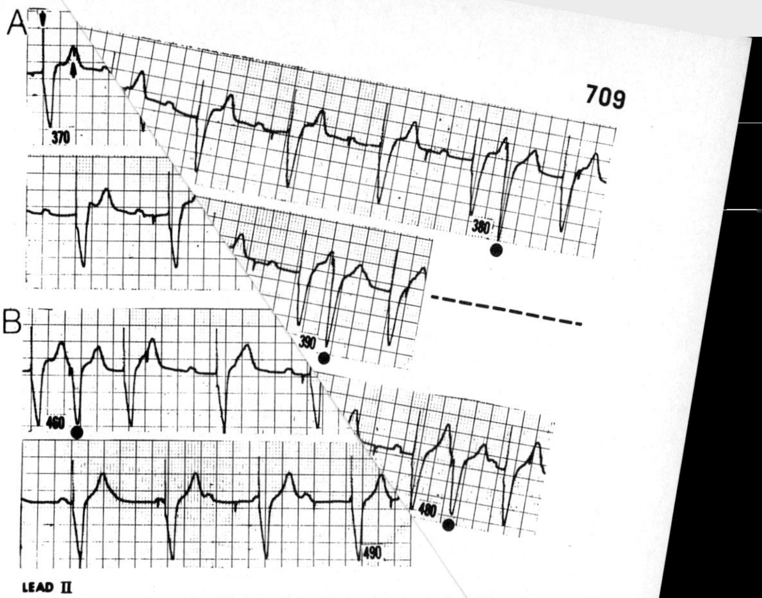

FIGURE 22–50. Supernormal excitation. Panels A noncontiguous portions of a continuous ECG recordin segment removed (dotted line). The patient presented pacemaker that had exceeded end-of-life and was no longe producing ventricular depolarization (small negative deflec cated by the upright arrow). A temporary pacemaker was and set at a fixed rate (asynchronous, V00; see Chap. 23). The deflections are indicated by the inverted arrow. The numbers in indicate the interval between the onset of the QRS complex and following subthreshold pacemaker stimulus. At intervals of 370 msec (beginning panel A) and 490 msec (end, panel B), the subthreshold stimulus fails to produce a propagated ventricular response. However, at intervals between 380 and 480 msec ventricular depolarizations result (filled circles). Thus, the period of supernormal excitation is 100 msec duration, from 380 to 480 msec after the onset of the QRS complex.

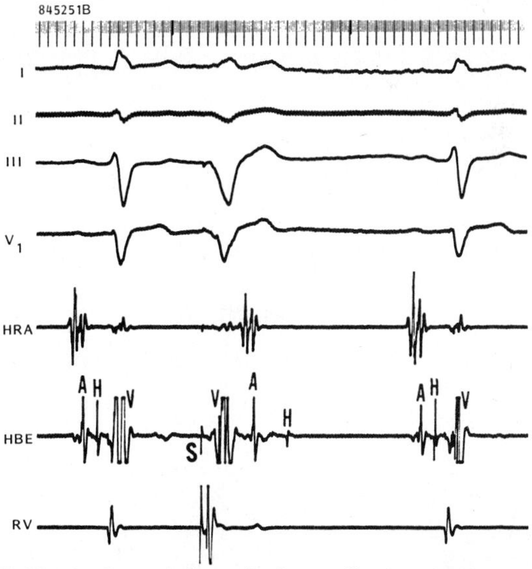

FIGURE 22–51. Concealed conduction. Following the first normally conducted sinus-initiated complex, a premature ventricular complex is stimulated (S). The next spontaneous sinus-initiated P wave blocks to produce a fully compensatory pause. The third sinus-initiated P wave conducts normally. From the His bundle recording it is obvious that the nonconducted sinus beat blocks distal to the His bundle recording site. Note that the A-H interval of the nonconducted sinus P wave beat is prolonged, suggesting that the premature ventricular complex retrogradely activated His and invaded the AV node, making it partially refractory to the next sinus beat. Since retrograde conduction into the AV node is not recorded, and can only be surmised on the basis of the increase in the following AH interval, it is an example of concealed conduction. Further, since retrograde His and AV node activation by the premature ventricular complex would not be apparent in the scalar ECG but is responsible for the compensatory pause, the blocked P wave is an example of concealed conduction.

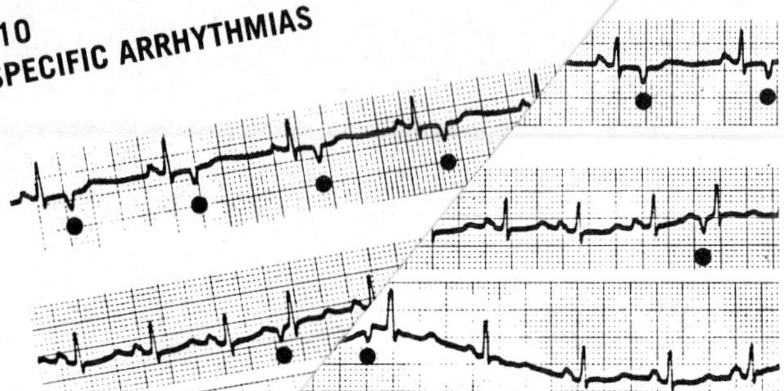

...asystole. *Top panel,* the atrial parasystolic ...nder the negative P waves) are present at a ... to the dominant sinus rhythm. The reason for ...s as follows: Each time the parasystolic impulse FIGURE...trium, it also discharges the sinus node. Diastolic impul... the sinus node begins at that point (reset) and results fix...ng sinus P wave (positive P wave). Thus, the constant ... discharge rate (interectopic interval approximately 960 ...setting of the sinus node, and constant phase 4 diastolic ...ization in the sinus node combine to result in fixed coupling. ...m *panel,* the sinus discharge rate is slightly faster. It is no longer ...charged by the parasystolic impulse which is still occurring ...t approximately 960 msec (slightly longer interval in the bottom tracing). Variable coupling, the usual presentation of parasystole, results. Lead 2.

These "classic" definitions of parasystole now need to be modified because it has been well established that the dominant sinus beats may modulate the discharge rate of the parasystolic rhythm despite entrance block (Fig. 20–19, p. 599).[367–372] Thus, wide variations in the modulated parasystolic cycle may occur. The "true" or unmodulated parasystolic cycle length can be determined by finding two consecutive parasystolic complexes without intervening beats. Phase response curves result. A triphasic phase-response curve has been suggested to account for apparent supernormal modulation.[368] Annihilation and entrainment of ventricular parasystolic rhythms also has been demonstrated.[370] Fixed coupling between the dominant and parasystolic rhythms can occur due to a variety of mechanisms, including entrainment.

Acknowledgments

The author thanks William M. Miles, M.D., for critical comments and Joan Zipes for secretarial assistance. Some of the illustrations were taken from records of patients studied by Eric N. Prystowsky, M.D. and William M. Miles, M.D.

REFERENCES

DIAGNOSTIC AND THERAPEUTIC CONSIDERATIONS

History

1. Sutherland, D. J., McPherson, D. D., Renton, K. W., Spencer, C. A., and Montague, T. J.: The effect of caffeine on cardiac rate, rhythm, and ventricular repolarization. Analysis of 18 normal subjects and 18 patients with primary ventricular dysrhythmia. Chest 87:319, 1985.
2. Thornton, J. R.: Atrial fibrillation in healthy nonalcoholic people after an alcoholic binge. Lancet 2:1013, 1984.
3. Engel, T. R., and Luck, J. C.: Effect on whiskey on atrial vulnerability and "holiday heart." J. Am. Coll. Cardiol. *1*:816, 1983.
4. Nordrehaug, J. E., Johannessen, K. A., and von der Lippe, G.: Serum potassium concentration as a risk factor of ventricular arrhythmias early in acute myocardial infarction. Circulation *71*:645, 1985.
5. Stewart, D. E., Ikram, H., Espiner, E. A., and Nicholls, M. G.: Arrhythmogenic potential of diuretic induced hypokalemia in patients with mild hypertension and ischemic heart disease. Br. Heart J. *54*:290, 1985.
6. Commerford, P. J., and Lloyd, E. A.: Arrhythmias in patients with drug toxicity, electrolyte and endocrine disturbances. Med. Clin. North Am. *68*:1051, 1984.

Physical Examination

7. Hess, D. S., Hanlon, T., Scheinman, M., Budge, R., and Desai, J.: Termination of ventricular tachycardia by carotid sinus massage. Circulation *65*:627, 1982.
8. Waxman, M. B., Wald, R. W., and Cameron, D.: Interactions between the autonomic nervous system and tachycardias in man. Cardiol. Clin. *1*:143, 1983.
9. Beal, M. F., Park, T. S., and Fisher, C. M.: Cerebral atheromatous embolism following carotid sinus pressure. Arch. Neurol. *38*:310, 1981.

Electrocardiography

10. Fisch, C.: The clinical electrocardiogram: A classic. Circulation *62* (Suppl. 3):1, 1980.
10a. Wellens, H. J. J.: The electrocardiogram. 80 years after Einthoven. J. Am. Coll. Cardiol. 7:484, 1986.
11. Hung J., Kelly, D. T., Hutton, B. F., Uther, J. B., and Baird, D. K.: Influence of heart rate and atrial transport on left ventricular volume and function: Relation to hemodynamic changes produced by supraventricular arrhythmia. Am. J. Cardiol. *48*:632, 1981.
12. Gillette, P. C., Smith, R. T., Garson, A., Jr., Mullins, C. E., Gutgesell, H. P., Goh, T. H., Cooley, D. A., and McNamara, D. G.: Chronic supraventricular tachycardia. A curable cause of congestive cardiomyopathy. J.A.M.A. *253*:391, 1985.
13. McLaran, C. J., Gersh, B. J., Sugrue, D. D., Hammill, S. C., Seward, J. B., and Holmes, D. R., Jr.: Tachycardia induced myocardial dysfunction. A reversible phenomenon? Br. Heart J. *53*:323, 1985.

Therapy

14. Chakko, C. S., and Gheorghiade, M.: Ventricular arrhythmias in severe heart failure: Incidence, significance, and effectiveness of antiarrhythmic therapy. Am. Heart J. *109*:497, 1985.

INDIVIDUAL CARDIAC ARRHYTHMIAS

Sinus Nodal Disturbances

15. Jalife, J.: Mitral entrainment and electrical coupling as mechanisms for synchronous firing of rabbit sino-atrial pace-maker cells. J. Physiol. *356*:221, 1984.
16. Salata, J. J., Gill, R. M., Gilmour, R. F., Jr., and Zipes, D. P.: Effects of sympathetic tone on vagally induced phasic changes in heart rate and AV nodal conduction in the anesthetized dog. Circ. Res. *58*:584, 1986.
17. Levy, M. N., and Martin, P. J.: Neural control of the heart. *In* Berne, R. M., et al. (eds.): Handbook of Physiology, The Cardiovascular System, Vol. I. Bethesda, Md., American Physiological Society, 1979, p. 581.
18. Boineau, J. P., Miller, C. B., Schnessler, R. B., Roeske, W. R., Autry, L. T., Wylde, A. C., and Hill, D. A.: Activation sequence and potential distribution maps demonstrating multi-centric atrial impulse origin in dogs. Circ. Res. *55*:532, 1984.
19. Crimm, A., Severance, H. W., Jr., Coffey, K., McKinnis, R., Wagner, G. S., and Califf, R. M.: Prognostic significance of isolated sinus tachycardia during the first three days of acute myocardial infarction. Am. J. Med. *76*:983, 1984.
20. Yee, R., Guiraudon, G. M., Gardner, M. J., Gulamhusein, S. S., and Klein, G.J.: Refractory paroxysmal sinus tachycardia: Management by subtotal right atrial exclusion. J. Am. Coll. Cardiol. 3:400, 1984.
21. Abdon, N. J., Landin, K., and Johansson, B. W.: Athlete's bradycardia as an embolising disorder? Symptomatic arrhythmias in patients aged less than 50 years. Br. Heart J. *52*:660, 1984.
22. Hilgard, J., Ezri, M. D., and Denes, P.: Significance of ventricular pauses of three seconds or more detected on twenty-four hour Holter recordings. Am. J. Cardiol. *55*:1005, 1985.
23. Guilleminault, C., Pool, P., Motta, J., and Gillis, A. M.: Sinus arrest during REM sleep in young adults. N. Engl. J. Med. *311*:1006, 1984.
24. Kerr, W. J., and Vance, J. P.: Oculocardiac reflex from the empty orbit. Anesthesia *38*:883, 1983.
25. Song, E., Segal, I., Hodkinson, J., and Kew, M. C.: Sinus bradycardia in obstructive jaundice—correlation with total serum bile acid concentrations. S. Afr. Med. J. *64*:548, 1983.
26. Weintraub, M., Hes, J. P., Rotmensch, H. H., Soferman, G., and Liron, M.: Extreme sinus bradycardia associated with lithium therapy. Isr. J. Med. Sci. *19*:353, 1983.
27. Mossuti, E., Rapisarda, A., Elia, F., Martello, G., Maltese, B., and Negro, R.: Conduction disorder caused by conjunctival installation of timolol. Description of a case. G. Ital. Cardiol. *13*:125, 1983.
28. Goldberg, S., Greenspon, A. J., Urban, P. L., Muza, B., Berger B., Walinsky, P., and Maroko, P. R.: Reperfusion arrhythmia: A marker of restoration of antegrade flow during intracoronary thrombolysis for acute myocardial infarction. Am. Heart J. *105*:26, 1983.
29. Myerburg, R. J., Estes, D., Zaman, L., Luceri, R. M., Kessler, K. M., Trohman, R. G., and Castellanos, A.: Outcome of resuscitation from bradyarrhythmic or asystolic prehospital cardiac arrest. J. Am. Coll. Cardiol. *4*:1118, 1984.
30. Dreifus, L. S., Michelson, E. L., and Kaplinsky, E.: Bradyarrhythmias: Clinical significance and management. J. Am. Coll. Cardiol. *1*:327, 1983.
31. Weiss, A. T., Rod, J. L., Gotsman, M. S., and Lewis, B. S.: Hydralazine in the management of symptomatic sinus bradycardia. Eur. J. Cardiol. *12*:261, 1981.
32. Benditt, D. G., Benson, D. W., Jr., Kreitt, J., Dunnigan, A., Pritzker, M. R., Crouse, L., and Scheinman, M. M.: Electrophysiologic effects of theophylline in young patients with recurrent symptomatic bradyarrhythmias. Am. J. Cardiol. 52:1223, 1983.

33. Rosenqvist, M., Brandt, J., and Schuller, H.: Atrial versus ventricular pacing in sinus node disease: A treatment comparison study. Am. Heart J. *111*:292, 1986.
34. Hrushesky, W. J., Fader, D., Schmitt, O., and Gilbertsen, V.: The respiratory sinus arrhythmia: The measure of cardiac age. Science *224*:1001, 1984.
35. Smith, S. A.: Reduced sinus arrhythmia in diabetic autonomic neuropathy: Diagnostic value of an age-related normal range. Br. Med. J. *285*:(6355):1599, 1982.
36. Coker, R., Koziell, A., Oliver, C., and Smith, S. E.: Does the sympathetic nervous system influence sinus arrhythmia in man? Evidence from combined autonomic blockade. J. Physiol. (Lond) *356*:459, 1984.
37. Gomes, J. A., Hariman, R. I., and Chowdry, I. A.: New application of direct sinus node recording in man: Assessment of sinus node recovery time. Circulation *70*:663, 1984.
38. Asseman, P., Berzin, B., Desry, D., Vilarem, D., Durand, P., Delmotte, C., Sarkis E. H., Lekieffre, J., and Thery, C.: Persistent sinus nodal electrograms during abnormally prolonged postpacing atrial pauses in sick sinus syndrome in humans: Sinoatrial block versus overdrive suppression. Circulation *68*:33, 1983.
39. Peretz, D. I., and Abdulla, A.: Management of cardioinhibitory hypersensitive carotid sinus syncope with permanent cardiac pacing—a 17-year prospective study. Can. J. Cardiol. *1*:86, 1985.
40. Ector, H., Rolies, L., and DeGeest, H.: Dynamic electrocardiography and ventricular pauses of 3 seconds and more: Etiology and therapeutic implications. PACE *6*:548, 1983.
41. Walter, P. F., Crawley, I. S., and Dorney, E. R.: Carotid sinus hypersensitivity and syncope. Am. J. Cardiol. *42*:396, 1978.
42. Merx, W., Effert, S., Hanrath, P., Pop, T., Rehder, W., and Schweizer, P.: Hyperactive carotid sinus reflex. Dtsch. Med. Wochenschr. *106*:135, 1981.
43. Davies, A. B., Stephens, M. R., and Davies, A. G.: Carotid sinus hypersensitivity in patients presenting with syncope. Br. Heart J. *42*:583, 1979.
44. Brown, K. A., Maloney, J. D., Smith, C. H., Hartzler, G. O., and Ilstup, D. M.: Carotid sinus reflex in patients undergoing coronary angiography: Relationship of degree and location of coronary artery disease in response to carotid sinus massage. Circulation *62*:697, 1980.
45. Morley, C. A., Dehn, T. C., Perrins, E. J., Chan, S. L., and Sutton, R.: Baroreflex sensitivity measured by the phenylephrine pressor test in patients with carotid sinus and sick sinus syndromes. Cardiovasc. Res. *18*:752, 1984.
46. Keating, E. C., Burks, J. M., and Calder, J. R., Jr.: Mixed carotid sinus hypersensitivity: Successful therapy with pacing, ephedrine, and propranolol. PACE *8*:356, 1985.
47. Wenger, T. L., Dohrmann, M. L., Strauss, H. C., Conley, M. J., Wechsler, A.S., and Wagner, G. S.: Hypersensitive carotid sinus syndrome manifested as cough syncope. PACE *3*:332, 1980.
48. Thorman, J., Neuss, H., Schlepper, M., and Mitrovic, V.: Effects of clonidine on sinus node function in man. Chest *80*:201, 1981.
49. Pick, A., and Langendorf, R.: Interpretation of Complex Arrhythmias. Philadelphia, Lea and Febiger, 1979, p. 127.
50. Surawicz, B., and Reddy, C. P.: Tachycardia-bradycardia syndrome. *In* Surawicz, B., et al. (eds.): Tachycardias. Boston, Martinus Nijhoff, 1984, p. 199.
50a. Crossen, K. J., and Cain, M. E.: Assessment and management of sinus node dysfunction. Mod. Concepts Cardiovasc. Dis. *55*:43, 1986.
51. Rosenqvist, M., Vallin, H., and Edhag, O.: Clinical and electrophysiologic course of sinus node disease: Five-year follow-up study. Am. Heart J. *109*:513, 1985.
52. Kang, P. S., Gomes, J. A., Kelen, G., and El-Sherif, N.: Role of autonomic regulatory mechanism in sinoatrial conduction and sinus nodal automaticity in sick sinus syndrome. Circulation *64*:832, 1981.
53. Desae, J. M., Scheinman, M. M., Strauss, H. C., Massie, B., and O'Young, J.: Electrophysiologic effects of combined autonomic blockade in patients with sinus node disease. Circulation *63*:953, 1981.
54. Simonsen, E., Nielsen, J. S., and Nielsen, B. L.: Sinus node dysfunction in 128 patients. A retrospective study with followup. Acta Med. Scand. *208*:343, 1980.
55. Duster, M. C., Bink-Boelkens, M. T., Wampler, D., Gillette, P. C., McNamara, D. G., and Cooley, D. A.: Long-term follow-up of dysrhythmias following the Mustard procedure. Am. Heart J. *109*:1323, 1985.
56. Hayes, C. J., and Gersony, W. M.: Arrhythmias after the Mustard operation for transposition of the great arteries: A long-term study. J. Am. Coll. Cardiol. 7:133, 1986.
57. Gillette, P. C., Wampler, D. G., Shannon, C., and Ott, D.: Use of cardiac pacing after the Mustard operation for transposition of the great arteries. J. Am. Coll. Cardiol. 7:138, 1986.
58. Mackintosh, A. F.: Sinoatrial disease in young people. Br. Heart J. *45*:62, 1981.
59. Beder, S. D., Gillette, P. C., Garson, A., Jr., Porter, C. B. J., and McNamara, D.G.: Symptomatic sick sinus syndrome in children and adolescents as the only manifestation of cardiac abnormality or associated with unoperated congenital heart disease. Am. J. Cardiol. *51*:1133, 1983.
60. Scott, O., Williams, G. J., and Fiddler, G. I.: Results of 24-hour ambulatory monitoring of electrocardiogram in 131 healthy boys age 10 to 13 years. Br. Heart J. *44*:304, 1980.
61. Kerr, C. R., Grant, A. O., Wenger, T. L., and Strauss, H. C.: Sinus node dysfunction. Cardiol. Clin. *1*:187, 1983.
62. Swiryn, S., McDonough, T., and Hueter, D. C.: Sinus node function and dysfunction. Med. Clin. North Am. *68*:935, 1984.
63. Bharati, S., Nordenberg, A., Bauernfeind, R., Varghese, J. P., Carvalho, A. G., Rosen, K. M., and Lev, M.: The anatomic substrate for the sick sinus syndrome in adolescents. Am. J. Cardiol. *46*:163, 1980.
64. Rossi, L.: The pathologic basis of cardiac arrhythmias. Cardiol. Clin. *1*:13, 1983.
65. Gomes, J. A., Kang, P. S., and El-Sherif, N.: Effects of digitalis on the human sick sinus node after pharmacologic autonomic blockade. Am. J. Cardiol. *48*:783, 1981.
66. Sung, R. J., Chang, M.S. and Chiang, B. N.: Clinical electrophysiology of supraventricular tachycardia. Cardiol. Clin. *1*:225, 1983.
67. Benditt, D. G., Benson, D. W., Jr., Dunnigan, A., Gornick, C. C., and Anderson, R. W.: Atrial flutter, atrial fibrillation and other primary atrial tachycardias. Med. Clin. North Am. *68*:895, 1984.

DISTURBANCES OF ATRIAL RHYTHM

68. Jalife, J., Michaels, D. C., and Langendorf, R.: Premature sinus complexes and modulation of automaticity. Circulation (abstract), *74*(Suppl II):471, 1986.
69. Chilson, D. A., Zipes, D. P., Heger, J. J., Browne, K. F., and Prystowsky, E.N.: Functional bundle branch block: Discordant response of right and left bundle branches to changes in heart rate. Am. J. Cardiol. *54*:313, 1984.
70. Zipes, D. P., Foster. P. R., Troup, P. J., and Pedersen, D. H.: Atrial induction of ventricular tachycardia: Reentry or triggered automaticity. Am. J. Cardiol. *44*:1, 1979.
71. Wellens, H. J. J., Bär, F. W., Farre, J., Ross, D. L., Wiener, I., and Vanagt, E. J.: Initiation and termination of ventricular tachycardia by supraventricular stimuli. Am. J. Cardiol. *46*:576, 1980.
72. Waldo, A. L.: Mechanisms of atrial fibrillation, atrial flutter, and ectopic atrial tachycardia—a brief review. Circulation (*in press*).
73. Robertson, C. E., and Miller, H. C.: Extreme tachycardia complicating the use of disopyramide in atrial flutter. Br. Heart J. *44*:602, 1980.
74. Boineau, J. P., Wylds, A. C., Autry, L. J., Schuessler, R. B., and Miller, C. B.: Mechanisms of atrial flutter as determined from spontaneous and experimental models. *In* Josephson, M. E., and Wellens, H.J.J. (eds.): Tachycardias: Mechanisms, Diagnosis and Treatment. Philadelphia, Lea & Febiger, 1984, p. 91.
75. Jackman, W. M., Prystowsky, E. N., Naccarelli, G. V., Heger, J. J., and Zipes, D. P.: Reevaluation of enhanced AV nodal conduction: Evidence to suggest a continuum of normal nodal physiology. Circulation *67*:441, 1983.
76. Moleiro, F., Mendoza, I. J., Medina-Ravell, V., Castellanos, A., and Myerburg, R. J.: One to one atrioventricular conduction during atrial pacing at rates of 300/min in absence of Wolff-Parkinson-White syndrome. Am. J. Cardiol. *48*:789, 1981.
77. Suarez, L. D., Kretz, A., Alvarez, J. A., Martinez, J. A., and Perosio, A. M.: Dissimilar atrial rhythms. A patient with triple right atrial rhythm. Am. Heart J. *100*:678, 1980.
78. Gomes, J. A., Kang, P. S., Matheson, M., Gough, W.B., Jr., and El-Sherif, N.: Coexistence of sick sinus rhythm and atrial flutter-fibrillation. Circulation *63*:80, 1981.
79. Simpson, R. J., Foster, J. R., and Gettes, L. S.: Atrial excitability and conduction in patients with interatrial conduction defects. Am. J. Cardiol. *50*:1331, 1982.
80. Dobmeyer, D. J., Stine, R. A., Leier, C. V., and Schaal, S.F.: Electrophysiologic mechanisms of provoked atrial flutter in mitral valve prolapse syndrome. Am. J. Cardiol. *56*:602, 1985.
81. Dunnigan, A., Benson, W., Jr., and Benditt, D. G.: Atrial flutter in infants: Diagnosis, clinical features, and treatment. Pediatrics *75*:725, 1985.
82. Silverman, N. H., Enderlein, M. A., Stanger, P., Teitel, D. F., Heymann, M. A., and Golbus, M. S.: Recognition of fetal arrhythmias by echocardiography. J. Clin. Ultrasound *13*:255, 1985.
83. Garson, A., Jr., Bink-Boelkens, M., Hesslein, P. S., Hordof, A. J., Keane, J. F., Neches, W. H., Porter, C. J., and other investigators of the pediatric electrophysiology society: Atrial flutter in the young: A collaborative study of 380 cases. J. Am. Coll. Cardiol. *6*:871, 1985.
84. Campbell, R. M., Dick, M., II, Jenkins, J. M., Spicer, R.L., Crowley, D. C., Rocchini, A. P., Snider, A. R., Stern, A.M., and Rosenthal, A.: Atrial overdrive pacing for conversion of atrial flutter in children. Pediatrics *75*:730, 1985.
85. Levy, S.: Role of pacing in treatment of supraventricular tachycardia (supraventricular tachycardia, Wolff-Parkinson-White, flutter). *In* Josephson, M. E., and Wellens, H.J.J. (eds.): Tachycardias: Mechanisms, Diagnosis Treatment. Philadelphia, Lea and Febiger, 1984, p. 223.
86. Camm, J., Ward, D., and Spurrell, R.: Response of atrial flutter to overdrive atrial pacing and intravenous disopyramide phosphate, singly and in combination. Br. Heart J. *44*:240, 1980.
87. Waxman, H. L., Myerburg, R. J., Appel, R., and Sung, R.J.: Verapamil for control of ventricular rate in paroxysmal supraventricular tachycardia and atrial fibrillation or flutter: A double-blind randomized cross-over study. Ann. Intern. Med. *94*:1, 1981.
88. Brandenburg, R. O., Jr., Holmes, D. R., Jr., Brandenburg, R. O., and McGoon, D. C.: Clinical follow up study of paroxysmal supraventricular tachyarrhythmias after operative repair of a secundum type atrial septal defect in adults. Am. J. Cardiol. *51*:273, 1983.
89. Ormerod, O. J., McGregor, C. G., Stone, D. L., Wisbey, C., and Petch, M. D.: Arrhythmias after coronary bypass surgery. Br. Heart J. *51*:618, 1984.
90. Douglas, P. S., Hirshfeld, J. W., Jr., and Edmunds, L. H., Jr.: Clinical correlates of atrial tachyarrhythmias after valve replacement for aortic stenosis. Circulation 72(Suppl. 2):159, 1985.
91. Spodick, D. H.: Frequency of arrhythmias in acute pericarditis determined by Holter monitoring. Am. J. Cardiol. 53:842, 1984.
92. Forfar, J. C., Miller, H. C., and Toft, A. D.: Occult thyrotoxicosis: A correctable cause of "idiopathic" atrial fibrillation. Am. J. Cardiol. *44*:9, 1979.
93. Takahashi, N., Seki, A., Imataka, K., and Fujii, J.: Clinical features of

paroxysmal atrial fibrillation: An observation of 94 patients. Jpn. Heart J. *22*:143, 1981.
94. Kannel, W. B., Abbott, R. D., Savage, D. D., and McNamara, P. M.: Epidemiologic features of chronic atrial fibrillation: The Framingham study. N. Engl. J. Med. *306*:1018, 1982.
95. Gajewski, J., and Singer, R. B.: Mortality in an insured population with atrial fibrillation. J.A.M.A. *245*:1540, 1981.
96. Olsson, S. B., Orndahl, G., Ernestrom, S., Eskielson, J., Persson, S., Grennert, M. L., and Johanson, B. W.: Spontaneous reversion from longlasting atrial fibrillation to sinus rhythm. Acta Med. Scand. *207*:5, 1980.
97. Wolf, P. A., Kannel, W. B., McGee, D. L., Meeks, S.L., Bharucha, N. E., and McNamara, P. M.: Duration of atrial fibrillation and imminence of stroke: The Framingham Study. Stroke *14*:664, 1983.
98. Hart, R. G., Coull, B. M., and Hart, D.: Early recurrent embolism associated with nonvalvular atrial fibrillation: A retrospective study. Stroke *14*:688, 1983.
99. Sherman, D. G., Goldman, L., Whiting, R. B., Jurgensen, K., Kaste, M., Easton, J. D.: Thromboembolism in patients with atrial fibrillation. Arch. Neurol. *41*:708, 1984.
100. Brand, F. N., Abbott, R. D., Kannel, W. B., and Wolf, P.F.: Characteristics and prognosis of lone atrial fibrillation. 30-year follow-up in the Framingham Study. J.A.M.A. *254*:3449, 1985.
101. Hunt, D., Sloman, G., and Penington, C.: Effects of atrial fibrillation on prognosis of acute myocardial infarction. Br. Heart J. *40*:303, 1978.
102. Sugiura, T., Iwasaka, T., Ogawa, A., Shiroyama, Y., Tsuji, H., Onoyama, H., and Inada, M.: Atrial fibrillation in acute myocardial infarction. Am. J. Cardiol. *56*:27, 1985.
103. Ewy, G. A., Ulfers, L., Hager, W. D., Rosenfeld, A.R., Roeske, W. R., and Goldman, S.: Response of atrial fibrillation to therapy: Role of etiology and left atrial diameter. J. Electrocardiol. *13*:119, 1980.
104. Hoglund, C., and Rosenhamer, G.: Echocardiographic left atrial dimension as a predictor of maintaining sinus rhythm after conversion of atrial fibrillation. Acta Med. Scand. *217*:411, 1985.
105. Meijler, F. L.: An "account" of digitalis and atrial fibrillation. J. Am. Coll. Cardiol. *5*:60A, 1985.
106. Halpern, S. W., Ellrodt, G., Singh, B. N., and Mandel, W. J.: Efficacy of intravenous procainamide infusion in converting atrial fibrillation to sinus rhythm. Relation to left atrial size. Br. Heart J. *44*:589, 1980.
106a. Horowitz, L. N., Spielman, S. R., Greenspan, A. M., Mintz, G. S., Morganroth, J., Brown, R., Brady, P. M., and Kay, H. R.: Use of amiodarone in the treatment of persistent and paroxysmal atrial fibrillation resistant to quinidine therapy. J. Am. Coll. Cardiol. *6*:1402, 1985.
107. Mancini, G. B. J., and Goldberger, A. L.: Cardioversion of atrial fibrillation: Consideration of embolization, anticoagulation, prophylactic pacemaker and long term success. Am. Heart J. *104*:617, 1982.
108. Akhtar, M.: Supraventricular tachycardias. Electrophysiologic mechanisms, diagnosis, and pharmacologic therapy. *In* Josephson, M. E., and Wellens, H.J.J. (eds.): Tachycardias: Mechanisms, Diagnosis Treatment. Philadelphia, Lea and Febiger, 1984, p. 137.
109. Rinkenberger, R. L., Prystowsky, E. N., Heger, J. J., Troup, P. J., Jackman, W. M., and Zipes, D. P.: Effects of intravenous and chronic oral verapamil administration in patients with supraventricular tachyarrhythmias. Circulation *62*:996, 1980.
110. Levine, J. H., Michael, J. R., and Guarnieri, T.: Multifocal atrial tachycardia: A toxic effect of theophylline. Lancet *1*(8419):12, 1985.
111. Bisset, G. S., Siegel, S. F., Gaum, W. E., and Kaplan, S.: Chaotic atrial tachycardia in childhood. Am. Heart J. *101*:268, 1981.
112. Levine, J. H., Michael, J. R., and Guarnieri, T.: Treatment of multifocal atrial tachycardia with verapamil. N. Engl. J. Med. *312*:21, 1985.
113. Iseri, L. T., Fairshter, R. D., Hardemann, J. L., and Brodsky, M. A.: Magnesium and potassium therapy in multifocal atrial tachycardia. Am. Heart J. *110*:789, 1985.

AV JUNCTIONAL RHYTHM DISTURBANCES

114. Wit, A. L., and Cranefield, P. F.: Mechanisms of impulse initiation in the atrioventricular junction and the effects of acetylstrophanthidin. Am. J. Cardiol. *49*:921, 1982.
115. Pick, A., and Dominguez, P.: Nonparoxysmal AV nodal tachycardias. Circulation *16*:1022, 1957.
116. Zipes, D. P., Gaum, W. E., Genetos, B. C., Glassman, R.D., Noble, R. J., and Fisch, C.: Atrial tachycardia without P wave masquerading as an AV junctional tachycardia. Circulation *55*:253, 1977.
117. Castellanos, A., Sung, R. J., and Myerburg, R. J.: His bundle electrocardiography in digitalis-induced atrioventricular junctional Wenckebach periods with irregular HH intervals. Am. J. Cardiol. *43*:653, 1979.
118. Rosen, M. R., Fisch, C., Hoffman, B. F., Danilo, P., Jr., Lovelace, D. E., and Knoebel, S. B.: Can accelerated atrioventricular junctional escape rhythms be explained by delayed afterdepolarizations? Am. J. Cardiol. *45*:1272, 1980.
119. Tenczer, J., Littmann, L., Rohla, M., and Fenyvesi, T.: The effects of overdrive pacing and lidocaine on atrioventricular junctional rhythms in man: The role of abnormal automaticity. Circulation *72*:480, 1985.
120. Palileo, E. V., Bauernfeind, R. A., Swiryn, S. P., Wyndham, C. R., and Rosen, K. M.: Chronic nonparoxysmal junctional tachycardia. Chest *80*:106, 1981.
121. Akhtar, M.: Atrioventricular nodal reentrant tachycardia. Med. Clin. North Am. *68*:819, 1984.
122. Brugada, P., and Wellens, H. J. J.: Electrophysiology, mechanisms, diagnosis, and treatment of paroxysmal recurrent atrioventricular nodal reentrant tachycardia. *In* Surawicz, B., et al. (eds.): Tachycardias. Boston, Martinus Nijhoff, 1984, p. 131.
123. Wu, D., Kou, H. C., Yeh, S. J., Lin, F. C., and Hung, J.S.: Determinants of tachycardia induction using ventricular stimulation in dual pathway atrioventricular nodal reentrant tachycardia. Am. Heart J. *108*:44, 1984.
124. Wah, J. Y. L., Friday, K., Sakurai, M., Lazzara, R., and Jackman, W.: Is the His bundle part of the AV nodal reentry circuit? Circulation *72*(Suppl. 3):271, 1985.
125. Bauernfeind, R. A., Swiryn, S., Strasberg, B., Palileo, E., Wyndham, C., Duffy, C., and Rosen, K. M.: Analysis of anterograde and retrograde fast pathway properties in patients with dual atrioventricular nodal pathways. Observations regarding the pathophysiology of the Lown-Ganong-Levine syndrome. Am. J. Cardiol. *49*:283, 1982.
126. Casta, A., Wolff, G. S., Mehta, A. V., Tamer, D., Garcia, O. L., Pickoff, A. S., Ferrer, P. L., Sung, R. H., and Gelband, H.: Dual atrioventricular nodal pathways: A benign finding in arrhythmia-free children with heart disease. Am. J. Cardiol. *46*:1013, 1980.
127. Brugada, P., Heddle, B., Green, M., and Wellens, H.J.J.: Initiation of atrioventricular nodal reentrant tachycardia in patients with discontinuous anterograde atrioventricular nodal conduction curves with and without documented supraventricular tachycardia: Observations on the role of a discontinuous retrograde conduction curve. Am. Heart J. *107*:685, 1984.
128. Garson, A., Jr., and Gillette, P. C.: Electrophysiologic studies of supraventricular tachycardia in children. I. Clinical-electrophysiologic correlations. Am. Heart J. *102*:233, 1981.
129. Swiryn, S., Bauernfeind, R. A., Palileo, E., Strasberg, B., Duffy, C. E., and Rosen, K. M.: Electrophysiologic study demonstrating triple antegrade AV nodal pathways in patients with spontaneous and/or induced supraventricular tachycardia. Am. Heart J. *103*:168, 1982.
130. Akhtar, M., Damato, A. N., Ruskin, J. N., Batsford, W.T., Reddy, C. P., Ticzon, A. R., Dhatt, M. S., Gomes, J.A.C., and Calon, A. H.: Antegrade and retrograde conduction characteristics in three patterns of paroxysmal atrioventricular junctional reentrant tachycardia. Am. Heart J. *95*:22, 1978.
131. Wu, D.: Dual atrioventricular nodal pathways: A reappraisal. PACE *5*:72, 1982.
132. Rosen, K. M., Bauernfeind, R. A., Swiryn, S., Strasberg, B., and Palileo, E. V.: Dual AV nodal pathways and AV nodal reentrant paroxysmal tachycardia. Am. Heart J. *101*:691, 1981.
133. Ko, P. T., Naccarelli, G. V., Gulamhusein, S., Prystowsky, E. N., Zipes, D. P., and Klein, G. J.: Atrioventricular dissociation during paroxysmal junctional tachycardia. PACE *4*:670, 1981.
134. Sung, B. J., Waxman, H. L., Saksena, S., and Juma, Z.: Sequence of retrograde atrial activation in patients with dual atrioventricular nodal pathways. Circulation *64*:1059, 1981.
135. Swiryn, S., Pavel, D., Byrom, E., Wyndham, C., Pietras, R., Bauernfeind, R., and Rosen, K. M.: Assessment of left ventricular function by radionuclide angiography during induced supraventricular tachycardia. Am. J. Cardiol. *47*:555, 1981.
136. Waxman, M. B., Sharma, A. B., Cameron, D. A., Huerta, F., and Wald, R. W.: Reflex mechanisms responsible for early spontaneous termination of paroxysmal supraventricular tachycardia. Am. J. Cardiol. *49*:259, 1982.
137. Tavsanoglu, S., and Ozenel, E.: Ice-water washcloth rather than facial emersion (diving reflex) for supraventricular tachycardia in adults (letter). Am. J. Cardiol. *56*:1003, 1985.
138. Sung, R. J., Elser, B., and McAllister, R. G., Jr.: Intravenous verapamil for termination of reentrant supraventricular tachycardias: Intracardiac studies correlated with plasma verapamil concentrations. Ann. Intern. Med. *93*:682, 1980.
139. Waxman, H. L., Myerburg, R. J., Appel, R., and Sung, R. J.: Verapamil for control of ventricular rate in paroxysmal supraventricular tachycardia and atrial fibrillation or flutter: A double-blind randomized cross-over study. Ann. Intern. Med. *94*:1, 1981.
140. Betriu, A., Chaitman, B. R., Bourassa, M. G., Brévers, G., Scholl, J., Bruneau, P., Gagne, P., and Chabot, M.: Beneficial effect of intravenous diltiazem in the acute management of paroxysmal supraventricular tachyarrhythmias. Circulation *67*:88, 1983.
141. Wu, D., Hung, J. S., Kuo, C. T., Hsu, K. S., and Shieh, W. B.: Effects of quinidine on atrioventricular nodal reentrant paroxysmal tachycardia. Circulation *64*:823, 1981.
142. Swiryn, S., Bauernfeind, R. A., Wyndham, C. R. C., Dhingra, R. C., Palileo, E., Strasberg, B., and Rosen, K.M.: Effects of oral disopyramide phosphate on induction of paroxysmal supraventricular tachycardia. Circulation *64*:169, 1981.
143. Bauernfeind, R. A., Wyndham, C. R., Dhingra, R. C., Swiryn, S. P., Palileo, E., Strasberg, B., and Rosen, K. M.: Serial electrophysiologic testing of multiple drugs in patients with atrioventricular nodal reentrant paroxysmal tachycardia. Circulation *62*:1341, 1980.
144. Zipes, D. P., DeJoseph, R. L., and Rothbaum, D. A.: Unusual properties of accessory pathways. Circulation *49*:1200, 1974.
145. Coumel, P., and Attuel, P.: Reciprocating tachycardia in overt and latent preexcitation. Influence of functional bundle branch block on the rate of the tachycardia. Eur. J. Cardiol. *1*:423, 1974.
146. Neuss, H., Schlepper, M., and Thormann, J.: Analysis of reentry mechanisms in three patients with concealed Wolff-Parkinson-White syndrome. Circulation *51*:75, 1975.
147. Slama, R., Coumel, P., and Bouvrain, Y.: Les syndromes de Wolff-Parkinson-White de type A inapparents ou latents en rythme sinusal. Arch. Mal. Coeur *66*:639, 1974.

148. Prystowsky, E. N., Miles, W. M., Heger, J. J., and Zipes, D. P.: Preexcitation syndromes. Mechanisms and management. Med. Clin. North Am. *68*:831, 1984.
149. Wellens, H. J. J., and Brugada, P.: Value of programmed stimulation of the heart in patients with the Wolff-Parkinson-White syndrome. *In* Josephson, M. E., and Wellens, H.J.J. (eds.): Tachycardias: Mechanisms, Diagnosis Treatment. Philadelphia, Lea and Febiger, 1984, p. 199.
150. Gallagher, J. J.: Accessory pathway tachycardia: Techniques of electrophysiologic study and mechanisms. Circulation (*in press*).
151. Ross, D. L., and Uther, J. B.: Diagnosis of concealed accessory pathways in supraventricular tachycardia. PACE 7:1069, 1984.
152. Kerr, C. R., Gallagher, J. J., and German, L. D.: Changes in ventriculoatrial intervals with bundle branch block aberration during reciprocating tachycardia in patients with accessory atrioventricular pathways. Circulation *66*:196, 1982.
153. Lehmann, M. H., Denker, S., Mahmud, R., Tchou, P., Dongas, J., and Akhtar, M.: Electrophysiologic mechanisms of functional bundle branch block at onset of induced orthodromic tachycardia in the Wolff-Parkinson-White syndrome. Role of stimulation method. J. Clin. Invest. *76*:1566, 1985.
154. Prystowsky, E. N., Heger, J. J., Jackman, W. M., Naccarelli, G. V., and Zipes, D. P.: Postmyocardial infarction incessant supraventricular tachycardia due to concealed accessory pathway. Am. Heart J. *103*:426, 1982.
155. Akhtar, M., Shenasa, M., and Schmidt, D. H.: Role of retrograde His-Purkinje block in the initiation of supraventricular tachycardia by ventricular premature stimulation in the Wolff-Parkinson-White syndrome. J. Clin. Invest. *67*:1047, 1981.
156. Przybylski, J, Chiale, P. A., Halpern, M. S., Nau, G.J., Elizari, M. V., and Rosenbaum, M. B.: Unmasking of ventricular preexcitation by vagal stimulation or isoproterenol administration. Circulation *61*:1030, 1980.

PREEXCITATION SYNDROME

157. Oehnell, R. F., Preexcitation, a cardiac abnormality. Acta Med. Scand. *151*(Suppl.):78, 1944.
158. Durrer, D., Schuilenburg, R. M., and Wellens, H. J. J.: Preexcitation revisited. Am. J. Cardiol. *25*:690, 1970.
159. Wolff, L., Parkinson, J., and White, P. D.: Bundle branch block with short P-R interval in healthy young people prone to paroxysmal tachycardia. Am. Heart J. 5:685, 1950.
160. Becker, A. H., and Anderson, R. H.: The Wolff-Parkinson-White syndrome and its anatomical substrates. Anat. Rec. *201*:169, 1981.
161. Kent, A. F. S.: Researches on the structure and function of the mammalian heart. J. Physiol. *14*:233, 1893.
162. Kent, A. F. S.: Observations on the auriculo-ventricular junction of the mammalian heart. Quart. J. Exp. Physiol. 7:193, 1913.
163. Hill, B. L., and Tilley, L. P.: Ventricular preexcitation in 7 dogs and 9 cats. J. Am. Vet. Med. Assoc. *187*:1026, 1985.
164. Boineau, J. P., and Moore, E. N.: Evidence for propagation of activation across an accessory atrioventricular connection in types A and B preexcitation. Circulation *41*:375, 1970.
165. Willems, J. L., Robles de Medina, E. O., Bernard, R., Coumel, P., Fisch, C., Krikler, D., Mazur, N. A., Meijler, F. L., Mogensen, L., Moret, P., Pisa, Z., Rautaharju, P. M., Surawicz, B., Watanabe, Y., and Wellens, H. J. J.: Criteria for intraventricular conduction disturbances and pre-excitation. J. Am. Coll. Cardiol. 5:1261, 1985.
166. Brechenmacher, C.: Atrio-His bundle tracts. Br. Heart J. *37*:853, 1975.
167. Lown, B., Ganong, W. F., and Levine, S. A.: The syndrome of short PR interval, normal QRS complex and paroxysmal rapid heart action. Circulation 5:693, 1952.
168. Mahaim, I: Kent's fibers and the AV paraspecific conduction through the upper connections of the bundle of His-Tawara. Am. Heart J. *33*:651, 1947.
169. Bardy, G. H., German, L. D., Packer, D. L., Coltorti, F., and Gallagher, J. J.: Mechanism of tachycardia using a nodofascicular Mahaim fiber. Am. J. Cardiol. *54*:1140, 1984.
170. Gallagher, J. J., Smith, W. M., Kasell, J. H., Benson, D.W., Jr., Sterba, R., and Grant, A. O.: Role of Mahaim fibers in cardiac arrhythmias in man. Circulation *64*:176, 1981.
171. Milstein, S., Scharma, A. D., Guiraudon, G. M., and Klein, G. J.: An algorithm for the electrocardiographic localization of accessory pathways in the Wolff-Parkinson-White syndrome (abstract). Circulation *74*(Suppl. II):300, 1986.
172. Durrer, D., Schoo, L., Schuilenberg, R. M., and Wellens, H. J. J.: The role of premature beats in the initiation and the termination of supraventricular tachycardia in the Wolff-Parkinson-White syndrome. Circulation *36*:644, 1967.
173. Kuck, K. H., Brugada, P., and Wellens, H. J. J.: Observations on the antidromic type of circus movement tachycardia in the Wolff-Parkinson-White syndrome. J. Am. Coll. Cardiol. 2:1003, 1983.
174. Bardy, G. H., Packer, D. L., German, L. D., and Gallagher, J. J.: Preexcited reciprocating tachycardia in patients with Wolff-Parkinson-White syndrome; incidence and mechanisms. Circulation *70*:377, 1984.
175. Morady, F., Scheinman, M. M., DiCarlo, L. A., Jr., Winston, S. A., Davis, J. C., Baerman, J. M., Krol, R. B., and Crevey, B. J.: Coexistent posteroseptal and right-sided atrioventricular bypass tract. J. Am. Coll. Cardiol. 5:640, 1985.
176. Wellens, H. J. J., Brugada, P., and Heddle, W. F.: Value of the 12 lead electrocardiogram in diagnosing type and mechanism of a tachycardia; a survey among 22 cardiologists. J. Am. Coll. Cardiol. *4*:176, 1984.
177. Bardy, G. H., Fedor, J. M., German, L. D., Packer, D.L., and Gallagher, J. J.: Surface electrocardiographic clues suggesting presence of a nodofascicular Mahaim fiber. J. Am. Coll. Cardiol. *3*:1116, 1984.
178. Ko, P. T., Naccarelli, G. V., Gulamhusein, S., Prystowsky, E. N., Zipes, D. P., and Klein, G. J.: Atrioventricular dissociation during paroxysmal junctional tachycardia. PACE *4*:670, 1981.
179. Gmeiner, R., Ng, C. K., Hammer, I., and Becker, A.E.: Tachycardia caused by an accessory nodoventricular tract: A clinico-pathologic correlation. Eur. Heart J. 5:223, 1984.
180. Critelli, G., Gallagher, J. J., Monda, V., Coltorti, F., Scherillo, M., and Rossi, L.: Anatomic and electrophysiologic substrate of the permanent form of junctional reciprocating tachycardia. J. Am. Coll. Cardiol. *4*:601, 1984.
181. Guarnieri, T., Sealy, W. C., Kasell, J. H., German, L.D., and Gallagher, J. J.: The nonpharmacologic management of the permanent form of junctional reciprocating tachycardia. Circulation *69*:269, 1984.
182. Wellens, H. J. J.: Observations in patients showing AV junctional echoes with a shorter PR than RP interval. Distinction between intranodal reentry or reentry using an accessory pathway with a long conduction time. Am. J. Cardiol. *48*:611, 1981.
182a. Smith, W. M., Broughton, A., Reiter, M. J., Benson, D. W., Jr., Grant, A. O., and Gallagher, J. J.: Bystander accessory pathway during AV node reentrant tachycardia. PACE *6*:537, 1983.
183. Sharma, A. D., Klein, G. J., Guiraudon, G. M., and Milstein, S.: Atrial fibrillation in patients with Wolff-Parkinson-White syndrome: Incidence after surgical ablation of the accessory pathway. Circulation *72*:161, 1985.
184. Klein, G. H., Bashore, T. M., Seller, T. B., Pritchett, E. L. C., and Gallagher, J. J.: Ventricular fibrillation in the Wolff-Parkinson-White syndrome. N. Engl. J. Med. *301*:1080, 1979.
185. Lloyd, E. A., Hauer, R. N., Zipes, D. P., Heger, J. J., and Prystowsky, E. N.: Syncope and ventricular tachycardia in patients with ventricular preexcitation. Am. J. Cardiol. *52*:79, 1983.
186. Milstein, S., Sharma, A. D., and Klein, G. J.: Nonclinical ventricular tachycardia in the Wolff-Parkinson-White syndrome. PACE *8*:678, 1985.
187. Hammil, S. C., Pritchett, E. L., Klein, G. J., Smith, W. M., and Gallagher, J. J.: Accessory atrioventricular pathways that conduct only in the antegrade direction. Circulation *62*:1335, 1980.
187a. Lerman, B. B., and Josephson, M. E.: Automaticity of the Kent bundle: Confirmation by phase 3 and phase 4 block. J. Am. Coll. Cardiol. *5*:996, 1985.
188. Guize, L., Soria, R., Chaouat, J. C., Cretien, J. M., Woue, D., and LeHeuzey, J. Y.: Prevalence and course of Wolff-Parkinson-White syndrome in a population of 138,048 subjects. Ann. Med. Interne (Paris) *136*:474, 1985.
189. Smith, W. M., Gallagher, J. J., Kerr, C. R., Sealy, W. C., Kasell, J. H., Benson, D. W., Jr., Reiter, M. J., Sterba, R., and Grant, A. O.: The electrophysiologic basis and management of symptomatic recurrent tachycardia in patients with Ebstein's anomaly of the tricuspid valve. Am. J. Cardiol. *49*:1223, 1982.
190. Drake, C. E., Hodsden, J. E., Sridharan, M. R., and Flowers, N. C.: Evaluation of the association of mitral valve prolapse in patients with Wolff-Parkinson-White type ECG and its relationship to the ventricular activation pattern. Am. Heart J. *109*:83, 1985.
190a. Vidaillet, H. J., Jr., Pressley, J. C., Gilbert, M. R., and German, L. D.: Multiple accessory pathways: A marker for familial preexcitation. Circulation *74*(Suppl. II):301, 1986.
191. Klein, G. J., and Gulamhusein, S. S.: Intermittent preexcitation in the Wolff-Parkinson-White syndrome. Am. J. Cardiol. *52*:292, 1983.
192. Bricker, J. T., Porter, C. J., Garson, A., Jr., Gillette, P. C., McVey, P., Traweek, M., and McNamara, D. G.: Exercise testing in children with Wolff-Parkinson-White syndrome. Am. J. Cardiol. *55*:1001, 1985.
193. Critelli, G., Gallagher, J. J., Perticone, F., Coltorti, F., Monda, V., and Condorelli, M.: Evaluation of noninvasive tests for identifying patients with preexcitation syndrome at risk of rapid ventricular response. Am. Heart J. *108*:905, 1984.
194. Akhtar, M., Gilbert, C. J., and Shenasa, M.: Effect of lidocaine on atrioventricular response via the accessory pathway in patients with Wolff-Parkinson-White syndrome. Circulation *63*:435, 1981.
195. Gulamhusein, S., Ko, P., Carruthers, S. G., and Klein, G. J.: Acceleration of the ventricular response during atrial fibrillation in the Wolff-Parkinson-White syndrome after verapamil. Circulation *65*:348, 1982.
196. Brugada, P., Facchini, M., and Wellens, H. J. J.: Effects of isoproterenol and amiodarone and the role of exercise in initiation of circus movement tachycardia in the accessory atrioventricular pathway. Am. J. Cardiol. *57*:146, 1986.
197. Wellens, H. J. J., Bär, F. W., Dassen, W. R., Brugada, P., Vanagt, E. J., and Farre, J.: Effect of drugs in the Wolff-Parkinson-White syndrome. Importance of initial length of effective refractory period of the accessory pathway. Am. J. Cardiol. *46*:665, 1980.

VENTRICULAR RHYTHM DISTURBANCES

198. Rosenberg, M. J., Uretz, E., and Denes, P.: Sleep and ventricular arrhythmias. Am. Heart J. *106*:703, 1983.
199. Guilleminault, C., Connolly, S. J., and Winkle, R. A.: Cardiac arrhythmia and conduction disturbances during sleep in 400 patients with sleep apnea syndrome. Am. J. Cardiol. *52*:490, 1983.
200. Suwa, M., Hirota, Y., Nagao, H., Kino, M., and Kawamura, K.: Incidence of the coexistence of left ventricular false tendons and premature ventricular contractions in apparently healthy subjects. Circulation *70*:793, 1984.
201. Shepard, J. W., Jr., Garrison, M. W., Grither, D. A., Evans, R., and Schweitzer, P. K.: Relationship of ventricular ectopy to nocturnal oxygen desaturation in patients with chronic obstructive pulmonary disease. Am. J. Med. *78*:28, 1985.
202. Winkle, R. A.: The relationship between ventricular ectopic beat frequency and heart rate. Circulation *66*:439, 1982.
203. Herlitz, J., Hjalmarson, A., Swedberg, K., Waagstein, F., Holmberg, S., and

Waldenstrom, J.: Relationship between infarct size and incidence of severe ventricular arrhythmias in a double-blind trial with metoprolol in acute myocardial infarction. Int. J. Cardiol. *6*:47, 1984.
204. Grande, P., and Pedersen, A.: Myocardial infarct size: Correlation with cardiac arrhythmias and sudden death. Eur. Heart J. *5*:622, 1984.
205. Uther, J. B., Richards, D. A. B., Dennis, A. R., and Ross, D. L.: The prognostic significance of programmed ventricular stimulation after myocardial infarction: A review. Circulation, in press.
206. Bhandari, A. K., and Rahimtoola, S. H.: Indications for intracardiac electrophysiological testing in survivors of acute myocardial infarction. Circulation, in press.
207. Gomes, J. A. C., Hariman, R. I., Kang, P., El-Sherif, N., Chowdhry, I., and Lyons, J.: Programmed electrical stimulation in patients with high-grade ventricular ectopy: Electrophysiologic findings and prognosis for survival. Circulation *70*:43, 1984.
208. Olsson, G., and Rehnqvist, N.: Ventricular arrhythmias during the first year after acute myocardial infarction: Influence of long-term treatment with metoprolol. Circulation *69*:1129, 1984.
209. Miller, J. M., Kienzle, M. G., Harken, A. H., and Josephson, M. E.: Morphologically distinct sustained ventricular tachycardias in coronary artery disease: Significance and surgical results. J. Am. Coll. Cardiol. *4*:1073, 1984.
210. Waspe, L. E., Brodman, R., Kim, S. G., Matos, J. A., Johnston, D. R., Scavin, G. M., and Fisher, J. D.: Activation mapping in patients with coronary artery disease with multiple ventricular tachycardia configurations: Occurrence and therapeutic implications of widely separate apparent sites of origin. J. Am. Coll. Cardiol. *5*:1075, 1985.
211. Buxton, A. E., Marchlinski, F. E., Waxman, H. L., Flores, B. T., Cassidy, D. M., and Josephson, M. E.: Prognostic factors in nonsustained ventricular tachycardia. Am. J. Cardiol. *53*:1275, 1984.
212. Naccarelli, G. V., Prystowsky, E. N., Jackman, W. M., Heger, J. J., Rahilly, G. T., and Zipes, D. P.: Role of electrophysiologic testing in managing patients who have ventricular tachycardia unrelated to coronary artery disease. Am. J. Cardiol. *50*:165, 1982.
213. Rinkenberger, R. L., Prystowsky, E. N., Jackman, W. M., Heger, J. J., and Zipes, D. P.: Conversion of nonsustained ventricular tachycardia to sustained ventricular tachycardia during drug therapy as determined by serial electrophysiology studies. Am. Heart J. *103*:177, 1982.
214. Spielman, S. R., Greenspan, A. M., Kay, H. R., Discigil, K. F., Webb, C. R., Sokoloff, N. M., Rae, A. P., Morganroth, J., and Horowitz, L. N.: Electrophysiologic testing in patients at high risk for sudden cardiac death. I. Nonsustained ventricular tachycardia and abnormal ventricular function. J. Am. Coll. Cardiol. *6*:31, 1985.
215. Schoenfeld, M. H., McGovern, B., Garan, H., Kelly, E., Grant, G., and Ruskin, J. N.: Determinants of the outcome of electrophysiologic study in patients with ventricular tachyarrhythmias. J. Am. Coll. Cardiol. *6*:298, 1985.
216. Akhtar, M.: Electrophysiologic bases for wide QRS complex tachycardia. PACE *6*:81, 1983.
217. Wellens, J. H. H., Bär, F. W. H. M., and Lie, K. I.: The value of the electrocardiogram in the differential diagnosis of a tachycardia with a widened QRS complex. Am. J. Med. *64*:27, 1978.
218. Miles, W. M., Prystowsky, E. N., Heger, J. J., and Zipes, D. P.: Evaluation of the patient with wide QRS tachycardia. Med. Clin. North Am. *68*:1015, 1984.
219. Gulamhusein, S., Yee, R., Ko, P. T., and Klein, G. J.: Electrocardiographic criteria for differentiating aberrancy and ventricular extrasystole in chronic atrial fibrillation: Validation by intracardiac recordings. J. Electrocardiol. *18*:41, 1985.
220. Dongas, J., Lehmann, M. H., Mahmud, R., Denker, S., Soni, J., and Akhtar, M.: Value of preexisting bundle branch block in the electrocardiographic differentiation of supraventricular from ventricular origin of wide QRS tachycardia. Am. J. Cardiol. *55*:717, 1985.
221. Josephson, M. E., Horowitz, L. N., Farshidi, A., and Kastor, J. A.: Recurrent sustained ventricular tachycardia. I. Mechanisms. Circulation *57*:431, 1978.
222. Morady, F., Scheinman, M. M., Gonzalez, R., and Hess, E.: His-ventricular dissociation in a patient with reciprocating tachycardia and a nodoventricular bypass tract. Circulation *64*:839, 1981.
223. Ruffy, R., Kim, S. S., and Lal, R.: Paroxysmal fascicular tachycardia: Electrophysiologic characteristics and treatment by catheter ablation. J. Am. Cardiol. *5*:1008, 1985.
224. Morady, F., DiCarlo, L., Winston, S., Davis, J. C., and Scheinman, M. M.: A prospective comparison of triple extrastimuli and left ventricular stimulation in studies of ventricular tachycardia induction. Circulation *70*:52, 1984.
225. Gomes, J. A., Kang, P. S., Khan, R., Kelen, G., and El-Sherif, N.: Repetitive ventricular response: Its incidence, inducibility, reproducibility, mechanism and significance. Br. Heart J. *46*:159, 1981.
226. Prystowsky, E. N., Naccarelli, G. V., Rahilly, G. T., Jr., Heger, J. J., and Zipes, D. P.: Electrophysiologic and anatomic characteristics associated with ventricular tachycardia induced at the right ventricular outflow tract but not at the apex. Am. J. Cardiol. *49*:959, 1982.
227. Naccarelli, G. V., Zipes, D. P., Rahilly, G. T., Heger, J. J., and Prystowsky, E. N.: Influence of tachycardia cycle length and antiarrhythmic drugs on pacing termination and acceleration of ventricular tachycardia. Am. Heart J. *105*:1, 1983.
228. Josephson, M. E., Horowitz, L. N., Farshidi, A., Spielman, S. R., Michaelson, E. L., and Greenspan, A. M.: Sustained ventricular tachycardia: Evidence for protected localized reentry. Am. J. Cardiol. *42*:416, 1978.
229. Josephson, M. E., Horowitz, L. N., Waxman, H. L., Cain, M. E., Spielman, S. R., Greenspan, A. M., Marchlinski, F. E., and Ezri, M. D.: Sustained ventricular tachycardia: Role of the 12-lead electrocardiogram in localizing site of origin. Circulation *64*:257, 1981.
230. Swiryn, S., Pavel, T., Byrom, M. E., Bauernfeind, R. A., Strasberg, B., Palileo, E., Lam, W., Wyndham, C. R., and Rosen, K. M.: Sequential regional phase mapping of radionuclide gated biventriculograms in patients with sustained ventricular tachycardia: Close correlation with electrophysiologic characteristics. Am. Heart J. *103*:319, 1982.
231. Bashore, T. M., Stine, R. A., Shaffer, P. B., Bush, C. A., Leier, C. V., and Schaal, S. F.: The non-invasive localization of ventricular pacing sites by radionuclide phase imaging. Circulation *70*:681, 1984.
232. Raichlen, J. S., Links, J. M., and Reid, P. R.: Effect of electrical activation site on left ventricular performance in ventricular tachycardia patients with coronary heart disease. Am. J. Cardiol. *55*:84, 1985.
233. Scrutinio, D., De Toma, L., Mangini, S. G., Lagioia, R., Accettura, D., Ricci, A., and Rizzon, P.: Ischemia related ventricular arrhythmias in patients with variant angina pectoris. Eur. Heart J. *5*:1013, 1984.
234. Gabliani, G. I., Winniford, M. D., Fulton, K. L., Johnson, S. M., Mauritson, D. R., and Hillis, L. D.: Ventricular ectopic activity with spontaneous variant angina: Frequency and relation to transient ST segment elevation. Am. Heart J. *110*:40, 1985.
235. Kerin, N. Z., Rubenfire, M., Willens, H. J., Rao, P., and Cascade, P. N.: The mechanism of dysrhythmias in variant angina pectoris: Occlusive versus reperfusion. Am. Heart J. *106*:1332, 1983.
236. Araki, H., Koiwaya, Y., Nakagaki, O, and Nakamura, M.: Diurnal distribution of ST-segment elevation and related arrhythmias in patients with variant angina. A study by ambulatory ECG monitoring. Circulation *67*:995, 1983.
237. Hess, O. M., Graf, C., Frey, R., Dettli, R., and Siegenthaler, W.: Coronary artery spasm with normal coronary arteries as the cause of recurrent ventricular fibrillation. Schweiz. Med. Wochenschr. *111*:755, 1981.
238. Rubin, D. A., Nieminski, K. E., Monteferrante, J. C., Magee, T., Reed, G. E., and Herman, M. V.: Ventricular arrhythmias after coronary artery bypass graft surgery: Incidence, risk factors, and long-term prognosis. J. Am. Coll. Cardiol. *6*:307, 1985.
239. Topol, E. J., Lerman, B. B., Baughman, K. L., Platia, E. V., and Griffith, L. S.: De novo refractory ventricular tachyarrhythmias after coronary revascularization. Am. J. Cardiol. *57*:57, 1986.
240. Ruskin, J. N., DiMarco, J. P., and Garan, H.: Out-of-hospital cardiac arrest: Electrophysiologic observations and selection of long-term antiarrhythmic therapy. N. Engl. J. Med. *303*:607, 1980.
241. Josephson, M. E., Horowitz, L. N., Spielman, S. R., and Greenspan, A. M.: Electrophysiologic and hemodynamic studies in patients resuscitated from cardiac arrest. Am. J. Cardiol. *46*:948, 1980.
242. Winkle, R. A., Derrington, D. C., and Schroeder, J. S.: Characteristics of ventricular tachycardia in ambulatory patients. Am. J. Cardiol. *39*:487, 1977.
243. Bigger, J. T., Jr., Fleiss, J. L., Kleiger, R., Miller, J. P., Rolnitzky, L. M., and the Multicenter Post-Infarction Research Group: The relationships among ventricular arrhythmias, left ventricular dysfunction and mortality in the 2 years after myocardial infarction. Circulation *69*:250, 1984.
244. Pedersen, D. H., Zipes, D. P., Foster, P. R., and Troup, P. J.: Ventricular tachycardia and ventricular fibrillation in a young population. Circulation *60*:988, 1979.
245. Vetter, V. L., Josephson, M. E., and Horowitz, L. N.: Idiopathic recurrent sustained ventricular tachycardia in children and adolescents. Am. J. Cardiol. *47*:315, 1981.
246. Reisch, P., DeSilva, R. A., Lown B., and Murawski, B. J.: Acute psychological disturbance preceding life-threatening ventricular arrhythmias. J.A.M.A. *246*:233, 1981.
247. Waxman, M. B., Wald, R. W., Finley, J. P., Bonnet, J. F., Downar, E., and Sharma, A. B.: Valsalva termination of ventricular tachycardia. Circulation *62*:843, 1980.
248. Sclarovsky, S., Kracoff, O., Arditi, A., Strasberg, B., Zafrir, N., Lewin, R. F., and Agmon, J.: Ventricular tachycardia. "Pleomorphism" induced by chest thump. Chest *81*:97, 1982.
249. Krijne, R.: Rate acceleration of ventricular tachycardia after a precordial chest thump. Am. J. Cardiol. *53*:964, 1984.
250. Molajo, A. O., Summers, G. D., and Bennett, D. H.: Effect of percutaneous transluminal coronary angioplasty on arrhythmias complicating angina. Br. Heart J. *54*:375, 1985.
251. Webster, M. W., Fitzpatrick, M. A., Nicholls, M. G., Ikram, H., and Wells, J. E.: Effect of enalapril on ventricular arrhythmias in congestive heart failure. Am. J. Cardiol. *56*:566, 1985.
252. Parmley, W. W., and Chatterjee, K.: Congestive heart failure and arrhythmias: An overview. Am. J. Cardiol. *57*:334B, 1986.
253. Belhassen, B., Pelleg, A., Parades, A., and Laniado, S.: Simultaneous AV nodal reentrant and ventricular tachycardias. PACE *7*:325, 1984.
254. Lerman, B. B., Belardinelli, L., West, A., Berne, R. M., and DiMarco, J. P.: Adenosine-sensitive ventricular tachycardia: Evidence suggesting cyclic AMP-mediated triggered activity. Circulation *74*:270, 1986.
255. Ward, D. E., Nathan, A. W., and Camm, A. J.: Fascicular tachycardia sensitive to calcium antagonists. Eur. Heart J. *5*:896, 1984.
256. Sung, R. J., Shapiro, W. A., Shen, E. N., Morady, F., and Davis, J.: Effects of verapamil on ventricular tachycardias possibly caused by reentry, automaticity and triggered activity. J. Clin. Invest. *72*:350, 1983.
257. Friedman, L. M., Byington, R. P., Capone, R. J., Furberg, C. D., Goldstein, S., and Lichstein, E.: Effect of propranolol in patients with myocardial infarction and ventricular arrhythmia. J. Am. Coll. Cardiol. *7*:1, 1986.
258. Myerburg, R. J., Kessler, K. M., Kiem, I., Pefkaros, K. C., Conde, C. A., Cooper, D., and Castellanos, A.: Relationship between plasma levels of procainamide, suppression of premature ventricular complexes and prevention of recurrent ventricular tachycardia. Circulation *64*:280, 1981.

259. Fontaine, G., Frank, R., Tonet, J. L., Guiraudon, G., Cabrol, C., Chomette, G., and Grosgogeat, Y.: Arrhythmogenic right ventricular dysplasia: A clinical model for the study of chronic ventricular tachycardia. Jpn. Circ. J. *48*:515, 1984.
260. Marcus, F. I., Fontaine, G. H., Guiraudon, G., Frank, R., Laurenceau, J. L., Malergue, C., and Grosgogeat, Y.: Right ventricular dysplasia: A report of 24 adult cases. Circulation *65*:384, 1982.
261. Dungan, W. T., Garson, A., Jr., and Gillette, P. C.: Arrhythmogenic right ventricular dysplasia. A cause of ventricular tachycardia in children with apparently normal hearts. Am. Heart J. *102*:745, 1981.
262. Robertson, J. H., Bardy, G. H., German, L. D., Gallagher, J. J., and Kisslo, J.: Comparison of two-dimensional echocardiographic and angiographic findings in arrhythmogenic right ventricular dysplasia. Am. J. Cardiol. *55*:1506, 1985.
263. Dunnigan, A., Pritzker, M. R., Benditt, D. G., and Benson, D. W., Jr.: Life-threatening ventricular tachycardias in late survivors of surgically corrected tetralogy of Fallot. Br. Heart J. *52*:198, 1984.
264. Harken, A. H., Horowitz, L. N., and Josephson, M. E.: Surgical correction of recurrent sustained ventricular tachycardia on complete repair of tetralogy of Fallot. J. Thorac. Cardiovasc. Surg. *80*:779, 1980.
265. Deanfield, J., McKenna, W., and Rowland, E.: Local abnormalities of right ventricular depolarization after repair of tetralogy of Fallot. A basis for ventricular arrhythmia. Am. J. Cardiol. *55*:522, 1985.
266. Kavey, R. W., Thomas, F. D., Byrum, C. J., Blackman, M. S., Sondheimer, H. M., and Bove, E. L.: Ventricular arrhythmias and biventricular dysfunction after repair of tetralogy of Fallot. J. Am. Coll. Cardiol. *4*:126, 1984.
267. Garson, A., Jr., Randall, D. C., Gillette, P. C., Smith, R. T., Moak, J. P., McVey, P., and McNamara, D. G.: Prevention of sudden death after repair of tetralogy of Fallot: Treatment of ventricular arrhythmias. J. Am. Coll. Cardiol. *6*:221, 1985.
268. VonOlshausen, K., Schafer, A., Mehmel, H. C., Schwartz, F., Senges, J., and Kubler, W.: Ventricular arrhythmias in idiopathic dilated cardiomyopathy. Br. Heart J. *51*:195, 1984.
269. McKenna, W. J., Oakley, C. M., Krikler, D. M., and Goodwin, J. F.: Improved survival with amiodarone in patients with hypertrophic cardiomyopathy and ventricular tachycardia. Br. Heart J. *53*:412, 1985.
270. Frank, M. J., Watkins, L. O., Prisant, L. M., Stefadouros, M. A., and Abdulla, A. M.: Potentially lethal arrhythmias and their management in hypertrophic cardiomyopathy. Am. J. Cardiol. *53*:1608, 1984.
271. Kowey, P. R., Eisenberg, R., and Engel, T. R.: Sustained arrhythmias in hypertrophic obstructive cardiomyopathy. N. Engl. J. Med. *315*:1566, 1984.
272. Borggrefe, M., Kuhn, H., Koniger, H. H., Stoter, H., Breithardt, G., Loogen, F., Schulte, H. D., and Bircks, W.: Arrhythmias in hypertrophic obstructive and non-obstructive cardiomyopathy. Eur. Heart J. *4*(Suppl F):245, 1983.
273. Meinertz, T., Hofmann, T., Kasper, W., Treese, N., Bechtold, H., Stienen, U., Pop, T., Leitner, E. V., Andresen, D., and Meyer, J.: Significance of ventricular arrhythmias in idiopathic dilated cardiomyopathy. Am. J. Cardiol. *53*:902, 1984.
274. Poll, D. S., Marchlinski, F. E., Buxton, A. E., Doherty, J. U., Waxman, H. L., and Josephson, M. E.: Sustained ventricular tachycardia in patients with idiopathic dilated cardiomyopathy: Electrophysiologic testing and lack of response to antiarrhythmic drug therapy. Circulation *70*:451, 1984.
275. Rosenthal, M. E., Hamer, A., Gang, E. S., Oseran, D. S., Mandel, W. J., and Peter, T.: The yield of programmed ventricular stimulation in mitral valve prolapse patients with ventricular arrhythmias. Am. Heart J. *110*:970, 1985.
276. Morady, F., Shen, E., Bhandari, A., Schwartz, A., and Scheinman, M. M.: Programmed ventricular stimulation in mitral valve prolapse: Analysis of 36 patients. Am. J. Cardiol. *53*:135, 1984.
277. Rahilly, G. T., Prystowsky, E. N., Zipes, D. P., Naccarelli, G. V., Jackman, W. M., and Heger, J. J.: Clinical and electrophysiologic findings in patients with otherwise normal electrocardiograms. Am. J. Cardiol. *50*:459, 1982.
278. Naccarelli, G. V., Prystowsky, E. N., Jackman, W. M., Heger, J. J., Rahilly, G. T., and Zipes, D. P.: Role of electrophysiologic testing in managing patients who have ventricular tachycardia unrelated to coronary artery disease. Am. J. Cardiol. *50*:165, 1982.
279. Strain, J. E., Grose, R. M., Factor, S. M., and Fisher, J. D.: Results of endomyocardial biopsy in patients with spontaneous ventricular tachycardia but without apparent structural heart disease. Circulation *68*:1171, 1983.
280. Sugrue, D. D., Holmes, D. R., Jr., Gersh, B. J., Edwards, W. D., McLaran, C. J., Wood, D. L., Osborn, M. J., and Hammill, S. C.: Cardiac histologic findings in patients with life-threatening ventricular arrhythmias of unknown origin. J. Am. Coll. Cardiol. *4*:952, 1984.
281. Fulton, D. R., Chung, K. J., Tabakin, B. S., and Keane, J. F.: Ventricular tachycardia in children without heart disease. Am. J. Cardiol. *55*:1328, 1985.
282. Coumel, P., Rosengarten, M. D., Leclercq, J. F., and Attuel, P.: Role of sympathetic nervous system in nonischemic ventricular arrhythmias. Br. Heart J. *47*:137, 1982.
283. Cercek, B., and Horvat, M.: Arrhythmias with brief, high-dose intravenous streptokinase infusion in acute myocardial infarction. Eur. Heart J. *6*:109, 1985.
284. Dessertenne, F.: Considerations sur l'electrocardiogramme de la fibrillation ventriculaire. Arch. Mal. Coeur 57:1421, 1964.
285. Fontaine, G., Frank, R., and Grosgogeat, Y.: Torsades de pointes: Definition and management. Mod. Conc. Cardiovasc. Dis. *51*:103, 1982.
286. Kay, G. N., Plumb, V. J., Arciniegas, J. G., Henthorn, R. W., and Waldo, A. L.: Torsade de pointes: The long-short initiating sequence and other clinical features. Observations in 32 patients. J. Am. Coll. Cardiol. 2:806, 1983.
287. Baroy, J. H., Ungerleider, R. M., Smith, W. M., and Ideker, R. E.: A mechanism of torsades de pointes in a canine model. Circulation *67*:52, 1983.
288. Bonatti, V., Rolli, A., and Botti, G.: Monophasic action potential studies in human subjects with prolonged ventricular repolarization and long QT syndromes. Eur. Heart J. *6*(Suppl. D):131, 1985.
289. Schechter, E., Freeman, C. C., and Lazzara, R.: Afterdepolarizations as a mechanism for the long QT syndrome: Electrophysiologic studies of a case. J. Am. Coll. Cardiol. *3*:1556, 1984.
290. Smith, W. M., and Gallagher, J. J.: "Les torsades de pointes": An unusual ventricular arrhythmia. Ann. Intern. Med. *93*:578, 1980.
291. Keren, A., Tzivoni, D., Gavish, D., Levi, J., Gottleib, S., Benhorin, J., and Stern, S.: Etiology warning signs and therapy of torsades de pointes—a study of ten patients. Circulation *64*:1167, 1981.
292. Tzivoni, D., Keren, A., Cohen, A. M., Loebel, H., Zahavi, I., Chenzbraun, A., and Stern, S.: Magnesium therapy for torsades de pointes. Am. J. Cardiol. *53*:528, 1984.
293. Khan, M. M., Logan, K. R., McComb, J. M., and Adgey, A. A.: Management of recurrent ventricular tachyarrhythmias associated with QT prolongation. Am. J. Cardiol. *47*:1301, 1981.
294. Kastor, J. A., Horowitz, L. N., Harken, A. H., and Josephson, M. E.: Clinical electrophysiology of ventricular tachycardia. N. Engl. J. Med. *304*:1004, 1981.
295. Browne, K. F., Zipes, D. P., Heger, J. J., and Prystowsky, E. N.: The influence of the autonomic nervous system on the QT interval. Am. J. Cardiol. *49*:898, 1982.
296. Surawicz, B., and Knoebel, S. B.: Long QT: Good, bad or indifferent? J. Am. Coll. Cardiol. *4*:398, 1984.
297. Bonatti, V., Rolli, A., and Botti, G.: Monophasic action potential studies in human subjects with prolonged ventricular repolarization and long QT syndromes. Eur. Heart J. *6*(Suppl D):131, 1985.
298. Jackman, W. M., Clark, M., Friday, K. J., Aliot, E. M., Anderson, J., and Lazzara, R.: Ventricular tachyarrhythmias in the long QT syndromes. Med. Clin. North Am. *68*:1079, 1984.
299. Bhandari, A. K., and Scheinman, M.: The long QT syndrome. Mod. Concepts Cardiovasc. Dis. *54*:45, 1985.
300. Jervell, A., and Lange-Nielsen, F.: Congenital deaf-mutism, functional heart disease with prolongation of the QT interval and sudden death. Am. Heart J. *54*:59, 1957.
301. Romano, C., Gemme, G., and Pongiglione, R.: Aritmie cardiache rare dell'eta pediatrica. II. Accessi sincopali per fibrillazione ventricolare parossistica. La Clinic. Paed. *45*:656, 1963.
302. Ward, O. C.: New familial cardiac syndrome in children. J. Irish Med. Assoc. *54*:103, 1964.
303. Selzer, A., and Wray, H. W.: Quinidine syncope: Paroxysmal ventricular fibrillation occurring during treatment of chronic atrial arrhythmias. Circulation *30*:17, 1964.
304. Tzivoni, D., Keren, A., Stern, S., and Gottlieb, S.: Disopyramide-induced torsades de pointes. Arch. Intern. Med. *141*:946, 1981.
305. Siegel, R. J., Cabeen, W. R., Jr., and Roberts, W. C.: Prolonged QT interval–ventricular tachycardia syndrome from massive rapid weight loss utilizing the liquid protein modified fast diet. Sudden death with sinus node ganglionitis and neuritis. Am. Heart J. *102*:121, 1981.
306. Pringle, T. H., Scobie, I. N., Murray, R. G., Kesson, C. M., and Maccuish, A. C.: Prolongation of the QT interval during therapeutic starvation: A substrate for malignant arrhythmias. Int. J. Obes. 7:253, 1983.
307. Taylor, G. J., Crampton, R. S., Gibson, R. S., Stebbins, P. T., Waldman, M. T., and Beller, G. A.: Prolonged QT interval at onset of acute myocardial infarction in predicting early phase ventricular tachycardia. Am. Heart J. *102*:16, 1981.
308. Mitsutake, A., Takeshita, A., Kuroiwa, A., and Nakamura, M.: Usefulness of the Valsalva maneuver in management of the long QT syndrome. Circulation *63*:1029, 1981.
309. Bhandari, A. K., Shapiro, W. A., Morady, F., Shen, E. N., Mason, J., and Scheinman, M. M.: Electrophysiologic testing in patients with the long QT syndrome. Circulation *71*:63, 1985.
310. Bharati, S., Dreifus, L., Bucheleres, G., Molthan, M., Covitz, W., Isenberg, H. S., and Lev, M.: The conduction system in patients with a prolonged QT interval. J. Am. Coll. Cardiol. *6*:1110, 1985.
311. Moss, A. J., Schwartz, P. J., Crampton, R. S., Locati, E., and Carleen, E.: The long QT syndrome: A prospective international study. Circulation *71*:17, 1985.
312. Levy, S., Hilaire, J., Clementy, J., Bartolin, R., Besse, P., Gerard, R., and Bricaud, H.: Bidirectional tachycardia. Mechanism derived from intracardiac recordings and programmed electrical stimulation. PACE *5*:633, 1982.
313. Buxton, A. E., Marchlinski, F. E., Doherty, J. U., Cassidy, D. M., Vassallo, J. A., Flores, B. T., and Josephson, M. E.: Repetitive, monomorphic ventricular tachycardia: Clinical and electrophysiologic characteristics in patients with and without organic heart disease. Am. J. Cardiol. *54*:997, 1984.
314. Slama, R., Leclercq, J. F., and Coumel, P.: Paroxysmal ventricular tachycardia in patients with apparently normal hearts. *In* Zipes, D. P., and Jalife, J. (eds.): Cardiac Electrophysiology and Arrhythmias. Orlando, FL, Grune and Stratton, 1985, p. 545.
315. Lloyd, E. A., Zipes, D. P., Heger, J. J., and Prystowsky, E. N.: Sustained ventricular tachycardia due to bundle branch reentry. Am. Heart J. *104*:1095, 1982.
316. Welch, W. J., Strasberg, B., Coelho, A., and Rosen, K. M.: Sustained macroreentrant ventricular tachycardia. Am. Heart J. *104*:166, 1982.
317. Touboul, P., Kirkorian, G., Atallah, G., and Moleur, P.: Bundle branch reentry: A possible mechanism of ventricular tachycardia. Circulation *67*:674, 1983.
318. Weaver, W. D., Cobb, L. A., Dennis, D., Ray, R., Hallstrom, A. P., and Copass, M. K.: Amplitude of ventricular fibrillation waveform and outcome after cardiac arrest. Ann. Intern. Med. *102*:53, 1985.
319. Surawicz, B.: Ventricular fibrillation. J. Am. Coll. Cardiol. 5(Suppl 6):43B, 1985.

320. Ornato, J. P., Gonzales, E. R., Morkunaus, A. R., Coyne, M. R., and Beck, C. L.: Treatment of presumed asystole during pre-hospital cardiac arrest: Superiority of electrical countershock. Am. J. Emerg. Med. 3:395, 1985.
321. Panidis, I. P., and Morganroth, J.: Sudden death in hospitalized patients: Cardiac rhythm disturbances detected by ambulatory electrocardiographic monitoring. J. Am. Coll. Cardiol. 2:798, 1983.
322. Ewy, G. A.: Ventricular fibrillation masquerading as asystole. Ann. Emerg. Med. *13*:811, 1984.
323. Thompson, B. M., Brooks, R. C., Pionkowski, R. S., Aprahamian, C., and Mateer, J. R.: Immediate countershock treatment of asystole. Ann. Emerg. Med. *13*:827, 1984.
324. Cobb, L. A., Werner, J. A., and Trobaugh, G. B.: Sudden cardiac death. I. A decade's experience with out-of-hospital resuscitation. Mod. Concepts Cardiovasc. Dis. *49*:31, 1980.
325. Adgey, A. A.: The Belfast experience with resuscitation ambulances. Am. J. Emerg. Med. 2:193, 1984.
326. Ritchie, J. L., Hallstrom, A. P., Troubaugh, G. B., Caldwell, J. H., and Cobb, L. A.: Out-of-hospital sudden coronary death: Rest and exercise radionuclide left ventricular function in survivors. Am. J. Cardiol. *55*:645, 1985.
327. Garson, A., Jr., and McNamara, D. G.: Sudden death in a pediatric cardiology population, 1958 to 1983: Relation to prior arrhythmias. J. Am. Coll. Cardiol. 5(Suppl 6):134B, 1985.
328. Stevenson, W. G., Brugada, P., Waldecker, B., Zehender, M., and Wellens, H. J. J.: Clinical, angiographic, and electrophysiologic findings in patients with aborted sudden death as compared with patients with sustained ventricular tachycardia after myocardial infarction. Circulation *71*:1146, 1985.
329. Schwartz, P. J., Zaza, A., Grazi, S., Lombardo, M., Lotto, A., Sbressa, C., and Zappa, P.: Effect of ventricular fibrillation complicating acute myocardial infarction on long-term prognosis: Importance of the site of infarction. Am. J. Cardiol. *56*:384, 1985.
329a. Standards and guidelines for cardiopulmonary resuscitation (CPR) and emergency cardiac care (FMC). J.A.M.A. *255*:2905, 1986.
329b. Hughes, W. G., and Ruedy, J. R.: Should calcium be used in cardiac arrest? Am. J. Med. *81*:285, 1986.
330. Norris, R. M., Barnaby, P. F., Brown, M. A., Geary, G. G., Clarke, E. D., Logan, R. L., and Sharpe, D. N.: Prevention of ventricular fibrillation during acute myocardial infarction by intravenous propranolol. Lancet 2:883, 1984.

HEART BLOCK

331. Inoue, T., Kobayashi, K., and Fukuzaki, H.: Ventriculo-atrial conduction in patients with normal and impaired atrioventricular conduction. Jpn. Heart J. *26*:707, 1985.
332. Zipes, D. P.: Second degree atrioventricular block. Circulation *60*:465, 1979.
333. Langendorf, R., and Pick, A.: Atrioventricular block, type II (Mobitz). Its nature and clinical significance. Circulation *38*:819, 1968.
334. Shaw, D. B., Kekwick, C. A., Veale, D., Gowers, J., and Whistance, T.: Survival in second degree atrioventricular block. Br. Heart J. *53*:587, 1985.
335. Braat, S. H., DeZwaan, C., Brugada, P., Coenegracht, J. M., and Wellens, H. J. J.: Right ventricular involvement with acute inferior wall myocardial infarction identifies high risk of developing atrioventricular nodal conduction disturbances. Am. Heart J. *107*:1183, 1984.
336. Feigel, D., Ashkenazy, J., and Kishon, Y.: Early and late atrioventricular block in acute inferior myocardial infarction. J. Am. Coll. Cardiol. *4*:35, 1984.
337. Strasberg, B., Pinchas, A., Arditti, A., Lewin, R. F., Sclarovsky, S., Hellman, C., Zafrir, N., and Agmon, J.: Left and right ventricular function in inferior acute myocardial infarction and significance of advanced atrioventricular block. Am. J. Cardiol. *54*:985, 1984.
338. Salata, J. J., Gill, R. M., Gilmour, R. F., Jr., and Zipes, D. P.: Effects of sympathetic tone on vagally-induced phasic changes in heart rate and atrioventricular node conduction in the anesthetized dog. Circ. Res. *58*:584, 1986.
339. Mangiardi, L. M., Bonamini, R., Conte, M., Gaita, F., Orzan, F., Presbitero, P., and Brusca, A.: Bedside evaluation of atrioventricular block with narrow QRS complexes: Usefulness of carotid sinus massage and atropine administration. Am. J. Cardiol. *49*:1136, 1982.
340. Markel, M., Miles, W. M., Zipes, D. P., and Prystowsky, E. N.: The effects of autonomic blockade on Mobitz II heart block. Circulation (abst), *74*(Suppl. II):31, 1986.
341. Southall, D. P., Johnston, F., Shinebourne, E. A., and Johnston, P. G.: 24-hour electrocardiograph study of heart rate and rhythm patterns in population of healthy children. Br. Heart J. *45*:281, 1981.
342. Zeppilli, P., Fenici, R., Sassara, M., Pirrami, M. M., and Caselli, G.: Wenckebach second degree AV block in top ranking athletes: An old problem revisited. Am. Heart J. *100*:281, 1980.
343. Vitasalo, M. T., Kala, R., and Eisalo, A.: Ambulatory electrocardiographic recording in endurance athletes. Br. Heart J. *47*:213, 1982.
344. Strasberg, B., Amat-y-Leon, F., Dhingra, R. C., Palileo, E., Swiryn, S., Bauernfeind, R., Wyndham, C., and Rosen, K. M.: Natural history of chronic second degree atrioventricular nodal block. Circulation *63*:1043, 1981.
345. Wald, R. W., and Waxman, M. B.: Depression of distal AV conduction following ventricular pacing. PACE *4*:84, 1981.
346. Takahashi, N., Gilmour, R. F., Jr., and Zipes, D. P.: Overdrive suppression of conduction in the canine His-Purkinje system after occlusion of the anterior septal artery. Circulation *70*:495, 1984.
347. Strasberg, B., Lam, W., Swiryn, S., Bauernfeind, R., Scagliotti, D., Palileo, E., and Rosen, K. M.: Symptomatic spontaneous paroxysmal AV nodal block to localized hyperresponsiveness of the AV node to vagotonic reflexes. Am. Heart J. *103*:795, 1982.
348. Ginks, W., Sutton, R., Siddons, H., and Leatham, A.: Unsuspected coronary artery disease as a cause of chronic atrioventricular block in middle age. Br. Heart J. *44*:699, 1980.
349. Ohkawa, S., Sugiura, M., Itoh, Y., Kitano, K., Hiraoka, K., Ueda, J., and Murakama, M.: Electrophysiologic and histologic correlates in chronic complete atrioventricular block. Circulation *64*:215, 1981.
350. Huhta, J. C., Maloney, J. D., Ritter, D. G., Ilstrup, D. M., and Feldt, R. H.: Complete atrioventricular block in patients with atrioventricular discordance. Circulation *67*:1374, 1983.
351. Litsey, S. E., Noonan, J. A., O'Connor, W. N., Cottrill, C. M., and Mitchell, B.: Maternal connective tissue disease and congenital heart block. Demonstration of immunoglobulin in cardiac tissue. N. Engl. J. Med. *312*:98, 1985.
352. Scott, J. S., Maddison, P. J., Taylor, P. V., Esscher, E., Scott, O., and Skinner, R. P.: Connective-tissue disease, antibodies to ribonucleoprotein, and congenital heart block. N. Engl. J. Med. *309*:209, 1983.
353. Ho, S. Y., Esscher, E., Anderson, R. H., and Michaelsson, M.: Anatomy of congenital complete heart block and relation to maternal anti-Ro antibodies. Am. J. Cardiol. *58*:291, 1986.
353a. Taylor, P. V., Scott, J. S., Gerlis, L. M., Esscher, E., and Scott, O.: Maternal antibodies against fetal cardiac antigens in congenital complete heart block. N. Engl. J. Med. *315*:667, 1986
354. Besley, D. C., McWilliams, G. J., Moodie, D. S., and Castle, L. W.: Long-term followup of young adults following permanent pacemaker placement for complete heart block. Am. Heart J. *103*:332, 1982.
355. Esscher, E.: Congenital complete heart block. Acta Pediatr. Scand. *70*:131, 1981.
356. Karpawich, P. P., Gillette, P. C., Garson, A., Jr., Hesslein, P. S., Porter, C. B., and McNamara, D. G.: Congenital complete atrioventricular block: Clinical and electrophysiologic predictors of need for pacemaker insertion. Am. J. Cardiol. *48*:109, 1981.
357. Benson, D. W., Jr., Spach, M. S., Edwards, S. B., Sterba, R., Serwer, G. A., Armstrong, B. E., and Anderson, P. A.: Heart block in children. Evaluation of subsidiary ventricular pacemaker recovery times and ECG tape recordings. Pediatr. Cardiol. 2:39, 1982.
358. Mond, H. G.: The bradyarrhythmias: Current indications for permanent pacing (Part I). PACE *4*:432, 1981.
359. Mond, H. G.: The bradyarrhythmias: Current indications for permanent pacing (Part II). PACE *4*:538, 1981.

OTHER ELECTROPHYSIOLOGIC ABNORMALITIES LEADING TO CARDIAC ARRHYTHMIAS

360. Rosenbaum, M. B., Levi, R. J., Elizari, M. V., Vetulli, H. M., and Sanchez, R. A.: Supernormal excitability and conduction. Cardiol. Clin. *1*:75, 1983.
361. Gilmour, R. F., Jr., Salata, J. J., and Zipes, D. P.: Rate related suppression and facilitation of conduction in isolated canine cardiac Purkinje fibers. Circ. Res. *57*:35, 1985.
362. Gilmour, R. F., Jr., Salata, J. J., and Davis, J. R.: Effects of 4-aminopyridine on rate-related depression of cardiac action potentials. Am. J. Physiol. *251*:H297, 1986.
362a. Moe, G. K., Childers, R. W., and Meredith, J.: An appraisal of "supernormal" AV conduction. Circulation *38*:5, 1968.
363. Fisch, C.: Concealed conduction. Cardiol. Clin. *1*:63, 1983.
364. Lehmann, M. H., Mahmud, R., Denker, S., Soni, J., and Akhtar, M.: Retrograde concealed conduction in the atrioventricular node: Differential manifestations related to level of intranodal penetration. Circulation *70*:392, 1984.
365. Klein, G. J., Yee, R., and Scharma, A. D.: Concealed conduction in accessory atrioventricular pathway: An important determinant of the expression of the arrhythmias in patients with Wolff-Parkinson-White syndrome. Circulation *70*:402, 1984.
366. Miller, J. M., Vassallo, J. A., Hargrove, W. C., and Josephson, M. E.: Intermittent failure of local conduction during ventricular tachycardia. Circulation 72:1286, 1985.
367. Nau, G. J., Aldariz, A. E., Acunzo, R. S., Halpern, M. S., Davidenko, J. M., Elizari, M. V., and Rosenbaum, M. B.: Modulation of parasystolic activity by non-parasystolic beats. Circulation *66*:462, 1982.
368. Oreto, G., Satullo, G., Luzza, F., Consolo, F., and Schamroth, L.: Supernormal modulation of ventricular parasystole: The triphasic phase-response curve. Am. J. Cardiol. *57*:283, 1986.
369. Castellanos, A., Luceri, R. M., Moleiro, F., Kayden, D. S., Trohman, R. G., Zamar, L., and Myerburg, R. J.: Annihilation, entrainment, and modulation of ventricular parasystolic rhythms. Am. J. Cardiol. *54*:317, 1984.
370. Antzelevitch, C., Bernstein, M. J., Feldman, H. N., and Moe, G. K.: Parasystole, reentry, and tachycardia: A canine preparation of cardiac arrhythmias occurring across inexcitable segments of tissue. Circulation *68*:1101, 1983.
371. Kinoshita, S., Nakagawa, K., Kato, N., Nishino, T., and Tanabe, Y.: Mechanism of supraventricular parasystole. Circulation *65*:208, 1982.
372. Antzelvitch, C., Jalife, J., and Moe, G. K.: Electrotonic modulation of pacemaker activity. Further biological and mathematical observations on the behavior of modulated parasystole. Circulation *66*:1225, 1982.

23 CARDIAC PACEMAKERS

by DOUGLAS P. ZIPES, M.D., and
EDWIN G. DUFFIN, Ph.D.

The artificial cardiac pacemaker is an electronic device that delivers electrical stimuli to the heart to treat bradycardias and tachycardias. Essential elements include a power source, usually a battery, which supplies energy for the stimuli and circuitry; an electronic circuit to regulate the timing and characteristics of the stimuli; and a lead composed of electrodes on a catheter or wire to connect the battery and circuit to the heart. The electrode is the uninsulated portion of the lead in contact with the body. At first, pacemakers were external units that provided temporary pacing by delivering stimuli to the skin[1] or to the heart through a lead, with the electronic device and power source remaining outside the body.[2] For many clinical situations, temporary pacemakers are still needed. The first totally implantable devices were reported in the late 1950s.[3-5] Today, an estimated one million patients worldwide are equipped with implanted pacemakers (500,000 in the United States). Advances in technology have been applied rapidly to pacemaker systems, and pacemakers themselves have changed dramatically from the 250-gram, asynchronous devices of the early 1960's. Present-day systems provide single- and dual-chamber pacemakers that can be programmed noninvasively, weigh between 23 and 75 gm, last an estimated 6 to 10 years, and are highly reliable.

INDICATIONS FOR CARDIAC PACING

Pacemakers are employed to treat patients who have symptomatic bradycardias and tachycardias. (The use of pacing as a diagnostic tool is discussed in Chapter 21.) The nature of the arrhythmia and the likelihood that it will persist or recur determine whether pacing, either temporary or permanent, is indicated (Table 23–1). As a general rule, in patients who have symptomatic bradycardias, drugs do not successfully and reliably speed up the heart rate or improve atrioventricular (AV) conduction for longer than several hours to several days without producing intolerable side effects. Therefore, regardless of the arrhythmia causing the bradycardia (e.g., sinus bradycardia or AV block), pacing may be indicated in such cases. In addition, pacing may be used both to terminate and to prevent a recurrence of some forms of tachycardia. The type of tachycardia and clinical setting determine whether pacing should be employed. Most often, other therapeutic approaches, particularly drugs and electrical cardioversion, are tried before pacing is instituted. The choice between temporary and permanent pacing is based on whether the rhythm disturbance is likely to be transient or permanent.

TEMPORARY PACING FOR BRADYCARDIAS. Temporary pacing is indicated in a variety of circumstances in which a symptomatic bradycardia is present or is likely to occur, such as after some forms of cardiac surgery,[6] during right heart catheterization in patients with preexisting left bundle branch block, during administration of some drugs that might inappropriately slow the heart rate, and prior to implanting a permanent pacemaker in patients with symptomatic bradycardia. Temporary pacing may also be useful in some patients who have symptoms of heart failure associated with reduced cardiac output secondary to a slow rate (Table 23–1).

Temporary Pacing During Acute Myocardial Infarction (See also p. 1266). The role of temporary pacing during acute myocardial infarction in patients who develop AV conduction disturbances is controversial because the risk-to-benefit ratio is unclear. For untreated patients who develop AV block in this situation the mortality rate is not well established, often because reported studies are spuriously influenced by forms of AV block that do not require pacing. Furthermore, causes of death not directly related to the conduction disturbance, such as ventricular fibrillation, may lead to sudden death in these patients. Such a death may be incorrectly reported as being due to complete heart block. However, it appears that the extent of myocardial involvement and resultant degree of heart failure are the most important prognostic factors in patients in whom AV conduction disturbances develop during acute myocardial infarction.[7]

First degree AV block during acute myocardial infarction has been reported to be associated with an increased incidence of progression to high-degree AV block.[7, 8] Although P-R prolongation occurs in patients in whom high-degree AV block follows, abrupt complete heart block frequently occurs without demonstrable prior P-R prolongation. First degree AV block that develops before or during acute myocardial infarction as an isolated finding is not an indication for temporary pacing.

Type I second degree AV block (p. 703) most commonly occurs during acute inferior myocardial infarction, presumably owing to transient ischemia or increased vagal tone in the region of the AV node, while *type II second degree AV*

TABLE 23–1 INDICATIONS FOR CARDIAC PACING

	Definitely Indicated	Probably Indicated	Probably Not Indicated	Definitely Not Indicated
Complete AV Block				
Congenital (AV nodal)				
Asymptomatic				X
Symptomatic	T,P			
Acquired (His-Purkinje)				
Asymptomatic		T,P		
Symptomatic	T,P			
Surgical (persistent)				
Asymptomatic	T	P		
Symptomatic	T,P			
Second Degree AV Block				
Type I (AV nodal)				
Asymptomatic				X
Symptomatic	T,P			
Type II (His-Purkinje)				
Asymptomatic		T,P		
Symptomatic	T,P			
First Degree AV Block				
AV Nodal				
Asymptomatic				X
Symptomatic			X	
His-Purkinje				
Asymptomatic				X
Symptomatic			X	
Bundle Branch Block				
Asymptomatic				X
Symptomatic				
Normal H-V		P‡		
Prolonged H-V	P			
Distal His block at paced atrial rates <130/min	P			
LBBB during right heart catheterization	T			
Acute Myocardial Infarction				
Newly acquired bifascicular BBB	T			
Preexisting BBB				X
Newly acquired BBB plus transient complete AV block	T	P		
Second degree AV block				
Type I (asymptomatic)				X
Type II	T	P		
Complete AV block	T	P		
Atrial Fibrillation with Slow Ventricular Response				
Asymptomatic				X
Symptomatic	T,P			
Sick Sinus Syndrome				
Asymptomatic			X	
Symptomatic	T,P			
Hypersensitive Carotid Sinus Syndrome				
Asymptomatic			X	
Symptomatic	T,P			
Bradycardia-Tachycardia Syndrome				
Asymptomatic			X	
Symptomatic	T,P			
Bradycardia-Miscellaneous				
Asymptomatic			X	
Symptomatic	T,P			

T = Temporary pacing; P = permanent pacing; X = pacing not indicated
BBB = Bundle branch block; LBBB = Left bundle branch block
HV = Measure of His-Purkinje conduction time
Δ = Site and rate of stimulation may influence success
Π = Atrial fibrillation with a rapid ventricular response may be a complication
** = Prove efficacy with temporary pacing
ss = May accelerate VT
‡ = No other cause found for symptoms

Table continued on opposite page

TABLE 23–1 INDICATIONS FOR CARDIAC PACING *Continued*

	Definitely Indicated	Probably Indicated	Probably Not Indicated	Definitely Not Indicated
Tachycardia Prevention$^{\Delta}$				
Associated with bradycardia	T,P			
Associated with long Q-T, torsades de pointes	T	P		
Not associated with bradycardia, long Q-T, torsades de pointes (after drug failure)		T	P**	
Tachycardia Termination (after drug failure)$^{**\Delta}$				
Atrial flutter	T,P			
Atrial fibrillation				X
AV nodal reentry	T,P			
Reciprocating tachycardia in WPW syndrome	T,P$^{\Pi}$			
Ventricular tachycardia	Tss	Pss		

block (p. 703) commonly occurs during acute anterior myocardial infarction, resulting from a large infarction that includes the interventricular septum.[9–11] Type I second degree AV block generally is transient, blocks in the AV node, is not associated with symptoms, and does not require pacing. On the other hand, type II second degree AV block is most commonly due to block in the His-Purkinje system, occurs in the setting of a bundle branch block, may progress to complete AV block, and requires temporary pacing.[12] Whether or not pacing is attempted, type II AV block is associated with a high mortality rate because of the concomitant large myocardial infarction.[13]

Patients who develop first degree or type I second degree AV block with a normal QRS complex and only axis deviation generally do not require prophylactic pacing. Uncommonly, acute inferior myocardial infarction results in a bradycardia that does require pacing. This may be a sinus bradycardia, or second-degree or complete AV block that is not transient and does not respond satisfactorily to atropine.[8] AV sequential pacing may provide important hemodynamic advantages, particularly if right ventricular infarction complicates the inferior myocardial infarction.

Available data on the significance of H-V interval prolongation as an indicator of progression to high degree AV block in acute myocardial infarction have led to controversial conclusions. Most patients studied who progress to complete heart block do demonstrate H-V interval prolongation during acute myocardial infarction. However, this finding does not necessarily imply that complete heart block is imminent, particularly if the H-V interval prolongation preceded the onset of acute myocardial infarction—a fact not always known. Thus, the clinical usefulness of recording the H-V interval to predict subsequent development of complete AV block as well as survival during acute myocardial infarction is still not settled.[7]

Development of complete AV block should be considered in the same manner as type II second degree AV block. It is important not to confuse the diagnosis of complete AV dissociation with complete AV block (Ch. 22). Mortality is influenced in large measure by the severity of the underlying heart disease. However, patients who develop type II second degree or complete AV block without pulmonary edema or shock still have a higher mortality rate than patients who do not have advanced AV block, with many deaths due to the abrupt development of AV block.[13] Therefore, temporary pacing is clearly indicated in this group of patients.

Temporary pacing is warranted in patients with acute myocardial infarction who develop new evidence of bifascicular block that may present as alternating right and left bundle branch block, right bundle branch block with left axis deviation, right bundle branch block with right axis deviation, and perhaps left bundle branch block with P-R interval prolongation. Most of these patients have acute anterior myocardial infarction and appear to be at increased risk of developing high-degree AV block.[7, 8, 13] Left bundle branch block with P-R prolongation is included in this group because, while these findings may represent bifascicular block in association with AV nodal disease, the majority of these patients have a prolonged H-V interval and probably trifascicular disease. The new development of left anterior fascicular block during acute myocardial infarction does not necessarily indicate left anterior descending coronary arery involvement or more extensive coronary disease.[14]

The role of prophylactic pacing in the setting of acute anterior myocardial infarction with new right bundle branch block and a normal axis or with new left bundle branch block and a normal P-R interval is more controversial; however, some evidence of decreased morbidity associated with pacing seems to justify its use in patients who do not have heart failure, provided that the complication rate of inserting a temporary pacing catheter is low.[7] It appears that preexisting, stable right bundle branch block or left bundle branch block with or without axis deviation is *not* an indication for prophylactic pacing, whether the block is present in a patient who has an acute infarction or in other situations, such as in patients undergoing surgery. While the development of bifascicular block is associated with a higher incidence of progression to advanced AV block, the mortality among patients who develop new bundle branch block alone and acute myocardial infarction is similar to that among patients who had bundle branch block prior to the infarction. The picture is confused by more recent data suggesting that prophylactic pacing is indicated in patients with preexisting bifascicular block and acute anterior infarction.[15]

In *summary*, prophylactic temporary pacing appears warranted in patients who have an acute myocardial infarction and who develop type II second or third degree AV block or bifascicular block of recent onset. Most of these patients have acute anterior myocardial infarction. Bundle branch block complicating acute myocardial infarction identifies the individual at significant risk for congestive heart failure, with death often secondary to myocardial failure or refractory ventricular arrhythmias. The presence of high-degree AV block per se appears to increase mortality in patients without pump failure, and immediate survival may be enhanced by prophylactic pacing in patients at high risk for developing abrupt complete heart block complicating acute myocardial infarction but without evidence of heart failure. The assumption that prophylactic pacing improves survival in patients with bundle branch block and significant heart failure complicating acute myocardial infarction remains speculative. Finally, patients with myocardial infarction who develop symptomatic bradycardia of any type that responds poorly to drug therapy should be considered as candidates for pacing.

TEMPORARY PACING FOR TACHYCARDIAS. Temporary pacing may be useful to terminate a variety of tachycardias, including atrial flutter, reciprocating tachycardias involving the sinus or AV node or an accessory pathway, and some sustained ventricular tachycardias. Isolated examples of other tachycardias terminated by pacing have been reported. Pacing does not terminate atrial or ventricular fibrillation. It is used generally when drug therapy has been ineffective and/or electrical cardioversion is contraindicated (as, for example, when digitalis toxicity is suspected), when repeated cardioversion is required owing to frequent recurrence of the tachycardia, or when a pacing catheter is already in place. A lead designed for low-energy transvenous cardioversion may be used to terminate ventricular tachycardia.[16] Transcutaneous, esophageal, or intracardiac pacing may be used.

Pacing can prevent several types of tachycardias, such as those associated with significant bradycardias (e.g., complete AV block) or with a prolonged Q-T interval that results in torsades de pointes[17, 18] (p. 698). Patients with the bradycardia-tachycardia syndrome may require pacing after termination of the tachycardia to prevent the bradycardia. Use of rapid pacing rates may suppress premature beats and prevent some tachycardias from recurring. Paired or coupled atrial pacing may reduce the ventricular rate if the premature atrial complex blocks in the AV junction; paired or coupled ventricular stimulation may reduce the effective ventricular rate if the premature ventricular complex results in electrical without mechanical systole. However, such premature stimulation risks precipitation of fibrillation.

PERMANENT PACING FOR BRADYCARDIAS. As for temporary pacing, permanent pacing is indicated in patients with symptomatic bradycardia regardless of the nature of the arrhythmia as long as it is likely to be permanent or recurrent, i.e., it is not associated with a transient condition such as acute myocardial infarction or drug toxicity.[19] The most common indications for permanent pacing are fixed or intermittent complete third degree AV block[20] (with sclerotic degeneration of the AV conducting system being the primary etiology) and the sick sinus syndrome,[20] manifest as sinus arrest or block, severe sinus bradycardia, or alternating periods of bradycardia and supraventricular tachycardia. In North America, sick sinus syndrome (see p. 667) accounts for 46 per cent of pacemaker implants and third degree AV block accounts for 31 per cent; in Europe, these rates are reversed, being 30 and 45 per cent, respectively. In patients with sick sinus syndrome (p. 667) drugs used to treat the tachycardia may aggravate the bradycardia, requiring permanent pacing for the latter. Patients symptomatic from sinus bradycardia or AV block caused by hypersensitive carotid sinus syndrome[21] or slow ventricular rates during chronic atrial fibrillation are also candidates for pacemakers. Sometimes asystole or bradycardia occurs only at the termination of a tachycardia and may be responsible for the patient's symptoms.

Major questions arise when one is considering *prophylactic* permanent pacing. There is general—although not complete—agreement that permanent pacing is indicated in asymptomatic patients with acquired complete AV block or well-documented type II second degree AV block (used here to include patients with His-Purkinje block [p. 704]), since the natural history appears to be one of progression to the point of symptoms. Although patients with documented transient high-degree AV block are at a substantial risk for sudden death, one could argue against permanently pacing a sedentary elderly individual who has complete AV block but has been totally asymptomatic.

The *prognosis* for patients who have chronic bundle branch block depends to a large extent on the presence and etiology as well as the severity of the associated heart disease. In most patients, the terminal event is usually one of heart failure or the complications of coronary artery disease. In the absence of clinically detectable heart disease, the long-term prognosis for this group of patients is good without pacing. Ventricular arrhythmias occur more often in patients who have chronic bundle branch block than in the normal population, but the mechanism of sudden death in any given patient is speculative. Most patients who die suddenly, especially those who have coronary artery disease, probably develop ventricular fibrillation (p. 745). No clinical variable (such as age, syncope, angina, or shortness of breath), physical finding (such as an S_3 gallop, cardiomegaly, or heart failure), or electrocardiographic finding (such as right bundle branch block with left axis deviation, right bundle branch block with right axis deviation, or P-R interval prolongation) is useful in predicting progression to complete heart block. All the above variables occur frequently in patients who have bundle branch block, yet the progression to complete heart block is relatively infrequent.

Patients who have chronic bifascicular block with a prolonged H-V interval develop AV block more readily than do patients who have a normal H-V interval (4.5 versus 0.6 per cent), but the risk of developing trifascicular block is still small, and *routine* permanent pacing is not warranted.[22] In a similar study of patients with bundle branch block, the incidence of progression to second or third degree AV block over 30 months was 3.5 per cent in those with a normal H-V interval compared with 12 and 25 per cent for those with an H-V interval greater than or equal to 70 msec or 100 msec, respectively. The incidence of all deaths and cardiac deaths was greater in the groups with a prolonged H-V interval.[23] Development of His-Purkinje block during atrial pacing at rates less than 130 beats/min may be a possible marker for development of complete heart block, although this criterion needs further validation. Data for patients with unexplained recurrent syncope or presyncope (p. 887) and bundle branch block suggest that permanent pacing is reasonable therapy only after an effort has been made to exclude noncardiac and other cardiac causes for the symptoms. However, in one study of patients with neurological symptoms and a prolonged H-V interval, prophylactic pacemaker insertion did not relieve symptoms or prolong life.[23] Some of these patients may have symptoms due to ventricular tachyarrhythmias, not bradyarrhythmias. Stressing AV conduction with intravenous disopyramide has been suggested as a means to predict patients prone to subsequent AV block.[24]

Finally, it has been conjectured that permanent prophylactic pacing helps prevent sudden death in survivors of acute myocardial infarction complicated by bundle branch block and transient high-degree AV block. However, the number of patients studied is small and the data are not conclusive.[8, 13, 25, 26]

PERMANENT PACING FOR TACHYCARDIAS. Preventing tachycardia is an important therapeutic application of pacing in selected subgroups of patients. Tachycardias that occur only in the setting of bradycardias can be prevented by pacing at normal rates. In general, pacing at accelerated rates to prevent recurrence of tachycardias in patients who otherwise have normal heart rates and rhythms is not successful over the long term. Therefore, except for bradycardia-related tachycardia, the most successful application of antitachycardia pacing to date is to terminate tachycardias after they start[6, 27] rather than to prevent their occurrence[27–30] (see page 728 for pacing for tachycardias).

PACEMAKER MODALITIES

Pacemakers perform two basic functions: (1) they all stimulate the heart and (2) most can sense impulses as well—i.e., they are equipped with amplifiers that register or recognize (sense) a spontaneous cardiac electrical event and then use that information to modulate the timing of the electrical stimulus delivered (pace). These two functions can be carried out in the atrium, the ventricle, or both.[31, 32] Sensing and stimulation are accomplished with pairs of electrodes directly in contact with the myocardium (a bipolar system) or with one electrode located at the heart and a second electrode, usually the pacemaker case, located remotely (a unipolar system).

Because pacemakers operate in a variety of complex combinations, a letter code—originally three positions[32] and now five[33] has been devised as a shorthand notation to identify the different types of pacemakers (Table 23–2). Symbols placed in the first two positions indicate the chambers in which the pacemaker paces (first position) and in which it senses (second position). "A" or "V" indicates that the device paces or senses the atrium or the ventricle; "D" indicates that it paces or senses in both chambers. "S" indicates a single-chamber unit designed to be suitable for either atrial or ventricular pacing, depending on how its parameters are programmed. The third position signifies in what manner the pacemaker responds to spontaneous electrical activity. "O" indicates that the pacemaker does not sense spontaneous electrical activity and therefore discharges at a fixed rate and is not influenced by cardiac events. "I" indicates that the pacemaker is inhibited from delivering a stimulus for a certain period of time in response to sensed electrical activity; i.e., its discharge cycle is "reset" by the spontaneous event. "T" indicates that a stimulus is discharged in response to sensed activity, while "D" in the third position indicates that the pacemaker responds to sensed atrial activity by delivering a stimulus to the ventricle; i.e., it acts as an artificial AV node but responds to sensed ventricular activity by inhibiting its ventricular stimulus (it is reset). "R" indicates the response mode of a special type of pacemaker used to treat patients who have certain kinds of tachycardias. It discharges stimuli when the sensed heart rate *exceeds* a preset value and is quiescent at normal heart rates. Thus, it functions in reverse relative to most pacemakers, which are usually quiescent when the heart rate exceeds a particular value and discharge when the patient's rate falls below that preset value.

The fourth and fifth positions have been newly added. Position four indicates whether and to what extent pacemaker function can be reversibly changed noninvasively ("programmed"). "P" indicates that only the rate and/or output can be altered, while "M" designates that other functions—such as sensitivity, duration of amplifier refractoriness, and so forth—can also be programmed. Recently, a "C" has been added to indicate a "communicating" feature, i.e., telemetry, with programmable functions assumed to be present. The fifth position is reserved for pacemakers used to treat tachycardias. Stimuli may be delivered as a burst, "B" (a short train of generally rapid sequential stimuli); at a normal rate, "N," in fixed-rate competition with the tachycardia; or at various intervals that automatically scan the cardiac cycle, "S," in an effort to find the appropriate premature interval that will successfully terminate the tachycardia.

The most commonly implanted pacemaker today is the demand ventricular pacemaker. It paces the ventricle (V), senses ventricular activity (V), and is inhibited from discharging (I) by sensed ventricular events—hence, the VVI pacemaker.

Each pacing modality has different functional capabilities (Table 23–3) and therefore specific indications and contraindications (Table 23–4).

ATRIAL AND VENTRICULAR ASYNCHRONOUS PACEMAKERS (AOO, VOO). The original pacemakers simply stimulated the myocardium at a constant rate independent of the underlying cardiac rhythm; used for pacing only, these devices could not sense any spontaneous activity.

TABLE 23–2 FIVE-POSITION PACEMAKER CODE

I. CHAMBER PACED	II. CHAMBER SENSED	III. MODE OF RESPONSE	IV. PROGRAMMABILITY	V. TACHYARRHYTHMIA FUNCTIONS*
V = Ventricle	V = Ventricle	I = Inhibited	P = Programmable rate and/or output	B = Burst
A = Atrium	A = Atrium	T = Triggered	M = Multiprogrammable	N = Normal rate competition
D = Atrium and ventricle	D = Atrium and ventricle	D = Atrial triggered and ventricular inhibited	O = None	S = Scanning
	O = None	R = Reverse		E = Externally activated
S = single chamber	S = single chamber	O = None		O = None

This table provides a "shorthand" description of pacemaker operation. Symbols placed in the first two positions indicate chambers in which the pacemaker functions; a symbol in the third position, the mode of operation of the pacemaker; in the fourth position, its programmable characteristics; and in the fifth position, its antitachycardia features. For example, if the pacing lead were inserted into the ventricle and the pulse generator were a ventricular demand inhibited unit, the chamber paced would be ventricle and the first letter in the five-position code would be "V." The chamber sensed would be ventricle and, therefore, the second letter in the five-position code would also be "V." The mode of response of the pacemaker would be to inhibit a pacing spike when spontaneous electrical activity were sensed and, therefore, "I" would be in the third position. If only the rate and/or output of the pulse generator could be programmed externally, "P" would be in the fourth position. If the pacemaker were used to treat tachycardias, the tachyarrhythmia function would be indicated in the fifth position. Pulse generators that pace or sense in both atrium and ventricle are indicated by the designation "D," meaning dual. If the pacemaker does not have a function in one of the classifications, "O" is used. Finally, some pacemakers have a "reverse" function in that they discharge when the rate becomes too fast (and are thus used to terminate tachycardias). These pacemakers are indicated by the letter "R" in the third position. The different types of tachyarrhythmia functions are discussed in the chapter. Recently, the letter "C" has been suggested for the fourth position to indicate a "communicating" function, i.e., telemetry, with programmable features assumed.

An "S" may be used as a manufacturer's designation to label multiprogrammable single-chamber pacemakers adaptable for either atrial or ventricular use.

*The fourth and fifth positions are optional, as is a comma separating the third and fourth positions.

TABLE 23–3 SENSING AND PACING CAPABILITIES OF AVAILABLE PACING MODES

Pacemaker Type	ICHD Code	Atrium	Ventricle	Response to Sensed Activity
Atrial Asynchronous	AOO	P		None
Ventricular Asynchronous	VOO		P	None
Atrial Demand	AAI AAT	S,P S,P		Inhibited Triggered
Ventricular Demand	VVI VVT		S,P S,P	Inhibited Triggered
Atrial Synchronous	VAT	S	P	Triggered
Atrial Synchronous, Ventricular Inhibited	VDD	S	S,P	Triggered (A) Inhibited (V)
AV Sequential	DVI	P	S,P	Inhibited
AV Sequential	DDI	S,P	S,P	Inhibited (A&V)
AV Universal	DDD	S,P	S,P	Inhibited on channel sensed (A&V); triggered on alternate channel (A&V)

P = Pacing; S = Sensing.

When the electrode is placed in the atrium, the pacemaker is called an asynchronous atrial pacemaker; in the ventricle, it is an asynchronous ventricular pacemaker. Asynchronous pacemakers are rarely used today except under special circumstances, generally to initiate or terminate tachycardias. Magnet application converts most pacemakers to their asynchronous mode.

ATRIAL AND VENTRICULAR DEMAND PACEMAKERS (AAI, AAT, VVI, VVT). In the early 1970's, sensing circuits were added to pacemakers so that they stimulated only on demand when no appropriate underlying spontaneous rhythm was detected by the pacemaker. This sensing function prevented competitive pacing and the attendant risk of inducing ventricular fibrillation. Such a risk is small in general and greater in patients with conditions such as myocardial ischemia. Demand pacemakers may operate in inhibited (I) or triggered (T) mode. Inhibited devices withhold the stimulus and reset their timing upon sensing spontaneous cardiac activity. Triggered devices are designed to deliver a stimulus into the absolute refractory period of the tissue immediately upon sensing spontaneous depolarization, and simultaneously to reset their timing cycle. Both types deliver a stimulus at the end of their timing cycle (pacemaker escape interval) if no spontaneous cardiac activity is detected (Figs. 23–1 and 23–2). The sensing circuits of these pacemakers are turned off for a period of time after delivery of a stimulus or sensing of spontaneous activity to avoid recognition of inappropriate signals such as T waves. This time interval is called the *pacemaker refractory period.*

The triggered mode was proposed to address concerns that unipolar inhibited devices might allow a patient to become asystolic if sensed extracardiac signals (e.g., pectoral muscle potentials, electrical signals from radio transmitters or power lines) were erroneously interpreted to be cardiac signals and thus inhibited pacemaker output. Modern circuitry has reduced the likelihood of such occurrences. The disadvantages of stimulating when it is not really necessary, such as distorting the ECG waveform and draining more power from the pacemaker, have resulted

ATRIAL DEMAND

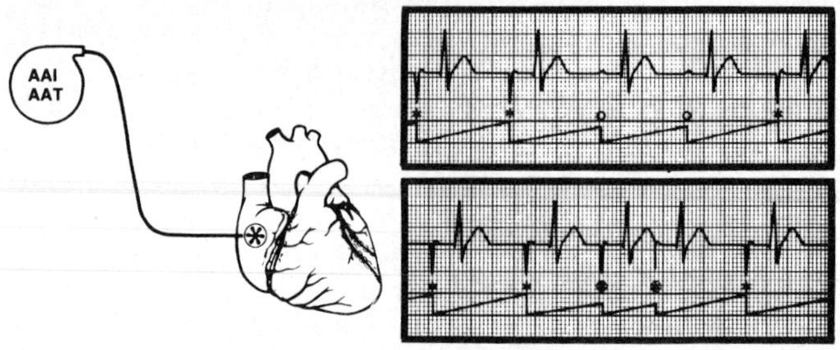

FUNCTION: PACES, SENSES ATRIUM

FIGURE 23–1. Atrial demand pacemakers (AAI, AAT). *Left,* The atrial demand pacemaker is connected to the right atrium. The lead termination is marked with a circle to indicate that the pacemaker senses atrial cardiac activity and an asterisk to indicate that it stimulates in the atrium. *Right,* Representative ECGs produced by atrial inhibited (AAI, upper tracing) and atrial triggered (AAT, lower tracing) pacing, with associated ladder diagrams, which are used to depict pacemaker timing. The slanted lines connecting a pair of horizontal parallel bars represent pacemaker escape interval timing; vertical lines indicate resetting of escape interval timing. After it is reset, the pacemaker escape interval begins and a pacing pulse occurs whenever the sloping line intersects a ladder bar. If the upper bar is intersected, atrial escape was in progress so atrial pacing occurs; if the lower bar is intersected, ventricular escape was in progress so ventricular pacing occurs. Note that sensing causes pacing in triggered devices (AAT, VVT) even though escape interval timing is not completed, so the diagrams show a sensing symbol (circle) with a pacing symbol (asterisk) superimposed. Some sensing modes (e.g., DDI [Fig. 23–5]) do not reset timing of escape intervals but prevent pacing function at the end of an escape interval. In the ladder diagrams this is indicated by dotting the post-sensing portion of the escape interval ramp and omitting the pacing symbol.

In the upper tracing, the first, second, and fifth atrial complexes are pacemaker-induced; the third and fourth atrial complexes are spontaneous and reset pacemaker timing while inhibiting delivery of the stimulus. In the lower tracing, the first, second, and fifth atrial complexes are pacemaker-induced; the third and fourth atrial complexes are spontaneous and reset pacemaker timing while triggering delivery of the stimulus into refractory atrial tissue. Note that the stimulus is delivered *after* the onset of the third and fourth P waves but initiates the other P waves.

VENTRICULAR DEMAND

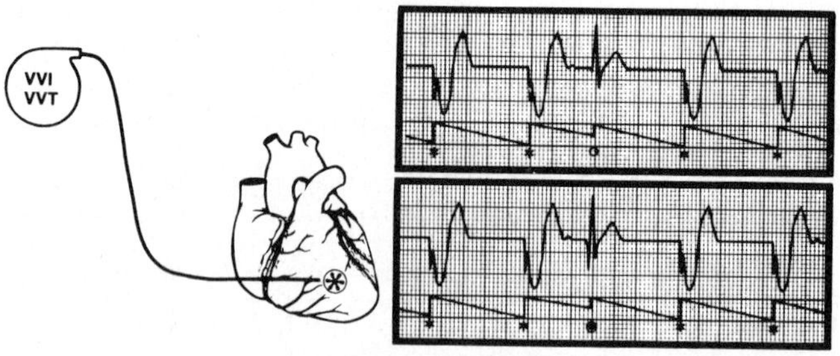

FUNCTION: PACES, SENSES VENTRICLE

FIGURE 23–2. Ventricular demand pacemakers (VVI, VVT). *Left,* The ventricular demand pacemaker is connected to the right ventricle, with a circle and an asterisk at the lead termination to indicate that the pacemaker senses ventricular cardiac activity and stimulates in the ventricle. *Right,* Representative ECG's produced by ventricular inhibited (VVI, upper tracing) and ventricular triggered (VVT, lower tracing) pacing, with associated ladder timing diagrams to indicate sensing (circle) and pacing (asterisk) functions and escape interval timing. In the upper tracing, the first, second, fourth, and fifth ventricular complexes are pacemaker-induced; the third ventricular complex results from normally conducted sinus activity. This ventricular complex resets the pacemaker timing and inhibits delivery of the ventricular stimulus. In the lower tracing, the first, second, fourth, and fifth ventricular complexes are pacemaker-induced; the third ventricular complex results from normally conducted sinus activity. This ventricular complex resets pacemaker timing and triggers delivery of the stimulus into the refractory ventricular tissue. Note that the stimulus is delivered *after* the onset of the third QRS complex but initiates the other QRS complexes.

TABLE 23–4 INDICATIONS AND CONTRAINDICATIONS FOR AVAILABLE PACING MODES

Mode	Indications	Contraindications	Advantages	Disadvantages
AOO	• Obsolete			
VOO	• Obsolete			
AAI, AAT	• SSS with normal AV conduction	• Atrial inexcitability • High atrial threshold • Abnormal AV conduction	• Simplest system providing properly timed sequential AV contraction; requires only one lead	• Ventricle not paced should AV block develop
AAI-RR	• Chronotropic incompetence with normal AV conduction	• Atrial inexcitability • High atrial threshold • Abnormal AV conduction	• Simplest system providing properly timed sequential AV contraction and variable rate in response to physiologic need; requires only one lead	• Ventricle not paced should AV block develop
VVI, VVT	• SSS without retrograde AV conduction • SSS with no hemodynamic benefit of atrial pacing • Chronic atrial fibrillation or flutter with AV block and a slow ventricular rate	• Hemodynamic insufficiency due to loss of AV synchrony ("pacemaker syndrome")	• Historical inertia • Relative simplicity	• Does not provide AV synchronous contraction • Rate does not change in response to external demands
VVI-RR	• Chronic atrial fibrillation or flutter with AV block and a slow ventricular rate • Atrial bradyarrhythmias • Normal sinus node function with impaired AV conduction	• Hemodynamic insufficiency due to loss of AV synchrony	• Simple system providing variable rate in response to physiologic need; requires only one lead	• Does not provide AV synchronous contraction
VAT VDD	• Normal sinus node function with impaired AV conduction	• Inappropriate atrial tachycardia or bradycardia • Retrograde atrial activation following ventricular stimulation of PVC's	• Maintains atrial transport and normal sinus control of ventricular rate when atrial rate is within tracking limits of pacemaker	• Does not maintain synchronous contractions during atrial bradycardia, since it does not pace the atria • Requires 2 leads
DVI	• Atrial bradyarrhythmias with or without impaired AV conduction	• Extended periods of atrial fibrillation/flutter	• Maintains sequential AV contraction during sinus bradycardia	• Does not alter rate in response to physiologic demands • Does not maintain AV synchronous contractions during periods of normal sinus rhythm and AV block • Competitive atrial pacing during normal sinus rhythm • Requires 2 leads
DDI	• Atrial bradyarrhythmias with or without impaired AV conduction	• Extended periods of atrial fibrillation/flutter	• Maintains AV contraction during sinus bradycardia	• Does not alter rate in response to physiological demands • Does not maintain AV synchronous contractions during periods of normal sinus rhythm and AV block • Requires 2 leads
DDD	• Atrial bradyarrhythmias with or without impaired AV conduction • Normal sinus node function with impaired AV conduction	• Retrograde atrial activation following ventricular stimulation or PVC's • Extended periods of atrial fibrillation/flutter • Frequent atrial tachycardias	• Maintains sequential AV contraction and sinus control of ventricular rate during normal sinus rhythm and during sinus bradycardia	• Requires 2 leads

SSS = sick sinus syndrome; RR = rate-responsive.

in relatively limited use of the triggered mode, although this mode can be valuable occasionally as an alternative to VVI pacing in patients experiencing myopotential inhibition of unipolar pacemakers or as a method to initiate and terminate some tachycardias noninvasively. For example, since the implanted unit senses electrical activity, it can be triggered to pace the heart in response to chest wall stimulation from an external pacemaker, replicating pacing cadences generally reserved for the electrophysiology laboratory. Also, triggered units are helpful diagnostically to determine when or if the pacemaker senses a spontaneous event, since in essence it "marks" that sensed event by delivering a triggered stimulus. Triggered function, therefore, is generally available in modern programmable pacemakers as an option for either permanent or temporary (diagnostic) purposes.

ATRIAL SYNCHRONOUS VENTRICULAR PACEMAKERS (VAT, VDD). To approximate normal cardiac function more closely, sophisticated dual-chamber (atrium and ventricle) "physiological" pacemakers were developed. The atrial synchronous ventricular pacemaker (VAT) (Fig. 23–3) was designed for use in patients with normal sinus node function but impaired AV conduction.[35] This device senses atrial activity by means of an electrode in the atrium and, after a suitable delay, paces the ventricles; it does not pace the atrium. This method of atrial sensing and ventricular pacing preserves the atrial contribution to ventricular filling and maintains sinus control over the ventricular rate. Thus, exercise that induces acceleration of the sinus rate concomitantly increases the paced ventricular rate. This pacemaker functions differently when lower and upper rate boundaries are reached. During atrial bradycardia below a

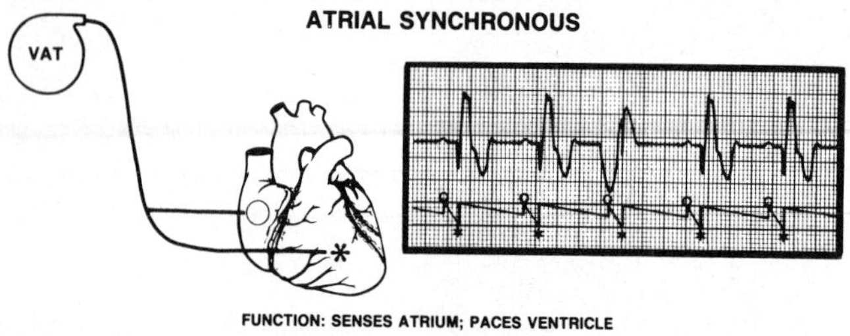

FIGURE 23–3. Atrial synchronous pacemaker (VAT). ***Left,*** **The VAT pacemaker leads are connected to the right atrium and ventricle. The circle at the atrial lead termination indicates that the pacemaker senses atrial activity and the asterisk at the ventricular lead termination indicates that it stimulates in the ventricle.** ***Right,*** **Representative ECG produced by atrial synchronous ventricular pacing, with associated ladder timing diagrams to indicate atrial sensing (circle above upper bar) and ventricular pacing (asterisk beneath lower bar) functions and escape interval timing. The first, second, fourth, and fifth ventricular complexes are stimulated by the pacemaker in response to pacemaker sensing of spontaneous atrial activity. The third ventricular complex is a premature ventricular contraction (PVC) that occurs simultaneously with a sinus-initiated atrial event. Since the pacemaker does not sense ventricular activity, it is triggered by the P wave (obscured by the PVC) and delivers a ventricular stimulus into the ST segment of the PVC.**

particular rate, the unit paces as an asynchronous ventricular pacemaker at a predetermined backup rate. During atrial tachycardia above a particular rate, the pacemaker paces no faster than its upper rate limit, yielding an AV response to sensed atrial activity that is typically 2:1, or similar to type I second degree AV block. The VAT device has been refined by the addition of a ventricular sensing amplifier, resulting in a pacemaker called the atrial synchronous ventricular inhibited pacemaker[36] (VDD) (Fig. 23–4). Addition of the ventricular sensing amplifier is important because it provides a VVI demand mode for backup pacing during sinus bradycardia. It also prevents the atrial amplifier from triggering a ventricular stimulus in the event that a premature ventricular complex (PVC) produces a strong enough signal to be detected at the atrial electrode. To prevent such undesirable triggering, the system is designed to ensure that ventricular amplifier sensing takes precedence. Finally, ventricular sensing prevents competitive pacing when a PVC occurs during the AV interval while the device is tracking normal sinus activity.

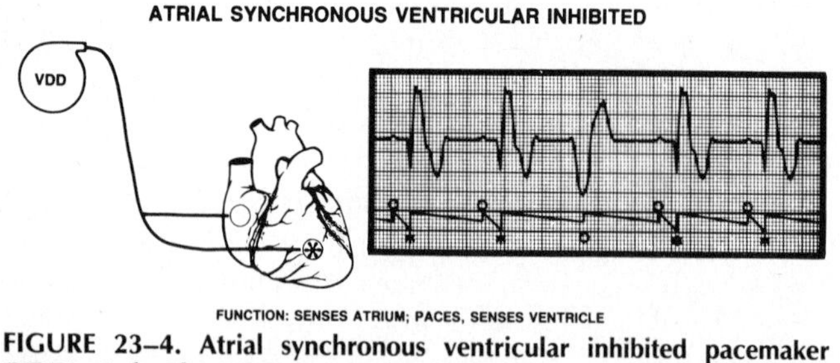

FIGURE 23–4. Atrial synchronous ventricular inhibited pacemaker (VDD). ***Left,*** **The VDD pacemaker leads are connected to the right atrium and ventricle. The circle at the atrial lead termination indicates that the pacemaker senses atrial activity and the circle and asterisk at the ventricular lead termination indicate that it senses spontaneous ventricular activity and stimulates in the ventricle.** ***Right,*** **Representative ECG produced by VDD pacing, with associated ladder timing diagrams to indicate atrial sensing (circles above upper bar), ventricular sensing (circle beneath lower bar), and ventricular pacing (asterisks beneath lower bar) functions and escape interval timing. This recording is identical to the VAT pacemaker ECG shown in Figure 23–3 except that the PVC is sensed by the ventricular amplifier and prevents the pacemaker from synchronizing to the sinus P wave (obscured by the PVC) and pacing into the ST segment of the PVC.**

Like the VAT pacemaker, the VDD pacemaker still does not pace the atrium, but it does sense and pace the ventricle. During sinus bradycardia, VAT and VDD pacemakers function in the VOO and VVI modes, respectively, and therefore, under such circumstances, do not maintain sequential AV contraction. Contraindications to VDD pacing include the presence of atrial tachycardias and bradycardias and the occurrence of retrograde conduction to the atria with a long V-A interval during ventricular pacing or PVC's. Should such retrograde activation occur after completion of the atrial refractory period of the VDD pacemaker (i.e., a portion of the pacemaker timing cycle during which atrial signals are not permitted to trigger ventricular pacing), atrial activity will be sensed, triggering a ventricular stimulus and initiating a *pacemaker-mediated tachycardia* (Fig. 23–20, p. 737).

AV SEQUENTIAL PACEMAKERS (DVI, DDI). For patients with abnormal sinus node function (sinus bradycardia, sinus arrest, and so forth) as well as impaired AV conduction, the atrial contribution to ventricular filling can be preserved by means of an AV sequential pacemaker[37] (DVI) (Fig. 23–5). This pacemaker senses only ventricular activity but is capable of stimulating both the atrium and the ventricle. Following ventricular sensed or paced events, this device monitors the ventricular electrogram. If ventricular activity is not detected within a prescribed pace-

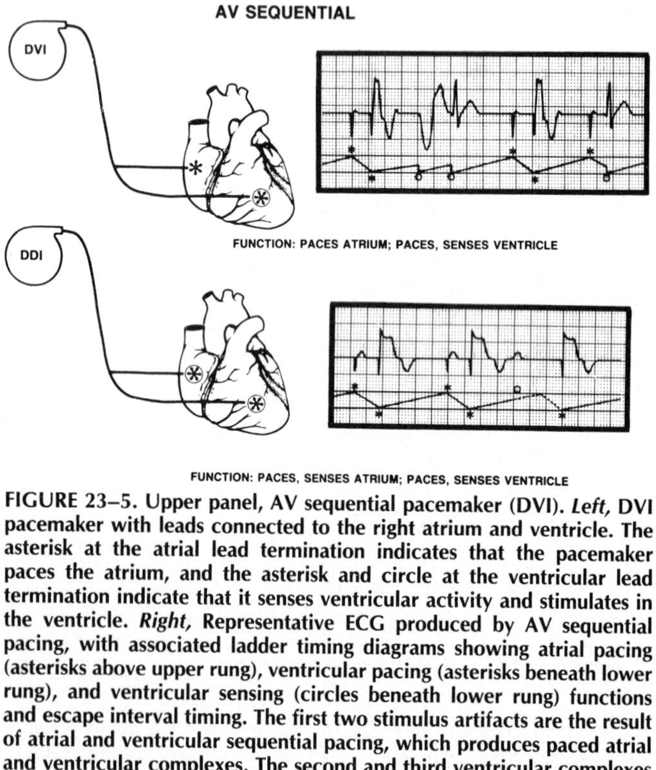

FIGURE 23–5. Upper panel, AV sequential pacemaker (DVI). ***Left,*** **DVI pacemaker with leads connected to the right atrium and ventricle. The asterisk at the atrial lead termination indicates that the pacemaker paces the atrium, and the asterisk and circle at the ventricular lead termination indicate that it senses ventricular activity and stimulates in the ventricle.** ***Right,*** **Representative ECG produced by AV sequential pacing, with associated ladder timing diagrams showing atrial pacing (asterisks above upper rung), ventricular pacing (asterisks beneath lower rung), and ventricular sensing (circles beneath lower rung) functions and escape interval timing. The first two stimulus artifacts are the result of atrial and ventricular sequential pacing, which produces paced atrial and ventricular complexes. The second and third ventricular complexes are a PVC and a normally conducted QRS following spontaneous atrial activity. These ventricular complexes (sensed only by the ventricular amplifier) inhibit both the atrial and ventricular stimuli. The third and fourth stimulus artifacts are again atrial and ventricular sequential pacing, occurring because no additional spontaneous ventricular activity took place within the pacemaker's escape interval. The final stimulus artifact, an atrial stimulus, produced an atrial complex that conducted normally to the ventricles. This conducted ventricular activity inhibited the ventricular stimulus and reset all pacemaker timing.**

Lower panel, The operation of the DDI AV sequential pacemaker is identical to that of the DVI device except that atrial sensing is provided and allows inhibition of atrial stimulation if atrial activity is sensed within the V-A escape interval. This is illustrated by the spontaneous P wave after the second paced QRS. Note that atrial sensing with DDI pacemakers does not trigger ventricular stimulation, so that the pacemaker rate does not change in response to atrial rhythms.

maker escape interval, the device stimulates the atrium. The pacemaker then waits long enough to allow passage of a normal A-V interval and, if no ventricular activity occurs, paces in the ventricle. Sensed spontaneous ventricular activity inhibits the ventricular stimulus and resets all pacemaker timing. If the ventricular rate is sufficiently rapid, atrial stimuli from the pacemaker are also inhibited. It is important to reemphasize that the DVI pacemaker does *not* sense spontaneous atrial activity and therefore cannot alter the paced rate in response to the physiologic needs. Some AV sequential pacemakers are of the "committed" type, i.e., they do not wait for normal AV conduction to occur but instead always stimulate the ventricles following delivery of an atrial stimulus.[38, 39]

A variant of the DVI pacemaker, the DDI pacemaker (Fig. 23–5) behaves identically except for the added ability to sense in the atrium and withhold atrial stimulation should a P wave be detected within the pacemaker's VA escape sequence. In this device, atrial sensing is used only to avoid competitive atrial stimulation, not for triggering ventricular stimulation.

FULLY AUTOMATIC OR UNIVERSAL PACEMAKER (DDD). The fully automatic or universal pacemaker (DDD)[40] combines features of the AAI, VDD, and DVI pacemakers by functioning as an atrial demand pacemaker (AAI) during normally conducted sinus bradycardia, as an atrial synchronous pacemaker (VDD) during normal sinus rates that block or conduct with AV delay to the ventricle, and as an AV sequential pacemaker (DVI) during sinus bradycardia characterized by blocked or prolonged AV conduction. During normally conducted sinus impulses, the pacemaker is totally inhibited (Fig. 23–6). Thus, this pacemaker most closely approaches the normal electrophysiology of the heart in order to preserve the optimal hemodynamic relationships between atrial and ventricular contraction.

Current contraindications to the use of a DDD pacemaker are (1) the presence of atrial tachycardias that are inappropriate for governing ventricular rate (since the DDD pacemaker senses the atrial rate and paces the ventricle accordingly, subject to upper rate limits as with the VDD pacemaker), and (2) as with the VDD units, retrograde conduction to the atrium with a long V-A conduction time following paced ventricular beats (i.e., the retrograde atrial response is sensed, triggers a paced ventricular beat, and thus creates an iatrogenic pacemaker-

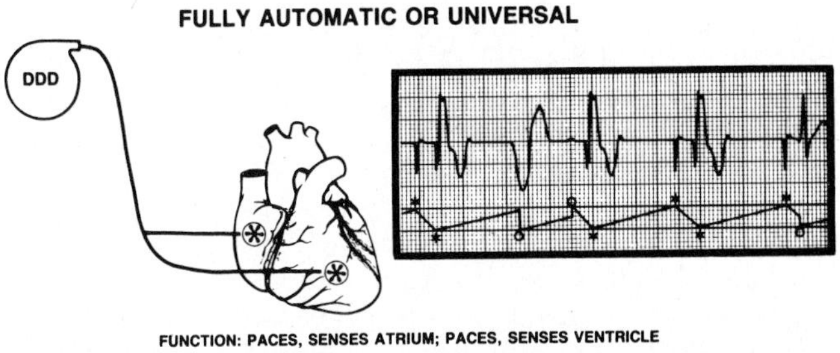

FIGURE 23–6. Fully automatic or universal pacemaker (DDD). *Left,* DDD pacemaker with leads connected to the right atrium and ventricle. Asterisks and circles at the atrial and ventricular lead terminations indicate that the pacemaker paces and senses in both atrium and ventricle. *Right,* Representative ECG produced by DDD pacing, with associated ladder timing diagrams showing atrial sensing and pacing functions (circles and asterisks above upper bar), ventricular sensing and pacing functions (circles and asterisks beneath lower bar), and escape interval timing. The first and fourth cardiac cycles, each preceded by two stimulus artifacts, are produced by atrial and ventricular sequential stimulation. The second QRS complex is a PVC, which resets all pacemaker timing and inhibits pacing. The third QRS complex is the result of ventricular pacing triggered by the pacemaker's sensing of the preceding sinus atrial event. The fifth QRS complex is the normally conducted result of atrial pacing.

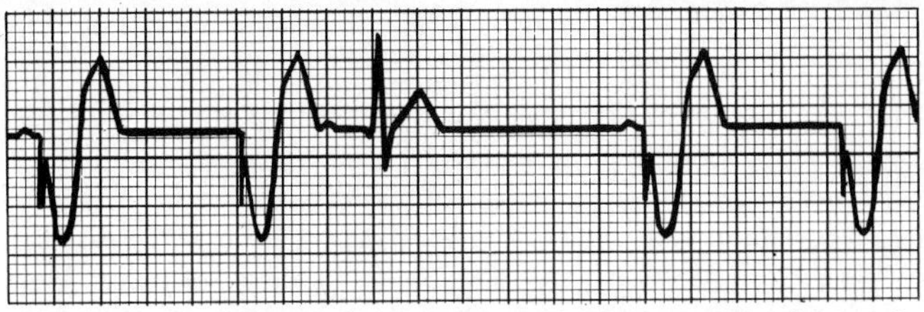

FIGURE 23–7. Operation of a VVI pacemaker incorporating hysteresis. Following two paced ventricular complexes, a sinus beat conducts to the ventricles and inhibits the pacemaker. When no additional spontaneous ventricular activity occurs, the pacemaker "escapes" at an interval of 1200 msec, with subsequent pacing intervals of 857 msec. Thus, the escape interval of the pacemaker exceeds the pacing interval, thereby allowing the patient to remain in a normally conducted rhythm for as much time as possible.

mediated tachycardia). Ultimately, the latter contraindication will be eliminated as improved designs allow atrial tracking devices to handle abnormal atrial signals appropriately.

HYSTERESIS. Pacemakers with the property of hysteresis are designed to operate as follows: the pacemaker escape interval (the interval between the last sensed spontaneous activity and the first paced beat) exceeds the interval between subsequent consecutive pacing cycles, so that normal sinus rhythm can be maintained over a wide range of rates (pacemaker-inhibited) while ensuring an adequate pacing rate when needed. This type of operation is displayed in Figure 23–7.

Although not generally described as hysteresis, the variation in the A-V interval offered by some dual-chamber pacemakers represents a similar function. In such devices the pacemaker's electrical A-V interval is shortened following sensed atrial events to compensate for the conduction time from the sinus node to the site of the atrial electrode. During AV sequential pacing, these devices generate a longer AV delay. Properly programmed, such operation presumably provides hemodynamically equivalent A-V intervals for both paced and sensed atrial events, although confirmatory data are scant.

It is important to recognize the different rate capabilities offered by the various pacemakers. Conventional AAI, AAT, VVI, VVT, DVI, and DDI pacemakers have a fixed rate that can be changed by reprogramming the pacemaker. The AAI and AAT pacemakers (assuming normal AV conduction) ensure that both atrial and ventricular rates do not drop below a minimal constant value while the VVI and VVT devices maintain a minimal constant ventricular rate. The DVI and DDI pacemakers behave like the AAI pacemaker except that they also pace the ventricle to maintain the ventricular rate equal to the atrial rate. The VDD pacemaker "tracks" the atrial rate between the lower escape interval of the pacemaker, at which it functions at a constant rate in the VVI mode, and an upper rate limit, at which the pacemaker induces second degree block (between the sensed atrial signals and the paced ventricular response) to maintain a fairly constant ventricular rate. The DDD pacemaker functions as a VDD pacemaker through the normal and fast rates but maintains a constant rate for atria and ventricles in the lower range by functioning in the AAI or DVI mode. Naturally, each of these pacemakers can be inhibited by spontaneous rhythm changes that increase the heart rate. These rate behaviors can be modified by the use of additional circuitry and sensors, as described in the next section.

RATE-RESPONSIVE PACEMAKERS. The benefits of automatic rate variability[41, 42] could be provided—even to patients who cannot increase their rates with exercise because of sinus node dysfunction—if an appropriate physiologic parameter, independent of sinus node function, could be measured and used to set the pacemaker rate. Various approaches are being explored, although most remain investigational. These include central venous temperature–sensing devices,[43, 44] oxygen saturation–sensing devices,[45] pH-responsive systems,[46] stroke volume,[47] and ventricular pressure–controlled devices.[48] Substantial clinical experience has been acquired with three single-chamber ventricular pacemaker designs that vary pacing rate in response to changes in the "Q-T" interval,[49–51] changes in respiratory rate,[52] or sensed mechanical activity of the body.[53]

The *Q-T sensing pacemaker* uses a conventional electrode system to sense and pace but has circuitry designed to determine the interval between stimulation and the peak of the intracardiac T wave. Increased sympathetic tone in response to the body's need for an accelerated heart rate shortens the Q-T interval, which in turn increases the pacemaker rate. Conversely, an increase in the Q-T interval slows the pacing rate. The device responds to *changes* in the Q-T interval rather than to absolute values, so that the rates do not reflect long-term shifts in the Q-T interval such as would be seen with electrolyte imbalance or chronic drug therapy. Advantages of this pacemaker include use of a stable, rugged sensor (the standard pacing lead) that requires no change in implant technique and the fact that the device responds to a parameter reflecting metabolic demand. Disadvantages include relatively slow response times, nonsustained rate changes, and some difficulty in ensuring reliable T-wave sensing without noise effects.

The *respiratory rate–dependent pacemaker* currently requires placement of two leads: a conventional cardiac pacing lead in the ventricle and an auxiliary lead in the subcutaneous tissue of the thorax. Variations in electrical impedance between the thoracic electrode and the pacemaker's indifferent electrode (generator case) reflect the patient's respiratory rate, which is processed to control the pacemaker rate. This approach uses a simple, reliable sensor and is responsive to exercise and metabolic needs. Drawbacks include the need for placement of an extra lead (although this may not be necessary in future versions),[54] potentially inappropriate response in patients with pulmonary disease or heart failure, and the fact that the patient can voluntarily alter the pacing rate.

The *activity-sensing pacemaker* uses a conventional lead system for sensing and pacing and incorporates a microphone-like sensor inside the pacemaker pulse generator case. This sensor responds to mechanical vibrations of the body, producing electrical signals proportional to the patient's physical activity level. These "activity" signals then determine the appropriate pacing rate. This approach affords a rapid response to patient needs, uses a sensor that is hermetically sealed within the pulse generator for reliable long-term service, and requires no change in implant technique. Disadvantages include its inability to respond to nonexercise-induced metabolic demands and the potential for minor rate increases in the presence of infrasonic environmental noises.

Although the rate-responsive devices commercially available at present are single-chamber pacemakers, these concepts can be readily adapted to dual-chamber applications, and such systems are now undergoing clinical evaluation.[54a] Future systems will probably incorporate multiple sensors, allowing compensation for the deficits of specific individual approaches.

HEMODYNAMIC CONSEQUENCES OF SEQUENTIAL AV CONTRACTION AND RATE VARIABILITY

Ventricular (VVI) pacing provides symptomatic improvement for the vast majority of patients who have sick sinus syndrome or impaired AV conduction by establishing a basal ventricular rate that ensures adequate cardiac output. There is evidence that some patients are not well served by fixed-rate ventricular pacing[55–63] (1) because this pacing mode only partially restores appropriate cardiac function (i.e., a minimal ventricular rate) to meet the demands of normal daily activity; (2) because the unnatural mechanical and electrical cardiac activation sequence associated with VVI pacing interferes with effective cardiac pumping; and (3) because the incidence of atrial fibrillation and congestive heart failure is reportedly increased in ventricular-paced patients with sinus node disease.[63] During ventricular pacing, atrial contraction may be absent, dissociated from ventricular activity, or improperly coupled to ventricular events by retrograde conduction. Inappropriately timed atrial systole effectively eliminates the booster pump action of the atrium present during normal sinus rhythm and impairs valve function.

A consistent ventriculoatrial activation sequence may be associated with greater hemodynamic compromise than is random AV dissociation because of significant decreases in systemic and left ventricular blood pressure and cardiac output along with concomitant increases in right atrial, ventricular, and pulmonary pressures. In some patients, congestive heart failure may result.[56, 63] Patients who have cannon *a* waves during ventricular pacing frequently experience hypotension due to a vasodepressor reflex initiated by the large left atrial pressure waves.[64] Numerous acute studies have shown gains in cardiac output that vary from 2 to 67 per cent after AV sequential or atrial asynchronous ventricular pacing is substituted for ventricular pacing.[65, 66] Sustained maintenance of hemodynamic gains has been shown in more recent studies.[67–69] In one series ventricular demand and atrial synchronous ventricular pacing were compared using measurements obtained invasively from exercising patients.[67, 68] Patients were first paced for 3-month intervals in either the VDD or the VVI mode and were then switched to the other mode. Invasive hemodynamic studies at rest and during exercise after each 3-month interval revealed that during the heaviest workload, VDD pacing increased cardiac output an average of 3.8 liters/min compared with VVI pacing despite the substantial compensatory increase in stroke volume that occurred with VVI pacing. Arteriovenous oxygen concentration differences during the heaviest workload and arterial lactate levels were lower during VDD pacing. Mean working capacity increased 23 per cent and was statistically the same in patients both below and above 65 years of age. A progressive decrease in long-term performance with VVI pacing was evidenced by decreased work capacity, increased heart size, and increased pulmonary artery pressure, while the significant gains resulting from VDD pacing were maintained chronically. The general conclusions of these studies have since been corroborated in a double-blind crossover study.[70]

The hemodynamic benefits of dual-chamber pacing accrue from AV synchrony and rate variability. The relative contribution of each of these factors is of particular interest in light of the introduction of single-chamber, sensor-driven, rate-responsive pacemakers. In a study of 10 patients, the results of atrial synchronous ventricular pacing were compared with those with fixed-rate ventricular pacing.[71] During atrial synchronous ventricular pacing, rates were determined by spontaneous sinus discharge rate. During ventricular pacing, rates were changed to equal the rates achieved during atrial synchronous pacing at comparable work levels. In these patients who were healthy except for complete AV block, atrial synchronous pacing at rest increased cardiac output by 11 per cent compared with ventricular pacing. With exercise carried out at 50 and 80 per cent of maximal aerobic tolerance, atrial synchronous and asynchronous ventricular pacing at matched rates produced no significant differences in cardiac output and stroke volume. These results indicate that rate increase is of major importance for increasing cardiac output with exercise, at least in patients without myocardial disease, while preserved AV synchrony seems much less important. These findings complement those of another study[72] in which 14 patients with symptomatic high-degree AV block were tested for exercise capacity with atrial synchronous ventricular pacing, matched-rate ventricular pacing, and fixed-rate ventricular pacing. Working capacity increased 24 per cent with atrial synchronous pacing and 20 per cent with matched-rate ventricular pacing, showing comparable improvements for either mode compared with fixed-rate ventricular pacing.

It should be noted that these findings do not address the issue of the appropriateness of rate increases achieved from sources other than the sinus node (e.g., the Q-T interval, pH, temperature, or activity), since the pacemaker rates were programmed at various exercise levels to match the rates obtained with the atrial synchronous mode—and therefore the sinus-determined rate—at corresponding exercise levels.

MODE SELECTION

Selection of the appropriate pacemaker modality for a given patient requires knowledge of the electrophysiological performance of the sinus node, AV conduction, and hemodynamic status. When available, these data can be used with the algorithm illustrated in Figure 23–8 to select the most suitable type(s) of device. One can begin by considering whether sinus node function is normal or abnormal. If it is normal (right branch of Figure 23–8), an atrial tracking pacemaker (VDD, DDD) may be appropriate, with suitable programming of upper rate limits to prevent angina and judicious selection of atrial refractory periods to prevent induction of pacemaker-mediated tachycardia in patients with retrograde conduction. If sinus node function is abnormal (left branch of Figure 23–8), with frequent periods of atrial fibrillation or flutter, a rate-responsive ventricular demand pacemaker would be chosen. Alternatively, a fixed-rate ventricular pacemaker (VVI, VVT) could be used if the patient's hemodynamic needs can be met without rate variability. If atrial flutter or fibrillation is not present and AV conduction is normal, a rate-responsive atrial demand pacemaker (or a conventional AAI/AAT unit) can be implanted unless the patient has hypersensitive carotid sinus syndrome. An atrial pacemaker alone is inappropriate therapy for patients with this syndrome, since AV conduction is frequently blocked by the excessive vagal tone (although this response is often veiled by concomitant sinus arrest (Fig. 22–21, p. 684). In patients with hypersensitive carotid sinus syndrome, a rate-responsive VVI pacemaker is preferred, although a DVI, DDI, or DDD pacemaker may also prove satisfactory. If the predominant atrial rhythm is normal with infrequent or brief episodes of atrial bradyarrhythmia, it is likely that an atrial tracking pacemaker (VDD, DDD) may be suitable. Finally, if sinus node function and AV conduction are both abnormal and the patient has extended periods of bradycardia, a rate-responsive VVI pacemaker would be ideal. Alternatively, a DVI or DDI pacemaker may be used if rate variability is not needed.

A concise summary of pacemaker mode selection based on the algorithm presented in Figure 23–8 can be found in Table 23–5.

TABLE 23–5 CONCISE SUMMARY OF INDICATIONS AND PREFERRED PACING MODES

	Atrial Rhythm		
AV Conduction	**Normal**	**Bradycardia**	**Bradycardia/ Tachycardia**
Normal	—	AAI-RR	AAI-RR
AV block without prolonged retrograde conduction time	DDD	DDD or VVI-RR	VVI-RR or DDI
AV block with prolonged retrograde VA conduction time	VVI-RR or DVI	VVI-RR or DVI	VVI-RR or DDI

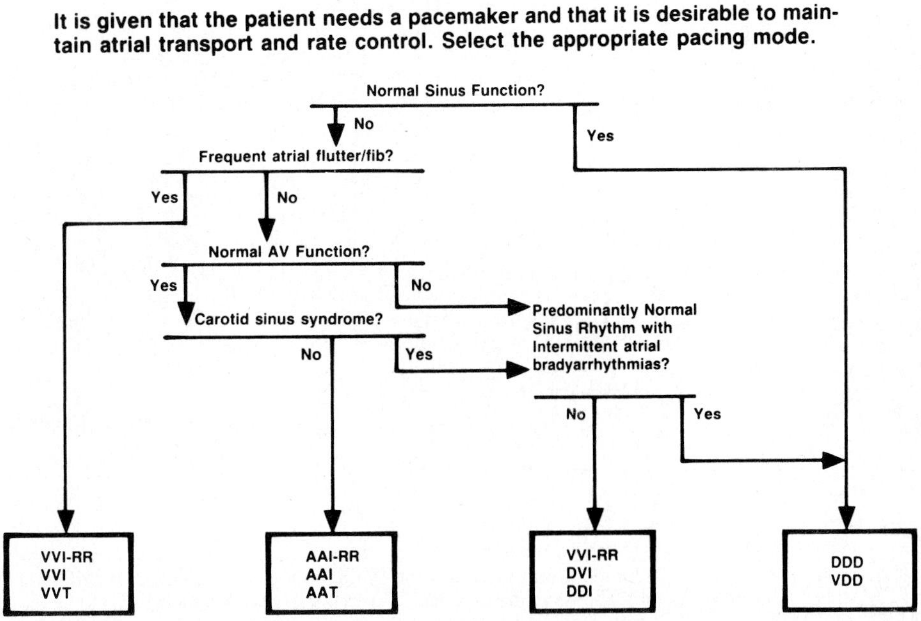

FIGURE 23–8. A flow chart providing an algorithm for selection of an appropriate pacemaker modality. This decision tree is described in detail in the text. (VVI-RR and AAI-RR refer to rate-responsive ventricular or atrial demand inhibited pacing.)

PACING FOR TACHYCARDIAS

Pacing to treat patients with tachycardias can be divided into four categories: (1) the need to maintain a normal rate when a required antiarrhythmic regimen produces bradycardia, (2) slowing the ventricular rate, (3) preventing recurrence of tachycardia, and (4) terminating tachycardia already present.[27]

In the first category, drugs such as digitalis, beta-adrenergic blockers (e.g., propranolol), clonidine, verapamil, and amiodarone (see Chap. 21) may result in symptomatic bradycardias that require some form of pacing to maintain normal heart rates. Similarly, ablation of the His bundle to interrupt AV conduction in a patient with drug-resistant supraventricular tachycardia with a rapid ventricular rate results in a bradycardia (due to the AV block) that requires pacing.[73] Classically, VVI pacemakers have been used for this purpose, although dual-chamber devices programmed to appropriate upper rate limits may be more desirable under specific circumstances in which the patient may be capable of achieving sustained periods of AV synchrony. Rate-responsive devices may be used to provide rate increases without the problems of atrial tracking during the supraventricular tachycardia.

An infrequently used alternative approach to slow the ventricular rate in patients with uncontrollable supraventricular tachycardia is the use of rapid atrial stimulation, which may initiate a rapid atrial tachycardia or atrial fibrillation that increases the degree of AV block owing to repetitive concealed conduction (see p. 202) and thus reduces the ventricular response.[74] Coupled or paired atrial pacing has also been used to reduce ventricular rate in drug-resistant atrial tachycardia,[75] because the second of the two atrial impulses blocks in the AV junction. Paired or coupled ventricular pacing for supraventricular or ventricular tachycardias reduces the effective ventricular rate by producing an electrical but not a mechanical response. The closely coupled premature ventricular stimulation intervals required may produce atrial or ventricular fibrillation.

Pacing successfully prevents recurrence of tachycardia only in selected circumstances. In 1960 Zoll and Linenthal demonstrated that ventricular pacing at slightly elevated but generally normal rates usually eliminated ventricular tachyarrhythmias in patients with advanced AV block and slow heart rates punctuated by bouts of ventricular tachycardias.[76] The occurrence of ventricular tachyarrhythmias in association with bradycardia may be related in part to a greater disparity between action potential duration and refractory period at slow heart rates. This temporal dispersion of recovery of excitability may be accentuated by a premature extrasystole, causing heterogeneous areas of conduction delay and block that may lead to reentry. Pacing at faster rates in the absence of ischemia may improve the synchrony of recovery and alleviate the ventricular arrhythmias (Fig. 23–9) (see Long Q-T Interval, Torsades de Pointes, p. 698).

It is important to note that accelerating the heart rate in the presence of ischemia may increase the degree of conduction delay within the ischemic area as well as the temporal dispersion of refractoriness. These changes may result in ventricular tachycardia and ventricular fibrillation. When one is pacing the hearts of patients who have had a myocardial infarction, care should be taken to find an optimal heart rate that will alleviate the arrhythmias but will not exacerbate the ischemia or produce new arrhythmias.

In some cases simply improving the patient's hemodynamic status[28] or restoring normal AV synchrony by means of an appropriate standard pacemaker[29, 77] will prevent the development of tachycardia. In others, pacing at moderately elevated rates suppresses ectopy and the recurrence of tachycardias. This effect must be well documented before a permanent pacemaker is implanted, because permanent pacing often fails to prevent recurrence of tachycardia over the long term. Also, the site of pacing—atrial or ventricular—may make a difference in efficacy. Short-term, temporary rapid pacing may effectively suppress ventricular tachycardias associated with torsades de pointes and Q-T prolongation. The mechanism by which this pacing mode is successful in some instances may relate to the phenomenon of overdrive suppression (p. 593). In patients who have accessory AV pathways, an atrial synchronous or DDD pacemaker with a suitably short AV interval may preclude development of a reciprocating tachycardia while preserving normal sinus control of ventricular rate.[78]

Selected drug-resistant tachycardias not amenable to surgical therapy can sometimes be terminated by a pace-

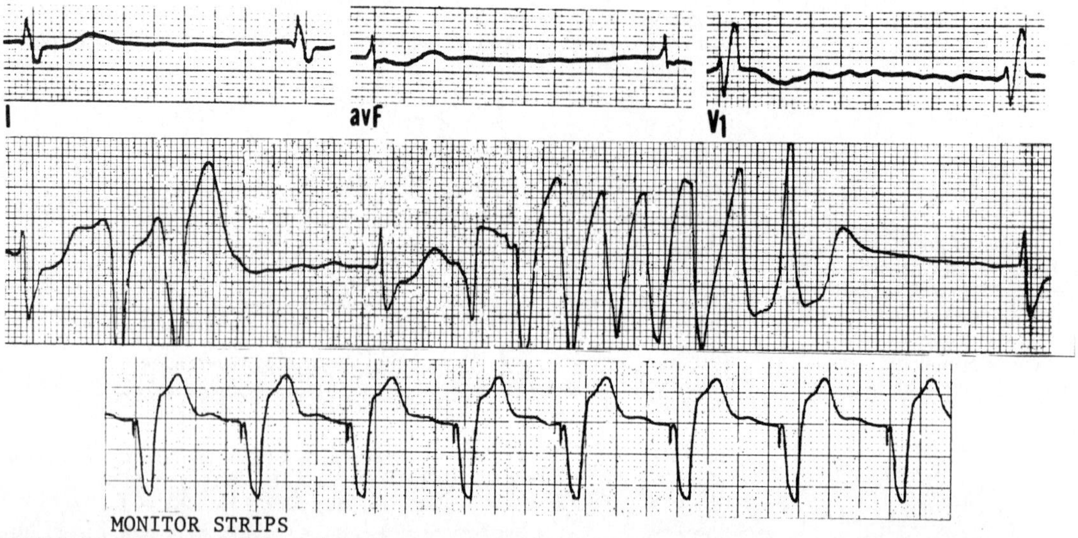

FIGURE 23–9. Electrocardiogram showing runs of ventricular tachycardia consequent to an inadequate ventricular escape rate in a patient with chronic atrial fibrillation and complete AV block (upper panels). Ventricular pacing at a rate of 85 ppm abolished the ventricular arrhythmia (lower panel).

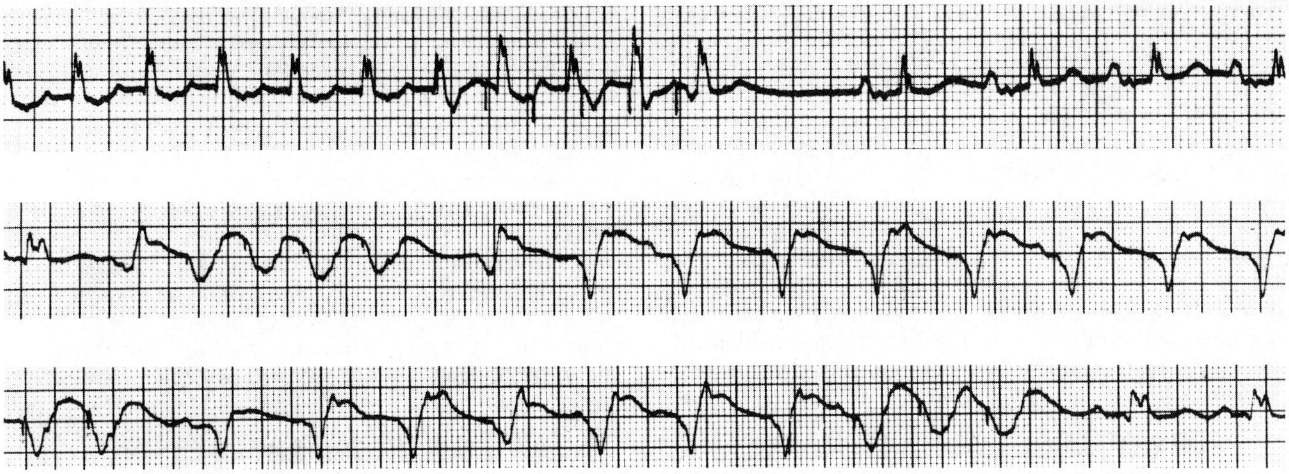

FIGURE 23–10. In the top tracing, a burst of pacing stimuli delivered from a patient-activated radiofrequency transmitter-receiver pacemaker terminates an episode of paroxysmal supraventricular tachycardia. In the middle tracing, a burst from a similar unit initiates an episode of a rather slow ventricular tachycardia, which is then terminated by a second burst of three stimuli (bottom tracing).

maker designed to produce an appropriate sequence of electrical stimuli.[79] Some of the pacemakers are activated by the patient when he notes the presence of a tachyarrhythmia,[80, 81] while others automatically discharge when the pacemaker senses that a tachycardia is present.[82, 83] For these latter pacemakers, accurate automatic detection and recognition of tachycardia remain a challenge.[84] Various cadences of stimuli can be delivered,[85, 86] including short bursts at high rates (Fig. 23–10), stimuli that scan the cardiac cycle and automatically change rate or shift the timing of one or more premature stimuli,[87] and coupled or paired stimuli. A "dual-demand" pacemaker automatically delivers stimuli at a fixed but relatively slow rate (e.g., 70 beats/min) when it senses the presence of a bradycardia (e.g., rates less than 70 beats/min) or a tachycardia (e.g., rates greater than 150 beats/min).[88] The tachycardia is terminated when an appropriately timed stimulus occurs during a particular part of the tachycardia cycle; this is called "underdrive termination" when the rate of pacing is less than the rate of the tachycardia. Overdrive pacing employs a pacing rate that exceeds the rate of the tachycardia. Dual-chamber (DVI) pacemakers can be made to operate in the dual-demand mode and pace with short AV intervals in patients who have AV nodal reentry or reciprocating tachycardia with accessory pathways.[89, 90] Unique "custom-built" devices with characteristics tailored for specific patients can also be applied. A self-adapting autodecremental overdrive pacing mode during which an increasing number of stimuli are delivered at progressively shorter cycle lengths seems to be a particularly safe and effective means of terminating tachycardias with pacing.[91, 92]

Single stimuli often fail to terminate a tachycardia because they fail to invade the circuit during the excitable gap, and pairs or bursts of stimuli must be used. While the use of multiple stimuli increases the success rate for termination, it also increases the likelihood of accelerating the tachycardia to flutter or fibrillation.[93] Naturally, this is not acceptable for a ventricular tachycardia,[94] so that pacing in this situation must be used conservatively and not without backup defibrillation capabilities. Also, initiation of atrial fibrillation in patients who have an accessory pathway with a short refractory period may result in unacceptably fast ventricular rates.

To solve some of these problems, the principles of transthoracic cardioversion have been adapted for use with implantable devices that can deliver synchronized cardioversion shocks to terminate sustained ventricular tachyarrhythmias.[16, 95–100] These systems can sometimes also terminate supraventricular tachyarrhythmias (Fig. 23–11). The most dramatic advance in electrical therapy of arrhythmias has been the introduction of the *fully implantable automatic cardioverter-defibrillator*[101, 102] capable of delivering 25- to 40-joule shocks directly to the myocardium.[101, 103–106] This device has substantially improved the prognosis for patients with malignant ventricular arrhythmias, demonstrating about a 2 per cent mortality from arrhythmias in the first year and 4 per cent in the second year.[104, 105] Although there are complications with these devices,[106] such pacemaker advances will significantly increase the

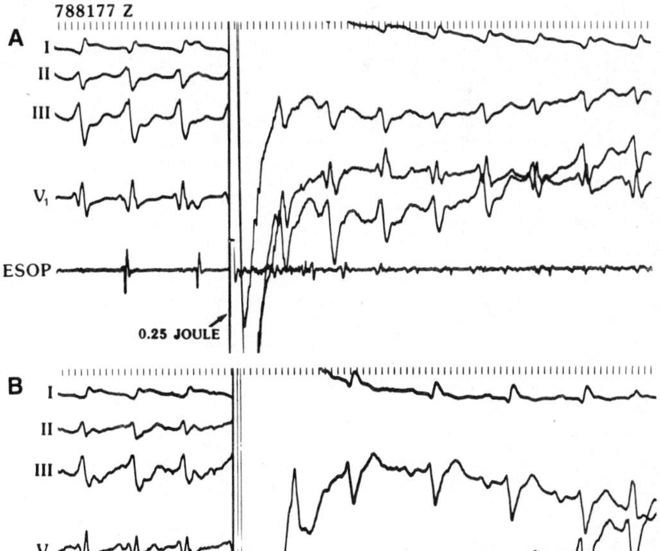

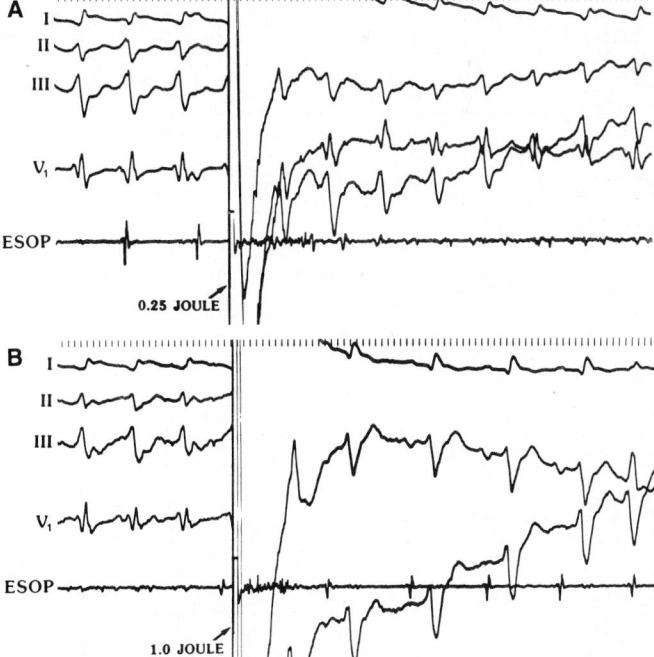

FIGURE 23–11. Electrocardiogram of a patient with ventricular tachycardia. *A,* A 0.25-joule shock is delivered synchronously into the QRS complex through a transvenous catheter. The stimulus fails to convert the ventricular rhythm but induces atrial fibrillation. *B,* A shock of 1.0 joule is delivered synchronously into the QRS complex, and the atrial fibrillation and ventricular tachycardia are both terminated to restore normal sinus rhythm. I, II, III, V_1 = scalar leads; esop = esophageal lead. (Study performed with the help of Eric N. Prystowsky, M.D., and James J. Heger, M.D.)

application of electrical devices for long-term treatment of tachycardias. Currently, pacing for tachycardia control accounts for less than 3 per cent of all pacemaker implantations. Interaction between the device and the environment will become increasingly important as combinations of therapy evolve. For example, drugs may decrease[107] or increase[108, 109] cardioversion-defibrillation thresholds. Preliminary reports suggest that quinidine, procainamide, bretylium, and digoxin do not affect internal defibrillation thresholds, while encainide and lidocaine elevate defibrillation thresholds. Amiodarone produces mixed results.[109]

PROGRAMMABILITY OF PACEMAKERS

Almost all permanent pacemaker implants today employ a programmable pacemaker. Programmability can be defined as noninvasive, reversible alteration of the electronically controlled performance of an implantable device such as a pacemaker. Use of a simple magnet to convert a demand pacemaker to its asynchronous mode is generally excluded from this definition, although it is in reality a simple form of programming. In the most advanced pacemakers, many performance characteristics are programmable, including rate, stimulus output, amplitude or duration, amplifier sensitivity, amplifier refractory period, hysteresis, pacing mode (e.g., sensor-determined rate-responsive behavior, unipolar/bipolar, VVI/VVT/VOO), and operation of channels that transfer special information (telemetry of intracardiac electrograms, programmed settings, measured performance data, device operation indicators such as a "marker channel," battery status, lead impedance). In addition, in dual-chamber pacemakers it is generally possible to program AV intervals, atrial rate tracking limits, rate-limiting behavior, and pacing mode (e.g., DDD to DVI or VVI).

Programmability benefits the patient by optimizing pacemaker function for specific patient needs, minimizing the need for invasive procedures to correct malfunctions or to revise the system to meet changing patient needs,[110–113] and facilitating troubleshooting procedures. Table 23–6 indicates applications for many of the commonly available programmable parameters. It should be emphasized that programmability must be used with care, since it presents the risk of establishing inappropriate parameter settings (e.g., insufficient output energy to maintain capture, dangerously high or low rates) and imposes a greater need for maintaining accurate records to prevent erroneous decisions when a clinician is unfamiliar with the rationale for the current programmed settings in a given patient.

POWER SOURCES

Nearly all pacemakers are battery-powered. External pacemakers typically have standard alkaline or mercury batteries of the type used in common household appliances (e.g., transistor radios, flashlights), although an occasional external device employs a rechargeable or lithium battery. Implantable pacemakers are generally powered by lithium batteries; a very small number are powered by nuclear batteries or radiofrequency energy broadcast to the pacemaker from an external device called a transmitter.[114]

In the early 1970's nuclear batteries were developed for implantable pacemakers. The most commonly employed nuclear battery converted the heat generated by decay of radioisotopic plutonium into electrical energy. Pacemakers using these batteries have demonstrated the greatest actual longevity of any pacemaker to date, surpassing in performance even the lithium battery as a pacemaker power source. Unfortunately, regulatory requirements associated with the use of a nuclear system make it inconvenient for the implanting physicians and unattractive from a commercial standpoint, although such units are still available from one manufacturer.

Virtually all current pacemakers are powered by some form of lithium battery. Lithium battery chemistries share certain characteristics that make them especially suitable for implantation, yet they exhibit significant differences.[115] Each of the lithium systems offers high-energy density and low internal losses due to self-discharge. Most of the systems can be hermetically sealed to prevent ingress of body fluids

TABLE 23–6 APPLICATIONS OF PROGRAMMABLE PACEMAKER PARAMETERS

Parameter	Patient/Pacemaker Optimization	Diagnostic Applications	Correction of Malfunctions
• Rate	• Improve cardiac output by allowing greater range of conducted sinus activity • Minimize angina by keeping the rate below that which produces pain • Suppress arrhythmias • Adapt pulse generator to pediatric needs (faster rates) • Terminate tachycardias with short rapid bursts of stimuli • Minimize "pacemaker syndrome" due to AV dissociation by selecting low rate	• Suppress pacing to assess underlying rhythm by ECG • Test AV conduction with an atrial pacemaker by determining rates at which AV block occurs • Test sinus function with an atrial pacemaker by using periods of rapid pacing to determine sinus node recovery times • Confirm atrial capture by altering pacemaker rate and observing concomitant ventricular rate change	
• Output Amplitude or Duration	• Maximize pulse generator longevity by selecting output energy that provides the minimal level of stimulation consistent with reliable maintenance of pacing • Provide increased energy for high-threshold patients • Avoid extracardiac stimulation (pectoral muscle, phrenic nerve)	• Evaluate pacing threshold	• Regain capture following threshold increases due to effects of infarcts, electrolyte disturbances, drugs • Eliminate diaphragmatic and pectoral muscle stimulation
• Amplifier Sensitivity	• Establish appropriate sensitivity to detect intracardiac electrogram while avoiding sensing of extraneous signals (pectoral muscle potentials, electromagnetic interference)	• Alter sensitivity to evaluate possible sources of oversensing or undersensing	• Compensate for changes in intracardiac electrogram amplitude • Resolve oversensing of T waves, muscle potentials, electromagnetic interference

Table continued on opposite page

TABLE 23–6 APPLICATIONS OF PROGRAMMABLE PACEMAKER PARAMETERS *Continued*

Parameter	Patient/Pacemaker Optimization	Diagnostic Applications	Correction of Malfunctions
• Refractory Period	• Extend duration for atrial pacing to avoid sensing conducted QRS complex • Shorten duration in ventricular pacing to detect closely coupled ventricular complexes	• Alter duration to evaluate possible causes of over- or undersensing	• Lengthen duration to avoid T-wave sensing • Shorten duration to eliminate failure to sense closely coupled ventricular complexes • Lengthen duration of atrial amplifier refractory period in VDD or DDD device to avoid sensing retrogradely conducted atrial activity
• Hysteresis	• Minimize pacemaker syndrome by allowing sinus rhythm to be maintained over widest possible rate range while establishing adequately high pacing rate when needed		
• Unipolar/Bipolar		• Evaluate lead fracture (bipolar → unipolar) • Enhance stimulus artifact visibility on ECG (bipolar → unipolar) • Evaluate oversensing (unipolar → bipolar)	• Convert to unipolar function to regain capture in case of lead fracture • Change mode to adapt to altered electrogram causing sensing failure • Convert to bipolar to eliminate sensing of myopotentials • Convert to bipolar to avoid extracardiac stimulation
• Mode	• Select optimum mode (e.g., VDD for patients who have normal sinus function and impaired AV conduction) • Alter mode if patient's needs change (e.g., VDD to DVI if patient develops sinus bradycardia)	• Establish triggered mode to enable external control of pacemaker from chest electrodes and external stimulator to perform noninvasive electrophysiological studies of sinus function. AV conduction, tachycardia initiation, efficacy of antiarrhythmic agents, and so forth; tachycardia can be terminated in a similar fashion • Confirm oversensing signal source by selecting triggered mode	• Change to backup mode (e.g., VVI) if atrial portion of dual-chamber system is nonfunctional (e.g., lead displacement) • Prevent oversensing by selecting asynchronous mode
• AV Delay	• Maximize hemodynamic efficacy • Control/prevent tachyarrhythmias		
• Atrial Rate Tracking Limit	• Maintain widest range of sinus rate control without incurring angina • Control ventricular response to atrial arrhythmias • Prevent synchronization to atrial activity at short R-P intervals during ventricular escape pacing in VDD mode that results in AV dissociation with pacemaker captures • Reduce the long delay between the sensed P wave and the resultant rate limit-delayed stimulus in the ventricle to minimize the occurrence of retrograde atrial activity	• Select high rate limit for stress testing	• Reduce tracking rate limit if pectoral muscle activity triggers rapid pacing
• Activity Threshold	• Ensure sensing of physical activity without undue sensitivity to infrasonic noise by selecting threshold for detection of activity signals		• Adjust threshold to higher value if environmental noise triggers pacing; reduce threshold if rate does not vary with exercise
• Rate Response	• Ensure sufficient rate increase for a given level of physical activity by setting relationship between sensed activity and associated rate	• An externally placed activity sensing pacemaker can be used to trigger an implanted VVT or AAT pacemaker to evaluate benefits of rate-responsive pacing prior to replacement of the implanted unit	
• Telemetry		• Compare programmed settings to actual device operation • Use marker channel indicators to determine which events pacemaker is causing and which events are being sensed • Use electrogram to evaluate causes of under- or oversensing • Use electrogram to evaluate drug effects on myocardium	

and egress of damaging battery materials. Each system offers unique electrical characteristics and varying degrees of reliability.[116–118] The most commonly used lithium batteries contain lithium iodide and lithium cupric sulfide.

Reported performance characteristics of the major power sources clearly show the substantial progress made toward creating a pacemaker that will be sufficiently long-lived to obviate replacement in the majority of patients. In 1986, survival probabilities associated with a large number of pacemakers using lithium power sources were reported: 7,641 lithium iodide–powered pacemakers showed a cumulative survival probability of 69 per cent at 9 years, while 3,071 lithium cupric sulfide–powered pacemakers exhibited a survival probability of 75 per cent at 9 years.[119] These data reflect actual clinical results and clearly demonstrate the longevity advantages of lithium power sources.

A small group of special-purpose antitachycardia pacemakers is powered by radiofrequency energy transmitted through the body to the implantable device. This is practical, because these pacemakers are not required to pace constantly but are used to generate short bursts of rapid asynchronous stimuli to terminate episodes of tachycardia.

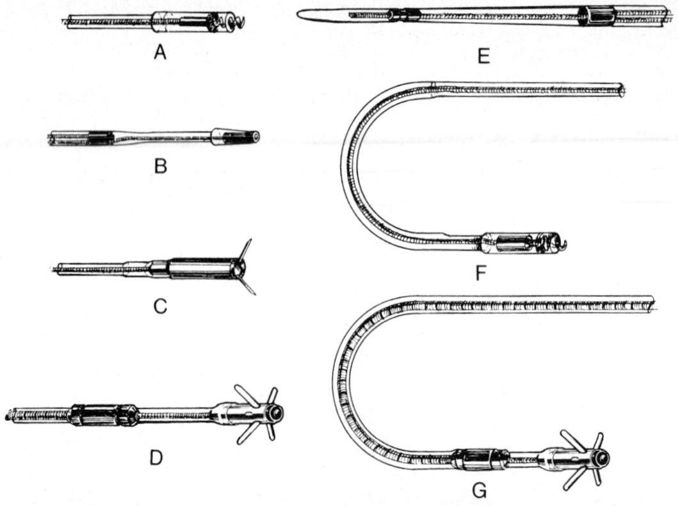

FIGURE 23–12. Examples of atrial and ventricular transvenous pacemaker electrodes. *A,* Unipolar endocardial urethane lead with a screw-in tip electrode for active fixation to the atrial or ventricular endocardial surface. *B,* Bipolar ventricular electrode utilizing flanged Silastic tip for positioning stability. *C,* Unipolar ventricular electrode with extensible metallic barb that provides active fixation to the ventricular myocardium. *D,* Bipolar urethane ventricular electrode with flexible tines adjacent to the tip electrode. The tines provide passive lead fixation by lodging within the trabecular structure of the ventricle. *E,* Bipolar Silastic lead designed for stable placement in the coronary sinus. The electrodes are shaped for atrial pacing applications. *F,* Unipolar urethane lead with J shape and screw-in tip electrode for active fixation to the atrial endocardial surface. *G,* Bipolar urethane atrial lead with J shape and flexible tines adjacent to the tip electrode. The J shape and tines provide passive fixation of the electrode within the atrium.

PACEMAKER ELECTRODE SYSTEMS ("LEADS")[120, 121]

The pulse generator is connected electrically to the heart by means of a wire and electrode system referred to as a *lead.* Electrodes may be unipolar or bipolar. In bipolar systems, the positive (anode) and negative (cathode) electrodes are both located within the cardiac chamber and are in contact with the endocardium, epicardium, or (screwed into) the myocardium. In unipolar systems, only the cathode is in the heart and a large area anode electrode, usually the metallic housing of the pulse generator, is at a remote location. Either approach is clinically acceptable. A common misconception is that unipolar leads provide larger signals for sensing purposes; however, there is in fact no statistical difference in signal amplitude or slew rate of electrograms generated from unipolar and bipolar records.[122] Pacing thresholds are also similar, although bipolar systems are less susceptible to extraneous electromagnetic interference (e.g., electrical signals generated by nearby power lines, automobile spark plugs, radio transmitters), extracardiac myopotential interference, unwanted extracardiac stimulation, or threshold changes due to tissue trauma at the pacemaker electrode site following external cardiac defibrillation. Permanent pacing leads are designed for either transvenous or epicardial placement. More than 90 to 95 per cent of implants are by the transvenous route.

TRANSVENOUS LEADS. These are usually implanted within the right ventricular apex for ventricular pacing and within the right atrial appendage or rarely the coronary sinus for atrial application. Leads are typically inserted via the cephalic, subclavian, or jugular veins, using fluoroscopy for visualization and stiff wires (stylets) inserted within the lumen of the lead to facilitate control during positioning. The stylets must be removed after lead placement to avoid damaging the lead. A rapid technique for placing the lead in the subclavian vein with minimal trauma involves a single venipuncture using a special percutaneous lead introducer. Risk is minimal with this approach, although there is the possibility of causing a pneumothorax or subclavian arterial injury. The use of urethane insulated leads with reduced diameters and a decreased coefficient of friction makes it possible to pass an atrial and a ventricular lead through a single vein, facilitating implantation of dual-chamber pacemaker systems.[123, 124] Transvenous leads come in a variety of designs, each purporting to insure stable permanent positioning of the electrodes[125–128] (Fig. 23–12). Many atrial leads also incorporate a "J" shape to aid in proper positioning within the atrial appendage. The transvenous approach is associated with low morbidity and, with current lead designs, a low rate of displacement.

EPICARDIAL LEADS. These are used far less frequently than transvenous systems, usually only in patients undergoing unrelated cardiac surgery. The placement approach depends on the type of epicardial electrode used. A transthoracic approach (thoracotomy) is used to apply electrodes that are sutured to the myocardium. More commonly, for ventricular applications, a sutureless corkscrew electrode or barbed-hook electrode is used, since these devices can be applied via a transmediastinal approach, avoiding entrance into the pleural cavity and reducing morbidity and discomfort[129] (Fig. 23–13).

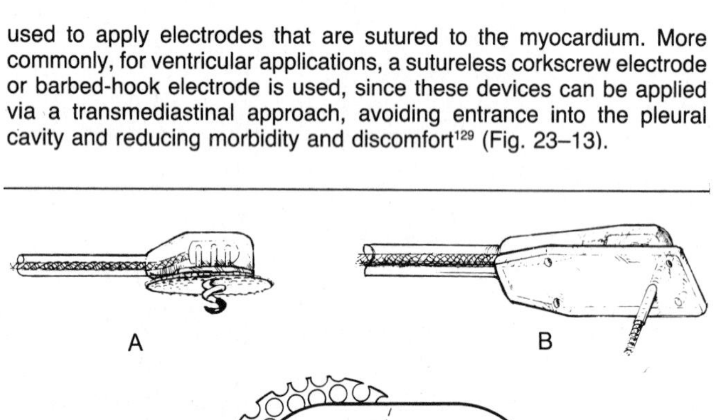

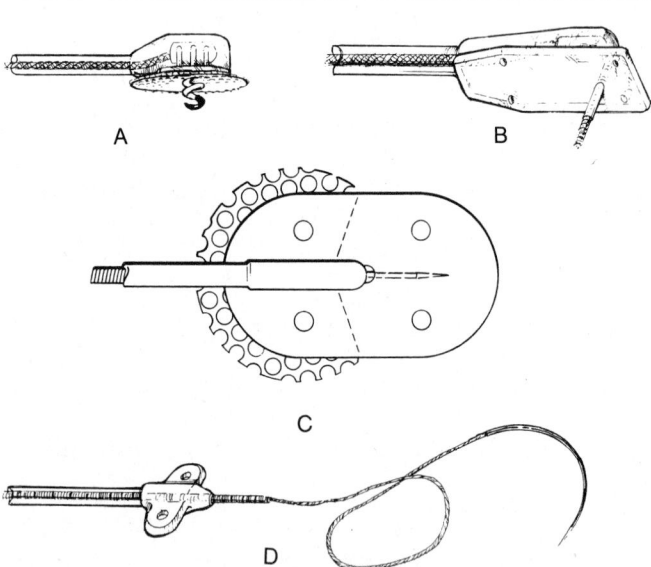

FIGURE 23–13. Examples of atrial and ventricular epicardial electrodes. *A,* Silastic sutureless unipolar ventricular electrode with corkscrew tip. Positive fixation is achieved by screwing the electrode into the myocardium. *B,* Silastic unipolar epicardial electrode designed to be sutured to either atrial or ventricular myocardium. *C,* Urethane unipolar epicardial barbed hook electrode providing positive fixation (without sutures) to either atrial or ventricular myocardium. *D,* Silastic unipolar electrode for atrial or ventricular use. The needle and suture material extending from the exposed stainless-steel electrode are used to fasten the electrode directly to the myocardium.

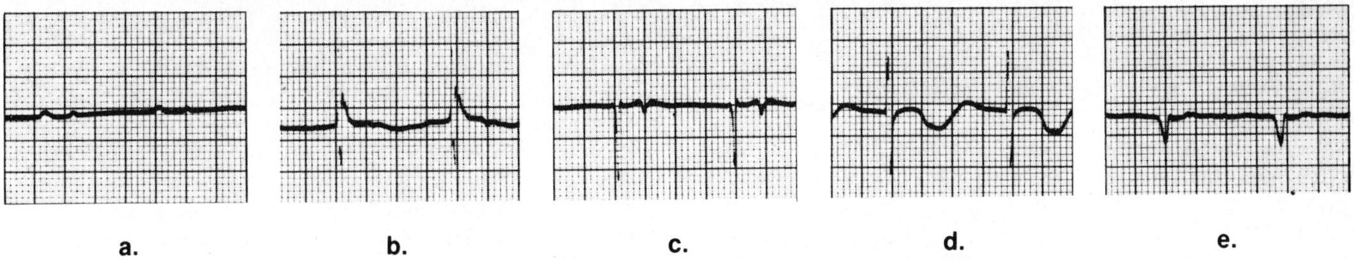

FIGURE 23–14. Electrograms obtained when bipolar electrode is located in the high superior vena cava (*a*), superior vena cava/right atrium (*b*), right atrium (*c*), right ventricle (*d*), and pulmonary artery (*e*). All tracings were calibrated at 1 mV/cm except *d*, which is recorded at one-half standard.

TEMPORARY PACING LEADS. These include transvenous catheter electrodes, wire electrodes, and precordial skin electrodes.[130] The technique for placing temporary transvenous catheter electrodes is similar to that used for permanent leads. Placement is facilitated by designing the catheters stiffer than would be acceptable for permanent use and by sometimes incorporating additional aids such as inflatable balloons or cuffs that "float" the catheter in the venous return of the bloodstream to the right ventricle. In the absence of fluoroscopy, ECG recordings from the catheter enable the user to determine the location of the electrodes (Fig. 23–14). Temporary wires frequently are placed in the atria and ventricles of patients at the time of open-heart surgery. These stainless-steel wires are used during the surgical procedure and during the postoperative recovery phase to help control the cardiac rhythm. Electrograms recorded from these electrodes aid in the diagnosis of complex arrhythmias.[6] In emergency situations, wire electrodes can be inserted percutaneously into the heart using a pericardiocentesis (or similar) needle. Also, during emergencies, surface skin electrodes placed on the chest wall can be stimulated with very high (and painful) voltages to achieve cardiac pacing transthoracically. Such an approach should be used only until a transvenous catheter electrode can be positioned. An improved transcutaneous pacing technique reported to cause minimal discomfort and to be suitable for prolonged use requires special large surface area electrodes and external pulse generators that provide stimuli of very long duration (about 40 msec).[131] This may offer a viable alternative approach to transvenous pacing.

ELECTRODE POSITION. For temporary and permanent pacing it is important to place the electrodes in a position that provides acceptably low stimulation thresholds and sufficiently large intracardiac signals to be sensed by the pulse generator. Generally this requires acute thresholds for the atrium or ventricle of less than 2 mA and 1.25 V, with stimuli 0.5 msec in duration, and ventricular electrograms greater than 4 mV or atrial electrograms exceeding 2 mV. Thresholds generally rise after acute positioning of the leads, reach a peak two to four times the acute values within the first 2 to 6 weeks, and then fall to intermediate values.[132] The electrogram typically decreases in amplitude by 15 per cent; its rate of rise with respect to time (slew rate) decreases as much as 50 per cent with maturation of the implant.[133] These factors must be considered when one is evaluating the acceptability of a given lead position.

PACEMAKER FOLLOW-UP

Despite the reliability of modern pacemakers, it is important to examine the patient and the pacemaker system regularly after implantation. Such followup has four major goals: (1) evaluation of the electrical function of the pacing system to detect malfunctions or imminent power-source depletion; (2) inspection of the implant site for possible difficulties, such as erosion or infection; (3) evaluation of the patient's cardiac status so that reprogramming or revision of the pacing system or of the concomitant drug regimen can be accomplished; and (4) maintenance of the physician-patient interaction to evaluate other problems or health needs, provide reassurance of progress, and offer an opportunity to discuss concerns that may arise.

The followup schedule should be arranged to allow close monitoring during the immediate postimplant period, moderately frequent observation during the routine service life of the system, and increased surveillance as the system nears completion of its service life. A suggested schedule for visits would be 6 and 12 weeks after implantation; twice annually, beginning 6 months after implantation; and monthly once the first signs of power-source depletion are observed. (In almost all pacemakers, power-source depletion appears as a rate decrease when the system is monitored with a magnet placed over the pulse generator.) Given the longevity of modern systems, it may be counterproductive to attempt to stretch out the last few months of service through frequent monitoring, since this will probably add only 5 to 10 per cent to the total service life while increasing monitoring costs by 30 to 40 per cent.

Followup visits should be scheduled in the physician's office or in a special pacemaker clinic where the patient can be seen in person. Telephone monitoring of the patient's electrocardiogram, pacing rate, and duration of the pulse generator stimulus carried out between personal evaluations can be of value as a supplement but should not replace office visits. Each visit should include a 12-lead ECG recording with a rhythm strip showing that the pacemaker appropriately captures and senses; measurement of pacemaker parameters using appropriate equipment to measure rate and pulse width; and a general physical examination, including careful scrutiny of the pacemaker pocket. Results of the followup procedure should be carefully recorded,[134] since much of the required analysis depends on changes in operation rather than absolute values of measured parameters. This record is especially important when following patients who have programmable pacemakers,[135] since changes may be totally innocuous if intentional (e.g., if a rate change is programmed to improve cardiac output) or may signify problems in performance of the device (e.g., if the rate is decreased owing to battery depletion).

Care should be exercised in selecting followup equipment, and data must be analyzed with full understanding and knowledge of the idiosyncrasies of the equipment used. For example, digital monitoring and recording systems frequently do not register the pacemaker stimulus or artifact reliably and reproducibly because of its extremely short duration.[136] As a result, the artifact may not always be recorded even though present, or its polarity and amplitude may vary markedly throughout the recording. Alternatively, such systems may substitute a standardized artifact for the real signal and eliminate diagnostic information in the process. Some followup clinics perform waveform analysis using an oscilloscope or special ECG machine to display the morphology of the pacemaker stimulus. One must be fully aware of the correct stimulus waveshape for each pacemaker to be evaluated. Modern pacemakers frequently produce much more complex stimulus pulse shapes than the traditional "square wave," and it is not unusual for such waveforms to be misread as signs of malfunction.

An often underestimated benefit of followup is a reduction in patient anxiety. A clear answer to a simple question can be extremely important to a patient's quality of life. In recognition of this, some clinics have formed pacemaker clubs that allow patients to meet periodically to compare notes and provide mutual support.

PACEMAKER MALFUNCTION

Complex systems involving electrical, mechanical, and physiological interactions inevitably malfunction, and pacemakers are no exception. Fortunately, the detection and correction of such problems are relatively straightforward when one uses the appropriate equipment.[137, 138]

EVALUATION PROCEDURES AND EQUIPMENT. Accurate patient records that include full descriptions of the pacemaker, the implantation procedure, and followup information are mandatory. Next, one must recognize that the most useful troubleshooting tool is a 12-lead ECG machine. This permits evaluation of pacemaker sensing, capture, and approximate rate; evaluation of electrode positioning by vectorial analysis of the stimulus artifact and of the pacemaker-generated QRS complex or P wave;[139] and confirmation of appropriate function for the mode of pacing employed. A digital counter is necessary for an accurate evaluation of changes in pacing rate and pulse width due to battery depletion, component failure, or reprogramming. A magnet placed over the pacemaker converts nearly all units to asynchronous (i.e., non-sensing) operation, which enables capture to be evaluated when the patient's intrinsic rhythm inhibits the pacemaker, and can be useful in diagnosing oversensing by disabling all sensing function. Magnets should be employed with care, since some pacemakers can be programmed by application of a suitable magnet, and there is always a slight risk of inducing tachyarrhythmias when one is pacing asynchronously.

Carotid sinus massage or the Valsalva maneuver may slow a patient's intrinsic rhythm and induce pacing, while exercise may be used to speed the patient's spontaneous rate to evaluate sensing capability. Chest-wall stimulation with an external stimulator connected to precordial skin electrodes can be utilized to test sensing function and to determine rate tracking limits for atrial tracking or triggered pacemakers (VAT, VDD, DDD, VVT, AAT). Manipulation of the pulse generator in its pocket can sometimes elicit electrocardiographic signs of a loose connection or damaged lead close to the generator site. Multiple radiographic or fluoroscopic views of the chest and pacemaker system will help determine lead position and detect gross lead fractures or disconnection from the generator. After implantation and before patient discharge from the hospital, an overpenetrated baseline chest x-ray (in posteroanterior and lateral views) should be obtained to establish lead configuration. An oscilloscope or special ECG recorder designed to display the waveshape of the pacemaker stimulus is used by some centers to evaluate lead problems or unusual component failures.

Use of a *pacemaker programmer*, by allowing one to vary stimulus strength, amplifier sensitivity, rates, refractory period, and pacing modes, enables noninvasive evaluation of multiple functions. In some of the new systems, such a programmer permits the user to obtain noninvasive intracardiac electrograms to evaluate sensing operation. Some systems provide telemetry of pacing lead impedance, a useful feature to evaluate lead system integrity, clearly revealing conductor fractures and disruption of insulation. Lead impedance is high with lead fracture but low with insulation break. Many systems include digital telemetry of the programmed settings and internally measured performance, allowing actual performance to be compared with expected performance. The most sophisticated systems provide a "marker channel," a noninvasively telemetered tracing that clearly identifies pacemaker sensing and pacing operations in conjunction with a surface ECG recording (Fig. 23–15).[138a]

Electrocautery, transthoracic electrical cardioversion or defibrillation can "program" DDD pacemakers to new settings; therefore, the pacemakers should be checked after such events.

Invasive procedures are necessary if noninvasive approaches fail to uncover and correct the problem. A *pacing system analyzer* is used to assess implantable pulse generator function (sensitivities, refractory periods, rates, pulse widths, and amplitudes), to evaluate lead integrity and positioning, and to provide electrophysiological data such as stimulation thresholds, electrogram amplitudes, or responses to pacing.[138b] Pacemaker-related problems fall into five broad categories: failure to pace, failure to sense, oversensing, pacing at an altered rate, and undesirable patient/pacemaker interactions.

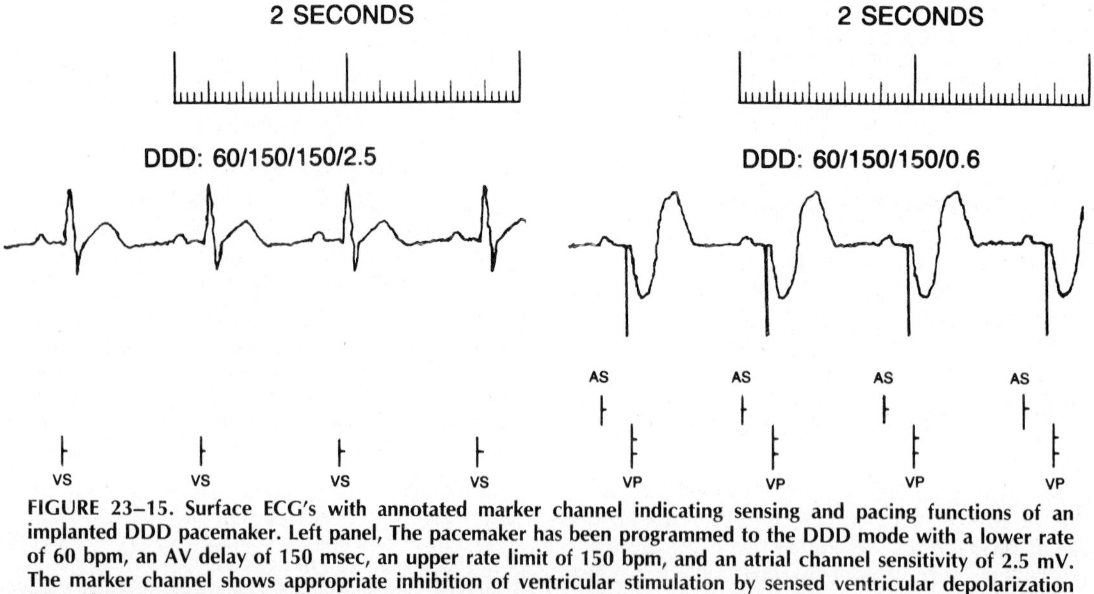

FIGURE 23–15. Surface ECG's with annotated marker channel indicating sensing and pacing functions of an implanted DDD pacemaker. Left panel, The pacemaker has been programmed to the DDD mode with a lower rate of 60 bpm, an AV delay of 150 msec, an upper rate limit of 150 bpm, and an atrial channel sensitivity of 2.5 mV. The marker channel shows appropriate inhibition of ventricular stimulation by sensed ventricular depolarization (VS). Absence of a marker channel indicating atrial sensing confirms loss of atrial sensing function. (Atrial pacing is inhibited by the conducted QRS complex.) Right panel, Atrial sensitivity has been increased from 2.5 mV to 0.6 mV. The pacemaker now synchronizes ventricular pacing to appropriately sensed atrial depolarization, and the marker channel confirms atrial sensing (AS) and ventricular pacing (VP).

FAILURE TO PACE. Failure to pace occurs when the pacemaker fails to deliver a stimulus when one should occur or when it delivers a stimulus that fails to depolarize the myocardium at a time when the tissue is fully excitable. Failure to deliver a stimulus can be due to (1) improper connection of the lead to the generator (e.g., set screws not tightened); (2) broken lead wires with no insulation defect; (3) "cross talk" between atrial and ventricular portions of dual-chamber pacemakers (discussed below); (4) pulse generator component failure; (5) power-source depletion; or (6) oversensing (discussed below). Delivery of an ineffective stimulus, resulting in loss of capture, may be due to (1) lead dislodgment (the most common cause); (2) myocardial perforation, migration of the lead to an extracardiac position; (3) defective lead insulation and/or wire fracture; (4) an increased stimulation threshold due to infarct, effects of cardioactive drugs such as flecainide, electrolyte imbalances such as hyperkalemia, or fibrosis at the electrode site; or (5) inappropriate programming of pacemaker stimulus strength. Lack of capture when a stimulus is delivered during the myocardial refractory period is a frequent source of misdiagnosis.

FAILURE TO SENSE. Failure to sense intracardiac signals may be due to lead dislodgment (the most common cause); inadequate amplitude or waveshape of the intracardiac electrogram due to inappropriate lead placement, fibrosis, infarct, drugs, or electrolyte disturbances; inappropriate programming of amplifier sensitivity, refractory periods, or mode (e.g., AOO, VOO); lead fracture or insulation defect; connector defect; or component failure (e.g., jammed magnetic reed switch).

Occasionally sensing failure is misdiagnosed when spontaneous cardiac electrical activity occurs simultaneously with the pacemaker stimulus and causes a fusion beat, which is the simultaneous activation of the ventricle (or atrium) by the intrinsic cardiac impulse (e.g., sinus initiated beat) and the pacemaker stimulus. If cardiac depolarization begins before the local electrogram reaches the electrode site to reset the pacemaker escape interval and prevent pacemaker discharge, a "pseudofusion" beat occurs. In this instance, the pacemaker stimulus becomes superimposed on the inscription of the spontaneous QRS complex (or P wave). Thus the QRS complex (or P wave) originates from a single activation site. Electrocardiographically the QRS complex or P wave begins well in advance of the pacemaker stimulus. Although this appears to be failure to sense, it is in fact perfectly normal operation. Similar electrocardiographic patterns occur when stimuli are delivered into refractory tissue, as in AAT or VVT pacing. In both situations the pacemaker stimulus does not alter the electrical activation sequence of the tissue and it is characterized on the ECG by a stimulus that merely distorts inscription of the P wave or QRS complex.

Another cause of apparent sensing failure is reversion to asynchronous operation in the presence of electromagnetic interference—also a normal mode of operation for many pacemakers. Finally, closely coupled intracardiac signals may occur within the pacemaker refractory period and may not be sensed. This is frequently seen with certain AV sequential (DVI) pacemakers that initiate the refractory period of the ventricular sense amplifier upon stimulation in the atrium. If the atrial response propagates to the ventricles, the pacemaker will not sense this conducted ventricular activity, but will stimulate into the refractory tissue. This is normal operation of such "committed" DVI devices (Fig. 23–16).

OVERSENSING. Occasionally, a pacemaker senses signals other than the cardiac signals it is designed to detect—a phenomenon referred to as "oversensing." Ventricular sensing pacemakers (DVI, DDI, VVI, VVT, VDD, DDD) may sense T waves if the pacemaker amplifier is too sensitive, if its refractory period is too short, or if the patient has unusually large or delayed intracardiac T waves. A dislodged ventricular lead resting near the right ventricular inflow tract may cause inappropriate sensing of atrial activity. Conversely, atrial sensing pacemakers (AAI, AAT, VAT, VDD, DDD) may inappropriately sense ventricular activity if the atrial amplifier refractory period is too short or if the atrial signals are too small to be sensed, with consequent failure to initiate appropriate atrial refractory periods. The ventricular amplifier in some dual-chamber pacemakers (DVI, DDI, DDD) may sense delivery of an atrial stimulus and inhibit the ventricular stimulus ("cross talk") if the ventricular blanking period (i.e., the period of time when ventricular sensing is disabled to prevent inappropriate sensing of atrial stimuli) is too short. Unipolar pacemakers may sense skeletal muscle potentials generated by contraction of the rectus abdominus or pectoralis major muscles (depending on implantation site), resulting in inappropriate inhibition (AAI, VVI, DVI, DDI, VDD, DDD) or triggering (AAT, VVT, VDD, VAT, DDD) of stimuli. Rarely, unipolar or bipolar pacemakers may sense diaphragmatic potentials. All pacemakers, except asynchronous devices, sense voltage changes that are produced when a lead with a hairline fracture or loose connection makes intermittent contact (make-break signals) (Fig. 23–17) or when two endocardial leads come into contact. Erratic pacemaker behavior with pauses of varying length should raise the possibility of electrode or lead problems rather than pulse generator malfunction. In all cases of suspected oversensing, placing the pacemaker in an asynchronous mode (with application of a magnet if the pacemaker is permanent or turning off the sensitivity if it is an external device) will abolish the symptoms caused by the pacemaker malfunction and confirm the diagnosis.

Electromagnetic interference (EMI) from power lines, radio or television transmitters, and other electrical noise sources occasionally may be sensed, especially by unipolar pacemakers, because the large separation between electrodes enhances EMI detection. Sometimes this results in inhibition or triggering, but more commonly it produces reversion to the asynchronous mode, which provides the patient with continued pacing support. Microwave ovens and weapons detection

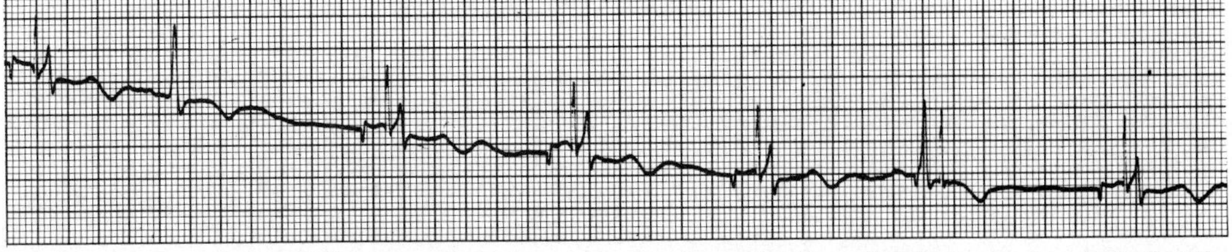

FIGURE 23–16. Surface ECG demonstrating an example of a "committed" mode DVI pacemaker. Note that the first, third, fourth, fifth, and seventh complexes are initiated by an atrial spike (small negative deflection) that paces the atrium and then a ventricular spike (large upright deflection) that paces the ventricle. The second QRS complex occurs sufficiently early to inhibit pacemaker discharge. However, the sixth QRS complex occurs early but not early enough to inhibit the atrial discharge. Following the atrial spike (seen as the initial negative deflection preceding the onset of the QRS complex, after the P wave), a conducted QRS complex occurs. However, this complex is not sensed by the pacemaker, which is, by design, committed to deliver a ventricular stimulus (large upright spike following the QRS complex in the ST segment) after stimulating the atrium, regardless of spontaneous ventricular activity. (Monitor lead.)

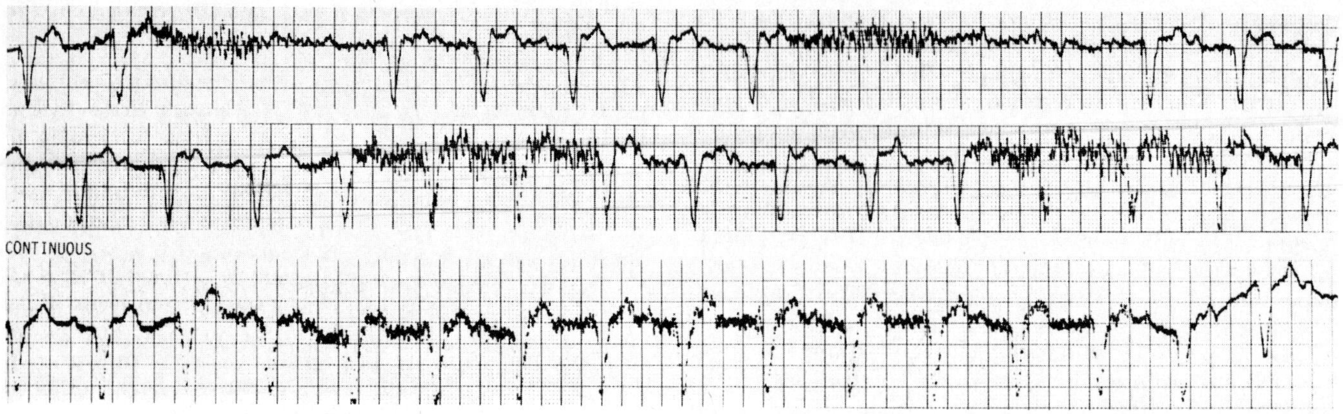

FIGURE 23–17. Electrocardiograms demonstrating inhibition of a bipolar demand pacemaker by make-break potentials created by intermittent contact at the pulse generator/lead connection. Make-break potentials were generated when the patient flexed the pectoralis major muscles ("noisy" portions of recordings). *Top,* Pacemaker in demand mode. Pulse generator discharge inhibited during isometric pectoralis muscle activity. *Middle,* Pacemaker converted to continuously discharging (asynchronous) mode by external application of magnet. Pulse generator discharges at normal rate during isometric exercise. *Bottom,* Pacemaker in demand mode following correction of improperly seated electrode terminal at the pulse generator connector block. Isometric pectoralis exercise has no effect on pulse generator discharge rate. (Monitor leads, 25 mm/sec paper speed.)

equipment no longer pose significant threats as a result of changes in pacemaker design. Very rarely, a pacemaker may sense the after-potentials remaining on a lead after delivery of a stimulus. Most often this is the result of using very wide pulse widths or excessively short refractory periods. Intrinsic EMI sources from muscle artifacts present more troublesome clinical problems than do extrinsic EMI sources from the environment.

PACING AT AN ALTERED RATE. Causes of unexpected pacing at an altered rate include oversensing that induces rate slowing due to inhibition or rate acceleration due to triggering; rate drift, a gradual benign shift of the pacing rate due to component aging or temperature effects (most commonly found in older pacemakers that do not use digital timing circuits); rate reduction built into most pacemakers to indicate approaching power-source depletion; and component failure (usually causing either no stimulus output or a rapid stimulation that is typically limited to less than 180 ppm by "runaway" protection circuits).

Frequent misdiagnoses of pacing at an altered rate include presence of rate hysteresis that produces a long escape interval following sensed activity; errors in paper drive speed or ambulatory monitor speed; reprogramming a programmable pacemaker without proper notation of the change in the patient's record; tracking spontaneous intrinsic cardiac rate accelerations with VVT, AAT, VAT, VDD, or DDD pacemakers; misinterpretation of nonpacemaker artifacts such as rapid spike potentials generated by muscle fasciculation or electrical noise in the ECG recording system. Lack of familiarity with operation of the device may lead to misdiagnosis. For example, a DVI pacemaker perceived to be pacing the ventricles at a rate equivalent to its V-A interval may, in fact, be delivering stimuli to the atrium and appropriately inhibiting ventricular stimuli in response to conducted ventricular activity (Fig. 23–18).

UNDESIRABLE PATIENT/PACEMAKER INTERACTIONS. Occasionally, undesirable patient/pacemaker system interactions develop. The pacemaker pocket may become infected, a hematoma may develop, or the generator may erode through the pocket site. These problems occur less frequently with the current small, light-weight generators. Some patients exhibit "twiddler's syndrome," in which they toy with their pulse generators and rotate them within the pocket, which could result in lead retraction and total system failure (Fig. 23–19).

Some forms of therapy may adversely affect operation of a pacemaker system. For example, defibrillation with the paddles placed too near the pulse generator may damage pacemaker components or may induce large currents in the pacing lead sufficient to elevate pacing thresholds or impair electrogram characteristics, particularly with unipolar pacemakers. Similarly, therapeutic levels of irradiation may adversely affect pacing function. Direct contact between an electrocautery probe and the pulse generator may damage pacemaker circuits or cause programmable devices to switch from programmed values of operation to a set of backup values (sometimes referred to as a "power-on reset").

Extracardiac stimulation of the pectoralis muscles or diaphragm may be observed. Decreasing the pulse width, voltage, or current of the stimulus usually eliminates or reduces such extracardiac stimulation.

Incorrect pacing mode selection for a given patient or changes in a patient's clinical status after implantation can have serious consequences. For example, atrial tracking pacemakers (VAT, VDD, DDD) may detect retrograde atrial activity conducted with a long R-P interval following ventricular stimulation and may induce "pacemaker-mediated tachycardia" with a rate equal to the pacemaker's upper rate limit (Fig. 23–20) or a rate equivalent to the sum of the retrograde conduction time plus the programmed A-V interval, whichever is slower. This problem can be avoided by programming the pacemaker atrial refractory period to a value that insures that retrograde events occur within the refractory period and therefore do not trigger ventricular pacing. Patients with an AAI pacemaker implanted to treat sinus node dysfunction or hypersensitive carotid sinus syndrome may develop AV block (Fig. 23–21). Patients may respond poorly to other specific pacing modes depending on their underlying hemodynamic and electrophysiological substrates. In many such cases, multiprogrammable pacemakers allow alteration of pacing system characteristics without resorting to invasive procedures.

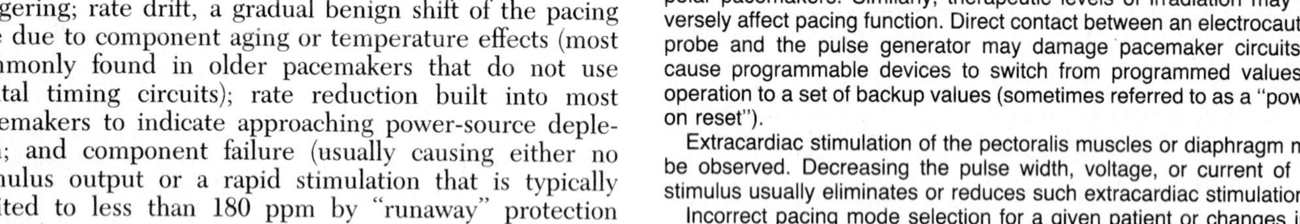

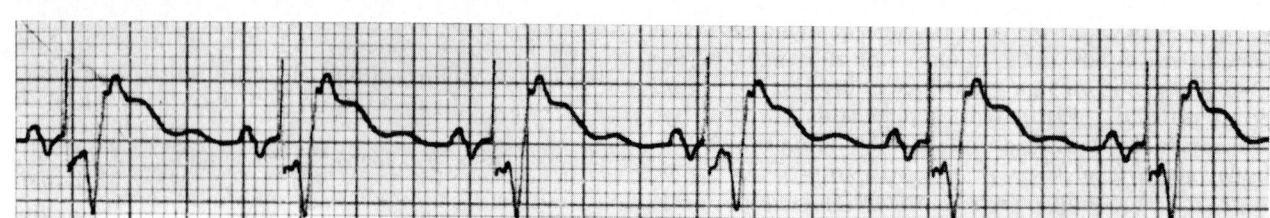

FIGURE 23–18. Electrocardiogram of a patient with a normally functioning noncommitted DVI pacemaker. In this recording, the pacemaker's atrial escape interval is completed shortly after the occurrence of spontaneous atrial activity (which is not sensed because DVI pacemakers have no atrial sensing circuits). The atrial stimulus, therefore, occurs immediately prior to the ventricular complex, which results from normal conduction of atrial activity. The pacemaker's ventricular stimulus is appropriately inhibited by sensing the conducted ventricular complex. Such records sometimes lead to a misdiagnosis of ventricular pacing at an accelerated rate when, in fact, the record indicates normal DVI pacemaker operation with delivery of atrial stimuli only. (Monitor lead.)

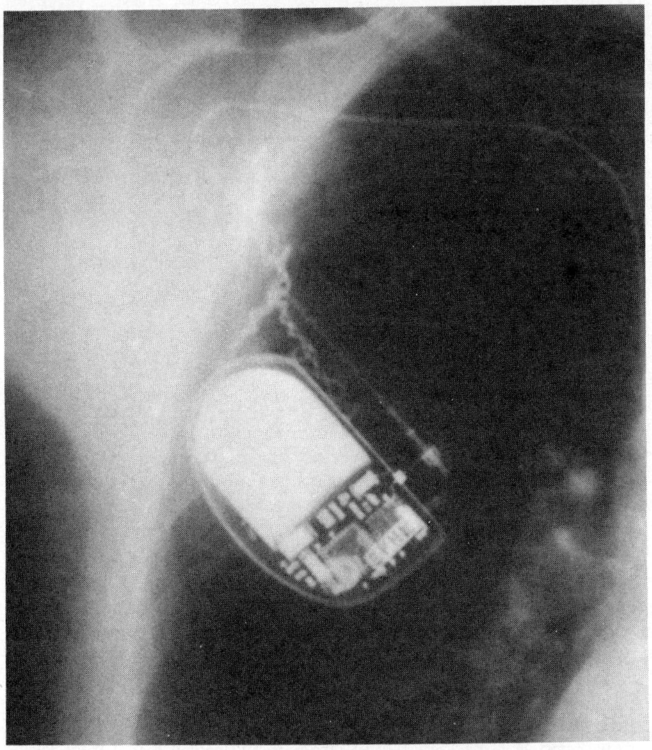

FIGURE 23–19. Radiograph of lead and pulse generator in patient who exhibited "twiddler's syndrome." Continual rotation of the pacemaker can result in twisting of the lead and eventual dislocation or fracture.

ILLUSTRATIVE APPROACHES

Two examples will demonstrate how one might approach problems of pacemaker malfunction.

INTERMITTENT LOSS OF CAPTURE AND FAILURE TO SENSE SPONTANEOUS VENTRICULAR ACTIVITY (Fig. 23–22). This patient had a ventricular demand (VVI) pacemaker implanted one year ago. The first step in troubleshooting is to list the likely causes of the problem. Since there are two malfunctions in this example (failure to sense and failure to pace), it is highly probable—although not absolutely certain—that there is a common cause. The most likely etiologies are as follows:

Lack of Capture:
Lead dislodgment, perforation.
Lead wire fracture.
Lead insulation failure.
Pulse generator failure.
Inappropriate programming of output energy.
High threshold.
Misread ECG ("loss of capture" seen only when stimulus occurs during cardiac refractory period).

Lack of Sensing:
Lead dislodgment, perforation.
Lead wire fracture.
Lead insulation failure.
Pulse generator failure.
Inappropriate programming of amplifier sensitivity or refractory period.
Inadequate electrogram amplitude (due to infarct, electrolyte disturbance, myocardial disease).
Electromagnetic interference–induced reversion to asynchronous mode.
Jammed-reed switch.
Misread ECG (fusion beats).

Analysis should begin by comparing a recent 12-lead ECG to a baseline tracing that predates the problem. The current tracing should be carefully reviewed to exclude misinterpretation of fusion or pseudofusion beats (p. 694) as sensing failure or of pacing stimuli occurring during the cardiac refractory period as lack of capture. Reversion to the asynchronous mode due to electromagnetic interference usually can be eliminated as a cause of non-sensing if a 12-lead ECG shows no signs of electrical interference. A comparison of the current and baseline ECGs should establish the presence or absence of lead position changes, including perforation, as evidenced by shifts in the vectors of the paced QRS complexes and pacing artifacts. It is important to remember that digital ECG systems with low sampling rates are not reliable for determining the vector fo the pacemaker stimulus because they are unable to reproduce the artifact without introducing severe distortion. An x-ray or fluoroscopy is used to help diagnose lead dislodgment. Insulation defects in the lead result in vector changes in the pacing artifact but not in the paced QRS complex.

Applying a magnet results in pacing without sensing. In most pacemakers, magnet application alters the pacing rate (sometimes by only a few milliseconds) in order to confirm that the reed switch is functioning and to eliminate the possibility of non-sensing due to a jammed reed switch.

Inappropriate programming can be evaluated by reprogramming the amplifier sensitivity and refractory period to restore sensing and to increase the stimulus intensity to restore capture. If such reprogramming failed to resolve the problem, or if the parameter settings required are not within normally accepted values, inappropriate programming can be excluded.

Wire fracture can produce non-sensing and lack of capture, but it is generally accompanied by random resetting of the escape interval as the broken wire ends touch intermittently. An x-ray pinpoints some

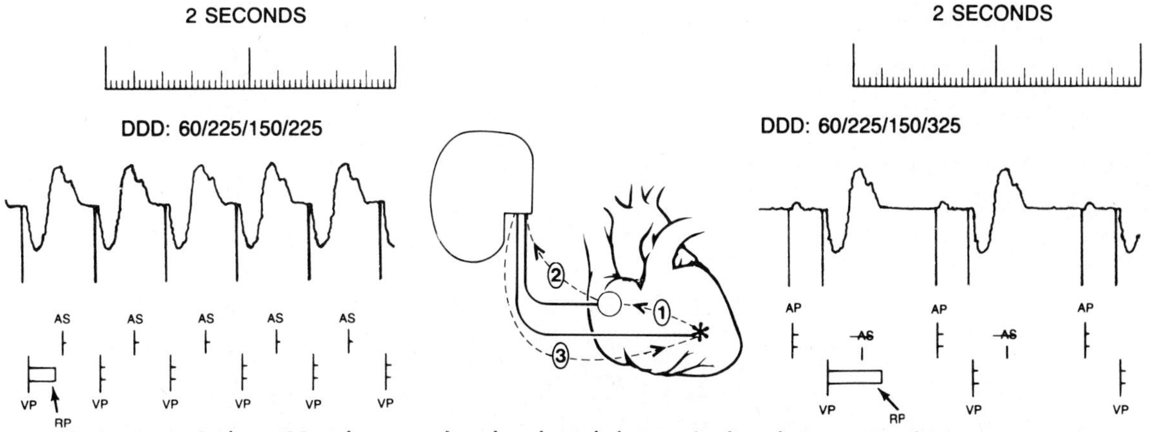

FIGURE 23–20. Surface ECG and annotated marker channels from an implanted DDD pacemaker. Left panel, The pacemaker is programmed in the DDD mode with a lower rate of 60 beats/min, an AV delay of 225 msec, an upper rate limit of 150 beats/min, and an atrial refractory period of 225 msec. Each ventricular stimulus (indicated in the marker channel as VP) results in retrograde atrial activation (dotted pathway 1 in center diagram), which is sensed by the pacemaker (dotted pathway 2 and indicated in the marker channel as AS), in turn triggering yet another ventricular stimulus (dotted pathway 3) and creating a pacemaker-mediated tachycardia. Right panel, The pacemaker atrial refractory period has been lengthened to 325 msec. Again, each ventricular stimulus produces a retrograde P wave, but these now occur during the pacemaker refractory period and do not trigger ventricular stimulation. Each retrograde P wave is indicated in the marker channel as having been sensed but not used as a trigger (AS). Thus, appropriate selection of the pacemaker atrial refractory period prevents pacemaker-mediated tachycardia.

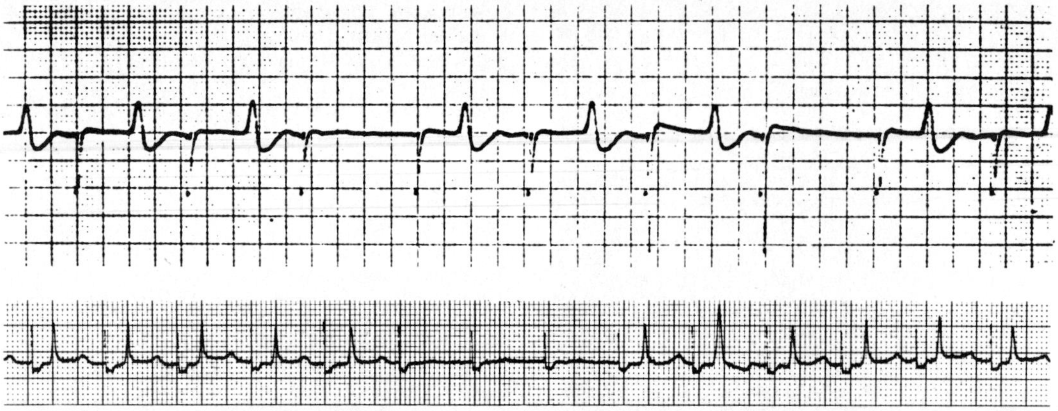

FIGURE 23–21. The top electrocardiogram illustrates inappropriate use of an atrial demand pacemaker (AAI) in a patient with type I second degree AV block. P waves cannot be seen clearly in this lead (monitor) but follow each atrial pacing stimulus. In the lower recording, carotid sinus massage during atrial pacing in a patient with hypersensitive carotid sinus syndrome results in a series of nonconducted P waves. (Monitor lead.)

fractures, but not all. In this example (Fig. 23–22), the regularity of the escape intervals probably excludes wire fractures as the cause of the problem, because such fractures generally produce erratic resetting of pacemaker timing and escape intervals of random duration.

At this point, noninvasive procedures have been explored to evaluate most potential causes for the reported malfunctions. Threshold elevation, inadequate electrogram characteristics, and pulse generator failure all require invasive evaluation, although some noninvasive determinations can be made if the patient has a sophisticated multiprogrammable pulse generator. Some of these devices can telemeter the intracardiac electrogram, facilitating evaluation of sensing problems. They also allow the user to obtain noninvasive threshold measurements. Nevertheless, correction of sensing and pacing failures due to any of these causes will require invasive procedures.

In the example cited, ECG evidence (shown in Figure 23–23) is most consistent with lead dislodgment. Note the axis shift in the pacemaker-stimulus artifact and in the paced QRS complexes. Lead displacement is the most common cause of sensing and capture failures.

TROUBLESHOOTING DUAL-CHAMBER SYSTEMS. A second example will be described and the electrocardiograms of Figure 23–24 will be analyzed. These records are taken from a patient with a bipolar noncommitted AV sequential pacemaker (DVI) programmed to an A-V interval of 150 msec. ECG exhibited variable A-V intervals up to 200 msec (Fig. 23–24, upper panel) with no evidence of ventricular pacing. If the pacing system were functioning normally, no A-V interval would exceed the programmed 150 msec. Potential causes for failure to pace include a broken lead, a defective pacemaker-lead connection, "cross talk" between atrial and ventricular channels of dual-chamber pacemakers, component failure, battery depletion, or oversensing. Oversensing could be due to sensing of P or T waves, myopotentials, electromagnetic interference, lead polarization afterpotentials, and cross talk (sensing of the atrial stimulus by the ventricular amplifier of a dual-chamber device) as well as detection of make-break potentials created by intermittent contact of broken electrode wires or loose connections at the pulse generator (Fig. 23–17).

As shown in the lower tracing of Figure 23–24, placement of the magnet over the pulse generator restored normal AV sequential pacing. This strongly suggests a problem due to oversensing. Myopotential inhibition can be excluded, since the generator is bipolar (muscle inhibition of bipolar generators is exceedingly rare) and because the atrial stimuli continue to occur without prolonged pauses. Electromagnetic interference can also be excluded because the generator is bipolar and there is no evidence of interference on the ECG. T-wave sensing is not a possible cause because the T waves occur after the point in the pacemaker timing cycle when a ventricular stimulus should have been generated. A loose connection can be excluded if manipulating the generator in the pocket produces no pacemaker rate changes. Lead fractures are relatively uncommon; there was no evidence of pacing failure with the magnet in place, and x-ray examination showed no evidence of conductor failure. Measurement of the A-V intervals in the upper panel of Figure 23–24 reveals that the third, fifth, seventh, and ninth atrial stimuli were timed from the preceding QRS complexes (the V-A interval for this pacemaker is programmed to 600 msec). The remaining stimuli were timed from their preceding occurrence rather than from the preceding QRS complexes. Thus, it is fairly evident that this pacemaker is being affected by "cross talk" between its atrial and ventricular channels. Each atrial stimulus is sensed by the ventricular amplifier that inhibits delivery of a ventricular stimulus. When the spontaneous QRS complex occurs sufficiently late after the atrial stimulus so that the QRS falls outside the ventricular amplifier refractory period (200 msec), the pacemaker timing is reset for a second time by the ventricular complex. Consequently, the atrial pacing rate is variable and the A-V interval is not controlled by the pacemaker. The patient's ventricular escape rhythm maintains the cardiac rhythm.

After the pacemaker pocket was opened, it was found that a 4.5-volt pacing stimulus delivered to the atrial lead reset the ventricular amplifier, thus confirming the diagnosis. Lead impedance measurements indicated a defect in the atrial lead insulation, which was found at the curvature on its J portion after removal of the lead. The insulation break allowed leakage currents from the atrial stimulus to create sufficient voltage at the ventricular lead to inhibit ventricular output. Replacement of the atrial lead corrected the problem.

These two examples were chosen to illustrate that pacing problems cover the range from being fairly simple to quite complex. The implanter's knowledge must be fairly sophisticated for appropriate selection, implantation, and management of these modern, multiprogrammable dual-chamber pacing devices.

PATIENT CONCERNS

A pacemaker can extend a patient's longevity and may greatly improve quality of life. Yet, if therapy is to provide maximal benefit, the

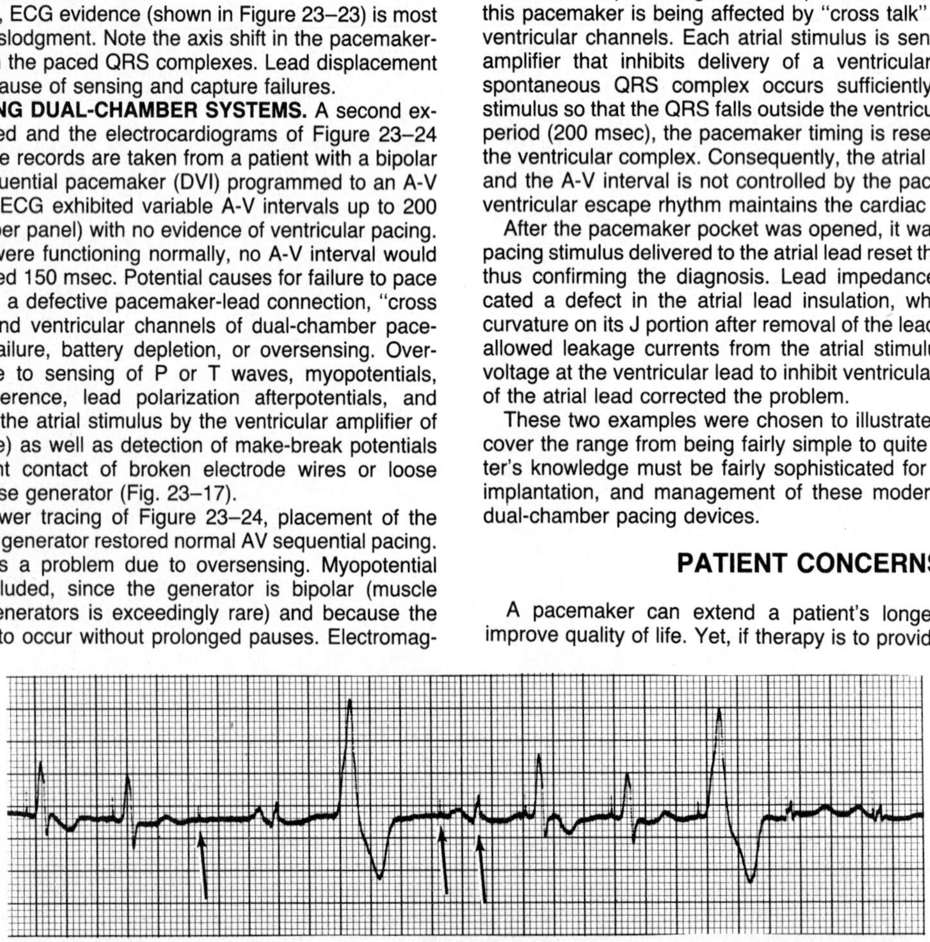

FIGURE 23–22. Failure of a VVI pacemaker. Note that pacing stimuli occasionally fail to elicit a paced QRS complex (first and second arrows), and the pacemaker occasionally fails to sense spontaneous ventricular activity (third arrow) even though it occurs after completion of the ventricular amplifier's 200 ms refractory period. (Monitor lead.)

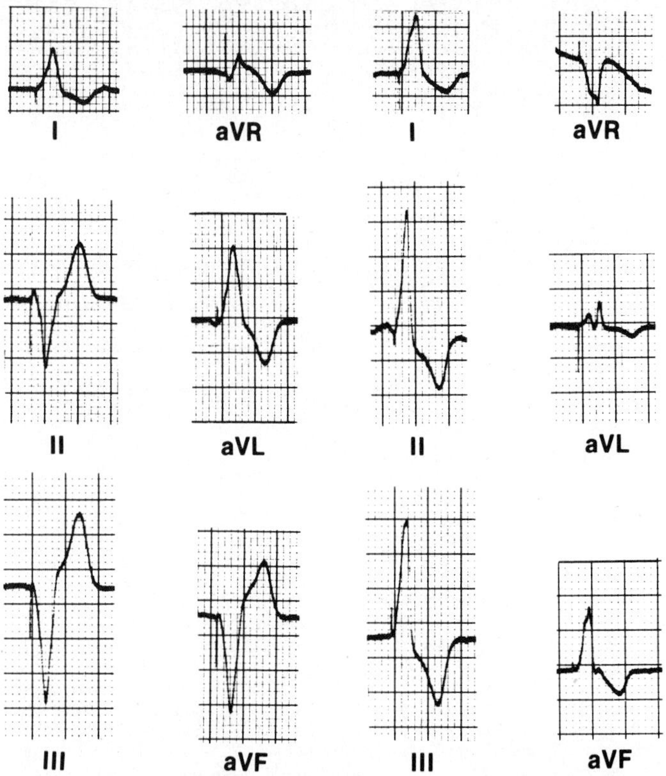

FIGURE 23–23. Leads I, II, III, aV_r, aV_l, and aV_f were recorded before (left panels) and after (right panels) this pacemaker developed the sensing and capture problems illustrated in Figure 23–22. Note that the vectors of the spikes and of the paced QRS complexes differ in the baseline ECG (left panel) from the vectors in the ECG recorded after the problem developed (right panel). This change in vectors is most consistent with migration of the electrode to a different position in the ventricle (right ventricular outflow tract), as was the case here.

patient's psychological needs must be considered as well. Patients should understand why they have a pacemaker, how it works (in simple terms), and what it will and will not do for them. (For example, many patients think that a pacemaker cures heart disease or makes the heart stronger.) They should be instructed about lifestyle restrictions, if any. If this is not explained, patients may become excessively apprehensive. The patient will be greatly concerned about dependency on the pacemaker, the risks of its failing, the anticipated longevity of the system, and the nature of the replacement procedure. If these issues are addressed with clear concise answers in lay terms, the patient with a pacemaker can fully enjoy the extension and better quality of life that this device offers.

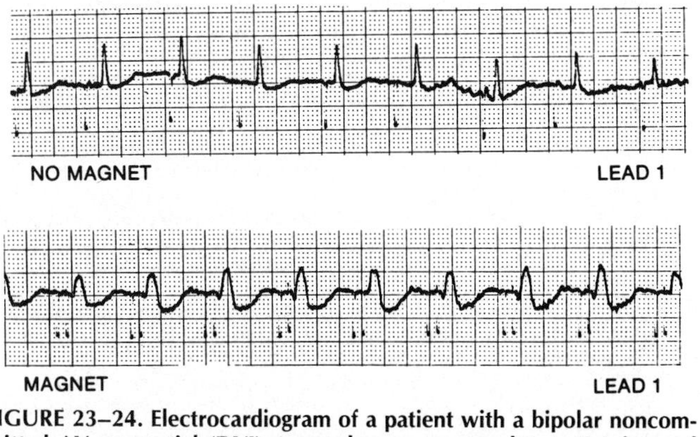

FIGURE 23–24. Electrocardiogram of a patient with a bipolar noncommitted AV sequential (DVI) pacemaker programmed to a V-A interval of 600 msec and an A-V interval of 150 msec. Upper panel, Tracing recorded without a magnet over the generator showing A-V intervals as long as 200 msec with no evidence of ventricular pacing. Placement of a magnet over the generator converts it to asynchronous pacing and restores the ventricular pacing function (lower panel). This is an example of "cross talk," a malfunction in which the ventricular stimulus is inhibited by inappropriate ventricular sensing of the atrial stimulus. In this case the cause was current leakage from damaged insulation on the atrial lead. (Lead I.)

Acknowledgment

The authors thank S. Serge Barold, M.D., for critical comments.

REFERENCES

Indications for Cardiac Pacing

1. Zoll, P.: Resuscitation of the heart in ventricular standstill by external electric stimulation. N. Engl. J. Med. *247*:768, 1952.
2. Lillehei, W., Gott, V. L., Hodges, P. C., Long, D. M., and Bakken, E.: Transistor pacemaker for treatment of complete atrioventricular dissociation. J.A.M.A. *172*:2006, 1960.
3. Elmquist, R., and Senning, A.: An implantable pacemaker for the heart. Proc. 2nd Int. Conf. Med. Elec. Eng., London, Iliffe and Sons, Ltd., 1959.
4. Zoll, P., and Linenthal, A.: Long-term electrical pacemakers for Stokes-Adams disease. Circulation *22*:341, 1960.
5. Chardack, W. M., Gage, A. A., and Greatbatch, W.: A transistorized self-contained implantable pacemaker for the long-term correction of complete heart block. Surgery *48*:643, 1960.
6. Waldo, A., Wells, J., Cooper, T., and MacLean, W.: Temporary cardiac pacing: Applications and techniques in the treatment of cardiac arrhythmias. Prog. Cardiovasc. Dis. *23*:451, 1981.
7. Fisch, G., Zipes, D., and Fisch, C.: Bundle branch block and sudden death. Prog. Cardiovasc. Dis. *23*:187, 1980.
8. Hindman, M. C., Wagner, G. S., JaRo, M., Atkins, J., DeSanctis, R., Hutter, A., Morris, J., Rubenfire, M., Scheinman, M., and Yeatmam. L.: The clinical significance of bundle branch block complicating acute myocardial infarction. II. Indications for temporary and permanent pacemaker therapy. Circulation *58*:689, 1978.
9. Langendorf, R., and Pick, A.: Atrioventricular block type II (Mobitz)—Its nature and clinical significance. Circulation *38*:819, 1968.
10. McNally, E., and Benchimol, A.: Medical and physiological considerations in the use of artificial cardiac pacing. Part 1. Am. Heart J. *75*:380, 1968.
11. Zipes, D.: Second degree atrioventricular block. Circulation *60*:465, 1979.
12. Dhingra, R., Denes, P., Wu, D., Chulquimia, R., and Rosen, K.: The significance of second degree atrioventricular block and bundle branch block. Observations regarding site and type of block. Circulation *49*:638, 1974.
13. Hindman, M., Wagner, G., Jaro, M., Atkins, J., Scheinman, M., DeSanctis, R., Hutter, H., Yeatman, L., Rubenfire, M., Pujura, C., Rubin, M., and Mars, J.: The clinical significance of bundle branch block complicating acute myocardial infarction. I. Clinical characteristics, hospital mortality, and one year follow-up. Circulation *58*:679, 1978.
14. Bosch, X., Theroux, T., Roy, D., Moise, A., and Waters, D D.: Coronary angiographic significance of left anterior fascicular block during acute myocardial infarction. J. Am. Coll. Cardiol. *5*:9, 1985.
15. Hollander, G., Nadiminti, V., Lichstein, E., Greengart, A., and Sanders, M.: Bundle branch block in acute myocardial infarction. Am. Heart J. *105*:738, 1983.
16. Zipes, D. P., Heger, J. J., and Prystowsky, E. N.: Synchronized low energy transvenous cardioversion. *In* Morganroth, J. (ed.): Sudden Cardiac Death. Orlando, FL., Grune and Stratton, 1986, pp. 285–300.
17. Keren, A., Tzivoni, D., Gavish, D., Levi, J., Gottlieb, S., BenHorin, J., and Stern, S.: Etiology, warning signs and therapy of torsades de pointes. Circulation *64*:1167, 1981.
18. Smith, W., and Gallagher, J.: "Les torsades de pointes": An unusual ventricular arrhythmia. Ann. Intern. Med. *93*:578, 1980.
19. Frye, R., Collins, J., DeSanctis, R., Dodge, H., Dreifus, L., Fisch, C., Gettes, L., Gillette, P., Parsonnet, V., Reeves, T. J., Weinberg, S.: Guidelines for permanent cardiac pacemaker implantation, May, 1984. Report of the Joint American College of Cardiology/American Heart Association Task Force on Assessment of Cardiovascular Procedures Subcommittee on Pacemaker Implantation. J. Am. Coll. Cardiol. *4*:434, 1984.
20. Feruglio, G. A., and Steinbach, R.: Pacing in the world today. World survey on cardiac pacing for the year 1979–1981. Proc. VIIth World Symposium on Cardiac Pacing. Steinbach, K. (ed.) Darmstadt, Steinkopff Verlag, 1983.
21. Sutton, R., Perrins, J., and Citron, P.: Physiological cardiac pacing. PACE *3*:207, 1980.
22. Dhingra, R., Palileo, E., Strasberg, B., Swiryn, S., Bauernfeind, R., Wyndham, C., and Rosen, K.: Significance of the HV interval in 517 patients with chronic bifascicular block. Circulation *64*:1265, 1981.
23. Scheinman, M. M., Peters, R. W., Morady, F., Sauve, M. J., Malone, T., and Modin, G.: Electrophysiologic studies in patients with bundle branch block. PACE *6*:1157, 1983.
24. Bergfeldt, L., Rosenqvist, M., Vallin, H., and Edhag, O.: Disopyramide-induced second and third degree atrioventricular block in patients with bifascicular block. An acute stress test to predict atrioventricular block progression. Br. Heart J. *53*:328, 1985.
25. Edhag, O., Bergfeldt, L., Edvardsson, N., Holmberg, S., Rosenqvist, M., and Vallin, H.: Pacemaker dependence in patients with bifascicular block during acute anterior myocardial infarction. Br. Heart J. *52*:408, 1984.
26. Watson, R. D., Glover, D. R., Page, A. J., Littler, W. A., Davies, P., deGiovanni, J., and Pentecost, B. L.: The Birmingham Trial of permanent pacing in patients with intraventricular conduction disorders after acute myocardial infarction. Am. Heart J. *108*:496, 1984.

27. Citron, P., and Duffin, E.: Implantable pacemakers for management of tachyarrhythmias. Herz *4*:269, 1979.
28. Hyman, A.: Permanent programmable pacemakers in the management of recurrent tachycardias. PACE *2*:28, 1979.
29. Khan, M., Logan, K., McComb, J., and Adgey, A.: Management of recurrent ventricular tachyarrhythmias associated with QT prolongation. Am. J. Cardiol. *47*:1301, 1981.
30. Leclercq, J., Rosengarten, M., Delcourt, P., Attuel, P., Coumel, P., and Slama, R.: Prevention of intraatrial reentry by chronic atrial pacing. PACE 3:163, 1980.

PACEMAKER MODALITIES

31. Harthorne, J. W.: Indications for pacemaker insertion: Types and modes of pacing. Prog. Cardiovasc. Dis. *23*:393, 1981.
32. Sutton, R., and Citron, P.: Electrophysiological and hemodynamic basis for application of new pacemaker technology in sick sinus syndrome and atrioventricular block. Br. Heart J. *41*:600, 1979.
33. Parsonnet, V., Furman, S., and Smyth, N. P. D.: Implantable cardiac pacemakers: Status report and resource guideline. Circulation *50*:A21, 1974.
34. Parsonnet, V., Furman, S., and Smyth, N. P. D.: A revised code for pacemaker identification. PACE *4*:400, 1981.
35. Nathan, D., Center, S., and Wu, C.: An implantable synchronous pacemaker for the long-term correction of complete heart block. Am. J. Cardiol. *11*:362, 1963.
36. Kruse, I., Ryden, L., and Duffin, E.: Clinical evaluation of atrial synchronous ventricular inhibited pacemakers. PACE *3*:641, 1980.
37. Berkovits, B., Castellanos, A., and Lemberg, L.: Bifocal demand pacing. Circulation *39*:44, 1969.
38. Barold, S., Falkoff, M., Ong, L., and Heinle, R.: Committed and uncommitted A-V sequential DVI pulse generators. Arrhythmias and electrocardiographic manifestations of normal function. Stimucoeur 9:353, 1981.
39. Barold, S., Falkoff, M., Ong,L., and Heinle, R.: Characterization of pacemaker arrhythmias due to normally functioning A-V demand (DVI) pulse generators. PACE 3:712, 1980.
40. Funke, H. D.: Three years' experience in optimized sequential cardiac pacing. Stimucoeur 9:26, 1981.
41. Fananapazir, L., Bennett, D. H., and Monks, P.: Atrial synchronized ventricular pacing: Contribution of the chronotropic response to improved exercise performance. PACE *6*:601, 1983.
42. Beyersdorf, F., Kreuzer, J., Happ, J., Zegelman, M., and Satter, P.: Increase in cardiac output with rate-responsive pacemaker. Ann. Thorac. Surg. *42*:201, 1986.
43. Alt, E., Hirgstetter, C., Heinz, M., and Blomer, H.: Rate control of physiologic pacemakers by central venous blood temperature. Circulation *73*:1206, 1986.
44. Fearnot, N. E., Jolgren, D. L., Tackes, W. A., Nelson, J. P., and Geddes, L. A.: Increasing cardiac rate by measurement of right ventricular temperature. PACE 7:1240, 1984.
45. Wirtzfeld, A., Heinze, R., Stanzl, K., Hockstein, K., Alt, E., and Liess, H. D.: Regulation of pacing rate by variations of mixed venous oxygen saturation. PACE 7:1257, 1984.
46. Camilli, L., Alcidi, L., Shapland, E., and Obina, S.: Results, problems, and perspectives with the auto-regulating pacemaker. PACE *6*:488, 1983.
47. Salo, R. W., Pederson, B. D., Olive, A. L., Lincoln, W. C., and Wallner, T. G.: Continuous ventricular volume assessment for diagnosis and pacemaker control. PACE 7:1267, 1984.
48. Bennett, T., Olson, W. H., Bornzin, G. A., and Baudino, M. D.: Alternative modes for physiologic pacing. *In* Gomez, F. (ed.): Cardiac Pacing. Mt. Kisco, N.Y., Futura Publishing Co., 1985, pp. 577–587.
49. Fananapazir, L., Rademaker, M., and Bennett, D. H.: Reliability of the evoked response in determining the paced ventricular rate and performance of the QT or rate responsive (TX) pacemaker. PACE *8*:701, 1985.
50. Goicolea de Ore, A., Ayza, M. W., Ramiro de la Llana, Morales, J. A., Diez, J. R. G., and Alvarez, J. G.: Rate responsive pacing: Clinical experience. PACE *8*:322, 1985.
51. Hedman, A., Nordlander, R., Pehrsson, S. K., and Astrom, H.: Clinical experience with rate responsive pacing by the evoked QT. Stimucoeur *14*:22, 1986.
52. Rossi, P., Aina, F., Rognoni, G., Occhetta, E., Plicchi, G., and Prando, M. D.: Increasing cardiac rate by tracking the respiratory rate. PACE 7:1246, 1984.
53. Humen, D., Kostuk, W. J., and Klein, G. J.: Activity-sensing rate-responsive pacing: Improvement in myocardial performance with exercise. PACE *8*:52, 1985.
54. Simmons, T., Maloney, J. D., Abi-Samra, F., Valenta, H., Napholtz, T., Castle, L., and Morant, V.: Exercise-responsive intravascular impedance changes as a rate controller for cardiac pacing. PACE 9:285, 1986.
54a. Kappenbergh, L. J., and Herpers, L.: Rate responsive dual chamber pacing. PACE 9:987, 1986.
55. Alicandri, C., Fouad, F., Tarazi, F., Castle, L., and Morant, V.: Three cases of hypotension and syncope with ventricular pacing: Possible role of atrial reflexes. Am. J. Cardiol. *42*:137, 1978.
56. Davidson, D., Braak, C., Preston, T., and Judge, R.: Permanent ventricular pacing: Effect of long-term survival, congestive heart failure, and subsequent myocardial infarction and stroke. Ann. Intern. Med. *77*:345, 1972.
57. Gamal, M., and Van Gelder, L.: Chronic ventricular pacing with ventriculoatrial conduction versus atrial pacing in three patients with symptomatic sinus bradycardia. PACE *4*:100, 1981.
58. Miller, M., Fox, S., Jenkins, R., Schwartz, J., and Toonder, F.: Pacemaker syndrome: A noninvasive means to its diagnosis and treatment. PACE *4*:503, 1981.
59. Patel, A., Yap, V., and Thomsen, J.: Adverse effects of right ventricular pacing in a patient with aortic stenosis. Chest 72:103, 1977.
60. Nishimura, R.,, Gersh, B., Holmes, D., Vlietstra, R., and Broadbent, J.: Outcome of dual-chamber pacing for the pacemaker syndrome. Mayo Clin. Proc. *58*:452, 1983.
61. Kag, R., Ambrose, J., Schek, L., Blake, J., Rubin, D., and Herman, M.: Pacemaker-induced pseudotricuspid regurgitation. Chest *83*:282, 1983.
62. Rabinovitch, M. A., Stewart, J., Chan, W., Dunlap, T. E., Kalff, V., Clare, J., Thrall, J. H., and Pitt, B.: Scintigraphic demonstration of ventriculo-atrial conduction in the ventricular pacemaker syndrome. J. Nucl. Med. *23*:795, 1982.
63. Rosenqvist, M., Brandt, J., and Schuller, H.: Atrial versus ventricular pacing in sinus node disease: A treatment comparison study. Am. Heart J. *111*:292, 1986.
64. Erlebacher, J., Danner, R., and Stelzer, P.: Hypotension with ventricular pacing: An atrial vasodepressor reflex in human beings. J. Am. Coll. Cardiol. *4*:550, 1984.
65. Videen, J. S., Huang, S. K., Bazgan, I. D., Mechling, E., and Patton, D. D.: Hemodynamic comparison of ventricular pacing and atrial synchronous ventricular pacing using radionuclide ventriculography. Am. J. Cardiol. *57*:1305, 1986.
66. Iwase, M., Sotobatta, I., Yokota, M., Takagi, S., Jing, H. X., Kawai, N., Hayashi, H., and Murase, M.: Evaluation of pulsed Doppler echocardiography of the atrial contribution to left ventricular filling in patients with DDD pacemakers. Am. J. Cardiol. *58*:104, 1986.
67. Kruse, I., Arnman, K., Conradson, T., and Ryden, L.: A comparison of acute and long-term hemodynamic effects of ventricular inhibited and atrial synchronous ventricular inhibited pacing. Circulation *65*:846, 1982.
68. Kruse, I., and Ryden, L.: A comparison of physical work capacity and systolic time intervals with ventricular inhibited and atrial synchronous ventricular inhibited pacing. Br. Heart J. *46*:129, 1981.
69. Sutton, R., Perrins, E., Morley, C., and Chan, S.: Sustained improvement in exercise tolerance following physiological cardiac pacing. Eur. Heart J. *4*:781, 1983.
70. Kristensson, B., Arnman, K., Smedgard, P., and Ryden, L.: Physiological versus single-rate ventricular pacing: A double-blind cross-over study. PACE *8*:85, 1985.
71. Kristensson, B., Arnman, K., and Ryden, L.: The hemodynamic importance of atrioventricular synchrony and rate increase at rest and during exercise. Eur. Heart J. *6*:773, 1985.
72. Pehrsson, S. K.: Influence of heart rate and atrioventricular synchronization and maximal work tolerance in patients treated with artificial pacemakers. Acta Med. Scand. *214*:311, 1983.

PACING FOR TACHYCARDIAS

73. Gallagher, J., Svenson, R., Kasell, J., German, L., Bardy, G., Broughton, A., and Critelli, G.: Catheter technique for closed-chest ablation of the atrioventricular conduction system: A therapeutic alternative for the treatment of refractory supraventricular tachycardia. N. Engl. J. Med. *306*:194, 1982.
74. Preston, T., Haynes, R., Gavin, W., and Hessel, E.: Permanent rapid atrial pacing to control supraventricular tachycardia. PACE *2*:331, 1979.
75. Arbel, E., Cohen, H., Langendorf, R., and Glick, G.: Successful treatment of drug-resistant atrial tachycardia and intractable congestive heart failure with permanent coupled atrial pacing. Am. J. Cardiol. *41*:336, 1978.
76. Zoll, P. M., Linenthal, A. J., and Zarsky, L. R.: Ventricular fibrillation: Treatment and prevention by external electric currents. N. Engl. J. Med. *262*:105, 1960.
77. Levy, S., Gerard, R., Jausseran, J., Boyer, C., Clementy, J., Baudet, E., and Bricaud, H.: Long-term results of permanent atrioventricular sequential demand pacing. PACE *2*:175, 1979.
78. Leclercq, J. F., Attuel, P., and Coumel, P.: Les stimulateurs cardiaques destines à traiter les tachycardies paroxystiques. Stimucoeur *7*:8, 1979.
79. Seger, J. J., and Griffin, J. C.: Electrical treatment of cardiac arrhythmias. Prog. Cardiovasc. Dis. (*in press*).
80. Hartzler, G., Holmes, D., and Osborn, M.: Patient-activated transvenous cardiac stimulation for the treatment of supraventricular and ventricular tachycardia. Am. J. Cardiol. *47*:903, 1981.
81. Ruskin, J., Garan, H., Poulin, F., and Harthorne, J. W.: Permanent radio frequency ventricular pacing for management of drug-resistant ventricular tachycardia. Am. J. Cardiol. *46*:317, 1980.
82. Griffin, J., Mason, J., and Calfee, R.: Clinical use of an implantable automatic tachycardia-terminating pacemaker. Am. Heart J. *100*:1093, 1980.
83. Neumann, G., Funke, H. D., Bakels, N., Kirchof, P. G., and Schaede, A.: A new atrial demand pacemaker for the management of supraventricular tachycardias. Proc. VIth World Symp. Cardiac Pacing, 27–7, 1979.
84. Slocum, J., Byrom, E., McCarthy, L., Sahakian, A., and Swiryn, S.: Computer detection of atrioventricular dissociation from surface electrocardiograms during wide QRS complex tachycardias. Circulation 72:1028, 1985.
85. Nathan, A. W., Spurrell, R. A., and Camm, A. J.: Steps toward the development of a safe and effective tachycardia terminating pacemaker. Eur. Heart J. 5:993, 1984.

86. Waldecker, B., Brugada, P., Zehender, M., Stevenson, W., denDulk, K., and Wellens, H. J. J.: Importance of modes of electrical termination of ventricular tachycardia for the selection of implantable antitachycardia devices. Am. J. Cardiol. 57:150, 1986.
87. Camm, A., Nathan, A., Hellestrand, K., Ward, D., and Spurrell, R.: The clinical evaluation of tachycardia termination by utilizing autodecremental atrial pacing. PACE *4*:A-84, 1981.
88. Curry, P., Rowland, E., and Krikler, D.: Dual-demand pacing for refractory atrioventricular reentry tachycardia. PACE *2*:137, 1979.
89. Castellanos, A., Waxman, M., Maleiro, F., Berkovits, B., and Sung, R.: Preliminary studies with an implantable multimodal A-V pacemaker for reciprocating atrioventricular tachycardias. PACE *3*:257, 1980.
90. Maloney, J., Medina-Ravell, V., Pieretti, O., Portillo, B., Maduro, C., Castellanos, A., and Berkovits, B.: Follow-up assessment of dual-demand, dual-chamber DVI-DVO pacing for automatic conversion, control, and prevention of refractory paroxysmal supraventricular tachycardia. PACE *4*:A-57, 1981.
91. Charos, G. S., Haffajee, C. I., Gold, R. L., Bishop, R. L., Berkovits, B. V., and Alpert, J. S.: A theoretically and practically more effective method for interruption of ventricular tachycardia: Self-adapting autodecremental overdrive pacing. Circulation 73:309, 1986.
92. denDulk, K., Kersschot, I. E., Brugada, P., and Wellens, H. J. J.: Is there a universal antitachycardia pacing mode? Am. J. Cardiol. *57*:950, 1986.
93. Waldecker, B., Brugada, P., denDulk, K., Zehender, M., and Wellens, H. J. J.: Arrhythmias induced during termination of supraventricular tachycardia. Am. J. Cardiol. *55*:412, 1985.
94. Peters, R. W., Scheinman, M. M., Morady, F., and Jacobson, L.: Long-term management of recurrent paryxosmal tachycardia by cardiac burst pacing. PACE *8*:35, 1985.
95. Jackman, W. M., and Zipes, D. P.: Low energy synchronous cardioversion of ventricular tachycardia using a catheter electrode in a canine model of subacute myocardial infarction. Circulation *66*:187, 1982.
96. Zipes, D. P., Jackman, W., Heger, J., Chilson, D., Browne, K., Nacarelli, G., Rahilly, G., and Prystowsky, E.: Clinical transvenous cardioversion of recurrent life-threatening ventricular tachyarrhythmias: Low-energy synchronized cardioversion of ventricular tachycardia and termination of ventricular fibrillation in patients using a catheter electrode. Am. Heart J. *103*:789, 1982.
97. Yee, R., Zipes, D. P., Galamhusein, S., Kallok, M. J., and Klein, G. J.: Low-energy countershock using an intravascular catheter in an acute care setting. Am. J. Cardiol. *50*:1124, 1982.
98. Miles, W. M., Prystowsky, E. N., Heger, J. J., and Zipes, D. P.: The implantable transvenous cardioverter: Long-term efficacy and reproducible ventricular tachycardia induction. Circulation *74*:518, 1986.
99. Zipes, D. P., Heger, J. J., Miles, W. M., Mahomed, Y., Brown, J. W., Spielman, S. R., and Prystowsky, E. N.: Early experience with an implantable cardioverter. N. Engl. J. Med. *311*:485, 1984.
100. Saksena, S., Chandran, P., Shah, Y., Boccadamo, R., Pantopoulos, D., and Rothbart, S. T.: Comparative efficacy of transvenous cardioversion and pacing in patients with sustained ventricular tachycardia: A prospective, randomized, cross-over study. Circulation 72:153, 1985.
101. Mirowski, M.: The automatic implantable cardioverter/defibrillator: An overview. J. Am. Coll. Cardiol. *6*:461, 1985.
102. Mirowski, M., Reid, P. R., Mower, M. M., Watkins, L., Platia, E. V., Griffith, L. S. C., and Juanteguy, J. M.: The automatic implantable cardioverter-defibrillator. PACE 7:534, 1984.
103. Platia, E. V., Griffith, L. S., Watkins, L., Jr., Mower, M. M., Guarnieri, T., Mirowski, M., and Reid, P. R.: Treatment of malignant ventricular arrhythmias with endocardial resection and implantation of the automatic cardioverter/defibrillator. N. Engl. J. Med. *314*:213, 1986.
104. Mirowski, M., Reid, P. R., Mower, M. M., Watkins, L., Jr., Platia, E. V., Griffith, L. S., Guarnieri, T., Thomas, A., and Juanteguy, J. M.: Clinical performance of the implantable cardioverter-defibrillator. PACE *7*:1345, 1984.
105. Echt, D. S., Armstrong, K., Schmidt, P., Oyer, P. E., Stinson, E. B., and Winkle, R. A.: Clinical experience, complications, and survival in 70 patients with the automatic implantable cardioverter/defibrillator. Circulation *71*:289, 1985.
106. Marchlinski, F. E., Flores, B. T., Buxton, A. E., Hargrove, W. C., III, Addonizio, V. P., Stephenson, L. W., Harken, A. H., Doherty, J. U., Grogan, E. W., Jr., and Josephson M. E.: The automatic implantable cardioverter-defibrillator: Efficacy, complications, and device failures. Ann. Intern. Med. *104*:481, 1986.
107. Ruffy, R., Schechtman, K., Monje, E., and Sandza, J.: Adrenergically mediated variations in the energy required to defibrillate the heart: Observations in closed-chest, nonanesthetized dogs. Circulation 73:374, 1986.
108. Troup, P. J., Chapman, P. D., Olinger, G. N., and Kleinman, L. H.: The implanted defibrillator: Relation of defibrillating lead configuration and clinical variables to defibrillation threshold. J. Am. Coll. Cardiol. *6*:1315, 1985.
109. Dorian, P., Fain, E. S., Davy, J., and Winkle, R. A.: Lidocaine causes a reversible concentration-dependent increase in defibrillation energy requirements. J. Am. Coll. Cardiol. *8*:327, 1986.
110. Furman, S., and Pannizzo, F.: Output programmability and reduction of secondary intervention after pacemaker implantation. J. Thorac. Cardiovasc. Surg. *81*:713, 1981.
111. Hayes, D. L., Maloney, J. D., Merideth, J., Holmes, D. R., Gersh, B., Broadbent, J. C., Osborn, M. J., and Fetter J.: Initial and early follow-up assessment of the clinical efficacy of a multiparameter-programmable pulse generator. PACE *4*:417, 1981.
112. Parsonnet, V., and Rodgers, T.: The present status of programmable pacemakers. Prog. Cardiovasc. Dis. *23*:401, 1981.
113. Eagle, K. A., Mulley, A. G., Singer, D. E., Schoenfeld, D., Harthorne, J. W., and Thibault, G. E.: Single-chamber and dual-chamber cardiac pacemakers: A formal cost comparison. Ann. Intern. Med. *105*:264, 1986.
114. Parsonnet, V.: Cardiac pacing and pacemakers. VII. Power sources for implantable pacemakers. Part 1. Am. Heart J. *94*:517, 1977.
115. Owens, B.: The role of solid electrolytes in lithium pacemaker batteries. Solid State Ionics *3*:273, 1981.
116. Bilitch, M., Hauser, R. G., Goldman, B. S., Furman, S., and Parsonnet, V.: Performance of cardiac pacemaker pulse generators. PACE *8*:276, 1985.
117. Hurzeler, P., Morse, D., Leach, C., Sands, B. S., Milton, J., Pennock, R., and Zinberg, A.: Longevity comparisons among lithium anode power cells for cardiac pacemakers. PACE *3*:555, 1980.
118. Owens, B., Brennen, K., and Kim, J.: Lithium pacemaker reliability. Stimucoeur 9:371, 1981.
119. Bilitch, M., Hauser, R. G., Goldman, B. S., Furman, S., and Parsonnet, V.: Performance of implantable cardiac rhythm management devices. PACE *9*:256, 1986.
120. Greatbatch, W.: Metal electrodes in bioengineering. CRC Crit. Rev. Bioeng. *5*(1):1, 1981.
121. Smyth, N. P. D.: Techniques of implantation: Atrial and ventricular, thoracotomy and transvenous. Prog. Cardiovasc. Dis. *23*(6):435, 1981.
122. DeCaprio, V., Hurzeler, P., and Furman, S.: A comparison of unipolar and bipolar electrograms for cardiac pacemaker sensing. Circulation *56*:750, 1977.
123. Parsonnet, V.: Routine implantation of permanent transvenous pacemaker electrodes in both chambers. A technique whose time has come. PACE *4*(1):109, 1981.
124. Parsonnet, V., Werres, R., Atherley, T., and Littleford, P.: Transvenous insertion of double sets of permanent electrodes. J.A.M.A. *243*:62, 1980.
125. Bisping, H., Kruezer, J., and Birkenheier, H.: Three years' clinical experience with a new endocardial screw-in lead with introduction protection for use in the atrium and ventricle. PACE *3*:424, 1980.
126. Furman, S., Pannizzo, F., and Campo, I.: Comparison of active and passive adhering leads for endocardial pacing–II. PACE *4*:78, 1981.
127. Messenger, J., Castellanet, M., Ellestadt, M., Greensberg, P., Wilson, W., and Stephenson, N.: New permanent endocardial atrial J lead: Implantation techniques and clinical performance. PACE *4*:A-59, 1981.
128. Mond, H., and Sloman, G.: Small tined ventricular pacemaker leads—reduction of lead complications. PACE *4*:A-60, 1981.
129. deFeyter, P., Majid, P., Hoitsma, H., Stroes, W., and Roos, J.: Permanent cardiac pacing with sutureless myocardial electrodes: Experience in first one hundred patients. PACE *3*:144, 1980.
130. Falk, R. H., Zoll, P. M., and Zoll, R. H.: Safety and efficacy of noninvasive cardiac pacing. A preliminary report. N. Engl. J. Med. *309*:1166, 1983.
131. Zoll, P., Zoll, R., and Belgard, A.: External noninvasive electric stimulation of the heart. Crit. Care Med. *9*(5):393 1981.
132. Furman, S., Hurzeler, P., and Mehra, R.: Cardiac pacing and pacemakers. IV. Threshold of cardiac stimulation. Am. Heart J. *94*:115, 1977-E.
133. Furman, S., Hurzeler, P., and DeCaprio, V.: Cardiac pacing and pacemakers. III. Sensing the cardiac electrogram. Am. Heart J. *93*:794, 1977-D.
134. MacGregor, D., Correy, H., Noble, E., Smardon, S., Wilson, G., Goldman, B., and Wigle, E.: Computer assisted reporting system for the follow-up of patients with cardiac pacemakers. PACE *3*:568, 1980.
135. Zipes, D. P.: Pacing 1980. PACE *4*:182, 1981.
136. Murdock, D., Morna, J., Stafford, J., King, L., Loeb, M., and Scanlon, P.: Pacemaker malfunction: Fact or artifact? Heart Lung *15*:150, 1986.
137. Cook, A. M., and Webster, J. G.: Therapeutic Medical Devices. Englewood Cliffs, N.J., Prentice-Hall, 1981.
138. Furman, S.: Cardiac pacing and pacemakers. VI. Analysis of pacemaker malfunction. Am. Heart J. *94*:378, 1977.
138a. Duffin, E. G.: The marker channel: A telemetric diagnostic aid. PACE 7:1165, 1984.
138b. Duffin, E. G., Rueter, J., and Anderson, K.: A dual chamber pacing system analyzer, the Medtronic model 5311. Prog. Pacing Clin. Electrophysiol. *4*:449, 1986.
139. Kaul, J., Macfarlane, P., Thomson, R., and Bain, W.: An anaysis of electrocardiographic, radiographic, and vector cardiographic findings in patients with implanted cardiac pacemakers. Am. Heart J. *99*:686, 1980.

24 CARDIAC ARREST AND SUDDEN CARDIAC DEATH

by ROBERT J. MYERBURG, M.D., and AGUSTIN CASTELLANOS, M.D.

DEFINITION

Sudden cardiac death (SCD) is natural death due to cardiac causes, heralded by abrupt loss of consciousness within one hour of the onset of acute symptoms, in an individual with or without known preexisting heart disease, but in whom the time and mode of death are unexpected. This definition reflects a view of the event which incorporates the key elements of "natural," "rapid," and "unexpected." It has been derived from past definitions in the literature[1–20] which have conflicted, mainly because the most useful operational definition of SCD differs for the clinician, the cardiovascular epidemiologist, the pathologist, and the scientist attempting to define pathophysiological mechanisms.

Four elements must be considered in the construction of a definition of SCD in order to satisfy medical, scientific, legal, and social disciplines: (1) prodromes, (2) onset, (3) cardiac arrest, and (4) biological death (Fig. 24–1). Since the proximate cause of all SCD is a disturbance of cardiac function incompatible with maintaining consciousness resulting from abrupt loss of cerebral blood flow, any definition must include the concept that a brief time interval exists between the onset of the mechanism directly responsible for cardiac arrest and the consequent loss of consciousness (Fig. 24–1*C*). However, the 1-hour definition refers to the duration of the "terminal event" (Fig. 24–1*B*), which is the interval between the onset of symptoms signaling the presence of a pathophysiological disturbance which will lead to the cardiac arrest and the onset of the cardiac arrest itself (Fig. 24–1*B* and 1*C*).

Premonitory signs and symptoms, which may occur over a period of weeks before a cardiac arrest,[17] tend to be nonspecific for the impending event.[8] However, *prodromes*

	A	B	C	D
EVENT	PRODROME: NEW OR WORSENING CARDIO-VASCULAR SYMPTOMS	ONSET OF TERMINAL EVENT	CLINICAL CARDIAC ARREST	PROGRESSION TO BIOLOGICAL DEATH
SYMPTOMS AND SIGNS	CHEST PAIN, DYSPNEA, PALPITATIONS, WEAKNESS	ABRUPT CHANGE IN SYMPTOMS, ELECTRICAL AND MECHANICAL DISTURBANCES, HYPOTENSION, LIGHTHEADEDNESS	LOSS OF EFFECTIVE CIRCULATION; LOSS OF CONSCIOUSNESS	FAILURE OF RESUSCITATION -OR- FAILURE OF ELECTRICAL, MECHANICAL, OR CNS IMPROVEMENT AFTER SUCCESSFUL INITIAL RESUSCITATION
INTERVAL BETWEEN EVENTS		SECONDS – 24 HOURS	INSTANTANEOUS TO 1 HOUR	4 – 6 MINUTES TO WEEKS

FIGURE 24–1. The definition of sudden death is divided into four temporal components: (A) prodromes, (B) onset of the terminal event, (C) the cardiac arrest itself, and (D) progression to biological death. Individual variability of the components influence the clinical expression: some have no prodromes with onset leading almost instantaneously to cardiac arrest, others may have an onset which lasts up to 1 hour before clinical cardiac arrest; some patients may live weeks after the cardiac arrest before progression to biological death if there has been irreversible brain damage and life support systems are used. These modifying factors influence application of the 1-hour definition. From the perspective of the clinician, the two most relevant factors are the onset of the terminal event (B), and the clinical cardiac arrest itself (C). In contrast, legal and social definitions focus on the time of biological death (D).

(Fig. 24–1A) which may be specific for an imminent cardiac arrest are relatively abrupt changes beginning during an arbitrarily defined period of up to 24 hours before the cardiac arrest.[4, 21] The fourth element, biological death (Fig. 24–1D), is not necessarily an immediate consequence of the clinical event of cardiac arrest. The latter point has been highlighted since the development of community-based intervention systems, in that patients may now remain biologically alive for a long period of time after the onset of a pathophysiological process which has caused irreversible damage and will ultimately lead to death.[18–20, 22] In this circumstance, the causative pathophysiological and clinical event is the cardiac arrest itself rather than the factors proximate to the delayed biological death. However, in legal, forensic, and certain social circumstances biological death must continue to be used as the most relevant event. Finally, the pathologist and the epidemiologist studying *unwitnessed deaths* may use the definition of sudden death for an individual known to be alive and functioning normally 24 hours before,[4] and this remains appropriate within its obvious limits because unwitnessed death cannot be ignored in their studies.[23] Thus, the generally accepted clinical-pathophysiological definition of up to 1 hour between onset of the terminal event and biological death requires qualifications for specific circumstances and uses.

The development of community-based intervention systems has also led to inconsistencies in the use of terms considered absolute. *Death* is defined biologically, legally, and literally as an absolute and irreversible event. Thus, SCD may be aborted, or a patient may survive cardiac arrest or cardiovascular collapse; however, survival after (sudden) death is a contradiction in terms. Table 24–1 provides definitions for events and terms related to the concept of SCD—death, cardiac arrest, and cardiovascular collapse.

TABLE 24–1 DEFINITION OF TERMS RELATED TO SUDDEN DEATH

Term	Definition	Qualifiers or Exceptions
Death	Irreversible cessation of all biological functions	None
Cardiac Arrest	Abrupt cessation of cardiac pump function which may be reversible by a prompt intervention but will lead to death in its absence	Rare spontaneous reversions; likelihood of successful intervention relates to mechanism of arrest and clinical setting
Cardiovascular Collapse	A (sudden) loss of effective blood flow due to cardiac and/or peripheral vascular factors which may reverse spontaneously (e.g., vasodepressor syncope) or only with interventions (e.g., cardiac arrest)	Nonspecific term which includes cardiac arrest and its consequences and also events which characteristically revert spontaneously

EPIDEMIOLOGY AND CAUSES OF SUDDEN DEATH

EPIDEMIOLOGY

The worldwide incidence of SCD is difficult to estimate because it varies largely as a function of coronary heart disease prevalence in different cultures.[24–27] Estimates for the United States range from 200,000 to nearly 400,000 SCD's annually,[28] the variation based in part upon the definition of sudden death used in individual studies.[5, 16] Most surveys and studies currently use the estimate of 300,000 SCD's annually,[29] a figure which represents nearly 50 per cent of all cardiovascular deaths in the United States.[24, 28, 29]

The influence of the temporal definition of sudden death on epidemiological data[4] is demonstrated by data derived from a retrospective death certificate study in a large metropolitan area in the United States reported by Kuller et al.[4] When the temporal definition was restricted to death less than 2 hours after the onset of symptoms, 12 per cent of all natural deaths were sudden, and 88 per cent of the sudden natural deaths were due to cardiac causes. This estimate is similar to observations in a large prospective cohort study—the Framingham study—in which 13 per cent of all deaths observed during a 26-year period were "sudden," defined as death within an hour of the onset of symptoms.[30, 31] In contrast to deaths occurring less than 2 hours after the onset of symptoms, the application of the 24-hour definition of sudden death to the data from Kuller et al.[4] increased the fraction of all natural deaths falling into the "sudden" category to 32 per cent but reduced the proportion of all sudden natural deaths which were cardiac deaths to 75 per cent.

More recent prospective studies demonstrate that approximately 50 per cent of all coronary heart disease deaths are sudden and unexpected, occurring shortly (instantaneous to 1 hour) after the onset of symptoms. In the prospective combined Albany-Framingham study of 4120 males, sudden death defined as death within 1 hour of an observed collapse was analyzed for a population of men dying between 45 and 74 years of age.[9] During a 16-year follow-up, there were 234 total coronary deaths/1000 population observed, of which 109 (47 per cent) were sudden and unexpected. Since coronary heart disease dominates sudden and total cardiac deaths in the United States, the fraction of total cardiac deaths which are sudden is similar to the fraction of coronary heart disease deaths which are sudden. This may not apply to other nations or to subcultures which have a lower prevalence of coronary heart disease. It is also of interest that the recent decline in coronary heart disease mortality in the United States[32] has not changed the fraction of coronary deaths that are sudden and unexpected.[33]

AGE, HEREDITY, GENDER, AND RACE

AGE. There are two ages of peak incidence of sudden death: between birth and 6 months of age (the sudden infant death syndrome) and between 45 and 75 years of age.[3] In the adult population, the *incidence* of sudden death due to coronary heart disease increases as a function of advancing age,[33–35] in parallel with the age-related increase in incidence of total coronary heart disease deaths.[32] However, the *proportion* of deaths due to coronary heart disease that are sudden and unexpected decreases with advancing age.[9, 33–35] Kuller et al.[36] reported that 76 per cent of coronary heart disease deaths in the 20 to 39 year age group were sudden and unexpected, and the Framingham data demonstrated that 62 per cent of all coronary heart disease deaths were sudden in the 45 to 54 year age group in men. The proportion fell progressively to 58 per cent in the 55 to 64 year age group and to 42 per cent in the 65 to 74 year age group.[34, 35] Age also influences the proportion of cardiovascular causes among all causes of natural sudden death in that the proportion of coronary deaths and of all cardiac causes of death which are sudden is highest in the younger age groups, while the fraction of total sudden natural deaths which are due to any cardiovascular cause is higher in the older age groups[37, 38] (Fig. 24–2). In their study of sudden death in children and

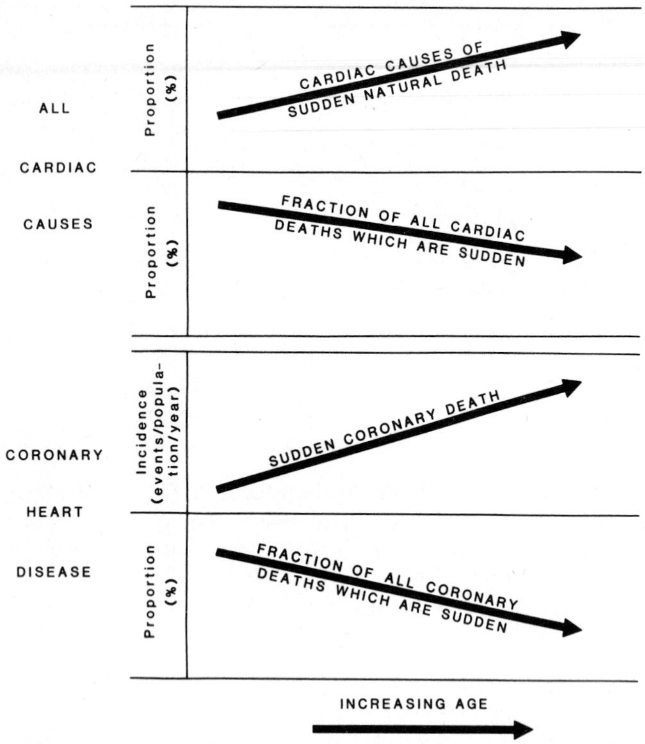

FIGURE 24–2. Sudden death as a function of age. Cardiac causes of sudden natural death increase as a function of increasing age from childhood to advanced age, while the proportion of all cardiac deaths which are sudden tends to decrease toward a plateau in the fifth, sixth, and seventh decades. In adults, the incidence of sudden coronary deaths increases as a function of age, but the proportion of all coronary deaths which are sudden decrease with age (see text for details).

young adults, Neuspiel and Kuller[37] reported that only 19 per cent of sudden natural deaths in children between 1 and 13 years of age were cardiac deaths; the proportion increased to 30 per cent in the 14- to 21-year age group. All of these studies on age factors used a 24-hour definition of sudden death.

HEREDITY. To the extent that SCD is an expression of underlying coronary heart disease, hereditary factors that contribute to coronary heart disease risk operate nonspecifically for the SCD syndrome.[39–44]

Among the less common causes of SCD, hereditary patterns have been reported for some specific syndromes. Such patterns are described for some forms of congenital and hereditary Q-T Interval prolongation,[45–47] (p. 699) hypertrophic obstructive cardiomyopathy,[48, 49] and familial SCD in children and young adults.[50] Although stable congenital conducting system abnormalities have a good prognosis,[51] progressive familial conducting system disease, which appears to have a hereditary pattern, carries a risk of SCD.[52–54] Familial sudden death associated with cardiac ganglionitis has been reported,[55] but an inheritance pattern has not been demonstrated in the reports to date.

GENDER. The SCD syndrome has a huge preponderance in males compared with females because of the protection females enjoy from coronary atherosclerosis prior to advanced years.[30, 31, 35] During the first 14 years of follow-up in the Framingham study, 59 of 66 (89 per cent) of sudden unexpected coronary deaths (<1 hour) occurred in men.[6] The Framingham study at 20 years of follow-up demonstrated a 3.8-fold excess incidence of sudden coronary death in men compared to women.[35] This male:female ratio is similar to data recorded in three prospective studies of prehospital cardiac arrest in which the percentages of males observed were 75 per cent (mean age, 63 years),[18] 85 per cent (mean age, 60 years),[19] and 89 per cent (mean age, 58 years),[56] respectively. In the study by Kuller et al.,[4] 75 per cent of all SCD's (using the 24-hour definition) in a 40- to 64-year-old population were in males. When the data in another study by Kuller et al. were analyzed for survival of less than 2 hours, the proportion of men increased to 80 per cent.[57] In the Framingham study,[35] the excess risk in men peaked at 6.75:1 in the 55- to 64-year age group, and then fell to 2.17:1 in the 65- to 74-year age group. Even though the overall risk is so much lower in women, the classic coronary risk factors are expressed in them.[30, 31, 58, 59] Cigarette smoking, diabetes, use of oral contraceptives,[60] and reduced vital capacity[31] are particularly strong factors.

RACE. A number of studies comparing racial differences and relative risk of SCD in whites and blacks with coronary heart disease in the United States have yielded inconclusive data.[4, 29, 61] However, data on the prevalence of coronary heart disease in Japanese men living in the United States have demonstrated that the low rates reported in those living in Japan tend to increase toward, but do not reach, levels observed in white men in the United States.[27, 62] Thus, an interplay between race and cultural factors may be operative.

BIOLOGICAL CORONARY RISK FACTORS AND SUDDEN DEATH

In general, the known coronary risk factors cannot be used to distinguish the patients at risk for SCD from those at risk for other manifestations of coronary heart disease.[9, 34] Using a multivariate analysis of selected risk factors (i.e., age, systolic blood pressure, heart rate, ECG abnormalities, vital capacity, relative weight, cigarette consumption, and serum cholesterol) from the population in the Framingham data, Kannel and Schatzkin[33] determined that 53 per cent of the SCD's in men and 42 per cent of those in women occurred among the 10 per cent of the population in the highest risk decile (Fig. 24–3). The comparison of risk factors in the victims of SCD to those in persons who developed any manifestations of coronary artery disease did not provide useful patterns, by either univariate or multivariate analyses, to distinguish victims of SCD from the overall pool.[9] Hypertension is a clearly established risk factor for coronary heart disease and also emerges as a highly significant risk factor for incidence of SCD.[9] However, there is no influence of increasing systolic blood pressure levels on the ratio of sudden deaths to total coronary heart disease deaths.[34] No relationship has been observed between cholesterol concentration and the proportion of coronary deaths that were sudden.[35] Neither the ECG pattern of left ventricular hypertrophy nor nonspecific ST-T wave abnormalities influence the proportion of total coronary deaths that are sudden and unexpected[34]; *only intraventricular conduction abnormalities are suggestive of a disproportionate number of SCD's.*[35] A low vital capacity also suggested a disproportionate risk for sudden versus total coronary deaths.[35] This is of interest because such a relationship was particularly striking in the analysis of data on women in the Framingham study who had died suddenly.[30, 31] A high hematocrit was also predictive in women.[31]

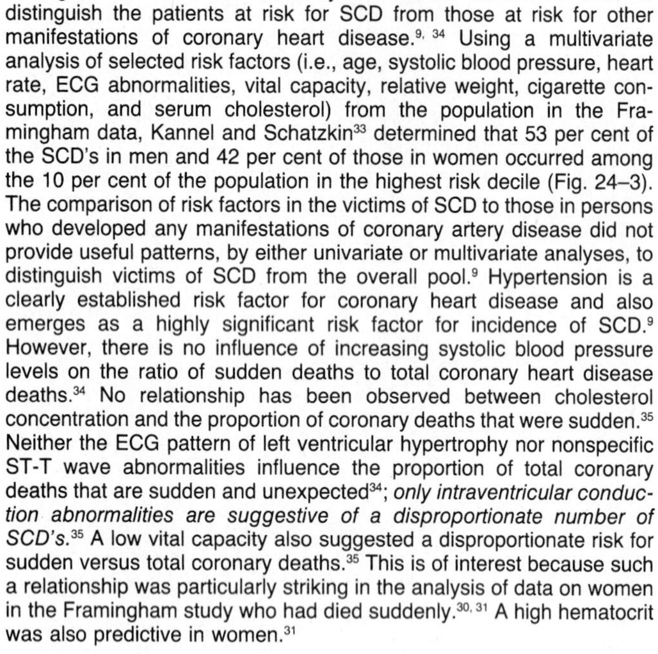

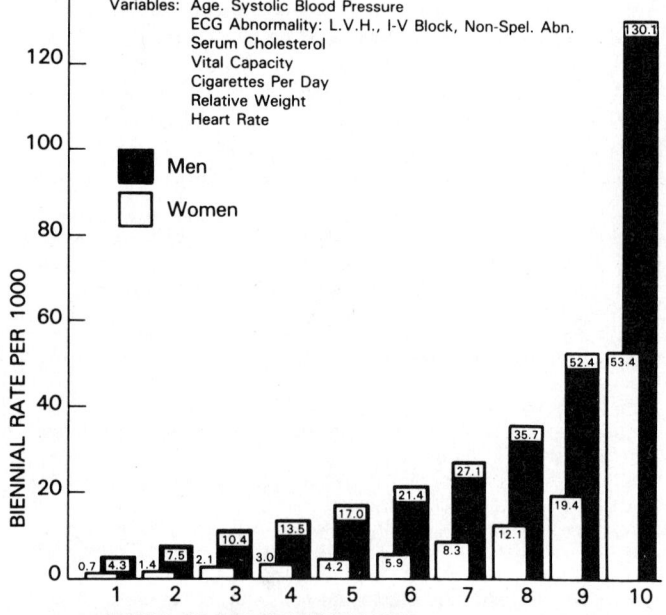

FIGURE 24–3. Risk of sudden death by decile of multivariant risk: 26-year follow-up, the Framingham Study. ECG = electrocardiographic; IV = intraventricular; LVH = left ventricular hypertrophy; Non-Spec Abn = nonspecific abnormality. (From Kannel, W. B., and Shatzkin, A.: Sudden death: Lessons from subsets in population studies. Reprinted by permission of the American College of Cardiology. J. Am. Coll. Cardiol. 5[Suppl 6]:141B, 1985.)

LIFE STYLE, PSYCHOSOCIAL, AND ENVIRONMENTAL FACTORS

LIFE STYLE. There is a strong association between *cigarette smoking* and all manifestations of coronary heart disease. The Framingham study demonstrates that cigarette smokers have a 2- to 3-fold increase in sudden death risk in each decade of life at entry between 30 and 59 years, and that this is one of the few risk factors in which the proportion of coronary heart disease deaths that are sudden increases in association with the risk factor.[35] In addition, in a study of 310 survivors of out-of-hospital cardiac arrest, Hallstrom et al.[63] observed a 27 per cent incidence of recurrent cardiac arrest at 3 years in those who continued to smoke after their index event, compared to 19 per cent in those who stopped ($p < 0.04$) Obesity is a second factor which appears to influence the proportion of coronary deaths occurring suddenly.[31, 35] With increasing relative weight, the percentage of coronary heart disease deaths that were sudden in the Framingham study increased linearly from a low of 39 per cent to a high of 70 per cent. Of course, total coronary heart disease deaths increased with increasing relative weight as well.

Epidemiological observations suggest a relationship between *low levels of physical activity* and increased coronary heart disease death risk.[64] The Framingham study, however, showed an *insignificant* relationship between low levels of physical activity and incidence of sudden death but a high proportion of sudden to total cardiac deaths at *higher* levels of physical activity.[35]

PSYCHOSOCIAL FACTORS. These appear to influence the risk for sudden cardiac deaths. Rahe and coworkers[65] recorded recent life changes in the realms of health, work, home and family, and personal and social factors, relating the magnitude of such changes to myocardial infarction and SCD. There was an association between significant elevations of life-change scores during the 6 months before a coronary event (p. 000), and the association was particularly striking in victims of SCD. In a study of sudden death in women, those who died suddenly were less often married, had fewer children, and had greater educational discrepancies with their spouses than did age-related controls living in the same neighborhood as the sudden death victims. A history of psychiatric treatment, cigarette smoking, and greater quantities of alcohol consumption than the controls also characterized the sudden death group.[66] Ruberman and coworkers reported on the influences of psychosocial factors on sudden and total death after myocardial infarction in 2320 male survivors of myocardial infarction.[67] Controlling for other major prognostic factors, including frequency of premature ventricular contractions, a greater than 4-fold increase in risk of sudden and total deaths was predicted by *social isolation* and a *high level of life stress*. These psychosocial factors were inversely related to levels of education. In an earlier study, a more than 3-fold increase of sudden death risk during follow-up after myocardial infarction had been reported in men who had complex ventricular ectopy and low levels of education compared with better-educated men with the same arrhythmias.[68] Interestingly, there was no relation between educational level and recurrent myocardial infarction.

In a survey of life style, it was found that persons with lower educational levels smoked more cigarettes, drank more alcohol, exercised less, and were more overweight.[69] The studies by Friedman and Rosenman[70] on the time-oriented, aggressive *type A personality* characteristics (p. 000) have suggested an increased incidence of all manifestations of coronary heart disease in such patients, including the incidence of sudden cardiac death.

FUNCTIONAL CLASSIFICATION AND SUDDEN DEATH. The Framingham study demonstrated a striking relationship between functional classification and death during a 2-year follow-up period. However, the proportion of deaths that were sudden did not vary with functional classification, ranging from 50 to 57 per cent in all groups, ranging from those free of clinical heart disease to those in functional class IV.[35]

SUDDEN DEATH AND PREVIOUS CORONARY HEART DISEASE

Although SCD is the first clinical manifestation of coronary heart disease to 20 to 25 per cent or more of all coronary heart disease patients,[9, 16, 23, 29] a previous myocardial infarction can be identified in as many as 75 per cent of patients who die suddenly. The high incidence of both clinical and unrecognized prior myocardial infarction in victims of SCD has led to a search for predictors of SCD in survivors of myocardial infarction, as well as in patients with other clinical manifestations of coronary heart disease.

VENTRICULAR ECTOPY IN CHRONIC ISCHEMIC HEART DISEASE. Most forms of ventricular ectopic activity (PVC's) in the absence of heart disease[71] are prognostically benign. However, when present in persons over the age of 30, PVC's select a subgroup with a higher probability of coronary artery disease and of SCD.[72] In addition, the occurrence of PVC's in survivors of myocardial infarction,[73, 73a] particularly if frequent and of complex forms such as multiform or repetitive PVC's,[74–83] predicts an increased risk of SCD on long-term follow-up. The majority of these studies have identified both *frequency* and *forms* of ventricular ectopic activity as indicators of risk, but uniformity of such classifications is lacking.[84] Although most studies cite a frequency cutoff of 10 PVC's/hour as a threshold level for increased risk, some have identified frequency cutoffs in the range of 1 to 9 PVC's/hour, 10 PVC's/1000 sinus beats, and more than 20 PVC's/hour. Forms suggested as high risk include multiform PVC's, bigeminy, short coupling intervals (R-on-T phenomenon), and salvos of three or more ectopic beats.[84] Several investigators have recently emphasized that the most powerful predictor among the various forms of PVC's is salvos of three or more complexes.[80–83, 85, 86] In hierarchical classification of chronic PVC's used for the purpose of expressing prognostic implications, the Lown classification of ventricular arrhythmias has been employed generally.[87] However, the validity of the application of this classification for risk stratification has been questioned[81, 88] and alternative systems have been proposed.[84, 89]

Many of the reported studies have been based on a single ambulatory monitor sample recorded 1 week to several months after the onset of acute myocardial infarction, and the duration of the samples has ranged from 1 hour to 48 hours. Ruberman et al.[85] reported that repeated short-term (1-hour) ambulatory recordings at 6-month intervals beginning 1 month after myocardial infarction reestablished the increased risk imparted by complex forms of PVC's for the ensuing 3½-year interval as long as complex forms remained on the interval recordings (Fig.

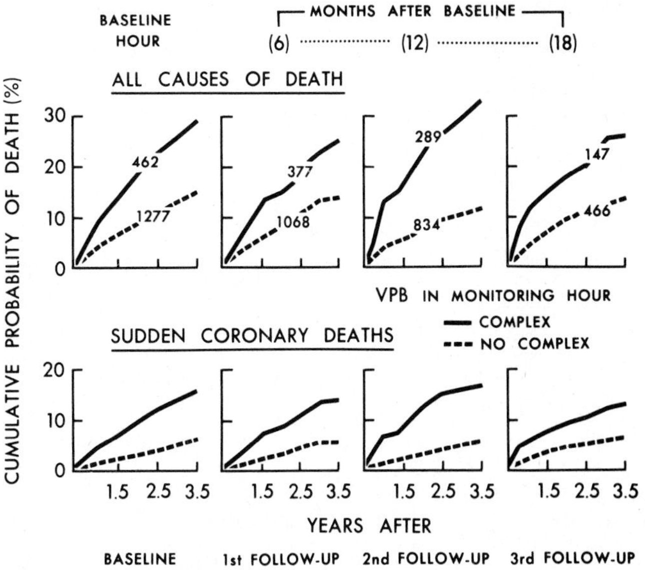

FIGURE 24–4. Complex PVC's and sudden and total death during sequential 3½ year follow-up periods among survivors of myocardial infarction. The four separate monitoring periods at 6-month intervals used demonstrate that the significance of complex VPB's as a predictor of sudden and total mortality does not change as a function of time up to 18 months after the infarction. (Modified from Ruberman, W., et al.: Repeated 1-hour electrocardiographic monitoring of survivors of myocardial infarction at 6-month intervals: Arrhythmia detection and relation to prognosis. Reprinted by permission of the American College of Cardiology. Am. J. Cardiol. *47*:1197, 1981.)

TABLE 24–2 CAUSES AND CONTRIBUTING FACTORS IN SUDDEN CARDIAC DEATH

I. CORONARY ARTERY ABNORMALITIES
- A. Coronary atherosclerosis
  - 1. Chronic ischemic heart disease with transient supply/demand imbalance—thrombosis, spasm, physical stress
  - 2. Acute myocardial infarction
  - 3. Chronic atherosclerosis with change in myocardial substrate
- B. Congenital abnormalities of coronary arteries
  - 1. Anomalous origin from pulmonary artery
  - 2. Other coronary AV fistula
  - 3. Origin of left coronary artery from right sinus of Valsalva
  - 4. Origin of right coronary artery from left sinus of Valsalva
  - 5. Hypoplastic or aplastic coronary arteries
  - 6. Coronary-intracardiac shunt
- C. Coronary artery embolism
  - 1. Aortic or mitral endocarditis
  - 2. Prosthetic aortic or mitral valves
  - 3. Abnormal native valves or LV mural thrombus
  - 4. Platelet embolism
- D. Coronary arteritis
  - 1. Polyarteritis nodosa, progressive systemic sclerosis, giant cell arteritis
  - 2. Mucocutaneous lymph node syndrome (Kawasaki's disease)
  - 3. Syphilitic coronary ostial stenosis
- E. Miscellaneous mechanical obstruction of coronary arteries
  - 1. Coronary artery dissection in Marfan syndrome
  - 2. Coronary artery dissection in pregnancy
  - 3. Prolapse of aortic valve myxomatous polyps into coronary ostia
  - 4. Dissection or rupture of sinus of valsalva
- F. Functional obstruction of coronary arteries
  - 1. Coronary artery spasm with or without atherosclerosis
  - 2. Myocardial bridges

II. HYPERTROPHY OF VENTRICULAR MYOCARDIUM
- A. Left ventricular hypertrophy associated with coronary atherosclerosis
- B. Hypertensive heart disease without significant coronary atherosclerosis
- C. Hypertrophic myocardium secondary to valvular heart disease
- D. Hypertrophic cardiomyopathy
  - 1. Obstructive
  - 2. Nonobstructive
- E. Primary or secondary pulmonary hypertension
  - 1. Advanced chronic right ventricular overload
  - 2. Pulmonary hypertension in pregnancy

III. MYOCARDIAL DISEASES AND HEART FAILURE
- A. Chronic congestive heart failure
  - 1. Ischemic cardiomyopathy
  - 2. Idiopathic congestive cardiomyopathy
  - 3. Alcoholic cardiomyopathy
  - 4. Hypertensive cardiomyopathy
  - 5. Post-myocarditis cardiomyopathy
  - 6. Postpartum cardiomyopathy
- B. Acute cardiac failure
  - 1. Massive acute myocardial infarction
  - 2. Acute myocarditis
  - 3. Acute alcoholic cardiac dysfunction
  - 4. Ball-valve embolism in aortic stenosis or prosthesis
  - 5. Mechanical disruptions of cardiac structures
    - (a) Rupture of ventricular free wall
    - (b) Disruption of mitral apparatus
      - (1) Papillary muscle
      - (2) Chordae tendineae
      - (3) Leaflet
    - (c) Rupture of interventricular septum
  - 6. Acute pulmonary edema in noncompliant ventricles

IV. INFLAMMATORY, INFILTRATIVE, NEOPLASTIC, AND DEGENERATIVE PROCESSES
- A. Acute viral myocarditis with or without ventricular dysfunction
- B. Myocarditis associated with the vasculitides
- C. Sarcoidosis
- D. Progressive systemic sclerosis
- E. Amyloidosis
- F. Hemochromatosis
- G. Idiopathic giant cell myocarditis
- H. Chagas' disease
- I. Cardiac ganglionitis
- J. Arrhythmogenic right ventricular dysplasia
- K. Neuromuscular diseases (e.g., muscular dystrophy, Friedreich's ataxia, myotonic dystrophy)
- L. Intramural tumors
  - 1. Primary
  - 2. Metastatic
- M. Obstructive intracavitary tumors
  - 1. Neoplastic
  - 2. Thrombotic

V. DISEASES OF THE CARDIAC VALVES
- A. Valvular aortic stenosis/insufficiency
- B. Mitral valve disruption
- C. Mitral valve prolapse
- D. Endocarditis
- E. Prosthetic valve dysfunction

VI. CONGENITAL HEART DISEASE
- A. Congenital aortic or pulmonic valve stenosis
- B. Right-to-left shunts with Eisenmenger's physiology
  - 1. Advanced disease
  - 2. During labor and delivery
- C. After surgical repair of congenital lesions; e.g., tetralogy of Fallot

VII. ELECTROPHYSIOLOGIC ABNORMALITIES
- A. Abnormalities of the conducting system
  - 1. Fibrosis of the His-Purkinje system
    - (a) Primary degeneration (Lenègre's disease)
    - (b) Secondary to fibrosis and calcification of the "cardiac skeleton" (Lev's disease)
    - (c) Post-viral conducting system fibrosis
    - (d) Hereditary conducting system disease
  - 2. Anomalous pathways of conduction
- B. Prolonged Q-T interval syndrome
  - 1. Congenital
    - (a) With deafness
    - (b) Without deafness
  - 2. Acquired
    - (a) Drug effect
    - (b) Electrolyte abnormality
    - (c) Toxic substances
    - (d) Hypothermia
    - (e) CNS injury
- C. Idiopathic ventricular fibrillation
  - 1. Absence of identifiable structural or functional causes
  - 2. Sleep-death in Southeast Asians
    - (a) Bangungut
    - (b) Pokkuri
    - (c) Nonlaitai

VIII. ELECTRICAL INSTABILITY RELATED TO NEUROHUMORAL AND CENTRAL NERVOUS SYSTEM INFLUENCES
- A. Catecholamine-dependent lethal arrhythmias
- B. Central nervous system related
  - 1. Psychic stress, emotional extremes
  - 2. Auditory related
  - 3. "Voodoo" death in primitive cultures
  - 4. Diseases of the cardiac nerves
  - 5. Congenital Q-T interval prolongation

IX. SUDDEN INFANT DEATH SYNDROME AND SUDDEN DEATH IN CHILDREN
- A. Sudden infant death syndrome
  - 1. Immature respiratory control functions
  - 2. Susceptibility to lethal arrhythmias
  - 3. Congenital heart disease
  - 4. Myocarditis
- B. Sudden death in children
  - 1. Eisenmenger syndrome, aortic stenosis, hypertrophic cardiomyopathy, pulmonary atresia

Table continued on following page

TABLE 24–2 CAUSES AND CONTRIBUTING FACTORS IN SUDDEN CARDIAC DEATH *Continued*

IX. SUDDEN INFANT DEATH SYNDROME *Continued*
   2. After corrective surgery for congenital heart disease
   3. Myocarditis
   4. Unexplained

X. MISCELLANEOUS
   A. Sudden death during extreme physical activity
   B. Mechanical interference with venous return
      1. Acute cardiac tamponade
      2. Massive pulmonary embolism
      3. Acute intracardiac thrombosis
   C. Dissecting aneurysm of the aorta
   D. Toxic/metabolic disturbances
      1. Electrolyte disturbances
      2. Metabolic disturbances
      3. Proarrhythmic effects of antiarrhythmic drugs
      4. Proarrhythmic effects of noncardiac drugs
   E. Mimics of sudden cardiac death
      1. "Cafe coronary"
      2. Acute alcoholic states ("holiday heart")
      3. Acute asthmatic attacks
      4. Air or amniotic fluid embolism

24–4). Although the question of whether intervention with antiarrhythmic drugs alters risk of SCD in such patients has not yet been satisfactorily answered, it is the subject of intensive research. All of the studies reported to date have been limited by design features which make it impossible to answer the question of therapeutic efficacy.[90]

It has also been suggested that *left ventricular dysfunction* is a major co-factor for the risk implied by chronic PVC's after myocardial infarction,[82] and that both complex forms of PVC's and left ventricular dysfunction are independent predictors which exert lethal expressions most powerfully in different time periods after myocardial infarction. The risk of death indicated by post-myocardial infarction PVC's is therefore enhanced by the presence of left ventricular dysfunction, which appears to exert its influence most strongly in the first 6 months after infarction.[83] Finally, there are data suggesting that the risk associated with post-infarction complex PVC's is higher in patients who have non-Q wave infarctions than whose with transmural infarctions.[91]

CAUSES OF SUDDEN CARDIAC DEATH

Coronary heart disease and its consequences are the disease processes underlying at least 80 per cent of SCD's in Western cultures. It is also the most common cause in many of those areas of the world in which the prevalence of coronary heart disease is lower. Despite this established relationship between coronary heart disease and SCD,[92] a complete understanding of the problem of SCD requires the recognition of other etiologies which, although less common and often quite rare (Table 24–2), may be recognizable before death, may have therapeutic implications, and may provide broad insight into the sudden death problem.

CORONARY ARTERY ABNORMALITIES. Although structural abnormalities of coronary arteries other than coronary atherosclerosis are infrequent causes of SCD, the relative risk of SCD may be quite high for specific abnormalities. Nonatherosclerotic coronary artery abnormalities include congenital lesions, coronary artery embolism, coronary arteritis, and mechanical abnormalities of the coronary arteries. Among the congenital lesions, *anomalous origin of a left coronary artery from the pulmonary artery* (p. 927) is relatively common[93, 94] and has a high early death rate if not surgically treated.[95] The risk for SCD is not excessively high,[93] however, except in patients who survive to adulthood without surgical intervention.[94, 95] Other forms of coronary AV fistulas are much less frequent and have a low incidence of SCD. In contrast, *anomalous origin of a left coronary artery from the right or noncoronary aortic sinus of Valsalva* (p. 929) is a rare anomaly which appears to have a higher risk of SCD,[96–102] particularly when the anomalous artery passes between the aortic and pulmonary artery roots. *Anomalous origin of the right coronary artery from the left sinus of Valsalva* (p. 929) has also been reported in association with SCD,[98–102] but may not have the same risk as origin of the left coronary from the right sinus of Valsalva. Congenitally hypoplastic, stenotic, or atretic left coronary arteries are uncommon abnormalities which have a high risk of myocardial infarction but not of SCD.[93, 101]

Embolism to the coronary arteries occurs most commonly in aortic valve endocarditis and from thrombotic material on diseased or prosthetic aortic or mitral valves.[103] Emboli may also originate from left ventricular mural thrombi or iatrogenically as a consequence of surgery or cardiac catheterization. Symptoms of myocardial ischemia, and symptoms and signs of myocardial infarction, are the most common manifestations. However, in each of these categories SCD is a risk resulting from the electrophysiological consequences of the embolic ischemic event. Although embolism of platelet aggregates is a pathophysiological mechanism which has not clearly been demonstrated to be associated with SCD in clinical settings, some observations have recently focused attention on the feasibility of such a mechanism.[104, 105]

The mucocutaneous lymph node syndrome (Kawasaki's disease)[106, 107] (p. 1014) carries a risk of SCD in association with coronary arteritis. Polyarteritis nodosa and related vasculitis syndromes (p. 1722) can cause SCD presumably because of coronary arteritis,[108] as can coronary ostial stenosis in syphilitic aortitis[51] (p. 1566). The latter has become a very rare manifestation of syphilis.[109]

Several types of mechanical obstruction to coronary arteries must be listed among causes of SCD. Coronary dissection, with or without dissection of the aorta, occurs in the Marfan syndrome[110, 111] (p. 1725) and has also been reported in the peripartum period of pregnancy.[112] Among the rare mechanical causes of SCD are prolapse of myxomatous polyps from the aortic valve into coronary ostia[113] as well as dissection or rupture of a sinus of Valsalva aneurysm, with involvement of the coronary ostia and proximal coronary arteries.[114]

Coronary artery spasm (p. 294) may cause serious arrhythmias and SCD[115, 116] with or without concomitant coronary atherosclerotic lesions.[115] Painless myocardial ischemia,[117] associated with either spasm or fixed lesions, may be a cause of heretofore unexplained sudden death.[118, 119] Finally, deep *myocardial bridges* over coronary arteries (p. 284) have been reported in association with SCD during strenous exercise.[120]

VENTRICULAR HYPERTROPHY. Hypertrophic muscle is a common denominator among many causes of SCD,[121] has been identified as an independent risk factor for SCD,[6] and may be a factor in propensity to potentially lethal arrhythmias.[121–123] The underlying states resulting in hypertrophy include hypertensive heart disease with or without atherosclerosis, valvular heart disease, obstructive and nonobstructive hypertrophic cardiomyopathy, primary pulmonary hypertension with right ventricular hypertrophy, and advanced right ventricular overload secondary to congenital heart disease. Each of these conditions is associated with risk of SCD, and it has been suggested that patients with severely hypertrophic ventricles are particularly susceptible to arrhythmic death.[121]

Hypertrophic Obstructive Cardiomyopathy (p. 1418). A risk of SCD in hypertrophic obstructive cardiomyopathy was identified in the early clinical and hemodynamic studies of this entity.[48] Two subsequent large series have yielded similar data on the magnitude of this risk. Goodwin[124] observed 48 deaths, of which 32 (67 per cent) were sudden, among a cohort of 254 patients followed for a mean of 6 years, while Shah et al.[125] reported that 26 of 49 deaths (55 per cent) among 190 patients were sudden. Specific clinical markers have not been especially predictive of SCD in individual patients, although young age,[124, 126] strong family history,[49, 124] and worsening symptoms[124] appear to indicate higher risk. In one study, however, 54 per cent of the sudden deaths occurred in patients without any functional limitations.[126] The mechanism of SCD in patients with hypertrophic obstructive cardiomyopathy was initially thought to involve outflow tract obstruction, possibly as a consequence of catecholamine stimulation, but more recent data have focused on cardiac arrhythmias as a probable mechanism of sudden death in this disease.[121, 127–130] These studies have demonstrated a high prevalence of high-risk or potentially lethal arrhythmias on ambulatory monitoring[127, 129] or the inducibility of potentially lethal arrhythmias during invasive electrophysiological testing.[130, 131] The question of whether the pathogenesis of the arrhythmias represents an interaction between electrophysiological and hemodynamic abnormalities or is a consequence of electrophysiological derangement of hypertrophied muscle[121–123] is unanswered as of this writing. The observation that patients with nonobstructive hypertrophic cardiomyopathy have high-risk arrhythmias and are at increased risk for SCD[127] suggests that an electrophysiological mechanism secondary to the hypertrophied muscle itself plays some role. Stafford and colleagues[132] reported exercise-related cardiac arrest in nonobstructive hypertrophic cardiomyopathy. Ventricular fibrillation (VF) was reproduced during electrophysiological testing after induction of atrial fibrillation with a rapid ventricular response. In athletes under 35 years of age, hypertrophic cardiomyopathy is the most common cause of SCD, in contrast to athletes over the age of 35 among whom ischemic heart disease is the most common cause.[100, 102, 133–135]

HEART FAILURE AND SUDDEN DEATH. The advent of therapeutic interventions which provide better long-term control of the symptoms of congestive heart failure has not yet resulted in improved long-term survival of such patients. However, the proportion of heart failure patients with stable hemodynamics who die suddenly appears to be increasing.[136] In reports to date, as many as 47 per cent of deaths in heart failure patients are categorized as SCD's.

The interaction between post-myocardial infarction ventricular arrhythmia and depressed ejection fraction in determining risk for SCD has been described.[82, 83] The majority of studies addressing the relationship between chronic congestive heart failure and SCD focused on patients with ischemic idiopathic and alcoholic congestive cardiomyopathy.[86, 136–140] A chronic myopathic syndrome after myocarditis has been cited as an infrequent but well-documented cause of SCD.[141] Postpartum cardiomyopathy (p. 1866) may also cause SCD.

Acute Heart Failure. All causes of acute cardiac failure, in the absence of prompt interventions, may result in SCD resulting from either the circulatory failure itself or secondary arrhythmias. The electrophysiological mechanisms involved have been proposed to be related to acute stretching of myocardial fibers and/or the His-Purkinje system, with its experimentally demonstrated arrhythmogenic effect,[142] but the roles of neurohumoral mechanisms and acute electrolyte shifts have not been fully evaluated.[136] Among the causes of acute cardiac failure which are associated with SCD are massive acute myocardial infarction, acute myocarditis, acute alcoholic cardiac dysfunction, and a number of mechanical causes of heart failure such as massive pulmonary embolism, mechanical disruption of intracardiac structures secondary to infarction or infection, and ball valve embolism to the outflow tract in aortic or mitral stenosis (Table 24–2).

INFLAMMATORY, INFILTRATIVE, NEOPLASTIC, AND DEGENERATIVE DISEASES OF THE HEART. Almost all diseases in this category have been associated with SCD, with or without concomitant cardiac failure. Acute viral myocarditis with left ventricular dysfunction (p. 1442) is commonly associated with cardiac arrhythmias, including potentially lethal arrhythmias: It is now recognized that serious ventricular arrhythmias or SCD can occur in myocarditis in the absence of clinical evidence of left ventricular dysfunction.[51, 141, 143] Viral carditis also may cause damage isolated to the specialized conducting system and result in a propensity to arrhythmias; the rare association of this process with SCD has been reported.[144–146] The risk of potentially lethal arrhythmias is not limited to the acute phase of the disease.[141]

Myocardial involvement in collagen vascular disorders, tumors, chronic granulomatous diseases, infiltrative disorders, and protozoan infestations varies widely, but in all instances, SCD may be the initial or terminal manifestation of the disease process. Among the granulomatous diseases, *sarcoidosis* (p. 1434) stands out because of the frequency of SCD. Roberts et al.[147] reported that SCD was the terminal event in 67 per cent of sarcoid heart disease deaths; the occurrence of SCD has been related to the extent of cardiac involvement.[148] In a report on the pathological findings in nine patients who died of *progressive systemic sclerosis* (p. 1723), eight who died suddenly had evidence of transient ischemia and reperfusion histologically, suggesting that this might represent Raynaud-like involvement of coronary vessels.[149] In contrast, *arrhythmogenic right ventricular dysplasia* (p. 697) is associated with a high incidence of arrhythmias, particularly recurrent ventricular tachycardia, but the frequency of SCD appears to be relatively low.[150] *Amyloidosis* of the heart (p. 1431) may also cause sudden death. An incidence of 30 per cent has been reported[151]; diffuse involvement of ventricular muscle or of the specialized conducting system may be associated with SCD.[152–154]

DISEASES OF THE CARDIAC VALVES. Prior to the advent of surgery for valvular heart disease, *aortic stenosis* was one of the more common noncoronary causes of SCD. Campbell reported in 1968 that 44 of 70 (73 per cent) deaths in patients with aortic stenosis were sudden.[155] The advent of safe and effective procedures for aortic valve replacement has reduced the incidence of this cause of sudden death,[156] but patients with prosthetic or heterograft aortic valve replacements remain at some risk for SCD due to arrhythmias, prosthetic valve dysfunction, or coexistent coronary heart disease.[157] SCD has been reported to be the second most common mode of death after valve replacement surgery, accounting for 62 of 298 deaths (21 per cent).[158] The incidence peaked 3 weeks after operation and then plateaued after 8 months. Nonetheless, the risk is appreciably lower than in those patients who had not had the advantage of valvular surgery in prior years. A high incidence of ventricular arrhythmia has been observed during follow-up of patients with valve replacement, especially in those who had aortic stenosis, multiple valve surgery, or cardiomegaly.[159] Sudden death during follow-up was associated with ventricular arrhythmias and thromboembolism. Hemodynamic variables were less predictive. Although all valvular stenotic lesions are associated with some risk for SCD, valvular regurgitation, particularly chronic aortic regurgitation and acute mitral regurgitation, may also be associated with SCD.

Mitral valve prolapse (p. 1045) is prevalent and is associated with a high incidence of cardiac arrhythmias; however, the incidence of SCD is quite low.[160, 161] This complication appears to correlate with nonspecific ST-T wave changes in the inferior leads on the electrocardiogram.[162] In data reviewed from 17 reported instances of

SCD in mitral valve prolapse patients, these nonspecific ST-T wave changes were present in 6 of 8 who had had antemortem electrocardiograms.[163] An association with redundancy of mitral leaflets on echocardiogram has also been suggested.[164] Reported associations between Q-T interval prolongation or preexcitation and SCD in mitral prolapse syndrome are less consistent.[161]

Endocarditis of the aortic and mitral valves (see Chap. 34) may be associated with rapid death resulting from acute disruption of the valvular apparatus, coronary embolism, or abscesses of valvular rings or the septum; however, such deaths are rarely true sudden deaths as conventionally defined.

CONGENITAL HEART DISEASE. The congenital lesions most commonly associated with SCD are aortic stenosis[143, 165, 166] (pp. 932 and 937) and communications between the left and right sides of the heart with Eisenmenger syndrome[167] (pp. 932 and 937). In the latter, the risk of SCD is a function of pulmonary vascular disease severity; also, there is an extraordinarily high risk of maternal mortality during labor and delivery in the pregnant patient with Eisenmenger syndrome (p. 1856).[168] Potentially lethal arrhythmias and SCD have been described as late complications after surgical repair of complex congenital lesions, particularly tetralogy of Fallot[169] (p. 946), transposition of the great arteries,[170] and atrioventricular canal.[171] These patients should be followed closely and treated aggressively when cardiac arrhythmias are identified.[171]

ELECTROPHYSIOLOGICAL ABNORMALITIES. Acquired disease of the AV node and His-Purkinje system and the presence of accessory pathways of conduction are two groups of structural abnormalities of specialized conduction which may be associated with SCD. Epidemiological studies have suggested that intraventricular conduction disturbances in coronary heart disease are one of the few factors that may increase the proportion of SCD in coronary heart disease.[35] A specific clinical example is the risk of VF during the first 30 days after myocardial infarction in patients with anterior infarctions and bundle branch block. Lie et al.[172] reported that 47 per cent of patients who had late hospital VF had had anteroseptal infarcts with bundle branch block, and that these 14 were from a total pool of only 40 patients with the combination of bundle branch block and anterior myocardial infarction. Thus, there was a 35 per cent incidence of VF in this subgroup, which represented only 4.1 per cent of a total of 966 myocardial infarctions. This risk persists for 6 weeks after the infarction and then abates.[173] AV block or intraventricular conduction abnormalities were found in 9 of 10 patients who had recurrent VF during hospitalization after resuscitation from prehospital cardiac arrest.[20]

Primary fibrosis (Lenegre's disease)[174] or secondary mechanical injury (Lev's disease)[175] of the His-Purkinje system is commonly associated with intraventricular conduction abnormalities and symptomatic AV block, and less commonly with SCD. The identification of individuals at risk and efficacy of pacemakers for preventing SCD, rather than only ameliorating symptoms, has been the subject of debate.[176, 177] Survival may depend more on the nature and extent of the underlying disease than on the conduction disturbance itself.[178] Patients with congenital AV block (Chap. 30) or nonprogressive congenital intraventricular block generally have a low risk of SCD.[179, 180] Progressive congenital intraventricular blocks predict a high risk,[52–54, 180] and a hereditary form has been reported in association with a familial propensity to SCD.[53, 54, 180]

The anomalous pathways of conduction, bundles of Kent in the Wolff-Parkinson-White syndrome, and Mahaim fibers are commonly associated with nonlethal arrhythmias. However, when the anomalous pathways of conduction have very short refractory periods, the occurrence of atrial fibrillation may allow the induction of VF during very rapid conduction across the bypass tract.[181–183] The incidence of SCD in patients with short refractory period bypass tracts is not yet known. Patients who have multiple pathways appear to be at higher risk of SCD.[181]

Q-T PROLONGATION (See also p. 699). The prolonged Q-T interval syndrome is a functional abnormality, perhaps associated with neurogenic influences, that may cause lethal arrhythmias.[184] In the hereditary *congenital form* two varieties have been reported, those with autosomal recessive inheritance and associated deafness, the Jervell and Lange-Nielsen syndrome,[45, 185] and those without deafness, the Romano-Ward syndrome).[46, 47] Some patients have prolonged Q-T intervals throughout life without any manifest arrhythmias, while others are highly susceptible to ventricular arrhythmias, particularly the torsades de pointes form of ventricular tachycardia[186]; SCD is a risk of the abnormality in these patients. Patients at higher risk are characterized by deafness, female gender, syncope, and documented torsades de pointes or prior ventricular fibrillation, and they require aggressive medical or surgical interventions.[187, 188]

The *acquired form* of prolonged Q-T interval may be due to drug idiosyncrasies (particularly antiarrhythmics and psychotropic drugs), electrolyte abnormalities, hypothermia, toxic substances, and central nervous system injury.[188] It has also been reported in both intensive weight reduction programs involving the use of liquid protein diets[189–191] and in anorexia nervosa.[192] Lithium carbonate may prolong the Q-T interval and has been reported to be associated with an increased incidence of SCD in cancer patients with preexisting heart disease.[193] Acquired prolonged Q-T intervals generally carry a risk of serious arrhythmias and SCD, but the risk is abolished when the inciting factor is removed. In acquired prolonged Q-T syndrome, as in the congenital form, the torsades de pointes form of VT is commonly the specific arrhythmia triggering or degenerating into lethal VF.

ELECTRICAL INSTABILITY DUE TO NEUROHUMORAL AND CENTRAL NERVOUS SYSTEM INFLUENCES. Catecholamine-dependent lethal arrhythmias in the absence of Q-T interval prolongation with control by beta-adrenoreceptor blocking agents have been described.[194] Several central nervous system–related interactions with cardiac electrical stability have been suggested. The hereditary forms of prolonged Q-T interval syndrome, discussed above, appear to have a relationship to sympathetic nervous system imbalance.[184, 195, 196] Lown and coworkers identified psychic stress as a mediating factor for advanced cardiac arrhythmias and perhaps SCD.[197–199] Epidemiological data also suggest an association between behavioral abnormalities and the risk of SCD, particularly in women,[66, 67] and emotional extremes have been suggested as a triggering mechanism for SCD.[3, 200–202] Associations between auditory stimulation[143, 203] and auditory auras[204] and SCD have been reported.[143, 203] The auditory abnormalities in some forms of congenital Q-T prolongation have already been cited.[45, 185]

The syndrome of so-called "voodoo deaths" in underdeveloped cultures was studied extensively.[205, 206] There appears to be an association between isolation from the tribe, a sense of hopelessness, severe bradyarrhythmias, and sudden death. With cultural changes in these areas the syndrome is less amenable to observation and study; however, there do remain pockets of cultural isolation in which the syndrome no doubt still exists.

SUDDEN INFANT DEATH SYNDROME AND SCD IN CHIL-

DREN. The sudden infant death syndrome occurs between birth and 6 months of age, more commonly in males, and has an incidence of 0.1 to 0.3 per cent of live births.[207] Because of its abrupt nature, a cardiac mechanism had been sought for many years.[208–210] but a variety of causes, with respiratory dysfunction playing a major role, are considered likely.[211] It is believed that many cases of the sudden infant death syndrome represent a form of "sleep apnea" which, if prolonged, may lead to hypoxia, cyanosis, and cardiac arrhythmias. Experience with "near-misses" and the results of respiratory monitoring, in conjunction with the propensity of the syndrome to occur in premature infants, all suggested impaired central nervous system respiratory control reflexes, possibly due to immaturity.[207, 211–214] However, recently there has been interest in the possibility of obstructive apnea as another possible mechanism.[211] Identification of individual infants at risk is difficult, but it is clear that the risk does not persist beyond the first 6 months of life.

Despite the current focus on the respiratory mechanisms involved in the syndrome, their role has not yet been explicity established.[212] Furthermore, the question of whether or not an identifiable subset of infants who have apneic spells are particularly prone to genesis of cardiac arrhythmias remains conjectural.[213–215] A primary cardiac etiology is still considered as the basis in some victims of this syndrome.[211, 215] Thus, Marino and Kane[216] observed either accessory pathways (two cases) or dispersed or immature AV nodal or bundle branch cells in the annulus fibrosis (four cases) among a group of seven sudden infant death syndrome victims studied by detailed histopathology.

SCD in children beyond the age group at risk for sudden infant death syndrome is often associated with identifiable heart disease,[142, 217] although one study identified cardiac causes in only 25 per cent of sudden natural death victims between the ages of 1 and 21 years.[37] Approximately 25 per cent of SCD's in children occur in those who have undergone previous surgery for congenital cardiac disease. Of the remaining 75 per cent, over one-half occur in children who have one of four lesions: congenital aortic stenosis, Eisenmenger syndrome, pulmonary stenosis or atresia, and obstructive hypertrophic cardiomyopathy.[217] Neuspiel and Kuller[37] observed 14 cases of myocarditis among 51 SCD's in children (27 per cent).

Other Causes of Sudden Death

SCD in athletes during or after extreme physical activity is infrequent but receives a great deal of attention when it does occur. The majority of such individuals have a previously unrecognized cardiac abnormality, with hypertrophic cardiomyopathy with or without obstruction, valvular aortic stenosis, and occult coronary artery disease as the most common etiologies identified after death.[101, 102, 133–135, 218, 219] However, a small group of such victims have neither previously determined functional abnormality nor structural abnormalities at postmortem examination.[20, 100, 102, 141, 142]

There are rare instances of idiopathic VF causing SCD in the absence of any identifiable structural or functional abnormality of the heart.[220] Such syndromes are of concern because the individual patient remains at risk for recurrence after surviving an initial event. In addition, these events tend to occur in young, otherwise healthy individuals. A specific variation of this syndrome has been observed in southeast Asians. Many years ago, syndromes referred to as *Bangungut* in young Filipino males,[221] *Pokkuri* in young Japanese males,[222] and *Nonlaitai* in young Laotian males[223] were reported. In each, there was a tendency for sudden death to occur during sleep, and at one time a toxic cause was suspected.[221, 222] However, documented cases have now been reported in Laotians who came to the United States after the Vietnam War. The mechanism was identified to be VF in some of these cases; in at least one instance, electrophysiological study demonstrated inducible VT by programmed electrical stimulation.[224] The fact that these cases continue to occur in a new cultural setting suggests that there may be a hereditary predisposition.

There are also a number of noncardiac conditions which *mimic SCD.* These include the so-called *cafe coronary,*[225, 226] in which food, usually an unchewed piece of meat, lodges in the oropharynx and causes an abrupt obstruction at the glottis. The classical description of a cafe coronary is sudden cyanosis and collapse in a restaurant, with lively conversation usually accompanying the meal. The *holiday heart syndrome* is characterized by cardiac arrhythmias, most commonly atrial, and other cardiac abnormalities associated with acute alcoholic states.[227] It has not been determined whether potentially lethal arrhythmias occurring in such settings account for reported sudden deaths associated with acute alcoholic states.[3] *Massive pulmonary embolism* (Chap. 47) may cause acute cardiovascular collapse and sudden death; sudden death in severe acute asthmatic attacks, without prolonged deterioration of the patient's condition, is well recognized.[228] Air or amnionic fluid embolism at the time of labor and delivery may cause sudden death on rare occasions, with the clinical picture mimicking sudden cardiac death.[229] Peripartum air embolism caused by an unusual sexual practice has been reported as a cause of such sudden deaths.[230]

Proarrhythmic effects of antiarrhythmic drugs have received particular attention,[231, 232] but psychotropic drugs, arrhythmogenic effects of toxic substances, and electrolyte disturbances—particularly hypokalemia, hypocalcemia, and hypomagnesemia—have also been implicated.[188] The proarrhythmic effects resulting in worsening of arrhythmias is more commonly associated with normal than with prolonged Q-T intervals, and therefore is difficult to predict.[231, 232]

Finally, a number of abnormalities not directly involving the heart may cause SCD or mimic it. These include aortic dissection (p. 1554), acute cardiac tamponade (p. 1492), and rapid exsanguination (Chap. 45).

PATHOLOGY AND PATHOPHYSIOLOGY OF SUDDEN DEATH

Pathological observations in SCD victims reflect the epidemiological and clinical preponderance of coronary heart disease as the major structural predisposing factor.[233] Liberthson and coworkers[234] reported that 81 per cent of 220 autopsied victims of SCD had pathological findings of coronary heart disease as the major etiological factor, i.e., more than one coronary vessel with more than 75 per cent stenosis. At least one vessel with more than 75 per cent stenosis was found in 94 per cent of victims, acute coronary occlusion in 58 per cent, healed myocardial infarction in 44 per cent, and acute myocardial infarction in 27 per cent. These observations are consistent with many other studies of the frequency of coronary disease in sudden death victims. The numerous other specific causes of SCD collectively account for no more than 10 to 20 per cent of cases, but they have provided a large base of enlightening pathological data.[51, 141]

THE PATHOLOGY OF SUDDEN DEATH DUE TO CORONARY HEART DISEASE

THE CORONARY ARTERIES. Extensive atherosclerosis is the most common pathological finding in the coronary arteries of victims of SCD (Table 24–3). In postmortem

TABLE 24–3 PATHOLOGICAL FINDINGS IN SUDDEN DEATH DUE TO CORONARY HEART DISEASE

The Coronary Arteries	Ventricular Myocardium
A. Chronic atherosclerosis	A. Healed myocardial infarction
B. Acute lesions	B. Left ventricular hypertrophy
1. Plaque fissuring	C. Ventricular aneurysm
2. Platelet aggregates	D. Acute myocardial infarction
3. Acute thrombus	
4. Organizing thrombus	
5. Coronary artery spasm	

examinations of 169 hearts, sites of 75 per cent or more stenosis were present in 3 or 4 of the major vessels in 61 per cent of the hearts studied; 2 vessels with 75 per cent or more stenosis were found in 15 per cent, and 24 per cent of the hearts had either single-vessel disease or no vessels having lesions producing 75 per cent stenosis.[235] A distinctly higher proportion of hearts having 3 or 4 vessels with 75 per cent stenotic lesions occurred in white males (70 per cent) compared with white females (34 per cent). In contrast, 58 per cent of the hearts of both black males and black females had 3 or 4 vessels with 75 per cent or more stenoses. Consistent with clinical findings in survivors of prehospital cardiac arrest,[20] there was no special predilection of disease distribution for any coronary artery, and there was no quantitative difference between proximal and distal distribution of disease. Kuller et al.[57] pointed out that 90 per cent or greater narrowing of at least one coronary artery was found in 77 per cent of autopsied victims of sudden *coronary* death, compared with 8 per cent of victims of other causes of sudden death. Davies[51] reported that 61 per cent of patients dying suddenly due to coronary heart disease had 3 vessels with 75 per cent or more stenosis at any one point; an additional 18 (23 per cent) had 2 vessels with 75 per cent or more stenosis. Among 100 age- and sex-matched controls who died of trauma or cerebral tumors, only 27 per cent had 2- or 3-vessel disease, and 52 per cent had no vessels with lesions of 75 per cent or more. In the same study, the majority of sudden deaths due to coronary heart disease were associated with at least one point of more than 85 per cent stenosis (Fig. 24–5), and Davies suggested that this parameter provided the best discrimination between hearts of SCD victims and controls.

Roberts and colleagues[236, 237] have quantitated coronary artery narrowing at postmortem examination of sudden coronary death victims and controls. Thirty-six per cent of 5 mm segments of the coronary arteries from the SCD group had 76 to 100 per cent cross-sectional area reductions compared with 3 per cent in the controls. An additional 34 per cent of the sections from the SCD group had 51 to 75 per cent reductions in cross-sectional areas. Only 7 per cent of the sections from the SCD patients had 0 to 25 per cent reductions in cross-sectional areas. The *distribution* of the lesions causing greater than 75 per cent narrowing was similar in the three major coronary arteries, but quantitative differences between proximal and distal halves of the vessels were inconsistent.[236, 237] Similar conclusions resulted from pathological observations of prehospital cardiac arrest victims who were not successfully resuscitated.[234] These studies, taken together, lead to the conclusions that extensive coronary artery disease is the pathological hallmark for the large percentage of SCD's due to coronary heart disease and that there is no specific anatomical pattern of distribution of the disease which preselects SCD victims.

The role of acute *coronary artery thrombosis* as a factor in precipitating SCD is less clear.[238–250] In one study of 100 consecutive sudden coronary death victims, 44 per cent had major (more than 50 per cent luminal occlusion) recent coronary thrombi, 30 per cent had minor occlusive thrombi, and 21 per cent had plaque fissuring.[241] Only 5 per cent had no acute coronary artery changes; 65 per cent of the thrombi occurred at sites of preexisting high-grade stenoses, and an additional 19 per cent were found at sites of more than 50 per cent stenosis. An overview of the major studies on the incidence of acute thrombotic occlusions, in which the definition of sudden death ranges from 15 minutes to 24 hours, reveals wide variation in the reported frequency of recent coronary thrombosis in sudden death. It ranged from 15 to 64 per cent, but the majority of studies which used 6 hours or less as the definition of "sudden" had frequencies of less than 40 per cent.[105, 233, 234, 238–250] Factors which confound the analysis of such data include relationships between platelet aggregates and thrombus formation and the spontaneous lysis of clots.

Baba et al.[247] reported the presence of *organizing* thrombus in approximately 31 per cent of 121 sudden coronary heart disease deaths. They were commonly associated with sites of more than 75 per cent chronic obstruction and with concomitant acute lesions at the same sites, leading to the speculation that clinical events 5 to 7 days before death might create a substrate for fatal acute coronal events. *Coronary artery spasm*, an established cause of acute ischemia, may also cause SCD, and is recognizable in rare instances at postmortem examination.[251]

THE MYOCARDIUM. Myocardial pathology in SCD due to coronary heart disease reflects the extensive chronic atherosclerosis which is usually present. Studies in nonsurvivors of prehospital cardiac arrest, from epidemiological sources, and medical examiner studies indicate that healed myocardial infarction is a common finding in sudden coronary death victims, with most investigators reporting

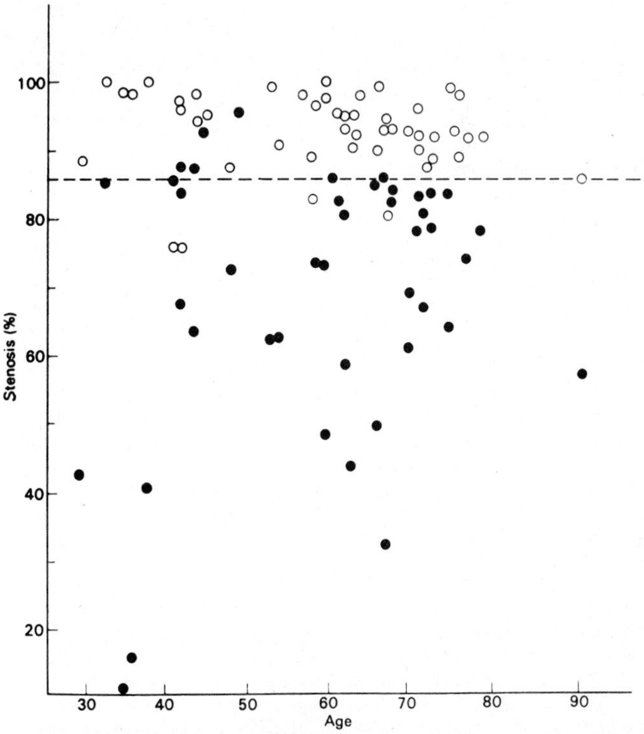

FIGURE 24–5. Comparison of the degree of stenosis of the worst single segment at any site in the main coronary arteries, right, left anterior descending, and left circumflex in males. Solid circles = control subjects, open circles = ischemic sudden death. The data suggest that over 85 per cent stenosis is found in most cases of sudden ischemic deaths; less than 75 per cent stenosis is not associated with sudden death. (From Davies, M. J., and Popple, A. W.: Sudden unexpected cardiac death—a practical approach to the forensic problem. Histopathology *3*:255, 1979.)

frequencies ranging from 40 to more than 70 per cent.[8, 220, 242, 252–256] For example, Newman and coworkers[252, 253] reported that 72 per cent of males in a 25 to 44 year age group who died suddenly (24 or fewer hours) with no previous clinical history of coronary heart disease had scars of large (63 per cent) or small (less than 1 cm cross-sectional area, 9 per cent) areas of healed myocardial necrosis. The incidence of acute myocardial infarction is considerably less, with pathological evidence of recent myocardial infarction averaging approximately 20 per cent. Even though the problem of pathological recognition of early acute myocardial infarction confounds some of these observations, the figures fit quite well with studies in out-of-hospital cardiac arrest survivors which suggest that the incidence of evolution of new myocardial infarction is in the range of 20 to 30 per cent.

VENTRICULAR HYPERTROPHY AND SUDDEN DEATH

Myocardial hypertrophy may interact with acute or chronic ischemia, but the nature of the interaction in SCD is incompletely understood.[257] The correlation between increased heart weight and severity of coronary heart disease in SCD victims is not close[235]; heart weights are higher in SCD victims than in those with non-sudden death despite similar prevalence of history of hypertension prior to death.[8] Anderson[121] interprets these observations to suggest that LV hypertrophy itself may be a predisposing factor to SCD. Although there are data to suggest increased susceptibility to potentially lethal ventricular arrhythmias in patients with left ventricular hypertrophy of many etiologies,[122, 258–260] the study by Roberts and Podolak[261] on massively enlarged hearts (i.e., more than 1000 gm) did not indicate an excess incidence of SCD in such patients. However, the underlying pathology in that study was dominated by lesions producing volume overload.

SPECIALIZED CONDUCTING SYSTEM IN SCD

Pathological data on the specialized conducting system of victims of SCD are surprisingly sparse. Lie[262] studied the specialized conducting system of 49 of 120 SCD patients with no previous history of coronary heart disease who died within 6 hours of onset of symptoms. Thirty-nine patients had acute myocardial infarction and 10 did not. Two patients with acute anteroseptal infarctions had hemorrhage and/or infarction involving the AV node and peripheral bundle branches. Luminal narrowing of the artery to the AV node was present in 50 per cent, but there were no thromboses of vessels to the specialized conducting system. Evidence of ischemic injury was present to an equal frequency in SCD[262] and myocardial infarction patients.[263]

Fibrosis of the specialized conducting system is a common but nonspecific endpoint of multiple etiologies. While this process is associated with AV block or intraventricular conduction abnormalities, its role in SCD is uncertain. Both Lev's and Lenegre's diseases, ischemic injury due to small vessel disease, and numerous infiltrative or inflammatory processes all may result in such changes (Table 24–4). In addition, active inflammatory processes such as myocarditis and infiltrative processes such as amyloidosis, scleroderma, hemochromatosis, and morbid obesity all may damage or destroy the AV node and/or bundle of His and result in AV block.[264] Focal diseases such as sarcoidosis, Whipple's disease, and rheumatoid arthritis may also involve the conducting system. These various categories of conducting system disease have been considered as possible pathological substrates for SCD which may be overlooked because of the difficulty in doing careful postmortem examinations of the conducting system routinely.[264] Focal involvement of conducting tissue by tumors (especially mesothelioma of the AV node but also lymphoma, carcinoma, rhabdomyoma, and fibroma) has also been reported,[246] and rare cases of SCD have been associated with these lesions. It has been suggested that abnormal postnatal morphogenesis of the specialized conducting system may be a significant factor in some SCD's in infants and children.[264]

TABLE 24–4 PATHOLOGICAL CHANGES IN THE CARDIAC NERVE IN SUDDEN CARDIAC DEATH

SPECIALIZED CONDUCTION SYSTEM

A. Chronic fibrosis
   1. Primary
   2. Secondary
B. Acute ischemic injury
C. Inflammatory and infiltrative diseases
D. Focal diseases—granulomas, tumors
E. Arteritis
F. Abnormal postnatal morphogenesis

CARDIAC NERVES

A. Cardiac plexus disruption
B. Neural depletion in cardiomyopathy
C. Viral neuropathy
D. Neural ganglionitis
E. Neurotoxic injury
F. Hereditary neuropathy
G. Extrinsic nerve abnormalities

CARDIONEUROPATHY AND SCD

Diseases of cardiac nerves have recently received attention for their possible role in SCD.[265, 266] Cardiac neural involvement may be the result of random damage to neural elements within the myocardium (i.e., "secondary" cardioneuropathy), or may be "primary" such as in a selective cardiac viral neuropathy.[266] Secondary involvement may be a consequence of ischemic neural injury in coronary heart disease and has been postulated to result in autonomic destabilization, enhancing the propensity to arrhythmias. There is some experimental data in support of this hypothesis.[267–269] Involvement of neural plexes, with or without conducting system involvement, has been observed at necropsy in 54 per cent of patients who died within 24 hours of onset of myocardial infarction.[265] Specific etiologies for primary cardioneuropathies are less obvious. Viral, neurotoxic, and hereditary causes (e.g., progressive muscular dystrophy and Friedreich's ataxia) have been emphasized.

Disordered extrinsic neural involvement of the heart is generally considered to be functional, such as in prolonged Q-T interval syndrome; however, stellate ganglion inflammation has been observed in some tissues removed surgically for symptomatic Q-T prolongation in hereditary Q-T syndrome[270] or after myocardial infarction.[271] The possible significance of such extrinsic cardiac neural involvement is not yet clear.[271]

MECHANISMS AND PATHOPHYSIOLOGY OF CARDIAC ARREST

The occurrence of potentially lethal tachyarrhythmias, or of severe bradyarrhythmia or asystole, is the end of a cascade of pathophysiological abnormalities which result from complex interactions between coronary vascular events, myocardial injury, variations in autonomic tone, and/or the metabolic and electrolyte state of the myocardium. There is no uniform hypothesis regarding mechanisms by which these elements interact to lead to the final pathway of lethal arrhythmias, and it is likely that multiple combinations and permutations of dysfunction lead to the same endpoint.

Pathophysiological Mechanisms of Lethal Tachyarrhythmias

CORONARY ARTERY STRUCTURE AND FUNCTION. In that large majority of SCD's associated with coronary atherosclerosis, the distribution of chronic arterial narrowing has been well defined by pathological studies.[51, 233, 234, 236, 238] However, the specific mechanisms by which these lesions lead to potentially lethal disturbances of electrical stability are poorly understood. Steady-state reductions in regional myocardial blood flow, in the absence of superimposed acute lesions, may create a setting in which alterations in the metabolic or electrolyte state of the myocardium, or neural fluctuations will result in loss of electrical stability.[136] Increased myocardial oxygen demand with a fixed supply may be the mechanism of exercise-induced arrhythmias and sudden death during intense physical activity in athletes or others whose heart disease had not previously become clinically manifested.[100, 102, 133–135, 218, 219, 272] Vasoactive events leading to acute reduction in regional myocardial blood flow in the presence of a normal or previously compromized circulation constitute a common cause of transient ischemia, angina pectoris, arrhythmias, and perhaps SCD.[115, 119, 273] Coronary artery spasm or modulation of coronary collateral flow exposes the myocardium to the double hazard of transient ischemia and reperfusion.[274] The mechanism of production of spasm is unclear, although sites of endothelial disease appear to predispose.[275] A role of the autonomic nervous system, particularly mechanisms related to alpha-adrenoceptor activity, has been suggested[276–281]; vagal activity may also be involved in the production of spasm.[278, 282] However, neurogenic influences do not appear to be a sine qua non for the production of spasm. Vessel susceptibility and humoral factors, particularly those related to platelet activation and aggregation,[283] must also be considered.

Recent studies have refocused attention on platelet aggregation or thrombosis or both as key events in the initiation of lethal arrhythmias.[105, 233, 241, 246, 284] Chronic stable atherosclerotic plaques appear to undergo endothelial damage, with plaque fissuring, leading to platelet activation and aggregation, followed by thrombosis. In addition to initiating the thrombus, platelet activation produces a series of biochemical alterations which may enhance or retard susceptibility to VF via vasomotor modulation.[285] The frequency of VF induced by acute coronary occlusion in dogs has been markedly reduced by prostacyclin at doses sufficient to prevent platelet aggregation.[286] Hammon and Oates studied the effects of thromboxane synthetase inhibitors[285] and demonstrated protection against the induction of experimental VF, presumably by blocking conversion of PGH_2 to thromboxane A_2, which theoretically shunts accumulated PGH_2 to metabolic pathways favoring conversion to prostacyclin. Inhibition of cyclooxygenase by concurrent indomethacin administration gave further support to the hypothesis that PGH_2 shunting to other prostaglandin pathways might protect against VF by prostacyclin production. The possibility that inhibition of prostacyclin production might enchance the risk of VF[285] is supported by the finding from the Aspirin-Myocardial Infarction Study that the incidence of recurrent myocardial infarction is reduced by aspirin, but the relative and perhaps absolute numbers of SCD tended to increase.[287]

A number of pieces of indirect evidence support the possibility that more than the mechanical consequences to flow is involved in platelet-activated thrombosis of coronary arteries in SCD. Davies and Thomas[241] pointed out that 95 of 100 subjects who died suddenly (fewer than 6 hours after the onset of symptoms) had acute coronary thrombi, plaque fissuring, or both. This incidence was considerably higher than in many previous reports, but it is noteworthy that only 44 per cent of the patients had the largest thrombus occluding 51 per cent or more of the cross-sectional area of the involved vessel, and only 18 per cent of the patients had more than 75 per cent occlusion. This raises questions whether mechanical obstruction to flow was dominant, or whether the high incidence of nonoccluding thrombi simply reflected the state of activation of the platelets. The discrepancy between the relatively high incidence of acute thrombi in postmortem studies and the low incidence of evolution of new myocardial infarction among survivors of out-of-hospital VF[18–20, 288] highlights this question. Spontaneous thrombolysis or a dominant role of spasm induced by platelet products, or a combination, may explain this discrepancy.

THE UNSTABLE MYOCARDIUM AND INITIATION OF LETHAL ARRHYTHMIAS. The onset of acute ischemia produces immediate electrical, mechanical, and biochemical dysfunction of cardiac muscle. The specialized conducting tissue is more resistant to acute ischemia than is working myocardium, and therefore the electrophysiological consequences are less intense and delayed in onset in this tissue.[289] Experimental studies have also provided data on the long-term consequences of left ventricular hypertrophy and healed experimental myocardial infarction. Tissue exposed to chronic stress produced by long-term left ventricular pressure overload[290] and tissue which has healed after ischemic injury[291, 292] both show lasting cellular electrophysiological abnormalities, including regional changes in transmembrane action potentials and refractory periods, which may establish a propensity to chronic lethal arrhythmias. In fact, these studies have demonstrated that acute ischemic injury or acute myocardial infarction in the presence of healed myocardial infarction is more arrhythmogenic than is the same extent of acute ischemia in previously normal tissue.[292, 293] In addition to the direct effect of ischemia on normal or previously abnormal tissue, it is possible that reperfusion after transient ischemia may cause lethal arrhythmias.[294–296] Reperfusion of ischemic areas may occur by three mechanisms: (1) spontaneous thrombolysis, (2) collateral flow from other coronary vascular beds to the ischemic bed, and (3) reversal of vasospasm.

ELECTROPHYSIOLOGICAL EFFECTS OF ACUTE ISCHEMIA. Within the first minutes after experimental coronary ligation, there is a propensity to ventricular arrhythmias which abates after 30 minutes and reappears after several hours.[297] The initial 30 minutes of arrhythmias is divided into two periods, the first of which lasts for approximately 10 minutes and is presumably directly related to the initial ischemic injury. The second period (20 to 30 minutes) may be related either to reperfusion of ischemic areas or to the evolution of differing injury patterns in the epicardial and endocardial muscle.[298, 299] At a myocardial cellular level, the immediate consequences of ischemia, which include loss of integrity of cell membranes with efflux of K^+, influx of Ca^{++}, acidosis, reduction of transmembrane resting potentials, and enhanced automaticity in some tissues, are followed by a separate series of changes during reperfusion. Those of particular current interest are the possible continued influx of Ca^{++} which may produce electrical instability,[296, 300] responses to alpha- and/or beta-adrenoceptor stimulation,[267, 268, 301–303] and neurophysiologically induced afterdepolarization as triggering responses for Ca^{++}-dependent arrhythmias.[300, 307] Other possible mechanisms studied experimentally include formation of superoxide radicals in reperfusion arrhythmias,[304, 305] a direct or indirect role of angiotensin-converting enzyme activity in potentially lethal arrhythmias,[306] and differential responses of endocardial and epicardial muscle activation times and refractory periods during ischemia or reperfusion.[298, 308–310]

The importance of the myocardial response to the onset of ischemia has been emphasized, on the basis of the demonstration of dramatic cellular electrophysiological changes during the first 30 seconds after coronary occlusion.[311] However, the state of the myocardium at the time of onset of ischemia is a critical additional factor. Tissue healed after previous injury appears to be more susceptible to the electrical destabilizing effects of acute ischemia, as is chronically hypertrophied muscle. Of more direct clinical relevance is the suggestion that K^+ depletion by diuretics, and clinical hypokalemia, may make ventricular myocardium more susceptible to potentially lethal arrhythmias.[312–314] The association of metabolic and electrolyte abnormalities, as well as neurophysiological and neurohumoral changes[136, 198, 269, 307, 315–318] with SCD, emphasize the importance of changes in the myocardial substrate in the propensity to lethal arrhythmias. Most direct among myocardial metabolic changes in response to ischemia are acute increase in interstitial K^+ levels to values exceeding 15 mM, a fall in tissue pH to below 6.0, changes in adrenoceptor activity, and alterations in autonomic nerve traffic,[142] all of which tend to create and maintain electrical instability, especially if regional in distribution. Other metabolic changes such as cyclic AMP elevation, accumulation of free fatty acids and their metabolites, lysophosphoglycerides, and impaired myocardial glycolysis also have been suggested as myocardial destabilizing influences.[319]

THE TRANSITION FROM MYOCARDIAL INSTABILITY TO POTENTIALLY LETHAL ARRHYTHMIAS. *The combination of a triggering event and a susceptible myocardium is evolving as a fundamental electrophysiological concept for the mechanism of initiation of potentially lethal arrhythmias.* The endpoint of their interaction is disorganization of patterns of myocardial activation, usually by premature impulses (i.e., the "trigger"), into multiple uncoordinated reentrant pathways (i.e., ventricular fibrillation). Clinical,[84, 320] experimental,[239] and pharmacological[291] data all suggest that triggering events and the myocardial instability permitting the evolution of lethal arrhythmias may be dissociated from one another. In the absence of myocardial vulnerability, many triggering events, such as frequent and complex PVC's, may be innocuous.

The onset of ischemia is accompanied by abrupt reduction in transmembrane resting potential, amplitude, and duration of the action potential in the affected area,[311] with little change in remote areas. When ischemic cells depolarize to resting potentials less than −60 mV, they may become inexcitable and of little electrophysiological importance. However, as they are depolarizing to that range, or repolarizing as a consequence of reperfusion, the membranes pass through ranges of reduced excitability, upstroke velocity, and time courses of repolarization; these characteristics result in slow conduction and electrophysiological instability. These events occurring regionally in ischemic myocardium, adjacent to nonischemic tissue, create a setting for the key elements of reentry—slow conduction and unidirectional block—which makes them vulnerable to reentrant arrhythmias. When premature impulses are generated in this environment, they may further alter the dispersion of recovery between ischemic tissue, chronically abnormal tissue, and normal cells,[292, 293] ultimately leading to complete disorganization and VF. VF is probably not a consequence only of reentry.[142] Rapid-enhanced automaticity due to ischemic injury to the specialized conducting tissue, or slow-channel–triggered activity in partially depolarized tissue, may result in rapid bursts of automatic activity which could also lead to failure of coordinated conduction and VF.

The dispersion of refractory periods produced by acute ischemia, which provides the substrate for reentrant tachycardias and VF, may be further enhanced by a healed ischemic injury. The time course of repolarization is lengthened after healing of ischemic injury[291, 292] and shortened by acute ischemia.[292, 296, 311] The coexistence of the two appears to make the ventricle more susceptible to sustained arrhythmias in some experimental models.[292]

Bradyarrhythmias and Asystolic Arrest

The basic electrophysiological mechanism in this form of arrest is failure of normal subordinate automatic activity to assume pacemaking function of the heart in the absence of normal function of the sinus node and/or AV junction. Bradyarrhythmic and asystolic arrests are more common in severely diseased hearts, and probably represent diffuse involvement of subendocardial Purkinje fibers. Systemic influences which increase extracellular K^+ concentration, such as anoxia, acidosis, shock, renal failure, trauma, and hypothermia, may result in partial depolarization of normal or already diseased pacemaker cells in the His-Purkinje system, with a decrease in the slope of spontaneous phase 4 depolarization, and ultimate loss of automaticity.[321, 322] Generally, these are processes which produce global dysfunction of automatic cell activity, in contrast to the regional dysfunction more common in acute ischemia. Functionally depressed automatic cells (e.g., due to increased extracellular K^+ concentration) are more susceptible to overdrive suppression. Under these conditions, brief bursts of tachycardia may be followed by prolonged asystolic periods, with further depression of automaticity by the consequent acidosis and increased local K^+ concentration or by changes in adrenergic tone. The ultimate consequence may be degeneration into VF or persistent asystole.

Electromechanical Dissociation

This is among the least common of the mechanisms of SCD. Fozzard[323] has separated electromechanical dissociation into *primary* and *secondary* forms. The common denominator in both is continued electrical rhythmicity of the heart in the absence of effective mechanical function. The secondary form includes those causes which result from an abrupt cessation of cardiac venous return, such as massive pulmonary embolism, acute malfunction of prosthetic valves, exsanguination, and cardiac tamponade from hemopericardium. The primary form is the more familiar; in it none of these obvious mechanical factors are present, but ventricular muscle fails to produce an effective contraction despite continued electrical activity—i.e., *failure of electromechanical coupling.* Although this generally occurs as an end-stage event in advanced heart disease, it may occasionally be seen in patients with acute ischemic events or more commonly after electrical resuscitation from a prolonged cardiac arrest. Although not thoroughly understood, it appears that global ischemia or diffuse disease or both provide the pathophysiological substrate and that the proximate mechanism for failure of electromechanical coupling may be abnormal intracellular Ca^{++} metabolism, intracellular acidosis, and perhaps ATP depletion.

CLINICAL CHARACTERISTICS OF THE PATIENT WITH CARDIAC ARREST

Prior to the development of coronary care units, the in-hospital mortality due to acute myocardial infarction was in the range of 25 to 30 per cent.[324–326] The current in-hospital mortality rate (see Chap. 39) is lower in large part because of prevention of in-hospital sudden deaths, now that acute potentially lethal arrhythmias in this setting are preventable or reversible.[327, 328] However, the prior relationship between acute myocardial infarction and SCD in the in-hospital setting ingrained the concept of the association between the two, which was then extrapolated to the setting of out-of-hospital cardiac arrests. With the advent of community-based emergency rescue systems, leading to cohorts of survivors of out-of-hospital cardiac arrest, it rapidly became apparent that the majority of these cardiac arrests were, in fact, not associated with the evolution of a new transmural myocardial infarction. Studies from Seattle[19] and Miami[288] both demonstrated that only a minority of survivors of out-of-hospital VF had clinical evidence indicating that a new transmural myocardial infarction was associated with the cardiac arrest. In the Seattle study, only one of five survivors had new transmural infarctions.[19] These studies led to the conclusion that in the majority of such patients, transient pathophysiological events were responsible for cardiac arrest. That this conclusion is reasonable and has clinical relevance is suggested by the fact that the recurrence rate in survivors of prehospital cardiac arrest is low in the subgroup of patients who had documentation of a new transmural myocardial infarction. However, it was found to be 30 per cent at 1 year and 45 per cent at 2 years in those survivors who did not have a new transmural myocardial infarction.[18, 19] These recurrence rates have decreased more recently,[56] possibly due to long-term interventions (Ch. 38).

Clinical cardiac arrest and SCD are best described in the framework of the same four phases of the event used to establish definitions (see Fig. 24–1): prodromes, onset of the terminal event, the cardiac arrest, and progression to biological death or survival.

PRODROMAL SYMPTOMS

Patients at risk for SCD may have prodromes such as chest pain, dyspnea, weakness or fatigue, palpitations, and a number of nonspecific complaints. Several epidemiological and clinical studies demonstrated that such symptoms may presage coronary events, particularly myocardial infarction and SCD,[8, 57, 329, 330] and result in contact with the medical system weeks to months before SCD.[329] In a prospective study in Edinburgh, Scotland, however, only 12 per cent of victims of SCD had consulted a physician because of new or worsening angina pectoris during periods of up to 6 months before death.[331] In contrast, 33 per cent of myocardial infarction patients had consulted their physicians for this complaint. Nonetheless, 46 per cent of victims of SCD had seen a physician within 4 weeks prior to death, but three-fourths of them had sought medical help for complaints which appeared to be unrelated to the heart. Liberthson et al.,[18] in a study of patients successfully resuscitated after prehospital cardiac arrest, noted that 28 per cent reported retrospectively that they had had new or changing angina pectoris or dyspnea in the 4 weeks before arrest, and that 31 per cent had seen a physician during this time but only 12 per cent because of these symptoms. Attempts to identify prospectively early prodromal symptoms which are more specific for the patient at risk for SCD have not yet been successful. Fatigue has been a particularly common symptom in the days or weeks before SCD in a number of studies,[329] but this symptom is nonspecific. The prodromata occurring within the last hours or minutes before cardiac arrest are more specific for heart disease and may include symptoms of arrhythmias, ischemia, or heart failure.[21, 332, 333] Liberthson et al.[234] reported specific cardiac symptoms at a mean interval of about 3.8 hours before collapse in 24 per cent of victims of SCD. However, most studies have reported such symptoms even less commonly, particularly when victims whose deaths were instantaneous are included.[8]

ONSET OF THE TERMINAL EVENT

The period of 1 hour or less between acute changes in cardiovascular status and the cardiac arrest itself, which has been defined as the "onset of the terminal event," is a subject about which there is limited information. Reports from ambulatory monitor recordings fortuitously obtained at the time of unexpected cardiac arrest indicate dynamic change in cardiac electrical activity during the minutes or hours before the onset of cardiac arrest.[332, 334–336] These reports suggest that increasing heart rate and advancing grades of ventricular ectopy—including R-on-T phenomenon and VT—are common antecedents of VF. Although these recordings suggest transient electrophysiological destabilization of the myocardium, the extent to which these objective observations are paralleled by clinical symptoms is less well documented. SCD's due to either arrhythmias or acute circulatory failure mechanisms involve a high incidence of acute myocardial disorders at the onset of the terminal event: such disorders are more likely to be ischemic when the death is due to arrhythmias and to be associated with low output states or myocardial anoxia when the deaths are due to circulatory failure.[21, 336a]

Abrupt, unexpected loss of effective circulation may be caused by cardiac arrhythmias or mechanical disturbances, but the majority of such events that terminate in SCD are arrhythmic in origin. Hinkle and Thaler[336a] classified cardiac deaths among 142 subjects who died during a follow-

TABLE 24–5 DIFFERENCES IN CLINICAL STATUS IMMEDIATELY BEFORE DEATH IN PATIENTS DYING OF ARRHYTHMIA AND CIRCULATORY FAILURE

Clinical Status Immediately Before Death	Arrhythmic Deaths (N = 82) (Class I)	Circulatory Failure Deaths (N = 59) (Class II)
Comatose	0/82 (0%)	56/59 (95%)
Standing or actively moving	39/82 (48%)	0/59 (0%)
Terminal arrhythmia		
• Ventricular fibrillation	15/18 (83%)	3/9 (33%)
• Asystole	3/18 (17%)	6/9 (67%)
Duration of terminal illness		
• <1 hour	53/82 (65%)	4/59 (7%)
• >24 hours	17/82 (21%)	48/59 (81%)
Nature of terminal illness		
• Acute cardiac events	80/82 (98%)	8/59 (14%)
• Noncardiac events	1/82 (1%)	51/59 (86%)

Modified from Hinkle, L. E. and Thaler, H. T.: Clinical classification of cardiac deaths. Circulation. 65:457, 1982.

up of 5 to 10 years. Class I was labeled arrhythmic death and class II was death due to circulatory failure. The distinction between the two classes was based upon whether circulatory failure preceded (class II) or followed (class I) the disappearance of the pulse. Among deaths which occurred less than 1 hour after the onset of the terminal illness, 93 per cent were due to arrhythmias; in addition, 90 per cent of deaths due to heart disease were initiated by arrhythmic events rather than circulatory failure. Table 24–5 demonstrates that deaths due to circulatory failure occurred predominantly in patients who could be identified as having terminal illnesses (95 per cent were comatose), were associated more frequently with bradyarrhythmias than with VF as the terminal arrhythmias, and were dominated by noncardiac events as the terminal illness. In contrast, 98 per cent of the arrhythmic deaths were associated primarily with cardiac disorders.

CLINICAL FEATURES OF CARDIAC ARREST

The cardiac arrest itself is an event characterized by abrupt loss of consciousness due to failure of adequate cerebral blood flow. It is an event which will uniformly lead to death in the absence of an active intervention, although spontaneous reversions occur rarely. The most common cardiac mechanism is VF, followed by bradyarrhythmias or asystole, and sustained VT.[20] Other less frequent mechanisms include electromechanical dissociation, rupture of the ventricle,[337] cardiac tamponade, acute mechanical obstruction to flow, and acute disruption of a major blood vessel.[3, 51, 141]

The potential for successful resuscitation is a function of the setting in which cardiac arrest occurs, the mechanism of the arrest, and the underlying clinical status of the victim.[338, 338a] Closely related to the potential for successful resuscitation is the decision of whether or not to attempt to resuscitate.[339, 340]

At present there are fewer low-risk patients with otherwise uncomplicated myocardial infarctions than heretofore to influence in-hospital cardiac arrest statistics[327, 341, 342] In a recent study, Bedell and coworkers[343] reported that only 14 per cent of in-hospital CPR patients were discharged from the hospital alive, and that 20 per cent of these died within the ensuing 6 months. Although 41 per cent of the patients had suffered an acute myocardial infarction, 73 per cent had a history of congestive heart failure, and 20 per cent had had prior cardiac arrests. The mean age of 70 years (10 years older than the populations in several major prehospital cardiac arrest studies[18, 19, 56]) may have influenced the outcome statistics, but the patient population at risk for in-hospital cardiac arrest was heavily influenced by patients with high-risk complicated myocardial infarction or patients with other high-risk markers. Noncardiac clinical diagnoses were dominated by renal failure, pneumonia, sepsis, diabetes, and a history of cancer. The strong male dominance consistently reported in out-of-hospital cardiac arrest studies is not present in in-hospital patients, but the better prognosis of VT or VF mechanisms, compared to bradyarrhythmic or asystolic mechanisms, persists (27 per cent survival versus 8 per cent survival). However, the proportion of arrests which are due to VT or VF in-hospital is considerably less (33 per cent), with the combination of respiratory arrest, asystole, and electromechanical dissociation dominating the statistics (61 per cent).

The significant risk factors for death after CPR are listed in Table 24–6. The facts that the fraction of out-of-hospital cardiac arrest survivors who are discharged from the hospital alive may now equal or exceed the fraction of in-hospital cardiac arrest victims who are discharged alive,[343, 344] and that the post-discharge mortality rate for in-hospital cardiac arrest survivors is higher than that for out-of-hospital cardiac arrest survivors,[56, 343, 345, 346] are telling clinical statistics. Not only do they emphasize the success of preventive measures for cardiac arrest in low-risk in-hospital patients, causing those statistics to be dominated by higher risk patients, but they also emphasize the improvement in prehospital and in-hospital care of out-of-hospital cardiac arrest victims.

TABLE 24–6 PREDICTORS OF MORTALITY AFTER IN-HOSPITAL CARDIOPULMONARY RESUSCITATION

Before arrest
Hypotension (systolic BP <100 mm Hg)
Pneumonia
Renal failure (BUN >50 mg/dl)
Cancer
Homebound life style
During arrest
Arrest duration >15 minutes
Intubation
Hypotension (systolic BP <100 mm Hg)
Pneumonia
Homebound life style
After resuscitation
Coma
Need for pressors
Arrest duration >15 minutes

Modified from Bedell, S. E., et al: Survival after cardiopulmonary resuscitation in the hospital. N. Engl. J. Med. 309:569, 1983.

Cardiac arrest associated with coronary heart disease in the hospitalized elderly patient has a similar outcome. Gulati et al.[347] reported that 14 of 52 (27 per cent) elderly patients (mean age, 76 years) were successfully resuscitated, although only 9 (17 per cent) remained alive after 1 week. Coronary heart disease was the etiology in 48 patients (92 per cent); 5 of 22 patients (23 per cent) with VF arrests survived and only 1 of 19 (5 per cent) with asystole survived.

PROGRESSION TO BIOLOGICAL DEATH

The time course for progression from cardiac arrest to biological death relates to the mechanism of the cardiac arrest, the nature of the underlying disease process, and the delay between onset and resuscitative efforts. Unattended VF characteristically leads to the onset of irreversible brain damage within 4 to 6 minutes, and biological death follows within a matter of minutes thereafter. In large series, however, it has been demonstrated that a limited number of victims may remain biologically alive for longer periods and may be resuscitated after delays in excess of 8 minutes before beginning basic life support and in excess of 16 minutes before advanced life support.[348] Despite these exceptions, it clear that the statistical probability for a favorable outcome deteriorates rapidly as a function of time after unattended cardiac arrest; younger patients with less severe disease and the absence of coexistent multisystem disease appear to have a higher probability of a favorable outcome after such delays. Irreversible injury of the central nervous system generally occurs before biological death, and the interval may extend to a period of weeks in those patients who are resuscitated during the temporal gap between brain damage and biological death. Such events have led to the discrepancy between the cardiac arrest itself and biological death in individuals whose fate is cast by the cardiac arrest (see Definition, p.

742). In-hospital cardiac arrest due to VF is less likely to have a protracted course between the arrest and biological death, with patients either surviving after a prompt intervention or succumbing rapidly because of inability to stabilize cardiac rhythm or hemodynamics.[343]

Those patients whose cardiac arrest is due to sustained VT with cardiac output inadequate to maintain consciousness may remain in VT for considerably longer periods, with flow which is marginally sufficient to maintain viability. This allows a longer interval between the onset of cardiac arrest and the end of the period which will allow successful resuscitation. The lives of such patients usually terminate in VF or an asystolic arrest if the VT is not actively or spontaneously reverted. Once the transition from VT to VF or to a bradyarrhythmia occurs, the subsequent course to biological death is similar to that in patients in whom VF or bradyarrhythmias is the initiating event.

The progression in patients with asystole or bradyarrhythmias as the initiating event is more rapid. Such patients, whether in an in-hospital[343] or out-of-hospital[20, 349, 350] environment, have a very poor prognosis because of advanced heart disease or coexistent multisystem disease. They tend to respond poorly to interventions, even if the heart is successfully paced.[351] Although a small subgroup of patients with bradyarrhythmias associated with electrolyte or pharmacological abnormalities may respond well to interventions, the majority progress rapidly to biological death.[349] The infrequent cardiac arrests due to mechanical factors such as tamponade, structural disruption, and impedance to flow by major thromboembolic obstructions to right or left ventricular outflow are reversible only in those instances in which the mechanism is recognized and an intervention is feasible. The vast majority of these events lead to rapid biological death, although prompt relief of tamponade may save some lives.

HOSPITAL COURSE OF SURVIVORS OF CARDIAC ARREST

The hospital course of survivors of cardiac arrest is characterized by an initial period of instability, followed by clinical features which are determined by the electrical and hemodynamic status of the patient, and the consequence of central nervous system injury occurring during the cardiac arrest.[20, 22] The conditions of patients who are resuscitated immediately from *primary* VF associated with acute myocardial infarction generally stabilize promptly, and they require no special management after the early phase of the infarction (Ch. 38). The management after *secondary cardiac arrest in myocardial infarction* is dominated by the hemodynamic status of the patient. In survivors of *prehospital cardiac arrest*, the initial 24 to 48 hours of hospitalization are characterized by a tendency to ventricular arrhythmias, which generally respond well to antiarrhythmic therapy.[20, 288, 333] The overall rate of recurrent cardiac arrest is low, approximately 10 to 20 per cent, but the mortality rate in patients who have recurrent cardiac arrests is approximately 50 per cent.[18–20] Only 5 to 10 per cent of in-hospital deaths after prehospital resuscitation are due to recurrent cardiac arrhythmias.[20, 22] Patients who have recurrent cardiac arrest have a high incidence of either new or preexisting A-V or intraventricular conduction abnormalities.[20]

The most common *cardiac* cause of delayed death during hospitalization after prehospital cardiac arrest is hemodynamic deterioration, which accounts for approximately one-third of deaths in-hospital.[20, 22] However, noncardiac events related to central nervous system injury which occurred during the cardiac arrest itself are the most common cause of death in hospitalized survivors of out-of-hospital cardiac arrest. These include anoxic encephalopathy and sepsis related to prolonged intubation and hemodynamic monitoring lines.[20, 22] Fifty-nine per cent of deaths during index hospitalization after prehospital resuscitation have been reported to be due to such causes.[20] It has been reported that 39 per cent of 457 consecutive patients in coma never awakened after admission to the hospital and died after a median survival of 3.5 days.[352] Two-thirds of the 61 per cent who awakened had no gross deficits, and an additional 21 per cent had persisting cognitive deficits only. Of the patients who were to awaken, 25 per cent had done so by admission, 71 per cent by the first hospital day, and 92 per cent by the third day. However, a small number of patients awakened after prolonged hospitalization. Of the 206 hospital deaths (45 per cent of the 457 patients), 80 per cent had not awakened before death. Among all deaths, those occurring within the first 48 hours of hospitalization were usually due to hemodynamic deterioration or arrhythmias, regardless of the neurological status; later deaths were related to neurological complications. Admission characteristics most predictive of subsequent awakening included motor response, pupillary light response, spontaneous eye movement, and blood sugar below 300 mg/dl.[353]

CLINICAL PROFILE OF SURVIVORS OF OUT-OF-HOSPITAL CARDIAC ARREST

The clinical features of survivors of cardiac arrest not associated with acute myocardial infarction are dominated by the underlying coronary heart disease present in the vast majority. Complex PVC's have been reported in 84 per cent of survivors of prehospital cardiac arrest who had serial ambulatory monitor recordings.[288, 354, 355] These arrhythmias are difficult to suppress during a long-term antiarrhythmic drug management program[355] and show only a statistically nonsignificant trend to higher grades of ventricular ectopy in victims of recurrent cardiac arrest compared with long-term survivors.[56] Unifocal PVC's have been observed in 90 per cent of survivors and complex forms in 67 per cent.[356] Complex forms were strongly associated with a history of congestive heart failure or previous myocardial infarction. Frequent complex forms were observed in 56 per cent of the patients who had recurrent cardiac arrests compared with 28 per cent who did not. Goldstein et al.[346] carried out ambulatory monitor recordings within 3 months of the cardiac arrest event; complex PVC's were found in 89 per cent of the survivors, couplets or repetitive forms in approximately 60 per cent, and salvos in 30 per cent. The strongest predictors of subsequent mortality were use of digitalis, elevated BUN, cerebrovascular accident, previous myocardial infarction, and age; however, the presence of complex PVC's or frequent ectopy ($\geq$ 25 PVC's/hour) added strongly to risk.

Studies of left ventricular function in out-of-hospital cardiac arrest survivors have shown a wide variation, ranging from severe dysfunction to as many as 50 per cent of the survivors having normal or near-normal measurements[56] (Fig. 24–6*A*). The author found that the ejection fraction of those who died during follow-up was lower than that of the long-term survivors (38 versus 45 per cent, respectively).[20, 56] However, patients who died of recurrent cardiac arrest had higher ejection fractions than those who died non-sudden cardiac deaths (43 versus 25 per cent) (Fig. 24–6*B*). Ritchie et al.[357] reported on studies of left ventricular function by radionuclide techniques in 154 survivors of out-of-hospital VF, 91 of whom had both rest and exercise studies. The mean ejection fraction at

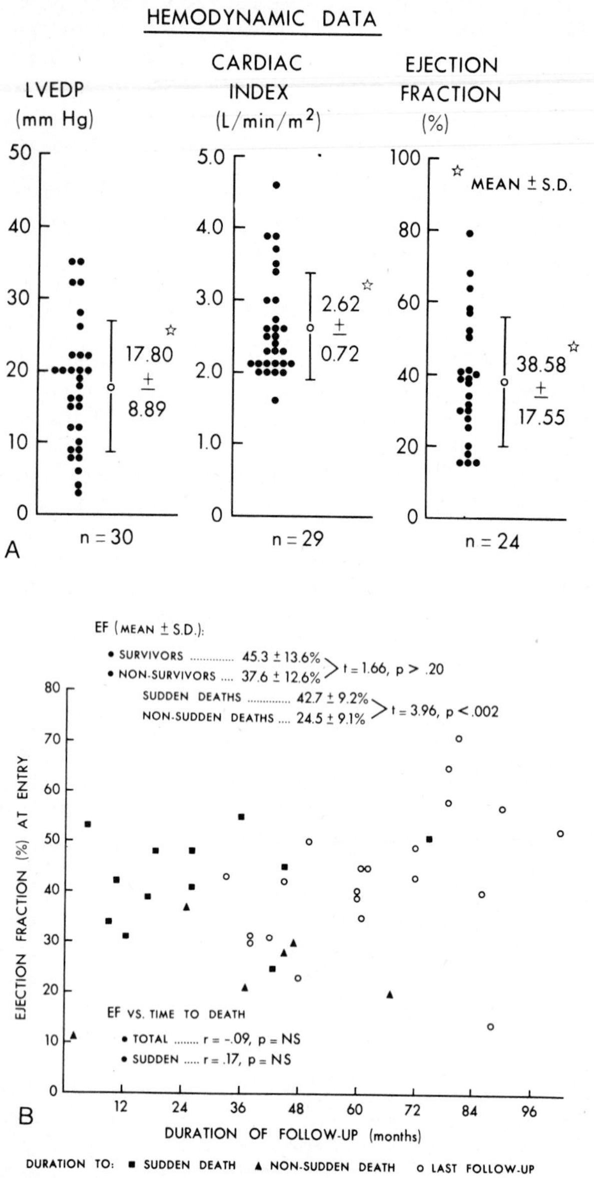

FIGURE 24–6. *A*, Hemodynamic data from prehospital cardiac arrest victims studied during initial post-arrest hospitalization, and *B*, the relationship between ejection fraction (EF) at initial study and long-term outcome. These data indicate a broad range of cardiac function (*A*), and a statistically insignificant difference between EF at entry in long-term survivors and in recurrent cardiac arrest victims (*B*). Severity of decreased EF was more predictive of non-sudden deaths. (*A*, From Myerburg, R. J., et al.: Clinical, electrophysiologic, and hemodynamic profile of patients resuscitated from prehospital cardiac arrest. Am. J. Med. *68*:568, 1980. *B*, From Myerburg, R. J., et al.: Long-term survival after prehospital cardiac arrest: Analysis of outcome during an 8-year study. Circulation *70*:538, 1984, by permission of the American Heart Association, Inc.)

rest was 40 per cent, with 29 per cent having values greater than 50 per cent. Only 3 of 91 patients (3 per cent) studied had a normal increase (> +5 per cent) in ejection fraction during exertion. Only 18 per cent had normal resting wall motion. The ejection fraction at rest was the best predictor of death during follow-up.[357] Fifty per cent of survivors studied by cardiac catheterization and angiography had ejection fractions below 50 per cent, and 30 per cent had LV end diastolic pressures greater than 15 mm Hg[358]; in this study, ejection fraction and severity of wall motion abnormality correlated with risk of recurrent cardiac arrest.

Coronary angiographic studies in survivors of out-of-hospital cardiac arrest have shown that, as a group, this population tends to have extensive disease but no specific pattern of abnormalities. Moderate-to-severe stenosis of the left main coronary artery was present in only 8 per cent of the patients in one series,[358] and only 9 per cent in another,[20] frequencies not different from those in the overall population of coronary heart disease patients. Significant lesions in two or more vessels were present in 74 per cent of the patients who had any coronary lesions in one study,[20] and 94 per cent of the patients in another had 70 per cent or less stenosis in one or more arteries.[358] Among patients who had recurrent cardiac arrests, the incidence of triple vessel disease was higher than among those who did not.

Exercise testing is commonly used to evaluate the need for and response to antiischemic therapy in survivors of prehospital cardiac arrest. However, the incidence of positive tests related to ischemia is relatively low, although termination of testing because of fatigue is common.[288, 355, 359] Mortality during follow-up is greater in patients who had angina or failure of a normal rise in systolic blood pressure occurring during exercise.[359]

Electrocardiographic observations in survivors of out-of-hospital cardiac arrest have proved of value only for discriminating risk of recurrence between those whose arrest was associated with new transmural myocardial infarction from all others. Patients who develop documented new Q waves in association with cardiac arrest are at much lower risk for recurrence.[18, 288, 360] A higher incidence of repolarization abnormalities (ST-segment depression, flat T waves, prolonged QTc) occurs in out-of-hospital cardiac arrest survivors than in post-myocardial infarction patients, and these might be markers for increased risk.[361]

Lower serum K^+ levels were observed in survivors of cardiac arrest than in patients with acute myocardial infarction or stable coronary heart disease.[362] However, the investigators concluded that this was a consequence of resuscitation interventions, rather than a preexisting state

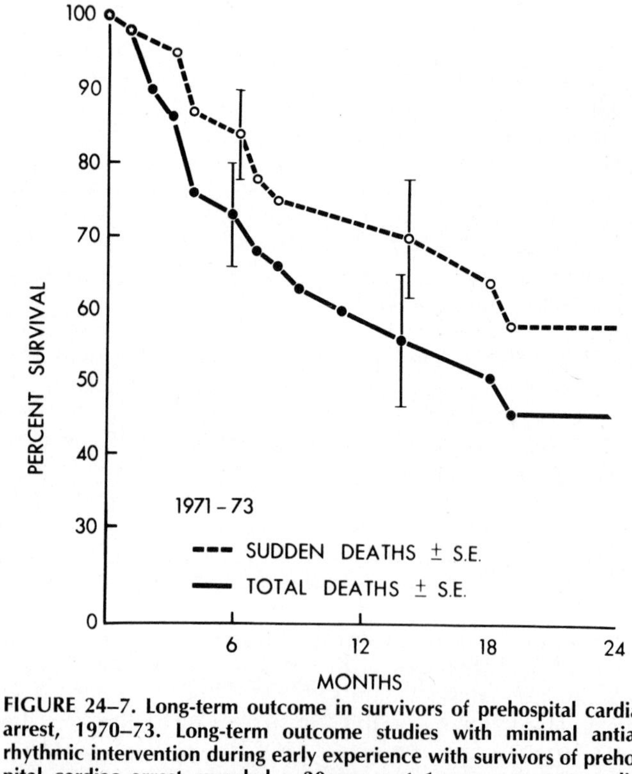

FIGURE 24–7. Long-term outcome in survivors of prehospital cardiac arrest, 1970–73. Long-term outcome studies with minimal antiarrhythmic intervention during early experience with survivors of prehospital cardiac arrest revealed a 30-per cent 1-year recurrent cardiac arrest rate, and 45-per cent 2-year cumulative rate. Total mortality at 2 years was nearly 60 per cent.

due to chronic diuretic use. Higher resting lactate levels have been reported in prehospital cardiac arrest survivors than in normal subjects.[363] Lactate levels correlated inversely with ejection fractions and directly with PVC frequency and complexity.

Studies from the early 1970's in both Miami[18] and Seattle[19] indicated that the risk of recurrent cardiac arrest in the first year after surviving an initial event was approximately 30 per cent and at 2 years was 45 per cent. Total mortality at 2 years was approximately 60 per cent in both studies (Fig. 24–7). In both of these studies, less than half of the patients followed were being treated with long-term antiarrhythmic therapy; beta-adrenoceptor blocker therapy was in its infancy, and Ca^{++}-entry blockers were not yet available. Thus, these figures appear to be as close to valid natural history figures as possible. However, they can serve only as historical control figures for current observations.

MANAGEMENT OF CARDIAC ARREST

COMMUNITY-BASED INTERVENTIONS IN OUT-OF-HOSPITAL CARDIAC ARREST

Systems for intervention in out-of-hospital cardiac arrest have their roots in the development of the coronary care unit (CCU) approach to the management of potentially lethal arrhythmias.[364, 365] Prior to that, cardiac arrest in the setting of acute coronary events was almost uniformly fatal, wherever it occurred. With the development of the key elements of the CCU, i.e., continuous monitoring, cardiopulmonary resuscitation, effective acute drug therapy, and electrical management of tachycardias, bradycardias, and VF, there was a dramatic reduction in the immediate in-hospital mortality from potentially lethal arrhythmias occurring in the course of acute coronary events.[342] The next step toward the development of community-based intervention for cardiac arrest was the concept of the mobile coronary care unit,[366] which was based on the rationale of providing a CCU environment during the high-risk prehospital phase of acute myocardial infarction. Only a small extension in concept led to the development of community-based intervention systems designed to respond routinely to out-of-hospital cardiac arrests. The systems as developed in the United States are largely integrated into fire departments as emergency rescue systems. They employ paramedical personnel or emergency medical technicians trained in cardiopulmonary resuscitation (CPR) and the use of telemetered monitoring equipment, defibrillators, and specific intravenous drug therapy. Although the initial prehospital intervention experience in Miami and Seattle[18, 19] in the early 1970's yielded only 14 and 10 per cent survivals to discharge, respectively, current statistics indicate that such systems are becoming increasingly effective in saving lives.[344, 360] By the mid 1970's, both had increased survival rates to about 25 per cent,[20, 344] and by the early 1980's to 30 per cent or more.[344]

IMPORTANCE OF ELECTRICAL MECHANISM. The electrical mechanism of out-of-hospital cardiac arrest, as defined by the initial rhythm recorded by emergency rescue personnel, has a powerful impact on success of initial resuscitation and outcome, the latter measured in terms of patients discharged from the hospital alive. The subgroup of patients who are in sustained VT at the time of first contact, although it is the smallest group statistically, has the best outcome (Fig. 24–8). The author reported that 88 per cent of patients in cardiac arrest due to VT were successfully resuscitated and admitted to the hospital alive, and 67 per cent were ultimately discharged alive.[20] However, this relatively low-risk group represents only 7 to 10 per cent of all cardiac arrests in studies reported to date. Because of the inherent time lag between collapse and initial recordings, it is possible that many more cardiac arrests begin as rapid sustained VT and degenerate into VF before arrival of emergency rescue personnel.

Patients who are in a bradyarrhythmia or asystole at initial contact have the worst prognosis; only 9 per cent of such patients in the Miami study were admitted to the hospital alive and none were discharged.[20] In a later experience there was some improvement in outcome, although it was strictly limited to those patients in whom the initial bradyarrhythmia recorded was an idioventricular rhythm which responded promptly to chronotropic agents in the field.[349] Bradyarrhythmias also have adverse prognostic implications after defibrillation from VF in the field. Patients who were defibrillated to an initial heart rate less than 60 beats/min, regardless of the specific bradyarrhythmic mechanism, had a poor prognosis, with 95 per cent of such patients dying either before hospitalization or in the hospital (Fig. 24–9).[18, 367] In contrast, an initial heart rate in excess of 100 beats/min yielded a 43 per cent rate of discharge from hospital, with only 17 per cent of such patients dying before hospitalization, and 40 per cent during hospitalization. Heart rates between 60 and 100 beats/min after defibrillation yield intermediate results.

The outcome in the largest group of patients, those in whom VF is the initial rhythm recorded, is intermediate between sustained VT and bradyarrhythmia and asystole. Figure 24–8 demonstrates that 40 per cent of such patients were successfully resuscitated and admitted to the hospital alive, and 23 per cent were ultimately discharged alive.[20]

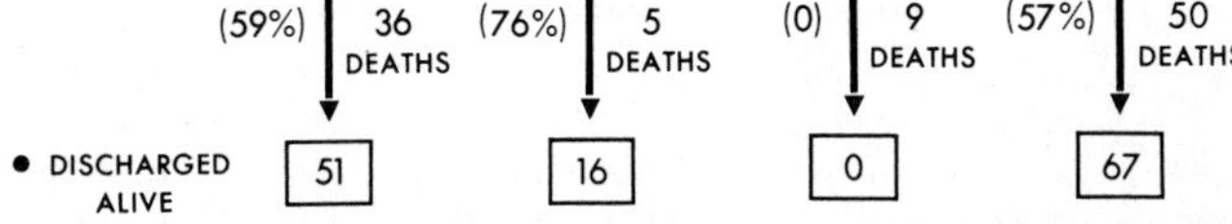

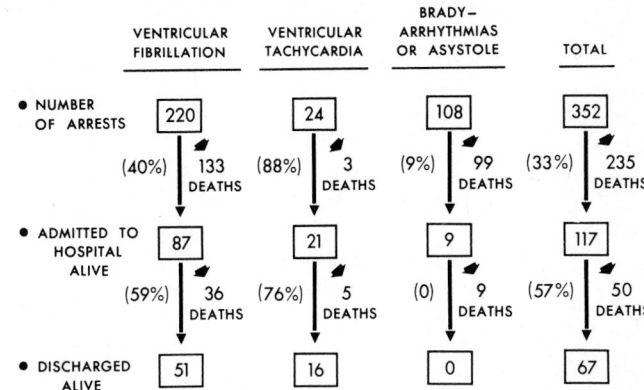

FIGURE 24–8. Survival related to initial electrophysiological mechanisms recorded during prehospital cardiac arrest. The figures highlighted by the boxes indicate the number of patients in each of three mechanism categories (ventricular fibrillation, ventricular tachycardia, and brady-arrhythmia/asystole), plus totals. In each category, the data indicate the number of prehospital cardiac arrests (*top*), the number of patients successfully resuscitated in the field and transferred to the hospital alive (*middle*), and the number of patients who survived hospitalization and were discharged (*bottom*). The percentages in parentheses indicate survivals at each level of care for each category. (From Myerburg, R. J., et al.: Clinical, electrophysiologic, and hemodynamic profile of patients resuscitated from prehospital cardiac arrest. Am. J. Med. *68*:568, 1980.)

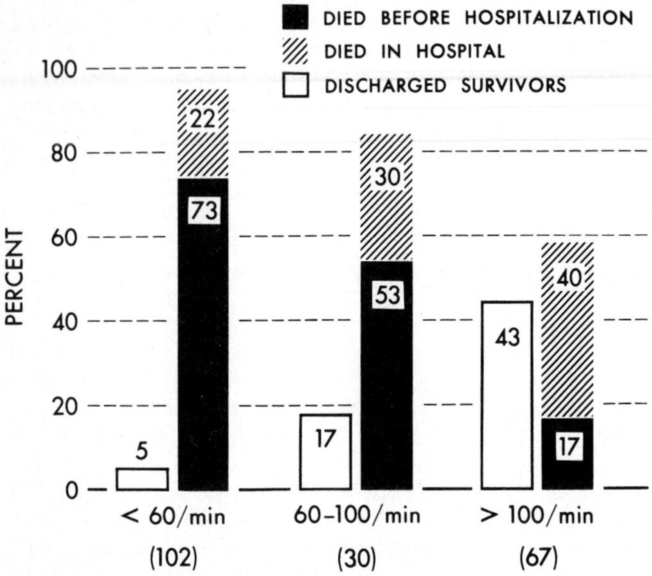

FIGURE 24–9. Prognostic implication of initial heart rate after prehospital defibrillation. Prehospital and in-hospital deaths, and long-range survival (i.e., discharged survivors), are compared to the initial post-defibrillation heart rate, <60 beats/min, 60 to 100 beats/min, or > 100 beats/min. (Modified from Liberthson, R. R., et al.: Prehospital ventricular fibrillation: Prognosis and follow-up course. Reprinted by permission of N. Engl. J. Med. *291*:317, 1974.)

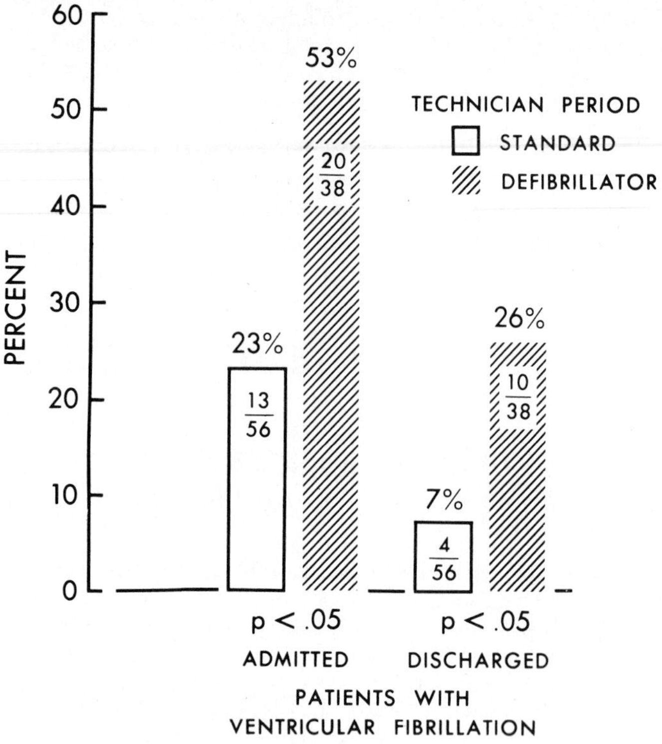

FIGURE 24–10. Standard CPR by emergency medical technicians versus immediate defibrillation in the prehospital setting. Survival to admission and discharge with standard care versus early defibrillation (see text). (Modified from Eisenberg, M. S., et al.: Treatment of out-of-hospital cardiac arrests with rapid debrillation by emergency medical technicians. Reprinted by permission of N. Engl. J. Med. *302*:1379, 1980.)

More recent data indicate continued improvement in outcome. The proportion of each of the electrophysiological mechanisms responsible for cardiac arrest varies among the studies, with VF ranging from 65 to greater than 90 per cent of the study populations, and bradyarrhythmia and asystole ranging from 10 to 30 per cent.[20, 333, 344, 350, 360]

The factors which contribute to improving outcome are incompletely understood. Both improved prehospital care and improvements in in-hospital technology and practices may contribute. Of these two general factors, the influence of prehospital care has been studied in more detail. Eisenberg and coworkers[368] compared initial resuscitation and ultimate discharge alive in two subgroups of patients, those who had standard CPR continuously from the arrival of emergency rescue personnel through transport to an emergency room where defibrillation took place, and another group in whom paramedics or emergency rescue personnel trained to defibrillate were allowed to do so at the scene of the cardiac arrest. The standard CPR technique resulted in only 23 per cent of patients arriving at the hospital alive and 7 per cent discharged alive, in contrast to the immediate defibrillation group in which 53 per cent arrived at the hospital alive and 26 per cent were discharged alive (Fig. 24–10). Subsequent data continue to support the concept that early defibrillation is a key element in improving survival rates.[344, 348, 369] Immediate defibrillation by ambulance technicians is especially important in rural communities, where it yields a 19 per cent survival, compared with only 3 per cent from standard CPR.[370]

A second element in prehospital care which appears to contribute to outcome is the role of bystander CPR by lay persons awaiting the arrival of emergency rescue personnel. It has been reported that although there was no significant difference in the percentage of patients successfully resuscitated and admitted to the hospital alive with (67 per cent) or without (61 per cent) bystander intervention, almost twice as many prehospital cardiac arrest victims were ultimately discharged alive when they had had

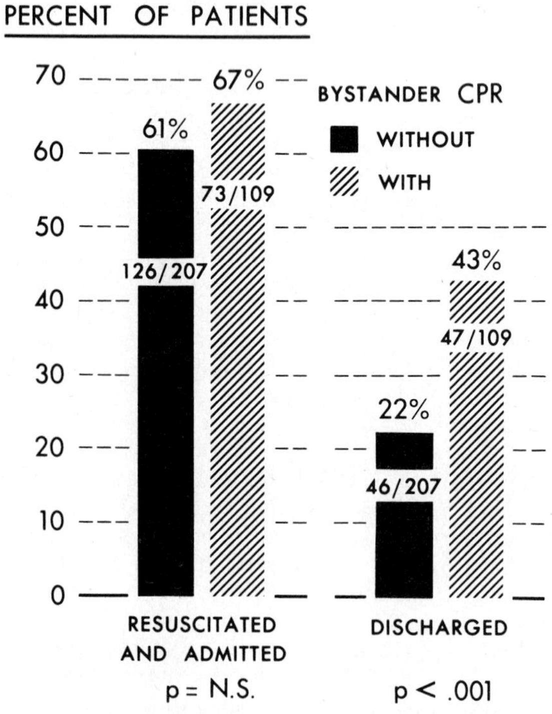

FIGURE 24–11. Influence of lay bystander cardiopulmonary resuscitation (CPR) on outcome after prehospital cardiac arrest. There was no influence of bystander intervention on the proportion of victims resuscitated and admitted to the hospital alive, but those with bystander CPR had a significantly higher survival and rate of discharge than did those without bystander CPR. (From Myerburg, R. J., et al.: Survivors of prehospital cardiac arrest. J.A.M.A. *247*:1485, 1982. Copyright 1982, American Medical Association.)

bystander CPR (43 per cent) than when such support was not provided (22 per cent) (Fig. 24–11).[22] Central nervous system protection, expressed as early regaining of consciousness, appears to be the major protective element of bystander CPR.[22] The rationale for bystander intervention is further highlighted by the relationship between time to defibrillation and survival, when analyzed as a function of time to initiation of basic CPR. It has been reported that more than 40 per cent of victims whose defibrillation and other advanced life support activities were instituted more than 8 minutes after collapse survived if basic CPR had been initiated less than 2 minutes after onset of the arrest. A delay of more than 5 minutes to basic CPR was associated with no survivors.[344]

The time from onset of cardiac arrest to advanced life support influences outcome statistics. Mayer[371] reported improved short-term (to hospital admission) and long-term (to hospital discharge) survival rates for prehospital VF victims with short paramedic response times compared with those with long response times. Improvement in both early neurological status and survival occurs in the patients defibrillated by first responders, even if they are minimally trained emergency technicians allowed to carry out defibrillation as part of basic life support, compared with delays incorporated by awaiting more highly trained paramedics.[372] Thus the time to defibrillation plays a central role in determining outcome in cardiac arrest due to VF.

The success of lidocaine for preventing primary VF in acute myocardial infarction in coronary care units[373] (p. 763) also led to the concept that routine prehospital administration of the drug might reduce prehospital cardiac arrests in these patients.[374] On the basis of encouraging results, its use by not only physicians and paramedics but also by high-risk patients themselves has been suggested.[375]

MANAGEMENT OF THE INDIVIDUAL PATIENT

The management of cardiac arrest is divided into five elements: (1) the initial response, (2) basic life support, (3) advanced life support and definitive resuscitative efforts, (4) post-cardiac arrest care, and (5) long-term management. The first of these can be applied by a broad population base, which includes physicians and nurses as well as paramedical personnel, emergency rescue technicians, and lay persons educated in bystander intervention. The requirements for specialized knowledge and skills become progressively more focused as the patient moves through post-cardiac arrest management and into long-term follow-up care.

INITIAL RESPONSE

This activity includes both diagnostic maneuvers and elementary interventions. The first action of the person(s) in attendance when an individual collapses unexpectedly must be *confirmation that collapse is due to a cardiac arrest*. A few seconds of observation for respiratory movements and skin color and simultaneous palpation of major arteries for the presence or absence of a pulse yields sufficient information to determine whether a life-threatening incident is in progress. The absence of carotid or femoral pulses, particularly if confirmed by the absence of an audible heartbeat, is the primary diagnostic criterion and can be performed accurately by trained lay persons. Skin color may be pale or intensely cyanotic. Absence of respiratory efforts, or the presence of only agonal respiratory efforts, in conjunction with an absent pulse, is diagnostic of cardiac arrest; however, respiratory efforts may persist for a minute or more after the onset of the arrest. In contrast, absence of respiratory efforts or severe stridor with persistence of a pulse suggests a primary respiratory arrest which will lead to a cardiac arrest in a short time. In the latter circumstance, initial efforts should include exploration of the oropharynx in search of a foreign body and the Heimlich maneuver, particularly if this occurs in a setting in which aspiration is likely (e.g., restaurant death or "cafe coronary.")[225, 226]

THUMPVERSION. Once the diagnosis of cardiac arrest is established, two immediate initial efforts are carried out: a blow to the chest (precordial thump, "thumpversion") and clearing the airway so that proper CPR can be carried out. Although the American Heart Association now recommends the use of precordial thumps only in monitored patients because of concern about converting VT to VF,[338, 338a] Caldwell and coworkers urged its continued use on the basis of a prospective study in 5000 patients.[376] In their study, precordial thumps successfully reverted VF in 5 events, VT in 11, asystole in 2, and undefined cardiovascular collapse in 2 others in whom the electrical mechanism was unknown. In no instance was conversion of VT to VF observed. Since the latter is the major concern of the precordial thump technique, and electrical activity can be initiated by mechanical stimulation in the asystolic heart,[377, 378] the technique may be used in the absence of monitoring when the diagnosis is clear and no other option is available. For attempted thumpversion in cardiac arrest, one or two blows should be delivered firmly to the junction of the middle and lower third of the sternum from a height of 8 to 10 inches, but the effort should be abandoned if the patient does not immediately develop a spontaneous pulse and begin breathing. Another mechanical method, which requires that the patient still be conscious, is "cough-induced cardiac compression"[379] or "cough-version."[376, 380] In the former, a conscious act of forceful coughing by the patient in VF may support forward flow by cyclic increases in intrathoracic pressure[379]; the same act during sustained ventricular tachycardia may cause conversion.[376, 380]

AIRWAY. The next step is clearing the airway. This includes tilting the head backward and lifting the chin, in addition to seeking foreign bodies—including dentures—and removing them. The Heimlich maneuver should be performed if there is reason to suspect a foreign body lodged in the oropharynx. This entails wrapping the arms around the victim from the back and delivering a sharp thrust to the upper abdomen with a closed fist.[381] If it is not possible for the person in attendance to carry out the maneuver because of insufficient physical strength, mechanical dislodgment of the foreign body can sometimes be achieved by abdominal thrusts with the unconscious patient in a supine position. The Heimlich maneuver is not entirely benign: ruptured abdominal viscera in the victim have been reported,[382] as has an instance in which the rescuer has disrupted his own aortic root and died.[383]

If there is strong suspicion that respiratory arrest precipitated cardiac arrest, particularly in the presence of a mechanical airway obstruction, a second precordial thump should be delivered after the airway is cleared.

BASIC LIFE SUPPORT

The goal of this activity is to maintain viability of the central nervous system, heart, and other vital organs until definitive intervention can be achieved. The activities included within basic life support encompass both the initial responses outlined above and their natural flow into establishing ventilation and perfusion.[384] This range of activities can be carried out not only by professional and paraprofessional personnel but also by trained emergency technicians and lay persons. Time is the key issue, and there should be no delay between the diagnosis and preparatory efforts in the initial response and the institution of basic life support.

MOUTH-TO-MOUTH RESPIRATION. With the head properly placed and the oropharynx clear, mouth-to-mouth respiration can be initiated if no specific rescue equipment is available. To a large extent, the procedure used for establishing ventilation is dependent upon the site at which the cardiac arrest occurs. A variety of devices are available, including plastic oropharyngeal airways, esophageal obturators, the masked AMBU bag, and endotracheal tubes. The latter is the preferred procedure, but time should not be sacrificed even in the in-hospital setting while awaiting an endotracheal tube or a person trained to insert it quickly and properly. Thus, in the in-hospital setting, temporary support with AMBU bag ventilation is the usual method until endotracheal intubation can be carried out, and in the out-of-hospital setting mouth-to-mouth resuscitation is used while awaiting emergency rescue personnel. The effect of the acquired immune deficiency syndrome and hepatitis B transmission on attitudes toward mouth-to-mouth resuscitation by bystanders and even professional personnel in hospitals is an area of concern,[338a] but there are at present no data to assess the impact of this problem on outcome of resuscitative efforts.

Conventional CPR techniques require that the lungs be inflated once every 5 seconds when two persons are available for the resuscitative effort and twice every 15 seconds when only one person is present to carry out both ventilation and chest wall compression.[384] A new technique of CPR, which is based upon increased intrathoracic pressure as the prime mover of blood rather than cardiac compression itself,[369, 385] is currently being evaluated; the cyclic ventilatory techniques are altered in this procedure (see below).

CHEST COMPRESSION (Fig. 24–12). The second element of basic life support, chest compression, is intended to maintain blood flow until definitive steps can be taken. The rationale as originally developed was based on the hypothesis that cardiac compression allows the heart to maintain an externally driven pump function by sequential emptying and filling of its chambers, with competent valves favoring the forward direction of flow. In fact, the application of this technique has proved successful when used as recommended.[384] The palm of one hand is placed over the lower sternum and the heel of the other rests on the dorsum of the lower hand. The sternum is then depressed with the resuscitator's arms straight at the elbows to provide a less tiring and more forceful fulcrum at the junction of the shoulders and back (Fig. 24–12). Using this technique, sufficient force is applied to depress the sternum approximately 3 to 5 cm, with abrupt relaxation, and the cycle is carried out at a rate of approximately 80 to 100/min.[338a] Despite the fact that this conventional technique produces measurable carotid artery flow and a record of successful resuscitations, the absence of a pressure gradient across the heart in the presence of an extrathoracic arterial-venous pressure gradient has lead to a concept that it is not cardiac compression per se but rather a pumping action produced by pressure changes in the entire thoracic cavity that optimizes systemic blood flow during resuscitation.[369, 385–387] Experimental work in which the chest is compressed during ventilations rather than between them (simultaneous compression-ventilation, SCV) demonstrate better extrathoracic arterial flow.[385, 387–389] However, increased carotid artery flow does not necessarily equate with improved cerebral perfusion,[369, 390, 391] and the reduction in coronary blood flow caused by elevated intrathoracic pressures by certain techniques[369, 392] may be too high a price for the improved peripheral flow. In addition, a high thoracoabdominal gradient has been demonstrated during experimental SCV[393] which could divert flow from the brain in the absence of concomitant abdominal binding. Studies of comparative efficacy of the conventional CPR and the SCV techniques in clinical settings are under way.

ADVANCED LIFE SUPPORT AND DEFINITIVE RESUSCITATION

This next step in the sequence of resuscitative efforts is designed to achieve definitive support and stabilization of the patient.[384] The implementation of advanced life support does not indicate abrupt cessation of basic life support activities but rather a transition from one level of activity to the next. In the past, advanced life support required judgments and technical skills which removed it from the realm of activity of lay bystanders and even emergency

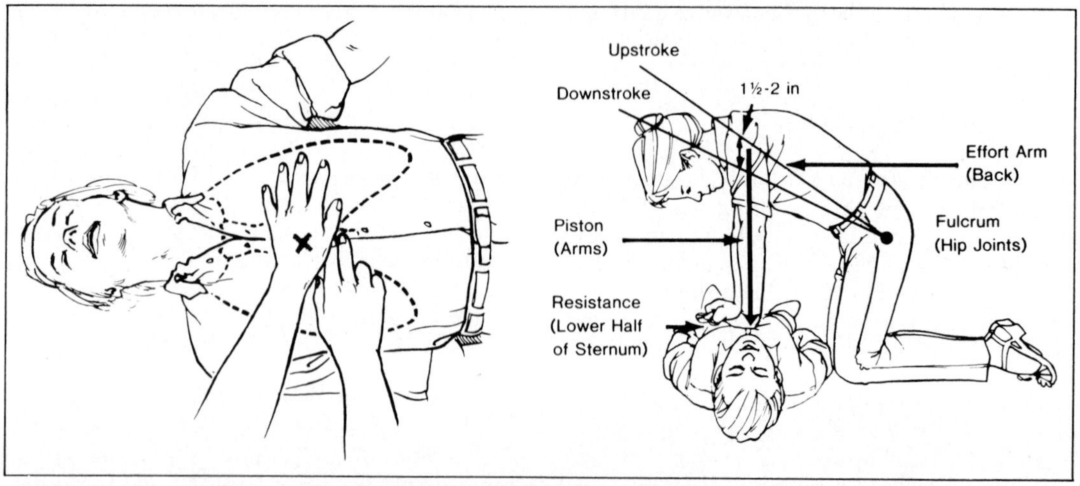

FIGURE 24–12. External chest compression. *Left,* Locating the correct hand position on the lower half of the sternum. *Right,* Proper position of the rescuer, with shoulders directly over the victim's sternum and elbows locked. (From Standard and guidelines for cardiopulmonary resuscitation [CPR] and emergency cardiac care [ECC]. J.A.M.A. *255*:2905, 1986. Copyright 1986, American Medical Association.)

medical technicians, limiting these activities to specifically trained paramedical personnel, nurses, and physicians. With further education of emergency technicians, many community-based CPR programs now permit them to carry out advanced life support activities.[348, 368] In addition, the development and testing of equipment which has the ability to sense and analyze air flow, sense cardiac electrical activity, and provide definitive electrical intervention[394, 395] may eventually provide a limited role for lay bystanders in advanced life support.

The general goals of advanced life support are to optimize ventilation, revert the cardiac rhythm to one which is hemodynamically effective, and maintain and support the restored circulation. Thus, during advanced life support, the patient (1) will be intubated and well oxygenated, (2) will be defibrillated, cardioverted, or paced, and (3) will have an intravenous line established to deliver necessary medications. After intubation, the goal of ventilation is to reverse hypoxemia and not merely achieve a high alveolar pO_2. Thus, oxygen rather than room air should be used to ventilate the patient; if possible, the arterial pO_2 should be monitored. Respirator support in hospital and AMBU bag via an endotracheal tube or face mask in the out-of-hospital setting are generally used.

DEFIBRILLATION-CARDIOVERSION (Fig. 24–13). Rapid conversion to an effective cardiac electrical mechanism is a key step for successful resuscitation.[344, 360] Delay should be minimal, even when conditions for cardiopulmonary resuscitation are optimal. When VF or a rapid VT is recognized on a monitor or by telemetry, defibrillation should be carried out immediately with a shock of 200 joules. Up to 90 per cent of VF victims weighing up to 90 kg can be resuscitated successfully with a 200-joule shock,[396–398] and a 300- or 360-joule shock may be used if this is not successful. High-energy defibrillation has been suggested by some,[399] but not in excess of 360 joules; others have expressed caution about the use of high energies.[400] Failure of the initial one or two shocks to cardiovert successfully to an effective rhythm is a poor prognostic sign;[338, 384] however, resuscitative efforts should not be abandoned. At this point, the focus should be on ventilation and correcting the biochemistry of the blood, efforts which will render the heart more likely to reestablish a stable rhythm—i.e., improved oxygenation, reversal of acidosis, and improvement of the underlying electrophysiological condition. Although adequate oxygenation of the blood is crucial in managing the metabolic acidosis of cardiac arrest, additional correction may be achieved if necessary by intravenous administration of sodium bicarbonate. However, it is important to recognize that much less sodium bicarbonate than was previously recommended is adequate for treatment of acidosis in this setting[401, 402] and that excessive quantities can be deleterious.[402–404] While some investigators question the use of sodium bicarbonate at all because risks of alkalosis, hypernatremia, and hyperosmolality related to its use may outweigh its benefits,[405] the acidotic patient (particularly if resistant to defibrillation) may benefit from administration of 1 mEq/kg of sodium bicarbonate while CPR is being carried out. Up to 50 per cent of this dose may be repeated every 10 to 15 minutes during the course of cardiopulmonary resuscitation.[406] When possible, arterial pH, pO_2, and pCO_2 should be monitored during the resuscitation.

PHARMACOTHERAPY. Electrical stability of the heart may be achieved by intravenous administration of *lidocaine* during resuscitation. As a matter of routine, all patients should receive a bolus of 1 mg/kg of lidocaine (p. 627) intravenously, with the dose repeated in 2 minutes in those in whom resuscitation remains unsuccessful or unstable

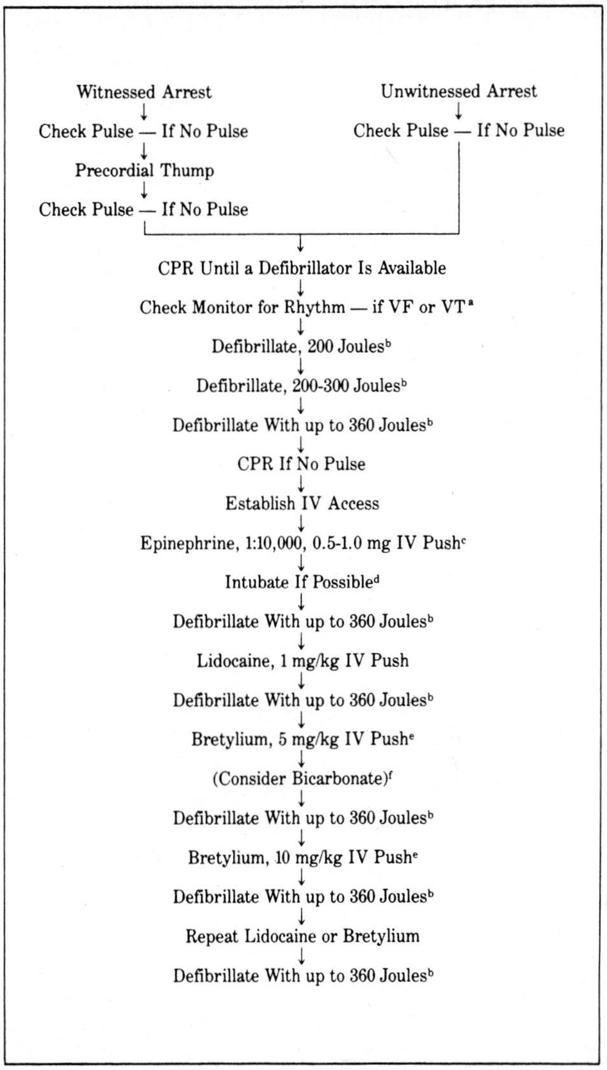

FIGURE 24–13. Algorithm for treatment of VF (and pulseless VT). This sequence was developed to assist in teaching how to treat a broad range of patients with VF and VT. Some patients may require care not specified herein; this algorithm should not be construed as prohibiting such flexibility. Flow of algorithm presumes that VF is continuing. CPR indicates cardiopulmonary resuscitation.

[a]Pulseless VT should be treated identically to VF.

[b]Check pulse and rhythm after each shock. If VF recurs after transiently converting (rather than persists without ever converting), use whatever energy level has previously been successful for defibrillation.

[c]Epinephrine should be repeated every 5 minutes.

[d]Intubation is preferable. If it can be accomplished simultaneously with other techniques, the earlier the better. However, defibrillation and epinephrine are more important initially if the patient can be ventilated without intubation.

[e]Some may prefer repeated doses of lidocaine, which may be given in 0.5 mg/kg boluses every 8 minutes to a total dose of 3 mg/kg.

[f]Value of sodium bicarbonate is questionable during cardiac arrest, and it is not recommended for routine cardiac arrest sequence. Consideration of its use in a dose of 1 mEq/kg is appropriate at this point. Half of original dose may be repeated every 10 minutes if it is used. (From Standard and guidelines for cardiopulmonary resuscitation [CPR] and emergency cardiac care [ECC]. J.A.M.A. *255*:2905, 1986. Copyright 1986, American Medical Association.)

electrical activity persists. A continuous infusion of lidocaine follows, at a rate of 1 to 4 mg/min, depending upon the patient's age, size, and other factors.[407] The patient who remains in VF after these initial efforts should be given *epinephrine*, 0.5 to 1.0 mg (5 to 10 ml of a 1:10,000 solution) intravenously, and attempts at defibrillation should be repeated. This dose of epinephrine can be repeated every 5 minutes during the resuscitation. It may be given by the intracardiac route only in the absence of or inaccessibility of intravenous or endotracheal routes of administration.[338a] Continued failure is an indication for other antiarrhythmic drugs, the most widely used at this time being *procainamide hydrochloride* (p. 630)[408] and *bretylium tosylate* (p. 635).[409, 410] Procainamide is administered as a series of 100 mg boluses every 5 minutes to a total dose of 500 to 1000 mg, followed by a constant infusion of 2 to 4 mg/min. Bretylium tosylate given in an initial dose of 5 mg/kg intravenously is followed by another attempt at defibrillation. Additional doses can be given every 15 minutes, to a maximum of 25 mg/kg. Intravenous amiodarone (p. 637), given as a 150 to 500 mg bolus and a 10 mg/kg/day infusion, has also been suggested for refractory VT and VF.[411] In patients in whom acute hyperkalemia is the triggering event for resistant VF, or who are hypocalcemic or toxic from Ca^{++}-entry blocking drugs, 10 per cent calcium gluconate, 5 to 20 ml infused at a rate of 2 to 4 ml/min, may be helpful.[338a] Calcium should *not* be used routinely during resuscitation.[411a]

BRADYARRHYTHMIC AND ASYSTOLIC ARREST. The approach to the patient with bradyarrhythmic or asystolic arrest differs (Fig. 24–14). Once this form of cardiac arrest is recognized, efforts should focus on those activities which are likely to favor the emergence of a stable spontaneous rhythm, or attempts should be made to pace the heart. Epinephrine (0.5 to 1.0 mg) and atropine 0.6 to 2.0 mg intravenously, are commonly used in an attempt to elicit a spontaneous electrical activity or increase the rate of a bradycardia. These have had only limited success, as has intravenous isoproterenol infusions in doses up to 15 to 20 μg/min. In the absence of an intravenous line, epinephrine (1 mg—i.e., 10 ml of a 1:10,000 solution) may be given by the intracardiac route, but the dangers of coronary or myocardial laceration should be recognized.

If Rhythm Is Unclear and Possibly Ventricular Fibrillation, Defibrillate as for VF. If Asystole is Present[a]
↓
Continue CPR
↓
Establish IV Access
↓
Epinephrine, 1:10,000, 0.5 - 1.0 mg IV Push[b]
↓
Intubate When Possible[c]
↓
Atropine, 1.0 mg IV Push (Repeated in 5 min)
↓
(Consider Bicarbonate)[d]
↓
Consider Pacing

FIGURE 24–14. Approach to the treatment of asystole (cardiac standstill). This sequence was developed to assist in teaching how to treat a broad range of patients with asystole. Some patients may require care not specified herein; this algorithm should not be construed to prohibit such flexibility. Flow of algorithm presumes asystole is continuing. VF = ventricular fibrillation; IV = intravenous.

[a]Asystole should be confirmed in two leads.

[b]Epinephrine should be repeated every 5 minutes.

[c]Intubation is preferable; if it can be accomplished simultaneously with other techniques, the earlier the better. However, cardiopulmonary resuscitation (CPR) and use of epinephrine are more important initially if patient can be ventilated without intubation.

[d]Value of sodium bicarbonate is questionable during cardiac arrest and it is not recommended for the routine cardiac arrest sequence. Consideration of its use in a dose of 1 mEq/kg is appropriate at this point. Half of original dose may be repeated every 10 minutes if it is used. (From Standard and guidelines for cardiopulmonary resuscitation [CPR] and emergency cardiac care [ECC]. J.A.M.A. *255*:2905, 1986. Copyright 1986, American Medical Association.)

Continue CPR
↓
Establish IV Access
↓
Epinephrine, 1:10,000, 0.5 - 1.0 mg IV Push[a]
↓
Intubate When Possible[b]
↓
(Consider Bicarbonate)[c]
↓
Consider Hypovolemia,
Cardiac Tamponade,
Tension Pneumothorax,
Hypoxemia,
Acidosis,
Pulmonary Embolism

FIGURE 24–15. Electromechanical dissociation. This sequence was developed to assist in teaching how to treat a broad range of patients with electromechanical dissociation. Some patients may require care not specified herein. This algorithm should not be construed to prohibit such flexibility. Flow of algorithm presumes that electromechanical dissociation is continuing.

[a]Epinephrine should be repeated every 5 minutes.

[b]Intubation is preferable. If it can be accomplished simultaneously with other techniques, the earlier the better. However, epinephrine is more important initially if the patient can be ventilated without intubation.

[c]Value of sodium bicarbonate is questionable during cardiac arrest, and it is not recommended for routine cardiac arrest sequence. Consideration of its use in a dose of 1 mEq/kg is appropriate at this point. Half of original dose may be repeated every 10 minutes if it is used. (From Standard and guidelines for cardiopulmonary resuscitation [CPR] and emergency cardiac care [ECC]. J.A.M.A. *255*:2905, 1986. Copyright 1986, American Medical Association.)

Pacing of the bradyarrhythmic or asystolic heart has been limited in the past by the availability of personnel capable of carrying out such procedures at the scene of cardiac arrests. With the development of more effective external pacing systems in recent years[412] the role of pacing and its influence on outcome must now be reevaluated. Unfortunately, all data to date suggest that the *asystolic* patient continues to have a very poor prognosis, despite new techniques.[343, 349, 412a]

A recently published update on standards for cardiopulmonary resuscitation and emergency cardiac care[338a] included a series of teaching algorithms to be used as guides to appropriate care. Figures 24–13 to 24–15 are the algorithms for ventricular fibrillation and pulseless ventricular tachycardia, asystole (or cardiac standstill), and electromechanical dissociation, respectively. These general teaching guides are not to be interpreted as inclusive of all possible approaches or contingencies. The special circumstance of cardiopulmonary resuscitation in pregnant women requires additional attention to effects of drugs on the gravid uterus and the fetus, mechanical and physiological influences of pregnancy on efficacy of cardiopulmonary resuscitation, and risk of complications such as ruptured uterus and lacerated liver.[412b]

When electrical stability is achieved, the focus of attention shifts to maintaining the hemodynamic status of the electrically resuscitated patient. Catecholamines are used in cardiac arrest not only in an attempt to achieve better electrical stability (e.g., conversion from fine to coarse ventricular fibrillation, or increase the rate of spontaneous contraction during bradyarrhythmias) but also for their inotropic and peripheral vascular effects. Epinephrine is the first choice among the catecholamines for use in cardiac arrest because it increases myocardial contractility, elevates perfusion pressure, may convert electromechanical dissociation to electromechanical coupling, and improves chances for defibrillation. Because of its adverse effects on renal and mesenteric flow, norepinephrine is a less desirable agent despite its inotropic effects. When the chronotropic effect of epinephrine is undesirable, dopamine or dobutamine is preferable to norepinephrine for inotropic effect. Isoproterenol may be used for the treatment of primary or postdefibrillation bradycardia when heart rate control is the primary goal of therapy to improve cardiac output. Calcium chloride, 2 to 4 mg/kg, is commonly given in an attempt to enhance the contractile state of the myocardium in patients with hypotension or to reverse electromechanical dissociation which persists after administration of catecholamines. The efficacy of this intervention is uncertain. Stimulation of alpha-adrenoceptors may be important during definitive resuscitative efforts.[413–417] For instance, the alpha-adrenoceptor stimulating effects of epinephrine and higher dosages of dopamine, producing elevation of aortic diastolic pressures by peripheral vasoconstriction[413, 414] with increased cerebral[415] and myocardial flow,[417] have been reemphasized recently.[369, 415] In addition, the relative importance of alpha-adrenoceptors on defibrillation in experimental VF has also been suggested.[414]

POST-CARDIAC ARREST CARE

For successfully resuscitated cardiac arrest victims, whether the event occurred in- or out-of-hospital, post-cardiac arrest care includes admission to an intensive care unit and continuous monitoring for a minimum of 48 to 72 hours. Some elements of post-arrest management are common to all resuscitated patients, but prognosis and certain details of management are specific for the clinical setting in which the cardiac arrest occurred. The major management categories include: (1) primary cardiac arrest in acute myocardial infarction, (2) secondary cardiac arrest in acute myocardial infarction, (3) cardiac arrest associated with noncardiac disorders, and (4) survivors of out-of-hospital cardiac arrest.

PRIMARY CARDIAC ARREST IN ACUTE MYOCARDIAL INFARCTION (See also p. 1249). VF in the absence of preexisting hemodynamic complications (i.e., primary VF) is currently less common in hospitalized patients than the 15 to 20 per cent incidence, which existed before availability of coronary care units. Early aggressive antiarrhythmic treatment is probably responsible,[418] and those events which do occur involve a high success rate of reversibility with prompt interventions in properly equipped emergency rooms or coronary care units.[419] After resuscitation, patients are maintained on a lidocaine infusion at 2 to 4 mg/min. Antiarrhythmic support is discontinued after 48 to 72 hours if arrhythmias do not persist (p. 1262). The occurrence of VF in the early phase of myocardial infarction is not an indication for late hospital or long-term antiarrhythmic therapy.[76] Rapid VT producing the clinical picture of cardiac arrest in acute myocardial infarction is treated similarly; its intermediate and long-term implications are the same as VF. Cardiac arrest due to bradyarrhythmias or asystole in acute inferior wall myocardial infarction, in the absence of primary hemodynamic consequences, is very uncommon and may respond to either atropine or pacing. The prognosis is good, with no special long-term care required in most instances. Rarely, symptomatic bradyarrhythmias that require permanent pacemakers persist in survivors. In contrast to inferior myocardial infarction, bradyarrhythmic cardiac arrest associated with large anterior wall infarctions (and atrioventricular or intraventricular block) has a very poor prognosis (p. 1263).

SECONDARY CARDIAC ARREST IN ACUTE MYOCARDIAL INFARCTION. The immediate mortality among patients in this setting ranges from 59 to 89 per cent, depending upon severity of the hemodynamic abnormalities and size of the myocardial infarction.[341] Resuscitative efforts commonly fail in such patients, and when they are successful the post-cardiac arrest management is often difficult. When secondary cardiac arrest occurs by the mechanisms of VT or VF, lidocaine in standard dosages is employed, although the dose may have to be reduced in the presence of severe heart failure.[407] Other antiarrhythmics may have to be used in addition to or instead of lidocaine if complex arrhythmias persist or cardiac arrest recurs. The success of interventions and prevention of recurrent cardiac arrest relate closely to the outcome of managing the hemodynamic status. The incidence of cardiac arrest due to bradyarrhythmias or asystole, or to electromechanical dissociation, is higher in the secondary form of cardiac arrest in acute myocardial infarction.[420] Such patients generally have large myocardial infarctions, major hemodynamic abnormalities, and may be acidotic and hypoxemic. Even with aggressive therapy the prognosis after a bradyarrhythmic or asystolic arrest in such patients is very poor, and patients are resuscitated only rarely from electromechanical dissociation. All patients in circulatory failure at the onset of arrest are in a high-risk category, with only a 2 per cent survival rate of hypotensive patients in one extensive study.[343]

CARDIAC ARREST IN IN-HOSPITAL PATIENTS WITH NONCARDIAC ABNORMALITIES. These patients fall into two major categories: (1) those with life-limiting diseases such as malignancies, sepsis, organ failure, end-stage pulmonary disease, and advanced central nervous system disease; and (2) those with acute toxic or proarrhythmic states which are potentially reversible. In the former category, the ratio of tachyarrhythmic to bradyarrhythmic cardiac arrest is low, with a higher percentage of the arrests associated with bradyarrhythmias or asystole,[343] and the prognosis is poor. Although the data may be somewhat skewed by the practice of assigning "do not resuscitate" orders to patients with end-stage disease, available data for attempted resuscitations show a poor outcome. Bedell et al.[343] reported that only 7 per cent of resuscitated cancer patients, 3 per cent of renal failure patients, and no patients with sepsis or acute central nervous system disease were successfully resuscitated and discharged from the hospital alive. For the few successfully resuscitated patients in these categories, post-arrest management is dictated by the underlying precipitating factors with supportive cardiac care directed to stabilizing hemodynamics, respiratory, and cardiac electrical states.

Almost all antiarrhythmic drugs,[186, 188, 231, 232] a number of drugs used for noncardiac purposes which have proarrhythmic effects,[188, 193] and electrolyte disturbances may precipitate potentially lethal arrhythmias and cardiac arrest. Quinidine and the other class I–A antiarrhythmic drugs, the newer class I–C drugs, and perhaps class III drugs are the best recognized in the antiarrhythmic category.[186, 188, 231, 232] Among other categories of drugs,[188, 193] the phenothiazines, tricyclic antidepressants, lithium,[193] and cardiovascular drugs which are not antiarrhythmics—such as phenylamine and lidoflazin—are recognized causes. Hypokalemia and hypomagnesemia, and perhaps hypocalcemia, are the electrolyte disturbances most closely associated with cardiac arrest. Acidosis and hypoxia may potentiate the vulnerability associated with electrolyte disturbances. Proarrhythmic effects may be foreshadowed by prolongation of the Q-T interval, although this electrocardiographic change is often not present.[191] The torsades des pointes form of VT is a common manifestation of proarrhythmic effects. This arrhythmia is usually unstable and self-limiting and may terminate spontaneously, degenerate to VF, or evolve into a sustained VT. Cardiac arrest due to this mechanism is managed by pacing, isoproterenol, and removal of the offending agent.[231] When the patient's condition can be stabilized until the offending factor is removed (e.g., proarrhythmic drugs) or corrected (e.g., electrolyte imbalances, hypothermia), the prognosis is excellent.[343] The recognition of torsades de pointes (p. 698) and the identification of its risk by prolongation of the Q-T interval in association with the offending agent are helpful in managing these patients. No long-term prophylaxis is required in most patients. In contrast, beta-adrenoceptor blocking drugs or stellate ganglionectomy are required for long-term management of patients with the congenital form of Q-T interval prolongation who have been resuscitated after life-threatening arrhythmias.

POST-CARDIAC ARREST CARE IN SURVIVORS OF PREHOSPITAL CARDIAC ARREST. The initial management of survivors of out-of-hospital cardiac arrest centers on stabilizing the cardiac electrical status, supporting hemodynamics, and providing supportive care for reversal of organ damage which has occurred as a consequence of the cardiac arrest. Frequent complex ventricular arrhythmias are common during the first 48 to 72 hours after resuscitation;[20] however, they are often manageable by conventional treatment. The risk of recurrent cardiac arrest is relatively low, and arrhythmias account for only 10 per cent of in-hospital deaths after successful prehospital resuscitation.[20, 368] However, since the mortality rate among those who do have recurrent cardiac arrest during the index hospitalization is 50 per cent, antiarrhythmic therapy is used in all patients during the first 48 hours of post-arrest hospitalization in an attempt to prevent recurrent cardiac arrest. Lidocaine is the drug of choice for initial management, followed by intravenous procainamide or bretylium if initial drug therapy fails. Patients who have either preexisting or new atrioventricular or intraventricular conduction disturbances are at particularly high risk for recurrent cardiac arrest.[20] The routine use of temporary pacemakers has been evaluated in such patients but was not found to be useful for preventing early recurrent cardiac arrest. Invasive techniques for hemodynamic monitoring are used in unstable patients but not routinely for those who are stable on admission.

Respiratory support by conventional methods is used as necessary. During the convalescent period, attention to central nervous system status, including physical rehabilitation, is of primary importance to an optimal outcome. Bass[421] has recently summarized the neurological sequelae to cardiac arrest, including a review of various interventions. Preliminary data which suggested a beneficial effect of barbituate loading for reversal of ischemic brain injury during and after cardiac arrest[422] have not been supported by a multicenter study of thiopental loading in comatose post-arrest patients.[423] Management of other organ system injury (e.g., renal, hepatic) as well as early recognition and treatment of infectious complications, also contributes to ultimate survival.

LONG-TERM MANAGEMENT OF SURVIVORS OF OUT-OF-HOSPITAL CARDIAC ARREST. When the survivor of prehospital cardiac arrest has passed through the early convalescent period (5 to 7 days), has awakened, and has stable cardiopulmonary dynamics, decisions must be made regarding the nature and extent of the work-up required to establish a long-term management strategy. The goals of the work-up are to identify the specific etiology of the cardiac arrest (if not already evident), clarify the functional status of the patient's cardiovascular system, establish long-term therapy, and determine endpoints of both antiarrhythmic and antiischemic therapy. The extent of the work-up is dictated largely by the degree of central nervous system recovery and the factors already known to have contributed to the cardiac arrest. For instance, patients who have limited return of central nervous system function generally do not undergo extensive work-ups, and patients whose cardiac arrests were triggered by an acute transmural myocardial infarction have a work-up no different from that of any other patient with acute myocardial infarction.

Survivors of prehospital cardiac arrest not associated with acute myocardial infarction who have good return of neurological function undergo extensive diagnostic work-ups and carefully designed long-term therapy. The work-up generally includes cardiac catheterization with coronary angiography, an evaluation of functional significance of coronary lesions by stress-imaging techniques, and estimation of baseline susceptibility to life-threatening arrhythmias and of the expected response to long-term therapy.

GENERAL MANAGEMENT. The general care of survivors of cardiac arrest is determined by the specific etiology and the pathophysiology of the underlying process. For patients with ischemic heart disease (who form the vast majority of this population), control of episodes of myocardial ischemia, optimization of therapy for left ventricular dysfunction, and attention to general medical status are all addressed. Antiischemic therapy may be medical or surgical, depending upon the anatomy and physiology of the disease process. Although there are limited data suggesting that coronary bypass surgery may improve the recurrence rate and total mortality rates after survival from prehospital cardiac arrest,[424] no properly controlled prospective studies have validated this impression. Therefore, indications for surgery are limited to two groups of patients: (1) those who have a conventional indication for surgery such as left main coronary artery disease or uncontrolled angina pectoris,[288] and (2) those who meet specific criteria for surgery directed to arrhythmia control (e.g., discrete ventricular aneurysms, and inducible potentially lethal arrhythmias not controlled by medical therapy).[425]

Medical antiischemic therapy includes nitrates, beta-adrenoceptor blocking agents, and Ca^{++}-entry blockers. Beta-adrenoceptors may have both an anti-anginal effect and also influence the role of sympathetic nervous system activity on the genesis of potentially lethal arrhythmias. Although two studies could not establish a difference in long-term outcome between survivors receiving and those not receiving beta blockers,[56, 345] Morady and colleagues[116] recently suggested that medical or surgical antiischemic therapy, rather than antiarrhythmic therapy, should be the primary approach to long-term management of the subgroup of prehospital cardiac arrest survivors in whom transient myocardial ischemia was the inciting factor. In a report from the Coronary Artery Surgery Study (CASS), Holmes et al.[425a] compared sudden death rates in medically and surgically treated patients in the CASS registry. This study did not address directly the issue of surgery in survivors of out-of-hospital cardiac arrest, but there was a significant difference at 5 years, with a 98 per cent sudden death–free survival in the surgical group versus 94 per cent in the medical group ($p < .0001$). The differences were minimal in the groups with one- or two-vessel disease and no history of heart failure, but expanded to 91 and 69 per cent, respectively, in patients with three-vessel disease and a history of heart failure. The question of how to apply these data to indications for surgery for cardiac arrest survivors remains unanswered at this time. The problem is further confounded by the fact that assignment of the 13,476 analyzable patients to medical versus surgical groups was not randomized (i.e., based on clinical judgment). Further evaluation of the specific role of coronary surgery *after* out-of-hospital cardiac arrest is needed.

The long-term management of the consequences of left ventricular dysfunction by conventional means such as digitalis preparations and chronic diuretic use has recently been evaluated in several studies. Data from the Multiple Risk Factor Intervention Trial (MRFIT) suggested a higher mortality rate in the special intervention group,[426] presumably related to diuretic use and K^+ depletion, and other data regarding the relationship between K^+ depletion and arrhythmias have focused attention on routine use of such drugs. Although the facts are far from conclusive at present,[312] use of such drugs should be accompanied by careful monitoring of electrolytes. Similar concerns have been raised in respect to digitalis use in high-risk patients following acute myocardial infarction.[427–431] As of this writing, use of digoxin in survivors of prehospital cardiac arrest should be tailored to specific indications for left ventricular dysfunction.

Prevention of Recurrent Cardiac Arrest

Long-term therapeutic strategies intended to prevent recurrences of potentially lethal arrhythmias have been based on several medical approaches, on antiarrhythmic surgery, and on the use of implantable devices. Historically, the first of the medical approaches proposed was plasma level monitored antiarrhythmic therapy,[354, 355] then therapy guided by suppression of arrhythmias identified by ambulatory monitoring and exercise testing,[432, 433] and more recently suppression of inducibility of high-risk arrhythmias by electrophysiological programmed stimulation (EPS) protocols.[434–440] Antiarrhythmic surgery[425, 441, 442] evolved in parallel with programmed stimulation approaches to management, and most recently antitachycardiac and antifibrillatory devices[441, 443, 444] have been developed and studied in subgroups of these patients. A problem which impinges upon all long-term strategies is the lack of a reliable current natural history denominator against which to compare the results of any intervention.

LONG-TERM ANTIARRHYTHMIC THERAPY. The antiarrhythmic approach to long-term management of survivors of prehospital cardiac arrest was devised on two assumptions: (1) that the high frequency of chronic PVC's identified in cardiac arrest survivors constitutes a triggering mechanism for potentially lethal arrhythmias, and (2) that electrophysiological instability of the myocardium predisposing to potentially lethal arrhythmias can be modified by antiarrhythmic drugs.[320, 355] In an 8-year follow-up study of 61 survivors of prehospital cardiac arrest whose management was based upon empirical dose titration to achieve stable high therapeutic plasma concentrations of antiarrhythmic agents, the recurrent cardiac arrest rate was 10 per cent at 1 year and 15 per cent at 2 years (Fig. 24–16), with 31 per cent of the recurrences occurring in patients whose drug has been stopped or changed without monitoring of the levels of the new drug.[56] With the development of more detailed methods of analysis of ambulatory monitoring recordings[432, 433] and electrophysiologic stimulation (EPS) for testing inducibility of clinically significant arrhythmias, attention focused on these more specific and individualized means of evaluating drug therapy. Graboys et al.[433] reported the outcome in a group of 123 patients with malignant ventricular arrhythmias who had survived one or more cardiac arrests. Suppression of specific forms of ventricular ectopy (salvos of three or more ectopic beats and early cycle PVC's) identified on ambulatory monitoring or exercise testing was accompanied by a significantly reduced mortality rate, compared to those in whom such suppression was not achieved. The mortality rate was more than 80 per cent at 3 years in patients whose complex forms could not be suppressed, compared to a nearly 90 per cent survival of those whose complex PVC's were suppressed.

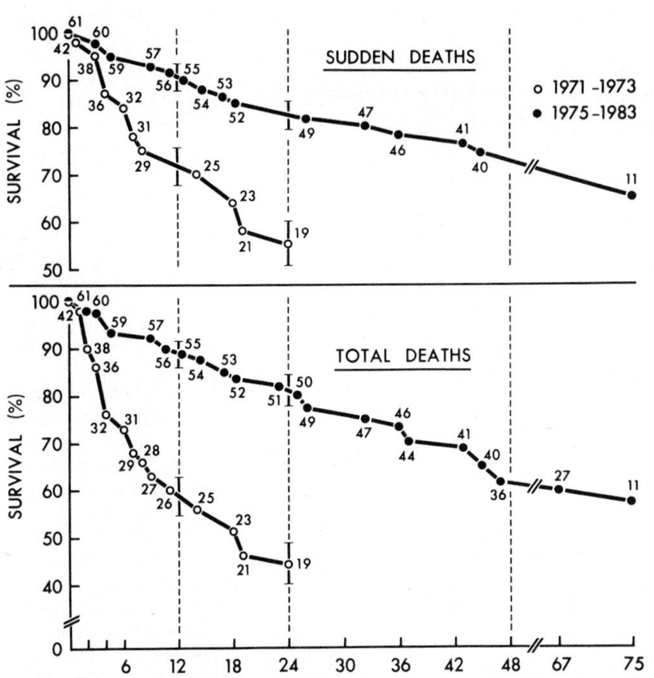

FIGURE 24–16. Sudden deaths and total deaths in survivors of prehospital cardiac arrest during an 8-year follow-up period (closed circles). Compared to 1970–73 historical experience during the initial Miami studies (open circles). The more recent experience indicates a 67 per cent reduction in recurrent cardiac arrest rate in the first year of follow-up. Whether this was due to aggressive antiarrhythmic therapy or other factors in the patient populations or their management cannot be determined from comparison to historic controls. However, the 10-per cent 1-year mortality rate is similar to outcome with other forms of antiarrhythmic intervention in recent years. (From Myerburg, R. J., and Kessler, K. M.: Management of patients who survive cardiac arrest. Mod. Concepts Cardiovasc. Dis. *55*:61, 1986.)

The use of programmed electrophysiological stimulation for guiding therapy in survivors of prehospital cardiac arrest is more complex because of problems related to sensitivity and specificity of the various pacing protocols[445] and serious concerns about the extent to which the myocardial status at the time of electrophysiologic stimulation reflects that at the time of the cardiac arrest. Imponderables such as the extent to which electrode catheter–stimulated extrasystoles mimic spontaneous PVC's, and the ischemic, autonomic, and biochemical status of the heart at the time of the study, may influence the data.[446] Nonetheless, among a series of 5 studies,[434–439] induction of sustained VT or VF at baseline study ranged from 31 to 58 per cent, and successful suppression of inducibility ranged from 18 to 78 per cent. The mortality rate during follow-up of those patients in whom inducibility was suppressed by antiarrhythmic therapy ranged from 0 to 22 per cent (mean, 9 per cent), compared to a range of 22 to 78 per cent (mean, 43 per cent) in those patients in whom VT or VF was still inducible on any antiarrhythmic therapy.

The evaluation of these data is significantly influenced by definitions of inducibility and noninducibility and also by the clinical details of the patient population in each of the studies, which varied considerably. In most reports VF or sustained VT could not be induced in 25 to 30 per cent of the patients. The greater discrepancies were in the numbers of patients in whom these were inducible into sustained versus nonsustained arrhythmias. It is probable that differences are determined in part by the numbers of patients who have anatomically discrete ventricular aneurysms in various referral populations. Careful attention to protocol details, anatomy of the disease processes, and definitions of inducibility may help clarify these discrepancies in the future. For the present, however, in approximately 40 per cent of *unselected* survivors of cardiac arrest VF or sustained VT can be anticipated to be inducible into sustained arrhythmias. For the subgroup with discrete ventricular aneurysms, as many as 80 per cent may show this inducibility.[288, 436]

It is generally agreed that inducibility into a *sustained* clinical arrhythmia provides an indication of risk and its prevention is an endpoint for therapy, but the induction of *nonsustained* forms is more controversial. Most data suggest that induction of nonsustained rhythms may indicate risk, but it is often nonspecific if a quite aggressive protocol is used.[445] The use of the suppression of nonsustained arrhythmias as an endpoint of therapy is not considered valid at present. The significance of *noninducibility* at baseline EPS testing in relation to risk and long-term management is also a controversial issue. Opinions range from the assumption that patients showing noninducibility are not electrophysiologically unstable and require no long-term antiarrhythmic therapy[116, 434, 439, 440] to the other extreme that such patients remain at risk but do not provide an objective endpoint of therapy by this method, and therefore must be treated by complex PVC suppression or other techniques.[56, 288, 355, 432, 433] While some patients in this category have had cardiac arrest based upon transient ischemia and require control with antiischemic therapy,[116] the difficulty of identifying patients who are best managed by antiischemic rather than antiarrhythmic therapy is considerable. Many clinicans use the two modes of treatment concomitantly. In the 5 EPS studies, 24-month mortality in patients who had noninducibility ranged from 3 to 38 per cent, higher than in patients in whom inducibility could be suppressed by antiarrhythmic therapy (average, 9 per cent) but lower than those in whom inducibility could not be suppressed (average, 43 per cent).

SURGICAL MANAGEMENT (p. 648). Techniques initially conceived for control of recurrent sustained VT, map-guided endocardial resection,[447] and encircling endocardial ventriculotomy[448] are also used for survivors of out-of-hospital cardiac arrest. This approach is limited largely to those patients who have inducibility into sustained VT and VF during electrophysiological testing, are unresponsive to drug therapy, and have suitable ventricular and coronary artery anatomy. Unfortunately, data available on this approach to management of cardiac arrest survivors are derived from broader studies of either mixed populations (i.e., recurrent VT and cardiac arrest survivors) or mixed therapeutic approaches (i.e., surgery after medical failure). Nonetheless, it appears that surgical intervention is successful in selected patients in whom medical therapy does not produce an acceptable endpoint,[422, 438, 439] even though statistics limited to out-of-hospital cardiac arrest survivors are difficult to derive from published data.

IMPLANTABLE DEVICES (Ch. 23). The development of a reliable implantable defibrillator has added a new dimension to the management of patients at high risk of cardiac arrest.[449] Mirowski and coworkers[443] evaluated the results in 52 patients who had survived an arrhythmic cardiac arrest plus at least one recurrence not associated with acute myocardial infarction. Other forms of preventive management had failed in all these patients, and the group had a mean of 3.9 cardiac arrests per patient. The analysis is complicated by the fact that concomitant cardiovascular surgical procedures were carried out in 15 patients, and approximately the same number had previous surgery, plus pacemaker implantation in 9. Although 12 of these 52 very high-risk patients died during a 14-month mean follow-up period producing a 23 per cent 1-year total mortality rate, the 1-year sudden death rate was 8.5 per cent. Devices were triggered 62 times in 17 patients. Assuming death would have followed in these patients without the device, the total 1-year mortality rate would have been 48 per cent. Subsequently, Echt and colleagues[444] reported their experience in 70 patients. Since 35 of their patients (50 per cent) had had no previous cardiac arrests (14 patients with uncontrollable recurrent ventricular tachycardia) or only 1 previous arrest (21 patients), this population may have been less "unstable" than Mirowski's group.[443] There was a mean of 1.9 ± 1.7 cardiac arrests/patient, 3.1 ± 2.3 arrhythmic episodes/patient, and 4.0 ± 2.1 drug failures/patient. During an average follow-up period of 8.9 months (range, 1 to 33 months), 37 patients (53 per cent) received one or more shocks. The 12-month total death rate was 10 per cent, the sudden death rate was less than 2 per cent, and the complication rate was acceptably low. Finally, Platia et al.[441] evaluated the concomitant use of the device with ventricular endocardial resection for refractory ventricular arrhythmias. During a mean 25-month follow-up, 4 of 25 patients (16 per cent) had recurrent tachycardia which was successfully reverted by the device, but 1 patient died because the device malfunctioned.

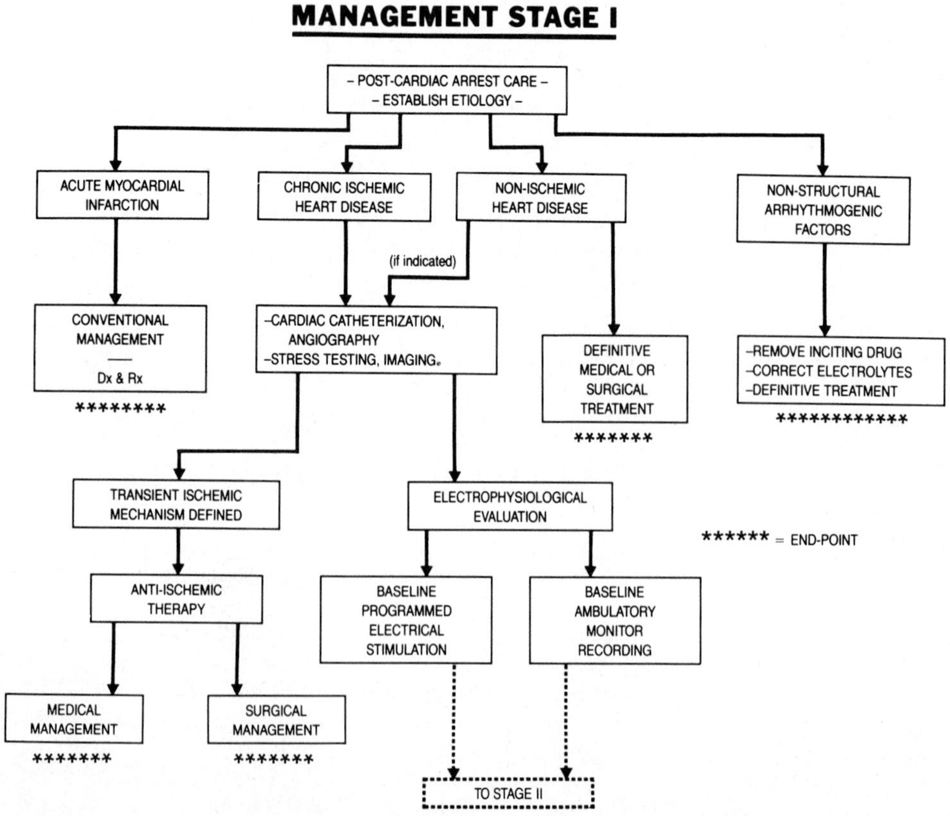

FIGURE 24–17. Management algorithm—stage I. Flow diagram for initial management and diagnostic activities in survivors of prehospital cardiac arrest. Patients whose arrests were associated with new acute transmural myocardial infarction or nonstructural arrhythmogenic factors are managed by conventional techniques. All patients with chronic ischemic heart disease, and many with nonischemic heart disease, enter a pathway which leads to advanced electrophysiological study and management. (From Myerburg, R. J., and Kessler, K. M.: Management of patients who survive cardiac arrest. Mod. Concepts Cardiovasc. Dis. *55*:61, 1986.)

Management Algorithm

The options for diagnostic evaluation and long-term management of cardiac arrest survivors are complex, with specific problems unique both to patient subgroups and to the various therapeutic strategies. A two-tiered algorithm has been developed as a guide to management on the basis of current information and limitations.[450] Management stage I (Fig. 24–17) addresses diagnostic evaluation and general management, and stage II (Fig. 24–18) is oriented to advanced strategies for control of potentially lethal arrhythmias. Endpoints of management are reached in stage I for those patients in whom cardiac arrest was precipitated by acute myocardial infarction, those who have some forms of noncoronary heart disease or cardiac arrest clearly related to transient ischemia, and those who have cardiac arrest due to proarrhythmic factors, such as adverse drug effect or electrolyte imbalances. Patients with life-limiting concurrent morbid states and those who have major post-arrest residual damage of the central nervous system also reach their management endpoints in stage I.

Among the remainder, who constitute the majority of survivors and most commonly have chronic ischemic heart disease, electrophysiological stimulation should be performed (Fig. 24–18). In that subgroup of patients in whom sustained VT with or without degeneration to VF is inducible (*pathway A*), the primary endpoint of therapy is prevention of inducibility by an appropriate antiarrhythmic agent or drug combination. Once identified, the plasma concentration required to achieve noninducibility should be noted and monitored periodically during follow-up. In those patients in whom this approach is not feasible because of noninducibility of sustained VT or VF, another objective approach should be employed—specifically, the evaluation of response of complex PVC's on ambulatory monitoring to antiarrhythmic agents (*pathway B*, Fig. 24–18). Those patients who have salvos or nonsustained VT on ambulatory monitoring are titrated with antiarrhythmic drugs singly or in combination in an attempt to suppress repetitive forms.[433] If this is successful, it is used as the endpoint of therapy.[450a] In those patients who have neither inducibility by electrophysiological stimulation nor complex forms on ambulatory monitoring, antiischemic therapy,[116] usually with additional antiarrhythmic therapy[56, 320] should be employed. This approach also has been used in some patients in whom inducibility in the laboratory is not preventable or whose ambulatory monitor repetitive forms are not suppressible, as has the empirical use of amiodarone or other new or experimental drugs. However, the promising statistics on antiarrhythmic surgical procedures[425, 441, 442, 448] and implantable antitachycardia and antifibrillatory devices[441, 443, 444] now appear to warrant their use in lieu of empiric therapy in many patients in this category (Fig. 24–18, *pathway C*).

Surgical intervention is preferred in patients who have discrete ventricular aneurysms, have inducibility into sustained VT or VF, and cannot be managed by antiarrhythmic drugs. The results of surgery in such patients have been encouraging.[425] Implantable devices are the method of choice for patients who have survived a *recurrence on therapy predicted to be successful by one of the other endpoints*, and in many of those who fail the EPS or

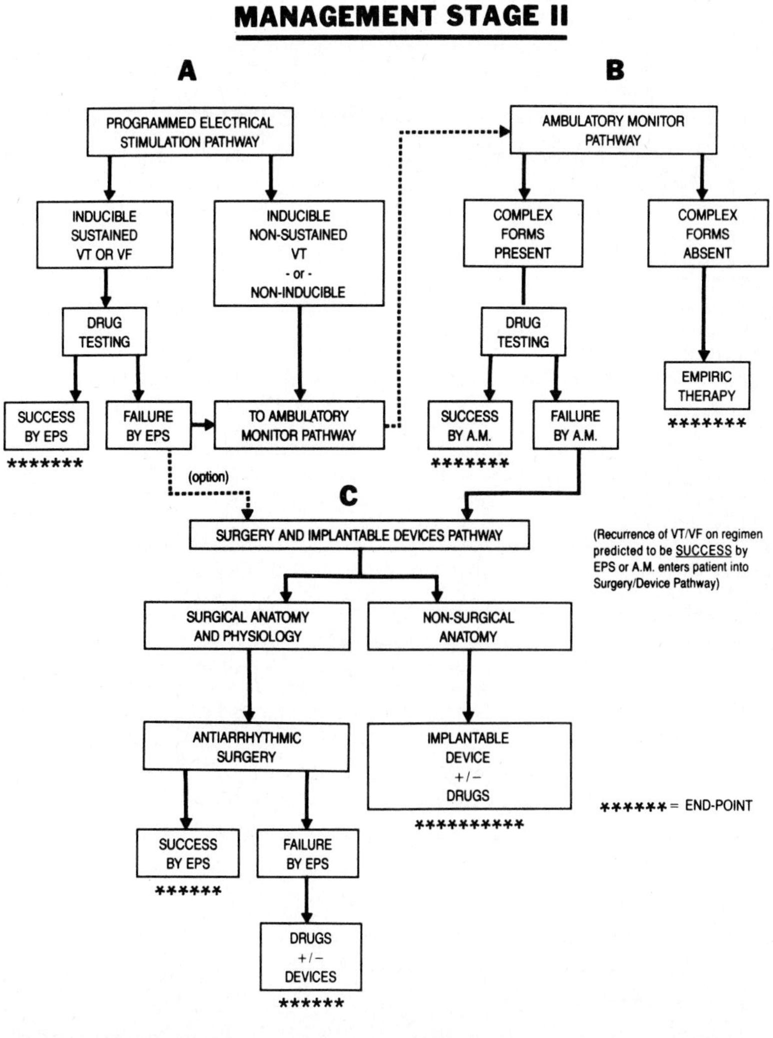

FIGURE 24–18. Management algorithm—Stage II. Advanced electrophysiological evaluation of survivors of prehospital cardiac arrest. Patients generally enter *pathway A*—programmed electrical stimulation (EPS), and if inducible into sustained VT or VT/VF, they are managed by drug testing using this technique. If successful, this becomes the endpoint. If the patient fails EPS, or if patients are inducible into nonsustained VT or noninducible at baseline study, they enter the ambulatory monitor (A.M.) pathway (*pathway B*). Some patients who fail EPS, if unstable, might enter directly to *pathway C*—surgery or implantable devices. The route through pathways B and C is explained in the text. (From Myerburg, R. J., and Kessler, K. M.: Management of patients who survive cardiac arrest. Mod. Concepts Cardiovasc. Dis., *55*:61, 1986.)

ambulatory monitoring legs of the algorithm and are considered to be at high risk. Concomitant antiarrhythmic therapy after a device is implanted may reduce the number of shocks delivered.[444] Implantable devices may also have a role in conjunction with antiarrhythmic surgery, especially in those in whom inducibility into high-risk arrhythmias remains postoperatively.[441, 442]

The recent statistics for each of the approaches outlined above are intriguing. Each method has now been recognized to yield a 1-year survival rate of up to 90 per cent or better, compared with the 70 per cent survival cited earlier. Whether this means that each of the methods is equally effective or that some other uncontrolled factor is influencing outcome has not been defined and requires further evaluation. One fact which is clear, however, is the high risk attendant upon indiscriminant changes in pharmacological therapy which has been determined appropriate by any of the endpoints used. Swerdlow et al.[422] and Myerburg et al.,[56] using very different therapeutic approaches, have both reported that arbitrary cessation, or changes in therapy without retesting for the endpoint used to establish the initial therapy, is accompanied by a high risk of recurrent cardiac arrest.

SUDDEN DEATH AND PUBLIC SAFETY

The unexpectedness of SCD has raised questions concerning secondary risk to the public created by persons in the throes of a cardiac arrest. There are no controlled data available to guide public policy regarding individuals at high risk for potentially lethal arrhythmias and for abrupt incapacitation. Myerburg and Davis[451] reported observations on 1348 sudden deaths due to coronary heart disease in persons 65 years of age or less during a 7-year period in Dade County, Florida. One hundred and one (7.5 per cent) of these deaths occurred in individuals engaged in activities at the time of death which were potentially hazardous to the public (e.g., 56 driving private automobiles or taxis, 15 driving trucks, 10 working at altitude, 2 piloting aircraft) and 122 (9.1 per cent) of the victims had occupations which could create potential hazards to others if an abrupt loss of consciousness had occurred while at work (e.g., 57 taxi and truck drivers, 8 aircraft pilots, 9 bus drivers, 9 policemen and firemen). However, there were no catastrophic events as a result of these cardiac arrests, only minor property damage in 19 and minor injuries in 5. Levy et al.[452] reported a case of a bus driver with a strong history of coronary heart disease who caused the deaths of himself and several others, but they did not conclusively demonstrate that unexpected cardiac arrest was the proximate cause of the accident. Furthermore, Waller et al.[453] studied an elderly population and demonstrated that cardiac disease alone was not responsible for a significant increase in accident risk: *senility, or senility plus cardiovascular disease, was much more important.* Several other studies also have led to the conclusion that risk to the public is small.[454–456] In specific reference to private automobile drivers, most of the data show that sudden death at the wheel usually involves enough of a prodrome to allow the driver to get to the roadside before losing consciousness.[451, 454–456] Therefore, although there are likely to be isolated instances in which cardiac arrest causes public hazards in the future, the risk appears to be small, and since it is difficult to identify specific individuals at risk, sweeping restrictions to avoid such risks appear unwarranted. The exceptions are persons with multisystem disease, particularly senility, and individual circumstances requiring specific consideration, such as high-risk patients who have special responsibilities—school bus drivers, aircraft pilots, trainmen, and truck drivers.

REFERENCES

DEFINITION

1. Weiss, S.: Instantaneous "physiologic" death. N. Engl. J. Med. 223:793, 1940.
2. Spain, D. M., Bradess, V. A., and Mohr, C.: Coronary atherosclerosis as a cause of unexpected and unexplained death: An autopsy study from 1949–1959. J.A.M.A. *174*:384, 1960.
3. Burch, G. E., and DePasquale, N. P.: Sudden, unexpected, natural death. Am. J. Med. Sci. *249*:86, 1965.
4. Kuller, L., Lilienfeld, A., and Fisher, R.: An epidemiological study of sudden and unexpected deaths in adults. Medicine *46*:341, 1967.
5. Paul, O., and Schatz, M.: On sudden death. Circulation *43*:7, 1971.
6. Gordon, T., and Kannel, W. B.: Premature mortality from coronary heart disease. The Framingham Study. J.A.M.A. *215*:1617, 1971.
7. Biorck, C., and Wikland, B.: Sudden death—what are we talking about? Circulation *45*:256, 1972.
8. Friedman, M., Manwaring, J. H., Rosenman, R. H., Donlon, G., Ortega, P., and Grube, S. M.: Instantaneous and sudden deaths: Clinical and pathological differentiation in coronary artery disease. J.A.M.A. *225*:1319, 1973.
9. Kannel, W. B., Doyle, J. T., McNamara, P. M., Quickenton, P., and Gordon, T.: Precursors of sudden coronary death: Factors related to the incidence of sudden death. Circulation *51*:606, 1975.
10. Helmers, C., Lundman, T., Maasing, R., and Wester, P. O.: Mortality pattern among initial survivors of acute myocardial infarction using a life-table technique. Acta Med. Scand. *200*:469, 1976.
11. Mitchell, J. R. A., and Schwartz, C. J.: Arterial Disease. Oxford, Blackwell, 1965.
12. Ruberman, W., Weinblatt, E., Goldberg, J. D., Frank, C. W., and Shapiro, S.: Ventricular premature beats and mortality after myocardial infarction. N. Engl. J. Med. *297*:750, 1977.
13. Myerburg, R. J.: Sudden death. J. Cont. Ed. Cardiol. *14*:15, 1978.
14. Lovegrove, T., and Thompson, P.: The role of acute myocardial infarction in sudden cardiac death—a statistician's nightmare. Am. Heart J. *96*:711, 1978.
15. Thomas, A. C., Davies, M. J., and Popple, A. W.: A pathologist's view of sudden cardiac death. *In* Kulbertus, H. E., and Wellens, H. J. J. (eds.): Sudden Death. The Hague, Netherlands, Martinus Nijhoff, 1980, pp. 34–48.
16. Goldstein, S.: The necessity of a uniform definition of sudden coronary death: Witnessed death within 1 hour of the onset of acute symptoms. Am. Heart J. *103*:156, 1982.
17. Kuller, L. H.: Prodromata of sudden death and myocardial infarction. Adv. Cardiol. *25*:61, 1978.
18. Liberthson, R. R., Nagel, E. L., Hirschman, J. C., and Nussenfeld, S. R.: Prehospital ventricular fibrillation: Prognosis and follow-up course. N. Engl. J. Med. *291*:317, 1974.
19. Baum, R. S., Alvarez, H., and Cobb, L. A.: Survival after resuscitation from out-of-hospital ventricular fibrillation. Circulation *50*:1231, 1974.
20. Myerburg, R. J., Conde, C. A., Sung, R. J., Mayorga-Cortes, A., Mallon, S. M., Sheps, D. S., Appel, R. A., and Castellanos, A.: Clinical, electrophysiologic, and hemodynamic profile of patients resuscitated from prehospital cardiac arrest. Am. J. Med. *68*:568, 1980.
21. Hinkle, L. E: The immediate antecedents of sudden death. Acta Med. Scand. *210*:207, 1981.
22. Thompson, R. G., Hallstrom, A. P., and Cobb, L. A.: Bystander-initiated cardiopulmonary resuscitation in the management of ventricular fibrillation. Ann. Intern. Med. *90*:737, 1979.
23. Kuller, L. H.: Sudden death: Definition and epidemiologic considerations. Prog. Cardiovasc. Dis. *23*:1, 1980.

EPIDEMIOLOGY AND CAUSES OF SUDDEN DEATH

24. Epstein, F. H., and Pisa, Z.: International comparisons in ischemic heart disease mortality. Proc. Conf. on the Decline in Coronary Heart Disease Mortality. DHEW, NIH Publication No. 79–1610, Washington, D.C., U.S. Government Printing Office, 1979, pp. 58–88.
25. Kagan, A. R., Sternby, N. H., Vermura, K., Vanecek, R, Vilhert, A. M., Lifsic, A. M., Matova, E. E., Zahor, Z., and Zdanov, V. S.: Atherosclerosis of the aorta and coronary arteries in 5 towns. Bull. W.H.O. *53*:485, 1976.
26. McGill, H. C. (ed): The Geographic Pathology of Atherosclerosis. Baltimore, Williams and Wilkins, 1968.
27. Gordon, T., Garcia-Palmieri, M. R., Kagan, A., Kannel, W. B., and Schiffman, J.: Differences in coronary heart disease in Framingham, Honolulu, and Puerto Rico. J. Chronic Dis. *27*:329; 1974.
28. Report of the Working Group on Arteriosclerosis of the National Heart, Lung, and Blood Institute (Volume 2): Patient Oriented Research–Fundamental and Applied, Sudden cardiac death. DHEW, NIH Publication No. 82-2035, Washington, D.C., U.S. Government Printing Office, 1981, pp. 114–122.
29. Goldstein, S.: Sudden Death and Coronary Heart Disease. Mt. Kisco, N.Y., Futura Publishing Co., 1974.
30. Schatzkin, A., Cupples, L. A., Heeren, T., Morelock, S., Mucatel, M., and Kannel, W. B.: The epidemiology of sudden unexpected death: Risk factors for men and women in the Framingham Heart Study. Am. Heart J. *107*:1300, 1984.
31. Schatzkin, A., Cupples, L. A., Heeren, T., Morelock, S., and Kannel, W. B.: Sudden death in the Framingham Heart Study: Differences in incidence and risk factors by sex and coronary disease status. Am. J. Epidemiol. *120*:888, 1984.
32. Rosenberg, H. M., and Klebbs, A. J.: Trends in cardiovascular mortality with a focus on ischemic heart disease: United States, 1950–1976. Proc. Conf. Decline in Coronary Heart Disease Mortality. DHEW NIH Publication No. 79-1610, Washington, D.C., U.S. Government Printing Office, 1979, pp. 11–41.
33. Kannel, W. B., and Schatzkin, A.: Sudden death: Lessons from subsets in population studies. J. Am. Coll. Cardiol. *5*(Suppl 6):141B, 1985.
34. Doyle, J. T., Kannel, W. B., McNamara, P. M., Quickenton, P., and Gordon, T.: Factors related to suddenness of death from coronary disease: Combined Albany-Framingham studies. Am. J. Cardiol. 37:1073, 1976.
35. Kannel, W. B., and Thomas, H. E.: Sudden coronary death: The Framingham study. Ann. N.Y. Acad. Sci., *382*:3, 1982.

36. Kuller, L., Lilienfeld, A., and Fischer, R.: Sudden and unexpected deaths in young adults: An epidemiologic study. J.A.M.A. *198*:158, 1966.
37. Neuspiel, D. R., and Kuller, L. H.: Sudden and unexpected natural death in childhood and adolescence. J.A.M.A. *254*:1321, 1985.
38. Luke, J. L., and Helpern, M.: Sudden unexpected deaths from natural causes in young adults. Arch. Pathol. *85*:10, 1968.
39. Slack, J., and Evans, K. A.: The increased risk of death from ischemic heart disease in first-degree relatives of 121 men and 96 women with ischemic heart disease. J. Med. Genet. *3*:239, 1966.
40. Falconer, D. S.: The inheritance of liability to certain diseases, estimated from the incidence among relatives. Ann. Hum. Genet. *29*:51, 1965.
41. Slack, J.: Genetic influences on coronary heart disease in young women. *In* Oliver, M. J., (ed.): Coronary Heart Disease in Young Women. New York, Churchill Livingstone, 1978, pp. 24–34.
42. Harvald, B., and Hauge, M.: Coronary occlusion in twins. Acta Med. Genet. Gemellol. *19*:248, 1970.
43. Brown, M. S., and Goldstein, J. L.: Familial hypercholesterolemia: A genetic defect in the low-density lipoprotein receptor. N. Engl. J. Med. *294*:1386, 1976.
44. Neufeld, H. N., and Goldbourt, V.: Coronary heart disease: Genetic aspects. Circulation *67*:943, 1983.
45. Jervell, A., and Lange-Neilsen, F.: Congenital deaf-mutism, functional heart disease with prolongation of the Q-T interval, and sudden death. Am. Heart J. *54*:59, 1957.
46. Ward, O. C.: A new familial cardiac syndrome in children. J. Irish Med. Assoc. *54*:103, 1964.
47. Garza, L. A., Vick, R. L., Nora, J. J., and McNamara, D. G.: Heritable Q-T prolongation without deafness. Circulation *41*:39, 1970.
48. Braunwald, E., Morrow, A. G., Cornell, W. P., Aygen, M. M., and Hilbish, T. F.: Idiopathic hypertrophic subaortic stenosis: Clinical, hemodynamic, and angiographic manifestations. Am. J. Med. *29*:924, 1960.
49. Clark, C. E., Henry, W. L., and Epstein, S. E.: Familial prevalence and genetic transmission of idiopathic hypertrophic subaortic stenosis. N. Engl. J. Med. *289*:709, 1973.
50. Green, J. R., Krovetz, M. J., Shanklin, D. R., DeVito, J. J., and Taylor, W. J.: Sudden unexpected death in three generations. Arch. Intern. Med. *124*:359, 1969.
51. Davies, M. J.: Pathological view of sudden cardiac death. Br. Heart J. *45*:88, 1981.
52. Gazes, P. C., Culer, R., Taber, E., and Kelly, R. E.: Congenital familial cardiac conduction defects. Circulation *32*:32, 1965.
53. Gault, J. H., Cantwell, J., Lev, M., and Braunwald, E.: Fatal familial cardiac arrhythmias. Histologic observations on the cardiac conduction system. Am. J. Cardiol. *29*:548, 1972.
54. Lynch, H. T., Mohiuddin, S., Moran, J., Kaplan, A., Sketch, M., Zencka, A., and Runco, V.: Heredity progressive atrioventricular conduction defect. Am. J. Cardiol. *36*:297, 1975.
55. James, T. N., and MacLean, W. A. H.: Paroxysmal ventricular arrhythmias and familial sudden death associated with neural lesions in the heart. Chest *78*:24, 1980.
56. Myerburg, R. J., Kessler, K. M., Estes, D., Conde, C. A., Luceri, R. M., Zaman, L., Kozlovskis, P. L., and Castellanos, A.: Long-term survival after prehospital cardiac arrest: Analysis of outcome during an 8-year study. Circulation *70*:538, 1984.
57. Kuller, L., Cooper, M., and Perper, J.: Epidemiology of sudden death. Arch. Intern. Med. *129*:714, 1972.
58. Krueger, D. E., Ellenberg, S. S., Bloom, S., Calkins, B. M., Jacyna, R., Nolan, D. C., Phillips, R., Rios, J. C., Sobieski, R., Shekelle, R. B., Spector, K. M., Stadel, B. V., Stolley, P. D., and Terris, M.: Risk factors for fatal heart attack in young women. Am. J. Epidemiol. *113*:357, 1981.
59. Wenger, N. K.: Coronary disease in women. Am. Rev. Med. *36*:285, 1985.
60. Jick, H., Dinan, B., Herman, R., and Rothman, K. J.: Myocardial infarction and other vascular diseases in young women: Role of estrogens and other factors. J.A.M.A. *240*:2548, 1978.
61. Hagstrom, R. M., Federspiel, C. F., and Ho, Y. C.: Incidence of myocardial infarction and sudden death from coronary heart disease in Nashville, Tennessee. Circulation *44*:884, 1971.
62. Marmot, M. E., Syme, S. L., Kagan, A., Kato, H., Cohen, J. B., and Belsky, J.: Epidemiologic studies of coronary heart disease and stroke in Japanese men living in Japan, Hawaii, and California: Prevalence of coronary and hypertensive heart disease and associated risk factors. Am. J. Epidemiol. *102*:514, 1975.
63. Hallstrom, A. P., Cobb, L. A., and Ray, R.: Smoking as a risk factor for recurrence of sudden cardiac arrest. N. Engl. J. Med. *314*:271, 1986.
64. Paffenbarger, R. S., Hale, W. E., Brand, R. J., and Hyde, R. T.: Work energy level, personal characteristics, and fatal heart attack: A birth-cohort effect. Am. J. Epidemiol. *105*:200, 1977.
65. Rahe, R. H., Romo, M., Bennett, L., and Siltman, P.: Recent life changes, myocardial infarction, and abrupt coronary death. Arch. Intern. Med. *133*:221, 1974.
66. Talbott, E., Kuller, L. H., Petre, K., and Perper, J.: Biologic and psychosocial risk factors of sudden death from coronary disease in white women. Am. J. Cardiol. *39*:858, 1977.
67. Ruberman, W., Weinblatt, E., Goldberg, J. D., and Chaudhary, B. S.: Psychosocial influences on mortality after myocardial infarction. N. Engl. J. Med. *311*:552, 1984.
68. Weinblatt, E., Ruberman, W., Goldberg, J. D., Frank, C. N., Shapiro, S., and Chaudhary, B. S.: Relation of education to sudden death after myocardial infarction. N. Engl. J. Med. *299*:60, 1978.
69. Lambert, C. A., Netherton, D. R., Finison, L. J., Hyde, J. N., and Spaight, S. J.: Risk factors and life style: A statewide health-interview survey. N. Engl. J. Med. *306*:1048, 1982.
70. Friedman, M., and Rosenman, R. H.: Association of specific overt behavior pattern with blood and cardiovascular findings. J.A.M.A. *169*:1286, 1959.
71. Kennedy, H. L., Whitlock, J. A., Sprague, M. K., Kennedy, L. J., Buckingham, T. A., and Goldberg, R. J.: Long-term follow-up of asymptomatic healthy subjects with frequent and complex ventricular ectopy. N. Engl. J. Med. *312*:193, 1985.
72. Chiang, B. N., Perlman, L., Ostrander, L. D., and Epstein, F.: Relation of premature systole to coronary heart disease and sudden death in the Tecumseh epidemiologic study. Ann. Intern. Med. *70*:1159, 1969.
73. Coronary Drug Project Research Group: Prognostic importance of premature beats following myocardial infarction: Experience in the coronary drug project. J.A.M.A. *223*:1116, 1973.
73a. Pratt, C. M., Theroux, P., Slymen, D., Riordan-Bennett, A., Morisette, D., Galloway, A., Seals, A. A., and Hallstrom, A.: Spontaneous variability of ventricular arrhythmias in patients at increased risk for sudden death after acute myocardial infarction: Consecutive ambulatory electrocardiographic recordings of 88 patients. Am. J. Cardiol. *59*:278, 1987.
74. Moss, A. J., Schnitzler, R., Green, R., and DeCamilla, J.: Ventricular arrhythmias 3 weeks after acute myocardial infarction. Ann. Intern. Med. *75*:837, 1971.
75. Kotler, M. N., Tabatznik, B., Mower, M. M., and Tominaga, S.: Prognostic significance of ventricular ectopic beats with respect to sudden death in the late post-infarction period. Circulation *47*:959, 1973.
76. Vismara, L. A., Amsterdam, B. A., and Mason, D. T.: Relation of ventricular arrhythmias in the late-hospital phase of acute myocardial infarction to sudden death after hospital discharge. Am. J. Med. *59*:6, 1975.
77. Moss, A. J., Davis, H. T., DeCamilla, J., and Bayer, L. W.: Ventricular ectopic beats and their relation to sudden and non-sudden cardiac death after myocardial infarction. Circulation *60*:998, 1979.
78. Moss, A. J., DeCamilla, J., and David, H.: Factors associated with cardiac death in the post-hospital phase of myocardial infarction. *In* Kulbertus, H. E., and Wellens, H. J. J. (eds.): Sudden Death. The Hague, Netherlands, Martinus Nijhoff, 1980, pp. 237–247.
79. Ruberman, W., Weinblatt, E., Goldberg, J. D., Frank, C. W., and Shapiro, S.: Ventricular premature beats and mortality after myocardial infarction. N. Engl. J. Med. *297*:750, 1977.
80. Ruberman, W., Weinblatt, E., Goldberg, J. D., Frank, C. W, Chaudhary, B. S., and Shapiro, S.: Ventricular premature complexes and sudden death after myocardial infarction. Circulation *64*:297, 1981.
81. Bigger, J. T., and Weld, F. M.: Analysis of prognostic significance of ventricular arrhythmias after myocardial infarction: Shortcomings of Lown grading system. Br. Heart J. *45*:717, 1981.
82. Schulze, R. A., Strauss, H. W., and Pitt, B.: Sudden death in the year following myocardial infarction: Relationship of ventricular premature contractions in the late hospital phase and left ventricular ejection fraction. Am. J. Med. *62*:192, 1977.
83. Bigger, J. T., Fleiss, J. L., Kleiger, R., Miller, J. P., Rolnitzky, L. M., and the Multicenter Post-Infarction Research Group: The relationships among ventricular arrhythmias, left ventricular dysfunction, and mortality in the 2 years after myocardial infarction. Circulation *69*:250, 1984.
84. Myerburg, R. J., Kessler, K. M., Luceri, R. M., Zaman, L., Trohman, R. G., Estes, D., and Castellanos, A.: Classification of ventricular arrhythmias based on parallel hierarchies of frequency and form. Am. J. Cardiol. *54*:1355, 1984.
85. Ruberman, W., Weinblatt, E., Frank, C. W., Goldberg, J. D., and Shapiro, S.: Repeated 1-hour electrocardiographic monitoring of survivors of myocardial infarction at 6-month intervals: Arrhythmia detection and relation to prognosis. Am. J. Cardiol. *47*:1197, 1981.
86. Follansbee, W. P., Michelson, E. L., and Morganroth, J.: Non-sustained ventricular tachycardia in ambulatory patients. Characteristics and association with sudden cardiac death. Ann. Intern. Med. 92:741, 1980.
87. Lown, B., and Wolf, M.: Approaches to sudden death from coronary heart disease. Circulation *44*:130, 1971.
88. Bigger, J. T., Weld, F. M., and Rolnitzky, L. N.: Problems with the Lown grading system for observational and experimental studies in ischemic heart disease. *In* Harrison, D. C. (ed.): Cardiac Arrhythmias: A Decade of Progress. Boston, G. K. Hall, 1981, pp. 653–670.
89. Campbell, R. W. F.: Evaluation of antiarrhythmic drugs: Should the Lown classification be used as a measure of efficacy? *In* Morganroth, J., Moore, E. N., Dreifus, L. S., and Michelson, E. L. (eds.): The Evaluation of New Antiarrhythmic Drugs. The Hague, Netherlands, Martinus Nijoff, 1981, pp. 113–121.
90. Myerburg, R. J., Zaman, L., Luceri, R., Kessler, K. M., Kayden, D., and Castellanos, A.: Antiarrhythmic drug therapy after myocardial infarction. *In* Kulbertus, H. E., and Wellens, H. J. J. (eds.): The First Year After Myocardial Infarction. Mt. Kisko, N.Y., Futura Publishing Co., 1983, pp. 321–339.
91. Maisel, A. S., Scott, N., Gilpin, E., Ahnve, S., LeWinter, M., Henning, H., Collins, D., and Ross, J.: Complex ventricular arrhythmias in patients with Q wave versus non-Q wave myocardial infarction. Circulation *72*:963, 1985.
92. Cobb, L. A., Baum, R. S., Alvarez, H., and Schaffer, W. A.: Resuscitation from out-of-hospital ventricular fibrillation: 4-year follow-up. Circulation *52*(Suppl 3):223, 1975.
93. Levin, D. C., Fellows, K. E., and Abrams, H. L.: Hemodynamically significant primary anomalies of the coronary arteries: Angiographic aspects. Circulation *58*:25, 1978.
94. Weisselhoeft, H., Fawcett, J. S., and Johnson, A. L.: Anomalous origin of the left coronary artery from the pulmonary trunk. Circulation *38*:403, 1968.
95. Harthorne, J. W., Scannell, J. G., and Dinsmore, R. E.: Anomalous origin of

the left coronary artery: Remedial cause of sudden death in adults. N. Engl. J. Med. *275*:660, 1966.
96. Kimbiris, D., Iskandrian, A. S., Segal, B. L., and Bemis, C. E.: Anomalous aortic origin of coronary arteries. Circulation *58*:606, 1978.
97. Cheltlin, M.D., Decastro, C. M., and McAllister, H. A.: Sudden death as a complication of anomalous left coronary origin from the anterior sinus of Valsalva: A not-so-minor congenital anomaly. Circulation *50*:780, 1974.
98. Benge, W., Martins, J. B., and Funk, D. C.: Morbidity associated with anomalous origin of the right coronary artery from the left sinus of Valsalva. Am. Heart J. *99*:96, 1980.
99. Roberts, W. C., Siegel, R. J., and Zipes, D. P.: Origin of the right coronary artery from the left sinus of Valsalva and its functional consequences: Analysis of 10 necropsy patients. Am. J. Cardiol. *49*:863, 1982.
100. Maron, B. J., Epstein, S. E., and Roberts, W. C.: Causes of sudden death in competitive athletes. J. Am. Coll. Cardiol. 7:204, 1986.
101. Jokl, E., and McClellan, J. T.: Exercise and cardiac death: Asymptomatic cardiac disease causing sudden death in association with physical activity. Med. Sport 5:1, 1971.
102. Waller, B. F.: Exercise-related sudden death in young (age ≤ 30 years) and old (age > 30 years) conditioned subjects. *In* Wenger, N. K. (ed.): Exercise and the Heart. Philadelphia, F. A. Davis Co., 1985, pp. 9–73.
103. Roberts, W. C.: Coronary embolism: A review of causes, consequences, and diagnostic considerations. Cardiovasc. Med. *3*:699–710, 1978.
104. El Maraghi, N., and Genton, E.: The relevance of platelet and fibrin thromboembolism of the coronary microcirculation, with special reference to sudden cardiac death. Circulation *62*:936, 1980.
105. Haerem, J. W.: Mural platelet microthrombi and major acute lesions of main epicardial arteries in sudden coronary death. Atherosclerosis *19*:529, 1974.
106. Kawasaki, T., Kosaki, S., and Okawa, S.: A new infantile acute febrile mucocutaneous lymph node syndrome prevailing in Japan. Pediatrics *54*:271, 1974.
107. Kegel, S. M., Dorsey, T. J., Rowen, M., and Taylor, W. F.: Cardiac death in mucocutaneous lymph node syndrome. Am. J. Cardiol. *40*:282, 1977.
108. Thiene, G., Valente, M., and Rossi, L.: Involvement of the cardiac conduction system in panarteritis nodosa. Am. Heart J. 95:716, 1978.
109. Heggveit, H. A.: Syphilitic aortitis—a clinicopathological autopsy of 100 cases. Circulation *29*:346, 1964.
110. Guthrie, W., and Maclean, H.: Dissecting aneurysms of arteries other than the aorta. J. Pathol. *108*:219, 1972.
111. Roberts, W. C., and Honig, H. S.: The spectrum of cardiovascular disease in the Marfan syndrome. Am. Heart J. *104*:115, 1982.
112. Shaver, P. J., Carrig, T. F., and Baker, W. P.: Postpartum coronary artery dissection. Br. Heart J. *40*:83, 1978.
113. Harris, L. S., and Adelson, L.: Fatal coronary embolism from a myxomatous polyp of the aortic valve. An unusual cause of sudden death. Am. J. Clin. Pathol. *43*:61, 1965.
114. Roberts, W. C.: Pathology of arterial aneurysms. *In* Bergan, J. J., and Yao, S. T. (eds.): Aneurysms, Diagnosis and Treatment. New York, Grune and Stratton, 1982, pp. 17–43.
115. Miller, D. D., Waters, D. D., Szlachcic, J., and Theroux, P.: Clinical characteristics associated with sudden death in patients with variant angina. Circulation *66*:588, 1982.
116. Morady, F., DiCarlo, L., Winston, S., Davis, J. C., and Scheinman, M. M.: Clinical features and prognosis of patients with out-of-hospital cardiac arrest and a normal electrophysiologic study. J. Am. Coll. Cardiol. *4*:39, 1984.
117. Cohn, P. F.: Silent myocardial ischemia in patients with a defective anginal warning system. Am. J. Cardiol. *45*:697, 1980.
118. Sharma, B., Francis, G., Hodges, M., and Asinger, R.: Demonstration of exercise-induced ischemia without angina in patients who recover from out-of-hospital ventricular fibrillation. Am. J. Cardiol. *47*:445, 1981 (Abstract).
119. Maseri, A., Severi, S., and Marzullo, P.: Role of coronary arterial spasm in sudden coronary ischemic death. Ann. N.Y. Acad. Sci. *382*:204, 1982.
120. Morales, A. R., Romanelli, R., and Boucek, R. J.: The mural left anterior descending coronary artery, strenuous exercise, and sudden death. Circulation *62*:230, 1980.
121. Anderson, K. P.: Sudden death, hypertension, and hypertrophy. J. Cardiovasc. Pharmacol. *6*(Suppl 3):S498, 1984.
122. Anderson, K. P.: Hypertension and sudden cardiac death. N.Z. Med. J. *95*:33, 1982.
123. Messerli, F. H., Ventura, H. O., Elizardi, D. J., Dunn, F. G., and Frohlich, E. D.: Hypertension and sudden death: Increased ventricular ectopic activity in left ventricular hypertrophy. Am. J. Med. 77:18, 1984.
124. Goodwin, J. F.: The frontiers of cardiomyopathy. Br. Heart J. *48*:1, 1982.
125. Shah, P. M., Adelman, A. G., Wigle, E. D., Gobel, F. L., Burchell, A. B., Hardarson, T., Curiel, L., de la Calzade, C., Oakley, C. M., and Goodwin, J. F.: The natural (and unnatural) history of hypertrophic obstructive cardiomyopathy. Circ. Res. *35*(Suppl 2):179, 1974.
126. Maron, B. J., Roberts, W. C., and Epstein, S. E.: Sudden death in hypertrophic cardiomyopathy: A profile of 78 patients. Circulation *65*:1388, 1982.
127. Savage, D. D., Seides, S. F., Maron, B. J., Myers, D. J., and Epstein, S. E.: Prevalence of arrhythmias during 24-hour electrocardiographic monitoring and exercise testing in patients with obstructive and non-obstructive hypertrophic cardiomyopathy. Circulation *59*:866, 1979.
128. Goodwin, J. F., and Krikler, D. M.: Arrhythmia as a cause of sudden death in hypertrophic cardiomyopathy. Lancet 2:937, 1976.
129. Maron, B. J., Savage, D. D., Wolfson, J. K., and Epstein, S. E.: Prognostic significance of 24 hour ambulatory electrocardiographic monitoring in patients with hypertrophic cardiomyopathy: A prospective study. Am. J. Cardiol. *48*:252, 1981.
130. Anderson, K. P., Stinson, E. B., Derby, G. C., Oyer, P. E., and Mason, J. W.: Vulnerability of patients with obstructive hypertrophic cardiomyopathy to ventricular arrhythmia induction in the operating room. Am. J. Cardiol. *51*:811, 1983.
131. Kowey, P. R., Eisenberg, R., and Engel, T. R.: Sustained arrhythmias in hypertrophic obstructive cardiomyopathy. N. Engl. J. Med. *310*:1566, 1984.
132. Stafford, W. J., Trohman, R. G., Bilsker, M., Zaman, L., Castellanos, A., and Myerburg, R. J.: Cardiac arrest in an adolescent with atrial fibrillation and hypertrophic cardiomyopathy. J. Am. Coll. Cardiol 7:701, 1986.
133. Maron, B. J., Epstein, S. E., and Roberts, W. C.: Hypertrophic cardiomyopathy: A common cause of sudden death in the young competitive athlete. Eur. Heart J. *4*(Suppl F):135, 1983.
134. Waller, B. F.: Sudden death in midlife. Cardiovasc. Med. *10*:55, 1985.
135. Northcote, R. J., Flannigan, C., and Ballantyne, D.: Sudden death and vigorous exercise: A study of 60 deaths associated with squash. Br. Heart J. *55*:198, 1986.
136. Packer, M.: Sudden unexpected death in patients with congestive heart failure: A second frontier. Circulation *72*:681, 1985.
137. Schugoll, G. I., Bowen, P. J., Moore, J. P., and Lenkin, M. L.: Follow-up observations and prognosis in primary myocardial disease. Arch. Intern. Med. *129*:67, 1972.
138. Huang, S. K., Messer, J. V., and Denes, P.: Significance of ventricular tachycardia in idiopathic dilated cardiomyopathy: Observations in 35 patients. Am. J. Cardiol. *51*:507, 1983.
139. Meinertz, T., Hoffmann, T., Kasper, W., Treese, N., Bechtold, H., Steinen, V., Pop, T., Leitner, E.-R.V., Andresen, D., and Meyer, J.: Significance of ventricular arrhythmias in idiopathic dilated cardiomyopathy. Am. J. Cardiol. *53*:902, 1984.
140. Poll, D. S., Marchinski, F. E., Buxton, A. E., Doherty, J. V., Waxman, H. L., and Josephson, M. E.: Sustained ventricular tachycardia in patients with idiopathic dilated cardiomyopathy: Electrophysiologic testing and lack of response to antiarrhythmic drug therapy. Circulation *70*:451, 1984.
141. Warren, J. V.: Unusual sudden death. Cardiol. Ser. *8*(4):5, 1984.
142. Surawicz, B.: Ventricular fibrillation. J. Am. Coll. Cardiol. *51*(Suppl B):43, 1985.
143. Topaz, O., and Edwards, J. E.: Pathologic features of sudden death in children, adolescents, and young adults. Chest *87*:476, 1985.
144. Sevy, S., Kelly, J., and Ernst, H.: Fatal paroxysmal tachycardia associated with focal myocarditis of the Purkinje system in a 14-month-old child. J. Paediatr. 27:796, 1968.
145. Robboy, S. J.: Atrioventricular node inflammation: Mechanisms of sudden death in protracted meningococcemia. N. Engl. J. Med. *286*:1091, 1972.
146. Morales, A. R., Adelman, S., and Fine, G.: Varicella myocarditis—A case of sudden death. Arch. Pathol. *91*:29, 1971.
147. Roberts, W. C., McAllister, H. A., and Farrans, V. J.: Sarcoidosis of the heart: A clinicopathologic study of 35 necropsy patients (group I) and review of 78 previously described necropsy patients (group II). Am. J. Med. *63*:86, 1977.
148. Silverman, K. J., Hutchins, G. M., and Bulkley, B. H.: Cardiac sarcoid: A clinicopathologic study of 84 unselected patients with systemic sarcoidosis. Circulation *58*:1204, 1978.
149. Bulkley, B. H., Klacsman, P. G., and Hutchins, G. M.: Angina pectoris, myocardial infarction and sudden cardiac death with normal coronary arteries: A clinicopathological study of nine patients with progressive systemic sclerosis. Am. Heart J. *95*:563, 1978.
150. Marcus, F. L., Fontaine, G. H., Guiraudon, G., Frank, R., Laurenceau, J. L., Malergue, C., and Grosgogeat, Y.: Right ventricular dysplasia: A report of 24 adult cases. Circulation *65*:384, 1982.
151. Wright, J. R., and Calkins, E.: Clinical-pathologic differentiation of common amyloid syndromes. Medicine *60*:429, 1981.
152. Buja, L. M., Khoi, N. B., and Roberts, W. C.: Clinically signficant cardiac amyloidosis: Clinicopathologic findings in 15 patients. Am. J. Cardiol. *26*:394, 1970.
153. Ridolfi, R. L., Bulkley, B. H., and Hutchins, G. M.: The conduction system in cardiac amyloidosis: Clinical and pathologic features of 23 patients. Am. J. Med. *62*:677, 1977.
154. James, T. N.: Pathology of the cardiac conduction system in amyloidosis. Ann. Intern. Med. *65*:28, 1966.
155. Campbell, M.: Calcific aortic stenosis and congenital bicuspid aortic valves. Br. Heart J. *30*:606, 1968.
156. Smith, N., McAnulty, J. G., and Rahimtoola, S. H.: Severe aortic stenosis with impaired left ventricular function and clinical heart failure: Results of valve replacement. Circulation *58*:255, 1978.
157. Rahimtoola, S. H.: Valvular heart disease: A perspective. J. Am. Coll. Cardiol. *1*:199, 1983.
158. Blackstone, E. H., and Kirklin, J. W.: Death and other time-related events after valve replacement. Circulation *72*:753, 1985.
159. Konishi, Y., Matsuda, K., Nishiwaki, N., Shimada, I., Kitas, Y., Ban, T., Tatsuda, N., Minami, K., Konishi, T., and Ikeguchi, S.: Ventricular arrhythmias late after aortic and/or mitral valve replacement. Jpn. Cir. J. *49*:576, 1985.
160. Devereux, R. B., Perloff, J. K., Reichek, N., and Josephson, M. E.: Mitral valve prolapse. Circulation *54*:3, 1976.
161. Chesler, E., King, R. A., and Edwards, J. E.: The myxomatous mitral valve and sudden death. Circulation *67*:632, 1983.
162. Campbell, R. W. F., Godman, M. G., Fiddler, G. I., Marquis, R. M., and Julian, D. G.: Ventricular arrhythmias in the syndrome of balloon deformity

of mitral valve: Definition of possible high-risk group. Br. Heart J. *38*:1053, 1976.

163. Pocock, W. A., Bosman, C. K., Chesler, E., Barlow, J. E., and Edwards, J. E.: Sudden death in primary mitral valve prolapse. Am. Heart J. *107*:378, 1984.
164. Nishimura, R. A., McGoon, M. D., Shub, C., Miller, F. A., Ilstrup, D. M., and Tajik, A. J.: Echocardiographically documented mitral valve prolapse: Long-term follow-up of 237 patients. N. Engl. J. Med. *313*:1305, 1985.
165. Glew, R. H., Varghese, P. J., Krovetz, L. J., Dorst, J. P., and Rowe, R. D.: Sudden death in congenital aortic stenosis: A review of 8 cases with an evaluation of premonitory clinical features. Am. Heart J. *78*:615, 1969.
166. Hoffman, J. I. E.: The natural history of congenital isolated pulmonic and aortic stenosis. Ann. Rev. Med. *20*:15, 1969.
167. Young, D., and Marks, H.: Fate of the patient with the Eisenmenger syndrome. Am. J. Cardiol. *28*:658, 1971.
168. Jones, A. M., and Howitt, G.: Eisenmenger syndrome in pregnancy. Br. Med. J. *1*:1627, 1965.
169. Garson, A., Nihill, M. R., McNamara, D. G., and Cooley, D. A.: Status of the adult and adolescent after repair of tetralogy of Fallot. Circulation *59*:1232, 1979.
170. Gillette, P. C., Kugler, J. D., Garson, A., Gutgesell, H. P., Duff, D. F., and McNamara, D. G.: The mechanism of cardiac dysrhythmia after Mustard operation for transposition of the great arteries. Am. J. Cardiol. *45*:1225, 1980.
171. Garson, A., and McNamara, D. G.: Sudden death in a pediatric cardiology population, 1958 to 1983: Relation to prior arrhythmias. J. Am. Coll. Cardiol. *5*(Suppl B):134B, 1985.
172. Lie, K.I., Leim, K. L., Schuilenberg, R. M., David, G. K., and Durrer, D.: Early identification of patients developing late in-hospital ventricular fibrillation after discharge from the coronary care unit. Am. J. Cardiol. *41*:674, 1978.
173. Hauer, R. N. W., Lie, K. I., Liem, K. L., and Durrer, D.: Long-term prognosis in patients with bundle branch block complicating acute anteroseptal infarction. Am. J. Cardiol. *49*:1581, 1982.
174. Lenegre, J.: The pathology of complete atrioventricular block. Prog. Cardiovasc. Dis. *6*:317, 1964.
175. Lev, M.: Anatomic basis for atrioventricular block. Am. J. Med. *37*:742, 1964.
176. Denes, P., Dhingra, R. C., Wu, D., Wyndham, C. R., Amat-y-Leon, F., and Rosen, K. M.: Sudden death in patients with chronic bifascicular block. Arch. Intern. Med. *137*:1005, 1977.
177. McAnulty, J. H., Rahimtoola, S. H., Murphy, E. S., Kaufman, S., Ritzmann, L. W., Kanarek, P., and DeMots, H.: A prospective study of sudden death in "high risk" bundle branch block. N. Engl. J. Med. *299*:209, 1978.
178. McAnulty, J. H., Rahimtoola, S. H., Murphy, E., DeMots, H., Ritzmann, L., Kanarek, P. E., and Kauffman, S.: Natural history of "high-risk" bundle-branch block: Final report of a prospective study. N. Engl. J. Med. *307*:137, 1982.
179. Anderson, R. H., Wenick, A. C. G., Losekoot, T. G., and Becker, A. E.: Congenitally complete heart block. Circulation *56*:90, 1977.
180. Stephan, E.: Hereditary bundle branch system defect. Survey of a family with four affected generations. Am. Heart J. *95*:89, 1978.
181. Kline, G. J., Bashore, T. M., Sellers, T. D., Pritchett, E. L. C., Smith, W. M., and Gallagher, J. J.: Ventricular fibrillation in the Wolff-Parkinson-White syndrome. N. Engl. J. Med. *301*:1080, 1979.
182. Wellens, H. J. J., and Durrer, D.: Wolff-Parkinson-White syndrome and atrial fibrillation: Relation between refractory period of accessory pathway and ventricular rate during atrial fibrillation. Am. J. Cardiol. *34*:777, 1974.
183. Castellanos, A., Myerburg, R. J., Craparo, K., Befeler, B., and Agha, A.: Factors regulating ventricular rates during atrial flutter and fibrillation in pre-excitation (Wolff-Parkinson-White) syndrome. Br. Heart J. *35*:811, 1973.
184. Schwartz, P. J., Periti, M., and Malliani, A.: The long Q-T syndrome. Am. Heart J. *89*:378, 1975.
185. Fraser, G. R., Froggatt, P., and James, T. N.: Congenital deafness associated with electrocardiographic abnormalities, fainting attacks and sudden death. Q. J. Med. *33*:362, 1964.
186. Smith, W. M., and Gallagher, J. J.: Les torsades de pointes. Ann. Intern. Med. *93*:578, 1980.
187. Moss, A. J., Schwartz, P. J., Crampton, R. S., Locati, E., and Carleen, E.: The long-QT syndrome: A prospective international study. Circulation *71*:17, 1985.
188. Bhandari, A. K., and Scheinman, M.: The long QT syndrome. Mod. Concepts Cardiovasc. Dis. *54*:45, 1985.
189. Singh, B. N., Gaarder, T. D., Kanegae, T., Goldstein, M., Montgomerie, J., and Mills, H.: Liquid protein diets and torsades de pointes. J.A.M.A. *240*:115, 1978.
190. Michiel, R. R., Sneider, J. S., Dickstein, R. A., Hayman, H. H., and Eich, R. H.: Sudden death in a patient on a liquid protein diet. N. Engl. J. Med. *298*:1005, 1978.
191. Isner, J. M., Sours, H. E., Paris, A. L., Ferrans, V. J., and Roberts, W. C.: Sudden, unexpected death in avid dieters using the liquid-protein-modified-fast diet: Observations in 17 patients and the role of the prolonged QT interval. Circulation *60*:1401, 1979.
192. Isner, J. M., Roberts, W. C., Heymsfield, S. B., and Yager, J.: Anorexia nervosa and sudden death. Ann. Intern. Med. *102*:49, 1985.
193. Lyman, G. H., Williams, C. C., Dinwoodie, W. R., and Schocken, D. D.: Sudden death in cancer patients receiving lithium. J. Clin. Oncol. *2*:1270, 1984.
194. Coumel, P., Rosengarten, M. D., Leclercq, J. F., and Attuel, P.: Role of sympathetic nervous system in non-ischemic ventricular arrhythmias. Br. Heart J. *47*:137, 1982.
195. Schwartz, P. J.: The idiopathic long Q-T syndrome. Ann. Intern. Med. *99*:561, 1982.
196. Crampton, R. S.: Stellate ganglion block and stimulation in long QT syndrome, sympathetic dystrophy of the arm, and normals. *In* Schwartz, P. J., Brown, A. M., Malliani, A., and Zanchetti, A. (eds.): Neural Mechanisms in Cardiac Arrhythmias. New York, Raven Press, 1978, pp. 55–74.
197. Lown, B., Temte, J. V. C., Reich, P., Gaughan, C., Regestein, Q., and Hal, H.: Basis for recurring ventricular fibrillation in the absence of coronary heart disease and its management. N. Engl. J. Med. *294*:623, 1976.
198. Lown, B., and Verrier, R.: Neural activity and ventricular fibrillation. N. Engl. J. Med. *294*:1165, 1976.
199. Lown, B., DeSilva, R. A., and Lenson, R.: Role of psychologic stress and autonomic nervous system changes in provocation of ventricular premature complexes. Am. J. Cardiol. *41*:979, 1977.
200. Engel, G. L.: Sudden and rapid death during psychological stress. Ann. Intern. Med. *74*:771, 1971.
201. Dimsdale, J. E.: Emotional causes of sudden death. Am. J. Psychiatr. *134*:1361, 1977.
202. Engel, G. L.: Psychologic stress, vasodepressor, vasovagal, syncope, and sudden death. Ann. Intern. Med. *89*:403, 1978.
203. Wellens, H. J. J., Vermeulen, A., and Durrer, D.: Ventricular fibrillation occurring on arousal from sleep by auditory stimuli. Circulation *46*:661, 1972.
204. Sheps, D. S., Conde, C. A., Mayorga-Cortes, A., Mallon, S. M., Sung, R. J., Castellanos, A., and Myerburg, R. J.: Primary ventricular fibrillation: Some unusual features. Chest *72*:235, 1977.
205. Cannon, W. B.: "Voodoo" death. Psychosom. Med. *19*:182, 1957.
206. Burrell, R. J. W.: The possible bearing of curse death and other factors in Bantu culture on the etiology of myocardial infarction. *In* James, T. N., and Keyes, J. W. (eds.): The Etiology of Myocardial Infarction. Boston, Little, Brown, 1963.
207. Baba, N., Quattrochi, J. J., Reiner, C. B., Adrion, W., McBride, P. T., and Yates, A. J.: Possible role of the brain stem in sudden infant death syndrome. J.A.M.A. *249*:2789, 1983.
208. Fraser, G. R., and Frogatt, P.: Unexpected cot deaths. Lancet *2*:56, 1966.
209. Schwartz, P. J.: Cardiac sympathetic innervation and the sudden infant death syndrome: A possible pathogenetic link. Am. J. Med. *60*:167, 1976.
210. Valdes-Dapena, M. A.: Sudden infant death syndrome: A review of the medical literature. Pediatrics *66*:597, 1980.
211. Valdes-Dapena, M. A.: Are some sudden crib deaths sudden cardiac deaths? J. Am. Coll. Cardiol. *5*(Suppl B):113B, 1985.
212. Avery, M. E., and Frantz, I. D.: To breathe or not to breathe: What have we learned about apneic spells and sudden infant death? N. Engl. J. Med. *309*:107, 1983.
213. Brooks, J. G.: Apnea of infancy and sudden infant death syndrome. Am. J. Dis. Child. *136*:1012, 1982.
214. Hodgman, J. E., Hoppenbrouwers, T., Geidel, S., Hadeed, A., Sterman, M. B., Harper, R., and McGinty, D.: Respiratory behavior in near-miss sudden infant death syndrome. Pediatrics *69*:785, 1982.
215. Southall, D. P., Richard, J. M., de Swiet, M., Arrowsmith, W. A., Creed, J. E., Fleming, P. J., Franklin, A. J., Orme, R. L., Radford, M. J., Wilson, A. J., Shannon, D. C., Alexander, J. R., Brown, N. J., and Shinebourne, E. A.: Identification of infants destined to die unexpectedly during infancy: Evaluation of predictive importance of prolonged apnea and disorders of cardiac rhythm or conduction. Br. Med. J. *286*:1092, 1983.
216. Marino, T. A., and Kane, B. M.: Cardiac atrioventricular junctional tissues in hearts from infants who died suddenly. J. Am. Coll. Cardiol. *5*:1178, 1985.
217. Lambert, E. C., Menon, V. A., Wagner, H. R., and Viad, P.: Sudden unexpected death from cardiovascular disease in children. Am. J. Cardiol. *34*:89, 1974.
218. Roberts, W. C., and Maron, B. J.: Sudden death while playing professional football. Am. Heart J. *102*:1061, 1981.
219. Waller, B. F., Csere, R. S., Baker, W. P., and Roberts, W. C.: Running to death. Chest *79*:346, 1981.
220. Reichenbach, D. D., Moss, N. S., and Meyer, E.: Pathology of the heart in sudden cardiac death. Am. J. Cardiol. *39*:865, 1977.
221. Aponte, C.: The enigma of "bangungut." Ann. Intern. Med. *52*:1259, 1960.
222. Sugai, M.: A pathologic study on sudden and unexpected death, especially on the cardiac death autopsied by medical examiners in Tokyo. Acute Pathol. Jpn. *9*:723, 1959.
223. Baron, R. C., Thacker, S. B., Gorelkin, L., Vernon, A. A., Taylor, W. R., and Chol, K.: Sudden death among Southeast Asian refugees: An unexplained nocturnal phenomenon. J.A.M.A. *250*:2947, 1983.
224. Otto, C. M., Tauxe, R. V., Cobb, L. A., Greene, L., Gross, B. W., Werner, J. A., Burroughs, R. W., Samson, W. E., Weaver, W. D., and Trobaugh, C. B.: Ventricular fibrillation causes sudden death in Southeast Asian immigrants. Ann. Intern. Med. *101*:45, 1984.
225. Haugen, R. K.: The cafe coronary: Sudden deaths in restaurants. J.A.M.A. *186*:142, 1963.
226. Eller, W. C., and Haugen, R. K.: Food asphyxiation—restaurant rescue. N. Engl. J. Med. *289*:81, 1973.
227. Ettinger, P. O., Wu, C. F., De La Cruz, C., Weisse, A. B., Ahmed, S. S., and Regan, T. J.: Arrhythmias and the "holiday heart": Alcohol-associated cardiac rhythm disorders. Am. Heart J. *95*:555, 1978.
228. Benatar, S. R.: Fatal asthma. N. Engl. J. Med. *314*:243, 1986.
229. Morgan, M.: Amniotic fluid embolism. Anaesthesia *34*:20, 1979.
230. Aronson, M. E., and Nelson, P. K.: Fatal air embolism in pregnancy resulting from an unusual sexual act. Obstet. Gynecol. *30*:127, 1967.
231. Velebit, V., Podrid, P., Lown, B., Cohen, B. H., and Graboys, T. B.: Aggravation and provocation of ventricular arrhythmia by antiarrhythmic drugs. Circulation *65*:886, 1982.
232. Ruskin, J. N., McGovern, B., Garan, H., DiMarco, J. P., and Kelly, E.: Antiarrhythmic drugs: A possible cause of out-of-hospital cardiac arrest. N. Engl. J. Med. *309*:1302, 1983.

PATHOLOGY AND PATHOPHYSIOLOGY OF SUDDEN DEATH

233. Baroldi, G., Falzi, G., and Mariani, F.: Sudden coronary death: A postmortem study in 208 selected cases compared to 97 "control" subjects. Am. Heart J. 98:20, 1979.
234. Liberthson, R. R., Nagel, E. L., Hirschman, J. C., Nussenfeld, S. R., Blackbourn, B. D., and Davis, J. R.: Pathophysiologic observations in prehospital ventricular fibrillation and sudden cardiac death. Circulation *49*:790, 1974.
235. Perper, J. A., Kuller, L. H., Cooper, M.: Arteriosclerosis of coronary arteries in sudden, unexpected deaths. Circulation 52(Suppl 3):27, 1975.
236. Roberts, W. C., and Jones, A. A.: Quantitation of coronary arterial narrowing at necropsy in sudden coronary death. Analysis of 31 patients and comparison with 25 controls. Am. J. Cardiol. *44*:39, 1979.
237. Warnes, C. A., and Roberts, W. C.: Sudden coronary death: Relation of amount and distribution of coronary narrowing at necropsy to previous symptoms of myocardial ischemia, left ventricular scarring, and heart weight. Am. J. Cardiol. *54*:65, 1984.
238. Friedman, M., Manwaring, J. H., Rosenman, R. H., Donlon, G., Ortego, P., and Grube, S. M.: Instantaneous and sudden deaths: Clinical and pathological differentiation in coronary artery disease. J.A.M.A. *225*:1319, 1973.
239. Spain, D. M., and Bradess, V. A.: Sudden death from coronary heart disease. Survival time, frequency of thrombi and cigarette smoking. Chest 58:107, 1970.
240. Roberts, W. C., and Buja, L. M.: The frequency and significance of coronary arterial thrombi and other observations in fatal acute myocardial infarction: A study of 107 necropsy patients. Am. J. Med. 52:425, 1972.
241. Davies, M. J., and Thomas, A.: Thrombosis and acute coronary artery lesions in sudden cardiac ischemic death. N. Engl. J. Med. *310*:1137, 1984.
242. Lie, J. T., and Titus, J. L.: Pathology of the myocardium and the conduction system in sudden coronary death. Circulation 52(Suppl 3):41, 1975.
243. Baroldi, G., Falzi, A., Mariani, F., and Baroldi, L. A.: Morphology, frequency, and significance of intramural arterial lesions in sudden coronary death. G. Ital. Cardiol. *10*:644, 1980.
244. Titus, J. L., Oxman, H. A., Connolly, D. C., and Hobrego, F. T.: Sudden unexpected death as the initial manifestation of coronary heart disease. Clinical and pathological observations. Singapore Med. J. *14*:291, 1973.
245. Myers, A., and Dewar, H. A.: Circumstances attending 100 sudden deaths from coronary artery disease with coroner's necropsies. Br. Heart J. 37:1133, 1975.
246. Davies, M. J., and Popple, A. W.: Sudden unexpected cardiac death—a practical approach to the forensic problem. Histopathology 3:255, 1979.
247. Baba, N., Bashe, W. J., Jr., Keller, M. D., Geer, J. C., and Anthony, J. R.: Pathology of atherosclerotic heart disease in sudden death. I. Organizing thrombus and acute coronary vessel lesions. Circulation 52(Suppl 3):53, 1975.
248. Rissanen, V., Romo, M., and Siltanen, P.: Prehospital sudden death from ischaemic heart disease—a postmortem study. Br. Heart J. *40*:1025, 1978.
249. Scott, R. G., and Briggs, R. S.: Pathological findings in prehospital deaths due to coronary atherosclerosis. Am. J. Cardiol 29:782, 1972.
250. Crawford, T., Dexter, D, and Teare, R. D.: Coronary artery pathology in sudden death from myocardial ischaemia. Lancet *1*:181, 1961.
251. Roberts, W. C., Currey, R. C., Isner, J. M., Waller, B. F., McManus, B. M., Mariani-Constantini, R., and Ross, A. M.: Sudden death in Prinzmetal's angina with coronary spasm documented by angiography. Analysis of three necropsy patients. Am. J. Cardiol. 50:203, 1982.
252. Newman, W. P., Strong, J. P., Johnson, W. D., Oalmann, M. C., Tracy, R. E., and Rork, W. A.: Community pathology of atherosclerosis and coronary heart disease in New Orleans: Morphologic findings in young black and white men. Lab. Invest. *44*:496, 1981.
253. Newman, W. P., Tracy, R. E., Strong, J. P., Johnson, W. D., and Oalmann, M. C.: Pathology of sudden cardiac death. N.Y. Acad. Sci. 382:39, 1982.
254. Bashe, W. J., Baba, N., Keller, M. D. Geer, J. C., and Anthony, J. R.: Pathology of atherosclerotic heart disease in sudden death: The significance of myocardial infarction. Circulation 52(Suppl 3):63, 1975.
255. Schwartz, C. J., and Gerrity, R. G.: Anatomical pathology of sudden unexpected cardiac death. Circulation 52(Suppl 3):18, 1975.
256. Kuller, L. H., Cooper, M., Perper, J., and Fisher, R.: Myocardial infarction and sudden death in an urban community. Bull. N.Y. Acad. Med. *49*:532, 1973.
257. James, T. N.: Morphologic substrates of sudden death: Summary. J. Am. Coll. Cardiol. 5(Suppl B):81B, 1985.
258. Simon, A. B., and Zioto, A. E.: Coarctation of the aorta: Longitudinal assessment of operated patients. Circulation *50*:456, 1974.
259. Wagner, H. R., Ellison, R. C., Keane, J. F., Humphries, J. O., and Nadas, A. S.: Clinical course in aortic stenosis. Circulation 56(Suppl 1):47, 1972.
260. Anderson, K. P.: Sudden death in hypertrophic cardiomyopathy. Cardiovasc. Rev. 5:363, 1984.
261. Roberts, W. C., and Podolak, N. J.: The king of hearts: Analysis of 23 patients with hearts weighing 1,000 grams or more. Am. J. Cardiol. 55:485, 1985.
262. Lie, J. T.: Histopathology of the conduction system in sudden death from coronary heart disease. Circulation *51*:446, 1975.
263. Lie, J. T., and Hunt, D.: The cardiac conduction system in acute myocardial infarction. Aust. N.Z. J. Med. *4*:331, 1974.
264. James, T. N.: Neural variations and pathologic changes in structure of the cardiac conduction system and their functional significance. J. Am. Coll. Cardiol. 5(Suppl):71B, 1985.
265. Rossi, L.: Pathologic changes in the cardiac conduction and nervous system in sudden coronary death. Ann. N.Y. Acad. Sci. *382*:50, 1982.
266. James, T. N.: Primary and secondary cardioneuropathies and their functional significance. J. Am. Coll. Cardiol. 2:983, 1983.
267. Barber, M. J., Mueller, T. M., Henry, D. P., Felten, S. Y., and Zipes, D. P.: Transmural myocardial infarction in the dog produces sympathectomy in non-infarcted myocardium. Circulation *67*:787, 1982.
268. Gaide, M. S., Myerburg, R. J., Kozlovskis, P. L., and Bassett, A. L.: Elevated sympathetic response of epicardium proximal to healed myocardial infarction. Am. J. Physiol. *14*:646, 1983.
269. Corr, P. B., and Gillis, R. A.: Autonomic neural influences on the dysrhythmias resulting from myocardial infarction. Circ. Res. *43*:1, 1978.
270. Diederick, K., Djoniagic, H., Schreiner, W. B., and Bos, I.: Hereditares QT syndrom: ein weiterer Fall mit Grenzstrang Ganglionitis. Herz-Kreis *3*:149, 1982.
271. Rossi, L.: Cardioneuropathy and extracardiac neural disease. J. Am. Coll. Cardiol. *5*(Suppl):66B, 1985.
272. Cobb, L. A., and Weaver, W. D.: Exercise: A risk for sudden death in patients with coronary heart disease. J. Am. Coll. Cardiol. *7*:215, 1986.
273. Maseri, A., Saveri, S., DeNes, M., L'Abbate, A., Chierchia, S., Marzilli, M., Ballestra, A. M., Parodi, O., Biagini, A., and Distante, A.: "Variant" angina: One aspect of a continuous spectrum of vasospastic myocardial ischemia. Am. J. Cardiol. *42*:1019, 1978.
274. Schamroth, L.: Mechanism of lethal arrhythmias in sudden death. Possible role of vasospasm and release. Pract. Cardiol. *7*:105, 1981.
275. MacAlpin, R. N.: Relation of coronary arterial spasm to sites of organic stenosis. Am. J. Cardiol. *46*:143, 1980.
276. Ricci, D. R., Orlick, A. E., Cipriano, P. R., Guthaner, D. F, and Harrison, D. C.: Altered adrenergic activity in coronary arterial spasm: Insight into mechanism based on study of coronary hemodynamics and the electrocardiogram. Am. J. Cardiol. *43*:1073, 1979.
277. Luchi, R. J., Chahine, R. A., and Raizner, A. E.: Coronary artery spasm. Ann. Intern. Med. *91*:441, 1979.
278. Yasue, H., Touyama, M., Shimamoto, M., Kato, H., Tanaka, S., and Akiyama, F.: Role of the autonomic nervous system in the pathogenesis of Prinzmetal's variant form of angina. Circulation *50*:534, 1974.
279. Yasue, H., Touyama, M., Kato, H., Tanaka, S., and Akiyama, F.: Prinzmetal's variant form of angina as a form of alpha-adrenergic receptor-mediated coronary artery spasm: Documentation by coronary arteriography. Am. Heart J. *91*:148, 1976.
280. Robertson, D., Robertson, R. M., Nies, A. S., Oates, J. A., and Freisinger, G. C.: Variant angina pectoris: Investigation of indexes of sympathetic nervous system function. Am. J. Cardiol. *43*:1080, 1979.
281. Mudge, G. H., Grossman, W., Millis, R. M., Lesch, M., and Braunwald, E.: Reflex increase in coronary vascular resistance in patients with ischemic heart disease. N. Engl. J. Med. 295:1333, 1976.
282. Endo, M., Hirosawa, K., Kaneko, N., Hase, K., Inoue, Y., and Konno, S.: Prinzmetal's variant angina. Coronary arteriogram and left ventriculogram during angina attack induced by methacholine. N. Engl. J. Med. *294*:252, 1976.
283. Buda, A. J., Fowles, R. E., Schroeder, J. S., Hunt, S. A., Cipriano, P. R., Stinson, E. D., and Harrison, D. C.: Coronary artery spasm in the denervated transplanted human heart. A clue to underlying mechanisms. Am. J. Med. *70*:1144, 1981.
284. Mehta, J., and Mehta, P.: Role of platelets and prostaglandins in coronary artery disease. Am. J. Cardiol. *48*:366, 1981.
285. Hammon, J. W., and Oates, J. A.: Interaction of platelets with the vessel wall in the pathophysiology of sudden cardiac death. Circulation *73*:224, 1986.
286. Starnes, V. A., Primm, R. K., Woosley, R. L., Oates, J. A., and Hammon, J. W.: Administration of prostacyclin prevents ventricular fibrillation following coronary occlusion in conscious dogs. J. Cardiovasc. Pharmacol. *4*:765, 1982.
287. Aspirin-Myocardial Infarction Study Research Group: A randomized controlled trial of aspirin in persons recovered from myocardial infarction. J.A.M.A. *243*:661, 1980.
288. Myerburg, R. J., Kessler, K. M., Zaman, L., Conde, C. A., and Castellanos, A.: Survivors of prehospital cardiac arrest. J.A.M.A. *247*:1485, 1982.
289. Cox, J. L., Daniel, T. M., and Boineau, J. P.: The electrophysiologic time-course of acute myocardial ischemia and the effects of early coronary artery reperfusion. Circulation *48*:971, 1973.
290. Cameron, J. S., Myerburg, R. J., Wong, S. S., Gaide, M. S., Epstein, K., Alvarez, R., Gelband, H., Guse, P. A., and Bassett, A. L.: Electrophysiologic consequences of chronic experimentally induced left ventricular pressure overload. J. Am. Coll. Cardiol. 2:481, 1983.
291. Myerburg, R. J., Bassett, A. L., Epstein, K., Gaide, M. S., Kozlovskis, P., Wong, S. S., Castellanos, A., and Gelband, H.: Electrophysiologic effects of procainamide in acute and healed experimental ischemic injury of cat myocardium. Circ. Res. *50*:386, 1982.
292. Myerburg, R. J., Epstein, K., Gaide, M. S., Wong, S. S., Castellanos, A., Gelband, H., and Bassett, A. L.: Electrophysiologic consequences of experimental acute ischemia superimposed upon healed myocardial infarction in cats. Am. J. Cardiol. *49*:323, 1982.
293. Myerburg, R. J., Epstein, K., Gaide, M. S., Wong, S. S., Castellanos, A., Gelband, H., and Bassett, A. L.: Cellular electrophysiology in acute and healed experimental myocardial infarction. Ann. N.Y. Acad. Sci. *382*:90, 1982.
294. Corbalan, R., Verrier, R. L., and Lown, B.: Differing mechanisms for ventricular vulnerability during coronary artery occlusion and release. Am. Heart J. *92*:223, 1976.
295. Kaplinsky, E., Ogawa, S., Michelson, E. L., and Dreifus, L. S.: Instantaneous and delayed ventricular arrhythmias after reperfusion of acutely ischemic myocardium: Evidence for multiple mechanisms. Circulation 63:333, 1981.

296. Kimura, S., Bassett, A. L., Saoudi, N. C., Cameron, J. S., Kozlovskis, P. L., and Myerburg, R. J.: Cellular electrophysiological changes and "arrhythmias" during experimental ischemia and reperfusion in isolated cat ventricular myocardium. J. Am. Coll. Cardiol. *7*:833, 1986.
297. Harris, A. S.: Delayed development of ventricular ectopic rhythms following experimental coronary occlusion. Circulation *1*:1318, 1950.
298. Kimura, S., Bassett, A. L., Kohya, T., Kozlovskis, P. L., and Myerburg, R. J.: Simultaneous recording of action potentials from endocardium and epicardium during ischemia in the isolated cat ventricle: Relation of temporal electrophysiological heterogeneities to arrhythmias. Circulation *74*:401, 1986.
299. Janse, M. J., van Capelle, F. J. L., Morsink, H., Kleber, A. G., Wilms-Schopman, F. J. L., Cardinal, R., Naumann d'Alnoncourt, C., and Durrer, D.: Flow of "injury" current and patterns of excitation during early ventricular arrhythmias in acute regional myocardial ischemia in isolated porcine and canine hearts. Evidence for two different arrhythmogenic mechanisms. Circ. Res. *47*:151, 1980.
300. Sharma, A. D., Saffitz, J. E., Lee, B. L., Sobel, B. E., and Corr, P. B.: Alpha adrenergic-mediated accumulation of calcium in reperfused myocardium. J. Clin. Invest. *72*:802, 1982.
301. Corr, P. B., Shayman, J. A., Kramer, J. B., and Kipnis, R. J.: Increased alpha-adrenergic receptors in ischemic cat myocardium. J. Clin. Invest. *67*:1232, 1981.
302. Sheridan, D. J., Penkoske, P. A., Sobel, B. E., and Corr, P. B.: Alpha-adrenergic contributions to dysrhythmia during myocardial ischemia and reperfusion in cats. J. Clin. Invest. *65*:161, 1980.
303. Schwartz, P. J., and Stone, H. L.: Left stellectomy in the prevention of ventricular fibrillation caused by acute myocardial ischemia in conscious dogs with anterior myocardial infarction. Circulation *62*:1256, 1980.
304. Gaudel, Y., and Duvelleroy, M.: Role of oxygen radicals in cardiac injury due to reoxygenation. J. Mol. Cell Cardiol. *16*:459, 1984.
305. Manning, A. S., Coltart, D. J., and Hearse, D. J.: Ischemia and reperfusion-induced arrhythmias in the rat: Effects of xanthine oxidase inhibition with allopurinol. Circ. Res. *55*:545, 1984.
306. van Gilst, W. H., de Graeff, P. A., Kingma, J. H., Wesseling, H., and de Langen, C. D. J.: Captopril reduces purine loss and reperfusion arrhythmias in the rat heart after coronary artery occlusion. Eur. J. Pharmacol. *100*:113, 1984.
307. Verrier, R. L., Hagestad, E. L.: Role of the autonomic nervous system in sudden death. *In* Josephson, M. E. (ed.): Sudden Cardiac Death. Philadelphia, F. A. Davis Co., 1985, pp. 41–63.
308. Kaplinsky, E., Ogawa, S., and Dreifus, L. S.: Central role of subendocardial activation in the genesis of malignant ventricular tachycardia and fibrillation. Am. J. Cardiol. *41*:427, 1978.
309. Klein, G. J., Idelser, R. E., Smith, W. M., Harrison, L. A., Kasell, J., Wallace, A. G., and Gallagher, J. J.: Epicardial mapping of the onset of ventricular tachycardia initiated by programmed stimulation in the canine heart with chronic infarction. Circulation *60*:1375, 1979.
310. Chilson, D. A., Peigh, P., Mahomed, Y., and Zipes, D. P.: Encircling endocardial ventriculotomy interrupts vagal-induced prolongation of endocardial and epicardial refractoriness in the dog. J. Am. Coll. Cardiol. *5*:290, 1985.
311. Janse, M. J., and Downer, E.: The effect of acute ischaemia on transmembrane potentials in the intact heart. Relation to re-entry mechanisms. *In* Kulbertus, H. E. (ed.): Re-entrant Arrhythmias. Lancaster, MTP Press, 1977, pp. 195–209.
312. Kuller, L. H., Hulley, S. B., Cohen, J. D., and Neaton, J.: Unexpected effects of treating hypertension in men with electrocardiographic abnormalities: A critcal analysis. Circulation *73*:114, 1986.
313. Cooper, W. D., Kuan, P., Reuben, S. R., and VandenBurg, M. J.: Cardiac arrhythmias following acute myocardial infarction: Associations with the serum potassium level and prior diuretic therapy. Eur. Heart J. *5*:464, 1984.
314. Struthers, A. D., Whitesmith, R., and Reid, J. L.: Prior thiazide diuretic treatment increases adrenaline-induced hypokalaemia. Lancet *1*:1358, 1983.
315. Skinner, J. E.: Regulation of cardiac vulnerability by the cerebral defense system. J. Am. Coll. Cardiol. *5*(Suppl B):88, 1985.
316. Schwartz, P. J., Billman, G. E., and Stone, H. L.: Autonomic mechanisms in ventricular fibrillation induced by myocardial ischemia during exercise in dogs with healed myocardial infarction. Circulation *69*:790, 1984.
317. Verrier, R. L., and Lown, B.: Experimental studies of psychophysiological factors in sudden cardiac death. Acta Med. Scand. *660*(Suppl):57, 1982.
318. Schwartz, P. J., and Stone, H. L.: The role of autonomic nervous system in sudden coronary death. Ann. N.Y. Acad. Sci. *382*:162, 1982.
319. Opie, L. H.: Products of myocardial ischemia and electrical instability of the heart. J. Am. Coll. Cardiol. *5*(Suppl B):162, 1985.
320. Myerburg, R. J., Kessler, K. M., Kiem, I., Pefkaros, K. C., Conde, C. A., Cooper, D., and Castellanos. A.: The relationship between plasma levels of procainamide, suppression of premature ventricular contractions, and prevention of recurrent ventricular tachycardia. Circulation *64*:280, 1981.
321. Vassalle, M.: Cardiac pacemaker potentials at different extra- and intracellular K+ concentrations. Am. J. Physiol. *208*:770, 1965.
322. Vassalle, M.: On the mechanisms underlying cardiac standstill: Factors determining success or failure of escape pacemakers in the heart. J. Am. Coll. Cardiol. *5*(Suppl B):35, 1985.
323. Fozzard, H. A.: Electromechanical dissociation and its possible role in sudden cardiac death. J. Am. Coll. Cardiol. *5*(Suppl B):31, 1985.

CLINICAL CHARACTERISTICS OF THE PATIENT WITH CARDIAC ARREST

324. Russek, H. I., and Zohman, B. L.: Prognosis in the "uncomplicated" first attack of acute myocardial infarction. Am. J. Med. Sci. *224*:496, 1952.
325. Pell, S., and D'Alonzo, C. A.: Immediate mortality and five-year survival of employed men with a first myocardial infarction. N. Engl. J. Med. *270*:915, 1964.
326. Ball, C. O. T., Billings, F. T., Furman, R. H., Brothers, G. B., Thomas, J., and Meneely, G. R.: The functional circulatory consequences of myocardial infarction: A biostatistical analysis following Wiggers' schema. Circulation *11*:749, 1955.
327. Lown, B., Fakhro, A. M., Hood, W. B., and Thorn, G. W.: The coronary care unit: New perspectives and directions. J.A.M.A. *199*:156, 1967.
328. Kimball, J. J., and Killip, T.: Aggressive treatment of arrhythmias in acute myocardial infarction: Procedures and results. Prog. Cardiovasc. Dis. *10*:483, 1968.
329. Feinlieb, M., Simon, A. B., Gillum, J. R., and Margolis, J. R.: Prodromal symptoms and signs of sudden death. Circulation *52*(Suppl 3):155, 1975.
330. Simon, A. B., and Alonzo, A. A.: Sudden death in non-hospitalized cardiac patients. Arch. Intern Med. *132*:163, 1973.
331. Fulton, M., Lutz, W., Donald, K. W., Kirby, B. J., Duncan, B., Morrison, S. L., Kerr, F., Julian, D. G., and Oliver, M. F.: Natural history of unstable angina. Lancet *1*:860, 1972.
332. Hinkle, L. E., Argyros, D. C., Hayes, J. C., Robinson, T., and Alonso, D. R.: Pathogenesis of an unexpected sudden death: Role of early cycle ventricular premature contractions. Am. J. Cardiol. *39*:873, 1977.
333. Goldstein, S., Landis, J. R., Leighton, R., Ritter, G., Vasu, C. M., Lantis, A., and Serokman, R.: Characteristics of the resuscitated out-of-hospital cardiac arrest victim with coronary heart disease. Circulation *64*:977, 1981.
334. Nikolic, G., Bishop, R. L., and Singh, J. B.: Sudden death recorded during Holter monitoring. Circulation *66*:218, 1982.
335. Pratt, C. M., Francis, M. J., Luck, J. C., Wyndham, C. R., Miller, R. R., and Quinones, M. A.: Analysis of ambulatory electrocardiograms in 15 patients during spontaneous ventricular fibrillation with special reference to preceding arrhythmic events. J. Am. Coll. Cardiol. *2*:789, 1983.
336. Panidis, I. P., and Morganroth, J.: Holter monitoring and sudden cardiac death. Cardiovasc. Rev. *5*:283, 1984.
336a. Hinkle, L. E., and Thaler, H. T.: Clinical classification of cardiac deaths. Circulation *65*:457, 1982.
337. Bates, R. J., Beutler, S., Resnekov, L., and Anagnostopoulos, C. E.: Cardiac rupture: Challenge in diagnosis and management. Am. J. Cardiol. *40*:429, 1977.
338. Creed, J. D., Packard, J. M., Lambrew, C. T., and Lewis, A. J.: Defibrillation and synchronized cardioversion. *In* McIntyre, K. M., and Lewis, A. J. (eds.): Textbook of Advanced Cardiac Life Support, Dallas, American Heart Association, Inc., 1983, pp. 89–96.
338a. Standard and guidelines for cardiopulmonary resuscitation (CPR) and emergency cardiac care (ECC). J.A.M.A. *255*:290, 1986.
339. Lo, B., and Jonsen, A. R.: Clinical decisions to limit treatment. Ann. Intern. Med. *93*:764, 1980.
340. Lo, B., and Steinbrook, R. L.: Deciding whether to resuscitate. Arch. Intern. Med. *143*:1561, 1983.
341. Robinson, J. S., Sloman, G., Mathew, T. H., and Goble, A. J.: Survival after resuscitation from cardiac arrest in acute myocardial infarction. Am. Heart J. *69*:740, 1965.
342. Killip, T., and Kimball, J. T.: Treatment of myocardial infarction in a coronary care unit: A two-year experience with 250 patients. Am. J. Cardiol. *20*:457, 1967.
343. Bedell, S. E., Delbanco, T. L., Cook, E. F., and Epstein, F. H.: Survival after cardiopulmonary resuscitation in the hospital. N. Engl. J. Med. *309*:569, 1983.
344. Cobb, L. A., and Hallstrom, A. P.: Community-based cardiopulmonary resuscitation: What have we learned? Ann. N.Y. Acad. Sci. *382*:330, 1982.
345. Cobb, L. A., Hallstrom, A. P., Weaver, W. D., Trobaugh, G. B., and Greene, H. L.: Considerations in the long-term management of survivors of cardiac arrest. Ann. N.Y. Acad. Sci. *432*:247, 1984.
346. Goldstein, S., Landis, J. R., Leighton, R., Ritter, R., Vasu, S. M., Wolfe, R. A., Acheson, A., and Medendorp, S. V.: Predictive survival models for resuscitated victims of out-of-hospital cardiac arrest with coronary heart disease. Circulation *71*:873, 1985.
347. Gulati, R. S., Bhan, G. L., and Horan, M. A.: Cardiopulmonary resuscitation of old people. Lancet *2*:267, 1983.
348. Eisenberg, M. S., Bergner, L., and Hallstrom, A. P.: Cardiac resuscitation in the community: Importance of rapid provision and implications of program planning. J.A.M.A. *241*:1905, 1979.
349. Myerburg, R. J., Estes, D., Zaman, L., Luceri, R. M., Kessler, K. M., Trohman, R. G., and Castellanos, A.: Outcome of resuscitation from bradyarrhythmic or asystolic prehospital cardiac arrest. J. Am. Coll. Cardiol. *4*:1118, 1984.
350. Iseri, L. T., Humphrey, S. B., and Siner, E. J.: Prehospital brady-asystole cardiac arrest. Ann. Intern. Med. *88*:741, 1978.
351. Jaggarao, N. S. V., Heber, M., Grainger, R., Vincent, R., Chamberlain, D. A., and Aronson, A. L.: Use of an automated external defibrillator-pacemaker by ambulance staff. Lancet *2*:73, 1982.
352. Longstreth, W. T., Inui, T. S., Cobb, L. A., and Copass, M. K.: Neurologic recovery after out-of-hospital cardiac arrest. Ann. Intern. Med. *98*:588, 1983.
353. Longstreth, W. T., Diehr, P., and Inui, T. S.: Prediction of awakening after out-of-hospital cardiac arrest. N. Engl. J. Med. *308*:1378, 1983.
354. Myerburg, R. J., Briese, F. R., Conde, C. A., Mallon, S. B., Liberthson, R. B., and Castellanos, A.: Long-term antiarrhythmic therapy in survivors of prehospital cardiac arrest: Initial 18 months' experience. J.A.M.A. *238*:2621, 1977.
355. Myerburg, R. J., Conde, C. A., Sheps, D. S., Appel, R. A., Kiem, I., Sung, R. J., and Castellanos, A.: Antiarrhythmic drug therapy in survivors of

prehospital cardiac arrest: Comparison of effects on chronic ventricular arrhythmias and on recurrent cardiac arrest. Circulation *59*:855, 1979.
356. Weaver, W. D., Cobb, L. A., and Hallstrom, A. P.: Ambulatory arrhythmia in resuscitated victims of cardiac arrest. Circulation *66*:212, 1982.
357. Ritchie, J. L., Hallstrom, A. P., Troubaugh, G. B., Caldwell, J. H., and Cobb, L. A.: Out-of-hospital sudden coronary death: Rest and exercise radionuclide left ventricular function in survivors. Am. J. Cardiol. *55*:645, 1985.
358. Weaver, W. D., Lorch, G. S., Alvarez, H. A., and Cobb, L. A.: Angiographic findings and prognostic indicators in patients resuscitated from sudden cardiac death. Circulation *54*:895, 1976.
359. Weaver, W. D., Cobb, L. A., and Hallstrom, A. P.: Characteristics of survivors of exertion- and nonexertion-related cardiac arrest: Value of subsequent exercise testing. Am. J. Cardiol. *50*:671, 1982.
360. Cobb, L. A., Werner, J. A., and Trobaugh, G. B.: Sudden cardiac death: I. A decade's experience with out-of-hospital resuscitation; and II. Outcome of resuscitation, management, and future directions. Mod. Concept Cardiovasc. Dis. *49*:31–37, 1980.
361. Haynes, R. E., Hallstrom, A. P., and Cobb, L. A.: Repolarization abnormalities in survivors of out-of-hospital ventricular fibrillation. Circulation *57*:654, 1978.
362. Thompson, R. G., and Cobb, L. A.: Hypokalemia after resuscitation from out-of-hospital cardiac arrest. J.A.M.A. *248*:2860, 1982.
363. Sheps, D. S., Conde, C., Cameron, B., Lo, W. C., Appel, R., Castellanos, A., Harkness, D. R., and Myerburg, R. J.: Resting peripheral blood lactate elevation in survivors of prehospital cardiac arrest: Correlation with hemodynamic, electrophysiologic, and oxyhemoglobin dissociation indexes. Am. J. Cardiol. *44*:1276, 1979.

MANAGEMENT OF CARDIAC ARREST

364. Lown, B., Fakhro, A. M., Hood, W. B., Jr., and Thorn, G. W.: The coronary care unit: New perspectives and directives. J.A.M.A. *199*:188, 1967.
365. Goldman, L.: Coronary care units: A perspective on their epidemiologic impact. Int. J. Cardiol. 2:284, 1982.
366. Pantridge, J. F., and Adgey, A. A. J.: Pre-hospital coronary care. The mobile coronary care unit. Am. J. Cardiol. *24*:666, 1969.
367. Nagel, E. L., Liberthson, R. R., Hirschman, J. C., and Nussenfeld, S. R.: Emergency care. Circulation 52(Suppl 3):216, 1975.
368. Eisenberg, M. S., Copass, M. K., Hallstrom, A. P., Blake, B., Bergner, L., Short, F. A., and Cobb, L. A.: Treatment of out-of-hospital cardiac arrests with rapid defibrillation by emergency medical technicians. N. Engl. J. Med. *302*:1379, 1980.
369. Ewy, G. A.: Current status of cardiopulmonary resuscitation. Mod. Concepts Cardiovasc. Dis. *53*:43, 1984.
370. Stults, K. R., Brown, D. D., Schug, V. L., and Bean, J. A.: Prehospital defibrillation performed by emergency medical technicians in rural communities. N. Engl. J. Med. *310*:219, 1984.
371. Mayer, J. D.: Paramedic response time and survival from cardiac arrest. Soc. Sci. Med. *13D*:267, 1979.
372. Weaver, W. D., Copass, M. K., Bufi, D., Ray, R., Hallstrom, A. P., and Cobb, L. A.: Improved neurologic recovery and survival after early defibrillation. Circulation *69*:943, 1984.
373. Lie, K. I., Wellens, H. J. J., van Capelle, F. J., and Durrer, D.: Lidocaine in the prevention of primary ventricular fibrillation. N. Engl. J. Med. *291*:1324, 1974.
374. Valentine, P. A., Frew, J. L., Mashford, M. L., and Sloman, J. G.: Lidocaine in the prevention of sudden death in the prehospital phase of acute infarction. N. Engl. J. Med. *291*:1327, 1974.
375. Koster, R. W., and Dunning, R. J.: Intramuscular lidocaine for prevention of lethal arrhythmias in the prehospitalization phase of acute myocardial infarction. N. Engl. J. Med. *313*:1105, 1985.
376. Caldwell, G., Miller, G., Quinn, E., Vincent, R., and Chamberlain, D. A.: Simple mechanical methods for cardioversion: Defense of the precordial thump and cough version. Br. Med. J. *291*:627, 1985.
377. Theorell, T.: Electrokinetic considerations of mechanoelectrical transduction. Ann. N.Y. Acad. Sci. *137*:950, 1966.
378. Lown, B., and Taylor, J.: "Thumpversion" (Editorial). N. Engl. J. Med. *283*:1223, 1970.
379. Criley, J. M., Blaufuss, A. N., and Kissel, J. L.: Cough-induced cardiac compression: Self-administered form of cardiopulmonary resuscitation. J.A.M.A. *263*:1246, 1976.
380. Wei, J. Y., Greene, H. L., and Weisfeldt, M. L.: Cough-facilitated conversion of ventricular tachycardia. Am. J. Cardiol. *45*:174, 1980.
381. Heimlich, H. J.: A life-saving maneuver to prevent food-choking. J.A.M.A. *234*:398, 1975.
382. Visintine, R. E., and Baick, C. H.: Ruptured stomach after Heimlich maneuver. J.A.M.A. *234*:415, 1975.
383. Feldman, T., Mallon, S. M., Bolooki, H., Trohman, R. G., Guzman, P., and Myerburg, R.: Fatal acute aortic regurgitation in a person performing the Heimlich maneuver (letter). N. Engl. J. Med., *315*:1613, 1986.
384. Standards and guidelines for cardiopulmonary resuscitation (CPR) and emergency cardiac care (ECC). J.A.M.A. *244*:453, 1980.
385. Weisfeldt, M. L., and Chandra, N.: Physiology of cardiopulmonary resuscitation. Ann. Rev. Med. *32*:435, 1981.
386. Weisfeldt, M. L., Chandra, N., and Tsitlik, J. E.: Increased intrathoracic pressure–not direct heart compression–causes the rise in intrathoracic vascular pressures during CPR in dogs and pigs. Crit. Care Med. 9:377, 1981.
387. Rudikoff, M. T., Maughan, W. L., Effrom, M., Freund, P., and Weisfeldt, M. L.: Mechanisms of blood flow during cardiopulmonary resuscitation. Circulation *61*:345, 1980.
388. Niemann, J. T., Rosborough, J. P., Hausknecht, M., Garner, D., and Criley, J. M.: Pressure-synchronized cineangiography during experimental cardiopulmonary resuscitation. Circulation *4*:985, 1981.
389. Chandra, N., Rudikoff, M., and Weisfeldt, M. L.: Simultaneous chest compression and ventilation at high airway pressure during cardiopulmonary resuscitation. Lancet *1*:175, 1980.
390. Ditchey, R. V., and Lindenfeld, J.: Potential adverse effects of volume loading on perfusion of vital organs during closed-chest resuscitation. Circulation *69*:181, 1984.
391. Michael, J. R., Guerci, D., Koehler, R. C., Shi, A.-Y, Tsitlik, J., Chandra, N., Niedermeyer, E., Rogers, M. C., Traystman, R. J., and Weisfeldt, M. L.: Mechanisms by which epinephrine augments cerebral and myocardial perfusion during cardiopulmonary resuscitation in dogs. Circulation *69*:822, 1984.
392. Sanders, A. B., Ewy, G. A., Alferness, A., Taft, T., and Zimmerman, M.: Failure of one method of simultaneous chest compression, ventilation, and abdominal binding during CPR. Crit. Care Med. *120*:509, 1982.
393. Ducas, J., Roussos, C. H., Karsaidis, C., and Magder, S.: Thoracoabdominal mechanisms during resuscitation maneuvers. Chest *84*:446, 1983.
394. Heber, M.: Out-of-hospital cardiac arrest using the "Heart Aid," an automated external defibrillator-pacemaker. Int. J. Cardiol. *3*:456, 1983.
395. Cummins, R. O., Eisenberg, M., Bergner, L., and Murray, J. A.: Sensitivity, accuracy, and safety of an automatic external defibrillator. Lancet *2*:318, 1984.
396. Pantridge, J. F., Adgey, A. A. J., Webb, S. W., and Anderson, J.: Electrical requirements for ventricular defibrillation. Br. Med. J. 2:313, 1975.
397. Adgey, A. A. J., Patton, N. J., Campbell, N. P. S., and Webb, S. W.: Ventricular defibrillation: Appropriate energy levels. Circulation *60*:219, 1979.
398. Gascho, J. A., Crampton, R. S., Cherwek, M. L., Siper, J. N., Cohen, F. P., and Obren, W. M.: Determinants of ventricular defibrillation in adults. Circulation *60*:231, 1979.
399. Tacker, W. A., and Ewy, G. A.: Emergency defibrillation dose, recommendation and rationale. Circulation *60*:223, 1979.
400. Lown, B., Crampton, R. S., and DeSilva, R. A.: The energy for ventricular defibrillation: Too little or too much? N. Engl. J. Med. *298*:1252, 1978.
401. Bishop, R. L., and Weisfeldt, M. L.: Sodium bicarbonate administration during cardiac arrest. Effect on arterial pH, PCO_2, and osmolality. J.A.M.A. *235*:506, 1976.
402. Sodium bicarbonate in cardiac arrest (Editorial). Lancet *1*:946, 1976.
403. Mattar, J. A., Weil, M. H., Shubin, H., and Stein, L.: Cardiac arrest in the critically ill: Hyperosmolal states following cardiac arrest. Am. J. Med. *56*:162, 1974.
404. Berenyi, K. J., Wolk, M., and Killip, T.: Cerebrospinal fluid acidosis complicating therapy of experimental cardiopulmonary arrest. Circulation *52*:319, 1975.
405. Weil, M. H., Trevino, R. P., and Rackow, E. C.: Sodium bicarbonate during CPR: Does it help or hinder? Chest *88*:487, 1985.
406. White, R. D.: Cardiovascular Pharmacology: Part I. *In* McIntyre, K. M., and Lewis, A. J. (eds.): Textbook of Advanced Life Support. Dallas, American Heart Association, Inc., 1983, pp. 99–114.
407. Thompson, P. D., Melmon, K. L., Richardson, J. A., Cohn, K., Cudihee, R., Steinbrunn, W., and Rowland, M.: Lidocaine pharmacokinetics in advanced heart failure, liver disease, and renal failure in humans. Ann. Intern. Med. *78*:499, 1973.
408. Giardina, E. G., Heissenbuttel, R. H., and Bigger, J. T.: Intermittent intravenous procainamide to treat ventricular arrhythmias. Correlation of plasma concentration with effect on arrhythmia, electrocardiogram, and blood pressure. Ann. Intern. Med. *78*:183, 1973.
409. Holder, D. A., Sniderman, A. D., Fraser, G., and Fallen, E. L.: Experience with bretylium tosylate by a hospital cardiac arrest team. Circulation *55*:541, 1977.
410. Haynes, R. E., Chinn, T. L., Copass, M. K., and Cobb, L. A.: Comparison of bretylium tosylate and lidocaine in the resuscitation of patients from out-of-hospital ventricular fibrillation: A randomized clinical trial. Am. J. Cardiol. *487*:353, 1981.
411. Kutalek, S. P., Horowitz, L. N., Spielman, S. R., and Greenspan, A. M.: Emergent use of intravenous amiodarone for refractory ventricular tachyarrhythmias. Circulation 72(Suppl 3):274, 1985 (Abstract).
411a. Hughes, W. G., and Ruedy, J. R.: Should calcium be used in cardiac arrest? Am. J. Med. *81*:285, 1986.
412. Zoll, P. M., Zoll, R. H., Clinton, J. E., Eitel, D. R., and Antman, E. M.: External non-invasive temporary cardiac pacing: Clinical trials. Circulation *71*:937, 1985.
412a. Knowlton, A. A., and Falk, R. H.: External cardiac pacing during in hospital cardiac arrest. Am. J. Cardiol. *51*:1295, 1986.
412b. Lee, R. V., Rogers, B. D., White, L. M., and Harvey, R. C.: Cardiopulmonary resuscitation of pregnant women. Am. J. Med. *81*:311, 1986.
413. Redding, J. S., and Pearson, J. W.: Evaluation of drugs for cardiac resuscitation. Anesthesiology *24*:203, 1963.
414. Yakaitis, R. W., Otto, C. W., Blitt, C. D.: Relative importance of alpha and beta-adrenergic receptors during resuscitation. Crit. Care Med. *7*:293, 1979.
415. Holmes, H. R., Babbs, C. F., Voorhees, W. D., Tacker, W. A., and deGaravilla, B.: Influence of adrenergic drugs upon vital organ perfusion during CPR. Crit. Care Med. *8*:137, 1980.
416. Otto, C. W., Yakaitis, R. W., Redding, J. S., and Blitt, C. D.: Comparison

of dopamine, dobutamine, and epinephrine in CPR. Crit. Care Med. 9:366, 1981.

417. Ralston, S. H., Voorhees, W. D., and Babbs, C. F.: Intrapulmonary epinephrine during prolonged cardiopulmonary resuscitation: Improved regional blood flow and resuscitation in dogs. Ann. Emerg. Med. *13*:79, 1984.
418. Wyman, M. G., and Hammersmith, L.: Comprehensive treatment plan for the prevention of primary ventricular fibrillation in acute myocardial infarction. Am. J. Cardiol. *33*:661, 1974.
419. Conley, M. J.. McNeer, J. F., Lee, K. L., Wagner, G. S., and Rosati, R. A.: Cardiac arrest complicating acute myocardial infarction: Predictability and prognosis. Am. J. Cardiol. *39*:7, 1977.
420. Norris, R. M., and Mercer, C. J.: Significance of idioventricular rhythms in acute myocardial infarction. Prog. Cardiovasc. Dis. *16*:455, 1974.
421. Bass, E.: Cardiopulmonary arrest: Pathophysiology and neurologic complications. Ann. Intern. Med. *103*:920, 1985.
422. Breivik, H., Safar, P., Sands, P., Fabritius, R., Lin, B., Lust, P., Mullie, A., Orr, M., Renck, H., and Synder, J. V.: Clinical feasibility trials of barbiturate therapy after cardiac arrest. Crit. Care Med. *6*:228, 1978.
423. Brain Resuscitation Clinical Trial I Study Group: Randomized clinical study of thiopental loading in comatose survivors of cardiac arrest. N. Engl. J. Med. *314*:397, 1986.
424. Cobb, L. A., Hallstrom, A. P., Zia, M., Trobaugh, G. B., Greene, H. L., and Weaver, W. D.: Influence of coronary revascularization on recurrent suddent cardiac death syndrome. J. Am. Coll. Cardiol. *1*:688, 1983 (Abstract).
425. Harken, A. H., Wetstein, L., and Josephson, M. E.: Mechanisms and surgical management of ventricular tachyarrhythmias. *In* Josephson, M. E. (ed.): Sudden Cardiac Death. Philadelphia, F.A. Davis Co., 1985, pp. 287–300.
425a. Holmes, D. R., Davis, K. B., Mock, M. B., Fisher, L. B., Gersh, R. J., Killip, T., Pettinger, M., and Participants in the Coronary Artery Surgery Study: The effect of medical and surgical treatment on subsequent sudden cardiac death in patients with coronary artery disease: A report from the Coronary Artery Surgery Study. Circulation 73:1254, 1986.
426. Multiple Risk Factor Intervention Trial Research Group: Baseline rest electrocardiographic abnormalities, antihypertensive treatment, and mortality in the Multiple Risk Factor Intervention Trial. Am. J. Cardiol *55*:1, 1985.
427. Moss, A. J., Davis, H. T., Conard, D. L., DeCamilla, J. J., and Odoroff, C. L.: Digitalis-associated cardiac mortality after myocardial infarction. Circulation *64*:1150, 1981.
428. Bigger, J. T., Fleiss, J. L., Rolnitzky, L. M., Merab, J. P., and Ferrick, K. L.: Effect of digitalis treatment on survival after acute myocardial infarction. Am. J. Cardiol. *55*:623, 1985.
429. Ryan, T. J., Bailey, K. R., McCabe, C. H., Luk, S., Fisher, L. D., Mock, B. M., and Killip, T.: The effects of digitalis on survival in high risk patients with coronary artery disease: The Coronary Artery Surgery Study (CASS). Circulation *67*:735, 1983.
430. Madsen, E. G., Gilpin, E., Henning, H., Ahnve, S., LeWinter, M., Mazur, J., Shabetai, R., Collins, D., and Ross, J.: Prognostic importance of digitalis after acute myocardial infarction. J. Am. Coll. Cardiol. *3*:681, 1984.
431. Muller, J. E., Turi, Z. G., Stone, P. H., Rude, R. E., Raabe, D. S., Jaffe, A. S., Gold, H. K., Gustafson, N., Poole, W. K., Passamani, E., Smith, T. M., Braunwald, E., and the MILIS Study Group: Digoxin therapy and mortality after myocardial infarction: Experience in the MILIS study. N. Engl. J. Med. *314*:265, 1986.
432. Lown, B., and Graboys, T. B.: Management of patients with malignant ventricular arrhythmias. Am. J. Cardiol. *39*:910, 1977.
433. Graboys, T. B., Lown, B., Podrid, P. J., and DeSilva, R.: Long-term survival of patients with malignant ventricular arrhythmias treated with antiarrhythmic drugs. Am J. Cardiol. *50*:437, 1982.
434. Ruskin, J. N., DiMarco, J. P., and Garan, H.: Out-of-hospital cardiac arrest: Electrophysiologic observations and selection of long-term antiarrhythmic therapy. N. Engl. J. Med. *303*:607, 1980.
435. Josephson, M. E., Horowitz, L. N., Spielman, S. C., and Greenspan, A. M.: Electrophysiologic and hemodynamic studies in patients resuscitated from cardiac arrest. Am. J. Cardiol. *46*:948, 1980.
436. Roy, D., Waxman, H. L., Kienzle, M. G., Buxton, A. F., Marchlinski, F. E., and Josephson, M. E.: Clinical characteristics and long-term follow-up in 119 survivors of cardiac arrest: Relation to inducibility at electrophysiologic testing. Am. J. Cardiol. *52*:969, 1983.
437. Benditt, D. G., Benson, D. W., Jr., Klein, G. J., Pritzker, M. C., Kriett, J. M., and Anderson, R. W.: Prevention of recurrent sudden cardiac arrest: Role of provocative electropharmacologic testing. J. Am. Coll. Cardiol. *2*:418, 1983.
438. Morady, F., Scheinman, M. M., Hess, D. S., Sung, R. J., Shen, E., and Shapiro, W.: Electrophysiologic testing in the management of survivors of out-of-hospital cardiac arrest. Am. J. Cardiol. *51*:85, 1983.
439. Skale, B. T., Miles, W. M., Heger, J. J., Zipes, D. P., and Prystowsky, E. N.: Survivors of cardiac arrest: Prevention of recurrence by drug therapy as predicted by electrophysiologic testing or electrocardiographic monitoring. Am. J. Cardiol. *57*:113, 1986.
440. Kehoe, R. F., Moran, J. M., Zheutlin, T., Tommaso, C., and Lesch, M.: Electrophysiologic study to direct therapy in survivors of prehospital ventricular fibrillation. (Abstr) Am. J. Cardiol. *49*:928, 1982.
441. Platia, E. V., Griffith, L. S. C., Watkins, L., Mower, M. M., Guarnieri, T., Mirowski, M., and Reid, P. R.: Treatment of malignant ventricular arrhythmias with endocardial resection and implantation of the automatic cardioverter-defibrillator. N. Engl. J. Med. *314*:213, 1986.
442. Swerdlow, C. R., Winkle, R. A., and Mason, J. W.: Determinants of survival in patients with ventricular tachycardia. N. Engl. J. Med. *308*:1436, 1983.
443. Mirowski, M., Reid, P. R., Winkle, R. A., Mower, M. M., Watkins, L., Stinson, G. B., Griffith, L. S. C., Kallman, C. H., and Weisfeldt, M. L.: Mortality in patients with implanted automatic defibrillators. Ann. Intern. Med. *98*:585, 1983.
444. Echt, D. S., Armstrong, K., Schmidt, P., Oyer, P. E., Stinson, E. B., and Winkle, R. A.: Clinical experience, complications, and survival in 70 patients with the automatic implantable cardioverter/defibrillator. Circulation *71*:289, 1985.
445. Wellens, H. J. J., Brugada, P., and Stevenson, W. G.: Programmed electrical stimulation of the heart in patients with life-threatening ventricular arrhythmias: What is the significance of induced arrhythmias and what is the correct stimulation protocol? Circulation 72:1, 1985.
446. Myerburg, R. J., and Zaman, L.: Discussion of indications for intracardiac electrophysiologic studies in survivors of prehospital cardiac arrest. Circulation (Suppl) (*in press*).
447. Josephson, M. E., Harken, A. H., and Horowitz, L. N.: Endocardial excision: A new surgical technique for the treatment of recurrent ventricular tachycardia. Circulation *60*:1430, 1979.
448. Guiradon, G., Fontaine, G., Frank, R., Escarde, G., and Etievant, P.: Encircling endocardial ventriculotomy: A new surgical treatment for life-threatening ventricular tachycardias resistant to medical treatment following myocardial infarction. Ann. Thorac. Surg. *26*:438, 1978.
449. Mirowski, M., Reid, P. R., Mower, M. M., Watkins, L., Gott, V. L., Schauble, J. F., Langer, A., Heilman, M. S., Kolenik, S. A., Fischell, R. E., and Weisfeldt, M. L.: Termination of malignant ventricular arrhythmias with an implanted automatic defibrillator in human beings. N. Engl. J. Med. *303*:322, 1980.
450. Myerburg, R. J., and Kessler, K. M.: Management of patients who survive cardiac arrest. Mod. Concepts Cardiovasc. Dis. *55*:61, 1986.
450a. Kim, S. O., Seiden, S. W., Felder, S. D., Waspe, L. E., and Fisher, J. D.: Is programmed stimulation of value in predicting the long-term success of antiarrhythmic therapy for ventricular tachycardia? N. Engl. J. Med. *315*:356, 1986.
451. Myerburg, R. J., and Davis, J. H.: The medical ecology of public safety. I. Sudden death due to coronary heart disease. Am. Heart J. *68*:586, 1964.
452. Levy, R. L., De La Chapelle, C. E., and Richards, D. W.: Heart disease in drivers of public motor vehicles as a cause of highway accidents. J.A.M.A. *184*:143, 1963.
453. Waller, J. A.: Cardiovascular disease, aging, and traffic accidents. J. Chron. Dis. *20*:615, 1967.
454. Peterson, B. J., and Petty, C. S.: Sudden natural death among automobile drivers. J. Forensic Sci. *7*:274, 1962.
455. Baker, S. P., and Spitz, W. U.: An evaluation of the hazard created by natural death at the wheel. N. Engl. J. Med. *283*:405, 1970.
456. Kerwin, A. J.: Sudden death while driving. Can. Med. Assoc. J. *131*:312, 1984.

25 HIGH–CARDIAC OUTPUT STATES

by WILLIAM GROSSMAN, M.D., and
EUGENE BRAUNWALD, M.D.

METABOLIC DETERMINANTS OF CARDIAC OUTPUT

Discussion of high–cardiac output states should begin with a definition of normal cardiac output and a brief review of the factors that determine cardiac output. The quantity of blood delivered to the systemic circulation per unit of time is termed the *cardiac output*, generally expressed in liters per minute. For a normal adult weighing 70 kg, resting cardiac output is approximately 6.25 liters/min.[1] Since the total volume of blood contained in the vascular system is approximately 75 ml/kg body weight in normal subjects,[2] or 5.2 liters in a 70-kg man, it is apparent that the total blood volume is moved around the circulation in a little less than 1 minute. Transient but substantial increases in cardiac output normally occur in response to changing metabolic demands, such as with exercise. However, a sustained increase in cardiac output—the subject of this chapter—is distinctly abnormal and contributes significantly to the symptoms and clinical presentation of several disease states.

The blood pumped by the heart delivers oxygen and a variety of substrates to the metabolizing tissues and removes carbon dioxide and other products of metabolism. In addition, blood transfers the heat generated by metabolic activity from the internal organs to the cutaneous bed, where it is dissipated. Derangement of any of the homeostatic mechanisms by which these functions are regulated can result in sustained deviations of the cardiac output (either increases or decreases) from its normal value.

OXYGEN REQUIREMENTS OF THE TISSUES

The average normal adult consumes approximately 110 to 150 (mean, 128) ml/sq meter of oxygen each minute, delivered by the blood to metabolically active tissues. If arterial blood normally contains 190 ml O_2/liter (95 per cent saturation if oxygen-carrying capacity equals 200 ml O_2/liter), and if cardiac output equals 3.2 liters/min/sq meter, then by Fick's principle (p. 252) the mixed venous blood returning from metabolically active tissue will have an oxygen content of approximately 150 ml/liter, i.e., an oxygen saturation of 75 per cent. The arteriovenous oxygen difference of 40 ml/liter represents the average normal extraction of oxygen by the body's tissues in the basal state. This average extraction represents a heterogeneity of metabolic activities, with skin, kidney, and skeletal muscle extracting relatively little oxygen in the basal state, whereas the heart extracts approximately 120 ml O_2/liter at rest.

As tissue metabolism increases, the arteriovenous oxygen difference rises and if cardiac output remains constant is limited by a factor termed the *extraction reserve*. The normal extraction reserve for oxygen is 3, which means that given the augmented metabolic demand, the tissues can extract three times the normal quantity of oxygen, i.e., 3×40 ml O_2/liter $=$ 120 ml O_2/liter.[3] Thus, if arterial saturation remains constant at 95 per cent, full utilization of the extraction reserve results in a mixed venous oxygen content of 70 ml/liter (190 − 120 ml/liter), or 35 per cent saturation, which corresponds to the pulmonary arterial oxygen saturation found in normal subjects studied at maximal exercise.

It is of interest that this value of 3 for the extraction reserve of oxygen predicts that in progressive cardiac decompensation, in order to meet the basal oxygen requirements of the body, oxygen extraction will increase until the arteriovenous oxygen difference has tripled, i.e., until the limit of extraction reserve has been reached and cardiac output has fallen to one-third its normal value. Further reduction of cardiac output results in systemic hypoxia, anaerobic metabolism, metabolic acidosis, and, eventually, circulatory collapse. It has been repeatedly observed that a persistent fall in resting cardiac output to below one-third of normal resting values is incompatible with life. However, long before the cardiac output has declined to this low level, the heart will be unable to meet the augmented requirements of the metabolizing tissues during activity or in resting patients with a hyperkinetic state, such as pregnancy or hyperthyroidism.

MECHANISMS FOR INCREASED CARDIAC OUTPUT. Under basal or near-basal conditions in the intact subject, most changes in cardiac output can be accounted for by changes in the capacity of the peripheral vascular bed to return blood to the heart, which, in turn, causes alterations in the preload. Conditions that lower peripheral vascular resistance are among the most important factors augmenting the venous return and therefore elevating cardiac output. These include anemia, arteriovenous fistulas, beriberi, thyrotoxicosis, pregnancy, and Paget's disease. A reduction in vascular resistance also occurs in (1) muscular exercise, in which dilatation occurs in the arterioles supplying the exercising muscles; (2) fever, in which there is reduced vascular resistance as a consequence of dilated cutaneous vessels; and (3) severe anoxia, in which generalized vascular dilatation also often occurs. These reductions in vascular resistance increase cardiac output not only by lowering ventricular afterload, but also by reducing the impedance to venous return, thus tending to increase ventricular preload.

Guyton has properly emphasized the significance of venous return in the regulation of cardiac output.[3] He has pointed out that the ratio of blood volume to capacitance of the systemic circulation determines the level of peripheral venous pressure and that this ratio is a prime determinant of the venous pressure gradient (i.e., the pressure difference between the small veins and the right atrium), which is closely related to the force that returns blood to the heart. According to this formulation, an augmentation of blood volume or reduction of venous capacitance will raise this gradient, augment venous return, and, in the presence of normal cardiac function, increase cardiac output.

As pointed out in Chapter 14, cardiac output depends on the interactions of intrinsic myocardial contractility with the prevailing conditions of myocardial loading. Figure 25–1 describes this interaction in terms of the resting and active left ventricular pressure-volume relationships; the same physiological control mechanisms are operative for the right ventricle. According to this formulation,[4–6] ACDE represents the control cardiac cycle (Fig. 25–1). End-diastolic pressure and volume are indicated by point A, isovolumetric contraction by line ABC, ejection by line CD, isovolumetric relaxation by line DE, and diastolic filling by segment EA. This type of construction is based on the concept that at constant contractility, ventricular pressure and volume at end systole (point D) always return to the active pressure-volume relationship (upper curve) (Fig. 13–29, p. 407). When ventricular *afterload* is decreased, as occurs with the reduction of systemic or pulmonary vascular resistance or a decline in blood viscosity (characteristic of most of the conditions discussed in this chapter[7]), the resultant cardiac cycle is denoted by ABFG, which has a considerably larger stroke volume (SV_Y) than the control stroke volume for cycle ABCDE (SV_X). If ventricular *preload* now rises, as occurs with an arteriovenous fistula and many of the other conditions to be discussed, the resultant cardiac cycle would be denoted by HIFG, with stroke volume SV_Z rising further still. Thus, the reduction of afterload and increase in preload act in concert to augment stroke volume, in some instances quite strikingly. With no change in heart rate, these changes in afterload and preload will be translated into an increase in cardiac output.

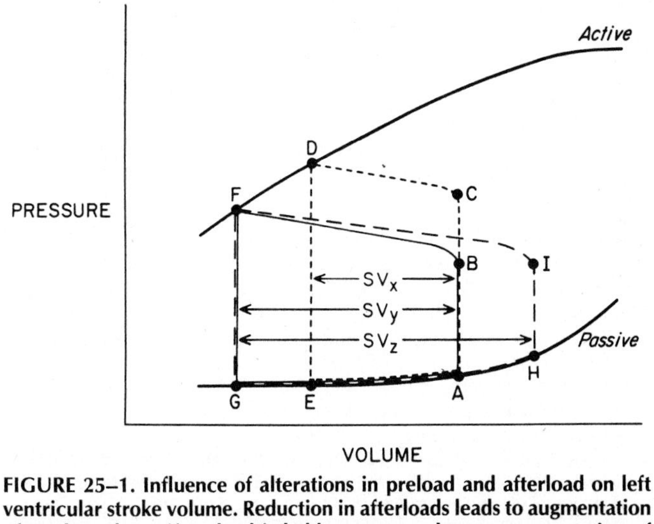

FIGURE 25–1. Influence of alterations in preload and afterload on left ventricular stroke volume. Reduction in afterloads leads to augmentation of stroke volume if preload is held constant, whereas augmentation of preload increases stroke volume if afterload is constant. In most conditions associated with a high–cardiac output state, both afterload reduction and preload augmentation are present. The control cardiac cycle is inscribed by points ABCDE; pure afterload reduction leads to cycle ABFG; a cycle demonstrating both afterload reduction and preload augmentation is indicated by HIFG. SV_X represents the stroke volume of the control cycle, SV_Y the augmented stroke volume effected by afterload reduction alone, and SV_Z the stroke volume with combined afterload reduction and preload augmentation, as might be seen with an arteriovenous fistula.

Left ventricular afterload is influenced by a number of variables, including the tone of the systemic arterioles, the elasticity of the aorta and large arteries, the viscosity of the blood, the obstruction to left ventricular outflow, and the size and thickness of the left ventricle (Chap. 15). Left ventricular preload is a function of the condition of the mitral valve, compliance of the left ventricle, blood volume, venous tone, and strength and timing of left atrial contraction. Most important, it is a function of the venous return to the left atrium; this in turn is determined by the pressure gradient responsible for the return of blood from the systemic veins to the right atrium and by the function of the right side of the heart as well as the pulmonary vascular resistance. When the latter two parameters are normal, the venous return pressure gradient becomes the principal determinant of left ventricular preload.

Increases in *contractility*, not illustrated in Figure 25–1, shift the active pressure-volume relationship curve upward and to the left, so that at any given preload and afterload left ventricular ejection would proceed to a smaller end-systolic volume, thereby delivering a larger stroke volume. *Tachycardia* is also an important mechanism for increasing cardiac output, because the minute cardiac output is the product of stroke volume and heart rate.

HEAT DISSIPATION AND CONSERVATION

Body temperature and its regulation are important determinants of cardiac output. Hypothermia lowers cardiac output and hyperthermia raises it in an exponential relationship. Temperature elevation raises cardiac output by means of two distinct mechanisms: (1) Cellular metabolism, and therefore oxygen consumption, and the production of vasodilator metabolites are a function of body temperature. With increased oxygen consumption and production of vasodilator metabolites, cardiac output rises as a consequence of reduced afterload and increased venous return, as described above. (2) Cutaneous blood flow is the principal means available to the body for temperature regulation. When total body metabolism is augmented or body temperature rises or both, marked increases in cutaneous blood flow to dissipate heat may be sufficient to increase total cardiac output substantially. The importance of this mechanism is evident in patients with the common forms of low-output congestive heart failure who are unable to increase cardiac output, cannot augment cutaneous blood flow, and therefore exhibit considerable difficulty with heat dissipation.

Substantial increases in cardiac output normally occur in response to increased environmental heat and humidity. Burch and associates reported that in the humid tropical summer weather of New Orleans, measurements of cardiac output were 57 per cent greater than in an air-conditioned ward.[8] Because oxygen consumption was higher in the hot, humid environment, it was not possible to determine whether the increased output was simply a response to increased metabolic demand. However, the arterial–mixed venous oxygen difference either remained unchanged or fell, suggesting that the rise in cardiac output exceeded the oxygen requirement and reflected the body's attempt to increase the effectiveness of heat dissipation. Systemic arteriolar resistance falls in a hot and humid environment,[8] presumably reflecting dilatation of the cutaneous bed, and the resultant reduction in ventricular afterload and augmentation of venous return may be an important mechanism in mediating cardiac output.

MYOCARDIAL RESPONSE TO SUSTAINED INCREASES IN CARDIAC OUTPUT

Just as the normal heart can increase its activity to meet the augmented peripheral demands imposed by muscular exertion, so can it tolerate the sustained higher demands imposed by hypermetabolic states (e.g., fever, pregnancy, and hyperthyroidism) and hyperkinetic, nonhypermetabolic conditions (e.g., anemia, arteriovenous fistula, and beriberi) in which reduction of afterload and augmentation of venous return and preload lead to a sustained increase in flow load. Relying on hypertrophy and dilatation as its principal long-term compensatory mechanisms, the heart can maintain normal tissue oxygenation and normal ventricular filling pressures for many years. On the other hand, when imposed on a heart whose function is intrinsically impaired, these increased demands either cannot be met or can be met only by using compensatory mechanisms to the point that the physiological and clinical manifestations of heart failure appear.

Obviously there are exceptions to these basic principles: (1) Extreme anemia (hematocrit <15 per cent), (2) the combination of severe anemia (hematocrit = 15 to 20 per cent) and arteriovenous fistula, as occurs in patients with renal failure with placement of an external shunt for hemodialysis (p. 1839), and (3) the rapid development of severe hyperthyroidism (e.g., thyroid storm) or a large arteriovenous fistula (e.g., aortocaval) may overwhelm even a normal heart and result in heart failure.

Adaptation of the heart to an abnormal burden depends not only on the baseline state of myocardial function and on the magnitude of the additional circulatory burden imposed but also on the *rate* at which the new burden is added. Thus, severe anemia, thyrotoxicosis, or an arteriovenous fistula is far more likely to lead to cardiac decompensation when it develops suddenly rather than slowly. For this reason, conditions such as Paget's disease and Albright's syndrome, in which volume overload develops slowly, seldom, if ever, cause heart failure.

HIGH-OUTPUT HEART FAILURE

DEFINITIONS. The definition of heart failure (p. 426) will be reviewed here in order to explain more fully the special circumstance of high-output failure. Heart failure may be said to exist when the heart *fails* to perform its primary functions, which include both diastolic and systolic components. The former (diastolic) consists of receiving deoxygenated blood at low pressure (<8 mm Hg) from the systemic veins into the right atrium and ventricle and of receiving oxygenated blood at low pressure (<10 mm Hg) from the pulmonary veins into the left atrium and ventricle. The latter (systolic) involves the propelling of blood into the pulmonary artery and aorta at appropriate pressures and in a quantity sufficient to meet the metabolic needs of the body. From a physiological point of view, the diastolic or recipient functions of the heart are as essential as its systolic or contractile functions. Diastolic heart failure may occur in a variety of conditions (e.g., constrictive pericarditis, mitral stenosis, restrictive cardiomyopathy, acute aortic or mitral regurgitation, hypertrophic cardiomyopathy) in which myocardial contractility and the end-systolic pressure-volume relation (Fig. 25–1) are normal, but left and/or right heart filling pressures are increased and cause signs and symptoms of congestive failure.

PHYSIOLOGICAL CONSIDERATIONS. In high-output states, the venous return is substantially increased. If this increase occurs suddenly, an acute volume overload of left and right heart chambers ensues. The resultant acute increase in ventricular preload or end-diastolic volume (Fig. 25–1*A* through *H*) is associated with higher ventricular diastolic pressures, and if this rise in filling pressure is of sufficient magnitude, symptoms of congestive heart failure will occur even though myocardial contractile function is normal. Eccentric or volume overload hypertrophy develops in response to a sustained increase in ventricular end-diastolic wall stress (Fig. 14–8, p. 432). This pattern of ventricular hypertrophy is characterized by addition of new sarcomeres in series, lengthening of the myocardial fibers that compose the ventricular walls, and an increase in *ventricular diastolic capacity*. With this adaptation, the higher venous return can be accommodated in the enlarged ventricle without any increase in diastolic pressure, and symptoms of congestive heart failure are absent. *Tachycardia* is an acute mechanism for blunting the rise in ventricular diastolic pressure associated with sudden onset of a high–cardiac output state. For example, if the cardiac output (and hence the venous return per minute) rises abruptly from 6 to 12 liters/min, as might occur with the sudden development of a large arteriovenous fistula, a rise in heart rate from 60 to 120 beats/min will keep the venous return *per beat* unchanged. With development of volume overload hypertrophy, the tachycardia will gradually diminish.

Although volume overload hypertrophy will often permit adequate cardiac function in patients with a sustained high-output state, myocardial dysfunction may develop gradually, so that the hypertrophied myocardium exhibits depressed contractility. Myocardial failure in such patients may manifest itself as *high-output heart failure*, since the cardiac output tends to remain elevated above normal in such patients (albeit lower than before development of the high output failure state). This development of myocardial contractile dysfunction is similar to what is observed in patients with chronic, severe valvular regurgitation (e.g., aortic or mitral regurgitation) or with a large patent ductus arteriosus.

In addition to myocardial contractile dysfunction developing gradually in response to the sustained volume overload of a high-output state, thyrotoxicosis and beriberi may impair myocardial metabolism directly, and severe anemia may interfere with myocardial function by producing myocardial hypoxia, as discussed below.

High-output heart failure often results when a patient with preexisting heart disease and limited cardiac reserve has the need for a sustained increase in cardiac output, as in the development of anemia, thyrotoxicosis, or pregnancy. Patients with a mild cardiomyopathy or prior myocardial infarction may develop high ventricular filling pressures when cardiac output doubles.

DIFFERENTIATION BETWEEN HIGH- AND LOW-OUTPUT HEART FAILURE. Sometimes it is difficult to distinguish between low-output and high-output heart failure. The normal range of cardiac output in the basal state is wide (2.6 to 4.0 liters/min/sq meter), and in many patients with so-called low-output heart failure, the cardiac output *at rest* may be within normal limits. On the other hand, in patients with high-output failure, cardiac output may not be excessive, but rather may be close to the upper limit of normal, particularly when heart failure is severe.

In the usual forms of low-output heart failure, the characteristically inadequate delivery of oxygen to the metabolizing tissues is reflected in an abnormally widened arterial–mixed venous oxygen difference (Chap. 15). In mild cases, this abnormality may become evident only during the stress of increased activity. In patients with high-output heart failure, the arterial–mixed venous oxygen difference is usually normal or may even be abnormally low, as in arteriovenous fistula, because the mixed venous oxygen saturation is raised by the admixture of blood that has been shunted away from some of the metabolizing tissues. In such cases delivery of oxygen to these tissues is reduced, despite the low arterial–mixed venous oxygen difference. When heart failure occurs in patients with high cardiac output, the arterial–mixed venous oxygen difference still exceeds the level that existed after the level of cardiac output rose but *before* the development of heart failure, and therefore the cardiac output, as stated above, although high in the normal range or elevated, is nonetheless lower than it was before heart failure developed.

CONDITIONS ASSOCIATED WITH SUSTAINED INCREASES IN CARDIAC OUTPUT

ANEMIA

PHYSIOLOGICAL MECHANISMS. Anemia is most commonly responsible for a sustained increase in cardiac output, which occurs consistently when the hematocrit falls below 25 per cent. However, when the anemia is associated with a condition that produces a marked rise in blood viscosity (which increases afterload), such as multiple myeloma or macroglobulinemia, cardiac output may fail to rise even in the absence of heart disease. A number of studies have supported a role for the lowered viscosity of blood in the high cardiac output of anemia.[7] In addition, it has been found that when exchange transfusions were carried out in dogs with methemoglobinemia using blood in which viscosity was unaltered, cardiac output remained unchanged.[9] However, when a reduction of oxygen-carrying capacity similar to that in methemoglobinemia was produced by an exchange transfusion with low-viscosity dextran, cardiac output rose. In an important experiment the effects of acute anemia produced in dogs by exchange transfusion with low-molecular-weight (70,000 daltons) or high-molecular-weight (500,000 daltons) dextran were compared.[10] The former produced a 93 per cent increase in cardiac output and the latter only a 43 per cent increase. Because the severity of the anemia was the same in both groups (hematocrit = 18 per cent), they concluded that the difference in cardiac output probably reflected the substantial differences in viscosity. Because an increase in cardiac output still occurred in the dogs with normal blood viscosity who received high-molecular-weight dextran, it is clear that lowered viscosity, although important, cannot be the sole cause of increased cardiac output. The reduced left ventricular afterload in anemia results from a reduction not only in blood viscosity, but in systemic arteriolar tone as well. The mechanism responsible for the latter change is unclear, but local tissue hypoxia, lactic acidemia, and the accumulation of vasodilator metabolites such as adenosine and possibly of bradykinin may all play a role.

To investigate the adjustment of the peripheral circulation to severe anemia, anemia was induced in conscious dogs by progressive phlebotomy and volume replacement over a period of 2 to 4 weeks.[11] At a hematocrit of 22 per cent, heart rate was elevated and resistance to flow in the coronary and iliac beds was strikingly reduced, whereas resistance in the mesenteric and the renal beds remained essentially constant. In the presence of severer anemia (hematocrit = 14 per cent), resistance in the mesenteric and the renal beds also declined. During exercise, both coronary and iliac blood flow rose further, but in contrast to nonanemic dogs, in which the mesenteric and the renal flow remained constant during exercise, both the mesenteric and the renal blood flow fell markedly (Fig. 25–2). Thus in resting, conscious dogs, reduction in visceral flow is *not* a feature of the cardiovascular response to severe anemia, although some redistribution of blood flow does occur; however, the added stress of exercise during severe anemia results in substantial reductions in flow in at least the mesenteric and the renal vascular beds.

There is evidence that the autonomic nervous system plays a key role in the circulatory adaptation to anemia.

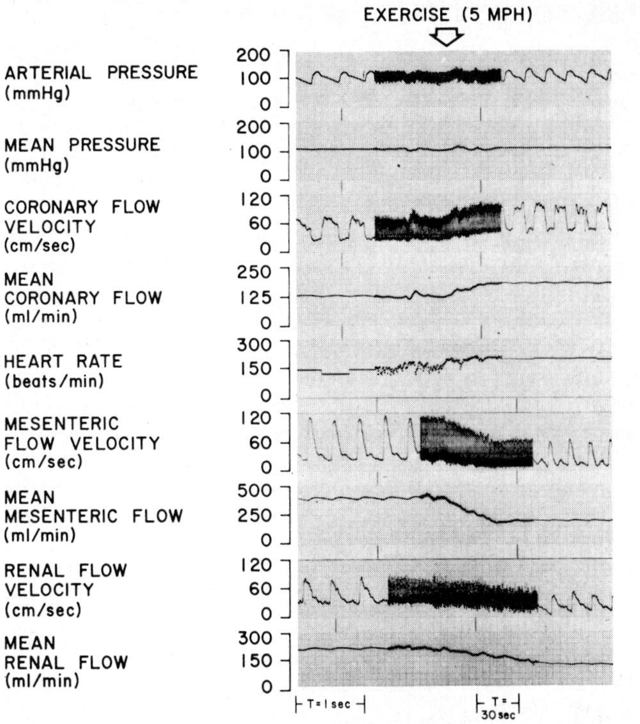

FIGURE 25–2. Response of an anemic dog to exercise. Phasic and mean arterial pressures and phasic and mean blood flows in the coronary, mesenteric, and renal beds are shown along with heart rate. In each case regional flow was initially recorded simultaneously with arterial pressure. (From Vatner, S. F., et al.: Regional circulatory adjustments to moderate and severe chronic anemia in conscious dogs at rest and during exercise. Circ. Res. *30*:731, 1972, by permission of the American Heart Association, Inc.)

The responses to severe isovolemic anemia in intact dogs were compared with those in dogs subjected to chronic cardiac denervation. The elevation of cardiac output was significantly greater in the intact animals than in the denervated ones. In intact dogs the increase in cardiac output stemmed predominantly from a rise in heart rate, whereas elevations in stroke volume played a less important role. In contrast, in the cardiac-denervated dogs, the increase in cardiac output tended to result from an augmented stroke volume.[12] In this connection the finding that tissue hypoxia can lead to an autonomic reflex response resulting in reduced arteriolar resistance is of considerable interest.[13] Thus, it may be concluded that an intact autonomic nervous system is necessary for mediation of a portion of the normal circulatory response to acutely induced anemia.

In a study of patients with chronic anemia (iron deficiency or megaloblastic), it was found that with corrective treatment, the cardiac index fell to normal (from 4.7 to 3.4 liters/min/sq meter), heart rate decreased (from 83 to 70 beats/min), and systemic vascular resistance rose (from 1017 to 1526 dynes-sec-cm^{-5}).[14] These changes could be reproduced acutely while the subjects were still anemic by infusion of methoxamine or assumption of the upright posture, suggesting that a combination of vasodilatation and a redistribution of blood volume might be responsible for mediating the hyperkinetic circulatory response to chronic anemia.

Clinical Findings

The consequences of anemia depend, to an important extent, on its rate of development. When it occurs rapidly, as in hemorrhage, blood volume is not maintained, and the picture of hypovolemic shock predominates (Chap. 19). If anemia develops more slowly, so that blood volume is maintained, cardiac output rises—predominantly as a result of tachycardia—with little change in stroke volume. In chronic severe anemia, heart rate is usually normal or only minimally elevated, and cardiac output is therefore elevated principally as a consequence of augmented stroke volume; the latter is associated with cardiac dilatation and hypertrophy. Not only is the cardiac output elevated at rest, but the augmentation of output during exercise tends to be excessive, often exceeding 1000 ml/100 ml increase in oxygen consumption per minute (normal = 550 to 800 ml).[15] Sometimes this excessive response is seen in patients with only mild anemia (hematocrit = 30 per cent) who have normal resting cardiac outputs.[16] Because cardiac output is elevated while pulmonary artery pressure is normal, calculated pulmonary vascular resistance (like calculated systemic vascular resistance) is often reduced, and this variable declines further during exercise.[17] Left ventricular end-diastolic pressure remains within normal limits even in severe anemia, unless heart failure supervenes.[18]

The effect of *acute* anemia on cardiac function was studied in anesthetized dogs in which left ventricular function became depressed when the hematocrit was reduced below 24 per cent.[19] However, the otherwise normal human heart can tolerate moderately severe anemia (hematocrit = 20 to 25 per cent) for many years without showing any impairment of function; when heart failure occurs in patients with this degree of anemia, *it usually signifies the presence of underlying heart disease that had been compensated until the burden of an augmented cardiac output was added.* Similar considerations apply to the development of angina pectoris and other manifestations of myocardial ischemia. However, two important exceptions should be noted: (1) patients with severe anemia (hematocrit ≤ 15 per cent), in whom clinical evidence of impaired cardiac function can exist even in the absence of apparent underlying heart disease; and (2) patients with sickle cell anemia (p. 1736), who do *not* exhibit a reduction of viscosity and therefore lose this hemodynamic benefit imparted by other forms of anemia.[20, 21] Also, in these patients small thrombi characteristically develop in the pulmonary and coronary vessels, thereby impairing both systemic and cardiac oxygenation and leading to pulmonary hypertension, cor pulmonale, and perhaps even myocardial fibrosis secondary to ischemia. In addition, there may be arterial oxygen desaturation secondary to pulmonary venous-arterial shunting. Such patients exhibit hyperventilation, an increased alveolar-arterial oxygen tension gradient, abnormal ventilation of the dead space during exercise, and a disturbance of pulmonary perfusion with venous-arterial shunting. The most likely basis for these changes is the sickling phenomenon within the pulmonary vascular bed.[22] Arterial hypoxemia, produced by the pulmonary shunt, probably accounts for some of the exercise hyperpnea, partly by increasing chemoreceptor drive and by augmenting lactic acidemia.[23]

HISTORY. Chronic anemia produces surprisingly few symptoms, which may consist of easy fatigability, mild exertional dyspnea, and occasionally palpitations and cardiac awareness (p. 788). If heart failure or angina pectoris is present, it is likely that the high cardiac output is superimposed on some specific cardiac abnormality, such as valvular stenosis or regurgitation, or coronary artery disease. Patients with sickle cell anemia and hemoglobin sickle cell (SC) disease may complain of chest pain and unexplained dyspnea owing to in situ pulmonary thrombosis and infarction.[22]

PHYSICAL EXAMINATION. The anemic patient generally has a pale "pasty" appearance; in black, brown, or tanned persons in whom examination of the skin color is of little help, the finding of paleness of the conjunctivae, mucous membranes, and palmar creases is helpful. Arterial pulses are bounding, "pistol shot" sounds can be heard over the femoral arteries (Duroziez's sign), and subungual capillary pulsations (Quincke's pulse) are present as in patients with aortic regurgitation. A medium-pitched, midsystolic murmur along the left sternal border, generally Grade 1/6 to 3/6 in intensity (seldom accompanied by a thrill), is common. Heart sounds are accentuated, and the pulmonic component of the second heart sound may be particularly prominent in patients with sickle cell anemia and pulmonary hypertension; in such patients a right ventricular lift can usually be palpated. Elevation of the cardiac output and the physical findings characteristic of anemia are present in patients with sickle cell anemia and hemoglobin SC disease at *higher* hemoglobin levels than in patients with other forms of anemia.[18] A middiastolic flow murmur secondary to augmented blood flow across the mitral valve orifice, holosystolic murmurs resulting from tricuspid and mitral regurgitation secondary to ventricular dilatation, and rarely diastolic murmurs resulting from aortic and pulmonic valve incompetence secondary to dilatation of these vessels may be heard. Occasionally a third heart sound is audible at the cardiac apex. Jugular venous distention is uncommon, and although peripheral edema and hepatomegaly are occasionally present, they may be due not only to heart failure, but also to accompanying abnormalities such as hypoproteinemia and nutritional deficiency.

Laboratory findings in patients with severe anemia usually include mild to moderate cardiomegaly on chest roentgenogram. The electrocardiogram usually does not show any specific changes, but may show T-wave inversions in lateral precordial leads. The echocardiogram generally shows a modest and symmetrical increase in size of all chambers, with large systolic excursions of the septal and posterior left ventricular walls and a normal ejection fraction. Hematological and blood chemical findings reflect the specific type of anemia present.

MANAGEMENT. Treatment of heart failure associated with severe anemia should be specific for the anemia (e.g., iron, folate, vitamin B_{12}, and so forth). When congestive heart failure is present, diuretics and cardiac glycosides are advisable, although some clinicians believe that the latter drugs are not helpful in this condition. Because many patients with heart failure and anemia have significant underlying heart disease, the administration of glycosides may be desirable, particularly if there is evidence for depressed myocardial contractility.

When both heart failure and anemia are severe, treatment must be carried out on an urgent basis and presents a difficult challenge. On the one hand, correction of the anemia is desirable to increase oxygen delivery to metabolizing tissues and thereby decrease the need for a sustained high cardiac output. On the other hand, a too-rapid expansion of the blood volume could intensify the manifestations of heart failure, and an increase in hematocrit will potentially depress cardiac output because of increased blood viscosity. The diagnostic steps for determining the etiology of the anemia should be taken immediately (e.g., blood drawn for serum iron, folate, and vitamin B_{12} measurements). The patient should be placed at bed rest and given supplementary oxygen. *Packed red blood cells* should then be transfused slowly (250 to 500 ml/24 hr), preceded or accompanied by vigorous diuretic therapy (e.g., furosemide, 20 to 40 mg IV immediately followed by 40 mg orally every 8 hours), and the patient should be observed *closely* for the development or exacerbation of dyspnea and pulmonary rales, so that the transfusion can be discontinued immediately to avoid precipitating pulmonary edema. Vasodilator therapy is seldom helpful, since impedance to left ventricular emptying is already markedly reduced in most cases.

HYPERTHYROIDISM (See also p. 1805)

PHYSIOLOGICAL MECHANISMS. Substantial increases in cardiac output commonly occur in hyperthyroidism, and cardiac indexes of 5 to 7 liters/min/sq meter are common,[24] generally resulting from increases in both stroke volume and heart rate. At least five mechanisms have been thought to contribute to this high-output state:

1. Augmented metabolic rate that causes vasodilation as seen with muscular exercise. It has been well documented that systemic vascular resistance is decreased in hyperthyroidism.[24]

2. Increased heat production consequent to the augmented metabolism characteristic of hyperthyroidism results in elevation of cardiac output owing to cutaneous dilatation. This latter mechanism is particularly important in patients with thyroid storm, in whom hyperthermia—with temperatures occasionally as high as 106° F (41° C)—is associated with an intense cardiac drive to maintain an elevated cardiac output, occasionally resulting in high-output failure and circulatory collapse.

3. Despite the foregoing, Goldman and associates[25] showed that the high-output state associated with thyrotoxicosis is not solely dependent on a low systemic vascular resistance. These investigators produced thyrotoxicosis in calves and administered phenylephrine to increase systemic vascular resistance back to euthyroid levels; despite this elimination of systemic vasodilatation, cardiac output remained markedly elevated. The high-output state appeared to be primarily due to increases in blood volume, in mean circulatory filling pressure, and in the pressure gradient for venous return.

4. Thyroid hormone has a direct, stimulating effect on myocardial contractility,[27–30] which augments stroke volume at any preload and afterload. This effect has been clearly documented in animal experiments[27, 29, 30] as well as in humans[28, 31] and may involve a fundamental alteration in myocardial contractile proteins, such as increased activity of myosin ATPase,[32–34] or in the function of the sarcoplasmic reticulum.[35]

5. There is still an undefined relationship between the hyperthyroid state and the sympathoadrenal system, characterized by suppression of the manifestations of the hyperthyroid state by administration of antiadrenergic agents. Beta-adrenoceptor stimulation potentiates certain biochemical changes induced at the cell membrane level by triiodothyronine.[36] The tachycardia, widened pulse pressure, and shortened circulation time all return toward normal with beta-receptor blockade,[26, 37] indicating that adrenergic influences play a role in maintaining the high-output state in hyperthyroid patients. However, the tachycardia of thyrotoxicosis is due not only to the *direct* effects of thyroid hormone and adrenergic influences on the sinoatrial node but also to a reduction in the cholinergic restraint. This does not appear to result from decreased responsiveness of the end organ or impaired release of the cholinergic nerve transmitter, but from a reduction in cholinergic discharge in the thyrotoxic state, which may result from an abnormality in central or afferent mechanisms.[38]

CLINICAL FINDINGS. Symptoms may include nervousness, diaphoresis, heat intolerance, personality disorder, fatigue, and weight loss despite increased appetite. Palpitations are common, and atrial fibrillation is occasionally the presenting manifestation. Symptoms of congestive heart failure are uncommon and, as discussed below, suggest underlying cardiac disease of a different nature.

The principal *physical findings* of hyperthyroidism include tremor; widened palpebral fissures with resultant "stare"; lid lag; exophthalmos; warm, moist, smooth skin; and hyperactive deep tendon reflexes. *Cardiovascular examination* often reveals tachycardia, a widened pulse pressure, and brisk carotid and peripheral arterial pulsations. On palpation the cardiac apex is hyperkinetic. The first heart sound is loud, and the third and fourth sounds are occasionally present. A midsystolic murmur along the left sternal border, secondary to increased flow, is common; occasionally this murmur has an unusual scratchy component (the so-called Means-Lerman scratch) thought to be due to the rubbing together of normal pleural and pericardial surfaces as a consequence of hyperkinetic heart action. Rarely, systolic murmurs of mitral and tricuspid regurgitation, presumably secondary to papillary muscle dysfunction, may occur in thyrotoxicosis and disappear with the establishment of the euthyroid state.

Laboratory findings are those of hyperthyroidism and include elevated levels of thyroxine or triiodothyronine, mild normochromic normocytic anemia, occasional relative lymphocytosis, low serum cholesterol levels, and occasional elevation of serum alkaline phosphatase.

The *chest roentgenogram* is usually normal, although the echocardiogram may show increased left ventricular wall thickness and chamber dimensions and a normal or increased ejection fraction and velocity of shortening.[31] Systolic time intervals may show a low value for the ratio of the preejection period to left ventricular ejection time (PEP/LVET ratio), consistent with increased myocardial contractility.

The *electrocardiogram* often shows widespread but nonspecific ST-segment elevation and upward coving, with terminal T-wave inversion in about one-fourth of patients and shortening of the Q-T interval.[38a] ST-segment depression is uncommon in the absence of coronary artery disease. Atrial fibrillation may occur and is often associated with an unusually rapid ventricular response (i.e., 170 to 220 beats/min) as a consequence of the markedly shortened refractory period of the atrioventricular conduction system. There is relative resistance to slowing of the ventricular rate with digitalis.[39] Spontaneous reversion to sinus rhythm is common. Varying degrees of atrioventricular block,[40] presumably secondary to inflammatory changes in the atrioventricular node induced by hyperthyroidism, are occasional manifestations.

The *echocardiogram* demonstrates evidence of increased myocardial contractility and elevated cardiac output. The latter finding may be manifested by a normal or slightly increased left ventricular stroke volume in association with a substantial tachycardia (Fig. 25–3).

TREATMENT. Management of the cardiovascular manifestations of hyperthyroidism depends primarily on treatment of the endocrine abnormality, as outlined in Chap. 55. However, the elevated heart rate, systolic pressure, pulse pressure, and cardiac output, palpitations, and other manifestations of cardiac hyperactivity, as well as tremor, lid lag, hyperreflexia, and widened palpebral fissures can be reduced by administering antiadrenergic agents.[28, 37, 41, 42] The rapid ventricular rate of atrial fibrillation responds particularly well to intravenous propranolol, which may be administered in 1-mg increments every 5 minutes until the ventricular rate is controlled; sometimes sinus rhythm

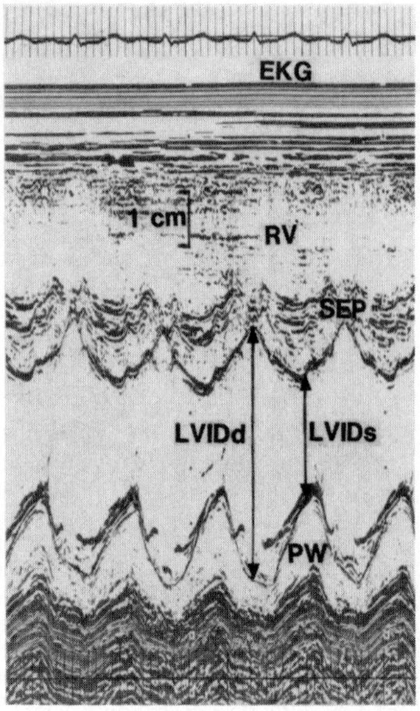

FIGURE 25–3. M-mode echocardiographic study of the left ventricle from a young woman with hyperthyroidism. Left ventricular internal dimension in diastole (LVIDd) is normal at 4.6 cm, while end-systolic dimension (LVIDs) is reduced at 2.25 cm. The percent fractional shortening is increased at 51 per cent (normal greater than 28 to 30 per cent), indicating increased contractility. Heart rate is 128 beats/min. Using standard formulae, stroke volume was estimated to be 80 ml and cardiac output was calculated at 10.2 liters/min. EKG = electrocardiogram; 1 cm = 1 centimeter; RV = right ventricle; SEP = septum; PW = posterior wall. (Courtesy of Patricia Come, M.D., Beth Israel Hospital, Boston, Massachusetts.)

is restored. Oral beta-adrenoceptor blockers in doses ordinarily used in the treatment of chronic stable angina are useful in controlling ventricular rate and other cardiovascular manifestations of hyperthyroidism over longer periods of time, until the euthyroid state is achieved. It must be appreciated, however, that despite the salutary effects of beta-blocking agents, they are only adjunctive measures and do not affect the underlying disease process. Indeed, they do not reduce the elevated metabolic rate.[41] *Thyroid storm* with hyperpyrexia, marked tachycardia, and pulmonary edema also responds to propranolol, 1 to 2 mg administered intravenously as above, together with sodium iodide (to prevent further release of stored thyroid hormones), and adrenal glucocorticoids, cooling blankets, aspirin, and intravenous fluids.[43]

Thyrotoxic Heart Disease

As in many other high-output states, the hyperkinetic state of hyperthyroidism does not usually lead to heart failure or angina pectoris in the absence of underlying cardiac or coronary artery disease; the normal heart appears capable of tolerating the burden imposed by hyperthyroidism simply by means of dilatation and hypertrophy. A rare exception is the development of heart failure in patients with neonatal thyrotoxicosis without underlying heart disease.[44] However, when the elevated flow load of hyperthyroidism is superimposed on a reduced cardiovascular reserve (i.e., asymptomatic or only mildly symptomatic heart disease), congestive heart failure is likely to ensue. Similarly, in patients with obstructive coronary artery disease who are asymptomatic or who have only mild evidence of ischemia in the euthyroid state, the demand for increased coronary blood flow with hyperthyroidism frequently leads to an exacerbation of angina.

Beta-adrenoceptor blockade may be both helpful and harmful in patients with thyrotoxic heart disease and *heart failure*. Although it may be beneficial by lowering the ventricular rate, particularly by prolonging the refractory period of the atrioventricular conduction system in patients with atrial fibrillation, it may also diminish myocardial contractility by blocking the adrenergic support of the heart. Therefore it must be administered cautiously to the patient with thyrotoxic heart disease and heart failure and only after treatment with a digitalis glycoside, with the patient at rest and under careful observation. The initial dose should be small (e.g., propranolol, 0.5 mg IV or 10 mg orally), and the patient should be observed after the administration to be sure that heart failure is not intensified. In contrast to the situation in heart failure, beta-adrenoceptor blockers are particularly useful in the management of angina pectoris associated with hyperthyroidism and coronary artery disease, and in this condition larger doses are usually well tolerated.

The association of thyrotoxicosis and anginal pain has been demonstrated in the presence of normal coronary vessels on arteriography.[45] These patients showed ischemia in that pacing resulted in lactate production. The possibility of thyrotoxicosis should therefore be considered in the differential diagnosis of patients having anginal pain and normal coronary arteriograms (Chap. 39).

It is particularly important to recognize so-called *apathetic hyperthyroidism*, a condition in which the usual clinical manifestations of thyrotoxicosis, such as palpitations, tachycardia, and moist skin, are not present. In such patients the first clinical signs of hyperthyroidism may be unexplained heart failure, an exacerbation of angina pectoris, or unexplained atrial fibrillation, usually but not always with a rapid ventricular rate. Hence it is important to consider the diagnosis of hyperthyroidism in all patients, particularly those over the age of 55 years, who present in this fashion.

SYSTEMIC ARTERIOVENOUS FISTULAS

Systemic arteriovenous fistulas may be congenital or acquired; the latter are either post-traumatic or iatrogenic. Increased cardiac output associated with such fistulas depends on the size of the communication and the magnitude of the resultant reduction in systemic vascular resistance. An increased right atrial pressure does not seem to be necessary to maintain the high-output state, although plasma volume is generally increased.

The *physical findings* depend in part on the underlying disease and the location of the shunt. In general, a widened pulse pressure, brisk carotid and peripheral arterial pulsations, and mild tachycardia are present. *Branham's sign* (also called Nicaladoni-Branham's sign), which consists of slowing of the heart after manual compression of the fistula,[46, 47] is present in the majority of cases; this maneuver also raises arterial and lowers venous pressure. The tachycardia associated with arteriovenous fistula has been studied in an experimental preparation,[48] and the results suggest the operation of a cardioaccelerator reflex with both afferent and efferent pathways in the vagus nerves.

The skin overlying the fistula is warmer than normal, and a continuous "machinery" murmur and thrill are usually present over the lesion. Third and fourth heart sounds are commonly heard, as well as a precordial midsystolic murmur secondary to increased cardiac output. The electrocardiographic changes of left ventricular hypertrophy are often seen. Rarely, the fistula may become infected, leading to bacterial endarteritis.

CONGENITAL ARTERIOVENOUS FISTULAS. Congenital

TABLE 25–1 CONGENITAL ARTERIOVENOUS ANOMALIES

COMMON COMPLAINTS	
Disfigurement	20%
Swelling	19%
Pain	15%
Other (pulsation, ulceration, increased length of limb)	20%
PHYSICAL SIGNS	
Hemangioma, varices, bruit, or swelling, alone or in combination	100%
Color changes	
Erythema	40%
Cyanosis	12%

Adapted from Szilagyi, D. E., et al.: Congenital arteriovenous anomalies of the limbs. Arch. Surg. *111*:423, 1976. Copyright 1976, American Medical Association.

arteriovenous fistulas result from arrest of the normal embryonic development of the vascular system and are structurally similar to embryonic capillary networks. They range from barely noticeable strawberry birthmarks to enormous clusters of engorged vascular channels that may deform an entire extremity. Most frequently, the vessels of the lower extremities are involved (i.e., femoral, iliac, and popliteal), and the resultant clinical manifestations vary enormously.[49] When fistulas are large, patients generally complain of disfigurement as well as of swelling and pain in the limb (Table 25–1). On examination, erythema and cyanosis are usually apparent, as are venous varices, a continuous murmur, and a thrill. Left heart failure occurs, particularly in patients with larger lesions that involve the pelvis as well as the extremities.[50, 51] Physical examination shows hemangiomatous changes associated with venous distention, deformity, and increased limb length. The fistulous connection may involve any vascular bed, including an internal mammary artery–pulmonary artery connection. Angiography is useful in confirming the diagnosis and in determining the physical extent of the anomaly.

Surgical excision is the ideal treatment, but in many instances the lesions are not sufficiently localized to permit this. The results of ligation and excision have been unsatisfactory in the majority of cases, since the congenital arteriovenous communications are usually not confined to a single anatomical segment or to a circumscribed anatomical region. Complete cure of these lesions is possible in only a few instances. Embolization of Gelfoam pellets delivered through a catheter has been reported to obliterate multiple systemic arteriovenous fistulas and thereby diminish high-output heart failure.[52]

Hereditary Hemorrhagic Telangiectasia. Also known as Osler-Weber-Rendu disease, this condition may be associated with arteriovenous fistulas, particularly in the lungs and liver; the latter condition can produce a hyperkinetic circulation,[53, 54] as well as hepatomegaly with abdominal bruits. Because of the presence of oxygenated blood in the inferior vena cava and right atrium, this condition may be misdiagnosed as atrial septal defect.[55]

The congenital arteriovenous communication resulting from *hemangioendothelioma of the liver* is commonly associated with marked increases in cardiac output, sometimes as high as 10.5 liters/min/sq meter, and congestive heart failure.[56, 57] These lesions, which are extremely difficult to treat surgically, may be quite large, increase in size with time, and lead to heart failure even in infancy. They are often associated with sizable cutaneous hemangiomas, which should alert the clinician to the possibility of their presence. Hepatic hemangioendotheliomas have been reported to respond to prednisone in the newborn[56] or to hepatic artery ligation.[58]

ACQUIRED ARTERIOVENOUS FISTULAS. Naturally acquired arteriovenous fistulas occur most frequently after such injuries as gunshot wounds and stab wounds and may involve any part of the body, most frequently the thigh.[59] Blood flow in the affected limb distal to the fistula diminishes after the creation of the fistula but then returns to normal and often increases with the passage of time. As a consequence, the affected limb is usually larger than its opposite member, and the overlying skin is warmer; cellulitis, venostasis, edema, and dermatitis with pigmentation frequently occur, in part as a consequence of chronically elevated venous pressure. Surgical repair or excision is generally advisable in fistulas that develop after gunshot wounds or trauma. An arteriovenous fistula may be produced by inadvertent damage to blood vessels during an operation (most frequently a nephrectomy, laminectomy,[60]

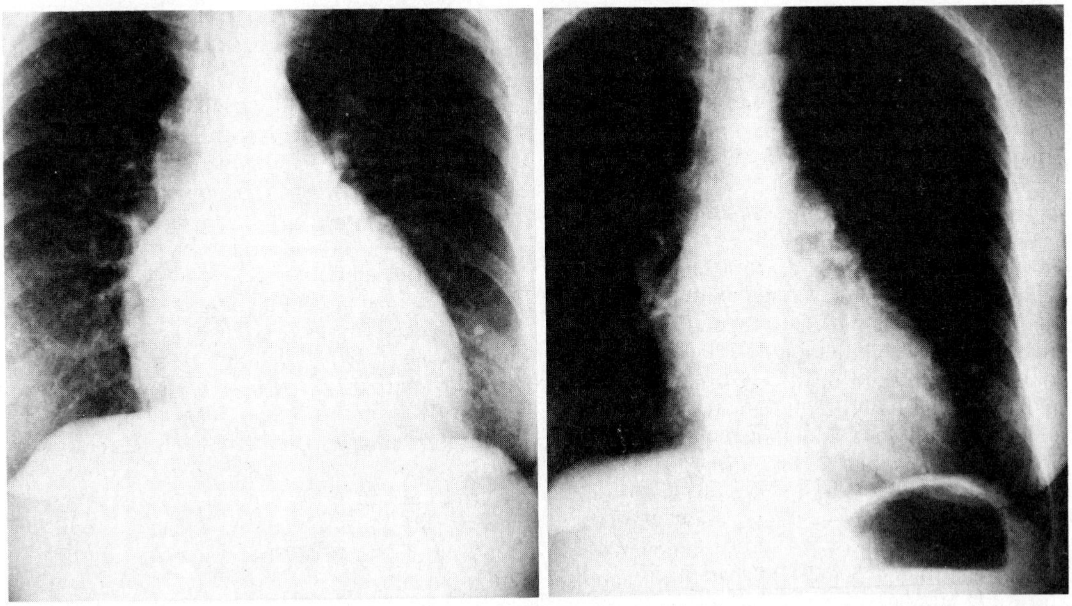

FIGURE 25–4. *Left,* Chest roentgenogram demonstrating cardiomegaly and pulmonary vascular congestion in patient with high-output cardiac failure attributable to end-to-side cephalic vein–radial artery fistula in wrist. *Right,* One month after banding of vein, cardiomegaly has decreased and pulmonary vascular congestion has improved. (From Anderson, C. B., et al.: Cardiac failure and upper extremity arteriovenous dialysis fistulas. Arch. Intern. Med. *136*:292, 1976. Copyright 1976, American Medical Association.)

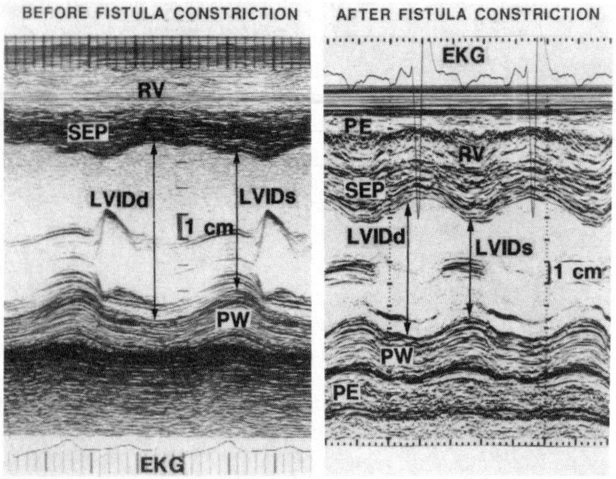

FIGURE 25–5. M-mode echocardiograms of the left ventricle from a 31-year-old woman in heart failure with chronic renal failure and a surgically constructed radial arteriovenous fistula, treated with hemodialysis. The left panel shows that left ventricular internal dimension at end-diastole (LVIDd = 7.0 cm) and at end systole (LVIDs = 5.3 cm) are markedly increased. Also, fractional shortening was reduced. Using standard formulae, cardiac output was estimated to be 9.9 liters/min. Following surgical constriction of the fistula (right panel), echocardiographic study revealed LVIDd and LVIDs of 6.0 cm and 4.5 cm, respectively. Cardiac output was estimated to be 7.2 liters/min. Per cent fractional shortening (26 per cent) and estimated left ventricular ejection fraction (49 per cent) remained slightly depressed, consistent with some underlying myocardial depression. EKG = electrocardiogram; RV = right ventricle; SEP = septum; 1 cm = 1 centimeter; PW = posterior wall; PE = pericardial effusion. (Courtesy of Patricia Come, M.D., Beth Israel Hospital, Boston, Massachusetts.)

or cholecystectomy) or a percutaneous vascular catheterization procedure.

A rare form of acquired arteriovenous fistula results from spontaneous rupture of an aortic aneurysm into the inferior vena cava. This usually produces an enormous arteriovenous shunt and rapidly progressive left ventricular failure. On physical examination a pulsating mass can be readily palpated superficially in the abdomen, and a continuous bruit is audible.

Massive fistulas may be associated with Wilms' tumor of the kidney, and these have, on rare occasions, caused high-output cardiac failure in children.[61]

High-output congestive heart failure resulting from the arteriovenous shunts surgically constructed for vascular access in patients on chronic hemodialysis are not uncommon.[62–65] Cardiac outputs as high as 10 liters/min/sq meter, which decrease substantially during temporary occlusion of the shunt, have been found in such patients. These values undoubtedly also reflect the chronic anemia present in many of these patients, but it is clear that it is the added hemodynamic burden imposed by the shunt that precipitates heart failure in patients who had previously tolerated chronic anemia without apparent impairment of cardiac function. It is usually possible to revise or band the fistula to reduce it to the appropriate size for dialysis without compromising cardiac function (Fig. 25–4).[62] Echocardiography demonstrates fairly dramatic findings in patients with high-output failure in association with a surgically constructed shunt for hemodialysis (Fig. 25–5).

As is the case with other hyperkinetic lesions, the rapidity of the onset of the load and its size, as well as the presence and severity of the underlying heart disease, determine whether or not heart failure will develop.

BERIBERI HEART DISEASE

PATHOGENESIS AND CLINICAL CONSIDERATIONS. This condition is due to severe thiamine deficiency persisting for at least 3 months. Clinical beriberi is found most frequently in the Far East, although even in that part of the world it is far less prevalent now than in the past. It occurs predominantly in those individuals whose staple diet consists of polished rice, which is deficient in thiamine but high in carbohydrates. The presence of thiamine in the enriched flour used in white bread has virtually eradicated this disease in the United States and Western Europe, where beriberi is found most commonly in diet faddists and alcoholics; like polished rice, alcohol is low in vitamin B_1 but has a high carbohydrate content. In the West, alcoholics become thiamine-deficient not only because of a low intake of the vitamin but also because they eat "junk" foods or drink large quantities of beer, with their high carbohydrate content and therefore their great demand for thiamine. A reappearance of beriberi heart disease has been reported in Japan, mainly in teenagers, and has been attributed to the recent tendency for teenagers to ingest excessive amounts of sweet carbonated drinks, instant noodles, and polished rice.[66] Most cases presented in the summer months and were believed to be precipitated by strenuous exertion with a resultant sudden increase in thiamine requirements. All of the patients presented with edema ("wet beriberi") with general malaise and fatigue. Neurological manifestations were uncommon. Hemodynamic findings in those studied before and after treatment with thiamine are presented in Figure 25–6. Since their original description by Wenckebach,[67] the hemodynamic abnormalities associated with beriberi

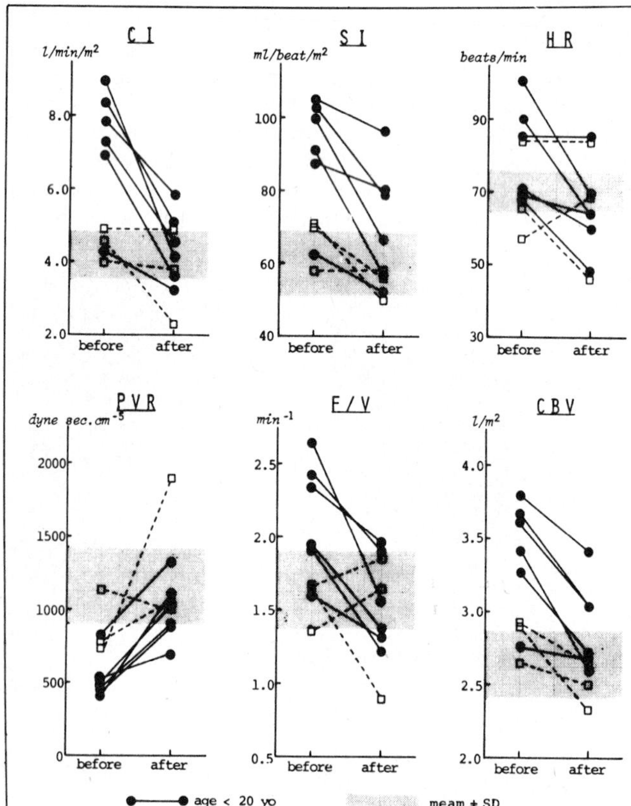

FIGURE 25–6. Changes in cardiac index (CI), stroke index (SI), heart rate (HR), peripheral vascular resistance (PVR), blood turnover rate (F/V), and circulatory blood volume (CBV) in patients treated for beriberi in Kyoto, Japan. (From Kawai, C., et al.: Reappearance of beriberi heart disease in Japan. Am. J. Med. 69:383, 1980.)

heart disease have gained considerable attention.[68–71] The elevation of cardiac output is presumably secondary to the reduced systemic vascular resistance and augmented venous return, and it is suspected that these are caused by lesions of the sympathetic nuclei.

The role of thiamine diphosphate as a coenzyme is well established. In mammals, thiamine diphosphate is required for a variety of reactions that have in common the cleavage of carbon-carbon bonds—the oxidative decarboxylation of alpha-keto acids (pyruvate and alpha-ketoglutarate) and keto analogs of leucine, isoleucine, and valine and the transketolase reaction in the pentose phosphate pathway. Thiamine triphosphate is important in the binding of thiamine diphosphate to its various apoenzymes. The entire spectrum of changes in thiamine deficiency can be explained by the inhibition of these key enzymatic reactions and, in some instances, by the accumulation of proximal metabolites.

Physical findings in most cases presenting in Western countries are those of the high-output state and usually of severe generalized malnutrition and vitamin deficiency. Evidence of peripheral neuropathy with sensory and motor deficits is common (so-called dry beriberi), as is the presence of nutritional cirrhosis characterized by paresthesias of the extremities, decreased or absent knee and ankle jerks, painful glossitis, the anemia of combined iron and folate deficiency, and hyperkeratinized skin lesions. However, the cases in Japanese teenagers[66] were not characterized by other signs of vitamin or nutritional deficiency, and it is possible that similar cases (wet beriberi above) may occur in Western teenagers indulging in similar dietary fads.

Beriberi heart disease[71–74] is characterized by evidence of biventricular failure, sinus rhythm, and marked edema (so-called wet beriberi). There is arteriolar vasodilatation, and the cutaneous vessels may be dilated, or in later cases with congestive heart failure, they may be constricted. Therefore, the absence of warm hands does not discount the diagnosis of beriberi. A third heart sound and an apical systolic murmur are heard almost invariably, and there is a wide pulse pressure characteristic of the hyperkinetic state.

The electrocardiogram characteristically exhibits low voltage of the QRS complex prolongation of the Q-T interval, and low voltage or inversion of T waves. The chest roentgenogram usually shows biventricular enlargement, pulmonary congestion, and pleural effusions. In alcoholics with beriberi heart disease, the left ventricular ejection fraction and peak left ventricular dP/dt are usually reduced.[71] The role played by alcoholic cardiomyopathy (p. 1417) in this hemodynamic picture is not clear. The cardiac output falls, and the peripheral resistance rises acutely when thiamine is administered in the catheterization laboratory.[72]

Laboratory diagnosis can be made by demonstration of increased serum pyruvate and lactate levels in the presence of a low transketolase level.[75] Thiamine concentration may be determined in biological fluids,[76–78] and the blood thiamine level furnishes an index of thiamine availability, whereas transketolase activity indicates the ability to convert thiamine into metabolically active forms. The most reliable test of thiamine deficiency is the augmentation of whole blood or erythrocyte transketolase (ETK) activity with treatment (the absolute levels being of little aid). Thiamine functions as a coenzyme for transketolase in the pentose phosphate pathway of glucose metabolism. An increase of circulating ETK activity with treatment or when thiamine diphosphate is added to the patient's blood in vitro (the so-called TPP [thiamine pyrophosphate] effect) is helpful in the diagnosis. In the in vitro test, the normal TPP effect is a 0 to 14 per cent increase of ETK activity; a 15 to 24 per cent increase is a borderline response, and a 25 per cent or more increase is evidence of clinical thiamine deficiency.[79] Leukocyte transketolase activity may prove to be a more sensitive index of the thiamine deficiency than the erythrocyte activity.

At *postmortem examination* the heart usually shows simple dilation without other changes. On microscopic examination, there is sometimes edema and hydropic degeneration of the muscle fibers. Nonspecific but abnormal histological and electron microscopic changes have been found in cardiac biopsy specimens.

Heart failure may develop explosively in beriberi, and some patients succumb to the illness within 48 hours of the onset of symptoms. So-called "Shoshin" beriberi, seen most frequently in the Orient, is a fulminating form of the disease[80] characterized by hypotension, tachycardia, and lactic acidosis; if left untreated, the patients die in pulmonary edema. Thus, since the course of the disease may advance rapidly, treatment must be begun immediately once the diagnosis has been established. In the Western world this fulminant form of the disease is uncommon.

TREATMENT. Akbarian and coworkers have reported careful hemodynamic studies which suggest that vasomotor depression or paralysis may be responsible for the depressed vascular resistance.[70] They studied four patients in whom ethanol excess was responsible for the thiamine deficiency. All had increased heart rate and cardiac output (averaging 6 liters/min/sq meter) and reduced arterial–mixed venous oxygen difference and systemic vascular resistance. Right and left ventricular filling pressures and blood volume were also elevated. In one patient intravenous thiamine led to a reduction in cardiac output (from 8.0 to 3.9 liters/min) and an elevation of systemic vascular resistance (from 969 to 1863 dynes-sec-cm^{-5}). Because ouabain then led to substantial improvement, the investigators concluded that the thiamine had converted high-output failure to low-output failure. In other studies they found that the low systemic vascular resistance did not respond to methoxamine infusion until after correction of the thiamine deficiency.

Patients with beriberi heart disease fail to respond adequately to digitalis and diuretics alone. However, improvement after the administration of thiamine (up to 100 mg IV followed by 25 mg per day orally for 1 to 2 weeks) may be dramatic. Marked diuresis, decrease in heart rate and size, and clearing of pulmonary congestion may occur within 12 to 48 hours.[70, 80, 81] However, the acute reversal of the vasodilatation induced by correction of the deficiency may cause the unprepared left ventricle to go into low-output failure. Therefore, patients should receive a glycoside and diuretic therapy along with thiamine.

Latent beriberi deficiency may occur in conditions such as alcoholic cardiomyopathy and in other forms of refractory congestive heart failure. The possibility of thiamine deficiency should be considered in many patients with heart failure of obscure origin. It should be pointed out that the development of thiamine deficiency has been reported in patients receiving prolonged treatment with furosemide.[82] Thus patients with heart failure from other etiologies could develop superimposed beriberi heart disease unless adequate thiamine intake is maintained.

PAGET'S DISEASE

PATHOGENESIS. Paget's disease of bone is an asymmetrical process characterized by extremely rapid bone formation and resorption of the involved areas. Histologically, this excessive formation and resorption of bone is mediated by osteoblasts and is followed by replacement of normal marrow by vascular fibrous connective tissue, increases in the vascularity of the diseased bones, and an increase in the size of the vessels originating from the periosteal plexus with an augmentation of periosteal vascularity. Increased blood flow occurs through extremities involved by Paget's disease and may be as high as nine times the normal level.[83–84a] Because of the increased vascularity of bone affected by Paget's disease, it has been assumed that this high flow occurred through the involved bone.[85] However, studies with radioactive technetium-labeled microspheres injected into the femoral arteries of patients with Paget's disease have shown no evidence of arteriovenous shunting.[86] Instead, it appears that the additional blood flow through an affected, resting limb passes through the *cutaneous tissue* overlying the involved bone, possibly secondary to local heat production resulting from the increased metabolic activity of affected bone.[83]

CLINICAL FINDINGS. These are a function of the extent of the disease and the specific bones involved. Involvement of at least 15 per cent of the skeleton by Paget's disease in an active stage, accompanied by a high alkaline phosphatase level, is necessary before a clinically significant augmentation of cardiac output is observed.

A recent study[87] compared 20 control subjects with two groups of patients with Paget's disease. The two groups of patients with Paget's disease were defined by the extent of skeletal involvement (less than or greater than 15 per cent skeletal involvement by radiographic criteria). The patients with minimal (<15 per cent) skeletal involvement had normal cardiac function on the basis of echocardiographic and systolic time interval analysis. In contrast, patients with more extensive skeletal involvement showed abnormal cardiovascular function. Four of the seven patients in this latter group had markedly increased cardiac outputs; also, increased left ventricular diastolic dimension and increased left ventricular mass indicative of cardiac hypertrophy were found in these patients. Finally, calcification of the mitral annulus and aortic valve was more common in the patients with extensive skeletal involvement.

An example of echocardiographic findings in a patient with severe Paget's disease is shown in Figure 25–7. Such a high-output state may be well tolerated for years with the patient remaining asymptomatic. However, if a specific cardiac disorder (e.g., valvular disease, coronary stenosis) is present, the combination may cause rapid clinical deterioration.

The physical findings are those of Paget's disease of bone with swelling or deformity of one or more long bones, enlargement of the skull, facial pain, headache, backache or pain, and an elevated blood alkaline phosphatase level. The cardiovascular findings are not distinguishable from those in other conditions with high-output states. In addition, metastatic calcifications are characteristic. If they involve the heart, they may lead to sclerosis and calcification of the valve rings, with extension into the interventricular septum, and may produce abnormalities of atrioventricular or interventricular conduction.

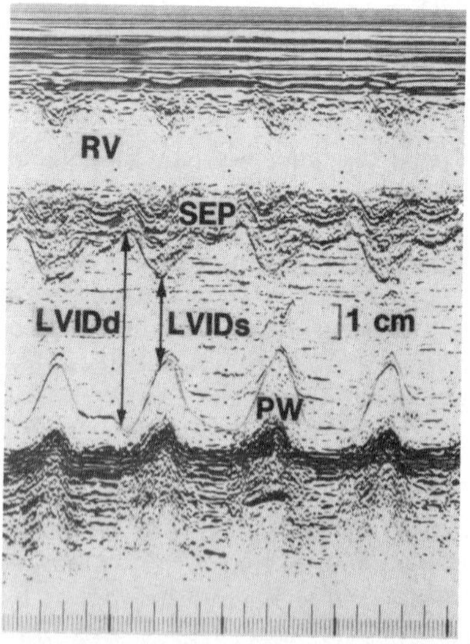

FIGURE 25–7. M-mode echocardiographic study of the left ventricle in a 57-year-old man with a 25-year history of severe Paget's disease. The left ventricular internal diameter at end-diastole (LVIDd) is increased at 5.9 cm. Fractional shortening is increased at 56 per cent, and ejection fraction was calculated to be 86 per cent. Stroke volume was estimated to be 148 ml, and given a heart rate of 61 beats/min, cardiac output was calculated at 9.0 liters/min. RV = right ventricle; SEP = septum; 1 cm = 1 centimeter; PW = posterior wall. (Courtesy of Patricia Come, M.D., Beth Israel Hospital, Boston, Massachusetts.)

TREATMENT. Treatment is generally unsatisfactory, although the long-term use of salmon calcitonin may be beneficial; however, the reported effects of such treatment on the high-output state are mixed.[88] Oral etidronate disodium has been used in the treatment of Paget's disease. In one report etidronate disodium provided symptomatic relief, including reduced bone pain, and in two-thirds of patients the elevated cardiac output returned to normal within 3 months.[89]

Cytotoxic drugs, including actinomycin D and mithramycin, have also been found to be useful in lowering the elevated cardiac output in Paget's disease, but these potent agents have serious toxic side effects.

FIBROUS DYSPLASIA (ALBRIGHT'S SYNDROME)

This condition, in which there is proliferation of fibrous tissue in bone, may also be associated with an elevated cardiac output.[90–93] Fibrous dysplasia has the appearance typical of fibromas, in which are embedded areas of coarse fiber bone with wide osteoid seams, prominent cement lines, and many thin-walled sinusoids; it has been postulated that these sinusoids act as multiple minute arteriovenous fistulas, leading to deformity and fractures. There is abnormal cutaneous pigmentation (i.e., dark brown macules) on one side of the midline and sexual precocity in females. Multiple bones are involved, and the cardiac output may be elevated, as in patients with Paget's disease of bone.

PREGNANCY

(See also Chap. 60)

The effects of pregnancy on the normal circulation and the relationship between pregnancy and cardiovascular disease are discussed in detail in Chap. 60. Here it should be pointed out that in pregnancy, cardiac output rises slowly to a peak averaging 40 per cent above control and is accompanied by an increase in blood volume and a reduction in systemic vascular resistance. The elevation of cardiac output is related only in part to the augmented total metabolism characteristic of pregnancy because the output reaches a peak between the twentieth and twenty-fourth weeks of gestation, yet the combined oxygen needs of mother and fetus continue to climb to reach a peak at term; hormonal effects appear to be responsible in part. This physiological increase in cardiac output does not lead to congestive failure, except when, as is the case for other chronic high–cardiac output states, the pregnancy is superimposed on underlying cardiac disease or is added to another major cardiovascular burden.

HYPERKINETIC HEART SYNDROME

Gorlin and coworkers described a group of patients with increased cardiac output of no discernible cause; cardiac indices averaged 6.4 liters/min/sq meter, with slightly elevated systolic and pulse pressures, normal mean arterial pressure, and low systemic vascular resistance.[94, 95] Most were young men with a hyperkinetic precordium, often with third and fourth heart sounds, systolic ejection clicks, midsystolic murmurs along the left sternal border, electrocardiograms suggestive of left ventricular hypertrophy, and radiological evidence of plethoric lung fields. The high value for oxygen consumption (177 ml/min/sq meter) in Gorlin's early report suggested that anxiety contributed to the elevated cardiac output. Indeed, it has been pointed out earlier that anxiety can lead to significant increases in oxygen consumption and cardiac output.[96] However, it is now clear that in some patients with this syndrome, cardiac output is elevated even after sedation and in the presence of normal oxygen consumption.

Such patients generally receive medical attention because of palpitations, tachycardia, cardiac awareness, atypical chest pain, an unconvincing history of fatigue, dyspnea, or tachypnea.[97, 98] Various diagnoses have been attached to some patients with the hyperkinetic heart syndrome, including neurasthenia, anxiety neurosis, Da Costa syndrome, effort syndrome, and soldier's heart[99]; however, some patients with the hyperkinetic heart syndrome do not have manifestations associated with these syndromes, while others with these nonspecific syndromes do not have a chronically elevated cardiac output. A condition which is similar or identical to the hyperkinetic heart syndrome has been described by Frohlich and coworkers as "hyperdynamic beta-adrenergic circulatory state," since treatment with propranolol resulted in improvement.[100]

The elevated systolic arterial pressure and cardiac output and lowered systemic vascular resistance characteristic of this condition are restored to normal by beta-adrenoceptor blockade. Therapy with a beta-adrenoceptor blocking agent has been effective in some patients; indeed, cardiac output has been maintained at normal levels for 2 years with propranolol at doses of 80 to 160 mg/day and promptly returned to the previously elevated levels when the drug was discontinued (Fig. 25–8).[101, 102]

There has been some speculation that the hyperkinetic heart syndrome is related to hypertrophic obstructive cardiomyopathy, in that a hyperkinetic precordium, systolic murmur, and elevated cardiac output are present in both conditions (Chap. 42). However, the resemblance between these two conditions is only superficial, and no definitive link between them has been proved. Although it has been proposed that hypertrophic obstructive cardiomyopathy may be a complication of the hyperkinetic syndrome, the authors have not encountered any patient in whom this transition occurred, nor has it been satisfactorily documented by others.

A number of studies have been reported describing the long-term follow-up of patients who had been diagnosed as having the hyperkinetic heart syndrome.[102, 103] In one,[102] 14 patients were observed for 5 years. Half the group received propranolol and the remaining seven patients received placebo. There was symptomatic improvement in the treated group, and symptoms recurred when the beta-adrenoceptor blocker was discontinued. However, neither propranolol-treated nor placebo-treated patients developed echocardiographic evidence of left ventricular hypertrophy. In a second study,[103] 19 patients initially diagnosed as having hyperkinetic heart syndrome were followed for periods of 11 to 25 years. One patient died of complicating severe mitral stenosis. Of the remaining patients, in general, the initial physical findings had disappeared or decreased. Two patients developed sustained hypertension. It was concluded that the long-term prognosis of the condition is excellent, and beta blockade was recommended only for those with significant symptoms or hypertension.[104]

An abnormally elevated cardiac output at rest may be responsible for the elevation of arterial pressure in some patients with essential hypertension (Chap. 27). Although this is generally associated with early or labile hypertension,[105] an elevated cardiac output has been observed in some patients with fixed, severe hypertension as well.[106] Presumably, the augmented sympathetic drive to the heart and vascular bed is responsible for both elevated cardiac output and elevated vascular resistance in this subset of patients.

HEPATIC DISEASE

Increased cardiac output has been reported to occur in patients with cirrhosis of the liver,[107–113] and it has been speculated that it may represent the effect of arteriovenous shunting (e.g., vascular spiders) within the liver and other organs. Microarteriovenous fistulas in the lung are usually responsible for arterial hypoxemia and the shunting in the lung[108–112]; less commonly, collateral vessels between the portal and pulmonary veins are responsible for the right-to-left shunting and cyanosis. In some cases pulmonary arteriovenous shunting may result in 10 to 20 per cent of mixed venous blood traversing the lungs without gas exchange.[108]

Hepatocellular failure, regardless of etiology, induces systemic vasodilatation and increases the cardiac output. The increase in cardiac output may be striking, with elevations of two to four times the normal value at rest.[107] In patients with acute hepatitis the hyperkinetic state reverses when the hepatitis subsides. The mechanism responsible for the widespread arteriolar dilatation and the resulting hyperkinetic state is not clear. Hypoxemia can contribute to the high cardiac output but does not appear to be a sufficient explanation. Diminished deactivation of vasodilator substances and estrogens may be important.

RENAL DISEASE (See also Chap. 59)

Cardiac output has been reported to increase in some[114–115a] but not all[116] patients with acute glomerulonephritis. In a report of six patients with acute glomerulonephritis,[115a] cardiac output was increased to an

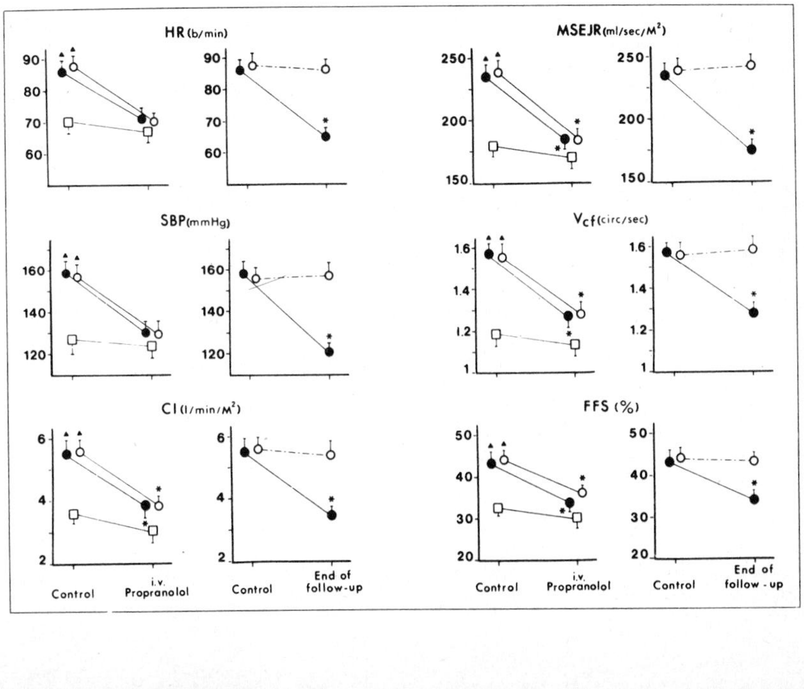

FIGURE 25–8. The first and the third columns show the averages (± SD) of heart rate (HR), systolic blood pressure (SBP), cardiac index (CI); left ventricular mean rate of systolic ejection (MSEJR), mean velocity of circumferential fiber shortening (V_{cf}) and per cent fiber fractions shortening (FFS) in 9 normal subjects (squares) and in 14 hyperkinetic patients (circles) before and after intravenous propranolol. Values in hyperkinetic subjects to receive long-term oral propranolol and those to be untreated are indicated by full and open circles, respectively. The second and fourth columns show the averages (± SD) of the same circulatory variables in the control state and at the end of 5-year follow-up in the treated (full circles, 7 cases) and untreated group (open circles, 7 cases). * indicates differences from control value significant at $p < 0.01$. (From Fiorentini, C., Olivari, M. T., Moruzzi, P., and Guazzi, M. D.: Long-term follow-up of the primary hyperkinetic heart syndrome. Am. J. Med. *71*:225, 1981.)

average of 5.4 liters/min/sq meter. Oxygen consumption also increased, as did mean arterial and pulmonary wedge pressures, whereas systemic vascular resistance was normal and the arterial–mixed venous oxygen difference was reduced. Because the patients were in the oliguric stage of their disease, it appears that the combination of hypervolemia, resulting from abnormal salt and water retention, and the increased metabolic rate (high oxygen consumption) was responsible for the high–cardiac output state.

The *pulmonary edema* that occurs in some patients with acute nephritis is not usually a reflection of left ventricular failure, but may be a consequence of the hypervolemia. In addition, left ventricular work may be strikingly elevated as a consequence of the augmentation of cardiac output and arterial pressure; this is associated with an elevation of left ventricular end-diastolic pressure as the ventricle moves up to the steep portion of its diastolic pressure-volume curve (Chap. 15). This condition has been termed the *congested state* by Eichna to contrast it with heart failure, in which a true abnormality of cardiac function occurs.[117]

As has already been pointed out, elevated cardiac output secondary to anemia is common in chronic renal failure and the arteriovenous fistula created for a vascular access site in patients on hemodialysis often contributes to this high-output state (p. 1839).

PULMONARY DISEASE (See also Chap. 48)

Although some investigators have reported elevated values for cardiac output at rest in patients with chronic pulmonary disease,[118] most have failed to show this consistently[119, 120]; in fact, some have reported finding unexplained left ventricular dysfunction and a low cardiac output in such patients.[120, 121] It appears that in some patients with chronic pulmonary disease who exhibit a predominance of obstructive bronchitis with marked hypoxemia (Type B, "blue bloaters," p. 1606), cardiac output is normal or increased, probably reflecting a response to the lowered arterial oxygen tension and the augmented blood volume resulting from secondary polycythemia. Cardiac output is generally depressed in patients with classic cor pulmonale.

POLYCYTHEMIA VERA (See also Chap. 55)

This condition is also frequently associated with increased cardiac output,[122] despite the added resistance to ventricular ejection imposed by the increased viscosity; right and left atrial pressures are usually normal, and the elevated cardiac output returns to normal with appropriate treatment of the polycythemia. The marked hypervolemia in this condition may be responsible for the high cardiac output despite the elevated blood viscosity.[122] The most serious cardiovascular consequence of polycythemia vera is the high risk of developing intravascular thromboses.

CARCINOID SYNDROME (See also p. 1439)

This syndrome, characterized by cutaneous flushing, telangiectasia, diarrhea, and bronchial constriction, results from the release of serotonin and other mediators by carcinoid tumors.[123] These tumors vary in their synthesis of indoles and may elaborate chemically unrelated agents, including histamine, bradykinin, and adrenocorticotrophic hormone. In addition to the endocardial disease, described in Chap. 42, an elevated cardiac output in the resting state accompanied by a reduced arterial–mixed venous oxygen difference is common.[124] It results from the reduction of vascular resistance, presumably owing to continuous release of mediator(s) and/or to excessive blood flow through metastatic tumors, the latter producing an arteriovenous fistula–like effect.

DERMATOLOGICAL DISORDERS

Cardiac output is increased in certain erythrodermic skin diseases, such as psoriasis and exfoliative dermatitis,[125, 126] as well as in Kaposi's sarcoma.[127] Increased flow of blood through the skin or tumor, producing the hemodynamic equivalent of multiple arteriovenous fistulas, appears to be responsible, and cardiac output returns to normal with appropriate treatment of the cutaneous disorder.[128]

OBESITY (See also p. 1819)

Massive obesity is characterized by marked increases in blood volume, cardiac output, and stroke volume. Left ventricular filling pressure is elevated, owing to the combination of increased preload and reduced ventricular distensibility.[129, 130] Arterial pressure is often elevated as a result of the raised cardiac output in the presence of a relatively restricted arterial capacity caused by the low vascularity of adipose tissue.[131] The combination of increased stroke volume and arterial pressure results in marked elevations of stroke work. The left ventricle dilates, and left ventricular function, as reflected in the relation between left ventricular end-diastolic pressure and stroke work, as well as in V_{max}, is depressed, particularly in the extremely obese.[129]

Weight loss results in normalization of oxygen consumption, cardiac output, and systemic arterial pressure, but ventricular filling pressures may remain elevated.[132] When obesity persists, as is usually the case, systemic hypertension often becomes severe, and the combination of excessive preload and afterload and the resultant left ventricular hypertrophy and dilatation may lead to congestive heart failure.

REFERENCES

METABOLIC DETERMINANTS OF CARDIAC OUTPUT

1. Barratt-Boyes, B. G., and Wood, E. H.: Cardiac output and related measurements and pressure values in the right heart and associated vessels together with an analysis of the hemodynamic response to the inhalation of high oxygen mixtures in healthy subjects. J. Lab. Clin. Med. *51*:72, 1958.
2. Sjostrand, T.: Blood volume, *In* Hamilton, S. F., and Dow, P. (eds.): Handbook of Physiology. Section 2. Circulation. Volume II, Washington D. C., American Physiological Society, 1962, p. 53.
3. Guyton, A. C.: The relationship of cardiac output to arterial pressure control. Circulation *64*:1079, 1981.
4. Sagawa, K.: The end-systolic pressure-volume relation of the ventricle: Definition, modifications, and clinical use. Circulation *63*:1223, 1981.
5. Borow, K. M., Green, L. H, Grossman, W., and Braunwald, E.: Left ventricular end-systolic stress-shortening and stress-length relations in humans. Am. J. Cardiol. *50*:1301, 1982.
6. McKay, R. G., Aroesty, J. M., Heller, G. V., Royal, H. D., Als, A. V., and Grossman, W.: Assessment of the end-systolic pressure-volume relationship in human beings with the use of a time varying elastance model. Circulation *74*:97, 1986.
7. Richardson, T. Q., and Guyton, A. C.: Effects of polycythemia and anemia on cardiac output and other circulatory factors. Am. J. Physiol. *197*:1167, 1959.
8. Burch, G. E., DePasquale, N., Hyman, A., and DeGraff, A. C.: Influence of tropical weather on cardiac output, work, and power of right and left ventricles of man resting in hospital. Arch. Intern. Med. *104*:553, 1959.
9. Murray, J. F., and Escobar, E.: Circulatory effects of blood viscosity: Comparison of methemoglobinemia and anemia. J. Appl. Physiol. *25*:594, 1968.

CONDITIONS ASSOCIATED WITH SUSTAINED INCREASES IN CARDIAC OUTPUT

10. Fowler, N. O., and Holmes, J. C.: Blood viscosity and cardiac output in acute experimental anemia. J. Appl. Physiol. *39*:453, 1975.
11. Vatner, S. F., Higgins, C. B., and Franklin, D.: Regional circulatory adjustments to moderate and severe chronic anemia in conscious dogs at rest and during exercise. Circ. Res. *30*:731, 1972.
12. Glick, G., Plauth, W. H., Jr., and Braunwald, E.: Role of the autonomic nervous system in the circulatory response to acutely induced anemia in unanesthetized dogs. J. Clin. Invest. *43*:2112, 1964.
13. Liang, C., and Huckabee, W. E.: Mechanisms regulating the cardiac output response to cyanide infusion: A model of hypoxia. J. Clin. Invest. 52:3115, 1973.
14. Duke, M., and Abelmann, W. H.: The hemodynamic response to chronic anemia. Circulation *39*:503, 1969.
15. Sproule, B. J., Mitchell, J. H., and Miller, W. F.: Cardiopulmonary physiological responses to heavy exercise in patients with anemia. J. Clin. Invest. *39*:378, 1960.
16. Graettinger, J. S., Parsons, R. L., and Campbell, J. A.: A correlation of clinical and hemodynamic studies in patients with mild and severe anemia with and without congestive failure. Ann. Intern. Med. 58:617, 1963.
17. Kumar, A. E., Gupta, G. D., Kumar, R., and Singh, M. M.: Pulmonary vascular adaptation to the hyperkinetic state of severe anemia. Clin. Res. *17*:578, 1969.
18. Varat, M. A., Adolph, R. J., and Fowler, N. O.: Cardiovascular effects of anemia. Am. Heart J. *83*:415, 1972.
19. Case, R. B., Berglung, E., and Sarnoff, S. J.: Ventricular function. VII. Changes in coronary resistance and ventricular function resulting from acutely induced anemia and the effect thereon of coronary stenosis. Am. J. Med. *18*:397, 1955.
20. Balfour, I. C., Covitz, W., Davis, H., Rao, P. S., Strong, W. B., and Alpert, B. S.: Cardiac size and function in children with sickle cell anemia. Am. Heart. J. *108*:345, 1984.
21. Denenberg, B. S., Criner, G., Jones, R., and Spann, J. F.: Cardiac function in sickle cell anemia. Am. J. Cardiol. *51*:1674, 1983.
22. Moser, K. M., and Shea, J. G.: The relationship between pulmonary infarction, cor pulmonale and the sickle states. Am. J. Med. *22*:561, 1957.
23. Miller, G. J., Serjeant, G. R., Sivapraqasam, S., and Petch, M. C.: Cardi-

opulmonary responses and gas exchange during exercise in adults with homozygous sickle-cell disease. Clin. Sci. *44*:113, 1973.
24. Merillon, J. P., Passa, P., Chastre, J., Wolf, A., and Gourgon, R.: Left ventricular function and hyperthyroidism. Br. Heart J. *46*:137, 1982.
25. Goldman, S., Olajos, M., and Morkin, E.: Control of cardiac output in thyrotoxic calves. J. Clin. Invest. *73*:358, 1984.
26. Wiener, L., Stout, B. D., and Cox, J. W.: Influence of beta sympathetic blockade on the hemodynamics of hyperthyroidism. Am. J. Med. *46*:227, 1969.
27. Buccino, R. A., Spann, J F., Jr., Pool, P. E., Sonnenblick, E. H., and Braunwald, E.: Influence of thyroid state on intrinsic contractile properties and energy stores of the myocardium. J. Clin. Invest. *46*:1669, 1967.
28. Grossman, W., Robin, N. I., Johnson, L. W., Brooks, H. L., Selenkow, H. A., and Dexter, L.: The enhanced myocardial contractility of thyrotoxicosis. Ann. Intern. Med. *74*:869, 1971.
29 Goldman, S., Olajos, M., Friedman, H., Roeske, W. R., and Morkine, E.: Left ventricular performance in conscious thyotoxic calves. Am. J. Physiol. *242*:H113, 1982.
30. Feldman, T., Borow, K. M., Sarne, D. H., Neumann, A., and Lang, R. M.: Myocardial mechanics in hyperthyroidism· Importance of left ventricular loading conditions, heart rate and contractile state. J. Am. Coll. Cardiol. 7:967, 1986.
31. Lewis, B. S., Ehrenfelk, E. N., Lewis, N., and Gotsman, M. S.: Echocardiographic left ventricular function in thyrotoxicosis. Am. Heart J. *97*:460, 1979.
32. Banerjee, S. K. Flink, I. L., and Morkin, E.: Enzymatic properties of native and *N*-ethylmaleimide modified cardiac myosin from normal and thyrotoxic rats. Circ. Res. *39*:319, 1976.
33. Rovetto, M. J., Hjalmarson, A. C., Morgan, H. E., Barrett, M. J., and Goldstein, R. A.: Hormonal control of cardiac myosin ATPase in the rat. Circ. Res. *31*:397, 1972.
34. Izumo, S., Nadal-Ginard, B., and Mahdavi, V.: All members of myosin heavy chain multigene family are regulated by thyroid hormone in a highly tissue specific manner. Science *231*:597, 1986.
35. Takacs, I. E., Szabo, J., Noszray, K., Szentmiklosi, A. J., Cseppento, A., and Szegi, J.: Alterations of contractility and sarcoplasmic reticulum function of rat heart in experimental hypo- and hyperthyroidism. Gen. Physiol. Biophys. *4*:271, 1985.
36. Etzkorn, J., Hopkins, P., Gray, J., Segal, J., and Ingbar, S. H.: Beta-adrenergic potentiation of the increased in vitro accumulation of cytoleucine by rat thymocytes induced by triiodothyronine. J. Clin. Invest. *63*:1172, 1979.
37. Clozel, J. P., Danchin, N., Genton, P., Thomas, J. L., and Cherrier, F.: Effects of propranolol and of verapamil on heart rate and blood pressure in hyperthyroidism. Clin. Pharmacol. Ther. *36*:64, 1984.
38. White, C. W., and Zimmerman, T. J.: Reduced cholinergic sinus node restraint in hyperthyroidism. Circulation *54*:890, 1976.
38a. Hoffman, I., and Lowrey, R. D.: The electrocardiogram in thyrotoxicosis. Am. J. Cardiol. *8*:893, 1960.
39. Braunwald, E., Mason, D. T., and Ross, J., Jr.: Studies on the cardiocirculatory actions of digitalis. Medicine (Balt.) *44*:233, 1965.
40. Muggia, A. L., Stjernholm, M., and Houle, T.: Complete heart block with thyrotoxic myocarditis. N. Engl. J. Med. *283*:1099, 1970.
41. Grossman, W., Robin, N. I., Johnson, L. W., Brooks, H. L., Selenkow, H. A., and Dexter, L.: Effects of beta blockade on the peripheral manifestations of thyrotoxicosis. Ann. Intern. Med. *74*:875, 1971.
42. Gaffney, T. E., Braunwald, E., and Kahler, R. L.: Effects of guanethidine on tri-iodothyroxine induced hyperthyroidism in man. N. Engl. J. Med. *265*:16, 1961.
43. Newmark, S. R., Himathonekum, T., and Shane, J. M.: Hyperthyroid crises. J.A.M.A. *230*:592, 1974.
44. Shapiro, S., Steiner, M., and Dimich, I.: Congestive heart failure in neonatal thyrotoxicosis. A curable cause of heart failure in the newborn. Clin. Pediatr. *14*:1155, 1975.
45. Resnekov, L., and Falicov, R. E.: Thyrotoxicosis and lactate-producing angina pectoris with normal coronary arteries. Br. Heart J. *39*:51, 1977.
46. Nicoladoni, C.: Phlebarteriectasie der rechten oberen Extremitat. Arch. Klin. Chri. *18*:252, 1875.
47. Branham, H. H.: Aneurysmal varix of the femoral artery ana vein following a gunshot wound. Int. J. Surg. *3*:250, 1890.
48. Gupta, P. D., and Singh, M.: Neural mechanism underlying tachycardia induced by non-hypotensive A-V shunt. Am. J. Physiol. *236*:H35, 1979.
49. Szilagyi, D. E., Smith, R. F., Elliott, J. P., and Hageman, J. H.: Congenital arteriovenous anomalies of the limbs. Arch Surg. *111*:423, 1976.
50. Becker, D. G., Fish, C. R., and Juergen, S. J. L.: Arteriovenous fistulas of the female pelvis. Obstet. Gynecol. *31*:799, 1968.
51. Price, A. C., Coran, A. G., and Mattern, A. L.: Hemangioendothelioma of the pelvis: A cause of cardiac failure in the newborn. N. Engl. J. Med. *286*:647, 1972.
52. Coel, M. N., and Alksne, J. F.: Embolization to diminish high output failure secondary to systemic angiomatosis (Ullman's syndrome). Vasc. Surg. *12*:336, 1978.
53. Burckhardt, D., Stalder, G. A., Ludin, H., and Bianchi, L.: Hyperdynamic circulatory state due to Osler-Weber-Rendu disease with intrahepatic arteriovenous fistulas. Am. Heart J. *85*:797, 1973.
54. Baranda, M. M., Perez, M., DeAndres, J., De La Hoz, C., Merino, J., and Aguirre, C.: High-output congestive heart failure as first manifestation of Osler-Weber-Rendu disease. J. Vasc. Dis. *35*:568, 1984.
55. Radtke, W. E., Smith, H. C., Fulton, R. E., and Adson, M. R.: Misdiagnosis of atrial septal defect in patients with hereditary telangiectasis (Osler-Weber-Rendu disease) and hepatic arteriovenous fistulas. Am. Heart J. *95*:235, 1978.
56. Rocchini, A. P., Rosenthal, A., Issenberg, H. J., and Nadas, A. S.: Hepatic hemangioendothelioma: Hemodynamic observations and treatment. Pediatrics *57*:131, 1976.
57. Zavota, L., Bini, F., Carano, N., Agnetti, A., and Squarcia, U.: Hepatic hemangiomatosis with congestive cardiac failure and development into a cholostatic hepatopathy. Pediatr. Med. Chir. *6*:621, 1984.
58. DeLorimer, A. A., Simpson, E. B., Baum, R., and Carlsson, E.: Hepatic artery ligation for hepatic hemangiomatosis. N. Engl. J. Med. *277*:333, 1967.
59. Dorney, E. R.: Peripheral AV fistula of fifty-seven years' duration with refractory heart failure. Am. Heart J. *54*:778, 1957.
60. Hildreth, D. H., and Turcke, D. A.: Postlaminectomy arteriovenous fistula. Surgery *81*:512, 1977.
61. Sanyal, S. K., Saldivar, V., Coburn, T. P., Wrenn, E. L., Jr., and Kumar, M.: Hyperdynamic heart failure due to A-V fistula associated with Wilms' tumqr. Pediatrics *57*:564, 1976.
62. Anderson, C. B., Codd, J. R., Graff, R. A., Groce, M. A., Harter, H. R., and Newton, W. T.: Cardiac failure and upper extremity arteriovenous dialysis fistulas. Arch. Intern. Med. *136*:292, 1976.
63. Ahearn, D. J., and Maher, J. F.: Heart failure as a complication of hemodialysis arteriovenous fistula. Ann. Intern. Med. *77*:201, 1972.
64. Anderson, C. B., and Groce, M. A.: Banding of arteriovenous dialysis fistulas to correct high-output cardiac failure. Surgery *78*:552, 1975.
65. Fee, H. J., Levisman, J., Doud, R. B., and Golding, A. L.: High output congestive failure from femoral arteriovenous shunts for vascular access. Ann. Surg. *183*:321, 1976.
66. Kawai, C., Wakabayashi, A., Matsumura, T., and Yui, Y.: Reappearance of beriberi heart disease in Japan; a study of 23 cases. Am. J. Med. *69*:383, 1980.
67. Aalsmeer, W. C., and Wenckebach, K. F.: Herz und Kreislauf, bei der Beriberi Krankheit. Wien. Arch. Int. Med. *16*:193, 1929.
68. Weiss, S., and Wilkinson, R. W.: The nature of the cardiovascular disturbances in nutritional deficiency states (beriberi). Ann. Intern. Med. *11*:104, 1937.
69. Burwell, C. S., and Dexter, L.: Beriberi heart disease. Trans. Assoc. Am. Phys. *60*:59, 1947.
70. Akbarian, M., Yankopoulos, N. A., and Abelmann, W. H.: Hemodynamic studies in beriberi heart disease. Am. J. Med. *41*:197, 1966.
71. Ayzenberg, O., Silber, M. H., and Bortz, D.: Beriberi heart disease. A case report describing the hemodynamic features. S. Afr. Med. J. *68*:263, 1985.
72. Akram, H., Maslowski, A. H., Smith, B. L., and Nichols, M. G.: The haemodynamic, histopathological and hormonal features of alcoholic beriberi. Q. J. Med. *50*:359, 1981.
73. Carson, P.: Alcoholic cardiac beriberi. Br. Med. J. *284*:1817, 1982.
74. Editorial: Cardiovascular beriberi. Lancet *1*:1287, 1982.
75. Akbarian, M., and Dreyfus, P. M.: Blood trans-ketolase activity in beriberi heart disease. J.A.M.A. *20*:77, 1968.
76. Baker, H., and Frank, O.: Clinical Vitaminology: Methods and Interpretation. New York, Wiley Interscience, 1968.
77. Baker, H., quoted in Saùberlich, H. E.: Biochemical alterations in thiamine deficiency—their interpretation. Am. J. Clin. Nutr. *20*:543, 1967.
78. Brin, M.: Erythrocyte transketolase in early thiamine deficiency. Ann. N.Y. Acad. Sci. *98*:528, 1962.
79. Brin, M.: The use of the erythrocyte in the functional evaluation of vitamin adequacy. *In* Bishop, L., and Surgenor, D. M. (eds.): The Red Blood Cell. New York, Academic Press, 1964, p. 45.
80. Jeffrey, F. E., and Abelmann, W. H.: Recovery of proved Shoshin beriberi. Am. J. Med. *50*:123, 1971.
81. Whittemore, R., and Caddell, J. L.: Metabolic and nutritional diseases. *In* Moss, A. J., et al. (eds.): Heart Disease in Infants, Children and Adolescents. 2nd ed. Baltimore, Williams and Wilkins Co., 1977, pp. 590 and 591.
82. Yui, Y., Fujiwara, H., Mitsui, H., et al.: Furosemide-induced thiamine deficiency. Jpn. Circ. J. *42*:744, 1978.
83. Heistad, D. D., Abboud, F. M., Schmid, P. G., Mark, A. L., and Wilson, W. R.: Regulation of blood flow in Paget's disease of the bone. J. Clin. Invest. *55*:69, 1975.
84. Arnalich, F., Plaza, I., Sobrino, J. A., Oliver, J., Barbado, J., Pena, J. M., and Vazquez, J. J.: Cardiac size and function in Paget's disease of bone. Int. J. Cardiol. *5*:491, 1984
84a. Miyazaki, T., Hirose, N., Kawamura, J., Kageyama, Y., Iikuni, K., and Yanagishita, T.: A case of generalized Paget's disease of bone complicating high output heart failure. Nippon Naika Gakkai Zasshi 72:47, 1983.
85. Woodhouse, N. J. Y., Crosbie, W. A., and Mohamedally, S. M.: Cardiac output in Paget's disease: Response to long-term salmon calcitonin therapy. Br. Med. J. *4*:686, 1975.
86. Rhodes, B. A., Gregson, N. D., and Hamilton, C. R., Jr.: Absence of anatomic arteriovenous shunts in Paget's disease of bone. N. Engl. J. Med. *287*:686, 1972.
87. Arnalich, A., Plaza, I., Sobrino, J. A., Oliver, J., Barbado, J., Peña, J. M., and Vazquez, J. J.: Cardiac size and function in Paget's disease of bone. Int. J. Cardiol. *5*:491, 1984.
88. Crosbie, W. A., Mohamedally, S. M., and Woodhouse, N. J. Y.: Effect of salmon calcitonin on cardiac output, oxygen transport, and bone turnover in patients with Paget's disease. Clin. Sci. Molec. Med. *48*:537, 1975.
89. Henley, J. W., Croxson, R. S., and Ibbertson, H. K.: The cardiovascular system in Paget's disease of bone—the response to therapy with calcitonin and diphosphonate. N. Z. Med. J. *84*(Abstr.):161, August, 1976.
90. Howarth, S.: Cardiac output in osteitis deformans. Clin. Sci. *12*:271, 1953.
91. Rutishauser, E., Veyrat, R., and Rouiller, C.: La vascularization de l'os pagé tique, e tude anatomo-pathologique. Presse Med. *62*:654, 1954.
92. Lequime, J., and Denolin, H.: Circulatory dynamics in osteitis deformans. Circulation *12*:215, 1955.
93. McIntosh, H. D., Miller, D. E., Gleason, W. L., and Goldner, J. L.: The circulatory dynamics of polyostotic fibrous dysplasia. Am. J. Med. *32*:393, 1962.

94. Gorlin, R., Brachfeld, N., Turner, J. O., Messer, J. V., and Salazar, E.: The idiopathic high cardiac output state. J. Clin. Invest. *38*:2144, 1959.
95. Gorlin, R.: The hyperkinetic heart syndrome. J.A.M.A. *182*:823, 1962.
96. Hickam, J. B., Cargill, W. H., and Golden, A.: Cardiovascular reactions to emotional stimuli. Effect on cardiac output, arteriovenous oxygen difference, arterial pressure, and peripheral resistance. J. Clin. Invest. *27*:290, 1947.
97. Guazzi, M. D.: Hyperkinetic heart syndrome. Primary Cardiol. *10*:94, 1984.
98. Meshkov, A. P.: Hyperkinetic heart syndrome in adolescence: Characteristics of the clinical course and methodological principles of diagnosis. Sov. Med. *4*:96, 1984.
99. Editorial: The hyperkinetic heart. Lancet *2*:967, 1982.
100. Frohlich, E. D., Tarazi, R. C., and Dustan, H. P.: Hyperdynamic beta adrenergic circulatory state: Increased beta receptor responsiveness. Arch. Intern. Med. *123*:1, 1969.
101. Guazzi, M., Polese, A., Magrini, F., Fiorentini, C., and Olivari, M. T.: Long-term treatment of the hyperkinetic heart syndrome with propranolol. Am. J. Med. Sci. *270*:465, 1975.
102. Fiorentini, C., Olivarai, M. T., Moruzzi, P., and Guazzi, M. D.: Long-term follow-up of the primary hypertrophic heart. Am. J. Med. *71*:221, 1981.
103. Gillum, R. F., Teicholz, L. E., Herman, M. V., and Gorlin, R.: The idiopathic hyperkinetic heart syndrome: Clinical course and long-term prognosis. Am. Heart J. *102*:728, 1981.
104. Gallo, G., and Foresti, A.: Use of sotalol in the hyperkinetic heart syndrome: Clinical and Holter dynamic electrocardiographic evaluation. Cardiologia *29*:237, 1984.
105. Julius, S., and Esler, M.: Autonomic nervous cardiovascular regulation in borderline hypertension. Am. J. Cardiol. *36*:685, 1975.
106. Ibrahim, M. M., Tarazi, R. C., Dustan, H. P., Bravo, E. L., and Gifford, R. W.: Hyperkinetic heart in severe hypertension: A separate clinical hemodynamic entity. Am. J. Cardiol. *35*:667, 1975.
107. Kowalski, J. J., and Abelmann, W. H.: The cardiac output at rest in Laennec's cirrhosis. J. Clin. Invest. *32*:1025, 1953.
108. Wechsler, R. L., Myers, J. D., Dekker, A., Carey, L., and Stilley, J. W.: Cardiovascular effects of severe liver disease. Am. J. Dig. Dis. *21*:114, 1976.
109. Wolfe, J. D., Tashkin, D. P. Holly, F. E. Brachman, M. B., and Genovesi, M. G.: Hypoxemia of cirrhosis. Am. J. Med. *63*:746, 1977.
110. Murray, J. F, Dawson, A. M., and Sherlock, S.: Circulatory changes in chronic liver disease. Am. J. Med. *24*:358, 1958.
110a. MacNee, W., Buist, T., Finlayson, N. D. C., Lamb, D., Miller, H. C., Muir, A. L., and Douglas, A. C.: Multiple microscopic pulmonary arteriovenous connections in the lungs presenting as cyanosis. Thorax *40*:316, 1985.
111. Kelbaek, H., Ericksen, J. Brynjolf, I., Raboel, A., Lund, J. O., Munck, O., Bonnevie, O., and Godtfredsen, J.: Cardiac performance in patients with asymptomatic alcoholic cirrhosis of the liver. Am. J. Cardiol. *54*:852, 1984.
111a. Hales, M.: Multiple small arteriovenous fistulae of the lungs. Am. J. Pathol. *32*:927, 1956.
112. Berthelot, P., Walker, M. B., Sherlock, S., and Reid, L.: Arterial changes in the lungs in cirrhosis of the liver: Lung spider nevi. N. Engl. J. Med. *274*:291, 1966.
113. Fischer, D. M. Casanova, R., and Aldi, M.: High-output heart failure in hepatic cirrhosis. G. Ital. Cardiol. *11*:1520, 1981.
114. McCrary, W. W.: The heart in glomerulonephritis. Pediatrics *69*:1176, 1966.
115. DeFanzio V., Christensen, R. C., Regan, T. J., Baer, L. M., Morita, Y., and Hellems, H. K.: Circulatory changes in acute glomerulonephritis. Circulation *20*:190, 1959.
115a. Binak, K., Sirmaci, N., Ucak, D., and Harmanci, N.: Circulatory changes in acute glomerulonephritis at rest and during exercise. Br. Heart J. *37*:833, 1975.
116. Eichna, L. W., Farber, S. T., Berger, A. R., Rader, B., Smith, W. W., and Albert, R. E.: Non-cardiac circulatory congestion simulating congestive heart failure. Trans. Assoc. Am. Phys. *67*:72, 1954.
117. Eichna, L. W.: Circulatory congestion and heart failure. Circulation *22*:864, 1960.
118. Harvey, R. M., Ferrer, M. I., Richards, D. W., and Cournand, A.: Influence of chronic pulmonary disease on the heart and circulation. Am. J. Med. *10*:719, 1951.
119. Burrows, B., Kettel, L. J., Niden, A. H., Rabinowitz, M., and Diener, C. F.: Patterns of cardiovascular dysfunction in chronic obstructive lung disease. N. Engl. J. Med. *286*:912, 1972.
120. Baum, G. L., Schwartz, A., Llamas, R. M., and Castillo, C.: Left ventricular function in chronic obstructive lung disease. N. Engl. J. Med. *285*:361, 1971.
121. Frank, M. J., Weisse, A. B., Moschos, C. B., and Levinson, G. E.: Left ventricular function, metabolism, and blood flow in chronic cor pulmonale. Circulation *47*:798, 1973.
122. Cobb, L. A., Kramer, R. J., and Finch, C. A.: Circulatory effects of chronic hypervolemia in polycythemia vera. J. Clin. Invest. *39*:1722, 1960.
123. Grahame-Smith, D. G.: The carcinoid syndrome. *In* Bondy, P. K., and Rosenberg, L. E. (eds.): Metabolic Control and Disease. 8th ed. Philadelphia, W. B. Saunders Co., 1980, p. 1703.
124. Schwaber, J. R., and Lukas, D. S.: Hyperkinemia and cardiac failure in the carcinoid syndrome. Am. J. Med. *32*:846, 1962.
125. Voight, G. C., Kronthal, H. L., and Crounse, R. G.: Cardiac output in erythroderma skin disease. Am. Heart J. *72*:615, 1966.
126. Shuster, S.: High output cardiac failure from skin disease. Lancet *1*:1338, 1963.
127. Hecht, H. H., Candiolo, B. M., Malkinson, F. D., Nair, K. G., and Saqueton, A. C.: On cardio-cutaneous syndromes. Trans. Assoc. Am. Phys. *80*:91, 1967.
128. Prens, E. P., and Smeenk, G.: Effect of photochemotherapy on the cardiovascular system. Dermatologica *167*:208, 1983.
129. DeVitiis, O., Fazio, S., Petito, M., Maddalena, G., Contaldo, F., and Mancini, M.: Obesity and cardiac function. Circulation *64*:477, 1981.
130. Messerli, F. H., Ventura, H. O., Reisin, E. Dreslinski, G. R., Dunn, F. G., MacPhee, A. A., and Frohlich, E. D.: Borderline hypertension and obesity: Two prehypertensive states with elevated cardiac output. Circulation *66*:55, 1982.
131. Messerli, F. H.: Cardiovascular effects of obesity and hypertension. Lancet *1*:1165, 1982.
132. Backman, L., Freyschuss, U., Hallberg, D., and Melcher, A.: Reversibility of cardiovascular changes in extreme obesity. Acta Med. Scand. *205*:367, 1979.

26 PULMONARY HYPERTENSION

by WILLIAM GROSSMAN, M.D., and
EUGENE BRAUNWALD, M.D.

NORMAL PULMONARY CIRCULATION

During the passage of blood through the lungs, hemoglobin molecules are normally oxygenated to nearly their full capacity and the blood is cleansed of much particulate matter and bacteria. The lungs, in addition to functioning as a blood oxygenator and filter, play a dominant role in achieving acid-base balance by excreting carbon dioxide, thereby helping to maintain an optimum blood pH.[1] Normally, the pulmonary vascular bed offers remarkably little resistance to flow. Pulmonary hypertension results when reductions in the caliber of the pulmonary vessels and/or increases in pulmonary blood flow occur.

PULMONARY BLOOD FLOW, PRESSURE, AND RESISTANCE

CIRCULATION IN THE NORMAL ADULT. *Pulmonary blood flow* refers to the volume of blood per unit of time that passes from the pulmonary artery through the capillary bed and into the pulmonary veins. However, it must be remembered that the lungs have a dual circulation and receive both systemic venous blood (the "pulmonary blood flow") through the pulmonary artery as well as arterial blood through the bronchial circulation. The bronchial arteries ramify normally into a capillary network drained by bronchial veins, some of which empty into the pulmonary veins, whereas the remainder empty into the systemic venous bed. Therefore the bronchial circulation constitutes a physiological "right-to-left" shunt. The function of the bronchial circulation is to provide nutrition to the airways. Normally blood flow through this system is quite low, amounting to approximately 1 per cent of cardiac output:[2] the resulting desaturation of left atrial blood is usually trivial. However, in some forms of pulmonary disease, e.g., severe bronchiectasis or cystic fibrosis, and in the presence of many congenital cardiovascular malformations that cause cyanosis, the blood flow through the bronchial circulation can increase significantly and account for nearly 30 per cent of the left ventricular output.[3] In pulmonary disease, significant right-to-left shunting through the bronchial circulation may result in arterial desaturation. In cyanotic congenital heart disease, bronchial blood flow may participate in gas exchange and improve systemic oxygenation.

The normal pulmonary artery pressure in an individual living at sea level has a peak systolic value of 18 to 25 mm Hg, an end-diastolic value of 6 to 10 mm Hg, and a mean value ranging from 12 to 16 mm Hg (Chap. 9).* Definite pulmonary hypertension is present when pulmonary artery systolic and mean pressures exceed 30 and 20 mm Hg, respectively. The normal mean pulmonary venous pressure is 6 to 10 mm Hg; therefore, the normal arteriovenous pressure difference, which moves the entire cardiac output across the pulmonary vascular bed, ranges from 2 to 10 mm Hg. This small pressure gradient is all the more remarkable when one considers that to move the same amount of blood per minute through the systemic vascular bed a pressure differential of approximately 90 mm Hg (systemic arterial mean pressure minus right atrial mean pressure) is required.

Thus, the normal pulmonary vascular bed offers less than one-tenth the *resistance* to flow offered by the systemic bed. *Vascular resistance* is generally quantified, by analogy to Ohm's law, as the ratio of pressure drop (ΔP in mm Hg) to mean flow (Q in liters/min) (p. 255). The ratio is commonly multiplied by 79.9 (or 80 for simplification) to express the results in dynes-seconds-centimeters^{-5}. This conversion to metric units may be avoided, i.e., resistance may be expressed in units of mm Hg/liter/min, which are sometimes referred to as hybrid units, PRU (peripheral resistance units), or Wood units. The calculated pulmonary vascular resistance in normal adults[4] is 67 ± 23 (S.D.) dynes-sec-cm^{-5}.

Vascular resistance reflects a composite of variables that includes, but is not limited to, the cross-sectional area of

*All pressures discussed here are in reference to atmospheric pressure at the level of the heart. True transmural pressures are more physiologically meaningful, especially when pulmonary parenchymal disease is present, but these are rarely measured.

small muscular arteries and arterioles. Other determinants are blood viscosity, the total mass of lung tissue (i.e., resistance is higher in infants and children than in adults), proximal vascular obstruction (e.g., pulmonary coarctation, pulmonary embolism, peripheral pulmonic stenosis), and extramural compression of vessels (perivascular edema).

Because the pulmonary vascular bed contains considerable elastic tissue, the cross-sectional area of the bed varies directly with transmural pressure and flow. Therefore, pulmonary vascular resistance decreases passively with increases in flow, as illustrated in Figure 48–7, p. 1604. The fall in resistance results in part from the increase in the radius of distensible vessels secondary to increased flow. From a consideration of the Poiseuille relationship—in which $R = \Delta P/Q = 8\eta\ell/\pi r^4$, where R = resistance, ΔP = pressure drop, Q = flow, η = viscosity of fluid, and ℓ and r = length and radius of the vessel, respectively—it is apparent that resistance can be effectively influenced by even small changes in the radius of the vessel. Recruitment of additional vascular channels will also contribute to the fall in resistance that characterizes increased flow through the pulmonary circuit. This phenomenon is particularly prominent in the upright position, when vessels in the upper parts of the lungs are in a partially collapsed state owing to low hydrostatic pressure (p. 547).

The reduction in resistance in a distensible vascular bed which occurs with increased flow has been offered as the explanation for the absence of pulmonary hypertension in many patients with large left-to-right intracardiac shunts, particularly of the pretricuspid variety (e.g., atrial septal defect). However, it must be pointed out that the increased distensibility of pulmonary vessels in such situations has developed over years and that this principle is not necessarily applicable to acute increases in pulmonary blood flow.[5] In this regard, the results of studies with unilateral occlusion of a pulmonary artery using a balloon catheter are relevant.[6] Figure 26–1 illustrates the relationship between the flow and pressure drop, ΔP, across the left lung during balloon occlusion of the right pulmonary artery, at rest and during exercise, and under both conditions together. It is apparent that acute increases in flow in the supine position were associated with increases in ΔP, so that vascular resistance of the lung (the slope of the line relating ΔP to flow) remained unchanged. In the upright position, however, blood vessels in the upper part of the lung are usually in a partially or fully collapsed state (Fig. 18–5, p. 548) and with an increase in flow, these vessels may be expanded, thereby reducing vascular resistance.[5]

The influence of blood viscosity on pulmonary vascular resistance is also important, particularly in the cyanotic patient with hematocrit in excess of 60 per cent or in the severely anemic patient with hematocrit less than 20 per cent. In experiments in dogs in which pulmonary pressure-flow curves were constructed at varying hematocrits and rates of flow, ΔP doubled when the hematocrit was increased from 43 per cent to 64 per cent at a normal flow, indicating a doubling of effective pulmonary vascular resistance.[7]

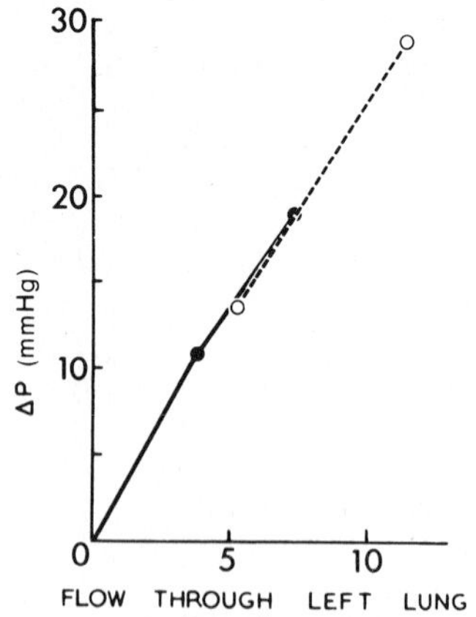

FIGURE 26–1. The relation between the drop in pressure (ΔP) and blood flow across the left lung in a supine normal human subject studied with and without occlusion of one pulmonary artery during rest (●—●) and exercise (○—○). In both states, rest and exercise, the lower circles indicate flow through both lungs and the upper circles flow through one lung. (From Harris, P., and Heath, D.: The Human Pulmonary Circulation. 2nd ed. New York, Churchill Livingstone, 1977.)

FETAL AND NEONATAL CIRCULATIONS

(See also p. 1598)

In the fetus, oxygenated blood enters the heart from the inferior vena cava and streams across the foramen ovale to the left atrium, left ventricle, ascending aorta, and cranial vessels. Desaturated blood returns from the superior vena cava and passes through the tricuspid valve into the right ventricle and pulmonary artery. Since the resistance of the pulmonary vascular bed in the collapsed fetal lung is extremely high, only 10 to 30 per cent of the total right ventricular output passes through the lungs, the remainder being shunted across the ductus arteriosus to the descending aorta and thence back to the placenta. At birth, there is an abrupt change in the pulmonary circulation. With the first breath of extrauterine life, expansion of the lungs and the abrupt rise in the P_{O_2} of blood lead to a release of pulmonary arteriolar vasoconstriction and a stretching and dilatation of muscular pulmonary arteries and arterioles, with a marked drop in vascular resistance.[8–10] This facilitates a large increase in pulmonary blood flow and results in an augmented left atrial volume and pressure. The latter closes the flap valve of the foramen ovale, so that interatrial right-to-left shunting ordinarily ceases within the first hour of life. Normally, the ductus arteriosus closes over the next 10 hours as a result of contraction of the thick smooth muscle bundles within its wall in response to a rising arterial oxygen tension and a change in the prostaglandin milieu.[11] Following the initial dramatic fall in pulmonary vascular resistance at birth, there is a continuous decline over the first few months of life associated with thinning of the media of muscular pulmonary arteries and arterioles until the normal adult pattern is achieved.[2, 12]

RESPONSE TO ANOXIA, DRUGS, AND NEURAL, HORMONAL, AND ENVIRONMENTAL FACTORS

It is well established that acute *hypoxia* elicits pulmonary vasoconstriction,[13–16] and there is general agreement that this response is part of a self-regulatory mechanism for adjusting capillary perfusion to alveolar ventilation. There appears to be an age dependency and a considerable species variability in the magnitude of this vasoconstrictor response, which is quite intense in cattle, intermediate in humans and the pig, and comparatively mild in dogs and sheep[17]; hypoxic vasoconstriction is more profound in the infant or young mammal than in the adult. Variability exists within a given species as well, and there is strong evidence for a genetic determination of individual reactivity to hypoxia in animals.[17, 18] This finding, if it is applicable to humans, may be relevant to the occasional familial occurrence of primary pulmonary hypertension in humans (p. 808).

The mechanism of the acute pulmonary vasoconstriction that occurs in response to hypoxia is uncertain (Fig. 26–2). There is some evidence that hypoxia-induced local release of histamine may play an important role, with pulmonary vasoconstriction secondary to stimulation of pulmonary vascular H_1-receptors (cf. discussion of histamine below). A role for increased calcium entry into vascular smooth muscle (Fig. 26–3) in mediating hypoxic pulmonary vasoconstriction is suggested by the observation that the Ca^{++} antagonist verapamil inhibits hypoxic pulmonary vasoconstriction.[19] The clinical relevance of this observation is supported by a study of the pulmonary vascular effects of nifedipine in 13 patients with acute respiratory failure, studied in a respiratory care unit.[20] In this study, the Ca^{++} antagonist nifedipine produced a reduction in pulmonary vascular resistance dependent on the severity of hypoxia.

The effects of chronic hypoxia on pulmonary hemodynamics and histology have been studied in the rat.[21] Mean pulmonary artery pressure rose substantially after 3 days of hypoxia and had doubled by day 14. These hemodynamic

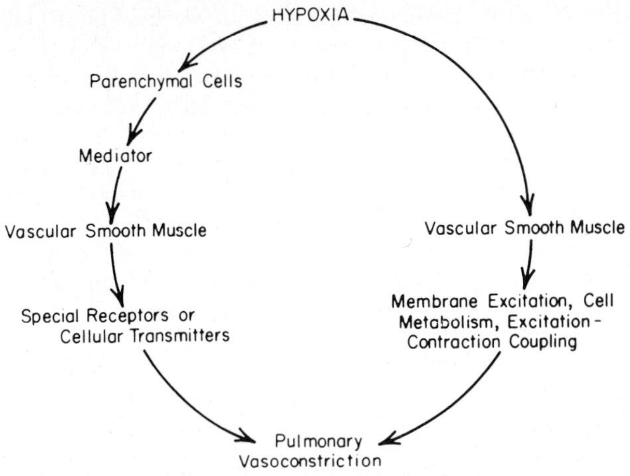

FIGURE 26–2. Alternate hypotheses to explain pulmonary vasoconstriction during hypoxia. *Left,* Indirect mechanism—mediator released by nonmuscle (parenchymal) cells of the lungs diffuses to vascular smooth muscle, where it engages cellular receptors and mechanisms to activate the contractile process. *Right,* Direct mechanism—the effects of hypoxia are exerted directly on vascular smooth muscle by affecting one or more stages in the contractile process; excitation, contraction, or the coupling of the two. (From Fishman, A. P.: Hypoxia on the pulmonary circulation; how and where it acts. Circ. Res. *38*:221, 1976, by permission of the American Heart Association, Inc.)

changes were associated with (1) abnormal extension of muscle into peripheral arteries where it is not normally present, (2) increased wall thickness of the muscular arteries, and (3) reduction in the number of arteries expressed as an increase in the ratio of alveoli to arteries. In a follow-up study,[22] it was found that these hypoxia-induced chronic vascular changes were more extensive in infants than in adult rats. Furthermore, after recovery under normoxic conditions for 3 months, residual vascular changes were present in all animals studied, but again were more marked in the younger rats.

Changes in alveolar oxygenation affect the oxygenation of blood in small pulmonary arteries and arterioles by

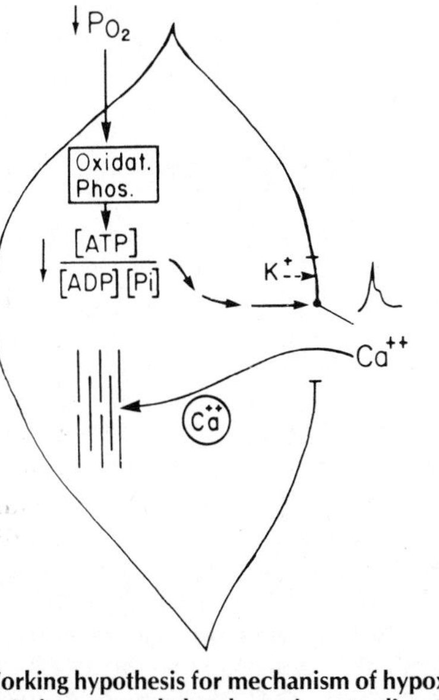

FIGURE 26–3. Working hypothesis for mechanism of hypoxic pulmonary vasoconstriction. It is proposed that hypoxia acts directly on smooth muscle of small, peripheral arteries reducing the rate of mitochondrial oxidative phosphorylation and the cytosolic (ATP)/(ADP) (Pi). The decrease in phosphate potential (or change in level of some other metabolite) then leads to membrane depolarization, calcium influx, and contraction. (From McMurtry, I. F., Stanbrook, H. S., and Rounds, S.: The mechanism of hypoxic pulmonary vasoconstriction: A working hypothesis. *In* Loeppky, J. A., and Riedesel, M. L. (eds.): Oxygen Transport to Human Tissues. New York, Elsevier-North Holland, 1982, pp. 77–89.)

direct gaseous diffusion from the alveoli, respiratory bronchioles, and alveolar ducts in the pulmonary arterioles,[23–25] even though the latter are "upstream" in relation to the alveoli. This fact, taken together with evidence for a reduction in pulmonary arterial blood volume during hypoxia,[26] supports the view that the small pulmonary arteries and arterioles are the main sites of vasoconstriction and increased resistance during hypoxia.[26, 27] While alveolar oxygen tension is a major physiological determinant of pulmonary arteriolar tone, a reduction in the oxygen tension in the mixed venous blood flowing through the small pulmonary arteries and arterioles may also lead to pulmonary arterial vasoconstriction.[15, 28] *Acidemia* appears to potentiate the effects of hypoxemia (Fig. 48–4, p. 1601), whereas alkalosis may be protective.[29–31] Thus, two potent stimuli for vasodilatation in the systemic arteriolar bed cause vasoconstriction of pulmonary arteries and arterioles. Although *hypercapnia* can be shown to increase pulmonary vascular resistance in some experimental preparations, the effects are variable and probably not important in humans.[15]

Morphological studies have demonstrated that the media and adventitia of the large elastic pulmonary arteries and of the large pulmonary veins are supplied by nerve fibers that may influence the distensibility of these capacitance vessels.[2, 13] Although *neural regulation* of pulmonary vascular resistance can be demonstrated[32] and may be particularly important in fetal life, its importance in the normal human adult is uncertain. *Chemical and hormonal regulation* of pulmonary vascular resistance is a complex and as yet incompletely understood subject, with roles having been reported for catecholamines, acetylcholine, prostaglandins, histamine, bradykinin, serotonin, and angiotensin.[2, 13, 23, 33–60] The exact site of action of these agents within the pulmonary vascular tree (i.e., arterioles, venules, capillaries, and so on) is uncertain at present.

There is controversy concerning the effects of *alpha-adrenergic agonists* on the pulmonary vascular bed. Several studies have shown that norepinephrine causes increases in pulmonary arterial and wedge pressures with no change in pulmonary blood flow or pulmonary vascular resistance.[48–51] Systemic arterial pressure increases markedly, and this presumably accounts for the increase in pulmonary venous pressure. In one study an increase in pulmonary vascular resistance with norepinephrine was reported,[52] and there is experimental evidence for alpha-adrenergic–mediated constriction of small pulmonary arteries and veins induced by either the injection of norepinephrine or the stimulation of sympathetic nerves.[53]

Both the alpha blocker phentolamine and tolazoline (Priscoline), which also exhibits alpha-adrenergic blocking action, have been shown to lower pulmonary vascular resistance.[54] Tolazoline was first reported in the pharmacological literature as a vasodepressor agent having effects comparable to those of histamine. Subsequently, it was shown to antagonize the actions of alpha-adrenergic agonists. Like phentolamine, it is an imidazoline compound, and both these agents have vasodepressor effects independent of their alpha-adrenergic antagonistic properties. In fact, there is some evidence that the pulmonary vasodilator effect of tolazoline is mediated through histamine-2 receptors.[55] Tolazoline has been reported to produce a transient fall in pulmonary vascular resistance in patients with pulmonary hypertension having a major reversible component, including primary pulmonary hypertension.[56–58]

Beta-adrenergic stimulation with isoproterenol has been shown repeatedly to cause pulmonary *vasodilatation.*[6] In contrast, beta-adrenergic blockade does not produce any change in pulmonary vascular resistance, suggesting that there is no tonic activation of beta receptors for maintenance of the normal low pulmonary vascular resistance. *Acetylcholine* is also a potent relaxant of pulmonary arteries and arterioles[33–35] and transiently lowers pulmonary vascular resistance in patients with elevated pulmonary vascular resistance with a major reversible component.

Lung tissue is particularly active in the synthesis, metabolism, and release of a number of the *prostaglandins*, some of which may play a role in the regulation of pulmonary vascular resistance. Prostaglandins I_2 and E are active pulmonary vasodilators, whereas $F_2\alpha$ and A_2 are pulmonary vasoconstrictors.[36] The role of these prostaglandins and their precursors in the regulation of pulmonary vascular tone in humans is uncertain at present. However, the prostaglandin synthesis inhibitor (indomethacin) produced a substantial increase in pulmonary vascular resistance and a decline in cardiac output.[37] If inhibition of prostaglandin synthesis leads to an *increase* in pulmonary vascular resistance, it might be expected that specific prostaglandin infusion might have a vasodilatory effect on the pulmonary vasculature. This was examined in two studies of patients with pulmonary hypertension (primary in nine cases and secondary to thromboembolism and obstructive airway disease in the other two cases) who received an intravenous infusion of PGI_2 (prostacyclin).[38, 39] Pulmonary arterial pressure and pulmonary vascular resistance fell toward normal; however, systemic vascular resistance decreased as well (with resultant systemic hypotension in three of the four cases), and the ratio of pulmonary to systemic vascular resistance remained unchanged or increased in all cases. This suggests that PGI_2 acted as a general vasodilator, without selective pulmonary vascular action.

Histamine, a vasodilator in the systemic circulation, is primarily a vasoconstrictor in the pulmonary vascular bed. Since large doses of histamine receptor blockers or histamine depletors attenuate the hypoxia-induced pulmonary vasoconstrictor response, it has been suggested that histamine may actually be the chemical mediator of hypoxia-induced vasoconstriction in animals.[40–44] This suggestion is supported by the observation that the periarterial mast cells in the rat and guinea pig lung lose their granules and apparently release histamine during hypoxia.[27] However, other experimental findings are contradictory,[13] and as a consequence, the role of histamine in the regulation of the pulmonary circulation in man remains unclear. Perhaps this confusion can be resolved by the finding that histamine may have both pulmonary vasoconstrictor (H_1-receptor) and vasodilator (H_2-receptor) actions.[59–61] In at least one study, histamine acted as a pulmonary vasoconstrictor in the presence of normal oxygenation and as a vasodilator under hypoxic conditions.[59] As mentioned above, tolazoline may act through stimulation of the H_2-receptors.[55]

Serotonin is a potent pulmonary vasoconstrictor in experimental animals[46] but apparently has little or no effect in humans.[47] In this regard, it should be noted that in patients with hepatic metastases of malignant carcinoid of the bowel, large quantities of serotonin are produced and changes in the endocardium and valves of the right side of the heart may occur, but these patients do not exhibit pulmonary hypertension. *Angiotensin II*, generated in the lung by means of enzymatic conversion of angiotensin I, is thought to be a potent pulmonary vasoconstrictor.[27] However, its role in the normal regulation of pulmonary vascular resistance in humans is unknown.

HIGH ALTITUDE. Life at high altitudes is associated with pulmonary hypertension of variable severity, reflecting the range of reactivities of different persons to the pulmonary vasoconstrictive effect of hypoxia.[15, 62–64] As discussed earlier, pulmonary arterial pressure normally declines rapidly following birth at sea level. However, the fall in pulmonary artery pressure of infants born at high altitude may be slower in onset and of lesser magnitude.[65] Mean pulmonary arterial pressure in normal adults living 10,000 feet above sea level is approximately 25 mm Hg[66] and increases to over 50 mm Hg with exercise. The relationship between *cigarette smoking* and chronic obstructive lung diseases is clear.[67–69] Since many patients with chronic obstructive lung diseases exhibit pulmonary hypertension (Chap. 49),[70, 71] cigarette smoking may be considered an indirect stimulus to the development of pulmonary hypertension.

SECONDARY PULMONARY HYPERTENSION

Pulmonary hypertension results when there is increased resistance to blood flow at any of a number of sites within the circulation, the pulmonary vascular bed itself representing only one of these potential sites (Table 26–1). In addition to increased resistance to blood flow, markedly increased flow alone may cause pulmonary hypertension, even when resistance to flow is normal at every point in the circulation. Hypoventilation and its various causes have been listed as a separate category of conditions associated with pulmonary hypertension, although this is somewhat arbitrary, and it might well be argued that these conditions all produce pulmonary hypertension by hypoxic pulmonary vasoconstriction and thus represent a subcategory of increased resistance to flow through the pulmonary vascular bed.

INCREASED RESISTANCE TO PULMONARY VENOUS DRAINAGE

PATHOPHYSIOLOGY. Increased resistance to pulmonary venous drainage is a mechanism common to several conditions of diverse etiology in which pulmonary arterial hypertension occurs. Altered resistance to pulmonary venous drainage may be the result of diseases affecting the left ventricle or pericardium, mitral or aortic valvular disease, or rare entities such as cor triatriatum, left atrial myxoma, or pulmonary veno-occlusive disease (see below).

The magnitude of pulmonary hypertension depends, in part, on the performance of the right ventricle. In response to an acute stress, such as pulmonary embolism, the normal right ventricle of an adult living at sea level can develop systolic pulmonary pressures of 45 to 50 mm Hg, above which right ventricular failure supervenes. Systolic pressures of 80 to 100 mm Hg can be generated only by a hypertrophied right ventricle that is normally perfused. If right ventricular infarction or ischemia has occurred,[72–74] or if the right and left ventricles are both affected by a myopathic process, right ventricular failure will occur at lower levels of pulmonary vascular pressures, and significant pulmonary hypertension may not develop despite an increase in pulmonary vascular resistance.

In the presence of a healthy, nonischemic right ventricle, an increase in left atrial pressure from subnormal levels

TABLE 26–1 CLASSIFICATION OF PULMONARY HYPERTENSION

I. Increased Resistance to Pulmonary Venous Drainage
  A. Elevated left ventricular diastolic pressure
    1. Left ventricular failure
    2. Reduced left ventricular compliance
    3. Constrictive pericarditis
  B. Left atrial hypertension
    1. Mitral valve disease
    2. Cor triatriatum
    3. Left atrial myxoma or thrombus
  C. Pulmonary venous obstruction
    1. Congenital stenosis of pulmonary veins
    2. Anomalous pulmonary venous connection with obstruction
    3. Pulmonary veno-occlusive disease
    4. Mediastinal fibrosis

II. Increased Resistance to Flow Through Pulmonary Vascular Bed
  A. Decreased cross-sectional area of pulmonary vascular bed secondary to parenchymal diseases
    1. Chronic obstructive pulmonary disease
    2. Restrictive lung disease
    3. Collagen-vascular diseases (scleroderma, systemic lupus erythematosus [SLE], rheumatoid arthritis)
    4. Fibrotic reactions (Hamman-Rich syndrome, desquamative interstitial pneumonitis, pulmonary hemosiderosis)
    5. Sarcoidosis
    6. Neoplasm
    7. Pneumonia
    8. Status post pulmonary resection
    9. Congenital pulmonary hypoplasia (Down syndrome)
  B. Decreased cross-sectional area of pulmonary vascular bed secondary to Eisenmenger syndrome
  C. Other conditions associated with decreased cross-sectional area of the pulmonary vascular bed
    1. Primary pulmonary hypertension
    2. Hepatic cirrhosis and/or portal thrombosis
    3. Chemically induced—aminorex fumarate, *Crotalaria* alkaloids
    4. Persistent fetal circulation in the newborn

III. Increased Resistance to Flow Through Large Pulmonary Arteries
  A. Pulmonary thromboembolism
  B. Peripheral pulmonic stenosis
  C. Unilateral absence or stenosis of a pulmonary artery

IV. Hypoventilation
  A. Obesity-hypoventilation syndromes
  B. Pharyngeal-tracheal obstruction
  C. Neuromuscular disorders
    1. Myasthenia gravis
    2. Poliomyelitis
    3. Damage to central respiratory center
  D. Disorders of the chest wall
  E. Pulmonary parenchymal disorders associated with hypoventilation

V. Miscellaneous Causes of Pulmonary Hypertension
  A. Residence at high altitude
  B. Isolated partial anomalous pulmonary venous drainage
  C. Tetralogy of Fallot
  D. Hemoglobinopathies
  E. Intravenous drug abuse
  F. Alveolar proteinosis
  G. Takayasu's disease

up to 7 mm Hg results in a fall in both pulmonary vascular resistance and the pressure gradient across the lungs.[5] These reductions may reflect distention of a population of compliant small vessels or recruitment of additional vascular channels or both. With further increases in left atrial pressure, pulmonary arterial pressure rises along with pulmonary venous pressure, i.e., at a constant pulmonary blood flow, the pressure gradient between the pulmonary artery and veins and the pulmonary vascular resistance remains constant.[5] Finally, when pulmonary venous pressure approaches or exceeds 25 mm Hg on a chronic basis, a disproportionate elevation of pulmonary artery pressure occurs, i.e., the pressure gradient between the pulmonary artery and veins rises while pulmonary blood flow remains constant or falls, indicating an elevation in pulmonary vascular resistance that is due, in part, to pulmonary vasoconstriction. The latter occurs to a variable extent in response to passive elevations of pulmonary venous pressure and probably reflects the reactivity of the pulmonary vasculature, which may be variable between and within species.

In the dog, for example, experimental production of pulmonary venous hypertension rarely results in vasoconstrictive pulmonary hypertension.[75, 76] This probably reflects the low reactivity of the canine vascular bed, since in this species even acute hypoxia fails to elicit a consistent substantial pulmonary vasoconstrictor response. In contrast, the bovine pulmonary vascular bed is more reactive; pulmonary venous constriction in the calf results in substantial and progressive pulmonary arterial vasoconstriction.[77] In the human there is considerable variability in pulmonary arterial vasoconstriction in response to pulmonary venous hypertension. Marked reactive pulmonary hypertension, with pulmonary artery systolic pressures in excess of 80 mm Hg, occurs in somewhat less than one-third of patients with pulmonary venous pressures elevated chronically in excess of 25 mm Hg. The fact that less than one-third of patients with severe mitral stenosis develop severe reactive pulmonary hypertension also argues in favor of a spectrum of variability in pulmonary vascular reactivity to chronic increases in pulmonary venous pressure. This is similar to the marked variability in pulmonary vascular reactivity to hypoxia, discussed earlier. The mechanism involved in elevating pulmonary vascular resistance is unclear. There may be a neural component; also, an elevation of pulmonary venous pressure may narrow or close airways, which may diminish ventilation and lead to hypoxia and, in turn, elevate pulmonary artery pressure. Finally, interstitial pulmonary edema secondary to pulmonary venous hypertension may encroach on the vascular lumen and contribute to the pulmonary arterial hypertension.

Transient, unilateral balloon occlusion of one pulmonary artery in patients with increased pulmonary venous pressure and disproportionate pulmonary arterial hypertension increases the flow through the contralateral lung and produces a substantial fall in vascular resistance.[78] This finding is in contrast to that in normal subjects, in whom increased flow through one lung is not associated with a fall in resistance[5] (Fig. 26–1), and indicates that the increased resistance in patients with pulmonary venous hypertension and markedly elevated pulmonary vascular resistance cannot be due entirely to fixed anatomical changes. Finally, pulmonary vasodilatation in response to the injection of acetylcholine into the pulmonary arteries in some patients with mitral stenosis and severe pulmonary hypertension also supports the concept of a pulmonary arterial vasoconstrictor contribution to the pulmonary hypertension in these patients with chronic increases in pulmonary venous pressure.[33, 35, 79]

The *pulmonary blood volume* is an additional determinant of pulmonary artery pressure in patients with increased resistance to pulmonary venous drainage. The volume of blood in the lungs obviously reflects a balance between inflow and outflow and is therefore influenced by the output of the two ventricles and the relative distensibilities of the pulmonary vascular bed and the left side of the heart. If the output of the left ventricle decreases transiently while that of the right ventricle remains constant, pulmonary blood volume and therefore pulmonary vascular pressures will tend to rise until the outputs of the two ventricles again equalize. Similarly, if the distensibility of the left heart decreases (as may occur in left ventricular hypertrophy, fibrosis, acute ischemia, or constrictive pericarditis) relative to that of the pulmonary vascular bed, pulmonary vascular pressures and blood volume will increase. Obviously, recruitment (i.e., opening of previously unperfused vessels by increasing vascular distensibility) will limit the rise in pulmonary vascular pressure for any given increase in pulmonary blood volume.

PATHOLOGY. *Structural changes* in the pulmonary vascular bed develop in association with chronic pulmonary venous hypertension, irrespective of its etiology. At the ultrastructural level, these changes include swelling of the pulmonary capillary endothelial cells, thickening of their basal lamina, and wide separation of groups of connective tissue fibrils, indicative of interstitial edema. With persistence of the edema, there is proliferation of reticular and elastic fibrils, so that the alveolar capillaries become embedded in dense connective tissue.[5] The permeability of interendothelial junctions depends on pulmonary capillary pressure, with leakage of large molecules (40,000 to 60,000 daltons) occurring at capillary pressures in excess of approximately 30 mm Hg.[80, 81]

Light microscopic examination of the lungs of patients with pulmonary venous hypertension shows distention of pulmonary capillaries, thickening and rupture of the basement membranes of endothelial cells, and transudation of erythrocytes through these ruptured membranes into the alveolar spaces, which contain fragments of disintegrating erythrocytes. Pulmonary hemosiderosis is commonly observed (Fig. 6–26A, p. 155), and may progress to extensive fibrosis. In the late stages of pulmonary venous hypertension, areas of hemorrhage may be scattered throughout the lungs, edema fluid and coagulum may collect in the alveolar spaces, and there may be widespread organization and fibrosis of pulmonary alveoli. Membranous pneumocytes are absent from the alveolar walls, having been replaced by granular pneumocytes and giving rise to what is termed "cuboidal metaplasia." Occasionally, particularly in patients with chronic pulmonary venous hypertension due to mitral valve disease, ossification of alveolar spaces will occur[82, 83] (Fig. 6–26B, p. 155). Pulmonary lymphatics may become markedly distended, giving the appearance of lymphangiectasis, particularly when the pulmonary venous pressure chronically exceeds 30 mm Hg.

Anatomical changes in the pulmonary arteries in pulmonary hypertension secondary to increased resistance to pulmonary venous drainage depend on whether the pulmonary venous hypertension is the result of a congenital malformation (in which case the alterations are present at birth) or acquired. When pulmonary venous (and therefore arterial) hypertension is *congenital*, the elastic tissue in the main pulmonary artery resembles that of the fetal pulmonary artery and the adult aorta, i.e., the elastic fibrils are long, uniform, unbranched, and parallel to one another. When the pulmonary hypertension is acquired, the elastic tissue in the pulmonary trunk is of the adult pulmonary variety, i.e., the elastic fibrils are short, irregular, and branched and form a loosely arranged network. Structural alterations in the small pulmonary arteries, arterioles, and venules (Fig. 26–4) include medial hypertrophy and intimal fibrosis and, rarely, necrotizing arteritis. However, vasodilatation and plexiform lesions are not seen. As discussed subsequently (p. 802), the latter lesions characterize the "irreversible" forms of pulmonary arterial hypertension, and their absence in that form of pulmonary hypertension associated with chronic pulmonary venous pressure elevation correlates with the reversibility of the pulmonary hypertension.

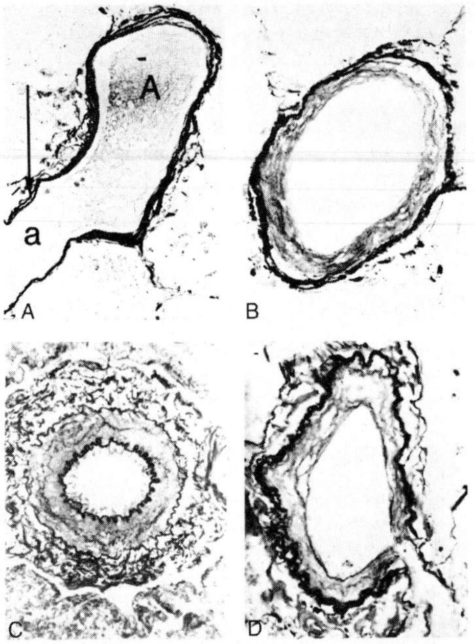

FIGURE 26–4. *A,* Oblique section through a muscular pulmonary artery, A, showing the characteristic thin media bounded by inner and outer elastic laminae. An arteriolar branch, a, arises from the parent vessel and passes downwards and to the left. Its wall consists of a single elastic lamina except near its origin from its parent artery where the remains of a thin media bounded by two elastic laminae can still be seen (arrow) (E, VG × 284). *B,* Transverse section of a normal pulmonary venule. The wall consists of a single elastic lamina. There is considerable intimal fibrosis due to age change. (E. VG × 375). Muscular pulmonary artery (C) and venule (D) in a young woman with severe mitral stenosis. Note the marked hypertrophy in the artery, and the crenated internal elastic lamina, suggesting constriction. The venule shows severe intimal fibrosis. (Adapted by permission from Harris, P., and Heath, D.: The Human Pulmonary Circulation. 3rd ed. New York, Churchill Livingstone, 1986, pp. 338 and 341.)

Morphological changes in pulmonary blood vessels have correlated with the hemodynamic findings in patients with mitral stenosis who underwent both hemodynamic assessment and lung biopsy. Medial hypertrophy in the small muscular pulmonary arteries and muscularization of arterioles occurred only when pulmonary vascular resistance exceeded 260 dynes-sec-cm^{-5} · M^2,[84] but a linear relationship did not exist between the degree of medial hypertrophy and the level of pulmonary vascular resistance, suggesting that factors in addition to medial hypertrophy caused the pulmonary hypertension. Pulmonary lymphangiectasis occurred only with marked elevations of pulmonary venous pressure, and the presence of pulmonary hemosiderosis did not correlate well with the level of the pulmonary artery wedge pressure.

PULMONARY HYPERTENSION SECONDARY TO ELEVATION OF LEFT VENTRICULAR DIASTOLIC PRESSURE

Left ventricular systolic failure resulting from ischemic heart disease, hypertension, left-sided valvular heart disease, or cardiomyopathy will result in (1) increased left ventricular end-systolic volume, (2) higher ventricular end-diastolic pressure, and (3) passive elevations of left atrial, pulmonary venous, and pulmonary arterial pressures. Since chronic increases in mean left ventricular filling pressure exceeding 25 mm Hg are uncommon, the resultant pulmonary arterial hypertension will be only moderate, unless increases in pulmonary vascular resistance occur. In the absence of an increase in the latter, a normal pulmonary artery mean pressure of 15 mm Hg may rise to approximately 30 mm Hg as a result of severe left ventricular failure, characterized by an increase of 15 mm Hg in left ventricular mean diastolic pressure (e.g., from 10 to 25 mm Hg). Since cardiac output is usually reduced in such patients, the mean pulmonary artery pressure would be considerably less than 30 mm Hg if pulmonary vascular resistance remained unchanged. However, many patients with left ventricular failure exhibit increased pulmonary vascular resistance (i.e., in the range of 200 to 300 dynes-sec-cm^{-5}) and moderately severe pulmonary hypertension (pulmonary artery systolic and mean pressures exceeding 60 and 40 mm Hg, respectively).

Decreased left ventricular distensibility resulting from a variety of causes may be associated with increased resistance to left ventricular filling, elevation of left ventricular end-diastolic pressure, and passive increases in left atrial, pulmonary venous, and pulmonary arterial pressures.[85] Specific conditions associated with decreased left ventricular distensibility include concentric left ventricular hypertrophy from a variety of causes,[85–87] diffuse fibrosis as a consequence of ischemic disease,[88] and restrictive cardiomyopathy of various etiologies.[89–91] These causes of pulmonary arterial hypertension should be distinguished from those secondary to left ventricular systolic failure, since they do not respond to digitalis or other inotropic drugs. Usually, the levels of pulmonary hypertension in such patients are only moderate, and increases in pulmonary vascular resistance are less marked than with other causes of elevated pulmonary venous pressure.

Constrictive pericarditis (Chap. 44) is also associated with increased pulmonary artery pressures as a result of an increase in the resistance to pulmonary venous drainage into the left side of the heart. Pulmonary artery systolic pressure is usually only mildly increased in this condition, ranging from 35 to 45 mm Hg at rest,[91] but commonly exceeding 50 to 60 mm Hg in such patients during exertion.[92]

PULMONARY HYPERTENSION SECONDARY TO LEFT ATRIAL HYPERTENSION

Mitral Stenosis (See also Chap. 33)

This valvular lesion represents an important cause of pulmonary hypertension.[93] While this is initially a result of an increase in resistance to pulmonary venous drainage, many patients subsequently exhibit marked pulmonary vasoconstriction and anatomical changes in vessels, so that the pulmonary hypertension is "reactive" as well as "passive." The elevation of pulmonary vascular resistance and the associated pulmonary hypertension may come to dominate the clinical picture in mitral stenosis (Fig. 26–5).[94–97] Thus, patients with mitral stenosis often develop what might be considered to be a more proximal obstruction at the level of the pulmonary arterioles and small muscular arteries (the "second stenosis"), with resultant pulmonary hypertension equal to or exceeding systemic arterial pressure. The clinical picture in such patients is characterized by right ventricular failure with distended neck veins, hepatomegaly, and ascites (p. 1026). Patients exhibit marked fatigue, occasionally a more serious complaint than dyspnea. The murmur of mitral stenosis may be soft or even inaudible, and the opening snap of the stenotic mitral valve may be indistinguishable from a loud pulmonic component of S_2, owing to narrowing of the S_2–opening snap interval. Pulmonary congestion and edema may not be prominent clinically. Cardiac output is usually markedly reduced. This constellation of findings may obscure the underlying diagnosis of mitral stenosis and suggest instead either primary pulmonary hypertension or pulmonary hypertension secondary to some other disorder, such as chronic recurrent pulmonary embolism.

DIAGNOSTIC STUDIES.[98] These usually permit identification of the cause of the severe pulmonary hypertension. The echocardiogram shows left atrial enlargement and other features characteristic of mitral stenosis (p. 1030). At cardiac catheterization, the pulmonary arterial hypertension is associated with substantial elevations of the pulmonary wedge pressure, and there is generally a sizable (> 10 mm Hg) pressure gradient between pulmonary capillary wedge and left ventricular diastolic pressures. The latter finding is of key importance in distinguishing mitral stenosis from primary pulmonary hypertension, a condition in which left atrial size and the wedge pressure are normal and in which there is no diastolic pressure gradient between the wedge and left ventricular pressures (p. 810).

In general, acute elevations of pulmonary venous pressure equal to or greater than 25 mm Hg result in the formation of pulmonary edema. However, pulmonary venous pressure may rise gradually to levels of 35 mm Hg or more without the development of gross pulmonary edema.[95, 99–101]

PROTECTION AGAINST PULMONARY EDEMA. At least three mechanisms that tend to protect against pulmonary edema formation are operative in patients with mitral stenosis and chronic elevations of pulmonary venous pressure in excess of 25 mm Hg (Chap. 18). First, lymphatic drainage of the pulmonary interstitium increases abruptly when pulmonary venous pressure is increased to 25 mm Hg.[102, 103] Acute increases in pulmonary lymph flow of up to eight times the resting level will occur when pulmonary venous pressure is raised to 30 mm Hg for a 10-minute interval, and the increased lymphatic flow will persist at high levels for 30 to 60 minutes after pulmonary venous pressure has returned to normal.[102] In models of *chronic* pulmonary venous pressure elevation, increases in pulmonary lymph flow of up to 28 times normal have been observed.[103] Histological evidence of marked dilatation of the pulmonary lymphatics has been observed in some patients with chronic left atrial pressure overload.[2, 5, 104] Thus, despite the imbalance of Starling forces at the capillary level, the edema fluid may be drained away as rapidly as it is formed, and as a result chronic elevation of pulmonary venous pressure to levels exceeding 30 to 35 mm Hg may not lead to clinical evidence of pulmonary edema.

Diminished permeability of the capillary alveolar barrier is a second protective mechanism that might be operative in patients with *chronic* pulmonary venous hypertension in excess of 25 mm Hg. There is morphological evidence of thickening of the layer between the capillary lumen and the alveolar space.[105–108] A third mechanism operating in patients with chronic increased resistance to pulmonary venous drainage is the reactive constriction of small muscular pulmonary arteries and arterioles (Fig. 26–4). This constriction, which results in considerable elevation of pulmonary artery pressure, is usually associated with a significant decline in right ventricular output (and therefore pulmonary blood flow). The lower pulmonary blood flow tends to diminish the formation of pulmonary edema, since it results in substantially lower left atrial and pulmonary venous pressures at any given size of the mitral valve orifice[109] or for any given impairment of left ventricular

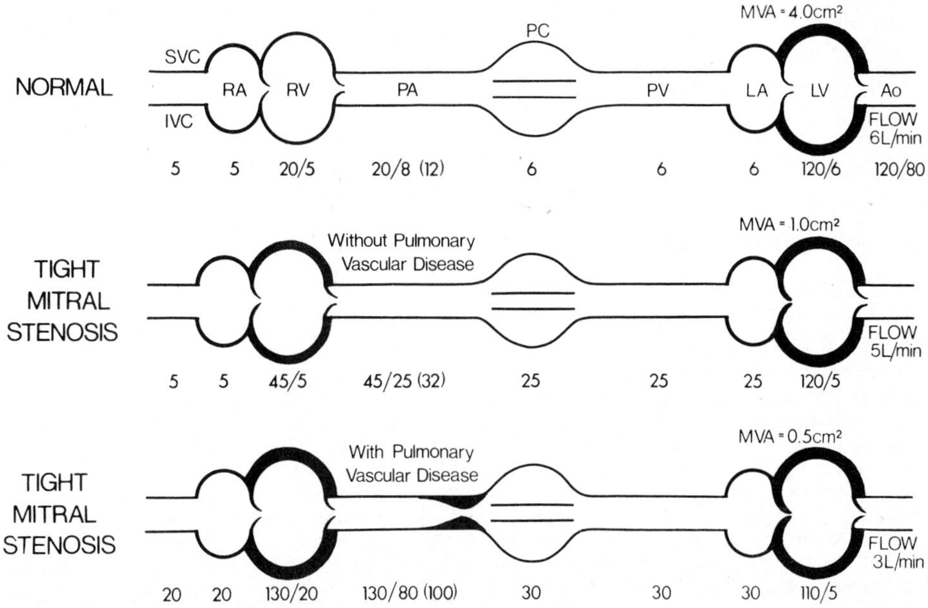

FIGURE 26–5. Schematic diagram of cardiopulmonary circulation in patients with tight mitral stenosis with and without pulmonary vascular disease. Pressures (in mm Hg) are listed for the superior and inferior venae cavae (SVC and IVC), right atrium (RA), right ventricle (RV), pulmonary arteries (PA), capillaries (PC), veins (PV), left atrium (LA), left ventricle (LV), and aorta (Ao) for the normal circulation (*upper panel*) and for the two types of mitral stenosis (*middle and lower panels*). Note that with pulmonary vascular disease (the "second stenosis") severe pulmonary hypertension occurs, and right ventricular failure develops. (Modified from the data of Dexter[95] and Schlant.[96])

function. Despite this protective effect of pulmonary vasoconstriction, pulmonary hypertension is often tolerated poorly in these patients, who commonly show prominent signs of right ventricular failure. Thus, the patient trades pulmonary for peripheral edema and the symptom of dyspnea for the fatigue and lethargy of low cardiac output.

After corrective surgery on the mitral valve, both pulmonary vascular resistance and pulmonary hypertension decline,[110–112] the major extent of which is noted within the first postoperative week. Factors involved in this improvement include reduction of reactive vasoconstriction resulting from (1) distention of the pulmonary vascular bed (i.e., from relief of myogenic vasoconstriction); (2) the resolution of edema within the walls of small arteries and arterioles; and (3) reversal of the morphological changes in Heath-Edwards Grades I to III (p. 802) seen commonly in mitral stenosis.

PULMONARY HYPERTENSION SECONDARY TO PULMONARY VENOUS OBSTRUCTION

Obstruction to pulmonary venous drainage also occurs in association with unusual conditions, such as cor triatriatum, stenosis of pulmonary veins, obstructive forms of anomalous pulmonary venous connection, and pulmonary veno-occlusive disease.

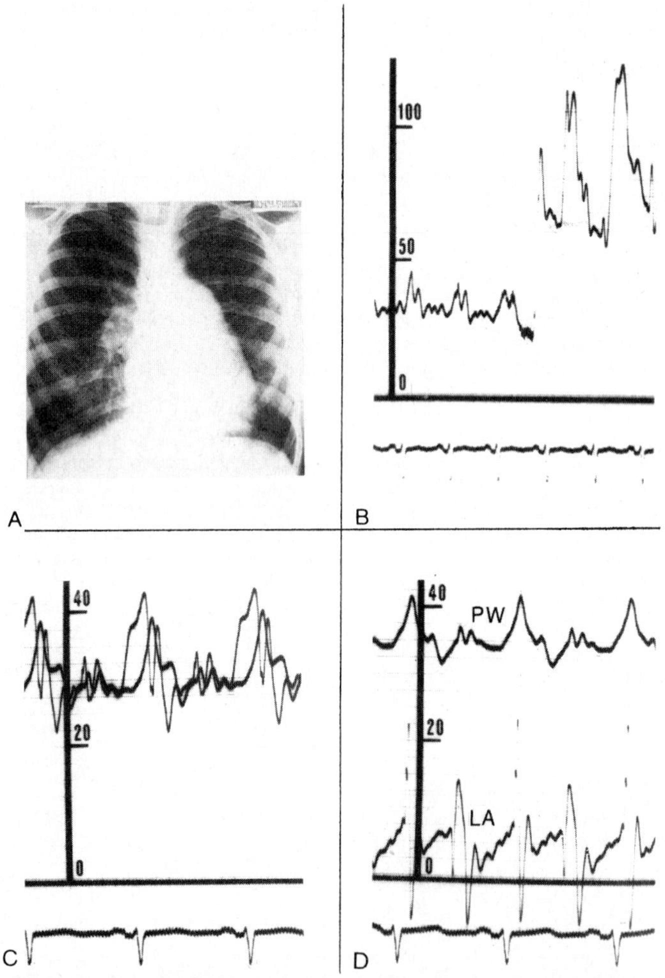

FIGURE 26–6. Findings in a 10-year-old boy with congenital cor triatriatum. The plain chest roentgenograph (*Panel A*) shows very large pulmonary arteries as well as evidence of pulmonary venous hypertension. Catheter pullback (*Panel B*) from pulmonary artery wedge to proximal pulmonary artery indicates that a substantial component of the pulmonary hypertension resides in the pulmonary arteriolar bed. *Panel C* demonstrates equality of pulmonary wedge and pulmonary venous pressures, both of which are considerably elevated compared to pressure low in the left atrium (*Panel D*). (From Harris, P., and Heath, D.: The Human Pulmonary Circulation. 3rd ed. New York, Churchill Livingstone, 1986, p. 356.)

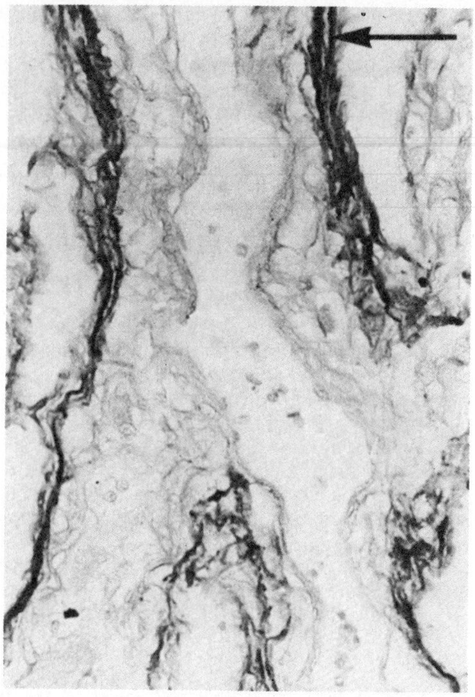

FIGURE 26–7. Longitudinal section of a small pulmonary vein, receiving two venules, from a girl of 16 years with pulmonary veno-occlusive disease. Both the vein and its tributaries show extensive blockage by loose, basophilic fibrous tissue. The remaining lumen, much reduced in size, passes through the vein and one of its tributaries. There is some "arterialization" of the venous media (arrow). (E. VG × 375.) (From Harris, P., and Heath, D.: The Human Pulmonary Circulation. 3rd ed. New York, Churchill Livingstone, 1986, p. 438.)

COR TRIATRIATUM. This is a malformation in which partitioning of the left atrium creates two left atrial subchambers (p. 940). The posterior subchamber receives the pulmonary venous inflow, which then drains through an opening in the partition into the anterior subchamber and thence through the mitral orifice into the left ventricle. When the opening in the partition separating the two left atrial subchambers is small, severe pulmonary venous and pulmonary arterial hypertension result.[113] Findings in a representative case are shown in Figure 26–6. In this patient, pulmonary artery pressure was 120/60 mm Hg, while pulmonary artery wedge and pulmonary venous pressures were equal at more than 30 mm Hg. However, pressure in the anterior subchamber was normal at less than 10 mm Hg. The diagnosis is established by cardiac catheterization, and operative correction may be curative.

PULMONARY VENO-OCCLUSIVE DISEASE. This is an uncommon condition characterized by progressive fibrotic obstruction of the veins and particularly the venules of both lungs.[5] Histological examination may reveal the veins to be blocked by loose fibrous tissue (Fig. 26–7). Later, there may be intimal fibrosis in many veins resembling organization of a thrombus, with a central luminal channel surrounded by a rim of collagenous tissue or with recanalization of a number of wide luminal channels, separated by septa. However, the histological picture in some cases demonstrates extensive blockage of pulmonary venules by basophilic fibrous tissue[5] and intimal proliferation[114] without any evidence of a thrombotic process. The lungs show pulmonary edema with congestion and areas of interstitial fibrosis and hemosiderosis. The involvement of veins and lungs may be diffuse, but in some instances the most severe lesions are focal and not equally distributed. The condition usually affects children or young adults and is characterized clinically by exertional dyspnea, orthopnea, and cyanosis. The pulmonary artery pressure is usually markedly elevated (frequently ≥ 70 mm Hg systolic), and right ventricular failure may be present.

The pathogenesis of the obstructive changes is unknown, and it is debated regarding whether this condition represents a distinct entity or a syndrome of various causes.[115] Since it has been observed that a febrile, influenza-like illness sometimes precedes pulmonary veno-occlusive disease,[5, 114] it has been proposed that a viral infection may deplete the pulmonary venous endothelium of its plasminogen activator, thus leading to in situ thrombosis.[116] In pulmonary veno-occlusive disease, in contrast to primary pulmonary hypertension, the radiographic changes are suggestive of pulmonary venous hypertension with Kerley B lines (Fig. 6–40, p. 164) and sometimes interstitial and alveolar pulmonary edema. However, in some cases there is no radiological evidence of increased pulmonary venous pressure. If the pulmonary veno-occlusive disease affects large veins, the wedge pressure will be elevated, and this measurement will then serve to distinguish this condition from primary pulmonary hypertension.[5] However, if the disease affects primarily the smaller veins, the wedge pressure may not reflect the level of the pressure within the pulmonary capillaries and may even be normal. The explanation for this discrepancy depends on the heterogeneity of pulmonary venular involvement; a theoretical explanation is presented by Harris and Heath.[5]

INCREASED RESISTANCE TO FLOW THROUGH THE PULMONARY VASCULAR BED

PULMONARY PARENCHYMAL DISEASE

Pulmonary hypertension is a common sequel to chronic bronchitis and emphysema (Chap. 49).[70] It had long been believed that the elevated pulmonary artery pressures in patients with emphysema resulted from destruction of the pulmonary vascular bed. Current views minimize this pathogenic pathway, since no direct correlation exists between the severity of the emphysema and the degree of right ventricular hypertrophy.[117, 118]

PATHOPHYSIOLOGY. Hypoxia-induced vasoconstriction probably plays a major role in producing pulmonary hypertension in patients with chronic bronchitis and emphysema.[2, 119–121] There is also evidence for a pulmonary vasoconstrictive action by hydrogen ions, particularly in the presence of hypoxia. In this regard, in patients with chronic obstructive lung disease, pulmonary artery pressure correlates inversely with arterial oxygen saturation and directly with arterial P_{CO_2},[122–125] providing indirect evidence for a role for hypoxia and hypercapnia in the production of pulmonary hypertension. When patients with chronic bronchitis and emphysema inspire high concentrations of oxygen acutely, there is only a modest decrease in pulmonary artery pressure and vascular resistance,[123, 126–128] both of which remain considerably elevated. This suggests that muscular hypertrophy of pulmonary arterioles may in itself be of importance in maintaining the hypoxic pulmonary hypertension.

TRIALS WITH OXYGEN THERAPY. However, the results of two large trials designed to assess the role of long-term oxygen therapy in cor pulmonale due to chronic bronchitis and emphysema have been disappointing.[129, 130] Long-term domiciliary oxygen therapy in one study was associated with no change in mean pulmonary artery pressure after 500 days of oxygen treatment, compared with a 3-mm Hg increase in the control group.[129] In another study, nocturnal oxygen administration was associated with a 7 per cent increase in pulmonary vascular resistance after 6 months, as compared to an 11 per cent decrease in patients receiving continuous oxygen.[130] However, the efficacy of oxygen in prolonging life was greatest in patients with a low pulmonary vascular resistance, and the authors concluded that changes in pulmonary vascular resistance were not the cause of the lower mortality in patients on continuous oxygen therapy.[130] These findings and others[5] suggest that factors other than simple hypoxemic pulmonary hypertension are operative in producing the cor pulmonale of chronic bronchitis and emphysema.

Blood volume and red cell mass, in particular, increase during acute respiratory failure and may contribute to the development of elevated pulmonary arterial pressures. By increasing blood viscosity, increases in hematocrit to within the range commonly seen in chronic bronchitis and emphysema (i.e., 50 to 55 per cent) result in 30 to 50 per cent increases in the transpulmonary arteriovenous pressure gradient at constant blood flow.

SPECIFIC DISORDERS. In patients with *chronic obstructive lung disease*, the extent of destruction of alveoli and the accompanying reductions in alveolar surface area do not correlate closely with the degree of pulmonary hypertension. Thus, the decrease in the cross-sectional area of the pulmonary capillary bed in such patients plays a minor role in elevating pulmonary vascular resistance. A particular association exists between centrilobular (as opposed to panacinar) emphysema and pulmonary hypertension. Right ventricular hypertrophy may occur when only 10 to 15 per cent of the lung is involved in centrilobular emphysema, in contrast to 40 to 70 per cent involvement in patients with panacinar emphysema. This difference may reflect poorer gas exchange in the former circumstance. In patients with advanced bullous emphysema, physical compression of or encroachment on pulmonary capillary beds may play a role, and reduction of pulmonary artery pressure following resection of bullae has been reported[131]; this may be related to reduced compression of the vessel and in part to the associated improvement of gas exchange.

Progressive interstitial pulmonary fibrosis may be associated with pulmonary hypertension. The latter occurs particularly in patients with *progressive systemic sclerosis* (p. 1723), in whom the fibrotic process leads to major reduction in the cross-sectional area of the pulmonary vascular bed due to obliteration of alveolar capillaries and narrowing and obliteration of many small arteries and arterioles.[2, 5] Moreover, a marked elevation of pulmonary artery pressure (≥ 100 mm Hg systolic) and resistance (≥ 2000 dynes-sec-cm^{-5}) in patients with a variant of scleroderma, the *CREST syndrome* (calcinosis, Raynaud's phenomenon, esophageal dysmotility, sclerodactyly, and telangiectasia), has been reported[132] (p. 1723). In patients with the CREST form of *scleroderma*, marked right ventricular dysfunction may be present with right ventricular ejection fractions less than 30 per cent, presumably reflecting systolic overload of the right ventricle due to severe pulmonary vascular disease,[133] and in some instances sclerodermatous narrowing of coronary arteries.

Fibrous obliteration of the pulmonary vascular bed and pulmonary hypertension have also been described in patients with various forms of pulmonary vasculitis (Table 26–2). These include isolated Raynaud's phenomenon,[134–136] dermatomyositis,[137] rheumatoid arthritis,[138] and systemic lupus erythematosus.[136, 139, 140] In the latter a *lupus anticoagulant* may be present in the IgG or IgM fractions of the serum; this may cause a paradoxical hypercoagulable state, intrapulmonary microthrombi, and pulmonary hypertension.[141] Pulmonary hypertension is an uncommon accompaniment of the Hamman-Rich syndrome,[142] desquamative

TABLE 26–2 PULMONARY VASCULITIDES

Vasculitides in which lung is the major organ involved:
Wegener's granulomatosis
Lymphomatoid granulomatosis
Lymphocytic angiitis and granulomatosis
Churg-Strauss syndrome
Overlap vasculitis
Necrotizing sarcoid granulomatosis
Vasculitides in which lung may be involved:
Henoch-Schönlein syndrome
Disseminated leukocytoclastic vasculitis
Cryoglobulinemia
Disseminated giant cell arteritis
Behçet's disease
Takayasu's disease
Polyarteritis nodosa
Diseases in which pulmonary vasculitis may be part of the spectrum of pathology:
Collagen-vascular disorders
Rheumatoid arthritis
Systemic lupus erythematosus
Progressive systemic sclerosis
Eosinophilic pneumonias
Sarcoidosis
Immunoblastic lymphadenopathy
Organic dust diseases (hypersensitivity pneumonitides)
Bronchocentric granulomatosis
Ulcerative colitis
Ankylosing spondylitis
Hughes-Stovin syndrome

From Fulmer, J. D., and Kaltreider, H. B.: The pulmonary vasculitides. Chest 82:615, 1982.

interstitial pneumonia, idiopathic pulmonary hemosiderosis,[143] and sarcoidosis.[5, 144] It is not clear whether significant pulmonary hypertension may result from pulmonary fibrosis due to radiation therapy.

Diffuse lymphatic spread of carcinoma may cause pulmonary hypertension and right heart failure.[145] In many cases tumor microemboli and the attendant thrombotic and fibrotic reaction lead to vascular obstruction. Obstruction of the major pulmonary arteries by tumor (usually sarcoma) may be a cause of right ventricular and main pulmonary artery hypertension.[2, 146] Congenital pulmonary aplasia or hypoplasia, the latter often observed in Down syndrome,[146a] may be responsible for an elevation of pulmonary vascular resistance and pulmonary hypertension.

EISENMENGER SYNDROME

(See also pp. 921 and 999)

Decreased cross-sectional area of the pulmonary arteriolar bed with irreversible pulmonary hypertension characterizes the so-called Eisenmenger syndrome. This term was used by Wood[147] to refer to patients with congenital cardiac lesions and severe pulmonary hypertension in whom reversal of a left-to-right shunt has occurred. Left-to-right shunts are due usually to congenital cardiovascular malformations[148–154] (e.g., atrial and ventricular septal defects, patent ductus arteriosus). Much less commonly they result from acquired lesions (e.g., ventricular septal defect secondary to acute myocardial infarction).

PATHOPHYSIOLOGY (p. 796). Pulmonary hypertension in congenital heart disease may occur simply because of increased pulmonary blood flow. When chronic, the increased pulmonary flow is often associated with a passive reduction in pulmonary resistance and little elevation of pulmonary vascular pressures. In a normal adult with a pulmonary blood flow (PBF) of 5 liters/min, a pulmonary vascular resistance (PVR) of 60 dynes-sec-cm^{-5}, and a mean left atrial pressure (LA) of 6 mm Hg, the pulmonary artery mean pressure (PA) may be calculated from the expression

$$PVR = \frac{(PA - LA)80}{PBF} = \frac{(PA - 6)80}{5} = 60 \text{ dynes-sec-cm}^{-5}$$

$$PA = \frac{60 \times 5}{80} + 6 = 10 \text{ mm Hg}$$

If PBF is doubled, a reduction in PVR to 30 dynes-sec-cm^{-5} will maintain PA mean pressure at a normal level of 10 mm Hg. However, if PBF is increased four- to sixfold, the reserve capacity of the pulmonary vascular bed will be exceeded, and pulmonary artery pressure will rise. Thus, if the PVR is 30 dynes-sec-cm^{-5}, a PBF of 30 liters/min will be associated with a mean PA pressure that is only minimally elevated at 17 mm Hg, although the high right ventricular stroke volumes associated with the augmentation in pulmonary blood flow result in considerably higher values (40 to 45 mm Hg) for pulmonary artery and right ventricular systolic pressures. If the capacity of the pulmonary vascular bed to accommodate extra blood flow is diminished owing to mild parenchymal lung disease that results in a higher, albeit normal, PVR of 90 dynes-sec-cm^{-5}, the mean PA pressure in the patient with a PBF of 30 liters/min will approximate 40 mm Hg; systolic PA and right ventricular pressures may exceed 60 mm Hg. If no underlying arteriolar vascular disease exists, abolition of the shunt by corrective operation restores pulmonary blood flow and PA pressure to normal.

Commonly, an increase in pulmonary vascular resistance makes a variable contribution to the pulmonary hypertension associated with congenital heart disease. The increase in vascular resistance may have both a functional and a fixed component. The former—the "Bayliss" or myogenic theory—is thought to be related to pulmonary arteriolar vasoconstriction stimulated by distention of muscular pulmonary arteries and arterioles. According to this concept, distention of the vessel acts as a stimulus to vasoconstriction, which leads to increased work of the vascular smooth muscle and in turn to hypertrophy of the smooth muscle in the vessel wall.[5]

If a congenital cardiovascular defect causes pulmonary hypertension from the time of birth, the small, muscular arteries of the fetal lung may ndergo delayed or only partial involution, resulting in persistently high levels of pulmonary vascular resistance (p. 905). This is true especially of those lesions in which a left-to-right shunt enters the right ventricle or pulmonary artery directly (i.e., a post–tricuspid valve shunt, such as ventricular septal defect or patent ductus arteriosus); these patients experience a higher incidence of severe and irreversible pulmonary vascular damage than those in whom the shunt is proximal to the tricuspid valve (pre-tricuspid shunts, as in atrial septal defect and partial anomalous pulmonary venous drainage). In the latter category, pulmonary pressures fall after birth, and the fetal vascular pattern usually regresses; later in life, however, pulmonary hypertension may result from a large pre-tricuspid left-to-right shunt, which enhances the risk of pulmonary vascular damage.

PATHOLOGY. The extent of reversibility of pulmonary vascular obstructive disease in the presence of congenital heart disease varies. From an anatomical point of view, reversible conditions are those in which the decreased pulmonary arteriolar cross-sectional area is the result of medial hypertrophy and vasoconstriction; irreversibility is associated with the presence of necrotizing arteritis and plexiform lesions in these small vessels.[2, 148–154] The classification by Heath and Edwards[155] of six grades of structural change is widely employed to assess the potential reversibility of pulmonary vascular disease and is summarized as follows: *Grade I* is characterized by hypertrophy of the media of small muscular pulmonary arteries and arterioles. In *Grade II*, intimal cellular proliferation is added to the medial hypertrophy. *Grade III* is characterized by advanced medial thickening with hypertrophy and hyperplasia, together with progressive intimal proliferation and concentric fibrosis that results in obliteration of many arterioles and small arteries. In *Grade IV*, dilatation and so-called "plexiform lesions" of the muscular pulmonary arteries and arterioles are observed (Fig. 26–8). The latter consist of a plexiform network of capillary-like channels within a dilated segment of a muscular pulmonary artery. The channels are separated by proliferating endothelial cells, which often contain thrombi; indeed, the network of capillary channels may constitute recanalization of a throm-

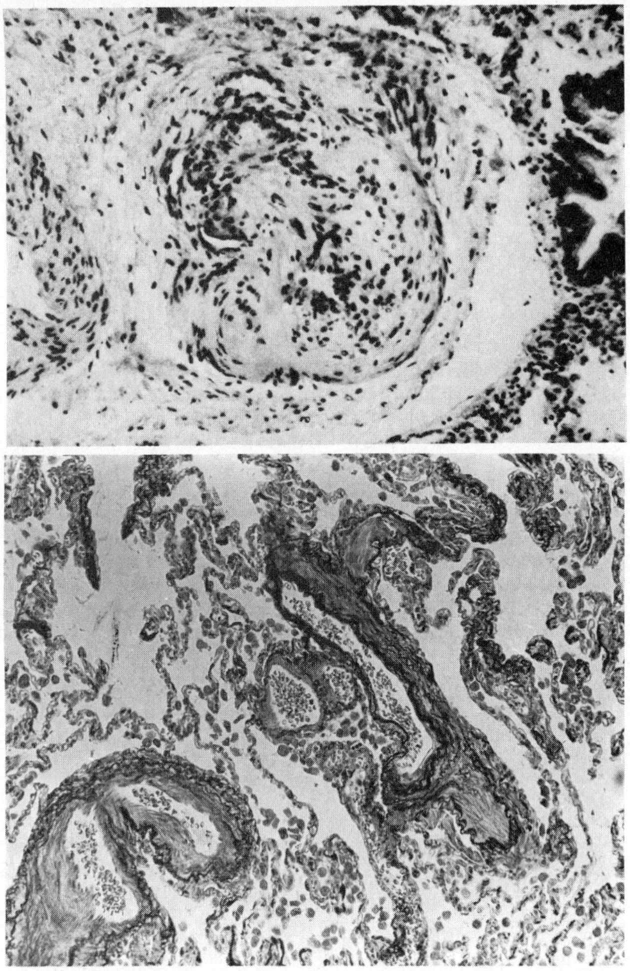

FIGURE 26–8. *Top*, Histological section from the lung of a 3-year-old boy with a common atrioventricular canal and severe pulmonary hypertension. A muscular pulmonary artery with an early plexiform lesion is seen as well as fibrinoid necrosis of the media and active proliferation of intimal cells. (From Wagenvoort, C. A., and Wagenvoort, N.: Pathology of Pulmonary Hypertension. 2nd ed. New York, John Wiley and Sons, 1977.) *Bottom*, Photomicrograph of a lung biopsy specimen from a 35-year-old man with a patent ductus arteriosus and systemic pulmonary hypertension. A predominance of advanced changes is seen, including plexiform and dilatation lesions.

bus. *Grade V* changes include complex plexiform, angiomatous, and cavernous lesions and hyalinization of intimal fibrosis (Fig. 26–9). Finally, *Grade VI* is characterized by the presence of necrotizing arteritis.

The Heath and Edwards classification implies that the morphological alterations are sequential, with Grade I being the earliest stage and Grade VI being the "end stage" of pulmonary vascular obliterative disease. That such an orderly progression may not in fact occur is suggested by the findings of Wagenvoort, which indicate that plexiform lesions develop gradually in areas affected by necrotizing arteritis. They have suggested that fibrinoid necrosis of a small segment of a pulmonary arterial branch leads to medial destruction and subsequent aneurysmal dilatation of the vessel as well as the formation of a fibrin clot in the lumen, often with admixture of platelets.[2, 148] Organization of the fibrin clot by strands of intimal cells leads to formation of the plexus; the small capillary-like channels within the plexus (Fig. 26–8) provide continuity to the distal portion of the artery, which undergoes post-stenotic dilatation. With time, the inflammatory component of the process subsides, fibrin disappears, and the strands of intimal cells become fibrotic. Wagenvoort's view is supported by animal experiments in which end-to-end systemic-pulmonary anastomoses resulted in arteritis and fibrinoid necrosis prior to the appearance of plexiform lesions.[155a, 156] Thus, although Heath-Edwards Grades I, II, and III may represent chronological progression, evidence exists that Grade VI (necrotizing arteritis) changes appear next, followed by Grades IV and V end-stage alterations.

CLINICAL CONSIDERATIONS. As mentioned above, *Eisenmenger syndrome* is the term used by Wood to refer to patients with congenital central communications with severe pulmonary hypertension, in whom reversal of a left-to-right shunt has occurred across the pulmonary-systemic communication.[147] The patients described originally by Eisenmenger had ventricular septal defects, and the term *Eisenmenger complex* is applied to patients with severe pulmonary hypertension and right-to-left shunt through such a defect. The term *Eisenmenger syndrome* is applied to any anomaly in which the pathophysiological process leads to obliterative pulmonary vascular disease, including pre- and post-tricuspid shunts. Heath-Edwards Grades IV to VI changes are usual in these patients; occasionally, lesser anatomical changes predominate and may be reversible after successful corrective operation.

When the pulmonary vascular resistance has increased to equal (or exceed) systemic resistance, and the anatomical changes of the pulmonary vessels are predominantly those of Grades IV to VI, surgical closure of the intracardiac communication will fail to relieve pulmonary hypertension and will be associated with a prohibitive immediate risk.

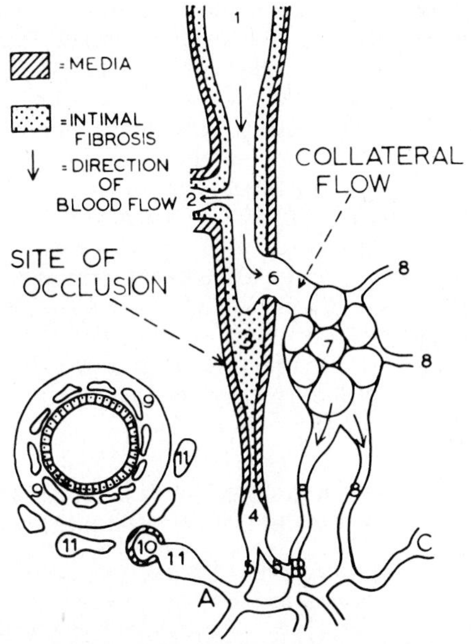

FIGURE 26–9. Diagram to show the origin and probable connections of small thin-walled blood vessels in the lung in grade 5 hypertensive pulmonary vascular disease. 1 = Dilated muscular pulmonary artery with thin media and intimal fibrosis: this is part of the generalized dilatation proximal to the site of vascular occlusion. 2 = Hypertrophied muscular pulmonary artery arising as a side branch of 1 with heaped-up intimal fibrous tissue at the site of origin. 3 = Terminal muscular pulmonary artery totally occluded by fibrous tissue: the media may be thick, as shown, or abnormally thin. 4 = Terminal dilated pulmonary arteriole. 5 = Capillaries in alveolar walls arising from pulmonary arteriole. 6 = Dilated, thin-walled, vein-like branch of hypertrophied parent muscular pulmonary artery. 7 = Localized "dilatation lesion:" an angiomatoid lesion is shown. 8 = Capillaries in alveolar walls arising from dilatation lesions. 9 = Dilated thin-walled vessel in submucosa of small bronchus. 10 = Small bronchial artery in fibrous coat of small bronchus giving rise to thin-walled branches shown as 11. A = Bronchopulmonary anastomosis at capillary level. B = Anastomosis between capillaries arising from parent muscular pulmonary artery and from "dilatation lesions." C = Possible anastomosis between thin-walled vessels derived from pulmonary artery and those derived from pulmonary vein. (From Harris, P., and Heath, D.: The Human Pulmonary Circulation. 3rd ed. New York, Churchill Livingstone, 1986, p. 255.)

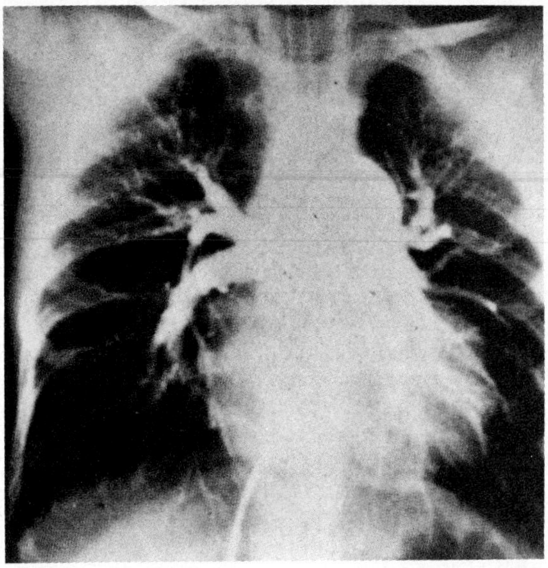

FIGURE 26–10. Pulmonary arteriogram of a boy aged 4 years with a ventricular septal defect and patent ductus arteriosus and reversed shunt. The narrowness of the peripheral branches of the pulmonary artery contrasts with the dilation of its main branches. Pulmonary arterial pressure, 90/60 mm Hg; wedge pressure, 4 mm Hg. Pulmonary blood flow, 1.6 l · min⁻¹; systemic flow 3.2 l · min⁻¹. (From Harris, P., and Heath, D.: The Human Pulmonary Circulation. 3rd ed. New York, Churchill Livingstone, 1986, p. 317.)

Operation will, in fact, hasten death in most survivors who had either balanced shunts or predominant right-to-left shunts, since closure of the right-to-left communication merely increases the load on an already overburdened right ventricle. Structural changes in the pulmonary vascular bed are evident in pulmonary arteriograms, which reveal dilated main branches and narrowing of the peripheral branches (Fig. 26–10). These changes can be evaluated by means of quantitative analysis of the pulmonary wedge angiogram.[157] This technique has been employed successfully by Rabinovitch, Reid, and coworkers, who have demonstrated progressively more abrupt tapering of the pulmonary arteries in patients with increasingly abnormal hemodynamics and increasingly severe structural changes in lung biopsy tissue (Fig. 26–11).[157]

Other Conditions Associated With Decreased Cross-sectional Area of the Pulmonary Vascular Bed

PRIMARY PULMONARY HYPERTENSION. This condition has been more recently called "unexplained pulmonary hypertension" by a working committee of the World Health Organization[158] and is discussed in detail beginning on the next page.

HEPATIC CIRRHOSIS AND PORTAL VEIN THROMBOSIS. These conditions have been occasionally associated with pulmonary hypertension and obliterative changes in the pulmonary arteriolar bed.[158–161] Fishman has speculated that there is a common pathophysiological mechanism to these cases and others in which pulmonary hypertension is associated with ingestion of a variety of substances (*Crotalaria* alkaloids, aminorex[162]), and he has termed this "dietary pulmonary hypertension."[163] According to this concept, certain metabolites of ingested foods or drugs may induce pulmonary hypertension if they gain access to the pulmonary circulation or, if by damaging the liver, they lead to release of vasoactive substances that subsequently reach the lungs and injure pulmonary vessels.

PERSISTENT FETAL CIRCULATION IN THE NEWBORN. This condition has been reported as a cause of severe pulmonary hypertension.[164–166] Affected infants exhibit cyanosis, tachypnea, acidemia, normal pulmonary parenchymal markings on chest x-ray, and anatomically normal hearts. Cyanosis is the result of right-to-left shunting across the foramen ovale and through a patent ductus arteriosus.[164] The condition may be due to persistence of extremely muscular small pulmonary arteries, a diminution in the absolute number of these resistance vessels, or a combination of the two.[166]

Increased Resistance to Flow Through Large Pulmonary Arteries

PULMONARY THROMBOEMBOLISM (Chap. 47). This condition may cause pulmonary hypertension by impeding blood flow through the major pulmonary arteries and their branches. Generally, a single episode of pulmonary embolism resolves, and follow-up studies reveal normal pulmonary vasculature and pressure in the majority of patients.[167, 168] Occasionally, chronic pulmonary hypertension results when repeated, multiple emboli fail to resolve.

PERIPHERAL PULMONIC STENOSIS. This is a congenital lesion that occurs particularly in association with supravalvular aortic stenosis or as a sequela of the rubella syndrome (p. 941). Hypertension in the proximal pulmonary arteries depends on the extent, location, and severity of the stenotic lesions.[2, 169, 170]

UNILATERAL ABSENCE OF EITHER THE RIGHT OR THE LEFT PULMONARY ARTERY. This is a rare congenital anomaly.[171] Often the condition is associated with a ventricular septal defect or patent ductus arteriosus, and the incidence of pulmonary hypertension is high. Pulmonary hypertension may also be observed in the absence of associated abnormalities, presumably because the thick-walled fetal pulmonary arterial bed is stimulated to constrict and undergo anatomical obliterative changes when the total cardiac output flows through only one lung from birth onward. The same mechanism may operate in patients with unilateral pulmonary artery stenosis in whom elevated pressure is observed in the main and uninvolved pulmonary arteries. Relief of the obstructive lesion by operation has been associated with marked improvement.[172]

Hypoventilation

As discussed earlier in this chapter, conditions associated with hypoxia may cause pulmonary hypertension, particularly if there is

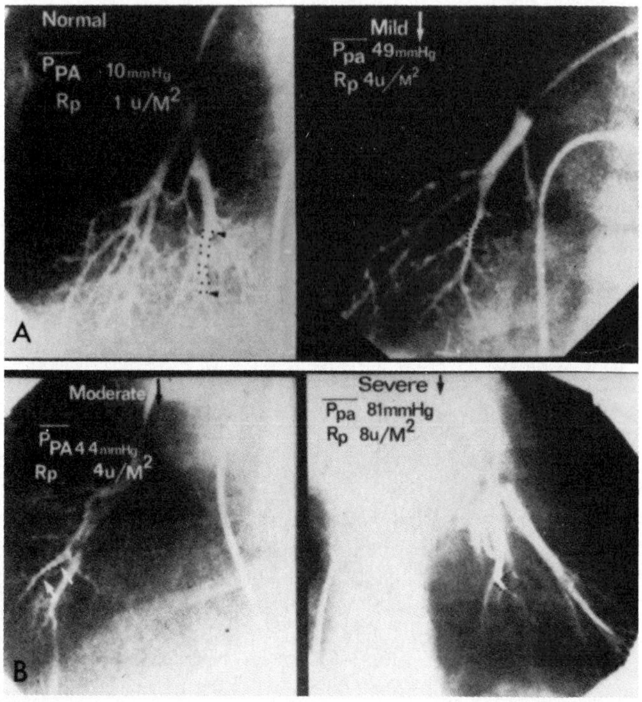

FIGURE 26–11. ***A,*** **The left panel is a wedge angiogram from a patient with normal mean pulmonary artery pressure ($\bar{P}_{pa}$). There is gradual tapering of the arteries (arrows indicate luminal diameters of 2.5 mm and 1.5 mm) and dense background haze. The right-hand panel is a wedge angiogram from a patient with elevated $\bar{P}_{pa}$ and mild elevation of pulmonary vascular resistance (Rp); the arteries taper more abruptly (see arrows), and the background haze is mildly decreased.** ***B,*** **The left panel is a wedge angiogram from a patient with elevated Rp in whom the arteries taper abruptly (see arrows at luminal diameters of 2.5 mm and 1.5 mm), and the background haze is moderately decreased. The right-hand panel is a wedge angiogram from a patient with severe elevation in RP in whom the arteries taper very abruptly (see arrows), and the background haze is severely reduced. (From Rabinovitch, M., Keane, J. F., Fellows, K. E., et al.: Quantitative analysis of the pulmonary wedge angiogram in congenital heart defects. Circulation *63*:152, 1981, by permission of the American Heart Association, Inc.)**

associated acidemia.[29-31] A number of disorders that affect the upper airways, neuromuscular control, or pulmonary parenchyma lead to hypoventilation and (in the setting of a reactive pulmonary vascular bed) pulmonary hypertension.

THE OBESITY-HYPOVENTILATION SYNDROME[173, 174] (See also p. 1610). Also called the pickwickian syndrome, this condition may lead to substantial pulmonary hypertension (mean pulmonary artery pressure ≥ 50 mm Hg), which correlates with the presence of hypoxemia and acidosis (Fig. 48–4, p. 1601). *Pharyngeal-tracheal obstruction* occurs in the presence of hypertrophied tonsils and adenoids[175, 176] and may cause reversible pulmonary hypertension.

NEUROMUSCULAR DISORDERS. These include myasthenia gravis, poliomyelitis, and damage to the central respiratory center.[177] They may cause hypoventilation of sufficient severity to result in pulmonary hypertension (p. 1609). *Disorders of the chest wall* (kyphoscoliosis, pectus excavatum) may also cause hypoventilation and pulmonary hypertension (p. 1610).

The pulmonary hypertension in all of these conditions subsides with restoration of normal respiration and correction of the hypoxia. It should also be recognized that hypoxia may intensify pulmonary hypertension of other causes. For example, severe pulmonary hypertension occurring in children with a left-to-right shunt who reside at high altitude is often due to the combination of high pulmonary blood flow and superimposed hypoxic pulmonary vasoconstriction; pulmonary pressures may fall rapidly toward normal when residence is established at sea level.

Other Causes of Pulmonary Hypertension

HIGH-ALTITUDE PULMONARY EDEMA (See also p. 551). This entity is associated with reversible pulmonary hypertension. It is observed particularly in individuals acclimatized to high altitudes who, after a stay of some days or weeks at sea level, return to high altitude.[178] The finding of high-altitude pulmonary edema in four persons without a right pulmonary artery has been reported,[179] giving support to speculation concerning the combined role of hypoxia and hyperperfusion in patients with this anomaly.[180]

OTHER CONDITIONS. Severe pulmonary hypertension is an occasional but unusual finding in patients with *isolated partial anomalous pulmonary venous drainage*.[181] Speculation exists that the cause may be the increase in pulmonary blood flow associated perhaps with a reflex pulmonary arterial vasoconstriction secondary to distention of the right atrium.

The cause of the pulmonary hypertension that occasionally develops following surgical correction of *tetralogy of Fallot* is unclear. In the patient with tetralogy of Fallot, pulmonary vascular thrombotic lesions are common and, if extensive, may predispose to pulmonary hypertension when operation—either complete correction or creation of a left-to-right shunt—causes a sudden increase in pulmonary blood flow.[2, 182]

Sickle cell anemia may be complicated by in situ pulmonary thrombosis and infarction (p. 1736), although this does not usually lead to pulmonary hypertension. There are two case reports of cor pulmonale associated with hemoglobin SC disease,[183, 184] but the prevalence of pulmonary hypertension in individuals with this condition is unknown.

Intravenous drug abuse may lead to diffuse pulmonary vascular occlusion and pulmonary hypertension, as in the case of a 25-year-old man who intravenously injected himself with crushed, dissolved pentazocine.[185] After 1 month he developed chest pain, shortness of breath, and fatigue and was found to have a pulmonary artery pressure of 72/30 mm Hg (mean 46 mm Hg) with a right atrial pressure of 14 mm Hg. Analysis of lung biopsy material implicated embolization of the cellulose filter material in the tablet with subsequent severe tissue reaction and granuloma formation. Prednisone therapy led to improvement in the clinical state and gradual lowering of the pulmonary artery pressure.

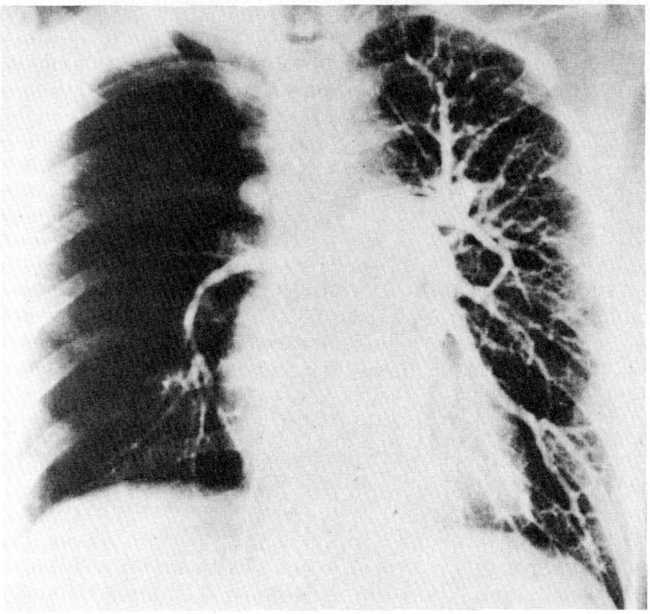

FIGURE 26–12. Pulmonary angiogram from a 27-year-old Japanese woman with Takayasu's disease and pulmonary hypertension. There is marked narrowing of the right pulmonary artery and no appearance of its branches. (Reprinted with permission from Kawai, C.: Pulmonary pulseless disease: Pulmonary involvement in so-called Takayasu's disease. Chest *73*:651, 1978.)

A patient in whom moderately severe pulmonary hypertension developed in association with *alveolar proteinosis* has been reported.[186] Hypoxemia seemed to be the mediating factor, and the patient showed substantial reduction in pulmonary artery pressure (60/25 mm Hg to 32/14 mm Hg) in response to oxygen inhalation. Pulmonary arterial involvement with pulmonary hypertension has been reported to occur in approximately 25 per cent of patients with *Takayasu's disease*.[187-189] The pulmonary pressure elevations are usually only moderate, but striking abnormalities may be present on lung scan or pulmonary angiogram (Fig. 26–12). Histological changes include thickening of the intima and hypertrophy of the media of the small pulmonary arteries.

PRIMARY (UNEXPLAINED) PULMONARY HYPERTENSION

In some patients with pulmonary hypertension, no cause is discernible, in which case the pulmonary hypertension is termed idiopathic, essential, unexplained,[158] or, most frequently, *primary*.[190-192] In contrast to systemic hypertension, in which the etiology is primary (essential) in a large percentage of patients (Chap. 27), primary hypertension in the pulmonary circuit is uncommon. Primary pulmonary hypertension (PPH) is often readily suspected on clinical examination, but the diagnosis should be made only after detailed examination of the heart and lungs, i.e., ordinarily after cardiac catheterization and pulmonary angiography have revealed no specific cause for the pulmonary hypertension.

ETIOLOGY

Although a number of theories have been advanced to explain the origin of PPH, none has as yet gained clear ascendancy. Indeed, were the etiology of the pulmonary hypertension clear, the designation "primary" would not be appropriate.

Recurrent occult systemic venous thrombosis with pulmonary embolism may be extremely difficult to exclude as the cause of pulmonary hypertension.[190-192] A number of patients with chronic, recurrent thromboembolic disease develop pulmonary hypertension and cor pulmonale slowly, with no overt clinical manifestation of pulmonary embolism (p. 1612). Early in their course, such patients may exhibit pulmonary angiographic findings characteristic of emboli, but late in the course such findings may be absent. Therefore, it has been argued that PPH may result from recurrent episodes of asymptomatic pulmonary embolism.[191, 192] In support of this theory is the common autopsy finding of clinically unrecognized organizing or recanalizing pulmonary emboli in patients considered during life to have had PPH.[191–194] Moreover, one can produce experimental pulmonary arterial lesions in animals resembling those seen in patients with PPH by intravenous injection of autologous thrombi or other material (e.g., plant spores or polystyrene beads).[195–197] The fact that PPH occasionally develops or worsens post partum also supports a thromboembolic or an amniotic fluid embolic etiology.

An alternative explanation relates the development of PPH to *thrombosis* in situ in small pulmonary arteries, with resultant widespread pulmonary vascular obstruction. In support of this theory, various defects in coagulation, including abnormal platelet function and defective fibrinolysis, have been demonstrated in patients with PPH.[193, 198–203] A relationship between microangiopathic hemolytic anemia, thrombocytopenia, and PPH has also been suggested. The development of PPH in young women taking contraceptive pills has been thought to be related to the hypercoagulable state that these agents induce.

On the other hand, some pathological studies have demonstrated important morphological differences in the pulmonary vascular bed of patients with thromboembolic or thrombotic pulmonary hypertension, compared with changes noted in patients with PPH (Table 26–3). These findings argue *against* recurrent pulmonary thromboembolism or in situ thrombosis as the unique etiology of PPH.[193, 194, 199, 200] In patients with thromboembolic or thrombotic pulmonary hypertension, thrombi of varying sizes and in various stages of organization can generally be demonstrated in pulmonary arteries and arterioles. By contrast, in many patients with PPH, pulmonary arterioles exhibit intimal fibrosis of the onionskin type, medial hypertrophy, fibrinoid necrosis and arteritis, dilatation, and plexiform lesions (Figs. 26–13 and 26–14); thrombi in pulmonary arteries and arterioles, when present, are small and of recent origin. Although recent studies[191, 192] confirm that perhaps half or more of patients considered on clinical grounds to be suffering from PPH may be found at autopsy to have had chronic thromboembolism, a sizable percentage of patients with a clinical diagnosis of PPH have the pathological picture of plexogenic pulmonary arteriopathy,[190, 192] suggesting a role for intense vasoconstriction with resultant fibrinoid necrosis of the muscular pulmonary arteries.[190]

CONGENITAL DEFECTS. Several of these have been proposed as causes of PPH. A deficiency in the media of the pulmonary arterial bed resulting in intimal thickening and proliferation with consequent obstruction of small pulmonary vessels has been suggested as the underlying defect.[204] Persistence of the fetal pulmonary arterial architecture,[205] increased systemic-pulmonary arterial collaterals,[206–208] and a generalized degenerative pulmonary arteriopathy[209] have also been proposed, although the latter two lesions are felt to be secondary to the pulmonary hypertension itself,[194, 199, 200] and none has been found in the systemic arteries of patients with PPH.

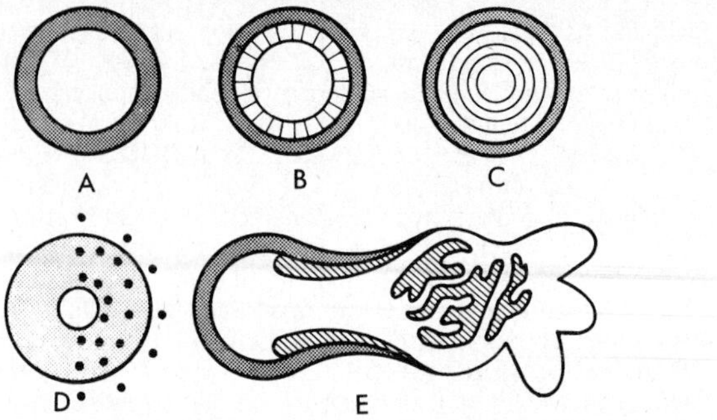

FIGURE 26–13. Plexogenic pulmonary arteriopathy. Arteries with (*A*) medial hypertrophy, (*B*) cellular intimal proliferation, (*C*) concentric-laminar intimal fibrosis, (*D*) fibrinoid necrosis with or without arteritis, and (*E*) plexiform lesions. (From Wagenvoort, C. A., and Wagenvoort, N.: Pathology of Pulmonary Hypertension. New York, copyright 1977, reprinted by permission of John Wiley and Sons, Inc.)

COLLAGEN-VASCULAR DISEASE. The occurrence of an arteritis and of fibrinoid necrosis in the walls of the smaller pulmonary arteries, and the frequent presence of Raynaud's phenomenon in patients with PPH, has led some authorities to suggest that PPH may be a form of collagen-vascular or autoimmune disease.[210, 211] Since Raynaud's phenomenon is an expression of vasospasm in digital arteries, its presence in 10 to 30 per cent of patients with PPH suggests that vasospasm in pulmonary arteries may be present as well. Interestingly, in families of patients with PPH, other members not affected by the disease may exhibit Raynaud's phenomenon. Pulmonary hypertension occurs frequently in patients with the so-called CREST syndrome[132, 133] (p. 801), a variant of scleroderma. The histological changes in the pulmonary vessels in patients with this syndrome resemble those seen in patients with PPH and are similar to those seen in the pulmonary vessels of about 10 per cent of patients with the more usual forms of progressive systemic sclerosis.[132]

TAKAYASU'S (GIANT CELL) ARTERITIS. This frequently involves the pulmonary vessels (Fig. 26–12), but the pathological changes resemble those seen in systemic arteries (p. 802). In the vast majority of these patients, the aorta and major arch vessels are involved as well. This condition can also be distinguished from PPH by the fact that the occlusive changes occur in the large and intermediate vessels rather than in the more distal vessels characteristic of PPH.[188]

OTHER ETIOLOGICAL FACTORS. A number of cases of PPH coexisting with postnecrotic *hepatic cirrhosis* have been reported,

TABLE 26–3 HISTOPATHOLOGICAL DIFFERENTIATION BETWEEN THREE DISEASES WHICH MAY PRESENT CLINICALLY AS "UNEXPLAINED PULMONARY HYPERTENSION"

	Muscular Pulmonary Arteries					Pulmonary Veins and Venules	
Disease	Type of Intimal Proliferation	Medial Hypertrophy	Plexiform Lesions	Fibrinoid Necrosis	Arteritis	Intimal Fibrosis	State of Media
Primary pulmonary hypertension	Concentric onion-skin type; occasional thrombi near fibrinoid necrosis	Severe in early stages; less severe in late stages	Common	Frequent	Frequent	Age change only	Normal
Recurrent pulmonary thromboembolism	Fresh, organizing and recanalized thrombi; eccentric pads of intimal fibroelastosis	Slight, except at site of thrombus	Absent	Absent	Very rare (only with infected emboli)	Age change only	Normal
Pulmonary veno-occlusive disease	Usually absent or slight	Slight	Absent	Very rare	Very rare	Loose fibrosis leading to widespread pronounced occlusion; recanalization common	Mimics that of muscular pulmonary artery

From Harris, P., and Heath, D.: The Human Pulmonary Circulation. 3rd ed. New York, Churchill Livingstone, 1986, p. 415.

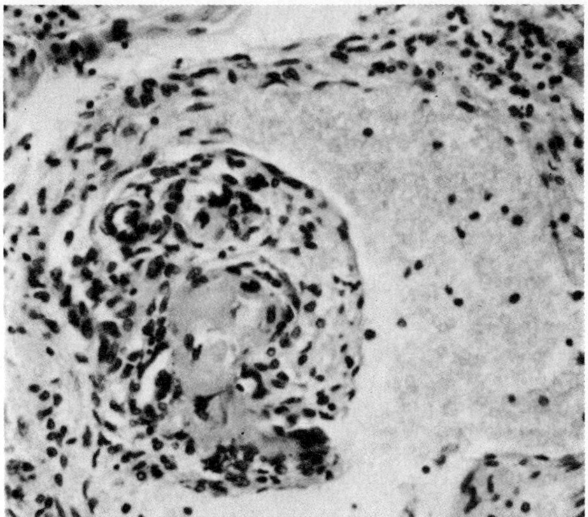

A

B

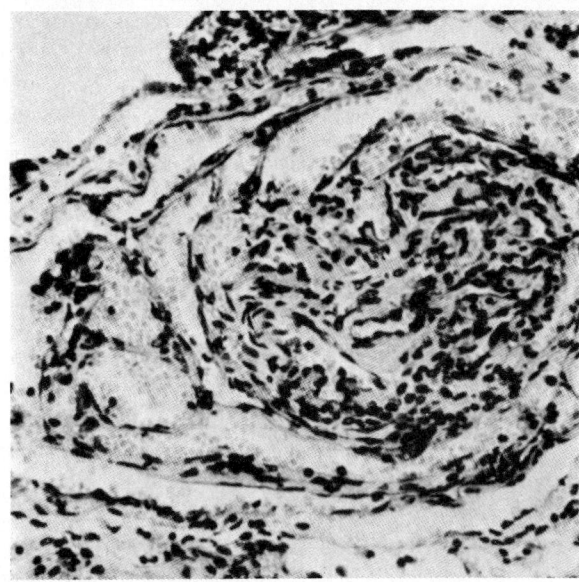

FIGURE 26–14. *A*, Early plexiform lesion of muscular pulmonary artery in a 13-year-old girl with unexplained plexogenic pulmonary arteriopathy. There is active proliferation of cells in a fibrin clot (hematoxylin and eosin, × 225). *B*, Full-grown plexiform lesion in muscular pulmonary artery in a 28-year-old woman with unexplained plexogenic pulmonary arteriopathy (hematoxylin and eosin, × 225). (From Wagenvoort, C. A., and Wagenvoort, N.: Pathology of Pulmonary Hypertension. New York, copyright 1977, reprinted by permission of John Wiley and Sons, Inc.)

suggesting that a vasculitis might be responsible for the pulmonary hypertension.[212–216] *Polyarteritis nodosa* and *hypersensitivity to a variety of drugs*, including penicillin, chloramphenicol, and the sulfonamides, have also been suggested as etiologies for PPH,[200, 217] although allergic vasculitis is unlikely to affect only the pulmonary vasculature.[194] Occasionally a patient with PPH has been erroneously diagnosed as suffering from polyarteritis nodosa limited to the lungs.[194, 218]

AMINOREX FUMARATE. Pulmonary hypertension has developed in a number of individuals who had ingested this anorexigenic drug.[219–221] The clinical course of these patients was similar to that of patients with PPH, although in some instances regression of pulmonary hypertension upon withdrawal of the drug was reported.[222] Although causation has not been demonstrated definitively, the circumstantial evidence in favor of this relationship is impressive.[190] Since only 0.2 per cent of individuals ingesting the drug develop pulmonary hypertension, some other factor such as a genetic predisposition or an idiosyncratic reaction must be involved.

MONOCROTALINE. Severe pulmonary hypertension can be produced in rats by the administration of *monocrotaline* or other pyrrolizidine alkaloids derived from the seeds of the plant *Crotalaria spectabilis* or of *fulvine*, an alkaloid derived from *Crotalaria fulva*.[223, 224] Severe necrotizing pulmonary arteritis and luminal obstruction in small venules develops in these animals.

Monocrotaline-induced pulmonary vascular disease appears to follow activation of lung ornithine decarboxylase, an important enzyme in the biosynthesis of polyamines, such as spermidine and spermine.[225] A role for platelets in the production of pulmonary hypertension following monocrotaline lung injury has been suggested by recent work[226] using antiplatelet antiserum to induce thrombocytopenia. When given 3 to 6 days after monocrotaline administration, the antiplatelet serum substantially blunted the development of pulmonary hypertension.[226] Although natives of the West Indies who ingest *Crotalaria fulva* in "bush tea" may develop veno-occlusive disease of the liver,[227] no instances of pulmonary hypertension in humans have been attributed to *Crotalaria*.

FEMALE HORMONES. The following observations suggest that *female hormones* may be involved in the genesis of PPH: (1) This condition occurs most frequently in pubertal females, (2) there is a tendency for exacerbations to occur in the postpartum period, and (3) there may be an association between the use of oral contraceptives and the development of PPH.[228] The manner in which this endocrine effect may operate on the pulmonary vascular bed is obscure.

Thus, in most patients considered on clinical grounds to have PPH, no evidence can be adduced to support the etiological importance of thromboembolism, congenital or immunological abnormalities, collagen-vascular disease, or drug ingestion. Although pulmonary hypertension can truly be said to be primary in such patients, a number of factors have been identified that may shed some light on the mechanisms underlying the development of pulmonary hypertension, even in these patients. It is well known that there is considerable interindividual variation in the reactivity of the pulmonary vascular bed. Vasoconstrictive stimuli, such as hypoxia or acidosis, can produce marked pulmonary hypertension in one person and be essentially without effect in another. The pulmonary arterial pressor response to hypoxia is particularly great in individuals with blood group A.[13, 15] This variability in the responsivity of the pulmonary vascular bed undoubtedly accounts for the fact that only a minority of individuals develop pulmonary edema on exposure to high altitude (p. 796). In addition, the severity of pulmonary hypertension and the level of pulmonary vascular resistance vary considerably among individuals with congenital heart disease and comparably sized ventricular septal defects. Presumably, there is a *genetic basis for these differences in pulmonary vascular reactivity*, just as there appears to be a genetic basis for the increased reactivity of the systemic vascular bed in essential systemic hypertension (p. 829).

The finding of increased pulmonary vascular reactivity and pulmonary vasoconstriction in patients with PPH, suggests that a marked *vasospastic or constrictive tendency* underlies the development of PPH in predisposed individuals.[190, 194] The autonomic nervous system has been considered a factor in the development of PPH through stimulation of the pulmonary vascular bed by either neuronally released or circulating catecholamines. In some patients with PPH, the response to pulmonary vasodilators such as tolazoline, acetylcholine, or isoproterenol is a reduction in both pulmonary artery pressure and pulmonary vascular resistance,[56, 57, 191, 229–231] supporting the notion of the importance of the autonomic nervous system in maintaining an elevated level of pulmonary vascular resistance. Other patients, however, are unresponsive to pulmonary vasodilating agents. Samet and Bernstein reported an interesting case of a patient with PPH who, when examined initially, exhibited marked pulmonary vasodilatation in response to an infusion of acetylcholine.[232] Three years later, on repeat catheterization, the pulmonary hypertension was more severe, and the patient did not respond to acetylcholine infusion. This observation suggests that patients with PPH initially may have increased pulmonary vasomotor tone.

As the disease progresses, functional changes give way to fixed, anatomical lesions unaffected by pharmacological intervention.

FAMILIAL PPH. Such cases have been reported with autosomal dominant inheritance[233–236]; other than from a positive family history, there is no way to distinguish these patients from those with the sporadic form of the disease. They may represent instances of the genetic transmission of extreme pulmonary vascular reactivity. The interplay between certain environmental factors such as hypoxia and a genetic predisposition for pulmonary vascular reactivity may also underlie the development of PPH. The reactivity of the pulmonary vascular bed of cattle to hypoxia has been shown clearly to be genetically determined.[18] In addition, it has been reported that the incidence of PPH increases at high altitude and that children with this condition improve when they move to lower altitudes[194]; conversely, the condition of patients with PPH may become worse if they ascend to higher altitudes.

PATHOLOGICAL FINDINGS

Several pathological findings (Table 26–3) are common to almost all patients with PPH (Figs. 26–14 and 26–15): (1) intimal thickening of the smaller pulmonary arteries and arterioles with fibrosis, producing a characteristic "onionskin" configuration (Fig. 26–16); (2) increased thickness of the media of muscular pulmonary arteries and muscularization of arterioles; (3) necrotizing arteritis in the walls of muscular pulmonary arteries with fibrinoid necrosis of the media of such vessels[194, 195]; and (4) *plexiform lesions*, i.e., dilated, thin-walled side branches of muscular pulmonary arteries probably resulting from endothelial proliferation (Figs. 26–13 and 26–14). These lesions are responsible for the term *plexogenic pulmonary arteriopathy*, which is now frequently used to characterize the pathological changes in this condition. Although characteristic of PPH, these anatomical changes are not pathognomonic of the disease and are also found in patients with pulmonary hypertension secondary to cardiac shunts (p. 802).

The pathological diagnosis of PPH can be made when the above-mentioned features, particularly the plexiform lesions, occur in the absence of congenital cardiac shunts

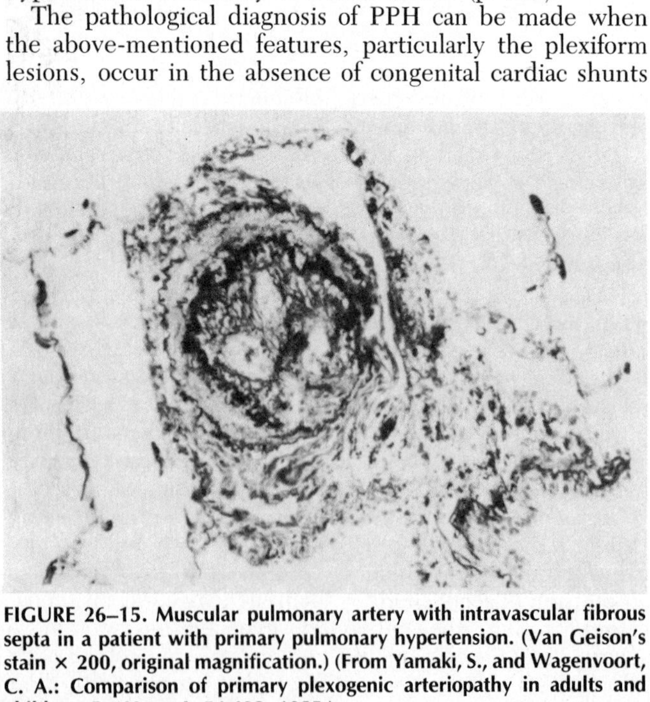

FIGURE 26–15. Muscular pulmonary artery with intravascular fibrous septa in a patient with primary pulmonary hypertension. (Van Geison's stain × 200, original magnification.) (From Yamaki, S., and Wagenvoort, C. A.: Comparison of primary plexogenic arteriopathy in adults and children. Br. Heart J. *54*:432, 1985.)

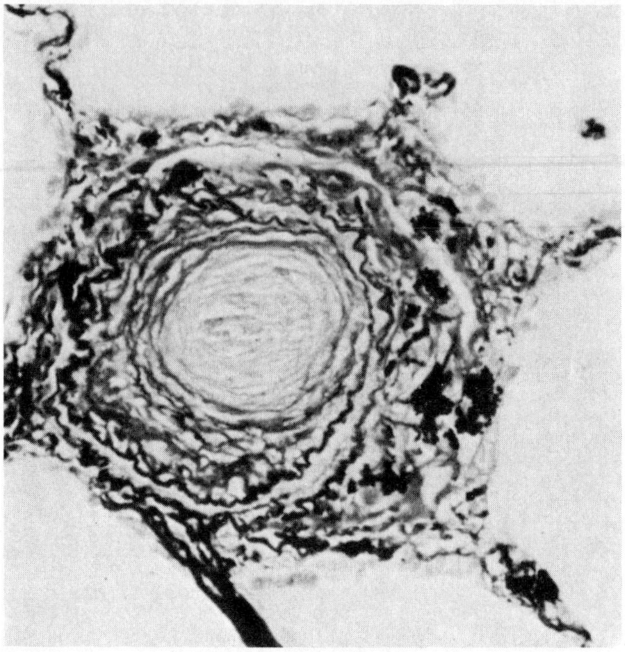

FIGURE 26–16. Transverse section of muscular pulmonary artery from a case of primary pulmonary hypertension in a man 50 years of age. There is intimal fibroelastosis of the "onionskin" type, with atrophy and disruption of the underlying media (elastic/van Gieson, × 375.) (From Harris, P., and Heath, D.: The Human Pulmonary Circulation, 3rd ed. New York, Churchill Livingstone, 1986.)

and when there is no evidence of old or fresh pulmonary emboli, such as eccentric intimal proliferation, recanalizing channels, and intraluminal fibrous webs. The pattern of elastic tissue of the pulmonary trunk is of the adult variety in PPH, consistent with the belief that the pulmonary hypertension was acquired during adult life.[237] A number of pathological findings are *secondary* to the pulmonary hypertension itself, i.e., in situ thromboses in small pulmonary arteries, atherosclerosis of the major pulmonary arterial trunks, and marked right ventricular hypertrophy.

Reid and coworkers examined the lungs of a number of patients with PPH using quantitative pathological techniques and electron microscopy.[199, 238] These investigators noted thickening of the basement membranes and of the endothelial cells of small (< 40 μm), nonmuscular pulmonary arterioles. The endothelial cells also contained increased numbers of organelles and pinocytotic vesicles, suggesting heightened metabolic activity; indeed, in some nonmuscular pulmonary arterioles, proliferation of endothelial cells obliterated the vascular lumen.[238] Quantitative analysis of the vessels in patients with PPH demonstrated a distinct reduction in the number of small, nonmuscular pulmonary arterioles. Residual, nonfunctioning "ghost vessels" seemed to remain in place of these small arterioles. At more proximal levels of the pulmonary vascular bed, there was considerable hypertrophy of smooth muscle of the media of small muscular pulmonary arteries.[199]

A *tentative* pathophysiological scheme for PPH consistent with the observed findings, but not yet firmly established, is presented in Figure 26–17. In an individual who is susceptible–whether on a genetic or an acquired basis–stimuli for pulmonary vasoconstriction result in excessive responses and transient pulmonary hypertension. Frequent episodes of pulmonary vasoconstriction and the resultant pulmonary hypertension eventually cause hypertrophy of the smooth muscle in the media of these vessels and perhaps thickening and proliferation of the endothelial cells in the nonmuscular vessels. Intense vasoconstriction may lead to fibrinoid necrosis of the arteriolar wall, with subsequent development of plexiform lesions. Ultimately,

Vasoconstriction or vasospasm in susceptible individuals
↓
Decreased flow in small pulmonary arterioles and reactive pulmonary hypertension
↓
Damage to and eventual loss of small pulmonary arterioles (replaced by ghost vessels)
↓ ↑
Pulmonary hypertension
↓
Decreased cross-sectional area in pulmonary vascular bed at level of small pulmonary arterioles
↑
Development of plexiform lesions with further reduction of vascular cross-sectional area

FIGURE 26–17. Possible pathogenesis of primary pulmonary hypertension.

the vessels are reduced in number, and the residua of these destroyed vessels can be seen histologically as "ghost vessels." Destruction of large numbers of pulmonary arterioles reduces the cross-sectional area of the pulmonary vascular bed, thus producing a permanent increase in pulmonary vascular resistance and fixed pulmonary hypertension. The latter, in turn, damages other blood vessels and initiates a vicious circle, with progressively rising pulmonary arterial pressure.

CLINICAL FEATURES

NATURAL HISTORY AND SYMPTOMATOLOGY. One of the largest studies on the natural history of PPH was reported from the Mayo Clinic.[192] This study consisted of a long-term follow-up of 120 patients in whom PPH was diagnosed by clinical and hemodynamic criteria. Seventy-three per cent of the patients were female, and the mean age at diagnosis was 34 years (3 to 64 years). The median interval from initial clinical manifestation to the time of clinical and hemodynamic diagnosis was 1.9 years. The four most frequent clinical features at the time of diagnosis were exertional dyspnea (75 per cent), loud second heart sounds (98 per cent), roentgenographic abnormalities (95 per cent) including cardiomegaly and prominent central pulmonary arteries, and electrocardiographic abnormalities (95 per cent) such as right ventricular hypertrophy, right axis deviation, and large P waves. Less frequent clinical features included exertional dizziness or syncope (30 per cent), exertional chest pain (8 per cent), and peripheral edema (8 per cent). Ten per cent of the study population had Raynaud's phenomenon, 7 (6 per cent) had chronic liver disease, and 5 (4 per cent) had a history of superficial thrombophlebitis. In two families, PPH affected two brothers.

The *prognosis* of PPH in the Mayo Clinic series[192] is illustrated in Figure 26–18. As can be seen from this figure, survival is poor in patients with PPH, with only 21 per cent surviving to 5 years. However, patients who received anticoagulants clearly had a better survival rate than did those who did not receive anticoagulants. This was not a randomized study, and the choice to administer anticoagulants was determined by individual physicians using their clinical judgment for each case. However, the utilization of anticogulant therapy in patients with a clinical and hemodynamic diagnosis of PPH is supported by the findings at autopsy in the Mayo Clinic series. Fifty-six patients of their total group underwent autopsy, and lung tissue in these patients revealed two major pathological types: thromboembolic pulmonary hypertension in 32 patients (57 per cent) and plexogenic pulmonary arteriopathy in 18 patients (32 per cent). Thus, thromboembolism without any evidence of plexiform lesions was the major pathological feature in more than half the patients autopsied. As a result of these findings, Fuster and coworkers[192] recommend anticoagulation as standard therapy for patients with a clinical and hemodynamic diagnosis of PPH.

The mode of death in patients with PPH is variable, and in the Mayo Clinic series contributing factors included right heart failure (63 per cent), pneumonia (7 per cent), sudden death (7 per cent), death related to cardiac catheterization (5 per cent), pulmonary artery dissection with tamponade (1 per cent), and death during a minor operation (1 per cent). In 15 per cent of cases, the contributing factors or cause of death could not be determined.

Some patients with PPH, followed by means of serial catheterization over a number of years, exhibit some hemodynamic improvement if they are given pulmonary vasodilating agents when they are first seen.[229] During later stages of the disease, however, such drugs have no effect on the pulmonary vascular bed.[229, 232] Late in the course of the disease, patients develop right ventricular failure, and exertional syncope may occur, presumably because of a low fixed cardiac output and hypoxemia. PPH is a fatal disease in almost all instances; the duration of symptoms varies, but on the average death occurs approximately 3 years after the onset of symptoms. The course may be more precipitous in some patients, particularly in children, whereas a few patients have lived for as long as 30 years after the onset of symptoms.[2, 239] In one reported case, PPH appeared to regress.[240]

Patients with PPH commonly complain of exertional

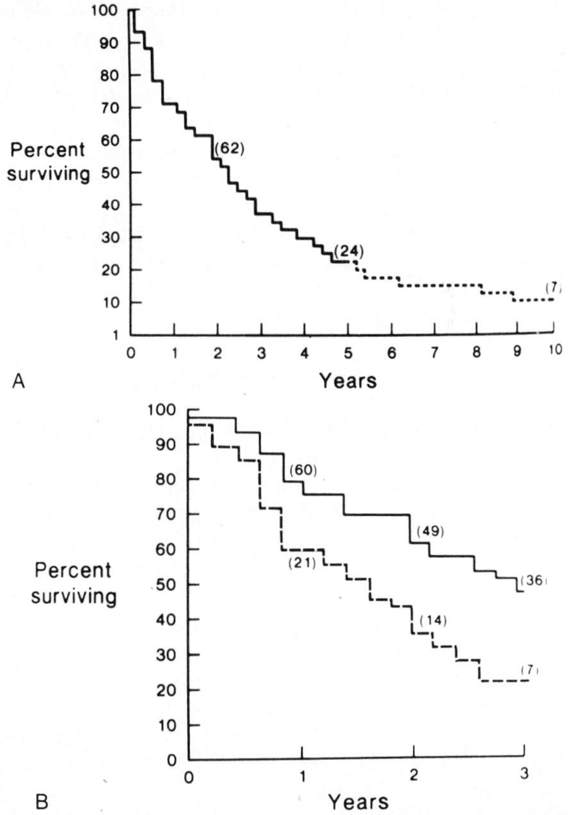

FIGURE 26–18. Prognosis in patients with a clinical and hemodynamic diagnosis of primary pulmonary hypertension. *Panel A*, the observed survival for the entire group (115 patients who survived diagnostic cardiac catheterization). *Panel B*, the observed survival with (solid line) and without (dashed line) anticoagulant treatment in these same patients. Treatment with anticoagulants was not randomized but was based on clinical preference of the primary physician caring for the patient. As can be seen, survival was substantially better in the patients who received anticoagulants. (From Fuster, V., et al.: Primary pulmonary hypertension: Natural history and the importance of thrombosis. Circulation *70*:580, 1984, by permission of the American Heart Association, Inc.)

dyspnea, syncope, precordial chest pain, weakness, and, later, dyspnea at rest.[191, 192, 241] These symptoms probably all result from low cardiac output or hypoxemia or both. Precordial chest pain may also be secondary to ischemia of the right ventricular subendocardium or distention of the major pulmonary arteries or both.[242, 243] The pain may radiate to the neck but not characteristically to the arms. Palpitations are also common and may be caused by ventricular tachyarrhythmias, which occur not infrequently in the late stages of PPH. Occasionally, cough and hemoptysis occur. These latter symptoms may be due to rupture of dilated plexiform lesions, to in situ pulmonary arterial thromboses, or to episodes of pulmonary embolism occurring late in the course of the disease.

PHYSICAL EXAMINATION. Examination of patients with PPH discloses findings consistent with pulmonary hypertension and right ventricular pressure overload: a large *a* wave in the jugular venous pulse; a low-volume carotid arterial pulse with a normal upstroke; a left parasternal (right ventricular) heave; a systolic pulsation produced by a dilated, tense pulmonary artery in the second left interspace; an ejection click and flow murmur in the same area; a closely split second heart sound with a loud pulmonic component; a fourth heart sound of right ventricular origin; and, late in the course, signs of right ventricular failure (hepatomegaly, peripheral edema, and ascites) may be present. Patients with severe pulmonary hypertension may also have prominent *v* waves in the jugular venous pulse, owing to tricuspid regurgitation; a third heart sound of right ventricular origin; a high-pitched early diastolic murmur of pulmonic regurgitation; and a holosystolic murmur of tricuspid regurgitation.[191, 192, 241] Cyanosis is a late finding in PPH and may be due to a patent foramen ovale with a right-to-left shunt occurring secondary to elevation of right atrial pressure. Other causes for cyanosis include a markedly reduced cardiac output with systemic vasoconstriction, intrapulmonary right-to-left shunting via vascular anastomoses, and ventilation-perfusion mismatches in the lung itself.[241] Uncommonly, the left laryngeal nerve becomes paralyzed as a consequence of compression by a dilated pulmonary artery.[244]

LABORATORY FINDINGS

HEMATOLOGICAL AND CHEMICAL STUDIES. Results of these studies are usually normal in patients with PPH. If there is arterial oxygen desaturation, polycythemia may be present. A number of investigators have reported hypercoagulable states, abnormal platelet function, defects in fibrinolysis, and other abnormalities of coagulation in patients with PPH.[193, 198, 202] Abnormal liver function tests can indicate right ventricular failure with resultant systemic venous hypertension.

ELECTROCARDIOGRAPHY. The electrocardiogram in PPH will exhibit right atrial and right ventricular enlargement, and a direct correlation between the magnitude of the QRS-T angle and the level of pulmonary arterial pressure has been reported.[193]

ROENTGENOGRAPHY. X-ray examination of the chest in patients with PPH shows enlargement of the main pulmonary artery and its major branches, with marked tapering of peripheral arteries.[245, 246] The right ventricle and atrium may also be enlarged. Fluoroscopic examination may disclose exaggerated pulsations of secondary pulmonary arterial branches, reflecting an elevation in pulmonary arterial pulse pressure. However, in contrast to the plethoric peripheral lung fields in patients with left-to-right shunts, oligemia is noted in these lung regions in patients with PPH (Fig. 26–19). It has been suggested that survival in PPH correlates inversely with the size of the main pulmonary artery[246]—a reasonable suggestion, since the latter correlates with the height of the pulmonary arterial pressure. The diameter of the pulmonary artery may be determined from computed tomographic (CT) scans, and thereby used to estimate pulmonary artery pressures.[246a]

PULMONARY FUNCTION TESTS. Pulmonary function tests are usually normal; rarely, a defect in diffusion capacity is present and may be the result of increased capillary-to-alveolar distance secondary to hypertrophy of vascular endothelial cells. Some patients have increased residual volumes and reduced maximum voluntary ventilation. Arterial blood gas analysis usually reveals evidence of hyperventilation with low P_{CO_2} and elevated pH, whereas arterial P_{O_2} is normal or slightly reduced.

ECHOCARDIOGRAPHY. This technique demonstrates enlargement of the right atrium and ventricle, small or normal left ventricular dimensions, and a thickened interventricular septum. The septal/posterior left ventricular wall ratio may be abnormally increased, as in hypertrophic obstructive cardiomyopathy (Chap. 5), but the other echocardiographic signs characteristic of that condition are not present. The E-F slope of the anterior mitral valve leaflet is reduced, presumably because of the diminished flow rate across the mitral valve, whereas the diastolic motion of the posterior mitral leaflet is normal. Systolic prolapse of the mitral valve is frequently present, as is abnormal septal motion of the ventricular septum, presumably due to right ventricular dilatation or tricuspid and pulmonic regurgitation or both.[246b] Doppler echocardiographic evidence of right ventricular systolic hypertension may be obtained by measuring the velocity of the tricuspid regur-

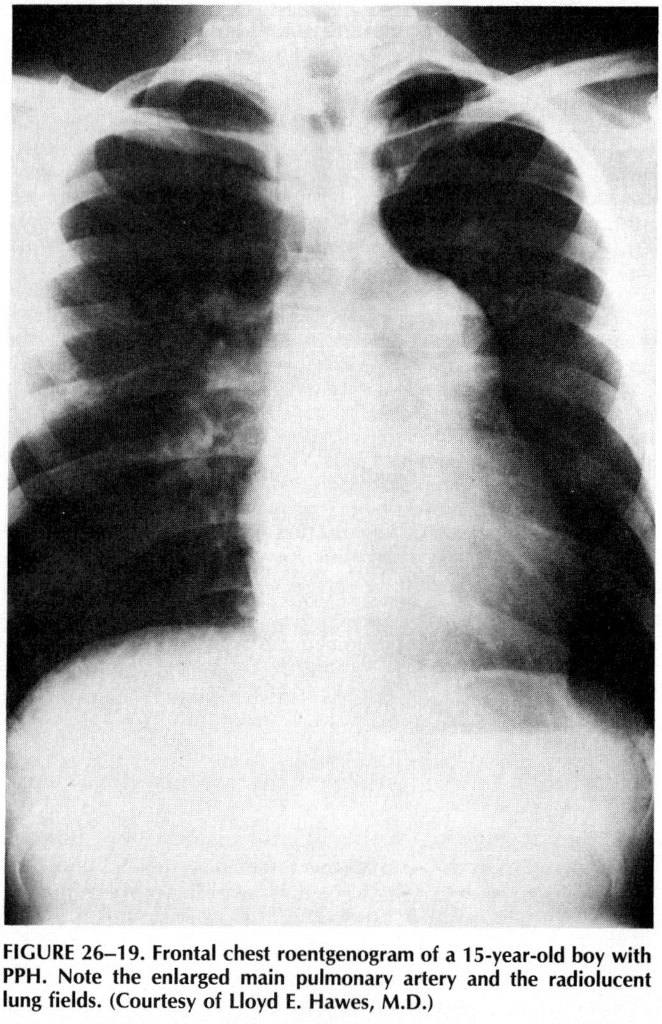

FIGURE 26–19. Frontal chest roentgenogram of a 15-year-old boy with PPH. Note the enlarged main pulmonary artery and the radiolucent lung fields. (Courtesy of Lloyd E. Hawes, M.D.)

gitant jet and using the Bernouilli formula (p. 1201). In addition, the pulmonary valve echogram[246c] and assessment of right-sided systolic time intervals[247] may be helpful in this regard as well.

LUNG SCAN. Perfusion lung scans in patients with PPH are usually either normal or demonstrate small, nonspecific, subsegmental defects. Lung scanning may be hazardous late in the course of the disease because the macroaggregated albumin particles employed in scanning may significantly reduce the already critically narrowed cross-sectional area of the pulmonary vascular bed.[248]

CARDIAC CATHETERIZATION AND ANGIOGRAPHY (Table 26–4). The diagnosis of PPH cannot be confirmed without performing cardiac catheterization and pulmonary angiography. Some patients may be too ill for one or both of these procedures (see below), and in such individuals, the diagnosis must remain tentative and be based primarily on exclusion, following clinical evaluation and noninvasive tests. Right-heart catheterization reveals elevated pulmonary arterial and right-ventricular systolic pressures that may approach, equal, or sometimes even exceed systemic arterial levels; right atrial pressure may also be increased. The calculated pulmonary vascular resistance is extremely high, approaching or sometimes even exceeding systemic vascular resistance. When tricuspid regurgitation is absent, the *a* wave in the right atrial pressure tracing is predominant; when it is present, the height of the *v* wave may equal or exceed that of the *a* wave. Left ventricular, left atrial, and pulmonary capillary wedge pressures are low or normal, but it is often difficult to record the pulmonary capillary wedge pressure. A patent foramen ovale with a small right-to-left shunt may be present.

TABLE 26–4 APPLICATIONS OF CATHETERIZATION IN ESTABLISHING ETIOLOGIC DIAGNOSIS OF PULMONARY HYPERTENSION

CONDITION	TEST APPLIED	FINDING
Congenital heart disease	Step up in O_2 saturation in right heart, H_2 electrode studies in the right heart	Left to right shunt and location of shunt
	Cardiogreen injection in right heart with sampling in systemic artery	Right to left shunt and location of shunt
	Cardiac angiography	
Peripheral pulmonary artery stenoses	Intrapulmonary arterial pressure	Intrapulmonary arterial pressure gradients
	Pulmonary angiograph	Pulmonary arterial branch stenoses
Major pulmonary arterial occlusion by clot, or tumor*	Continuous pressure recording from distal pulmonary artery to main pulmonary artery	Focal pressure gradient in a lobar or larger pulmonary artery, intravascular filling defect or narrowing
	Selective or main pulmonary angiography	
Mitral stenosis Cor triatriatum Supravalvar mitral ring	Simultaneous wedge and left ventricular pressure recording	An elevated wedge pressure and mean mitral valve diastolic pressure gradient $>$ 3 mm Hg at rest, both of which increase with exercise
Mitral regurgitation	Simultaneous wedge and left ventricular pressure recording	Large systolic pressure wave in wedge tracing. Regurgitation of contrast from left ventricular angiogram into the left atrium.
Left ventricular dysfunction or diastolic overload	Left ventricular pressure	Left ventricular end diastolic pressure $>$ 15 mm Hg
	Left ventricular angiogram	Left ventricular contraction abnormality and/or ejection fraction $<$ 50%

*Ventilation and perfusion lung scans precede catheterization.

From Reeves J. T., and Groves, B. M.: Approach to the patient with pulmonary hypertension. *In* Weir, E. K., and Reeves, J. T.: Pulmonary Hypertension. Mt. Kisco, NY, Futura Publishing Co., 1984, p. 20.

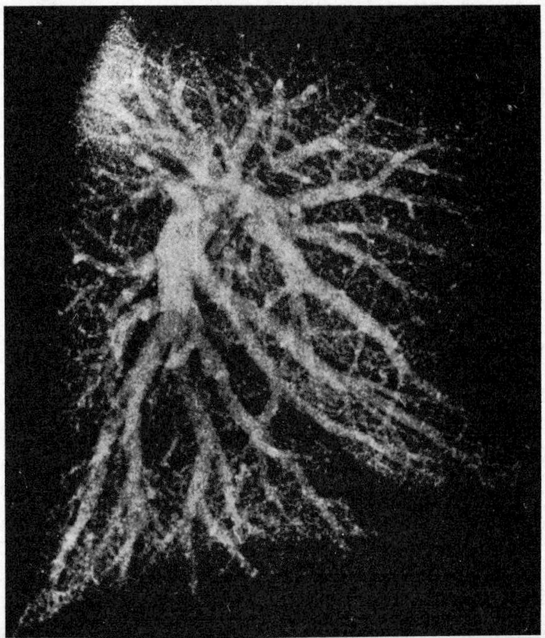

A

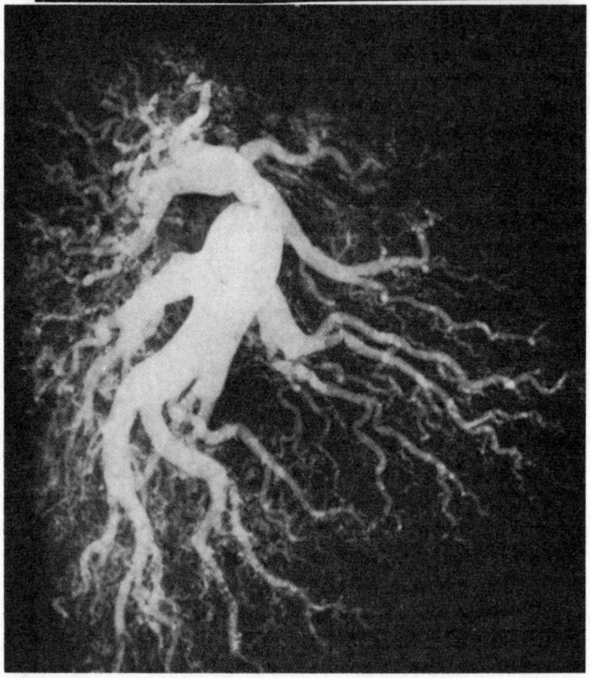

B

FIGURE 26–20. *A*, Postmortem pulmonary arteriogram of a normal lung in a 22-year-old man. The caliber of the pulmonary arteries tapers down gradually, and there is a rather dense background filling of vessels. *B*, Postmortem pulmonary arteriogram from an 18-year-old man with unexplained plexogenic pulmonary arteriopathy (primary pulmonary hypertension). The main branches are dilated. (From Wagenvoort, C. A., and Wagenvoort, N.: Pathology of Pulmonary Hypertension. New York, copyright 1977, reprinted by permission of John Wiley and Sons, Inc.)

Pulmonary angiography demonstrates large central pulmonary arteries with marked peripheral tapering. Postmortem arteriograms demonstrate absence of "background haze" secondary to the loss of small, nonmuscular pulmonary arterioles (Fig. 26–20).[199] Right ventriculography usually demonstrates a thick-walled chamber, sometimes with delayed emptying, i.e., elevated right ventricular end-diastolic and end-systolic volumes and a reduced ejection fraction, a result of the markedly elevated pulmonary vascular resistance.

Cardiac catheterization and angiography carry an increased risk in patients with PPH. In the Mayo Clinic series,[192] five deaths were related to cardiac catheterization in the study cohort of 120 patients. Interestingly, pulmonary angiography had been performed in only one of these patients. Maintenance of adequate oxygenation by administration of supplemental oxygen and avoidance of vasovagal reactions (and rapid treatment of those that occur) should reduce the risk of invasive studies in this patient group. The risk of inducing atrial and/or ventricular arrhythmias can be minimized by the use of balloon flotation catheters and avoidance of prolonged attempts at catheterization by inexperienced operators. Pulmonary angiography can be performed safely using a segmental angiographic technique with hand injection of small amounts of radiographic contrast through the terminal lumen of a balloon-flotation catheter, while the balloon is inflated.[249] The new nonionic contrast agents appear to be better tolerated in these patients.

TABLE 26–5 CAUSES OF PULMONARY HYPERTENSION IN WHICH CATHETERIZATION DOES NOT ESTABLISH ETIOLOGIC DIAGNOSIS

Condition	Procedure Needed to Establish Etiology	Result
Pulmonary parenchymal disease	Chest x-ray	Radiographic abnormality
	Pulmonary function tests such as spirometry, volumes, compliance, DLCO, A-aO_2 gradient	Airflow obstruction, pulmonary restriction and/or decreased compliance and diffusion capacity with altered gas exchange
	Bronchoscopy if indicated	
Recurrent pulmonary microembolism or microarterial thrombosis	Lung biopsy	Eccentric intimal fibrosis, fibrous strands
Pulmonary venous thrombosis or fibrosis	Lung biopsy	Pulmonary venous occlusion and fibrosis
Primary pulmonary hypertension	Lung biopsy	Pulmonary arterial medial hypertrophy and/or concentric intimal fibrosis
Pulmonary vasculitis	Clinical and laboratory evidence of collagen vascular disease	
	Lung biopsy	Perivascular inflammation
Drug induced dietary pulmonary hypertension	History of intake	
Pulmonary hypertension of newborn		

From Reeves, J. T., and Groves, B. M.: Approach to the patient with pulmonary hypertension. *In* Weir, E. K., and Reeves, J. T.: Pulmonary Hypertension. Mt. Kisco, NY, Futura Publishing Co., 1984, p. 21.

TABLE 26–6 DIAGNOSTIC STUDIES USEFUL FOR ELUCIDATING CAUSES OF PULMONARY HYPERTENSION

Potential Cause of Pulmonary Hypertension	Possible Diagnostic Studies
a) Pulmonary embolic disease	ventilation/perfusion scans and/or selective, lobar pulmonary angiography (preferably biplane)
b) Pulmonary venous thrombosis or obstruction	chest x-ray, angiography, lung biopsy
c) Congenital intra-cardiac shunts causing increased pulmonary blood flow	indicator dilution studies
d) Increased left atrial pressure; secondary to mitral or aortic valve disease, left ventricular dysfunction or systemic hypertension	pulmonary artery wedge pressure or left atrial pressure (via patent foramen ovale) (> 15 mm Hg)
e) Pulmonary airways disease (e.g., chronic bronchitis and emphysema)	respiratory function tests (FVC/FEV_1)
f) Hypoxic pulmonary hypertension associated with (i) impaired ventilation; either central (CNS) or peripheral (chest wall problems or upper airway obstruction). (ii) residence at high altitude	sleep apnea studies and respiratory tests
g) Interstitial lung disease, pneumoconioses and fibrosis (e.g., silicosis, rheumatoid disease and sarcoidosis)	chest x-ray, spirometry and carbon monoxide diffusion, rheumatoid factor, lymph node biopsy
h) Collagen disease (e.g., SLE, polyarteritis nodosa, scleroderma)	LE cells, skin, muscle, or other tissue biopsy, esophageal motility studies
i) Parasitic disease (schistosomiasis or filariasis)	rectal biopsy, complement fixation, skin tests, blood smears
j) Cirrhosis or portal vein thrombosis	liver function tests
k) Peripheral pulmonary artery stenosis (including Takayasu's disease and fibrosing mediastinitis)	selective pulmonary angiography, or pressure gradient at catheterization
l) Sickle cell disease	erythrocyte morphology, hemoglobin electrophoresis
m) Choriocarcinoma and hydatidiform mole	serum or urinary beta subunit of chorionic gonadotrophin
n) Intravenous injection of pulverized pills	lung biopsy

From Weir, E. K.: Diagnosis and management of primary pulmonary hypertension. *In* Weir, E. K., and Reeves, J. T.: Pulmonary Hypertension. Mt. Kisco, NY, Futura Publishing Co., 1984, p. 141.

DIAGNOSIS

It is essential that diagnostic efforts (Tables 26–5, 26–6) be vigorously pursued in patients with severe pulmonary hypertension in order to insure that no patient with secondary pulmonary hypertension is erroneously classified as having PPH. Secondary pulmonary hypertension is often treatable in that the cause can be attacked directly; even when it cannot, the prognosis is usually not as grave as it is in PPH. However, it must be appreciated that patients with PPH may tolerate diagnostic procedures poorly. These individuals can experience sudden cardiovascular collapse and even death during or shortly after the induction of general anesthesia for surgical procedures, during cardiac catheterization and angiography, and even following arterial puncture or radioisotopic lung scanning.[248] Although the mechanism responsible for the cardiovascular collapse and sudden death has not been defined clearly, it may be presumed that these interventions act as stimuli to further constriction of the already narrowed pulmonary vascular bed, followed by the sudden development or exacerbation of right heart failure or arrhythmias or both.

The *differential diagnosis* of PPH includes a number of causes of secondary pulmonary hypertension. Indeed, a definitive diagnosis of PPH can be established post mortem only after careful histological examination of the pulmonary vasculature. Exclusion of mitral stenosis, congenital cardiac defects (including cor triatriatum), pulmonary embolism, and pulmonary venous obstruction by means of catheterization and angiography is imperative. *"Silent" mitral stenosis*, i.e., without the characteristic diastolic murmur, can be excluded by means of echocardiographic visualization of the motion of the mitral valve and the absence of a transvalvular pressure gradient (Chap. 33). *Congenital heart defects* with Eisenmenger syndrome can be ruled out if significant left-to-right or right-to-left shunts are absent. The use of indicator-dilution curves (p. 253) and angiography is useful in this regard. *Cor triatriatum* (p. 940) is recognized by appropriate hemodynamic studies (Fig. 26–6) and angiographic visualization of the left atrial membrane. This entity presents a characteristic left atrial echocardiogram with normal mitral valve motion. Cardiac catheterization reveals a hemodynamic pattern similar in some ways to mitral stenosis, i.e., a diastolic pressure gradient between the left ventricle and the chamber proximal to the membrane. *Pulmonary embolism* (Chap. 47) can be excluded by means of pulmonary angiography, and *sickle cell disease with in situ pulmonary vascular thrombosis* (Chap. 55) can be evaluated by hemoglobin electrophoresis. The presence of severe *pulmonary parenchymal disease* can be recognized by the characteristic physical findings, chest roentgenogram, and pulmonary function tests (Chap. 48). *Collagen vascular disease* is suggested by the involvement of other organ systems or the presence of abnormal immunological phenomena, such as antinuclear antibodies and LE cells (Chap. 54). *Pulmonary veno-occlusive disease* is characterized by progressive narrowing of nearly all small pulmonary veins and venules, many of which exhibit complete occlusion by fibrous tissue. It is suggested clinically by the finding of a normal pulmonary artery "wedge" pressure together with chest x-ray evidence of Kerley B lines and pulmonary edema. However, the pulmonary artery wedge pressure is elevated in some cases.[5]

TREATMENT OF PULMONARY HYPERTENSION

Treatment of pulmonary hypertension (Table 26–7) will be most successful when it is possible to identify the inciting cause and remove it before irreversible damage has been done to the pulmonary vasculature. Thus, closure of central shunts while they are still predominantly left-to-right, and before extensive plexiform and angiomatoid lesions have developed in the lungs, will usually correct pulmonary hypertension in the setting of congenital heart disease with central left-to-right shunt. Patients with hypoventilation secondary to hypertrophied tonsils and adenoids will experience cure of associated pulmonary hypertension with tonsillectomy.[175, 176]

In patients in whom removal of the inciting cause is not possible (or where the cause is unknown, as in PPH), therapy for pulmonary hypertension is directed at decreasing resistance to pulmonary blood flow and improving the cardiocirculatory response to right ventricular pressure overload.

Decreasing resistance to pulmonary blood flow can be accomplished only when the site of the increased resistance (Table 26–1) is identified. Thus, when left ventricular failure with secondary left atrial hypertension is the cause of increased resistance to pulmonary blood flow, relief of left ventricular failure (Chap. 17) will lead to lowering of pulmonary artery pressure. When decreased cross-sectional area of the pulmonary vascular bed is causing pulmonary hypertension, *pulmonary vasodilators* may be tried; it is likely that they will be effective only in cases in which active vasoconstriction of small muscular arteries or arterioles is contributing significantly to the pulmonary hypertension.

In recent years, there has been considerable interest in the use of pulmonary vasodilators as chronic therapy for PPH.[37–39, 250–285] This approach is based on the observation that muscular hypertrophy, rather than intimal hyperplasia, is the earliest finding in patients developing primary pulmonary hypertension. Because of the difficulty in predicting or interpreting the results of vasodilator therapy in patients with unexplained pulmonary hypertension, lung biopsy has been recommended whenever possible before starting pulmonary vasodilator therapy.[158, 254] There is much to recommend this approach, including the possibility of uncovering a specific but unexpected cause of the pulmonary hypertension, such as pulmonary thromboembolism or a collagen-vascular disorder, as well as assessing the reversibility or irreversibility of the vascular changes prior to treatment. This latter point is all the more important, since vasodilator therapy may be hazardous in some patients with advanced pulmonary hypertension.[37, 250, 251, 256, 261, 262, 265]

VASODILATORS. Vasodilator agents that have been used for either the acute or the chronic treatment of pulmonary hypertension include oxygen,[71, 120, 121, 278] hydralazine,[252, 256, 258, 270, 271] phentolamine,[272, 285] sublingual isoproterenol,[273, 274, 283] diazoxide,[275–277] nifedipine,[20, 252, 253, 255–257, 259–261, 280–282] prostacyclin,[38, 39, 258, 279] tolazoline,[37, 56] verapamil,[261–264] nitroglycerin,[265, 266] and captopril.[267] Effectiveness of these agents has been quite variable. In one report of 10 women with acute PPH, only sublingual isoproterenol (alone or combined with isosorbide dinitrate) produced a fall in pulmonary vascular resistance: diazoxide, hydralazine, phentolamine, and tolazoline were ineffective.[37] In contrast, hydralazine was found to be effective in each of 4 patients with primary pulmonary hypertension by one group[270] and in 6 of 12 patients with PPH by a second group.[271] Similar conflicting results have been reported for diazoxide.[37, 275–277] Prostacyclin (PGI_2) has been reported to reverse completely the pulmonary vasoconstriction in a neonate with persistent fetal circulation[279] but was less impressive in four adult patients with pulmonary hypertension of diverse etiology.[38] The hemodynamic effects of prostacyclin on the pulmonary circulation have been reported to resemble those of hydralazine, and the suggestion has been made that acute effects of prostacyclin administration may predict the response to hydralazine.[258] Nifedipine has been reported to prevent the acute pulmonary vasoconstriction associated with hypoxia,[20] and preliminary reports suggest that it may have therapeutic value in pulmonary hypertension of various etiologies.[252, 255–257, 259, 260]

Conflicting results are not surprising, since most institutions have been able to study only small numbers of patients, and the underlying pathological condition (re-

TABLE 26–7 TREATMENT OF PULMONARY HYPERTENSION

I. Remove Inciting Cause (when possible)
Examples: Surgical correction of mitral stenosis[110–112] or cor triatriatum,[113] closure of anatomical site of predominant left-to-right shunt, removal of massively hypertrophied tonsils and adenoids,[175] avoidance of offending drug or agent (aminorex, *Crotalaria* alkaloids, intravenous drug abuse)

II. Decrease Resistance to Pulmonary Blood Flow
- A. Lower left atrial or left ventricular diastolic pressure, when these are elevated
- B. Pulmonary vasodilators
  1. Oxygen[71, 120, 121, 278]
  2. Hydralazine[252, 256, 258, 270, 271]
  3. Phentolamine[272, 285]
  4. Isoproterenol[273, 274, 283]
  5. Diazoxide[275–277]
  6. Nifedipine[20, 252, 253, 255–257, 259–261, 280–282]
  7. Prostaglandins[38, 39, 258, 279]
  8. Tolazoline[37, 56]
  9. Verapamil[261–264]
  10. Nitroglycerin[265, 266]
  11. Captopril[267]
- C. Heart-lung transplantation[286–290]
- D. Anticoagulation: recurrent pulmonary embolism,[167] pulmonary veno-occlusive disease, ?PPH[192]

III. Improve Cardiocirculatory Response to Right Ventricular Pressure Overload
- A. Appropriate pulmonary toilet to maximize alveolar ventilation and oxygenation
- B. Prophylaxis (vaccines) for influenza and pneumonia; prompt, vigorous treatment of any pulmonary infection
- C. Diuretics (spironolactone and furosemide or a thiazide) with low-salt diet
- D. Pulmonary vasodilators (see IIB)
- E. Inotropic agents (digitalis glycosides, newer oral beta agonists, etc.)

versible vs. irreversible pulmonary vascular changes) has been unknown for the majority of patients in nearly all published reports on vasodilation therapy for pulmonary hypertension. Despite these shortcomings, there appears to be a heterogeneity in individual responsiveness to various pulmonary vasodilators, and there is some evidence that the findings on acute drug testing predict long-term results of treatment for individual patients.[255, 259, 263, 266, 270–272, 278] Accordingly, it seems reasonable to assess the acute hemodynamic response to a variety of agents in the patient with severe pulmonary hypertension and to use the results of this assessment to design chronic therapy. As already mentioned, it is essential to determine the underlying cause of the patient's pulmonary hypertension whenever possible, since this may affect therapy in a fundamental way: An aggressive diagnostic approach, including lung biopsy, may be necessary in many cases.

HEART-LUNG TRANSPLANTATION. This procedure has been performed as therapy for advanced, otherwise untreatable pulmonary vascular disease.[286–290] The largest experience with combined heart and lung transplantation is at Stanford University, where 40 such transplants have been performed between March 9, 1981 and June 1, 1987.[286–290a] Sixty-seven per cent of these patients survived for 1 year and 57 per cent for 2 years after transplantation. Early mortality has improved over the time of their total experience, with only one early death occurring in the last eight patients. Two late deaths occurred in patients undergoing combined heart and lung transplantation at 14 and 15 months after operation. One death was sudden and apparently the result of an acute myocardial infarction, while the other represented progressive respiratory failure. At autopsy, both patients had severe proliferative coronary atherosclerosis, which has been noted previously in patients undergoing heart transplantation alone. In addition, however, obliterative bronchiolitis affected the lungs of both patients. A third patient required repeat heart and lung transplantation at 37 months following the initial procedure because of progressive respiratory failure from obliterative bronchiolitis. His heart also showed severe coronary artery disease. Thus, although progress has been made in improving the results of combined heart and lung transplantation, major problems still exist. With advances in immunosuppressive therapy and surgical technique, it is likely that additional numbers of patients will be treated with lung or combined heart-lung transplantation.

ANTICOAGULATION. This is clearly indicated in pulmonary hypertension associated with recurrent pulmonary emboli.[167] Its role in other forms of pulmonary hypertension (e.g., veno-occlusive disease) is conjectural and rests on postmortem or biopsy studies showing thrombi in large and small pulmonary veins or arteries.[2, 5, 114, 182] However, as described earlier (p. 809), the Mayo Clinic group[191, 192] has reported clinical evidence that anticoagulants may improve the prognosis in at least some patients with severe pulmonary hypertension (Fig. 26–20).

Even when pulmonary hypertension can be neither cured nor improved, the cardiocirculatory response to right ventricular pressure overload can often be improved with amelioration of right heart failure and an increase in forward cardiac output. The elements of a program designed to accomplish these goals is given in Table 26–6, III, A to E.

REFERENCES

NORMAL PULMONARY CIRCULATION

1. Comroe, J. H., Jr.: The main functions of the pulmonary circulation. Circulation *33*:146, 1966.
2. Wagenvoort, C. A., and Wagenvoort, N.: Pathology of Pulmonary Hypertension. 2nd ed. New York, John Wiley and Sons, 1977.
3. Fritts, H. W., Harris, P., Chidsey, C. A., Clauss, R. H., and Cournand, A.: Estimation of flow rate through bronchial-pulmonary vascular anastomoses with use of T-1824 dye. Circulation *23*:390, 1961.
4. Barratt-Boyes, B. G., and Wood, E. H.: Cardiac output and related measurements and pressure values in the right heart and associated vessels, together with an analysis of the hemodynamic response to the inhalation of high oxygen mixtures in healthy subjects. J. Lab. Clin. Med. *51*:72, 1958.
5. Harris, P., and Heath, D.: The Human Pulmonary Circulation. 3rd ed. New York, Churchill Livingstone, 1986, 702 pp.
6. Harris, P., Segel, N., and Bishop, J. M.: The relation between pressure and flow in the pulmonary circulation in normal subjects and in patients with chronic bronchitis and mitral stenosis. Cardiovasc. Res. *1*:73, 1968.
7. Nihill, M. R., McNamara, D. G., and Vick, R. L.: The effects of increased blood viscosity on pulmonary vascular resistance. Am. Heart J. 92:65, 1976.
8. Dawes, G. S., Mott, J. C., Widdicombe, J. G., and Wyatt, D. G.: Changes in the lungs of the newborn lamb. J. Physiol. *121*:141, 1953.
9. Adams, F. H., and Lind, J.: Physiologic studies on the cardiovascular status of normal newborn infants. Pediatrics *19*:431, 1957.
10. Rudolph, A. M.: The changes in the circulation after birth. Their importance in congenital heart disease. Circulation *41*:343, 1970.
11. Friedman, W. F., Molony, D. A., and Kirkpatrick, S. E.: Prostaglandins: Physiological and clinical correlations. Adv. Pediatr. *25*:151, 1978.
12. Naeye, R. L.: Arterial changes during the perinatal period. Arch. Pathol. *71*:121, 1961.
13. Fishman, A. P.: Hypoxia on the pulmonary circulation: How and where it acts. Circ. Res. *38*:221, 1976.
14. Von Euler, U. S., and Liljestrand, G.: Observations on the pulmonary arterial blood pressure in the cat. Acta Physiol. Scand. *12*:301, 1946.
15. Silove, E. D., Inoue, T., and Grover, R. F.: Comparison of hypoxia, pH, and sympathomimetic drugs on bovine pulmonary vasculature. J. Appl. Physiol. *24*:355, 1968.
16. Haneda, T., Nakajima, T., Shirato, K., Onodera, S., and Takisima, T.: Effects of oxygen breathing on pulmonary vascular input impedance in patients with pulmonary hypertension. Chest 83:520, 1983.
17. Grover, R. F., Vogel, J. H. K., Averill, K. H., and Blount, S. G.: Pulmonary hypertension. Individual and species variability relative to vascular reactivity. Am. Heart J. *66*:1, 1963.
18. Weir, E. K., Tucker, A., Reeves, J. T., and Will, D. H.: Pulmonary hypertension in cattle at high altitude. Cardiovasc. Res. *8*:745, 1975.
19. McMurty, I. F., Davidson, A. B., Reeves, J. T., and Grover, R. F.: Inhibition

of hypoxic pulmonary vasconstriction by calcium antagonist in isolated rat lungs. Circ. Res. *38*:99, 1960.

20. Simonneau, G., Escourron, P., Duroux, P., and Lockhart, A.: Inhibition of hypoxic pulmonary vasoconstriction by nifedipine. N. Engl. J. Med. *304*:1582, 1981.
21. Rabinovitch, M., Gamble, W., Nadas, A. S., Miettinen, O. S., and Reid, L.: Rat pulmonary circulation after chronic hypoxia: Hemodynamic and structural features. Am. J. Physiol. *236*:H818, 1979.
22. Rabinovitch, M., Gamble, W. J., Miettinen, O. S., and Reid, L.: Age and sex influence on pulmonary hypertension of chronic hypoxia and on recovery. Am. J. Physiol. *240*:H62, 1981.
23. Sobel, B. J., Bottex, G., Emirgil, C., and Gissen, H.: Gaseous diffusion from alveoli to pulmonary vessels of considerable size. Circ. Res. *13*:71, 1963.
24. Staub, N. C.: Gas exchange vessels in the cat lung. Fed. Proc. *20*:107, 1961.
25. Jameson, A. G.: Gaseous diffusion from alveoli into pulmonary arteries. J. Appl. Physiol. *19*:448, 1964.
26. Glazier, J. B., and Murray, J. F.: Sites of pulmonary vasomotor reactivity in the dog during alveolar hypoxia and serotonin and histamine infusion. J. Clin. Invest. *50*:2550, 1971.
27. Bergofsky, E. H.: Mechanisms underlying vasomotor regulation of regional pulmonary blood flow in normal and disease states. Am. J. Med. *57*:378, 1974.
28. Hauge, A.: Hypoxia and pulmonary vascular resistance: The relative effects of pulmonary arterial and alveolar Po_2. Acta Physiol. Scand. *76*:121, 1969.
29. Liljestrand, G.: Chemical control of the distribution of the pulmonary blood flow. Acta Physiol. Scand. *44*:216, 1958.
30. Enson, Y., Giuntini, C., Lewis, M. L., Morris, T. Q., Ferrer, M. I., and Harvey, R. M.: The influence of hydrogen ion concentration and hypoxia on the pulmonary circulation. J. Clin. Invest. *43*:1146, 1964.
31. Vogel, J. G. K., and Blount, G., Jr.: The role of hydrogen ion concentration in the regulation of pulmonary arterial pressure: Observations in a patient with hypoventilation and obesity. Circulation *32*:788, 1965.
32. Kadowitz, P. J., Joiner, P. D., and Hyman, A. L.: Effect of sympathetic nerve stimulation on pulmonary vascular resistance in the intact spontaneously breathing dog. Proc. Soc. Exp. Biol. Med. *147*:68, 1974.
33. Harris, P.: Influence of acetylcholine on the pulmonary arterial pressures. Br. Heart J. *29*:272, 1957.
34. Fritts, H. W., Harris, P., Clauss, R. H., Odell, J. E., and Cournand, A.: The effect of acetylcholine on the human pulmonary circulation under normal and hypoxic conditions. J. Clin. Invest. *37*:99, 1958.
35. Wood, P., Besterman, E. M., Towers, M. K., and McIlroy, M. B.: The effect of acetylcholine on pulmonary vascular resistance and left atrial pressure in mitral stenosis. Br. Heart J. *19*:279, 1957.
36. Kadowitz, P. J., and Hyman, A. L.: Differential effects of prostaglandins A_1 and A_2 on pulmonary vascular resistance in the dog. Proc. Soc. Exp. Biol. Med. *149*:282, 1975.
37. Hermiller, J. B., Bambach, D., Thompson, M. J., Huss, P., Fontana, M. E., Magorien, M. D., Unverferth, D. V., and Leier, C. V.: Vasodilators and prostaglandin inhibitors in primary pulmonary hypertension. Ann. Intern. Med. *97*:480, 1982.
38. Guadagni, D. N., Ikram, H., and Maslowski, A. H.: Haemodynamic effects of prostacyclin (PGI_2) in pulmonary hypertension. Br. Heart J. *45*:385, 1981.
39. Rubin, L. J., Groves, B. M., Reeves, J. T., Frosdono, M., Handel, F., and Cato, A. E.: Prostacyclin-induced acute pulmonary vasodilation in primary pulmonary hypertension. Circulation *66*:334, 1982.
40. Kay, J. M., Waymire, J. C., and Grover, R. F.: Lung mast cell hyperplasia and pulmonary histamine forming capacity in hypoxic rats. Am. J. Physiol. *226*:178, 1974.
41. Haas, F., and Bergofsky, E. H.: Role of the mast cell in the pulmonary pressor response to hypoxia. J. Clin. Invest. *51*:3154, 1972.
42. Hauge, A.: Role of histamine in hypoxic pulmonary hypertension in the rat. I. Blockade or potentiation of endogenous amines, kinins, and ATP. Circ. Res. *22*:371, 1968.
43. Hauge, A., and Melmon, K. L.: Rise of histamine in hypoxic pulmonary hypertension in the rat. II. Depletion of histamine, serotonin, and catecholamines. Circ. Res. *22*:385, 1968.
44. Susmano, A., and Carleton, R. A.: Prevention of hypoxic pulmonary hypertension by chlorpheniramine. J. Appl. Physiol. *31*:531, 1971.
45. Altura, B. M., and Zweifach, B. W.: Pharmacologic properties of antihistamines in relation to vascular reactivity. Am. J. Physiol. *209*:550, 1965.
46. Shepherd, J. T., Donald, D. E., Linder, E., and Swan, H. J. C.: Effect of small doses of 5-hydroxytryptamine (serotonin) on pulmonary circulation in the closed chest dog. Am. J. Physiol. *197*:963, 1959.
47. Harris, P., Fritts, H. W., and Cournand, A.: Some circulatory effects of 5-hydroxytryptamine in man. Circulation *21*:1134, 1960.
48. Luchsinger, P. C., Seipp, H. W., and Patel, D. V.: Relationship of pulmonary artery wedge pressure to left atrial pressure in man. Circulation *11*:315, 1962.
49. Regan, T. J., DeFazio, V., Binak, K., and Hellems, H. K.: Norepinephrine induced pulmonary congestion in patients with aortic valve regurgitation. J. Clin. Invest. *38*:1564, 1959.
50. Fowler, N. O., Westcott, R. N., Scott, R. C., and McGuire, J.: The effect of norepinephrine upon pulmonary arteriolar resistance in man. J. Clin. Invest. *30*:517, 1951.
51. Goldring, R. M., Turino, G. M., Cohen, G., Jameson, A. G., Bass, B. G., and Fishman, A. P.: The catecholamines in the pulmonary arterial pressor response to acute hypoxia. J. Clin. Invest. *41*:1211, 1962.
52. Patel, D. J., Lange, R. L., and Hecht, H. H.: Some evidence for active constriction in the human pulmonary vascular bed. Circulation *18*:19, 1958.
53. Kadowitz, P. J., Joiner, P. D., and Hyman, A. L.: Influence of sympathetic stimulation and vasoactive substances on the canine pulmonary veins. J. Clin. Invest. *56*:354, 1975.
54. Yoshida, Y.: Studies on the pathologic physiology of pulmonary hypertension in mitral valve disease. I. The role of sympathetic nervous system on the increment of pulmonary vascular resistance. Jpn. Circ. J. *33*:359, 1969.
55. Sanders, J., Miller, D. D., and Patil, P. N.: Alpha adrenergic and histaminergic effects of tolazoline-like imidazolines. J. Pharmacol. Exp. Ther. *195*:362, 1975.
56. Rudolph, A. M., Paul, M. H., Sommer, L. S., and Nadas, A. S.: Effects of tolazoline hydrochloride (Priscoline) on circulatory dynamics of patients with pulmonary hypertension. Am. Heart J. *55*:424, 1958.
57. Dresdale, D. T., Michton, R. J., and Schultz, M.: Recent studies in primary pulmonary hypertension including pharmacodynamic observations on pulmonary vascular resistance. Bull. N.Y. Acad. Med. *30*:195, 1954.
58. Vogel, J. H. K., Grover, R. F., Jamieson, G., and Blount, S. G., Jr.: Long-term physiologic observations in patients with ventricular septal defect and increased pulmonary vascular resistance. Adv. Cardiol. *11*:108, 1974.
59. Tucker, A., Hoffman, E. A., and Weir, E. K.: Histamine receptor antagonism does not inhibit hypoxic pulmonary vasoconstriction in dogs. Chest *71*(Suppl):261, 1977.
60. Okpako, D. T.: A dual action of histamine on guinea pig lung vessels. Br. J. Pharmacol. *45*:311, 1972.
61. Tucker, A., Weir, E. K., Reeves, J. T., and Grover, F.: Histamine H_1 and H_2 receptors in pulmonary and systemic vasculature of the dog. Am. J. Physiol. *229*:1008, 1975.
62. Moret, P., Covarrubias, E., Coudert, J., and Duchosall, F.: Cardiocirculatory adaptation to chronic hypoxia. Acta Cardiol. (Brux.) *27*:596, 1972.
63. Penazola, D., Sime, F., Banchero, N., Gamboa, R., Cruz, J., and Marticorena, E.: Pulmonary hypertension in healthy men born and living at high altitudes. Am. J. Cardiol. *11*:150, 1963.
64. Hecht, H. H., and McClement, J. H.: A case of chronic mountain sickness in the United States: Clinical, physiologic, and electrocardiographic observations. Am. J. Med. *25*:470, 1968.
65. Penazola, D., Sime, F., Banchero, N., and Gamboa, R.: Pulmonary hypertension in healthy men born and living at high altitudes. Med. Thorac. *19*:449, 1962.
66. Vogel, J. H. K., Weaver, W. F., Rose, R. L., Blount, S. G., Jr., and Grover, R. F.: Pulmonary hypertension on exertion in normal men living at 10,150 feet (Leadville, Colorado). Med. Thorac. *19*:461, 1962.
67. Niewoehner, D. E., Kleinerman, J., and Rice, D. B.: Pathologic changes in the peripheral airways of young cigarette smokers. N. Engl. J. Med. *291*:755, 1974.
68. United States Department of Health, Education, and Welfare: The health consequences of smoking: A report of the Surgeon General, 1972. DHEW publication No. v72 (HSM) 72-7516. Washington, D.C., U.S. Government Printing Office, 1972.
69. Spain, D. M., Siegel, H., and Bradess, V. A.: Emphysema in apparently healthy adults: smoking, age, and sex. J.A.M.A. *224*:322, 1973.
70. Burrow, B., Kettel, L. J., Niden, A. H., Rabinowitz, M., and Diener, C. F.: Patterns of cardiovascular dysfunction in chronic obstructive lung disease. N. Engl. J. Med. *286*:912, 1972.
71. Neff, T. A., and Petty, T. L.: Long-term continuous oxygen therapy in chronic airway obstruction. Ann. Intern. Med. *72*:621, 1970.

SECONDARY PULMONARY HYPERTENSION

72. Brooks, H. L., Kirk, E. S., Vokonas, P. S., Urschel, C. W., and Sonnenblick, E. H.: Performance of the right ventricle under stress. J. Clin. Invest. *50*:2176, 1971.
73. Berman, J. L., Green, L. G., and Grossman, W.: Right ventricular diastolic pressure in coronary artery disease. Am. J. Cardiol. *44*:1263, 1979.
74. Lorell, B. H., Leinbach, R. C., Pohost, G. M., Gold, H. K., Dinsmore, R. E., Hutter, A. M., Jr., Pastore, J. D., and DeSanctis, R. W.: Right ventricular infarction. Am. J. Cardiol. *43*:463, 1979.
75. Vasco, J. S., Elkins, R. C., Fogarty, T. J., and Morrow, A. G.: The experimental production of chronic mitral valvular obstruction. J. Thorac. Cardiovasc. Surg. *53*:875, 1967.
76. Haddy, F. J., Ferrin, A. L., Hannon, D. W., Alden, J. F., Adams, W. L., and Baronofsky, I. D.: Cardiac function in experimental mitral stenosis. Circ. Res. *1*:219, 1953.
77. Silove, E. D., Tavernor, W. D., and Berry, C. L.: Reactive pulmonary arterial hypertension after pulmonary venous constriction in the calf. Cardiovasc. Res. *6*:36, 1972.
78. Charms, B. L., Brofman, B. L., and Adicoff, A.: Differential pulmonary artery occlusion in patients with chronic pulmonary disease. Am. J. Med. *26*:527, 1959.
79. Soderholm, B., and Werko, L.: Acetylcholine and the pulmonary circulation in mitral valvular disease. Br. Heart J. *21*:1, 1959.
80. Kay, J. M., and Edwards, F. R.: Ultrastructure of the alveolar-capillary wall in mitral stenosis. J. Pathol. *111*:239, 1973.
81. Szidon, J. P., Pietra, G. G., and Fishman, A. P.: The alveolar-capillary membrane and pulmonary edema. N. Engl. J. Med. *286*:1200, 1972.
82. Hicks, J. D.: Acute arterial necrosis in the lungs. J. Pathol. Bacteriol. *65*:333, 1953.
83. Whitaker, W., Black, A., and Warrack, A. J. N.: Pulmonary ossification in patients with mitral stenosis. J. Fac. Radiol. (Lond.) *7*:29, 1955.
84. Jordan, S. C., Hicken, P., Watson, D. A., Heath, D., and Whitaker, W.: Pathology of the lungs in mitral stenosis in relation to respiratory function and pulmonary haemodynamics. Br. Heart J. *28*:101, 1966.
85. Grossman, W., and Lorell, B. H.: Diastole. Boston, Martinus Nijhoff, 1987.
86. Grossman, W., McLaurin, L. P., and Stefadouros, M. A.: Left ventricular stiffness associated with chronic pressure and volume overloads in man. Circ. Res. *35*:793, 1974.

87. Grossman, W., McLaurin, L. P., Moos, S. P., Stefadouros, M. A., and Young, D. T.: Wall thickness and diastolic properties of the left ventricle. Circulation *49*:129, 1974.
88. Dodek, A., Kassebaum, D. G., and Bristow, J. D.: Pulmonary edema in coronary artery disease without cardiomegaly: Paradox of the stiff heart. N. Engl. J. Med. *286*:1347, 1972.
89. Benotti, J. R., Grossman, W., and Cohn, P. F.: The clinical profile of restrictive cardiomyopathy. Circulation *61*:1206, 1980.
90. Kern, M. J., Lorell, B. H., and Grossman, W.: Cardiac amyloidosis masquerading as constrictive pericarditis. Cathet. Cardiovasc. Diagn. *8*:629, 1982.
91. Lorell, B. H., and Grossman, W.: Profiles in constrictive pericarditis, restrictive cardiomyopathy and cardiac tamponade. *In* Grossman, W. (ed.): Cardiac Catheterization and Angiography. 3rd ed. Philadelphia, Lea and Febiger, 1986.
92. Sawyer, C. G., Burwell, C. S., Dexter, L., Eppinger, E. C., Goodale, W. T., Gorlin, R., Harken, D. E., and Haynes, F. W.: Chronic constrictive pericarditis: Further consideration of the pathologic physiology of the disease. Am. Heart J. *44*:207, 1952.
93. Alpert, J. S., Irwin, R. S., and Dalen, J. E.: Pulmonary hypertension. Curr. Probl. Cardiol. *5*:39H, 1981.
94. Grossman, W.: Profiles in valvular heart disease. *In* Grossman, W. (ed.): Cardiac Catheterization and Angiography. 3rd ed. Philadelphia, Lea and Febiger, 1986.
95. Dexter, L.: Physiologic changes in mitral stenosis. N. Engl. J. Med. *254*:829, 1986.
96. Schlant, R. C.: Altered cardiovascular function of rheumatic heart disease and other acquired valvular disease. *In* Hurst, J. L., and Logue, R. B. (eds.): The Heart. 4th ed. New York, McGraw-Hill Book Co., 1978, p. 971.
97. Wood, P.: An appreciation of mitral stenosis. I. Clinical features; II. Investigation and results. Br. Med. J. *1*:1051 and 1131, 1954.
98. McLaurin, L. P., Gibson, T., Waider, W., Grossman, W., and Craige, E.: An appraisal of mitral valve echocardiograms mimicking mitral stenosis in conditions with right ventricular pressure overload. Circulation *48*:801, 1973.
99. Araujo, J., and Lukas, D. S.: Interrelationships among pulmonary capillary pressure, blood flow and valve size in mitral stenosis: Limited regulatory effects of the pulmonary vascular resistance. J. Clin. Invest. *31*:1082, 1952.
100. Wood, P.: Pulmonary hypertension with special reference to the vasoconstrictive factor. Br. Heart J. *20*:557, 1958.
101. Davies, L. G., Goodwin, J. F., and VanLeuven, B. D.: The nature of pulmonary hypertension in mitral stenosis. Br. Heart J. *16*:440, 1954.
102. Robin, E. R., and Meyer, E. C.: Cardiopulmonary effects of pulmonary venous hypertension with special reference to pulmonary lymphatic flow. Circ. Res. *8*:324, 1960.
103. Uhley, H. N., Leeds, S. E., Sampson, J. J., and Friedman, M.: Role of pulmonary lymphatics in chronic pulmonary edema. Circ. Res. *11*:966, 1962.
104. Parker, F., and Hicken, P.: The relation between left atrial hypertension and lymphatic distention in lung biopsies. Thorax *15*:54, 1960.
105. Parker, F., and Weiss, S.: The nature and significance of the structural changes in the lungs in mitral stenosis. Am. J. Pathol. *12*:573, 1936.
106. Coalson, J. J., Jacques, W. E., Campbell, G. S., and Thompson, W. M.: Ultrastructure of the alveolar capillary membrane in congenital and acquired heart disease. Arch. Pathol. *83*:377, 1967.
107. Kay, J. M., and Edwards, F. R.: Ultrastructure of the alveolar capillary wall in mitral stenosis. J. Pathol. *111*:239, 1973.
108. Heath, D., and Edwards, J. E.: Histological changes in the lung in diseases associated with pulmonary venous hypertension. Br. J. Dis. Chest *53*:8, 1959.
109. Carabello, B. A., and Grossman, W.: Calculation of stenotic valve orifice area. *In* Grossman, W. (ed.): Cardiac catheterization and angiography. 3rd ed. Philadelphia, Lea and Febiger, 1986.
110. Braunwald, E., Braunwald, N. S., Ross, J., Jr., and Morrow, A. G.: Effects of mitral valve replacement on pulmonary vascular dynamics of patients with pulmonary hypertension. N. Engl. J. Med. *273*:509, 1965.
111. Dalen, J. E., Matloff, J. M., Evans, G. L., Hoppin, F. G., Bhardwaj, P., Harken, D. E., and Dexter, L.: Early reduction of pulmonary vascular resistance after mitral valve replacement. N. Engl. J. Med. *277*:387, 1967.
112. Zener, J. C., Hancock, E. W., Shumway, N. E., and Harrison, D. C.: Regression of extreme pulmonary hypertension after mitral valve surgery. Am. J. Cardiol. *30*:820, 1972.
113. Magidson, A.: Cor triatriatum. Severe pulmonary arterial hypertension and pulmonary venous hypertension in a child. Am. J. Cardiol. *9*:603, 1962.
114. Stoler, M. H., Anderson, N. M., and Stuard, I. D.: A case of pulmonary veno-occlusive disease in infancy. Arch. Pathol. Lab. Med. *106*:645, 1982.
115. Wagenvoort, C. A.: Pulmonary veno-occlusive disease: Entity or syndrome. Chest *69*:82, 1976.
116. Liebow, A. A., McAdam, A. J., Carrington, C. B., and Vigmonte, M.: Intrapulmonary veno-obstructive disease. Circulation *36* (Suppl. II):172, 1967.
117. Cromie, J. B.: Correlation of anatomic pulmonary emphysema and right ventricular hypertrophy. Am. Rev. Respir. Dis. *84*:657, 1961.
118. Hicken, P., Heath, D., and Brewer, D.: The relation between the weight of the right ventricle and the percentage of abnormal air space in the lung in emphysema. J. Pathol. Bacteriol. *92*:519, 1966.
119. Harvey, R. M., Ferrer, M. I., Richards, D. W., and Cournand, A.: Influence of chronic pulmonary disease on the heart and circulation. Am. J. Med. *10*:719, 1951.
120. Abraham, A. S., Cole, R. B., Green, I. D., Hedworth-Whitty, R. B., Clarke, S. W., and Bishop, J. M.: Factors contributing to the reversible pulmonary hypertension in patients with acute respiratory failure studied by serial observation during recovery. Circ. Res. *24*:51, 1969.
121. Abraham, A. S., Cole, R. B., and Bishop, J.: Effects of prolonged oxygen administration on the pulmonary hypertension of patients with chronic bronchitis. Circ. Res. *23*:147, 1968.
122. Segel, N., and Bishop, J. M.: The circulation in patients with chronic bronchitis and emphysema at rest and during exercise with special reference to the influence of changes in blood viscosity and blood volumes on the pulmonary circulation. J. Clin. Invest. *45*:1555, 1966.
123. Horsfield, K., Segel, N., and Bishop, J. M.: The pulmonary circulation in chronic bronchitis at rest and during exercise breathing air and 80% oxygen. Clin. Sci. *34*:473, 1968.
124. Harvey, R. M., Ferrer, M. I., Richards, D. W., Jr., and Cournand, A.: Influence of chronic pulmonary disease on the heart and circulation. Am. J. Med. *10*:719, 1951.
125. Yu, P. N., Lovejoy, F. W., Joos, H. A., Nye, R. E., and McCann, W. S.: Studies of pulmonary hypertension. I. Pulmonary circulatory dynamics in patients with pulmonary emphysema at rest. J. Clin. Invest. *32*:130, 1953.
126. Kitchin, A. H., Lowther, C. P., and Matthews, M. B.: The effect of exercise and of breathing oxygen-enriched air on the pulmonary circulation in emphysema. Clin. Sci. *21*:93, 1961.
127. Wilson, R. H., Hoseth, W., and Dempsey, M. E.: The effects of breathing 99.6% oxygen on pulmonary vascular resistance and cardiac output in patients with pulmonary emphysema and chronic hypoxia. Ann. Intern. Med. *42*:629, 1955.
128. Aber, G. M., Harris, A. M., and Bishop, J. M.: The effect of acute changes in inspired oxygen concentration of cardiac, respiratory and renal function in patients with chronic obstructive airways disease. Clin. Sci. *26*:133, 1964.
129. Stuart-Harris, C., Bishop, J. M., Clark, T. J. H., Dornhorst, A. C., Cotes, J. E., Flenley, D. C., Howard, P., and Oldham, P. H.: Long-term domiciliary oxygen therapy in chronic hypoxic cor pulmonale complicating chronic bronchitis and emphysema. Lancet *1*:681, 1981.
130. Nocturnal Oxygen Therapy Trial Group: Continuous or nocturnal oxygen therapy in hypoxic chronic obstructive airways disease? Ann. Intern. Med. *93*:391, 1980.
131. Foreman, S., Weill, H., Duke, R., George, R., and Ziskind, M.: Bullous disease of the lung: Physiologic improvement after surgery. Ann. Intern. Med. *69*:757, 1968.
132. Salerni, R., Rodnan, G. P., Leon, D. F., and Shaver, J. A.: Pulmonary hypertension in the CREST syndrome variant of progressive systemic sclerosis (scleroderma). Ann. Intern. Med. *86*:394, 1977.
133. Follansbee, W. P., Curtiss, E. I., Medsger, T. A., Owens, G. R., Steen, V. D., and Rodnan, G. P.: Myocardial function and perfusion in the CREST syndrome variant of progressive systemic sclerosis. Am. J. Med. *77*:489, 1984.
134. Seldin, D. W., Ziff, M., and DeGraff, A. V., Jr.: Raynaud's phenomenon associated with pulmonary hypertension. Tex. State J. Med. *58*:654, 1962.
135. Winters, W. L., Jr., Joseph, R. R., and Lerner, N.: "Primary" pulmonary hypertension and Raynaud's phenomenon. Arch. Intern. Med. *114*:821, 1964.
136. Kanemoto, N., Gonda, N., Katsu, M., and Fukada, J.: Two cases of pulmonary hypertension with Raynaud's phenomenon: Primary pulmonary hypertension and systemic lupus erythematosus. Jpn. Heart J. *16*:354, 1975.
137. Caldwell, I. W., and Aitchison, J. D.: Pulmonary hypertension in dermatomyositis. Br. Heart J. *18*:273, 1956.
138. Walker, W. C., and Wright, V.: Pulmonary lesions and rheumatoid arthritis. Medicine *47*:501, 1968.
139. Gladman, D. D., and Sternberg, L.: Pulmonary hypertension in systemic lupus erythematosus. J. Rheumatol. *12*:2, 1985.
140. Santini, D., Fox, D., Kloner, R. A., Konstam, M., Rude, R. E., and Lorell, B. H.: Pulmonary hypertension in systemic lupus erythematosus: Hemodynamics and effects of vasodilator therapy. Clin. Cardiol. *3*:406, 1980.
141. Asherson, R. A., Mackworth-Young, C. G., Boey, M. L., Hull, R. G., Saunders, A., Gharavi, A. E., and Hughes, G. R. V.: Pulmonary hypertension in systemic lupus erythematosus. Br. Med. J. *287*:1024, 1983.
142. Muschenheim, C.: Some observations on the Hamman-Rich disease. Am. J. Med. Sci. *241*:279, 1961.
143. Soergel, K. H., and Sommers, S. C.: Idiopathic pulmonary hemosiderosis and related syndromes. Am. J. Med. *32*:499, 1962.
144. Manglo, A., Fisher, J., Libby, D. M., and Saddekni, S.: Sarcoidosis, pulmonary hypertension, and acquired peripheral pulmonary artery stenosis. Cathet. Cardiovasc. Diagn. *11*:69, 1985.
145. Kane, R. D., Hawkins, H. K., Miller, J. A., and Noce, P. S.: Microscopic pulmonary tumor emboli associated with dyspnea. Cancer *36*:1473, 1975.
146. Jacques, J. E., and Barclay, R.: The solid sarcomatous pulmonary artery. Br. J. Dis. Chest *11*:123, 1974.
146a. Cooney, T. P., and Thurlbeck, W. M.: Pulmonary hypoplasia in Down's syndrome. N. Engl. J. Med. *307*:1170, 1982.
147. Wood, P.: The Eisenmenger syndrome, or pulmonary hypertension with reversed central shunt. Br. Med. J. *2*:755, 1958.
148. Yamaki, S., and Wagenvoort, C. A.: Comparison of primary plexogenic arteriopathy in adults and children. A morphometric study in 40 patients. Br. Heart J. *54*:428, 1985.
149. Haworth, S. G.: Pulmonary vascular disease in different types of congenital heart disease. Implications for interpretation of lung biopsy findings in early childhood. Br. Heart J. *52*:557, 1984.
150. Rabinovitch, M., Keane, J. F., Norwood, W. I., Castaneda, A. R., and Reid, L.: Vascular structure in lung tissue obtained at biopsy correlated with pulmonary hemodynamic findings after repair of congenital heart defects. Circulation *69*:655, 1984.
151. Haworth, S. G.: Pulmonary vascular disease in secundum atrial septal defect in childhood. Am. J. Cardiol. *51*:265, 1983.
152. Davies, N. J. H., Shinebourne, E. A., Scallan, M. J., Sopwith, T. A., and Denison, D. M.: Pulmonary vascular resistance in children with congenital heart disease. Thorax *39*:895, 1984.
153. Juaneda, E., and Haworth, S. G.: Pulmonary vascular disease in children with truncus arteriosus. Am. J. Cardiol. *54*:1314, 1984.

154. Takahashi, T., Wagenvoort, C. A.: Density of muscularized arteries in the lung. Arch. Pathol. Lab. Med. *107*:23, 1983.
155. Heath, D., and Edwards, J. E.: The pathology of hypertensive pulmonary vascular disease. A description of six grades of structural changes in the pulmonary arteries with special reference to congenital cardiac septal defects. Circulation *18*:533, 1958.
155a. Harley, R. A., Friedman, P. J., Saldana, M., Liebow, A. A., and Carrington, C. B.: Sequential development of lesions in experimental extreme pulmonary hypertension. Am. J. Pathol. *52*:52A, 1968.
156. Saldana, M. E., Harley, R. A., Liebow, A. A., and Carrington, C. B.: Extreme experimental pulmonary hypertension in relation to polycythemia. Am. J. Pathol. *52*:935, 1968.
157. Rabinovitch, M., Keane, J. F., Fellows, K. E., Castaneda, A. R., and Reid, L.: Quantitative analysis of the pulmonary wedge angiogram in congenital heart defects. Circulation *63*:152, 1981.
158. Fishman, A. P.: Unexplained pulmonary hypertension. Circulation *65*:651, 1982.
159. Senior, R. M., Britton, R. C., Turino, G. M., Wood, J. A., Langer, G. A., and Fishman, A. P.: Pulmonary hypertension associated with cirrhosis of the liver and portacaval shunts. Circulation *37*:88, 1968.
160. Levine, O. R., Harris, R. C., Blanc, W. A., and Mellins, R. B.: Progressive pulmonary hypertension in children with portal hypertension. J. Pediatr. *83*:964, 1973.
161. Segel, N., Kay, J. M., Bayley, T. J., and Paton, A.: Pulmonary hypertension with hepatic cirrhosis. Br. Heart J. *30*:575, 1968.
162. Kay, J. M., Smith, P., and Heath, D.: Aminorex and the pulmonary circulation. Thorax *26*:262, 1971.
163. Fishman, A. P.: Dietary pulmonary hypertension. Circ. Res. *35*:657, 1974.
164. Levin, D. E., Heymann, M. A., Kitterman, J. A., Gregory, G. A., Phibbs, R. H., and Rudolph, A. M.: Persistent pulmonary hypertension of the newborn infant. J. Pediatr. *89*:626, 1976.
165. Finn, M. C., Williams, L. C., and King, T. D.: Persistent fetal circulation in the newborn. J. La. State Med. Soc. *129*:169, 1977.
166. Haworth, S. G., and Reid, L.: Persistent fetal circulation: Newly recognized structural features. J. Pediatr. *88*:614, 1976.
167. Paraskos, J. A., Adelstein, S. J., Smith, R. E., Rickman, F. D., Grossman, W., Dexter, L., and Dalen, J. E.: Late prognosis of acute pulmonary embolism. N. Engl. J. Med. *289*:55, 1973.
168. Dalen, J. E., Banas, J. S., Jr., Brooks, H. L., and Dexter, L.: Resolution rate of acute pulmonary embolism in man. N. Engl. J. Med. *280*:1194, 1969.
169. Delaney, T. B., and Nadas, A. S.: Peripheral pulmonic stenosis. Am. J. Cardiol. *13*:451, 1964.
170. McCue, C. M., Robertson, L. W., Lester, R. G., and Mauck, H. P.: Pulmonary artery coarctations. J. Pediatr. *67*:222, 1965.
171. Pool, P. E., Vogel, J. H. K., and Blount, S. G., Jr.: Congenital unilateral absence of a pulmonary artery. Am. J. Cardiol. *10*:706, 1962.
172. Cohn, L. H., Sanders, J. H., Jr., and Collins, J. J., Jr.: Surgical treatment of congenital unilateral pulmonary arterial stenosis with contralateral pulmonary hypertension. Am. J. Cardiol. *38*:257, 1976.
173. Burwell, C. S., Robin, E. D., Whaley, R. D., and Bickelmann, A. G.: Extreme obesity associated with alveolar hypoventilation. Am. J. Med. *21*:811, 1956.
174. James, T. N., Frame, B., and Coates, E. D.: De subitaneis mortibus. III. Pickwickian syndrome. Circulation *48*:1311, 1973.
175. Noonan, A. J.: Reversible cor pulmonale due to hypertrophied tonsils and adenoids: Studies in two cases. Circulation 32(Suppl. II):164, 1965.
176. Menashe, V. D., Farrchi, C., and Miller, M.: Hypoventilation and cor pulmonale due to chronic upper airway obstruction. J. Pediatr. *57*:198, 1965.
177. Naeye, R. L.: Alveolar hypoventilation and cor pulmonale secondary to damage to the respiratory center. Am. J. Cardiol. *8*:416, 1961.
178. Hultgren, H. N., Lopez, C. E., Lundberg, E., and Miller, H.: Physiologic studies of pulmonary edema at high altitude. Circulation *29*:393, 1964.
179. Hackett, P. H., Creagh, C. E., Grover, R. F., Honigman, B., Houston, C. S., Reeves, J. T., Sophocles, A. M., and Van Hardenbroek, M.: High altitude pulmonary edema in persons without the right pulmonary artery. N. Engl. J. Med. *302*:1070, 1980.
180. Staub, N. C.: Pulmonary edema—Hypoxia and overperfusion. N. Engl. J. Med. *302*:1085, 1980.
181. Saaluke, M. G., Shapiro, S. R., Perry, L. W., and Scott, L. P.: Isolated partial anomalous pulmonary vascular obstructive disease. Am. J. Cardiol. *39*:439, 1977.
182. Heath, D., DuShane, J. W., Wood, E. H., and Edwards, J. E.: The etiology of pulmonary thrombosis in cyanotic congenital heart disease with pulmonary stenosis. Thorax *13*:213, 1958.
183. Durant, J. R., and Cortes, F. M.: Occlusive pulmonary vascular disease associated with hemoglobin SC disease. Am. Heart J. *71*:100, 1966.
184. Rowley, P. T., and Enlander, D.: Hemoglobin SC disease presenting as acute cor pulmonale. Am. Rev. Respir. Dis. *98*:494, 1968.
185. Houck, R. J., Bailey, G. L., Daroca, P. J., Brazda, F., Johnson, F. B., and Klein, R. C.: Pentazocine abuse: Report of a case with pulmonary arterial cellulose granulomas and pulmonary hypertension. Chest *77*:2, 1980.
186. Oliva, P. B., and Vogel, J. H. K.: Reactive pulmonary hypertension in alveolar proteinosis. Chest *58*:167, 1970.
187. Kawai, C., Ishikawa, K., Kato, M., Ishii, Y., and Nakao, K.: Pulmonary pulseless disease: Pulmonary involvement in so-called Takayasu's disease. Chest *73*:651, 1978.
188. Lande, A., and Bard, R.: Takayasu's arteritis: An unrecognized cause of pulmonary hypertension. Angiography *27*:114, 1976.
189. Rose, A. G., Halper, J., and Factor, S. M.: Primary arteriopathy in Takayasu's disease. Arch. Pathol. Lab. Med. *108*:644, 1984.
190. Haworth, S. G.: Primary pulmonary hypertension. Br. Heart J. *49*:517, 1983.
191. McGoon, M. D., and Edwards, W. D.: Primary pulmonary hypertension: current status. Mod. Concepts Cardiovasc. Dis. *54*:29, 1985.
192. Fuster, V., Steele, P. M., Edwards, W. D., Gersh, B. J., McGoon, M. D., and Frye, R. L.: Primary pulmonary hypertension: Natural history and the importance of thrombosis. Circulation *70*:580, 1984.
193. Trell, E., and Lindstrom, C.: Primary and chronic thromboembolic pulmonary hypertension. Acta Med. Scand. *534* (Suppl.):1, 1972.
194. Wagenvoort, C. A., and Wagenvoort, N.: Primary pulmonary hypertension. A pathologic study of the lung vessels in 156 clinically diagnosed cases. Circulation *42*:1163, 1970.
195. Edwards, W. D., and Edwards, J. E.: Clinical primary pulmonary hypertension—three pathological types. Circulation *56*:884, 1977.
196. Harrison, C. V.: Experimental pulmonary arteriosclerosis. J. Pathol. Bacteriol. *60*:289, 1948.
197. Bernard, P. J.: Pulmonary arteriosclerosis and cor pulmonale due to recurrent-thromboembolism. Circulation *10*:343, 1954.
198. Inglesby, T. V., Singer, J. W., and Gordon, D. S.: Abnormal fibrinolysis in familial pulmonary hypertension. Am. J. Med. *55*:5, 1973.
199. Anderson, E. G., Simon, G., and Reid, L.: Primary and thrombo-embolic pulmonary hypertension: a quantitative pathological study. J. Pathol. *110*:273, 1973.
200. Trell, E.: Primary and chronic thromboembolic pulmonary hypertension. Angiology *23*:558, 1972.
201. Stuard, I. D., Heusinkveld, R. S., and Moss, A. J.: Microangiopathic hemolytic anemia and thrombocytopenia in primary pulmonary hypertension. N. Engl. J. Med. *287*:869, 1972.
202. Franz, R. C., Ziady, F., Coetzee, W. J. C., and Hugo, N.: A possible causal relationship between defective fibrinolysis and pulmonary hypertension. S. Afr. Med. J. *55*:170, 1979.
203. Tubbs, R. R., Levin, R. D., Shirey, E. K., and Hoffman, G. C.: Fibrinolysis in familial pulmonary hypertension. Am. J. Clin. Pathol. *71*:384, 1979.
204. Evans, W., Short, D. S., and Bedford, D. E.: Solitary pulmonary hypertension. Br. Heart J. *19*:93, 1957.
205. Goodale, F., Jr., and Thomas, W. A.: Primary pulmonary arterial disease. Arch. Pathol. *58*:568, 1954.
206. Wade, G., and Ball, J.: Unexplained pulmonary hypertension. Q. J. Med. *26*:83, 1957.
207. Wood, D. A., and Miller, M.: The role of the dual pulmonary circulation in various pathologic conditions of the lungs. J. Thorac. Surg. *7*:649, 1938.
208. Brinton, W. D.: Primary pulmonary hypertension. Br. Heart J. *12*:305, 1950.
209. James, T. N.: Degenerative arteriopathy with pulmonary hypertension: a revised concept of so-called primary pulmonary hypertension. Henry Ford Hosp. Med. Bull. *9*:271, 1961.
210. Walcott, G., Burchell, H. B., and Brown, A. L.: Primary pulmonary hypertension. Am. J. Med. *49*:70, 1970.
211. Farrar, J. F., Reye, R. D. K., and Stuckey, D.: Primary pulmonary hypertension in childhood. Br. Heart J. *23*:605, 1961.
212. Naeye, R. L.: "Primary" pulmonary hypertension with coexisting portal hypertension. A retrospective study of six cases. Circulation *22*:376, 1960.
213. Segel, N., Kay, J. M., Bayley, T. J., and Paton, A.: Pulmonary hypertension with hepatic cirrhosis. Br. Heart J. *30*:575, 1968.
214. Lal, S., and Fletcher, E.: Pulmonary hypertension and portal venous system thrombosis. Br. Heart J. *30*:723, 1968.
215. Senior, R. M., Britton, R. C., Turino, G. M., Wood, J. A., Langer, G. A., and Fishman, A. P.: Pulmonary hypertension associated with cirrhosis of the liver and with portacaval shunts. Circulation *37*:88, 1968.
216. Chun, P. K. C., San Antonio, R. P., and Davia, J. E.: Laennec's cirrhosis and primary pulmonary hypertension. Am. Heart J. *99*:779, 1980.
217. Barnard, P. J., and Davel, J. G. A.: Primary pulmonary vascular disease with cor pulmonale: Report of three cases in children, one with congenital hypertension and two siblings with allergic vasculitis and disorders of skeletal epiphyses. Am. J. Dis. Child. *92*:115, 1956.
218. Braunstein, H.: Periarteritis nodosa limited to the pulmonary circulation. Am. J. Pathol. *31*:837, 1955.
219. Gurtner, H. P., Gertsch, M., Salzmann, C., Scherrer, M., Stucki, P., and Wyss, F.: Häufen sich die primär vaskulären Forem des Cor Pulmonale? Schweiz. Med. Woenschr. *98*:1579, and 1695; 1968.
220. Gahl, von K., Fabel, H., Freiser, E., Harmjanz, D., Ostertag, H., and Stender, H. S.: Primäre vaskuläre pulmonale Hypertonie. Z. Kreislaufforsch. *59*:868, 1970.
221. Gurtner, H. P.: Pulmonary hypertension, "plexogenic pulmonary arteriopathy" and the appetite depressant drug aminorex: Post or propter? Bull. Eur. Physiopathol. Resp. *15*:897, 1979.
222. Gertsch, M., and Stucki, P.: Weitgehend reversibele primär vaskuläre pulmonale Hypertonie bei einem Patienten mit Menocil-Einnahme. Z. Kreislaufforsch. *59*:902, 1970.
223. Meyrick, B., and Reid, L.: Development of pulmonary arterial changes in rats fed *Crotalaria spectabilis*. Am. J. Pathol. *94*:37, 1979.
224. Wagenvoort, C. A., Wagenvoort, N., and Dijk, H. J.: Effect of fulvine on pulmonary arteries and veins of the rat. Thorax *29*:522, 1974.
225. Olson, J. W., Hacker, A. D., Altiere, R. J., and Gillespie, M. N.: Polyamines and the development of monocrotaline-induced pulmonary hypertension. Am. J. Physiol. *247*:H682, 1984.
226. Hilliker, K S., Bell, T. G., Lorimer, D., and Roth, R. A.: Effects of thrombocytopenia on monocrotaline pyrrole-induced pulmonary hypertension. Am. J. Physiol. *246*:H747, 1984.

227. Stuart, K. L., and Bras, G.: Veno-occlusive disease of the liver. Q. J. Med. *26*:291, 1957.
228. Kleiger, R. E., Boxer, M., Ingham, R. E., and Harrison, D. C.: Pulmonary hypertension in patients using oral contraceptives. A report of six cases. Chest *69*:143, 1976.
229. Daoud, F. S., Reeves, J. T., and Kelly, D. B.: Isoproterenol as a potential pulmonary vasodilator in primary pulmonary hypertension. Am. J. Cardiol. *42*:817, 1978.
230. Shepherd, J. T., Edwards, J. E., Burchell, H. B., Swan, H. J. C., and Wood, E. H.: Clinical, physiological and pathological considerations in patients with idiopathic pulmonary hypertension. Br. Heart J. *19*:70, 1957.
231. Marshall, R. J., Helmholz, H. F., and Shepherd, J. T.: Effect of acetylcholine on pulmonary vascular resistance in a patient with idiopathic pulmonary hypertension. Circulation *20*:391, 1959.
232. Samet, P., and Bernstein, W. H.: Loss of reactivity of the pulmonary vascular bed in primary pulmonary hypertension. Am. Heart J. *66*:197, 1963.
233. Robertson, B., Rosenhamer, G., and Lindberg, J.: Idiopathic pulmonary hypertension in two siblings. Acta Med. Scand. *186*:569, 1969.
234. Melmon, K. L., and Braunwald, E.: Familial pulmonary hypertension. N. Engl. J. Med. *269*:770, 1963.
235. Rogge, J. D., Mishkin, M. E., and Genovese, P. D.: The familial occurrence of primary pulmonary hypertension. Ann. Intern. Med. *65*:672, 1966.
236. Kingdon, H. S., Cohen, L. S., Roberts, W. C., and Braunwald, E.: Familial occurrence of primary pulmonary hypertension. Arch. Intern. Med. *118*:422, 1966.
237. Heath, D., and Edwards, J. E.: Configuration of elastic tissue of pulmonary trunk in idiopathic pulmonary hypertension. Circulation *21*:59, 1960.
238. Meyrick, B., Clarke, S. W., Symons, C., Woodgate, D. J., and Reid, L.: Primary pulmonary hypertension—A case report including electron microscopic study. Br. J. Dis. Chest *68*:11, 1974.
239. Suarez, L. D., Sciandro, E. E., Llera, J. J., and Perosio, A. M.: Long-term followup in primary pulmonary hypertension. Br. Heart J. *41*:702, 1979.
240. Bourdillon, P. D. V., and Oakley, C. M.: Regression of primary pulmonary hypertension. Br. Heart J. *38*:264, 1976.
241. Sleeper, J. C., Orgain, E. S., and McIntosh, H. D.: Primary pulmonary hypertension. Review of clinical features and pathologic physiology with a report of pulmonary hemodynamics derived from repeated catheterization. Circulation *26*:1358, 1962.
242. Ross, R. S.: Right ventricular hypertension as a cause of precordial pain. Am. Heart J. *61*:134, 1961.
243. Viar, W. N., and Harrison, T. R.: Chest pain in association with pulmonary hypertension; its similarity to the pain of coronary disease. Circulation *5*:1, 1952.
244. Wilmshurst, P. T., Webb-Peploe, M. M., and Corker, R. J.: Left recurrent laryngeal nerve palsy associated with primary pulmonary hypertension and recurrent pulmonary embolism. Br. Heart J. *49*:141, 1983.
245. Kanemoto, N., Furuya, H., Etoh, T., Sasamoto, H., and Matsuyama, S.: Chest roentgenograms in primary pulmonary hypertension. Chest *76*:45, 1979.
246. Anderson, G., Reid, L., and Simon, G.: The radiographic appearances in primary and in thromboembolic pulmonary hypertension. Clin. Radiol. *24*:113, 1973.
246a. Kuriyama, K., Gamsu, G., Stern, R. G., Cann, C. E., Herfkens, R. J., and Brundage, B. H.: CT-determined pulmonary artery diameters in predicting pulmonary hypertension. Invest. Radiol. *19*:16, 1984.
246b. Goodman, D. J., Harrison, D. C., and Popp, R. L.: Echocardiographic features of primary pulmonary hypertension. Am. J. Cardiol. *33*:438, 1974.
246c. Marin-Garcia, J., Moller, J. H., and Mirvis, D. M.: The pulmonic valve echogram in the assessment of pulmonary hypertension in children. Pediatr. Cardiol. *4*:209, 1983.
247. Kosturakis, D., Goldberg, S. J., Allen, H. D., and Loeber, C.: Doppler echocardiographic prediction of pulmonary arterial hypertension in congenital heart disease. Am. J. Cardiol. *53*:1110, 1984.
248. Child, J. S., Wolfe, J. D., Tashkin, D., and Nakano, F.: Fatal lung scan in a case of pulmonary hypertension due to obliterative pulmonary vascular disease. Chest *67*:308, 1975.
249. Benotti, J. R., and Grossman, W.: Pulmonary angiography. *In* Grossman, W. (ed.): Cardiac Catheterization and Angiography. 3rd ed. Lea and Febiger, Philadelphia, 1986.
250. Oakley, C. M.: Management of primary pulmonary hypertension. Br. Heart J. *53*:1, 1985.
251. Packer, M.: Vasodilator therapy for primary pulmonary hypertension. Limitations and Hazards. Ann. Intern. Med. *103*:258, 1985.
252. Rich, S., Brundage, B. H., and Levy, P. S.: The effect of vasodilator therapy on the clinical outcome of patients with primary pulmonary hypertension. Circulation *71*:1191, 1985.
253. Berkenboom, G., Sobolski, J., and Stoupel, E.: Failure of nifedipine treatment in primary pulmonary hypertension. Br. Heart J. *47*:511, 1982.
254. Fishman, A. P.: Primary pulmonary hypertension: More light or more tunnel? (editorial) Ann. Intern. Med. *94*:815, 1981.
255. Rubin, L. J., Nicod, P., Hillis, L. D., and Firth, B. G.: Treatment of primary pulmonary hypertension with nifedipine. A hemodynamic and scintigraphic evaluation. Ann. Intern. Med. *99*:433, 1983.
256. Fisher, J., Borer, J. S., Moses, J. W., Goldberg, H. L., Niarchos, A. P., Whitman, H. H., III, and Mermelstein, M.: Hemodynamic effects of nifedipine versus hydralazine in primary pulmonary hypertension. Am. J. Cardiol. *54*:646, 1984.
257. Ocken, S., Reinitz, E., and Strom, J.: Nifedipine treatment of pulmonary hypertension in a patient with systemic sclerosis. Arthritis Rheum. *86*:794, 1983.
258. Groves, B. M., Rubin, L. J., Frosolono, M. F., Cato, A. E., and Reeves, J. T.: A comparison of the acute hemodynamic effects of prostacyclin and hydralazine in primary pulmonary hypertension. Am. Heart J. *110*:1200, 1985.
259. Lunde, P., and Rasmussen, K.: Long-term beneficial effect of nifedipine in primary pulmonary hypertension. Am. Heart J. *108*:415, 1984.
260. Saito, D., Haraoka, S., Yoshida, H., Kusachi, S., Yasuhara, K., Nishihara, M., Fukuhara, J., and Hagashima, H.: Primary pulmonary hypertension improved by long-term oral administration of nifedipine. Am. Heart J. *105*:1041, 1983.
261. Packer, M., Medine, N., and Yushak, M.: Adverse hemodynamic and clinical effects of calcium channel blockade in pulmonary hypertension secondary to obliterative pulmonary vascular disease. J. Am. Coll. Cardiol. *4*:890, 1984.
262. Packer, M., Medina, N., Yushak, M., and Wiener, I.: Detrimental effects of verapamil in patients with primary hypertension. Br. Heart J. *52*:106, 1984.
263. Malcic, I., and Richter, D.: Verapamil in primary pulmonary hypertension. Br. Heart J. *53*:345, 1985.
264. O'Brien, J. T., Hill, J. A., and Pepine, C. J.: Sustained benefit of verapamil in pulmonary hypertension with progressive systemic sclerosis. Am. Heart J. *109*:380, 1985.
265. Hoit, B., Gregoratos, G., and Shabetai, R.: Paradoxical pulmonary vasoconstriction induced by nitroglycerin in idiopathic pulmonary hypertension. J. Am. Coll. Cardiol. *6*:490, 1985.
266. Pearl, R. G., Rosenthal, M. H., Schroeder, J. S., and Ashton, J. P. A.: Acute hemodynamic effects of nitroglycerin in pulmonary hypertension. Ann. Intern. Med. *99*:9, 1983.
267. Niarchos, A. P., Whitman, H. H., Goldstein, J. E., and Laragh, J. H.: Hemodynamic effects of captopril in pulmonary hypertension of collagen vascular disease. Am. Heart J. *104*:834, 1982.
268. Rich, S., Martinez, J., Lam, W., Levy, P. S., and Rosen, K. M.: Reassessment of the effects of vasodilator drugs in primary pulmonary hypertension: Guidelines for determining a pulmonary vasodilator response. Am. Heart J. *105*:119, 1983.
269. Reeves, J. T.: Hope in primary pulmonary hypertension? N. Engl. J. Med. *302*:112, 1980.
270. Rubin, L. J., and Peter, R. H.: Oral hydralazine therapy for primary pulmonary hypertension. N. Engl. J. Med. *302*:69, 1980.
271. Lupi-Herrera, E., Sandoval, J., Seoane, M., and Bialostozky, D.: The role of hydralazine therapy for pulmonary arterial hypertension of unknown cause. Circulation *65*:645, 1982.
272. Ruskin, J. N., and Hutter, A. M.: Primary pulmonary hypertension treated with oral phentolamine. Ann. Intern. Med. *90*:772, 1979.
273. Shettigar, U. R., Hultgren, H. N., Specter, M., Martin, R., and Davies, D. H.: Primary pulmonary hypertension: favorable effect of isoproterenol. N. Engl. J. Med. *295*:1414, 1978.
274. Summer, W. R.: Primary pulmonary hypertension. *In* Fortuin, N. J. (ed.): Current Therapy in Cardiovascular Disease-2. Philadelphia, B. C. Decker, 1987, p. 282.
275. Wang, S. W. S., Pohl, J. E. F., Rowlands, D. J., and Wade, E. G.: Diazoxide in the treatment of primary pulmonary hypertension. Br. Heart J. *40*:572, 1978.
276. Klinke, W. P., and Gilbert, J. A. L.: Diazoxide in primary pulmonary hypertension. N. Engl. J. Med. *302*:91, 1980.
277. Buch, J., and Wennevold, A.: Hazards of diazoxide in pulmonary hypertension. Br. Heart J. *46*:401, 1981.
278. Nagasaka, Y., Akuisu, H., Lee, Y. S., Fugimoto, S., and Chikamori, J.: Long-term favorable effects of oxygen administration on a patient with primary pulmonary hypertension. Chest *74*:299, 1978.
279. Lock, J. E., Olley, P. M., Coceani, P. M., Swyer, P. R., and Rowe, R. D.: Use of prostacyclin in persistent fetal circulation. Lancet *1*:1343, 1979.
280. DeFeyter, P. J., Kerkkamp, H. J. J., and deJong, J. P.: Sustained beneficial effect of nifedipine in primary pulmonary hypertension. Am. Heart J. *105*:333, 1983.
281. Melot, C., Naeije, R., Mols, P., Vandenbossche, J-L., and Denolin, H.: Effects of nifedipine on ventilation/perfusion matching in primary pulmonary hypertension. Chest *83*:203, 1983.
282. Olivari, M. T., Cohn, J. N., Carlyle, P., and Levine, T. B.: Beneficial hemodynamic and exercise response to nifedipine in primary pulmonary hypertension. J. Am. Coll. Cardiol. *1*:735, 1983.
283. Lupi-Herrera, E., Bialostozky, D., and Sobrino, A.: The role of isoproterenol in pulmonary artery hypertension of unknown etiology (primary). Chest *79*:292, 1981.
284. Fyler, D. C.: Can vasodilators ameliorate pulmonary hypertension? J. Cardiovasc. Med. *8*:237, 1983.
285. Cohen, M. L., and Kronzon, I.: Adverse hemodynamic effects of phentolamine in primary pulmonary hypertension. Ann. Intern. Med. *95*:591, 1981.
286. Schroeder, J.: Personal communication, 1987.
287. Jamieson, S. W., Stinson, E. B., Oyer, P. E., Theodore, J., Hunt, S., Dawkins, K., Billingham, M., and Shumway, N. E.: Heart and lung transplantation for pulmonary hypertension. Am. J. Surg. *147*:740, 1984.
288. Dawkins, K. D., Jamieson, S. W., Hunt, S. A., Baldwin, J. C., Burke, C. M., Morris, A., Billingham, M. E., Theodore, J., Oyer, P. E., Stinson, E. B., and Shumway, N. E.: Long-term results, hemodynamics, and complications after combined heart and lung transplantation. Circulation *71*:919, 1985.
289. Jamieson, S. W., Stinson, E. B., Oyer, P. E., Reitz, B. A., Baldwin, J., Modry, D., Dawkins, K., Theodore, J., Hunt, S., and Shumway, N. E.: Heart-lung transplantation for irreversible pulmonary hypertension. Ann. Thorac. Surg. *38*:554, 1984.
290. Dawkins, K. D., Haverich, A., Derby, G. C., Scott, W. G., Reitz, B. A., Stinson, E. B., Jamieson, S. W., and Shumway, N. E.: Long-term hemodynamics following combined heart and lung transplantation in primates. J. Thorac. Cardiovasc. Surg. *89*:55, 1985.

27 SYSTEMIC HYPERTENSION: Mechanisms and Diagnosis

by NORMAN M. KAPLAN, M.D.

DEFINITIONS, INCIDENCE, AND CONSEQUENCES OF HYPERTENSION

Despite significant advances in its recognition and control, hypertension remains the major risk factor for coronary, cerebral, and renal vascular diseases, which cause over half of all deaths in the United States. In the Framingham cohort, the risk of developing coronary disease was twice as high among hypertensive compared with normotensive subjects and the risk for stroke was eight times higher[1] (Fig. 27–1). The number of people identified as having hypertension continues to increase. Based on data from the 1976–1980 National Health and Examination Survey, the number of hypertensives in the United States in 1983 was estimated to be 57.7 million[2]—more than double the estimate made in 1960–1962. This rise reflects both the greater population at risk (including more elderly patients) and the use of a lower level of blood pressure as a criterion for diagnosis (i.e., 140/90 rather than 160/95 mm Hg). Lowering this criterion has been justified because of the increased risk for eventual cardiovascular disease associated with systolic blood pressure levels above 140 mm Hg and diastolic levels above 90[3]. However, because these numbers are based on only one set of readings, the number of persons whose blood pressure is persistently elevated is probably overestimated by as much as one-third.[4]

The greater awareness of the dangers of elevated blood pressure along with the availability of safer and more effective antihypertensive agents has led to a therapeutic explosion. *In the United States, hypertension has become the most frequent reason for visits to physicians*[5] *as well as the leading indication for prescription drugs.*[6] These statistics reflect the extension of treatment to more people with mild hypertension, defined as diastolic pressures of 90 to 104 mm Hg, who make up almost 80 per cent of the hypertensive population (Fig. 27–2). Many enthusiastically applaud this therapeutic explosion, attributing to it the decline in cardiovascular morbidity and mortality rates in

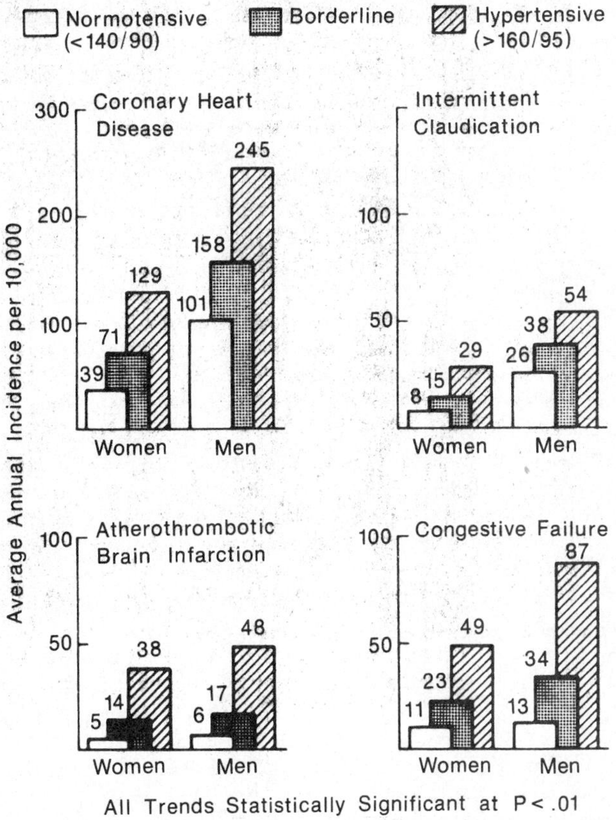

FIGURE 27–1. Age-adjusted risk of cardiovascular morbidity according to hypertensive status at each biennial examination in men and women aged 45 to 74 years (Framingham Heart Study cohort, 18-year follow-up). (From Castelli, W. P., and Anderson, K.: A population at risk. Prevalence of high cholesterol levels in hypertensive patients in the Framingham study. Am. J. Med. *80*[Suppl. 2A]:23, 1986.)

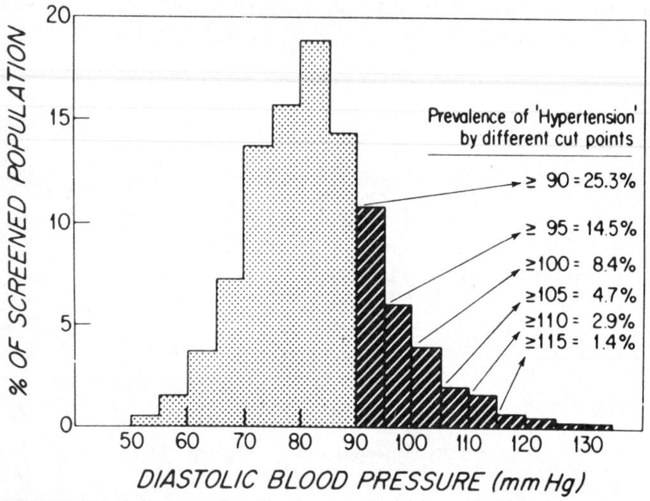

FIGURE 27–2. Frequency distribution of diastolic blood pressure at home screen of 158,906 persons, 30 to 69 years of age, HDFP, 1974. (From Hypertension Detection and Follow-up Program Cooperative Group: The Hypertension Detection and Follow-up Program. A Progress Report. Circ. Res. *40*[Suppl. I]:106, 1977, by permission of the American Heart Association, Inc.)

the U.S. and elsewhere since 1968.[7] However, objective assessments suggest that treatment of hypertension has played only a minor role in this decline and that cessation of smoking and a reduction in cholesterol levels have had a much greater effect.[8] The issue as to the role played by expanded antihypertensive therapy could be viewed as irrelevant if it were not for the growing concern that such therapy, *as it has been practiced*, may add to cardiovascular risk or at least cause bothersome side effects. This important issue is considered on page 862.

DEFINITION OF HYPERTENSION

Since more adults in the U.S. are having their blood pressure measured (74 per cent in 1985),[9] a greater number of asymptomatic hypertensives are being identified. The question of which levels are considered sufficiently elevated to justify therapy has increasingly become a problem in clinical practice. Blood pressure varies widely throughout the day and night, whether the person usually has normal or unusually high levels. Since everyone exhibits such swings, the designation *labile hypertension* is neither useful nor meaningful.[10] In some patients, this variability can be attributed to physical activity or emotional stress, while in others it is without obvious cause.

In a few patients, markedly elevated levels clearly indicate serious disease requiring immediate treatment. However, in most cases, initial readings are not high enough to indicate immediate danger, and the diagnosis of hypertension should be substantiated by repeated readings. The reason for such caution is obvious: the diagnosis of hypertension imposes psychological and socioeconomic burdens on an individual and usually *implies the need for a commitment to lifelong therapy.*

Ambulatory recordings are used both to establish the diagnosis and to monitor the patient's response to therapy. These measurements are usually lower than office readings, in one study averaging 28/15 mm Hg lower than those recorded in a clinic by physicians.[11] Since these measurements appear to be more accurate in predicting the development of cardiovascular disease,[12] it is likely that they will be used more often as the technique becomes more readily available.

DOCUMENTATION OF HYPERTENSION. For routine sphygmomanometry, the following guidelines are offered:

1. Multiple readings should be obtained using appropriate techniques (pp. 20 to 21, Table 27–1).
2. Although the logical approach would be to calculate the average values from multiple readings when deciding whether or not hypertension is present, even a single high measurement should not be disregarded. In large populations, single, casual measurements have been found to predict a greater likelihood of subsequent cardiovascular disease.[1] This increased risk applies to women as well as men and to blacks as well as whites.[13] However, such elevated measurements do not necessarily predict fixed hypertension in each case. For example, in one study, only 10.8 per cent of 719 men ages 18 to 30 with initial systolic values of 140 to 170 began to exhibit systolic pressures persistently above 140 over the next 12 to 15 years.[14] Nonetheless, persistently elevated pressures were found 2.3 times more often among those with initially high readings, obviously placing them at higher risk.
3. Systolic elevations pose a risk that is equal to or greater than that posed by diastolic elevations.[1] Isolated systolic hypertension, as is commonly seen among the elderly, presents a risk, particularly for stroke.[15] With regard to the management of such patients, the need for greater certainty is obvious, since as many as one-third of people over 65 have isolated systolic hypertension.[2]
4. The elderly often have sclerotic brachial arteries that may not become occluded until very high pressures are exerted by the balloon;

TABLE 27–1 GUIDELINES IN MEASURING BLOOD PRESSURE

- I. Conditions for patient
  - A. Posture
    1. For initial reading, patient should be supine for 5 min; take blood pressure in both arms and, in patients below age 20, one leg. Thereafter, take readings immediately and 2 min after patient stands. If pressure differs between arms, use arm with higher pressure.
    2. For routine followup, patient should sit quietly for 5 min and arm should be supported at level of heart.
    3. In patients who are diabetic or receiving antihypertensive therapy, occasionally check for postural changes.
  - B. Circumstances
    1. No caffeine for preceding hour.
    2. No smoking for preceding 15 min.
    3. No exogenous adrenergic stimulants (phenylephrine in nasal decongestants, eye drops for pupillary dilation).
    4. Quiet, warm setting.
    5. Home readings under varying circumstances and, to an even greater degree, 24-hour ambulatory recordings may be preferable and more accurate in predicting subsequent cardiovascular disease.
- II. Equipment
  - A. Cuff size: Preferably the bladder should encircle and cover two-thirds of the length of the arm; if not, place bladder over the brachial artery; if bladder is too small, spuriously high readings may result.
  - B. Manometer: Aneroid gauges should be calibrated every 6 months against a mercury manometer.
  - C. For infants, use equipment employing ultrasound, e.g., Doppler method.
- III. Technique
  - A. Number of readings
    1. Initially take 3, separated by as much time as is practical, on 3 different days.
    2. Thereafter, or with higher initial readings, take at least 2 readings.
    3. Anticipate considerable variability; if results vary by more than 10 mm Hg, take additional readings.
  - B. Performance
    1. Inflate bladder quickly to a pressure of 20 mm Hg above systolic, as recognized by disappearance of radial pulse.
    2. Deflate bladder 3 mm Hg every second.
    3. Record Korotkoff phase V (disappearance) except in children, in whom use of phase IV (muffling) is advocated.
    4. If Korotkoff sounds are weak, have patient raise the arm and open and close the hand 5 to 10 times, after which bladder should be inflated quickly.

therefore, cuff diastolic levels may be considerably higher than those measured intraarterially.[16] In patients with high cuff readings but little or no hypertensive retinopathy, cardiac hypertrophy, or other evidence of longstanding hypertension, particularly when the radial arteries remain palpable after occlusion by the cuff,[17] "pseudohypertension" should be suspected and ruled out before treatment is begun. In a few patients, a direct intraarterial pressure measurement may be needed to protect against the inadvertent induction of hypotension with antihypertensive therapy.

5. Elderly persons with elevated systolic pressure should be monitored carefully for significant falls in pressure either with sudden upright posture[18] or after meals.[19] These changes probably reflect a progressive loss of baroreceptor responsiveness with age, making the elderly particularly susceptible to marked orthostatic hypotension after even small decreases in vascular volume.[20]

For the individual patient, hypertension can be definitively diagnosed when most readings are at a level known to be associated with a significantly higher cardiovascular risk without treatment. The recommendations of the Third Joint National Committee are shown in Table 27–2.[21] Notice that diastolic levels of 85 to 89 mm Hg are classified as *high normal blood pressure*, a recommendation stemming from a prospective 8.6-year observation of over 7,000 white American men ages 40 to 59. A 52 per cent increase in relative risk for coronary disease was noted among those in the middle quintile, whose diastolic pressures were between 80 and 87, compared with patients with diastolic pressures below 80 mm Hg.[22] On the basis of these findings, persons with diastolic pressures persistently above 85 mm Hg should be advised that they may be at increased risk and counseled to follow better health habits, hopefully to lessen the progression toward definite hypertension.

BORDERLINE HYPERTENSION. As already mentioned, in view of the usual variability in blood pressure levels, the term "labile" is inappropriate for describing diastolic pressures that only occasionally exceed 90 mm Hg. Instead, the term "borderline" should be used. In many patients, the initial diastolic measurement may exceed 90 mm Hg but repeat readings taken soon after may be well below this value. In the Hypertension Detection and Follow-up Program, 29 per cent of blacks and 39 per cent of whites displayed this pattern.[23] Such patients should be advised that their blood pressure level is "borderline elevated" and should be checked annually while they follow general hygienic measures. Long-time tracking of patients with borderline hypertension has not been sufficient to provide firm data regarding the likelihood that persistent hypertension will develop.

HYPERTENSION IN CHILDREN AND ADOLESCENTS (see also pp. 852 and 1016). The caution advised in dealing with adults with borderline hypertension is even more necessary with regard to children. Based on blood pressure measurements in large numbers of normal children, readings above the 95th percentile may be considered to be abnormal.[24]

TABLE 27–2 THIRD JOINT NATIONAL COMMITTEE CLASSIFICATION OF BLOOD PRESSURE

RANGE (mm Hg)	CATEGORY*
Diastolic:	
< 85	Normal blood pressure
85 to 89	High normal
90 to 104	Mild hypertension
105 to 114	Moderate hypertension
≥ 115	Severe hypertension
Systolic, when diastolic is <90:	
< 140	Normal blood pressure
140 to 159	Borderline isolated systolic hypertension
≥ 160	Isolated systolic hypertension

*A classification of borderline isolated systolic hypertension (systolic BP = 140 to 159 mm Hg) or isolated systolic hypertension (systolic BP > 160 mm Hg) takes precedence over a classification of high normal BP (diastolic BP = 85 to 89 mm Hg) when both occur in the same person. A classification of high normal BP (diastolic BP = 85 to 89 mm Hg) takes precedence over a classification of normal BP (systolic BP < 140 mm Hg) when both occur in the same person.

From the 1984 report of the Joint National Committee on Detection, Evaluation, and Treatment of High Blood Pressure. Arch. Intern. Med. *144*:1045, 1984.

TABLE 27–3 SUGGESTED UPPER LIMITS OF NORMAL BLOOD PRESSURE IN CHILDREN BY AGE, SUGGESTED BY THIRD JOINT NATIONAL COMMITTEE

AGE (yr)	ARTERIAL BLOOD PRESSURE (SYSTOLIC/DIASTOLIC) (mm Hg)
14 to 18	< 135/90
10 to 14	< 125/85
6 to 10	< 120/80
< 6	< 110/75

From the 1984 report of the Joint National Committee on Detection, Evaluation, and Treatment of High Blood Pressure. Arch. Intern. Med. *144*:1045, 1984.

Although upper limits of normal in children of various ages were proposed in the Third Joint National Committee report[21] (Table 27–3), premature labeling of such children as hypertensive should be avoided, since long-time tracking is only now being carried out.[25] Appropriate management for asymptomatic children with sustained elevations in blood pressure has not been established. Although many maintain similarly high readings over 3- to 4-year periods, most become normotensive. Of 256 white 10- to 14-year-olds initially in the upper quintile of blood pressure, only 38 per cent remained so classified 4 years later.[26] Such patients should be followed carefully, with particular emphasis placed on weight reduction in those who are overweight in the hope of preventing progression of the disease. If nondrug therapies are not successful, antihypertensive agents should probably be prescribed for those with sustained hypertension.

FREQUENCY OF HYPERTENSION

Since we now know that variability in blood pressure levels is usual and often considerable, we have come to appreciate the wisdom of Pickering, who repeatedly warned against artificially classifying patients as "normotensive" or "hypertensive" on the basis of a single reading.[27] As noted previously, the diagnostic criterion chosen to divide the population greatly affects the number of people considered hypertensive: the prevalence almost doubles when a level of 140/90 instead of 160/95 mm Hg is used. Most surveys prior to 1980 using single measurements assigned a level of 160/95 mm Hg as the minimum blood pressure denoting hypertension for adults. The levels used to define hypertension shown in Table 27–2 are lower, but if the diagnosis is based on multiple measurements taken under reasonably controlled circumstances (as it should be), these lower levels seem appropriate. With the lower numbers, hypertension is common, and its frequency increases with the age of the population[28] (Fig. 27–3). The incidence of hypertension among blacks is greater at every age beyond adolescence, and a given level of hypertension tends to induce more vascular damage in blacks than in whites, even though systemic hemodynamics are affected similarly in the two races.

SECONDARY HYPERTENSION. Among the large number of people with hypertension, it would be helpful to know whether some secondary process—perhaps curable by operation or more easily controlled by a specific drug—is likely to be present (Table 27–4), so that the clinician can determine whether more definitive diagnostic testing is in order. Often when hypertension occurs secondary to some other disease, it is obviously related to the underlying disease and therefore of little diagnostic or therapeutic concern. Our attention will be directed toward those secondary processes more frequently considered in the differential diagnosis of hypertension because of their frequency or lack of readily apparent distinguishing features.

TABLE 27–4 TYPES OF HYPERTENSION

I. *Systolic and Diastolic Hypertension*
  A. Primary, essential, or idiopathic
  B. Secondary
    1. Renal
      a. Renal parenchymal disease
        (1) Acute glomerulonephritis
        (2) Chronic nephritis
        (3) Polycystic disease
        (4) Connective tissue diseases
        (5) Diabetic nephropathy
        (6) Hydronephrosis
      b. Renovascular
      c. Renin-producing tumors
      d. Renoprival
      e. Primary sodium retention (Liddle syndrome, Gordon syndrome)
    2. Endocrine
      a. Acromegaly
      b. Hypothyroidism
      c. Hypercalcemia
      d. Hyperthyroidism
      e. Adrenal
        (1) Cortical
          (a) Cushing's syndrome
          (b) Primary aldosteronism
          (c) Congenital adrenal hyperplasia
        (2) Medullary: Pheochromocytoma
      f. Extraadrenal chromaffin tumors
      g. Carcinoid
      h. Exogenous hormones
        (1) Estrogen
        (2) Glucocorticoids
        (3) Mineralocorticoids: Licorice
        (4) Sympathomimetics
        (5) Tyramine-containing foods and monoamine oxidase inhibitors
    3. Coarctation of the aorta
    4. Pregnancy-induced hypertension
    5. Neurological disorders
      a. Increased intracranial pressure
        (1) Brain tumor
        (2) Encephalitis
        (3) Respiratory acidosis
      b. Sleep apnea
      c. Quadriplegia
      d. Acute porphyria
      e. Familial dysautonomia
      f. Lead poisoning
      g. Guillain-Barré syndrome
    6. Acute stress, including surgery
      a. Psychogenic hyperventilation
      b. Hypoglycemia
      c. Burns
      d. Pancreatitis
      e. Alcohol withdrawal
      f. Sickle cell crisis
      g. Postresuscitation
      h. Postoperative
    7. Increased intravascular volume
    8. Ethanol, drugs, and other substances
II. *Systolic Hypertension*
  A. Increased cardiac output
    1. Aortic valvular insufficiency
    2. Arteriovenous fistula, patent ductus
    3. Thyrotoxicosis
    4. Paget's disease of bone
    5. Beriberi
    6. Hyperkinetic circulation
  B. Rigidity of aorta

Most surveys to determine the relative proportion of various secondary diseases are biased as a result of the selection process, with only the increasingly suspect population "funneled" to an investigator interested in a particular disease. Thus, estimates as high as 20 per cent for certain secondary forms of hypertension have been reported; however, these do not necessarily reflect the incidence in the population at large. Estimates more likely to be indicative of the situation in usual clinical practice are shown in Table 27–5.[29–31] Berglund et al. surveyed a random sample of the 47- to 54-year-old men in Göteborg, Sweden, whose blood pressures were above 175/115 mm Hg, so that both women and milder hypertensives were excluded.[29] Even though secondary forms are more common among those with more severe hypertension, 94 per cent of these patients with diastolic levels above 115 mm Hg had primary (essential) hypertension. A closer approximation of the case in usual medical practice is the survey by Rudnick et al. in which patients were middle-class whites seen in a family practice in Hamilton, Canada, from 1965 to 1974.[30] In this, as in the other three surveys, many of the patients underwent intravenous pyelography in addition to providing a history and undergoing a physical examination and routine urine and blood tests. Although a few patients with secondary diseases may have been

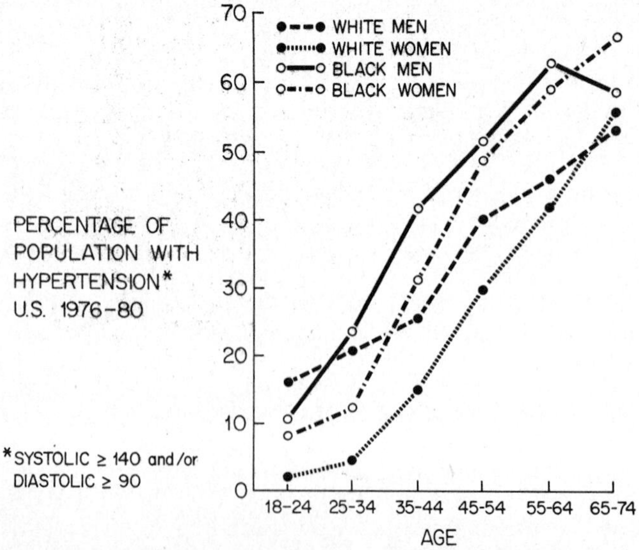

FIGURE 27–3. The prevalence of hypertension among white and black men and women in the United States, defined as systolic of 140 and/or diastolic of 90 or higher, from the National Health and Nutrition Examination Survey II, 1976–1980.

TABLE 27–5 FREQUENCY OF VARIOUS DIAGNOSES IN HYPERTENSIVE SUBJECTS

Diagnosis	Berglund et al.[29]	Rudnick et al.[30]	Danielson et al.[31]
Essential hypertension	94%	94%	95.3%
Chronic renal disease	4%	5%	2.4%
Renovascular disease	1%	0.2%	1.0%
Coarctation of aorta	0.1%	0.2%	
Primary aldosteronism	0.1%		0.1%
Cushing's syndrome		0.2%	0.1%
Pheochromocytoma			0.2%
Oral contraceptive–induced	(Men only)	0.2%	0.8%
No. of patients	689	665	1,000

Adapted from Berglund, G., et al.: Br. Med. J. 2:554, 1976; Rudnick, K. V., et al.: Canad. Med. Assoc. J. *117*:492, 1977; Danielson, M., and Dammstrom, B.: Acta Med. Scand. *209*:451, 1981.

missed, the similarity of data strongly supports the view that in 95 per cent of all hypertensives there will be no recognizable cause.

THE CHANGING NATURE OF CHILDHOOD HYPERTENSION. Even among children, secondary hypertension is less common than indicated by previous surveys of hospital-based populations. As more apparently normal children are being screened and more are found to be hypertensive, the clinical presentation of childhood hypertension is changing from that of a rare and serious disease, usually related to renal damage, to a more common and usually asymptomatic process, in most cases without recognizable cause.[25] Many prepubertal hypertensive children do not have recognizable secondary diseases, whereas most identified after puberty have idiopathic hypertension.

Selective Screening

Because of the relatively low frequency of the various secondary diseases, the clinician should be selective in carrying out various screening and diagnostic tests. The presence of features "inappropriate" for hypertension indicates the need for additional tests (Table 27–6). However, for the nine out of 10 hypertensive patients without these features, a hematocrit, urine analysis, automated blood biochemical profile (including plasma glucose, potassium, creatinine, and cholesterol), and an electrocardiogram are all that is required. Although some would include other tests, an inordinate number of screening tests for relatively rare diseases will increase the likelihood of a false-positive result. For example, according to Bayes' theorem (p. 235), using a prevalence rate of 2 per cent for renovascular hypertension, the predictive value of an intravenous pyelogram (IVP) suggestive of this diagnosis is only 10 per cent.[32]

Thus, screening tests should be reserved for those relatively few patients with suspicious features on initial history, physical examination, and laboratory testing, so that the predictive value of a positive test will justify their use. Even among children, in whom renal hypertension is much more prevalent, the addition of an IVP to "routine" testing is difficult to defend.[25] Certainly, in adults without features suggestive of renovascular hypertension (i.e., young age, severe hypertension, abdominal bruit), an abnormal IVP is more likely to be a false-positive result than a true-positive one indicative of a specific diagnosis.[4]

NATURAL HISTORY OF UNTREATED HYPERTENSION

Knowledge about the natural history of the disease must be gleaned from previous reports. Since the efficacy of antihypertensive therapy has been proved, it is no longer ethical simply to observe large numbers of hypertensives for prolonged periods without instituting suitable therapy. However, recently completed trials of therapy for mild hypertension have provided useful information about the shorter-term effects of untreated hypertension (3 to 5 years) based on results in placebo-treated controls.

TABLE 27–6 FEATURES OF "INAPPROPRIATE" HYPERTENSION

1. Onset before age 20 or after age 50
2. Level of blood pressure > 180/110 mm Hg
3. Organ damage
   a. Funduscopic findings of Grade 2 or higher
   b. Serum creatinine > 1.5 mg/100 ml
   c. Cardiomegaly (on x-ray or echocardiogram) or left ventricular hypertrophy (on electrocardiogram)
4. Features indicative of secondary causes
   a. Unprovoked hypokalemia
   b. Abdominal bruit
   c. Variable pressures with tachycardia, sweating, tremor
   d. Family history of renal disease
5. Poor response to therapy that is usually effective

SYMPTOMS AND SIGNS. Because uncomplicated hypertension is almost always asymptomatic, a person may be unaware of the consequent progressive cardiovascular damage for as long as 10 to 20 years. Only if blood pressure is measured frequently and people are made aware that hypertension is harmful even if asymptomatic will the remaining 50 per cent of Americans with unrecognized or inadequately treated hypertension be managed effectively. Symptoms often attributed to hypertension—i.e., headache, nosebleed, tinnitus, dizziness, and fainting—may be observed just as commonly in the normotensive population.[33] Headache is usually considered the most frequent and bothersome symptom. Some attribute it to the presence of hypertension,[34] while others believe that it is largely nonspecific, often psychogenic, and more likely to be identified among hypertensive patients because they are more likely to be asked about the symptom.[35] Nocturia and postural unsteadiness were the only other commonly noted symptoms among untreated hypertensives.[34]

COURSE OF UNTREATED HYPERTENSION. As noted in Figure 27–1, even minimal hypertension is accompanied by significant increases in coronary and other cardiovascular diseases. However, these figures may be misleading, since they seem to imply that most hypertensives, including those with minimally elevated pressures, will experience adverse consequences of hypertension, and rather quickly. The issue is well identified in the data from the so-called Pooling Project, which includes part of the Framingham cohort displayed in Figure 27–1. As noted previously, these data indicate that those white men with

TABLE 27–7 RISK FOR MAJOR CORONARY EVENTS AT 8.6 YEARS IN 7054 WHITE MEN BY DIASTOLIC BLOOD PRESSURE AT ENTRY

DIASTOLIC BP AT ENTRY*	MAJOR CORONARY EVENTS/1000 (ADJUSTED RATE)	RELATIVE RISK	ABSOLUTE EXCESS RISK/1000
Below 80 (Quintiles 1 and 2)	66.0	1.0	—
80 to 87 (Quintile 3)	100.6	1.52	34.6
88 to 95 (Quintile 4)	109.4	1.66	43.4
Above 95 (Quintile 5)	143.3	2.17	77.3

*Blood pressure (BP) ranges varied slightly for various 5-year age groups: 40 to 44, 45 to 49, and so on.
Data from The Pooling Project Research Group. J. Chronic Dis. *31*:201, 1978.

diastolic pressures of 80 to 87 mm Hg had a 52 per cent greater relative risk of having a major coronary event over an 8.6-year period than did those with diastolic pressures below 80 (Table 27–7). However, this increased relative risk translates to an absolute excess risk of 3.5 men per 100 over the 8.6-year interval. Obviously the majority of those with even higher diastolic pressures did not suffer a major coronary event. Nonetheless, because there are so many individuals with hypertension, the fact that even a minority of them will suffer a premature cardiovascular event in the course of their disease makes hypertension a major societal problem. In fact, when the death rates for various levels of diastolic blood pressure are multiplied by the proportion of people in the population who have these various levels, the majority of excess deaths attributable to hypertension are found to occur among those with minimally elevated pressures.[36]

As the public and the medical profession have become aware of the overall societal consequences of even "mild" hypertension, enthusiasm for its early recognition and aggressive treatment has continued to mount. This enthusiasm for therapy was apparent even before definitive evidence was available that treatment would relieve some of these risks. In 1977, prior to publication of the results of any large-scale trials of therapy for mild hypertension, 76 per cent of a representative sample of U.S. physicians indicated that they would prescribe antihypertensive drugs to asymptomatic 45-year-old male patients with diastolic pressures of 90 to 99 mm Hg.[37] A closer look at the issue of deciding upon the need for therapy is provided in Chapter 28. However, further consideration of the natural course of hypertension, as it applies to the individual patient, is needed in order to answer a basic question: Are the blood pressure and the consequent risk high enough to justify medical intervention? Unless the risk is high enough to mandate some form of intervention, there seems to be no need to identify and label the person as hypertensive, since psychological and socioeconomic burdens accompany this label; unless risks clearly outweigh these burdens, caution is obviously advised. A cogent view of this issue has been offered by Geoffrey Rose:[38]

> As doctors we are trained to feel responsible for patients—that is, to care for the sick; and from that position accepting responsibility for those with major risk factors is not too difficult a transition. They are almost patients. A general practitioner, say, makes a routine measurement of a man's blood pressure and finds it raised. Thereafter both the man and the doctor will say that he 'suffers' from high blood pressure. He walked in a healthy man but he walks out a patient, and his newfound status is confirmed by the giving and receiving of tablets. An inappropriate label has been accepted because both public and professional felt that if the man were not a patient the doctor would have no business treating him. In reality the care of the symptomless hypertensive person is preventive medicine, not therapeutics.

Rose would certainly not deny the benefits of preventive medicine but goes on to emphasize the need for great caution in applying preventive measures to large groups of people:

> If a preventive measure exposes many people to a small risk, the harm it does may readily . . . outweigh the benefits, since these are received by relatively few . . . . We may thus be unable to identify that small level of harm to individuals from long-term intervention that would be sufficient to make that line of prevention unprofitable or even harmful. Consequently we cannot accept long-term mass preventive medication.

We are thus left with a dilemma: for hypertensive individuals as a whole, even those with the least elevated pressures, risk is increased; for the individual hypertensive, the risk may not justify the labeling or treatment of the condition.

ASSESSMENT OF INDIVIDUAL RISK

Guidelines are available to help practitioners resolve this dilemma in dealing with the individual patient. These guidelines are based upon the overall assessment of cardiovascular risk and the biological aggressiveness of the hypertension. They are intended to apply only to those with *mild* hypertension, as defined in the Hypertension Detection and Follow-up Program as diastolic pressure between 90 and 104 mm Hg; those with diastolic levels persistently above 105 mm Hg have been shown to be at high enough risk from the hypertension per se to justify immediate intervention.

OVERALL CARDIOVASCULAR RISK. The Framingham Study and other epidemiological surveys have clearly defined certain risk factors for premature cardiovascular disease in addition to hypertension (see Chap. 36). For varying levels of blood pressure, the Framingham data (available in the Coronary and Stroke Risk Handbooks published by the American Heart Association and in slide rules provided by pharmaceutical companies) show the increasing likelihood of a vascular event over the next eight years for both men and women at various ages as more and more risk factors are added. For example, a 40-year-old man with a systolic blood pressure of 195 mm Hg who is otherwise at low risk would have a 4.6 per cent chance of a vascular event in the next eight years. A man of the same age with the same pressure but with all the additional risk factors (elevated serum cholesterol, cigarette smoking, glucose intolerance, and left ventricular hypertrophy on the electrocardiogram) has a 70.8 per cent chance. Obviously the higher the overall risk, the more intensive the interventions should be.

An interesting—and disturbing—connection between untreated hypertension and *hypercholesterolemia* has been found in reports from Framingham[1] and Australia.[39] In the large-scale Multiple Risk Factor Intervention Trial (MRFIT), hypertensive men showed an increased risk for coronary disease with every increment in serum cholesterol, from levels of 182 mg/dl.[40] Thus hypertensives may be burdened with an even greater risk than their blood pressure would impose. This issue is examined further in Chapter 28.

TARGET ORGAN DAMAGE. The biological aggessiveness of a given level of hypertension varies between individuals. This inherent propensity to induce vascular damage can be ascertained best by examination of the eyes, heart, and kidney.

Funduscopic Examination. As described by Keith, Wagener, and Barker in 1939, vascular changes in the fundus reflect both hypertensive neuroretinopathy and arteriosclerotic retinopathy.[41] The two processes first induce narrowing of the arteriolar lumen (Grade 1) and then sclerosis of the adventitia and/or thickening of the arteriolar wall, visible as arteriovenous nicking (Grade 2). Progressive hypertension induces rupture of small vessels, seen as hemorrhages and exudates (Grade 3) and eventually papilledema (Grade 4) (see Fig. 2–1, p. 16). Among 855 50-year-old men followed for 12.5 years, attenuated arterioles and focal narrowing were found to be closely related to the presence of hypertension and subsequent mortality from strokes, whereas crossing defects (arteriovenous "nicking") were more predictive of mortality from arteriosclerotic disease.[42]

Cardiac Involvement

1. *Left ventricular hypertrophy on electrocardiography,* based on increased voltage of QRS complexes, intrinsicoid deflection over leads V_5 or V_6 greater than 0.06 sec, and ST-segment depression greater than 0.5 mm (p. 191).

2. *Left ventricular enlargement on x-ray* (p. 142) *or echocardiography* (p. 121). Echocardiograms are more sensitive in recognizing early cardiac involvement. Using as evidence for hypertrophy a left ventricular mass index of 110 g/m^2 or greater for women and 134 g/m^2 or greater for men, 12 per cent of 145 patients with borderline hypertension (i.e., 140/90 to 159/94) had left ventricular hypertrophy as did 20 per cent of 316 patients with mild, uncomplicated hypertension (i.e., 160/95 or higher)[43] (Fig. 27–4).

3. *Abnormalities in left ventricular filling and ejection:* (1) a decreased filling rate in early diastole, implying increased myocardial stiffness, accompanied by an increased contribution of atrial systole to left ventricular filling,[44] and (2) in longstanding hypertension, a reduction in global ejection fraction, as measured in one study by radionuclide ventriculography after the volume challenge of passive leg elevation.[45]

4. *Severe diastolic dysfunction:* Early in the course, systolic function is usually normal or even supernormal.[46] In some elderly patients with severe concentric hypertrophy and a small ventricular cavity, left ventricular emptying may be so excessive and diastolic filling so prolonged as to induce dyspnea that mimics systolic heart failure.[47]

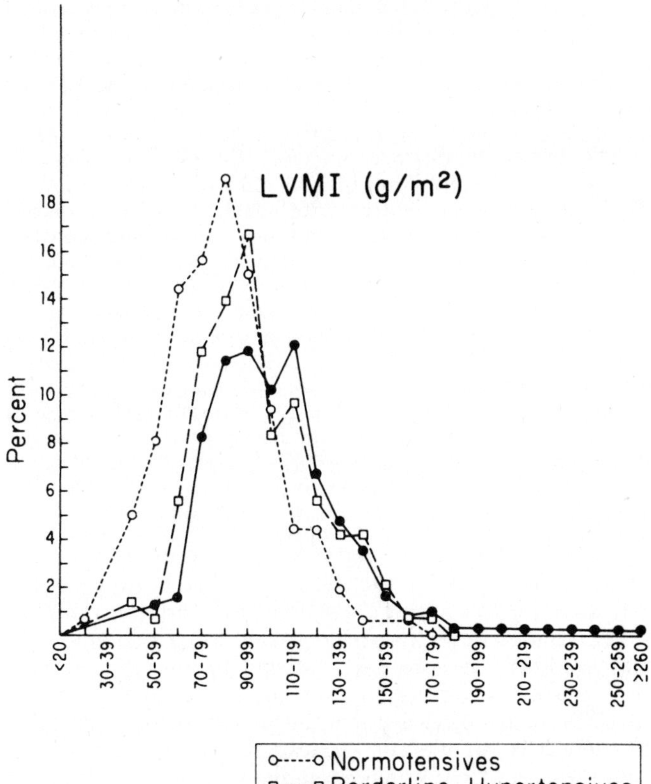

FIGURE 27–4. Distribution of values for echocardiographic measurement of left ventricular mass index (LVMI) in the three patient groups. (From Hammond, I. W., Devereux, R. B., Alderman, M. H., Lutas, E. M., Spitzer, M. C., Crowley, J. S., and Laragh, J. H.: The prevalence and correlates of echocardiographic left ventricular hypertrophy among employed patients with uncomplicated hypertension. Reprinted with permission from the American College of Cardiology. J. Am. Coll. Cardiol. *7*:639, 1986.)

5. *Changes indicative of coronary artery disease.*

6. *Clinical manifestations of left ventricular failure.*

Additional observations of the natural progression and induced regression of left ventricular hypertrophy as well as the above-mentioned cardiac findings are needed to understand their meaning and significance. But the presence of hypertrophy on echocardiography has been found to be a risk factor for death, independent of blood pressure and other risk factors.[48]

Renal Function. Renal dysfunction, too subtle to be recognized, may be responsible for the development of most cases of essential hypertension. As discussed on p. 840, increased renal retention of salt and water may be a mechanism initiating idiopathic hypertension, but the increase is so small that it escapes detection. With detailed study, both structural damage and functional derangement can be found in almost all hypertensive individuals, even in those with apparently early, mild disease.[49] In patients with longstanding hypertension, a loss of concentrating ability may be manifested by nocturia, creatinine clearance may be decreased, and albumin may be found in the urine even to within the nephrotic range.[50] As hypertension-induced nephrosclerosis proceeds, the plasma creatinine level begins to rise, and eventually renal insufficiency with uremia develops in 10 to 20 per cent of patients. Prognosis is closely related to the degree of renal damage.[51]

Cerebral Involvement. Hypertension, particularly systolic, is a major risk factor for stroke and for transient ischemic attacks caused by extracranial atherosclerosis.[52] Cerebral function should be tested, but it is not possible to relate subtle cerebral dysfunction to the severity of the blood pressure.

PLASMA RENIN ACTIVITY AS A PROGNOSTIC GUIDE. In 1972, Brunner et al. published data showing that a group of hypertensives with low levels of plasma renin activity (PRA) had a more benign course, with no heart attacks or strokes uncovered on retrospective analysis.[53] Subsequently, many investigators have examined the relationship between renin levels and cardiovascular complications and found that with few exceptions, patients with low PRA have no more benign a course than do those with normal PRA.[54] Indeed, in a 5-year prospective study, patients with initially low renin levels suffered as many heart attacks and strokes as those with normal levels, although when a cardiovascular complication appeared, initially low renin levels tended to rise.[55] This sequence may provide a rational explanation for the finding in Brunner's study, since patients whose initially low renin levels rose after a complication would not have been recognized retrospectively.

Based on the above described assessments of overall cardiovascular risk and severity of hypertension, it should be possible to determine the approximate risk status and prognosis for individual patients. This can most easily be accomplished with the Framingham data, as described on page 824.

SHORT-TERM COURSE OF LOW-RISK HYPERTENSION. Data on the 4-year experiences of over 1600 "low-risk" hypertensives who served as controls in the Australian Therapeutic Trial document the validity of this assessment.[56] To enter this placebo-versus-drug trial, the patients had to be free of all identifiable cardiovascular disease, with the second set of diastolic pressures between 95 and 109 mm Hg. Thus, they could be considered "low-risk" hypertensives. Over the next 4 years, in the majority of these patients, who were given placebo tablets but neither nondrug nor drug therapy, blood pressures *dropped progressively,* from an average of 157/102 to 144/91 mm Hg. Diastolic pressure was below 95 mm Hg in 47.5 per cent at the end of the trial. The fall in blood pressure was not related to any recognizable change in the patient's status; similar decreases occurred independent of changes in or stability of body weight. Of great interest was the lack of excess morbidity or mortality among those whose diastolic pressures remained below 100 mm Hg.

These results strongly support the view that certain patients can be characterized as being at relatively low risk and can therefore safely do without drug therapy long enough for the clinician to monitor both their blood pressure levels over time and the effectiveness of nondrug therapies, if indicated. The large number of patients whose pressures fell and the high average degree of fall may seem surprising, but none of these patients started with any identifiable cardiovascular disease or complications due to hypertension. Moreover, placebo may be more effective than no therapy. Similar results were observed in the even larger Medical Research Council (MRC) trial in England, in which over 18,000 patients with pretreatment diastolic pressures between 95 and 109 mm Hg were randomly assigned to antihypertensive drugs or placebo.[57] At the end of 5 years, these pressures had dropped to below 90 mm Hg in 43 per cent of the men and 50 per cent of the women on placebo.

THE POTENTIAL FOR PROGRESSION. Although these data reflect the benign nature of "low-risk" hypertension over the short term, it should be noted that the diastolic blood pressure rose above 110 mm Hg in 12 per cent of the nondrug-treated patients in both the Australian and English trials. Therefore, continued monitoring of the blood pressure levels is obviously needed for all patients with even the mildest "low-risk" hypertension.

A SYNTHESIS OF RISK. In the MRC trial, age, male sex, hypercholesterolemia, and cigarette smoking, along with the level of systolic blood pressure at entry, were related significantly to the subsequent development of cardiovascular complications.[57] The ability to discriminate between those who did and did not suffer a coronary or cerebrovascular event in this 5-year trial was not precise; however, the degree of risk from hypertension can be categorized with reasonable accuracy, taking into account (1) the level of blood pressure; (2) the biological nature of the hypertension, based on target organ function; and (3) the coexistence of other risks. Although risk is increased for the hypertensive population as a whole, problems are more likely in those with higher levels of pressure (diastolic above 100 mm Hg), considerable target organ damage (retinopathy, cardiomegaly, renal damage), and other risk factors (hypercholesterolemia, cigarette smoking, diabetes). For them, immediate and "aggressive" reduction of pressure seems indicated. But for the majority, who are at relatively low risk, the more reasonable approach would be to continue to monitor the blood pressure while encouraging healthful habits, such as weight control, moderate sodium restriction, isotonic exercise, and relaxation, in hopes of slowing progression of the disease (Chap. 28).

This approach justifies the screening and identification of all persons with elevated blood pressure. Since there is no certain way to predict the course of the blood pressure, all hypertensives should be followed, and recognition of their hypertension should motivate them to follow good health habits. In this way, no harm should be done and the potential benefit may be considerable if progression of the disease can be slowed by nondrug therapies.

COMPLICATIONS OF HYPERTENSION

The higher the level of blood pressure, the more likely various cardiovascular diseases will develop prematurely through acceleration of atherosclerosis—the pathological hallmark of uncontrolled hypertension. If untreated, about 50 per cent of hypertensive patients die of coronary heart disease, about 33 per cent of stroke, and 10 to 15 per cent of renal failure. Those with rapidly accelerating hypertension die more frequently of renal failure, as do those who are diabetic, once proteinuria or other evidence of nephropathy develops.[58] It is easy to underestimate the role of hypertension in producing the underlying vascular damage that leads to these cardiovascular catastrophes. Death is usually attributed to stroke or myocardial infarction instead of to the hypertension that was largely responsible. Moreover, hypertension may not persist after a myocardial infarction or stroke.

TABLE 27–8 VASCULAR COMPLICATIONS OF HYPERTENSION

HYPERTENSIVE	ATHEROSCLEROTIC
Malignant phase	Coronary heart disease
Hemorrhagic stroke	Sudden death
Congestive heart failure	Other arrhythmias
Nephrosclerosis	Atherothrombotic stroke
Aortic dissection	Peripheral vascular disease

Adapted from Smith, W. M.: Treatment of mild hypertension. Results of a ten-year intervention trial. Circ. Res. 25(Suppl. I):98, 1977, by permission of the American Heart Association, Inc.

In general, the vascular complications of hypertension can be considered as either "hypertensive" or "atherosclerotic" (Table 27–8). The former are more directly caused by the increased blood pressure per se and can be prevented by lowering this level; the latter have more multiple causations (Chap. 36), and although hypertension may represent the most significant of the known risk factors in quantitative terms, lowering blood pressure may not, by itself, halt the atherosclerotic process.

The path from hypertension to vascular disease likely involves two interrelated processes: *pulsatile flow* and *smooth muscle cell replication.* O'Rourke has stated

> The physiologically important changes in contour of the arterial pressure wave in hypertension...include rise in mean pressure, increase in pulse pressure, increase in maximal dP/dt, increase in mean systolic pressure, and variable change in mean diastolic pressure. Principally because of the earlier return of wave reflection during systole, there is a greater difference between mean systolic and mean diastolic pressure. The primary change in hypertension is in mean pressure; the other consequences follow. Ill effects of hypertension are attributable to these secondary consequences....Tension in the arterial wall is dependent on arterial pressure and caliber according to the law of Laplace. Such tension is placed on lamellar units of collagen and elastin in the wall. These are the units that are damaged in the complications of hypertension—medionecrosis, aneurysm formation, atherosclerosis, rupture, and hemorrhage. These stresses that cause such damage can be related to mean arterial pressure, pulse pressure, and maximal dP/dt....Hypertension per se is probably not as important a factor in causing arterial complications as is the resulting altered distensibility and accelerated reflection that lead to increased pulse pressure and maximal dP/dt, with resulting fatigue, degeneration, and ultimate rupture.[59]

The second process responsible for atheromatous vascular damage, i.e., a specific connection between these mechanical forces and the reaction by the arterial wall, has been demonstrated in tissue taken from patients with coarctation of the aorta: arterial smooth muscle cells previously exposed to high pressure in vivo have a shorter in vitro life span, suggesting that they have already undergone an increased number of replications in response to the high pressure.[60] The connection likely involves endothelial injury, interference with synthesis of endothelium-derived relaxing factor,[61] and adherence of platelets with subsequent release of growth factors[62] (p. 1178) (Fig. 27–5).

Whatever the mechanism of the damage, hypertension is a major factor in cardiovascular disease. Let us examine more closely these various cardiovascular diseases, the incidence of which is so clearly increased by hypertension.

CORONARY HEART DISEASE (See also p. 1173). Hypertension increases left ventricular wall tension, leading to structural, biochemical,

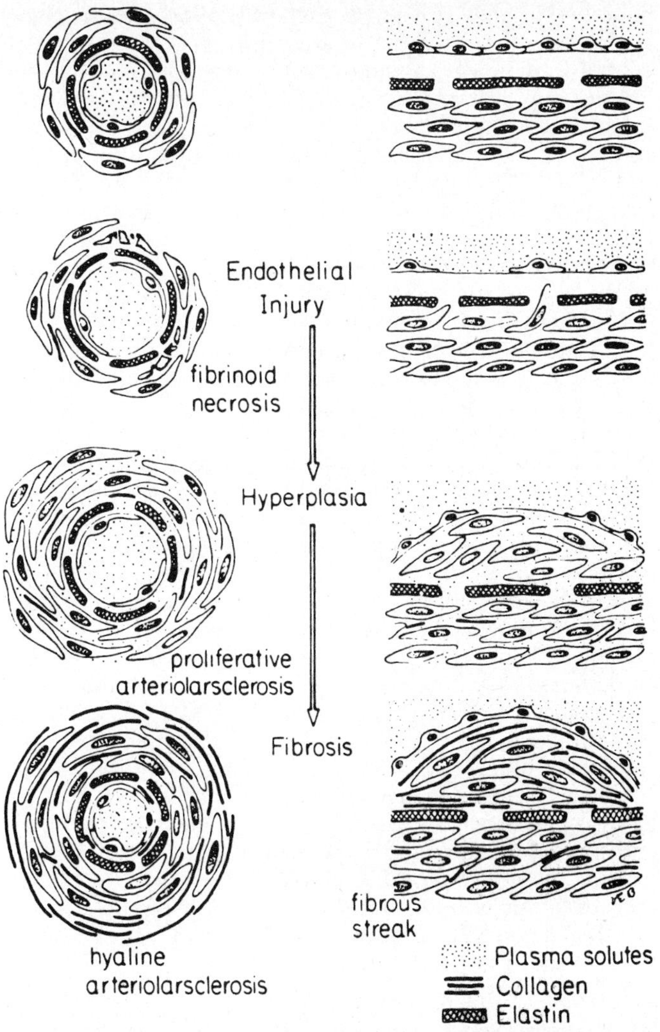

FIGURE 27–5. Small-vessel arteriosclerosis, or arteriolarsclerosis, has many features in common with large-vessel atherosclerosis. This diagram outlines mechanisms whereby both lesions might originate from a common source, endothelial injury, which leads to entry of serum factors that stimulate replication of smooth muscle cells. In the large vessel, the result is accumulation of smooth muscle cells in the intima and formation of an atherosclerotic plaque. In small vessels, the result is hypertrophy, hyperplasia, and fibrosis of the vascular media. (From Schwartz, S. M., and Ross, R.: Cellular proliferation in atherosclerosis and hypertension. Prog. Cardiovasc. Dis. *26*:355, 1984.)

and physiological changes in the myocardium. In concert with accelerated atherosclerosis in coronary vessels, these lead to coronary heart disease manifested as angina, myocardial infarction, and sudden death. As noted earlier, left atrial and ventricular enlargement and dysfunction are increasingly being recognized in patients with uncomplicated hypertension, particularly by means of echocardiography.[43–46] When such overt abnormalities appear, risk of a coronary event sharply increases.[48]

The association between hypertension and coronary disease may be obscured. In the Framingham cohort, the incidence of myocardial infarction was twice as high among hypertensive compared with normotensive persons.[63] However, the proportion of myocardial infarcts not clinically recognized but identified only on routine biennial ECG's was twofold higher among those with hypertension. Moreover, after myocardial infarction, hypertension may recede and never return to its previous level. In 37 of 58 hypertensive patients, blood pressure returned to normal and remained normal for up to 8 weeks.[64] Interestingly, participants in the Coronary Drug Project whose blood pressure decreased after recurrent myocardial infarction had a higher mortality rate, probably reflecting severe pump dysfunction.[65] On the other hand, if hypertension persists, it too poses a major risk of death.[66]

CONGESTIVE HEART FAILURE. The relationships between hypertension and congestive heart failure were clearly demonstrated in the Framingham Study.[67] Hypertension was present in 75 per cent of all patients with congestive heart failure, and the incidence of failure increased in both men and women at all ages as systolic or diastolic pressure increased. Despite treatment, 50 per cent of those who developed congestive heart failure died within 5 years. The increased systemic vascular resistance responsible for the elevated blood pressure may be both the cause of congestive heart failure and the reason it may worsen through activation of compensatory responses to the reduction in cardiac output[68] (Fig. 27–6).

LARGE-VESSEL DISEASE. Occlusive vascular disease of both proximal and peripheral arteries is increased in patients with hypertension (Fig. 27–1). Presumably by accentuating atherosclerosis and medial necrosis, hypertension is also a predisposing factor for aortic aneurysm and dissection.[69]

CEREBROVASCULAR DISEASE. Hypertension is an even more potent risk factor for cerebrovascular accidents than for coronary or renal vascular disease. In Framingham, the incidence of brain infarcts was 5 to 30 times greater in hypertensive than in normotensive subjects[1] (Fig. 27–1). Systolic pressures are even more predictive than are diastolic pressures,[52] and isolated systolic hypertension, so commonly seen in the elderly, is associated with an incidence of strokes two to four times greater than that in normotensive persons of the same age.[70]

In hypertensive patients, strokes most commonly arise from atherothrombotic infarcts of smaller penetrating branches of the middle cerebral and basilar arteries. Intracerebral hemorrhage, although less common, is more lethal. Subarachnoid bleeding also occurs more commonly in hypertensives. Transient ischemic attacks (TIA's), which are temporary episodes of focal cerebral dysfunction, develop more commonly on the background of hypertension; when they occur in concert with carotid bruits, the risk of stroke is increased.[52]

Lowering of the blood pressure will prevent initial and recurrent strokes.[56, 57] However, transient and spontaneously reversible hypertension may appear immediately after the stroke,[71] so unless the pressure is very high and causing immediate damage, a gradual reduction of longstanding hypertension is wise, allowing cerebral autoregulation to maintain normal perfusion. Rapid reduction of chronically elevated pressures to levels well tolerated by normal individuals may invoke cerebral hypoperfusion, which may cause ischemic brain damage.[72] Elderly patients are particularly susceptible because the mechanism of cerebral autoregulation becomes sluggish with age.

RENAL DAMAGE. Hypertension is the most common cause of progressive renal insufficiency,[73] and some evidence of renal damage is common in patients with hypertension. This evidence, reflecting nephrosclerosis, includes an elevated serum uric acid level, which is present in one-third of untreated hypertensives.[74] Levels of a lysosomal enzyme, *N*-acetyl-beta-D-glucosaminidase, thought to be of renal origin, are frequently elevated in both serum and urine of patients with mild hypertension.[49]

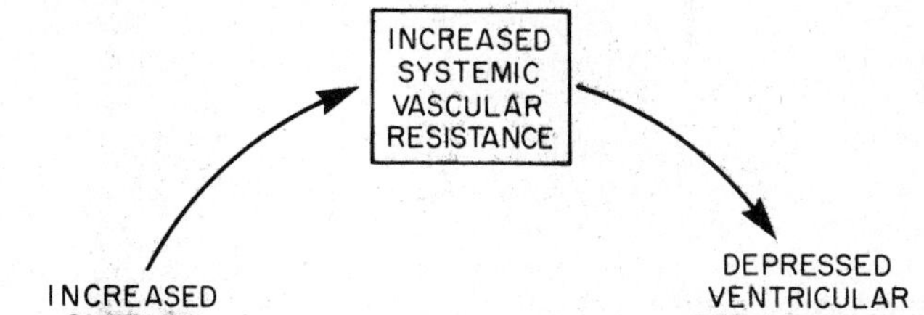

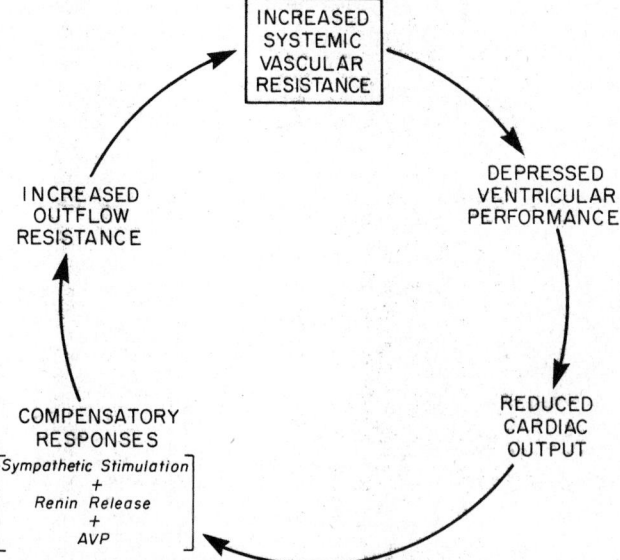

FIGURE 27–6. A unifying hypothesis for congestive heart failure. Severe and/or longstanding hypertension impairs left ventricular function, ultimately causing heart failure. Heart failure results in decreased flow, which activates several biologic systems leading to excessive peripheral vasoconstriction. The failing left ventricle reacts to this as a further impedance to ejection, setting the stage for a vicious cycle. AVP = arginine vasopressin. (Modified from Francis, G. S., Goldsmith, S. R., Levine, T. B., Olivari, M. R., and Cohn, J. N.: The neurohumoral axis in congestive heart failure. Ann. Intern. Med. *101*:370, 1984.)

The course of the relationship between hypertension and the kidneys is often uncertain: as primary renal diseases progress, they frequently cause hypertension. As we shall see, renal dysfunction, although not clinically evident, may be the basic defect in primary hypertension, and the degree of renal dysfunction is closely related to prognosis. Antihypertensive treatment may protect the kidneys, allowing some patients with even far-advanced renal insufficiency to survive for many years.[75]

RISK OF HYPERTENSION IN SPECIAL GROUPS

BLACKS. Although blood pressure in blacks is not higher than that in whites during adolescence,[24] adult blacks have hypertension more frequently, producing higher rates of morbidity and mortality. In particular, they suffer more renal damage, leading to a significantly greater prevalence of end-stage disease requiring chronic dialysis.[73] Hypertension in blacks has been characterized as having a relatively greater component of fluid volume excess, including a higher prevalence of low plasma renin activity and a greater responsiveness to diuretic therapy.[76] These and other features suggestive of volume excess may reflect larger degrees of one or more of the abnormalities in sodium transport across cell membranes that are described on p. 833. For now, we need only mention the presence of various differences in cellular transport in blacks compared with whites, such as a lower reaction velocity of the Na^+,K^+-ATPase pump in red cells, which is associated with higher intracellular sodium concentrations.[77]

Perhaps blacks evolved the physiological machinery that would offer protection in their original habitat, i.e., hot, arid climates in which avid sodium conservation was necessary for survival. Because their diet was relatively low in sodium,[78] they are more susceptible to "sodium overload" when they migrate to areas where sodium intake is excessive. This view is supported by the experience of the Xhosa people in Southern Africa: when they migrated to urban areas, their blood pressures began to rise in association with their increased dietary intake of sodium.[79] In addition to the exposure to sodium, blacks may also be more susceptible to hypertension because they tend to ingest less potassium.[80]

WOMEN. In general, women suffer less cardiovascular morbidity and mortality than men for any degree of hypertension (Fig. 27–1). Moreover, before menopause, hypertension is less common in women than in men (Fig. 27–3). Perhaps the lower frequency and severity of hypertension reflect the lower blood volume afforded women by their monthly menses.

THE ELDERLY. As more people live longer, more predominantly systolic and combined systolic and diastolic hypertension will be seen. Earlier, we noted the high frequency and risks of systolic hypertension among the elderly, a population that may have certain special needs. To a large extent, the progressive rise in systolic pressure reflects a loss of compliance within the major arteries due to permanent sclerosis; therapy may be either ineffectual, since vasodilation may not be possible, or poorly tolerated, since a shrinkage of fluid volume or decrease in cardiac output may diminish blood flow to the brain.[20] Baroreceptor sensitivity often decreases with age, so that the buffering effect of this reflex with changes in posture and the like may be lost; old people may experience a greater fall in blood pressure upon standing[18] as well as a propensity for postprandial hypotension.[19] In many elderly patients with significant hypertension of recent onset, chronic renal disease or atherosclerotic renovascular disease will be a cause of the elevated blood pressure.

MECHANISMS OF PRIMARY (ESSENTIAL) HYPERTENSION

When the specific cause of hypertension is unknown, we can begin by considering those factors known to affect blood pressure (Fig. 27–7). Although other forces may be involved, cardiac output and peripheral resistance are the primary determinants of arterial pressure. The interplay of various derangements in factors affecting cardiac output and peripheral resistance may precipitate the disease, and these may differ in both type and degree in different patients. Looking for a single defect in all patients with essential hypertension may be a mistake. The following sage advice was presented in an editorial in *The Lancet:*

> Blood pressure is a measurable end-product of an exceedingly complex series of factors including those which control blood-vessel caliber and responsiveness, those which control fluid volume within and outside the vascular bed, and those which control cardiac output. None of these factors is independent; they interact with each other and respond to changes in blood pressure. It is not easy, therefore, to dissect out cause and effect. Few factors which play a role in cardiovascular control are completely normal in hypertension: indeed, normality would require explanation, since it would suggest a lack of responsiveness to increased pressure.[81]

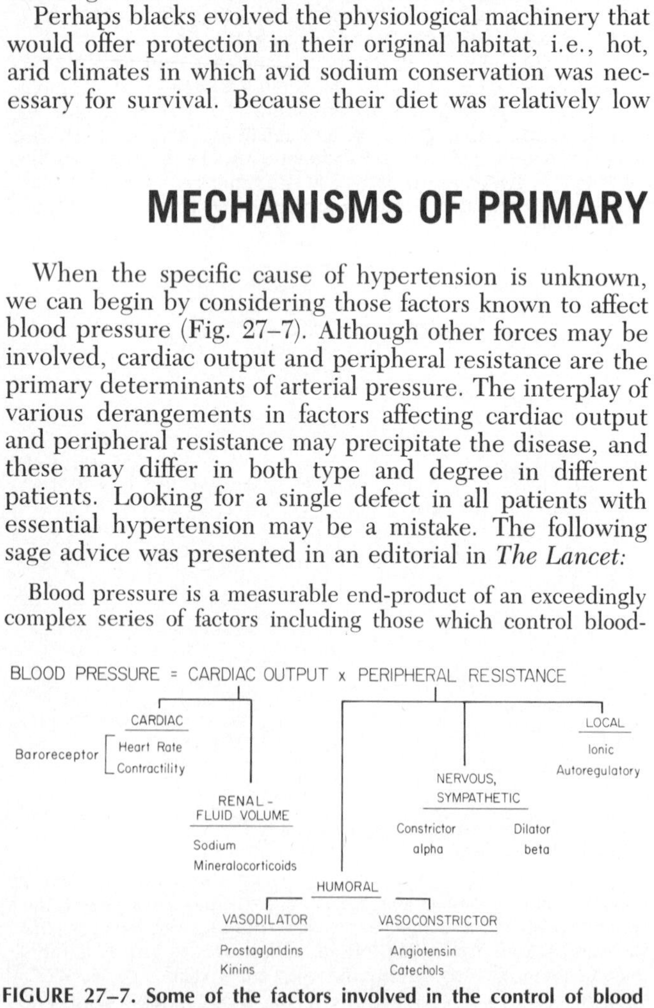

FIGURE 27–7. Some of the factors involved in the control of blood pressure that affect the basic equation: blood pressure = cardiac output × peripheral resistance.

The search for such defects to unravel the pathogenesis of essential hypertension may be misguided for another reason—it may not be a distinct disease caused by specific abnormalities. Pickering advocated the concept that essential hypertension was only a quantitative deviation from the norm, so that people were arbitrarily called "hypertensive" if they were on the higher portion of a unimodal distribution curve, rather than being on a separate portion of a biomodal curve.[27] The distribution of blood pressure in large populations is, in fact, unimodal (Fig. 27–2), but such curves do not exclude the possibility that those who become hypertensive are qualitatively different.

HEMODYNAMIC PATTERNS

Before presenting a specific hypothesis that includes such qualitative differences, let us examine the hemodynamic patterns of cardiac output and peripheral resistance that have been measured in patients with hypertension.

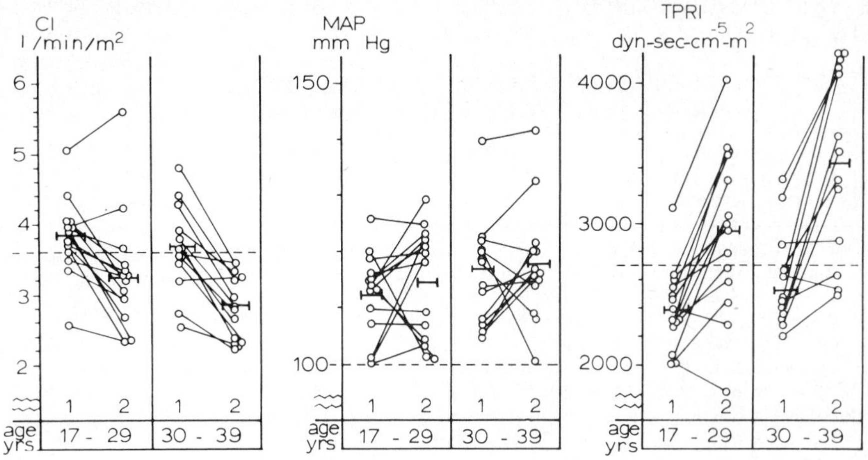

FIGURE 27–8. A 10-year follow-up study of the hemodynamics at rest in 28 untreated patients with essential hypertension. Cardiac index (CI), mean arterial pressure (MAP), and total peripheral resistance index (TPRI) at first (1) and second (2) study. Values between brackets ([—]) are mean values. The broken horizontal lines represent the upper limits of normal. (From Lund-Johansen, P.: Hemodynamic alterations in hypertension—spontaneous changes and effects of drug therapy. Acta Med. Scand. *603*[Suppl.]:1, 1977.)

One caution is needed: the pathogenesis of the disease is probably a slow and gradual process. By the time blood pressure becomes elevated, the initiating factors may no longer be apparent, since they may have been "normalized" by the compensatory interactions alluded to above. Nonetheless, when a group of untreated, young hypertensive patients was initially studied, cardiac output was normal or slightly increased and peripheral resistance was normal[82] (Fig. 27–8). Over the next 10 years, cardiac output fell and peripheral resistance rose. Although this pattern may be common, it may not occur invariably. In a few patients a high-output state may persist, perhaps because of increased sympathetic and decreased parasympathetic drive.[83] In others, peripheral resistance is abnormally high, even in the presence of high output.[84] Regardless of how hypertension begins, the eventual primacy of increased resistance can be shown even in models of hypertension that feature an initial increase in fluid volume and cardiac output. For example, patients in whom primary aldosteronism was completely controlled with the aldosterone antagonist spironolactone were followed after this drug was discontinued and the syndrome was allowed to recur in its natural manner.[85] Initially, plasma volume was expanded; however, it returned toward normal as peripheral resistance rose progressively.

AUTOREGULATION. The pattern of high output changing to high resistance does occur in some instances. How does the change come about? One possible mechanism is the process of autoregulation, a property intrinsic to resistance vessels, in which an increase in blood flow beyond the needs of the tissue leads to vasoconstriction (p. 884). As this decreases blood flow and brings supply and demand into balance, peripheral resistance increases. Folkow has shown that this functional change leads quickly to structural alterations that thicken the vessel walls.[86] In concert or independently, an increase in vascular reactivity to pressor stimuli may also be involved. In experimental models, this increased sensitivity appears before blood pressure rises and may thus be a primary mechanism in increased peripheral resistance.[87] To summarize the observational data, cardiac output and fluid volume may be elevated initially, but hypertension is maintained by an increased peripheral resistance that may reflect first functional changes (i.e., vasoconstriction) and then vessel wall thickening.

GENETIC PREDISPOSITION

(See also p. 1179)

Familial correlations relative to blood pressure levels have been noted in infants as young as 6 months, supporting a genetic mechanism.[88] In studies of twins and family members in which the degree of familial aggregation of blood pressure levels is compared with the closeness of genetic sharing, the genetic contributions have been estimated to range from 30 to 60 per cent.[89] In other populations, shared genes could explain about 25 per cent of the variability in blood pressure—a much larger contribution than shared environment (about 5 per cent) but less than age and sex (about 30 to 40 per cent), leaving another 30 to 40 per cent unexplained.[90] Unquestionably, environment plays some role: the significant correlation between blood pressures of spouses has no other recognizable explanation.[91] Although the debate concerning the roles of heredity and environment may be largely academic, it could have important practical implications. First, children and siblings of hypertensives should be more carefully screened. Second, they should be vigorously advised to avoid environmental factors known to aggravate hypertension and increase cardiovascular risks (e.g., smoking, inactivity, and sodium).

THE INHERITED DEFECT. If heredity does indeed play a role, what is inherited? A number of possibilities have been suggested, including a heightened sympathetic ner-

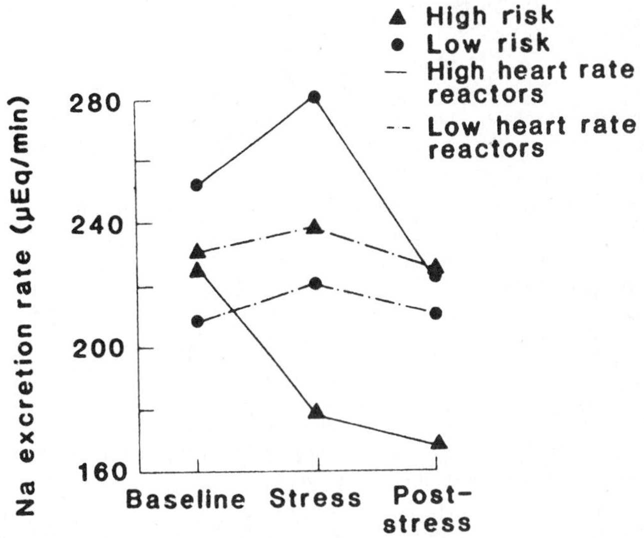

FIGURE 27–9. Rates of sodium excretion during baseline, the stress of competitive mental tasks, and the poststress periods, each of 1-hour duration, in 40 young males. The high-risk subjects had occasional systolic blood pressures above 140 mm Hg or a parental history of hypertension, whereas the low risk subjects had neither. The high heart rate reactors had mean increases of 13 beats/min during the stress, the low reactors less than that. (From Light, K. C., Koepke, J. P., Obrist, P. A., and Willis, P. W.: Psychological stress induces sodium and fluid retention in men at high risk for hypertension. Science *220*:429, 1983. Copyright 1983 by the American Association for the Advancement of Science.)

TABLE 27–9 EVIDENCE FOR A ROLE OF SODIUM IN PRIMARY (ESSENTIAL) HYPERTENSION

1. In large populations, prevalence of hypertension tends to increase with increasing levels of sodium intake.
2. Multiple, scattered groups who consume little sodium (less than 50 mmol/day) have little or no hypertension. When they consume more sodium, hypertension appears.
3. Animals given sodium loads, if genetically predisposed, develop hypertension.
4. Some people, when given large sodium loads over short periods, develop an increase in vascular resistance and blood pressure.
5. An increased concentration of sodium is present in the vascular tissue and blood cells of most hypertensives.
6. Sodium restriction, to a level of 60 to 90 mmol per day, will lower blood pressure in most people. The antihypertensive action of diuretics requires an initial natriuresis.

vous response to stress,[92] a defect in renal excretion of sodium,[93] and a defect in the transport of sodium across cell membranes.[94] These will be discussed later in this chapter. One study that may connect all these factors should be mentioned before we discuss these possibilities (Fig. 27–9).[95] When two groups of normotensive young men underwent an hour of mental stress, nine of the 13 whose parents were hypertensive (the high-risk group) showed a fall in sodium excretion, whereas sodium excretion rose slightly among those with normotensive parents (the low-risk group). The fall in sodium excretion was greater in those whose heart rate increased during the mental stress (the high reactors), suggesting a common pathway of the genetic influence on renal sodium excretion through the sympathetic nerves.

DIETARY SODIUM EXCESS

Evidence *for the role of excessive dietary sodium intake in the pathogenesis of hypertension* is summarized in Table 27–9. Most individuals consume more sodium than necessary and probably a great deal more than our ancestors consumed. The change probably occurred when food sources began to be harvested, stored, and processed instead of grown or caught and eaten fresh. Although the evidence in the table is impressive, some remain unconvinced and believe that it does not justify recommending any modification of current dietary sodium intake.[96] It seems clear that no direct relationship between sodium intake and blood pressure exists.[97] Furthermore, the massive long-term interventional studies that would be needed to prove a causal connection between sodium and the development of hypertension in man will almost certainly not be feasible, although in one study halving sodium intake in newborn infants for 6 months reduced blood pressure levels by a small but significant degree.[98]

The primary hypothesis to be developed here considers excess dietary sodium as a *necessary* though certainly *not sufficient* mechanism in the development of hypertension. It proposes that a genetic abnormality exposes some of the population to the pro-hypertensive effects of one or more environmental factors. A person predisposed because of an inherited defect might not develop hypertension if the environmental influence is avoided. *Both the genetic defect and the environmental influence are needed.* Similarly, the degree of hypertension that develops could reflect varying degrees of exposure to the environmental influence(s). Homozygotes might also develop more hypertension than heterozygotes, or there may be more than one genetic defect, so that the end result could vary markedly depending on the interplay of multiple genetic and environmental factors.

As complicated as the eventual situation may be, the hypothesis to be developed proposes only one of two possible genetic defects involving sodium and calcium transport and two major environmental factors. The genetic defects involve the renal excretion of sodium and the transport of sodium and calcium across cell membranes; the environmental factors are excess dietary sodium intake and stress. It is recognized that this hypothesis is based on evidence that is still incomplete and may turn out to be inaccurate or limited; however, at this time it seems both logical and parsimonious.

SYMPATHETIC NERVOUS ACTIVATION

Evidence for an increased level of sympathetic nervous activation in hypertensives is summarized in Table 27–10. Increased sympathetic nervous activity could raise blood pressure in a number of ways—either alone or in concert with stimulation of renin release by catecholamines—by causing arteriolar and venous constriction, by increasing cardiac output, or by altering the normal renal pressure-volume relationship[99] (Fig. 27–10). In addition to cardiac stimulation by sympathetic activity, vagal inhibitory responses to baroreceptor and other stimuli may also be important.[83] In humans with denervated transplanted hearts, both pulse and blood pressures fail to display the usual nocturnal fall, and hypertension is frequent.[100] The transient increase in epinephrine during stress reactions may invoke a more prolonged pressor response by facilitating the release of norepinephrine from sympathetic neurons.[101]

In addition to the data shown in Figure 27–9, numerous studies have shown that normotensives whose parents are hypertensive tend to show a greater rise in pulse and blood pressure after various mental stresses. This presumably inherited cardiovascular hyperreactivity is particularly prominent in those who exhibit denial behavior and suppress their emotions.[102] Normotensive subjects with a positive family history of primary hypertension have also shown an increased blood pressure response to a stepwise infusion of norepinephrine, with a significant shift to the left of a plot relating changes in blood pressure and plasma norepinephrine.[103] The subjects did *not* display a similar hyperresponsiveness to infused angiotensin II with regard to either blood pressure or aldosterone secretion.

In whatever manner it comes about, increased sympathetic nervous activation may be responsible for a change in the normal relationship between blood pressure and sodium excretion, i.e., pressure-natriuresis. This effect of sympathetic activation likely involves the recruitment of increased renin-angiotensin activity, which may then assume the major role in the resetting of pressure-natriuresis.

TABLE 27–10 EVIDENCE FOR SYMPATHETIC NERVOUS ACTIVATION IN PRIMARY (ESSENTIAL) HYPERTENSION

1. In animals, acute hypertension can be induced by release of catecholamines in response to discrete brain lesions.
2. In rats bred to become hypertensive spontaneously, alerting stimuli invoke greater discharges from central autonomic centers.
3. Some hypertensive people have high plasma catecholamine levels that correlate with blood pressure.
4. Hypertensives with high plasma catechols (and high plasma renin levels) display greater suppressed hostility on psychometric testing.
5. Some hypertensives overrespond to stress, and hypertension occurs more often in persons exposed to high levels of psychogenic stress.
6. Drugs that inhibit adrenergic nervous activity lower blood pressure.

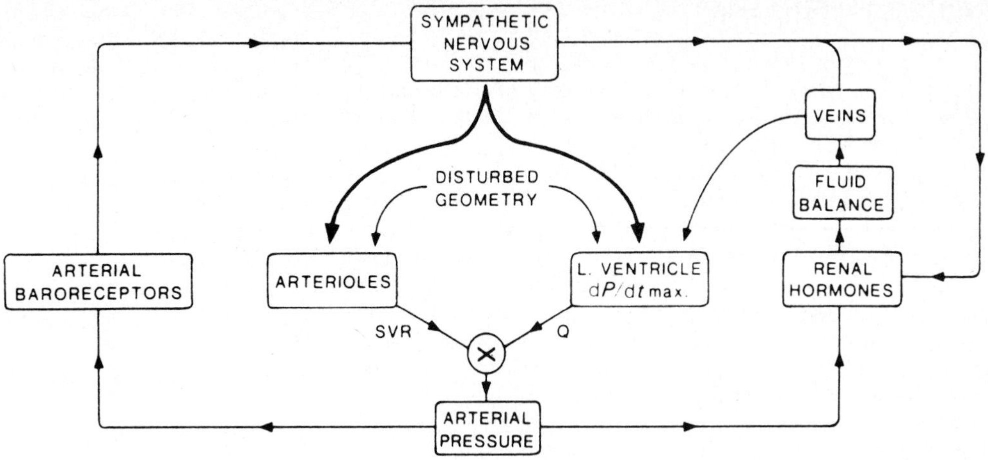

FIGURE 27–10. Schema of the hemodynamic perturbations induced in the hypertensive patient, demonstrating the interactions of adaptive hypertrophy of the arteriolar media, and of the left ventricle, with sympathetic nervous activity. (From Prys-Roberts, C.: Anaesthesia and hypertension. Br. J. Anaesth. *56*:711, 1984.)

PRESSURE-NATRIURESIS

When the normal kidney is exposed to higher arterial pressure, it quickly excretes extra sodium and water. Guyton and coworkers have long argued that this process of pressure-natriuresis must be reset in a hypertensive, because if it were not, whatever caused the pressure to rise would be countered by enhanced natriuresis, which would shrink fluid volume and restore normal pressure.[104] This resetting of the pressure-natriuresis curve can arise from increased resistance within the renal efferent arterioles, which could be due to exposure to increased concentrations of or increased sensitivity to angiotensin II or catecholamines.[105] The greater degree of efferent arteriolar constriction would increase the fraction of blood filtered (filtration fraction), increasing the peritubular oncotic pressure and thereby exerting a greater force for reabsorption of tubular sodium.

Both human[106] and animal[107] data have shown increased renal efferent arteriolar constriction early in the course of hypertension. Studies in humans, using radioxenon to measure renal blood flow, indicate excessive sympathetically mediated, reversible intrarenal vasoconstriction in early hypertension and, to a lesser degree, in normotensives with a positive family history for hypertension (Fig. 27–11).[106] In animals, direct visualization of renal tissue in hypertensive hamsters demonstrated a greater degree of constriction of efferent than of afferent arterioles upon exposure to either norepinephrine or angiotensin.[107]

FAILURE OF RENAL BLOOD FLOW MODULATION. In an intriguing series of observations, Hollenberg, Williams, and coworkers have identified a *failure to modulate renal blood flow in response to sodium loads* in about half the 80 per cent of hypertensives with normal or high levels of plasma renin activity.[108] These patients, identified as "nonresponders" or "nonmodulators" because PRA levels do not decrease after saline infusion, fail to excrete the sodium load as readily as do the "responders" (Fig. 27–12). This decreased natriuretic response is restored to normal by pretreatment with an angiotensin converting-enzyme (ACE) inhibitor, suggesting that the pre-ACE inhibitor failure to modulate renal blood flow reflects high or fixed levels of angiotensin within the renal efferent arterioles.

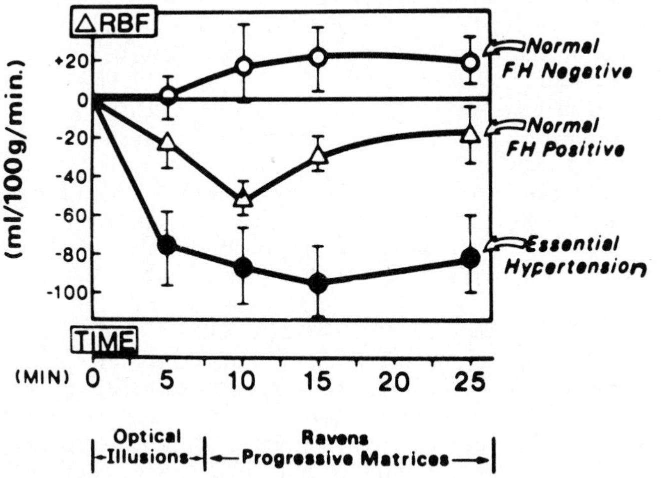

FIGURE 27–11. The response of renal blood flow (RBF) to the mild emotional stress provoked by performing a nonverbal IQ test, Ravens Progressive Matrices, in normotensives with either a negative or a positive family history and in patients with essential hypertension. (From Hollenberg, N. K., Williams, G. H., and Adams, D. F.: Essential hypertension: Abnormal renal vascular and endocrine responses to a mild psychological stimulus. Hypertension *3*:11, 1981, by permission of the American Heart Association, Inc.)

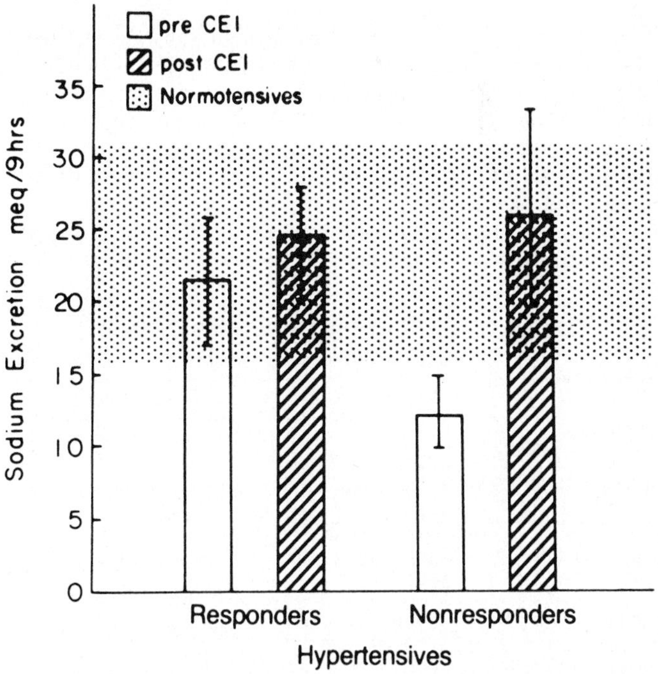

FIGURE 27–12. Sodium excretion during the 9 hours after a sodium load in the responders (n = 9) and nonresponders (n = 7) with normal renin essential hypertension. Note that converting enzyme inhibition (CEI) corrected the blunted natriuresis in the nonresponders and did not influence the responders' rate of sodium excretion significantly. The 95 per cent confidence interval for the normotensive subjects is depicted by the hatched area. (From Rydstedt, L. L., Williams, G. H., and Hollenberg, N. K.: Renal and endocrine response to saline infusion in essential hypertension. Hypertension *8*:217, 1986, by permission of the American Heart Association, Inc.)

In addition, adrenal secretion of aldosterone in response to sodium deprivation is blunted.[109] This lower level of aldosterone would lead to increased renin release in order to close the renin-angiotensin-aldosterone-volume feedback loop. Therefore, with a low-sodium intake, they would have angiotensin-mediated hypertension. However, under the more usual circumstances of a high sodium intake, nonresponders would tend to have volume-mediated hypertension, since they do not excrete sodium loads in a normal manner. Thus, their failure to increase renal blood flow in order to excrete sodium loads would translate into a resetting or blunting of pressure-natriuresis.

FLUID VOLUME. The proposed reset pressure-natriuresis curve should result in a relatively greater volume within the circulation for a given level of blood pressure. Plasma volume that is *relatively* (though not absolutely) expanded has been measured in at least 80 per cent of hypertensives compared with the expected and observed progressive decrease in volume with increasing blood pressure among normotensive subjects.[110] Moreover, total body exchangeable sodium was found to be positively correlated with levels of systolic blood pressure in 132 men with primary hypertension.[111] However, in this study and in others,[112] the *absolute* level of blood volume and body sodium are *not* increased in most people with established hypertension, even though, as stated above, the volume relative to the level of pressure is elevated. This *relatively* increased body fluid volume (inappropriately high for the level of blood pressure) would tend to distend the vascular bed, which may be reduced in response to the vasoconstrictive action of the high levels of catecholamines and angiotensin.

NATRIURETIC HORMONES. When plasma volume is expanded, renal excretion of sodium is increased, in part by the action of one or more circulating natriuretic hormones. One, arising from the atria, has been totally synthesized and intensively studied since its recognition by deBold and coworkers in 1981.[113] Although increased levels of circulating *atrial natriuretic peptide* (ANP) have been reported in patients with essential hypertension,[114] the role of this hormone in hypertension remains uncertain. (For further discussion, see p. 1831.)

Although the existence of another natriuretic hormone has been postulated for over 30 years, it remains neither isolated nor characterized, despite a great deal of work (Table 27–11).[115] In animals, the hormone appears to come from the hypothalamus.[116] Increased circulating levels of an endogenous inhibitor of Na^+,K^+-ATPase, which shares immunological determinants with the cardiac glycoside digoxin and which has been called *endoxin*, have been measured in volume-expanded hypertensive animals[117] and humans.[118] Some have found increased levels of such a circulating ouabain-like factor in essential hypertensives,[119] while others have not.[120] Some are able to show that such a natriuretic factor from the hypothalamus acts on renal cells as a potent regulator of Na^+,K^+-ATPase activity[121]; others report that the Na^+,K^+-ATPase inhibitor in human plasma is not an endogenous glycoside at all but that the phenomena attributed to it are accounted for by physiological concentrations of nonesterified fatty acids and lysophospholipids.[122] The current situation is confusing, but ongoing research should clarify the issue.

In the meantime, many believe in the existence of such a hormone, arising in response to volume expansion and inducing natriuresis by inhibiting renal Na^+,K^+-ATPase, thereby reducing active sodium reabsorption. In the hypothesis being developed, the natriuresis provoked by inhibition of renal Na^+,K^+-ATPase would counter the forces that initially increased renal sodium reabsorption at the onset of the process which eventually leads to hypertension. Thereby the tendency toward continually expanding fluid volume would be thwarted. However, in addition to its inhibitory effect on the renal Na^+,K^+-ATPase pump, the putative natriuretic hormone has been postulated to inhibit the same pump present in vascular smooth muscle.[123] This ouabain-sensitive pump is the major physiological regulator of the marked gradient of sodium and potassium concentrations across cell membranes, extracellular sodium being 140 mmol/liter and intracellular sodium being less than 10, whereas extracellular potassium is 4 mmol/liter and intracellular potassium is around 100 mmol/liter. Inhibition of this pump would inhibit sodium efflux from cells and thus increase intracellular sodium concentration.

Sodium concentration within vascular tissue of hypertensive patients was shown to be increased by Tobian and Binion in 1952.[124] Since then, most measurements of intracellular sodium content have used more readily accessible red and white blood cells. The sodium content of white cells from hypertensives has been uniformly found to be increased, with convincing evidence that the increase reflects an abnormality of the sodium pump.[125] The use of non-nucleated red cells, with a much less active pumping mechanism, has provided rather ambiguous results. Only recently, has active sodium pumping, as assessed by the ouabain-sensitive sodium efflux rate constants, been found to be significantly correlated in leukocytes and resistance vessels from 18 subjects, supporting the use of the white cells as appropriate surrogates for what happens in vascular tissue.[126]

OTHER TRANSPORT MECHANISMS. Other cellular transport mechanisms have also been recognized and studied in experimental and human hypertension (Fig. 27–13). In brief, lithium-sodium countertransport in red cells has almost uniformly been increased in essential hypertension, with most studies finding a genetic linkage.[125] Reduced rates of sodium-potassium cotransport, on the other hand, have not been shown as consistently, perhaps because of methodological differences or failure to control various patient variables.[127] Increased red cell lithium-sodium countertransport has also been shown to correlate with reduced renal lithium clearance, which is considered to be a marker of increased proximal renal tubular reabsorption

TABLE 27–11 CHARACTERISTICS OF TWO NATRIURETIC FACTORS

	DIGOXIN-LIKE	ATRIAL PEPTIDE
Source	Plasma Hypothalamus (?)	Atria
Effect	Acute natriuresis and diuresis Unknown duration	Acute natriuresis and diuresis Short duration
Chemical nature	Molecular weight <500 daltons Resists proteolysis Contains no amino acids Inhibits Na^+, K^+-ATPase Binds to digoxin antibodies	Molecular weight >5,000 daltons Destroyed by proteolytic enzymes Contains 24 to 28 amino acids No effect on Na^+, K^+-ATPase
Vascular response	Vasoconstrictor Raises arterial blood pressure	Vasodilator Lowers arterial blood pressure

Adapted from Grantham, J. J., and Edwards, R. M.: Natriuretic hormones: At last, bottled in bond? J. Lab. Clin. Med. *103*:333, 1984.

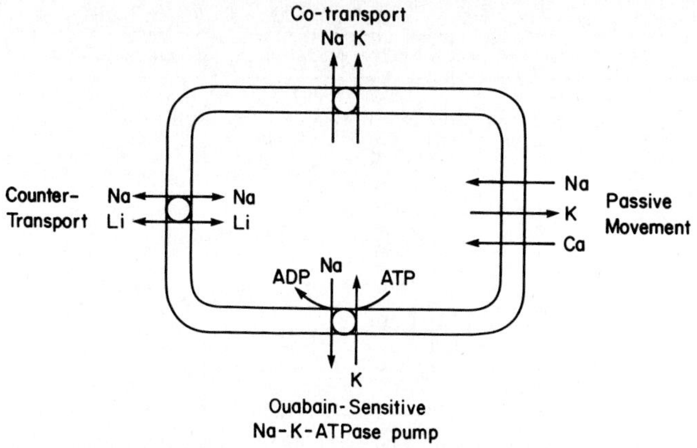

FIGURE 27–13. Schematic representation of four sodium transport mechanisms that have been demonstrated in red blood cells.

of sodium.[128] As noted earlier, such reabsorption is held by some to be a primary event in the pathogenesis of hypertension, so Na-Li countertransport may turn out to be a useful marker for both the genetic linkage and the basic mechanism of primary hypertension.

Beyond these alterations in active transport mechanisms, passive inward sodium movement may also be increased in cells from hypertensive subjects.[129] This increased intracellular concentration would, in turn, stimulate the Na^+,K^+-ATPase pump to extrude more sodium in an attempt to maintain normal levels. Despite the earlier hypothesized reduction of sodium pump activity by the putative natriuretic hormone, numerous studies in experimental hypertension have shown increased sodium pump activity.[130, 131] Thus, an increase in passive inward transport with a secondary increase in pump activity may turn out to be the basic mechanism responsible for higher intracellular sodium concentrations in primary hypertension.[129]

INCREASED INTRACELLULAR SODIUM AND CALCIUM

Regardless of the mechanism involved, intracellular sodium is likely to be increased in primary hypertension. The manner by which intracellular sodium levels induce hypertension may involve inhibition of a sodium-calcium exchange mechanism, leading to an increase in intracellular calcium. Blaustein calculated that a rise of 0.5 mmol/liter in intracellular sodium could cause an increase in intracellular calcium of 4 to 40 μmol/liter—enough to increase the resting tone of vascular smooth muscle by 50 per cent.[132] The increase in intracellular calcium is, in turn, translated into an increase in vascular resistance by its binding to a myofilament regulatory protein and stimulation of myosin phosphorylation.[133] Indirect support for such calcium-mediated vasoconstriction in patients with primary hypertension comes from their increased dilator response to calcium entry-blocking drugs but not to nitroprusside, which induces vasodilation by other mechanisms.[134]

A "COMPLETE" HYPOTHESIS OF THE GENESIS OF ESSENTIAL HYPERTENSION. The "complete" hypothesis incorporates much of what is known about experimental and clinical primary hypertension. This hypothesis was formulated predominantly by deWardener and coworkers, who proposed that the increased fluid volume that stimulates natriuretic hormone was induced by an inherited defect in renal sodium excretion acting in concert with excessive dietary sodium intake.[135] Their proposal was based on experimental evidence obtained during kidney transplantation involving Dahl sodium-sensitive hypertensive rats, which showed that blood pressure "follows the kidney." When a kidney was transplanted from a hypertensive donor rat into a normotensive host rat, the blood pressure of the host rose. The reverse also occurred, i.e., a kidney implanted from a normotensive rat lowered the blood pressure of a hypertensive host.[136] This proposal, however, disregards the rather convincing evidence of a resetting of the pressure-natriuresis curve and does not require mediation of stress-induced activation of the sympathetic nervous system. Therefore, although less parsimonious, the scheme depicted in Figure 27–14 is a more complete representation of currently available clinical and experimental evidence for the pathogenesis of essential hypertension.

Most of the steps in this schema can be bypassed by the direct insertion of a defect in membrane permeability to sodium or calcium. As described earlier, genetic linkages with one or more of the sodium transport pathways have been found in hypertensive patients and in some of their normotensive children,[125] which could, in the manner

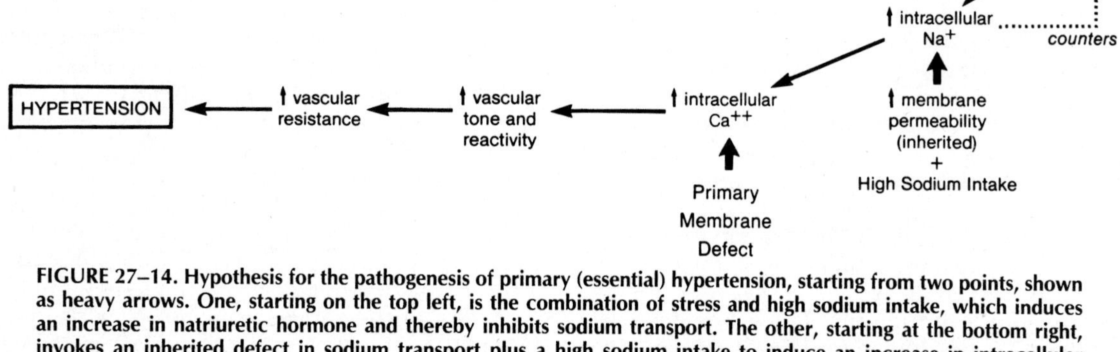

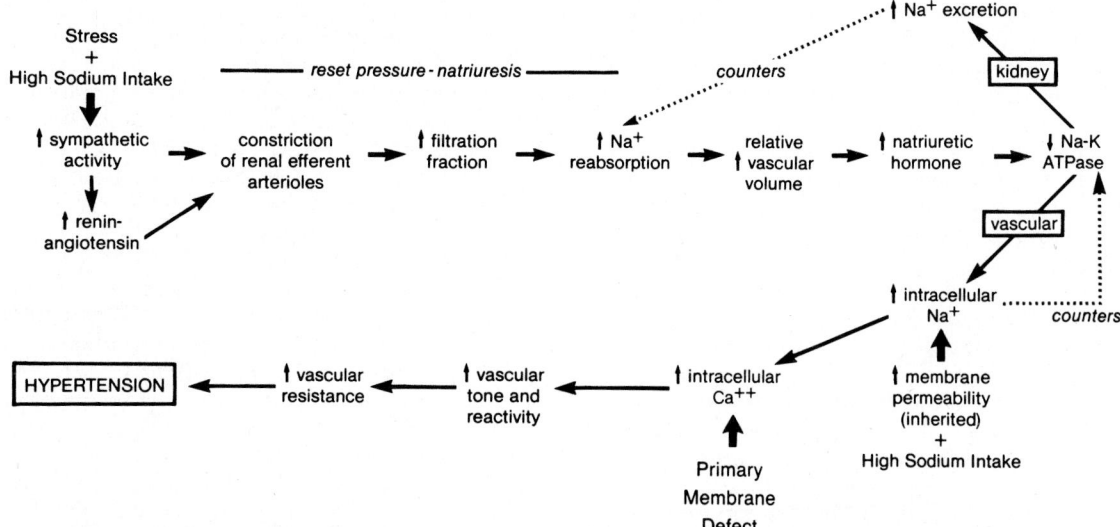

FIGURE 27–14. Hypothesis for the pathogenesis of primary (essential) hypertension, starting from two points, shown as heavy arrows. One, starting on the top left, is the combination of stress and high sodium intake, which induces an increase in natriuretic hormone and thereby inhibits sodium transport. The other, starting at the bottom right, invokes an inherited defect in sodium transport plus a high sodium intake to induce an increase in intracellular sodium.

proposed by Blaustein,[132] secondarily increase intracellular calcium.

DIRECT INCREASE IN INTRACELLULAR CALCIUM. A rapidly expanding and in some ways even more impressive body of evidence supports a *primary defect in calcium transport*, which could bypass most of the preceding hypothetical construct.[137-139] First, an increase in free cytosolic calcium has been measured in fat cells[137] and platelets[140] from patients with primary hypertension, possibly owing to impaired removal of calcium or an increased delivery of calcium to the cytosol. In spontaneously hypertensive rats, calcium influx is increased but the removal rate is not.[141] Second, high-affinity binding of calcium to the inner aspect of cell membranes is reduced in hypertensive rats and humans.[137] Altered metabolism of phosphoinositides, a class of membrane lipids involved in calcium transport, has been found in red cell membranes in hypertensive rats and humans and could be responsible for changes in calcium movement and binding.[142] It has been postulated that the same defect responsible for the decrease in membrane affinity for calcium may also reduce activity of the sodium pump. At the same time, increased membrane permeability to sodium might stimulate the sodium pump. According to this hypothesis, sodium pump activity could then be either reduced or elevated, both effects having been reported in studies of cells from hypertensive patients. The primary problem is considered to be within the structure of the membrane, with increases in intracellular calcium and sodium secondary to the membrane abnormality.

OTHER ABNORMALITIES OF CALCIUM METABOLISM. Hypertension may be associated with a number of other abnormalities in calcium metabolism, including (1) decreased dietary calcium intake[143]; (2) increased urinary calcium excretion,[144] which may be attributable largely to increased intake and excretion of sodium[145]; (3) decreased serum ionized calcium but normal total serum calcium[146]; (4) slightly increased serum parathyroid hormone levels, postulated to rise in response to the lower ionized calcium levels subsequent to an increase in urinary calcium excretion[144]; (5) reduction in blood pressure in about half of patients given 1 to 2 gm of supplemental calcium per day.[147] These findings are the components of a "calcium deficiency" hypothesis for primary hypertension.[143] Despite its attraction, however, this hypothesis lacks a theoretical foundation, and an equally impressive body of evidence can be marshaled against it.[148, 149]

As the author and others have noted,[150] at least three defects in calcium metabolism may be involved in hypertension, all of which could lead to increased intracellular calcium and, thereby, vasoconstriction (Fig. 27–15). In scheme 1, a decrease in membrane binding of calcium might lead to an increase in free intracellular calcium levels and be associated with impaired renal tubular reabsorption of calcium. In scheme 2, the increase in calcium is secondary to the primary increase in intracellular sodium. In scheme 3, renal hypercalciuria would be secondary to high sodium intake, with a subsequent fall in serum calcium and a secondary rise in parathyroid hormone, which could induce vasoconstriction. Obviously, none of these schemes has been proved to be involved in the majority of hypertensives. Calcium supplements could either worsen or improve the situation, sometimes lowering but other times raising blood pressure levels unpredictably. For this reason, they should not be used indiscriminately as antihypertensive agents.

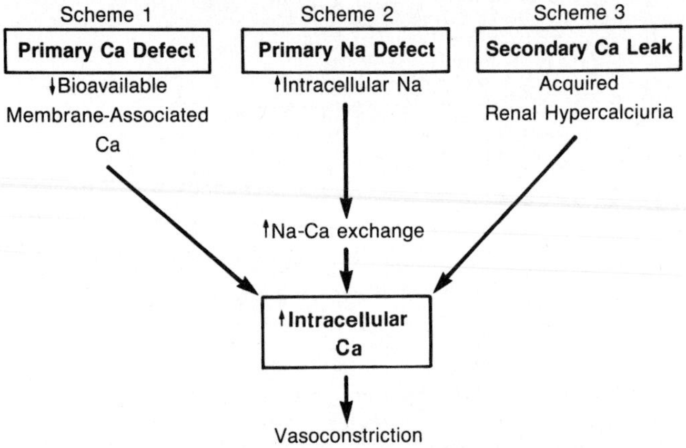

FIGURE 27–15. Three possible defects in calcium metabolism, all of which could eventuate in increased intracellular calcium. (From Pak, C.: Calcium and hypertension. *In* Horan, M. J., et al. [eds.] NIH Workshop on Nutrition and Hypertension: Proceedings from a Symposium. Bethesda, March 12–14, 1984.)

THE RENIN-ANGIOTENSIN-ALDOSTERONE SYSTEM

Despite their overall attractions, theories concerning sodium and calcium in the genesis of essential hypertension have not been established. Other mechanisms, involving in particular the renin-angiotensin system, deserve consideration.

Renin is synthesized primarily in the juxtaglomerular cells and is secreted in both active and inactive forms, the latter in much larger amount. Release of renin may be stimulated by at least five mechanisms: (1) pressure within the renal afferent arteriole (i.e., the baroreceptor mechanism), (2) the concentration of sodium or chloride within the macula densa, (3) stimulation of renal sympathetic nerves, (4) circulating angiotensin II, and (5) plasma electrolyte concentration.

Although the function of *inactive renin* and the manner of its conversion to the active form remain unknown, it is extracted largely during one passage through the coronary circulation, suggesting that it could exert cardiotropic effects.[151] It is also present in large quantity in the ovary, where it may play a role in reproductive function.[152] The *active form of renin* acts as a proteolytic enzyme, cleaving a substrate protein to liberate the decapeptide angiotensin I. This inactive prohormone is in turn converted into the potent octapeptide hormone angiotensin II by a converting enzyme. Angiotensin II has two major actions: (1) control of blood pressure through constriction of arterial vessels and (2) control of body fluid volume through an increase in renal retention of salt and water (Fig. 27–16). In addition, a direct connection between angiotensin and the previously described sodium transport hypothesis has been shown in cultured smooth muscle cells from rat aorta.[153] When angiotensin II was added to these cells, their permeability to sodium was increased threefold and intracellular sodium concentration rose proportionally. Angiotensin may thereby shortcircuit part of the scheme shown in Figure 27–14 and induce hypertension through a direct effect on sodium transport.

Increases in renin-angiotensin are directly responsible for renovascular hypertension and are associated with a variety of other hypertensive diseases discussed subsequently. As noted earlier, inappropriately high and fixed tissue levels of angiotensin may be one of the switches that turn on the pathogenetic mechanism for primary (essential) hypertension, at least in the 40 per cent of hypertensives

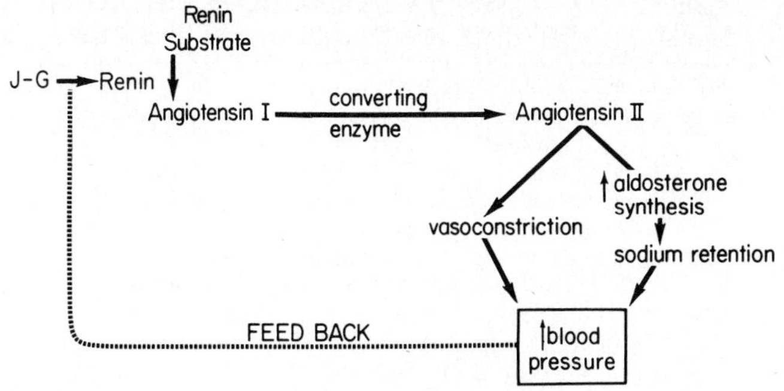

FIGURE 27–16. Overall scheme of the renin-angiotensin mechanism.

who are "nonmodulators."[109] Measuring plasma renin activity (PRA) may also provide a marker for different elements of the hypertensive spectrum.

USE OF RENIN ASSAYS. Clinicians who use renin assays must be aware that various physiological or pharmacological maneuvers can affect the level of PRA (Table 27–12). Since renin release is controlled by multiple systems, various conditions can influence renin levels by means of more than one mechanism. For example, upright posture may increase renin by decreasing effective plasma volume and renal perfusion pressure and increasing catecholamine levels. The lesson to be learned here is that renin secretion and PRA levels can be altered by a multitude of factors, some easily recognized and avoided and others not yet identified. Even when the same assay procedure and testing conditions are used in the same patients with no recognizable changes in clinical conditions, PRA may change. The prudent clinician will take as many of the known variables into account as possible and recognize the vagaries of PRA, taking care neither to ascribe more certainty to a given level than is justified nor to make important diagnostic, prognostic, or therapeutic decisions based upon small differences.

TABLE 27–12 CLINICAL CONDITIONS AFFECTING RENIN LEVELS

DECREASED PRA	INCREASED PRA
Expanded fluid volume	*Shrunken fluid volume*
Salt loads, oral or IV	Salt deprivation
Primary salt retention (Liddle syndrome, Gordon syndrome)	Fluid losses
Mineralocorticoid excess	Diuretic-induced
Primary aldosteronism	Gastrointestinal losses
Congenital adrenal hyperplasia	Hemorrhage
Cushing's syndrome	Salt-wasting renal disease
Licorice excess	Decreased effective plasma volume
Deoxycorticosterone (DOC), 18-hydroxy-DOC excess	Upright posture
	Adrenal insufficiency
Catecholamine deficiency	Cirrhosis with ascites
Autonomic dysfunction	Nephrotic syndrome
Therapy with adrenergic neuronal blockers	*Decreased renal perfusion pressure*
Therapy with beta-adrenoceptor blockers	Therapy with peripheral vasodilators
Hyperkalemia	Renovascular hypertension
Decreased renin substrate (?)	Accelerated-malignant hypertension
Androgen therapy	Chronic renal disease (renin-dependent)
Decrease of renal tissue	Juxtaglomerular hyperplasia (Bartter syndrome)
Hyporeninemic hypoaldosteronism	
Chronic renal disease (volume-dependent)	*Catecholamine excess*
Anephric state	Pheochromocytoma
Increasing age	Stress: Hypoglycemia, trauma
	Exercise
Unknown	Hyperthyroidism
Low-renin essential hypertension	Caffeine
	Hypokalemia
	Increased renin substrate
	Pregnancy
	Estrogen therapy
	Autonomous renin hypersecretion
	Renin-secreting tumors
	Acute damage to juxtaglomerular cells
	Acute renal failure
	Acute glomerulonephritis
	Unknown
	High-renin essential hypertension

From Kaplan, N. M.: Clinical Hypertension. 4th ed. Baltimore, © by Williams and Wilkins, 1986, p. 104.

RENIN LEVELS IN ESSENTIAL HYPERTENSION. Many studies have reaffirmed Helmer's original findings that among patients with uncomplicated essential hypertension, renin values are low in about 30 per cent, normal in 60 per cent, and high in 10 per cent.[154] The percentage of cases of low-renin hypertension increases progressively with the age of the population. Although this may represent a different underlying hypertensive process, more likely it simply reflects a progressive decline in functioning juxtaglomerular cells or in their responsiveness, a process that occurs in normal subjects as well but is accentuated in hypertensive individuals, in whom nephrosclerosis is usually more advanced.

The separation of patients into low, normal, and high renin categories is in large part artifactual. The dividing line between low and normal is arbitrary and depends upon the type of analysis applied to the data. Renin levels in essential hypertension follow a continuous distribution curve, with a predominance of lower values because of the larger proportion of blacks and older people in the hypertensive population.[155] As shown in Figure 27–17, PRA measurements can be useful for recognizing certain hypertensive syndromes with distinctly low or high levels. For the majority of patients with essential hypertension, little seems to be gained from a determination of their renin status.

ROLE OF RENIN IN ESSENTIAL HYPERTENSION. As we have seen, most patients with essential hypertension have normal levels of PRA. Since high pressure in the renal afferent arterioles should suppress the release of renin from juxtaglomerular cells through the baroreceptor mechanism, the presence of normal renin levels may be considered to be inappropriately elevated. Thus, the normal negative feedback between blood pressure and renin release may be imperfect in hypertension, resulting in inappropriately high renin levels that may contribute to the condition. Recall the studies of Hollenberg et al. in which

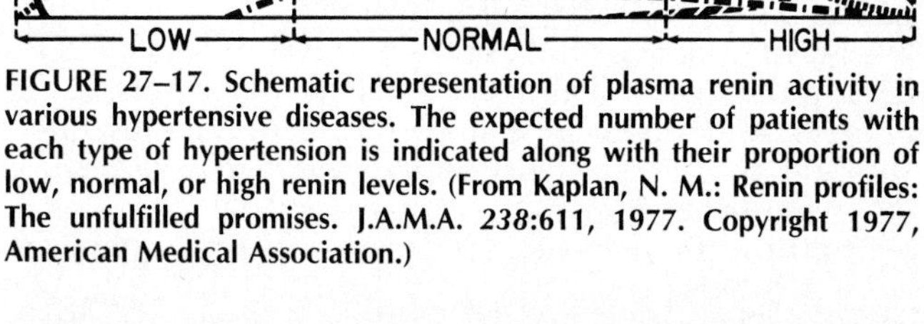

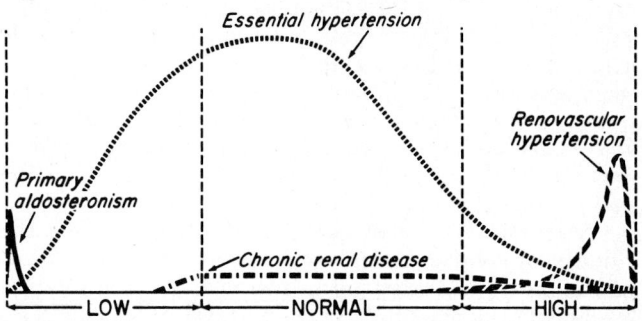

FIGURE 27–17. Schematic representation of plasma renin activity in various hypertensive diseases. The expected number of patients with each type of hypertension is indicated along with their proportion of low, normal, or high renin levels. (From Kaplan, N. M.: Renin profiles: The unfulfilled promises. J.A.M.A. *238*:611, 1977. Copyright 1977, American Medical Association.)

as many as half of patients with high or normal PRA levels appeared to have fixed, high tissue levels of angiotensin II that may have been responsible for their hypertension.[108,109] On the other hand, low renin levels, which seem more appropriate to primary hypertension, may be due to increased sensitivity of adrenal cortical receptors to angiotensin, so that less angiotensin (and therefore renin) would be needed to maintain fluid volume; when given exogenous angiotensin, patients with low renin show a supernormal rise in plasma aldosterone.[156]

Thus, we are left with no clear definition of the role of the renin-angiotensin system in essential hypertension. In patients with natural or induced high renin levels, renin-angiotensin probably has a considerable influence, whereas in the majority of hypertensive patients, i.e., those with normal or low renin levels, its effect is probably minimal. Drugs that inhibit the activity of this mechanism, specifically the converting enzyme inhibitors, lower blood pressure in about half of patients with primary hypertension, possibly indicating a specific pathogenetic role for renin-angiotensin. More likely, this reflects a nonspecific response to the removal of one of the body's major pressor mechanisms. An analogous situation would be the lowering of blood pressure by drugs that inhibit the sympathetic nervous system in about the same proportion of hypertensive patients.

LOW-RENIN ESSENTIAL HYPERTENSION. Low or suppressed renin levels in 30 per cent of the hypertensive population, as previously argued, most likely represents a portion of the gaussian distribution curve that is shifted toward the low side because of the larger proportion of blacks and older people and is not indicative of a peculiar form of hypertension. In fact, whenever blood pressure is raised, renin suppression would be expected via the renal baroreceptor mechanism. Nonetheless, the known presence of low renin levels in other hypertensive diseases associated with mineralocorticoid excess or volume expansion has prompted an extensive search for such a mechanism in low-renin essential hypertension. In addition, some believe that patients with low renin levels may have a better prognosis and special therapeutic needs.

Diagnosis. Possible mechanisms underlying low-renin hypertension go beyond volume expansion with or without mineralocorticoid excess (Table 27–13), although an expanded body fluid volume would be a logical explanation. Even though such expansion has been reported, the majority of careful analyses have failed to indicate any abnormality.[157] If volume expansion were responsible for low-renin hypertension, a logical mechanism would be an excess in one or another mineralocorticoid hormone. Despite repeated claims to this effect, subsequent study has failed to document either the excess or the mineralocorticoid potency of the putative hormone.[158] A subtle deficiency of the adrenal enzyme 11-hydroxylase, associated with increased levels of deoxycorticosterone and deoxycortisol has been reported in hypertensive patients, but this finding remains to be validated.[159]

Prognosis. As already noted (p. 825), one retrospective study showed that patients with low-renin hypertension had no myocardial infarcts or strokes over a 7-year interval, whereas 11 per cent of those with normal renin and 14 per cent of those with high renin levels had experienced one of these cardiovascular complications.[53] Several subsequent studies have failed to document an improved prognosis in low-renin hypertension.[54]

Therapy. In keeping with their presumed volume excess, patients with low-renin essential hypertension have been found by some to exhibit a greater fall in blood pressure with diuretic therapy than do those with normal-renin hypertension.[160] If this is true, the better response does not necessarily indicate a greater volume load; by definition, patients with low renin are less responsive to stimuli that increase renin levels, including diuretics, so that they experience a lower rise in PRA with such therapy. Less renin and angiotensin could result in less compensatory vasoconstriction and aldosterone secretion, so that volume depletion would proceed and blood pressure would fall further in low-renin hypertensive patients given a diuretic.

In the aggregate, the evidence that patients with low renin are unique in the spectrum of essential hypertension seems slim. For now, the prudent clinician may assume that the routine determination of renin status is not needed in decisions about how to manage patients with essential hypertension.

TABLE 27–13 POSSIBLE MECHANISMS FOR LOW-RENIN HYPERTENSION—CLINICAL EXPRESSION

I. "Physiological" inhibition of renin release
  A. Increased pressure at the juxtaglomerular apparatus and/or increased sodium load at macula densa
    1. Elevated perfusion pressure: Primary hypertension
    2. Expanded effective plasma volume
      a. Renal sodium retention
        Primary: Liddle and Gordon syndromes
        Secondary to increased mineralocorticoid activity
          Aldosterone: Primary aldosteronism
          DOC: Congenital adrenal hyperplasia, adrenal tumors
          18-hydroxy-DOC and other steroids
          Glycyrrhizic acid: Licorice, carbenoxolone
      b. Prolonged excessive salt intake in genetically predisposed
      c. Increased natriuretic hormone
    3. Decreased capacity of vascular bed
  B. Decreased sympathetic nervous system activity: Diabetes mellitus, adrenergic blocking drugs, (?) primary hypertension
  C. Increased potassium intake
  D. Increased systemic or intrarenal angiotensin II
II. Derangement of juxtaglomerular apparatus
  A. Inability to produce or release active renin: Chronic renal disease, (?) primary hypertension
  B. Defect in sensing mechanism: (?) Primary hypertension
III. Interference with generation of angiotensin II in vitro or enhanced generation of angiotensin II in vivo
IV. Increased adrenal sensitivity to angiotensin II: (?) Primary hypertension

From Kaplan, N. M.: Clinical Hypertension. 4th ed. Baltimore, © by Williams and Wilkins, 1986, p. 107.

OTHER HYPOTHETICAL MECHANISMS IN ESSENTIAL HYPERTENSION

VASOPRESSIN. High endogenous levels of the hormone vasopressin have been incriminated in certain experimental models of hypertension, but measurements in humans do not substantiate a relation between even very high plasma vasopressin levels and hypertension.[161]

VASODEPRESSOR DEFICIENCY. In addition to an excess of the various vasopressor hormones, a deficiency of one or more of these hormones may be involved in experimental and clinical hypertension.

Bradykinin. This nonapeptide is cleaved from a protein substrate, kininogen, by the action of the enzyme kallikrein. No evidence has been found of a systemic deficiency of kallikrein or bradykinin in patients with essential hypertension.[162]

Prostaglandins. These ubiquitous fatty-acid derivatives have profound pharmacological effects, but their involvement in human disease remains unproved. Prostaglandins (PG) that act at their site of synthesis have been shown to produce physiologically important effects, so that the search for *circulating* prostaglandins may be futile.[163] Prostacyclin, synthesized within the vessel wall, is vasodilatory; thromboxane A, released from platelets, is vasoconstrictive.

The major site of PG action relative to hypertension may be in the kidney. PGE_2 is synthesized mainly in the renal medulla by medullary interstitial cells. When PGE_2 or its precursor, arachidonic acid, is infused into the renal artery, renal vasodilation, increased renal blood flow, and natriuresis follow. Thus, PGE_2 may protect against ischemia. When renal blood flow is compromised, both renin and PG are released. By this mechanism the kidney can raise systemic blood pressure via the renin-angiotensin system without diminishing renal blood flow, since intrarenal PG could counteract the effects of intrarenal angiotensin.[164] A deficiency of PGE_2 might then lead to hypertension by impairing renal function and causing fluid retention as well as by accentuating the effects of renin-angiotensin. A major clinical problem has been the use of nonsteroidal antiinflammatory drugs, which inhibit renal PG production. In patients with borderline renal function, PG may precipitate renal failure[165] and may raise blood pressure even in patients with normal renal function.[164]

Renomedullary Lipids. In addition to the acidic prostaglandins, two lipids from renomedullary interstitial cells have been identified that exert definite antihypertensive effects in animals.[166] One is neutral, the other highly polar. The polar vasodepressor substance appears to be an alkyl ether analog of phosphatidylcholine. The role of these renomedullary lipids in human pathophysiology is not yet known.

OTHER POSSIBLE MECHANISMS. The foregoing does not exhaust the list of suggested mechanisms underlying essential hypertension. Excesses of various minerals, particularly lead,[167] and changing ratios among dietary sodium, calcium, and potassium have also been postulated. Although a possible role for endogenous opioid peptides in the regulation of blood pressure has been noted in animals,[168] there are no data pertaining to humans. Support for these and other postulated mechanisms is meager, and the overall schemes involving intracellular sodium and calcium discussed earlier (p. 833) seem more than adequate to explain the pathogenesis of essential hypertension. However, a number of associations between hypertension and other conditions have been noted and may offer additional insights into the potential causes and possible prevention of the disease. For example, when associations among 35 anthropometric, biochemical, and life style characteristics and nine different blood pressure measurements in 618 adults were examined by multiple regression analysis, certain correlations were found to be significant—body size and psychological stress were associated with systolic blood pressure, while obesity, smoking, alcohol, and plasma sodium were associated with diastolic blood pressure. Urine sodium and potassium excretion could not be correlated with any blood pressure measure.[169] Such correlations do not prove causality, but suggest that those features associated with hypertension may be involved in its pathogenesis.

ASSOCIATION OF HYPERTENSION WITH OTHER CONDITIONS

OBESITY. Despite the possible overestimation of blood pressure levels in the obese because of the use of sphygmomanometric cuffs that are too small (p. 21), true hypertension is more common among these individuals and probably adds to their risk of developing ischemic heart disease. In the Framingham offspring study, adiposity, as measured by subscapular skinfold thickness, was the major controllable contributor to hypertension, with estimates of 78 per cent of hypertension in men and 64 per cent in women attributable to obesity.[170] The *distribution* of body fat also seems important, since blood pressure as well as blood triglyceride and glucose levels tend to be highest in those with central or upper body obesity.[171] Although some report that the degree of cardiovascular risk for any level of blood pressure is lower in obese subjects than in nonobese,[172] others do not.[173]

The mechanism by which obesity leads to hypertension likely involves increases in blood volume, stroke volume, and cardiac output.[174] A common thread among hypertension, obesity, and glucose intolerance has been identified in a large population sample of Israelis.[175] Among the hypertensives, 83.4 per cent had either glucose intolerance or obesity. The authors postulate that insulin resistance, associated with both glucose intolerance and obesity, may be responsible for the hypertension, and they provide suggestive evidence that this involves an increase in intracellular sodium concentration.

Children seem particularly vulnerable to the hypertensive effects of weight gain.[25] Therefore, avoidance of childhood obesity seems important, with the hope of avoiding subsequent hypertension. The evidence that weight reduction will lower established hypertension is discussed on p. 1018.

PHYSICAL INACTIVITY. Physical fitness may help prevent hypertension, and persons who are already hypertensive may lower their blood pressure by means of regular isotonic exercise.[176] Preventing hypertension may be one of the ways exercise seems to protect against the development of cardiovascular disease. Among 14,998 Harvard male alumni followed for 16 to 50 years, those who did not engage in vigorous sports play were at 35 per cent greater risk for developing hypertension, whether or not they had higher blood pressures while at Harvard, a family history of hypertension, or obesity—factors that also increased the risk of hypertension.[177]

ALCOHOL INTAKE. The role of alcohol in amounts consumed by a large segment of the population demands special emphasis. Even in small quantities alcohol may raise blood pressure; in larger quantities alcohol may be responsible for a significant number of cases of hypertension. In all studies of this problem, the relationship between alcohol and blood pressure has been found to be independent of all other known variables. Some have found a linear, progressively increasing level of blood pressure with increasing consumption of alcohol[178]; others report a threshold effect, often with lower levels of blood pressure among those who drink 1 to 2 ounces of ethanol a day than among those who drink none at all.[179] The latter pattern more clearly parallels the association with total and coronary mortality.[180] The reduction in coronary disease in persons who ingest small amounts of alcohol, beyond any effect on blood pressure, may reflect a greater mobilization of tissue-free cholesterol for hepatic removal and excretion.[181]

The pressor effect of alcohol primarily reflects an increase in cardiac output and heart rate, probably the consequence of a rapid rise in plasma epinephrine and cortisol levels and a slower rise in plasma norepinephrine, as measured in young men with light to moderate drinking habits.[182] In animals, ethanol initially increases the permeability of the plasma membrane to sodium and suppresses Na^+,K^+-ATPase pump activity.[183] Such changes would increase free intracellular calcium levels[184] (Fig. 27–18).

SMOKING. Cigarette smoking raises blood pressure, probably through the nicotine-induced release of norepinephrine from adrenergic nerve endings.[185] Yet when smokers quit, a trivial rise in blood pressure may occur, probably reflecting a gain in weight.

DIABETES MELLITUS (See also p. 1816). Hypertension is present in about two-thirds of patients with longstanding diabetes with the associated intercapillary glomerulosclerosis described by Kimmelstiel and Wilson, and the prevalence of essential hypertension in the overall diabetic population is somewhat increased.[186] The coexistence of diabetes and hypertension almost redoubles the already high rate of cardiovascular mortality seen in nondiabetic hypertensives.[187]

When they are hypertensive, patients with diabetes mellitus may confront some interesting problems. With progressive renal insufficiency and autonomic neuropathy, they may have few functional juxtaglomerular cells and a reduced ability to stimulate the release of renin. As a result, very low renin levels are often observed, with a tendency toward development of the syndrome of hyporeninemic hypoaldosteronism. If hypoglycemia develops because of too much insulin or other drugs, severe hyper-

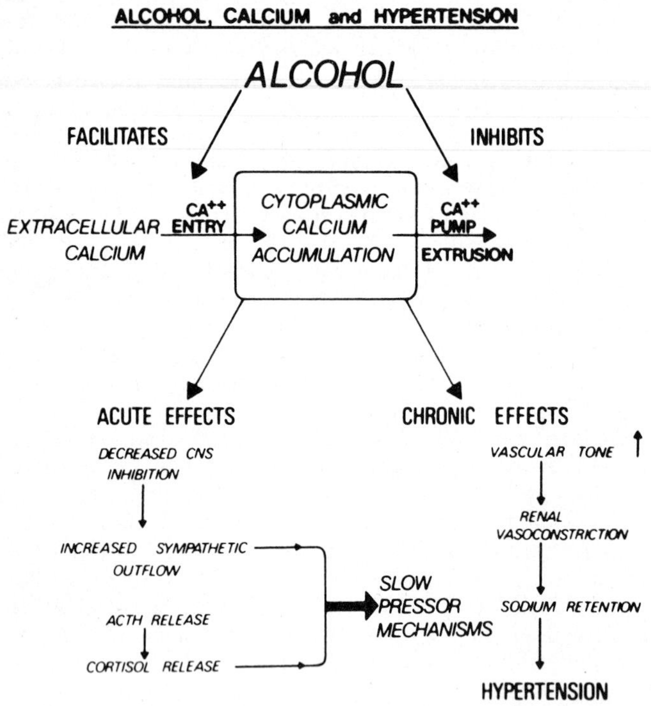

FIGURE 27–18. Schema by which chronic alcohol consumption may lead to hypertension in susceptible individuals. (From Arkwright, P., Beilin, L. J., Vandongen, R., Rouse, I. L., and Masarei, J. R.: Plasma calcium and cortisol as predisposing factors to alcohol related blood pressure elevation. J. Hypertension 2:387, 1984.)

tension may occur as a result of stimulated sympathetic nervous activity.

Diabetics are also susceptible to special problems associated with antihypertensive therapy. Diuretics may exacerbate the carbohydrate intolerance, probably by inducing potassium deficiency. Those who are brittle and prone to hypoglycemia may have difficulties with beta-adrenoceptor blocking agents, since these drugs would blunt their protective catecholamine response, and severe hypoglycemia might develop without warning. On the other hand, successful reduction of their blood pressure may protect them from the otherwise inexorable progress of diabetic nephropathy.[188] Converting enzyme inhibitors may be especially effective in reducing the high intraglomerular pressures that are probably responsible for the progressive glomerulosclerosis of diabetes.[189]

Polycythemia (See also p. 1742). Polycythemia vera is frequently associated with hypertension. More common is a "pseudo-" or "stress" polycythemia with a high hematocrit and increased blood viscosity but contracted plasma volume as well as normal red cell mass and serum erythropoietin levels. Such patients may also have elevated plasma fibrinogen levels.[190]

Gout. Hyperuricemia is present in 25 to 50 per cent of individuals with untreated essential hypertension; this is about five times the frequency among normotensive persons. In 71 male hypertensives, asymptomatic hyperuricemia was associated with decreased renal blood flow, presumably a reflection of nephrosclerosis.[74] When diuretics are used, the uric acid level rises further; however, even after prolonged exposure, patients with diuretic-induced hyperuricemia do not seem to develop urate deposition, so that treatment for the elevated uric acid level is usually unnecessary.[191] Nonetheless, gout may be precipitated by diuretic-induced hyperuricemia in those who are genetically susceptible.

Other Diseases. Other diseases and conditions have been found more commonly in patients with essential hypertension, including uterine fibromyoma, color blindness, and increased intraocular pressure.[4] In addition, several diseases actually induce hypertension, i.e., cause secondary hypertension.

SECONDARY FORMS OF HYPERTENSION

(See Tables 27–4 and 27–5, p. 822)

ORAL CONTRACEPTIVE USE

The use of estrogen-containing oral contraceptive pills may be the most common cause of secondary hypertension. Most women who take them experience a slight rise in blood pressure, and about 5 per cent will develop hypertension (i.e., blood pressure above 140/90 mm Hg) within 5 years of oral contraceptive use. This is more than twice the incidence seen among women of the same age who do not use these agents.[192] Although the hypertension is usually mild, it may persist after the oral contraceptive is discontinued, may be severe, and is almost certainly a factor in the increased cardiovascular mortality seen among young women who take these agents.[193] Despite these facts, these drugs have provided effective and safe birth control for millions of women and the need for oral contraceptives remains.

The dangers of oral contraceptives should be kept in proper perspective. While it is true that use of these drugs is associated with increased morbidity and mortality, overall mortality from cardiovascular disease has been progressively declining among women in the United States at a rate equal to that noted among American men. Although the relative rates of coronary and cerebral vascular diseases are increased three- to seven-fold among users of oral contraceptives, and much of this effect persists even after they are stopped, the absolute number of women affected is small, particularly among those below age 35 who do not smoke.[193] The excess annual death rate attributable to oral contraceptive use for women who do not smoke is 1 per 77,000, whereas for women 35 to 44 who smoke this rate is 1 per 2000. Thus, for most, these agents—particularly the currently used low-estrogen and progesterone forms—seem safe for the purposes of temporary birth control.

In addition to hypertension, the major contributors to the cardiovascular complications of oral contraceptive use include an increased tendency for the blood to clot, changes in lipid and carbohydrate metabolism, an increase in coronary artery smooth muscle tone, and proliferation of fibroblasts and smooth muscle cells in vessel walls.[194]

INCIDENCE. The best data on the incidence of oral contraceptive-induced hypertension have come from a large, ongoing study by the Royal College of General

Practitioners. The incidence of hypertension was 2.6 times greater among 23,000 pill users compared with 23,000 nonusers, resulting in a 5 per cent incidence over 5 years of oral contraceptive use.[193] In addition, this incidence increased with long duration of pill use, being only slightly higher than that among controls during the first year but rising to almost three times higher by the fifth year. In a much smaller but more carefully performed prospective study of 186 Scottish women, systolic pressure rose in 164 (by more than 25 mm Hg in 8) and diastolic pressure rose in 150 (by more than 20 mm Hg in 2) during the first 2 years of oral contraceptive use. After 3 years, the mean rise in 83 of these women was 9.2 mm Hg.[195] The current use of smaller amounts of estrogen (20 to 35 μg) rather than the 50 μg taken by most of these women may induce less hypertension.[196]

CLINICAL FEATURES. Hypertension may develop in any woman taking estrogens, but the likelihood is much greater among those who are over age 35 or obese or who drink large quantities of alcohol.[197] The presence of hypertension during a prior pregnancy increases this likelihood but not enough to preclude pill use in such women who require contraception. In most women, the hypertension is mild; however, in some it may accelerate rapidly and cause severe renal damage.[198] When the pill is discontinued, blood pressure falls to normal within 3 to 6 months in about half the cases. Whether the pill caused permanent hypertension in the other half or just uncovered essential hypertension at an earlier time is not clear.

MECHANISMS OF HYPERTENSION. Oral contraceptives probably cause hypertension by renin-aldosterone–mediated volume expansion. Increases in body weight, plasma volume, and cardiac output were measured in 30 women given an oral contraceptive for 2 to 3 months, even though their blood pressure rose little over this short interval.[199] Estrogens and the synthetic progestogens used in oral contraceptive pills both cause sodium retention. This probably results from the following sequence (Fig. 27–19): (1) Estrogen increases the hepatic synthesis of renin substrate. (2) In the presence of increased substrate, more angiotensin is generated from whatever level of renin is present in the circulation. As a result of the increased level of angiotensin II, renin release is partially inhibited, so that its concentration in peripheral blood is lowered back to normal.[200] (3) The increased levels of angiotensin stimulate adrenal synthesis of aldosterone, which causes sodium retention. At the same time, systemic and renal vasoconstriction is induced by the angiotensin, and renal blood flow is reduced.[201] Significant elevations of blood pressure may occur

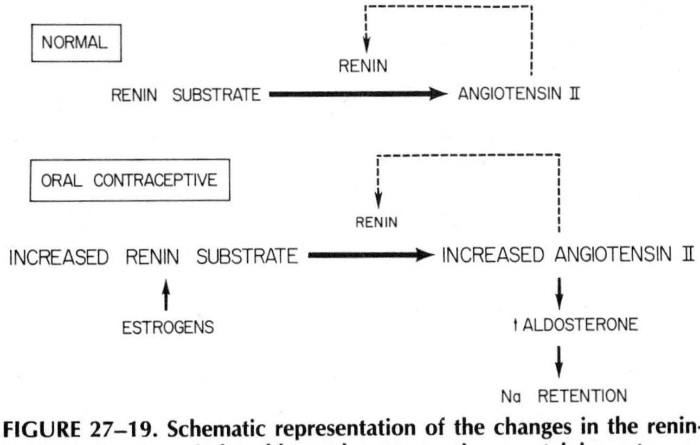

FIGURE 27–19. Schematic representation of the changes in the renin-angiotensin system induced by oral contraceptives containing estrogen. The dotted lines show the feedback inhibition of renin release by angiotensin II. (From Kaplan, N. M.: Clinical Hypertension. 4th ed. Baltimore, © by Williams and Wilkins, 1986, p. 370.)

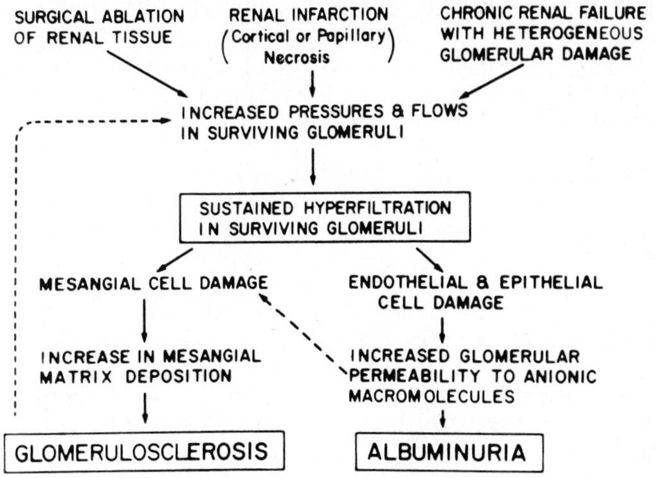

FIGURE 27–20. The hypothetical scheme relating compensatory glomerular hemodynamic changes in surviving glomeruli to pathologic changes in those nephron units. (From Hostetter, T. H.: The hyperfiltering glomerulus. Med. Clin. North Am. *68*:387, 1984.)

only in those persons with the greatest degree of vascular sensitivity to the increased levels of angiotensin. The amount of progestogen may also be important; more vascular disease has been noted with the use of 250 μg of levonorgestrel than with 150 μg of this progestogen.[202]

MANAGEMENT. The use of estrogen-containing oral contraceptives should be restricted in women over age 35, particularly if they smoke or are hypertensive or obese. Women given the pill should be properly monitored as follows: (1) the supply should be limited initially to 3 months and thereafter to 6 months; (2) they should be required to return for a blood pressure check before an additional supply is provided; and (3) if blood pressure has risen, an alternative contraceptive should be offered. If the pill remains the only acceptable contraceptive, the elevated blood pressure can be reduced with appropriate therapy. In view of the probable role of aldosterone, use of a diuretic-spironolactone combination seems appropriate. In those who stop taking oral contraceptives, evaluation for secondary hypertensive diseases should be postponed for at least 3 months to allow the renin-aldosterone changes to remit. If the hypertension does not recede, additional workup and therapy may be needed.

POSTMENOPAUSAL ESTROGEN USE. Millions of women use estrogen for its potential benefits after menopause. It does not appear to induce hypertension,[203] even though it does induce various changes in the renin-aldosterone mechanism seen with oral contraceptives. Moreover, the majority of case-control studies have shown a significantly *lower* mortality rate from coronary heart disease among postmenopausal estrogen users than nonusers.[204–206]

PARENCHYMAL RENAL DISEASE

(See also Chap. 59)

After oral contraceptives, renal parenchymal disease (mainly chronic glomerulonephritis) is the most common cause of secondary hypertension, responsible for 2 to 4 per cent of cases seen in unselected adult populations (Table 27–5). As chronic renal disease worsens, hypertension usually appears and contributes further to the deterioration of renal function[207–209] (Fig. 27–20). In addition, primary hypertension is a common cause of progressive renal damage. In the United States, it is responsible for at least one of every six cases of end-stage renal disease (ESRD) leading to chronic dialysis or renal transplantation.[73] The higher prevalence of hypertension among American blacks is probably responsible for their significantly higher rate of ESRD, with hypertension as the underlying cause in one-third to one-half of these patients.

Not only does hypertension cause renal failure and renal failure cause hypertension, but more subtle renal dysfunction may be involved in patients with primary (essential) hypertension. As discussed earlier (p. 831), the kidneys may initiate the hemodynamic cascade eventuating in primary hypertension. As that disease progresses, some renal dysfunction is demonstrable in most patients; progressive renal damage is the end result and is the cause of death in at least 10 per cent of hypertensives. As will be documented further (p. 869), early treatment of hypertension will protect against nephrosclerosis, so that there is hope that the control of hypertension will slow the progression and reduce the frequency of ESRD.

In hypertension with renal parenchymal disease the sequence of progressively worsening renal damage is: (1) Acute renal diseases that are often reversible. (2) Unilateral and bilateral diseases without renal insufficiency. (3) Chronic renal disease with renal insufficiency. (4) Hypertension in the anephric state and after renal transplantation.

ACUTE RENAL DISEASES. Hypertension may appear with any sudden, severe insult to the kidneys that either markedly impairs the excretion of salt and water, which leads to volume expansion, or reduces renal blood flow, which sets off the renin-angiotensin mechanism. Bilateral ureteral obstruction is an example of the former; sudden bilateral renal artery occlusion, as by emboli, is an example of the latter. Relief of either may dramatically reverse severe hypertension. Some of the collagen diseases may also produce rapidly progressive renal damage. The more common acute processes are glomerulonephritis and oliguric renal failure.

Acute Glomerulonephritis. Although the classic syndrome of type-specific poststreptococcal nephritis appearing after pharyngitis has become much less common, glomerular lesions of various types may be associated with hypertension.[210] Moreover, although the epidemic post-streptococcal disease is usually self-limited, some patients follow a progressive, smoldering course that may lead to renal insufficiency.[211] Patients with sporadic disease may have underlying, previously unrecognized chronic disease, and they frequently have progressive renal disease with hypertension. Typically, hypertension accompanies the oliguria and fluid retention of acute renal injury. The presence of renal damage in acute glomerulonephritis is usually obvious, with abnormalities of the urinary sediment; however, these may be minimal, and severe hypertension may be the presenting feature.

Hypertension is best relieved by fluid and sodium restriction and by appropriate doses of potent diuretics such as furosemide. Dialysis and parenteral antihypertensive drugs may be needed if encephalopathy supervenes. In milder cases, the hypertension recedes as the edema is relieved. However, some patients have a rapidly progressive course, often with prolonged anuria.

Acute Oliguric Renal Failure. Acute renal failure occurs after shock develops, particularly in patients in whom renin levels are already high, such as cirrhotics with ascites or at the end of pregnancy. The release of even more renin by decreased blood pressure and effective circulating blood volume may flood the renal vasculature and cause such intense renal vasoconstriction that renal function shuts down.[212] Hypertension in this setting is usually not an important problem and can be controlled by preventing volume overload. High doses of furosemide may be helpful, but dialysis is often needed. When acute renal failure occurs on the background of accelerated or malignant hypertension, aggressive therapy, including dialysis, may be followed by sustained recovery of renal function.[213]

Vasculitis. Rapidly progressive renal deterioration with severe hypertension occurs not infrequently during the course of scleroderma and other forms of vasculitis (p. 1723). Therapy with antihypertensives, particularly angiotensin-converting enzyme inhibitors, may reverse the process.[214]

RENAL DISEASE WITHOUT RENAL INSUFFICIENCY. Although an entire kidney may be removed without obvious effect and no rise in blood pressure,[215] hypertension may be associated with unilateral and bilateral renal parenchymal diseases in the absence of significant renal insufficiency. Such hypertension may reflect other unrecognized processes, but most likely it is caused by activation of the renin-angiotensin mechanism. However, in some patients whose hypertension has been relieved by correction of a renal defect, the levels of renin have not been found to be high.

Unilateral Parenchymal Renal Disease. A variety of unilateral kidney diseases may be associated with hypertension, and in some of these the affected kidney may appear shrunken. Most small kidneys do not cause hypertension, and when they are indiscriminately removed, hypertension is relieved in only about 25 per cent of patients.[216] Of that 25 per cent, most have arterial occlusive disease, either as the primary cause of the renal atrophy or secondary to irregular scarring of the parenchyma.[217]

In many of these cases, high levels of renin can be found in the venous blood from the shrunken kidney, while in some, renal vein renin activity levels have been falsely normal.[218] Forms of unilateral kidney disease associated with curable hypertension include hypoplasia, reflux nephropathy, hydronephrosis, radiation and traumatic injury, cysts and tumors, including Wilms' tumors and hypernephromas as well as the rare juxtaglomerular cell tumors.[217]

Polycystic Kidney Disease. Although patients with adult polycystic kidney disease usually progress to renal insufficiency, some retain reasonably normal glomerular filtration rates (GFR) and display no azotemia. Hypertension, although more common in those with renal failure, is present in perhaps half of those with a normal GFR and probably reflects variable degrees of both renin excess and fluid retention.[219]

Chronic Pyelonephritis. The relationship between pyelonephritis and hypertension is multifaceted: pyelonephritis, either unilateral or bilateral, may cause hypertension; hypertensive individuals may be more susceptible to renal infection. In patients with hypertension but fairly normal renal function, renin levels are high,[220] probably from interstitial scarring with obstruction of intrarenal vessels.

CHRONIC RENAL DISEASES WITH RENAL INSUFFICIENCY. As dialysis and transplantation prolong the lives of more patients with renal insufficiency, their hypertension must be dealt with over much longer periods. Hypertension in most patients with renal insufficiency is predominantly caused by volume overload due to the inability of the reduced functioning renal mass to handle the usual sodium and water intake. With proper attention to sodium and water intake and, if needed, adequate dialysis, control of blood pressure may not be particularly difficult. Unfortunately, some patients are much more fragile, alternating between low and high pressures, and some are much more resistant, presumably because of a greater contribution of high renin levels to the hypertension. With judicious use of available therapy, hypertension should not be a major problem for most patients with renal insufficiency.

In view of increasing evidence that glomerular capillary hypertension is responsible for the progressive loss of renal function once renal insufficiency appears,[207–209] aggressive reduction of this type of hypertension in order to prevent further renal loss is being actively studied. Preliminary experimental evidence suggests that converting enzyme inhibitors may be particularly effective in this regard.[221]

Mechanisms for Hypertension. Volume excess, either absolute[222] or relative,[223] is the predominant mechanism for hypertension in renal insufficiency. This may involve increases in pressor sensitivity to sodium,[224] redistribution of more fluid into the intravascular space,[224] and inhibition of sodium transport via Na^+,K^+-ATPase pumps.[225] Some degree of renin-mediated vasoconstriction is probably also involved in many patients and may be unmasked by the administration of angiotensin-converting enzyme inhibitors.[226] Adrenergic hyperactivity may also contribute, although this too may be apparent only after therapy.[227] The possibility of reversible bilateral renovascular disease among patients with renal insufficiency and severe hypertension should be noted. In one series of 21 such patients, 10 appeared to have renovascular hypertension that was often made worse by medical therapy but helped by revascularization.[228] Use of antihypertensive therapy for patients with renal disease is discussed in Chapter 28.

Diabetic Nephropathy. Hypertension often accompanies the syndrome of diabetic nephropathy caused by intercapillary glomerulosclerosis and may reflect both advancing renal insufficiency with the inability to handle volume loads and extensive structural narrowing of the peripheral vasculature—the hallmark of longstanding diabetes. Moreover, intrarenal hypertension probably accelerates the progress of the glomerulosclerosis,[207–209] and antihypertensive therapy has been shown to slow the progression of renal failure[188] (Fig. 27–21). More effective relief of glomerular capillary hypertension may be possible with converting enzyme inhibitors,[229] which have been shown to reduce the heavy proteinuria that often supervenes in diabetic nephropathy.[230] As common as it is, hypertension may not be as severe or as likely to progress to an accelerated-malignant phase in diabetics with nephropathy for two reasons: first, these patients often have a diminished intravascular volume due to the hypoalbuminemia of the nephrotic syndrome; second, they have low renin levels, presumably owing to hyalinization of juxtaglomerular cells.

Hyporeninemic Hypoaldosteronism. Renin levels may become so low that the syndrome of hyporeninemic hypoaldosteronism develops. Although this pattern may accompany other forms of chronic renal disease, it is found most commonly among diabetics, since they are unable to mobilize either the aldosterone or the insulin needed to transfer potassium from the blood to the tissues and are thus particularly vulnerable to hyperkalemia.[231] Whether diabetic or not, patients with this syndrome are usually recognized by a degree of hyperkalemia out of proportion to the degree of renal damage. The low renin levels are inadequate to stimulate aldosterone, and renal potassium excretion falls. Renin suppression in these patients may also reflect the expansion of fluid volume so common in advanced renal disease.[232] Caution is obviously needed in treating such patients with either supplemental potassium or potassium-sparing diuretics.

Analgesic Nephropathy. Reversible renal insufficiency

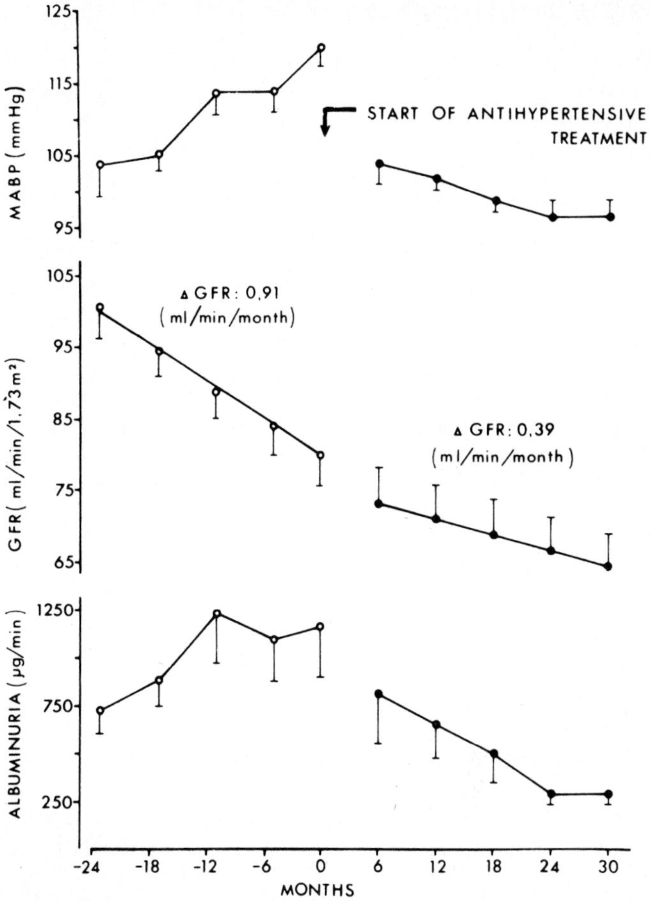

FIGURE 27–21. Average course of mean arterial blood pressure (MABP), glomerular filtration rate (GFR), and albuminuria before (o) and during (~) effective antihypertensive treatment in 10 patients. (From Parving, H-H., Andersen, A. R., Smidt, U. M., and Svendsen, P. A.: Early aggressive antihypertensive treatment reduces rate of decline in kidney function in diabetic nephropathy. Lancet *1*:1175, 1983.)

may accompany the inhibition of renal prostaglandins by nonsteroidal antiinflammatory agents,[165] and permanent renal damage may supervene after prolonged exposure to analgesics, particularly phenacetin. In some countries, notably Australia, this is a common form of chronic renal disease.[233] Until late in their course, these patients have a greater propensity for salt-wasting and therefore may have less severe hypertension. However, in Australians, severe hypertension has been noted in 50 to 86 per cent of patients with analgesic nephropathy. Among those with malignant hypertension, a higher prevalence of renal artery stenosis and, at times, active sloughing of renal papillae was observed.[233] Although aspirin alone rarely seems to cause renal dysfunction, it may reversibly depress glomerular filtration if given to patients with underlying renal disease or during sodium restriction, presumably because of the increased dependency of renal perfusion upon renal prostaglandins under these circumstances.[234]

HYPERTENSION DURING CHRONIC DIALYSIS AND AFTER RENAL TRANSPLANTATION. In patients with ESRD, blood pressure depends mainly upon body fluid volume. With neither the vasoconstrictor effects of renal renin nor the vasodepressor actions of various renal hormones, blood pressure may be particularly labile and sensitive to changes in adrenergic activity.[235] Among patients receiving maintenance hemodialysis every 48 hours, elevated blood pressures tend to fall progressively after dialysis is completed, remain depressed during the remainder of the first 24 hours, and rise again during the second day.[236] Thus, antihypertensive therapy may only be needed on the days between dialyses.

Successful renal transplantation may cure primary (essential) hypertension,[237] but various problems may result in about half the recipients becoming hypertensive within one year.[238] These problems include stenosis of the renal artery at the site of anastomosis, rejection reactions, high doses of adrenal steroids, and excess renin derived from the retained diseased kidneys. Removal of the native diseased kidneys may relieve hypertension caused by their persistent secretion of renin.[239] The source of the donor kidney may also play a role in the subsequent development of hypertension in the recipient: more hypertension has been observed when donors had a family history of hypertension[240] or when the donors had died of subarachnoid hemorrhage and had probably been hypertensive.[241, 242]

RENOVASCULAR HYPERTENSION

The diagnosis and therapy of renovascular hypertension have changed dramatically recently. These changes are most welcome since this, more than all the other more common secondary forms of hypertension, has proved difficult to diagnose and treat.

Less than 2 per cent of adults with hypertension have renovascular hypertension, the prevalence in different series varying from less than 1 to as high as 20 per cent, depending on patient selection.[4] Higher prevalence figures sometimes reflect the inclusion of patients with renovascular disease in whom the hypertension is not caused by renal ischemia. As people grow older, atherosclerotic disease of the renal arteries becomes increasingly common. The diagnosis must be based upon evidence that the renovascular lesion is the cause of the hypertension.

The highest prevalence of renovascular hypertension is among patients with severe, accelerated hypertension. In one group of 123 such patients, 23 per cent or more had renovascular hypertension.[243] Similarly, patients with severe hypertension and renal insufficiency have a high incidence of bilateral renovascular disease.[228] Renovascular hypertension in children is usually a result of congenital dysplasia of the renal arteries.[25] Infants have been found to develop the syndrome owing to thrombosis of the renal artery after catheterization of the umbilical artery.[244]

CLASSIFICATION. In adults, the two major types of renovascular disease tend to appear at different times and in different sexes[245] (Table 27–14). Atherosclerotic disease affecting mainly the proximal third of the main renal artery is seen mostly in older men. Fibroplastic disease involving mainly the distal two-thirds and branches of the renal arteries appears most commonly in younger women. Overall, about two-thirds of cases are caused by atherosclerotic disease and one-third by fibroplastic disease. The nonatherosclerotic stenoses involve all layers of the renal artery, but the most common is medial fibroplasia. In addition, there are a number of other intrinsic and extrinsic causes of renovascular hypertension, including emboli within the renal artery or compression of this vessel by nearby tumors.[4] An interesting association has been noted between increased mobility of the right kidney and fibroplastic involvement of the right renal artery.[246] With repeated stretching of the renal artery, structural changes might be produced, leading to renal artery stenosis sufficient to cause renovascular hypertension.

Among blacks, less atherosclerosis develops in the main renal arteries and the incidence of renovascular hypertension is lower.[247] Among diabetic hypertensive individuals, despite their greater propensity for vascular disease, the incidence of atherosclerotic renal artery stenosis is not increased.[248]

Most renovascular hypertension develops from partial obstruction of one main renal artery, although only a branch need be involved; segmental disease was found in 11 per cent of cases in one large series.[249] On the other hand, if apparent complete occlusion of the renal artery is slow in developing, enough collateral flow will become available to preserve the viability of the kidney. In this way, the seemingly nonfunctioning kidney may be responsible for continued renin secretion and hypertension. If recognized, such totally occluded vessels can sometimes be repaired, with return of renal function and relief of hypertension.[250]

Renovascular stenosis is often bilateral, although usually one side is clearly predominant. In the Cooperative Study on Renovascular Hypertension, 25 per cent of the subjects had bilateral atherosclerotic or fibroplastic disease.[251] The possibility should be suspected in those with renal insufficiency, particularly if rapidly progressive oliguric renal failure develops without evidence of obstructive uropathy.

MECHANISMS. Since Goldblatt produced renovascular hypertension in the dog in 1934, the pathophysiology of this disease has been studied extensively. Confusion has arisen because of the use of one-kidney models, which are more appropriate to the study of renal parenchymal hypertension. The sequence of changes in the two-kidney (one-clip) model and in patients with renovascular hypertension almost certainly starts with the release of greater amounts of renin when sufficient ischemia is induced to diminish pulse pressure in the renal afferent arterioles. A reduction of renal perfusion pressure by 50 per cent leads to an immediate and persistent increase in renin secretion from the ischemic kidney, with suppression of secretion from the contralateral one.[252] With time, renin levels fall

TABLE 27–14 FEATURES OF ATHEROSCLEROTIC AND FIBROUS RENAL ARTERY DISEASE

Renal Artery Disease	Incidence (%)	Age (yr)	Location of Lesion in Renal Artery	Natural History
Atherosclerosis	60	>50	Proximal 2 cm; branch disease rare	Progression in 50%, often to total occlusion
Fibrous dysplasias:				
Intimal fibroplasia	4 to 5	Children, young adults	Mid-main renal artery and/or branches	Progression, dissection, and/or thrombosis common
Medial fibroplasia	30	25 to 50	Distal main renal artery and/or branches	Progression in 33%, dissection and/or thrombosis rare
Periarterial fibroplasia	4 to 5	15 to 30	Mid-to-distal main renal artery or branches	Progression, dissection, and/or thrombosis common
Fibromuscular hyperplasia	<1	Children, young adults	Mid-renal artery or branches	Progression in most cases

From Novick, A. C.: The case for surgical therapy. *In* Narins, R. G. (ed.): Controversies in Nephrology and Hypertension. New York, Churchill Livingstone, 1984, p. 182.

(but not to the low levels expected based on the elevated blood pressure), accompanied by an expanded body fluid volume and increased cardiac output.[253]

In patients with proved renovascular hypertension of many years' duration, excess renin secretion persists, so that the experimental data are confirmed clinically. However, when renovascular hypertension induces extensive nephrosclerosis in the contralateral kidney, a different picture may evolve. Relief of the stenosis may not relieve the hypertension; rather, the contralateral kidney becomes the culprit, with the stenotic kidney's vessels having been protected from the high pressure. With removal of the contralateral kidney, the hypertension may recede.[254]

DIAGNOSIS. The presence of certain clinical features indicates the need for a screening test for renovascular hypertension in perhaps 10 per cent of all hypertensives. A positive screening test, or very strong clinical features, calls for more definitive confirmatory tests.

Clinical Features. Renovascular hypertension may be suspected on the following clinical grounds:

• Presence of an abdominal bruit, particularly if a diastolic component is present and if the bruit is heard lateral to the midline. Bruits confined to systole and heard mostly in older patients and that are loudest in the midepigastrium usually reflect atherosclerosis in the abdominal aorta.

• Onset of hypertension before age 30, particularly in white women who are slender.

• Onset of hypertension after renal trauma.

• Severe, rapidly accelerating hypertension that is difficult to control.

• Evidence of rapidly deteriorating renal function, particularly after therapy is begun with a converting enzyme inhibitor.[255]

The differing clinical picture of the two major forms of renovascular disease was clearly delineated by the Cooperative Study on Renovascular Hypertension:[256] "Patients with atherosclerotic lesions were older, had a higher systolic blood pressure and more frequent arterial disease in areas outside of the kidney, and were more likely to develop target-organ damage than were patients with essential hypertension. In contrast, patients with fibromuscular hyperplasia were young, predominantly female, more likely to have no family history of hypertension, and less prone to develop cardiomegaly."

Some patients have renovascular hypertension but may have none of the clinical features described above and clinically resemble patients with mild essential hypertension. Nonetheless, these features should be used to exclude the majority of hypertensives from additional workup and to identify the 10 per cent or so who should undergo a complete evaluation. In the past, routine performance of intravenous pyelography or other screening tests with a high percentage of false-positive results in all hypertensives resulted in more false-positive than true-positive results,[32] mandating even more unnecessary examinations, with their attendant costs and risks. Initial results with the plasma renin *response to oral captopril,*[257] described below, look very promising, and this may turn out to be a screening test that can be applied to a larger population to find the disease in those who do not have the more classic clinical features. Nonetheless, those who present with rapidly accelerating hypertension with Grade 3 or 4 retinopathy should be highly suspect.

Diagnostic Tests. Until recently, various screening tests were advocated for those with suspicious clinical features, including intravenous pyelography, isotopic renography, and peripheral plasma renin activity assays. However, each of these is relatively nonspecific and not highly sensitive, so that many false-positive and false-negative results were obtained.[258] Increasingly, the diagnostic approach has become more direct: arteriography is recommended as the first and definitive test when renovascular hypertension is suspected.

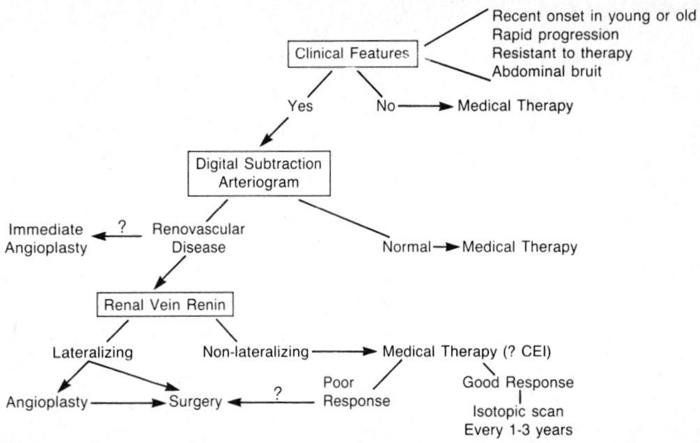

FIGURE 27–22. A scheme for the evaluation and management of renal vascular hypertension. (From Kaplan, N. M.: Clinical Hypertension. 4th ed. Baltimore, © by Williams and Wilkins, 1986, p. 327.)

The scheme shown in Figure 27–22 suggests that *digital subtraction arteriography* (p. 303), be carried out first followed by renal vein renin assays to confirm the functional significance of lesions seen on arteriography. Digital subtraction causes less morbidity for the patient but, with currently available equipment, is not as effective as selective direct arteriography for visualizing small and peripheral lesions. Venous angiography seems unlikely to be useful, since it often misses major lesions and requires an even larger dye load.[259]

In the future, if a lesion is seen, immediate angioplasty may be performed. Most prefer to obtain evidence of the functional significance of the lesion, which usually involves looking for higher levels of renin activity in venous blood from the affected kidney than from the nonaffected side and the inferior vena cava below the renal veins. However, overall results with the lateralizing test of renal vein renin have not clearly indicated surgical curability: in a review of all published data, the sensitivity of this test was 80 per cent and the specificity only 62 per cent, and surgery led to improvement in 92 per cent of those with positive tests but also in 65 per cent of those with negative tests.[260]

Even though arteriography is increasingly available and relatively safe, it cannot be used as a screening test except in those who seem very likely to have the disease, such as a young woman with recent onset of severe hypertension and a diastolic bruit over one kidney. For screening among populations with an expected prevalence of perhaps 5 per cent (taking only those with clinical features suggestive of renovascular hypertension), an easy and safe procedure that results in few false-negatives is needed. A certain number of false-positive results must be expected; considering that about 20 per cent of all adults will have primary (essential) hypertension, at least 20 per cent of patients with renovascular hypertension would be expected to have positive screening tests but would not be cured through repair of the stenosis, so that these results would be classified as "false-positives."

The initial report of a large experience with measurement of peripheral blood renin activity (PRA) before and one hour after a single 50-mg dose of the converting enzyme inhibitor captopril suggests that this approach may provide an easy, noninvasive way to establish the functional significance of a lesion, either after or preferably before arteriography[257] (Fig. 27–23). The procedure requires only that the patient be on a normal sodium intake and off

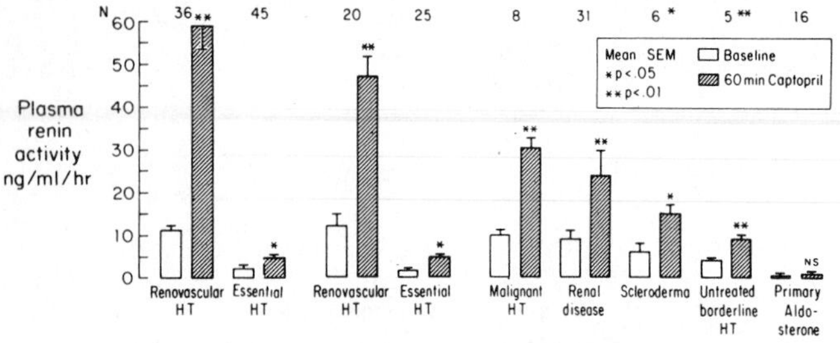

FIGURE 27–23. Plasma renin response 60 minutes after an oral dose of captopril in groups of various types of treated and untreated hypertensive patients. N = number in each group. (From Muller, F. B., Sealey, J. E., Case, D. B., Atlas, S. A., Pickering, T. G., Pecker, M. S., Preibisz, J. J., and Laragh, J. H.: The captopril test for identifying renovascular disease in hypertensive patients. Am. J. Med. *80*:633, 1986.)

diuretics; if possible, other antihypertensive medications should be withdrawn for 3 weeks, although the test was almost equally valid among those examined while on therapy. After the patient sits for 30 minutes, venous blood is obtained for basal PRA, and 50 mg of captopril is given orally. At 60 minutes, another blood sample for stimulated PRA is obtained. The criteria for a positive test for renovascular hypertension is a stimulated PRA of 12 ng/ml/hr or more, an absolute increase in PRA of 10 ng/ml/hr or more, and a 150 per cent or greater increase in PRA or, if baseline PRA is below 3 ng/ml/hr, a 400 per cent increase. Among the 112 patients with essential hypertension tested, only two showed false-positive results; among the 40 with renovascular hypertension, there were no false-negative results.

The test was accurate in patients with good renal function, but it gave both false-positive and false-negative results in a considerable portion of those with impaired renal function. This procedure may turn out to be generally useful as a screening test for renovascular disease. The authors recommend it as a way to identify the process in many patients who would not otherwise be screened. This seems increasingly to be a good idea, since relief of renovascular hypertension by either angioplasty or surgery is being reported in a larger proportion of patients, including many who would not have been candidates for repair only a few years ago. At the same time, problems with the most effective form of medical therapy, converting enzyme inhibitors, have surfaced.

MANAGEMENT. Unfortunately, little is known about the natural history of untreated renovascular disease so it is difficult to assess the results of therapy. No properly controlled study comparing medical versus surgical treatment is available, although one is now in progress at Vanderbilt Medical School.[261] Advances in medical therapy have made it easier to control the hypertension and the availability of transluminal angioplasty offers another "curative" approach, but current evidence supports surgical repair as being more likely to provide relief of hypertension and preserve renal function. Among 41 patients randomly allocated to medical therapy in the ongoing Vanderbilt trial, 17 showed deterioration of renal function or loss of renal size, despite acceptable blood pressure control in 15 of the 17.

These results were obtained prior to availability of converting enzyme inhibitors, which may be considered a two-edged sword; one edge provides better control of renovascular hypertension than may be possible with other antihypertensive medications,[262] while the other edge exposes the already ischemic kidney to a further loss of blood flow by removing the high levels of angiotensin II that were supporting its circulation.[255] Despite the generally excellent control of hypertension with converting enzyme inhibitors, the recommendation has been made by members of the MRC Blood Pressure Unit that "in patients who are candidates for operation, enalapril should usually be given for no more than one month before proceeding to corrective surgery, to allow maximum blood pressure reduction without endangering the stenotic kidney for too long."[263] Other converting enzyme inhibitors would share enalapril's potential for mischief, but the statement ends with the recommendation that "enalapril can nevertheless be given effectively long-term in patients unsuitable for corrective surgery."

Angioplasty. As experience builds with angioplasty, it has been shown to cure or improve 60 to 90 per cent of patients, more with fibromuscular disease than with atherosclerosis, as is also the case for surgery.[264] It will likely be done more and more frequently as the initial procedure, particularly in patients who are poor candidates for major surgery.

Surgery. Despite the availability of better medical therapy and angioplasty, surgical repair is being shown to relieve renovascular hypertension in an increasing number of patients, including the elderly[265] and those with renal insufficiency.[228] Overall guidelines for surgery remain unsettled, depending in part on the local availability and aggressiveness of angioplasters and vascular surgeons. However, most agree that surgery is indicated in patients whose hypertension is not well controlled or whose renal function deteriorates on medical therapy as well as in those with only a transient response to angioplasty or when lesions are not amenable to that procedure. Nevertheless, easier ways to recognize and relieve renovascular hypertension have been developed. Of the 5 to 10 per cent of hypertensive patients most likely to have this condition, we should be able to diagnose and successfully treat most.

RENIN-SECRETING TUMORS

Made up of juxtaglomerular cells or hemangiopericytomas, these tumors have been found mostly in young patients with severe hypertension, very high renin levels in both peripheral blood and the kidney harboring the tumor, and secondary aldosteronism manifested by hypokalemia.[266] The tumor can usually be recognized by selective renal angiography, usually performed for suspected renovascular hypertension. More commonly, children with Wilms' tumors may have hypertension and high renin levels that revert to normal after nephrectomy.[267]

ADRENAL CAUSES OF HYPERTENSION

(See Chap. 58)

Three adrenal causes of hypertension will now be considered—primary excesses of aldosterone, cortisol, and catecholamines. Together these constitute less than 1 per cent of all hypertensive diseases. In addition, congenital adrenal hyperplasia will be discussed. Each can usually be recognized with relative ease, and patients suspected of having these disorders can be screened by means of readily available tests.

More of a problem than the diagnosis of these adrenal disorders is the need to exclude their presence because of the increasing identification of incidental adrenal masses when abdominal computed tomography (CT) is done to diagnose intraabdominal pathology. Unsuspected adrenal tumors were found in 25 of 3,600 abdominal CT scans (0.7 per cent) obtained for reasons unrelated to the adrenal gland.[268, 269] As known from prior autopsy studies, most of these adrenal tumors were nonfunctioning. Only 1 of the 25 turned out to be a functioning tumor, a pheochromocytoma that was obvious on appropriate testing.

PRIMARY ALDOSTERONISM

(See p. 1810)

First recognized in 1954, this disease is relatively rare in unselected populations (Table 27–5), although it may be found in 1 to 2 per cent of patients referred to centers for special study.[270, 271]

PATHOPHYSIOLOGY. Primary aldosterone excess usually arises from solitary benign adenomas. As diagnostic tests improved and became more readily available, larger numbers of patients with minimal features were recognized and many were found to have bilateral adrenal hyperplasia, the number averaging about 25 per cent of all cases of aldosteronism. The validity of defining the condition in these patients with bilateral hyperplasia as "idiopathic hyperaldosteronism" has been questioned by investigators from the MRC Blood Pressure Unit who argued that "idiopathic hyperaldosteronism is at the upper end of a wider-than-normal distribution of aldosterone [secretion] in essential hypertension, from which it has been separated wrongly."[272] Nonetheless, there is some evidence that patients with bilateral adrenal hyperplasia may be responding to an aldosterone-stimulating factor,[273] and they often exhibit some features of aldosterone excess.[274] Even more difficult to explain are a few instances of unilateral hyperplasia.[275]

Some other variants of primary aldosterone excess have been described. A few patients have familial glucocorticoid-suppressible hyperaldosteronism[276]; a few extraadrenal tumors may hypersecrete aldosterone[277]; exogenous mineralocorticoids may cause "pseudoaldosteronism," including the glycyrrhizinic acid in licorice from candy or extract[278] or chewing tobacco.[279]

Whatever the source, excess aldosterone causes hypertension and hypokalemia, here defined as a plasma potassium level below 3.2 mEq/liter (Fig. 27–24). Very rarely, the syndrome has been recognized in normotensive individuals.[280] Not so rarely, hypokalemia may be absent or only intermittent, but in most patients with adenomas, persistent hypokalemia is observed.[271]

The hypertension begins as a volume overload but soon converts, as do apparently all forms of hypertension, to increased peripheral resistance.[85] Nonetheless, high levels of atrial natriuretic peptide are present in the plasma, and the assay may prove to be a helpful diagnostic test.[281] Hypertension may be severe, with a mean pressure in one group of 136 patients of 205/123 mm Hg and four of the patients showing histological evidence of malignant hypertension on renal biopsy.[282] Furthermore, 23 per cent of these patients had a serious vascular complication such as stroke or myocardial infarction. In association with the increased pressure and expanded blood volume, renin secretion is suppressed. Although this finding has been almost invariable with hyperaldosteronism, the overwhelming majority of hypertensive patients with suppressed renin do not have this syndrome (Table 27–12).

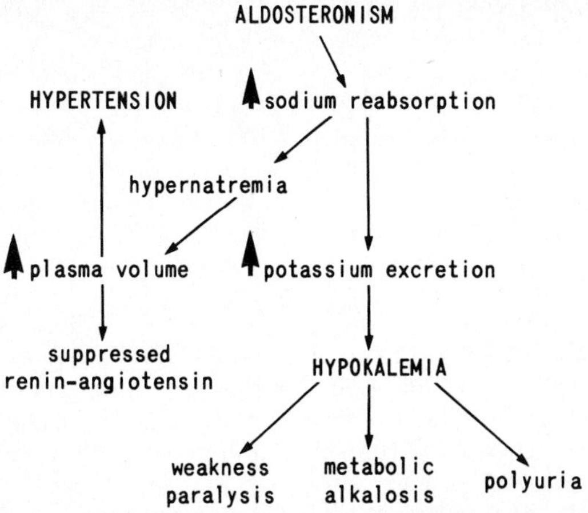

FIGURE 27–24. Pathophysiology of primary aldosteronism. (From Kaplan, N. M.: Clinical Hypertension. 4th ed. Baltimore, © by Williams and Wilkins, 1986, p. 402.)

Hypokalemia results from the aldosterone-mediated increase in renal potassium excretion. Although hypokalemia may not be recognized until diuretics or salt loads are ingested, the effects may be striking, with muscular weakness, polyuria, metabolic alkalosis, impaired carbohydrate tolerance, and blunting of circulatory reflexes.

DIAGNOSIS. Serious consideration should be given to the diagnosis of primary aldosteronism when hypertension and hypokalemia coexist. If the rare normokalemic patient with the disease is thereby missed, little will be lost as long as the patient is protected by appropriate treatment of the hypertension. Since this is likely to include a diuretic, significant hypokalemia will soon become manifest, making the diagnosis obvious.

Potassium-Wasting. The first step in evaluating the hypokalemic hypertensive should be to determine potassium excretion in a 24-hour urine sample collected while

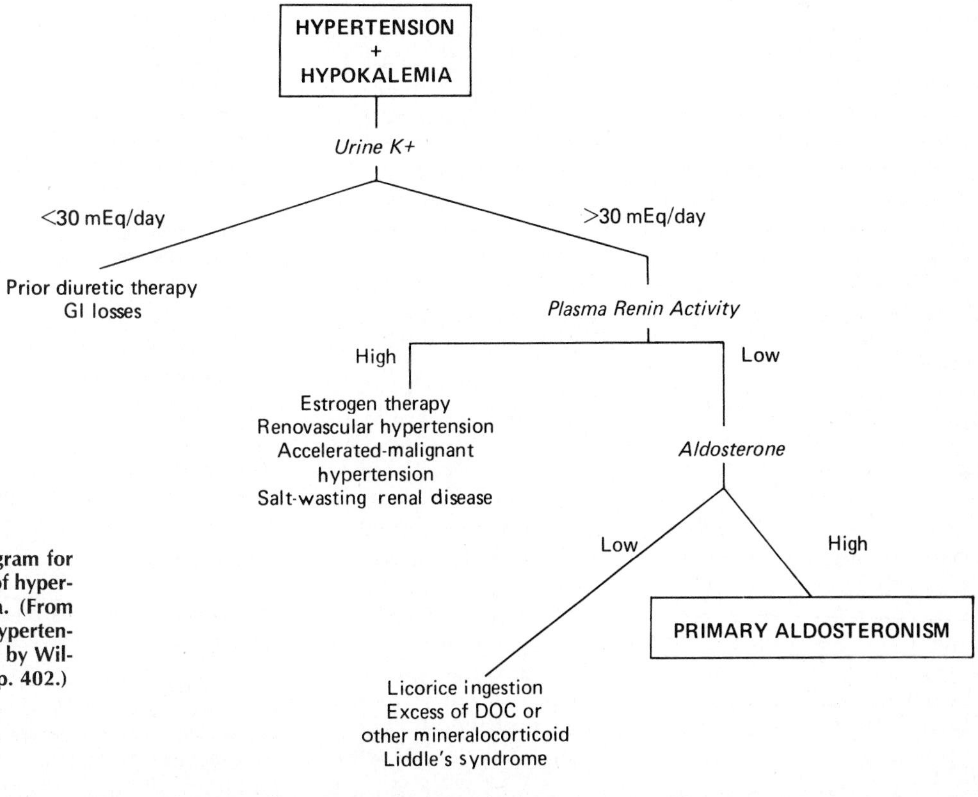

FIGURE 27–25. Flow diagram for the differential diagnosis of hypertension with hypokalemia. (From Kaplan, N. M.: Clinical Hypertension. 4th ed. Baltimore, © by Williams and Wilkins, 1986, p. 402.)

the patient is hypokalemic, receiving no supplemental potassium or diuretic, and ingesting a normal sodium intake (i.e., urinary sodium excretion is above 100 mEq/day) (Fig. 27–25). If, under these circumstances, urinary potassium is less than 30 mEq/day, mineralocorticoid excess is highly unlikely, and the workup can be aborted; if the value is greater than this, further evaluation is warranted. In most hypertensive patients hypokalemia is caused by the prior use of diuretics. Losses may be large and may require prolonged potassium supplementation. On the other hand, severe hypokalemia appearing soon after the initiation of diuretic therapy may presage primary aldosteronism.

Renin Suppression. If urinary potassium-wasting has been documented, the patient should receive potassium supplementation for a period of 3 to 6 weeks to bring the plasma potassium level within the normal range and maintain it, so that subsequent studies will be unaffected by hypokalemia. One or another mild stimulus to renin secretion should be applied to demonstrate suppression. By whatever technique, renin levels are usually significantly suppressed in patients with primary aldosteronism, although a few have normal levels.[271]

Aldosterone Excess. Increased levels of aldosterone can be found in urine or blood. When urine is analyzed, the 24-hour collection should contain over 100 mEq of sodium to insure that high aldosterone levels are not simply secondary to sodium restriction. Various techniques to suppress endogenous aldosterone secretion have been used to insure further that the aldosterone excess is primary. These include high-sodium diets, infusions of saline, injections of DOCA, and oral administration of fludrocortisone (Florinef).

A high aldosterone-to-renin ratio in plasma, either on single or integrated samples, is a useful screening test.[283] More reliable documentation of high and nonsuppressible aldosterone levels can be obtained with the saline suppression test of plasma aldosterone, in which 2 liters of normal saline are infused over a 4-hour interval.[284] The plasma aldosterone level remains elevated in patients with primary aldosteronism but is suppressed to below 10 ng/dl in patients with essential hypertension or secondary aldosteronism. Patients with bilateral hyperplasia often exhibit intermediate levels (between 5 and 10 ng/dl). Once the diagnosis of hyperaldosteronism has been established, the response to high doses of the aldosterone antagonist spironolactone may be used to prepare the patient for surgery and to predict the response to operation.[285]

Bilateral Adrenal Hyperplasia. Various maneuvers are available to differentiate patients with apparent aldosterone excess due to bilateral adrenal hyperplasia from those with an adrenal adenoma.[4] The differential diagnosis should be made, and only those patients with a tumor should be subjected to operation, since it may not be possible to determine the type of pathological condition at operation without removing both adrenal glands.

Computerized axial tomography is capable of identifying adrenal lesions smaller than 1.0 cm, and this procedure is the best initial test to identify the type of adrenal disease.[286] If it fails to define an adrenal adenoma when the clinical situation is strongly suggestive, either an adrenal scintillation scan with an iodinated cholesterol derivative[287] or bilateral adrenal vein catheterization with venography and analysis of venous steroid levels may be utilized.[288] Rather than false-negative tests, there will probably be more problems with false-positive CT scans, i.e., finding nonfunctioning adrenal tumors, which are present in a considerable number of both normotensive and hypertensive persons.[268, 269]

THERAPY. Once the diagnosis of primary aldosteronism is made and the type of adrenal disorder has been established, the choice of therapy is fairly easy: patients with a solitary adenoma require resection of the tumor; those with bilateral hyperplasia should be treated with spironolactone (p. 1811) and a thiazide diuretic (p. 513).[285] Fortunately, the doses of spironolactone required for chronic therapy are usually low enough to avoid bothersome side effects. Triamterene[289] and amiloride[290] will also control the disease if spironolactone is poorly tolerated. When an adenoma is resected, about 75 per cent of patients will become normotensive, while the other 25 per cent remain hypertensive, either from preexisting essential hypertension or from renal damage due to prolonged secondary hypertension.

CUSHING'S SYNDROME

(See p. 1810)

Hypertension occurs in about 80 per cent of patients with Cushing's syndrome. If left untreated, it can cause congestive heart failure and death.[291] As with hypertension of other endocrine causes, the longer it is present, the less likely it is to disappear when the underlying cause is relieved.

MECHANISM OF HYPERTENSION. Blood pressure may increase for a number of reasons.[292] The secretion of a mineralocorticoid, DOC or aldosterone, or another hypertension-producing steroid may also be increased along with cortisol. The excess cortisol exerts a sufficient intrinsic salt-retaining effect to expand volume and lead to hypertension. Cortisol stimulates the synthesis of renin substrate, which in turn causes more angiotensin to be generated. Vascular reactivity to pressor substances, including norepinephrine, increases.

DIAGNOSIS. The syndrome should be suspected in patients with central obesity, thin skin, muscle weakness, and osteoporosis. If clinical features are suggestive, the diagnosis can be either ruled out or virtually assured by the simple, overnight *dexamethasone suppression test*.[293] In normal subjects, the level of plasma cortisol in a sample drawn at 8 a.m. after a bedtime dose of 1 mg of dexamethasone should be below 7 μg/100 mg. If the level is higher, additional workup is in order to establish both the diagnosis of cortisol excess and the pathological type. Patients who are under stress or depressed may fail to show suppression and may be distinguished from those with Cushing's disease by their attenuated response to corticotropin-releasing hormone.[294] Measurement of urine free cortisol levels is almost as good a screening test: most patients who do not have Cushing's syndrome excrete less than 100 μg/24 hours. Measurement of cortisol in one-hour urine samples may serve as well as plasma measurements for basal levels and suppression tests.[295]

If screening tests are abnormal, a longer dexamethasone suppression test should be done, using 0.5 mg every 6 hours and then 2.0 mg every 6 hours, each for 2 days. Urinary 17-hydroxycorticoid (17-HOCS) or free cortisol excretion and plasma cortisol levels should be measured on the second day of each dose. Patients with Cushing's syndrome fail to suppress urinary 17-HOCS to below 4.0 mg/day or urine free cortisol to below 25 μg/day on the 0.5-mg dose; if Cushing's syndrome is caused by excess pituitary ACTH drive with bilateral adrenal hyperplasia, urinary 17-HOCS or free cortisol will be suppressed to below 40 per cent of the control value on the 2.0-mg dose.[293] As plasma ACTH assays become more reliable, they will provide an additional means of differentiating pituitary and ectopic ACTH excess from adrenal tumors with ACTH suppression.[296]

THERAPY. In about two-thirds of patients with Cushing's syndrome, the process begins with overproduction of ACTH by the pituitary, which leads to bilateral adrenal hyperplasia.[297] Although pituitary hyperfunction may reflect a hypothalamic disorder, the majority of patients have discrete pituitary adenomas that can usually be resected by selective transsphenoidal microsurgery.[298] High-voltage pituitary irradiation is often curative. Only rarely is bilateral adrenalectomy necessary. Medical therapy is almost never curative.

If an adrenal tumor is present, it should be surgically removed. With earlier diagnosis and more selective surgical therapy, it is hoped that more patients with Cushing's syndrome will be cured without the need for lifelong glucocorticoid replacement therapy and with permanent relief of their hypertension.

PHEOCHROMOCYTOMA

(See also p. 1812)

The wild fluctuations in blood pressure and dramatic symptoms of pheochromocytoma usually alert both the patient and the physician to the possibility of this diagnosis. However, such fluctuations may be missed or, as occurs in half the patients, the hypertension may be persistent. The symptoms may be incorrectly ascribed to psychoneurosis by practitioners not sensitized to "spells," which usually represent menopausal hot flushes or anxiety-induced hyperventilation. Unfortunately, if the diagnosis is missed, severe complications may arise from exceedingly high blood pressure and damage to the heart by catecholamines. Stroke and hypertensive crises with encephalopathy and retinal hemorrhages may occur, probably because blood pressure levels soar in vessels unprepared by a chronic hypertensive condition. Fortunately, a simple and inexpensive test will detect the disease with virtual certainty, so that diagnostic indecision may be minimized.

PATHOPHYSIOLOGY. Pheochromocytomas may arise wherever the sympathogonia from the primitive neural crest come to lie. These cells differentiate into ganglion cells, neuroblasts, and chromaffin cells. Tumors develop from each of these cell types; ganglioneuromas and neuroblastomas usually occur in children and are recognized by the presence of large amounts of the precursor of catecholamines, dihydroxyphenylalanine.[299] Paragangliomas may arise in chemoreceptor tissue, where they are called chemodectomas, at multiple sites along the sympathetic chain,[300] including the organ of Zuckerkandl; and in the urinary bladder. Pheochromocytomas are often found in patients with neurofibromatosis and hypertension.[301]

About 90 per cent of pheochromocytomas arise in the adrenal medulla; 10 per cent are bilateral and another 10 per cent are malignant. Multiple adrenal tumors are particularly common in patients with simple familial pheochromocytoma and multiple endocrine neoplasia Type II in association with medullary carcinoma of the thyroid (Sipple's syndrome) or with mucosal ganglioneuromas in addition (Type IIB or III). Diffuse medullary hyperplasia may precede the development of tumors, and the tumors may, in fact, reflect extreme degrees of nodular hyperplasia.[302] The recognition of various peptide-producing endocrine tumors, including those with multiple endocrine neoplasias, may be aided by the finding of high levels of plasma chromogranin A, a protein that is co-stored and co-released with peptide hormones.[303]

Secretion from nonfamilial pheochromocytomas varies considerably, with small tumors tending to secrete larger proportions of active catecholamines. If the predominant secretion is epinephrine, which is formed only in the adrenal medulla, the symptoms reflect its effects—mainly systolic hypertension due to increased cardiac output, tachycardia, sweating, flushing, and apprehension. If norepinephrine is predominantly secreted, as from some of the adrenal tumors and from almost all the extraadrenal tumors, the symptoms include both systolic and diastolic hypertension from peripheral vasoconstriction but less tachycardia, palpitations, and anxiety.

DIAGNOSIS. Many more hypertensive patients have variable blood pressures and "spells" than the 0.1 per cent or so who harbor a pheochromocytoma. Spells with paroxysmal hypertension may occur with a number of stresses and a large number of conditions may involve transient catecholamine release (Table 27–15). A pheochromocytoma should be suspected in patients with hypertension that is either paroxysmal or persistent and accompanied by certain symptoms and signs, as listed in Table 27–16. In addition, children and patients with rapidly accelerating hypertension should be screened. Those whose tumors secrete predominantly epinephrine are prone to postural hypotension from a contracted blood volume and blunted sympathetic reflex tone. Suspicion should be heightened if activities such as bending over, exercise, smoking or dipping snuff, or palpation of the abdomen cause repetitive spells that begin abruptly, advance rapidly, and subside within minutes.[304]

High levels of catecholamines may induce myocarditis (Chap. 42), which may progress to cardiomyopathy and left ventricular failure.[305] In the patient described by Baker et al., the decreased cardiac output that resulted from myocardial damage kept the blood pressure normal. Acute myocardial infarction also occurs with increased frequency.[306] Opiates given to such patients may raise the pressure through release of catecholamines.[307]

LABORATORY CONFIRMATION. The easiest and best procedure is either a 24-hour or spot urine assay for total metanephrines. This catecholamine metabolite is least affected by various interfering substances including antihypertensive drugs. The ranges and sensitivities for the three urinary tests reported in multiple series are shown in Table 27–17, showing the superiority of the metanephrine assay.[308] Urinary metanephrine excretion will be increased if patients are taking sympathomimetic drugs, monoamine oxidase inhibitors, or the alpha- and beta-adrenoceptor blocker labetalol.[309] It will be decreased for the next few days after use of x-ray contrast media containing methylglucamine (e.g., Renografin, Hypaque). Therefore, the urine should be collected before an IVP or other such procedure is done.

Plasma catecholamine assays may provide a way to confirm the diagnosis.[310] If plasma levels are equivocal, measurement of a plasma norepinephrine level 3 hours after a single 0.3-mg oral dose of the adrenergic inhibitor clonidine has been shown to separate the nonpheochromocytoma patients, whose levels are suppressed, from those with the disease, whose levels are not suppressed.[311] Failure of normal suppression with clonidine has been noted in patients without this tumor who are taking a diuretic.[312]

LOCALIZATION OF THE TUMOR. Once the diagnosis has been made, medical therapy should be started and the tumor localized by CT scan, which usually demonstrates these typically large tumors with ease. Radioisotopes that localize in chromaffin tissue are available and are of additional help in the few patients in whom localization is not possible by CT.[313]

TABLE 27–15 CONDITIONS THAT MAY SIMULATE PHEOCHROMOCYTOMA

Cardiovascular
- Hyperdynamic, labile hypertension
- Paroxysmal tachycardia
- Angina, coronary insufficiency
- Acute pulmonary edema
- Eclampsia
- Hypertensive crisis during or after surgery
- Hypertensive crisis with monoamine oxidase inhibitors
- Rebound after abrupt cessation of clonidine and other antihypertensives

Psychoneurological
- Anxiety with hyperventilation
- Migraine and cluster headaches
- Brain tumor
- Stroke
- Diencephalic seizures
- Porphyria
- Lead poisoning
- Familial dysautonomia
- Acrodynia
- Autonomic hyperreflexia, as with quadriplegia

Endocrinological
- Menopause
- Thyrotoxicosis
- Diabetes mellitus
- Hypoglycemia
- Carcinoid
- Mastocytosis

Factitious: Ingestion of sympathomimetics

From Kaplan, N. M.: Clinical Hypertension. 4th ed. Baltimore, © by Williams and Wilkins, 1986, p. 381.

TABLE 27–16 FEATURES SUGGESTIVE OF PHEOCHROMOCYTOMA

Hypertension: Persistent or paroxysmal
- Markedly variable blood pressures (± orthostatic hypotension)
- Sudden paroxysms (± subsequent hypertension) in relation to:
  - Stress: Anesthesia, angiography, parturition
  - Pharmacological provocation: Histamine, nicotine, caffeine, beta blockers, saralasin, glucocorticoids, tricyclic antidepressants
  - Manipulation of tumors: Abdominal palpation, urination
- Rare patients persistently normotensive
- Unusual settings: Childhood, pregnancy, familial
  - Multiple endocrine adenomas: Medullary carcinoma of thyroid (MEN-2), mucosal neuromas (MEN-3)
  - Neurocutaneous lesions: Neurofibromatosis

Associated Symptoms:
- Sudden spells with headache, sweating, palpitations, nervousness, nausea, and vomiting
- Pain in chest or abdomen

Associated Signs:
- Sweating, tachycardia, arrhythmia, pallor, weight loss

From Kaplan, N. M.: Clinical Hypertension. 4th ed. Baltimore, © by Williams and Wilkins, 1986, p. 386.

TABLE 27–17 URINARY TESTS FOR PHEOCHROMOCYTOMA

Compound	Urinary Excretion (mg/day or μg/mg creatinine) Normal Adults	Pheochromocytoma	No. of Patients With Tumor	% Patients With Tumor Correctly Identified*
Free catecholamines	<0.1	0.1 to 10.0	179	85
Metanephrine + normetanephrine	<1.2	1.0 to 100.0	282	96
Vanillylmandelic acid	<6.5	5 to 600	294	84

From Manu, P., and Runge, L. A.: Biochemical screening for pheochromocytoma: Superiority of urinary metanephrines measurements. Am. J. Epidemiol. *120*:788, 1984.

THERAPY. Once diagnosed and localized, pheochromocytomas should be resected. Great care should be taken in preparing patients for operation and managing them through the procedure.[314] The most important part of their preoperative management is adrenoceptor blockade sufficient to overcome vasoconstriction and allow the reduced blood volume to reexpand. If the tumor is unresectable, chronic medical therapy with the alpha blocker phenoxybenzamine (Dibenzyline) or the inhibitor of catechol synthesis α-methyl-tyrosine (Demser) can be used.

CONGENITAL ADRENAL HYPERPLASIA

Two distinct enzymatic defects may induce hypertension: (1) *11-hydroxylase deficiency,* which leads to virilization (from excessive androgens) and hypertension with hypokalemia (from excessive DOC). A partial deficiency has been recognized in 15 patients with what appeared to be ordinary primary hypertension[159] and in women with only hirsutism[315] or menstrual irregularities.[316] (2) *17-Hydroxylase deficiency,* which also causes hypertension from excess DOC, but, in addition, causes failure of secondary sexual development because sex hormones are also deficient.[317] Affected children are hypertensive, but the defect in sex hormone synthesis may not become obvious until after puberty. Thereafter, affected males display ambiguity of sexual development and fail to mature.

OTHER CAUSES OF HYPERTENSION

A host of other causes of hypertension are known (see Table 27–4). One that is likely becoming more common is ingestion of various drugs—prescribed (e.g., cyclosporine[318]), over-the-counter (e.g., phenylpropanolamine[319]), and illicit (e.g., cocaine).

COARCTATION OF THE AORTA

(See pp. 929 and 994)

Congenital narrowing of the aorta may occur at any level of the thoracic or abdominal aorta. It is usually found just beyond the origin of the left subclavian artery or distal to the insertion of the ligamentum arteriosum. The coarctation may be localized or more diffuse. Other cardiac anomalies usually accompany the latter, and over half of those afflicted die during the first year of life, although operative treatment of both the coarctation and associated anomalies may reduce this mortality rate. With less severe postductal lesions, damage is more insidious, and symptoms may not appear until the teenage years or later.

Hypertension in the arms and weak or absent femoral pulses are the classic features of coarctation. The pathogenesis of the hypertension may be more complicated than simple mechanical obstruction: a generalized vasoconstrictor mechanism is likely involved, which may be either renin-angiotensin or sympathetic nervous activity.[320] The lesion may be detected by two-dimensional echocardiography (Fig. 31–15, p. 996), and aortography proves the diagnosis (Fig. 30–30, p. 931). To diminish the development of congestive heart failure, endocarditis, and stroke, the obstruction should be corrected in early childhood.[321] Immediately after surgical repair, the blood pressure may transiently rise even further, and mesenteric arteritis may develop. These changes may reflect very high levels of renin-angiotensin and catecholamines and can be prevented by the prophylactic use of beta blockers.[322]

HYPERPARATHYROIDISM

(See p. 1814)

As noted earlier (p. 1814), calcium may be intimately involved in the pathogenesis of primary hypertension, and increased levels of parathyroid hormone may be present as a response to a urinary calcium leak.[144] In addition, hypertension occurs in one-fourth to one-half of patients with hyperparathyroidism and is found commonly in patients with other hypercalcemic states.[323] As more patients are found to be hypertensive and undergo routine testing of serum calcium, asymptomatic hypercalcemia associated with hyperparathyroidism is not infrequently recognized. Moreover, thiazide diuretics—the most frequently used drugs in the treatment of hypertension—may accentuate previously borderline hypercalcemia.

The mechanism by which hypercalcemia elevates blood pressure probably involves a direct increase in the contractility of vascular smooth muscle and activation of the sympathetic nervous system.[323] After surgical correction of hyperparathyroidism, hypertension often persists.[324]

HYPERTENSION AFTER HEART SURGERY

Transient hypertension may develop postoperatively for various reasons: pain, physical and emotional excitement, hypoxia, hypercapnia, and excessive volume loads[325] (Table 27–18). More severe hypertension has been noted to follow a number of cardiovascular surgical procedures:

1. *Coronary bypass surgery.* The incidence, exceeding 33 per cent, is far higher than after other major cardiac or noncardiac surgery. The problem appears more commonly on the background of preexisting hypertension, greater than 50 per cent obstruction of the left main coronary artery, or the preoperative use of beta blockers.[326] The hemodynamic pattern of increased peripheral resistance can be explained by the markedly high plasma catecholamine and renin activity measured in such patients. In those patients who had previously received beta blocker therapy, the postoperative hypertension may also reflect a rebound phenomenon. Therefore, continuation of beta

TABLE 27–18 HYPERTENSION ASSOCIATED WITH CARDIAC SURGERY

Preoperative
- Anxiety, angina, and the like
- Discontinuation of antihypertensive therapy
- "Rebound" from discontinuing beta-adrenoceptor blocking agents in patients with coronary artery disease

Intraoperative
- Induction of anesthesia
  - Specific drugs
  - Hypertension due to tracheal intubation and nasopharyngeal, urethral, or rectal manipulation
- Precardiopulmonary bypass (during sternotomy and chest retraction)
- Cardiopulmonary bypass
- Postcardiopulmonary bypass (during surgery)

Postoperative
- Early (within 2 hours)
  - Obvious cause: Hypoxia, hypercarbia, ventilatory difficulties, hypothermia, shivering, arousal from anesthesia
  - No obvious cause: After myocardial revascularization; less frequently after valve replacement; early (Sealy type I) hypertension after resection of aortic coarctation
- Intermediate (12 to 36 hours after surgery): Sealy type II after repair of aortic coarctation
- Late (weeks to months): After aortic valve replacement by homografts

From Estafanous, F. G., and Tarazi, R. C.: Systemic arterial hypertension associated with cardiac surgery. Am. J. Cardiol. *46*:685, 1980.

blocker therapy through the perioperative period is likely to reduce the frequency of the problem. If it occurs, therapy is often required: intravenous nitroglycerin[327] and calcium antagonists[328] are effective, as is stellate ganglion or thoracic epidural block.[325]

2. *Aortic valve replacement.* Transient hypertension may give way to more permanent hypertension. In one series, 53 per cent of 116 patients were hypertensive 5 years after surgery, and hypertension was a major determinant of late failure of the homograft valve.[329]

3. *Closure of an atrial septal defect.*[330]

4. *Cardiac transplantation.*[100]

SLEEP APNEA. Increasing recognition has been given to the association between sleep apnea and various cardiovascular complications.[331] Sleep apnea has been recognized in as many as 30 per cent of hypertensive patients, many without gross obesity, and hypertension has been noted in as many as 80 per cent of patients with sleep apnea.[332, 333] The mechanism probably involves activation of numerous central vasomotor reflexes during hypoxia, but the exact manner by which recurrent apnea leads to permanent hypertension is unknown. Nevertheless, elevations in blood pressure have been reduced upon relief of sleep apnea.[334]

SPECIAL TOPICS IN HYPERTENSION

PREGNANCY-INDUCED HYPERTENSION

(See p. 1859)

A small percentage of women enter pregnancy with hypertension, but a larger number develop hypertension while pregnant. With a diastolic blood pressure exceeding 84 mm Hg at any time during gestation, fetal mortality increases, more so if accompanied by proteinuria.[335] More than 10,000 fetal deaths and one-sixth of all maternal deaths in the United States every year are attributable to hypertension.[336] Although the cause of pregnancy-induced hypertension is unknown, it can be recognized early and managed with relative ease. Most instances of serious hypertensive complications during pregnancy are associated with poor or absent obstetrical care.[337] Since blood pressure falls during the course of normal pregnancy[338] (Fig. 27–26), different criteria are needed for diagnosis of hypertension. In most cases, these involve a rise in blood pressure of 30/15 mm Hg or more, or an absolute level greater than 140/90 mm Hg on two or more occasions at least 6 hours apart. As with other forms of hypertension, blood pressure may vary by 20 to 40 mm Hg within short intervals for no apparent reason.[339]

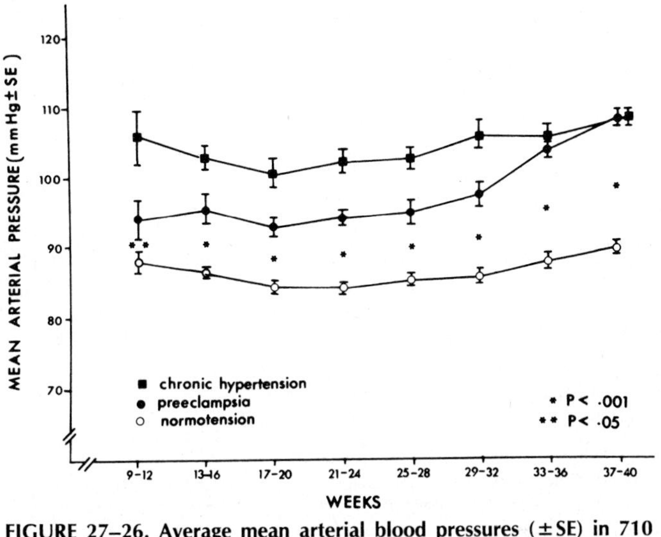

FIGURE 27–26. Average mean arterial blood pressures (±SE) in 710 women who remained normotensive throughout pregnancy, in 46 who developed preeclampsia, and in 37 with chronic hypertension. (From Moutquin, J. M., Rainville, C., Giroux, L., Raynauld, P., Amyot, G., Bilodeau, R., and Pelland, N.: A prospective study of blood pressure in pregnancy: Prediction of preeclampsia. Am. J. Obstet. Gynecol. *151*:191, 1985.)

Several types of hypertension are seen: (1) Pregnancy-induced hypertension: Hypertension developing after the 20th week of gestation. If proteinuria or edema accompanies the hypertension, the term preeclampsia is applicable. Figure 27–26 shows that the blood pressures of those who developed preeclampsia were higher during the first half of pregnancy compared with those who remained normotensive throughout.[338] (2) Eclampsia: The above, plus convulsions not caused by coincidental neurological disease. (3) Chronic hypertension of whatever cause: Most of these patients have essential hypertension that may not have been recognized prior to pregnancy and that is often masked by the usual fall in blood pressure during the midtrimester (Fig. 27–26). (4) Preeclampsia superimposed on chronic hypertension.

MECHANISMS

The hemodynamic changes of normal pregnancy are described in Chapter 60. When pregnancy-induced hypertension begins, peripheral resistance rises, vascular reactivity to pressor agents increases, plasma volume falls, and renal function diminishes.[340] A failure of the normal expansion of blood and body fluid volume may lead to hypertension by reducing uteroplacental perfusion. The frequency with which pregnancy-induced hypertension develops has been found to increase progressively with the initial maternal hemoglobin (Hb) value, rising from 7 per cent with initial values under 10.5 gm/dl to 42 per cent at Hb concentrations over 14.5 gm/dl.[341] This observation has been explained by the assumption that the higher the Hb level, the higher the blood viscosity, which would reduce uteroplacental perfusion. Hemoconcentration with hypovolemia is a feature of pregnancy-induced hypertension and is probably caused by hypoalbuminemia, which reduces colloid osmotic pressure and thereby leads to a loss of fluid from the vascular compartment,[342] further reducing uteroplacental circulation.

Whether these hemodynamic changes are cause or effect, the basic problem seems to be an imbalance between placental mass and blood flow.[343] In some women predisposed to preeclampsia, placental blood flow is impaired, as in those with diabetes or preexisting chronic hypertension. In others, placental mass is increased, as in those with multiple births and hydatidiform moles. In those most predisposed, i.e., young primigravidas, both a relatively greater placental mass and an inadequately developed blood supply may be involved.

Whatever the basic reason, when the uteroplacental

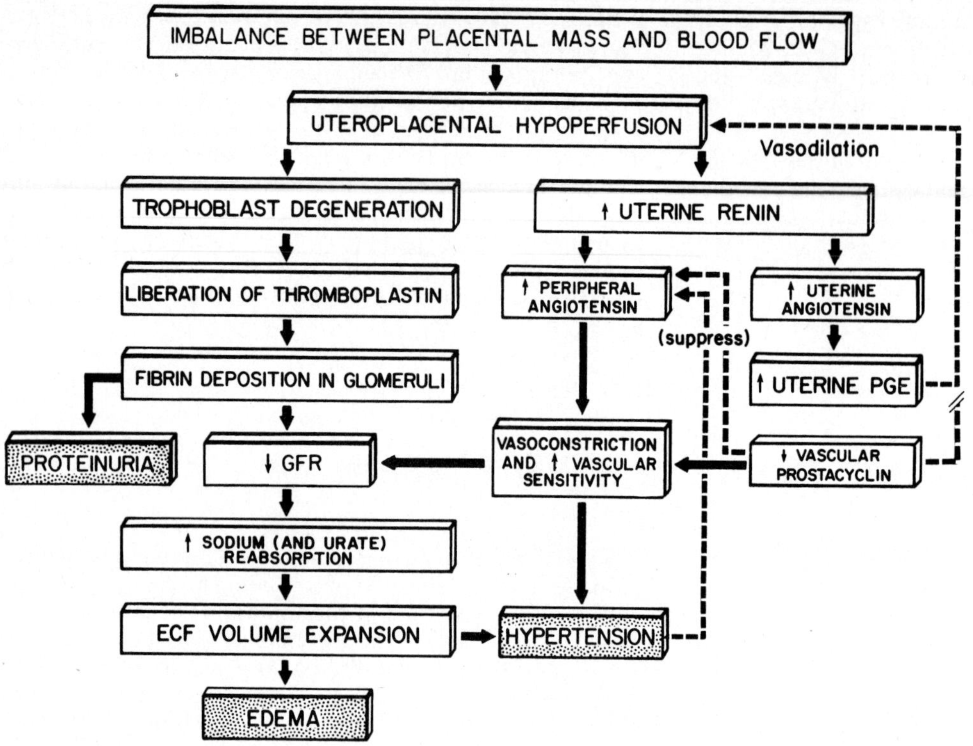

FIGURE 27–27. A unified working hypothesis for the pathophysiology of pregnancy-induced hypertension. The solid lines lead to the three primary manifestations: proteinuria, edema, and hypertension. The dotted lines indicate attempts to counteract the underlying defect of uteroplacental hypoperfusion. (From Kaplan, N. M.: Clinical Hypertension. 4th ed. Baltimore, © by Williams and Wilkins, 1986, p. 367.)

structure is hypoperfused, the cascade of events shown in Figure 27–27 may be set into motion; events shown on the left are well documented, while those on the right are less so. The scheme suggests that when the uterus is hypoperfused, it secretes more renin, which generates more angiotensin within the placental circulation. In response to moderately increased levels of angiotensin, uteroplacental blood flow increases, possibly as a result of the action of angiotensin to liberate increased amounts of vasodilatory prostaglandins, particularly prostacyclin. The vasodilation provides an appropriate compensatory response to hypoperfusion, but this compensation may be inadequate in the patient with pregnancy-induced hypertension; prostacyclin levels in various fluids and in both fetal and maternal blood vessels are lower in those with pregnancy-induced hypertension than in normal pregnancy, whereas excess amounts of the vasoconstrictor thromboxane have been measured in placental tissue from patients with pregnancy-induced hypertension.[344]

The mounting evidence for this imbalance has been well summarized:[345]

> These observations have been linked to those suggesting that changes in prostaglandin metabolism cause preeclamptic hypertension. Increased sensitivity to the pressor effects of infused angiotensin II is an early feature of the disorder.[346] The pressor response to angiotensin II in pregnant women is blunted by infusing prostaglandin E_2[347] or prostacyclin[348] and is augmented by giving inhibitors of prostaglandin synthetase,[349] including aspirin. These observations suggest, but do not prove, that an imbalance of vasoconstrictor and vasodilator prostaglandins, either circulating or in the arterial wall, may alter arterial tone in preeclampsia. Most attractive is the concept that the vasoconstricting factor is thromboxane release by circulating platelets, although prostaglandins produced by the placenta itself cannot be excluded. It is therefore logical to consider using antiplatelet agents to prevent or treat preeclampsia.

Wallenburg et al. have reported that 60 mg a day of aspirin, started at 28 weeks' gestation, significantly reduced the frequency of pregnancy-induced hypertension in women judged to be at high risk because of their increased sensitivity to angiotensin infusion.[350] These results amplify those of Beaufils et al., who also reported protection by aspirin, 150 mg a day, plus dipyridamole, 300 mg a day, given from the end of the first trimester.[351] Obviously, larger controlled clinical trials are needed. In the meantime, however, the evidence for a prostaglandin imbalance as an important factor in the pathogenesis of pregnancy-induced hypertension looks increasingly impressive. As attractive as this scheme appears, some favor other theories, including (1) a primary alteration in platelet function leading to slow intravascular coagulation with fibrin deposition[352]; and (2) an immunogenetic basis, which could explain the increased incidence of preeclampsia in first pregnancies, its familial tendency, and its association with an enlarged placenta.[353] In addition, an increase in sodium transport across red cells[354] and higher sodium concentration in white cells[355] have been reported in pregnancy-induced hypertension, along with an increase in an ouabain-like sodium pump inhibitor in the amniotic fluid.[356] Whether these changes are primary or secondary to other hemodynamic changes is not known.

CLINICAL FEATURES

The distinction between preeclampsia and chronic hypertension should be made, since the former is a self-limited disease that should be treated more conservatively. In most patients the distinction can be made (Table 27–19), but sometimes only after delivery. As noted, the absolute level of blood pressure elevation need not be great to increase fetal mortality. The mother may be particularly vulnerable to encephalopathy because of her previously normal blood pressure. As is described in more detail under Hypertensive Crises (p. 853), cerebral blood flow is normally kept constant over a fairly narrow range of mean arterial pressure, roughly between 60 and 100 mm Hg in normotensive individuals. In a previously normotensive young woman, an acute rise in blood pressure to 150/100 mm Hg may exceed the upper limit of autoregulation, resulting in a "breakthrough" of cerebral blood flow (acute dilatation) that leads to cerebral edema, convulsions, and all of the clinical manifestations of eclampsia.

TABLE 27–19 DIFFERENCES BETWEEN PREECLAMPSIA AND CHRONIC HYPERTENSION

	PREECLAMPSIA	CHRONIC HYPERTENSION
Age	Young (<20)	Older (>30)
Parity	Primigravida	Multipara
Onset	After 20 weeks of pregnancy	Before 20 weeks of pregnancy
Weight gain and edema	Sudden	Gradual
Systolic blood pressure	<160	>160
Funduscopic findings	Spasm, edema	Arteriovenous nicking, exudates
Proteinuria	Present	Absent
Plasma uric acid	Increased	Normal
Blood pressure after delivery	Normal	Elevated

Even traces of *proteinuria* add significantly to the seriousness of the clinical situation. *Renal damage* may be reflected in a falling creatinine clearance rate and a rising plasma uric acid concentration. Some pedal edema is seen in over half of normal pregnant women, but a sudden weight gain of more than 2 pounds in one week and the subsequent appearance of more *generalized edema* commonly forewarns of preeclampsia. On funduscopic examination, sequential constriction of the retinal arterioles is seen first, followed by *retinal edema* causing a retinal sheen. The presence of *arteriovenous nicking and exudates* suggests a chronic hypertensive process. If any one of the following clinical features is present and does not improve, delivery within 24 hours should be considered: diastolic blood pressure above 100 mm Hg, headaches, visual scotomas, proteinuria 2+ or greater, or epigastric pain.

MANAGEMENT

Primigravidas should be followed carefully for the presence or development of hypertension, particularly if they are young or diabetic or have a family history of preeclampsia. A simple test to predict subsequent preeclampsia has been found to have fair specificity and sensitivity.[357] The supine pressor test, or "roll-over" test, involves measuring the blood pressure first in the left lateral recumbent position and then in the supine position. A rise in the diastolic pressure of 20 mm Hg or greater within 2 to 5 minutes is considered positive. If the test is carried out in a normotensive primigravida at about the 28th week of pregnancy and if the result is positive, the patient should be instructed to restrict her activity and be seen frequently. Neither diuretics nor sodium restriction has been found to be helpful[358] and, in view of the evidence that pregnancy-induced hypertension is associated with reduced uteroplacental flow, the prudent course is not to reduce body fluid volume.

Once the blood pressure rises, the patient's physical activity should be restricted, preferably by admission to a high-risk pregnancy unit where she can be observed carefully. In one report, remarkable results were achieved in such a low-cost hospital setting.[359] Most women became normotensive without medication and safely carried the fetus to maturity. As a result, perinatal mortality fell to 9 per 1000—lower than that noted among infants born to women without preeclampsia on the general obstetrical ward at the same hospital.

ANTIHYPERTENSIVE THERAPY. Antihypertensive drug therapy is used only if diastolic pressure does not fall below 110 mm Hg on modified bedrest. Diuretics and salt restriction are avoided. Methyldopa (Aldomet) (p. 872) or hydralazine (Apresoline) (p. 876) is usually chosen, the former for more chronic oral use[360] and the latter for more acute parenteral use. Beta blockers were initially thought to be contraindicated in preeclampsia, owing to scattered reports of fetal hypoglycemia, bradycardia, and respiratory depression. However, a properly controlled prospective study showed that therapy with atenolol was effective in reducing the blood pressure, with no adverse effects on the mother or fetus.[361] Metoprolol has also been shown to be safe.[362]

Chronic Hypertension. If pregnancy begins during antihypertensive drug therapy, including diuretics, medications are usually continued, based on the belief that the mother should be protected and that the fetus will not suffer from any sudden hemodynamic shifts such as occur when therapy is first begun. Among women with chronic hypertension who were not undergoing treatment, therapy with either hydralazine or methyldopa significantly reduced the incidence of preeclampsia when compared with a placebo-treated group.[363] However, despite treatment with drugs, the incidence of fetal growth retardation remains higher in patients with chronic hypertension.[364] Those with severe hypertension during the first trimester, despite intensive therapy, often progress to superimposed preeclampsia and have a high perinatal mortality and morbidity.[365]

MANAGEMENT OF ECLAMPSIA. With appropriate care of preeclampsia, eclampsia hardly ever supervenes; when it does, however, maternal mortality may reach 14 per cent and fetal mortality 27 per cent.[366] Among those women who die, contraction band necrosis of the myocardium, indicative of coronary artery spasm, is frequently noted and may be a contributing factor.[367] In 245 consecutive cases in which the following approach was taken, only one maternal death occurred and fetal survival was excellent[368]: Susceptible patients are given magnesium sulfate ($MgSO_4$) prophylactically, and blood pressure is brought under control with antihypertensive agents. If convulsions have already occurred, they are halted with $MgSO_4$, and delivery is delayed until the blood pressure is controlled and fluid and electrolyte balance is achieved. Patients with severe eclampsia who have persistent oliguria after a fluid challenge should undergo hemodynamic monitoring, since management may require additional volume or a reduction in preload or afterload.[369]

CONSEQUENCES OF PREGNANCY-INDUCED HYPERTENSION

The long-term prognosis of women with pregnancy-induced hypertension is excellent. When 200 women with eclampsia were followed for up to 44 years, the distribution of blood pressures was identical to that in the general population.[370] Chesley concludes that "eclampsia neither is a sign of latent essential hypertension nor causes hypertension." The long-term mortality rate in black women having eclampsia and of white women having eclampsia as multiparas is increased, probably because they had underlying but previously unrecognized chronic hypertension or renal disease.

After delivery, women may develop transient or persistent hypertension. In many, early essential hypertension may have been masked by the hemodynamic changes of pregnancy. Some women develop postpartum heart failure that may be an idiopathic cardiomyopathy but is usually related to hypertension, preexisting heart disease, or complications of pregnancy[371] (p. 1858). A small number develop rapidly progressive acute oliguric renal failure associated with severe hypertension.

HYPERTENSION IN CHILDREN AND ADOLESCENTS

(See also Ch. 32)

The linkage between hypertension in children and adolescents and that in adults is being strengthened, but long-term tracking studies are not available to document the natural history of the process. As an example, taken from the description of abnormal sodium transport in the pathogenesis of primary hypertension (Chap. 27), half the normotensive children of hypertensive parents have the abnormality,[94] but it will take another 20 or more years to determine whether the abnormality presages the development of hypertension. Nevertheless, a great deal of work is being carried out to define the frequency, mechanisms, natural history, and treatment of hypertension in childhood.

The grids published in 1977 by a task force of the NHLBI, have been widely accepted as the "official" new standards for the distribution of blood pressure levels in normal male and female children, ages 2 to 17 years. However, other surveys have found the normal levels to be lower by an average of 5 to 10 mm Hg and few children to be definitely hypertensive.[25] The most obvious reason for these lower levels is the use of repeated blood pressure measurement in most of these other surveys. The need to take more than one reading is obvious: in the Dallas survey, 8.9 per cent of 10,641 eighth-graders had levels at or above the 95th percentile on the first screening but only 1.2 per cent had hypertension on reexamination.[372] In a number of studies, repeated measurements are being taken to assess the tracking of blood pressure levels. Correlations as high as 0.7 are noted over one year but these decrease considerably over longer periods of time. For example, after 4 years of followup of a random sample of 596 Dutch children, only 25 per cent of the boys and 22 per cent of the girls who were in the upper 10 per cent of the diastolic blood pressure distribution at the time of the first examination were in the same percentile 4 years later.[373]

Children who have the highest pressures tend to be larger and more mature, with higher levels of adrenal androgen secretion.[374] In a study of 2165 children examined 4 years apart, those who maintained their blood pressure in the upper quintile also tended to be of greater size and maturity than did those in the lower quintiles of blood pressure.[375] Obesity is associated with higher levels of pressure,[376] but children who are thin and in the upper range of blood pressure levels tend to remain at that high level, more than do those who are obese.[26] Prevention of childhood obesity is being increasingly advocated, along with a reduction in high levels of sodium intake.[377] Additional factors related to blood pressure levels are listed in Table 27–20. Interestingly, blood pressures among healthy black children are not higher—and may be lower—than those seen among white children.[24] Thus, the reason for the much greater incidence of hypertension in black adults must be sought among factors that are active mainly beyond adolescence or that have a long "incubation."

TABLE 27–20 EPIDEMIOLOGICAL FACTORS RELATED TO BLOOD PRESSURE LEVELS IN CHILDREN AND ADOLESCENTS

Genetic
Parental and sibling blood pressure levels
Erythrocyte sodium flux
Urinary kallikrein level
Environmental
Socioeconomic status
Rural vs. urban residence
Migration from developing to developed area
Pulse rate
Mixed genetic and environmental
Body mass and muscular development
Salt
Stress

From Lieberman, E.: *In* Kaplan, N. M. (ed.): Clinical Hypertension. 4th ed. Baltimore, © by Williams and Wilkins, 1986, p. 453.

PRIMARY (ESSENTIAL) HYPERTENSION. When asymptomatic children with persistently elevated pressures are studied, most turn out to have no recognizable secondary cause. In the Muscatine survey, 23 of the 41 with high pressures were obese; of the 18 lean subjects, 13 had essential hypertension.[375] The *hemodynamic profile* in children with primary hypertension is similar to that of adults in that an elevated peripheral vascular resistance is the major finding.[378] Thus, hypertension in children does not usually fit a "hyperdynamic" pattern, with high cardiac output and fast pulse rates. The role of the sympathetic nervous and angiotensin mechanisms in blood pressure elevation among children remains unknown. Plasma renin and aldosterone levels tend to be low in those with the higher levels of blood pressure, and plasma catecholamine levels are usually normal,[379] but children may show a greater cardiovascular response to mental and other types of stress than do normotensive children.[92]

Cardiac effects of even relatively small elevations in blood pressure may be found in careful studies of heart size and function. In 114 hypertensive high school students, heart size and contractile functions as determined by echocardiography were significantly increased in comparison to findings in normotensive subjects of the same age.[380] Abnormal patterns of left ventricular filling have been noted on pulsed Doppler examinations in children with only mildly elevated blood pressures.[381] Whether these changes are a cause or an effect of the elevated pressures remains uncertain, as does their relationship to the subjects' subsequent cardiovascular status.

SECONDARY HYPERTENSION IN CHILDREN. As more experience is gained, the need for extensive laboratory workup for the majority of postpubertal children with relatively mild hypertension continues to be deemphasized.[25] Only those with moderate or severe hypertension (i.e., 10 mm Hg or more above the 95th percentile for their age and sex) or an abnormality on initial laboratory screening studies (i.e., elevated serum creatinine) need to undergo additional testing, including intravenous pyelography. Most instances of hypertension in children have no apparent cause, but when diastolic pressure exceeds 120 mm Hg, approximately 95 per cent will have secondary hypertension. Thus, it seems appropriate to investigate more thoroughly only those hypertensive children with abnormalities on the physical examination or on urine analysis and those with a blood pressure level 10 mm Hg or more above the 95th percentile. The proper therapy for children with hypertension remains uncertain. In general, the guidelines for adult hypertension provided in Chapter 28 are appropriate for the young, although a longer trial of weight reduction and sodium restriction seems indicated before drug treatment is begun. The long-term effects of various antihypertensive agents need to be more carefully assessed.

HYPERTENSIVE CRISES

DEFINITIONS. A number of clinical circumstances may require rapid reduction of the blood pressure (Table 27–21). These may be separated into *emergencies*, which require immediate reduction of blood pressure (within one hour) and *urgencies*, which can be treated more slowly. Unfortunately, in some conditions classified as emergencies, tissue ischemia may occur if blood pressure is reduced too much too rapidly, whereas some classified as "urgencies" may suffer tissue damage if blood pressure is lowered too slowly. Therefore, in practice, all patients with diastolic blood pressures above 130 mm Hg should be treated, some more rapidly with parenteral drugs, others more slowly with oral agents, as described on p. 880.

Hypertensive Crisis. In this condition—a true medical emergency—the blood pressure level is so high that immediate vascular damage is impending. A mean arterial pressure above 150 mm Hg is enough to produce vascular damage within hours in experimental animals.[382] In humans, a persistent diastolic pressure exceeding 140 mm Hg is often associated with acute vascular damage; some patients may suffer vascular damage from lower levels of pressure, while others manage to withstand even higher levels without apparent harm. As discussed below, the rapidity of the rise may be more important than the absolute level in producing acute vascular damage.

When the rise in pressure causes acute damage to retinal vessels, the term *accelerated-malignant hypertension* is used. The separation has been based upon the presence of retinal hemorrhages or exudates (accelerated) and papilledema (malignant). The clinical features and survival rates of those with or without papilledema are so similar that there is no reason to separate the two.[383] "Accelerated-malignant" hypertension is the preferred name, although just "malignant" may do.

TABLE 27–21 CIRCUMSTANCES REQUIRING RAPID TREATMENT OF HYPERTENSION

Hypertensive Emergencies:
Cerebrovascular
Hypertensive encephalopathy (any cause)
Intracerebral hemorrhage
Subarachnoid hemorrhage
Atherothrombotic brain infarction with severe hypertension
Malignant hypertension (some cases)
Cardiac
Acute aortic dissection
Acute left ventricular failure
Acute coronary insufficiency
After coronary bypass surgery
Others
Excessive circulating catecholamines:
Pheochromocytoma crisis
Food or drug interactions with monoamine oxidase inhibitors
Head injury
Postoperative bleeding from vascular suture lines
Severe epistaxis
Hypertensive Urgencies:
Accelerated and malignant hypertension
Rebound hypertension after sudden cessation of antihypertensive drugs
Surgical
Severe hypertension in patients requiring immediate surgery
Postoperative hypertension
Severe hypertension after kidney transplantation
Severe body burns

From Kaplan, N. M.: Clinical Hypertension. 4th ed. Baltimore, © by Williams and Wilkins, 1986, p. 274.

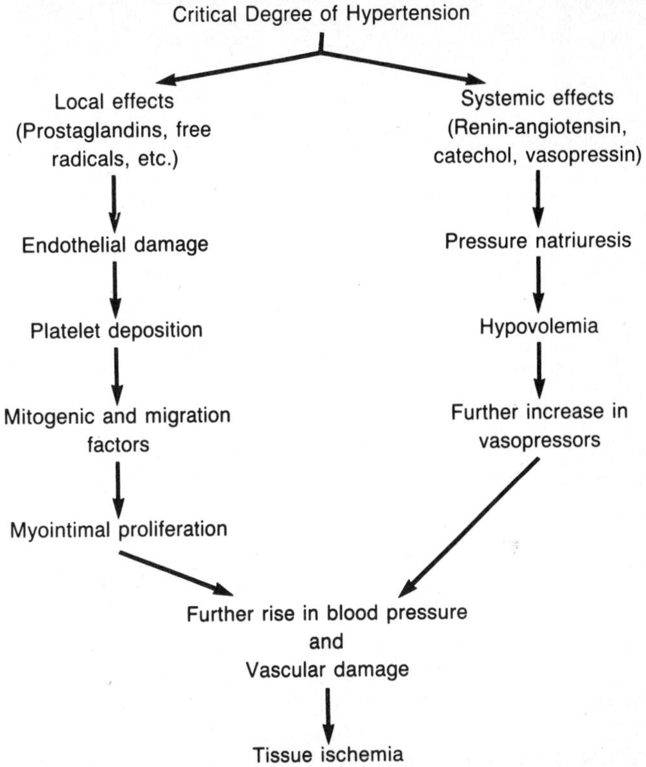

FIGURE 27–28. A scheme for the initiation and progression of malignant hypertension. (From Kaplan, N. M.: Clinical Hypertension. 4th ed. Baltimore, © by Williams and Wilkins, 1986, p. 274.)

Hypertensive Encephalopathy. This condition is characterized by headache, irritability, alterations in consciousness, and other manifestations of central nervous dysfunction with sudden and marked elevations in blood pressure. Symptoms can be reversed by a reduction in the pressure.

INCIDENCE. In about 1 per cent of patients with essential hypertension, the disease progresses to an accelerated-malignant phase. Presumably, if left untreated, many more patients would follow this pattern, since the incidence had been higher before effective therapies became available and seems to be decreasing steadily.[384]

Any hypertensive disease can initiate a crisis. Some, including pheochromocytoma and renovascular hypertension, do so at a higher rate than does essential hypertension. However, since hypertension is idiopathic in over 90 per cent of all patients, most hypertensive crises appear in the setting of preexisting essential hypertension.

PATHOPHYSIOLOGY. Whenever blood pressure rises and remains above a critical level, various processes set off a series of local and systemic effects that cause further rises in pressure and vascular damage[385] (Fig. 27–28). Two distinct but usually concurrent processes are involved in the pathogenesis of hypertensive encephalopathy. One is *functional*, i. e., dilatation of cerebral arterioles, allowing excessive cerebral blood flow that leads to hypertensive encephalopathy. The other is *structural*, i. e., acute damage to the arteriolar wall, resulting in increased permeability. Both processes are most likely the consequences of high blood pressure and may develop without apparent involvement of the renin-angiotensin or other hormonal mechanisms.[382]

Studies in animals and man by Strandgaard and associates have elucidated the mechanism of encephalopathy. First, they directly measured the caliber of pial arterioles over the cerebral cortex in cats whose blood pressures

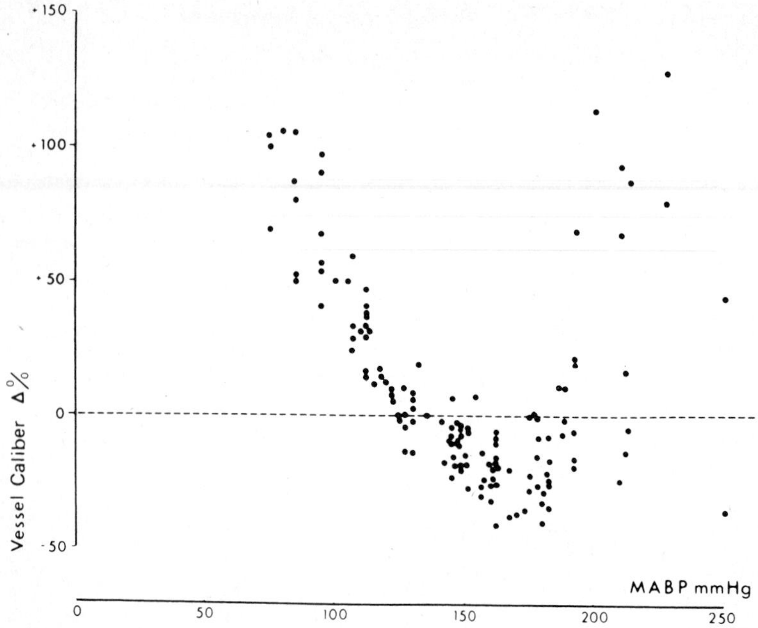

FIGURE 27–29. Changes observed in the caliber of pial arterioles with a caliber less than 50 μ in 8 cats when blood pressure was raised by intravenous infusion of angiotensin II. Calculation is based on the percentage of change from the caliber at a mean arterial blood pressure (MABP) of 135 mm Hg. (From MacKenzie, E. T., Strandgaard, S., Graham, D. I., Jones, J. V., Harper, A. M., and Farrar, J. K.: Effects of acutely induced hypertension in cats on pial arteriolar caliber, local cerebral blood flow, and the blood-brain barrier. Circ. Res. *39*:33, 1976, by permission of the American Heart Association, Inc.)

were varied over a wide range by infusion of vasodilators or angiotensin II[386] (Fig. 27–29). As the pressure fell, the arterioles became dilated; as the pressure rose, they became constricted. Thus, a constant cerebral blood flow was maintained by means of autoregulation, which is dependent upon the cerebral sympathetic nerves.[387] However, when mean arterial pressure rose above 180 mm Hg, the tightly constricted vessels could no longer withstand the pressure and suddenly dilated. This began in an irregular manner, first in areas with less muscle tone and then diffusely, producing generalized vasodilatation. This "breakthrough" of cerebral blood flow hyperperfuses the brain under high pressure, causing leakage of fluid into the perivascular tissue and resulting in cerebral edema and the syndrome of hypertensive encephalopathy. The vessel walls, in reaction to this excessive pressure, probably contribute to the injury by generating toxic superoxide anion radicals from accelerated arachidonate metabolism.[388]

In human subjects, cerebral blood flow was measured repetitively by an isotopic technique while blood pressure was lowered or raised with vasodilators or vasoconstrictors in a manner similar to that employed in the animal studies.[389] Curves depicting cerebral blood flow as a function of arterial pressure demonstrated autoregulation with a constancy of flow over mean pressures in normotensive persons from about 60 to 120 mm Hg and in hypertensive patients from about 110 to 180 mm Hg. This "shift to the right" in hypertensive patients is the result of structural thickening of the arterioles as an adaptation to the chronically elevated pressures. When pressures were raised beyond the upper limit of autoregulation, the same "breakthrough" with hyperperfusion occurred as was seen in the animal studies. In previously normotensive persons whose vessels have not been altered by prior exposure to high pressure, breakthrough occurred at a mean arterial pressure of about 120 mm Hg; in hypertensive patients, the breakthrough occurred at about 180 mm Hg.

These studies confirm clinical observations. In previously normotensive persons, severe encephalopathy occurs with relatively little hypertension. In children with acute glomerulonephritis and in women with eclampsia, convulsions may occur owing to hypertensive encephalopathy with blood pressures as low as 150/100 mm Hg. Obviously, chronically hypertensive patients withstand such pressures without difficulty; however, when pressures increase significantly, they too may develop encephalopathy.

MANIFESTATIONS AND COURSE. The symptoms and signs of hypertensive crises are usually dramatic (Table 27–22). However, some patients may be relatively asymptomatic, despite markedly elevated pressures and extensive organ damage. Young black men are particularly prone to hypertensive crisis with severe renal insufficiency but little obvious prior distress.

When the blood pressure is so high as to induce encephalopathy or accelerated-malignant hypertension, the following clinical features are frequently present:

1. Renal insufficiency with protein and red cells in the urine and azotemia; acute oliguric renal failure may also develop.
2. Elevated levels of PRA from the diffuse intrarenal ischemia, resulting in secondary aldosteronism, often manifested by hypokalemia. Although not causal, the secondarily elevated renin and aldosterone levels most likely exacerbate the hypertensive process.
3. Microangiopathic hemolytic anemia with red cell fragmentation and intravascular coagulation.
4. Cardiac size and function may *not* be particularly abnormal in those who suddenly develop malignant hypertension.[390]

If left untreated, patients die quickly from brain damage or more gradually from renal damage. Before effective therapy was available, less than 25 per cent of patients with malignant hypertension survived one year and only 1 per cent survived 5 years. With therapy, over 70 per cent survive one year and about 50 per cent survive 5 years.[383] Death in patients with severe hypertension is usually from stroke or renal failure if it occurs in the first few years after onset. If therapy keeps patients alive for longer than 5

TABLE 27–22 CLINICAL CHARACTERISTICS OF HYPERTENSIVE CRISIS

Blood pressure:	Usually > 140 mm Hg diastolic
Funduscopic findings:	Hemorrhages, exudates, papilledema
Neurological status:	Headache, confusion, somnolence, stupor, visual loss, focal deficits, seizures, coma
Cardiac findings:	Prominent apical impulse, cardiac enlargement, congestive failure
Renal:	Oliguria, azotemia
Gastrointestinal:	Nausea, vomiting

From Kaplan, N. M.: Clinical Hypertension, 4th ed. Baltimore, © by Williams and Wilkins, 1986, p. 278.

TABLE 27–23 DISEASES TO BE DIFFERENTIATED FROM A HYPERTENSIVE CRISIS

Acute left ventricular failure
Uremia from any cause, particularly with volume overload
Cerebral vascular accident
Subarachnoid hemorrhage
Brain tumor
Head injury
Epilepsy (postictal)
Collagen diseases, particularly lupus, with cerebral vasculitis
Encephalitis
Overdose and withdrawal from narcotics, amphetamines, and so on
Hypercalcemia
Acute anxiety with hyperventilation syndrome

years, death will likely be due to coronary artery disease, in which factors other than the high pressure per se are probably also involved.

DIFFERENTIAL DIAGNOSIS. The presence of hypertensive encephalopathy or accelerated-malignant hypertension demands immediate, aggressive therapy to lower blood pressure effectively. Except in pregnancy or in catecholamine excess, therapy may be instituted before the specific cause is known. However, certain serious diseases as well as psychogenic problems, i. e., acute anxiety with hyperventilation or panic attacks,[391] can mimic a hypertensive crisis (Table 27–23), and management of these conditions obviously requires different diagnostic and therapeutic approaches. In particular, blood pressure should not be lowered too abruptly in a patient with a stroke.

Specific therapy of hypertensive crises is described on p. 880.

REFERENCES

DEFINITIONS, INCIDENCE, AND CONSEQUENCES OF HYPERTENSION

1. Castelli, W. P., and Anderson, K.: A population at risk: Prevalence of high cholesterol levels in hypertensive patients in the Framingham Study. Am. J. Med. *80*(Suppl. 2A):23, 1986.
2. Subcommittee on Definition and Prevalence of the 1984 Joint National Committee: Hypertension prevalence and the status of awareness, treatment, and control in the United States. Hypertension 7:457, 1985.
3. Working Group on Risk and High Blood Pressure: An epidemiological approach to describing risk associated with blood pressure levels. Hypertension 7:641, 1985.
4. Kaplan, N. M.: Clinical Hypertension. 4th ed. Baltimore, Williams and Wilkins, 1986.
5. National Center for Health Statistics, Lawrence, L., and McLemore, T. (eds.): 1981 Summary: National Ambulatory Medical Care Survey. Advance Data From Vital and Health Statistics, No. 88. DHHS Pub. No. (PHS)83-1250. Hyattsville, Md., Public Health Service, March 16, 1983.
6. Baum, C., Kennedy, D. L., Forbes, M. B., and Jones, J. K.: Drug use and expenditures in 1982. J.A.M.A. 253:382, 1985.
7. Moser, M., Black, H., and Stair, D.: The dilemma of mild hypertension. Drugs *31*:279, 1986.
8. Goldman, L., and Cook, E. F.: The decline in ischemic heart disease mortality rates: An analysis of the comparative effects of medical interventions and changes in lifestyle. Ann. Intern. Med. *101*:825, 1984.
9. National Center for Health Statistics, Thornberry, O. T., Wilson, R. W., and Golden, P. (eds.): Health promotion and disease prevention. Provisional data from the National Health Interview Survey, United States, January–June 1985. Advance Data From Vital and Health Statistics, No. 119. DHHS Pub. No. (PHS)86-1250. Hyattsville, Md., Public Health Service, May 14, 1986.
10. Horan, M. J., Kennedy, H. L., and Padgett, N. E.: Do borderline hypertensive patients have labile blood pressure? Ann. Intern. Med. *94*:466, 1981.
11. Porchet, M., Bussien, J. P., Waeber, B., Nussberger, J., and Brunner, H. R.: Unpredictability of blood pressures recorded outside the clinic in the treated hypertensive patient. J. Cardiovasc. Pharmacol. *8*:332, 1986.
12. Perloff, D., Sokolow, M., and Cowan, R.: The prognostic value of ambulatory blood pressures. J.A.M.A. *249*:2792, 1983.
13. Johnson, J. L., Heineman, E. F., Heiss, G., Hames, C. G., and Tyroler, H. A.: Cardiovascular disease risk factors and mortality among black women and white women aged 40–64 years in Evans County, Georgia. Am. J. Epidemiol. *123*:209, 1986.
14. Froom, P., Bar-David, M., Ribak, J., Van Dky, D., Kallner, B., and Benbassat, J.: Predictive value of systolic blood pressure in young men for elevated systolic blood pressure 12 to 15 years later. Circulation *68*:467, 1983.
15. Zanchetti, A., and Leonetti, G.: Hypertension in the elderly: Special considerations. *In* Butler, R. N., and Bearn, A.G. (eds.): The Aging Process: Therapeutic Implications. New York, Raven Press, 1985, p. 175.
16. Finnegan, T. P., Spence, J. D., Wong, D. G., and Wells, G. A.: Blood pressure measurement in the elderly: Correlation of arterial stiffness with difference between intra-arterial and cuff pressures. J. Hypertension *3*:231, 1985.
17. Messerli, F. H., Ventura, H. O., and Amodeo, C.: Osler's maneuver and pseudohypertension. N. Engl. J. Med. *312*:1548, 1985.
18. Lipsitz, L. A., Storch, H. A., Minaker, K. L., and Rowe, J. W.: Intra-individual variability in postural blood pressure in the elderly. Clin. Sci. *69*:337, 1985.
19. Lipsitz, L. A., Nyquist, R. P., Jr., Wei, J. Y., and Rowe, J. W.: Postprandial reduction in blood pressure in the elderly. N. Engl. J. Med. *309*:81, 1983.
20. Shannon, R. P., Wei, J. Y., Rosa, R. M., Epstein, F. H., and Rowe, J. W.: The effect of age and sodium depletion on cardiovascular response to orthostasis. Hypertension *8*:438, 1986.
21. Joint National Committee on Detection, Evaluation, and Treatment of High Blood Pressure: The 1984 report of the Joint National Committee on Detection, Evaluation, and Treatment of High Blood Pressure. Arch. Intern. Med. *144*:1045, 1984.
22. The Pooling Project Research Group: Relationship of blood pressure, serum cholesterol, smoking habit, relative weight and ECG abnormalities to incidence of major coronary events: Final report of the pooling project. J. Chronic Dis. *31*:201, 1978.
23. Hypertension Detection and Follow-up Program Cooperative Group: Blood pressure studies in 14 communities. A two-stage screen for hypertension. J.A.M.A. *237*:2385, 1977.
24. Baron, A. E., Freyer, B., and Fixler, D. E.: Longitudinal blood pressures in blacks, whites, and Mexican Americans during adolescence and early adulthood. Am. J. Epidemiol. *123*:809, 1986.
25. Lieberman, E.: Hypertension in childhood and adolescence. *In* Kaplan, N.M. (ed.): Clinical Hypertension. 4th ed. Baltimore, Williams and Wilkins, 1986, p. 447.
26. Burke, G. L., Freedman, D. S., Webber, L. S., and Berenson, G. S.: Persistence of high diastolic blood pressure in thin children: The Bogalusa Heart Study. Hypertension *8*:24, 1986.
27. Pickering, G.: Hypertension: Definitions, natural histories and consequences. Am. J. Med. *52*:570, 1972.
28. National Center for Health Statistics, Rowland, W., and Roberts, J. (eds.): Blood Pressure Levels and Hypertension in Persons Ages 6–74 Years: United States, 1976–80. Advance Data From Vital and Health Statistics, No. 84, DHHS Pub. No. (PHS)82-1250. Hyattsville, Md., Public Health Service, October 8, 1982.
29. Berglund, G., Andersson, O., and Wilhelmsen, L.: Prevalence of primary and secondary hypertension: Studies in a random population sample. Br. Med. J. *2*:554, 1976.
30. Rudnick, K. V., Sackett, D. L., Hirst, S., and Holmes, C.: Hypertension in family practice. Can. Med. Assoc. J. *3*:492, 1977.
31. Danielson, M., and Dammstrom, B.: The prevalence of secondary and curable hypertension. Acta Med. Scand. *209*:451, 1981.
32. Møller-Petersen, J.: Nomogram for predictive values and efficiencies of tests. Lancet *1*:348, 1985.
33. Weiss, N. S.: Relation of high blood pressure to headache, epistaxis, and selected other symptoms. N. Engl. J. Med. *287*:631, 1972.
34. Bulpitt, C. J., Doller, C. T., and Carne, S.: Change in symptoms of hypertensive patients after referral to hospital clinic. Br. Heart J. *38*:121, 1976.
35. Bauer, G. E.: Hypertension and headache. Aust. N.Z. J. Med. *6*:492, 1976.
36. Hypertension Detection and Follow-Up Program Cooperative Group: The Hypertension Detection and Follow-Up Program. A progress report. Circ. Res. *40*:1–106, 1977.
37. Cloher, T. P., and Whelton, P. K.: Physician approach to the recognition and initial management of hypertension: Results of a statewide survey of Maryland physicians. Arch. Intern. Med. *146*:529, 1986.
38. Rose, G.: Strategy of prevention: Lessons from cardiovascular disease. Br. Med. J. *282*:1847, 1981.
39. MacMahon, S. W., and Macdonald, G. J.: Antihypertensive treatment and plasma lipoprotein levels: The associations in data from a population study. Am. J. Med. *80*(Suppl. 2A):40, 1986.
40. Stamler, J., Wentworth, D., and Neaton, J. D.: Prevalence and prognostic significance of hypercholesterolemia in men with hypertension: Prospective data on the primary screenees of the Multiple Risk Factor Intervention Trial. Am. J. Med. *80*(Suppl. 2A):33, 1986.
41. Sapira, J. D.: An internist looks at the fundus oculi. Disease-A-Month *30*:1, 1984.
42. Svardsudd, K., Wedel, H., Aurell, E., and Tibblin, G.: Hypertensive eye ground changes. Acta Med. Scand. *204*:159, 1978.
43. Hammond, I. W., Devereux, R. B., Alderman, M. H., Lutas, E. M., Spitzer, M.C., Crowley, J. S., and Laragh, J. H.: The prevalence and correlates of echocardiographic left ventricular hypertrophy among employed patients with uncomplicated hypertension. J. Am. Coll. Cardiol. *7*:639, 1986.
44. Ruddy, T. D., Zusman, R. M., Dighero, R. H., Miller, D. D., Christensen, D., Federman, E. B., Strauss, H. W., and Boucher, C. A.: Increased contribution of atrial systole to left ventricular diastolic filling in hypertensive patients. Abstract. Clin. Res. *34*:485A, 1986.
45. Marmor, A. T., Frankel, A., Plich, M., Satinger, A., and Front, D.: Decrease in global ejection fraction after volume challenge in long-standing hypertension. Am. Heart J. *111*:746, 1986.
46. Wikstrand, J.: Left ventricular function in early primary hypertension: Functional consequences of cardiovascular structural changes. Hypertension *6*(Suppl. III):III–108, 1984.

47. Topol, E. J., Traill, T. A., and Fortuin, N. J.: Hypertensive hypertrophic cardiomyopathy of the elderly. N. Engl. J. Med. *312*:277, 1985.
48. Kannel, W. B., and Abbott, R. D.: A prognostic comparison of asymptomatic left ventricular hypertrophy and unrecognized myocardial infarction: The Framingham Study. Am. Heart J. *111*:391, 1986.
49. Simon, G., and Altman, S.: Increased serum *N*-acetyl-β-D-glucosaminidase activity in human hypertension. Clin. Exp. Hyper. Theory Practice *A4*(3):355, 1982.
50. Mujais, S. K., Emmanouel, D. S., Kasinath, B. S., and Spargo, B. H.: Marked proteinuria in hypertensive nephrosclerosis. Am. J. Nephrol. *5*:190, 1985.
51. Bauer, G. E., and Humphrey, T. J.: The natural history of hypertension with moderate impairment of renal function. Clin. Sci. Molec. Med. *45*:191s, 1973.
52. Inzitari, D., Bianchi, F., Pracucci, G., Albanese, V., Argentino, C., Bono, G., Brambilla, G. L., Candelise, L., De Zanche, L., Mariani, F., Passero, S., Prencipe, M., and Fiesche, C.: The Italian multicenter study of reversible cerebral ischemic attacks: IV-blood pressure components and atherosclerotic lesions. Stroke *17*:185, 1986.
53. Brunner, H. R., Laragh, J. H., Baer, L., Newton, M. A., Goodwin, F. T., Krakoff, L. R., Bard, R. H., and Buhler, F. R.: Essential hypertension: Renin and aldosterone, heart attack and stroke. N. Engl. J. Med. *286*:441, 1972.
54. Kaplan, N. M.: The prognostic implications of plasma renin in essential hypertension. J.A.M.A. *231*:167, 1975.
55. Birkenhager, W. H., Kho, T. L., Schalekamp, M.A.D.H., Kolsters, G., Wester, A., and De Leeuw, P. W.: Renin levels and cardiovascular morbidity in essential hypertension. A prospective study. Acta Clin. Belg. *32*:168, 1977.
56. Management Committee: Untreated mild hypertension. Lancet *1*:185, 1982.
57. Medical Research Council Working Party: MRC trial of treatment of mild hypertension: Principal results. Br. Med. J. *291*:97, 1985.
58. Nyberg, G., Blohme, G., and Norden, G.: Constant glomerular filtration rate in diabetic nephropathy: Correlation to blood pressure and blood glucose control. Acta Med. Scand. *219*:67, 1986.
59. O'Rourke, M. F.: Basic concepts for the understanding of large arteries in hypertension. J. Cardiovasc. Pharmacol. 7:S14, 1985.
60. Bierman, E. L., Brewer, C., and Baum, D.: Hypertension decreases replication potential of arterial smooth muscle cells: Aortic coarctation in humans as model. Proc. Soc. Exp. Biol. Med. *166*:335, 1981.
61. Vanhoutte, P. M., Rubanyi, G. M., Miller, V. M., and Houston, D. S.: Modulation of vascular smooth muscle contraction by the endothelium. Ann. Rev. Physiol. *438*:307, 1986.
62. Schwartz, S. M., and Ross, R.: Cellular proliferation in atherosclerosis and hypertension. Prog. Cardiovasc. Dis. *26*:355, 1984.
63. Kannel, W. B., Dannenberg, A. L., and Abbott, R. D.: Unrecognized myocardial infarction and hypertension: The Framingham Study. Am. Heart J. *109*:581, 1985.
64. Astrup, J., Bisgaard-Frantzen, H. O., Nielsen, S. L., and Rossing, N.: Blood pressure-lowering effect of acute myocardial infarction. Lancet *2*:903, 1976.
65. Coronary Drug Project Research Group: Blood pressure in survivors of myocardial infarction. J. Am. Coll. Cardiol. *4*:1135, 1984.
66. Kannel, W. B., Sorlie, P., Castelli, W. P., and McGee, D.: Blood pressure and survival after myocardial infarction: The Framingham Study. Am. J. Cardiol. *45*:326, 1980.
67. McKee, P. A., Castelli, W. P., McNamara, P. M., and Kannel, W. B.: The natural history of congestive heart failure: The Framingham Study. N. Engl. J. Med. *285*:1441, 1971.
68. Francis, G. S., Goldsmith, S. R., Levine, T. B., Olivari, M. R., and Cohn, J.N.: The neurohumoral axis in congestive heart failure. Ann. Intern. Med. *101*:370, 1984.
69. Cooke, J. P., and Safford, R. E.: Progress in the diagnosis and management of aortic dissection. Mayo Clin. Proc. *61*:147, 1986.
70. Dyken, M. L., Wolf, P. A., Barnett, H. J. M., Bergan, J. J., Hass, W. K., Kannel, W.B., Kuller, L., Kurtzke, J. F., and Sundt, T. M.: Risk factors in stroke: A statement for physicians by the Subcommittee on Risk Factors and Stroke of the Stroke Council. Stroke *15*:1105, 1984.
71. Wallace, J. D., and Levy, L. L.: Blood pressure after stroke. J.A.M.A. *246*:2177, 1981.
72. Johansson, B. B.: Cerebral vascular bed in hypertension and consequences for the brain. Hypertension *6*(Suppl. III):III–81, 1984.
73. Sugimoto, T., and Rosansky, S. J.: The incidence of treated end stage renal disease in the Eastern United States: 1973–1979. Am. J. Public Health *74*:14, 1984.
74. Messerli, F. H., Frohlich, E. D., Dreslinski, G. R., Suarez, D. H., and Aristimuno, G. G.: Serum uric acid in essential hypertension: An indicator of renal vascular involvement. Ann. Intern. Med. *93*:817, 1980.
75. Bergstron, J., Alvestrand, A., Bucht, H., Gutierrez, A.: Progession of chronic renal failure in man is retarded with more frequent clinical follow-ups and better blood pressure control. Clin. Nephrol. *25*:1, 1986.
76. Holland, O. B., and Fairchild, C.: Renin classification for diuretic and beta-blocker treatment of black hypertensive patients. J. Chronic Dis. *35*:179, 1982.
77. Lasker, N., Hopp, L., Grossman, S., Bamforth, R., and Aviv, A.: Race and sex differences in erythrocyte Na^+, K^+, and Na^+-K^+-adenosine triphosphatase. J. Clin. Invest. *75*:1813, 1985.
78. Wilson, T. W.: History of salt supplies in West Africa and blood pressures today. Lancet *1*:784, 1986.
79. Sever, P. S., Peart, W. S., Gordon, D., and Beighton, P.: Blood pressure and its correlates in urban and tribal Africa. Lancet 2:60, 1980.
80. Barlow, R. J., Connel, M. A., and Milne, F. J.: A study of 48-hour faecal and urinary electrolyte excretion in normotensive black and white South African males. J. Hypertension *401*:197, 1986.

MECHANISMS OF PRIMARY (ESSENTIAL) HYPERTENSION

81. Editorial: Catecholamines in essential hypertension. Lancet 1:1088, 1977.
82. Lund-Johansen, P.: Hemodynamic alterations in hypertension—spontaneous changes and effects of drug therapy. Acta Med. Scand. Suppl. *603*:1, 1977.
83. Julius, S., Weder, A. B., and Egan, B. M.: Pathophysiology of early hypertension: Implication for epidemiologic research. *In* Gross, F., and Strasser, T. (eds.): Mild Hypertension: Recent Advances. New York, Raven Press, 1983, p. 219.
84. Korner, P. H.: Circulatory regulation in hypertension. Br. J. Clin. Pharmacol. *13*:95, 1982.
85. Wenting, G. J., Man In'T Veld, A. J., and Schalekamp, M.A.D.H.: Time-course of vascular resistance changes in mineralocorticoid hypertension of man. Clin. Sci. *61*:97, 1981.
86. Folkow, B.: Physiological aspects of primary hypertension. Physiol. Rev. *62*:347, 1982.
87. Hermsmeyer, K., Abel, P. W., and Trapani, A. J.: Norepinephrine sensitivity and membrane potentials of caudal arterial muscle in DOCA-salt, Dahl, and SHR hypertension in the rat. Hypertension *4*(Suppl. II):II–49, 1982.
88. Levine, R. S., Hennekens, C. H., Duncan, R. C., Robertson, E. G., Gourley, J., Cassady, J. C., and Gelband, H.: Blood pressure in infant twins: Birth to 6 months of age. Hypertension *2*(Suppl. I):I–29, 1980.
89. Havlik, R. J., and Feinleib, M.: Epidemiology and genetics of hypertension. Hypertension *4*(Suppl. III):III–121, 1982.
90. Longini, I. M., Higgins, M. W., Hinton, P. C., Moll, P. P., and Keller, J. B.: Environmental and genetic sources of familial aggregation of blood pressure in Tecumseh, Michigan. Am. J. Epidemiol. *120*:131, 1984.
91. Speers, M. A., Kasl, S. V., Freeman, D. H., and Ostfeld, A. M.: Blood pressure concordance between spouses. Am. J. Epidemiol. *123*:818, 1986.
92. Falkner, B., Onesti, G., and Hayes, P.: The role of sodium in essential hypertension in genetically hypertensive adolescents. *In* Onesti, G., and Kim, K.E., (eds.): Hypertension in the Young and the Old. New York, Grune and Stratton, 1981, p. 29.
93. Grim, C. E., Luft, F. C., Weinberger, M. H., Miller, J. Z., Rose, R. J., and Christian, J. C.: Genetic, familial and racial influences on blood pressure control systems in man. Aust. N.Z. J. Med. *14*:453, 1984.
94. Meyer, P., Garay, R. P., Nazaret, C., Dagher, G., Bellet, Z. M., Broyer, M., and Feingold, J.: Inheritance of abnormal erythrocyte cation transport in essential hypertension. Br. Med. J. *282*:1114, 1981.
95. Light, K. C., Koepke, J. P., Obrist, P. A., and Willis, P. W.: Psychological stress induces sodium and fluid retention in men at high risk for hypertension. Science *220*:429, 1983.
96. Brown, J. J., Lever, A. F., Robertson, J. I. S., Semple, P. F., Bing, R. F., Heagerty, A. M., Swales, J. D., Thurston, H., Ledingham, J. G. G., Laragh, J.H., Hansson, L., Nicholls, M. G., and Espiner, A. E.: Salt and hypertension. Lancet 2:456, 1984.
97. Bulpitt, C. J., Broughton, P. M. G., Markowe, H. L. J., Marmot, M. G., Rose, G., Semmence, A., and Shipley, M. J.: The relationship between both sodium and potassium intake and blood pressure in London civil servants: A report from the Whitehall department of environmental study. J. Chronic Dis. *39*:211, 1986.
98. Hofman, A., Hazebroek, A., and Valkenburg, H. A.: A randomized trial of sodium intake and blood pressure in newborn infants. J.A.M.A. *250*:370, 1983.
99. Prys-Rroberts, C.: Anaesthesia and hypertension. Br. J. Anaesth. *56*:711, 1984.
100. Reeves, R. A., Shapiro, A. P., Thompson, M. E., and Johnsen, A.- M.: Loss of nocturnal decline in blood pressure after cardiac transplantation. Circulation *73*:401, 1986.
101. Vincent, H. H., Boomsma, F., Man in'T Veld, A. J., and Schalekamp, M.A.D.H.: Stress levels of adrenaline amplify the blood pressure response to sympathetic stimulation. J. Hypertension *4*:255, 1986.
102. Jorgensen, R. S., and Houston, B. K.: Family history of hypertension, personality, patterns, and cardiovascular reactivity to stress. Psychosomatic Med. *48*:102, 1986.
103. Bianchetti, M. G., Beretta-Piccoli, C., Weidmann, P., and Ferrier, C.: Blood pressure control in normotensive members of hypertensive families. Kidney Int. *29*:882, 1986.
104. Guyton, A. C., Coleman, T. G., Cowley, A. W., Jr., Scheel, K. W., Manning, R. D., Jr., and Norman, R. A., Jr.: Arterial pressure regulation: Overriding dominance of the kidneys in long-term regulation and in hypertension. Am. J. Med. *52*:584, 1972.
105. Kaplan, N. M.: The Goldblatt Memorial Lecture. Part II: The role of the kidney in hypertension. Hypertension *1*:456, 1979.
106. Hollenberg, N. K., Williams, G. H., and Adams, D. F.: Essential hypertension: Abnormal renal vascular and endocrine responses to a mild psychological stimulus. Hypertension 3:11, 1981.
107. Click, R. L., Joyner, W. L., and Gilmore, J. P.: Reactivity of glomerular afferent and efferent arterioles in renal hypertension. Kidney Int. *15*:109, 1979.
108. Rydstedt, L. L., Williams, G. H., and Hollenberg, N. K.: Renal and endocrine response to saline infusion in essential hypertension. Hypertension *8*:217, 1986.
109. Williams, G. H., and Hollenberg, N. K.: Are non-modulating patients with essential hypertension a distinct subgroup? Implications for therapy. Am. J. Med. *79*(Suppl. 3C):3, 1985.
110. London, G. M., Safer, M. E., Weiss, Y. A., Corvol. P. L., Lehner, J. P.,

Menard, J.M., Simon, A. C., and Milliez, P. L.: Volume-dependent parameters in essential hypertension. Kidney Int. *11*:204, 1977.

111. Beretta-Piccoli, C., Weidmann, P., Brown, J. J., Davies, D. L., Lever, A. F., and Robertson, J. I. S.: Body sodium blood volume state in essential hypertension: Abnormal relation of exchangeable sodium to age and blood pressure in male patients. J. Cardiovasc. Pharmacol. *6*(Suppl. 1):s134, 1984.
112. Beretta-Piccoli, C., Fischbacher, A., Rothenbuhler, A., Gerber, A., and Weidmann, P.: Body sodium/blood volume state in normotensive members of normotensive and hypertensive families. J. Hypertension *4*:229, 1986.
113. Needleman, P., and Greenwald, J. E.: Atriopeptin: A cardiac hormone intimately involved in fluid, electrolyte, and blood-pressure homeostasis. N. Engl. J. Med. *314*:828, 1986.
114. Sagnella, G. A., Shore, A. C., Markandu, N. D., and MacGregor, G. A.: Raised circulating levels of atrial natriuretic peptides in essential hypertension. Lancet *1*:179, 1986.
115. Grantham, J. J., and Edwards, R. M.: Natriuretic hormones: At last, bottled in bond? J. Lab. Clin. Med. *103*:333, 1984.
116. Haupert, G. T., Carilli, C. T., and Cantley, L. C.: Hypothalamic sodium-transport inhibitor is a high-affinity reversible inhibitor of Na^+-K^+-ATPase. Am. J. Physiol. *247*:F919, 1984.
117. Haddy, F. J., and Pamnani, M. B.: Evidence for a circulating endogenous Na^+-K^+ pump inhibitor in low-renin hypertension. Fed. Proc. *44*:2789, 1985.
118. Hamlyn, J. M., Levinson, P. D., Ringel, R., Levin, P. A., Hamilton, B. P., Blaustein, M. P., and Kowarski, A. A.: Relationships among endogenous digitalis-like factors in essential hypertension. Fed. Proc. *44*:2782, 1985.
119. Sagnella, G. A., Jones, J. C., Shore, A. C., Markandu, N. D., and MacGregor, G.A.: Evidence for increased levels of a circulating ouabainlike factor in essential hypertension. Hypertension *8*:433, 1986.
120. Boon, N. A., Harper, C., Aronson, J. K., and Grahame-Smith, D. G.: Cation transport functions in vitro in patients with untreated essential hypertension: A comparison of erythrocytes and leucocytes. Clin. Sci. *68*:511, 1985.
121. Haupert, G. T., Chen, E., Ray, S., and Cantiello, H.: Hypothalamic factor (HF) regulates Na^+-pump activity in cultured renal tubular epithelial cells (LLC-PK1) [Abstract]. Clin. Res. *34*:597A, 1986.
122. Kelly, R. A., O'Hara, D. S., Mitch, W. E., and Smith, T. W.: Identification of NaK-ATPase inhibitors in human plasma (Abstract). Clin. Res. *34*:480A, 1986.
123. Allen, J. C., Navran, S. A., and Kahn, A. M.: Na^+-K^+-ATPase in vascular smooth muscle. Am. J. Physiol. *250*:C536, 1986.
124. Tobian, L., Jr., and Binion, J. T.: Tissue cations and water in arterial hypertension. Circulation *5*:754, 1952.
125. Hilton, P. J.: Cellular sodium transport in essential hypertension. N. Engl. J. Med. *314*:222, 1986.
126. Aalkjaer, C., Parvin, S. D., Bing, R. F., Heagerty, A. M., Bell, P. R. F., and Swales, J. D.: Cell membrane sodium transport: A correlation between human resistance vessels and leucocytes. Lancet *1*:649, 1986.
127. Canessa, M., Spalvins, A., Laski, C., and Williams, G. H.: The effect of reduced Na intake on red cell (RBC) Na transport in normotensive (NT) and essential hypertensive (HT) subjects (Abstract). Clin. Res. *34*:476A, 1986.
128. Weder, A. B.: Red-cell lithium-sodium countertransport and renal lithium clearance in hypertension. N. Engl. J. Med. *314*:198, 1986.
129. Heagerty, A. M., Riozzi, A., Brand, S. C., Bing, R. F., Thurston, H., and Swales, J. D.: Membrane transport of ions in hypertension: A review. Scand. J. Clin. Lab. Invest. *46*(Suppl. 180):54, 1986.
130. Friedman, S. M.: Evidence for an enhanced transmembrane sodium (Na^+) gradient induced by aldosterone in the incubated rat tail artery. Hypertension *4*:230, 1982.
131. Moreland, R. S., Major, T. C., and Webb, R. C.: Contractile responses to ouabain and K^+-free solution in aorta from hypertensive rats. Am. J. Physiol. *250*:H612, 1986.
132. Blaustein, M. P.: Sodium transport and hypertension: Where are we going? Hypertension *6*:445, 1984.
133. Rasmussen, H.: The calcium messenger system. N. Engl. J. Med. *314*:1094, 1986.
134. Robinson, B. F., Dobbs, R. J., and Bayley, S.: Response of forearm resistance vessels to verapamil and sodium nitroprusside in normotensive and hypertensive men: Evidence for a functional abnormality of vascular smooth muscle in primary hypertension. Clin. Sci. *63*:33, 1982.
135. DeWardener, H. E., and Clarkson, E. M.: Concept of natriuretic hormone. Physiol. Rev. *65*:658, 1985.
136. Dahl, L. K., and Heine, M.: Primary role of renal homografts in setting chronic blood pressure levels in rats. Circ. Res. *36*:692, 1975.
137. Postnov, Y. V., and Orlov, S. N.: Ion transport across plasma membrane in primary hypertension. Physiol. Rev. *65*:904, 1985.
138. Swales, J. D.: Abnormal ion transport by cell membranes in hypertension. *In* Robertson, J.I.S. (ed.): Handbook of Hypertension, Vol. 1. Clinical Aspects of Essential Hypertension. New York, Elsevier Science Publishers, 1983, p. 239.
139. Robinson, B. F.: Sodium and calcium handling. *In* Kaplan, N. M., Brenner, B., and Laragh, J. (eds.): Perspectives in Hypertension. Vol. 1. The Kidney in Hypertension. New York, Raven Press, 1986.
140. Erne, P., Bolli, P., Burgisser, E., and Buhler, F. R.: Correlation of platelet calcium with blood pressure. N. Engl. J. Med. *310*:1084, 1984.
141. Bruschi, G., Bruschi, M. E., Orlandini, G., Cavatorta, A., Borghetti, A., Ferrandi, M., and Bianchi, G.: Why is $[Ca^{2+}]_i$ increased in blood cells in primary hypertension? J. Hypertension *3*(Suppl. 3):S45, 1985.
142. Marche, P., Koutouzov, S., Girard, A., Elghozi, J.-L., Meyer, P., and Ben-Ishay, D.: Phosphoinositide turnover in erythrocyte membranes in human and experimental hypertension. J. Hypertension *3*:25, 1985.
143. McCarron, D. A.: Is calcium more important than sodium in the pathogenesis of essential hypertension? Hypertension *7*:607, 1985.
144. McCarron, D. A., Pingree, P. A., Rubin, R. J., Gaucher, S. M., Molitch, M., and Krutzik, S.: Enhanced parathyroid function in essential hypertension: A homeostatic response to a urinary calcium leak. Hypertension *2*:162, 1980.
145. Breslau, N. A., McGuire, J. L., Zerwekh, J. E., and Pak, C. Y. C.: The role of dietary sodium on renal excretion and intestinal absorption of calcium and on vitamin D metabolism. J. Clin. Endocrinol. Metab. *55*:369, 1982.
146. Mcarron, D. A.: Low serum concentrations of ionized calcium in patients with hypertension. N. Engl. J. Med. *307*:226, 1982.
147. McCarron, D. A., and Morris, C. D.: Blood pressure response to oral calcium in persons with mild to moderate hypertension. Ann. Intern. Med. *103*:,825, 1985.
148. Lau, K., and Eby, B.: The role of calcium in genetic hypertension. Hypertension *7*:657, 1985.
149. Kaplan, N. M., and Meese, R. B.: The calcium deficiency hypothesis of hypertension: A critique. Ann. Intern. Med. *105*:947, 1986.
150. Pak, C. Y. C.: Calcium and hypertension. *In* Horan, M. J., Blaustein, M., Dunbar, J. B., Kachadorian, W., Kaplan, N. M., and Simopoulos, A.P. (eds.): NIH Workshop on Nutrition and Hypertension: Proceedings from a Symposium. Bethesda, Maryland, March 12–14, 1984. New York, Biomedical Information Corporation, 1985, p. 155.
151. Skinner, S. L., Thatcher, R. L., Whitworth, J. A., and Horowitz, J. D.: Extraction of plasma prorenin by human heart. Lancet *1*:995, 1986.
152. Glorioso, N., Atlas, S. A., Laragh, J. H., Jewelewicz, R., and Sealey, J. E.: High concentrations of prorenin in human ovarian follicular fluid [Abstract]. Endocrinol *118*(Suppl.):222, 1986.
153. Brock, T. A., Lewis, L. J., and Smith, J. B.: Angiotensin increases Na^+ entry and Na^+/K^+ pump activity in cultures of smooth muscle from rat aorta. Proc. Natl. Acad. Sci. USA *79*:1438, 1982.
154. Helmer, O. M.: Renin activity in blood from patients with hypertension. Can. Med. Assoc. J. *90*:221, 1964.
155. Kaplan, N. M.: Renin profiles: The unfulfilled promises. J.A.M.A. *238*:611, 1977.
156. Wisgerhof, M., and Brown, R. D.: Increased adrenal sensitivity to angiotensin II in low-renin essential hypertension. J. Clin. Invest. *61*:1456, 1978.
157. Lebel, M., Brown, J. J., Kremer, D., Robertson, J. I. S., Schalekamp, M., Davies, D. L., Lever, A. F., Tree, M., Beevers, D. G., Frazier, R., Morton, J.J., and Wilson, A.: Sodium and the renin-angiotensin system in essential hypertension and mineralocorticoid excess. Lancet *2*:308, 1974.
158. Gomez-Sanchez, C. E., Holland, O. B., and Upcavage, R.: Urinary free 19-nor-deoxycorticosterone and deoxycorticosterone in human hypertension. J. Clin. Endocrinol. Metab. *60*:234, 1985.
159. De Simone, G., Tommaselli, A. P., Rossi, R., Valentino, R., Lauria, R., Scopacasa, F., and Lombardi, G.: Partial deficiency of adrenal 11-hydroxylase: A possible cause of primary hypertension. Hypertension *7*:204, 1985.
160. Vaughan, E. D., Jr., Laragh, J. H., Gavras, I., Buhler, F. E., Gavras, H., Brunner, H. R., and Baer, L.: Volume factor in low and normal renin essential hypertension. Am. J. Cardiol. *32*:523, 1973.
161. Padfield, P. L., Brown, J. J., Lever, A. F., Morton, J. J., and Robertson, J. I. S.: Blood pressure in acute and chronic vasopressin excess. N. Engl. J . Med. *304*:1067, 1981.
162. Holland, O. B., Chud, J. M., and Braunstein, H.: Urinary kallikrein excretion in essential and mineralocorticoid hypertension. J. Clin. Invest. *65*:347, 1980.
163. Smith, W. L.: Prostaglandin biosynthesis and its compartmentation in vascular smooth muscle and endothelial cells. Ann. Rev. Physiol. *48*:251, 1986.
164. Stoff, J. S.: Prostaglandins and hypertension. Am. J. Med. *80*(Suppl. 1A):56, 1986.
165. Adams, D. H., Michael, J., Bacon, P. A., Howie, A. J., McConkey, B., and Adu, D.: Non-steroidal anti-inflammatory drugs and renal failure. Lancet *1*:57, 1986.
166. Muirhead, E. E., and Pitcock, J. A.: The renal antihypertensive hormone. J. Hypertension *3*:1, 1985.
167. Weiss, S. T., Munoz, A., Stein, A., Sparrow, D., and Speizer, F. E.: The relationship of blood lead to blood pressure in a longitudinal study of working men. Am. J. Epidemiol. *123*:800, 1986.
168. Lang, R. E., Bruckner, U. B., Kempf, B., Rascher, W., Sturm, V., Unger, T., Speck, G., and Ganten, D.: Opioid peptides and blood pressure regulation. Clin. Exper. Hyper. Theory Practice *A4*:249, 1982.
169. Jorde, L. B., Williams, R. R., and Kuida, H.: Factor analysis suggesting contrasting determinants for different blood pressure measurements. Hypertension *8*:243, 1986.
170. Garrison, R. J., Kannel, W. B., Stokes, J. III, and Castelli, W. P.: Incidence and precursors of hypertension in young adults: The Framingham offspring study. Abstract, 25th Conference Cardiovascular Epidemiology, CVD Epid. Newsletter 37, American Heart Association (Abstr. 50), 1985, Vol. 3, pp. 7–9.
171. Stern, M. P., and Haffner, S. M.: Body fat distribution and hyperinsulinemia as risk factors for diabetes and cardiovascular disease. Arteriosclerosis *6*:123, 1986.
172. Barrett-Connor, E., and Khaw, K.-T.: Is hypertension more benign when associated with obesity? Circulation *72*:53, 1985.
173. Bloom, E., Reed, D., Yano, K., and MacLean, C.: Does obesity protect hypertensives against cardiovascular disease? J.A.M.A. *256*:2972, 1986.
174. Raison, J., Achimastos, A., Asmar, R., Simon, A., and Safar, M.: Extracellular and interstitial fluid volume in obesity with and without associated systemic hypertension. Am. J. Cardiol. *57*:223, 1986.
175. Modan, M., Halkin, H., Almog, S., Lusky, A., Eshkol, A., Shefi, M., Shitrit, A., and Fuchs, Z.: Hyperinsulinemia: A link between hypertension obesity and glucose intolerance. J. Clin. Invest. *75*:809, 1985.
176. Jennings, G., Nelson, L., Nestel, P., Esler, M., Korner, P., Burton, D., and Bazelmans, J.: The effects of changes in physical activity on major cardiovascular risk factors, hemodynamics, sympathetic function, and glucose utilization in man: A controlled study of four levels of activity. Circulation *73*:30, 1986.

177. Paffenbarger, R. S., Jr., Wing, A. L., Hyde, R. T., and Jung, D. L.: Physical activity and incidence of hypertension in college alumni. Am. J. Epidemiol. *117*:245, 1983.
178. Klatsky, A. L., Friedman, G. D., and Armstrong, M.A.: The relationships between alcoholic beverage use and other traits to blood pressure: a new Kaiser-Permanente study. Circulation *73*:628, 1986.
179. Jackson, R., Stewart, A., Beaglehole, R., and Scragg, R.: Alcohol consumption and blood pressure. Am. J. Epidemiol. *122*:1037, 1985.
180. Moore, R. D., and Pearson, T. A.: Moderate alcohol consumption and coronary artery disease. Medicine *65*:242, 1986.
181. Karsenty, C., Baraona, E., Savolainen, M. J., and Lieber, C. S.: Effects of chronic ethanol intake on mobilization and excretion of cholesterol in baboons. J. Clin. Invest. *75*:976, 1985.
182. Ireland, M. A., Vandongen, R., Davidson, L., Beilin, L. J., and Rouse, I. L.: Acute effects of moderate alcohol consumption on blood pressure and plasma catecholamines. Clin. Sci. *66*:643, 1984.
183. Blachley, J. D., Johnson, J. H., and Knochel, J. P.: The harmful effects of ethanol on ion transport and cellular respiration. Am. J. Med. Sci. *289*:22, 1985.
184. Arkwright, P. D., Beilin, L. J., Vandongen, R., Rouse, I. L., and Masarei, J. R.: Plasma calcium and cortisol as predisposing factors to alcohol related blood pressure elevation. J. Hypertension *2*:387, 1984.
185. Benowitz, N. L., Kuyt, F., and Jacob, P. III: Influence of nicotine on cardiovascular and hormonal effects of cigarette smoking. Clin. Pharmacol. Ther. *36*:74, 1984.
186. Klein, R., Klein, B. E. K., Moss, S. C., and DeMets, D. L.: Blood pressure and hypertension in diabetes. Am. J. Epidemiol. *122*:75, 1985.
187. Aromaa, A., Reunanen, A., and Pyorala, K.: Hypertension and mortality in diabetic and non-diabetic Finnish men. J. Hypertension *2*(Suppl. 3):205, 1984.
188. Parving, H. H., Anderson, A. R., Smidt, U. M., and Svendsen, P. A.: Early aggressive antihypertensive treatment reduced rate of decline in kidney function in diabetic nephropathy. Lancet *2*:1175, 1983.
189. Ando, K., Fujita, T., Ito, Y., Noda, H., and Yamashita, K.: The role of renal hemodynamics in the antihypertensive effect of captopril. Am. Heart J. *111*:347, 1986.
190. Letcher, R. L., Chien, S., Pickering, T. G., Sealey, J. E., and Laragh, J. H.: Direct relationship between blood pressure and blood viscosity in normal and hypertensive subjects. Role of fibrinogen concentration. Am. J. Med. *70*:1195, 1981.
191. Breckenridge, A.: Hypertension and hyperuricaemia. Lancet *1*:15, 1966.

SECONDARY FORMS OF HYPERTENSION

192. Stadel, B. V.: Oral contraceptives and cardiovascular disease. N. Engl. J. Med. *305*:672, 1981.
193. Royal College of General Practitioners' Oral Contraception Study: Further analyses of mortality in oral contraceptive users. Lancet *1*:541, 1981.
194. Chilvers, E., and Rudge, P.: Cerebral venous thrombosis and subarachnoid haemorrhage in users of oral contraceptives. Br. Med. J. *292*:524, 1986.
195. Weir, R. J.: Effect on blood pressure of changing from high to low dose steroid preparation in women with oral contraceptive induced hypertension. Scott. Med. J. *27*:212, 1982.
196. Tsai, C. C., Williamson, O., Kirkland, B. H., Braun, J. O., and Lam, C. F.: Low-dose oral contraception and blood pressure in women with a past history of elevated blood pressure. Am. J. Obstet. Gynecol. *151*:28, 1985.
197. Wallace, R. B., Barrett-Connor, E., Criqui, M., Wahl, P., Hoover, J., Hunninghake, D., and Heiss, G.: Alteration in blood pressures associated with combined alcohol and oral contraceptive use—the Lipid Research Clinics Prevalence Study. J. Chronic Dis. *35*:251, 1982.
198. Petitti, D. B., and Klatsky, A. L.: Malignant hypertension in women aged 15 to 44 years and its relation to cigarette smoking and oral contraceptives. Am. J. Cardiol. *52*:297, 1983.
199. Walters, W. A. W., and Lim, Y. L.: Haemodynamic changes in women taking oral contraceptives. J. Obstet. Gynecol. Br. Commonw. *77*:1007, 1970.
200. Goldhaber, S. Z., Hennekens, C. H., Spark, R. F., Evans, D. A., Rosner, B., Taylor, J. O., and Kass, E. H.: Plasma renin substrate renin activity, and aldosterone levels in a sample of oral contraceptive users from a community survey. Am. Heart J. *107*:119, 1984.
201. Hollenberg, N. K., Williams, G. H., Burger, B., Chenitz, W., Hooshmand, I., and Adams, D. F.: Renal blood flow and its response to angiotensin II. Circ. Res. *38*:35, 1976.
202. Kay, C. R.: Progestogens and arterial disease—Evidence from the Royal College of General Practitioners' study. Am. J. Obstet. Gynecol. *141*:762, 1982.
203. Pfeffer, R. I., Kurosaki, T. T., and Charlton, S. K.: Estrogen use and blood pressure in later life. Am. J. Epidemiol. *110*:469, 1979.
204. Bush, T. L., and Barrett-Connor, E.: Noncontraceptive estrogen use and cardiovascular disease. Epidemiol. Rev. *7*:80, 1985.
205. Wilson, P. W. F., Garrison, R. J., and Castelli, W. P.: Postmenopausal estrogen use, cigarette smoking, and cardiovascular morbidity in women over 50: The Framingham Study. N. Engl. J. Med. *313*:1038, 1985.
206. Stampfer, M. J., Willett, W. C., Colditz, G. A., Rosner, B., Speizer, F. E., and Hennekens, C. H.: A prospective study of postmenopausal estrogen therapy and coronary heart disease. N. Engl. J. Med. *313*:1044, 1985.
207. Hostetter, T. H.: The hyperfiltering glomerulus. Med. Clin. N. Am. *68*:387, 1984.
208. Anderson, S., Meyer, T. W., Rennke, H. G., and Brenner, B. M.: Control of glomerular hypertension limits glomerular injury in rats with reduced renal mass. J. Clin. Invest. *76*:612, 1985.
209. Dworkin, L. D., and Feiner, H. D.: Glomerular injury in uninephrectomized spontaneously hypertensive rats. A consequence of glomerular capillary hypertension. J. Clin. Invest. *77*:797, 1986.
210. Guidi, E., Magni, M., di Belgiojoso, G. B., Minetti, L., and Bianchi, G.: Blood pressure in patients with four different primary glomerulopathies. Clin. Exper. Hyper. Theory Practice *A6*:1357, 1984.
211. Garcia, R., Rubio, L., and Rodriguez-Iturbe, B.: Long-term prognosis of epidemic poststreptococcal glomerulonephritis in Maracaibo: Follow-up studies 11 to 12 years after the acute episode. Clin. Nephrol. *15*:291, 1981.
212. Levinsky, N. G.: Pathophysiology of acute renal failure. N. Engl. J. Med. *296*:1453, 1977.
213. Bakir, A. A., Bazilinski, N., and Dunea, G.: Transient and sustained recovery from renal shutdown in accelerated hypertension. Am. J. Med. *80*:172, 1986.
214. Traub, Y. M., Shapiro, A. P., Rodnan, G. P., Medsger, T. A., McDonald, R. H., Jr., Steen, V. D., Osial, T. A., Jr., and Tolchin, S. F.: Hypertension and renal failure (scleroderma renal crisis) in progressive systemic sclerosis: Review of a 25-year experience with 68 cases. Medicine *62*:335, 1983.
215. Anderson, C. F., Velosa, J. A., Frohnert, P. P., Torres, V. E., Offord, K. P., Vogel, J. P., Donadio, J. V., Jr., and Wilson, D. M.: The risks of unilateral nephrectomy: Status of kidney donors 10 to 20 years postoperatively. Mayo Clin. Proc. *60*:367, 1985.
216. Smith, H. W.: Unilateral nephrectomy in hypertensive disease. J. Urol. *76*:685, 1956.
217. Lüscher, T. F., Wanner, C., Hauri, D., Siegenthaler, W., and Vetter, W.: Curable renal parenchymatous hypertension: Current diagnosis and management. Cardiology 72(Suppl. 1):33, 1985.
218. Lambertson, R. P., Noth, R. H., and Glickman, M.: Frequent falsely negative renal vein renin tests in unilateral renal parenchymal disease. J. Urol. *125*:477, 1981.
219. Calabrese, G., Vagelli, G., Cristofano, C., and Barsotti, G.: Behaviour of arterial pressure in different stages of polycystic kidney disease. Nephron *32*:207, 1982.
220. Siamopoulos, K., Sellars, L., Mishra, S. C., Essenhigh, D. M., Robson, V., and Wilkinson, R.: Experience in the management of hypertension with unilateral chronic pyelonephritis: Results of nephrectomy in selected patients. Q. J. Med. *207*:349, 1983.
221. Anderson, S., Rennke, H. G., and Brenner, B. M.: Therapeutic advantage of converting enzyme inhibitors in arresting progressive renal disease associated with systemic hypertension in the rat. J. Clin. Invest. *77*:1993, 1986.
222. Brod, J., Bahlmann, J., Cachovan, M., and Pretschner, P.: Development of hypertension in renal disease. Clin. Sci. *64*:141, 1983.
223. Danielsen, H., Pedersen, E. B., and Christensen, J. N.: Relationship of angiotensin II, aldosterone, arginine vasopressin, adrenaline and noradrenaline in plasma, blood and extracellular volumes to blood pressure in chronic glomerulonephritis. Eur. J. Clin. Invest. *16*:85, 1986.
224. Koomans, H. A., Roos, J. C., Boer, P., Geyskes, G. G., and Mees, E. J. D.: Salt sensitivity of blood pressure in chronic renal failure. Evidence for renal control of body fluid distribution in man. Hypertension *4*:190, 1982.
225. Swaminathan, R., Glegg, G., Cumberbatch, M., Zareian, Z., and McKenna, F.: Erythrocyte sodium transport in chronic renal failure. Clin. Sci. *62*:489, 1982.
226. Brunner, H. R., Wauters, J., McKinstry, D., Waeber, B., Turini, G., and Gavras, H.: Inappropriate renin secretion unmasked by captopril (SQ14 225) in hypertension of chronic renal failure. Lancet *2*:704, 1978.
227. Henrich, W. L., Mitchell, H., Anderson, S., Cronin, R., and Pettinger, W. A.: Effect of antihypertensive therapy on plasma catecholamines in renal failure patients. Clin. Nephrol. *16*:131, 1981.
228. Ying, C. Y., Tifft, C. P., Gavras, H., and Chobanian, A. V.: Renal revascularization in the azotemic hypertensive patients resistant to therapy. N. Engl. J. Med. *311*:1070, 1984.
229. Zatz, R., Dunn, B. R., Meyer, T. W., Anderson, S., Rennke, H. G., and Brenner, B. M.: Prevention of diabetic glomerulopathy by pharmacological amelioration of glomerular capillary hypertension. J. Clin. Invest. *77*:1925, 1986.
230. Taguma, Y., Kitamoto, Y., Futaki, G., Ueda, H., Monma, H, Ishizaki, M., Takahashi, H., Sekino, H., and Sasaki, Y.: Effect of captopril on heavy proteinuria in azotemic diabetics. N. Engl. J. Med. *313*:1617, 1985.
231. Perez, G. O., Lespier, L., Knowles, R., Oster, J. R., and Vaamonde, C. A.: Potassium homeostasis in chronic diabetes mellitus. Arch. Intern. Med. *137*:1018, 1977.
232. Gordon, R. D.: Syndrome of hypertension and hyperkalemia with normal glomerular filtration rate. Hypertension *8*:93, 1986.
233. Kincaid-Smith, P.: Analgesic abuse and the kidney. Kidney Int. *17*:250, 1980.
234. Muther, R. S., Potter, D. M., and Bennett, W. M.: Aspirin-induced depression of glomerular filtration rate in normal humans: Role of sodium balance. Ann. Intern. Med. *94*:317, 1981.
235. Textor, S. C., Gavras, H., Tifft, C. P., Bernard, D. B., Idelson, B., and Brunner, H.: Norepinephrine and renin activity in chronic renal failure. Evidence for interacting roles in hemodialysis hypertension. Hypertension *3*:294, 1981.
236. Battle, D. C., von Riotte, A., and Lang, G.: Delayed hypotensive response to dialysis in hypertensive patients with end-stage renal disease. Am. J. Nephrol. *6*:14, 1986.
237. Curtis, J. J., Luke, R. G., Dustan, H. P., Kashgarian, M., Whelchel, J. D., Jones, P., and Diethelm, A. G.: Remission of essential hypertension after renal transplantation. N. Engl. J. Med. *309*:1009, 1983.
238. Waltzer, W. C., Turner, S., Frohnert, P., and Rapaport, F. T.: Etiology and pathogenesis of hypertension following renal transplantation. Nephron *42*:102, 1986.

239. Curtis, J. J., Luke, R. G., Diethelm, A. G., Whelchel, J. D., and Jones, P.: Benefits of removal of native kidneys in hypertension after renal transplantation. Lancet 2:739, 1985.
240. Guidi, E., Bianchi, G., Rivolta, E., Ponticelli, C., di Palo, F. Q., Minetti, L., and Polli, E.: Hypertension in man with a kidney transplant: Role of familial versus other factors. Nephron *41*:14, 1985.
241. Strandgaard, S., and Hansen, U.: Hypertension in renal allograft recipients may be conveyed by cadaveric kidneys from donors with subarachnoid haemorrhage. Br. Med. J. *292*:1041, 1986.
242. Adams, H. P., Jr., Dawson, G., Coffman, T. J., and Corry, R. J.: Stroke in renal transplant recipients. Arch. Neurol. *43*:113, 1986.
243. Davis, B. A., Crook, M. E., Vestal, R. E., and Oates, J. A.: Prevalence of renovascular hypertension in patients with grade III or IV hypertensive retinopathy. N. Engl. J. Med. *301*:1273, 1979.
244. Plumer, L. B., Kaplan, G. W., and Mendoza, S. A.: Hypertension in infants—A complication of umbilical arterial catheterization. J. Pediatr. *89*:802, 1976.
245. Novick, A. C.: The case for surgical therapy. *In* Narins, R.G. (ed.): Controversies in Nephrology and Hypertension. New York, Churchill Livingstone, 1984, p. 181.
246. de Zeeuw, D., Burema, J., Donker, A. J. M., van der Hem, G. K., and Mandema, E.: Nephroptosis and hypertension. Lancet *1*:213, 1977.
247. Keith, T.A. III: Renovascular hypertension in black patients. Hypertension *4*:438, 1982.
248. Munichoodappa, C., d'Elia, J. A., Libertino, J. A., Gleason, R. E., and Christlieb, A. R.: Renal artery stenosis in hypertensive diabetics. J. Urol. *121*:555, 1979.
249. Bookstein, J. J.: Segmental renal artery stenosis in renovascular hypertension. Radiology *90*:1073, 1968.
250. Zinman, L., and Libertino, J. A.: Revascularization of the chronic totally occluded renal artery with restoration of renal function. J. Urol. *118*:517, 1977.
251. Bookstein, J. J., Abrams, H. L., Buenger, R. E., Reiss, M. D., Lecky, J. W., Franklin, S. S., Bleifer, K. W., Varady, P. D., and Maxwell, M. H.: Radiologic aspects of renovascular hypertension. Part 3. Appraisal of arteriography. J.A.M.A. *21*:368, 1972.
252. Fiorentini, C., Guazzi, M. D., Olivari, M. T., Bartorelli, A., Necchi, G., and Magrini, F.: Selective reduction in renal perfusion pressure and blood flow in man: Humoral and hemodynamic effects. Circulation *63*:973, 1981.
253. Buggy, J., Fink, G. D., Johnson, A. K., and Brody, M. J.: Prevention of the development of renal hypertension by anteroventral third ventricular tissue lesions. Circ. Res. *40*(Suppl. 1):110, 1977.
254. Thal, A. P., Grage, T. B., and Vernier, R. L.: Function of the contralateral kidney in renal hypertension due to renal artery stenosis. Circulation *27*:36, 1963.
255. Wenting, G. J., Tan-tjiong, H. L., Derkx, F. H. M., de Bryun, J. H. B., Man In't Veld, A. J., and Schalekamp, M.A.D.H.: Split renal function after captopril in unilateral renal artery stenosis. Br. Med. J. *288*:886, 1984.
256. Simon, N., Franklin, S. S., Bleifer, K. W., and Maxwell, M.H.P: Clinical characteristics of renovascular hypertension. J.A.M.A. *220*:1209, 1972.
257. Muller, F. B., Sealey, J. E., Case, D. B., Atlas, S. A., Pickering, T. G., Pecker, M.S., Prebisz, J. J., and Laragh, J. H.: The captopril test for identifying renovascualar disease in hypertensive patients. Am. J. Med. *80*:633, 1986.
258. Carmichael, D. J. S., Mathias, C. J., Snell, M. E., and Peart, S.: Detection and investigation of renal artery stenosis. Lancet *1*:667, 1986.
259. Hillman, B. J.: Digital radiology of the kidney. Radiol. Clin. North Am. *23*:211, 1985.
260. Rudnick, M. R., and Maxwell, M. H.: Limitations of renin assays. *In* Narins, R.G. (ed.): Controversies in Nephrology and Hypertension. New York, Churchill Livingstone, 1984, p. 123.
261. Dean, R. H., Kieffer, R. W., Smith, B. M., Oates, J. A., Nadeau, J. H. J., Hollifield, J. W., and DuPont, W. D.: Renovascular hypertension. Arch. Surg. *116*:1408, 1981.
262. Reams, G. P., Bauer, J. H., and Gaddy, P.: Use of the converting enzyme inhibitor enalapril in renovascular hypertension: Effect on blood pressure, renal function, and the renin-angiotensin-aldosterone system. Hypertension 8:290, 1986.
263. Tillman, D. M., Malatino, L. S., Cumming, A. M. M., Hodsman, G. P., Leckie, B.J., Lever, A. F., Morton, J. J., Webb, D. J., and Robertson, J. I. S.: Enalapril in hypertension with renal artery stenosis: Long-term follow-up and effects on renal function. J. Hypertension *2*(Suppl. 2):93, 1984.
264. Kuhlmann, U., Greminger, P., Grüntzig, A., Schneider, E., Puliadis, G., Luscher, T., Steurer, J., Siegenthaler, W., and Vetter, W.: Long-term experience in percutaneous transluminal dilatation of renal artery stenosis. Am. J. Med. *79*:692, 1985.
265. Olin, J. W., Vidt, D. G., Gifford, R. W., Jr., and Novick, A. C.: Renovascular disease in the elderly. An analysis of 50 patients. J. Am. Coll. Cardiol. *5*:1232, 1985.
266. Conn, J. W., Cohen, E. L., Lucas, C. P., McDonald, W. J., Blough, W. M., Jr., Eveland, W. C., Bookstein, J. J., and Lapides, J.: Primary reninism. Hypertension, hyperreninemia, and secondary aldosteronism due to renin-producing juxtaglomerular cell tumors. Arch. Intern. Med. *130*:682, 1972.
267. Sheth, K. J., Tang, T. T., Blaedel, M. E., and Good, T. A.: Polydipsia, polyuria, and hypertension associated with renin-secreting Wilms' tumor. J. Pediatr. *92*:921, 1978.
268. Glazer, H. S., Weyman, P. J., Sagel, S. S., Levitt, R. G., and McClennan, B. L.: Nonfuctioning adrenal masses: Incidental discovery on computed tomography. Am. J. Roentgenol. *139*:81, 1982.
269. Prinz, R. A., Brooks, M. H., Churchill, R., Graner, J. L., Lawrence, A. M., Palozan, E., and Sparagana, M.: Incidental asymptomatic adrenal masses detected by computed tomographic scanning: Is operation required? J.A.M.A. *248*:701, 1982.
270. Weinberger, M. H., Grim, C. E., Hollifield, J. W., Kem, D. C., Ganguly, A., Kramer, N. J., Yune, H. Y., Wellman, H., and Donohue, J. P.: Primary aldosteronism. Ann. Intern. Med. *90*:386, 1979.
271. Bravo, E. L., Tarazi, R. C., Dustan, H. P., Fouad, F. M., Textor, S. C., Gifford, R.W., and Vidt, D. G.: The changing clinical spectrum of primary aldosteronism. Am. J. Med. *74*:641, 1983.
272. McAreavey, D., Murray, G. D., Lever, A. F., and Robertson, J. I. S.: Similarity of idiopathic aldosteronism and essential hypertension. Hypertension *5*:116, 1983.
273. Griffing, G. T., Berelowitz, B., Hudson, M., Salzman, R., Manson, J. A. E., Aurrechia, S., Melby, J. C., Pedersen, R. C., and Brownie, A. C.: Plasma immunoreactive gamma melanotropin in patients with idiopathic hyperaldosteronism, aldosterone-producing adenomas, and essential hypertension. J. Clin. Invest. *76*:163, 1985.
274. Banks, W. B., Kastin, A. J., Biglieri, E. D., and Ruiz, A. E.: Primary adrenal hyperplasia: A new subset of primary hyperaldosteronism. J. Clin. Endocrinol. Metab. *58*:783, 1984.
275. Oberfield, S. E., Levine, L. S., Firpo, A., Lawrence, D., Stoner, E., Levy, D.J., Sem, S., and New, M. I.: Primary hyperaldosteronism in childhood due to unilateral macronodular hyperplasia: Case report. Hypertension *6*:75, 1984.
276. Gomez-Sanchez, C. E., Montgomery, M., Ganguly, A., Holland, O. B., Gomez-Sanchez, E. P., Grim, C. E., and Weinberger, M. H.: Elevated urinary excretion of 18-oxycortisol in glucocorticoid-suppressible aldosteronism. J. Clin. Endocrinol. Metabol. *59*:1022, 1984.
277. Ferriss, J. B., Brown, J. J., Fraser, R., Lever, A. F., and Robertson, J. I. S.: Primary aldosterone excess: Conn's syndrome and similar disorders. *In* Robertson, J. I. S. (ed.): Handbook of Hypertension. Vol. 2. Clinical Aspects of Secondary Hypertension. New York, Elsevier Science Publishers, 1983, p. 132.
278. Cereda, J. M., Trono, D., and Schifferli, J.: Liquorice intoxication caused by alcohol-free pastis. Lancet *1*:1442, 1983.
279. Blachley, J. D., and Knochel, J. P.: Tobacco chewer's hypokalemia: Licorice revisited. N. Engl. J. Med. *302*:784, 1980.
280. Matsunaga, M., Hara, A., Song, T. S., Hashimoto, M., Tamori, S., Ogawa, K., Morimoto, K., Pak, C. H., Kawai, C., and Yoshida, O.: Asymptomatic normotensive primary aldosteronism: Case report. Hypertension *5*:240, 1983.
281. Tunny, T. J., and Gordon, R. D.: Plasma atrial natriuretic peptide in primary aldosteronism (before and after treatment) and in Bartter's and Gordon's syndromes. Lancet *1*:272, 1986.
282. Ferriss, J. B., Beevers, D. G., Brown, J. J., Davies, D. L., Fraser, R., Lever, A.F., Mason, P., Neville, A. M., and Robertson, J. I. S.: Clinical, biochemical and pathological features of low renin ("primary") hyperaldosteronism. Am. Heart J. 95:375, 1978.
283. Zadik, Z., Levin, P. A., Hamilton, B. P., and Kowarski, A. A.: Detection of primary aldosteronism by the 6-hour integrated aldosterone/renin ratio. Hypertension *8*:285, 1986.
284. Holland, O. B., Brown, H., Kuhnert, L. V., Fairchild, C., Risk, M., and Gomez-Sanchez, C. E.: Further evaluation of saline infusion for the diagnosis of primary aldosteronism. Hypertension *6*:717, 1984.
285. Ferriss, J. B., Beevers, D. G., Brody, K., Brown, J. J., Davies, D. L., Fraser, R., Kremer, D., Lever, A. F., and Robertson, J. I. S.: The treatment of low-renin ("primary") hyperaldosteronism. Am. Heart J. *96*:97, 1978.
286. Abrams, H. L., Siegelman, S. S., Adams, D. F., Sanders, R., Feinberg, H. J., Hessel, S. J., and McNeil, B. J.: Computed tomography versus ultrasound of the adrenal gland: A prospective study. Radiology *143*:121, 1982.
287. Gross, M. D., Shapiro, B., Grekin, R. J., Freitas, J. E., Glazer, G., Beierwaltes, W.H., and Thompson, N. W.: Scintigraphic localization of adrenal lesions in primary aldosteronism. Am. J. Med. *77*:839, 1984.
288. Vaughan, N.J.A., Jowett, T.P., Slater, J.D.H., Wiggins, R.C., Lightman, S.L., Ma, J.T.C., and Payne, N.N.: The diagnosis of primary hyperaldosteronism. Lancet *1*:120, 1981.
289. Ganguly, A., and Weinberger, M.H.: Triamterene-thiazide combination: Alternative therapy for primary aldosteronism. Clin. Pharmacol. Ther. *30*:246, 1981.
290. Griffing, G.T., Cole, A.G., Aurecchia, S.A., Sindler, B.A., Komanicky, P., and Melby, J.C.: Amiloride in primary hyperaldosteronism. Clin. Pharmacol. Ther. *31*:56, 1982.
291. Ross, E.J., and Linch, D.C.: Cushing's syndrome—killing disease: Discriminatory value of signs and symptoms aiding early diagnosis. Lancet *2*:646, 1982.
292. Gomez-Sanchez, C.E.: Cushing's syndrome and hypertension. Hypertension *8*:258, 1986.
293. Crapo, L.: Cushing's syndrome: A review of diagnostic tests. Metabolism *28*:955, 1979.
294. Gold, P.W., Loriaux, D.L., Roy, A., Kling, M.A., Calabrese, J.R., Kellner, C.H., Nieman, L.K., Post, R.M., Pickar, D., Gallucci, W., Avgerinos, P., Paul, S., Oldfield, E.H., Cutler, G.B., Jr., and Chrousos, G.P.: Responses to corticotropin-releasing hormone in the hypercortisolism of depression and Cushing's disease: Pathophysiologic and diagnostic implications. N. Engl. J. Med. *314*:1329, 1986.
295. Contreras, L.N., Hane, S., and Tyrrell, J.B.: Urinary cortisol in the assessment of pituitary-adrenal function: Utility of 24-hour and spot determinations. J. Clin. Endocrinol. Metab. *62*:965, 1986.
296. Atkinson, A.B., Chestnutt, A., Crothers, E., Woods, R., Weaver, J.A., Kennedy, L., and Sheridan, B.: Cyclical Cushing's disease: Two distinct rhythms in a patient with a basophil adenoma. J. Clin. Endocrinol. Metab. *60*:328, 1985.
297. White, F.E., White, M.C., Drury, P.L., Fry, I.K., and Besser, G.M.: Value of computed tomography of the abdomen and chest in investigation of Cushing's syndrome. Br. Med. J. *284*:771, 1982.

298. Carpenter, P.C.: Cushing's syndrome: Update of diagnosis and management. Mayo Clin. Proc. *61*:49, 1986.
299. Goldstein, D.S., Stull, R., Eisenhofer, G., Sisson, J.C., Weder, A., Averbuch, S.D., and Keiser, H.R.: Plasma dihydroxyphenylalanine in neuroblastoma and pheochromocytoma. Ann. Intern. Med. *105*:887, 1986.
300. Dunn, G.D., Brown, M.J., Sapsford, R.N., Mansfield, A.O., Hemingway, A.P., Sever, P.S., and Allison, D.J.: Functioning middle mediastinal paraganglioma (phaeochromocytoma) associated with intercarotid paragangliomas. Lancet *1*:1061, 1986.
301. Kalff, V., Shapiro, B., Lloyd, R., Sisson, J.C., Holland, K., Nakajo, M., and Beierwaltes, W.H.: The spectrum of pheochromocytoma in hypertensive patients with neurofibromatosis. Arch. Intern. Med. *142*:2092, 1982.
302. Valk, T.W., Frager, M.S., Gross, M.D., Sisson, J.C., Wieland, D.M., Swanson, D.P., Mangner, T.J., and Beierwaltes, W.H.: Spectrum of pheochromocytoma in multiple endocrine neoplasia. A scintigraphic portrayal using ^{131}I-metaiodobenzylguanidine. Ann. Intern. Med. *94*:762, 1981.
303. O'Connor, D.T., and Deftos, L.J.: Secretion of chromogranin A by peptide-producing endocrine neoplasms. N. Engl. J. Med. *314*:1145, 1986.
304. McPhaul, M., Punzi, H.A., Sandy, A., Borganelli, M., Rude, R., and Kaplan, N.M.: Snuff-induced hypertension in pheochromocytoma. J.A.M.A. 252:2860, 1984.
305. Baker, G., Zeller, N.H., Weitzner, S., and Leach, J.K.: Pheochromocytoma without hypertension presenting as cardiomyopathy. Am. Heart J. *83*:688, 1972.
306. Gupta, K.K.: Phaeochromocytoma and myocardial infarction. Lancet *1*:281, 1975.
307. Chaturvedi, N.C., Walsh, M.J., Boyle, D.M., and Barber, J.M.: Diamorphine-induced attack of paroxysmal hypertension in phaeochromocytoma. Br. Med. J. 2:538, 1974.
308. Manu, P., and Runge, L.A.: Biochemical screening for pheochromocytoma: Superiority of urinary metanephrines measurements. Am. J. Epidemiol. *120*:788, 1984.
309. Bouloux, P.-M.G., and Perrett, D.: Interference of labetalol metabolites in the determination of plasma catecholamines by HPLC with electrochemical detection. Clin. Chim. Acta *150*:111, 1985.
310. Young, M.J., Shapiro, B., and Domechowski, C.: Comparison of diagnostic tests for pheochromocytoma (Abstract). Clin. Res. *34*:387A, 1986.
311. Bravo, E.L., Tarazi, R.C., Fouad, F.M., Vidt, D.G., and Gifford, R.W., Jr.: Clonidine-suppression test. A useful aid in the diagnosis of pheochromocytoma. N. Engl. J. Med. *305*:623, 1981.
312. Hui, T.P., Krakoff, L.R., Felton, K., and Yeager, K.: Diuretic treatment alters clonidine suppression of plasma norepinephrine. Hypertension *8*:272, 1986.
313. Chatal, J.F., and Charbonnel, B.: Comparison of iodobenzylguanidine imaging with computed tomography in locating pheochromocytoma. J. Clin. Endocrinol. Metab. *61*:769, 1985.
314. Manger, W.M., and Gifford, R.W., Jr.: Hypertension secondary to pheochromocytoma. Bull. N.Y. Acad. Med. *58*:139, 1982.
315. Lucky, A.W., Rosenfield, R.L., McGuire, J., Rudy, S., and Helke, J.: Adrenal androgen hyperresponsiveness to adrenocorticotropin in women and acne and/or hirsutism: Adrenal enzyme defects and exaggerated adrenarche. J. Clin. Endocrinol. Metab. *62*:840, 1986.
316. Cathelineau, G., Brerault, J., Fiet, J., Julien, R., Dreux, C., and Canivet, J.: Adrenocortical 11β-hydroxylation defect in adult women with postmenarchal onset of symptoms. J. Clin. Endocrinol. Metab. *51*:287, 1980.
317. Dean, J.H., Shackleton, C.H.L., and Winter, J.S.D.: Diagnosis and natural history of 17-hydroxylase deficiency in a newborn male. J. Clin. Endocrinol. Metab. *59*:513, 1984.
318. Textor, S.C., Forman, S.J., Borer, W.Z., Bravo, E.L., and Carlson, J.: Blood pressure, hormonal and renal changes during cyclosporine (CYA) administration in normotensive bone marrow transplant (BMT) recipients with normal renal function (Abstract). Clin. Res. *34*:487A, 1986.
319. Pentel, P.R., Asinger, R.W., and Benowitz, N.L.: Propranolol antagonism of phenylpropanolamine-induced hypertension. Clin. Pharmacol. Ther. *37*:488, 1985.
320. Liard, J.-F., and Spadone, J.-C.: Regional circulations in experimental coarctation of the aorta in conscious dogs. J. Hypertension *3*:281, 1985.
321. Clarkson, P.M., Nicholson, M.R., Barratt-Boyes, B.G., Neutze, J.M., and Whitlock, R.M.: Results after repair of coarctation of the aorta beyond infancy: A 10 to 28 year follow-up with particular reference to late systemic hypertension. Am. J. Cardiol. *51*:1481, 1983.
322. Gidding, S.S., Rocchini, A.P., Beekman, R., Szpunar, C.A., Moorehead, C., Behrendt, D., and Rosenthal, A.: Therapeutic effect of propranolol on paradoxical hypertension after repair of coarctation of the aorta. N. Engl. J. Med. *312*:1224, 1985.
323. Vlachakis, N.D., Frederics, R., Velasquez, M., Alexander, N., Singer, F., and Maronde, R.F.: Sympathetic system function and vascular reactivity in hypercalcemic patients. Hypertension *4*:452, 1982.
324. Posen, S., Clifton-Bligh, P., Reeve, T.S., Wagstaffe, C., and Wilkinson, M.: Is parathyroidectomy of benefit in primary hyperparathyroidism? Q. J. Med. *54*:241, 1985.
325. Estafanous, F.G., and Tarazi, R.C.: Systemic arterial hypertension associated with cardiac surgery. Am. J. Cardiol. *46*:685, 1980.
326. Whelton, P.K., Flaherty, J.T., MacAllister, N.P., Watkins, L., Potter, A., Johnson, D., Russel, R.P., and Walker, W.G.: Hypertension following coronary artery bypass surgery. Role of preoperative propranolol therapy. Hypertension 2:291, 1981.
327. Flaherty, J.T., Magee, P.A., Gardner, T.L., Potter, A., and MacAllister, N.P.: Comparison of intravenous nitroglycerin and sodium nitroprusside for treatment of acute hypertension developing after coronary artery bypass surgery. Circulation *65*:1072, 1982.
328. Hess, W., Schulte-Sasse, U., and Tarnow, J.: Nifedipine versus nitroprusside for controlling hypertensive episodes during coronary artery bypass surgery. Eur. Heart J. *5*:140, 1984.
329. Layton, C., Brigden, W., McDonald, L., Monro, J., McDonald, A., and Weaver, J.: Systemic hypertension after homograft aortic valvar replacement. A cause of late homograft failure. Lancet *2*:1343, 1973.
330. Cockburn, J.S., Benjamin, I.S., Thompson, R.M., and Bain, W.H.: Early systemic hypertension after surgical closure of atrial septal defect. J. Thorac. Cardiovasc. Surg. *16*:1, 1975.
331. Stradling, J.R., and Phillipson, E.A.: Breathing disorders during sleep. Q. J. Med. *58*:3, 1986.
332. Kales, A., Bixler, E.O., Cadieux, R.J., Schneck, D.W., Shaw, L.C. III, Locke, T.W., Vela-Bueno, A., and Soldatos, C.R.: Sleep apnoea in a hypertensive population. Lancet *2*:1005, 1984.
333. Williams, A.J., Houston, D., Finberg, S., Lam, C., Kinney, J.L., and Santiago, S.: Sleep apnea syndrome and essential hypertension. Am. J. Cardiol. *55*:1019, 1985.
334. Burack, B.: The hypersomnia-sleep apnea syndrome: Its recognition in clinical cardiology. Am. Heart J. *107*:543, 1984.

SPECIAL TOPICS IN HYPERTENSION

335. Friedman, E.A., and Neff, R.K.: Hypertension-hypotension in pregnancy. Correlation with fetal outcome. J.A.M.A. *239*:2249, 1978.
336. Kaunitz, A.M., Hughes, J.M., Grimes, D.A., Smith, J.C., Rochat, R.W., and Kafrissen, M.E.: Causes of maternal mortality in the United States. Obstet. Gynecol. *65*:605, 1985.
337. Sibai, B.M., Abdella, T.N., Spinnato, J.A., and Anderson, G.D.: The incidence of nonpreventable eclampsia. Am. J. Obstet. Gynecol. *154*:581, 1986.
338. Mountquin, J.M., Rainville, C., Giroux, L., Raynauld, P., Amyot, G., Bilodeau, R., and Pelland, N.: A prospective study of blood pressure in pregnancy: Prediction of preeclampsia. Am. J. Obstet. Gynecol. *151*:191, 1985.
339. Sawyer, M.M., Lipshitz, J., Anderson, G.D., Dilts, P.V., and Halperin, L.: Diurnal and short-term variation of blood pressure: Comparison of preeclamptic, chronic, hypertensive, and normotensive patients. Obstet. Gynecol. *58*:291, 1981.
340. Gallery, E.D.M.: Pregnancy-associated hypertension: Interrelationships of volume and blood pressure changes. Clin. Exper. Hyper.—Hyper. Pregnancy *B1*:39, 1982.
341. Murphy, J.F., O'Riordan, J., Newcombe, R.G., Coles, E.C., and Pearson, J.F.: Relation of haemoglobin levels in first and second trimesters to outcome of pregnancy. Lancet *1*:992, 1986.
342. Øian, P., Maltau, J.M., Noddeland, H., and Fadnes, H.O.: Transcapillary fluid balance in pre-eclampsia. Br. J. Obstet. Gynaecol. *93*:235, 1986.
343. Lunnell, N.O., Nylund, L.E., Lewander, L.E., and Sarby, B.: Uteroplacental blood flow in pre-eclampsia measurements with indium-113m and a computer-linked gamma camera. Clin. Exper. Hyper.—Hyper. Pregnancy *B1*:105, 1982.
344. Walsh, S.W.: Preeclampsia: An imbalance in placental prostacyclin and thromboxane production. Am. J. Obstet. Gynecol. *152*:335, 1985.
345. Editorial: Aspirin and pre-eclampsia. Lancet *1*:18, 1986.
346. Nakamura, T., Ito, M., Matsui, K., Yoshimura, T., Kawasaki, N., and Maeyama, M.: Significance of angiotensin sensitivity test for prediction of pregnancy-induced hypertension. Obstet. Gynecol. *67*:388, 1986.
347. Broughton Pipkin, F.B., Hunter, J.C., Turner, S.R., and O'Brien, P.M.S.: Prostaglandin E_2 attenuates the pressor response to angiotensin II in pregnant subjects but not in nonpregnant subjects. Am. J. Obstet. Gynecol. *142*:168, 1982.
348. Broughton Pipkin, F.B., Morrison, R., and O'Brien, P.M.S.: Prostacyclin blunts the pressor response to angiotensin II in human pregnancy. Proc. IV World Cong. Int. Soc. Study Hypertension Preg. 1984, p. 64.
349. Everett, R.B., Worley, R.J., MacDonald, P.C., and Gant, N.F.: Effect of prostaglandin synthetase inhibitors on pressor response to angiotensin II in human pregnancy. J. Clin. Endocrinol. Metab. *46*:1007, 1978.
350. Wallenburg, H.C.S., Dekker, G.A., Markovitz, J.W., and Rotmans, P.: Low-dose aspirin prevents pregnancy-induced hypertension and pre-eclampsia in angiotensin-sensitive primigravidae. Lancet *1*:1, 1986.
351. Beaufils, M., Uzan, S., Donsimoni, R., and Colau, J.C.: Prevention of pre-eclampsia by early antiplatelet therapy. Lancet *1*:840, 1985.
352. Vaziri, N.D., Toohey, J., Powers, D., Keegan, K., Gupta, A., Alikhani, S., Mashood, M., and Barbari, A.: Activation of intrinsic coagulation pathway in pre-eclampsia. Am. J. Med. *80*:103, 1986.
353. Alderman, B.W., Sperling, R.S., and Daling, J.R.: An epidemiological study of the immunogenetic aetiology of pre-eclampsia. Br. Med. J. *292*:372, 1986.
354. Weissberg, P.L., Weaver, J., Woods, K.L., West, M.J., and Beevers, D.G.: Pregnancy induced hypertension: Evidence for increased cell membrane permeability to sodium. Br. Med. J. *287*:709, 1983.
355. McMurray, J.A., and Morgan, D.B.: The sodium content of lymphocytes and mixed leucocytes in pregnancy and pregnancy induced hypertension. Clin. Exper. Hyper.—Hyper. Pregnancy *B3*:23, 1984.
356. Graves, S.W., and Williams, G.H.: An endogenous ouabain-like factor associated with hypertensive pregnant women. J. Clin. Endocrinol. Metab. *59*:1070, 1984.
357. Oney, T., and Kaulhausen, H.: The value of the angiotensin sensitivity test in the early diagnosis of hypertensive disorders in pregnancy. Am. J. Obstet. Gynecol. *142*:17, 1982.

358. Collins, R., Yusuf, S., and Peto, R.: Overview of randomised trials of diuretics in pregnancy. Br. Med. J. *290*:17, 1985.
359. Cunningham, F.G., and Pritchard, J.A.: How should hypertension during pregnancy be managed? Experience at Parkland Memorial Hospital. Med. Clin. North Am. *68*:505, 1984.
360. Cockburn, J., Ounsted, M., Moar, V.A., and Redman, C.W.B.: Final report of study on hypertension during pregnancy: The effects of specific treatment on the growth and development of the children. Lancet *1*:647, 1982.
361. Rubin, P.C., Butters, L., Clark, D., Sumner, D., Belfield, A., Pledger, D., Low, R.A.L., and Reid, J.L.: Obstetric aspects of the use in pregnancy-associated hypertension of the beta-adrenoceptor antagonist atenolol. Am. J. Obstet. Gynecol. *150*:389, 1984.
362. Wichman, K., Ryden, G., and Karlberg, B.E.: A placebo controlled trial of metoprolol in the treatment of hypertension in pregnancy. Scand. J. Clin. Lab. Invest. *44*(Suppl. 169):90, 1984.
363. Welt, S.I., Dorminy, J.H., Jelovsek, F.R., Crenshaw, M.C., and Gall, M.D.: The effect of prophylactic management and therapeutics on hypertensive disease in pregnancy: Preliminary studies. Obstet. Gynecol. *57*:557, 1981.
364. Mabie, W.C., Pernoll, M.L., and Biswas, M.K.: Chronic hypertension in pregnancy. Obstet. Gynecol. *67*:197, 1986.
365. Sibai, B.M., and Anderson, G.D.: Pregnancy outcome of intensive therapy in severe hypertension in first trimester. Obstet. Gynecol. *67*:517, 1986.
366. Lopez-Llera, M.: Complicated eclampsia. Fifteen years' experience in a referral medical center. Am. J. Obstet. Gynecol. *142*:28, 1982.
367. Bauer, T.W., Moore, G.W., and Hutchins, G.M.: Morphologic evidence for coronary artery spasm in eclampsia. Circulation *65*:255, 1982.
368. Pritchard, J.A., Cunningham, F.G., and Pritchard, S.A.: The Parkland Memorial Hospital protocol for treatment of eclampsia. Evaluation of 245 cases. Am. J. Obstet. Gynecol. *148*:951, 1984.
369. Clark, S.L., Greenspoon, J.S., Aldahl, D., and Phelan, J.P.: Severe preeclampsia with persistent oliguria: Management of hemodynamic subsets. Am. J. Obstet. Gynecol. *154*:490, 1986.
370. Chesley, L.C.: Hypertension in pregnancy: Definitions, familial factor, and remote prognosis. Kidney Int. *18*:234, 1980.
371. Cunningham, F.G., Pritchard, J.A., Hankins, G.D.V., Anderson, P.L., Lucas, M.J., and Armstrong, K.F.: Peripartum heart failure: Idiopathic cardiomyopathy or compounding cardiovascular events? Obstet. Gynecol. *67*:157, 1986.
372. Fixler, D.E., Laird, W.P., Fitzgerald, V., Stead, S., and Adams, R.: Hypertension screening in schools: Results of the Dallas study. Pediatrics *63*:32, 1979.
373. Hofman, A., Valkenburg, H.A., Maas, J., and Groustra, F.N.: The natural history of blood pressure in childhood. Int. J. Epidemiol. *14*:91, 1985.
374. Katz, S.H., Hediger, M.L., Zemel, B.S., and Parks, J.S.: Blood pressure, body fat, and dehydroepiandrosterone sulfate variation in adolescence. Hypertension *8*:277, 1986.
375. Lauer, R.M., Anderson, A.R., Beaglehole, R., and Burns, T.L.: Factors related to tracking of blood pressure in children: U.S. National Center for Health Statistics Health Examination Surveys Cycles II and III. Hypertension *6*:307, 1984.
376. Wilson, S.L., Gaffney, F.A., Laird, W.P., and Fixler, D.E.: Body size, composition, and fitness in adolescents with elevated blood pressures. Hypertension *7*:417, 1985.
377. Hofman, A., and Grobbee, D. E.: Non-pharmacological intervention in primary hypertension in childhood. Clin. Exp. Hypertens. (A) *8*:813, 1986.
378. Hofman, A., Ellison, R.C., Newburger, J., and Miettinen, O.S.: Blood pressure and haemodynamics in teenagers. Br. Heart J. *48*:377, 1982.
379. Sinaiko, A.R., Gillum, R.F., Jacobs, D.R., Sopko, G., and Prineas, R.J.: Renin-angiotensin and sympathetic nervous system activity in grade school children. Hypertension *4*:299, 1982.
380. Goldring, D., Hernandez, A., Choi, S., Lee, J.Y., Londe, S., Lindgren, F.T., and Burton, R.M.: Blood pressure in a high school population. II. Clinical profile of the juvenile hypertensive. J. Pediatr. *95*:298, 1979.
381. Snider, A.R., Gidding, S.S., Rocchini, A.P., Rosenthal, A., Dick, M. II, Crowley, D.C., and Peters, J.: Doppler evaluation of left ventricular diastolic filling in children with systemic hypertension. Am. J. Cardiol. *56*:921, 1985.
382. Beilin, L.J., and Goldby, F.S.: High arterial pressure versus humor factors in the pathogenesis of the vascular lesions of malignant hypertension. Clin. Sci. Molec. Med. *52*:111, 1977.
383. Ahmed, M.E.K., Walker, J.M., Beevers, D.G., and Beevers, M.: Lack of difference between malignant and accelerated hypertension. Br. Med. J. *292*:235, 1986.
384. Lee, T.H., and Alderman, M.H.: Malignant hypertension: Declining mortality rate in New York City, 1958 to 1974. N.Y. State J. Med. *778*:1389, 1978.
385. Kincaid-Smith, P.: Understanding malignant hypertension. Aust. N.Z. J. Med. *11*:64, 1981.
386. MacKenzie, E.T., Strandgaard, S., Graham, D.I., Jones, J.V., Harper, A.M., and Farrar, J.K.: Effects of acutely induced hypertension in cats on pial arteriolar caliber, local cerebral blood flow, and the blood-brain barrier. Circ. Res. *39*:33, 1976.
387. Heistad, D.D.: Protection of the blood-brain barrier during acute and chronic hypertension. Fed. Proc. *43*:205, 1984.
388. Kontos, H.A.: Oxygen radicals in cerebral vascular injury. Circ. Res. *57*:508, 1985.
389. Strandgaard, S., Olesen, J., Skinhoj, E., and Lassen, N.A.: Autoregulation of brain circulation in severe arterial hypertension. Br. Med. J. *1*:507, 1973.
390. Shapiro, L.M., and Beevers, D.G.: Malignant hypertension: Cardiac structure and function at presentation and during therapy. Br. Heart J. *49*:477, 1983.
391. White, W.B., and Baker, L.H.: Episodic hypertension secondary to panic disorder. Arch. Intern. Med. *146*:1129, 1986.

28 SYSTEMIC HYPERTENSION: Therapy

by NORMAN M. KAPLAN, M.D.

INDICATIONS FOR THERAPY

The treatment of most patients with hypertension is relatively easy. Current therapy will lower the blood pressure in the majority of patients with hypertension, most of whom start with only minimally elevated pressures; a residue of perhaps 20 per cent of patients remain who are difficult to control.[1] The active drug therapy of patients with mild hypertension, defined as diastolic blood pressure (DBP) between 90 and 104 mm Hg, has expanded markedly in the past few years as a result of the confluence of three events: (1) even minimally elevated pressures have been shown to increase the overall risk for premature cardiovascular disease; (2) trials have shown that progression of hypertension, strokes, and, probably, heart failure can be reduced by drug therapy; and (3) medications that are easier to take have become available and been intensively marketed.

Because of these factors and the inherent desire for patients and physicians to take direct action against perceived dangers, millions of asymptomatic persons are now being treated with antihypertensive drugs. Although more individuals have been immunized against infectious diseases, the number of people worldwide now being *continuously treated* for hypertension represents the largest use of long-term drug therapy. The use of such therapy is more "aggressive" in the United States than anywhere else; indeed, treatment of hypertension is now the most common reason for patient visits to doctors and the most common indication for prescribing drugs. These statistics reflect the practice of more than two-thirds of U.S. physicians to institute drug therapy at levels of DBP between 90 and 100 mm Hg in asymptomatic patients.[2] In Canada, England, and elsewhere, most physicians institute drug therapy only at DBP levels above 100 mm Hg.

Such aggressive therapy has been vigorously defended, and credited for at least some of the reduction in coronary and stroke mortality seen in the United States since 1968.[3] Others question the wisdom of such therapeutic activism. In the words of an English practitioner, "in the U.S., the threshold for diagnosis is the threshold for treatment. The question 'to treat or not to treat' need no longer be asked. A free-fire zone has been created above diastolic 90, in which we simply shoot everything that moves."[4]

The wisdom of "simply shooting everything that moves," i.e., the aggressive treatment of hypertension, has been questioned for two principal reasons: (1) the awareness that the risks of relatively mild hypertension, although apparent for the aggregate, are not shared by all[5]; (2) the inability to show clear protection against coronary disease by drug therapy in six clinical trials involving more than 20,000 patients[6–12] (Table 28–1). Mainly as a result of this apparent inability to protect against coronary disease, concerns have risen about biochemical changes induced by the drugs used in these trials, changes which may have, at the same time they reduced risk by lowering blood pressure, increased risk in various ways, such as by lowering potassium, raising lipids, or altering glucose tolerance.

THE VARIABLE RISK. For the population at large, every increment of blood pressure increases the risk for cardiovascular disease. However, as noted on page 824, the *absolute* increase in risk is relatively small for those with

TABLE 28–1 TRIALS OF DRUG VS. PLACEBO THERAPY FOR MILD-TO-MODERATE HYPERTENSION

		Mortality Rates per 1,000 Person-Years					
		Cerebrovascular Disease			Coronary Heart Disease		
Trials (Reference)	No. of Patients	*Placebo*	*Drug*	*Difference (%)*	*Placebo*	*Drug*	*Difference (%)*
VA, 1970[7]	380	11.2	1.6	−86	17.5	9.6	−45
USPHS, 1977[8]	389	0.0	0.0	—	1.5	1.5	—
Australian, 1980[9]	3,427	0.9	0.4	−56	1.6	0.7	−56
Oslo, 1980[10]	785	1.0	0.0	−100	1.0	2.7	+170
MRC, 1985[11]	17,354	0.6	0.4	−33	2.3	2.5	+9
EWPHBP, 1985[12]	840	16.0	11.0	−32	24.0	15.0	−38

MRC, Medical Research Council; EWPHBP, European Working Party on High Blood Pressure in the Elderly Trial.

only minimally elevated pressures, who constitute the largest portion of the hypertensive population, approximately 75 per cent having DBP between 90 and 104 mm Hg. Moreover, elevated blood pressure may not pose the direct risk for coronary disease that it does for stroke, renal damage, and congestive failure, the forms of cardiovascular disease which are "hypertensive" or pressure-related (Table 27–8, p. 826). Coronary disease, in particular, may primarily reflect atherosclerosis whose cause is multifactorial (see Chap. 35), with the acceleration imposed by *mild* hypertension playing only a minor role.

RESULTS OF CLINICAL TRIALS

Thus the inability to show clear protection against coronary disease by reduction of the blood pressure in the six controlled clinical trials which compared active therapy with placebo (Table 28–1) may not reflect a failure of the therapy, but a misguided attempt. Nonetheless, in some of these six controlled trials and in two other large trials wherein therapy was given to all, but more to one half than to the other half, a greater reduction of the blood pressure did protect some of the participants[13, 14] (Table 28–2). In both of the large trials, carried out in the United States, those patients who had normal electrocardiograms at entry were protected by more intensive therapy, whereas those with abnormal entry electrocardiograms suffered higher coronary mortality with more therapy. Because high doses of diuretics were used in these trials and most of the excess coronary mortality was due to sudden death from arrhythmias, the possibility of diuretic-induced hypokalemia as being responsible has been raised.[15]

Whatever the reasons, antihypertensive therapy, *as used in these eight trials*, has not been found clearly to protect against coronary disease, the major cause of morbidity and mortality among hypertensive patients. A diuretic, often in relatively high doses, was the first, and often the only, drug in all of the trials except for half of the treated patients in the Medical Research Council (MRC) trial.

A different approach, specifically the use of a beta blocker as first drug, was used in the other half of the treated patients in the MRC trial. It, too, failed to provide overall protection against coronary disease, other than in the men who did not smoke. A similar selective protection by beta blockers against coronary disease only in nonsmoking males was noted in another large trial,[16] so there may be reason to choose that approach among such patients. More about the choice of drug for therapy will be provided later in this chapter. For now, note should simply be taken that the overall failure to show protection against coronary disease by drug treatment of mild hypertension may not reflect a fault of reduction of the blood pressure, but a fault of the manner by which it was lowered.

One point should be recognized that may bias the results against the demonstration of protection. In most cases the results were analyzed on all subjects who entered the trials, rather than on just those who remained in them. This analysis by "intention to treat" has been defended as giving a more correct answer to the basic question addressed in such trials: "Will those who are started on active therapy benefit more than those who are not?" But the placebo-treated patients whose blood pressure rose to what was defined as too high a level to allow them to remain off active therapy, some 10 per cent to 15 per cent of the placebo group, and who probably would have suffered a high rate of cardiovascular events if left on placebo, were then placed on active therapy. The overall experience in the placebo group, including those removed into active therapy, would thereby look better than it was, and it could therefore be more difficult to show benefit from active therapy.

TABLE 28–2 CORONARY MORTALITY RATES PER 1000 PERSON-YEARS IN PATIENTS WITH OR WITHOUT ECG ABNORMALITIES AT ENTRY

Trial (Reference)	No. of Subjects	Coronary Heart Disease Rate per 1000 Person-Years: Less Therapy	More Therapy	Difference (%)
HDFP[13]*				
Normal ECG	3210	3.1	2.0	−35
Abnormal ECG	1963	3.5	4.3	+23
MRFIT[14]				
Normal ECG	5593	3.4	2.6	−24
Abnormal ECG	2418	2.9	4.9	+70

*The HDFP (Hypertension and Follow-up Program) patients were those men with diastolic blood pressure of between 90 and 104 mm Hg not on antihypertensive therapy at baseline, who were therefore similar to those in the MRFIT (Multiple Risk Factor Intervention Trial) population.

GUIDELINES FOR TREATMENT

Despite these qualifications, the sum of current evidence supports the view that the risks of mild hypertension are not so great and the benefits of active therapy are not so large as to mandate that all be treated. A more aggressive course could be justified if there were no risks or problems associated with active therapy but, in all trials, 20 per cent to 40 per cent of patients given drug therapy experienced some adverse effects, seldom life-threatening but often enough to interfere with the quality of life.

In view of the legitimate concerns arising from the evidence now available, a reconsideration of the common practice of "shooting everything that moves" seems appropriate. The need for active drug therapy for those with moderate or severe hypertension, i.e., DBP above 105 mm Hg, is incontrovertible. Nonetheless, there is a need to insure that their pressure is persistently elevated: Among the patients enrolled in the Australian trial whose DBP was between 105 and 109 after two sets of readings 4 weeks apart, 11 per cent of those given only placebo pills had DBP persistently below 90 mm Hg for the next 4 years. Their blood pressure fell mostly during the first 4 months. Therefore, unless there is an obvious need for the more immediate institution of drug therapy, such as progressive target organ damage or blood pressures so high as to threaten immediate danger, all patients should be given the opportunity to achieve a spontaneous reduction of their initially high pressures over a 4- to 6-month interval. During that time they should have their pressures carefully monitored, since if it goes up—as it did in 10 per cent to 15 per cent of the placebo-treated patients in the six trials shown in Table 28–1—immediate institution of drug therapy may be indicated.

The monitoring logically can be done at home and, perhaps in the near future, with ambulatory 24-hour monitoring, which may provide, in a condensed manner, better prognostic evidence than multiple blood pressure measurements taken in the office.[17] While the blood pressure is being monitored, the use of appropriate non-drug therapies may help lower the pressure even more, without risk and with relatively little inconvenience. Such non-drug therapies may not only lower the blood pressure, but also reduce overall cardiovascular risk by relief of such conditions as hyperlipidemia, glucose intolerance, and alcohol abuse (p. 866).

THE LEVEL OF BLOOD PRESSURE TO TREAT

Uncertainty remains as to the ability of drug therapy to protect against coronary disease in those with mild hypertension. Nonetheless, successful reduction of elevated blood pressure will protect against progression of hypertension, stroke, and, probably, congestive heart failure and renal damage. Therefore, drug therapy is indicated in *all* with DBP persistently above 100 mm Hg, in many with DBP above 95 mm Hg, and in some with DBP above 90 mm Hg or an even lower level.

The risk associated with elevations of systolic pressure has been shown to be even more linear and equally strong than with elevations of diastolic pressure (p. 820). Unfortunately, most trials have mainly considered DBP levels, so that there is less evidence concerning the levels of systolic blood pressure that mandate therapy. This is particularly true among the large segment of elderly people with predominant or pure systolic hypertension. A trial to determine whether therapy will protect them has been begun,[18] but it will probably be 1994 or later before the results are known. Meantime, elevations of systolic pressure above 170 mm Hg, at any age, deserve gradual reduction by appropriate non-drug and drug therapies.

Rationale for Use of Different Levels

The benefit of treating all patients with persistent DBP above 100 mm Hg seems well established on the basis of the clinical trials shown in Table 28–1. The evidence for benefit of those with DBP above 95 mm Hg is less certain but reasonably strong (Fig. 28–1). These curves[16] show progressive falls in both cardiac events and stroke when blood pressures were reduced from above 110 to below 95 mm Hg. Below 95 mm Hg no significant falls in the already quite low event rates were observed. Similar protection in those whose initial readings were above 95 mm Hg was demonstrated in the Australian[9] and the MRC[11] trials. In the latter, overall protection was not shown for women, probably because the event rates among the nontreated women with DBP below 100 mm Hg was so low that little protection could be demonstrated.

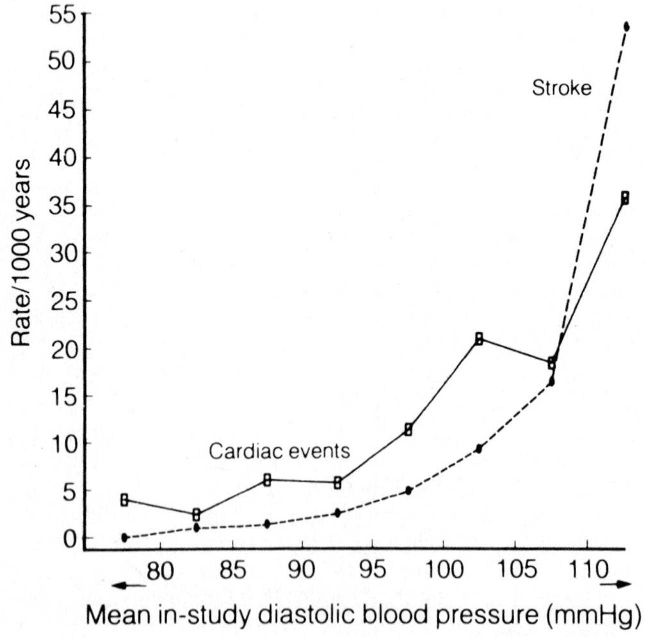

FIGURE 28–1. Absolute rate of cardiac events and stroke related to diastolic blood pressure during antihypertensive treatment. The extremes of the diastolic pressure scale include all values at or below 80 and above 110 mm Hg. Square = cardiac events; Circle = stroke. (From IPPPSH Collaborative Group: Cardiovascular risk and risk factors in a randomized trial of treatment based on the beta-blocker oxprenolol: The International Prospective Primary Prevention Study in Hypertension [IPPPSH]. J. Hypertension 3:388, 1985.)

Those with DBP between 90 and 95 mm Hg, who constitute 40 per cent of the entire hypertensive population, have not been found to benefit from drug therapy in the controlled trials shown in Table 28–1. Part of this failure may reflect the finding that many of the patients in these trials were not, in fact, hypertensive: None of the trials required more than a 2-month run-in period before randomization to active or placebo therapy, and it has been shown that as many as one-third to one-half of patients with DBP above 95 will be persistently below 90 after 4 to 6 months *on no therapy.*

In addition, the risks are relatively small at such low levels of elevated blood pressure, and the trials, despite their size and duration, may not have been adequate to show protection with so little preexisting risk. Moreover, the trials mainly involved low-risk, otherwise healthy patients, unlike many seen in clinical practice. In the Hypertension Detection and Follow-up Program (HDFP) trial those patients with initial DBP between 90 and 95 mm Hg whose pressures were lowered more aggressively (the stepped-care group) had fewer cardiovascular events than did those whose pressures were lowered less. Because HDFP was not a placebo-controlled trial, some argue that the lower event rate reflected better general medical care rather than more reduction in blood pressure,[19] but the latter probably played a significant role.[20]

However, the more intensively treated (Special Intervention) half of the patients in the Multiple Risk Factor Intervention trial (MRFIT) whose initial DBP was between 90 and 94 mm Hg had a *higher* total and coronary death rate than did those given less therapy (Usual Care), so the evidence from the two large non-placebo-controlled trials done in the United States remains contradictory.

There is, then, legitimate cause for the disagreement among the experts as to at what level to institute active drug therapy, some believing that drug therapy should be given to all with DBP above 90 mm Hg, others believing that it should be given only to those with DBP above 100 mm Hg. The disagreement is not only of academic interest. As many as 40 million persons in the United States alone are in that 90 to 100 mm Hg range, so obviously the issue has great clinical relevance.

On the basis of available data, the position presented by participants in a conference sponsored by the World Health Organization and the International Society of Hypertension seems to be an appropriate compromise[21] (Fig. 28–2). In substance, it states that after 3 to 6 months of observation, 95 mm Hg DBP should be used as the level for institution of active drug therapy. Some patients who are at high overall risk should probably be treated even if they have lower levels of DBP. Included in this group are diabetics who have early evidence of glomerulosclerosis that will surely progress if untreated. For such patients, active drug therapy may even be indicated at DBP levels below 90 mm Hg. More clinical trials are needed among such patients, but those at high risk may need the benefits potentially available from a lower blood pressure, despite the risks attendant to the therapy used to achieve the lower pressure.

Although it has not been possible to predict with certainty which patients will develop complications, the larger the number of other cardiovascular risk factors present,

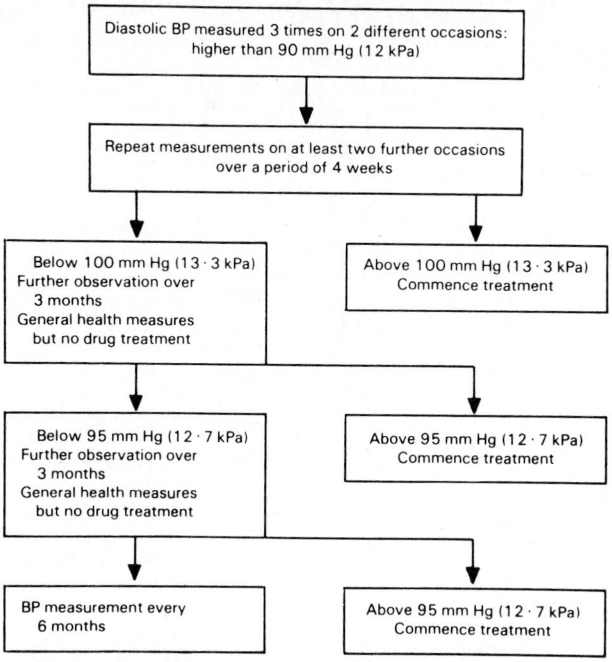

FIGURE 28–2. Definition, blood pressure (BP) measurement, and management of mild hypertension. (From WHO/ISH: 1986 guidelines for the treatment of hypertension: Memorandum from a WHO/ISH meeting. Bull. WHO *64*:293, 1986.)

the larger the number of complications observed.[22] The importance of cigarette smoking has been particularly emphasized.[11] Because of their relatively lower degree of risk at every level of pressure, women are relatively less in need of therapy than are men. The level for instituting therapy in most women may appropriately be a DBP of 100 mm Hg, rather than the level of 95 for most men.

THE LEVEL OF BLOOD PRESSURE TO REACH

Once having decided to treat, the clinician should aim for as low a blood pressure as can be reached with reasonable amounts of medication and with minimal side

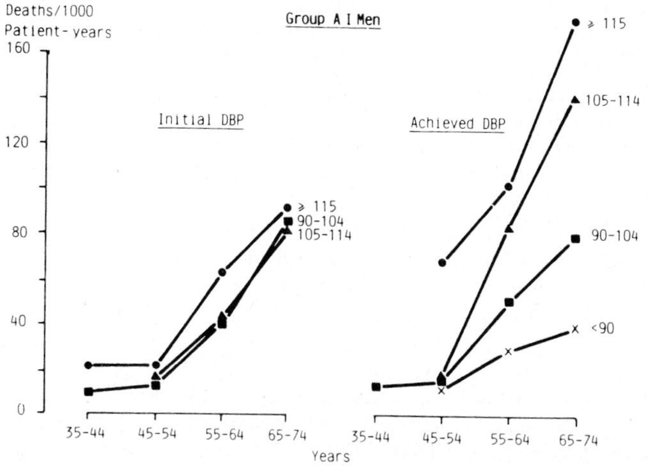

FIGURE 28–3. Age-specific mortality rates (death/1000 patient-years) for a subset of 1162 men not initially on therapy whose blood pressures were measured both at entry to the clinic and thereafter during treatment. At all ages the influence of achieved blood pressure on mortality was greater than that of initial blood pressure. DBP = diastolic blood pressure. (From Isles, C. G., Walker, L. M., Beevers, G. D., Brown, I., Cameron, H. L., Clarke, J., Hawthorne, V., Hole, D., Lever, A. F., Robertson, J. W. K., and Wapshaw, J. A.: Mortality in patients of the Glasgow Blood Pressure Clinic. J. Hypertension 4:146, 1986.)

effects. As found in the Australian,[9] MRC,[11] and the International Prospective Primary Prevention Study in Hypertension (IPPPSH)[16] trials and documented further by clinical experience,[1, 23] mortality rates in patients receiving therapy are little affected by the initial pretreatment level of blood pressure but are closely related to the level of blood pressure achieved during therapy (Fig. 28–3); the lower the level achieved, the less the mortality.

It appears, then, that the lower the blood pressure on therapy the better, even if many with equally low blood pressures without therapy may not be at enough risk to mandate the institution of therapy. This suggests that there are risks associated with therapy and, in order to overcome them, the pressure must be lowered to levels below what would ordinarily be needed. Other explanations for the higher mortality noted among treated hypertensives may clarify the apparent inability to reduce risk to the degree observed at the same levels of blood pressure without therapy. These include inadequate control of the blood pressure, risks inherently related to hypertension that cannot be overcome, and inclusion of more "high-risk" subjects in clinical trials.

Regardless, risks from therapy cannot be discounted, emphasizing the need for care in deciding to institute therapy, in choosing the drugs to be used, and in monitoring the patient's progress. Once therapy is started, the blood pressure should be reduced to below 140/90 mm Hg and, if feasible, to near 120/80. Despite the attraction of this approach, some patients may suffer if blood pressures are lowered to "normal" levels. Some of these adverse effects are related to overly aggressive therapy, with precipitous falls to hypotensive levels.[24] However, some are not so easily explained,[25] so that one must be willing to accept less than ideal control for some patients. The development of impotence in men may be a fairly common reflection of lowering of the blood pressure to levels that do not seem to be too low but that may be insufficient to maintain adequate blood flow through vessels which are already partially occluded by atherosclerosis.

Once having achieved good control, it may be possible to reduce or withdraw drug therapy. Perhaps one-fourth of patients with initially mild hypertension who achieve good control with therapy will remain normotensive for at least 1 year after their therapy is stopped.[26] Such patients need to remain under observation.

There is no single answer to the question of whom to treat with drugs for mild hypertension. Each patient must be considered separately, taking various factors into account. The foregoing discussion should indicate the wisdom of withholding drug therapy from many of these patients, at least until the effects of time and non-drug therapies have been given a chance.

NON-DRUG THERAPY

Interest in the use of various non-drug therapies for the treatment of hypertension, particularly diet and exercise, has risen markedly in the past few years. Yet many practitioners either do not use them or use them in a casual, perfunctory manner. This hesitant attitude can be attributed both to the sparsity of firm evidence indicating that these therapies succeed and to the difficulty many have faced in convincing patients to adhere to them. This situation is likely to change: Evidence for the effectiveness of these approaches is growing, techniques for improving adherence are being popularized, and patients seem increasingly willing to adopt changes in life style. These changes come at a propitious time, when many more people are being identified as hypertensive and are considered in need of lowering their blood pressure. Although most have turned first to drugs, the evidence presented in the previous section suggests that these can be safely withheld from many hypertensives to allow non-drug therapies a chance to be effective.

In part, the underuse of non-drug therapies is due to the excitement over newly available drugs and the massive advertising campaigns to promote their use. Without commercial advocates, non-drug therapies have been unable to compete. Moreover, when physicians decide to treat a condition, they expect immediate results with virtual certainty. Such expectations were clearly justified when the majority of patients had fairly severe hypertension; however, as the large number of patients with mild hypertension enter the picture, a more relaxed, gradual approach to their management seems more appropriate.

Just as the increased awareness of the problem of patients' frequent poor adherence to drug therapy has led to attempts to improve the situation,[27] similar attention toward adherence to non-drug therapies will probably improve their effectiveness. These measures should be introduced gradually and gently. Too many and too drastic changes in life style may discourage patients from accepting needed care. Eventually, however, all hypertensive patients should benefit from mild restriction of dietary salt, reduction of excess body weight, and moderation of alcohol intake.[28] Although high blood lipid levels and cigarette smoking have little, if any, direct effect on blood pressure, patients with hypertension should be encouraged to eliminate their risk factors that predispose to cardiovascular disease (see Chap. 36).

WEIGHT REDUCTION. In most published studies, weight loss has been shown to reduce blood pressure.[29] In two of the better-controlled studies, performed by the same investigators, overweight hypertensives were randomly assigned to a placebo pill, a beta blocker, or a diet reduced by 1,000 kcal per day for 21 weeks; those on the diet had a great fall in blood pressure, a reduction in left ventricular mass, and an improvement in blood lipids (Table 28–3).[30, 31]

These studies are among the best published to document the antihypertensive efficacy of weight reduction; however, there may be a floor below which further weight loss may not be accompanied by further falls in blood pressure.[32] Although the rate of recidivism among obese people may be high, an attempt at weight reduction in all obese hypertensive patients should be made, using whatever

TABLE 28–3 EFFECTS OF 21 WEEKS OF THERAPY IN THREE GROUPS OF OBESE HYPERTENSIVES

	Weight Reduction	Metoprolol	Placebo
Weight (kg)	−8.3	+2.5	+0.5
Systolic blood pressure (mm Hg)	−14.2	−12.4	−8.9
Diastolic blood pressure (mm Hg)	−12.7	−7.5	−4.4
Left ventricular mass index (gm/m²)	−14.8	−1.3	−1.5
Total cholesterol (% change)	−6%	−4%	+3%
HDL-cholesterol (% change)	+6%	−10%	+2%

From MacMahon, S. W., et al.: Comparison of weight reduction with metoprolol in treatment of hypertension in young overweight patients. Lancet *1*:1233, 1985; and MacMahon, S. W., et al.: The effect of weight reduction on left ventricular mass. A randomized controlled trial in young, overweight hypertensive patients. N. Engl. J. Med. *314*:334, 1986.

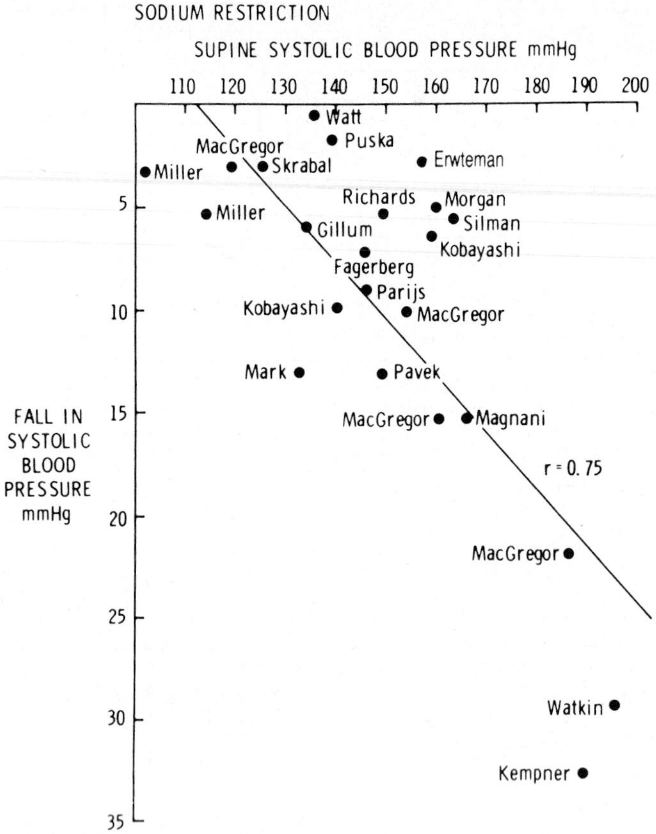

FIGURE 28–4. Fall in supine systolic blood pressure with sodium restriction plotted against pretreatment supine systolic blood pressure in data from published studies whose first author is indicated. (From MacGregor, G. A.: Sodium is more important than calcium in essential hypertension. Hypertension 7:633, 1985 by permission of the American Heart Association, Inc.)

level of caloric restriction the patient is able to maintain. The discovery that they have hypertension may be a strong motivation for patients to reduce. A further incentive may be the knowledge that if weight reduction succeeds in lowering blood pressure, the need for taking medications may be delayed or even avoided.

DIETARY SODIUM RESTRICTION. On page 830 evidence was presented incriminating the typically high sodium content of the diet of people living in acculturated, industrialized societies as a cause of hypertension. Once hypertension is present, modest salt restriction may help lower the blood pressure. In common with all forms of therapy, both drug and non-drug, the extent of the fall in blood pressure observed with varying degrees of sodium restriction tends to increase with increasing pretreatment levels of pressure (Fig. 28–4).[33]

Not all hypertensives will respond to the moderate degree of sodium restriction used in most of these studies, to a level of 70 to 100 mmol sodium, or approximately 2 gm, per day. The varying responsiveness may reflect one or more observed differences among patients on lower sodium intakes, including (a) variable degrees of activation of counterregulatory mechanisms, such as the renin-aldosterone system[34] and catecholamines[35]; (b) variable changes in the activity of the sodium-potassium pump and other membrane transport systems[36, 37]; and (c) variable degrees of underlying modulation of adrenal, renal, or other vascular responses.[38]

More rigid degrees of sodium restriction are not only difficult for patients to achieve, but may also be counterproductive: The marked stimulation of renin-aldosterone that accompanies rigid sodium restriction may prevent the blood pressure from falling and increase the amount of potassium wastage if diuretics are concomitantly used.[39] In animals, low sodium intake, down to levels of only 1:100 of usual intake, may stunt growth,[40] but this hardly seems to be a legitimate concern in humans.

Even if the blood pressure does not fall with moderate degrees of sodium restriction, the patient may still benefit: Improved arterial distensibility,[41] increased antihypertensive effectiveness of other drugs, with the apparent exception of slow-channel calcium blockers,[42] and less diuretic-induced potassium wastage[39] have all been reported among patients on moderate sodium restriction. Although there is no assurance that moderate sodium restriction will help, there is no evidence that it will hurt. Therefore, the author considers it to be useful for all persons, as a preventive measure in those who are normotensive and, more certainly, as partial therapy in those who are hypertensive.

The easiest way to accomplish moderate sodium restriction is to substitute natural foods for processed foods, since natural foods are low in sodium and high in potassium, whereas most processed foods have had sodium added and potassium removed. Additional guidelines include the following:

1. Add no sodium chloride to food during cooking or at the table.
2. If a salty taste is desired, use a half sodium and half potassium chloride preparation, such as Morton's Lite Salt, or a pure potassium chloride substitute.
3. Avoid or minimize the use of "fast" foods, many of which have high sodium content.
4. Recognize the sodium content of some antacids and proprietary medications. Whereas Alka-Seltzer contains more than 500 mg of sodium, Rolaids are virtually salt free.

In order to insure adherence to the diet, occasionally measuring the sodium content of an overnight urine collection may be helpful, particularly if the patient is given immediate feedback as to its content so that if additional instruction is needed, it can be provided at that visit.[43]

POTASSIUM SUPPLEMENTATION. Some of the advantages of a lower sodium intake may relate to its tendency to increase body potassium content, both by a coincidental increase in dietary potassium intake and by a decrease in potassium wastage if diuretics are being used. Although potassium deficiency clearly exerts multiple effects that may increase the blood pressure,[44] evidence that correction of hypokalemia[45] or addition of dietary potassium to normokalemics will lower the blood pressure is skimpy.[46, 47] Nonetheless, diuretic-induced hypokalemia may be more of a danger than many suspect, so that, for various reasons, hypertensive patients should be protected from potassium depletion.

MAGNESIUM SUPPLEMENTATION. The only well-controlled trial found no effect on the blood pressure of giving 15 mmol per day of magnesium to normomagnesemic hypertensives.[48] However, those who are magnesium depleted may not be able to replete concomitant potassium deficiency.[49]

CALCIUM SUPPLEMENTATION. As noted on page 834, an increase in free intracellular calcium may be a final step in the pathogenesis of essential hypertension. Nonetheless, hypertensive patients may have a lower calcium intake and higher urinary calcium excretion than do normotensives.[50] In short-term studies about half of hypertensives given 1 gm of supplemental calcium per day have a fall in blood pressure.[51, 52] Because others given calcium supplements may have a rise in blood pressure, the best course is to insure that calcium intake is not inadvertently reduced by reduction of milk and cheese in an attempt to reduce saturated fat and sodium intake but not to give supplemental calcium unless an antihypertensive effect is substantiated.

OTHER DIETARY CHANGES. Some lowering of the blood pressure has been noted in studies of a lacto-ovo-vegetarian diet,[53] a high-fiber, low-fat, low-sodium diet,[54] and a diet high in fish oil.[55] Such diets may be helpful in various other ways to reduce cardiovascular risk and may be particularly useful in hypertensive diabetics.[56]

When consumed by non-coffee drinkers, caffeine equivalent to the amount in three cups of coffee will raise the blood pressure, probably by activation of the sympathetic nervous system.[57] However, chronic caffeine ingestion is not associated with significant rises in blood pressure because of tolerance to the hemodynamic effects.

MODERATION OF ALCOHOL. Moderate alcohol consumption, less than 1 oz of ethanol per day, does not increase the prevalence of hypertension. Heavier drinking clearly exerts a pressor effect that makes *alcohol abuse the most common cause of reversible hypertension.*[58] One to two portions of alcohol-containing beverages a day, containing 0.5 to 1.0 oz of ethanol, need not be prohibited, particularly since fewer coronary events have been noted in those who consume that amount.[59] Such protection from coronary disease was demonstrable in subjects who consumed a moderate amount of alcohol in a regular, consistent pattern but not among binge drinkers of similar amounts of alcohol.[60]

ISOTONIC EXERCISE. Isometric exercise, such as weight-lifting, pushing, and pulling, may be harmful to the hypertensive patient. During an isometric contraction, blood pressure rises often to high levels by a reflex mechanism. On the other hand, in well-controlled studies, regular isotonic exercise has resulted in a 5 to 10 mm Hg reduction in blood pressure, accompanied by, and probably related to, a fall in sympathetic nervous activity.[61, 62]

RELAXATION TECHNIQUES. Various forms of relaxation—transcendental meditation, yoga, biofeedback, psychotherapy—have reduced the blood pressure of some hypertensives, at least transiently.[63] Most studies have been poorly controlled, but an impressive effect was observed by Patel et al.[64] They randomly assigned half of a group of newly identified hypertensives to a biofeedback-aided relaxation program for 8 weeks, while the other half served as controls, being seen as often but not given the relaxation therapy. Both at the end of the active program and 4 years later (during which time the subjects had been asked to continue to practice relaxation but had not been seen), blood pressures among the treated group were significantly lowered.

THE POTENTIAL OF NON-DRUG THERAPY

Part of the antihypertensive effect reported with these and other non-drug therapies may be attributable to the nonspecific fall in blood pressure so often seen when repeated readings are taken. Such decreases may reflect a statistical regression toward the mean, a placebo effect, or a relief of anxiety and stress with time. The same phenomenon is probably also responsible for much of the initial response to drug therapy, so that success may be attributed to both drugs and non-drugs when it is deserved by neither.

Few long-term studies of the effectiveness of non-drug therapies have been carried out. Two are now in progress, involving former participants in the HDFP trial who have been taken off their antihypertensive therapy and followed on various non-drug regimens, including sodium restriction or weight reduction, to see how many remain normotensive compared with those on no therapy.[65, 66] Preliminary results show that about one-third more remain normotensive on non-drug therapy than on no therapy.

Whether such success can be achieved by individual practitioners is uncertain. However, because help is available, including various educational materials for patients, professional assistants such as dietitians and psychologists, and groups organized for weight reduction, exercise, and relaxation therapies, the effort seems both increasingly easy and likely to be successful in lowering blood pressure.

ANTIHYPERTENSIVE DRUG THERAPY

If the non-drug therapies described above are not followed or turn out to be ineffective, or if the level of hypertension at the onset is so high that immediate drug therapy is deemed necessary, the general guidelines listed in Table 28–4 should be helpful in improving patient adherence to lifelong treatment. More detailed guidance is also available.[67]

GENERAL GUIDELINES

Most of the points listed in Table 28–4 are rather obvious, but a few deserve additional comment. Item 5E, "Use the fewest daily doses needed," has not been found to influence adherence significantly, but patients prefer to take medications less frequently.[68] At present, most antihypertensive medications can be given to most patients either once or twice a day. Although a few patients may be better controlled with more frequent doses, even patients with end-organ damage and resistant hypertension can often be managed by once-a-day therapy. In 55 such patients, a once-a-day regimen of diuretic, minoxidil, and nadolol controlled 46 for almost a year, although 6 had intolerable side effects.[69]

PHARMACOLOGICAL PRINCIPLES. Item 6b in Table 28–4 suggests starting with small doses of medication, aiming for a reduction of 5 to 10 mm Hg in blood pressure at each step. Some physicians, by nature and training, desire to control a patient's hypertension rapidly and completely. Regardless of which drugs are used, this approach often leads to easy fatigability, weakness, and postural dizziness, a feeling of being washed out, which many patients find intolerable, particularly when they felt well before therapy was begun. Although hypokalemia and other electrolyte abnormalities may be responsible for some of these symptoms, a more likely explanation has been provided by the studies of Strandgaard and Paulson.[70] As shown in the top half of Figure 28–5, they reconfirmed the constancy of cerebral blood flow by autoregulation over a range of mean arterial pressures from about 60 to 120 mm Hg in normal subjects and from 110 to 180 mm Hg in patients with hypertension. This shift to the right protects the hypertensive patient from a surge of blood flow, which could cause cerebral edema. However, the shift also predisposes the hypertensive patient to cerebral ischemia when blood pressure is lowered.

TABLE 28–4 GENERAL GUIDELINES TO IMPROVE PATIENT ADHERENCE TO ANTIHYPERTENSIVE THERAPY

1. Be aware of the problem and be alert to signs of patient nonadherence.
2. Establish the goal of therapy: to reduce blood pressure to normotensive levels with minimal or no side effects.
3. Educate the patient about his disease and its treatment.
4. Maintain contact with the patient.
   a. Encourage visits and calls to allied health personnel.
   b. Allow the pharmacist to monitor therapy.
   c. Make contact with patients who do not return.
5. Keep care inexpensive and simple.
   a. Do the least work-up needed to rule out secondary causes.
   b. Obtain follow-up laboratory data only yearly unless indicated more often.
   c. Use home blood pressure readings.
   d. Use non-drug, no-cost therapies.
   e. Use the fewest daily doses of drugs needed.
   f. If appropriate, use combination tablets.
6. Prescribe according to pharmacological principles.
   a. Add one drug at a time.
   b. Start with small doses, aiming for 5 to 10 mm Hg reductions at each step.
   c. Prevent volume overload with adequate diuretic and sodium restriction.
   d. Be willing to stop unsuccessful therapy and try a different approach.
   e. Anticipate side effects.
   f. Adjust therapy to ameliorate side effects that do not spontaneously disappear.
   g. Continue to add drugs, stepwise, in sufficient doses to achieve the goal of therapy.

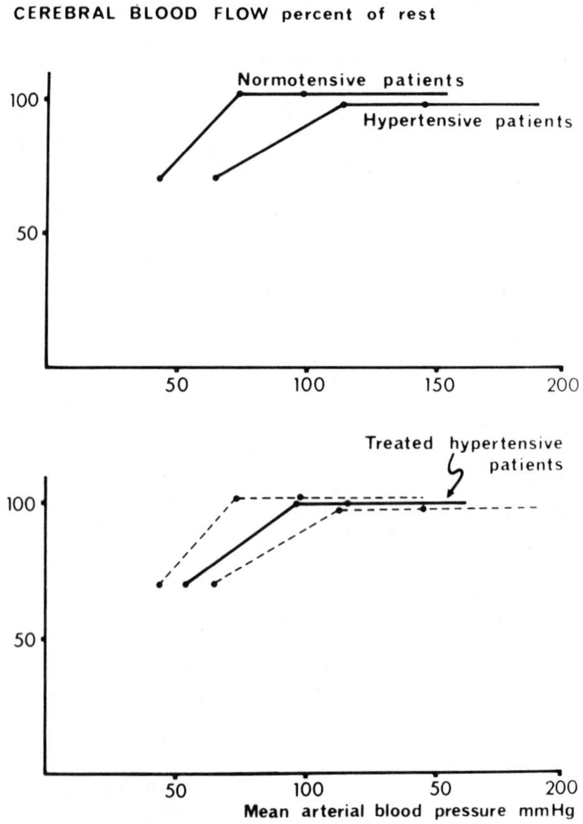

FIGURE 28–5. Idealized curves of cerebral blood flow showing the range of autoregulation in normotensive and hypertensive patients (upper graph) and the shift back toward normal after antihypertensive therapy (lower graph). The lower limit of autoregulation maintaining a normal cerebral blood flow is a mean arterial blood pressure of about 60 mm Hg in normotensive and 110 in hypertensive individuals. (From Strandgaard, S.: Autoregulation of cerebral blood flow in hypertensive patients. Circulation *53*:720, 1976, by permission of the American Heart Association, Inc.)

The lower limit of autoregulation necessary to preserve a constant cerebral blood flow in hypertensive patients is a mean of about 110 mm Hg. Thus acutely lowering the pressure from 160/110 (mean = 127) to 140/85 (mean = 102) may induce cerebral hypoperfusion, although hypotension in the accepted sense has not been produced. This provides an explanation for what many patients experience at the start of antihypertensive therapy, i.e., manifestations of cerebral hypoperfusion, even though blood pressure levels do not seem inordinately low.

These observations suggest the need for a gradual approach to antihypertensive therapy in order to avoid symptoms related to overly aggressive blood pressure reduction. Fortunately, as shown in the bottom of Figure 28–5, if therapy is continued for a period of time, the curve of cerebral autoregulation shifts back toward normal, allowing patients to tolerate greater reductions in blood pressure without experiencing symptoms. Recent work points to differences in the effects of different types of antihypertensive drugs on cerebral blood flow: Both alpha blockers and converting enzyme inhibitors (CEIs) appear to improve autoregulation, whereas direct vasodilators do not.[70, 71]

STEPPED CARE. Item 6 in Table 28–4 refers to the addition of drugs, stepwise, in sufficient doses to achieve the goal of therapy. Over the past 30 years the purely empirical basis for the use of antihypertensive drugs has gradually been replaced by a more rational and effective stepped-care approach,[72] which involves use of a diuretic or an adrenergic blocking drug first and stepwise addition of other drugs as needed.

Attempts have been made to provide an even more scientific basis for selecting the drug, an approach that more closely fits a patient's hemodynamic disturbance.[73] This approach, based on the renin profile, divides hypertensive patients into those with lower renin levels, i.e., "volume" or "wet" hypertension, or higher renins, i.e., "vasoconstriction" or "dry" hypertension, and advocates the use of diuretics, calcium channel blockers, or postsynaptic alpha blockers for the lower renin portion and CEI's or beta blockers for those with high renin levels. The concept is attractive, but as detailed on page 829, almost all hypertension is associated with increased peripheral resistance and the actual measurements of volume and vasoconstriction do not uphold use of the plasma renin levels as a simple indicator for these hemodynamic variables. Moreover, a single renin measurement may not be a certain indicator of a patient's long-term status. Fortunately, simple demographics may serve as well: Younger and white patients (who generally have higher renin levels) tend to respond better to CEI's and beta blockers; older and black patients (who generally have lower renin levels) respond better to diuretics, calcium channel blockers, and, perhaps, alpha blockers.

Rather than always starting with a diuretic, the preference of 90 per cent of U.S. physicians in a recent survey,[2] the more rational approach would be to pick one or another drug on the basis of various patient features: age, race, concomitant diseases, propensity to side effects. If the first choice works poorly or causes side effects, a drug from another class would logically be substituted. Thereby, the patient should receive the least number of drugs with the greatest likelihood of a "tailored" response.

Some continue to advocate a diuretic as the first drug because of its relative ease of use, long-term effectiveness, and low cost.[74] However, problems with diuretics continue to surface.[75] These problems may explain the higher mortality rate observed in those with preexisting electrocardiographic abnormalities who were more intensively treated in the HDFP and MRFIT trials.[13, 14] Therefore, the use of other drugs as an alternative to a diuretic as the first step in therapy is likely to become more common practice.

For those with severer hypertension, in whom the first choice can be expected to be only partially effective, the stepped-care approach makes good scientific sense. A diuretic will enhance the effectiveness of most other drugs used, preventing the "pseudotolerance" that develops because of the fluid retention that frequently follows the use of some adrenergic blocking drugs and vasodilators.[76] In addition, supplemental use of a vasodilator as the third drug, required in about 10 per cent of patients whose hypertension is not controlled by a diuretic and adrenergic blocking drug, has been shown to be eminently sound on pharmacological grounds as well.[77]

DIURETICS

Diuretics useful in the treatment of hypertension may be divided into four major groups by their primary site of action within the tubule, starting in the proximal portion and moving to the collecting duct:[78] (1) agents acting on the proximal tubule, such as carbonic anhydrase inhibitors, which have limited antihypertensive efficacy; (2) loop diuretics; (3) thiazides and related sulfonamide compounds; and (4) potassium-sparing agents (Fig. 17–12, p. 514). A thiazide is the usual choice, often in combination with a potassium-sparing agent. Loop diuretics should be reserved for those patients with renal insufficiency or resistant hypertension.

MODE OF ACTION. All diuretics initially lower the blood pressure by increasing urinary sodium excretion and by reducing plasma volume, extracellular fluid volume, and cardiac output. Within 6 to 8 weeks the lowered plasma, extracellular fluid volume, and cardiac output return toward normal. At this point and beyond the lower blood pressure is related to a fall in peripheral resistance, thereby improving the underlying hemodynamic defect of hypertension. The mechanism responsible for the lowered peripheral resistance is unknown, but there is a need for an initial diuresis, since diuretics fail to lower the blood pressure in chronic dialysis patients with nonfunctioning kidneys.[79] With the shrinkage in volume and lower blood pressure, increased secretion of renin and aldosterone retard the continued sodium diuresis. Both renin-induced vasoconstriction and aldosterone-induced sodium retention prevent continued diminution of body fluids and progressive fall in blood pressure while diuretic therapy is continued.

CLINICAL EFFECTS. With continuous diuretic therapy, blood pressure usually falls about 10 mm Hg, although the degree depends on various factors, including the initial height of the pressure, the quantity of sodium ingested, the adequacy of renal function, and the intensity of the counterregulatory renin–aldosterone response. As with other antihypertensive agents, the reduction of pressure may be much greater in severer than in milder hypertension: In 227 hypertensive patients treated for up to 12 years with diuretics alone, mean blood pressure fell from 203/121 to 162/97; in 50 per cent, DBP was reduced to below 100 mm Hg.[80] As shown in this study, the antihypertensive effect of the diuretic persists indefinitely, although it may be overwhelmed by dietary sodium intake above 8 gm per day.

If other drugs are used, a diuretic may also be needed. Without a concomitant diuretic, antihypertensive drugs that do not block the renin–aldosterone mechanism may cause sodium retention. This mechanism probably reflects the success of the drugs in lowering the blood pressure and may involve the abnormal renal pressure–natriuresis relationship that is presumably present in primary hypertension (p. 831). Just as it takes more pressure to excrete a given load of sodium in the hypertensive individual, so does a lowering of pressure toward normal incite sodium retention. The hypertensive kidney is consistent: High pressure is needed for normal sodium excretion; normal pressure is considered to be too low, so sodium is retained.

The critical need for adequate diuretic therapy to keep intravascular volume diminished has been repeatedly documented.[76] Therefore, diuretics are likely to continue to be widely used in antihypertensive therapy. Newer agents, however, such as calcium blockers and CEI's, may continue to maintain lower blood pressure without inducing sodium retention, so that diuretics may not be needed when they are used.

DOSAGE AND CHOICE OF AGENT. Most patients with mild to moderate hypertension and reasonably intact renal function, i.e., serum creatinine below 2.0 mg/dl, will respond to the lower doses of the various diuretics listed in Table 28–5. An amount equivalent to 25 mg of hydrochlorothiazide is usually adequate; larger doses will have some additional antihypertensive effect but at the price of additional potassium wastage.[81] For uncomplicated hypertension, a moderately long-acting thiazide is a logical choice and a single morning dose of hydrochlorothiazide will provide a 24-hour antihypertensive effect.[82] When a short-acting drug (furosemide, 40 mg given twice daily) was compared with a longer-acting drug (hydrochlorothiazide, 50 mg give twice daily), blood pressure was lowered significantly only with the longer-acting drug.[83]

With renal insufficiency, manifested by a serum creatinine level above 2.5 mg/dl or creatinine clearance below 25 ml/min, thiazides are usually not effective, and multiple doses of furosemide or a single dose of metolazone will be needed.[84]

TABLE 28–5 DIURETICS AND POTASSIUM-SPARING AGENTS AVAILABLE IN 1987

	Daily Dosage (mg)	Duration of Action (hours)
Thiazides		
Bendroflumethiazide (Naturetin)	2.5–5.0	More than 18
Benzthiazide (Aquatag, Exna)	12.5–50	12–18
Chlorothiazide (Diuril)	250–500	6–12
Cyclothiazide (Anhydron)	1–2	18–24
Hydrochlorothiazide (Esidrix, HydroDiuril, Oretic)	12.5–50	12–18
Hydroflumethiazide (Saluron)	12.5–50	18–24
Methyclothiazide (Enduron)	2.5–5.0	More than 24
Polythiazide (Renese)	1–4	24–48
Trichlormethiazide (Metahydrin, Naqua)	1–4	More than 24
Related sulfonamide compounds		
Chlorthalidone (Hygroton)	12.5–50	24–72
Indapamide (Lozol)	2.5	24
Metolazone (Zaroxolyn, Diulo)	1.0–5.0	24
Quinethazone (Hydromox)	50–100	18–24
Loop diuretics		
Bumetanide (Bumex)	1–10	4–6
Ethacrynic acid (Edecrin)	50–200	12
Furosemide (Lasix)	40–480	4–6
Potassium-sparing agents		
Amiloride (Midamor)	5–10	24
Spironolactone (Aldactone)	25–100	8–12
Triamterene (Dyrenium)	50–100	12

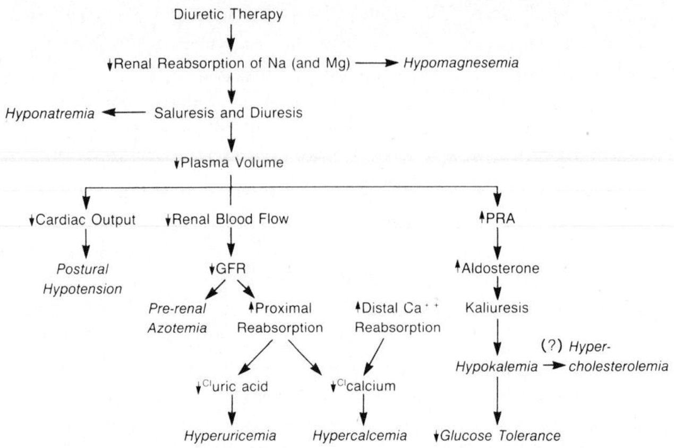

FIGURE 28–6. The mechanisms by which chronic diuretic therapy may lead to various complications. The mechanism for hypercholesterolemia remains in question, although it is shown as arising via hypokalemia. (From Kaplan, N. M.: Clinical Hypertension, 4th ed. Baltimore, © by Williams and Wilkins, 1986, p. 192.)

SIDE EFFECTS. A number of biochemical changes often accompany successful diuresis, including a decrease in plasma potassium and increases in glucose and cholesterol (Fig. 28–6).

Hypokalemia. Serum potassium falls an average of 0.67 mmol/liter after institution of continuous, daily diuretic therapy for hypertension.[85] Among 158 hypertensives given diuretics for 2 years, plasma potassium levels fell to between 3.0 and 3.3 mmol/liter in 29 per cent and to between 2.6 and 2.9 mmol/liter in 7 per cent.[86] This fall in serum concentration may not reflect a significant decrease in total body potassium, nor may it progress after the initial increase in lumen flow rate.[87] Nonetheless, it may precipitate potentially hazardous ventricular ectopic activity, even in patients not known to be susceptible because of concomitant digitalis therapy or myocardial irritability.[88] The arrhythmogenic effect of diuretic-induced hypokalemia may become manifest only at times of stress, when catecholamines may lower the plasma potassium level another 0.5 to 1.0 mmol/liter.[89] Although not all believe that patients with diuretic-induced hypokalemia have an increased propensity to cardiac arrhythmias,[90] increased frequencies of ventricular ectopic activity have been documented in hypokalemic patients with ischemic heart disease[91] or after an acute myocardial infarction.[92]

Most patients are unaware of mild diuretic-induced hypokalemia, although it may contribute to leg cramps, polyuria, and muscle weakness. But subtle interference with antihypertensive therapy may accompany even mild hypokalemia, and correction of hypokalemia may result in a fall in blood pressure.[45] In addition to increasing the propensity to ventricular ectopic activity, hypokalemia may be responsible for the occasional loss of carbohydrate tolerance and the frequent rise in plasma lipids seen with diuretic use.

Prevention of hypokalemia is preferable to correction of potassium deficiency. The following maneuvers should help prevent diuretic-induced hypokalemia:

- Use the smallest amount of diuretic needed.
- Use a moderately long-acting (12- to 18-hour) diuretic, such as hydrochlorothiazide, since longer-acting drugs (e.g., chlorthalidone) may increase potassium loss.[39]
- Restrict sodium intake to less than 100 mmol per day (i.e., 2 gm sodium).
- Increase dietary potassium intake.
- Restrict concomitant use of laxatives.
- Use a combination of a thiazide with a potassium-

sparing agent.[81] If the latter is prescribed, avoid supplemental potassium, since dangerous hyperkalemia may supervene if these drugs are given together.

• The concomitant use of a beta blocker or a CEI may diminish potassium loss, presumably by blunting the diuretic-induced rise in renin–aldosterone.

If hypokalemia is to be treated, the above maneuvers should be instituted, along with some form of supplemental potassium. Potassium chloride is preferred for correction of the associated alkalosis. Despite the occasional appearance of mucosal lesions in the stomach after large doses, slow-release formulations of potassium chloride are both safe and effective, and most patients prefer them to liquid preparations. If tolerated, granular potassium chloride can be given as a salt substitute; thereby, extra potassium will be provided while sodium intake is reduced. Caution is necessary when supplemental potassium chloride is given to older patients with borderline renal function in whom hyperkalemia may be induced.

Hypomagnesemia. In some patients concomitant diuretic-induced magnesium deficiency will prevent the restoration of intracellular deficits of potassium,[49] so that hypomagnesemia should be corrected. Magnesium deficiency may also be responsible for some of the arrhythmias ascribed to hypokalemia.[93]

Hyperuricemia. The serum uric acid level is elevated in as many as one-third of untreated hypertensive patients, particularly in those who are obese. With chronic diuretic therapy, hyperuricemia appears in another third of patients, probably as a consequence of increased proximal tubular reabsorption accompanying volume contraction. Diuretic-induced hyperuricemia only seldom precipitates acute gout or chronic nephropathy, and most agree that it need not be treated. If therapy is used, a uricosuric drug, such as probenecid, should be given. Although allopurinol is often used, it is more likely to cause side effects and is a less rational choice, since the problem is a failure to excrete uric acid and not its overproduction.

Hyperlipidemia. Serum cholesterol levels often rise after diuretic therapy.[75, 94] Although the rise in lipids can be prevented by a diet low in saturated fat,[95] the propensity to worsen the lipid profile may reduce the potential for diuretic therapy to reduce the incidence of coronary disease while it lowers blood pressure.

Hypercalcemia. A slight rise in serum calcium, less than 0.5 mg/dl, is frequently seen with thiazide diuretic therapy, at least in part because increased calcium reabsorption accompanies the increased sodium reabsorption in the proximal tubule induced by contraction of extracellular fluid volume.[96] The rise is of little clinical importance except in patients with previously unrecognized hyperparathyroidism, who may experience a much more marked rise.

Hyperglycemia. Diuretics may impair glucose tolerance and rarely may precipitate diabetes mellitus, perhaps by direct suppression of insulin secretion from the diuretic-induced hypokalemia.[97]

Other Problems. A surprisingly high rate of impotence (22.6 per cent) was found among men taking 10 mg of bendroflumethiazide per day, compared with a rate of 10.1 per cent among those on placebo and 13.2 per cent among those on propranolol in the large MRC trial.[98] This high rate may reflect the rather large dose of the diuretic and perhaps the resultant hypokalemia.

Nonsteroidal antiinflammatory drugs (NSAID's) may inhibit the antihypertensive effects of both thiazides and loop diuretics, presumably by inhibiting the synthesis of vasodilatory prostaglandins in the kidney. Most find that the NSAID agent sulindac, which is less active in the kidney, has less of a tendency to interfere with diuretic action.[99]

OTHER DIURETICS

LOOP DIURETICS. As described on page 870, loop diuretics are usually needed in the treatment of hypertensive patients with renal insufficiency, defined as a serum creatinine above 2.5 mg/dl. Furosemide has been most widely used, although metolazone may work as well and requires only a single daily dose.[84] Many use furosemide in the management of uncomplicated hypertension, but as noted earlier, this drug seems to provide less antihypertensive effect when given once or twice a day than do longer-acting diuretics.

POTASSIUM-SPARING AGENTS. These drugs are normally used in combination with a diuretic. Of the three currently available, one (spironolactone) is an aldosterone antagonist, while the other two (dyrenium and amiloride) are direct inhibitors of potassium secretion. In combination with a thiazide diuretic, they will diminish the amount of potassium wasting.[81] Although they are more expensive than thiazides alone, they may decrease the total cost of therapy by reducing the need to monitor and treat potassium depletion.

AN OVERVIEW OF DIURETICS IN HYPERTENSION

Diuretics have been effective for the treatment of millions of hypertensive patients during the past 30 years. They reduce DBP and maintain it below 90 mm Hg in about half of all hypertensive patients, providing the same degree of effectiveness as most other antihypertensive drugs.[100] In two groups that constitute a rather large portion of the hypertensive population, the elderly[101] and blacks,[102] diuretics may be particularly effective. One diuretic tablet per day is usually all that is needed, minimizing cost and maximizing adherence to therapy.

The side effects of diuretic therapy are usually not overtly bothersome, but the hypokalemia, hypercholesterolemia, and worsening of glucose tolerance that often accompany prolonged diuretic therapy have given rise to increasing concerns about their long-term benignity. This concern has been fueled by the failure of diuretic-based therapy to reduce coronary mortality in the six major trials of the therapy of mild hypertension (Table 28–1). Therefore, the author believes that diuretics will be less commonly used as first drug in the future. When they are used, more care will be taken to monitor and prevent the various biochemical changes they may induce.

ADRENOCEPTOR BLOCKING DRUGS

A number of adrenoceptor blocking drugs are available, including some that act centrally on vasomotor center activity, peripherally on neuronal catecholamine discharge, or by blocking alpha- and/or beta-adrenoceptors (Table 28–6); some act at multiple sites. Figure 28–7, a schematic view of the ending of an adrenergic nerve and the effector cell with its receptors, depicts how some of these drugs act. When the nerve is stimulated, norepinephrine, which is synthesized and stored in granules, is released into the synaptic cleft. It binds to postsynaptic alpha- and beta-adrenoceptors and thereby initiates various intracellular processes. In vascular smooth muscle, alpha stimulation causes constriction and beta stimulation causes relaxation.

TABLE 28–6 ADRENERGIC INHIBITORS USED IN TREATMENT OF HYPERTENSION

1. Peripheral neuronal inhibitors
   a. Reserpine
   b. Guanethidine (Ismelin)
   c. Guanadrel (Hylorel)
   d. Bethanidine (Tenathan)
2. Central adrenergic inhibitors
   a. Methyldopa (Aldomet)
   b. Clonidine (Catapres)
   c. Guanabenz (Wytensin)
3. α-Receptor blockers
   a. α_1- and α_2-receptor
      (1) Phenoxybenzamine (Dibenzyline)
      (2) Phentolamine (Regitine)
   b. α_1-receptor: Prazosin (Minipress)
4. β-Receptor blockers
   a. Acebutolol (Sectral)
   b. Atenolol (Tenormin)
   c. Metoprolol (Lopressor)
   d. Nadolol (Corgard)
   e. Pindolol (Visken)
   f. Propranolol (Inderal)
   g. Timolol (Blocadren)
5. α- and β-receptor blocker: Labetalol (Normodyne, Trandate)

In the central vasomotor centers, sympathetic outflow is inhibited by alpha stimulation; the effect of beta stimulation is unknown.

An important aspect of sympathetic activity involves the feedback of norepinephrine to alpha- and beta-adrenoceptors located on the neuronal surface, i.e., presynaptic receptors.[103] Presynaptic alpha-adrenoceptor activation inhibits release, whereas presynaptic beta-adrenoceptor activation stimulates further norepinephrine release. These presynaptic receptors probably play a role in the action of some of the drugs to be discussed.

Elucidation and quantitation of the various actions of these drugs remain incomplete. The listing in Table 28–6 is based on the predominant site of action according to currently available data. The action of beta-adrenoceptor blockers probably depends on a peripheral effect but then almost certainly also act on central vasomotor mechanisms.

DRUGS THAT ACT WITHIN THE NEURON

Reserpine, guanethidine, and related compounds act to inhibit the release of norepinephrine from peripheral adrenergic neurons, each in a different manner.

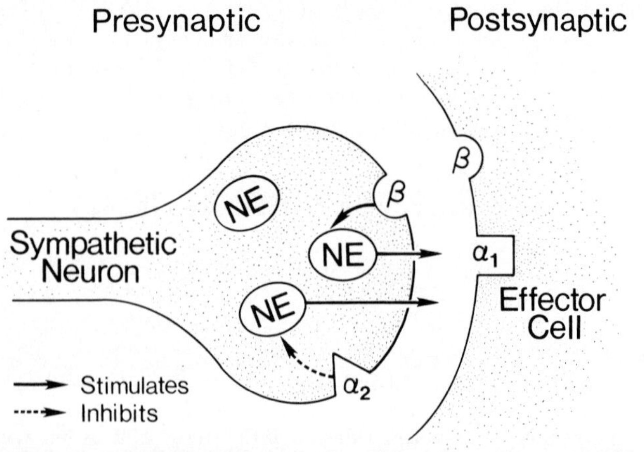

FIGURE 28–7. Simplified schematic view of the adrenergic nerve ending showing that norepinephrine (NE) is released from its storage granules when the nerve is stimulated and enters the synaptic cleft to bind to alpha$_1$ and beta receptors on the effector cell (postsynaptic). In addition, a short feedback loop exists, in which NE binds to alpha$_2$ and beta receptors on the neuron (presynaptic), to inhibit or to stimulate further release, respectively.

RESERPINE. Reserpine, the most active and widely used of the derivatives of the rauwolfia alkaloids, depletes the postganglionic adrenergic neurons of norepinephrine by inhibiting its uptake into storage vesicles, exposing it to degradation by cytoplasmic monoamine oxidase. The peripheral effect is predominant, although the drug enters the brain and depletes central catecholamine stores as well. This probably accounts for the sedation and depression seen with reserpine use. The drug has certain advantages: Only one dose a day is needed; in combination with a diuretic, the antihypertensive effect is significant, greater than that noted with propranolol in one comparative study[104]; little postural hypotension is noted; and many patients experience no side effects. The drug has a relatively flat dose–response curve, so that a dose of only 0.05 mg per day will give almost as much antihypertensive effect as 0.125 or 0.25 mg per day but fewer side effects.[105] However, the psychological depression that occurs in perhaps 2 per cent of patients may be severe but difficult to recognize and treat. The specter of breast cancer associated with reserpine raised in 1974 has not been substantiated.[106] Although it remains popular in some places, the use of reserpine has declined progressively.

GUANETHIDINE. Guanethidine and a series of related guanidine compounds, including guanadrel, bethanidine, and debrisoquine, act by inhibiting the release of norepinephrine from the adrenergic neurons, perhaps by a local anesthetic-like effect on the neuronal membrane. In order to act, the drug must be actively transported into the nerve through an amine pump. Various drugs, in particular tricyclic antidepressants, amphetamines, and ephedrine, competitively block the uptake of guanethidine into the nerves and thereby antagonize its effects.

Their low lipid solubility prevents these drugs from entering the brain, so that sedation, depression, and other side effects on the central nervous system are not seen. Initially, the predominant hemodynamic effect is to decrease cardiac output; after continued use, peripheral resistance declines. Blood pressure is reduced further when the patient is upright, owing to gravitational pooling of blood in the legs, since compensatory sympathetic nervous system-mediated vasoconstriction is blocked. This results in the most common side effect, postural hypotension. Patients should be advised to arise slowly, sleep with the head of the bed elevated, and wear elastic hose to minimize this potential problem. Unlike reserpine, guanethidine has a steep dose–response curve, so that it can be successfully used in treating hypertension of any degree in daily doses of 10 to 300 mg. Like reserpine, it has a long biological half-life and may be given once daily. As other drugs have become available, guanethidine has been mainly relegated to the treatment of severe hypertension unresponsive to all other agents.

Guanadrel, *bethanidine*, and *debrisoquin* are similar to guanethidine but have a shorter duration of action and perhaps fewer side effects.[107]

DRUGS THAT ACT UPON RECEPTORS

Predominantly Central Alpha Agonists

From the late 1960's until recently, methyldopa was the most widely used of the adrenoceptor blockers, but its use has fallen off as beta blockers and other drugs have become more popular. In addition, two other drugs—clonidine and guanabenz—which act similarly to methyldopa but have fewer serious side effects have become available.

METHYLDOPA (ALDOMET). The primary site of action of methyldopa, in common with the other central alpha agonists, is within the central nervous system, where alpha-methylnorepinephrine, synthesized from methyldopa, is released from adrenoceptor neurons and stimulates central alpha adrenoreceptors, reducing the sympathetic outflow from the central nervous system.[108] The blood pressure mainly falls from a decrease in peripheral resistance with little effect on cardiac output. However, as is true with all adrenoceptor blockers, patients with borderline cardiac function may develop congestive failure by removal of adrenoceptor support. On the other hand, methyldopa, probably in concert with other antihypertensive agents that decrease sympathetic activity, may reduce the degree of left ventricular hypertrophy as noted by echocardiography.[109] Renal blood flow is well maintained, and significant postural hypotension is unusual. Therefore, the drug has been widely used in hypertensive patients with renal insufficiency or cerebrovascular disease; smaller doses are needed in the presence of renal insufficiency. Renin levels usually decrease, but the reduction in blood pressure is dependent neither on initially high plasma renin activity nor on a subsequent fall in this level.

Methyldopa need be given no more than twice daily. The dosage range is from 250 to 3,000 mg per day, with most patients responding to 750 to 1,500 mg. As in the case of the other adrenoceptor blockers and peripheral vasodilators that may cause reactive fluid retention, methyldopa is best used in combination with a diuretic.

Side effects include some that are common to centrally acting drugs that reduce sympathetic outflow: sedation, dry mouth, orthostatic hypotension, impotence, and galactorrhea. However, methyldopa causes some unique side effects that are probably of an autoimmune nature, since a positive antinuclear antibody test is seen in about 10 per cent of patients who take the drug and red cell autoantibodies in about 20 per cent. Clinically apparent hemolytic anemia is quite rare, probably because methyldopa also impairs reticuloendothelial function so that antibody-sensitized cells are not removed from the circulation and hemolyzed.[110] Inflammatory diseases in various organs have been reported, most commonly involving the liver with diffuse parenchymal injury similar to viral hepatitis.[111]

CLONIDINE (CATAPRES). Although of different structure, clonidine shares many features with methyldopa: It probably acts at the same central sites, has similar antihypertensive efficacy, and causes many of the same bothersome but less serious side effects (e.g., sedation, dry mouth). It does not, however, induce the autoimmune and inflammatory side effects.

As an alpha-adrenoreceptor agonist, the drug also acts on presynaptic alpha receptors and inhibits norepinephrine release (Fig. 28–7), and plasma catecholamine levels fall.[108] The drug has a fairly short biological half-life, so that when it is discontinued, the inhibition of norepinephrine release disappears within about 12 to 18 hours, and plasma catecholamine levels rise. This is probably responsible for the rapid rebound of the blood pressure to pretreatment levels and the occasional appearance of withdrawal symptoms, including tachycardia, restlessness, and sweating. Rarely, the blood pressure increases beyond the pretreatment level. Similar overshoots have been reported after the discontinuation of a variety of other antihypertensives.[112] If the rebound requires treatment, clonidine may be reintroduced or alpha adrenoreceptor antagonists given. By itself, clonidine often induces fluid retention, so that it should generally be used with a diuretic. After control has been achieved with two daily doses of clonidine and a diuretic, it may be maintained with a single bedtime dose.

Clonidine is available in a *transdermal* preparation which may provide smoother blood pressure control for as long as 7 days with fewer side effects.[113] However, bothersome skin rashes preclude its use in perhaps one-fourth of patients.

Clonidine has been used to treat severe hypertension with hourly doses of 0.1 and 0.2 mg.[114] In addition, it suppresses withdrawal symptoms from opiates and may have wider use in various psychiatric disorders.[115]

GUANABENZ. This drug differs in structure but shares many characteristics with both methyldopa and clonidine, acting primarily as a central alpha agonist. It may differ, however, in not causing reactive fluid retention,[116] so that it may turn out to be effective without the need for a concomitant diuretic. Moreover, unlike diuretics, the use of guanabenz has been found to reduce serum cholesterol.[117]

LOFEXIDINE AND GUANFACINE. These drugs, similar to clonidine, are under clinical investigation.[118, 119]

Alpha-Adrenoceptor Antagonists

Before 1977 the only alpha blockers used to treat hypertension were phenoxybenzamine (Dibenzyline) and phentolamine (Regitine). These drugs are effective in acutely lowering blood pressure, but their effects are offset by an accompanying increase in cardiac output, and side effects are frequent and bothersome. Their limited effect may reflect their blockade of presynaptic alpha-adrenoceptors, which interferes with the feedback inhibition of norepinephrine release (Fig. 28–7). Increased catecholamine release would then blunt the action on postsynaptic alpha-adrenoceptors. Their use has largely been limited to the treatment of patients with pheochromocytoma.

PRAZOSIN (MINIPRESS). Prazosin is the first of a group of selective antagonists of the postsynaptic $alpha_1$ receptors. Although prazosin was introduced as a peripheral vasodilator, subsequent study has clearly shown the primary effect of this group of drugs to be that of a postsynaptic alpha blocker.[120] By blocking alpha-mediated vasoconstriction, prazosin induces a fall in peripheral resistance with both venous and arteriolar dilation. Because the presynaptic alpha adrenoceptor is left unblocked, the feedback loop for the inhibition of norepinephrine release is intact, an action which is also certainly responsible for the greater antihypertensive effect of the drug and the absence of concomitant tachycardia, tolerance, and renin release. The inhibition of norepinephrine release may also account for the propensity toward postural hypotension. Because this is mainly noted with the first dose and in patients with lower plasma renin levels, it has been attributed to the presence of increased alpha tone or blunted renin reactivity.[121] This problem can be mitigated by limiting the first dose to 1 mg and withholding diuretic therapy for a few days on either side of the start of prazosin.

Prazosin is as effective as other first-line antihypertensives and is similarly aided by concomitant use of a diuretic. When added to patients poorly controlled on standard triple therapy (diuretic, beta blocker, and vasodilator, prazosin may reduce blood pressure even more than anticipated.[122] It can be safely and effectively used in patients with renal insufficiency. The favorable hemodynamic changes—a fall in peripheral resistance with maintenance of cardiac output—make prazosin an attractive choice for patients who wish to remain physically active. Patients who may have trouble with beta blockers, including those with asthma or peripheral vascular disease, should be able to tolerate alpha blockade. In addition, blood lipids are not adversely altered and may actually improve with alpha blockers, unlike the adverse effects observed with diuretics and beta blockers.[123]

Side effects, beyond first-dose postural hypotension, include the nonspecific effects of lower blood pressure, such as dizziness, weakness, fatigue, and headaches. Most patients, however, find the drug easy to take, with little sedation, dry mouth, or impotence.

OTHER ALPHA BLOCKERS. At least three other alpha blockers have been extensively studied and will probably become available: doxazosin,[124] indoramin,[125] and trimazosin.[126] Beyond longer duration of action, they appear to differ little from prazosin.

Beta-Adrenoceptor Antagonists

(See also p. 1330)

In the past few years beta-adrenoceptor blockers have been used increasingly, becoming the most popular form of antihypertensive therapy after diuretics. Their popularity reflects their relative effectiveness and freedom from bothersome side effects. However, they are no more effective in lowering blood pressure than are other adrenoceptor blocking agents, such as reserpine,[104] and side effects occur in up to 20 per cent of hypertensive patients.[11] Some of these side effects, including fatigue, bronchospasm, peripheral vasospasm, and depression, may be quite bothersome. For the majority of patients who do not develop such side effects, beta blockers are usually easy to take, since somnolence, dry mouth, and impotence are seldom encountered. Because beta blockers have been found to reduce mortality after acute myocardial infarction (p. 1288), i.e., secondary prevention,[127] it was assumed that they might offer special protection against initial coronary events, i.e., primary prevention. In large clinical trials propranolol[11] and oxprenolol[16] reduced the incidence of coronary events or mortality in men who did not smoke cigarettes. Among the remainder, these beta blockers offered no special protection.

THE VARIETY OF BETA BLOCKERS. The beta blockers now available in the United States are listed in Table 39–2 (p. 1331), and others are available in other countries. Pharmacologically, they differ considerably with respect to degree of absorption, protein binding, and bioavailability. But the three most important differences affecting their clinical use are cardioselectivity, intrinsic sympathomimetic activity, and lipid solubility. Despite these differences, they all seem to be about equally effective as antihypertensives.

Cardioselectivity. As seen in Figure 28–8, acebutolol, atenolol, and metoprolol are relatively cardioselective, having a greater blocking effect on the $beta_1$ adrenoceptors in the heart than on the $beta_2$ adrenoceptors in the bronchi, peripheral blood vessels, and elsewhere. Such cardioselectivity can be easily shown using small doses in acute

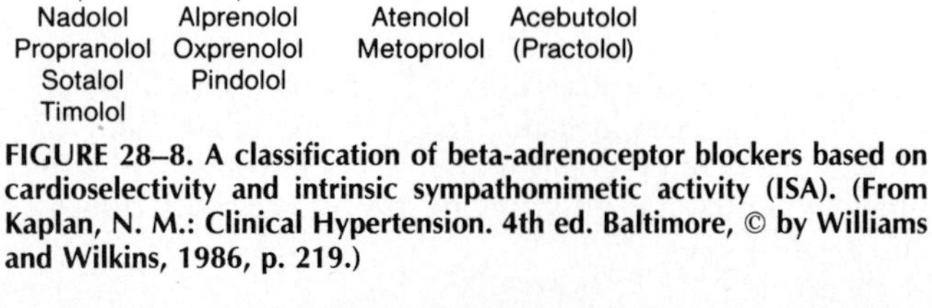

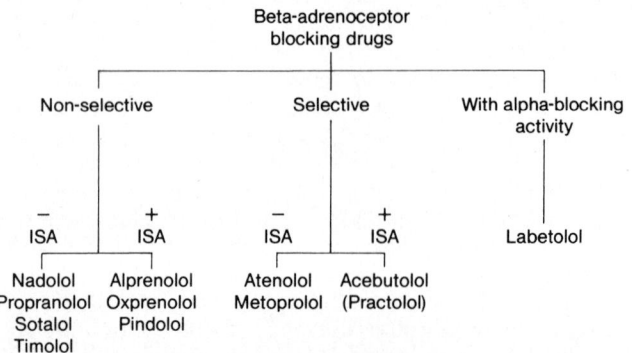

FIGURE 28–8. A classification of beta-adrenoceptor blockers based on cardioselectivity and intrinsic sympathomimetic activity (ISA). (From Kaplan, N. M.: Clinical Hypertension. 4th ed. Baltimore, © by Williams and Wilkins, 1986, p. 219.)

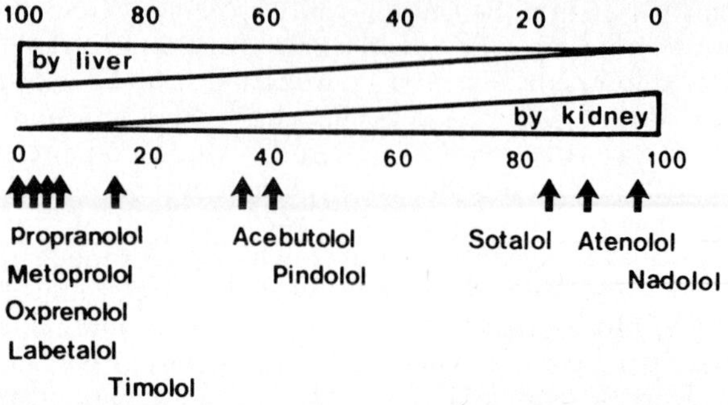

FIGURE 28–9. The relative degree of clearance by hepatic uptake and metabolism (liver) and renal excretion (kidney) of 10 beta-adrenoceptor blocking agents. The differences largely reflect differences in lipid solubility, which progressively diminishes from left to right. (From Meier, J.: Beta-adrenoceptor-blocking agents: Pharmacokinetic differences and their clinical implications illustrated on pindolol. Cardiology *64*[Suppl 1]:1, 1979.)

studies; with the rather high doses used to treat hypertension, much of this effect is lost.

Intrinsic Sympathomimetic Activity (ISA). Pindolol and acebutolol have ISA, interacting with beta receptors to cause a measurable agonist response but at the same time blocking the greater agonist effects of endogenous catecholamines. As a result, while in usual doses they lower the blood pressure to about the same degree as other beta blockers, pindolol and acebutolol cause a smaller decline in heart rate, cardiac output, and renin levels. A drug with ISA may prove useful when a beta blocker is needed for patients in whom bradycardia or peripheral vascular disease is a problem. During exercise the influence of ISA is reduced, so that similar hemodynamic effects are noted as with non-ISA beta blockers.[128] As noted under Side Effects, ISA blunts the adverse effects on lipid metabolism seen with non-ISA beta blockers.[129]

Lipid Solubility. Atenolol and nadolol are the least lipid-soluble of the beta blockers (Fig. 28–9). This could translate into two clinically important advantages: (1) Because they escape hepatic inactivation, they remain as active drugs in the plasma much longer, allowing once-a-day dosage; and (2) because they do not enter the brain as readily, they may cause fewer central nervous system (CNS) side effects. However, with the relatively large doses used to treat hypertension, once-a-day administration is effective with most, if not all, beta blockers. No properly controlled comparative study on CNS side effects has been published, but in view of the reported high rate of depression with propranolol,[130] this could be a major advantage of less lipid-soluble agents.

Mode of Action. Despite these and other differences, the various beta blockers now available seem about equipotent as antihypertensive agents. How they lower the blood pressure remains uncertain, although a number of possible mechanims are likely to be involved. In those without ISA, cardiac output falls 15 to 20 per cent and renin release is reduced about 60 per cent. Central nervous beta-adrenoceptor blockade may reduce sympathetic discharge, but similar antihypertensive effects are seen with those drugs that are more lipid soluble, and therefore in high concentration within the CNS, and those that are less lipid soluble.[131] Recall, too, that blockade of presynaptic beta adrenoceptors should inhibit catecholamine release (Fig. 28–7). In addition, beta blockers have been reported to reduce free calcium within red cells.[132] If this happens elsewhere, it could contribute to their antihypertensive effect.

At the same time that beta blockers lower blood pressure through various means, their blockade of peripheral beta adrenoceptors inhibits vasodilation, leaving alpha adrenoceptors open to catecholamine-mediated vasoconstriction. As a result, peripheral resistance rises.[133] A decrease in peripheral blood flow is a common problem with beta blocker therapy in cold climates.

Clinical Effects. Even in small doses, beta blockers begin to lower the blood pressure within a few hours, although their maximal effect may not be noted for some weeks. Even though progressively higher doses have usually been given, careful study has shown a near-maximal effect from smaller doses: in a double-blind crossover study involving 24 patients, 40 mg of propranolol twice a day provided the same antihypertensive effects as 80, 160, or 240 mg twice a day.[134] The degree of blood pressure reduction is at least comparable to that noted with other antihypertensive drugs. By itself, a beta blocker will lower the DBP to below 90 mm Hg in about half the patients with mild to moderate hypertension; when combined with a diuretic, the percentage rises to about 80.[104] Duration of action is well beyond the drugs' plasma half-life so that most can be used once daily. One of the attractions of these drugs is the constancy of their antihypertensive action, altered little by changes in activity, posture, or temperature. Because the sympathetic nervous system is blocked, the hemodynamic responses to stress are reduced, probably enough to interfere with athletic performance.[128]

Beta blockers have been proposed as initial monotherapy.[72] This approach may be effective for many younger, white hypertensives but may not be suitable for many older or black patients. As noted before, both blacks[102] and patients over age 50[135] have been found to respond less well to beta blocker monotherapy. It should be noted that others find that the response in the elderly is as good to a beta blocker as to a diuretic.[136]

SPECIAL USES FOR BETA BLOCKERS

Coexisting Ischemic Heart Disease. Even without evidence that beta blockers protect patients from initial coronary events, the antiarrhythmic and antianginal effects of these drugs make them especially valuable in hypertensive patients with coexisting coronary disease.

Patients Needing Antihypertensive Vasodilator Therapy. If a diuretic and an adrenoceptor blocker are inadequate to control blood pressure, the addition of a vasodilator is a logical third step. When used alone, direct vasodilators induce reflex sympathetic stimulation of the heart. The simultaneous use of beta blockers prevents this undesirable increase in cardiac output, which not only bothers the patient, but also dampens the antihypertensive effect of the vasodilator.

Patients with Hyperkinetic Hypertension. Some hypertensive patients have increased cardiac output that may persist for many years. Beta blockers are particularly effective in such patients, but a reduction in exercise capacity may restrict their use in young athletes.

Patients with Marked Anxiety. The somatic manifestations of anxiety—tremor, sweating, and tachycardia—can be helped,[137] without the undesirable effects of methods commonly used to control anxiety, such as alcohol and tranquilizers.

SIDE EFFECTS. Most of the side effects of beta blockers relate to their major pharmacologic action, the blockade of beta adrenoceptors. Patients with certain concomitant problems may have them worsen when beta adrenoceptors are blocked. These include peripheral vascular disease, bronchospasm, and congestive heart failure.

Diabetics may have additional problems with beta blockers, more so with nonselective ones. The responses to hypoglycemia, both the symptoms and the counterregulatory hormonal changes that raise blood sugar levels, are partially dependent on sympathetic nervous activity. Diabetics who are susceptible to hypoglycemia may not be aware of the usual warning signals and may not rebound as quickly. The majority of noninsulin-dependent diabetics can take the drugs without difficulty, although their diabetes may be exacerbated, probably from beta blocker interference with insulin secretion.[138]

The most common side effects are fatigue and depression. Fatigue may reflect the decrease in cerebral blood flow that may accompany successful lowering of the blood pressure by any drug (Fig. 28–5). More direct effects on the CNS—depression, insomnia, nightmares, and hallucinations—occur in some patients. In one large series the use of antidepressant medications increased 50 per cent more among patients prescribed propranolol than among patients prescribed hydralazine or oral hypoglycemic agents.[130] Although the diagnosis of depression was not substantiated, this report suggests that this may be a common problem with beta blocker use. Of all the side effects, CNS ones are most dose dependent. The remainder are likely to develop, if at all, with small doses and do not tend to increase in frequency with higher doses, presumably because smaller doses provide as much beta blockade as will occur in most tissues. The more common side effects of central agonists—sedation, depression, dry mouth—are rare.

When a beta blocker is discontinued suddenly, angina pectoris may appear for the first time or, if previously present, may be intensified. Patients with hypertension are more susceptible to coronary disease, so they should be weaned gradually. Perturbations of lipoprotein metabolism may accompany the use of non-ISA beta blockers.[94] A review of published data indicates that nonselective agents may cause greater falls in cardioprotective high-density lipoprotein–cholesterol levels, whereas ISA agents cause less or no effect. Patients with renal insufficiency may take beta blockers without additional hazard, although modest falls in renal blood flow and glomerular filtration rate have been measured, presumably from renal vasoconstriction.[139] Dosage of the lipid-insoluble atenolol and nadolol should be reduced in patients with renal insufficiency.

Caution is advised in the use of beta blockers in patients suspected of having pheochromocytoma (p. 1814), since unopposed alpha-adrenoceptor action may precipitate a serious hypertensive crisis if this disease is present. The use of beta blockers during pregnancy has been clouded by scattered case reports of various fetal problems. However, prospective studies have found that the use of beta blockers to treat hypertension during pregnancy did not lead to an increase in fetal morbidity.[140]

Various systemic reactions have been reported with even the small amounts of beta blocker absorbed from topic ophthalmic use.[141]

AN OVERVIEW OF BETA BLOCKERS IN HYPERTENSION. Beta blockers are likely to continue to be popular in the treatment of hypertension. They may be particularly effective in patients with higher renin levels. If a beta blocker is chosen, those that have ISA, that are more cardioselective and lipid-insoluble, offer the likelihood of less perturbations of lipid and carbohydrate metabolism and greater patient adherence to therapy, since only one dose a day will be needed and side effects are likely be minimized.

Alpha- and Beta-Adrenoceptor Antagonists

The combination of an alpha and a beta blocker in one molecule is available in the form of labetalol, which combines both alpha and beta blocking actions, in a ratio between 1:3 and 1:7. The fall in pressure mainly results from a decrease in peripheral resistance, with little or no fall in cardiac output.[142] The most bothersome side effects are related to postural hypotension. Intravenous labetolol has been used successfully to treat hypertensive emergencies, particularly those resulting from catecholamine excess.[143]

VASODILATORS

Until recently, direct-acting arteriolar vasodilators were mainly used as third drugs, when a diuretic and adrenergic blocker did not control the blood pressure. However, with the availability of vasodilators of different types that can be easily tolerated when used as first or second drugs, a wider and earlier application of vasodilators in therapy of hypertension has begun (Table 28–7).

DIRECT VASODILATORS

Hydralazine (Apresoline) is the only agent of this type now available for routine use. Minoxidil is more potent but is usually reserved for patients with severe, refractory hypertension associated with renal insufficiency. Diazoxide and nitroprusside are given intravenously for hypertensive crises and are discussed on pages 519 and 876.

HYDRALAZINE. First introduced in 1953, hydralazine has regained popularity since it was recognized that beta blockers could be used to prevent its side effects and enhance its efficacy. Since the early 1970's hydralazine, in combination with a diuretic and a beta blocker, has been used increasingly to treat severer hypertension. The drug acts directly to relax the smooth muscle in precapillary resistance vessels with little or no effect on postcapillary venous capacitance vessels. As a result, blood pressure falls by a reduction in peripheral resistance, but in doing so a number of reactive processes are activated by the arterial baroreceptor arc that blunt the decrease in pressure and cause side effects.[144] These involve a rise in both plasma norepinephrine and epinephrine, which increase venous return, heart rate, and contractility, causing a rise in cardiac output and stroke volume, unlike the hemodynamic responses to the venoarteriolar dilator nitroprusside, which reduces venous return and thereby cardiac output, without an effect on peripheral resistance (Fig. 28–10).

With hydralazine, when a diuretic is used to overcome the tendency for fluid retention and a beta blocker is used to prevent the reflex increase in sympathetic activity and rise in renin, the vasodilator is more effective and causes few, if any, side effects.

TABLE 28–7 VASODILATOR DRUGS USED TO TREAT HYPERTENSION

Drug	Relative Action on Arteries (A) or Veins (V)
Direct	
Hydralazine	A >> V
Minoxidil	A >> V
Nitroprusside	A = V
Diazoxide	A > V
Nitroglycerin	V > A
Calcium antagonists	
Diltiazem	A >> V
Nifedipine	A >> V
Verapamil	A >> V
Converting enzyme inhibitors	
Captopril	A > V
Enalapril	A > V
Alpha blockers	A = V

1A,B

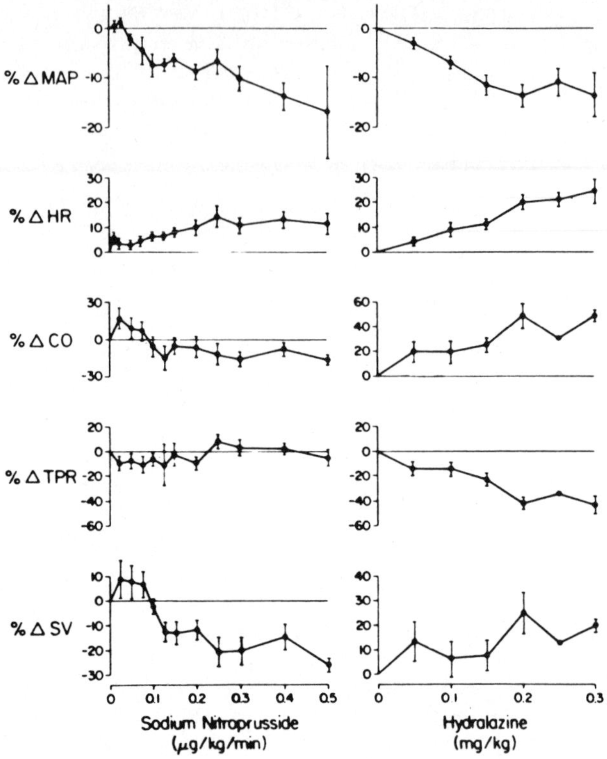

FIGURE 28–10. Percentage changes in mean arterial pressure (%ΔMAP), heart rate (%ΔHR), cardiac output (%ΔCO), total peripheral resistance (%ΔTPR), and stroke volume (%ΔSV) caused by sodium nitroprusside and hydralazine. (From Shepherd, A. M. M., and Irvine, N. A.: Differential hemodynamic and sympathoadrenal effects of sodium nitroprusside and hydralazine in hypertensive subjects. J. Cardiovasc. Pharmacol. *8*:529, 1986.)

The drug need be given only twice a day. Its daily dosage should be kept below 400 mg to prevent the lupus-like syndrome that appears in 10 to 20 per cent of patients who receive more. This reaction, although uncomfortable to the patient, is almost always reversible. In fact, lower subsequent blood pressure and improved survival were noted among 42 patients with this toxic reaction when compared with matched patients given hydralazine who did not experience the reaction.[145] The reaction is uncommon with daily doses of 200 mg or less and is more common in slow acetylators of the drug.

Without the protection conferred by concomitant use of an adrenoceptor blocker, numerous other side effects—tachycardia, flushing, headache, and precipitation of angina—are seen; with the combination, most patients experience few or no side effects. Older patients, with reduced baroreceptor responsiveness, may be able to tolerate hydralazine without adrenergic blockade. Concomitant intake of a nonsteroidal antiinflammatory drug may blunt its hypotensive action.[146]

MINOXIDIL. This drug, unrelated to other vasodilators, acts in a manner similar to hydralazine but is even more effective and may be used once a day. It has been found to be particularly useful in managing patients with severe hypertension and renal insufficiency.[147] Even more than with hydralazine, diuretics and adrenoceptor blockers must be used with minoxidil to prevent the reflex increase in cardiac output and fluid retention. The drug also causes hair to grow profusely, and the facial hirsutism discourages some women from taking the drug. Previous concerns that the drug leads to pulmonary hypertension and causes right atrial lesions, as it does in dogs, have been shown to be unfounded.[147] However, pericardial effusions have appeared in about 3 per cent of those given minoxidil and are probably related to the renal insufficiency that is usually present. However, they are sometimes seen in patients without renal or cardiac failure.[148]

Calcium Antagonists

(See also p. 1332)

Calcium antagonists are likely to be widely used in the treatment of hypertension. They differ in both their sites and their mode of action[149]; nifedipine and other dihydropyridine derivatives have the most attractive hemodynamic profile: They have the greatest peripheral vasodilatory action with little effect on cardiac conduction. However, comparative trials have shown verapamil[150] and diltiazem[151] to also be effective antihypertensives, and they may cause fewer side effects.

Calcium antagonists may cause at least an initial natriuresis, probably by causing renal vasodilation,[152] which may obviate the need for concurrent diuretic therapy. In fact, they, unlike all other antihypertensive agents, may have their effectiveness reduced rather than enhanced by concomitant dietary sodium restriction.[153] Calcium antagonists may be particularly effective in elderly[135] and black[154] hypertensives. Concerns about their possible effects on various hormonal and other secretory processes that involve calcium entry seem largely unfounded.[155] Renin and aldosterone secretion may be impaired,[156] which may contribute to the lack of fluid retention seen with their use. Nifedipine has been effectively used to reduce high levels of blood pressure quickly. Doses of 10 to 20 mg provide almost uniform reduction of blood pressure by 25 per cent within 30 minutes.[157]

Renin-Angiotensin Blockers

Activity of the renin-angiotensin system may now be inhibited in four ways (Fig. 28–11), three of which can be applied clinically. The first, use of adrenergic blockers to inhibit the release of renin, was discussed earlier in this chapter. The second, direct inhibition of renin activity by antirenin antibodies, is not now clinically feasible. The fourth, blockade of angiotensin's actions by a competitive blocker, is feasible, in the form of saralasin, which requires intravenous administration. The third, inhibition of the enzyme that converts the inactive decapeptide angiotensin I to the active octapeptide angiotensin II, is now being widely practiced with the use of the orally effective converting enzyme inhibitors (CEI) captopril (Capoten) and enalapril (Vasotec). Captopril was originally introduced for use, in fairly large doses, only in patients resistant or intolerant to other medications. It and enalapril, in small doses, have now been found to be both effective in and well tolerated by patients with mild hypertension.[158, 159] In these patients, as in those with severe hypertension, a diuretic may be needed to achieve an adequate response.

MODE OF ACTION. *Captopril* was synthesized as a specific inhibitor of the converting enzyme that breaks the peptidyldipeptide bond in angiotensin I. It binds to three sites on the converting enzyme, thereby preventing the enzyme from attaching to and splitting the angiotensin I structure. Because angiotensin II cannot be formed and angiotensin I is inactive, the CEI paralyzes the renin-angiotensin system, thereby removing the effects of endogenous angiotensin II as both a vasoconstrictor and a stimulant to aldosterone synthesis. Enalapril, differing primarily by the absence of a sulfhydryl group, works in a similar manner. It is a prodrug which is hydrolyzed after absorption to form the active CEI enalaprilat, the process slowing the onset but prolonging the duration of its action.

The same enzyme which converts angiotensin I to angiotensin II is also responsible for inactivation of the vasodepressor hormone bradykinin. By inhibiting the breakdown of bradykinin, CEI may increase the concentration of a vasodepressor hormone while it decreases the concentration of a vasoconstrictor hormone.[160] Levels of vasodilatory prostaglandins may be increased simultaneously. In whatever manner it works, CEI lowers blood pressure mainly by reducing peripheral resistance, with little, if any, effect on heart rate, cardiac output, or body fluid volumes. The lack of a rise in heart rate despite a significant fall in blood pressure has been explained by resetting of the baroreceptor reflex,[161] although other mechanisms may also be involved.[162]

CLINICAL USE. The antihypertensive response to CEI is greatest in those patients whose hypertension is being generated by high levels of angiotensin II, such as those with renovascular hypertension. Similarly, the response in those with lesser contributions by angiotensin II will be enhanced by concomitant use of a diuretic, which will raise endogenous angiotensin II levels. In patients with uncomplicated primary hypertension, a CEI will provide a similar antihypertensive effect as a diuretic or a beta blocker.[100] CEI's are less effective in blacks,[158] perhaps because blacks tend to have lower renin levels. Despite the repeated observation that diuretics enhance the effectiveness of CEI's, the CEI itself may induce a considerable natriuresis, presumably in renal vasodilation.[163]

The initial dose of CEI may precipitate a rather dramatic but transient fall in blood pressure, but the full effect may not be seen for 7 to 10 days.[164] The initial dosage may be as little as 12.5 mg b.i.d. of captopril or 5 mg once a day of enalapril. Because much of the drug is excreted by the kidneys, smaller doses are usually adequate in patients with renal insufficiency. The response to CEI is usually

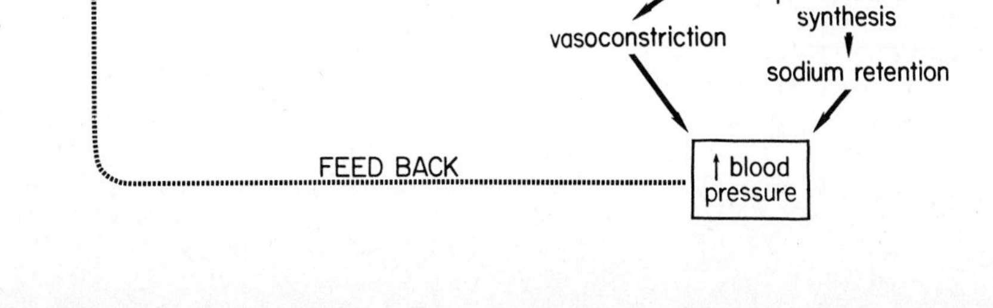

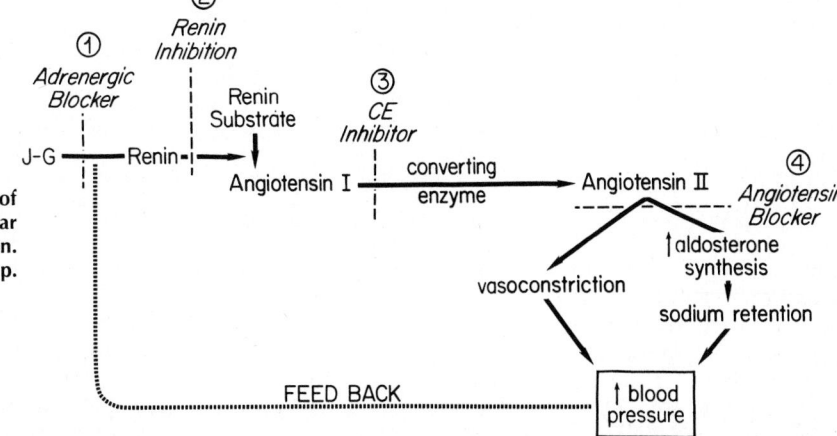

FIGURE 28–11. The four sites of action of inhibitors of the renin-angiotensin system. (J-G = juxtaglomerular apparatus.) (From Kaplan, N. M.: Clinical Hypertension. 4th ed. Baltimore, © by Williams and Wilkins, 1986, p. 101.)

well maintained, perhaps because its suppression of aldosterone mitigates the tendency toward volume expansion that often antagonizes the effects of other antihypertensives.

CEI's may find wider use if the inability to modulate adrenal and renal responses to different levels of sodium intake, ascribed to fixed high angiotensin II levels, turns out to be a common defect in normal and high-renin hypertensives.[38] The defect appears to be corrected by CEI therapy, holding the promise for a more specific form of therapy for a large portion of the hypertensive population.

These drugs have been a mixed blessing for patients with renovascular hypertension. On the one hand, the plasma renin response to a single dose of captopril may provide a simple diagnostic test for the disease (p. 843).[165] More important, they usually control the blood pressure effectively.[166] On the other hand, their removal of the high levels of angiotensin II may deprive the stenotic kidney of the hormonal drive to its blood flow, thereby causing a marked fall of renal perfusion.[167] Those with solitary kidneys or bilateral disease may develop renal failure.[166]

Patients with intraglomerular hypertension, specifically those with diabetic nephropathy or reduced renal functional mass, may especially benefit from the reduction in efferent arteriolar resistance that follows reduction in angiotensin II. The experimental evidence for this protection is strong.[168, 169] The clinical evidence, although now limited, is supportive.[170]

SIDE EFFECTS. Most patients who take a CEI experience no side effects. In controlled studies patients have significantly fewer adverse effects from a CEI than from a diuretic or a beta blocker[100] or from a beta blocker or methyldopa.[171] The major advantages are related to the absence of effects intimately involved in the sites of action of other drugs: no CNS side effects, no reduction in cardiac output, no interference with sympathetic activity. Beyond the decrease in bothersome overt side effects, CEI therapy does not produce biochemical changes that may be of even more concern, even though they are not so obvious: neither rises in lipids, glucose, or uric acid nor falls in potassium levels are seen.

To be sure, CEI's may cause both specific and nonspecific adverse effects. Among the specific ones are rash, loss of taste, glomerulopathy manifested by proteinuria, and leukopenia. These seem to be less common with enalapril, presumably because it does not have a sufhydryl group in its structure.[160] In addition, these drugs may cause a hypersensitivity reaction with angioneurotic edema or a persistent cough. As indicated earlier, there is a tendency for "first-dose" hypotension and progressive loss of renal perfusion, particularly in patients who start with high endogenous angiotensin II levels. In addition, there is at least a potential problem for those on a CEI who coincidentally develop volume depletion, as from gastroenteritis. They may be unable to marshal the compensatory homeostatic responses that involve increased angiotensin II and aldosterone. Lastly, patients on potassium supplements or sparing agents may not be able to excrete potassium loads, and therefore may develop hyperkalemia.

AN OVERVIEW OF CEI THERAPY. These drugs may be widely used for all degrees and forms of hypertension, if their relative freedom from adverse effects commonly seen with other agents is as true as it appears and their particular ability to decrease intrarenal hypertension is translated into greater protection from progressive renal damage. Despite these attractions, for most patients, they are no more effective than other drugs and they have the potential for some adverse effects.

OTHER DRUGS. A variety of other forms of antihypertensive therapy are under investigation. The only one that currently appears to hold promise is the serotonin antagonist ketanserin.[172]

SPECIAL CONSIDERATIONS IN THERAPY

CHOICE OF DRUGS. As noted earlier in this chapter, the stepped-care approach, now widely followed, has been broadened to include a beta blocker along with a diuretic as first choice.[72] The author believes that the choices should be broadened even further, since other effective and well-tolerated agents are now available, including alpha blockers, calcium-entry blockers, and CEI's. There is little overall difference in their effectiveness, but younger patients tend to respond better to beta blockers and CEI's, older ones to calcium blockers and diuretics. The choice is then logically made on the basis of ease of administration, freedom from side effects, and, it is hoped, the likelihood of protection from coronary disease. Certain trade-offs may be required: Reserpine or a thiazide may be given in only one dose per day at little cost, but the side effects may be excessive; methyldopa, despite its efficacy, may cause some unique and serious problems and is increasingly seen as a poor choice; if poor patient adherence is likely, clonidine should be avoided; prazosin may provide more "physiological" control of the blood pressure but may cause bothersome postural hypotension; beta blockers are probably acceptable for most patients but may commonly cause CNS problems and rarely serious side effects, even after careful exclusion of patients known to be susceptible. CEI's will probably be increasingly used, as will calcium blockers, particularly when they are available in once- and twice-a-day formulations.

If a second drug is needed, a diuretic may be used, if it was not the first choice. If a third drug is needed, hydralazine will often be added, although prazosin or a CEI may also be effective if a beta blocker is the second drug. The logical process is to substitute a drug from another class if the first choice does not work and to choose drugs of different classes if more than one is needed.

REASONS FOR INADEQUATE RESPONSES. Often patients do not respond well because they do not take their medications. On the other hand, what appears to be a poor response based on office readings of blood pressure may turn out to be an adequate response when home readings are used. However, a number of factors may be responsible for a poor response even if the appropriate medication is taken regularly (Table 28–8). Perhaps most common is volume overload owing to either inadequate diuretic or excessive dietary sodium intake. Larger doses or more potent diuretics may bring resistant hypertension under control.[76] On the other hand, there are a few patients whose blood pressure is resistant to therapy because of overly vigorous diuresis, which contracts vascular volume and activates both renin and catecholamines. This is most likely to occur in patients with obligatory salt-wasting resulting from interstitial renal disease.

ANESTHESIA IN HYPERTENSIVE PATIENTS (See also p. 1698). In the absence of significant cardiac dysfunction, hypertension does not add to the cardiovascular risks of surgery.[173] Most anesthesiologists suggest that hypertensive patients should be well controlled by means of medications before anesthesia and surgery. Patients receiving beta blockers have slightly lower blood pressure during surgery and even lower pressures during intubation and after extubation, with no adverse effects on hemodynamic

TABLE 28–8 CAUSES OF POOR RESPONSE TO ANTIHYPERTENSIVE DRUGS

1. Inadequate drugs
   a. Doses too low
   b. Inappropriate combinations, e.g., two centrally acting adrenergic inhibitors
   c. Rapid inactivation, e.g., hydralazine
   d. Incomplete absorption related to food intake
   e. Antagonism from other drugs
      (1) Sympathomimetics
      (2) Antidepressants
      (3) Adrenal steroids
      (4) Nonsteroidal antiinflammatory drugs
2. Associated conditions
   a. Alcohol intake above 2 oz/day
   b. Renal insufficiency
   c. Renovascular hypertension
   d. Pheochromocytoma
3. Volume overload
   a. Inadequate diuretic
   b. Excessive sodium intake
   c. Fluid retention from reduction of blood pressure
   d. Progressive renal damage
4. Volume depletion → increased renin → vasoconstriction
   a. Renal salt-wasting
   b. Overly aggressive diuretic therapy

measures.[174] Patients receiving calcium antagonists may occasionally manifest adverse effects with inhalation agents such as halothane, enflurane, and isoflurane, either because their cardiovascular effects are similar or because they may increase the plasma levels of the calcium antagonists.[175]

Hypertension is often observed during and immediately after coronary bypass surgery. Nitroglycerin and nifedipine are equally effective during surgery.[176] Nitroprusside is the usual choice during the postoperative period, but toxicity, often in the form of loss of consciousness and cyanide or thiocyanate toxicity, may develop in those who are critically ill and given the drug for prolonged periods.[177]

HYPERTENSIVE CHILDREN. Almost nothing is known about the effects of various antihypertensive medications given to children over long periods. Because most of the adrenoceptor blockers act on the CNS, their effects on growth hormone, gonadotropins, and other hormones involved in maturation and growth should be ascertained. However, in the absence of adequate data, an approach similar to that advocated for adults is advised.[178] The doses of drugs are shown in Table 32-3, p. 1019. Emphasis has been placed on the need for weight reduction in hypertensive children who are obese, thereby attempting to control hypertension without the need for drug therapy.

HYPERTENSION DURING PREGNANCY. This topic is discussed in Chapter 60.

THE ELDERLY WITH SYSTOLIC HYPERTENSION. Here again, almost no long-term controlled data are available as to the indications for therapy and the appropriate choice of drugs. If both systolic and diastolic pressures are elevated, elderly patients should be treated in a manner similar to that for younger persons; they seem to respond as well and have no more problems with medications.[12] In view of the reduced effectiveness of the baroreceptor reflex[179] and the failure of cerebral autoregulation that may occur in the elderly, drugs with a propensity to cause postural hypotension should be avoided, and all drugs should be given in slowly increasing doses to prevent excessive lowering of the pressure.

Isolated systolic hypertension in the elderly presents a risk, particularly for strokes.[180] It is likely that judicious lowering of the pressure will protect against and not precipitate cardiovascular catastrophes. Admittedly, most isolated elevations of systolic pressure are due to structural hardening of the arterial walls, and the vessels may not be able to dilate as well as the functionally constricted, more pliant vessels of young people. The goals of therapy should not be rigid; a systolic pressure of 160 mm Hg seems reasonable for people over 60 years of age. It is hoped that data on the effectiveness of therapy for isolated systolic hypertension will be forthcoming from the Systolic Hypertension in the Elderly Program (SHEP) trial. The preliminary data from this trial show that the systolic pressures of most will respond to a small dose of a diuretic, without inordinate side effects.[18] Low-sodium diets,[181] calcium blockers,[135] and alpha blockers[182] may be especially effective in the elderly. Despite the observation that elderly patients respond less well to beta blockers than do younger patients,[135] the response to a beta blocker was equal to that of a diuretic in a large, controlled study of elderly patients.[136]

As noted on page 821, some elderly people may have high blood pressure as measured by the sphygmomanometer but may have less or no hypertension when direct intraarterial readings are made. Presumably their pseudohypertension is related to the failure of the sphygmomanometer cuff to collapse the rigid artery beneath the cuff. For those patients with vessels that feel rigid and who have few retinal or cardiac findings of hypertension, as would be expected with high sphygmomanometer readings, direct intraarterial measurements should be made before therapy is begun in order to avoid inordinately lowering blood pressures which are not, in fact, elevated.

HYPERTENSION WITH RENAL INSUFFICIENCY (See also p. 839). In the presence of renal insufficiency, hypertension is usually predominantly caused by volume excess, and most patients can be successfully treated with salt restriction and diuretics. When serum creatinine exceeds 2.5 mg/dl, thiazides are usually relatively ineffective, and either metolazone or high doses of furosemide are required.[84] A few patients with chronic renal disease have a more resistant form of hypertension, usually associated with—and perhaps caused by—high levels of plasma renin activity. Medical therapy has been increasingly effective, not only in controlling the hypertension, but also in halting the deterioration of renal function.[183] With appropriate therapy, which may include hemodialysis for some time, hypertension can be controlled in most patients and the deterioration of renal function slowed.[184] Experimental evidence suggests that CEI's may be even more effective in preserving residual renal function,[168] particularly when diabetic nephropathy is responsible.[169]

HYPERTENSION WITH CONGESTIVE HEART FAILURE. Cardiac output may fall so markedly in hypertensive patients who are in heart failure that their blood pressure is reduced, obscuring the degree of hypertension; often, however, the diastolic pressure is raised by intense vasoconstriction while the systolic pressure falls as a result of the reduced stroke volume. Lowering the blood pressure may, by itself, relieve the heart failure. Chronic unloading has been most efficiently accomplished with CEI's (p. 877).[185] Antihypertensive drugs that primarily decrease cardiac output, particularly beta blockers, which remove the heart's needed sympathetic support, may be dangerous in the presence of heart failure.

HYPERTENSION WITH ISCHEMIC HEART DISEASE. The coexistence of ischemic heart disease makes antihypertensive therapy even more essential, since relief of the hypertension may ameliorate the coronary disease. Beta blockers and calcium-entry blockers are particularly useful if angina or arrhythmias are present.

The often markedly high levels of blood pressure during

TABLE 28–9 DRUGS FOR HYPERTENSIVE CRISES

Drug	Dosage	Onset of Action	Adverse Effects
Vasodilators			
Nitroprusside (Nipride, Nitropress)	0.5–10 μg/kg/min as I.V. infusion	Instantaneous	Nausea, vomiting, muscle twitching, sweating, thiocyanate intoxication
Nitroglycerin	5–100 μg/min as I.V. infusion	2–5 min	Bradycardia, tachycardia, flushing, headache, vomiting, methemoglobinemia
Diazoxide (Hyperstat)	50–100 mg/IV bolus, repeated or 15–30 mg/min by I.V. infusion	2–4 min	Nausea, hypotension, flushing, tachycardia, chest pain
Hydralazine (Apresoline)	10–20 mg I.V. 10–50 mg I.M.	10 min 20–30 min	Tachycardia, flushing, headache, vomiting, aggravation of angina
Adrenoceptor inhibitors			
Phentolamine (Regitine)	5–15 mg I.V.	1–2 min	Tachycardia, flushing
Trimethaphan (Arfonad)	1–4 mg/min as I.V. infusion	5–10 min	Paresis of bowel and bladder, orthostatic hypotension, blurred vision, dry mouth
Labetalol (Normodyne, Trandate)	20–80 mg I.V. bolus every 10 min 2 mg/min I.V. infusion	5–10 min	Vomiting, scalp tingling, burning in throat and groin, postural hypotension, dizziness, nausea
Methyldopa (Aldomet)	250–500 mg I.V. infusion	2–3 hours	Drowsiness

the early phase of an acute myocardial infarction may reflect sympathetic nervous hyperreactivity to pain. The combined alpha and beta blocker labetalol has been found to be effective and apparently safe in this setting.[186] Nifedipine has also been successfully used.[187]

HYPERTENSION WITH DIABETES MELLITUS. Diuretics may worsen diabetic control, probably because they induce potassium depletion. Brittle diabetics on insulin should not be given nonselective beta blockers, since these drugs may prevent the outpouring of catecholamines that counteracts a precipitous fall in blood sugar levels, thereby preventing the recognition of impending hypoglycemia and delaying the rebound rise in the blood sugar.

HYPERTENSION WITH PSYCHIATRIC ILLNESS. Patients who are anxious and emotionally labile may benefit from the calming effects of beta blockers on the somatic manifestations of anxiety.[137] However, caution is advised in using beta blockers, particularly the lipid-soluble ones,[130] which may induce depression, insomnia, and nightmares. If antidepressant or antipsychotic medications are needed, they will not blunt the effects of beta blockers or CEI's as they may those of guanethidine, methyldopa, or clonidine.

THERAPY FOR HYPERTENSIVE CRISES

When diastolic blood pressure exceeds 140 mm Hg, rapidly progressive damage to the arterial vasculature is demonstrable experimentally, and a surge of cerebral blood flow may rapidly lead to encephalopathy (see Fig. 28–5). Previously normotensive patients may develop encephalopathy at much lower levels of blood pressure. If such high pressures persist or there are any signs of encephalopathy, the pressures should be lowered using parenteral agents in those considered to be in immediate danger, or with oral agents in those who are alert and in no other acute distress.

A number of drugs for this purpose are now available (Table 28–9). If DBP exceeds 140 mm Hg, and the patient has any complications, such as a stroke or congestive heart failure, a constant infusion of nitroprusside is most effective and will almost always lower the pressure to the desired level. Constant monitoring, preferably with an intraarterial line, is mandatory; a slightly excessive dose may abruptly lower the pressure to levels that will induce shock. The potency and rapidity of action of nitroprusside make it the treatment of choice for life-threatening hypertension. As seen in Figure 28–11, nitroprusside acts as a venous and arteriolar dilator, so that venous return and cardiac output are lowered. With prolonged infusions, cyanide toxicity is rare, whereas thiocyanate toxicity may develop more insidiously.[188]

Those patients needing parenteral therapy but with less serious hypertension can be given small bolus injections or a constant infusion of diazoxide, intravenous labetalol, or hydralazine.[189] The latter drug is widely used to treat preeclampsia. With any of these agents, intravenous furosemide is often needed to lower the blood pressure further and prevent retention of salt and water. Diuretics should not be given if volume depletion is initially present.

For patients in less immediate danger, oral therapy may be used. Almost every drug has been used and most will, with repeated doses, reduce high pressures.[190] Clonidine, 0.1 to 0.2 mg every hour, has been successfully used,[114] but the current preference of many is nifedipine, 10 mg by mouth or sublingually repeated in 30 minutes if needed.[157] The pressure almost always falls about 25 per cent within the first 30 minutes. Rarely, and not unexpectedly, a few patients may suffer tissue ischemia with such rapid and marked falls in pressure. In some patients, particularly if their current high pressures are simply a reflection of stopping previously effective oral medication, that medication may be restarted. If their nonadherence to therapy was caused by side effects, appropriate changes should be made.

Fortunately, fewer patients in a hypertensive crisis are being seen, presumably because more hypertensive patients are being recognized and treated before the disease enters this malignant course. It is hoped that the continued successful treatment of many more hypertensives will lead to similar increases in prevention of the other, subtler, but more frequent, long-range sequelae of hypertension.

REFERENCES

INDICATIONS FOR THERAPY

1. Isles, C. G., Walker, L. M., Beevers, G. D., Brown, I., Cameron, H. L., Clarke, J., Hawthorne, V., Hole, D., Lever, A. F., Robertson, J. W. K., and Wapshaw, J. A.: Mortality in patients of the Glasgow Blood Pressure Clinic. J. Hypertension *4*:141, 1986.
2. Cloher, T. P., and Whelton, P. K.: Physician approach to the recognition and initial management of hypertension. Arch. Intern. Med. *146*:529, 1986.
3. Moser, M., Black, H., and Stair, D.: The dilemma of mild hypertension. Drugs *31*:279, 1986.
4. Hart, J. T.: The practitioner's view. *In* Gross, F., and Strasser, T. (eds.): Mild Hypertension: Recent Advances. New York, Raven Press, 1983, p. 365.
5. Working Group on Risk and High Blood Pressure: An epidemiological approach to describing risk associated with blood pressure levels. Final report of the Working Group on Risk and High Blood Pressure. Hypertension 7:641, 1985.
6. Kaplan, N. M.: Clinical Hypertension. 4th ed. Baltimore, Williams and Wilkins, 1986, p. 166.
7. Veterans Administration Cooperative Study Group on Antihypertensive Agents: Effects of treatment on morbidity in hypertension. II. Results in

patients with diastolic blood pressure averaging 90 through 114 mm Hg. J.A.M.A. *213*:1143, 1970.

8. U. S. Public Health Service Hospitals Cooperative Study Group, Smith, W. M.: Treatment of mild hypertension. Results of a ten-year intervention trial. Circ. Res. *40*(Suppl. 1):1–98, 1977.
9. Management Committee: The Australian therapeutic trial in mild hypertension. Lancet *1*:1261, 1980.
10. Helgeland, A.: Treatment of mild hypertension: A five year controlled drug trial. The Oslo Study. Am. J. Med. *69*:725, 1980.
11. Medical Research Council Working Party: MRC trial of treatment of mild hypertension: Principal results. Br. Med. J. *291*:97, 1985.
12. Amery, A., Birkenhager, W., Brixko, P., Blupitt, C., Clement, D., Deruyttere, M., Dollery, D., Fagard, R., Forette, F., Forte, J., Hamdy, R., Henry, J. F., Joossens, J. V., Leonetti, G., Lund-Johansen, P., O'Malley, K., Petrie, J., Strasser, T., and Tuomilehto, J.: Mortality and morbidity results from the European Working Party on high blood pressure in the elderly trial. Lancet *1*:1349, 1985.
13. Hypertension Detection and Follow-up Program Cooperative Research Group: The effect of antihypertensive drug treatment on mortality in the presence of resting electrocardiographic abnormalities at baseline: The HDFP experience. Circulation *70*:996, 1984.
14. Multiple Risk Factor Intervention Trial Research Group: Baseline rest electrocardiographic abnormalities, antihypertensive treatment, and mortality in the Multiple Risk Factor Intervention Trial. Am. J. Cardiol. *55*:1, 1985.
15. Kaplan, N. M.: Therapy of mild hypertension: An overview. Am. J. Cardiol. *53*:2A, 1984.
16. IPPPSH Collaborative Group: Cardiovascular risk and risk factors in a randomized trial of treatment based on the beta-blocker oxprenolol: The International Prospective Primary Prevention Study in Hypertension (IPPPSH). J. Hypertension 3:379, 1985.

GUIDELINES FOR TREATMENT

17. Perloff, D., Sokolow, M., and Cowan, R.: The prognostic value of ambulatory blood pressures. J.A.M.A. *249*:2792, 1983.
18. Hulley, S. B., Furberg, C. D., Gurland, B., McDonald, R., Perry, H. M., Schnaper, H. W., Schoenberger, J. A., Smith, W. M., and Vogt, T. M.: Systolic hypertension in the elderly program (SHEP); Antihypertensive efficacy of chlorthalidone. Am. J. Cardiol. *56*:913, 1985.
19. Heyden, S., Schneider, K., and Fodor, J. G.: Comprehensive health care and noncardiovascular mortality: An unlikely explanation of the findings from the Hypertension Detection and Follow-up Program Editorial. Circulation 72:692, 1985.
20. Hardy, R. J., and Hawkins, C. M.: The impact of selected indices of antihypertensive treatment on all-cause mortality. Am. J. Epidemiol. *117*:566, 1983.
21. WHO/ISH: 1986 guidelines for the treatment of mild hypertension: memorandum from a WHO/ISH meeting. Bull. W.H.O. *64*:31, 1986.
22. Samuelsson, O., Wilhelmsen, L., Elmfeldt, D., Pennert, K., Wedel, H., Wikstrand, J., and Berglund, G.: Predictors of cardiovascular morbidity in treated hypertension: Results from the Primary Preventive Trial in Goteborg, Sweden, J. Hypertension 3:167, 1985.
23. Bulpitt, C. J., Beevers, D. G., Butler, A., Coles, E. C., Hunt, D., Munro-Faure, A. D., Newson, R. B., O'Riordan, P. W., Petrie, J. C., Rajagopalan, B., Rylance, P. B., Twallin, G., Webster, J., and Dollery, C. T.: The survival of treated hypertensive patients and their causes of death: A report from the DHSS Hypertensive Care Computing Project (DHCCP). J. Hypertension *4*:93, 1986.
24. Ledingham, J. G. G., and Rajagopalan, B.: Cerebral complications in the treatment of accelerated hypertension. Q. J. Med. *48*:25, 1979.
25. Stewart, I. M. G.: Relation of reduction in pressure to first myocardial infarction in patients receiving treatment for severe hypertension. Lancet *1*:861, 1979.

NON-DRUG THERAPY

26. Alderman, M. H., Davis, T. K., Gerber, L. M., and Robb, M.: Antihypertensive drug therapy withdrawal in a general population. Arch. Intern. Med. *146*:1309, 1986.
27. Greenfield, S., Kaplan, S., and Ware, J. E. Jr.: Expanding patient involvement in care. Ann. Intern. Med. *102*:520, 1985.
28. Subcommittee on Nonpharmacologic Therapy of the 1984 Joint National Committee on Detection, Evaluation, and Treatment of High Blood Pressure: Nonpharmacologic approaches to the control of high blood pressure. Hypertension 8:444, 1986.
29. Kaplan, N. M.: Non-drug treatment of hypertension. Ann. Intern. Med. *102*:359, 1985.
30. MacMahon, S. W., Macdonald, G. J., Bernstein, L., Andrews, G., and Blacket, R. B.: Comparison of weight reduction with metoprolol in treatment of hypertension in young overweight patients. Lancet *1*:1233, 1985.
31. MacMahon, S. W., Wilcken, D. E. L., and Macdonald, G. J.: The effect of weight reduction on left ventricular mass. A randomized controlled trial in young, overweight hypertensive patients. N. Engl. J. Med. *314*:334, 1986.
32. Cohen, N., and Flamenbaum, W.: Obesity and hypertension. Demonstration of a "floor effect." Am. J. Med. *80*:177, 1986.
33. MacGregor, G. A.: Sodium is more important than calcium in essential hypertension. Hypertension 7:628, 1985.
34. Richards, A. M., Nicholls, M. G., Espiner, E. A., Ikram, H., Hamilton, E. J., Wells, J. E., Maslowski, A. H., and Yandle, T. G.: Endogenous angiotensin-aldosterone-pressure relationships during sodium restriction. Hypertension 7:681, 1985.
35. Andersson, O. K., Persson, B., Hedner, T., Aurell, M., Berglund, G., and Fagerberg, B.: Central haemodynamics, baroreceptor sensitivity and alpha$_1$ adrenoceptor-mediated vascular reactivity during weight-stable sodium restriction in obese men with hypertension. J. Hypertension *4*:101, 1986.
36. Poston, L., Johnson, V. E., Gray, H. H., Hilton, P. J., Markandu, N. D., and MacGregor, G. A.: The effect of dietary sodium restriction on leucocyte sodium transport in normotensive subjects and in patients with essential hypertension. Klin. Wochenschr. *63*(Suppl. 3):136, 1985.
37. Stokes, G. S., Monaghan, J. C., Middleton, A. T., Shirlow, M., and Marwood, J. F.: Effects of dietary sodium deprivation or erythrocyte sodium concentration and cation transport in normotensive and untreated hypertensive subjects. J. Hypertension *4*:35, 1986.
38. Rydstedt, L. L., Williams, G. H., and Hollenberg, N. K.: Renal and endocrine response to saline infusion in essential hypertension. Hypertension *8*:217, 1986.
39. Ram, C. V. S., Garrett, B. N., and Kaplan, N. M.: Moderate sodium restriction and various diuretics in the treatment of hypertension. Arch. Intern. Med. *141*:1015, 1981.
40. Toal, C. B., and Leenen, F. H. H.: Dietary restriction and development of hypertension in spontaneous hypertensive rats. Am. J. Physiol. *245*:H1081, 1983.
41. Avolio, A. P., Clyde, K. M., Beard, T. C., Cooker, H. M., Ho, K. K. L., and O'Rourke, M. F.: Improved arterial distensibility in normotensive subjects on a low salt diet. Arteriosclerosis *6*:166, 1986.
42. Morgan, T., Anderson, A., Wilson, D., Myers, J., Murphy, J., and Nowson, C.: Paradoxical effect of sodium restriction on blood pressure in people on slow-channel calcium blocking drugs. Lancet *1*:793, 1986.
43. Kaplan, N. M., Simmons, M., McPhee, C., Carnegie, A., Stefanu, C., and Cade, S.: Two techniques to improve adherence to dietary sodium restriction in the treatment of hypertension. Arch. Intern. Med. *42*:1638, 1982.
44. Anonymous: Dietary potassium and hypertension (Editorial). Lancet *1*:1308, 1985.
45. Kaplan, N. M., Carnegie, A., Raskin, P., Heller, J. A., and Simmons, M.: Potassium supplementation in hypertensive patients with diuretic-induced hypokalemia. N. Engl. J. Med. *312*:746, 1985.
46. Richards, A. M., Nicholls, M. G., Espiner, E. A., Ikram, H., Maslowski, A. H., Hamilton, E. J., and Wells, J. E.: Blood pressure response to moderate sodium restriction and to potassium supplementation in mild essential hypertension. Lancet *1*:757, 1984.
47. Svetkey, L. P., Yarger, W. E., Feussner, J. R., Delong, E., and Klotman, P. E.: Placebo-controlled trial of oral potassium in the treatment of mild hypertension. Clin. Res. *34*(Abs.):487A, 1986.
48. Cappuccio, F. P., Markandu, N. D., Beynon, G. W., Shore, A. C., Sampson, B., and MacGregor, G. A.: Lack of effect of oral magnesium on high blood pressure: A double-blind study. Br. Med. J. *291*:235, 1985.
49. Whang, R., Flink, E. B., Dyckner, T., Wester, P. O., Aikawa, J. K., and Ryan, M. P.: Magnesium depletion as a cause of refractory potassium repletion. Arch. Intern. Med. *145*:1686, 1985.
50. McCarron, D. A.: Is calcium more important than sodium in the pathogenesis of essential hypertension? Hypertension 7:607, 1985.
51. McCarron, D. A., and Morris, C. D.: Blood pressure response to oral calcium in persons with mild to moderate hypertension. Ann. Intern. Med. *103*:825, 1985.
52. Grobbee, D. E., and Hofman, A.: Effect of calcium supplementation on diastolic blood pressure in young people with mild hypertension. Lancet *2*:703, 1986.
53. Rouse, I. L., Beilin, L. J., Mahoney, D. P., Margetts, B. M., Armstrong, B. K., Record, S. J., Vandongen, R., and Barden, A.: Nutrient intake, blood pressure, serum and urinary prostaglandins and serum thromboxane B_2 in a controlled trial with a lacto-ovo-vegetarian diet. J. Hypertension *4*:241, 1986.
54. Dodson, P. M., Pacy, P. J., and Cox, E. V.: Long-term follow-up of the treatment of essential hypertension with a high-fibre, low-fat and low-sodium dietary regimen. Hum. Nutr. Clin. Nutr. *39C*:213, 1985.
55. Herold, P. M., and Kinsella, J. E.: Fish oil consumption and decreased risk of cardiovascular disease: A comparison of findings from animal and human feeding trials. Am. J. Clin. Nutr. *43*:566, 1986.
56. Pacy, P. J., Dodson, P. M., ad Fletcher, R. F.: Effect of a high carbohydrate, low sodium and low fat diet in type 2 diabetics with moderate hypertension. Int. J. Obesity *10*:43, 1986.
57. Robertson, D., Hollister, A. S., Kincaid, D., Workman, R., Goldberg, M. R., Tung, C., and Smith, B.: Caffeine and hypertension. Am. J. Med. *77*:54, 1984.
58. Jackson, R., Stewart, A., Beaglehole, R., and Scragg, R.: Alcohol consumption and blood pressure. Am. J. Epidemiol. *122*:1037, 1985.
59. Moore, R. D., and Pearson, T. A.: Moderate alcohol consumption and coronary artery disease. Medicine *65*:242, 1986.
60. Gruchow, H. W., Hoffman, R. G., Anderson, A. J., and Barboriak, J. J.: Effects of drinking patterns on the relationship between alcohol and coronary occlusion. Atherosclerosis *43*:393, 1982.
61. Duncan, J. J., Farr, J. E., Upton, S. J., Hagan, R. D., Oglesby, M. E., and Blair, S. N.: The effects of aerobic exercise on plasma catecholamines and blood pressure in patients with mild essential hypertension. J.A.M.A. *254*:2609, 1985.
62. Jennings, G., Nelson, L., Nestel, P., Esler, M., Korner, P., Burton, D., and Bazelmans, J.: The effects of changes in physical activity on major cardiovascular risk factors, hemodynamics, sympathetic function, and glucose utilization in man: A controlled study of four levels of activity. Circulation *73*:30, 1986.
63. Health and Public Policy Committee: Biofeedback of hypertension. Ann. Intern. Med. *102*:709, 1985.
64. Patel, C., Marmot, M. G., Terry, D. J., Carruthers, M., Hunt, B., and Patel,

M.: Trial of relaxation in reducing coronary risk: 4-year follow-up. Br. Med. J. *290*:1103, 1985.

65. Langford, H. G., Blaufox, M. D., Oberman, A., Hawkins, C. M., Curb, J. D., Cutter, G. R., Wassertheil-Smoller, S., Pressel, S., Babcock, C., Abernethy, J. D., Hotchkiss, J., and Tyler, M.: Dietary therapy slows the return of hypertension after stopping prolonged medication. J.A.M.A. *253*:657, 1985.
66. Stamler, R., Stamler, J., Grimm, R., Dyer, A., Gosch, F. C., Berman, R., Elmer, P., Fishman, J., Van Heel, N., Civinelli, J., and Hoeksema, R.: Nonpharmacological control of hypertension. Prev. Med. *14*:336, 1985.

ANTIHYPERTENSIVE DRUG THERAPY

67. Haynes, R. B., Mattson, M. E., Garrity, T. F., Chobanian, A. V., Leventhal, H., Dunbar, J. M., Levine, R. J., Engebretson, T. O., and Levy, R. L.: Management of patient compliance in the treatment of hypertension. Report of the NHLBI Working Group. Hypertension *4*:415, 1982.
68. Asplund, J., Danielson, M., and Ohman, P.: Patients compliance in hypertension—the importance of number of tablets. Br. J. Clin. Pharmacol. *17*:547, 1984.
69. Spitalewitz, S., Porush, J. G., and Reiser, I. W.: Minoxidil, nadolol, and a diuretic. Once-a-day therapy for resistant hypertension. Arch. Intern. Med. *146*:882, 1986.
70. Strandgaard, S., and Paulson, O. B.: Cerebral autoregulation. Stroke *15*:413, 1984.
71. Barry, D. I.: Cerebral blood flow in hypertension. J. Cardiovasc. Pharmacol. *7* (Suppl.):S94, 1985.
72. Joint National Committee on Detection, Evaluation, and Treatment of High Blood Pressure: The 1984 report of the Joint National Committee on Detection, Evaluation, and Treatment of High Blood Pressure. Arch. Intern. Med. *144*:1045, 1984.
73. Laragh, J. H.: Potential of alpha-blockade in treating human hypertension: A role of indoramin. J. Cardiovasc. Pharmacol. *8* (Suppl. 2):S37, 1986.
74. Freis, E. D.: The cardiovascular risks of thiazide diuretics. Clin. Pharmacol. Ther. *39*:239, 1986.
75. Johnson, B. F., Saunders, R., Hickler, R., Marwaha, R., and Johnson, J.: The effects of thiazide diuretics upon plasma lipoproteins. J. Hypertension *4*:235, 1986.
76. Dustan, H. P., Tarazi, R. C., and Bravo, E. L.: Dependence of arterial pressure on intravascular volume in treated hypertensive patients. N. Engl. J. Med. *286*:861, 1972.
77. Zacest, R., Gilmore, E., and Koch-Weser, J.: Treatment of essential hypertension with combined vasodilation and beta-adrenergic blockade. N. Engl. J. Med. *286*:617, 1972.
78. Lant, A.: Diuretics. I. Clinical pharmacology and therapeutic use. Drugs *29*:57, 1985.
79. Bennett, W. M., McDonald, W. J., Kuehnel, E., Hartnett, M. N., and Porter, G. A.: Do diuretics have antihypertensive properties independent of natriuresis? Clin. Pharmacol. Ther. *22*:499, 1977.
80. Beevers, D. G., Hamilton, M., and Harpur, J. E.: The long-term treatment of hypertension with thiazide diuretics. Postgrad. Med. J. *47*:639, 1971.
81. Ridgeway, N. A., Ginn, D. R., and Alley, K.: Outpatient conversion of treatment to potassium-sparing diuretics. Am. J. Med. *80*:785, 1986.
82. Lutterodt, A., Nattel, S., and McLeod, P. J.: Duration of antihypertensive effect of a single daily dose of hydrochlorothiazide. Clin. Pharmacol. Ther. *27*:324, 1980.
83. Anderson, J. Godfrey, B. E., Hill, D. M., Munro-Faure, A. D., and Sheldon, J.: A comparison of the effects of hydrochlorothiazide and of furosemide in the treatment of hypertensive patients. Quart. J. Med. *40*:541, 1971.
84. Dargie, H. J., Allison, M. E. M., Kennedy, A. C., and Gray, M. J. B.: High dosage metolazone in chronic renal failure. Br. Med. J. *4*:196, 1972.
85. Morgan, D. B., and Davidson, C.: Hypokalemia and diuretics: An analysis of publications. Br. Med. J. *280*:905, 1980.
86. Sandor, F. F., Pickens, P. T., and Crallan, J.: Variations of plasma potassium concentrations during long-term treatment of hypertension with diuretics without potassium supplements. Br. Med. J. *284*:711, 1982.
87. Velazquez, H., and Wright, F. S.: Control by drugs of renal potassium handling. Annu. Rev. Pharmacol. Toxicol. *26*:293, 1986.
88. Holland, O. B.: Ventricular ectopic activity with diuretic-induced hypokalemia. Clin. Res. *34*(Abs.):480A, 1986.
89. Struthers, A. D., Whitesmith, R., and Reid, J. L.: Prior thiazide diuretic treatment increases adrenaline-induced hypokalemia. Lancet *1*:1358, 1983.
90. Papademetriou, V.: Diuretics, hypokalemia, and cardiac arrhythmias: A critical analysis (Editorial). Am. Heart J. *111*:1217, 1986.
91. Stewart, D. E., Ikram, H., Espiner, E. A., and Nicholls, M. G.: Arrhythmogenic potential of diuretic induced hypokalemia in patients with mild hypertension and ischaemic heart disease. Br. Heart J. *54*:290, 1985.
92. Johansson, B. W.: Effect of beta blockade on ventricular fibrillation- and ventricular tachycardia-induced circulatory arrest in acute myocardial infarction. Am. J. Cardiol. *57*:34F, 1986.
93. Rasmussen, H. S., McNair, P., Norregard, P., Backer, V., Lindeneg, O., and Balslev, S.: Intravenous magnesium in acute myocardial infarction. Lancet *1*:234, 1986.
94. Weidmann, P., Uehlinger, D. E., and Gerber, A.: Antihypertensive treatment and serum lipoproteins. J. Hypertension *3*:297, 1985.
95. Grimm, R. H., Leon, A. S., Hunninghake, D. B., Lenz, K., Hanna, P., and Blackburn, H.: Effects of thiazide diuretics on plasma lipids and lipoproteins in mildly hypertensive patients. Ann. Intern. Med. *94*:7, 1981.
96. Stier, C. T., Jr., and Itskovitz, H. D.: Renal calcium metabolism and diuretics. Annu. Rev. Pharmacol. Toxicol. *26*:101, 1986.
97. Veterans Administration Cooperative Study Group on Antihypertensive Agents: Propranolol or hydrochlorothiazide alone for the initial treatment of hypertension. IV. Effect on plasma glucose and glucose tolerance. Hypertension 7:1008, 1985.
98. Medical Research Council Working Party on Mild to Moderate Hypertension: Adverse reactions to bendrofluazide and propranolol for the treatment of mild hypertension. Lancet *2*:539, 1981.
99. Wong, D. G., Spence, J. D., Lamki, L., Freeman, D., and McDonald, J. W. D.: Effect of nonsteroidal anti-inflammatory drugs on control of hypertension by beta-blockers and diuretics. Lancet *1*:997, 1986.
100. Helgeland, A., Strømmen, R., Hagelund, C. H., and Tretli, A.: Enalapril, atenolol, and hydrochlorothiazide in mild to moderate hypertension. Lancet *1*:872, 1986.
101. Management Committee: Treatment of mild hypertension in the elderly. Med. J. Aust. *2*:398, 1981.
102. Veterans Administration Cooperative Study Group on Antihypertensive Agents: Comparison of propranolol and hydrochlorothiazide for the initial treatment of hypertension. I. Results of short-term titration with emphasis on racial differences in response. J.A.M.A. *248*:1996, 1982.
103. Rosendorf, C.: α-Adrenoreceptors in hypertension. J. Cardiovasc. Pharmacol. *8* (Suppl. 2):S3, 1986.
104. Veterans Administration Cooperative Study Group on Antihypertensive Agents: Propranolol in the treatment of essential hypertension. J.A.M.A. *237*:2303, 1977.
105. Participating Veterans Administration Medical Centers: Low dose vs. standard dose of reserpine. J.A.M.A. *248*:2471, 1982.
106. Horwitz, R. I., and Feinstein, A. R.: Exclusion bias and the false relationship of reserpine and breast cancer. Arch. Intern. Med. *145*:1873, 1985.
107. Finnerty, F. A., Jr., and Brogden, R. N.: Guanadrel: A review of its pharmacodynamic and pharmacokinetic properties and therapeutic use in hypertension. Drugs *30*:22, 1985.
108. Struthers, A. D., Brown, M. J., Adams, E. F., and Dollery, C. T.: The plasma noradrenaline and growth hormone response to α-methyldopa and clonidine in hypertensive subjects. Br. J. Clin. Pharmacol. *19*:311, 1985.
109. Fouad, F. M., Nakashima, Y., Tarazi, R. C., and Salcedo, E. E.: Reversal of left ventricular hypertrophy in hypertensive patients treated with methyldopa. Am. J. Cardiol. *49*:795, 1982.
110. Kelton, J. G.: Impaired reticuloendothelial function in patients treated with methyldopa. N. Engl. J. Med. *313*:596, 1985.
111. Kaplowitz, N., Aw, T. Y., Simon, F. R., and Stolz, A.: Drug-induced hepatotoxicity. Ann. Intern. Med. *104*:826, 1986.
112. Houston, M. C.: Abrupt cessation of treatment in hypertension: Consideration of clinical features, mechanisms, prevention and management of the discontinuation syndrome. Am. Heart J. *102*:415, 1981.
113. Weber, M. A., Drayer, J. I. M., McMahon, F. G., Hamburger, R., Shah, A. R., and Kirk, L. N.: Transdermal administration of clonidine for treatment of high blood pressure. Arch. Intern. Med. *144*:1211, 1984.
114. Houston, M. C.: Treatment of hypertensive emergencies and urgencies with oral clonidine loading and titration. Arch. Intern. Med. *146*:586, 1986.
115. Bond, W. S.: Psychiatric indications for clonidine: the neuropharmacologic and clinical basis. J. Clin. Psychopharmacol. *6*:81, 1986.
116. Gehr, M., MacCarthy, E. P., and Goldberg, M.: Natriuretic and water diuretic effects of central α_2-adrenoceptor agonists. J. Cardiovasc. Pharmacol. *6*:S781, 1984.
117. Kaplan, N. M.: Effects of guanabenz on plasma lipid levels in hypertensive patients. J. Cardiovasc. Pharmacol. *6*:S841, 1984.
118. Lopez, L. M., and Mehta, J. L.: Comparative efficacy and safety of lofexidine and clonidine in mild to moderately severe systemic hypertension. Am. J. Cardiol. *53*:787, 1984.
119. Sorkin, E. M., and Heel, R. C.: Guanfacine. A review of its pharmacodynamic and pharmacokinetic properties, and therapeutic efficacy in the treatment of hypertension. Drugs *31*:301, 1986.
120. Beretta-Piccoli, C., Ferrier, C., and Weidmann, P.: α_1-Adrenergic blockade and cardiovascular pressor responses in essential hypertension. Hypertension *8*:407, 1986.
121. Nicholson, J. P., Resnick, L. M., Pickering, T. G., Marion, R., Sullivan, P., and Laragh, J. H.: Relationship of blood pressure response and the renin-angiotensin system to first-dose prazosin. Am. J. Med. *78*:241, 1985.
122. Heagerty, A. M., Russell, G. I., Bing, R. F., Thurston, H., and Swales, J. D.: The addition of prazosin to standard triple therapy in the treatment of severe hypertension. Br. J. Clin. Pharmacol. *13*:539, 1982.
123. Sacks, F. M., and Dzau, V. J.: Adrenergic effects on plasma lipoprotein metabolism. Speculation and mechanisms of action. Am. J. Med. *80* (Suppl. 2A):71, 1986.
124. Lund-Johansen, P., Omvik, P., and Haugland, H.: Acute and chronic haemodynamic effects of doxazosin in hypertension at rest and during exercise. Br. J. Clin. Pharmacol. *21*:45S, 1986.
125. Bishop, N., Mackintosh, A. F., Stoker, J. B., Mary, D. A. S. G., and Linden, R. J.: The effect of indoramin on exercise performance in mild hypertension. J Cardiovasc. Pharmacol. *8* (Suppl. 2):S30, 1986.
126. Vincent, J., Elliott, H. L., Meredith, P. A., and Reid, J. L.: Racial differences in drug responses—a comparative study of trimazosin and α_1-adrenoceptor responses in normotensive Caucasians and West Africans. Br. J. Clin. Pharmacol. *21*:401, 1986.
127. Pedersen, T. R., for the Norwegian Multicenter Study Group: Six-year follow-up of the Norwegian multicenter study on timolol after acute myocardial infarction. N. Engl. J. Med. *313*:1055, 1985.
128. Choong, C. Y. P., Roubin, G. S., Harris, P. J., Tokuyasu, Y., Shen, W.-F., Bautovich, G. J., and Kelly, D. T.: A comparison of the effects of β-blockers with and without intrinsic sympathomimetic activity on hemodynamics and left ventricular function at rest and during exercise in patients with coronary artery disease. J. Cardiovasc. Pharmacol. *8*:441, 1986.
129. Johnson, B. F., Weiner, B., Marwaha, R., and Johnson, J.: The influence of

pindolol and hydrochlorothiazide on blood pressure, and plasma renin and plasma lipid levels. J. Clin. Pharmacol. *26*:258, 1986.
130. Avorn, J., Everitt, D. E., and Weiss, S.: Increased antidepressant use in patients prescribed β-blockers. J.A.M.A. *255*:357, 1986.
131. van Zwieten, P. A., and Timmermans, P. B. M. W. M.: Brain levels and acute antihypertensive activity of β-blockers. Eur. J. Clin. Pharmacol. *28* (Suppl.):13, 1985.
132. Baumgart, P., Zidek, W., Schmidt, W., Haecker, W., Dorst, K. G., and Vetter, H.: Intracellular calcium in hypertension: Effect of treatment with β-adrenoreceptor blockers. J. Cardiovasc. Pharmacol. 8:559, 1986.
133. Fagan, T. C., Gourley, L. A., Sawyer, P. R., Lee, J. T., Walle, T., and Gaffney, T. E.: Acute hypotensive effects of oral and intravenous propranolol: Early alterations in peripheral resistance. J. Clin. Hypertension. *1*:21, 1986.
134. Serlin, M. M. Orme, M. L'E., Baber, N. A., Sibeon, R. G., Laws, E., and Breckenridge, A.: Propranolol in the control of blood pressure: A dose-response study. Clin. Pharmacol. Ther. 27:586, 1980.
135. Muller, F. B., Bolli, P., Erne, P., Kiowski, W., and Buhler, F. R.: Use of calcium antagonists as monotherapy in the management of hypertension. Am. J. Med. 77:11, 1984.
136. Wikstrand, J., Westergren, G., Berglund, G., Bracchetti, D., Van Couter, A., Feldstein, C. A., Ming, K. S., Kuramoto, K., Landahl, S., Meaney, E., Pedersen, E. B., Rahn, K. H., Shaw, J., Smith, A., and Waal-Manning, H.: Antihypertensive treatment with metoprolol or hydrochlorothiazide in patients aged 60 to 75 years. Report from a double-blind international multicenter study. J.A.M.A. *255*:1304, 1986.
137. Sherwood, A., Allen, M. T., Obrist, P. A., and Langer, A. W.: Evaluation of beta-adrenergic influences on cardiovascular and metabolic adjustments to physical and psychologic stress. Psychophysiology 23:89, 1986.
138. Chap, Z., Ishida, T., Chou, J., Michael, L., Hartley, C., Entman, M., and Field, J. B.: Effects of alpha and beta adrenergic blockade on hepatic glucose balance before and after oral glucose. J. Clin. Invest. 77:1357, 1986.
139. Bauer, J. H.: Adrenergic blocking agents and the kidney. J. Clin. Hypertension *3*:199, 1985.
140. De Swiet, M.: Antihypertensive drugs in pregnancy. Br. Med. J. *291*:365, 1985.
141. Fraunfelder, F. T.: Ocular β-blockers and systemic effects. Arch. Intern. Med. *146*:1073, 1986.
142. Lund-Johansen, P.: Pharmacology of combined α-β-blockade II. Haemodynamic effects of labetalol. Drugs *28* (Suppl. 2):35, 1984.
143. Lebel, M., Langlois, S., Belleau, L. J., and Grose, J. H.: Labetalol infusion in hypertensive emergencies. Clin. Pharmacol. Ther. *37*:615, 1985.
144. Shepherd, A. M. M., and Irvine, N. A.: Differential hemodynamic and sympathoadrenal effects of sodium nitroprusside and hydralazine in hypertensive subjects. J. Cardiovasc. Pharmacol. 8:527, 1986.
145. Perry, H. M., Jr., Camel, G. H., Carmody, S. E., Ahmed, K. A., and Perry, E. F.: Survival in hydralazine-treated hypertensive patients with and without late toxicity. J. Chronic Dis. *30*:519, 1977.
146. Cinquegrani, M. P., and Liang, C.: Indomethacin attenuates the hypotensive action of hydralazine. Clin. Pharmacol. Ther. *39*:564, 1986.
147. Hagstam, K., Lundgren, R., and Wieslander, J.: Clinical experience of long-term treatment with minoxidil in severe arterial hypertension. Scand. J. Urol. Nephrol. *16*:57, 1982.
148. Houston, M. C., McChesney, J. A., Chatterjee, K.: Pericardial effusion associated with minoxidil therapy. Arch. Intern. Med. *141*:69, 1981.
149. Hurwitz, L.: Pharmacology of calcium channels and smooth muscle. Annu. Rev. Pharmacol. Toxicol. *26*:225, 1986.
150. Agabiti-Rosei, E., Muiesan, M. L., Romanelli, G., Castellano, M., Beschi, M., Corea, L., and Muiesan, G.: Similarities and differences in the antihypertensive effect of two calcium antagonist drugs, verapamil and nifedipine. J. Am. Coll. Cardiol. 7:916, 1986.
151. Halperin, A. K., and Cubeddu, L. X.: The role of calcium channel blockers in the treatment of hypertension. Am. Heart J. *111*:363, 1986.
152. Sunderrajan, S., Reams, G., and Bauer, J. H.: Renal effects of diltiazem in primary hypertension. Hypertension 8:238, 1986.
153. Nicholson, J. P., Resnick, L. M., James, G. D., Jennis, R., and Laragh, J. H.: Sodium restriction and the antihypertensive effect of nitrendipine. Clin. Res. *34* (Abs.):404A, 1986.
154. Fadayomi, M. O., Akinroye, K. K., Ajao, R. O., and Awosika, L. A.: Monotherapy with nifedipine for essential hypertension in adult blacks. J. Cardiovasc. Pharmacol. 8:466, 1986.
155. Veldhuis, J. D., Borges, J. L. C., Drake, C. R., Rogol, A. D., Kaiser, D. L., and Thorner, M. O.: Divergent influences of the structurally dissimilar calcium entry blockers, diltiazem and verapamil, on thyrotropin- and gonadotropin-releasing hormone-stimulated anterior pituitary hormone secretion in man. J. Clin. Endocrinol. Metab. *60*:144, 1985.
156. Marone, C., Luisoli, S., Bomio, F., Beretta-Piccoli, C., Bianchetti, M. G., and Weidmann, P.: Body sodium-blood volume state, aldosterone, and cardiovascular responsiveness after calcium entry blockade with nifedipine. Kidney Int. 28:658, 1985.
157. Houston, M. C.: Treatment of hypertensive urgencies and emergencies with nifedipine. Am. Heart J. *111*:963, 1986.
158. Weinberger, M. H.: Blood pressure and metabolic responses to hydrochlorothiazide, captopril, and the combination in black and white mild-to-moderate hypertensive patients. J. Cardiovasc. Pharmacol. 7:S52, 1985.
159. Reams, G. P., and Bauer, J. H.: Long-term effects of enalapril monotherapy and enalapril/hydrochlorothiazide combination therapy on blood pressure, renal function, and body fluid composition. J. Clin. Hypertension *1*:55, 1986.
160. Todd, P. A., and Heel, R. C.: Enalapril. A review of its pharmacodynamic and pharmacokinetic properties, and therapeutic use in hypertension and congestive heart failure. Drugs *31*:198, 1986.
161. Giudicelli, J. F., Berdeaux, A., Edouard, A., Richer, C., and Jacolot, D.: The effect of enalapril on baroreceptor-mediated reflex function in normotensive subjects. Br. J. Clin. Pharmacol. *20*:211, 1985.
162. Ajayi, A. A., and Reid, J. L.: The effect of enalapril on baroreceptor mediated reflex function in normotensive subjects. Br. J. Clin. Pharmacol. *21*:338, 1986.
163. Navis, G. J., de Zeeuw, D., and de Jong, P. E.: Enalapril and the kidney: renal vasodilation and natriuresis due to the inhibition of angiotensin II formation. J. Cardiovasc. Pharmacol. 8: (Suppl. 1):S30, 1986.
164. Atlas, S. A., Case, D. B., Sealey, J. E., Laragh, J. H., and McKinstry, D. N.: Interruption of the renin-angiotensin system in hypertensive patients by captopril induces sustained reduction in aldosterone secretion, potassium retention and natriuresis. Hypertension *1*:274, 1979.
165. Muller, F. B., Sealey, J. E., Case, D. B., Atlas, S. A., Pickering, T. G., Pecker, M. S., Preibisz, J. J., and Laragh, J. H.: The captopril test for identifying renovascular disease in hypertensive patients. Am. J. Med. *80*:633, 1986.
166. Reams, G. P., Bauer, J. H., and Gaddy, P.: Use of the converting enzyme inhibitor enalapril in renovascular hypertension. Hypertension 8:290, 1986.
167. Wenting, G. J., Tan-Tjiong, H. L., Derkx, F. H. M., de Bruyn, J. H. B., Man in't Veld, A. J., and Schalekamp, M. A. D. H.: Split renal function after captopril in unilateral renal artery stenosis. Br. Med. J. *288*:886, 1984.
168. Raij, L., Chiou, X-C., Owens, R., and Wrigley, B.: Therapeutic implications of hypertension-induced glomerular injury. Am. J. Med. 79 (Suppl. 3C):37, 1985.
169. Zatz, R., Dunn, B. R., Meyer, T. W., Anderson, S., Rennke, H. G., and Brenner, B. M.: Prevention of diabetic glomerulopathy by pharmacological amelioration of glomerular capillary hypertension. J. Clin. Invest. 77:1925, 1986.
170. Taguma, Y., Kitamoto, K., Futaki, G., Ueda, H., Monma, H., Ishizaki, M., Takahashi, H., Sekino, H., and Sasaki, Y.: Effect of captopril on heavy proteinuria in azotemic diabetics. N. Engl. J. Med. *313*:1617, 1985.
171. Croog, S. H., Levine, S., Testa, M. A., Brown, B., Bulpitt, C. J., Jenkins, C. D., Klerman, G. L., and Williams, G. H.: The effects of antihypertensive therapy on the quality of life. N. Engl. J. Med. *314*:1657, 1986.
172. Houston, D. S., and Vanhoutte, P. M.: Serotonin and the vascular system. Role in health and disease, and implications for therapy. Drugs *31*:149, 1986.

SPECIAL CONSIDERATIONS IN THERAPY

173. Goldman, L.: Cardiac risks and complications of noncardiac surgery. Ann. Intern. Med. 98:504, 1983.
174. Magnusson, J., Thulin, T., Werner, O., Jarhult, J., and Thomson, D.: Haemodynamic effects of pretreatment with metoprolol in hypertensive patients undergoing surgery. Br. J. Anaesth. *58*:251, 1986.
175. Rogers, K., Hysing, E. S., Merin, R. G., Taylor, A., Hartley, C., and Chelly, J. E.: Cardiovascular effects of and interaction between calcium blocking drugs and anesthetics in chronically instrumented dogs. II. Verapamil, enflurane, and isoflurane. Anesthesiology *64*:568, 1986.
176. van Wezel, H. B., Bovill, J. G., Schuller, J., Gielen, J., and Hoeneveld, M. H.: Comparison of nitroglycerine, verapamil and nifedipine in the management of arterial pressure during coronary artery surgery. Br. J. Anaesth. *58*:267, 1986.
177. Patel, C. B., Laboy, V., Venus, B., Mathru, M., and Wier, D.: Use of sodium nitroprusside in post-coronary bypass surgery. A plea for conservatism. Chest *89*:663, 1986.
178. Lieberman, E.: Hypertension in childhood and adolescence. *In* Kaplan, N. M. (ed.): Clinical Hypertension. 4th ed. Baltimore, Williams and Wilkins, 1986, p. 447.
179. Shimada, K., Kitazumi, T., Ogura, H., Sadakane, N., and Ozawa, T.: Differences in age-independent effects of blood pressure on baroreflex sensitivity between normal and hypertensive subjects. Clin. Sci. *70*:489, 1986.
180. Curb, J. D., Borhani, N. O., Entwisle, G., Tung, B., Kass, E., Schnaper, H., Williams, W., and Berman, R.: Isolated systolic hypertension in 14 communities. Am. J. Epidemiol., *121*:362, 1985.
181. Niarchos, A. P., Weinstein, D. L., and Laragh, J. H.: Comparison of the effects of diuretic therapy and low sodium intake in isolated systolic hypertension. Am. J. Med. 77:1061, 1984.
182. Ram, C. V. S., Kaplan, N. M., Devous, M. D., Sr., and Bonte, F. J.:Cerebral blood flow and blood pressure response to prazosin therapy in the elderly hypertensive patients. Clin. Res. *34* (Abs.): 485A, 1986.
183. Bergstrom, J., Alvestrand, A., Bucht, H., and Gutierrez, A.: Progression of chronic renal failure in man is retarded with more frequent clinical follow-ups and better blood pressure control. Clin. Nephrol. 25:1, 1986.
184. Bakir, A. A., Bazilinski, N., and Dunea, G.: Transient and sustained recovery from renal shutdown in accelerated hypertension. Am. J. Med. *80*:172, 1986.
185. Kromer, E. P., Riegger, G. A. J., Liebau, G., and Kochsiek, K.: Effectiveness of converting enzyme inhibition (enalapril) for mild congestive heart failure. Am. J. Cardiol. *57*:459, 1986.
186. Renard, M., Jacobs, Ph., Liebens, I., Abou Hamdam, B., and Bernard, R.: A comparison of the effects of combined or separate alpha- and beta-blockade in the treatment of hypertension in the acute stage of myocardial infarction. Int. J. Cardiol. *10*:149, 1986.
187. Majid, P. A., Niznick, J., Nishizaki, S., and Haq, A.: Hemodynamic effects of nifedipine in acute myocardial infarction with observations in infarct size. J. Cardiovasc. Pharmacol. 8:262, 1986.
188. Cetnarowski, A. B., and Conti, D. R.: Nitroprusside toxicity and low-dose infusion. Ann. Intern. Med. *104*:895, 1986.
189. Ferguson, R. K., and Vlasses, P. H.: Hypertensive emergencies and urgencies. J.A.M.A. 255:1607, 1986.
190. Anderson, R. J., and Reed, W. G.: Current concepts in treatment of hypertensive urgencies. Am. Heart J. *111*:211, 1986.

29 HYPOTENSION AND SYNCOPE

by BURTON E. SOBEL, M.D., and
ROBERT ROBERTS, M.D.

The *sudden* development of hypotension, particularly when it occurs in a recumbent patient, is usually associated with impaired systemic perfusion and may be an important feature of shock, as discussed in detail in Chapter 19. In contrast, *chronic hypotension*, with systolic pressure in the range of 85 to 110 mm Hg, is not pathological and may actually be associated with a longer life expectancy than a "normal" arterial pressure. This chapter deals with a variety of syndromes responsible for *episodic hypotension* and its cardinal clinical manifestation, syncope.

REGULATION OF ARTERIAL PRESSURE

(See also page 562)

Systemic arterial pressure is closely related to the product of cardiac output and systemic vascular resistance. *Cardiac output* is the product of heart rate and stroke volume, the latter being determined by interactions between preload, afterload, and contractility, as described in Chapter 15. Thus, the cardiac causes of sudden hypotension relate to abrupt reductions in ventricular rate, as occurs with atrioventricular block, or in stroke volume, as may occur in hypovolemia (reduced preload); massive pulmonary embolism (augmented afterload); or to massive myocardial infarction (impaired ventricular function). *Vascular resistance* varies inversely with the fourth power of the radius of the resistance vessels, the arterioles, and therefore is determined by the intrinsic physical characteristics of these vessels, i.e., the ratio of lumen to wall thickness; the degree of extravascular support and compression; and the extent of contraction of the smooth muscle in the vascular wall.

Contraction of vascular smooth muscle is in turn influenced by (1) metabolic and mechanical autoregulatory mechanisms that act to maintain *nearly* constant perfusion of each vascular bed—there is substantial evidence that adenosine is a principal metabolic mediator of vascular resistance (p. 1198); (2) neurogenic vasoconstrictor influences, operating through the action of adrenergic neurotransmitter norepinephrine on alpha-adrenoceptors in vascular smooth muscle; (3) neurogenic vasodilator influences, operating through the action of acetylcholine on muscarinic receptors, or norepinephrine on $beta_2$ receptors, and perhaps of histamine, serotonin, and other transmitters; and (4) circulating and locally released vasoactive substances, including catecholamines, angiotensin II, bradykinin, and prostaglandins. The vascular causes of hypotension may involve any of these four mechanisms (Table 29–1).

The autonomic nervous system plays a major role in the maintenance of arterial pressure because it influences both cardiac output and the degree of constriction of the vessels of resistance (arterioles) and capacitance (venules and veins). The afferent limbs of the autonomic reflex arcs that acutely regulate arterial pressure arise in stretch receptors in the aortic arch, the carotid sinuses, ventricles, and atria. Impulses are transmitted along afferent fibers in the glossopharyngeal and vagus nerves to extensive central connections in the medulla. Synapses connect not only the sympathetic and parasympathetic nuclei and efferent arcs but also the cerebral cortex and hypothalamic nuclei, which control hormonal secretion via the pituitary gland (Fig. 29–1).

A sudden reduction of arterial and intraventricular pressure diminishes the stimulation of pressoreceptors, which in turn reflexly activates sympathetic outflow and inhibits parasympathetic activity. As a result, vascular smooth muscle in arterioles and veins constricts, whereas heart rate and myocardial contractility are augmented. In addition, as arterial pressure falls, adrenal medullary secretion increases, along with the output of antidiuretic hormone (ADH), adrenocorticotropic hormone (ACTH), renin, and aldosterone; all these effects tend to restore the arterial pressure toward control levels. Opposite changes occur if arterial pressure rises suddenly. Thus, the operation of these baroreceptors and a number of hormonal systems normally serve to buffer the body from a variety of influences that would otherwise produce marked alterations in arterial pressure.

In a resting supine adult, the level of sympathetic discharge to the vasculature is low.[1] Assumption of the upright posture is accompanied by venous pooling of approximately 700 ml of blood in the legs.[1,2] Systemic arterial pressure is maintained by venous and arterial constriction mediated by sympathetic stimulation. Even modest reflex changes of this type markedly facilitate maintenance of venous return and stroke volume.[1] The initial gravitational effects associated with upright posture are compensated not only by reflex arteriolar and venous constriction but also by acceleration of heart rate and by mechanical factors that limit venous pooling in the lower extremities, including venous valves, "milking" of veins in the lower extremities by contractions of the leg musculature, and reduced intrathoracic pressure that facilitates venous return. The increased sympathetic activity is reflected in a rise in concentration of plasma catecholamines.[3] As a consequence of these compensatory mechanisms, when a normal person assumes the upright posture, there is only a transient decline in systolic arterial blood pressure, generally of 5 to 15 mm Hg. Diastolic pressure tends to rise, and mean arterial pressure remains essentially unchanged; cardiac output and stroke volume decline; and there is reflex tachycardia and vasoconstriction, the latter reflected in a rise in systemic vascular resistance. In patients with orthostatic hypotension, by definition the decline in arterial pressure with assumption of the upright posture is more profound and persistent. Depending on the severity and duration of the hypotension, it may be accompanied by symptoms of impaired cerebral perfusion such as dizziness, presyncope, or syncope.

Hypotension may be a manifestation of impairment of any element in (1) the afferent limb, including the carotid,

TABLE 29–1 IMPORTANT CAUSES OF PROLONGED OR INTERMITTENT HYPOTENSION

1. Cardiac dysfunction
   a. Disturbances of rate and rhythm
      (1) Conduction abnormalities
      (2) Diverse dysrhythmias, including severe bradycardias and paroxysmal tachycardias
   b. Obstruction to flow
      (1) Aortic or pulmonary subvalvular, valvular, or supravalvular stenosis
      (2) Hypertrophic obstructive cardiomyopathy
      (3) Atrial myxoma or thrombus
      (4) Primary pulmonary hypertension
      (5) Pulmonary peripheral branch stenosis
      (6) Pulmonary emboli
      (7) Cardiac tamponade
      (8) Mitral or tricuspid stenosis
      (9) Malfunctioning prosthetic aortic or mitral valve
      (10) Cor triatriatum
      (11) Tetralogy of Fallot
      (12) Eisenmenger's syndrome
   c. Impaired ventricular function
      (1) Myocardial infarction
      (2) Cardiomyopathy
2. Decreased effective circulating blood volume
   a. Hemorrhage
   b. Dehydration
   c. Diabetes insipidis
   d. Severe burn
   e. Hemodialysis
   f. Third trimester pregnancy
   g. Arteriovenous shunt or venous insufficiency
3. Vascular or neurological dysfunction
   a. Vasovagal
   b. Postural hypotension
      (1) Idiopathic
      (2) Acquired
      (3) Familial
      (4) Deconditioning with prolonged bed rest or space flight
      (5) Heat stroke
      (6) Fever
      (7) Anorexia nervosa
      (8) Pregnancy
   c. Hyperventilation
   d. Carotid sinus hypersensitivity
   e. Glossopharyngeal neuralgia, micturition, deglutition, or post-tussive syncope
   f. Syncope migraine
   g. Acute or chronic autonomic neuropathy
   h. Guillain-Barré syndrome
4. Metabolic and endocrine disturbances
   a. Pheochromocytoma
   b. Serotonin-secreting tumors
   c. Hyperbradykininemia
   d. Adrenal insufficiency
   e. Electrolyte disturbance, especially hypokalemia
5. Drug toxicity
   a. Vasodilators
   b. Adrenergic antagonists
   c. Diuretics
   d. Phenothiazines
   e. Antidepressants
   f. Nitrates
   g. Calcium channel blockers
   h. Barbiturates and other CNS depressants
   i. Vincristine and other neuropathic drugs
   j. Quinidine and other drugs with negative chronotropic effects
   k. Digitalis
   l. Marijuana
   m. Alcohol
   n. Cocaine
   o. Insulin

aortic, ventricular, and atrial baroreceptors; (2) the central vasomotor centers; (3) the cortical or spinal outflow efferent tracts; (4) the peripheral sympathetic or parasympathetic nerves; (5) mechanical factors that normally limit pooling in the peripheral veins; (6) intravascular blood volume; and (7) the heart's ability to maintain cardiac output.

CAUSES OF ORTHOSTATIC HYPOTENSION

Clinically, the causes of orthostatic hypotension may be classified as follows:[3a, 4]

1. *Chronic idiopathic hypotension*, a primary degenerative disorder impairing the function of the autonomic nervous system (discussed below).

2. *Vasoactive drugs*, including essentially all antihypertensive but particularly ganglionic blocking agents (rarely used in ordinary practice); depletors of catecholamines such as reserpine; and drugs that block the neuronal release of catecholamines, such as guanethidine (Chap. 28). In patients with hypertension who are treated too vigorously with antihypertensive drugs, particularly when the treatment is accompanied by dehydration and hypovolemia, postural hypotension is common. Other drugs not used in the treatment of hypertension, such as tranquilizers, sedatives, hypnotics, or antidepressants, may also induce

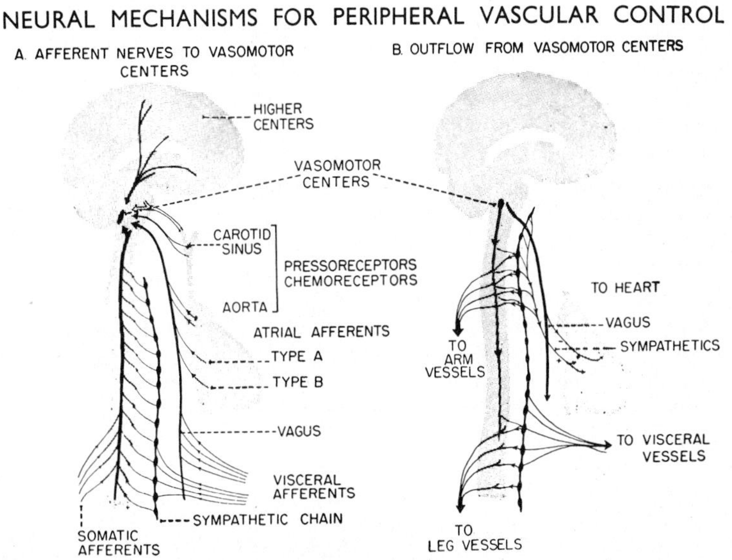

FIGURE 29–1. The vasomotor centers in the medulla receive afferent impulses from many different areas of the body, including the higher centers of the nervous system, heart, blood vessels, viscera, and somatic pain receptors. Efferent impulses descend via the spinal cord in the intermediolateral column and initiate sympathetic impulses to the blood vessels throughout the organism. (From Rushmer, R. F.: Cardiovascular Dynamics. Philadelphia, W. B. Saunders Company, 1961, p. 153.)

hypotension by depressing the vasomotor center. Orthostatic hypotension, although rarely seen with judicious use of calcium antagonists, may be encountered more frequently as these drugs are employed more widely in the treatment of angina, particularly when they are used in combination with nitrates and other vasodilators (p. 1327). Postural hypotension may occur in association with administration of numerous other agents, such as bromocriptine.[5]

3. *Disorders of the peripheral, autonomic, or central nervous system,* including diabetes mellitus, alcoholism, uremia, pyridoxine deficiency, multiple sclerosis, tabes dorsalis, pernicious anemia, Parkinson's disease, vascular lesions in the brain stem, neoplasms, and cysts (particularly in the parasellar region and in the posterior fossa), Wernicke's encephalopathy, syringomyelia, and a number of demyelinating disorders.

4. *Cardiovascular deconditioning* after any prolonged illness with prolonged recumbency, especially in elderly patients.

5. *Diseased or varicose veins* causing pooling of blood in the lower extremities.

6. *The supine hypotensive syndrome of pregnancy* (p. 1850), resulting from obstruction of the inferior vena cava with reduction in venous return and decline in cardiac output.

7. *Infiltration of vessel walls,* which may preclude a physiological response to sympathetic stimulation, e.g., amyloidosis.

8. *Surgically induced sympathectomy* with abolition of vasopressor reflex responses.

9. *Idiopathic hypovolemia* associated with reduction of blood volume without apparent cause and responsive to expansion of plasma volume acutely with intravenously administered colloid and chronically with long-term administration of mineralocorticoids.[6]

CHRONIC IDIOPATHIC ORTHOSTATIC HYPOTENSION

This syndrome, the *Bradbury-Eggleston syndrome,* which most often occurs in older men, has also been termed *primary autonomic insufficiency* and is characterized by postural hypotension without a compensatory tachycardia, hypohidrosis, impotence, and disturbed sphincter control.[7] Hypertension in the supine position and postprandial hypotension are relatively common. Dizziness, visual disturbances, presyncope, and syncope accompanying standing or walking are typical signs and occur with distressing regularity, especially when the upright posture is assumed suddenly and during the early morning hours; the course is usually progressive. The *Shy-Drager syndrome* (also known as multiple system atrophy) is a somewhat similar disorder but exhibits prominent degeneration of the central nervous system, with involvement of the extrapyramidal tracts and basal ganglia.[8-10] The degeneration involves the dorsal nucleus of the vagus and pigmented brain stem nuclei, intermediate and lateral columns of the spinal cord, and sympathetic ganglia[11, 12]; in a variant form the pathological findings resemble those of Parkinson's disease, with dementia, extrapyramidal signs, loss of facial expressions, and tremor. *Secondary orthostatic hypotension* occurs in a number of neurological disorders that involve the autonomic nervous system, including alcoholic and diabetic neuropathy, subacute combined sclerosis, spinal cord transection, syringomyelia, and tabes dorsalis.

The postural hypotension in chronic idiopathic orthostatic hypotension and in many of the forms of secondary orthostatic hypotension[13] is due primarily to impairment of peripheral vasoconstriction, acceleration of heart rate, and maintenance of cardiac output in response to the assumption of the upright posture.[3, 14-16] There is a greater than normal decline in arterial pressure during the Valsalva maneuver, with a reduced or absent arterial pressure overshoot following release, as well as a paradoxical decline in arterial pressure during exercise.

Kontos et al. found that patients with idiopathic orthostatic hypotension do not exhibit the normal vasoconstriction in the forearm and hands in response to intraarterial administration of tyramine, whereas the vasoconstrictor responses to intraarterial administration of norepinephrine are augmented. These findings strongly suggest that sympathetic nerve endings are depleted of and unable to take up norepinephine. Depletion of norepinephrine from sympathetic nerve endings was confirmed by histochemical demonstration of the absence of catecholamine-specific fluorescence in sympathetic vasomotor nerves.[17, 18]

Excretion of norepinephrine and its synthesis from precursors are reduced in this condition.[19-22] Plasma renin release and aldosterone secretion in response to assumption of the erect posture or to salt restriction are also blunted,[17, 19-21] possibly contributing to the difficulty in augmenting plasma volume to compensate adequately for the impaired reflex control of vasomotor tone. Thus, blood volume in patients with these disorders is normal or only slightly increased.

Patients with idiopathic orthostatic hypotension and multiple central nervous system defects have *normal* plasma levels of norepinephrine while recumbent that fail to increase normally after standing or exertion. In contrast, patients with peripheral autonomic insufficiency *without* signs of central nervous system defects have *low* levels of plasma norepinephrine while recumbent that also fail to increase normally after standing or exercise. Both groups have low levels of plasma dopamine beta-hydroxylase. These findings are consistent with other pathological and pharmacological observations. This suggests that patients with idiopathic orthostatic hypotension and central nervous system disease are unable to activate appropriately an otherwise intact sympathetic nervous system, whereas in patients without signs of central nervous system disease, the defect affects peripheral sympathetic nerves.[12]

Since the fundamental disorder is not amenable to therapy, the *treatment* of patients with chronic idiopathic hypotension and the Shy-Drager syndrome must be symptomatic[23] and may involve a combination of measures. These include: (1) a high-salt diet and judicious and monitored administration of mineralocorticoids such as fludrocortisone to expand plasma volume; (2) hydroxyamphetamine, dihydroergotamine,[24, 25] L-dopa,[9] or other directly or indirectly acting sympathomimetic agents; combined with (3) caffeine[25a]; (4) a monoamine oxidase inhibitor, such as tranylcypromine, to augment norepinephrine concentration at nerve endings[20, 26-28]; (5) propranolol, a nonselective beta blocker that may prevent adrenergically mediated vasodilation and result in unopposed vasoconstriction[9, 29]; (6) indomethacin, which acts presumably by inhibiting synthesis of vasodilatory prostaglandins[9]; (7) mechanical support by elastic stockings or, in severe cases, an antigravity suit (Fig. 29–2); (8) paradoxically, clonidine can increase blood pressure in some patients with severe idiopathic orthostatic hypotension.[30] Its action is often prolonged and it should be used carefully. When orthostatic hypotension is mild, clonidine is contraindicated because it may exacerbate the hypotension; and (9) programmed atrial pacing is an alternative means for treatment of severely affected patients with an inadequate heart rate response to hypotension.[31, 31a] Twenty-four–hour automated and ambulatory monitoring of blood pressure is

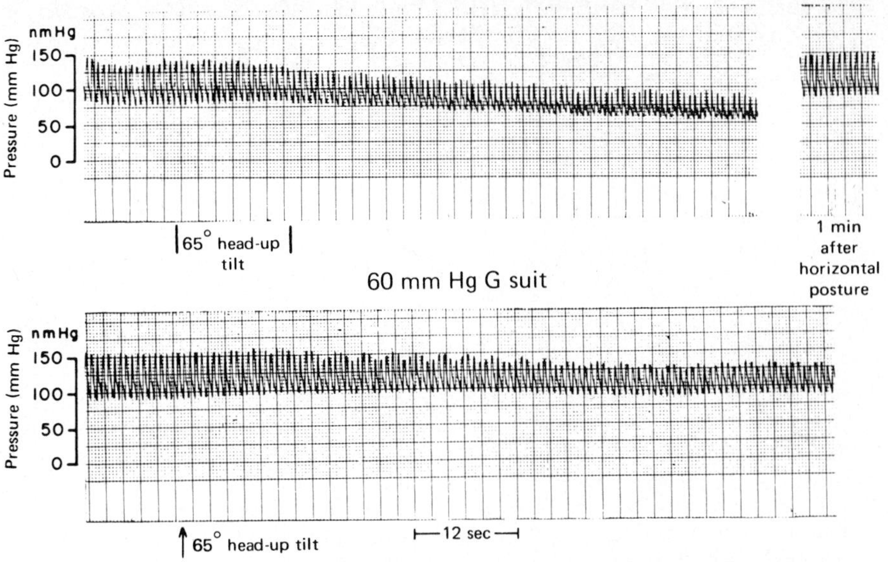

FIGURE 29–2. Direct recording of intraarterial blood pressure in a patient with orthostatic hypotension. *Top panel,* Drop in blood pressure accompanying a change from horizontal to head-up tilt position (140/85 to 85/65 mm Hg), with recovery accompanying return to the horizontal position. *Bottom panel,* Minimal change in blood pressure (155/90 to 125/90 mm Hg) with the same postural changes but with the patient wearing an antigravity suit. (From Fowler, N. O.: Cardiac Diagnosis and Treatment. 3rd ed. Hagerstown, Md., Harper and Row, 1980, p. 1210.)

helpful for assessment of all of these forms of treatment.[32] The *prognosis* for survival is approximately 10 years following the development of symptoms in patients without other evident neurological disease, but it is only about 5 years in patients with associated abnormalities of the central nervous system.

FAMILIAL DYSAUTONOMIA. Familial dysautonomia (Riley-Day syndrome) is a progressive disorder inherited in a pattern consistent with an autosomal recessive trait limited primarily to Ashkenazi Jews.[33] It is characterized by the appearance at or soon after birth of autonomic instability with both postural hypotension and hypertensive episodes due to defective reflex control of vascular tone. Other features include fever; impaired perception of pain, temperature, and taste; lack of fungiform papillae on the tongue; impaired lacrimation; diminished or absent deep tendon reflexes; ataxia; loss of the histamine-flare response; feeding difficulties; and susceptibility to viral pneumonia in infancy.[33, 34]

Tissue norepinephrine stores are normal or elevated[35]; the concentrations of plasma catecholamines are normal in patients who are recumbent and at rest but fail to increase normally with exercise or assumption of the upright posture. Plasma dopamine beta-hydroxylase activity and the excretion of vanillylmandelic acid (VMA) are often reduced, consistent with impaired release of catecholamines from sympathetic nerve endings.[35] The cardiovascular response to infused norepinephrine is exaggerated, suggesting receptor hypersensitivity or reduced uptake of the neurotransmitter by nerve endings or both.

Patients with familial dysautonomia synthesize and store norepinephrine in sympathetic nerve endings and release catecholamines from the adrenal medulla in response to stress induced by hypoglycemia.[36] Thus, the hypertensive episodes that frequently accompany even mild anxiety and are associated with increases in plasma norepinephrine may, like the response to infused catecholamines, reflect increased reactivity of vascular receptors to released adrenal catecholamines.

Although the specific abnormality responsible for familial dysautonomia remains unidentified,[33, 34] defective release of norepinephrine from the nerve endings is a prominent pathophysiological component. Although it may reflect abnormalities in the afferent or efferent sympathetic system, demonstrable degeneration in the reticular formation of the brain stem suggests a primary abnormality in the central nervous system. However, in some patients the defect may be confined to the peripheral autonomic nervous system. In these patients at rest and in the recumbent position, circulating concentrations of catecholamines are low and do not rise in response to stress.[12]

Unfortunately, no specific treatment is available, and the disease progresses to death in early adult life. Symptomatic treatment involves the general measures described previously for management of postural hypotension as well as the administration of parasympathomimetic agents, such as bethanechol chloride (Urecholine), to facilitate lacrimation, reduce gastric distention and vomiting, improve esophageal motility, and improve bladder control.

A similar disorder is manifested by severe orthostatic hypotension and ptosis but otherwise apparently normal parasympathetic and sympathetic cholinergic function.[37] Concentrations of norepinephrine in plasma are less than 10 per cent of normal. In contrast, concentrations of dopamine are increased markedly. Dopamine release is elicited rapidly by assumption of an upright posture or administration of yohimbine, and dopamine beta-hydroxylase activity is undetectable in plasma. Thus, the disorder appears to reflect dysfunction or deficiency of dopamine beta-hydroxylase, the enzyme that is responsible for the conversion of dopamine to norepinephrine. In contrast to familial dysautonomia this disorder is mild and compatible with prolonged life into adulthood. Lacrimation, corneal and deep tendon reflexes, taste, olfaction, and sweating remain intact. Meiosis does not occur after topical administration of methacholine.

METABOLIC ABNORMALITIES RESPONSIBLE FOR ORTHOSTATIC HYPOTENSION. Metabolic or endocrine disturbances leading to reduction of plasma volume, altered adrenergic function, or vasodilatation may underlie persistent or episodic hypotension. These include diabetes mellitus, primary systemic amyloidosis, and acute porphyria. The hypovolemia seen with adrenocortical insufficiency, hypoaldosteronism, and salt-wasting nephritis is the primary cause of hypotension in these conditions, although altered vascular responses to catecholamines may contribute in Addison's disease, and diminished levels of angiotensin may play a role in conditions in which plasma renin activity is low.[38, 39]

Depletion of plasma volume is characteristically associated with pheochromocytoma and is a primary cause of postural hypotension in this disorder (p. 1812). However, epinephrine-induced vasodilatation contributes in some patients with epinephrine-secreting tumors. Rarely, circulatory instability results from high concentrations of circulating bradykinia. Hyperbradykininemia, a disorder that is sometimes familial, is characterized by severe tachycardia and a narrowed pulse pressure. The cause is an enzyme deficiency resulting in impaired destruction of the circulating peptides.[40] Kinins may also play a role in the hypotension and syncope sometimes seen with the carcinoid syndrome.

SYNCOPE

Syncope refers to loss of consciousness due to the impairment (usually temporary) of cerebral perfusion.[41] The metabolism of the brain, in contrast to that of many other organs, is exquisitely dependent on perfusion. In contrast to skeletal muscle, for example, storage of high-energy phosphate in the brain is limited, and energy supply depends largely on the oxidation of glucose extracted from the blood. Consequently, cessation of cerebral flow leads to loss of consciousness within approximately 10 seconds (Table 29–2).[42]

A typical syncopal episode is characterized by hypotension, pallor, diaphoresis, and loss of consciousness in a motionless patient with depressed, shallow respirations and intact sphincter tone. If postural hypotension is the cause, cerebral blood flow is usually restored promptly, and consciousness is regained when the patient falls or is placed in a horizontal position. Although syncope is most often associated with the upright posture because it is frequently a manifestation of postural hypotension, it may result from conduction disturbances or other arrhythmias

TABLE 29–2 FACTORS POTENTIALLY AFFECTING CEREBRAL PERFUSION SELECTIVELY

1. Metabolic causes
Hypercapnia
Hypotension
2. Decreased effective perfusion pressure
Cerebral vascular disease (usually atherosclerotic)
Arterial spasm
Increased intracranial pressure
Cerebral venospasm
Transient ischemic attacks
Subclavian steal

causing profound, sudden reductions in cardiac output in which case postural associations may be lacking.

Faintness or presyncope, a less severe but etiologically similar phenomenon, is characterized by sudden weakness, the inability to stand, visual difficulty, and the sensation of impending loss of consciousness. At this stage, frank loss of consciousness can often be averted if cerebral perfusion is restored, as by the assumption of the supine posture.

REFLEX-MEDIATED VASOMOTOR INSTABILITY

Inappropriate or excessive activation of vasomotor reflexes may initiate syncope in syndromes such as *carotid sinus hypersensitivity*. Under physiological conditions, afferent impulses from the carotid sinuses are transmitted via the glossopharyngeal nerve to vasomotor and cardioinhibitory centers in the medulla. The efferent limb of the carotid sinus reflex comprises vagal and cervical sympathetic fibers (Fig. 29–3).[43, 44] Afferent impulses from the carotid sinus impinge on the medulla with a frequency dependent on the pressure and rate of change of pressure in the walls of the vessel. Increased pressure leads to an increased frequency of afferent stimulation of the central vasomotor (pressor) center. Consequently, parasympathetic outflow increases, sympathetic outflow is reduced, and systemic vasodilatation and bradycardia ensue.

A clinical syndrome, the hypersensitive carotid sinus syndrome, has been recognized as a cause of hypotension, bradycardia, dizziness, presyncope, and syncope.[44, 45] Two major forms of hypersensitive carotid sinus syndromes have been well delineated.[46] The most common, the *vagal* or *cardioinhibitory* type, occurring in approximately 70 per cent of patients with this syndrome, is manifested by sinus bradycardia, sinus arrest, atrioventricular block, a combination of these disturbances, or even asystole (Fig. 29–4). The second, or *vasodepressor type*, is manifested by marked hypotension without significant bradycardia or atrioventricular (AV) block. Many patients exhibit a combination of both the cardioinhibitory and the vasodepressor syndromes.[47] Carotid sinus hypersensitivity usually occurs in the elderly[47a] and is more frequent in men than in women. Arteriosclerosis, hypertension, diabetes mellitus, and local pathological changes such as scars, lymph nodes, and tumors involving the carotid body[46] predispose to a hyperactive carotid sinus. Episodes are often precipitated by turning the head or pressure on the carotid sinus area, such as during shaving. Attacks can be initiated and the diagnosis thereby confirmed by manual pressure on the carotid sinus. Occasionally, cervical lymphadenopathy, scar tissue, or a carotid body tumor may be responsible.[46] Usually, however, the underlying increased sensitivity of the carotid sinus to pressure accompanying specific movements of the neck or a tight collar is not associated with an overt anatomic lesion.[48, 49] Electrophysiological study usually reveals normal intrinsic function of the sinoatrial node and atrioventricular conduction system.

Diagnosis is confirmed by applying manual pressure to the carotid artery in the region of the carotid sinus with the patient supine and the head in a neutral position.[50] Pressure should be applied only lightly at first on *one* side and for a maximum of 20 seconds at a time while the electrocardiogram and blood pressure are monitored. Normal subjects exhibit mild sinus bradycardia, sometimes with first-degree atrioventricular block. Ventricular asystole with a duration of 3 seconds or more or a decrease in systolic arterial blood pressure exceeding 50 mm Hg is a definitively abnormal response. Complications of carotid sinus stimulation are rare but potentially catastrophic and include cardiac standstill and hemiplegia.[51] The risk is greatest in elderly, hypertensive patients with cerebral or extracranial vascular occlusive disease. Emergency treatment with closed chest cardiac compression, intravenous atropine, epinephrine, and norepinephrine is indicated.

Other coexisting causes of syncope or episodes mimicking syncope must be excluded, since documentation of a hypersensitive carotid sinus does not prove that it is responsible for the syncopal episode in an individual case.[51] Impaired cerebral perfusion due to cerebral vascular disease may also be responsible for syncope associated with extrinsic pressure on the vessels of the neck,[47] and this condition must be differentiated from the hypersensitive carotid sinus syndrome.

If the syndrome is caused by an anatomically identifiable lesion, such as a carotid sinus tumor, excision is required.

CAROTID SINUS REFLEXES

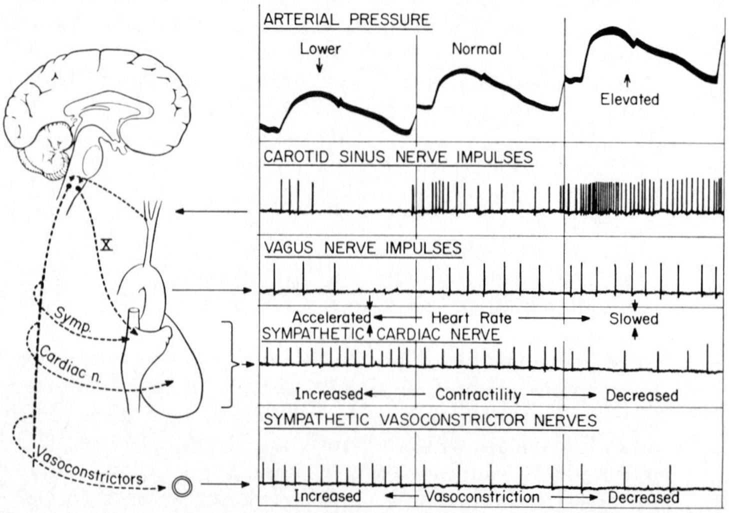

FIGURE 29–3. Relationship between carotid sinus discharge and arterial blood pressure. With a drop in blood pressure (first panel), the frequency of baroreceptor impulses decreases, afferent vagal impulses decrease, and efferent sympathetic nerve impulses increase. The sympathetic vasoconstrictor fiber impulse traffic is active, and an increase in peripheral resistance occurs, resulting in a rise in blood pressure. With an increase in blood pressure, the opposite occurs, resulting in vasodilatation and a drop in blood pressure. (From Rushmer, R. F.: Cardiovascular Dynamics. Philadelphia, W. B. Saunders Company, 1961, p. 150.)

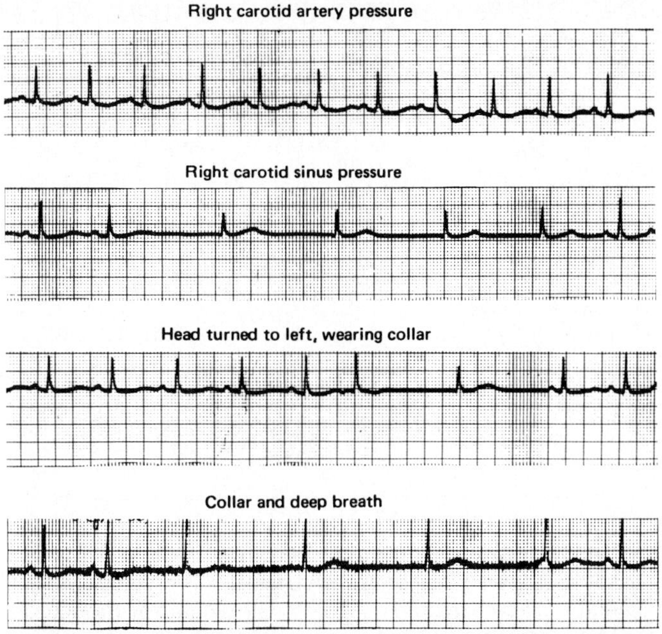

FIGURE 29–4. Electrocardiographic tracings obtained from a patient with the hypersensitive carotid sinus syndrome who presented with attacks of dizziness associated with wearing a tight collar (cardioinhibitory type). Right carotid pressure or sudden turning of the head while wearing a tight collar produced suppression of the sinoatrial node with a junctional escape rhythm. (From Fowler, N. O.: Cardiac Diagnosis and Treatment. 3rd ed. Hagerstown, Md., Harper and Row, 1980, p. 1208.)

In the usual case in which no anatomical cause is recognizable and when symptoms are infrequent, reassurance, precautions to avoid rapid movements, and avoidance of tight collars usually constitute effective therapy.[49, 51] Frequent symptoms should be evaluated by ambulatory electrocardiographic monitoring. If associated with severe bradycardia, they may be ameliorated by ventricular[47] or atrioventricular pacing,[48] administration of alpha-adrenergic agonists such as ephedrine, anticholinergic drugs, or a combination.[48a] Surgical resection[47] or denervation[52] of the hypersensitive carotid sinus may be required for refractory cases, particularly when syncope is due to vasodilatation rather than to bradycardia. Irradiation of the carotid sinus is not effective.[46]

OTHER CAUSES OF SYNCOPE SECONDARY TO AFFERENT STIMULATION. Afferent impulses associated with pain in the ear, soft palate, larynx, or pharynx are transmitted centrally via the glossopharyngeal and vagal nerves and may also give rise to reflex hypotension and syncope[53, 54] associated with sinus bradycardia, sinus arrest, or heart block.[55] *Glossopharyngeal neuralgia* is characterized by paroxysmal pain usually localized to the posterior pharynx or external auditory canal. It may be accompanied by syncope, secondary to bradycardia and systemic vasodilatation. It may be caused by tumor invasion of the glossopharyngeal nerve and may be treated by intracranial section of the glossopharyngeal nerve.[56–56b] Syncope, often with associated severe vertigo, which follows pleural or peritoneal taps and prostatic massage, may be responsible for similar cardiovascular changes.

Syncope[57–60] or occasionally severe bradycardia without syncope[59] may be provoked by swallowing, usually in association with esophageal tumor,[57] diverticulum,[58] or spasm,[59] but sometimes occurs in patients without overt esophageal disease (*deglutition syncope*).[60] Attacks can be reproduced by inflation of a balloon at the level of an esophageal diverticulum in some patients and in others can be prevented by administration of atropine or by local anesthesia of the vagus nerve in the neck with procaine.[61, 62] In some cases afferent impulses may be transmitted via the glossopharyngeal nerve, which also supplies the posterior pharynx and a portion of the esophagus. Treatment requires correction of overt esophageal disease. Palliation and reduction of recurrent syncope may be achieved with the use of an artificial pacemaker in selected patients.

Another reflex-mediated syndrome, *postmicturition syncope*, occurs typically in healthy young to middle-aged men, usually when the patient arises from bed to void. Syncope occurs during or immediately after micturition, and recovery is rapid and complete. Recurrent episodes are rare. Predisposing factors include ingestion of alcohol, diminished food intake, fatigue, and upper respiratory tract infection.[63] Increased vagal stimulation at night, vagal sensory input from the bladder during micturition and the standing position during voiding represent the most common triggering factors of this syndrome.[64]

Paroxysms of coughing may be accompanied by giddiness, vertigo, or syncope, particularly in short, stocky, middle-aged men with chronic lung disease (*post-tussive syncope*). Syncope may occur even with patients in the recumbent position. Sequelae are rare.[65] Syncope in this syndrome may result not only from reflex-mediated mechanisms but also from hydraulic factors, particularly when it follows a paroxysm of coughs, in which case it may result from increased intracranial pressure, which can sometimes be relieved by surgery of the spine.[65, 66] In syncope associated with paroxysms of coughing, the intrathoracic, intraarterial, and cerebrospinal fluid pressures increase to levels as high as 300 mm Hg. During the paroxysm, pressure within the cerebral vessels declines because of the diminished cardiac output resulting from inhibition of venous return due to the elevated intrathoracic pressure and secondary to the increased intracranial pressure reflecting the rise in cerebrospinal fluid pressure. Accordingly, cerebral perfusion declines precipitously (Table 29–2).

VASOVAGAL HYPOTENSION AND SYNCOPE (VASODEPRESSOR SYNCOPE, THE COMMON FAINT). This type of syncope is the most frequently encountered form, accounting for more than 55 per cent of cases in some series.[67] It is often precipitated by the sight of blood; the sudden loss of blood, such as that occurring with phlebotomy; a sudden stressful or painful experience, such as arterial puncture or venipuncture; surgical manipulation; or severe trauma. Vasodepressor syncope is most likely to occur in association with hunger, fatigue, or crowding, particularly in a hot room. Premonitory signs and symptoms are common, including pallor, yawning, sighing, hyperventilation, epigastric discomfort, nausea, diaphoresis, blurred vision, impaired hearing, a vague feeling of unawareness, mydriasis, and sometimes a rapid heart rate. It generally occurs with the patient in an upright position, and if the patient sits or lies down promptly, frank syncope may be aborted.[68]

Vasovagal syncope can be differentiated generally from other, more serious derangements on the basis of knowledge of onset, the setting in which syncope occurs, dependence on posture, appearance of the patient at the time of and after the episode, and the presence or absence of residual manifestations (Table 29–3).[69]

PATHOPHYSIOLOGY. Despite intensive study of vasodepressor syncope, its etiology has not been elucidated definitively.[70–73] Early in the process, peripheral vasodilatation appears to predominate. Blood pressure declines modestly while blood flow to the limbs, cardiac output, and heart rate remain essentially constant.[71–73] Later, resistance in the skeletal muscular beds is reduced, and skeletal blood flow rises markedly while flow through other vascular beds such as the cutaneous, mesenteric, renal, and cerebral declines as arterial pressure falls rapidly. Although cardiac output does not usually decline markedly in vasodepressor syncope, the pathophysiological mechanism must involve more than arteriolar dilation (or failure of normal arteriolar constriction in the upright position), since in normal individuals the fall in peripheral vascular resistance induced by vasodilatation would be compensated for by a compensatory increase in heart rate and cardiac output, which would limit the reduction of arterial pressure. In patients with vasodepressor syncope, however, cardiac output and heart rate fail to rise, presumably owing to some impairment of venous return, perhaps because of venous dilatation or failure of normal venous constriction. In addition, there appears to be a diminished rise in plasma renin, and presumably this reduces angiotensin-mediated vasoconstriction.

The marked vasodilatation in skeletal muscle beds may be mediated, in part, by reflexes triggered by stimulation of intracardiac receptors[74, 75] in a cycle that may involve hypotension due to peripheral vasodilatation, reflex-increased sympathetic stimulation of the heart, increased intramyocardial wall tension and stimulation of intracardiac receptors, and reflex-potentiated vasodilatation.[76] The vasodilatation may also be exacerbated by efferent cholinergic sympathetic stimulation of the

TABLE 29–3 DIFFERENTIATING VASOVAGAL SYNCOPE FROM SEIZURE OR CARDIAC SYNCOPE

	Vasovagal Syncope	Seizure	Cardiac Syncope
Onset	Prodromal weakness, nausea, and diaphoresis lasting seconds to minutes	Sudden onset, or brief aura; déjà vu; olfactory, gustatory, or visual hallucinations	Sudden onset or onset preceded by cardiac signs and symptoms such as tightness, dyspnea, diaphoresis, or palpitations
Typical setting	Emotional upset, prolonged standing, uncomfortable surroundings, or when the patient first arises in the morning with a full urinary bladder	Any setting including sleep, blinking lights, or monotonous music	Any setting
Posture at time of occurrence	Upright	Upright or supine	Upright or supine
Appearance of patient	Pallor. A weak pulse may be noted by observers.	Cyanotic; stertorous breathing	Pallor. Irregular pulse may be noted by observers.
Residua	Rapid recovery is typical. Syncope may recur with assumption of upright position. Occasional brief clonic movements or urinary incontinence may occur.	Slow recovery with postictal state and Todd's paresis	Recovery may be sudden or gradual. If cardiac arrest occurs, seizure activity or other signs of cerebral hypoxia may be evident.

Modified from Branch, W. T., Jr.: Approach to syncope. J. Gen. Intern. Med. *1*:49, 1986.

arterioles in skeletal muscle.[72] With syncope the electroencephalogram shows slow wave activity of large amplitude.

The hyperventilation that generally precedes and accompanies vasodepressor syncope results in a decline in arterial pCO_2, which in turn produces cerebral vasoconstriction, thereby further impairing cerebral perfusion. Later, heart rate, arterial pressure, central venous pressure, and cardiac output decline precipitously.

During the recovery period, oliguria is common, mediated by increased secretion of antidiuretic hormone (ADH).[77] This finding suggests that some of the other clinical features of the syndrome, including pallor and nausea, may be mediated in part by posterior pituitary hormones.[78]

Management. Vasovagal syncope appearing for the first time demands a thorough diagnostic evaluation, since the syncope may be caused by conditions such as valvular or subvalvular aortic stenosis, hypertrophic obstructive cardiomyopathy, carotid sinus hypersensitivity, or another unrecognized cardiac or neurological abnormality. Therapy consists of placing the patient in the recumbent position with the lower extremities elevated (reverse Trendelenburg). Removal of the offending stimuli, inhalation of spirits of ammonia, and stimulation of the face with cold water usually suffice in treatment of the acute episode. Treatment with vasopressors is not usually required. Consciousness is usually regained rapidly, with a somewhat slower regression of bradycardia. Rarely, if recovery is delayed, atropine may be helpful.

CARDIAC CAUSES OF SYNCOPE

The common denominator in syncope of cardiac cause is a transient, marked diminution of cardiac output due to an arrhythmia or reduced stroke volume.[79, 80] The association of syncope and bradycardia, first described by Gerbezius in 1719 and later by Morgagni in 1769[81] and by Adams in 1827,[82] was clarified by Stokes in 1846, who recognized the etiological connections between a change in heart rate and cerebral manifestations.[83] The mechanism underlying syncope even among patients with complete heart block is often a superimposed arrhythmia (such as transient asystole or ventricular fibrillation)[84] at the time of loss of consciousness[84] rather than the heart block per se. Thus, the generic term "arrhythmia-induced syncope" may be more useful.[85]

The prognosis of syncope is often difficult to establish because of the lack of a specific etiological diagnosis. Despite vigorous search, identification of etiology is accomplished in less than 50 per cent of patients[86] in part because of the episodic nature of the problem. When a specific cause can be identified, the diagnosis is most often established by history, physical examination, or analysis of the electrocardiogram.[86–90] Extensive testing has a low diagnostic yield.[68] However, in elderly patients, in-depth cardiac evaluations are justified.[91] Patients in whom cardiac causes can be excluded exhibit lower mortality than that seen when cardiac causes are implicated because of an incidence of sudden cardiac death as high as 24 per cent in the first year after syncope attributable to cardiac causes.

More than 50, 000 new cases of complete heart block occur annually in the United States,[85] and approximately 50 per cent of patients with acquired, complete heart block experience syncope. The causes of complete heart block are listed in Table 30–4 and discussed in detail in Chapter 23.

ARRHYTHMIAS CAUSING SYNCOPE. Arrhythmia-induced syncope may result from asystole, severe bradycardia, or tachyarrhythmia and generally conforms to one of the following categories:

1. Transitory, complete interruption of atrioventricular conduction with asystole during the "preautomatic pause" or "pacemaker warm-up" interval.
2. Asystole developing in the presence of persistent complete heart block, owing to failure of the intra- or infranodal pacemaker, accompanied by a preautomatic pause in other potential pacemakers.
3. Paroxysmal ventricular tachycardia or fibrillation precipitated by ischemia due to the slow heart rate in patients with complete heart block.

TABLE 29–4 CAUSES OF COMPLETE HEART BLOCK

1. Structural abnormalities of the conduction system
   a. Congenital heart block
   b. Infectious diseases such as diphtheria, syphilis, toxoplasmosis, mumps, rheumatic fever
   c. Collagen diseases
   d. Valvular heart disease
   e. Degenerative disease (Lev's disease, Lenegre's disease, Friedreich's ataxia, progressive muscular dystrophy, myotonic dystrophy, Duchenne's dystrophy)
   f. Coronary artery disease with or without infarction
   g. Tumors
   h. Endocrine and metabolic disorders (gout with urate deposition in the conduction system, hypo- and hyperthyroidism, hemochromatosis, Addison's disease)
   i. Trauma
   j. Diseases of unknown etiology (Reiter's syndrome, sarcoidosis, amyloidosis, Paget's disease)
2. Electrolyte disturbances such as hyperkalemia, acidosis, hypomagnesemia
3. Drug toxicity: Examples include digitalis, quinidine, lidocaine, aprindine, phenytoin (Dilantin), and amitriptyline (Elavil)

4. Paroxysmal ventricular tachycardia or fibrillation in patients with normal atrioventricular conduction, recognized with the use of ambulatory electrocardiographic monitoring.

5. Supraventricular tachy- or bradyarrhythmias leading to decreased cardiac output secondary to the rate itself or to the deleterious effects of the arrhythmia on myocardial perfusion already compromised by coronary artery disease.

6. Asystole due to atrial standstill with failure of automaticity in subsidiary pacemakers, commonly seen in patients with the sick sinus syndrome.[92]

7. Combinations of conduction disturbances and supraventricular arrhythmia, commonly associated with the sick sinus syndrome (p. 667).

HEMODYNAMIC ABNORMALITIES PREDISPOSING TO SYNCOPE. During exercise systemic vascular resistance ordinarily declines as a consequence of arteriolar dilatation secondary to the accumulation of vasodilator metabolites. Normally, this vasodilatation is more than compensated for by the augmentation of cardiac output and arterial pressure during heavy exertion (Chap. 8). However, in those severe forms of heart disease in which cardiac output rises proportionately less than vascular resistance falls, arterial pressure declines, sometimes to hazardous levels. Thus, exertional hypotension and syncope are characteristic features of virtually all forms of heart disease in which cardiac output is relatively fixed and fails to rise normally or even declines during exertion. It is most characteristic of severe valvular aortic stenosis and other forms of obstruction to left ventricular outflow and of coronary artery disease in which global ischemia occurs during exertion.

The mechanism responsible for exertional hypotension and syncope in patients with lesions producing right or left outflow tract obstruction probably involves peripheral vasodilatation as well as decreased cardiac output, the former reflexes resulting from high intraventricular pressure acting on ventricular baroreceptors with blunting of the compensatory carotid and aortic baroreceptor-mediated reflexes.[93, 94] Patients with aortic valvular stenosis have been shown to exhibit an excessive reduction of forearm vascular resistance with exertion, with a return of the physiological vasoconstrictor response after correction of the aortic valve lesion.[93] In patients in whom syncope can be ascribed to obstruction to left ventricular outflow, surgical intervention is ordinarily necessary. Syncope in patients with prosthetic cardiac valves is an ominous phenomenon, often indicative of the need for urgent reoperation to relieve a mechanical obstruction caused by serious dysfunction of the prosthetic valve or formation of a thrombus.

When left ventricular outflow tract obstruction is dynamic, as in hypertrophic obstructive cardiomyopathy (p. 1418), it is exacerbated by increased contractility, decreased chamber dimensions, or decreased afterload and distending pressure. Thus, drugs with positive inotropic effects such as digitalis or arterial or venous vasodilators such as nitroglycerin may precipitate hypotension.[95]

Sustained hypotension associated with ischemic heart disease is usually due to severely impaired ventricular function, but episodic hypotension or syncope often results from conduction disturbances or arrhythmia. Sometimes, marked hypotension accompanies angina pectoris or acute myocardial infarction, owing to increased parasympathetic activity, particularly with ischemia of the inferior wall (Chap. 38). Afferent reflexes from atrial and ventricular myocardium or from the coronary vessels themselves elicit increased parasympathetic outflow, bradycardia, and hypotension, which, coupled with the decreased contractility resulting from ischemia, may precipitate syncope.[15, 96, 97]

Pedunculated left atrial myxoma (p. 1471) or a large thrombus may obstruct the left ventricular inflow tract and suddenly reduce cardiac output. An important clinical clue to the diagnosis is the association of syncope with specific postures (such as sitting or leaning forward) because of movement of a pedunculated or migratory tumor or clot into the left ventricular inflow tract.

Systemic hypotension may be a critical complication in patients with *congenital heart disease* characterized by right-to-left shunting (Chaps. 30 and 31). When pulmonary blood flow is reduced with right-to-left shunting through an intracardiac communication associated with obstruction to right ventricular outflow or severe pulmonary hypertension, marked arterial hypoxemia occurs; this serves as a potent vasodilatory stimulus.

Hypotension may also result from obstruction to outflow due to lesions *extrinsic* to the heart, such as massive pulmonary embolus (Chap. 47), Takayasu's disease (Chap. 46), and supravalvular aortic stenosis (Chaps. 30 and 31), all of which interfere with ventricular emptying. Syncope is a manifestation of primary pulmonary hypertension (Chap. 26) and rarely of pulmonary valvular stenosis (Chaps. 30 and 31); it may accompany cardiac tamponade (Chap. 44).

DIFFERENTIAL DIAGNOSIS OF SYNCOPE

Syncope and presyncope must be differentiated from a variety of other acute episodes. It is critical, for example, to distinguish syncopal episodes from epileptic seizures, particularly the akinetic type. In general, syncope due to vasomotor failure or impaired cardiac output occurs when the patient is in the upright position, although syncopal episodes secondary to cardiac arrhythmia may occur in any position. Syncope occurs most commonly in young women or elderly men and, in contrast to epilepsy, in most instances (1) is of gradual onset *without* aura; (2) is *not* associated with injury from falling; (3) is *not* associated with convulsive movements, biting of the lips, or urinary incontinence; (4) is *brief*, with a rapid return to consciousness; and (5) is *not* followed by a state of confusion.

Epileptic seizures, in contrast, can occur with the patient in any position and are sudden in onset; the warning aura, if it occurs at all, lasts only a few seconds. Injury from falling is frequent, as are convulsive movements with the eyes upturned. The period of unconsciousness usually lasts for minutes, and there is often urinary incontinence, biting of the lips, and a prolonged postictal state of mental confusion and drowsiness.

Attacks of *cerebral ischemia* due to cerebral arteriosclerosis may produce transient ischemic attacks characterized by neurological deficits that tend to resemble each other from attack to attack. These are often visual disturbances, hemiparesis, hemianesthesia, slurred speech, and impaired consciousness.

Anxiety attacks may produce dizziness but not frank syncope. They are usually characterized by, and can be reproduced by, hyperventilation, which results in reduction of cerebral blood flow; are not accompanied by cardiac arrhythmia; and are not relieved by recumbency. *Hysterical fainting* occurs most frequently in persons with hysterical personalities and is not accompanied by any changes in blood pressure, heart rate, or skin color. *Hypoglycemia* is manifested by confusion, sinus tachycardia, jitteriness, and other symptoms of sympathetic stimulation, ultimately leading to loss of consciousness. Loss of consciousness with this entity proceeds gradually but is often prolonged, constituting frank coma. When caused by a tumor of the islets of Langerhans, it occurs with and can be reproduced by prolonged fasting, but when hypoglycemia is reactive, it tends to occur 3 to 5 hours after meals. The diagnosis is confirmed by the finding of reduced blood glucose.

APPROACH TO DIAGNOSIS OF POSTURAL HYPOTENSION AND SYNCOPE

The cause of postural hypotension or syncope is often obvious, after a thorough history and physical examination and laboratory tests selected on the basis of positive findings have been done.[97a] In taking the patient's history, the examiner must determine the onset, frequency, and duration of premonitory symptoms; circumstances surrounding the attacks (such as relationship to meals, alcohol ingestion, cough, micturition, defecation, or movements of the head and neck); associated symptoms such as nausea, vomiting, chest pain, or dyspnea; medications utilized; the presence of potentially predisposing disorders such as diabetes mellitus, chronic illness with weight loss, prolonged bed rest, blood loss, or plasma volume depletion. Exclusion of the simple faint is important, since this condition usually requires no treatment and only minor investigation.

Physical examination should focus on the following:

1. Evaluation of blood pressure with the patient recumbent and standing after the patient has been recumbent for at least 3 minutes;
2. Evaluation of blood pressure in both arms and legs;
3. Recognition of bruits in the carotid, subclavian, supraorbital, and temporal vessels;
4. Detection of cyanosis, clubbing, and other signs of congenital heart disease; and
5. Assessment of the heart rate and blood pressure response to carotid sinus pressure and simulated movements precipitating syncope.

Accurate measurement of blood pressure with the patient recumbent and standing is all that is required to detect postural hypotension. The patient should be recumbent for at least 3 minutes before assuming an upright posture. If acceleration of heart rate accompanies postural hypotension, the syncope is more likely to be drug-induced, secondary to prolonged deconditioning, or due to old age rather than because of degenerative or familial orthostatic hypotension. Detection of bruits in the vessels of the neck may suggest vascular obstruction. Since hypotensive episodes due to congenital heart disease in adults are usually caused by intracardiac shunts, cyanosis and clubbing may be important clues. Carotid hypersensitivity is established by maneuvers that reproduce the patient's symptoms and by simulation of movements potentially precipitating syncope in a given case, such as turning movements of the head. Assessment of the blood pressure in both arms and legs is particularly helpful in detecting differences due to obstructive vascular disease such as Takayasu's disease.

Test of autonomic function may be particularly helpful (Table 28–5). The response to the Valsalva maneuver is often diagnostic (Fig. 30–5). In addition, assessment of the following may be useful:

1. Twenty-four–hour (ambulatory) electrocardiographic recordings (p. 609): Many patients with underlying cardiac causes of syncope have normal electrocardiograms between attacks, although some exhibit abnormalities such as premature ventricular contractions, atrial arrhythmias, or minor conduction defects. These abnormalities in themselves do not confirm the cause of syncope. Often it is necessary to monitor patients for 24 hours, preferably during their usual activities. Short runs of ventricular tachycardia, transient complete heart block, or asystole may be demonstrable. If the patient develops syncope or presyncope during the recording, and the electrocardiogram reveals an arrhythmia that can account for the symptoms, appropriate treatment is instituted; this usually consists of drugs for tachyarrhythmias and permanent pacing for bradyarrythmias. If, on the other hand, the recording is normal even though the patient concurrently develops syncope, arrhythmias can be excluded as a cause of symptoms. The increased diagnostic yield from multiple compared with single 24-hour recordings is marginal.[98, 99] Nevertheless, in patients with recurrent syncope potentially attributable to coronary artery disease, extensive monitoring should be implemented. Availability of transmitter systems with built-in memory makes long-term monitoring via telephonic transmission feasible. Patients can activate such systems when an episode of presyncope or syncope begins and transmit the recorded electrocardiographic information later, after recovery.

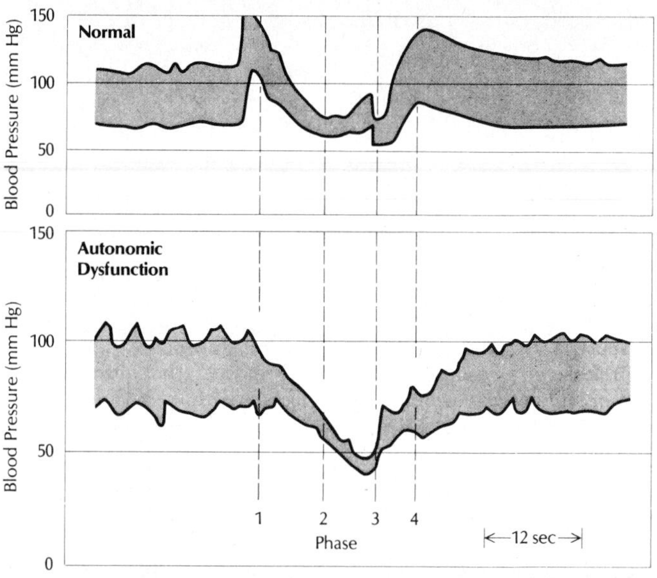

FIGURE 29–5. With a normal Valsalva response (*top*), exhaling against pressure causes compression of the aorta and thus an increase in blood pressure during phase 1. During phase 2, reduced left ventricular filling causes the pulse pressure to decline; reflex vasoconstriction soon reverses the downward shift. Phase 3 occurs after the strain is released; the blood pressure again declines briefly. In phase 4, continuing vasoconstriction causes blood pressure overshoot, widened pulse pressure, and baroreceptor-mediated bradycardia. In autonomic disorders, defective vasoconstriction and baroreceptors cause downward drift of blood pressure during phase 2. In addition, neither overshoot nor bradycardia occurs during phase 4. (From Schatz, I. J.: Orthostatic Hypotension: Diagnosis and Treatment. Hosp. Pract., p. 59, April, 1984.)

2. Electrophysiologic evaluation with programmed atrial and ventricular stimulation may be useful for detection of occult cardiac causes of syncope.[102] As many as 80 per cent of patients with coronary artery disease, 39 per cent of those with valvular heart disease, and 27 per cent of those without structural heart disease manifest diagnostic abnormalities evident with invasive testing.[102–107] Among patients with structural heart disease, electrophysiologic testing is helpful for guiding treatment for underlying tachy- or bradyarrhythmias.[108–110] When the cause of syncope is obscure, inducibility of recurrent atrial or ventricular tachycardia accompanied by syncope or presyncope strongly suggests that the arrhythmia occurs spontaneously and is responsible for the syncope.[106–108] The presence of uni- or bifascicular block with stress-induced complete heart block by atrial pacing, a prolonged His-ventricular

(HV) interval on His bundle recordings, or the demonstration of prolonged sinoatrial node recovery in patients with symptoms of hypotension or syncope may implicate conduction system disease, requiring a permanent artificial pacemaker.[111]

3. Determination of levels of plasma electrolytes, catecholamines (with the patient supine and upright), dopamine beta-hydroxylase, and urinary vanillylmandelic acid (VMA): Under physiological conditions, plasma catecholamine concentrations increase several-fold with assumption

TABLE 29–5 EVALUATION OF AUTONOMIC FUNCTION

Procedure	Mechanism and Normal Pathway Tested	Normal Response	Usual Clinical Implications of Abnormal Response
Standing (sometimes simulated in the laboratory with the use of a tilt table)	Systemic venous pooling of blood leads to a reduction of cardiac output, decreased baroreceptor discharge, and consequent vasomotor center stimulation in the central nervous system, sympathetic discharge, and end-organ response and vasoconstriction	≤ 20 mm Hg decrease of systolic arterial blood pressure associated with modest tachycardia and an increase of ≥ 140 pg/ml of plasma norepinephrine	Exaggerated hypotension suggests the presence of a lesion affecting the afferent, central, or efferent adrenal system or end-organ unresponsiveness
Deep breathing	Afferent, central, and efferent vagal system	≥ 10 beat/min variation in heart rate or R-R interval measured electrocardiographically	Impaired vagal function due to afferent, central, or efferent component lesions or end-organ unresponsiveness
Valsalva maneuver	Increased intrathoracic pressure diminishes systemic venous return to the heart after transitory augmentation of pulmonary venous return. Cardiac output declines, eliciting systemic hypotension, decreased baroreceptor discharge, and afferent, central, and efferent sympathoadrenal discharge with tachycardia. Sustained sympathoadrenal discharge results in a post-Valsalva overshoot of blood pressure and consequent modest bradycardia	A 4-phase response, including transitory initial blood pressure elevation, ≥50% decrease of systemic arterial blood pressure with tachycardia during the maneuver, and a blood pressure overshoot with modest tachycardia after release of Valsalva	Sympathetic lesion (afferent, central, efferent) or end-organ unresponsiveness
Hyperventilation	Vasomotor center responsivity and efferent sympathoadrenal system	A decrease of arterial pressure of 10 to 20 mm Hg	A central lesion
Cold pressor test (immersion of an extremity in ice water for 1 to 3 minutes)	Centrally mediated sympathoadrenal discharge as well as afferent pain fiber stimulation, spinal cord reflex arcs, efferent sympathetic discharge, and end-organ response	≥ 15 mm Hg increase in both systolic and diastolic blood pressure	A central or efferent sympathetic lesion
Inhalation of amyl nitrite	Systemic arterial vasodilatation leads to reduction of systemic arterial blood pressure, decreased baroreceptor discharge, afferent and central nervous system stimulation, and efferent sympathetic discharge	Tachycardia in response to systemic arterial hypotension	Central or efferent sympathetic lesion
Induction of hyperthermia	Augmentation of core temperature by 1°C leads to centrally mediated sympathetic stimulation involving cholinergic postganglionic neurons	Sweating	Central or efferent sympathetic lesions. End-organ unresponsiveness can be excluded with a direct sweat test with 5 to 15 mg of pilocarpine HCl or electrical stimulation
Administration of atropine (0.02 mg/kg)	Efferent parasympathetic fibers, including vagal fibers	An increase of heart rate by ≥ 20% or resting rate	Central or efferent parasympathetic impairment
Administration of tyramine (200 to 6000 μg doses incrementally)	Release of catecholamine stores from adrenergic nerves	Increased systemic blood pressure by ≤ 20 mm Hg/1000 μg bolus	Postganglionic sympathetic lesion
Norepinephrine bitartrate (0.05 to 0.07 μg/kg/min)	End-organ response (peripheral vasculature)	An increase of systolic and diastolic blood pressures of approximately 20 mm Hg	Exaggerated hypertension implies the presence of a postganglionic sympathetic lesion or denervation hypersensitivity
Responses of the pupil to conjunctival sac instillations of 1 to 2 drops of epinephrine HCl (1:1000) or 4% phenylephrine or indirect-acting agents such as hydroxyamphetamine (1%) or cocaine (4%)	End-organ response	No effect with dilute solutions of direct-acting agents; mydriasis with indirect-acting agents	Exaggerated response to epinephrine implies the presence of a postganglionic sympathetic lesion (denervation hypersensitivity). Absence of mydriasis to indirect-acting agents but not to cocaine implies a preganglionic or central lesion. A sympathetic lesion can be confirmed by absence of mydriasis induced by homatropine (5%), a cholinergic antagonist

Modified from Henrich, W. L.: Autonomic insufficiency. Arch. Intern. Med. *142*:339, 1982.

of the upright position. In contrast, among patients with idiopathic orthostatic hypotension or diabetic neuropathy, the response is markedly blunted or absent. In these patients, basal plasma dopamine beta-hydroxylase levels are low, and values do not increase with assumption of an upright posture. Urinary VMA and plasma catecholamines are elevated markedly in patients with pheochromocytoma; rarely, the tumor may predominantly secrete epinephrine, eliciting paradoxical hypotension.

4. Determination of plasma aldosterone and mineralocorticoids: Among patients with primary or secondary adrenal cortical insufficiency or hypoaldosteronism, concentrations of plasma and urinary mineralocorticoids are low.

5. Glucose tolerance test: A normal glucose tolerance test with normal plasma insulin responses will exclude functional hypoglycemia, an insulin-secreting tumor, and diabetes mellitis, which is an important cause of orthostatic hypotension (p. 1816).

6. Electroencephalography: This test frequently detects abnormalities in patients with epilepsy, even when performed between attacks.

7. Ophthalmotonometry and cerebral angiography: These tests are sometimes necessary to identify a cerebral or extracranial vascular lesion.

8. Physiological stress tests, such as carotid sinus stimulation and tilt-table tests, with evaluation of the plasma catecholamine response: In patients with orthostatic hypotension or recurring vasovagal fainting episodes without obvious cause, it may be necessary to assess the hemodynamic and catecholamine responses to tilting, since hypotension without a physiological compensatory elaboration of catecholamines is common in this entity.

A combined approach that employs meticulous acquisition of historical data, thorough physical examination, and judicious utilization of selected laboratory procedures will generally delineate even the most obscure causes of recurrent hypotension and syncope.

REFERENCES

REGULATION OF ARTERIAL PRESSURE

1. Folkow, B.: Nervous control of the blood vessels. Physiol. Rev. *35*:629, 1955.
2. Hickam, J. B, and Pryor, W. W.: Cardiac output in postural hypotension. J. Clin. Invest. *30*:410, 1951.
3. Cryer, P. E., and Weiss, S.: Reduced plasma norepinephrine response to standing in autonomic dysfunction. Arch. Neurol. *33*:275, 1976.

CAUSES OF ORTHOSTATIC HYPOTENSION

3a. Streeten, D. H. (ed.): Orthostatic Disorders of the Circulation: Mechanisms, Manifestations and Treatment. New York, Plenum Press, 1987, 272 pp.
4. Hines, S., and Houston, M.: The clinical spectrum of autonomic dysfunction. Am. J. Med. *70*:1091, 1981.
5. Linch, D. C., Shaw, K. M., Mohleman, M. F., and Ross, E. J.: Bromocriptine induced postural hypotension in acromegaly. Lancet 2:320, 1978.
6. Fouad, F. M., Tadena-Thome, L., Bravo, E. L., and Tarazi, R. C.: Idiopathic hypovolemia. Arch. Intern. Med. *104*:298, 1986.
7. Bradbury, S., and Eggleston, C.: Postural hypotension: A report of three cases. Am. Heart J. *1*:73, 1925.
8. Shy, G. M., and Drager, G. A.: A neurological syndrome associateed with orthostatic hypotension. A clinical pathological study. Arch. Neurol. 2:511, 1960.
9. Schatz, I. J.: Orthostatic hypotension: Diagnosis and treatment. Hosp. Pract. p. 59, April 1984.
10. Imaizumi, T., Takeshita, A., Ashihara, T., Nakamura, M., Tsuji, S., and Shibazaki, H.: Increase in reflex vasoconstriction with indomethacin in patients with orthostatic hypotension and central nervous system involvement. Br. Heart J. *52*:581, 1984.
10a. Pastakia, B., Polinsky, R., DiChiro, G., Simmons, J. T., Brown, R., and Wener, L.: Multiple system atrophy (Shy-Drager syndrome): MR imaging. Radiology *159*:499, 1986.
11. Bannister, R.: Degeneration of the autonomic nervous system. Lancet 2:175, 1971.
12. Ziegler, M. G., Lake, C. R., and Kopin, I. J.: The sympathetic nervous system defect in primary orthostatic hypotension. N. Engl. J. Med. *296*:293, 1977.
13. Hilsted, J., Parving, H.-H., Christensen, N. J., Benn, J., and Galbo, H.: Hemodynamics in diabetic orthostatic hypotension. J. Clin. Invest. *68*:1427, 1981.
14. Schatz, I. J.: Orthostatic hypotension. I. Functional and neurogenic causes. Arch. Intern. Med. *144*:773, 1984.
15. Abboud, F. M., Heistad, D. D., Mark, A. L., and Schmid, P. G.: Reflex control of the peripheral circulation. Prog. Cardiovasc. Dis. *18*:371, 1976.
16. Kopin, I. J., Polinsky, R. J., Oliver, J. A., Oddershede, I. R., and Ebert, M. H.: Urinary catecholamine metabolites distinguish different types of sympathetic neuronal dysfunction in patients with orthostatic hypotension. J. Clin. Endocrinol. Metab. *57*:632, 1983.
16a. Tantengco, M. V., Onrot, J., Robertson, D., Robertson, R. M., and Light, R. T.: Orthostatic hypotension: Clinical spectrum and approach to treatment. Compr. Ther. *12*:41, 1986.
17. Kontos, H. A., Richardson, D. W., and Norvell, J. E.: Norepinephrine depletion in idiopathic orthostatic hypotension. Ann. Intern. Med. *82*:336, 1975.
18. Bannister, R., Crowe, R., Eames, R., and Brunstock, G.: Adrenergic innervation in autonomic failure. Neurology *31*:1501, 1981.
19. Luft, R., and von Euler, U. S.: Two cases of postural hypotension showing a deficiency in release of norepinephrine and epinephrine. J. Clin. Invest. *32*:1065, 1953.
20. Onrot, J., Goldberg, M. R., Hollister, A. S., Giaggioni, I., Robertson, R. M., and Robertson, D.: Management of chronic orthostatic hypotension. Am. J. Med. *80*:454, 1986.
21. Goodall, M., Harlan, W. R., Jr., and Alton, H.: Noradrenaline release and metabolism in orthostatic (postural) hypotension. Circulation *36*:489, 1967.
22. Goodall, M. C. C., Harlan, W. R., Jr., and Alton, H.: Decreased noradrenaline (norepinephrine) synthesis in neurogenic orthostatic hypotension. Circulation *38*:592, 1968.
23. Onrot, J., Goldberg, M. R., Hollister, A. S., Biaggioni, I., Robertson, R. M., and Robertson, D.: Management of chronic orthostatic hypotension. Am. J. Med. *80*:454, 1986.
24. Fouad, F. M., Tarazi, R. C., and Bravo, E. L.: Dihydroergotamine in idiopathic orthostatic hypotension: Short-term intramuscular and long-term oral therapy. Clin. Pharmacol. Ther. *30*:782, 1981.
25. Chobanian, A. V. Tifft, C. P., Faxon, D. P., Creager, M. A., and Sackel, H.: Treatment of chronic orthostatic hypotension with ergotamine. Circulation *67*:602, 1983.
25a. Hoeldtke, R. D., Cavanaugh, S. T., Hughes, J. D., and Polansky, M.: Treatment of orthostatic hypotension with dihydroergotamine and caffeine. Ann. Intern. Med. *105*:168, 1986.
26. Wieling, W., Borst, C., Van Brederode, J. F. M., Van Dongen Torman, M. A., Van Montfrans, G. A., and Dunning, A. J.: Testing for autonomic neuropathy: Heart rate changes after orthostatic manoeuvres and static muscle contraction. Clin. Sci. *64*:581, 1983.
27. Nogues, M. A., Newman, P. K., Male, V. J., and Foster, J. B.: Cardiovascular reflexes in syringomyelia. Brain *105*:835, 1982.
28. Nanda, R. N., Johnson, R. H., and Keogh, H. J.: Treatment of neurogenic orthostatic hypotension with a monoamine oxidase inhibitor and tyramine. Lancet 2:1164, 1976.
29. Brevetti, G., Chiariello, M., Giudice, P., De Michele, G., Mansi, D., and Campanella, G.: Effective treatment of orthostatic hypotension by propranolol in the Shy-Drager syndrome. Am. Heart J. *102*:938, 1981.
30. Robertson, D., Goldberg, M. R., Hollister, A. S., Wade, D., and Robertson, R. M.: Clonidine raises blood pressure in severe idiopathic orthostatic hypotension. Am. J. Med. *74*:193, 1983.
31. Kristinsson, A.: Programmed atrial pacing for orthostatic hypotension. Acta Med. Scand. *214*:79, 1983.
31a. Kenny, R. A., Bayliss, J., Ingram, A., and Sutton, R.: Head-up tilt: A useful test for investigating unexplained syncope. Lancet *1*:1352, 1986.
32. Brevetti, G., Chiariello, M., Bonaduce, D., Canonico, V., Breglio, R., and Condorelli, M.: 24-Hour blood pressure recording in patients with orthostatic hypotension. Clin. Cardiol. 8:406, 1985.
33. Riley, C. M., Day, R. L., Greeley, D. M., and Langford, W. E.: Central autonomic dysfunction with defective lacrimation. I. Report of 5 cases. Pediatrics 3:468, 1949.
34. Dancis, J., and Smith, A. A.: Familial dysautonomia. N. Engl. J. Med. *274*:207, 1966.
35. Ziegler, M. G., Lake, C. R., and Kopin, I. J.: Deficient sympathetic nervous response in familial dysautonomia. N. Engl. J. Med. *294*:630, 1976.
36. Smith, A. A., and Dancis, J.: Catecholamine release in familial dysautonomia. N. Engl. J. Med. 277:61, 1967.
37. Robertson, D., Goldberg, M. R., Onrot, J., Hollister, A. S., Wiley, R., Thompson, J. G., Jr., and Robertson, R. M.: Isolated failure of autonomic noradrenergic neurotransmission. Evidence for impaired beta-hydroxylation of dopamine. N. Engl. J. Med. *314*:1494, 1986.
38. Williams, G. H., Cain, J. P., Dluhy, R. G., and Underwood, R. H.: Studies of the control of plasma aldosterone concentration in normal man. I. Response to posture, acute and chronic volume depletion, and sodium loading. J. Clin. Invest. *51*:1731, 1972.
39. Axelrod, F. B., and Pearson, J.: Congenital sensory neuropathies: Diagnostic distinction from familial dysautonomia. Am. J. Dis. Child. *138*:947, 1984.
40. Streeten, D. H. P., Kerr, L. P., Prior, J. C., Kerr, C., and Dalakos, T. G.: Hyperbradykininism: A new orthostatic syndrome. Lancet 2:1048, 1972.

SYNCOPE

41. McHenry, L. C., Jr., Fazekas, J. F., and Sullivan, J. F.: Cerebral hemodynamics of syncope. Am. J. Med. Sci. *241*:173, 1961.
42. Rossen, R., Kabat, H., and Anderson, J. P.: Acute arrest of cerebral circulation in man. A.M.A. Arch. Neurol. Psychiatry *50*:510, 1943.

43. Hering, H. E.: Die Sinus Reflexe vom Sinus Caroticus werden durch einen Nerven (Sinusvert) vermittelt, der ein Ast des Nervus glossopharyngeus ist. Munch. Med. Wschr. *71*:1265, 1924.
44. Weiss, S., and Baker, J. P.: The carotid sinus reflex in health and disease: Its role in the causation of fainting and convulsions. Medicine *12*:297, 1933.
45. Leatham, A.: Carotid sinus syncope. Br. Heart J. *47*:409, 1982.
46. Gardner, R. S., Magovern, G. J., Park, S. B., Cushing, W. J., Liebler, G. A., and Hughes, R.: Carotid sinus syndrome: New surgical considerations. Vasc. Surg. *9*:204, 1975.
47. Almquist, A., Gornick, C., Benson, W., Jr., Dunnigan, A., and Benditt, D. G.: Carotid sinus hypersensitivity: Evaluation of the vasodepressor component. Circulation *71*:927, 1985.
47a. Murphy, A. L., Rowbothan, B. J., Boyle, R. S., Thew, C. M., Fardoulys, J. A., and Wilson, K.: Carotid sinus hypersensitivity in elderly nursing home patients. Aust. NZ J. Med. *16*:24, 1986.
48. Morley, C. A., Dehn, T. C. B., Perrins, E. J., Chan, S. L., and Sutton, R.: Baroreflex sensitivity measured by the phenylephrine pressor test in patients with carotid sinus and sick sinus syndromes. Cardiovasc. Res. *18*:752, 1984.
48a. Sugrue, D. D., Gersh, B. J., Holmes, D. R., Wood, D. L., Osborn, M. J., and Hammill, S. C.: Symptomatic "isolated" carotid sinus hypersensitivity: Natural history and results of treatment with anticholinergic drugs or pacemaker. J. Am. Coll. Cardiol. 7:158, 1986.
49. Sugrue, D. D., Wood, D. L., and McGoon, M. D.: Carotid sinus hypersensitivity and syncope. Mayo Clin. Prac. *59*:637, 1984.
50. Lown, B., and Levine, S. A.: The carotid sinus: Clinical value of its stimulation. Circulation *23*:766, 1961.
51. Coplan, N. L., and Schweitzer, P.: Carotid sinus hypersensitivity. Case report and review of the literature. Am. J. Med. *77*:561, 1984.
52. Trout, H. H., III, Brown, L. I., and Thompson, J. E.: Carotid sinus syndrome: Treatment by carotid sinus denervation. Am. Surg. *189*:575, 1979.
53. Lee, Y. T., Lee, T. K., and Tsai, H. C.: Glossopharyngeal neuralgia as the cause of cardiac syncope: A case report with a review of literature. J. Formosan Med. Assoc. *4*:103, 1975.
54. Khero, B. A., and Millins, C. B.: Cardiac syncope due to glossopharyngeal neuralgia. Arch. Intern. Med. *128*:806, 1971.
55. Kong, Y., Heyman, A., Entman, M. L., and McIntosh, H. D.: Glossopharyngeal neuralgia associated with bradycardia, syncope, and seizures. Circulation *30*:109, 1964.
56. Dykman, T. R., Montgomery, E. B., Gerstenberger, P. D., Zeiger, H. E., Clutter, W. E., and Cryer, P. E.: Glossopharyngeal neuralgia with syncope secondary to tumor: Treatment and pathophysiology. Am. J. Med. *71*:165, 1981.
56a. Barbash, G. I., Keren, G., Korczyn, A. D., Sharpless, N. S., Chayen, M., Copperman, Y., and Laniado, S.: Mechanisms of syncope in glossopharyngeal neuralgia. Electroencephalogr. Clin. Neurophysiol. *63*:231, 1986.
56b. Weinstein, R. E., Herec, D., and Friedman, J. H.: Hypotension due to glossopharyngeal neuralgia. Arch. Neurol. 43:90, 1986.
57. Waddington, J. K. B., Matthews, H. R., Evans, C. C., and Ward, D. W.: Carcinoma of the esophagus with swallow syncope. Br. Med. J. 3:232, 1975.
58. Wik, B., and Hillestead, L.: Deglutition syncope. Br. Med. J. *3*:747, 1975.
59. Tolman, K. G., and Ashworth, W.: Syncope induced by dysphagia correction by esophageal dilatation. Am. J Dig. Dis. *16*:1026, 1971.
60. St. John, J. N.: Swallow syncope: A form of glossopharyngeal neuralgia? Can. Med. Assoc. J. *134*:309, 1986.
61. Weiss, S., and Ferris, E. B.: Adams-Stokes syndrome with transient complete heart block of vasovagal reflex origin. Arch. Intern. Med. *54*:931, 1934.
62. James, A. H.: Cardiac syncope after swallowing. Lancet *1*:771, 1958.
63. Haldane, J. H.: Micturition syncope. Can. Med. Assoc. J. *101*:712, 1969.
64. Godec, C. J., and Cass, A. S.: Micturition syncope. J. Urol. *126*:551, 1981.
65. Larson, S. J., Sances, A., Baker, J. B., and Reigel, D.: Herniated cerebellar tonsils and cough syncope. J. Neurosurg. *40*:524, 1974.
66. Corbett, J. J., Butler, A. B., and Kaufman, B.: Sneeze syncope, basilar invagination and Arnold-Chiari type I malformation. J. Neurol. Neurosurg. Psychiatry 39:381, 1976.
67. Wayne, H. H.: Syncope, physiological considerations, and an analysis of the clinical characteristics of 510 patients. Am. J. Med. *30*:418, 1961.
68. Day, S. C., Cook, F., Funkenstein, H., and Goldman, L.: Evaluation and outcome of emergency room patients with transient loss of consciousness. Am. J. Med. 73:15, 1983.
69. Branch, W. T., Jr.: Approach to syncope. J. Gen. Intern. Med., *1*:49, 1986.
70. Barcroft, H., Edholm, O. G., McMichael, J., and Sharpey-Schafer, E. P.: Posthemorrhagic fainting: Study by cardiac output and forearm flow. Lancet *1*:489, 1944.
71. Weissler, A. M., Warren, J. V., Estes, E. H., Jr.: McIntosh, H. D., and Leonard, J. J.: Vasopressor syncope: Factors influencing cardiac output. Circulation *15*:875, 1957.
72. Glick, G., and Yu, P. N.: Hemodynamic changes during spontaneous vasovagal reactions. Am. J. Med. *34*:42, 1963.
73. Epstein, S. E., Stampfer, M., and Beiser, G. D.: Role of the capacitance and resistance vessels in vasovagal syncope. Circulation 37:524, 1968.
74. Aviado, D. M., Jr., and Schmidt, C. F.: Cardiovascular and respiratory reflexes from the left side of the heart. Am. J. Physiol. *196*:726, 1959.
75. Friedberg, C. K.: Syncope: Pathological physiology: Differential diagnosis and treatment (II). Mod. Concepts Cardiovasc. Dis. *40*:61, 1971.
76. Martin, A. K., Hackel, D. B., and Sieber, H. O.: Intraventricular pressure changes in dogs during hemorrhagic shock. Fed. Proc. *22*:252, 1963.
77. Brun, C., Knudsen, E. O. E., and Raaschou, F.: Kidney function and circulatory collapse, postsyncopal oliguria. J. Clin. Invest. *25*:568, 1946.
78. Stead, E. A., Jr., Kunkel, P., and Weiss, S.: Effect of pitressin in circulatory collapse induced by sodium nitrate. J. Clin. Invest. *18*:673, 1939.
79. Wright, K. E., Jr., and McIntosh, H. D.: Syncope: A review of pathophysiological mechanisms. Progr. Cardiovasc. Dis. *13*:580, 1971.
80. MacMurray, F. G.: Stokes-Adams disease: A historical review. N. Engl. J. Med. *256*:643, 1957.
81. Morgagni, J. B.: The seats and causes of disease. *In* Major, H. H. (ed.): Classic Descriptions of Disease. Oxford, Blackwell Scientific Publications, 1948, p. 346.
82. Adams, R.: Cases of diseases of the heart, accompanied with pathological observations. Dublin Hosp. Rep. *4*:353, 1827.
83. Stokes, W.: Observations on some cases of permanently slow pulse. Dublin Q. J. Med. Sci. *2*:73, 1846.
84. Parkinson, J., Papp, C., and Evans, W.: The electrocardiogram of the Stokes-Adams attack. Br. Heart J. *3*:171, 1941.
85. Pomerantz, B., and O'Rourke, R. A.: The Stokes-Adams syndrome. Am. J. Med. *46*:941, 1969.
86. Kapoor, W. N., Karpf, M., Wieand, S., Peterson, J., and Levey, G. S.: A prospective evaluation and follow-up of patients with syncope. N. Engl. J. Med. *309*:197, 1983.
87. Silverstein, M. D., Singer, D. E., Mulley, A. G., Thibault, G. E., and Barnett, G. O.: Patients with syncope admitted to medical intensive care units. J.A.M.A. *248*:1185, 1982.
88. Kapoor, W. N., Peterson, J. R., and Karpf, M.: Micturition syncope: A reappraisal. J.A.M.A. *253*:796, 1985.
89. Schatz, I. J.: Orthostatic hypotension. Arch. Intern. Med. *144*:773 and 1037, 1984.
90. Kapoor, W., Karpf, M., and Levey, G. S.: Issues in evaluating patients with syncope. Ann. Intern. Med. *100*:755, 1984.
91. Lipsitz, L. A.: Syncope in the elderly. Ann. Intern. Med. 99:92, 1983.
92. Moss, A. J., and Davis, R. J.: Brady-tachy syndrome. Prog. Cardiovasc. Dis. *16*:439, 1974.
93. Mark, A. L., Kioschos, J. M., Abboud, F. M., Heistadt, D., and Schmid, P. G.: Abnormal vascular responses to exercise in patients with aortic stenosis. J. Clin. Invest. 52:1138, 1973.
94. Richards, A. M., Nicholls, M. G., Ikram, H., Hamilton, E. J. and Richards, R. D.: Syncope in aortic valvular stenosis. Lancet *2*:1113, 1984.
95. Braunwald, E., Brockenbrough, E. D. and Frye, R. J.: Studies on digitalis. V. Comparison of the effects of ouabain on left ventricular dynamics in valvular aortic stenosis and hypertrophic subaortic stenosis. Circulation *26*:166, 1962.
96. Jarisch, A., and Zotterman, Y.: Depressor reflexes from the heart. Acta Physiol. Scand. *16*:31, 1948.

APPROACH TO DIAGNOSIS

97. Eckberg, D. L., Dabinsky, M., and Braunwald, E.: Defective cardiac parasympathetic control in patients with heart disease. N. Engl. J. Med. *285*:877, 1971.
97a. Radack, K. L.: Syncope: Cost-effective patient workup. Postgrad. Med. *80*:169, 1986.
98. Johansson, B. E.: Evaluation of alteration of consciousness and palpitations. *In* Wenger, N. K., Mock, M. B., and Ringvist, I. (eds.): Ambulatory Electrocardiographic Recording. Chicago, Year Book Medical Publishers, Inc., 1981, p. 321.
99. Sharma, A. D., Klein, G. J., and Milstein, S.: Diagnostic assessment of recurrent syncope. PACE *7*:749, 1984.
100. Pratt, C. M., Francis, M. J., Stone, C. L., Young, J. B., and Griffin, J. C.: Transtelephonic electrocardiographic monitoring: Reliability in detecting the ischemic ST segment response during exercise. Am. Heart J. *108*:967, 1984.
101. Pratt, C. M., Slymen, J. D., Wierman, A., Francis, M. J., English, L., Thornton, B., Stone, C., Young, J. B., and Roberts, R.: Can asymptomatic telephone electrocardiographic transmissions serve as a surveillance system to detect unsuspected increases in complex ventricular arrhythmias? J. Am. Col. Cardiol. 7(abs):190A, 1986.
102. Hess, D. S., Morady, F., and Scheinman, M. M.: Electrophysiologic testing in the evaluation of patients with syncope of undetermined origin. Am. J. Cardiol. *50*:1309, 1982.
103. DiMarco, J. P., Garan, H., Ruskin, J. N.: Approach to the patient with recurrent syncope of unknown cause. Mod. Concepts Cardiovasc. Dis. 52:11, 1983.
104. Akhtar, M., Shenasa, M., Denker S., Gilbert, C., and Rizwi, N.: Role of cardiac electrophysiologic studies in patients with unexplained recurrent syncope. PACE *6*:192, 1983.
105. Morady, F., and Scheinman, M. M.: The role and limitations of electrophysiologic testing in patients with unexplained syncope. Int. J Cardiol. *4*:229, 1983.
106. Morady, F., Shen, E., Schwartz, A., Hess, D., Bhandari, A., Sung, R. J., and Scheinman, M. M.: Long-term follow-up of patients with recurrent unexplained syncope evaluated by electrophysiologic testing. J. Am. Coll. Cardiol. 2:1053, 1983.
107. Teichman, S. L., Felder, S. D., Matos, J. A., Kim, S. G., Waspe, L. E., and Fisher, J. D.: The value of electrophysiologic studies in syncope of undetermined origin: Report of 150 cases. Am. Heart J. *110*:469, 1985.
108. DiMarco, J. P., Garan, H., Harthorne, W., and Ruskin, J. N.: Intracardiac electrophysiologic techniques in recurrent syncope of unknown cause. Ann. Intern. Med. 95:542, 1981.
109. Josephson, M. D., and Seides, S. F.: Clinical Cardiac Electrophysiology: Techniques and Interpretations. Philadelphia, Lea and Febiger, 1979, p. 44.
110. Kapoor, W. N., Karpf, M., Maher, Y., Miller, R. A., and Levey, G. S.: Syncope of unknown origin: The need for a more cost-effective approach to its diagnostic evaluation. J.A.M.A. *247*:2687, 1982.
111. Hauer, R. N. W., Lie, K. I., Liem, K. L., and Durrer, D.: Long term prognosis in patients with bundle branch block complicating acute anteroseptal infarction. Am. J. Cardiol. *49*:1581, 1982.

PART III DISEASES OF THE HEART, PERICARDIUM, AORTA, AND PULMONARY VASCULAR BED

30 CONGENITAL HEART DISEASE IN INFANCY AND CHILDHOOD

by WILLIAM F. FRIEDMAN, M.D.

GENERAL CONSIDERATIONS

DEFINITION

Congenital cardiovascular disease is defined as an *abnormality at birth in cardiocirculatory structure or function.* Congenital cardiovascular malformations result generally from altered embryonic development of a normal structure or failure of such a structure to progress beyond an early stage of embryonic or fetal development. The aberrant patterns of flow created by an anatomical defect may, in turn, significantly influence the structural and functional development of the remainder of the circulation. For instance, the presence in utero of mitral atresia may not permit normal development of the left ventricle, aortic valve, and ascending aorta. Similarly, constriction of the fetal ductus arteriosus may result directly in right ventricular dilatation and tricuspid regurgitation in the fetus and newborn, contribute importantly to the development of pulmonary arterial aneurysms in the presence of ventricular septal defect and absent pulmonic valve, or, further, result in an alteration in the number and caliber of fetal and newborn pulmonary vascular resistance vessels. In this same regard, postnatal events may markedly influence the clinical presentation of a specific "isolated" malformation. The infant with Ebstein's malformation of the tricuspid valve may improve dramatically as the magnitude of tricuspid regurgitation diminishes with normal fall in pulmonary vascular resistance after birth; the infant with hypoplastic left heart syndrome or interrupted aortic arch may not exhibit circulatory collapse, and the baby with pulmonic atresia or severe stenosis may not become cyanotic until normal spontaneous closure occurs of a patent ductus arteriosus. Ductal constriction many days after birth may also be a central factor in some infants in the development of coarctation of the aorta. Still later in life the patient with a ventricular septal defect may experience spontaneous closure of the abnormal communication, or develop right ventricular outflow tract obstruction and/or aortic regurgitation, or pulmonary vascular obstructive disease. These selected examples serve to emphasize that anatomical and physiological changes in the heart and circulation may continue indefinitely from prenatal life in association with any specific congenital cardiocirculatory lesion.

It should be recognized further that certain congenital defects are not apparent on gross inspection of the heart or circulation. Examples include the electrophysiological pathways for ventricular preexcitation or interruptions in the cardiac conduction system giving rise to paroxysmal supraventricular tachycardia or congenital complete heart block, respectively. Similarly, abnormalities in the development of myocardial autonomic innervation or in the ultrastructure of myocardial cells may ultimately prove to contribute to asymmetrical septal hypertrophy and left ventricular outflow tract obstruction. These examples make clear that occasional difficulties arise in distinguishing between congenital anomalies that are readily apparent at or shortly after birth and lesions that may have as their basis a subtle or undetectable abnormality that is present at birth.

INCIDENCE

The true incidence of congenital cardiovascular malformations is difficult to determine accurately, partly because of the difficulties in definition discussed above. It has been estimated that approximately 0.8 per cent of live births are complicated by a cardiovascular malformation.[1] This figure does not take into account what may be the two most common cardiac anomalies: the congenital, nonstenotic bicuspid aortic valve[2] and the leaflet abnormality associated with mitral valve prolapse.[3] Moreover, the widely quoted 0.8 per cent incidence figure fails to include small preterm

TABLE 30–1 FREQUENCY OF OCCURRENCE OF CARDIAC MALFORMATIONS AT BIRTH

Disease	Percentage
Ventricular septal defect	30.5
Atrial septal defect	9.8
Patent ductus arteriosus	9.7
Pulmonic stenosis	6.9
Coarctation of the aorta	6.8
Aortic stenosis	6.1
Tetralogy of Fallot	5.8
Complete transposition of the great arteries	4.2
Persistent truncus arteriosus	2.2
Tricuspid atresia	1.3
All others	16.5

Data based on 2310 cases.

infants, almost all of whom have persistent patent ductus arteriosus, or the prevalence of cardiovascular abnormalities in stillborn infants. Thus, it is clear that past statistical analyses have seriously underestimated the incidence of congenital heart disease.

Precise data concerning frequency of individual congenital lesions are also lacking, and the results of many analyses differ, depending upon the source (living or dead) and the selection of the study population.[4] Table 30–1 is a compilation from both clinical and pathological studies that approximates the frequency of occurrence of specific cardiovascular malformations.[5, 6]

Taken in toto, children with congenital heart disease are predominantly male. Moreover, specific defects may show a definite sex preponderance; patent ductus arteriosus and atrial septal defect are more common in *females*, whereas valvular aortic stenosis, congenital aneurysm of the sinus of Valsalva, coarctation of the aorta, tetralogy of Fallot, and transposition of the great arteries are more common in *males*.

Extracardiac anomalies occur in approximately 25 per cent of infants with significant cardiac disease,[7] and their presence may significantly increase mortality. Often the extracardiac anomalies are multiple, in part involving the musculoskeletal system; one third of infants with both cardiac and extracardiac anomalies have some established syndrome.

ETIOLOGY

Malformations appear to result from an interaction between multifactorial genetic and environmental systems too complex to allow a single specification of etiology.[8, 8a] In most instances, a causal factor cannot be identified. Maternal rubella, ingestion of thalidomide early during gestation, and chronic maternal alcohol abuse are environmental insults known to interfere with normal cardiogenesis in man.[9–12] *Rubella syndrome* consists of cataracts, deafness, microcephaly, and, either singly or in combination, patent ductus arteriosus, pulmonic valvular and/or arterial stenosis, and atrial septal defect. *Thalidomide* is associated with major limb deformities and occasionally with cardiac malformations without predilection for a specific lesion. The *fetal alcohol syndrome* consists of microcephaly, micrognathia, microphthalmia, prenatal growth retardation, developmental delay, and cardiac defects. The latter—often defects of the ventricular septum—occur in approximately 45 per cent of affected infants. *Maternal lupus erythematosus* during pregnancy has been linked to congenital complete heart block (p. 967). Animal experiments have incriminated hypoxia, deficiency or excess of several vitamins, intake of several categories of drugs, and ionizing irradiation as teratogens capable of causing cardiac malformations.[10] The precise relationship of these animal teratogens to human malformations is not clear.

The genetic aspects of congenital heart disease are discussed extensively in Chapter 49. A single gene mutation may be causative in the familial forms of atrial septal defect with prolonged AV conduction, mitral valve prolapse, ventricular septal defect, congenital heart block, situs inversus, pulmonary hypertension, the combination of supravalvular aortic stenosis and peripheral pulmonary arterial stenosis, and the syndromes of Noonan, LEOPARD, Holt-Oram, Ellis–van Creveld, and Kartagener. Table 30–2 provides a partial list of syndromes in which cardiovascular anomalies may be manifestations of the pleiotropic effects of single genes or examples of gross chromosomal defects. Less than 5 to 10 per cent of all cardiac malformations can be accounted for by chromosomal aberrations or genetic mutations or transmission.

The finding that, with some exceptions, only one of a pair of monozygotic twins is affected by congenital heart disease indicates that the vast majority of cardiovascular malformations are not inherited in a simple manner.[13] Family studies indicate a two- to ten-fold increase in the incidence of congenital heart disease in siblings of affected patients or in the offspring of an affected parent. Malformations are often concordant or partially concordant within families.[14] Because the incidence of congenital heart disease in the offspring or siblings of an index patient is only 2 to 10 per cent, it is rarely wise to discourage the parents of one affected child from having additional children if either parent is free of a cardiovascular anomaly.[15] Moreover, the low recurrence rate and the increasing possibilities for effective treatment for nearly all cardiac lesions usually justify a positive approach to family counseling. When two or more members of the family are affected, the recurrence risk may be quite high, and a pedigree should be obtained before further counseling. If a dominant or recessive mendelian pattern is established, the mendelian laws apply, and the risk of recurrence in each pregnancy is equal.

PREVENTION

The feasibility of preventive programs will depend upon what is learned in the future about the cause of the 90 per cent or more of cardiovascular anomalies for which no cause is currently known. Strict testing in animals of new drugs that may be teratogenic when taken during pregnancy may be expected to reduce the chances of another thalidomide tragedy. In this regard, the dictum cannot be emphasized too strongly that no medication should be taken during pregnancy without prior consultation with a physician. Physicians dealing with pregnant women should be aware of known teratogens as well as of drugs that may have a functional rather than a structural damaging influence on the fetal and newborn heart and circulation and should recognize that drugs abound for which there is inadequate information concerning their teratogenic potential. Similarly, appropriate use of radiological equipment and techniques for reducing gonadal and fetal radiation exposure should always be employed to reduce the potential hazards of this likely cause of birth defects.

Detection of abnormal chromosomes in fetal cells obtained from amniotic fluid or chorionic villus biopsy (Chap. 49) may occasionally predict cardiac malformation as one component of the multiple system involvement that may exist in such syndromes as Down, Turner, or trisomy 13–15 (D1) and 16–18 (E). Similarly, identification in such cells of the enzyme disorders observed in the mucopolysaccharidoses, homocystinuria, or type II glycogen storage disease may allow one to predict the ultimate presence of cardiac disease. Lastly, immunization of children with rubella vaccine will avoid the effects of maternal rubella and its cardiac consequences.

EMBRYOLOGY

NORMAL CARDIAC DEVELOPMENT. Correlation of anatomical features of malformed hearts and embryonic cardiac morphology allows a developmental analysis of various anomalies. Detailed accounts of

TABLE 30–2 SYNDROMES WITH ASSOCIATED CARDIOVASCULAR INVOLVEMENT

Syndrome	Major Cardiovascular Manifestations	Major Noncardiac Abnormalities
Heritable and Possibly Heritable		
Ellis–van Creveld	Single atrium or atrial septal defect	Chondrodystrophic dwarfism, nail dysplasia, polydactyly
TAR (thrombocytopenia-absent radius)	Atrial septal defect, tetralogy of Fallot	Radial aplasia or hypoplasia, thrombocytopenia
Holt-Oram	Atrial septal defect (other defects common)	Skeletal upper limb defect, hypoplasia of clavicles
Kartagener	Dextrocardia	Situs inversus, sinusitis, bronchiectasis
Laurence-Moon-Biedl-Bardet	Variable defects	Retinal pigmentation, obesity, polydactyly
Noonan	Pulmonic valve dysplasia, cardiomyopathy (usually hypertrophic)	Webbed neck, pectus excavatum, cryptorchidism
Tuberous sclerosis	Rhabdomyoma, cardiomyopathy	Phakomatosis, bone lesions, hamartomatous skin lesions
Multiple lentigenes (LEOPARD)	Pulmonic stenosis	Basal cell nevi, broad facies, rib anomalies
Rubinstein-Taybi	Patent ductus arteriosus (others)	Broad thumbs and toes, hypoplastic maxilla, slanted palpebral fissures
Familial deafness	Arrhythmias, sudden death	Sensorineural deafness
Weber-Osler-Rendu	Arteriovenous fistulas (lung, liver, mucous membranes)	Multiple telangiectasias
Apert	Ventricular septal defect	Craniosynostosis, midfacial hypoplasia, syndactyly
Incontinentia pigmenti	Patent ductus arteriosus	Irregular pigmented skin lesions, patchy alopecia, hypodontia
Alagille (arteriohepatic dysplasia)	Peripheral pulmonic stenosis, pulmonic stenosis	Biliary hypoplasia, vertebral anomalies, prominent forehead, deep-set eyes
DiGeorge	Interrupted aortic arch, tetralogy of Fallot, truncus arteriosus	Thymic hypoplasia or aplasia, parathyroid aplasia or hypoplasia, ear anomalies
Friedreich's ataxia	Cardiomyopathy and conduction defects	Ataxia, speech defect, degeneration of spinal cord dorsal columns
Muscular dystrophy	Cardiomyopathy	Pseudohypertrophy of calf muscles, weakness of trunk and proximal limb muscles
Cystic fibrosis	Cor pulmonale	Pancreatic insufficiency, malabsorption, chronic lung disease
Sickle cell anemia	Cardiomyopathy, mitral regurgitation	Hemoglobin SS
Conradi-Hünermann	Ventricular septal defect, patent ductus arteriosus	Asymmetrical limb shortness, early punctate mineralization, large skin pores
Cockayne	Accelerated atherosclerosis	Cachectic dwarfism, retinal pigment abnormalities, photosensitivity dermatitis
Progeria	Accelerated atherosclerosis	Premature aging, alopecia, atrophy of subcutaneous fat, skeletal hypoplasia
Connective Tissue Disorders		
Cutis laxa	Peripheral pulmonic stenosis	Generalized disruption of elastic fibers, diminished skin resilience, hernias
Ehlers-Danlos	Arterial dilatation and rupture, mitral regurgitation	Hyperextensible joints, hyperelastic and friable skin
Marfan	Aortic dilatation, aortic and mitral incompetence	Gracile habitus, arachnodactyly with hyperextensibility, lens subluxation
Osteogenesis imperfecta	Aortic incompetence	Fragile bones, blue sclerae
Pseudoxanthoma elasticum	Peripheral and coronary arterial disease	Degeneration of elastic fibers in skin, retinal angioid streaks
Inborn Errors of Metabolism		
Pompe's disease	Glycogen storage disease of heart	Acid maltase deficiency, muscular weakness
Homocystinuria	Aortic and pulmonary artery dilatation, intravascular thrombosis	Cystathionine synthetase deficiency, lens subluxation, osteoporosis
Mucopolysaccharidoses: Hurler; Hunter	Multivalvular and coronary and great artery disease, cardiomyopathy	Hurler: Deficiency of α-L-iduronidase, corneal clouding, coarse features, growth and mental retardation Hunter: Deficiency of L-idurano-sulfate sulfatase, coarse facies, clear cornea, growth and mental retardation
Morquio; Scheie; Maroteaux-Lamy	Aortic incompetence	Morquio: Deficiency of N-acetylhexosamine sulfate sulfatase, cloudy cornea, normal intelligence, severe bone changes involving vertebrae and epiphyses Scheie: Deficiency of α-L-iduronidase, cloudy cornea, normal intelligence, peculiar facies Maroteaux-Lamy: Deficiency of arylsulfatase B, cloudy cornea, osseous changes, normal intelligence
Chromosomal Abnormalities		
Trisomy 21 (Down syndrome)	Endocardial cushion defect, atrial or ventricular septal defect, tetralogy of Fallot	Hypotonia, hyperextensible joints, mongoloid facies, mental retardation
Trisomy 13 (D)	Ventricular septal defect, right ventricle patent ductus arteriosus, double-outlet right ventricle	Single midline intracerebral ventricle with midfacial defects, polydactyly, nail changes, mental retardation
Trisomy 18 (E)	Congenital polyvalvular dysplasia, ventricular septal defect, patent ductus	Clenched hand, short sternum, low arch dermal ridge pattern on fingertips, mental retardation
Cri du chat (short-arm deletion-5)	Ventricular septal defect	Cat cry, microcephaly, antimongoloid slant of palpebral fissures, mental retardation

Table continued on opposite page

TABLE 30–2 SYNDROMES WITH ASSOCIATED CARDIOVASCULAR INVOLVEMENT *Continued*

Syndrome	Major Cardiovascular Manifestations	Major Noncardiac Abnormalities
XO (Turner)	Coarctation of aorta, biscuspid aortic valve, aortic dilatation	Short female, broad chest, lymphedema, webbed neck
XXXY and XXXXX	Patent ductus arteriosus	XXXY: Hypogenitalism, mental retardation, radial-ulnar synostosis XXXXX: Small hands, incurving of fifth fingers, mental retardation
Sporadic Disorders		
VATER association	Ventricular septal defect	Vertebral anomalies, anal atresia, tracheo-esophageal fistula, radial and renal anomalies
CHARGE association	Tetralogy of Fallot (other defects common)	Colobomas, choanal atresia, mental and growth deficiency, genital and ear anomalies
Williams	Supravalvar aortic stenosis, peripheral pulmonic stenosis	Mental deficiency, elfin facies, loquacious personality, hoarse voice
Cornelia de Lange	Ventricular septal defect	Micromelia, synophrys, mental and growth deficiency
Shprintzen (velocardiofacial)	Ventricular septal defect, tetralogy of Fallot, right aortic arch	Cleft palate, prominent nose, slender hands, learning disability
Teratogenic Disorders		
Rubella	Patent ductus arteriosus, pulmonic valvular and/or arterial stenosis, atrial septal defect	Cataracts, deafness, microcephaly
Alcohol	Ventricular septal defect (other defects)	Microcephaly, growth and mental deficiency, short palpebral fissures, smooth philtrum, thin upper lip
Dilantin	Pulmonic stenosis, aortic stenosis, coarctation, patent ductus arteriosus	Hypertelorism, growth and mental deficiency, short phalanges, bowed upper lip
Thalidomide	Variable	Phocomelia
Lithium	Ebstein's anomaly, tricuspid atresia	None

Modified from Friedman, W. F.: Congenital heart disease. *In* Braunwald, E., et al. (eds.): Harrison's Principles of Internal Medicine. 11th ed. New York, McGraw-Hill Book Co., 1987, p. 940.

the normal development of the cardiovascular system are provided elsewhere.[16–18] In brief, during the first month of gestation the primitive, straight cardiac tube is formed, comprising the sinuatrium, the primitive ventricle, the bulbus cordis, and the truncus arteriosus in series (Fig. 30–1). In the second month of gestation this tube doubles over on itself to form two parallel pumping systems, each with two chambers and a great artery. The two atria develop from the sinuatrium; the atrioventricular canal is divided by the endocardial cushions into tricuspid and mitral orifices; and the right and left ventricles develop from the primitive ventricle and bulbus cordis. Differential growth of myocardial cells causes the straight cardiac tube to bear to the right, and the bulboventricular portion of the tube doubles over on itself, bringing the ventricles side by side (Fig. 30–2). Migration of the atrioventricular canal to the right and of the ventricular septum to the left serves to align each ventricle with its appropriate atrioventricular valve. At the distal end of the cardiac tube the bulbus cordis divides into a subaortic muscular conus and a subpulmonic muscular conus; the subpulmonic conus elongates and the subaortic conus reabsorbs, allowing the aorta to move posteriorly and connect with the left ventricle.

ABNORMAL DEVELOPMENT. A host of anomalies may result from defects in this basic developmental pattern. Thus, double-inlet left ventricle (p. 965) is observed if the tricuspid orifice does not align over the right ventricle. The various types of persistent truncus arteriosus (p. 925) result from failure of the truncus to divide into main pulmonary artery and aorta. Double-outlet anomalies of the right ventricle (p. 960) are produced by failure of either the subpulmonic or subaortic conus to resorb, whereas resorption of the subpulmonic instead of the subaortic conus may be central to transposition of the great arteries (p. 953).

The Atria. The primitive sinuatrium is separated into right and left atria by the downgrowth from its roof of the septum primum toward the atrioventricular canal, thereby creating an inferior intraatrial ostium primum opening (Fig. 30–3). Multiple perforations form in the anterosuperior portion of the septum primum as the septum secundum begins to develop to the right of the former. The coalescence of these perforations forms the ostium secundum. The septum secundum completely separates the atrial chambers except for a central opening—the fossa ovalis—which is covered by tissue of the septum primum forming the valve of the foramen ovale. Fusion of the endocardial cushions anteriorly and posteriorly divides the atrioventricular canal into tricuspid and mitral inlets (Fig. 30–4). The inferior portion of the atrial septum, the superior portion of the ventricular septum, and portions of the septal leaflets of both the tricuspid and mitral valves are formed from the endocardial cushions. The integrity of the atrial septum depends on growth of the septum primum and septum secundum and proper fusion of the endocardial cushions. Atrial septal defects (p. 915) and varying degrees of endocardial cushion defect (p. 917) are the result of developmental deficiencies of this process.

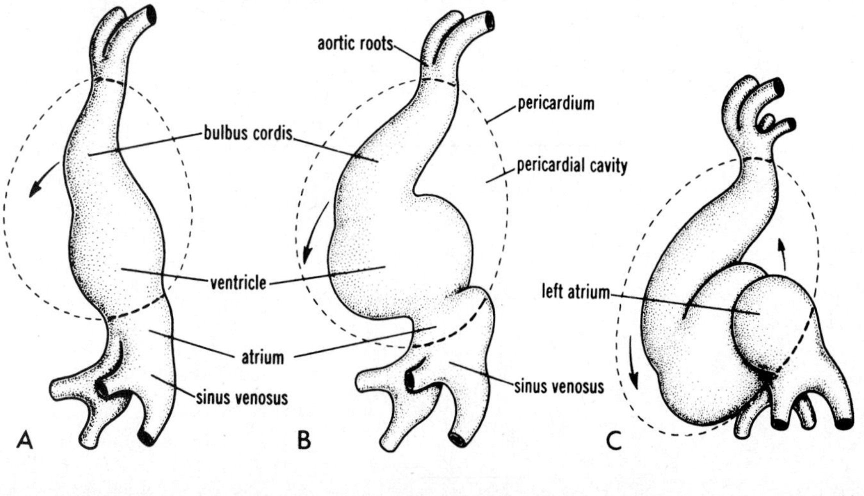

FIGURE 30–1. Formation of the cardiac loop as seen from the left side at 32 days (*A*), 34 days (*B*), and 38 days (*C*). Dashed line indicates parietal pericardium. The atrium gradually assumes an intrapericardial position. (From Langman, J., and van Mierop, L. H. S.: Development of the cardiovascular system. *In* Moss, A. J., and Adams, F. H. [eds.]: Heart Disease in Infants, Children and Adolescents. Baltimore, Williams and Wilkins, 1968.)

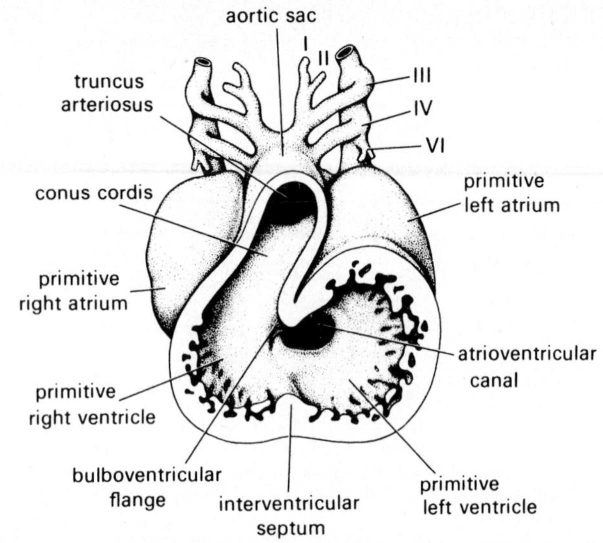

FIGURE 30–2. Frontal section through the heart of 5-mm embryo showing the side-by-side primitive ventricles and the single opening of the atrium into the ventricles. (From Langman, J., and van Mierop, L. H. S.: Development of the cardiovascular system. *In* Moss, A. J., and Adams, F. H. [eds.]: Heart Disease in Infants, Children and Adolescents. Baltimore, Williams and Wilkins, 1968.)

The Ventricles. Partitioning of the ventricles occurs as cephalad growth of the main ventricular septum results in its fusion with the endocardial cushions and the infundibular or conus septum. Defects in the ventricular septum may occur owing to a deficiency of septal substance; malalignment of septal components in different planes, preventing their fusion; or an overly long conus, keeping the septal components apart. Isolated defects (p. 920) probably result from the former mechanism, while the latter two appear to generate the ventricular defects seen in tetralogy of Fallot (p. 946) and transposition complexes (p. 952).

The Lungs. These structures arise from the primitive foregut and are drained early in embryogenesis by channels from the splanchnic plexus to the cardinal and umbilicovitelline veins. An outpouching from the posterior left atrium forms the common pulmonary vein, which communicates with the splanchnic plexus, establishing pulmonary venous drainage to the left atrium. The umbilicovitelline and anterior cardinal vein communications atrophy as the common pulmonary vein is incorporated into the left atrium. Anomalous pulmonary venous connections (p. 961) to the umbilicovitelline (portal) venous system or to the cardinal system (superior vena cava) result from failure of the common pulmonary vein to develop or establish communications to the splanchnic plexus. Cor triatriatum (p. 940) results from a narrowing of the common pulmonary vein–left atrial junction.

The Great Arteries. The truncus arteriosus is connected to the dorsal aorta in the embryo by six pairs of aortic arches. Partition of the truncus arteriosus into two great arteries is a result of the fusion of tissue arising from the back wall of the vessel and the truncus septum. Rotation of the truncus coils the aorticopulmonary septum and creates the normal spiral relationship between aorta and pulmonary artery. Semilunar valves and their related sinuses are created by absorption and hollowing out of tissue at the distal side of the truncus ridges. Aorticopulmonary septal defect (p. 925) and persistent truncus arteriosus (p. 925) represent varying degrees of partitioning failure.

Although the six aortic arches appear sequentially, portions of the arch system and dorsal aorta disappear at different times during embryogenesis (Fig. 30–5). The first, second, and fifth sets of paired arches regress completely. The proximal portions of the sixth arches become the right and left pulmonary arteries and the distal left sixth arch becomes the ductus arteriosus. The third aortic arch forms the connection between internal and external carotid arteries, while the left fourth arch becomes the arterial segment between left carotid and subclavian arteries; the proximal portion of the right subclavian artery forms from the right fourth arch. An abnormality in regression of the arch system in a number of sites can produce a wide variety of arch anomalies, whereas a failure of regression results generally in a double aortic arch malformation.

FETAL AND TRANSITIONAL CIRCULATIONS

Although the illness created by the presence of a cardiac malformation is almost always recognized only after an affected baby is born, important effects on the circulation have existed from early in pregnancy until the time of delivery.[19] Thus, knowledge of the changes in cardiocirculatory structure, function, and metabolism that accompany development is central to a systematic comprehension of congenital heart disease.

FETAL CIRCULATORY PATHWAYS. Dynamic alterations occur in the circulation during the transition from fetal to neonatal life when the lungs, rather than the placenta, take over the function of gas exchange. The single fetal circulation consists of parallel pulmonary and systemic pathways (Fig. 30–6) in contrast to the two-circuit system in the newborn and adult in whom the pulmonary vasculature exists in series with the systemic circulation. Prenatal survival is not endangered by major cardiac anomalies as long as one side of the heart can drive blood from the great veins to the aorta; in the fetus, blood can bypass the nonfunctioning lungs both proximal and distal to the heart. Oxygenated blood returns from the placenta through the umbilical vein and enters the portal venous system. A variable amount of this stream bypasses the hepatic microcirculation and enters the inferior vena cava via the ductus venosus. Inferior vena caval blood is composed of flow from the ductus venosus, hepatic vein, and lower body venous drainage, which is summarily deflected to a significant extent across the foramen ovale into the left atrium. Almost all superior vena caval blood passes directly through the tricuspid valve entering the right ventricle. Most of the blood that reaches the right ventricle bypasses the high-resistance, unexpanded lungs and passes through the ductus arteriosus into the descending aorta. The right ventricle contributes approximately 55 per

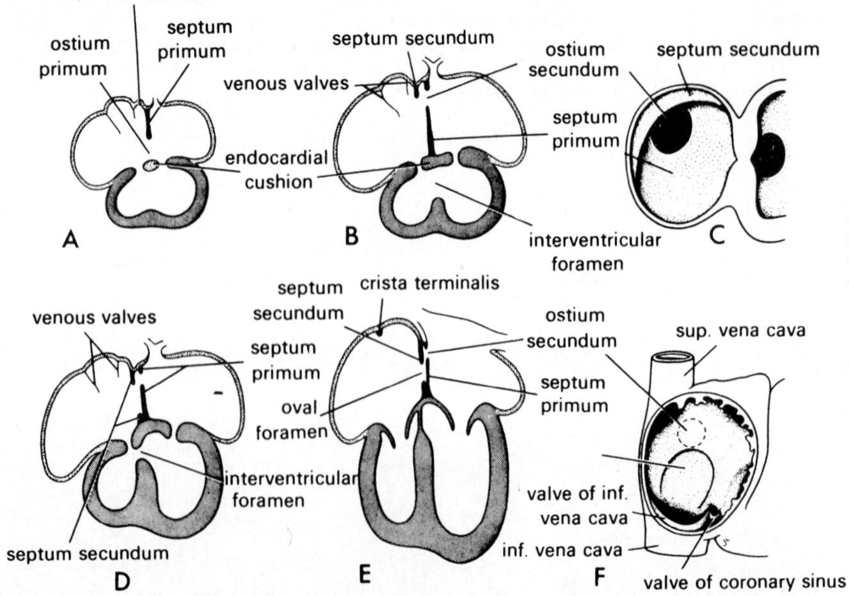

FIGURE 30–3. Diagrammatic representation of the atrial septa at 30 days (*A*), at 33 days (*B*), at 33 days (seen from the right side) (*C*), at 37 days (*D*), and in the newborn (*E*); the newborn atrial septum viewed from the right (*F*). (From Langman, J., and van Mierop, L. H. S.: Development of the cardiovascular system. *In* Moss, A. J., and Adams, F. H. [eds.]: Heart Disease in Infants, Children and Adolescents. Baltimore, Williams and Wilkins, 1968.)

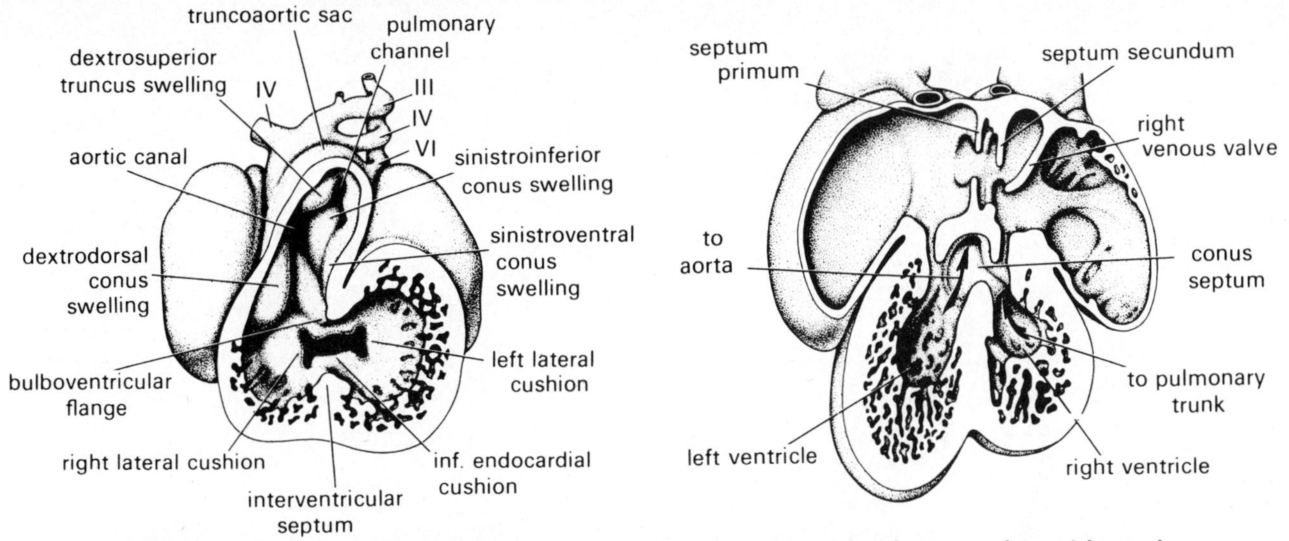

FIGURE 30–4. Frontal section through the heart of a 9-mm embryo (*left panel*) and 15-mm embryo (*right panel*). At 9 mm, development is noted of the cushions in the atrioventricular canal, and the truncus and conus swellings are visible. At 15 mm, the conus septum is completed; note the septation in the atrial region. (From Langman, J., and Van Mierop, L. H. S.: Development of the cardiovascular system. *In* Moss, A. J., and Adams, F. H. [eds.]: Heart Disease in Infants, Children and Adolescents. Baltimore, Williams and Wilkins, 1968.)

cent and the left 45 per cent to the total fetal cardiac output. The major portion of blood ejected from the left ventricle supplies the brain and upper body, with lesser flow to the coronary arteries; the balance passes across the aortic isthmus to the descending aorta where it joins with the large stream from the ductus arteriosus before flowing to the lower body and placenta.

FETAL PULMONARY CIRCULATION. In fetal life pulmonary arteries and arterioles are surrounded by a fluid medium, have relatively thick walls and small lumina, and resemble comparable arteries in the systemic circulation. The low pulmonary blood flow in the fetus (7 to 10 per cent of the total cardiac output) is the result of high pulmonary vascular resistance. Fetal pulmonary vessels are highly reactive to changes in oxygen tension or in the pH of blood perfusing them as well as to a number of other physiological and pharmacological influences.

EFFECTS OF CARDIAC MALFORMATIONS ON THE FETUS. Although fetal somatic growth may be unimpaired, the hemodynamic effects in utero of many cardiac malformations may alter the development and structure of the fetal heart and circulation.[19] Thus, total anomalous pulmonary venous connection in utero may result in underdevelopment of the left atrium and left ventricle (p. 938), and premature closure of the foramen ovale may result in hypoplasia of the left ventricle. Moreover, postnatally the caliber of the aortic isthmus may be reduced (p. 930) in the presence of lesions in utero that create left ventricular hypertrophy and impede filling because of reduced compliance of that chamber or that interfere with left ventricular filling directly (e.g., mitral stenosis) or indirectly by diverting a proportion of left ventricular output away from the ascending aorta while increasing right ventricular output and ductus arteriosus flow (e.g., endocardial cushion defect with left ventricular–right atrial shunt or aortic or subaortic stenosis with ventricular septal defect). Similarly, obstruction in utero to right ventricular outflow is associated with an increase in proximal aortic flow and diameter and almost never with aortic coarctation (p. 930). In these and other examples it is important to recognize that malformations compatible with fetal survival may nonetheless result in abnormal development of the circulation in utero and also affect circulatory adjustments after birth.

FUNCTION OF THE FETAL HEART. Compared to the adult heart, the fetal and newborn heart is unique with respect to its ultrastructural appearance,[20] its mechanical and biochemical properties,[21–23] and its autonomic innervation.[22–25] During late fetal and early neonatal development there is maturation of the excitation-contraction coupling process or the biochemical composition of the heart's energy-utilizing myofibrillar proteins and of ATP and creatine phosphate energy-producing proteins.[23] Moreover, fetal and neonatal myocardial cells are small in diameter and reduced in density, so that the young heart contains relatively more noncontractile mass (primarily mitochondria, nuclei, and surface membranes) than later in postnatal life. As a result, force generation and the extent and velocity of shortening are decreased, and stiffness and water content of ventricular myocardium are increased in the fetal and early newborn periods. The diminished function of the young heart is reflected in its limited ability to increase cardiac output in the presence of either a volume load or a lesion that increases resistance to emptying.[26] Although functional integrity exists of efferent and afferent cardiac autonomic pathways early in life, fetal and newborn myocardium lacks the complete development of sympathetic but not cholinergic innervation. Thus, adaptation to cardiocirculatory stress in fetal or early newborn life may be less effective than in the adult.

CHANGES AT BIRTH. Normally, the fundamental change that occurs at birth is a division of the single parallel fetal circulation into separate, independent circulations. Inflation of the lungs at the first inspiration produces a marked reduction in pulmonary vascular resistance owing partly to the sudden suspension in air of fetal pulmonary vessels previously supported by fluid media. The reduced extravascular pressure assists new vessels to open and already patent vessels to enlarge. The rapid decrease in pulmonary vascular resistance is related more

FIGURE 30–5. *A*, Aortic arches and dorsal aortas before transformation into the definitive vascular pattern. *B*, Aortic arches and dorsal aortas after transformation. The obliterated components are indicated by broken lines. (From Langman, J., and van Mierop, L. H. S.: Development of the cardiovascular system. *In* Moss, A. J., and Adams, F. H. [eds.]: Heart Disease in Infants, Children and Adolescents. Baltimore, Williams and Wilkins, 1968.)

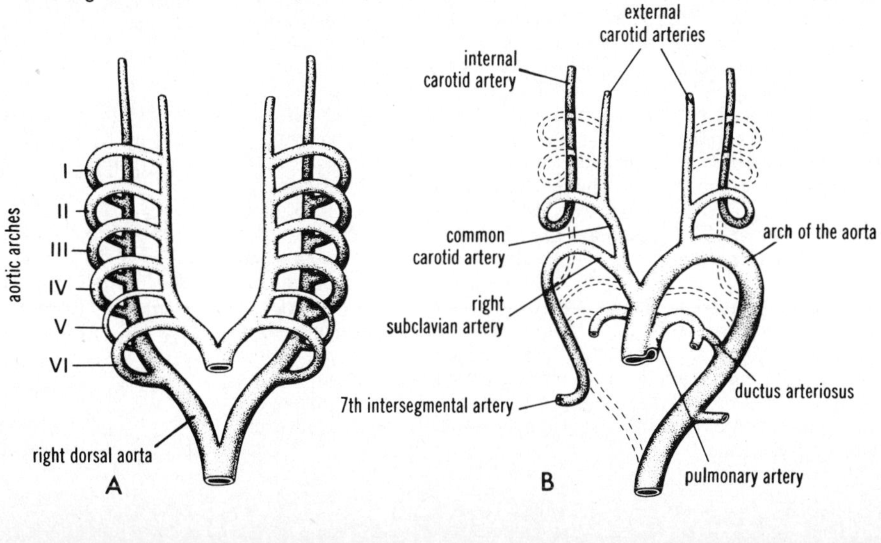

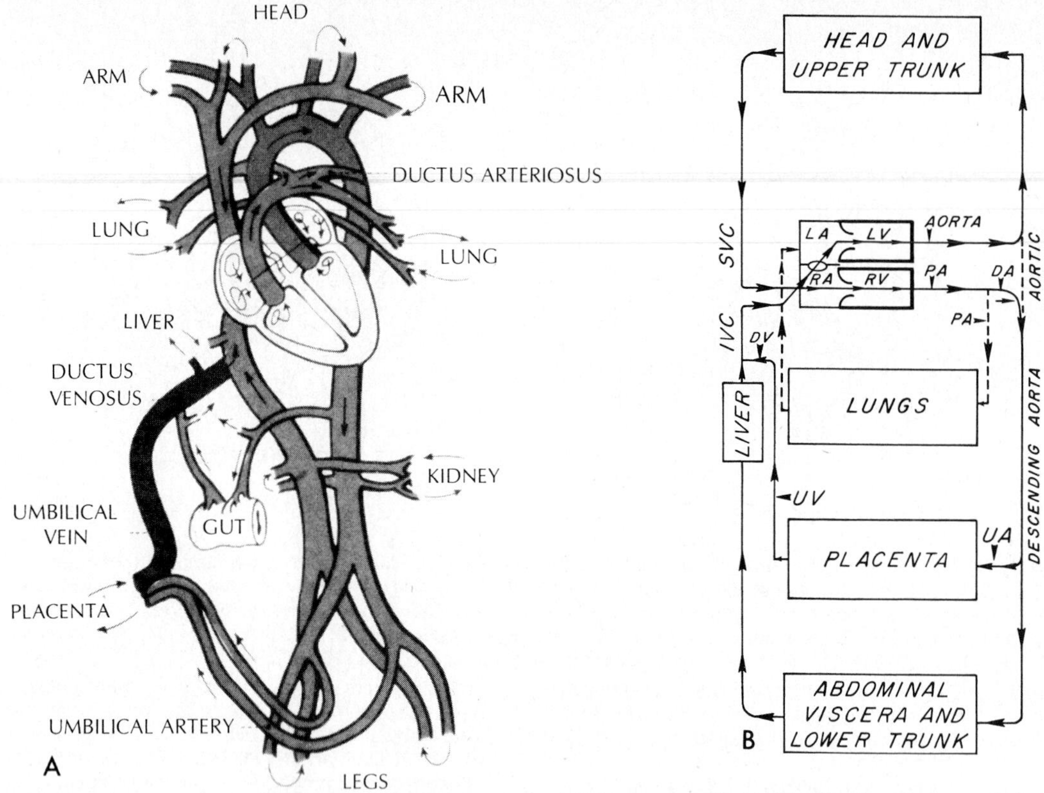

FIGURE 30–6. ***A,*** **The fetal circulation. Shading shows the relative oxygenation of the blood, and arrows indicate its direction of flow.** ***B,*** **Prenatally, a fraction of umbilical venous (UV) blood enters the ductus venosus (DV) and bypasses the liver. This relatively well-oxygenated blood flows across the foramen ovale to the left heart, preferentially perfusing the coronary arteries, head, and upper trunk. Superior vena caval (SVC) blood is ejected by the right heart into the pulmonary artery (PA) and ductus arteriosus (DA). This stream circulates to the placenta as well as to the abdominal viscera and lower trunk. Dashed lines indicate diminished blood flow to and from the lungs and across the aortic isthmus. IVC = inferior vena cava, RA = right atrium, LA = left atrium, RV = right ventricle, LV = left ventricle, PA = pulmonary artery. (From Kaplan, S.: Congenital heart disease.** ***In*** **Vaughan, V. C., and McKay, R. J. [eds.]: Nelson Textbook of Pediatrics. 10th ed. Philadelphia, W. B. Saunders Company, 1975.)**

importantly to vasodilatation due to the increase in oxygen tension to which pulmonary vessels are exposed than to physical expansion of alveoli with gas. Pulmonary arterial pressure falls, and pulmonary blood flow increases greatly. Systemic vascular resistance rises when clamping of the umbilical cord removes the low-resistance placental circulation. Increased pulmonary blood flow increases the return of blood to the left atrium and raises left atrial pressure, which in turn closes the foramen ovale. The shift in oxygen dependence from the placenta to the lungs produces a sudden increase in arterial blood oxygen tension, which, in concert with alterations in the local prostaglandin milieu, initiates constriction of the ductus arteriosus.[27] Pulmonary pressure falls further as the ductus constricts. In mature infants the ductus arteriosus is closed functionally within 10 to 15 hours, with total anatomical closure following within a few weeks by a process of thrombosis, intimal proliferation, and fibrosis. A high incidence exists in preterm infants of persistent patency of the ductus arteriosus, because of an immaturity of those mechanisms responsible for constriction (p. 923). In surviving preterm infants the ductus arteriosus spontaneously closes within 4 to 12 months of birth.

The ductus venosus, ductus arteriosus, and foramen ovale remain potential channels for blood flow after birth, Thus, persistent patency of the ductus venosus may mask the most marked signs of pulmonary venous obstruction in infants with total anomalous pulmonary venous connection below the diaphragm (p. 961). Similarly, lesions producing right or left atrial volume or pressure overload may stretch the foramen ovale and render incompetent the flap valve mechanism for its closure. Anomalies that depend on patency of the ductus arteriosus for preserving pulmonary or systemic blood flow remain latent until the ductus arteriosus constricts. A common example is the sudden intensification of cyanosis observed in the infant with tetralogy of Fallot when the magnitude of pulmonary hypoperfusion is unmasked by spontaneous closure of the ductus arteriosus. Moreover, there is increasing evidence that ductal constriction is a key factor in the postnatal development of coarctation of the aorta (p. 930). Lastly, it should be recognized that because the ductus arteriosus is potentially patent after birth and the pulmonary resistance vessels are hyperreactive, hypoxic pulmonary vasoconstriction of diverse etiologies may result in a right-to-left shunt through the ductus.

PATHOLOGICAL CONSEQUENCES OF CONGENITAL CARDIAC LESIONS

CONGESTIVE HEART FAILURE

Although the basic mechanisms of cardiac failure, as outlined in Chapter 14, are the same for all ages, the pediatric cardiologist should recognize clearly that the common causes, time of onset, and often the approach to treatment vary with age.[28–30] Recently, the advent of fetal echocardiography has allowed the diagnosis of intrauterine cardiac failure. The cardinal findings of fetal heart failure are scalp edema, ascites, pericardial effusion, and decreased fetal movements. Although abnormalities in several organ systems may result in nonimmunological fetal hydrops, cardiac causes include a host of structural, functional, rhythm, and metabolic disturbances of the heart. Infants under one year of age with cardiac malformations account for 80 to 90 per cent of pediatric patients who develop congestive failure. Moreover, cardiac decompensation in the infant is a medical emergency necessitating immediate treatment if the patient is to be saved.

In the preterm infant, especially under 1500 grams birthweight, persistent patency of the ductus arteriosus is the most common cause of cardiac decompensation, and other forms of structural heart disease are rare. In the full-term newborn the earliest important causes of heart failure are the hypoplastic left heart and coarctation of the aorta syndromes, paroxysmal atrial tachycardia, cerebral or hepatic arteriovenous fistula, and myocarditis. Among the lesions commonly producing heart failure beyond age 1 to 2 weeks, when diminished pulmonary vascular resistance allows substantial left-to-right shunting, are ventricular septal and atrioventricular septal defects, transposition of the great arteries, truncus arteriosus, and total anomalous pulmonary venous connection, often with pulmonary venous obstruction. Although heart failure is most usually the result of a structural defect or of myocardial disease, it should be recognized that the newborn myocardium may be depressed severely by such abnormalities as hypoxemia and acidemia, anemia, septicemia, marked hypoglycemia, hypocalcemia, and polycythemia. In the older child, heart failure is often due to acquired disease (Chap. 32) or is a complication of open-heart surgical procedures. In the acquired category are rheumatic and endomyocardial diseases, infective endocarditis, hematological and nutritional disorders, and severe cardiac arrhythmias.

CLINICAL MANIFESTATIONS IN THE INFANT. The clinical expression of cardiac decompensation in the infant consists of distinctive signs of pulmonary and systemic venous congestion and altered cardiocirculatory performance that resemble, but often are not identical to, those of the older child or adult (Table 30–3).[31] These reflect the interplay between the hemodynamic burden and adaptive responses. Common symptoms and signs are feeding difficulties and failure to gain weight and grow, tachypnea, tachycardia, pulmonary rales and rhonchi, liver enlargement, and cardiomegaly. Less frequent manifestations include peripheral edema, ascites, pulsus alternans, gallop rhythm, and inappropriate sweating. Pleural and pericardial effusions are exceedingly rare. The distinction between left and right heart failure is less obvious in the infant than it is in the older child or adult, since most lesions that create a left ventricular pressure or volume overload also result in left-to-right shunting of blood through the foramen ovale and/or patent ductus arteriosus as well as pulmonary hypertension due to elevated pulmonary venous pressures. Conversely, augmented filling or elevated pressure of the right ventricle in the infant reduces left ventricular compliance disproportionately when compared to the older child or adult and gives rise to signs of both systemic and pulmonary venous congestion.[22]

Fatigue and dyspnea on exertion express themselves as a feeding problem in the infant. Characteristically, the respiratory rate in heart failure is rapid (50 to 100 breaths/min). In the presence of left ventricular failure, interstitial pulmonary edema reduces pulmonary compliance and results in tachypnea and retractions. Excessive pulmonary blood flow via significant left-to-right shunts may further decrease lung compliance. Moreover, upper airway obstruction may be produced by selective enlargement of cardiovascular structures. In patients with large left-to-right shunts and left atrial and main pulmonary artery enlargement, the left main stem bronchus may be compressed, resulting in emphysematous expansion of the left upper or lower lobe or left lower lobe collapse.[32] Respiratory distress with grunting, flaring of the alae nasi, and intercostal retractions is observed when failure is severe and especially when pulmonary infection precipitates cardiac decompensation, which is often the case. Under these circumstances pulmonary rales may be due to the infection or failure or both. A resting heart rate with little variability is characteristic of heart failure. Hepatomegaly is seen regularly in infants in failure, although liver tenderness is uncommon. Cardiomegaly may be assessed roentgenographically, but it must be recognized that in the normal newborn infant the cardiac diameter may be as much as 60 per cent of the thoracic diameter, and the large thymus gland in infants interferes occasionally with evaluation of heart size. Echocardiography provides a good estimate of cardiac performance and chamber dimensions, and values may be compared to data derived from normal infants.[33–36]

TABLE 30–3 FEATURES OF HEART FAILURE IN INFANTS

Poor feeding and failure to thrive
Respiratory distress—mainly tachypnea
Rapid heart rate (160 to 180 beats/min)
Pulmonary rales or wheezing
Cardiomegaly and pulmonary edema on x-ray
Hepatomegaly (peripheral edema unusual)
Gallop sounds
Color—ashen pale or faintly cyanotic
Excessive perspiration
Diminished urine output

Cardiac decompensation may progress with extreme rapidity in the first hours and days of life, producing a clinical picture of advanced cardiogenic shock and a profoundly obtunded infant. The presence of marked hepatomegaly and gross cardiomegaly usually allows distinction from noncardiac causes of diminished systemic perfusion.

CYANOSIS

(See also page 6)

Cyanosis is produced by an increased amount of reduced hemoglobin in cutaneous vessels in excess of 3 gm/dl. Peripheral cyanosis usually reflects an abnormally great extraction of oxygen from normally saturated arterial blood, commonly the result of peripheral cutaneous vasoconstriction. Central cyanosis is a result of arterial blood oxygen unsaturation, most often in patients with congenital heart disease caused by shunting of systemic venous blood into the arterial circuit. Infants especially may appear cyanotic when in heart failure because of both peripheral and central factors; the latter may include severe impairment of pulmonary function that commonly exists with alveolar hypoventilation, ventilation-perfusion inequality, or impaired oxygen diffusion. In patients with central cyanosis due to arterial oxygen unsaturation, the degree of cutaneous discoloration depends upon the absolute amount of reduced hemoglobin, the magnitude of the right-to-left shunt relative to systemic flow, and the oxyhemoglobin saturation of venous blood. The last of these depends in turn upon the tissue extraction of oxygen. Commonly, cyanosis appears or intensifies with physical activity or exercise as the saturation of systemic venous blood declines concurrent with an increase in right-to-left shunting across a defect as peripheral vascular resistance decreases. Oxygen transfer to the tissues is affected by shifts in the oxygen-hemoglobin dissociation relationship, which may be altered by blood pH and levels of red blood cell 2,3-diphosphoglycerate concentration.[37]

CLUBBING AND POLYCYTHEMIA. Prominent accompaniments of arterial hypoxemia are polycythemia and clubbing of the digits. The latter is associated with an increased number of capillaries with increased blood flow through extensive arteriovenous aneurysms and an increase of connective tissue in the terminal phalanges of the fingers and toes. Polycythemia is a physiological response to chronic hypoxemia that stimulates erythrocytosis. The extremely high hematocrits observed in patients with arterial oxygen unsaturation cause a progressive increase in blood viscosity, especially beyond packed red blood cell volumes of 60 per cent. Both the hematocrit and the circulating whole blood volume are increased in polycythemia accompanying cyanotic congenital heart disease; the hypervolemia is the result of an increase in red cell volume. The augmented red blood cell volume provoked by hypoxemia provides an increased oxygen-carrying capacity and enhanced oxygen supply to the tissues. The compensatory polycythemia is often of such severity that it becomes a liability and produces adverse physiological effects such as thrombotic lesions in diverse organs and a hemorrhagic diathesis.[38] In this regard, oral steroid contraceptives are contraindicated in the adolescent cyanotic female because of the enhanced risk of cerebral thrombosis. Red cell volume reduction and replacement with plasma or albumin (erythrophoresis) lowers blood viscosity and increases systemic blood flow and systemic oxygen transport and thus may be helpful in the management of patients with severe hypoxic polycythemia (hematocrit ≥ 65 per cent). A final hematocrit of 55 to 63 per cent should be achieved; the higher level is necessary in patients with low initial oxygen saturation in order to avoid a severe reduction in arterial oxygen content. Acute phlebotomy without fluid replacement is contraindicated.

CEREBRAL AND PULMONARY COMPLICATIONS. Cerebral vascular accidents and brain abscesses occur particularly in cyanotic patients with substantial arterial desaturation.[39–41] *Cerebral thrombosis* is most common under age 2 years in severely cyanotic children, even in the presence of relatively low hematocrits, and occurs especially in a clinical setting in which oxygen requirements are raised by fever or, if blood viscosity is increased, by dehydration.

Brain abscesses are an important complication of cyanotic heart disease.[40, 41] They are rare under 18 months of age and commonly are of insidious onset marked by headache, low-grade fever, vomiting, and a change in personality. Seizures or paralysis less frequently heralds the onset of a brain abscess. Abscess must be suspected in any cyanotic child with focal neurological signs. Morbidity and mortality are related inversely to oxygen saturation levels. Brain abscess is thought to occur in approximately 2 per cent of the population with cyanotic congenital heart disease; a mortality rate of 30 to 40 per cent is often related to delay in diagnosis and treatment.

Paradoxical embolus is a rare complication of cyanotic heart disease, usually observed only at necropsy.[42] Emboli arising in systemic veins may pass directly to the systemic circulation, since right-to-left intracardiac shunts allow venous blood to bypass the normal filtering action of the lungs.

Retinopathy, consisting of dilated tortuous vessels progressing to papilledema, and retinal edema is occasionally observed in cyanotic patients and appears to be related to decreased arterial oxygen saturation and/or to erythrocytosis but not to hypercapnea.

Hemoptysis is an uncommon but major complication in cyanotic patients with congenital heart disease and occurs most often in the presence of pulmonary vascular obstructive disease or in patients with an extensive bronchial collateral circulation or pulmonary venous congestion.[43] Massive hemoptysis almost always represents rupture of a dilated bronchial artery.

SQUATTING. After exertion, patients with cyanotic heart disease, especially tetralogy of Fallot, typically assume a squatting posture in order to obtain relief from breathlessness.[44] Squatting appears to improve arterial oxygen saturation by increasing systemic vascular resistance, thereby diminishing the right-to-left shunt, and also by the pooling of markedly desaturated blood in the lower extremities. In addition, systemic venous return and therefore pulmonary blood flow may increase.

HYPOXIC SPELLS. Hypercyanotic or hypoxemic spells commonly complicate the clinical course in younger children with certain types of cyanotic heart disease, especially tetralogy of Fallot (p. 946).[44, 45] The spells are characterized by anxiety, hyperpnea, and a sudden marked increase in cyanosis; they are the result of an abrupt reduction in pulmonary blood flow. Unless terminated, the hypercyanotic episodes may lead to convulsions and may even be fatal. The sudden reduction in pulmonary blood flow may be precipitated by fluctuations in arterial pCO_2 and pH, a sudden fall in systemic or increase in pulmonary vascular resistance, or an acute increase in the severity of right ventricular outflow tract obstruction either by augmented contraction of the hypertrophied muscle in the right ventricular outflow tract or by a decrease in right ventricular cavity volume due to tachycardia. *Treatment* consists of oxygen administration, placing the child in the knee-chest position, and administration of morphine sulfate. Additional medications that may prove of value include the intravenous administration of sodium bicarbonate to correct the accompanying acidemia, alpha-adrenoceptor stimulants such as neosynephrine or methoxamine to raise peripheral resistance and diminish right-to-left shunting, and beta-adrenoceptor blocking agents that reduce cardiac sympathetic tone and depress cardiac contractility directly and that increase ventricular volume by reducing heart rate.

ACID-BASE IMBALANCE

Disturbances in blood gas and acid-base equilibrium are noted particularly in infants with either congestive heart failure or cyanosis.[46] Large-volume left-to-right shunts, especially with pulmonary edema, may be associated with moderate respiratory acidemia and a lowering of arterial oxygen tensions, reflecting an increase in the alveolar-arterial oxygen tension gradient and ventilation-perfusion imbalance. Interference with carbon dioxide transport implies moderate to severe failure in these infants. Lesions associated with a reduced systemic cardiac output, such as severe coarctation of the aorta or critical aortic stenosis in infancy, present often with cardiac failure complicated by a severe metabolic acidemia and relatively high values of arterial oxygen tension. The latter finding, even in the presence of right-to-left shunting across a patent ductus arteriosus, is a result of diminished systemic perfusion and an elevated pulmonary-to-systemic blood flow ratio. Respiratory acidemia and depressed levels of oxygen tension are observed in infants with obstruction to pulmonary venous return and right-to-left atrial shunting. Infants with severe hypoxemia due to lesions such as transposition of the great arteries or pulmonic atresia often show metabolic acidemia and marked reductions in carbon dioxide tension secondary to hyperventilation resulting from hypoxic stimulation of peripheral chemoreceptors.

IMPAIRED GROWTH

Impaired growth and physical development and delayed onset of adolescence are common features of many cyanotic and, to a lesser extent, acyanotic forms of congenital heart disease.[47] Mental development is rarely affected. In general, the severity of growth disturbance depends upon the anatomical lesion and its functional effect. Most children with mild defects grow normally. Weight gain is commonly slower than linear growth in acyanotic patients with large left-to-right shunts, whereas in cyanotic congenital heart disease height and weight usually parallel each other. Boys appear to be more retarded in growth than girls, especially in the second decade. Skeletal maturity (i.e., bone age) is delayed in cyanotic children in relation to the severity of hypoxemia. In some children, prenatal factors such as intrauterine infection and chromosomal or other hereditary and nonhereditary syndromes are responsible for growth retardation. In other patients, extracardiac malformations may contribute to poor weight gain and linear growth. Additional explanations for the mechanisms of growth interference have implicated malnutrition as a result of anorexia and inadequate nutrients and caloric intake, hypermetabolic state, acidemia and cation imbalance, tissue hypoxemia, diminished peripheral blood flow, chronic cardiac decompensation, malabsorption or protein loss, recurrent respiratory infections, and endocrine or genetic factors. In some instances, the underdevelopment is influenced little by operative correction of the underlying cardiac anomaly. Among factors that may be responsible for persistent growth retardation postoperatively are age at operation, hemodynamically significant residual lesions, and sequelae or complications of operation. As a general rule, it is unwise preoperatively to guarantee to the parents of a child with heart disease that surgery will result in accelerated growth and development.

PULMONARY HYPERTENSION

(See also Chap. 26)

Pulmonary hypertension is a common accompaniment of many congenital cardiac lesions, and the status of the pulmonary vascular bed is often the principal determinant of the clinical manifestations, course, and whether surgical treatment is feasible.[48] Increases in pulmonary arterial pressure result from elevations of pulmonary blood flow and/or resistance, the latter due sometimes to an increase in vascular tone, but usually the result of underdevelopment and/or obstructive, obliterative structural changes within the pulmonary vascular bed.[49]

Normally, pulmonary vascular resistance falls rapidly immediately after birth owing to onset of ventilation and subsequent release of hypoxic pulmonary vasoconstriction. Subsequently the medial smooth muscle of pulmonary arterial resistance vessels thins gradually.[50] This latter process is delayed often by several months in infants with large aorticopulmonary or ventricular communications, at which time levels of pulmonary vascular resistance are still somewhat elevated. In patients with high pulmonary arterial pressure from birth, failure of normal growth of the pulmonary circulation may occur, and anatomical changes in the pulmonary vessels in the form of proliferation of intimal cells and intimal and medial thickening often progress, so that in the older child or adult vascular resistance may ultimately become fixed by obliterative changes in the pulmonary vascular bed. The causes of pulmonary vascular obstructive disease remain unknown, although increased pulmonary blood flow, increased pulmonary arterial blood pressure, elevated pulmonary venous pressure, polycythemia, systemic hypoxia, acidemia, and the nature of the bronchial circulation have all been implicated. There are many patients with pulmonary vascular obstruction whose cardiac anomaly places them at particular risk quite early in life, precluding survival to adulthood. Patients at particularly high risk for the development of significant pulmonary vascular obstruction are those with certain forms of cyanotic congenital heart disease, such as complete transposition of the great arteries with or without ventricular septal defect or patent ductus arteriosus, single ventricle without pulmonary stenosis, double outlet right ventricle, and truncus arteriosus. Other conditions in which pulmonary vascular obstruction appears to progress rapidly include large ventricular septal defect, as well as the less common conditions of unilateral pulmonary artery absence, congenital left-to-right shunts in an environment of high altitude or in association with the Down syndrome of trisomy 21, and complete atrioventricular canal defects, even unassociated with a chromosomal anomaly.

MECHANISMS OF DEVELOPMENT OF PULMONARY HYPERTENSION. Intimal damage appears to be related to shear stresses, since endothelial cell damage occurs at high-flow shear rates. A reduction in pulmonary arteriolar lumen size due to either thickened medial muscle or vasoconstriction increases the velocity of flow. Shear stress also increases as blood viscosity rises; therefore, infants with hypoxemia and high hematocrits as well as increased pulmonary blood flow are at increased risk of developing pulmonary vascular disease. In patients with left-to-right shunts, pulmonary arterial hypertension, if not present in infancy or childhood, may never occur or may not develop until the third or fourth decade or later. Once developed, intimal proliferative changes with hyalinization and fibrosis are not reversible by repair of the underlying cardiac defect. In severe pulmonary vascular obstructive disease, arteriovenous malformations may develop and predispose to massive hemoptysis.

Most vexing is the variability among patients with the same or similar cardiac lesions in both the time of appearance and rate of progression of their pulmonary vascular obstructive process. While genetic influences may be operative (an example is the apparent acceleration of pulmonary vascular disease in patients with congenital heart disease and trisomy 21), evidence is now accumulating for important pre- and postnatal modifiers of the pulmonary vascular bed that appear, at least in part, to be lesion-dependent. Thus, a quantitative variability exists in the pulmonary vascular bed related to the *number*, not just the size and wall structure, of arterial vessels within the pulmonary circulation.[51,52] Modeling of the blood vessels occurs proximal to and within terminal bronchioles (pre- and intraacinar vessels, respectively) continuously from before birth. The intraacinar vessels, in particular, increase in size and number from late fetal life throughout childhood with minimal muscularization of their walls. The ensuing increase in the cross-sectional area of the pulmonary arterial circulation allows the cardiac output to rise substantially without an increase in pulmonary arterial pressure. If, however, the presence of a cardiac lesion interferes with the normal growth and multiplication of these most peripheral arteries, the resulting elevation of pulmonary vascular resistance may first be related to failure of the intraacinar pulmonary circulation to develop fully, and then secondarily to the morphological changes of obliterative vascular disease—medial thickening, intimal proliferation, hyalinization and fibrosis, and angiomatoid and plexiform lesions, and, ultimately, arterial necrosis.[49]

In essence, the morphometric framework adds an important dimension, that of growth and development of the pulmonary circulation, to the traditional view of pulmonary vascular obstructive disease occurring primarily as a result of anatomical changes in the individual pulmonary arterioles. The biologic basis of pulmonary hypertension is the subject of a recent, extensive review.[52]

ASSESSMENT OF PATIENT WITH PULMONARY HYPERTENSION. It is important to understand the difficulties that exist with standard methods of assessing the severity of pulmonary vascular obstructive disease. Clinical, electrocardiographic, and echocardiographic observations do not distinguish between reversible and irreversible elevations in pulmonary vascular resistance. Hemodynamic measurements at cardiac catheterization are the mainstay in assessing the pulmonary vascular bed, especially its reactivity. The premium on accuracy is high, because the presence, degree, and reactivity of pulmonary vascular obstruction determine the feasibility and long-term outcome of operation. Surgery must not be offered to patients with severe, fixed pulmonary vascular obstruction even when the cardiac defect is anatomically correctable. Such patients either do not survive operation or, if they do, are not benefited and more often than not are harmed.

The aims of hemodynamic study are to quantify and compare the pulmonary and systemic flows and resistances and to determine the reactivity of the pulmonary vascular bed in patients with pulmonary hypertension. Because resistance to pulmonary blood flow cannot be measured directly, it is calculated from the ratio of pressure gradient to flow across the pulmonary bed according to Poiseuille's equation, which refers to steady flow of a Newtonian fluid through straight, rigid tubes. There are potential errors in applying the equation and errors inherent in the methods of measurement. Furthermore, it is not possible in every patient to catheterize the pulmonary artery; when this is the case pulmonary venous wedge pressures may be used but they are not always reliable indicators of pulmonary artery pressure, and the moment of hemodynamic evaluation may not be representative of potentially variable states of the pulmonary circulation. Nonetheless, a practical index of pulmonary vascular resistance can be established from measurements of pulmonary and systemic arterial pressures and calculated flows. One can then determine whether administration of drugs or oxygen reduces the pulmonary vascular resistance, implying that the resistance is not fixed and therefore may decrease or at least not progress after successful operation. A reduction in calculated pulmonary vascular resistance in response to oxygen inhalation or pharmacological intervention does not exclude coexisting anatomical pulmonary vascular disease, but does imply that there is a component of potentially reversible vasoconstriction contributing to the high resistance.

Other Diagnostic Methods. Because of the aforementioned shortcomings, additional methods have been developed to study the morphology of the small pulmonary arteries in patients with pulmonary hypertension. An example is the use of high-resolution magnification for *pulmonary wedge angiography* to determine the presence and extent of obstructive pulmonary vascular changes.[53] Pulmonary wedge angiograms, assessed quantitatively, appear to correlate well with both hemodynamic findings and histological observations of the structural state of the pulmonary vascular bed. Of additional interest is the current practical application of morphometric structural analyses that attempt to identify for operation patients whose postoperative pulmonary hemodynamics might be expected to improve, if not normalize.[54] Thus, *lung biopsy* at surgery has been proposed in patients with equivocal hemodynamic data to aid in determining whether to proceed with operation in reasonable anticipation of postoperative regression of elevated pulmonary vascular resistance.

THE MORPHOMETRIC APPROACH. Decisions on optimal timing of operations are often difficult because of the varying rates of development of pulmonary vascular disease in different patients with the same anomaly and because the evaluation of pulmonary vascular resistance and reactivity in the catheterization laboratory is a less than perfect science. Preoperative lung biopsy employing the Heath-Edwards criteria has enjoyed little popularity, especially because sampling errors may result from the scatter of different grades of lesions in different parts of the lung. Accordingly, it is attractive to seek an alternative method that would obviate these problems. In this regard, application of a morphometric approach holds promise, because the described changes in pulmonary vessel morphological characteristics are more uniformly distributed throughout the lung and, importantly, lend themselves to quantification.

Three abnormalities have been identified as anatomical markers of elevated pulmonary vascular resistance: (1) an excessive and premature extension of vascular smooth muscle into intraacinar pulmonary arteries, (2) failure of preacinar arterial wall thickness to regress normally, and (3) failure of pulmonary arteries to grow and proliferate normally during postnatal development. Frozen-section lung biopsy provides a firmer basis for judgment of whether reparative or palliative operation should proceed. The technique has proved useful in patients with univentricular hearts or tricuspid atresia in determining the feasibility of a Fontan procedure (p. 950) and in patients with lesions known to exhibit early and rapidly progressive pulmonary vascular disease, such as complete transposition of the great arteries, complete atrioventricular canal defect, and nonrestrictive ventricular septal defect.

CLINICAL MANIFESTATIONS OF PULMONARY HYPERTENSION. When this condition is associated with a large left-to-right shunt, the clinical manifestations reflect the specific malformation responsible. When pulmonary vascular resistance is elevated and a significant right-to-left shunt exists, the patient is cyanotic, and polycythemia and clubbing are noted. A dominant *a* wave in the jugular venous pulse may be seen reflecting vigorous right atrial contraction due to diminished compliance of the right ventricle. In some instances there are large systolic *c-v* waves, which suggest tricuspid regurgitation. A prominent right ventricular parasternal lift and palpable systolic expansion of the pulmonary artery are present. A soft pulmonary systolic ejection murmur preceded by an ejection sound and followed by a markedly accentuated pulmonic component of the second heart sound are often audible on auscultation; an early diastolic decrescendo blowing murmur of pulmonary regurgitation may be heard. If right ventricular failure and dilatation supervene, the systolic murmur of tricuspid regurgitation may be audible at the lower left sternal border. Right ventricular enlargement may be evident on the chest roentgenogram and electrocardiogram. The former examination also reveals a conspicuously enlarged pulmonary artery, prominent hilar pulmonary vascular markings, and attenuated peripheral vessels. The site of the underlying defect may be localized by means of two-dimensional and Doppler echocardiography and/or cardiac catheterization and angiocardiography. Pressures in the right side of the heart are essentially identical to systemic pressures in cyanotic patients if the shunt is at the ventricular or aorticopulmonary levels, but they are usually lower than systemic pressures in patients with an intraatrial shunt. No specific treatment has proved beneficial for obstructive pulmonary vascular disease.

This fact underscores the importance of efforts to define the optimal age of operation in order to provide the highest probability of postoperative normalization of the pulmonary vascular bed. It is important to emphasize that almost all congenital cardiovascular defects are amenable to surgical repair in infancy, and it is likely that the surgical art will progress to the point that virtually all patients with lesions associated with pulmonary hypertension will be operated on within the first 6 months to 2 years of life. When this goal is reached without increased operative mortality, the incidence of postoperative pulmonary vascular obstruction may well achieve the status of a bygone concern.

OTHER CONSEQUENCES OF CONGENITAL HEART DISEASE

INFECTIVE ENDOCARDITIS (See also Chap. 34). Infective endocarditis is uncommon under age 2 years and thereafter most often affects children with tetralogy of Fallot (especially after systemic-pulmonary anastomosis), ventricular septal defect, aortic stenosis, and patent ductus arteriosus. Postsurgical patients with prosthetic heterograft or homograft valves or conduits are at particular risk. A causative organism can be isolated in approximately 90 per cent of children, usually either alpha-streptococci (usually *Strep. viridans*) or *Staphylococcus aureus*.[55, 56] Fungal endocarditis is quite rare in the pediatric age group. Mortality appears to be highest when coagulase-positive *Staphylococcus* is the offending organism and when the endocarditis involves the left, rather than the right, side of the heart. Most recent data suggest 75 to 80 per cent overall survival.[55] Factors predisposing to endocarditis may be identified in approximately one-third of cases. These include cardiovascular surgery with infection during the perioperative period; respiratory tract infections; and ear, nose, throat, and dental procedures. Less often, contamination during a surgical procedure or cardiac catheterization or an infection involving the skin, genitourinary tract, or other organ system has been the cause.

Although routine antimicrobial prophylaxis is recommended for all children with congenital heart disease and for the majority of patients after operative repair of the lesion, it should be recognized that many

TABLE 30–4 PROPHYLACTIC ANTIBIOTICS FOR PROTECTION FROM BACTERIAL ENDOCARDITIS

For Dental Procedures and Upper Respiratory Tract Surgery	
I. For most patients: **oral penicillin**	*Adults:* 2 gm of penicillin V 1 hour before procedure and then 1 gm 6 hours after initial dose. *Children less than 60 pounds:* 1 gm of penicillin V 1 hour before procedure and then 500 mg 6 hours after initial dose.
II. For those *allergic to penicillin* (may also be selected for those receiving oral penicillin as continuous rheumatic fever prophylaxis): **erythromycin**	*Adults:* 1 gm orally 1 hour before procedure and then 500 mg 6 hours after initial dose. *Children:* 20 mg/kg orally 1 hour before procedure and then 10 mg/kg 6 hours after initial dose.
III. For those patients at *higher risk* of infective endocarditis (especially those with prosthetic heart valves) who are not allergic to penicillin: **ampicillin** plus **gentamicin**	*Adults:* 1–2 gm plus gentamicin 1.5 mg/kg IM or IV, both given 30 minutes before procedure; then penicillin V 1 gm orally 6 hours after initial dose. *Children:* Timing of doses is same as for adults. Dosages are ampicillin 50 mg/kg and gentamicin 2 mg/kg.
IV. For *higher risk* patients (especially those with prosthetic heart valves) who are *allergic to penicillin:* **vancomycin**	*Adults:* Vancomycin 1 gm IV over 60 min, begun 60 min before procedure; no repeat dose is necessary. *Children:* Vancomycin 20 mg/kg IV over 60 min, begun 60 min before procedure; no repeat dose is necessary.
For Gastrointestinal and Genitourinary Tract Surgery and Instrumentation	
I. For most patients: **ampicillin** plus **gentamicin**	*Adults:* 2 gm ampicillin IM or IV plus gentamicin 1.5 mg/kg IM or IV given 30 min before procedure. May repeat once 8 hours later. *Children:* Same timing of medications as adult schedule. Dosages are ampicillin 50 mg/kg and gentamicin 2 mg/kg.
II. For patients *allergic to penicillin:* **vancomycin** plus **gentamicin**	*Adults:* 1 gm vancomycin IV given over 60 min plus 1.5 mg/kg gentamicin IM or IV, each given 60 min before procedure. Doses may be repeated once 8–12 hours later. *Children:* Timing as above. Doses are vancomycin 20 mg/kg and gentamicin 2 mg/kg.
III. Oral regimen for minor or repetitive procedures in low-risk patients: **amoxicillin**	*Adults:* 30 gm amoxicillin one hour before procedure and 1.5 gm 6 hours after inital dose. *Children:* Same timing of doses: 50 mg/kg initial dose and 25 mg/kg follow-up dose.

Adapted from The Report of the Committee on Rheumatic Fever and Infective Endocarditis, American Heart Association, 1984.

different microbes are responsible for the disease and that an effective preventive approach may center ultimately on active immunization rather than antibiotics. Currently, antibiotic prophylaxis is recommended for all dental procedures except minor readjustments of braces, oral trauma, and other procedures such as tonsillectomy, gastrointestinal surgery, and genitourinary surgery, or diagnostic procedures such as proctosigmoidoscopy and cystoscopy (Table 30–4).[56] The risk of endocarditis is undoubtedly related both to the magnitude of bacteremia and to the type of underlying heart disease. Since infection on a prosthetic heart valve or conduit may be devastating, combinations of antibiotics given parenterally are advisable in these patients.

CHEST PAIN (See also pages 3 and 1316). *Angina pectoris* is an uncommon symptom of cardiac disease in infants and children, occurring in association with anomalous pulmonary origin of a coronary artery or occasionally in association with severe aortic stenosis, pulmonic stenosis, or pulmonary hypertension due to pulmonary vascular obstruction. Cardiac pain in the infant with anomalous coronary artery (p. 927) most usually takes the form of irritability and crying during feeding or straining at bowel movement. In children with severe left or right ventricular outflow tract obstruction chest pain commonly follows effort and is identical to angina observed in adults. Cardiac pain associated with *pulmonary vascular obstruction* may be anginal in nature but often is evanescent and pleuritic in type. Atypical forms of chest pain associated with the syndrome of *mitral valve prolapse* are much less usual in children than adults. A sensation of chest discomfort or cardiac awareness is frequently interpreted as pain by the parents of children with cardiac arrhythmias. Careful questioning serves to identify palpitations rather than pain as the symptom and often elicits an additional history of anxiety, pallor, and sweating. Pain due to *pericarditis* is commonly of acute onset, is associated with fever, and can be identified by specific physical, roentgenographic, and echocardiographic findings.

Most commonly, chest pain in children is *musculoskeletal* in origin and may be reproduced upon upper extremity movement or by palpation; often, chest wall pain is the result of *costochondritis*. Lastly, children, like adults, may suffer chest pain of nonspecific pattern owing to *anxiety* in the presence or absence of hyperventilation; often a history is elicited of a family member or friend who had died recently or suffered myocardial infarction.

SYNCOPE (See also Chap. 29). Syncope is an unusual feature of heart disease in children; its presence suggests specific diagnoses, the most common being an arrhythmia. The symptom is observed in children with complete atrioventricular block that is less often of congenital origin than a sequela of cardiac operation. Syncope due to abrupt episodes of either bradycardia or tachycardia occurs in association with the sick sinus syndrome. The latter is most commonly produced in children after surgical procedures involving the region of the sinoatrial node, e.g., atrial septal defect closure or Mustard's procedure for transposition of the great arteries (p. 956). Syncope is an occasional but ominous symptom if associated with severe aortic stenosis, pulmonary vascular obstruction, or a left atrial myxoma that transiently occludes left ventricular inflow.

SUDDEN DEATH (See also Chap. 24). In contrast to adults, children seldom die suddenly and unexpectedly from cardiovascular disease. Arrhythmias, hypoxemia, and coronary insufficiency secondary to left ventricular outflow tract obstruction are the most frequent causes of death.[57] Sudden death is most often reported in patients with aortic stenosis or hypertrophic obstructive cardiomyopathy, the Eisenmenger syndrome of pulmonary vascular obstruction, myocarditis, congenital complete heart block, primary endocardial fibroelastosis, anomalies of the coronary arteries, and cyanotic congenital heart disease with pulmonic stenosis or atresia. A relationship exists between strenuous exercise and sudden death in patients with aortic stenosis or obstructive cardiomyopathy, thus providing justification for restricting patients with these lesions from gymnastic activities and strenuous competitive sports.

APPROACH TO THE HIGH-RISK INFANT WITH CONGENITAL HEART DISEASE

Approximately one-third of all infants born with congenital heart disease will die in the first months of life without prompt recognition, accurate diagnosis, or treatment of their life-threatening anomaly. Heart failure and cyanosis are the two cardinal signs of the high-risk infant with heart disease, and this section will provide an approach for the management of each.

HEART FAILURE (See also Chap. 17)

Care of the infant with heart failure must include careful consideration of the underlying structural or functional disturbance. The general aims of treatment are to achieve an increase in cardiac performance, augment peripheral perfusion, and decrease pulmonary and systemic venous congestion. It must be emphasized, however, that under many conditions medical management cannot control the effects of the abnormal loads imposed by a host of congenital cardiac lesions. Under these circumstances cardiac catheterization and operative intervention may be urgently required.[58] Thus, initial therapy is aimed at stabilizing the infant's condition for diagnostic hemodynamic and angiocardiographic study as soon as possible. In almost all situations the decision to intervene surgically or to continue medical management requires a definitive anatomical diagnosis.

Reserve Mechanisms in the Neonatal Heart

Pediatricians, in particular, should be aware of the important concept of cardiac reserve, because it is in this regard that important differences exist between the young heart (the preterm or newborn infant) and the fully developed heart of the older child, adolescent, and adult (Fig. 30–7).

Clinicians have long recognized the unique fragility and lability of the neonatal circulation in response to disease states and various physiological stimuli. Moreover, it is often apparent that newborns may exhibit suboptimal therapeutic responses to drugs such as digitalis, which directly stimulate cardiac contractility. The reasons for the age dependency of these observations have their basis in the reduced ability of the hearts of premature and full-term newborns, when compared with the heart and circulation of the older child or adult, to call upon a functional reserve capacity in order to adapt to stress.[28, 58]

Studies from the author's and other laboratories have shown that structural, functional, biochemical, and pharmacological properties of the young heart differ considerably from those of its older counterpart. The young heart contains fewer myofilaments with which to generate force and shorten during contraction. In addition, the chamber stiffness of the young heart's ventricles is also greater than that seen later in life. This means that any increase in ventricular filling or volume in the small, young heart results in a disproportionately greater rise in ventricular wall tension or stress. Similarly, it takes a smaller increase in ventricular filling to reach the limits of assistance given to cardiac pump and muscle function by stretching the myofilaments—that is, *preload or diastolic reserve is limited.* The young heart generates relatively less force and shortens less; that is, it cannot generate the same ventricular systolic pressures or wall tensions, or obtain the same stroke volume augmentation from any initial stretch, when compared with the older heart. With these facts in mind, it must be remembered that the oxygen consumption of the normal newborn is considerably higher than later in life; accordingly, the newborn at rest has a much higher cardiac output/m^2 than the child or adult. Thus, even in the absence of stress, the young heart must function near peak performance just to satisfy the normal demands of the peripheral tissues. Since newborn cardiac performance at rest is so close to its ceiling, or limits of function, there is very little *systolic reserve* that may be called upon in order to adapt to an acute or chronic stress such as asphyxia or a pressure or volume load from an obstructive lesion or left-to-right circulatory shunt, respectively.

In addition to *preload reserve* available to the heart from the Frank-Starling mechanism, and *systolic reserve* available through direct stimulation of cardiac contractility or through decreasing afterload to mechanically augment systolic emptying, there is a third, *heart rate reserve,* mechanism. The latter consists of the ability of the heart to change its rate of pumping to raise the level of cardiac output. In this regard the newborn is also limited, since its own intrinsic heart rate is normally quite high. In addition, heart failure per se will raise the frequency of contraction even further, primarily as a result of high circulating levels of catecholamines. In this sense, the newborn's heart rate is also closer than the child or adult's to its ceiling or upper limits of effectiveness. Furthermore, increases in heart rate occur largely at the expense of diastolic filling time. Thus, at very rapid heart rates, there is a disproportionately diminished diastolic time, and, therefore, diminished time for perfusion of the myocardium via its own coronary arterial system. In addition, rapid heart rates result in elevated myocardial energy expenditure and increased myocardial demand for oxygen. The sum of these considerations indicates that newborn *heart rate reserve* is reduced.

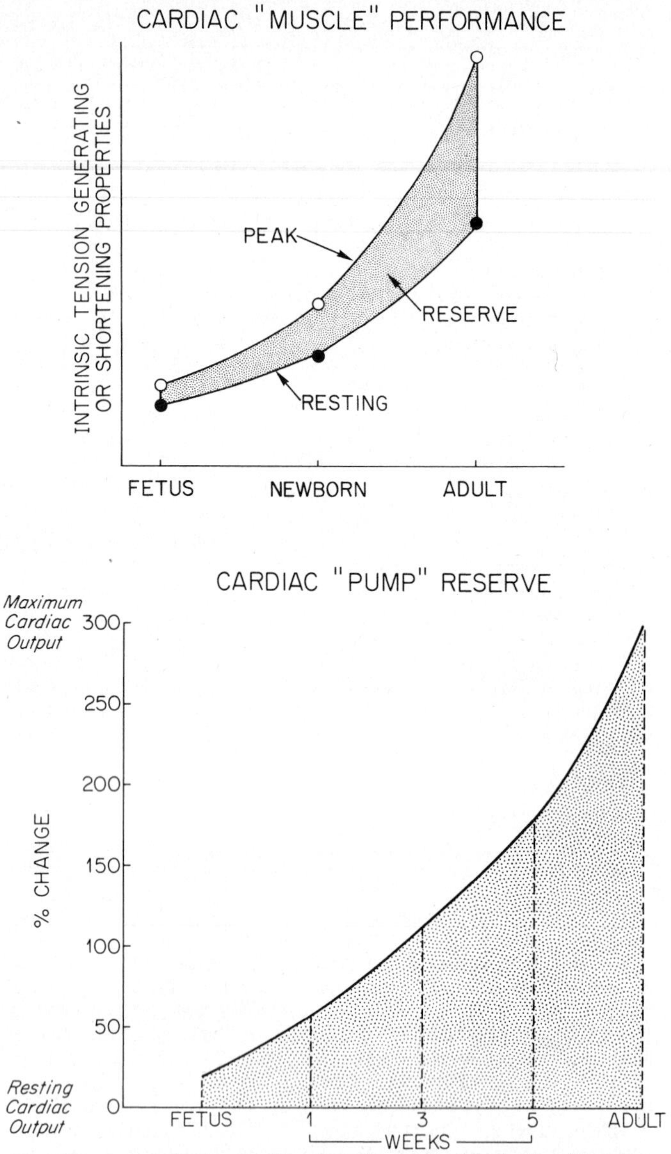

FIGURE 30–7. Schema of reduced cardiac reserve in fetal and newborn hearts compared with the adult. In the newborn infant, resting cardiac muscle performance (*top panel*) is close to the peak of ventricular function because of limitations in diastolic, systolic, and heart rate reserve. Similarly, pump reserve (*bottom panel*) early in life is limited by these factors, as well as by a much higher resting cardiac output relative to body weight, compared with the adult.

TREATMENT OF HEART FAILURE (See also Chap. 17). Table 30–5 lists supportive and pharmacological measures in the treatment of the newborn with heart failure. The supportive measures are designed to increase tissue oxygen supply, decrease tissue oxygen consumption, and correct metabolic abnormalities. Digitalis glycosides and certain diuretic agents provide the most important elements of medical therapy, but it is important to recognize that the dosage regimen of drugs administered to young patients must be adjusted to take into account the age and size of the patient and the maturity-dependent pharmacological properties of cardioactive drugs.[58] Since this is especially true in early infancy, Table 30–6 provides the dosages of digoxin and diuretics commonly employed. Digoxin is the glycoside used exclusively to treat pediatric patients in most cardiac centers, since it is readily absorbed, is available in convenient dosage form, and is excreted rapidly from the body. Premature infants are more sensitive to digitalis than are full-term newborns who, in turn, are more sensitive than older infants. Infants absorb and excrete digoxin as well as adults do, and the relative

TABLE 30–5 TREATMENT OF CONGESTIVE HEART FAILURE

I. Rest (occasional sedation)
    Semi-Fowler position
    Temperature and humidity control
    Oxygen
II. Diet—Decrease NaCl load, recognize danger of aspiration
III. Medications
    Correct hypoglycemia, anemia, or acidemia, if present
    Treat infection, if contributing factor
    Diuretics
    Digitalis
    Occasional need for catecholamine infusion, mechanical ventilation, peritoneal dialysis, afterload reduction, prostaglandin infusion or blocker
IV. Surgery

distribution of the glycoside to different body tissues is also similar. The prevailing dose schedules for digoxin produce higher serum concentrations in infants than would be considered optimal for adults.[59] The basis for the higher digitalis requirement in infancy is unclear, although it may relate to an age-dependent alteration in the sensitivity of the myocardium per se to the glycosides. In this regard, infants tolerate higher serum digoxin concentrations than adults without developing signs of toxicity. In the adult, the usual therapeutic concentrations of digoxin are less than 2 ng/ml blood, and toxicity commonly occurs above that level. In contrast, in infants, therapeutic levels of digoxin range from 1 to 5 ng/ml (mean = 3.5), while toxicity is associated with concentrations in excess of 3 ng/ml. Older children have therapeutic and toxic levels similar to those of adults.

A restricted fluid intake (65 ml/kg/day) and a low-sodium diet (1 to 2 mEq/kg/day) should accompany diuretic therapy in the most seriously ill infants with heart failure. Furosemide is the agent of choice when the rapid elimination of excess salt and water is needed. Hydrochlorothiazide, occasionally in conjunction with spironolactone or triamterene to reduce potassium loss and sodium retention, is convenient for long-term therapy.

Other pharmacological approaches may prove to be of significant benefit in selected instances in which digitalis and diuretics are relatively ineffective. In situations in which cardiac decompensation is not the result of an obstructive lesion, catecholamines may be employed temporarily to alleviate cardiac failure while the patient is awaiting more definitive operative treatment (Table 30–7).[18] In infants with the coarctation of the aorta syndrome, in whom ductal constriction unmasks the aortic branch point producing aortic narrowing (p. 930), or aortic arch interruption, heart failure may be reversed dramatically by the intravenous infusion of prostaglandin E_1 (0.03–0.1 mg/kg/min), which results in dilatation of the ductus arteriosus and relief of the obstruction.[60, 61] Conversely, in preterm infants in whom patent ductus arteriosus is responsible for profound cardiopulmonary deterioration, constriction for the ductus arteriosus may be accomplished by inhibition of prostaglandin synthesis with the nonsteroidal anti-inflammatory agent indomethacin (0.2 mg/kg IV).[27, 62, 63] Vasodilator therapy is also employed in infants or children with heart disease in whom preload or afterload alterations may be expected to improve cardiac performance (Table 30–8).[28, 29, 58] Moreover, treatment of severe cardiac failure often requires combining inotropic and afterload-reducing agents (p. 524). The combination of dopamine and nitroprusside has been used extensively and effectively in the pediatric population, primarily in the setting of low cardiac output after open heart surgery.[28] Use of oral afterload-reducing agents, e.g., hydralazine or captopril, in association with digoxin is worthwhile in the long-term therapy of outpatients with congestive cardiomyopathy and/or with significant mitral or aortic regurgitation.

CYANOSIS

Cyanosis in the infant often presents as a diagnostic emergency, necessitating prompt detection of the underlying cause. The schema in Figure 30–8 outlines a general approach to diagnosis. The cardiologist must distinguish between three types of cyanosis—peripheral, differential, and central—while recognizing that cyanosis may accompany diseases of the central nervous, hematological, respiratory, and cardiac systems.

PERIPHERAL CYANOSIS. Peripheral cyanosis (normal ar-

TABLE 30–6 DIURETIC AND DIGITALIS DOSAGES FOR INFANTS

PREPARATION	DOSAGE AND ROUTE OF ADMINISTRATION
Furosemide	IV, 1 mg/kg/dose; oral, 2 to 6 mg/kg/day
Ethacrynic acid	IV, 1 mg/kg/dose; oral, 2 to 3 mg/kg/day
Hydrochlorothiazide	Oral, 2 to 5 mg/kg/day
Spironolactone	Oral, 1 to 3 mg/kg/day
Triamterene	Oral, 2 to 4 mg/kg/day
Digoxin	
Elixir	0.05 mg/ml
Parenteral	0.10 mg/ml

AGE AND WEIGHT	DOSE AND ROUTE*	
	Acute Digitalization	Maintenance
Prematures <1.5 kg	10–20 μg/kg IV Total Digitalizing Dose (TDD): ½, ¼, ¼ of dose q 8h	4 μg/kg/day IV (may increase to 4 μg/kg q 12h at age 1 month)
1.5–2.5 kg	Same as above	4 μg/kg q 12h IV
Full-term newborns	30 μg/kg IV, TDD	4–5 μg/kg q 12h IV
Infants (1–12 months)	35 μg/kg IV, TDD	5–10 μg/kg q 12h IV
>12 months	40 μg/kg IV, TDD (maximum 1.0 mg)	5–10 μg/kg q 12h IV
Older children (over 20 kg)	1.0–2.0 mg IV, TDD over 48 hours	0.125–0.250 mg IV q day

*P.O. dose approximately 20% greater than IV dose except in "older children." In older children, IV = P.O.
TDD = Total digitalizing dose.

TABLE 30–7 DOSAGE REGIMENS: INOTROPIC AGENTS

Drug	Dose	Comments
Epinephrine (Adrenalin)	0.05–1.0 μg/kg/min IV	May cause hypertension and cardiac arrhythmias; inactivated in alkaline solution
Isoproterenol (Isuprel)	0.05–0.5 μg/kg/min IV	May decrease coronary blood flow; results in peripheral and pulmonary vasodilation
Norepinephrine (Levophed)	0.05–0.5 μg/kg/min IV	Causes significant vasoconstriction
Dobutamine (Dobutrex)	2–10 μg/kg/min IV (Max 40 μg/kg/min)	No direct effect on renal perfusion, little or no peripheral vasodilatation or tachycardia
Dopamine (Intropin)	2–20 μg/kg/min IV (Max 50 μg/kg/min)	
	2–5 μg/kg/min	Significant renal vasodilatation
	5–8 μg/kg/min	Inotropic ± heart rate acceleration
	>8 μg/kg/min	Significant heart rate acceleration
	>10 μg/kg/min	± Vasoconstriction
	15–20 μg/kg/min	Significant vasoconstriction
	(Above dose/effect relations speculative in neonates)	
Amrinone	Dose schedule not established for Pediatrics	May cause thrombocytopenia, hepatic and GI disturbance, fever, and arrhythmias
	Adults: 40 μg/kg/min IV for 1 hr, then 6–10 μg/kg/min; 50–450 mg/day po divided TID	

From Friedman, W. F., and George, B. L.: New concepts and drugs in the treatment of congestive heart failure. Pediatr. Clin. North Am. *31*:1197, 1984.

terial oxygen saturation and widened arteriovenous oxygen differences) usually indicates stasis of blood flow in the periphery. The level of reduced hemoglobin in the capillaries of the skin usually exceeds 3 gm/100 ml. The most prominent causes of peripheral cyanosis in the newborn are autonomically controlled alterations in the cutaneous distribution of capillary blood flow (acrocyanosis) and septicemia associated with evidence of a low cardiac output, i.e., hypotension, weak pulse, and cold extremities. In many instances peripheral cyanosis is clearly the result of a cold environment or high hemoglobin content. When caused by the former, vasodilatation produced by immersing the extremity in warm water for several minutes will reverse the cyanosis.

CENTRAL CYANOSIS. Oxygen unsaturation in central cyanosis may result from inadequately oxygenated pulmonary venous blood, in which case inhalation of 100 per cent oxygen may diminish or clear the discoloration (see below). Conversely, in instances in which cyanosis is due to an intra- or extracardiac right-to-left shunt, pulmonary venous blood is fully saturated, and inhalation of 100 per cent oxygen generally will not improve the infant's color. It is necessary to qualify the latter statement because oxygen may act directly in infants with elevated pulmonary vascular resistance to dilate the pulmonary blood vessels and thus reduce the magnitude of the venoarterial shunt. Central cyanosis may also be due to the replacement of normal by abnormal hemoglobin, as in methemoglobinemia.

Several factors influence the oxygen saturation produced at any given arterial pO_2. These include temperature, pH, ratio of fetal-to-adult hemoglobin, and erythrocyte concentration of 2,3-diphosphoglycerate. For example, fetal hemoglobin has a higher affinity for oxygen than does adult hemoglobin and therefore would be more highly saturated at any given pO_2. Thus, determination of the systemic arterial oxygen tension may provide a more accurate picture of the underlying pathophysiology than simply measuring the oxygen saturation.

DIFFERENTIAL CYANOSIS. Differential cyanosis virtually always indicates the presence of congenital heart disease, often with patency of the ductus arteriosus and coarctation of the aorta as components of the abnormal anatomical complex. If the upper part of the body is pink and the lower part of the body blue, coarctation of the aorta or interruption of the aortic arch is probable, with oxygenated blood supplying the upper body and desaturated blood supplying the lower body via right-to-left flow through the ductus arteriosus. The latter occurs also in patients with patent ductus arteriosus and markedly elevated pulmonary vascular resistance. A patient with transposition of the great arteries and coarctation of the aorta with retrograde flow through a patent ductus arteriosus demonstrates the reverse situation, i.e., the lower part of the body is pink

TABLE 30–8 DOSAGE REGIMENS: VASODILATORS

Drug	Dose and Route of Administration	Comments
Nitroglycerin	0.5–20 μg/kg/min IV (Max 60 μg/kg/min IV)	Dosage schedule for IV and other routes of administration not well established for children
Hydralazine (Apresoline)	0.5 mg/kg/day po q6–8h (Max 200 mg/day or 7 mg/kg/day) 1.5 μg/kg/min IV or 0.1–0.5 mg/kg/dose IV q6h (Max 2 mg/kg–q6h)	May cause tachycardia, GI symptoms, neutropenia, lupus-like syndrome
Captopril (Capoten)	0.1–0.4 mg/kg/dose po given q6–24h as needed	May cause neutropenia/proteinuria
Nitroprusside (Nipride)	0.5–8 μg/kg/min IV	May result in thiocyanate or cyanide toxicity if used in high doses or for prolonged periods of time; light sensitive
Prazosin (Minipress)	1st dose: 5 μg/kg po (Max 25 μg/kg/dose q6h)	Initial dose used to elevate hypotensive effects; orthostatic hypotension, attenuation of hemodynamic effects may occur

From Friedman, W. F., and George, B. L.: New concepts and drugs in the treatment of congestive heart failure. Pediatr. Clin. North Am. *31*:1197, 1984.

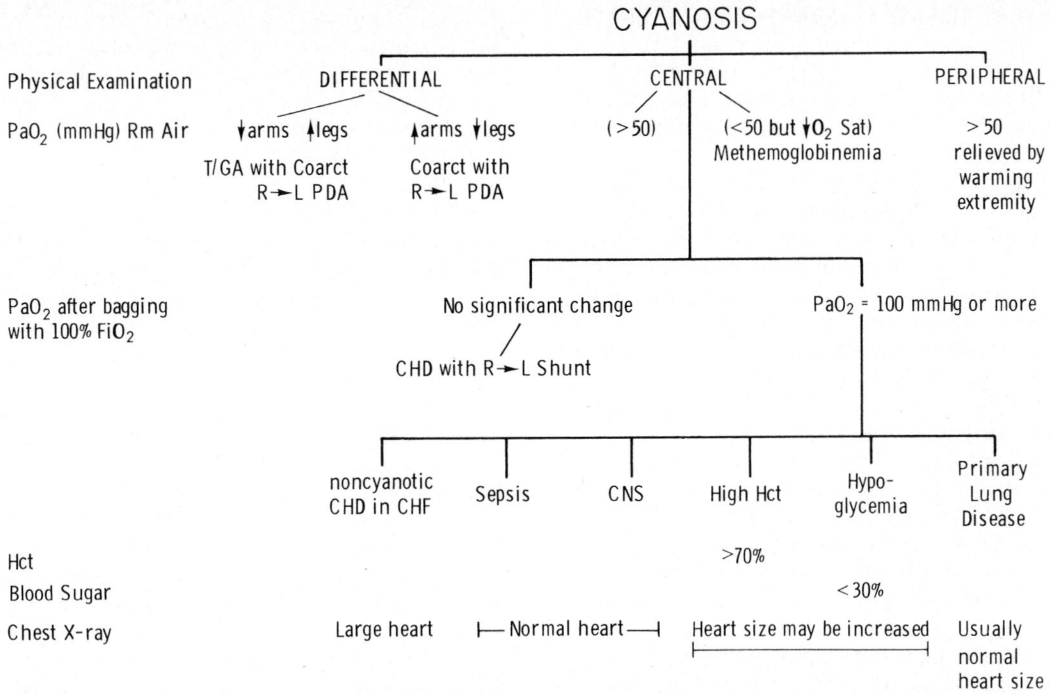

FIGURE 30–8. Flow chart for the evaluation of cyanotic infants. Tests to be done are listed at the left. The response to each of these tests leads along the line to the proper diagnostic category. CHD = congenital heart disease, CHF = congestive heart failure, CNS = central nervous system, Hct = hematocrit, PDA = patent ductus arteriosus, T/GA = transposition of great arteries. (From Kirkpatrick, S. E., et al.: Differential diagnosis of congenital heart disease in the newborn—University of California, San Diego, School of Medicine, and University Hospital, San Diego [Specialty Conference]. West. J. Med. *128*:127, 1978.)

and the upper part blue. Simultaneous determinations of oxygen saturation in the temporal or right brachial artery and the femoral artery are helpful in confirming the presence of differential cyanosis.

CENTRAL NERVOUS SYSTEM AND HEMATOLOGICAL CAUSES OF CYANOSIS. Irregular, shallow breathing secondary to central nervous system depression results in reduced alveolar ventilation and an abnormally low alveolar oxygen tension. Alveolar arterial pCO_2 becomes elevated, and arterial pO_2 is reduced. Sedatives and hypnotics administered to the mother during labor cause central nervous system depression in the newborn and intracranial hemorrhage secondary to birth trauma, accounting for most cases.

Methemoglobinemia, either congenital or acquired, is a rare cause of cyanosis in the newborn, with recognizable cyanosis occurring in affected babies when 15 per cent or more of the total hemoglobin is replaced by methemoglobin. Venous blood exposed to room air normally becomes pink but remains dark in infants with methemoglobinemia. Arterial blood with a normal partial pressure of oxygen but a low oxygen saturation should suggest the diagnosis, which may be established conclusively by spectrophotometry.

DIFFERENTIATING BETWEEN PULMONARY AND CARDIAC CAUSES OF CYANOSIS. The distinction between respiratory signs and symptoms arising from cyanotic cardiac disease and those associated with a primary pulmonary disorder is an important challenge to the cardiologist.[31] Upper airway obstruction precipitates cyanosis by producing alveolar hypoventilation due to reduced pulmonary ventilation. Mechanical obstruction may occur from the nares to the carina, and the important diagnostic possibilities among congenital abnormalities are choanal atresia, vascular ring, laryngeal web, and tracheomalacia. Acquired causes include vocal cord paresis, obstetrical injury to the cricothyroid cartilage, and foreign body. Structural abnormalities in the lungs due to intrapulmonary disease are more frequently a basis for cyanosis among newborns than is upper airway obstruction. Hyaline membrane disease, atelectasis, or pneumonitis causing inflammation, collapse, and fluid accumulation in the alveoli results in incompletely oxygenated blood reaching the systemic circulation.

Successfully distinguishing between these various causes of cyanosis depends upon interpretation of the respiratory pattern, the cardiac physical examination, evaluation of arterial blood gases (Table 30–9), and interpretation of the electrocardiogram, chest x-ray, and echocardiogram.

RESPIRATORY PATTERNS. The key to differential diagnosis at the bedside is commonly the proper evaluation of the pattern of respiration. Normally, term infants exhibit a progressive reduction in respiratory rate during the first day of life from 60 to 70/minute to 35 to 55/minute. Moreover, mild intercostal retractions and minimal expiratory grunting disappear within several hours of birth. An increased depth of respiration in the presence of cyanosis, but without other signs of respiratory distress, is often

TABLE 30–9 ARTERIAL BLOOD GASES IN VARIOUS DISORDERS CAUSING CYANOSIS IN INFANTS

Pattern	pH	pO_2	pCO_2	Response to O_2	Venous pH	Suggested Condition
1	↓	↓↓	↑	↑↑	↓	Hyaline membrane or other pulmonary parenchymal disease
2	↓	↓	↑↑↑	↑	↓	Hypoventilation
3	—	↓	—	↑	—	Venous admixture
4	↓	↓↓	—	—	↓	Decreased or ineffective pulmonary blood flow
5	↓↓↓	↓	—↑	—↑	↓↓↓↓	Systemic hypoperfusion

associated with congenital cardiac disease in which inadequate pulmonary blood flow is the most important functional component.

The most important variations from normal respiratory patterns are apnea and bradypnea, and tachypnea. Intermittent apneic episodes are common in premature infants with central nervous system immaturity or disease. In addition, higher centers may be depressed as a result of severe hypoxemia, acidemia, or the administration of pharmacological agents to mother or baby. The association of apneic episodes, lethargy, hypotonicity, and a reduction in spontaneous movements most often point to intracranial disease as an underlying cause.

Diverse conditions result in tachypnea in the newborn period. Tachypnea in the presence of intrinsic pulmonary disease with upper or lower airway obstruction is usually accompanied by flaring of the alae nasi, chest wall retractions, and grunting. In contrast, tachypnea associated with intense cyanosis in the absence of obvious respiratory distress suggests the presence of cyanotic congenital heart disease. In general, highest respiratory rates (80 to 110/min) are seen in association with primary lung, and not heart, disease. Frequently, an initial chest x-ray is diagnostic, especially if the problem is aspiration, mucous plug, adenomatoid malformation, lobar emphysema, diaphragmatic hernia, pneumothorax, lung agenesis, pulmonary hemorrhage, or an abnormal thoracic cage configuration. Choanal atresia may be excluded by passing a feeding tube through the nares, and the more common types of esophageal atresia and tracheoesophageal fistula may be excluded by passing the tube farther into the stomach.

CARDIAC EXAMINATION. Specific findings upon cardiovascular examination may direct attention to a cardiac etiology for cyanosis. Peripheral perfusion is poor in the presence of severe primary myocardial disease or the hypoplastic left heart syndrome. In contrast, peripheral pulses are bounding and the dorsalis pedis and palmar pulses are easily palpable in infants with patent ductus arteriosus, truncus arteriosus, or aorticopulmonary window. A marked discrepancy between upper and lower extremity blood pressures helps identify the infant with coarctation of the aorta. Inspection and palpation of the precordium allows an overall estimate of cardiac activity. A suprasternal notch and precordial thrill may occasionally be felt in the infant with patent ductus arteriosus, critical aortic stenosis, or coarctation of the aorta. Characterization of the second heart sound may be of help, since it is often single in infants with a hypoplastic left heart complex, pulmonary atresia with or without an intact ventricular septum, and truncus arteriosus. Wide splitting of the second heart sound may occur in infants with total anomalous pulmonary venous return. Ejection sounds are often detectable in infants with persistent truncus arteriosus and occasionally with critical aortic or pulmonic stenosis. The presence of a third heart sound is normal, but a gallop rhythm may provide a clue to myocardial failure. Wide splitting of the first and second heart sounds and prominent third and fourth heart sounds may produce the characteristically rhythmic auscultatory cadence of Ebstein's anomaly of the tricuspid valve (p. 951). The presence of a cardiac murmur may point clearly to underlying cardiac disease, but the absence of a murmur does not exclude the presence of a cardiac malformation. Moreover, cardiac murmurs of specific anomalies are often atypical in the newborn period. However, certain cardiac murmurs such as the decrescendo holosystolic murmur of tricuspid regurgitation in Ebstein's anomaly or transient tricuspid regurgitation of infancy may point clearly to a proper diagnosis. Auscultation of the head and abdomen may detect the murmur of an arteriovenous malformation at those sites in infants who present with findings of severe heart failure.

BLOOD GAS AND pH PATTERNS. Arterial blood gases may be a reliable method of evaluating cyanosis, suggesting the type of altered physiology, and assessing responses to therapeutic maneuvers.[46] Blood gases should be obtained in room air and in 100 per cent oxygen. Stick capillary samples from the patient's warmed heel may be employed, although determinations obtained by arterial puncture are preferable for evaluation of oxygenation, since they are less susceptible to alterations in regional blood flow in the critically ill infant. Sampling of right radial or temporal arterial blood is preferable, since these sites are proximal to flow through a ductus arteriosus and do not reflect right-to-left ductal shunting, as would a sample from the descending aorta obtained via an umbilical artery catheter. A trial of continuous positive airway pressure may improve oxygenation in infants with either hyaline membrane disease or pulmonary edema. Arterial blood gas patterns in various pathophysiological conditions are listed in Table 30–9. Pattern 1 is typically observed in infants with ventilation-perfusion abnormalities on the basis of primary respiratory disease often associated with elevated pulmonary vascular resistance and venoarterial shunting across a patent foramen ovale or patent ductus arteriosus. Pulmonary hypoventilation with CO_2 retention produces pattern 2. In the presence of a lesion causing obligatory venous admixture, such as total anomalous pulmonary venous connection (pattern 3), the response to oxygen may reflect an increase in pulmonary venous return secondary to a fall in pulmonary vascular resistance. Pattern 4 is seen typically in infants with a cardiac malformation that results in reduced pulmonary blood flow. Oxygen administration in these infants does not alter the arterial pO_2. The alterations of pattern 5 are observed when systemic hypoperfusion is the principal hemodynamic problem. In these babies the arteriovenous oxygen difference is high, and the acidemia may be progressive and unrelenting.

ELECTROCARDIOGRAM. The electrocardiogram is less helpful in suggesting a diagnosis of heart disease in the premature and newborn infant than in the older child. Right ventricular hypertrophy is a normal finding in the neonate, and the range of normal voltages is wide. However, specific observations may offer major clues to the presence of a cardiovascular anomaly. A counterclockwise, superiorly oriented frontal QRS loop with absent or reduced right ventricular forces suggests the diagnosis of tricuspid atresia (p. 949). In contrast, when the QRS axis is normal but left ventricular forces predominate, the diagnosis of pulmonic atresia must be considered (p. 945). The counterclockwise, superior QRS orientation is also observed in infants with an endocardial cushion defect (p. 917) and in some with double-outlet right ventricle (p. 960); right ventricular forces in these babies are increased. The initial septal vector should be assessed from the electrocardiogram. Often Q waves are not clearly seen in the lateral precordial leads in the first 72 hours of life. A leftward, posteriorly directed septal vector giving rise to Q waves in the right precordial leads is abnormal and suggests the presence of marked right ventricular hypertrophy, single ventricle (p. 965), or inversion of the ventricles (p. 957). T-wave alterations may be seen in a normal neonatal electrocardiogram and may be of no specific consequence. However, by 72 hours of age the T waves should be inverted in V_3 and V_1 and upright in the lateral precordium; persistently upright T waves in the right precordial leads are a sign of right ventricular hypertrophy. Depressed or flattened T waves in the lateral precordium may suggest subendocardial ischemia and a left heart outflow tract obstructive lesion, electrolyte disturbance, acidosis, or hypoxemia. An electrocardiographic pattern of myocardial infarction suggests a diagnosis of anomalous pulmonary origin of the coronary artery (p. 927). Lastly, rhythm disturbances such as complete heart block or supraventricular tachycardia can be detected readily by electrocardiography.

RADIOGRAPHIC EXAMINATION (See also pp. 157 to 162). The chest x-ray is often the single most useful examination in differentiating between respiratory and cardiac causes of cyanosis in the newborn period. Determination of a normal cardiac and abdominal situs aids in ruling out several kinds of complex cyanotic cardiac malformations associated with asplenia or polysplenia with abdominal heterotaxy and dextrocardia (p. 964). The distinct appearance of pulmonary parenchymal disease such as the classic reticulogranular pattern of hyaline membrane disease may allow a specific radiological diagnosis. In those premature infants with a large ductus arteriosus the x-ray appearance often evolves from the typical findings of hyaline membrane disease to increased pulmonary vascular markings and finally to perihilar and generalized pulmonary edema. Most importantly, the pediatric cardiologist depends heavily on the evaluation of pulmonary vascular markings to categorize congenital cardiac malformations in the newborn infant according to function. In the presence of cyanosis, diminished pulmonary vascular markings call attention to the group of anomalies that includes tetralogy of Fallot, pulmonic stenosis with intact ventricular septum, pulmonic atresia, tricuspid atresia, and Ebstein's malformation of the tricuspid valve. Reduced pulmonary blood flow is responsible for the systemic arterial desaturation in these babies. Increased pulmonary vascular markings in the cyanotic infant are associated with lesions in which an obligatory admixture of systemic venous and pulmonary venous blood occurs. The more common anomalies in this category include transposition of the great arteries, hypoplastic left heart syndrome, truncus arteriosus, and total anomalous pulmonary venous drainage.

As mentioned earlier, overall heart size in the normal newborn infant is greater than in the older child, and cardiothoracic ratios up to 0.60 are within normal limits. Occasionally, the thymus shadow obscures the cardiac silhouette and prohibits accurate estimation of heart size. An enlarged heart on x-ray examination suggests a cardiac disorder. However, in the presence of severe respiratory difficulties with an increase in carbon dioxide tension and a decrease in both pH and arterial oxygen tension, cardiomegaly may be only moderate. A right aortic arch suggests the presence of either tetralogy of Fallot or persistent truncus arteriosus. An ovoid heart with a narrow base associated with increased pulmonary vascular marking is typical of transposition of the great arteries. A boot-shaped heart with concavity of the pulmonary outflow tract suggests tetralogy of Fallot, pulmonic atresia, or tricuspid atresia.

ECHOCARDIOGRAPHY (See also pp. 113 to 119). **Fetal Echocardiography.** Ultrasound technology now allows examination of human fetal cardiac development and function in utero. Diagnostic-quality images of the fetal heart in utero can be obtained as early as 16 weeks of gestation. Cardiac structures are imaged primarily by cross-sectional echocardiography and augmented by a combination of range-gated pulse Doppler ultrasonography and M-mode echocardiography.[64–66] The analysis of the structure and function of the fetal heart during the second and third trimesters of pregnancy has allowed cardiologists to counsel prospective parents, and in a number of instances to formulate management plans for pregnancy, delivery, and the immediate postnatal period. Using fetal echocardiography, major forms of congenital heart disease have been diagnosed in utero, and cardiac rhythm abnormalities have been detected, permitting direct efforts at transplacental therapy. In particular, it has been established that a high incidence exists of cardiac pathology in the presence of nonimmune fetal hydrops. It appears clear that hydrops fetalis often represents end-stage fetal cardiac decompensation (Fig. 30–9). Atrioventricular valve insufficiency often causes fetal right ventricular volume overload and systemic venous hypertension leading to hydrops fetalis.

Pulsed Doppler ultrasound examination of the fetus importantly supplements the echocardiographic findings in identifying the responsible defects, such as Ebstein's malformation of the tricuspid valve, atrial isomerism with atrioventricular septal defects, and the absent pulmonary valve and hypoplastic left heart syndromes.

Fetal cardiac ultrasound is of especial importance in analyzing disturbances of fetal cardiac rhythm, which are usually first suspected on the basis of auscultatory findings. Transabdominal electrocardiography cannot distinguish atrial depolarization, and is of limited value in the analysis of cardiac arrhythmias in utero. However, M-mode recordings of cardiac motion versus time allow conclusions regarding electrical events in the fetal heart, as they are reflected by the mechanical responses that are recorded echocardiographically. Supraventricular tachyarrhythmias are a common cause of nonimmune fetal hydrops (Fig. 30–10). Detection is of practical use in the management of these patients because the problem is treatable with use of various antiarrhythmic drugs, such as digoxin, procainamide, propranolol, and digoxin combined with verapamil, administered to the mother and reaching the fetus transplacentally.

Echocardiography is of immense value in distinguishing heart disease from lung disease in the newborn.[36] Echocardiographic diagnoses that can often be made with cer-

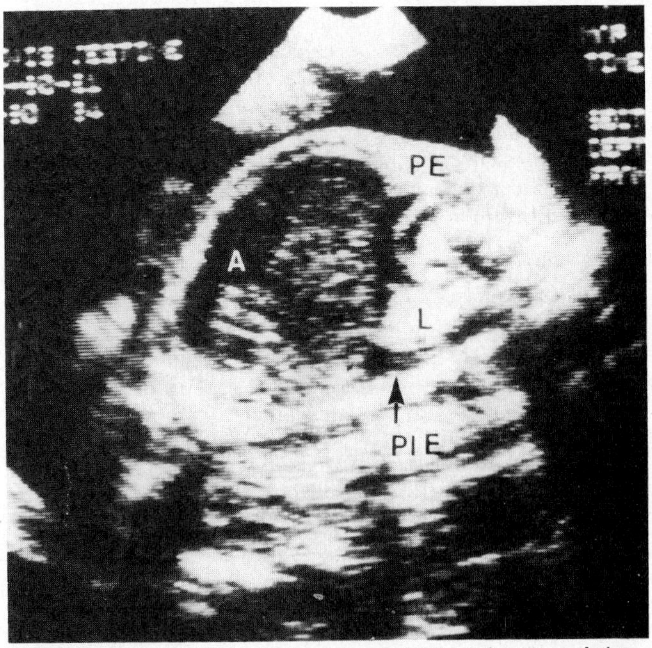

FIGURE 30–9. Abdominal ultrasound examination of a 28-week fetus with nonimmunological fetal hydrops fetalis. A = ascites, PE = pericardial effusion, L = lung, PIE = pleural effusion. The fetal heart is to the right and inferior of the white arrow showing the pericardial effusion.

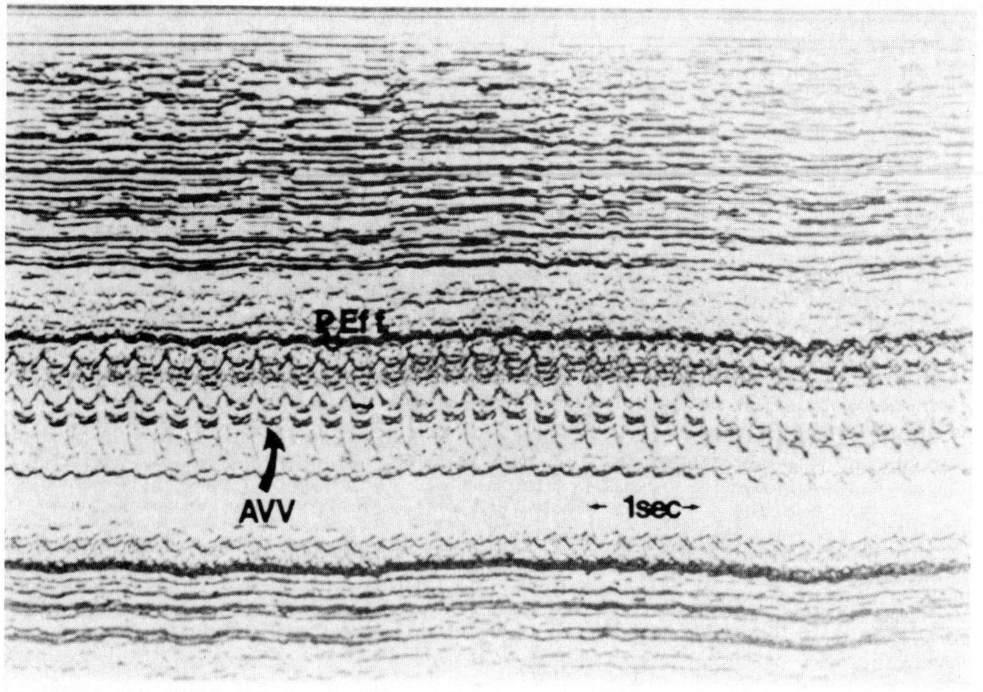

FIGURE 30–10. M-mode echocardiogram at 35 weeks' gestation, showing fetal supraventricular tachycardia and pericardial effusion (PEff). The tracing, taken at the midventricular level, allows the heart rate to be calculated from atrioventricular valve (AVV) motion (250 beats/min). (Courtesy of Charles Kleinman, M.D.)

tainty include hypoplastic left heart syndrome, aortic valve stenosis, membranous and fibromuscular subvalvar aortic stenosis, aortic coarctation, hypertrophic cardiomyopathy, cor triatriatum, atrial septal defect, tricuspid atresia, Ebstein's anomaly of the tricuspid valve, valvar pulmonic stenosis, atrioventricular septal defect, single ventricle, double-outlet right ventricle, transposition of the great arteries, and patent ductus arteriosus. The echocardiogram provides suggestive and occasionally conclusive evidence for tetralogy of Fallot, truncus arteriosus, total anomalous pulmonary venous connection, and pulmonary atresia with an intact ventricular septum.

Doppler ultrasonography (p. 87) has supplemented the two-dimensional echocardiographic examination by its ability to quantify valve gradients, cardiac output, blood flow patterns in the cardiac chambers and great arteries, and often shunt size.[67] For example, the pulmonary or systemic blood flow (ml/sec) can be calculated by multiplying the mean velocity (cm/sec) measured by Doppler ultrasound in the pulmonary artery or aorta, and multiplied by the cross-sectional area (cm^2) of the vessel. The coupling of Doppler ultrasonographic techniques with the two-dimensional echocardiogram, and the representation in color of abnormalities in flow, volume, and direction (p. 88), greatly improves diagnostic accuracy.

CARDIAC CATHETERIZATION (See also Chap. 9). If a cardiac anomaly is identified by noninvasive studies or if a clear-cut differentiation cannot be made between cardiac and pulmonary disease, heart catheterization and angiocardiography are required to define the underlying state precisely. Hemodynamic study of the newborn infant carries a small but distinct risk.[68] As a general rule, cardiac catheterization is not performed unless the information sought is central to the management of the infant. Infants with serious heart disease usually require therapeutic intervention, and thus catheterization should be performed only when surgical support is readily available. Cardiac catheterization is indicated in most newborns who experience congestive heart failure in the first days after birth if the cause is an anatomical abnormality rather than an arrhythmia or a metabolic disturbance. Preferably, medical measures will have been instituted to stabilize the clinical state before a hemodynamic study is performed.

It is generally agreed that almost all newborns with cyanotic congenital heart disease require immediate cardiac catheterization, since there is considerable risk of rapid deterioration.[58] Under these circumstances hemodynamic and angiographic study may not only provide the anatomical diagnosis required prior to emergency operation but may also allow the opportunity for therapeutic maneuvers such as balloon atrial septostomy to facilitate intercirculatory mixing in patients with complete transposition of the great arteries or to augment interatrial shunting in patients with a restrictive patent foramen ovale and either tricuspid, pulmonic, or mitral atresia, or total anomalous pulmonary venous connection. In addition, the selective infusion of low doses of prostaglandin E_1 (0.05–0.1 μg/kg/min) intravenously has been employed at cardiac catheterization for the emergency palliation of ductus-dependent cardiac lesions such as pulmonary atresia, aortic coarctation and interruption of the aortic arch.[60] Since a patent ductus arteriosus maintains pulmonary and systemic blood flow, respectively, in these infants, dilatation of the ductus with vasodilatory prostaglandins may retard their clinical deterioration. Thus, prostaglandin E_1 infusion has been shown to be an effective short-term measure to correct hypoxemia and acidemia and to improve the pre- and intraoperative status of infants requiring surgical relief of the congenital cardiac lesion that is causing pulmonary or systemic hypoperfusion.

Therapeutic Catheterization (See also Ch. 9). Balloon atrial septostomy was the first catheter intervention proven useful to treat congenital heart disease, and remains the standard initial palliation in infants with complete transposition of the great arteries.[69] Recently, additional transcatheter techniques have been employed successfully to treat congenital heart disease.[69, 70] These include knife blade atrial septostomy, umbrella closure of the patent ductus arteriosus,[70a] and balloon and coil embolization of large systemic pulmonary artery collateral vessels and arteriovenous fistulas. Other procedures that have expanded the role of the cardiac catheter from a diagnostic tool to a therapeutic instrument include transvenous or transarterial pacemaker insertion and retrieval of foreign bodies from the cardiovascular system. Transluminal balloon angioplasty is currently used principally in pediatrics for dilation of pulmonic valve stenosis, recoarctation of the aorta, and peripheral pulmonary artery stenosis. Still unproven are transluminal angioplasty approaches to native coarctation and congenital aortic and mitral stenosis.

Electrophysiological Studies (See also Ch. 9). The cardiac catheterization laboratory is also being used with increasing frequency to define the anatomical and physiological diagnoses of arrhythmias, in order to enable an accurate prognosis and to provide a rational basis for treatment.[70b] The invasive electrophysiological approach provides unique information that cannot be obtained noninvasively. These include determination of conduction times of individual components of the conducting system and measurement of refractory periods for structures such as the atrioventricular node, HIS bundle, and bundle branches. In addition, one can determine the initiating features, sustaining mechanisms, and possible perturbations that terminate the arrhythmia. This latter maneuver is particularly important since it may enable the planning of effective drug treatment. It may also determine the advisability of catheter ablation, pacemaker control, or surgical treatment of the rhythm disturbance.

SPECIFIC CARDIAC DEFECTS

Many classifications of congenital cardiovascular lesions have been proposed on the basis of hemodynamic, anatomical, and radiographic factors. Although there is overlapping between groups, the following arrangement of cardiac anomalies is used in this chapter: (1) communications between the systemic and pulmonary circulations without cyanosis (left-to-right shunts), (2) obstructing valvular and vascular lesions with or without associated right-to-left shunt, (3) abnormalities in the origins of the great arteries and veins (the transposition complexes), (4) malpositions of the heart and cardiac apex, and (5) miscellaneous anomalies.

LEFT-TO-RIGHT SHUNTS

ATRIAL SEPTAL DEFECT (See also p. 982)

MORPHOLOGY. Atrial septal defect is one of the most commonly recognized congenital cardiac anomalies in adults but is very rarely diagnosed and even less commonly results in disability in infants.[71] The anatomical sites of interatrial defects are depicted in Figure 30–11. Defects of the sinus venosus type are high in the atrial septum near the entry of the superior vena cava and are frequently associated with, and may be a consequence of, anomalous connection of pulmonary veins from the right lung to the junction of the superior vena cava and right atrium.[72] Most often the atrial septal defect involves the fossa ovalis, is midseptal in location, and is of the ostium secundum type. This type of defect is a true deficiency of the atrial septum and should not be confused with a patent foramen ovale. Embryologically the left side of the atrial septum is derived from the septum primum, which possesses an opening—the interatrial ostium secundum (Fig. 30–3). The ostium secundum lies forward and superior to the position of the foramen ovale. The latter is formed by the septum secundum and occupies the right side of the atrial septum. Tissue of the septum primum lying to the left of the foramen ovale serves as a flap valve that usually becomes fused postnatally with the side of the foramen ovale yielding an anatomically closed or sealed foramen. "Probe patency," or an incomplete seal of the foramen ovale, occurs in approximately 25 per cent of adults. A widely patent foramen ovale may be considered an acquired form of atrial septal defect that occurs especially when a disproportion exists between the size of the foramen ovale and the effective length of its valve. Enlargement of the foramen ovale per se is commonly associated with obstructive lesions of the right side of the heart, whereas a short valve relative to the size of the foramen is often seen in large-volume left-to-right shunts in which left atrial dilatation is prominent.

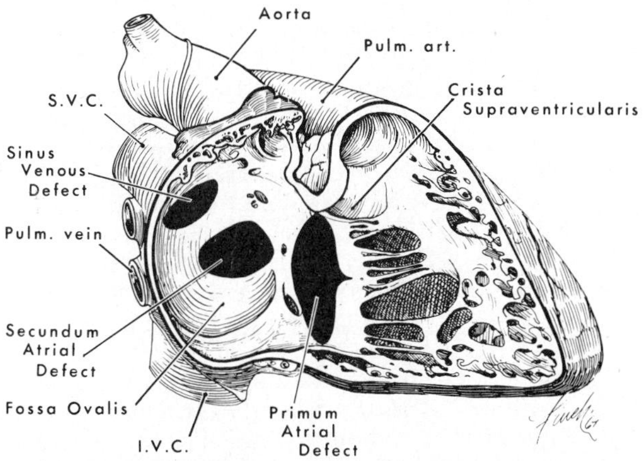

FIGURE 30–11. Composite locations of atrial defects. S.V.C. = superior vena cava, I.V.C. = inferior vena cava.

Ostium primum atrial septal anomalies are a form of atrioventricular septal defect and will be dealt with in the following section. Lutembacher's syndrome is a designation applied to the rare combination of atrial septal defect and mitral stenosis, which is almost invariably the result of acquired rheumatic valvulitis. Ten to 20 per cent of patients with ostium secundum atrial septal defect also have prolapse of the mitral valve as an associated anomaly.[73]

HEMODYNAMICS. The magnitude of the left-to-right shunt through an atrial septal defect depends on the size of the defect and the relative compliance of the ventricles, and the relative resistance in the pulmonary and in the systemic circulation.[74] In patients with a small atrial septal defect or patent foramen ovale, the left atrial pressure may exceed the right by several mm Hg, whereas the mean pressure in both atria is nearly identical when the defect is large. Left-to-right shunting occurs predominantly in late ventricular systole and early diastole with some augmentation during atrial contraction. The shunt results in diastolic overloading of the right ventricle and increased pulmonary blood flow. During the first few days and weeks of life pulmonary resistance falls and systemic resistance rises, facilitating right ventricular emptying and impeding left ventricular emptying; the left-to-right shunt rises. Early in infancy left-to-right flow through even a large interatrial communication is commonly limited by both the reduced chamber compliance of thickened neonatal right ventricle and the elevated pulmonary and reduced systemic vascular resistance of the neonate. The pulmonary vascular resistance is commonly normal or low in the older infant or child with atrial septal defect, and the volume load is usually well tolerated, even though pulmonary blood flow may be two to five times greater than systemic. A transient and small right-to-left shunt occurring with the onset of left ventricular contraction and especially during respiratory periods of decreasing intrathoracic pressure is common in patients with ostium secundum defect, even in the absence of pulmonary hypertension.

CLINICAL FINDINGS. Patients with atrial septal defect are usually asymptomatic in early life, although occasional reports exist of congestive heart failure and recurrent pneumonia in infancy.[71] Children with atrial septal defect may experience easy fatigability and exertional dyspnea. They tend to be somewhat underdeveloped physically and prone to respiratory infection. Atrial arrhythmias, pulmonary arterial hypertension, development of pulmonary vascular obstruction, and heart failure are exceedingly uncommon in the pediatric age range, in contrast to their common appearance in adults with atrial septal defect. In the former group, diagnosis is entertained often after detection of a heart murmur on routine physical examination prompts a more extensive cardiac evaluation.

Common findings on *physical examination* include a prominent right ventricular cardiac impulse and palpable pulmonary artery pulsation. The first heart sound is normal or split, with accentuation of the tricuspid valve closure sound. Increased flow across the pulmonic valve is responsible for a midsystolic pulmonary ejection murmur. After the normal postnatal drop in pulmonary vascular resistance, the second heart sound is split widely and is relatively fixed in relation to respiration in patients with normal pulmonary pressures and low pulmonary vascular impedance because of a delay in pulmonic valve closure. With pulmonary hypertension the splitting interval is a function of the electromechanical intervals of each ventricle; wide splitting occurs with shortening of the left and/or lengthening of the right ventricular electromechanical interval.[75] If the shunt is large, increased blood flow across the tricuspid valve is responsible for a middiastolic rumbling murmur at the lower left sternal border. In patients with associated prolapse of the mitral valve an apical holosystolic or late systolic murmur radiating to the axilla is often heard, but a midsystolic click may be difficult to discern. Moreover, left ventricular precordial overactivity is usually absent because mitral regurgitation is mild in most patients.

In the teenage patient, the physical findings may be altered when an increase in pulmonary vascular resistance results in diminution of the left-to-right shunt. Both the pulmonary and tricuspid murmurs decrease in intensity, whereas the pulmonic component of the second heart sound becomes accentuated and the two components of the second heart sound may fuse; a diastolic murmur of pulmonic incompetence appears. Cyanosis and clubbing accompany development of a right-to-left shunt.

The *electrocardiogram* in patients with an ostium secundum defect usually shows right-axis deviation, right ventricular hypertrophy, and rSR′ or rsR′ pattern in the right precordial leads with a normal QRS duration (Fig. 30–12; also see Fig. 31–5, p. 983). It is not clear whether the delay in right ventricular activation is a manifestation of right ventricular volume overload or a true conduction delay in the right bundle branch and peripheral Purkinje system.[76] Left-axis deviation of the P wave in the frontal plane (manifested by a negative P wave in lead III) suggests the presence of a sinus venosus rather than an ostium secundum type of atrial septal defect. Left-axis deviation and superior orientation and counterclockwise rotation of

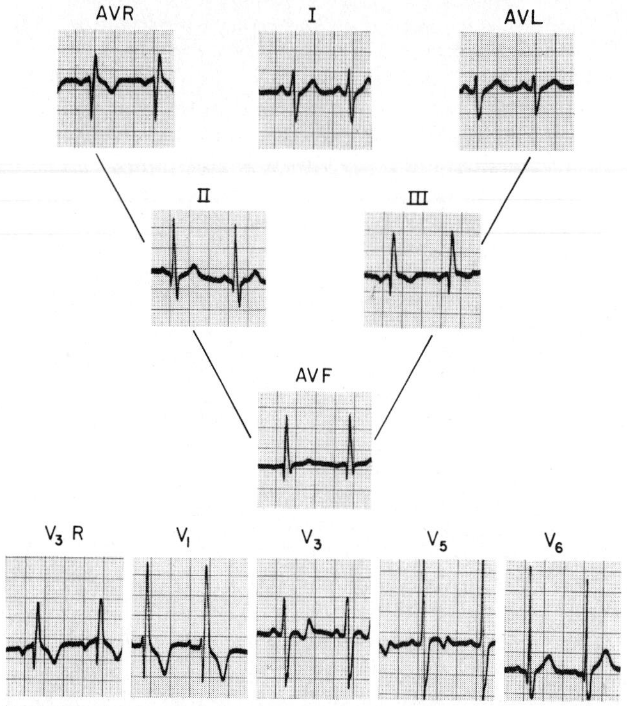

FIGURE 30–12. Typical electrocardiographic tracing in secundum atrial septal defect showing right axis deviation, rSR′ in the right precordial leads and right ventricular hypertrophy. (Courtesy of Delores A. Danilowicz, M.D.)

the QRS loop in the frontal plane suggests the presence of either an ostium primum defect or a secundum atrial septal defect in association with mitral valve prolapse. Prolongation of the P-R interval may be seen with all types of atrial septal defects; the prolonged internodal conduction time may be related to both the increased size of the atrium and the increased distance for internodal conduction produced by the defect itself.[76] *Chest roentgenograms* (Figs. 6–28, 6–29, and 6–30, pp. 157, 158) reveal enlargement of the right atrium and ventricle, dilatation of the pulmonary artery and its branches, and increased pulmonary vascular markings. Dilatation of the proximal portion of the superior vena cava is noted occasionally in patients with a sinus venosus defect. Left atrial dilatation is extremely rare but may be observed when significant mitral regurgitation exists. Echocardiographic features include pulmonary arterial and right ventricular dilatation and anterior systolic (paradoxical) or "flat" interventricular septal motion if significant right ventricular volume overload is present.[34] The defect may be visualized directly by two-dimensional echo imaging, particularly from a subcostal view of the interatrial septum[34] (Fig. 30–13; also see Fig. 5–76, p. 116). Mitral valve prolapse may also be identified by echocardiographic examination (Figs. 5–50–52, p. 106).

In many institutions, two-dimensional echocardiography, supplemented by conventional or color-coded Doppler flow and/or contrast echocardiography, has supplanted cardiac catheterization as the confirmatory test for atrial septal defect.[77–79] Cardiac catheterization is then employed if inconsistencies exist in the clinical data or if significant pulmonary hypertension is suspected.

Diagnosis may be readily confirmed at *cardiac catheterization* by passage of the catheter across the atrial defect. The site at which the catheter crosses, if high in the cardiac silhouette, may suggest a sinus venosus defect; if midseptal, a patent foramen ovale or ostium secundum defect; or, if low, a primum defect.[80] Serial determinations of the oxygen saturation or indicator dilution curve techniques may be used to estimate the magnitude of the shunt. In young patients, pressures on the right side of the heart

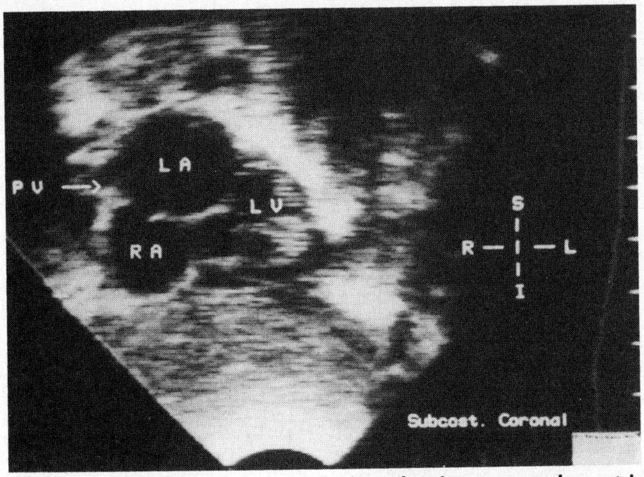

FIGURE 30–13. Subcostal coronal view showing a secundum atrial septal defect between the left atrium (LA) and the right atrium (RA). The right upper pulmonary vein (PV) is seen entering the left atrium. This view is posterior to the major portion of the ventricles; the left ventricle (LV) is seen, but only a small portion of the right ventricle (unlabeled) is apparent. I = inferior, L = left, R = right, S = superior. (Courtesy of Norman Silverman, M.D.)

are often normal, despite a large shunt. When a high oxygen saturation is found in the superior vena cava or when the catheter enters pulmonary veins directly from the right atrium, a sinus venosus defect is likely, and indicator dilution curves and selective angiography will aid in identifying the number and location of the anomalous veins. Partial anomalous pulmonary venous connection, although generally associated with sinus venosus defect, may occasionally accompany secundum defects. Selective left ventricular angiography will identify prolapse of the mitral valve and allow assessment of the magnitude of mitral regurgitation that may be present in such patients.

In contrast to adults, children with sinus venosus or secundum types of atrial septal defect rarely require treatment for heart failure or antiarrhythmic medications for atrial fibrillation or supraventricular tachycardia. Respiratory tract infections should be treated promptly. Although the risk of infective endocarditis is low, antibiotics should be administered prophylactically prior to dental procedures.

MANAGEMENT. *Operative repair*, ideally in patients 2 to 4 years of age, should be advised for all patients with uncomplicated atrial septal defects in whom there is evidence of significant left-to-right shunting, i.e., with pulmonary to systemic flow ratios exceeding approximately 1.5:1.0. The defect is closed by suture or with a patch of prosthetic material with the patient on cardiopulmonary bypass. Earlier surgical repair is definitive treatment for the small number of infants and young children with significant symptoms or congestive failure. The surgical mortality rate is less than 1 per cent, and results are generally excellent. While the mitral valve may be examined directly at operation, it is rarely necessary in childhood to attempt plication or replacement of a ballooning or prolapsing mitral valve. Operation should not be carried out in patients with small defects and trivial left-to-right shunts (pulmonary-to-systemic flow ratio $\leq$ 1.5:1.0) or in those with severe pulmonary vascular disease (pulmonary-to-systemic resistance ratio $\geq$ 0.7:1.0) without a significant left-to-right shunt. Subtle evidence of left ventricular dysfunction may be observed preoperatively at cardiac catheterization in children with isolated large atrial septal defects but without overt left or right ventricular failure.[81] Thus, decreased left ventricular stroke volume and cardiac output have been observed in children with both low and normal left ventricular end-diastolic volumes. In routine catheterization studies carried out on patients whose atrial septal defects were closed during preadolescence or later a residual reduced cardiac output response to intense upright exercise in the absence of residual shunts, arrhythmias, or pulmonary arterial hypertension has been observed.[81, 82] However, normal myocardial function is preserved in patients in whom the defects were closed in early childhood.

Intracardiac electrophysiological studies reveal a high incidence of intrinsic dysfunction of the sinoatrial and atrioventricular nodes, which persists after surgical repair. These intrinsic nodal abnormalities are more common in sinus venosus than in ostium secundum defects,[83] but occur in both varieties.

ATRIOVENTRICULAR SEPTAL DEFECTS

Atrioventricular (AV) septal defects comprise a range of malformations characterized by varying degrees of incomplete development of the inferior portion of the atrial septum, the inflow portion of the ventricular septum, and the atrioventricular valves (Fig. 30–3). These anomalies have also been called endocardial cushion defects and atrioventricular canal defects. The basic defect is a deficiency of the atrioventricular septum which separates the left ventricular inlet from the right atrium; it causes anomalies which range in severity from a small ostium primum atrial septal defect to a complete AV canal, which involves also defects in the interventricular septum and the mitral and tricuspid valves. The latter are often abnormal to varying degrees, with five or six leaflets present of variable size, and variability also in the completeness of their commissures. Often AV septal defects are encountered in association with other congenital abnormalities such as asplenia or polysplenia syndromes, trisomy 21 (Down syndrome), and Ellis–van Creveld syndrome of ectodermal dysplasia and polydactyly.

OSTIUM PRIMUM DEFECT (PARTIAL ATRIOVENTRICULAR CANAL). Ostium primum atrial septal defects lie immediately adjacent to the atrioventricular valves, either of which may be deformed and incompetent. Most often, only the anterior or septal leaflet of the mitral valve is displaced and is commonly cleft; the tricuspid valve is usually not involved. A cleft is often considered to be present in the mitral valve, although it is likely that the valve is in fact a trileaflet structure with the cleft representing an abnormal commissure. The interatrial defect is often large, and the size of the left-to-right interatrial shunt in these patients is controlled by the same factors that exist in patients with ostium secundum atrial septal defect. Moreover, the clinical features are quite similar and consist principally of right ventricular precordial hyperactivity, a wide and persistently split second heart sound, a right ventricular outflow tract systolic ejection murmur, and a middiastolic tricuspid flow rumble. The murmurs of AV valve regurgitation may be audible if either valve is significantly abnormal; usually, however, serious AV valve regurgitation is absent. In the occasional patient, mitral regurgitation is substantial and creates prominent signs of left ventricular overload.

Chest roentgenography usually reveals right atrial and ventricular cardiomegaly, prominence of the right ventricular outflow tract, and increased pulmonary vascular markings. The *electrocardiogram* is characteristic and shows a right ventricular conduction defect accompanied by left-axis deviation and by superior orientation and counterclockwise rotation of the QRS loop in the frontal plane (Fig. 31–5, p. 983).[84] Hemodynamic factors do not appear to be important in producing the characteristic electrocardiogram. Rather, the superior QRS vector in patients with a shortened H-V interval appears to be related to early activation of the posterobasal left ventricular wall; in other patients with a normal conduction time between the bundle of His and the ventricles, the counterclockwise superior inscription of the frontal plane vector appears to be related to late activation of the anterolateral left ventricular wall.[85, 86] A prolonged P-R interval is observed in many patients with an ostium primum atrial septal defect; prolonged internodal conduction may be related to displacement of the AV node in a posteroinferior direction in some patients or to the enlarged right atrium, or both.[87]

Echocardiographic features include enlargement of both the right ventricle and the pulmonary artery, systolic anterior ventricular septal motion, prolonged mitral-septal apposition in diastole, and various abnormalities in mitral valve motion.[88–90] The defect is easily visualized from the precordial apical and subxiphoid positions, with the latter views best demonstrating the relationship between the atrial defect, AV valves, and the interventricular septum (Figs. 30–14 and 5–83, color plate No. 2). Interatrial septal tissue is absent in the region of the crest of the interventricular septum; the trileaflet configuration of the mitral valve may also be identified. The subxiphoid long-axis view of the left ventricular outflow tract exhibits the "gooseneck" deformity in a fashion similar to a right anterior oblique left ventricular angiogram (see Fig. 30–16). The *angiographic features* resemble those in the complete form or atrioventricular canal defect and are discussed below.

COMPLETE ATRIOVENTRICULAR CANAL DEFECT. The complete form of the atrioventricular (AV) septal defect includes, in addition to the ostium primum atrial septal defect, a ventricular septal defect in the posterior basal inlet portion of the ventricular septum and a common AV orifice. The common AV valve usually has six leaflets, left superior and inferior, left and right lateral, and right superior and inferior. The left and right superior leaflets together are often referred to as the "anterior" bridging leaflet. No attachment exists between the left superior and inferior leaflets and the right superior and inferior leaflets. The left superior leaflet may cross the crest of the ventricular septum to reside partially on the right ventricular side. A classification of complete AV canal defect into types A, B, and C reflects the variability and the degree of left superior leaflet bridging of the ventricular septum. Thus, in type A the left superior leaflet is entirely over the left ventricle, and together with the right superior leaflet is attached by chordae tendineae to the crest of the ventricular septum. In type C there is marked rightward displacement of the left superior leaflet, which floats freely over the crest of the ventricular septum and is not attached to it by chordae tendineae. In type B, chordal attachments extend medially to an anomalous papillary muscle adjacent to the septum in the right ventricle.

A high incidence exists (approximately 35 per cent) of additional cardiovascular lesions in patients with common AV canal. Principal among these are tetralogy of Fallot, double-outlet right ventricle, transposition of the great arteries, total anomalous pulmonary venous connection, variable sites of left ventricular outflow tract obstruction, pulmonic stenosis, and persistent left superior vena cava. Moreover, the complete AV canal anomaly is seen commonly in patients with Down syndrome.

Diagnosis. Patients with common AV canal defects present clinically under age one year with a history of frequent respiratory infections and poor weight gain. Heart failure in infancy is extremely common. The *physical findings* are similar to those observed in patients with ostium primum atrial septal defect but may include as well the holosystolic, lower left sternal border murmur of an interventricular communication and/or the decrescendo, holosystolic apical murmur of mitral regurgitation. The *electrocardiographic features* of complete AV canal defects resemble those in the partial ostium primum variety of atrioventricular septal anomalies (Fig. 31–5, p. 983). *Radiographically*, the usual findings are generalized cardiomegaly and engorged pulmonary vessels. Two-dimensional echocardiography is diagnostic (Fig. 30–15).[90] The atrial defect appears as a dropout of echoes from the leftmost portion of the interatrial septum immediately above the AV valves. AV leaflet morphology is best seen from the parasternal and subxiphoid short-axis views, with simultaneously visualized superior and inferior leaflets. The ventricular defect lies beneath the AV valve leaflets. On *hemodynamic study*, patients with persistent common AV canal invariably have elevated pulmonary arterial pressures; beyond age 2 years a significant number of these patients have progressively severe pulmonary vascular obstructive disease. Echocardiographic features are shown in Figure 5–78 (p. 117).

Diagnosis is also established reliably by selective left ventricular *angiocardiography* using rapid injection of relatively large quantities of contrast material. The findings include an absence of the AV septum and a deficiency of the inlet portion of the ventricular septum, with elongation of the left ventricular outflow tract in relationship to the inflow tract. The leaflets of the left AV valve may often be

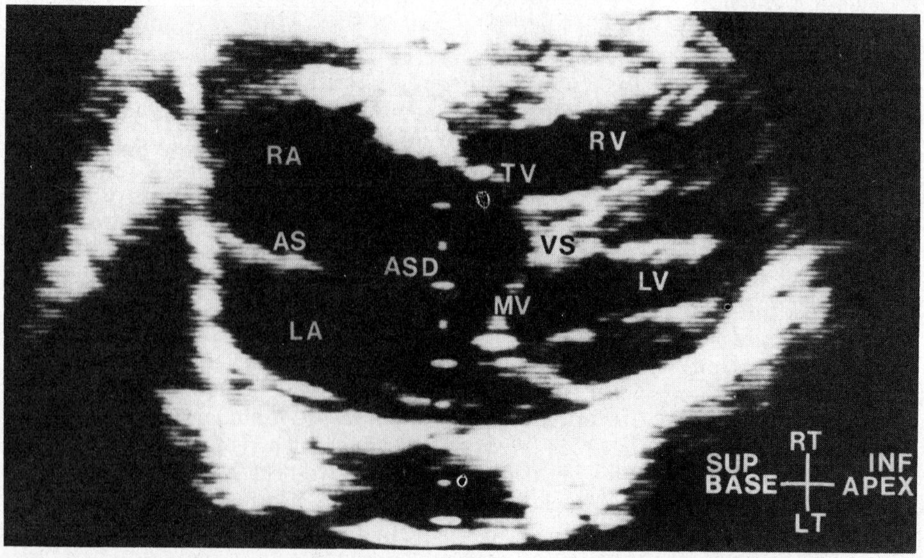

FIGURE 30–14. Subcostal four-chamber view showing an ostium primum atrial septum defect (ASD). There is echo dropout in the inferior portion of the atrial septum (AS). RA = right atrium, LA = left atrium, TV = tricuspal valve, MV = mitral valve, VS = ventricular septum, RV = right ventricle, LV = left ventricle. (Courtesy of Thomas DiSessa, M.D.)

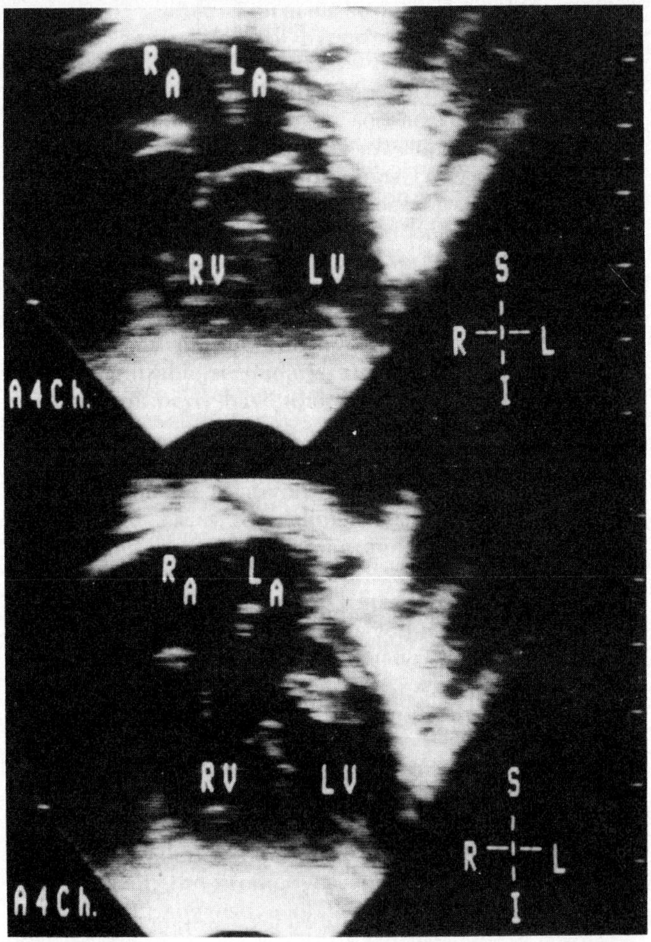

FIGURE 30–15. Apical four-chamber views of a common atrioventricular canal defect. The images are oriented anatomically. In systole, shown in the top panel, the atrioventricular valve leaflet is closed, with no apparent attachment of the atrioventricular valve to the ventricular septum. The interatrial and interventricular septal defects are represented by echo dropout above and below the common AV valve. In diastole, shown in the bottom panel, the AV valve is open, showing the valve resting on the crest of the ventricular septum and the entire defect allowing communication between all four cardiac chambers. RA = right atrium, LA = left atrium, RV = right ventricle, LV = left ventricle. (Courtesy of Norman Silverman, M.D.)

visualized to determine the location and magnitude of valvar incompetence. The aortic valve is elevated and displaced anteriorly relative to the AV valves, changing the relationship between the anterior components of the left AV valve and the aorta which produces a pathognomonic "gooseneck" deformity seen angiographically in diastole (Fig. 30–16). Additional findings include a jet of contrast material from left ventricle directly to right atrium or via mitral regurgitation and left-to-right atrial shunting. Conventional anteroposterior and lateral left ventricular angiographic views may not always differentiate between the partial and complete types of AV canal defects because all have the characteristic "gooseneck" left ventricular outflow tract deformity and because mitral regurgitation into the right atrium may obscure the presence or absence of a defect in the ventricular septum. Axial cine angiography, however, permits a more accurate distinction between types of atrioventricular septal defects, since the hepatoclavicular view helps greatly in separating a left ventricular–right atrial communication and shunt from left ventricular–left atrial regurgitation with subsequent left-to-right atrial shunt. In addition, the long axial oblique view portrays the atrioventricular portion of the ventricular septum.[91]

Management. The complete form of AV canal cardiac decompensation should be controlled initially. If an adequate response to medical therapy occurs early in life, hemodynamic study is indicated at approximately age 3 to 6 months to determine the level of pulmonary vascular resistance, since infants with the complete form of the AV canal defect are at high risk of obstructive pulmonary vascular disease. The level of major shunting should be determined during the initial hemodynamic and angiographic study, since, if it is mainly at the ventricular level, pulmonary artery banding may occasionally be advised for intractable heart failure and failure to thrive. Often, however, there is a significant left ventricular–right atrial shunt either directly or indirectly via mitral regurgitation and left-to-right interatrial shunting, which will be unaffected by pulmonary artery banding and requires complete surgical correction. In most centers primary repair in patients who have intractable heart failure, growth failure, or severe pulmonary hypertension is the preferred approach at any age.[92, 93, 93a] Mild to moderate mitral regurgitation often persists after surgical repair, particularly if significant AV valve incompetence existed preoperatively. Rarely, if left AV leaflet tissue is remarkably deficient or deformed, mitral valve replacement may be required. Recent advances in the surgical approach to complex forms of AV canal defects have greatly improved the outlook for patients born with this malformation. These include a more precise preoperative detection of such anatomical features as additional muscular ventricular septal defects, malalignment of the complete AV canal, and left ventricular hypoplasia.[92] Operative improvement is related primarily to a clearer understanding of the anatomy of this complex lesion and to the ability to reconstruct the left AV valve, often by splitting of papillary muscles and shortening of chordae tendineae, with or without annuloplasty. Most surgeons prefer to close the septal defects with a single patch rather than to separate ventricular and atrial patches. Suture placement is avoided in the region of the AV node and the bundle of His.

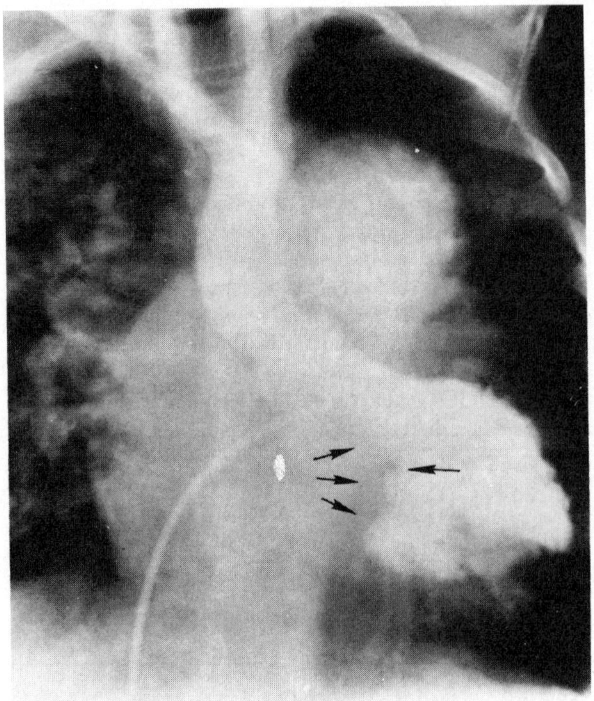

FIGURE 30–16. Left ventriculogram in systole in a patient with an endocardial cushion defect. The concavity of the right border of the left ventricle (left arrows) is caused by the abnormal position of the mitral orifice.

VENTRICULAR SEPTAL DEFECT (VSD)

(See also p. 985)

Among the most prevalent of cardiac malformations, defects of the ventricular septum occur commonly, both as isolated anomalies and in combination with other anomalies. The ventricular septum consists of a fibrous component, the membranous septum, and a muscular portion; the latter has three components—the inlet, trabecular, and outlet parts (Fig. 30–4). Defects result when a deficiency of growth or a failure of alignment or fusion exists of component parts. Most often there is a single opening in the perimembranous portion of the septum, although, as Figure 30–17 shows, a defect may occur anywhere in the interventricular septum. Defects vary in size from barely visible openings to almost complete absence of the interventricular septum. In the extremely common type of perimembranous ventricular septal defect that lies below the infundibular septum, the bundle of His is contiguous with the posterior-inferior aspect of the defect, while the proximal right bundle branch is close to the inferior edge. Supracristal (subpulmonic) ventricular septal defects lie beneath the pulmonic valve and are remote from the conduction system. These are also referred to as anterior malalignment, conal, subaortic outflow, and infundibular defects. They may occur as isolated lesions but more often are combined with other malformations related to defects in truncal development, such as persistent truncus arteriosus, transposed aorta with overriding pulmonary artery (Taussig-Bing variety of double-outlet right ventricle), and complete transposition of the great arteries. If the ventricular defect is posteriorly located in the inlet region just beneath the tricuspid septal leaflet, it is referred to as AV canal type septal defect. Muscular defects, when single, are usually located in the posterior portion of the ventricular septum; they are often multiple, however, and have no predilection for a particular site.[98]

Two-dimensional echocardiography may often identify the type of defect in the ventricular septum.[94–97] Perimembranous ventricular septal defects are identified by septal dropout in the area behind the septal leaflet of the tricuspid valve and below the right border of the aortic annulus. The supracristal or anterior malalignment type of ventricular septal defect appears just below the posterior semilunar valve cusps, entirely superior to the tricuspid valve. The subpulmonary ventricular septal defect appears as echo dropout within the outflow septum, which extends to the pulmonary annulus. One or two of the aortic cusps may be visualized protruding through the defect into the right ventricular outflow tract. The isolated AV canal type of ventricular septal defect extends from the fibrous annulus of the tricuspid valve into the muscular septum, and is often entirely beneath the septal tricuspid leaflet. Muscular defects may appear anywhere throughout the ventricular septum, and may be either single and large, or small and multiple. Anatomical localization of all ventricular septal defects is facilitated by coupling two-dimensional ultrasound images with a Doppler system, and also by superimposing a color-coded direction and velocity of blood flow on the real-time images (Figs. 31–8 and 31–9, color plate No. 4).[95]

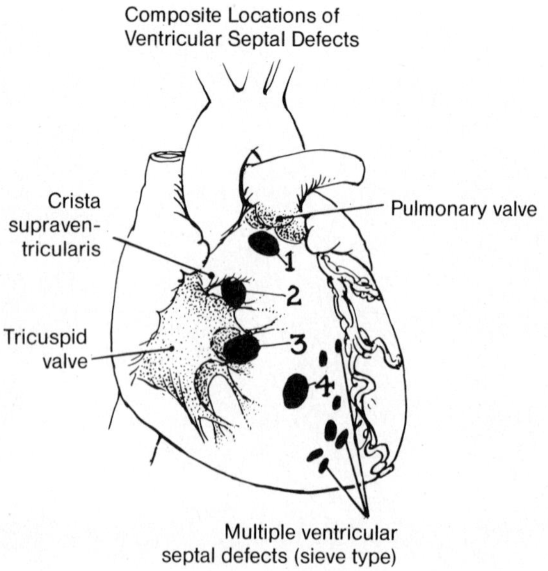

FIGURE 30–17. Anatomical classification of defects of the interventricular septum. Type 1 defects are superoanterior to the crista supraventricularis; Type 2 defects are posteroinferior to the crista supraventricularis; Type 3 defects are located under the septal leaflet of the tricuspid valve; Type 4 defects are multiple and involve the muscular septum. (From Friedman, W. F., et al.: Multiple muscular ventricular septal defects. Circulation *32*:35, 1965, by permission of the American Heart Association, Inc.)

In general, the functional disturbance caused by a ventricular septal defect depends primarily on its size and the status of the pulmonary vascular bed rather than on the location of the defect. A small ventricular septal defect with high resistance to flow permits only a small left-to-right shunt. A large interventricular communication allows a large left-to-right shunt only if there is no pulmonic stenosis or high pulmonary vascular resistance, since these factors also determine shunt flow. Resistance to left ventricular emptying also affects shunt flow because it is an important factor in determining left ventricular pressure. Large defects allow both ventricles to function hemodynamically as a single pumping chamber with two outlets, equalizing the pressure in the systemic and pulmonary circulations. In such patients the magnitude of the left-to-right shunt varies inversely with pulmonary vascular resistance.

A wide spectrum exists in the natural history of ventricular septal defects, ranging from spontaneous closure to congestive cardiac failure and death in early infancy. Within this spectrum are possible development of pulmonary vascular obstruction, right ventricular outflow tract obstruction, aortic regurgitation, and infective endocarditis.[98–107]

INFANCY. It is unusual for a ventricular septal defect to cause difficulties in the immediate postnatal period, although congestive heart failure during the first 6 months of life is a frequent occurrence. Early diagnosis is helpful in order to insure more careful observation of the affected infant.[104] The examining physician usually suspects the diagnosis because of a harsh systolic murmur at the lower left sternal border. The electrocardiogram and chest roentgenogram are within normal limits in the immediate neonatal period because appreciable left-to-right shunting occurs only after the pulmonary vascular resistance decreases as the pulmonary vessels lose their fetal characteristics. It is desirable to follow these infants closely. A ventricular septal defect that either decreases in size or closes completely during the first year of life presents no problems to the practicing physician. Spontaneous closure occurs by age 3 years in approximately 40 per cent of patients born with ventricular septal defect; occasional patients, however, do not experience spontaneous closure until age 8 to 10 years.[100] Closure is more common in patients born with a small ventricular septal defect; nonetheless, approximately 7 per cent of infants with a large defect and congestive heart failure early in life may also experience spontaneous closure. Partial rather than complete closure is common in patients with both large and small ventricular septal defects. Anatomically, reduction of the ventricular septal defect is often based on adherence of the tricuspid valve to the defect, hypertrophy of septal muscle, or ingrowth of fibrous tissue. Rarely, closure of the ventricular septal defect is the result of prolapse of an aortic cusp[105] or infective endocarditis.[106] Some defects close when an aneurysm forms in the ventricular septum.[103] On auscultation a click may be heard in early systole as the aneurysm tenses toward the right; the septal aneurysm may be detected by echocardiography as an anterior systolic bulge in the right ventricular outflow tract. A persistent minute ventricular septal defect is not life-threatening unless infective endocarditis develops. With proper precautions the incidence of this complication is less than 1 per cent.

If a moderate or large defect maintains its size after birth, the net left-to-right shunt increases during the first month of life as pulmonary vascular resistance falls. *Physical examination* during this time usually reveals a thrill along the lower left sternal border, and the holosystolic murmur of flow across the interventricular defect is accompanied by a low-pitched diastolic rumble at the apex, reflecting increased flow across the mitral valve. *Chest roentgenograms* reveal increased pulmonary vascular markings; evidence of left or biventricular hypertrophy may be observed on the electrocardiogram. Infants with a large left-to-right shunt tend to do poorly, with recurrent upper and lower respiratory tract infections, failure to gain weight, and congestive heart failure. Congestive heart failure may be severe and intractable despite intensive medical management.

Management. For these infants we currently recommend primary intracardiac repair of the ventricular septal defect rather than surgical banding of the pulmonary artery[107] in order to reduce pulmonary blood flow and alleviate heart failure. An exception is made for the rare infant with multiple ventricular septal defects and a sieve-like septum who is at higher risk for operative repair. Operation is usually deferred, along with debanding of the pulmonary artery, until the child reaches 3 to 5 years. Primary closure of the ventricular septal defect, preferably through the right atrium, may be performed in infancy employing cardiopulmonary bypass, profound hypothermia and cardiocirculatory arrest, or a combination of the two techniques. Mortality is less than 10 per cent if the defect is isolated and uncomplicated but approaches 25 per cent if multiple anomalies are present.[108]

Fortunately, medical treatment often is successful in controlling congestive heart failure. Nevertheless, these infants should be referred for cardiac catheterization to evaluate pulmonary vascular resistance and to detect associated defects that may require operation, such as patent ductus arteriosus and coarctation of the aorta.

It is of utmost importance to identify patients who may develop irreversible pulmonary vascular obstructive disease (the Eisenmenger reaction).[108–110] Retrospective analyses of children who develop this complication indicate that infants with systemic or near systemic pressures in the pulmonary artery at the time of initial hemodynamic study are most at risk. Recatheterization before age 18 months and a second determination of pulmonary vascular resistance should be performed in these patients in order to decide whether surgical intervention is necessary to prevent development of fixed obliterative changes in the pulmonary vessels. It is likely that multiple factors are involved in the development of pulmonary vascular disease (Ch. 26 and p. 905). The anatomically large ventricular septal defect allows some or all of the systemic pressure to be transmitted to the pulmonary arteries, thereby retarding regression of their muscular media. Medial hypertrophy in the first months of life is responsible for higher pulmonary vascular resistance than would be anticipated for the amount of pulmonary blood flow. The shearing forces created by the high velocity of flow through narrowed pulmonary arterioles cause endothelial damage that is progressive. While an elevation in left atrial pressure may contribute to the rise in pulmonary vascular resistance, it is not an essential factor, since pulmonary venous pressures can be low in patients who later develop pulmonary vascular disease. Nonetheless, pulmonary venous hypertension may also contribute to pulmonary arterial vasoconstriction and thus to increased shear forces. In this same regard, pulmonary vasoconstriction enhancing the risk of pulmonary vascular obstruction may also be caused by hypoxia due to either high altitude or lung disease. At high altitude, large ventricular septal defects have higher pulmonary vascular resistances and smaller shunts than at low altitude.

CHILDHOOD. Beyond the first year of life a variable clinical picture emerges in children with ventricular septal defect.[98–107] If a small defect is present, the child is usually asymptomatic, the electrocardiogram is generally normal, and the chest roentgenogram shows normal or only a mild increase in pulmonary vascular markings. Effort intolerance and fatigue are associated with moderate left-to-right shunts. These children exhibit cardiomegaly with a forceful left ventricular impulse and a prominent systolic thrill along the lower left sternal border. The second heart sound is normally split, with moderate accentuation of the pulmonic component; a third heart sound and rumbling diastolic murmur that reflects increased flow across the mitral valve are audible at the cardiac apex. The characteristic murmur resulting from flow across the defect is harsh and holosystolic, is best heard along the third and fourth interspaces to the left of the sternum, and is widely transmitted over the precordium. A basal midsystolic ejection murmur due to increased flow across the pulmonic valve may also be heard. The electrocardiogram reveals left or combined ventricular hypertrophy, and the chest roentgenogram shows cardiomegaly, left atrial enlargement, and vascular engorgement.

RIGHT VENTRICULAR OUTFLOW TRACT OBSTRUCTION. With time, the clinical picture changes in 5 to 10 per cent of patients with ventricular septal defect and a moderate to large left-to-right shunt early in life. It begins to resemble more closely the tetralogy of Fallot (p. 946), i.e., subvalvular right ventricular outflow tract obstruction due to progressive hypertrophy of the crista supraventricularis develops. Depending on the severity of the latter process, it may result ultimately in reduced blood flow and a right-to-left shunt across the ventricular septal defect. As right ventricular outflow tract obstruction develops, the holosystolic murmur is replaced by the crescendo-decrescendo ejection systolic murmur of pulmonic stenosis, and the pulmonary closure sound becomes softer. Right ventricular hypertrophy is evident on the electrocardiogram, while the chest x-ray shows a reduction in pulmonary vascular markings and a smaller heart size with a right ventricular configuration. Infundibular hypertrophy may progress quite rapidly within the first year of life, but the typical evolution to a clinical picture of cyanotic tetralogy of Fallot often takes 1 to 4 years. In those infants who develop right ventricular outflow obstruction the incidence of spontaneous closure or reduction in size of a ventricular septal defect is low.

AORTIC REGURGITATION (AR). This is a well-described complication of ventricular septal defect that occurs in approximately 5 per cent of patients.[111, 112] It is usually noted after age 5 years when a physician detects the early diastolic blowing murmur and wide pulse pressure of aortic regurgitation while following a patient with a ventricular septal defect. The diagnosis is confirmed readily by Doppler echocardiography. In such patients, aortic regurgitation may become the predominant hemodynamic abnormality. It is of interest that ventricular septal defect with aortic regurgitation is rare in Europe and the United States, with an incidence of approximately 4 per cent of all cases of isolated ventricular septal defect, whereas in Japan the incidence is substantially higher (approximately 10 per cent). In the Japanese, in particular, aortic regurgitation is the result of herniation of an aortic leaflet (usually the right coronary) through a subpulmonic supracristal ventricular septal defect. In these patients, closure of the ventricular septal defect may be all that is required to relieve aortic regurgitation. In many patients, however, especially in the western world, the ventricular septal defect is below the infundibular septum (crista supraventricularis). While aortic leaflet herniation, especially of the right or noncoronary cusp, may occur in some of these patients, quite often aortic regurgitation results from a primary abnormality of the valve, usually one defective commissure. In the latter situation, plication of the elongated leaflet may lessen, but not abolish, the aortic regurgitation; in some patients prosthetic aortic valve replacement may be necessary to provide hemodynamic relief. In most patients with ventricular septal defect and aortic regurgitation, the ventricular septal defect is small to moderate in size, and mild right ventricular outflow tract obstruction exists. The latter is caused either by subpulmonic infundibular stenosis or projection of the herniated aortic cusp into the right ventricular outflow tract. The distinction between types of ventricular septal defect with aortic regurgitation can usually be made by selective left ventricular angiocardiography to define the site of the interventricular communication in combination with retrograde aortography to assess the anatomy and competence of the aortic valve (Fig. 30–18).

Management. Treatment of the patient with ventricular septal defect and aortic regurgitation is controversial. In patients with a large, hemodynamically significant left-to-right shunt, repair of the ventricular septal defect is indicated, but aortic regurgitation is repaired only if at least moderate aortic regurgitation exists. If a supracristal ventricular septal defect without aortic regurgitation is identified at cardiac catheterization in early childhood, a sensible argument for prophylactic closure of the ventricular septal defect can be put forth to prevent the potential complication of aortic valve incompetence. In the presence of moderate or severe aortic regurgitation, valvuloplasty is preferred to valve replacement, in recognition of the fact that the severity of aortic regurgitation may increase in subsequent years and that reoperation with valve replacement may be necessary. Operation should probably be deferred in asymptomatic patients with a subcristal ventricular septal defect and an insignificant left-to-right shunt in whom aortic regurgitation is not severe. If the defect is supracristal in the same clinical setting, its closure may not alleviate the mild degree of aortic incompetence but may retard its progression.

It is rarely necessary to restrict the activities of a child with an isolated ventricular septal defect in any way. Infective bacterial endocarditis is always a threat, and antibiotic prophylaxis for dental procedures and minor surgery is indicated.[113] Respiratory infections require prompt evaluation and treatment. These children should be seen at least once or twice yearly to detect changes in the clinical picture that suggest the development of pulmonary vascular obliterative changes.

PULMONARY VASCULAR OBSTRUCTION. If a child who previously had a loud murmur and thrill associated with poor growth suddenly has a growth spurt, fewer respiratory infections, and a diminution of the intensity of the cardiac murmur and disappearance of the thrill, he or she may be developing severe obliterative changes in the pulmonary vascular bed. An increase in intensity of the pulmonic component of the second heart sound, a reduction in heart size on chest roentgenograms, and more pronounced right ventricular hypertrophy on the electrocardiogram are also noted. These changes occur because the increased pulmonary vascular resistance causes a decrease in the left-to-right shunt. If these changes are suspected, cardiac catheterization should be repeated; if they are confirmed, prompt surgical repair is indicated before an inoperable predominant right-to-left shunt ensues. If operation is performed under age 2 years, pulmonary vascular resistance may be expected to fall to normal levels (Fig 30–19).[110] In older patients the degree to which pulmonary vascular resistance is elevated before operation is a critical factor determining prognosis. If the pulmonary vascular resistance is one-third or less of the systemic value, progressive pulmonary vascular disease after operation is unusual. However, if a moderate-to-severe increase in pulmonary vascular resistance exists preoperatively, either no change or progression of pulmonary vascular disease is common postoperatively. Moreover, the presence of increased pulmonary vascular resistance results in a higher immediate postoperative mortality rate for closure of ventricular septal defect. These observations make it clear that a large ventricular septal defect should be approached surgically very early in life when pulmonary vascular disease is still reversible or has not yet developed.

MISCELLANEOUS VENTRICULAR DEFECTS. Unusual forms of ventricular septal defect include multiple muscular defects and left ventricular–right atrial communications. Defects in the muscular ventricular septum frequently are multiple small fenestrations that produce a large net left-to-right shunt.[98] Their recognition is a necessary preliminary to successful operation, since incomplete repair may result in postoperative cardiac failure and death. A shunt from the left ventricle to right atrium may occur with a ventricular septal defect in the most superior portion of the ventricular septum, since the tricuspid valve is lower than the mitral valve. The clinical, electrocardiographic, and radiological findings in these patients do not differ appreciably from

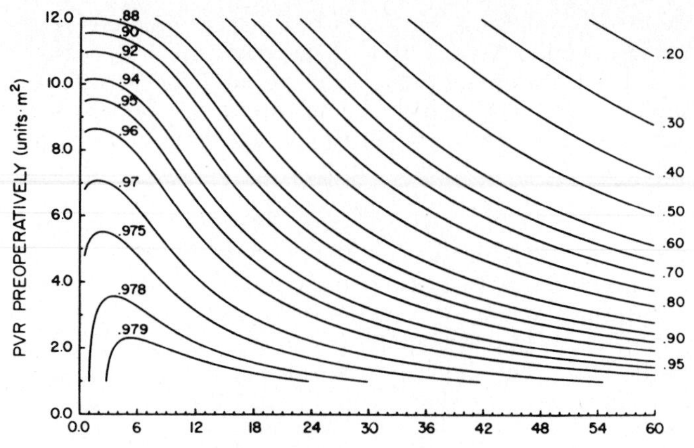

FIGURE 30–19. Probability of overall surgical "cure" after repair of a single large ventricular septal defect; cure is defined as 5 or more years postoperative survival and pulmonary artery mean pressure less than 25 mm Hg. The contour lines are constructed according to the combined effect of age at operation and preoperative pulmonary vascular resistance, e.g., 95 per cent cure is anticipated if operation is performed in the first year with pulmonary vascular resistance (PVR) of 6 units. (From Kirklin, J. W., and Barratt-Boyes, B. G.: Cardiac Surgery. New York, John Wiley & Sons, 1986, p. 649.)

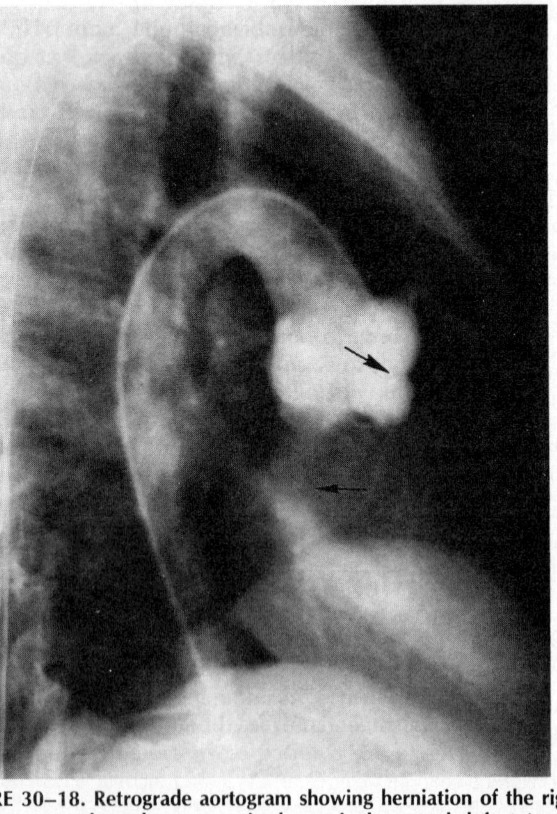

FIGURE 30–18. Retrograde aortogram showing herniation of the right coronary cusp through a supracristal ventricular septal defect (upper arrow) and the jet of aortic regurgitation (lower arrow). (Courtesy of Robert White, M.D.)

those of a simple ventricular septal defect, although right atrial enlargement may provide a clue to correct diagnosis of left ventricular–right atrial communication. The pathophysiology of single or common ventricle (p. 965) may resemble that of a large ventricular septal defect, although these defects are dissimilar embryologically. The single chamber frequently is the morphological left ventricle; malposition of the great arteries is quite common. There may be no detectable cyanosis if selective streaming and increased pulmonary blood flow rather than complete mixing occurs. Pulmonary hypertension invariably is present unless pulmonic stenosis exists. It is imperative to differentiate a single ventricle from a large ventricular septal defect by echocardiography[95, 96] and angiography[91] because the operative approaches to the former malformation require a complex septation technique or the atriopulmonary Fontan connection.

MANAGEMENT OF VENTRICULAR SEPTAL DEFECT. When clinical findings suggest a moderate shunt but no pulmonary hypertension, elective hemodynamic evaluation should be advised between ages 3 and 6 years. Of prime importance in the hemodynamic evaluation is a determination of pressure and blood flow in the pulmonary artery.[114] Surgical treatment is not recommended for children who have normal pulmonary arterial pressures with small shunts (pulmonary-systemic flow ratios of less than 1.5 to 2.0:1). In such patients the remaining risk of infective endocarditis[114] does not exceed the risk of operation. Moreover, although the inherent risk of operation is small, the possibility of postoperative heart block, infection, or other complications of operation and cardiopulmonary bypass dictates a conservative approach when the cardiac defect may be well tolerated for life.

With larger shunts, elective operation may be advised before the child enters school, thus minimizing any subsequent distinction of these patients from their normal classmates (Fig. 30–19). A total assessment of the psychosocial dynamics of the family and child is obviously helpful in determining the proper age for elective operation in each patient.

Complete heart block is the most significant surgically induced conduction system abnormality, occurring immediately following surgery in less than 1 per cent of patients. Late-onset complete heart block is occasionally a problem, especially in the 10 to 25 per cent of patients whose postoperative electrocardiographic findings show complete right bundle branch block with left anterior hemiblock.[115] When the latter electrocardiographic pattern is observed in patients with transient complete heart block in the early postoperative period, electrophysiological studies should be conducted at postoperative cardiac catheterization. It would appear that patients presenting postoperatively with right bundle branch block and left anterior hemiblock fall into two different populations, defined by either peripheral damage to the conduction system or damage to the bundle of His or its proximal branches.[116] The former has not been associated with transient postoperative complete heart block, and these patients have been found to have a generally benign course. Trifascicular damage may be demonstrated in the latter population by a prolonged H-V interval, which implies a higher risk of complete heart block later in life. Although the prophylactic use of permanent pacemakers in asymptomatic patients with evidence of trifascicular damage is not currently recommended, this group certainly requires careful follow-up and continued study.

Treadmill exercise studies in patients who preoperatively had normal or only moderately elevated pulmonary vascular resistance and essentially normal postoperative cardiac catheterization data may uncover late abnormalities in circulatory function.[117, 118] Despite normal cardiac output at rest, an impaired cardiac output response to exercise is noted in some. Moreover, despite a normal pulmonary arterial pressure at rest, markedly abnormal increases in pulmonary arterial pressure may be noted during exercise. These findings may be related to abnormal left ventricular function after closure of the ventricular septal defect and/or to persistent pathological changes in the pulmonary arterioles or to abnormal pulmonary vascular reactivity.[119] A direct relationship exists between age at operation and the magnitude of the pulmonary arterial pressure response to intense exercise, suggesting that early operation may prevent permanent impairment of the functional capacity of the myocardium and pulmonary vascular bed.

Occasionally a child may come to medical attention who has already developed pulmonary vascular obstruction and a net right-to-left shunt across the ventricular septal defect. Symptoms may consist of exertional dyspnea, chest pain, syncope, and hemoptysis; the right-to-left shunt leads to cyanosis, clubbing, and polycythemia. At present there is little to offer this group of patients other than continuing support to the patient and family.

PATENT DUCTUS ARTERIOSUS

(See also p. 993)

The ductus arteriosus exists normally in the fetus as a widely patent vessel connecting the pulmonary trunk and the descending aorta just distal to the left subclavian artery (Fig. 30–5). In the fetus most of the output of the right ventricle bypasses the unexpanded lungs via the ductus arteriosus and enters the descending aorta where it travels to the placenta, the fetal organ of oxygenation. Until recently it was assumed that during fetal life the ductus arteriosus was a passively open channel that constricted postnatally by means of undefined molecular mechanisms in response to the abrupt rise in arterial pO_2 accompanying the first breath of life.[120] Even in utero the lumen of the ductus arteriosus may be influenced by vasoactive substances, particularly prostaglandins.[62, 63, 121–123] Thus, inhibition of prostaglandin synthesis causes profound constriction of the ductus arteriosus in the mammalian fetus that may be reversed by administration of vasodilatory E-type prostaglandins. Initial contraction and functional closure of the ductus arteriosus immediately after birth is related both to the sudden increase in arterial oxygen saturation that accompanies ventilation and to changes in the synthesis and metabolism of vasoactive eicosanoids. Intimal proliferation and fibrosis proceed more gradually, so that anatomical closure may take as long as several weeks for completion.

The ductus arteriosus is a unique structure after birth, since its patency may, on the one hand, result in cardiac decompensation but may, on the other hand, provide the only life-sustaining conduit to preserve systemic or pulmonary arterial blood flow in the presence of certain cardiac malformations.[60] Appreciable left-to-right shunting across the patent ductus arteriosus frequently complicates the clinical course of infants born prematurely.[27] The ductal shunt has been implicated specifically in the deterioration of pulmonary function in infants with the respiratory distress syndrome in whom severe congestive heart failure is often unresponsive to digitalis and diuretics.[63]

A distinction should be made between patency of the ductus arteriosus in the *preterm* infant, who lacks the normal mechanisms for postnatal ductal closure because of immaturity, and the full-term newborn, in whom patency of the ductus is a true congenital malformation, related most likely to a primary anatomical defect of the elastic tissue within the wall of the ductus.[124] In the former circumstance, delayed spontaneous closure of the ductus may be anticipated if the infant does not succumb to the cardiopulmonary difficulties caused by the ductus itself or to some lethal complication of prematurity, such as hyaline membrane disease, intraventricular hemorrhage, or necrotizing enterocolitis. In similar fashion, some full-term newborns have persistent patency of the ductus arteriosus for weeks or months because their relative hypoxemia contributes to vasodilatation of the channel. In the latter category are infants born at high altitude; those born with congenital malformations causing hypoxemia, such as pulmonic atresia with and without ventricular septal defect; or malformations in which ductal flow supplies the systemic circulation, such as hypoplastic left heart syndrome, interruption of the aortic arch, or some examples of coarctation of the aorta syndrome. In the clinical settings in which the ductus preserves pulmonary blood flow, the essentially inevitable spontaneous closure of the vessel is associated with profound clinical deterioration. The latter may be reversed medically within the first 4 to 5 days of life by infusion of prostaglandin E_1 intravenously. By dilating the constricted ductus arteriosus, this results in a temporary increase in arterial blood oxygen tension and oxygen saturation and correction of acidemia.[60] These infants can then undergo operative repair or a palliative systemic-pulmonary anastomosis, under more optimal circumstances. Pharmacological dilation of the ductus arteriosus is also effective in the preoperative restoration of systemic blood flow and the alleviation of heart failure, especially in infants with aortic coarctation, and in infants with complete transposition of the great arteries in whom intercirculatory mixing is augmented.[59]

PREMATURE INFANTS. In most, if not all, preterm infants under 1500 grams birthweight, persistence of a patent ductus arteriosus is prolonged, and in approximately one-third of these infants a large aorticopulmonary shunt is responsible for significant cardiopulmonary deterioration.[63] Radiographic, echocardiographic, and Doppler ultrasound signs of significant left-to-right shunting usually precede the appearance of physical findings suggesting ductal patency. A significant increase in the cardiothoracic ratio is seen on sequential radiographs as well as increased pulmonary arterial markings progressing to perihilar and generalized pulmonary edema. Serial echocardiographic evaluations that demonstrate increases in left ventricular enddiastolic and left atrial dimensions, especially when correlated with the aforementioned radiographic signs, are highly accurate in detecting a large shunt.[125, 126] The clinical findings include bounding peripheral pulses, an infraclavicular and interscapular systolic murmur (occasionally a continuous murmur), precordial hyperactivity, hepatomegaly, and either multiple episodes of apnea and bradycardia or respirator dependency. Cardiac catheterization carries a high risk in the preterm infant and is rarely indicated unless the diagnosis is obscure.

Management of the preterm infant with a patent ductus arteriosus varies, depending upon the magnitude of shunting and the severity of hyaline membrane disease, since the ductus may contribute importantly to mortality in the respiratory distress syndrome. Intervention in an asymptomatic infant with a small left-to-right shunt is unnecessary, since the patent ductus arteriosus will almost invariably undergo spontaneous closure and will not require late surgical ligation and division. Those infants who demonstrate unmistakable signs of a significant ductal left-to-right shunt during the course of the respiratory distress syndrome are often unresponsive to medical measures to control congestive heart failure and require closure of the patent ductus arteriosus in order to survive. These infants are best managed within the first 2 to 7 days of life by pharmacological inhibition of prostaglandin synthesis with indomethacin to constrict and close the ductus[127–131]; surgical ligation is required in the approximately 10 per cent of infants unresponsive to indomethacin.[132] Early intervention is advised in order to reduce the likelihood of bronchopulmonary dysplasia related to prolonged respirator and oxygen dependency. Less often, indications for pharmacological or surgical closure of the ductus consist of life-threatening episodes of apnea and bradycardia or a prolonged failure to gain weight and grow.

FULL-TERM INFANTS AND CHILDREN. In full-term newborns and older infants and children, patency of the ductus arteriosus occurs particularly in females and in the offspring of pregnancies complicated by first-trimester rubella. Although most frequent in isolated form, the anomaly may coexist with other malformations, particularly coarctation of the aorta, ventricular septal defect, pulmonic stenosis, and aortic stenosis. Flow across the ductus is determined by the pressure relationship between the aorta and the pulmonary artery and by the cross-sectional area and length of the ductus itself.[133] Most commonly, pulmonary pressures are normal, and a persistent gradient and shunt from aorta to pulmonary artery exist throughout the cardiac cycle. Physical examination reveals a characteristic thrill and a continuous "machinery" murmur with a late systolic accentuation at the upper left sternal border. The left atrium and left ventricle enlarge to accommodate the increased pulmonary venous return, and flow murmurs across the mitral and aortic valves may be detected. With significant left-to-right shunting, the runoff of blood through the ductus causes a widened systemic pulse pressure and bounding peripheral pulses. The hemodynamic abnormality is reflected electrocardiographically by left ventricular and occasionally left atrial hypertrophy, and radiologically by left atrial hypertrophy, and radiologically by left atrial and ventricular enlargement, and prominent ascending aorta and pulmonary artery, and pulmonary vascular engorgement. The clinical diagnosis may be difficult when the findings do not conform to the classic presentation.[134] As mentioned above, disappearance of the diastolic component of the murmur is common in premature infants because higher pulmonary arterial diastolic pressures exist at that age. In older patients both heart failure and pulmonary hypertension are associated with a reduction in the pressure gradient across the ductus arteriosus and result in atypical systolic murmurs. When severe pulmonary vascular obstructive disease results in reversal of flow through the ductus and preferential shunting of unoxygenated blood to the descending aorta, the toes, rather than the fingers, may show cyanosis and clubbing.

The full-term infant with patent ductus arteriosus may survive for a number of years, although occasionally a large defect results in heart failure and pulmonary edema early in life. The leading causes of death in older children are infective endocarditis and heart failure. Beyond the third decade severe pulmonary vascular obstruction has been known to cause aneurysmal dilatation, calcification, and rupture of the ductus.[134]

The patent ductus can usually be visualized directly by two-dimensional echocardiography (Figs. 30–20 and 5–81 and 5–82, p. 118); range-gated pulse Doppler echocardiography shows the characteristic flow abnormalities across the ductus, as well as a continuous flow disturbance in the pulmonary artery.[126] Cardiac catheterization may be indicated when additional lesions or pulmonary vascular obstruction is suspected. In the absence of severe pulmonary vascular disease with predominant right-to-left shunting

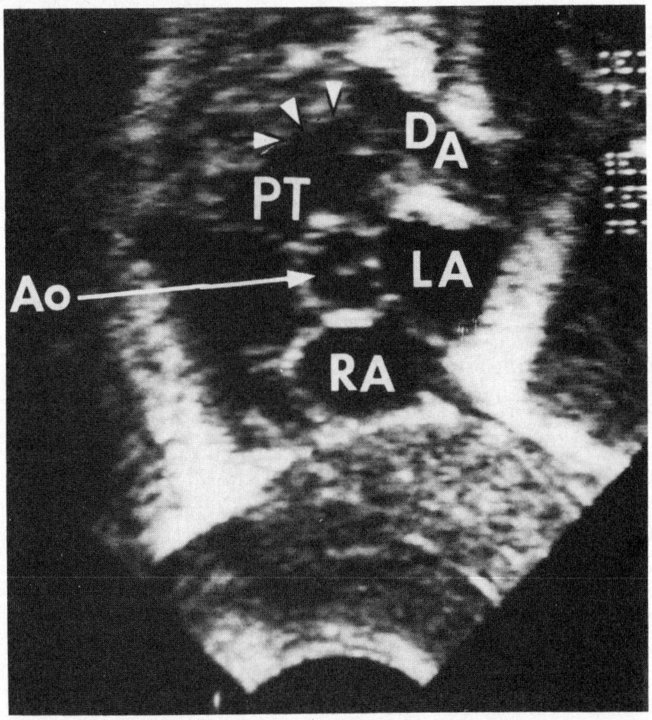

FIGURE 30–20. Parasternal short-axis view of a patent ductus arteriosus (arrowheads) in an infant. The pulmonic valve is the linear echo just beneath the pulmonary trunk (PT). AO = aortic valve, DA = descending aorta, RA = right atrium, LA = left atrium. (From Perloff, J.: The Clinical Recognition of Congenital Heart Disease, 3rd ed. Philadelphia, W. B. Saunders Company, 1986.)

the anatomical presence of a patent ductus is generally considered sufficient indication for operation. Ligation or division of the ductus carries a low risk, whether performed electively in the asymptomatic child or at any age if symptoms are present. The operative risk is reduced if heart failure can be compensated by medical measures before surgery. Operation should be deferred for several months in patients treated successfully for infective endarteritis because the ductus may remain somewhat edematous and friable. Rarely, when the infection will not subside with intensive antibiotic treatment, surgical ligation may be necessary to eradicate the infection.

AORTICOPULMONARY SEPTAL DEFECT

Aorticopulmonary window or fenestration, partial truncus arteriosus, and aortic septal defect are other designations applied to this relatively uncommon anomaly. Septation of the aortopulmonary trunk occurs by fusion of the conotruncal ridges (Fig. 30–4). The right and left sixth aortic arches, destined to become the pulmonary arteries, join the pulmonary artery to complete great artery development (Fig. 30–5). Congenital defects between the ascending aorta and the pulmonary artery result from faulty development of this area during embryonic life. The typical aortopulmonary septal defect results because of incomplete fusion of the distal aortal-pulmonary septum.[134a, 135] Malalignment of the conotruncal ridges results in unequal partitioning of the aortopulmonary trunk, which may result in partial or complete fusion of the right pulmonary artery to the aorta. The usual defect consists of a communication between the aorta and pulmonary artery just above the semilunar valves. Persistent patency of the ductus arteriosus is an associated lesion in 10 to 15 per cent of cases. Less common accompanying cardiovascular lesions include ventricular septal defect, aortic origin of the right pulmonary artery, coarctation of the aorta, and right aortic arch. Aorticopulmonary septal defects are usually large and are accompanied by severe pulmonary arterial hypertension.

PHYSICAL EXAMINATION. The pulses are typically bounding, like those of a large patent ductus arteriosus. However, the murmur is rarely continuous, and a basal systolic murmur is most common.[136] Cardiomegaly is present, and pulmonary hypertension is reflected in a loud and palpable sound of pulmonary valve closure. Aorticopulmonary septal defect should be suspected whenever a large shunt into the pulmonary artery is demonstrated at catheterization. Diagnosis of the anomaly and its distinction from patent ductus and persistent truncus arteriosus can usually be done by two-dimensional echocardiography, but definitive identification of the AP window and associated malformations requires hemodynamic study and selective angiocardiography with the injection of contrast material into the left ventricle and/or the root of the aorta (Fig. 30–21). Although occasional patients may survive to adulthood with uncorrected aorticopulmonary septal defect, most will die early in life unless surgical treatment is undertaken. Operative correction is indicated in all symptomatic infants when the diagnosis is made. Elective repair is advised at 3 to 6 months. Profound hypothermic total circulatory arrest or total cardiopulmonary bypass is required, and the defect is closed via a transaortic approach, usually with a prosthetic patch.[137]

PERSISTENT TRUNCUS ARTERIOSUS

Persistent truncus arteriosus is a rare but serious anomaly in which a single vessel forms the outlet of both ventricles and gives rise to the systemic, pulmonary, and coronary arteries.[138, 139] The defect results from failure of septation of the embryonic truncus by the infundibular truncal ridges (Fig. 30–4). It is always accompanied by a ventricular septal defect and frequently by a right-sided aortic arch. The ventricular septal defect is due to the absence or underdevelopment of the distal portion of the pulmonary infundibulum. The truncal valve is usually tricuspid but is quadricuspid in approximately one-third of patients and, rarely, bicuspid. Truncal valve regurgitation and truncal valve stenosis are each seen in 10 to 15 per cent of patients. There may be a single coronary artery, displacement of the coronary ostia (usually the left ostium posteriorly), or a single posterior descending coronary artery arising from the right coronary or, less often, from the left circumflex artery, especially in patients with a single coronary artery.[140]

Truncus malformations may be classified either anatomically according to the mode of origin of pulmonary vessels from the common trunk or from a functional point of view, based on the magnitude of blood flow to the lungs.[141] In the common type (type I) of truncus arteriosus malformation a partially separate pulmonary trunk of varying length exists because of the presence of an incompletely formed aorticopulmonary septum (Fig. 30–22). The pulmonary trunk is usually very short and gives rise to left and right pulmonary arteries. When the aorticopulmonary septum is absent, there is no discrete main pulmonary artery component, and both pulmonary artery branches arise

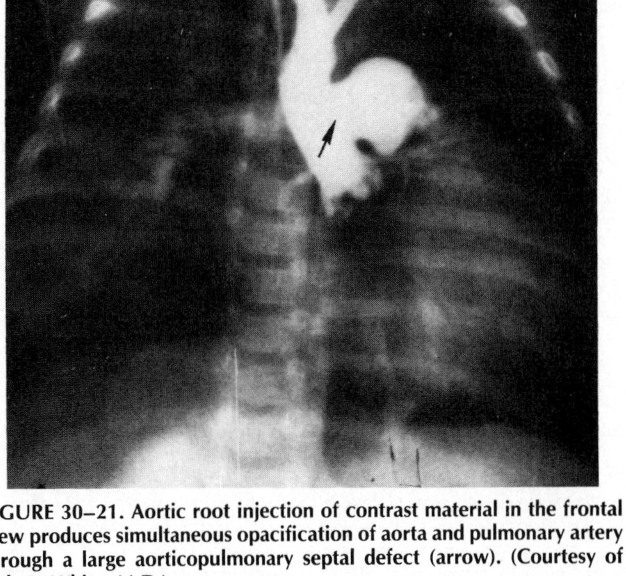

FIGURE 30–21. Aortic root injection of contrast material in the frontal view produces simultaneous opacification of aorta and pulmonary artery through a large aorticopulmonary septal defect (arrow). (Courtesy of Robert White, M.D.)

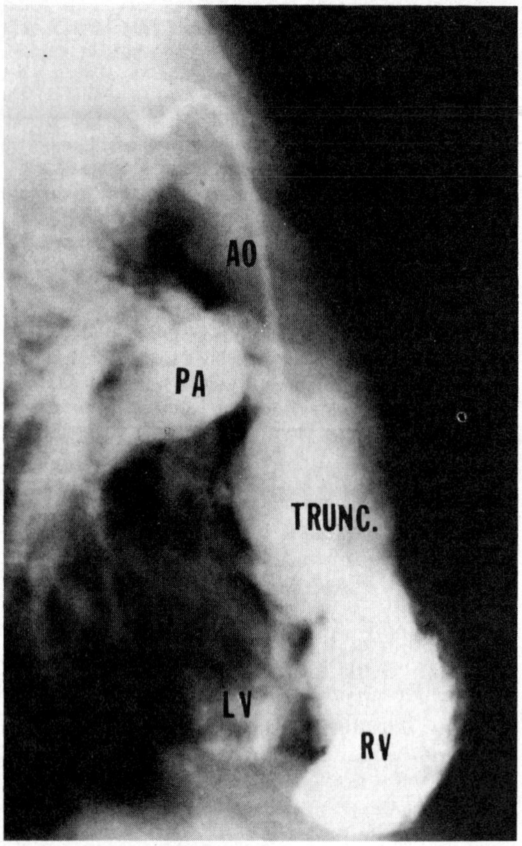

FIGURE 30–22. Right ventriculogram in the lateral view in a patient with type I truncus arteriosus. The contrast agent enters the left ventricle (LV) across a ventricular septal defect. The pulmonary artery (PA) arises directly from the persistent truncus arteriosus (TRUNC). AO = aorta, RV = right ventricle. (Courtesy of Robert White, M.D.)

directly from the truncus. In type II, each pulmonary artery arises separately but close to the other from the posterior aspect of the truncus. In type III, each pulmonary artery arises from the lateral aspect of the truncus. Less commonly, one pulmonary artery branch may be absent, with collateral arteries supplying the lung that does not receive a pulmonary artery branch from the truncus. Truncus arteriosus malformation should not be confused with "pseudotruncus arteriosus," which is the severe form of tetralogy of Fallot with pulmonary atresia in which the single aorta arises from the heart accompanied by a remnant of atretic pulmonary artery (p. 946).

Pulmonary blood flow is governed by the size of the pulmonary arteries and the pulmonary vascular resistance. In infancy, pulmonary blood flow is usually excessive, since pulmonary vascular resistance is not greatly increased. Thus, despite an obligatory admixture of systemic and pulmonary venous blood in the common trunk, only minimal cyanosis is present. Rarely, pulmonary blood flow is restricted by hypoplastic or stenotic pulmonary arteries arising from the truncus. Pulmonary vascular obstruction usually does not restrict pulmonary blood flow before 1 year of age.[142] Hence, the infant with truncus arteriosus usually presents with mild cyanosis coexisting with the cardiac findings of a large left-to-right shunt. Symptoms of heart failure and poor physical development usually appear in the first weeks or months of life. The most frequent physical findings include cardiomegaly, a systolic ejection sound accompanied by a thrill, a loud single second heart sound, a harsh systolic murmur, and a low-pitched middiastolic rumbling murmur and bounding pulses.

Truncal valve incompetence is suggested by the presence of a diastolic decrescendo murmur at the base of the heart.[143] The physical findings are quite different if pulmonary blood flow is restricted by either high pulmonary vascular resistance or pulmonary arterial stenosis: cyanosis is prominent, congestive failure is rare, and only a short systolic ejection may be audible accompanied occasionally by continuous murmurs posteriorly of bronchial collateral flow. Left ventricular hypertrophy alone or in combination with right ventricular hypertrophy is present electrocardiographically when a prominent left-to-right shunt exists; right ventricular hypertrophy is observed in patients with restricted pulmonary blood flow. The radiographic findings depend upon the hemodynamic circumstances. Gross cardiomegaly with left or combined ventricular enlargement, left atrial enlargement, and a small or absent main pulmonary artery segment with pulmonary vascular engorgement are the usual radiographic features. A right aortic arch is common (25 to 30 per cent of patients). When pulmonary blood flow is reduced, both heart size and pulmonary vascular markings are less prominent.

The *echocardiographic* features of truncus arteriosus (Fig. 30–23) include the detection of a large truncal root overriding the ventricular septum, truncal valve abnormalities, an increase in the right ventricular dimension, and mitral valve–truncal root continuity. The dimension of the left atrium determined echocardiographically provides a good index of pulmonary flow. Differentiation between truncus arteriosus and tetralogy of Fallot by ultrasound may be difficult unless the separate origin can be identified of pulmonary arteries or via a single trunk from the ascending portion of a single arterial root (Fig. 30–27). Diagnosis should be suspected at cardiac catheterization if the catheter fails to enter the central pulmonary arteries from the right ventricle. Selective angiocardiography and retrograde aortography are necessary to establish a precise diagnosis and to reveal the common trunk arising from the heart and the origin of the pulmonary arteries from the truncus.

The early fatal course as well as early development of pulmonary vascular obstructive disease in patients surviving infancy is responsible for the poor prognosis associated with truncus arteriosus. In infants and young children with large left-to-right shunts, surgical banding of one or both pulmonary arteries to reduce pulmonary flow has been employed with little success. Corrective operation is preferred before age 3 to 6 months to avoid the development of severe pulmonary vascular obstructive disease.[144, 145]

SURGICAL TREATMENT. Operation consists of closure of the ventricular septal defect, leaving the aorta arising from the left ventricle; the pulmonary arteries are excised from their truncus origin and a valve-containing prosthetic conduit or aortic homograft valve conduit is used to establish continuity between the right ventricle and the pulmo-

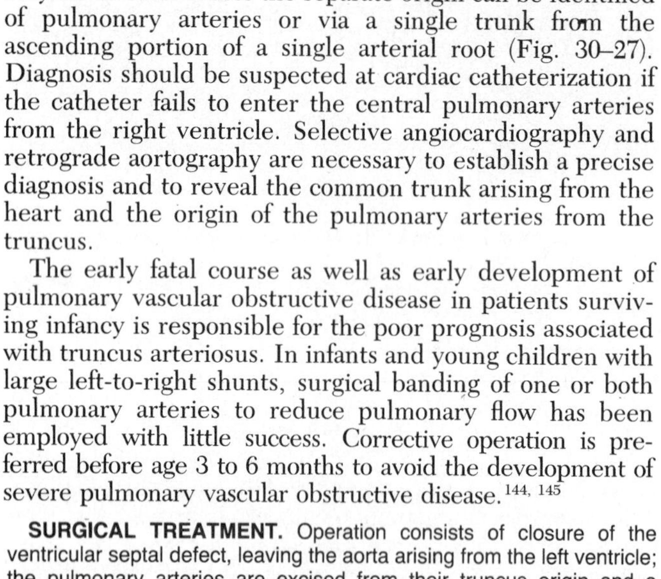

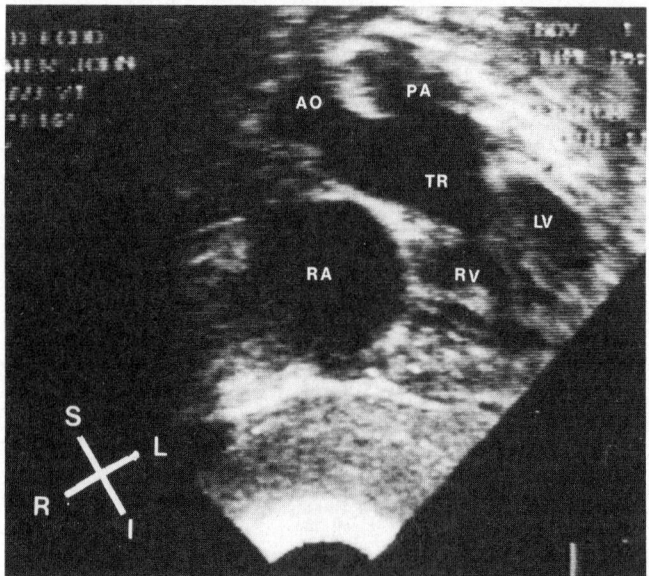

FIGURE 30–23. Truncus arteriosus, shown by a subcostal view with superior angulation of the transducer to image the truncal root (TR). The tricuspid valve is closed in ventricular systole. The truncal root sits above both the right ventricle (RV) and left ventricle (LV). The pulmonary artery (PA) arises directly from the truncus. AO = aorta, RA = right atrium.

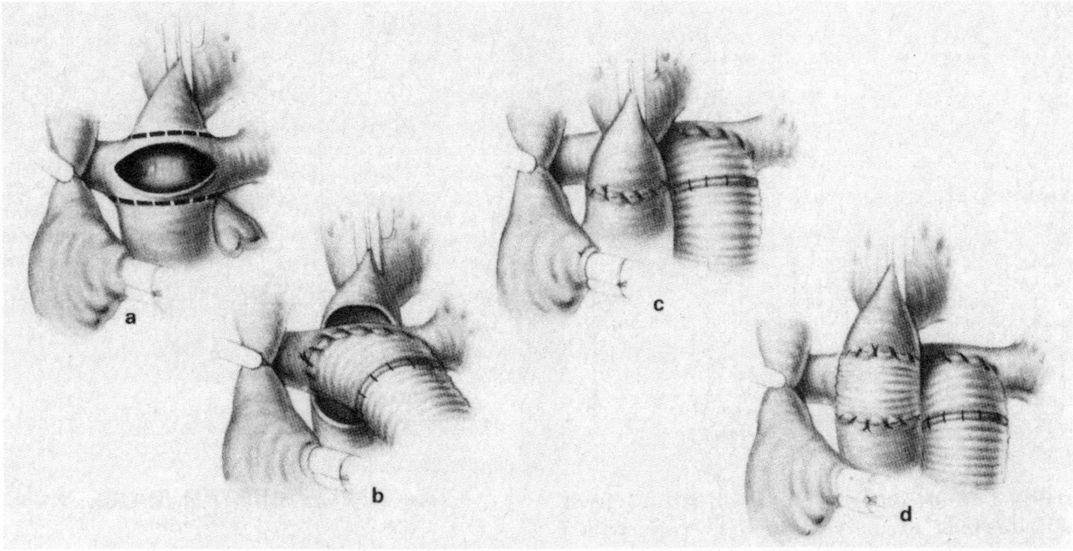

FIGURE 30–24. Operative correction of truncus arteriosus, type III. The pulmonary arteries arise separately from the truncus. An anterior incision is made and a segment of aorta containing the orifices of both pulmonary arteries is excised from the truncus (a). The cuff of tissue containing the two pulmonary arteries is anastomosed to an extracardiac valved conduit (b). Aortic continuity is restored by direct suture (c), or by interposing a preclotted graft (d). The diagram does not show closure of the ventricular septal defect. (From Stark, J., and DeLeval, M.: Surgery for Congenital Heart Defects. New York, Grune and Stratton, 1983, p. 420.)

nary arteries (Fig. 30–24). Truncal valve regurgitation significantly enhances the risk of corrective surgery, since valve replacement is associated with significantly increased surgical mortality. Patients with only one pulmonary artery are especially prone to early development of severe pulmonary vascular disease but otherwise are not at increased risk from surgery. With truncus arteriosus defects, the possible inequalities of pressure and flow between the two pulmonary arteries often make precise calculation of pulmonary resistance difficult. Corrective operation may be performed in patients with at least one adequate pulmonary artery having low distal pressure or arteriolar resistance. Conversely, significant systemic arterial desaturation in a patient with two pulmonary arteries and with neither pulmonary artery stenosis nor a previous pulmonary artery band signifies that high pulmonary vascular resistance exists and that the condition is probably inoperable. It is not yet clear how often and at what age the conduit between the right ventricle and pulmonary artery must be replaced with a larger prosthesis either because of growth of the patient in whom a small conduit causes eventual obstruction, heterograft valve degeneration, or obstruction created by neointimal proliferation within a prosthetic conduit. When operation is carried out with a conduit in the first year of life, conduit replacement is often required within 3 to 5 years.

CORONARY ARTERIOVENOUS FISTULA

(See also p. 1001)

Coronary arteriovenous fistula is an unusual anomaly that consists of a communication between one of the coronary arteries.[146] The right coronary artery, or its branches, is the site of the fistula in approximately 55 per cent of the cases; the left coronary artery is involved in about 35 per cent, and both coronary arteries in 5 per cent. Connections between the coronary system and a cardiac chamber appear to represent persistence of embryonic intertrabecular spaces and sinusoids. The majority of these fistulas drain into the right ventricle, right atrium, or coronary sinus; fistulous communication to the pulmonary artery, left atrium, or left ventricle is much less frequent. Most often the shunt through the fistula is of small magnitude, and myocardial blood flow is not compromised.[147] Potential complications include pulmonary hypertension and congestive heart failure if a large left-to-right shunt exists, bacterial endocarditis, rupture or thrombosis of the fistula or an associated arterial aneurysm, and myocardial ischemia distal to the fistula due to decreased coronary blood flow.

The majority of patients are asymptomatic and are referred because of a cardiac murmur that is loud, superficial, and continuous at the lower or midsternal border. The site of maximal intensity of the murmur is related to the site of drainage and is usually different from the second left intercostal space—the classic site of the continuous murmur of persistent ductus arteriosus—except when the fistula drains into the pulmonary artery or right ventricle. In the latter situation the murmur is louder in diastole than in systole because of compression of the fistula by contracting myocardium. The electrocardiogram and chest x-ray are quite often normal and rarely show selective chamber enlargement or myocardial ischemia. Significantly enlarged coronary arteries may be detected by two-dimensional echocardiography, and the actual diagnosis of an arteriovenous fistula can occasionally be made by combining two-dimensional echocardiography and Doppler techniques to detect the entrance site of the shunt, which is characterized typically by a continuous turbulent systolic and diastolic flow pattern.[148, 149]

Retrograde thoracic aortography or coronary arteriography can be employed reliably to identify the size and anatomical features of the fistulous tract, which may be closed by suture obliteration in most cases.[150] In the presence of a large left-to-right shunt and symptoms of heart failure, the decision to operate is clearly justified. Most often the fistula is closed in asymptomatic patients in order to prevent future symptoms or complications such as infective endocarditis. The prognosis following successful closure of a coronary artery–cardiac chamber fistula is excellent.

ANOMALOUS PULMONARY ORIGIN OF THE CORONARY ARTERY (See also p. 1000)

This rare malformation occurs in approximately 0.4 per cent of patients with congenital cardiac anomalies. In almost all patients the left coronary artery originates from the posterior sinus of the pulmonary artery.[150]

Unusual cases have been reported in which the right coronary artery, or the entire coronary artery system, originates from the main pulmonary trunk. Embryologically the distal coronary artery system is formed by 9 weeks from solid angioblastic buds that extend throughout the epicardium to form the major coronary artery branches. Proximally the coronary network forms a ring around the truncus arteriosus, joining with coronary buds from the primitive aortic sinuses as the truncus

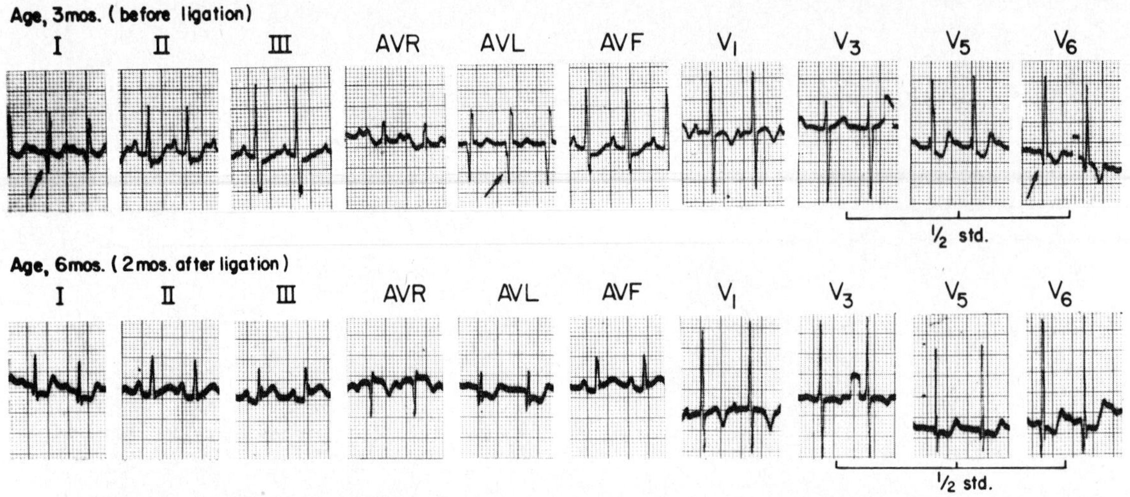

FIGURE 30–25. Typical electrocardiogram of an infant with anomalous left coronary artery before (*above*) and after (*below*) ligation of the anomalous left coronary artery. Arrows point to the abnormal Q waves. (Courtesy of Delores A. Danilowicz, M.D.)

partitions to form the great arteries. The varieties of anomalous pulmonary origin of the coronary artery are the result of displacement in this proximal process.

During fetal life pulmonary artery pressure is slightly greater than aortic pressure, and perfusion of the left coronary artery is antegrade. After birth, when pulmonary artery pressure falls below aortic pressure, perfusion of the left coronary artery from the pulmonary artery ceases, and the direction of flow in the anomalous vessel reverses. Blood flows from the aorta to the right coronary artery, then through collateral channels to the left coronary artery, and finally to the pulmonary artery. In effect, the left coronary artery behaves as a fistulous communication between the aorta and pulmonary artery. If adequate collateral channels exist or develop between the two coronary artery circulations, total myocardial perfusion through the right coronary artery increases. In 10 to 15 per cent of patients myocardial ischemia never develops because extensive intercoronary collaterals allow survival to adolescence or adulthood. In fact, if collateral blood flow is considerable, the patient may develop the clinical manifestations of a large arteriovenous shunt and a continuous or diastolic murmur. Older children or adults usually present with a continuous murmur or with mitral regurgitation resulting from dysfunction of ischemic or infarcted papillary muscles. In some instances the coronary anomaly is unsuspected until a previously well adolescent or adult experiences angina, heart failure, or sudden death.

By far the most common clinical presentation are those infants who suffer a myocardial infarction and develop congestive heart failure. The infant syndrome usually becomes manifested at age 2 to 4 months with angina-like symptoms that may occasionally be misinterpreted as colic. Feeding and defecation are often accompanied by dyspnea, irritability and crying, pallor, diaphoresis, and occasional loss of consciousness. The diagnosis of anomalous origin of the coronary artery is supported by the electrocardiographic demonstration of deep Q waves in association with ST-segment alterations and T-wave inversions in leads I, aV_L, V_5, and V_6 (Fig. 30–25). Chest roentgenograms show moderate to severe enlargement of the left atrium and ventricle. Occasionally, the origin of the anomalous left coronary artery may be visualized echocardiographically from long- or short-axis views of the pulmonary artery. Absence of the left coronary artery from its usual origin in the left sinus of Valsalva does not distinguish this lesion from single coronary artery. Doppler examination reveals continuous turbulent flow in the pulmonary artery near the coronary orifice, and may also disclose associated mitral regurgitation. Ischemia or infarction is suggested by the echocardiographic findings of segmental wall motion abnormalities, particularly involving the anterolateral free wall of the left ventricle. Stress thallium scintigraphy shows a characteristic defect of the anterolateral wall of the left ventricle (Fig. 31–20, p. 1001).

Aortography or coronary angiography is the definitive diagnostic procedure and demonstrates the retrograde drainage of the coronary vessel into the pulmonary artery (Fig. 30–26). It should be recognized that ventricular arrhythmias may complicate the course of hemodynamic study. Management of these infants depends, in part, upon the magnitude of shunting into the pulmonary artery, which may be determined by oximetry, indicator dilution curves, or angiography.

MANAGEMENT. *Medical treatment* is indicated in all infants with myocardial infarction for congestive heart failure, arrhythmias, and cardiogenic shock. In patients with a small left-to-right shunt or no shunt at all, the prognosis is exceedingly poor with conservative management, justifying an attempt to reestablish a two coronary artery system. The *operations* that have been employed include reimplanting the left coronary artery into the aortic root, surgically creating an aortopulmonary window and a tunnel to convey blood from the window across the back of the pulmonary trunk to the origin of the anomalous left

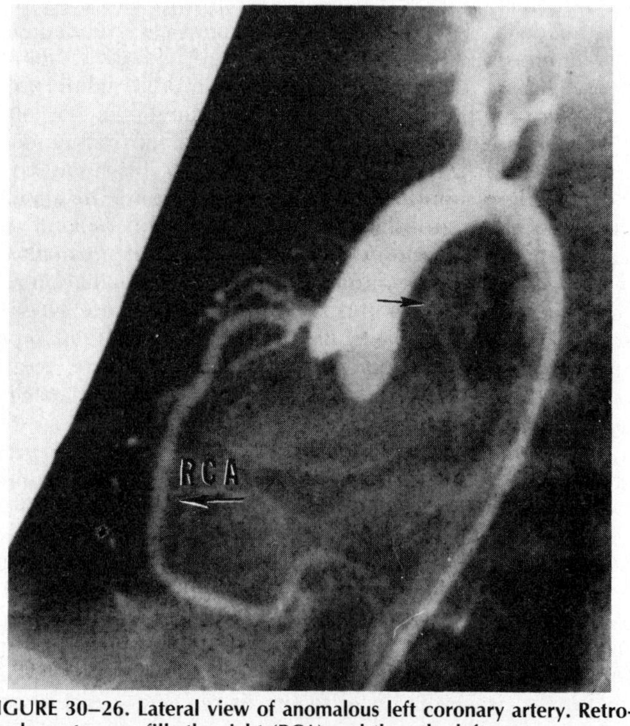

FIGURE 30–26. Lateral view of anomalous left coronary artery. Retrograde aortogram fills the right (RCA) and then the left coronary artery through collateral channels. The left coronary artery enters the main pulmonary artery (upper arrow). (Courtesy of Robert Freedom, M.D.)

coronary artery, with reconstruction of the anterior wall of the pulmonary trunk, or anastomosis of the left coronary artery with the subclavian artery or with the aorta via a graft.[151, 152] If clinical deterioration occurs in infants in whom a sizable left-to-right shunt exists into the pulmonary artery, simple ligation of the left coronary artery at its origin prevents retrograde flow and allows perfusion of the left ventricle with blood supplied through anastomoses with the right coronary artery. If medical management stabilizes the infant with significant intercoronary collaterals, operation should be postponed to allow the patient to grow, since increased size of the vessels enhances the likelihood of successful reimplantation or coronary arterial bypass surgery. The outcome of surgery and ultimate prognosis are influenced significantly by the degree of myocardial damage suffered preoperatively. Uncommonly, it is necessary to consider aneurysmectomy or mitral valve replacement.

AORTIC SINUS ANEURYSM AND FISTULA

(See also p. 1002)

Congenital aneurysm of an aortic sinus of Valsalva, particularly the right coronary sinus, is an uncommon anomaly occurring more often in males. The malformation consists of a separation, or lack of fusion, between the media of the aorta and the annulus fibrosis of the aortic valve.[153] The receiving chamber of the aorticocardiac fistula usually is the right ventricle, but occasionally, when the noncoronary cusp is involved, the fistula drains into the right atrium.

Five to 15 per cent of aneurysms originate in the posterior or noncoronary sinus; rarely is the left aortic sinus involved. Associated anomalies are common and include bicuspid aortic valve, ventricular septal defect, and coarctation of the aorta.

It is not clear whether the aneurysm itself is present at birth, although the deficiency in the aortic media would appear to be congenital. Reports in children are infrequent, since progressive aneurysmal dilatation of the weakened area develops but may not be recognized until the third or fourth decade of life when rupture into a cardiac chamber occurs.

The *unruptured aneurysm* generally does not produce a hemodynamic abnormality, although pressure on the intracardiac conduction system by an unruptured aneurysm may be a rare cause of complete atrioventricular block; myocardial ischemia may rarely be caused by coronary arterial compression. Rupture often is of abrupt onset, causes chest pain, and creates continuous arteriovenous shunting and volume loading of both right and left heart chambers, which results in heart failure.[154] An additional complication is bacterial endocarditis, which may originate either on the edges of the aneurysm or on those areas in the right side of the heart that are traumatized by the jetlike stream of blood flowing through the fistula.

The presence of this anomaly should be suspected in a patient with a history of chest pain of recent onset, symptoms of diminished cardiac reserve, bounding pulses, and a loud superficial continuous murmur accentuated in diastole when the fistula opens into the right ventricle as well as a thrill along the right or left lower parasternal border. The *physical findings* may occasionally be difficult to distinguish from those produced by a coronary arteriovenous fistula. *Electrocardiography* shows biventricular hypertrophy, and chest roentgenography demonstrates generalized cardiomegaly. Two-dimensional and pulsed Doppler *echocardiographic* studies may detect the walls of the aneurym and disturbed flow within the aneurysm or at the site of perforation, respectively.[155] *Cardiac catheterization* reveals a left-to-right shunt at the ventricular or, less commonly, the atrial level; the diagnosis may be established definitively by retrograde thoracic aortography (Fig. 30–27). Preoperative medical management consists

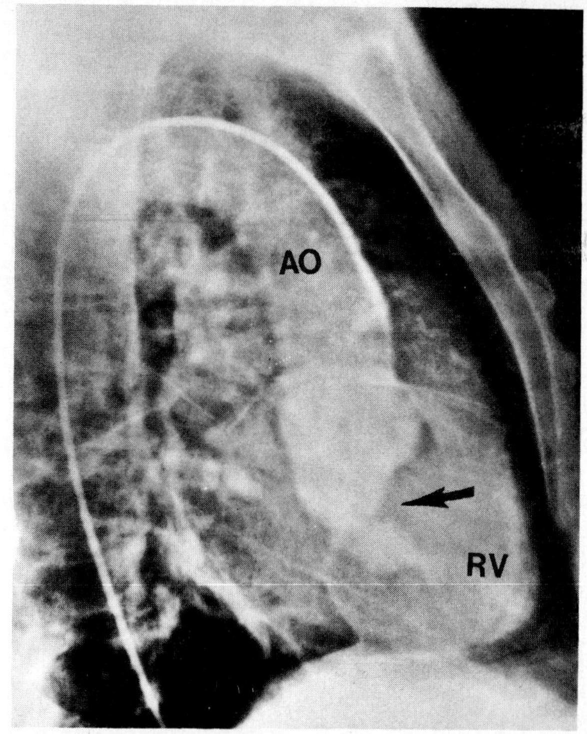

FIGURE 30–27. A retrograde aortogram shows the fistulous connection between the noncoronary sinus of Valsalva and the right ventricle (RV) (arrow). AO = aorta. (Courtesy of Robert White, M.D.)

of measures to relieve cardiac failure and to treat coexistent arrhythmias or endocarditis, if present. At operation the aneurysm is closed and amputated, and the aortic wall is reunited with the heart, either by direct suture or with a prosthesis.[154] Every effort should be made to preserve the aortic valve in children, since patch closure of the defect combined with prosthetic valve replacement greatly enhances the risk of operation in small patients.

VALVULAR AND VASCULAR LESIONS WITH OR WITHOUT RIGHT-TO-LEFT SHUNT

AORTIC ARCH OBSTRUCTION

The conventional anatomical and clinical division into pre- and postductal coarctation or infantile and adult types, respectively, is misleading, since the anatomical localization is inaccurate and the age-dependency of clinical presentation does not hold true (i.e., the adult type is seen often in the first weeks of life). A spectrum of anatomical lesions exists, causing obstruction of the aortic arch or proximal portion of the descending aorta. These range from a localized coarctation or constriction of the lumen, most commonly located just distal to the origin of the left subclavian artery and related closely to the attachment of the ductus arteriosus with the aorta, to diffuse narrowing or interruption of a portion of the aortic arch. In this chapter, aortic arch obstruction is divided into three types: (1) localized juxtaductal coarctation, (2) hypoplasia of the aortic isthmus, and (3) aortic arch interruption. *Pseudocoarctation* is a term used synonymously with "kinking," or "buckling," of the aorta, which is a subclinical form of localized juxtaductal coarctation of the aorta.[156]

LOCALIZED JUXTADUCTAL COARCTATION

(See also p. 994)

MORPHOLOGY. This lesion consists of a localized shelf-like thickening and infolding of the media of the posterolateral aortic wall opposite the ductus arteriosus; the wall of the aorta into which the ductus or ligamentum arteriosum inserts is not involved.[157] Juxtaductal coarctation occurs two to five times more commonly in males than in females, and there is a high degree of association with gonadal dysgenesis (Turner syndrome) and bicuspid aortic valve. Other common associated anomalies include ventricular septal defect and mitral stenosis or regurgitation. The most important extracardiac anomaly is aneurysm of the circle of Willis.

Juxtaductal coarctation is most likely related to an abnormality in the pattern of ductus arteriosus blood flow in utero, which, in turn, may be the result of associated intracardiac anomalies.[157, 158] Thus, in fetal life, blood flow through the aortic isthmus constitutes only 12 to 17 per cent of the total cardiac output, while blood flow through the ductus arteriosus exceeds that across the aortic valve. The dorsal aortic wall directly opposite the ductus arteriosus will resemble morphologically the apex of a normal branch point of the aorta if ductal flow pathways in utero diverge, with some flow directed cephalad into the aortic isthmus and the remainder proceeding into the descending aorta. The aortic branch point is identical histologically to the posterior shelf of juxtaductal aortic coarctation. A divergence of ductal flow is fostered by the presence of lesions in the fetus that create an imbalance between left and right ventricular outputs, with right-sided flow predominating (e.g., bicuspid aortic valve, mitral valve anomaly). In the absence of an anomaly fostering augmented ductal flow, a branch point may be created by an alteration in the angle at which the ductus arteriosus meets the aorta, pointing the ductal stream directly against the posterior aortic wall rather than obliquely down into the descending aorta. Cardiac anomalies that cause augmented ascending aortic blood flow (e.g., pulmonic atresia or stenosis, tetralogy of Fallot) prevent development of a branch point and, indeed, are almost never seen in association with juxtaductal coarctation of the aorta.

During fetal life the posterior aortic shelf is not obstructive, since blood may pass readily from the ascending aorta to the descending aorta by traversing the anterior aortic segment and the aortic end of the ductus arteriosus. Postnatally, however, when the ductus undergoes obliteration at its aortic end, the shelflike projection of the posterior aortic wall unmasks the obstruction to aortic flow (Fig. 30–28). Following pharmacological interventions that dilate the ductus arteriosus (prostaglandin E_1 infusion) the pressure difference may be obliterated across the site of coarctation, since the fetal flow pattern is reestablished.[60, 159]

The *pathogenesis* of juxtaductal coarctation described above explains the prevalence of associated intracardiac anomalies that foster reduced ascending aortic and augmented ductus arteriosus flow in utero, and the absence of associated intracardiac anomalies in which the converse flow conditions exist in utero. The dependence of aortic obstruction on constriction of the ductus arteriosus postnatally explains the variable onset after birth of the clinical manifestations of coarctation, as well as the dramatic alleviation of obstruction produced pharmacologically by dilatation of the ductus arteriosus.

CLINICAL FINDINGS. The manifestations of juxtaductal coarctation of the aorta depend upon the prominence of the posterolateral aortic shelf, which determines the intensity of obstruction, and on the rapidity with which obstruction develops. Rapid, severe obstruction in infancy is a prominent cause of left ventricular failure and systemic hypoperfusion. Substantial left-to-right shunting across a patent foramen ovale and pulmonary venous hypertension secondary to heart failure cause pulmonary arterial hypertension. Because little or no aortic obstruction existed during fetal life, the collateral circulation in the newborn period is often poorly developed. Characteristically in these infants, peripheral pulses are weak throughout the body until left ventricular function is improved with medical management; a significant pressure difference then develops between the arms and the legs, allowing detection of a pulse discrepancy. Cardiac murmurs are nonspecific in infancy and commonly are derived from associated lesions. The electrocardiogram shows right-axis deviation and right ventricular hypertrophy; the chest x-ray shows generalized cardiomegaly and pulmonary arterial and venous engorgement. Hemodynamic study allows delineation of the site and extent of aortic obstruction and the detection of associated cardiac malformations. Most infants with early-onset severe heart failure respond poorly to medical management, and surgical excision of the coarctation or a subclavian flap angioplasty is often required.[160, 161]

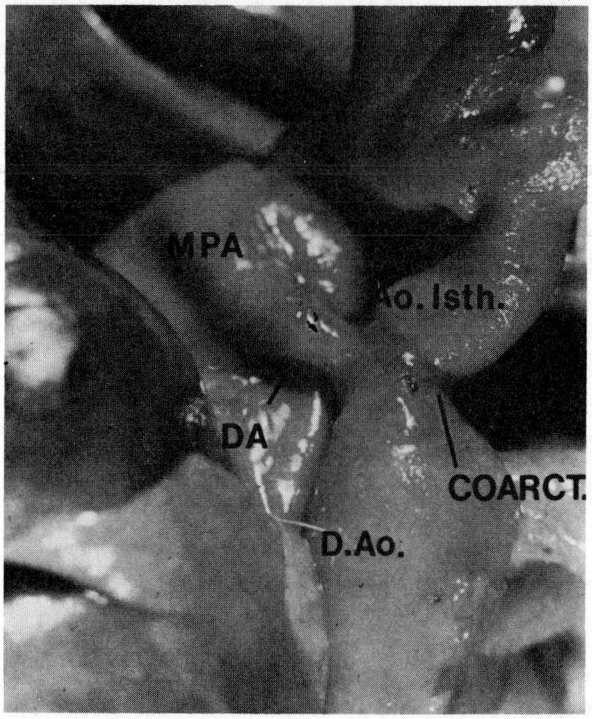

FIGURE 30–28. Juxtaductal coarctation (COARCT) unmasked by constriction of the ductus arteriosus (DA). MPA = main pulmonary artery, D.Ao. = descending aorta, Ao.Isth. = aortic isthmus. (Courtesy of Norman Talner, M.D.)

Aortic obstruction may develop slowly in infants in whom the posterolateral aortic shelf is not prominent at birth and in whom ductus arteriosus constriction is gradual. In these babies compensatory myocardial hypertrophy and an extensive collateral circulation have time to develop. If the obstruction does not intensify and cardiac failure does not occur by age 6 to 9 months, circulatory compensation is likely until adult life.

The majority of children with isolated juxtaductal coarctation are asymptomatic. Complaints of headache, cold extremities, and claudication with exercise may be noted, although attention is usually directed to the cardiovascular system by detection of a heart murmur or upper extremity hypertension on routine physical examination. Mechanical factors rather than those of renal origin play the primary role in the production of hypertension. Absent, markedly diminished, or delayed pulsations in the femoral arteries and a low or unobtainable arterial pressure in the lower extremities with hypertension in the arms are the basic clues to the diagnosis. A midsystolic murmur over the anterior chest, back, and spinous processes is most frequent, becoming continuous if the lumen is narrowed sufficiently to result in a high-velocity jet across the lesion throughout the cardiac cycle (Fig. 31–14, p. 995). Additional systolic and continuous murmurs over the lateral thoracic wall may reflect increased flow through dilated and tortuous collateral vessels. *Electrocardiography* reveals left ventricular hypertrophy of varying degrees, depending on the height of arterial pressure above the obstruction and the patient's age. Combined with right ventricular hypertrophy, this usually implies a complicated lesion. *Chest roentgenograms* may show a dilated left subclavian artery high on the left mediastinal border and

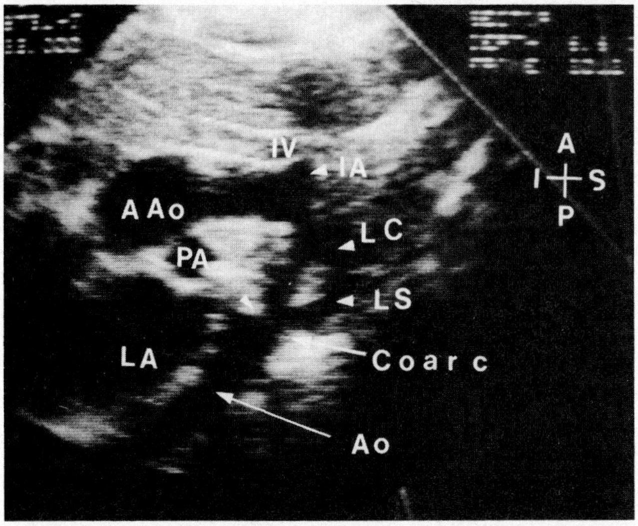

FIGURE 30–29. Aortic coarctation (Coarc) is visualized from the suprasternal notch. The aorta (Ao) can be traced from the ascending aorta (AAo). The aortic arch is somewhat narrowed and the relationship of the left subclavian artery (LS) to the coarctation is identified clearly. LA = left atrium, PA = pulmonary artery, IA = innominate artery, LC = left carotid artery. (Courtesy of Norman Silverman, M.D.)

a dilated ascending aorta. Indentation of the aorta at the site of coarctation and pre- and poststenotic dilatation (the "3" sign) along the left paramediastinal shadow is almost pathognomonic. Poststenotic dilatation may also be detected by indentation of the barium-filled esophagus. Notching of the ribs, an important radiographic sign, is due to erosion by dilated collateral vessels, increases with age, and usually becomes apparent between the fourth and twelfth years of life. The aortic coarctation may be visualized directly by two-dimensional echocardiography from high parasternal or suprasternal notch views with short focused transducers, and from the subxiphoid window with extended focal range transducers (Figs. 30–29 and 31–15, p. 996). Doppler examination reveals a flow disturbance and high velocity jet at the site of obstruction.[162] Computed tomography,[163] magnetic resonance imaging (Fig. 12–35, p. 374) or cardiac catheterization and aortography (Fig. 30–30) are indicated to localize accurately the site of obstruction, determine the length of the coarctation, and, particularly, to identify associated malformations.

MANAGEMENT. Subclavian flap aortoplasty (Fig. 30–31), particularly in neonates and infants, or surgical resection and end-to-end anastomosis of uncomplicated juxtaductal coarctation of the aorta can be accomplished with excellent results in most patients[161]; some surgeons prefer an on-lay patch across the site of obstruction. In children who are

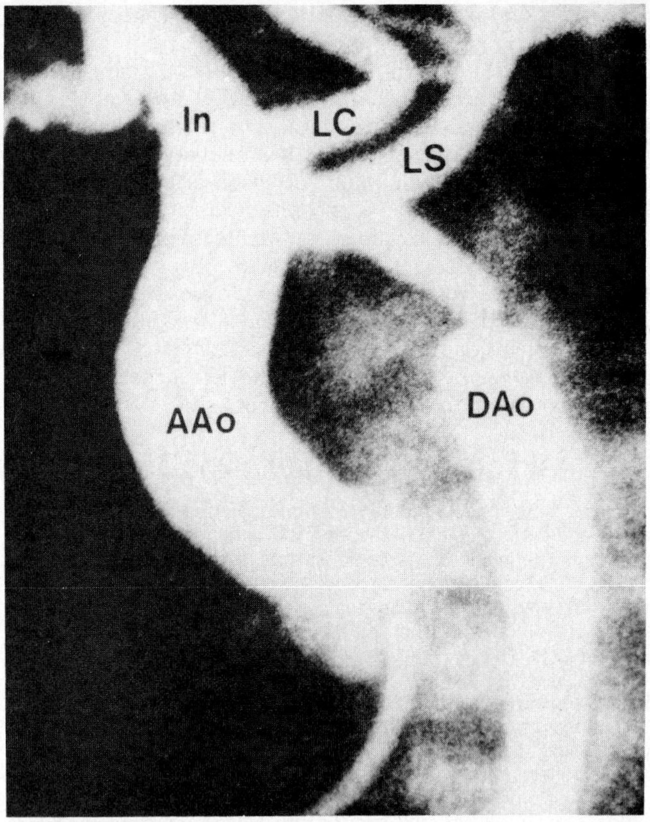

FIGURE 30–30. Retrograde aortogram demonstrates the discrete site of coarctation of the aorta, hypoplasia of the aortic isthmus, and poststenotic dilation of the descending aorta (DAo). AAo = ascending aorta, In = innominate artery, LC = left common carotid artery, LS = left subclavian artery.

asymptomatic it is preferable to delay surgery until age 4 to 6 years, at which time coarctation rarely recurs.[164] Paradoxical hypertension of short duration is often noted in the immediate postoperative period. A resetting of carotid baroreceptors and increased catecholamine secretion appear to be responsible for the initial phase of systemic hypertension with a later, second phase of prolonged elevation of systolic and particularly diastolic blood pressure related to activation of the renin-angiotensin system.[165–167] Occasionally, a necrotizing panarteritis of the small vessels of the gastrointestinal tract of uncertain cause complicates the course of recovery.

A 5 to 10 per cent risk of recurrent narrowing exists after repair of coarctation in infancy.[168] This problem is treated most effectively by transcutaneous balloon angioplasty,[168a] which may be expected to reduce markedly, but

FIGURE 30–31. Subclavian flap aortoplasty repair of aortic coarctation. *A*, The left subclavian artery has been ligated and divided; the aorta is incised from below the coarctation ridge of tissue, which is carefully excised. *B*, The distal end of the subclavian artery forms a flap, which is sutured to the aortotomy. (From Stark, J., and DeLaval, M.: Surgery for Congenital Heart Defects. New York, Grune and Stratton, 1983, p. 216.)

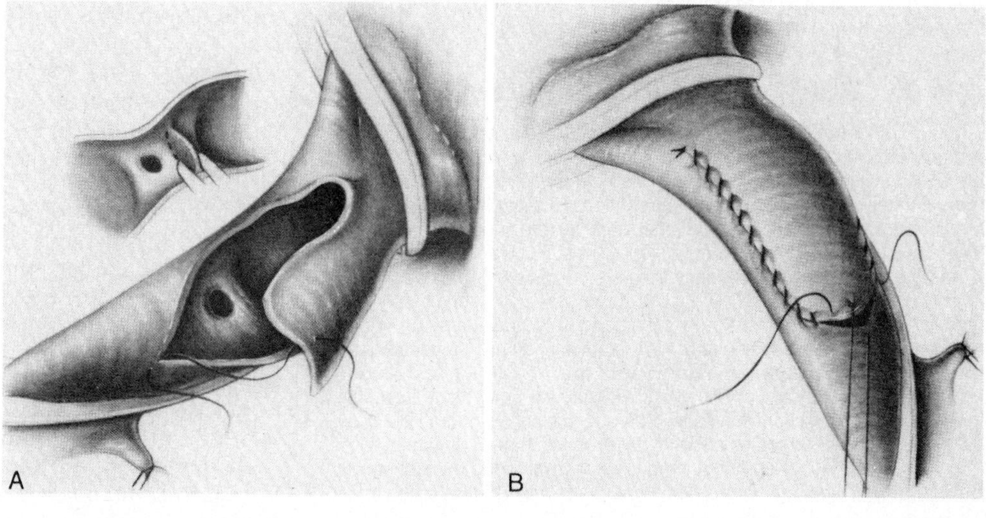

not abolish entirely, the pressure difference across the site of recoarctation.[169]

In those patients who survive the first 2 years of life, complications of juxtaductal coarctation are uncommon before the second or third decade. The chief hazards to patients with coarctation result from severe hypertension and include the development of cerebral aneurysms and hemorrhage, hypertensive encephalopathy, rupture of the aorta, left ventricular failure, and infective endocarditis. Systemic hypertension in the absence of residual coarctation has been observed in resting or exercise-stressed patients postoperatively and appears to be related to the duration of preoperative hypertension.[170, 171] Lifelong observation is desirable because of the late onset of hypertension in some postoperative patients.

HYPOPLASIA OF THE AORTIC ARCH

The aorta isthmus, the portion of aorta between the left subclavian artery and the ductus arteriosus, normally is narrowed in the fetus and newborn. The lumen of the aortic isthmus is approximately two-thirds that of the ascending and descending aorta until age 6 to 9 months, when the physiological narrowing disappears.[172] Pathological tubular hypoplasia of the aortic arch is usually noted in the aortic isthmus and is referred to often as preductal or infantile coarctation of the aorta.[173] Associated major cardiac malformations occur in virtually all such infants and include large ventricular septal defect, atrioventricular septal defect, transposition of the great arteries, Taussig-Bing anomaly, and double-outlet right ventricle. The ventricular septal defect is most often subpulmonary, lying within the substance of the infundibular septum. Thus, muscle persists between the aortic and pulmonary valve leaflets, which, when displaced leftward, produces subaortic stenosis. Persistent patency of the ductus arteriosus commonly coexists, and right-to-left flow across the ductus arteriosus usually provides filling of the descending aorta. The adequacy of blood flow to the lower body depends upon the degree of aortic hypoplasia, the caliber of the ductus arteriosus, and the relationship between pulmonary and systemic vascular resistance. Substantial right-to-left shunting through a wide open ductus arteriosus minimizes the arterial blood pressure difference between the upper and lower body. Differential cyanosis of the toes and feet with normal color of the fingers and hands may be difficult to discern because intracardiac left-to-right shunting and pulmonary edema attenuate the differences in oxygen saturation in the ascending and descending aorta. Clinical deterioration is associated with ductal constriction or a fall in pulmonary vascular resistance. Moreover, the clinical presentation is often dictated by the hemodynamic effects of complex associated intracardiac malformations. Infants most often present with findings of a large left-to-right intracardiac shunt, pulmonary hypertension, and marked cardiac decompensation. Although tubular hypoplasia is detectable by two-dimensional echocardiography, cardiac catheterization is required to evaluate the full extent of the intra- and extracardiac lesions.[174] Surgical repair of aortic arch hypoplasia must usually be accompanied by operative palliation or correction of associated intracardiac lesions. Aortic angioplasty incorporating the subclavian-aortic anastomosis, and a tubular prosthetic conduit are among the operative approaches to correct long segment narrowing. Recoarctation is common and often necessitates transcatheter balloon aortoplasty and/or a second operation later in life to relieve anastomotic stenosis.

AORTIC ARCH INTERRUPTION

Aortic arch interruption is a rare and usually lethal anomaly; unless treated surgically almost all infants die within the first month of life.[175] Interruptions distal to the left subclavian artery (Type A) occur with approximately equal frequency to interruptions distal to the left common carotid artery (Type B); interruptions distal to the innominate artery (Type C) are extremely uncommon. The right subclavian artery is often of variable origin, arising frequently from the descending aortic segment distal to the interruption.[176] The clinical presentation resembles that seen in tubular hypoplasia or severe juxtaductal coarctation of the aorta with a patent ductus arteriosus. In almost all patients a ventricular septal defect and patent ductus arteriosus coexist with the arch interruption. Since the ductus arteriosus provides lower body blood flow, its spontaneous constriction results in profound clinical deterioration. The latter may be ameliorated temporarily by prostaglandin E_1 infusion.[27, 60, 159] The VSD is most often subpulmonary, lying within the substance of the infundibular septum. Thus, muscle persists between the aortic and pulmonary valve leaflets, which, when displaced leftward, produces subaortic stenosis. Other complex intracardiac malformations, such as transposition of the great arteries, aortopulmonary window, and truncus arteriosus are common.[177] An association is frequent with DiGeorge syndrome of thymic hypoplasia or aplasia and the accompanying immunological and hypocalcemia problems. The major clinical problem is severe congestive heart failure as a consequence of volume overload of the left ventricle due to an associated intracardiac left-to-right shunt and of pressure overload imposed by systemic hypertension. Operation is rarely possible by direct anastomosis, and reconstitution usually necessitates interposition of a tubular synthetic graft or a direct anastomosis between the aorta and one of its major brachiocephalic vessels.[175, 176]

CONGENITAL VALVULAR AORTIC STENOSIS (See also p. 978)

MORPHOLOGY. Congenital valvular aortic stenosis is a relatively common anomaly, estimated to occur in 3 to 6 per cent of patients with congenital cardiovascular defects. However, it must be appreciated that the true incidence of the malformation is probably grossly underestimated because the congenital bicuspid aortic valve may be undetected in early life, and becomes stenotic and of clinical significance only in adult life, at a time when it may be indistinguishable from the acquired forms of aortic stenosis. Congenital valvular aortic stenosis occurs much more frequently in males than in females, with the sex ratio approximating 4:1. Associated cardiovascular anomalies have been noted in as many as 20 per cent of patients.[178] Patent ductus arteriosus and coarctation of the aorta occur most frequently with valvular aortic stenosis; all three of these lesions may coexist.

The basic malformation consists of thickening of valve tissue with varying degrees of commissural fusion. Most commonly, the valve is bicuspid with a single fused commissure and an eccentrically placed orifice. A third commissure, incomplete or rudimentary, may sometimes be apparent. Less commonly, the valve has three fused cusps with a stenotic central orifice. In some patients the stenotic aortic valve is unicuspid and dome-shaped with no or one lateral attachment to the aorta at the level of the orifice. In infants and young children with severe aortic stenosis the aortic valve ring may be relatively underdeveloped. This lesion forms a continuum with the hypoplastic left heart syndrome and the aortic atresia and hypoplasia complexes. Secondary calcification of the valve is extremely rare in childhood, but the dynamics of blood flow associated with the congenitally deformed aortic valve lead ultimately to thickening of the cusps and calcification in adult life. When the obstruction is hemodynamically significant, concentric hypertrophy of the left ventricular wall and dilatation of the ascending aorta occur.

HEMODYNAMICS. The hemodynamic abnormalities produced by obstruction to left ventricular outflow are discussed on p. 900. A peak systolic gradient exceeding 75 mm Hg in association with a normal cardiac output or an effective aortic orifice less than 0.5 cm^2/m^2 body surface area is considered to reflect critical obstruction to left ventricular outflow.[178–180] The normal outflow orifice approximates 2.0 cm^2/m^2 body surface area; areas of 0.5 to 0.8 cm^2/m^2 signify moderate obstruction. When the area is larger than 0.8 cm^2/m^2, the obstruction is considered to be mild; when less than 0.4 cm^2/m^2, it is severe.

Generally, the resting cardiac output and stroke volume are within normal limits. During exercise, most children with critical stenosis show an elevation of the cardiac output and an associated elevation in the transvalvular pressure gradient.[181] When left ventricular failure occurs, the cardiac output decreases, and the left atrial, left ventricular end-diastolic, and pulmonary vascular pressures increase.

The blood supply to the myocardium may be compromised significantly in infants and children with aortic stenosis, despite normal patency of the coronary arteries.[182] Coronary blood flow and arterial oxygen content are critical determinants of oxygen supply to the myocardium. Since intramyocardial compressive forces are greatest in the subendocardium, blood flow to that region of left ventricle is entirely diastolic in the presence of elevated left ventricular systolic pressure. In patients with left ventricular outflow tract obstruction, coronary vasodilatation may give an inadequate response to an increase in the demands of the myocardium for oxygen at rest or with exercise. When subendocardial vessels are dilated maximally the coronary artery driving pressure and the duration of diastole determine the magnitude of subendocardial flow. When the duration of systolic ejection lengthens across the stenotic orifice, diastole is shortened, especially at high heart rates. Moreover, a reduction occurs in coronary driving pressure if left ventricular end-diastolic pressure is high or if aortic diastolic pressure is low, e.g., with aortic regurgitation or heart failure. In patients with severe aortic stenosis the redistribution of flow away from the subendocardium and the ischemia that results to that portion of ventricular muscle may be estimated by relating the diastolic pressure time index (DPTI) (i.e., the area between the aortic and left ventricular pressures in diastole) to the systolic pressure time index (SPTI) (a measure of myocardial oxygen demands). Inadequate subendocardial oxygen delivery has been shown to exist when the ratio [DPTI × arterial oxygen content/SPTI] falls below 10.[182]

INFANCY. Special comment concerning this malformation as it is seen in infants is warranted, in view of the unique problems presented by patients in this age group.[183, 185a] Fortunately, isolated aortic valvular stenosis seldom causes symptoms in infancy. Occasionally, however, this lesion may be responsible for profound and intractable heart failure. Despite normal coronary arterial anatomy, infarction of left ventricular papillary muscles may occur, resulting in an acquired form of mitral valvular regurgitation that intensifies the heart failure state. In addition, endocardial fibroelastosis may result from limited subendocardial oxygen delivery and myocardial degeneration may be significant.[185] The symptomatic infant with isolated valvular aortic stenosis is irritable, pale, and hypotensive and presents with tachycardia, cardiomegaly, and pulmonary congestion manifested by dyspnea, tachypnea, subcostal retractions, and diffuse rales. Cyanosis may be observed secondary to pulmonary venous desaturation. The systolic murmur in infants is often atypical; it is best heard at the apex or along the lower left sternal border and may be confused with that caused by a ventricular septal defect. Occasionally, in infants with heart failure, the murmur may be absent or extremely soft, becoming louder when myocardial contractility is improved with digitalis and other medical measures. Frequently, the response to medical management of the infant with heart failure is poor.

The electrocardiographic findings may not be characteristic; left ventricular hypertrophy and/or strain as well as right atrial enlargement and right ventricular hypertrophy may be detected shortly after birth.[183] The latter signs of right heart involvement result from both pulmonary hypertension secondary to elevated left ventricular diastolic and left atrial pressures and from volume loading of the right ventricle due to left-to-right shunting across the foramen ovale. Survival past the early neonatal period does not preclude subsequent difficulties, and clinical deterioration may recur with the onset of physiological anemia.

Congenital aortic stenosis must be considered a medical emergency in the seriously ill newborn, and echocardiography, and sometimes cardiac catheterization and angiocardiography may be indicated in the first 24 hours of life. Two-dimensional echocardiographic long-axis views of the left ventricular outflow tract demonstrate doming of the aortic valve (Fig. 5–57, p. 108). The parasternal short-axis view bisects the face of the valve, demonstrating the anatomy of the commissures.[186, 187] M-mode recordings best demonstrate wall thickness and motion. Doppler echocardiography provides an accurate estimate of the pressure gradient across the site of obstruction[186–190] (Fig. 5–58, p. 109). Commonly, hemodynamic findings include left-to-right shunting at the atrial level, elevated left atrial and left ventricular end-diastolic pressures, and a small pressure drop across the aortic valve as a result of a markedly reduced cardiac output. Occasionally, right-to-left shunting across a patent ductus arteriosus is encountered. The presence of a normal or enlarged left ventricular cavity and normal or dilated ascending aorta allows distinction of aortic stenosis from the hypoplastic left heart syndrome angiographically. Because prolonged periods of stabilization are uncommon with medical therapy, early and definitive establishment of the diagnosis and prompt valvulotomy are usually justified. Poor myocardial performance resulting from endocardial fibroelastosis, subendocardial ischemia, and reduced left ventricular compliance, and inadequate relief of obstruction with or without significant aortic regurgitation are among the factors accounting for high operative mortality and morbidity. Open repair under direct vision is the preferred type of operation.[184, 191]

CHILDHOOD. Congenital aortic stenosis may be responsible for severe obstruction to left ventricular outflow in the absence of the clinical symptoms of diminished cardiac reserve that are so frequent in other forms of congenital heart disease.[192] Most children with congenital aortic stenosis grow and develop normally and are asymptomatic. Attention is usually called to these children when a murmur is detected on routine examination. When symptoms occur, those noted most commonly are fatigability, exertional dyspnea, angina pectoris, and syncope. Less often described are abdominal pain, profuse sweating, and epistaxis. Generally, the symptomatic child has critical stenosis. Sudden death poses a distinct threat to patients with severe obstruction.[180] Although the precise cause is poorly understood, ventricular arrhythmias, perhaps initiated by acute myocardial ischemia, are probably the most common inciting event. Speculation exists that an abrupt rise in intracavity left ventricular systolic pressure elicits a reflex hypotensive syncope that promotes acute ischemia and ventricular fibrillation.[193] Bacterial endocarditis occurs in approximately 4 per cent of patients with congenital valvular aortic stenosis.

DIAGNOSIS. Physical Findings. When the magnitude of obstruction is significant, a left ventricular lift is usually palpable, and a precordial systolic thrill is often palpated over the base of the heart with transmission to the jugular notch and along the carotid arteries; presystolic expansion is often palpable. Usually the obstruction is mild if neither a left ventricular lift nor a thrill is present.

Opening of the aortic valve produces a systolic aortic ejection sound that is typically present at the cardiac apex when the valve is mobile, particularly in patients with mild to moderate stenosis. A delay in closure of the stenotic aortic valve leads to a single or a closely split second heart sound, and paradoxical splitting may be present. Generally, a fourth heart sound is associated with severe obstruction. A loud, harsh, rhomboid-shaped systolic murmur starts after completion of left ventricular isometric contraction and is best heard at the base of the heart. The murmur, like the thrill, radiates to the suprasternal notch and carotid vessels as well as to the apex. An early diastolic blowing murmur of aortic regurgitation is present in some patients, but unless the valve leaflets have been eroded by bacterial endocarditis, the regurgitation is usually not hemodynamically significant; uncommonly, in patients with a congenitally bicuspid valve, aortic regurgitation may be severe and may predominate.

Electrocardiography. There is a tendency for *electrocardiographic signs* of left ventricular hypertrophy to vary with the severity of obstruction, although a normal or near-normal electrocardiogram does not exclude severe aortic stenosis.[194] The presence of a left ventricular "strain pattern," consisting of left ventricular hypertrophy combined with ST-segment depressions and T-wave inversion in the left precordial leads, generally indicates that severe aortic stenosis is present (Fig. 30–32).

In patients under 10 years of age the *electrocardiogram* is a more reliable guide in indicating the severity of the stenosis than in older patients.[192] Findings in the younger age group that often accompany severe obstruction are T-wave vectors in the frontal plane to the left of −40°, widening of the angle between the mean QRS and T forces in the frontal plane in excess of 100°, an S wave in V_1 greater than 16 mm, and an R wave in V_5 exceeding 20 mm. Nonetheless, it is important to recognize that these voltages may be excessive in patients who do not have severe stenosis. A good relationship appears to exist between exercise-induced electrocardiographic changes and the severity of obstruction; ischemic ST-segment changes have been observed in patients with normal resting cardiac indices and transvalvular pressure differences in excess of 50 mm Hg or an abnormal left ventricular oxygen supply-demand ratio.[181]

Roentgenography. Overall heart size is normal or the degree of enlargement is slight in most children with congenital valvular aortic stenosis. Concentric left ventricular hypertrophy accompanies moderate or severe obstruction and is manifested by rounding of the cardiac apex in the frontal projection and posterior displacement in the lateral view.

Echocardiography. The M-mode echocardiographic findings that may suggest a diagnosis of aortic valve stenosis include multiple diastolic closure lines, or a single eccentrically placed diastolic closure line in the aortic lumen; left ventricular posterior wall and septal thickening; reduced separation of thickened aortic valve leaflets; and aortic root dilation (p. 113). Two-dimensional echocardiography demonstrates impaired mobility of cusp tissue, altered phasic movement of the aortic valve with increased superior and reduced lateral excursions of valve echoes, and an increase in the internal aortic root dimension distal to the level of the valve annulus.[188] The parasternal short-axis view of the valve demonstrates the leaflet anatomy (Fig. 30–33).

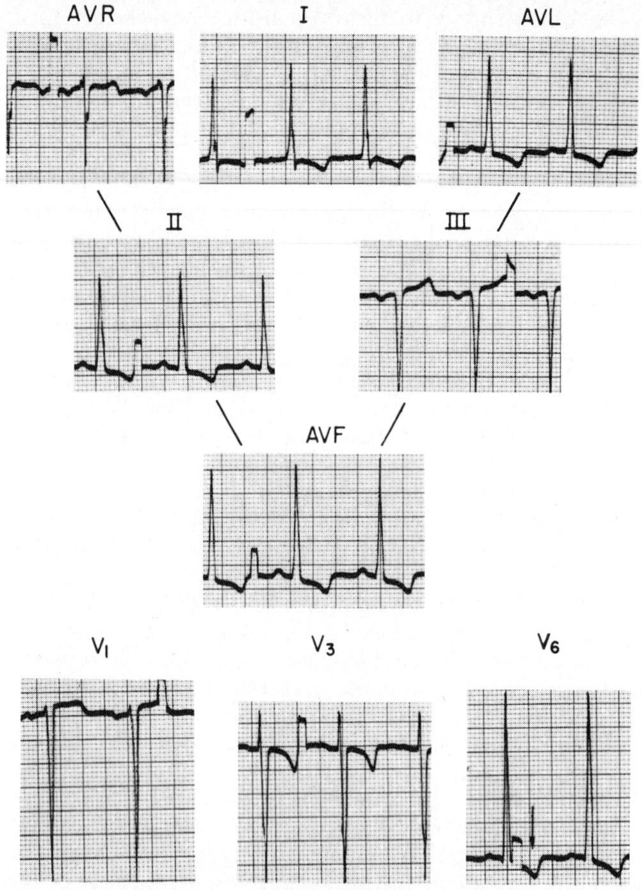

FIGURE 30–32. Congenital aortic stenosis. This tracing shows left ventricular hypertrophy and the typical left ventricular "strain" pattern (V_6, arrow). (Courtesy of Delores A. Danilowicz, M.D.)

The most accurate noninvasive approach to quantify the severity of obstruction combines continuous-wave Doppler flow analysis with the two-dimensional echocardiographic determination of the area of the orifice[186–190] (p. 99). A simple estimate of the transvalvular gradient (in mm Hg) may be calculated as 4 times the square of the peak Doppler velocity (meters/sec).

In patients without cardiac decompensation, a consistent relationship has been shown to exist between peak left ventricular systolic pressure and left ventricular wall thick-

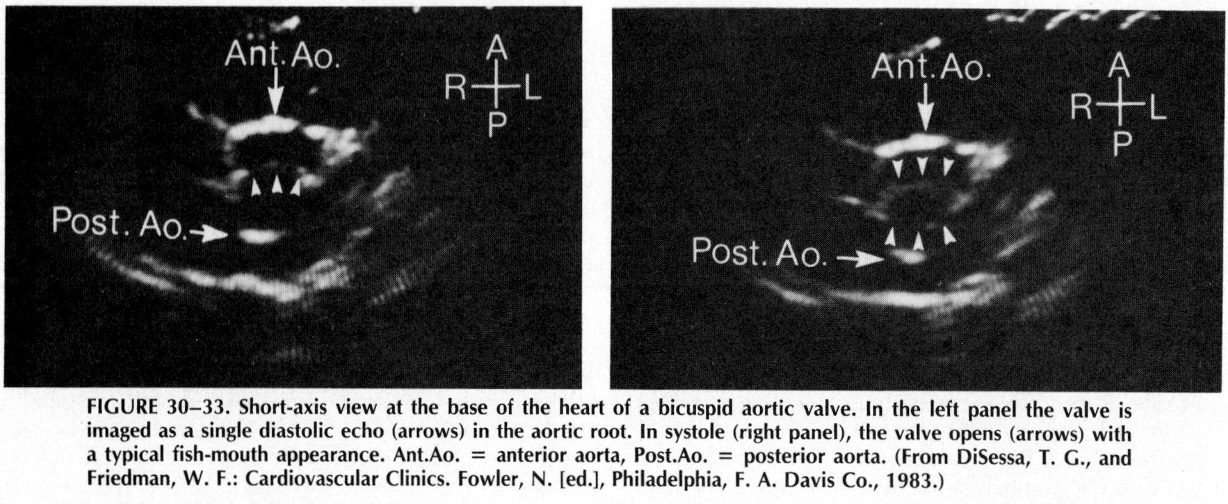

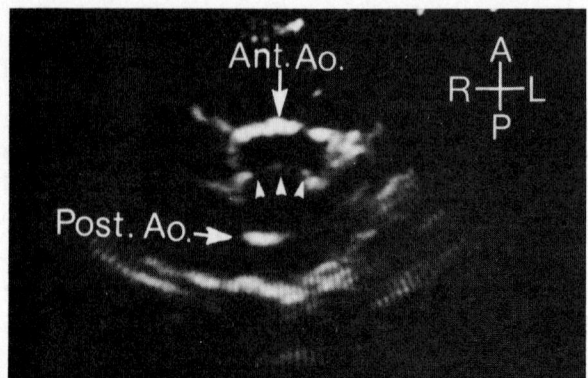

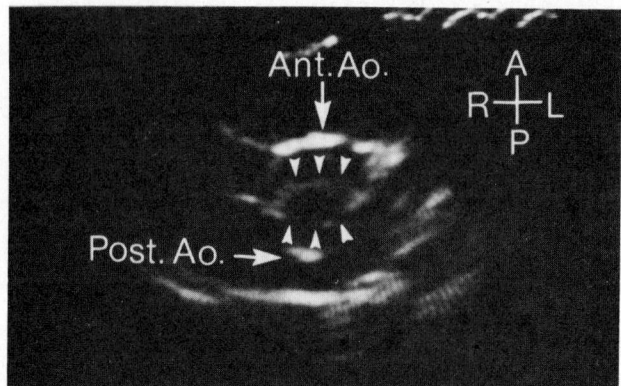

FIGURE 30–33. Short-axis view at the base of the heart of a bicuspid aortic valve. In the left panel the valve is imaged as a single diastolic echo (arrows) in the aortic root. In systole (right panel), the valve opens (arrows) with a typical fish-mouth appearance. Ant.Ao. = anterior aorta, Post.Ao. = posterior aorta. (From DiSessa, T. G., and Friedman, W. F.: Cardiovascular Clinics. Fowler, N. [ed.], Philadelphia, F. A. Davis Co., 1983.)

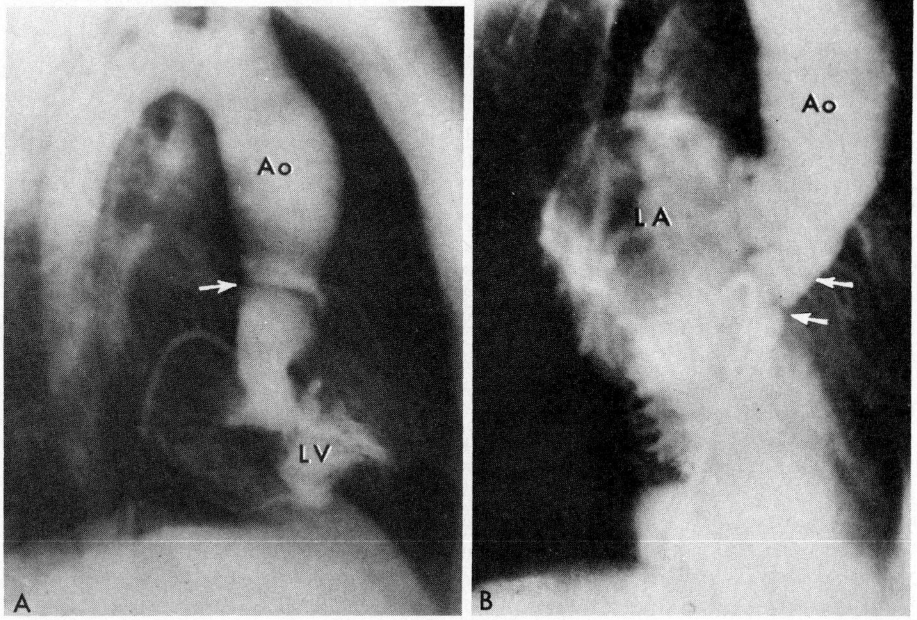

FIGURE 30–34. *A*, Left ventricular angiocardiogram obtained by the transseptal method in a patient with congenital valvular aortic stenosis. Ao = post-stenotic dilatation of the aorta; LV = left ventricle. Arrow denotes the thickened valve cusp. *B*, Selective angiocardiogram in a patient with discrete subvalvular stenosis (bottom arrow). Associated mitral regurgitation is evident from the reflux of contrast into an enlarged left atrium (LA). The aorta valve (top arrow) is normal, and the right coronary artery is visualized. (From Friedman, W. F., and Kirkpatrick, S. E.: Congenital aortic stenosis. *In* Moss, A. J., Adams, F. H., and Emmanouilides, G. C. [eds.]: Heart Disease in Infants, Children and Adolescents. 2nd ed. Baltimore, Williams and Wilkins, 1977.)

ness measured by ultrasound. A good correlation has been shown between the echocardiographically obtained end-systolic left ventricular posterior wall thickness–to–minor axis ratio. The relationship is expressed as left ventricular pressure (mm Hg) = 225 × systolic wall thickness/systolic internal diameter.[195] The presence of aortic regurgitation may reduce the predictive accuracy of this determination. Pulse Doppler echocardiography detects the altered and disturbed turbulence of flow.

Cardiac catheterization is more important for establishing the site and severity rather than the presence of aortic stenosis, since the malformation is usually diagnosed readily by clinical examination. Catheterization is indicated in any child with a clinical diagnosis of aortic stenosis in whom the clinical examination, roentgenogram, resting or exercise electrocardiogram, or echocardiogram suggests the possibility of severe obstruction.[180] Even in the absence of such findings, hemodynamic study should be performed if symptoms exist that might be related to aortic stenosis.

The site and severity of obstruction are established at cardiac catheterization, and associated malformations are identified. Typically, the angiocardiographic features of valvular stenosis are thickening of the aortic cusps and of the left ventricular wall with slight or no dilatation of the left ventricular cavity, poststenotic dilatation of the ascending aorta, and occasionally a jet of contrast material entering the ascending aorta through a narrowed valve orifice that is central or eccentric (Fig. 30–34). The leaflets of the bicuspid valve are domed in systole; a central jet corresponds to the orifice of the stenotic valve. In contrast, the stenotic orifice of the unicommissural valve may be visualized by the systolic jet in contact with the posterior wall of the aorta, with leaflet tissue and valve motion seen only anteriorly.

Congenital aortic stenosis is frequently a progressive disorder, even early in life, in a significant fraction of patients presenting initially with mild obstruction (Fig. 30–35).[196–202] Thus, clinical deterioration may be anticipated because of an intensification in the severity of stenosis rather than the development of significant aortic regurgitation. Progression of obstruction is usually the result of the increase in cardiac output that occurs concurrent with increased body growth. Less often, a decrease in the area of the orifice is an added factor in the intensification of obstruction. The onset of symptoms or changes in the phonocardiogram or graphic pulse tracings, chest roentgenograms, electrocardiograms, or vectorcardiograms cannot be depended upon to indicate progressive obstruction in the individual patient; Doppler echocardiography is most reliable.

MANAGEMENT. The malformed aortic valve is a potential site of bacterial infection; antibiotic prophylaxis is recommended for all patients, regardless of the severity of obstruction. Strict avoidance of strenuous physical activity is advised if severe aortic stenosis is present. Participation

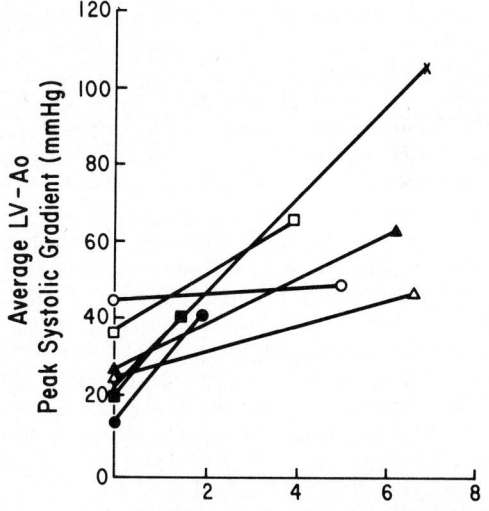

REFERENCE	NUMBER OF PATIENTS	AVERAGE AGE (yrs.) 1st CATH	2nd CATH
■ HOHN et al.	4	6,10,10,45	N.A.
● BENTIVOGLIO et al.	1	27	29
□ EL-SAID et al.	18	7	11
○ HURWITZ	19	9	14
▲ FRIEDMAN et al.	9	6.8	13.1
△ COHEN et al.	15	8.5	15.1
X BANDY and VOGEL	1	5	12

FIGURE 30–35. Composite of serial hemodynamic studies from seven medical centers showing the relationships between time and the left ventricular (LV)–aortic (Ao) pressure gradients in patients with congenital aortic stenosis. (From Friedman, W. F., et al.: Congenital aortic stenosis in adults. *In* Roberts, W. C. [eds.]: Congenital Heart Disease in Adults. Philadelphia, F. A. Davis, 1979, p. 235.)

in competitive sports should probably also be restricted in patients with milder degrees of obstruction. Digitalis should be administered to patients who have symptoms of diminished cardiac reserve and should also be considered in patients with left ventricular hypertrophy, even if they are not in heart failure.

The most important decision concerns the advisability of *surgical treatment.* Among the factors influencing the indications, techniques, and results of operation are the patient's age, the nature of the valvular deformity, and the experience of the surgical team.[180] The recommendation that operation is indicated depends more often on the presence of severe obstruction than on the symptoms described by the patient. At the present time, operation is advised for any child with critical stenosis (i.e., a peak systolic pressure gradient exceeding 75 mm Hg, measured in the basal state when the cardiac output is normal) or a calculated effective orifice less than 0.5 cm^2/m^2 body surface area. In the presence of clinical symptoms, a left ventricular strain pattern on the electrocardiogram, or an abnormal exercise electrocardiogram, operation may be recommended with less rigid regard to the hemodynamic assessment of the severity of stenosis. After severe stenosis has been established hemodynamically, the potential hazard of sudden death dictates that surgical treatment not be postponed unnecessarily. Operation is carried out under direct vision after institution of cardiopulmonary bypass; judicious incision of the fused commissures enlarges the valve orifice and does not result in significant aortic regurgitation. A mortality rate less than 2 per cent can be expected when operation is performed by an experienced surgeon. Substantial relief of obstruction occurs in the majority of patients unless the valve ring is hypoplastic. The role of percutaneous balloon aortic valvuloplasty is currently being studied.[203, 204]

Long-term follow-up studies have provided evidence that aortic valvulotomy is a safe and effective means of treatment with excellent relief of symptoms that were present preoperatively.[205] In some patients, aortic regurgitation may be progressive and require prosthetic valve replacement. Moreover, following commissurotomy the valve leaflets remain somewhat deformed, and it is quite possible that further degenerative changes, including calcification, will lead to significant stenosis in later years.[206, 207] Thus, prosthetic valve replacement is required in approximately 35 per cent of patients within 15 to 20 years of the original operation. Since the valves are not rendered anatomically normal, antibiotic prophylaxis is indicated in all patients postoperatively, even if the systolic pressure gradient has been abolished completely.

DISCRETE SUBAORTIC STENOSIS

This malformation accounts for 8 to 10 per cent of all cases of congenital aortic stenosis and occurs twice as frequently in males as in females. The lesion consists of a membranous diaphragm or fibromuscular ring encircling the left ventricular outflow tract just beneath the base of the aortic valve.

Distinction of subvalvular from valvular aortic stenosis is extremely difficult by means of clinical findings alone.[178] A systolic ejection sound is rarely heard, and the diastolic murmur of aortic regurgitation is more common than it is in valvular aortic stenosis. Dilatation of the ascending aorta is common, but valvular calcification is not observed.

Echocardiography is useful in the differentiation between valvular and subvalvular stenosis.[208, 209] (Figs. 5–72 and 5–73, p. 115). Two-dimensional echo studies from the apical two-chamber and left parasternal and subxiphoid long-axis views demonstrate persistent, prominent echoes in the subaortic left ventricle in both systole and diastole (Fig. 30–36). Doppler sampling proximal to the aortic valve shows increased flow velocity.[209] Most importantly, echocardiography can also identify hypertrophic subaortic stenosis when it coexists with fixed subaortic stenosis and for differentiating between the two forms of obstruction.[210]

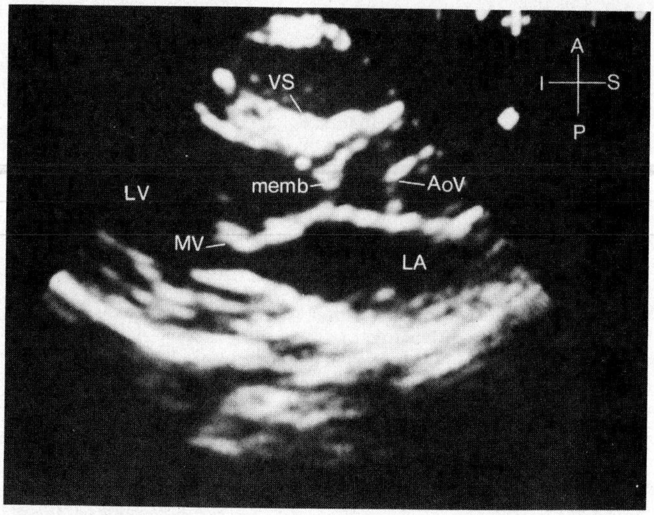

FIGURE 30–36. Long-axis view of discrete membranous subaortic stenosis. A discrete membrane (memb) is imaged in the left ventricular (LV) outflow tract beneath and parallel to the aortic valve (AoV), extending from the ventricular septum (VS) to the anterior leaflet of the mitral valve (MV). LA = left atrium.

Definitive distinction between valvular and subvalvular obstruction is provided by recording pressure tracings as a catheter is withdrawn across the outflow tract and valve or by localizing the site of obstruction with selective left ventricular angiocardiography (Fig. 30–34).

Mild degrees of aortic valvular regurgitation are commonly observed in patients with discrete subaortic stenosis and appear to be caused by thickening of the valve and impaired mobility of the cusps secondary to the trauma created by the high-velocity jet passing through the subaortic diaphragm. Further deformation of these abnormal valve cusps by the vegetations of bacterial endocarditis often results in severe aortic regurgitation.

Because of the likelihood of both progressive obstruction and aortic regurgitation, the presence of even mild or moderate subaortic stenosis warrants consideration of elective operation.[211] The risks of operation in patients with discrete subaortic stenosis and valvular aortic stenosis are essentially the same. Surgical correction is accomplished by excising the membrane or fibrous ridge. Operation may be expected to improve the hemodynamic state substantially; frequently it is totally curative.[212, 213] In a small number of patients, secondary muscular hypertrophy of the outflow tract and a pressure gradient may persist following the operative relief of valvular or discrete subvalvular aortic stenosis.[214] Balloon dilatation has also been reported to be a successful mode of therapy.[214a]

UNCOMMON FORMS OF SUBAORTIC STENOSIS

In some patients, valvular and subvalvular aortic stenosis coexist, with hypoplasia of the aortic valve ring and thickened valve leaflets, producing a tunnel-like narrowing of the left ventricular outflow tract.[215] Additional findings often include a small ascending aorta. The subvalvular fibrous process usually extends onto the aortic valve cusps and almost always makes contact with the ventricular aspect of the anterior mitral leaflet at its base. The presence of "tunnel stenosis" may be suspected echocardiographically and angiographically from the appearance of the outflow tract and the aortic root. Operative treatment is often complicated by the necessity for prosthetic or homograft replacement of the aortic valve as well as for enlarging the aortic annulus, proximal aorta, and left ventricular outlet tract (the Konno operation). Operation is controversial utilizing a prosthetic, valve-containing conduit between the left ventricular apex and descending aorta.[216]

Various anatomical lesions other than a discrete membrane or ridge may produce subaortic stenosis.[217, 218] Among these are abnormal adherence of the anterior leaflet of the mitral valve to the left septal surface, and the presence in the left ventricular outflow tract of accessory endocardial cushion tissue. In some patients with atrioventricular canal, the part of the ventricular septum that contributes to the wall of the left ventricular outflow tract is deficient, and the ventricular aspect of the anterior leaflet of the common atrioventricular valve is adherent to the posterior edge of the deficient septum, resulting in a narrow left ventricular outflow tract. Malalignment of the conoventricular septum, resulting in an inferior ventricular septal defect, produces a leftward superior deviation and insertion of the conal septum obstructing left ventricular outflow.[217] In patients with single ventricle and an outflow chamber, the bulboventricular foramen serves as a potential site of aortic outflow obstruction. Additional, rarer causes of subaortic stenosis include redundant dysplastic left atrioventricular valve tissue in patients with congenitally corrected transposition of the great arteries and anomalous muscle bundles of the left ventricular outflow tract.[218] A muscular type of subaortic stenosis may result from a convergence of all the mitral chordae into one or two fused papillary muscles; a "parachute" deformity of the mitral valve is produced that is often seen in association with supravalvular stenosis of the left atrium and coarctation of the aorta. In some of these patients, discrete membranous subvalvular aortic obstruction has also been noted.

In patients with ventricular septal defect, muscular subaortic stenosis has been shown to develop after surgical banding of the pulmonary artery, possibly as a result of hypertrophy of the conal septum or crista supraventricularis encroaching on the left ventricular outflow tract above the septal defect.

Subaortic muscular hypertrophy secondary to diffuse involvement of the myocardium by glycogen storage disease (Pompe's disease) is an extremely rare cause of obstruction to left ventricular outflow. A positive family history, symptoms of muscular weakness, heart failure in infancy, and the characteristic electrocardiographic findings of a short PR interval, high-voltage QRS and T waves, and left ventricular hypertrophy warrant skeletal muscle biopsy or fibroblast culture, permitting a premortem diagnosis.

The last relatively uncommon form of subaortic stenosis to be mentioned occurs infrequently in patients with congenitally corrected transposition of the great arteries in whom an anomalous muscle bundle in the subaortic area of the arterial ventricle obstructs outflow.

SUPRAVALVULAR AORTIC STENOSIS

Supravalvular aortic stenosis is a congenital narrowing of the ascending aorta that may be localized or diffuse, originating at the superior margin of the sinuses of Valsalva just above the levels of the coronary arteries.

The clinical picture of supravalvular obstruction usually differs in major respects from that observed in the other forms of aortic stenosis. Chief among these differences is the association of supravalvular aortic stenosis with idiopathic infantile hypercalcemia, a disease that may be related to deranged vitamin D metabolism.[219–223] The designation "supravalvular aortic stenosis syndrome" or "Williams' syndrome" is applied to the distinctive clinical picture produced by coexistence of the cardiac and multiple system disorder. Additional manifestations of this syndrome include a peculiar elfin facies (Fig. 30–37), mental retardation, auditory hyperacusis, narrowing of peripheral systemic and pulmonary arteries, inguinal hernia, strabismus, and abnormalities of dental development. In some patients, moderate thickening of the aortic cusps and valvular pulmonary stenosis may occur in association with peripheral pulmonary artery stenosis. Rarely, patients have mitral valve abnormalities with prolapse and mitral regurgitation.

Experimental hypervitaminosis D produced in the pregnant rabbit has caused craniofacial abnormalities and malformations resembling those of supravalvular aortic stenosis in the offspring.[219, 220] In humans, with one exception, chromosome studies have consistently revealed normal karyotypes. Most often supravalvular aortic stenosis is a feature of the distinctive syndrome described above. However, peripheral pulmonary artery stenosis and the aortic anomaly are also seen in familial and sporadic forms unassociated with the other features of the syndrome.[224] Genetic studies suggest that the familial anomaly is transmitted as an autosomal dominant with variable expression. Some family members may have supravalvular pulmonic stenosis either as an isolated lesion or in combination with the supravalvular aortic anomaly. Unlike the other forms of aortic stenosis, there appears to be no sex predilection.

Three anatomical types of supravalvular aortic stenosis are recognized, although some patients may have findings of more than one type. Most common is the hourglass type, in which marked thickening and disorganization of the aortic media produce a constricting annular ridge at the superior margin of the sinuses of Valsalva. The membranous type is the result of fibrous or fibromuscular semicircular diaphragm with a small central opening stretched across the lumen of the aorta. Uniform hypoplasia of the ascending aorta characterizes the hypoplastic type.

Because the coronary arteries arise proximal to the site of outflow

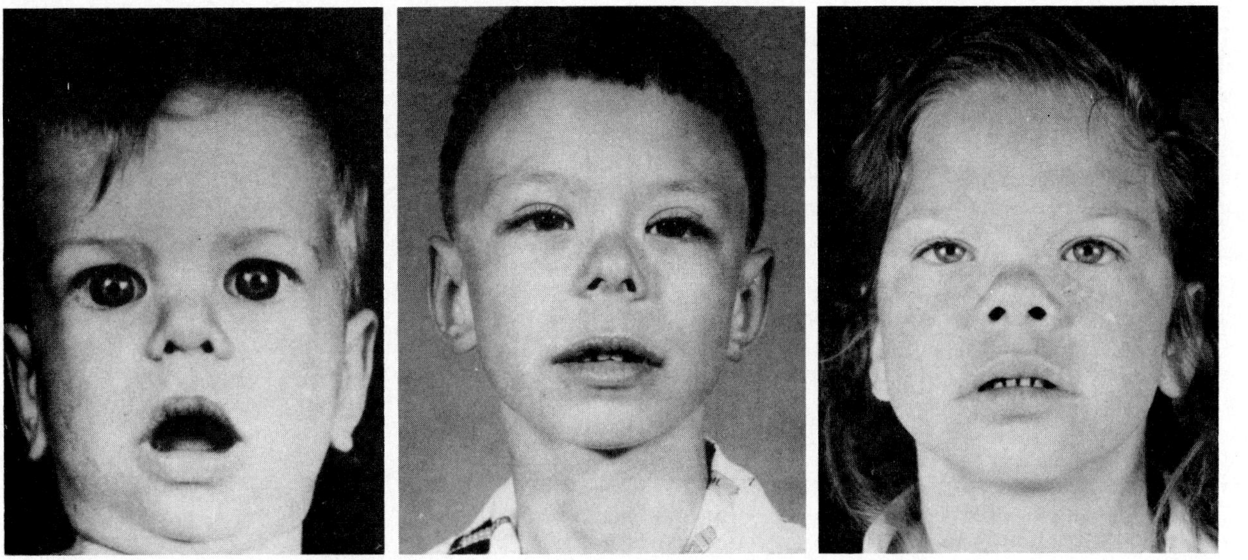

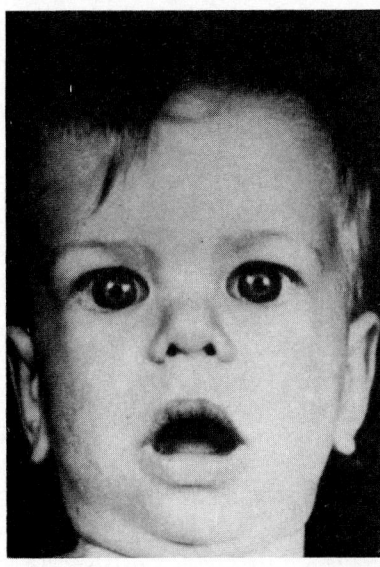

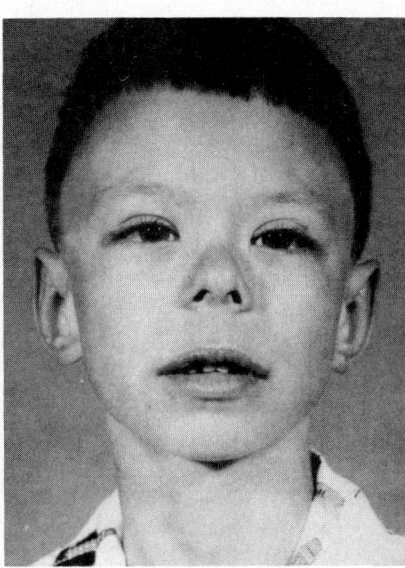

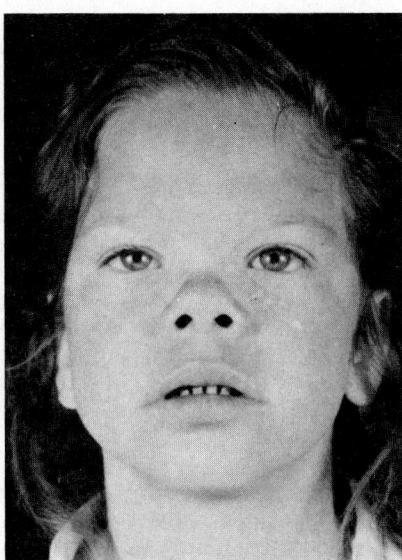

FIGURE 30–37. Typical elfin facies in three patients with supravalvular aortic stenosis. (From Friedman, W. F., and Kirkpatrick, S. E.: Congenital aortic stenosis. *In* Moss, A. J., Adams, F. H., and Emmanouilides, G. C. [eds.]: Heart Disease in Infants, Children and Adolescents. 2nd ed. Baltimore, Williams and Wilkins, 1977.)

obstruction in supravalvular aortic stenosis, they are subjected to the elevated pressure that exists within the left ventricle. These vessels are often dilated and tortuous, and premature coronary arteriosclerosis has been observed. Moreover, if the free edges of some or all of the aortic cusps adhere to the site of supravalvular stenosis, coronary artery inflow may be reduced. The formation of thoracic aortic aneurysms has been described in several patients.

Most often, patients with supravalvular aortic stenosis syndrome are mentally retarded and resemble one another in their facial features. The typical appearance is similar to the elfin facies observed in the severe form of idiopathic infantile hypercalcemia and is characterized by a high prominent forehead, epicanthal folds, underdeveloped bridge of the nose and mandible, overhanging upper lip, strabismus, and anomalies of dentition (Fig. 30–37). Recognition of this distinctive appearance, even in infancy, should alert the physician to the possibility of underlying multiple system disease. In addition, a positive family history in a patient with a normal appearance and clinical signs suggesting left ventricular outflow obstruction should lead to the suspicion of either supravalvular aortic stenosis or hypertrophic obstructive cardiomyopathy.[224] Patients with supravalvular aortic obstruction appear to be subject to the same risks of unexpected sudden death and infective endocarditis as those with valvular aortic stenosis.

With few exceptions, the major *physical findings* resemble those observed in patients with valvular aortic stenosis. Among these exceptions are accentuation of aortic valve closure due to elevated pressure in the aorta proximal to the stenosis, an infrequent systolic ejection sound, and the especially prominent transmission of a thrill and murmur into the jugular notch and along the carotid vessels. Uncommonly, there is an early diastolic, decrescendo, blowing murmur of aortic regurgitation due to the fusion of one or more cusps to the area of stenosis. The narrowing of the peripheral pulmonary arteries that often coexists in these patients frequently produces a late systolic or continuous murmur that may help distinguish this anomaly from valvular aortic stenosis. This differentiation is reinforced by the frequent finding of a significant disparity between the arterial pressures in the upper extremities in supravalvular aortic stenosis; the systolic pressure in the right arm tends to be the higher of the two and occasionally exceeds that in the femoral arteries. The disparity in pulses may relate to the tendency of a jet stream to adhere to a vessel wall (Coanda effect) and selective streaming of blood into the innominate artery.[225, 226]

Electrocardiography generally reveals left ventricular hypertrophy when obstruction is severe. However, biventricular, or even right ventricular, hypertrophy may be found if significant narrowing of peripheral pulmonary arteries coexists. Radiographically, in contrast to valvular and discrete subvalvular aortic stenosis, poststenotic dilation of the ascending aorta is rarely seen. Usually the sinuses of Valsalva are dilated and ascending aorta and the aortic arch are of normal size or appear small.

Echocardiography is the most valuable technique for localizing the site of obstruction to the supravalvular area (Fig. 30–38) and Doppler examination and retrograde aortic catheterization can determine the degree of hemodynamic abnormality.

The supravalvular aortic lumen may be widened by the insertion of an oval- or diamond-shaped fabric patch in those patients with a normal ascending aorta.[227] If the aorta is markedly hypoplastic, this operation merely displaces the pressure gradient distally without abolishing the obstruction. Under these circumstances, repair may require

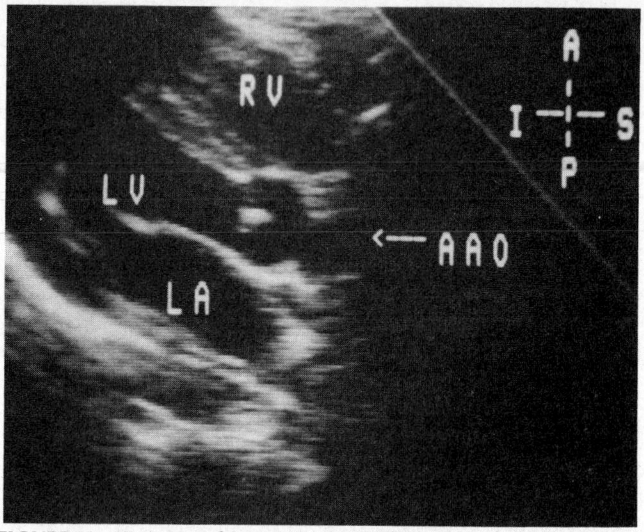

FIGURE 30–38. Supravalvar aortic stenosis is seen in a parasternal long-axis view. The constriction is distal to the sinuses of Valsalva in the ascending aorta (AAO). RV = right ventricle, LV = left ventricle, LA = left atrium. (Courtesy of Norman Silverman, M.D.)

replacement or widening of the entire hypoplastic aorta with an appropriate prosthesis. Operation may be recommended when relatively little hypoplasia of the ascending aorta and arch exists and when the obstruction is discrete and significant, i.e., with a systolic gradient exceeding 50 mm Hg.

HYPOPLASTIC LEFT HEART SYNDROME

This designation is used to describe a group of closely related cardiac anomalies characterized by underdevelopment of the left cardiac chambers, atresia or stenosis of the aortic and/or the mitral orifices, and hypoplasia of the aorta.[228] These anomalies are an especially common cause of heart failure in the first week of life. The left atrium and ventricle often exhibit *endocardial fibroelastosis*. Pulmo-

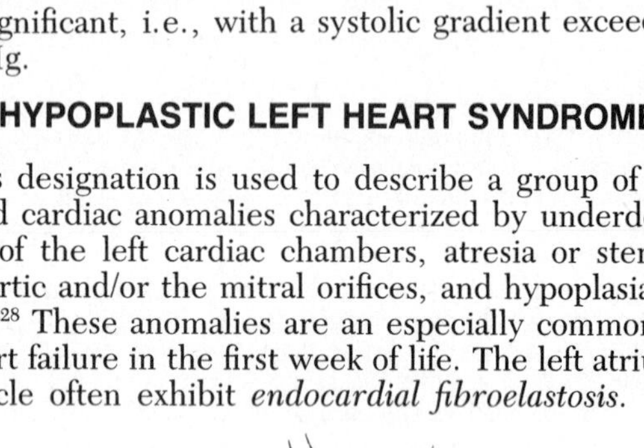

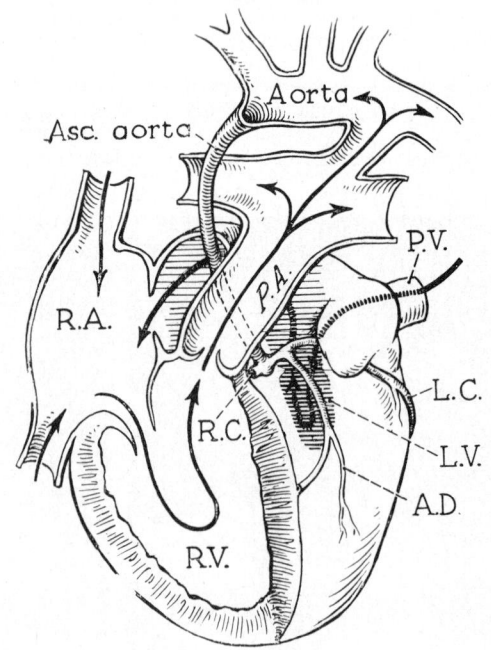

FIGURE 30–39. Hypoplastic left heart with aortic hypoplasia, aortic valve atresia, and a hypoplastic mitral valve and left ventricle. R.A. = right atrium, R.V. = right ventricle, R.C. = right coronary artery, P.A. = pulmonary artery, P.V. = pulmonary vein, L.C. = left coronary artery, L.V. = left ventricle, A.D. = anterior descending coronary artery. (From Neufeld, H. N., et al.: Diagnosis of aortic atresia by retrograde aortography. Circulation *25*:278, 1962, by permission of the American Heart Association, Inc.)

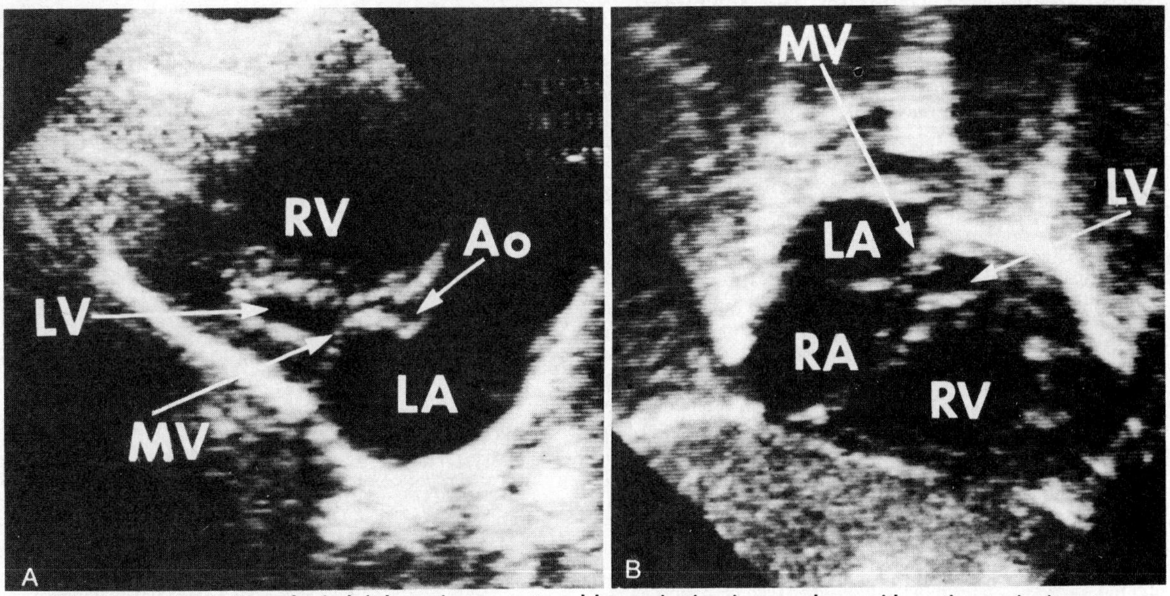

FIGURE 30–40. *A,* Hypoplastic left heart in a parasternal long-axis view in a newborn with aortic atresia, intact ventricular septum and patent but hypoplastic mitral valve (MV). The left ventricular (LV) cavity is diminutive and the ascending aorta (Ao) is hypoplastic. Right ventricular (RV) dilation is noted. *B,* In the subcostal four-chamber view dilatation of the right atrium (RA) and right ventricle (RV) is noted. The endocardial echoes are very bright due to fibroelastosis. (From Perloff, J.: The Clinical Recognition of Congenital Heart Disease. 3rd ed. Philadelphia, W. B. Saunders Company, 1986.)

nary venous blood traverses a patent foramen ovale and a dilated and hypertrophied right ventricle acts as the systemic, as well as the pulmonary, ventricle; the systemic circulation receives blood via a patent ductus arteriosus (Fig. 30–39). The diagnosis should be considered in infants, particularly males, with the sudden onset of heart failure, systemic hypoperfusion, and nonspecific murmur. Electrocardiography frequently reveals right axis deviation, right atrial and ventricular enlargement, and ST and T-wave abnormalities in the left precordial leads. Chest roentgenography may show only slight enlargement shortly after birth, but with clinical deterioration there is marked cardiomegaly and increased pulmonary venous and arterial vascular markings.

The echocardiographic findings are usually diagnostic (Fig. 30–40) and include a diminutive aortic root and left ventricular cavity and absence or poor visualization of aortic and mitral valve echoes, which, when seen, are of diminished amplitude and mobility.[229] Retrograde aortography shows hypoplasia of the ascending aorta (Fig. 30–41).

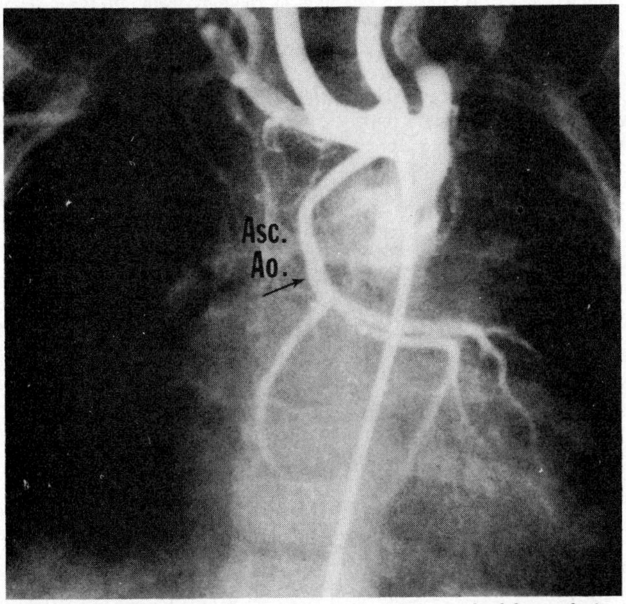

FIGURE 30–41. Retrograde aortogram showing marked hypoplasia of the ascending aorta (Asc. Ao.) (arrow) in an infant with hypoplastic left heart syndrome. (From Freedom, R. M., et al.: Aortic atresia with normal left ventricle: Distinctive angiocardiographic findings. Cath. Cardiovasc. Diag. *3*:283, 1977.)

Medical therapy directed at cardiac decompensation, hypoxemia, and metabolic acidemia rarely allows survival beyond the first days of life. Constriction of the patent ductus arteriosus and limited flow through a restrictive patent foramen ovale are the principal factors responsible for early death. Prostaglandin E_1 infusion is effective in maintaining ductal patency. Some centers are attempting staged surgical management in an effort to provide long-term palliation.[228, 230] The first stage, often referred to as the Norwood procedure, consists of creating an unobstructed communication between the right ventricle and aorta, and enlargement of the ascending aorta. The right ventricular–aortic connection has been accomplished with homograft or prosthetic conduits from the right ventricle or pulmonary trunk to the descending aorta, or by direct connection between the proximal pulmonary trunk and ascending aorta, which also enlarges the ascending aorta. Pulmonary blood flow and pressure are controlled by a tubed interposition systemic pulmonary shunt to the distal pulmonary artery. The patent ductus arteriosus is ligated. A large interatrial communication must also be assured in stage 1 to allow free access of pulmonary venous blood to the tricuspid valve. In stage II, an interatrial baffle is created to provide continuity between left atrium and tricuspid valve; the pulmonary arterial circulation is provided by direct anastomosis of the right atrium to the pulmonary arteries (the Fontan connection). In some centers, the preferred operation is human cardiac transplantation. Although cardiac xenotransplantation has been attempted, it is a highly controversial approach.[231, 232]

CONGENITAL AORTIC REGURGITATION

Congenital aortic valve regurgitation is an extremely rare isolated congenital cardiac lesion.[232a] Most often aortic regurgitation occurs in association with congenital valvular aortic stenosis in which the valve commissures are fused inhibiting cusp mobility, subvalvular aortic stenosis in which the aortic ring is dilated and the valve cusps are deformed, coarctation of the aorta when the aortic ring is dilated and the aortic valve is bicuspid, ventricular septal defect (p. 920), and endocardial fibroelastosis. Aortic valve regurgitation may also accompany aortic sinus aneurysm or be secondary to dilatation of the ascending aorta in patients with Marfan syndrome, Turner syndrome, cystic medial necrosis, or osteogenesis imperfecta in which the aortic lesions are manifestations of the underlying connective tissue disorder (Chap. 54).

Severe aortic regurgitation may also occur through channels other than the aortic valve.[232b, 233] Thus, aortico–left ventricular tunnel is a rare anomaly that must be distinguished from congenital aortic valve regurgitation, since the approach to management of the former does not usually include consideration for prosthetic valve replacement. The aortico–left ventricular tunnel is an abnormal channel beginning in the ascending aorta above the right coronary orifice and ending in the left ventricle below the right aortic cusp. The channel usually passes behind the right ventricular infundibulum and through the ventricular septum.

Echocardiography, Doppler interrogation, and aortography combine to establish a precise diagnosis. Exercise testing is useful to assess the severity of the lesion.[234] In infants and children with congenital aortic regurgitation the severity of regurgitation increases with time, and valve replacement, rather than plication, is almost always necessary to correct the lesion. Operation should be deferred until symptoms, signs, and noninvasive assessment dictate its necessity. Conversely, closure of an aortico–left ventricular communication is advisable before progressive dilation of the aortic annulus creates secondary changes in the aortic valve itself which may necessitate aortic valve replacement.

PULMONARY VEIN ATRESIA AND STENOSIS

Pulmonary vein atresia is a quite rare anomaly in which the pulmonary veins do not connect with the heart or with a major systemic vein.[235] The lesion is incompatible with life, but infants may survive for days, probably because communications exist between the pulmonary veins and the bronchial or esophageal veins that allow limited egress for pulmonary venous blood. Pulmonary vein stenosis may occur as a focal stenosis at the atrial junction or generalized hypoplasia of one or more pulmonary veins. There is an extremely high incidence of associated cardiac malformations, including atrial septal defect, tetralogy of Fallot, tricuspid and mitral atresia, and endocardial cushion defect. The severe pulmonary vein obstruction imposed by pulmonary vein abnormalities causes severe cyanosis, congestive cardiac failure, and early death. Focal stenosis of one or more pulmonary veins at the atrial junction, recognized by two-dimensional echocardiography or angiography, may be relieved surgically.[236, 237] Results of transcutaneous balloon angioplasty have been disappointing.

COR TRIATRIATUM

(See also p. 985)

In this malformation failure of resorption of the common pulmonary vein results in a left atrium divided by an abnormal fibromuscular diaphragm into a posterosuperior chamber receiving the pulmonary veins and an anteroinferior chamber giving rise to the left atrial appendage and leading to the mitral orifice.[238] The communication between the divided atrial chambers may be large, small, or absent depending on the size of the opening(s) in the subdividing diaphragm, which determines the degree of obstruction to pulmonary venous return. Elevations of both pulmonary venous pressure and pulmonary vascular resistance result in severe pulmonary artery hypertension.

The diagnosis is established by two-dimensional echocardiography; cardiac catheterization and angiography are only necessary if major associated cardiac anomalies are suspected.[239] The obstructive membrane is visualized in the parasternal long- and short-axis and four-chamber (Fig. 30–42) views, and can be distinguished from a supravalvular mitral ring by its position superior to the left atrial appendage, which forms a part of the distal chamber. Also present are diastolic fluttering of the mitral leaflets and

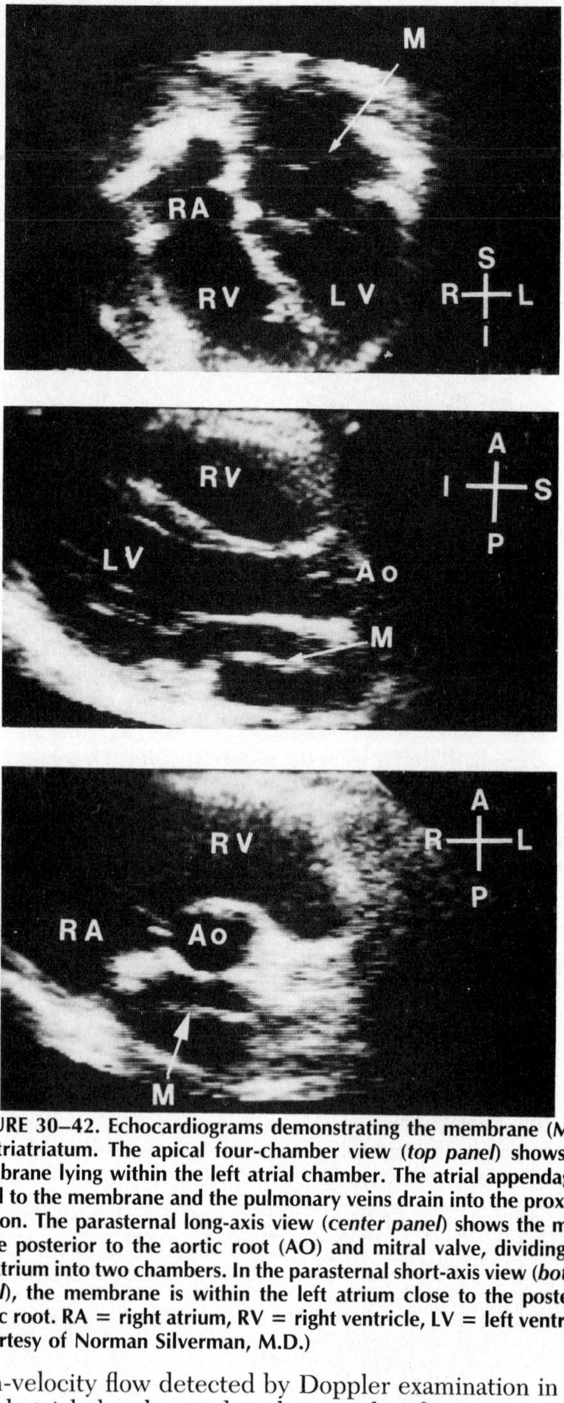

FIGURE 30–42. Echocardiograms demonstrating the membrane (M) of cor triatriatum. The apical four-chamber view (*top panel*) shows the membrane lying within the left atrial chamber. The atrial appendage is distal to the membrane and the pulmonary veins drain into the proximal portion. The parasternal long-axis view (*center panel*) shows the membrane posterior to the aortic root (AO) and mitral valve, dividing the left atrium into two chambers. In the parasternal short-axis view (*bottom panel*), the membrane is within the left atrium close to the posterior aortic root. RA = right atrium, RV = right ventricle, LV = left ventricle. (Courtesy of Norman Silverman, M.D.)

high-velocity flow detected by Doppler examination in the distal atrial chamber and at the mitral orifice.

The diagnosis should be suspected at cardiac catheterization if the pulmonary arterial wedge pressure is higher than a simultaneous left atrial pressure. The diagnosis may also be established by visualizing the obstructing lesion angiographically. Although rare, it is important to recognize the malformation because it may be easily correctable at operation.[240]

CONGENITAL MITRAL STENOSIS

Anatomical types of mitral stenosis include the parachute deformity of the valve, in which shortened chordae tendineae converge and insert into a single large papillary muscle; thickened leaflets with shortening and fusion of the chordae tendineae; an anomalous arcade of obstructing papillary muscles; accessory mitral valve tissue; and a supravalvular circumferential ridge of connective tissue arising at the base of the atrial aspect of the mitral leaflets.[241, 242] Associated cardiac defects are common, including endocardial fibroelastosis, coarctation of the aorta, patent ductus arteriosus, and left ventricular outflow tract obstruction. Two-dimensional echocardiography, combined with Doppler studies, often provides a complete analysis of the anatomy and function of congenital left ventricular inflow lesions.[243, 244] The clinical and hemodynamic consequences of isolated congenital mitral stenosis are similar to those of acquired mitral obstruction with modifications imposed by coexisting anomalies.

The prognosis is poor; symptoms attributable to pulmonary vein obstruction begin usually in infancy and the majority of patients expire before age one year unless successfully operated upon. Conduit bypass of the mitral valve and prosthetic valve replacement are required if a reparative operation is not possible.[245, 246] The use of a porcine bioprosthesis is contraindicated because of its rapid degeneration in the infant or young child. Transcatheter balloon angioplasty may prove to be an alternative to surgical mitral commissurotomy in selected patients beyond infancy.[247]

CONGENITAL MITRAL REGURGITATION

The syndrome of *mitral valve prolapse* is discussed on p. 1045. This condition is generally quite benign in children. However, occasional difficulties exist with infective endocarditis, arrhythmias, atypical chest pain, and sudden death.

Isolated congenital mitral regurgitation of hemodynamic significance is an unusual lesion in infants and children. Most often, congenital malformations of the mitral valve producing insufficiency are encountered in association with endocardial cushion defect, congenitally corrected transposition of the great arteries, endocardial fibroelastosis, anomalous pulmonary origin of the coronary artery, congenital subaortic stenosis, hypertrophic obstructive cardiomyopathy, and coarctation of the aorta. Mitral valve dysfunction is also seen commonly in a variety of metabolic disorders (e.g., the mucopolysaccharidoses), primary and secondary cardiomyopathies, connective tissue disease (e.g., rheumatoid arthritis, Marfan syndrome, Ehlers-Danlos syndrome, pseudoxanthoma elasticum), and rheumatic and nonrheumatic inflammatory diseases of the myocardium[248] (see Chap. 54).

The various anatomical lesions that result in isolated congenital mitral regurgitation include prolapse of one or both mitral leaflets, cleft or perforated mitral leaflet, inadequate leaflet tissue, double orifice of the mitral valve, anomalous insertion of chordae tendineae (anomalous mitral arcade), redundant leaflet tissue, displacement inferiorly of the ring of the inferior leaflet into the left ventricle, and abnormal length of chordae tendineae.[249] The clinical and hemodynamic findings in patients with isolated congenital mitral incompetence resemble those observed in acquired mitral regurgitation. Mitral annuloplasty (which is preferred) and prosthetic valve replacement are procedures reserved for infants or children who are at least moderately symptomatic despite comprehensive medical management, often with repeated episodes of pulmonary infection, or cardiac failure with anorexia and retarded growth and development.[249, 250] Operative candidates are shown by echocardiographic, Doppler, hemodynamic, and angiographic studies to have pulmonary hypertension, a regurgitant fraction in excess of 50 per cent, and a marked increase in left ventricular end-diastolic volume.

PULMONARY ARTERIOVENOUS FISTULA

(See also p. 1002)

Abnormal development of the pulmonary arteries and veins in a common vascular complex is responsible for this rare congenital anomaly. A variable number of pulmonary arteries communicate directly with branches of the pulmonary veins; in some cases the fistula receives systemic arterial branches.[251, 252] The majority of patients have an associated Weber-Osler-Rendu syndrome; additional associated problems include bronchiectasis and other malformations of the bronchial tree, and absence of the right lower lobe. Venoarterial shunting depends upon the extent of the fistulous communications and may result in cyanosis and secondary polycythemia. Patients with hereditary hemorrhagic telangiectasis are often anemic owing to repeated blood loss and may have less obvious cyanosis. Systolic and continuous murmurs are audible over areas of the fistula(s). Rounded opacities of variable size in one or both lungs on chest roentgenogram may suggest the presence of the lesion. Pulmonary angiography reveals the site and extent of the abnormal communication. Unless the lesions are widespread throughout both lungs, surgical treatment aimed at removing the lesions with preservation of healthy lung tissue is commonly indicated to avoid the complications of massive hemorrhage, bacterial endocarditis, and rupture of arteriovenous aneurysms.

Transcatheter balloon or plug or coil occlusion embolotherapy may prove to be the therapeutic procedure of choice.[251, 253]

PERIPHERAL PULMONARY ARTERY STENOSIS (See also p. 992)

Stenosis of the pulmonary artery may be single or multiple and occur anywhere from the main pulmonary trunk to the smaller peripheral arterial branches.[254] Associated defects are observed in the majority of patients and include pulmonic valvular stenosis, ventricular septal defect, tetralogy of Fallot, and supravalvular aortic stenosis.

The most important cause of significant pulmonary artery stenoses producing symptoms in the newborn is intrauterine rubella infection.[255] Diagnosis is facilitated in these infants by finding elevations of the IgM fraction and rubella antibody titer. Other cardiovascular malformations seen commonly in association with congenital rubella include patent ductus arteriosus, pulmonic valve stenosis, and atrial septal defect. Generalized systemic arterial stenotic lesions may also be a feature of the rubella embryopathy, often involving large and medium-sized vessels such as the aorta and coronary, cerebral, mesenteric, and renal arteries. Cardiovascular lesions are but one manifestation of intrauterine rubella infection, since cataracts, microphthalmia, deafness, thrombocytopenia, hepatitis, and blood dyscrasias are also common. Thus, the clinical picture in infants with rubella syndrome depends upon the severity of the cardiovascular lesions and the associated abnormalities of other organs and systems.

Obstruction within the pulmonary arterial tree may be classified into four types: (1) stenosis of the main pulmonary trunk or the main left or right branch; (2) narrowing at the bifurcation of the pulmonary artery, extending into both right and left branches; (3) multiple sites of peripheral branch stenosis; and (4) a combination of main and peripheral stenosis. Pulmonary artery obstruction may be produced by localized narrowing, diffuse constrictions, or rarely, by a membrane or diaphragm. Poststenotic dilatation is usual when the stenosis is localized, but may be absent or minimal with elongated constriction. It should be recognized that a physiological branch pulmonary artery stenosis is often present in the normal newborn in whom both right and left main pulmonary arteries are small and arise almost perpendicular from a large main pulmonary artery.[256] The branch vessels increase in size with growth and become less angulated in their take-off from the main pulmonary artery.

The degree of obstruction is the principal determinant of clinical severity; the type of obstruction determines the feasibility of direct surgical relief. The clinical features vary; most infants and children are asymptomatic.[257] An ejection systolic murmur at the upper left sternal border that is well transmitted to the axillae and back is most common. The presence of an ejection sound suggests that pulmonic valve stenosis coexists. The pulmonic component of the second heart sound may be slightly accentuated, but occasionally is extremely loud if multiple peripheral stenoses exist. A continuous murmur is audible, especially in patients with main or branch stenosis, and particularly if an associated cardiovascular anomaly produces increased pulmonary blood flow. Electrocardiography shows right ventricular hypertrophy when obstruction is severe; left axis deviation with counterclockwise orientation of the frontal QRS vector is common in the rubella syndrome and when the lesion coexists with supravalvular aortic stenosis. Mild or moderate stenosis usually produces a normal chest roentgenogram; detectable differences in vascularity between regions of the lungs or dilated pulmonary artery segments are uncommon. When obstruction is bilateral and severe, right atrial and ventricular enlargement may be observed.

Diagnosis is confirmed by observing pressure gradients within the pulmonary arterial system at cardiac catheteri-

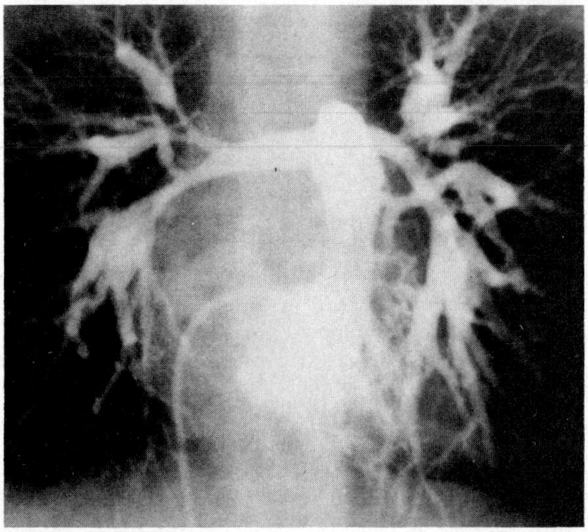

FIGURE 30–43. Right ventricular angiocardiogram showing multiple sites of peripheral pulmonic stenosis and poststenotic dilatation of the peripheral pulmonic arteries.

zation; digital subtraction and/or selective pulmonary angiography defines the exact location, extent, and distribution of the lesion (Fig. 30–43). Mild to moderate unilateral or bilateral stenosis does not require surgical relief; numerous stenotic areas are not amenable to correction, even with intraoperative balloon angioplasty.[258–260] Well-localized obstruction of severe degree in the main pulmonary artery or its major branches may be alleviated by percutaneous transcatheter balloon angioplasty (p. 1336) or with a patch graft or bypassed with a tubular conduit. The natural history of peripheral pulmonary stenosis is not clear. Obstruction may increase by discrepant growth between a stenotic area and normal portions of the pulmonary artery tree, or as a result of an increase in cardiac output, especially during adolescence. Rarely, hypertrophy is progressive of right ventricular infundibular muscle and results in hypercyanotic spells.

PULMONIC STENOSIS WITH INTACT VENTRICULAR SEPTUM (See also p. 991)

Valvular pulmonic stenosis, resulting from fusion of the valve cusps during mid to late intrauterine development, is the most common form of isolated right ventricular obstruction and occurs in approximately 7 per cent of patients with congenital heart disease. Hypertrophy of the septal and parietal bands narrowing the right ventricular infundibulum often accompanies the pulmonic valve lesion, especially if it is severe. Fused cusps of varying thickness and rigidity form a fibrous dome in the most severe forms. Pulmonic valve dysplasia, especially common in patients with Noonan syndrome (p. 1625), produces obstruction in the absence of adherent leaflets because leaflets are thickened, rigid, and myxomatous and are limited in their lateral movement because of the presence of tissue pads within the pulmonic valve sinuses.[261]

INFANCY. The clinical presentation and course of circulation in the newborn with pulmonic stenosis depends on the severity of obstruction and the degree of development of the right ventricle and its outflow tract, the tricuspid valve, and the pulmonary arterial tree.[262] The greater the degree of pulmonic valve stenosis, the more closely the manifestations resemble those observed with pulmonary atresia and intact ventricular septum (see p. 944). Severe pulmonic stenosis is characterized by cyanosis due to right-to-left shunting through the foramen ovale, cardiomegaly, and diminished pulmonary blood flow in the absence of persistent patency of the ductus arteriosus. Hypoxemia and metabolic acidemia, rather than right ventricular failure, are the main clinical disturbances in the symptomatic neonate and can be alleviated temporarily by infusion of prostaglandin E_1 to dilate the ductus arteriosus and increase pulmonary blood flow. Distinction of these babies from those with tetralogy of Fallot or tricuspid or pulmonary atresia is usually possible, since infants with tetralogy generally do not have roentgenographic evidence of cardiomegaly; infants with tricuspid and pulmonary atresia show a preponderance of left ventricular forces by electrocardiography in contrast to the right ventricular hypertrophy observed usually with critical pulmonic stenosis in the absence of right ventricular hypoplasia. Combined two-dimensional echocardiographic and continuous-wave Doppler examination (Figs. 5–68, p. 113, and 5–69, p. 114) characterize the anatomical valve abnormality and its severity, and have importantly reduced the requirement for cardiac catheterization and angiographic studies to establish a precise diagnosis (Fig. 30–44).[263–265] Pulmonary valvotomy is often the therapeutic procedure of choice, but a systemic-to-pulmonary arterial shunt may also be necessary in infants with underdevelopment of the right ventricular cavity.[265a] Transcatheter balloon valvuloplasty may be expected to reduce, but not abolish, the pressure difference in neonates with mobile doming valves but not in those with dysplastic valves.[266, 267]

CHILDHOOD. The clinical profile of patients with valvular pulmonic stenosis beyond infancy is generally distinctive.[268] The severity of obstruction is the most important determinant of the clinical course. In the presence of a normal cardiac output a peak systolic transvalvular pressure gradient between 50 and 80 mm Hg or a peak systolic right ventricular pressure between 75 and 100 mm Hg is considered to be moderate stenosis; levels below and above that range are classified as mild and severe, respectively. Patients with mild pulmonic stenosis are generally asymptomatic and the condition is discovered during routine examination. In patients with more significant obstruction the severity of stenosis may increase with time. Progression may be relative and reflect disproportionate physical growth of the patient, infundibular narrowing due to progressive hypertrophy of the right ventricular outflow tract, or fibrosis of the valve cusps. Symptoms, when present, vary from mild exertional dyspnea and mild cyanosis to signs and symptoms of heart failure depending upon the degree of obstruction and the level of myocardial compensation. Exertional fatigue, syncope, and chest pain are related to an inability to augment pulmonary blood flow during exercise in some patients with moderate or severe obstruction.

The severity of obstruction is often suggested by the physical findings. Right ventricular hypertrophy reduces compliance of that chamber and a forceful right atrial contraction is necessary to augment right ventricular filling. Prominent *a*-waves in the jugular venous pulse, a fourth heart sound, and, occasionally, presystolic pulsations of the liver reflect a vigorous atrial contraction and suggest the presence of severe stenosis. Cardiomegaly and a right ventricular parasternal lift accompany moderate or severe obstruction. A systolic thrill is palpable along the upper left sternal border in all but the mildest forms of stenosis. The first heart sound is normal and is followed by a systolic ejection sound at the upper left sternal edge produced by sudden opening of the stenotic valve; an ejection sound is

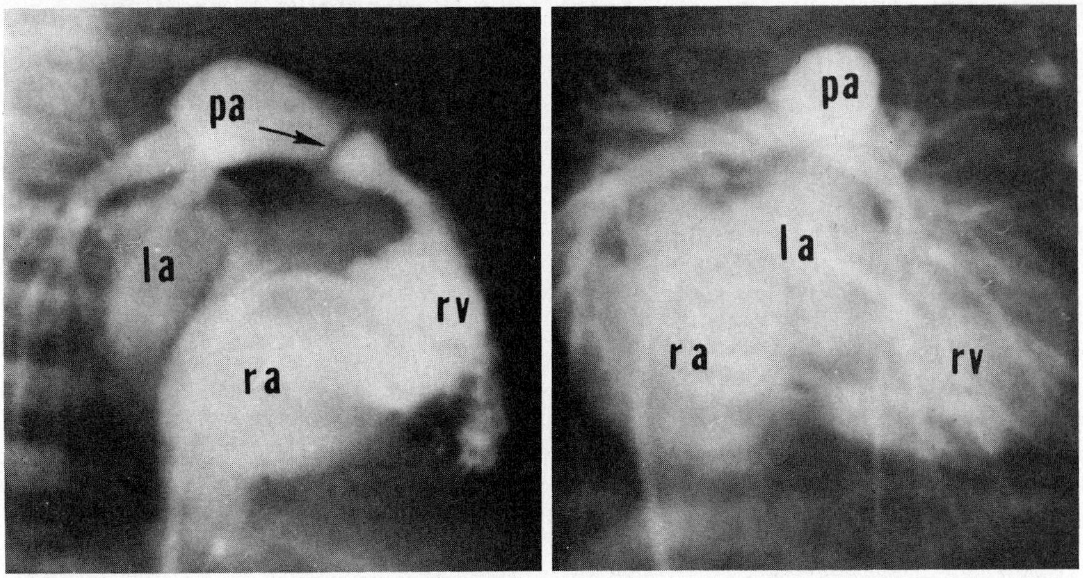

FIGURE 30–44. Right ventriculogram in an infant with critical pulmonic stenosis shows the thickened, nonmobile pulmonic valve (arrow) in the lateral projection (*left*). Both the lateral and frontal (*right*) projections show regurgitation of contrast material across the tricuspid valve into the right atrium (ra), with subsequent shunting across the foramen ovale to the left atrium (la). rv = right ventricle; pa = pulmonary artery. (Courtesy of Norman Talner, M.D.)

not heard in patients with pulmonic valve dysplasia. The ejection sound typically is louder during expiration; when it is inaudible or occurs less than 0.08 second from the onset of the Q wave on electrocardiogram, severe obstruction is suggested. Right ventricular ejection is prolonged in patients with moderate or severe stenosis and the sound of pulmonic valve closure is delayed and soft. The characteristic feature of valvular pulmonic stenosis on auscultation is a harsh, diamond-shaped systolic ejection murmur heard best at the upper left sternal border. The systolic murmur becomes louder and its crescendo occurs later in systole, obscuring the aortic component of the second sound with more severe degrees of valvular obstruction, since these patients have a greater prolongation of right ventricular systole. The holosystolic decrescendo murmur of tricuspid regurgitation may accompany severe pulmonic stenosis, especially in the presence of congestive heart failure. Cyanosis, reflecting venoarterial shunting through a patent foramen ovale, is absent with mild stenosis and infrequent with moderate obstruction. However, cyanosis may not be apparent in patients with severe obstruction if the atrial septum is intact.

Electrocardiography may be helpful in assessing the degree of obstruction to right ventricular output.[269] In mild cases the electrocardiogram is often normal, whereas moderate and severe stenoses are associated with right axis deviation and right ventricular hypertrophy. A tall QR wave in the right precordial leads with T-wave inversion and ST-segment suppression (right ventricular "strain") reflects severe stenosis. When an rSR′ pattern is observed in lead V_1 (20 per cent of patients) generally lower right ventricular pressures are found than in patients with a pure R wave of equal amplitude. High amplitude P waves in leads II and V_1 indicating right atrial enlargement are associated with severe stenosis. Chest roentgenography in patients with mild or moderate pulmonic stenosis often shows a heart of normal size and normal pulmonary vascularity (Figs. 6–32 and 6–33, pp. 159 and 160). Poststenotic dilatation of the main and left pulmonary arteries is often evident. Right atrial and right ventricular enlargement are observed in patients with severe obstruction and resultant right ventricular failure. The pulmonary vascularity may be reduced in patients with severe stenosis, right ventricular failure, and/or a venoarterial shunt at the atrial level (p. 162).

Reliable localization of the site of obstruction and assessment of its severity is obtained by combined continuous-wave Doppler and two-dimensional echocardiography.[263, 264] Parasternal and subcostal imaging are required to detect most accurately maximal pulmonary artery blood flow velocity, which is converted to a pressure difference across the valve utilizing a modified Bernoulli equation [pressure difference (mm HG) = 4 × the squared peak Doppler velocity (m/s)].

Cardiac catheterization and *angiocardiography* with right ventricular injection also localizes the site of obstruction, evaluates its severity, and documents the coexistence of additional cardiac malformations (Fig. 30–45). The resting cardiac output is usually normal, even in cases of severe stenosis, and most children show the ability to increase cardiac output with exercise.[270] Right ventricular dysfunction occurs especially when venoarterial shunting

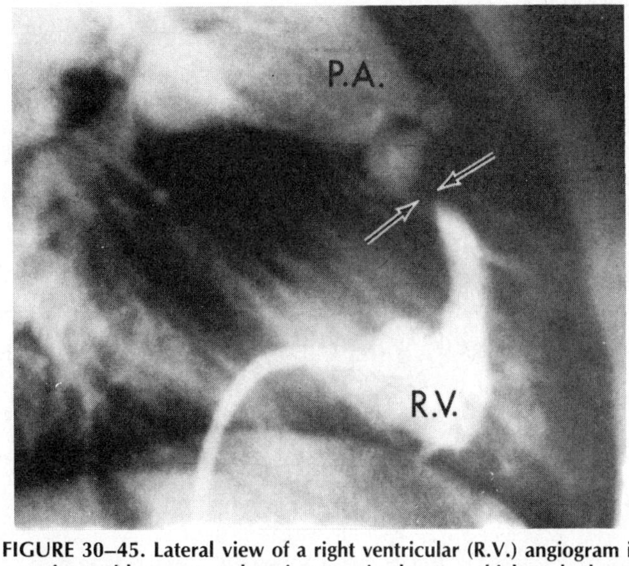

FIGURE 30–45. Lateral view of a right ventricular (R.V.) angiogram in a patient with severe pulmonic stenosis shows a thickened, domed pulmonic valve, below which exists marked hypertrophy of the right ventricular infundibulum (arrows). Poststenotic dilatation of the pulmonary artery (P.A.) is evident.

is significant and produces systemic arterial desaturation. In patients with critical stenosis, care must be taken during hemodynamic study that the cardiac catheter does not dangerously occlude the stenotic valve opening. The angiographic appearance of a typical valvular pulmonic stenosis differs from that of a dysplastic valve. The former is thickened and domes during systole, returning to a normal configuration in diastole. Poststenotic dilatation of the main pulmonary trunk and sometimes of the left pulmonary artery is observed often. The leaflets of the dysplastic valve are not fused anatomically, but are thickened and immobile, creating little change in the angiographic picture during the cardiac cycle. Moreover, a small annulus and narrow sinuses of Valsalva are common accompaniments of valve dysplasia. With either type of valve, systolic narrowing of the right ventricular infundibulum is usually associated with moderate or severe obstruction.

Mild and moderate pulmonic valve stenoses have a generally favorable course; uncommonly, progression occurs in the severity of obstruction.[271, 272] Serial hemodynamic studies reveal unchanged pressure gradients over 4- to 8-year intervals in three-fourths of patients. Equal percentages of the remainder have an increase or a decrease in the severity of obstruction; significant increases in the pressure gradient occur especially in children under age 4 years who have at least moderate obstruction at initial examination.

Percutaneous transluminal balloon valvuloplasty (p. 1336) is the initial procedure of choice in patients with typical valve pulmonary stenosis and moderate to severe degrees of obstruction.[266, 267] This approach provides palliative improvement; it is not yet clear if improvement is permanent. In these same patients *surgical relief* can also be accomplished at extremely low risk.[262] The valve is approached through an incision in the pulmonary arterial trunk, and resection of infundibular muscle, if necessary, may be accomplished through the pulmonic valve. In patients with a dysplastic valve, in whom transcatheter valvuloplasty is ineffective, the thickened valve tissue is removed and a patch is often required to widen the annulus and proximal main pulmonary artery. In children with mild pulmonic valve stenosis prophylaxis against infective endocarditis is recommended; these patients need not restrict their physical activities.

PULMONIC ATRESIA WITH INTACT VENTRICULAR SEPTUM

This anomaly is an uncommon and serious cause of cyanosis in the neonatal period that may respond well to aggressive medical and surgical treatment.[273] In almost all infants the pulmonic valve is atretic; in the majority both the valve ring and the main pulmonary artery are hypoplastic. Occasionally, the right ventricular infundibulum may be atretic or extremely narrowed. Although a spectrum exists in right ventricular cavity size and configuration, the lesion is often classified into two types: Type 1, with a diminutive right ventricular chamber, often with tricuspid stenosis, and Type 2, with a large right ventricle and frequently tricuspid regurgitation (Fig. 30–46). In most infants the right ventricle is hypoplastic and sinusoidal communications exist between the right ventricular cavity and the coronary circulation, presumably kept open by the high right ventricular pressure.[274] The desaturated blood carried through the sinusoids may compromise myocardial oxygen supply.

Since the pulmonic valve is imperforate and completely obstructed, systemic venous blood returning to the heart bypasses the right ventricle through an interatrial communication. Right ventricular output does not contribute to the effective cardiac output and is proportional to the magnitude of tricuspid regurgitation and the size and extent of the sinusoidal communications with the coronary arterial tree. The blood supply to the lungs is derived from the bronchial circulation and from flow through a persistently patent ductus arteriosus. The size and patency of the ductus arteriosus are critical determinants in postnatal survival; ductus closure results in death. Reduced pulmonary blood flow via a partially constricted ductus arteriosus results in profound hypoxemia, tissue hypoxia, and metabolic acidemia.

The diagnosis is suggested by roentgenographic findings of pulmonary hypoperfusion and the electrocardiographic observation of a normal QRS axis, absent or diminished right ventricular forces, and/or dominant left ventricular forces. In the minority of infants with marked tricuspid regurgitation, the right ventricle and right atrium are massively enlarged. The echocardiogram in the usual infant shows a small right ventricular cavity and diminutive or absent pulmonic valve echoes.[275] Doppler examination shows continuous retrograde flow to the pulmonary artery and/or its branches through a patent ductus arteriosus which is usually narrow and tortuous. Only if tricuspid valve echoes are imaged by ultrasound examination can tricuspid atresia be distinguished from pulmonic atresia. Contrast echocardiography showing filling of the right ventricle across the tricuspid valve in diastole may clarify the latter distinction.

Cardiac catheterization is performed usually on an emergency basis. Since survival depends upon patency of the

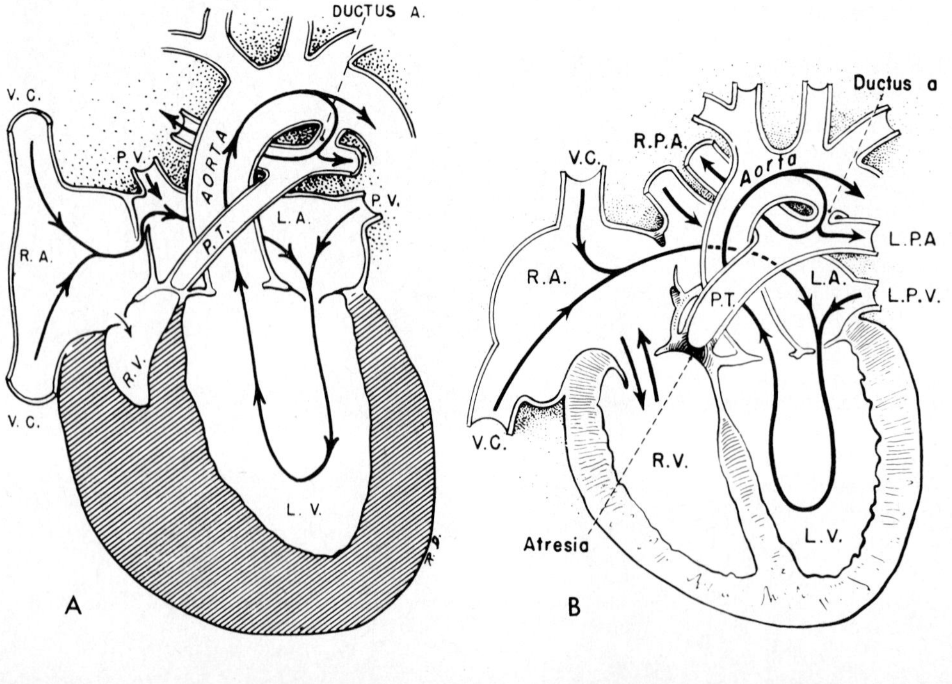

FIGURE 30–46. Pulmonic atresia with intact ventricular septum. With a competent tricuspid valve the right ventricular chamber is diminutive (*A*); significant tricuspid regurgitation is associated with a normal or large right ventricular cavity (*B*). V.C. = vena cava; R.A. = right atrium; R.V. = right ventricle; P.T. = pulmonary trunk; P.V. = pulmonary vein; L.A. = left atrium; L.V. = left ventricle; Ductus A. = ductus arteriosus; L.P.A. = left pulmonary artery; R.P.A. = right pulmonary artery; L.P.V. = left pulmonary vein. (From Edwards, J. E.: Congenital malformations of the heart and great vessels. *In* Gould, S. E. [ed.]: Pathology of the Heart. 2nd ed. Springfield, Ill., Charles C Thomas, 1960.)

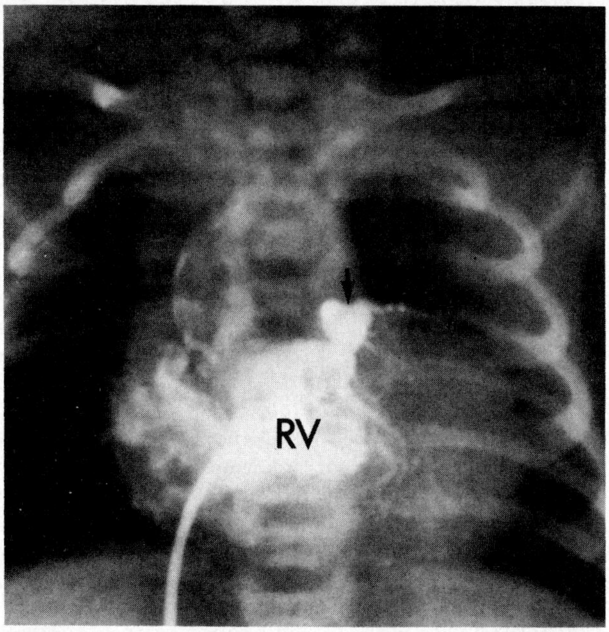

FIGURE 30–47. Right ventricular angiocardiogram in the frontal projection in a 1-day-old infant with an atretic pulmonic valve (arrow). The cavity of the right ventricle (RV) is small and eccentrically shaped. (Courtesy of Robert Freedom, M.D.)

ductus arteriosus, infusion of prostaglandin E_1 (0.05-0.1 μg/kg/min) intravenously may dramatically reverse clinical deterioration and improve arterial blood gases and pH.[60] The usual hemodynamic findings are right atrial and right ventricular hypertension, the latter often greater than systemic pressure, and a massive right-to-left interatrial shunt. Selective angiocardiography establishes the diagnosis and allows evaluation of the degree of separation between the right ventricular infundibular and pulmonary trunk, the size of the right ventricular cavity and of the pulmonary arteries (Fig. 30–47), and the anatomy and function of the tricuspid valve. In the majority of infants with a diminutive right ventricle, balloon atrial septostomy followed by a systemic-pulmonary artery shunt provides palliation. The ultimate prognosis is poor unless continuity can be established between the right ventricle and the pulmonary arteries by pulmonary valvotomy or prosthetic conduit at initial or second operation.[273–276] Decompression of the right ventricle permits that chamber to grow and both the tricuspid and pulmonary orifices to enlarge.[277] In some patients in whom systemic-pulmonary arterial shunt is not feasible for anatomical reasons, short-term palliation may be provided by formalin infiltration of the adventitia of the patent ductus arteriosus.[278] In other patients who are unsuitable candidates for a one- or two-stage complete correction, the Fontan right atrium–pulmonary anastomosis may be effective several years after shunt palliation in the newborn period.

INTRAVENTRICULAR RIGHT VENTRICULAR OBSTRUCTION

Infundibular pulmonic stenosis with an intact ventricular septum and the presence of anomalous muscle bundles are the principal causes of intraventricular right ventricular obstruction (Fig. 30–48).[279] Subpulmonic infundibular stenosis occurs usually at the proximal portion of the infundibulum and consists of a fibrous band at the junction of the right ventricular cavity and outflow tract. The clinical manifestations, course, and prognosis of patients with infundibular stenosis are similar to those with valvular stenosis, although the former diagnosis is suggested by the absence of a systolic ejection sound and a systolic murmur lower along the left sternal border. Doppler echocardiography, withdrawal pressure tracings, and selective right ventricular angiocardiography permit localization of the site of obstruction and assessment of its extent and severity. Surgical treatment consists of resection of the fibrotic narrowed area and hypertrophied muscle. Occasionally it may be necessary to widen the outflow tract with a pericardial or prosthetic patch.

A two-chambered right ventricle is formed by right ventricular obstruction due to anomalous muscle bundles; most of the patients have an associated malalignment or perimembranous ventricular septal defect, and approximately 5 per cent have subaortic stenosis.[279] Aberrant hypertrophied muscle bands traverse the right ventricular cavity, extending from its anterior wall to the crista supraventricularis and/or the portion of the adjacent interventricular septum. The anomalous pyramid-shaped muscle mass obstructs blood flow through the body of the right ventricle and produces a proximal high-pressure inflow chamber and a distal low-pressure chamber. Thus, this type of obstruction is distinguishable from that in tetralogy of Fallot, in which hypertrophied infundibular muscle protrudes into but does not cross the cavity of the right ventricle.

The clinical, electrocardiographic, and chest roentgenographic findings resemble those observed in pulmonic valvular or subvalvular infundibular obstruction, although the systolic thrill and murmur may be displaced lower along the left sternal border. Progressive obstruction occurs in some patients. The diagnosis may be established by two-dimensional echocardiography. Selective right ventricular angiocardiography is necessary for most accurate diagnosis and reveals a filling defect in the midportion of the right ventricle which does not often change significantly with systole and diastole. The treatment for anomalous muscle bundles consists of surgical removal.[280] In the

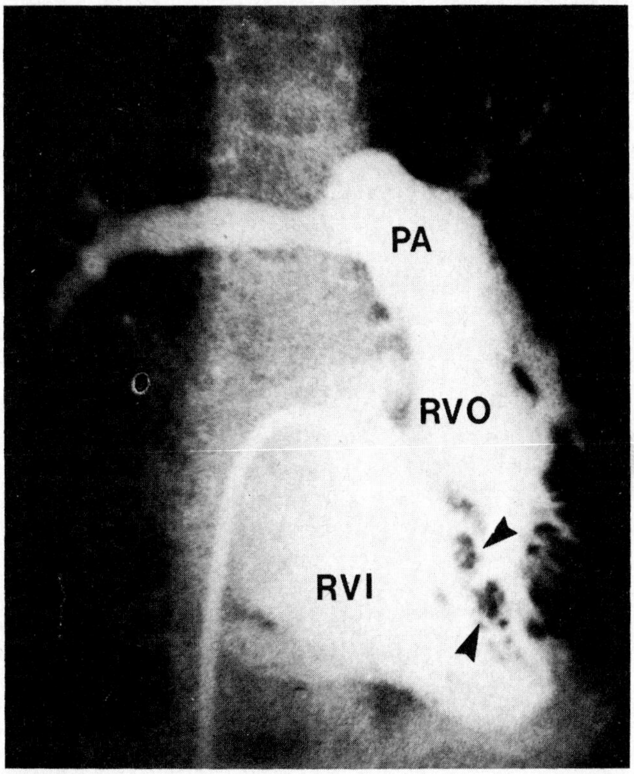

FIGURE 30–48. Intraventricular right ventricular obstruction. The right ventricular inflow (RVI) and outflow (RVO) tracts are separated by bands (arrows) creating intraventricular right ventricular obstruction. PA = pulmonary artery.

absence of preoperative recognition of the anomaly, the surgeon should be alerted to the correct diagnosis by the presence of a dimple on the ordinarily smooth anterior surface of the right ventricle and/or the inability to view the tricuspid valve through a longitudinal ventriculotomy because of the presence of the abnormal muscle mass.

TETRALOGY OF FALLOT (See also p. 988)

DEFINITION. The overall incidence of this anomaly approaches 10 per cent of all forms of congenital heart disease, and it is the most common cardiac malformation responsible for cyanosis after one year of age.[281, 282] The four components of this malformation are (1) ventricular septal defect, (2) obstruction to right ventricular outflow, (3) overriding of the aorta, and (4) right ventricular hypertrophy. The basic anomaly is the result of an anterior deviation of the septal insertion of the infundibular ventricular septum from its usual location in the normal heart between the limbs of the trabecular septum. The malalignment interventricular defect usually is large, approximating the aortic orifice in size, and is located high in the septum just below the right cusp of the aortic valve, separated from the pulmonic valve by the crista supraventricularis. The aortic root may be displaced anteriorly and straddle or override the septal defect, but, as in the normal heart, it lies to the right of the origin of the pulmonary artery. In the majority of cases no dextroposition of the aorta exists; the overriding aorta is a phenomenon secondary to the subaortic location of the ventricular septal defect.

HEMODYNAMICS. The degree of obstruction to pulmonary blood flow is the principal determinant of the clinical presentation. The site of obstruction is variable;[283] infundibular stenosis is the only major obstruction in approximately 50 per cent of patients and coexists with valvular obstruction in another 20 to 25 per cent (Fig. 30–49). Supravalvular and peripheral pulmonary arterial narrowing may be observed, and unilateral absence of a pulmonary artery (usually the left) is found in a small number of patients. Circulation to the abnormal lung is accomplished by bronchial and other collateral arteries.[284, 285] Atresia of the pulmonic valve, infundibulum, or main pulmonary artery is referred to occasionally as "pseudotruncus arteriosus." True truncus arteriosus with absent pulmonary arteries (Type 4) differs from Fallot's tetralogy, in which pulmonary artery branches are present but are fed by a patent ductus arteriosus and/or bronchial arteries[284, 285] (see Fig. 30–52). A right-sided aortic knob, arch, and descending aorta occur in approximately 25 per cent of patients with tetralogy of Fallot. The coronary arteries may have surgically important variations:[286] the anterior descending artery may originate from the right coronary artery; a single right coronary artery may give off a left branch that courses anterior to the pulmonary trunk; a single left coronary artery may give off a right branch that crosses the infundibulum of the right ventricle. Enlargement of the infundibular branch of the right coronary artery often presents a problem with respect to a right ventriculotomy. Associated cardiac anomalies exist in approximately 40 per cent of patients. Major associated cardiac anomalies include patent ductus arteriosus, multiple (usually muscular) ventricular septal defects, and complete atrioventricular septal defects. Localized single or multiple peripheral pulmonary arterial stenotic lesions are common; rarely, the right or left pulmonary artery may arise anomalously from the ascending aorta. Infrequently, aortic valve regurgitation results from aortic cusp prolapse. Associated extracardiac anomalies are present in 20 to 30 per cent of patients.

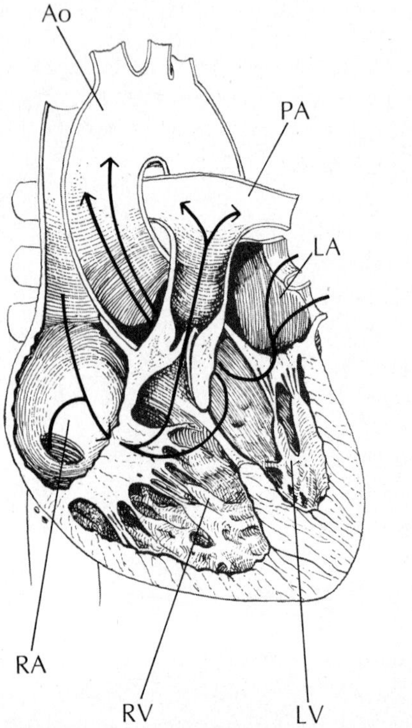

FIGURE 30–49. Tetralogy of Fallot with infundibular and valvular pulmonic stenosis. The arrows indicate direction of blood flow. A substantial right-to-left shunt exists across the ventricular septal defect. RA = right atrium; LA = left atrium; RV = right ventricle; LV = left ventricle; Ao = aorta; PA = pulmonary artery.

The relationship between the resistance to blood flow from the ventricles into the aorta and into the pulmonary vessels plays a major role in determining the hemodynamic and clinical picture.[282] Thus, the severity of obstruction to right ventricular outflow is of fundamental significance. When right ventricular outflow tract obstruction is severe, the pulmonary blood flow is reduced markedly, and a large volume of unsaturated systemic venous blood is shunted from right to left across the ventricular septal defect. Severe cyanosis and polycythemia occur, and symptoms and sequelae of systemic hypoxemia are prominent. At the opposite end of the spectrum, the terms "acyanotic" or "pink" tetralogy of Fallot are often used to describe an interventricular communication and a milder degree of obstruction to right ventricular outflow with little or no venoarterial shunting. In many infants and children the obstruction to right ventricular outflow is mild but progressive, so that early in life pulmonary exceeds systemic blood flow, and the symptoms resemble those produced by a simple ventricular septal defect.

CLINICAL MANIFESTATIONS. Few children with tetralogy of Fallot remain asymptomatic or acyanotic. Most are cyanotic from birth or develop cyanosis before age one year. In general, the earlier the onset of systemic hypoxemia, the more likely the possibility that severe pulmonary outflow tract stenosis or atresia exists. Dyspnea with exertion, clubbing, and polycythemia are common. When resting after exertion, children with tetralogy characteristically assume a squatting posture. The latter may be obvious even in infancy; many cyanotic infants prefer to lie in a knee-chest position. Spells of intense cyanosis related to a sudden increase in venoarterial shunting and a reduction in pulmonary blood flow have their onset most often between 2 and 9 months of age and constitute an important threat to survival.[287] The attacks are not restricted to patients with severe cyanosis; they are characterized by hyperpnea and increasing cyanosis that progresses to limpness and syncope and occasionally terminates in convulsions, a cerebrovascular accident, and death.

Physical examination reveals variable degrees of underdevelopment and cyanosis. Clubbing of the terminal digits may be prominent after the first year of life. The heart is not hyperactive or enlarged; a right ventricular impulse and systolic thrill are palpable often along the left sternal border. An early systolic ejection sound that is aortic in origin may be heard at the lower left sternal border and apex; the second heart sound is single, the pulmonic component rarely being audible. A systolic ejection murmur is produced by flow across the narrowed right ventricular infundibulum or pulmonic valve. The intensity and duration of the murmur vary inversely with the severity of obstruction—the opposite of the relationship that exists in patients with pulmonic stenosis and an intact ventricular septum. Polycythemia, decreased systemic vascular resistance, and increased obstruction to right ventricular outflow may all be responsible for a decrease in intensity of the murmur; with extreme outflow tract stenosis or pulmonic atresia and during an attack of paroxysmal hypoxemia, there may be no or only a very short, faint murmur. A continuous murmur faintly audible over the anterior or posterior chest reflects flow through enlarged bronchial collateral vessels. Occasionally, a loud continuous murmur of flow through a patent ductus arteriosus may be heard at the upper left sternal border.

LABORATORY EXAMINATION. The *electrocardiogram* ordinarily shows right ventricular and, less frequently, right atrial hypertrophy. In a patient with acyanotic tetralogy, combined ventricular hypertrophy may be noted initially, progressing to right ventricular hypertrophy as cyanosis develops. *Roentgenographic* examination characteristically reveals a normal-sized, boot-shaped heart (coeur en sabot) with prominence of the right ventricle and a concavity in the region of the underdeveloped right ventricular outflow tract and main pulmonary artery (Fig. 6–37, p. 162). The pulmonary vascular markings are typically diminished, and the aortic arch and knob may be on the right side; the ascending aorta is generally large. A uniform, diffuse, fine reticular pattern of vascular markings is noted in the presence of prominent collateral vessels. Single-crystal *echocardiographic* findings include aortic enlargement, aortic-septal discontinuity, and aortic overriding of the ventricular septum.[288] Two-dimensional echocardiography (Fig. 5–84, p. 119) shows the right ventricular outflow tract to be narrowed and in a more horizontal

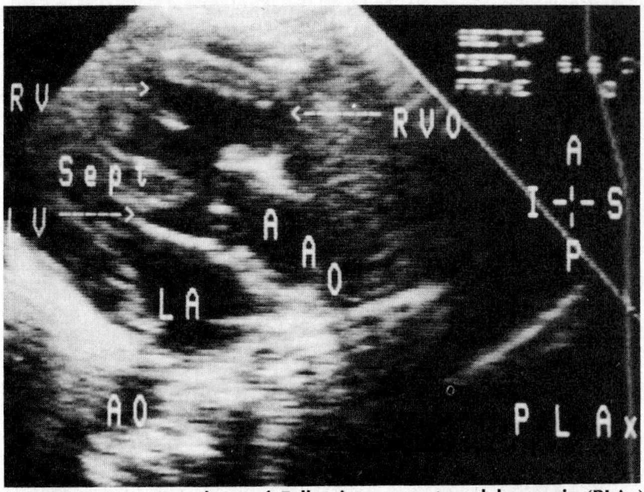

FIGURE 30–50. Tetralogy of Fallot in a parasternal long-axis (PLAx) view, which demonstrates the aorta overriding the ventricular septum (Sept). RV = right ventricle, RVO = right ventricular outflow tract, LV = left ventricle, LA = left atrium, AO = ascending aorta. (Courtesy of Norman Silverman, M.D.)

orientation than normal. The main pulmonary artery and its branches are mildly to severely hypoplastic. The usual malalignment ventricular septal defect lies superior to the tricuspid valve and immediately below the aortic valve cusps. These findings are best displayed in views of the long axis of the right ventricular outflow tract, which are the subxiphoid short axis and high transverse parasternal echo windows. Echo views which show the anteroposterior coordinates best indicate the overriding of the aorta; these are the parasternal long-axis, apical two-chamber, and subxiphoid views (Fig. 30–50). The echocardiographic examination also reveals the origin of the main pulmonary artery from the right ventricle, and continuity of the main pulmonary artery with its right and left branches. The demonstration of mitral-semilunar valve continuity helps distinguish tetralogy from double-outlet right ventricle with pulmonic stenosis, in which discontinuity of the mitral valve echo and the aortic cusp echo is a critical feature.

Cardiac catheterization and selective *angiocardiography* (Fig. 30–51) are necessary to confirm the diagnosis; assess the magnitude of right-to-left shunting; provide details of additional muscular ventricular septal defects, if present; evaluate the architecture of the right ventricular outflow tract, pulmonic valve, and annulus and the morphology and caliber of the main branches of the pulmonary arteries; and analyze the anatomy of the coronary arteries. *Axial cineangiography*, utilizing the sitting-up projection, greatly

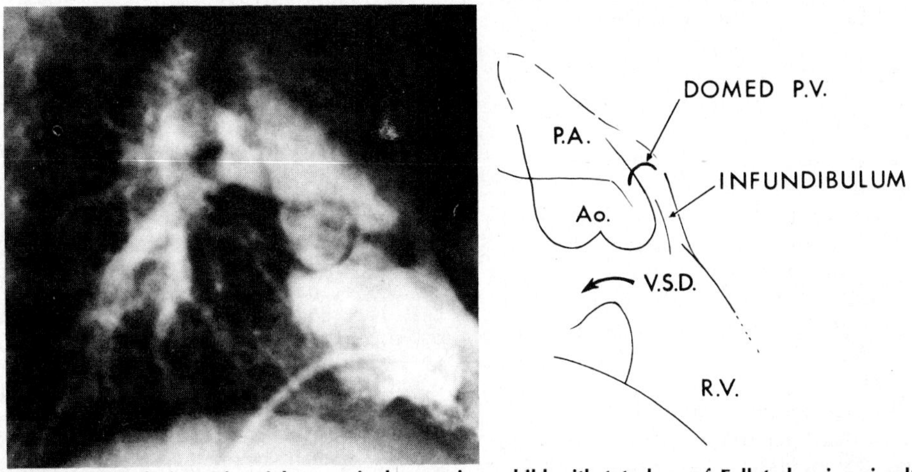

FIGURE 30–51. Lateral view of a right ventriculogram in a child with tetralogy of Fallot showing simultaneous opacification of the pulmonary artery (P.A.) and aorta (Ao.). P.V. = pulmonic valve; V.S.D. = ventricular septal defect; R.V. = right ventricle.

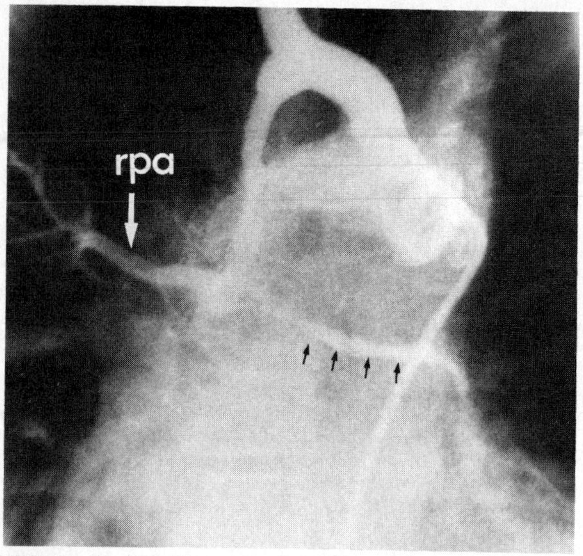

FIGURE 30–52. Selective systemic collateral bronchial arteriogram demonstrates "gull-wing" configuration of the hypoplastic right pulmonary artery (rpa) and left pulmonary artery (arrows) in a patient with tetralogy of Fallot and pulmonic atresia. (Courtesy of Robert Freedom, M.D.)

facilitates evaluation of the pulmonary outflow tract and arteries.[91, 289] The preoperative assessment of tetralogy with pulmonic atresia must include delineation of the arterial supply to both lungs by selective catheterization and visualization of bronchial collateral arteries with late serial filming; pulmonary arteries may be opacified only after the bronchial collateral arteries have cleared of contrast material (Fig. 30–52).[290, 291] A patient with pulmonic atresia should not be ruled out as a candidate for surgical correction unless an inadequate pulmonary arterial supply to the lungs is demonstrated clearly. Rarely, injection of contrast through a catheter in the pulmonary venous capillary wedge position is required to assess the possibility that anatomical pulmonary arteries are present.[292] Computer-assisted axial tomography may visualize central pulmonary arteries when conventional angiography cannot.[291]

MANAGEMENT. Among the factors that may complicate the management of patients with tetralogy are iron deficiency anemia, infective endocarditis, paradoxical embolism, polycythemia, coagulation disorders, and cerebral infarction or abscess. Paroxysmal hypercyanotic spells may respond quickly to oxygen, placing the child in the knee-chest position, and morphine. If the spell persists, metabolic acidosis will develop from prolonged anaerobic metabolism, and infusion of sodium bicarbonate may be necessary to interrupt the attack. Vasopressors, beta-adrenoceptor receptor blockade, or general anesthesia may occasionally be necessary.

Total correction is advisable ultimately for almost all patients with tetralogy of Fallot.[293–297] Early definitive repair, even in infancy, is currently advocated in most centers prepared properly for infant intracardiac surgery. Successful early correction appears to prevent the consequences of progressive infundibular obstruction and acquired pulmonic atresia, delayed growth and development, and complications secondary to hypoxemia and polycythemia with bleeding tendencies. The size of the pulmonary arteries, rather than the age or size of the infant or child, is the most important determinant in assessing candidacy for primary repair; marked hypoplasia of the pulmonary arteries is a relative contraindication for early corrective operation. When the latter exists, a palliative operation designed to increase pulmonary blood flow is recommended and consists usually in the smallest infants of a systemic-pulmonary arterial anastomosis.[293] A transventricular infundibulectomy or valvulotomy is an additional palliative procedure that may be considered. Total correction can then be carried out at a lower risk later in childhood or adolescence. The palliative procedures relieve hypoxemia due to diminished pulmonary blood flow and reduce the stimulus to polycythemia. Since pulmonary venous return is augmented, the left atrium and ventricle are stimulated to enlarge their capacity in anticipation of total correction. In the most severe forms of tetralogy of Fallot with pulmonic atresia, the goals of operation include establishment of nonstenotic continuity between the right ventricle and pulmonary arteries, closure of the intracardiac shunt(s), and interruption of surgically created shunts or major collateral arteries to the lungs.[282, 295] When atresia is confined to the infundibulum or pulmonic valve, repair may be accomplished by infundibular resection and reconstruction of the outflow tract with a pericardial patch. If a long segment exists of pulmonary arterial atresia, a valve-containing conduit is inserted from the right ventricle to the distal pulmonary artery. The presence of a single pulmonary artery in the hilus of either lung is a prerequisite for repair of pulmonic atresia. A conduit may also be necessary in less severe forms of right ventricular outflow tract obstruction when an anomalous coronary artery crosses the right ventricular outflow tract.

A variety of complications are common in the postoperative period after palliative or corrective operation. Mild-to-moderate left ventricular decompensation may be secondary to the sudden increase in pulmonary venous return; varying degrees of pulmonic valvular regurgitation increase right ventricular cavity size further.[298] Bleeding problems are seen frequently, especially in older polycythemic patients. Complete right bundle branch block or the pattern of left anterior hemiblock is seen often, but disabling dysrhythmias are infrequent.[299–301] Restricted pulmonary arterial flow is the greatest cause for early and late mortality and poor late results.[302] After convalescence from intracardiac repair, symptoms of hypoxemia and severe exercise intolerance are relieved even in the presence of some residual right ventricular outflow tract obstruction, pulmonic valve incompetence, and/or cardiomegaly.[303–306] However, cardiovascular performance at rest or during exercise may remain below normal, and major complications, such as trifascicular block, complete heart block, ventricular arrhythmias, and sudden death may rarely occur many years after surgical treatment.[299–305]

CONGENITAL ABSENCE OF THE PULMONIC VALVE

In the majority of cases of this rare malformation, the lesion is associated with a ventricular septal defect, a narrowed obstructive annulus of the pulmonic valve, and marked aneurysmal dilatation of the pulmonary arteries. The combination of anomalies is referred to often as tetralogy of Fallot with absent pulmonic valve. The obstructing lesion consists principally of underdeveloped, primitive valve tissue within a hypoplastic annulus; infundibular obstruction and the ventricular septal defect do not differ from classic tetralogy of Fallot. The massively dilated pulmonary arteries are often the major determinant of the clinical course, since they frequently result in upper airway obstruction and severe respiratory distress in infancy.[307] Poststenotic pulmonary artery aneurysms develop in utero, and their size and location appear to be related to the magnitude of pulmonic regurgitation in fetal life, the orientation of the right ventricular infundibulum to the right or left, and the size of the ductus arteriosus.[308] It has been suggested that the aneurysmal dilatation is related pathogenetically to agenesis of the ductus arteriosus.[309]

The *clinical features* are often distinctive, with an early onset of

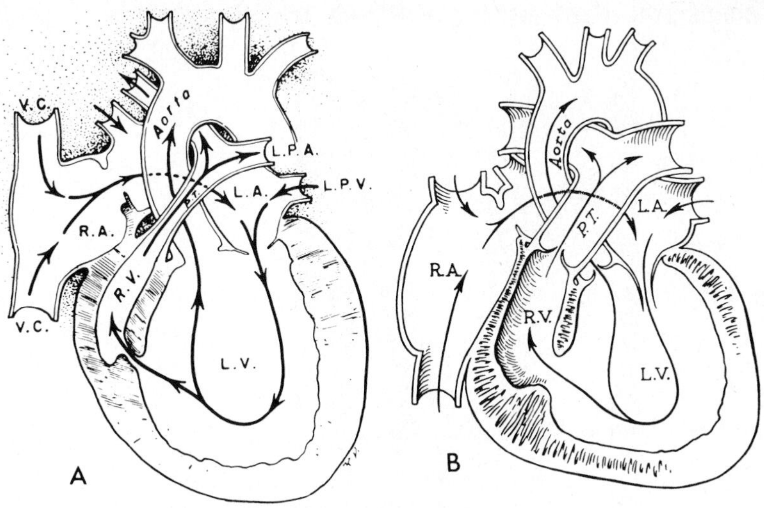

FIGURE 30–53. *A*, Tricuspid atresia with normally related great arteries, a small ventricular septal defect, diminutive right ventricular chamber, and narrowed outflow tract. *B*, An example of tricuspid atresia and complete transposition of the great arteries in which the left ventricular chamber is essentially a common ventricle, with the aorta arising from an infundibular component (R.V.) of the common ventricle. V.C. = vena cava; R.A. = right atrium; L.A. = left atrium; R.V. = right ventricle; L.V. = left ventricle; L.P.V. = left pulmonary vein; L.P.A. = left pulmonary artery. (From Edwards, J. E., and Burchell, H. B.: Congenital tricuspid atresia: Classification. Med. Clin. North Am. *33*:1177, 1949.)

severe respiratory distress due to tracheobronchial compression accompanied by a systolic ejection and a widely transmitted low-pitched, decrescendo diastolic murmur at the upper left sternal border. In the absence of pulmonary complications cyanosis is commonly mild. *Roentgenographically* the heart is moderately enlarged; hyperinflated lung fields are observed with large hilar densities representing the aneurysmally dilated pulmonary arteries. The *echocardiographic* features are similar to those seen in classic tetralogy of Fallot, in addition to massive dilatation of the main pulmonary artery and branch pulmonary arteries. Remnants of pulmonary cusps may be visible. Right ventricular dilatation is produced by significant pulmonary regurgitation; the latter is identified by retrograde diastolic flow in the pulmonary arteries and right ventricle at Doppler examination. Definitive diagnosis is established by cardiac catheterization and selective angiocardiography. Prognosis is related to the intensity of upper airway obstruction; pulmonary complications are the usual cause of death in infancy. If survival beyond infancy is accomplished the respiratory symptoms usually diminish, probably because of maturational changes in the structure of the tracheobronchial tree. The surgical approach in infancy is often unsatisfactory[310]; a variety of procedures have been attempted, ranging from aneurysmorrhaphy to pulmonary artery suspension to transection and reanastomosis of pulmonary artery segments. Also suggested are ligation of the main pulmonary artery and creation of a systemic-pulmonary shunt, and primary repair of the ventricular septal defect with pulmonary arterial plication. In older patients the stenotic annulus may be widened with a patch and the ventricular septal defect closed. It is rarely necessary to replace the pulmonic valve.

TRICUSPID ATRESIA

This anomaly is characterized by absence of the tricuspid orifice, an interatrial communication, hypoplasia of the right ventricle, and the presence of a communication between the systemic and pulmonary circulations, usually a ventricular septal defect.[311, 312] Thus, there is a univentricular atrioventricular connection, consisting of a left-sided mitral valve between the morphological left atrium and left ventricle. Unequal division of the atrioventricular canal by fusion of the right-sided endocardial cushions has been proposed as the embryological fault. Patients may be subdivided into those with normally related great arteries (60 to 70 per cent of cases) and those with D-transposition of the great arteries; further classification depends upon the presence of pulmonic stenosis or atresia and the absence or size of the ventricular septal defect (Fig. 30–53). Additional cardiovascular malformations are often present, especially in patients with D-transposition of the great arteries, and include persistent left superior vena cava, patent ductus arteriosus, coarctation of the aorta, and juxtaposition of the atrial appendages.

The association with other cardiac malformations determines whether or not pulmonary blood flow is decreased, normal, or increased and therefore the degree of systemic hypoxemia.[313] The clinical picture is dominated usually by symptoms resulting from greatly diminished pulmonary blood flow with severe cyanosis. Cyanosis results from an obligatory admixture of systemic and pulmonary venous blood in the left atrium and its intensity is dependent primarily upon the magnitude of pulmonary blood flow. Heart failure, rather than cyanosis, is the predominant problem in infants with torrential pulmonary blood flow, which results when D-transposition of the great arteries, a ventricular septal defect, and an unobstructed pulmonary outflow tract coexist. If the latter patients survive infancy, they are candidates for pulmonary vascular obstructive disease; a favorable response to pulmonary arterial banding is common early in life.

Clinical diagnosis is accurate in the vast majority of infants with tricuspid atresia and pulmonary hypoperfusion. The *electrocardiographic* findings of left-axis deviation, right atrial enlargement, and left ventricular hypertrophy in a cyanotic infant strongly suggest tricuspid atresia.[314] *Echocardiography* reveals a small or absent right ventricle, large left ventricle, and absent tricuspid valve echoes (Figs. 30–54 and 5–71, p. 115); further, it may demonstrate the relationship of the great arteries unless pulmonic atresia is present.[315] Contrast cross-sectional echocardiography reveals the abnormal flow patterns; apical and subxiphoid cross-sectional views best reveal the atretic tricuspid orifice. *Roentgenographically* there are diminished pulmonary vascular markings and a concavity in the region of the cardiac silhouette usually occupied by the main pulmonary artery. The right atrial shadow may be prominent unless left-sided juxtaposition of the atrial appendages exists, which produces a straight and flattened right heart border.

At *cardiac catheterization* the right ventricle cannot be entered directly from the right atrium. When the great arteries are related normally, pulmonary blood flow is found to be derived from shunting through a ventricular

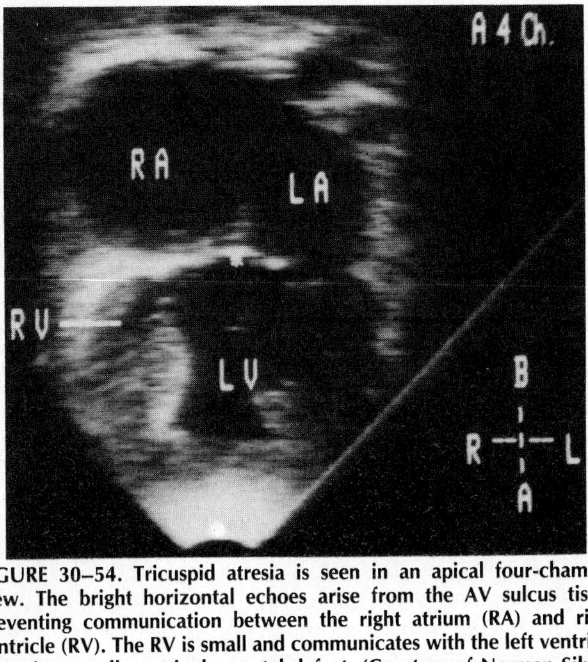

FIGURE 30–54. Tricuspid atresia is seen in an apical four-chamber view. The bright horizontal echoes arise from the AV sulcus tissue preventing communication between the right atrium (RA) and right ventricle (RV). The RV is small and communicates with the left ventricle (LV) via a small ventricular septal defect. (Courtesy of Norman Silverman, M.D.)

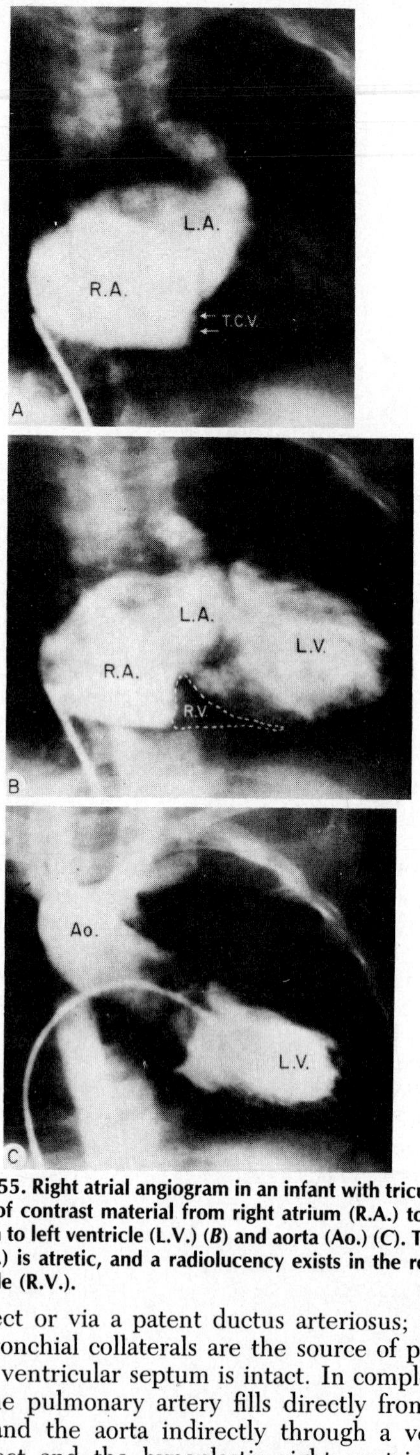

FIGURE 30–55. Right atrial angiogram in an infant with tricuspid atresia shows flow of contrast material from right atrium (R.A.) to left atrium (*A*), and then to left ventricle (L.V.) (*B*) and aorta (Ao.) (*C*). The tricuspid valve (T.C.V.) is atretic, and a radiolucency exists in the region of the right ventricle (R.V.).

septal defect or via a patent ductus arteriosus; the latter and the bronchial collaterals are the source of pulmonary flow if the ventricular septum is intact. In complete transposition the pulmonary artery fills directly from the left ventricle and the aorta indirectly through a ventricular septal defect and the hypoplastic right ventricle. Since complete admixture exists in the left atrium of pulmonary and systemic venous return, the degree of systemic arterial hypoxemia depends on the pulmonary:systemic flow ratio. Right atrial angiography does not opacify the right ventricle unless via a ventricular septal defect (Fig. 30–55). Selective left ventricular *angiography* permits identification of the hypoplastic right ventricle, the size and location of the ventricular septal defect, the type of pulmonary obstruction, the relationship between the great arteries, and the size of the distal pulmonary arterial tree.

Balloon atrial septostomy in those infants with a restrictive interatrial communication and palliative operations designed to increase pulmonary blood flow (systemic arterial–or venous–pulmonary artery anastomosis) are capable of producing clinical improvement of significant duration in patients with diminished blood flow.[313]

Functional correction of the anomaly has been accomplished by direct anastomosis of, or insertion of a nonvalved prosthetic conduit between, the right atrium and pulmonary artery and closure of the interatrial communication (Fontan procedure) (Fig. 30–56).[316–318a] If the right ventricle is not markedly hypoplastic, it may be utilized in the correction to generate forward flow into the pulmonary vascular bed. Also, if the right ventricle is not too hypoplastic, it may be used as a pumping chamber by anastomosis of the right atrial appendage to the right ventricle with the aid of a pericardial patch, leaving the outflow tract and pulmonic valve intact.[319, 320] A previously existing systemic artery–to–pulmonary artery anastomosis must be closed, but a systemic vein–to–pulmonary artery anastomosis may be left in place. Candidates for these corrective procedures must have normal pulmonary vascular resistance and a mean pulmonary artery pressure less than 20 mm Hg, pulmonary arteries of adequate size, and good left ventricular function.[316] The postoperative period is usually characterized transiently by a superior vena cava syndrome with right heart failure, edema, ascites, and hepatomegaly.[321]

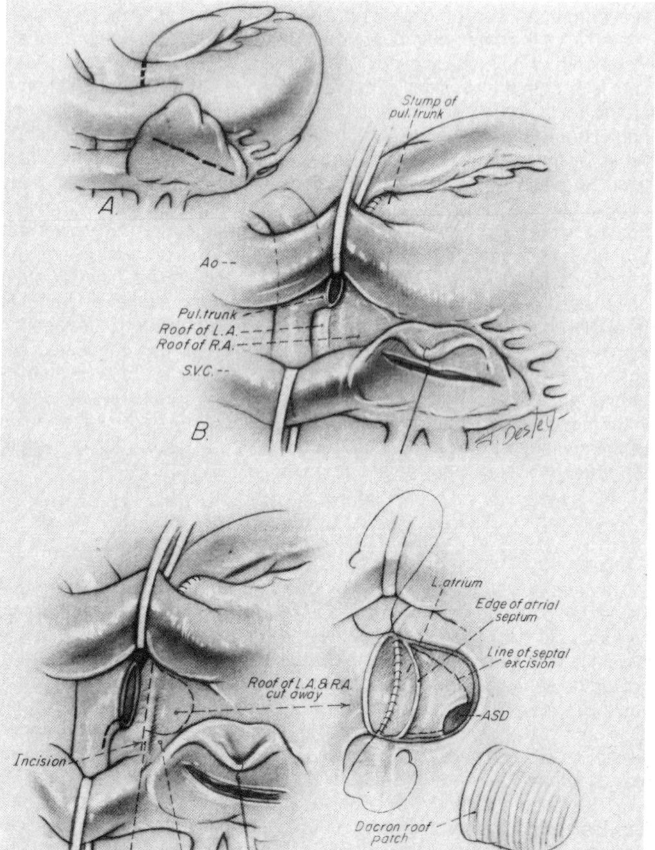

FIGURE 30–56. The Fontan operation with direct right atrial–pulmonary artery connection. *A*, The right atrium is opened through an oblique incision and the pulmonary artery transsected above the pulmonary valve. *B*, The proximal pulmonary trunk is closed and the distal end brought toward the right atrium beneath the aorta. *C*, The pulmonary artery is enlarged if a complex atrial septal baffle is required, the atrial septum is excised and a circular button of atrial roof removed. *D*, The posterior wall of the openings into the pulmonary artery and the atria are anastomosed; if the anterior wall of the right atrium and pulmonary artery cannot easily be brought together for direct anastomoses, a convex Dacron roof patch is employed. AO = aorta, RA = right atrium, LA = left atrium, ASD = atrial septal defect. (From Kirklin, J. W., and Barratt-Boyes, B. G.: Cardiac Surgery. John Wiley & Sons, 1986, p. 873.)

EBSTEIN'S ANOMALY OF THE TRICUSPID VALVE (See also p. 997)

This malformation is characterized by a downward displacement of the tricuspid valve into the right ventricle due to anomalous attachment of the tricuspid leaflets (Fig. 30–57).[322] Tricuspid valve tissue is dysplastic and a variable portion of the septal and inferior cusps adhere to the right ventricular wall some distance away from the atrioventricular junction.[323] The abnormally situated tricuspid orifice produces a portion of the right ventricle lying between the atrioventricular ring and the origin of the valve, which is continuous with the right atrial chamber. This proximal segment is "atrialized," and a distal, functionally small ventricular chamber exists. The degree of impairment of right ventricular function depends primarily on the extent to which the right ventricular inflow portion is atrialized and on the magnitude of tricuspid valve regurgitation.

CLINICAL MANIFESTATIONS. These are variable because the spectrum of pathology varies widely and because of the presence of associated malformations.[324] An interatrial communication consisting of a patent foramen ovale or an ostium secundum atrial septal defect is present in over half the cases. The most common important associated defect is pulmonic stenosis or atresia. Other coexistent anomalies may include an ostium primum type of atrial septal defect and ventricular septal defect alone or in combination with other lesions. The Ebstein's lesion is commonly observed in association with congenitally corrected transposition of the great arteries, in which the tricuspid valve is in the left atrioventricular orifice (p. 957). The usual manifestations in infancy are cyanosis, a cardiac murmur, and severe congestive heart failure. The magnitude of tricuspid regurgitation in the neonate is enhanced because the pulmonary vascular resistance is normally high early in life (Fig. 30–58).[325] In this regard it may be difficult in some newborn infants with Ebstein's anomaly and massive tricuspid regurgitation to distinguish between organic pulmonic atresia and the presence of elevated perinatal pulmonary vascular resistance.[326] In such infants retrograde aortography is quite likely to fill the pulmonary root and allow visualization of the pulmonic valve via a patent ductus arteriosus, serving to differentiate a normal from an abnormal pulmonary outflow tract. The tricuspid regurgitation in infants with Ebstein's anomaly may lessen substantially, and cyanosis may disappear early in life as pulmonary vascular resistance falls, only to recur at a later age when right ventricular dysfunction and/or paroxysmal arrhythmias develop. In some infants with Ebstein's malformation, cyanosis is intensified suddenly as the degree of pulmonary hypoperfusion is unmasked by spontaneous closure of a patent ductus arteriosus.

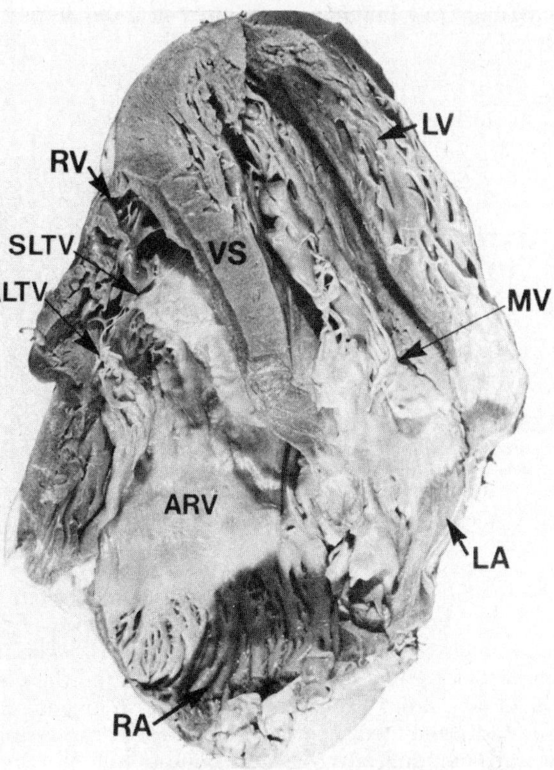

FIGURE 30–57. Anatomical specimen of Ebstein's anomaly of the tricuspid valve, cut in the same plane as an apical four-chamber echocardiographic view (Fig. 30–59). The septal and anterior leaflets of the tricuspid valve (SLTV, ALTV) are displaced into the right ventricle (RV), producing a large atrialized right ventricle (ARV). VS = ventricular septum, RA = right atrium, LA = left atrium, MV = mitral valve, LV = left ventricle. (Courtesy of Thomas DiSessa, M.D.)

Beyond infancy the onset of symptoms is insidious; the most common complaints are exertional dyspnea, fatigue, and cyanosis. Approximately 25 per cent of patients suffer episodes of paroxysmal atrial tachycardia. A prominent systolic pulsation of the liver and a large *v* wave in the jugular venous pulse accompany the systolic thrill and murmur of tricuspid regurgitation. Wide splitting of the first and second heart sounds and prominent third and fourth heart sounds may produce a characteristically rhythmic auscultatory cadence with a triple, quadruple, or quintuple combination of sounds.

The *electrocardiographic abnormalities* commonly fall into two categories: those with a right bundle branch block pattern and those with the Wolff-Parkinson-White syn-

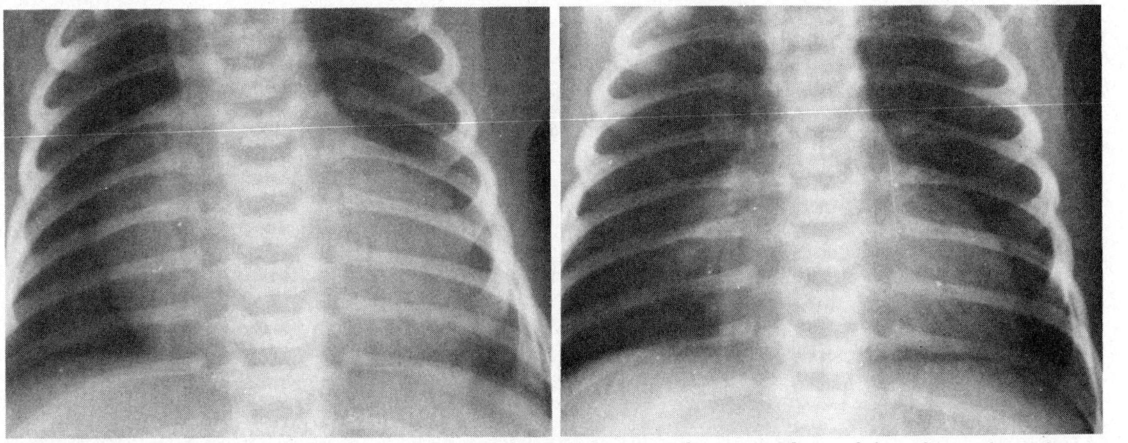

FIGURE 30–58. Chest roentgenograms in an infant with Ebstein's anomaly at ages 6 hours (*left*) and 2 weeks (*right*). The reduction in both overall heart size and right atrial prominence is a result of diminished tricuspid regurgitation as pulmonary vascular resistance falls postnatally. (Courtesy of Norman Talner, M.D.)

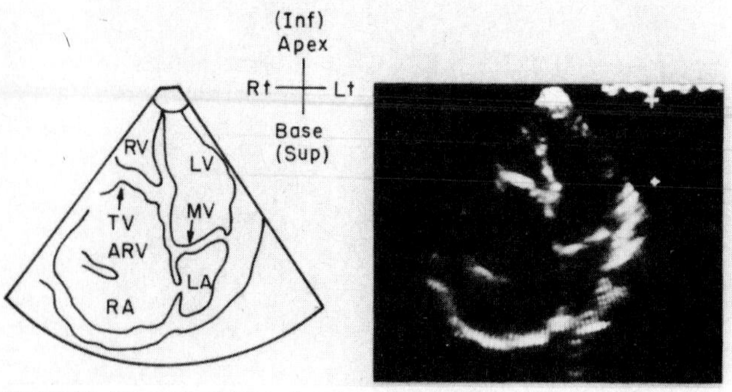

FIGURE 30–59. Apical four-chamber view of Ebstein's anomaly, corresponding to the anatomical specimen in Figure 30–57. RA = right atrium, LA = left atrium, MV = mitral valve, LV = left ventricle, TV = tricuspid valve, ARV = atrialized right ventricle, RV = right ventricle. (Courtesy of Thomas DiSessa, M.D.)

drome. The pattern in the latter is almost always type B, resembling left bundle branch block with predominant S waves in the right precordial leads. The presence of the Wolff-Parkinson-White pattern increases the risk of supraventricular paroxysmal tachycardia.[327] Most often the electrocardiogram shows giant P waves, a prolonged P-R interval, and prolonged terminal QRS depolarization, producing variable degrees of right bundle branch block. These distinctive findings help distinguish Ebstein's anomaly from other forms of right ventricular dysplasia whose presenting problem is often an arrhythmia. *Roentgenographic* and fluoroscopic studies usually demonstrate an enlarged right atrium, a small right ventricle, and a pulmonary artery with reduced pulsations; the pulmonary vascularity may be reduced if a large right-to-left shunt is present.

The principal M-mode *echocardiographic findings* observed in patients with this anomaly, as well as in those with other forms of right ventricular volume overload, are an increase in right ventricular dimension, paradoxical ventricular septal motion, an increase in tricuspid valve excursion, and an abnormal closing velocity of the tricuspid valve. More specific findings for Ebstein's anomaly include a delay in tricuspid valve closure relative to mitral closure and a decrease in the E-F slope of the tricuspid valve, an abnormal anterior position of the tricuspid valve during diastole, and the detection of tricuspid valve echoes with more lateral placement of the transducer than usual.[328] Cross-sectional echocardiographic techniques are superior for observation of the inferior and leftward displacement of the tricuspid valve and simultaneously demonstrate the abnormal positional relation between the tricuspid and mitral valves (Figs. 30–59, 5–70, p. 114, and 31–16, p. 998). Moreover, the boundaries of the atrialized right ventricle may be defined. Specific diagnosis requires identification, usually from an apical four-chamber view, of displacement of the septal tricuspid leaflet.[329] Tricuspid regurgitation, if present, is detected by Doppler examination.

At *cardiac catheterization* the intracavitary electrocardiogram recorded just proximal to the tricuspid valve shows a right ventricular type of complex, while the pressure recorded is that of the right atrium (Fig. 30–60). Usually a right-to-left atrial shunt is present. The hemodynamic findings depend upon the degree of tricuspid regurgitation. The heart is unusually irritable and a high incidence of significant arrhythmias exists during catheterization. Selective right ventricular *angiocardiography* shows the position of the displaced tricuspid valve, the size of the right ventricle, and the configuration of the outflow portion of the right ventricle.

Ebstein's anomaly may be compatible with a relatively long and active life, with most patients surviving into the third decade.[324] In some disabled patients moderate improvement has resulted from anastomosis of the superior vena cava to the right pulmonary artery (the Glenn procedure) to divert systemic venous return from the right atrium and to increase pulmonary blood flow. Benefit has resulted in older patients from replacement or repair of the tricuspid valve and closure of the atrial defect with or without ligation and marsupialization of the thin atrialized portion of the right ventricle.[330–332] In patients with a preexcitation syndrome (p. 604) that is producing life-threatening rhythm disturbances, the accessory conduction pathways should be divided. It should be recognized, however, that patients with Ebstein's anomaly are poor surgical risks at all ages.

TRANSPOSITION COMPLEXES

The term *transposition* identifies a group of malformations that have in common abnormal relationships between the cardiac chambers and great arteries. In this chapter the term is employed to include both anomalous insertion of the pulmonary veins and cardiac malpositions.

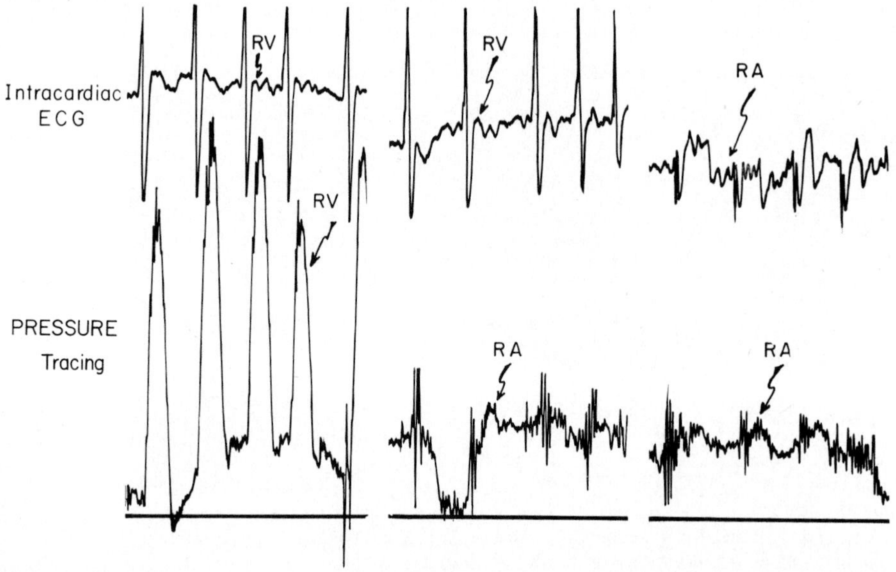

FIGURE 30–60. With a catheter in the "atrialized" portion of the right ventricle (RV), the intracardiac electrocardiogram in a patient with Ebstein's anomaly continues to show a ventricular complex, while right atrial pressure (RA) is recorded at the same site. (Courtesy of Delores A. Danilowicz, M.D.)

COMPLETE TRANSPOSITION OF THE GREAT ARTERIES

ANATOMICAL FINDINGS. This is a common and potentially lethal form of heart disease in newborns and infants.[333] The malformation consists of the aorta arising from the morphological right ventricle and the pulmonary artery from the morphological left ventricle. With rare exceptions there is no fibrous continuity between the aortic and mitral valve.[334] Usually the origin of the aorta is to the right and anterior to, but may be lateral to, the main pulmonary artery. Thus, dextro or D-transposition is a term often used interchangeably with complete transposition. The embryogenesis of complete transposition of the great arteries is controversial. There is consensus that the ventricular origins of the great arteries are reversed following development of a straight rather than a spiral infundibulotruncal septum. Transposition appears to result from a transfer of the pulmonary artery, instead of the aorta, from the heart tube's outlet zone to the left ventricle. The latter may result from maldevelopment of the infundibulum, or a combination of both infundibulum maldevelopment and truncal malseptation; the former results if the subpulmonary, rather than the subaortic infundibulum, is absorbed.

The anatomical arrangement results in two separate and parallel circulations. Some communication between the two circulations must exist after birth in order to sustain life; otherwise, unoxygenated systemic venous blood is directed inappropriately to the systemic circulation and oxygenated pulmonary venous blood is directed to the pulmonary circulation. Almost all patients have an interatrial communication (Fig. 30–61). Two-thirds have a patent ductus arteriosus, and about one-third have an associated ventricular septal defect. Complete transposition occurs more frequently in the offspring of diabetic mothers and more often in males than in females. Without treatment, approximately 30 per cent of these infants die within the first week of life; 50 per cent within the first month; 70 per cent within 6 months; and 90 per cent within the first year.[333] Those who live beyond infancy have, as a general rule, either an isolated large atrial septal defect or a single ventricle, or ventricular septal defect and pulmonic stenosis. Current aggressive medical and surgical approaches to this group of patients have transformed the prognosis for an infant with this malformation from hopeless to hopeful.

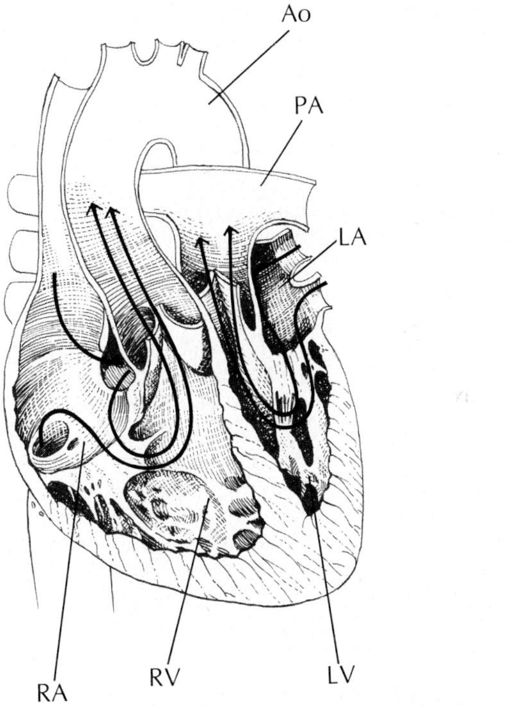

FIGURE 30–61. Complete transposition of the great arteries. Intercirculatory mixing occurs only at the atrial level. RA = right atrium; LA = left atrium; RV = right ventricle; LV = left ventricle; Ao = aorta; PA = pulmonary artery.

The *clinical course* is determined by the degree of tissue hypoxia, the ability of each ventricle to sustain an increased workload in the presence of reduced coronary arterial oxygenation, the nature of the associated cardiovascular anomalies, and the anatomical and functional status of the pulmonary vascular bed.[335] A bidirectional shunt is always present, because continuous unidirectional shunting would result in a progressive depletion of the circulating volume in either the pulmonary or the systemic vascular bed.

HEMODYNAMICS. A major determinant of the systemic arterial oxygen saturation is the amount of blood exchanged between the two circulations by intercirculatory shunts. The net volume of blood passing left-to-right from the pulmonary to the systemic circulation represents the anatomical left-to-right shunt and is, in fact, the effective systemic blood flow (i.e., the amount of oxygenated pulmonary venous return reaching the systemic capillary bed). Conversely, the volume of blood passing right-to-left from the systemic to the pulmonary circulation constitutes the anatomical right-to-left shunt and is, in fact, the effective pulmonary blood flow (i.e., the net volume of unsaturated systemic venous return perfusing the pulmonary capillary bed). The net volume exchange between the two circulations per unit time is equal. The magnitude of the intercirculatory mixing volume is modified by the number of intercirculatory communications that exist, the presence of associated obstructive intra- and extracardiac anomalies, the extent of the bronchopulmonary circulation, and the relationships between pulmonary and systemic vascular resistance. For example, in the newborn with an intact ventricular septum and a constricted or closed patent ductus arteriosus, inadequate mixing through a small patent foramen ovale is often the cause of severe hypoxemia. If a large interatrial communication or a ventricular septal defect exists, systemic arterial oxygen saturation is influenced more importantly by the pulmonary–systemic blood flow relationship than by the adequacy of mixing; augmented pulmonary blood flow produces a higher systemic arterial saturation if the left ventricle can sustain a high-output state without the intervention of congestive heart failure and pulmonary edema. The systemic arterial oxygen saturation will be quite low, despite adequate intercirculatory mixing sites, if pulmonary blood flow is reduced by left ventricular outflow tract obstruction or increased pulmonary vascular resistance.

Infants with complete transposition of the great arteries are particularly susceptible to the early development of *pulmonary vascular obstructive disease.*[336] Severe morphological alterations develop in the pulmonary vascular bed by the age of 1 or 2 years in almost all patients with an associated large ventricular septal defect or large patent ductus arteriosus in the absence of obstruction to left ventricular outflow. Advanced pulmonary vascular disease is seen also within this same time frame in 5 to 10 per cent of patients without a patent ductus arteriosus and with an intact ventricular septum. Systemic arterial hypoxemia, increased pulmonary blood flow, and pulmonary hypertension contribute to the development of pulmonary vascular obstruction in these patients as they do in other forms of congenital heart disease. Among the additional factors implicated in the accelerated and more widespread pulmonary vascular obstruction found in patients with complete transposition is the presence of extensive bronchopulmonary anastomotic channels, which enter the pulmonary vascular bed proximal to the pulmonary capillary bed; thus, oxygen tension is reduced at the precapillary level, causing pulmonary vasoconstriction.[337] Beyond the early neonatal period many patients have an abnormal distribution pattern of pulmonary blood flow, with preferential flow to the right lung.[338] The asymmetrical distribution of pulmonary blood flow in these individuals results from an abnormal rightward inclination of the main pulmonary artery in the transposition malformation that favors flow from the main to the right pulmonary artery. Persistently increased pulmonary blood flow to the right lung would be expected to contribute to pulmonary vascular obstructive changes within the lung; in the left pulmonary vascular bed, thrombotic changes may occur because of the combination of reduced flow and polycythemia. Finally, it should be recognized that a prenatal alteration in pulmonary vascular smooth muscle may exist, since blood perfusing the fetal lungs in complete transposition of great arteries has a higher than normal pO_2 and may serve to dilate pulmonary vessels in utero. Postnatally such vessels may have an enhanced capacity to constrict in response to vasoactive stimuli and suffer anatomical, obliterative changes.

CLINICAL FINDINGS. Average birthweight and size of infants born with complete transposition of the great arteries are greater than normal. The usual clinical manifestations are dyspnea and cyanosis from birth, progressive hypoxemia, and congestive heart failure. Early in postnatal life the clinical manifestations and course are influenced principally by the magnitude of intercirculatory mixing. The most severe cyanosis and hypoxemia are observed in infants with only a small patent foramen ovale or ductus arteriosus and an intact ventricular septum in whom mixing is inadequate, or in those infants with relatively reduced pulmonary blood flow because of left ventricular outflow tract obstruction.[339, 340] With a large persistent patent ductus arteriosus or a large ventricular septal defect, cyanosis may be minimal and heart failure is the usual dominant problem after the first few weeks of life.[341] It should be recognized that a patent ductus arteriosus is present in about half of newborn infants with transposition, although it closes functionally and anatomically soon after birth in almost all cases. If the ductus arteriosus remains open, better mixing of the venous and arterial circulations is usually at the expense of pulmonary artery hypertension.

Cardiac murmurs are of little diagnostic significance and are absent or insignificant in approximately 30 to 50 per cent of infants with complete transposition of the great arteries and an intact ventricular septum. In infants with a large persistent patent ductus arteriosus, less than half exhibit physical signs typical of ductus arteriosus, such as continuous murmur, bounding pulses, or a prominent mid-diastolic rumble. Moreover, *differential cyanosis* due to reversed pulmonary-to-systemic shunting across the ductus arteriosus is difficult to detect because of generalized arterial desaturation. In those infants with a large ventricular septal defect, a pansystolic murmur emerges usually within the first 7 to 10 days of life. In newborns with transposition and severe pulmonic stenosis or atresia, the clinical findings are similar to those in the infant with tetralogy of Fallot.

The most usual *electrocardiographic findings* include right-axis deviation, right atrial enlargement, and right ventricular hypertrophy, reflecting that the right ventricle is the systemic pumping chamber. Combined ventricular hypertrophy may be present in those patients with a large ventricular septal defect and elevated pulmonary blood flow. Isolated left ventricular hypertrophy is encountered rarely in patients with a ventricular septal defect and a hypoplastic right ventricle, in many of whom the tricuspid valve is displaced abnormally and straddles a ventricular septal defect. In the first days of life the chest x-ray may appear normal, particularly in infants with an intact ventricular septum. Thereafter, roentgenographic findings are often highly suggestive of the diagnosis[342] and consist of (1) progressive cardiac enlargement in early infancy; (2) a characteristic oval or egg-shaped cardiac configuration in the anteroposterior view, and a narrow vascular pedicle created by superimposition of the aortic and pulmonary artery segments; and (3) increased pulmonary vascular markings (Fig. 30–62). A right aortic arch is seen in approximately 4 per cent of infants with an intact ventricular septum and 11 per cent of infants with a ventricular septal defect.

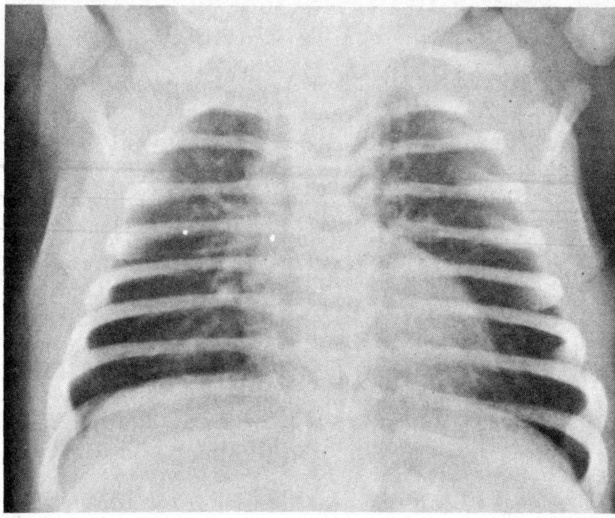

FIGURE 30–62. Chest roentgenogram in a 4-day-old infant with complete transposition of the great arteries showing an oval-shaped heart with a narrow base and increased pulmonary vascular markings.

ECHOCARDIOGRAPHY. Two-dimensional echocardiography is extremely useful in the diagnosis of complete transposition of the great arteries.[343–346] In sagittal cross sections the aorta is observed to ascend retrosternally in contrast to the normal posterior sweep of the pulmonary artery. With transverse short-axis cross-sectional imaging, the diagnosis is confirmed by demonstrating that the anterior great artery (the aorta) is to the right of the posterior great artery (pulmonary) or that the two arteries are visualized side by side (Fig. 30–63). Moreover, from this plane the course of the two great arteries may be traced in order to delineate their ventricle of origin, demonstrating that the anterior rightward vessel (aorta) originates from the right ventricle and the posterior leftward vessel (pulmonary artery) originates from the left ventricle (Fig. 30–64). Echocardiography may also assist in identifying associated defects. Ventricular septal defects may be localized to the membranous, atrioventricular, and trabecular muscular septa, and malalignment types of ventricular septal defects may be identified if the infundibular septum is shifted either anteriorly or posteriorly. A subaortic obstruction may be created by anterior shifting of the infundibular septum, whereas a posterior shift may narrow the subpulmonary area. The nature of left ventricular outflow tract obstruction may be further identified as a fixed obstruction caused by a fibromuscular ridge or as a dynamic obstruction caused by deviation of the interventricular septum toward the left ventricular cavity and the

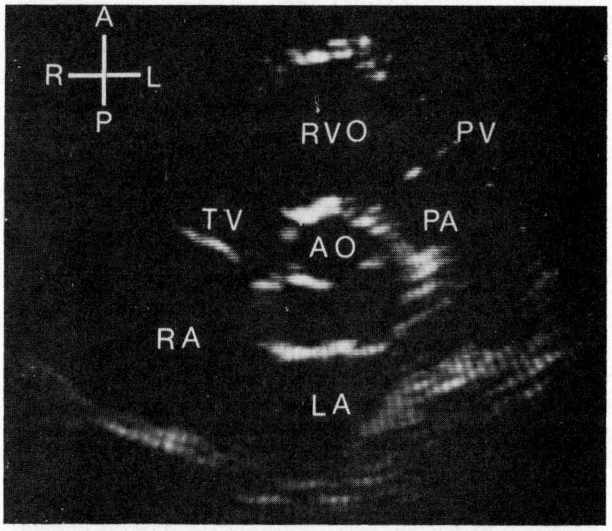

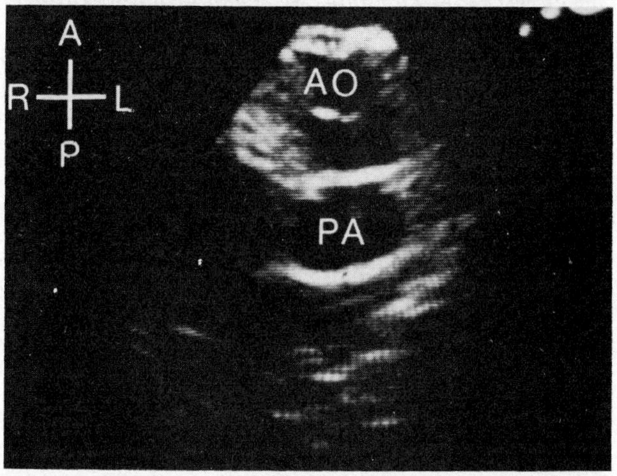

FIGURE 30–63. *Top*, A two-dimensional echocardiographic short-axis scan demonstrates normal great artery relationships. The right ventricular outflow tract (RVO) wraps around the aorta (AO) in a clockwise fashion. The pulmonic valve (PV) is to the left of the aortic valve. *Bottom*, Short-axis scan shows the abnormal great artery relationships in an infant with transposition of the great arteries. The aorta (AO) is directly anterior and slightly to the right of the pulmonary artery (PA). The clockwise partial encirclement of the aorta by the right ventricular outflow tract is no longer observed. A = anterior, L = left, P = posterior, R = right, LA = left atrium, RA = right atrium, TV = tricuspid valve.

apposition between a thickened interventricular septum and systolic anterior motion of the mitral valve.[347]

CARDIAC CATHETERIZATION AND ANGIOCARDIOGRAPHY. The diagnostic portion of the cardiac catheterization allows confirmation of the anatomical derangement of the great arteries and establishes the presence of associated lesions; in the newborn it should always be accompanied by a palliative balloon atrial septostomy, which serves to enlarge the interatrial communication and improve oxygenation. In the older neonate, usually beyond age 3 weeks, thickening of the atrial septum may preclude satisfactory balloon septostomy. In these instances, transcatheter blade septostomy is the preferred approach to palliation. Two-dimensional echocardiography, with or without fluoroscopy, may be used as the imaging mode for both balloon and blade creation of an atrial septal defect.[348] Subcostal four-chamber and sagittal views image cardiac anatomy and catheter position during the procedure, substantially reducing radiation dosage.

Both the diagnostic and palliative procedures can be performed by percutaneous entry into the femoral vein, umbilical vein catheterization, or direct cutdown into the femoral or saphenous vein. The catheter passes easily across the foramen ovale into the left atrium and left ventricle and may be manipulated into the pulmonary artery by means of a flow-directed balloon-guided catheter or by manipulation of a standard catheter bent in the form of a J loop within the left ventricle, with the tip pointed posteriorly to the pulmonary artery. When a large ventricular septal defect is present, a catheter can often be manipulated directly across it from the right ventricle into the pulmonary artery.

The major abnormal hemodynamic findings include right ventricular pressure at systemic levels and either a high or low left ventricular pressure, depending on pulmonary blood flow, pulmonary vascular resistance, and the presence or absence of left ventricular outflow tract obstructive lesions. Oxygen saturation in the aorta is lower than that in the pulmonary artery. Application of the Fick principle to the calculation of pulmonary and systemic blood flow in these patients is an important source of error. Assumed values of oxygen consumption are unreliable in the severely hypoxemic infant. Moreover, because systemic and particularly pulmonary arteriovenous oxygen differences may be quite reduced, small errors in oxygen saturation values result in large errors in flow calculations. Furthermore,

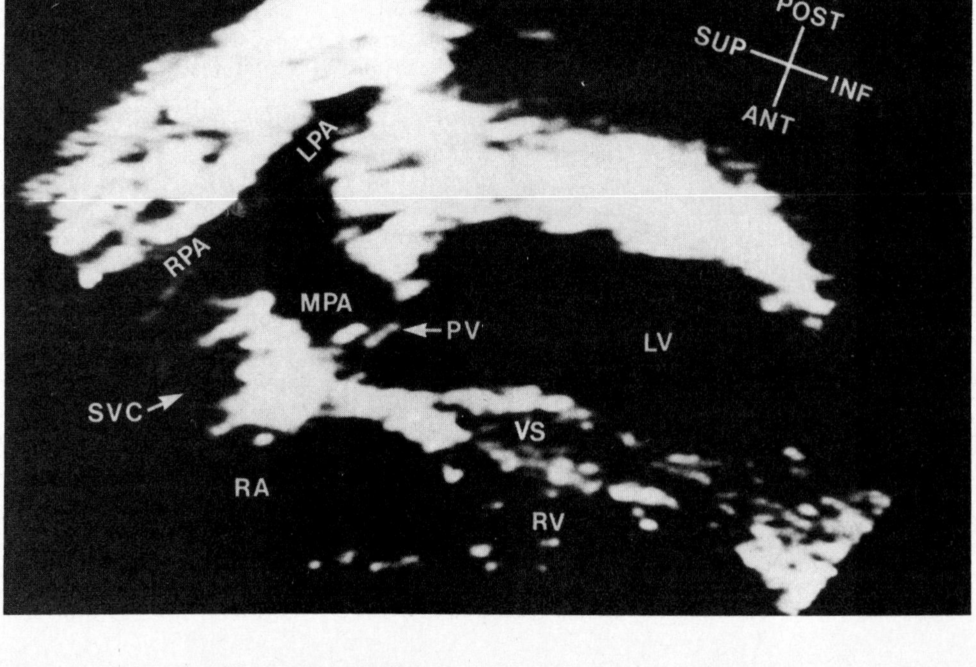

FIGURE 30–64. Complete transposition of the great arteries in a subcostal long-axis view with anterior transducer tilt. The main pulmonary artery (MPA) is seen exiting the left ventricle (LV) and bifurcating into its right and left branches (RPA, LPA). SVC = superior vena cava, RA = right atrium, RV = right ventricle, VS = ventricular septum, PV = pulmonary valve. (Courtesy of Thomas DiSessa, M.D.)

because bronchial collaterals enter the pulmonary circuit at the precapillary level, a true mixed pulmonary artery saturation cannot be sampled; pulmonary blood flow is therefore overestimated when one uses a sample from the central pulmonary artery, and pulmonary vascular resistance values are often underestimated.

Selective ventricular angiography is diagnostic and demonstrates that the anteriorly placed aorta arises from the right ventricle and the posteriorly placed pulmonary artery in continuity with the mitral valve arises from the left ventricle. The status of the ductus arteriosus and the site and size of a ventricular septal defect can be well visualized by angiography (Fig. 30–65). Interventricular defects posterior and inferior to the crista supraventricularis occur in approximately half of these patients; less often the defects are anterior and superior to the crista supraventricularis or are of the atrioventricular canal type.[349] A variety of lesions may be identified as the cause of left ventricular outflow tract obstruction, including ventricular septal hypertrophy with systolic anterior movement of the mitral valve, discrete or tunnel fibromuscular subpulmonic stenosis, valvular and supravalvular stenosis, and rarely, an aneurysm of the membranous ventricular septum or redundant tricuspid valve tissue protruding through a ventricular septal defect.

A number of coronary arterial patterns are seen in patients with complete transposition of the great arteries.[333] In the majority, the left coronary artery originates in the left sinus and the right coronary artery originates in the posterior sinus, with single ostium above both the left and the posterior sinus. In almost 20 per cent of patients the left circumflex artery arises as a branch of the right coronary artery; a single coronary artery is present in approximately 6 per cent; in 3 to 4 per cent of patients either the right coronary and anterior descending arteries originate in the left sinus with the left circumflex originating in the posterior sinus, or two ostia are present above one sinus, one giving rise to the right and the other to the left coronary artery.

MANAGEMENT. Medical treatment is often of limited help but should be vigorous now that functional correction of the malformation has become a possibility. Conservative measures include the use of oxygen, digitalis, diuretics, iron (if an associated iron-deficiency anemia is present), and intravenous sodium bicarbonate for severe hypoxemic metabolic acidosis. Dilatation of the ductus arteriosus by prostaglandin E_1 in the early neonatal period both augments pulmonary blood flow and enhances intercirculatory mixing.[60] The creation or enlargement of an interatrial communication is the simplest procedure for providing increased intracardiac mixing of systemic and pulmonary venous blood; preferably this is achieved by rupturing the valve of the foramen ovale by balloon catheter during transseptal catheterization of the left side of the heart (Rashkind's procedure), or by blade septostomy. Surgical atrial septectomy is rarely required. The balloon should be inflated to a diameter of approximately 15 mm before pullback to the right atrium. Salutary results consist of a fall in left atrial pressure, equalization of mean left and right atrial pressures, and an increase in the systemic arterial oxygen saturation. When the foramen ovale is stretched by the balloon without accomplishing rupture of the septum primum valve of the fossa ovalis, the improvement in oxygenation is short-lived. Infusion or reinfusion intravenously of prostaglandin E_1 (0.05 to 0.1 mg/kg/min) has been shown to improve systemic oxygenation temporarily in the latter situation, by dilating the ductus arteriosus and thereby facilitating intercirculatory mixing.[60] Although balloon atrial septotomy is usually successful in stabilizing the infant's condition[60] and allowing survival in the neonatal period, the initial rise in systemic arterial oxygen saturation to 65 to 75 per cent is often not sustained beyond 6 to 9 months of age.

Surgical Treatment. The development of *corrective operations* for infants born with transposition of the great arteries has greatly improved prognosis.[350–354] Intraatrial correction by the *Mustard* technique is accomplished by excision of the interatrial septum and creation of a new interatrial septum with a pericardial baffle diverting the systemic venous return into the left ventricle through the mitral valve and thence to the left ventricle and pulmonary artery, while the pulmonary venous blood is diverted through the tricuspid valve and right ventricle to the aorta. The Senning procedure is based upon a similar principle and consists of diversion of left pulmonary venous blood by a coronary sinus flap and rerouting of caval flow by the use of an atrial wall flap. In most major medical centers intraatrial corrective operation is performed at any age in patients with an intact ventricular septum who do not improve after balloon atrial septotomy. If palliative septostomy provides adequate relief of hypoxemia, the atrial rerouting operation is performed routinely in most infants with transposition of the great arteries and intact ventricular septum by 3 to 9 months of age with a surgical mortality less than 5 per cent. Clinical improvement is usually quite dramatic. In some patients postoperative complications are observed that are directly related to the

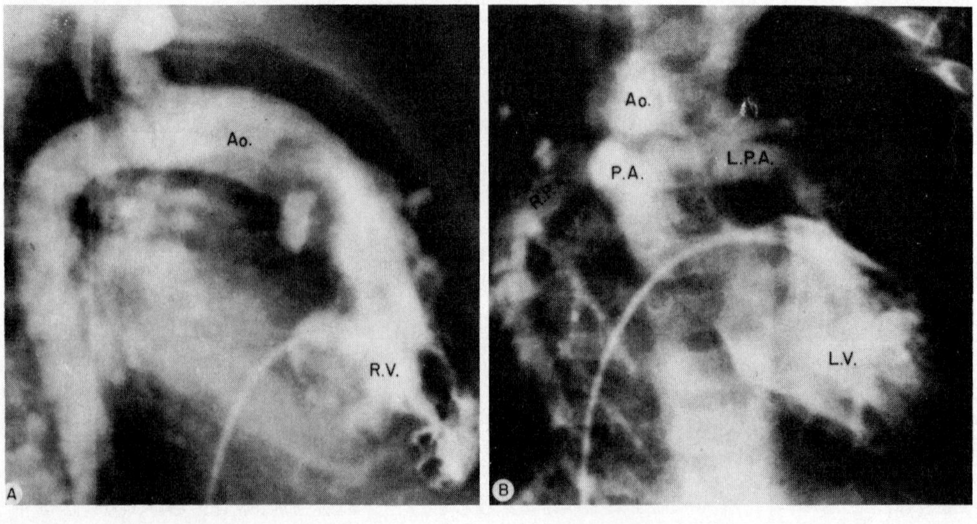

FIGURE 30–65. Lateral (*A*) and frontal (*B*) views of selective ventriculograms in a child with complete transposition of the great arteries and a ventricular septal defect (V.S.D.). Ao. = aorta, R.V. = right ventricle, P.A. = pulmonary artery, L.V. = left ventricle, R.P.A. = right pulmonary artery, L.P.A. = left pulmonary artery. (Courtesy of Delores A. Danilowicz, M.D.)

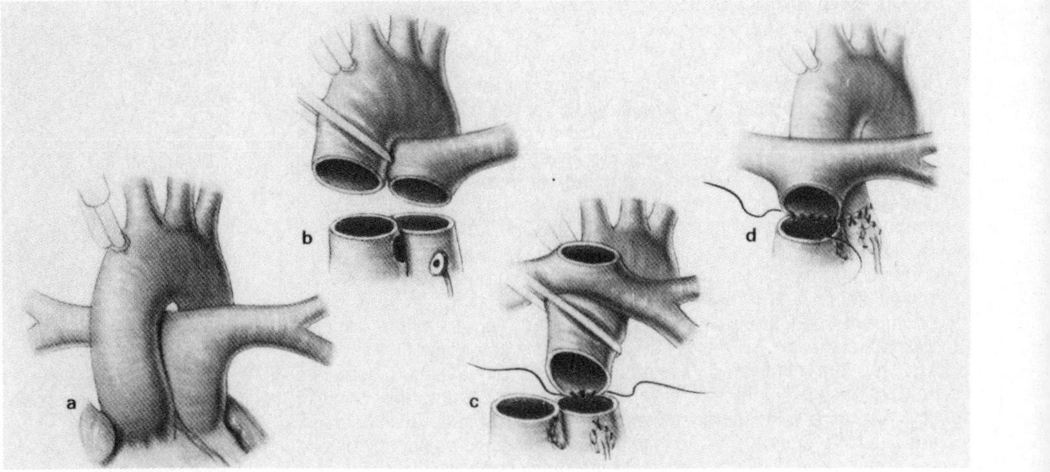

FIGURE 30–66. Complete transposition of the great arteries, corrected by a modified arterial switch operation. The aorta and pulmonary artery are transected and the orifices of the coronary arteries are excised with a rim of adjacent aortic wall (b). The aorta is brought under the bifurcation of the pulmonary artery, and the proximal pulmonary artery and the aorta are anastomosed without necessitating graft interposition. The coronary arteries are transferred to the pulmonary artery (c). The mobilized pulmonary artery is directly anastomosed to the proximal aortic stump (d). (From Stark, J., and deLaval, M.: Surgery for Congenital Heart Defects. New York, Grune and Stratton, 1983, p. 379.)

intraatrial repair (shunts across the intraatrial patch and obstruction to either systemic or pulmonary venous return or both.[355, 356] There is a high incidence of early and late postoperative dysrhythmias that are more likely to have their basis in injury to the sinoatrial node and/or its arterial supply than in disruption of internodal tracts or damage to the atrioventricular node.[357–359] Tricuspid regurgitation is a less common complication of operation and may be related in some patients to a preexisting abnormality of the tricuspid valve,[360] whereas in most it is related to right ventricular dysfunction. Although the assessment of right ventricular contractility is difficult, it would appear that the right ventricular pump function is impaired prior to Mustard operation and does not return to normal following successful surgery.[361, 362] It seems unlikely that the right ventricle can perform as a systemic pumping chamber for the duration of a normal life span.[363] Experience is accumulating with a one-stage anatomical correction in which both coronary arteries are transposed to the posterior artery; the aorta and pulmonary arteries are transsected, contraposed, and anastomosed (Jatene operation) (Fig. 30–66).[354] Although intermediate and long-term follow-up studies are limited, the arterial switch anatomical correction may be complicated by coronary ostial stenosis, acquired supravalvular aortic and/or pulmonary stenosis, and aortic incompetence.

Within the first month of life the arterial switch operation may be performed as a single-stage repair. In older infants it appears necessary to prepare the left ventricle to withstand the systemic pressure which is produced after switching the great arteries, since, if the ventricular septum is intact, left ventricular pressure and left ventricular wall thickness fall normally in relation to the postnatal reduction in pulmonary artery pressure.[365] In these infants a two-stage approach is employed, the first of which consists of banding the pulmonary artery; the arterial switch is performed 4 to 5 months later.

In the unusual infant with an intact ventricular septum and a significant patent ductus arteriosus, an early intraatrial corrective operation with closure of the ductus is indicated at 4 to 6 months of age to prevent the likely progression of pulmonary vascular disease. Debate exists concerning the optimal management of patients with a large ventricular septal defect.[351, 352] In some centers pulmonary artery banding is advocated early in life, followed by definitive intracardiac repair at 1 to 2 years of age. Others favor a one-stage intraatrial repair with patch closure of the ventricular septal defect prior to age 3 to 6 months. Still others perform an arterial switch anatomical correction within the first 3 to 4 months of age, unless the coronary arterial anatomy is considered unfavorable at operation. Infants with transposition of the great arteries plus a ventricular septal defect and left ventricular outflow tract obstruction may require a systemic–pulmonary artery anastomosis when a pronounced diminution in pulmonary blood flow exists. A later corrective procedure for these patients bypasses the left ventricular outflow obstruction and employs an intracardiac ventricular baffle connecting the left ventricle to the aorta and an extracardiac prosthetic conduit between the right ventricle and the distal end of a divided pulmonary artery (Rastelli procedure).[364] In patients with significant pulmonary vascular obstructive disease the risk of definitive repair (anatomical correction or intraatrial baffle and closure of the ventricular septal defect) is great. In this group of patients a "palliative" Mustard or Senning procedure leaving the ventricular septal defect open often provides good, short-term, symptomatic improvement by increasing arterial oxygen tension and reducing the stimulus to progressive polycythemia.[366]

CONGENITALLY CORRECTED TRANSPOSITION OF THE GREAT ARTERIES

This term is applied to two distinctly different anomalies, anatomically corrected transposition or malposition of the great arteries and physiologically corrected, levo- or L-transposition of the great arteries.

MORPHOLOGY. Anatomically corrected malposition of the great arteries is a rare form of congenital heart disease in which the great arteries are abnormally related to each other and to the ventricles but arise, nonetheless, above the anatomically correct ventricles.[367, 368] Because of this, the term *malposition*, rather than *transposition*, is preferable. The anomaly results from either leftward looping of the ventricular segment of the embryonic heart tube in the situs solitus heart, or rightward looping in the situs inversus heart. In this unusual malformation the aorta is anterior and to the left (levo- or L-malposition) and the pulmonary artery is posteromedial and to the right, presumably because of a subaortic conus which causes mitral/aortic discontinuity. When no other defect exists, the circulation proceeds normally. When an associated lesion prompts echocardiographic examination, the diagnosis is indicated by the finding of atrioventricular concordance in association with wide mitral/aortic discontinuity with an anteriorly placed aorta. At cardiac catheterization, the diagnosis of the abnormal relationships between the great arteries may be made by biplane angiocardiography. Anomalies commonly associated with anatomically corrected malposition of the great arteries include ventricular septal defect, left juxtaposition of the atrial appendages, tricuspid atresia or stenosis, and valvular and subvalvular pulmonic stenosis.

Invariably, the term *congenitally corrected transposition* is applied to the patient in whom a functional correction of the circulation exists by virtue of the relationships between the ventricles and great arteries.[369, 370] Corrected or L-transposition occurs when the primitive cardiac tube loops to the left, instead of to the right, during embryogenesis.[371] The anatomical right ventricle comes to lie on the left and receives oxygenated blood from the left atrium; this blood is ejected into an anteriorly placed, left-sided aorta. The anatomical left ventricle lies to the right and connects the right atrium to a posteriorly placed pulmonary artery. Thus, there is both a ventriculoarterial and an atrioventricular discordant connection, with ventricular inversion. This arrangement of the great arteries and ventricles (in contrast to the uncorrected, complete, or D-transposition) permits functional correction, so that systemic venous blood passes into the pulmonary trunk while arterialized pulmonary venous blood flows into the aorta. In the heart with congenitally corrected transposition, the venae cavae and coronary sinus drain into a right atrium that is normal in position and structure. Venous blood flows from the right atrium, designated as the "venous atrium," across an atrioventricular valve that has the structure of a normal mitral valve and into the right-sided "venous ventricle." The venous ventricle, however, has the morphological characteristics of a normal left ventricle, i.e., its interior lining is trabeculated, it has no crista supraventricularis, and the atrioventricular valve is in continuity with the posteriorly placed semilunar valve. It ejects blood into the pulmonary trunk, which arises posterior to the ascending aorta. Oxygenated blood returns from the lungs to the left atrium, which is normal in position and structure; from here it flows into the left-sided "arterial ventricle" across an atrioventricular valve that has the structure of a normal tricuspid valve. The interior lining of the arterial ventricle has the morphological characteristics of a normal right ventricle (i.e., it has coarse trabeculations and a crista supraventricularis), and the tricuspid atrioventricular valve is not in continuity with the anteriorly placed semilunar valve. The arterial ventricle ejects blood into the aorta, which arises anterior to the pulmonary trunk. In addition to inversion of the cardiac ventricles, there is inversion of the conduction system and coronary arteries. Commonly associated anatomical lesions include atrial and ventricular septal defects, often accompanied by valvular or subvalvular pulmonary stenosis; single ventricle with an outlet chamber with or without pulmonic stenosis; left atrioventricular valve regurgitation, usually because of an Ebstein's malformation of the left-sided tricuspid valve; and abnormalities of visceral and atrial situs.[372]

CLINICAL MANIFESTATIONS. The clinical presentation, course, and prognosis of patients with congenital functionally corrected transposition vary, depending on the nature and severity of the complicating intracardiac anomalies.[373] Patients in whom corrected transposition exists as an isolated anomaly present no functional alterations and have no symptoms. Asymptomatic children with an increase in the size of the systemic ventricle, owing to significant left to right shunting or tricuspid regurgitation usually develop symptoms of systemic ventricular dysfunction by the third or fourth decade.[372]

The physical findings in congenitally corrected transposition are those of the associated lesions with two exceptions: (1) a single accentuated second heart sound is usually present in the second left intercostal space, representing closure of the aortic valve lying lateral and anterior to the pulmonic valve; and (2) there is a high incidence of cardiac dysrhythmias. Because of the inversion of the heart's conduction system the electrocardiogram may provide important clues in the diagnosis. An abnormal direction of initial (septal) depolarization from right to left causes leftward, anterior, and superior orientation of the initial QRS forces and reversal of the precordial Q-wave pattern (Q waves are present in the right precordial leads and absent in the left).

LABORATORY EXAMINATION. In addition to inversion of the conduction system, the His bundle is elongated because of the greater distance between the atrioventricular node and the base of the ventricular septum.[374] The His bundle is located beneath the pulmonic valve in the position of mitral pulmonary continuity; thus, it is subject to significant excursions during mitral valve closure. This arrangement may be a causal factor in the arrhythmias and atrioventricular conduction disturbances commonly observed in these patients. First-degree atrioventricular (AV) block occurs in about 50 per cent, and complete AV block

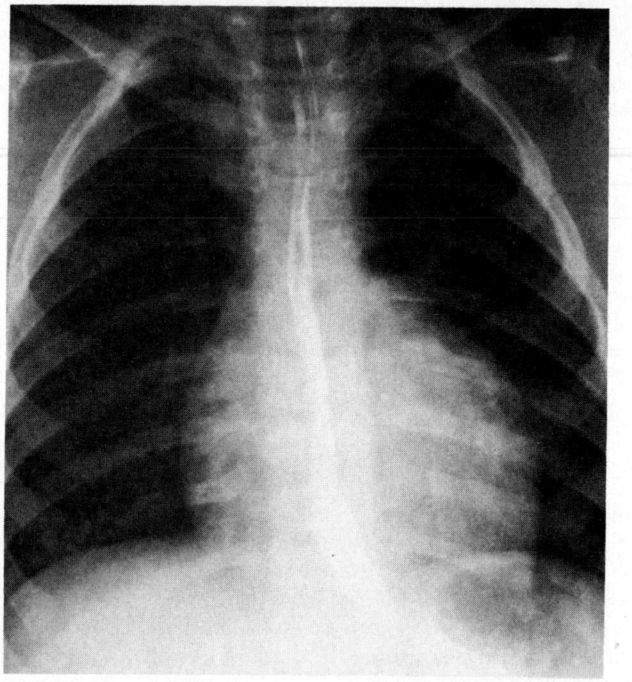

FIGURE 30–67. Chest roentgenogram in a child with congenitally corrected transposition of the great arteries. The smooth convexity of the left superior cardiac border is formed by the displaced ascending aorta. The main pulmonary artery is medially displaced and absent from the cardiac silhouette.

occurs in 10 to 15 per cent of patients. Other degrees of AV dissociation may be observed as well as paroxysmal supraventricular tachycardia and ventricular extrasystoles. In some patients, Kent bundle connections provide the anatomical substrate for preexcitation.[375] Roentgenographic examination characteristically reveals absence of the normal pulmonary artery segment and a smooth convexity of the left supracardiac border produced by the displaced ascending aorta (Fig. 30–67). The latter may be visualized by radionuclide scintillation scans of the central circulation. The main pulmonary trunk is medially displaced and absent from the cardiac silhouette; the right pulmonary hilus is often prominent and elevated compared to the left, producing a right-sided "waterfall" appearance.

Two-dimensional echocardiography seeks to identify the morphology of each ventricle by defining the characteristics of the inflow and outflow tracts and papillary and trabecular muscle morphology, ventricular shape, and great artery position.[376] By tracing the great arteries back to their ventricles of origin in subxiphoid and parasternal short-axis planes, one would find that the anterior leftward great artery (the aorta) arises from the left-sided ventricle and is not in continuity with the left-sided atrioventricular valve. The great arteries exit the heart in parallel fashion; the position, origin, and branching pattern of the great arteries are observed in subxiphoid and suprasternal views, while the anteroposterior and right-left positions of the great arteries can be seen from the parasternal short-axis position. Because the ventricular septum lies in the anteroposterior plane parallel to the echo beam, it may not be visualized from a left parasternal view. In apical-basal or subxiphoid, four-chamber echo views, the right and left ventricular morphology and the inverted atrioventricular valves may be ascertained correctly. The latter views also demonstrate the level of attachment of the atrioventricular valves and allow detection of inferior displacement of the left-sided tricuspid valve when Ebstein's anomaly coexists.

At *cardiac catheterization* the diagnosis should be sus-

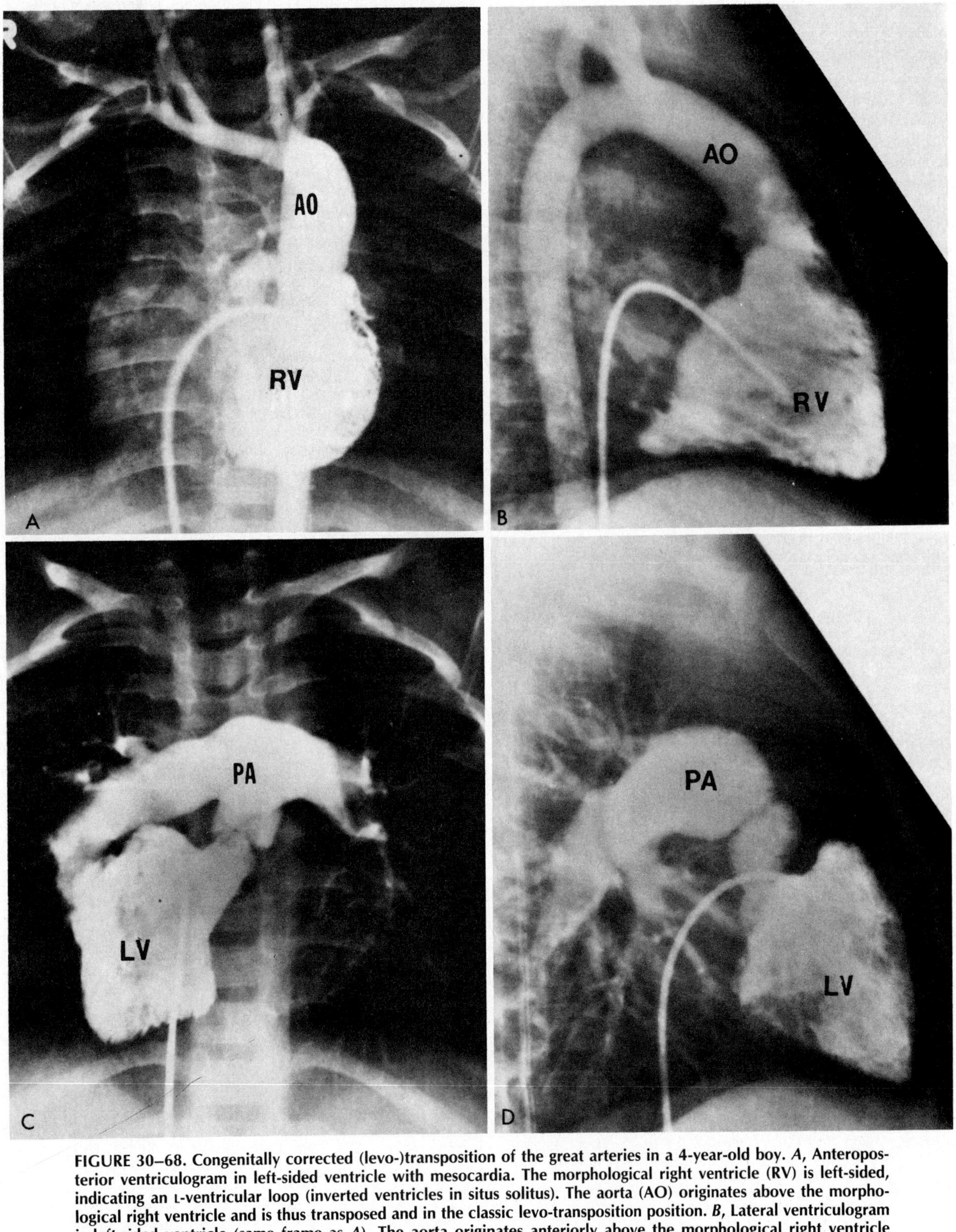

FIGURE 30–68. Congenitally corrected (levo-)transposition of the great arteries in a 4-year-old boy. *A*, Anteroposterior ventriculogram in left-sided ventricle with mesocardia. The morphological right ventricle (RV) is left-sided, indicating an L-ventricular loop (inverted ventricles in situs solitus). The aorta (AO) originates above the morphological right ventricle and is thus transposed and in the classic levo-transposition position. *B*, Lateral ventriculogram is left-sided ventricle (same frame as *A*). The aorta originates anteriorly above the morphological right ventricle (RV). *C*, Anteroposterior ventriculogram in right-sided morphological left ventricle (LV). The transposed pulmonary artery (PA) arises from this ventricle, and the ventricular septum appears intact. Pulmonic valve thickening is also evident. The aorta (*A*) is to the left of the pulmonary artery. Note that the ventricular septum in the L-ventricular loop is visualized best in the anteroposterior views. *D*, Lateral ventriculogram in right-sided ventricle (same frame as *C*). The pulmonary artery is posterior to the aorta, and supravalvular pulmonic narrowing is seen. (From Freedom, R. M., et al.: The differential diagnosis of levo-transposed or malposed aorta. An angiocardiographic study. Circulation *50*:1040, 1974, by permission of the American Heart Association, Inc.)

pected when the venous catheter enters a posterior and midline main pulmonary trunk. Retrograde arterial catheter passage establishes the typical position of the ascending aorta at the upper left cardiac border. Hemodynamic abnormalities depend upon the lesions associated with corrected transposition. Selective *angiocardiography* allows visualization of the transposed great arteries and morphological differentiation of the two ventricles (Fig. 30–68). The ventricles tend to lie side by side, with the ventricular septum oriented in an anteroposterior direction. Selective aortography demonstrates the inverted coronary arterial pattern that is invariably present in corrected transposition. The competence of the left atrioventricular valve may be determined by injection of contrast material into the arterial ventricle.[377] When a left-sided Ebstein's malformation exists, the leaflets are displaced distal to the true valve annulus. The level of the annulus may be determined by visualization of the circumflex branch of the left coronary artery, which courses posteriorly in the AV groove.

Specific problems have attended operative repair of the lesions associated with congenitally corrected transposition, owing primarily to the course of the AV conduction system and the coronary arterial pattern.[378] Intraoperative electrophysiological mapping of the course of the conduction system has been proposed to reduce, but not abolish, the risk of surgically induced heart block. The AV bundle is located anteriorly and in relation to the anterolateral quadrant of the pulmonary outflow tract. Thus, when a ventricular septal defect is present, the bundle is usually related to the anterior and superior margins of the defect and lies beneath the pulmonic valve. In corrected transposition, the coronary arteries have a course appropriate to their ventricles, i.e., the anterior descending and circumflex arteries supply the morphological left ventricle, and the right coronary artery supplies the morphological right ventricle. However, because the great arteries are transposed, the noncoronary sinus is the anterior sinus of the aortic valve. Occasionally, the inversion of the coronary arterial system may limit and preclude an incision into the venous ventricle, thereby interfering with exposure of intracardiac defects in the usual manner. The disadvantage in approaching intracardiac anomalies using an incision in the morphological right ventricle is that this is the systemic ventricle. When significant pulmonary stenosis exists with a ventricular septal defect, a valved extracardiac conduit is often a required part of the surgical repair. Surgical risks are especially high in patients in whom significant regurgitation exists from the arterial ventricle to the arterial atrium. In these patients, annuloplasty, or more usually valve replacement, is required. In all operative approaches, if complete heart block has been present intermittently or permanently pre- or intraoperatively, permanent epicardial atrial and ventricular pacemaker leads are implanted.

DOUBLE-OUTLET RIGHT VENTRICLE

MORPHOLOGY. Other designations applied to this lesion include origin of both great arteries from the right ventricle, partial transposition, complete transposition of the aorta and levo-position of the pulmonary artery, complete dextroposition of the aorta, and the Taussig-Bing complex. This is an extremely heterogeneous category of malformations in which an abnormal relationship exists between the aorta and the pulmonary trunk, which arise wholly or in large part from the right ventricle.[379, 380]

Currently, a uniform definition or classification does not exist of double-outlet right ventricle. To some, double-outlet right ventricle means origin of one great artery and at least 50 per cent of the other over the right ventricle; others require the presence of conus muscle between both great arteries and the atrioventricular annulus. One or both great arteries may arise from an infundibular chamber; there may be considerable variability in the amount of subarterial conus muscle. Thus, the semilunar valves may lie side by side, or with the pulmonary valve more anterior and superior, or with a more anterior and superior aortic valve. A malalignment type of ventricular septal defect is almost always present in double-outlet right ventricle because the infundibular septum is positioned abnormally. When the amount of conus muscle beneath the two great arteries varies, the ventricular septal defect is commonly positioned beneath the more posterior semilunar valve, which, in fact, usually overrides the interventricular septum through this ventricular septal defect. The amount of conus muscle underneath the valve determines the position of the semilunar root in relation to the ventricles below. Thus, double-outlet right ventricle resides within the spectrum of conotruncal abnormalities ranging from tetralogy of Fallot to transposition of the great arteries. Occasionally, the ventricular septal defect extends beneath both great arteries and is referred to as doubly committed. In some instances, the ventricular septal defect is remote to both great arteries, or is considered uncommitted, in which case the defect often lies in the inlet or muscular portion of the interventricular septum.

More than half of patients with double-outlet right ventricle have associated anomalies of the atrioventricular valves.[381] Mitral atresia associated with a hypoplastic left ventricle is common; less often observed are tricuspid stenosis, Ebstein's anomaly of the tricuspid valve, complete atrioventricular septal defect, and overriding or straddling of either atrioventricular valve. Aortic coarctation may be associated with double-outlet right ventricle, particularly when the subaortic area is narrowed by malalignment of the infundibular septum. Double-outlet right ventricle may also be a component of the multiple cardiovascular anomalies of the splenic dysgenesis or heterotaxy syndromes. An increased incidence of the anomaly occurs in infants with the trisomy 18 syndrome.

The pathological features in most patients include side-by-side pulmonic and aortic valves and discontinuity between the mitral and aortic valves. The latter exists because muscular infundibulum is usual beneath both semilunar valves. The ventricular septal defect may be remote from or related closely to one or both semilunar valves (Fig. 30–69).[381] When the interventricular defect is subpulmonic, with or without a straddling pulmonary trunk, the complex is designated "Taussig-Bing." In most patients the interventricular septal defect is below the crista supraventricularis and is subaortic in location. Least often the

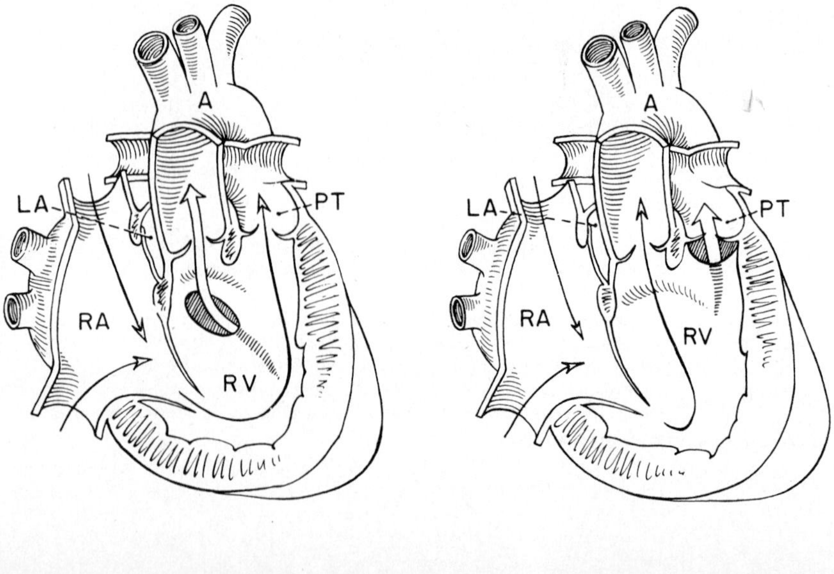

FIGURE 30–69. Double-outlet right ventricle (RV) with side-by-side relation of great arteries is illustrated in both panels. A subaortic ventricular septal defect (VSD) below the crista supraventricularis (*left*) favors delivery of left ventricular blood to the aorta (A). Location of the VSD above the crista (*right*) favors streaming to the pulmonary trunk (PT). LA = left atrium; RA = right atrium; PT = pulmonary trunk. (From Sridaromont, S., et al.: Double outlet right ventricle: Hemodynamic and anatomic correlations. Am. J. Cardiol. *38*:85, 1976.)

defect is either remote from both semilunar valves ("uncommitted") or underlies both ("doubly committed").

CLINICAL MANIFESTATIONS. The clinical and physiological picture is determined by the size and location of the ventricular septal defect and the presence or absence of pulmonic stenosis. In the Taussig-Bing form of double-outlet right ventricle, the malformation resembles physiologically and clinically complete transposition with ventricular septal defect and pulmonary hypertension. When the ventricular septal defect is subaortic, the stream of blood from the left ventricle is directed preferentially to the aorta. Thus, there may be little or no detectable cyanosis, and these patients usually clinically resemble those with an isolated, large ventricular septal defect and pulmonary hypertension. The most important determinant of the natural history in both these types of double-outlet right ventricle is the progression of pulmonary vascular obstruction. In contrast, when there is pulmonary outflow tract obstruction, which is often severe and found commonly in those patients in whom the ventricular septal defect is subaortic, clinical findings are similar to those of cyanotic tetralogy of Fallot. In some patients, especially without pulmonic stenosis, the electrocardiogram shows a superiorly oriented counterclockwise frontal plane QRS loop in addition to right ventricular hypertrophy.[382] The pattern appears to result from relative hypoplasia of the anterosuperior left bundle and preferential activation of the posteroinferior left ventricular wall. The presence of the latter electrocardiographic pattern in patients with double-outlet right ventricle should raise the possibility of a coexistent atrioventricular septal defect or abnormality of the mitral valve.[381]

DIAGNOSIS. Two-dimensional *echocardiography* may reliably distinguish double-outlet right ventricle from other lesions causing cyanosis, such as tetralogy of Fallot and transposition of the great arteries.[383] The relative anteroposterior positions of the great arteries can be determined from the parasternal short-axis view. The parasternal long-axis view shows the position of the more posterior semilunar root relative to the interventricular septum and anterior mitral leaflet, and is the best view for demonstrating the presence of subarterial conus muscle. Subxiphoid views best demonstrate the position of both great arteries over the ventricles. Each great artery is displayed on long- and short-axis subxiphoid sweeps. In reporting echocardiographic results, it is imperative to state each component anatomical feature, i.e., the position of both great arteries, the presence and amount of infundibulum under each semilunar valve, the anatomy of both subpulmonary and subaortic outflow tracts, the position and size of the associated ventricular septal defect, and the presence of all other associated lesions, particularly atrioventricular valve anomalies and coarctation of the aorta.

In each of the different types of double-outlet right ventricle, precise delineation of the malformation also depends on careful angiocardiographic analysis. The diagnosis can be established with confidence when the angiographic findings include simultaneous opacification of both great vessels from the right ventricle, aortic and pulmonic valves at the same transverse level, and separation of the aortic valve from the aortic leaflet of the mitral valve by the crista supraventricularis (Fig. 30–70).[384] The position of the ventricular septal defect and the relationships between the great arteries must be defined in order to plan surgical procedures appropriately.

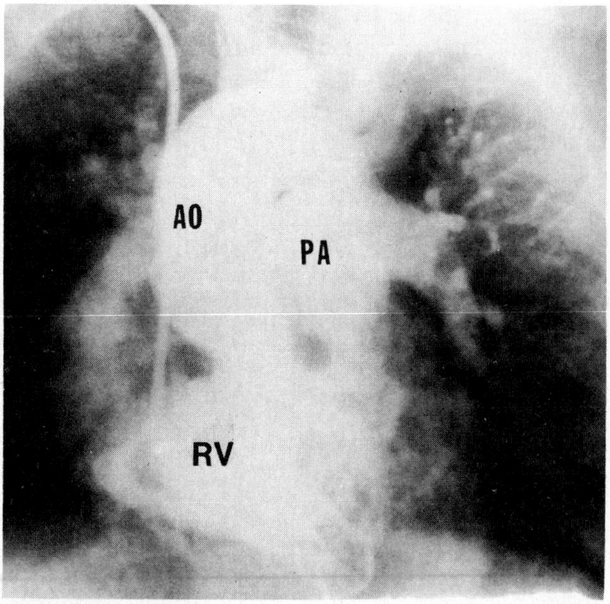

FIGURE 30–70. Simultaneous opacification of both great arteries from a right ventricular injection of contrast material in a patient with double-outlet right ventricle (RV). The aortic and pulmonic valves are at the same transverse level. AO = aorta, PA = pulmonary artery. (Courtesy of Robert White, M.D.)

SURGICAL TREATMENT. In double-outlet right ventricle with subaortic ventricular septal defect, repair is accomplished by creating an intraventicular baffle that conducts left ventricular blood to the aorta.[380] When the ventricular septal defect is subpulmonic, repair is accomplished by use of one of three procedures: by creating an intraventricular conduit that conducts left ventricular blood to the pulmonary arteries and performing the Mustard or Senning procedure, by creating an intraventricular baffle directing left ventricular blood to the aorta and connecting the right ventricle to the pulmonary artery by use of a valve-containing conduit, or by closure of the ventricular septal defect and arterial switch.[379, 380, 385–387] When the ventricular septal defect is doubly committed, i.e., both subaortic and subpulmonic, operation consists of creating an intraventricular baffle that conducts left ventricular blood to the aorta. The type of double-outlet right ventricle in which the ventricular septal defect is remote and uncommitted to either semilunar orifice has infrequently been repaired successfully.

DOUBLE-OUTLET LEFT VENTRICLE

One of the rarest cardiac anomalies consists of both great arteries arising from the morphological left ventricle. Usually, conal musculature or an infundibulum is absent or deficient beneath the orifices of both semilunar valves.[388] A broad spectrum of associated malformations exists. A ventricular septal defect and valvular or subvalvular pulmonic stenosis have been present in most patients. Angiocardiographic assessment of the spatial relations of the origins of the great arteries is essential to an accurate diagnosis and to evaluating the possibility of operative repair.[389]

TOTAL ANOMALOUS PULMONARY VENOUS CONNECTION

This anomaly has been estimated to account for 1 to 3 per cent of all cases of congenital heart disease and 2 per cent of deaths therefrom in the first year of life.[390, 391] The anomaly is the result of persistence during embryogenesis of communications between the pulmonary portion of the foregut plexus and the cardinal or umbilicovitelline system of veins, resulting in the connection of all the pulmonary veins either to the right atrium directly or to the systemic veins and their tributaries. Since all venous blood returns to the right atrium, an interatrial communication is an integral part of this malformation. Additional major cardiac malformations occur in about 30 per cent of patients.[235] Among these are common atrium, single ventricle, truncus arteriosus, and anomalies of the systemic veins. Extracardiac malformations, particularly of the alimentary, endocrine, and genitourinary systems, are present in 25 to 30 per cent of cases.

The *anatomical varieties* of total anomalous pulmonary venous connection may be subdivided depending upon the level of the abnormal drainage (Fig. 30–71). Table 30–10 provides average figures of the distribution of the sites of anomalous connection.[235] The anomalous connection is usually supradiaphragmatic and to the left brachiocephalic vein, right atrium, coronary sinus, or superior vena cava. In approximately 13 per cent, particularly in males, the distal site of connection is below the diaphragm. In this situation a common trunk originates from the confluence of pulmonary veins and descends in front of the esophagus, penetrating the diaphragm through the esophageal hiatus. The anomalous trunk then connects the portal vein or one of its tributaries, ductus venosus, or, rarely, to one of the hepatic veins. In rare cases various combinations of anomalous connection occur in which drainage is to multiple levels.

HEMODYNAMICS. The physiological consequences and, accordingly, the clinical picture depend upon the size of the interatrial communication and on the magnitude of the pulmonary vascular resistance.[390] When the interatrial communication is small, systemic blood flow is markedly limited.[391] Right atrial and systemic venous pressures are

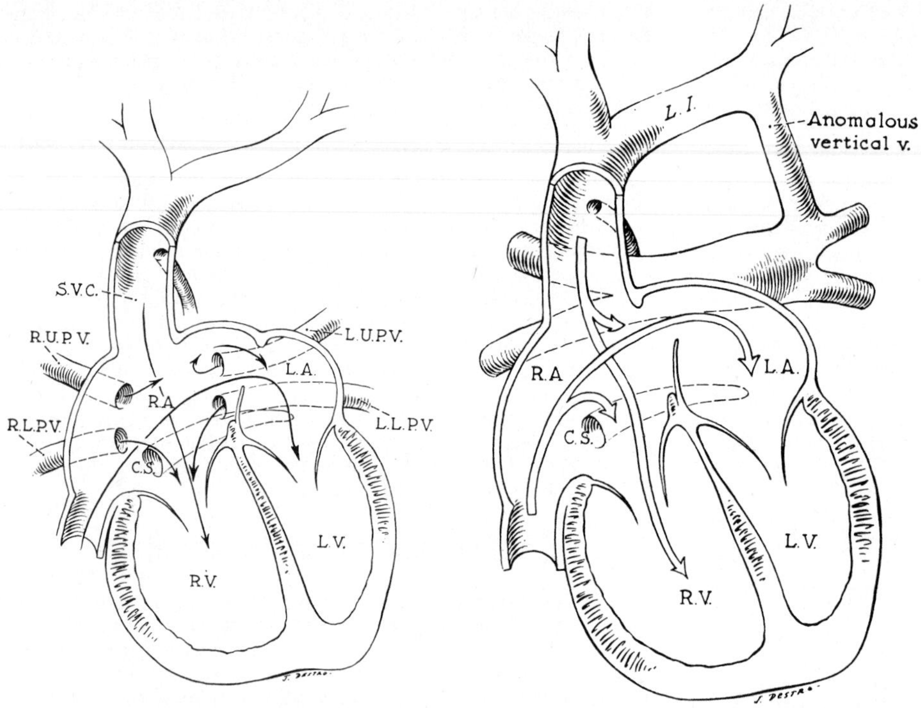

FIGURE 30–71. Two common types of total anomalous pulmonary venous connection are illustrated. These are connections to the right atrium (*left*) and to the left innominate vein (*right*). S.V.C. = superior vena cava; I.V.C. = inferior vena cava; R.A. = right atrium; L.A. = left atrium; C.S. = coronary sinus; R.V. = right ventricle; L.V. = left ventricle; R.U.P.V. = right upper pulmonary veins; L.U.P.V. = left upper pulmonary veins; R.L.P.V. = right lower pulmonary veins; L.L.P.V. = left lower pulmonary veins; R.H. = right hepatic vein; L.H. = left hepatic vein; L.P.V. = left portal vein; R.P.V. = right portal vein; L.I. = left innominate vein. (From Wagenvoort, C. A., et al.: Pathology of the Pulmonary Vasculature. Springfield, Ill., Charles C Thomas, 1964.)

elevated, and hepatic enlargement and peripheral edema are present. The size of the interatrial communication is also an important determinant in the development in utero and postnatally of the left atrium and left ventricle. Left atrial cavity size is usually somewhat reduced, whereas left ventricular volumes may be reduced or normal. The magnitude of pulmonary blood flow and therefore the ratio of oxygenated to unoxygenated blood that returns to the right atrium are a function of pulmonary vascular resistance. The arterial oxygen saturation, which ranges from markedly reduced to normal values, is inversely related to the pulmonary vascular resistance. In this regard, in most patients the principal determinant of pulmonary pressures and resistance is less related to augmented pulmonary blood flow and pulmonary arteriolar vascular obstruction than to the presence and intensity of pulmonary venous obstruction.[391, 392] Obstruction to pulmonary venous return and pulmonary venous hypertension are invariably present in patients with infradiaphragmatic anomalous pulmonary venous connection and in many with a supradiaphragmatic pathway. In the former type, pulmonary venous obstruction results from the length and narrowness of the common pulmonary venous trunk, compression at the esophageal hiatus of the diaphragm, constriction at the subdiaphragmatic site of insertion, or pulmonary venous return that must pass first through the portal-hepatic circulation before returning to the right atrium. When venous obstruction occurs in supradiaphragmatic types of drainage, constriction may exist at the entrance site of the anomalous veins into the systemic venous circulation, and/or the anomalous venous channel may be kinked or situated abnormally and compressed between the left pulmonary artery and left bronchus.[393] Occasionally the presence of a small, restrictive patent foramen ovale results in pulmonary venous obstruction. Pulmonary vascular obstructive disease is rare during infancy, although exceptions have been reported.[394] In patients without pulmonary venous obstruction the risk of developing the Eisenmenger reaction is comparable to that in patients with an atrial septal defect.

CLINICAL MANIFESTATIONS. The majority of patients with total anomalous pulmonary venous connection have symptoms during the first year of life, and 80 per cent will die before age one year if left untreated.[390] The few who remain asymptomatic have a relatively good prognosis; once the condition is detected, operation may be elected later in childhood. Symptomatic infants with total anoma-

TABLE 30–10 SITE OF CONNECTION IN TOTAL ANOMALOUS PULMONARY VENOUS CONNECTION

1. Connection to right atrium	15%
2. Connection to common cardinal system	
a. (Right) superior vena cava	11%
b. Azygos vein	1%
3. Connection to left common cardinal system	
a. Left innominate vein	36%
b. Coronary sinus	16%
4. Connection to umbilicovitelline system	
a. Portal vein	6%
b. Ductus venosus	4%
c. Inferior vena cava	2%
d. Hepatic vein	1%
5. Multiple sites	7%
6. Unknown	1%

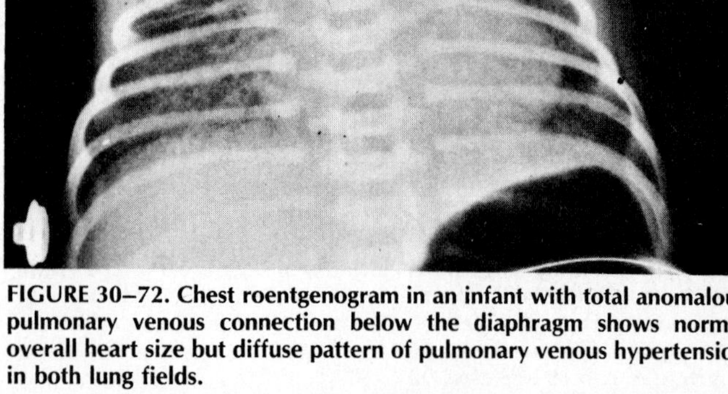

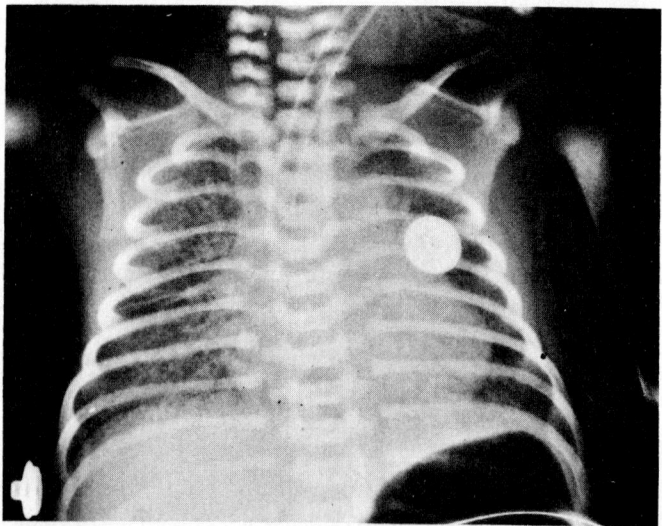

FIGURE 30–72. Chest roentgenogram in an infant with total anomalous pulmonary venous connection below the diaphragm shows normal overall heart size but diffuse pattern of pulmonary venous hypertension in both lung fields.

lous pulmonary venous connection present with signs of heart failure and/or cyanosis. Infants with pulmonary venous obstruction present with the early onset of severe dyspnea, pulmonary edema, cyanosis, and right heart failure. Cardiac murmurs are often not prominent. In the unobstructed forms of total anomalous pulmonary venous connection the characteristic physical findings include right ventricular precordial overactivity and minimal cyanosis unless congestive heart failure intervenes. Multiple heart sounds are often audible, consisting of a first heart sound followed by an ejection sound; a fixed, widely split second heart sound with an accentuated pulmonic component; and a third and often a fourth heart sound. A soft systolic ejection murmur is usual along the left sternal border, and a middiastolic murmur of flow across the tricuspid valve is commonly audible at the lower left sternal border.

Laboratory Findings. The *electrocardiogram* shows right-axis deviation and right atrial and right ventricular hypertrophy. *Roentgenograms* of the chest reveal increased pulmonary blood flow; the right atrium and ventricle are dilated and hypertrophied, and the pulmonary artery segment is enlarged[395] (Fig. 30–72). In addition, the specific site of anomalous connection may result in a characteristic appearance of the cardiac silhouette. Thus, in patients with total anomalous pulmonary venous connection to the left brachiocephalic vein, the superior vena cava on the right, left brachiocephalic vein superiorly, and vertical vein on the left produce a cardiac shadow that resembles a "snowman" or "figure of eight." The upper right cardiac border may be prominent when the anomalous connection is to the right superior vena cava.

Echocardiography demonstrates marked enlargement of the right ventricle and a small left atrium.[396] Occasionally, an echo-free space representing the common pulmonary venous chamber may be seen to lie behind the left atrium on ultrasound examination.[35] Diagnostic echo findings include an absence of pulmonary vein connections to a small left atrium in the presence of right to left bulging of the septum primum at the foramen ovale. Positive diagnosis is made by identifying pulmonary venous connection to the systemic veins, coronary sinus, or right atrium, rather than to the left atrium. All four pulmonary veins and their connections must be identified to diagnose mixed types accurately. There is no standard echocardiographic method for tracing pulmonary venous pathways because of their diverse anatomical positions.

At *cardiac catheterization* those patients found to have systemic arterial saturations below 70 to 75 per cent and with pulmonary artery pressure at or above systemic levels are likely to have pulmonary venous obstruction. Variations in oxygen saturation in the systemic venous circulation may be helpful. In the subdiaphragmatic type, a step-up may not be apparent in inferior vena caval oxygen saturations obtained via femoral vein cannulation because of the contribution of highly oxygenated renal venous blood to the caval stream. In contrast, sampling of the hepatic or portal vein via a catheter inserted through the umbilical vein will yield diagnostically higher oxygen saturations, indicating anomalous return to those vessels. Selective pulmonary arteriography and *indicator dilution* studies at cardiac catheterization are especially helpful in determining the drainage pathways of the pulmonary veins. Indicator dye injected into the right ventricle or pulmonary artery takes longer to reach the peripheral arterial sampling site than does dye injected into the vena cava or right atrium. The contours of dilution curves obtained from a peripheral artery after injection into both the right atrium and a pulmonary vein are identical and show a large right-to-left shunt, while the left atrial curve is normal. If the cardiac catheter can be manipulated directly into the anomalous trunk through its site of connection, selective injection of contrast material into the common channel provides anatomical definition of the pulmonary venous tree. If the pulmonary veins cannot be entered directly, selective right and left main pulmonary artery injection of contrast material is often more helpful than is injection into a main pulmonary artery, since many infants have a persistent patent ductus arteriosus through which the contrast agent flows right to left. Moreover, the drainage from both lungs must be outlined clearly in order to exclude a mixed type of anomalous venous drainage. Pulmonary venous obstruction may be detected by noting a pressure difference between the pulmonary artery wedge pressure and the right atrium.

TREATMENT. Balloon atrial septotomy may provide dramatic palliation for the infant in whom the small size of an interatrial communication limits the amount of blood reaching the left side of the heart and systemic circulation.[391] Unless pulmonary vascular disease is present, results of operation for total anomalous pulmonary venous connection in patients beyond infancy are generally good.[397–399] The procedure consists of creating an anastomosis between the common pulmonary venous channel and left atrium and closing the atrial defect and the anomalous venous pathway. Improved results of operation in infancy require that postoperative pulmonary venous hypertension be averted by construction of a generally large anastomosis with or without enlargement of the left atrium. Normal hemodynamics and cardiac function have been demonstrated after surgical correction.[400]

PARTIAL ANOMALOUS PULMONARY VENOUS CONNECTION

(See also p. 985)

In this condition one or more of the pulmonary veins, but not all, are connected to the right atrium or to one or more of its venous tributaries. An atrial septal defect, particularly one of the sinus venosus type, commonly accompanies this anomaly; the usual connection involves the veins of the right upper and middle lobe and the superior vena cava.[235] Exclusive of atrial septal defects, major additional cardiac malformations occur in approximately 20 per cent of patients; these include ventricular septal defect, tetralogy of Fallot, and a variety of complex anomalies.

In the absence of associated anomalies, the physiological disturbance is determined by the number of anomalous veins and their site of connection, the presence and size of an atrial septal defect, and the state of the pulmonary vascular bed.[401] In the usual patient with isolated partial pulmonary venous connection, the hemodynamic state and physical findings are similar to those in atrial septal defect. Rarely, venous drainage of the right lung is into the inferior vena cava. This condition is often associated with hypoplasia of the right lung, dextroposition of the heart, pulmonary parenchymal abnormalities, and anomalous systemic supply to the lower lobe of the right lung from the abdominal aorta or its main branches.[402] This complex has been designated the "scimitar syndrome" because of the characteristic roentgenographic finding of a crescent-like shadow in the right lower lung field that is produced by the anomalous venous channel.

At *cardiac catheterization*, partial anomalous pulmonary venous connection to the coronary sinus, azygos vein, or superior vena cava may be identified by careful and frequent oximetry sampling. Oximetry is of limited value when the anomalous connection is to the inferior vena cava, because of both reduced flow through the right lung and the contribution to the vena caval stream of highly oxygenated blood from the renal veins. Selective angiography is most helpful the farther away from the right atrium the anomalous veins connect. Surgical repair offers definitive therapy at low risk if pulmonary vascular obliterative disease has not yet developed.

MALPOSITIONS OF THE HEART AND CARDIAC APEX

Positional anomalies of the heart refer to conditions in which the cardiac apex is located in the right side of the chest (dextrocardia) or is centrally located (mesocardia) or in which there is a normal location of the heart in the left side of the chest but abnormal position of the viscera (isolated levocardia). Commonly, such hearts are abnormal with respect to chamber localization and great artery attachments; associated complex intra- and extracardiac lesions are common.

Problems of terminology abound in the literature describing these complex cardiac anomalies, although sensible and uniform systems of classification are available.[403, 404]

ANATOMICAL FEATURES. Defining the cardiac anatomy in instances of cardiac malposition requires a description of three cardiac segments—the visceroatrial situs, the ventricular loop, and the conotruncus (the atria, ventricles, and great arteries, respectively). In addition to defining positional interrelationships, the description of the malposed heart must also include the connections of the ventricles to the atria and great arteries as well as chamber identification, both morphologically and functionally.

To accomplish accurate diagnosis often requires a synthesis of findings from noninvasive tests such as two-dimensional echocardiography, computed tomography, magnetic resonance imaging (when available), as well as hemodynamic and cineangiographic findings obtained at cardiac catheterization.[405, 406]

In general, the determination of the body situs indicates the position of the atria. The visceral situs can usually be determined by the location of the stomach bubble and liver on a routine roentgenogram and of the inferior vena cava by means of echocardiography or the position of a cardiac catheter, or by means of a computed axial tomogram or venous or radioisotope angiocardiogram. Atrial anatomy is best investigated noninvasively by using subxiphoid long- and short-axis and apical four-chamber echocardiographic views. Venous contrast injections may be useful to define systemic venous connections.

Situs solitus is the normal arrangement of viscera and atria, with the right atrium right-sided, and the left atrium left-sided. Situs solitus is further characterized by a trilobed right lung and eparterial bronchus (i.e., the right upper lobe bronchus that passes above the right pulmonary artery), a bilobed left lung and hyparterial bronchus (i.e., the left bronchus that passes below the left pulmonary artery), the major lobe of the liver on the right, a left-sided stomach and spleen, and right-sided venae cavae. Situs inversus is a mirror image of normal. Situs ambiguous or visceral heterotaxy refers to an anatomically uncertain or indeterminant body configuration. The latter is seen often in association with congenital asplenia, which resembles bilateral right-sidedness, and congenital polysplenia, which resembles bilateral left-sidedness.[407]

Asplenia. Cardiac anomalies associated commonly with asplenia include anomalous systemic venous connection, atrial septal or complete endocardial cushion defect, common ventricle, transposition of the great arteries, severe pulmonic stenosis or atresia, and anomalous pulmonary venous connection. Polysplenia is associated commonly with absence of the hepatic portion of the inferior vena cava with azygos continuation, bilateral superior venae cavae, anomalous pulmonary venous connection, and atrial septal defect (either ostium secundum or endocardial cushion). Pulmonic stenosis and double-outlet right ventricle are each observed in approximately 25 per cent of cases. It is important to recognize these complex syndromes in order to distinguish them from forms of cyanotic heart disease that may be amenable to corrective surgical therapy. Diagnosis is suggested by a symmetrical liver shadow roentgenographically and, in asplenia, by the presence of Howell-Jolly and Heinz bodies in red blood cells demonstrated on blood smear, and it is confirmed by a negative or abnormal radioactive spleen scan.

Once the type of visceral situs is defined, it is necessary to describe the bulboventricular loop. Normally, the primitive cardiac tube bends to the right (D-loop), which brings the anatomical right ventricle to the right of the anatomical left ventricle. An L-loop brings the morphological right ventricle left-sided relative to the morphological left ventricle. The L-loop is normal in the presence of situs inversus, but in situs solitus it is synonymous with inverted ventricles.

VENTRICULAR MORPHOLOGY. The number, morphology, and size of the ventricle can be ascertained by using a variety of echocardiographic views. The morphological features of each ventricle can also be identified angiographically. The anatomical right ventricle is equipped with a tricuspid valve, is highly trabeculated, and contains the septal band of the single papillary muscle; its infundibulum lies anterior to and superiorly beyond the outlet of the left ventricle. The anatomical right ventricle generally connects with whichever of the two great arteries is the more anterior. The anatomical left ventricle is smooth-walled and contains an outlet that lies posterior to the right ventricular infundibulum; its entrance is guarded by a bicuspid mitral valve, the anterior leaflet of which is normally in continuity with elements of the semilunar valve at its outlet.

GREAT ARTERIES. The great arteries are described in terms of their positional interrelationships and their ventricular connections. Each outflow tract and semilunar valve should be examined in both long- and short-axis echocardiographic views.[406] The ventriculoarterial alignments may be determined by direct visualization from the subxiphoid window. The relation between the great arteries can best be demonstrated noninvasively using parasternal short-axis echocardiographic views, which display the semilunar roots. The aortic arch and brachiocephalic arteries are seen well using suprasternal notch views. The pulmonary artery is seen from high parasternal or suprasternal notch short-axis sections. The ventricular attachments may be normal or may form the anomalies of double-outlet right or left ventricle or transposition. The arterial interrelationships are described as D (dextro), in which the ascending aorta sweeps toward the right and lies to the right of the main pulmonary artery; L (levo), in which the ascending aorta sweeps toward the left and lies to the left of the main pulmonary artery; or A (antero), which is the rare situation in which the aorta lies directly in front of the pulmonary artery. The D, L, and A descriptions of the aorticopulmonary artery interrelationships should not be confused with the D-or L-loop designation of the ventricular interrelationships.[404]

Employing segmental sets composed of descriptive units of visceroatrial situs/ventricular loop/great artery relationships greatly simplifies expression of the type of cardiac anatomy present in cardiac malposition.[404] For example, the normal heart in a patient with situs inversus and dextrocardia is referred to as inversus/L loop/L normal; complete transposition of the great arteries in a patient with situs inversus is referred to as inversus/L loop/L transposition; functionally corrected transposition in a patient with situs solitus is referred to as solitus/L loop/L transposition; dextrocardia and functionally corrected transposition is designated solitus/D loop/D transposition with dextrocardia.

After the cardiac chambers are diagnosed functionally (arterial and venous), the positional and morphological relationships are understood, and the presence of associated anomalies has been established, the principles of medical and surgical treatment apply to these cardiac malpositions as they do to normally located hearts.

OTHER CONDITIONS

Congenital Pericardial Defects

(See also p. 1525)

Isolated pericardial defects are rare. They occur most commonly in males and are usually left-sided, although they may be right-sided, diaphragmatic, or total.[408] The anomaly is produced by deficient formation of the pleuropericardial membrane, or, if diaphragmatic, defective formation of the septum transversum. Associated congenital anomalies of the heart and lungs occur in approximately 30 per cent of cases. Most patients with the isolated defect are asymptomatic. Nonspecific anterior chest pain may be the result of torsion of the great arteries due to absence of the stabilizing forces of the left pericardium.[409]

With complete absence of the left pericardium a conspicuous apical impulse may be noted shifted leftward to the anterior or midaxillary line. Electrocardiographic changes may be related to levo-position of the heart; a leftward displacement of the QRS transition in the precordial leads and vertical or right-axis deviation are usual. The diagnosis may be suggested by chest roentgenograms.[410] With complete left pericardial absence, the heart is levo-posed, and the aortic knob, pulmonary artery, and ventricles form three prominent left heart border convexities.

A partial left pericardial defect may be suspected by varying degrees of prominence of the pulmonary artery and/or the left atrial appendage. Echocardiographic findings often mimic those observed in patients with right ventricular volume overload (enlarged right ventricle and abnormal ventricular septal motion), probably owing to the altered cardiac position and motion within the thorax.[411, 412] Other echocardiographic clues include lateral extension of the left atrial appendage as it herniates through the pericardial defect; this is best seen in short-axis views. The anomaly can be diagnosed definitively by computed tomography, magnetic resonance imaging, angiocardiography, or by inducing a left pneumothorax and observing air under the right pericardium when the patient is placed in the right lateral decubitus position.[413]

Complete absence of the left pericardium requires no treatment. However, partial defects may impose serious risks, including herniation and strangulation of the ventricles or left atrial appendage with left-sided defects, or the possibility of a superior vena cava obstructive syndrome with right-sided defects.[414] In the diaphragmatic type, cardiac compression by abdominal contents requires surgical repair.[415] Partial left or right defects may be closed with a patch of mediastinal pleura.

Single Atrium

Single or common atrium is a rare isolated defect. The anomaly consists of an absent atrial septum, usually with a cleft in the anteromedial leaflet of the mitral valve, and occasionally, with a cleft tricuspid valve as well. The lesion may be seen as one component of the Ellis–van Creveld syndrome (Table 30–2) or of the complex cardiac anomalies seen in patients with asplenia or polysplenia.

Single atrium may be suspected clinically by the presence of cardiac murmurs of an atrial septal defect and mitral regurgitation associated with mild cyanosis, roentgenographic evidence of cardiac enlargement and increased pulmonary blood flow, and electrocardiographic features of atrioventricular septal defect.[416] An absence of echoes from any part of the atrial septum is the essential feature of two-dimensional echocardiographic examination, which also may show a cleft anterior mitral leaflet, increased right ventricular end-diastolic dimension, paradoxical ventricular septal motion, and dilated, pulsatile pulmonary trunk. Angiographically, the absence of the atrial septum produces a large, globular shaped, single atrial structure. Selective left ventricular angiocardiography shows the characteristic gooseneck appearance seen in the various forms of atrioventricular septal defect. In the absence of pulmonary vascular obstructive disease surgical correction is indicated by means of a prosthetic patch.

Univentricular Atrioventricular Connection (Single Ventricle)

Hearts with univentricular atrioventricular connection comprise a family of complex lesions in which both atrioventricular valves, or a common atrioventricular valve, open into a single ventricular chamber.[417] Terminology is varied and the anomaly is often referred to as single or common ventricle, which is imprecise but useful shorthand for the entity. The definition excludes examples of tricuspid or mitral atresia. Single ventricle is almost always accompanied by abnormal great artery positional relationships; the incidence of L-malposition of the great arteries is approximately equal to that of D-malposition.[418] Associated anomalies are common and include, in particular, pulmonic valvular or subvalvular stenosis, subaortic stenosis, total or partial anomalous pulmonary venous connection, and coarctation of the aorta.

MORPHOLOGY. In approximately 80 per cent of patients the single ventricle morphologically resembles a left ventricular chamber that is separated from an infundibular outlet chamber by a bulboventricular septum.[419] The opening is variously called the bulboventricular foramen or ventricular septal defect. The infundibular chamber is considered to represent developmentally the outflow tract of the right ventricle. When the great arteries are malposed, the infundibulum lying anterior at the basal position of the single ventricle communicates with the aorta and may be in one of two positions: noninverted (D-malposition), when it is situated at the right basal aspect of the heart, or inverted (L-malposition), when it is located at the left base of the heart. In the unusual situation in which the great arteries are related normally, the infundibulum communicates with the pulmonary trunk.[418] *Double-inlet left ventricle* is a term used synonymously to describe the most frequently encountered single ventricular chamber that has the anatomical characteristics of the left ventricle. Less commonly the single ventricular chamber resembles a right ventricle (double-inlet right ventricle) or contains features suggestive of both or neither ventricle; the latter two situations have occasionally been designated common ventricle and single ventricle of the primitive type, respectively.[418]

CLINICAL FINDINGS. Depending upon the associated anomalies, the clinical presentation of single ventricle mimics other conditions in which cyanosis and decreased (or increased) pulmonary blood flow coexist, e.g., tetralogy of Fallot or tricuspid atresia in the former instance, and complete transposition of the great arteries and double-outlet right ventricle in the latter. The electrocardiogram in double-inlet left ventricle without inversion of the infundibulum (D-malposition) usually shows features of left ventricular hypertrophy. With infundibular inversion (L-malposition) the electrical forces are directed anteriorly and rightward, as they are in ventricular inversion without associated defects. In patients with the more primitive types of common or single ventricle there is a repetitious rS pattern in all the precordial electrocardiographic leads. Chest roentgenographic findings resemble those observed in patients with complete (dextro-) transposition of the great arteries or functionally corrected (levo-) transposition of the great arteries without features distinctive for single ventricle.

In those patients in whom two separate atrioventricular valves communicate with the single ventricular chamber, echocardiography suggests the correct diagnosis when echoes are visualized from the two valves without an intervening interventricular septum.[419, 420] In the absence of ventricular septal echoes when the two valves are not visualized simultaneously, they may be identified separately with a careful long-axis sweep of the ventricle. It is possible to detect the presence of a small outflow chamber anterior to the atrioventricular valves by using subxiphoid or parasternal short-axis views, and a plane orthogonal to the long-axis plane (Fig. 30–73). The single ventricle with a single atrioventricular valve is suspected when the excursion of echoes from the single valve located posteriorly in the ventricular chamber is of large amplitude. Enhanced assessment of the atrioventricular valve(s) in patients with single ventricle is provided by saline contrast echocardiography.[421] In the presence of two atrioventricular valves, a peripheral or central venous injection of saline results in a cloud of echoes that appear in the tricuspid valve orifice during ventricular diastole and anterior to the mitral valve in the same cardiac cycle. The echo cloud appears within the ventricle during diastole after

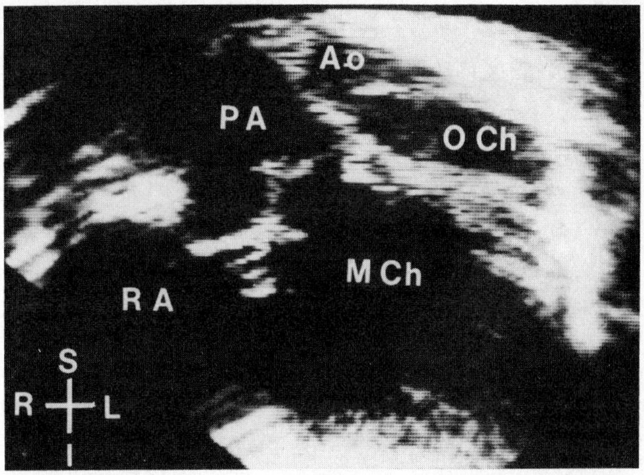

FIGURE 30–73. Single ventricle imaged in a subcostal coronal view. The pulmonary (PA) arises from a main chamber (MCh) of left ventricular type. The right atrioventricular valve is seen in part between the main chamber and the right atrium (RA). The ascending aorta (AO) arises anteriorly from a small outlet chamber (OCh). The bulboventricular foramen or ventricular septal defect is not identified in this plane. (Courtesy of Norman Silverman, M.D.)

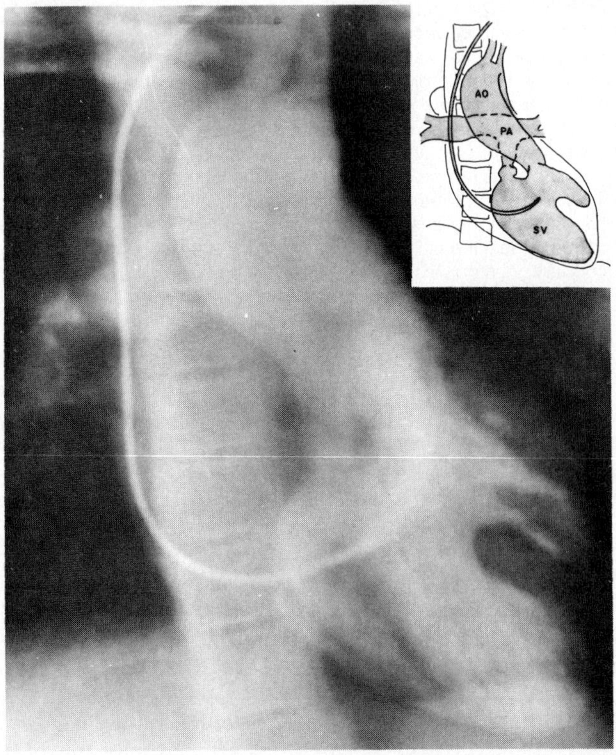

FIGURE 30–74. Selective ventriculogram in a child with single ventricle (SV). There is levo-malposition of the great arteries with the aorta (AO) communicating with a small outflow chamber. The pulmonary artery (PA) arises from a single ventricular chamber, which has the anatomical characteristics of a left ventricle. There is moderate pulmonic stenosis.

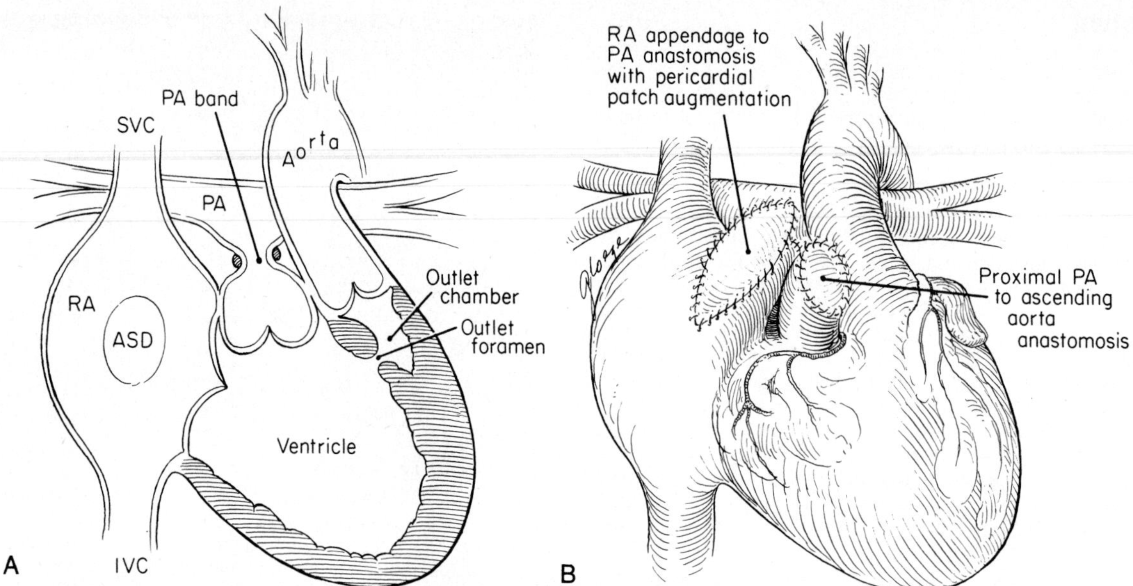

FIGURE 30–75. *A*, The preoperative anatomy of a univentricular heart of the left ventricular type with left anterior subaortic outlet chamber, ventricular arterial discordance, left atrioventricular valve atresia, atrial septal defect (ASD), and subaortic stenosis caused by a restrictive bulboventricular outlet foramen. *B*, The physiologic operative repair. The proximal pulmonary artery (PA) anastomosed to the ascending aorta (augmented by a prosthetic patch) and a modified Fontan procedure created (right atrial to the pulmonary artery anastomosis). Not shown is the interatrial baffle committing the pulmonary venous return to the right atrioventricular valve. (From Lin, A. E., et al.: Subaortic obstruction in complex heart disease. Reprinted with permission from the American College of Cardiology. J. Am. Coll. Cardiol. 7:617, 1986.)

complete opening of the mitral valve (after the mitral valve E point). In most patients with a common atrioventricular valve, the cloud of echoes enters the ventricle during ventricular diastole, from behind the echoes of the only identifiable atrioventricular valve. Occasionally, the contrast technique may identify the outflow chamber; the echo cloud appears initially in the common ventricular chamber during the rapid filling phase of ventricular diastole and arrives later in the outflow chamber during subsequent ventricular systole. Selective ventriculography is necessary to delineate with certainty the anatomical type of single ventricle and to diagnose the associated great artery interrelationships and the presence or absence of additional lesions (Fig. 30–74).

Attempts to partition the single ventricle with a Dacron or Teflon prosthetic patch have met with modest success as well as a high incidence of postoperative complete heart block.[422, 423] The septation operation is best performed in patients with double-inlet left ventricle, a rudimentary right ventricular outflow chamber which is anterior and leftward, and a discordant ventriculoarterial connection, with either absent or mild pulmonary stenosis. Creation of an atriopulmonary conduit (the Fontan procedure) and closure of the tricuspid orifice is a technique best applied to patients with severe pulmonary stenosis or previous pulmonary artery band procedure (Fig. 30–75).[318, 423] Palliative procedures designed to either increase pulmonary blood flow (systemic-pulmonary anastomosis) or limit pulmonary blood flow (pulmonary artery banding) often allow survival to adolescence in patients with a single ventricle.

VASCULAR RINGS

MORPHOLOGY. The normal development of the aortic arch system is described on page 900 (Fig. 30–5). The term *vascular ring* is employed for those aortic arch or pulmonary artery malformations that exhibit an abnormal relationship with the esophagus and trachea, causing compression, dysphagia, and/or respiratory symptoms.[424] The most common and serious vascular ring is produced by a double aortic arch in which both the right and left fourth embryonic aortic arches persist. In the most common type of double aortic arch there is a left ligamentum arteriosum or ductus arteriosus, and both arches are patent, the right being larger than the left. A right aortic arch with a left ductus or ligamentum arteriosum connecting the left pulmonary artery and the upper part of the descending aorta and with an anomalous right subclavian artery arising from the left descending aorta are additional important vascular ring arrangements.[425] The latter anomaly exists frequently in cases of tetralogy of Fallot and otherwise uncomplicated coarctation of the aorta. An unusual cause of tracheal compression is the "vascular sling" created by an anomalous left pulmonary artery that arises from a rightward, elongated pulmonary trunk and courses between the trachea and esophagus before it branches normally within the left lung.[426] This arrangement is commonly associated with other cardiac and extracardiac anomalies.

CLINICAL FINDINGS. The symptoms produced by vascular rings depend upon the tightness of anatomical constriction of the trachea and esophagus and consist principally of respiratory difficulties, cyanosis (associated especially with feeding), stridor, and dysphagia. The electrocardiogram is normal unless associated cardiovascular anomalies are present. The barium esophagogram is a useful screening procedure. Prominent posterior indentation of the esophagus is observed in the common vascular ring arrangements, although the pulmonary artery "vascular sling" produces an anterior indentation. Unusual and rare aortic arch anomalies may create rings that impinge on the trachea but do not compress the esophagus and that will not be suspected by this simple radiographic procedure but rather by bronchoscopy. CT examination is helpful in the diagnosis of this malformation (Fig. 12–14, p. 366). Selective contrast angiography is usually required to delineate the anatomy of the aorta and its branches or the course of the main pulmonary arteries. Computed axial tomography and magnetic resonance imaging offer excellent imaging alternatives.[427, 428]

MANAGEMENT. The severity of symptoms and the anatomy of the malformation are the most important factors in determining treatment. Patients, particularly infants, with respiratory obstruction require prompt surgical intervention. Operative repair of the double aortic arch requires division of the minor arch (usually the left).[429] A reported 20 to 30 per cent operative mortality is related, in part, to problems in postoperative respiratory care, especially when there is coexistent residual anatomical tracheal narrowing. Patients with a right aortic arch and a left ductus or ligamentum arteriosum require division of the ductus or ligamentum and/or ligation and division of the left subclavian artery, which is the posterior component of the ring. Operation is rarely indicated for patients with an aberrant right subclavian artery derived from a left aortic arch and left descending aorta. In patients with a pulmonary artery vascular sling, operation consists of detachment of the left pulmonary artery at its origin and anastomosis to the main pulmonary artery directly or via a conduit of its proximal end brought anterior to the trachea.[429]

CONGENITAL ARRHYTHMIAS

This classification refers to arrhythmias present in infancy, whose causes, when known, relate to a structural malformation or defect of the conduction system or to an acquired prenatal condition such as myocarditis, hypoxia, acidosis, and transplacental passage of a drug or substance from mother to fetus. In these latter examples, the substrate for the postnatal expression of the rhythm disturbance existed before birth and the arrhythmia is therefore designated "congenital." Complete heart block and supraventricular and ventricular tachycardias are the most common important congenital arrhythmias.[430] The electrophysiological and electrocardiographic features of these arrhythmias are discussed elsewhere in the text (Chaps. 22 and 23).

CONGENITAL COMPLETE HEART BLOCK

The atrioventricular node and the His bundle originate during fetal development as separate structures and later join together. Anatomical studies have shown the basic lesion in congenital complete heart block to consist of discontinuity between the atrial musculature and the AV node or the His bundle, if the AV node is absent. Occasionally, the anatomical interruption may be situated between the AV node and the main His bundle, or within the bundle itself.[431] No known etiology exists for the vast majority of cases of congenital heart block in infants who usually have otherwise anatomically normal hearts. However, fetal myocarditis, idiopathic hemorrhage and necrosis involving conduction tissue, and degeneration and fibrosis related in some instances to the transplacental passage of immune complexes from mothers with systemic lupus erythematosus are all entities capable of causing congenital heart block.[432] Less often, congenital heart block may be associated with various forms of congenital heart disease, the most common malformation being congenitally corrected transposition of the great arteries.

Detection of consistent fetal bradycardia (heart rate 40 to 80 beats/min) by auscultation, fetal echocardiography (Fig. 30–76), or electronic monitoring allows anticipation of the correct diagnosis. The newborn, especially with a ventricular rate less than 50 beats/min and atrial rate in excess of 150 beats/min, is at highest risk; the presence of an associated cardiovascular anomaly greatly lessens the chances of survival.[433] Treatment is not required for the asymptomatic infant. Digitalization is recommended for the baby in congestive heart failure, irrespective of complete heart block. Isoproterenol and other sympathomimetic drugs and atropine do not have permanent or beneficial effects. Congestive heart failure and Stokes-Adams attacks require pacemaker treatment at any age.[430, 434] Initial management of the child in whom permanent epicardial pacemaker insertion is indicated usually involves preoperative insertion of a transvenous intracardiac electrode into the right ventricle in order to protect the patient from serious arrhythmias during the induction of anesthesia.[434–436] A variety of problems may be anticipated after pacemaker implantation related to growth of the patient, which stresses the lead system; the fragility of the lead system in a physically active young patient; and the limited life span of the pulse generator. Patients with congenital complete heart block who survive infancy usually remain asymptomatic until late in childhood or adolescence.[437]

SUPRAVENTRICULAR TACHYCARDIA

Paroxysmal tachycardia of supraventricular origin may have its origin in utero or in the immediate postnatal period.[438] The most frequent arrhythmias producing symptoms are paroxysmal atrial tachycardia with or without ventricular preexcitation, atrial flutter, and junctional tachycardia. The arrhythmia may cause intrauterine cardiac failure; its detection and persistence prenatally should prompt consideration of administration of digitalis, or if that fails, of propranolol or verapamil, to the mother if amniocentesis indicates surfactant deficiency and fetal lung

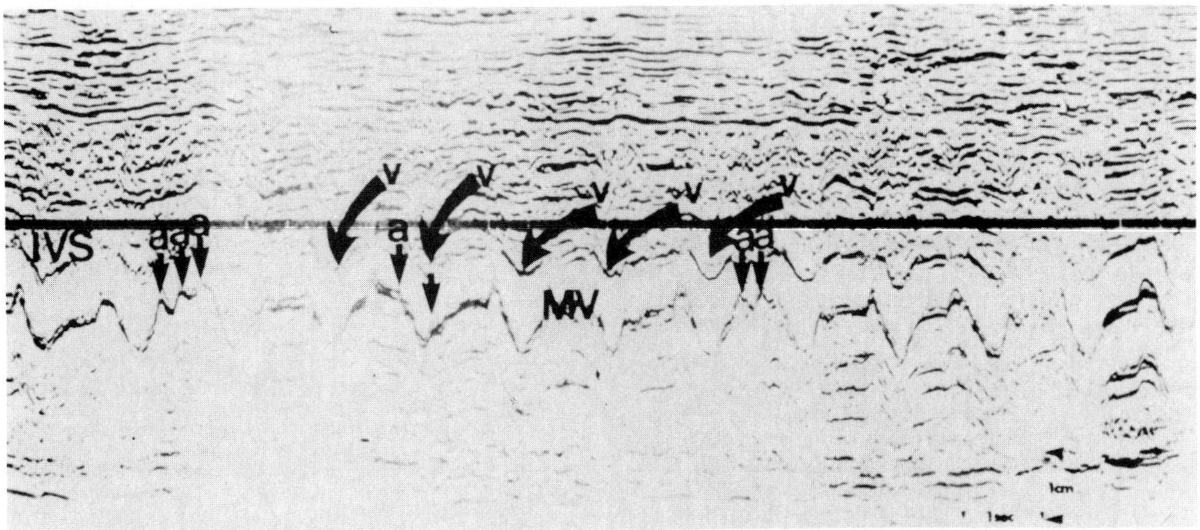

FIGURE 30–76. Fetal M-mode echocardiogram of complete heart block at 28 weeks' gestation. A slow ventricular rate of 45 to 50 beats/min is seen by the undulations (v, curved arrows) of the interventricular septum (IVS). Atrial contractions (a, straight vertical arrows) cause regular undulations of the mitral valve (MV) at a rate of 120–130/min. The atrial activity has no fixed relationship to the idioventricular rhythm. (Courtesy of Charles Kleinman, M.D.)

immaturity, since early delivery is not indicated if the baby will have hyaline membrane disease, or cesarean section or induced labor may be indicated if the fetus is close to term. No recognizable cause exists for the disorder in the vast majority of infants. The transplacental passage of long-acting thyroid-stimulating (LATS) and immune gamma 2 globulin from hyperthyroid mothers, hypoglycemia, and Ebstein's anomaly of the tricuspid valve are occasionally causative.[439] Wolff-Parkinson-White syndrome (p. 202) is present in 10 to 50 per cent of infants with supraventricular tachycardia.[440] Symptoms produced by the tachyarrhythmia after birth are subtle and often go undetected until signs of heart failure have been present for 24 to 36 hours. Conversion to normal sinus rhythm is usually accomplished by administration of digitalis, direct-current cardioversion, transesophageal atrial pacing, or eliciting a diving reflex by covering the face with an ice-cold wet washcloth for 4 to 5 seconds.[438, 441] Conversion should be followed by digitalization on a prophylactic basis. Common practice consists of digitalis treatment for 9 to 12 recurrence-free months followed by its abrupt cessation. Recurrence of tachycardia, particularly in those infants with ventricular preexcitation, is not uncommon; maintenance of normal rhythm may require the administration, alone or in combination, of digitalis, phenytoin sodium, verapamil, and propranolol.[438] The rate of recurrence falls substantially between ages 2 and 10 years, with a slight rise during adolescence. In general, the prognosis is excellent.

ELECTROPHYSIOLOGICAL STUDIES. Beyond infancy, patients whose condition is refractory to medical treatment are candidates for electrophysiological catheter evaluation, which facilitates differentiation of a causative ectopic anatomical focus within the atria from accessory conduction pathways.[440, 442] Endocardial mapping is performed to specifically localize the site of earliest activation in the atrium, or to identify multiple foci of ectopic impulses. Electrophysiological studies should include measurement of resting intervals and sinus and atrioventricular node function, including recovery times, effective refractory period, and Wenckebach conduction. Premature atrial stimulation may be used to interrupt tachycardia. Premature ventricular stimulation is employed to measure retrograde conduction and localize the site of earliest atrial activation, and to assess the effective refractory period of the accessory pathway. Coronary sinus and right atrial catheters provide localization of the site of earliest atrial activation during tachycardia, and allow measurement of the antegrade effective refractory period of the accessory pathway.

If the tachyarrhythmia is refractory to pharmacological therapy or catheter ablative techniques, it may be treated definitively with intraoperative mapping and a variety of operative maneuvers, including cryoablation, surgical division of accessory conduction pathways, subendocardial excision of the ectopic focus, and atrial disconnection.[443, 444]

ATRIAL FLUTTER. Uncommonly, atrial flutter is the cause of supraventricular tachycardia,[445] especially in the setting of newborn infants with hydrops fetalis, whose intrauterine tachyarrhythmia is an alternation between supraventricular tachycardia with Wolff-Parkinson-White syndrome and atrial flutter. Another common clinical setting for atrial flutter is the infant under age 6 months with an otherwise normal heart, who shows frequent premature atrial contractions. In infants, classic flutter waves may not be present on a surface electrocardiogram or rhythm strip; detection may require recordings of transesophageal atrial electrograms. Acute treatment with electrical conversion or overdrive pacing, either through the esophagus or with an intracardiac atrial catheter, effectively terminates the rhythm disturbance.[445, 446] If synchronized direct current electrocardioversion is employed, standby pacing should be available; if overdrive pacing is utilized the same pacing catheter can be used to pace the heart in the event of a systole. Uncommonly, chronic drug treatment with digitalis, digitalis plus quinidine, or amiodarone may be required.

Junctional automatic tachycardia is characterized by a narrow QRS complex and AV dissociation, with the ventricular rate faster than the normal atrial rate. Ventricular dysfunction and congestive heart failure occur early, and the rhythm disturbance is generally not convertible to sinus rhythm by any medical treatment.[438] Since sudden death occurs commonly, pacemaker implantation is recommended with a subsequent effort at either catheter or surgical ablation.

VENTRICULAR TACHYCARDIA. Ventricular tachycardia is defined as three or more consecutive premature ventricular contractions. The definition, however, fails to identify a high-risk group. Infants or children who meet this criterion but seldom require treatment and seem to be at little risk have no symptoms and no evidence of anatomical heart disease. Potentially serious ventricular tachycardia in the newborn is associated with Q-T prolongation, mitral valve prolapse, and Marfan syndrome. In these settings the tachycardia is potentially life-threatening and always merits treatment.[438]

The cause of long Q-T syndrome (p. 699) is unknown; proposed are regional abnormalities of ventricular repolarization on the basis of an imbalance of right and left sympathetic innervation of the heart. The two most effective treatments are beta blockade and high thoracic left sympathectomy, which reduce the incidence of syncope and sudden death without affecting the QT interval.

The treatment of ventricular tachycardia (p. 694) consists of intravenous administration of lidocaine, followed by direct current electrical cardioversion. In the absence of Q-T prolongation, but in the presence of mitral prolapse or other cardiac abnormalities, chronic treatment should be undertaken of multiform premature ventricular contractions, couplets, or ventricular tachycardia, as described on p. 699. In infants and children unresponsive to conventional or investigative antiarrhythmic drugs, surgical treatment—by either cryoablation or excision—may be life-saving.[447]

REFERENCES

GENERAL CONSIDERATIONS

1. Mitchell, S. C., Korones, S. B., and Berendes, H. W.: Congenital heart disease in 56,109 births. Incidence and natural history. Circulation *43*:323, 1971.
2. Roberts, W. C.: Anatomically isolated aortic valvular disease: The case against its being of rheumatic etiology. Am. J. Cardiol. *49*:151, 1970.
3. Warth, D. C., King, M. E., Cohen, J. M., Tesoriero, V. L., Marcus, E., and Weyman, A. E.: Prevalence of mitral valve prolapse in normal children. J. Am. Coll. Cardiol. *5*:1173, 1985.
4. Fyler, D. C.: Report of the New England regional infant cardiac program. Pediatrics *65*(Suppl.):375, 1980.
5. Fontana, R. S., and Edwards, J. E.: Congenital Cardiac Disease: A Review of 357 Cases Studied Pathologically. Philadelphia, W. B. Saunders Company, 1962.
6. Bankl, H.: Congenital malformations of the heart and great vessels: Synopsis of pathology, embryology and natural history. Baltimore-Munich, Urban and Schwarzenberg, 1977.
7. Greenwood, R. D.: Cardiovascular malformations associated with extracardiac anomalies and malformation syndromes. Clin. Pediatr. *23*:145, 1984.
8. Rose, V., Gold, R. J. M., Lindsay, G., and Allen, M.: A possible increase in the incidence of congenital heart defects among the offspring of affected parents. J. Am. Coll. Cardiol. *6*:376, 1985.
8a. Nora, J. J., and Nora, A. H.: Maternal transmission of congenital heart diseases: New recurrence risk figures and the questions of cytoplasmic inheritance and vulnerability to teratogens. Am. J. Cardiol. *59*:459, 1987.
9. de la Cruz, M. V., Munoz-Castellanos, L., and Nadal-Ginard, S.: Extrinsic factors in the genesis of congenital heart disease. Br. Heart J. *33*:203, 1971.
10. Wilson, J. G., and Warkeny, J.: Teratology: Principles and Techniques. Chicago, University of Chicago Press, 1965.
11. Ruttenberg, H. D.: Concerning the etiology of congenital cardiac disease. Am. Heart J. *84*:437, 1972.
12. Ouelette, E. M., Rossett, H. L., Rossman, M. P., and Wiener, L.: Adverse effects on offspring of maternal alcohol abuse during pregnancy. N. Engl. J. Med. *297*:528, 1977.
13. Noonan, J.: Twins, conjoined twins, and cardiac defects. Am. J. Dis. Child. *132*:17, 1978.
14. Corone, P., Bonaiti, C., Feingold, J., Fromont, S., and Berthet-Bondet, D.: Familial congenital heart disease: How are the various types related? Am. J. Cardiol. *51*:942, 1983.
15. Nora, J. J., and Nora, A. H.: The evolution of specific genetic environmental counseling in congenital heart diseases. Circulation 57:205, 1978.
16. Anderson, R. H., and Ashley, G. T.: Anatomic development of the cardiovascular system. *In* Davies, J., and Dobbing, J. (eds.): Scientific Foundations of Paediatrics. London, Heinemann, 1974, p. 165.
17. Langman, J., and van Mierop, L. H. S.: Development of the cardiovascular

system. *In* Moss, A. J., and Adams, F. H. (eds.): Heart Disease in Infants, Children and Adolescents. Baltimore, Williams and Wilkins, 1968, p. 3
18. Los, J. A.: Embryology. *In* Watson, H. (ed.): Paediatric Cardiology. London, Lloyd Luke Ltd., 1968, p. 1.
19. Rudolph, A. M.: Congenital Diseases of the Heart. Chicago, Year Book Medical Publishers, 1974.
20. Sheldon, C. A., Friedman, W. F., and Sybers, H. D.: Scanning electron microscopy of fetal and neonatal lamb cardiac cells. J. Molec. Cell. Cardiol. *8*:853, 1976.
21. McPherson, R. A., Kramer, M. F., Covell, J. W., and Friedman, W. F.: A comparison of the active stiffness of fetal and adult cardiac muscle. Pediatr. Res. *10*:660, 1976.
22. Friedman, W. F.: The intrinsic physiologic properties of the developing heart. Progr. Cardiovasc. Dis. *15*:87, 1972.
23. Ingwall, J. S., Kramer, M. F., Woodman, D., and Friedman, W. F.: Maturation of energy metabolism in the lamb: Changes in myosin ATPase and creatine kinase activities. Pediatr. Res. *15*:1128, 1981.
24. Friedman, W. F.: Physiological properties of the developing heart. Paediatric Cardiology. Vol. 6. New York, Churchill Livingstone, 1986, p. 3.
25. Geis, W. P., Tatooles, C. J., Priola, D. V., and Friedman, W. F.: Factors influencing neurohumoral control of the heart and newborn. Am. J. Physiol. *228*:1685, 1975.
26. Romero, T. E., and Friedman, W. F.: Limited left ventricular response to volume overload in the neonatal period. Pediatr. Res. *13*:910, 1979.
27. Friedman, W. F., Fitzpatrick, K. M., Merritt, T. A., and Feldman, B. H.: The patent ductus arteriosus. Clin. Perinatol. *5*:411, 1978.

PATHOLOGICAL CONSEQUENCES

28. Friedman, W. F., and George, B. L.: Medical progress—Treatment of congestive heart failure by altering loading conditions of the heart. J. Pediatr. *106*:697, 1985.
29. Friedman, W. F., and George, B. L.: Treatment of cardiac failure in infants. Compr. Ther. *12*:8, 1986.
30. Artman, M., Parrish, M. D., and Graham, T. P., Jr.: Congestive heart failure in childhood and adolescence: Recognition and management. Am. Heart J. *105*:471, 1983.
31. Sahn, D. J., and Friedman, W. F.: Difficulties in distinguishing cardiac from pulmonary disease in the neonate. Pediatr. Clin. North Am. *20*:293, 1973.
32. Stanger, P., Lucas, R. V., Jr., and Edwards, J. E.: Anatomic factors causing respiratory distress in acyanotic congenital cardiac disease: Special reference to bronchial obstruction. Pediatrics *43*:760, 1969.
33. DiSessa, T. G., and Friedman, W. F.: Echocardiographic evaluation of cardiac performance. Cardiol. Clin. *1*:487, 1983.
34. DiSessa, T. G., and Friedman, W. F.: Echocardiographic evaluation of cardiac performance. *In* Friedman, W. F., and Higgins, C. B. (eds.): Pediatric Cardiac Imaging. Philadelphia, W. B. Saunders Company, 1984, p. 219.
35. Mercier, J. C., DiSessa, T. G., Jarmakani, J., and Friedman, W. F.: Two dimensional echocardiographic assessment of left ventricular volumes and ejection fraction. Circulation *65*:962, 1982.
36. Gutgesell, H. P.: Echocardiographic assessment of cardiac function in infants and children. J. Am. Cardiol. *5*:95S, 1985.
37. Teitel, D., and Rudolph, A. M.: Perinatal oxygen delivery and cardiac function. Adv. Pediatr. *32*:321, 1985.
38. Rosenthal, A., Nathan, D. G., Marty, A. T., Button, L. N., Miettinen, O. S., and Nadas, A. S.: Acute hemodynamic effects of red cell volume reduction, polycythemia of cyanotic congenital heart disease. Circulation *42*:297, 1970.
39. Voigt, G. C., and Wright, J. R.: Cyanotic congenital heart disease and sudden death. Am. Heart J. *87*:773, 1974.
40. Fischbein, C. A., Rosenthal, A., Fischer, E. G., Nadas, A. S., and Welch, K.: Risk factors for brain abscess in patients with congenital heart disease. Am. J. Cardiol. *34*:97, 1974.
41. Shaher, R. M., and Deuchard, D. C.: Hematogenous brain abscess in cyanotic congenital heart disease. Am. J. Med. *52*:349, 1972.
42. Corrin, C.: Paradoxical embolism. Br. Heart J. *26*:549, 1964.
43. Haroutunian, L. M., and Neill, C. A.: Pulmonary complications of congenital heart disease: Hemoptysis. Am. Heart J. *84*:540, 1972.
44. Guntheroth, W. G., Morgan, B. C., and Mullens, G. L.: Physiologic studies of paroxysmal hyperpnea in cyanotic congenital heart disease. Circulation *31*:70, 1965.
45. Bonchek, L. I., Starr, A., Sunderland, C. O., and Menashe, V. D.: Natural history of tetralogy of Fallot in infancy. Circulation *48*:392, 1973.
46. Talmer, N. S.: Congestive heart failure in the infant. Pediatr. Clin. North Am. *18*:1011, 1971.
47. Rosenthal, A., and Castaneda, A. R.: Growth and development after cardiovascular surgery in infants and children. *In* Rosenthal, A., Sonnenblick, E. H., and Lesch, M. (eds.): Postoperative Congenital Heart Disease. New York, Grune and Stratton, 1975, p. 119.
48. Friedman, W. F., Heiferman, M. F., and Perloff, J. K.: Late postoperative pulmonary vascular disease—Clinical concerns. *In* Engle, M. A., and Perloff, J. K. (eds.): Congenital Heart Disease After Surgery. New York, Yorke Medical Publishers, 1983, p. 151.
49. Heath, D., and Edwards, J. E.: The pathology of hypertensive pulmonary vascular disease. Circulation *18*:533, 1958.
50. Levin, D. L., Rudolph. A. M., Heymann, M. A., and Phibbs, R. H.: Morphological development of the pulmonary vascular bed in the fetal lamb. Circulation *53*:144, 1976.
51. Rabinovitch, M., and Reid, L. M.: Quantitative structural analysis of the pulmonary vascular bed in congenital heart defects. *In* Engle, M. A. (ed.): Pediatric Cardiovascular Disease. Philadelphia, F. A. Davis, 1981, p. 149.
52. Friedman, W. F.: Proceedings of the National Heart, Lung and Blood Institute Pediatric Cardiology Workshop: Pulmonary Hypertension. Pediatr. Res. *20*:8, 1986.
53. Rabinovitch, M., Keane, J. F., Fellows, K. E., Castaneda, A. R., and Reid, L.: Quantitative analysis of the pulmonary wedge angiogram in congenital heart defects. Circulation *63*:152, 1981.
54. Rabinovitch, M., Castaneda, A. R., and Reid, L.: Lung biopsy with frozen section as a diagnostic aid in patients with congenital heart defects. Am. J. Cardiol. *47*:77, 1981.
55. Van Hare, G. F., Ben-Shachar, G., Liebman, J., Boxerbaum, B., and Riemenschneider, T. A.: Infective endocarditis in infants and children during the past 10 years: A decade of change. Am. Heart J. *107*:1235, 1984.
56. Dajani, A. S.: Prevention of bacterial endocarditis. Pediatr. Infect. Dis. *4*:349, 1985.

APPROACH TO THE HIGH-RISK INFANT

57. Driscoll, D. J., and Edwards, W. D.: Sudden unexpected death in children and adolescents. J. Am. Coll. Cardiol. *5*:118B, 1985.
58. Friedman, W. F., and George, B. L.: New concepts and drugs in the treatment of congestive heart failure. Pediatr. Clin. North Am. *31*:1197, 1984.
59. Park, M. K.: Use of digoxin in infants and children, with specific emphasis on dosage. J. Pediatr. *108*:871, 1986.
60. Freed, M. D., Hegmann, M. A., Lewis, A. B., Roehl, S. L., and Kensey, R. C.: Prostaglandin E_1 in infants with ductus arteriosus dependent congenital heart disease. Circulation *64*:899, 1981.
61. Lewis, A. B., Freed, M. D., Hegmann, M. A., Roehl, S. L., and Kensey, R. C.: Side effects of therapy with prostaglandin E_1 in infants with critical congenital heart disease. Circulation *64*:893, 1981.
62. Friedman, W. F., Kurlinski, J., Jacob, J., DiSessa, T. G., Gluck, L., Merritt, T. A., and Feldman, B. H.: Inhibition of prostaglandin and prostacyclin synthesis in clinical management of PDA. Semin. Perinatol. *4*:125, 1980.
63. Friedman, W. F.: Patent ductus arteriosus in respiratory distress syndrome. Pediatr. Cardiol. *4*(Suppl 2):3, 1983.
64. Kleinman, C. S., and Donnerstein, R. L.: Ultrasonic assessment of cardiac function in the intact human fetus. J. Am. Coll. Cardiol. *5*:84S, 1985.
65. Silverman, N. H., Kleinman, C. S., Rudolph, A. M., Copel, J. A., Weinstein, E. M., Enderlein, B. S., and Golbus, M.: Fetal atrioventricular valve insufficiency associated with nonimmune hydrops: A two-dimensional echocardiographic and pulsed Doppler ultrasound study. Circulation *72*:825, 1985.
66. Kleinman, C. S., Donnerstein, R. L., Talner, N. S., and Hobbins, J. C.: Fetal echocardiography for evaluation of in utero congestive heart failure. N. Engl. J. Med. *306*:568, 1982.
67. Goldberg, S. J.: A review of pediatric Doppler echocardiography. Am. J. Dis. Child. *138*:1003, 1984.
68. Stanger, P., Heymann, M. A., Tarnoff, H., Hoffman, J. I. E., and Rudolph, A. M.: Complications of cardiac catheterization of neonates, infants and children. Circulation *50*:595, 1974.
69. Rashkind, W. J., Tait, M. A. S., and Gibson, R. J., Jr.: Interventional cardiac catheterization in congenital heart disease. Int. J. Cardiol. *7*:1, 1985.
70. Lock, J. E., Keane, J. F., and Fellows, K. E.: The use of catheter intervention procedures for congenital heart disease. J. Am. Coll. Cardiol. *7*:1420, 1986.
70a. Rashkind, W. J., Mullins, C. E., Hellenbrand, W. E., and Tait, M. A.: Nonsurgical closure of patent ductus arteriosus: Clinical application of the Rashkind PDA occluder system. Circulation *75*:583, 1987.
70b. Kugler, J. D., Bansal, A. M., Cheatham, J. P., Pinsky, W. W., Mooring, P. K., and Hofschire, P. J.: Drug-electrophysiology studies in infants, children and adolescents. Am. Heart J. *110*:144, 1985.

SPECIFIC CARDIAC DEFECTS

71. Hunt, C. E., and Lucas, R. V., Jr.: Symptomatic atrial septal defect in infancy. Circulation *42*:1042, 1973.
72. Davea, J. E., Cheitlin, M. D., and Bedynek, J. L.: Sinus venosus atrial septal defect. Am. Heart J. *85*:177, 1973.
73. Leachman, R. D., Cokkinos, D. V., and Cooley, D. A.: Association of ostium secundum atrial septal defects with mitral valve prolapse. Am. J. Cardiol. *38*:167, 1976.
74. Levin, A. R., Spach, M. S., Boineau, J. P., Canent, R. V., Jr., Capp, M. P., and Jewett, P. H.: Atrial pressure flow dynamics and atrial septal defects (secundum type). Circulation *37*:476, 1968.
75. O'Toole, J. D., Reddy, I., Curtiss, E. I., and Shaver, J. A.: The mechanism of splitting of the second heart sound in atrial septal defect. Circulation *41*:1047, 1977.
76. Clark, E. B., and Kugler, J. D.: Preoperative secundum atrial septal defect with coexisting sinus node and atrioventricular node dysfunction. Circulation *65*:976, 1982.
77. Shub, C., Tajik, A. J., Seward, J. B., Hagler, D. J., and Danielson, G. K.: Surgical repair of uncomplicated atrial septal defect without "routine" preoperative cardiac catheterization. J. Am. Coll. Cardiol. *6*:49, 1985.
78. Freed, M. D., Nadas, A. S., Norwood, W. I., and Castaneda, A. R.: Is routine preoperative cardiac catheterization necessary before repair of secundum and sinus venosus atrial septal defects? J. Am. Coll. Cardiol. *4*:333, 1984.
79. Suzuki, Y., Kambara, H., Kadota, K., Tamaki, S., Yamazato, A., Nohara, R., Osakada, G., Kawai, C., Kubo, S., and Karaguchi, T.: Detection of intracardiac shunt flow in atrial septal defect using a real-time two-dimensional color-coded Doppler flow imaging system and comparison with contrast two-dimensional echocardiography. Am. J. Cardiol. *56*:347, 1985.
80. Taketa, R. M., Sahn, D. J., Simon, A. L., Pappelbaum, S. J., and Friedman, W. F.: Catheter positions in congenital cardiac malformations. Circulation *51*:749, 1975.

81. Levin, A. R., Liebson, P. R., Ehlers, K. H., and Daimant, B.: Assessment of left ventricular function in atrial septal defect. Pediatr. Res. 9:894, 1975.
82. Epstein, S. E., Beiser, G. D., Goldstein, R. E., Rosing, D. R., Redwood, D. R., and Morrow, A. G.: Hemodynamic abnormalities in response to mild and intense upright exercise following operative correction of an atrial septal defect or tetralogy of Fallot. Circulation *42*:1065, 1973.
83. Karpawich, P. P., Antillon, J. R., Cappola, P. R., and Agarwal, K. C.: Pre- and postoperative electrophysiologic assessment of children with secundum atrial septal defect. Am. J. Cardiol. *55*:519, 1985.
84. Borkon, A. M., Pieroni, D. R., Varghese, P. J., Ho, C. S., and Rowe, R. D.: The superior QRS axis in ostium primum ASD. Am. Heart J. 92:15, 1975.
85. Goodman, D. J., Harrison, D. C., and Cannom, D. S.: Atrioventricular conduction in patients with incomplete endocardial cushion defect. Circulation *49*:630, 1974.
86. Jacobsen, J. R., Gillette, P. C., Corbett, B. N., Rabinovitch, M., and McNamara, D. G.: Intracardiac electrography in endocardial cushion defects. Circulation *54*:599, 1976.
87. Waldo, A. L., Kaiser, G. A., Bowman, F. O., Jr., and Malm, J. R.: Etiology of prolongation of the PR interval in patients with an endocardial cushion defect. Circulation *43*:19, 1973.
88. Bierman, F. Z., and Williams, R. G.: Subxyphoid two-dimensional imaging of the interatrial septum in infants and neonates with congenital heart disease. Circulation *60*:80, 1979.
89. Lange, L. W., Sahn, D. J., Allen, H. D., and Goldberg, S. J.: Subxyphoid cross-sectional echocardiography in infants and children with congenital heart disease. Circulation *59*:513, 1979.
90. Smallhorn, J. F., Tommasini, G., and Anderson, R. H.: Assessment of atrioventricular septal defects by two-dimensional echocardiography. Br. Heart J. *47*:109, 1982.
91. Elliott, L. P., Bargeron, L. M., Jr., and Green, C. E.: Angled angiography: General approach and findings. *In* Friedman, W. F., and Higgins, C. B. (eds.): Pediatric Cardiac Imaging. Philadelphia, W. B. Saunders Company, 1984, p. 1.
92. Castaneda, A. R., Mayer, J. E., and Jonas, R. A.: Repair of complete atrioventricular canal in infancy. World J. Surg. *9*:590, 1985.
93. Santos, A., Boucek, M., Ruttenberg, H., Veasy, G., Orsmond, G., and McGough, E.: Repair of atrioventricular septal defects in infancy. J. Thorac. Cardiovasc. Surg. *91*:505, 1986.
93a. Clapp, S. K., Perry, B. L., Farooki, Z. Q., Jackson, W. L., Karpawich, P. P., Hakimi, M., Arciniegas, E., and Green, E. W.: Surgical and medical results of complete atrioventricular canal: A ten-year review. Am. J. Cardiol. *59*:454, 1987.
94. Beerman, L. B., Park, S. C., Fischer, D. R., Fricker, F. J., Mathews, R. A., Neches, W. H., Lenox, C. C., and Zuberbuhler, J. R.: Ventricular septal defect associated with aneurysm of the membranous septum. J. Am. Coll. Cardiol. *5*:118, 1985.
95. Ortiz, E., Robinson, P. J., Deanfield, J. E., Franklin, R., Macartney, F. J., and Wyse, R. K. H.: Localisation of ventricular septal defects by simultaneous display of superimposed colour Doppler and cross sectional echocardiographic images. Br. Heart J. *54*:53, 1985.
96. Hagler, D. J., Edwards, W. D., Seward, J. B., and Tajik, A. J.: Standardized nomenclature of the ventricular septum and ventricular septal defects, with applications for two-dimensional echocardiography. Mayo Clin. Proc. *60*:741, 1985.
97. Murphy, D. J., Ludomirsky, A., and Huhta, J. C.: Continuous-wave Doppler in children with ventricular septal defect: Noninvasive estimation of interventricular pressure gradient. Am. J. Cardiol. *57*:428, 1986.
98. Friedman, W. F., Mehrizi, A., and Pusch, A. L.: Multiple muscular ventricular septal defects. Circulation *32*:35, 1964.
99. Dickinson, D. F., Arnold, R., and Wilkinson, J. L.: Ventricular septal defects in children born in Liverpool. Evaluation of natural course and surgical implications in an unselected population. Br. Heart J. *46*:47, 1981.
100. Weidman, W. H., Blount, S. G., Jr., DuShane, J. W., Gersony, W. M., Hayes, C. J., and Nadas, A. S.: Clinical course in ventricular septal defect. Natural history study. Circulation *56*(Suppl.):I-56, 1977.
101. Lister, G., Hellenbrand, W. E., Kleinman, C. S., and Talner, N. S.: Physiologic effects of increasing hemoglobin concentration in left to right shunting in infants with ventricular septal defects. N. Engl. J. Med. *306*:502, 1982.
102. Beekman, R. H., Rocchini, A. P., and Rosenthal, A.: Hemodynamic effects of hydralazine in infants with a large ventricular septal defect. Circulation *65*:523, 1982.
103. Ramaciotti, C., Keren, A., and Silverman, N. H.: Importance of (perimembranous) ventricular septal aneurysm in the natural history of isolated perimembranous ventricular septal defect. Am. J. Cardiol. *57*:268, 1986.
104. Friedman, W. F., and Pitlick, P. T.: Ventricular septal defect in infancy—University of California, San Diego (Specialty Conference). West. J. Med. *120*:295, 1974.
105. Alpert, B. S., Cook, D. H., Varghese, P. J., and Rowe, R. D.: Spontaneous closure of small ventricular septal defects: A ten-year follow-up. Pediatrics *63*:204, 1979.
106. Blumenthal, S., Griffiths, S. P., and Morgan, B. C.: Bacterial endocarditis in children with heart disease. (A review based on the literature and experience with 58 cases.) Pediatrics *26*:993, 1960.
107. Yeager, S. B., Freed, M. D., Keane, J. F., Norwood, W. I., and Castaneda, A. R.: Primary surgical closure of ventricular septal defect in the first year of life: results in 128 infants. J. Am. Coll. Cardiol. *3*:1269, 1984.
108. Friedli, B., Kidd, B. S. L., Mustard, W. T., and Keith, J. D.: Ventricular septal defect with increased pulmonary vascular resistance. Am. J. Cardiol. *22*:403, 1974.
109. Hislop, A., Haworth, S. G., Shinebourne, E. A., and Reid, L.: Quantitative structural analysis of pulmonary vessels in isolated ventricular septal defect in infancy. Br. Heart J. *37*:1014, 1975.
110. DuShane, J. W., and Kirklin, J. W.: Late results of the repair of ventricular septal defect on pulmonary vascular disease. *In* Kirklin, J. W. (ed.): Advances in Cardiovascular Surgery. New York, Grune and Stratton, 1973, p. 9.
111. Kawashima, Y., Danno, M., Shimizu, Y., Matsuda, H., Miyamoto, T., Fugita, T., Kozuka, T., and Manabe, H.: Ventricular septal defects associated with aortic insufficiency. Anatomic classification and method of operation. Circulation *47*:1057, 1973.
112. Keane, J. F., Plauth, W. H., Jr., and Nadas, A. S.: Ventricular septal defect with aortic regurgitation. Natural history study. Circulation *56*(Suppl.):I-72, 1977.
113. Gersony, W. M., and Hayes, C. J.: Bacterial endocarditis in patients with pulmonary stenosis, aortic stenosis, or ventricular septal defect. Natural history study. Circulation *56*(Suppl.):I-84, 1977.
114. deLeval, M.: Ventricular septal defects. *In* Stark, J., and deLeval, M. (eds.): Surgery for Congenital Heart Defects. New York, Grune and Stratton, Inc., 1983, p. 271.
115. Godman, M. J., Roberts, N. K., and Izukawa, T.: Late postoperative conduction disturbances after repair of ventricular septal defect in tetralogy of Fallot. Circulation *49*:214, 1974.
116. Okarama, E. O., Guller, B., Molony, J. D., and Weidman, W. H.: Etiology of right bundle-branch block pattern after surgical closure of ventricular-septal defects. Am. Heart J. *90*:14, 1975.
117. Otterstad, J. E., Simonsen, S., and Erikssen, J.: Hemodynamic findings at rest and during mild supine exercise in adults with isolated uncomplicated ventricular septal defects. Circulation *71*:650, 1985.
118. Maron, B. J., Redwood, D. R., Hirschfield, J. W., Jr., Goldstein, R. E., Morrow, A. G., and Ebstein, S. E.: Postoperative assessment of patients with ventricular septal defect and pulmonary hypertension. Response to intense upright exercise. Circulation *48*:864, 1973.
119. Graham, T. P., Jr., Atwood, G. F., Boucek, R. J., Jr., Cordell, D., and Boerth, R. C.: Right ventricular volume characteristics in ventricular septal defect. Circulation *54*:800, 1976.
120. Heymann, M. A., and Rudolph, A. M.: Control of the ductus arteriosus. Physiol. Rev. *55*:62, 1975.
121. Friedman, W. F., Printz, M. P., Kirkpatrick, S. E., and Hoskins, E. J.: The vasoactivity of the fetal lamb ductus arteriosus studied in utero. Pediatr. Res. *17*:331, 1983.
122. Skidgel, R. A., Friedman, W. F., and Printz, M. P.: Prostaglandin biosynthetic activities of the fetal lamb ductus arteriosus, other blood vessels and fetal lung. Pediatr. Res. *18*:12, 1984.
123. Printz, M. P., Skidgel, R. A., and Friedman, W. F.: Studies of pulmonary prostaglandin biosynthetic and catabolic enzymes as factors in ductus arteriosus patency and closure: Evidence for a shift in products with gestational age. Pediatr. Res. *18*:19, 1984.
124. Gittenberger-DeGroot, A. C.: Persistent ductus arteriosus: Most probably a primary congenital malformation. Br. Heart J. *39*:610, 1977.
125. Sahn, D. J., Vaucher, Y., Williams, D. E., Allen, H. D., Goldberg, S. E., and Friedman, W. F.: Echocardiographic detection of large left to right shunts and cardiomyopathies in infants and children. Am. J. Cardiol. *38*:73, 1976.
126. Vick, G. W., III, Huhta, J. C., and Gutgesell, H. P.: Assessment of the ductus arteriosus in preterm infants utilizing suprasternal two-dimensional/Doppler echocardiography. J. Am. Coll. Cardiol. *5*:973, 1985.
127. Friedman, W. F., Hirschklau, M. J., Printz, M. P. Pitlick, P. T., and Kirkpatrick, S. E.: Pharmacologic closure of patent ductus arteriosus in the premature infant. N. Engl. J. Med. *295*:526, 1976.
128. Jacob, J., Gluck, L., DiSessa, T. G., Kulovich, M., Kurlinski, J., Merritt, T., and Friedman, W. F.: The contribution of PDA in the neonate with severe RDS. J. Pediatr. *96*:79, 1980.
129. Merritt, T. A., Harris, J. P., and Roghmann, K.: Early closure of the patent ductus arteriosus in very low birth weight infants: A controlled trial. J. Pediatr. *99*:281, 1981.
130. Gersony, W. M., Peckham, G. J., Ellison, R. C., Miettinen, O. S., and Nadas, A. S.: Effects of indomethacin in premature infants with patent ductus arteriosus: Results of a national collaborative study. J. Pediatr. *102*:895, 1983.
131. Reller, M. D., Lorenz, J. M., Kotagal, U. R., Meyer, R. A., and Kaplan, S.: Hemodynamically significant PDA: An echocardiographic and clinical assessment of incidence, natural history, and outcome in very low birth weight infants maintained in negative fluid balance. Pediatr. Cardiol. *6*:17, 1985.
132. Wagner, H. R., Ellison, R. C., Zierler, S., Lang, P., Purohit, D. M., Behrendt, D., and Waldhausen, J. A.: Surgical closure of patent ductus arteriosus in 268 preterm infants. J. Thorac. Cardiovasc. Surg. *87*:870, 1984.
133. Jarmakani, M. M., Graham, T. P., Jr., Canent, R. V., Jr., Spach, M. S., and Capp, M. P.: Effect of site of shunt on left heart volume characteristics in children with ventricular septal defect and patent ductus arteriosus. Circulation *40*:411, 1969.
134. Bessenger, F. B., Jr., Blieden, L. C., and Edwards, J. E.: Hypertensive pulmonary vascular disease associated with patent ductus arteriosus. Circulation *52*:157, 1975.
134a. Kutsche, L. M., and Van Mierop, L. H. S.: Anatomy and pathogenesis of aorticopulmonary septal defect. Am. J. Cardiol. *59*:443, 1987.
135. Neufeld, H. N., Lesser, R. G., Adams, P., Jr., Anderson, R. C., Lillehiei, C. W., and Edwards, J. E.: Aorticopulmonary septal defect. Am. J. Cardiol. *9*:12, 1962.
136. Parker, B. M., Burford, T. H., Carlsson, E. C., and Buchner, E. F.: The diagnosis of aortico-pulmonary septal defect. Am. Heart J. *65*:534, 1963.
137. Stark, J.: Aorto-pulmonary window. *In* Stark, J., and deLeval, M. (eds.): Surgery for Congenital Heart Defects. New York, Grune and Stratton, Inc., 1953, p. 483.
138. Van Praagh, R.: Classification of truncus arteriosus communis. Am. Heart J. *92*:129, 1976.

139. Crupi, G., Macartney, F. J., and Anderson, R. H.: Persistent truncus arteriosus: A study of 66 autopsy cases with special reference to definition and morphogenesis. Am. J. Cardiol. *40*:569, 1977.
140. Shrivastava, F., and Edwards, J. E.: Coronary arterial origin and persistent truncus arteriosus. Circulation *55*:551, 1977.
141. Calder, L., Van Praagh, R., Sears, W. P., Corwin, R., Levy, A., Keith, J. D., and Paul, M. H.: Truncus arteriosus communis. Am. Heart J. *92*:23, 1976.
142. Juaneda, E., and Haworth, S. G.: Pulmonary vascular disease in children with truncus arteriosus. Am. J. Cardiol. *54*:1314, 1984.
143. Gelband, H., Van Meter, S., and Gersony, W. M.: Truncal valve abnormalities in infants with persistent truncus arteriosus. Circulation *45*:397, 1972.
144. Di Donato, R. M., Fyfe, D. A., Puga, F. J., Danielson, G. K., Ritter, D. G., Edwards, W. D., and McGoon, D. C.: Fifteen-year experience with surgical repair of truncus arteriosus. J. Thorac. Cardiovasc. Surg. *89*:414, 1985.
145. deLeval, M.: Persistent truncus arteriosus. *In* Stark, J., and deLeval, M. (eds.): Surgery for Congenital Heart Defects. New York, Grune and Stratton, Inc., 1983, p. 417.
146. Morgan, J. R., Forker, A. D., O'Sullivan, M. J., and Fosburg, R. G.: Coronary arterial fistulas. Am. J. Cardiol. *34*:32, 1972.
147. Liberthson, R. R., Sagar, K., Berkoben, J. P., Weintraub, R. M., and Levine, F. H.: Congenital coronary arteriovenous fistula. Circulation *59*:849, 1979.
148. Cooper, M. J., Bernstein, D., and Silverman, N. H.: Recognition of left coronary artery fistula to the left and right ventricles by contrast echocardiography. J. Am. Coll. Cardiol. *6*:923, 1985.
149. Miyatake, K., Okamoto, M., Kinoshita, N., Fusejima, K., Sakakibara, H., and Nimura, Y.: Doppler echocardiographic features of coronary arteriovenous fistula. Complementary roles of cross sectional echocardiography and the Doppler technique. Br. Heart J. *51*:508, 1984.
150. Ruttenhouse, E. A., Doty, D. B., and Ehrenhaft, J. L.: Congenital coronary artery-cardiac chamber fistula. Review of operative management. Ann. Thorac. Surg. *20*:468, 1975.
151. Midgley, F. M, Watson, D. C., Jr., Scott, L. P., III, Kuehl, K. S., Perry, L. W., Galioto, F. M., Jr., Ruckman, R. N., and Shapiro, S. R.: Repair of anomalous origin of the left coronary artery in the infant and small child. J. Am. Coll. Cardiol. *4*:1231, 1984.
152. Stephenson, L. W., Edmunds, L. H., Jr., Friedman, S., Meijboon, E., Gewitz, M., and Weinberg, P.: Subclavian-left coronary artery anastomosis for anomalous origin of the left coronary artery from the pulmonary artery. Circulation *64* (Suppl. 2):130, 1981.
153. Boutefeu, J. M., Morat, P. R., Hahn, C., and Hauf, E.: Aneurysms of the sinus of Valsalva. Report of seven cases in review of the literature. Am. J. Med. *65*:18, 1978.
154. Drummer, E. M., Moodie, D. S., Hobbs, R. E., and Fitzgerald, R.: Aneurysm of the aortic sinuses of Valsalva: Hemodynamics and long-term prognosis after surgery. Vasc. Surg. *18*:273, 1984.
155. Engle, P. J., Held, J. S., Bel-Kahn, J. V. D., and Spitz, H.: Echocardiographic diagnosis of congenital sinus of Valsalva aneurysm. Circulation *63*:705, 1981.
156. Smyth, P. T., and Edwards, J. E.: Pseudocoarctation, kinking or buckling of the aorta. Circulation *46*:1027, 1972.
157. Hutchins, G. M.: Coarctation of the aorta explained as a branch point of the ductus arteriosus. Am. J. Pathol. *63*:203, 1971.
158. Talner, N. S., and Berman, M. A.: Postnatal development of obstruction in coarctation of the aorta: Role of the ductus arteriosus. Pediatrics *56*:562, 1975.
159. Heymann, M. A., Berman, W., Jr., Rudolph, A. M., and Whitman, V.: Dilatation of the ductus arteriosus by prostaglandin E_1 in aortic arch abnormalities. Circulation *59*:169, 1979.
160. Goldman, S., Hernandez, J., and Pappas, G.: Results of surgical treatment of coarctation of the aorta in the critically ill neonate. J. Thorac. Cardiovasc. Surg. *91*:732, 1986.
161. Kopf, G. S., Hellenbrand, W., Kleinman, C., Lister, G., Talner, N., and Laks, H.: Repair of aortic coarctation in the first three months of life: Immediate and long-term results. Ann. Thorac. Surg. *41*:425, 1986.
162. Shaddy, R. E., Snider, A. R., Silverman, N. H., and Lutin, W.: Pulsed Doppler findings in patients with coarctation of the aorta. Circulation *73*:82, 1986.
163. Godwin, G. D., Herfkens, R. L., Brundage, D. H., and Lipton, N. J.: Evaluation of coarctation of the aorta by computed tomography. J. Comput. Assist. Tomogr. *5*:153, 1981.
164. Beekman, R. H., Rocchini, A. P., Behrendt, D. M., and Rosenthal, A.: Reoperation for coarctation of the aorta. Am. J. Cardiol. *48*:1108, 1981.
165. Igler, F. O., Boerboom, L. E., Werner, P. H., Donegan, J. H., and Kampine, J. P.: Coarctation of the aorta and narrow receptor resetting. Circulation Res. *48*:365, 1981.
166. Gidding, S. S., Rocchini, A. P., Beekman, R., Szpunar, C. A., Moorehead, C., Behrendt, D., and Rosenthal, A.: Therapeutic effect of propranolol on paradoxical hypertension after repair of coarctation of the aorta. N. Engl. J. Med. *312*:1224, 1985.
167. Gidding, S. S., Rocchini, A. P., Moorehead, C., Schork, M. A., Rosenthal, A.: Increased forearm vascular reactivity in patients with hypertension after repair of coarctation. Circulation *71*:495, 1985.
168. Johnson, R. G., Williams, G. R., Razook, J. D., Thompson, W. M., Lane, M. M., and Elkins, R. C.: Reoperation in congenital aortic stenosis. Ann. Thorac. Surg. *40*:156, 1985.
168a. Isner, J. M., Donaldson, R. F., Fulton, D., Bhan, I., Payne, D. D., and Cleveland, R. J.: Cystic medial necrosis in coarctation of the aorta: A potential factor contributing to adverse consequences observed after percutaneous balloon angioplasty of coarctation sites. Circulation *75*:689, 1987.
169. Hess, J., Mooyaart, E. L., Busch, H. J., Bergstra, A., and Landsman, M. L. J.: Percutaneous transluminal balloon angioplasty in restenosis of coarctation of the aorta. Br. Heart J. *55*:459, 1986.
170. Maron, B. J., Humphries, J., Rowe, R. D., and Mellits, E. D.: Prognosis of surgically corrected coarctation of the aorta. Circulation *47*:119, 1973.
171. Freed, M. D., Rocchini, A., Rosenthal, A., Nadas, A. S., and Castaneda, A. R.: Exercise-induced hypertension after surgical repair of coarctation of the aorta. Am. J. Cardiol. *43*:253, 1979.
172. Van Woezik, E. V. M., Kline, H. W., and Krediet, P.: Normal internal calibers of ostia, great arteries and aortic isthmus in children. Br. Heart J. *39*:860, 1977.
173. Bharati, S., and Lev, M.: The surgical anatomy of the heart in tubular hypoplasia of the transverse aorta (preductal coarctation). J. Thorac. Cardiovasc. Surg. *91*:79, 1986.
174. Graham, T. P., Jr., Atwood, G. F., Boerth, R. C., Boucek, R. J., Jr., and Smith, C. W.: Right and left heart size and function in infants with symptomatic coarctation. Circulation *56*:641, 1977.
175. Hammon, J. W., Jr., Merrill, W. H., Prager, R. L., Graham, T. P., Jr., and Bender, H. W., Jr.: Repair of interrupted aortic arch and associated malformations in infancy: Indications for complete or partial repair. Ann. Thorac. Surg. *42*:17, 1986.
176. Norwood, W. I., Lang, P., Castaneda, A. R., and Hougen, T. J.: Reparative operations for interrupted aortic arch with ventricular septal defect. J. Thorac. Cardiovasc. Surg. *86*:832, 1983.
177. Dekker, A. O., Gittenberger-de-Groot, A. C., and Roozendaal, H.: The ductus arteriosus and associated cardiac anomalies in interruption of the aortic arch. Pediatr. Cardiol. *2*:185, 1982.
178. Friedman, W. F., and Benson, L. B.: Congenital aortic stenosiis. *In* Adams, F. H., and Emmanouilides, G. C. (eds.): Moss' Heart Disease in Infants, Children and Adolescents. 3rd ed. Baltimore, Williams and Wilkins, 1983.
179. Donner, R., Carabello, B. A., Black, I., and Spann, J. F.: Left ventricular wall stress in compensated aortic stenosis in children. Am. J. Cardiol. *51*:946, 1983.
180. Friedman, W. F., and Pappelbaum, S. J.: Indications for hemodynamic evaluation and surgery in congenital aortic stenosis. Pediatr. Clin. North Am. *18*:1207, 1971.
181. Kveselis, D. A., Rocchini, A. P., Rosenthal, A., Crowley, D. C., Dick, M., Snider, A. R., and Moorhead, C.: Hemodynamic determinants of exercise-induced ST-segment depression in children with valvar aortic stenosis. Am. J. Cardiol. *55*:1133, 1985.
182. Lewis, A. L., Heymann, M. A., Stanger, P., Hoffman, J. I. E., and Rudolph, A. M.: Evaluation of subendocardial ischemia in valvar aortic stenosis in children. Circulation *49*:978, 1974.
183. Lakier, J. B., Lewis, A. B., Heymann, M. A., Stanger, P., Hoffman, J. I. E., and Rudolph, A. M.: Isolated aortic stenosis of the neonate: Natural history and hemodynamic considerations. Circulation *50*:801, 1974.
184. Sink, J. D., Smallhorn, J. F., Macartney, F. J., Taylor, J. F. N., Stark, J., and De Leval, M. R.: Management of critical aortic stenosis in infancy. J. Thorac. Cardiovasc. Surg. *87*:82, 1984.
185. Broderick, T. W., Higgins, C. B., and Friedman, W. F.: Critical aortic stenosis in neonates. Radiology *129*:393, 1978.
185a. Huhta, J. C., Carpenter, R. J., Jr., Moise, K. J., Jr., Deter, R. L., Ott, D. A., and McNamara, D. G.: Prenatal diagnosis and postnatal management of critical aortic stenosis. Circulation *75*:573, 1987.
186. Skjaerpe, T., Hegrenaes, L., and Hatle, L.: Noninvasive estimation of valve area in patients with aortic stenosis by Doppler ultrasound and two-dimensional echocardiography. Circulation *72*:810, 1985.
187. Ohlsson, J., and Wranne, B.: Noninvasive assessment of valve area in patients with aortic stenosis. J. Am. Coll. Cardiol. *7*:501, 1986.
188. Robinson, P. J., Wyse, R. K. H., Deanfield, J. E., Franklin, R., and Macartney, F. J.: Continuous wave Doppler velocimetry as an adjunct to cross sectional echocardiography in the diagnosis of critical left heart obstruction in neonates. Br. Heart J. *52*:552, 1984.
189. Zoghbi, W. A., Farmer, K. L., Soto, J. G., Nelson, J. G., and Quinones, M. A.: Accurate noninvasive quantification of stenotic aortic valve area by Doppler echocardiography. Circulation *73*:452, 1986.
190. Smith, M. D., Dawson, P. L., Elion, J. L., Wisenbaugh, T., Kwan, O. L., Handshoe, S., and DeMaria, A. N.: Systematic correlation of continuous-wave Doppler and hemodynamic measurements in patients with aortic stenosis. Am. Heart J. *111*:245, 1986.
191. Edmunds, L. H., Jr., Wagner, H. R., and Heymann, M. A.: Aortic valvulotomy in neonates. Circulation *61*:421, 1980.
192. Braunwald, E., Goldblatt, A., Aygen, M. M., Rockoff, S. D., and Morrow, A. G.: Congenital aortic stenosis. I. Clinical and hemodynamic findings in 100 patients. Circulation *27*:426, 1963.
193. Johnson, A. M.: Aortic stenosis, sudden death, and the left ventricular baroreceptors. Br. Heart J. *33*:1, 1971.
194. Wagner, H. R., Weidman, W. H., Ellison, R. C., and Miettinen, O. S.: Indirect assessment of severity in aortic stenosis. Natural history study. Circulation *56* (Suppl.):I–20, 1977.
195. Hagan, A. D., DiSessa, T. G., and Friedman, W. F.: Reliability of echocardiography in diagnosing and quantitating valvular aortic stenosis. J. Cardiovasc. Med. *5*:391, 1980.
196. Hohn, A. R., Van Praagh, S., Moore, A. A. D., Vlad, P., and Lambert, E. C.: Aortic stenosis. Circulation *31* (Suppl. III):4, 1965.
197. Bentivoglio, L. G., Sagarminaga, J., and Uricchio, J.: Congenital bicuspid aortic valve: A clinical and hemodynamic study. Br. Heart J. *22*:321, 1960.
198. El-Said, G., Gallioto, F. J., Mullens, C. E., and McNamara, D. G.: Natural hemodynamic history of congenital aortic stenosis in childhood. Am. J. Cardiol. *30*:6, 1972.
199. Hurwitz, R. A.: Aortic valve stenosis in childhood: Clinical and hemodynamic history. J. Pediatr. *82*:228, 1973.
200. Friedman, W. F., Modlinger, J., and Morgan, J.: Serial hemodynamic observations in asymptomatic children with valvar aortic stenosis. Circulation *43*:91, 1971.
201. Cohen, L. S., Friedman, W. F., and Braunwald, E.: Natural history of mild congenital aortic stenosis elucidated by serial hemodynamic studies. Am. J. Cardiol. *30*:1, 1972.

202. Bandy, G. E., and Vogel, J. H. K.: Progressive congenital valvular aortic stenosis. Chest *60*:189, 1971.
203. Rupprath, G., and Neuhaus, K-L.: Percutaneous balloon valvuloplasty for aortic valve stenosis in infancy. Am. J. Cardiol. *56*:1655, 1985.
204. Walls, J. T., LaBabidi, Z., Curtis, J. J., and Silver, D.: Assessment of percutaneous balloon pulmonary and aortic valvuloplasty. J. Thorac. Cardiovasc. Surg. *88*:352, 1984.
205. Bisset, G. S., III, Meyer, R. A., Hirschfeld, S. S., James, F. W., Schwartz D. C., and Kaplan, S.: Aortic valve replacement in childhood: Evaluation of left ventricular function by electrocardiography, echocardiography and graded exercise testing. Am. J. Cardiol. *52*:568, 1983.
206. Presbitero, P., Sommerville, J., Chion, R. R., and Ross, D.: Open aortic valvulotomy for congenital aortic stenosis. Last results. Br. Heart J. *47*:26, 1982.
207. Friedman, W. F., Novak, V., and Johnson, A. D.: Congenital aortic stenosis in adults. *In* Roberts, W. C. (ed.): Congenital Heart Disease in Adults. Philadelphia, F. A. Davis, 1979, p. 235.
208. DiSessa, T. G., Hagan, A. D., Isabel-Jones, J. B., and Friedman, W. F.: Two-dimensional echocardiographic evaluation of discrete subaortic stenosis from the apical long axis view. Am. Heart J. *101*:774, 1981.
209. Kinney, E. L., Machado, H., Cortada, X., and Galbut, D. L.: Diagnosis of discrete subaortic stenosis by pulsed and continuous wave echocardiography. Am. Heart J. *110*:1069, 1985.
210. Bloom, K. R., Meyer, R. A., Bove, K. E., and Kaplan, S.: The association of fixed and dynamic left ventricular outflow obstruction. Am. Heart J. *89*:586, 1975.
211. Newfeld, E. A., Muster, A. J., Paul, M. H., Idriss, F. S., and Riker, W. L.: Discrete subvalvular aortic stenosis in childhood. Am. J. Cardiol. *38*:53, 1976.
212. Brown, J., Stevens, L., Lynch, L., Caldwell, R. Girod, D., Hurwitz, R., Mahony, L., and King, H.: Surgery for discrete subvalvular aortic stenosis: Actuarial survival, hemodynamic results, and acquired aortic regurgitation. Ann. Thorac. Surg. *40*:151, 1985.
213. Moses, R. D., Barnhart, G. R., and Jones, M.: The late prognosis after localized resection for fixed (discrete and tunnel) left ventricular outflow tract observation. J. Thorac. Cardiovasc. Surg. *87*:410, 1984.
214. Somerville, J., Stone, S., and Roth, D.: Fate of patients with fixed subaortic stenosis after surgical removal. Br. Heart J. *43*:629, 1980.
214a. Lababidi, Z., Weinhaus, L., Stoeckle, H., Jr., and Walls, J. T.: Transluminal balloon dilatation for discrete subaortic stenosis. Am. J. Cardiol. 59:423, 1987.
215. Maron, B. J., Redwood, D. R., Roberts, W. C., Henry, W. L., Morrow, A. G., and Epstein, S. E.: Tunnel subaortic stenosis. Circulation *54*:404, 1976.
216. Ergin, M. A., Cooper, R., LaCourte, M., Golinko, R., and Griepp, R. B.: Experience with left ventricular apicoaortic conduits for complicated left ventricular outflow obstruction in children and young adults. Ann. Thorac. Surg. *32*:369, 1981.
217. Waldman, J. D., Schneeweiss, A., Edwards, W. D., Lamberti, J. J., Shem-Tov, A., and Neufeld, H. N.: The obstructive subaortic conus. Circulation *70*:339, 1984.
218. Edwards, J. E.: Pathology of left ventricular outflow tract obstruction. Circulation *31*:586, 1965.
219. Friedman, W. F., and Roberts, W. C.: Vitamin D and the supravalvular aortic stenosis syndrome: The transplacental effects of vitamin D on the aorta of the rabbit. Circulation *34*:77, 1966.
220. Friedman, W. F.: Vitamin D embryopathy. Adv. Teratol. *3*:85, 1968.
221. Friedman, W. F., and Mills, L. F.: The relationship between vitamin D and the craniofacial and dental anomalies of the supraventricular aortic stenosis syndrome. Pediatrics *43*:12, 1969.
222. Garcia, R. C., Friedman, W. F., Kaback, M. M., and Rowe, R. D.: Idiopathic hypercalcemia and supravalvular aortic stenosis: Documentation of a new syndrome. N. Engl. J. Med. *271*:117, 1964.
223. Taylor, A. B., Stern, P. H., and Bell, N. H.: Abnormal regulation of circulating 25-hydroxy vitamin D in the Williams syndrome. N. Engl. J. Med. *306*:972, 1982.
224. Kahler, R. L., Braunwald, E., Plauth, W. H., Jr., and Morrow, A. G.: Familial congenital heart disease. Am. J. Med. *40*:384, 1966.
225. French, J. W., and Guntheroth, W. G.: An explanation of asymmetric upper extremity blood pressure in supravalvular aortic stenosis: The Coanda effect. Circulation *42*:31, 1970.
226. Goldstein, R. E., and Epstein, S. E.: Mechanism of elevated innominate artery pressures in supravalvular aortic stenosis. Circulation *42*:23, 1970.
227. Flaker, G., Teske, D., Kilman, J., Hosier, D., and Wooley, C.: Supravalvular aortic stenosis. A 20-year clinical perspective and experience with patch aortoplasty. Am. J. Cardiol. *15*:256, 1983.
228. Sade, R. M., Crawford, F. A., Jr., and Fyfe, D. A.: Symposium on hypoplastic left heart syndrome. J. Thorac. Cardiovasc. Surg. *91*:937, 1986.
229. Bash, S. E., Huhta, J. C., Vick, G. W., III, Gutgesell, H. P., and Ott, D. A.: Hypoplastic left heart syndrome: Is echocardiography accurate enough to guide surgical palliation? J. Am. Coll. Cardiol. *7*:610, 1986.
230. Norwood, W. I., Lang, P., and Hansen, D. D.: Physiologic repair of aortic atresia-hypoplastic left heart sydrome. N. Engl. J. Med. *308*:23, 1983.
231. Bailey, L. L., Nehlsen-Cannarella, S. L., Concepcion, W., and Jolley, W. B.: Baboon-to-human cardiac xenotransplantation in a neonate. J.A.M.A. *254*:3321, 1985.
232. Caplan, A. L.: Ethical issues raised by research involving xenografts. J.A.M.A. *254*:3339, 1985.
232a. Frahm, C. J., Braunwald, E., and Morrow, A. G.: Congenital aortic regurgitation. Am. J. Med. *31*:63, 1961.
232b. Levy, M. J., Schachner, A., and Blieden L. C.: Aortico-left ventricular tunnel. J. Thorac. Cardiovasc. Surg. *84*:102, 1982.
233. Grant, P., Abrams, L. D., De Giovanni, J. V., Shah, K. J., and Silove, E. D.: Aortico-left ventricular tunnel arising from the left aortic sinus. Am. J. Cardiol. *55*:1657, 1985.
234. Goforth, D., James, F. W., Kaplan, S., and Donner, R.: Maximal exercise in children with aortic regurgitation: An adjunct to noninvasive assessment of disease severity. Am. Heart J. *108*:1306, 1984.
235. Lucas R. V., Jr.: Anomalous venous connection, pulmonary and systemic. *In* Adams, F. H., and Emmanouilides, G. C. (eds.): Moss' Heart Disease in Infants, Children and Adolescents. 3rd ed. Baltimore, Williams and Wilkins, 1983, p. 458.
236. Bini, R. M., Cleveland, D. C., Ceballos, R., Bargeron, L. M., Pacifico, A. D., and Kirklin, J. W.: Congenital pulmonary vein thrombosis. Am. J. Cardiol. *54*:369, 1984.
237. Pacifico, A. D., Mandke, N. V., McGrath, L. B., Colvin, E. V., Bini, R. M., and Bargeron, L. M., Jr.: Repair of congenital pulmonary venous thrombosis with living autologous atrial tissue. J. Thorac. Cardiovasc. Surg. *89*:604, 1985.
238. Marin-Garcia, J., Tandon, R., Lucas, R. V., Jr., and Edwards, J. E.: Cor triatriatum: Study of 20 cases. Am. J. Cardiol. *35*:59, 1975.
239. Jacobstein, M. D., and Hirschfeld, S. S.: Concealed left atrial membrane: Pitfalls in the diagnosis of cor triatriatum and supravalvular mitral stenosing ring. Am. J. Cardiol. *49*:780, 1982.
240. Oglietti, J., Cooley, D. A., Izquierdo, J. P., Ventemiglia, R., Muasher, I., Hallman, G. L., and Reul, G. J.: Cor triatriatum: Operative results in 25 patients. Ann. Thorac. Surg. *35*:415, 1983.
241. Ruckman, R. N., and Van Praagh, R.: Anatomic types of congenital mitral stenosis: Report of 49 autopsy cases with consideration of diagnosis and surgical implications. Am. J. Cardiol. *42*:592, 1978.
242. Parr, G. V. S., Fripp, R. A., Whitman, V., Bharati, S., and Lev, M.: Anomalous mitral arcade: Echocardiographic and angiographic reception. Pediatr. Cardiol. *4*:163, 1983.
243. Glaser, J., Yakirevich, V., and Vidine, B. A.: Preoperative echographic diagnosis of supravalvular stenosing ring of the left atrium. Am. Heart J. *108*:169, 1984.
244. Smallhorn, J., Tommasini, G., Deanfield, J., Douglas, J., and Macartney, F.: Congenital mitral stenosis. Anatomical and functional assessment by echocardiography. Br. Heart J. *45*:527, 1981.
245. Midgley, F. M., Perry, L. W., and Potter, B. M.: Conduit bypass of mitral valve: A palliative approach to congenital mitral stenosis. Am. J. Cardiol. *56*:493, 1985.
246. Antunes, M. J.: Bioprosthetic valve replacement in children—long-term follow-up of 135 isolated mitral valve implantations. Eur. Heart J. *5*:913, 1984.
247. Kveselis, D. A., Rocchini, A. P., Beekman, R., Snider, A. R., Crowley, D., Dick, M., and Rosenthal, A.: Balloon angiography for congenital and rheumatic mitral stenosis. Am. J. Cardiol. *57*:348, 1986.
248. Perloff, J. K.: Evolving concepts of mitral valve prolapse. N. Engl. J. Med. *307*:369, 1982.
249. Carpentier, A.: Congenital malformations of the mitral valve. *In* Stark, J., and deLeval, M. (eds.): Surgery for Congenital Heart Defects. New York, Grune and Stratton, Inc., 1983, p. 467.
250. Carpentier, A., Branchini, B., Cour, J. C., Asfaou, E., Villani, M., Deloche, A., Relland, J., D'Allaines, C., Blondeau, P., Piwnica, A., Parenzan, L., and Brom, G.: Congenital malformations of the mitral valve in children: Pathology and surgical treatment. J. Thorac. Cardiovasc. Surg. *72*:854, 1976.
251. White, R. I., Jr., Mitchell, S. E., Barth, K. H., Kaufman, S. L., Kadir, S., Chang, R., and Terry, P. B.: Angioarchitecture of pulmonary arteriovenous malformations: An important consideration before embolotherapy. Am. J. Radiol. *140*:681, 1983.
252. Vincent, R. N., Casiro, O. G., Pelech, A. N., and Collins, G. F. N.: Evaluation of pulmonary vascular resistance in the presence of a large pulmonary arteriovenous malformation. J. Am. Coll. Cardiol. *7*:1104, 1986.
253. Gonzalez, V. R., Pieper, W. M., and Kap-herr, S. H.: Pulmonary arteriovenous fistula in childhood. Z. Kinderchir. *40*:101, 1985.
254. D'Cruz, I. A., Agustssou, M. M., Bicoff, J. P., Weinberg, M., Jr., and Arcilla, R. A.: Stenotic lesions of the pulmonary arteries. Clinical hemodynamic findings in 84 cases. Am. J. Cardiol. *13*:441, 1964.
255. Venables, A. W.: The syndrome of pulmonary stenosis complicating maternal rubella. Br. Heart J. *27*:49, 1965.
256. Danilowicz, D. A., Rudolph, A. M., Hoffman, J. I. E., and Heymann, M. A.: Physiologic pressure differences between main and branch pulmonary arteries in infants. Circulation *45*:410, 1972.
257. Eldredge, W. J., Tingelstad, J. B., Robertson, L. W., Mauck, H. P., and McCue, C. M.: Observations on the natural history of pulmonary artery coarctation. Circulation *45*:404, 1972.
258. Edwards, B. S., Lucas, R. V., Jr., Lock, J. E., and Edwards, J. E.: Morphologic changes in the pulmonary arteries after percutaneous balloon angioplasty for pulmonary arterial stenosis. Circulation *71*:195, 1985.
259. Rocchini, A. P., Kveselis, D., Dick, M., Crowley, D., Snider, A. R., and Rosenthal, A.: Use of balloon angioplasty to treat peripheral pulmonary stenosis. Am. J. Cardiol. *54*:1069, 1984.
260. Ring, J. C., Bass, J. L., Marvin, W., Fuhrman, B. P., Kulik, T. J., Foker, J. E., and Lock, J. E.: Management of congenital stenosis of a branch pulmonary artery with balloon dilation. J. Thorac. Cardiovasc. Surg. *90*:35, 1985.
261. Koretzky, E., Moller, J. H., Korns, M E., Schwartz, C. J., and Edwards, J. E.: Congenital pulmonary stenosis resulting from dysplasia of valve. Circulation *40*:43, 1969.
262. Polansky, D. B., Clark, E. B., and Doty, D. B.: Pulmonary stenosis in infants and young children. Ann. Thorac. Surg. *39*:159, 1985.
263. Trowitzsch, E., Colan, S. D., and Sanders, S. P.: Two-dimensional echocardiographic evaluation of right ventricular size and function in newborns with severe right ventricular outflow tract obstruction. J. Am. Coll. Cardiol. *6*:388, 1985.
264. Hagler, D. J., Tajik, A. J., Seward, J. B., and Ritter, D. G.: Noninvasive assessment of pulmonary valve stenosis, aortic valve stenosis and coarctation of the aorta in critically ill neonates. Am. J. Cardiol. *57*:369, 1986.

265. Johnson, G. L., Kwan, O. L., Handshoe, S., Noonan, J. A., and DeMaria, A. N.: Accuracy of combined two-dimensional echocardiography and continuous wave Doppler recordings in the estimation of pressure gradient in right ventricular outlet obstruction. J. Am. Coll. Cardiol. 3:1013, 1984.
265a. Srinivasan, V., Konyer, A., Broda, J. J., and Subramanian, S.: Critical pulmonary stenosis in infants less than three months of age: A reappraisal of closed transventricular pulmonary valvotomy. Ann. Thorac. Surg. *34*:46, 1982.
266. Kan, J. S., White, R. I., Jr., Mitchell, S. E., Anderson, J. H., and Gardner, T. J.: Percutaneous transluminal balloon valvuloplasty for pulmonary valve stenosis. Circulation *69*:554, 1984.
267. Miller, G. A. H.: Balloon vavuloplasty and angioplasty in congenital heart disease. Br. Heart J. *54*:285, 1985.
268. Mody, M. R.: The natural history of uncomplicated valvular pulmonary stenosis. Am. Heart J. *90*:317, 1975.
269. Ellison, R. C., and Miettinen, O. S.: Interpretation of rSR′ in pulmonic stenosis. Am. Heart J. *88*:7, 1974.
270. Krabill, K. A., Wang, Y., Einzig, S., and Moller, J. H.: Rest and exercise hemodynamics in pulmonary stenosis: Comparison of children and adults. Am. J. Cardiol. *56*:360, 1985.
271. Danilowicz, D., Hoffman, J. I. E., and Rudolph, A. M.: Serial studies of pulmonary stenosis in infancy and childhood. Br. Heart J. *37*:808, 1975.
272. Wennevold, A., and Jacobsen, J. R.: Natural history of valvular pulmonary stenosis in children below the age of two years: Long-term follow-up with serial heart catheterizations. Eur. J. Cardiol. *8*:371, 1978.
273. Rao, P. S.: Comprehensive management of pulmonary atresia with intact ventricular septum. Ann. Thorac. Surg. *40*:409, 1985.
274. Zuberbuhler, J. R., and Anderson, R. H.: Morphological variations in pulmonary atresia with intact ventricular septum. Br. Heart J. *41*:281, 1979.
275. Trowitzsch, E., Colan, S. D., and Sanders, S. P.: Two-dimensional echocardiographic evaluation of right ventricular size and function in newborns with severe right ventricular outflow tract obstruction. J. Am. Coll. Cardiol. *6*:388, 1985.
276. Joshi, S. V., Brawn, W. J., and Mee, R. B. B.: Pulmonry atresia with intact ventricular septum. J. Thorac. Cardiovasc. Surg. *91*:192, 1986.
277. Milliken, J. C., Laks, H., Hellenbrand, W., George, B., Chin, A., and Williams, R. G.: Early and late results in the treatment of patients with pulmonary atresia and intact ventricular septum. Circulation 72:II–61, 1985.
278. Larson, J. E., Fleming, W. H., Sarafian, L. B., Rogler, W. C., Hofschire, P. J., and McManus, B. M.: Combined prostaglandin therapy and ductal formalin infiltration in neonatal pulmonary oligemia. J. Thorac. Cardiovasc. Surg. *90*:907, 1985.
279. Danilowicz, D., and Ishmael, R.: Anomalous right ventricular muscle bundle: Clinical pitfalls and extracardiac anomalies. Clin. Cardiol. *4*:146, 1981.
280. Kveselis, D., Rosenthal, A., Ferguson, P., Behrendt, D., and Sloan, H.: Long-term prognosis after repair of double-chamber right ventricle with ventricular septal defect. Am. J. Cardiol. *54*:1292, 1984.
281. Kirklin, J. W., and Karp, R. B.: The tetralogy of Fallot: From a surgical viewpoint. Philadelphia, W. B. Saunders Company, 1970.
282. Perloff, J. K., Friedman, W. F., Laks, H., and Child, J. S.: From the cyanotic infant to the acyanotic adult—the odyssey of the blue baby. UCLA School of Medicine Interdisciplinary Conference. West. J. Med. *139*:673, 1983.
283. Rayo, B. N., Anderson, R. C., and Edwards, J. E.: Anatomic variations in tetralogy of Fallot. Am. Heart J. *81*:361, 1971.
284. Liao, P. K., Edwards, W. D., Julsrud, P. R., Puga, F. J., Danielson, G. K., and Feldt, R. H.: Pulmonary blood supply in patients with pulmonary atresia and ventricular septal defect. J. Am. Coll. Cardiol. *6*:1343, 1985.
285. Johnson, R. J., Sauer, U., Buhlmeyer, K., and Haworth, S. G.: Hypoplasia of the intrapulmonary arteries in children with right ventricular overflow tract obstruction, ventricular septal defect, and major aortopulmonary collateral arteries. Pediatr. Cardiol. *6*:137, 1985.
286. Fellows, K. E., Freed, M. D., Keane, J. F., Van Praagh, R., Bernard, W. R., and Castaneda, A. C.: Results of routine preoperative coronary angiography and tetralogy of Fallot. Circulation *51*:561, 1977.
287. Morgan, B. C., Guntheroth, W. G., Blume, R. S., and Fyler, D. C.: A clinical profile of paroxysmal hyperpnea in cyanotic congenital heart disease. Circulation *31*:66, 1965.
288. Ueda K., Nojima, K., Saito, A., Nakano, H., Yokota, M., and Muraoka, R.: Modified Blalock-Taussig shunt operation without cardiac catheterization: Two-dimensional echocardiographic preoperative assessment in cyanotic infants. Am. J. Cardiol. *54*:1296, 1984.
289. Freedom, R. M.: Axial angiocardiography in the critically ill infant. *In* Friedman, W. F., and Higgins, C. B. (eds.): Pediatric Cardiac Imaging. Philadelphia, W. B. Saunders Company, 1984, p. 26.
290. Benson, L. N., Laks, H., Lois, J., Dajee, H., Child, J., and Perloff, J. K.: Surgical correction of pulmonary atresia and ventricular septal defect with large systemic-pulmonary collaterals. Ann. Thorac. Surg. *38*:522, 1984.
291. Sondheimer, H. M., Oliphant, M., Schneider, B., Kavey, R. E. W., Blackman, M. S., and Parker, F. B.: Computerized axial tomography of the chest for visualization of absent pulmonary arteries. Circulation *65*:1020, 1982.
292. Nihill, M. R., Mullins, C. E., and MacNamara, D. G.: Visualization of the pulmonary arteries in pseudo-truncus by pulmonary vein wedge angiography. Circulation *58*:140, 1978.
293. Kirklin, J. W., Blackstone, E. H., Kirklin, J. K., Pacifico, A. D., Aramendi, J., and Bargeron, L. M., Jr.: Surgical results and protocols in the spectrum of tetralogy of Fallot. Ann. Surg. *198*:251, 1983.
294. Pacifico, A. D. Allen, R. H., and Colvin, E. V.: Direct reconstruction of pulmonary artery arborization anomaly and intracardiac repair of pulmonary atresia with ventricular septal defect. Am. J. Cardiol. *55*:1647, 1985.
295. Kirklin, J. K., Pacifico, A. D., and Kirklin, J. W.: Tetralogy of Fallot: Principles of surgical management. Mod. Probl. Paediatr. *22*:139, 1983.
296. Hammon, J. W., Jr., Henry, C. L., Jr., Merrill, W. H., Graham, T. P., Jr., and Bender, H. W., Jr.: Tetralogy of Fallot: Selective surgical management to minimize operative mortality. Ann. Thorac. Surg. *40*:280, 1985.
297. Zhao, H. X., Miller, D. C., Reitz, B. A., and Shumway, N. E.: Surgical repair of tetralogy of Fallot. J. Thorac. Cardiovasc. Surg. *89*:204, 1985.
298. Naito, Y., Fujita, T., Yagihara, T., Isobe, F., Yamamoto, F., Tanaka, K., Manabe, H., Takahashi, O., and Kamiya, T.: Usefulness of left ventricular volume in assessing tetralogy of Fallot for total correction. Am. J. Cardiol. *56*:356, 1985.
299. Kobayashi, J., Hirose, H., Nakano, S., Matsuda, H., Shirakura, R., and Kawashima, Y.: Ambulatory electrocardiographic study of the frequency and cause of ventricular arrhythmia after correction of Fallot. Am J. Cardiol. *54*:1310, 1984.
300. Garson, A., Jr., Randall, D. C., Gillette, P. C., Smith, R. T., Moak, J. P., McVey, P., and McNamara, D. G.: Prevention of sudden death after repair of tetralogy of Fallot: Treatment of ventricular arrhythmias. J. Am. Coll. Cardiol. *6*:221, 1985.
301. Dunnigan, A., Pritzker, M. R., Benditt, D. G., Benson, D. W., Jr.: Life threatening ventricular tachycardias in late survivors of surgically corrected tetralogy of Fallot. Br. Heart J. *52*:198, 1984.
302. Garson, A., Jr., and McNamara, D. G.: Post-operative tetralogy of Fallot. *In* Engle, M. A. (ed.): Pediatric Cardiovascular Disease. Philadelphia, F. A. Davis, 1981, p. 407.
303. Oku, H., Shirotani, H., Sunakawa, A., and Yokoyama, T.: Postoperative long-term results in total correction of tetralogy of Fallot: Hemodynamics and cardiac function. Ann. Thorac. Surg. *41*:413, 1986.
304. Kavey, R. W., Thomas, F. D., Byrum, C. J., Blackman, M. S., Sondheimer, H. M., and Bove, E. L.: Ventricular arrhythmias and biventricular dysfunction after repair of tetralogy of Fallot. J. Am. Coll. Cardiol. *4*:126, 1984.
305. Rosenthal, A., Behrendt, D., Sloan, H., Ferguson, P., Snedecor, S. M., and Schork, M. A.: Long-term prognosis (15 to 26 years) after repair of tetralogy of Fallot: I. Survival and symptomatic status. Ann. Thorac. Surg. *38*:151, 1984.
306. Ilbawi, M. N., Idriss, F. S., DeLeon, S. Y., Muster, A. J., Berry, T. E., and Paul, M. H.: Long-term results of porcine valve insertion for pulmonary regurgitation following repair of tetralogy of Fallot. Ann. Thorac. Surg. *41*:478, 1986.
307. Ilbawi, M. N., Fedorchik, J., Muster, A. J., Idriss, F. S., DeLeon, S. Y., Gidding, S. S., and Paul, M. H.: Surgical approach to severely symptomatic newborn infants with tetralogy of Fallot and absent pulmonary valve. J. Thorac. Cardiovasc. Surg. *91*:584, 1986.
308. Fischer, D. R., Neches, W. H., Beerman, L. B., Fricker, F. J., Siewers, R. D., Lenox, C. C., and Park, S. C.: Tetralogy of Fallot with absent pulmonic valve: Analysis of 17 patients. Am. J. Cardiol. *53*:1433, 1984.
309. Emmanouilides, G. C., Thanopoulos, B., Siassi, B., and Fishbein, M: Agenesis of ductus arteriosus associated with the syndrome of tetralogy of Fallot and absent pulmonary valve. Am. J. Cardiol. *37*:403, 1976.
310. Dunnigan, A., Oldham, H. N., and Benson, D. W.: Absent pulmonary valve syndrome in infancy: Surgery reconsidered. Am. J. Cardiol. *48*:117, 1981.
311. Anderson, R. H., Wilkerson, J. L, Gerlis, L. M., Smyth, A., and Becker, A. E.: Atresia of the right atrioventricular orifice. Br. Heart J. *39*:414, 1977.
312. Rao, P. S. (ed.): Tricuspid Atresia. Mt. Kisco, N.Y., Futura Publishing Co., Inc., 1982.
313. Dick, M., Fyler, D. C., and Nadas, A. S.: Tricuspid atresia, clinical course in 101 patients. Am. J. Cardiol. *36*:327, 1975.
314. Bharati, S., and Lev, M.: Conduction system in tricuspid atresia with and without regular D-transposition. Circulation *56*:423, 1977.
315. Koiwaya, Y., Watanabe, K., and Hirata, T.: Contrast two-dimensional echocardiography in diagnosis of tricuspid atresia. Am. Heart J. *101*:507, 1981.
316. Fontan, F., Deville, C., Quaegebeur, J., Ottenkamp, J., Sourdille, N., Choussat, A., and Brom, G. A.: Repair of tricuspid atresia in 100 patients. J. Thorac. Cardiovasc. Surg. *85*:647, 1983.
317. Alboliras, E. T., Porter, C. J., Danielson, G. K., Puga, F. J., Schaff, H. V., Rice, M. J., and Driscoll, D. J.: Results of the modified Fontan operation for congenital heart lesions in patients without preoperative sinus rhythm. J. Am. Coll. Cardiol. *6*:228, 1985.
318. Kirklin, J. K., Blackstone, E. H., Kirklin, J. W., Pacifico, A. D., and Bargeron, L. M., Jr.: The Fontan operation: Ventricular hypertrophy, age, and date of operation as risk factors. J. Thorac. Cardiovasc. Surg. (*in press*).
318a. Girod, D. A., Fontan, F., Deville, C., Ottenkamp, J., and Choussat, A.: Long-term results after the Fontan operation for tricuspid atresia. Circulation *75*:605, 1987.
319. Girod, D. A., Rice, M. J., Mair, D. D., Julsrud, P. R., Puga, F. J., and Danielson, G. K.: Relationship of pulmonary artery size to mortality in patients undergoing the Fontan operation. Circulation 72:II–93, 1985.
320. Ottenkamp, J., Wenink, A. C. G., Quaegebeur, J. M., Rohmer, J., Gittenberger-de-Groot, A. C., Brom, A. G., and Fontan, F.: Tricuspid atresia—morphology of the outlet chamber with special emphasis on surgical implications. J. Thorac. Cardiovasc. Surg. *89*:597, 1985.
321. DiSessa, T. G., Child, J. S., Perloff, J. K., Wu, L., Williams, R. G., Laks, H., and Friedman, W. F.: Systemic venous and pulmonary arterial flow patterns after Fontan's procedure for tricuspid atresia or single ventricle. Circulation *70*:898, 1984.
322. Ehren, B. L., Mills, M., and Lower, R. R.: Congenital tricuspid insufficiency: Definition and review. Chest *69*:637, 1976.
323. Gussenhoven, E. J., Stewart, P. A., Becker, A. E., Essed, C. E., Ligtvoet, K. M., and De Villeneuve, V. H.: "Offsetting" of the septal tricuspid leaflet in normal hearts and in hearts with Ebstein's anomaly. Am. J. Cardiol. *53*:172, 1984.
324. Guiliani, E. R., Fuster, V., Brandenberg, R. O., and Mair, D. D.: Ebstein's anomaly: The clinical features and natural history of Ebstein's anomaly of the tricuspid valve. Mayo Clin. Proc. *54*:163, 1979.
325. Boucek, R. J., Jr., Graham, T. P., Jr., Morgan, J. P., Atwood, G. F., and Boerth, R. C.: Spontaneous resolution of massive congenital tricuspid insufficiency. Circulation *54*:795, 1976.
326. Freedom, R. M., Culham, J. A. G., Olley, P. M., Moes, C. A. F., and Rowe,

R. D.: The differentiation of functional from organic pulmonary atresia: The role of aortography. Am. J. Cardiol. *41*:914, 1978.
327. Kastor, J. A., Goldreier, B. N., Josephson, M. E., Perloff, J. K., Scharf, D. L., Manchester, J. H., Schelbourne, J. C., and Hirshfield, J. W., Jr.: Electrophysiologic characteristics of Ebstein's anomaly of the tricuspid valve. Circulation *52*:987, 1975.
328. Gussenhoven, W. J., Spitaels, S. E. C., Bom, N., and Becker, A. E.: Echocardiographic criteria for Ebstein's anomaly of tricuspid valve. Br. Heart J. *43*:31, 1980.
329. Hirschklau, M. J., Sahn, D. J., Hagan, A. D., Williams, D. E., and Friedman, W. F.: Cross-sectional echocardiographic features of Ebstein's anomaly of the tricuspid valve. Am. J. Cardiol. *40*:400, 1977.
330. Oh, J. K., Holmes, D. R., Jr., Hayes, D. L., Porter, C. J., and Danielson, G. K.: Cardiac arrhythmias in patients with surgical repair of Ebstein's anomaly. J. Am. Coll. Cardiol. *6*:1351, 1985.
331. Mair, D. D., Seward, J. B., Driscoll, D. J., and Danielson, G. K.: Surgical repair of Ebstein's anomaly: Selection of patients and early and late operative results. Circulation 72:11–70, 1985.
332. Prajbehl, A. B.: Ebstein's anomaly: Sixteen years' experience with valve replacement without plication of the right ventricle. Thorax 39:8, 1984.
333. Paul, M. H.: D-Transposition of great arteries. *In* Adams, F. H., and Emmanouilides, G. C. (eds.): Moss' Heart Disease in Infants, Children and Adolescents, 3rd ed. Baltimore, Williams and Wilkins, 1983, p. 296.
334. Thiene, G., Razzolini, R., and Dalla-Volta, S.: Aorto-pulmonary relationship, arterio-ventricular alignment, and ventricular septal defects in complete transposition of the great arteries. Eur. J. Cardiol. *4*:13, 1976.
335. Mair, D. D., and Ritter, D. G.: Factors influencing systemic arterial oxygen saturation in complete transposition of the great arteries. Am. J. Cardiol. *31*:742, 1973.
336. Lakier, J. B., Stanger, P., Heymann, M. A., Hoffman, J. I. E., and Rudolph, A. M.: Early onset of pulmonary vascular obstruction in patients with aortopulmonary transposition and intact ventricular septum. Circulation *51*:875, 1975.
337. Aziz, K. U., Paul, M. H., and Rowe, R. D.: Bronchopulmonary circulation in D-transposition of the great arteries: Possible role and genesis of accelerated pulmonary vascular disease. Am. J. Cardiol. *39*:432, 1977.
338. Muster, A. J. Paul, M. H., Van Grondell, E. A., and Conway, J. J.: Asymmetric distribution of the pulmonary blood flow between the right and left lungs in D-transposition of the great arteries. Am. J. Cardiol. *38*:352, 1976.
339. Sansa, M., Tonkin, I. L., Bargeron, L. M., and Elliott, L. P.: Left ventricular outflow tract obstruction in transposition of the great arteries. Am. J. Cardiol. *44*:88, 1979.
340. Chiu, I., Anderson, R. H., Macartney, F. J., De Leval, M. R., and Startk, J.: Morphologic features of an intact ventricular septum susceptible to subpulmonary obstruction in complete transposition. Am. J. Cardiol. *53*:1633, 1984.
341. Waldman, J. D., Paul, M. H., Newfeld, E. A., Muster, A. J., and Idriss, F. S.: Transposition of the great arteries with intact ventricular septum and patent ductus arteriosus. Am. J. Cardiol. *39*:232, 1977.
342. Tonkin, I. L., Kelley, M. J., Bream, P. R., and Elliott, L. P.: The frontal chest film as a method of suspecting transposition complexes. Circulation *53*:1016, 1976.
343. Chin, A. J., Yeager, S. B., Sanders, S. P., Williams, R. G., Bierman, F. Z., Burger, B. M., Norwood, W. I., and Castaneda, A. R.: Accuracy of prospective two-dimensional echocardiographic evaluation of left ventricular outflow tract in complete transposition of the great arteries. Am. J. Cardiol. 55:759, 1985.
344. Deal, B. J., Chin, A. J., Sanders, S. P., Norwood, W. I., and Castaneda, A. R.: Subxiphoid two-dimensional echocardiographic identification of tricuspid valve abnormalities in transposition of the great arteries with ventricular septal defect. Am. J. Cardiol. *55*:1146, 1985.
345. Marino, B., de Simone, G., Pasquini, L., Giannico, S., Marcelletti, C., Ammirati, A., Guccione, P., Boldrini R., and Ballerini, L.: Complete transposition of the great arteries: Visualization of left and right outflow tract obstruction by oblique subcostal two-dimensional echocardiography. Am. J. Cardiol. *55*:1140, 1985.
346. Chin, A. J., Yeager, S. B., Sanders, S. P., Williams, R. G., Bierman, F. Z., Burger, B. M., Norwood, W. I., and Castaneda, A. R.: Accuracy of prospective two-dimensional echocardiographic evaluation of left ventricular outflow tract in complete transposition of the great arteries. Am. J. Cardiol. *55*:759, 1985.
347. DiSessa, T. G., Childs, W., Ti, C. C., and Friedman, W. F.: Systolic anterior motion of the mitral valve in a one day old infant with transposition of the great vessels. J. Clin. Ultrasound *6*:186, 1978.
348. Lin, A. E., Di Sessa, T. G., Williams, R. G., Leighton, J., Gross, K., and Wong, A. L.: Balloon and blade atrial septostomy facilitated by two-dimensional echocardiography. Am. J. Cardiol. *57*:273, 1986.
349. Moene, R. J., Oppenheimer-Dekker, A., Wenink, A. C. G., Bartelings, M. M., and De Groot, G.: Morphology of ventricular septal defect in complete transposition of the great arteries. Am. J. Cardiol. *55*:1566, 1985.
350. Graham, T. P., Burger, J. Bender, H. W., Hammon, J. W., Boucek, R. J., Jr., and Appleton, S.: Improved right ventricular function after intra-atrial repair of transposition of the great arteries. Circulation 72:II-45, 1985.
351. Pacifico, A. D., Stewart, R. W., and Bargeron, L. M., Jr.: Repair of transposition of the great arteries with ventricular septal defect by an arterial switch operation. Circulation *68*:II-49, 1983.
352. Kanter, K. R., Anderson, R. H., Lincoln, C., Rigby, M. L., and Shinebourne, E. A.: Anatomic correction for complete transposition and double-outlet right ventricle. J. Thorac. Cardiovasc. Surg. *90*:690, 1985.
353. Mahony, L., Turley, K., Ebert, P., and Heymann, M. A.: Long-term results after atrial repair of transposition of the great arteries in early infancy. Circulation *66*:253, 1982.
354. Castaneda, A. R., Norwood, W. I., Jonas, R. A., Colon, S. D., Sanders, S. P., and Lang, P.: Transposition of the great arteries and intact ventricular septum: Anatomical repair in the neonate. Ann. Thoracic Surg. *38*:438, 1984.
355. Graham, T. P., Jr.: Hemodynamic residua and sequelae following intraatrial repair of transposition of the great artery. A review. Pediatr. Cardiol. *2*:203, 1982.
356. Smallhorn, J. F., Gow, R., Freedom, R. M., Trusler, G. A., Olley, P., Pacquet, M., Gibbons, J., and Vlad, P.: Pulsed Doppler echocardiographic assessment of the pulmonary venous pathway after the Mustard or Senning procedure for transposition of the great arteries. Circulation *73*:765, 1986.
357. Gillette, P. C., Wampler, D. G., Shannon, C., and Ott, D.: Use of cardiac pacing after the Mustard operation for transposition of the great arteries. J. Am. Coll. Cardiol. *7*:138, 1986.
358. Gillette, P. C., Kuglar, J. D., Garson, A., Jr., Gutgesell, H. P., Duff, D. F., and McNamara, D. G.: Mechanisms of cardiac arrhythmias after the Mustard operation for transposition of the great arteries. Am. J. Cardiol. *45*:1225, 1980.
359. Duster, M. C., Bink-Boelkens, M. T. E., Wampler, D., Gillette, P. C., McNamara, D. G., and Cooley, D. A.: Long-term follow-up of dysrhythmias following the Mustard procedure. Am. Heart J. *109*:1323, 1985.
360. Huhta, J. C., Edwards, W. D., Danielson, G. K., and Feldt, R. H.: Abnormalities of the tricuspid valve in complete transposition of the great arteries with ventricular septal defect. J. Thorac. Cardiovasc. Surg. *83*:569, 1982.
361. Borow, K. M., Keane, J. F., Castaneda, A. R., and Fried, M. D.: Systemic ventricular function in patients with tetralogy of Fallot, ventricular septal defect and transposition of the great arteries repaired during infancy. Circulation *64*:878, 1981.
362. Okuda, H., Nakazawa, M., Imai, Y., Kurosawa, H., Takanashi, Y., Hoshino, S., and Takao, A.: Comparison of ventricular function after Senning and Jatene procedures for complete transposition of the great arteries. Am. J. Cardiol. *55*:530, 1985.
363. Benson, L. N., Bonet, J., Olley, P. M., Trusler, G., Rowe, R. D., and Morch, J.: Assessment of right ventricular function during supine bicycle exercise after Mustard's operation. Circulation *65*:1052, 1982.
364. Moulton, A. L., De Leval, M. R., Macartney, F. J., Taylor, J. F. N., and Stark, J.: Rastelli procedure for transposition of the great arteries, ventricular septal defect, and left ventricular outflow tract obstruction. Early and late results in 41 patients. Br. Heart J. *45*:20, 1981.
365. Danford, D. A., Huhta, J. C., and Gutgesell, H. P.: Left ventricular wall stress and thickness in complete transposition of the great arteries. J. Thorac. Cardiovasc. Surg. *89*:610, 1985.
366. Dhasmana, J. P., Stark, J., De Leval, M., Macartney, F. J., Rees, P. G., and Taylor, J. F. N.: Long-term results of the "palliative" Mustard operation. J. Am. Coll. Cardiol. *6*:1138, 1985.
367. Colli, A. M., De Leval, M., and Somerville, J.: Anatomically corrected malposition of the great arteries. Am. J. Cardiol. *55*:1367, 1985.
368. Kirklin, J. W., Pacifico, A. D., Bargeron, L. M., Jr., and Soto, B.: Cardiac repair and anatomically corrected malposition of the great arteries. Circulation *48*:153, 1973.
369. Berry, W. B., Roberts, W. C., Morrow, A. G., and Braunwald, E.: Corrected transposition of the aorta and pulmonary trunk: Clinical, hemodynamic, and pathologic findings. Am. J. Med. *36*:35, 1964.
370. Freedberg, D. Z., and Nadas, A. S.: Clinical profile of patients with congenital corrected transposition of the great arteries. N. Engl. J. Med. *282*:1053, 1970.
371. Allwork, S. P., Bentall, H. H., Becker, A. E., Cameron, H., Gerlis, L. M., Wilkinson, J. L., and Anderson, R. H.: Congenitally corrected transposition of the great arteries. Morphologic study of 32 cases. Am. J. Cardiol. *38*:910, 1976.
372. Bjarke, B. B., and Kidd, B. S. L.: Congenitally corrected transposition of the great arteries: A clinical study of 101 cases. Acta Paediatr. Scand. *65*:153, 1976.
373. Huhta, J. C., Danielson, G. K., Ritter, D. G., and Ilstrup, D. M.: Survival in atrioventricular discordance. Pediatr. Cardiol. *6*:57, 1985.
374. Waldo, A. L., Pacifico, A. D., Bargeron, L. M., Jr., James, T. N., and Kirklin, J. W.: Electrophysiological delineation of specialized AV conduction system in patients with corrected transposition of the great vessels and ventricular septal defect. Circulation 52:435, 1975.
375. Bharati, B., Rosen, K., Steinfield, L., Miller, R. A., and Lev, M.: The anatomic substrate for pre-excitation in corrected transposition. Circulation *62*:831, 1980.
376. Meissner, M. D., Panidis, I. P., Eshaghpour, E., Mintz, G. S., and Ross, J.: Corrected transposition of the great arteries: Evaluation by two-dimensional and Doppler echocardiography. Am. Heart J. *111*:599, 1986.
377. Freedom, R. M., Harrington, D. P., and White, R. I., Jr.: The differential diagnosis of levotransposed or malposed aorta: An angiocardiographic study. Circulation *50*:1040, 1974.
378. McGrath, L. B., Kirklin, J. W., Blackstone, E. H., Pacifico, A. D., Kirklin, J. K., and Bargeron, L. M., Jr.: Death and other events after cardiac repair in discordant atrioventricular connection. J. Thorac Cardiovasc. Surg. *90*:711, 1985.
379. Piccoli, G., Pacifico, A. D., Kirklin, J. W., Blackstone, E. H., Kirlin, J. K., and Bargeron, L. M., Jr.: Changing results and concepts in the surgical treatment of double-outlet right ventricle: Analysis of 137 operations in 126 patients. Am. J. Cardiol. 52:549, 1983.
380. Kirklin, J. W., Pacifico, A. D., Blackstone, E. H., Kirklin, J. K., and Bargeron, L. M., Jr.: Current risks and protocols for surgery for double outlet right ventricle: Derivation from an 18-year experience. J. Thorac. Cardiovasc. Surg. (*in press*).
381. Sondheimer, H. M., Freedom, R. M., and Olley, P. M.: Double outlet right ventricle: Clinical spectrum and prognosis. Am. J. Cardiol. *39*:709, 1977.

382. Goitein, K. J., Neches, W. H., Park, S. C., Matthews, R. A., Lennox, C. C., and Zuberbuhler, J. R.: Electrocardiogram in double chamber right ventricle. Am. J. Cardiol. *45*:604, 1980.
383. Macartney, F. J., Rigby, M. L., Anderson, R. H., Stark, J., and Silverman, N. H.: Double outlet right ventricle. Cross-sectional echocardiographic findings, their anatomical explanation and surgical relevance. Br. Heart J. *52*:164, 1984.
384. Sridaromont, S., Ritter, D. G., Feldt, R. H., Davis, G. D., and Edwards, J. E.: Double outlet right ventricle: Anatomic and angiocardiographic correlations. Mayo Clin. Proc. *53*:555, 1978.
385. Kanter, K., Anderson, R., Lincoln, C., Firmin, R., and Rigby, M.: Anatomic correction of double-outlet right ventricle with subpulmonary ventricular septal defect (the "Taussig-Bing" anomaly). Ann. Thorac. Surg. *41*:287, 1986.
386. Doty, D. B.: Correction of Taussig-Bing malformation by intraventricular conduit. J. Thorac. Cardiovasc. Surg. *91*:133, 1986.
387. Stark, J.: Double-outlet ventricles. *In* Stark, J., and deLeval, M. (eds.): Surgery for Congenital Heart Defects. New York, Grune and Stratton, 1983, p. 397.
388. Van Praagh, R., and Weinberg, P. M.: Double outlet left ventricle. *In* Adams, F. H., and Emmanouilides, G. C. (eds.): Moss' Heart Disease in Infants, Children and Adolescents. 3rd ed. Baltimore, Williams and Wilkins, 1983, p. 370.
389. Murphy, E. A., Gillis, D. A., and Sridhara, K. S.: Intraventricular repair of double outlet left ventricle. Ann. Thor. Surg. *31*:364, 1981.
390. Gathman, G. E., and Nadas, A. S.: Total anomalous pulmonary venous connection: Clinical and physiologic observations in 75 pediatric patients. Circulation *42*:143, 1970.
391. Ward, K. E., Mullins, C. E., Huhta, J. C., Nihill, M. R., McNamara, D. G., and Cooley, D. A.: Restrictive interatrial communication in total anomalous pulmonary venous connection. Am. J. Cardiol. *57*:1131, 1986.
392. Turley, K., Tucker, W. Y., Ullyot, D. J., and Ebert, P. A.: Total anomalous pulmonary venous connection in infancy. Influence of age and type of lesion. Am. J. Cardiol. *45*:92, 1980.
393. Elliott, L. P., and Edwards, J. E.: The problem of pulmonary venous obstruction in total anomalous pulmonary venous connection to the left innominate vein. Circulation *25*:913, 1962.
394. Newfeld, E. A., Wilson, A., Paul, M. H., and Reisch, J. S.: Pulmonary vascular disease in total anomalous pulmonary venous drainage. Circulation *61*:103, 1980.
395. Haworth, S. G., Reid, L., and Simon, G.: Radiological features of the heart and lungs in total anomalous pulmonary venous return in early infancy. Clin. Radiol. *28*:561, 1977.
396. Huhta, J. C., Gutgesell, H. P., and Nihill, M. R.: Cross sectional echocardiographic diagnosis of total anomalous pulmonary venous connection. Br. Heart J. *53*:525, 1985.
397. Galloway, A. C., Campbell, D. N., and Clarke, D. R.: The value of early repair for total anomalous pulmonary venous drainage. Pediatr. Cardiol. *6*:77, 1986.
398. Reardon, M. J., Cooley, D. A., Kubrusly, L., Ott, D. A., Johnson, W., Kay, G. L., and Sweeney, M. S.: Total anomalous pulmonary venous return: Report of 201 patients treated surgically. Texas Heart Inst. J. *12*:131, 1985.
399. Stark, J.: Anomalies of the pulmonary venous return. *In* Stark, J., and deLeval, M. (eds.): Surgery for Congenital Heart Defects. New York, Grune and Stratton, Inc., 1983, p. 235.
400. Matthew, R., Thilenius, O. G., Replogle, R. L., and Arcilla, R. A.: Cardiac function in total anomalous pulmonary venous return before and after surgery. Circulation *55*:361, 1977.
401. Healey, J. E.: An anatomic survey of anomalous pulmonary veins.: Their clinical significance. J. Thorac. Cardiovasc. Surg. *23*:433, 1952.
402. Gikonyo, D. K., Tandon, R., Lucas, R. V., Jr., and Edwards, J. E.: Scimitar syndrome in neonates: Report of four cases and review of the literature. Pediatr. Cardiol. *6*:193, 1986.
403. Stanger, P., Rudolph, A. M., and Edwards, J. E.: Cardiac malpositions: An overview based on a study of 65 necropsy specimens. Circulation *56*:159, 1977.
404. Van Praagh, R.: Diagnosis of complex congenital heart disease: Morphologic-anatomic method and terminology. Cardiovasc. Intervent. Radiol. *7*:115, 1984.
405. Tonkin, I. L. D.: The definition of cardiac malpositions with echocardiography and computed tomography. Pediatr. Cardiac Imaging 157, 1984.
406. Silverman, N. H.: An ultrasonic approach to the diagnosis of cardiac situs, connections, and malpositions. Pediatr. Cardiac Imaging 188, 1984.
407. Peoples, W. M., Moller, J. H., and Edwards, J. E.: Polysplenia: A review of 146 cases. Pediatr. Cardiol. *4*:129, 1983.
408. Nasser, W. K.: Congenital absence of the left pericardium. Am. J. Cardiol. *26*:466, 1970.
409. Morgan, J. R., Rogers, A. K., and Forker, A. D.: Congenital absence of the left pericardium: Clinical findings. Ann. Intern. Med. *74*:370, 1971.
410. Pernot, C., Hoeffel, J. C., and Henry, M.: Radiologic patterns of congenital malformation of the pericardium. Radiol. Clin. (Basel) *44*:505, 1975.
411. Nicolosi, G. L., Borgioni, L., Alberti, E., Burelli, C., Maffesanti, M., Marion, P., Slavich, G., and Zanuttini, D.: M-mode and two-dimensional echocardiography in congenital absence of the pericardium. Chest *81*:610, 1982.
412. Rowland, T. W., Twible, E. A., Norwood, W. I., Jr., and Keane, J. F.: Partial absence of the left pericardium diagnosis by two-dimensional echocardiography. Am. J. Dis. Child. *136*:628, 1982.
413. Schiavone, W. A., and O'Donnell, J. K.: Congenital absence of the left portion of parietal pericardium demonstrated by nuclear magnetic resonance imaging. Am. J. Cardiol. *55*:1439, 1985.
414. Jones, J. W., and McManus, B. M.: Fatal cardiac strangulation by congenital partial pericardial defect. Am. Heart J. *107*:183, 1984.
415. Rowland, T. W., Twible, E. A., Norwood, W. J., Jr., and Keane, J. F.: Partial absence of the left pericardium. Am. J. Dis. Child. *136*:628, 1982.
416. Rastelli, G., Kirklin, J. W., and Titus, J. L.: Anatomic observations on complete form of persistent common atrioventricular canal with special reference to atrioventricular valves. Mayo Clin. Proc. *41*:296, 1966.
417. Anderson, R. H., Macartney, F. J., Tynan, M., Becker, A. E., Freedom, R. M., Godman, M. J., Hunter, S., Quero-Jimenez, M., Rigby, M. L., Shinebourne, E. A., Sutherland, G., Smallhorn, J. G., Soto, G., Gaetano, T., Wilkinson, J. L., Wilcox, B. R., and Zuberbuhler, J. R.: Univentricular atrioventricular connection: The single ventricle trap unsprung. Pediatr. Cardiol. *4*:273, 1983.
418. Thies, W. R., Soto, B., Diethelm, E., Bargeron, L. M., Jr., and Pacifico, A. D.: Angiographic anatomy of hearts with one ventricular chamber: The true single ventricle. Am. J. Cardiol. *55*:1363, 1985.
419. Huhta, J. C., Seward, J. B., Tajik, A. J., Hagler, D. J., and Edwards, W. D.: Two-dimensional echocardiographic spectrum of univentricular atrioventricular connection. J. Am. Coll. Cardiol. *5*:149, 1985.
420. DiSessa, T. G., Isabel-Jones, J. G., Heins, H., Hernandez, J. G., Bloor, C., and Friedman, W. F.: Two-dimensional echocardiographic features of the univentricular heart. Cardiovasc. Ultrason. *3*:89, 1984.
421. Seward, J. B., Tajik, A. J., Haggler, D. J., and Ritter, D. G.: Contrast echocardiography in single or common ventricle. Circulation *55*:513, 1977.
422. Stefanelli, G., Kirklin, J. W., Naftel, D. C., Blackstone, E. H., Pacifico, A. D., Kirklin, J. K., Soto, B., and Bargeron, L. M., Jr.: Early and intermediate-term (10-year) results of surgery for univentricular atrioventricular connection ("single ventricle"). Am. J. Cardiol. *54*:811, 1984.
423. Pacifico, A. D., Kirklin, J. K., and Kirklin, J. W.: Surgical management of double inlet ventricle. World J. Surg. *9*:579, 1985.
424. Stevenson, O., Soderlund, S., Thoren, C., and Wallgren, G.: Arterial anomalies causing compression of the trachea and/or the esophagus. Acta Paediatr. Scand. *60*:81, 1971.
425. Park, C. D., Waldhausen, J. A., Friedman, S., Aberdeen, I., and Jamson, J.: Tracheal compression by the great arteries in the mediastinum: Report of 39 cases. Arch. Surg. *103*:626, 1971.
426. Koopot, R., Nikaido, H., and Idriss, F. S.: Surgical management of anomalous left pulmonary artery causing tracheobronchial obstruction: Pulmonary artery sling. J. Thorac. Cardiovasc. Surg. *69*:239, 1975.
427. Baron, R. L., Gutierrez, F. R., and McKnight, R. C.: Computed tomographic evaluation of the great arteries and aortic arch malformations. *In* Friedman, W. F., and Higgins, C. B. (eds.): Pediatric Cardiac Imaging. Philadelphia, W. B. Saunders Company, 1983, p. 135.
428. Biancaniello, T. M., and Heneghan, M. A.: Cardiac imaging with nuclear magnetic resonance: Technical considerations and potential clinical application. *In* Friedman, W. F., and Higgins, C. B. (eds): Pediatric Cardiac Imaging. Philadelphia, W. B. Saunders Company, 1983, p. 270.
429. deLeval, M.: Vascular rings. *In* Stark, J., and deLeval, M. (eds.): Surgery for Congenital Heart Defects. New York, Grune and Stratton, Inc., 1983, p. 227.
430. Garson, A., Jr.: Arrhythmias in pediatric patients. Med. Clin. North Am. *68*:1171, 1984.
431. Anderson, R. H., Wenick, A. C. G., Losekoot, T. G., and Becker, A. E.: Congenitally complete heart block. Circulation *56*:90, 1977.
432. Litsey, S. E., Noonan, J. A., O'Connor, W. N., Cottrill, C. M., and Mitchell, B.: Maternal connective tissue disease and congenital heart block. N. Engl. J. Med. *312*:98, 1985.
433. Thilenius, O. G., Chiemmongkoltip, P., Cassels, D. E., and Arcilla, R. A.: Hemodynamic studies in children with congenital atrioventricular block. Am. J. Cardiol. *30*:13, 1972.
434. Mahoney, L. T., Marvin, W. J., Jr., Atkins, D. L., Clark, E. B., and Lauer, R. M.: Pacemaker management for acute onset of heart block in childhood. J. Pediatr. *107*:207, 1985.
435. Beder, S. D., Hanisch, D. G., Cohen, M. H., Van Heeckeren, D., Ankeney, J. L., and Riemenschneider, T. A.: Cardiac pacing in children: A 15-year experience. Am. Heart J. *109*:152, 1985.
436. Epstein, M. L., Knauf, D. G., and Alexander, J. A.: Long-term follow-up of transvenous cardiac pacing in children. Am. J. Cardiol. *57*:889, 1986.
437. Michaelsson, M., and Engle, M. A.: Congenital complete heart block: An international study of the natural history. Cardiovasc. Clin. *4*:85, 1982.
438. Kleinman, C. S., Donnerstein, R. L., DeVore, G. R., Jaffee, C. C., Lynch, D. C., Berkowitz, R. L., Talner, N. S., and Hobbins, J. C.: Fetal echocardiography for evaluation of in utero congestive heart failure. N. Engl. J. Med. *306*:568, 1982.
439. Radford, D. J., Izukawa, T., and Rowe, R. D.: Congenital paroxysmal atrial tachycardia. Arch. Dis. Child. *51*:613, 1976.
440. Deal, B. J., Keane, J. F., Gillette, P. C., and Gardon, A., Jr.: Wolff-Parkinson-White syndrome and supraventricular tachycardia during infancy: Management and follow-up. J. Am. Coll. Cardiol. *5*:130, 1985.
441. Benson, D. W., Jr., Dunnigan, A., Benditt, D. G., Thompson, T. R., Narayan, A., and Boros, S.: Prediction of digoxin treatment failure in infants with supraventricular tachycardia: Role of transesophageal pacing. Pediatrics *75*:288, 1985.
442. Gillette, P. C.: Supraventricular arrhythmias in children. J. Am. Coll. Cardiol. *5*:122B, 1985.
443. Ott, D. A., Garson, A., Cooley, D. A., and McNamara, D. G.: Definitive operation for refractory cardiac tachyarrhythmias in children. J. Thorac. Cardiovasc. Surg. *90*:681, 1985.
444. Holmes, D. R., Jr., Danielson, G. K., Gersh, B. J., Osborn, M. J., Wood, D. L., McLaran, C., Sugrue, D. D., Porter, C. J., and Hammill, S. C.: Surgical treatment of accessory atrioventricular pathways and symptomatic talchycardia in children and young adults. Am. J. Cardiol. *55*:1509, 1985.
445. Garson, A., Jr., Bink-Boelkens, M., Hesslein, P. S., Hordof, A. J., Keane, J. F., Neches, W. H., and Porter, C. J.: Atrial flutter in the young: A collaborative study of 380 cases. J. Am. Coll. Cardiol. *6*:871, 1985.
446. Dunnigan, A., Benson, W., Jr., and Benditt, D. G.: Atrial flutter in infancy: Diagnosis, clinical features and treatment. Pediatrics *75*:725, 1985.
447. Garson, A., Jr., Gillette, P. C., Titus, J. L., Hawkins, E., Kearney, D., Ott, D., Cooley, D. A., and McNamara, D. G.: Surgical treatment of ventricular tachycardia in infants. N. Engl. J. Med. *310*:1443, 1984.

31 CONGENITAL HEART DISEASE IN THE ADULT

by KENNETH M. BOROW, M.D., and
EUGENE BRAUNWALD, M.D.

GENERAL PRINCIPLES

During the past 25 years, more than 500,000 patients with functionally important cardiac malformations have attained adulthood. As a consequence, the adult with congenital heart disease, often after complete or partial surgical correction, represents a growing challenge to the cardiologist treating adults.[2, 3] The magnitude of this success is due primarily to the medical and surgical advances achieved since the early 1960's. For years, cardiac catheterization was the study of choice for diagnosis of intracardiac and extracardiac defects and was appropriately considered the gold standard. Recently, with two-dimensional echocardiographic imaging, especially in conjunction with quantitative Doppler echocardiography, invasive studies have been avoided in many adults with congenital heart disease.[3a] These procedures supply highly accurate anatomical and physiological information at low cost and minimal patient discomfort. For the first time, multiple serial assessments are easily possible in patients with congenital heart disease. In the future, even more noninvasive delineation of cardiac anatomy may be possible, using magnetic resonance imaging and rapid acquisition computerized tomographic techniques[3b] (Chap. 12).

At present, palliative or corrective surgical procedures have been developed for almost all congenital cardiac anomalies. With recent advances in cardiac as well as heart-lung transplantation techniques, and their application to infants and children, the day may soon arrive when *all* cardiac anomalies are amenable to surgery. The net result will be further increases in the number of patients born with congenital heart disease who survive to adulthood. Such patients, in nearly all cases, have residual or potential problems that require close medical follow-up.[4, 4a, 5] This task will fall increasingly on the adult cardiologist. It is therefore of great importance that clinicians understand the anatomy, pathophysiology, clinical presentation, diagnostic approaches, and medical as well as surgical natural histories of those congenital cardiac defects in which survival to adulthood is relatively common.

RELATIVE INCIDENCE IN ADULTS AND CHILDREN. The relative incidence of the various congenital heart lesions in adults differs from that in children. Complex congenital lesions are considerably more common in children than in adults. Ventricular septal defect is the most common cardiovascular malformation diagnosed in children, whereas stenosis of a congenital bicuspid aortic valve and atrial septal defect are the lesions most frequently found in adults. In infants the most common cardiac lesion producing cyanosis is transposition of the great arteries, whereas in the adult population it is tetralogy of Fallot.

Occasionally congenital heart disease remains undetected until the patient reaches adulthood. Two factors contribute to this delay in diagnosis: First, in children, a cardiovascular malformation may go unrecognized or may be mistaken for a functional murmur because of the subtle manner in which it becomes manifested. The classic example of this situation is the small or moderate-sized isolated atrial septal defect. Second, medical attention may be inadequate, particularly for children who grow up in medically underserved areas, and as a consequence cardiovascular anomalies of even moderate severity may go undetected.

GENETICS AND CONGENITAL HEART DISEASE (See also pp. 897 and 1624). As an increasing number of women with congenital heart disease reach childbearing age, the need for detailed information regarding the etiology, as well as the risk of recurrence, of congenital lesions becomes more apparent. Nora and Nora reported that the cause of congenital heart disease is predominantly genetic in 8 per cent of cases and predominantly environmental in 2 per cent. In the remaining 90 per cent, a complex interaction between genetic and environmental factors is thought to exist.[5a] Not surprisingly, the greater the number of affected first-degree relatives with congenital heart disease within the family, the greater the risk of recurrence. The recurrence risk is somewhat higher if the affected first-degree relative is a parent rather than a sibling. When two first-

TABLE 31–1 RECURRENCE RISK IN SIBLINGS IF A PATIENT HAS A SPECIFIC FORM OF CONGENITAL HEART DISEASE

	Nora	Anderson	Allen
Aortic valve atresia	1.1%	—	3.6%
Coarctation of the aorta	1.8%	0.8%	6.6%
Tetralogy of Fallot	3.0%	2.1%	1.6%
Transposition of the great arteries	1.7%	0%	0%
Truncus arteriosus	1.1%	—	7.7%
Complex congenital heart disease	—	1.2%	8.9%
Simple lesions	3.4%	2.1%	3.5%
Pulmonary stenosis			
Ventricular septal defect			
Persistent ductus arteriosus			
Atrial septal defect			

Modified from Allan, L. D., et al.: Familial recurrence of congenital heart disease in a prospective series of mothers referred for fetal echocardiography. Am. J. Cardiol. 58:334, 1986.

degree relatives are affected, the recurrence risk for the next child becomes two to three times as great compared with the case when only one first-degree relative is affected.[5a–7]

Fetal echocardiography performed at an early stage in pregnancy has been used as a screening procedure for recurrences of cardiac anomalies in mothers with a family history of congenital heart disease.[7–9] Allan and coworkers reported on 1021 such mothers.[7] The overall recurrence rate was 2 per cent with a previously affected child and 10 per cent with two previously affected children. These results may reflect more complete collection of data than was previously possible in studies based solely on postnatal information. As seen in Table 31–1, certain forms of congenital heart disease recur much more frequently than others.

PSYCHOSOCIAL EFFECTS OF CONGENITAL HEART DISEASE ON THE YOUNG ADULT. The functional capabilities and self-image of children with congenital heart disease may influence their subsequent level of performance as adults. Wright and coworkers addressed this issue in 188 young adult patients ranging in age from 16 to 23 years.[10] The diagnoses were divided fairly evenly between isolated valvular aortic stenosis, isolated valvular pulmonary stenosis, and tetralogy of Fallot. Subjects were interviewed and evaluated by a psychologist, given tests of physical endurance, including a treadmill exercise electrocardiogram, and questioned about their history by both a cardiologist and a rehabilitation medicine specialist. Overall, physical function scores were slightly below average. Childhood activities had been affected in 30 per cent of the patients but seriously disrupted in only 17 per cent. School experiences had been positive, with two-thirds of patients seeking post-high school-level education; antisocial activities were uncommon. Subjects had few specific health concerns, although many wanted more information about life style implications of their heart disease. These young adults are similar to most older patients with congenital heart disease in that they are socially adaptable, capable of living productive lives, and often aided by counseling.[10a]

INSURABILITY OF PATIENTS WITH CONGENITAL HEART DISEASE. Most patients with congenital heart disease can purchase life insurance. However, in most cases the premium rates they must pay are increased. In general, only patients with very simple lesions are insured at regular rates. Such lesions include mild valvular pulmonary stenosis as well as uncomplicated, surgically corrected atrial and ventricular septal defects, persistent ductus arteriosus, and valvular pulmonary stenosis. Table 31–2 provides a general guideline for insurability of young patients with congenital heart disease.[11] Note that the actuarial survival statistics for most lesions after surgery are not available past early adult life. Not until this data base becomes more complete will a uniform standard of insurability be available for older patients with congenital heart disease.

TABLE 31–2 GENERAL GUIDELINE FOR INSURABILITY OF YOUNG PATIENTS WITH CONGENITAL HEART DISEASE

	Standard Rates	Increased Rates	Not Insurable
Aortic regurgitation			
a. Mild or moderate		X	
b. Severe			X
Aortic stenosis			
a. Mild or moderate		X	
b. Postoperative		X	
c. Subvalvular, mild		X	
d. Subvalvular, postoperative		X	
e. Supravalvular, postoperative		X	
Atrial septal defect			
a. Large	X		
b. Postoperative			X
c. Postoperative with sinus node dysfunction			X
Coarctation of the aorta			
a. Mild		X	
b. Moderate or severe			X
c. Postoperative with normal BP		X	
d. Postoperative with residual hypertension			X
Congenital complete heart block		X	
D-Transposition of the great arteries			
a. Preoperative			X
b. Postoperative		X	
Ebstein's anomaly			
a. Mild			X
b. Moderate			X
Persistent ductus arteriosus			
a. Preoperative			X
b. Postoperative	X		
Pulmonic stenosis			
a. Mild	X		
b. Moderate or severe			X
c. Postoperative	X		
Tetralogy of Fallot			
a. Preoperative			X
b. Postoperative		X	
Tricuspid atresia			X
Truncus arteriosus			X
Ventricular septal defect			
a. Small or moderate		X	
b. Postoperative			
1. Uncomplicated	X		
2. Residual shunt		X	
3. Residual pulmonary vascular obstructive disease			X

Modified from Truesdell, S. C., et al.: Life Insurance in Children with Cardiovascular Disease. Pediatrics 77:687, 1986.

SPECIFIC MALFORMATIONS

CONGENITAL ABNORMALITIES OF THE LEFT VENTRICULAR OUTFLOW TRACT

(See also p. 932)

Congenital abnormalities of the left ventricular outflow tract can occur at valvular, subvalvular, or supravalvular levels. Because of the high survival rate of surgery for left ventricular outflow tract obstruction in childhood, many of the patients, when seen as adults, will have already undergone at least one surgical procedure.

ANATOMY. Congenital malformations of the aortic valve are present in 1 to 2 per cent of the total adult population and are much more common in males than in females. The common cause of congenital valvular aortic stenosis (AS) is the bicuspid valve, with peripheral fusion of the leaflets and diminished effective orifice size[11a] (Fig. 31–1). A raphe or ridge is frequently present on the larger of the cusps.[12] Much less common are unicuspid, quadricuspid, or congenitally stenotic trileaflet aortic valves. Perhaps most frequent is a bicuspid valve that is functionally normal early in life; it may become thickened, fibrotic, calcified, and stenotic during adulthood.[12a] Congenital valvular AS may be associated with coarctation of the aorta and, less frequently, ventricular septal defect or isolated pulmonic stenosis.[13] In the young or middle-aged adult, isolated valvular AS is usually congenital rather than rheumatic in origin.[13, 14] By age 45, approximately 50 per cent of all bicuspid valves show some degree of stenosis.[13, 15] The frequency and severity of valvular narrowing increase with age, in part reflecting progressive calcium deposition within the leaflets.[16] Aortic valve prolapse in association with bicuspid aortic valve may also occur.[12, 17, 18] The degree of prolapse is unrelated to patient age or cusp asymmetry. Aortic regurgitation requiring valve replacement may occur on the basis of valve prolapse, intrinsic abnormalities in leaflet coaptation, or valve infection. All patients with congenital abnormalities of the aortic valve require antibiotic prophylaxis against infective endocarditis.

In adults, subvalvular AS can be discrete (so-called membranous or diaphragmatic) or more fibromuscular (i.e., ridge-like).[19] Some dynamic component can be present in either type. Subaortic stenosis is more common in males than in females. Whether it is truly a congenital lesion in all cases remains uncertain, since severe and rapid progression of subvalvular obstruction has been demonstrated during early infancy.[20, 21] Aortic regurgitation, which commonly accompanies congenital subaortic stenosis, may reflect repeated trauma to the undersurface of the aortic valve leaflets, leading to fibrosis and thickening. The regurgitation may be progressive even after surgical relief of the subaortic obstruction. In rare cases, combined stenosis at the valvular and subvalvular levels may occur.[22]

Two types of *supravalvular AS* are seen in adults.[23] Most frequently encountered is an hourglass deformity with segmental narrowing of the ascending aorta just above the aortic valve. The aortic arch and descending aorta are of normal caliber. In the less common hypoplastic form, there is diffuse or tubular narrowing of the entire ascending aorta, aortic arch, and descending aorta. In either type, there may be some degree of attachment between the aortic valve cusps and anterior supravalvular tissue. Supravalvular aortic stenosis may be familial, sporadic, or, rarely, the result of congenital rubella infection. When combined with mental retardation and "elfin facies" (Fig. 30–37, p. 937), the diagnosis of Williams' syndrome can be made.[24] All forms of supravalvular AS may be associated with peripheral pulmonary artery stenosis. Because the coronary arteries are proximal to the level of obstruction, they are exposed to abnormally elevated systolic pressures. This results in hypertrophy of the vessel walls and predisposes to premature coronary arteriosclerosis. Congenital supravalvular AS should be distinguished from its acquired counterpart, which is usually due to atherosclerotic lesions of the aortic root and coronary ostia in patients with familial hypercholesterolemia[25] (see p. 1179).

PATHOPHYSIOLOGY. Regardless of the etiology or level of left ventricular outflow tract obstruction, left ventricular

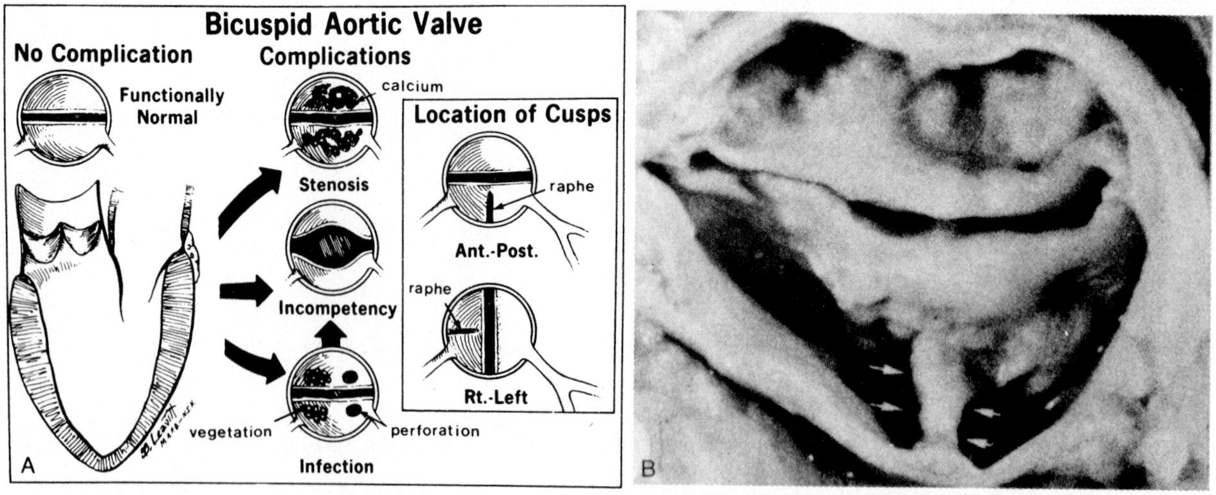

FIGURE 31–1. *A,* The congenitally bicuspid aortic valve. The location of the cusps and raphes and the acquired complications of the congenital malformation are depicted. *B,* Calcified, stenotic, congenitally bicuspid aortic valve. The cusps are situated anteriorly and posteriorly, and the commissures right and left respectively. The valve has a raphe (white arrows) in the anterior cusp. Valve of a 61-year-old man. At catheterization 2 years before his death, the peak systolic gradient across the valve was 45 mm Hg when the cardiac index was 2.6 liters/min/m^2. He had complete heart block secondary to destruction of the atrioventricular bundle by calcium. (From Roberts, W. C.: Congenital cardiovascular abnormalities usually silent until adulthood, *In* Roberts, W. C. [ed.]: Adult Congenital Heart Disease. Philadelphia, F. A. Davis Co., 1987, pp. 646 and 647.)

systolic hypertension is present and acts as a stimulus for the development of concentric hypertrophy. Left ventricular compliance is frequently decreased, resulting in elevations of left ventricular end-diastolic and left atrial mean pressures and resulting symptoms of pulmonary congestion. Because of increased left ventricular muscle mass and high intracavitary systolic pressure, left ventricular ischemia may occur even in the absence of significant coronary artery disease. Ischemia is uncommon in supravalvular AS because coronary arterial pressure rises pari passu with left ventricular systolic pressure. In some patients with severe stenosis, cardiac output may not increase appropriately during exercise, reflecting severe mechanical obstruction of the outflow tract and/or left ventricular dysfunction. This can result in exercise-induced syncope or presyncope.

SYMPTOMS. The major symptoms of congenital left ventricular outflow tract obstruction in the adult include angina pectoris, syncope, and congestive heart failure.[14] Sudden death during exercise can occur in patients with severe stenosis but is seldom the presenting event in a previously undiagnosed or asymptomatic adult.[26] In patients with valvular AS, hemodynamic and clinical compensation are common until middle age. However, from the time of onset of symptoms, the average survival in patients with unrepaired severe valvular AS is less than 5 years.[26]

PHYSICAL EXAMINATION. The predominant physical finding in the adult with congenital valvular AS is a harsh systolic ejection murmur, loudest along the right upper sternal edge and radiating along the carotid arteries (Figs. 3–22, p. 56, and 4–4, p. 67). In mild to moderate valvular AS, an ejection click caused by abrupt cessation of movement of the thickened, doming leaflets is frequently present (Fig. 3–11, p. 48). In contrast to the click found in pulmonic stenosis, the aortic click does *not* vary in intensity with respiration. As the severity of the valvular AS increases, the murmur becomes longer and louder and peaks later during systole. The carotid pulse demonstrates the characteristic findings of a delayed upstroke and systolic shudder. The apical precordial impulse is often heaving and sustained, with a palpable atrial presystolic lift. In subvalvular AS (Fig. 4–5, p. 67), the early systolic ejection click is absent and a murmur of aortic regurgitation is more common. In supravalvular AS, a prominent thrill and systolic murmur are frequently present over the right upper precordial, suprasternal notch and carotid areas. The arterial pressure is 10 to 15 mm Hg higher in the right than in the left arm.

NONINVASIVE STUDIES. The *electrocardiogram* shows a variable degree of left ventricular hypertrophy (p. 191). Approximately three-fourths of adult patients with severe valvular AS (left ventricular to aortic pressure gradient greater than 75 mm Hg) exhibit left ventricular hypertrophy with strain. This finding is less common in patients with mild to moderate obstruction (Table 31–3).

On *chest roentgenography*, poststenotic dilatation of the ascending aorta is common in patients with valvular AS. However, this finding does not correlate well with the severity of the obstruction. Calcification of the aortic valve becomes evident with increasing frequency during the third decade of life. Overall heart size is usually normal until left ventricular failure occurs, although the left ventricle may be prominent in patients with only moderate

TABLE 31–3 ELECTROCARDIOGRAPHIC PATTERNS ASSOCIATED WITH CONGENITAL HEART DISEASE

	Electrocardiographic Pattern																
Cardiac Defect	Atrial Flutter/Fibrillation	Supraventricular Tachycardia	Ventricular Arrhythmia	Atrioventricular Block	Preexcitation Syndrome	Abnormal P-wave Orientation	Right Atrial Overload	Left Atrial Overload	Left Bundle Branch Block	Left Axis Deviation	Right Bundle Branch Block	Right Ventricular Volume Overload	Right Ventricular Pressure Overload	Left Ventricular Volume Overload	Left Ventricular Pressure Overload	Biventricular Overload	Abnormal Q Waves or Myocardial Infarction Pattern
Atrial septal defect (secundum)	++	+	0	+	0	+	++	+	0	0	+	+++	+	0	0	0	0
Prolapsed mitral valve syndrome	+	+	+	0	+	0	0	+	0	0	0	0	0	+	0	0	0
Aortic stenosis	0	0	+	+	0	0	0	+	+	+	0	0	0	0	+++	0	0
Idiopathic hypertrophic subaortic stenosis	+	0	++	0	+	0	0	++	++	++	0	0	0	0	+++	0	++
Pulmonary stenosis	0	0	0	0	0	0	++	0	0	0	+	+	+++	0	0	0	0
Ventricular septal defect	+	0	0	0	0	0	0	+	+	0	0	0	0	+++	0	+	0
Patent ductus arteriosus	+	0	0	0	0	0	0	++	+	+	0	0	0	+++	0	+	0
Tetralogy of Fallot	0	0	+	0	0	0	++	0	+	0	+	0	+++	0	0	+	0
Coarctation of aorta	+	0	0	0	0	0	0	+	+	0	0	0	0	0	++	0	0
Eisenmenger syndrome	+	0	+	0	0	0	++	0	0	0	+	0	+++	0	0	+	0
Atrial septal defect (primum)	++	+	0	++	0	0	+	+	+++	0	+	+++	+	+	0	+	0
Corrected transposition*	+	+	0	+++	+	0	+	+	+	0	0	0	0	+	+	+	+++
Ebstein's anomaly	++	+++	0	+	++	0	+++	0	+	0	+++	+	0	0	0	0	0
Tricuspid atresia	+	+	+	0	0	0	+++	+	+++	+	0	0	0	+	+	0	+
Congenital anomalies of coronary arteries	+	0	++	0	0	0	0	++	++	+	0	0	0	+	+	0	+++
Transposition of great arteries (postop)	+	++	0	+	0	0	+	0	0	0	0	0	+++	0	0	0	0

+ + + = Almost always seen (characteristic of defect).
+ + = Commonly seen with defect.
+ = Sometimes seen with defect (especially with associated defects or advancing age).
0 = Rarely seen with defect.

*The precordial QRS progression in corrected transposition may mimic left ventricular hypertrophy, usually with ST-segment abnormalities. True hypertrophy of the left-sided ventricle can occur in corrected transposition from associated left atrioventricular valvular regurgitation, ventricular septal defect, and so on.

From Ellison, R. C., and Sloss, L. J.: Electrocardiographic features of congenital heart disease in the adult. *In* Roberts, W. C. (ed.): Congenital Heart Disease in Adults. Philadelphia, F. A. Davis Co., 1987, pp. 168–169.

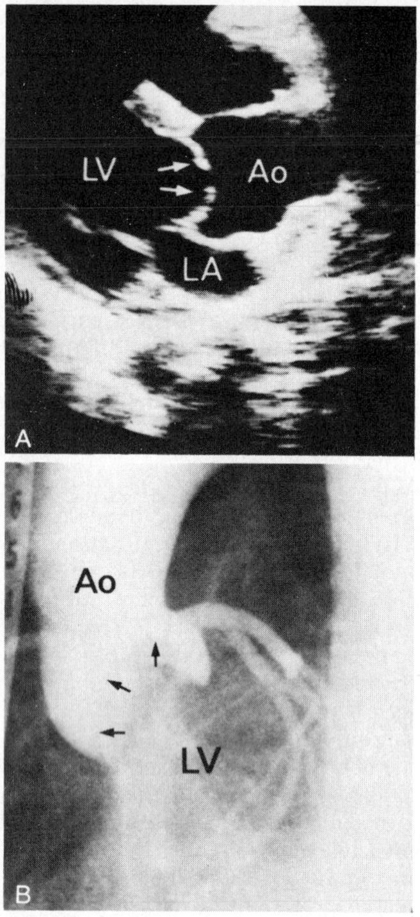

FIGURE 31–2. Valvular aortic stenosis. Echocardiographic and angiographic findings in a young adult. *A,* Two-dimensional echocardiographic study with the transducer in the long-axis parasternal position demonstrating leaflet doming and thickening (arrows). *B,* Aortogram from the same patient showing doming of the aortic valve leaflets. The negative shadow in the proximal aortic root (Ao) is caused by a jet of nonopacified blood from the left ventricle (LV) as it exits through the stenotic aortic valve. LA = left atrium.

obstruction (gradient of approximately 50 mm Hg) even without failure. In neither subvalvular nor supravalvular AS is dilatation of the proximal aorta present.

Echocardiography. This has become the noninvasive technique of choice for the diagnosis and physiological assessment of left ventricular outflow tract obstruction in adults (p. 108). By M-mode echocardiography, the bicuspid aortic valve is often thickened with an eccentric closure line, reflecting the asymmetry of the valve leaflets. Rather than opening fully with ventricular systole, the leaflets frequently show a doming pattern. When this occurs, leaflet excursion seen by M-mode study may not accurately reflect the severity of the stenosis. This problem can be solved in part by the use of two-dimensional echocardiography to demonstrate leaflet doming on the long-axis parasternal view and the presence of only two leaflets on the short-axis parasternal view (Fig. 31–2; also see Figs. 5–67, p. 113, and 30–33, p. 934). Using this technique, Brandenburg and coworkers demonstrated a sensitivity, specificity, and diagnostic accuracy for bicuspid aortic valve of 78, 96, and 93 per cent, respectively.[12] Two-dimensional echocardiography is also useful in diagnosing the presence of associated intracardiac anomalies.[17, 21, 27] In subvalvular AS, M-mode echocardiography in conjunction with two-dimensional imaging demonstrates the presence and type of obstruction.[19] Supravalvular AS is well assessed using two-dimensional echocardiography, with which the extent and type of narrowing involving the ascending aorta can be determined (Fig. 30–38, p. 938). Magnetic resonance imaging (Chap. 12) has also been used successfully to diagnose this lesion (Fig. 31–3).[28]

Doppler echocardiography acts synergistically with ultrasound imaging (two-dimensional echocardiography) to provide a noninvasive estimate of pressure gradients in patients with obstruction to left ventricular outflow. The *pulsed* Doppler technique allows *localization* of the level of obstruction.[29] This is particularly important in differentiating between subvalvular, valvular, and supravalvular stenoses. *Continuous-wave* Doppler allows accurate *quantitation* of peak instantaneous and mean systolic gradients across the level of obstruction[30–35] (p. 99). When continuous-wave Doppler and calibrated carotid pulse tracings are recorded simultaneously, accurate estimates of left ventricular instantaneous pressures over the course of ventricular ejection are possible.[36] Finally, color flow Doppler mapping (p. 88) permits assessment of the direction and magnitude of aortic regurgitation, a common complication in adults with congenitally bicuspid valves, as well as the detection of associated intracardiac shunts.

NATURAL HISTORY—MEDICAL. Results of studies on the natural history of congenital valvular AS depend largely on the bias introduced into patient selection. This is true

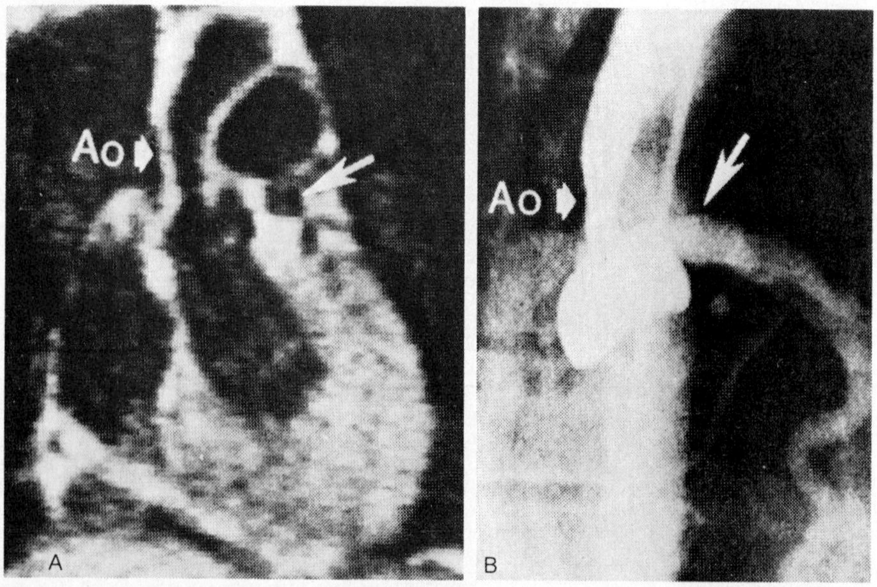

FIGURE 31–3. Supravalvular aortic stenosis. *A,* Left anterior oblique magnetic resonance image from a young woman revealing severe left ventricular hypertrophy, tubular stenosis of the ascending aorta (Ao) (short arrow), and dilated left main coronary artery (long arrow). *B,* Aortogram from the same patient demonstrating diffuse supravalvular aortic stenosis (short arrow) and a dilated left coronary artery (long arrow). (From Boxer, R. A., et al.: Diagnosis and postoperative evaluation of supravalvular aortic stenosis by magnetic resonance imaging. Am. J. Cardiol. *58*:368, 1986.)

because the time of onset of symptoms and the severity of obstruction can vary dramatically among patients. For example, in Campbell's classic study of patients with unoperated congenital AS, only 70 per cent survived to age 25 years.[37] Similarly, Reid and Coleman reported that 34 per cent of their 128 patients with congenital AS required surgical intervention before the age of 20 years.[38] In contrast, patients with bicuspid aortic valves, many of which are nonstenotic at birth, can reach old age before requiring surgery.[39] The decision of when to operate for congenital valvular AS in adults depends on multiple factors, including the severity and type of symptoms, the calculated aortic valve area, and the state of left ventricular function.[26, 40] Interestingly, symptoms caused by left ventricular systolic dysfunction are uncommon in patients under 40 years of age; in fact, left ventricular performance may be hyperkinetic in children and young adults.[41] However, pressure overload hypertrophy in valvular AS is often associated with abnormal early diastolic relaxation and filling, particularly in adults. This raises left ventricular diastolic and pulmonary capillary pressures and may be responsible for dyspnea in patients with AS.[42, 43]

The level of acceptable physical activity in young adult patients with AS is frequently a controversial issue. According to the Task Force for Congenital Heart Disease of the American College of Cardiology,[44] patients with mild AS (<20 mm Hg peak systolic gradient at rest) and normal left ventricular performance can participate in all competitive sports. Patients with moderate AS (gradient at rest between 20 and 40 mm Hg) can participate in low-intensity sports if mild or no left ventricular hypertrophy or strain is present on the electrocardiogram and if the exercise tolerance test is normal and no serious arrhythmias are present on the 24-hour ambulatory ECG. Patients with greater than 40 mm Hg peak systolic pressure gradient at rest should not participate in competitive sports.

In general, criteria used in the selection of patients for surgical treatment include a peak systolic ejection gradient in excess of 75 mm Hg and a mean systolic gradient exceeding 40 to 50 mm Hg, in association with a normal forward cardiac output and an aortic valve area less than approximately 0.7 cm^2 (0.4 cm^2/m^2 body surface area). In patients with reduced forward cardiac output, the peak and mean systolic ejection gradients may be low, reflecting underlying myocardial dysfunction or afterload mismatch. In such patients, calculation of the aortic valve area is vital for determining the hemodynamic significance of the left ventricular outflow tract obstruction.

NATURAL HISTORY—INTERVENTIONAL THERAPY. *Percutaneous balloon valvuloplasty* (p. 1059) may become the procedure of choice in young adult patients with congenital valvular AS. Early reports in adults suggest that balloon valvuloplasty can result in significant improvement in ventricular performance and valvular function without the production of life-threatening complications[45–49] (Figs. 31–4 and 40–22, p. 1391). The mechanisms by which balloon angioplasty causes improvement of valvular function include separation of fused commissures, fracture of nodular calcification, and stretching of rigid leaflets.

Surgery. The young adult with severe valvular AS but *without* calcification of the valve may be a candidate for aortic valvulotomy. However, residual or recurrent stenosis as well as valvular incompetence are frequent complications of this procedure.[26, 50, 51] The palliative nature of this procedure was emphasized by the study of Hsieh et al.[52] The clinical courses of 59 patients who underwent valvotomy for AS after 1 year of age were reviewed. Mean follow-up period was 17.7 years. Actuarial analysis indicated that the probability of survival was 94 per cent at 5 years and 77 per cent at 22 years. Thirteen patients died, seven of whom did so suddenly. The probability of being free of serious events (defined as death, reoperation, and endocarditis) was 92 per cent at 5 years but only 39 per cent at 22 years after valvotomy. In the older patient, aortic valve replacement is often necessary, owing to leaflet calcification and fibrosis.

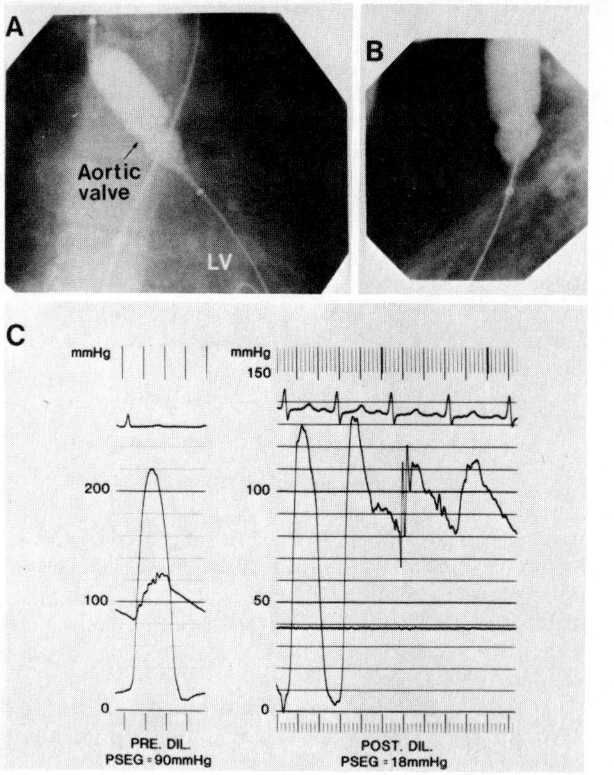

FIGURE 31–4. Valvular aortic stenosis. *A* and *B*, angiographic views of the indentation produced in an inflated balloon by a stenotic aortic valve in a young adult. *C*, Left ventricular and aortic pressure tracing in the same patient demonstrating a reduction in peak systolic ejection gradient (PSEG) from 90 mm Hg pre-dilation (pre dil) to 18 mm Hg immediately post-dilation (post dil). (Courtesy of James Lock, M.D.)

In patients with subaortic stenosis, resection of the obstructing lesion is performed through the proximal aortic root. In some cases, septal myectomy or myotomy is required. In symptomatic patients with left ventricular outflow tract obstruction that is not readily amenable to repair by conventional methods, a left ventricular to aortic conduit may be necessary.[53] Such patients most often have severe annular AS or severe long-segment fibromuscular stenosis. Finally, patients with supravalvular AS are most successfully treated with patch aortoplasty.[23] Although this effectively reduces the supravalvular obstruction, residual abnormalities remain, including AS and aortic insufficiency.

Long-Term Surgical Follow-up. Late results of operations performed for relief of left ventricular outflow tract obstruction in young patients are increasingly important to the adult cardiologist. In a large cumulative study,[50] patients operated on between the ages of 1 and 18 years were evaluated between 5 and 14 years postoperatively. The operative mortalities for the 522 patients with valvular AS and for the 222 patients with fixed valvular AS were 1.9 per cent and 6 per cent, respectively. Late survival rates were 90 per cent (472 of 522) and 86 per cent (190 of 222), respectively. Fifty-three per cent of those patients operated on for valvular and 54 per cent of those operated on for subvalvular stenosis had satisfactory late results, defined as freedom from residual or recurrent left ventricular outflow tract obstruction, clinically significant aortic regurgitation, reoperation, endocarditis, or late death. Thus it appears that operations performed during childhood for many patients with left ventricular outflow tract obstruction are palliative rather than curative. The long-term implications of this situation in an emerging population of young adults remain undefined. It is likely that reoperation with aortic valve replacement during adult life will be necessary in a large proportion of patients in whom aortic valvulotomy or balloon angioplasty was carried out during infancy or childhood.

ATRIAL SEPTAL DEFECT

(See also p. 915)

Atrial septal defect (ASD) accounts for 7 per cent of all congenital heart disease and for 30 per cent of congenital heart disease in adults, in whom it is second only to bicuspid aortic valve in frequency of occurrence. Failure to suspect this lesion is the most common cause of clinical misdiagnosis.

ANATOMY. ASD's can be divided into three anatomical types (Fig. 30–11, p. 915).[53a] The most common is the *ostium secundum* defect, which accounts for approximately 70 per cent of all ASD's. It is located in the region of the fossa ovalis and may be either single or fenestrated. Secundum ASD is three times more common in females than in males and is particularly common in the Holt-Oram syndrome. Approximately 20 to 30 per cent of patients with secundum ASD will have associated mitral valve prolapse (p. 1045) or findings suggestive of myxomatous abnormality of the mitral valve.[54, 55] This may explain the high incidence of mitral regurgitation in patients with ASD's over 50 years of age. Other lesions associated with secundum ASD include pulmonic and mitral valve stenoses. The combination of ASD and rheumatic mitral stenosis (Lutembacher syndrome) is now rare.[56] Patients with Lutembacher syndrome have peripheral edema, exertional dyspnea, and fatigue in the absence of significant orthopnea and paroxysmal nocturnal dyspnea. The lack of symptoms of pulmonary venous hypertension is due to decompression of left atrial pressures through the ASD. If the ASD is repaired without relief of the mitral stenosis, pulmonary edema may occur.

The second category of ASD is the *sinus venosus* type, accounting for approximately 15 per cent of all ASDs. This defect is usually located in the upper portion of the interatrial septum near the orifice of the superior vena cava.[57, 58] It is most often crescent-shaped and may be associated with partial anomalous pulmonary venous drainage of the right upper lobe or other right-sided pulmonary veins. The right middle and right lower lobes are almost never involved without involvement of the right upper lobe.

The third type is the *ostium primum* ASD. This also accounts for about 15 per cent of the total. It results from a defect in the lower portion of the atrial septum, the area of the ostium primum.[59] It is often associated with a "cleft" anterior leaflet of the mitral valve as well as abnormal attachments of rudimentary chordae tendineae to the upper rim of the ventricular septum. The septal leaflet of the tricuspid valve may be similarly cleft. Atrioventricular valvular regurgitation may be present from birth. The AV node is frequently displaced posteriorly and the left anterior fascicle of the conduction system may be hypoplastic. This results in early activation of the posterobasal aspect of the left ventricle and the ECG finding of marked left-axis deviation.

PATHOPHYSIOLOGY. Blood flow through the ASD occurs primarily during late systole, early ventricular diastole, and atrial systole. The magnitude of the left-to-right shunt depends on the size of the defect, the relationship of the right and left ventricular compliances, and the ratio of the pulmonary-to-systemic vascular resistance.[60–61a] The net result in an uncomplicated ASD is volume overload and enlargement of the right atrium and right ventricle without dilatation of the left-sided cardiac chambers. Because the right ventricle is more compliant than the left, blood preferentially enters the right-sided chambers of the heart.[60] If pulmonary artery hypertension occurs, associated with right ventricular hypertrophy and diminished ventricular compliance, the magnitude of the left-to-right shunt decreases. In some cases, pulmonary vascular obstructive disease with subsequent right-to-left shunting across the ASD may occur.[62] Elevations in pulmonary artery pressures may also be caused by high transpulmonary flow rather than by increased pulmonary vascular resistance. Prolonged exposure of the pulmonary bed to increased blood flow does not invariably result in pulmonary vascular obstructive disease.[63] In sinus venosus ASD, even without pulmonary hypertension, a right-to-left shunt may be the result of blood streaming from the superior vena cava directly into the left atrium.

SYMPTOMS. Dyspnea, fatigue, respiratory illness, and supraventricular arrhythmias are the most common presenting problems.[63, 64] While more than two-thirds of patients 1 to 10 years of age with secundum ASD will have no symptoms, only 4 per cent of those over 40 years of age will be totally asymptomatic.[65–67] Chest pain similar to angina pectoris may occur. It usually has no hemodynamic correlate, is relieved by closure of the defect, and may be due to right ventricular ischemia when right ventricular hypertrophy is present.

PHYSICAL EXAMINATION. The patient with an uncomplicated ASD often has a prominent *v* wave in the jugular venous pulse, reflecting left atrial venous events. The *v* wave is even more prominent when mitral regurgitation is present.[60] Cyanosis and clubbing are sometimes evident in patients with right-to-left shunting. On auscultation, the tricuspid closure sound is usually loud, with prominence of the first heart sound. In a patient with a large ASD and left-to-right shunting, *fixed* splitting of the second heart sound occurs, reflecting a relatively constant ratio of right ventricular to left ventricular stroke volumes and ejection times (Fig. 2–16, p. 30, and Fig. 3–9, p. 47). A right-sided atrial gallop (S_4) is often present. There is almost always a midsystolic flow murmur across the pulmonic valve orifice. A murmur louder than grades 3 to 4 out of 6 or a murmur associated with a thrill suggests the presence of associated valvular pulmonic stenosis. In patients with large shunts, a soft mid-diastolic tricuspid flow rumble as well as a tricuspid valve opening snap may be present along the lower left sternal border (Fig. 4–21, p. 77). A small number of patients have a low-pitched murmur of pulmonic regurgitation secondary to dilatation of the pulmonary valve annulus. This is in contrast to the high-pitched diastolic decrescendo pulmonic regurgitant murmur often heard with pulmonary hypertension. Patients with ostium secundum ASD and pulmonary vascular obstructive disease may have a loud, often palpable pulmonary component of the second heart sound, a short systolic ejection murmur, a pulmonary ejection sound, and a murmur of tricuspid regurgitation.[64] An apical holosystolic murmur owing to mitral regurgitation may be present with

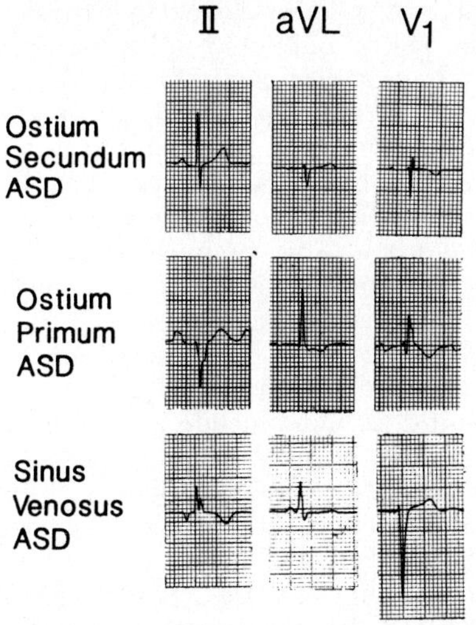

FIGURE 31–5. Electrocardiograms typical of ASD. ***Top,*** **Tracing from a young woman with secundum ASD demonstrates incomplete right bundle branch block and right-axis deviation.** ***Middle,*** **A patient with primum ASD shows first-degree AV block, complete right bundle branch block, and left-axis deviation.** ***Bottom,*** **Junctional rhythm as commonly seen in sinus venosus ASD, here associated with right bundle branch block. All recordings are at standard voltage. (From Feldman, T., and Borow, K. M.: ASD in adults—Diagnosis and management. Cardiovasc. Med. *11*:21, 1986.)**

an ostium primum defect and, less commonly, a secundum ASD.

NONINVASIVE STUDIES. The *electrocardiogram* is characterized by incomplete or, less frequently, complete right bundle branch block (Figs. 31–5 and 30–12, p. 916).[68] Right ventricular hypertrophy with strain suggests the presence of pulmonary hypertension or pulmonic stenosis. Two-thirds of patients with secundum ASD have right axis deviation, and less than one-third have an abnormal frontal plane QRS axis. Patients with secundum ASD experience atrial fibrillation or flutter, which occurs with higher incidence with increasing age and degree of pulmonary hypertension.[63, 69] Sinus venosus ASD is often associated with low atrial and junctional rhythms. Ostium primum as well as long-standing ostium secundum defects may be associated with first-degree AV block, which probably reflects prolonged conduction through the atria.[70] Ostium primum defects are associated with marked left-axis deviation and a superior frontal plane QRS vector loop[70, 71] (Fig. 7–25, p. 197).

More than 80 per cent of adult patients with ostium secundum ASD and a large left-to-right shunt have an enlarged cardiac silhouette on *chest roentgenogram*[68] (Fig. 6–28, p. 157). With an uncomplicated large defect, pulmonary plethora may be present (Fig. 6–30*A*, p. 158), as well as enlargement of the pulmonary arteries, right atrium, and right ventricle. With the development of pulmonary vascular obstructive disease, there is enlargement of the proximal branches of the pulmonary artery, with tapering and "pruning" of the peripheral pulmonary arteries (Fig. 6–29, p. 158). Calcification of the pulmonary arteries may also become evident.

Echocardiography. The M-mode *echocardiogram* in an uncomplicated ASD (Fig. 5–79, p. 117) shows right ventricular dilatation. During diastole, the septum bulges in a right-to-left direction and behaves as if it were part of the right ventricle. During systole, the septum contracts with the left ventricle. This results in geometric changes associated with the appearance of flattened or paradoxical motion of the interventricular septum on the M-mode echocardiogram. The left ventricular end-diastolic dimension has been reported to be decreased in ASD, a finding which may reflect diminished left ventricular preload as well as an alteration in left ventricular geometry.[72] Mitral valve prolapse is often present, especially with ostium secundum defects.[54, 73] Two-dimensional echocardiography may be helpful in the diagnosis of ASD (Figs. 5–76, and 5–77, p. 116; 30–13, p. 917; and 30–14, p. 918).[68, 74–77] Artifactual dropout of echoes from the interatrial septum may occur when ultrasound imaging is performed from the precordial and apical transducer positions. With the subcostal approach, the echo beam is perpendicular to the septum and will more accurately demonstrate atrial septal anatomy. Transesophageal two-dimensional echocardiography may be more sensitive than transthoracic imaging but requires esophagoscopy.[78] Regardless of the two-dimensional approach and technique used, ostium secundum defects are visualized as centrally located, whereas ostium primum defects are imaged in the lower part of the septum. Two-dimensional echocardiographic study in ostium primum ASD will demonstrate the abnormal mitral valve attachment to the interventricular septum. Short-axis parasternal view of the mitral valve may also demonstrate the cleft anterior leaflet (Fig. 31–6). The sensitivity of two-dimensional echocardiography for detecting ASD's of the ostium secundum, ostium primum, and sinus venosus varieties is 90 per cent, virtually 100 per cent, and 45 per cent, respectively.[79] Estimates of systemic and pulmonary blood flow, pulmonary-to-systemic flow ratio ($\dot{Q}_p/\dot{Q}_s$), and pulmonary artery systolic pressure can be performed with Doppler blood flow velocity measurements.[80–83] Noninvasive determination of the magnitude of left-to-right shunts by Doppler examination correlates well with determinations made by the Fick method as long as outflow tract obstruction, semilunar valve regurgitation, and persistent ductus arteriosus are not present. Color flow Doppler mapping will frequently demonstrate both the anatomical position and direction of blood flow through an ASD[68, 84, 84a] (Fig. 5–83, Color plate No. 2).

Radionuclide ventriculography (p. 315) is useful in the evaluation of right ventricular ejection fraction and wall motion, and for the estimation of $\dot{Q}_p/\dot{Q}_s$ by first-pass study.[85, 86] Contrast-enhanced fast CT imaging (Fig. 12–15, p. 366) and magnetic resonance imaging may also be useful for detecting ASD's.[87–89]

CARDIAC CATHETERIZATION. This procedure is unnecessary in many patients with ASD who have typical clinical as well as characteristic echocardiographic and Doppler findings.[90–92] Catheterization and angiography should be performed in patients suspected of having an ASD who

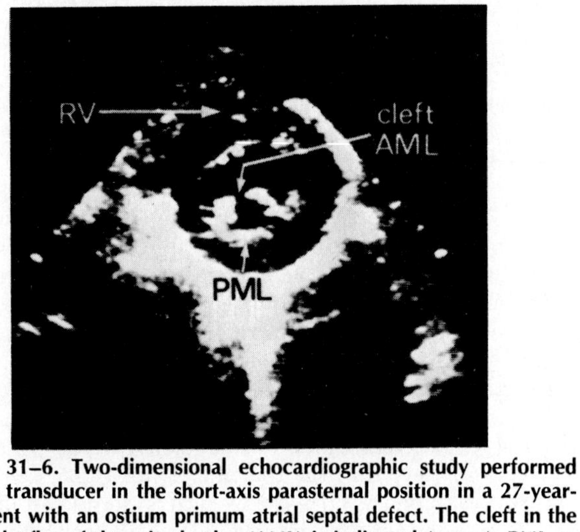

FIGURE 31–6. Two-dimensional echocardiographic study performed with the transducer in the short-axis parasternal position in a 27-year-old patient with an ostium primum atrial septal defect. The cleft in the anterior leaflet of the mitral valve (AML) is indicated (arrow). PML = posterior mitral leaflet; RV = right ventricle.

have atypical physical findings, evidence of severe pulmonary hypertension, cyanosis, right heart failure, or associated anatomical lesions. When right heart catheterization is performed from the femoral vein, it is almost always possible to cross the ASD and enter the left atrium. Because many patients have a probe patent foramen ovale, proof of a significant defect depends on hemodynamic, angiographic, and oximetric data. With a large ASD, the right atrial *v* wave is increased and may equal or exceed the *a* wave, normally the dominant wave in the right atrial pressure pulse. A difference in mean pressures of more than 5 mm Hg between the two atria is strong evidence against the presence of a large ASD. Usually, right ventricular systolic pressure is less than 50 mm Hg and pulmonary vascular resistance is normal. When pulmonary blood flow is markedly increased, a systolic pressure gradient of up to 20 mm Hg may exist across the pulmonary valve and branch bifurcation without the presence of anatomical pulmonic stenosis. Some patients with elevated pulmonary artery pressures will have reactive pulmonary vasculature, as noted by a fall in pulmonary vascular resistance after inhalation of 100 per cent oxygen. In other patients with more marked elevations of pulmonary vascular resistance, a decreasing left-to-right shunt and eventual right-to-left shunting across the ASD are possible. Operative risk is highest in such patients.

A secundum ASD may be demonstrated by angiography. Left anterior oblique rotation with cranial angulation places the atrial septum perpendicular to the x-ray beam and allows direct visualization of the ASD after contrast injection in the left atrium. Left-to-right shunting of contrast material may be seen during the levo phase of a right ventriculogram or pulmonary arteriogram. Left ventriculography in the anteroposterior plane will show the typical "gooseneck" deformity of the left ventricle outflow tract in ostium primum ASD (Figs. 6–54, p. 176, and 30–16, p. 919). Mitral regurgitation as well as the cleft itself may be visualized (Fig. 31–6). Selective injection into one of the right pulmonary veins may outline the upper portion of the interatrial septum or further identify the level of the ASD.

NATURAL HISTORY—MEDICAL. The clinical diagnosis of ASD's may be difficult in some patients because of subtle physical findings and the relative paucity of symptoms. Moreover, ASD's may not be recognized in adults because of the presence of associated conditions, such as coronary artery disease or chronic obstructive pulmonary disease. One characteristic of ASD that sets it apart from many other congenital heart lesions is the prolonged period during which the patient experiences few symptoms.[57, 67] In the preoperative era, patients with large secundum ASD had an average life span of 40 to 50 years.[67] Those with unrepaired primum ASD had a mean life span of 30 years. In patients with low or normal pulmonary vascular resistance, symptoms of fatigue, dyspnea on exertion, atrial arrhythmias, and right ventricular failure are uncommon before the fourth decade but become increasingly common and severe thereafter. The frequency of pulmonary artery hypertension can be expected to increase with age; as many as 30 per cent of adult patients with ASD have this finding.[61] The onset of atrial arrhythmias (frequent atrial premature depolarization, atrial tachycardia, flutter and fibrillation) is often the harbinger of right ventricular failure. Pulmonary and paradoxical systemic emboli are relatively common in adult patients with atrial fibrillation and right heart failure.[93] With long-standing pulmonary hypertension, right ventricular hypertrophy, dilatation, and failure as well as pulmonic and tricuspid regurgitation are common findings. Hypoxia, hemoptysis, low forward cardiac output, arrhythmias, and death may follow. Other fatal complications include pulmonary infection, brain abscess, and rupture of the pulmonary artery.[68]

The issue of whether left ventricular performance is normal in patients with uncomplicated ASD is an interesting one. Older studies suggested that intrinsic abnormalities of left ventricular function do exist in some patients,[94, 95] but these findings have been questioned.[65, 76, 96] Bonow et al. demonstrated that left ventricular ejection fraction at rest measured by radionuclide angiography was normal in adults with ASD without evidence of hemodynamically severe right or left ventricular failure.[96] However, the response of the ejection fraction to exercise was frequently abnormal. Impairment of the left ventricular response to exercise resolved after operative closure of the defect. This study suggests that left ventricular dysfunction in patients with ASD may result from reversible mechanical factors. These would include right ventricular volume overload with abnormal displacement of the ventricular septum and perhaps diminished left ventricular preload rather than intrinsic, irreversible impairment of left ventricular contractility. The two-dimensional echocardiographic study of Takahashi and coworkers[65] and the invasive study of Carabello et al.[76] support this conclusion.

Pregnancy is usually well tolerated when uncomplicated ASD is present [97] (p. 1854). Few patients, especially those with pulmonary artery hypertension, will experience paradoxical emboli after delivery. Marked elevation of pulmonary vascular resistance is associated with maternal mortality approaching 50 per cent during pregnancy, especially at the time of delivery.[97] The risk does not diminish until after the first postpartum week. Pregnancy should therefore be avoided in patients with severe pulmonary artery hypertension. The risk of thromboembolism in cyanotic patients with ASD is an absolute contraindication to the use of oral contraceptives. Intrauterine devices are relatively contraindicated because of the risk of infection. Tubal ligation may be considered, and injectable medroxyprogesterone acetate (Depo-Provera) has been used.[98]

Prophylaxis for infective endocarditis is generally considered unnecessary before or after repair of an uncomplicated secundum ASD, even when a patch is used. However, associated lesions, such as mitral valve prolapse or cleft mitral or tricuspid leaflet, may require prophylaxis.

NATURAL HISTORY—INTERVENTIONAL THERAPY. *Transcatheter closure* of ASD's has been attempted in a small number of children and adults with a moderate level of success.[48, 99–101] This involves the use of either a single- or a double-disc prosthesis, which is introduced from the femoral vein and advanced across the defect to the left atrium. After proper placement, the prosthesis is released and the defect closed (Fig. 40–23, p. 1392).

SURGERY. In general, uncomplicated ASD's should be closed in all adults under the age of 45 when there is a left-to-right shunt with $\dot{Q}_p/\dot{Q}_s$ greater than 1.5:1.0. Spontaneous closure is uncommon in adults.[102] Operative mortality is under 1 per cent in young to middle-aged adult patients with secundum or sinus venous defects. Patients over age 60 years have a 6 per cent operative mortality.[63] Primum ASD is more difficult to repair and carries a slightly higher operative mortality. In nearly all cases, life expectancy is improved after surgery.[63] This includes the older patient with an ASD and chronic right heart failure without severe pulmonary vascular obstructive disease.[63] The pulmonic flow murmur may persist postoperatively, but the tricuspid diastolic flow murmur usually resolves.

At the present time, heart-lung transplantation is the only potential viable surgical alternative for the patient with a net right-to-left shunt and Eisenmenger syndrome.[103, 104] In contrast, adult patients with ASD, cyanosis, pulmonary hypertension, increased pulmonary vascular resistance, and a net left-to-right shunt have survived surgery and become acyanotic with marked symptomatic and hemodynamic improvement.[105] Unlike younger patients, the elderly have little or no reduction in pulmonary vascular resistance. With restoration of normal $\dot{Q}_p/\dot{Q}_s$, there is a decrease in pulmonary resistance.[68] In some patients, pulmonary vascular resistance may continue to increase postoperatively, presumably owing to pulmonary thrombosis.[106]

LONG-TERM SURGICAL FOLLOW-UP. If the ASD is corrected during childhood, right atrial and right ventricular size will usually return to normal.[107] Right heart enlargement commonly persists when defects are closed after age 25 years.[68] Right ventricular ejection fraction is usually normal, despite the presence of pulmonary hypertension. A decrease in the right ventricular ejection fraction may occur after repair because of the reduction in right ventricular preload accompanying ASD closure.[108] Cardiac index response to exercise may remain abnormal after operation, possibly the result of persistent right ventricular dysfunction. Electrocardiographic evidence of right ventricular hypertrophy and radiographic prominence of the main pulmonary artery may also persist. More than half of the patients undergoing repair after the fifth decade have either persistent or new atrial fibrillation or other postoperative atrial tachyarrhythmias. Appearance of these rhythm disturbances may be delayed for months to years after surgery.[109] Patients with preoperative atrial fibrillation or flutter are more likely to sustain postoperative atrial arrhythmias.[110] Early or late complete heart block may follow repair of primum ASD. Although cardiac rhythm, AV conduction, and right ventricular hypertrophy do not substantially improve after operation, there is clear-cut improvement in heart size and symptoms, with a majority of patients asymptomatic 1 year after operation.[68]

PATENT FORAMEN OVALE

Patent foramen ovale (PFO) is the most common feature of the fetal circulation that is retained into adult life.[111] In a recent study of 965 human autopsy specimens, the overall incidence of PFO was 27 per cent.[111] The frequency declined progressively with increasing age from 34 per cent during the first three decades of life to 25 per cent during the fourth through eighth decades, to 20 per cent during the ninth and tenth decades. The mean size of the PFO was 4.9 mm (range, 1 to 10 mm in 98 per cent of cases). No abnormalities on physical examination, electrocardiogram, or chest roentgenogram are associated with PFO. Left-to-right shunts do not usually occur. Interestingly, a PFO may provide access to the left side of the heart from the right atrium at the time of cardiac catheterization. The defect is significant only in that it is a potential route for paradoxical embolism.[111] Any condition resulting in higher right atrial than left atrial pressure may cause right-to-left shunting through the PFO. This can occur with (1) the Valsalva maneuver, (2) use of positive end-expiratory pressure, (3) pulmonary embolism, (4) pulmonary artery hypertension, (5) chronic obstructive pulmonary disease, (6) valvular pulmonic stenosis, and (7) right ventricular myocardial infarction.[111]

ANEURYSM OF THE INTERATRIAL SEPTUM

This abnormality may be either primary (i.e., caused by redundancy of the fossa ovale membrane) or secondary (i.e., associated with significant long-standing right or left atrial hypertension). In adults, two-dimensional echocardiography has shown that the primary type of aneurysm of the interatrial septum associated with bulging into the right atrium is much more common than was previously suspected.[112–117] On ultrasound imaging, the aneurysm has an echolucent appearance with a persistent interruption or echo dropout of the atrial septum.[115] The presence of an accompanying ASD must be excluded. Mitral valve prolapse is a common associated finding.[114, 118, 119] The clinical significance of these aneurysms lies in the potential for right atrial outflow tract obstruction or as a source of left atrial thrombus and subsequent peripheral embolization. The differential diagnosis of an aneurysm of the interatrial septum includes right atrial thrombus, atrial myxoma, prominent eustachian valve, remnants of the Chiari network, and hematoma of the atrial septum.[112, 113, 115] On physical examination, a midsystolic click may be present. A mid-diastolic murmur may be audible in the presence of impairment to blood flow through the tricuspid valve. There are no data to suggest that in the asymptomatic patient anticoagulant therapy or surgical aneurysmectomy is beneficial.

COR TRIATRIATUM

(See also p. 940)

In this uncommon cardiac anomaly, a membrane separates the atrium (usually the left) into two compartments.[119a] The proximal chamber contains the site of entry of the pulmonary veins, while the distal chamber is associated with the mitral valve and left atrial appendage. In its classic presentation, dyspnea, frequent respiratory infections, and limited exercise capacity are present. Although symptoms most often occur during childhood, a number of patients have been asymptomatic into the third decade of life.[120, 121] When obstruction to blood flow from the proximal (i.e., accessory) chamber to the left atrium is present, signs and symptoms of pulmonary venous hypertension occur. On *physical examination*, an increased intensity of the pulmonary component of the second heart sound as well as murmurs of pulmonary and/or tricuspid regurgitation are common. Two-dimensional echocardiography is particularly useful in diagnosing this lesion[120, 122] (Fig. 30–42, p. 940).

In the *adult patient*, the differential diagnosis includes rheumatic mitral stenosis, left atrial tumor, and left atrial thrombus. Surgical correction of cor triatriatum is indicated if symptoms of pulmonary venous hypertension are present.

PARTIAL ANOMALOUS PULMONARY VENOUS CONNECTION

(See also p. 963)

This anomaly occurs when one or more (but not all) of the pulmonary veins drain into the right atrium or systemic venous circulation rather than into the left atrium.[123, 124] This malformation is often associated with an ASD of the sinus venosus type. When partial anomalous venous return is associated with an ASD, the natural history, physical examination, electrocardiogram, and chest roentgenogram are usually indistinguishable from those of patients with isolated ASD. Patients with partial anomalous pulmonary venous drainage and an intact atrial septum usually exhibit respiratory phasic variation of the second heart sound and can thereby be distinguished from patients with associated ASD, in which fixed splitting is present (Fig. 3–9, p. 47). Systolic flow murmurs across the pulmonary outflow tract and diastolic murmurs across the tricuspid orifice are common. Electrocardiographic and roentgenographic findings are identical to those in patients with ASD. When the entire right lung drains into the inferior vena cava (the "scimitar syndrome"), the anomalous vein can sometimes be identified on the plain chest roentgenogram as well as on two-dimensional echocardiographic study.[125] Techniques that have been successful in establishing this diagnosis at the time of cardiac catheterization include (1) differential indicator-dye dilution curves from the right and left main pulmonary arteries, (2) careful probing of the atrial septum with a catheter, (3) assessment of the levo phase of a pulmonary angiogram, and (4) selective injection of contrast media into an anomalous pulmonary vein that has been entered by a catheter.[123] Right heart pressures are usually normal. In most patients with anomalous pulmonary venous return and an intact atrial septum, the left-to-right shunt is usually modest in size (i.e., pulmonary-to-systemic blood flow ratio less than 2:1). Pulmonary hypertension seldom develops in such patients. Surgical correction consists of incorporating the site of drainage of the anomalous vein into the left atrium and closing the ASD, if it is present. Operation is usually indicated when the pulmonary-to-systemic blood flow ratio exceeds 1.5:1.0.

Total anomalous pulmonary venous return (p. 961) is seldom seen in adults.

VENTRICULAR SEPTAL DEFECT

(See also p. 920)

Ventricular septal defect (VSD) is the most common congenital malformation reported in infants and children.

However, in adults, it is surpassed in frequency by ASD, a change that can be related to three factors[126, 127]: First—and most important—a significant number of VSD's (even those with large left-to-right shunts) close spontaneously during infancy or childhood; occasionally spontaneous closure occurs during adulthood.[128] Second, patients with VSD may die of heart failure early in life. Finally, many patients with VSD now undergo surgical closure of the defect during childhood.[128a]

ANATOMY (Fig. 30–17, p. 920). There are four major anatomical types of VSD.[126–130a] The most common, accounting for 75 per cent of all cases, is the membranous variety, which is located inferior to the crista supraventricularis in the region of the membranous septum, in proximity to the septal leaflet of the tricuspid valve. In some patients, the membranous VSD permits communication between the left ventricle and the right atrium (Gerbode defect).[131, 132] Second is the muscular type, which may be either single or multiple and accounts for 10 per cent of all such lesions. They may become smaller or even close during late ventricular systole as the muscle surrounding the defect contracts. Spontaneous closure by growth of muscle borders is common. Third are defects of the atrioventricular (AV) canal type (p. 918). These occur most frequently in patients with trisomy 21 and make up about 10 per cent of all VSD's. AV canal defects occupy the posterior ventricular septum near the junction of the mitral and tricuspid valve annuli and the lower interatrial septum. They are often large and are frequently associated with clefts of the anterior leaflet of the mitral valve and of the septal leaflet of the tricuspid valve. There may be abnormal chordal attachments to the rim of the ventricular septum. The fourth type is the supracristal VSD. This anomaly, which constitutes about 5 per cent of all VSD's, is located above and anterior to or within the crista supraventricularis, and may underlie the annulus of the aortic valve in the region of the right and noncoronary cusps. These defects are generally small and of little hemodynamic significance. However, they may result in progressive aortic regurgitation because of extensive prolapse of the aortic valve leaflet into the defect[129] (Fig. 30–18, p. 922). With time, the aortic valve leaflet may actually seal off the defect; thus the only finding is aortic regurgitation, which usually develops during childhood and becomes more severe by middle age.

PATHOPHYSIOLOGY. The physiological consequences of a VSD are determined by the size of the defect, the relative ratio of pulmonary to systemic vascular resistance, and associated lesions. Pathophysiology is influenced more by the defect's size than by its location.[133] A small restrictive defect results in little or no increased cardiac or pulmonary workload. A large nonrestrictive VSD permits equilibration of systolic pressures in the two ventricles, with pulmonary blood flow determined by the relationship between systemic and pulmonary vascular resistance.[134] These patients are at great risk for the development of pulmonary vascular obstructive disease and Eisenmenger syndrome, with right or biventricular hypertrophy, reversal of the shunt flow, and systemic arterial desaturation. Those with large defects plus acquired pulmonary stenosis can present with physiology similar to that seen in patients with tetralogy of Fallot.

SYMPTOMS. Patients with moderate or large VSD's without pulmonary vascular obstructive disease have significant left-to-right shunting, with volume overload of the left atrium and ventricle.[128, 135] However, left ventricular failure is generally not part of the natural history of this congenital defect in patients over 2 years of age, unless aortic regurgitation or infective endocarditis supervenes.[136]

PHYSICAL EXAMINATION. An adult patient with a small VSD has normal jugular venous and carotid pulse configurations. There is often an abrupt, forceful apical impulse. On palpation of the precordium, a thrill may be present along the left lower or midsternal border areas.[128, 136] The first and second heart sounds are often obscured by a prominent high-frequency holosystolic murmur. Some patients with small membranous VSD's will have a systolic click best heard along the left sternal border during expiration, owing to an aneurysm at the site of the defect.[127] In the case of small muscular defects, the murmur may decrease or end before the second heart sound, owing to complete closure of the defect during late systole. The cardiac examination in a patient with a large VSD is characterized by a holosystolic or ejection murmur (Fig. 4–14, p. 72) plus a mid-diastolic mitral flow rumble and a prominent third heart sound.[135] If pulmonary vascular resistance is elevated, as is relatively common in the adult, there is shortening and softening of the systolic murmur, and increased intensity of the pulmonary component of the second heart sound.[137, 138] A pulmonary ejection sound and diastolic murmur of pulmonic regurgitation may also be present (Fig. 4–15, p. 72).

NONINVASIVE STUDIES. The *electrocardiogram* in the adult with a small, uncomplicated VSD is usually normal.[128] When a large defect is present, left atrial and left ventricular enlargement occur. Left ventricular hypertrophy, usually with diastolic volume overload pattern, is present in uncomplicated, moderately large defects. The presence of right-axis deviation or a progressive rightward shift of the QRS axis in the frontal plane suggests right ventricular hypertrophy secondary to either acquired infundibular obstruction or pulmonary vascular obstructive disease.

The *chest roentgenogram* is usually normal in the adult patient with a small VSD. Large defects are characterized by increased pulmonary vascular markings in association with pulmonary arterial, left atrial, and left ventricular enlargement. With the development of pulmonary vascular obstructive disease, marked central pulmonary artery dilatation occurs with "pruning" of the peripheral arterial vessels.

The M-mode *echocardiogram* is generally not diagnostic of VSD, frequently showing only left atrial and left ventricular dilatation. Two-dimensional echocardiography can often provide a definitive diagnosis of VSD and can demonstrate the position of the defect, chamber size, as well as wall thicknesses, and ventricular shortening characteristics[130, 139] (Fig. 31–7). Pulsed-wave Doppler echocardiography can be used to localize the position of the VSD[140] (Fig. 5–80, p. 118). Continuous-wave Doppler has the additional advantage of allowing accurate estimation of right ventricular and pulmonary artery systolic pressures as well as the ratio of pulmonary to systemic arterial blood flow ($\dot{Q}_p/\dot{Q}_s$).[141–143] Color flow Doppler mapping will frequently demonstrate the position and size of a defect, the timing and direction of blood flow between the ventricles, and associated cardiac lesions (Figs. 31–8 and 31–9). Contrast-enhanced cine CT imaging (Fig. 12–16, p. 366) and magnetic resonance imaging have also been successful in diagnosing the size and position of ventricular septal defects (Fig. 31–10).[89]

CARDIAC CATHETERIZATION. This is useful for measurements of systemic and pulmonary arterial resistances and blood flows. Angiography allows delineation of the defect's size, location, and number as well as assessment of associated cardiac anomalies (Fig. 31–7).

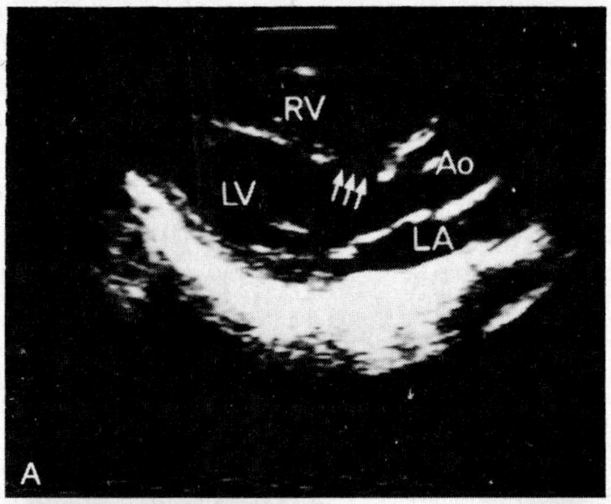

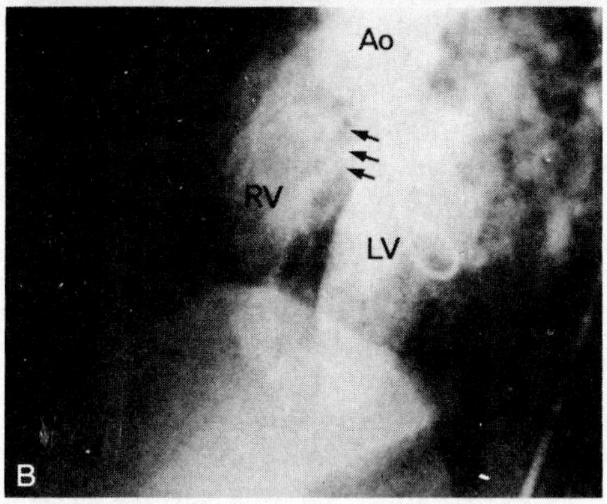

FIGURE 31–7. Two-dimensional echocardiogram (A) and cineangiogram (B) from a 34-year-old woman with a ventricular septal defect (VSD) and a grade 3/6 holosystolic murmur, loudest along the left and right lower sternal borders. *A,* The long-axis parasternal view of the heart shows a high VSD, probably in the membranous septum (arrows). *B,* The left ventriculogram demonstrates the presence of a membranous VSD (arrows). The pulmonary-to-systemic flow ratio was 2.3 to 1.0; pulmonary artery pressures were mildly elevated. LV = left ventricle; LA = left atrium; RV = right ventricle; Ao = aorta.

NATURAL HISTORY—MEDICAL. The natural history of VSD in adults differs depending on the size of the defect and the magnitude of the pulmonary vascular resistance. Patients with small defects are generally asymptomatic and not at risk for the development of pulmonary vascular obstructive disease. However, they are at increased risk for the development of infective endocarditis, which occurs in almost 4 per cent of patients with VSD,[128, 135] usually by the third or fourth decade of life. Most often the infection occurs on the "jet" lesion (Fig. 34–7, p. 1101), a traumatic endocardial deposit in the right ventricle that results from the impact of the high-velocity blood across a restricted defect.[144] The risk of endocarditis after spontaneous closure of a VSD is extremely low.

Simple, small VSD's with normal pulmonary artery pressure and pulmonary-to-systemic flow ratios less than 1.5:1.0 in asymtomatic persons generally do not require surgical closure. Women with such defects tolerate pregnancy without difficulty. Adult patients with large VSD's and low pulmonary vascular resistance are uncommon. Although these patients may develop left ventricular dysfunction and symptoms of congestive heart failure, they generally do not develop pulmonary vascular obstructive abnormalities.[135]

Aortic regurgitation was noted in 5.5 per cent of all patients with a VSD followed in the Natural History Study of Congenital Heart Disease.[145] In most cases, the VSD was either membranous or supracristal. No patient under 2 years of age had this combination of lesions, supporting the impression that the aortic regurgitation is an acquired problem. Of the 34 patients over 11 years of age with VSD's and aortic regurgitation, the latter was of at least moderate severity in 20 (59 per cent). Because most of the younger patients had only mild disease, it appears that the aortic regurgitation may be a progressive lesion. In another study, Corone et al.[135] noted the presence of aortic regurgitation in 6.3 per cent of 790 patients with VSD. In 15 per cent of these patients, aortic regurgitation developed as a consequence of infective endocarditis. In a third study, Momma and coworkers reported on 395 patients with supracristal VSD.[129] Aortic valvular deformities included prolapse without aortic regurgitation in 19 per cent, prolapse and aortic regurgitation in 24 per cent, and aneurysm of the sinus of Valsalva in 9 per cent. From this study it was evident that a wide spectrum of hemodynamic abnormalities may occur, ranging from a large VSD with trivial aortic regurgitation to a small VSD with severe regurgitation. If not operated on during childhood, most patients with VSD and aortic regurgitation survive to adult life, at which time they usually develop left ventricular dysfunction and require surgical treatment.

Progressive pulmonary vascular disease is one of the most feared complications in patients with VSD.[146] Adults with pulmonary hypertension and a left-to-right shunt may develop progressively severer obliterative pulmonary vascular disease, with eventual reversal of their shunt (i.e., Eisenmenger complex) (p. 999).[146] This usually appears before the end of the second or during the third decade of life.[147] Sudden death, hemoptysis, chest pain resembling angina pectoris, cerebral abscess, and paradoxical emboli are complications of VSD with pulmonary hypertension and right-to-left shunt. Once symptoms appear, the ultimate prognosis is poor, although the patient may survive for 5 to 10 years of sedentary life style, death usually occurs by the fourth decade of life.

Infundibular pulmonic stenosis, which is gradually progressive, may develop in an occasional adult patient with isolated VSD. Left-to-right shunts may reverse in such patients when obstruction to right ventricular outflow becomes sufficiently severe.[135]

Women with a VSD resulting in a small or moderate-

FIGURE 31–8. See color plate 4.

FIGURE 31–9. See color plate 4.

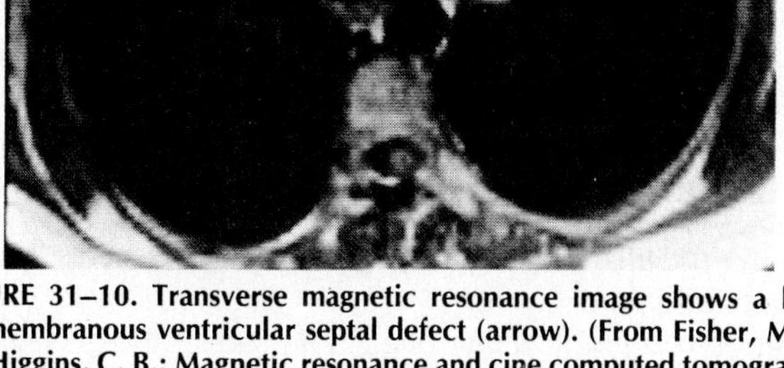

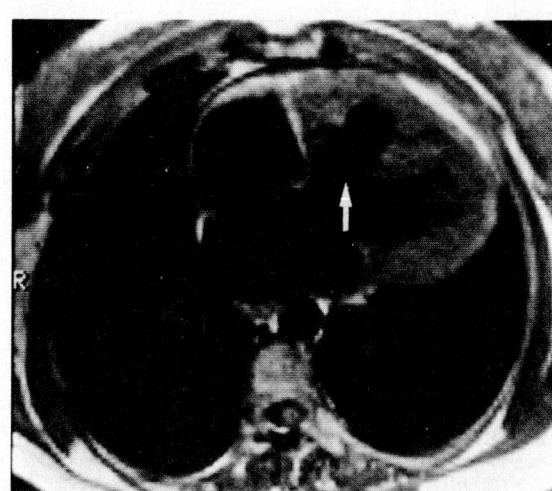

FIGURE 31–10. Transverse magnetic resonance image shows a large perimembranous ventricular septal defect (arrow). (From Fisher, M. R., and Higgins, C. B.: Magnetic resonance and cine computed tomography. *In* Roberts, W. C. [ed.]: Adult Congenital Heart Disease. Philadelphia, F. A. Davis Co., 1987, p. 231.)

sized left-to-right shunt (i.e., pulmonary-to-systemic flow ratios less than 2:1) and only modest pulmonary hypertension (i.e., pulmonary artery systolic pressure less than 50 mm Hg) can generally tolerate pregnancy well (Ch. 60). In women with larger left-to-right shunts, left ventricular failure may occur, while those with more severe pulmonary hypertension may have further elevation of pulmonary arterial pressure during pregnancy. Pregnancy is poorly tolerated by patients with Eisenmenger's complex.

NATURAL HISTORY—SURGERY. In most cases, closure of a VSD is recommended during childhood. However, some adult patients do present with this lesion. In the absence of Eisenmenger complex and a trivial left-to-right shunt ($Q_p/Q_s < 1.5:1.0$) closure of the VSD is usually indicated and it is carried out through the right atrium and tricuspid orifice. Depending on the size of the defect, primary closure or closure with a patch is used. In patients with normal pulmonary vascular resistance, operative mortality is less than 2 per cent. Adult patients with the combination of VSD and aortic regurgitation frequently require either aortic valvuloplasty or aortic valve replacement at the time of VSD closure. Cardiac transplantation alone is contraindicated, since the fixed elevated pulmonary vascular resistance would result in acute right ventricular dysfunction in the transplanted heart. Therefore, combined heart-lung transplantation is the only potentially "curative" therapy for patients with VSD and Eisenmenger complex.[103, 104] Initial results are encouraging.[103]

Long-Term Surgical Follow-up. After VSD closure, most patients demonstrate improvement in symptoms.[148] Residual pulmonary artery hypertension may persist, even in the asymptomatic patient. A postoperative pulmonary flow murmur as well as systolic murmur suggestive of a residual VSD are common. However, less than 10 per cent of patients have hemodynamically important residual shunts.

It remains controversial whether long-term ventricular performance is normal in patients who undergo VSD closure after childhood. To investigate this issue, Maron et al.[149] as well as Lueker et al.[150] used exercise testing to evaluate postoperative cardiovascular function in adult patients with surgically closed VSD's. In several patients, hemodynamic measurements were normal at rest but abnormal with vigorous exercise. This suggests that postoperative left ventricular function may be abnormal in patients who undergo closure of a large VSD at an older age. However, both of these studies assessed left ventricular function in patients whose defects were repaired during the 1960's, when the myocardial preservation techniques used were inferior to those currently available. The net effect of intraoperative myocardial ischemia on postoperative left ventricular performance in such patients is unknown. More recently, ventricular performance at rest and during exercise was compared using equilibrium gated radionuclide angiography in 34 patients (mean age, 27 years) with hemodynamically documented VSD.[151] The response of left ventricular ejection fraction to dynamic exercise was abnormal in patients who previously underwent surgical closure of VSD as well as in patients with residual defects. This again raises the issue of whether chronic left ventricular volume overload may be detrimental to myocardial function and argues for surgical correction during childhood.

Complications that can occur long term after VSD surgery include aortic regurgitation, infective endocarditis, pulmonary hypertension, infundibular pulmonic stenosis, and heart failure.[136, 147] In theory, the risk of infective endocarditis is small in patients in whom the VSD has been completely closed. However, when small residual defects and/or valvular abnormalities are present, endocarditis prophylaxis is indicated.

VENTRICULAR SEPTAL DEFECT WITH OBSTRUCTION TO RIGHT VENTRICULAR OUTFLOW (TETRALOGY OF FALLOT)

(See also p. 940)

The combination of a VSD and right ventricular outflow tract obstruction results in very different pathophysiology, clinical course, and physical signs, depending on whether the VSD is proximal or distal to the level of the obstruction, and when it is proximal, on the severity of obstruction to right ventricular outflow.[151a]

ANATOMY. In classic tetralogy of Fallot, a large VSD (malalignment type) is associated with infundibular and/or valvular pulmonic stenosis, right ventricular hypertrophy, and an overriding aorta (Fig. 30–49, p. 946).[151b] In such patients, right and left ventricular pressures are usually equal. The VSD is located proximal to the level of the right ventricular outflow tract obstruction and is therefore associated with high right ventricular systolic pressures. Right-to-left shunting of blood through the VSD is usual. In the past, many adult patients diagnosed clinically as having "pink" or acyanotic tetralogy of Fallot had a high membranous VSD associated with hypertrophy of subinfundibular anomalous muscle bundles.[152] These bundles separated the right ventricle into a high-pressure proximal chamber and a low-pressure distal chamber (so-called double-chamber right ventricle).[152–154]

PATHOPHYSIOLOGY. In patients with tetralogy of Fallot, the pathophysiology is determined by the severity of the right ventricular outflow tract obstruction, the size of the VSD, and the relationship between systemic vascular resistance and overall impedance to blood flow from the right ventricle. In all cases, the VSD communicates with the right ventricle in a region *proximal* to the outflow tract obstruction. In contrast, in patients with a double-chambered right ventricle and a membranous VSD, the septal defect communicates with the low-pressure distal portion of the right ventricle. The resultant physiology resembles that of a simple VSD rather than tetralogy of Fallot, and the patients remain acyanotic. In fact, pulmonary blood flow may be increased rather than decreased, as in patients with tetralogy of Fallot.

SYMPTOMS AND PHYSICAL EXAMINATION. When the obstruction to right ventricular outflow is mild, a left-to-right shunt is predominant, despite the equality of pressures in the two ventricles. The patient is acyanotic, the lung fields are plethoric, and there may be two separate systolic murmurs, i.e., a holosystolic murmur resulting from the VSD and a midsystolic murmur secondary to the obstruction to right ventricular outflow. Cyanotic patients with severe obstruction to right ventricular outflow are usually recognized during infancy or early childhood, at which time they undergo a palliative surgical procedure or, more likely, total surgical repair. Survival of patients with tetralogy of Fallot into adult life usually reflects mild to at most moderate obstruction to right ventricular outflow in association with relatively well-preserved pulmonary blood flow. Adults with tetralogy of Fallot may give a history of cyanosis of delayed onset. This is due to the gradual and progressive development of obstruction to pulmonary outflow. Some patients will become noticeably cyanotic only under conditions of decreased systemic vascular resistance, i.e., exercise, sedation, fever, or general anesthesia. These situations are characterized by increased right-to-left flow of blood across the VSD. As the severity of the right ventricular outflow tract obstruction increases, the systolic ejection murmur, which is due to turbulent blood flow across the outflow tract, peaks earlier in systole and decreases in intensity. If the obstruction to right ventricular outflow is complete, a large obligatory right-to-left shunt occurs, the lungs are perfused through systemic collateral vessels, and there is severe cyanosis and usually no systolic murmur. Instead, there is a continuous murmur originating from bronchial collaterals. This variant of tetralogy of Fallot is termed *pseudotruncus arteriosus.*

Congestive heart failure is unusual in patients with tetralogy of Fallot. The large VSD allows decompression of the right ventricle, no matter how severe the stenosis, and prevents the right ventricular systolic pressure from exceeding that in the aorta (i.e., nonrestrictive VSD). However, diminished cardiac reserve is not uncommon in adults with tetralogy of Fallot. Exertional dyspnea and poor exercise tolerance have been reported in approximately one-third of individuals with unoperated tetralogy of Fallot who survived into the third decade of life.[155] An occasional patient may complain of orthopnea and/or paroxysmal nocturnal dyspnea.

NONINVASIVE STUDIES. The *electrocardiogram* in tetralogy of Fallot is characterized by right-axis deviation, right ventricular hypertrophy, and, in older patients, a right ventricular conduction abnormality. By middle age the patient with uncorrected tetralogy may develop atrial fibrillation or flutter. Patients with double-chambered right ventricle and membranous VSD frequently have right ventricular conduction abnormalities or subtle evidence of right ventricular hypertrophy.

The *chest roentgenogram* in tetralogy of Fallot, which is classic in infants and children (i.e., a small boot-shaped heart and decreased pulmonary blood flow), is less typical in adults. On posteroanterior view, the heart is often of normal size. The aortic arch is right-sided in approximately 30 per cent of cases. On lateral view, right ventricular enlargement is frequently noted. Pulmonary vascularity is normal or even increased in almost half the adult patients, particularly those who are acyanotic.[155] These patients usually have well-developed systemic-to-pulmonary collateral vessels that can be visualized during angiography. It is this collateral blood flow to the lungs that accounts for the long survival of some adults who do not undergo palliative or corrective surgical procedures for this defect.[155, 156]

On M-mode *echocardiography*, the abnormal relationship between the aortic annulus and the interventricular septum can usually be demonstrated. The VSD can occasionally be recognized as dropout of septal echoes. A two-dimensional echocardiographic examination (Figs. 5–84, p. 119, and 30–50, p. 947) gives information regarding the presence and degree of aortic overriding, the extent and location of the infundibular obstruction, the size of the pulmonic valve and main pulmonary artery, the degree of right ventricular hypertrophy, and the location of the VSD.[157, 158] Pulsed Doppler study is useful for qualitative assessment of blood flow through the VSD or across a regurgitant tricuspid and/or pulmonary valve. Continuous-wave Doppler allows quantitation of right ventricular outflow tract systolic gradients (Fig. 31–11) as well as pressure gradients in patients with palliative aortic-pulmonary shunts.[159] Color flow Doppler mapping assists in quantifying the magnitude and direction of pulmonary regurgitant flow, especially in patients who have undergone corrective surgery (Fig. 31–12). It is also useful for detection of a residual VSD after surgical correction. Magnetic resonance imaging has been used to assess and diagnose intracardiac and extracardiac anatomy in tetralogy of Fallot[89] (Fig. 31–13).

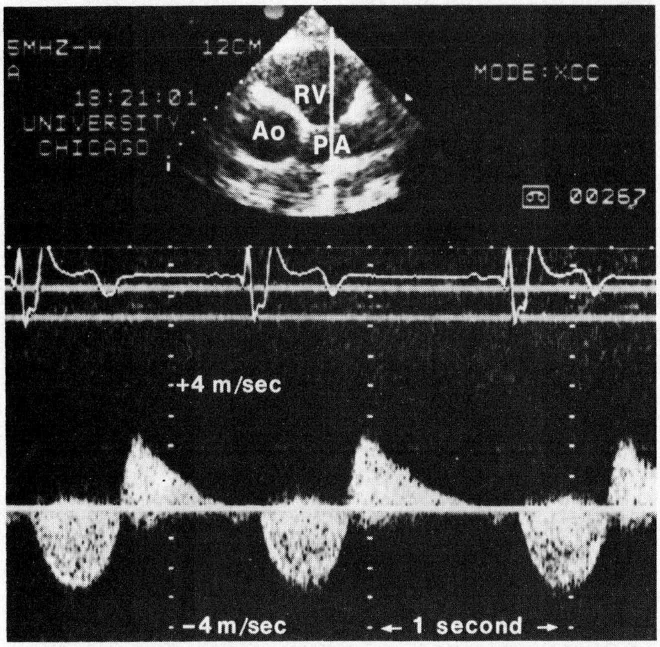

FIGURE 31–11. Continuous-wave Doppler tracings acquired from a 23-year-old woman who underwent total surgical correction of tetralogy of Fallot at age 6 years. The small two-dimensional echocardiographic sector at the top of the figure demonstrates the position of the ultrasound beam through the right ventricular (RV) outflow tract, pulmonary valve, and pulmonary artery (PA). There is a 2.8 m/sec peak gradient across the RV outflow area. This is equivalent to a residual peak instantaneous ejection gradient of 31 mm Hg. Evidence also exists for pulmonary regurgitation which lasts well into diastole and is probably of moderate severity.

The major information to be obtained at *cardiac catheterization and angiography* includes the size of the pulmonary annulus and pulmonary arteries, the severity of right ventricular outflow tract obstruction, and the exact location and size of the VSD. In some patients with tetralogy of Fallot, the coronary artery to the anterior interventricular groove originates from the right coronary system and crosses the infundibulum. It is important to look for this anomaly, since corrective surgery frequently requires an incision through the infundibular area. In patients with prior surgical systemic-to-pulmonary shunts, kinking of the pulmonary artery may occur at the anastomotic site, resulting in peripheral pulmonic stenosis. Angiography is also useful in locating collateral vessels and determining the significance of associated or acquired anomalies.

NATURAL HISTORY—MEDICAL. Tetralogy of Fallot is the most common cyanotic congenital heart anomaly in the adult. Since the advent of palliative and later corrective operations, it has become uncommon to see adults with tetralogy who have not undergone at least one cardiac surgical procedure. Data from the pre-surgical era suggest that approximately 10 per cent of patients with this lesion survive to the third decade, and only 3 per cent to the fourth.[160, 161] Infrequently, survival over age 60 years has occurred.[161] In two reports encompassing 172 adults with

FIGURE 31–12. See color plate 4.

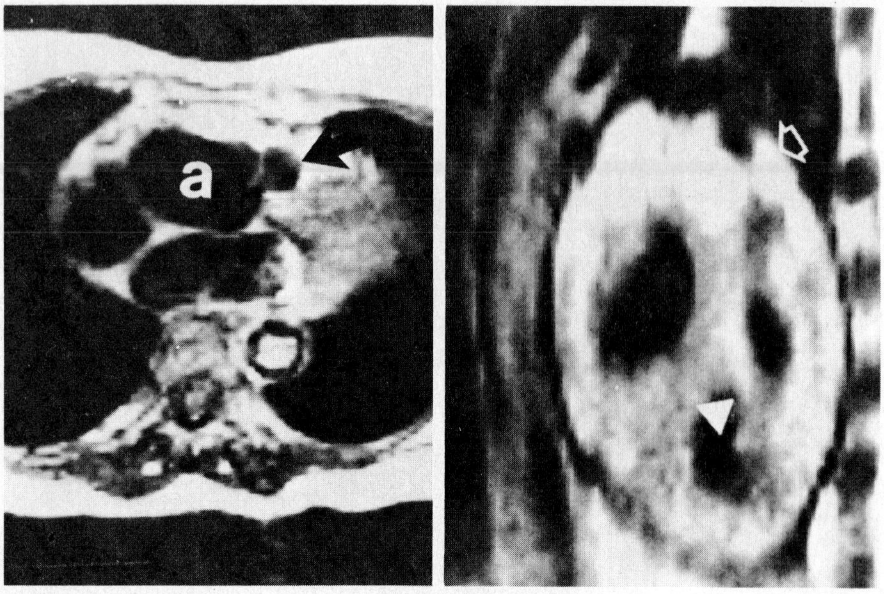

FIGURE 31–13. Transverse (left) and sagittal (right) magnetic resonance images of an adult patient with tetralogy of Fallot. Transverse image shows the disparity in diameter of the enlarged root of the aorta (a) and the hypoplastic pulmonary annulus (arrow). The sagittal image reveals narrowing of the right ventricle by a hypertrophied muscle band (arrowhead), infundibulum, and annulus (open arrow). (From Fisher, M. R., and Higgins, C. B.: Magnetic resonance and cine computed tomography. *In* Roberts, W. C. [ed.]: Adult Congenital Heart Disease. Philadelphia, F. A. Davis Co., 1987, p. 229.)

tetralogy of Fallot, congestive heart failure and cardiomegaly were present in approximately one-third of all patients.[155, 156] Adults with tetralogy complain frequently of severe headaches, dizziness, and episodes of exertional chest pain that resembles that of angina pectoris in character.[155] Their chronic hypoxemia stimulates release of increased quantities of erythropoietin, resulting in polycythemia. A hematocrit exceeding 65 per cent is associated with marked increases in blood viscosity and resistance to blood flow and substantially increases the possibility of intravascular thrombosis, thrombotic strokes, and paradoxical emboli. These patients are also at risk for infective endocarditis, brain abscesses, and attacks of acute gouty arthritis, the latter resulting from a high turnover of erythrocyte nucleic acid and subsequent hyperuricemia. Maternal and fetal mortality rates are high among patients with uncorrected tetralogy of Fallot. As is the case with other forms of cyanotic congenital heart disease, the offspring tend to be small for their gestational age.

SURGICAL THERAPY. *Palliative surgery* for tetralogy of Fallot was common before the advent of low-risk corrective surgery. Palliative operations were aimed at relieving hypoxia by increasing pulmonary blood flow. This was usually accomplished by surgically creating a communication between the systemic and pulmonary arterial circulations. The most commonly performed procedure was the *Blalock-Taussig* shunt (i.e., end-to-side anastomosis of a subclavian artery to the pulmonary artery). This shunt was of moderate size and seldom caused heart failure or pulmonary vascular obstructive disease. In contrast, the *Pott's procedure* (i.e., anastomosis of the descending aorta to the pulmonary artery) was often complicated by pulmonary vascular obstruction and congestive heart failure and was difficult to take down at the time of total correction. The *Waterston* shunt (i.e., anastomosis between the ascending aorta and the pulmonary artery), although associated with fewer complications than the Pott's procedure, still could lead to heart failure and pulmonary vascular obstruction. In addition, kinking, aneurysm formation, and even obstruction have been reported at the anastomosis site. Other potential risks of palliative procedures include continued right-to-left shunting at the ventricular level, with paradoxical emboli and infective endocarditis. In a retrospective study of 350 patients with tetralogy of Fallot conducted 10 to 25 years after palliative surgery, 38 per cent of patients were alive without any further cardiac operation, 30 per cent had undergone total correction, and 32 per cent had died.[162] Actuarial survival at 25 years of the patients who had palliation was 50 per cent compared with 83 per cent for the group who subsequently had complete correction. As a general rule, the adult patient with tetralogy of Fallot and a palliative shunt should undergo total surgical repair.[163]

Total surgical repair of tetralogy of Fallot can be undertaken in adults with a mortality rate comparable to that reported in children.[160, 163–166] For example, in the Mayo Clinic experience from 1960 to 1982, in which 30 patients between 40 and 60 years of age underwent total repair, only one (3 per cent) early postoperative death occurred.[160] Surgery includes takedown of any prior palliative shunts, patch closure of the VSD, and relief of the right ventricular outflow tract obstruction. The latter is accomplished using one or a combination of the following: infundibular resection, pulmonary valvotomy, and patch enlargement of the right ventricular outflow tract and possibly main pulmonary artery. In rare cases, an extracardiac conduit from the right ventricular outflow tract to the main pulmonary artery may be required. Postoperative bleeding from extensive collateral vessels may pose special problems in adults.

Whenever possible, total correction should be performed early in life. In a study comparing left ventricular function in patients with tetralogy of Fallot whose defects were repaired during infancy versus those repaired in late childhood or adolescence, left ventricular dysfunction was present only in patients with surgical correction after the age of 4 years.[167] An age-related comparison of the ultrastructural appearance of infundibular muscle resected at operative repair demonstrates that severe interstitial fibrosis, myofibrillar lysis, and other intracellular degenerative changes are common in adults but are absent from samples obtained from children with tetralogy of Fallot.[168] It is possible that such degenerative changes in the myocardium affect cardiac function adversely and are, in part, the cause of heart failure and arrhythmias in older patients with tetralogy of Fallot.[169, 170] Operative repair in patients with double-chambered right ventricle and VSD seldom requires reconstruction or patching of the right ventricular outflow tract and infrequently requires a ventricular septal patch.

In general, *long-term surgical follow-up* for tetralogy of Fallot has been quite favorable. Obstruction to right ventricular outflow and/or pulmonary regurgitation as well as residual VSD are the most common anatomical problems after repair.[160, 162, 166, 171] Electrophysiological abnormalities include (1) right bundle branch block, (2) left anterior hemiblock, (3) prolonged intraatrial, AV nodal, and His-Purkinje conduction times, and (4) complete heart block.[169, 172–174] Several studies have shown a correlation between resting or exercise-induced ventricular arrhythmias, abnormal hemodynamics, and sudden death.[166, 173, 175, 176] Ventricular ectopic activity may be a late-developing phenomenon and may increase in severity with longer postoperative intervals.[174, 176] Repaired tetralogy of Fallot patients who have ventricular arrhythmias should be treated aggressively with antiarrhythmic drugs.[174, 176] In the report of Rosenthal and coworkers on 182 patients with tetralogy of Fallot repaired 15 to 26 years earlier, the cumulative survival at 25 years postoperatively was 94.4 per cent.[152] Forty-seven per cent of patients were New York Heart Association (NYHA) functional class 1, while 29 per cent, 3 per cent, and 0 per cent were functional classes 2, 3, and 4, respectively. There were nine late deaths. These findings are similar to data reported from several other major surgical centers.[164, 165, 174] Pregnancy after successful total correction of tetralogy of Fallot seems to pose little threat to either mother or child.

One fact is clear as the number of long-term surgical survivors of tetralogy of Fallot increases: It should be expected that acquired problems (such as myocardial infarction owing to coronary arteriosclerosis and sclerocalcific aortic valve disease) will be added to the list of postoperative problems in this population.

PULMONIC STENOSIS

(See also p. 942)

Pulmonic stenosis (PS) is one of the more common congenital cardiac malformations that allow survival to adulthood.[177–179]

ANATOMY. Approximately 80 per cent of all cases of right ventricular outflow tract obstruction occur at the valvular level. *Valvular PS* is due to partial fusion and variable thickening of a tricuspid or, less commonly, a bicuspid pulmonic valve. The valve usually has a domed "fish mouth" appearance with a central or eccentric orifice, but may be dysplastic, with thick, rigid, shortened cusps lacking commissural fusion. Marked dilatation of the main and left pulmonary arteries is common.[180] Pulmonic valve atresia has physiological consequences very different from those of valvular PS[181, 182] and is discussed elsewhere (p. 944). *Subvalvular PS* seldom occurs as an isolated lesion. It may be diffuse or discrete and consists of fibrous or fibromuscular tissue. In patients with valvular PS, hypertrophy of the right ventricular infundibulum may occur with age and contribute to the degree of right ventricular outflow tract obstruction. Occasionally there are muscle bundles that insert into the right ventricular inflow tract, resulting in midcavity narrowing and a systolic pressure gradient. This creates the so-called double-chambered right ventricle, with a high proximal and a low distal pressure area.[154]

PATHOPHYSIOLOGY. Regardless of the level of obstruction, right ventricular systolic pressure overload and hypertrophy are nearly universal findings in PS. In the absence of right ventricular failure, ventricular systolic hypertension varies directly with the significance of the stenosis.[178] Diminished right ventricular compliance is a common finding in patients with moderate to severe right ventricular outflow tract obstruction.

SYMPTOMS. Most adult patients with mild PS are asymptomatic. In adults with severe stenosis, dyspnea and fatigue secondary to an inadequate response of cardiac output to exercise are the most common symptoms.[183–185] Orthopnea does not occur in such patients, since their pulmonary venous pressure is normal; a small right-to-left shunt through a patent foramen ovale is common. Eventually, patients with severe grades of PS develop tricuspid regurgitation and frank right ventricular failure. The latter may ultimately become intractable and fatal. Exertional syncope or light-headedness occasionally occurs in patients with severe PS, but sudden death is extremely uncommon.[183] Chest pain resembling that of angina pectoris occasionally develops in children but is observed most frequently in adults with severe PS in whom right ventricular oxygen requirements are greatly increased.[183, 184] Patchy fibrosis of the hypertrophied right ventricle is a common finding with such patients at postmortem examination.

PHYSICAL EXAMINATION. On palpation, a systolic thrill is often present along the left upper sternal border of the chest. This is especially true in severe valvular PS, in which case a sustained right ventricular heave in the mid to lower left sternal area may also be present. These findings should be distinguished from the hyperdynamic right ventricular precordial impulse found with an ASD and a moderate to large left-to-right shunt. The murmur in valvular PS is loudest at the left upper sternal border and is often associated with an ejection click (Fig. 4–10, p. 70). In contrast to the inspiratory increase of most right-sided cardiac sounds, the intensity of the click *decreases* with inspiration.[178] The murmur of mild PS is relatively short and soft. As the severity of the stenosis increases, the murmur becomes longer and louder and peaks later in systole, finally engulfing the aortic component of the second heart sound. A murmur less than grade 4 out of 6 intensity with a normal pulmonic component of the second heart sound suggests a gradient less than 80 mm Hg. A right-sided atrial systolic sound is common in severe PS; it is usually accentuated with inspiration. The major ascultatory differences between valvular and subvalvular PS are the absence of an ejection click and the left mid to lower sternal border position of the maximal intensity of the systolic ejection murmur in the subvalvular lesion.

NONINVASIVE STUDIES. The *electrocardiogram* in patients with mild to moderate PS is either normal or shows only a right ventricular conduction abnormality. In severe PS, right-axis deviation, right ventricular hypertrophy with strain, and right atrial enlargement are commonly present. A QR complex in V_1 (Fig. 7–16, p. 193) correlates with a right ventricular to pulmonary artery peak systolic pressure gradient exceeding 80 mm Hg. Right ventricular hypertrophy is present in 80 per cent of patients with severe stenosis, and those without it are unlikely to have critical obstruction. If the right ventricle is somewhat hypoplastic, right ventricular hypertrophy may not be evident. When present, P pulmonale suggests severe PS.

The *chest roentgenogram* in mild to moderate PS shows a normal or nearly normal cardiac silhouette (Fig. 6–32, p. 159), whereas in the severe form, right ventricular and right atrial enlargement may be present (Fig. 6–33, p. 160). Poststenotic dilatation of the main and left pulmonary arteries occurs in nearly all patients with valvular PS and helps distinguish it from the other types of right ventricular outflow tract obstruction. However, the degree of prominence of the main pulmonary artery segment does not correlate with the severity of the obstruction. In most patients, the pulmonary vascular markings are normal.

Echocardiography can usually define both the anatomy and physiological importance of PS. On M-mode study, an exaggerated diastolic pulmonic valve leaflet excursion associated with cuspal thickening may be evident in valvular PS. Two-dimensional imaging through the right ventricular outflow tract area frequently demonstrates the domed, stenotic valve and thickened leaflets (Fig. 5–68, p. 113). This technique is particularly useful for assessing the presence of associated intracardiac lesions.[154, 186] Continuous-wave Doppler echocardiography allows accurate estimation of the total gradient between the right ventricle and pulmonary artery.[178, 187–190] In this manner, noninvasive assessment of the severity of valvular PS before and after intervention can be performed. Pulsed Doppler and especially color flow Doppler mapping are useful for determining the severity of preoperative as well as postoperative (or post balloon valvuloplasty) pulmonic regurgitation.

CARDIAC CATHETERIZATION. Cineangiography with right ventriculography demonstrates a discrete jet of blood exiting through the valve, with leaflet doming and poststenotic pulmonary artery dilatation (Fig. 6–50, p. 173; 6–52, p. 175; 30–44 and 30–45, p. 943). Cardiac catheterization is unnecessary in asymptomatic patients who have typical findings of mild PS. In the symptomatic older patient, such study is helpful for clarifying the degree of right ventricular dysfunction, the level of obstruction, and the presence of any associated lesion.[185]

NATURAL HISTORY—MEDICAL. In patients with normal forward cardiac output, the severity of PS may be grouped according to the peak systolic pressure gradient between the right ventricle and the pulmonary artery. In general, up to 25 mm Hg is considered trivial, 25 to 49 mm Hg mild, 50 to 79 mm Hg moderate, and greater than 80 mm Hg severe. Data from a multicenter study on nonoperated valvular PS showed that among 184 patients aged 4 to 28 years who underwent two catheterizations 4 to 8 years apart, the peak systolic pressure remained within 10 mm Hg of the original value in 72 per cent of the cases while increasing in 14 per cent and decreasing in 14 per cent.[191] Thus, in most patients, valvular PS is a relatively stable, or at most slowly progressive, disease.

The clinical course of PS varies, depending on the severity of obstruction. Most adults with mild to moderate disease are asymptomatic. In severe right ventricular outflow tract obstruction, overt right ventricular failure may occur by the fourth to fifth decade of life, along with tricuspid regurgitation and subsequent edema and ascites. Adults with severe PS in general exhibit a lower than normal cardiac index at rest and during exercise in conjunction with significant elevations in right ventricular end-diastolic pressure.[185] When compared with children with similar severity of stenosis, an age-dependent abnormality in both right ventricular systolic and diastolic performance is evident. Thus severe PS, if untreated, adversely affects the right ventricular myocardium. Infective endocarditis is less common in patients with PS than in those with VSD, valvular AS, or coarctation of the aorta. Antibiotic prophylaxis for dental and surgical procedures is often given for uncorrected valvular PS as well as after valvulotomy.

NATURAL HISTORY–INTERVENTIONAL THERAPY. *Percutaneous balloon valvuloplasty* for typical valvular PS has been performed worldwide and appears to be a safe and effective procedure.[48, 192–198] Successful balloon valvuloplasty has been reported in patients as old as 60 years.[101, 194, 196] In these cases, 40 to 95 mm Hg reductions in right ventricular to pulmonary artery peak systolic pressure gradients have occurred. In adults, this procedure can generally be performed without general anesthesia and is now considered by many to be the treatment of choice for typical (i.e., nondysplastic) valvular PS.[192–198] Several studies in which follow-up catheterizations have been performed have shown no restenosis in patients who were initially treated successfully.[194, 195]

Surgery. It is generally agreed that symptomatic adults with PS should undergo either surgical valvulotomy or percutaneous balloon valvuloplasty. More controversial is whether or not to intervene invasively in asymptomatic adults with moderate or severe PS. Currently, the role of percutaneous balloon valvuloplasty vs. surgical valvulotomy for treatment of valvular PS is unclear. Preliminary results suggest that balloon valvuloplasty provides excellent palliative, if not permanent, improvement. If this is true, most patients with severe valvular PS, regardless of symptoms, would improve from interventional therapy. Patients with significant subvalvular PS require surgical resection of the obstructing lesion.

Long-Term Follow-up for Interventional Therapy. As noted earlier, there are no significant long-term follow-up data for balloon valvuloplasty in adults. However, surgical valvulotomy has been performed for more than 35 years. There are few reports of late complications of surgery. Electrocardiographic and roentgenographic evidence of right ventricular hypertrophy may persist after surgical repair. However, lack of improvement on the electrocardiogram within 3 years suggests significant residual PS. Children usually show a normal hemodynamic response to exercise after valvulotomy, but many adults show a persistently abnormal one. Restenosis after valvulotomy is uncommon.

PULMONARY ARTERY STENOSIS

(See also p. 941)

Stenosis of the pulmonary artery (the main vessel or a branch, single or multiple) is commonly associated with other congenital malformations, including atrial or ventricular septal defects, supravalvular aortic stenosis, Noonan's syndrome, persistent ductus arteriosus, tetralogy of Fallot, and the congenital rubella syndrome. Occasionally the malformation occurs in an isolated form. Because pulmonary arterial stenosis is usually not lethal, an increasing number of patients with peripheral pulmonary artery stenosis are being recognized in adult life. The principal complication is right ventricular pressure overload. Poststenotic dilation of peripheral pulmonary arterial branches occasionally leads to the formation of thin-walled aneurysms that can rupture and produce significant hemoptysis.[199] If the pulmonic valve is normal in such patients, pulmonic ejection sounds are absent and splitting of the second heart sound is usually normal. The systolic murmurs are typically crescendo-decrescendo and are widely distributed over the thorax. Stenosis in a pulmonary arterial branch occasionally gives rise to a continuous murmur. This occurs most frequently when moderate to severe pulmonary artery hypertension is present proximal to the area of narrowing and reflects the existence of a pressure gradient across the stenotic site throughout the cardiac cycle.

The diagnosis is usually established by selective angiography (Fig. 30–43, p. 942).

If stenosis of either pulmonary arterial branch is sufficiently close to the main pulmonary artery, or if there are no further peripheral branch stenoses, a graft can be constructed to bypass the obstruction from the main pulmonary artery to the branch distal to the stenosis. Alternatively, patch grafts may be placed to enlarge the lumen at sites of obstruction. If the area of peripheral pulmonary artery stenosis extends into the lung parenchyma, effective surgical repair may not be possible. Percutaneous balloon angioplasty for relief of stenotic pulmonary arteries in children has met with moderately good success.[48, 192] The place of balloon angioplasty for such lesions in the adult is yet to be defined.[199a]

IDIOPATHIC DILATATION OF THE PULMONARY ARTERY

This malformation is characterized by congenital dilatation of the main pulmonary artery and its branches in the absence of any apparent anatomical or physiological cause.[192a] It may be the result of a defect in the normal development of the pulmonary arterial elastic tissue. Patients with this disorder are asymptomatic. *Physical examination* may reveal a palpable pulmonary arterial impulse in the second left intercostal space, a pulmonic ejection sound, and a midsystolic murmur heard best in the second left intercostal space. In most cases, the second heart sound is normally split, although wide splitting with normal respiratory variation has been reported. The *electrocardiogram* is normal. *Chest roentgenogram* as well as two-dimensional *echocardiogram* reveals a dilated pulmonary artery without cardiac chamber enlargement. Although idiopathic dilatation of the pulmonary artery has no clinical significance, it is important to distinguish this lesion from ASD or PS, with which it can be confused.

PERSISTENT DUCTUS ARTERIOSUS

(See also p. 923)

In utero, the ductus arteriosus diverts blood flow away from the high resistance pulmonary circuit and into the descending aorta. In this manner, relatively desaturated blood is directed away from the coronary and cerebral circulations and toward the low resistance placental circulation. Failure of the ductus to completely close in postnatal life leads to an abnormal communication between the systemic and pulmonary vascular beds.

ANATOMY. The persistent ductus arteriosus extends from the aortic isthmus near the origin of the left subclavian artery to the left pulmonary artery just distal to the pulmonary branch bifurcation. It can vary in length, shape, and cross-sectional area.

PATHOPHYSIOLOGY AND SYMPTOMS. The physiological consequences of a persistent ductus arteriosus (PDA) are determined by the caliber of the ductal lumen and by the ratio of the pulmonary-to-systemic vascular resistance. In the case of a large umcomplicated PDA, blood flows through the ductus into the lungs throughout the cardiac cycle, reflecting the persistent pressure gradient that exists between the aorta and the pulmonary artery. The result is increased pulmonary blood flow and enlargement of the pulmonary arteries, left atrium, left ventricle, and ascending aorta. Such patients are at high risk for the eventual development of congestive heart failure.[200–203a] If pulmonary artery hypertension is present, pulmonary vascular obstructive disease with bidirectional or reversed shunting through the ductus may develop.[203, 204] Differential cyanosis characterized by a relatively pink right upper extremity and cyanotic lower extremities is quite specific for a PDA with Eisenmenger's physiology. Eventually, when the pulmonary vascular disease becomes severe, generalized cyanosis occurs. In the adult patient with PDA, the most common symptoms include exercise intolerance and dyspnea.[203, 204b]

PHYSICAL EXAMINATION. The patient with a large ductus associated with low pulmonary vascular resistance has a wide arterial pulse pressure, bounding peripheral arterial pulses, and a hyperdynamic left ventricular apical impulse.[202] Such patients are generally normal in appearance unless the ductus is part of the congenital rubella syndrome. The characteristic auscultatory finding in a PDA is a high-pitched continuous murmur[200, 203] (Fig. 4–26, p. 80). The murmur is loudest at the infraclavicular or left upper sternal border area, begins after the first heart sound, peaks around the second heart sound, and extends variably into diastole. If a large left-to-right shunt is present, a middiastolic flow rumble across the mitral valve may be audible at the left ventricular apex. If the pulmonary vascular resistance becomes elevated, which is more common in adults than in infants and children, the left-to-right shunt is diminished, and the typical continuous murmur is replaced by a rough systolic murmur with an accentuated pulmonary component of the second heart sound.[203] Eventually, the pulmonary vascular resistance may equal or exceed the systemic vascular resistance, resulting in a palpable right ventricular systolic impulse, a loud pulmonary component of the second heart sound, a pulmonary ejection click, and a murmur of pulmonary regurgitation (Fig. 4–24, p. 79). Although clinical signs of pulmonary artery hypertension are present, the cause may be difficult to determine, since the characteristic continuous murmur is now absent.

NONINVASIVE STUDIES. The patient with a small persistent ductus may have a normal *electrocardiogram.* If the anomaly is large, left ventricular hypertrophy with a diastolic overload pattern is common.[202, 203] Normal sinus rhythm is usual until the development of congestive heart failure, at which time atrial fibrillation frequently occurs. Right ventricular hypertrophy usually reflects the Eisenmenger physiology.

On *chest roentgenogram,* a PDA with a large left-to-right shunt is characterized by pulmonary plethora as well as dilatation of the proximal pulmonary arteries, left atrium, and left ventricle. The area between the aortic knob and the pulmonary artery on the anteroposterior projection may appear filled. The ascending aorta and aortic knob are often prominent, findings that may help distinguish a PDA from ventricular and atrial septal defects. In the adult, calcification of the ductus may occasionally be noted[203] (Fig. 6–31, p. 159). If Eisenmenger physiology develops, the central pulmonary arteries enlarge and become dilated with attenuated peripheral vessels.

The M-mode *echocardiogram* is nonspecific in PDA, and shows left atrial, left ventricular, and aortic root enlargement. On two-dimensional study, the ductus itself may be visualized if large (Fig. 30–20, p. 925). Doppler echocardiography is often helpful in quantifying the magnitude of the left-to-right shunt, detecting pulmonary artery hypertension, and assessing the presence of turbulent blood flow within the main pulmonary artery[205, 206] (Figs. 5–81 and 5–82, p. 118). Color-flow Doppler mapping may also be useful for visualization of blood flow into the pulmonary artery.[206a]

CARDIAC CATHETERIZATION. In an adult patient with an uncomplicated PDA, the typical finding at cardiac catheterization is an oxygen saturation step-up at the pulmonary artery level. Cardiac catheterization is useful in determining the magnitude of the shunt, evaluating the degree of pulmonary artery hypertension, and testing the reactivity of the pulmonary vasculature to pharmacologic interventions. The catheter can usually be passed from the main pulmonary artery through the ductus into the descending aorta. Angiocardiography will detect a right-to-left shunt with opacification of the descending aorta (Fig. 6–46, p. 170). Aortography with the patient in the left lateral position will frequently delineate the PDA and differentiate it from other causes of a continuous precordial murmur, including (1) pulmonary and systemic atrioventricular fistulae, (2) rupture of a sinus of Valsalva aneurysm, (3) the combination of VSD and aortic regurgitation, (4) coronary artery fistula to either the right atrium, right ventricle, or coronary sinus, (5) anomalous origin of the left coronary artery from the pulmonary trunk, (6) severe peripheral pulmonic stenosis, or (7) aortopulmonary window.

NATURAL HISTORY—MEDICAL. The three major complications observed in adults with PDA include ventricular dysfunction, infective endarteritis, and obliterative pulmonary vascular disease.[200–204] Patients with small left-to-right shunts from a PDA seldom, if ever, develop heart failure or pulmonary vascular obstructive disease. However, they are at risk of developing infective endarteritis. This most often occurs on the "jet" lesion that appears in the intima of the pulmonary artery opposite the orifice of the ductus. On occasion, endarteritis develops within the ductus itself. Patients with large left-to-right shunts may develop left ventricular failure, particularly during infancy and again after the age of 20 years.[200, 202, 203] In very rare cases, survival to old age occurs in the presence of a PDA with a large left-to-right shunt.[207] Right ventricular failure is common in patients with pulmonary vascular obstructive disease and reversed shunting.

As is the case for VSD, pulmonary vascular disease in patients with PDA is either present from birth (in individuals who retain the high pulmonary vascular resistance of fetal life) or develops gradually with time (in adolescence or early adult life).[200] A large left-to-right shunt with left ventricular failure and elevation of pulmonary venous pressure may accelerate the development of obliterative pulmonary vascular disease. Exertional dyspnea and/or fatigue occurs commonly in patients with pulmonary vascular disease and is unusual in patients with normal or near-normal pulmonary vascular resistance.[203] Dilatation of the main pulmonary artery in patients with severe pulmonary vascular obstruction may compress the recurrent laryngeal nerve and cause hoarseness. Since most of the desaturated blood is shunted into the descending aorta, cyanosis and clubbing may be overlooked if the patient's feet are not inspected carefully (differential cyanosis). Most of the right-to-left shunt is directed to the legs, and this is primarily responsible for the complaint by some patients of marked leg fatigue in the absence of dyspnea.[203] The continuous murmur of a persistent ductus disappears as pulmonary vascular resistance rises, often to be replaced by the early diastolic blowing murmur of pulmonic regurgitation.

Paradoxical embolism occurs on occasion through a PDA with reversal of flow. Pulmonary hypertension secondary to pulmonary embolism may diminish or even reverse a previously present left-to-right shunt, thereby predisposing the patient to paradoxical embolism. Ductal aneurysms can occur in adults, and these may rupture or dissect with catastrophic outcome.[208–210]

INTERVENTIONAL THERAPY. *Surgery* for closure of a PDA in childhood is generally considered to be the simplest cardiothoracic operative procedure currently performed.[211] In the adult patient, however, ligation and/or division of a PDA may present a number of difficulties not present in children.[207, 208] Because the ductus in older patients may be calcified and brittle as well as aneurysmally dilated, it can rupture during closure. The results of such a catastrophic event may be minimized by performing the procedure with cardiopulmonary bypass standby. Operation is usually beneficial in adult patients with large left-to-right shunts regardless of age, presence of congestive heart failure, or cardiomegaly on chest x-ray.[202, 203] In patients with marked elevation of the pulmonary vascular resistance, operative closure of a PDA may not substantially improve the patient's prognosis or result in a significant fall in pulmonary artery pressures.[211] Both the morbidity and mortality of surgery are increased in such patients.

Catheter closure of a PDA using various techniques has been proposed.[99, 209, 212, 213] The most promising is the double-disc device developed by Rashkind.[99] Although little experience using this technique has been acquired in adults, it does represent an exciting possibility for nonsurgical closure of a PDA in the older patient.

COARCTATION OF THE AORTA

(See also pp. 848 and 929)

Coarctation of the aorta is one of the causes of surgically correctable hypertension. While it may cause left ventricular failure in infancy,[214] adult patients with this anomaly are usually asymptomatic and are frequently discovered during a search for the etiology of hypertension.[215, 215a] In the study by Glancy and coworkers, diagnosis in 65 per cent of patients with isolated coarctation was made on routine physical examination or chest roentgenogram.[216] In 17 of 22 adults, there was a delay of 10 to 33 years between the initial discovery of a murmur and/or systemic hypertension and referral of the patient for surgical correction. This emphasizes the fact that consideration of the diagnosis is the key factor in identifying adult patients with coarctation. Males with this malformation outnumber females by more than 2:1.

ANATOMY. In most cases of coarctation in the adult, there is an abnormal ridge of posterior aortic wall media protruding into the aortic lumen opposite the insertion of the ligamentum arteriosum.[216a] This results in an eccentric narrowing of the thoracic aortic lumen just distal to the origin of the frequently dilated left subclavian artery[215] (Fig. 30–28, p. 930). Occasionally the coarctation is proximal to or involves the origin of the left subclavian artery.[217] In rare cases, the right subclavian artery is aberrant and originates from the right side of the descending thoracic aorta distal to the site of the coarctation. Cases have also been reported in which the coarcted segment occurs in the ascending or more distal descending thoracic aorta or even in the abdominal aorta. Extensive arterial collaterals, usually involving the internal mammary and intercostal arteries, develop between the proximal high-pressure zone and the distal low-pressure area.

Coarctation is frequently associated with other congenital malformations, including bicuspid aortic valve, PDA, VSD, and mitral valve abnormalities.[215, 218–220] Berry aneurysms of the circle of Willis, which are more common in patients with coarctation, are probably acquired rather than congenital.[221]

PATHOPHYSIOLOGY. Despite intensive investigation, the mechanism of systemic hypertension remains incompletely defined in patients with coarctation. Mechanical effects of the narrowed aortic lumen were emphasized in early studies. It was suggested that in the face of a normal forward cardiac output, a significant narrowing in the thoracic aorta produced an obligate pressure gradient across the coarcted segment and elevated pressures proximal to the stenosis. However, since the renal vascular bed lies distal to the coarctation site in the low-perfusion-pressure zone, it may be an important contributor to the pathophysiology of coarctation. This would occur through the operation of the renin-angiotensin system. In addition, actual structural differences exist in the aorta, with the precoarctational wall being more rigid than the postcoarctational wall.[222] This may have long-term influence on baroreceptors in the upper vascular bed, thus explaining a portion of the preoperative proximal hypertension and the frequent lack of normalization of blood pressure postoperatively.[222, 223]

SYMPTOMS. The most common complaints are headaches, intermittent claudication, and leg fatigue. Patients frequently seek medical attention because of symptoms associated with left ventricular failure, endarteritis, aortic rupture or dissection, or cerebral hemorrhage owing to rupture of an aneurysm of the circle of Willis. Aortic rupture usually occurs in the ascending aorta or just distal to the coarctation in a poststenotic aortic aneurysm. Endocarditis occurs most commonly on an associated bicuspid valve; endarteritis of the coarctation is less common.[215, 224]

PHYSICAL EXAMINATION. Patients with coarctation usually have a normal physical appearance. However, coarctation is the most common anomaly associated with Turner's syndrome and should be specifically searched for in this condition.

Blood pressure must be measured in both arms and at least one leg with cuffs of appropriate size; this is best accomplished by Doppler ultrasound. Eighty per cent of patients under 19 years of age and 84 per cent of patients older than 19 years are hypertensive. Typically, the systolic blood pressure is elevated disproportionately to the diastolic blood pressure, resulting in a wide pulse pressure and bounding pulses proximal to the coarctation. In the most common cases of coarctation, the systolic pressure in one arm is within 10 mm Hg of that in the other and is significantly higher than the systolic pressure in either leg. A systolic blood pressure in the right arm exceeding that in the left arm by more than 15 mm Hg implies that the site of narrowing is at, or proximal to, the origin of the left subclavian artery. If the systolic blood pressure in the right arm is more than 10 mm Hg lower than that in the left, an aberrant origin of the right subclavian artery from a low-pressure zone distal to the site of coarctation should be suspected.

In most cases, simultaneous palpation of upper- and lower-extremity pulses is diagnostic, revealing a diminished and delayed femoral (compared with right radial) artery pulse. When only a small difference exists between systolic pressures in the arm and leg, dynamic exercise exacerbates the difference and accentuates the physical findings.

On *precordial examination*, thrills in the suprasternal notch are common; rarely, a patient will have visible subcutaneous collaterals between the scapulae or on the other side of the sternum. Auscultation usually reveals an ejection-type murmur (which can be generated by the coarctation itself, an associated bicuspid aortic valve, or arterial collaterals). When generated by the coarctation itself, the murmur is usually best heard over the posterior thorax between the scapulae. The presence of a bicuspid aortic valve frequently produces a constant ejection click as well as murmurs of aortic stenosis and/or regurgitation. Murmurs generated by collateral vessels *typically* begin after the first heart sound and extend beyond the aortic component of the second heart sound (Fig. 31–14).

NONINVASIVE STUDIES. The *electrocardiogram* of coarctation patients is nonspecific. In one study[225] in which there were 48 patients with isolated coarctation, increased

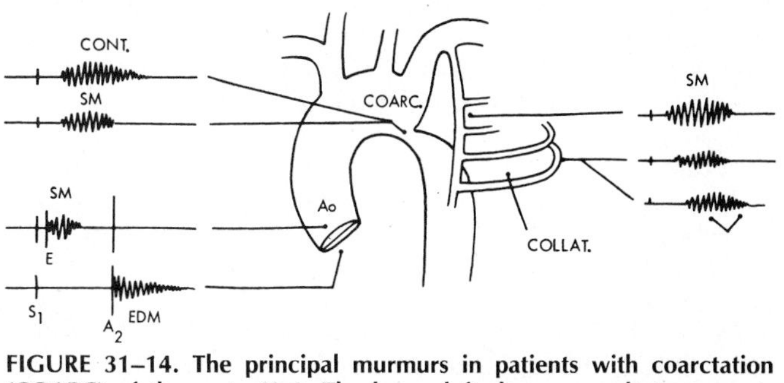

FIGURE 31–14. The principal murmurs in patients with coarctation (COARC) of the aorta (Ao). The lower left shows auscultatory events associated with a bicuspid aortic valve, namely, an aortic ejection sound (E), a short midsystolic murmur (SM), and an early diastolic murmur (EDM) of aortic regurgitation. On the upper left are shown the continuous (CONT) and the delayed systolic murmurs (SM) that originate in the coarctation itself and are best heard posteriorly over the thoracic spine. On the right are shown collateral (COLLAT) arterial murmurs that are crescendo-descrescendo in shape and delayed in onset and termination because of origin in vessels some distance from the heart. Collateral murmurs are, as a rule, bilateral and are here shown on one side as a matter of convenience. (S_1 = first heart sound; A_2 = aortic second sound). (From Perloff, J. K.: The Clinical Recognition of Congenital Heart Disease, 3rd ed. Philadelphia, W. B. Saunders Company, 1987, p. 139.)

QRS voltage was the most common abnormality. Even so, the electrocardiogram can be entirely within normal limits. This is especially true in adolescent or young adult male patients in whom large QRS voltages across the precordium are common even in normal subjects. Left ventricular strain pattern is not invariably present.

Most adult patients with significant coarctation have abnormal *chest roentgenograms* (Figs. 6–34 and 6–35, p. 160). Nonspecific findings that can be present include cardiomegaly and a dilated ascending aorta. More specific findings usually consist of poststenotic dilation of the descending thoracic aortic shadow and rib notching. The dilated left subclavian artery usually produces a convex shadow proximal to the coarcted segment. In association with the poststenotic dilation, this produces a characteristic "3" sign. An oral dose of barium demonstrates a "reverse 3" image for the same reasons. Rib notching is caused by erosion of the costal grooves owing to dilated tortuous collateral intercostal arteries. It is uncommon in patients under the age of 6 years but is present among most adults with this anomaly. In typical coarctation, notching involves the third to eighth ribs bilaterally and is usually only present posteriorly, since anterior intercostal arteries do not run in costal grooves. If the coarctation is proximal to, or involves the origin of, the left subclavian artery, there is no stimulus for collateral development on the left side, and rib notching will be limited to the right hemithorax. Similarly, if the right subclavian artery arises aberrantly in the low-pressure zone distal to the site of coarctation, rib notching is limited to the left posterior ribs.

Noninvasive imaging of the heart and extracardiac structures is often clinically useful in patients with coarctation. M-mode and two-dimensional echocardiography are helpful in diagnosing associated lesions (e.g., a bicuspid aortic valve) as well as in assessing the degree of left ventricular hypertrophy. Using a suprasternal or infraclavicular transducer position, the coarctation site and take-off of the left subclavian artery can occasionally be visualized (Figs. 31–15 and 30–29, p. 931). In many cases, pulsed Doppler echocardiography can localize the level of the coarctation, while continuous-wave Doppler can estimate closely the pressure gradient across the narrowed aortic segment.[226–230] Other imaging techniques, including digital subtraction angiography, rapid-acquisition computerized tomography, and magnetic resonance imaging (Fig. 12–35, p. 374), are also useful in defining the anatomy of coarctation.[229]

Cardiac catheterization and angiography may be indicated in an individual patient to demonstrate the severity of the coarctation (Fig. 30–30, p. 931), to define the anatomy of the arch and collateral vessels, to assess the coronary arteries for stenosis, and to evaluate the hemodynamic importance of associated cardiac lesions. Depending on the results of long-term follow-up studies, balloon dilatation angioplasty may be another indication for cardiac catheterization in such patients.

NATURAL HISTORY—MEDICAL. Liberthson and coworkers reviewed 234 cases of unoperated coarctation of the aorta evaluated at Massachusetts General Hospital between 1948 and 1978.[221] Only 4 per cent of patients between the ages of 1 and 40 years had symptoms of congestive heart failure compared with 67 per cent of patients older than 40 years. In this same series, 6 per cent of patients experienced cerebrovascular events, 3 per cent suffered myocardial infarction, 2 per cent developed bacterial endocarditis, and 2 per cent developed aortic dissection or rupture. In Campbell's review of 304 autopsy cases of unrepaired coarctation, 25 per cent of the patients died before age 20, 50 per cent by age 32, 75 per cent by age 46, and 90 per cent by age 58.[224] The mean age at death

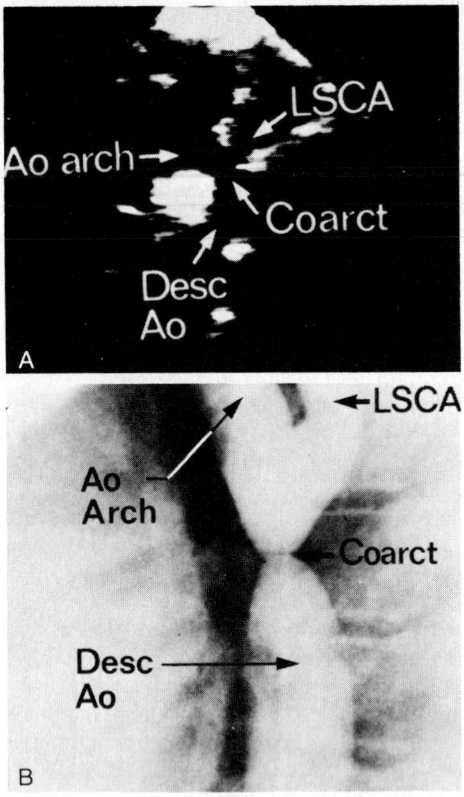

FIGURE 31–15. *A,* **Two-dimensional echocardiogram obtained using the infraclavicular transducer position in a patient with coarctation of the aorta. A discrete area of narrowing in the aorta can be seen just distal to the takeoff of the left subclavian artery (LSCA).** *B,* **Aortography confirmed a discrete coarctation of the aorta. Areas of pre- and poststenotic dilatation are present. Coarct = coarctation of the aorta; Ao arch = aortic arch; Desc Ao = descending aorta.**

for patients with coarctation was 34 years, compared with a normal life expectancy of 71 years. Major causes of death in patients under age 30 years included aortic rupture, endocarditis, and cerebrovascular events. The major cause of death after age 30 years was congestive heart failure. Campbell estimated that the incidence of endocarditis (or endarteritis) was between 0.6 and 1.3 per cent a year. The infection most commonly involved a bicuspid aortic valve, the coarctation site itself, or associated collateral vessels. Aortic rupture usually occurred between ages 20 and 30 years and most commonly involved the proximal ascending aorta. Patients who developed intracranial hemorrhage were usually hypertensive, with most events related to the presence of berry aneurysms. Most complications that arose among patients with coarctation resulted from hypertension that occurred proximal to the coarcted segment.

The high incidence of congestive heart failure in older patients with coarctation of the aorta may be explained by the complex pathophysiology of the lesion itself. In a recent study using load-independent indices of left ventricular contractility, all patients with unrepaired coarctation over age 20 years were found to have left ventricular contractile dysfunction.[230] This could reflect several hemodynamic derangements, including (1) higher myocardial oxygen requirements secondary to the chronically elevated ventricular afterload; (2) abnormalities in early ventricular diastolic function, reflecting elevated late systolic load and the consequent reduction in left ventricular systolic performance; and (3) impaired function of the aorta relative to its ability to accept pulsatile blood flow from the left ventricle. This reflects problems caused by increased aortic wall thickness proximal to the site of coarctation and reduced central aortic capacitance leading to alterations in the pulsatile properties of the proximal aorta and upper body arteries.

Medical management of the pregnant woman with coarctation of the aorta can be challenging (p. 1855). In a review of the obstetrical experience of 28 women with unrepaired coarctation of the aorta, there was no maternal mortality; however, the spontaneous abortion rate was 25 per cent.[231] Most of the remaining pregnancies were uncomplicated and the infants were normal. Because of the increased cardiac output associated with the second and third trimesters of pregnancy, patients with unrepaired coarctation of the aorta may experience a significant increase in systolic arterial pressure. In many cases, antihypertensive therapy may be required. Nitroprusside infusion is often useful in treating acute elevations in blood pressure during delivery and the immediate postpartum period. In a small fraction of patients with coarctation of the aorta, aortic dissection or rupture occurs during pregnancy. However, it is likely that in such cases intrinsic disease of the ascending aorta with cystic necrosis was present before pregnancy. Fortunately, this complication is so uncommon in women with unrepaired coarctation of the aorta followed in modern obstetrical practice that there seems to be little rationale for elective coarctation repair during pregnancy.[211, 231] The bacteremia that accompanies labor seldom results in endocarditis or endarteritis in patients with coarctation.

NATURAL HISTORY—INTERVENTIONAL

Balloon Dilation Angioplasty. This procedure is a reliable method of treating *recurrent* narrowing after repair of coarctation in infancy.[192, 232–239] Despite case reports of successful balloon dilation of sites of coarctation in adults, this procedure currently remains experimental.[236, 239, 240] Most worrisome is the potential for aneurysm formation in the area of the old coarctation.[192] In some instances, the angiographic appearance of such a lesion has prompted prophylactic excision of the affected area.

Surgery. Operative correction of coarctation is performed through a left thoracotomy. In infants and young children, subclavian patch angioplasty is the favored repair (Fig. 30–31, p. 931). For adults, correction usually entails resection of the coarcted segment and interposition of a graft between the proximal and distal ends.[237–245] After surgical correction, the risk of vegetative endocarditis or endarteritis does not appreciably decrease; thus the patient should continue to receive antibiotic prophylaxis.

During the first week after operation for coarctation, significant systemic hypertension is frequently present, even in patients with an adequate repair.[216, 246–249] In the immediate postoperative period (i.e., the first 12 to 24 hours), a rise in systolic pressure may occur, followed on the second or third day by a rise in diastolic pressure.[246] The hypertension that occurs within 24 hours of repair is associated with evidence of hyperactivity of the sympathetic nervous system, such as a decreased response to cold pressor stimuli[246] and markedly elevated plasma norepinephrine levels.[247] The paradoxical hypertension that occurs 2 to 3 days postoperatively is associated with a marked transient rise in plasma renin activity and is probably best treated with either a converting enzyme inhibitor or with beta-blockade therapy.[246, 248–250]

Long-Term Surgical Follow-up. It is important to realize that in patients with coarctation of the aorta, surgery offers repair or relief but not total correction of cardiovascular abnormalities.[243] Although overall left ventricular performance is usually well preserved,[251, 252] long-term problems may include persistent systemic hypertension, restenosis at the coarctation site, and complications from associated intracardiac and extracardiac anomalies. The mechanism of persistent postoperative hypertension is unclear, but proposed possibilities include resetting of the carotid baroreceptors, hypoplasia of the distal arterial tree, and activation of the renin-angiotensin system. The development of persistent postoperative hypertension appears to be a function of the timing of surgical repair. In one review, only 6 per cent of patients receiving surgical correction between the ages of 1 and 5 years were left with residual hypertension, whereas 50 per cent of patients undergoing surgery after the age of 40 years suffered from persistent hypertension despite successful abolition of the pressure difference between upper and lower extremities.[221] In a retrospective assessment of 248 patients 11 to 25 years after repair, Maron and associates found that 12 per cent of the patients had died, 78 per cent had evidence of cardiovascular disease, and 40 per cent had persistent hypertension despite the fact that surgical repair was adequate in most.[253] The experience at the Green Lane Hospital in New Zealand is quite similar. In that report, 160 patients operated on for coarctation of the aorta between the ages of 1 and 54 years were evaluated 10 to 28 years postoperatively.[147] Most patients were hypertensive before operation. The frequency of hypertension decreased markedly in the first postoperative years. Blood pressure was normal in most patients 5 to 10 years after operation, but when followed-up for longer periods, the proportion of patients with hypertension increased. Hypertension was more common in patients operated on after 20 years of age than in those aged 5 to 19 years at operation. The likelihood of being alive without complications and with a normal blood pressure was 69 per cent at 10 years, 55 per cent at 15 years, and 20 per cent at 25 years postoperatively.

The need for reoperation for coarctation may occur because of either residual coarctation or recurrent narrowing at the original coarctation site.[241] The two most common causes of residual coarctation are a technically inadequate repair that limits the aortic lumen by 50 per cent or more and hypoplasia of the aortic arch proximal to the repair site. In general, recurrent coarctation is thought to exist if a resting systolic pressure gradient greater than 10 mm Hg across the aortic repair site develops over a period after operation. Suggested mechanisms include failure of adequate growth of the anastomosis, active scarring with fibrosis and aortic narrowing at the site of repair, thrombosis on the suture line, and retention in the vascular repair of ductal tissue that can proliferate to narrow the aortic lumen.[241]

In addition to patients who have residual resting hypertension, there are patients with no or only mild elevations of blood pressure and no residual gradient at rest who have an exaggerated exercise-induced rise in systolic blood pressure. This is frequently associated with development of a significant difference in pressures between the upper and lower extremities, and may signify the presence of a mild to moderately narrowed coarctation repair site.[147, 241, 244, 254–256] Accurate measurement of pressure gradients between the right arm and legs, both at rest and during exercise, is considered an integral part of the follow-up examination in patients with repaired coarctation. Reoperation should be considered in a symptomatic patient with an arm-to-leg pressure gradient greater than 35 mm Hg in whom the coarctation site has been visualized at cardiac catheterization.[262]

In most cases, patients with significant residual or recurrent aortic narrowing benefit from either balloon angioplasty or surgery. The key to improved long-term survival is early recognition and treatment as well as continued medical supervision for an indefinite postoperative period.

EBSTEIN'S ANOMALY OF THE TRICUSPID VALVE

(See also p. 951)

ANATOMY. Ebstein's anomaly of the tricuspid valve comprises a wide variety of anatomical derangements. The principal abnormality is downward displacement of a malformed tricuspid valve into an underdeveloped right ventricle with reduced pumping capacity[257, 258] (Fig. 30–57, p. 951). The presence of a portion of the right ventricle between the atrioventricular groove and the downward displaced origin of the septal and posterior leaflets of the tricuspid valve results in a direct communication between the right atrium and the "artrialized" right ventricle. In some cases, the septal leaflet of the tricuspid is absent. Typically, the anterior leaflet of the tricuspid valve is abnormally elongated with whip-like redundant motion during each cardiac cycle. This valve leaflet may also be thickened and tethered.[259, 260] Commonly associated anatomical defects include secundum atrial septal defect, patent foramen ovale, ventricular septal defect, pulmonary stenosis or atresia, and mitral valve prolapse.

PATHOPHYSIOLOGY. The degree of hemodynamic compromise to right ventricular function depends on the amount of right ventricular tissue above the tricuspid valve, as well as the extent of adherence of the valve tissue to the right ventricular wall. The atrialized portion of the right ventricle is usually hypokinetic, contributing little to the ventricle's forward stroke volume. Tricuspid regurgitation, a problem frequently associated with Ebstein's anomaly, further compromises effective right ventricular output.[261, 262] Many patients with Ebstein's anomaly have a concomitant interatrial communication (an atrial septal defect or patent foramen ovale) that allows right-to-left shunting of blood.

Cyanosis occurs in one-half to three-fourths of adult patients with this malformation and may appear or worsen with exercise, fatigue, or exposure to cold. In the other one-fourth, right ventricular pumping capacity is almost normal. In nearly all cases of anatomically uncomplicated Ebstein's anomaly, left ventricular systolic performance is normal.

PHYSICAL EXAMINATION. Although most patients with Ebstein's anomaly are phenotypically normal, they may demonstrate central cyanosis and clubbing of the digits. The first heart sound is typically loud and widely split. This is due predominantly to the abnormally large size and increased excursion of the anterior tricuspid leaflet[263] (Fig. 3–5, p. 45). Multiple systolic clicks owing to vibrations of this frequently sail-like leaflet may be present. Loud third and fourth heart sounds are common in older patients. The most common murmur is that of tricuspid regurgitation. Occasionally a diastolic murmur of tricuspid stenosis may be present.

NONINVASIVE STUDIES. The *electrocardiogram* frequently demonstrates peaked P waves as well as right ventricular conduction delay or complete right bundle branch block. Right ventricular hypertrophy is not associated with Ebstein's anomaly. Wolff-Parkinson-White syndrome (usually type B) occurs in 10 to 25 per cent of patients with this malformation.[261, 264–266] The *chest roentgenogram* generally shows cardiomegaly owing predominantly to a markedly dilated right atrium (Fig. 30–58). If significant right-to-left shunting across an ASD is present, there may be diminished pulmonary blood flow. *Echocardiography* has recently been shown to be the diagnostic procedure of choice in patients with Ebstein's anomaly.[259–261, 267] On M-mode study, a large anterior leaflet of the tricuspid valve is recorded from almost any anterior precordial transducer position. In conjunction with this finding is delayed closure of the tricuspid, occurring 30 to 70 msec after mitral valve closure. Two dimensional echocardiography is, however, much more sensitive and specific for making the diagnosis of Ebstein's anomaly. The apical four-chamber view allows simultaneous visualization of the atrioventricular ring, the displaced tricuspid valve leaflets, the true and atrialized right ventricles, the anatomical right atrium, and the left-sided cardiac chambers (Fig. 31–16) (Figs. 5–70, p. 114, and 30–59, p. 952). Morphological anbormalities detected by two-dimensional echocardiography that correlate well with diminished functional capacity and clinical well-being include (1) a small true right ventricle and large atrialized right ventricle, (2) extreme septal leaflet displacement, (3) absent septal leaflet, (4) displaced and tethered anterior leaflet, and (5) aneurysmal dilation of the right ventricular outflow tract.[259, 260] The combination of two-dimensional and Doppler echocardiography allows careful anatomical and physiological assessment of associated lesions. Color flow Doppler mapping is particularly useful for defining the magnitude and direction of tricuspid regurgitant jets.[206a] Recently, rapid-acquisition computerized tomography has also been shown to be a reliable imaging technique for diagnosing Ebstein's anomaly of the tricuspid valve (Fig. 31–17).[268]

Cardiac catheterization carries a higher than normal risk in patients with Ebstein's anomaly. In an international cooperative study reported

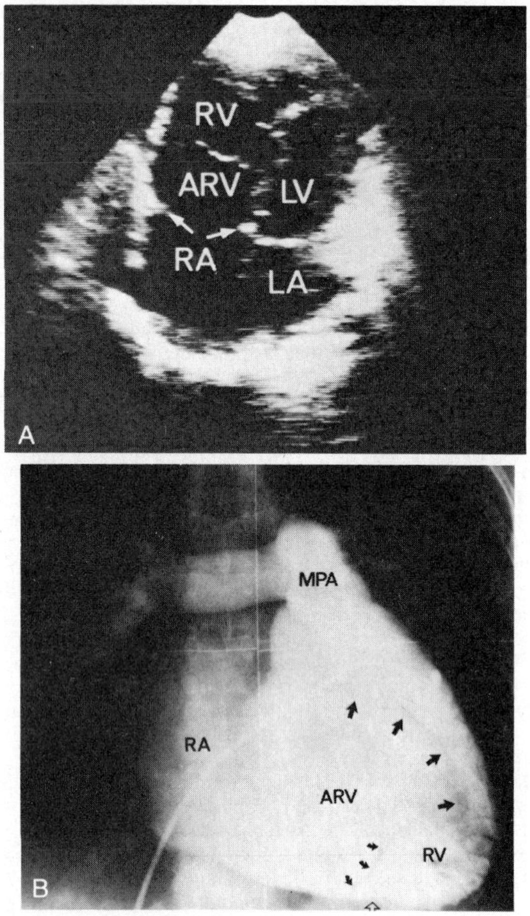

FIGURE 31–16. Ebstein's anomaly of the tricuspid valve. *A,* Systolic frame from a two-dimensional echocardiographic study obtained using the apical transducer position in a mildly cyanotic 25-year-old woman with a holosystolic murmur and multiple systolic clicks. Portions of the tricuspid valve are displaced downward into the right ventricle (RV) diagnostic of Ebstein's anomaly. The arrows delineate the level of the atrioventricular (AV) groove. The portion of the RV between the AV groove and the downward displaced origin of the tricuspid valve leaflets is termed the atrialized right ventricle (ARV), an area that is hemodynamically right atrium (RA) but electrophysiologically RV. The true RA is enlarged. Both the left atrium (LA) and the left ventricle (LV) are decreased in size. Mitral valve prolapse is present. In other panels, right-to-left bowing of the interatrial septum was present, suggesting an atrial septal defect that was relatively small. Pulsed Doppler echocardiographic study confirmed the presence of tricuspid regurgitation. *B,* Right ventriculogram from the same patient demonstrating downward displacement of the large, sail-like anterior (straight solid arrows) and smaller posterior (curved solid arrows) leaflets of the tricuspid valve. A notch (open arrow) is apparent at the site of the anomalous insertion of the tricuspid valve. The RV is moderately hypoplastic. Pulmonic stenosis is absent. MPA = main pulmonary artery.

by Watson, 90 of 363 patients undergoing cardiac catheterization experienced atrial arrhythmias.[265] In addition, there were 13 deaths. Because of the high degree of reliability of echocardiographic techniques for evaluating Ebstein's anomaly, cardiac catheterization in the adult patient should be reserved for cases with unresolved hemodynamic questions or unclear anatomy of associated lesions.

NATURAL HISTORY—MEDICAL. The severity of the anatomical abnormalities associated with Ebstein's anomaly is variable, with a considerable proportion of these patients surviving into adult life.[261] Many patients remain asymptomatic until the third or fourth decade. Patients with milder forms of Ebstein's anomaly may even have a normal life expectancy. Right ventricular failure, characterized by dyspnea, fatigue, weakness, and peripheral edema, usually marks the beginning of a downhill course for the adult patient with Ebstein's anomaly; heart failure is the most common cause of death.[261] Syncope secondary to atrial and ventricular arrhythmias and precordial discomfort are also ominous signs. Palpitations are common, since patients with Ebstein's anomaly are prone to atrial and ventricular arrhythmias. Sudden death, presumably secondary to arrhythmias, occurs in as many as 20 per cent of adults with Ebstein's anomaly.[264, 266] The derangements in right heart morphology and function in Ebstein's anomaly contribute to significant alterations in left ventricular geometry. These geometric alterations are associated frequently with mild left ventricular hypokinesis and are probably the result of diminished left ventricular preload.[268a] Paradoxical embolism and brain abscess are other common complications. Women who are not cyanotic and have mild Ebstein's anomaly may safely and successfully complete a normal pregnancy.[262]

SURGICAL THERAPY. Surgery for Ebstein's anomaly has met with variable success. It has been generally reserved for patients who are NYHA functional class 3 or 4. Operative approaches have included annuloplasty or replacement of the tricuspid valve, plication of the free wall of the atrialized portion of the right ventricle, right atrial reduction, and closure of the ASD.[269–274] If the right ventricle has sufficient capacity to accept the entire cardiac output, operative results may be salutary. Because of the rapid clinical deterioration that usually commences after the onset of right ventricular failure, surgical intervention should be considered for patients with this complication. However, if the functional right ventricular cavity is small and has a low compliance and pumping capacity, replacement of the tricuspid valve and closure of the interatrial communication results in a severe low-output state.

Long-Term Surgical Follow-up. Surgical treatment of Ebstein's anomaly has been characterized by improvement in clinical symptoms and decrease in cardiac size. Symptomatic arrhythmias continue to be a problem postoperatively in many cases.[271, 273, 274] In some cases, ablation of accessory atrioventricular pathways can eliminate postoperative tachyarrhythmias. Patients who experienced perioperative ventricular tachycardia or fibrillation are at particularly high risk of sudden death.[274]

RIGHT VENTRICULAR DYSPLASIA

(See also p. 697)

Right ventricular dysplasia is a pathological condition in which there is partial or total replacement of a portion of right ventricular musculature

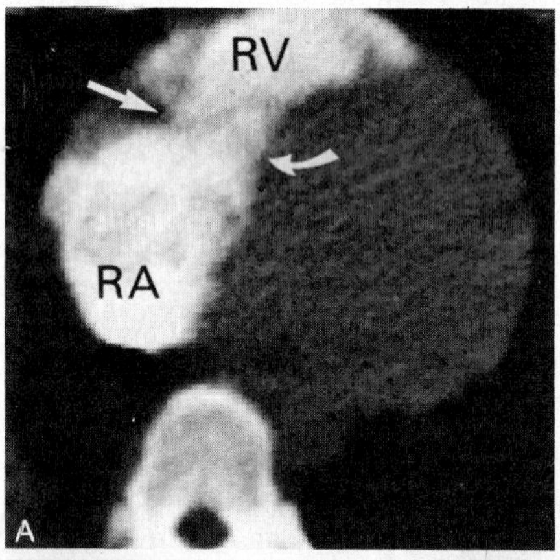

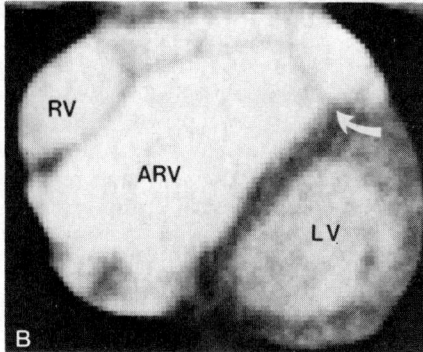

FIGURE 31–17. Contrast-enhanced ultrafast computerized tomographic (CT) images. *A,* Normally positioned anterior (straight arrow) and septal (curved arrow) leaflets of the tricuspid valve in an adult woman without cardiac disease. *B,* Study from a 42-year-old woman with Ebstein's anomaly of the tricuspid valve. There is downward displacement of the septal leaflet (curved arrow) as well as a large "sail" anterior leaflet. The functional right ventricle (RV) is small while the atrialized right ventricle (ARV) is markedly dilated. (Courtesy of Bruce Brundage, M.D.)

with adipose and fibrous tissue.[275–280] In its extreme, called *Uhl's anomaly*, there is apposition of endocardial and epicardial layers of the affected areas.[281–284] Right ventricular dysplasia is more common in males and may be associated with mitral valve prolapse.[275] In some cases, a familial predisposition may exist.[282, 284] Three clinical forms of right ventricular dysplasia have been described.[280] These include (1) patients with signs and symptoms of right ventricular failure, (2) patients who present with either ventricular tachycardia with a left bundle branch configuration[275, 276, 280, 285] or supraventricular tachyarrhythmias,[285, 286] and (3) asymptomatic patients with cardiomegaly on chest roentgenogram or right ventricular dilatation at autopsy. In a report of 24 patients with right ventricular dysplasia, mean age at the time of hospitalization was 39 years.[275]

The *physical examination* in adults with right ventricular dysplasia is often normal except for the right-sided fourth heart sound. Two dimensional *echocardiography*, which usually demonstrates right ventricular enlargement with normal left ventricular chamber size, can be helpful in distinguishing right ventricular dysplasia from other lesions, such as Ebstein's anomaly of the tricuspid valve, ASD, partial anomalous pulmonary venous drainage, congenital absence of the left pericardium,[275, 287] right ventricular infarction, or tricuspid regurgitation.[275, 279, 280] At *cardiac catheterization*, angiography shows increased right ventricular size.[279, 280] In some cases, segmental motion abnormalities with systolic expansion of the infundibular area may be present.[275, 279, 280]

The pathogenesis and *natural history* of right ventricular dysplasia are unknown. While right ventricular dysfunction predominates, latent left ventricular performance abnormalities may be elicited by exercise stress testing.[277] The importance of this observation is suggested by a patient with right ventricular dysplasia followed for 16 years in whom progressive dilatation and functional deterioration of the right ventricle followed by the left ventricle occurred.[278] In most cases, symptoms depend on the rate of the patient's tachyarrhythmia. Many patients with ventricular tachycardia respond to antiarrhythmic drug treatment; some require surgery. Because the entire right ventricle is potentially arrhythmogenic, ablating a single site of ventricular tachycardia may not eliminate the arrhythmia. An operation which prevents arrhythmic activity arising from the right ventricle from spreading to the left ventricle has been developed. This is accomplished by dissecting the right ventricular free wall from its left ventricular attachments. When subsequently resutured, the fibrous scar that forms with healing confines right ventricular arrhythmias to that chamber. Initial results in a small number of patients have been promising.[288] Fortunately, death resulting from ventricular fibrillation is uncommon in this lesion.[289]

LESS COMMON FORMS OF CYANOTIC CONGENITAL HEART DISEASE IN THE ADULT

In general, adults with less common forms of cyanotic congenital heart disease can be divided into two physiological categories. These include patients with obligatory right-to-left shunts and patients with Eisenmenger syndrome. They can also be classified into three broad groups according to how frequently they are encountered (Table 31–4).[290]

OBLIGATORY RIGHT-TO-LEFT SHUNTS. In these patients, cyanosis commences during infancy. In most cases, a two-stage surgical approach is pursued. This includes palliative surgery early in life, followed later by physiological correction. The result has been an increasing number of patients who survive long term. An example of physiological correction is the Fontan procedure for tricuspid atresia (p. 950). This involves patch closure of the ASD in conjunction with a conduit to direct systemic venous blood from the right atrium or right atrial appendage to the hypoplastic right ventricle or, more commonly, the right or main pulmonary artery.[290–294] This operation results in long-term improvement in exercise duration and cardiorespiratory response.[286, 287] Not surprisingly, a negative correlation between age at "repair" and postoperative exercise capacity has been reported.[294]

Another congenital malformation with potential for physiological correction and subsequent survival into adulthood is dextro-transposition of the great arteries (p. 953). Such patients are cyanotic from birth. In the past, the results of surgery using either the Mustard or the Senning procedure[295–297] have been encouraging. Recently, anatomical correction of dextro-transposition (i.e., switch procedure) has been possible. Short-term evaluations suggest that conversion of the left ventricle from the pulmonary to the systemic pumping chamber is well tolerated if surgery is performed early in life.[298]

Rarely, patients with anomalies such as pulmonary atresia (p. 944), truncus arteriosus (p. 925), or univentricular hearts (p. 965) survive to adult life.[299–301] Surgical treatment of such patients with synthetic right heart conduits may result in markedly improved quality of life and long-term survival.[290] No significant data are currently available regarding the use of cardiac transplantation in patients with complex cyanotic heart disease.

TABLE 31–4 CYANOTIC CONGENITAL HEART DISEASE ENCOUNTERED IN ADULTS

I. Anomalies relatively frequently encountered
  A. With reduced pulmonary blood flow and normal pulmonary vascular resistance
    1. Tetralogy of Fallot
    2. Pulmonary atresia with ventricular septal defect
    3. Pulmonary stenosis with atrial right-to-left shunt
  B. With increased pulmonary vascular resistance
    1. Ventricular septal defect with Eisenmenger reaction
    2. Patent ductus arteriosus with Eisenmenger reaction
    3. Atrial septal defect with Eisenmenger reaction
II. Anomalies less frequently encountered
  A. With reduced pulmonary blood flow and normal pulmonary vascular resistance
    1. Single ventricle with pulmonary stenosis or atresia
    2. Tricuspid atresia with pulmonary stenosis, atresia, or small ventricular septal defect
    3. Transposition with pulmonary stenosis or atresia
    4. Double-outlet right ventricle with pulmonary stenosis or atresia
  B. With increased pulmonary vascular resistance
    1. Single ventricle with Eisenmenger reaction
    2. Transposition with Eisenmenger reaction
    3. Truncus arteriosus with Eisenmenger reaction
    4. Double-outlet right ventricle with Eisenmenger reaction
III. Anomalies rarely encountered
  A. Congenital pulmonary arteriovenous fistula
  B. Congenital vena caval to left atrial communication
  C. Mitral atresia
  D. Double-outlet right ventricle
  E. Asplenia or polysplenia syndrome
  F. Total anomalous pulmonary venous return

From Roberts, W. C.: Adult Congenital Heart Disease. Philadelphia, F. A. Davis Co., 1987, p. 542.

EISENMENGER SYNDROME. The term *Eisenmenger complex* is used to specifically refer to the anatomical physiological combination of a ventricular septal defect, pulmonary vascular disease, and right-to-left shunting of blood.[146a, 302] The more general term *Eisenmenger syndrome* is used to describe any communication between the systemic and pulmonary circulations that produces pulmonary vascular disease of such severity that bidirectional or predominantly right-to-left shunting occurs (Table 31–5). Most of these patients become cyanotic in adolescence or early in adult life. The cyanosis, along with digital clubbing and polycythemia, is generally progressive.[303] Death often occurs suddenly, although symptomatic arrhythmias do not usually pose a problem until late in the natural history of the disease. Symptoms

TABLE 31–5 CONGENITAL CARDIAC LESIONS THAT CAN BE COMPLICATED BY THE EISENMENGER REACTION

Aortic shunts
- Persistent ductus arteriosus
- Aorticopulmonary septal defect
- Truncus arteriosus
- Pulmonic atresia, ventricular septal defect, and large "bronchial" collateral vessels

Ventricular shunts
- Ventricular septal defect
- Single ventricle
- Transposition of the great arteries with ventricular septal defect
- Double-outlet right ventricle
- Tricuspid atresia and ventricular septal defect without pulmonic stenosis
- Mitral atresia and ventricular septal defect or single ventricle
- Atrioventricular canal

Atrial shunts
- Atrial septal defect: secundum, primum, sinus venosus
- Common atrium
- Total anomalous pulmonary venous return
- Partial anomalous pulmonary venous return
- Transposition with atrial septal defect

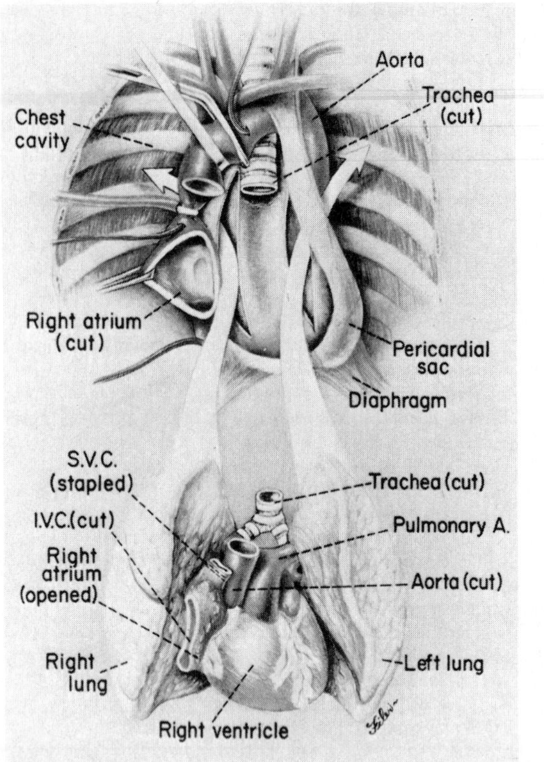

FIGURE 31–18. Drawing of a heart-lung transplant procedure in which the recipient heart and lungs have been removed and the donor heart and lungs prepared for implantation. IVC = inferior vena cava; SVC = superior vena cava; Pulmonary A = pulmonary artery. (From Griffith, B. P., et al.: Cardiopulmonary Transplantation. Surgical Rounds, 17, 1985.)

of heart failure are common in adults with Eisenmenger syndrome. In most cases, these can be controlled by medical therapy and are not severely disabling. In general, chest pain, syncopal attacks, and hemoptysis are considered to be ominous prognostic signs.

Pregnancy is contraindicated in women with severe pulmonary vascular disease.[304] If early termination of the pregnancy is not possible, close fetal and maternal monitoring, as well as judicious medical care, is required throughout the prenatal period. Maternal and fetal risk become maximal during labor and delivery. Uterine contractions, especially when associated with the application of forceps, may have an adverse effect on pulmonary and systemic hemodynamics.[305] Management of such patients should include inhalation of high concentrations of oxygen and epidural anesthesia. Serial arterial blood gas determinations may be useful in detecting changes in shunt flow associated with an acute increase in pulmonary vascular resistance or a sudden fall in systemic vascular resistance. Increased maternal risk extends at least several days into the immediate postpartum period.

Conventional surgical treatment carries an excessively high operative and postoperative risk in patients with Eisenmenger syndrome. This reflects persistence or even worsening of elevations in pulmonary vascular resistance after surgical closure of the defect.[103, 302, 303] The continued abnormality in right ventricular afterload frequently leads to worsening of the signs and symptoms of right heart failure. While the long-term outlook for patients with Eisenmenger syndrome is guarded, it is often true that they may lead reasonably active and productive lives through early adulthood.

Organ transplant surgery is potentially the only curative therapy for patients with Eisenmenger's syndrome. Cardiac transplantation alone is inadequate, since the unprepared donor right ventricle invariably fails when acutely confronted with exceedingly high pulmonary vascular resistance. Similarly, single lung transplantation does not provide adequate relief of the underlying disease process. Therefore, combined heart-lung transplantation must be performed. This has the major advantage of removing all of the diseased cardiopulmonary tissue and replacing it with anatomically, physiologically, and immunologically matched organs (Fig. 31–18).[103]

CORONARY ARTERY ANOMALIES AND CORONARY ARTERIOVENOUS FISTULA

Primary congenital anomalies of the coronary circulation occur in isolation from major malformations of the cardiovascular system. Their hemodynamic significance varies, depending on the specific anatomy. For example, when both the right and the left coronary arteries originate from the pulmonary artery, death occurs during the early neonatal period.[306] In contrast, certain anomalies allow long-term survival, with the diagnosis made only as an incidental finding at autopsy. Four categories of coronary artery anomalies are of particular importance in the adult population. These include (1) origin of one coronary artery from the pulmonary artery, (2) origin of both coronary arteries from the right sinus of Valsalva, (3) origin of both coronary arteries from the left sinus of Valsalva, and (4) coronary arteriovenous fistula.

ORIGIN OF ONE CORONARY ARTERY FROM THE PULMONARY ARTERY. *Anomalous origin of the left coronary artery (LCA) from the pulmonary artery* (Bland-White-Garland syndrome, p. 927) is the most common of these anomalies. Approximately 10 per cent of the patients survive to adulthood.[306–308a] The pathophysiology of this type of anomalous origin of the LCA is complex. During the early neonatal period, ascending aortic and pulmonary artery pressures are similar. This results in antegrade perfusion of the LCA with blood from the pulmonary trunk. By 1 year of age, the pulmonary vascular resistance is much lower than the systemic vascular resistance. This leads to preferential flow of blood in the direction of lower vascular resistance. The net result is a "coronary steal" phenomenon in which oxygenated blood from the ascending aorta enters the LCA by way of collateral vessels from the right coronary artery, with eventual exit through the main LCA into the pulmonary artery. Long-term survival is totally dependent on the development of these large collateral channels between the normally and abnormally located coronary arteries.[306–309]

By adulthood, the right coronary artery and its branches are dilated and tortuous, while the LCA is much smaller, with thinner, more friable vessel walls.[307] As a consequence of the large left-to-right shunt that occurs, the ventricular cavities dilate, cardiac mass increases, and oxygenated blood is diverted from the myocardium to the pulmonary artery. Moodie and coworkers have suggested that "coronary steal,"

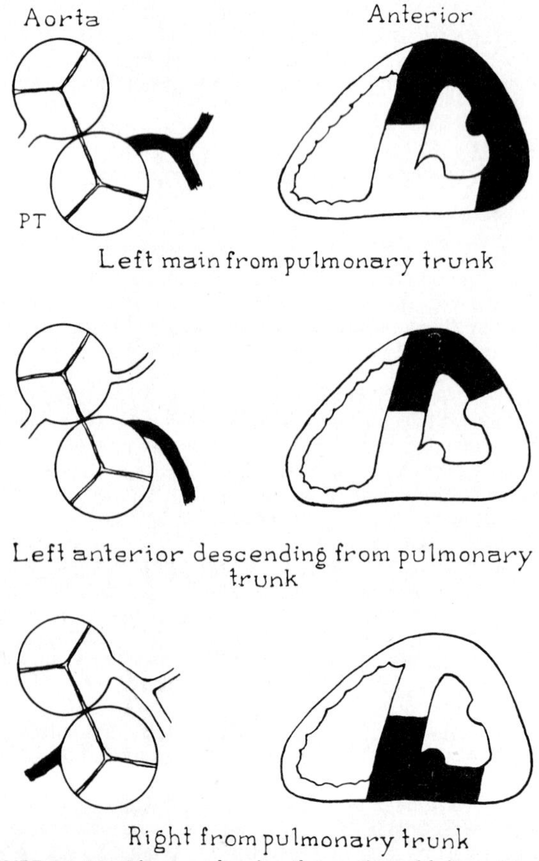

FIGURE 31–19. Diagram showing the portion of left ventricular myocardium at risk of ischemia or necrosis when the left main, left anterior descending, or right coronary artery arises from the pulmonary trunk (PT). (From Roberts, W. C.: Major anomalies of coronary arterial origin seen in adulthood. Am. Heart J. *111*:944, 1986.)

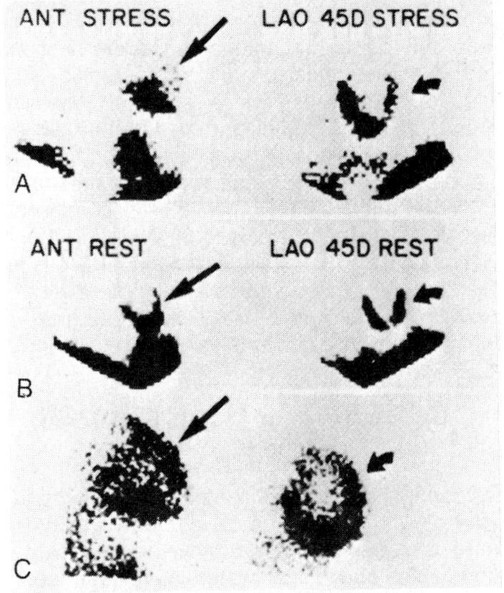

FIGURE 31–20. *A,* Preoperative stress thallium study from a 22-year-old woman with anomalous origin of the left coronary artery from the pulmonary artery. The arrow points to a region of decreased activity anterolaterally on the left anterior oblique (LAO) view. *B,* Preoperative resting thallium study in the same patient demonstrating relatively homogenous uptake anterolaterally (straight arrow) and posterolaterally on the LAO view (curved arrow). *C,* Postoperative stress thallium study in the same patient demonstrating normal homogenous uptake in the anterior view in the region supplied by the left anterior descending coronary artery (straight arrow), and on the LAO view (curved arrow) in the region supplied by the left circumflex artery. (From Moodie, D. S., et al.: Anomalous origin of the left coronary artery from the pulmonary artery [Bland-White-Garland syndrome] in adult patients: Long-term followup after surgery. Am. Heart J. *106*:383, 1983.)

rather than limitations of collateral blood flow, results in myocardial ischemia and sudden death in these patients (Fig. 31–19).[307, 310] In some cases, few or no symptoms are present until the occurrence of some catastrophic event. Other patients experience exertional chest pain, dyspnea with exercise, and syncope. Physical examination is most often remarkable for a continuous murmur along either sternal border or at the base of the heart. This is due to flow through the collateral vessels or reversal of flow in the anomalous LCA. A mitral regurgitation murmur secondary to ischemic injury to the papillary muscles may also be present.[307, 308] The electrocardiogram usually shows ischemic abnormalities with poor R wave progression over the anterior precordium (Fig. 30–25, p. 928). In most instances, no actual clinical events associated with myocardial infarction have occurred.

In infants, two-dimensional and Doppler echocardiography have correctly diagnosed this lesion. In adults, however, visualization of the coronary arteries may be difficult.[306, 311, 312] The definitive diagnosis of the anomaly is made by angiographic injection of contrast material into the lumen of the right coronary artery (or aortic root), with visualization of collateral filling of the LCA and subsequent emptying into the pulmonary artery (Figs. 10–28, p. 289, and 30–26, p. 928).[306, 313] Thallium-201 myocardial imaging at rest and during exercise has been proposed as a useful method of assessing coronary perfusion in such patients (Fig. 31–20).[307, 310]

In the adult, the natural history of untreated anomalous LCA from the pulmonary artery is noteworthy for a high incidence of sudden death. This is usually associated with physical exertion and may be the initial clinical manifestation of the anomaly. The surgical approach involves either (1) reimplantation of the anomalous coronary artery from the pulmonary artery to the aorta, (2) ligation of the anomalous LCA from inside the pulmonary artery alone, or (3) ligation in conjunction with a saphenous vein bypass graft to the left main coronary artery.[308] Although the superiority of one surgical method over another has not been demonstrated, many centers favor the ligation and bypass approach. Long-term surgical follow-up is often impressive, with improvement in symptoms and resolution of myocardial perfusion abnormalities on thallium-201 study (Fig. 31–20).

Anomalous Origin of the Right Coronary Artery (RCA) from the Pulmonary Artery. This uncommon anomaly is usually noted at necropsy.[306, 314] Patients may be asymptomatic or minimally symptomatic (i.e., dyspnea and exertional angina) as long as right ventricular oxygen demands are not excessive. However, as might be anticipated, pulmonary hypertension of any etiology is poorly tolerated in such individuals. The electrocardiogram does not usually show ischemic abnormalities or ventricular hypertrophy. Two-dimensional echocardiography and color flow Doppler mapping have proved useful for evaluating such patients.[315] Definitive diagnosis is usually made by angiography, with injection into the main LCA and subsequent visualization of collateral flow to the RCA and emptying into the pulmonary artery (Fig. 31–19). Sudden death has been reported with this anomaly.[306, 315] Therefore, even in asymptomatic patients, transsection of the RCA from the pulmonary artery and direct anastomosis of the RCA to the aorta is recommended.

Anomalous Origin of the Left Anterior Descending (LAD) Coronary Artery from the Pulmonary Artery. This anomaly, too, is uncommon. In such patients, the main LCA and RCA have normal origins. Roberts and Robinowitz summarized data on seven adult patients (age range, 18 to 55 years) with this anomaly.[316] Six patients were symptomatic, with angina pectoris secondary to myocardial ischemia and/or mitral regurgitation from papillary muscle dysfunction (Fig. 31–19). The average age at onset of symptoms was 27 years. Most patients had either systolic or continuous precordial murmurs. The electrocardiogram showed myocardial ischemia; diagnosis was made by means of coronary arteriography. In general, operative treatment is recommended to relieve symptoms and possibly prolong life.[306, 316]

ORIGIN OF BOTH CORONARY ARTERIES FROM THE RIGHT SINUS OF VALSALVA (Figs. 10–29, p. 289, and 10–30, p. 290). This anomaly is physiologically important when the left main coronary artery courses between the aorta and the pulmonary trunk.[306, 317, 317a] Barth and Roberts reviewed the necropsy data of 43 such patients and found that in 34 cases (79 per cent), death was of coronary origin. Of these 34 patients (31 males, 3 females), 26 (76 per cent) died before age 20 years and the other 8 (24 per cent) died between the ages of 49 and 82 years. Ninety-six per cent of those who died before 20 years of age did so suddenly in association with vigorous exertion. Many of these patients had exertional syncope, angina pectoris, or exertional dyspnea before their demise. Of the eight older patients, four died of consequences of acute myocardial infarction. Although the exact cause of exertional myocardial ischemia in these patients remains controversial, it is clear that blood flow through the LCA becomes limited. This may occur when increased cardiac output results in dilation of the aorta and pulmonary artery, thereby stretching and compressing the LCA. This is particularly important, since the proximal portion of the vessel is frequently narrowed because of the acute angle it has to make in its leftward passage behind the pulmonary artery. In addition, coronary ostial narrowing may be present. The diagnosis of origin of both coronary arteries from the right sinus of Valsalva is difficult to make ante mortem. Resting and stress electrocardiography, echocardiography, and thallium-201 perfusion studies have not always identified which patients with this coronary anatomy are at risk for sudden death.[317] Once the diagnosis is made and confirmed by angiography, operative intervention is probably indicated for the prevention of sudden death and for relief of exercise-induced symptoms of myocardial ischemia.[306] Saphenous vein or mammary artery bypass grafts to the left anterior descending and left circumflex coronary arteries have relieved symptoms in some patients. Other surgical approaches that have demonstrated some success include enlargement of the narrowed left main coronary ostium and reestablishment of the normal anatomical location of the origin of the left main coronary artery to the left sinus of Valsalva.

ORIGIN OF BOTH CORONARY ARTERIES FROM THE LEFT SINUS OF VALSALVA. This anomaly may result in compression of the proximal right coronary artery by a mechanism similar to that described for the LCA when it arises from the right sinus of Valsalva. Until recently, this anomaly was considered to be of little clinical importance. However, it is now known that such patients may experience angina pectoris, syncope, ventricular fibrillation, and, occasionally, sudden death.[306, 318, 319] Brandt and coworkers suggested that in addition to a slit-like ostium in the anomalous vessel and compression of the anomalous vessel between the aorta and the pulmonary artery, there may be a 50 per cent decrease in coronary reserve in the abnormal vascular segment.[318] This latter abnormality has been reversed by placement of a bypass graft beyond the anomalous segment of the RCA. Because sudden death as the presenting manifestation of this coronary artery anomaly is uncommon, it has been suggested that operative intervention may be able to be reserved until the patient has developed clinical signs and symptoms of myocardial ischemia.[306]

CONGENITAL CORONARY ARTERIOVENOUS FISTULA (See p. 927). Fistulas may occur between either the right or the left coronary artery and the right atrium, coronary sinus, or right ventricle.[320, 320a] The right coronary artery is involved more frequently than the left, but both can be affected.[321] Hemodynamic disturbances consist of a left-to-right shunt of variable magnitude and myocardial ischemia. Most patients with this anomaly not treated surgically survive to adulthood, although their life expectancy is usually reduced.[321] The majority of patients are asymptomatic until the fifth or sixth decade, when signs and symptoms of left ventricular failure occur secondary to the left-to-right shunt.[320, 321] The development of heart failure is related to the duration and magnitude of the left-to-right shunt; the latter may increase as the fistula increases in size over a period of time.

The continuous murmur characteristic of this anomaly may change to a systolic murmur in those adults who develop congestive heart failure with elevated right heart pressures. Adults with this malformation may demonstrate ischemic ST-segment changes in the precordial leads. Two-dimensional and pulsed Doppler echocardiographic studies have been able to image coronary artery fistulas and identify their site of drainage.[322–328] Diagnosis is usually made by aortography (Fig. 30–27, p. 929) or by coronary arteriography (Fig. 10–27, p. 288). Surgical closure of the fistula is indicated in patients with moderately large left-to-right shunts (pulmonary-to-systemic blood flow ratios exceeding 1.5:1.0). This procedure generally relieves manifestations of diminished cardiac reserve.[306]

CONGENITAL PULMONARY ARTERIOVENOUS FISTULAS

(See also p. 941)

Pulmonary arteriovenous fistulas arise through abnormal development of pulmonary arteries or veins.[329, 329a] The fistula replaces the normal capillary bed and usually consists of a tangle of tortuous vessels or several large and, on occasion, aneurysmal vascular trunks.[329] They usually involve the lower lobes or the right middle lobe and can be solitary or multiple and of varying size.[330, 331] Pulmonary arteriovenous fistulas may coexist with systemic telangiectasias as part of the Osler-Weber-Rendu disease,[329] in which there are multiple small telangiectasias in the skin, oral (Fig. 2–3, p. 17) and nasal mucosa, gastrointestinal tract, liver, central nervous system, and kidneys. The physiological consequences of pulmonary arteriovenous fistulas depend principally on the quantity of venous blood that is shunted into the systemic circulation; if this amount is sufficiently large, cyanosis can result.[332] Usually only a modest increase in cardiac output occurs in contrast to the marked increase that may occur with a systemic arteriovenous fistula. Complications include rupture of the fistulous vessels, with resultant hemoptysis or hemothorax, paradoxical embolism, cerebral abscess, and infectious endarteritis.[329] Cardiac failure seldom, if ever, occurs in adults with this malformation. Pulmonary arteriovenous fistulas are usually discovered during routine chest roentgenography in asymptomatic individuals. A solitary fistula or multiple fistulas confined to one lobe can be treated by means of lobectomy; patients with fistulas in multiple lobes are usually not considered to be surgical candidates.[331] Catheter embolization using mechanical occluding devices can also be employed in selected cases to obliterate a pulmonary arteriovenous fistula.[330] Isolated varicose dilatation of one or more of the pulmonary veins without an arteriovenous communication is an uncommon malformation. Hemoptysis is the principal complication.

CONGENITAL ANEURYSMS OF THE SINUS OF VALSALVA

(See also p. 924)

Congenital absence of the media in the aortic wall behind a sinus of Valsalva may result in aneurysmal dilatation of the sinus.[333, 334] This dilatation may enlarge over a period of years. Nonruptured aneurysms usually cause no cardiac dysfunction. However, coronary insufficiency and occlusion, with infarction secondary to the expanding sinus of Valsalva, have been described. In most cases, the right coronary artery is compressed over the large aneurysm. Conduction abnormalities are also relatively common because of the proximity of the right coronary and noncoronary cusps to the common bundle of His and proximal portions of the right bundle and left anterior fascicle.[335] Rupture of an aneurysm of the sinus of Valsalva occurs more commonly in males than in females and is usually to the right atrium and/or right ventricle.[336–338] This complication, which usually develops between the ages of 18 and 30 years, may present as sudden onset of chest pain and dyspnea.[333, 334] These symptoms may persist or may gradually resolve, even without specific therapy.

On *physical examination*, a loud, continuous murmur accompanied by a thrill along the low sternum is commonly found.[334] Classically, rupture results in a hyperdynamic cardiovascular system with resultant biventricular dilatation. Associated aortic regurgitation, thought to be secondary to aneurysm-induced displacement of the aortic valve leaflets, may be present whether or not rupture has occurred. Electrocardiographic findings are variable, with a right ventricular strain pattern common, especially when rupture is into the right atrium.[337] Chest roentgenogram may be normal, may demonstrate pulmonary plethora, or may be remarkable for enlargement of the cardiac silhouette.

In recent years, aneurysms of the sinus of Valsalva have been diagnosed with increasing frequency owing to the high sensitivity and specificity of two-dimensional and pulsed Doppler echocardiography.[338–342] In addition, these techniques have been useful in demonstrating right ventricular outflow tract obstruction secondary to unruptured sinus of Valsalva aneurysms[339–341] and in localizing the exit chamber when rupture has occurred.[337, 338] Medical management is recommended for isolated unruptured aneurysms. When rupture does occur, early surgical intervention is indicated.[336] Successful surgical obliteration of a ruptured aneurysm of the sinus of Valsalva results in dramatic relief of symptoms.[336]

CONGENITAL HEART BLOCK

(See also p. 967)

Criteria for congenital heart block include a slow heart rate present from birth (or noted at an early age) without a history of myocarditis, ischemic heart disease, cardiomyopathy, or prior cardiac surgery.[342] Multiple lesions of the conduction system have been reported, including (1) absence of a myocardial connection between atrial conduction tissue and the atrioventricular node, (2) failure of development of the atrioventricular node, and (3) degeneration of previously developed AV nodal tissue with replacement by fibrous tissue.[342, 343] Adults with congenital heart block without associated malformations may be asymptomatic for many years. This is due to the presence of a stable accelerated junctional pacemaker under autonomic control, which allows for some increase in heart rate during exercise. Thus a reasonably normal hemodynamic response to exercise and other stresses may occur.[344] A 95 per cent 20-year survival has been reported for patients with congenital heart block.[342]

Familial congenital heart block, inherited as an autosomal dominant trait, has been noted in some families.[345] It is of considerable interest that mothers with systemic lupus erythematosus and other connective tissue diseases give birth to children with a surprisingly high incidence of congenital heart block.[342, 346, 347] In general, patients with familial congenital heart block with wide QRS complexes and/or associated cardiac malformations have a poorer prognosis than do patients without these features.

A number of serious complications have been noted in adults with congenital heart block, including malignant ventricular tachyarrhythmias (both with exercise testing and on Holter monitoring), Stokes-Adams attacks, and decreased cardiac output.[348, 349] Exercise stress testing and Holter monitoring should be carried out in such patients, since they may disclose an indication for antiarrhythmic therapy and/or permanent pacing (e.g., tachyarrhythmias, prolonged asystole, or marked ventricular slowing). Exercise intolerance secondary to bradycardia is also an indication for permanent pacing. Most patients with congenital complete heart block do not require pacing in childhood. However, the frequency of symptoms related to rhythm abnormalities increases with patient age. By age 50 years, nearly all patients have had placement of a permanent pacemaker.

Women with congenital heart block tolerate pregnancy without difficulty, although Stokes-Adams attacks have been reported to commence shortly after delivery.[348] Insertion of a temporary transvenous pacemaker may be helpful for maintaining stable hemodynamics at the time of delivery in women with marked bradycardia owing to congenital heart block. In patients with permanent pacemakers inserted for either congenital or acquired complete heart block, improved hemodynamics may be achieved if the pacing rate is increased immediately before labor and delivery.

REFERENCES

GENERAL PRINCIPLES

1. Manning, J. A.: Insurability and employability of young cardiac patients. *In* Engle, M. A. (ed.): Pediatric Cardiovascular Disease. Philadelphia, F. A. Davis Co., 1981, p. 117.
2. Roberts, W. C. (ed.): Adult Congenital Heart Disease. Philadelphia, F. A. Davis Co., 1987.
3. Perloff, J. K.: The Clinical Recognition of Congenital Heart Disease. 3rd ed. Philadelphia, W. B. Saunders Company, 1987.

3a. Henry, W. L., and Takenaka, K.: Evaluation of older children and adults with congenital heart disease by M-mode, 2-dimensional, and Doppler echocardiography. *In* Roberts, W. C. (ed.): Adult Congenital Heart Disease. Philadelphia, F. A. Davis Co., 1987, pp. 243–286.

3b. Fisher, M. R., and Higgins, C. B.: Magnetic resonance and cine computed tomography. *In* Roberts, W. C. (ed.): Adult Congenital Heart Disease. Philadelphia, F. A. Davis Co., 1987, pp. 221–242.

4. Graham, T. P.: Assessing the results of surgery for congenital heart disease—A continuing process. Circulation 65:1049, 1982.

4a. Cheitlin, M. D.: Congenital heart disease in the adult. Mod. Concepts Cardiovasc. Dis. *55*:20, 1986.
5. Perloff, J. K.: Adults with surgically treated congenital heart disease. J.A.M.A. *250*:2033, 1983.
5a. Nora, J. J., and Nora, A. H.: The evolution of specific genetic and environmental counseling in congenital heart disease. Circulation *57*:205, 1978.
6. Anderson, R. C.: Fetal and infant death, twinning, and cardiac malformations in families of 2000 children with and 500 without cardiac defects. Am. J. Cardiol. *38*:218, 1976.
7. Allan, L. D., Crawford, D. C., Chita, S. K., Anderson, R. H., and Tynan, M. J.: Familial recurrence of congenital heart disease in a prospective series of mothers referred for fetal echocardiography. Am. J. Cardiol. *58*:334, 1986.
8. Allan, L. D.: Prenatal cardiology. Curr. Opinions Cardiol. *1*:107, 1986.
9. Huhta, J. C.: Uses and abuses of fetal echocardiography: A pediatric cardiologist's view. J. Am. Coll. Cardiol. *8*:451, 1986.
10. Wright, M., Jarvis, S., Wannamaker, E., and Cook, D.: Congenital heart disease: Functional abilities in young adults. Arch. Phys. Med. Rehabil. *66*:289, 1985.
10a. Canobbio, M. M.: Counseling the adult with congenital heart disease. *In* Roberts, W. C. (ed.): Adult Congenital Heart Disease. Philadelphia, F. A. Davis Co., 1987, pp. 733–740.
11. Truesdel, S. C., Skorton, D. J., and Lauer, R. M.: Life insurance for children with cardiovascular disease. Pediatrics *77*:687, 1986.

SPECIFIC MALFORMATIONS

11a. Friedman, W. F., and Johnson, A. D.: Congenital aortic stenosis. *In* Roberts, W. C. (ed.): Adult Congenital Heart Disease. Philadelphia, F. A. Davis Co., 1987, pp. 357–374.
12. Brandenburg, R. O., Tajik, A. J., Edwards, W. D., Reeder, G. S., Shub, C., and Seward, J. B.: Accuracy of 2-dimensional echocardiographic diagnosis of congenitally bicuspid aortic valve—Echocardiographic-anatomic correlation in 115 patients. Am. J. Cardiol. *51*:1469, 1983.
12a. Perloff, J. K.: Congenital aortic stenosis; congenital aortic regurgitation. *In* The Clinical Recognition of Congenital Heart Disease. 3rd ed. Philadelphia, W. B. Saunders Company, 1987, pp. 84–124.
13. Roberts, W. C.: The congenitally bicuspid aortic valve. A study of 85 autopsy patients. Am. J. Cardiol. *26*:72, 1970.
14. Borow, K. M.: Congenital aortic stenosis in the adult. J. Cardiovasc. Med. *8*:1163, 1983.
15. Fenoglio, J. J., McAllister, H. A., DeCastro, C. M., Davia, J. E., and Cheitlin, M. D.: Congenital bicuspid aortic valve after age 20. Am. J. Cardiol. *39*:164, 1977.
16. Wagner, S., and Selzer, A.: Patterns of progression of aortic stenosis—A longitudinal hemodynamic study. Circulation *65*:709, 1982.
17. Shapiro, L., Thwaites, B., Westgate, C., and Donaldson, R.: Prevalence and clinical significance of aortic valve prolapse. Br. Heart J. *54*:179, 1985.
18. Arvan, S.: Aortic valve prolapse in congenital and acquired systemic disease. Arch. Intern. Med. *145*:1601, 1985.
19. Motro, M., Schneeweiss, A., Shen-Tov, A., Vered, Z., Hegesh, J., Neufeld, H. N., and Rath, S.: Two-dimensional echocardiography in discrete subaortic stenosis. Am. J. Cardiol. *53*:896, 1984.
20. Freeman, R. M., Pelech, A., Brand, A., Vogel, M., Olley, P. M., Smallhorn, J., and Rowe, R. D.: The progressive nature of subaortic stenosis in congenital heart disease. Int. J. Cardiol. *8*:137, 1985.
21. Somerville, J.: Fixed subaortic stenosis—A frequently misunderstood lesion. Int. J. Cardiol. *8*:145, 1985.
22. Schneeweiss, A., Motro, M., Stem-Tov, A., Blieden, L. C., and Neufeld, H. N.: Discrete subaortic stenosis associated with congenital valvular aortic stenosis—A diagnostic challenge. Am. Heart J. *106*:55, 1983.
23. Flaker, G., Teske, D., Kilman, J., Hosier, D., and Wooley, C.: Supravalvular aortic stenosis—A 20-year-clinical perspective and experience with patch aortoplasty. Am. J. Cardiol. *51*:256, 1983.
24. Williams, J. C. P., Barrett-Boyes, B. G., and Lowe, J. B.: Supravalvular aortic stenosis. Circulation *24*:1311, 1961.
25. Beppu, S., Minura, Y., Sakakibara, H., Nagata, S., Park, Y. D., Nambu, S., and Yamamoto, A.: Supravalvular aortic stenosis and coronary ostial stenosis in familial hypercholesterolemia: Two-dimensional echocardiographic assessment. Circulation. *67*:878, 1983.
26. Hossack, K. F., Heutze, J. M., Iowe, J. B., and Barratt-Boyes, B. G.: Congenital valvular aortic stenosis—Natural history and assessment of operation. Br. Heart J. *43*:561, 1980.
27. Stewart, W. J., King, M. E., Gillam, L. D., Guyer, D. E., and Weyman, A. E.: Prevalence of aortic prolapse with bicuspid aortic valve and its relation to aortic regurgitation: A cross-sectional echocardiographic study. Am. J. Cardiol. *54*:1277, 1984.
28. Boxer, R. A., Fishman, M. C., LaCorte, M. A., Singh, S., and Parnell, V. A.: Diagnosis and postoperative evaluation of supravalvular aortic stenosis by magnetic resonance imaging. Am. J. Cardiol. *58*:367, 1986.
29. Ciobanu, M., Abbasi, A. S., Allen, M., Herman, A., and Spellberg, R.: Pulsed Doppler echocardiography in the diagnosis and estimation of severity of aortic insufficiency. Am. J. Cardiol. *49*:339, 1982.
30. Hegrenaes, L., and Hatle, L.: Aortic stenosis in adults, non-invasive estimation of pressure by continuous wave Doppler echocardiography. Br. Heart J. *54*:396, 1985.
31. Teirstein, P., Yock, P., and Popp, R.: The accuracy of Doppler ultrasound measurement of pressure gradients across irregular, dual, and tunnellike obstructions to blood flow. Circulation *72*:577, 1985.
32. Snider, A. R., Stevenson, J. G., French, J. W., Rocchini, A. P., Dick, M., Rosenthal, A., Crowley, D. C., and Beekman, R.: Comparison of high pulse repetition frequency and continuous wave Doppler echocardiography for velocity measurement and gradient prediction in children with valvular and CHD. J. Am. Coll. Cardiol. *7*:873, 1986.
33. Richards, K. L., Cannon, S. R., Miller, J. F., and Crawford, M. H.: Calculation of aortic valve area by Doppler echocardiography: A direct application of the continuity equation. Circulation *73*:964, 1986.
34. Smith, M., Dawson, P., Elion, J., Wisenbaugh, T., Kwan, O., Handshoe, S., and DeMaria, A.: Systematic correlation of continuous-wave Doppler and hemodynamic measurements in patients with aortic stenosis. Am. Heart J. *111*:245, 1986.
35. Smith, M., Kwan, O., and DeMaria, A.: Value and limitations of continuous-wave Doppler echocardiography in estimating severity of valvular stenosis. J.A.M.A. *255*:3145, 1986.
36. Borow, K. M., Neumann, A., Briller, R., Spencer, K. T., and Werth, D.: Can the modified Bernoulli equation be used to accurately determine intraventricular pressures throughout systole in patients with valvular aortic stenosis? J. Am. Coll. Cardiol. (*in press*).
37. Campbell, M.: The natural history of congenital aortic stenosis. Br. Heart J. *30*:514, 1968.
38. Reid, J. M., and Coleman, E. N.: The management of congenital aortic stenosis. Thorax *37*:902, 1982.
39. Nylander, E., Ekman, I., Marklund, T., Sinnerstad, B., Karlsson, E., and Wranne, B.: Severe aortic stenosis in elderly patients. Br. Heart J. *55*:480, 1986.
40. Stark, J., and DeLeval, M. (eds.): Surgery for Congenital Heart Defects. Orlando, Fla., Grune and Stratton, 1983, p. 71.
41. Borow, K. M., Colan, S. D., and Neumann, A.: Altered left ventricular mechanics in patients with valvular aortic stenosis and coarctation of the aorta: Effects on systolic performance and late outcome. Circulation *72*:515, 1985.
42. Eichhorn, P., Gremm, J., Koch, R., Hess, O., Carroll, J., and Krayenbuehl, H. P.: Left ventricular relaxation in patients with left ventricular hypertrophy secondary to aortic valve disease. Circulation *65*:1395, 1982.
43. Fifer, M., Borow, K. M., Colan, S., and Lorell, B.: Early diastolic left ventricular function in children and adults with aortic stenosis. J. Am. Coll. Cardiol. *5*:1147, 1985.
44. McNamara, D. G., Bricker, J. T., Galioto, F. M., Graham, T. P., James, F. W., and Rosenthal, A.: Task Force I: Congenital heart disease. J. Am. Coll. Cardiol. *6*:1200, 1985.
45. Lababidi, Z., Wu, J., and Walls, J. T.: Percutaneous balloon aortic valvuloplasty: Results in 23 patients. Am. J. Cardiol. *53*:194, 1984.
46. Walls, J. T., Lababidi, Z., Curtis, J. J., and Silver, D.: Assessment of percutaneous balloon pulmonary and aortic valvuloplasty. J. Thorac. Cardiovasc. Surg. *88*:352, 1984.
47. McKay, R., Safiam, R., Lock, J., Mandell, V., Thurer, R., Schnitt, S., and Grossman, W.: Balloon dilatation of calcific aortic stenosis in elderly patients: Postmortem, intraoperative, and percutaneous valvuloplasty studies. Circulation *74*:119, 1986.
48. Baker, E. J.: Interventional catheterization. Curr. Opinions Cardiol. *1*:93, 1986.
49. McKay, R. G., Safiam, R. D., Lock, J. E., Diver, D. J., Berman, A. D., Warren, S. E., Come, P. C., Baim, D. S., Mandell, V. E., Royal, H. D., and Grossman, W.: Assessment of left ventricular and aortic valve function after aortic balloon valvuloplasty in adult patients with critical aortic stenosis. Circulation *75*:192, 1987.
50. Jones, M., Barnhart, G. R., and Morrow, A. G.: Late results after operation for left ventricular outflow tract obstruction. Am. J. Cardiol. *50*:569, 1982.
51. Prebiterc, P., Sommerville, J., Revel-Chion, R., and Ross, D.: Open aortic valvotomy for congenital aortic stenosis—Late results. Br. Heart J. *47*:26, 1982.
52. Hsieh, K. S., Keane, J. F., Nadas, A. S., Bernhard, W. F., and Castaneda, A. R.: Long-term followup of valvotomy before 1968 for congenital aortic stenosis. Am. J. Cardiol. *58*:338, 1986.
53. Rocchini, A. P., Brown, J., Crowley, D. C., Girod, D. A., Bernhardt, D., and Rosenthal, A.: Clinical and hemodynamic follow-up of left ventricular to aortic conduits in patients with aortic stenosis. J. Am. Coll. Cardiol. *1*:1135, 1983.
53a. Perloff, J. K.: Atrial septal defect. *In* The Clinical Recognition of Congenital Heart Disease. 3rd ed. Philadelphia, W. B. Saunders Company, 1987, pp. 272–349.
54. Nagata, S., Nimura, Y., Sakakibara, H., Beppu, S., Yung-Dae, P., Kawazoe, K., and Fijita, T.: Mitral valve lesion associated with secundum atrial septal defect—Analysis by realtime two-dimensional echocardiography. Br. Heart J. *49*:51, 1983.
55. Ballester, M., Presbitero, P., Foale, R., Rickards, A., and McDonald, L.: Prolapse of the mitral valve in secundum atrial septal defect: A functional mechanism. Eur. Heart J. *4*:472, 1983.
56. Steinbrunn, W., Cohn, D. E., and Selzer, A.: Atrial septal defect associated with mitral stenosis: The Lutembacher syndrome revisited. Am. J. Med. *48*:295, 1970.
57. Bates, E. R.: Survival for 88 years with sinus venous atrial septal defect. J. Am. Geriatr. Soc. *33*:151, 1986.
58. Davia, J. E., Chietlin, M. D., and Bedynek, J. L.: Sinus venosus atrial septal defect: Analysis of fifty cases. Am. Heart J. *85*:177, 1973.
59. Meljboom, E. J., Ebels, T., Anderson, R. H., Leenwen, M. J. M., Deanfield, J. E., Eijgelaar, A., and Heide, J. N. H.: Left atrioventricular valve after surgical repair in atrioventricular septal defect with separate valve orifices ("Ostium primum atrial septal defect"): An echo-Doppler study. Am. J. Cardiol. *57*:433, 1986.
60. Joffe, H. S.: Effect of age on pressure-flow dynamics in secundum atrial septal defect. Br. Heart J. *51*:469, 1984.
61. Galve, E., Angel, J., Evangelista, A., Anivarro, I., Permanyer-Miralda, G.,

and Soler-Soler, J.: Bidirectional shunt in uncomplicated atrial septal defect. Br. Heart J. *51*:480, 1984.

61a. Hamilton, W. T., Haffajee, C. I., Dalen, J. E., Dexter, L., and Nadas, A. S.: Atrial septal defect secundum: Clinical profile with physiologic correlates. *In* Roberts, W. C. (ed.): Adult Congenital Heart Disease. Philadelphia, F. A. Davis Co., 1987, pp. 395–408.

62. Schofield, P., Barber, P., and Kingston, T.: Preoperative and postoperative pulmonary function tests in patients with atrial septal defect and their relation to pulmonary artery pressure and pulmonary:systemic flow ratio. Br. Heart J. *54*:577, 1985.

63. St. John Sutton, M. G., Tajik, A. J., and McGoon, D. C.: Atrial septal defect in patients aged 60 years or older: Operative results and long-term postoperative followup. Circulation *64*:402, 1981.

64. Fisher, J., Platia, E. V., Weiss, J. L., and Brinker, J. A.: Atrial septal defect in the adult: Clinical findings before and after surgery. Cardiovasc. Rev. Rep. *4*:396, 1983.

65. Carabello, B. A., Gash, A., Mayers, D., and Spann, J. F.: Normal left ventricular systolic function in adults with atrial septal defect and left heart failure. Am. J. Cardiol. *49*:1868, 1982.

66. Liberthson, R. R., Boucher, C. A., Fallon, J. T., and Buckley, M. J.: Severe mitral regurgitation—A common occurrence in the aging patient with secundum atrial septal defect. Clin. Cardiol. *4*:229, 1981.

67. Perloff, J. K.: Ostium secundum atrial septal defect—survival for 87 and 94 years. Am. J. Cardiol. 53:388, 1984.

68. Feldman, T., and Borow, K. M.: Atrial septal defect in adults: Diagnosis and management. Cardiovasc. Med. *11*:19, 1986.

69. Vetter, V. L., and Horowitz, L. N.: Electrophysiologic residual and sequelae of surgery for congenital heart defects. Am. J. Cardiol. *50*:588, 1982.

70. Ellison, R. C., and Sloss, L. J.: Electrocardiographic features of congenital heart disease in the adult. *In* Roberts, W. C. (ed.): Congenital Heart Disease in Adults. Philadelphia, F. A. Davis Co., 1979, p. 267.

71. Hynes, J. K., Tajik, A. J., Seward, J. B., Fuster, V., Ritter, D. G., Brandenburg, R. O., Puga, F. J., Danielson, G. K., and McGoon, D. C.: Partial atrioventricular canal defect in adults. Circulation *66*:284, 1982.

72. Weyman, A. E., Wann, S., Feigenbaum, H., and Dillon, J. C.: Mechanisms of abnormal septal motion in patients with right ventricular volume overload. Circulation *54*:179, 1976.

73. Davies, M. J.: Mitral valve in secundum atrial septal defects. Br. Heart J. *46*:126, 1981.

74. Nasser, F. N., Tajik, A. J., Seward, J. B., and Hagler, D. J.: Diagnosis of sinus venosus atrial septal defect by two-dimensional echocardiography. Mayo Clin. Proc. *56*:568, 1981.

75. Forfar, J. C., and Godman, M. J.: Functional and anatomical correlates in atrial septal defect: an echocardiographic analysis. Br. Heart J. *54*:193, 1985.

76. Takahashi, H., Sakamoto, T., Hada, Y., Amano, K., Hasegawa, I., Takahashi, T., and Suzuki, J.: Left ventricular function in atrial septal defect by two-dimensional echocardiography. J. Cardiovasc. Ultrasonogr. *4*:283, 1985.

77. Shub, C., Tajik, J., and Seward, J. B.: Clinically "silent" atrial septal defect: Diagnosis by two-dimensional and Doppler echocardiography. Am. Heart J. *110*:665, 1985.

78. Hanrath, P., Schluter, M., Langenstein, B. A., Polster, J., Engel, S., and Krebber, H. J.: Detection of ostium secundum atrial septal defects by transesophageal cross-sectional echocardiography. Br. Heart J. 49:350, 1983.

79. Shub, C., Dimopoulos, I. N., Seward, J. B., Callahan, J. A., Tancredi, R. G., Schattenberg, T. T., Reeder, G. S., Hagler, D. J., and Tajik, A. J.: Sensitivity of two-dimensional echocardiography in the direct visualization of atrial septal defects utilizing the subcostal approach; experience with 154 patients. J. Am. Coll. Cardiol. *2*:127, 1983.

80. Kitabatake, A., Inoue, M., Asao, M., Ito, H., Masuyama, T., Tanouchi, J., Morita, T., and Hori, M.: Noninvasive evaluation of the ratio of pulmonary to systemic flow in atrial septal defect by duplex Doppler echocardiography. Circulation 69:73, 1984.

81. Valdes-Cruz, L. M., Horowitz, S., Mesel, E., Sahn, D. J., Fisher, D. C., and Larson, D.: A pulsed Doppler echocardiographic method for calculating pulmonary and systemic blood flow in atrial level shunts: Validation studies in animals and initial human experience. Circulation 69:80, 1984.

82. Isobe, M., Yazaki, Y., Takaku, F., Kolzumi, K., Hara, K., Tsuneyoshi, H., Yamaquchi, T., and Machii, K.: Prediction of pulmonary arterial pressure in adults by pulsed Doppler echocardiography. Am. J. Cardiol. 57:316, 1986.

83. Martin-Duran, R., Larman, M., Trugeda, A., Vazquezde Prada, J. A., Ruano, J., Torres, A., Figuerosa, A., Pajaron, A., and Nistol, F.: Comparison of Doppler determined elevated pulmonary arterial pressure with pressure measured at cardiac catheterization. Am. J. Cardiol. 57:859, 1986.

84. Suzuki, Y., Kambara, H., Kadota, K., Tamaki, S., Yamazato, A., Nohara, R., Osakada, G., and Kawai, C.: Detection of intracardiac shunt flow in atrial septal defect using a real-time two-dimensional color-coded Doppler flow imaging system and comparison with contrast two-dimensional echocardiography. Am. J. Cardiol. *56*:347, 1985.

84a. Sherman, F. S., Sahn, D. J., Valdes-Cruz, L. M., Chung, K. J., Elias, W., and Swensson, R. E.: Two-dimensional Doppler color flow mapping for detecting atrial and ventricular septal defects. Echocardiography *3*:527, 1986.

85. Liberthson, R. R., Boucher, C. A., Strauss, H. W., Dinsmore, R. E., McKusick, K. A., and Pohost, G. M.: Right ventricular function in adults with atrial septal defect—Preoperative and postoperative assessment and clinical implications. Am. J. Cardiol. *47*:56, 1981.

86. Ginzton, L. E., Frech, W., and Mena, I.: Combined contrast echocardiographic and radionuclide diagnosis of atrial septal defect: Accuracy of the technique and analysis of erroneous diagnoses. Am. J. Cardiol. 53:1639, 1984.

87. Von Schultess, G. K., Fisher, M. R., and Higgins, C. B.: Pathologic blood flow in pulmonary vascular disease as shown by gated magnetic resonance imaging. Ann. Intern. Med. *108*:317, 1985.

88. Lowell, D., Turner, D., Smith, S., Bucheleres, G., Santucci, B., Gresick, R., and Monson, D.: The detection of atrial and ventricular septal defects with electrocardiographically synchronized magnetic resonance imaging. Circulation 73:89, 1986.

89. Higgins, C. B., Byrd, B. F., Farmer, D. W., Osaki, L., Silverman, N. H., and Cheitlin, M.: Magnetic resonance imaging in patients with congenital heart disease. Circulation *70*:851, 1984.

90. Borow, K. M.: Under what circumstances can cardiac surgery be undertaken without catheterization? J. Cardiovasc. Med. *8*:84, 1983.

91. Freed, M. D., Nadas, A. S., Norwood, W. I., and Castaneda, A. R.: Is routine preoperative cardiac catheterization necessary before the repair of secundum and sinus venosus atrial septal defects? J. Am. Coll. Cardiol. *4*:333, 1984.

92. Shub, C., Tajik, J., Seward, J. B. V., Hagler, D. J., and Danielson, G. K.: Surgical repair of uncomplicated atrial septal defect without "routine" preoperative cardiac catheterization. J. Am. Coll. Cardiol. *6*:49, 1985.

93. Jones, H. R., Caplan, L. R., Come, P. C., Swinton, N. W., and Breslin, D. J.: Cerebral emboli of paradoxical origin. Ann. Neurol. *13*:314, 1983.

94. Dexter, L.: Atrial septal defect. Br. Heart J. *18*:208, 1956.

95. Popio, K. A., Gorlin, R., Teichholz, L. E., Cohn, P. F., Bechtel, D., and Herman, M. V.: Abnormalities of left ventricular function and geometry in adults with an atrial septal defect: Ventriculographic, hemodynamic and echocardiographic studies. Am. J. Cardiol. *36*:302, 1975.

96. Bonow, R. O., Borer, J. S., Rosing, D. R., Bacharach, S. L., Green, M. V., and Kent, K. M.: Left ventricular functional reserve in adult patients with atrial septal defect: Pre- and postoperative studies. Circulation *63*:1315, 1981.

97. Whittemore, R.: Congenital heart disease: Its impact on pregnancy. Hosp. Pract. *18*:65, 1983.

98. McAnulty, J. H., Metcalfe, J., and Ueland, K.: General guidelines in the management of cardiac disease. Clin. Obstet. Gynecol. *24*:773, 1981.

99. Rashkind, W. J.: Transcatheter treatment of congenital heart disease. Circulation 67:711, 1983.

100. Rashkind, W. J.: Interventional cardiac catheterization in congenital heart disease. Int. J. Cardiol. *7*:1, 1985.

101. Baker, E. J.: Valvoplasty, angioplasty, and embolotherapy in congenital heart disease. Int. J. Cardiol. *12*:139, 1986.

102. Cockerham, J. T., Martin, T. C., Gutierrez, F. R., Hartmann, A. F., Goldring, D., and Strauss, A. W.: Spontaneous closure of secundum atrial septal defect in infants and young children. Am. J. Cardiol. *52*:1267, 1983.

103. McGregor, C. G. A., Jamieson, S. W., Baldwin, J. C., Burke, C. M., Dawkins, K. D., Stinson, E. B., Oyer, P. E., Billingham, M. E., Zusman, D. R., Reitz, B. A., Morris, A., Yousem, S., Hunt, S. A., and Shumway, N. E.: Combined heart-lung transplantation for end-stage Eisenmenger's syndrome. J. Thorac. Cardiovasc. Surg. *91*:443, 1986.

104. Kapelanski, D. P.: Cardiopulmonary transplantation. Pulm. Clin. Update *2*:1, 1987.

105. DiSesa, V. J., Cohn, L. H., and Grossman, W.: Management of adults with congenital bidirectional cardiac shunts, cyanosis, and pulmonary vascular obstruction; successful operative repair in three patients. Am. J. Cardiol. *51*:1495, 1983.

106. Friedman, W. F., and Heiferman, M. F.: Clinical problems of postoperative pulmonary vascular disease. Am. J. Cardiol. *50*:631, 1982.

107. Graham, T. P.: Ventricular performance in adults after operation for congenital heart disease. Am. J. Cardiol. *50*:612, 1982.

108. Konstam, M. A., Idoine, J., Wynne, J., Grossman, W., Cohn, L., Beck, J. R., Kozlowski, J., and Holman, B. L.: Right ventricular function in adults with pulmonary hypertension with and without atrial septal defect. Am. J. Cardiol. *51*:1144, 1983.

109. Perloff, J. K.: Adults with surgically treated congenital heart disease. J.A.M.A. *250*:2033, 1983.

110. Brandenberg, R. O., Jr., Holmes, D. R., Brandenberg, R. O., and McGoon, D. C.: Clinical followup study of paroxysmal supraventricular tachyarrhythmias after operative repair of a secundum type atrial septal defect in adults. Am. J. Cardiol. *51*:273, 1983.

111. Hagen, P. T., Scholz, D. G., and Edwards, W. D: Incidence and size of patent foramen ovale during the first 10 decades of life: An autopsy study of 965 normal hearts. Mayo Clin. Proc. 59:17, 1984.

112. Hanley, P., Tajik, J., Hynes, J., Edwards, W., Reeder, G., Hagler, D., and Seward, J.: Diagnosis and classification of atrial septal aneurysm by two-dimensional echocardiography: Report of 80 consecutive cases. J. Am. Coll. Cardiol. *6*:1370, 1985.

113. Wysham, D. G., McPherson, D. D., and Kerber, R. E.: Asymptomatic aneurysm of the interatrial septum. J. Am. Coll. Cardiol. *4*:1311, 1984.

114. Roberts, W. C.: Aneurysm (redundancy) of the atrial septum (fossa ovale membrane) and prolapse (redundancy) of the mitral valve. Am. J. Cardiol. *54*:1153, 1984.

115. Hauser, A. M., Timmis, G. C., Stewart, J. R., Ramos, R. G., Gangadharan, V., Westveer, D. C., and Gordon, S.: Aneurysm of the atrial septum as diagnosed by echocardiography: Analysis of 11 patients. Am. J. Cardiol. 53:1402, 1984.

116. Belkin, R. N., Waugh, R. A., and Kisslo, J.: Interatrial shunting in atrial septal aneurysm. Am. J. Cardiol. 57:310, 1986.

117. Longhini, C., Brunazzi, C., Musacci, G., Caneva, M., Bandello, A., Bolomini, L., Barbiero, M., Toselli, T., and Barbaresi, F.: Atrial septal aneurysm: Echopolycardiographic study. Am. J. Cardiol. *56*:653, 1985.

118. Iliceto, S., Papa, A., Sorino, M., and Rizzon, P.: Combined atrial septal aneurysm and mitral valve prolapse: Detection by two-dimensional echocardiography. Am. J. Cardiol. *54*:1151, 1984.

119. Arvan, S.: Incidental interatrial septal aneurysm associated with mitral valve prolapse. Am. Heart J. *111*:603, 1986.

119a. Perloff, J. K.: Congenital mitral stenosis; cor triatriatum; congenital pulmonary vein stenosis. *In* The Clinical Recognition of Congenital Heart Disease. 3rd ed. Philadelphia, W. B. Saunders Company, 1987, pp. 161–178.
120. Ostman-Smith, I., Silverman, N. H., Oldershaw, P., Lincoln, C., and Shinebourne, E. A.: Cor triatriatum sinistrum diagnostic features on cross sectional echocardiography. Br. Heart J. *51*:211, 1984.
121. Fuster-Siebert, M., Llorens, R., Arcas-Meca, R., Rubio-Alvarez, J., Prieto-Galan, F., and Gengochea, J. B.: Cor triatriatum with mitral valve disease in adults. Tex. Heart Inst. J. *9*:363, 1982.
122. Jacobstein, M. D., and Hirschfeld, S. S.: Concealed left atrial membrane: Pitfalls in the diagnosis of cor triatriatum and supravalvular mitral ring. Am. J. Cardiol. *49*:780, 1982.
123. Alpert, J. S., Dexter, L., Vieweg, W. V. R., Haynes, F. W., and Dalen, J. E.: Anomalous pulmonary venous return with intact atrial septum: Diagnosis and pathophysiology. Circulation *56*:870, 1977.
124. Bauer, A., Korfer, R., and Bircks, W.: Left-to-right shunt of atrial level due to anomalous venous connection of the left lung. J. Thorac. Cardiovasc. Surg. *84*:626, 1982.
125. Oakley, D., Naik, D., Verel, D., and Rajan, S.: Scimitar vein syndrome: Report of nine new cases. Am. Heart J. *107*:596, 1984.
126. Anderson, R. H., Lenox, C. C., and Zuberbuhler, J. R.: Mechanisms of closure of perimembranous ventricular septal defect. Am. J. Cardiol. 52:341, 1983.
127. Ramaciotti, C., Keren, A., Silverman, N. H.: Importance of (perimembranous) ventricular septal aneurysm in the natural history of isolated perimembranous ventricular septal defect. Am. J. Cardiol. *57*:268, 1986.
128. Weidman, W. H., DuShane, J. W., and Ellison, R. C.: Clinical course in adults with ventricular septal defect. Circulation *56*:178, 1977.
128a. Engle, M. A., Kline, S. A., and Borer, J. S.: Ventricular septal defect. *In* Roberts, W. C. (ed.): Adult Congenital Heart Disease. Philadelphia, F. A. Davis Co., 1987, pp. 409–442.
129. Momma, K., Toyama, K., Takao, A., Ando, M., Nakazawa, M., Hirosawa, K., and Imai, Y.: Natural history of subarterial infundibular ventricular septal defect. Am. Heart J. *108*:1312, 1984.
130. Capelli, H., Andrade, J. L., and Somerville, J.: Classification of the site of ventricular septal defect by two-dimensional echocardiography. Am. J. Cardiol. *51*:1474, 1983.
130a. Perloff, J. K.: Ventricular septal defect. *In* The Clinical Recognition of Congenital Heart Disease. 3rd ed. Philadelphia, W. B. Saunders Company, 1987, pp. 365–403.
131. Burrows, P. E., Fellows, K. E., and Keane, J. F.: Cineangiography of the perimembranous ventricular septal defect with left ventricular–right atrial shunt. J. Am. Coll. Cardiol. *1*:1129, 1983.
132. Grenadier, E., Shem-Tov, A., Motro, M., and Palant, A.: Echocardiographic diagnosis of left ventricular-right atrial comunication. Am. Heart J. *106*:407, 1983.
133. Nakazawa, M., Takao, A., Shimizu, T., and Chon, Y.: Afterload reduction treatment for large ventricular septal defects: dependence of hemodynamic effects of hydralazine on pretreatment systemic blood flow. Br. Heart J. *49*:461, 1983.
134. Nakazawa, M., Takao, A., Chon, Y., Shimizu, T., Kanaya, M., and Momma, K.: Significance of systemic vascular resistance in determining the hemodynamic effects of hydralazine on large ventricular septal defects. Circulation *68*:420, 1983.
135. Corone, P., Doyon, F., Gaudeau, S., Guerin, F., Vernant, P., Ducam, H., Rumeau-Rouquette, C., and Gaudeau, P.: Natural history of ventricular septal defect: A studying involving 790 cases. Circulation *55*:908, 1977.
136. Otterstad, J. E., Erikssen, J., Froysaker, T., and Simonsen, S.: Longterm results after operative treatment of isolated ventricular septal defect in adolescents and adults. Acta Med. Scand. *1*:708, 1986.
137. Warnes, C. A., Boger, J. E., and Roberts, W. C.: Eisenmenger ventricular septal defect with prolonged survival. Am. J. Cardiol. *54*:460, 1984.
138. Gould, L., and Gopalaswamy, C.: Late survival of a patient with ventricular septal defect and Eisenmenger syndrome. Angio. J. Vascu. Dis. *33*:769, 1982.
139. Andrade, J. L., Serino, W., Deleval, M., and Somerville, J.: Two-dimensional echocardiographic assessment of surgically closed ventricular septal defect. Am J. Cardiol. *52*:325, 1983.
140. Stevenson, J. G., Kawabori, I., Stamm, S. J., Bailey, W. W., Hall, D. G., Mansfield, P. B., and Rittenhouse, E. A.: Pulsed Doppler echocardiographic evaluation of ventricular septal defect patches. Circulation *70* (Suppl. 1):1, 1984.
141. Otterstad, J. E., Simonsen, S., Vatne, K., and Myhre, E.: Doppler echocardiography in adults with isolated ventricular septal defect. Eur. Heart J. *5*:332, 1984.
142. Murphy, D. J., Ludomirsky, A., and Huhta, J. C: Continuous-wave Doppler in children with ventricular septal defect: Noninvasive estimation of interventricular pressure gradient. Am. J. Cardiol. *57*:428, 1986.
143. Silbert, D. R., Brunson, S. C., Scheff, R., and Diament, S.: Determination of right ventricular pressure in the presence of a ventricular septal defect using continuous-wave Doppler ultrasound. J. Am. Coll. Cardiol. *8*:379, 1986.
144. Agathangelou, N. E., Dos Santos, L. A., and Lewis, B. S.: Real-time 2-dimensional echocardiographic imaging of right-sided cardiac vegetations in ventricular septal defect. Am. J. Cardiol. *52*:420, 1983.
145. Keane, J. F., Plauth, W. H., and Nadas, A. S.: Ventricular septal defect with aortic regurgitation. Circulation *56*:172, 1977.
146. Friedman, W. F., and Heiferman, M. F.: Clinical problems of postoperative pulmonary vascular disease. Am. J. Cardiol. *50*:631, 1982.
146a. Graham, T. P., Jr.: The Eisenmenger syndrome. *In* Roberts, W. C. (ed.): Adult Congenital Heart Disease. Philadelphia, F. A. Davis Co., 1987, pp. 567–582.
147. Clarkson, P. M., Nicholson, M. R., Barratt-Boyes, B. G., Neutze, J. M., and Whitlock, R. M.: Results after repair of coarctation of the aorta beyond infancy: A 10 to 28 year followup with particular reference to late systemic hypertension. Am. J. Cardiol. *51*:1481, 1983.
148. McNamara, D. G., and Latson, L. A.: Long-term followup of patients with malformations for which definitive surgical repair has been available for 25 years or more. Am. J. Cardiol. *50*:560, 1982.
149. Maron, B. J., Redwood, D. R., Hirshfeld, J. W., Jr., Goldstein, R. E., Morrow, A. G., and Epstein, S. E.: Postoperative assessment of patients with ventricular septal defect and pulmonary hypertension. Response to intense upright exercise. Circulation *48*:864, 1973.
150. Lueker, R. D., Vogel, J. H. K., and Blount, S. G.: Cardiovascular abnormalities following surgery for left-to-right shunts. Circulation *40*:785, 1969.
151. Jablonsky, G., Hilton, J. D., Liu, P. P., March, J. E., Druck, M. N., Bar-Shlomo, B., and McLaughlin, P. R.: Rest and exercise ventricular function in adults with congenital ventricular septal defects. Am. J. Cardiol. *51*:293, 1983.
151a. Perloff, J. K.: Ventricular septal defect with pulmonic stenosis. *In* The Clinical Recognition of Congenital Heart Disease. 3rd ed. Philadelphia, W. B. Saunders Company, 1987, pp. 404–442.
151b. Garson, A., Jr., McNamara, D. G., and Cooley, D. A.: Tetralogy of Fallot. *In* Roberts, W. C. (ed.): Adult Congenital Heart Disease. Philadelphia, F. A. Davis Co., 1987, pp. 493–520.
152. Rosenthal, A., Behrendt, D., Sloan, H., Ferguson, P., Snedecor, S. M., and Schork, A.: Long-term prognosis (15–26 years) after repair of tetralogy of Fallot: I. Survival and symptomatic status. Ann. Thorac. Surg. *38*:151, 1984.
153. Matina, D., van Doesburg, N. H., Fouron, J., Guerin, R., and Davignon, A.: Subxiphoid two-dimensional echocardiographic diagnosis of double-chambered right ventricle. Circulation *67*:885, 1983.
154. Von Doenhoff, L. J., and Nanda, N. C.: Obstruction within the right ventricular body: Two-dimensional echocardiographic features. Am. J. Cardiol. *51*:1498, 1983.
155. Higgins, C. B.., and Mulder, D. G.: Tetralogy of Fallot in the adult. Am. J. Med. *29*:837, 1972.
156. Abraham, K. A., Cherian, G., Rao, V. D., Sukumar, I. P., Krishnaswami, S., and John, S.: Tetralogy of Fallot in adults: A report of 147 patients. Am. J. Med. *66*:811, 1979.
157. Issaz, K., Cloez, J. L., Marcon, F., Worms, A. M., and Pernot, C.: Is the aorta truly dextroposed in tetralogy of Fallot? A two-dimensional echocardiographic answer. Circulation *73*:892, 1986.
158. Oberhansli, I., and Frieli, B.: Cross sectional echocardiographic assessment of left ventricular volume and ejection fraction in patients with tetralogy of Fallot comparison with biplane angio measurements. Br. Heart J. *52*:191, 1984.
159. Marx, G. R., Allen, H. D., and Goldberg, S. J.: Doppler echocardiographic estimation of pulmonary artery pressure in patients with aortic-pulmonary shunts. J. Am. Cardiol. *7*:880, 1986.
160. Hu, D. C. K., Seward, J. B., Puga, F. J., Fuster, V., and Tajik, A.: Total correction of tetralogy of Fallot at age 40 years and older: Long-term followup. J. Am. Coll. Cardiol. *5*:40, 1985.
161. Chin, J., Bashour, T., and Kabbani, S.: Tetralogy of Fallot in the elderly. Clin. Cardiol. *7*:453, 1984.
162. Presbitero, P., D'Antonio, P., Brusca, A., and Morea, M.: Prognosis of Fallot's tetralogy after palliative operations: 10–25 year follow-up. Pediatr. Cardiol. *4*:175, 1983.
163. Mattila, S., Luosto, R., Ketonen, P., Nieminen, M., Merikallio, E., and Kyllonen, K. E. J.: Total correction of tetralogy of Fallot in adults. Scand. J. Thorac. Cardiovasc. Surg. *18*:23, 1984.
164. Fuster, V., McGoon, D. C., Kennedy, M. A., Ritter, D. G., and Kirklin, J. W.: Long-term evaluation (12 to 22 years) of open heart surgery for tetralogy of Fallot. Am. J. Cardiol. *46*:635, 1980.
165. Katz, N. M., Blackstone, E. H., Kirklin, J. W., Pacifico, A. D., and Bargeron, L. M.: Late survival and symptoms after repair of tetralogy of Fallot. Circulation *65*:403, 1982.
166. Tamer, D., Wolff, G. S., Ferrer, P., Pickoff, A. S., Casta, A., Mehta, A. V., Garcia, O., and Gelband, H.: Hemodynamics and intracardiac conduction after operative repair of tetralogy of Fallot. Am. J. Cardiol. *51*:552, 1983.
167. Borow, K. M., Green, L. H., Castaneda, A. R., and Keane, J. F.: Left ventricular function after repair of tetralogy of Fallot and its relationship to age at surgery. Circulation *61*:1150, 1980.
168. Jones, M., and Ferrans, V. J.: Myocardial degeneration in congenital heart disease: Comparison of morphologic findings in young and old patients with congenital heart disease associated with muscular obstruction to right ventricular outflow. Am. J. Cardiol. *39*:1051, 1977.
169. Deanfield, J. E., Ho, S. Y., Anderson, R. H., McKenna, W. J., Allwork, S. P., and Hallidie-Smith, K. A.: Late sudden death after repair of tetralogy of Fallot: A clinicopathologic study. Circulation *67*:626, 1983.
170. DeLorgeril, M., Friedli, B., and Assimacopoulos, A.: Factors affecting left ventricular function after correction of tetralogy of Fallot. Br. Heart J. *52*:536, 1984.
171. Bove, E. L., Byrum, C. J., Thomas, D., Kavey, R. W., Sondheimer, H. M., Blackman, M. S., and Parker, F. B.: The influence of pulmonary insufficiency on ventricular function following repair of tetralogy of Fallot. J. Thorac. Cardiovasc. Surg. *85*:69, 1983.
172. Tamer, D., Wolff, G. S., Ferrer, P., Pickoff, A. S., Casta, A., Mehta, A. V., Garcia, O., and Gelband, H.: Hemodynamics and intracardiac conduction after operative repair of tetralogy of Fallot. Am. J. Cardiol. *51*:552, 1983.
173. Burns, R. J., Lui, P. P., Druck, M. N., Seawright, S. J., Williams, W. G., McLaughlin, P. R.: Analysis of adults without complex ventricular arrhythmias after repair of tetralogy of Fallot. J. Am. Coll. Cardiol. *4*:226, 1984.
174. Garson, A., Randall, D. C., Gillette, P. C., Smith, R. T., Moak, J. P., McVey, P., and McNamara, D. G.: Prevention of sudden death after repair

of tetralogy of Fallot: Treatment of ventricular arrhythmias. J. Am. Coll. Cardiol. 6:221, 1985.
175. Deanfield, J. E., McKenna, W. J., and Hallidie-Smith, K. A.: Detection of late arrhythmia and conduction disturbance after correction of tetralogy of Fallot. Br. Heart J. 44:248, 1980.
176. Garson, A., Gillette, P. C., Gutgesell, H. P., and McNamara, D. G.: Stress-induced ventricular arrhythmia after repair of tetralogy of Fallot. Am. J. Cardiol. 46:1006, 1980.
177. Hoffman, J. E., and Christianson, R.: Congenital heart disease in a cohort of 19,502 births with long-term followup. Am. J. Cardiol. 42:641, 1978.
178. Feldman, T., and Borow, K. M.: Adults with pulmonic stenosis: Management. Cardiovasc. Med. 9:711, 1984.
179. Kaplan, S., Adolph, R. J., and Murphy, D. J.: Pulmonic valve stenosis. *In* Roberts, W. C. (ed.): Adult Congenital Heart Disease. Philadelphia, F. A. Davis Co., 1987, pp. 477–492.
180. Perloff, J. K.: Congenital pulmonic stenosis. *In* The Clinical Recognition of Congenital Heart Disease. 3rd ed. Philadelphia, W. B. Saunders Company, 1987, pp. 188–219.
181. Barber, G., Danielson, G. K., Puga, F. J., Herse, C. T., and Driscoll, D. J.: Pulmonary atresia with ventricular septal defect: Preoperative and postoperative responses to exercises. J. Am. Coll. Cardiol. 7:630, 1986.
182. Fyfe, D. A., Edwards, W. D., and Driscoll, D. J.: Myocardial ischemia in patients with pulmonary atresia and intact ventricular septum. J. Am. Coll. Cardiol. 8:402, 1986.
183. Johnson, L. W., Grossman, W., Dalen, J. E., and Dexter, L.: Pulmonic stenosis in the adult: Long-term followup results. N. Engl. J. Med. 287:1159, 1972.
184. Covarrubias, E. A., Sheikh, M. U., Isner, J. M., Gomes, M., Hufnagel, C. A., and Roberts, W. C.: Calcific pulmonic stenosis in adulthood. Chest 75:399, 1979.
185. Krabill, K. A., Wang, Y., Einzig, S., and Moller, J. H.: Rest and exercise hemodynamics in pulmonary stenosis: Comparison of children and adults. Am. J. Cardiol. 56:360, 1985.
186. Tajik, A. J., Seward, J. B., Hagler, D. J., Mair, D. D., and Lie, J. T.: Two-dimensional realtime ultrasonic imaging of the heart and great vessels: Technique, image orientation, structure identification, and validation. Mayo Clin. Proc. 53:271, 1978.
187. Johnson, G. L., Kwan, I. L., Handshoe, S., Noonan, J. A., and DeMaria, A. N.: Accuracy of combined two-dimensional echocardiography and continuous wave recordings in the estimation of pressure gradient in right ventricular outlet obstruction. J. Am. Coll. Cardiol. 3:1013, 1984.
188. Houston, A. B., Simpson, I. A., Sheldon, C. D., Doig, W. B., and Coleman, E. N.: Doppler ultrasound in the estimation of the severity of pulmonary infundibular stenosis in infants and children. Br. Heart J. 55:381, 1986.
189. Goldberg, S. J., Vasko, S. D., Allen, H. D., and Marx, G. R.: Can the technique of Doppler estimate of pulmonary stenosis gradient be simplified? Am. Heart J. 111:709, 1986.
190. Sullivan, I. D.: Doppler echocardiography. Curr. Opinions Cardiol. 1:102, 1986.
191. Nugent, E. W., Freddom, R. M., Nora, J. J., Ellison, R. C., Rowe, R. D., and Nadas, A. S.: Clinical course in pulmonary stenosis. Circulation 56:1, 1977.
192. Lock, J., Keane, J., and Fellows, K.: The use of catheter intervention procedures for congenital heart disease. J. Am. Coll. Cardiol. 7:1420, 1986.
192a. Perloff, J. K.: Idiopathic dilatation of the pulmonary trunk. *In* The Clinical Recognition of Congenital Heart Disease. 3rd ed. Philadelphia, W. B. Saunders, 1987, pp. 220–225.
193. Lababidi, Z., and Wu, J.: Percutaneous balloon pulmonary valvuloplasty. Am. J. Cardiol. 52:560, 1983.
194. Kan, J. S., White, R. I., Mitchell, S. E., Anderson, J. H., and Gardner, T. J.: Percutaneous transluminal balloon valvuloplasty for pulmonary valve stenosis. Circulation 69:554, 1984.
195. Tynan, M., Baker, E. J., Rohmer, J., Johnes, O. D. H., Reidy, J. F., Joseph, M. C., and Ottenkamp, J.: Percutaneous balloon pulmonary valvuloplasty. Br. Heart J. 53:520, 1985.
196. Gibbs, J. L., Stanley, C. P., and Dickenson, D. F.: Pulmonary balloon valvoplasty in late adult life. Int. J. Cardiol. 11:237, 1986.
197. Rocchini, A. P., Kveselis, D. A., Crowley, D., Dick, M., and Rosenthal, A.: Percutaneous balloon valvuloplasty for treatment of congenital pulmonary valvular stenosis in children. J. Am. Coll. Cardiol. 3:1005, 1984.
198. Kveselis, D. A., Rocchini, A. P., Snider, R., Rosenthal, A., Crowley, D. C., and Dick, M.: Results of balloon valvuloplasty in the treatment of congenital valvular pulmonary stenosis in children. Am. J. Cardiol. 56:527, 1985.
199. Roberts, N., and Moes, C. A. F.: Supravalvular pulmonic stenosis. J. Pediatr. 82:838, 1973.
199a. Hoekenga, D. E., Stevens, G. F., and Ball, W. S.: Percutaneous angioplasty for peripheral pulmonary stenosis in an adult. Am. J. Cardiol. 59:188; 1987.
200. Campbell, M.: Natural history of patent ductus arteriosus. Br. Heart J. 30:4, 1968.
201. Woodruff, W. W., Gabliani, G., and Grant, A. O.: Patent ductus arteriosus in the elderly. South. Med. J. 76:1436, 1983.
202. Marquis, R. M., Miller, H. C., McCormack, R. J. M., Matthews, M. B., and Kitchin, A. H.: Persistence of ductus arteriosus with left to right shunt in the older patient. Br. Heart J. 48:469, 1982.
203. Fisher, R. G., Moodie, D. S., Sterba, R., and Gill, C. C.: Patent ductus arteriosus in adults—Long term followup: Nonsurgical versus surgical treatment. J. Am. Coll. Cardiol. 8:280, 1986.
203a. Perloff, J. K.: Patent ductus arteriosus. *In* The Clinical Recognition of Congenital Heart Disease. 3rd ed. Philadelphia, W. B. Saunders Company, 1987, pp. 467–497.
204. McManus, B. M., Hahn, P. F., Smith, J. A., Roberts, W. C., and Jackson, J. H.: Eisenmenger ductus arteriosus with prolonged survival. Am. J. Cardiol. 54:462, 1984.
204b. McManus, B. M.: Patent ductus arteriosus. *In* Roberts, W. C. (ed.): Adult Congenital Heart Disease. Philadelphia, F. A. Davis Co., 1987, pp. 455–476.
205. Wilson, N., Dickinson, D. F., Goldbert, S. J., and Scott, O.: Pulmonary artery velocity patterns in ductus arteriosus. Br. Heart J. 52:462, 1984.
206. Perez, J. E., Nordlicht, S. M., and Geltman, E. M.: Patent ductus arteriosus in adults: Diagnosis by suprasternal and parasternal pulsed Doppler echocardiography. Am. J. Cardiol. 53:1473, 1984.
206a. Reeder, G. S., Seward, J. B., Hagler, D. J., and Tajik, A. J.: Color-flow imaging in congenital heart disease. Echocardiography 3:533, 1986.
207. John, S., Muralidharan, S., Mani, G. K., Krishnaswmai, S., and Sukumar, I. P.: The adult ductus. J. Thorac. Cardiovasc. Surg. 82:314, 1981.
208. Borow, K. M., Hessel, S. J., and Sloss, L. J.: Fistulous aneurysm of ductus arteriosus. Br. Heart J. 45:467, 1981.
209. Danza, F. M., Fusco, A., Breda, M., Bock, E., Lemmo, G., and Colavita, N.: Ductus arteriosus aneurysm in an adult. Am. J. Radiol. 143:131, 1984.
210. Fripp, R. R., Whitman, V., Waldhausen, J. A., and Boad, D. K.: Ductus arteriosus aneurysm presenting as pulmonary artery obstruction: Diagnosis and management. J. Am. Coll. Cardiol. 6:234, 1985.
211. Whittemore, R., Hobbins, J. C., and Engle, M. A.: Pregnancy and its outcome in women with and without surgical treatment of congenital heart disease. Am. J. Cardiol. 50:641, 1982.
212. Wernly, J. A., and Ameriso, J. L.: Intra-aortic closure of the calcified patent ductus. J. Thorac. Cardiovasc. Surg. 80:206, 1980.
213. Sato, K., Fujino, M., Kozuka, T., Naito, Y., Kitamura, S., Nakanom S., Ohyama, C., and Kawashima, Y.: Transfemoral plug closure of patent ductus arteriosus. Experience in 61 cases treated without thoracotomy. Circulation 51:337, 1975.
214. Hesslain, P. S., Gutgesell, H. P., and McNamara, D. G.: Prognosis of symptomatic coarctation of the aorta in infancy. Am. J. Cardiol. 51:299, 1983.
215. Serfas, D., and Borow, K. M.: Coarctation of the aorta: Anatomy, pathophysiology, and natural history. J. Cardiovasc. Med. 8:575, 1983.
215a. Maron, B. J.: Aortic isthmic coarctations. *In* Roberts, W. C. (ed.): Adult Congenital Heart Disease. Philadelphia, F. A. Davis Co., 1987, pp. 443–454.
216. Glancy, D. L., Morrow, A. G., Simon, A. L., and Roberts, W. C.: Juxtaductal aortic coarctation—analysis of 84 patients studied hemodynamically, angiographically, and morphologically after age 1 year. Am. J. Cardiol. 51:537, 1983.
216a. Perloff, J. K.: Coarctation of the aorta. *In* The Clinical Recognition of Congenital Heart Disease. 3rd ed. Philadelphia, W. B. Saunders Company, 1987, pp. 125–160.
217. Elzenga, N. J., and Gittensberger-Degroot, A.: Localized coarctation of the aorta and age dependent spectrum. Br. Heart J. 49:317, 1983.
218. Anderson, R. H., Lenox, C. C., and Zuberbuhler, J. R.: Morphology of ventricular septal defect associated with coarctation of aorta: Br. Heart J. 50:176, 1983.
219. Smallhorn, J. F., Anderson, R. H., and Macartney, F. J.: Morphological characterization of ventricular septal defects associated with coarctation of aorta by cross-sectional echocardiography. Br. Heart J. 49:485, 1983.
220. Duncan, W. J., Ninomiya, K., Cook, D. H., and Rowe, R. D.: Noninvasive diagnosis of neonatal coarctation and associated anomalies using two-dimensional echocardiography. Am. Heart J. 106:63, 1983.
221. Liberthson, R. R., Pennington, D. G., Jacobs, M. L., and Dagget, W. M.: Coarctation of the aorta—Review of 234 patients and clarification of management problems. Am. J. Cardiol. 43:835, 1979.
222. Shested, J., Baandrup, U., and Mikkelsen, E.: Different reactivity and structure of the prestenotic and poststenotic aorta in human coarctation—Implications for baroreceptor function. Circulation 65:1060, 1982.
223. Simon, A. B., and Zloto, A. E.: Coarctation of the aorta. Longitudinal assessment of operated patients. Circulation 50:456, 1974.
224. Campbell, M.: Natural history of coarctation of the aorta. Circulation 41:1067, 1970.
225. Glancy, D. L., Morrow, A. G., Simon, A. L., and Roberts, W. C.: Juxtaductal aortic coarctation—analysis of 84 patients studied hemodynamically, angiographically, and morphologically after 1 year. Am. J. Cardiol. 51:537, 1983.
226. Shaddy, R. E., Snider, A. R., Silverman, N. H., and Lutin, W.: Pulsed Doppler findings in patients with coarctation of the aorta. Circulation 73:82, 1986.
227. Sanders, S. P., MacPherson, D., and Yeager, S. B.: Temporal flow velocity profile in the descending aorta in coarctation. J. Am. Coll. Cardiol. 7:603, 1986.
228. Marx, G. R., and Allen, H. D.: Accuracy and pitfalls, of Doppler evaluation of the pressure gradient in aortic coarctation. J. Am. Coll. Cardiol. 7:1379, 1986.
229. Boxer, R. A., LaCorte, M. A., Singh, S., Cooper, R., Fishman, M. C., Goldman, M., and Stein, H. L.: Nuclear magnetic resonance imaging in evaluation and follow-up of children treated for coarctation of the aorta. J. Am. Coll. Cardiol. 7:1095, 1986.
230. Borow, K. M., Colan, S. D., and Neumann, A.: Altered left ventricular mechanics in patients with valvular aortic stenosis and coarctation of the aorta: Effects on systolic performance and late outcome. Circulation 72:515, 1985.
231. Deal, K., and Wooley, C. F.: Coarctation of the aorta and pregnancy. Ann. Intern. Med. 78:706, 1973.
232. Lock, J. E., Bass, J. L., Amplatz, K., Fuhrman, B. P., and Castaneda-Zuniga, W.: Balloon dilation angioplasty of aortic coarctations in infants and children. Circulation 68:109, 1983.
233. Sperling, D. R., Dorsey, T. J., Rowen, M., and Gazzaniga, A. B.: Percutaneous transluminal angioplasty of congenital coarctation of the aorta. Am. J. Cardiol. 51:562, 1983.
234. Kan, J. S., White, R. I., Mitchell, S. E., Farmlett, E. J., Donahoo, J. S.,

and Gardner, T. J.: Treatment of restenosis of coarctation by percutaneous transluminal angioplasty. Circulation *68*:1087, 1983.

235. Finley, J. P., Beaulieu, R. G., Nanton, M. A., and Roy, D. L.: Balloon catheter dilatation of coarctation of the aorta in young infants. Br. Heart J. *50*:411, 1983.
236. Lababidi, Z. A., Daskalopoalos, D. A., and Stoeckle, H.: Transluminal balloon coarctation angioplasty: Experience with 27 patients. Am. J. Cardiol. *54*:1288, 1984.
237. Lock, J. E.: Now that we can dilate, should we? Am. J. Cardiol. *54*:1360, 1984.
238. Hess, J., Mooyaart, E. L., Busch, H. J., Bergstra, A., and Landsman, M. L.: Percutaneous transluminal balloon angioplasty in restenosis of coarctation of the aorta. Br. Heart J. *55*:459, 1986.
239. Allen, H. D., Marx, G. R., Ovitt, T. W., and Goldberg, S. J.: Balloon dilation angioplasty for coarctation of the aorta. Am. J. Cardiol. *57*:828, 1986.
240. Lababidi, Z., Madigan, N., Wu, J. R., and Murphy, T. J.: Balloon coarctation angioplasty in an adult. Am. J. Cardiol. *53*:350, 1984.
241. Foster, E. D.: Reoperation for aortic coarctation. Ann. Thorac. Surg. *38*:81, 1984.
242. Clarkson, P. M., Brandt, P. W., Barratt-Boyes, B. G., Rutherford, J. D., Kerr, A. R., and Neurtze, J. M.: Prosthetic repair of coarctation of the aorta with particular reference to dacron onlay patch grafts and late aneurysm formation. Am. J. Cardiol. *56*:342, 1985.
243. Engle, M. A.: A long look at surgery for coarctation of aorta. J. Am. Coll. Cardiol. *6*:887, 1985.
244. Smith, R. T., Sade, R. M., Riopel, D. A., Taylor, A. B., Crawford, F. A., and Hohn, A. R.: Stress testing for comparison of synthetic patch aortoplasty with resection and end to end anastomosis for repair of coarctation in childhood. J. Am. Coll. Cardiol. *4*:765, 1986.
245. Berendes, J. N., Bredee, J. J., Schipperheyn, J. J., and Mashhour, Y. A. S.: Mechanism of spinal cord injury after cross-clamping of the descending thoracic aorta. Circulation *66*(Suppl. I):112, 1982.
246. Rocchini, A. P., Rosenthal, A., and Barger, C. A.: Pathogenesis of paradoxical hypertension after coarctation resection. Circulation *54*:382, 1976.
247. Benedict, C. R., Grahame-Smith, D. G., and Fisher, A.: Changes in plasma catecholamine and dopamine beta-hydroxylase after corrective surgery for coarctation of the aorta. Circulation *57*:598, 1978.
248. Gidding, S. S., Rocchini, A., Beekman, R., Szpnar, C. A., Moorehead, C., Behrendt, D., and Rosenthal, A.: Therapeutic effect of propranolol on paradoxical hypertension after repair of coarctation of the aorta. N. Engl. J. Med. *312*:1124, 1985.
249. Farrell, B. G., Parker, F. B., Poirier, R. A., Anderson, G., Streeter, D. H. P., and Blackman, M.: Angiotensin blockade in postoperative paradoxical hypertension of coarctation of the aorta. Surg. Forum *30*:189, 1979.
250. Casta, A., Conti, V. R., Talabi, A., and Brouhard, B. H.: Effective use of captopril in postoperative paradoxical hypertension of coarctation of the aorta. Clin. Cardiol. *5*:551, 1982.
251. Kimball, B. P., Shurvell, B. L., Houle, S., Fulop, J. C., Rakowski, H., and McLaughlin, P. R.: Persistent ventricular adapations in postoperative coractation of the aorta. J. Am. Coll. Cardiol. *8*:172, 1986.
252. Carpenter, M. A., Dammann, J. F., Watson, D. D., Jedeikin, R., Tompkins, D. G., and Beller, G. A.: Left ventricular hyperkinesia at rest and during exercise in normotensive patients 2 to 27 years after coarctation repair. J. Am. Coll. Cardiol. *6*:879, 1985.
253. Maron, B. J., Humphries, J. O., and Rowe, R. D.: Prognosis of surgically corrected coarctations of the aorta: A 20 year postoperative appraisal. Circulation *47*:119, 1973.
254. Freed, M. D., Rocchini, A., and Rosenthal, A.: Exercise-induced hypertension after surgical repair of coarctation of the aorta. Am. J. Cardiol. *43*:253, 1979.
255. James, F. W., and Kaplan S: Systolic hypertension during submaximal exercise after correction of coarctation of aorta. Circulation *49* and *50*(Suppl. 2):II-27, 1974.
256. Markel, H., Rocchini, A. P., Beekman, R. H., Martin, J., Moorehead, C., and Rosenthal, A.: Exercise-induced hypertension after repair of coarctation of the aorta: Arm versus leg exercise. J. Am. Coll. Cardiol. *8*:165, 1986.
257. Anderson, K. R., Zuberbuhler, J. R., Anderson, R. H., Becker, A. E., and Lie, J. T.: Morphologic spectrum of Ebstein's anomaly of the heart. Mayo Clin. Proc. *54*:174, 1979.
258. Anderson, K. R., and Lie, J. T.: Pathologic anatomy of Ebstein's anomaly of the heart revisited. Am. J. Cardiol. *41*:739, 1978.
259. Shiina, A., Seward, J. B., Tajik, A. J., Hagler, D. J., and Danielson, G. K.: Two-dimensional echocardiographic-surgical correlation in Ebstein's anomaly: Preoperative determination of patients requiring tricuspid valve plication vs. replacement. Circulation *68*:534, 1983.
260. Shiina, A., Seward, J. B., Edwards, W. D., Hagler, D. J., and Tajik, A. J.: Two-dimensional echocardiographic spectrum of Ebstein's anomaly: Detailed anatomic assessment, J. Am. Coll. Cardiol. *3*:356, 1984.
261. Giuliani, E. R., Fuster, V., Brandenburg, R. O., and Mair, D. D.: Ebstein's anomaly: The clinical features and natural history of Ebstein's anomaly of the tricuspid valve. Mayo Clin. Proc. *54*:163, 1979.
262. Radford, D. J., Graff, R. F., and Neilson, G. H.: Diagnosis and natural history of Ebstein's anomaly. Br. Heart J. *54*:517, 1985.
263. Willis, P. W., and Craige, E.: First heart sound in Ebstein's anomaly: Observations on the cause of wide splitting by echophonocardiographic studies before and after operative repair. J. Am. Coll. Cardiol. *2*:1165–8, 1983.
264. Hansen, J. F., Leth, A., Dorph, S., and Wennevold, A.: The prognosis in Ebstein's disease of the heart—Long-term followup of 22 patients. Acta Med. Scand. *201*:331, 1977.
265. Watson, H.: Natural history of Ebstein anomaly of tricuspid valve in childhood and adolescence. An international cooperation study of 505 cases. Br. Heart J. *36*:417, 1974.
266. Rossi, L., and Thiene, G.: Mild Ebstein's anomaly associated with supraventricular tachycardia and sudden death. Am. J. Cardiol. *53*:332, 1984.
267. Gussenhoven, E. J., Steward, P. A., Becker, A. E., Essed, C. E., Ligtvoet, K. M., and DeVilleneuve, V. H.: "Offsetting" of the septal tricuspid leaflet in normal hearts and in hearts with Ebstein's anomaly: Anatomic and echographic correlation. Am. J. Cardiol. *53*:172, 1984.
268. Brundage, B. H., and Chomaka, E.: Clinical applications of cardiac CT imaging. Mod. Concepts Cardiovasc. Dis. *54*:39, 1985.
268a. Benson, L. N., Child, J. S., Schwaiger, M., Perloff, J. K., and Schelbert, H. R.: Left ventricular geometry and function in adults with Ebstein's anomaly of the tricuspid valve. Circulation *75*:353, 1987.
269. Caralps, J. M., Aris, A., Bonnin, J. O., Solanes, H., and Torner, M: Ebstein's anomaly: Surgical treatment with tricuspid valve replacement without right ventricular plication. Ann. Thorac. Surg. *31*:277, 1981.
270. Danielson, G. K., and Fuster, V.: Surgical repair of Ebstein's anomaly. Ann. Surg. *196*:499, 1982.
271. Abe, T., and Komatsu, S.: Valve replacement for Ebstein's anomaly of the tricuspid valve: early and long-term result of eight cases. Chest *84*:414, 1983.
272. Behl, P. R., and Blesovsky, A.: Ebstein's anomaly: Sixteen years experience with valve replacement without plication of the right ventricle. Thorax *39*:8, 1984.
273. Silver, M. A., Cohen, S. R., McIntosh, C. L., Cannon, R. O., and Roberts, W. C.: Late (5 to 132 months) clinical and hemodynamic results after either tricuspid valve replacement or annuloplasty for Ebstein's anomaly of the tricuspid valve. Am. J. Cardiol. *54*:627, 1984.
274. Ok, J. K., Holmes, D. R., Hayes, D. L., Porter, C. J., and Danielson, G. K.: Cardiac arrhythmias in patients with surgical repair of Ebstein's anomaly. J. Am. Coll. Cardiol. *6*:1351, 1985.
275. Marcus, F. I., Fontaine, G. H., Guiraudon, G., Frank, R., Laurenceau, J. L., Marlergue, C., and Grosgogeat, Y.: Right ventricular dysplasia—A report of 24 adult cases. Circulation *65*:384, 1982.
276. Olsson, S. B., Edvardsson, N., Emanuelsson, H., and Enestrom, S.: A Case of arrhythmogenic right ventricular dysplasia with ventricular fibrillation. Clin. Cardiol. *5*:591, 1982.
277. Manyari, D. E., Klein, G. J., GulamHusein, S., Goughner, K., Guiraudon, G. M., Wyse, G., and Mitchell, L. B.: Arrhythmogenic right ventricular dysplasia: A generalized cardiomyopathy? Circulation *68*:251, 1983.
278. Higuchi, S., Caglar, N. M., Shimada, R., Yamada, A., Takeshita, A., and Nakamura, M.: 16-year follow-up of arrhythmogenic right ventricular dysplasia. Am. Heart J. *108*:1363, 1984.
279. Robertson, J. H., Bardy, G. H., German, L. D., Gallaghner, J. J., and Kisslo, J.: Comparison of two-dimensional echocardiographic and angiographic findings in arrhythmogenic right ventricular dysplasia. Am. J. Cardiol. *55*:1506, 1985.
280. Manyari, D. E., Duff, H. J., Kostuk, W. J., Belenkie, I., Klein, G. J., Wyse, G., Mitchell, L. B., Boughner, D., Guiraudon, G., and Smith, E. R.: Usefulness of noninvasive studies for diagnosis of right ventricular dysplasia. Am. J. Cardiol. *57*:1147, 1986.
281. Gaffney, F. A., Nicod, P., Lin, J. C., and Rude, R. E.: Noninvasive recognition of the parchment right ventricle (Uhl's anomaly arrhythmogenic right ventricular dysplasia) syndrome. Clin. Cardiol. *6*:235, 1983.
282. Diggelmann, U., and Baur, H. R.: Familial Uhl's anomaly in the adult. Am. J. Cardiol. *53*:1402, 1984.
283. Bewick, D. J., Chandler, B. M., and Montague, T. J.: Dilated right ventricular cardiomyopathy: Uhl's disease. Chest *90*:300, 1986.
284. Child, J. S., Perloff, J. K., Francoz, R., Yeatman, L. A., Henze, E., Schelbert, H. R., and Laks, H.: Uhl's anomaly (parchment right ventricle): Clinical echocardiographic, radionuclear, hemodynamic and angiocardiographic features in 2 patients. Am. J. Cardiol. *53*:635, 1984.
285. Morady, F., Shen, E. N., and Scheinman, M. M.: Unusual features of arrhythmogenic right ventricular dysplasia: Am. J. Cardiol. *53*:639, 1984.
286. Frais, M. A., Manyari, D. E., Duff, H. J., Wyse, D. G., White, A. V. M., and Mitchell, L. B.: Coexistent arrhythmogenic right ventricular dysplasia and Wolff-Parkinson-White syndrome. Am. J. Cardiol. *53*:632, 1984.
287. Candan, I., Erol, C., and Sonel, A.: Cross-sectional echocardiographic appearance in presumed congenital absence of the left pericardium. Br. Heart J. *55*:405, 1986.
288. Guiraudon, G. M., Klein, G. J., Gulamhusein, S. S., Painvin, G. A., Delcampo, C., Gonzales, J. C., and Ko, P. T.: Total disconnection of the right ventricular free wall: Surgical treatment of right ventricular tachycardia associated with right ventricular dysplasia. Circulation *67*:464, 1983.
289. Olsson, S. B., Edvardsson, N., Emanuelsson, H., and Enestrom, S.: A case of arrhythmogenic right ventricular dysplasia with ventricular fibrillation. Clin. Cardiol. *5*:591, 1982.
290. Graham, T. P., Jr., and Friesinger, G. C.: Complex cyanotic congenital heart disease. *In* Roberts, W. C. (ed.): Adult Congenital Heart Disease. Philadelphia, F. A. Davis Co., 1987, pp. 541–566.
291. Hagler, D. J., Seward, J. B., Tajik, A. J., and Ritter, D. J.: Functional assessment of the Fontan operation combined m-mode, two-dimensional and Doppler echocardiographic studies. J. Am. Coll. Cardiol. *4*:756, 1984.
292. Mair, D., Rice, M., Hagler, D., Puga, F., McGoon, D., and Danielson, G.: Outcome of the Fontan procedure in patients with tricuspid atresia. Circulation *73* (Suppl. 2):II-88, 1985.
293. Nakazawa, M., Nakanisih, T., Okuda, H., Satomi, G., Nakae, S., Imai, Y., and Tarao, A.: Dynamics of right heart flow in patients after Fontan procedure. Circulation *69*:306, 1984.
294. Driscoll, D., Danielson, G., Puga, F., Schaff, H., Heise, C., and Staats, B.: Exercise tolerance and cardiorespiratory response to exercise after the Fontan operation for tricuspid atresia or functional single ventricle. J. Am. Coll. Cardiol. *7*:1084, 1986.
295. Park, S. C., Necxhes, W. H., Mathews, R. A., Fricker, F. J., Beerman, L.

B., Rischer, D. R., Lenox, C. C., and Zuberbuhler, J. R.: Hemodynamic function after the mustard operation for transposition of the great arteries. Am. J. Cardiol. *51*:1514, 1983.

296. Carceller, A., Fouron, J., Smallhorn, J., Cloez, J., VanDoesburg, N., Mauran, P., Ducharme, G., Pernot, C., and Davignon, A.: Wall thickness, cavity dimensions, and myocardial contractility of the left ventricle in patients with simple transposition of the great arteries. Circulation *73*:622, 1986.

297. Smallhorn, J., Gow, R., Freedom, R., Trusler, G., Olley, P., Pacquet, M., Gibbons, J., and Vlad, P.: Pulsed Doppler echocardiographic assessment of the pulmonary venous pathway after the mustard or Senning procedure for transposition of the great arteries. Circulation *73*:765, 1986.

298. Borow, K. M., Arensman, F. W., Webb, C., Radley-Smith, R., and Yacoub, M. H.: Assessment of the left ventricular contractile state after anatomic correction of transposition of the great arteries. Circulation *69*:106, 1984.

299. Graham, T. P., and Freisinger, G. C.: Complex cyanotic congenital heart disease in adults. *In* Roberts, W. C. (ed.): Congenital Heart Disease in Adults. Philadelphia, F. A. Davis Co., 1979, p. 383.

300. Piccoli, G., Pacifico, A. D., Kirklin, J. W., Blackstone, E. H., Kirklin, J. K., and Bargeron, L. M.: Changing results and concepts in the surgical treatment of double-outlet right ventricle: Analysis of 137 operations in 126 patients. Am. J. Cardiol. *52*:549, 1983.

301. Freedom, R., Benson, L., Smallhorn, J., Williams, W., Trusler, G., and Rowe, R.: Subaortic stenosis, the univentricular heart, and banding of the pulmonary artery: An analysis of the courses of 43 patients with univentricular heart palliated by pulmonary artery banding. Circulation *73*:758, 1986.

302. Graham, T. P.: The Eisenmenger reaction and its management. *In* Roberts, W. C. (ed.): Congenital Heart Disease in Adults. Philadelphia, F. A. Davis Co., 1979, p. 531.

303. Friedman, W. F., and Heiferman, M. F.: Clinical problems of postoperative pulmonary vascular disease. Am. J. Cardiol. *50*:631, 1982.

304. Pirlo, A., and Herren, A. L.: Eisenmenger's syndrome and pregnancy. A case report and review of the literature. Anesth. Rev. *6*:9, 1979.

305. Midwall, J., Jaffin, H., Herman, M. V., and Kupersmith, J.: Shunt flow and pulmonary hemodynamics during labor and delivery in the Eisenmenger's syndrome. Am. J. Cardiol. *42*:299, 1978.

306. Roberts, W. C.: Major anomalies of coronary arterial origin seen in adulthood. Am. Heart J. *111*:941, 1986.

307. Moodie, D. S., Fyfe, D., Gill, C. C., Cook, S. A., Lytle, B. W., Taylor, P. C., Fitzgerald, R., and Sheldon, W. C.: Anomalous origin of the left coronary artery from the pulmonary artery (Bland-White-Garland syndrome) in adult patients: Long-term followup after surgery. Am. Heart J. *106*:381, 1983.

308. Westaby, S., Davies, G. J.: Successful mitral valve replacement and myocardial revascularization in an adult with anomalous origin of the left coronary artery from the pulmonary artery. J. Thorac. Cardiovasc. Surg. *91*:188, 1986.

308a. Perloff, J. K.: Anomalous origin of the left coronary artery from the pulmonary trunk. *In* The Clinical Recognition of Congenital Heart Disease. 3rd ed. Philadelphia, W. B. Saunders Company, 1987, pp. 498–510.

309. Cottrill, C. M., Cafis, D., McMillen, M., O'Conner, W. N., Noonan, J. A., and Todd, E. P.: Anomalous left coronary artery from the pulmonary artery: Significance of associated intracardiac defects. J. Am. Coll. Cardiol. *6*:237, 1985.

310. Moodie, D. S., Cook, S. A., Gill, C. C., and Napoli, C. A.: Thallium-201 myocardial imaging in young adults with anomalous left coronary artery arising from the pulmonary artery. J. Nucl. Med. *21*:1076, 1980.

311. Caldwell, R. L., Hurwitz, R. A., Girod, D. A., Weyman, A. E., and Feigenbaum, H.: Two-dimensional echocardiographic differentiation of anomalous left coronary artery from congestive cardiomyopathy. Am. Heart J. *106*:710, 1983.

312. Ryan, T., Armstrong, W. F., and Feigenbaum, H.: Prospective evaluation of the left main coronary artery using digital two-dimensional echocardiography. J. Am. Coll. Cardiol. *7*:807, 1986.

313. Shem-Tov, A. A., Hegesh, J., Schneeweiss, A., and Neufeld, H. N.: Visualization of left coronary artery in anomalous origin of left coronary artery from pulmonary artery. Am. Heart J. *108*:621, 1984.

314. Worsham, C., Sanders, S. P., Burger, B. M.: Origin of the right coronary artery from the pulmonary trunk: Diagnosis by two-dimensional echocardiography. Am. J. Cardiol. *55*:232, 1985.

315. Shah, R. M., Nanda, N. C., Hsiung, M. C., Moos, S., and Roitman, D.: Identification of anomalous origin of the right coronary artery from pulmonary trunk by Doppler color flow mapping. Am. J. Cardiol. *57*:366, 1986.

316. Roberts, W. C., and Robinowitz, M.: Anomalous origin of the left anterior descending coronary artery from the pulmonary trunk with origin of the right and left circumflex coronary arteries from the aorta. Am. J. Cardiol. *54*:1381, 1984.

317. Barth, C., III, and Roberts, W.: Left main coronary artery originating from the right sinus of Valsalva and coursing between the aorta and pulmonary trunk. J. Am. Coll. Cardiol. *7*:366, 1986.

317a. Perloff, J. K.: Congenital anomalies of the coronary circulation. *In* The Clinical Recognition of Congenital Heart Disease. 3rd ed. Philadelphia, W. B. Saunders Company, 1987, pp. 663–674.

318. Brandt, G., Martins, J. B., and Marcus, M. L.: Anomalous origin of the right coronary artery from the left sinus of Valsalva. N. Engl. J. Med. *309*:596, 1983.

319. Isner, J. M., Shen, E. M., Martin, E. T., and Fortin, R. V.: Sudden unexpected death as a result of anomalous origin of the right coronary artery from the left sinus of Valsalva. Am. J. Med. *76*:155, 1984.

320. Hobbs, R. E., Millit, H. D., Raghavan, R. V., Moodle, D. S., and Sheldon, W. C.: Coronary artery fistulae: A 10-year review. Cleve. Clin. Q. *49*:191, 1982.

320a. Perloff, J. K.: Congenital coronary artery fistula. *In* The Clinical Recognition of Congenital Heart Disease. 3rd ed. Philadelphia. W. B. Saunders Company, 1987, pp. 511–525.

321. Liberthson, R. R., Sagar, K., Berkoben, J. P., Weintraub, R. M., and Levine, R. H.: Congenital coronary arteriovenous fistula: Report of 13 patients, reviews of the literature and delineation of management. Circulation *59*:849, 1979.

322. Chia, B. L., Ee, B., Tan, A., Choo, M., and Tan, L.: Two-dimensional and pulsed Doppler echocardiographic abnormalities in coronary artery-pulmonary artery fistula. Chest *86*:901, 1984.

323. Miyatake, K., Okamoto, M., Kinoshita, N., Fusejima, K., Sakakibara, H., and Nimura, Y.: Doppler echocardiographic features of coronary arteriovenous fistula: Complementary roles of cross sectional echocardiography and the Doppler technique. Br. Heart J. *51*:508, 1984.

324. Agatston, A. S., Chapman, E., Hildner, F. J., and Samet, P.: Diagnosis of a right coronary artery-right atrial fistula using two-dimensional and Doppler echocardiography. Am. J. Cardiol. *54*:238, 1984.

325. Slater, J., Lighty, G. W., Winer, H. E., Kahn, M. L., Kronzon, I., Isom, O. W.: Doppler echocardiography and computed tomography in diagnosis of left coronary arteriovenous fistula. J. Am. Coll. Cardiol. *4*:1290, 1984.

326. Chenn, C. C., Hwang, B., Hsiung, M. C., Chaing, B. N., Meng, L. C., Wang, D. J., and Wang, S. P.: Recognition of coronary arterial fistula by Doppler 2-dimensional echocardiography. Am. J. Cardiol. *53*:392, 1984.

327. Friedman, D., and Rutkowski, M.: Coronary artery fistula: A pulsed Doppler/two-dimensional echocardiographic study. Am. J. Cardiol. *55*:1652, 1985.

328. Cooper, M. J., Berstein, D., and Silverman, N. H.: Recognition of left coronary artery fistula to the left and right ventricles by contrast echocardiography. J. Am. Coll. Cardiol. *6*:923, 1985.

329. Dines, D. E., Seward, J. B., and Bernatz, P. E.: Pulmonary arteriovenous fistulas. Mayo Clin. Proc. *58*:176, 1983.

329a. Perloff, J. K.: Congenital pulmonary arteriovenous fistula. *In* The Clinical Recognition of Congenital Heart Disease. 3rd ed. Philadelphia, W. B. Saunders Company, 1987, pp. 641–652.

330. Mittila, S., Meurala, H., Jarvinen, A., and Ketonen, P.: Pulmonary arteriovenous fistulas. Scand. J. Thorac. Cardiovasc. Surg. *16*:165, 1982.

331. White, R. I., Mitchell, S. E., Barth, K. H., Kaufman, S. L., Kadir, S., Chang, R., and Terry, P. B.: Angioarchitecture of pulmonary arteriovenous malformations: An important consideration before embolotherapy. Am. J. Radiol. *140*:681, 1983.

332. Vincent, R., Casiro, O., Pelech, A., and Collins, G.: Evaluation of pulmonary vascular resistance in the presence of a large pulmonary arteriovenous malformation. J. Am. Coll. Cardiol. 7:1104, 1986.

333. Boutefeu, J. M., Moret, P. R., Hahn, C., and Hauf, E.: Aneurysms of the sinus of Valsalva. Report of seven cases and review of the literature. Am. J. Med. *65*:18, 1983.

334. Atoy, A. E., Alpert, M. A., Bertuso, J. R., and Lawson, D. L.: Right sinus of Valsalva aneurysm presenting as an echocardiographic right atrial mass. Am. Heart J. *112*:169, 1986.

335. Metras, D., Coulibalty, A. O., Outtra, K.: Calcified unruptured aneurysm of sinus of Valsalva with complete heart block and aortic regurgitation. Br. Heart J. *48*:507, 1982.

336. Mayer, E. D., Ruffmann, K., Saggau, W., Butzmann, B., Bernhardt-Mayer, K., Schatton, N., and Schmitz, W.: Ruptured aneurysms of the sinus of Valsalva. Ann. Thorac. Surg. *42*:81, 1986.

337. Przybojewski, J. Z., Blake, R. S., and DeWett Lubbe, J. J.: Rupture of sinus of Valsalva aneurysm into both right atrium and right ventricle. S. Afr. Med. J. *63*:616, 1983.

338. Perloff, J. K.: Congenital aneurysms of the sinuses of Valsalva. *In* The Clinical Recognition of Congenital Heart Disease. 3rd ed. Philadelphia, W. B. Saunders Company, 1987, pp. 526–539.

339. Desai, A. G., Sharma, M. O., Kumar, D. M., Hansoti, R. C., and Kalke, M. S.: Echocardiographic diagnosis of unruptured aneurysms of right sinus of Valsalva: An unusual cause of right ventricular outflow obstruction. Am. Heart J. *109*:363, 1985.

340. Gibbs, K., Reardon, M., Strickman, N., DeCastro, C., Gerard, J., Rycyna, J., Hall, R., and Cooley, D.: Hemodynamic compromise (tricuspid stenosis and insufficiency) caused by an unruptured aneurysm of the sinus of Valsalva. J. Am. Coll. Cardiol. 7:1177, 1986.

341. Kiefaber, R., Tabakin, B., Coffion, L., and Gibson, T.: Unruptured sinus of Valsalva aneurysm with right ventricular outflow obstruction diagnosed by two-dimensional and Doppler echocardiography. J. Am. Coll. Cardiol. *7*:438, 1986.

342. Ohkawa, S., Sugiura, M., Itoh, Y., Kitano, K., Hiraoka, K., Veda, K., and Murakami, M.: Electrophysiologic and histologic correlations in chronic complete atrioventricular block. Circulation *64*:215, 1981.

343. Corne, R. A., and Mathewson, F. A. L.: Congenital complete atrioventricular heart block: A 25-year followup study. Am. J. Cardiol. *29*:412, 1972.

344. Vetter, V. L., and Rashkind, W. J.: Congenital complete heart block and connective tissue disease. N. Engl. J. Med. *309*:236, 1983.

345. Lynch, H. T., Mohiuddin, S., Moran, J., Kaplan, A., Sketch, M., Zencka, A., and Runco, V.: Hereditary progressive atrioventricular conduction defect. Am. J. Cardiol. *36*:297, 1975.

346. Scott, J. S., Maddison, P. J., Taylor, P. V., Esscher, E., Scott, O., and Skinner, R. P.: Connective-tissue disease, antibodies to ribonucleoprotein and congenital heart block. N. Engl. J. Med. *309*:209, 1983.

347. Clauvel, J. P., and Danon, F.: Antibodies to ribonucleoprotein and congenital heart block. N. Engl. J. Med. *309*:1583, 1983.

348. Reid, J. M., Coleman, E. N., and Doig, W.: Complete congenital heart block—Report of 35 cases. Br. Heart J. *48*:236, 1982.

349. Winkler, R. B., Freed, M. D., and Nadas, A. S.: Exercise-induced ventricular ectopy in children and young adults with complete heart block. Am. Heart J. *99*:87, 1980.

32 ACQUIRED HEART DISEASE IN INFANCY AND CHILDHOOD

by WILLIAM F. FRIEDMAN, M.D.

Since many of the topics discussed in this chapter are given more substantial coverage elsewhere in this text, the emphasis herein will be placed on features of acquired heart disease that are relatively unique or common in infancy and childhood, although the disease processes per se may not recognize age-related boundaries. Acute rheumatic fever and rheumatic heart disease, connective tissue disorders, and the mucopolysaccharidoses are discussed in Chapter 54. The hyperlipidemias are discussed in Chapters 36 and 49.

NONRHEUMATIC INFLAMMATORY DISEASE

INFECTIVE MYOCARDITIS

(See also Chapter 42)

Infectious processes causing inflammatory disease of the heart may occur at any age, even during fetal life. Etiological agents include bacteria, viruses, fungi, protozoa, helminths, rickettsia, and spirochetes. As a general rule, very few of the generalized illnesses caused by these agents feature significant involvement of the heart. Myocardial involvement may be demonstrated histologically, but in most cases little or no expression of cardiac inflammation will be detected clinically. Important exceptions are infections due to certain viruses, diphtheria, and trypanosomes; these are discussed individually below.

VIRAL MYOCARDITIS. Coxsackie B and rubella viruses are the most common causative agents in infective myocarditis of the newborn. The rubella embryopathy and its associated cardiovascular malformations are discussed on page 897. Active *rubella myocarditis* occurs in utero and may cause varying degrees of myocardial damage.[1] Invariably, however, other cardiovascular manifestations of the rubella syndrome dominate the clinical picture.

Coxsackie B typically causes outbreaks of epidemic myocarditis but may occur in the isolated infant in the newborn nursery, commonly with a fatal outcome.[2, 3] The illness is of sudden onset and is characterized by fever, tachycardia, signs of systemic hypoperfusion, cyanosis, and occasionally cardiac failure. In some infants signs and symptoms of encephalomyelitis and hepatitis predominate. The diagnosis is suggested by electrocardiographic findings of atrial and/or ventricular arrhythmias, generalized ST-segment and T-wave changes, and low-voltage QRS complexes, accompanied by the appearance of marked generalized cardiomegaly and pulmonary vascular congestion on the chest roentgenogram. Echocardiography reveals dilatation of both ventricles and depressed indices of cardiac performance. Echocardiography is especially helpful in excluding congenital cardiac structural anomalies. The diagnosis is strongly suggested or confirmed when the virus can be isolated from pericardial fluid, pharyngeal secretions, or feces, and elevations occur in type-specific–neutralizing, hemagglutination-inhibiting, or complement-fixing antibody.[4] Digitalis, diuretics, and general supportive measures are of limited benefit. Although increased sensitivity to the toxic effects of the glycosides is common, digitalis should be administered cautiously and continued until heart size is normal, since cardiac failure may recur when the drug is discontinued.

Numerous viral agents have been identified as a cause of myocarditis in childhood beyond infancy.[5–7] The most common are Coxsackie A and B (Fig. 32–1), influenza, adenovirus, and ECHO virus. Moreover, myocarditis, usually of mild degree, may be associated with the common viral infectious diseases of childhood, including mumps, measles, infectious mononucleosis, varicella, and variola. Although the diagnosis is generally one of exclusion, it may be suggested by the presence of sustained tachycardia out of proportion to fever, cardiomegaly without significant murmurs, poor-quality heart sounds, a gallop rhythm, an unexplained arrhythmia, and the electrocardiographic findings already mentioned. Important differential diagnostic possibilities include endocardial fibroelastosis, glycogen storage disease with cardiac involvement, anomalous pulmonary origin of a coronary artery, critical aortic stenosis in infancy, and coarctation of the aorta or hypoplastic left heart syndromes.

The vast majority of these children recover from the acute episode of myocarditis with few or no sequelae. On occasion patients may retain a permanent conduction defect or mild cardiac enlargement as a result of the acute illness. Morever, a child may progress from the acute

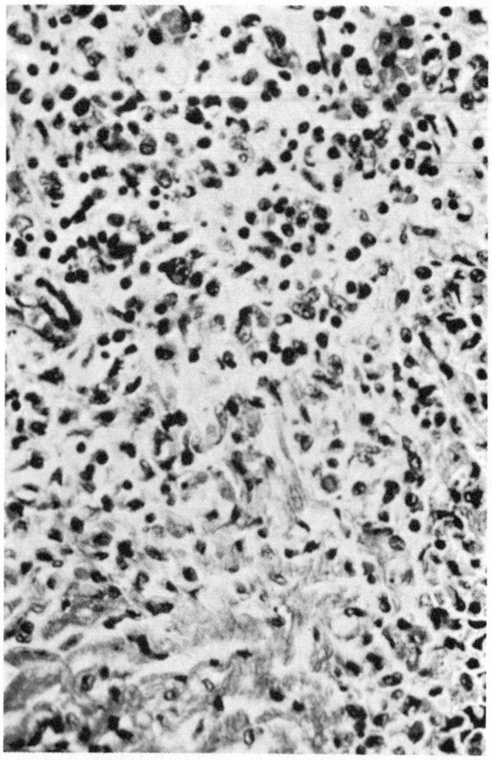

FIGURE 32–1. Photomicrograph of Coxsackie B_2 viral myocarditis. The major features are myocardial necrosis, edema, and heavy infiltrate of lymphocytes and large mononuclear cells. (× 400.) (From Gore, I., and Kline, I. K.: Pericarditis and myocarditis. *In* Gould, S. E. [ed.]: Pathology of the Heart and Blood Vessels. 3rd ed. Springfield, Ill., Charles C Thomas, 1968, p. 740.)

episode to a chronic dilated cardiomyopathy, characterized by signs of left ventricular dysfunction and mitral valve insufficiency. Unfortunately, there are no predictive criteria to identify the latter situation.[8] Cardiac transplantation has been successful in some of these children with cardiomyopathy and a chronic, relentless, and refractory course of heart failure. However, cardiac transplantation in children, and especially in infants or very young children, is complicated by growth suppression related to the required corticosteroid doses, and the complexity and severity of the immunosuppression in these infection-prone age groups.

DIPHTHERITIC CARDIOMYOPATHY. Diphtheria usually occurs in unimmunized children, especially in the western United States. Cardiac involvement is the result of the bacterial endotoxin rather than cardiac invasion by the bacillus.[9] Cardiac dysfunction appears to be related to abnormal fat metabolism since diphtheria toxin causes marked depletion of myocardial carnitine, a cofactor required for the beta-oxidation of fats.[10] Thus, what was formerly designated a form of myocarditis is now considered an acute metabolic cardiomyopathy. The pathology includes extensive intracellular fat vacuolization and glycogen depletion.

Cardiac involvement occurs in approximately 10 per cent of affected patients and is the most common cause of death from this disease. Heart disease is most reliably indicated by electrocardiographic changes, which range from ST-segment and T-wave changes to arrhythmias and conduction disturbances, including complete heart block.[11] Occasionally, the electrocardiographic pattern of myocardial infarction may emerge. The electrocardiogram is a fair indicator of the extent of myocardial involvement and of prognosis. The latter is generally favorable if only ST-segment and T-wave changes are observed in the absence of conduction system disturbances. Right or left bundle branch block and complete atrioventricular block are associated with mortality rates of 50 to 80 per cent. The electrocardiographic findings may be accompanied by evidence of myocardial dysfunction and ventricular chamber dilatation on cardiac ultrasound.

Treatment for diphtheritic cardiomyopathy is generally unsatisfactory. All patients should receive diphtheria antitoxin and intravenous penicillin after appropriate skin testing. Although corticosteroids have been used in the treatment of the myocardial problem, their value is debatable. Digitalis, diuretics, and antiarrhythmic medications are usually indicated. Recently, parenteral administration of carnitine has been found to partially reverse diphtheritic cardiac dysfunction and reduce the risk of cardiac death.[12] If the child recovers from the acute episode of diphtheritic cardiomyopathy, the prognosis is quite good.

MYOCARDITIS DUE TO TRYPANOSOMAL INFECTION. Chagas' disease (p. 1445) is a chronic parasitosis caused by *Trypanosoma cruzi*, transmitted to humans by the bite of insects in the reduviid family. In the United States the disease is seen mostly in the southern states; endemic infection occurs in Latin America. Its most important clinical manifestation is a late-developing, chronic myocarditis and, much less frequently, an early acute myocarditis that is fatal in up to 10 per cent of cases.[13] In patients surviving the acute stage, cardiomyopathy may occur after an interval of 10 to 30 years.[14] Diagnosis of the acute illness is supported by findings of edema and adenitis in the region of the insect bite, associated with low-grade intermittent fever, sweating, muscular pain, and at times, diarrhea and vomiting; weeks or months later, cardiomegaly, gallop rhythm, and conduction disturbances may be noted. Xenodiagnosis (examination of the excreta of laboratory-bred insects fed on the patient) or complement-fixation tests provide confirmation. There is no satisfactory treatment. Prophylaxis consists of control of the carrier of the parasites, reduvid bugs, by benzene hexachloride. A nitrofuran compound, nifurtinox, appears effective in the acute stage of infection, but not during the intracellular parasitic infection period.[15, 16]

Trypanosoma rhodesiense, which causes African sleeping sickness, may also produce myocardial hemorrhage, interstitial edema, mononuclear infiltration, and myocardial degeneration.[17] Cardiac involvement is usually relatively mild, and the clinical picture is dominated by evidence of encephalitis.

INFECTIVE PERICARDITIS

(See also p. 1508)

Numerous infectious agents may be responsible for infective pericarditis. Viral and tuberculous inflammatory pericardial disease is discussed in detail in Chapter 44. Of special concern in infancy and childhood is disease due to pyogenic bacteria.[18, 19] Purulent pericarditis occurs most often in the first two decades of life and is especially common in children under 6 years of age. Acute bacterial pericarditis is usually fatal if misdiagnosed or improperly treated. The most common pathogens are *Staphylococcus aureus*, *Streptococcus pneumoniae*, *Hemophilus influenzae*, and *Neisseria meningitides*. Unusual organisms causing purulent pericarditis include *Escherichia coli*, *Pseudomonas*, *Salmonella*, *Klebsiella*, *Proteus*, and *Bacteroides*. *Hemophilus influenzae*, in particular, affects infants and young children, usually in association either with upper respiratory infection and croup, with lower respiratory pneumonia, bronchitis, or occasionally with meningitis.

Presenting clinical signs and symptoms vary depending on the age of the patient, the responsible organism, and the site(s) of associated infection. The latter two require identification if therapy is to be effective. Fever, tachycardia, dyspnea, and chest pain are invariably present. Pericardial exudate resulting from the acute suppurative process commonly produces signs of life-threatening cardiac tamponade. Physical findings suggestive of purulent pericarditis include neck vein distention and hepatomegaly, pulsus paradoxicus, and/or systemic hypotension with a narrow pulse pressure, muffled and distant heart sounds, marked cardiomegaly, and a point of maximal cardiac impulse well within the area of percussed dullness. Although the presence of a pericardial friction rub points clearly to pericardial involvement, this sign occurs infrequently.

An enlarged, globular cardiac configuration on chest x-ray and electrocardiographic findings of diminished QRS amplitude and abnormalities of the ST segment (usually elevated) and T waves (often inverted) usually focus attention on the pericardium. Echocardiographic evaluation (p. 127) is reliable for establishing the diagnosis of significant pericardial effusion and for directing and guiding pericardiocentesis.[20] Culture and examination of pericardial fluid obtained by pericardiocentesis are essential for diagnosis and treatment. Unless effective surgical drainage is combined with antibiotic treatment the mortality rate is high. Operation should consist of creation of a subxiphoid pericardial window with placement of a drainage tube, or anterior pericardiectomy with tube drainage.[21] Early aggressive diagnosis and treatment reduce the risk of death substantially (10 to 20 per cent). Pericardial constriction is uncommon, but all patients should be followed carefully for this complication.

POSTPERICARDIOTOMY SYNDROME

In the first year after cardiac operation in which the pericardium is opened, and rarely in the second or third postoperative year, a febrile illness may occur, consisting of a pericardial and pleural inflammatory reaction with effusion and often with pulmonary parenchymal involvement. The illness occurs in approximately 35 per cent of children undergoing pericardiotomy and is usually self-limiting; infants undergoing open-heart surgery are affected rarely. It is characterized by fever; chest, neck, or shoulder pain that becomes worse with inspiration; anorexia; and laboratory findings of leukocytosis and an elevated erythrocyte sedimentation rate.[22] Recurrences are uncommon and usually mild. Physical, electrocardiographic, and roentgenographic signs of pericardial involvement vary with the magnitude of the effusion. Echocardiographic detection of the effusion is common between 4 to 10 days postoperatively.[23] Cardiac tamponade, while not usual, occurs with sufficient frequency to warrant careful observation of the patient.

Viral infection and an autoimmume reaction have been implicated in the pathogenesis. Serum antibodies and a rise in titer are found frequently against adenovirus, Coxsackie virus, and cytomegalovirus. Elevations in levels of heart-reactive antibody are common.

The syndrome must be distinguished from infective endocarditis and the postperfusion syndrome of atypical lymphocytosis and hepatomegaly, which occurs approximately 3 to 6 weeks after extracorporeal circulation and is caused by cytomegalovirus infection.[24]

Treatment of the postpericardiotomy syndrome depends upon the degree of patient discomfort and the magnitude of pericardial and/or pleural effusion. In some patients signs of cardiac tamponade will require pericardiocentesis. Bed rest and salicylates or indomethacin lessen patient discomfort and diminish the production of pleural or pericardial fluid. Corticosteroids are indicated for severe illness and promptly relieve fever and symptoms. Antibiotics are not useful in the treatment. Prolonged therapy is rarely necessary because of the self-limited nature of this postoperative complication. However, late or recurrent tamponade, although rare, may require reinstitution of treatment.[25]

PRIMARY CARDIOMYOPATHIES

Obstructive cardiomyopathies are discussed in Chapter 42. The important nonobstructive cardiomyopathies, of special concern in infants and children, are the familial and nonfamilial forms of endocardial fibroelastosis,[26–29b] which afflict many of the patients also designated as having *primary congestive cardiomyopathy.*[30] By definition, this diagnostic term excludes patients whose myocardial dysfunction is caused by infection, a cardiac anomaly, or increased preload or afterload.[31] Congestive cardiomyopathy is mainly a disease of infants, with most cases becoming manifested before the age of one year, with a history of respiratory or diarrheal illness preceding the onset of cardiac symptoms. The overall mortality exceeds 30 per cent, the vast majority of fatal cases occurring during the first episode of cardiac failure. Most severely ill patients probably have endocardiac fibroelastosis, although the latter can only be confirmed definitively after myocardial biopsy or autopsy. Myocardial biopsy is a risky procedure, not commonly performed in infancy.[32] The focus of discussion in this chapter is on endocardial fibroelastosis.

ENDOCARDIAL FIBROELASTOSIS. Various designations have been applied to this condition, including endocardial sclerosis, fetal endocarditis, fetal endomyocardial fibrosis, and elastic tissue hyperplasia.[26] In recent years familial cases have been encountered more commonly than has the isolated form. The data provided by family studies fit neither an autosomal recessive nor a multifactorial mode of inheritance. Although the reasons are obscure, a marked reduction has been observed in the past decade of isolated, nonfamilial, endocardial fibroelastosis. No definite cause for this condition has been established, although a host of theories have been proposed; inadequate subendocardial blood flow and/or pre- or postnatal inflammation or infection are currently considered the most likely pathogenetic pathways.[28]

Pathologically, both primary and secondary forms of endocardial fibroelastosis (EFE) have been recognized.[29] In the *secondary* variety, focal areas of opaque fibroelastotic thickening of the mural endocardium or cardiac valves are observed in association with other types of cardiac malformations. Underlying cardiovascular anomalies are almost always obstructive lesions, particularly of the left side of the heart, and these create cardiac hypertrophy and an imbalance in the myocardial oxygen supply-demand relationship. Thus, secondary EFE occurs quite commonly in aortic stenosis, coarctation of the aorta, and hypoplastic left heart syndrome.

This discussion focuses on the *primary* form of EFE, which invariably involves the left ventricle and mitral and aortic valves without significant associated cardiac defects. Primary EFE commonly produces a marked dilatation of the left ventricle; rarely, a "contracted" type of primary EFE is observed, in which the left ventricle is relatively hypoplastic or normal in size. In the latter situation the right and left atrium and the right ventricle are markedly enlarged and hypertrophied, with minimal or no endocardial sclerosis. In the common, dilated type of primary EFE, microthrombi may be found adherent to the endocardium. The diffuse endocardial hyperplasia may be several millimeters thick (Fig. 32–2). The aortic and mitral valve leaflets are thickened and distorted; mitral regurgitation is especially common. The papillary muscles and chordae tendineae are involved in the fibroelastic process and are shortened and distorted.

Primary EFE is a disease of infancy; symptoms develop usually between 2 and 12 months of age, although rarely they may be present shortly after birth. Clinical features reflect left ventricular dysfunction and congestive heart failure.[33, 34] Noted initially are fatigue and breathlessness during feeding, failure to thrive, irritability, pallor, increased sweating, peripheral cyanosis, cough, wheezing, or grunting. Symptoms are usually rapidly progressive. Examination of the infant reveals tachycardia, cardiomegaly, a gallop rhythm, and hepatosplenomegaly. Cardiac murmurs may be absent; approximately 40 per cent of infants have the characteristic apical systolic murmur of mitral regurgitation.

Chest roentgenography reveals marked, generalized cardiomegaly with normal or congested pulmonary vascular markings. A typical electrocardiographic finding is left ventricular hypertrophy with inverted T waves in the left precordial leads; less usual are tracings suggestive of myocardial infarction, varying degrees of atrioventricular block, or arrhythmias. Echocardiographic features include an increase in left atrial and left ventricular dimensions, reduced left ventricular septal and posterior wall motion, reduced ejection fraction,[34a] and abnormal mitral valve motion. The diagnosis of primary EFE is usually made easily by the characteristic clinical findings but is, nonetheless, one of exclusion. Differential diagnosis includes anomalous pulmonary origin of the left coronary artery, myocarditis, hypertrophic obstructive cardiomyopathy, anomalies causing left ventricular outflow tract obstruction, and glycogen storage disease of the heart. In general, the first four of these entities differ appreciably from fibroelastosis in their electrocardiographic or echocardiographic features; the skeletal muscle biopsy in glycogen storage disease is diagnostic.

Hemodynamic studies reveal evidence of left ventricular dysfunction.[35] This includes elevations in left ventricular end-diastolic and left atrial pressures, moderate pulmonary hypertension, widened arteriovenous oxygen differences, and reduced left ventricular stroke volume and cardiac output. Angiography usually demonstrates a markedly dilated left ventricle, a reduced ejection fraction, and varying degrees of mitral regurgitation. The configuration of the left ventricular chamber is usually globular or spherical; dyskinetic or akinetic patterns of contraction are uncommon. Endomyocardial catheter biopsy techniques (p. 262) are difficult to use in infants but, when employed, will show a diagnostic invasion of the endocardium and subendocardium by fibroelastic tissue.[36] The *contracted form* of primary EFE produces a clinical picture of left-sided obstructive disease, particularly if the mitral valve is small. Left atrial pressure is elevated, with pulmonary artery pressures at or near systemic arterial levels.

The optimal management of patients with primary EFE consists of early and prolonged treatment with digitalis. Glycoside therapy should be continued for many years after the disappearance of symptoms, since cessation of the drug may result in acute cardiac failure, even when the heart size has returned to normal. The results of pericardial poudrage and mitral valve replacement in seriously afflicted infants have been disappointing.

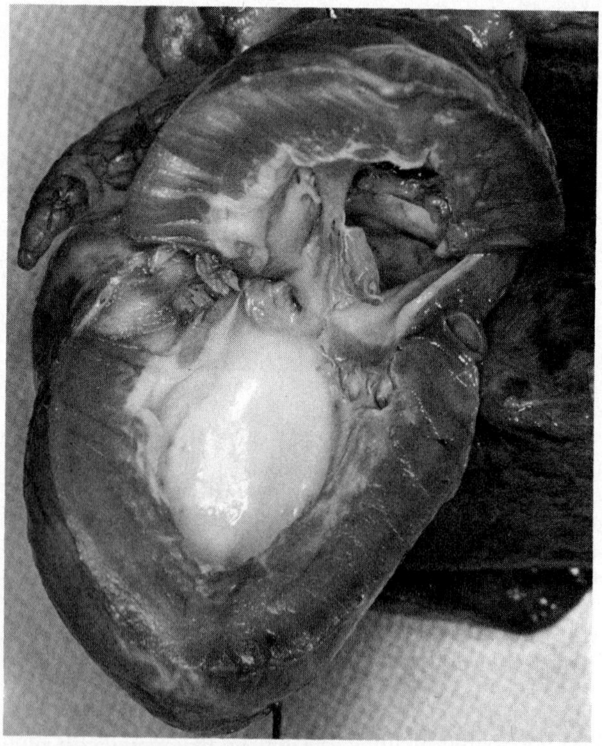

FIGURE 32–2. Diffuse left ventricular endocardial fibroelastosis. There is myocardial hypertrophy and obliteration of the papillary muscles as well as encroachment of the sclerotic subendocardial process onto the base of the aortic cusps. (From Tingelstaad, J. B., et al.: The electrocardiogram in the contracted type of primary endocardial fibroelastosis. Am. J. Cardiol. *27*:304, 1971.)

SECONDARY CARDIOMYOPATHIES

The designation "secondary" cardiomyopathy refers to intrinsic myocardial disease that is secondary to or associated with systemic disease or diseases of other organs or in other systems. Myocardial disease coexisting with collagen vascular disorders (Chap. 54), neuromuscular disorders (Chap. 57), neoplasms (Chap. 55), acute glomerulonephritis (Chap. 59), and thalassemia (Chap. 55) is discussed elsewhere in this text. Additional secondary cardiomyopathies of special interest to those caring for infants and children are those seen in infants of diabetic mothers, and associated with glycogen storage disease, neonatal thyrotoxicosis, infantile beriberi, protein-calorie malnutrition, tropical endomyocardial fibrosis, anthracycline toxicity, and the mucocutaneous lymph node syndrome. Attention is directed to each of these latter disorders.

CARDIOMYOPATHY IN INFANTS OF DIABETIC MOTHERS

Infants born of diabetic mothers are exposed to chronic hyperinsulinism in utero and to reactive hypoglycemia after birth. Such infants occasionally display two basic forms of cardiomyopathy, both of which are usually transient.[37–39] It has been suggested that suboptimal metabolic control of maternal diabetes during pregnancy increases the incidence of these abnormalities.[40] In some of these infants, hypertrophy and hyperplasia of myocardial cells constitute a diffuse process, producing reversible signs and symptoms that resemble those of congestive cardiomyopathy. In other infants, the clinical findings are indistinguishable from hypertrophic obstructive cardiomyopathy. The natural history in this latter group has, in general, been one of gradual spontaneous regression within 1 to 12 months of obstructive murmurs, cardiomegaly, and electrocardiographic and echocardiographic abnormalities typical of hypertrophic obstructive cardiomyopathy.

GLYCOGEN STORAGE DISEASE

Glycogen storage disease is the result of a deficiency of one or more of the enzymes involved in the biosynthesis and degradation of glycogen. The heart is importantly involved in type II (Pompe's disease), which results from a deficiency of alpha-1,4-glucosidase (acid maltase), a lysosomal enzyme that hydrolyzes glycogen into glucose.[41] This disease is a hereditary error of metabolism transmitted through a single recessive autosomal gene. Generalized glycogenosis takes place but occurs especially in the heart, the skeletal muscles, and the liver. The glycogen within cardiac muscle cells is biochemically normal but is present in excessive amounts, both within lysosomes and free in the cytoplasm.[41] As a result, the heart enlarges, often to a marked degree, and congestive heart failure supervenes. Usually glycogen deposition within the myocardium is uniform, although occasionally the interventricular septum is especially involved, producing subpulmonic obstruction or a constellation of features indistinguishable from hypertrophic obstructive cardiomyopathy. Selective angiography has revealed a distinctive trabeculation of the left ventricle in some infants.[42]

Clinical signs of type II glycogen storage disease usually become prominent in the early neonatal period.[41a] Characteristic symptoms include failure to thrive, progressive hypotonia, lethargy, and a weak cry. Prominent early features include nonspecific cardiac murmurs, cardiomegaly, signs of congestive heart failure, macroglossia, poor skeletal muscle tone, and weakness. The electrocardiogram shows extremely tall, broad QRS complexes with a short P-R interval (commonly less than 0.09 sec) (Fig. 32–3).

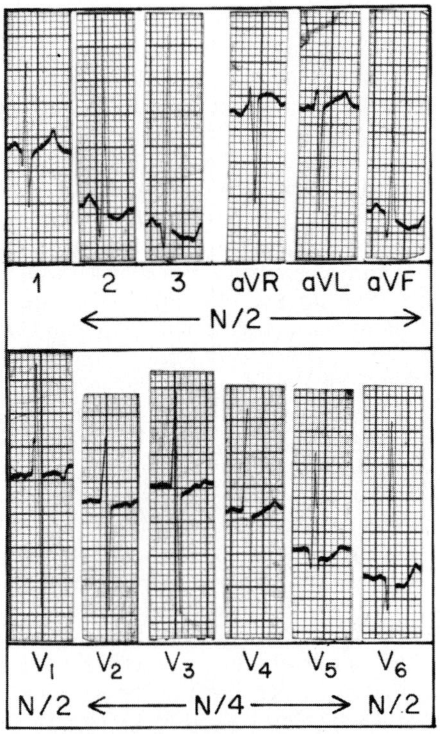

FIGURE 32–3. Electrocardiogram in an infant with glycogen storage disease showing a short PR interval and left ventricular hypertrophy.

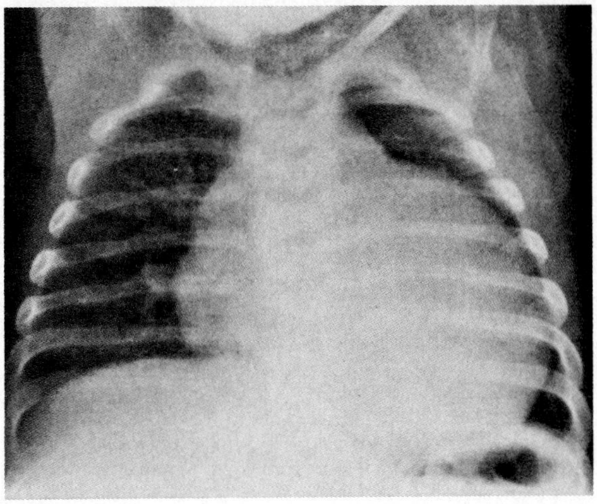

FIGURE 32–4. Chest roentgenogram of an infant with glycogen storage disease showing massive cardiomegaly and pulmonary edema. (From Taussig, H.: Congenital Malformations of the Heart. Vol. 2. 2nd ed. Commonwealth Fund, Harvard University, Boston, 1960, p. 901.)

The short P-R interval may be the result of facilitated atrioventricular conduction due to myocardial glycogen deposition. Less often, deep Q waves are observed over the mid or left precordium as well as T-wave inversion and ST-segment elevation. Chest roentgenograms show an enlarged globular heart associated with pulmonary vascular congestion (Fig. 32–4). In rare patients with cardiac glycogenosis the cardiac murmur suggests left ventricular outflow tract obstruction and/or mitral regurgitation; the echocardiographic, hemodynamic, and angiographic features in this subgroup are indistinguishable from those in infants with hypertrophic obstructive cardiomyopathy. Diagnosis is confirmed by demonstrating the enzymatic deficiency in lymphocytes, skeletal muscle, or liver. Skeletal muscle biopsy reveals histological and histochemical evidence of glycogen deposition.

Cardiac glycogenosis may be confused with other entities that cause cardiac failure in the early months of life, including endocardial fibroelastosis, anomalous pulmonary origin of the left coronary artery, fixed and dynamic forms of left ventricular outflow tract obstruction, coarctation of the aorta, and myocarditis. The short P-R interval and the skeletal muscle hypotonia in glycogen storage disease help distinguish this disorder from *endocardial fibroelastosis*. Infants with an anomalous pulmonary origin of the *left coronary artery* usually have a distinctive electrocardiographic pattern of anterolateral myocardial infarction. In infants with *coarctation of the aorta* the pulse and blood pressure discrepancies between the upper and lower extremities point to the proper diagnosis (p. 929). *Myocarditis* is usually of abrupt onset in a previously healthy child and is not associated with marked hypotonia; the generally low-voltage electrocardiogram does not show the short P-R interval. Occasionally the skeletal muscle hypotonia and the macroglossia in infants with glycogen storage disease raise the possibilities of amyotonia congenita and cretinism or mongolism, respectively.

Cardiac glycogenosis leads to progressive impairment of myocardial function; Pompe's disease is uniformly fatal usually within the first year of life. Death is quite often the result of either cardiac failure or complications of respiratory management such as pneumonia or aspiration.

NEONATAL THYROTOXICOSIS

Thyroid-stimulating immunoglobulin traverses the placental barrier and stimulates the fetal thyroid gland when maternal hyperthyroidism exists.[43] Infants are often born prematurely or are small for gestational age. Jitteriness and irritability are noted early. Cardiac findings include tachycardia, bounding pulses, systolic hypertension, and a precordial systolic murmur. Frequently, congestive heart failure is present, and occasionally, the presenting finding is an episode of paroxysmal atrial tachycardia. A neonatal goiter may be observed, especially if the mother received iodine therapy during pregnancy.

Diagnosis should be anticipated whenever a history of hyperthyroidism exists in the mother. Neonatal thyrotoxicosis occurs in the offspring of about 1 to 2 per cent of these women. A maternal level of thyroid-stimulating immunoglobulin should be obtained before delivery in anticipation of the problem arising in the newborn infant, since high levels are often observed in both mother and offspring. The serum levels of thyroxine are increased in the newborn.

The infant who has heart failure may be treated with digitalis and propylthiouracil or carbamizole. However, the latter two drugs will not be completely effective for many weeks; a beta blocker is usually helpful in addition to these agents. Supportive measures such as sedation and minimal stimulation may be helpful. Exchange transfusion or corticosteroid treatment is of no proven benefit.

Infants usually improve between the second and third month of life, although lack of attention to the problem or inadequate therapy may result in a fatal outcome.

INFANTILE BERIBERI

(See also p. 786)

Thiamine (vitamin B_1) deficiency occurs mainly in regions of southeast Asia, India, Brazil, and Africa, in which the dietary staple is polished rice or cassava. Thiamine functions as a coenzyme in decarboxylation of alpha-keto acids and in the utilization of pentose in the hexose monophosphate shunt. A reduction in myocardial energy production causes symptoms in the infant, usually between 1 and 4 months of age, who is breastfed by a thiamine-deficient mother.[44] Such infants are usually edematous, irritable, pale, and anorectic. Hoarseness or aphonia is common, owing to involvement of the recurrent laryngeal nerve; blepharoptosis occurs in one-third of infants. Typically, cardiac involvement manifests as dilatation of the right ventricle and prominent signs of systemic venous congestion. Electrocardiographic findings are nonspecific, and radiological findings consist principally of right ventricular dilatation. Infantile beriberi may be rapidly fatal but responds quickly and well to administration of thiamine (25 to 50 mg intravenously initially, with reduction of the dose to 10 mg/day for several days, and then orally for several weeks). Dramatic amelioration occurs within a few days of the cardiac findings. Cure is complete with no known sequelae.

PROTEIN-CALORIE MALNUTRITION

(See also p. 1821)

This is a major public health problem in underdeveloped areas of the tropics.[45, 46] In infants, inadequate diet results in a state of emaciation termed "marasmus"; "kwashiorkor" is a designation applied to this syndrome in children beyond one year of age. The disease results from a deficiency of protein relative to calories, although the latter and other essential nutrients are often lacking as well. General muscle wasting, loss of subcutaneous fat, and atrophy of most organs, including the heart, are typical in marasmic infants. In both marasmus and kwashiorkor, thinning and atrophy of cardiac muscle fibers and interstitial edema or vacuolization of the myocardial fibers are noted.[47] As the condition progresses, listlessness becomes prominent. Cardiovascular collapse is precipitated easily in these infants by the stress of infection.

In both infancy and childhood the principal physical findings reflect systemic hypoperfusion and consist principally of hypothermia, hypotension, tachycardia, and low-amplitude peripheral arterial pulsations. Peripheral usually nonpitting edema is prominent, as are wasting of the skeletal musculature, exfoliative dermatitis, and gray or reddish discoloration of the hair. Changes seen on electrocardiogram and on radiographic examination are nonspecific.

Treatment should be directed at correction of fluid and electrolyte imbalance, eradication of infection, and management of such associated problems as anemia and parasitic infestation. Care is required in the correction of dehydration or severe anemia, since volume overload of the heart is easily produced. Supplements of potassium and magnesium are often required, and because of deficiencies in these elements, digitalis should probably be avoided or used with extreme caution. If the infant or child survives the initial phase, a well-balanced diet will effect an impressive recovery over several months' duration.

TROPICAL ENDOMYOCARDIAL FIBROSIS

Endomyocardial fibrosis is a rare, acquired, progressive disease, usually involving children and young adults from Africa, Southeast Asia, and South America. This cardiomyopathy of unknown etiology is characterized by focal endocardial fibrosis of one or rarely both ventricles.[48] Controversy exists as to whether or not tropical endomyocardial fibrosis, which is not associated with eosinophilia, and Löffler's endocarditis with eosinophilia (Chap. 42) are the same disorders described from tropical and temperate climates, respectively.[49] Endocardial fibrosis is located almost exclusively in the inflow tracts of the ventricles and commonly involves one or the other atrioventricular valve. Partial obliteration of either cardiac chamber results in reduced ventricular compliance with impairment of filling. The fibrotic process often involves the chordae tendineae, resulting in mitral and/or tricuspid regurgitation. Plaques of heaped-up fibrous tissue without elastic fibers are especially common within the left ventricle. Endomyocardial fibrosis involving the right ventricle may have to be differentiated from Ebstein's anomaly of the tricuspid valve (p. 951), and endomyocardial fibrosis involving the left ventricle may have to be differentiated from rheumatic mitral regurgitation.

When left ventricular disease predominates, the clinical findings often resemble those of mitral stenosis or regurgitation. When endocardial involvement of the right ventricle is more severe than that of the left ventricle, the patient usually presents with findings of markedly elevated systemic venous pressure and tricuspid regurgitation.

Treatment is supportive, and survival usually depends on the extent of endocardial and valvular involvement and is better when right ventricular disease predominates. Mean survival after the onset of symptoms is approximately 24 months. Specific treatment does not exist, and corticosteroid therapy has not proved efficacious. Surgical excision (decortication) of affected tissue with prosthetic valve replacement has been associated with clinical improvement.[50, 51] However, children most severely affected by this disease reside in regions of the tropics and subtropics where cardiac surgery is not readily available.

MUCOCUTANEOUS LYMPH NODE SYNDROME (KAWASAKI'S DISEASE)

The mucocutaneous lymph node syndrome in infancy (Kawasaki's disease) was first described in Japan in 1967. Many thousands of cases from Japan have been reported and the disorder is being recognized with increasing frequency in North America and Europe.[52, 52a]

The syndrome presents as a febrile illness in children that occurs before the age of 10 and usually before the age of 2 years. They commonly have fever and ocular and oral manifestations followed in 5 days by a rash and indurative edema of the hands and feet, with palmar and plantar erythema. Finally, after about 2 weeks, cutaneous desquamation occurs. Diagnostic criteria include (1) a fever lasting 5 days or more that is unresponsive to antibiotics; (2) bilateral congestion of the ocular conjunctiva; (3) peripheral limb changes that include an indurative peripheral edema and erythema of the palms and feet, followed later in the course of the illness by a membranous desquamation of the fingertips; (4) changes in the lips and mouth, including dry, erythematous, and fissured lips, injected oropharyngeal mucosa, and a strawberry tongue; and (5) a polymorphous exanthema of the trunk without crusts or vesicles. Diagnosis is accepted when the first criterion and at least three of the remainder are present.

In addition to the mucous membrane and cutaneous effects, multiple organ system involvement has been noted. Noncardiovascular complications of the illness include arthritis, cerebrospinal fluid pleocytosis, pulmonary infiltrates, and hydrops of the gallbladder. The illness is often accompanied by cervical adenopathy, diarrhea, leukocytosis with a predominance of neutrophils, thrombocytosis, sterile pyuria and proteinuria, elevated liver transaminases, an elevation in the erythrocyte sedimentation rate and alpha-2-globulin, and a positive C-reactive protein.

An extensive search for the etiology of Kawasaki's disease has been unproductive. Most recently, however, high retrovirus-associated reverse transcriptase levels of activity in peripheral blood mononuclear cells of patients implicate a lymphotropic retrovirus as a direct cause of the vasculitis, or indirectly via immune mechanisms.[52b]

On the basis of pathological data, progression of the disease may be divided into four stages.[53] In stage I, lasting 1 to 9 days, acute perivasculitis of the small arteries is evident and involves the vasa vasorum of the major coronary arteries. Pericarditis, interstitial myocarditis, and endocardial inflammation are also seen; these changes consist chiefly of neutrophilic, eosinophilic, and lymphocytic infiltrations. In stage II, of 12 to 25 days' duration, panvasculitis involves the major coronary arteries. It affects the intima, media, and adventitia and results in aneurysm and thrombus formation.[53a] In stage III, of 28 to 31 days' duration, granulating thrombi and marked intimal thickening cause partial or total occlusion of the major coronary arteries. Stage IV follows and may be of many years' duration, in which healing occurs, consisting of myocardial scarring, calcification, and recanalization of occluded arteries.

The syndrome has an associated acute mortality of 1 to 3 per cent, secondary to complications from coronary artery involvement, myocarditis, or pericarditis, with a majority of deaths occurring in the third or fourth week of the illness.[54] Other children may die later in life as a result of myocardial infarction[54a]. Autopsy examination has almost uniformly demonstrated coronary arterial aneurysms, with occlusion due to thromboendarteritis (Fig. 32–5). The spectrum of cardiovascular involvement is outlined in Table 32–1.

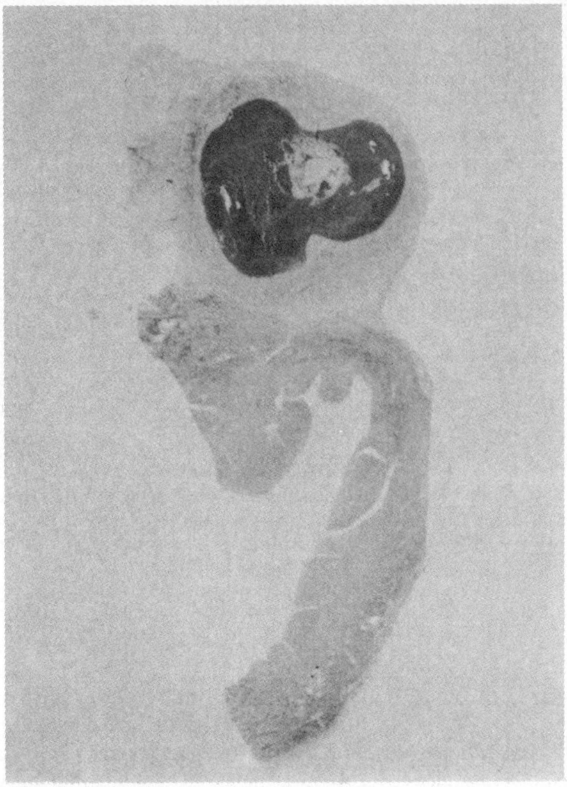

FIGURE 32–5. Low-power photomicrograph of a coronary artery aneurysm with recent occlusive thrombosis in a patient with mucocutaneous lymph node syndrome. (From Landing, B. H., and Larson, E. J.: Are infantile periarteritis nodosa with coronary artery involvement and fatal mucocutaneous lymph node syndrome the same? Comparison of 20 patients from North America with patients from Hawaii and Japan. Pediatrics *59*:651, 1977. Copyright American Academy of Pediatrics, 1977.)

The disease has often been misdiagnosed in the United States as scarlet fever, Stevens-Johnson syndrome, Rocky Mountain spotted fever, rheumatoid arthritis, scleroderma, or lupus erythematosus.

Infants and children with this syndrome should be watched closely for signs of cardiac involvement. A significant number of patients show evidence of myocarditis or pericarditis, or both, in the early phases of the disease.[55, 56] Electrocardiographic evidence of myocarditis with low voltage and nonspecific ST-T wave changes is seen in 45 per cent of patients, echocardiographic evidence of poor left ventricular function in 25 per cent, pericardial effusion in 9 per cent, cardiomegaly on chest radiographs in 25 per cent, and a gallop rhythm in 12 per cent. Aneurysms of the coronary arteries with narrowing, tortuosity, and ob-

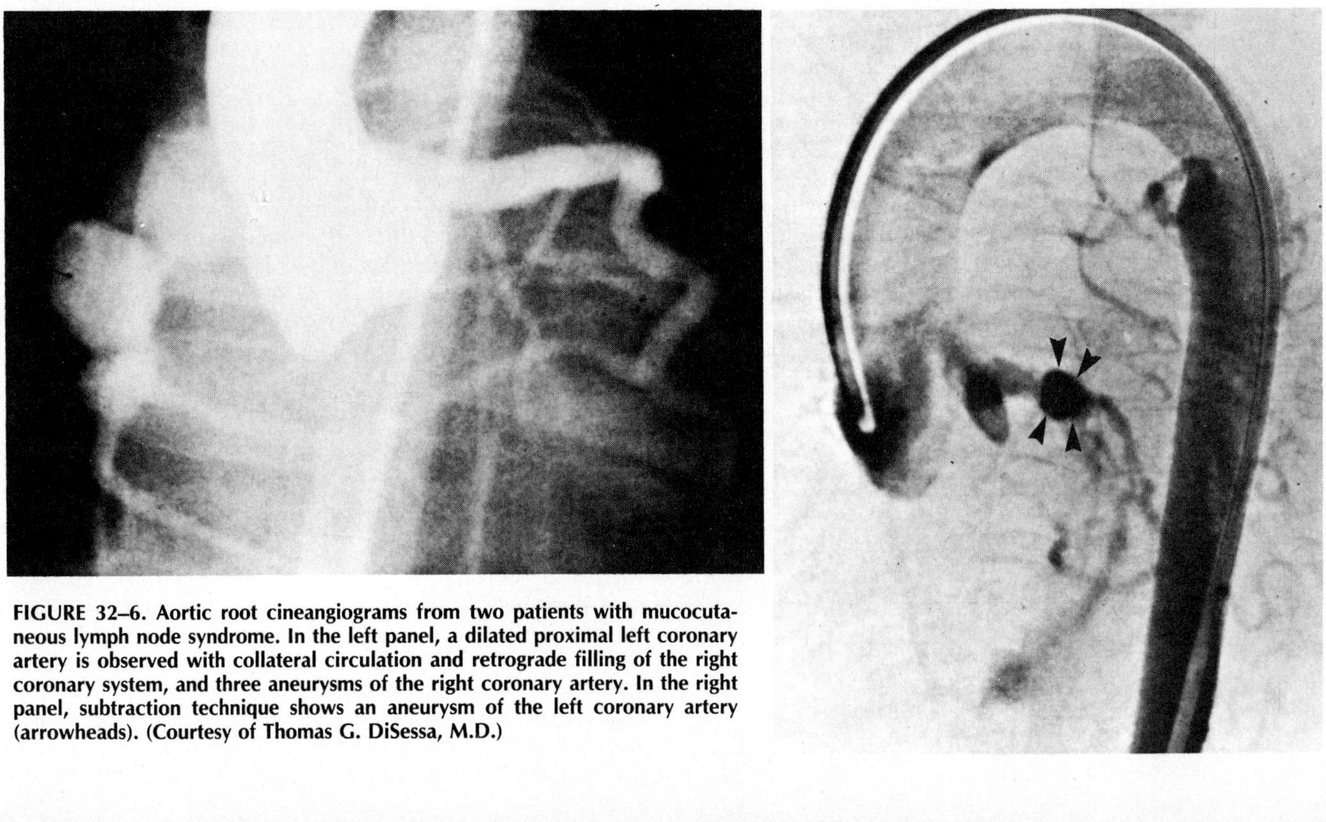

FIGURE 32–6. Aortic root cineangiograms from two patients with mucocutaneous lymph node syndrome. In the left panel, a dilated proximal left coronary artery is observed with collateral circulation and retrograde filling of the right coronary system, and three aneurysms of the right coronary artery. In the right panel, subtraction technique shows an aneurysm of the left coronary artery (arrowheads). (Courtesy of Thomas G. DiSessa, M.D.)

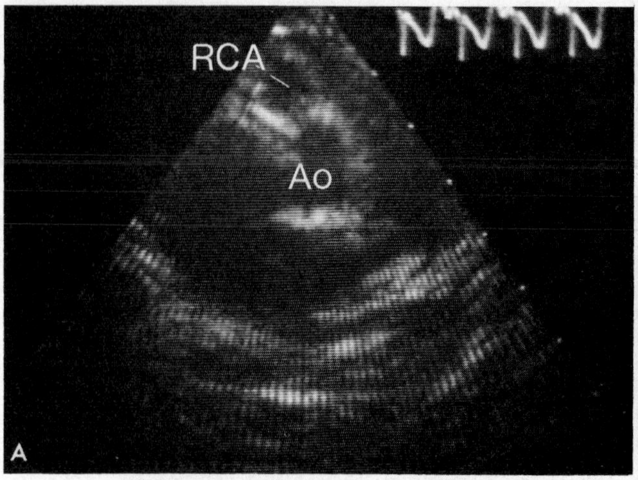

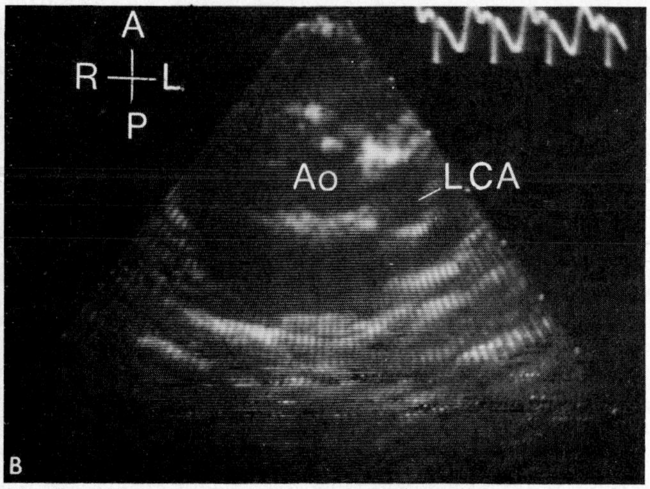

FIGURE 32–7. Short-axis cross-sectional echocardiographic views of aneurysms of the proximal right coronary artery (RCA) (*A*) and proximal left coronary artery (LCA) (*B*) in a 3-year-old boy with mucocutaneous lymph node syndrome. The right ventricular outflow tract is anterior (A) to the aorta (Ao) and the left atrium is posterior (P). R = right; L = left.

struction are almost invariably present on aortography and coronary angiography[57–59a] (Fig. 32–6). Excellent success has been achieved in visualizing aneurysmal coronary lesions with two-dimensional cross-sectional echocardiography (Fig. 32–7).[59–60a] Approximately half of the children with coronary aneurysms diagnosed shortly after the acute phase of the disease subsides have normal-appearing vessels by angiography 1 or 2 years later.[61–64] In those patients with residual cardiac abnormalities following recovery from the acute illness phase, associated findings may include impairment of left ventricular function secondary to the coronary arterial involvement and papillary muscle dysfunction with mitral regurgitation.[64b]

No treatment has been proven effective, to date, to prevent the formation of coronary artery aneurysms. It appears that corticosteroid therapy is *detrimental* during the acute illness. High-dose salicylate treatment (50 to 100 mg/kg/day) is advisable for all patients in the acute phase of the illness, and later in low doses (3–5 mg/kg/day) to inhibit platelet aggregation in the hope of preventing subsequent thrombus formation and occlusion of the coronary arteries. In many children with Kawasaki's disease, there is failure to achieve therapeutic serum concentrations of salicylate despite high oral doses because of impaired gastrointestinal absorption of salicylate.[65] Therefore, regular monitoring of serum salicylate levels is advisable. In children who have no evidence of coronary artery disease and in whom the platelet count has returned to normal, the aspirin may be discontinued after 2 to 6 months. In patients who develop coronary arterial involvement, aspirin therapy should be maintained indefinitely (3 to 5 mg/kg/day). Recently, investigators in Japan have empirically treated children with Kawasaki's disease with intravenous gamma globulin (400 mg/kg/day × 4), together with high-dose salicylates (to achieve a serum salicylate level of 18 to 30 mg/dl).[66] Data from randomized, controlled trials of this therapy in the United States show a substantial reduction in the formation of coronary arterial aneurysms.[67]

Two-dimensional echocardiography is indicated in all children with a diagnosis of Kawasaki's disease, with or without evidence of significant cardiac involvement. Coronary angiography is recommended for those patients with severe symptoms of cardiovascular involvement, persistence of cardiomegaly or heart failure, ischemic ST-T wave changes or an ECG pattern of myocardial infarction, signs of mitral insufficiency, or cardiac calcification by chest x-ray. The prognosis for chidren with vascular involvement should be guarded;[68, 69] some will be candidates for coronary arterial bypass surgery.[70, 71]

TABLE 32–1 SPECTRUM OF CARDIOCIRCULATORY FINDINGS IN KAWASAKI'S DISEASE

Carditis (myocarditis, pericarditis)
Congestive heart failure
Arrhythmias
Coronary Angiitis
Thromboendarteritis—aneurysms
Regression
Thrombosis—recanalization
Obstruction—stenosis
Collaterals
Rupture
Myocardial ischemia or infarction
Ventricular aneurysm
Papillary muscle dysfunction—mitral regurgitation
Arterial involvement
Pulmonary/renal angiitis—pulmonary/renal hypertension
Arteritis, aneurysms: femoral, iliac, brachial, cerebral, hepatic, etc.

ANTHRACYCLINE TOXICITY

(See also p. 1748)

Anthracycline drugs such as doxorubicin and daunomycin, used as cancer chemotherapeutic agents, cause a dose-related cardiomyopathy.[72] The risk of cardiac involvement increases significantly with doses in excess of 500 mg/m^2.[73] The onset of cardiac symptoms is often delayed, occurring 2 to 3 months after the anthracycline dose. Cardiac dysfunction usually presents first as unexplained tachycardia, progressing to dyspnea, congestive heart failure, hepatomegaly, and often death. The cardiomyopathy is most often reversible only in its early stages. Later, it is usually poorly responsive to digitalis, diuretics, and afterload reduction agents. Quite often patients are in remission from their neoplasm when the drug's cardiotoxicity proves lethal.

SYSTEMIC HYPERTENSION

(See also p. 853)

Unfortunately, many physicians usually consider hypertension a disease of adults and not of children. Thus, all too frequently, blood pressure is not recorded during the pediatric physical examination. It should be emphasized that elevations in systemic blood pressure may occur in as much as 2 per cent of the pediatric population, and that

TABLE 32–2 CONDITIONS ASSOCIATED WITH HYPERTENSION IN INFANTS AND CHILDREN

Congenital

Coarctation of the aorta
Gonadal dysgenesis (Turner syndrome)
Rubella syndrome
Pseudoxanthoma elasticum (Ehlers-Danlos syndrome)
Ask-Upmark syndrome (segmental renal artery dysplasia)
Renal arterial abnormalities
Multiple systemic and pulmonary artery stenoses
Solitary renal cyst
Hydronephrosis

Genetic

Diabetes mellitus
Neurofibromatosis (von Recklinghausen's disease)
Adrenogenital syndrome
Pheochromocytoma
Polycystic kidney disease (infantile and adult forms)
Familial nephritis (Alport's syndrome)
Little's syndrome
Fabry's disease (angiokeratoma corporis diffusum)
Familial dysautonomia (Riley-Day syndrome)
Essential hypertension
Tuberous sclerosis with angiolipomas
Primary hyperparathyroidism
Porphyria

Pharmacological

Sympathomimetics: ephedrine, epinephrine, isoproterenol
Adrenal steroids
Heavy metals: mercury, lead
Licorice

Acquired, renal

Unilateral hydronephrosis
Unilateral pyelonephritis
Renal trauma
Renal tumors
Unilateral multicystic kidney
Unilateral ureteral occlusion
Renal artery stenosis
Renal arteritis
Fibromuscular dysplasia of the renal artery
Renal fistula
Renal artery aneurysm
Chronic pyelonephritis superimposed on abnormal kidneys
Nephritis: shunt nephritis, acute poststreptococcal disease, anaphylactoid purpura, disseminated lupus erythematosus
Renal tuberculosis
Renal cortical necrosis: hemolytic uremic syndrome; sepsis
Renal vein thrombosis
Radiation nephritis
Postrenal transplantation

Acquired, other than renal

Hyperthyroidism
Retrosternal goiter
Guillain-Barré syndrome or poliomyelitis
Cerebral edema
Stevens-Johnson syndrome
Neuroblastoma
Hypercalcemia or hypernatremia
Adrenal adenoma or hyperplasia: primary aldosteronism or Cushing's syndrome
Hyperuricemic nephropathy
Burns

Modified from Lieberman, E.: Diagnostic evaluation of hypertensive children. Pediatr. Ann. *6*:390, 1977.

undetected or untreated hypertension may lead to well-documented unfortunate consequences.[74–76] Three points in particular require recognition:

1. Causes of hypertension in infants and children differ markedly from those in adults. Most children have secondary rather than essential forms of hypertension (Table 32–2); therefore, a premium must be placed on searching for a remedial cause.
2. Offspring of hypertensive parents are known to have an increased susceptibility to blood pressure elevation.
3. Children with elevated blood pressure require the same surveillance and treatment as do adults.

Accurate blood pressure measurements require cuffs of different sizes because of the variation in arm size from infancy through adolescence. To measure blood pressure correctly, the inner rubber bag should be wide enough to cover two-thirds of the length and three-fourths of the circumference of the upper arm or thigh while leaving the antecubital or popliteal fossa free. A cuff that is too small is likely to produce spuriously high readings. In infants under age 2 years the flush technique may be used, although a Doppler instrument is preferred.[77, 78] Since disappearance of the Korotkoff sound may cause underestimation of the diastolic pressure, both muffling (the fourth Korotkoff sound) and the disappearance of the sound (the fifth Korotkoff sound) should be recorded. The fourth Korotkoff sound is the more accurate measure of diastolic pressure in most prepubertal children; beyond adolescence the fifth sound more closely reflects diastolic pressure.[79, 80]

The normal ranges of blood pressure relative to age are illustrated in Figures 32–8 to 32–10 and serve as a guide in judging unsafe levels. The accuracy and precision of these blood pressure grids are limited because of differences in the study population in skeletal growth, body weight, sexual maturity, race, and socioeconomic status.[81, 82] Also, since considerable variation exists in most children's pressures, it should be recognized that a single blood pressure recording at, or higher than, the 90th percentile at a single point in time may not be an abnormal finding. In an apparently healthy child measurements should be repeated serially; further investigation is warranted if the blood pressure persists at or above the 90th percentile. In contrast, definite or severe hypertension, i.e., pressures well beyond the broad limits of normal, require prompt investigation and treatment.[83] Particularly urgent attention must be paid to those children whose systolic and diastolic pressures are remarkably high, i.e., equal to or greater than 180 and 110 mm Hg, respectively. Other findings identifying the patient at acute risk include

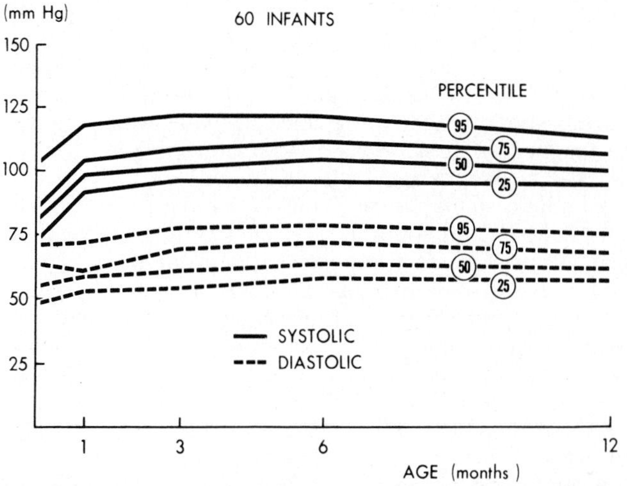

FIGURE 32–8. Percentile distributions of blood pressure in infancy. (From Levine, R. S., et al.: Tracking correlations of blood pressure levels in infancy. Pediatrics *61*:121, 1978. Copyright American Academy of Pediatrics, 1978.)

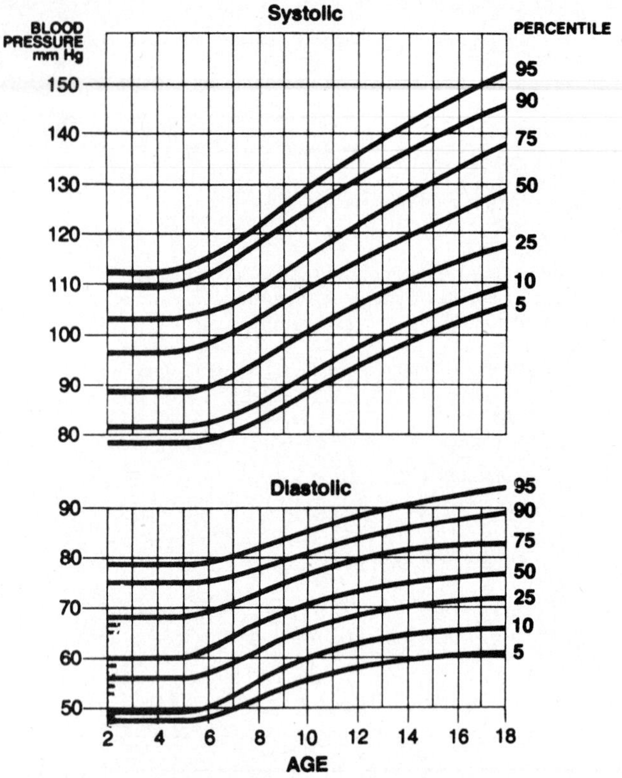

FIGURE 32–9. Percentile distribution of blood pressure in boys (right arm, seated). (From Blumenthal, S., et al.: Report of the task force on blood pressure control in children. Pediatrics 59[Suppl.]:797, 1977. Copyright American Academy of Pediatrics, 1977.)

localized neurological signs and/or local or generalized seizures; blurred vision or such eye ground changes are retinal hemorrhage, exudate, papilledema, or retinal arterial constriction; renal or abdominal pain; evidence of left ventricular hypertrophy or cardiac decompensation; renal dysfunction; palpation of an abdominal mass or enlargement of the kidneys; or auscultation of an abdominal bruit.

Evaluation of the asymptomatic child or adolescent with a blood pressure level above the 90th percentile on three or more occasions includes a careful history focusing on conditions or drugs known to be associated with or to predispose to high blood pressure. These include oral contraceptives (p. 838), use of glucocorticoids, renal disease (p. 839), and symptoms suggesting aldosteronism (p. 845), i.e., spells, weakness, polyuria, muscle cramps, or pheochromocytoma (p. 847), i.e., excessive sweating, palpitations. The family history should be reviewed for eclampsia during the mother's pregnancy as well as any familial occurrence of hypertension, premature coronary artery disease, stroke, or renal failure.

Common *symptoms* in hypertensive children are headache, nausea and vomiting, loss of appetite, epistaxis, and palpitation. A dietary history should be obtained with an emphasis on sodium intake. The *physical examination* is directed at detecting conditions associated with secondary hypertension (Table 32–2) and finding evidence of target organ damage on funduscopic and cardiac examination. Typically, the physical findings in hypertensive disorders in children reflect the underlying cause of the elevated pressure; distinctive physical findings accompany many of the conditions listed in Table 32–1 (see also Chap. 27).

Laboratory studies are aimed primarily at identifying secondary causes of hypertension.[84] The minimal laboratory tests required are a urinalysis, complete blood count, serum electrolytes, blood urea nitrogen, serum creatinine, echocardiogram, electrocardiogram, and chest roentgenogram. Since the most common cause of secondary hypertension in children is renal disease, evaluation often proceeds to include plasma renin activity with 24-hour urinary sodium excretion, rapid-sequence intravenous pyelogram, and isotopic or angiographic analysis of the kidneys and/or their blood supply. Fortunately, most identifiable causes of correctable hypertension in children and adolescents are associated with clinical findings that direct attention to a particular organ system (renal, endocrine, central nervous, and cardiovascular). Less often, hypertension may result from tumors (ganglioneuroma, pheochromocytoma, Wilms', and neuroblastoma) or collagen vascular disease. Laboratory studies should be as specific as possible in order to avoid an unselected analysis of every organ system theoretically associated with hypertension. In general, the younger the child and the higher the blood pressure elevation, the more vigorous should be the laboratory evaluation. It should be recognized that although essential hypertension is often a diagnosis by exclusion in prepubertal children, it is a viable diagnosis, particularly in adolescents.[84] In the author's opinion the need for extensive laboratory investigations has been overemphasized in children or adolescents with mild sustained elevations in blood pressure.

Asymptomatic children and adolescents with borderline or only mildly elevated blood pressure (< 5 to 10 mm Hg beyond the 90th percentile values for age) may not require antihypertensive pharmacological agents but should receive counseling regarding weight control, salt abuse, and avoidance of agents with pressor effects (e.g., caffeine, some bronchoconstrictors, nicotine, and so on). These patients should be encouraged to be active physically, especially in exercises improving cardiovascular fitness. Isometric or static exercise such as wrestling and weight

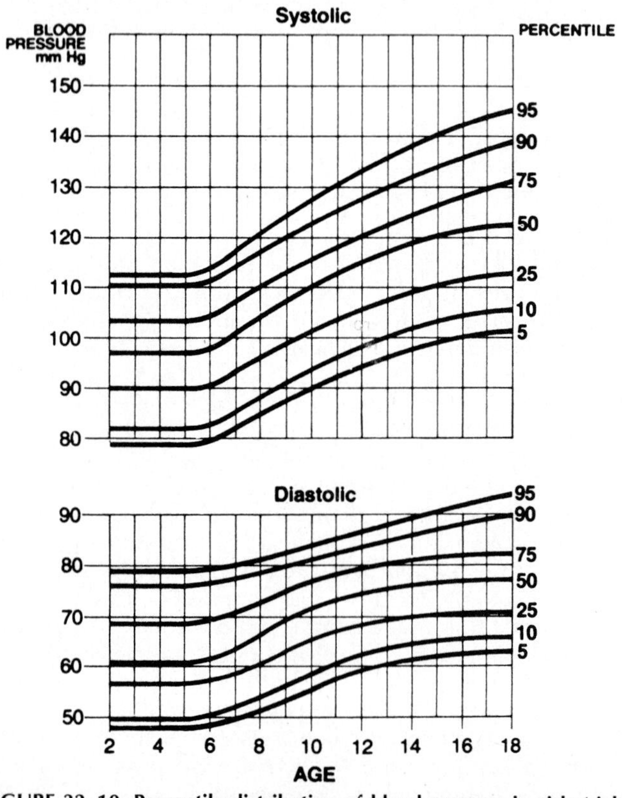

FIGURE 32–10. Percentile distribution of blood pressure in girls (right arm, seated). (From Blumenthal, S., et al.: Report of the task force on blood pressure control in children. Pediatrics 59[Suppl.]:797, 1977. Copyright American Academy of Pediatrics, 1977.)

TABLE 32–3 DRUGS COMMONLY USED IN PEDIATRIC CARDIOLOGY

Drug	Route of Administration	Dosage
Acetaminophen (Tylenol)	PO or PR	<1 year 60 mg (q4h); 1 to 3 years 120 mg (q4h); >3 years 120 to 240 mg (q4h)
Acetylsalicylic acid (Aspirin)	PO or PR	30 to 100 mg/kg/day (q4h)
ε-Aminocaproic acid (Amicar)	IV	Total 100 mg/kg; ¼ total dose (q1h)
Aminophylline	PO, PR, or IV	12 mg/kg/day (q6h)
Ammonium chloride	PO	75 mg/kg/day (q6h)
Atropine	IV, SC, or PO	0.01 to 0.03 mg/kg (q4–6h)
Bicarbonate sodium	IV	1 to 2 mEq/kg/5 min
Bishydroxycoumarin (Dicumarol)	PO	Loading dose: 50 to 100 mg Maintenance: 10 to 50 mg/day (Regulate according to prothrombin times)
Bretylium	IV	5 mg/kg/dose over 10 minutes, then 50 to 100 μg/kg/min
Calcium chloride	IV	1 to 4 ml of 10% solution; for cardiac arrest, 10 mg/kg/dose
Calcium gluconate	IV	2 to 6 ml of 10% solution; for cardiac arrest, 10 mg/kg/dose
	PO	500 mg/kg/day (q6h)
Captopril	PO	0.1 to 0.4 mg/kg/dose (q6–24h)
Chlorothiazide (Diuril)	PO	20 to 40 mg/kg/day (q12h)
Chlorthalidone	PO	1 to 2 mg/kg/day (q12h)
Cholestyramine (Questran)	PO	250 to 1500 mg/kg/day (q6–12h)
Clofibrate (Atromid S)	PO	0.5 to 1.5 mg/day in divided doses
Clonidine (Catapres)	PO	0.002 to 0.008 mg/kg/day in divided doses
Codeine	PO	0.5 to 1.5 mg/kg/dose (q3h)
Dexamethasone (Decadron)	IV	0.2 to 0.4 mg/kg/dose (q6h) for cerebral edema
Diazoxide	IV	3 to 5 mg/kg/dose over 30 sec (q2–6h) (careful of severe hypotension)
Digitalis (Digoxin)		Loading dose: Premature infants 0.01–0.02 mg/kg IV or IM Term infants Parenteral: Up to 4 wk: 0.03 mg/kg; 4 wk to 12 mo: 0.035 mg/kg; Over 12 mo: 0.040 mg/kg; Beyond 2 yr: 0.03 mg/kg Oral: approximately 20% greater than IV dose Maintenance: ⅓ to ¼ of loading dose, given in two divided doses/24 hr
Dobutamine	IV	2 to 10 μg/kg/min
Dopamine	IV	1 gm in 250 ml D_5W; 2 to 20 μg/kg/min
Edrophonium chloride (Tensilon)	IV	0.05 to 0.2 mg/kg/dose
Ephedrine sulfate	IM or PO	0.8 to 1.6 mg/kg/day (q6h)
Epinephrine (Adrenalin)	IV	For cardiac arrest: single dose: 0.1 to 1.0 ml of 1:1000; 0.1 to 1.0 μg/min infusion
Ethacrynic acid (Edecrin)	IV	1.0 mg/kg/day
Ethylenediaminetetraacetic acid (EDTA) disodium salt	IV	20 mg/ml: 10 to 50 mg/kg (q12h)
Furosemide (Lasix)	IV or IM	1 to 2 mg/kg/dose
	PO	1 to 4 mg/kg/day
Glucagon	IV	0.05 to 0.10 mg/kg/hr
Glucose 50%	IV	1 mg/kg/dose
Glucose 50% + Insulin	IV	1 gm glucose/kg (50% solution) with insulin, 1 unit/3 gm glucose
Guanethidine sulfate (Ismelin)	PO	0.2 to 1.0 mg/kg/day (q6h)
Heparin	IV	100 units/kg (q4h)
Hydralazine hydrochloride (Apresoline)	IV	0.8 to 3.0 mg/kg/day (q4–6h)
	PO	0.75 to 7.5 mg/kg/day (q6–8h)
Hydrochlorothiazide	PO	1 to 3 mg/kg/day (q12h)
Hydrocortisone sodium succinate (Solu-Cortef)	IV	For shock: 50 to 75 mg/kg (q6h)
Indomethacin	IV	0.2 mg/kg/dose
Innovar (Fentanyl citrate & Droperidol)	IV	0.01 to 0.02 ml/kg
Isoproterenol hydrochloride (Isuprel hydrochloride)	IV	0.05 to 0.25 μg/kg/min
Lidocaine (Xylocaine hydrochloride)	IV	Single dose: 1 mg/kg; 20 to 50 μg/kg/min infusion
Magnesium sulfate, 3%	IV	For neonatal seizure: single dose: 2 to 6 ml
Mannitol	IV	For cerebral edema: 1 to 2 gm/kg Repeated doses: 250 mg/kg (q4h) For hemoglobinuria: single dose: 0.5 gm/kg; 5% solution infusion if necessary
Meperidine hydrochloride (Demerol)	IM or IV	1 mg/kg/dose (q3h)
Meralluride (Mercuhydrin)	IM	<1 yr: single dose: 0.1 to 0.3 ml; 1 to 5 yr: single dose: 0.3 to 0.7 ml; >5 yr: single dose: 1 ml
Mercaptomerin sodium (Thiomerin sodium)	IM	Same as Meralluride
Metaraminol (Aramine metaraminol bitartrate)	IV	Single dose: 0.1 mg/kg or 50 mg/500 ml; titrate to effect infusion
Methyldopa (Aldomet)	PO or IV	10 to 40 mg/kg/day (q6–8h)
Methylprednisolone (Solu-Medrol)	IV	For shock: 30 mg/kg/dose; For cerebral edema: 4 to 5 mg/kg/dose
Minoxidil	PO	0.05 to 2.0 mg/kg/day
Morphine sulfate	SC	0.1 to 0.2 mg/kg/dose (q3h)
Naloxone hydrochloride (Narcan)	IM or IV	0.01 mg/kg/dose
Nitroprusside, sodium	IV	0.5 to 8.0 μg/kg/min initial rate; titrate to effect
Norepinephrine (Levophed bitartrate)	IV	0.1 to 1.0 μg/kg/min
Pentobarbital (Nembutal)	PO or IM	2 to 3 mg/kg/dose
Phenobarbital	PO or IM	3 to 5 mg/kg/day (q8h)

Table continued on following page

TABLE 32–3 DRUGS COMMONLY USED IN PEDIATRIC CARDIOLOGY *Continued*

Drug	Route of Administration	Dosage
Phenoxybenzamine	IV	0.5 to 1.0 mg/kg
Phentolamine	IV	0.05 to 0.10 mg/kg
Phenylephrine (Neo-Synephrine hydrochloride)	IV	10 mg/100 ml D_5W; 1 to 10 μg/kg/min, titrate to effect
Phenytoin (Dilantin)	PO or IV	For seizures: 5 to 10 mg/kg/day (q8h); For arrhythmias: 1 to 5 mg/kg/5 min
Potassium chloride	PO	1 to 2 mEq/kg/day
	IV	0.5 mEq/kg/hr not to exceed 2 mEq/kg, as 40 to 80 mEq/l solution
Potassium gluconate (Kaon) and Potassium triplex	PO	1 to 2 mEq/kg/day
Procainamide hydrochloride (Pronestyl)	PO	40 to 60 mg/kg/day (q4–6h)
	IM	5 to 8 mg/kg (q6h)
	IV	1 mg/kg/dose over 5 min
Propranolol hydrochloride (Inderal)	PO	1.0 to 6.0 mg/kg/day (divided q6h)
	IV	0.01 to 0.15 mg/kg (q6–8h)
	IM	0.5 to 1.0 mg/kg (q4–6h)
Promethazine	PO	1 to 2 mg/kg/day (q6–8h)
Prostaglandin E_1	IV	0.1 μg/kg/min, reduce to 0.01 μg/kg/min to maintain effect
Protamine sulfate	IV	3 mg for every 200 units of heparin
Quinidine gluconate	PO	10 to 30 mg/kg/day (q4–8h)
	IM or IV	2 to 10 mg/kg/dose (q3–6h)
Quinidine sulfate	PO	3 to 12 mg/kg/dose (q3h)
Reserpine (Serpasil)	PO	0.01 to 0.02 mg/kg/day (q12h)
	IM	0.07 mg/kg (q12h)
Sodium polystyrene sulfonate (Kayexalate)	PR	1 gm/kg mixed with 70% sorbitol
Spironolactone	PO	1 to 3 mg/kg/day (q6–12h)
Succinylcholine chloride (Anectine chloride)	IM	2 mg/kg/dose
	IV	1 mg/kg/dose
Tolazoline (Prixoline)	IV	1 mg/kg/dose, then 1 to 3 mg/kg/hr
Triamterene	PO	2–4 mg/kg/day
Trimethaphan camsylate (Arfonad)	IV	50 mg in 100 ml D_5W, titrate to effect
Tris (Hydroxymethyl) aminomethane (THAM)	IV	(0.3M) weight (kg) × base deficit = dose in ml
Tubocurarine chloride (curare)	IM or IV	Initial dose: 0.3 to 0.5 mg/kg; Subsequent dose: 0.1 mg/kg
Verapamil	IV	0.1 to 0.2 mg/kg/dose over 2 min
Vitamin K (Aquamephyton)	IM or IV	Single dose (neonate): 1 mg
Warfarin sodium crystalline (Coumadin)	PO or IM	Initial dose: 0.5 mg/kg Maintenance: 1 to 5 mg/day (Regulate according to prothrombin times)

lifting should be avoided, especially in children with evidence of left ventricular hypertrophy. If the latter exists or if these conservative measures do not result in normalization of blood pressure, treatment with antihypertensive drugs is indicated.

Drug therapy (Table 32–3) is aimed at prescribing the least complex regimen with the fewest side effects (see also Chap. 28). Pharmacological management is generally undertaken if diastolic blood pressure is greater than 85 mm Hg in children less than age 12 years, and greater than 90 mm Hg in children older than 12 years. If left ventricular hypertrophy is evident by echocardiogram, drug treatment is advisable at lower diastolic pressures. An oral thiazide diuretic is usually the initial drug of choice and may be combined with a potassium-sparing drug or with a dietary regimen that provides adequate potassium. If blood pressure control is not achieved, the beta-adrenergic blocking agent propranolol or methyldopa may be added to the regimen. Occasionally it is necessary to employ the angiotensin enzyme blocker captopril or vasodilator agents such as hydralazine or minoxidil or the central sympathetic inhibitor clonidine in patient management.

Acute, life-threatening episodes of hypertension occur rarely and in a variety of clinical situations.[85] Encephalopathy is the most severe complication of an acute hypertensive crisis; its presence demands immediate lowering of the systemic arterial blood pressure. Diazoxide is the agent of choice as a first drug for the patient with encephalopathy. If diazoxide is ineffective, catecholamine-producing tumors must be suspected and consideration given to employing alpha-adrenergic blocking agents such as phentolamine or phenoxybenzamine. Sodium nitroprusside is generally considered the agent to be administered when all others have failed. If an etiology for sustained hypertension has been detected, medical and/or surgical treatment should be directed at the underlying disease process.

HYPERLIPIDEMIAS

(See also Chaps. 36 and 49)

The importance of prevention of arteriosclerosis in childhood has only recently become generally accepted.[86, 87] Hyperlipidemic children are likely to become hyperlipidemic adults and are therefore at greater risk of future atherosclerotic disease.[87, 88] Although opinions vary about the feasibility of maintaining low serum lipid levels in normal children by dietary modification, a consensus exists that children whose serum cholesterol or triglyceride levels are beyond the 95th percentile for their age and sex should be treated. Guidelines for abnormal levels in the first two decades of life are provided in Table 32–4.

Hyperlipidemia is defined as an increase in the plasma concentration of cholesterol or triglycerides, or both, above these normal values, but it should be recognized that the latter may be changed as a result of future studies. Diagnosis should be reserved for those children with elevated cholesterol or triglyceride levels on two or more separate determinations from venous blood samples after a 12-hour fast; the laboratory in which the tests are performed must be unquestionably accurate and reliable.

TABLE 32–4 FASTING LIPID LEVELS IN SCHOOL CHILDREN

A. Cholesterol

	Males				Females			
Age	*5%*	*50%*	*95%*	*N*	*5%*	*50%*	*95%*	*N*
5	109	150	189	60	120	155	200	58
6	121	154	200	193	119	154	198	197
7	122	154	199	194	125	159	202	164
8	125	159	194	188	117	161	203	165
9	125	158	213	165	122	161	206	202
10	129	163	206	187	125	159	205	197
11	122	159	202	198	126	161	204	194
12	119	159	213	221	116	158	210	222
13	116	153	205	184	125	158	200	181
14	117	150	187	168	120	157	203	182
15	113	148	190	146	121	157	203	188
16	118	148	192	108	121	151	200	134
17	108	145	189	91	118	164	209	110

B. Triglyceride

	Males				Females			
Age	*5%*	*50%*	*95%*	*N*	*5%*	*50%*	*95%*	*N*
5	23	46	99	60	26	48	92	58
6	26	47	95	193	27	47	94	197
7	27	43	102	194	26	50	106	164
8	24	43	91	188	26	50	97	165
9	25	49	92	165	29	52	110	202
10	23	46	108	187	30	51	110	197
11	24	48	103	198	29	61	140	194
12	28	53	119	221	33	61	123	222
13	26	52	113	184	34	61	127	181
14	30	50	106	168	33	56	123	182
15	26	52	111	146	33	58	111	188
16	31	63	108	108	34	59	112	134
17	31	58	132	91	34	65	140	110

N = Number of children studied.

From Carter, G. A., et al.: Coronary heart disease risk factors: Identification and management. *In* Shen, J. T. (ed.): Clinical Practice of Adolescent Medicine. New York, Appleton-Century-Crofts, 1979.

In the absence of mass screening programs or incorporation of this test as part of routine pediatric practice, serum lipid levels should be analyzed in all children at regular intervals from families with hyperlipidemia or with histories that include hypertension, myocardial infarction, stroke, or peripheral vascular disease among parents or grandparents before age 50 years.[87, 89, 90] Differentiation is necessary between acquired hyperlipidemia and one of the familial, and presumably genetic, hyperlipidemias.

Homozygous familial hypercholesterolemia causes severe atherosclerosis of the coronary arteries and myocardial infarction in childhood; rarely it causes atherosclerosis of the aortic valve, leading to critical aortic stenosis that requires surgical treatment.[91]

REFERENCES

NONRHEUMATIC INFLAMMATORY DISEASE

1. Ainger, L. E., Lawyer, N. G., and Fitch, C. W.: Neonatal rubella myocarditis. Br. Heart J. *28*:691, 1966.
2. Ayuthya, T. S. N., Jayavasu, J., and Pongpanich, B.: Coxsackie group B virus in primary myocardial disease in infants and children. Am. Heart J. *88*:311, 1974.
3. Suckling, P. V., and Vogelpoel, L.: Coxsackie myocarditis of the newborn. Lancet *2*:421, 1970.
4. Lerner, A. M., and Wilson, F. M.: Virus myocardiopathy. Progr. Med. Virol. *15*:63, 1973.
5. Oda, T., Hamamoto, K. and Morinaga, H.: Clinical aspects of non-rheumatic myocarditis in children. Jpn. Circ. J. *43*:443, 1979.
6. Wink, K., and Schmitz, H.: Cytomegalovirus myocarditis. Am. Heart J. *100*:667, 1980.
7. Arita, M., Ueno, Y., and Masuyama, Y.: Complete heart block in mumps myocarditis. Br. Heart J. *46*:342, 1981.
8. Taliercio, C. P., Seward, J. B., Driscoll, D. J., Fisher, L. D., Gersh, B. J., and Tajik, A. J.: Idiopathic dilated cardiomyopathy in the young: Clinical profile and natural history. J. Am. Coll. Cardiol. *6*:1126, 1985.
9. Wittels, B., and Bressler, R. J.: Biochemical lesions of diphtheria toxin in the heart. J. Clin. Invest. *43*:630, 1964.
10. Challoner, D. R., and Prols, H. G.: Free fatty acid oxidation and carnitine levels in diphtheritic guinea pig myocardium. J. Clin. Invest. *51*:2071, 1972.
11. Srivastava, S. C., Puri, D. S., and Lumba, S. T.: An electrocardiographic study of myocarditis and diphtheria. J. Assoc. Phys. India *14*:365, 1966.
12. Ramos, A., Elias, P., Barrucand, L., and DaSilva, J.: The protective effect of carnitine in human diphtheritic myocarditis. Pediatr. Res. *18*:815, 1984.
13. Prata, A.: Chagas' heart disease. Cardiologia *52*:79, 1968.
14. Rosenbaum, M. B.: Chagasic myocardiopathy. Progr. Cardiovasc. Dis. *7*:199, 1964.
15. Shipper, H., McClarty, B. M., McRuer, K. E., Nash, R. A., and Penney, C. J.: Tropical diseases encountered in Canada: Chagas' disease. Can. Med. Assoc. J. *122*:165, 1980.
16. Drugs for parasitic infections. *In* Abramowicz, M. (ed.): The Medical Letter of Drugs and Therapeutics, Vol. 28 (Issue 706). The Medical Letter, Inc., New Rochelle, January 1986.
17. Koten, J. W., and DeRaadt, P.: Myocarditis and *Trypanosoma rhodesiense* infections. Trans. R. Soc. Trop. Med. Hyg. *63*:485, 1969.
18. Okoroma, E. O., Terry, L. W., and Scott, L. T.: Acute bacterial pericarditis in children: Report of 25 cases. Am. Heart J *90*:709, 1975.
19. VanReken, D., Strauss, A., Hernandez, A., and Feigin, R. D.: Infectious pericarditis in children. J. Pediatr. *85*:165, 1974.
20. Callahan, J. A., Seward, J. B., Nishimura, R. A., Miller, R. A., Jr., Reeder, G. S., Shub, C., Callahan, M. J., Schattenberg, T. T., and Tajik, A. J.: Two dimensional echocardiographically guided pericardiocentesis: Experience in 117 consecutive patients. Am. J. Cardiol. *55*:476, 1985.
21. Lajos, T. Z., Black, H. E., Cooper, R. G., and Wanka, J.: Pericardial decompression. Ann. Thorac. Surg. *19*:47, 1975.
22. Engle, M. A., Ehlers, K. H., O'Laughlin, J. E., Linday, L. A., and Fried, R.: The post-pericardiotomy syndrome: Iatrogenic illness with immunologic and virologic components. *In* Engle, M. A. (ed.): Pediatric Cardiovascular Disease. Philadelphia, F. A. Davis Co., 1981, p. 381.
23. Clapp, S. K., Garson, J., Jr., Gutgesell, H. P., Cooley, D. A., and McNamara, D. G.: Postoperative pericardial effusion and its relation to post-pericardiotomy syndrome. Pediatrics *66*:585, 1980.
24. Paloheimo, J. A., Van Essen, R., Klemola, E., Kaarinen, L., and Siltanen, P.: Sub-clinical cytomegalovirus infections and cytomegalovirus mononucleosis after open heart surgery. Am. J. Cardiol. *22*:624, 1968.
25. Kron, I. L., Rheuban, K., and Nolan, S. P.: Late cardiac tamponade in children. Ann. Surg. *199*:173, 1984.

PRIMARY CARDIOMYOPATHIES

26. Greenwood, R. D., Nadas, A. S., and Fyler, D. C.: The clinical course of primary myocardial disease in infants and children. Am. Heart J. *92*:549, 1976.
27. Goodwin, J. F.: The frontiers of cardiomyopathy. Br. Heart J. *48*:1, 1982.
28. Schryer, M. J. P., and Karnauchow, P. N.: Endocardial fibroelastosis: Etiologic and pathogenic considerations in children. Am. Heart J. *88*:557, 1974.
29. Moller, J. N., Lucas, R. V., Adams, P., Anderson, R. C., Jorgens, J., and Edwards, J. R.: Endocardial fibroelastosis. A clinical and anatomic study of 47 patients with emphasis on its relationship to mitral insufficiency. Circulation *30*:759, 1964.

290a. Taliercio, C. P., Seward, J. B., Driscoll, D. J., Fisher, L. D., Gersh, B. J., and Tajik, A. J.: Idiopathic dilated cardiomyopathy in the young: Clinical profile and natural history. J. Am. Col. Cardiol. *6*:1126, 1985.

29b. Hanukoglu, A., Fried, D., and Somekh, E.: Inheritance of familial primary endocardial fibroelastosis. Clin. Pediatr. *25*:272, 1986.

30. Tripp, M. E.: Congestive cardiomyopathy of childhood. *In* Barness, L. A. (ed.): Advances in Pediatrics. Year Book Medical Publishers, Inc., Chicago, Illinois, pp. 179–203, 1984.
31. Brandenburg, R. O.: Report of the WHO/ISFC Task Force on definition and classification of cardiomyopathy. Circulation *64*:437a, 1971.
32. Lewis, A. B., Neustein, H. B., Takahashi, M., and Lurie, P. R.: Findings on endomyocardial biopsy in infants and children with dilated cardiomyopathy. Am. J. Cardiol. *55*:143, 1985.
33. Lambert, E. C., and Vlad, P.: Primary endomyocardial disease. Pediatr. Clin. North Am. *5*:1057, 1958.
34. Sellers, F. J., Keith, J. D., and Manning, J. A.: The diagnosis of primary endocardial fibroelastosis. Circulation *29*:49, 1964.

34a. Akiba, T., Yoshikawa, M., Kinoda, M., Otaki, S., Kobayashi, Y., and Sato, T.: Assessment of cardiac performance by first-pass radionuclide angiocardiography in infants and children with normal heart and endocardial fibroelastosis. Tohoku J. Exp. Med. *148*:15, 1986.

35. McLaughlin, T. G., Schiebler, G. L., and Krovetz, L. J.: Hemodynamic findings in children with endocardial fibroelastosis. Am. Heart J. *75*:162, 1968.
36. Neustein, H. B., Lurie, P. R., and Fugita, M.: Endocardial fibroelastosis found on transvascular endomyocardial biopsy in children. Arch. Pathol. Lab. Med. *103*:214, 1979.

SECONDARY CARDIOMYOPATHIES

37. Gutgesell, H. P., Speer, M. E., and Rosenberg, H. S.: Characterization of the cardiomyopathy in infants with diabetic mothers. Circulation *51*:441, 1980.
38. Trowitzsch, E., Bigalke, U., Gisbertz, R., and Kallfelz, H. C.: Echocardiographic profile of infants of diabetic mothers. Eur. J. Pediatr. *140*:311, 1983.
39. Walther, F. J., Siassi, B., King, J., and Wu, P. Y-K.: Cardiac output in infants of insulin-dependent diabetic mothers. J. Pediatr. *107*:109, 1985.

40. Dickenson, E. F., Houlsby, W. T., and Wilkinson, J. L.: Unusual angiographic appearance of the left ventricle in two cases of Pompe's disease (glycogenosis type 2). Br. Heart J. *41*:238, 1979.
41. Bordiuk, J. N., Logato, M. J., Lovelace, R. E., and Blumenthal, S.: Pompe's disease: Electron myographic, electron microscopic and cardiovascular aspects. Arch. Neurol. (Chicago) *23*:113, 1970.
41a. Hwang, G., Meng, C. C., Lin, C. Y., and Hsu, H. C.: Clinical analysis of five infants with glycogen storage disease of the heart—Pompe's disease. Jpn. Heart J. 27:25, 1986.
42. Miller, E., Hare, J. W., Cloherty, J. P., Dunn, P. J., Gleason, R. E., and Kitzmiller, J. L.: Elevated maternal hemoglobin A_{1C} in early pregnancy and major congenital anomalies in infants of diabetic mothers. N. Engl. J. Med. *304*:1331, 1981.
43. Caddell, J. L.: Metabolic and nutritional diseases. *In* Adams, F. H., and Emmanouilides, G. C. (eds.): Moss' Heart Disease in Infants, Children and Adolescents, 3rd. ed. Baltimore, Williams and Wilkins Co., 1983, pp. 596–626.
44. Sanstead, H. H.: Clinical manifestations of certain vitamin deficiencies. *In* Goodhart, M. S., and Shils, M. E. (eds.): Modern Nutrition in Health and Disease. 5th ed. Philadelphia, Lea and Febiger, 1973, p. 593.
45. Sanstead, H. H.: Mineral metabolism and protein malnutrition. *In* Olson, R. E. (ed.): Protein Calorie Malnutrition. New York, Academic Press, 1975, p. 213.
46. Cadell, J. L.: Diseases of the cardiovascular system. *In* Jelliffe, B. B. (ed.): Diseases of Children in the Subtropics and Tropics. London, Edward Arnold, Ltd., 1970. p. 398.
47. Nutter, D. O., Murray, T. G., Heymsfield, S. B., and Fuller, E. O.: The effect of chronic protein-calorie undernutrition in the rat on myocardial function and cardiac function. Circ. Res. *45*:144, 1979.
48. Roberts, W. C., and Ferrans, V. J.: Pathological aspects of certain cardiomyopathies. Circ. Res. *34*(Suppl. II):II–128, 1974.
49. Roberts, W. C., Buja, L. M., and Ferrans, V. J.: Löffler's fibroplastic parietal endocarditis, eosinophilic leukemia, and Davies' endomyocardial fibrosis: The same disease at different stages? Pathol. Microbiol. (Basel) 35:90, 1970.
50. Lepley, D., Jr., Aris, A., Korns, M. E., Walker, J. A., and D'Cunha, R. M.: Endomyocardial fibrosis: A surgical approach. Ann. Thorac. Surg. *18*:626, 1974.
51. Metras, D., Coulibaly, A. O., Schauvet, J., Ekra, A., Bertrand, E., and Castaneda, A. R.: Endomyocardial fibrosis. J. Thorac. Cardiovasc. Surg. *83*:52, 1982.
52. DiSessa, T. G., Klitzner, T., Hiraishi, S., Welsh, M., and Kangarloo, H.: Cardiovascular effects of Kawasaki's disease. J. Cardiovasc. Med. *6*:1159, 1981.
52a. Neches, W. H.: Kawasaki disease: A continuing puzzle. Int. J. Cardiol. *11*:1, 1986.
52b. Burns, J. C., Geha, R. S., Schneeberger, E. E., Newburger, J. W., Rosen, F. S., Glezen, L. S., Huang, A. S., Natale, J., and Leung, D. Y. M.: Pulmonary activity in lymphocyte culture supernatants from patients with Kawasaki disease. Nature 323–814, 1986.
53. Hiraishi, S., Yashiro, K., Oguchi, K., and Nakazawa, K.: Clinical course of cardiovascular involvement in the mucocutaneous lymph node syndrome. Am. J. Cardiol. *47*:323, 1981.
53a. Fujiwara, T., Fujiwara, H., and Hamashima, Y.: Frequency and size of coronary arterial aneurysm at necropsy in Kawasaki disease. Am. J. Cardiol. *59*:808, 1987.
54. Nakano, H., Saito, A., Ueda, K., and Nojima, K.: Clinical characteristics of myocardial infarction following Kawasaki disease: Report of 11 cases. J. Pediatr. 108:198, 1986.
54a. Kato, H., Ichinose, E., and Kawasaki, T.: Myocardial infarction in Kawasaki disease: Clinical analyses in 195 cases. J. Pediatr. *108*:923, 1986.
55. Meade, R. H., and Brandt, L.: Manifestation of Kawasaki disease in New England outbreak of 1980. J. Pediatr. *100*:558, 1982.
56. Onouchi, Z., Shimazu, S., Takamatsu, T., and Hamaoka, K.: Aneurysms of the coronary arteries in Kawasaki disease: An angiographic study of 30 cases. Circulation *66*:6, 1982.
57. Nakanishi, T., Takao, A., Nakazawa, M., Endo, M., Niwa, K., and Takahashi, Y.: Mucocutaneous lymph node syndrome: Clinical, hemodynamic, and angiographic features of coronary obstructive disease. Am. J. Cardiol. *55*:6662, 1985.
58. Chung, K., Brandt, L., Fulton, D. R., and Kreidberg, M. B.: Cardiac and coronary arterial involvement in infants and children with mucocutaneous lymph node syndrome. Am. J. Cardiol. *50*:136, 1982.
59. Yoshida, H., Maeda, T., and Taniguchi, N.: Subcostal two-dimensional echocardiographic imaging of peripheral right coronary artery in Kawasaki disease. Circulation *65*:956, 1982.
59a. Koren, G., Lavi, S., Rose, V., and Rowe, R.: Kawasaki disease. Review of risk factors for coronary aneurysms. J. Pediatr. *108*:388, 1986.
60. Anderson, T. M., Meyer, R. A., and Kaplan, S.: Long-term echocardiographic evaluation of cardiac size and function in patients with Kawasaki's disease. Am. Heart J. *110*:107, 1985.
60a. Fujiwara, T., Fujiwara, H., Ueda, T., Nishioka, K., and Hamashima, Y.: Comparison of macroscopic, postmortem, angiographic and two-dimensional echocardiographic findings of coronary aneurysms in children with Kawasaki disease. Am. J. Cardiol. 6:199, 1986.
61. Grenadier, E., Allen, H. D., Goldberg, S. J., Valdes-Cruz, L. M., Sahn, D. J., Lima, C. O., and Barron, J. V.: Left ventricular wall motion abnormalities in Kawasaki's disease. J. Am. Coll. Cardiol. *1*:714, 1983.
62. Kato, H., Ichinose, E., Matsunaga, S., Suzuki, K., and Rikatake, N.: Fate of coronary aneurysms in Kawasaki disease: Serial coronary angiography and long-term follow-up study. Am. J. Cardiol. *49*:1758, 1982.
63. Anderson, T., Meyer, R. A., and Kaplan, S.: Long term evaluation of cardiac size and function in patients with Kawasaki disease. J. Am. Coll. Cardiol. *1*:714, 1983.
64. Suma, K., Takeuchi, Y., Shiroma, K., Tsuji, T., Inoue, K., Yoshikawa, T., Koyama, Y., Narumi, J., Asai, T., and Kusakawa, S.: Early and late postoperative studies in coronary arterial lesions resulting from Kawasaki's disease in children. J. Thorac. Cardiovasc. Surg. *84*:224, 1982.
64a. Takahashi, M., Mason, W., and Lewis, A. B.: Regression of coronary aneurysms in patients with Kawasaki syndrome. Circulation 75:387, 1987.
64b. Gidding, S. S., Shulman, S. T., Ilbawi, M., Crussi, F., and Duffy, C. E.: Mucocutaneous lymph node syndrome (Kawasaki disease): Delayed aortic and mitral insufficiency secondary to active valvulitis. J. Am. Coll. Cardiol. 7:894, 1986.
65. Koren, G., and MacLaod, S. M.: Difficulty in achieving therapeutic serum concentrations of salicylate in Kawasaki's disease. J. Pediatr. *105*:991, 1984.
66. Furusho, K., Nakano, H., Shinomiya, K., Tamura, T., Manabe, Y., Kawarano, M., Baba, K., Kamiya, T., Kiyosawa, N., Hayashidera, T., Hirose, O., Yokoyama, T., Baba, K., and Mori, C.: High-dose intravenous gammaglobulin for Kawasaki's disease. Lancet 2:1055, 1984.
67. Newburger, J. W., Takahasi, M., Burns, J. C., Beiser, A. S., Chung, K. J., Duffy, C. E., Glode, M. P., Mason, W. H., Reddy, V., Sanders, S. P., Shulman, S. T., Wiggins, J. W., Hicks, R. V., Fulton, D. R., Lewis, A. B., Leung, D. Y. M., Colton, T., Rosen, F. S., and Melish, M. E.: The treatment of Kawasaki syndrome with intravenous gamma globulin. N. Engl. J. Med. *315*:341, 1986.
68. Ohyagi, A., Hirose, K., Tsujimoto, S., Doyama, K., Watanabe, Y., and Nakie, T.: Kawasaki's disease complicated by acute myocardial infarction nine years after onset. Am. Heart J. *110*:670, 1985.
69. Kohr, R. M.: Progressive asymptomatic coronary artery disease as a late fatal sequelae of Kawasaki's disease. J. Pediatr. *108*:256, 1986.
70. Kitamura, S., Kawachi, K., Harima, R., Sakakibara, T., Hirose, H., and Kawashima, Y.: Surgery for coronary heart disease due to mucocutaneous lymph node syndrome (Kawasaki disease). Am. J. Cardiol. *51*:444, 1983.
71. Sethi, S., Ott, D., and Nihill, M.: Surgical management of cardiovascular complications of Kawasaki's disease. Texas Heart Inst. J. *10*:343, 1983.
72. Seraydarian, M. W., Artaza, L., and Yang, J. J.: Metabolic involvement and adriamycin cardiotoxicity. *In* Tajaddin, M., Bhatrab, B., and Siddegue, H. H. (eds.): Advances in Myocardiology, Vol. 2. Baltimore, University Park Press, 1980.
73. Legha, S. S., Benjamin, R. S., and MacKay, H. J.: Reduction of doxorubicin cardiotoxicity by prolonged continuous intravenous infusion. Ann. Intern. Med. *96*:133, 1982.

SYSTEMIC HYPERTENSION

74. New, M. I., and Levine, L. S.: Hypertension in childhood and adolescence. Cardiovasc. Rev. 3:115, 1982.
75. Lieberman, E.: Diagnostic evaluation of hypertensive children. Pediatr. Ann. *6*:390, 1977.
76. McCrory, W. W.: What should blood pressure be in children? Pediatrics *70*:143, 1982.
77. Schachter, J., Kuller, L. H., and Perfepti, C.: Blood pressure during the first two years of life. Am. J. Epidemiol. *116*:29, 1982.
78. Colan, S. D., Fujii, A., Borow, K. M., MacPherson, D., and Sanders, S. P.: Noninvasive determination of systolic, diastolic and end-systolic blood pressure in neonates, infants, and young children: Comparison with central aortic measurements. Am. J. Cardiol. 52:867, 1983.
79. Berenson, G. S., Webber, L. S., and Voors, A. W.: Diagnosing hypertension in children. J. Cardiovasc. Med., *6*:273, 1982.
80. Blumenthal, S., Epps, R. P., Heavenrich, R., Lauer, R. M., Lieberman, E., Mirkin, B., Mitchell, S. C., Naito, V. B., O'Hare, D., Smith, W. McF., Tarazi, R. C., and Upson, D.: Report of the task force on blood pressure control in children. Pediatrics 59(Suppl.):797, 1977.
81. Lauer, R. M., Clarke, W. R., and Beaglehole, R.: Level, trend and variability of blood pressure during childhood: The Muscatine study. Circulation *69*:242, 1984.
82. Lauer, R. M., Burns, T. L., and Clarke, W. R.: Assessing children's blood pressure—considerations of age and body size: The Muscatine study. Pediatrics *75*:1081, 1985.
83. McLean, L. G.: Therapy of acute severe hypertension in children. J.A.M.A. *239*:755, 1978.
84. Rocchini, A. P.: Childhood hypertension: Etiology, diagnosis, and treatment. Pediatr. Clin. N. Am. *31*:1259, 1984.
85. Fleischmann, L. E.: Management of hypertensive crises in children. Pediatr. Ann. *6*:410, 1977.

HYPERLIPIDEMIAS

86. Lee, J., Lauer, R. M., and Clarke, W. R.: Coronary risk factors in children. *In* Engle, M. A., (ed.): Pediatric Cardiovascular Disease. Philadelphia, F. A. Davis Co., 1981, p. 1.
87. Schrott, H. G., Clark, W. R., Abrahams, P., Wiebe, D. A., and Lauer, R. M.: Coronary artery disease mortality in relatives of hypertriglyceridemic school children: The Muscatine study. Circulation *65*:300, 1982.
88. Berwick, D. M., Cretin, S., and Keeler, E.: Cholesterol, children, and heart disease: An analysis of alternatives. Pediatrics *68*:721, 1981.
89. Schaefer, E. J., and Levy, R. I.: Pathogenesis and management of lipoprotein disorders. N. Engl. J. Med. *312*:1300, 1985.
90. Neill, C. A., Ose, L., and Kwiterovich, P. O., Jr.: Hyperlipidemia: Clinical clues in the first two decades of life. Johns Hopkins Med. J. *140*:171, 1977.
91. Forman, M. B., Kinsley, R. M., DuPlessis, J. P., Dansky, R., Milner, S., and Levin, S. E.: Surgical correction of combined supravalvular and valvular aortic stenosis in homozygous familial hypercholesterolemia. SA Med. J. *1*:579, 1982.

33 VALVULAR HEART DISEASE

by EUGENE BRAUNWALD, M.D.

MITRAL STENOSIS

ETIOLOGY AND PATHOLOGY

The predominant cause of mitral stenosis (MS) is rheumatic fever[1] (p. 1706). Far less frequently, it is congenital, and this form is observed almost exclusively in infants and young children (p. 940). Rarely, mitral stenosis is a complication of malignant carcinoid (p. 1439), systemic lupus erythematosus,[2] rheumatoid arthritis,[3] and the mucopolysaccharidoses of the Hunter-Hurley phenotype.[4] It has been suggested, although without proof, that a number of viruses, especially Coxsackie virus, may be responsible for chronic valvular heart disease, including MS.[5] Amyloid deposits may occur on rheumatic valves and contribute to the obstruction to left atrial emptying.[6] Methysergide therapy is an unusual but documented cause of MS.[7] MS, generally on a rheumatic basis, may be associated with atrial septal defect in Lutembacher syndrome (p. 982). Left atrial tumor, particularly myxoma (p. 1473); ball valve thrombus in the left atrium; and a congenital membrane in the left atrium, i.e., cor triatriatum (p. 940), may also obstruct left atrial outflow and therefore simulate MS. Although calcification of the mitral annulus usually causes mitral regurgitation (MR) (p. 1035), when subvalvular or intravalvular extension is extensive, MS may result.[8] Approximately 25 per cent of all patients with rheumatic heart disease have pure MS, and an additional 40 per cent have combined MS and MR.[9] Two-thirds of all patients with rheumatic MS are female.

Rheumatic fever results in four forms of fusion of the mitral valve apparatus leading to stenosis: (1) commissural, (2) cuspal, (3) chordal, and (4) combined.[10] Thickening of the commissures alone occurs in 30 per cent, of the cusps alone in 15 per cent, and of the chordae alone in 10 per cent; in the remainder, thickening of more than one of these structures is involved. Characteristically, mitral valve cusps fuse at their edges, and fusion of the chordae results in thickening and shortening of these structures. The stenotic mitral valve is typically funnel-shaped, and the orifice is frequently shaped like a "fish mouth" or buttonhole, with calcium deposits in the valve leaflets sometimes extending to involve the valve ring, which may become quite thick[10] (Figs. 33–1 and 54–5, p, 1710). The thickened leaflets may be so adherent and rigid that they cannot open or shut, reducing or rarely even abolishing the first heart sound (S_1) and leading to combined MS and MR.[11] There is a rough correlation between the severity of calcification and the transvalvular gradient.[12] When rheumatic fever results exclusively or predominantly in contraction and fusion of the chordae tendineae, with little fusion of the valvular commissures, dominant MR results.[13]

It probably takes a minimum of 2 years after the onset of acute rheumatic fever for severe MS to develop, and most patients in temperate climates remain asymptomatic for at least a decade more.[14] Symptoms commence most commonly in the third or fourth decade, although mild MS in the aged is becoming a more frequent finding.[14a, 14b] In the tropics, particularly in underdeveloped areas, the disease advances more rapidly, and severe MS may be present in early adolescence.[15] The debate continues about whether the anatomical changes result from a smoldering rheumatic process or whether once the valve has been deformed by the initial episode, the constant trauma produced by the turbulent blood flow leads to progressive fibrosis, thickening, and calcification of the valve apparatus.[16, 17]

Enlargement of the left atrium and resultant elevation of the left main stem bronchus, calcification of the left

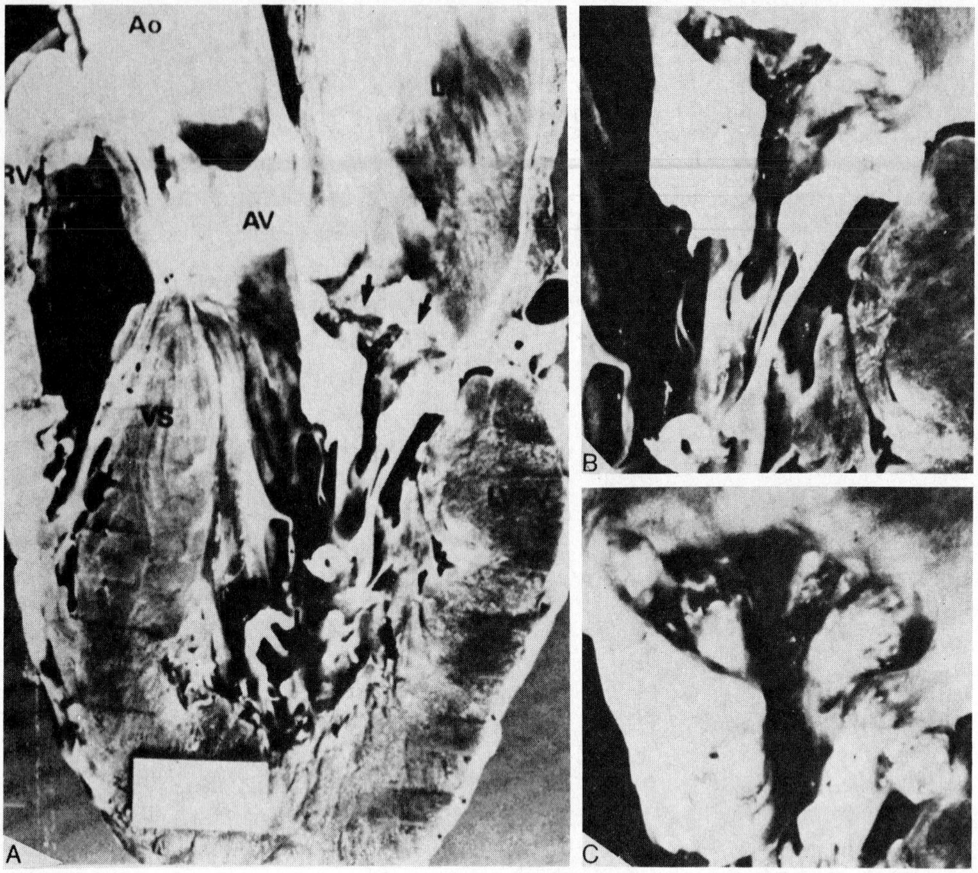

FIGURE 33–1. Rheumatic mitral stenosis in a 56-year-old man. *A*, The mitral valve leaflets are diffusely thickened by fibrous tissue and calcific deposits. Ao = aorta, AV = aortic valve, LA = left atrium, LV = left ventricle, RV = right ventricle, VS = ventricular septum. *B* and *C*, Close-ups of stenotic mitral valve showing fused chordae tenineae (arrows in *A*). LVFW = left ventricular free wall. (From Waller, B. F.: Rheumatic and nonrheumatic conditions producing valvular heart disease. *In* Frankl, W. S., and Brest, A. N. [eds.]: Cardiovascular Clinics. Valvular Heart Disease: Comprehensive Evaluation and Management. Philadelphia, F. A. Davis, 1986, p. 12.)

atrial wall, the development of mural thrombi, and obliterative changes in the pulmonary vascular bed (p. 799) may all result from chronic MS.

PATHOPHYSIOLOGY

In normal adults the mitral valve orifice is 4 to 6 cm^2. When the orifice is reduced to approximately 2 cm^2, which is considered mild MS, blood can flow from the left atrium to the left ventricle only if propelled by an abnormal pressure gradient. When the mitral valve opening is reduced to 1 cm^2, which is considered critical MS, a left atrioventricular pressure gradient of approximately 20 mm Hg (and therefore, in the presence of a normal left ventricular diastolic pressure, a mean left atrial pressure of approximately 25 mm Hg) is required to maintain normal cardiac output at rest (Figs. 33–2 and 33–3 and Fig. 9–10, p. 251). The elevated left atrial pressure in turn raises pulmonary venous and capillary pressures, resulting in exertional dyspnea (p. 476). The first bouts of dyspnea in patients with MS are usually precipitated by exercise, emotional stress, infection, or atrial fibrillation, all of which increase the rate of blood flow across the mitral orifice and result in further elevation of the left atrial pressure.[18, 19]

In order to assess the severity of obstruction of the mitral valve (and, for that matter, of any valve), it is essential to measure both the transvalvular pressure gradient and the flow rate. The latter depends not only on cardiac output but on heart rate as well. An increase in heart rate shortens diastole proportionately more than systole and diminishes the time available for flow across the mitral valve. Therefore, at any given level of cardiac output, tachycardia augments the transmitral valvular pressure gradient and elevates left atrial pressures further.[20, 21] This explains the sudden development of dyspnea and pulmonary edema in previously asymptomatic patients with MS who experience atrial fibrillation with a rapid ventricular rate[22] and the equally rapid improvement in these patients when the ventricular rate is slowed by means of cardiac glycosides and/or beta-adrenoceptor blocking agents, even when the cardiac output per minute remains constant. Hydraulic considerations dictate that at any given orifice size the transvalvular gradient is a function of the square of the transvalvular flow rate (p. 258 and Fig. 33–3).[23] Thus, a

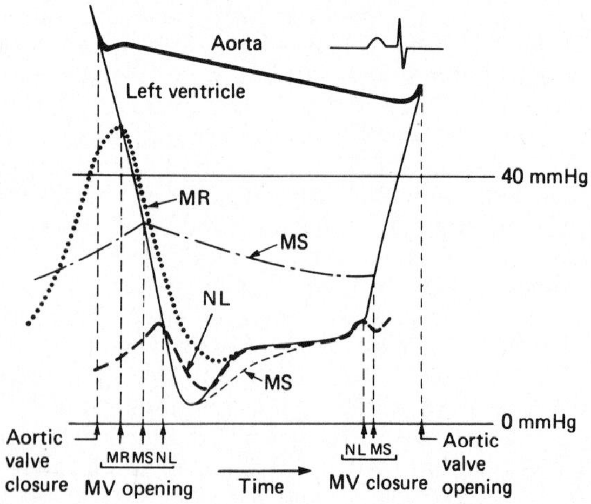

FIGURE 33–2. Schematic relationship of left ventricular (———), and aortic (▬▬▬) and pulmonary atrial wedge (PAW) pressures. Note that the higher the left atrial *v* wave, the earlier the pressure crossover, and the earlier the mitral valve (MV) opening. The higher left atrial end-diastolic pressure with severe mitral stenosis (MS) also results in later closure of the mitral valve. (PAW pressures in severe mitral regurgitation (···), mitral stenosis (— · — · — · —) and normal (– – – – – –).) The LV diastolic pressure in mitral stenosis (------) rises slowly, denoting the absence of a rapid filling wave. (From Braunwald, E., and Turi, Z. G.: Pathophysiology of mitral valve disease. *In* Ionescu, M. I., and Cohn, L. H. [eds.]: Mitral Valve Disease. London, Butterworths, 1985, p. 3.)

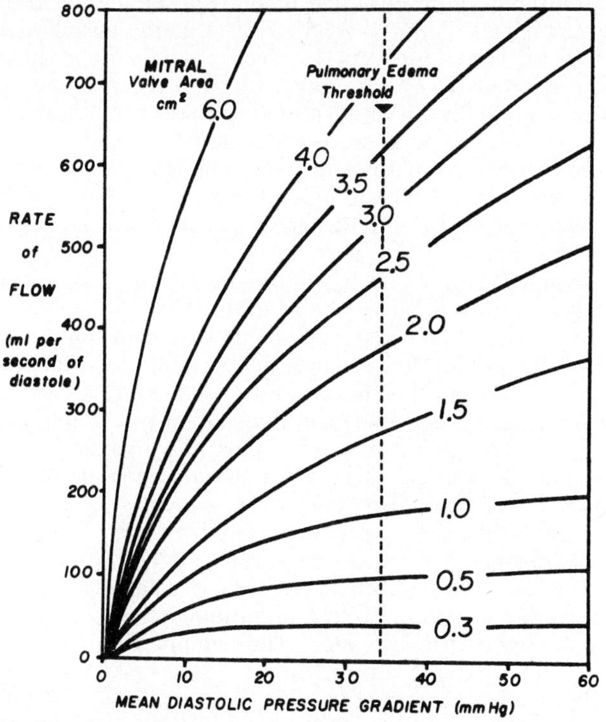

FIGURE 33–3. Chart illustrating the relation between mean diastolic gradient across the mitral valve and rate of flow across the mitral valve per second of diastole, as predicted by the Gorlin formula. Note that when the mitral valve area is 1.0 cm² or less, very little additional flow can be achieved by an increased pressure gradient. (From Wallace, A. G.: Pathophysiology of cardiovascular disease. *In* Smith, L. H., Jr., and Thier, S. O. [eds.]: Pathophysiology: The Biological Principles of Disease. The International Textbook of Medicine. Vol. 1. Philadelphia, W. B. Saunders Company, 1981, p. 1192.)

doubling of flow rate will quadruple the pressure gradient, so that a stress such as exercise in patients with moderate or severe MS will cause marked elevation of left atrial pressure.[24]

Atrial contraction augments the presystolic transmitral valvular gradient by approximately 30 per cent in patients with MS (Fig. 9–10, p. 251). Withdrawal of atrial transport when atrial fibrillation develops decreases cardiac output by about 20 per cent. The more rapid ventricular rate that is common in atrial fibrillation raises the transvalvular pressure gradient. Thus, hemodynamic considerations indicate the desirability of maintaining sinus rhythm in patients with MS.[25]

INTRACARDIAC AND INTRAVASCULAR PRESSURES

Left ventricular diastolic pressure is normal in patients with pure MS; coexisting MR, aortic valve lesions, systemic hypertension, ischemic heart disease, or cardiomyopathy may all be responsible for elevations of left ventricular diastolic pressure. In approximately 85 per cent of patients with pure MS, the end-diastolic volume is within the normal range, whereas it is reduced in the remainder.[26] In approximately one-fourth of patients with pure MS the ejection fraction and other ejection indices of systolic performance (p. 463) are below normal, most likely resulting from chronic reduction in preload and elevated afterload caused by reduced left ventricular thickness.[26a] Regional hypokinesis is common,[27] perhaps caused by extension of the scarring process from the mitral valve into the adjacent posterior basal myocardium[28] or by associated heart disease. The left ventricular mass is normal or slightly reduced.[26] Although it has long been postulated that persistent myocardial dysfunction, perhaps caused by smoldering rheumatic myocarditis, may be responsible for the poor results following surgical treatment of some patients with pure MS,[29] the bulk of available evidence suggests that myocardial *contractility* (as opposed to systolic performance) is normal or only slightly impaired in the majority of patients.[30] Associated ischemic heart disease may be responsible for myocardial dysfunction.[31] Most patients with MS show a normal elevation of ejection fraction and reduction of end-systolic volume during exercise.[32]

In MS and sinus rhythm, the *left atrial pressure pulse* generally exhibits a prominent atrial contraction (*a*) wave (Fig. 9–10, p. 251) and a gradual pressure decline after mitral valve opening (*y* descent) (Fig. 33–2); the mean left atrial pressure is elevated. In patients with mild to moderate MS without elevation of pulmonary vascular resistance, pulmonary arterial pressure may be normal or only slightly elevated at rest and rises only during exercise. However, in patients with severe MS and/or those in whom the pulmonary vascular resistance is significantly increased, pulmonary arterial pressure is elevated when the patient is at rest, and in rare cases of extreme elevation of the pulmonary vascular resistance it may exceed the systemic arterial pressure. Further elevations of left atrial and pulmonary vascular pressures occur during exercise (Fig. 9–10, p. 251) or tachycardia or both. With moderate elevation of pulmonary artery pressure, right ventricular performance is maintained.[33] An elevation of pulmonary arterial systolic pressure exceeding 70 mm Hg represents a serious impedance to emptying of the right ventricle, and when this level is exceeded in patients with rheumatic heart disease, right ventricular end-diastolic and right atrial pressures often rise. During exercise, patients with MS and pulmonary hypertension commonly fail to exhibit normal elevation of right ventricular ejection fraction.[32]

The *clinical and hemodynamic features* of MS of any given severity are dictated largely by the levels of cardiac output and pulmonary vascular resistance. The response to a given degree of mitral obstruction may be characterized on one end of the hemodynamic spectrum by a normal cardiac output and a high left atrioventricular pressure gradient or, at the opposite end of the spectrum, by a markedly reduced cardiac output and low transvalvular pressure gradient. In some patients with moderately severe stenosis (mitral valve area = 1.0 to 1.5 cm^2) cardiac output may be normal, not only at rest but during exertion as well. In these patients, marked elevation of left atrial and pulmonary capillary pressures leads to symptoms of severe pulmonary congestion. However, in the majority of patients with severe MS, cardiac output is subnormal at rest and rises subnormally during exertion, thus reducing the pulmonary venous pressure and the severity of symptoms of pulmonary congestion more than would be the case if the output rose normally. In patients with severe stenosis (mitral valve area < 1.0 cm^2), particularly when pulmonary vascular resistance is elevated, cardiac output is usually depressed at rest and fails to rise during exertion. These patients frequently have prominent symptoms secondary to a low cardiac output.

Pulmonary hypertension in patients with MS results from (1) passive backward transmission of the elevated left atrial pressure; (2) arteriolar constriction, which presumably is triggered by left atrial and pulmonary venous hypertension (reactive pulmonary hypertension); and (3) organic obliterative changes in the pulmonary vascular bed, which may be considered to be a complication of longstanding and severe MS (Chap. 26). (There is some evidence for reversible pulmonary vasoconstriction as well.[34]) In time, severe pulmonary hypertension results in right-sided failure and tricuspid and sometimes pulmonic regurgitation. However, it has been suggested that these changes in the pulmonary vascular bed may also be considered to exert a protective effect; the elevated precapillary resistance makes the development of symptoms of pulmonary congestion less likely by tending to prevent blood from surging into the pulmonary capillary bed and damming up behind the stenotic mitral valve, although this protection occurs at the expense of a decreased cardiac output.[21] Patients with severe MS manifest a marked reduction in lung compliance, an increase in the work of breathing, and a redistribution of pulmonary blood flow from the bases to the apices (p. 1873).

The combination of mitral valve disease and atrial inflammation secondary to rheumatic carditis causes left atrial dilatation, fibrosis of the atrial wall, and disorganization of the atrial muscle bundles. The last leads to disparate conduction velocities and inhomogeneous refractory periods. Premature atrial activation due either to an automatic focus or to reentry may stimulate the left atrium during the vulnerable period and may thus precipitate a bout of atrial fibrillation. Chronic atrial fibrillation results in turn in diffuse atrophy of the muscle, which causes further inhomogeneity of refractoriness and conduction and leads to irreversible atrial fibrillation.[35]

CLINICAL MANIFESTATIONS (Table 33–1)

HISTORY

The principal symptom of MS is dyspnea, largely the result of reduced compliance of the lungs (p. 1873). Vital capacity is reduced, presumably owing to the presence of engorged pulmonary vessels and interstitial edema. Patients with critical obstruction to left ventricular inflow and dyspnea upon ordinary activity (functional Class III) generally have orthopnea and are at risk of experiencing attacks of frank pulmonary edema. The latter may be precipitated by effort, emotional stress, respiratory infection, fever, sexual intercourse, pregnancy (p. 1854), or atrial fibrillation with a rapid ventricular rate or, indeed, by any condition that increases blood flow across the stenotic mitral valve, either by increasing total cardiac output or by reducing the time available for this flow of blood to occur. In patients with a markedly elevated pulmonary vascular resistance, right ventricular function is often impaired, and a rise in right ventricular output may be impossible. Therefore, they are less subject to sudden elevations of pulmonary capillary pressure and the accompanying attacks of pulmonary edema.[19, 36]

HEMOPTYSIS. Wood has differentiated between several kinds of *hemoptysis* complicating MS.[19]

1. Sudden hemorrhage (sometimes called pulmonary apoplexy), while often profuse, is rarely life-threatening.[37] This results from the rupture of thin-walled, dilated bronchial veins as a consequence of a sudden rise in left atrial pressure. After several years of pulmonary venous hypertension, the walls of these veins thicken appreciably, and this form of hemoptysis tends to disappear.
2. Blood-stained sputum associated with attacks of nocturnal dyspnea.
3. Pink, frothy sputum characteristic of acute pulmonary edema due to rupture of alveolar capillaries.
4. Pulmonary infarction, a late complication of MS associated with heart failure.
5. Blood-stained sputum complicating chronic bronchitis; the edematous bronchial mucosa in patients with chronic MS increases the likelihood of chronic bronchitis, a common complication of MS, particularly in Great Britain.

CHEST PAIN. A small fraction, perhaps 15 per cent, of patients with MS experience chest discomfort that is indistinguishable from angina pectoris.[18, 19] This symptom may be caused by right ventricular hypertension[38] or by coincidental coronary atherosclerosis,[31, 38a] or it may be secondary to coronary obstruction caused by coronary embolization.[39] In many such patients, however, a satisfactory explanation cannot be uncovered even after complete hemodynamic and angiographic studies.

THROMBOEMBOLISM. Prior to the advent of surgical treatment, this serious complication of MS[40, 41] developed in at least 20 per cent of patients at some time during the course of their disease, and in the past as many as 10 to 15 per cent of this group died as a consequence. Before the era of anticoagulant therapy and surgical treatment, approximately one-fourth of all fatalities in patients with

TABLE 33–1 DIAGNOSIS OF MITRAL VALVE DISEASE

	MITRAL STENOSIS	MITRAL REGURGITATION
Sex	Women > Men	Men > Women
Severity of rheumatic fever	Less severe	Often fulminating
Presystolic murmur	Present	Absent
First sound	Loud unless calcification	*Never loud*
Apical systolic murmur	Usually absent	Pansystolic or late
Mid-diastolic murmur	Long, not necessarily loud	*If present, short*
Opening snap of mitral valve	Present unless heavy calcification, pulmonary hypertension, or aortic regurgitation	Rarely present
Third sound	*Never present*	Commonly present and loud
Cardiac impulse	Tapping ("closing snap"); right ventricular type if pulmonary vascular resistance raised	Left ventricular type; right ventricular type if pulmonary vascular resistance raised
Radial pulse	Small volume	Small volume but collapsing
Systemic emboli	Common	Less common
Left atrial size	Enlarged but rarely aneurysmal	May be aneurysmal; systolic
Left ventricle	*Normal or poor filling,* aorta hypoplastic	*Enlarged, rapidly filling,* and hyperdynamic
Electrocardiogram	RVH if pulmonary vascular resistance raised	LVH; RVH if pulmonary vascular resistance raised
Hemodynamic data	a. LAP may be greatly raised b. Gradient across valve in diastole c. PVR may be severely raised	a. Less severely raised as a rule b. No gradient usually c. PVR not commonly greatly raised

RVH = right ventricular hypertrophy, LVH = left ventricular hypertrophy, LAP = left atrial pressure, PVR = pulmonary vascular resistance.
Modified from Oram, S.: Clinical Heart Disease. London, William Heinemann Medical Books, 1981, p. 335.

mitral valve disease were secondary to embolism. The tendency for embolization correlates inversely with cardiac output and directly with the patient's age and the size of the left atrial appendage; 80 per cent of patients in whom systemic emboli develop are in atrial fibrillation. When embolization occurs in patients in sinus rhythm, the possibility of transient atrial fibrillation and underlying infective endocarditis should be considered. There is no simple correlation between the incidence of embolism on one hand and the size of the mitral orifice or the level of pulmonary vascular resistance on the other. Indeed, embolism may be the first symptom of MS and may occur in patients with mild MS even before the development of dyspnea. Patients older than 35 with atrial fibrillation, especially with a low cardiac output and dilation of the left atrial appendage, are at the highest risk from emboli and therefore should be considered for prophylactic anticoagulant treatment.

Since thrombi are found in the left atrium at operation in only a minority of patients with a history of recent embolism, it is likely that only fresh clots are discharged. Approximately half of all clinically apparent emboli are found in the cerebral vessels. Coronary embolism may lead to myocardial infarction, angina pectoris, or both, and renal emboli may be responsible for the development of systemic hypertension. Emboli are recurrent and multiple in approximately 25 per cent of patients subject to this complication. Rarely, massive thrombosis develops in the left atrium, resulting in a pedunculated ball-valve thrombus, which may aggravate obstruction to left atrial outflow when a specific body position is assumed, or it may cause sudden death.[42]

INFECTIVE ENDOCARDITIS. This complication tends to occur less frequently on a rigid, thickened, calcified valve and is therefore more common in patients with mild than with severe MS.

OTHER SYMPTOMS. Compression of the left recurrent laryngeal nerve by a greatly dilated left atrium, enlarged tracheobronchial lymph nodes, and dilated pulmonary artery cause hoarseness (Ortner syndrome).[43] A history of repeated hemoptysis is common in patients with pulmonary hemosiderosis, and longstanding elevation of pulmonary venous pressure is present in patients with pulmonary ossification. Systemic venous hypertension, hepatomegaly, edema, ascites, and hydrothorax are all signs of severe MS with elevated pulmonary vascular resistance and right heart failure.

PHYSICAL EXAMINATION[44, 45]

Patients with severe MS, a low cardiac output, and systemic vasoconstriction often exhibit the so-called mitral facies, characterized by pinkish-purple patches on the cheeks.[19] The *arterial pulse* is usually normal, but in patients in whom the stroke volume is reduced, the pulse may be small in volume. The *jugular venous pulse* usually exhibits a prominent *a* wave in patients with sinus rhythm and elevated pulmonary vascular resistance (Fig. 3–35, p. 61). In atrial fibrillation, the *x* descent of the jugular pulse disappears, and there is only one crest, a prominent *v* or *c-v* wave, per cardiac cycle and a slow *y* descent. *Palpation* of the cardiac apex usually reveals an inconspicuous left ventricle; the presence of either a palpable presystolic expansion wave or an early diastolic rapid filling wave *excludes* significant MS. The presence of a readily palpable, tapping first heart sound (S_1) suggests that the anterior mitral valve leaflet is pliable. When the patient is in the left lateral recumbent position, the low-pitched diastolic rumbling murmur of MS is often palpable as a thrill at the apex. Often a right ventricular lift is palpable in the left parasternal region in patients with pulmonary hypertension. A markedly enlarged right ventricle may displace the left ventricle posteriorly and produce a prominent apex beat that can be confused with a left ventricular lift. A pulmonic closure sound (P_2) may be palpable in the second left intercostal space in patients with MS and pulmonary hypertension.

AUSCULTATION. The auscultatory (and phonocardiographic) features of MS (some of which are illustrated in Figs. 3–14, p. 50, and 33–4) include an accentuated S_1 with prolongation of the Q-S_1 interval, correlating with the level of the left atrial pressure.[11] Accentuation of S_1 occurs when the mitral valve is flexible[46] and is due in part to the rapidity with which left ventricular pressure rises at the time of mitral valve closure as well as to the wide closing excursion of the valve leaflets. Marked calcification or thickening of the mitral valve leaflets or both reduce the amplitude of S_1, probably because of diminished movement of the leaflets. As pulmonary artery pressure rises, P_2 at first becomes accentuated and widely transmitted and can often be readily heard and recorded at both the mitral and the aortic areas. With further elevation of pulmonary artery pressure, splitting of S_2 narrows because of reduced compliance of the pulmonary vascular bed, which shortens the "hang-out interval." Finally, S_2 becomes single and accentuated. Other signs of pulmonary hypertension include a nonvalvular pulmonic ejection sound (Fig. 3–13, p. 49) that diminishes during inspiration, owing to dilatation of the pulmonary artery; the systolic murmur of tricuspid regurgitation; a Graham Steell murmur of pulmonic regurgitation; and an S_4 originating from the right ventricle.[47] An S_3 originating from the left ventricle is absent, unless significant mitral or aortic regurgitation coexists.[48]

The *opening snap* (OS) of the mitral valve appears to be due to a sudden tensing of the valve leaflets by the chordae tendineae after the valve cusps have completed their opening excursion[44, 45] and is best heard at the apex and with the diaphragm of the stethoscope. It can usually be

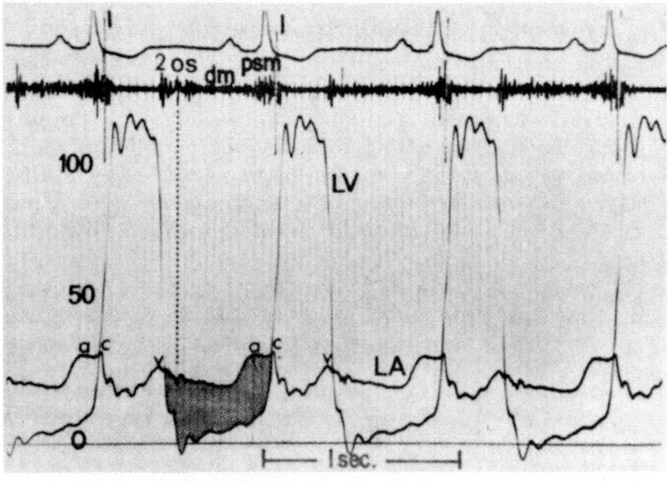

FIGURE 33–4. The auscultatory complex of mitral stenosis. An apical phonocardiogram demonstrates the accentuated first sound (1), opening snap (os), rumbling diastolic murmur (dm), and crescendo presystolic murmur (psm) in relation to simultaneous left ventricular (LV) and left atrial (LA) pressures. The first sound is coincident with the left atrial c wave, and the opening snap coincides with a notch (dotted line) on the downslope (*y* descent) of the left atrial *v* wave. The presystolic murmur exhibits a crescendo after the *a* wave peak, during a decline in the atrioventricular pressure gradient (shaded area). (Time lines = 0.04 sec.) (From Criley, J. M., et al.: Departures from the expected auscultatory events in mitral stenosis. *In* Likoff, W. [ed.]: Cardiovascular Clinics. Vol. 5, No. 2, Valvular Heart Disease. Philadelphia, F. A. Davis, 1973, p. 192.)

differentiated from P_2 because the OS occurs later, unless right bundle branch block is present. The mitral valve cannot be totally rigid if it produces an OS, which is usually accompanied by an accentuated S_1. Calcification confined to the tip of the mitral valve does not preclude an OS, although calcification of the body and tip does.[49] In patients with combined MS and regurgitation, the OS may be followed by an S_3. The mitral OS follows A_2 by 0.04 to 0.12 sec, and the A_2-OS interval varies inversely with left atrial pressure.[50] Although a short A_2-OS interval is a reliable indicator of severe MS, the converse is not necessarily the case, since the time interval between the actual opening of the mitral valve and the OS can be prolonged in the presence of valvular calcification and tight stenosis. The (Q-S_1)–(A_2-OS) correlates better with the height of the left atrial pressure than does either measurement alone.[51]

The diastolic murmur of MS is a low-pitched, rumbling murmur, best heard at the apex and with the bell of the stethoscope. When this murmur is soft, it is limited to the apex, but when louder, it may radiate to the axilla or the lower left sternal area. Although the intensity of the diastolic murmur is not closely related to the severity of stenosis, the *duration* of the murmur is a guide to the severity of mitral narrowing, and in patients with combined MS and MR, a long diastolic murmur always signifies the presence of significant stenosis and, in general, persists for as long as the gradient across the mitral valve exceeds approximately 3 mm Hg. The murmur usually commences immediately after the mitral OS. In mild MS, the early diastolic murmur is brief but commences again in presystole. In severe stenosis, the murmur is holodiastolic, with presystolic accentuation.

Although a *presystolic murmur* is usually present in patients with sinus rhythm in whom transvalvular blood flow is accelerated by atrial contraction, such a murmur may also occur in patients with atrial fibrillation, in whom it results from the increased velocity of blood flow across a mitral valve orifice that begins to narrow after the onset of left ventricular contraction[52, 53] (Fig. 4–18, p. 75). Since, in patients with atrial fibrillation, this murmur results from motion of the mitral valve leaflets, a flexible mitral valve is required for its generation; its absence in a patient with moderate or severe obstruction suggests either a rigid calcified valve or a markedly reduced cardiac output.

The *diastolic rumbling murmur* of MS may be masked by the presence of obesity, pulmonary emphysema, and a low cardiac output with a low flow rate across the mitral valve. The rumble may be sharply localized and thus missed unless palpation is used to detect the apex of the left ventricle and to pinpoint the area at which auscultation should be carried out. In so-called "silent" MS, there is usually marked right ventricular enlargement, so that the right ventricle occupies the cardiac apex, and cardiac output is reduced, so that the murmur either is not audible at all or can be heard only in the mid- or posterior axillary line.[54] Auscultation of the murmur is facilitated by placing the patient in the left lateral position and auscultating during expiration after a few sit-ups or other maneuvers described below.

Dynamic Auscultation. The diastolic murmur and OS of MS are often reduced during inspiration and augmented during expiration[44, 45, 55]—the opposite of what occurs when these findings are secondary to tricuspid stenosis. During inspiration the A_2-OS interval widens, and three sequential sounds (A_2, P_2, and OS) are frequently audible. Sudden standing and the resultant reduction of venous return lower left atrial pressure and widen the A_2-OS interval[56]; this maneuver is useful in distinguishing an A_2-OS combination from a split S_2, which narrows on standing. In contrast, A_2-OS is significantly narrowed during exercise as left atrial pressure rises. The diastolic rumbling murmur of MS is reduced during the strain of a Valsalva maneuver, and there is a delayed return to prestrain levels during the overshoot, six to eight beats after release. Amyl nitrite, coughing, isometric or isotonic exercise, and sudden squat-

TABLE 33–2 CONDITIONS OTHER THAN MITRAL STENOSIS THAT MAY SIMULATE AUSCULTATORY FINDINGS IN MITRAL STENOSIS

Auscultatory Event	Condition Other Than Mitral Stenosis	Explanation of Event
Loud and snapping first sound	Hyperkinetic states	High left ventricular dP/dt at time of mitral closure
Early diastolic opening snap	Myxoma of left atrium	Tumor movement into ventricle
		Abrupt checking of tumor (tumor plop)
	Constrictive pericarditis	Checking of ventricular filling by pericardium
	Tricuspid stenosis	Stenotic valve
Diastolic rumbling murmur	Aortic regurgitation	Preclosure of mitral valve
	(Austin Flint murmur)	(?) Regurgitant stream
		(?) Fluttering of mitral valve
	Dilated ventricle	Preclosure of mitral valve
	Myocarditis	(?) Centrifugal displacement of papillary muscles
	Cardiomyopathy	
	Hypertrophic, restrictive ventricle	Impaired filling of left ventricle
	Hypertrophic obstructive cardiomyopathy	(?) Impaired opening of mitral valve
	Aortic valve disease	
	Tricuspid stenosis	Narrow orifice
	Myxoma of left atrium	Narrow orifice
	Augmented atrioventricular flow	Preclosure of valve
	Mitral regurgitation	(?) Centrifugal displacement of papillary muscles
	Left-to-right shunts	
Crescendo presystolic murmur	Aortic regurgitation	Preclosure of mitral valve opposing atrial systole
	(Austin Flint murmur)	
	Hypertrophic, restrictive ventricle	Summation of S_4 and S_1 may simulate presystolic murmur
	Tricuspid stenosis	Narrow orifice
	Myxoma of left atrium	Narrow orifice

Modified from Criley, J. M., et al.: Departures from the expected auscultatory events in mitral stenosis. *In* Likoff, W. (ed.): Cardiovascular Clinics. Vol. 5, No. 2, Valvular Heart Disease. Philadelphia, F. A. Davis, 1973, p. 213.

ting are all useful in accentuating a faint or equivocal murmur of MS. Progressive narrowing of A_2-OS on serial examinations suggests an increase in the severity of stenosis, whereas widening of A_2-OS after mitral commissurotomy indicates that the severity of stenosis has been reduced significantly.

DIFFERENTIAL DIAGNOSIS. It is important to recognize that a variety of conditions other than MS may exhibit auscultatory findings that can be confused with MS, and these are summarized in Table 33–2. In addition to the findings listed in the table, the *Carey-Coombs* murmur of acute rheumatic fever (p. 1712) is a sign of active mitral valvulitis and can be confused with the murmur of MS. It is a soft, early diastolic murmur, usually varies from day to day, and is higher pitched than the diastolic rumbling murmur of established MS. In pure, severe MR—indeed, in any condition in which there is increased flow across a nonstenotic mitral valve—there may also be a short, diastolic murmur following an S_3. *Left atrial myxoma* may produce auscultatory findings similar to those in rheumatic valvular MS (p. 1472). A high-frequency early systolic murmur is audible along the lower left sternal border in one-third of patients with MS.[57] This should be distinguished from the apical (often holosystolic or late systolic murmur) of MR. In addition, a *pansystolic murmur of tricuspid regurgitation* and an S_3 originating from the right ventricle may be audible in the fourth intercostal space in the left parasternal region in patients with severe mitral stenosis. These signs, secondary to pulmonary hypertension, may be confused with the findings of MR.[58] However, the inspiratory augmentation of the murmur and of the S_3 and the prominent *v* wave in the jugular venous pulse aid in establishing that the murmur originates from the tricuspid valve. A decrescendo diastolic murmur along the left sternal border in patients with MS and pulmonary hypertension is usually due to aortic regurgitation and rarely represents a Graham Steell murmur of pulmonary regurgitation[59] (p. 79); the latter, when present, characteristically increases during inspiration.

LABORATORY EXAMINATION (Table 33–3)

ELECTROCARDIOGRAM. The ECG (and vectorcardiogram) are relatively insensitive techniques for the detection of mild MS, but they do show characteristic changes in patients with moderate or severe obstruction (Fig. 33–5). Left atrial enlargement (P-wave duration in lead II > 0.12 sec, terminal negative P force in lead V_1 > 0.003 mV/sec, P-wave axis between +45 and −30 degrees) is a principal electrocardiographic feature of MS (Fig. 7–11B, p. 189) and is found in 90 per cent of patients with significant MS and sinus rhythm.[60] The ECG signs of left atrial enlargement correlate more closely with left atrial volume than with left atrial pressure[61] and often regress following successful valvulotomy.[19] When atrial fibrillation is present, the fibrillatory waves are coarse, i.e., greater than 0.1 mV in amplitude in V_1, also suggesting the presence of atrial enlargement.[62] The development of atrial fibrillation correlates with the preexistent ECG diagnosis of left atrial enlargement and is related to the size and the extent of fibrosis of the left atrial myocardium,[34] the duration of atriomegaly, and the age of the patient.[63]

ECG evidence of right ventricular hypertrophy depends on the level

TABLE 33–3 SUMMARY OF FINDINGS FROM NONINVASIVE STUDIES IN MITRAL STENOSIS

ECG
- Left atrial enlargement ("P mitrale")
- Atrial fibrillation common
- Right ventricular hypertrophy
- Left ventricular hypertrophy only with coexistent valvular lesions or systemic hypertension

RADIOGRAPHY AND FLUOROSCOPY
- Left atrial enlargement seen as "double shadow" with displacement of barium on lateral film
- Straight left heart border
- Cardiomegaly (if any) due to RV enlargement
- Calcification of valve most easily seen on fluoroscopy

PHONOCARDIOGRAPHY AND PULSE TRACINGS
- Separation of aortic second sound and opening snap (A_2–OS interval) inversely related to degree of stenosis
- Apex cardiogram shows absence of a rapid left ventricular filling wave

M-MODE ECHOCARDIOGRAPHY
- Provides confirmation of diagnosis in virtually all patients in whom an adequate study can be performed
- Characteristic features
  - Left atrial enlargement
  - Thickening and limitation of motion of mitral valve leaflets
  - Concordant motion of anterior and posterior leaflets
  - Delayed rate of diastolic closure of mitral leaflets
  - Right ventricular enlargement in late stages
  - Left ventricular enlargement and hypertrophy only with coexistent valvular lesions or systemic hypertension
- Quantification of stenosis helpful but not definitive
- Based on:
  - Degree of opening and rate of diastolic apposition of leaflets
  - Rate of change of left atrial and left ventricular dimensions

TWO-DIMENSIONAL ECHOCARDIOGRAPHY
- Complementary to but no more sensitive than M-mode in confirming diagnosis
- Provides accurate *quantification* of mitral valve area by imaging entire valve orifice in diastole

DOPPLER ULTRASOUND
- Measures rate of flow across stenotic orifice, with higher rates of flow proportional to more severe degrees of mitral stenosis

NUCLEAR STUDIES
- Provide useful additional quantitative information about left ventricular function

From Bloomfield, P., et al.: Noninvasive investigations for the diagnosis of mitral valve disease. *In* Ionescu, M. I., and Cohn, L. H.: Mitral Valve Disease: Diagnosis and Treatment. London, Butterworths, 1985, p. 54.

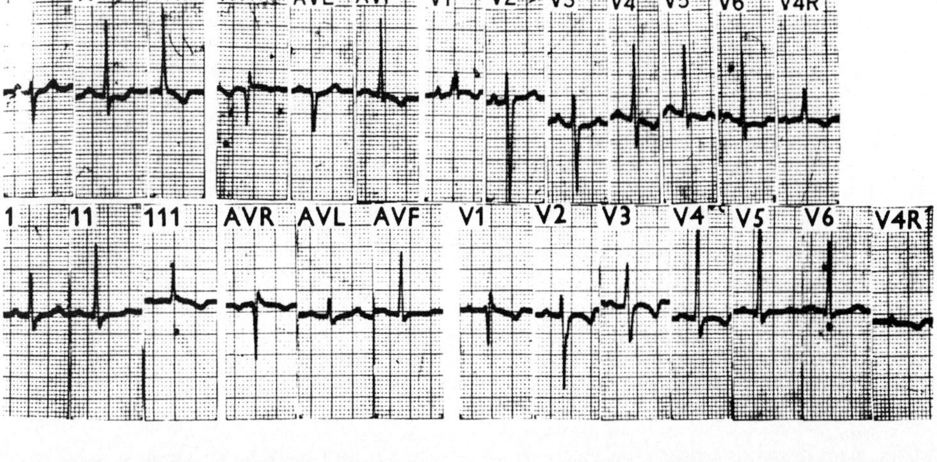

FIGURE 33–5. *Upper tracing,* ECG of a patient with tight mitral stenosis, pulmonary hypertension, right atrial enlargement, right axis deviation, and right ventricular hypertrophy. *Lower tracing,* Six months postcommissurotomy, the signs of right ventricular hypertrophy have regressed. (From Barlow, J. B.: Perspectives on the Mitral Valve. Philadelphia, F. A. Davis, 1987, p. 169.)

of right ventricular systolic pressure; this finding is infrequent in patients with right ventricular systolic pressures less than 70 mm Hg.[60] However, approximately half of all patients with right ventricular systolic pressures between 70 and 100 mm Hg manifest the electrocardiographic criteria for right ventricular hypertrophy, including both a mean QRS axis that is greater than 80 degrees in the frontal plane and an R:S ratio greater than 1.0 in V_1.[64] In other patients with this degree of pulmonary hypertension, there is no frank evidence of right ventricular hypertrophy, but the R:S ratio fails to increase from right to midprecordial leads. When right ventricular systolic pressures exceed 100 mm Hg, electrocardiographic evidence of right ventricular hypertrophy is found quite consistently. The mean QRS axis averages +150 degrees, and there is a Q-R morphology in the right precordial leads, accompanied by inverted or biphasic T waves.[65]

The *QRS axis in the frontal plane* often correlates with the severity of valve obstruction and with the level of pulmonary vascular resistance in pure MS; thus, a mean frontal axis between 0 and +60 degrees suggests that the mitral valve area exceeds 1.3 cm^2, whereas an axis greater than 60 degrees generally indicates that the valve area is less than 1.3 cm^2. In patients in whom pulmonary vascular resistance is greater than 650 dynes-sec-cm^{-5}, the mean axis usually exceeds +110 degrees.[64]

VECTORCARDIOGRAM. The characteristic *vectorcardiographic finding* in MS is right ventricular hypertrophy Type C (Fig. 7–10, p. 187) characterized by counterclockwise rotation in the horizontal plane and a terminal deflection directed to the right, posteriorly, and superiorly.[60, 64–66] In other patients with MS without frank right ventricular hypertrophy, QRS loops with posterior and rightward terminal appendages are evident without conduction delays.[60, 64] There is vectorcardiographic evidence of right ventricular hypertrophy Type A (Fig. 7–19, p. 194) in only 10 per cent of patients with MS, but when present it indicates that both the hypertrophy and the stenosis are severe. Vectorcardiograms showing right ventricular hypertrophy Type B (Fig. 7–19) are infrequent in MS.

Rotation of the P loop in the frontal plane, with superior orientation of the terminal P forces and a wide angle between the initial and terminal P vectors, occurs in about one-fourth of patients with pure mitral stenosis and may be the only evidence of left atrial enlargement.[67] The terminal portion of the P loop is usually directed posteriorly and inferiorly, and the T loop is often directed leftward and posterosuperiorly and is discordant with respect to the QRS loop, resulting in a diphasic T wave with initial negativity and terminal positivity in lead V_1.

RADIOLOGICAL FINDINGS (See also p. 154). Although the cardiac silhouette may be normal in the frontal projection, with the exception of an enlarged atrial appendage (Fig. 6–3*A*, p. 143) in patients with hemodynamically significant MS, left atrial enlargement is almost invariably evident on the lateral and left anterior oblique views.[68, 69] The size of the left atrium does *not* correlate with the severity of obstruction. However, extreme left atrial enlargement rarely occurs in pure MS; when it is present, MR is usually severe. Enlargement of the pulmonary artery, right ventricle, and right atrium (as well as the left atrium) is commonly seen in severe MS (Figs. 6–2, p. 142, and 6–13, p. 149). Occasionally, calcification of the mitral valve is evident on the chest roentgenogram (Fig. 6–9, p. 146), but, more commonly, fluoroscopy is required to detect valvular calcification.

Radiological changes in the lung fields (Fig. 6–26, p. 155) are useful in estimating the height of pulmonary venous pressure and thereby the severity of MS. Interstitial edema, an indication of severe obstruction, is manifest as Kerley B lines (dense, short, horizontal lines most commonly seen in the costophrenic angles).[70] This finding is present in 30 per cent of patients with resting pulmonary artery wedge pressures below 20 mm Hg and in 70 per cent of patients with pressures exceeding 20 mm Hg. Severe, longstanding mitral obstruction often results in Kerley A lines (straight, dense lines up to 4 cm in length and running toward the hilum) as well as the findings of pulmonary hemosiderosis[71] and rarely of parenchymal ossification.

Angiograms exposed in the right and left anterior oblique projections afford the best views of the mitral valve.[72] Although ideally contrast medium should be injected into the left atrium, it is often possible to achieve good visualization of the left side of the heart by injecting a large volume of contrast medium into the main pulmonary artery. Such left atrial or pulmonary angiograms provide an assessment of left atrial size, may demonstrate thickening and reduced motion of the valve leaflets (Fig. 6–53, p. 175), and may outline large intraluminal thrombi.[73] Left cine ventriculography is the primary (and often the sole) angiographic procedure for assessment of mitral valve motion. Although this technique allows visualization of only the ventricular aspect of the leaflet in patients with pure MS, it makes possible simultaneous assessment of left ventricular contractile function and of the subvalvular mitral apparatus.

ECHOCARDIOGRAPHY (See also p. 103). MS can ordinarily be readily diagnosed by M-mode echocardiography (Figs. 3–14, p. 50, and 5–44, p. 103), but this technique does not allow a precise determination of its severity. Echoes of a thickened, calcified stenotic rheumatic valve demonstrate increased acoustic impedance and fusion of the mitral valve leaflets and poor leaflet separation in diastole.[74] The leaflets fail to close in mid-diastole and may not reopen widely during atrial contraction. Normally, the posterior leaflet of the mitral valve moves posteriorly during early diastole, but in more than 90 per cent of

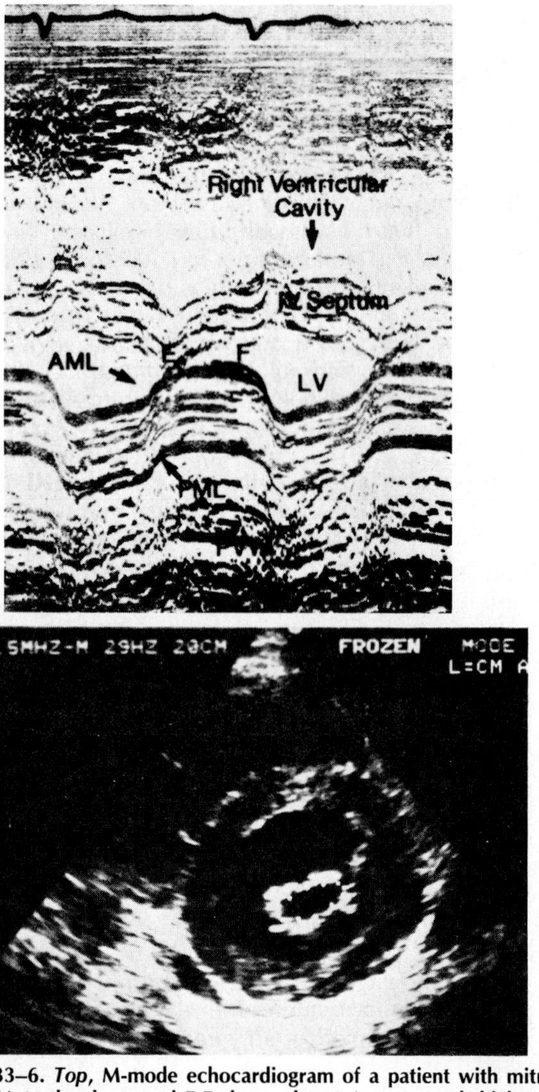

FIGURE 33–6. *Top,* M-mode echocardiogram of a patient with mitral stenosis. Note the decreased E-F slope, absent A wave, and thickened leaflets. The posterior mitral leaflet (PML) moves in an anterior direction with the anterior mitral leaflet (AML) during diastole. IV = interventricular septum, LV = left ventricle, PVW = posterior ventricular wall. (From Dalen, J. E.: Mitral stenosis. *In* Dalen, J. E., and Alpert, J. S. (eds.): Valvular Heart Disease. 2nd ed. Boston, Little, Brown and Company, 1987, p. 73.) *Bottom,* Two-dimensional parasternal short-axis view of the mitral valve orifice during diastole, demonstrating the echocardiographic method of mitral valve area calculation. The innermost border of the mitral orifice was planimetered with the use of a light-pen system to obtain the area (in cm^2). (From Smith, M. D., Handshoe, R., Handshoe, S., Kwan, O. L., and DeMaria, A. N.: Comparative accuracy of two-dimensional echocardiography and Doppler pressure half-time methods in assessing severity of mitral stenosis in patients with and without prior commissurotomy. Circulation *73*:102, 1986, by permission of the American Heart Association, Inc.)

patients with MS, both leaflets move anteriorly at this time (Fig. 33–6, *top*) and there is inadequate separation of the leaflets. The E–F slope is reduced,[75] but this finding is not pathognomonic of MS, since it may occur in other conditions in which left ventricular compliance and the velocity of left ventricular filling are reduced. However, in these other conditions the posterior leaflet of the mitral valve moves normally, emphasizing the importance of recording the motion of this structure in order to establish the diagnosis of MS by echocardiography. Reduction of the E–F slope does not correlate with the severity of obstruction. However, the maximal diastolic separation of the anterior and posterior leaflets,[76] their rate of diastolic apposition, and the slope of motion of the left ventricular posterior wall during diastole appear to correlate more closely with the mitral valve area.[75, 76] Two-dimensional echocardiography (Fig. 33–6, *bottom*) is more accurate than M-mode echocardiography in determining mitral orifice size[77, 77a, 78] (Fig. 5–45, p. 103). It reveals restricted motion and doming of the valve leaflets. The orifice can often be imaged directly and measured. This technique also provides information on the pliability and extent of calcification of the valve and its suitability for valvulotomy.

Other important echocardiographic findings in patients with pulmonary hypertension and MS include a small or absent *a* wave in the pulmonic valve echogram (Fig. 5–42, p. 102). The left atrium is usually enlarged, and the left ventricular cavity is normal or reduced in size. M-mode echocardiography is also useful in detecting mitral annular calcification, which may accompany MS and in which a band of dense echoes is present in the region of the mitral annulus, in contrast to the thin and delicate echoes recorded from the normal mitral annulus. Two-dimensional echocardiography may be helpful in the preoperative recognition of left atrial thrombus,[79] although the demonstration of a thrombus by the finding of neovascularity on coronary arteriography is probably a more accurate technique.

Doppler echocardiography is especially useful in quantifying the severity of MS[78, 80] (Figs. 5–46 and 5–47, p. 104). The peak velocity of transmitral flow is increased and the rate of decline of flow during early diastole is reduced. The time required for peak velocity to reach half its initial level correlates with the size of the mitral orifice. Doppler color flow imaging can be used to enhance the accuracy of the Doppler data by guiding the position of the beam.[80a]

MANAGEMENT

MEDICAL TREATMENT

Patients with rheumatic heart disease should receive penicillin prophylaxis for beta-hemolytic streptococcal infections, as outlined on page 1716, and prophylaxis for infective endocarditis, as summarized on page 1127. Anemia and infections should be treated promptly and aggressively in patients with valvular heart disease. Adolescents and young adults should be advised to avoid physically strenuous occupations.

In symptomatic patients with mitral valve disease, considerable improvement can be expected with oral diuretics and the restriction of sodium intake. Digitalis glycosides do not alter the hemodynamics and usually do not benefit patients with MS and sinus rhythm[81] but are helpful in the treatment of right-sided heart failure. However, as pointed out below, cardiac glycosides are of great value in slowing the ventricular rate in patients with atrial fibrillation. Measures designed to reduce pulmonary venous pressure, including sedation, assumption of the upright posture, and aggressive diuresis, are used to treat hemoptysis. If for any reason operation is not to be carried out, oral anticoagulants should be administered to patients with MS who have suffered systemic emboli, as well as patients who are at high risk of embolization, i.e., those who are in atrial fibrillation, especially if they are older than 40 years and have a greatly enlarged left atrium. Beta blockers may increase exercise capacity by reducing heart rate, even in patients with sinus rhythm.[81a]

In patients with rheumatic heart disease and heart failure and/or atrial fibrillation, anticoagulant therapy is helpful in preventing venous thrombosis and pulmonary embolism, in reducing the frequency of systemic embolism in patients who have experienced one or more previous embolic episodes, and in reducing the frequency of thromboembolism in patients with prosthetic heart valves. However, there is no firm evidence that anticoagulant therapy reduces the incidence of pulmonary or systemic embolism in patients in sinus rhythm in whom embolic episodes have not previously occurred and who are not in heart failure; consequently, these drugs are not administered under the aforementioned circumstances.

TREATMENT OF ARRHYTHMIAS. Frequent premature atrial contractions often presage atrial fibrillation, and the administration of antiarrhythmic drugs, as outlined on page 674, may be effective in preventing this complication. However, once atrial fibrillation has developed, these agents may be ineffective in restoring sinus rhythm or even in maintaining sinus rhythm following electrical cardioversion, because of pathological changes that occur in the atrium secondary to the arrhythmia itself. After electrical cardioversion, sinus rhythm can often be maintained with antiarrhythmic drugs in young patients with mild MS without marked left atrial enlargement who have been in atrial fibrillation less than 6 months and who have been treated with adequate doses of quinidine. In any event, if elective cardioversion (pharmacological or electrical) is to be attempted in the patient with MS and atrial fibrillation, a preparatory three-week course of anticoagulation should be given to minimize the risk of systemic embolism when sinus rhythm has resumed. Immediate treatment of atrial fibrillation should be directed toward reducing the ventricular rate by means of digitalis and, if possible, toward reestablishing sinus rhythm by a combination of pharmacological treatment and cardioversion. However, it must be appreciated that in 1 to 2 per cent of patients with MS, systemic embolism develops following electrical or pharmacological cardioversion. Paroxysmal atrial fibrillation and repeated conversions, spontaneous or induced, carry the risk of embolization.[82] Following reversion to sinus rhythm, administration of quinidine or a similar antiarrhythmic agent should be continued indefinitely in order to diminish the likelihood of recurrent fibrillation. In patients who cannot be converted or maintained in sinus rhythm, the ventricular rate at rest should be maintained at approximately 60 to 65 beats/min with digitalis. If this is not possible, small doses of a beta blocker, such as atenolol (25 mg daily), may be added. Repeat cardioversion is not indicated if the patient has not sustained sinus rhythm while on adequate doses of quinidine.

NATURAL HISTORY

The development of effective surgical treatment has obscured our understanding of the natural history of MS (Fig. 33–7) and, for that matter, of all valvular lesions.[83] Although few meaningful data are available, it appears that in temperate zones such as the United States and Europe, after a latent period of 20 to 25 years following an attack of rheumatic fever during which the patient is asymptomatic, it takes approximately 5 years for most patients to progress from mild disability (i.e., early Class II) to severe disability (i.e., Classes III or IV). The progression is much more rapid in patients with MS in subtropical areas such as India and the Philippines.[84] Polynesians, as well as Eskimos in Alaska and blacks in Alabama, also show an accelerated course. Economic conditions as well as genetic ones may play a role. In the presurgical era, Olesen found 62 per cent 5-year and 38 per cent 10-year survival among

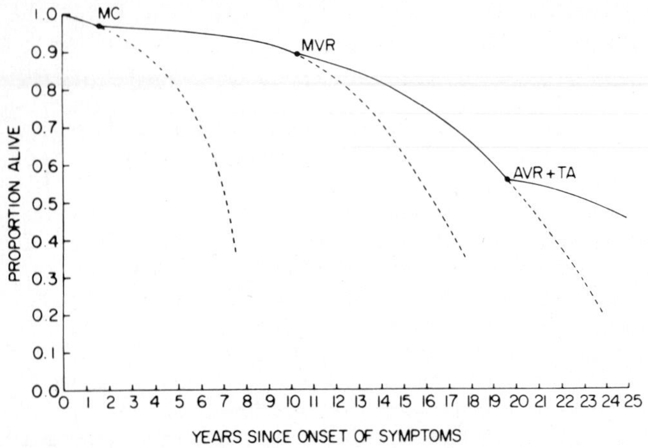

FIGURE 33–7. Schematic representation of the subsequent life history after the initial development of symptoms of a large group of patients with mitral stenosis. The solid circles indicate a surgical procedure. The dashed lines represent estimated survival of patients not receiving the surgical procedure. MC = mitral commissurotomy, MVR = mitral valve replacement, TA = tricuspid annuloplasty, AVR = aortic valve replacement. (From Kirklin, J. W., and Barratt-Boyes, B. G.: Cardiac Surgery. New York, John Wiley and Sons, 1986, p. 328.)

patients in New York Heart Association functional Class III but only a 15 per cent 5-year survival rate in patients in Class IV.[85] Among asymptomatic medically treated patients (Class I) with MS followed medically, 40 per cent had a worsened course or had died within 10 years. Among mildly symptomatic patients (Class II), the comparable number was 80 per cent.[86] In medically treated patients with MS or with combined MS and MR, Munoz et al. found a 45 per cent 5-year survival rate.[36] In a comparable group of patients subjected to mitral commissurotomy, the 5-year survival rate was substantially better. In an unselected mix of patients with MS of varying severity, 80 per cent were alive after 5 years and 60 per cent after 10 years of medical treatment.[87]

SURGICAL TREATMENT

INDICATIONS FOR OPERATION. Patients with MS who are asymptomatic or minimally symptomatic frequently remain so for years. However, once symptoms become more severe, the disease progresses relatively rapidly to death, and operation should therefore be carried out in symptomatic patients with moderate to severe MS (i.e., a mitral valve orifice size < 1.0 cm²/m² body surface area [BSA]).

There has been considerable debate concerning the need for routine cardiac catheterization in determining whether operation is indicated.[88–90] Although a careful clinical evaluation and noninvasive assessment, particularly using two-dimensional and Doppler echocardiography, can provide sufficient information to permit an informed decision in the majority of patients, the consequences of valvular surgery, particularly valve replacement, are so profound that I recommend preoperative catheterization and angiography in the following groups of patients with MS: (1) patients with heart murmurs and other findings suggesting the presence of valve lesions in addition to MS, (2) patients with associated chronic obstructive pulmonary disease, (3) patients in whom left atrial myxoma must be excluded, and (4) patients who have angina or angina-like chest pain in whom associated coronary artery disease must be excluded. Critical narrowing of one or more coronary vessels occurs in approximately one-fourth of all adults with severe MS. It is more common in men over 45 years who have angina and who have risk factors for coronary artery disease.[31, 91, 92] I believe that preoperative catheterization can be omitted in the young (< 40 years) patient without angina who has typical symptoms and classic findings of pure, severe MS on physical examination and by noninvasive tests, including two-dimensional and Doppler echocardiography.

Care of mildly symptomatic patients (Class II) must be individualized. It is necessary to consider and balance three important factors: (1) the size of the mitral orifice, (2) the degree to which the patient's life style is impaired by the mitral obstruction, (3) the operative risk, and (4) the history of complications, particularly systemic embolism. If there are no obvious contraindications to operation, left heart catheterization should be performed to determine the size of the valve orifice. In general, surgery can be deferred in patients with mild stenosis (i.e., mitral valve orifice size > 1.0 cm²/m² BSA), whereas it should be recommended for those with moderate or severe stenosis (i.e., mitral valve orifice size < 1.0 cm²/m² BSA). However, this plan is subject to qualification. For instance, operation might well be deferred in a retired woman in her seventies with modest needs for elevated cardiac output and a mitral valve orifice of 0.8 cm²/m² BSA. A 25-year-old laborer whose family's economic well-being depends on his continued physical exertion might be an excellent candidate for operation, although the mitral valve orifice size is 1.2 cm²/m² BSA.

Because of the high rate of recurrence, operation is also indicated in patients with MS in whom systemic embolism has previously occurred, even if they are otherwise asymptomatic and even though there is no definitive evidence that the incidence of recurrent emboli will be significantly reduced. In these cases, anticoagulants should be administered up to the time of operation. Although the risk of operation is higher in patients with advanced disease characterized by severe pulmonary hypertension and right-sided heart failure, surviving patients nearly always show striking clinical and hemodynamic improvement, with a marked reduction in pulmonary vascular pressures. In the pregnant patient with MS, operative treatment should be carried out only if serious pulmonary congestion occurs despite intensive medical treatment including bed rest (p. 1853).

There is no evidence that surgical treatment improves the prognosis of patients with no or only slight functional impairment. Therefore, valvulotomy is *not* indicated in patients who are entirely asymptomatic, except in unusual circumstances. For example, several years ago I saw a 33-year-old woman with moderately severe MS who had hemoptysis and pulmonary edema during the second trimester of a pregnancy at age 31. She then became asymptomatic but wished to have another child. Hemodynamic study showed a pulmonary wedge pressure of 17 mm Hg and a mitral orifice area of 1.7 cm²/m² BSA. Prophylactic mitral commissurotomy was undertaken in this patient, since it was virtually certain that another pregnancy would have resulted in serious heart failure.

SURGICAL TECHNIQUES. Three basically different operative approaches are available for the treatment of rheumatic MS (Fig. 33–8): (1) closed mitral commissurotomy[93, 94]; (2) open commissurotomy, i.e., commissurotomy carried out under direct vision with the aid of cardiopulmonary bypass; and (3) mitral valve replacement.[95] *Closed mitral commissurotomy*, performed with the aid of a transventricular dilator, is generally preferred to simple transatrial

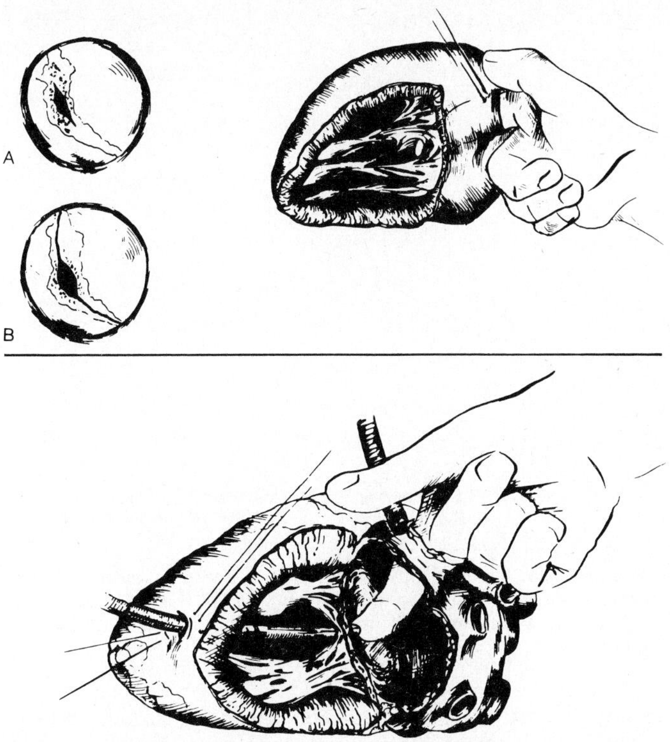

FIGURE 33–8. *Top*, Closed digital mitral commissurotomy. Mitral valve before (A) and after (B) valvotomy. *Bottom*, Transventricular closed mitral commissurotomy. Finger of the right hand in the left atrium. Tubbs dilator through the apex of the left ventricle in the ostium of the mitral valve. (From deVivie, E. R., and Hellberg, K.: Closed transventricular mitral commissurotomy. *In* Ionescu, M. I., and Cohn, L. H. [eds.]: Mitral Valve Disease: Diagnosis and Treatment. London, Butterworths, 1985, pp. 140 and 141.)

finger fracture.[93–95] It is an effective operation, provided that MR, atrial thrombosis, or valvular calcification is not serious and that chordal fusion and shortening are not severe. Unfortunately, few patients satisfy all these criteria, and they are difficult to identify preoperatively. In one large series,[93] hospital mortality was 1.5 per cent and 0.3 per cent of patients developed severe MR. Marked symptomatic improvement occurred in 86 per cent of survivors. Actuarial survival rate was 89.5 per cent after 18 years. Closed valvotomy for restenosis was carried out with a 6.7 per cent mortality. Long-term follow-up has shown that the results are best if the operation is carried out before chronic atrial fibrillation and/or heart failure have been established.[94] Therefore, closed mitral commissurotomy should be carried out with "pump standby"; if the surgeon is unable to achieve a satisfactory result, the patient is placed on cardiopulmonary bypass, and the commissurotomy is carried out under direct vision. Closed mitral commissurotomy is rarely used in the United States today, but is more popular in developing nations, where the expense of open-heart surgery is an important factor and where patients with mitral valve disease are younger. In any event, echocardiography is useful in selecting suitable candidates without valvular calcification or dense fibrosis.[96]

Most surgeons in the United States, Canada, and Western Europe now prefer to carry out *direct-vision* or *open commissurotomy*.[95–99a] Cardiopulmonary bypass is established, and in order to obtain a dry, quiet heart, body temperature is usually lowered, the heart is arrested, and the aorta is occluded intermittently (Chap. 51). Thrombi are removed from the atrium and its appendage, and the latter is often amputated in order to remove a potential source of postoperative emboli. The commissures are incised, and, when necessary, fused chordae are separated, the underlying papillary muscle is split, and the valves are debrided of calcium; mild or even moderate mitral regurgitation may be corrected with suture plication or annuloplasty. Left atrial and ventricular pressures are measured after bypass has been discontinued to confirm that the commissurotomy has, in fact, been effective. In patients with atrial fibrillation, conversion to sinus rhythm is carried out at the completion of the operation. In a series of open mitral valve reconstructive procedures for MS at the Brigham and Women's Hospital, the actuarial probability of survival at 10 years was 95 per cent; thromboemboli occurred in 9 of 120 patients. The annual reoperation rate was 1.7 per cent.[100]

The mortality rate after mitral commissurotomy, whether open or closed, ranges from 1 to 3 per cent, depending on the condition of the patient and the skill of the surgical team.[98–100] In general, open commissurotomy provides better hemodynamic relief of mitral valve obstruction than does the closed procedure,[101] and the risk of dislodging thrombi from the atrium or calcium from the mitral valve is also less.[98, 100] However, it must be recognized that mitral commissurotomy, whether open or closed, is a *palliative* rather than a curative operation, and even when successful, it merely "turns the clock back." Thus, it does not result in a normal mitral valve but, at best, in one resembling the valve as it existed perhaps a decade earlier. Since the valve is not normal postoperatively, turbulent flow may persist in the paravalvular region, and this may well play a role in restenosis. These changes are analogous to the development of obstruction in a congenitally bicuspid aortic valve and are not usually the result of recurrent rheumatic fever.

Mitral valve replacement is discussed on pages 1077 and 1081.

Although a contemporary control series of medically and surgically treated patients is not available (nor is it likely that it ever will be), appropriate surgical treatment appears to prolong survival substantially in patients with MS (Fig. 33–7).

Mitral Restenosis. This condition can be diagnosed with certainty only on the basis of three satisfactory hemodynamic or echocardiographic investigations: a preoperative study, a second study following a satisfactory operation in which an increase in the size of the valvular orifice can be demonstrated, and a third one after the reappearance of symptoms, when a reduction in size relative to the earlier postoperative study is noted. On the basis of clinical grounds alone, the incidence of "restenosis" has been estimated to range widely, from 2 to 60 per cent[102]; approximately 10 per cent of patients who have undergone mitral commissurotomy require reoperation within 5 years, but that fraction increases to 60 per cent by 10 years.[103] However, *the need for reoperation does not necessarily imply restenosis*. More often recurrent symptoms are due to one of four circumstances: (1) an inadequate first operation with residual stenosis; (2) the presence or development of MR, either at operation or as a consequence of infective endocarditis; (3) the progression of aortic valve disease; and (4) the development of ischemic heart disease. In a study in which the size of the mitral valve orifice was estimated using two-dimensional echocardiography in 18 patients who had undergone successful mitral commissurotomy, no change in the mitral valve area occurred over a 10- to 14-year period in 13 patients, whereas in 5 (28 per cent) true restenosis developed.[103] Approximately 10 per cent of patients returning to the hospital with persistent or recurrent symptoms 6 years after operation have true restenosis.[104]

Thus, in properly selected patients, mitral commissurotomy results in a significant increase in the size of the mitral orifice and, at a low risk, favorably alters the clinical course of an otherwise progressive disease. Pulmonary artery pressure falls promptly and decisively when mitral obstruction is effectively relieved.[105–107] Some patients maintain clinical improvement for many (10 to 15) years of follow-up. When a second operation is required because of symptomatic deterioration, the valve is usually calcified and more seriously deformed than at the time of the first operation, and adequate reconstruction may not be possible. Accordingly, mitral valve replacement is then usually necessary.[108] Also, in patients with combined MS and MR, and in those with extensive calcification involving the commissures of the valve, mitral replacement rather than commissurotomy is often required. The operative mortality following mitral valve replacement ranges from 4 to 8 per cent in most hospitals. As described below (p. 1079), the long-term fate of the prosthetic valves is not yet clear; also, the hazards of lifelong anticoagulant treatment in patients with mechanical prostheses cannot be neglected. Therefore, in patients in whom preoperative evaluation suggests that valve replacement may be required, the threshold for operation should be higher than in patients believed to require commissurotomy alone.

BALLOON MITRAL VALVULOPLASTY
(Fig. 40–21, p. 1390)

This represents an alternative to surgical treatment of MS. The technique consists of advancing a small balloon flotation catheter across the interatrial septum (after transseptal puncture), enlarging the opening and advancing one large (23 to 25 mm) or two smaller (12 to 18 mm) balloons across the mitral orifice, and inflating them within the orifice.[109–114] Commissural separation and fracture of nodular calcium appear to be the mechanisms responsible for improvement in valvular function. As of July 1, 1987, a total of 54 patients with MS have been treated by this technique at Boston's Beth Israel Hospital.[115] Forty-nine of these have been successful and the patients are either asymptomatic or have experienced a marked reduction of symptoms. The average calculated mitral valve area has doubled from 1.0 to 2.0 cm^2, the transvalvular gradients and wedge pressures have declined from averages of 15 to 8 mm Hg and 24 to 16 mm Hg, respectively (Fig. 33–9). Four complications have occurred: one perforation of the left atrium, one vagal reaction, one cerebral embolus, and one death during the procedure. Small left-to-right interatrial shunts may persist. There has been one death attributable to the procedure. Balloon valvuloplasty is a palliative procedure in that it does not correct the scarring or shortening of the chordae tendineae or other subvalvular structures.

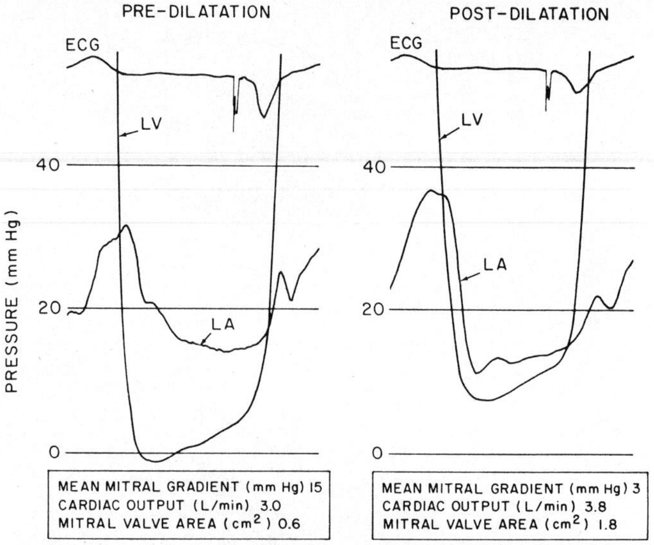

FIGURE 33–9. Simultaneous left atrial (LA) and left ventricular (LV) pressure before and after balloon valvuloplasty of the mitral valve in a patient with severe mitral stenosis. (Courtesy of Raymond G. McKay, M.D.)

While this technique is still in a developmental stage, it appears to be useful in patients who are unsuitable for surgery because of high risk. These may be very elderly patients with associated severe ischemic heart disease, as well as patients in whom MS is complicated by pulmonary, renal, or neoplastic disease. A second group consists of patients who refuse surgery. Also, it may be considered in women of childbearing age who may not accept a prosthesis with its attendant problems (p. 1080). If the risk associated with the procedure proves to be low, it may well be applicable for treating young patients with noncalcific MS in underdeveloped nations with limited facilities for open heart surgery.

MITRAL REGURGITATION

ETIOLOGY AND PATHOLOGY

The mitral valve apparatus involves the mitral annulus, the mitral leaflets per se, the chordae tendineae, and the papillary muscles. Abnormalities of any of these structures may cause mitral regurgitation (MR) (Table 33–4).[1, 10] The mitral valve prolapse syndrome, an important cause of MR, is discussed in this chapter (p. 1045).

ABNORMALITIES OF VALVE LEAFLETS. MR due to involvement of the valve *leaflets* occurs most commonly in chronic rheumatic heart disease and is more frequent in men than in women. It is a consequence of shortening, rigidity, deformity, and retraction of one or both cusps of the mitral valve as well as shortening and fusion of the chordae tendineae and papillary muscles.[116] Destruction of the mitral valve leaflets can also be a consequence of systemic lupus erythematosus,[117] penetrating and nonpenetrating trauma (p. 1542), and infective endocarditis (Chap. 34). Retraction of the mitral valve cusps during the healing phase of endocarditis can also cause MR.

ABNORMALITIES OF THE MITRAL ANNULUS

Dilatation. In a normal adult the mitral annulus measures approximately 10 cm in circumference. During systole, contraction of the surrounding left ventricular muscle causes the annulus to constrict, and this constriction contributes importantly to valve closure. MR secondary to dilatation of the mitral annulus (Fig. 33–10) can occur in any form of heart disease characterized by severe dilatation of the left ventricle.[118] It is often difficult to differentiate

TABLE 33–4 CAUSES OF ACUTE AND CHRONIC MITRAL REGURGITATION

TYPE	CONDITION
	Chronic Mitral Regurgitation
Inflammatory	Rheumatic heart disease
	Systemic lupus erythematosus
	Scleroderma
Degenerative	Myxomatous degeneration of mitral valve leaflets (Barlow's, click-murmur syndrome, prolapsing leaflet, mitral valve prolapse)
	Marfan syndrome
	Ehlers-Danlos syndrome
	Pseudoxanthoma elasticum
	Calcification of mitral valve annulus
Infective	Infective endocarditis on normal, abnormal, or prosthetic mitral valves
Structural	Ruptured chordae tendineae (spontaneous or secondary to myocardial infarction, trauma, mitral valve prolapse, endocarditis)
	Rupture or dysfunction of papillary muscle (ischemia or myocardial infarction)
	Dilatation of mitral valve annulus and left ventricular cavity (congestive cardiomyopathies, aneurysmal dilatation of the left ventricle)
	Hypertrophic cardiomyopathy
	Paravalvular prosthetic leak
Congenital	Mitral valve clefts or fenestrations
	Parachute mitral valve abnormality
	In association with
	Endocardial cushion defects
	Endocardial fibroelastosis
	Transposition of the great arteries
	Anomalous origin of the left coronary artery
	Acute Mitral Regurgitation
	Disorders of the mitral valve leaflets
	Infective endocarditis
	Trauma
	Left atrial myxoma
	Disorders of the chordae tendineae
	Infective endocarditis
	Rheumatic valvulitis
	Trauma
	Acute rheumatic fever
	"Spontaneous" rupture
	Disorders of the papillary muscles
	Dysfunction
	Ischemia
	Myocardial infarction
	Left ventricular dilatation
	Left ventricular aneurysm
	Rupture
	Trauma
	Acute myocardial infarct
	Myocardial abscess
	Prosthetic valve malfunction
	Deterioration of silastic disc
	Lodging of the ball or disc in the open position
	Dislodgement of the ball or disc
	Ring or strut fracture
	Paravalvular leak
	Suture or pledget dislodgement
	Deterioration of leaflets of tissue value
	Prosthetic valve endocarditis

Modified from Haffajee, C. I.: Chronic mitral regurgitation. *In* Dalen, J. E., and Alpert, J. S.: Valvular Heart Disease. 2nd ed. Boston, Little, Brown, and Company, 1987, p. 112 (top portion); and Rippe, J. M., and Howe, J. P., III: Acute mitral regurgitation. *In* Rippe, J. M., et al.: Intensive Care Medicine. Boston, Little, Brown, and Company, 1985 (bottom portion).

this secondary from the primary forms of MR, but it is notable that primary valvular regurgitation is often more severe than is regurgitation secondary to dilatation of the annulus.

Calcification. Idiopathic calcification of the mitral annulus is one of the most common cardiac abnormalities found at autopsy; in most hearts this degenerative change

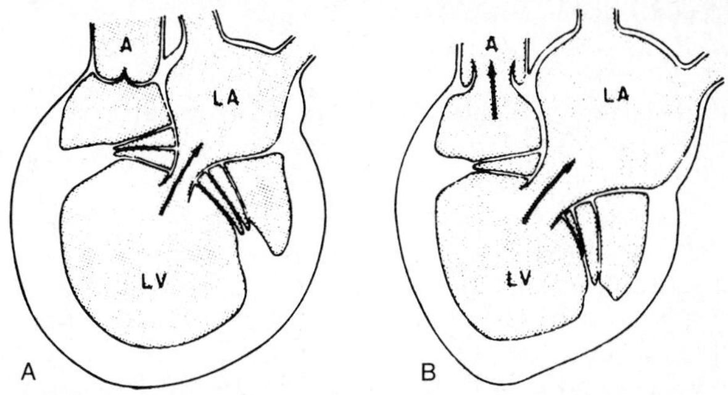

FIGURE 33–10. Proposed mechanism of regurgitation in left ventricular dilatation. The papillary muscles are displaced laterally and perhaps downward from the ring, permitting leaflet separation and regurgitation during early systole (*A*) and during ejection (*B*). (From Kremkau, E. L., et al.: Acquired, nonrheumatic mitral regurgitation: Clinical management with emphasis on evaluation of myocardial performance. Prog. Cardiovasc. Dis. *15*:414, 1973, by permission of Grune and Stratton, Inc.)

is of little functional consequence.[119] However, when it is severe it may be an important cause of MR in the elderly, and in contrast to MR secondary to rheumatic fever, this cause is more common in women than in men. In addition to the idiopathic form, degenerative calcification of the mitral annulus is accelerated by systemic hypertension, aortic stenosis, and diabetes, as well as by an intrinsic defect in the fibrous skeleton of the heart, such as occurs in the Marfan and Hurler syndromes. In these two conditions, the mitral annulus is not only calcified but also is dilated, further contributing to MR. The incidence of mitral annular calcification is also increased in patients with chronic renal failure with secondary hyperparathyroidism[120, 121] (Fig. 59–11, p. 1840). In the latter group it appears to be related to secondary hyperparathyroidism and an elevated calcium-phosphorus product.

When annular calcification is severe, a rigid, curved bar or ring of calcium encircles the mitral orifice (Fig. 6–20, p. 153), and calcific spurs may project into the adjacent left ventricular myocardium[122, 123]; the bulk of the calcium is located in the subvalvular region. The calcification may immobilize the basal portion of the mitral leaflets, preventing their normal excursion in diastole and coaptation in systole and aggravating the MR that results from loss of the normal sphincteric action of the mitral ring.[124, 125] Rarely, when severe calcification encroaches on or protrudes into the mitral orifice, obstruction to left ventricular filling may occur. Calcification of the aortic valve cusps is an associated finding in approximately 50 per cent of patients with severe annular calcification, but this rarely causes aortic stenosis. In patients with severe calcification the conduction system may be invaded by calcium, leading to atrioventricular and/or intraventricular conduction defects.[126] Occasionally, calcific deposits extend into the coronary arteries. The annulus may also become thick and rigid as a consequence of rheumatic involvement, and when this process is severe, it also can interfere with valve closure.

ABNORMALITIES OF THE CHORDAE TENDINEAE. These are important causes of MR. The chordae may be congenitally abnormal; rupture may be spontaneous ("primary")[127] or may occur as a consequence of infective endocarditis, trauma, rheumatic fever, myxomatous proliferation, or osteogenesis imperfecta.[128–132] In most cases no cause for chordal rupture is apparent, other than increased mechanical strain.[131] Chordae to the posterior leaflet rupture more frequently than to the anterior leaflets. Patients with idiopathic rupture of mitral chordae tendineae frequently exhibit pathological fibrosis of the papillary muscles. It is possible that the dysfunction of the papillary muscles may have caused stretching and ultimately rupture of the chordae. Chordal rupture may also result from acute left ventricular dilatation, regardless of etiology. Depending on the number and rate of chordal rupture, the resultant MR may be mild, moderate, or severe on the one hand or acute, subacute, or chronic on the other.

INVOLVEMENT OF THE PAPILLARY MUSCLES. Diseases of the left ventricular papillary muscles frequently cause MR.[133] Since these muscles are perfused by the terminal portion of the coronary vascular bed, they are particularly vulnerable to ischemia, and any disturbance in coronary perfusion may result in papillary muscle dysfunction (Figs. 33–11 and 33–12). When ischemia is transient, it results in temporary papillary muscle dysfunction and may cause transient episodes of MR during attacks of angina pectoris (p. 1321). When ischemia of papillary muscles is severe and persistent, as in acute myocardial infarction, it produces papillary muscle necrosis and chronic MR. The posterior papillary muscle, which is supplied by the posterior descending branch of the right coronary artery, becomes ischemic and infarcted more frequently than does the anterolateral papillary muscle, which is supplied by diagonal branches of the left anterior descending coronary artery and often by marginal branches from the left circumflex artery as well. Ischemia of the papillary muscle is caused most commonly by coronary artery disease, but it may also occur in severe anemia, shock, coronary arteritis of any etiology, and anomalous left coronary artery. In patients with healed myocardial infarcts, MR is frequent and is caused by dyskinesis of the left ventricular myocardium at the base of a papillary muscle.[135]

Left ventricular dilatation of any cause, including ischemia,[135] can alter the spatial relationships between the papillary muscles and the chordae tendineae and thereby result in MR (Fig. 33–10).[135a] Although *necrosis of a papillary muscle* is a frequent complication of myocardial infarction,[136] frank rupture of a papillary muscle is far less common. Total rupture of a papillary muscle is usually fatal because of the extremely severe MR that it produces.[137] However, rupture of one or two of the apical heads of a muscle, which results in a lesser degree of MR, makes survival possible, depending on the functional capacity of the left ventricle (Fig. 33–13).

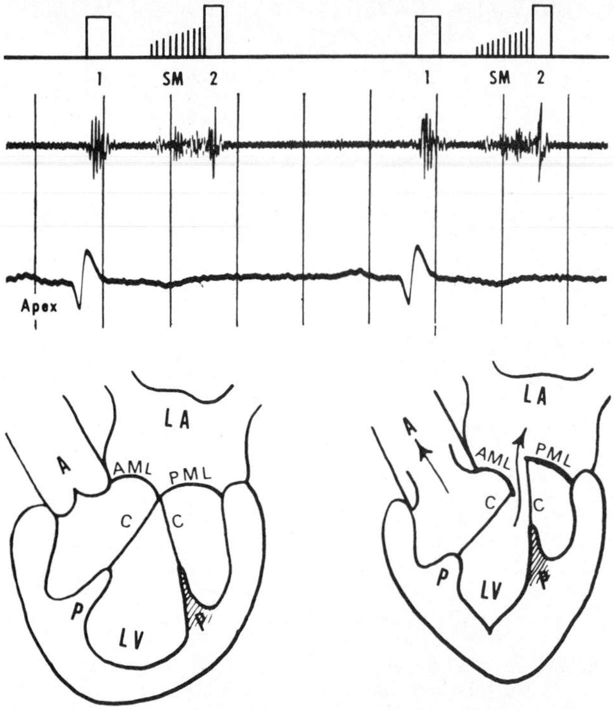

FIGURE 33–12. *Top,* Late systolic murmur (SM) that developed in a patient following an inferior myocardial infarction and is probably due to weakening of the posterior papillary muscle with prolapse of the mitral leaflet into the atrium during late systole. *Bottom,* Mitral regurgitation due to papillary muscle dysfunction. At the onset of systole (left), the anterior and posterior mitral valve leaflets (AML and PML) approximate. Later in systole (right), the anterior papillary muscle (P, nonhatched) contracts while the posterior papillary muscle (P, hatched) fails to contract because of ischemia or infarction. Part of the posterior leaflet is allowed to prolapse into the left atrium (LA) during systole, producing regurgitation. This process may involve either papillary muscle. C = chordae tendineae, LV = left ventricle, A = aorta. (From Ravin, A., et al.: Auscultation of the Heart. 3rd ed. Chicago, Year Book Medical Publishers, 1977, p. 99. Copyright © 1977 by Year Book Medical Publishers, Inc., Chicago.)

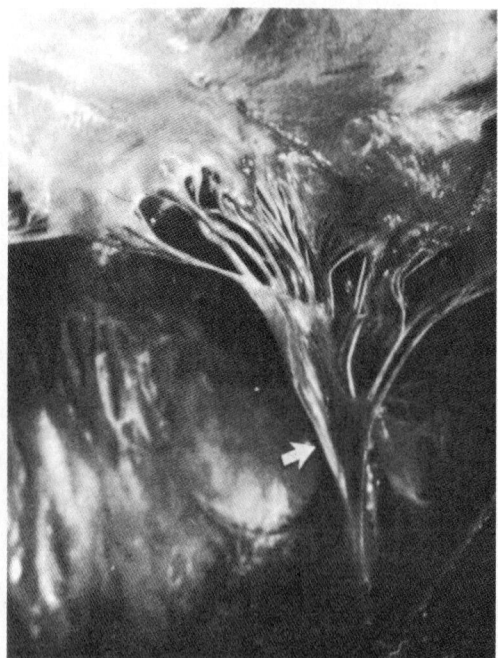

FIGURE 33–11. The posterior papillary muscle in a patient with chronic mitral regurgitation due to ischemic heart disease. The papillary muscle is thinned and replaced by fibrous tissue. The apical segment (arrows) is elongated and had undergone some calcification. (From Davies, M. J.: Aetiology and pathology of the diseased mitral valve. *In* Ionescu, M. I., and Cohn, L. H. [eds]: Mitral Valve Disease: Diagnosis and Treatment. London, Butterworths, 1985, p. 38.)

Some degree of MR is found in approximately 30 per cent of those patients with coronary artery disease who are being considered for coronary bypass surgery[135] and is secondary to ischemic damage of the papillary muscles or dilatation of the mitral valve ring or both.[138] The incidence and severity of regurgitation vary inversely with the left ventricular ejection fraction and directly with the left ventricular end-diastolic pressure.

A variety of other disorders of papillary muscles may also be responsible for the development of mitral regurgitation (Table 33–4).

These include congenital malposition; absence of one papillary muscle, resulting in the so-called parachute mitral valve syndrome (p. 941); and involvement or infiltration of papillary muscles by a variety of processes, including abscesses, granulomas, neoplasms, amyloidosis, and sarcoidosis.

Other causes of MR, discussed in greater detail elsewhere, include obstructive cardiomyopathy (p. 1418), pro-

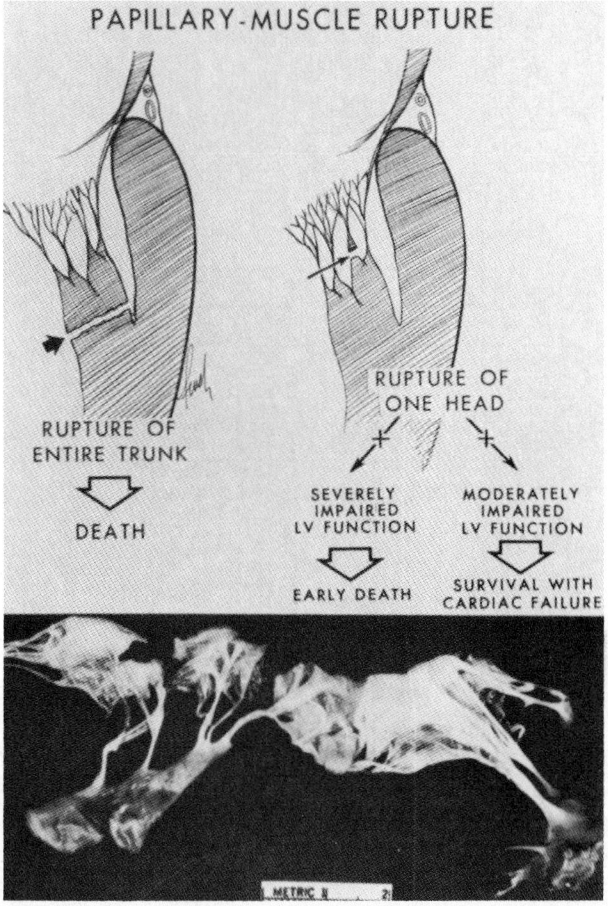

FIGURE 33–13. *Top*, Diagrammatic representation of the types of, and possible consequences of, papillary muscle rupture during acute myocardial infarction. It is likely that rupture of the entire trunk (*left*) is incompatible with survival in any patient, since a major portion of the support to both valve leaflets is destroyed. With rupture of an apical head (*right*), survival would appear to depend on the extent to which left ventricular function has been impaired by the infarct. With severe impairment, the additional burden of even modest mitral regurgitation may be intolerable, and death will ensue. If the left ventricle is less severely compromised, survival is possible for weeks or months, but congestive heart failure will invariably develop.

Bottom, Rupture of a portion of one papillary muscle during acute myocardial infarction in a 51-year-old man who underwent mitral valve replacement 3 months after the onset of infarction. Preoperatively, pulmonary arterial pressure was 60/28 mm Hg (mean = 40); pulmonary arterial wedge pressure, mean = 28, *v* = 42; left ventricular pressure = 74/17 mm Hg; and cardiac index = 1.7 liters/min/sq meter. The excised mitral valve shows the ventricular aspects of the leaflets. The leaflets are normal but the posteromedial papillary muscle is necrotic and fibrotic, and a portion of it is entwined in cordae tendineae at the margin of the anterior mitral leaflet. (From Roberts, W. C., et al.: Nonrheumatic valvular cardiac disease. A clinicopathologic survey of 27 different conditions causing valvular dysfunction. *In* Likoff, W. [ed.]: Cardiovascular Clinics. Vol. 5, No. 2, Valvular Heart Disease. Philadelphia, F. A. Davis, 1973, p. 395.)

lapse of the mitral valve (p. 1045), trauma affecting the leaflets[141] and/or papillary muscles,[142] a variety of congenital anomalies (p. 945) including cleft anterior leaflet[143] and ostium secundum atrial septal defect,[144] Kawasaki disease (p. 1014),[145] and left atrial myxoma (p. 1473).

PATHOPHYSIOLOGY

Since the regurgitant mitral orifice is in parallel with the aortic valve, the impedance to ventricular emptying is reduced in MR. Consequently, as the left ventricle decompresses into the left atrium—both during isometric contraction and early during ejection—the left ventricular volume declines. Almost half the regurgitant volume is ejected into the left atrium before the aortic valve opens.[146]

The volume of mitral regurgitant flow depends on the size of the regurgitant orifice as well as on the pressure gradient between the left ventricle and left atrium[147–151]; both of these factors—orifice size and pressure gradient—are labile. Left ventricular systolic pressure and therefore the left ventricular–left atrial gradient are dependent on systemic vascular resistance and forward stroke volume,[147] and in patients in whom the mitral annulus is not calcific or rigid, the cross-sectional area of the mitral annulus may be altered by many interventions. Thus, increases of both preload and afterload and depressions of contractility increase left ventricular size and enlarge the mitral annulus and thereby the regurgitant orifice.[151] In MR caused by conditions in which the mitral valve apparatus is not rigid, such as ventricular dilatation due to ischemic heart disease, hypertensive heart disease or cardiomyopathy, dysfunction of papillary muscles, and rupture of chordae tendineae, the volume of regurgitant flow is influenced significantly by left ventricular dimensions, which in turn affect the regurgitant orifice. When ventricular size is reduced by treatment with positive inotropic agents, diuretics and particularly vasodilators, the volume of regurgitant flow may become diminished, as reflected in the height of the *v* wave in the left atrial pressure pulse and in the intensity and duration of the systolic murmur. Conversely, left ventricular dilatation may increase MR.

In experiments in which the acute effects of equally severe MR and aortic regurgitation (AR) on the left ventricle were compared, left ventricular end-diastolic pressure, volume, and radius rose with both lesions, but far *less* so with MR.[152, 153] Peak left ventricular wall tension rose markedly when AR was induced but either did not change greatly or actually declined with MR. According to Laplace's law (p. 405), myocardial wall tension is related to the product of intraventricular pressure and ventricular radius. Since MR reduces both late systolic ventricular pressure and radius, left ventricular wall tension declines markedly (and proportionately to a greater extent than left ventricular pressure), permitting the velocity of myocardial fiber shortening to increase (Fig. 51–5*C*, p. 1668).

At any given left ventricular end-diastolic and aortic systolic pressures, MR reduces the tension developed by the left ventricular myocardium. The reduced load on the ventricle allows a greater proportion of the contractile energy of the myocardium to be expended in shortening than in tension development and explains how the left ventricle can adapt to the load imposed by chronic MR. Thus, it appears to be the reduction in left ventricular tension in MR that allows the left ventricle to increase its total output and ultimately accounts for the finding that patients with MR can sustain large regurgitant volumes for prolonged periods while maintaining forward cardiac output at normal levels for many years. Although the left ventricle initially compensates for the development of acute MR, in part by emptying more completely,[153] as regurgitation persists or increases, the function of the left ventricle deteriorates, and left ventricular end-diastolic volume increases progressively. This may enlarge the regurgitant orifice and thereby create a vicious circle in which "MR begets more MR."

A large volume of MR induced experimentally produces only slightly increased myocardial oxygen consumption,[154] because myocardial fiber shortening, which is elevated in MR, is not an important determinant of myocardial oxygen consumption[155] as are the three major factors (p. 1191).[159] One of these, tension, may be reduced, whereas the other two, contractility and heart rate, are little affected in this condition. In addition, the duration of left ventricular systolic tension is reduced in

MR. These experimental observations correlate with the low incidence of clinical manifestations of myocardial ischemia in patients with severe MR compared with that occurring in AS or AR or both, in which myocardial oxygen demands are augmented.

In patients with chronic MR, both left ventricular end-diastolic volume and mass are increased, with the degree of hypertrophy appropriate to the left ventricular dilatation, so that the ratio of left ventricular mass to end-diastolic volume is normal (Fig. 14–8, p. 432). In acute MR the left ventricle at first dilates rapidly. Before the myocardium becomes hypertrophied, the ratio of left ventricular mass to end-diastolic volume is reduced, i.e., the left ventricle is thin-walled.

Assessment of Myocardial Contractility in Mitral Regurgitation (See also p. 465)

Patients with severe MR often exhibit small elevations in ejection phase indices of myocardial contractility (p. 463), such as ejection fraction, extent, and velocity of circumferential fiber shortening (VCF) when they are in the compensated state as a consequence of reduced afterload.[156] However, by the time patients become symptomatic, peak and mean VCF have usually declined to normal levels. As MR persists, the tendency for a low impedance leak, which tends to increase myocardial shortening, is counteracted by the impairment of myocardial function characteristic of chronic overload. However, even in patients with overt heart failure secondary to MR, the ejection fraction and fractional fiber shortening may be only slightly reduced.[156, 157] Therefore, *normal* values for the ejection phase indices of myocardial performance in patients with severe MR may actually reflect impaired myocardial function, whereas a moderately reduced value (e.g., an ejection fraction of 40 to 50 per cent) generally signifies severe, not moderate, impairment of contractility. An ejection fraction under 40 per cent in patients with severe MR represents advanced myocardial dysfunction; such patients are high operative risks and may not experience marked improvement following mitral valve replacement, perhaps because of the increase in left ventricular afterload that occurs with abolition of the regurgitant leak.[158] In patients with chronic MR, there is often an increase in left ventricular compliance, so that ventricular end-diastolic volume may be increased with little or no elevation of end-diastolic pressure.[159] (Older patients with MR, however, exhibit an elevation of left ventricular end-diastolic pressure, probably as a consequence of a reduction of ventricular compliance.[160])

END-SYSTOLIC VOLUME. Preoperative myocardial contractility is an important determinant of the risk of operative death and of cardiac failure in the perioperative period and of the level of left ventricular function postoperatively. Therefore, it is not surprising that end-systolic pressure (or stress)/volume (or dimension) relation has emerged as a useful index for evaluating left ventricular function in patients with valvular regurgitation (p. 458).[160a, 161] Indeed, the simple measurement of end-systolic volume has been found to be more useful as a predictor of outcome than the ejection fraction, end-diastolic volume, or end-diastolic pressure.[162, 163, 163a] Patients with severe MR with a normal preoperative end-systolic volume (< 30 ml/m^2) retained normal left ventricular function postoperatively, whereas marked enlargement of the end-systolic volume (> 90 ml/m^2) signified a high perioperative mortality and residual left ventricular dysfunction. Patients with MR and modest enlargement of end-systolic volume (between 30 and 90 ml/m^2) usually tolerate operation satisfactorily but may have reduced left ventricular function postoperatively. For any level of end-systolic volume, patients with MR have more severe left ventricular dysfunction than do patients with aortic regurgitation.[161] This finding reflects the lower afterload in mitral regurgitation and correlates with the clinical observation that patients with mitral regurgitation have a less favorable response to surgical intervention than do those with aortic regurgitation.[162]

HEMODYNAMICS. Effective (forward) *cardiac output* is usually depressed in seriously symptomatic patients, whereas total left ventricular output (the sum of forward and regurgitant flow, which can be measured by radionuclide ventriculography)[163] is usually elevated. The atrial contraction (*a*) wave in the left atrial pressure pulse is usually not as prominent in MR as in MS, but the *v* wave is often much taller,[150] since it is inscribed during ventricular systole, when the left atrium is filled with blood from the pulmonary veins as well as from the left ventricle (Fig. 33–14). Indeed, backward transmission of the tall *v* wave into the pulmonary arterial bed may result in an early diastolic "pulmonary arterial *v* wave."[163b] During early diastole, as the distended left atrium suddenly empties; the *y* descent is particularly rapid. However, in patients with combined MS and MR, the *y* descent is gradual. Although a left atrioventricular pressure gradient persisting throughout diastole signifies the presence of significant associated MS, a brief early diastolic gradient may occur in patients with pure severe regurgitation as a result of the torrential flow of blood across a normal-sized mitral orifice (Fig. 33–2).

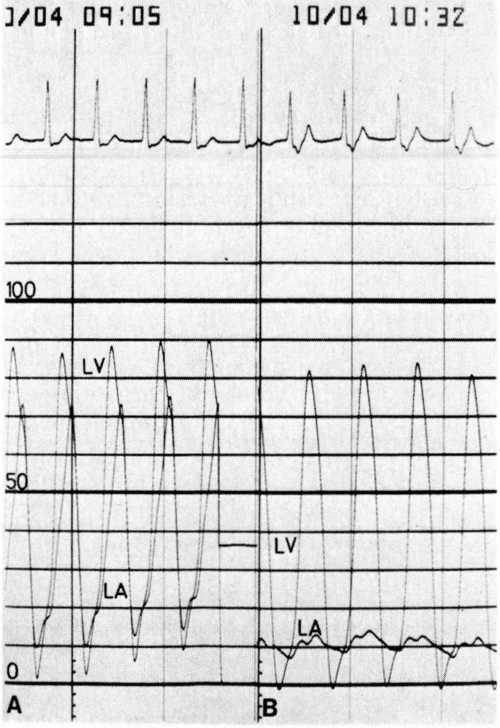

FIGURE 33–14. Intraoperative simultaneous left ventricular (LV) and left atrial (LA) pressures (mm Hg) before (*A*) and after (*B*) mitral valvuloplasty for correction of severe acute mitral regurgitation. Note the height of the *v* wave in the preoperative tracing. (From Barlow, J. B.: Perspectives on the Mitral Valve. Philadelphia, F. A. Davis, 1987, p. 257.)

LEFT ATRIAL COMPLIANCE. The compliance of the left atrium (and pulmonary venous bed) is an important determinant of the hemodynamic and clinical picture in MR. Three major subgroups of patients with severe MR based on left atrial compliance have been identified[153, 164, 165] (Figs. 33–15 and 33–16) and are characterized as follows:

1. Normal or Reduced Compliance. There is little enlargement of the left atrium but marked elevation of the mean left atrial pressure, particularly of the *v* wave,[166, 166a, 167, 167a] and pulmonary congestion is a prominent symptom. In most cases, severe MR has developed suddenly, as occurs with rupture of chordae tendineae, infarction of one of the heads of a papillary muscle, or perforation of a mitral leaflet as a consequence of trauma or endocarditis. Sinus rhythm is usually present; the left atrial wall frequently exhibits striking hypertrophy, is capable of contracting vigorously, and facilitates left ventricular filling. Thickening of the walls of the pulmonary veins and proliferative changes in the pulmonary arteries as well as marked elevation of pulmonary vascular resistance usually develop over the course of 6 to 12 months.

2. Markedly Increased Compliance. At the opposite end of the spectrum from patients in the first group are those with severe, longstanding MR with massive enlargement of the left atrium and normal or only slightly elevated

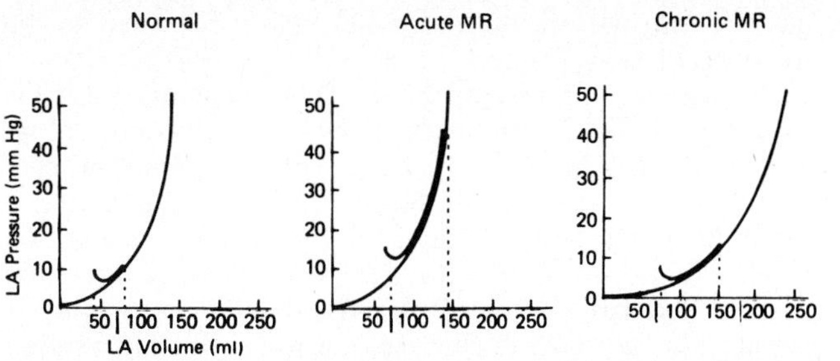

FIGURE 33–15. Schematic left atrial pressure-volume curves in a normal individual (*left*), a patient with acute mitral regurgitation (*center*), and a patient with chronic mitral regurgitation (*right*). The phasic increase in left atrial pressure and volume during left ventricular systole is indicated by the heavy trace superimposed on the left atrial pressure-volume curve. In the normal subject, there is an LA volume increase of 40 ml, due to return of blood from the pulmonary veins, during the period of time when the mitral valve is closed. This causes a peak *v* wave of 10 mm Hg. This valve acutely becomes insufficient (*center*), and the increase in LA volume during LV systole increases (in this example to 80 ml) because of the combination of the regurgitant volume and the pulmonary venous return, resulting in *v* waves to 45 mm Hg. In the same patient one year later (*right*) left atrial enlargement had occurred, so that the same degree of mitral regurgitation caused a much-reduced *v* wave because of increased left atrial compliance. (From Barry, W. H.: Invasive investigations for the diagnosis of mitral valve disease. *In* Ionescu, M. I., and Cohn, L. H. [eds.]: Mitral Valve Disease: Diagnosis and Treatment. London, Butterworths, 1985, p. 92.)

left atrial pressure. The atrial wall contains only a small remnant of muscle surrounded by a great deal of fibrous tissue. Longstanding MR in these patients has altered the physical properties of the left atrial wall and thereby displaced the atrial pressure-volume curve, allowing a normal or almost normal pressure to exist in a greatly enlarged left atrium. Pulmonary artery pressure and pulmonary vascular resistance are normal or only slightly elevated at rest. Atrial fibrillation and a low cardiac output are almost invariably present.[164]

3. Moderately Increased Compliance. This, the most common subgroup, consists of patients between the ends of the spectrum represented by groups 1 and 2; these patients have severe chronic MR and exhibit variable degrees of enlargement of the left atrium, associated with significant elevation of the left atrial pressure.

CLINICAL MANIFESTATIONS

(See Table 33–1, p. 1026)

HISTORY

The symptoms of patients with chronic MR are a function of the severity of regurgitation, its rate of progression, the level of pulmonary artery pressure, and the presence of associated valvular or coronary artery disease. Since symptoms do not usually develop in patients with chronic MR until the left ventricle fails, the time interval between the initial attack of rheumatic fever (when one has occurred) and the development of symptoms tends to be longer in MR than in MS and often exceeds 2 decades. Acute pulmonary edema occurs less frequently in chronic MR than in MS, presumably because sudden surges in left atrial pressure are less common.[18] Similarly, although hemoptysis and systemic embolization do occur in MR, they are less common than in MS. On the other hand, chronic weakness and fatigue secondary to a low cardiac output are more prominent features.

Patients with mild MR may remain asymptomatic for their entire lives.[55] The majority of patients with MR of rheumatic origin have only mild disability, unless regurgitation progresses as a result of chronic rheumatic activity, infective endocarditis, or rupture of chordae tendineae.[165] The development of atrial fibrillation affects the course adversely but not as dramatically as it does in MS, because the rapid ventricular rate often caused by this arrhythmia does *not* elevate left atrial pressure as markedly in mitral regurgitation. The course in patients with chronic MR tends to be less dramatic and punctuated with fewer acute complications than in patients with MS. However, this indolent course may, in fact, be deceptive. By the time that symptoms secondary to a reduced cardiac output and/or pulmonary congestion become apparent, serious and sometimes even irreversible left ventricular dysfunction may have developed.

In patients with severe chronic MR with a greatly enlarged left atrium and with relatively mild left atrial hypertension (group 2 with increased left atrial compliance, described above), pulmonary vascular resistance does not usually rise. Instead, the major symptoms, fatigue and exhaustion, are related to a low cardiac output. However, right heart failure, characterized by congestive hepatomegaly, ankle edema, and ascites, is observed both in patients

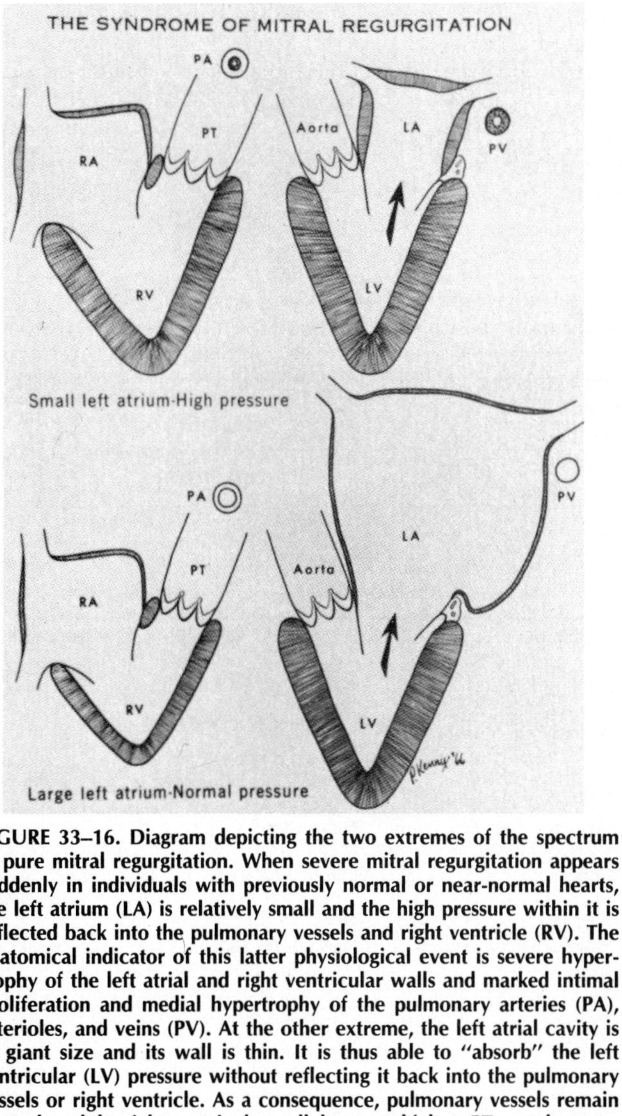

FIGURE 33–16. Diagram depicting the two extremes of the spectrum in pure mitral regurgitation. When severe mitral regurgitation appears suddenly in individuals with previously normal or near-normal hearts, the left atrium (LA) is relatively small and the high pressure within it is reflected back into the pulmonary vessels and right ventricle (RV). The anatomical indicator of this latter physiological event is severe hypertrophy of the left atrial and right ventricular walls and marked intimal proliferation and medial hypertrophy of the pulmonary arteries (PA), arterioles, and veins (PV). At the other extreme, the left atrial cavity is of giant size and its wall is thin. It is thus able to "absorb" the left ventricular (LV) pressure without reflecting it back into the pulmonary vessels or right ventricle. As a consequence, pulmonary vessels remain normal, and the right ventricular wall does not thicken. PT = pulmonary trunk; RA = right atrium. (From Roberts, W. C., et al.: Nonrheumatic valvular cardiac disease. A clinicopathologic survey of 27 different conditions causing valvular dysfunction. *In* Likoff, W. [ed.]: Cardiovascular Clinics. Vol. 5, No. 2, Valvular Heart Disease. Philadelphia, F. A. Davis, 1973, p. 403.)

with longstanding severe MR and in patients with acute regurgitation and elevated pulmonary vascular resistance. Angina pectoris is rare unless coronary artery disease coexists.

NATURAL HISTORY. This is variable and depends on a combination of the volume of regurgitation, the state of the myocardium, and the etiology of the underlying disorder. The condition in asymptomatic patients with mild MR usually remains stable for many years[166]; severe regurgitation develops in only a small percentage of these, in some cases because of intervening infective endocarditis[165] or rupture of chordae tendineae. Regurgitation tends to progress more rapidly in patients with connective tissue diseases, such as Marfan syndrome, than in those with chronic MR on a rheumatic basis. In an unselected group of patients with MR who were treated medically, approximately 80 per cent survived 5 years after the diagnosis and almost 60 per cent survived 10 years.[87] Patients with combined MS and MR had a poorer prognosis, with only 67 per cent surviving 5 years and 30 per cent surviving 10 years after diagnosis. Munoz et al., in studying a group of patients with greater disability, found that medically treated patients with severe MR had a 5-year survival rate of only 45 per cent.[36] Among medically treated patients with MR, the arteriovenous oxygen difference and ventricular end-diastolic volume were significant (inverse) predictors of survival.[166]

PHYSICAL EXAMINATION[168]

Palpation of the arterial pulse is helpful in differentiating aortic stenosis from MR, both of which may produce a prominent systolic murmur at the base of the heart. The carotid arterial upstroke is sharp in mitral regurgitation[168] and delayed in aortic stenosis; the volume of the pulse may be normal in both conditions or reduced in the presence of heart failure.

The cardiac impulse is brisk, hyperdynamic, and displaced to the left[18] (Fig. 3–28, p. 58), and a prominent left ventricular filling wave is frequently palpable in early diastole. Systolic expansion of the enlarged left atrium may result in a late systolic thrust in the parasternal region, which may be confused with right ventricular enlargement (p. 28).[169] Rarely, a greatly enlarged left atrium may be palpable in the third left intercostal space during systole.[18]

AUSCULTATION.[170] With severe, chronic MR due to defective valve cusps, S_1, produced by valve closure, is usually diminished.[120a] Wide splitting of S_2 is common and results from the shortening of left ventricular ejection and an earlier A_2 as a consequence of reduced resistance to left ventricular outflow. When pulmonary hypertension is present, P_2 is louder than A_2. The abnormal increase in the flow rate across the mitral orifice during the rapid filling phase is usually associated with an S_3, the auscultatory counterpart of a palpable rapid filling wave (Fig. 3–1, p. 43). A left ventricular S_3, i.e., one that is not augmented by inspiration, excludes predominant MS (unless aortic regurgitation, ischemic heart disease, or another cause of an S_3 is present).

The *systolic murmur* is the most prominent physical finding in MR; it must be differentiated from the systolic murmur heard in aortic stenosis, tricuspid regurgitation, ventricular septal defect and MS (Table 33–5). In most cases of severe MR the *systolic murmur* commences immediately after the soft S_1 and continues beyond and may obscure A_2 because of the persistence of the pressure difference between the left ventricle and left atrium (Fig. 4–2, p. 66). The holosystolic murmur of chronic mitral regurgitation is usually constant in intensity, blowing, high-pitched, and loudest at the apex (Fig. 4–11, p. 71) with radiation to the axilla and left infrascapular area; however, radiation toward the sternum or the aortic area may occur with abnormalities of the posterior leaflet. The murmur

TABLE 33–5 HELPFUL POINTS IN DIFFERENTIAL DIAGNOSIS OF MITRAL REGURGITATION, VENTRICULAR SEPTAL DEFECT, TRICUSPID REGURGITATION, AND AORTIC STENOSIS

Physical, Roentgenographic, or Electrocardiographic Feature	Mitral Regurgitation	Ventricular Septal Defect	Tricuspid Regurgitation	Aortic Stenosis
Systolic murmur	Harsh and pansystolic	Harsh and pansystolic	Pansystolic	Ejection, crescendo-decrescendo
Primary location of murmur	Apex	Left sternal border	Left sternal border	Base of heart; occasionally apical
Radiation of murmur	Axilla; occasionally base and neck	Left precordium	Little	Carotids
Thrill	Occasionally present at apex	Usually present at left sternal border	Rare	Occasionally present at base
Murmur with inspiration	No change	No change	Increases	No change
Valsalva maneuver	May increase	Increases or no change	No change	Decreases
Venous pressure	Often normal	Slightly elevated with prominent A and V waves	Elevated, with very prominent V waves	Usually normal
Pulsatile liver	No	No	Yes	No
Pulmonary component of S_2	Normal; occasionally increased	Normal or loud; usually delayed	Usually increased	Normal
Apical impulse	Hyperkinetic; occasional heaving	Hyperkinetic	Weak or normal	Forceful and sustained
ECG	Left ventricular hypertrophy; left atrial hypertrophy	Biventricular hypertrophy (Katz-Wachtel phenomenonon)	Right ventricular hypertrophy, occasional right atrial hypertrophy	Left ventricular hypertrophy with associated ST-T changes
Chest roentgenogram	Moderately enlarged heart, marked left atrial enlargement	Enlarged left and right ventricle	Enlarged right ventricle	Often normal heart size or left ventricular hypertrophy

From Haffajee, C. I.: Chronic mitral regurgitation. *In* Dalen, J. E., and Alpert, J. S.: Valvular Heart Disease. 2nd ed. Boston, Little, Brown and Company, 1987, p. 141.

TABLE 33–6 EFFECT OF VARIOUS INTERVENTIONS ON SYSTOLIC MURMURS

Intervention	Hypertrophic Obstructive Cardiomyopathy	Aortic Stenosis	Mitral Regurgitation	Mitral Prolapse
Valsalva	↑	↓	↓	↑ or ↓
Standing	↑	↑ or unchanged	↓	↑
Handgrip or squatting	↓	↓ or unchanged	↑	↓
Supine position with legs elevated	↓	↑ or unchanged	Unchanged	↓
Exercise	↑	↑ or unchanged	↓	↑
Amyl nitrite	↑ ↑	↑	↓	↑
Isoproterenol	↑ ↑	↑	↓	↑

↑ ↑ = Markedly increased.
Modified from Paraskos, J. A.: Combined valvular disease. *In* Dalen, J. E., and Alpert, J. S. (eds.): Valvular Heart Disease. Boston, Little, Brown and Company, 1981, p. 365.

shows little change even in the presence of large beat-to-beat variations of left ventricular stroke volume, as occur in atrial fibrillation, in contrast to most midsystolic (ejection) murmurs, such as in aortic stenosis, which vary greatly in intensity with stroke volume and therefore with the duration of diastole.[171] There is little correlation between the intensity of the systolic murmur and the severity of MR. Indeed, in patients with severe MR due to left ventricular dilatation or paraprosthetic valvular regurgitation or in those who have marked emphysema, obesity, or chest deformity, the systolic murmur may be barely audible or even absent.[172]

Pansystolic and late systolic murmurs (and pansystolic murmurs with late systolic accentuation) are characteristic of MR. When the murmur is confined to late systole, the regurgitation is usually mild and may be secondary to prolapse of the mitral valve or papillary muscle dysfunction, conditions that cause late systolic regurgitation. These causes of MR are frequently associated with a normal S_1 because initial closure of the mitral valve cusps may be unimpaired. The systolic murmur is usually of no more than Grade 3/6 intensity, is a mid to late diamond-shaped murmur, or exhibits late systolic accentuation and radiates more frequently to the lower left sternal border than to the axilla.[133] The murmur of papillary muscle dysfunction is particularly variable; it may become accentuated or holosystolic during acute myocardial ischemia and often disappears when ischemia is relieved.[173] The response of a mid- to late-systolic murmur to a number of maneuvers, as described on page 1049, helps to establish the diagnosis of prolapse of the mitral valve.

Dynamic Auscultation (Fig. 2–21, p. 38). The holosystolic murmur of rheumatic MR shows little variation during respiration. However, sudden standing and amyl nitrite inhalation usually diminish the murmur (Table 33–6), whereas squatting and methoxamine or phenylephrine augment it. The murmur is reduced during the strain of the Valsalva maneuver and shows a left-sided response, i.e., a transient overshoot, six to eight beats following release. The murmur is usually intensified by isometric exercise, differentiating it from the systolic murmurs of valvular aortic stenosis and hypertrophic obstructive cardiomyopathy, both of which are reduced by this intervention. The murmur of MR due to left ventricular dilatation decreases in intensity and duration with effective therapy with cardiac glycosides, diuretics, rest, and particularly vasodilators.

The holosystolic murmur of MR resembles that produced by a ventricular septal defect. However, the latter is usually loudest at the left sternal border rather than the apex and is often accompanied by a parasternal thrill. The murmur of MR may also be confused with that of tricuspid regurgitation, which is usually heard best along the left sternal border, is augmented during inspiration, and is accompanied by a prominent *v* wave and *y* descent in the jugular venous pulse.

When the chordae tendineae to the posterior leaflet of the mitral valve rupture, the regurgitant jet is often directed anteriorly, so that it impinges on the atrial septum adacent to the aortic root and causes a systolic murmur most prominent at the base of the heart, which can be confused with that of aortic stenosis. The acoustic energy derived from the mitral regurgitant jet may be transmitted to the aorta by the impact of the jet on the portion of the left atrial wall adjacent to the aortic root.[174] On the other hand, when the chordae to the anterior leaflet rupture, the jet is usually directed to the posterior wall of the left atrium, and the murmur may be transmitted to the spine or even to the top of the head.[175]

Patients with rheumatic disease of the mitral valve exhibit a spectrum of abnormalities, ranging from pure MS to pure MR. The presence of an S_3, a rapid left ventricular filling wave and left ventricular impulse on palpation, and a soft S_1 all favor predominant MR, whereas an accentuated S_1, a prominent OS with a short A_1-OS interval, and a soft short systolic murmur all point to predominant MS. Elucidation of the predominant valvular lesion may be complicated by the presence of a holosystolic murmur of tricuspid regurgitation in patients with pure MS and pulmonary hypertension; this murmur, as has already been noted, may sometimes be heard at the apex when the right ventricle is greatly enlarged and may therefore be mistaken for the murmur of MR. Many patients with severe tricuspid regurgitation have a low cardiac output and an inaudible or barely audible diastolic murmur of MS, further complicating the clinical diagnosis. An S_3 originating from the right ventricle in patients with MS and pulmonary hypertension may falsely suggest the presence of MR. On the other hand, systolic expansion of the left atrium, as occurs in severe MR, often produces a late systolic parasternal expansion that may be confused with right ventricular hypertrophy and falsely attributed to mitral stenosis.

LABORATORY EXAMINATION

(Table 33–7)

ELECTROCARDIOGRAM. The principal *electrocardiographic* findings in patients with mitral regurgitation are left atrial enlargement and atrial fibrillation.[60, 170, 176, 177] Electrocardiographic evidence of left ventricular enlargement occurs in about one-third of patients with severe MR. Approximately 15 per cent exhibit electrocardiographic evidence of right ventricular hypertrophy, a change which reflects the presence of pulmonary hypertension of sufficient severity to counterbalance not only the normally larger but actually hypertrophied left ventricle.

RADIOLOGICAL FINDINGS (See also p. 154). Cardiomegaly with left ventricular, and particularly with left atrial, enlargement is a common finding in patients with chronic severe MR.[72, 178] However, there is little correlation between left atrial size and pressure. Changes in the lung

TABLE 33–7 NONINVASIVE ASSESSMENT OF MITRAL REGURGITATION: COMPARISON OF FINDINGS IN ACUTE AND CHRONIC FORMS

ACUTE MITRAL REGURGITATION	CHRONIC MITRAL REGURGITATION
ECG	
Commonly normal unless acute ischemia is the cause of regurgitation	Left atrial enlargement (P mitrale) Atrial fibrillation common Left ventricular hypertrophy common with severe regurgitation
Radiology and fluoroscopy	
Heart size usually normal If regurgitation is severe may be pulmonary congestion and interstitial edema	Cardiomegaly common, mainly due to left ventricular enlargement Left atrial enlargement, especially with rheumatic mitral disease Fluoroscopy may demonstrate calcium in rheumatic mitral disease
Phonocardiography and pulse tracings	
Systolic murmur frequently terminates before S_2 S_3 common Apex cardiogram shows marked systolic impulse	Systolic murmur usually holosystolic S_3 occurs with more severe regurgitation Systolic impulse less marked than with acute severe mitral regurgitation
M-mode echocardiography	
Left atrium usually of normal size Left ventricle usually of normal size, may be vigorously hypercontractile Cause of acute regurgitation may be demonstrated; flail mitral leaflet, ruptured chordae or vegetations in infective endocarditis, etc.	Left atrium usually enlarged Left ventricle frequently dilated, with signs of volume overload Cause of chronic regurgitation may be defined; rheumatic disease, mitral valve prolapse, etc.
Two-dimensional echocardiography	
In both acute and chronic regurgitation more clearly defines severity of left ventricular volume overload and enhances assessment of left ventricular function. In majority of cases can define etiology of regurgitation, and is especially useful in elucidating difficult diagnostic problems in M-mode echocardiography	
Doppler ultrasound	
Facilitates detection of mitral regurgitation by identifying turbulent flow within left atrium in systole Aids quantification of degree of mitral regurgitation	
Nuclear cardiology	
Principal use is in quantitative assessment of ventricular performance, e.g., ejection fraction (EF). Quantitation of the degree of mitral regurgitation can be achieved by comparing left and right ventricular stroke volume. In acute regurgitation the EF is usually normal if increased. A decreased EF implies pre-existing regurgitation or severe ischemic damage to the left ventricle. In chronic regurgitation the EF is usually normal and may be decreased if long-standing volume overload leads to left ventricular dysfunction	

From Bloomfield, P., et al.: Noninvasive investigations for the diagnosis of mitral valve disease. *In* Ionescu, M. I., and Cohn, L. H.: Mitral Valve Disease: Diagnosis and Treatment. London, Butterworths, 1985, p. 63.

fields are less prominent in MR than in MS, but interstitial edema with Kerley B lines is frequently seen with acute regurgitation or with progressive left ventricular failure.

In patients with combined MS and MR, overall cardiac enlargement and particularly left atrial dilatation are prominent findings. However, it is often difficult to determine which lesion is predominant from the plain chest roentgenogram, since it may be difficult to distinguish between right and left ventricular enlargement. Predominant MS is suggested by relatively mild cardiomegaly, principally straightening of the left cardiac border with significant changes in the lung fields, whereas predominant MR is more likely when the heart is greatly enlarged and the changes in the lungs are relatively inconspicuous. When the left atrium is aneurysmally dilated chronic MR is almost always the dominant lesion. Calcification of the mitral valve occurs in patients with stenosis, regurgitation, or mixed lesions.

Calcification of the mitral annulus, an important cause of MR in the elderly, is most prominent in the posterior third of the cardiac silhouette[72] and is best visualized on films exposed in the lateral or right anterior oblique projection, in which it appears as a dense, coarse, C-shaped opacity (Fig. 6–24, p. 155).

The diagnosis of MR can be established definitively by means of left *ventricular angiocardiography*,[179] the prompt appearance of contrast material in the left atrium following its injection into the left ventricle indicating the presence of MR. The injection should be rapid enough to permit left ventricular opacification but slow enough to avoid the development of premature ventricular contractions, which can induce spurious regurgitation.

The regurgitant volume can be determined from the difference between the total left ventricular stroke volume, estimated angiocardiographically, and the simultaneous measurement of the effective forward stroke volume by Fick's method (p. 252). The results of such studies suggest that in patients with severe regurgitation, the regurgitant volume may approach and in rare instances may even exceed the effective forward stroke volume.

Qualitative but clinically useful estimates of the severity of MR may be made by cineangiographic observation of the degree of opacification of the left atrium and pulmonary veins following the injection of contrast material into the left ventricle. MR secondary to rheumatic heart disease is characterized angiographically by a central regurgitant jet and by thickened leaflets that exhibit reduced motion, whereas in regurgitation due to other causes, particularly dilatation of the mitral annulus or ruptured chordae and papillary muscles, the systolic jet may be eccentric, and the valves consist of thin filaments that display excessive motion. The etiology of the regurgitation, e.g., prolapse of the mitral valve, and a flail leaflet are often distinguishable angiographically.

ECHOCARDIOGRAPHY (See also p. 105). M-mode and two-dimensional echocardiography are more useful in determining the etiology and hemodynamic consequences of than in estimating the severity of MR.[181] Severe MR results in enlargement of the left atrium and left ventricle, with increased systolic motion of both of these chambers. The underlying cause of the regurgitation—e.g., rupture of chordae tendineae,[182] mitral valve prolapse (Figs. 5–50 to 5–52, p. 106), a flail leaflet (Fig. 5–53, p. 107), and vegetation, Fig. 5–53, p. 107)—can often be determined, and the echocardiogram may also show calcification of the mitral annulus as a band of dense echoes between the mitral apparatus and the posterior wall of the heart.[122, 183]

Two-dimensional echocardiography may be useful in the detection of significant MR by demonstrating failure of the leaflets to close; flail leaflets and valvular prolapse may also be identified by this technique (Figs. 5–51 and 5–52, p. 106). This technique is also useful for estimating the hemodynamic consequences of MR; with left ventricular dysfunction, end-diastolic and end-systolic volumes are increased.

Doppler echocardiography in MR reveals a high-velocity jet in the left atrium during systole. The severity of the regurgitation is a function of the distance from the valve that the jet can be detected and the size of the left atrium. Both color flow Doppler (Fig. 5–49, color plate No. 2) and pulsed techniques[184–186] have been found to correlate well with angiographic methods in estimating the severity of MR.

RADIOISOTOPE ANGIOGRAPHY. Gated pool imaging or first-pass angiography may reveal an increased end-diastolic volume; the regurgitant fraction can be estimated from the ratio of left ventricular to right ventricular stroke volume[163, 187]; in patients with mitral regurgitation and impaired left ventricular function, ejection fraction fails to rise normally during exercise.[188] Radionuclide angiograms are useful for interval follow-up of patients. Progressive increases in ventricular end-diastolic or end-systolic volumes often suggest that surgical treatment is necessary (see below).

ACUTE MITRAL REGURGITATION

The causes of acute MR are shown in Table 33–4 (*bottom*). They are diverse, however, as might be anticipated, they represent acute manifestations of disease processes which may, under other circumstances, cause chronic MR. Especially important causes of acute MR are infective endocarditis with disruption of valve leaflets or rupture of chordae tendinae, ischemic dysfunction or rupture of a papillary muscle, and malfunction of a prosthetic valve.

One major hemodynamic difference between acute and chronic MR derives from the differences in the compliance of the left atrium, as discussed on page 1039 and as illustrated in Figures 33–15 and 33–16. As shown in Table 33–8 (*top*), acute severe MR causes a marked reduction of forward stroke volume, a slight reduction of end-systolic volume, a small rise in end-diastolic volume, and an elevation of ejection fraction. The differences in the clinical features between acute and chronic MR are summarized in Table 33–8 (*bottom*). In patients with acute MR with a normal-sized left atrium (group 1 with normal or reduced left atrial compliance, described above), the left atrial pressure rises abruptly, possibly leading to pulmonary edema, marked elevation of pulmonary vascular resistance, and right-sided heart failure. Because the *v* wave is markedly elevated in acute MR, the pressure gradient between the left ventricle and atrium declines at the end of systole, and the murmur may not be holosystolic but decrescendo, ending well before A_2 (Fig. 4–16, p. 73). It is usually lower pitched and softer than the murmur of chronic MR. Pulmonary hypertension, common in acute MR, may increase the intensity of P_2 and the murmurs of pulmonary and tricuspid regurgitation, and a right-sided S_4 may develop. Rarely in patients with severe acute MR, a *v* wave (late systolic pressure rise) in the pulmonary artery pressure pulse may cause premature closure of the pulmonary valve, early P_2, and paradoxical splitting of S_2.[170] Acute MR, even if severe, often does not increase overall cardiac size on the chest roentgenogram and may produce only mild left atrial enlargement despite marked elevation of left atrial pressure. With acute MR, there may be little increase in the internal diameter of either of these chambers on the echocardiogram, but increased systolic motion of the ventricle is prominent.

ACUTE VS. CHRONIC MITRAL REGURGITATION

(See Table 33–8)

MANAGEMENT

MEDICAL TREATMENT

This includes all the measures used in the treatment of heart failure, as outlined in Chapter 17. Afterload reduction is of conspicuous benefit in the management of MR—both the acute and the chronic forms.[189, 189a, 190] By reducing the impedance to ejection into the aorta, the volume of blood regurgitating into the left atrium is reduced; it causes left atrial pressure and, in particular, the elevated *v* wave, to decline. Thus vasodilator therapy is actually directed at relieving the physiological abnormality rather than simply dealing with its consequences. In addition, decreasing left ventricular volume reduces the size of the mitral annulus and thereby the regurgitant orifice.[191] Afterload reduction with intravenous nitroprusside may be life-saving in acute MR due to rupture of the head of a papillary muscle occurring in the course of an acute myocardial infarction. It may permit stabilization of the patient's condition and thereby allow operation to be carried out with the patient in an optimal condition. When surgical treatment is contraindicated, chronic afterload reduction with an angiotensin inhibitor or oral hydralazine may improve the clinical state for months or even years in patients with severe, chronic MR. Digitalis glycosides play a more important role in the management of MR than of MS. Like diuretics, they are indicated in patients with MR, cardiomegaly, and sinus rhythm. Cardiac glycosides are particularly helpful in patients with established atrial fibrillation.

Antiarrhythmic therapy with quinidine or procainamide may be helpful in suppressing frequent atrial or ventricular premature contractions as well as in maintaining sinus

TABLE 33–8 CHARACTERISTICS OF ACUTE AND CHRONIC REGURGITATION

	End diastolic volume	End systolic volume	Forward stroke volume	Ejection fraction	Left atrial compliance	Left atrial pressure	LV muscle function
Acute MR	↑	↓	↓ ↓	↑	n	↑ ↑ ↑	n
Compensated chronic MR	↑ ↑ ↑	↓	n	↑	↑	n or ↑	n
Decompensated chronic MR	↑ ↑ ↑ ↑	↑ ↑	n or ↓	n or ↓	↑	↑ ↑	↓ ↓ ↓

CLINICAL FEATURES

Clinical feature	Chronic mitral regurgitation	Acute mitral regurgitation
Systolic murmur	Harsh, pansystolic	Softer, low pitched, decrescendo, ends before A_2
Primary location of murmur	Apex	Base of heart
Radiation of murmur	Axilla	Neck, spine, top of head
Thrill	Apex	Absent
Venous pressure	Normal	Increased with large V waves
Apical impulse	Hyperkinetic, heaving	Hyperkinetic, heaving until LV failure occurs
ECG	LVH, LAE	Normal or infarct pattern
Chest x-ray	Cardiomegaly, marked LA enlargement, Kerley B lines	Normal size heart, may show pulmonary edema

n = normal, LA = Left atrial, LAE = Left atrial enlargement, LVH = Left ventricular hypertrophy.

Modified from Kusiak, V., and and Brest, A. N.: Acute mitral regurgitation: Pathophysiology and management. *In* Frankl, W. S., and Brest, A. N. (eds.): Cardiovascular Clinics. Valvular Heart Disease: Comprehensive Evaluation and Management. Philadelphia, F. A. Davis, 1986, p. 273 (top portion); and Carabello, B. A., and Grossman, W.: Effects of acute and chronic mitral regurgitation on left ventricular mechanics and contractile muscle function. *In* Duran, C., et al. (eds.): Recent Progress in Mitral Valve Disease. London, Butterworths, 1984, p. 188 (bottom portion).

rhythm following electrical or pharmacological conversion from atrial fibrillation. Appropriate prophylaxis to prevent infective endocarditis (p. 1175) is indicated.

Left-heart catheterization, selective left ventricular angiocardiography, and coronary arteriography are indicated in patients with some functional disability despite optimal medical management. The objectives of these studies are to (1) confirm the presence of regurgitation and estimate its severity; (2) aid in the identification of patients with primary myocardial disease and relatively mild, functional MR secondary to ventricular dilatation who are not likely to benefit greatly from operation and in whom the operative risk is relatively high; (3) detect and assess the severity of any associated valve lesions; and (4) determine the presence and assess the extent of coronary artery disease. Because of the additional risks when surgical treatment is carried out in patients with left ventricular dysfunction, definitive diagnosis and characterization of left ventricular function and consideration of surgical treatment should not be deferred until the patient has developed severe heart failure.

SURGICAL TREATMENT

When operative treatment is under consideration, the chronic, often slowly progressive nature of MR must be weighed against the immediate risks and long-term uncertainties attendant upon surgery. Surgical mortality depends on the patient's hemodynamic and clinical state, particularly the function of the left ventricle, the presence of associated conditions such as renal, hepatic, or pulmonary disease, as well as on the experience of the surgical team. It does not appear to depend significantly on which of the currently widely used tissue or mechanical valve prostheses is employed. These are discussed on pages 1078 to 1081.

Reconstructive procedure (annuloplasty), often using a rigid or semirigid prosthetic ring (i.e., a Carpentier ring), (Fig. 33–17) or direct suture repair of the valve (Fig. 33–18), replacement reimplantation, elongation, or shortening of chordae tendineae has been successful in selected patients with pure or predominant MR. This includes patients who have severe noncalcific MR, a dilated mitral annulus, MR secondary to ruptured chordae to the posterior leaflet or perforation of a mitral leaflet due to infective endocarditis, absence of severe subvalvular chordal thickening, and no major loss of leaflet substance.[129, 192–201] A number of surgeons, particularly in Europe, have reported a relatively low operative mortality rate, in the range of 5 per cent, with long-term clinical improvement in the majority of survivors.[193] The results of these "plastic" operations have, in general, been more favorable in children and adolescents with pliable valves and in patients with severe coronary artery disease and MR secondary to annular dilatation, papillary muscle dysfunction or rupture, or chordal rupture. The advantage of repair of MR (as opposed to replacement with a prosthetic valve) are many; chronic anticoagulation and the hazards of bleeding and thromboembolism attendant upon implantation of a mechanical prosthesis are largely eliminated, as are the risks of late failure of a bioprosthesis. However, there is a distinct "learning curve" for mitral reconstructive procedures.[197] Furthermore, many regurgitant valves, particularly those which are thickened, severely deformed, calcified, and partly stenotic, do not lend themselves to reconstruction; mitral valve replacement is necessary. When severe MR is caused by myxomatous degeneration—especially when there is severe associated chordal disease—mitral valve replacement is usually required.[196]

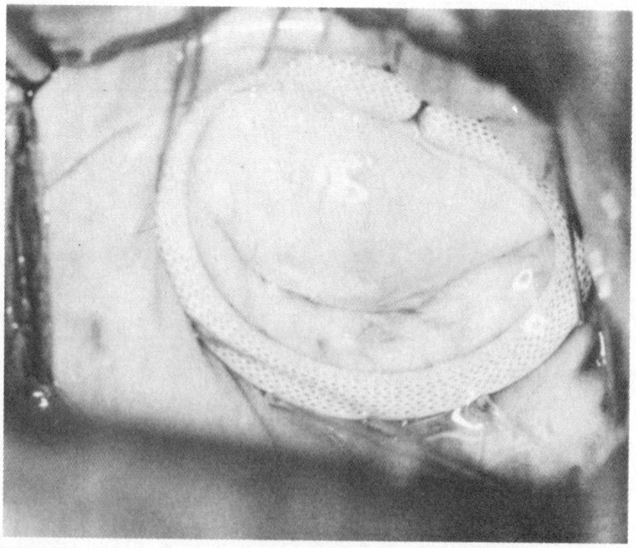

FIGURE 33–17. Intraoperative photograph of mitral valve after successful completion of valvuloplasty utilizing a Carpentier ring. Note that the apposition line between the anterior and posterior leaflets is regular and parallel to the posterior annulus of the mitral valve. (From Barlow, J. B.: Perspectives on the Mitral Valve. Philadelphia, F. A. Davis, 1987, p. 256.)

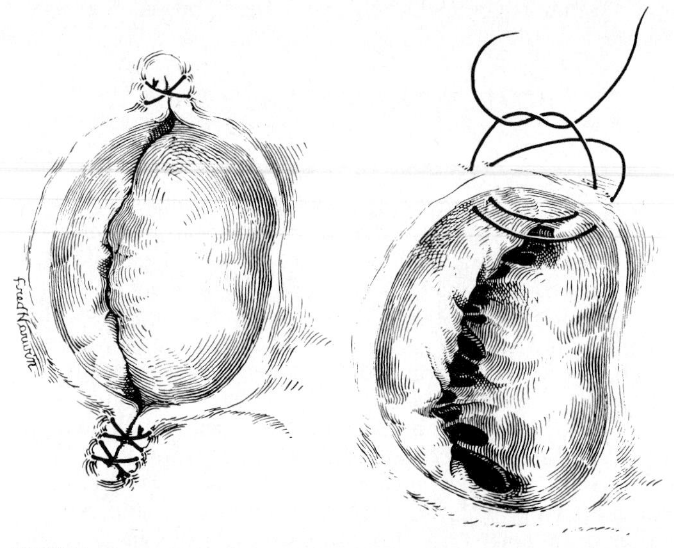

FIGURE 33–18. Commissural plication of the regurgitant mitral valve annulus. (From Starr, A., and Macmanus, Q.: Acquired valvular heart disease. *In* Effler, D. B. [ed.]: Blades' Surgical Diseases of the Chest. 4th ed. St. Louis, C. V. Mosby Co., 1978, p. 513.)

RESULTS. Mortality rates of 1 to 4 per cent in patients with predominant MS and of 2 to 7 per cent in patients with pure or predominant MR who undergo isolated mitral valve replacement operated upon electively in functional Class II or III are now common in many centers.[129, 202–211] Age per se is no barrier to successful surgery; mitral valve replacement can be carried out in patients older than 70 with the same or only slightly higher risk as in younger patients,[211] if their general health status is adequate. Surgical treatment substantially improves survival in patients with symptomatic MR. Factors such as an age of less than 60 years, a preoperative New York Heart Association functional Class of II, a cardiac index exceeding 2.0 liters/min/m^2, a left ventricular end-diastolic pressure less than 12 mm Hg, and a normal ejection fraction and end-systolic volume all correlate with improved immediate as well as long-term survival. Patients with moderate impairment of the ejection fraction (40 to 50 per cent) exhibit improved survival following surgical compared with medical treatment.[166] In other series, only age and preoperative ejection fraction predicted long-term survival following mitral valve replacement.[210]

In most patients with MR, the symptomatic state and thus the quality of life improve following valve replacement. Severe pulmonary hypertension is relieved almost uniformly,[105, 106] and left ventricular end-diastolic volume and mass are reduced. However, in contrast to patients with aortic or MS, whose cardiac function and cardiac symptoms generally improve following operation, patients with MR who had marked left ventricular dysfunction preoperatively sometimes remain symptomatic with a depressed ejection fraction[213] after a technically satisfactory operation. Furthermore, long-term survival in patients with predominant MR who undergo mitral valve replacement may be poorer than in those with pure stenosis or mixed stenotic and regurgitant lesions, presumably because left ventricular dysfunction may be quite advanced and largely irreversible by the time patients with pure regurgitation become seriously symptomatic.[214–219] Since, as indicated elsewhere, (p. 1027), MR reduces ventricular afterload, abolition of regurgitation raises afterload and thereby may interfere with left ventricular emptying, causing a reduction of the ejection fraction[159, 210] and an increase of end-systolic volume; these hemodynamic changes may be particularly troublesome during the early postoperative period, when vasodilator treatment may be effective. However, even though it is clearly desirable to operate on patients with MR before they develop marked left ventricular dysfunction, and despite these limitations of the results of surgical treatment in patients with severe left ventricular failure, operation is still indicated in the majority of these patients, since conservative therapy has little to offer.

The cause of the MR also plays an important role in the outcome following surgical treatment. In patients in whom mitral dysfunction is secondary to ischemic heart disease, the 5-year survival rate is about 30 per cent, whereas in rheumatic mitral regurgitation it is much better, approximately 70 per cent. Furthermore, occlusive coronary artery disease coexisting with, but not the primary cause of, mitral dysfunction is associated with decreased perioperative and long-term postoperative survival as well.[220] However, some improvement from mitral valve replacement can be expected even in patients with MR secondary to ischemic heart disease who are medically unresponsive and in congestive heart failure, as long as the cardiac index and ejection fraction exceed 1.5 liters/min/m^2 and 35 per cent, respectively. When left ventricular dysfunction is more severe, however, the risk of operative mortality becomes prohibitive.[221, 222]

Surgical Treatment of Acute Mitral Regurgitation. Emergency surgical treatment of acute left ventricular failure caused by acute MR due to myocardial infarction and rupture of the head of a papillary muscle, by trauma to the mitral valve, or by endocarditis is associated with higher mortality rate than is the elective surgical treatment of chronic MR. However, unless such patients with acute, severe MR and heart failure are treated aggressively, a fatal outcome is almost certain. If the condition of patients with MR secondary to acute infarction can be stabilized by medical treatment, it is preferable to defer operation until 4 to 6 weeks after infarction. Vasodilator treatment may be useful during this period. However, medical management should not be prolonged if multisystem (renal or pulmonary or both) failure occurs. Surgical mortality is also higher in patients with refractory heart failure (functional Class IV), in those in whom a previously implanted prosthetic valve must be replaced because of thromboembolism or valve dysfunction, and in those with active infective endocarditis (of a natural or prosthetic valve). Despite the higher surgical risks, the efficacy of early operation has been established in patients with infective endocarditis complicated by medically uncontrollable congestive heart failure, recurrent emboli, or both[216] (p. 1122). Since fungal endocarditis responds poorly to medical management, it is now the practice to recommend valve replacement in these cases *before* the onset of heart failure or embolization.

INDICATIONS FOR OPERATION. In view of advanced surgical techniques, reductions in operative mortality, improvements in mitral reconstructive procedures and artificial valves, as well as poor long-term results in many patients whose MR is corrected after a long history of heart failure, a more aggressive stance concerning the desirability of operation is in order. Only a few years ago I, along with many cardiologists, recommended operation for patients with chronic severe MR only if they were in functional Class III or IV,[223] i.e., with symptoms at rest or on ordinary activity despite intensive medical treatment. However, it is now my policy to recommend operation also for patients with severe MR who are in Class II, i.e., who become distinctly symptomatic only on heavy exertion, particularly if cardiomegaly and an elevated left ventricular end-systolic volume ($>$ 30 ml/m^2 BSA) persist despite aggressive medical therapy. Patients with severe MR who are asymptomatic or only mildly symptomatic and have normal ventricular function are considered to be candidates for surgical treatment only if it is likely that a reconstructive procedure will be sufficient. A useful approach is to follow the end-systolic wall stress/end-systolic volume index ratio (p. 463) using noninvasive techniques and to time operation when the index has begun to fall but before the patient becomes severely symptomatic. If valve replacement is likely to be necessary, a more cautious approach is indicated. Patients with moderate and even severe MR may live for many years with little deterioration of their condition.

THE MITRAL VALVE PROLAPSE SYNDROME

ETIOLOGY AND PATHOLOGY

The mitral valve prolapse (MVP) syndrome has been given many names, including the systolic click–murmur syndrome, Barlow syndrome, billowing mitral valve syndrome, ballooning mitral cusp syndrome, floppy valve syndrome, and redundant cusp syndrome.[224–231] It is a common but variable clinical syndrome resulting from diverse pathogenic mechanisms of the mitral valve apparatus. The MVP syndrome has become recognized as one of the most prevalent cardiac valvular abnormalities, affecting as much as 5 to 10 per cent of the population.[227, 232, 233] It had been thought for many years that midsystolic clicks and late systolic murmurs, the auscultatory hallmarks of this syndrome, were of extracardiac origin. However, in 1963 Barlow et al. demonstrated that

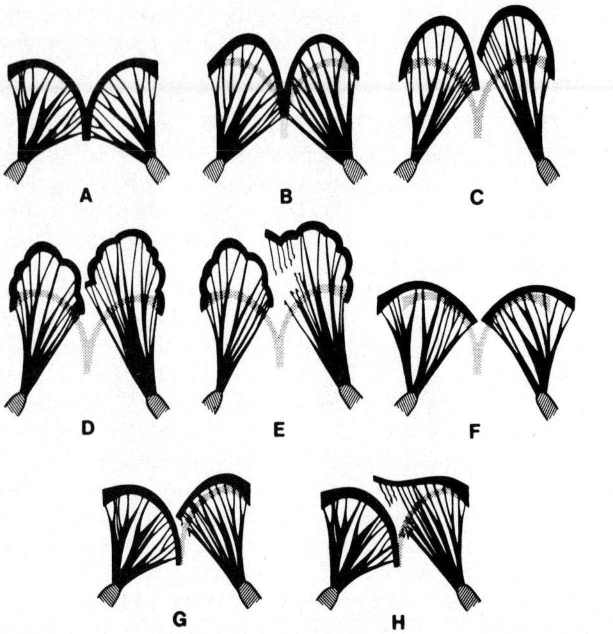

FIGURE 33–19. Diagrammatic representation of billowing (BML), floppy, prolapsed (MVP), and flail mitral valves. *A*, Normal mitral valve showing papillary muscles, chordae tendineae, and apposed leaflet edges. *B*, BML. The chordae are lengthened and the voluminous leaflets "billow" into the left atrium. In this and subsequent drawings, the positions of normal leaflets are superimposed with a stippled pattern. *C*, BML with MVP. The valve is incompetent. *D*, Floppy with MVP. *E*, Floppy and flail. Marked regurgitation is present. *F*, Recent-onset annular dilatation causes MVP with minimal BML, owing to loss of "keystone" effect. *G*, A ruptured minor chorda allows MVP without detectable BML. *H*, Flail with mild BML. (From Barlow, J. P., and Pocock, W. A.: Billowing, floppy, prolapsed or flail mitral valves? Am. J. Cardiol. *55*:501, 1985.)

these auscultatory findings are frequently associated with prolapse of the mitral valve, often with regurgitation.[234] Barlow and collaborators have distinguished between "billowing" and "prolapse" of the mitral valve.[224] Normally, the mitral valve billows slightly into the left atrium and an exaggeration should be termed "billowing mitral valve" (Fig. 33–19). A "floppy valve" is an extreme form of billowing. MVP occurs when the leaflet edges of the valve do not coapt, causing MR. With chordal rupture, the prolapsed mitral valve is "flail." Obviously, these conditions blend into one another, and it is often difficult to separate them sharply. Perloff et al. have proposed specific clinical criteria for the diagnosis of MVP.[226] They have divided the findings into three groups (Table 33–9): (1) major criteria, the presence of one or more of which establishes the diagnosis of MVP; (2) minor criteria, which cannot be discounted and which raise the suspicion of MVP but which by themselves are not sufficient to establish the diagnosis; and (3) nonspecific findings which, while often present in patients with MVP, are quite nonspecific. While they may alert the clinician, they do not aid in establishing the diagnosis. When rigorous two-dimensional echocardiography criteria (Fig. 33–20) (extension of leaflet tissue cephalad to the plane of the mitral annulus) were employed, only two of 100 healthy young women displayed MVP.[235] Such an approach may aid in avoiding overdiagnosis. This may occur with posterior bowing of the mitral valve on the M-mode echocardiogram which can be produced by incorrect transducer position.

The many causes of or conditions associated with prolapse of mitral valves into the left atrium during ventricular systole are shown in Table 33–10.[236–252] Prominent among these is myxomatous proliferation of the mitral valve, in which the spongiosa component of the valve, i.e., the middle layer of the leaflet composed of loose, myxomatous material, is unusually prominent[253, 254] and the quantity of acid mucopolysaccharide is increased secondary to a fundamental but as yet undefined abnormality of collagen metabolism.[242, 255] The concordance between inadequate production of type III collagen with echocardiographic findings of MVP in patients with type IV Ehlers-Danlos syndrome suggests that this abnormality of collagen is responsible.[256] Mucopolysaccharide infiltration and fragmentation of valvular collagen are common findings.[257] A reduction of type III and AB collagen has also been found in a patient with MVP without the Ehlers-Danlos syndrome.[258]

Electron microscopy has shown haphazard arrangement, disruption, and fragmentation of collagen fibrils. In mild cases, the valvular myxoid stroma is enlarged on histological examination but the leaflets are grossly normal. However, with increasing quantities of myxoid stroma, the leaflets become grossly abnormal and redundant (Fig. 33–21) and prolapse[259]; the severity of MR depends on the

TABLE 33–9 DIAGNOSTIC CRITERIA AND NONSPECIFIC FINDINGS IN MITRAL VALVE PROLAPSE

MAJOR CRITERIA

Auscultation
- Mid- to late systolic clicks and late systolic murmur or whoop alone or in combination at the cardiac apex

Two-dimensional echocardiogram
- Marked superior systolic displacement of mitral leaflets with coaptation point at or superior to annular plane
- Mild to moderate superior systolic displacement of mitral leaflets with
  - Chordal rupture
  - Doppler mitral regurgitation
  - Annular dilatation

Echocardiogram plus auscultation
- Mild to moderate superior systolic displacement of mitral leaflets with
  - Prominent mid to late systolic clicks at the cardiac apex
  - Apical late systolic or holosystolic murmur in the young
  - Late systolic "whoop"

MINOR CRITERIA

Auscultation
- Loud first heart sound with an apical holosystolic murmur

Two-dimensional echocardiogram
- Isolated mild to moderate superior systolic displacement of the posterior mitral leaflet
- Moderate superior systolic displacement of both mitral leaflets

Echocardiogram plus history
- Mild to moderate superior systolic displacement of mitral leaflets with
  - Focal neurologic attacks or amaurosis fugax in the young
  - First-degree relatives with major criteria

NONSPECIFIC FINDINGS

Symptoms
- "Atypical" chest pain, dyspnea, fatigue, lassitude, giddiness, dizziness, syncope
- Psychological disturbances

Physical appearance
- Thoracic bony abnormalities
- Hypomastia

Electrocardiogram
- T-wave inversions in inferior limb leads or lateral precordial leads
- Premature ventricular beats at rest, on exercise or on ambulatory ECG
- Supraventricular tachycardia

X-ray
- Scoliosis, pectus excavatum or carinatum, or loss of thoracic kyphosis

Two-dimensional echocardiogram
- Mild superior systolic displacement of anterior or anterior and posterior mitral leaflet

From Perloff, J. K., Child, J. S., and Edwards, J. E.: New guidelines for the clinical diagnosis of mitral valve prolapse. Am. J. Cardiol. 57:1124, 1986.

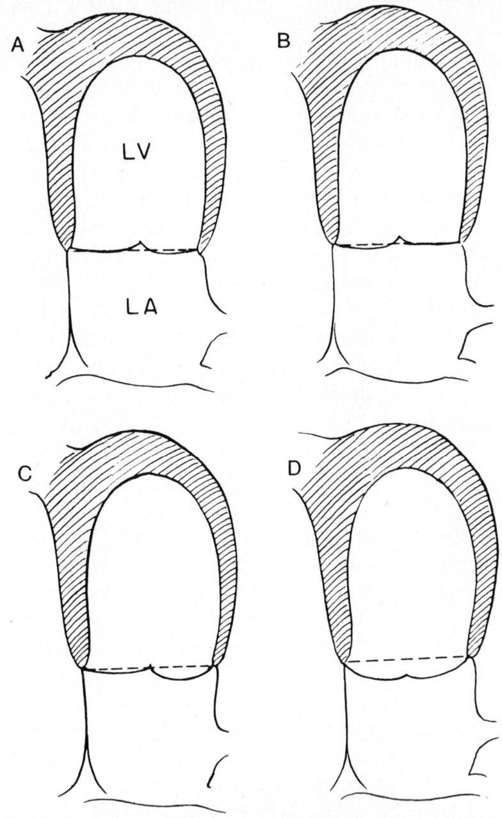

FIGURE 33–20. Schematic two-dimensional echocardiographic apical four-chamber views illustrating, in quantitative terms, mild, moderate and marked superior systolic displacement of mitral leaflets. Panels *A* and *B* show mild (1+) systolic displacement of (A) posterior and (B) anterior leaflets superior to the annular plane. The coaptation point is on the ventricular side of annulus. Panel *C* shows moderate (2+) superior systolic displacement of both leaflets with coaptation point at the level of the annular plane. Panel *D* shows marked (3+) superior systolic displacement of both leaflets above the annular plane together with the coaptation point. LA = left atrium, LV = left ventricle, RA = right atrium, RV = right ventricle. (From Perloff, J. K., Child, J. S., and Edwards, J. E.: New guidelines for the clinical diagnosis of mitral valve prolapse. Am. J. Cardiol. *57*:1127, 1986.)

extent of the prolapse. The cusps of the mitral valve, the chordae tendineae, and the annulus may all be affected by myxomatous proliferation. Degeneration of collagen within the central core of the chordae tendineae is primarily responsible for chordal rupture, which occurs commonly in this syndrome and may intensify the severity of MR (Fig. 33–19*E*), although increased chordal tension resulting from the enlarged area of the valve cusps may play a contributory role. Myxomatous changes in the annulus may result in annular dilatation and calcification—contributing to the severity of MR. Myxomatous proliferation, although most commonly affecting the mitral valve, is not limited to this valve but has been described in the tricuspid,[251] aortic, and pulmonic valves, particularly in patients with Marfan syndrome, and may lead to regurgitation of these valves. It has been proposed that cellular proliferation in response to repeated minor stress applies to the mitral valve apparatus during the cardiac cycle results in increased production of type III collagen. This concept is supported by the observation of an increase in prevalence of MVP in late adolescence and an increase in severity with age.[260] Hutchins et al. have proposed that the basic defect in MVP is a congenital separation between the junction of the atrial wall and the mitral valve and the left ventricular attachment. This causes hypermobility of the valve apparatus and leads, in time, to MVP.[260a]

The MVP syndrome appears to exhibit a strong hereditary component,[261–262a] transmitted as an autosomal dominant trait, and some cases of this syndrome appearing without any other obvious disorders may represent formes frustes of Marfan syndrome.[263] In an interesting report, MVP with transmission as an autosomal dominant was observed in 26 of a colony of 92 rhesus monkeys.[264] Although myxomatous proliferation of the mitral valve is idiopathic in most patients, it occurs in association with a variety of connective tissue disorders, including Marfan syndrome, Ehlers-Danlos syndrome,[264] osteogenesis imperfecta, pseudoxanthoma elasticum,[265] periarteritis nodosa, as well as with myotonic dystrophy,[241] Duchenne muscular dystrophy,[266] cardiomyopathy,[267] von Willebrand disease,[268] keratoconus,[269] hyperthyroidism,[246] and congenital malformations such as Ebstein's anomaly of the tricuspid valve, atrial septal defect of the ostium secundum variety,[236, 270] and the Holt-Oram syndrome (p. 1627). There appears to be a high incidence of MVP in patients with asthenic habitus[262a, 271] and a variety of congenital thoracic deformities, including a straight back, a pectus excavatum, or a shallow chest.[245, 248–250] The MVP syndrome may represent one manifestation of a number of systemic connective tissue disorders,[251] and thoracic abnormalities may represent another manifestation of the same disorders; frequently they coexist.

The MVP syndrome can coexist with rheumatic MS,[272] and it may develop following mitral commissurotomy for

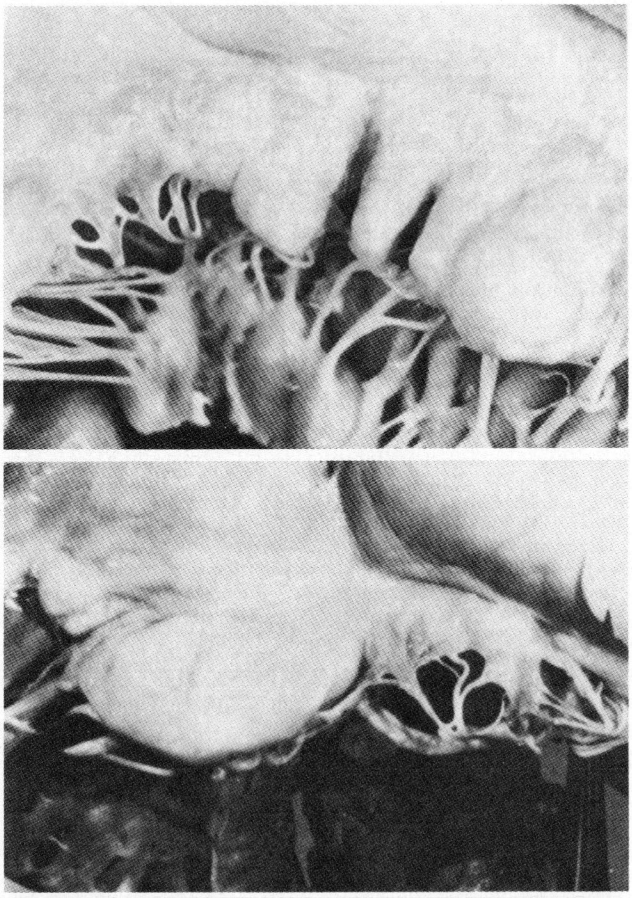

FIGURE 33–21. Typical scalloping, thickening, and bulging of posterior mitral leaflet in myxomatous mitral valve (*top*). Thickened bulging anterior mitral valve (*bottom*) demonstrates gross appearance of myxomatous change. (From Pape, L. A.: Pathogenesis and etiology of valvular heart disease. *In* Dalen, J. E., and Alpert, J. S. [eds.]: Valvular Heart Disease. 2nd ed. Boston, Little, Brown and Company, 1987, p. 12.)

TABLE 33–10 CONDITIONS CAUSING OR ASSOCIATED WITH MITRAL VALVE PROLAPSE OR NONEJECTION CLICK/MITRAL REGURGITANT SYSTOLIC MURMUR

Primary mitral valve prolapse	von Willebrand's syndrome
Marfan syndrome	Platelet abnormalities
Floppy valve syndrome	Migraine
Rheumatic endocarditis	Hypomagnesemia
Coronary artery disease	Osteogenesis imperfecta
Cardiomyopathy, congestive, hypertrophic	Inherited disorders of metabolism (Hunter-Hurler syndrome, Sanfilippo syndrome, Fabry's disease, Sandhoff's disease)
Myocarditis	
Trauma	
Left atrial myxoma	Anxiety neurosis, neurocirculatory asthenia, autonomic dysfunction
Polyarteritis nodosa, systemic lupus erythematosus	Congenital prolonged QT syndrome
Left ventricular aneurysm	
Ehlers-Danlos syndrome, pseudoxanthoma elasticum	Athlete's heart
	Turner syndrome
Pulmonary emphysema	Noonan syndrome
Relapsing polychondritis	Congenital heart disease (atrial septal defect, ventricular septal defect, patent ductus arteriosus, aorticopulmonary window, complete-absence left pericardium, membranous subaortic stenosis, supravalvular aortic stenosis, Ebstein's anomaly, corrected transposition of great vessels, infundibular pulmonary stenosis, Uhl's anomaly
Muscular dystrophy	
Wolff-Parkinson-White syndrome	
Straight back syndrome	
Thoracic skeletal abnormalities	
Neuro-ecto-mesodermal histodysplasia	
Hyperthyroidism	

From Barlow, J. B.: Perspectives on the Mitral Valve. Philadelphia, F. A. Davis, 1987, p. 61.

this lesion.[273] However, it is unlikely that rheumatic valvulitis, which is a proliferative process, causes myxomatous degeneration of the mitral valve. Rather it is more likely that the relationship between these two relatively common conditions is coincidental. In hypertrophic obstructive cardiomyopathy, prolapse of the posterior leaflet of the mitral valve may accompany the usual anterior displacement of the anterior mitral valve leaflet.[263, 274]

Ischemic heart disease and MVP are both common disorders and coexist not infrequently; MVP may also occur secondary to papillary muscle dysfunction. In some patients, MVP has been documented to develop for the first time *following* myocardial infarction.[275] Since MVP has also been reported in patients who have suffered acute myocardial infarction despite normal coronary arteriograms,[276] it is possible that coronary artery emboli are responsible for the infarction in this syndrome. MVP may cause myocardial ischemia by increasing tension on the base of the involved muscle.[274] It has also been proposed that coronary artery spasm occurs as a reflex response to prolapse of the posterior mitral leaflet and that the resultant ischemia may be responsible for angina or angina-like pain, myocardial infarction, arrhythmias, and sudden death in this syndrome.[277]

CLINICAL MANIFESTATIONS

The clinical presentations of the MVP syndrome are diverse. The condition has been observed in patients of all ages and in both sexes. It is a common syndrome; indeed, prolapse of the mitral valve has been reported to occur in 6 per cent of healthy young women surveyed by echocardiography.[232] One series of 100 presumably healthy young women revealed that 17 had a midsystolic click or late systolic murmur or both and that 10 of these 17 had evidence of prolapse of the mitral valve on echocardiography.[233] However, as noted above, since billowing of the mitral valve is a normal variant and M-mode echocardiographic findings may be nonspecific, it is likely that more rigorous criteria for diagnosis based on two-dimensional echocardiography will indicate a much lower prevalence.[226] In one series, about 20 per cent of patients who underwent mitral valve replacement had myxomatous proliferation of the valve on pathological examination.[278] Echocardiographic evidence of MVP has been found in more than 90 per cent of patients with Marfan syndrome[279] and in many of their first-degree relatives. MVP is now the most common cause of isolated regurgitation requiring mitral valve replacement.[280]

NATURAL HISTORY

The overwhelming majority of patients with MVP are asymptomatic. In many cases, otherwise asymptomatic patients with MVP suffer from undue anxiety, perhaps precipitated by their having been informed of the presence of heart disease. Patients may complain of palpitations, chest discomfort, and, when MR is severe, symptoms of diminished cardiac reserve. Chest discomfort may be typical of angina but most often is atypical in that it is prolonged, not clearly related to exertion, and punctuated by brief attacks of severe stabbing pain at the apex. The discomfort may be secondary to tension on papillary muscles and may be associated with abnormalities of wall motion or indentations of the wall of the left ventricle at the base of these muscles on angiography. It may be difficult to differentiate this discomfort from angina because of the coexistence of the MVP syndrome and true angina pectoris secondary to coronary artery disease.

Since MVP is sometimes associated with another form of heart disease, e.g., atrial septal defect, symptoms produced by the latter may predominate. It has been suggested that many of the symptoms are related to dysfunction of the autonomic nervous system, which occurs frequently in the MVP syndrome.[281–284] Patients with MVP have increased excretion and circulating concentrations of epinephrine and norepinephrine, presumably secondary to increased adrenergic tone, which may be responsible for many of the symptoms of the syndrome. Some exhibit excessive vasoconstriction, others striking orthostatic tachycardia.[282] Although many of the symptoms of MVP resemble those of neurocirculatory asthenia, the two conditions appear to be distinct and unrelated.[285]

PHYSICAL EXAMINATION

Palpation of the chest and of the carotid pulses reflects the severity of the existing MR, which may range from nonexistent to severe. The physical findings unique to the MVP syndrome are detected by auscultation and can be corroborated by phonocardiography.[224] The most important is a systolic click at least 0.14 sec after S_1 (Fig. 3–31, p. 59). This can be differentiated from a systolic ejection click, since it occurs distinctly *after* the beginning of the upstroke of the carotid pulse. Occasionally multiple mid- and late-systolic clicks are audible. They are most readily audible along the lower left sternal border and are believed to be produced by sudden tensing of the elongated chordae tendineae and of the prolapsing leaflets. The click is often, although not invariably, followed by a mid- to late-crescendo systolic murmur that continues to A_2. This murmur is similar to that produced by papillary muscle dysfunction, which is readily understandable, since both result from mid- to late-systolic MR. In general, the duration of the murmur is a function of the severity of the regurgitation, and when the murmur is confined to the latter portion of systole, regurgitation usually is not severe. However, as regurgitation becomes more severe, the murmur commences earlier and becomes holosystolic (Fig. 4–17, p. 74). It is important to emphasize the variability of these findings. Some patients exhibit both a midsystolic click and a mid- to late-systolic murmur; others present with one or the other of these two findings; still others have only a click on one occasion and only a murmur on another, both on a third examination, and no abnormality at all on a fourth. A loud mitral component of S_1 at the apex in patients with nonrheumatic MR suggests holosystolic MVP.[286] Conditions other than MVP cause midsystolic clicks; these include extracardiac causes and atrial septal aneurysms.[287] MVP may also cause an early diastolic sound or murmur, best heard at the apex or left sternal border 70 to 110 msec following A_2, at a time when the prolapsed posterior leaflet returned from the left atrium.[288]

DYNAMIC AUSCULTATION. The auscultatory and phonocardiographic findings are exquisitely sensitive to physiological and pharmacological interventions, and recognition of the changes induced by these interventions is of great value in the diagnosis of the MVP syndrome (Fig. 2–21, p. 38) (Table 33–6).[224, 263, 289] The mitral valve begins to prolapse when the reduction of left ventricular volume during systole reaches a critical point at which the mitral valve leaflets no longer coapt; at this instant, the click occurs and the murmur commences. Any maneuver that decreases left ventricular volume, such as a reduction of impedance to left ventricular outflow, a reduction in venous return, or an augmentation of contractility, will result in an earlier occurrence of prolapse during systole.[289] As a consequence, the click and onset of the murmur move closer to S_1. When prolapse is severe or left ventricular size is markedly reduced or both, prolapse may begin with the onset of systole, and as a consequence, the click may not be audible and the murmur may be holosystolic. On the other hand, when left ventricular volume is increased by an increase in venous return, a reduction of myocardial contractility, bradycardia, or an increase in the impedance to left ventricular emptying, both the click and the onset of the murmur will be delayed. Indeed, if the left ventricle becomes extremely large, prolapse may not occur at all, and the abnormal auscultatory features may disappear entirely.

During the straining phase of the Valsalva maneuver, upon sudden standing,[290] and early during the inhalation of amyl nitrite,[291] cardiac size decreases, and both the click and the onset of the murmur occur earlier in systole. In contrast, a sudden change from the standing to the prone position, leg-raising, prompt squatting, maximal isometric exercise, and, to a lesser extent, expiration will delay the click and the onset of the murmur. During the overshoot phase of the Valsalva maneuver (i.e., six to eight cycles following release) and with prolongation of the R-R interval either following a premature contraction or in atrial fibrillation, the click and onset of the murmur are usually delayed, and the intensity of the murmur is reduced.

In general, when the onset of the murmur is delayed, both its duration and its intensity are diminished, reflecting a reduction in the severity of MR. With some maneuvers, however, there is a discrepancy between changes in the intensity and duration of the murmur. Following amyl nitrite inhalation, for example, the reduced left ventricular size results in an earlier click and longer murmur, but the lower left ventricular systolic pressure diminishes regurgitation and the intensity of the murmur. Conversely, phenylephrine and methoxamine delay the click and the onset of the murmur, but the larger volume of regurgitation consequent to the elevated left ventricular systolic pressure increases regurgitation and the intensity of the murmur. A psychological stress may increase the intensity of the click and exacerbate arrhythmias in MVP,[292] a finding that might explain the intermittency of the auscultatory findings and arrhythmias in these patients. In the diagnosis of the MVP syndrome, it is generally more helpful to determine the effect of interventions on the timing of the click and murmur than on the intensity of the latter.

There may be confusion between the systolic murmurs of hypertrophic cardiomyopathy (HCM) and of MVP, particularly because midsystolic clicks and a late systolic murmur have been reported in HCM and because the murmur may increase in intensity and duration with standing and decrease with squatting in both conditions (p. 1423). However, the response to several interventions may be helpful in differentiating these two conditions. During the strain of the Valsalva maneuver, the murmur of HCM increases in intensity[293] in contrast to that in the syndrome, which becomes longer but usually not louder. The murmur of HCM becomes louder after amyl nitrite inhalation, whereas that of MVP does not. Following a premature beat, the murmur of HCM increases in intensity and duration, whereas that due to MVP usually remains unchanged or decreases.

LABORATORY EXAMINATION

ELECTROCARDIOGRAPHY

Most commonly, the electrocardiogram is within normal limits in asymptomatic patients with typical auscultatory and echocardiographic findings. In a minority of asymptomatic patients and in many symptomatic patients, the electrocardiogram characteristically shows inverted or biphasic T waves and nonspecific ST-segment changes in leads II, III, and aV_f and occasionally in the anterolateral leads as well.[224] The ST- and T-wave changes may become exaggerated during amyl nitrite inhalation and exercise. These electrocardiographic findings may be related to ischemia of the papillary muscles, or of the left ventricle at their bases, resulting from increased tension on these structures produced by the prolapsing valve. Alternatively, it is possible that the electrocardiographic abnormality reflects an underlying cardiomyopathy.

ARRHYTHMIAS. A spectrum of arrhythmias, including atrial and ventricular premature contractions and supraventricular and ventricular tachyarrhythmias[294–300] as well as bradyarrhythmias due to sinus node dysfunction or varying degrees of atrioventricular block,[301] have been observed in the MVP syndrome. Indeed, this syndrome should be considered in patients with otherwise unexplained arrhythmias. The mechanism of the arrhythmias is not clear. Diastolic depolarization of muscle fibers in the anterior mitral leaflet in response to stretch has been demonstrated experimentally,[302] and the abnormal stretch of the prolapsed leaflet may be of pathogenetic significance. Wit et al. have shown that mitral valve leaflets contain atrium-like muscle fibers in continuity with left atrial myocardium. It is possible that mechanical stimulation of these fibers generates slow-response action potentials and sustained rhythmic action that penetrates the cardiac chambers.[303] Although most of these arrhythmias are of little clinical importance, recurrent ventricular tachycardia, refractory to the usual agents, and even ventricular fibrillation have been reported. These serious ventricular arrhythmias are significantly more frequent in patients with ST-segment and T-wave abnormalities on the resting electrocardiogram.[304]

Paroxysmal supraventricular tachycardia is the most common sustained tachyarrhythmia in patients with the MVP syndrome and may be related to the high incidence of atrioventricular bypass tracts in this condition.[295] These bypass tracts are always left-sided and may be associated with the mitral valve abnormality. In the general population only 20 per cent of patients with paroxysmal supraventricular tachycardia have such bypass tracts, whereas the incidence in patients with MVP is three times as great. Conversely, there is evidence that there is a high incidence of MVP among patients with the Wolff-Parkinson-White syndrome.[305] However, the absence of electrocardiographic evidence of the Wolff-Parkinson-White syndrome should not be taken as evidence against the existence of bypass tracts in patients with the MVP syndrome who suffer attacks of supraventricular tachycardia. These considerations suggest that patients with the MVP syndrome who develop paroxysmal supraventricular tachycardia should be subjected to electrophysiological investigation. The outcome of such studies may be important, since digitalis or propranolol, which may be useful in reentry tachycardias, may be hazardous in the presence of antegrade conduction over an atrioventricular bypass tract. There is also an increased association between MVP and prolongation of the Q-T interval, and this association may play a role in the genesis of ventricular arrhythmias.[283, 306]

The relation between the MVP syndrome and sudden death is not clear.[307] Jeresaty collected 25 patients with MVP who died suddenly,[308] and Pocock et al. reviewed 17 patients.[309] But these are "numerators without denominators," and when the high incidence of both conditions is considered, it is difficult to interpret the coincidence. Considering the frequency of both conditions, these numbers are not very impressive. It is not clear how many, indeed if any, of these instances of sudden death were in fact caused by or related to the MVP syndrome. The immediate cause of the sudden, unexpected death is probably a tachyarrhythmia,[310] although complete heart block with prolonged asystole has also been reported in this syndrome and cannot be excluded.[311]

ECHOCARDIOGRAPHY (See also p. 105). Echocardiography plays a key role in the diagnosis of MVP and has been most useful in the delineation of this syndrome[312] (Fig. 3–31, p. 59; Fig. 4–17, p. 74; Figs. 5–50, 51, and 52, p. 106; and Fig. 33–20). The most common echocardiographic finding on M-mode echocardiography is abrupt posterior movement of the posterior leaflet or of both mitral leaflets in midsystole. A second finding is pansystolic posterior prolapse of one or both leaflets, giving rise to a "U"- or "hammock"-shaped configuration in the C-D segment (Fig. 5–50, p. 106) (the opposite of what is seen in hypertrophic obstructive cardiomyopathy, in which the anterior leaflet of the mitral valve moves toward the ventricular septum in midsystole): Holosystolic "hammocking" of less than 5 mm is not specific for MVP. Rarely, there is a sudden posterior collapse of the anterior mitral leaflet as it approaches the prolapsing posterior leaflet in early systole.[263, 313] All three of these echocardiographic patterns have in common the motion of the mitral valve posterior to the C-point. Although the systolic click usually occurs at the time of the abrupt posterior movement, there is considerable variability in the relationship between the auscultatory and echocardiographic events.

In studying patients with suspected MVP, it is important to direct the echo beam to the junction of the posterior walls of the left atrium and ventricle in order to visualize the posterior leaflet adequately. Since it is possible to establish a false-positive diagnosis from tracings obtained from the body of the leaflets, care must be taken to angulate the transducer in order to record valve motion from the free edge of the leaflet. M-mode echocardiography in some patients has missed MVP that was detected by two-dimensional echocardiography[314, 315] (Fig. 33–20). The apical four-chamber view has been proposed as the single best technique to define the syndrome, which is present when the mitral valve leaflets lie in the left atrium rather than in the left ventricle during systole.[316] Doppler echocardiography frequently reveals mild MR and is not always associated with an audible murmur. Moderate or severe MR is found in 10 per cent of patients, usually in men over the age of 50.[317]

The echocardiographic findings of MVP have been reported to occur in a large number of first-degree relatives of patients with established MVP,[318] but the variability in physical findings in this syndrome, already commented upon, extends to the echocardiogram.[319] Thus, some patients have a systolic click with or without a murmur and show no evidence of MVP on the echocardiogram. Conversely, the echocardiographic findings of MVP may be observed in patients without the click or murmur. Others have both the typical echocardiographic and auscultatory features.

Two-dimensional echocardiography has also revealed prolapse of the tricuspid and aortic valves in approximately one-fifth of patients with MVP.[320] Conversely, however, prolapse of the tricuspid and aortic valves[321] occurs uncommonly in patients without prolapse of the mitral valve; the latter echocardiographic finding is usually not associated with any aortic regurgitation.

Stress Scintigraphy

The differential diagnosis between two common conditions—MVP associated with atypical chest pain and electrocardiographic abnormalities, and primary coronary artery disease associated with MVP—may be aided by exercise electrocardiography[224] but myocardial scintigraphy using thallium-201 during exercise (p. 329) is probably more specific in this disorder. When findings are normal, i.e., when there is no evidence of exercise-induced regional myocardial ischemia, the diagnosis of MVP unrelated to ischemic heart disease is most likely.[322] However, the reverse is not always the case, since patients having MVP with or without associated coronary artery disease may exhibit myocardial perfusion defects—exercise-induced or following redistribution or both.[323]

ANGIOGRAPHY

The configuration of the left ventriculogram during systole is helpful in the diagnosis of MVP.[324] The right anterior oblique projection is most useful for defining the posterior leaflet of the mitral valve and the left anterior oblique projection for studying the anterior leaflet. The most helpful sign is extension of the mitral leaflet tissue inferiorly and posteriorly to the point of attachment of the mitral leaflets to the annulus fibrosis[325] (Fig. 33–22). Angiography may also reveal scalloped edges of the leaflets, reflecting redundancy of tissue.

Other abnormalities noted on angiography include dilatation, decreased systolic contraction, and calcification of the mitral annulus and poor contraction of the basal portion of the left ventricle.[326] There may be an indentation at the base of the posteromedial papillary muscle associated with prolapse of the posterior leaflet and resulting from abnormal traction on this muscle. With involvement of both papillary muscles, there may be an indentation of the anterior as well as the inferior wall of the left ventricle, giving the cardiac silhouette an hourglass appearance. These left ventricular contraction abnormalities are secondary to redundancy of the mitral valve leaflets and transmission of the abnormal tension on these leaflets to the papillary muscles and underlying left ventricle. Patients with MVP and little or no MR have normal left ventricular hemodynamics. An increased rate of circumferential fiber shortening may be observed in the presence of significant MR, as in patients with regurgitation of other etiologies.[326] Ejection fraction at rest determined by radionuclide angiography is normal in patients having MVP without associated MR. However, a subgroup of these patients do not exhibit a normal increase in ejection fraction during exercise, suggesting that a cardiomyopathic process may be responsible for the reduced cardiac reserve.[327]

NATURAL HISTORY

The outlook for MVP in children is excellent, a large majority remaining asymptomatic for many years without any change in clinical or laboratory manifestations.[328, 329, 329a]

Progressive MR occurs in about 15 per cent of patients over a 10- to 15-year period; the incidence of this complication is significantly greater in patients with both murmurs and clicks than in those with an isolated click. In many patients, rupture of chordae tendineae or infective endocarditis is responsible for the intensification of the mitral regurgitation.[224, 330] When MR is severe, valve replacement may be required[330a, 331]; indeed, MVP is an important cause

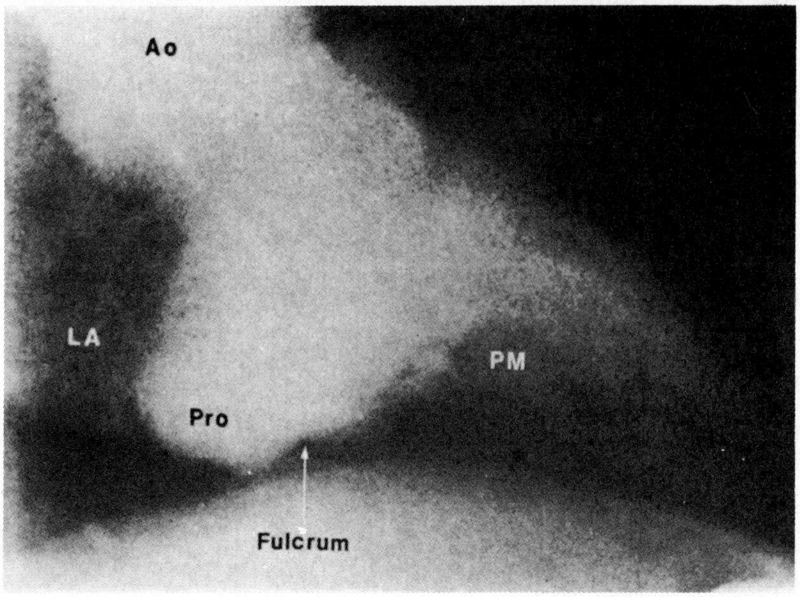

FIGURE 33–22. Systolic frame of left ventricular angiogram demonstrating prolapse (Pro) of the mitral valve. The posteromedial commissural scallop of the posterior mitral leaflet extends posteriorly and inferiorly to the fulcrum. PM = papillary muscle. (From Cohen, M. V., et al.: Angiographic-echocardiographic correlation in mitral valve prolapse. Am. Heart J. 97:46, 1979.)

of pure mitral regurgitation in patients requiring mitral valve replacement.[280] Patients with the MVP syndrome are also at risk of developing infective endocarditis,[330, 332–334] although the incidence appears to be extremely low in patients with a midsystolic click only.

Acute hemiplegia, transient ischemic attacks, cerebellar infarcts, amaurosis fugax, and retinal arteriolar occlusions all appear to occur more frequently in patients with the MVP syndrome, suggesting that cerebral emboli are unusually common in this condition.[335–341] These neurological complications are often associated with shortened platelet survival.[337] Loss of endothelial continuity and tearing of the endocardium overlying the myxomatous valve may initiate platelet aggregation and the formation of mural platelet-fibrin complexes.[338] The paroxysmal arrhythmias that occur in the MVP syndrome may contribute to the likelihood of embolization. Indeed, it is possible that cerebral embolization secondary to MVP may be a significant cause for unexplained strokes and other cerebral and retinal complications in young people with undetected cerebrovascular disease.[335] Similarly, myocardial infarction in patients with MVP and normal coronary arteries may be secondary to embolization.[341]

MANAGEMENT

Asymptomatic patients (or those whose principal complaint is anxiety) with no arrhythmias evident on a routine extended electrocardiographic tracing and on prolonged auscultation, with normal ST segments and without evidence of serious MR, should be reassured about the favorable prognosis but should have follow-up examinations every 2 to 4 years. This should include a two-dimensional echocardiogram, and if there is evidence of MR, a Doppler study. A Holter electrocardiogram is indicated in patients with a history of syncope or palpitations and serious arrhythmias on the routine ECG. Patients with a long systolic murmur may show progression of MR and should be examined more frequently, at intervals of approximately 12 months. Since infective endocarditis is a well-recognized complication of MVP,[332–334] *endocarditis prophylaxis* is advisable in patients with a typical systolic murmur and characteristic echocardiographic features. Although opinions on this point are not unanimous, prophylaxis is probably not necessary in patients with a midsystolic click without a systolic murmur.[333] Some, however, recommend prophylaxis when such patients are subjected to instrumentation of the upper respiratory or genitourinary tracts.[334]

Patients with a history of palpitations, lightheadedness, dizziness, or syncope or those who have arrhythmias on clinical examination or on a routine electrocardiogram should undergo ambulatory (24-hour) electrocardiographic monitoring or treadmill exercise testing or both. A beta-adrenoceptor blocker is the drug of choice for many ventricular arrhythmias, and either propranolol or phenytoin is useful in patients with prolongation of the Q-T interval. Beta-adrenoceptor blockade may also be useful in the treatment of chest discomfort, both in patients with associated coronary artery disease and in those with normal coronary vessels in whom the symptoms may be due to regional ischemia secondary to MVP.[342] Nitrates should be used with caution, since the reduction of cardiac size induced by these drugs may intensify the prolapse and the resultant ischemia of the base of the papillary muscles.

Patients with symptoms of reduced functional cardiac reserve should be treated like other patients with severe MR (p. 1043), and those with severe regurgitation who are not responsive to medical management may require mitral valve replacement. In patients with angina on effort and/or ischemic electrocardiographic changes and abnormalities on a thallium perfusion scan during exercise, coronary arteriography should be performed, and treatment should take into account the responsiveness of symptoms to medical management and the coronary anatomy, as outlined in Chapter 39. In patients with MVP who have had any of the aforementioned cerebral events and in whom no other etiology is apparent, anticoagulant therapy and/or drugs that interfere with platelet function, such as aspirin and dipyridamole, should be given.

Although this discussion has focused attention on complications of the MVP syndrome, it should not be forgotten that, on the whole, this is a benign condition and that the vast majority of patients with this syndrome remain asymptomatic for their entire lives and require, at most, observation every few years and reassurance.

AORTIC STENOSIS

ETIOLOGY AND PATHOLOGY

Obstruction to left ventricular outflow is localized most commonly at the aortic valve, discussed in this section. However, obstruction may also occur above the valve (supravalvular stenosis [p. 937]) or below the valve (discrete subvalvular aortic stenosis [p. 936]) or may be caused by hypertrophic obstructive cardiomyopathy (p. 1418). In an analysis of the hearts of 543 patients with valvular disease, Roberts found isolated aortic stenosis (AS) to be the most common lesion.[343] Valvular AS without accompanying mitral valve disease is more common in men and very rarely occurs on a rheumatic basis but instead is usually either congenital or degenerative in origin[10, 343a, 343b] (Fig. 33–23).

CONGENITAL AORTIC STENOSIS (See also pp. 932 and 978). Congenital malformations of the aortic valve may be unicuspid, bicuspid, or tricuspid or may be a dome-shaped diaphragm (Fig. 33–24).[10, 338] *Unicuspid valves* produce severe obstruction in infancy and are the most frequent malformations found in fatal valvular aortic stenosis in children under the age of one year.[344] Congenitally *bicuspid valves* may be stenotic with commissural fusion at birth, but more commonly they are not responsible for serious narrowing of the aortic orifice during childhood; their abnormal architecture induces turbulent flow, which traumatizes the leaflets and ultimately leads to fibrosis, increased rigidity, and calcification of the leaflets and narrowing of the aortic orifice[345] (Fig. 33–25). Infective endocarditis may develop on a congenitally bicuspid valve, which then becomes regurgitant. Rarely, a congenitally bicuspid valve is purely regurgitant in the absence of antecedent infection. It should be emphasized that in a majority of cases, a bicuspid valve is not stenotic at birth and that the changes causing stenosis resemble those occurring in senile, degenerative calcific stenosis of a tricuspid aortic valve except that in the congenitally bicuspid valve these changes occur several decades earlier.

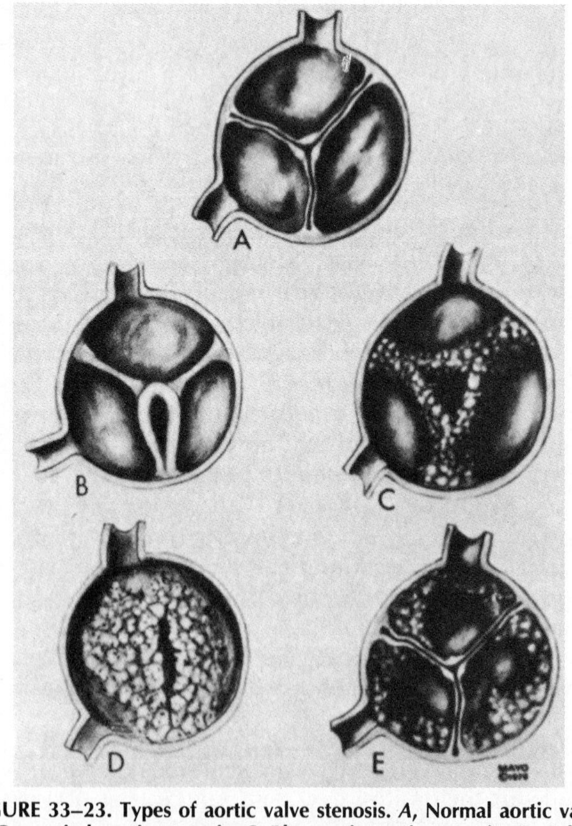

FIGURE 33–23. Types of aortic valve stenosis. *A*, Normal aortic valve. *B*, Congenital aortic stenosis. *C*, Rheumatic aortic stenosis. *D*, Calcific aortic stenosis. *E*, Calcific senile aortic stenosis. (From Brandenburg, R. O., et al.: Valvular heart disease—When should the patient be referred? Pract. Cardiol. *5*:50, 1979.)

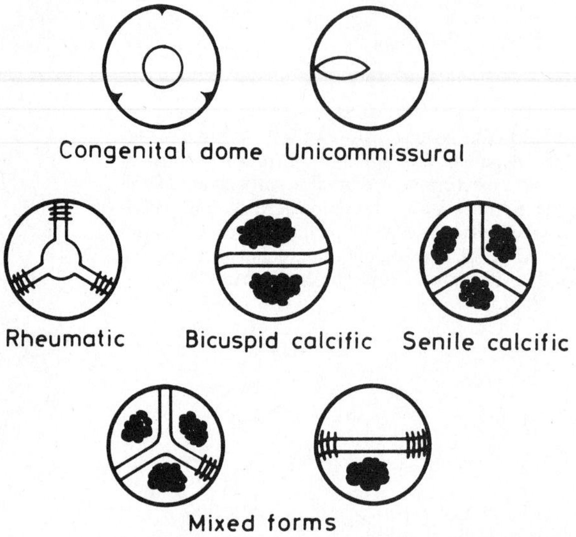

FIGURE 33–24. Schematic representation of the types of aortic valve stenosis, viewed from above. (From Davies, M. J.: Pathology of Cardiac Valves. London, Butterworths, 1980.)

A third form of a congenitally malformed valve is *tricuspid*, with the cusps of unequal size and some commissural fusion. Although many of these valves retain normal function throughout life, it has been postulated that the turbulent flow produced by the mild congenital architectural abnormality may lead to fibrosis and ultimately to calcification and stenosis. Tricuspid stenotic aortic valves in adults may be congenital, rheumatic, or degenerative in origin.

ACQUIRED AORTIC STENOSIS. Rheumatic AS results from adhesions and fusion of the commissures and cusps and vascularization of the leaflets and the valve ring, leading to retraction and stiffening of the free borders of the cusps, with calcific nodules present on both surfaces and an orifice that is reduced to a small round or triangular opening. As a consequence, the rheumatic valve is often regurgitant as well as stenotic (Figs. 33–24, 33–25, and 54–5*B*, p. 1710). The heart frequently exhibits other stigmata of rheumatic heart disease, especially mitral valve involvement. In degenerative (senile) calcific AS, the cusps are immobilized by a deposit of calcium along their flexion lines at their bases. This common cause of aortic stenosis in adults appears to result from years of normal mechanical stress on the valve. Although degenerative calcification may extend in the direction of the cusps, no commissural fusion is present. Degenerative "wear and tear" appears to be the most likely cause of this form of AS, which is commonly accompanied by calcifications of the mitral annulus and coronary arteries but rarely by aortic regurgitation. Both diabetes mellitus and hypercholesterolemia appear to be risk factors for the development of this lesion.[345a, 345b] The stenosis is produced by the calcific deposits that prevent the cusps from opening normally during systole (Fig. 33–25). In *atherosclerotic aortic valvular stenosis*,

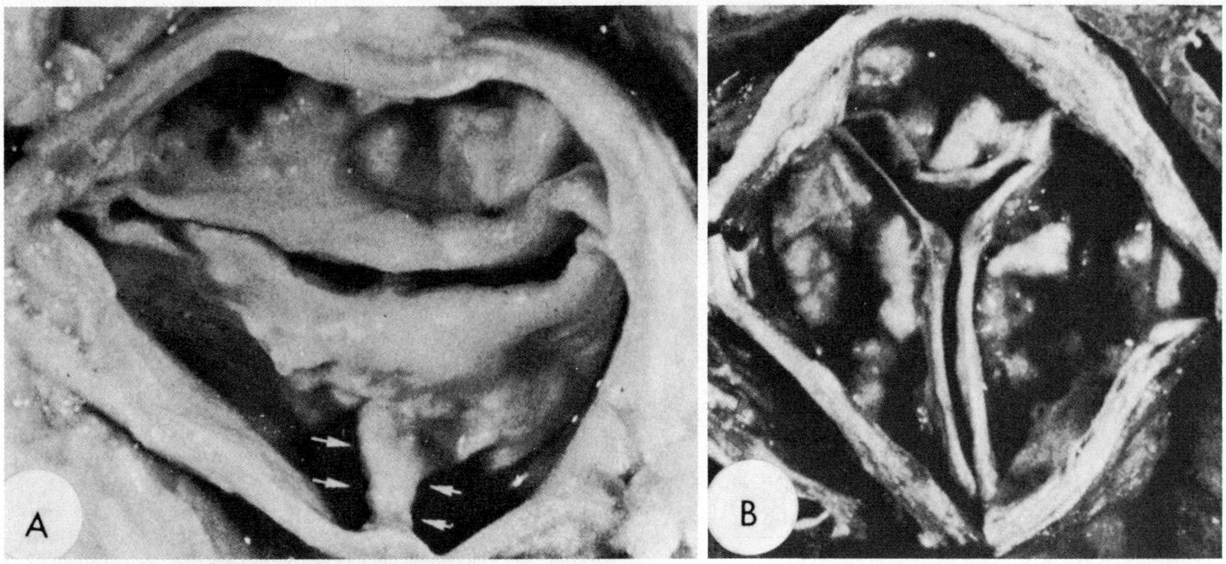

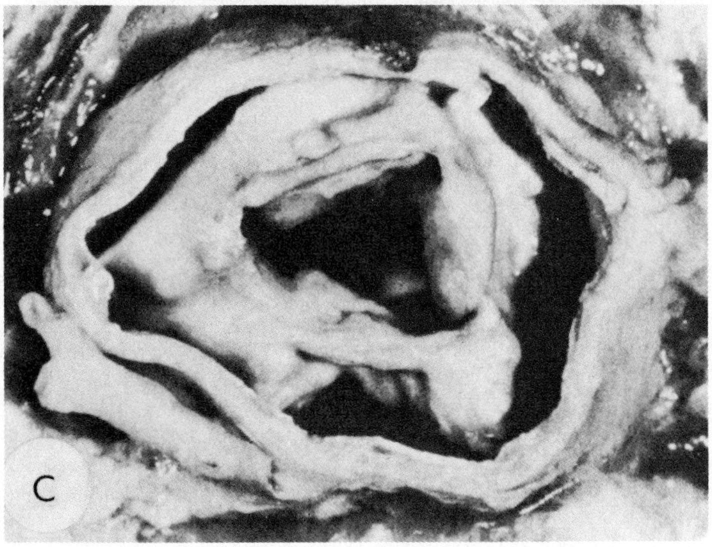

FIGURE 33–25. *A*, Calcified, stenotic, congenitally bicuspid aortic valve of a 59-year-old man. The cusps are situated anteriorly and posteriorly, with the commissures on the right and left. The valve has a raphe (white arrows) in the anterior cusp. Peak systolic gradient across the valve was 45 mm Hg, and the patient had complete heart block secondary to destruction of the atrioventricular bundle by calcium, which presumably had extended down from the aortic valvular cusps. *B*, Stenotic tricuspid aortic valve in A man of 81. Aortic stenosis in the elderly is characterized by calcific depositis on the aortic surfaces of the cusps and typically no or little commissural fusion. *C*, Stenotic tricuspid aortic valve in a 55-year-old man. Each of the three commissures is fused, producing a triangular fixed central orifice that is both stenotic and incompetent. (From Roberts, W. C.: Valvular, subvalvular and supravalvular aortic stenosis: Morphologic features. *In* Edwards, J. E. [ed]: Clinical-Pathologic Correlations #2. Philadelphia, F. A. Davis, 1973, pp. 100, 106, and 108.)

severe atherosclerosis involves the aorta and other major arteries; this form of AS occurs most frequently in patients with severe hypercholesterolemia and is observed in children with homozygous Type II hyperlipoproteinemia (p. 1640). *Rheumatoid involvement* of the valve is a rare cause of AS and results in nodular thickening of the valve leaflets and involvement of the proximal part of the aorta (p. 1719). *Ochronosis* is another rare cause of aortic stenosis.[346]

Roberts studied hearts with AS in patients between 15 and 65 years of age and found that almost 40 per cent were tricuspid. Since there was thickening of the mitral valve and a history of acute rheumatic fever in half of these cases, it is likely that the AS was rheumatic in etiology; in the remainder it was either congenital or degenerative in origin. In 90 per cent of hearts examined at autopsy in patients with AS who were older than 65 years, the valves were tricuspid, with nodular calcific deposits on the aortic aspects of the cusps, but without commissural fusion.[343]

Hemodynamically significant aortic stenosis leads to severe concentric left ventricular hypertrophy,[347] with heart weights as great as 1000 gm. The interventricular septum often bulges into and encroaches on the right ventricular cavity. When left ventricular failure supervenes, the left ventricle dilates,[347] the left atrium enlarges, and changes secondary to backward failure occur in the pulmonary vascular bed, right side of the heart, and systemic venous bed.

PATHOPHYSIOLOGY

The left ventricle responds to the sudden production of severe obstruction to outflow by dilatation and reduction of stroke volume. However, in adults with aortic stenosis, the obstruction usually develops and increases gradually over a prolonged period. In infants and children with congenital aortic stenosis, the valve orifice shows little change as the child grows, thereby intensifying obstruction quite gradually. Left ventricular function can be well maintained in experimentally produced, chronic, gradually developing subcoronary aortic stenosis.[348] Left ventricular output is maintained by the presence of left ventricular hypertrophy, which may sustain a large pressure gradient across the aortic valve for many years without a reduction in cardiac output, left ventricular dilatation, or the development of symptoms (Figs. 33–26 and 9–9, p. 251). A peak systolic pressure gradient exceeding 50 mm Hg in the presence of a normal cardiac output or an effective aortic orifice less than about 0.75 cm^2 in an average-sized adult, i.e., 0.4 cm^2/m^2 of body surface area (less than approximately one-fourth of the normal orifice) is generally considered to represent critical obstruction to left ventricular outflow.[349, 350]

As contraction of the left ventricle becomes progressively more isometric, the left ventricular pressure pulse exhibits a rounded, rather than flattened, summit. The elevated

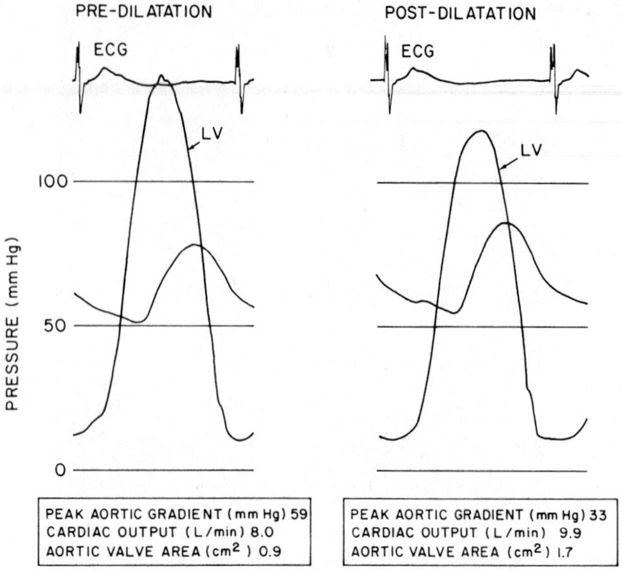

FIGURE 33–26. Simultaneous left ventricular (LV) and arterial pressure tracings recorded before and after balloon valvuloplasty in a patient with severe aortic stenosis. (Courtesy of Raymond G. McKay, M.D.)

left ventricular end-diastolic pressure, which is characteristic of severe AS, does not necessarily signify the presence of left ventricular dilatation or failure but often reflects diminished compliance of the hypertrophied left ventricular wall; usually it results from both processes.[351–354]

In patients with severe AS, large *a* waves usually appear in the left atrial pressure pulse because of the combination of enhanced contraction of a hypertrophied left atrium and diminished left ventricular compliance. Atrial contraction plays a particularly important role in filling of the left ventricle in AS.[25] It raises left ventricular end-diastolic pressure without producing a concomitant elevation of mean left atrial pressure.[355] This "booster pump" function of the left atrium prevents the pulmonary venous and capillary pressures from rising to levels that would produce pulmonary congestion, while at the same time maintaining left ventricular end-diastolic pressure at the elevated level necessary for effective left ventricular contraction. Loss of appropriately timed, vigorous atrial contraction, as occurs in atrial fibrillation or atrioventricular dissociation, may result in rapid clinical deterioration in patients with severe AS.

Although the *cardiac output* at rest is within normal limits in the majority of patients with severe AS,[350] it often fails to rise normally during exertion. Late in the course of the disease the cardiac output, stroke volume, and therefore the left ventricular–aortic pressure gradient all decline, whereas the mean left atrial, pulmonary capillary, pulmonary arterial, right ventricular systolic and diastolic, and right atrial pressures rise, sequentially. AS intensifies the severity of any existing mitral regurgitation by increasing the pressure gradient responsible for driving blood from the left ventricle to the left atrium. In addition, the dilatation of the left ventricle, which occurs late in the course of some patients with aortic valve disease, may produce mitral regurgitation, superimposing the hemodynamic changes associated with this lesion on those produced by AS. Also, as a consequence of pulmonary hypertension or bulging of the hypertrophied septum into the right ventricular cavity or both, the *a* wave in the right atrial pressure pulse becomes prominent.

Left ventricular end-diastolic volume usually remains normal until quite late in the course of the disease, but left ventricular mass increases in response to the chronic pressure overload, resulting in an increase in the mass/volume ratio. However, the increase in mass may not be as great as that seen with aortic regurgitation (AR) or combined AS and AR.

Myocardial Function in Aortic Stenosis

In experimental animals, when the aorta is suddenly constricted, left ventricular pressure rises, and there is a large increase in wall stress, whereas both extent and velocity of shortening decline. As pointed out in Chapter 14, the development of ventricular hypertrophy is one of the principal mechanisms by which the heart compensates for such an increased hemodynamic burden.[356, 357] The increased systolic wall stress induced by AS apparently leads to parallel replication of sarcomeres and concentric hypertrophy (Fig. 14–8, p. 432), and the increase in left ventricular wall thickness is often sufficient to counterbalance the increased pressure, so that peak systolic wall tension returns to normal or remains so if the obstruction develops slowly[358] (Fig. 14–9, p. 432). An inverse correlation between wall stress and ejection fraction exists in patients with AS. This suggests that the depressed ejection fraction and velocity of fiber shortening that occur in some patients are a consequence of inadequate wall thickening,[359] resulting in "afterload mismatch."[360] Patients having AS with compensated pressure overload as well as some with depressed left ventricular ejection fractions and overt congestive failure may have normal values for the rate of intraventricular stress ($d\sigma/dt$) and pressure (dP/dt) development.[361] In others, the lower ejection fraction is secondary to a depression of contractility (Fig. 14–11, p. 434); in the latter, the effectiveness of surgical treatment is reduced.[362] Thus, both altered contractility and increased afterload are operative in depressing left ventricular performance.[363]

From these considerations it is clear that in order to evaluate myocardial function in patients with AS, it is critical to relate the ejection phase indices to the existing wall tension (p. 453). Wall thickness is a critical determinant of ventricular performance in patients with AS; inadequate hypertrophy, an intrinsic depression of myocardial contractility, or a combination of these two defects may lead to a depression of ventricular performance.

DIASTOLIC STIFFNESS. Although ventricular hypertrophy is a key compensatory mechanism, to the pressure load imposed by AS it results in an adverse pathophysiological consequence, i.e., an increase in diastolic stiffness. As a result, greater intracavitary pressure is required for ventricular filling. Some patients with AS manifest an increase in chamber stiffness due simply to an increase in muscle mass but with no alteration in muscle stiffness; others exhibit increases in muscle stiffness as well as in chamber stiffness, both of which contribute to the elevation of ventricular diastolic filling pressure at any level of ventricular diastolic volume.[351–354, 364–366] Chamber stiffness may revert toward normal as hypertrophy regresses following relief of AS,[354] and at least in some patients muscle stiffness may also revert to normal. Whether this occurs in all patients is not clear. It is expected that this regression of stiffness would occur in patients with extensive myocardial fibrosis. Indeed, in some patients stiffness increases postoperatively as ventricular hypertrophy regresses, while interstitial fibrosis remains unchanged.[353]

A variety of changes in the *myocardial ultrastructure* have been documented in patients with severe AS. These include unusually large nuclei, loss of myofibrils, accumulation of mitochondria, large cytoplasmic areas devoid of contractile material, and proliferation of fibroblasts and collagen fibers in the interstitial space.[366a] The depression of cardiac function that occurs late in the course of the disease may well be related to these morphological alterations. In AS, coronary blood flow at rest is elevated in absolute terms but is normal when corrected for myocardial mass.[366b] There may be inadequate myocardial oxygenation in severe AS, even in the absence of coronary artery disease. The hypertrophied left ventricular muscle mass, the increased systolic pressure, and the prolongation of ejection all elevate myocardial oxygen requirements, and the abnormally heightened pressure compressing the coronary arteries exceeds the coronary perfusion pressure, thereby interfering with coronary blood flow.[367] Blood flow is also impaired by the elevation of left ventricular end-diastolic pressure, which lowers the diastolic aortic–left ventricular pressure (coronary perfusion pressure) gradient. Therefore, the subendocardium in severe aortic stenosis is susceptible to ischemia, and this underperfusion may be responsible for the development of myocardial ischemia.[367] Marcus et al. have demonstrated a reduction in the velocity of coronary blood flow during reactive hyperemia at the time of operation in patients with severe AS,[368] and this may be responsible for the angina commonly observed in these patients. Metabolic evidence of myocardial ischemia, i.e., lactate production, can be demonstrated when myocardial oxygen needs are stimulated by exercise or isoproterenol in patients with AS, in both the presence and the absence of coronary arterial narrowing.

CLINICAL MANIFESTATIONS

HISTORY

In the natural history of adults with AS, a long latent period exists during which there is gradually increasing obstruction and an increase in the pressure load on the myocardium while the patient remains asymptomatic. The cardinal symptoms of AS, which commence most commonly in the sixth decade of life, are angina pectoris, syncope, and heart failure.[337, 369] However, in patients in whom the obstruction remains unrelieved, once these symptoms become manifest, the prognosis is poor; survival curves show that the interval from the onset of symptoms to the time of death is approximately 2 years in patients with heart failure, 3 years in those with syncope, and 5 years in those with angina.[370, 371] *Angina* occurs in approximately two-thirds of patients with critical AS (about half of whom have significant coronary artery obstruction)[372] and usually resembles that observed in patients with coronary artery disease, in that it is commonly precipitated by exertion and relieved by rest. It results from the combination of increased oxygen needs by the hypertrophied myocardium and reduction of oxygen delivery secondary to the excessive compression of coronary vessels.[366, 368, 373] Rarely, it results from calcium emboli to the coronary vascular bed.[374] Angina may, of course, also result from coexisting coronary artery disease, and the absence of angina in a patient with severe AS suggests that serious obstructive coronary artery disease is not present.

Syncope is often orthostatic and is most commonly due to the reduced cerebral perfusion that occurs during exertion when arterial pressure declines consequent to systemic vasodilatation in the presence of a fixed cardiac output.[375] It may be preceded by premonitory symptoms and may be prolonged by arrhythmias.[376] Exertional hypotension may also be manifest as "graying out" spells or giddiness on effort. Syncope at rest may be due to transient ventricular fibrillation, from which the patient recovers spontaneously; transient atrial fibrillation with loss of the "atrial kick" and a precipitous decline in cardiac output; or transient atrioventricular block due to extension of the calcification of the valve into the conduction system. *Exertional dyspnea* with orthopnea, paroxysmal nocturnal dyspnea, and pulmonary edema reflect varying degrees of pulmonary venous hypertension. These are late symptoms in AS, and their presence for more than 5 years should suggest the possibility of associated mitral valvular disease. *Gastrointestinal bleeding*, idiopathic or due to angiodysplasia most commonly of the right colon or other vascular malformations, occurs more often than expected in patients with calcific AS; it may cease after aortic valve replacement.[377, 378] Infective endocarditis is a greater risk in younger patients with milder valvular deformity than in older patients with rock-like calcific aortic deformities. Cerebral emboli resulting in stroke or transient ischemic attacks may result from microthrombi on thickened bicuspid valves.[379] Calcific AS may cause embolization of calcium to a variety of organs, including the heart, kidney, and brain. Abrupt loss of vision has been reported when calcific emboli occluded the central retinal artery.[380]

Since cardiac output is usually well maintained for many years in patients with severe AS, marked fatigability, debilitation, peripheral cyanosis, and other manifestations of a low cardiac output are usually not prominent until quite late in the natural history of the disease. Atrial fibrillation, pulmonary hypertension, and systemic venous hypertension in patients with isolated aortic stenosis are often preterminal findings. Although AS may be responsible for sudden death (p. 748), this usually occurs in patients who had previously been symptomatic.

PHYSICAL EXAMINATION

The arterial pulse characteristically rises slowly and is small and sustained (pulsus parvus et tardus) (p. 23).[381, 382] In the advanced stage, systolic and pulse pressures are both reduced. However, in patients with mild stenosis with associated regurgitation and in older patients with an inelastic arterial bed, both systolic and pulse pressures may be normal or even increased. A systolic pressure exceeding 200 mm Hg is rare in patients with critical aortic stenosis.[381] The anacrotic notch and coarse systolic vibrations are felt most readily in the carotid arterial pulse, producing the so-called carotid shudder (Figs. 3–22, p. 56, and 4–4, p. 67). Simultaneous palpation of the apex and carotid arteries reveals a distinct lag in the latter in patients with severe AS.[382a] Although pulsus alternans occurs commonly in AS with left ventricular dysfunction[383] (Fig. 3–26, p. 57), obstruction of the aortic valve may prevent it from being recognized by examination of the peripheral arterial pulse. The jugular venous pulse usually shows prominent *a* waves (Fig. 4–8, p. 69), reflecting reduced right ventricular compliance consequent to hypertrophy of the ventricular septum.[384] With pulmonary hypertension and secondary right ventricular failure and tricuspid regurgitation, *v* or *c-v* waves may be prominent.

The cardiac impulse is sustained with left ventricular failure; it becomes displaced inferiorly and laterally. Presystolic distention of the left ventricle, i.e., a prominent precordial *a* wave, is often both visible and palpable. A hyperdynamic left ventricle suggests concomitant aortic or MR. A systolic thrill is usually best appreciated when the patient leans forward in full expiration. It is felt most readily in the second left intercostal space on either side of the sternum or in the suprasternal notch and is frequently transmitted along the carotid arteries.

Rarely, evidence of right ventricular failure with systemic venous congestion, hepatomegaly, and edema precedes left ventricular failure. Probably this is caused by the so-called Bernheim effect, which results from the hypertrophied ventricular septum bulging into and encroaching on the right ventricular cavity and leads to impairment of right ventricular filling. In such cases, the jugular venous pressure is elevated and the *a* wave is prominent.

AUSCULTATION (Tables 33–5, p. 1040, and 33–11 and 33–12). S_1 is normal or soft and S_4 is prominent, presumably because atrial contraction is vigorous and the mitral valve is partially closed during presystole.[385, 386] S_2 may be single because calcification and immobility of the aortic valve make A_2 inaudible, because P_2 is buried in the prolonged aortic ejection murmur, or because prolongation of left ventricular systole makes A_2 coincide with P_2. Paradoxical splitting of S_2, which suggests associated left ventricular dysfunction, may also occur. With left ventricular failure and secondary pulmonary hypertension, P_2 may become accentuated. When the valve is rigid, A_2 may be inaudible, but when the valve is flexible, A_2 may be snapping and accentuated (Fig. 3–22, p. 56).

An *aortic ejection sound* (p. 48) occurs simultaneously

TABLE 33–11 CONDITIONS FREQUENTLY CONFUSED WITH AORTIC STENOSIS

Condition	Distinguishing Features
Dilated aorta (hypertension, syphilis) with systolic murmur in second right intercostal space	No single or paradoxical S_2; A_2 normal or loud; murmur often short
Bruit arising in carotid or subclavian arteries (benign supraclavicular bruit, arterial occlusive disease)	Bruit louder in neck or supraclavicular fossae and may be obliterated by subclavian artery compression; bruit may be shorter; normal S_2
Pulmonic valvular stenosis	Murmur reaches A_2; more frequent systolic ejection click; P_2 faint and delayed; A_2 normal; right ventricular enlargement; occasional large jugular *a* wave
Severe aortic regurgitation	Widened pulse pressure; visible carotid pulse; A_2 may be normal
Minimal valvulitis or calcification	Normal A_2; normal respiratory motion of S_2; no left ventricular enlargement
Mitral regurgitation	Pansystolic or ejection murmur; normal respiratory variation of S_2; normal A_2; S_1 may be faint; S_3 gallop common if severe; aortic stenosis murmur often of grunting quality at cardiac apex; murmur usually well heard in left axilla, decreased by amyl nitrite inhalation (which increases murmur of aortic stenosis) and increased by administration of phenylephrine; no aortic valve calcification of fluoroscopy

From Fowler, N. O.: Aortic stenosis: Left ventricular outflow tract obstruction. *In* Fowler, N. O. (ed.): Cardiac Diagnosis and Treatment. 3rd ed. Hagerstown, Md., Harper and Row, 1980, p. 550.

with the halting upward movement of the aortic valve. It is dependent on mobility of the valve cusps and disappears when they become severely calcified. Thus, it is common in children with congenital AS but is rare in elderly adults with acquired calcific AS and rigid valves. This sound occurs approximately 0.06 sec after the onset of S_1, has a frequency similar to S_1, and is heard most readily with the diaphragm of the stethoscope along the left sternal border, although it is often well transmitted to the apex, where it may be confused with S_1 (and the S_1 may be mistaken for an S_4). In contrast to a pulmonic ejection sound, aortic ejection sounds usually do not vary with respiration and usually occur later.

The *systolic murmur* of AS is heard best at the base of the heart but is often well transmitted along the carotid vessels and to the apex. Cessation of the murmur before A_2 is usually helpful in differentiating it from a pansystolic mitral murmur, but it may be falsely considered to be a pansystolic murmur because it may end with S_2, which represents pulmonic valve closure, A_2 being soft or even inaudible (Figs. 3–22, p. 56, 4–1, p. 66, and 4–7, p. 68). In patients with calcified aortic valves, the murmur is harsh and rasping at the base, but high-frequency components selectively radiate to the apex (the so-called Gallavardin phenomenon), where it may actually be more prominent and where it may be mistaken for the murmur of mitral regurgitation. Frequently, there is a "quiet area" between the base and apex where the murmur is diminished in intensity, supporting the erroneous impression that the apical and basal murmurs have different origins. In general, the more severe the stenosis, the longer the duration of the murmur [387] and the more likely that it peaks in midsystole.[388] Spectral analysis has revealed high-frequency components in severe AS.[389, 390]

In patients with degenerative or atherosclerotic AS, there may be heavy valvular calcification, but obstruction may not be severe because the commissural fusion characteristic of congenital and rheumatic AS is absent. The nonfused calcified cusps vibrate freely, resulting in a softer, more musical murmur, more prominent at the apex than the murmur of congenital or rheumatic AS.[387] High-pitched decrescendo diastolic murmurs secondary to aortic regurgitation are common in many patients with dominant AS.

In hypertrophic cardiomyopathy (HCM), the murmur is delayed in onset and may continue up to A_2; the carotid artery characteristically rises sharply (Table 33–11) and is bisferiens. Palpation of the carotid pulse is also extremely helpful in differentiating between valvular AS on the one hand and HCM and MR on the other, because the arterial

TABLE 33–12 DIFFERENTIAL DIAGNOSIS OF AORTIC STENOSIS: PHYSICAL FINDINGS

Type of Stenosis	Maximum Murmur and Thrill	Aortic Ejection Sound	Aortic Component of Second Sound	Regurgitant Diastolic Murmur	Arterial Pulse
Acquired nonrheumatic	Second right sternal border to neck; may be at apex in the aged	Uncommon	Decreased or absent	Common	Delayed upstroke; anacrotic notch; ± small amplitude
Acquired rheumatic		Uncommon	Decreased or absent	Common	
Hypertrophic subaortic	Fourth left sternal border to apex (± regurgitant systolic murmur at apex)	Rare	Normal or decreased	Very rare	Brisk upstroke, sometimes bisferiens
Congenital valvular	Second right sternal border to neck (along left sternal border in some infants)	Very common in children, disappearing with decrease in valve mobility with age	Normal or increased in childhood; decreased with decrease in valve mobility with age	Uncommon in child; not uncommon in adult	Delayed upstroke; anacrotic notch; ± small amplitude
Congenital subvalvular	Discrete: like valvular; tunnel: left sternal border	Rare	Not helpful (normal, increased, decreased or absent)	Almost all	
Congenital supravalvular	First right sternal border to neck and sometimes to medial aspect of right arm; occasionally greater in neck than in chest	Rare	Normal or decreased	Uncommon	Rapid upstroke in right carotid, delayed in left carotid; right arm pulse pressure greater than left

From Levinson, G. E.: Aortic stenosis. *In* Dalen, J. E., and Alpert, J. S.: Valvular Heart Disease. 2nd ed. Boston, Little, Brown and Company, 1987, p. 202.

pulse generally rises slowly in AS but sharply in the other two conditions. However, confusion can arise in the young patient with congenital AS, in whom sudden upward displacement ("doming") of the pliant aortic leaflet or leaflets with ventricular systole may result in a brisk initial upstroke in the carotid pulse, coincident with the systolic ejection click.

When the left ventricle fails in AS and the cardiac output falls, the murmur becomes softer or disappears altogether, and the slowly rising pulse is more difficult to recognize. Stated simply, the clinical picture changes to that of severe left ventricular failure with a low cardiac output and pulmonary edema. Thus, occult AS may be a cause of intractable heart failure, and critical AS should be actively sought in patients with severe heart failure of unknown cause, since operative treatment may be life-saving and may result in substantial clinical improvement.[391, 392]

Dynamic Auscultation (Table 33–6). The murmur of valvular AS is augmented by the inhalation of amyl nitrite or with squatting or lying flat and is reduced in intensity during the Valsalva strain, which increases the murmur of HCM or that produced with vasopressors, moderate isometric exercise, or standing.[393] It varies in intensity from beat to beat when the duration of diastolic filling varies, as in atrial fibrillation or following a premature contraction, and this characteristic is helpful in differentiating AS from mitral regurgitation, in which the murmur is usually unaffected (Fig. 4–8, p. 69). An aortic diastolic murmur is frequently present in patients with valvular AS.

LABORATORY EXAMINATION

ELECTROCARDIOGRAM. The principal electrocardiographic change is left ventricular hypertrophy, which is found in approximately 85 per cent of patients with severe AS (Fig. 7–14*A*, p. 191). The absence of left ventricular hypertrophy does not exclude the presence of critical AS, and the relationship between the absolute voltages in precordial leads and the severity of obstruction, which is quite good in children with congenital AS, is not as good in adults. T-wave inversion and ST-segment depressions in leads having upright QRS complexes are common. ST-segment depressions greater than 0.3 mV in patients with AS suggest that severe ventricular hypertrophy is present. The progressive development of ST-segment and T-wave abnormalities suggests that hypertrophy has progressed. Occasionally, a "pseudoinfarction" pattern is present, characterized by a loss of r waves in the right precordial leads and an early vector directed posteriorly in the horizontal plane of the vectorcardiogram, simulating anteroseptal infarction. A good correlation has been reported between the sum of the QRS amplitude in 12 leads and the height of the left ventricular systolic pressure.[393a] There is evidence of left atrial enlargement in more than 80 per cent of patients with severe isolated AS[394]; the principal manifestation is prominent late negativity of the P wave in V_1 rather than an increased duration in lead II, suggesting that hypertrophy rather than dilatation is present. Atrial fibrillation is an uncommon and late sign of pure AS, and, when present in a patient who is not greatly disabled, should suggest the possibility of mitral valvular disease or ischemic heart disease.

The extension of calcific infiltrates from the aortic valve into the conduction system may cause various forms and degrees of atrioventricular and intraventricular block in 5 per cent of patients with calcific AS.[395–397] Conduction defects are more common in patients with mitral annular calcium.[397] Almost 10 per cent of all instances of left anterior hemiblock are secondary to aortic valvular disease.[398] Ambulatory electrocardiography frequently shows complex ventricular arrhythmias,[399] particularly in patients with myocardial dysfunction.[400]

VECTORCARDIOGRAM. In patients with severe AS, the vectorcardiogram usually shows an increase in the maximal spatial voltage and counterclock inscription of the loop in the transverse plane, with the major forces in the left posterior quadrant. In the left sagittal plane, the QRS loop is usually directed posteriorly and superiorly.[401]

GRAPHIC RECORDINGS. The indirect carotid, jugular, and apical pulse tracings, systolic time intervals, and phonocardiographic findings in AS are discussed in Chapters 3 and 4.

RADIOLOGICAL FINDINGS. Routine radiological examination may be entirely normal despite the presence of critical AS. The heart is usually of normal size or slightly enlarged, with a rounding of the left ventricular border and apex (Fig. 6–27, p. 156), unless regurgitation or left ventricular failure is present and causes substantial cardiomegaly. Poststenotic dilatation of the ascending aorta is a common finding. Calcification of the aortic valve is found in almost all adults with hemodynamically significant AS[402, 403]; it may have to be sought on fluoroscopy (or the echocardiogram) rather than on the roentgenogram. This is an important finding; indeed, the *absence* of calcium in the region of the aortic valve on careful fluoroscopic examination in a patient older than 35 essentially rules out severe AS. The converse is not true, however, and in patients over the age of 60, severe calcification of the aortic valve may occur with only mild obstruction. The left atrium may be slightly enlarged, and there may be radiological signs of pulmonary venous hypertension. However, when left atrial enlargement is marked, particularly if the atrial appendage is prominent, the presence of associated mitral valvular disease should be suspected.

Angiographic studies of the aortic valve are best performed by injecting contrast medium into the left ventricle and filming in the 30-degree right anterior oblique and 60-degree left anterior oblique projections. These examinations often make it possible to ascertain the number of cusps of the stenotic valve and to demonstrate doming of a thickened valve and a systolic jet. However, it must be appreciated that there is some hazard of the rapid injection of a large volume of contrast material into a high-pressure left ventricle, and this is ordinarily not indicated in patients with AS, critical obstruction, and/or left ventricular failure.

ECHOCARDIOGRAPHY (See also p. 108). The normal range of opening of the aortic valve is 1.6 to 2.6 cm, and normally the aortic valve leaflets are barely visible in systole. In patients with severe AS, thickened leaflets and a barely discernible aortic orifice in systole can often be recognized on the M-mode echocardiogram (Fig. 5–56, p. 108). However, a reduced aortic valve opening may also be seen in other conditions, such as heart failure, in which there is decreased blood flow across the aortic valve. In patients with a bicuspid aortic valve, the valve cusps are asymmetrical, resulting in their eccentric position within the aortic root. Dense, multiple echoes within the aortic root in the area of the aortic leaflets suggest valvular calcification and support the diagnosis of AS. Systolic vibrations of the interventricular septum are common in congenital AS.[404] Although M-mode echocardiography can be used to diagnose calcific AS, detect marked elevations in left ventricular end-diastolic pressure by prolongation of the A-C interval (Fig. 5–41, p. 101), detect dilatation of the aorta, and estimate the severity of left ventricular hypertrophy as well as assess left ventricular function, it cannot establish the severity of obstruction directly. Two-dimensional echocardiography may also be helpful in determining the severity of the stenosis, by imaging the orifice (Fig. 5–57, p. 108). Doppler echocardiography allows calculation of the left ventriculoaortic pressure gradient[405–408] using a modified Bernouilli equation (Figs. 5–58 and 5–59, p. 109). The noninvasively determined gradients correlate well with those determined by left heart catheterization (Fig. 33–27).

MANAGEMENT

MEDICAL TREATMENT

Patients with AS should be apprised of the hazards of endocarditis, and the necessity for endocarditis prophylaxis should be explained (p. 1127). Patients who are asymptomatic should be advised to report the development of any symptoms possibly related to AS to their physician. Noninvasive assessment of the severity of obstruction by Doppler echocardiography should be carried out. In patients with mild obstruction, this measurement should be repeated, because obstruction tends to become more severe over time.[409–412] There is a close correlation between the left ventricular–aortic systolic pressure gradient deter-

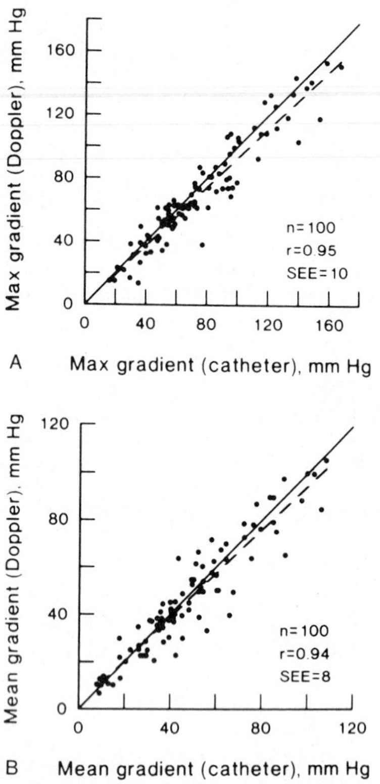

FIGURE 33–27. *A*, Correlation of simultaneous maximal (Max) Doppler and catheter pressure gradients in the 100 patients with aortic stenosis. The regression equation is: Doppler gradient = 0.5 + 0.93 × catheter gradient. *B*, Correlation of simultaneous mean Doppler and catheter pressure gradients in the 100 patients. The regression equation is: Doppler gradient = 1.8 + 0.93 × catheter gradient. The dotted lines represent the regression lines and the solid lines represent the lines of identity. (From Currie, P. J., et al.: Instantaneous pressure gradient: A simultaneous Doppler and dual catheter correlative study. Reprinted by permission of the American College of Cardiology. J. Am. Coll. Cardiol. *7*:803, 1986.)

mined by echocardiography and left heart catheterization (Fig. 33–27). Those with known or suspected critical obstruction should be cautioned to avoid vigorous athletic and physical activity. However, such restrictions do not apply to patients with mild obstruction. Because there is a tendency for the obstruction to become progressively more severe in patients with AS,[409, 410, 412] asymptomatic patients with AS should be followed carefully; in doing so, it is essential to look for signs of possible progression.[413] Repeated clinical examinations and electrocardiographic echocardiographic studies at intervals of 6 to 12 months are indicated in asymptomatic patients with significant AS.

There is no need to use digitalis glycosides unless evidence exists of an increase in ventricular volume or a reduced ejection fraction. Although diuretics are beneficial when there is abnormal accumulation of fluid, they must be used with caution, because hypovolemia may reduce the elevated left ventricular end-diastolic pressure, lower cardiac output, and produce orthostatic hypotension. Beta-adrenoceptor blockers can depress myocardial function and induce left ventricular failure and should be used only with great caution, if at all, in patients with AS.

Atrial arrhythmias occur in less than 10 per cent of patients with severe AS, perhaps because of the late occurrence of left atrial enlargement in this condition. When such an arrhythmia is observed in a patient with AS, the possibility of associated mitral valve disease should be considered. In light of the adverse hemodynamic effects of loss of atrial booster pump function with atrial fibrillation in patients with AS,[355] an effort should be made to prevent the development of this arrhythmia by pharmacological prophylaxis when premature atrial contractions are frequent. When atrial fibrillation does occur, the rapid ventricular rate may cause angina or electrocardiographic evidence of myocardial ischemia or both; in some cases, loss of the atrial "kick" and a sudden fall in cardiac output may cause serious hypotension. Therefore, this arrhythmia should be treated promptly (p. 672), and a search for previously unrecognized mitral valve disease should be undertaken.

Cardiac catheterization should be carried out in children in whom clinical examination and noninvasive tests suggest critical obstruction, regardless of whether or not symptoms are present. Adults considered to have severe AS should undergo catheterization if any symptoms develop. The purpose of catheterization in patients with AS is to localize the site and document the severity of the obstruction, to determine the state of left ventricular function, to ascertain the presence or absence of associated valvular disease, and, in patients with angina pectoris, to determine the status of the coronary circulation.

NATURAL HISTORY

In contrast to MS, which leads to symptoms almost immediately after its development, patients with severe AS may be asymptomatic for many years despite the presence of severe obstruction. The systolic pressure gradient can exceed 150 mm Hg, and the peak left ventricular systolic pressure can reach approximately 300 mm Hg with relatively little increase in overall heart size on radiographic examination, with normal left ventricular end-diastolic and end-systolic volumes. Patients with severe chronic AS tend to be free of cardiovascular symptoms until relatively late in the course of the disease. In Rapaport's series, 40 per cent of patients treated medically survived for 5 years and 20 per cent for 10 years after diagnosis.[87] In another series of patients with hemodynamically significant valvular AS treated medically, the 5-year survival rate was 64 per cent. However, once patients with AS become symptomatic with angina or syncope, the average survival is 2 to 3 years, whereas with congestive heart failure it is 1½ years[372] (Fig. 33–28). Sudden death, like syncope, in patients with severe AS may be due to cerebral hypoperfusion followed by arrhythmia. Among

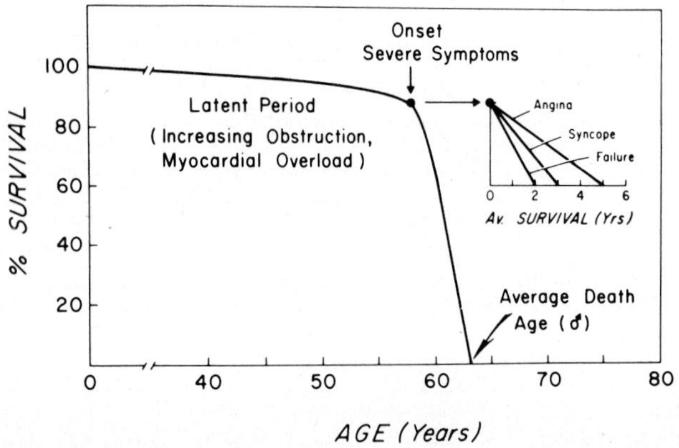

FIGURE 33–28. Natural history of aortic stenosis without operative treatment. (From Ross, J., Jr., and Braunwald, E.: Aortic stenosis. Circulation *38*[Suppl. V]:61, 1968, by permission of the American Heart Association, Inc.)

symptomatic patients with moderate or severe AS not subjected to operation, mortality rates from onset of symptoms were approximately 25 per cent at 1 year and 50 per cent at 2 years; more than half of the deaths were sudden. Asymptomatic patients have an excellent prognosis insofar as survival is concerned.[414] While severe AS is a potentially lethal disease, death, even when sudden, usually occurs in symptomatic patients. The obstruction tends to progress more rapidly in patients with degenerative calcific disease than in those with congenital or rheumatic disease.[415]

SURGICAL TREATMENT

INDICATIONS FOR OPERATION. The most critical decision in the management of patients with AS—indeed, of all patients with valvular heart disease—concerns the advisability and timing of surgical treatment. The indications for as well as the techniques and results of operation depend on the patient's age and the nature of the valvular deformity. In children and adolescents with noncalcific congenital AS, who most commonly have bicuspid aortic valves, simple commissural incision under direct vision usually leads to substantial hemodynamic improvement at a low risk, i.e., a mortality rate of less than 1 per cent (p. 936).[416] Therefore, this procedure is indicated not only in symptomatic patients but also in asymptomatic children and adolescents with critical aortic stenosis, i.e., a calculated effective orifice less than 0.75 cm^2/m^2 BSA. Despite the salutary hemodynamic results following this procedure, the valve is not rendered entirely normal anatomically, and the turbulent flow through it may lead to further deformation, calcification, the development of regurgitation, and restenosis after 10 to 20 years, probably requiring reoperation and valve replacement later.

In most adults with calcific AS, satisfactory valvular function *cannot* be restored, even by deliberate sculpturing procedures carried out under direct vision, and valve replacement is the surgical treatment of choice.[417] (Prosthetic valves are discussed on pp. 1078 to 1081.) The aortic valve should be replaced in patients with hemodynamic evidence of severe obstruction (aortic valve orifice < 0.75 cm^2 or < 0.4 cm^2/m^2 BSA) and symptoms believed to result from AS as well as in asymptomatic patients with serious left ventricular dysfunction and progressive cardiomegaly. Although a prospective randomized controlled study has not been carried out, the long-term mortality in patients undergoing operation in the latter group appears to be lower than that in medically treated patients without operation.[418] As artificial valves and surgical skills continue to improve, it is likely that patients with severe AS will become candidates for operation at earlier stages in the natural history of their disease. At the present time, I do not recommend prophylactic replacement of a critically narrow calcific aortic valve in totally asymptomatic patients without evidence of progressive left ventricular dysfunction.

RESULTS. Successful replacement of the aortic valve has resulted in substantial clinical and hemodynamic improvement in patients with AS, AR, or combined lesions.[417–423] In patients without frank left ventricular failure, the operative risk ranges from 2 to 8 per cent in most centers. Risk factors include New York Heart Association (NYHA) class, impairment of left ventricular function, age, and the presence of associated aortic regurgitation.[417] The 5-year actuarial survival rate of hospital survivors is approximately 85 per cent. Risk factors for late death include preoperative NYHA class, left ventricular function, preoperative ventricular arrhythmias, aortic regurgitation, older age, and concomitant untreated coronary artery disease.[417] Symptoms secondary to elevations of left atrial pressure and myocardial ischemia are relieved in virtually all patients. Hemodynamic results are equally impressive; elevated end-diastolic and end-systolic volumes show significant reductions. Ventricular performance often returns to normal more frequently in patients with AS than in those with aortic regurgitation.[424] The increased left ventricular mass is reduced toward (but not quite to) normal within 18 months following aortic valve replacement in patients with AS, AR, or mixed lesions.[365, 425]

When operation is carried out in patients with frank left ventricular failure or a depressed ejection fraction, the operative risk is higher, and the mortality ranges from 10 to 25 per cent, depending on the skill of the surgical team and the severity of depression of left ventricular function.[426] A depressed relation between ejection fraction and wall stress is a poor prognostic index (Fig. 14–11, p. 434), as is a depressed level of dP/dt max at any given left ventricular end-diastolic pressure.[419] Obviously, it is desirable to perform surgery before the development of heart failure, but even in the most desperate situations, such as cardiac arrest or pulmonary edema from AS, emergency operation sometimes may be life-saving. Certainly, in view of the extremely poor prognosis of such patients when they are treated medically, there is usually little choice but to advise immediate mechanical relief of obstruction, i.e., balloon angioplasty (see below) or emergency surgery.[427] Many symptomatic patients with calcific AS are elderly, and particular attention must be directed to the adequacy of their hepatic, renal, and pulmonary function. However, the results of aortic valve replacement are satisfactory in patients older than 70, and if the patient's general condition permits, age, per se, while adding to the risk, should not be considered a contraindication to operation.[428]

In patients with AS and obstructive coronary artery disease (a relatively common combination), aortic valve replacement and myocardial revascularization should be performed together. Although the risk of aortic valve surgery is increased by the association of coronary artery disease, the operative mortality in patients undergoing the combined procedure is not necessarily higher than that of isolated aortic valve replacement in this group.[417] Indeed, the surgical risk rises if severe coronary artery disease is left untreated. The ability to avoid serious myocardial ischemia in the perioperative period is a major factor that has served to reduce operative mortality. After the patient has been placed on cardiopulmonary bypass, the heart is protected by means of hypothermic cardiac arrest alone or combined with cardioplegia. The calcified valve must be removed with great care to avoid embolization of calcified fragments into the systemic circulation.

BALLOON VALVULOPLASTY

(See Fig. 40–22, p. 1391)

This new technique represents an increasingly attractive alternative to aortic valvotomy in children and adolescents with congenital AS and to aortic valve replacement in adults with calcific AS. A series of balloon dilatation catheters is advanced along a guidewire positioned at the left ventricular apex. In balloon dilatation carried out on postmortem specimens and in the operating room, fracture of calcified nodules and/or separation of fused commissures were found to be responsible for the relief of obstruction.[113, 429] There is considerable variation in patient response. However, this technique has resulted in relief of obstruction in most patients[430–433] (Fig. 33–26). Left ventricular ejection fraction tends to rise in patients with depressed left ventricular function.

As of July 1, 1987, 112 patients with calcific AS have undergone balloon valvuloplasty at Boston's Beth Israel Hospital[115]; their average age was 79 years and most were considered to be too ill or debilitated to be surgical candidates. The procedure was successful in 110 patients. Seventy-three patients have experienced striking clinical improvement which has lasted at least 6 months. Sixteen patients have died; five within 30 days of balloon valvuloplasty and 11 at an average of 3 months; 23 patients have developed restenosis. The procedure was unsuccessful in two patients. Complications include cardiac tamponade in two patients and the need for surgical vascular repair in 11 patients. Systemic embolization has not been observed although one patient developed aortic regurgitation.

Balloon aortic valvuloplasty, while still investigational, appears to be useful in patients with critical AS who decline surgical treatment or in whom surgical intervention is not advised because of an extremely high expected mortality. The procedure is also effective in young patients with noncalcific congenital AS. If with more experience the risk proves to be low, it is possible that balloon valvuloplasty may be utilized as an alternative in patients with calcific AS who are good candidates for surgical treatment.

AORTIC REGURGITATION

ETIOLOGY AND PATHOLOGY

Aortic regurgitation (AR) may be caused by primary disease of either the aortic valve leaflets or the wall of the aortic root or both (Table 33–13, Fig. 33–29). Among patients with pure AR coming to valve replacement, the percentage with aortic root disease has been increasing steadily during the past few decades and now accounts for more than one-third of all patients.[434]

VALVULAR DISEASE. *Rheumatic fever* is a common cause of primary disease of the valve leading to regurgitation.[10, 434, 435] The cusps become infiltrated with fibrous tissues and retract, a process that prevents cusp apposition during diastole and that usually leads to regurgitation into the left ventricle through a defect in the center of the valve. Often the associated fusion of the commissures may also restrict the opening of the valve, resulting in combined AS and AR (Fig. 33–30B); some associated mitral valve involvement is common. Other primary valvular causes of AR include *infective endocarditis* (Chap. 34), in which the infection may destroy the valve or cause a perforation of a leaflet, or the vegetations may interfere with proper coaptation of the cusps. *Trauma* (Fig. 45–8, p. 1542) resulting in a tear of the ascending aorta and loss of commissural support can cause prolapse of an aortic cusp. Although the most common complication of a *bicuspid valve* is stenosis in adult life, incomplete closure and/or prolapse of the larger of the two cusps of a congenitally *bicuspid valve* may cause regurgitation in childhood.[436] More commonly, progressive regurgitation of a congenitally bicuspid valve develops in the third and fourth decades[437, 438] (as may the aortic cusps in patients with Marfan syndrome, Ehlers-Danlos syndrome, cystic medionecrosis of the aorta, myxomatous proliferation of the aortic valve,[439, 439a] and related diseases of connective tissue). Less common causes of AR include a variety of forms of congenital AR (p. 1034); rupture of a congenitally fenestrated valve,[440] particularly in the presence of hypertension[441]; systemic lupus erythematosus[442]; rheumatoid arthritis[443] (p. 1719); ankylosing spondylitis[444] (p. 1717); and Whipple's disease.[445] Isolated congenital AR is an uncommon lesion on necropsy studies, but when present, it is usually associated with a bicuspid valve.[446]

AORTIC ROOT DISEASE. A variety of diseases produce aortic regurgitation by causing marked dilatation of the ascending aorta (Fig. 33–30C). These conditions, discussed in detail in Chapter 54, include annuloaortic ectasia, cystic medionecrosis of the aorta (either isolated or associated with classic Marfan syndrome), osteogenesis imperfecta, syphilitic aortitis, ankylosing spondylitis, Behçet syndrome,[447] psoriatic arthritis, arthritis associated with ulcerative colitis, relapsing polychondritis, Reiter syndrome, giant cell arteritis, osteogenesis imperfecta, and systemic hypertension.[441, 448–454]

Table 33–14 presents a comparison of the findings in four important conditions in which dilation of the aorta causes AR. In each of these, the aortic annulus may become greatly dilated, the aortic leaflets separate, and AR may ensue. Dissection of the diseased aortic wall may occur and may aggravate the AR. Dilatation of the aortic root may also have secondary effects on the aortic valve, since it results in tension and bowing of the individual cusps, which may thicken, retract, and become too short to close the aortic orifice. This leads to intensification of the AR, which increases left ventricular stroke volume, further dilating the ascending aorta and thus leading to a vicious circle.

AR, regardless of its etiology, produces dilatation and hypertrophy of the left ventricle, dilatation of the mitral valve ring, and sometimes hypertrophy and dilatation of the left atrium. Endocardial pockets frequently develop in

TABLE 33–13 MECHANISMS OF AORTIC REGURGITATION

1. Cusp abnormality	Perforation	Bacterial endocarditis
	Reduction in area	Rheumatic disease Rheumatoid disease Ankylosing spondylitis
2. Aortic root distortion (aortitis)		Ankylosing spondylitis Nonspecific urethritis Nonspecific aortitis Rheumatoid disease Syphilis
3. Loss of commissural support		Fallot-type VSD Dissection tears of aorta
4. Aortic root dilatation	Aortitis (inflammatory)	Syphilis All other aortitis
	"Aortopathy" (noninflammatory)	Marfan Familial Idiopathic Ehlers-Danlos Pseudoxanthoma elasticum

From Davies, M. J.: Pathology of Cardiac Valves. London, Butterworths, 1980.

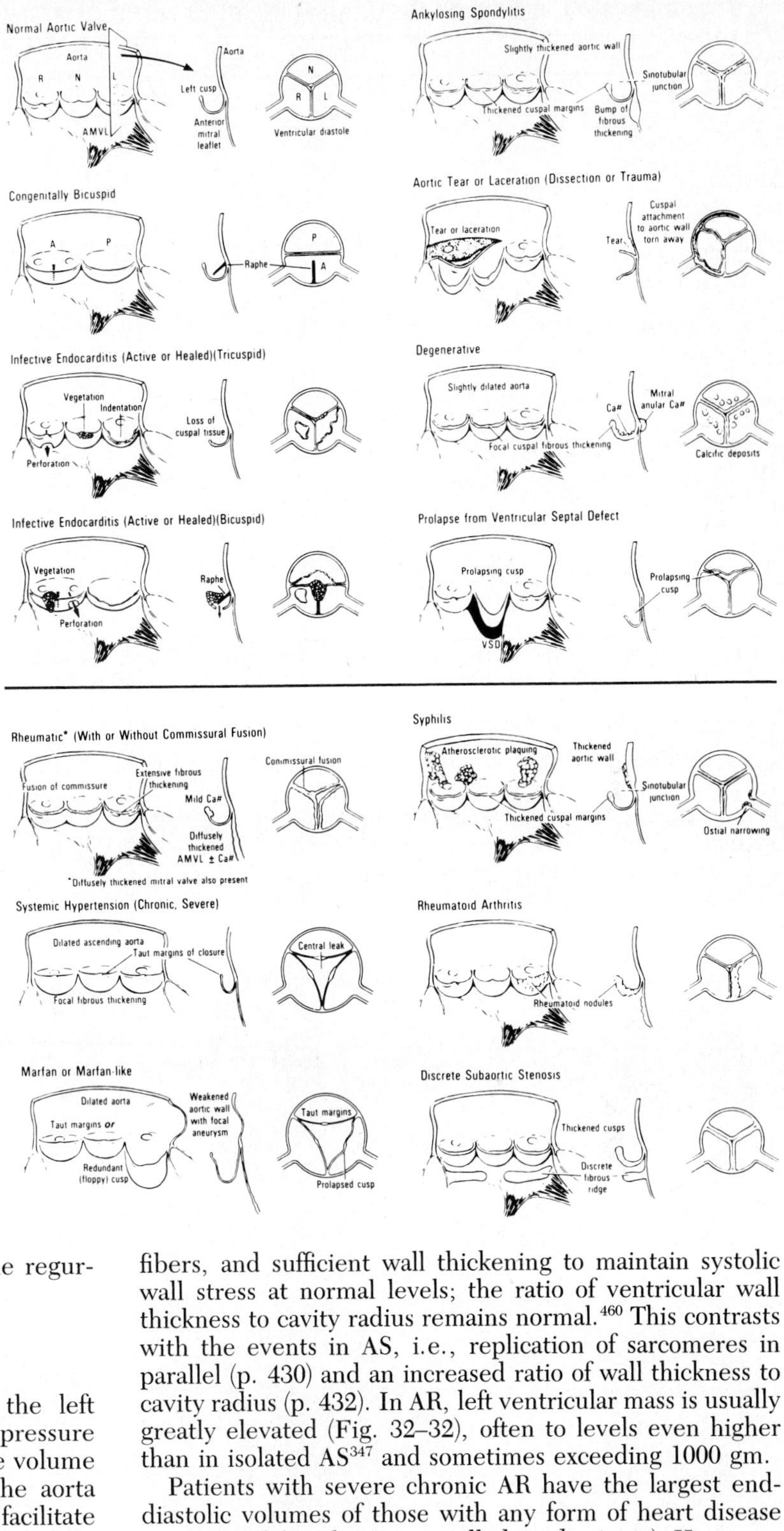

FIGURE 33–29. ***Top,*** **Diagram of various causes of pure aortic regurgitation.** ***Bottom,*** **Diagram of various causes of pure aortic regurgitation (continued). (From Waller, B. F.: Rheumatic and nonrheumatic conditions producing valvular heart disease.** ***In*** **Frankl, W. S., and Brest, A. N. [eds.]: Cardiovascular Clinics. Valvular Heart Disease: Comprehensive Evaluation and Management. Philadelphia, F. A. Davis, 1986, pp. 30 and 31.)**

the left ventricular cavity at sites of impact of the regurgitant jet.

PATHOPHYSIOLOGY

In contrast to MR, in which a fraction of the left ventricular stroke volume is ejected into the low-pressure left atrium, in AR the entire left ventricular stroke volume is ejected into a high-pressure chamber, i.e., the aorta (although the low aortic diastolic pressure does facilitate ventricular emptying during early systole). Whereas in MR the reduction of wall tension (i.e., reduced afterload) allows more complete systolic emptying, in AR the increase in left ventricular end-diastolic volume provides major hemodynamic compensation.[455–459]

Severe AR may occur with a normal effective forward stroke volume and a normal ejection fraction (total [forward plus regurgitant] stroke volume/end-diastolic volume), together with an elevated left ventricular end-diastolic pressure and volume (Figs. 33–31 and 33–32). In accord with Laplace's law (p. 405), left ventricular dilatation increases the left ventricular systolic tension required to develop any level of systolic pressure. The increased wall stress leads to replication of sarcomeres in series, elongation of fibers, and sufficient wall thickening to maintain systolic wall stress at normal levels; the ratio of ventricular wall thickness to cavity radius remains normal.[460] This contrasts with the events in AS, i.e., replication of sarcomeres in parallel (p. 430) and an increased ratio of wall thickness to cavity radius (p. 432). In AR, left ventricular mass is usually greatly elevated (Fig. 32–32), often to levels even higher than in isolated AS[347] and sometimes exceeding 1000 gm.

Patients with severe chronic AR have the largest end-diastolic volumes of those with any form of heart disease (Fig. 33–32) (resulting in so-called *cor bovinum*). However, end-diastolic pressure is not uniformly elevated (i.e., left ventricular compliance often becomes increased), and there is a wide scatter in the relationship between end-diastolic volume and end-diastolic pressure.[347] In the more severe cases of AR, the regurgitant flow may exceed 20 liters/min, so that the total left ventricular output approaches 25 liters/min, a level that can be achieved only by a trained endurance runner during maximal exercise. Thus, the adaptive response to chronic and gradually increasing AR permits the ventricle to function as an effective low-compliance pump, handling large end-diastolic and stroke volumes, often with little increase in filling pressure. During exercise, peripheral vascular resis-

TABLE 33–14 CARDIOVASCULAR MANIFESTATIONS OF CONDITIONS CAUSING AORTIC REGURGITATION

	Syphilis	Akylosing Spondylitis	Rheumatoid Arthritis	Marfan Syndrome
Average age	50	45	70	30
Predominant sex	Men	Men	Women	Men
Aortic regurgitation	+ + + +	+ + + +	+	+ + + +
Mitral regurgitation	0	+ +	+	+ + +
Conduction disturbances	+	+ + + +	+ +	+
Serology (STS)	+	0	0	0
Morphology of aorta				
Thickened adventitia	+ + + +	+ + + +	+	+
Degenerated media	+ + +	+ + +	0	+ + + +
Intimal proliferation	+ + +	+ + +	0	+
Vasa vasorum abnormal	+ + + +	+ + + +	0	0
Calcium	+ +	+	0	0
Aneurysms	+ + +	0	0	+ + +
Rupture	+	0	0	+
Dissection	0	0	0	+
Limited to sinuses	0	+	0	0
Morphology of aortic valve				
Cusp thickening				
Diffuse	0	+	0	0
Focal	+	0	+	+
Cusp calcification	0	0	0	0
Shortening	0	+	0	0
Commissural abnormality	+	+	0	0

From Roberts, W. C., et al.: Nonrheumatic valvular cardiac disease: A clinicopathologic survey of 27 different conditions causing valvular dysfunction. *In* Likoff, W. (ed.): Cardiovascular Clinics. Vol. 5, No. 2, Valvular Heart Disease. Philadelphia, F. A. Davis, 1973, p. 424.

tance declines, and with an increase in heart rate, diastole shortens and the regurgitation per beat decreases,[461–463] facilitating an increment in effective forward cardiac output without substantial increases in end-diastolic volume and pressure. The ejection fraction is often within normal limits, both at rest and during exercise when myocardial function, as reflected in the slope of the end-systolic pressure-volume relation is depressed.[464–466] Therefore, the latter is a more sensitive index of contractility than the former (p. 458).

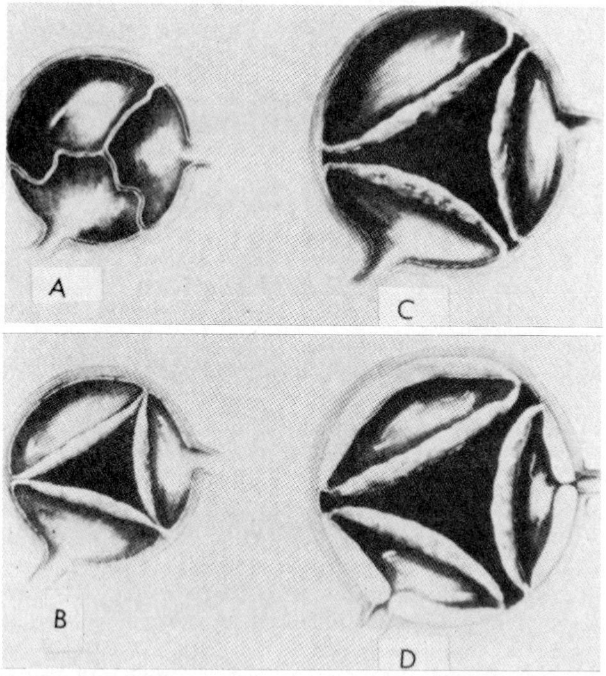

FIGURE 33–30. Variations in the aortic valve. ***A,*** **The normal valve.** ***B,*** **Shortening of the cusps characteristic of rheumatic aortic regurgitation. The caliber of the aorta is normal.** ***C,*** **Dilatation of the aorta, as occurs in syphilitic aortitis and other conditions in which dilatation is responsible for aortic regurgitation. The main feature results from bowing of the leaflets. Commissural separation is illustrated and may also be present.** ***D,*** **In addition to the features shown in** ***C,*** **there is atherosclerosis of the aorta, as occurs in syphilitic aortitis, with consequent coronary ostial narrowing. (From Roberts, W. C.: Valvular, subvalvular and supravalvular aortic stenosis: Morphologic features. In Edwards, J. E. [ed.]: Clinical-Pathologic Correlations #2. Philadelphia, F. A. Davis, 1973, p. 133.)**

As left ventricular function deteriorates, the end-diastolic volume increases without further elevation of the aortic regurgitant volume; the left ventricular end-diastolic radius/wall thickness ratio rises,[467] systolic tension rises, and afterload mismatch occurs[468] so that ejection fraction declines with any additional stress.[469] Ultimately the ejection fraction and forward stroke volume decline at rest, and ventricular emptying is impaired, i.e., end-systolic volume increases (Fig. 33–32). Many of these changes precede the development of symptoms. In advanced stages there may be considerable elevation of the left atrial, pulmonary artery wedge, pulmonary arterial, right ventricular, and right atrial pressures and lowering of the effective cardiac output, first during the stress of exercise[463] and then even at rest.

As is the case of MR (p. 1037), the end-systolic volume is a sensitive index of myocardial function in patients with AR and correlates with operative mortality and postoperative left ventricular dysfunction.[162] Both the immediate and the long-term results are excellent in patients with normal left ventricular end-systolic volumes (< 30 ml/m^2), poor in patients in whom this index is elevated (> 90 ml/m^2), and variable in patients with intermediate values. In general, however, for any given preoperative level of impairment of left ventricular function, the outlook for left ventricular function in the postoperative period is better in patients with AR than with MR..

When *acute* AR is induced experimentally, preload, wall tension, and myocardial oxygen consumption all rise substantially,[154, 456] a situation contrasting with that produced by acutely induced MR. In patients with chronic severe AR, myocardial oxygen requirements are also augmented by the increase in left ventricular mass. Since the major portion of coronary blood flow occurs during diastole, when arterial pressure is lower than normal, coronary perfusion pressure is reduced.[470] The result—a combination of increased oxygen demand and reduced supply—sets the

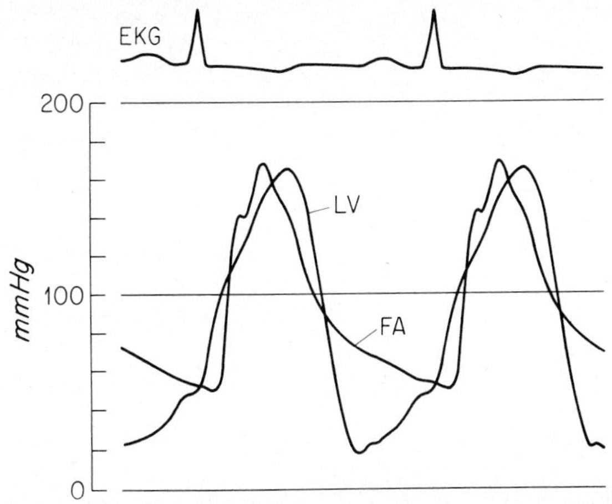

FIGURE 33–31. Pressure curves obtained from a 63-year-old man with symptoms of left ventricular failure and a loud decrescendo diastolic murmur. The femoral arterial (FA) pressure tracing demonstrates a widened pulse pressure of 115 mm Hg and equalization with left ventricular (LV) pressure late in diastole. The LV pressure curve exhibits a steady pressure increase throughout diastole, culminating in a markedly elevated end-diastolic pressure of 45 mm Hg. These findings are indicative of severe aortic regurgitation.

stage for the development of myocardial ischemia, especially during exercise.[471] The heightened activity of the adrenergic nervous system as a compensatory mechanism in patients with chronic AR is reflected in an abnormal increase in plasma catecholamine content during exercise, accompanied by a reduction in cardiac norepinephrine stores.[472] Symptomatic patients with severe chronic AR generally exhibit a depression of the relations between end-systolic pressure and stress and end-systolic volume. This depression of myocardial function, combined with the increased demands placed on the left ventricle, augments left ventricular end-diastolic volume and ultimately pressure causing symptoms of pulmonary congestion. These patients also demonstrate a failure of the normal decline in end-systolic volume or rise in ejection fraction during exercise, as determined by radionuclide angiography.[473] However, abnormal left ventricular function can be discerned even in subgroups of asymptomatic patients with normal ejection fractions; this dysfunction is reflected in failure of the normal increase in ejection fraction during exercise[474, 475] or a depressed end-systolic pressure-volume relation.[475] These techniques are likely to prove of great value in the identification of those patients with severe chronic aortic regurgitation, who, although asymptomatic or almost so, are at greater risk of developing left ventricular failure and therefore are candidates for consideration of surgical treatment.

ACUTE AORTIC REGURGITATION. In contrast to the pathophysiological events in chronic AR described above, in which the left ventricle has had the opportunity to adapt to the increased load, in *acute* regurgitation (caused most commonly by infective endocarditis, aortic dissection, and trauma) the regurgitant blood fills a ventricle of normal size that cannot accommodate the combined large regurgitant volume and inflow from the left atrium.[476, 477] Since total stroke volume cannot rise much acutely, forward stroke volume declines, left ventricular diastolic pressure rises rapidly to high levels,[455] and the left ventricle operates on a less compliant (steep) portion of its pressure-volume curve (Fig. 13–24, p. 402).[456]

The hemodynamic findings in acute AR contrast with those in chronic AR.[478] For a similarly severe degree of AR, the patient with acute regurgitation has a much smaller aortic pulse pressure and effective forward cardiac output, a smaller left ventricular volume, and a higher heart rate than the patient with chronic AR. In addition, as left ventricular pressure rises rapidly above left atrial pressure during early diastole, the mitral valve closes prematurely in diastole (Fig. 33–33).[479] This protects the pulmonary venous bed from backward transmission of the greatly elevated end-diastolic pressure. Premature closure of the mitral valve, together with the tachycardia that shortens diastole, reduces the time interval during which the mitral valve is open.[479] Left ventricular and aortic systolic pressures exhibit little change. Since aortic diastolic pressure cannot decline below the elevated left ventricular end-diastolic pressure, the systemic arterial pulse pressure widens relatively little.

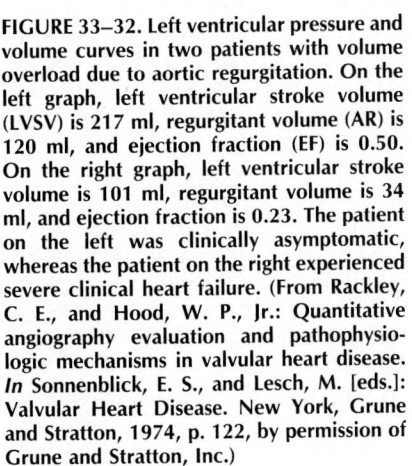

FIGURE 33–32. Left ventricular pressure and volume curves in two patients with volume overload due to aortic regurgitation. On the left graph, left ventricular stroke volume (LVSV) is 217 ml, regurgitant volume (AR) is 120 ml, and ejection fraction (EF) is 0.50. On the right graph, left ventricular stroke volume is 101 ml, regurgitant volume is 34 ml, and ejection fraction is 0.23. The patient on the left was clinically asymptomatic, whereas the patient on the right experienced severe clinical heart failure. (From Rackley, C. E., and Hood, W. P., Jr.: Quantitative angiography evaluation and pathophysiologic mechanisms in valvular heart disease. *In* Sonnenblick, E. S., and Lesch, M. [eds.]: Valvular Heart Disease. New York, Grune and Stratton, 1974, p. 122, by permission of Grune and Stratton, Inc.)

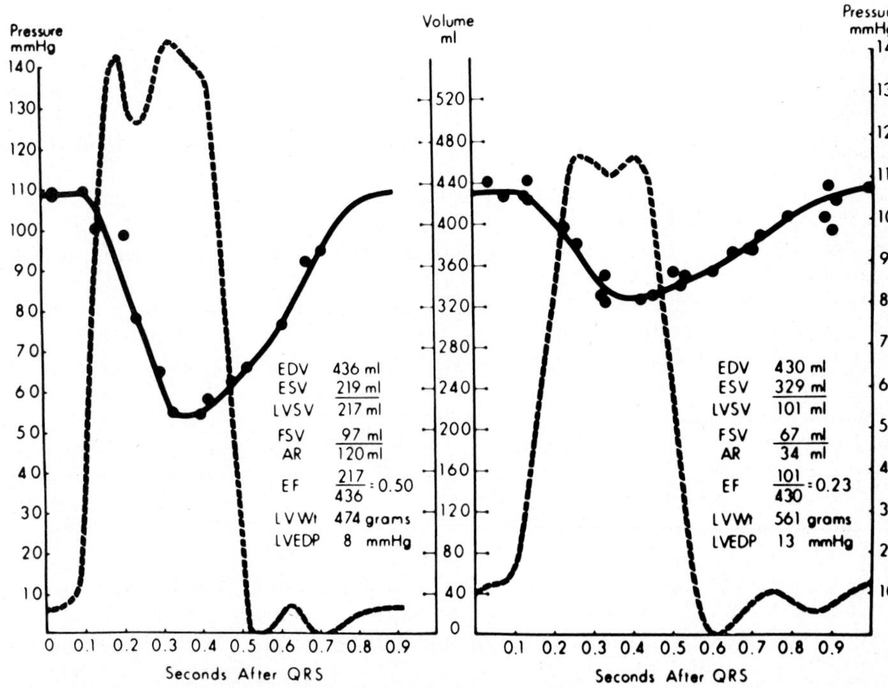

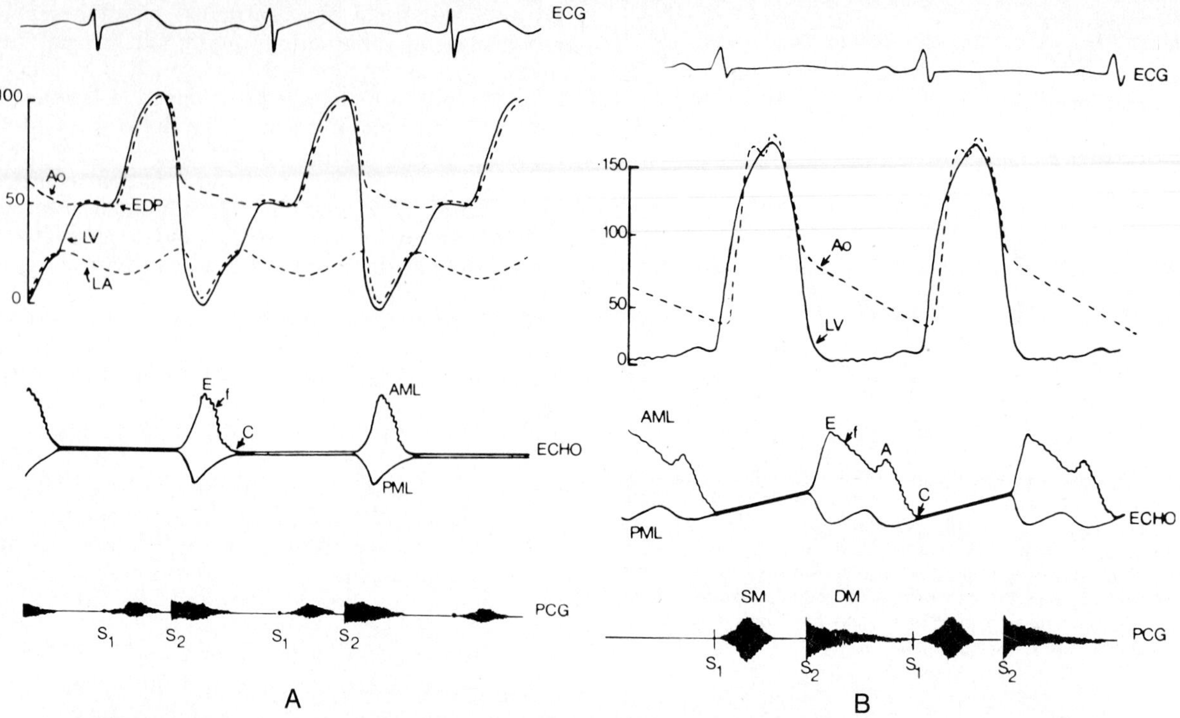

FIGURE 33–33. Schematic representations contrasting the hemodynamic, echocardiographic (ECHO), and phonocardiographic (PCG) manifestations of acute severe (*A*) and chronic severe (*B*) aortic regurgitation. Ao = aorta; LV = left ventricle; LA = left atrium; EDP = end-diastolic pressure; f = flutter of anterior mitral valve leaflet; AML = anterior mitral valve leaflet; PML = posterior mitral leaflet; SM = systolic murmur; DM = diastolic murmur; C = closure point of mitral valve. (From Morganroth, J., et al.: Acute severe aortic regurgitation. Ann. Intern. Med. *87*:225, 1977.)

CLINICAL MANIFESTATIONS

HISTORY

In patients with *chronic*, severe AR, there is a long period during which the left ventricle gradually undergoes enlargement while the patient remains asymptomatic or almost so.[435, 480] Symptoms of reduced cardiac reserve or myocardial ischemia develop, most often in the fourth or fifth decades and usually only after considerable cardiomegaly and myocardial dysfunction have occurred. When symptoms do develop, exertional dyspnea, orthopnea, and paroxysmal nocturnal dyspnea are the principal complaints. Syncope is rare, and although angina pectoris is less frequent than in patients with AS, nocturnal angina, often accompanied by diaphoresis, which occurs when the heart rate slows and arterial diastolic pressure falls to extremely low levels, may be particularly troublesome. These episodes may be accompanied by abdominal discomfort, presumably caused by splanchnic ischemia. Patients with severe AR often complain of an uncomfortable awareness of the heartbeat, especially on lying down, and disagreeable thoracic pain due to pounding of the heart against the chest wall. Tachycardia, occurring with emotional stress or exertion, may produce palpitations and head pounding; premature ventricular contractions are particularly distressing because of the great heave of the volume-loaded left ventricle during the postpremature beat. These complaints may be present for many years before symptoms of left ventricular dysfunction develop.

In light of the limited ability of the left ventricle to tolerate *acute* AR, patients with this valvular lesion often develop sudden clinical manifestations of cardiovascular collapse, with weakness, severe dyspnea, and hypotension; angina is uncommon.[478, 481]

PHYSICAL EXAMINATION

In patients with chronic severe AR, the head frequently bobs with each heartbeat (*de Musset's sign*),[482] and the pulses are of the water-hammer or collapsing type with abrupt distention and quick collapse (*Corrigan's pulse*) (p. 23). This pulse is readily visible in the carotid arteries and can be best appreciated by palpation of the radial artery with the patient's arm elevated. A bisferiens pulse may be present (Fig. 3–24, p. 56) and is more readily recognized in the brachial and femoral than in the carotid arteries. A variety of auscultatory findings provide confirmation of a wide pulse pressure. *Traube's sign* refers to booming systolic and diastolic sounds heard over the femoral artery, *Müller's sign* consists of systolic pulsations of the uvula, and *Duroziez's sign* consists of a systolic murmur heard over the femoral artery when it is compressed proximally and a diastolic murmur when it is compressed distally. Capillary pulsations, i.e., *Quincke's sign*, can be detected by pressing a glass slide on the patient's lip or by transmitting a light through the patient's fingertips.

Systolic arterial pressure is elevated, and diastolic pressure is abnormally low. *Hill's sign* refers to popliteal cuff systolic pressure exceeding brachial cuff pressure by more than 60 mm Hg. Korotkoff sounds often persist to zero even though intraarterial pressure rarely falls below 30 mm Hg. The point of change in intensity of the Korotkoff sounds, i.e., the muffling of these sounds in phase IV, correlates with the diastolic pressure. As heart failure develops, peripheral vasoconstriction may occur and arterial diastolic pressure may rise. However, this finding should not be interpreted as a reduction in the severity of the AR.

The apical impulse is diffuse and hyperdynamic and is displaced laterally and inferiorly; there may be systolic retraction over the parasternal region. A rapid ventricular filling wave is often palpable at the apex, as is a systolic thrill at the base of the heart or suprasternal notch and over the carotid arteries, resulting from the augmented stroke volume. In many patients, a carotid shudder is palpable or may be recorded.[483]

AUSCULTATION. In *chronic* severe AR, a soft S_1 and prolongation of the P-R interval frequently are present. A_2 is soft or absent, and P_2 may be obscured by the early diastolic murmur.[484] Thus, S_2 is variable; it may be absent or single or exhibit narrow or paradoxical splitting. A systolic ejection sound, presumably related to abrupt distention of the aorta by the augmented stroke volume, is frequently audible. An S_3 gallop correlates with an increased left ventricular end-systolic volume and has been suggested as a sign useful in considering patients with severe regurgitation for surgical treatment.[485]

The aortic regurgitant murmur is one of high frequency that begins immediately after A_2 (Figs. 4–22, p. 77, and 4–23, p. 78). It may be distinguished from the murmur of pulmonic regurgitation (p. 1076) by its earlier onset, i.e., immediately after A_2 rather than after P_2, and often by the presence of a widened pulse pressure. The murmur is heard best through the diaphragm of the stethoscope while the patient is sitting up and leaning forward, with the breath held in deep expiration. In severe AR, the murmur reaches an early peak and then has a dominant decrescendo pattern throughout diastole.

The severity of the regurgitation correlates better with the *duration* than with the *intensity* of the murmur. In mild AR, the murmur may be limited to the early phase of diastole and is typically high-pitched; in moderately severe and severe regurgitation, the murmur is holodiastolic and may have a rough quality. When the murmur is musical ("cooing dove" murmur), it usually signifies eversion or perforation of an aortic cusp. In severe AR and left ventricular decompensation, equilibration of aortic and left ventricular diastolic pressures in late diastole abolish this component of the regurgitant murmur. The murmur is best heard along the left sternal border in the third and fourth intercostal spaces when regurgitation is due to primary valvular disease, but it is often more readily audible along the right sternal border when it is due mainly to dilatation of the ascending aorta.[486] Murmurs in the latter position may be overlooked if auscultation along the right sternal border is not carried out routinely.

A mid- and late-diastolic apical rumble, the *Austin Flint murmur*, is common in severe AR and may occur in the presence of a normal mitral valve (Figs. 4–22, p. 77, and 33–34). This murmur appears to be created by rapid antegrade flow across a mitral orifice[461] that may be being narrowed by the rapidly rising left ventricular diastolic pressure caused by severe aortic reflux.[487] The Austin Flint murmur may be difficult to differentiate from that due to MS, but the presence of an opening snap and a loud S_1 in MS and the absence of these findings in AR are helpful clues (Table 33–15). As the left ventricular end-diastolic pressure rises, the Austin Flint murmur commences and terminates earlier, and in acute AR with premature diastolic closure of the mitral valve, the presystolic portion of the Austin Flint murmur is eliminated. A short, midsystolic murmur, grades 1 to 4/6, related to the increased ejection rate and stroke volume, may be audible at the base of the heart and transmitted to the carotid vessels. It may be higher pitched and less rasping than the murmur of aortic stenosis but is often accompanied by a thrill.

Dynamic Auscultation. The diastolic murmur of AR may be accentuated when the patient sits up and leans forward or by any intervention that raises the arterial pressure, such as infusion of a vasopressor drug, squatting, or isometric exercise. It is reduced by interventions that lower the systolic pressure, such as amyl nitrite inhalation and the strain of the Valsalva maneuver.[488] The Austin Flint murmur, like the murmur of AR, is augmented by isometric exercise and vasopressors and is reduced by amyl nitrite inhalation (Fig. 33–34).[488]

ACUTE AORTIC REGURGITATION. These patients often appear gravely ill, with tachycardia, severe peripheral vasoconstriction and cyanosis, and sometimes pulmonary congestion and edema (Table 33–16).[476, 478, 481] The peripheral signs of AR are often not impressive and certainly not as dramatic as in patients with chronic AR.[479] Duroziez's

TABLE 33–15 CHARACTERISTICS DISTINGUISHING THE MURMUR OF MITRAL STENOSIS FROM THE AUSTIN FLINT MURMUR

CLINICAL OR LABORATORY FINDING	MITRAL STENOSIS	AUSTIN FLINT MURMUR
Opening snap present	+	−
S_1 increased	+	−
S_3 present	−	+
Left ventricular enlargement and/or hypertrophy (physical examination, ECG, chest roentgenogram)	−	+
Right ventricular enlargement and/or hypertrophy (physical examination, ECG, chest roentgenogram)	+	−
Murmur decreases with amyl nitrite	−	+
Echocardiographic evidence of organic mitral stenosis	+	−
Presence of atrial fibrillation	+	−

From Alpert, J. S.: Chronic aortic regurgitation. *In* Dalen, J. E., and Alpert, J. S. (eds.): Valvular Heart Disease. 2nd ed. Boston, Little, Brown and Company, 1987, p. 291.

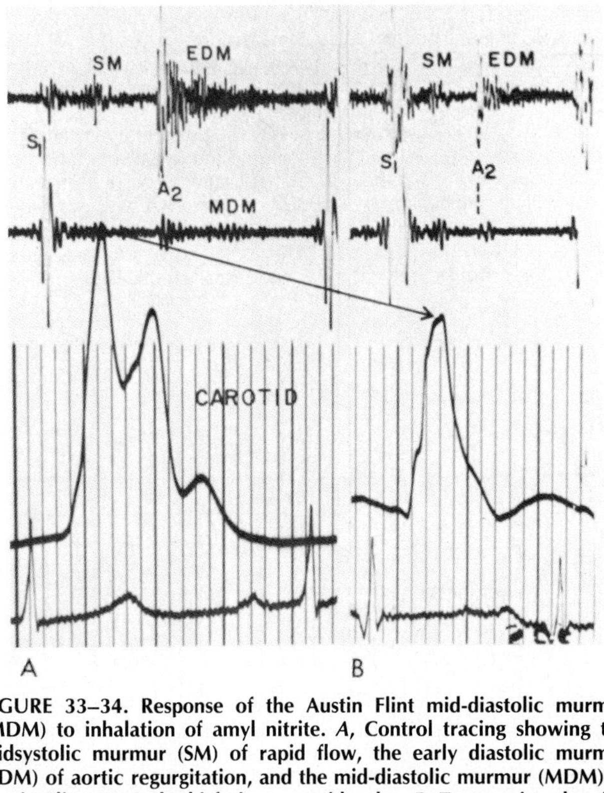

FIGURE 33–34. Response of the Austin Flint mid-diastolic murmur (MDM) to inhalation of amyl nitrite. *A*, Control tracing showing the midsystolic murmur (SM) of rapid flow, the early diastolic murmur (EDM) of aortic regurgitation, and the mid-diastolic murmur (MDM) of Austin Flint. Note the bisferiens carotid pulse. *B*, Test tracing showing loss of the bisferiens pulse as aortic regurgitation diminishes, together with a decrease in intensity of the early diastolic murmur and disappearance of the mid-diastolic Austin Flint murmur. (From Reichek, N., et al.: Clinical aspects of rheumatic valvular disease. Prog. Cardiovasc. Dis. *15*:521, 1973, by permission of Grune and Stratton.)

TABLE 33–16 MANIFESTATIONS OF SEVERE AORTIC REGURGITATION

	ACUTE	CHRONIC
CLINICAL FINDING		
Congestive heart failure	Early and sudden	Late and insidious
Arterial pulse		
Rate per minute	Increased	Normal
Rate of rise	Not increased	Increased
Systolic pressure	Normal to decreased	Increased
Diastolic pressure	Normal to decreased	Decreased
Pulse pressure	Near normal	Increased
Contour of peak	Single	Bisferiens
Pulsus alternans	Common	Uncommon
Left ventricular impulse	Near-normal to laterally displaced; not hyperdynamic	Laterally displaced, hyperdynamic
Auscultation		
First heart sound	Soft to absent	Normal
Aortic component of the second sound	Soft	Normal or decreased
Pulmonic component of the second sound	Normal or increased	Normal
Fourth heart sound	Consistently absent	Usually absent
Third heart sound	Common	Uncommon
Aortic systolic murmur	Grade 3 or less	Grade 3 or more
Aortic regurgitant murmur	Short, medium-pitched	Long, high-pitched
Austin Flint murmur	Mid-diastolic	Presystolic, mid-diastolic, or both
Peripheral arterial auscultatory signs	Absent	Present
ECG	Normal left ventricular voltage with minor repolarization abnormalities	Increased left ventricular voltage with major repolarization abnormalities
Chest roentgenogram		
Left ventricle	Normal to moderately increased	Markedly increased
Aortic root and arch	Usually normal	Prominent
Pulmonary venous pattern	Redistributed to upper lobes	Normal
ECHOCARDIOGRAPHIC VARIABLE		
Mitral valve		
Closure	Early	Normal
Opening	Late	Normal
Anterior leaflet E-F slope	Reduced	Normal
Diastolic fluttering	Yes	Yes
Septal wall motion	Normal	Hyperkinetic
Posterior wall motion	Normal	Hyperkinetic
End-diastolic dimension	Normal	Increased
Endsystolic dimension	Normal	Normal
Shortening fraction	Normal	Increased

Modified from Benotti, J. R.: Acute aortic insufficiency. *In* Dalen, J. E., and Alpert, J. S. (eds.): Valvular Heart Disease. 2nd ed. Boston, Little, Brown and Company, 1987, pp. 331 and 337.

murmur, pistol shot sounds over the peripheral arteries, and bisferiens pulses are absent. The arterial pulse may exhibit pulsus alternans. The normal pulse pressure may lead to serious underestimation of the severity of the valvular lesion. The left ventricular impulse is normal or nearly so, and the rocking motion of the chest characteristic of chronic AR is not apparent. S_1 may be soft or absent because of premature closure of the mitral valve.[489] Instead, the sound of mitral valve closure is heard occasionally in mid-diastole. However, closure of the mitral valve may be incomplete, and diastolic mitral regurgitation may occur.[490] Evidence of pulmonary hypertension, with an accentuated P_2 and an S_3 and S_4, is frequently present. The early diastolic murmur of acute AR is lower pitched and shorter than that of chronic AR, because as left ventricular end-diastolic pressure rises, the pressure gradient between the aorta and the left ventricle is rapidly reduced. The Austin Flint murmur, if present, is brief and ceases when left ventricular pressure exceeds left atrial pressure in diastole.

LABORATORY EXAMINATION

ELECTROCARDIOGRAM. *Chronic* AR results in left axis deviation and a pattern of left ventricular diastolic volume overload, characterized by an increase in initial forces (prominent Q waves in leads I, aV_1, and V_3 to V_6) and a relatively small r wave in V_1 (Fig. 33–35). With the passage of time, these initial forces diminish, but the total QRS amplitude increases. The T waves may be tall and upright in left precordial leads early in the course, but more commonly they are inverted, with ST-segment depressions.[491] Left intraventricular conduction defects occur late in the course and are usually associated with left ventricular dysfunction. When AR is caused by an inflammatory process, P-R prolongation may result.[492] However, the electrocardiogram is not an accurate predictor of the severity of AR or cardiac weight.[492] In *acute* AR, the electrocardiogram may or may not show left ventricular hypertrophy, despite the presence of left ventricular failure, depending upon the severity and duration of the regurgitation. However, nonspecific ST-segment and T-wave changes are common.

RADIOLOGICAL FINDINGS (See also p. 156). Cardiac size is a function of the duration and severity of regurgitation and the state of left ventricular function. In acute AR, there may be little cardiac enlargement, but marked enlargement is a common finding in chronic AR. Typically, the left ventricle enlarges in an inferior and leftward direction, causing a significant increase in the long axis (Fig. 6–4*A*, p. 143) but sometimes little or no increase in the transverse diameter of the heart. Calcification of the aortic valve is uncommon in patients with pure AR but is often present in patients with combined stenosis and regurgitation. As is the case with AS, the presence of distinct left atrial enlargement in the absence of heart failure should suggest the possibility of mitral valve disease. Dilatation of the ascending aorta is usually more marked than in AS and may involve the entire aortic arch, including the aortic knob. Severe, aneurysmal dilatation of the aorta should suggest that aortic root disease (e.g., Marfan syndrome, cystic medionecrosis, or annuloaortic ectasia) is responsible for the AR. Linear calcifications in the wall of the ascending aorta are seen in syphilitic aortitis but are nonspecific and observed in degenerative disease as well.

For angiographic assessment of AR, contrast material should be injected rapidly (i.e., 25 to 35 ml/sec) into the aortic root, and filming should be carried out in the right and left anterior oblique projections. Opacification may be improved by filming during a Valsalva maneuver. In acute AR, there is only a slight increase in ventricular end-diastolic volume, but with the passage of time both the end-diastolic volume and the thickness of the ventricular wall increase, usually in parallel.

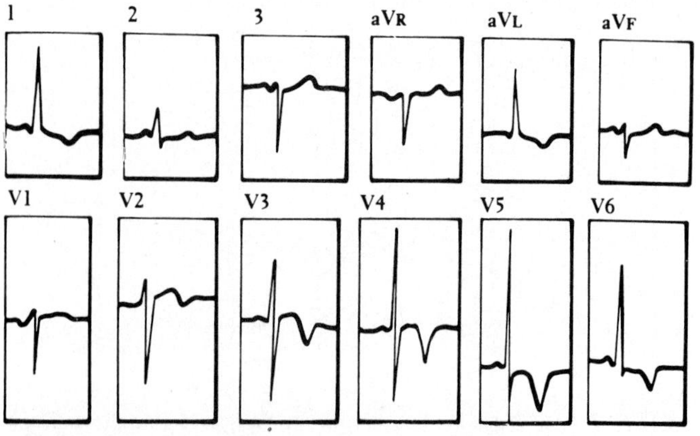

FIGURE 33–35. *Top,* **Diastolic overload pattern of left ventricular hypertrophy in the ECG. This pattern is commonly seen in younger patients with moderately severe to severe aortic regurgitation.** ***Bottom,*** **Left ventricular hypertrophy with associated ST-T changes in the ECG. This pattern is commonly seen in patients with severe, longstanding aortic regurgitation or in those with aortic regurgitation and associated arterial hypertension. (From Alpert, J. S.: Chronic aortic regurgitation.** ***In*** **Dalen, J. E., and Alpert, J. S. [eds.]: Valvular Heart Disease, 2nd ed. Boston, Little, Brown and Company, 1987, p. 295.)**

ECHOCARDIOGRAM (p. 109). The severity of regurgitation is reflected in increased motion of the septum and posterior wall, as recorded by M-mode echocardiography. In chronic AR, the left ventricular end-diastolic diameter and extent of systolic shortening are both augmented (Fig. 33–36*A*). There is increased motion of the interventricular septum and posterior left ventricular wall in compensated patients, but shortening is normal or reduced in patients with left ventricular failure. Serial studies, particularly with two-dimensional echocardiography, may detect early changes in left ventricular function, as reflected in increased end-diastolic and end-systolic diameters and reduced fractional shortening, which may be of assistance in selecting the optimal time for surgical intervention. Echocardiography is helpful in identifying the course of AR. It may show thickening of the valve cusps, prolapse of the valve, a flail leaflet (Fig. 33–36*A*), vegetations, or dilatation of the aortic root[493] (Fig. 33–37).

In acute AR (Table 33–15 and Fig. 33–33), the echocardiogram reveals a reduction in amplitude of the opening movement of the mitral valve, premature closure (Fig. 5–40, p. 101) and delayed opening of the mitral valve,[494] and a reduction in the E–F slope, indicating that the left ventricle is operating on the steep portion of its pressure-volume curve. Left ventricular end-diastolic dimensions are not markedly increased, and fractional shortening is normal. This contrasts with the findings in chronic AR, in which end-diastolic dimensions and wall motion are increased. Occasionally, with equilibration of aortic and left ventricular pressures in diastole, premature opening of the aortic valve may be detected.[495]

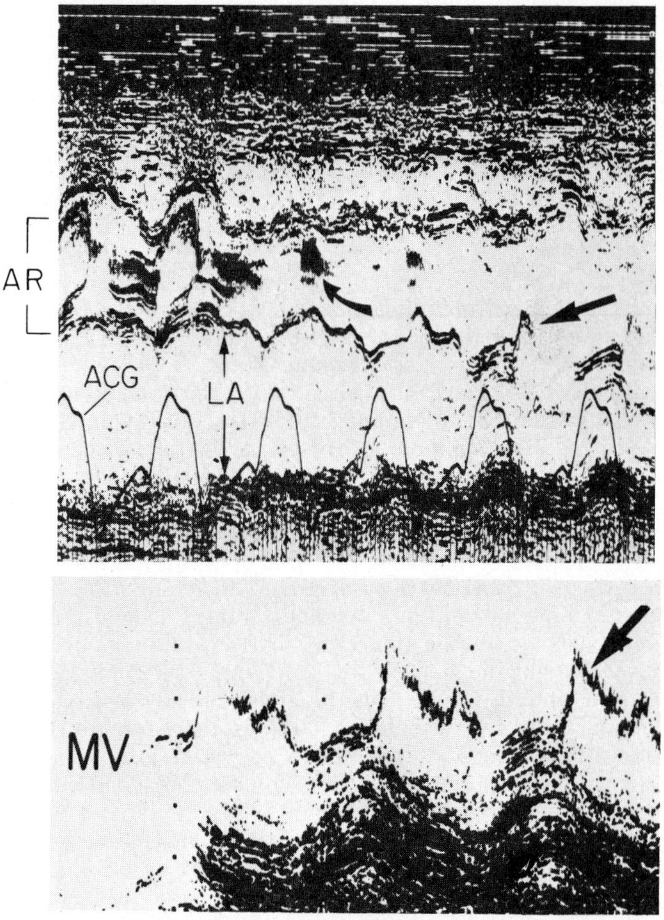

FIGURE 33–36. Top, Echocardiogram in severe aortic regurgitation. A markedly dilated aortic root (AR) is apparent on the left, appearing anterior to a slightly enlarged left atrium (LA). The left ventricle (at the right of the tracing) is dilated and demonstrates vigorous symmetrical contractile motion of the posterior wall and interventricular septum. Projecting anterior to the mitral valve is an abnormal diastolic echo (curved arrow) suggestive of a partially disrupted aortic valve cusp prolapsing into the left ventricular outflow tract. ACG = apexcardiogram. *Bottom,* Echocardiogram in aortic regurgitation. High-frequency diastolic vibrations (arrow) of the anterior mitral valve leaflet (MV) are typical of aortic regurgitation.

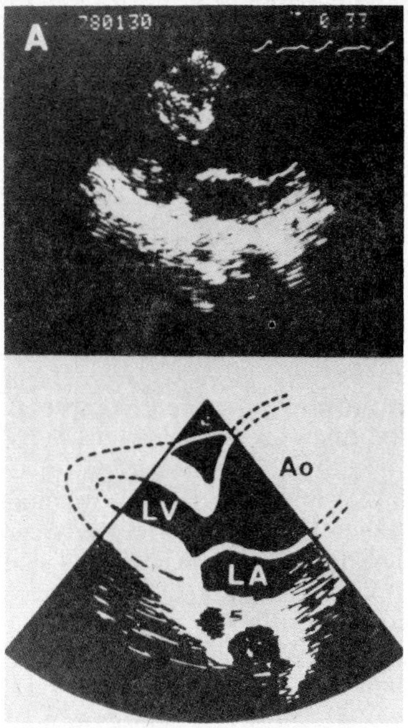

FIGURE 33–37. Panel *A*, Long-axis view of the aortic root (Ao) in end systole by two-dimensional echocardiography. The unusually dilated aortic root is visualized. (From Imaizumi, T., Orita, Y., Koiwaya, Y., et al.: Utility of two-dimensional echocardiography in the differential diagnosis of the etiology of aortic regurgitation. Am. Heart J. *103*:887, 1982.)

High-frequency, diastolic fluttering of the anterior leaflet of the mitral valve during diastole (Figs. 33–36*B* and 5–40, p. 101) is an important echocardiographic finding in both acute and chronic AR; it does not occur, however, when the mitral valve is rigid. This sign, which, unlike the Austin Flint rumble, occurs even in mild AR, results from the movement imparted to the anterior leaflet of the mitral valve by the jet of blood regurgitating from the aorta.

Doppler echocardiography (Figs. 5–60 and 5–61, p. 110) is the most sensitive and accurate technique in the detection of AR and is superior to the M-mode and two-dimensional techniques in this regard.[496] It readily detects mild degrees of AR that may be inaudible.[497] In addition, it provides an approach to the measurement of the regurgitation flow and the regurgitant orifice.[497–499]

RADIONUCLIDE TECHNIQUES. Radionuclide angiography, by allowing determination of the regurgitant fraction and of the left ventricular/right ventricular stroke volume ratio, provides an accurate noninvasive assessment of AR.[500, 501] This technique is nonspecific, because the ratio will be increased by associated MR and reduced by tricuspid or pulmonary regurgitation. However, in the absence of these complicating lesions, a left ventricular/right ventricular stroke volume ratio of 2.5 or more denotes severe AR. As indicated above, these techniques are of value in the assessment of left ventricular function in patients with AR.[473–475]

MANAGEMENT

ACUTE AORTIC REGURGITATION. Since early death due to left ventricular failure is frequent in patients with severe acute AR despite intensive medical management, prompt surgical intervention is indicated. Even a normal ventricle cannot sustain the burden of acute severe volume overload; therefore, the risk of *acute* AR is much greater than that of chronic AR.[476, 478, 479, 481] While the patient is being readied for surgery, intravenous treatment with a positive inotropic agent (dopamine or dobutamine) and/or vasodilator (nitroprusside) may be necessary. The agent and dosage should be selected on the basis of arterial pressure (Chap. 17). In patients with acute AR secondary to active infective endocarditis who are not compromised hemodynamically, operation may be deferred to allow 10 days to 2 weeks of intensive antibiotic therapy if the patient remains stable.[481] However, valve replacement should be undertaken at the earliest sign of hemodynamic instability if there is echocardiographic evidence of diastolic closure of the mitral valve,[502] or immediately upon completion of a 2-week course of antibiotics when acute, severe regurgitation has developed (p. 1122). The cautious use of vasodilators may be helpful in stabilizing the patient's condition but is no substitute for prompt surgery in the patients with pulmonary edema, severe pulmonary congestion, and/or an obvious low forward cardiac output state.

NATURAL HISTORY. Management of patients with chronic AR must take into account the natural history of the lesion.[503] Severe or moderately severe chronic AR is associated with a generally favorable prognosis for many years. Approximately 75 per cent of patients survive for 5 years and 50 per cent for 10 years after diagnosis.[87] However, as is the case for AS, once the patient becomes symptomatic, the condition often deteriorates rapidly. Without surgical treatment, death usually occurs within 4 years after the development of angina and within 2 years after the onset of heart failure. Even during the asymptomatic period gradual deterioration of left ventricular function may occur; it is important to intervene surgically before these changes have become irreversible.

MEDICAL TREATMENT

Patients with mild or moderate AR who are asymptomatic with normal or only minimally elevated cardiac dimensions require no therapy but should be followed clinically with echocardiography repeated yearly and with antibiotic prophylaxis for endocarditis. Patients with limitations of cardiac reserve and/or left ventricular dysfunction secondary to AR should not engage in vigorous sports or heavy exertion.[504] Cardiac glycosides should be employed in patients with severe AR, left ventricular dilatation, and sinus rhythm even in the absence of symptoms. If present, systemic arterial diastolic hypertension should be treated, since it increases the regurgitant flow; however, drugs that impair left ventricular function, such as propranolol, should be avoided. Atrial fibrillation and bradyarrhythmias are poorly tolerated and should be prevented if possible. Since these and other cardiac arrhythmias and infections are poorly tolerated in patients with severe AR, such complications must be treated promptly and vigorously. Even though nitroglycerin and other nitrates are not as helpful in relieving anginal pain as they are in patients with coronary artery disease or AS, they are worth a trial when this symptom occurs. Patients with AR secondary to syphilitic aortitis (p. 1567) should receive a full course of penicillin therapy. Although patients with left ventricular failure secondary to AR require surgical treatment, they also respond, as least temporarily, to treatment with digitalis glycosides, salt restriction, and diuretics. The response to vasodilator therapy is often impressive. Hemodynamic studies have shown beneficial effects of intravenous hydralazine,[505, 506] sublingual nifedipine,[507] and oral prazosin.[508] This form of therapy may be particularly helpful in stabilizing patients with acute lesions or those with decompensated chronic AR who are awaiting operation. Long-term (6 months) administration of hydralazine does not alter the severity of regurgitation but appears to improve systolic function.[509]

Asymptomatic patients with severe *chronic* AR and normal left ventricular function should be examined at intervals of approximately 6 months. In addition to clinical examination, x-ray, and electrocardiogram, serial noninvasive assessments of left ventricular size and performance should be carried out using echocardiography or radionuclide angiography or both.

SURGICAL TREATMENT

INDICATIONS FOR OPERATION. There is general agreement that operative correction is *not* indicated in patients with severe chronic AR who are asymptomatic, have good exercise tolerance, and have normal left ventricular function (as reflected in the ejection fraction determined by radionuclide angiography and left ventricular fractional shortening and end-systolic dimensions). Similarly, there is a consensus that surgical treatment is advisable generally in patients with severe AR who are symptomatic as a result of this lesion.[510–516]

Irreversible changes in left ventricular function are present in some symptomatic patients; even after successful surgical correction of AR, this subset of patients may develop congestive heart failure or have persistent cardiomegaly as well as depressed left ventricular function.[517–521] Patients whose ventricular function does not return to normal after aortic valve replacement often exhibit histological changes including massive fiber hypertrophy and increased interstitial fibrous tissue in the heart.[522] Postoperative left ventricular function is usually excellent in patients who have normal systolic function preoperatively.[520] In order to minimize the risk of postoperative left ventricular dysfunction, every effort should be made to operate on patients before serious left ventricular dysfunction occurs. Although quantitative biplane ventriculography is the most precise method for assessing left ventricular performance, it cannot be readily employed in serial fashion. Instead, serial echocardiograms, or radionuclide ventriculograms, should be obtained to detect changes in left ventricular size and function. These examinations can provide valuable information concerning progressive deterioration in left ventricular function at rest. Radionuclide angiography, in particular (p. 316), is a safe, simple, and noninvasive method that allows repeated evaluation of ejection fraction and end-systolic volume at rest and during exercise.

Patients with severely impaired left ventricular systolic function preoperatively are at high risk of developing irreversible left ventricular dysfunction and, indeed, of dying of congestive heart failure postoperatively. Some patients with impaired preoperative left ventricular function, on the other hand, improve postoperatively—both symptomatically and insofar as left ventricular function is concerned. Bonow et al. have reported that, after valve replacement, survival was excellent in patients with normal resting ejection fraction. However, patients with subnormal ejection fraction, preserved exercise tolerance, and only a brief (< 1 year) duration of left ventricular dysfunction also did well postoperatively. On the other hand, patients with subnormal ejection fraction and impaired tolerance and/or prolonged left ventricular dysfunction exhibited poor postoperative survival.[511, 522]

In *conclusion*, the decision to recommend aortic valve replacement in patients with severe AR is sometimes difficult. Operation should be deferred in asymptomatic patients with normal left ventricular function and should be recommended in symptomatic patients. Asymptomatic patients with impaired left ventricular function must be treated individually. A decision should not be based on a single abnormal measurement but rather on several observations of depressed ejection fraction and impaired exercise tolerance, carried out at intervals of approximately six months. If abnormalities are shown consistently and if any trend of deterioration is noted, operation should be carried out forthwith. If evidence of left ventricular dysfunction is borderline or is not consistent, the patient should be followed closely.

OPERATIVE PROCEDURES. The surgical treatment of AR and of combined AS and AR is valve replacement. (Prosthetic valves are discussed on pp. 1078 to 1081.) Since the aortic annulus in patients with severe AR is usually not as narrow as it is in patients with AS, a larger artificial valve can be inserted, and postoperative obstruction to left ventricular outflow is not a problem, as it may be in some patients with AS. Occasionally, when a leaflet has been torn from its attachments to the aortic annulus by trauma, surgical repair without valve replacement may be possible. In patients in whom AR is due to aneurysmal dilatation of the annulus and the ascending aorta, regurgitation may occasionally be reduced or eliminated by narrowing the annulus or by excising a portion of the aorta. More often, effective treatment in these patients requires replacement of the aortic valve and excision of the aneurysmal portion of the aorta and its replacement with a graft, sometimes with reimplantation of the coronary arteries. This more extensive procedure is associated with a higher operative risk than is aortic valve replacement alone.

Aortic valve replacement is discussed on page 1059. In general, results in patients with AR are similar to those in patients with AS, with a large percentage of patients exhibiting striking clinical improvement. Reductions in heart size and in left ventricular diastolic volume and mass occur in the majority of patients.[417, 523] However, as already indicated, the extent of improvement in left ventricular function may not be as salutary as in patients with aortic stenosis,[517, 521] perhaps reflecting the fact that ventricular dysfunction is more advanced in patients with AR by the time they become symptomatic and are referred for surgical treatment.[523a, 523b] As is the case for AS, the operative risk of aortic valve replacement in patients with AR depends on the general condition of the patient, the state of left ventricular function, and the skill of the surgical team; the mortality rate ranges from 3 to 8 per cent in most medical centers. A late mortality of approximately 5 per cent per year is observed in survivors in whom cardiac enlargement was marked and left ventricular dysfunction was prolonged preoperatively. By extending the indications for operation to symptomatic patients with normal left ventricular function as well as to asymptomatic patients with early left ventricular dysfunction, both early and late results are improving.[511, 512, 515, 522] It is likely that with the continued improvement of surgical techniques and results, it will become possible to extend the recommendation for operative treatment to asymptomatic patients with severe regurgitation and normal or nearly normal cardiac function. However, the risk of operation and the uncertainties of function of artificial valves suggests that the time for such a policy has not yet arrived.

TRICUSPID, PULMONIC, AND MULTIVALVULAR DISEASE

TRICUSPID STENOSIS

ETIOLOGY AND PATHOLOGY

Tricuspid stenosis (TS) is almost always rheumatic in origin. Other causes of obstruction to right atrial emptying are unusual and include tricuspid atresia (p. 949), right atrial tumors (which may produce a clinical picture suggesting rapidly progressive TS [p. 1472]), and the carcinoid syndrome (which more frequently produces tricuspid regurgitation [TR] [p. 1439] but which may occasionally produce TS). Rarely, obstruction to right ventricular inflow can be due to pericardial constriction, extracardiac tumors, and vegetations.

Rheumatic TS almost never occurs as an isolated lesion but generally accompanies mitral valve disease[524–528]; in many patients the aortic valve is also involved. TS is present at autopsy in about 15 per cent of patients with rheumatic heart disease but is of clinical significance in only about 5 per cent.[529]

Organic tricuspid valve disease is more common in India than in North America or Western Europe and has been reported to occur in the hearts of more than one-third of patients with rheumatic heart disease studied at autopsy in that country.[530] The anatomical changes of rheumatic TS resemble those of MS, with fusion and shortening of the chordae tendineae and fusion of the leaflets at their edges producing a diaphragm with a fixed central aperture.[10] As is the case for MS, TS is more common in women and, in the United States, is seen most commonly in persons between the ages of 20 and 60. Again, as in mitral valve disease, stenosis, regurgitation, or some combination of the two may exist.

The right atrium is often greatly dilated, and its walls are thickened. There may be evidence of severe passive congestion, with enlargement of the liver and spleen.

PATHOPHYSIOLOGY

A diastolic pressure gradient between the right atrium and ventricle—the hemodynamic expression of TS—is augmented when the transvalvular blood flow increases during exercise or inspiration and is reduced when flow declines during expiration. A mean diastolic pressure gradient exceeding 5 mm Hg is usually sufficient to elevate mean right atrial pressure to levels that result in systemic, venous congestion and, unless sodium intake has been restricted or diuretics have been given, is associated with jugular venous distention, ascites, and edema.

In patients with sinus rhythm, the right atrial *a* wave may be extremely tall (Fig. 33–38) and may even approach the level of the right ventricular systolic pressure. Resting

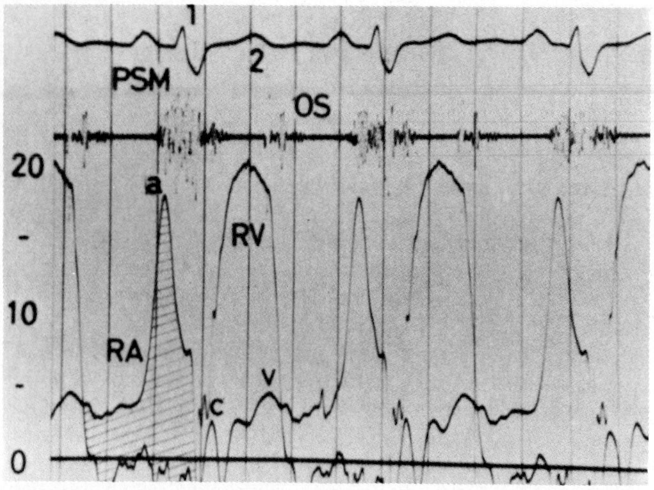

FIGURE 33–38. Phonocardiogram and right heart pressures in a patient with tricuspid stenosis. The giant right atrial *a* wave (a) nearly equals right ventricular (RV) systolic pressure and produces a large diastolic gradient (shaded area). A presystolic murmur (PSM), loud first heart sound (1), and early diastolic opening snap (OS) simulate the findings in mitral stenosis. (Time lines = 0.2 sec.) (From Criley, J. M., et al.: Departures from the expected auscultatory events in mitral stenosis. *In* Likoff, W. [ed.]: Valvular Heart Disease. Philadelphia, F. A. Davis, 1973, p. 214.)

cardiac output is usually markedly reduced and fails to rise during exercise, accounting for the normal or only slightly elevated left atrial, pulmonary arterial, and right ventricular systolic pressures, despite the presence of accompanying mitral valve disease.

A mean diastolic pressure gradient across the tricuspid valve as low as 2 mm Hg is sufficient to establish the diagnosis of TS. Therefore, whenever this diagnosis is suspected, right atrial and ventricular pressures should be recorded simultaneously, using two catheters or a single catheter with a double lumen, with one lumen opening on either side of the tricuspid valve. The effects of respiration on any pressure difference should be examined.

CLINICAL MANIFESTATIONS
(Table 33–17)

HISTORY. The low cardiac output characteristic of TS causes fatigue, and patients often complain of discomfort due to hepatomegaly, swelling of the abdomen, and anasarca. These symptoms, which are secondary to an elevated systemic venous pressure, are out of proportion to the degree of dyspnea.[525] Some patients complain of a fluttering discomfort in the neck, caused by giant *a* waves in the jugular venous pulse. Despite the coexistence of MS, the symptoms characteristic of this valve lesion, i.e., hemoptysis, paroxysmal nocturnal dyspnea, and acute pulmonary edema, are usually absent. Indeed, the absence of the symptoms of pulmonary congestion in a patient with obvious MS should suggest the possibility of TS.

PHYSICAL EXAMINATION. Because of the high frequency with which MS occurs in patients with TS, the diagnosis of the latter is commonly overlooked, since the physical findings are attributed to MS. Therefore, a high index of suspicion is required to detect the tricuspid valve lesion. In the presence of sinus rhythm (which is surprisingly common), the *a* wave in the jugular venous pulse is tall, sharp, and flicking and on first impression may be confused with an arterial pulsation; a presystolic hepatic pulsation is often palpable. The *y* descent is slow and barely appreciable, indicating the absence of normal rapid, early right ventricular filling. The lung fields are clear, and despite engorgement of the neck veins and the presence of ascites and anasarca, the patient is usually comfortable while lying flat. A parasternal (right ventricular) lift is inconspicuous, and pulmonic valve closure is not palpable, but occasionally the pulsations of a greatly enlarged right atrium may be felt to the right of the sternum. Thus, on inspection and palpation the combination of a prominent *a* wave in the jugular venous pulse in a patient with MS without the clinical signs of pulmonary hypertension or right ventricular enlargement should suggest the diagnosis of TS. This suspicion is strengthened when a diastolic thrill is felt at the lower left sternal edge, particularly during inspiration.[18]

The auscultatory findings of the accompanying MS are usually prominent and often overshadow the more subtle signs of TS. A tricuspid valvular opening snap (OS) may be audible but is often difficult to distinguish from a mitral OS. However, the tricuspid OS usually follows the mitral OS, and is localized to the lower left sternal border, whereas the mitral OS is usually most prominent at the apex and is more widely distributed. The diastolic murmur of TS is commonly heard best along the lower left parasternal border in the fourth intercostal space and is usually softer, higher pitched, and shorter in duration than the murmur of MS. The presystolic component has a scratchy quality, commences earlier (0.06 sec after the P wave in TS compared with 0.12 in MS), and has a crescendo-decrescendo configuration, diminishing before S_1.[526] The diastolic murmur and OS of TS are both augmented by inspiration, the Mueller maneuver, assumption of the right lateral decubitus position, leg-raising, inhalation of amyl nitrite, prompt squatting, and both isotonic and isometric exercise. They are reduced during expiration or the strain

TABLE 33–17 CLINICAL AND LABORATORY FEATURES OF RHEUMATIC TRICUSPID STENOSIS

History
Long history
Progressive fatigue, edema, anorexia
Minimal orthopnea, paroxysmal nocturnal dyspnea
Rheumatic fever in two-thirds of patients
Female preponderance
Orthopnea and paroxysmal nocturnal dyspnea are unusual
Pulmonary edema and hemoptysis are rare
Physical Findings
Signs of multivalvular involvement
Wasting
Peripheral cyanosis
Neck vein distension, with prominent V waves
Right ventricular lift
Associated murmurs of mitral and aortic valve disease
Holosystolic murmur maximal at left lower sternal border, accentuating with inspiration
Hepatic pulsation
Ascites, peripheral edema
Laboratory Findings
Normal sinus rhythm is frequently present with large A waves in the neck veins
Absent right ventricular life
Auscultation reveals a diastolic rumble at lower left sternal edge, increasing in intensity with inspiration
Electrocardiogram shows tall right atrial P waves and no right ventricular hypertrophy
Roentgenogram shows a dilated right atrium without an enlarged pulmonary artery segment

Modified from Ockene, I. S.: Tricuspid valve disease. *In* Dalen, J. E., and Alpert, J. S. (eds.): Valvular Heart Disease. 2nd ed. Boston, Little, Brown and Company, 1987, pp. 356 and 390.

of the Valsalva maneuver and return to control levels immediately (i.e., within two to three beats) after Valsalva release.

LABORATORY EXAMINATION

ELECTROCARDIOGRAM. In a patient with valvular heart disease in the absence of atrial fibrillation, TS is suggested by the presence of ECG evidence of right atrial enlargement disproportionate to the degree of right ventricular hypertrophy. The P-wave amplitude in leads II and V_1 exceeds 0.25 mV (p. 189), and there may be depression of the P-R segment resulting from increased magnitude of the atrial T wave. Since most patients with TS have mitral valve disease, the ECG signs of biatrial enlargement (p. 190) with abnormally tall, broad P waves in leads II, III, and aV_f and prominent positive and negative deflections in V_1 are commonly found. Right atrial dilatation may rotate the ventricular septum and affect QRS morphology in a manner so that the large volume of the right atrium between the exploring electrode and the ventricles reduces the amplitude of the QRS complex in lead V_1 (which often has a Q wave), whereas the QRS complex is much taller in V_2.

RADIOLOGICAL FINDINGS. The key radiological findings in TS are marked cardiomegaly, with conspicuous enlargement of the right atrium (i.e., prominence of the right heart border), which extends into a dilated superior vena cava and azygos vein, but without dilatation of the pulmonary artery. The vascular changes in the lungs characteristic of mitral valve disease may be masked, with little or no interstitial edema or vascular redistribution.

Angiography carried out following injection of contrast material into the right atrium and filming in the 30-degree right anterior oblique projection is useful for evaluating the appearance of the tricuspid valve. Thickening and decreased mobility of the leaflets, a jet through the constricted orifice, and thickening of the right atrial wall are characteristic findings.

ECHOCARDIOGRAM (See also p. 111). Although the motion of the normal tricuspid valve is similar to that of the normal mitral valve, it is more difficult to image. The changes in the echocardiogram in TS resemble those observed in MS. The M-mode echocardiogram usually shows thickening of the leaflets, a reduction in the E-F slope of the anterior leaflet, and paradoxical motion of the septal leaflet in diastole (Fig. 33–39).[531, 532] Calcification and thickening of the tricuspid valve often results in multiple and disorganized echoes. Two-dimensional echocardiography is more useful in the diagnosis of TS. It characteristically shows diastolic doming of the leaflets, thickening and restriction of excision of the other leaflets, and reduced separation of the tips of the leaflets[533–535] (Fig. 33–40).

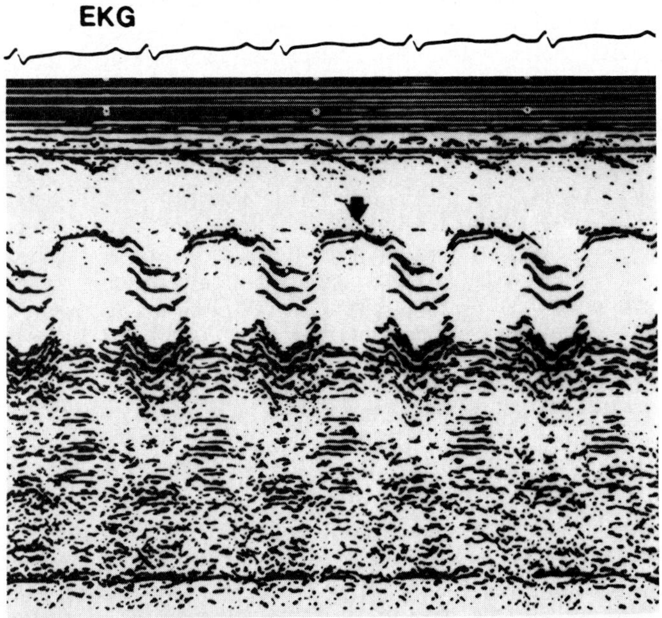

FIGURE 33–39. M-mode echocardiogram of a patient with carcinoid involvement of the tricuspid valve. The flat E-F slope (arrow) is consistent with tricuspid stenosis. (Reproduced with permission from Strickman, N. E., et al.: Carcinoid heart disease: A clinical, pathologic and therapeutic update. *In* Harvey, W. P., et al. [eds.]: Current Problems in Cardiology. Copyright © 1982 by Year Book Medical Publishers, Inc., Chicago.)

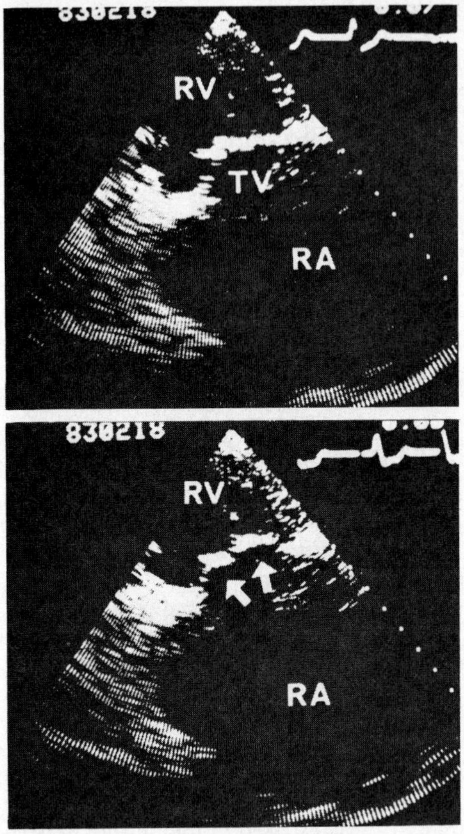

FIGURE 33–40. Two-dimensional echocardiograms in the long-axis view in a patient with tricuspid stenosis. *Top*, systolic frame. *Bottom*, diastolic frame that shows doming of both leaflets of the tricuspid valve (TV) (arrows). RA = right atrium; RV = right ventricle. (From Shimada, R., et al.: Diagnosis of tricuspid stenosis by M-mode and two-dimensional echocardiography. Am. J. Cardiol. *53*:164, 1984.)

MANAGEMENT

Although the fundamental approach to the management of severe TS is surgical treatment, intensive sodium restriction and diuretic therapy may diminish the symptoms secondary to the accumulation of excess salt and water. A prolonged preparatory period of diuresis may diminish hepatic congestion and thereby improve hepatic function sufficiently to diminish the risks of subsequent operation.

Surgical treatment of TS should be carried out at the time of mitral valvulotomy or valve replacement in patients with TS in whom mean diastolic pressure gradients exceed 5 mm Hg and tricuspid orifices are less than approximately 2.0 cm^2. Some patients with TS have coexisting valvular disease that requires surgery. The final decision concerning surgical treatment is made at the operating table. Since TS is almost always accompanied by some TR, simple finger fracture commissurotomy often does not result in significant hemodynamic improvement but may merely substitute severe regurgitation for stenosis. However, open valvulotomy in which the stenotic tricuspid valve is converted into a functionally bicuspid one may result in substantial improvement. The commissures between the anterior and septal leaflets and between the posterior and septal leaflets are opened; it is not advisable to open the commissure between the anterior and posterior leaflets for fear of producing severe regurgitation. If open commissurotomy does not restore reasonable normal valve function, the tricuspid valve may have to be replaced.[536, 537] A tissue valve (p. 1079) is preferred to a mechanical prosthesis in the tricuspid position because of the risk of thrombosis of the latter[538, 539] (p. 1081).

TRICUSPID REGURGITATION

ETIOLOGY AND PATHOLOGY (Table 33–18)

The most common cause of tricuspid regurgitation (TR) is not intrinsic involvement of the valve itself but *dilatation of the right ventricle* and of the tricuspid annulus, which may be complications of right ventricular failure of any cause (Fig. 33–41). Functional TR is observed in patients with right ventricular hypertension secondary to any form of cardiac and pulmonary vascular disease, most commonly mitral valve disease,[540–542] right ventricular infarction,[543] congenital heart disease (e.g., pulmonic stenosis and pulmonary hypertension secondary to Eisenmenger syndrome), primary pulmonary hypertension, and rarely in cor pulmonale. Severe TR has been reported to be the presenting manifestation in thyrotoxicosis.[544] In infants, TR may complicate right ventricular failure secondary to neonatal pulmonary diseases and pulmonary hypertension with persistence of the fetal pulmonary circulation.[545] In all of these cases, TR reflects the presence of, and in turn aggravates, severe right ventricular failure. TR results from

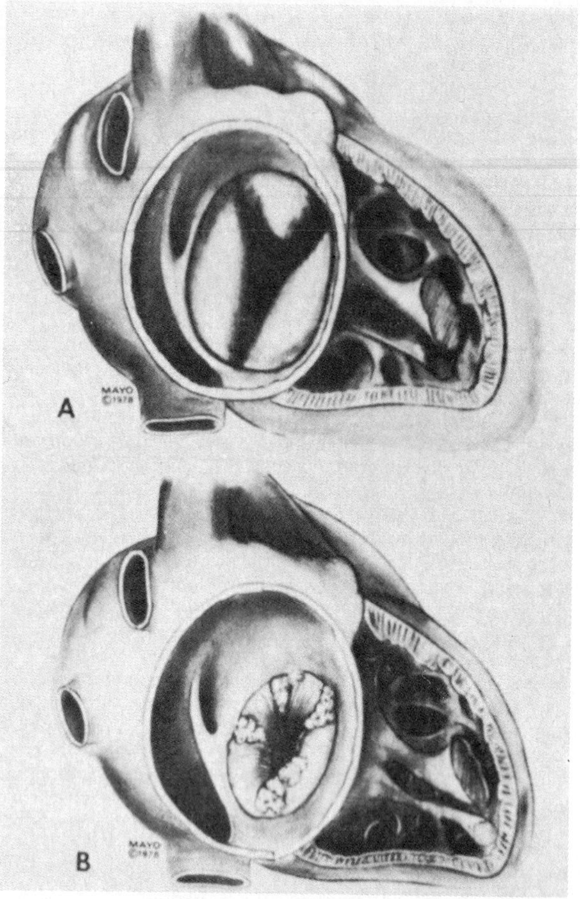

FIGURE 33–41. Types of tricuspid incompetence. *A*, Functional tricuspid incompetence secondary to dilatation of the right ventricle. *B*, Organic rheumatic tricuspid incompetence. (From Brandenburg, R. O., et al.: Valvular heart disease—When should the patient be referred? Pract. Cardiol. *5*:50, 1979.)

TABLE 33–18 CAUSES AND MECHANISMS OF PURE TRICUSPID REGURGITATION

CAUSES

I. Anatomically ABNORMAL valve
   A. Rheumatic
   B. Nonrheumatic
      1. Infective endocarditis
      2. Ebstein's anomaly
      3. Floppy (prolapse)
      4. Congenital (non-Ebstein's)
      5. Carcinoid
      6. Papillary muscle dysfunction
      7. Trauma
      8. Connective tissue disorders (Marfan)
      9. Rheumatoid arthritis
      10. Radiation
II. Anatomically NORMAL valve (functional)
   A. Elevated right ventricular systolic pressure (dilated annulus)

MECHANISMS

Condition	Leaflet Area	Annular Circumference	Leaflet Insertion
1. Floppy	$\uparrow$	$\uparrow$	Normal
2. Ebstein's anomaly	$\uparrow$	$\uparrow$	Abnormal
3. Pulmonary/right ventricular systolic hypertension	Normal	$\uparrow$	Normal
4. Papillary muscle dysfunction	Normal	Normal	Normal
5. Carcinoid	$\downarrow$/Normal	Normal	Normal
6. Rheumatic	$\downarrow$/Normal	Normal	Normal
7. Infective endocarditis	$\downarrow$/Normal	Normal	Normal

Modified from Waller, B. F.: Rheumatic and nonrheumatic conditions producing valvular heart disease. *In* Frankel, W. S., and Brest, A. N. (eds.): Cardiovascular Clinics. Valvular Heart Disease: Comprehensive Evaluation and Management. Philadelphia, F.A. Davis, 1986, pp. 35 and 95.

dilatation of the tricuspid annulus, reduction of the annulus during systole, and resultant failure of systolic valve coaptation of the tricuspid valve leaflets.[545a–547] Functional regurgitation may diminish or disappear as the right ventricle decreases in size. TR can also occur as a consequence of dilatation of the annulus in Marfan syndrome, in which it is not associated with right ventricular dilatation secondary to pulmonary hypertension.

A variety of disease processes can affect the tricuspid valve apparatus *directly* and lead to regurgitation. Thus, organic TR may occur on a congenital basis, as a part of Ebstein's anomaly (p. 951), common atrioventricular canal, when the tricuspid valve is involved in the formation of an aneurysm of the ventricular septum,[548] or as an isolated congenital lesion.[549] Rheumatic fever may attack the tricuspid valve directly,[540] and when it does so, it usually leads to both regurgitation and stenosis (Fig. 33–41*B*). Infarction, rupture, or ischemia of the papillary muscles of the right ventricle in coronary artery disease[543] and in perinatal asphyxia is an important cause of TR. TR may result from prolapse of the tricuspid valve caused by myxomatous changes in the valve and chordae tendineae; this condition usually, but not always, accompanies prolapse of the mitral valve[549a, 549b, 550] and may be associated with atrial septal defect.[551] Other causes include trauma[552] (p. 1542), infective endocarditis (Chap. 34),[553] particularly staphylococcal endocarditis in drug addicts, and surgical excision that has been necessary in patients with infective endocarditis unresponsive to medical management.[553]

TR can occur in the *carcinoid syndrome* (Fig. 33–42)

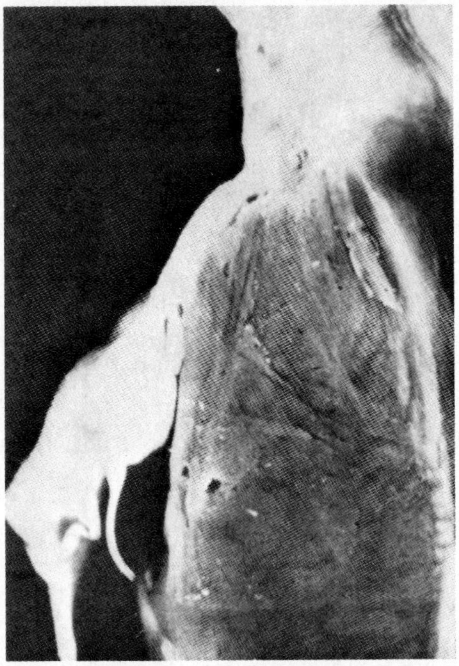

FIGURE 33–42. Septal tricuspid leaflet thickened by carcinoid plaques and fused to underlying ventricular septum. (From Callahan, J. A., et al.: Echocardiographic features of carcinoid heart Disease. Am. J. Cardiol. *50*:766, 1982.)

(p. 1439), which leads to focal or diffuse deposits of fibrous tissue on the endocardium of the valvular cusps and cardiac chambers and on the intima of the great veins and coronary sinus. The white, fibrous carcinoid plaques are most extensive on the right side of the heart, where they are usually deposited on the ventricular surfaces of the tricuspid valve and cause the cusps to adhere to the underlying right ventricular wall, thereby producing tricuspid regurgitation.[555, 556] Less common causes of tricuspid regurgitation include cardiac tumors, particularly right atrial myxoma (p. 1472); endomyocardial fibrosis (p. 1437); methysergide-induced valvular disease,[557] and systemic lupus erythematosus involving the tricuspid valve.[558]

CLINICAL MANIFESTATIONS (Table 33–17)

HISTORY. In the absence of pulmonary hypertension, TR is generally well tolerated. However, when pulmonary hypertension and TR coexist, cardiac output declines, and the manifestations of right-sided heart failure become intensified. Thus, the symptoms of TR result from a reduced cardiac output and from ascites, painful congestive hepatomegaly, and massive edema. Occasionally, patients complain of throbbing pulsations in the neck due to jugular venous distention, which intensify on effort,[18] and systolic pulsations of the eyeballs are sometimes noted.[559] In the many patients with TR who have mitral valve disease, the symptoms of the latter predominate. Symptoms of pulmonary congestion may abate as TR develops, but they are replaced by weakness, fatigue, and other manifestations of a depressed cardiac output.

PHYSICAL EXAMINATION (Figs. 3–32, p. 60, 4–13, p. 71, and 16–3, p. 480). Evidence of weight loss, cachexia, cyanosis, and jaundice is often present on inspection. Atrial fibrillation is common. There is jugular venous distention,[559a] the normal x and x' descents disappear, and a prominent systolic ("s") wave, i.e., a c-v wave, is apparent. The descent of this wave, the y descent, is sharp and becomes the most prominent event in the venous pulse (unless there is coexisting TS, in which case it is slowed). The v waves and y descents become more prominent during inspiration.[560] A venous systolic thrill and murmur in the neck may be present in severe TR.[561] The right ventricular impulse is hyperdynamic and thrusting in quality. Rarely, a right atrial systolic impulse may be observed or palpated along the right lower sternal edge.[18] In patients with combined mitral valve disease and TR, a relatively quiet zone may be present between the apex and the left sternal edge. Systolic pulsations of an enlarged tender liver are commonly present initially, but in chronic TR with congestive cirrhosis, the liver may be firm and nontender. Ascites and edema are frequent.

Auscultation (Table 33–5). This usually reveals an S_3 originating from the right ventricle, i.e., one which is accentuated by inspiration; when TR is associated with pulmonary hypertension, P_2 is accentuated as well. The murmur of TR is usually high-pitched, pansystolic, and loudest in the fourth intercostal space in the parasternal region but occasionally in the subxiphoid area. When TR is mild, the murmur may be short. With acute TR due to infective endocarditis or trauma, the murmur is usually of low intensity and limited to the first half of systole. When the right ventricle is greatly dilated and occupies the anterior surface of the heart, the murmur may be most prominent at the apex and difficult to distinguish from that produced by MR.

The response of the murmur to respiration and other maneuvers is of considerable aid in establishing the diagnosis of tricuspid regurgitation. It is usually augmented during inspiration[18, 562, 562a] (Rivero-Carvello's sign). However, when the failing ventricle can no longer increase its stroke volume, the inspiratory augmentation is lost. Under these circumstances, respiratory variation may be elicited by standing and thereby reducing venous return. The murmur also increases during inspiration, the Mueller maneuver (forced inspiration against a closed glottis), exercise, leg-raising, hepatic compresssion, and amyl nitrite inhalation as well as after a prolonged diastole, and it demonstrates an immediate overshoot after release of the Valsalva strain. It is reduced in intensity and duration in the standing position and during the strain of the Valsalva maneuver. Rarely, TR is silent except for the selective appearance of a soft systolic murmur during inspiration.[563]

Increased atrioventricular flow may cause a short early diastolic flow rumble in the left parasternal region following S_3.

LABORATORY EXAMINATION

RADIOLOGICAL FINDINGS. Marked cardiomegaly secondary to the condition responsible for the dilatation of the right ventricle is usually evident. The right atrium is prominent[560] (Fig. 6–2, p. 142). Evidence of elevated right atrial pressure may include distention of the azygos vein and the presence of pleural effusion. Ascites with upward displacement of the diaphragm may be present. Rarely, with prolonged elevation of right ventricular pressure, the tricuspid ring may calcify. The findings of pulmonary arterial and venous hypertension are common. Fluoroscopy may reveal systolic pulsations of the right atrium.

ELECTROCARDIOGRAM. This is usually nonspecific and characteristic of the lesion causing TR. Incomplete right bundle branch block, Q waves in lead V_1 (Fig. 7–12, p. 190), and atrial fibrillation are commonly found.

ECHOCARDIOGRAM (See also p. 111). In patients with TR secondary to dilation of the tricuspid annulus, the right atrium, right ventricle, and tricuspid annulus are usually dilated.[545–547] There is evidence of right ventricular diastolic overload, with paradoxical motion of the ventricular septum similar to that in atrial septal defect. Exaggerated motion and delayed closure of the tricuspid valve are evident in patients with Ebstein's anomaly. In patients with TR secondary to right ventricular dilatation and pulmonary hypertension, the pulmonic valve echogram shows a diminished or absent *a* deflection. *Prolapse of the tricuspid valve* may be evident on M-mode and two-dimensional echocardiography[549, 564] (Fig. 5–62, p. 111). Simultaneous echocardiographic studies of the tricuspid valve and phonocardiography may reveal a nonejection systolic click that occurs at the onset of prolapse, originating from the right side of the heart.

Contrast echocardiography involving rapid injection of saline or indocyanine green dye into an antecubital vein made while a two-dimensional echocardiogram is being recorded (p. 88) is both sensitive and specific for tricuspid regurgitation.[565] The injection produces microcavities that are readily visible on echocardiography and normally travel as a bolus through the circulation. In TR, these microcavities can be seen to travel back and forth across the tricuspid orifice and to pass into the inferior vena cava and hepatic veins during systole.[566] TR secondary to carcinoid heart disease shows thickened, retracted valve leaflets, fixed in a semiopen position throughout the cardiac cycle[555, 566a] whereas that due to endocarditis may reveal vegetations on the valve, or a flail valve.

Pulsed Doppler echocardiography revealing systolic flow from right ventricle to right atrium is an extremely sensitive technique for detecting TR.[567] A semiquantitative assessment can be made by measuring reverse velocity in the inferior vena cava[567a] and hepatic veins.[567b] Real-time two-dimensional color-coded Doppler imaging appears to be an extremely accurate, sensitive, and specific method for assessing TR.[568]

HEMODYNAMIC AND ANGIOGRAPHIC FINDINGS. The right atrial and right ventricular end-diastolic pressures are characteristically elevated in TR, whether the condition is due to organic disease of the tricuspid valve or is secondary to right ventricular systolic overload (e.g., pulmonary hypertension and pulmonic stenosis). The right atrial pressure tracing reveals absence of the *x* descent, a prominent *v* or *c-v* wave ("ventricularization" of the atrial pressure). Therefore, the right atrial pressure pulse increasingly resembles the right ventricular pressure pulse as the severity of tricuspid regurgitation increases (Fig. 33–43).[526]

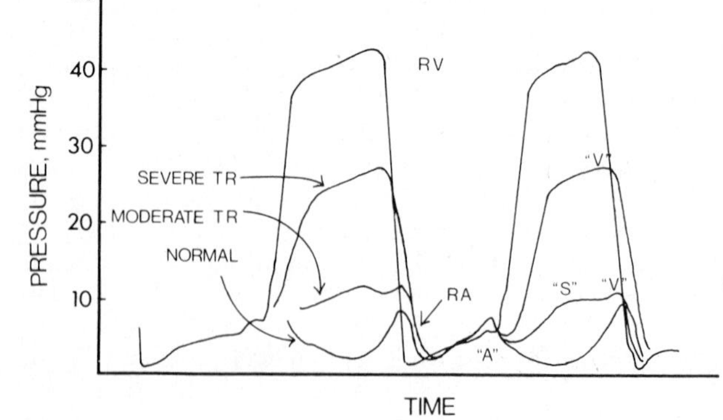

FIGURE 33–43. Appearance of right atrial (RA) pressure contour in patients with severe tricuspid regurgitation (TR), moderate TR, and no TR (normal). Note the regurgitant systolic (S) wave that blends with the normal filling (V) wave in severe TR. The resultant RA pressure waveform resembles a right ventricular (RV) pressure recording. (From Grossman, W. [ed.]: Cardiac Catheterization and Angiography. 3rd ed. Philadelphia, Lea and Febiger, 1986, p. 378.)

A rise or no change in right atrial pressure on deep inspiration, rather than the usual fall, is characteristic.[560, 569] Pulmonary artery (or right ventricular) systolic pressure may offer a rough guide as to whether the TR is primary (disease of the valve or its supporting structures) or secondary to right ventricular dilatation. A pulmonary artery or right ventricular systolic pressure less than 40 mm Hg favors a primary etiology, whereas a pressure greater than 60 mm Hg suggests that TR is secondary. A useful tool for assessing TR is the indicator dilution technique. Injection of indicator substance (e.g., indocyanine green) into the right ventricle with sampling in both the right atrium and a peripheral artery allows detection of the "early appearance" of indicator in the right atrium as well as quantitation of the relative magnitudes of forward versus regurgitant flows.

Diagnosis and quantitative assessment of TR can be aided in many instances by right ventriculography, but the fact that the catheter must be positioned across the tricuspid valve cannot exclude the possibility of a false-positive diagnosis of TR.[570] Modifications of previous angiographic techniques have been introduced in which a special, preformed catheter is positioned in the right ventricle, and angiography is carried out at low injection rates[571]; or a special balloon catheter is employed to minimize the induction of extrasystoles which can cause spurious regurgitation.[572]

MANAGEMENT

TR in the absence of pulmonary hypertension usually does not require surgical treatment. Indeed, both patients and experimental animals tolerate total excision of the tricuspid valve, as long as right ventricular systolic pressure is normal.[553] In some patients dilatation of the right side of the heart occurs months or years after valvulotomy, and insertion of a prosthetic valve can then be carried out after adequate sterilization of the valve ring.[573] *Surgical treatment* of acquired regurgitation secondary to annular dilatation was greatly improved when Carpentier introduced the concept of suturing the annulus to a nondeformable prosthetic ring of appropriate dimensions.[574] That portion of the annular circumference supported by the free ventricular wall may be shortened by a plicating suture.[575] Annuloplasty without insertion of a prosthetic ring (so-called DeVega annuloplasty) has also been found to be effective in patients with annular dilatation. This technique is now widely employed.[576, 577]

In patients with TR associated with mitral valve disease and pulmonary hypertension, the severity of the regurgitation should be assessed by palpation of the valve at the time of mitral commissurotomy or valve replacement. Patients with mild TR usually do not require surgical treatment; pulmonary vascular pressures decline following successful mitral valve surgery, and the mild TR tends to disappear. Excellent results have been reported in patients with moderate TR with the use of tricuspid annuloplasty,[574] often utilizing a Carpentier ring[575, 576, 576a] (Fig. 33–44). However, management of severe regurgitation is more controversial. It is not clear whether severe TR should be treated by annuloplasty or valve replacement, but most surgeons prefer the former approach. If it does not provide a good functional result, they resort to valve replacement.[578]

Organic disease of the tricuspid valve responsible for TR, as in Ebstein's anomaly[579, 580] or carcinoid heart disease,[581] usually requires valve replacement. The risk of thrombosis of valvular prostheses is greater in the tricuspid than in the mitral position, presumably because pressure

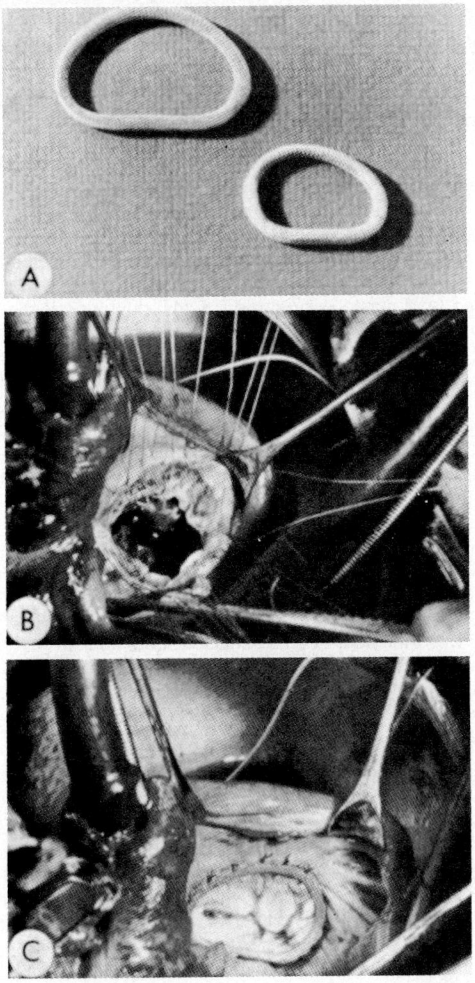

FIGURE 33–44. *A*, Carpentier rings. *B*, Ring being sutured into place. C, Completion of Carpentier ring annuloplasty. (From Starr, A.: Acquired disease of the tricuspid valve. *In* Sabiston, D. C., Jr., and Spencer, F. C. [eds.]: Gibbon's Surgery of the Chest. Philadelphia, W. B. Saunders Company, 1976, p. 1182.)

and flow rates are lower in the right side of the heart. For this reason, the artificial valve of choice for the tricuspid position in adults at present is a large porcine heterograft. Anticoagulants are not required, and a durability of up to 10 years has been established. In younger patients, a large diameter low-profile valve (St. Jude or Björk-Shiley[582]) is generally employed.

In treating the difficult problem of tricuspid valve endocarditis in heroin addicts, it has been noted that total excision of the tricuspid valve *without immediate replacement* can be tolerated. When antibiotic therapy is unsuccessful, valvular replacement frequently results in reinfection or continued infection. A diseased valvular tissue should be excised to eradicate the endocarditis, and antibiotic treatment can be continued. Most patients tolerate loss of the tricuspid valve without great difficulty. However, if medical management does not control the tricuspid regurgitation and the infection has been controlled, an artificial valve can be inserted later.[573]

PULMONIC VALVE DISEASE

ETIOLOGY AND PATHOLOGY. The congenital form is the most common cause of *pulmonic stenosis* (PS).[583] Its manifestations in children are discussed on page 942 and in adults on page 991. *Rheumatic* inflammation of the pulmonic valve is usually associated with involvement of other valves and rarely leads to serious deformity. However, a high incidence of significant pulmonic valve involvement secondary to rheumatic fever has been reported in Mexico City, perhaps related to the pulmonary hypertension that occurs at high altitudes and the resultant greater stress on the pulmonic valve.[584] *Carcinoid* plaques, similar to those involving the tricuspid valve (p. 1439), are often present in the outflow tract of the right ventricle in patients with malignant carcinoid and result in construction of the pulmonic valve ring, retraction and fusion of the valve cusps, and the combination of PS and pulmonic regurgitation (PR) (Fig. 33–45). Obstruction in the region of the pulmonic valve may be extrinsic to the valve apparatus and may be produced by cardiac tumors or aneurysm of the sinus Valsalva.[585]

By far the most common cause of PR is dilatation of the valve ring secondary to pulmonary hypertension (of any etiology) or to dilatation of the pulmonary artery, either idiopathic[586, 587] or consequent to a connective tissue disorder such as Marfan syndrome.[588] The second most common cause is infective endocarditis.[589–591] Less frequently, it is iatrogenic and is induced at the time of surgical treatment of congenital PS or tetralogy of Fallot. It may also result from a variety of lesions directly affecting the pulmonic valve. These include congenital malformations, such as absent, malformed, fenestrated, or supernumerary leaflets.[10] These anomalies may occur as isolated lesions[592] but more often are associated with other congenital anomalies, particularly tetralogy of Fallot, ventricular septal defect, and pulmonic valvular stenosis. Less common causes include carcinoid syndrome, rheumatic involvement,[593] injury produced by a pulmonary artery flow-directed catheter,[594] syphilis,[587] and chest trauma.[591]

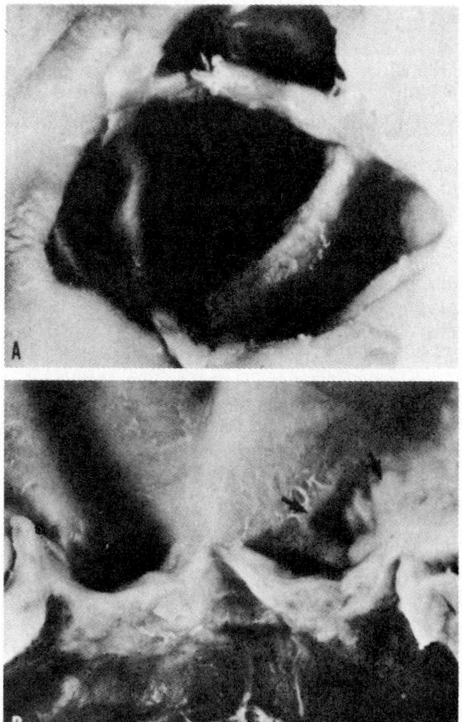

FIGURE 33–45. Carcinoid heart disease; pulmonary valve viewed from above (A) and opened (B). The thickened and retracted cusps result in valvular incompetence. The constricted annulus results in valvular stenosis. Carcinoid plaques (arrows) extend onto the pulmonary trunk. (From Callahan, J. A., et al.: Echocardiographic features of carcinoid heart disease. Am. J. Cardiol. *50*:767, 1982.)

CLINICAL MANIFESTATIONS

Like TR, isolated PR causes right ventricular volume overload and may be tolerated for many years without difficulty unless it complicates or is complicated by pulmonary hypertension, in which case it is usually accompanied by and aggravates right ventricular failure. Patients with PR caused by infective endocarditis who develop septic pulmonary emboli and pulmonary hypertension often exhibit severe right ventricular failure.[591] In most patients the clinical manifestations of the primary disease are severe and usually overshadow the PR, which often results only in incidental auscultatory findings. *Physical examination* reveals a hyperdynamic right ventricle, producing palpable systolic pulsations in the left parasternal area and an enlarged pulmonary artery that often results in palpable systolic pulsations in the second left intercostal space; sometimes systolic and diastolic thrills are felt in the same area. A tap reflecting pulmonic valve closure is usually easily palpable in the second intercostal space in patients with pulmonary hypertension and secondary PR.

AUSCULTATION. In patients with congenital absence of the pulmonic valve, P_2 is not audible, but this sound is accentuated in patients with PR secondary to pulmonary hypertension, particularly when the dilated pulmonary artery is near the chest wall. There may be wide splitting of S_2 due to prolongation of right ventricular ejection accompanying the augmented stroke volume.[593] A nonvalvular systolic ejection click due to the sudden expansion of the pulmonary artery by the augmented right ventricular stroke volume frequently initiates a midsystolic ejection murmur, most prominent in the second left intercostal space. An S_3 and S_4 originating from the right ventricle are often audible, most readily in the fourth intercostal space at the left parasternal area, and are augmented by inspiration.

In the absence of pulmonary hypertension, the diastolic murmur of PR is low-pitched and is usually heard best at the third and fourth left intercostal spaces adjacent to the sternum (Fig. 4–24, p. 79). The murmur commences when pressures in the pulmonary artery and right ventricle diverge, approximately 0.04 sec after P_2. It is diamond-shaped in configuration and brief, reaching a peak intensity when the gradient between these pressures is maximal and ending with equilibration of the pressures.[595] The murmur becomes louder during inspiration[596] and following inhalation of amyl nitrite.

When pulmonary artery systolic pressure exceeds approximately 70 mm Hg, dilatation of the pulmonic annulus results in a regurgitant jet of high velocity that is responsible for the so-called Graham Steell murmur of PR. This murmur is a high-pitched, blowing decrescendo murmur beginning immediately after P_2 and is most prominent in the left parasternal region in the second to fourth intercostal spaces (Fig. 4–24, p. 79). Thus, although it resembles the murmur of AR, it is usually accompanied by the findings of severe pulmonary hypertension, i.e., an accentuated P_2 or fused S_2, an ejection sound, and a systolic murmur of tricuspid regurgitation. Sometimes a low-frequency presystolic murmur is present, i.e., a right-sided Austin Flint murmur originating from the tricuspid valve that is analogous to the more common left-sided Austin Flint murmur originating from the mitral valve.[597]

The Graham Steell murmur of PR secondary to pulmonary hypertension usually increases in intensity with inspiration, exhibits little change after amyl nitrite inhalation or vasopressors, is diminished during the Valsalva strain, and returns to baseline intensity almost immediately after release of the Valsalva strain. This murmur resembles and may be confused with the diastolic blowing murmur of AR. However, indicator dilution studies[598] and aortography have established that a diastolic blowing murmur along the left sternal border in patients with rheumatic heart disease and pulmonary hypertension—even in the absence of peripheral signs of AR—is usually due to AR and not PR.

Laboratory Examination

ELECTROCARDIOGRAM. In the absence of pulmonary hypertension, PR often results in an ECG that reflects right ventricular diastolic overload, i.e., an rSr' (or rsR') configuration in the right precordial leads. PR secondary to pulmonary hypertension is usually associated with ECG evidence of right ventricular hypertrophy.

RADIOLOGICAL FINDINGS. Both the pulmonary artery and the right ventricle are usually enlarged,[599] but these signs are nonspecific. Fluoroscopy may demonstrate pronounced pulsation of the main pulmonary artery. PR can be diagnosed by observing opacification of the right ventricle following injection of contrast material into the main pulmonary artery (Fig. 33–46). The diagnosis is supported by noting superimposition of the pulmonary artery and right ventricular pressure curves during mid and late diastole. Indicator dilution techniques with injections into the pulmonary artery and sampling from the right ventricle,[600] as well as intracardiac phonocardiography,[587] can also be helpful in establishing the diagnosis in mild cases.

ECHOCARDIOGRAM. This shows right ventricular dilatation and, in patients with pulmonary hypertension, right ventricular hypertrophy as well. Diastolic fluttering of the tricuspid valve leaflets, similar to that of the mitral valve leaflets in AR, is often noted. Abnormal motion of the septum characteristic of volume overload of the right ventricle in diastole and/or septal flutter[601] may be evident. The motion of the pulmonic valve may point to the etiology of the pulmonic regurgitation.[602] Absence of *a* waves and systolic notching of the posterior leaflet suggest pulmonary hypertension; large *a* waves indicate pulmonic stenosis. PR can be detected by contrast echocardiography.[603] The pulsed Doppler technique is extremely accurate in detecting PR. Abnormal Doppler signals in the right ventricular outflow tract whose velocity is sustained throughout diastole are generally observed in patients in whom dilatation of the valve ring (functional regurgitation) is the cause. When the velocity falls during diastole, the pulmonary artery pressure is usually normal, and the regurgitation is caused by an abnormality of the valve itself.[602]

MANAGEMENT. PR per se is seldom severe enough to require specific treatment. Cardiac glycosides are useful in the management of right ventricular dilatation or failure. Treatment of the primary condition such as infective endocarditis or of the lesion responsible for the pulmonary hypertension, such as surgical treatment of mitral valvular disease, often ameliorates the PR. Surgical treatment of primary PR directed specifically at the pulmonic valve is required only occasionally because of intractable right heart failure, and under such circumstances valve replacement may be carried out.[604]

MULTIVALVULAR DISEASE

Multivalvular involvement is common, particularly in patients with rheumatic heart disease, and a variety of clinical and hemodynamic syndromes can be produced by different combinations of valvular abnormalities. Development of PR and TR secondary to dilatation of the pulmonic valve ring and tricuspid annulus, respectively, as a consequence of pulmonary hypertension secondary to disease involving the mitral or aortic valve or both, has already been discussed (pp. 1072 and 1075), as has the combination of *organic* rheumatic tricuspid and mitral valvular disease. In patients with multivalvular disease, the clinical manifestations depend on the relative severities of each of the lesions.[605] When the valvular abnormalities are of approximately equal severity, as a general rule, clinical manifestations produced by the more proximal (upstream) of two valvular lesions, i.e., the mitral valve in patients with

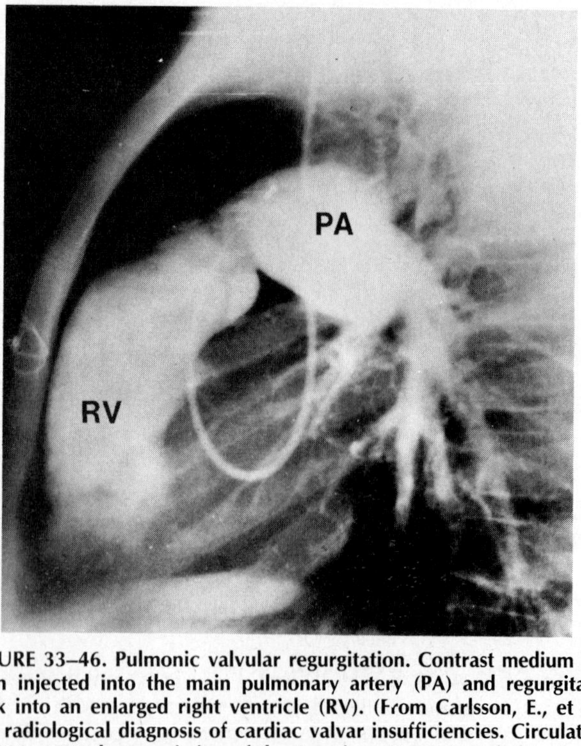

FIGURE 33–46. Pulmonic valvular regurgitation. Contrast medium has been injected into the main pulmonary artery (PA) and regurgitates back into an enlarged right ventricle (RV). (From Carlsson, E., et al.: The radiological diagnosis of cardiac valvar insufficiencies. Circulation 55:921, 1977, by permission of the American Heart Association, Inc.)

combined mitral and aortic valvular disease and the tricuspid valve in patients with combined tricuspid and mitral valvular disease, are more prominent than those produced by the distal lesion.

It is important to recognize multivalvular involvement preoperatively, since failure to correct all significant valvular disease at the time of operation increases mortality considerably. In patients with multivalvular disease, the relative severity of each lesion may be difficult to estimate by clinical examination and noninvasive techniques, because one lesion may mask the manifestations of the other. For this reason, patients suspected of multivalvular involvement and in whom surgical treatment is under consideration should undergo (in addition to careful clinical examination and noninvasive workup, with emphasis on two-dimensional and Doppler echocardiography), right- and left-heart catheterization and angiography. If there is any question concerning the presence of significant AS in patients undergoing an operation on the mitral valve, the aortic valve should be inspected, since overlooking this condition can lead to a high perioperative mortality. Similarly, it is useful to palpate the tricuspid valve at the time of operation on the mitral valve.

MITRAL STENOSIS AND AORTIC REGURGITATION

Approximately two-thirds of patients with severe MS have an early blowing diastolic murmur along the left sternal border with a normal pulse pressure; in 90 per cent of these the murmur is due to AR and is usually of little clinical importance. However, approximately 10 per cent of patients with MS have severe rheumatic AR,[606] which can usually be recognized by the peripheral signs of a widened pulse pressure, left ventricular dilatation and increased wall motion on echocardiography, and signs of left ventricular enlargement on radiological and electrocardiographic examinations.

In keeping with the general observation that a proximal lesion may mask a distal lesion, significant AR may be missed in patients with severe MS. The widened pulse pressure, in particular, may be absent in the latter. On clinical examination of patients with obvious AR, errors may be made in that MS may be missed or, conversely, may be falsely diagnosed. An accentuated S_1 and an opening snap in a patient with AR should suggest the possibility of mitral valvular disease. On the other hand, an Austin Flint murmur is often inappropriately considered to be the diastolic rumbling murmur of MS (Table 33–15, p. 1065). These two murmurs may be distinguished at the bedside by means of amyl nitrite inhalation, which diminishes the Austin Flint murmur (Fig. 33–34, p. 1065) but augments the murmur of MS; isometric handgrip and squatting augment both the diastolic murmur of AR and the Austin Flint murmur. Echocardiography, particularly pulsed Doppler echocardiography, is of decisive value in the detection of both lesions. Diastolic fluttering of the anterior leaflet of the mitral valve and of the ventricular septum is an important clue to the presence of AR in a patient with MS. Evidence of rapid left ventricular filling in diastole by apexcardiography or echocardiography should suggest the presence of associated AR.

Hemodynamic analysis reveals that MS reduces the left ventricular volume overload characteristic of AR.[607] This combination is relatively uncommon; only 10 of 150 patients with combined aortic and mitral valve disease had pure stenosis of both valves.[605]

MITRAL STENOSIS AND AORTIC STENOSIS

When severe MS and AS coexist, the former masks many of the clinical manifestations of the latter.[607a] The cardiac output tends to be reduced further than in patients with isolated AS, and the atrial booster pump mechanism, so important in filling the ventricle in AS (p. 1054), has little impact when MS is present. The reduction in cardiac output lowers both the transaortic valvular pressure gradient and the left ventricular systolic pressure, diminishes the incidence of angina, and retards the development of aortic calcification and left ventricular hypertrophy.[608] On the other hand, clinical manifestations associated with MS, such as pulmonary congestion and hemoptysis, atrial fibrillation, and systemic embolization, occur more frequently than in patients with isolated AS. On physical examination, presystolic distention of the left ventricle and an S_4, common in pure AS, are usually not present. The midsystolic murmur may be reduced in intensity and duration because of the reduced stroke volume. The *electrocardiogram* may fail to demonstrate left ventricular hypertrophy, but left atrial enlargement is common in patients in sinus rhythm. The *chest roentgenogram* is usually typical of MS except that calcium may be present in the region of the aortic valve. The two-dimensional and Doppler *echocardiograms* are of the greatest value because stenosis of both valves may be evident. However, the low cardiac output characteristic of this combination of lesions may reduce the transvalvular gradients estimated by Doppler echocardiography. The indirect *carotid pulse* tracing reveals a delayed upstroke.

It is vital to recognize the presence of hemodynamically significant aortic valvular disease (stenosis and/or regurgitation) preoperatively in patients who are to undergo surgical correction of MS, since isolated mitral valvulotomy may be hazardous in such patients; this operation can impose a sudden hemodynamic load on the left ventricle that may lead to acute pulmonary edema.

AORTIC STENOSIS AND MITRAL REGURGITATION

The combination of severe AS and MR is hazardous but fortunately relatively uncommon. Obstruction to left ventricular outflow, on the one hand, augments the volume of MR flow,[147] whereas the presence of MR, on the other, diminishes the ventricular preload necessary for maintenance of the left ventricular stroke volume in AS. The result is a reduced forward cardiac output and marked left atrial and pulmonary venous hypertension. The physical findings may be confusing because the delayed arterial pulse of AS may be counteracted by the sharp upstroke of MR, and it may be difficult to recognize two distinct systolic murmurs. Amyl nitrite tends to increase the intensity of the murmur of AS and to reduce that of MR. On echocardiography and roentgenography the left atrium and ventricle are usually larger than in isolated AS. Usually both valves must be treated surgically in patients with severe AS and MR.

AORTIC REGURGITATION AND MITRAL REGURGITATION

This relatively frequent combination of lesions[609] may be caused by rheumatic heart disease or by prolapse of both valves[610] or dilatation of both annuli in connective tissue disorders. The clinical features of AR usually predominate, and it may be difficult to determine whether the MR is due to organic involvement of this valve or dilatation of the mitral valve ring secondary to left ventricular enlargement. When both valvular leaks are severe, this combination of lesions is poorly tolerated. The normal mitral valve ordinarily serves as a "backup" to the aortic valve, and premature (diastolic) closure of the mitral valve limits the volume of reflux that occurs in patients with acute AR.[455] With combined regurgitant lesions, regardless of the etiology of the mitral lesion, blood may reflux from the aorta through both chambers of the left heart into the pulmonary veins. Physical and laboratory examination will usually show evidence of both lesions. Both lesions are frequently associated with an S_3 and a brisk arterial pulse. The relative severity of each lesion can be assessed best by contrast angiography.

When MR occurs in patients with AR secondary to left ventricular dilatation, it often regresses following aortic valve replacement. If severe, it may be corrected by annuloplasty at the time of aortic valve replacement. Replacement of an intrinsically normal mitral valve that is regurgitant due to a dilated annulus is neither necessary nor advisable.

SURGICAL TREATMENT OF MULTIVALVULAR DISEASE

Combined aortic and mitral valve replacement is usually associated with a higher risk and poorer survival than is replacement of one of these two valves.[611] Kirklin reported a 5-year survival rate of 70 per cent after double-valve replacement compared to 80 per cent for single-valve replacement.[612] The long-term survival is strongly dependent on the functional status preoperatively.[613] Also, patients operated on for the combination of AR and MR fared worse than did patients receiving double-valve replacement for any of the other combinations.[612]

Hemodynamically significant disease involving the mitral, aortic, and tricuspid valves is uncommon. Patients with these lesions often present in advanced heart failure with marked cardiomegaly, and surgical correction of all three valvular lesions is imperative. Attempts to shorten the duration of operation by leaving one severely impaired valve in place after a double valve replacement are usually unsatisfactory. However, triple valve replacement is a long and complex operation that has been reported to be associated with a mortality rate of 18 per cent in patients in functional Class III and 40 per cent in Class IV.[614] However, even this high risk must often be accepted because of the otherwise dismal prognosis in these patients.

Patients who survive triple-valve replacement usually show substantial clinical improvement in the early postoperative period,[615–617] and postoperative catheterization studies show marked reductions in pulmonary arterial and capillary pressures.[618] However, some patients succumb to arrhythmias[617] or congestive heart failure in the late postoperative period despite normally functioning prostheses. The cause of cardiac failure in this situation is not known, but it may be related to intraoperative myocardial ischemia, microemboli from the multiple prostheses, or continued subclinical episodes of rheumatic myocarditis.

When multiple prosthetic valves must be inserted, it is logical to select either two (or three) bioprostheses or mechanical prostheses in the same patient. If the patient is to be exposed to the hazards of anticoagulation for one mechanical prosthesis, it seem unreasonable to add the potential risks of early failure of a bioprosthesis.

ARTIFICIAL CARDIAC VALVES

The first successful replacements of the mitral and aortic valves were accomplished by Harken et al.[619] and Starr in 1960.[620] Two major groups of artificial (prosthetic) valves are currently available in models designed for both the atrioventricular (mitral and tricuspid) and the aortic positions: mechanical prostheses and bioprostheses (tissue valves).

MECHANICAL PROSTHESES

As of this writing, mechanical prosthetic valves fall into two groups: caged-ball and tilting-disc valves. The *Starr-Edwards* caged-ball valve (Fig. 33–47*A*), in which the sewing ring is cloth-covered to reduce the incidence of thromboembolism, is still widely used.[621–623] It has the longest record of predictable performance of any artificial valve. A disadvantage is its bulky cage design. It is therefore not suitable in patients with a small left ventricular cavity or a small aortic annulus, or in a valve–aortic arch composite graft. In a small number of patients it induces hemolysis, which may be greatly exaggerated and become of clinical importance if a perivalvular leak develops.

Several types of tilting-disc valves are widely employed; these are less bulky and have a lower profile than the caged-ball valve. The *Björk-Shiley* valve[624–627] (Fig. 33–47*B*) consists of a low-profile cobalt base alloy covered with a Teflon fabric sewing ring; its design allows an excellent ratio between the diameter of the valve orifice and tissue annulus. It contains a suspended tilting-disc occluder made of pyrolytic carbon (Pyrolyte). Two serious problems with this valve have been reported in a small number of patients: (1) sudden thrombosis and (2) strut fracture. Changes have been made to overcome these problems—the new disc is convexo-concave, its opening angle has been increased, and the outflow strut is fabricated as an integral part of the valve ring. These alterations appear to have greatly re-

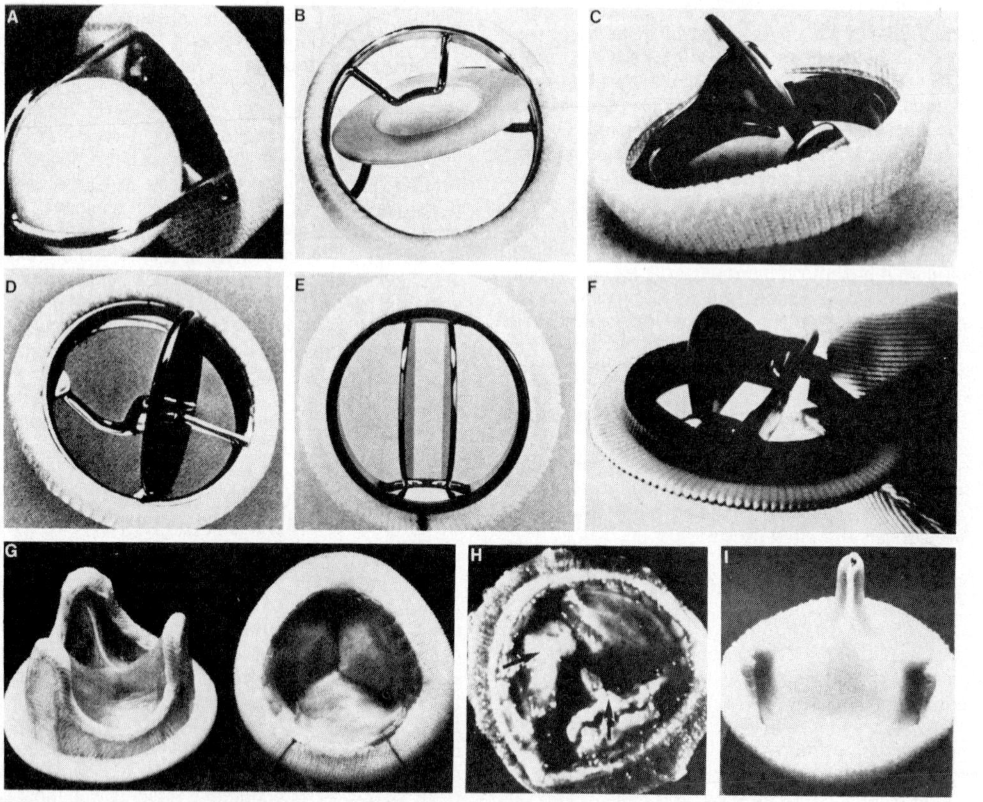

FIGURE 33–47. Prosthetic cardiac valves. *A*, Starr-Edwards caged ball valve with cloth sewing ring and bare struts. *B*, Björk-Shiley tilting disc valve. *C*, Omniscience tilting disc valve. *D*, Medtronic-Hall tilting disc valve. *E*, St. Jude medical bileaflet valve as viewed end on. Note the large size of the effective orifice area compared with the potential orifice area and the minimal obstruction to flow by the leaflets. *F*, Duromedics bileaflet valve. *G*, Carpentier-Edwards prosthetic valve. *H*, Porcine valve removed several years following implantation because of primary valve failure; arrows point to areas of calcification and destruction of leaflets. *I*, Ionescu-Shiley pericardial valve. (*A* from Starek, P. J. K., and *F* from Clark, R. E.; *In* Heart Valve Replacement and Reconstruction. Chicago, Year Book Medical Publishers, 1987, pp. 223 and 286. *B* from Björk, V.; *C* from Austin, E. H., III.; *E* from Crawford, F. A., Jr.; *G* and *H* from Magilligan, D. J., Jr.; and *I* from Crawford, F. A., Jr., in Crawford, F. A. [ed.]: Cardiac Surgery: Current Heart Valve Prostheses, Vol. 1. Philadelphia, Hanley and Belfus, 1987, pp. 184, 204, 252, 270, 271, and 286. *D* from Cobanoglu, A., Brockman, S. K., *In* Frankl, W. S., and Brest, A. N. [eds.]: Valvular Heart Disease: Comprehensive Evaluation and Management. Cardiovascular Clinics. Philadelphia, F. A. Davis, 1986, p. 404.)

duced the aforementioned problems, but it is not clear at the time of this writing whether they have been totally eliminated. The *Lillehei-Kaster* pivoting-disc valve consists of a titanium valve housing with a Teflon fabric sewing ring in which a Pyrolyte disc is suspended. In the open position, the disc swings to an angle of 80 degrees, providing a large central flow orifice. This valve is entirely satisfactory in the aortic position, but a relatively high incidence of thrombosis precludes its use in the mitral position.[628] Two adaptations of the Lillehei-Kaster tilting-disc valve, the *Omniscience*[628a, 628b] (Fig. 33–47*C*) and the *Omnicarbon*[628] valves, have been introduced in an effort to improve hemodynamics and decrease thrombogenicity. Early reports suggest that both of these goals may have been achieved, although there are some remaining concerns about thrombogenicity on the Omniscience valve in the mitral position.[629] A closely related valve is the *Medtronic-Hall* valve (Fig. 33–47*D*). Its pivoting disc has a central perforation that allows improved hemodynamics; thrombogenicity appears to be quite low, less than 1 per 100 patient-years in the aortic position and 1.5 per 100 patient-years in the mitral position.[630]

The *St. Jude* valve (Fig. 33–47*E*), constructed of pyrolytic carbon, has two semicircular discs that pivot between open and closed positions without the need for supporting struts. It appears to possess favorable flow characteristics and causes a lower transvalvular gradient at any outer diameter and cardiac output than the caged-ball or tilting-disc valves.[631–635] The St. Jude valve appears to have particularly favorable hemodynamic characteristics in the smaller sizes; therefore, it may be especially useful in children. Thrombogenicity in the mitral position *may* be less than for other prosthetic valves. A variation of the St. Jude valve, the *Duromedics* prosthesis (Fig. 33–47*F*), is also a bileaflet valve with curved leaflets and a hinge design, which supposedly enhances central flow and hemodynamic performance compared with the prototype. This valve appears to cause less regurgitation than other tilting-disc valves; the incidence of valve thrombosis and thromboembolism appears to be low.[628]

DURABILITY AND THROMBOGENICITY. All of these mechanical prosthetic valves have an excellent record of durability—up to 20 years in the case of the caged-ball valves. However, patients with any mechanical prosthesis, regardless of design or site of placement, require long-term anticoagulation because of the hazard of thromboembolism, which is greatest in the first postoperative year. Without anticoagulation the incidence of thromboembolism is three- to sixfold higher than with proper doses.[636, 636a] Anticoagulation with sodium warfarin should begin about 2 days after operation, and a prothrombin time in the range of 18 to 23 seconds should be achieved. This relatively conservative approach reduces the risk of anticoagulant hemorrhage, yet does not appear to be associated with a greater frequency of thromboembolism than a prothrombin time of 30 to 35 seconds. It must be recognized that the administration of warfarin carries its own mortality and morbidity, estimated at 0.2 and 2.2 per 100 patient-years, respectively. Despite treatment with anticoagulants, the incidence of thromboembolic complications with the best mechanical prostheses is still about 0.2 (fatal) and 1 to 2 (nonfatal) per 100 patient-years. This incidence tends to be slightly higher for prostheses in the mitral than in the aortic position; thrombosis of mechanical prostheses in the tricuspid position is quite high, and for this reason bioprostheses are preferred at this site. The incidence of embolization in patients who have experienced repeated emboli from a prosthetic valve despite anticoagulants may be reduced by replacement with a tissue valve.

TISSUE VALVES

Largely to overcome the risk of thromboembolism that is inherent in all mechanical prosthetic valves and the attendant hazards and inconvenience of permanent anticoagulant therapy, considerable effort has been devoted to the development of nonthrombogenic tissue valves.[637, 638] The first of these to be widely used were chemically sterilized homografts. Unfortunately, these exhibited a high incidence of breakdown within 3 years. Fresh antibiotic-treated cryopreserved frozen-irradiated homografts were then developed. These are more durable[639]; while they have many desirable properties, their use has been restricted by the problems inherent in their procurement.

PORCINE HETEROGRAFTS. To overcome this difficulty, porcine heterografts were developed and have been used clinically since 1965. At first, these valves were sterilized with formalin, which dissolved the collagen cross linkages in the valve cusps and resulted in a high failure rate. Then Carpentier et al. developed the process of fixation and sterilization of porcine heterografts using a dilute solution of glutaraldehyde, which appears to promote the stability of the collagen cross linkages. After their exposure to this agent, the valves become essentially inert collagen shells with little if any antigenicity. The valves are then mounted on semiflexible frames.[640]

Two porcine heterografts are widely used today[628a, 637, 638, 640–645]: (1) The *Hancock* valve is fixed with 0.2 per cent glutaraldehyde and is mounted on a Dacron cloth-covered flexible polypropylene strut. In the smaller aortic models, the right coronary cusp is replaced by a posterior cusp from another valve to reduce obstruction resulting from the septal shelf of the valve. (2) The *Carpentier-Edwards* valve (Fig. 33–47*G*) is pressure-fixed with 0.625 per cent glutaraldehyde and is mounted on a Teflon-covered Eljiloy strut in a manner to minimize the septal shelf. The hemodynamic profiles of the porcine heterografts are similar to those of comparably sized low-profile mechanical prostheses. In contrast to the latter, however, the valve orifice is blood-flow dependent, with greater orifice size as transvalvular flow increases.

During the first 3 postoperative months, while the sewing ring becomes endothelialized, the thromboembolic rate is high enough so that anticoagulation is extremely desirable. Thereafter, anticoagulants are not required for porcine valves in the aortic position, and the thromboembolic rate is approximately 1 to 2 per 100 patient-years without these drugs.[638, 642, 645] When these valves have been placed in the mitral position in patients who are in sinus rhythm, no preoperative thromboembolic episodes have occurred. No intraatrial thrombus has been seen at operation, anticoagulants are not needed (after the first 3 postoperative months), and the thromboembolic rate is also approximately 1 to 2 per 100 patient-years. This is comparable to that in patients with Björk-Shiley valves receiving (and therefore subject to the risks of) anticoagulants. In patients with the aforementioned risk factors (approximately one-third of all patients receiving mitral valve replacements), the hazard of thromboembolism persists. Indeed, in patients with atrial fibrillation the incidence of postoperative emboli following implantation of a porcine bioprosthesis into the mitral position is three times as high as in patients in sinus rhythm. Therefore, anticoagulants are required in these patients with these risk factors. However, this largely negates the principal advantage of the tissue valves. It is unlikely that any replacement of the mitral valve can be associated with a thromboembolism rate much below 0.5 per 100 patient years, since some of the emboli in patients with longstanding mitral disease are derived from the left atrium rather than from the valve itself.[646]

The major problem with porcine bioprostheses is their limited durability. Cuspal tears, degeneration, fibrin deposition, disruption of the fibrocollagenous structure, perforation, fibrosis, and calcification sufficiently severe to require reoperation (Fig. 33–47*H*) begin to appear in the fourth or fifth postoperative years, the rate increasing so that by 10 years the rate of primary tissue failure is approximately 20 per cent. In one report in which a 12-year follow-up is described,[643] the actuarial freedom from bioprosthetic primary tissue failure was only 61 per cent for valves in the mitral and 69 per cent for valves in the aortic position. It is likely that with the passage of time even more of these valves will fail and will require re-replacement. However, the valves usually do not fail suddenly, and the second operation can often be carried out on an elective basis, with a surgical mortality in the range of 10 to 15 per cent.[645] The time after implantation at which tissue valves fail varies inversely with age; it is prohibitively rapid in children and young adults. Bioprostheses also have extremely limited durability in patients with chronic renal failure and hypercalcemia related to secondary hyperparathyroidism.

PERICARDIAL XENOGRAFT. A second major type of bioprosthetic valve is the *Ionescu-Shiley pericardial xenograft* (Fig. 33–47*I*),[637, 638, 647–649] which consists of glutaraldehyde-treated bovine pericardium from which three leaflets are mounted on a Dacron, velour-covered titanium frame. This valve has the same low thrombogenicity as the porcine heterografts; the primary valve failure rate appears to be higher. However, the pericardial heterografts do appear to possess one modest advantage over the valve heterografts: they offer somewhat less resistance to blood flow and therefore may be useful in patients with a small aortic annulus.

Hemodynamics of Valve Replacements

It must be recognized that all valve replacements—mechanical prostheses as well as tissue valves—have an effective in vitro orifice size that is smaller than a normal human valve.[637, 638, 650] After implantation, tissue ingrowth and endothelialization reduce the in vivo effective orifice size further; therefore, most valve devices currently available must be considered to be mildly stenotic. However, postoperative hemodynamic measurements of the rigid prostheses show reasonably good function, with effective mitral valve orifice averaging 1.7 to 2.0 cm^2 and mitral valve gradients of 4 to 8 mm Hg at rest. Although definitive comparisons have not been carried out, the cloth-covered Starr-Edwards valve appears to be intrinsically slightly more stenotic than the tilting-disc valves. The St. Jude valve, in turn, may be slightly superior to the latter. In hemodynamic studies, the porcine and the bovine pericardial mitral valves behave in a fashion similar to that of an artificial prosthetic valve of the same diameter, although subtle, late hemodynamic deterioration with the porcine bioprosthesis has been reported.[650a] Serious hemodynamic obstruction of an artificial valve in the mitral position is quite uncommon, unless the valve is placed in a small left ventricular cavity or an unusually small mitral annulus or unless the prosthesis chosen is too large. However, this problem of intrinsic stenosis may be more serious in patients with aortic stenosis. In these the annulus into which the prosthesis is inserted is usually smaller than in patients with aortic regurgitation, and the surgeon may be forced to select an artificial valve of relatively small size. As a consequence, aortic valve replacement may not abolish obstruction but may merely convert severe to mild or moderate obstruction. When the smaller models of the porcine xenograft or mechanical prosthesis are placed into the aortic position, effective orifice areas of about 1.1 to 1.3 cm^2 are common. In such patients, peak transvalvular gradients as high as 40 mm Hg during exercise have been recorded. It is possible that the poor late results observed in a minority of patients may be the delayed effects of moderate stenosis of the prosthesis. In patients with aortic stenosis who do not exhibit clinical improvement postoperatively, it is important to evaluate the function of both the prosthetic valve and the left ventricle. Rarely, reoperation to correct a malfunctioning mechanical prosthesis may be necessary.

SELECTION OF AN ARTIFICIAL VALVE

Although there are significant differences between them, the overall advantages and disadvantages of tissue and prosthetic valves are almost evenly matched, and the choice between the two is often difficult. Most comparisons provide similar overall results, in terms of early and late mortality, prosthetic valve endocarditis and other complications, and the need for reoperation, at least for the first 5 or 6 years postoperatively. It is important that the relative advantages and disadvantages of the various valves be explained to the patient, who should be a participant in the final decision. As indicated, there appear to be no significant differences insofar as hemodynamics are concerned, except that in patients with an unusually small left ventricular cavity or mitral annulus, the low-profile (tilting-disc) prosthetic St. Jude or tissue valve may be superior to the more bulky caged-ball valve.[650, 651] Similarly, in patients with a small aortic annulus, the bileaflet mechanical St. Jude or Duromedics valve (among the mechanical prostheses) and the Ionescu-Shiley pericardial xenograft[652] appear to be preferable among the bioprostheses.

The major task is to weigh the advantage of durability and the disadvantage of the risk of thromboembolism and of anticoagulant treatment inherent in mechanical prostheses on the one hand with the advantage of low thrombogenicity and the disadvantage of abbreviated durability of the bioprostheses on the other. Therefore, tissue valves are preferred over mechanical prostheses in patients in whom anticoagulation is difficult to control, or in whom it is especially hazardous because they are prone to hemorrhage or are unreliable. Because of the uncertainties surrounding the long-term durability of bioprostheses, I believe that a mechanical prosthetic valve should be employed in patients under the age of approximately 65 to 70 years without any of the aforementioned contraindications to anticoagulants.[653] The following groups of patients should receive a bioprosthesis: (1) those with coexisting disease who are prone to hemorrhage, (2) those who are unreliable insofar as anticoagulant treatment is concerned, (3) those who are unwilling to take anticoagulants on a regular basis, and (4) those over the age of 65 to 70 in whom the question of valve durability may be less important and who by reason of their age may be at a greater risk of hemorrhage while taking anticoagulants.

Special Situations

Pregnancy. Females with artificial valves can tolerate the hemodynamic burden of pregnancy well, but the risk of thromboembolism is greatly increased in such patients with prosthetic valves when anticoagulation is interrupted and an increased risk of fatal fetal hemorrhage is seen in those in whom it is continued. There is also a risk of fetal malformation caused by the probable teratogenic effect of warfarin. These problems represent powerful arguments for the use of tissue valves in all women of childbearing age.[654–657] Women of childbearing age with a mechanical prosthesis should be counseled against pregnancy. When a woman in whom a mechanical prosthetic valve is already in place becomes pregnant, the risk to the fetus if the mother receives oral anticoagulants appears to be lower than the risk to the mother if anticoagulants are discontinued.[658] It is possible to use coumarin derivates safely during the second and third trimesters, but these agents are contraindicated between the 6th and 12th weeks. The appropriate heparin regimen during this period has yet to be worked out.[657]

Noncardiac Surgery. When this is required in patients with prosthetic mitral valves who are receiving anticoagulants, the risk is minimal when the drug regimen is stopped 1 to 3 days preoperatively and for a similar period postoperatively. It may be desirable, however, to protect the patient with low molecular weight dextran during the perioperative period.

Patients Who Are Destined to Receive Anticoagulants. In patients with earlier implantation of a mechanical prosthesis, chronic atrial fibrillation in the presence of an enlarged left atrium, a history of thromboembolism, or the presence of a thrombus in the left atrium at operation, I recommend a mechanical prosthesis because the potential advantage of a tissue valve is negated.

Children. The high incidence of bioprosthetic valve failure in children and adolescents[653] and in patients on chronic hemodialysis[202] prohibits their use in these groups. In young adults between the ages of 25 and 35, the failure of bioprosthetic valves is somewhat higher than it is in older adults; this serves as a relative, but not an absolute, contraindication to their use in this age group.

In children, a mechanical prosthesis—generally the St. Jude valve—with its favorable hemodynamics is preferred despite the disadvantages inherent in anticoagulants in this age group. Similarly, mechanical prostheses should be used in patients with chronic renal failure and/or hypercalcemia.

Tricuspid Position. The risk of thrombosis of all valves is highest in the tricuspid position because of the lower pressures and velocity of blood flow; this complication appears to be highest for tilting-disc valves, intermediate for caged-ball valves, and lowest for the bioprostheses, which are the valves of choice as tricuspid valve replacements.

DETECTION OF PROSTHETIC VALVE DYSFUNCTION. Artificial valves have characteristic auscultatory and phonocardiographic characteristics[659] (Fig. 3–19, p. 52). Echocardiography, phonocardiography, and cineradiography are extremely useful in the identification of artificial valve dysfunction.[659–662] Two-dimensional and Doppler echocardiography are particularly useful in the follow-up of patients who demonstrate clinical deterioration in the postoperative period following porcine heterograft implantation. These techniques may prove capable of distinguishing between failure of bioprosthesis (abnormal structure of valve motion) and left ventricular dysfunction.

REFERENCES

MITRAL STENOSIS

1. Roberts, W. C.: Morphologic features of the normal and abnormal mitral valve. Am. J. Cardiol. *51*:1005, 1983.
2. Evans, D. T. P., and Sloman, J. G.: Mitral stenosis and mitral incompetence due to Libman-Sacks endocarditis and mitral valve replacement. Aust. N. Z. J. Med. *11*:526, 1981.
3. Bortolotti, U., Valente, M., Agozzino, L., Mazzucco, A., and Thiene, G.: Rheumatoid mitral stenosis requiring valve replacement. Am. Heart J. *107*:1049, 1984.
4. Johnson, G. L., Vine, D. L., Cottrill, C. M., and Noonan, J. A.: Echocardiographic mitral valve deformity in the mucopolysaccharidoses. Pediatrics *67*:401, 1981.
5. Chandy, K. G., John, T. J., and Cherian, G.: Coxsackieviruses and chronic valvular heart disease. Am. Heart J. *100*:578, 1980.
6. Ladefoged, C., and Rohr, N.: Amyloid deposits in aortic and mitral valves. Virchows Arch. (A) *404*:301, 1984.
7. Misch, K. A.: Development of heart valve lesions during methysergide therapy. Br. Med. J. 2:365, 1974.
8. Osterberger, L. E., Goldstein, S., Khaja, F., and Lakier, J. B.: Functional mitral stenosis in patients with massive annular calcification. Circulation *64*:472, 1981.
9. Kumar, A., Sinha, M., and Sinha, D. N. P.: Chronic rheumatic heart diseases in Ranchi. Angiology *33*:141, 1982.
10. Waller, B. F.: Rheumatic and nonrheumatic conditions producing valvular heart disease. *In* Frankl, W. S., and Brest, A. N. (eds.): Cardiovascular Clinics. Valvular Heart Disease: Comprehensive Evaluation and Management. Philadelphia, F. A. Davis, 1986, pp. 3–104.
11. Wells, B.: The assessment of mitral stenosis by phonocardiography. Br. Heart J. *16*:261, 1954.
12. Lachman, A. S., and Roberts, W. C.: Calcific deposits in stenotic mitral valves. Circulation *57*:808, 1978.
13. Ionescu, M. I., and Cohn, L. H. (eds.): Mitral Valve Disease: Diagnosis and Treatment. London, Butterworths, 1985, 367 pp.
14. Bowe, J. C., Bland, F., Sprague, H. B., and White, P. D.: Course of mitral stenosis without surgery: 10 and 20 year perspectives. Ann. Intern. Med. 52:741, 1960.

14a. Somasundram, U., Euinton, H. A., and Williams, R. P.: Mitral valve stenosis in the elderly. Age Ageing *14*:285, 1985.

14b. Bell, M. H., and Mintz, G. S.: Mitral valve disease in the elderly. *In* Frankl, W. S., Brest, A. N. (eds.): Cardiovascular Clinics. Valvular Heart Disease: Comprehensive Evaluation and Management. Philadelphia, F. A. Davis, 1986, pp. 313–324.

15. Chopra, P., Tandon, H. D., Raizada, V., Gopinath, N., Butler, C., and Williams, R. C., Jr.: Comparative studies in mitral valves in rheumatic heart disease. Arch. Intern. Med. *143*:661, 1983.
16. Dalen, J. E., and Alpert, J. S. (eds.): Valvular Heart Disease. 2nd ed. Boston, Little, Brown and Company, 1987, 600 pp.
17. Hanson, T. P., Edwards, B. S., and Edwards, J. E.: Pathology of surgically excised mitral valves. Arch. Pathol. Lab. Med. *109*:823, 1985.
18. Reichek, N., Shelburne, J. D., and Perloff, J. R.: Clinical aspects of rheumatic valvular disease. Prog. Cardiovasc. Dis. *15*:491, 1973.
19. Wood, P.: An appreciation of mitral stenosis. Br. Med. J. *1*:1051 and 1113, 1954.
20. Arandi, D. T., and Carleton, R. A.: The deleterious role of tachycardia in mitral stenosis. Circulation *36*:511, 1967.
21. Dalen, J. E.: Mitral stenosis. *In* Dalen, J. E., and Alpert, J. S. (eds.): Valvular Heart Disease. 2nd ed. Boston, Little, Brown and Company, 1987, pp. 49–110.
22. Selzer, A.: Effects of atrial fibrillation upon the circulation in patients with mitral stenosis. Am. Heart J. *59*:518, 1960.
23. Gorlin, R., and Gorlin, S. G.: Hydraulic formula for calculation of the area of stenotic mitral valve, other cardiac valves and central circulatory shunts. Am. Heart J. *41*:1, 1951.
24. Nakhjavan, F. K., Katz, M. R., Maranhao, V., and Goldberg, H.: Analysis of influence of catecholamine and tachycardia during supine exercise in patients with mitral stenosis and sinus rhythm. Br. Heart J. *31*:753, 1969.
25. Stott, D. K., Marpole, D. G. F., Bristow, J. D., Kloster, F. E., and Griswold, H. E.: The role of left atrial transport in aortic and mitral stenosis. Circulation *41*:1031, 1970.
26. Kennedy, J. W.: The use of quantitative angiocardiography in mitral valve disease. *In* Duran, C., Angell, W. W., Johnson, A. D., and Oury, J. H. (eds.): Recent Progress in Mitral Valve Disease. London, Butterworths, 1984, pp. 149–159.

26a. Gash, A. K., Carabello, B. A., Cepin, D., and Spann, J. F.: Left ventricular ejection performance and systolic muscle function in patients with mitral stenosis. Circulation 67:148, 1983.

27. Colle, J. P., Rahal, S., Ohayon, J., Bonnet, J., Le Goff, G., Besse, P., and Bricaud, H.: Global left ventricular function and regional wall motion in pure mitral stenosis. Clin. Cardiol. *7*:573, 1984.
28. Heller, S. J., and Carleton, R. A.: Abnormal left ventricular contraction in patients with mitral stenosis. Circulation 42:1099, 1970.
29. Harvey, R. M., Ferrer, M. I., Samet, P., Bader, R. A., Bader, M. E., Cournand, A., and Richards, D. W.: Mechanical and myocardial factors in rheumatic heart disease in mitral stenosis. Circulation *11*:531, 1955.
30. Bolen, J. L., Lopes, M. G., Harrison, D. C., and Alderman, E. L.: Analysis of left ventricular function in response to afterload changes in patients with mitral stenosis. Circulation *52*:894, 1975.
31. Reis, R. N., and Roberts, W. C.: Amounts of coronary arterial narrowing by atherosclerotic plaques in clinically isolated mitral valve stenosis: Analysis of 76 necropsy patients older than 30 years. Am. J. Cardiol. *57*:1117, 1986.
32. Johnston, D. L., and Kostuk, W. J.: Left and right ventricular function during symptom-limited exercise in patients with isolated mitral stenosis. Chest *89*:186, 1986.
33. Wroblewski, E., Spann, J. F., and Bove, A. A.: Right ventricular performance in mitral stenosis. Am. J. Cardiol. *47*:51, 1981.
34. Halperin, J. L., Brooks, K. M., Rothlauf, E. B., Mindich, B. P., Ambrose, J. A., and Teichholz, L. E.: Effect of nitroglycerin on the pulmonary venous gradient in patients after mitral valve replacement. J. Am. Coll. Cardiol. 5:34, 1985.
35. Unverferth, D. V., Fertel, R. H., Unverferth, B. J., and Leier, C. V.: Atrial fibrillation in mitral stenosis: Histologic, hemodynamic, and metabolic factors. Int. J. Cardiol. 5:143, 1984.
36. Munoz, S., Gallardo, J., Diaz-Gorrin, J. R., and Medina, O.: Influence of

surgery on the natural history of rheumatic mitral and aortic valve disease. Am. J. Cardiol. *35*:234, 1975.
37. Scarlat, A., Bodner, G., and Liron, M.: Massive haemoptysis as the presenting symptom in mitral stenosis. Thorax *41*:413, 1986.
38. Ross, R. S.: Right ventricular hypertension as a cause of precordial pain. Am. Heart J. *61*:134, 1961.
38a. Saltups, A.: Coronary arteriography in isolated aortic and mitral valve disease. Aust. N. Z. J. Med. *12*:494, 1982.
39. Baxter, R. H., Reid, J. M., McGuiness, J. B., and Stevenson, J. G.: Relation of angina to coronary artery disease in mitral and aortic valve disease. Br. Heart J. *40*:918, 1978.
40. Nielson, G. H., Galea, E. G., and Hossack, K. F.: Thromboembolic complications of mitral valve disease. Aust. N. Z. J. Med. *8*:372, 1978.
41. Daley, R., Mattingly, T. W., Holt, C. L., Bland, E. F., and White, P. D.: Systemic arterial embolism in rheumatic heart disease. Am. Heart J. *42*:566, 1951.
42. Lie, J. T., and Entman, M. L.: "Hole-in-one" sudden death: Mitral stenosis and left atrial thrombus. Am. Heart J. *91*:798, 1976.
43. Sharma, N. G. K., Kapoor, C. P., Mahambre, L., and Borkar, M. P.: Ortner's syndrome. J. Indian Med. Assoc. *60*:427, 1973.
44. Horwitz, L. D., and Groves, B. M. (eds.): Signs and Symptoms in Cardiology. Philadelphia, J. B. Lippincott, 1985, 506 pp.
45. Abrams, J.: Mitral stenosis. *In* Essentials of Cardiac Physical Diagnosis. Philadelphia, Lea and Febiger, 1987, pp. 275–306.
46. McCall, B. W., and Price, J. L.: Movement of mitral valve cusps in relation to first heart sound and opening snap in patients with mitral stenosis. Br. Heart J. *29*:417, 1967.
47. Perloff, J. K.: Auscultatory and phonocardiographic manifestations of pulmonary hypertension. Prog. Cardiovasc. Dis. *9*:303, 1967.
48. Nixon, P. G. F.: The genesis of the third heart sound. Am. Heart J. *65*:712, 1963.
49. Chandraratna, P. A. N., Aronow, W. S., and Lurie, M.: Cross-sectional echocardiographic observations on the mechanism of preservation of the opening snap in calcific mitral stenosis. Chest *78*:822, 1980.
50. Ebringer, R., Pitt, A., and Anderson, S. T.: Haemodynamic factors influencing opening snap interval in mitral stenosis. Br. Heart J. *32*:350, 1970.
51. Craige, E.: Phonocardiographic studies in mitral stenosis. N. Engl. J. Med. *257*:650, 1957.
52. Criley, J. M., Chambers, R. D., Blaufuss, A. H., and Friedman, N. J.: Mitral stenosis: Mechanico-acoustical events. *In* Leon, D. F., and Shaver, J. A. (eds.): Physiological Principles of Heart Sounds and Murmurs. New York, American Heart Association Monograph No. 46, 1975, pp. 149–159.
53. Tavel, M. E., and Bonner, A. J., Jr.: Presystolic murmur in atrial fibrillation: Fact or fiction? Circulation *54*:167, 1976.
54. Harvey, W. P.: Silent valvular heart disease. *In* Likoff, W. (ed.): Cardiovascular Clinics. Vol. 5, No. 2, Valvular Heart Disease. Philadelphia, F. A. Davis, 1973, p. 77.
55. Stapleton, J. F.: Natural history of chronic valvular disease. *In* Frankl, W. S., and Brest, A. N. (eds.): Cardiovascular Clinics. Valvular Heart Disease: Comprehensive Evaluation and Management. Philadelphia, F. A. Davis, 1986, pp. 105–148.
56. Surawicz, B.: Effect of respiration and upright position on the interval between the two components of the second heart sound and that between the second sound and mitral opening snap. Circulation *16*:422, 1957.
57. Fuchs, R. M., Fisher, J., Schuster, E. H., and Fortuin, N. J.: The systolic murmur of mitral stenosis. Johns Hopkins Med. J. *151*:220, 1982.
58. Aravanis, C., and Michaelides, G.: Tricuspid insufficiency masquerading as mitral insufficiency in patients with severe mitral stenosis. Am. J. Cardiol. *20*:417, 1967.
59. McArthur, J. D., Sukumar, I. P., Munis, S. C., Krishnaswami, S., and Cherian, G.: Reassessment of Graham Steell murmur using platinum electrode technique. Br. Heart. J. *36*:1023, 1974.
60. Cooksey, J. D., Dunn, M., and Massie, E.: Clinical Vectorcardiography and Electrocardiography. 2nd ed. Chicago, Year Book Medical Publishers, 1977, p. 272.
61. Kasser, I., and Kennedy, J. W.: The relationship of increased left atrial volume and pressure to abnormal P waves on the electrocardiogram. Circulation *39*:339, 1969.
62. Mounsey, P.: The atrial electrocardiogram as a guide to prognosis after mitral valvulotomy. Br. Heart J. *21*:617, 1961.
63. Probst, P., Goldschlager, N., and Selzer, A.: Left atrial size and atrial fibrillation in mitral stenosis: Factors influencing their relationship. Circulation *48*:1281, 1973.
64. Cueto, J., Toshima, J., Armyo, G., Tuna, N., and Lillehei, C. W.: Vectorcardiographic studies in acquired valvular disease with reference to the diagnosis of right ventricular hypertrophy. Circulation *33*:588, 1967.
65. Taymor, R. C., Hoffman, I., and Henry, E.: The Frank vectorcardiogram in mitral stenosis. Circulation *30*:865, 1964.
66. Donoso, E., Jick, S., Braunwald, E., Lamelas, M., and Grishman, A.: The spatial vectorcardiogram in mitral valve disease. Am. Heart J. *53*:760, 1957.
67. Gooch, A. S., Calatayud, J. B., Gorman, P. A., Saunders, J. L., and Caceres, C. A.: Leftward shift of the terminal P forces in the ECG associated with left atrial enlargement. Am. Heart. J. *71*:727, 1966.
68. Chen, J. T. T., Behar, V. S., Morris, J. J., Jr., McIntosh, H. D., and Lester, R. G.: Correlation of roentgen findings with hemodynamic data in pure mitral stenosis. Am. J. Roentgenol. Radium Ther. Nucl. Med. *102*:280, 1968.
69. Amplatz, K.: The roentgenographic diagnosis of mitral and aortic valvular disease. Am. Heart J. *64*:556, 1962.
70. Melhem, R. E., Dunbar, J. D., and Booth, R. W.: "B" lines of Kerley and left atrial size in mitral valve disease: Their correlation with mean left atrial pressure as measured by left atrial puncture. Radiology *76*:65, 1961.
71. Fleischner, F. G., and Reiner, L.: Linear x-ray shadows in acquired pulmonary hemosiderosis and congestion. N. Engl. J. Med. *250*:900, 1954.
72. Van Houten, F. X., Adams, D. F., and Abrams, H. C.: Radiology of valvular heart disease. *In* Sonnenblick, E. H.,and Lesch, M. (eds.): Valvular Heart Disease. New York, Grune and Stratton, 1974, p. 1.
73. Parker, B. M., Friedenberg, M. J., Templeton, A. W. and Burford, T. H.: Preoperative angiocardiographic diagnosis of left atrial thrombi in mitral stenosis. N. Engl. J. Med. *273*:136, 1965.
74. Come, P. C.: Echocardiographic evaluation of valvular heart disease. *In* Come, P. C. (ed.): Diagnostic Cardiology. Philadelphia, J. B. Lippincott, 1985, pp. 407–458.
75. Fisher, M. L., Parisi, A. F., Plotnick, G. D., DeFelice, C. E., Carliner, N. H., and Fortuin, N. J.: Assessment of severity of mitral stenosis by echocardiographic leaflet separation. Arch. Intern. Med. *139*:402, 1979.
76. Egeblad, H., Berning, J., Saunamaki, K., Jacobsen, J. R., and Wennevold, A.: Assessment of rheumatic mitral valve disease: Value of echocardiography in patients clinically suspected of predominant stenosis. Br. Heart. J. *49*:38, 1983.
77. Thuillez, C., Theroux, P., Bourassa, M., Blanchard, M., Peronneau, P., Guermonprez, J.-L., Diebold, B., and Waters, D. D.: Pulsed Doppler echocardiographic study of mitral stenosis. Circulation *61*:381, 1980.
77a. Glover, M. U., Warren, S. E., Vieweg, W. V. R., Ceretto, W. J., Samtoy, L. M., and Hagan, A. D.: M-mode and two-dimensional echocardiographic correlation with findings at catheterization and surgery in patients with mitral stenosis. Am. Heart J. *105*:98, 1983.
78. Smith, M. D., Handshoe, R., Handshoe, S., Kwan, O. L., and DeMaria, A. N.: Comparative accuracy of two-dimensional echocardiography and Doppler pressure half-time methods in assessing severity of mitral stenosis in patients with and without prior commissurotomy. Circulation *73*:100, 1986.
79. Schweizer, P., Bardos, P., Erbel, R., Meyer, J., Merx, W., Messmer, B. J., and Effert, S.: Detection of left atrial thrombi by echocardiography. Br. Heart J. *45*:148, 1981.
80. Zoghbi, W. A., Farmer, K. L., Soto, J. G., Nelson, J. G., and Quinones, M. A.: Accurate noninvasive quantification of stenotic aortic valve area by Doppler echocardiography. Circulation *73*:452, 1986.
80a. Shandheria, B. K., Tajik, A. J., Reeder, G. S., Callahan, M. J., Nishimura, R. A., Miller, F. A., and Seward, J. B.: Doppler color flow imaging: A new technique for visualization and characterization of the blood flow jet in mitral stenosis. Mayo Clin. Proc. *61*:623, 1986.
81. Beiser, G. D., Epstein, S. E., Stampfer, M., Robinson, B., and Braunwald, E.: Studies on digitalis. XVIII. Effects of ouabain on the hemodynamic response to exercise in patients with mitral stenosis in normal sinus rhythm. N. Engl. J. Med. *278*:131, 1968.
81a. Klein, H. O., Sareli, P., Schamroth, C. L., Carim, Y. Epstein, M., and Marcus, B.: Effects of atenolol on exercise capacity in patients with mitral stenosis with sinus rhythm. Am. J. Cardiol. *56*:598, 1985.
82. Levine, H. J.: Which atrial fibrillation patients should be on chronic anticoagulation? J. Cardiovasc. Med. *6*:483, 1981.
83. Kloster, F. E., and Morris, C. D.: Natural history of valvular heart disease. Circulation *65*:1283, 1982.
84. Joswig, B. C., Glover, M. U., Handler, J. B., Warren, S. E., and Vieweg, W. V. R.: Contrasting progression of mitral stenosis in Malayans versus American-born Caucasians. Am. Heart J. *104*:1400, 1982.
85. Olesen, K. H.: The natural history of 271 patients with mitral stenosis under medical treatment. Br. Heart J. *24*:349, 1962.
86. Rowe, J. C., Bland, E. F., Sprague, H. B., and White, P. D.: The course of mitral stenosis without surgery: Ten- and twenty-year perspectives. Ann. Intern. Med. *52*:741, 1960.
87. Rapaport, E.: Natural history of aortic and mitral valve disease. Am. J. Cardiol. *35*:221, 1975.
88. Sutton, M. J. St.J., Oldershaw, P., Sacchetti, R., Paneth, M., Lennox, S. C., Gibson, R. V., and Gibson, D. G.: Valve replacement without preoperative cardiac catheterization. N. Engl. J. Med. *305*:1233, 1981.
89. Brandenburg, R. O.: No more routine catheterization for valvular heart disease? N. Engl. J. Med. *305*:1277, 1981.
90. O'Rourke, R. A.: Preoperative cardiac catheterization. Its need in most patients with valvular heart disease. J.A.M.A. *248*:745, 1982.
91. Chun, P. K. C., Gertz, E., Davia, J. E., and Cheitlin, M. D.: Coronary atherosclerosis in mitral stenosis. Chest *81*:36, 1982.
92. Ramsdale, D. R., Faragher, E. B., Bennett, D. H., Bray, C. L., Ward, C., and Beton, D. C.: Preoperative prediction of significant coronary artery disease in patients with valvular heart disease. Br. Med. J. *284*:223, 1982.
93. John, S., Bashi, V. V., Jairaj, P. S., Muralidharan, S., Ravikumar, E., Rajarajeswari, T., Krishnaswami, S., Sukumar, I. P., and Rao, P. S. S.: Closed mitral valvotomy: Early results and long-term follow-up of 3724 consecutive patients. Circulation *68*:891, 1983.
94. Gautam, P. C., Coulshed, N., Epstein, E. J., Llewellyn, M. J., Vargas, E., and Tallis, R. C.: Preoperative clinical predictors of long-term survival in mitral stenosis: Analysis of 200 cases followed for up to 27 years after closed mitral valvotomy. Thorax *41*:401, 1986.
95. de Vivie, E. R., and Hellberg, K.: Closed transventricular mitral commissurotomy. *In* Ionescu, M. I. and Cohn, L. H. (eds.): Mitral Valve Disease: Diagnosis and Treatment. London, Butterworths, 1985, pp. 139–152.
96. Dernevik, L., Brorsson, L., Wallentin, I., and William-Olsson, G.: Improved results of closed commissurotomy for mitral stenosis using ultrasonocardiography as selection ground. Acta Med. Scand. *210*:283, 1981.
97. Lower, R. R., and Ducey, K.: Open mitral valvotomy. *In* Ionescu, M. I., and Cohn, L. H. (eds.): Mitral Valve Disease: Diagnosis and Treatment. London, Butterworths, 1985, pp. 153–156.
98. Gross, R. I., Cunningham, J. N., Jr., Snively, S. L., Catinella, F. P., Nathan, I. M., Adams, P. X., and Spencer, F. C.: Long-term results of open radical

mitral commissurotomy: Ten year follow-up study of 202 patients. Am. J. Cardiol. *47*:821, 1981.
99. Duran, C.: Mitral reconstruction in predominant mitral stenosis. *In* Duran, C., Angell, W. W., Johnson, A. D., and Oury, J. H. (eds.): Recent Progress in Mitral Valve Disease. London, Butterworths, 1984, pp. 255–264.
99a. Smith, W. M., Neutze, J. M., Barratt-Boyes, B. G., and Lowe, J. B.: Open mitral valvotomy. Effect of preoperative factors on result. J. Thorac. Cardiovasc. Surg. *82*:738, 1981.
100. Cohn, L. H., Allred, E. N., Cohn, L. A., Disesa, V. J., Shemin, R. J., and Collins, J. J., Jr.: Long-term results of open mitral valve reconstruction for mitral stenosis. Am. J. Cardiol. *55*:731, 1985.
101. Aryanpur, I., Shakibi, J., Yazdanyar, A., Mehranpur, M., Paydar, M., Azar, H., Motlagh, F. A., Tarbiat, S., and Siassi, B.: Closed versus open mitral commissurotomy in children with rheumatic mitral stenosis. J. Thorac. Cardiovasc. Surg. *76*:223, 1978.
102. Aora, R., Khalilullah, M., Gupta, M. P., and Padmavati, S.: Mitral restenosis. Incidence and epidemiology. Indian Heart J. *30*:265, 1978.
103. Heger, J. J., Wann, L. S., Weyman, A. E., Dillon, J. C., and Feigenbaum, H.: Long-term changes in mitral valve area after successful mitral commissurotomy. Circulation *59*:443, 1979.
104. Higgs, L. M., Glancy, D. L., O'Brien, K. P., Epstein, S. E., and Morrow, A. G.: Mitral restenosis: An uncommon cause of recurrent symptoms following mitral commissurotomy. Am. J. Cardiol. *26*:34, 1970.
105. Braunwald, E., Braunwald, N. S., Ross, J., Jr., and Morrow, A. G.: Effects of mitral valve replacement on the pulmonary vascular dynamics of patients with pulmonary hypertension. N. Engl. J. Med. *273*:509, 1965.
106. Ward, C., and Hancock, B. W.: Extreme pulmonary hypertension caused by mitral valve disease. Natural history and results of surgery. Br. Heart J. *37*:74, 1975.
106a. Foltz, B. D., Hessel, E. A., and Ivey, T. D.: The early course of pulmonary artery hypertension in patients undergoing mitral valve replacement with cardioplegic arrest. J. Thorac. Cardiovasc. Surg. *88*:238, 1984.
107. Dalen, J. E., Matloff, J. M., Evans, G. L., Hoppin, F. G., Jr., Bhardwaj, P., Harken, D. E., and Dexter, L.: Early reduction of pulmonary vascular resistance after mitral valve replacement. N. Engl. J. Med. *277*:387, 1967.
108. Scott, W. C., Miller, D. C., Haverich, A., Mitchell, R. S., Oyer, P. E., Stinson, E. B., Jammieson, S. W., Baldwin, J. C., and Shumway, N. E.: Operative risk of mitral valve replacement: Discriminant analysis of 1329 procedures. Circulation *72*(Suppl. II):108, 1985.
109. Kaplan, J. D., Isner, J. M., Karas, R. H., Halaburka, K. R., Konstam, M. A., Hougen, T. J., Cleveland, R. J., and Salem, D. N.: In vitro analysis of mechanisms of balloon valvuloplasty of stenotic mitral valves. Am. J. Cardiol. *59*:318, 1987.
110. McKay, R. G., Lock, J. E., Safian, R. D., Come, P. C., Diver, D. J., Baim, D. S., Berman, A. D., Warren, S. E., Mandell, V. E., Royal, H. D., and Grossman, W.: Balloon dilation of mitral stenosis in adult patients: Postmorten and percutaneous mitral valvuloplasty studies. J. Am. Coll. Cardiol. *9*:723, 1987.
111. Al Zaibag, M., Ribeiro, P. A., Al Kasab, S., and Al Fagih, M. R.: Percutaneous double-balloon mitral valvotomy for rheumatic mitral valve stenosis. Lancet *1*:757, 1986.
112. Palacios, I. F., Lock, J. E., Keane, J. F., and Block, P. C.: Percutaneous transvenous balloon valvotomy in a patient with severe calcific mitral stenosis. J. Am. Coll. Cardiol. *7*:1416, 1986.
113. Rahimtoola, S. H.: Catheter balloon valvuloplasty of aortic and mitral valve stenosis in adults. Circulation *75*:895, 1987.
114. Kveselis, D. A., Rocchini, A. P., Beekman, R., Snider, A. R., Crowley, D., Dick, M., and Rosenthal, A.: Balloon angioplasty for congenital and rheumatic mitral stenosis. Am. J. Cardiol. *57*:348, 1986.
115. McKay, R. G.: Personal communication, 1987.

MITRAL REGURGITATION

116. Davies, M. J.: Aetiology and pathology of the diseased mitral valve. *In* Ionescu, M. I., and Cohn, L. H. (eds.): Mitral Valve Disease: Diagnosis and Treatment. London, Butterworths, 1985, pp. 27–42.
117. Dajee, H., Hurley, E. J., and Szarnicki, R. J.: Cardiac valve replacement in systemic lupus erythematosus. A review. J. Thorac. Cardiovasc. Surg. *85*:718, 1983.
118. Boltwood, C. M., Tei, C., Wong, M., and Shah, P. M.: Quantitative echocardiography of the mitral complex in dilated cardiomyopathy: The mechanism of functional mitral regurgitation. Circulation *68*:498, 1983.
119. Bloor, C. M.: Valvular heart disease in the elderly. J. Am. Geriatr. Soc. *30*:466, 1982.
120. Nestico, P. F., DePace, N. L., Kotler, M. N., Rose, L. I., Brezin, J. H., Swartz, C., Mintz, G. S., and Schwartz, A. B.: Calcium phosphorus metabolism in dialysis patients with and without mitral anular calcium. Analysis of 30 patients. Am. J. Cardiol. *51*:497, 1983.
121. Forman, M. B., Virmani, B., Robertson, R. M., and Stone, W. J.: Mitral anular calcification in chronic renal failure. Chest *85*:367, 1984.
122. Zanolla, L., Marino, P., Nicolosi, G. L., Peranzoni, P. F., and Poppi, A.: Two-dimensional echocardiographic evaluation of mitral valve calcification. Sensitivity and specificity. Chest *82*:154, 1982.
123. Mellino, M., Salcedo, E. E., Lever, H. M., Vasudevan, G., and Kramer, J. R.: Echographic-quantified severity of mitral anulus calcification: Prognostic correlation to related hemodynamic, valvular, rhythm, and conduction abnormalities. Am. Heart J. *103*:222, 1982.
124. Labovitz, A. J., Nelson, J. G., Windhorst, D. M., Kennedy, H. L., and Williams, G. A.: Frequency of mitral valve dysfunction from mitral anular calcium as detected by Doppler echocardiography. Am. J. Cardiol. *55*:133, 1985.
125. Nestico, P. F., Depace, N. L., Morganroth, J., Kotler, M. N., and Ross, J.: Mitral annular calcification: Clinical, pathophysiology, and echocardiographic review. Am. Heart J. *107*:989, 1984.
126. Takamoto, T., and Popp, R. L.: Conduction disturbances related to the site and severity of mitral anular calcification: A two-dimensional echocardiographic and electrocardiographic correlative study. Am. J. Cardiol. *51*:1644, 1983.
127. Scott-Jupp, W., Barnett, N. L., Gallagher, P. J., Monro, J. L., and Ross, J. K.: Ultrastructural changes in spontaneous rupture of mitral chordae tendineae. J. Pathol. *133*:185, 1981.
128. Oliveira, D. B. G., Dawkins, K. D., Kay, P. H., and Paneth, M.: Chordal rupture I: Aetiology and natural history. Br. Heart J. *50*:312, 1983.
129. Oliveira, D. B. G., Dawkins, K. D., Kay, P. H., and Paneth, M.: Chordal rupture II: Comparison between repair and replacement. Br. Heart J. *50*:318, 1983.
130. Hickey, A. J., Wilcken, D. E. L., Wright, J. S., and Warren, B. A.: Primary (spontaneous) chordal rupture: Relation to myxomatous valve disease and mitral valve prolapse. J. Am. Coll. Cardiol. *5*:1341, 1985.
131. Godley, R. W., Wann, L. S., Rogers, E. W., Feigenbaum, H., and Weyman, A. E.: Incomplete mitral leaflet closure in patients with papillary muscle dysfunction. Circulation *63*:565, 1981.
132. Gallagher, P. J., Caves, P. K., and Stinson, E. B.: Pathological changes in spontaneous rupture of chordae tendineae. Ann. Cir. Gynaecol. *66*:135, 1977.
133. Burch, G. E., DePasquale, N. P., and Phillips, J. H.: The syndrome of papillary muscle dysfunction. Am. Heart J. *75*:399, 1968.
134. Estes, E. H., Jr., Dalton, F. M., Entman, M. L., et al.: The anatomy and blood supply of the papillary muscle of the left ventricle. Am. Heart J. *71*:356, 1966.
135. Gahl, K., Sutton, R., Pearson, M., Caspari, P., Lairet, A., and McDonald, L.: Mitral regurgitation in coronary heart disease. Br. Heart J. *39*:13, 1977.
135a. Ballester, M., Jajoo, J., Rees, S., Rickards, A., and McDonald, L.: The mechanism of mitral regurgitation in dilated left ventricle. Clin. Cardiol. *6*:333, 1983.
136. Becker, A. E., and Anderson, R. H.: Mitral insufficiency complicating acute myocardial infarction. Eur. J. Cardiol. *2*:351, 1975.
137. Morrow, A. G., Cohen, L. S., Roberts, W. C., Braunwald, N. S., and Braunwald, E.: Severe mitral regurgitation following acute myocardial infarction and ruptured papillary muscle. Hemodynamic findings and results of operative treatment in four patients. Circulation *37*(Suppl. II):124, 1968.
138. Balu, V., Hershowitz, S., Masud, A. R. Z., Bhayana, J. N., and Dean, D. C.: Mitral regurgitation in coronary artery disease. Chest *81*:550, 1982.
139. Gottdiener, J. S., Maron, B. J., Schooley, R. T., Harley, J. B., Roberts, W. C., and Fauci, A. S.: Two-dimensional echocardiographic assessment of the idiopathic hypereosinophilis syndrome. Anatomic basis of mitral regurgitation and peripheral embolization. Circulation *67*:572, 1983.
140. Metras, D., Ouezzin-Coulibaly, A., Ouattara, K., Bertrand, E., and Chauvet, J.: Endomyocardial fibrosis masquerading as rheumatic mitral incompetence. A report of six surgical cases. J. Thorac. Cardiovasc. Surg. *86*:753, 1983.
141. Mazzucco, A., Rizzoli, G., Faggian, G., Aru, G., Bortolotti, U., Sorbara, C., and Chioin, R.: Acute mitral regurgitation after blunt chest trauma. Arch. Intern. Med. *143*:2326, 1983.
142. Jolly, D. T.: Traumatic rupture of a papillary muscle of the mitral valve due to blunt thoracic trauma. Can. Fam. Phys. *29*:1960, 1983.
143. DiSegni, E., and Edwards, J. E.: Cleft anterior leaflet of the mitral valve with intact septa. A study of 20 cases. Am. J. Cardiol. *51*:919, 1983.
144. Nagata, S., Nimura, Y., Sakakibara, H., Beppu, S., Park, Y-D., Kawazoe, K., and Fujita, T.: Mitral valve lesion associated with secundum atrial septal defect. Analysis of real-time two-dimensional echocardiography. Br. Heart J. *49*:151, 1983.
145. Gidding, S. S., Shulman, S. T., Ilbawi, M., Crussi, F., and Duffy, C. E.: Mucocutaneous lymph node syndrome (Kawasaki disease): Delayed aortic and mitral insufficiency secondary to active valvulitis. J. Am. Coll. Cardiol. *7*:894, 1986.
146. Eckberg, D. L., Gault, J. H., Bouchard, R. L., Karliner, J. S., and Ross, J., Jr.: Mechanics of left ventricular contraction in chronic severe mitral regurgitation. Circulation *47*:1252, 1973.
147. Braunwald, E., Welch, G. H., Jr., and Sarnoff, S. J.: Hemodynamic effects of quantitatively varied experimental mitral regurgitation. Circ. Res. *5*:539, 1957.
148. Pierpont, G. L., and Talley, R. C.: Pathophysiology of valvar heart disease. Arch. Intern. Med. *142*:998, 1982.
149. Spratt, J. A., Olsen, C. O., Tyson, G. S., Jr., Glower, D. D., Jr., Davis, J. W., and Rankin, J. S.: Experimental mitral regurgitation. Physiological effects of correction on left ventricular dynamics. J. Thorac. Cardiovasc. Surg. *86*:479, 1983.
150. Braunwald, E., and Turi, Z. G.: Pathophysiology of mitral valve disease. *In* Ionescu, M. I., and Cohn, L. H. (eds.): Mitral Valve Disease: Diagnosis and Treatment. London, Butterworths, 1985, pp. 3–10.
151. Yellin, E. L., Yoran, C., Frater, R. W. M., and Sonnenblick, E. H.: Dynamics of acute experimental mitral regurgitation. *In* Ionescu, M. I., and Cohn, L. H. (eds.): Mitral Valve Disease: Diagnosis and Treatment. London, Butterworths, 1985, pp. 11–26.
152. Urschel, C. W., Covell, J. W., Sonnenblick, E. H. Ross, J., Jr., and Braunwald, E.: Myocardial mechanics in aortic and mitral valvular regurgitation: The concept of instantaneous impedance as a determinant of the performance of the intact heart. J. Clin. Invest. *47*:867, 1968.
153. Braunwald, E.: Mitral regurgitation: Physiological, clinical and surgical considerations. N. Engl. J. Med. *281*:425, 1969.
154. Urschel, C. W., Covell, J. W., Graham, T. P., Clancy, R. L., Ross, J., Jr., Sonnenblick, E. H., and Braunwald, E.: Effects of acute valvular regurgitation on the oxygen consumption of the canine heart. Circ. Res. *23*:33, 1968.

155. Braunwald, E.: Control of myocardial oxygen consumption: Physiologic and clinical considerations. Am. J. Cardiol. *27*:416, 1971.
156. Ross, J., Jr.: Left ventricular function and the timing of surgical treatment in valvular heart disease. Ann. Intern. Med. *94*:498, 1981.
157. Vokonas, P. S., Gorlin, R., Cohn, P. F., Herman, M. V., and Sonnenblick, E. H.: Dynamic geometry of the left ventricle in mitral regurgitation. Circulation *48*:786, 1973.
158. Osbakken, M. D., Bove, A. A., and Spann, J. F.: Left ventricular regional wall motion and velocity of shortening in chronic mitral and aortic regurgitation. Am. J. Cardiol. *47*:1055, 1981.
159. Wong, C. Y. H., and Spotnitz, H. M.: Systolic and diastolic properties of the human left ventricle during valve replacement for chronic mitral regurgitation. Am. J. Cardiol. *47*:40, 1981.
160. Clancy, K. F., Iskandrian, A. S., Hakki, A-H., Nestico, P., and DePace, N. L.: Age-related changes in cardiovascular performance in mitral regurgitation: Analysis of 61 patients. Am. Heart J. *109*:442, 1985.
160a. Ramanathan, K. B., Knowles, J., Connor, M. J., Tribble, R., Kroetz, F. W., Sullivan, J. M., and Mirvis, D. M.: Natural history of chronic mitral insufficiency: Relation of peak systolic pressure/end-systolic volume ratio to morbidity and mortality. J. Am. Coll. Cardiol. *3*:1412, 1984.
161. Wisenbaugh, T., Spann, J. F., and Carabello, B. A.: Differences in myocardial performance and load between patients with similar amounts of chronic aortic versus chronic mitral regurgitation. J. Am. Coll. Cardiol. *3*:913, 1984.
162. Borow, K., Green, L. H., Mann, T., Sloss, L. J., Braunwald, E., Collins, J. J., Cohn, L., and Grossman, W.: End-systolic volume as a predictor of postoperative left ventricular performance in volume overload from valvular regurgitation. Am. J. Med. *68*:655, 1980.
163. Boucher, C. A., Bingham, J. B., Osbakken, M. D., Okada, R. D., Strauss, W. H., Block, P. C., Levine, F. H., Phillips, H. R., and Pohost, G. M.: Early changes in left ventricular size and function after correction of left ventricular volume overload. Am. J. Cardiol. *47*:991, 1981.
163a. Konstam, M. A., Wynne, J., Holman, B. L., Brown, E. J., Neil, J. M., and Kozlowski, J.: Use of equilibrium (gated) radionuclide ventriculography to quantitate left ventricular output in patients with and without left-sided valvular regurgitation. Circulation *64*:578, 1981.
163b. Grose, R., Strain, J., and Cohen, M. V.: Pulmonary arterial V waves in mitral regurgitation: Clinical and experimental observations. Circulation *69*:214, 1984.
164. Braunwald, E., and Awe, W. C.: The syndrome of severe mitral regurgitation with normal left atrial pressure. Circulation *27*:29, 1963.
165. Roberts, W. C., Braunwald, E., and Morrow, A. G.: Acute severe mitral regurgitation secondary to ruptured chordae tendineae. Clinical, hemodynamic and pathologic considerations. Circulation *33*:58, 1966.
166. Cohen, L. S., Mason, D. T., and Braunwald, E.: Significance of an atrial gallop sound in mitral regurgitation: A clue to the diagnosis of ruptured chordae tendineae. Circulation *35*:112, 1966.
166a. Gorlin, R.: Natural history, medical therapy and indications for surgery in mitral valve disease. *In* Ionescu, M. I., and Cohn, L. H. (eds.): Mitral Valve Disease: Diagnosis and Treatment. London, Butterworths, 1985, pp. 105–126.
167. Kusiak, V., and Brest, A. N.: Acute mitral regurgitation: Pathophysiology and management. *In* Frankl, W. S., and Brest, A. N. (eds.): Cardiovascular Clinics. Valvular Heart Disease: Comprehensive Evaluation and Management. Philadelphia, F. A. Davis, 1986, pp. 257–280.
167a. Rippe, J. M., and Howe, J. P. III.: Acute mitral regurgitation. *In* Dalen, J. E., and Alpert, J. S. (eds.): Valvular Heart Disease. 2nd ed. Boston, Little, Brown and Company, 1987, pp. 151–176.
168. Elkins, R. C., Morrow, A. G., Vasko, J. S., and Braunwald, E.: The effects of mitral regurgitation of the pattern of instantaneous aortic blood flow. Clinical and experimental observations. Circulation *36*:45, 1967.
169. Basta, L. L., Wolfson, P., Eckberg, D. L., and Abboud, F. M.: The value of left parasternal impulse recordings in the assessment of mitral regurgitation. Circulation *48*:1055, 1973.
170. Barlow, J. B.: Mitral regurgitation. *In* Perspectives on the Mitral Valve. Philadelphia, F. A. Davis, 1987, pp. 113–131.
170a. Haffajee, C. I.: Chronic mitral regurgitation. *In* Dalen, J. E., and Alpert, J. S. (eds.): Valvular Heart Disease. 2nd ed. Boston, Little, Brown and Company, 1987, pp. 111–150.
171. Karliner, J. S., O'Rourke, R. A., Kearney, D. J., and Shabetai, R.: Haemodynamic explanation of why the murmur of mitral regurgitation is independent of cycle length. Br. Heart J. *35*:397, 1973.
172. Aravanis, C.: Silent mitral insufficiency. Am. Heart J. *70*:620, 1965.
173. Dusall, J. C., Pryor, R., and Blount, S. G.: Systolic murmur following myocardial infarction. Am. Heart J. *87*:577, 1974.
174. Antman, E. M., Angoff, G. H., and Sloss, J. J.: Demonstration of the mechanism by which mitral regurgitation mimics aortic stenosis. Am. J. Cardiol. *42*:1044, 1978.
175. Merendino, K. A., and Hessel, E. A.: The murmur on top of the head in acquired mitral insufficiency. J.A.M.A. *199*:392, 1967.
176. Bentoviglio, L. G., Uricchio, J. F., Waldow, A., Likoff, W., and Goldberg, H.: An electrocardiographic analysis of mitral regurgitation. Circulation *18*:572, 1956.
177. Morris, J. J., Estes, E. H., Whalen, R. E., Thompson, H. K., and McIntosh, H. D.: P wave analysis in valvular heart disease. Circulation *29*:242, 1964.
178. Priest, E. A., Finlayson, J. K., and Short, D. S.: The x-ray manifestations in the heart and lungs of mitral regurgitation. Prog. Cardiovasc. Dis. *5*:219, 1962.
179. Wexler, L., Silverman, J. F., DeBusk, R. F., and Harrison, D. C.: Angiographic features of rheumatic and nonrheumatic mitral regurgitation. Circulation *44*:1080, 1971.
180. Mourant, A. J., Weaver, J., and Johnston, K.: Echocardiographic findings in rheumatic mitral valve disease with chordal rupture. J. Clin. Ultrasound *10*:79, 1982.
181. Pizzarello, R. A., Turnier, J., Goldman, M. A., Dworkin, P., Oka, M., Tortolani, A. J., and Padmanabhan, V. T.: Clinical and echocardiographic features of isolated severe pure mitral regurgitation. Clin. Cardiol. *7*:565, 1984.
182. Sweatman, T., Selzer, A., Kamageki, M., and Cohn, K.: Echocardiographic diagnosis of mitral regurgitation due to ruptured chordae tendineae. Circulation *46*:580, 1972.
183. Nair, C. K., Aronow, W. S., Sketch, M. H., Mohiuddin, S. M., Pagano, T., Esterbrooks, D. J., and Hee, T. T.: Clinical and echocardiographic characteristics of patients with mitral annular calcification. Am. J. Cardiol. *51*:992, 1983.
184. Wautrecht, J. C., Vandenbiossche, J. L., and Englert, M.: Sensitivity and specificity of pulsed Doppler echocardiography in detection of aortic and mitral regurgitation. Eur. Heart J. *5*:404, 1984.
185. Miyatake, K., Izumi, S., Okamoto, M., Kinoshita, N., Asonuma, H., Nakagawa, H., Yamamoto, K., Takamiya, M., Sakakibara, H., and Nimura, Y.: Semiquantitative grading of severity of mitral regurgitation by real-time two-dimensional Doppler flow imaging technique. J. Am. Coll. Cardiol. *7*:82, 1986.
186. Helmcke, F., Nanda, N. C., Hsiung, M. C., Soto, B., Adey, C. K., Goyal, R. G., and Gatewood, R. P., Jr.: Color doppler assessment of mitral regurgitation with orthogonal planes. Circulation *75*:175, 1987.
187. Thompson, R., Ross, I., and Elmes, R.: Quantification of valvular regurgitation by cardiac gated pool imaging. Br. Heart J. *46*:629, 1981.
188. Boucher, C. A., Okada, R. D., and Pohost, G. M.: Current status of radionuclide imaging in valvular heart disease. Am. J. Cardiol. *46*:1153, 1980.
189. Greenberg, B. H.: Mitral insufficiency: Use of vasodilators. Primary Cardiol. *10*:155, 1984.
189a. Chatterjee, K.: Vasodilator therapy for mitral regurgitation. *In* Duran, C., Angell, W. W., Johnson, A. D., and Oury, J. H. (eds.): Recent Progress in Mitral Valve Disease. London, Butterworths, 1984, pp. 138–148.
190. Schlant, R. C.: The management of chronic mitral regurgitation. Council on Clinical Cardiology Newsletter *12*:1, March 1986.
191. Yoran, C., Yellin, E. L., Becker, R. M., Gabbay, S., Frater, R. W. M., and Sonnenblick, E. H.: Mechanism of reduction of mitral regurgitation with vasodilator therapy. Am. J. Cardiol. *43*:773, 1979.
192. Orszulak, T. A., Schaff, H. V., Danielson, G. K., Piehler, J. M., Pluth, J. R., Frye, R. L., and McGoon, D. C.: Mitral regurgitation due to ruptured chordae tendineae. Early and late results of valve repair. J. Thorac. Cardiovasc. Surg. *89*:491, 1985.
193. Tandon, A. P., Silverton, N. P., and Ionescu, M. I.: Mitral valve repair (The Wooler annuloplasty). *In* Ionescu, M. I., and Cohn, L. H. (eds.): Mitral Valve Disease: Diagnosis and Treatment. London, Butterworths, 1985, pp. 171–178.
194. Spencer, F. C., Colvin, S. B., Culliford, A. T., and Isom, O. W.: Experiences with the Carpentier techniques of mitral valve reconstruction in 103 patients. J. Thorac. Cardiovasc. Surg. *90*:341, 1985.
195. Lessana, A., Viet, T. T., Ades, F., Kara, S. M., Ameur, A., Ruffenach, A., Guerin, F., Herreman, F., and Degeorges, M.: Mitral reconstructive operations. A series of 130 consecutive cases. J. Thorac. Cardiovasc. Surg. *86*:553, 1983.
196. Kirklin, J. W.: Mitral valve repair for mitral incompetence. Mod. Concepts Cardiovasc. Dis. *56*:7, 1987.
197. Antunes, M. J., Colsen, P. R., and Kinsley, R. H.: Mitral valvuloplasty: A learning curve. Circulation *68*(Suppl. II):70, 1983.
198. Carpentier, A.: Mitral reconstruction in predominant mitral incompetence. *In* Duran, C., Angell, W. W., Johnson, A. D., and Oury, J. H. (eds.): Recent Progress in Mitral Valve Disease. London, Butterworths, 1984, pp. 265–276.
199. Dawkins, K., Olivera, D., Kay, P., and Paneth, M.: Chordal rupture: Repair or replacement? *In* Duran, C., Angell, W. W., Johnson, A. D., and Oury, J. H. (eds.): Recent Progress in Mitral Valve Disease. London, Butterworths, 1984, pp. 428–435.
200. Kay, J. H. Carlish, R. A., and Dunne, E. F.: Mitral valve repair for mitral insufficiency. *In* Ionescu, M. I., and Cohn, L. H. (eds.): Mitral Valve Disease: Diagnosis and Treatment. London, Butterworths, 1985, pp. 157–170.
201. Duran, C. G.: Conservative surgery of the mitral valve: Ring annuloplasties. *In* Ionescu, M. I., and Cohn, L. H. (eds.): Mitral Valve Disease: Diagnosis and Treatment. London, Butterworths, 1985, pp. 179–190.
202. Cohn, L. H., Mudge, G. H., Pratter, F., and Collins, J. J., Jr.: Five- to eight-year followup of patients undergoing porcine heart-valve replacement. N. Engl. J. Med. *304*:258, 1981.
203. Bjork, V. O., Henze, A., and Lindblom, D.: The current status of prosthetic valves in the mitral position. *In* Duran, C., and Angell, W. W., Johnson, A. D., and Oury, J. H. (eds.): Recent Progress in Mitral Valve Disease. London, Butterworths, 1984, pp. 201–210.
204. Gore, J. M.: Prosthetic heart valves. *In* Dalen, J. E., and Alpert, J. S. (eds.): Valvular Heart Disease. 2nd ed. Boston, Little, Brown, and Company, 1987, pp. 509–528.
205. Cohn, L. H., Koster, J. K., VandeVanter, S., and Collins, J. J.: The in-hospital risk of rereplacement of dysfunctional mitral and aortic valves. Circulation *66*(Suppl. I):153, 1982.
206. Schuler, G., Peterson, K. L., Johnson, A., Francis, G., Dennish, G., Utley, J. R., Dailey, P. O., Ashburn, W., and Ross, J., Jr.: Temporal response of left ventricular performance to mitral valve surgery. Circulation *59*:1218, 1979.
207. Teply, J. F., Grunkemeier, G. L., Sutherland, H. D'A., Lambert, L. E., Johnson, V. A., and Starr, A.: The ultimate prognosis after valve replacement: An assessment at twenty years. Ann. Thorac. Surg. *32*:111, 1981.
208. Fuster, V., Pumphrey, C. W., McGoon, M. D., Chesebro, J. H., Pluth, J. R., and McGoon, D. C.: Systemic thromboembolism in mitral and aortic

Starr-Edwards prostheses: A 10- to 19-year followup. Circulation *66*(Suppl. I):157, 1982.

209. Zwart, H. H. J., Hicks, G., Schuster, B., Nathan, M., Tabrah, F., Wenzke, F., Ahmed, T., and DeWall, R. A.: Clinical experience with the Lillehei-Kaster valve prosthesis. Ann. Thorac. Surg. *28*:158, 1979.
210. Phillips, H. R., Levine, F. H., Carter, J. E., Boucher, C. A., Osbakken, M. D., Okada, R. D., Akins, C. W., Daggett, W. M., Buckley, M. J., and Pohost, G. M.: Mitral valve replacement for isolated mitral regurgitation: Analysis of clinical course and late postoperative left ventricular ejection fraction. Am. J. Cardiol. *48*:647, 1981.
211. Nicoloff, D. M., Emery, R. W., Arom, K. V., Northrup, W. F., Jorgensen, C. R., Wang, Y., and Lindsay, W. G.: Clinical and hemodynamic results with the St. Jude medical cardiac valve prosthesis. A three-year experience. J. Thorac. Cardiovasc. Surg. *82*:674, 1981.
212. Jamieson, W. R. E., Thompson, D. M., and Munro, A. I.: Cardiac valve replacement in elderly patients. Can. Med. Assoc. J. *123*:628, 1980.
213. Huikuri, H.: Effect of mitral valve replacement on left ventricular function in mitral regurgitation. Br. Heart J. *49*:328, 1983.
214. Schneider, R. M., and Helfant, R. H.: Timing of surgery in chronic mitral and aortic regurgitation. *In* Frankl, W. S., and Brest, A. N. (eds.): Cardiovascular Clinics. Valvular Heart Disease: Comprehensive Evaluation and Management. Philadelphia, F. A. Davis, 1986, pp. 361–374.
215. Carabello, B. A., and Grossman, W.: Effects of acute and chronic mitral regurgitation on left ventricular mechanics and contractile muscle function. *In* Duran, C., Angell, W. W., Johnson, A. D., and Oury, J. H. (eds.): Recent Progress in Mitral Valve Disease. London, Butterworths, 1984, pp. 181–192.
216. Smith, D. R.: Clinical diagnosis and evaluation of mitral valve disease. *In* Ionescu, M. I., and Cohn, L. H. (eds.): Mitral Valve Disease: Diagnosis and Treatment. London, Butterworths, 1985, pp. 43–52.
217. Cosgrove, D. M.: Valve reconstruction versus valve replacement. *In* Crawford, F. A. (ed.): Cardiac Surgery: Current Heart Valve Prostheses, Vol. 1. Hanley and Belfus, Philadelphia, 1987, pp. 143–158.
218. Peterson, K. L.: The timing of surgical intervention in chronic mitral regurgitation. Cathet. Cardiovasc. Diag. 9:433, 1983.
219. Peterson, K. L., and Tajimi, T.: The timing of surgical intervention in mitral regurgitation. *In* Duran, C., Angell, W. W., Johnson, A. D., and Oury, J. H. (eds.): Recent Progress in Mitral Valve Disease. London, Butterworths, 1984, pp. 171–180.
220. Bonchek, L. I.: Current status of cardiac valve replacement: Selection of a prosthesis and indications for operation. Am. Heart J. *101*:96, 1981.
221. Pinson, C. W., Cobanoglu, A., Metzdorff, M. T., Grunkemeier, G. L., Kay, P. H., and Starr, A.: Late surgical results for ischemic mitral regurgitation. Role of wall motion score and severity of regurgitation. J. Thorac. Cardiovasc. Surg. *88*:663, 1984.
222. Connolly, M. W., Gelbfish, J. S., Jacobowitz, I. J., Rose, D. M., Mendelsohn, A., Cappabianca, P. M., Acinapura, A. J., and Cunningham, J. N., Jr.: Surgical results for mitral regurgitation from coronary artery disease. J. Thorac. Cardiovasc. Surg. *91*:379, 1986.
223. Fowler, N. O., and van der Bel-Kahn, J. M.: Indications for surgical replacement of the mitral valve. With particular reference to common and uncommon causes of mitral regurgitation. Am. J. Cardiol. *44*:148, 1979.

THE MITRAL VALVE PROLAPSE SYNDROME

224. Pocock, W. A.: Mitral leaflet billowing and prolapse. *In* Barlow, J. B. (ed.): Perspectives on the Mitral Valve. Philadelphia, F. A. Davis, 1987, pp. 45–112.
225. Jeresaty, R. M.: Mitral valve prolapse: Definition and implications in athletes. J. Am. Coll. Cardiol. 7:231, 1986.
226. Perloff, J. K., Child, J. S., and Edwards, J. E.: New guidelines for the clinical diagnosis of mitral valve prolapse. Am. J. Cardiol. *57*:1124, 1986.
227. Savage, D. D., Garrison, R. J., Devereux, R. B., Castelli, W. P., Anderson, S. J., Levy, D., McNamara, P. M., Stokes, J., III, Kannel, W. B., and Feinleib, M.: Mitral valve prolapse in the general population. I. Epidemiologic features: The Framingham Study. Am. Heart J. *106*:571, 1983.
228. Savage, D. D., Devereux, R. B., Garrison, R. J., Castelli, W. P., Anderson, S. J., Levy, D., Thomas, H. E., Kannel, W. B., and Feinleib, M.: Mitral valve prolapse in the general population. 2. Clinical features: The Framingham Study. Am. Heart J. *106*:577, 1983.
229. Jeresaty, R. M.: Mitral Valve Prolapse. New York, Raven Press, 1979, 251 pp.
230. Abrams, J.: Mitral valve prolapse. *In* Essentials of Cardiac Physical Diagnosis. Philadelphia, Lea and Febiger, 1987, pp. 353–374.
231. Weiner, B. H., and Alpert J. S.: Mitral regurgitation: Mitral valve prolapse. *In* Dalen, J. E., and Alpert, J. S. (eds.): Valvular Heart Disease. 2nd ed. Boston, Little, Brown and Company, 1987, pp. 177–196.
232. Procacci, P. M., Savran, S. V., Schreiter, S. L., and Bryson, A. L.: Prevalence of clinical mitral valve prolapse in 1,169 young women. N. Engl. J. Med. *294*:1086, 1976.
233. Markiewicz, W., Stoner, J., London, E., Hunt, S. A., and Popp, R. L.: Mitral valve prolapse in one hundred presumably healthy young females. Circulation *53*:464, 1976.
234. Barlow, J. B., Pocock, W. A., Marchand, P., and Denny, M.: The significance of the late systolic murmurs. Am. Heart J. *66*:443, 1963.
235. Wann, L. S., Grove, J. R., Hess, T. R., Glisch, L., Ptacin, M. J., Hughes, C. V., and Gross, C. M.: Prevalence of mitral prolapse by two-dimensional echocardiography in healthy young women. Br. Heart J. *49*:334, 1983.
236. Ballester, M., Presbitero, P., Foale, R., Rickards, A., and McDonald, L.: Prolapse of the mitral valve in secundum atrial septal defect: A functional mechanism. Eur. Heart J. *4*:472, 1983.
237. Goldhaber, S. Z., Rubin, I. L., Brown, W., Robertson, N., Stubblefield, F., and Sloss, L. J.: Valvular heart disease (aortic regurgitation and mitral valve prolapse) among institutionalized adults with Down's syndrome. Am. J. Cardiol. *57*:278, 1986.
238. Zullo, M. A., Devereux, R. B., Kramer-Fox, R., Lutas, E. M., and Brown, W. T.: Mitral valve prolapse and hyperthyroidism: Effect of patient selection. Am. Heart J. *110*:977, 1985.
239. Margaliot, S. Z., Barzilay, J., Bar-David, M., Lewis, B. S., Froom, P., Forecast, D., and Gross, M.: Spontaneous pneumothorax and mitral valve prolapse. Chest *89*:93, 1986.
240. Jackson, A. C.: Neurologic disorders associated with mitral valve prolapse. Can. J. Neurol. Sci. *13*:15, 1986.
241. Streib, E. W., Meyers, D. G., and Sun, S. F.: Mitral valve prolapse in myotonic dystrophy. Muscle Nerve *8*:650, 1985.
242. Whittaker, P., Boughner, D. R., Perkins, D. G., and Canham, P. B.: Quantitative structural analysis of collagen in chordae tendineae and its relation to floppy mitral valves and proteoglycan infiltration. Brit. Heart J. *57*:264, 1987.
243. Johnson, G. L., Humphries, L. L., Shirley, P. B., Mazzoleni, A., and Noonan, J. A.: Mitral valve prolapse in patients with anorexia nervosa and bulimia. Arch. Intern. Med. *146*:1525, 1986.
244. Liberthson, R., Sheehan, D. V., King, M. E., and Weyman, A. E.: The prevalence of mitral valve prolapse in patients with panic disorders. Am. J. Psychiatry *143*:511, 1986.
245. Waite, P., and McCallum, C. A.: Mitral valve prolapse in craniofacial skeletal deformities. Oral Surg. Oral Med. Oral Pathol. *61*:15, 1986.
246. Bruman, A., Albom, M., Gilboa, Y., Ramot, Y., Golik, A., and Stryjer, D.: Mitral valve prolapse in hyperthyroidism of two different origins. Br. Heart J. *53*:374, 1985.
247. Sakuraba, H., Yanagawa, Y., Igarashi, T., Suzuki, Y., Suzuki, T., Watanabe, K., Ieki, K., Shimoda, K., and Yamanaka, T.: Cardiovascular manifestations of Fabry's disease. Clin. Genet. *29*:276, 1986.
248. Hirschfeld, S. S., Rudner, C., Nash, C. L., Jr., Nussbaum, E., and Brower, E. M.: Incidence of mitral prolapse in adolescent scoliosis and thoracic kyphosis. Pediatrics *70*:451, 1982.
249. Chan, F. L., Chen, W. W., Wong, P. H. C., and Chow, J. S. F.: Skeletal abnormalities in mitral valve prolapse. Clin. Radiol. *34*:207, 1983.
250. Chen, W. W., Chan, F. L., Wong, P. H. C., and Chow, J. S. F.: Familial occurrence of mitral valve prolapse: Is this related to the straight back syndrome? Br. Heart J. *50*:97, 1983.
251. Kalter, S., Fuentes, F., and Price, E.: Mitral and tricuspid valve prolapse in a patient with mixed connective tissue disease. South Med. J. *786*:794, 1983.
252. Lu-Li, S., Guang-Gen, C., and Ru-Lian, L.: Valve prolapse in Behçet's disease. Br. Heart J. *54*:100, 1985.
253. Olsen, E. G. J. and Al-Rufaie, H. K.: The floppy mitral valve. Study on pathogenesis. Br. Heart. J. *44*:674, 1980.
254. Pyeritz, R. E., and Wappel, M. A.: Mitral valve dysfunction in the Marfan syndrome. Am. J. Med. *74*:797, 1983.
255. Davies, M. J., Moore, B. P., and Braimbridge, M. V.: The floppy mitral valve. Study of incidence, pathology and complications in surgical, necropsy and forensic material. Br. Heart J. *40*:368, 1978.
256. Jaffe, A. S., Geltman, E. M., Rodey, G. E., and Uitto, J.: Mitral valve prolapse: A consistent manifestation of Type IV Ehlers-Danlos syndrome. The pathogenetic role of the abnormal production of Type III collagen. Circulation *64*:121, 1981.
257. King, B. D., Clark, M. A., Baba, N., Kilman, J. W., and Wooley, C. F.: "Myxomatous" mitral valves: Collagen dissolution as the primary defect. Circulation *66*:288, 1982.
258. Hammer, D., Leier, C. V., Baba, N., Vasko, J. S., Wooley, C. F., and Pinnell, S. R.: Altered collagen composition in a prolapsing mitral valve with ruptured chordae tendineae. Am. J. Med. *67*:863, 1979.
259. Gravanis, M. B., and Campbell, W. G., Jr.: The syndrome of prolapse of the mitral valve. Arch. Pathol. Lab. Med. *106*:369, 1982.
260. Hickey, A. J., and Wilcken, D. E. L.: Age and the clinical profile of idiopathic mitral valve prolapse. Br. Heart J. *55*:582, 1986.
260a. Hutchins, G. M., Moore, W., and Skoog, D. K.: The association of floppy mitral valve with disjunction of the mitral annulus fibrosus. N. Engl. J. Med. *314*:535, 1986.
261. Malcolm, A. D.: Mitral valve prolapse associated with other disorders. Causal coincidence, common link, or fundamental genetic disturbance? Br. Heart J. *53*:353, 1985.
262. Pader, E.: The familial incidence of mitral valve prolapse. A report of three generations in one family. N.Y. State J. Med. *84*:395, 1984.
262a. Schutte, J. E., Gaffney, F. A., Blend, L., and Blomoqvist, C. G.: Distinctive anthropometric characteristics of women with mitral valve prolapse. Am. J. Med. *71*:533, 1981.
263. O'Rourke, R. A., and Crawford, M. H.: The systolic click-murmur syndrome: Clinical recognition and management. Curr. Probl. Cardiol. *1*:1–60, 1976.
264. Cabeen, W. R., Jr., Reza, M. J., Kovick, R. B., and Stern, M. S.: Mitral valve prolapse and conduction defects in Ehlers-Danlos syndrome. Arch. Intern. Med. *137*:1227, 1977.
264a. Swindle, M. M., Blum, J. R., Lima, S. D., and Weiss, J. L.: Spontaneous mitral valve prolapse in a breeding colony of rhesus monkeys. Circulation *71*:146, 1985.
265. Lebwohl, M. G., Distefano, D., Prioleau, P. G., Uram, M., Yannuzzi, L. A., and Fleischmajer, R.: Pseudoxanthoma elasticum and mitral valve prolapse. N. Engl. J. Med. *307*:228, 1982.
266. Sanyal, S. K., Johnson, W. W., Dische, M. R., Pitner, S. E., and Beard, C.: Dystrophic degeneration of papillary muscle and ventricular myocardium. A basic for mitral valve prolapse in Duchenne's muscular dystrophy. Circulation *62*:430, 1980.
267. Mason, J. W., Koch, F. H., Billingham, M. E., and Winkle, R. A.: Cardiac

biopsy evidence for a cardiomyopathy associated with symptomatic mitral valve prolapse. Am. J. Cardiol. *42*:557, 1978.

268. Pickering, N. J., Brody, J. I., and Barrett, M. J.: Von Willebrand syndrome and mitral valve prolapse. Linked mesenchymal dysplasias. N. Engl. J. Med. *305*:131, 1981.
269. Beardsley, T. L., and Foulks, G. N.: An association of keratoconus and mitral valve prolapse. Ophthalmology *89*:35, 1982.
270. Rippe, J. M., Sloss, J. J., Angoff, G., and Alpert, J. S.: Mitral valve prolapse in adults with congenital heart disease. Am. Heart J. *97*:561, 1979.
271. Zema, M. J., Chiaramida, S., DeFilipp, G. J., Goldman, M. A., and Pizzarello, R. A.: Somatotype and idiopathic mitral valve prolapse. Cathet. Cardiovasc. Diagn. *8*:105, 1982.
272. Weinrauch, L. A., McDonald, D. G., DeSilva, R. A., Hawkins, E. T., Leland, O. S., and Shubrooks, S. J., Jr.: Mitral valve prolapse in rheumatic mitral stenosis. Chest *72*:752, 1977.
273. Gottdiener, J. S., Sherber, H. S., and Harvey, W. P.: Midsystolic click and mitral valve prolapse following mitral commissurotomy. Am. J. Med. *64*:295, 1978.
274. Barlow, J. B., Pocock, W. A., and Obel, I. W. P.: Mitral valve prolapse: Primary, secondary, both or neither? Am. Heart J. *102*:140, 1981.
275. Crawford, M. H.: Mitral valve prolapse due to coronary artery disease. Am. J. Med. *62*:447, 1977.
276. Imaizumi, T., Chandraratna, P. A. N., Whayne, T. F., Jr., Schechter, E., and Bhatia, S. K.: Transmural myocardial infarction. With the prolapsing mitral-leaflet syndrome and normal coronary arteries. Arch. Intern. Med. *138*:1354, 1978.
277. Sakuma, T., Kakihana, M., Togo, T., Matsuda, M., Ogawa, T., Sugishita, Y., Ito, I., and Kurusu, T.: Mitral valve prolapse syndrome with coronary artery spasm: A possible cause of recurrent ventricular tachyarrhythmia. Clin. Cardiol. *8*:306, 1985.
278. Tutassaura, H., Gerein, A. N., and Miyagishima, R. T.: Mucoid degeneration of the mitral valve. Clinical review, surgical management and results. Am. J. Surg. *132*:276, 1976.
279. Pan, C. W., Chen, C. C., Wang, S. P., Hsu, T., and Chiang, B. N.: Echocardiographic study of cardiac abnormalities in families of patients with Marfan's syndrome. J. Am. Coll. Cardiol. *6*:1016, 1985.
280. Guy, F. C., MacDonald, R. P. R., Fraser, D. B., and Smith, E. R.: Mitral valve prolapse as a cause of hemodynamically important mitral regurgitation. Can. J. Surg. *23*:166, 1980.
281. Davies, A. O., Mares, A., Pool, J. L., and Taylor, A. A.: Mitral valve prolapse with symptoms of beta-adrenergic hypersensitivity. $Beta_2$-adrenergic receptor supercoupling with desensitization on isoproterenol exposure. Am. J. Med. *82*:193, 1987.
282. Gaffney, F. A., Bastian, B. C., Lane, L. B., Taylor, W. F., Horton, J., Schutte, J. E., Graham, R. M., Pettinger, W., and Blomqvist, C. G.: Abnormal cardiovascular regulation in the mitral valve prolapse syndrome. Am. J. Cardiol. *52*:316, 1983.
283. Puddu, P. E., Pasternac, A., Tubau, J. F., Krol, R., Farley, L., and de Champlain, J.: QT Interval prolongation and increased plasma catecholamine levels in patients with mitral valve prolapse. Am. Heart J. *105*:422, 1983.
284. Boudoulas, H., Reynolds, J. C., Mazzaferri, E., and Wooley, C. F.: Metabolic studies in mitral valve prolapse syndrome. A neuroendocrine-cardiovascular process. Circulation *61*:1200, 1980.
285. Leor, R., and Markiewicz, W.: Neurocirculatory asthenia and mitral valve prolapse—Two unrelated entities? Isr. J. Med. Sci. *17*:1137, 1981.
286. Tei, C., Shah, P. M., Cherian, G., Wong, M., and Ormiston, J. A.: The correlates of an abnormal first heart sound in mitral valve prolapse syndromes. N. Engl. J. Med. *307*:334, 1982.
287. Alexander, M. D., Bloom, K. R., Hart, P., D'Silva, F., and Murgo, J. P.: Atrial septal aneurysm: A cause of midsystolic click. Report of a case and review of the literature. Circulation *63*:1186, 1981.
288. Wei, J. Y., and Fortuin, N. J.: Diastolic sounds and murmurs associated with mitral valve prolapse. Circulation *63*:559, 1981.
289. Delman, A. J., and Stein, E.: Mitral valve prolapse. *In* Dynamic Cardiac Auscultation and Phonocardiography. Philadelphia, W. B. Saunders Company, 1979, p. 888.
290. Towne, W.D., Patel, R., Cruz, J., Kramer, N., and Chawla, K. K.: Effects of gravitational stresses on mitral valve prolapse. I. Changes in auscultatory findings produced by progressive passive head-up tilt. Br. Heart J. *40*:482, 1978.
291. Winkle, R. A., Goodman, D. J., and Popp, R. L.: Simultaneous echocardiographic-phonocardiographic recordings at rest and during amyl nitrite administration in patients with mitral valve prolapse. Circulation *51*:522, 1975.
292. Combs, R. L., Shah, P. M., Klorman, R. S., and Klorman, R.: Effects of induced psychological stress on click and rhythm in mitral valve prolapse. Am. Heart J. *99*:714, 1980.
293. Braunwald, E., Oldham, H. N., Jr., Ross, J., Jr., Linhart, J. W., Mason, D. T., and Fort, L., III: The circulatory response of patients with idiopathic hypertrophic stenosis to nitroglycerin and to the Valsalva maneuver. Circulation, *29*:422, 1964.
294. Swartz, M. H., Teichholz, L. E., and Donoso, E.: Mitral valve prolapse. A review of associated arrhythmias. Am. J. Med. *62*:377, 1977.
295. Josephson, M. E., Horowitz, L. N., and Kastor, J. A.: Proximal supraventricular tachycardia in patients with mitral valve prolapse. Circulation *57*:111, 1978.
296. Wei, J. Y., Bulkley, B. H., Schaeffer, A. H., Greene, H. L., and Reid, P. R.: Mitral valve prolapse syndrome and recurrent ventricular tachyarrhythmias. Ann. Intern. Med. *89*:6, 1978.
297. Bharati, S., Granston, A. S., Liebson, P. R., Loeb, H. S., Rosen, K. M., and Lev, M.: The conduction system in mitral valve prolapse syndrome with sudden death. Am. Heart J. *101*:667, 1981.
298. Ware, J. A., Magro, S. A., Luck, J. C., Mann, D. E., Nielsen, A. P., Rosen, K. M., and Wyndham, C. R. C.: Conduction system abnormalities in symptomatic mitral valve prolapse: An electrophysiologic analysis of 60 patients. Am. J. Cardiol. *53*:1075, 1984.
299. Kavey, R-E. W., Blackman, M. S., Sondheimer, H. M., and Byrum, C. J.: Ventricular arrhythmias and mitral valve prolapse in childhood. J. Pediatrics *105*:885, 1984.
300. Kramer, H. M., Devereux, R. B., Savage, D. D., and Kramer-Fox, R.: Arrhythmias in mitral valve prolapse. Arch. Intern. Med. *144*:2360, 1984.
301. Gelfand, M. L., and Kloth, H.: Bradyarrhythmia in mitral valve prolapse treated with a pacemaker. Bull. N. Y. Acad. Med. *54*:889, 1978.
302. Wit, A. L., Fenoglio, J. J., Wagner, B. M., and Bassett, A. L.: Electrophysiological properties of cardiac muscle in the anterior mitral valve leaflet and the adjacent atrium in the dog. Possible implications for the genesis of atrial dysrhythmias. Circ. Res. *32*:731, 1973.
303. Wit, A. L., Fenoglio, J. J., Hordof, A. J., and Reemtsma, K.: Ultrastructure and transmembrane potentials of cardiac muscle in the human anterior mitral valve leaflet. Circulation *59*:1283, 1979.
304. Campbell, R. W. F., Godman, M. G., Fiddler, G. I., Marquis, R., and Julian, D. G.: Ventricular arrhythmias in syndrome of balloon deformity of mitral valve. Definition of possible high risk group. Br. Heart J. *38*:1053, 1976.
305. Gallagher, J. J., Gilbert, M., and Svenson, R. H.: Wolff-Parkinson-White syndrome. The problem, evaluation and surgical corection. Circulation *57*:767, 1975.
306. Bekheit, S. G., Ali, A. A., Deglin, S. M., and Jain, A. C.: Analysis of QT interval in patients with idiopathic mitral valve prolapse. Chest *81*:620, 1982.
307. Devereaux, R. B., Perloff, J. K., Reichek, N., and Josephson, M. D.: Mitral valve prolapse. Circulation *54*:3, 1976.
308. Jeresaty, R. M.: Mitral Valve Prolapse. New York, Raven Press, 1979, 251 pp.
309. Pocock, W. A., Bosman, C. K., Chesler, E., Barlow, J. B., and Edwards, J. E.: Sudden death in primary mitral valve prolapse. Am. Heart J. *107*:378, 1984.
310. Chesler, E., King, R. A., and Edwards, J. E.: The myxomatous mitral valve and sudden death. Circulation *67*:632, 1983.
311. Leichtman, D., Nelson, R., Gobel, F. L., Alexander, C. S., and Cohn, J. N.: Bradycardia with mitral valve prolapse: A potential mechanism of sudden death. Ann. Intern. Med. *85*:453, 1976.
312. Popp, R. L., Brown, O. R., Silverman, J. F., and Harrison, D. C.: Echocardiographic abnormalities in the mitral valve prolapse syndrome. Circulation *49*:428, 1974.
313. Waller, B. F., Maron, B. J., DelNegro, A. A., Gottdiener, J. S., and Roberts, W. C.: Frequency and significance of M-mode echocardiographic evidence of mitral valve prolapse in clinically isolated pure mitral regurgitation: Analysis of 65 patients having mitral valve replacement. Am. J. Cardiol. *53*:139, 1984.
314. Abbasi, A. S., DeCristofaro, D., Anabtawi, J., and Irwin, L.: Mitral valve prolapse: Comparative value of M-mode, two-dimensional and Doppler echocardiography. J. Am. Coll. Cardiol. *2*:1219, 1983.
315. Alpert, M. A., Carney, R. J., Flaker, G. C., Sanfelippo, J. F., Webel, R. R., and Kelly, D. L.: Sensitivity and specificity of two-dimensional echocardiographic signs of mitral valve prolapse. Am. J. Cardiol. *54*:792, 1984.
316. Morganroth, J., Mardelli, T. J., Naito, M., and Chen, C. C.: Apical cross-sectional echocardiography. Standard for the diagnosis of idiopathic mitral valve prolapse syndrome. Chest *79*:23, 1981.
317. Panidis, I. P., McAllister, M., Ross, J., and Mintz, G. S.: Prevalence and severity of mitral regurgitation in the mitral valve prolapse syndrome: A Doppler echocardiographic study of 80 patients. J. Am. Coll. Cardiol. *7*:975, 1986.
318. Sahn, D. J., Wood, J., Allen, H. D., Peoples, W., and Goldberg, S. J.: Echocardiographic spectrum of mitral valve motion in children with and without mitral valve prolapse: The nature of false-positive diagnosis. Am. J. Cardiol. *39*:422, 1977.
319. Arvan, S., and Tunick, S.: Relationship between auscultatory events and structural abnormalities in mitral valve prolapse: A two-dimensional echocardiographic evaluation. Am. Heart J. *108*:1298, 1984.
320. Ogawa, S., Hayashi, J., Sasaki, H., Tani, M., Akaishi, M., Mitamura, H., Sano, M., Hoshino, T., Handa, S., and Nakamura, Y.: Evaluation of combined valvular prolapse syndrome of two-dimensional echocardiography. Circulation *65*:174, 1982.
321. Rodger, J. C., and Morley, P.: Abnormal aortic valve echoes in mitral prolapse. Echocardiographic features of floppy aortic valve. Br. Heart J. *47*:337, 1982.
322. Klein, G. J., Kostuk, W. J., Boughner, D. R., and Chamberlain, M. J.: Stress myocardial imaging in mitral leaflet prolapse syndrome. Am. J. Cardiol. *42*:746, 1978.
323. Butman, S., Chandraratna, P. A. N., Milne, N., Olson, H., Lyons, K., and Aronow, W. S.: Stress myocardial imaging in patients with mitral valve prolapse: Evidence of a perfusion abnormality. Cathet. Cardiovasc. Diagn. *8*:243, 1982.
324. Ranganathan, N., Silver, M. D., Robinson, T. I., and Wilson, J. K.: Idiopathic prolapse mitral leaflet syndrome. Angiographic-clinical correlations. Circulation *54*:707, 1976.
325. Cohen, M. V., Shah, P. K., and Spindola-Franco, H.: Angiographic-echocardiographic correlation of mitral valve prolapse. Am. Heart J. *97*:43, 1979.
326. Cipriano, P. R., Kline, S. A., and Baltaxe, H. A.: An angiographic assessment of left ventricular function in isolated mitral valvular prolapse. Invest. Radiol. *15*:293, 1980.
327. Gottdiener, J. S., Borer, J. S., Bacharach, S. L., Green, M. V., and Epstein, S. E.: Left ventricular function in mitral valve prolapse: Assessment with radionuclide cineangiography. Am. J. Cardiol. *47*:7, 1981.
328. Bisset, G. S., III, Schwartz, D. C., Meyer, R. A., James, F. W., and Kaplan,

S.: Clinical spectrum and long-term followup of isolated mitral valve prolapse in 119 children. Circulation *62*:423, 1980.
329. Mills, P., Rose, J., Hollingsworth, J., Amara, I., and Craige, E.: Long-term prognosis of mitral valve prolapse. N. Engl. J. Med. *297*:13, 1977.
329a. Greenwood, R. D.: Mitral valve prolapse: Incidence and clinical course in a pediatric population. Clin. Pediatr. *23*:318, 1984.
330. Corrigall, D., and Popp, R.: Mitral valve prolapse and infective endocarditis. Am. J. Med. *63*:215, 1977.
330a. Koligash, A. J., Bush, C. A., Fontana, M. B., Ryan, J. M., Kilman, J., and Wooley, C. F.: Mitral valve prolapse syndrome: Analysis of 62 patients aged 60 years and older. Am. J. Cardiol. *52*:534, 1983.
331. Tresch, D. D., Doyle, T. P., Boncheck, L. I., Siegel, R., Keelan, M. H., Jr., Olinger, G. N., and Brooks, H. L.: Mitral valve prolapse requiring surgery. Clinical and pathologic study. Am. J. Med. *78*:245, 1985.
332. Clemens, J. D., Horwitz, R. I., Jaffe, C. C., Feinstein, A. R., and Stanton, B. F.: A controlled evaluation of the risk of bacterial endocarditis in persons with mitral valve prolapse. N. Engl. J. Med. *307*:776, 1981.
333. Hickey, A. J., MacMahon, S. W., and Wilcken, D. E. L.: Mitral valve prolapse and bacterial endocarditis: When is antibiotic prophylaxis necessary? Am. Heart J. *109*:431, 1985.
334. MacMahon, S. W., Hickey, A. J., Wilcken, D. E. L., Wittes, J. T., Feneley, M. P., and Hickie, J. B.: Risk of infective endocarditis in mitral valve prolapse with and without systolic murmurs. Am. J. Cardiol. *59*:105, 1987.
335. Barnett, H. J. M., Boughner, D. R., Taylor, D. W., Cooper, P. E., Kostuk, W. J., and Nichol, P. M.: Further evidence relating mitral-valve prolapse to cerebral ischemic events. N. Engl. J. Med. *302*:139, 1980.
336. Walsh, P. N., Kansu, T. A., Corbett, J. J., Savino, P. J., Goldburgh, W. P., and Schatz, N. J.: Platelets, thromboembolism and mitral valve prolapse. Circulation *63*:552, 1981.
337. Hanson, M. R., Conomy, J. P., and Hodgman, J. R.: Brain events associated with mitral valve prolapse. Stroke *11*:499, 1980.
338. Schnee, M. A., and Bucal, A. A.: Fatal embolism in mitral valve prolapse. Chest *83*:285, 1983.
339. Vared, Z., Oren, S., Rabinowitz, B., Meltzer, R. S., and Neufeld, H. N.: Mitral valve prolapse. Quantitative analysis and long-term followup. Isr. J. Med. Sci. *21*:644, 1985.
340. Barletta, G. A., Gagliardi, R., Benvenuti, L., and Fantini, F.: Cerebral ischemic attacks as a complication of aortic and mitral valve prolapse. Stroke *16*:219, 1985.
341. Makino, H., and Al-Sadir, J.: Myocardial infarction in patients with mitral valve prolapse and normal coronary arteries. J. Am. Coll. Cardiol. *1*:661, 1983.
342. Winkle, R. A., and Harrison, D.: Propranolol for patients with mitral valve prolapse. Am. Heart J. *93*:422, 1977.

AORTIC STENOSIS

343. Roberts, W. C.: Valvular, subvalvular and supravalvular aortic stenosis. Morphologic features. Cardiovasc. Clin. *5*:97, 1973.
343a. Panidis, I. P., and Segal, B. L.: Aortic valve disease in the elderly. *In* Frankl, W. S., and Brest, A. N. (eds.): Cardiovascular Clinics. Valvular Heart Disease: Comprehensive Evaluation and Management. Philadelphia, F. A. Davis, 1986, pp. 289–312.
343b. Levinson, G. E.: Aortic stenosis. *In* Dalen, J. E., and Alpert, J. S. (eds.): Valvular Heart Disease. 2nd ed. Boston, Little, Brown, and Company, 1987, pp. 197–282.
344. Moller, J. H., Nakib, A., Elliott, R. S., and Edwards, J. E.: Symptomatic congenital aortic stenosis in the first year of life. J. Pediatr. *67*:728, 1966.
345. Braunwald, E., Goldblatt, A., Aygen, M. M., Rockoff, S. D., and Morrow, A. G.: Congenital aortic stenosis: Clinical and hemodynamic findings in 100 patients. Circulation *27*:426, 1963.
345a. Narang, N. K., Andrew, A. M. R., Chaudhury, H. R., and Gaba, B. S.: Aortic stenosis due to familial hypercholesterolemic xanthomatosis. A case report with brief review of literature. Indian Heart J. *30*:189, 1978.
345b. Deutscher, S., Rockette, H. E., and Krishnaswami, V.: Diabetes and hypercholesterolemia among patients with calcific aortic stenosis. J. Chron. Dis. *37*:407, 1984.
346. Ptacin, M., Sebastian, J., and Bamrah, V. S.: Ochronotic cardiovascular disease. Clin. Cardiol. *8*:441, 1985.
347. Kennedy, J. W., Twiss, R. D., and Blackmon, J. R.: Quantitative angiocardiography. III. Relationships of left ventricular pressure volume and mass in aortic valve disease. Circulation *38*:838, 1968.
348. Carabello, B. A., Mee, R., Collins, J. J., Jr., Kloner, R. A., Levin, D., and Grossman, W.: Contractile function in chronic gradually developing subcoronary aortic stenosis. Am. J. Physiol. *240*:H80, 1981.
349. Morrow, A. G., Roberts, W. C., Ross, J., Jr., Fisher, D. R., Behrendt, D. M., Mason, D. T., and Braunwald, E.: Clinical staff conference. Obstruction to left ventricular outflow. Current concepts of management and operative treatment. Ann. Intern. Med. *69*:1255, 1968.
350. Grossman, W.: Profiles in valvular heart disease. *In* Cardiac Catheterization and Angiography. 3rd ed. Philadelphia, Lea and Febiger, 1986, pp. 359–381.
351. Diver, D. J., Royal, H. D., Aroesty, J. M., McKay, R. G., Ferguson, J. J., Warren, S. E., and Lorell, B. H.: Influence of left ventricular load on abnormal diastolic function in patients with aortic stenosis. J. Am. Coll. Cardiol. (*in press*).
352. Oldershaw, P. J., Dawkins, K. D., Ward, D. E., and Gibson, D. G.: Diastolic mechanisms of impaired exercise tolerance in aortic valve disease. Br. Heart J. *49*:568, 1983.
353. Hess, O. M., Ritter, M., Schneider, J., Grimm, J., Turina, M., and Krayenbuehl, H. P.: Diastolic stiffness and myocardial structure in aortic valve disease before and after valve replacement. Circulation *69*:855, 1984.
354. Murakami, T., Hess, O. M., Gage, J. E., Grimm, J., and Krayenbuehl, H. P.: Diastolic filling dynamics in patients with aortic stenosis. Circulation *73*:1162, 1986.
355. Braunwald, E., and Frahm, C. J.: Studies on Starling's law of the heart. IV. Observations on the hemodynamic functions of the left atrium in man. Circulation *24*:633, 1961.
356. Donner, R., Carabello, B. A., Black, I., and Spann, J. F.: Left ventricular wall stress in compensated aortic stenosis in children. Am. J. Cardiol. *51*:946, 1983.
357. DePace, N. L., Ren, J-F., Iskandrian, A. S., Kotler, M. N., Hakki, A-H., and Segal, B. L.: Correlation of echocardiographic wall stress and left ventricular pressure and function in aortic stenosis. Circulation *67*:854, 1983.
358. Sasayama, S., Ross, J., Jr., Franklin, D., Bloor, C. M., Bishop, S., and Dilley, R. B.: Adaptations of the left ventricle to chronic pressure overload. Circ. Res. *38*:172, 1976.
359. Gunther, S., and Grossman, W.: Determinants of ventricular function in pressure overload hypertrophy in man. Circulation *59*:679, 1979.
360. Ross, J., Jr.: Afterload mismatch and preload reserve: A conceptual framework for the analysis of ventricular function. Prog. Cardiovasc. Dis. *18*:255, 1976.
361. Fifer, M. A., Gunther, S., Grossman, W., Mirsky, I., Carabello, B., and Barry, W. H.: Myocardial contractile function in aortic stenosis as determined from the rate of stress development during isovolumic systole. Am. J. Cardiol. *44*:1318, 1979.
362. Carabello, B. A., Green, L. H., Grossman, W., Cohn, L. H., Koster, J. K., and Collins, J. J., Jr.: Hemodynamic determinants of prognosis of aortic valve replacement in critical aortic stenosis and advanced congestive heart failure. Circulation *62*:42, 1980.
363. Huber, D., Grimm, J., Koch, R., and Krayenbuehl, H. P.: Determinants of ejection performance in aortic stenosis. Circulation *64*:126, 1981.
364. Peterson, K. J., Tsuji, J., Johnson, A., DiDonna, J., and LeWinter, M.: Diastolic left ventricular pressure-volume and stress-strain relations in patients with valvular aortic stenosis and left ventricular hypertrophy. Circulation *58*:77, 1978.
365. Dineen, E., and Brent, B. N.: Aortic valve stenosis: Comparison of patients to those without chronic congestive heart failure. Am. J. Cardiol. *57*:419, 1986.
366. Fifer, M. A., Borow, K. M., Colan, S. D., and Lorell, B. H.: Early diastolic left ventricular function in children and adults with aortic stenosis. J. Am. Coll. Cardiol. *5*:1147, 1985.
366a. Schwarz, F., Flameng, W., Schaper, J., Langebartels, F., Sesto, M., Hehrlein, F., and Schlepper, M.: Myocardial structure and function in patients with aortic valve disease and their relation to postoperative results. Am. J. Cardiol. *41*:661, 1978.
366b. Bertrand, M. E., LaBlanche, J. M., Tilmant, P. Y., Thieuleux, F. P., Delforge, M. R., and Carre, A. G.: Coronary sinus blood flow at rest and during isometric exercise in patients with aortic valve disease. Mechanism of angina pectoris in presence of normal coronary arteries. Am. J. Cardiol. *47*:199, 1981.
367. Vinten-Johansen, J., and Weiss, H. R.: Oxygen consumption in subepicardial and subendocardial regions of the canine left ventricle—The effect of experimental acute valvular aortic stenosis. Circ. Res. *46*:139, 1980.
368. Marcus, M. L., Dot, D. B., Hiratzka, L. F., Wright, C. G., and Eastham, C. L.: Decreased coronary reserve. A mechanism for angina pectoris in patients with aortic stenosis and normal coronary arteries. N. Engl. J. Med. *307*:1362, 1982.
369. Contratto, A. W., and Levine, S. A.: Aortic stenosis with special reference to angina pectoris and syncope. Ann. Intern. Med. *10*:1636, 1936.
370. Ross, J., Jr., and Braunwald, E.: The influence of corrective operations on the natural history of aortic stenosis. Circulation *37*(Suppl. V):61, 1968.
371. Frank, S., Johnson, A., and Ross, J., Jr.,: Natural history of valvular aortic stenosis. Br. Heart J. *35*:41, 1973.
372. Hakki, A.-H:, Kimbiris, D., Iskandrian, A. S., Segal, B. L., Mintz, G. S., and Bemis, C. E.: Angina pectoris and coronary artery disease in patients with severe aortic valvular disease. Am. Heart J. *100*:441, 1980.
373. Lombard, J. T., and Selzer, A.: Valvular aortic stenosis: A clinical and hemodynamic profile of patients. Ann. Intern. Med. *106*:292, 1987.
374. Holley, K. E., Bahn, R. C., McGoon, D. C., and Mankin, H. T.: Spontaneous calcific embolization associated with calcific aortic stenosis. Circulation *27*:197, 1963.
375. Flamm, M. D., Braiff, B. A., Kimball, R., and Hancock, E. W.: Mechanism of effort syncope in aortic stenosis. Circulation *36*(Suppl. II):109, 1967.
376. Schwartz, L. S., Goldfischer, J., Sprague, G. J., and Schwartz, S. P.: Syncope and sudden death in aortic stenosis. Am. J. Cardiol. *23*:647, 1969.
377. Shoenfeld, Y., Eldar, M., Bedazovsky, B., Levy, M. J., and Pinkhas, J.: Aortic stenosis associated with gastrointestinal bleeding. A survey of 612 patients. Am. Heart J. *100*:179, 1980.
378. Love, J. W.: The syndrome of calcific aortic stenosis and gastrointestinal bleeding: Resolution following aortic valve replacement. J. Thorac. Cardiovasc. Surg. *83*:779, 1982.
379. Pleet, A. B., Massey, E. W., and Vengrow, M. E.: TIA, stroke, and the bicuspid aortic valve. Neurology *31*:1540, 1981.
380. Brockmeier, L. B., Adolph, R. J., Gustin, B. W., Holmes, J. C., and Sacks, J. G.: Calcium emboli to the retinal artery in calcific aortic stenosis. Am. Heart J. *101*:32, 1981.
381. Wood, P.: Aortic stenosis. Am. J. Cardiol. *1*:553, 1958.
382. Chun, P. K. C., and Dunn, B. E.: Clinical clue of severe aortic stenosis. Simultaneous palpation of the carotid and apical impulses. Arch. Intern. Med. *142*:2284, 1982.

382a. Abrams, J.: Aortic stenosis. *In* Essentials of Cardiac Physical Diagnosis. Philadelphia, Lea and Febiger, 1987, pp. 205–224.
383. Cooper, T., Braunwald, E., and Morrow, A. G.: Pulsus alternans in aortic stenosis: Hemodynamic observations in 50 patients studied by left heart catheterization. Circulation *18*:64, 1958.
384. Perloff, J. K.: Clinical recognition of aortic stenosis. The physical signs and differential diagnosis of the various forms of obstruction to left ventricular outflow. Prog. Cardiovasc. Dis. *10*:323, 1968.
385. Goldblatt, A., Aygen, M. M., and Braunwald, E.: Hemodynamic-phonocardiographic correlations of the fourth heart sound in aortic stenosis. Circulation *26*:92, 1962.
386. Caulfield, W. H., deLeon, A. C., Perloff, J. K., and Steelman, R. B.: The clinical significance of the fourth heart sound in aortic stenosis. Am. J. Cardiol. *28*:179, 1971.
387. Morton, B. C.: Natural history and management of chronic aortic valve disease. Can. Med. Assoc. J. *126*:477, 1982.
388. Forssell, G., Jonasson, R., and Orinius, E.: Identifying severe aortic valvular stenosis by bedside examination. Acta Med. Scand. *218*:397, 1985.
389. Johnson, G. R., Adolph, R. J., and Campbell, D. J.: Estimation of the severity of aortic valve stenosis by frequency analysis of the murmur. J. Am. Coll. Cardiol. *1*:1315, 1983.
390. Johnson, G. R., Myers, G. S., and Lees, R. S.: Evaluation of aortic stenosis by spectral analysis of the murmur. J. Am. Coll. Cardiol. *6*:55, 1985.
391. Morgan, D. J. R., and Hall, R. J. C.: Occult aortic stenosis as cause of intractable heart failure. Br. Med. J. *1*:784, 1979.
392. Dymond, D. S., Wolf, F. G., and Schmidt, D. H.: Severe left ventricular dysfunction in critical aortic stenosis—reversal following aortic valve replacement. Postgrad. Med. J. *59*:781, 1983.
393. Delman, A. J., and Stein, E.: Valvular aortic stenosis. *In* Dynamic Cardiac Auscultation and Phonocardiography. Philadelphia, W. B. Saunders Company, 1979, p. 795.
393a. Siegel, R. J. and Roberts, W. C.: Electrocardiographic observations in severe aortic valve stenosis: Correlative necropsy study to clinical, hemodynamic, and ECG variables demonstrating relation of 12-lead QRS amplitude to peak systolic transaortic pressure gradient. Am. Heart J. *103*:210, 1982.
394. Gooch, A. S., Calatayud, J. B., Rogers, P. A., and Garman, P. A.: Analysis of the P wave in severe aortic stenosis. Dis. Chest *49*:459, 1966.
395. Thompson, R., Mitchell, A., Ahmed, M., Towers, M., and Yacoub, M.: Conduction defects in aortic valve disease. Am. Heart J. 98:3, 1979.
396. Rasmussen, K., Thomsen, P. E. B., and Bagger, J. P.: H. V. interval in calcific aortic stenosis. Relation to left ventricular function and effect of valve replacement. Br. Heart J. 52:82, 1984.
397. Nair, C. K., Aronow, W. S., Stokke, K., Mohiuddin, S. M., Thomson, W., and Sketch, M. H.: Cardiac conduction defects in patients older than 60 years with aortic stenosis and without mitral annular calcium. Am. J. Cardiol. *53*:169, 1984.
398. Rosenbaum, M., Elizari, M., and Lazari, J.: Los Hemibloques. Buenos Aires, Paidos, 1968, p. 363.
399. Klein, R. C.: Ventricular arrhythmias in aortic valve disease: Analysis of 102 patients. Am. J. Cardiol. *53*:1079, 1984.
400. Olshausen, K. V., Schwarz, F., Apfelbach, J., Rohrig, N., Kramer, B., and Kubler, W.: Determinants of the incidence and severity of ventricular arrhythmias in aortic valve disease. Am. J. Cardiol. *51*:1103, 1983.
401. Bell, H., Pugh, D., and Dunn, M.: Vectorcardiographic evolution of left ventricular hypertrophy. Br. Heart J. *30*:70, 1968.
402. Siegel, R. J., Maurer, G., Navatpumin, T., and Shah, P. K.: Accurate noninvasive assessment of critical aortic valve stenosis in the elderly. J. Am. Coll. Cardiol. *1*:639, 1983.
403. Szamosi, A., and Wassberg, B.: Radiologic detection of aortic stenosis. Acta Radiol. Diagn. *24*:201, 1983.
404. Vukas, M., Wallentin, I., and Hjalmarson, A.: Analysis of systolic vibrations of interventricular septum in patients with aortic valvular stenosis. Acta Med. Scand. *210*:397, 1981.
405. Teinen, D., and Eriksson, P.: Quantification of transvalvular pressure differences in aortic stenosis by Doppler ultrasound. Int. J. Cardiol. 7:121, 1985.
406. Agatston, A. S., Chengot, M., Rao, A., Hildner, F., and Samet, P.: Doppler diagnosis of valvular aortic stenosis in patients over 60 years of age. Am. J. Cardiol. *56*:106, 1985.
407. Yeager, M., Yock, P. G., and Popp, R. L.: Comparison of Doppler-derived pressure gradient to that determined at cardiac catheterization in adults with aortic valve stenosis: Implications for management. Am. J. Cardiol. 57:644, 1986.
408. Currie, P. J., Hagler, D. J., Seward, J. B., Reeder, G. S., Fyfe, D. A., Bove, A. A., and Tajik, A. J.: Instantaneous pressure gradient: A simultaneous Doppler and dual catheter correlative study. J. Am. Coll. Cardiol. 7:800, 1986.
409. Jonasson, R., Jonsson, B., Nordlander, R., Orinius, E., and Szamosi, A.: Rate of progression of severity of valvular aortic stenosis. Acta Med. Scand. *213*:51, 1983.
410. Nestico, P. F., DePace, N. L., Kimbiris, D., Hakki, A-H., Khanderia, B., Iskandrian, A. S., and Segal, B.: Progression of isolated aortic stenosis. Analysis of 29 patients having more than one cardiac catheterization. Am. J. Cardiol. 52:1054, 1983.
411. Hoagland, P. M., Cook, E. F., Wynne, J., and Goldman, L.: Value of noninvasive testing in adults with suspected aortic stenosis. Am. J. Med. *80*:1041, 1986.
412. Cohen, L. S., Friedman, W. F., and Braunwald, E.: Natural history of mild congenital aortic stenosis elucidated by serial hemodynamic studies. Am. J. Cardiol. *30*:1, 1972.
413. Cheitlin, M. D., Gertz, E. W., Brundage, B. H., Carlson, C. J., Quash, J. A., and Bode, R. S., Jr.: Rate of progression of severity of valvular aortic stenosis in the adult. Am. Heart J. *98*:689, 1979.
414. Chizner, M. A., Pearle, D. L., and deLeon, A. C., Jr.: The natural history of aortic stenosis in adults. Am. Heart J. *99*:419, 1980.
415. Wagner, S., and Selzer, A.: Patterns of progression of aortic stenosis: A longitudinal hemodynamic study. Circulation *65*:709, 1982.
416. Kirklin, J. W., and Barratt-Boyes, B. G.: Congenital valvular aortic stenosis. *In* Cardiac Surgery. New York, John Wiley and Sons, 1986, pp. 972–988.
417. Kirklin, J. W., and Barratt-Boyes, B. G.: Aortic valve disease. *In* Cardiac Surgery. New York, John Wiley and Sons, 1986, pp. 374–420.
418. Copeland, J. B., Griepp, R. B., Stinson, E. B., and Shumway, N. E.: Long-term followup after isolated aortic valve replacement. J. Thorac. Cardiovasc. Surg. *74*:875, 1977.
419. Mirsky, I., Henschke, C., Hess, O. M., and Krayenbuehl, H. P.: Prediction of postoperative performance in aortic valve disease. Am. J. Cardiol. *48*:295, 1981.
420. Khanna, S. K., Ross, J. K., and Monro, J. L.: Homograft aortic valve replacement: Seven years' experience with antibiotic-treated valves. Thorax *36*:330, 1981.
421. DiSesa, V. J., Collins, J. J., Jr., and Cohn, L. H.: Valve replacement in the small annulus aorta: Performance of the Hancock modified-orifice bioprosthesis. *In* Cohn, L. H., and Gallucci, V.: Cardiac Bioprostheses. New York, Yorke Medical Books, 1982, p. 552.
422. Gill, C. C., King, H. C., Lytle, B. W., Cosgrove, D. M., Golding, L. A. R., and Loop, F. D.: Early clinical evaluation of aortic valve replacement with the St. Jude medical valve in patients with a small aortic root. Circulation *66*(Suppl. I):147, 1982.
423. Acar, J., Ducimetiere, P., Cadilhac, M., Jallut, H., and Vahanian, A.: Prognosis of surgically treated chronic aortic valve disease. Predictive indicators of early postoperative risk and long-term survival, based on 439 cases. J. Thorac. Cardiovasc. Surg. *82*:114, 1981.
424. Pantely, G., Morton, M., and Rahimtoola, S. H.: Effects of successful, uncomplicated valve replacement on ventricular hypertrophy, volume and performance in aortic stenosis and in aortic incompetence. J. Thorac. Cardiovasc. Surg. *75*:383, 1978.
425. Kennedy, J. W., Doces, J., and Stewart, D. K.: Left ventricular function before and following aortic valve replacement. Circulation *56*:944, 1977.
426. O'Tolle, J. D., Geiser, E. A., Reddy, S., Curtiss, E. I., and Landfair, R. M.: Effect of preoperative ejection fraction on survival and hemodynamic improvement following aortic valve replacement. Circulation *58*:1175, 1978.
427. Smith, N., McAnulty, J. H., and Rahimtoola, S. H.: Severe aortic stenosis with impaired left ventricular function and clinical heart failure: Results of valve replacement. Circulation *58*:255, 1978.
428. Kay, P. H., and Paneth, M.: Aortic valve replacement in the over seventy age group. J. Cardiovasc. Surg. *22*:312, 1981.
429. Safian, R. D., Mandell, V. S., Thurer, R. E., Hutchins, G. M., Schnitt, S. J., Grossman, W., and McKay, R. G.: Postmortem and intraoperative balloon valvuloplasty of calcific aortic stenosis in elderly patients: Mechanisms of successful dilation. J. Am. Coll. Cardiol. *9*:655, 1987.
430. McKay, R. G., Safian, R. D., Lock, J. E., Mandell, V. S., Thurer, R. L., Schnitt, S. J., and Grossman, W.: Balloon dilatation of calcific aortic stenosis in elderly patients: Postmortem intraoperative and percutaneous valvuloplasty studies. Circulation *74*:119, 1986.
431. Cribier, A., Savin, T., Berland, J., Rocha, P., Mechmeche, R., Saoudi, N., Behar, P., and Letac, B.: Percutaneous transluminal balloon valvuloplasty of adult aortic stenosis: Report of 92 cases. J. Am. Coll. Cardiol. *9*:381, 1987.
432. McKay, R. G., Safian, R. D., Lock, J. E., Diver, D. J., Berman, A. D., Warren, S. E., Come, P. C., Baim, D. S., Mandell, V. E., Royal, H. D., and Grossman, W.: Assessment of left ventricular and aortic valve function after aortic balloon valvuloplasty in adult patients with critical aortic stenosis. Circulation *75*:192, 1987.
433. Palacios, I., Block, P. C., Brandi, S., Blanco, P., Casal, H., Pulido, J. I., Munoz, S., D'Empaire, G., Ortega, M. A., Jacobs, M., and Vlahakes, G.: Percutaneous balloon valvotomy for patients with severe mitral stenosis. Circulation *75*:778, 1987.

AORTIC REGURGITATION

434. Olson, L. J., Subramanian, R., and Edwards, W.D.: Surgical pathology of pure aortic insufficiency: A study of 225 cases. Mayo Clin. Proc. *59*:835, 1984.
435. Alpert, J. S.: Chronic aortic regurgitation. *In* Dalen, J. E., and Alpert, J. S. (eds.): Valvular Heart Disease. 2nd ed. Boston, Little, Brown and Company, 1987, pp. 283–318.
436. Stewart, W. J., King, M. E., Gillam, L. D., Guyer, D. E., and Weyman, A. E.: Prevalence of aortic valve prolapse with bicuspid aortic valve and its relation to aortic regurgitation: A cross-sectional echocardiographic study. Am. J. Cardiol. *54*:1277, 1984.
437. Frahm, C. J., Braunwald, E., and Morrow, A. G.: Congenital aortic regurgitation. Clinical and hemodynamic findings in four patients. Am. J. Med. *31*:63, 1961.
438. Roberts, W. C., Morrow, A. G., McIntosh, C. L., Jones, M., and Epstein, S. E.: Congenitally bicuspid aortic valve causing severe, pure aortic regurgitation without superimposed infective endocarditis. Am. J. Cardiol. *47*:206, 1981.
439. Allen, W. M., Matloff, J. M., and Fishbein, M. C.: Myxoid degeneration of the aortic valve and isolated severe aortic regurgitation. Am. J. Cardiol. *55*:439, 1985.
439a. Shapiro, L. M., Thwaites, B., Westgate, C., and Donaldson, R.: Prevalence and clinical significance of aortic valve prolapse. Br. Heart J. *54*:179, 1985.

440. Morain, S. V., Casanegra, P., Maturana, G., and Dubernet, J.: Spontaneous rupture of a fenestrated aortic valve. Surgical treatment. J. Thorac. Cardiovasc. Surg. 73:716, 1977.
441. Waller, B. F., Kishel, J. C., and Roberts, W. C.: Severe aortic regurgitation from systemic hypertension. Chest *82*:365, 1982.
442. Thandroyen, F. T., Matisonn, R. E., and Weir, E. K.: Severe aortic incompetence caused by systemic lupus erythematosus. S.A. Med. J. *54*:166, 1978.
443. Kramer, P. H., Imboden, J. B., Jr., Waldman, F. M., Turley, K., and Ports, T. A.: Severe aortic insufficiency in juvenile chronic arthritis. Am. J. Med. *74*:1088, 1983.
444. Demoulin, J. C., Lespagnard, J., Bertholet, M., and Soumagne, D.: Acute fulminant aortic regurgitation in ankylosing spondylitis. Am. Heart J. *105*:859, 1983.
445. Bostwick, D. G., Bensch, K. G., Burke, J. S., Billingham, M. E., Miller, D. C., Smith, J. C., and Keren, D. F.: Whipple's disease presenting as aortic insufficiency. N. Engl. J. Med. *305*:995, 1981.
446. Darvill, F. R., Jr.: Aortic insufficiency of unusual etiology. J.A.M.A. *184*:753, 1963.
447. Rae, S. A., Vandenburg, M., and Scholtz, C. L.: Aortic regurgitation and false aneurysm formation in Behcet's disease. Postgrad. Med. J. *56*:438, 1980.
448. Emanuel, R., Ng, R. A. L., Marcomichelakis, J., Moores, E. C., Jefferson, K. E., Macfaul, P. A., and Withers, R.: Formes frustes of Marfan's syndrome presenting with severe aortic regurgitation. Clinicogenetic study of 18 families. Br. Heart J. *39*:190, 1977.
449. Roberts, W. C., Hollingsworth, J. F., Bulkley, B. H., Jaffe, R. B., Epstein, S. E., and Stinson, E. B.: Combined mitral and aortic regurgitation in ankylosing spondylitis: Angiographic and anatomic features. Am. J. Med. *56*:237, 1974.
450. Reid, G. D., Patterson, M. W. H., Patterson, A. C., and Cooperberg, P. L.: Aortic insufficiency in association with juvenile ankylosing spondylitis. J. Pediatr. *95*:78, 1979.
451. Paulus, H. E., Pearson, C. M., and Pitts, W., Jr.: Aortic insufficiency in five patients with Reiter's syndrome: A detailed clinical and pathologic study. Am. J. Med. *53*:464, 1972.
452. Hollingworth, P., Hall, P. J., Knight, S. C., and Newman, R.: Lone aortic regurgitation, sacroiliitis, and HLA B27: Case history and frequency of association. Br. Heart J. *42*:229, 1979.
453. Heppner, R. L., Babitt, H. I., Bianchine, J. W., and Warbasse, J. R.: Aortic regurgitation and aneurysm of sinus of Valsalva associated with osteogenesis imperfecta. Am. J. Cardiol. *31*:654, 1973.
454. Esdah, J., Hawkins, D., Gold, P., Freedman, S., and Duguid, W. P.: Vascular involvement in relapsing polychondritis. Can. Med. Assoc. J. *116*:1019, 1977.
455. Welch, G. H., Jr., Braunwald, E., and Sarnoff, S. J.: Hemodynamic effects of quantitatively varied experimental aortic regurgitation. Circ. Res. *5*:546, 1957.
456. Belenkie, I., and Rademaker, A.: Acute and chronic changes after aortic valve damage in the intact dog. Am. J. Physiol. *241*:H95, 1981.
457. Iskandrian, A. S., Hakki, A-H., Manno, B., Amenta, A., and Kane, S. A.: Left ventricular function in chronic aortic regurgitation. J. Am. Coll. Cardiol. *1*:1374, 1983.
458. Boucher, C. A., Wilson, R. A., Kanarek, D. J., Hutter, A. M., Jr., Okada, R. D., Liberthson, R. R., Strauss, H. W., and Pohost, G. M.: Exercise testing in asymptomatic or minimally symptomatic aortic regurgitation: Relationship of left ventricular ejection fraction to left ventricular filling pressure during exercise. Circulation *67*:1091, 1983.
459. Johnson, L. L., Powers, E. R., Tzall, W. R., Feder, J., Sciacca, R. R., and Cannon, P. J.: Left ventricular volume and ejection fraction response to exercise in aortic regurgitation. Am. J. Cardiol. *51*:1379, 1983.
460. Grossman, W., Jones, D., and McLaurin, L. P.: Wall stress and patterns of hypertrophy in the human left ventricle. J. Clin. Invest. *56*:56, 1975.
461. Laniado, S., Yellin, E. L., Yoran, C., Strom, J., Hori, M., Gabbay, S., Terdiman, R., and Frater, R. W. M.: Physiologic mechanism in aortic insufficiency. I. The effect of changing heart rate on flow dynamics. II. Determinants of Austin Flint murmur. Circulation *66*:226, 1982.
462. Kawanishi, D. T., McKay, C. R., Chandraratna, A. N., Nanna, M., Reid, C. L., Elkayam, U., Siegel, M., and Rahimtoola, S. H.: Cardiovascular response to dynamic exercise in patients with chronic symptomatic mild-to-moderate and severe aortic regurgitation. Circulation *73*:62, 1986.
463. Massie, B. M., Kramer, B. L., Loge, D., Topic, N., Greenberg, B. H., Cheitlin, M. D., Bristow, J. D., and Byrd, R. D.: Ejection fraction response to supine exercise in asymptomatic aortic regurgitation: Relation to simultaneous hemodynamic measurements. J. Am. Coll. Cardiol. *5*:847, 1985.
464. Mehmel, H. C., Olshausen, K. V., Schuler, G., Schwarz, F., and Kubler, W.: Estimation of left ventricular myocardial function by the ejection fraction in isolated, chronic, pure aortic regurgitation. Am. J. Cardiol. *54*:610, 1984.
465. Iskandrian, A. S., Hakki, A-H., and Kane-Marsch, S.: Left ventricular pressure/volume relationship in aortic regurgitation. Am. Heart J. *110*:1026, 1985.
466. Shen, W. F., Roubin, G. S., Choong, C. Y-P., Hutton, B. F., Harris, P. J., Fletcher, P. J., and Kelly, D. T.: Evaluation of relationship between myocardial contractile state and left ventricular function in patients with aortic regurgitation. Circulation *71*:31, 1985.
467. Scognamiglio, R., Roelandt, J., Fasoli, G., Marchese, D., Prandi, A. M., and Stritoni, P.: Relation between myocardial contractility, hypertrophy and pump performance in patients with chronic aortic regurgitation: An echocardiographic study. Int. J. Cardiol. *6*:473, 1984.
468. Ricci, D. R.: Afterload mismatch and preload reserve in chronic aortic regurgitation. Circulation *66*:826, 1982.
469. Greenberg, B., Massie, B., Thomas, D., Bristow, J. D., Cheitlin, M., Broudy, D., Szlachcic, J., and Krishnamurthy, G.: Association between the exercise ejection fraction response and systolic wall stress in patients with chronic aortic insufficiency. Circulation *71*:458, 1985.
470. Falsetti, H. L., Carroll, R. J., and Cramer, J. A.: Total and regional myocardial blood flow in aortic regurgitation. Am. Heart J. *97*:485, 1979.
471. Uhl, G. S., Boucher, C. A., Oliveros, R. A., and Murgo, J. P.: Exercise-induced myocardial oxygen supply-demand imbalance in asymptomatic or mildly symptomatic aortic regurgitation. Chest *80*:686, 1981.
472. Maurer, W., Ablasser, A., Tschada, R., Hausen, M., Saggau, W., and Kubler, W.: Myocardial catecholamine metabolism in patients with chronic aortic regurgitation. Circulation *66*(Suppl. I):139, 1982.
473. Dehmer, G. J., Firth, E. G., Hillis, L. D., Corbett, J. R., Lewis, S. E., Parkey, R. W., and Willerson, J. T.: Alterations in left ventricular volumes and ejection fraction at rest and during exercise in patients with aortic regurgitation. Am. J. Cardiol. *48*:17, 1981.
474. Lewis, S. M., Riba, A. L., Berger, H. J., Davies, R. A., Wackers, F. J. T., Alexander, J., Sands, M. J., Cohen, L., S., and Zaret, B. L.: Radionuclide angiographic exercise left ventricular performance in chronic aortic regurgitation: Relationship to resting echographic ventricular dimensions and systolic wall stress index. Am. Heart J. *103*:498, 1982.
475. Schuler, G., Olshausen, K. V., Schwarz, F., Mehmel, H., Hofmann, M., Hermann, H.-J., Lange, D., and Kubler, W.: Noninvasive assessment of myocardial contractility in asymptomatic patients with severe aortic regurgitation and normal left ventricular ejection fraction at rest. Am. J. Cardiol. *50*:45, 1982.
476. Benotti, J. R.: Acute aortic insufficiency. *In* Dalen, J. E., and Alpert, J. S. (eds.): Valvular Heart Disease. 2nd ed. Boston, Little, Brown and Company, 1987, pp. 319–352.
477. Dervan, J., and Goldberg, S.: Acute aortic regurgitation: Pathophysiology and management. *In* Frankl, W. S., and Brest, A. N. (eds.): Cardiovascular Clinics. Valvular Heart Disease: Comprehensive Evaluation and Management. Philadelphia, F. A. Davis, 1986, pp. 281–288.
478. Perloff, J. K.: Acute severe aortic regurgitation: Recognition and management. J. Cardiovasc. Med. *8*:209, 1983.
479. Mann, T., McLaurin, L. P., Grossman, W., and Craige, E.: Assessing the hemodynamic severity of acute aortic regurgitation due to infective endocarditis. N. Engl. J. Med. *293*:108, 1975.
480. Spagnuolo, M., Kloth, H., Taranta, A., Doyle, E., and Pasternack, B.: Natural history of rheumatic aortic regurgitation: Criteria predictive of death, congestive heart failure and angina in young patients. Circulation *44*:368, 1971.
481. Benotti, J. R., and Dalen, J. E.: Aortic valvular regurgitation: Natural history and medical treatment. *In* Cohn, L. H., and DiSesa, V. J. (eds.): Aortic Regurgitation: Medical and Surgical Management. New York, Marcel Dekker, 1986, pp. 1–54.
482. Sapira, J. D.: Quincke, deMusset, Duroziez and Hill: Some aortic regurgitations. South. Med. J. *74*:459, 1981.
483. Alpert, J. S., Veiweg, W. V. R., and Hagan, A. D.: Incidence and morphology of carotid shudders in aortic valve disease. Am. Heart J. *92*:435, 1976.
484. Sabbah, H. N., Khaja, F., Anbe, D. T., and Stein, P. D.: The aortic closure sound in pure aortic insufficiency. Circulation *56*:859, 1977.
485. Abdulla, A. M., Frank, M. J., Erdin, R. A., Jr., and Canedo, M. I.: Clinical significance and hemodynamic correlates of the third heart sound gallop in aortic regurgitation. A guide to optimal timing of cardiac catheterization. Circulation *64*:464, 1981.
486. Harvey, W., Corrado, M. A., and Perloff, J. K.: "Right-sided" murmurs of aortic insufficiency. Am. J. Med. Sci. *245*:53, 1963.
487. Fortuin, N. J., and Craige, E.: On the mechanism of the Austin Flint murmur. Circulation *45*:558, 1972.
488. Delman, A. J., and Stein, E.: Aortic regurgitation. *In* Dynamic Cardiac Auscultation and Phonocardiography. Philadelphia, W. B. Saunders Company, 1979, pp. 811–824.
489. Spring, D. A., Folts, J. D., Young, W. P., and Rowe, G. G.: Premature closure of the mitral and tricuspid valves. Circulation *45*:663, 1972.
490. Wong, M.: Diastolic mitral regurgitation. Hemodynamic and angiographic correlation. Br. Heart J. *31*:468, 1969.
491. Estes, E. H.: Left ventricular hypertrophy in acquired heart disease: A comparison of the vectorcardiogram in aortic stenosis and aortic insufficiency. *In* Hoffman, I. (ed.): Vectorcardiography. Amsterdam, North Holland Publishing Co., 1976.
492. Roberts, W. C., and Day, P. J.: Electrocardiographic observations in clinically isolated, pure, chronic, severe aortic regurgitation: Analysis of 30 necropsy patients aged 19 to 65 years. Am. J. Cardiol. *55*:431, 1985.
493. DePace, N. L., Nestico, P. F., Kotler, M. N., Mikntz, G. S., Kimbiris, D., Goel, I. P., Glazier-Laskey, E. E., and Ross, J.: Comparison of echocardiography and angiography in determining the cause of severe aortic regurgitation. Br. Heart J. *51*:36, 1984.
494. Meyer, T., Sareli, P., Pocock, W. A., Hadassah, D., Epstein, M., Barlow, J.: Echocardiographic and hemodynamic correlates of diastolic closure of mitral valve and diastolic opening of aortic valve in severe aortic regurgitation. Am. J. Cardiol. *59*:1144, 1987.
495. Weaver, W. F., Wilson, C. S., Rourke, T., and Caudill, C. C.: Mid-diastolic aortic valve opening in severe acute aortic regurgitation. Circulation *55*:112, 1977.
496. Grayburn, P. A., Smith, M. D., Handshoe, R., Friedman, B. J., and Demaria, A. N.: Detection of aortic insufficiency by standard echocardiography, pulsed Doppler echocardiography and auscultation. Ann. Intern. Med. *104*:599, 1986.
497. Veyrat, C., Lessana, A., Abitbol, G., Ameur, A., Benaim, R., and Kalmanson, D.: New indexes for assessing aortic regurgitation with two-dimensional Doppler echocardiographic measurements of the regurgitant aortic valvular ara. Circulation *68*:998, 1983.
498. Kitabatake, A., Ito, H., Inoue, M., Tanouchi, J., Ishihara, K., Morita, T.,

Fujii, K., Yhoshida, Y., Masuyama, T., Yoshima, H., Hori, M., and Kamad, T.: A new approach to noninvasive evaluation of aortic regurgitation fraction by two-dimensional Doppler echocardiography. Circulation *72*:523, 1985.

499. Masuyama, T., Kodama, K., Kitabatake, A., Nanto, S., Sato, H., Uematsu, M., Inoue, M. and Kamada, T.: Noninvasive evaluation of aortic regurgitation by continuous-wave Doppler echocardiography. Circulation *73*:460, 1986.

500. Manyari, D. E., Nolewajka, A. J., and Kostuk, W. J.: Quantitative assessment of aortic valvular insufficiency by radionuclide angiography. Chest *81*:170, 1982.

501. Steingart, R. M., Yee, C., Weinstein, L., and Scheuer, J.: Radio-nuclide ventriculographic study of adaptations to exercise in aortic regurgitation. Am. J. Cardiol. *51*:483, 1983.

502. Sareli, P., Klein, H. O., Schamroth, C. L., Goldman, A. P., Antunes, M. J., Pocock, W. A., and Barlow, J. B.: Contribution of echocardiography and immediate surgery to the management of severe aortic regurgitation from active infective endocarditis. Am. J. Cardiol. *57*:413, 1986.

503. Goldschlager, N., Pfeifer, J., Cohn, K., Pepper, R., and Selzer, A.: The natural history of aortic regurgitation. A clinical and hemodynamic study. Am. J. Med. *54*:577, 1973.

504. Cheitlin, M. D., Bonow, R. O., Parmley, W. W., Roberts, W. C., Swan, H. J. C., and Williams, J. F., Jr.: Task force II: Acquired valvular heart disease. J. Am. Coll. Cardiol. *6*:1209, 1985.

505. Greenberg, B. H., DeMots, H., Murphy, E., and Rahimtoola, S. H.: Mechanism for improved cardiac performance with arteriolar dilators in aortic insufficiency. Circulation *63*:263, 1981.

506. Elkayam, U., McKay, C. R., Weber, L., Eisenberg, D., and Rahimtoola, S. H.: Favorable effects of hydralazine on the hemodynamic response to isometric exercise in chronic severe aortic regurgitation. Am. J. Cardiol. *54*:1603, 1984.

507. Fioretti, P., Benussi, B., Scardi, S., Klugmann, S., Brower, R. W., and Camerini, F.: Afterload reduction with nifedipine in aortic insufficiency. Am. J. Cardiol. *49*:1728, 1982.

508. Jebavy, P., Koudelkova, E., and Henzlova, M.: Unloading effects of prazosin in patients with chronic aortic regurgitation. Am. Heart J. *105*:567, 1983.

509. Kleaveland, J. P., Reichek, N., McCarthy, D. M., Chandler, T., Priest, C., Muhammed, A., Makler, P. T., and Hirschfeld, J., Jr.: Effects of six-month afterload reduction therapy with hydralazine in chronic aortic regurgitation. Am. J. Cardiol. *57*:1109, 1986.

510. Hoshino, P. K., and Gaasch, W. H.: When to intervene in chronic aortic regurgitation. Arch. Intern. Med. *146*:346, 1986.

511. Bonow, R. O., Picone, A. L., McIntosh, C. L., Jones, M., Rosing, D. R., Maron, B. J., Lakatos, E., Clark, R. E., and Epstein, S. E.: Survival and functional results after valve replacement for aortic regurgitation from 1976 to 1983: Impact of preoperative left ventricular function. Circulation *72*:1244, 1985.

512. Turina, J., Turina, M., Rothlin, M., and Krayenbuehl, H. P.: Improved late survival in patients with chronic aortic regurgitation by earlier operation. Circulation *70*(Suppl. I):147, 1984.

513. Gee, D. S., Juni, J. E., Santinga, J. T., and Buda, A. J.: Prognostic significance of exercise-induced left ventricular dysfunction in chronic aortic regurgitation. Am. J. Cardiol. *56*:605, 1985.

514. Stone, P. H., Clark, R. D., Goldschlager, N., Selzer, A., and Cohn, K.: Determinants of prognosis of patients with aortic regurgitation who undergo aortic valve replacement. J. Am. Coll. Cardiol. *3*:1118, 1984.

515. Fioretti, P., Roelandt, J., Bos, R. J., Meltzer, R. S., van Hoogenhuijze, D., Serruys, P. W., Nauta, J., and Hugenholtz, P. G.: Echocardiography in chronic aortic insufficiency: Is valve replacement too late when left ventricular end-systolic dimension reaches 55 mm? Circulation *67*:216, 1983.

516. Louagie, Y., Brohet, C., Robert, A., Lopez, E., Jaumin, P., Schoevaerdts, J. C., and Chalant, C. H.: Factors influencing postoperative survival in aortic regurgitation. J. Thorac. Cardiovasc. Surg. *88*:225, 1984.

517. Kumpuris, A. G., Quinones, M. A., Waggoner, A. D., Kanon, D. J., Nelson, J. G., and Miller, R. R.: Importance of preoperative hypertrophy, wall stress and end-systolic dimension as echocardiographic predictors of normalization of left ventricular dilatation after valve replacement in chronic aortic insufficiency. Am. J. Cardiol. *49*:1091, 1982.

518. Henry, W. L., Bonow, R. O., Rosing, D. R., and Epstein, S. E.: Observations on the optimum time for operative intervention for aortic regurgitation. II. Serial echocardiographic evaluation of asymptomatic patients. Circulation *61*:484, 1980.

519. Toussaint, C., Cribier, A., Cazor, J. L., Soyer, R., and Letac, B.: Hemodynamic and angiographic evaluation of aortic regurgitation 8 and 27 months after aortic valve replacement. Circulation *64*:456, 1981.

520. Bonow, R. O., Rosing, D. R., Kent, K. M., and Epstein, S. E.: Timing of operation for chronic aortic regurgitation. Am. J. Cardiol. *50*:325, 1982.

521. O'Rourke, R. A., and Crawford, M. H.: Timing of valve replacement in patients with chronic aortic regurgitation (Editorial). Circulation *61*:493, 1980.

522. Bonow, R. O.: Noninvasive evaluation: Prognosis and timing of operation in symptomatic and asymptomatic patients with chronic aortic regurgitation. *In* Cohn, L. H., and DiSesa, V. J. (eds.): Aortic Regurgitation: Medical and Surgical Management. New York, Marcel Dekker, 1986, pp. 55–86.

523. Carroll, J. D., Gaasch, W. H., Naimi, S., and Levine, H. J.: Regression of myocardial hypertrophy: Electrocardiographic-echocardiographic correlations after aortic valve replacement in patients with chronic aortic regurgitation. Circulation *65*:980, 1982.

523a. Carroll, J. D., Gaasch, W. H., Zile, M. R., and Levine, H. J.: Serial changes in left ventricular function after correction of chronic aortic regurgitation. Dependence on early changes in preload and subsequent regression of hypertrophy. Am. J. Cardiol. *51*:476, 1983.

523b. Donaldson, R. M., Florio, R., Rickards, A. F., Bennett, J. G., Yacoub, M., Ross, D. N., and Olsen, E.: Irreversible morphological changes contributing to depressed cardiac function after surgery for chronic aortic regurgitation. Br. Heart J. *48*:589, 1982.

TRICUSPID, PULMONIC, AND MULTIVALVULAR DISEASE

524. Smith, J. A., and Levine, S. A.: Clinical features of tricuspid stenosis. Am. Heart J. *23*:739, 1942.

525. Perloff, J. K., and Harvey, W. P.: The clinical recognition of tricuspid stenosis. Circulation *22*:346, 1960.

526. Morgan, J. R., Forker, A. D., Coates, J. R., and Myers, W. S.: Isolated tricuspid stenosis. Circulation *44*:729, 1971.

527. Ockene, I. S.: Tricuspid valve disease. *In* Dalen, J. E., and Alpert, J. S. (eds.): Valvular Heart Disease. 2nd ed. Boston, Little, Brown and Company, 1987, pp. 353–402.

528. Wooley, C. F., Fontana, M. E., Kilman, J. W., and Ryan, J. M.: Tricuspid stenosis: Atrial systolic murmur, tricuspid opening snap and right atrial pressure pulse. Am. J. Med. *78*:375, 1985.

529. Kitchin, A., and Turner, R.: Diagnosis and treatment of tricuspid stenosis. Br. Heart J. *26*:354, 1964.

530. Mahapatra, R. K., Agarwal, J. B., and Wasir, H. S.: Rheumatic tricuspid stenosis. Indian Heart J. *30*:138, 1978.

531. Daniels, S. J., Mintz, G. S., and Kotler, M. N.: Rheumatic tricuspid valve disease. Two-dimensional echocardiographic, hemodynamic, and angiographic correlations. Am. J. Cardiol. *51*:492, 1983.

532. Pillai, M. G., Sharma, S., Munsi, S. C., Desai, A. G., and Panday, S. R.: Value of echocardiography in detecting rheumatic tricuspid stenosis. J. Cardiovasc. Ultrasonogr. *4*:185, 1985.

533. Guyer, D. E., Gillam, L. D., Foale, R. A., Clark, M. C., Dinsmore, R., Palacios, I., Block, P., King, M. E., and Weyman, A. E.: Comparison of the echocardiographic and hemodynamic diagnosis of rheumatic tricuspid stenosis. J. Am. Coll. Cardiol. *3*:1135, 1984.

534. Nanna, M., Chandraratna, A., Reid, C., Nimalasuriya, A., and Rahimtoola, S. H.: Value of two-dimensional echocardiography in detecting tricuspid stenosis. Circulation *67*:221, 1983.

535. Shimada, R., Takeshita, A., Nakamura, M., Tokunaga, K., and Hirata, T.: Diagnosis of tricuspid stenosis by M-mode and two-dimensional echocardiography. Am. J. Cardiol. *53*:164, 1984.

536. Péterffy, A., Jonasson, R., and Henze, A.: Haemodynamic changes after tricuspid valve surgery. Scand. J. Thorac. Cardiovasc. Surg. *15*:161, 1981.

537. Throburn, C. W., Morgan, J. J., Shanahan, M. X., and Chang, V. P.: Long-term results of tricuspid valve replacement and the problem of prosthetic valve thrombosis. Am. J. Cardiol. *51*:1128, 1983.

538. Boskovic, D., Elezovic, I., Boskovic, D., Simin, N., Rolovic, Z., and Josipovic, V.: Late thrombosis of the Bjork-Shiley tilting disc valve in the tricuspid position. J. Thorac. Cardiovasc. Surg. *91*:1, 1986.

539. Cobanoglu, A., and Starr, A.: Tricuspid valve surgery: Indications, methods, and results. *In* Frankl, W. S., and Brest, A. N. (eds.): Cardiovascular Clinics. Valvular Heart Disease: Comprehensive Evaluation and Management. Philadelphia, F. A. Davis, 1986, pp. 375–388.

540. Manoharan, S., Mohan, J. C., Arora, R., Sethi, K. K., and Khalilullah, M.: Organic tricuspid valve involvement in rheumatic heart disease: A prospective study by two-dimensional echocardiography. Indian Heart J. *38*:60, 1986.

541. Waller, B. F., Moriarty, A. T., Eble, J. N., Davey, D. M., Hawley, D. A., and Pless, J. E.: Etiology of pure tricuspid regurgitation based on anular circumference and leaflet area: Analysis of 45 necropsy patients with clinical and morphologic evidence of pure tricuspid regurgitation. J. Am. Coll. Cardiol. *7*:1063, 1986.

542. Shafie, M. Z., Hayat, N., and Majid, O. A.: Fate of tricuspid regurgitation after closed valvotomy for mitral stenosis. Chest *88*:870, 1985.

543. McAllister, R. G., Jr., Friesinger, G. C., and Sinclair-Smith, B. C.: Tricuspid regurgitation following inferior myocardial infarction. Arch. Intern. Med. *136*:95, 1976.

544. Dougherty, M. J., and Craige, E.: Apathetic hyperthyroidism presenting as tricuspid regurgitation. Chest *63*:767, 1973.

545. Scheck-Krejca, H., Zulstra, F., Roelandt, J., and Vletter-McGhie, J.: Diagnosis of tricuspid regurgitation: Comparison of jugular venous and liver pulse tracings with combined two-dimensional and Doppler echocardiography. Europ. Heart J. *7*:973, 1986.

545a. Come, P. C., and Riley, M. F.: Tricuspid anular dilatation and failure of tricuspid leaflet coaptation in patients with tricuspid regurgitation. Am. J. Cardiol. *55*:599, 1985.

546. Tei, C., Pilgrim, J. P., Shah, P. M., Ormiston, J. A., and Wong, M.: The tricuspid valve annulus: Study of size and motion in normal subjects and in patients with tricuspid regurgitation. Circulation *66*:665, 1982.

547. Mikami, T., Kudo, T., Sakurai, N., Sakamoto, S., Tanabe, Y., and Yasuda, H.: Mechanisms for development of functional tricuspid regurgitation determined by pulsed Doppler and two-dimensional echocardiography. Am. J. Cardiol. *53*:160, 1984.

548. Esaghpour, E., Kawai, N., and Linhart, J. W.: Tricuspid insufficiency associated with aneurysm of the ventricular septum. Pediatrics *61*:586, 1978.

549. Sakai, K., Inoue, Y., and Osawa, M.: Congenital isolated tricuspid regurgitation in an adult. Am. Heart J. *110*:680, 1985.

549a. Schlamowitz, R. A., Gross, S., Keating, E., Pitt, W., and Mazur, J.: Tricuspid valve prolapse: A common occurrence in the click-murmur syndrome. J. Clin. Ultrasound. *10*:435, 1982.

549b. Weinreich, D. J., Burke, J. F., Bharati, S., and Lev, M.: Isolated prolapse of the tricuspid valve. J. Am. Coll. Cardiol. *6*:475, 1985.

550. Jackson, D., Gibbs, H. R., and Zee-Cheng, C.-S.: Isolated tricuspid valve prolapse diagnosed by echocardiography. Am. J. Med. *80*.281, 1986.

551. Chandraratna, P. A. N., Littman, B. B., and Wilson, D.: The association between atrial septal defect and prolapse of the tricuspid valve. An echocardiographic study. Chest *73*:839, 1978.

552. Eskilsson, J.: Tricuspid insufficiency caused by nonpenetrating chest trauma. Acta Med. Scand. *218*:347, 1985.

553. Ginzton, L. E., Siegel, R. J., and Criley, J. M.: Natural history of tricuspid

valve endocarditis: A two-dimensional echocardiographic study. Am. J. Cardiol. *49*:1853, 1982.
554. Arbulu, A., and Asfaw, I.: Tricuspid valvulectomy without prosthetic replacement. Ten years of clinical experience. J. Thorac. Cardiovasc. Surg. *82*:684, 1981.
555. Callahan, J. A., Wroblewski, E. M., Reeder, G. S., Edwards, W. D., Seward, J. B., and Tajik, A. J.: Echocardiographic features of carcinoid heart disease. Am. J. Cardiol. *50*:762, 1982.
556. Gutman, J. M., and Schiller, N. B.: Carcinoid heart disease: Diagnostic usefulness of echocardiography. Primary Cardiol. *9*:130, 1983.
557. Mason, J. W., Billingham, M. E., and Friedman, J. P.: Methysergide-induced heart disease: A case of multivalvular and myocardial fibrosis. Circulation *56*:889, 1977.
558. Laufer, J., Frand, M., and Milo, S.: Valve replacement for severe tricuspid regurgitation caused by Libman-Sacks endocarditis. Br. Heart J. *48*:294, 1982.
559. Allen, S. J., and Naylor, D.: Pulsation of the eyeballs in tricuspid regurgitation. Can. Med. Assoc. J. *133*:119, 1985.
559a. Abrams, J.: Tricuspid regurgitation. *In* Essentials of Cardiac Physical Diagnosis. Philadelphia, Lea and Febiger, 1987, pp. 375–400.
560. Cha, S. D., and Gooch, A. S.: Diagnosis of tricuspid regurgitation: Current status. Arch. Intern. Med. *143*:1763, 1983.
561. Amidi, M., Irwin, J. M., Salerni, R., Lavine, S. J., Zuberbuhler, J. R., Shaver, J. A., and Leon, D. F.: Venous systolic thrill and murmur in the neck: A consequence of severe tricuspid insufficiency. J. Am. Coll. Cardiol. *7*:942, 1986.
562. Cha, S. D., Gooch, A. S., and Maranhao, V.: Intracardiac phonocardiography in tricuspid regurgitation: Relation to clinical and angiographic findings. Am. J. Cardiol. *48*:578, 1981.
562a. Maisel, A. S., Atwood, J. E., and Goldberger, A. L.: Hepatojugular reflux: Useful in the bedside diagnosis of tricuspid regurgitation. Ann. Intern. Med. *101*:781, 1984.
563. Sepulveda, G., and Lukas, D. S.: The diagnosis of tricuspid insufficiency: Clinical features in 60 cases with associated mitral valve disease. Circulation *11*:552, 1955.
563a. Brown, A. K., and Anderson, V.: The value of contrast cross-sectional echocardiography in the diagnosis of tricuspid regurgitation. Eur. Heart J. *5*:62, 1984.
564. Tei, C., Shah, P. M., Cherian, G., Trim, P. A., Wong, M., and Ormiston, J. A.: Echocardiographic evaluation of normal and prolapsed tricuspid valve leaflets. Am. J. Cardiol. *52*:796, 1983.
565. Meltzer, R. S., van Hoogenhuyze, D., Serruys, P. W., Haalebos, M. M. P., Hugenholtz, P. G., and Roelandt, J.: Diagnosis of tricuspid regurgitation by contrast echocardiography. Circulation *63*:1093, 1981.
566. Tei, C., Shah, P. M., and Ormiston, J. A.: Assessment of tricuspid regurgitation by directional analysis of right atrial systolic linear reflux echoes with contrst M-mode echocardiography. Am. Heart J. *103*:1025, 1982.
566a. Forman, M. B., Byrd, B. F., Oates, J. A., and Robertson, R. M.: Two-dimensional echocardiography in the diagnosis of carcinoid heart disease. Am. Heart J. *107*:492, 1984.
567. Curtius, J. M., Thyssen, M., Breuer, H. W. M., and Loogen, F.: Doppler versus contrast echocardiography for diagnosis of tricuspid regurgitation. Am. J. Cardiol. *56*:333, 1985.
567a. Diebold, B., Touati, R., Blanchard, D., Colonna, G., Guermonprez, J. L., Peronneau, P., Forman, J., and Maurice, P.: Quantitative assessment of tricuspid regurgitation using pulsed Doppler echocardiography. Br. Heart J. *50*:443, 1983.
567b. Pennestri, F., Loperfido, F., Salvatori, M. F., Mongiardo, R., Ferrazza, A., Guccione, P., and Manzoli, U.: Assessment of tricuspid regurgitation by pulsed Doppler ultrasonography of the hepatic veins. Am. J. Cardiol. *54*:363, 1984.
568. Suzuki, Y., Kambara, H., Kadota, K., Tamaki, S., Yamazato, A., Nohara, R., Osakada, G., Kawai, C., Kubo, S., and Karaguchi, T.: Detection and evaluation of tricuspid regurgitation using a real-time, two-dimensional, color-coded, Doppler flow imaging system: Comparison with contrast two-dimensional echocardiography and right ventriculography. Am. J. Cardiol. *57*:811, 1986.
569. Lingameni, R., Cha, S. D., Maranhao, V., Booch, A. S., and Goldberg, H.: Tricuspid regurgitation: Clinical and angiographic assessment. Cathet. Cardiovasc. Diagn. *5*:7, 1979.
570. Pepino, C. J., Nichols, W. W., and Selby, J. H.: Diagnostic tests for tricuspid insufficiency: How good? Cathet. Cardiovasc. Diagn. *5*:1, 1979.
571. Lingameni, R., Cha, S. D., Maranhao, V., Gooch, A. S., and Goldberg, H.: Tricuspid regurgitation: Clinical and angiographic assessment. Cathet. Cardiovasc. Diagn. *5*:7, 1979.
572. Ubago, J. L., Figueroa, A., Colman, T., Ochoteco, A., Rodriguez, M., and Duran, C. M. G.: Right ventriculography as a valid method for the diagnosis of tricuspid insufficiency. Cathet. Cardiovasc. Diagn. *7*:433, 1981.
573. Barbour, D. J., and Roberts, W. C.: Valve excision only versus valve excision plus replacement for active infective endocarditis involving the tricuspid valve. Am. J. Cardiol. *57*:475, 1986.
574. Carpentier, A., Deloche, A., and Dauptain, J.: A new reconstructive operation for correction of mitral and tricuspid insufficiency. J. Thorac. Cardiovasc. Surg. *61*:1, 1971.
575. Duran, C. M. G., Pomar, J. L., Colman, T., Figueroa, A., Revuelta, J. M., and Ubago, J. L.: Is tricuspid valve repair necessary? J. Thorac Cardiovasc. Surg. *80*:849, 1980.
576. Kirklin, J. W., and Barratt-Boyes, B. G.: Tricuspid valve disease. *In* Cardiac Surgery. New York, John Wiley and Sons, 1986, pp. 447–462.
576a. Chidambaram, M., Abdulali, S. A., Baliga, B. G., and Ionescu, M. I.: Long-term results of DeVega tricuspid annuloplasty. Ann. Thorac. Surg. *43*:185, 1987.
577. Stolf, N. A. G., Moreira, L. F. P., Costa, R., Grimberg, M., Bittencourt, D., Verginelli, G., Pillegi, F., and Zerbini, E. J.: The DeVega annuloplasty as surgical treatment for tricuspid incompetence. Int. J. Surg. *68*:201, 1983.
578. Kratz, J. M., Crawford, F. A., Stroud, M. R., Appleby, D. C., and Hanger, K. H.: Trends and results in tricuspid valve surgery. Chest *88*:837, 1985.
579. Abe, T., and Komatsu, S.: Valve replacement for Ebstein's anomaly of the tricuspid valve. Chest *84*:414, 1983.
580. Silver, M. A., Cohen, S. R., McIntosh, C. L., Cannon, R. O., III, and Roberts, W. C.: Late (5 to 132 months) clinical and hemodynamic results after either tricuspid valve replacement of annuloplasty for Ebstein's anomaly of the tricuspid valve. Am. J. Cardiol. *54*:627, 1984.
581. Miller, B. R., Vohr, F. H., Christian, F. V., and Singh, A. K.: Cardiac valvular replacement in carcinoid heart disease. Am. J. Med. *75*:896, 1983.
582. Mestres, C.-A., Igual, A., and Murtra, M.: The Bjork-Shiley tilting disc valve in the tricuspid position. Scand. J. Thorac. Cardiovasc. Surg. *17*:197, 1983.
583. Kirshenbaum, H. D.: Pulmonary valve disease. *In* Dalen, J. E., and Alpert, J. S. (eds.): Valvular Heart Disease. 2nd ed. Boston, Little, Brown and Company, 1987, pp. 403–438.
584. Vela, J. E., Conteras, R., and Sosa, F. R.: Rheumatic pulmonary valve disease. Am. J. Cardiol. *23*:12, 1969.
585. Seymour, J., Emanuel, R., and Patterson, N.: Acquired pulmonary stenosis. Br. Heart J. *30*:776, 1968.
586. Brayshaw, J. R., and Perloff, J. K.: Congenital pulmonary insufficiency complicating idiopathic dilatation of the pulmonary artery. Am. J. Cardiol. *10*:282, 1962.
587. Runco, V., and Levin, H. S.: The spectrum of pulmonic regurgitation. *In* Physiologic Principles of Heart Sounds and Murmurs. American Heart Association Monograph No. 46, 1975, p. 175.
588. Childers, R. W., and McCrea, P. C.: Absence of the pulmonary valve. A case occurring in the Marfan's syndrome. Circulation *29*:598, 1964.
589. Cassling, R. S., Rogler, W. C., and McManus, B. M.: Isolated pulmonic valve infective endocarditis: A diagnostically elusive entity. Am. Heart J. *109*:558, 1985.
590. Cremieux, A. C., Witchitz, S., Malergue, M. C., Wolff, M., Vittecocq, D., Vilde, J. L., Frottier, J., Valere, P. E., Gibert, C., and Saimot, A. G.: Clinical and echocardiographic observations in pulmonary valve endocarditis. Am. J. Cardiol. *56*:610, 1985.
591. DePace, N. L., Nestico, P. F., Iskandrian, A. S., and Morganroth, J.: Acute severe pulmonic valve regurgitation: Pathophysiology, diagnosis and treatment. Am. Heart J. *108*:567, 1984.
592. Collins, N. P., Braunwald, E., and Morrow, A. G.: Isolated congenital pulmonic valvular regurgitation. Am. J. Med. *28*:159, 1960.
593. Jacoby, W. J., Tucker, D. H., and Sumner, R. G.: The second heart sound in congenital pulmonary valvular insufficiency. Am. Heart J. *69*:603, 1965.
594. O'Toole, J. D., Wurtzbacher, J. J., Wearner, N. E., and Jain, A. C.: Pulmonary valve injury and insufficiency during pulmonary-artery catheterization. N. Engl. J. Med. *301*:1167, 1979.
595. Bousvaros, G. A., and Deuchar, D. C.: The murmur of pulmonary regurgitation which is not associated with pulmonary hypertension. Lancet *2*:962, 1961.
596. Enomoto, D., Fenster, P. E., Ewy, G. A., and Salomon, N.: Effect of mitral regurgitation on the murmur of pulmonic regurgitation. Chest *83*:822, 1983.
597. Green, E. W., Agruss, N. S., and Adolph, R. J.: Right-sided Austin Flint murmur. Documentation by intracardiac phonocardiography, echocardiography and postmortem findings. Am. J. Cardiol. *32*:370, 1973.
598. Braunwald, E., and Morrow, A. G.: A method for detection and estimation of aortic regurgitant flow in man. Circulation *17*:505, 1958.
599. Pernot, C., Hoeffel, J. C., Henry, M., Worms, A. M., Stehlin, H., and Louis, J. P.: Radiological patterns of congenital absence of the pulmonary valve in infants. Radiology *102*:619, 1972.
600. Collins, N. P., Braunwald, E., and Morrow, A. G.: Detection of pulmonic and tricuspid valvular regurgitation by means of indicator solutions. Circulation *20*:561, 1959.
601. Van Meurs-Van Woezik, H., McGhie, J., and Roelandt, J.: Septal flutter in pulmonary insufficiency. J. Cardiovasc. Ultrasonogr. *3*:159, 1984.
602. Miyatake, K., Okamoto, M., Kinoshita, N., Matsuhisa, M., Nagata, S., Beppu, S., Park, Y.-D., Sakakibara, H., and Nimura, Y.: Pulmonary regurgitation studied with the ultrasonic pulsed Doppler technique. Circulation *65*:969, 1982.
603. Meltzer, R. S., Vered, Z., Hegesh, T., Benjamin, P., Visser, C. A., Shem-Tov, A. A., and Neufeld, H. N.: Diagnosis of pulmonic regurgitation by contrast echocardiography. Am. Heart J. *107*:102, 1984.
604. Emery, R. W., Landes, R. G., Moller, J. H., and Nicoloff, D. M.: Pulmonary valve replacement with a porcine aortic heterograft. Ann. Thorac. Surg. *27*:148, 1979.
605. Paraskos, J. A.: Combined valvular disease. *In* Dalen, J. E., and Alpert, J. S. (eds.): Valvular Heart Disease. 2nd ed. Boston, Little, Brown and Company, 1987, pp. 439–508.
606. Segal, J., Harvey, W. P., and Hufnagel, C. A.: Clinical study of one hundred cases of severe aortic insufficiency. Am. J. Med. *21*:200, 1956.
607. Gash, A. K., Carabello, B. A., Kent, R. L., Frazier, J. A., and Spann, J. F.: Left ventricular performance in patients with coexistent mitral stenosis and aortic insufficiency. J. Am. Coll. Cardiol. *3*:703, 1984.
607a. Zitnik, R. S.: The masking of aortic stenosis by mitral stenosis. Am. Heart J. *69*:22, 1965.
608. Schattenberg, T. T., Titus, J. L., and Parkin, T. W.: Clinical findings in acquired aortic valve stenosis. Effect of disease of other valves. Am. Heart J. *73*:322, 1967.
609. Melvin, D. B., Tecklenberg, P. L., Hollingsworth, J. F., Levine, F. H., Glancy, D. L., Epstein, S. E., and Morrow, A. G.: Computer-based analysis

of preoperative and postoperative prognostic factors in 100 patients with combined aortic and mitral valve replacement. Circulation *48*(Suppl. III):58, 1973.

610. Rippe, J. M.: Multiple floppy valves. An echocardiographic syndrome. Am. J. Med. *66*:817, 1979.
611. Baxley, W. A., and Soto, B.: Hemodynamic evaluation of patients with combined mitral and aortic prostheses. Am. J. Cardiol. *45*:42, 1980.
612. Kirklin, J. W., and Barratt-Boyes, B. G.: Combined aortic and mitral valve disease with or without tricuspid valve disease. *In* Cardiac Surgery. New York, John Wiley and Sons, 1986, pp. 431–446.
613. Stephenson, L. W., Edie, R. N., Harken, A. H., and Edmunds, L. H.: Combined aortic and mitral valve replacement: Changes in practice and prognosis. Circulation *69*:640, 1984.
614. Stephenson, L. W., Kouchoukos, N. T., and Kirklin, J. W.: Triple valve replacement: An analysis of eight years' experience. Ann. Thorac. Surg. *23*:327, 1977.
615. MacManus, Q., Grunkemeier, G., and Starr, A.: Late results of triple valve replacement: A 14-year review. Ann. Thorac. Surg. *25*:402, 1978.
616. Péterffy, A., Jonasson, R., and Björk, V. O.: Ten years' experience of surgical management of triple valve disease. Early and late results in thirty-four consecutive cases. Scand. J. Thorac. Cardiovasc. Surg. *13*:191, 1979.
617. Vatterott, P. J., Gersh, B. J., Fuster, V., Schaff, H. V., Danielson, G. K., Pluth, J. R., and McGoon, D. C.: Long-term followup (2–20 years) of patients with triple valve replacement. J. Am. Coll. Cardiol. *1*:586, 1983 (Abstr).
618. Rhodes, G. R., McIntosh, C. L., Redwood, D. R., Itscoitz, S. B., and Epstein, S. E.: Clinical and hemodynamic results following triple valve replacement: Mechanical vs. porcine xenograft prostheses. Circulation *56*(Suppl. II):122, 1977.
619. Harken, D. E., Soroff, M. S., and Taylor, M. C.: Partial and complete prostheses in aortic insufficiency. J. Thorac. Cardiovasc. Surg. *40*:744, 1960.
620. Starr, A., and Edwards, M. L.: Mitral replacement: Clinical experience with a ball-valve prosthesis. Ann. Surg. *154*:726, 1961.
621. McGoon, M. D., Fuster, V., McGoon, D. C., Pumphrey, C. W., Pluth, J. R., and Elvebeck, L. R.: Aortic and mitral valve incompetence: Long-term followup (10 to 19 years) of patients treated with the Starr-Edwards prosthesis. J. Am. Coll. Cardiol. 3:930, 1984.
622. Starr, A.: The Starr-Edwards valve. J. Am. Coll. Cardiol. *6*:899, 1985.
623. Cobanoglu, A., and Starr, A.: Starr-Edwards silastic ball prosthesis: State of the art 25 years later. *In* Crawford, F. A. (ed.): Cardiac Surgery: Current Heart Valve Prostheses. Vol. 1. Hanley and Belfus, Philadelphia, 1987, pp. 171–182.
624. Björk, V. O., and Lindblom, D.: The monostrut Björk-Shiley heart valve. J. Am. Coll. Cardiol. *6*:1142, 1985.
625. Sethia, B., Turner, M. A., Lewis, S., Rodger, R. A., and Bain, W. H.: Fourteen years' experience with the Björk-Shiley tilting disc prosthesis. J. Thorac. Cardiovasc. Surg. *91*:350, 1986.
626. Boskovic, D., Elezovic, I., Boskovik, D., Simin, N., Rolovic, Z., and Josipovic, V.: Late thrombosis of the Björk-Shirley tilting disc valve in the tricuspid position. J. Thorac. Cardiovasc. Surg. *91*:1, 1986.
627. Björk, V. O.: The Björk-Shiley tilting disc valve: Past, present, and future. *In* Crawford, F. A. (ed.): Cardiac Surgery: Current Heart Valve Prostheses. Vol. 1. Hanley and Belfus, Philadelphia, 1987, pp. 183–202.
628. Austin, E. H., III: Other mechanical prostheses. *In* Crawford, F. A. (ed.): Cardiac Surgery: Current Heart Valve Prostheses. Vol. 1. Hanley and Belfus, Philadelphia, 1987, pp. 237–268.
628a. Cobanoglu, A., and Brockman, S. K.: Selection of a prosthetic heart valve. *In* Frankl, W. S., and Brest, A. N. (eds.): Cardiovascular Clinics. Valvular Heart Disease: Comprehensive Evaluation and Management. Philadelphia, F. A. Davis, 1986, pp. 399–414.
628b. Carrier, M., Martineau, J. P., Bonan, R., and Pelletier, L. C.: Clinical and hemodynamic assessment of the omniscience prosthetic heart valve. J. Thorac. Cardiovasc. Surg. *93*:300, 1987.
629. Cortina, J. M., Martinell, J., Artiz, V., Fraile, J., and Rabago, G.: Comparative clinical results with Omniscience (STMI), Medtronic-Hall, and Björk-Shiley convexo-concave (70 degrees) prostheses in mitral valve replacement. J. Thorac. Cardiovasc. Surg. *91*:174, 1986.
630. Starek, P. J. K., Beaudet, R. L., and Hall, K.-V.: The Medtronic-Hall valve: Development and clinical experience. *In* Crawford, F. A. (ed.): Cardiac Surgery: Current Heart Valve Prostheses. Vol. 1. Hanley and Belfus, Philadelphia, 1987, pp. 223–236.
631. Sezai, Y., Umeda, S., Okazaki, T., Okamoto, I., Rikukawa, H., and Shiono, M.: Hemodynamic and hemolytic features of the St. Jude medical valve prostheses. J. Cardiovasc. Surg. *25*:16, 1984.
632. Gray, R. J., Chaux, A., Matloff, J. M., DeRobertis, M., Raymond, M., Stewart, M., and Yoganathan, A.: Bileaflet, tilting disc and porcine aortic valve substitutes: In vivo hydrodynamic characteristics. J. Am. Coll. Cardiol. 3:321, 1984.
633. Horstkotte, D., Haerten, K., Seipel, L., Korfer, R., Budde, T., Bircks, W., and Loogen, F.: Central hemodynamics at rest and during exercise after mitral valve replacement with different prostheses. Circulation *68*(Suppl. II):161, 1983.
634. Baudet, E. M., Oca, C. C., Roques, X. F., Laborde, M. N., Hafez, A. S., Collot, M. A., and Ghidoni, I. M.: A 5½ year experience with the St. Jude medical cardiac valve prosthesis. J. Thorac. Cardiovasc. Surg. *90*:137, 1985.
635. Crawford, F. A.: The St. Jude valve. *In* Crawford, F. A. (ed.): Cardiac Surgery: Current Heart Valve Prostheses. Vol. 1. Hanley and Belfus, Philadelphia, 1987, pp. 203–222.
636. Harker, L. A.: Antithrombotic therapy following mitral valve replacement. *In* Duran, C., et al. (eds.): Recent Progress in Mitral Valve Disease. London, Butterworths, 1984, pp. 340–348.
636a. Edmunds, L. H., Jr.: Thromboembolic complications of current cardiac valvular prostheses. Ann. Thorac. Surg. *34*:96, 1981.
637. Cohn, L. H., and Callucci, V. (eds.): Cardiac Bioprostheses. New York, Yorke Medical Books, 1982, 591 pp.
638. Starek, P. J. K. (ed.): Heart Valve Replacement and Reconstruction. Chicago, Year Book Medical Publishers, 1985, 332 pp.
639. Sugimoto, J. T., and Karp, R. B.: Homografts and cyropreserved valves. *In* Crawford, F. A. (ed.): Cardiac Surgery: Current Heart Valve Prostheses. Vol. 1. Hanley and Belfus, Philadelphia, 1987, pp. 295–316.
640. Carpentier, A., Lemaigre, G., and Robert, L.: Biological factors affecting long-term results of valvular heterografts. J. Thorac. Cardiovasc. Surg. *58*:467, 1969.
641. Cohen, S. R., Silver, M. A., McIntosh, C. L., and Roberts, W. C.: Comparison of late (62 to 140 months) degenerative changes in simultaneously implanted and explanted porcine (Hancock) bioprostheses in the tricuspid and mitral valve positions in six patients. Am. J. Cardiol. *53*:1599, 1984.
642. Zussa, C., Ottino, G., diSumma, M., Poletti, G. A., Zattera, G. F., Pansini, S., and Morea, M.: Porcine cardiac bioprostheses: Evaluation of long-term results in 990 patients. Ann. Thorac. Surg. *39*:243, 1985.
643. Bortolotti, U., Milano, A., Mazzucco, A., Valfre, C., Talenti, E., Guerra, F., Thiene, G., and Gallucci, V.: Results of reoperation for primary tissue failure of porcine bioprostheses. J. Thorac. Cardiovasc. Surg. *90*:564, 1985.
644. Fawzy, M. E., Halim, M., Ziady, G., Mercer, E., Phillips, R., and Andaya, W.: Hemodynamic evaluation of porcine bioprostheses in the mitral position by Doppler echocardiography. Am. J. Cardiol. *59*:643, 1987.
645. Magilligan, D. J., Jr.: Porcine Bioprostheses. *In* Crawford, F. A. (ed.): Cardiac Surgery: Current Heart Valve Prostheses. Vol. 1. Hanley and Belfus, Philadelphia, 1987, pp. 269–284.
646. Janusz, M. T., Jamieson, W. R. E., Burr, L. H., Miyagishima, R. T., and Tyers, F. O.: Thromboembolic risks and role of anticoagulants in patients in chronic atrial fibrillation following mitral valve replacement with porcine bioprostheses. J. Am. Coll. Cardiol. *1*:587, 1983.
647. Crawford, F. A.: The Ionescu-Shiley pericardial xenograft. *In* Crawford, F. A. (ed.): Cardiac Surgery: Curent Heart Valve Prostheses. Vol. 1. Hanley and Belfus, Philadelphia, 1987, pp. 285–294.
648. Brais, M. P., Bedard, J. P., Goldstein, W., Koshal, A., and Keon, W. J.: Ionescu-Shiley pericardial xenografts: Followup of up to 6 years. Ann. Thorac. Surg. *39*:105, 1985.
648a. Gallo, I., Nistal, F., Revuelta, J. M., Garcia-Satue, E., Artinano, E., and Duran, C. G.: Incidence of primary tissue valve failure with the Ionescu-Shiley pericardial valve. J. Thorac. Cardiovasc. Surg. *90*:278, 1985.
649. Ionescu, M. I., Silverton, N. P., and Tandon, A. P.: The pericardial xenograft valve in the mitral position. *In* Ionescu, M. I., and Cohn, L. H. (eds.): Mitral Valve Disease: Diagnosis and Treatment. London, Butterworths, 1985, pp. 253–272.
650. Ubago, J. L., Figueroa, A., Colman, T., Ochoteco, A., and Duran, C. G.: Hemodynamic factors that affect calculated orifice areas in the mitral Hancock xenograft valve. Circulation *61*:388, 1980.
650a. DiSesa, V. J., Collins, J. J., Jr., and Cohn, L. H.: Mitral valve replacement with porcine bioprosthesis. *In* Ionescu, M. I., and Cohn, L. H. (eds.): Mitral Valve Disease: Diagnosis and Treatment. London, Butterworths, 1985, pp. 243–252.
651. Roberts, W. C.: Complications of cardiac valve replacement: Characteristic abnormalities of prostheses pertaining to any specific site. Am. Heart J. *103*:113, 1982.
652. Nashof, S. A. M., Sethia, B., Turner, M. A., Davidson, K. G., Lewis, S., and Baim, W. H.: Björk-Shiley and Carpentier-Edwards Valves: A comparative analysis. J. Thorac. Cardiovasc. Surg. *93*:394, 1987.
653. Hammond, G. L., Geha, A. S., Klopf, G. S., and Hashim, S. W.: Biological versus mechanical valves. Analysis of 1116 valves inserted in 1012 adult patients with a 4818 patient-year and a 5327 valve-year followup. J. Thorac. Cardiovasc. Surg. *93*:182, 1987.
654. Guidozzi, F.: Pregnancy in patients with prosthetic cardiac valves. S. Afr. Med. J. *64*:961, 1984.
655. Javares. T., Coto, E. O., Maiques, V., Rincon, A., Such, M., and Caffarena, J. M.: Pregnancy after heart valve replacement. Int. J. Cardiol. 5:731, 1984.
656. Salazar, E., Zajarias, A., Gutierrez, N., and Iturbe, I.: The problem of cardiac valve prostheses, anticoagulants, and pregnancy. Circulation *70*(Suppl. I):169, 1984.
657. Iturbe-Alessio, I., Fonesca, M. D. C., Mutchinik, O., Santos, M. A., Zajarias, A., and Salazar, E.: Risks of anticoagulant therapy in pregnant women with artificial heart valves. N. Engl. J. Med. *315*:1390, 1986.
658. Limet, R., and Grondin, C. M.: Cardiac valve prostheses, anticoagulation and pregnancy. Ann. Thorac. Surg. *23*:337, 1977.
659. Smith, N. D., Raizada, V., and Abrams, J.: Auscultation of the normally functioning prosthetic valve. Ann. Intern. Med. *95*:594, 1981.
660. Kotler, M. N., Mintz, G. S., Panidis, I., Morganroth, J., Segal, B. L., and Ross, J.: Noninvasive evaluation of normal and abnormal prosthetic valve function. J. Am. Col. Cardiol. 2:151, 1983.
661. Klein, H. O., Schamroth, C. L., Marcus, B. D., Hummel, D., Antunes, M., and Sareli, P.: Echo-phonocardiographic assessment of the Medtronic-Hall mitral valve prosthesis: Observations on normal and abnormal function. J. Cardiovasc. Ultrasonogr. *5*:115, 1986.
662. Come, P. C.: Pitfalls in the diagnosis of periprosthetic valvular regurgitation by pulsed Doppler echocardiography. J. Am. Coll. Cardiol (*in press*).

34 INFECTIVE ENDOCARDITIS

by LOUIS WEINSTEIN, M.D., Ph.D.

PATHOGENESIS OF INFECTIVE ENDOCARDITIS

MICROBIOLOGY

Infective endocarditis has been primarily classified as acute or subacute, according to the nature of the responsible organism. Thus, when *Staphylococcus aureus*, *Streptococcus pneumoniae*, *Neisseria meningitidis*, *Neisseria gonorrhoeae*, *Streptococcus pyogenes*, and *Hemophilus influenzae* are the causative agents, the endocarditis is considered acute. In contrast, when viridans streptococcus or *Staphylococcus epidermidis* is recovered from the blood, the infection is called subacute. This clinical differentiation remains important because the presenting manifestations, the duration of the course, the nature of the complications, and the final outcome differ greatly, even when appropriate antimicrobial therapy and other therapeutic modalities are applied. It has become clear, however, that there is an appreciable number of instances in which the clinical manifestations and course bear no relation to the invading organism. The differences between *acute* and *subacute* endocarditis are not fundamental, since, as Lerner and Weinstein have pointed out,[1] disease that is originally acute may be converted to subacute status by appropriate therapy, whereas subacute disease may suddenly become life-threatening when serious complications develop. In addition, they and others[2–4] have studied patients with valvular infections caused by *Staph. aureus* with a consistently subacute course, as well as other patients infected with *Streptococcus viridans* in whom clinical behavior was entirely acute; this has been true especially in some instances of enterococcal disease.

The microbiology of infective endocarditis is summarized in Table 34–1.[5–94]

MICROBIOLOGY OF PROSTHETIC VALVE ENDOCARDITIS. Infections of prosthetic valves have involved a large number of microbes, some of which have been associated only with this kind of disease.[95, 96] The bulk of microorganisms responsible for invasion of cardiac prostheses are, however, the same as those that cause infection of natural valves. *Staphylococcus* is the dominant cause of early prosthetic valve endocarditis, reflecting surgical contamination. The pathogenesis of late prosthetic valve endocarditis, like that of native valve endocarditis, is transient bacteremia and viridans streptococci. In addition, *Hemophilus*, *Brucella*, and *Candida* are known to invade prosthetic as well as natural valves. Among those that have been primarily involved in infection of valvular prostheses are gram-negative bacteria such as *Serratia*, *Acinetobacter calcoaceticus*, *Pseudomonas cepacia*, *Pseudomonas aeruginosa*, *Pseudomonas multophilia*, *Flavobacterium*, *Bacteroides*, *Edwardsiella tarda*, and *Eikenella corrodens*. Gram-positive organisms that invade prosthetic rather than natural valves include streptococci groups B, D, and L, (lactobacilli, *Legionella*, and mycobacteria). *S. epidermidis* affects patients with prostheses more often than it does those who have not had valves replaced, and it is the most common cause of disease early after operation. When prosthetic infection occurs late, both staphylococci and streptococci are commonly involved; however, *Staph. epidermidis* is much more common than *Staph. aureus*. Most instances of endocarditis due to *Propionibacterium acnes*, *Bacteroides*, and *E. corrodens* have occurred in patients with cardiac prostheses. Endocarditis caused by the atypical mycobacteria *Mycobacterium chelonei*, *Mycobacterium gordonae*, and *Mycobacterium fortuitum* complex has been observed only on cardiac bioprostheses (porcine valves [Table 34–1]).

The recent striking increase in the incidence of endocarditis caused by yeasts and fungi is attributable almost entirely to the presence of valvular prostheses, to the increased number of patients addicted to drugs administered intravenously, and to long-term antimicrobial therapy. The organisms most commonly involved are *Candida*, *Aspergillus*, and *Histoplasma*. Among the species of *Candida* recovered from infected prostheses have been *albicans*, *parapsilosis*, *tropicalis*, *stellatoidea*, and *krusei* (Table 34–1).

An appreciable number of infections involving prosthetic valves—especially those caused by unusual bacteria, yeasts, and fungi—are probably superinfections induced by antimicrobial chemoprophylaxis or therapy. Organisms may also be introduced into the bloodstream during intravenous injection of drugs in addicted persons.

Cumulative experience indicates that aortic valve prostheses are more frequently infected than prostheses

TABLE 34–1 MICROBIOLOGY OF ENDOCARDITIS

GRAM-POSITIVE COCCI	
Streptococci	**Group D Streptococci**[21]
Strep. viridans[5]	*Strep. faecalis*[8]
Strep. milleri[6]	*Strep. faecium*[8]
Strep. morbillum[7]	*Strep. durans*[8]
Strep. mitior[8]	*Strep. liquefaciens*[8]
Strep. constellatus[9]	*Strep. zymogenes*[8]
Strep. sanguis[8]	*Strep. equinus*[8]
Strep. mutans[10]	*Strep. bovis*[22]
Nutritionally deficient Strep.[11, 12]	**Staphylococcus**
Group A[13]	*Staph. aureus*[23]
Group B[14]	*Staph. epidermidis*[24, 25]
Group C[15]	*Staph. xylosus*[26]
Group G[16]	*Staph. salivarius*[8]
Group L[17]	*Staph. saprophyticus*[8]
Strep. pneumoniae[18]	*Staph. warneri*[27]
Stomatococcus[19]	
Aerococcus[20]	
GRAM-POSITIVE BACILLI	
C. diphtheriae[28]	*Legionella*[37]
Corynebacterium JK[29]	*Rothia dentocariosa*[38]
Corynebacterium, group 2[30]	*Erysipelothrix*[39]
Diphtheroids[31]	*Streptobacillus moniliformis*[40]
C. hemolyticum[32]	*B. subtilis*[41]
Lactobacillus[33]	*B. cereus*[42]
Listeria monocytogenes[34]	*Clostridium perfringens*[43]
Nocardia israelii[35]	
Actinomyces israelii (bovis)[36]	
GRAM-NEGATIVE BACILLI	
E. coli[44]	*Yersinia*[55]
K. pneumoniae[44]	*Campylobacter*[56]
Ps. aeruginosa[45]	*Brucella*[57]
Ps. cepacia[46]	*Citrobacter*[58]
Ps. multophilia[47]	*Edwardsiella*[59]
Ps. alcaligenes[48]	*Chromobacter*[60]
Serratia[49]	*Kingella kingae*[61]
Acinetobacter[44]	*Pasteurella multocida*[62]
A. actinomycetecomitans[50]	*Salmonella*[63]
H. influenzae[51]	*Eikenella corrodens*[64]
H. parainfluenzae[52]	*Bacteroides oralis*[65]
H. aphrophilus[53]	*Leptotrichia buccalis*[66]
Cardiobacterium hominis[54]	*H. aegyptius*[67]
GRAM-NEGATIVE COCCI	**MYCOBACTERIA**
N. gonorrhoeae[68]	*M. tuberculosis*[74]
N. meningitidis[69]	*M. chelonei*[75]
N. subflava[70]	*M. gordonae*[76]
N. mucosa[71]	*M. fortuitum*[77]
N. flava[8]	**NONBACTERIAL ORGANISMS**
N. sicca[72]	*Coxiella burnetii*[78]
N. catarrhalis[8]	*Chlamydia trachomatis*[79]
N. pharyngis[8]	*Chlamydia psittaci*[80]
Moraxella[73]	
YEAST AND FUNGI	
C. albicans[81]	*Saccharomyces*[8]
C. parapsilosis[82]	*Blastomyces*[81]
C. tropicalis[8]	*Aspergillus*[87]
C. stellatoidea[8]	*Mucor*[88]
C. krusei[8]	*Trichosporon*[89]
C. guilliermondi[8]	*Penicillium*[90]
Torulopsis glabrata[83]	*Petrillium*[91]
Cryptococcus neoformans[84]	*Paecilomyces*[92]
Histoplasma[85]	*Phialophora* (Wangiella)[93]
Coccidiodes[86]	*Chromosporium*[94]

Most of the references listed in this table are to papers describing not only the organisms but also the clinical features of the endocarditis with which they are associated.

replacing other valves. One study of prosthetic endocarditis demonstrated infection in 3 per cent of patients in whom the aortic valve was replaced versus 1 per cent of those with mitral valve prostheses.[97] Infection of combined mitral and aortic valve prostheses is not uncommon. Complications of infected prostheses include ruptured mycotic aneurysms, ruptured aorta, ruptured aneurysm of the sinus of Valsalva, perivalvular abscess, myocardial abscess, pericardio-mediastinal fistula, abscess of the atrioventricular ring, and thrombosis of the prosthesis.

PATHOLOGY

Vegetations are common to all types of infective endocarditis and are situated most frequently on the valvular leaflets and less often on the endocardium of the ventricles or of the left atrium (McCallum's patch of rheumatic carditis) and on pulmonary or other arteries. When fresh, the vegetations are pink, red, yellow, or green but change to gray as they heal. These lesions are usually larger and much more friable than those of rheumatic fever; small particles are easily broken off and embolize. The largest vegetations develop in the course of fungal infections of the valves; emboli that arise from these are large enough to occlude major arteries, a distinguishing characteristic of this type of endocarditis (Fig. 34–1). Occasionally, the vegetations formed during infection by *Staph. aureus* are larger than those associated with alpha-streptococci. In some instances of infection of prosthetic valves and, less often, when staphylococci or some gram-negative organisms are involved, valvular lesions may be of such size that they obstruct the valve orifice, sharply reduce cardiac output, and lead to congestive heart failure.

Infective endocarditis involves the left side of the heart much more frequently than the right, affecting the mitral, aortic, or both valves, in that order.[98] Endocarditis of the pulmonic and tricuspid valves is relatively uncommon; however, the latter has increased during the past 20 years with the rise in drug addiction. Although much more common in acute than in subacute valvular infections, vegetations on the mitral valve may extend along the chordae tendineae to the apex of the papillary muscles. This may lead to rupture of these structures, especially in acute infections. Rupture is rare in subacute endocarditis unless the infection has remained untreated for a prolonged period, when aortic valvular vegetations spread by contiguity along the ventricular endocardium or when ulcerated lesions appear on the ventricular surface of the anterior mitral cusp.

Necrosis of the affected valve may lead to aneurysms and/or perforation of the cusps. This occurs most often in acute infective endocarditis, especially that caused by *Staph. aureus*, but only rarely in subacute valvular infections. In addition to aneurysms of the sinus of Valsalva, these lesions, when present at the base of the aorta, may extend into the pericardial space between the aorta and pulmonary artery and produce a hemorrhagic, pyogenic, or fibrinous pericarditis (Fig. 34–2). The infectious process may invade the interventricular septum. Septal perforation may follow when endocarditis is acute. In a study of 45 cases of *active left-sided endocarditis*, as well as a review of autopsy reports, Buchbinder and Roberts[99] noted that myocardial lesions were present in 88 to 100 per cent of cases. Evidence of bacterial endocarditis involving previously normal valves was found in as many as 42 per cent of patients. Heart failure caused by valvular dysfunction occurred in 59 to 74 per cent of patients studied at autopsy. Papillary muscle necrosis that did not lead to mitral regurgitation was present in 58 per cent. Pericarditis produced by direct extension of inflammation into the pericardium was noted in 8 per cent of patients. Of 31 patients with infection of the aortic valve, 12 had ring abscesses, an indication of severe destruction of valvular cusps.

Studies of the gross pathology of *healed left-sided endocarditis* revealed that half had anatomical lesions readily attributable to healed infective endocarditis.[100] Unequivo-

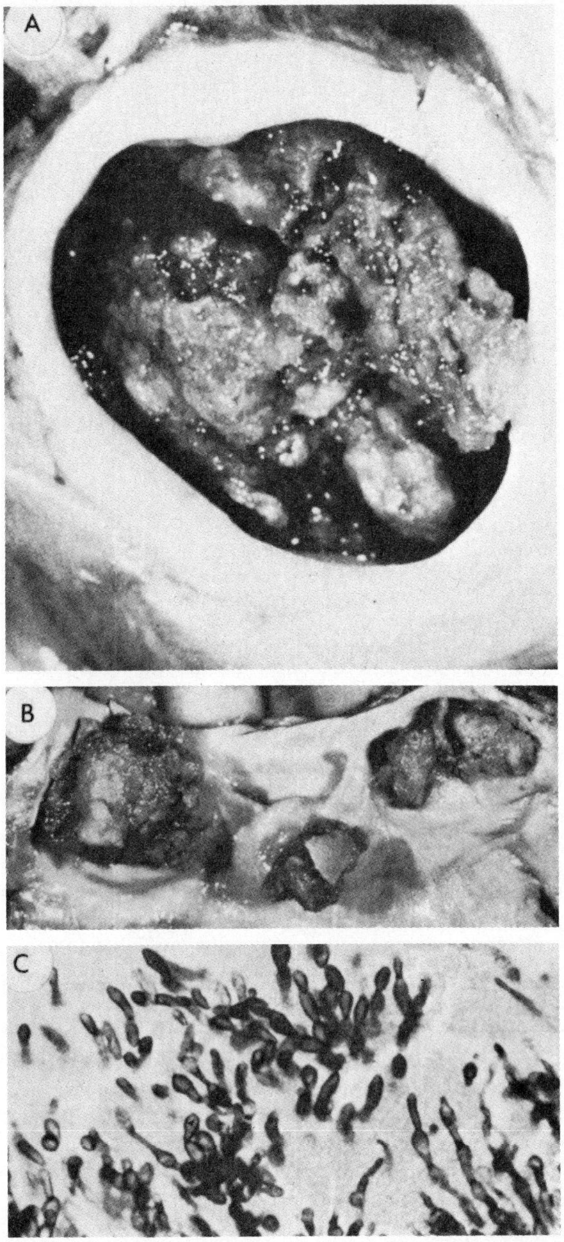

FIGURE 34–1. *Candida parapsilosis* **endocarditis involving the aortic valve led to an embolus to the left anterior descending coronary artery with a large transmural acute myocardial infarct two months before death.** ***A,*** **Aortic valve viewed from above. The large vegetations appear to obstruct the valve orifice.** ***B,*** **Opened valve showing vegetations on each cusp.** ***C,*** **Photomicrograph of vegetation showing pseudomycelia of** ***C. parapsilosis.*** **(Methenamine silver stain.) (From Roberts, W. C., and Buchbinder, N. A.: Healed left-sided infective endocarditis. A clinicopathological study of 59 patients. Am. J. Cardiol.** ***40*****:876, 1976.)**

cal residua of valvular infection were more common in purely incompetent than in stenotic or mixed valvular disease. Half of the patients had either cuspal perforation, probably secondary to ring abscesses, ruptured chordae tendineae, or aneurysms. The mitral or aortic valve or both were either stenotic or purely incompetent. Patients with valvular perforations and ruptured chordae tendineae usually had pure regurgitation. The stenotic valves were diffusely fibrotic; most contained calcific deposits. Diffuse or focal fibrosis was present in incompetent valves. Autopsy findings suggested that the left-sided valves had been anatomically normal in 15 per cent of patients prior to the development of endocarditis. Forty-one per cent of patients had underlying rheumatic heart disease and 29 per cent had a congenital cardiac lesion.

The pathoanatomy of *right-sided bacterial endocarditis* in 12 patients was reported by Roberts and Buchbinder.[101] Bacteria were present on the tricuspid or pulmonary valve in seven cases. Among the lesions observed were ruptured chordae tendineae, necrosis of the papillary muscles, and suppurative or nonsuppurative myocarditis. In 9 of 12 patients the vegetations in the right side of the heart did not extend to involve the basal attachments of the leaflets to the annuli. Mural lesions were observed in three cases; in two they were present on the right ventricular endocardium.

PATHOLOGY OF PROSTHETIC VALVE ENDOCARDITIS. In contrast to native valve endocarditis, in which the mitral valve predominates, the aortic valve is more prone to develop prosthetic valve endocarditis.[101a] The incidence of development of endocarditis is approximately equal for mechanical prostheses and bioprostheses. Excellent studies of the gross pathology of endocarditis involving *prosthetic valves* have been recorded by Arnett and Roberts[102] and Anderson et al.[103] The former studied 22 necropsied patients with infections of rigid-frame valvular prostheses replacing aortic valves in 15 and mitral valves in 7 cases (Fig. 34–3). Endocarditis developed within 2 months after operation in 8 patients, and 2 months or longer postoperatively in 14 patients. The infection was most often located behind the site of attachment of the prosthesis to the valve ring. It spread to adjacent structures in 13 patients, 11 of whom had aortic prostheses. In most cases the prosthetic valve was detached. Conduction defects, including left bundle branch or complete block, were present in seven patients. These were observed most often when aortic prostheses were present, suggesting that conduction abnormalities were related to the presence of abscess or necrosis in the upper area of the interventricular septum.

Among 22 patients with endocarditis involving valvular prostheses studied by Anderson et al. at autopsy, 95 per cent had cardiac hypertrophy and 73 per cent had dilated left ventricles.[103] Dysfunction of the prosthesis was present in 17 per cent and was due to ulceration or perforation of a cusp (Fig. 34–4), paravalvular leak, entrapment of the poppet by a thrombus, perforation of a ring abscess into the right ventricle, or mitral stenosis (most common). Fifty-seven per cent of patients experienced infection of the aortic annulus, while involvement of the mitral annulus was observed in 43 per cent. Fibrinous or purulent pericarditis, aortic stenosis due to exuberant vegetations, and embolic myocarditis (abscess and focal necrosis) were also noted. In two patients with first-degree block the atrioventricular node was extensively involved by the inflammatory

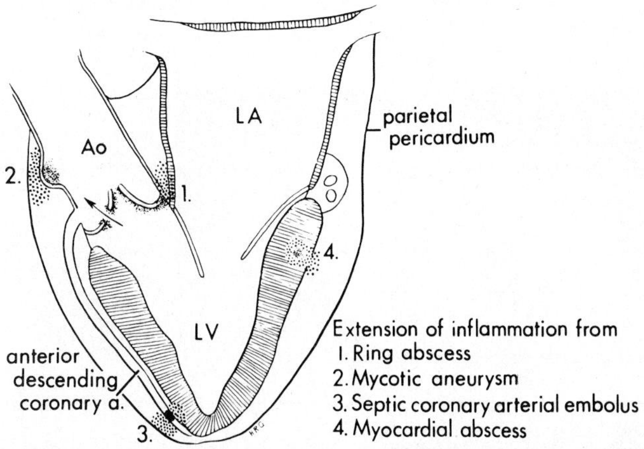

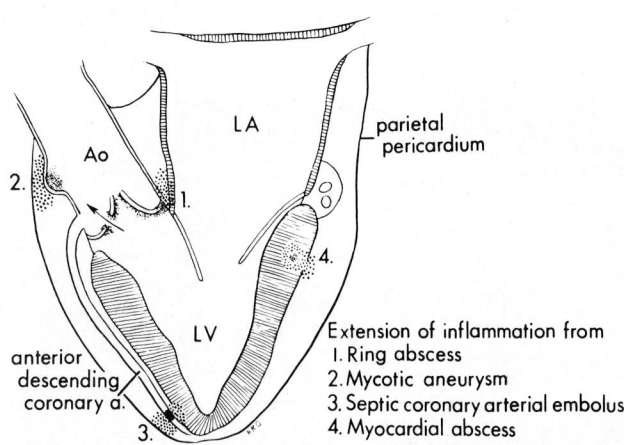

FIGURE 34–2. Schematic portrayal of the pathogenesis of pericarditis in infective endocarditis. Ao = aorta; LV = left ventricle; LA = left atrium. (From Roberts, W. C., and Buchbinder, N. A.: Healed left-sided infective endocarditis. A clinicopathological study of 59 patients. Am. J. Cardiol. ***40*****:876. 1976.)**

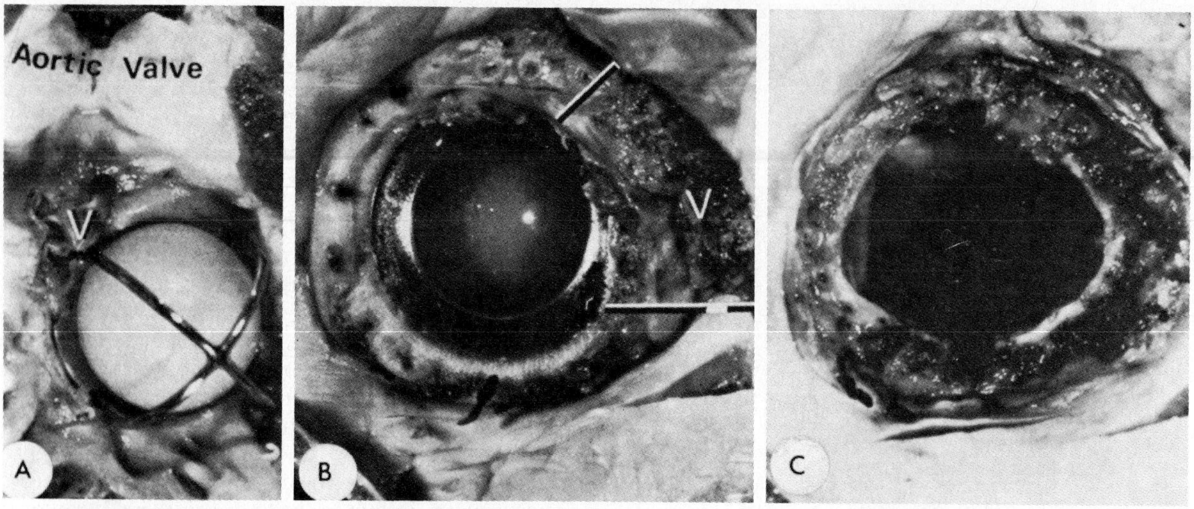

FIGURE 34–3. Prosthetic mitral valve endocarditis caused by *Staphylococcus epidermidis*. The infection appeared 10 years after replacement of both mitral and tricuspid valves. At necropsy, only the mitral prosthesis was infected. *A*, Infected mitral valve prosthesis viewed from the left ventricle. Vegetative material (V) is present on the prosthetic annulus just below the aortic valve. *B*, Prosthesis as viewed from the left atrium showing vegetations (V) at the junction of the prosthetic and natural valve annuli. *C*, Same view after removal of the prosthesis, showing even greater extension of the infection at the site of attachment of the prosthesis. (From Arnett, E. N., and Roberts, W. C.: Prosthetic valve endocarditis. Clinicopathological analysis of 22 necropsy patients with comparison of observations in 74 necropsy patients with active infective endocarditis involving natural left-sided cardiac valves. Am. J. Cardiol. *38*:281, 1976.)

process that had extended from an abscess of the aortic ring; the bundle of His was intact. Among the extracardiac findings were peripheral (85 per cent), splenic (59 per cent), renal (50 per cent), and cerebral (45 per cent) emboli.

The principal pathological finding in endocarditis associated with a mechanical prosthesis is valve ring abscess, the major cause of treatment failure. This leads to valvular dehiscence and paravalvular regurgitation. The pathological features of infected *porcine bioprostheses* have been described by Bartolloti et al.[104] The vegetations were friable, small to massive, and present on the inflow surface of the valve. Infected cusps were torn, frayed, or perforated (Fig. 34–4). Ring abscess or valvular calcification was uncommon. Among the histological findings were deposition of fibrin on the inflow surface of the valve and breakdown of collagen. Moderate to marked subendothelial inflammation was present in some instances. Macrophages, neutrophils, and clusters of bacteria within the tissue of the cusps were noted in all cases. Granulomas were present when fungi were involved. The following features that distinguish endocarditis involving porcine valves from that of infection of rigid-frame prostheses have been pointed out by Ferrans et al.[105]: (1) infection can involve the porcine valve itself as well as fibrin, organized thrombi, and fibrous tissue of the patient, and destroy the valve; (2) ring abscesses are uncommon; (3) perforation of cusps does not occur; (4) valvular stenosis is common; and (5) paravalvular leaks are uncommon.

Schoen and his colleagues at the Brigham and Women's Hospital[106–108] have contrasted the pathoanatomical features of endocarditis involving mechanical and bioprosthetic valves. The overall incidence of infection ranged from 1 to 4 per cent. In their autopsy series none of the 378 patients who died within 30 days of operation had endocarditis. Although dehiscence of mechanical prosthesis was common, infection of the prosthesis itself did not occur. The infectious process, however, often involved the sewing ring, spread to the annulus, and led to the development of an abscess. In contrast, endocarditis in patients with bioprostheses was localized to the valve cusps and led to valvular incompetence owing to cuspal tears, perforation, or partial or total destruction of the valve.

HISTOLOGICAL CHANGES. Histological abnormalities of subacute infective endocarditis were described by Libman and Friedberg. They noted that the vegetations consisted essentially of platelet-fibrin thrombi containing colonies of bacteria on and below the surface and suggested that the thrombus was derived from the inflamed valve that had undergone destructive change (Fig. 34–5). The inflammatory reaction consisted chiefly of mononuclear cells, lymphocytes, and histiocytes; few polymorphonuclear cells were present. Not uncommonly, giant cells

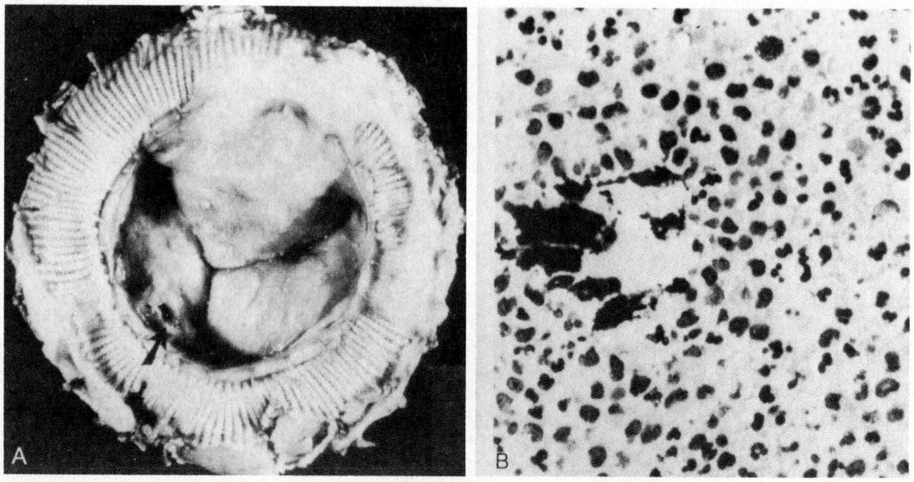

FIGURE 34–4. Bioprosthetic bacterial endocarditis involving cusps. *A*, gross photograph demonstrating cuspal perforation. *B*, histologic section of vegetation with focal calcifications (hematoxylin and eosin stain; magnification × 560). (From Schoen, F. J., Collins, J. J. Jr., and Cohn, L. H.: Long-term failure rate and morphologic correlations in porcine bioprosthetic heart valves. Am. J. Cardiol. *51*:957, 1983.)

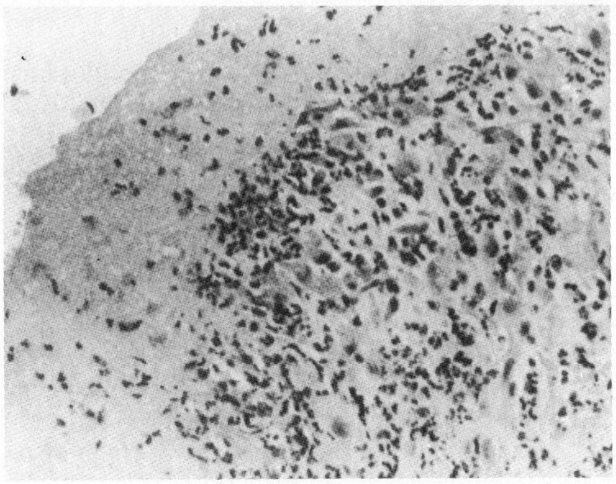

FIGURE 34–5. Endocarditis vegetation showing fibrin mesh on valve surface and dense interstitial infiltrate of inflammatory cells including mononuclear cells, polymorphonuclear leukocytes, and histiocytes (hematoxylin-eosin, × 300). (From Williams, R. C., and Kilpatrick, K.: Immunofluorescence studies of cardiac valves in infective endocarditis. Arch. Intern. Med. *145*:297, 1985.)

containing phagocytized bacteria were present. The cusp underlying the vegetation was the site of a destructive process that was either localized or extended to both surfaces. Healing was an early and prominent feature. At this stage, most of the bacteria had disappeared. In addition to inflammatory cells, the cusp contained numerous capillaries and fibroblasts. When healing was prolonged, the vegetations became calcified.

The myocardium may show a variety of lesions. These are usually diffuse or localized collections of lymphocytes and mononuclear cells and are the so-called Bracht-Wächter lesions that replace the muscle itself. Diffuse or localized collections of polymorphonuclear cells, with or without myocardial necrosis or miliary abscesses, are occasionally observed. Gross suppuration is absent. Muscle fibers may show degenerative changes, often with small scars in various stages of healing. The small coronary branches show swelling and proliferation of the endothelial cells of capillaries and arterioles, arteriolitis, or necrosis of the media or adventitia; perivascular cellular infiltrates and scars may be present. A large branch of a coronary artery may contain an embolus or reveal a mycotic aneurysm.

Among the lesions noted in cases of right-sided endocarditis have been myocardial abscesses containing colonies of bacteria, septic emboli (extramural or intramural) in one or more coronary arteries, foci of necrosis in the ventricular wall or papillary muscles, calcification of individual myocardial fibers, and acute pneumonia with pulmonary infarcts or abscesses.[101] The histopathological findings observed during necropsy of patients with left-sided infective endocarditis were foci of myocardial fibrosis in the ventricular papillary muscles, ventricular free wall, or both.[100]

The histology of acute bacterial endocarditis is entirely different from that of the subacute form of the disease. In the former, the histological picture is of a rapidly progressive destructive lesion, with no features that indicate any attempt at healing, such as the presence of fibroblasts or organization. In untreated cases, the fibrin-platelet thrombus contains only polymorphonuclear leukocytes and a large number of bacteria. The affected underlying valve is the site of necrosis. These features satisfy the criteria for the term *ulcerative endocarditis* that has been applied to this type of disease and explain the predisposition to tearing of the valvular leaflets, rupture of papillary muscles and chordae tendineae, the formation of aneurysms, and the frequency of intracardiac spread of infection—common complications of this type of disease.

PORTALS OF ENTRY OF ORGANISMS AND PREDISPOSING FACTORS

The primary event in the pathogenesis of infective endocarditis is the intrusion of organisms into the bloodstream. This is usually transient when the source of the organisms is the indigenous microflora of the skin, upper respiratory tract, oral cavity, intestinal tract, genitalia, and lower urinary tract, manipulation of which may lead to transient bacteremia.

Transient Bacteremias

DENTAL PROCEDURES. The incidence of transient bacteremia associated with extraction of teeth has been reported to range from 18 to 85 per cent. The organisms are most commonly streptococci. They are seldom present in the blood for longer than 15 to 20 minutes, but this may be prolonged when multiple teeth are removed. In addition, "diphtheroids," *Staph. epidermidis*, and anaerobic members of the normal oral microflora have also been recovered. Peterson and Peacock noted transient bacteremia in 35 per cent of 101 children who had nondiseased primary teeth removed, in 53 per cent of those in whom diseased primary and permanent teeth were extracted, and in 61 per cent undergoing removal of healthy permanent teeth.[109] Among dental procedures other than extraction associated with transient bacteremia are rocking of teeth, chewing of paraffin or hard candy, scaling of gums, brushing of teeth, periodontal operations, dental prophylaxis, use of unwaxed dental floss, and use of oral irrigation devices (Water-Pik). It must be emphasized that infective endocarditis may occur in edentulous persons.[110] An excellent review of the role of dental manipulations in the pathogenesis of infective endocarditis has been published by Bayliss et al.[111]

TONSILLOADENOIDECTOMY. This procedure involving the airway is most commonly associated with bacteremia; from 28 to 38 per cent of patients subjected to this operation experience transient bacterial invasion of the bloodstream. Other manipulations in this area that may lead to bacteremia are bronchoscopy (the rigid but not the fiberoptic instrument), orotracheal intubation, and nasal operations. Among the organisms present in the circulation have been *Staph. aureus*, streptococci, *Hemophilus* species, *Strep. pneumoniae*, and *Staph. epidermidis*.

OTHER PROCEDURES. *Barium enema* may be accompanied by transient bacteremia. LeFrock and his associates[112] reported that in 11.4 per cent of patients who underwent this study, bacteria appeared transiently in the blood. In another study 10 per cent of patients who underwent sigmoidoscopy had transient bacteremia; viridans streptococci were present in 90 per cent of these.[113] The first case of endocarditis after this procedure has been reported.[114] Shull et al. carried out fiberoptic gastroscopy in 50 patients; after the procedure, 4 exhibited bacteremia that lasted from 5 to 30 minutes.[115] This incidence is lower than that after colonoscopy.[116] Transient bacteremia also occurs with percutaneous biopsy of the liver.[117]

A large variety of *urological procedures* have resulted in transient bacterial invasion of the blood[118]; these include internal urethrotomy, urethral dilatation, prostatectomy, removal of indwelling catheter from patients with infected urine, retropubic prostatectomy, cystoscopy, and urethral catheterization. Gram-negative bacilli are the most common transient intruders. As anticipated, the incidence of bacteremia is higher in patients with infected urine.

Invasion of the bloodstream does not occur during parturition. However, about 85 per cent of patients who underwent a suction abortion experienced transient bacteremia. In a few instances, organisms were recovered from the blood after only suction abortion.[119]

Among other procedures that have been associated with transient bacteremia and, in some cases, endocarditis are nasal intubation,[120] injection sclerotherapy of esophageal varices,[121] bouginage for esophageal stricture,[122] anal dilation,[123] laparoscopy,[124] peritoneovenous shunting for ascites,[125] catheterization of the right heart,[126] central venous lines,[127] flow-directed pulmonary arterial catheterization,[128] replacement of prosthetic valves,[129] electrolysis,[130] acupuncture,[131] and vasectomy.[132]

CIRRHOSIS. Snyder et al. reported that infective endocarditis[133] among patients admitted to the hospital was 3.4 times more frequent when cirrhosis was present than when it was absent.

DRUG ADDICTION AND SURGERY. Addiction to the intravenous use of drugs has become an increasingly important factor predisposing to the development of infective endocarditis. Other risk factors include cardiac surgery, especially the insertion of prosthetic valves; the appearance of a paravalvular leak, probably because it produces hemodynamic abnormalities, favors the deposition of platelet-fibrin thrombi on which organisms may be implanted. Prolonged use of polyethylene catheters is associated with an increased risk of endocarditis related to either colonization of the tip of the catheter or entry of organisms at the site where the tube enters the skin.

BURNS. Burned patients appear to be more susceptible to infective endocarditis. In the study by Baskin et al., the infection involved the right side of the heart in 18 patients, the left in 9, and both sides in 8.[134] The disease was acute in 22 and subacute in 13. Murmurs were detectable in only two instances. The most common organism present on the valves was *Staph. aureus* (77 per cent).

PACEMAKERS. An uncommon source of infection of the heart is the transvenous cardiac pacemaker.[135] Sustained staphylococcal bacteremia (at least 12 hours) may develop 2 weeks to 10 months after insertion of the apparatus. Endocarditis has been associated with infection in the subcutaneous pocket into which the pacemaker is inserted.

OTHER PREDISPOSING FACTORS. A number of other infectious and noninfectious predisposing factors have been reported by Garvey and Neu.[136] Among these are neoplastic disease, nonmalignant hematological disorders, "collagen-vascular" disease, diabetes mellitus, chronic active viral hepatitis, preexisting renal failure, treatment with corticosteroids (50 per cent of patients), antitumor chemotherapy and radiation (20 per cent of cases), perinephric abscess, obstruction of the common bile duct, perforation of the bowel (*Clostridium perfringens* endocarditis), and infections of sternal wounds produced in the course of cardiac surgery. Hyperalimentation is also associated with an increased risk of fungal endocarditis.

Extracardiac Foci of Infection

Foci of infection *outside* the heart may serve as sources of bacteremia that lead to the development of endocarditis. Among such lesions are mild to severe infections of the skin ("pimple," boils), especially if they are mishandled by squeezing or inappropriate surgical incision. The organism most often responsible for disease in this situation is *Staph. aureus*. Disease of the lung caused by *Strep. pyogenes* and other highly invasive organisms, such as *H. influenzae*, may also serve as a source of bacteremia and subsequent infective endocarditis. The toxic shock syndrome[137] and syphilis may also predispose to the development of endocarditis.

Among other extracardiac lesions are acute hematogenous osteomyelitis, acute pyelonephritis, meningococcemia with or without meningitis, brucellosis, Q fever, rat-bite fever, and a variety of immunosuppressive disorders, including the vasculitides when they are complicated by bacteremia, and superinfection by bacteria or fungi induced by therapy with antibiotics. A significant number of the patients with infections of normal valves are immunosuppressed because of major underlying disease or treatment with corticosteroids or radiation.[136, 138] These persons were older, and involvement of the right side of the heart was more likely than in those who were immunologically competent. They were also more susceptible to invasion of the valves by gram-negative bacilli and fungi. In about one-third of cases, the presence of infective endocarditis was not suspected during life. The fatality rate was 57 per cent in this group and only 28 per cent in patients who were without immunological abnormalities. Aortic valvular infective endocarditis has been described in a patient with systemic lupus erythematosus who had Libman-Sacks endocarditis.[139]

Infective endocarditis is a subtle and often lethal complication of *hemodialysis*.[140] The source of the organisms has been infection or manipulation of access sites and dental procedures, most commonly involving *Staph. aureus*. The incidence of infection is lower in patients with arteriovenous fistulas that in those with arteriovenous cannulas. Although *P. aeruginosa* is a frequent cause of infection of access sites, it produces endocarditis uncommonly. Cure of the cardiac infection requires, in addition to antimicrobial therapy, removal of the shunt.

A rare predisposing factor in the pathogenesis of infective endocarditis is penetration of the heart by a foreign body.[141, 142] Cardiac catheterization may rarely be associated with a transient bacteremia that leads to the development of infective endocarditis.

UNDERLYING HEART DISEASE

RHEUMATIC HEART DISEASE. Although chronic rheumatic heart disease was the underlying lesion in from 80 to 90 per cent of cases of subacute bacterial endocarditis for many years,[3] this has not been so since antimicrobial agents have become available. This may be related to the decreased incidence of acute rheumatic fever and to the highly successful prevention of recurrences of the disease (p. 1707). At present, only about 40 to 60 per cent of instances of infective endocarditis are superimposed on preexisting rheumatic heart disease.[14] The long-held concept that patients with pure mitral stenosis, atrial fibrillation, and congestive heart failure were at extremely low risk of developing endocarditis does not appear to be as important as it was in the past.

Uncommonly, both infective endocarditis and acute rheumatic carditis may be present simultaneously. The differential diagnosis of acute rheumatic fever and infective endocarditis may, in some instances, be difficult because (1) blood cultures may occasionally be positive in the former and negative in the latter, (2) both conditions feature fever and leukocytosis, and (3) petechiae may be present in both. Blood cultures should be obtained in patients in whom fever persists despite treatment with adequate doses of salicylate. If four or more cultures yield an organism, the possibility of superimposed infective endocarditis must be seriously considered and appropriate antimicrobial therapy instituted.

CONGENITAL HEART DISEASE (See also p. 906). Although probably more frequently the basis for endocarditis in children, congenital heart disease is also important in adults.[143] Gelfman and Levine[144] reported in 1942 that endocarditis occurred in about 6.5 per cent of 453 youngsters over the age of 2 years with congenital heart disease studied at necropsy; the incidence has been recorded to be as high as 16 per cent.[145, 146] In patients younger than 2 years, valvular infection is less commonly superimposed on anatomical defects of the heart. In the first weeks or months of life, this disease is usually a complication of an episode of overwhelming sepsis; murmurs are usually absent, diagnosis is difficult, and the fatality rate is inordinately high.

Patent ductus arteriosus, ventricular septal defect, and tetralogy of Fallot are the congenital lesions most commonly associated with infective endocarditis[147]; aortic or pulmonic stenosis is less frequent. The frequency of infection in patients with ventricular septal defect (Fig. 34–6) has been estimated to be 1 in 470 patient years.[148] When ventricular septal defect and aortic regurgitation coexist, the incidence of endocarditis increases to about 24 per cent. In patients with the tetralogy of Fallot in whom an anastomosis has been created between the systemic and pulmonary circulations, infective endocarditis occurs more frequently than in any other form of congenital heart disease.

Atrial septal defects seldom become infected, probably because of the absence of large interatrial pressure gradients. However, endocarditis involving the mitral valve has occurred in patients with ostium primum defects. Endocarditis tends to develop most frequently in congenital lesions that produce significant pressure gradients.[149] In cases of coarctation of the aorta the infectious process is usually situated on the poststenotic side and on an accompanying bicuspid aortic valve.[150] The pulmonic valve is most often involved in infective endocarditis involving the tetralogy of Fallot.[151] The left pulmonary artery in the area of the ductal orifice is the site most often infected in patients with patent ductus arteriosus. Other congenital defects that predispose to endocarditis are a common atrioventricular valve, a rare accompaniment of complete endocardial cushion defect[152] and subdiaphragmatic subaortic stenosis.[153]

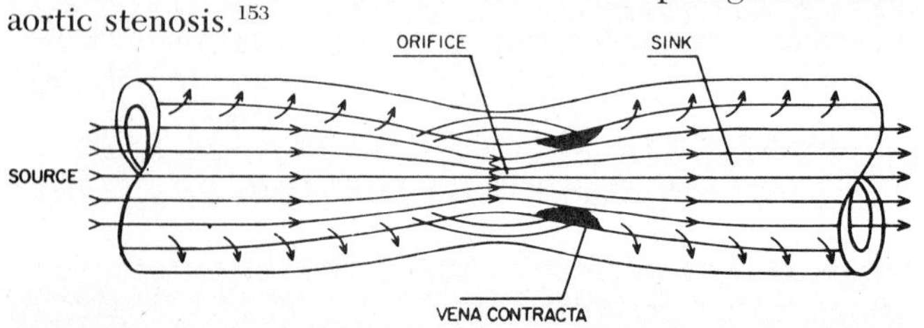

FIGURE 34–6. Venturi model of high-pressure source driving a bacterial aerosol into a low-pressure sink. Characteristic distribution of bacterial colonies is shown at the vena contracta. (From Rodbard, S.: Blood velocity in endocarditis. Circulation *27*:18, 1963, by permission of the American Heart Association, Inc.)

ATHEROSCLEROSIS AND CALCIFICATION. Kerr suggested that, as the population aged, atherosclerotic heart disease would probably become a significant lesion predisposing to the development of infective endocarditis.[4] It has since become clear that certain factors associated with aging play an important role in the pathogenesis of this infection and account for the increase in the incidence of bacterial disease of the heart in the older age group. Atheromatous deposits on the aortic valve have been noted at autopsy in 25 per cent of patients over 40 years of age who have succumbed to endocarditis. The incidence of valvular atheromas, excrescences, and nodules increases progressively with age; these lesions are most prominent in areas where the change in pressure and turbulence of flow are greatest, such as the left side of the heart, in general, and the aortic valve, in particular.[154] Watanakunakorn has described five older patients with calcification of the mitral valve annulus who developed endocarditis.[155] The organisms involved were gram-negative cocci and *Staph. aureus.*

SUBAORTIC STENOSIS. The incidence of infective endocarditis in patients with *hypertrophic obstructive cardiomyopathy* (p. 1418) is in the range of 5 to 10 per cent, but in one recent report it was as high as 50 per cent. The aortic valve is infected most often, followed by the mitral valve alone or both valves simultaneously.[156, 157] The infectious process originates on the ventricular aspect of the anterior portion of the anterior mitral leaflet which is frequently thickened and becomes susceptible to bacterial invasion as a result of the trauma produced by the abutting action of the anterior mitral leaflet against the thickened septum. Infection may then extend to the chordae tendineae and produce tears.

In ten patients with *discrete membranous subaortic stenosis* and endocarditis, the infection was noted to involve the aortic valve in all, the aorta above the aortic valve in six, the mitral valve in four, and the membranous ridge in three. The high incidence of endocarditis of the aortic valve and wall in this condition compared with valvular infection in hypertrophic cardiomyopathy suggested that there is a more prominent jet stream in discrete membranous stenosis than in hypertrophic cardiomyopathy, and that this causes more damage to the aortic leaflets and wall.

MITRAL VALVE PROLAPSE (See also p. 1045). Although it had been known for some time that patients with mitral valve prolapse (MVP) were susceptible to infective endocarditis,[158] it is only recently that the approximate risk of this complication has been defined. In a case-controlled echocardiographic study of hospitalized patients with MVP as the only risk for the development of endocarditis, Clements and his colleagues[159] found that 25 per cent of 51 persons with valvular infections had MVP. Only 7 per cent of 153 persons free of endocarditis had this lesion. The odds ratio was 8:2. This indicated a considerably greater risk of bacterial endocarditis in persons with MVP, especially in those with mitral insufficiency. This level of risk was considered too high by Retchin et al.[160] On the basis of a calculation of "attributable risk," they suggested that "even those individuals with mitral valve prolapse and hemodynamically significant murmurs would have only between one and three chances per year of developing endocarditis." Hickey and Wilcken[161] pointed out that "although the risk of bacterial endocarditis is greater in patients with MVP, the absolute risk remains low," and that this is associated with the presence of a preexisting systolic murmur.

MARFAN SYNDROME. Up until 1974, 21 cases of infective endocarditis occurring in patients with the *Marfan syndrome* (p. 1725) had been reported.[162] The mitral valve is infected most often. Although the aortic valve is commonly abnormal in this disease, it is seldom the site of infection.

CARDIAC SURGERY. Cardiac surgery represents an iatrogenic type of underlying heart disease that predisposes to the development of infective endocarditis.

A study of 122 cases of postcardiotomy endocarditis by Starkebaum et al. indicated that the disease appeared within 2 weeks in 27 per cent[163]; 70 per cent occurred within 2 months. The findings were consistent with the hypothesis that the incubation period of postcardiotomy endocarditis is short.

Eight cases of bacterial endocarditis after penetration of the heart by *foreign bodies* have been recorded.[141, 142]

Certain types of cardiac surgery impose a higher risk of infective endocarditis than does the implantation of a prosthesis. Kaplan et al. have reported that 8 per cent of patients with tetralogy of Fallot developed endocarditis after Pott's procedure (i.e., aortopulmonary shunt). Intracardiac infection also appears to be increased in patients operated on for tricuspid atresia.[164] The highest risk of infective endocarditis is associated with operative procedures on patients with transposition of the great arteries. Valvular infections have not been a notable complication in coronary bypass operations.

PROSTHETIC VALVES. Several studies have indicated that prosthetic valve endocarditis (PVE) may occur "early" (up to 60 days) or "late" (more than 60 days) after operation.[101a, 165] It has been suggested that the "early" appearance of infection usually indicates extracardiac infection as the source of the organisms and that the later fever develops the more likely PVE is present.[166] Staphylococci have been reported by Wilson and his associates[167] to be the most common (47.5 per cent) organisms involved in "early-onset" endocarditis of prosthetic valves; 27 per cent of the strains were *S. epidermidis.* Streptococci were predominant (42 per cent) in the "late-onset" cases. Karchmer et al.[168] noted that 87 per cent of infections of prosthetic valves occurring within 1 year after surgery were caused by methicillin-resistant *S. epidermidis*; this was true in only 2 per cent of cases of "late-onset" disease.

Wilson et al.[167] have recently made the following important comment concerning PVE: "Although the incidence of prosthetic valve endocarditis may be declining, the absolute number of cases of this infection is increasing. This increase has probably resulted from greater sophistication of cardiac surgical techniques, which has allowed more patients to undergo cardiac valve replacement and other complicated surgical procedures. Prosthetic valve endocarditis currently accounts for approximately 16 per cent of the total number of infective endocarditis seen at the Mayo Clinic." The overall incidence of endocarditis involving prosthetic valves is approximately 2 per cent. The frequency with which this occurs is related to the interval elapsing between the surgery and the development of infection. It is somewhat higher when the valvular infection occurs late. In a review of 12,000 reported instances of valve replacements, Mayer and Schoenbaum[169] found the incidence of PVE to have decreased from 3.2 per cent in the 1960's to 2.1 per cent in the 1970's. The case fatality did not change, however, over this period. "Late" aortic PVE occurred in 0.24 per cent of patients followed for 1 year and progressed to 2.2 per cent in patients studied for longer than 5 years. The case fatality rate was 78 per cent in "early-onset" PVE and 4.6 per cent in "late-onset" PVE. Risk factors that indicated a poor clinical response to medical therapy alone included the presence of congestive cardiac failure, infection by an organism other than a streptococcus, location in a nonhet-erograft, systemic emboli, early onset of PVE, and fever persisting for longer than 10 days.

Risk factors that play a role in the development of infection of prosthetic valves (PVE) have been evaluated by several investigators. The actuarial risk for the development of PVE was 3.1 per cent at 12 months and 5.7 per cent at 6 months after surgery in 2,462 patients studied by Calderwood et al.[170]; it was higher when more than one prosthetic valve was implanted. Mechanical valves were more prone to infection than porcine ones during the first 3 postoperative months; there was no difference after 5 years. The risk of late PVE after replacement of multiple or mitral, but not aortic, valves was increased in elderly persons. Endocarditis of native valves, black race, and longer cardiopulmonary bypass time were identified as additional risk factors.

The results of an actuarial analysis of the risk of PVE in almost 1600 patients who had undergone valve replacement have been reported by Rutledge et al.[171] The cumulative risk was 3 per cent at 5 years and 5 per cent at 10 years after surgery. In "early" PVE the risk of infection peaked 15 days postoperatively and was 45 episodes per 100,000 patient days. This then rapidly declined and remained stable at about one episode per 100,000 patient days from 150 days to 20 years after insertion of the prosthesis. There was no correlation between the specific type of valve, the model and position of the valve, the number of valves implanted, the incidence of PVE, or the fatality rate. Ivert et al.[172] have indicated that the risk factors for developing PVE were native endocarditis, black race, mechanical prostheses but not bioprostheses, male sex, and a longer period of time on cardiopulmonary bypass. The risk was greatest 3 weeks after valve replacement.

Among the complications of PVE are obstruction of the outlet of ball-type mechanical valves (Starr-Edwards), especially when fungi are responsible for infection, embolization of large arteries (fungal PVE), annular abscess, calcification and/or cuspal rupture of bioprostheses, and infection of various types of patches.

Among the conditions predisposing to invasion of prosthetic valves by organisms in the *early* postoperative period are infected surgical wounds in the chest and urinary catheters. Sources of infection include contamination of blood by the oxygenator and of the blood used to prime the pump; the connecting tubes on the large venous and arterial cannulas; direct contamination by hands, instruments, or room air; reactivation of latent infection in patients with episodes of endocarditis before placement of the prosthetic valve; and contamination of the prosthesis. Predisposing conditions in the convalescent period include bacteremia from sites of infection in the chest wound or at the cannulation site, infected pleural fluid, postoperative pneumonia, tracheostomy, contaminated indwelling catheters, and superinfections related to prophylaxis or therapy with antimicrobial agents. Conditions predisposing to *late* endocarditis are infections of the urinary tract, dental procedures, disease of the upper airway, ingrown toenails, use of the nasal cautery, and pilonidal cyst. The primary factor involved in both early and late convalescence is bacteremia resulting from dental, dermatological, gastrointestinal, and genitourinary procedures or minor surgical operations. In addition to these, Dismukes et al. reported that cystoscopy, excision of a carbuncle, uterine dilatation and curettage, paravalvular leaks that developed immediately postoperatively, and preexisting endocarditis (same organism) predisposed to infection of the prosthetic valves.[173]

NORMAL VALVES. There is an increasing number of instances of infective endocarditis involving otherwise *normal valves*, particularly in cases of the acute form of the disease. For example, 40 to 60 per cent of patients with infections caused by *Staph. aureus* have previously normal cardiac valves. This is also true in an appreciable number of instances in which *Strep. pyogenes*, *Strep. pneumoniae*, *N. meningitidis*, and *N. gonorrhoeae* are involved. In recent years endocarditis affecting normal valves has occurred more frequently because of the increase in the number of persons using intravenous illicit drugs.

MYOCARDIAL INFARCTION. Infective endocarditis may occur as a complication of myocardial infarction.[174] The location of the infection is determined by the site of necrosis of the muscle, and the predisposing factor is the development of a platelet-fibrin clot over the infarcted area. The infection may be situated on the left side of the septum in cases of anteroseptal infarction or on the endocardium over the site of damage in the left ventricle. In addition, development of an *aneurysm* in which a clot forms provides a potential area of invasion for organisms.

NONVALVULAR INFECTIVE ENDOCARDITIS. Nonvalvular infective endocarditis may occur in *ventricular septal defect*. Three sites are commonly involved. One is the point of impact of the jet stream on the right ventricular endocardium; the resulting injury leads to the formation of a small platelet-fibrin thrombus on which bacteria may be implanted. Infection may also develop on the right side of the septal opening; the Venturi effect created by the flow of blood from an area of high pressure (left ventricle) to one of lower pressure (right ventricle) leads to the deposition of a clot around the opening on the right side of the septum. Much less common is infection of the left ventricular side of the defect. The risk of infection is reduced when the septal opening is large because this does not produce an interventricular pressure gradient.

A rare form of nonvalvular infection of the heart is infected *atrial myxoma*. A patient described by Graham et al. is one of four similar cases, three of which had *Staph. aureus* infections.[175] Embolization to the central nervous system occurred in every instance. Infection of an atrial myxoma by *Histoplasma capsulatum* has been described.[176]

Single or multiple *myocardial abscesses* may develop in the course of bacteremias unrelated to valvular infection. *Staph. aureus* and *N. meningitidis* are among the most common organisms involved. Several instances of subacute bacterial endocarditis in patients with *rheumatic valvular disease* in which the infection did not involve any of the affected valves have been noted. In such cases the infectious process was superimposed on McCallum's patch, an area of endocardial injury in the left atrium induced by the acute rheumatic process.

LOCALIZATION OF ENDOCARDITIS

Subacute Endocarditis

Since Osler's[177] classic description of endocarditis, many investigators have tried to explain the fact that infected endocardial vegetations consistently occur in the same location. Four mechanisms are responsible for the initiation and localization of the *subacute* infection: (1) a previously damaged cardiac valve or a hemodynamic situation in which damage results from a jet effect, produced by blood flowing from a zone of high pressure to one of relatively low pressure, as in mitral regurgitation or ventricular septal defect (Table 34–2); (2) a sterile platelet-fibrin thrombus;

TABLE 34–2 LOCI OF LESIONS IN ENDOCARDITIS

Condition	High-Pressure Source	Orifice	Low-Pressure Sink	Location of Lesions	Satellite Lesions
Coarctation of aorta	Central aorta	Coarctation	Distal aorta	Downstream wall	Lateral wall of aorta peripheral to stenotic lesion
Patent ductus arteriosus	Aorta	Ductus	Pulmonary artery	Pulmonary artery	Pulmonic valve
Arteriovenous fistula	Artery	Fistula	Vein	Fistula and vein	
Ventricular septal defect	Left ventricle	Defect	Right ventricle	Right ventricular surface defect	Pulmonary artery
Aortic regurgitation	Aorta	Closed aortic valves	Left ventricle	Ventricular surface aortic valve	Mitral chordae
Mitral regurgitation	Left ventricle	Closed mitral valves	Left atrium	Atrial surface mitral valve	Atrium
Pulmonic regurgitation	Pulmonary artery	Closed pulmonic valves	Right ventricle	Ventricular surface pulmonic valve	
Tricuspid regurgitation	Right ventricle	Closed tricuspid valves	Right atrium	Atrial surface tricuspid valve	

Adapted from Rodbard, S.: Blood velocity and endocarditis. Circulation 27:18, 1963, by permission of the American Heart Association, Inc.

(3) bacteremia, often transient; and (4) a high titer of agglutinating antibody against the infecting organism.

THE JET AND VENTURI EFFECTS. Of 1024 patients with infective endocarditis studied by Lepeschkin at autopsy, mitral valves were involved in 86 per cent, aortic valves in 55 per cent, tricuspid valves in 19.6 per cent, and pulmonic valves in 1.1 per cent.[178] By correlating the impact of pressure on these valves with the frequency of involvement of the corresponding valves, Lepeschkin presented a strong argument for *mechanical stress* as a critical factor in the evolution of endocarditis.

By injecting a bacterial aerosol into the air stream passing through an agar Venturi tube, Rodbard elegantly demonstrated how high pressure drives an infected fluid into a low-pressure sink to establish a characteristic pattern of colony distribution; a collar of maximal deposition consistently appeared in the low-pressure sink immediately beyond the orifice (Fig. 34–6).[149] This model helps to explain the distribution of lesions often complicating various cardiac valvular and septal defects (Table 34–2). The early observation that in infective endocarditis the atrial side of the valve and adjacent segment of atrium are characteristically involved in patients with mitral regurgitation is also explained; a Venturi effect is produced when blood is driven from a high-pressure source (the left ventricle) through an orifice (the nearly closed but regurgitant mitral valve) into a low-pressure sink (the atrium). A jet effect on the atrial wall establishes the other site of potential involvement, McCallum's patch (Fig. 34–7).

The sites of aortic valvular infection are established in a similar way. Some degree of aortic regurgitation appears to be crucial. The high-pressure source is the aorta, and the low-pressure sink is the left ventricle. Vegetations are typically found on the ventricular surface of the aortic leaflets. Satellite lesions, which may be found on the chordae tendineae, are the result of a high-velocity regurgitant stream from an incompetent aortic valve—a situation analogous to the jet effect in mitral regurgitation. In a ventricular septal defect with a small orifice and left-to-right shunt, a Venturi effect often leads to the development of lesions around the orifice on the right ventricular side of the opening. Secondary lesions may be present on the right ventricular wall opposite the defect, the site of impact of the jet. Similar hemodynamic relations in tricuspid regurgitation, arteriovenous fistula, coarctation of the aorta, and patent ductus arteriosus can be used, in each instance, to predict the location of the endothelial lesions. Table 34–2 presents the distribution of endocardial infections in common cardiovascular disorders.

Attenuation of the jet and Venturi effects is seen in congestive heart failure and atrial fibrillation and helps to explain the long-recognized infrequency of infective endocarditis in these settings.[179] Likewise, defects with surface areas large enough to abolish a gradient and those in which smaller volumes minimize the gradient are not usually associated with endocarditis. These findings probably explain the rarity of endocarditis in isolated atrial septal defects and the greater threat of infection in small than in large ventricular septal defects. The lesion responsible for the initiation of endocarditis is occasionally too small to produce enough turbulence to create an audible murmur.

THE PLATELET-FIBRIN THROMBUS. Turbulence and the jet effect traumatize the endothelial surface and initiate a series of events that may lead to the establishment of an infected focus. Collagen is exposed, and platelet deposition occurs in a manner analogous to the formation of the primary platelet plug of normal hemostasis after vascular injury. Central to these events is the role of the sterile platelet-fibrin thrombus, or so-called nonbacterial thrombotic endocarditis. The nonspecific nature of the sterile platelet-fibrin thrombus is emphasized by the fact that it can be produced as a result of numerous types of stress or injury.

BACTEREMIA AND AGGLUTINATING ANTIBODIES. As already pointed out (p. 1097), transient bacteremias frequently occur in normal persons. They are usually without clinical importance, even when sterile platelet-fibrin thrombi have developed on areas of previously injured endocardium. In most cases the failure of implantation of organisms on such sites is related to the small number and low invasive capability of circulating organisms. A major factor, probably involved in initiating

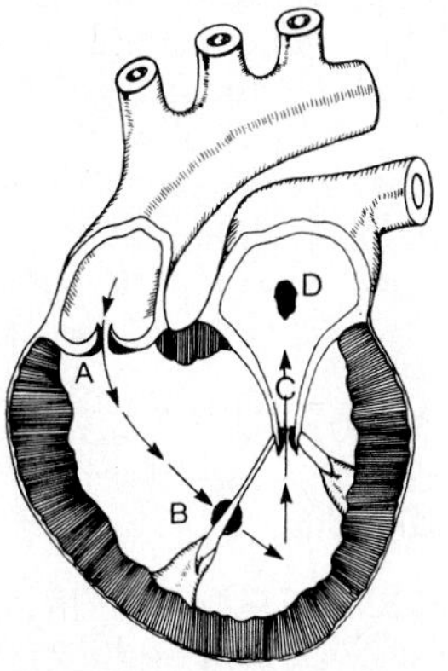

FIGURE 34–7. High-velocity streams in mitral and aortic regurgitation and sites of endocarditis lesions. Arrows at left indicate a high arterial pressure that generates regurgitant flow from aorta to ventricle. The endocarditic lesions appear at the ventricular surface of the aortic valve (A). The stream through the incompetent aortic valve may produce lesions on the chordae tendineae of the aortic leaf of the mitral valve (B). If the mitral valves cannot seat properly during ventricular systole, the regurgitant stream (arrows at right) will pass to the sink of the left atrium, and the endocarditic lesion will tend to become engrafted on the atrial surface of the mitral valve (C). The atrial endocardium in line with the regurgitant stream may produce a fibrous area, MacCallum's patch (D), which may become another site of endocarditic lesions. (Adapted from Rodbard, S.: Blood velocity in endocarditis. Circulation *27*:18, 1963, by permission of the American Heart Association, Inc.)

subacute valvular infection because it permits large numbers of bacteria to adhere to the sterile platelet-fibrin thrombus, is *circulating antibody*, especially agglutinins. By clumping the organisms, the antibody produces an inoculum large enough to induce bacterial multiplication and infection—a phenomenon much more important in the pathogenesis of subacute than of acute endocarditis.

Evidence of the importance of antibody may be found in studies of the development of endocarditis in horses[180] undergoing immunization with pneumococci. Infected vegetations appeared late in the course of immunization, coincidentally with the highest titers of antibody. The exact mechanism by which pathogens ultimately adhere to the platelet-fibrin thrombus is unknown. One possibility is that the platelet-covered lesion somehow provides a favorable sticky surface.

Acute Endocarditis

The pathoanatomical mechanisms involved in the development of acute bacterial endocarditis are quite different from those in the subacute form. In 50 to 60 per cent of acute cases, previously *normal* valves are the sites of infection. It appears, therefore, that the presence of a sterile platelet-fibrin thrombus is unnecessary in the pathogenesis of this form of the valvulitis. Because the organisms responsible for the acute infection (*Staph. aureus, Strep. pneumoniae, N. meningitidis* or *gonorrhoeae, Strep. pyogenes,* and *H. influenzae*) are highly invasive, only small numbers are required to establish infection. Thus the critical requirement in the pathogenesis of acute endocarditis is bacteremia caused by an invasive organism. It should be pointed out, however, that acute infective endocarditis may also occur in patients with underlying acquired or congenital valvular damage and that, in these patients, sterile platelet-fibrin thrombi may be present and facilitate infection just as is the case in subacute endocarditis.

The exact mechanism by which pathogenic bacteria invade normal valve leaflets has now been determined. Specific properties of various bacteria determine their ability to adhere to the surface of cardiac valves. Gould et al.[181] and Holmes and Ramirez-Ronda[182] examined the capacity of a number of organisms to adhere to canine and human valvular leaflets in vitro. The degree of adherence was found to vary with the type of organism studied, being highest with enterococci and *Staph. aureus*, followed by viridans streptococci, *Staph. epidermidis*, and *P. aeruginosa* and lowest with *Escherichia coli* and *Klebsiella pneumoniae*. These data are of potentially great clinical importance because they probably explain the relative frequency with which certain bacteria, especially *Staph. aureus*, infect previously normal valves. Of equal clinical interest is the demonstration of the poor adherence of *E. coli* and *K. pneumoniae*, which may very well account for the low incidence of endocarditis caused by these organisms, despite the well-known high frequency with which they produce bacteremia.

In subacute bacterial endocarditis the inducing bacteremia frequently originates not from an infectious process, but from trauma to areas in which the causative organisms normally reside as components of the indigenous flora, such as the teeth, urogenital tract, or intestine. In acute endocarditis the inducing bacteremia originates in an active infection, usually at a site remote from the heart, such as the skin, lungs, or genitourinary tract. In an appreciable number of instances, however, there is no demonstrable portal of entry of the organisms into the bloodstream; this may be the case when *Staph. aureus* is the causative agent.

CLINICAL MANIFESTATIONS

Four mechanisms may be involved in the pathogenesis of the clinical manifestations of infective endocarditis: (1) the infectious process on the involved valve, (2) embolization, (3) metastatic infection, and (4) deposition of abnormal globulins and circulating immune complexes at various sites remote from and in the heart. All four of these mechanisms are not present in every patient, and there are also striking qualitative and quantitative differences in their roles in the acute and subacute forms of the disease.[183]

MODES OF ONSET

Subacute Endocarditis

INCUBATION PERIOD. The exact "incubation period" of subacute infective endocarditis is difficult to define. However, an extensive review of the literature by Starkebaum et al.,[163] based on a study of the time elapsing between exposure to a situation that might induce transient bacteremia and the development of the first manifestations of valvular infection, suggested that the median "incubation period" is about 1 week. Symptoms appeared within 2 weeks in about 84 per cent of the patients. Thus the "incubation period" of subacute bacterial endocarditis is often shorter than realized. Procedures carried out more than 2 weeks before onset of symptoms are not likely to be causally related.

MANIFESTATIONS OF INFECTION. In many instances the onset of subacute infective endocarditis is characterized by the *general manifestations of infection* without any signs or symptoms suggesting disease of the heart or any other organ. Common complaints include persistent low-grade fever, lassitude, anorexia, fatigue, loss of weight, sleepiness, and a grippe-like syndrome. Subacute endocarditis may simulate a number of disorders that suggest involvement of extracardiac sites. These are: (a) headache, generalized pain, malaise, and respiratory symptoms resembling influenza; (b) fever, cough, loss of weight, weakness, pain in the chest, and even hemoptysis, suggesting the possibility of tuberculosis; (c) elevated temperature and arthralgia or arthritis suggestive of acute rheumatic fever; (d) diarrhea, fever, headache, and drowsiness, symptoms similar to those of typhoid fever; (e) intermittent chills and fever, resembling malaria (common in persons who are treated with salicylates intermittently to control fever and who experience rigor just before the temperature begins to rise); (f) dyspnea, precordial discomfort, palpitation, and, at times, peripheral edema (frequently in patients in whom valvular infection has been present for weeks or months and in whom congestive heart failure finally develops); (g) fever and pain in the right upper abdomen consistent with hepatic or subdiaphragmatic infection; (h) fever, abdominal pain, and urinary symptoms with or without hematuria; (i) a clinical picture suggesting carcinoma of the stomach, characterized by vomiting, postprandial distress, and anorexia, or a syndrome suggestive of appendicitis.[184]

DEVELOPMENT OF COMPLICATIONS. Other modes of onset of subacute infective endocarditis are related to the development of complications of the disease that often appear before therapy is initiated, especially when the infection has not been treated for weeks or months. Some of these are embolic, some are due to progressive involvement of the valve, while others result from the development and activity of immunological disorders.[185]

EMBOLIC COMPLICATIONS. Manifestations of this type of onset include (a) *sudden occlusion of the middle cerebral artery*, leading to hemiplegia; (b) a clinical picture of *acute meningitis*, in which the spinal fluid is sterile but contains an increased number of cells, concentration of protein, and a normal sugar content; (c) manifestations consistent with diffuse encephalitis; (d) sudden development of pain in either the right or left upper abdominal quadrant caused by gross infarction of either the kidney or the spleen; (e) hematuria without pain, caused by small, multiple infarcts of the kidney, interstitial nephritis, or diffuse proliferative glomerulonephritis; (f) unilateral blindness of acute onset caused by embolic occlusion of the retinal artery; and (g) myocardial infarction caused by embolic occlusion of one of the coronary arteries. The first manifestation of endocarditis involving the right side of the heart, particularly the tricuspid valve, may be the development of "pneumonia" which is actually an embolic pulmonary infarct. The appearance of multiple areas of infiltration in the lungs in a patient with fever and a murmur should alert the physician immediately to the possibility of infection of the right side of the heart.

PROGRESSIVE VALVULAR INVOLVEMENT. The modes of onset related to continued activity of an acute infectious process on the affected valve in untreated persons are a change in the character of a murmur and the development of progressive cardiac failure due to valvular dysfunction induced by slow destruction and fibrosis of the involved valve.

IMMUNOLOGICAL DISORDERS. An increasing number of patients with subacute infective endocarditis in whom the diagnosis is delayed for weeks or months may have, as the first manifestation, findings related to the development of immunological phenomena. Some persons may first come to medical attention because of the weakness, anorexia, and anemia associated with renal failure caused by interstitial nephritis or proliferative glomerulonephritis resulting from the deposition of immune complexes in the kidney. Others may complain of arthralgias or arthritis probably related to the presence of the same type of complexes in the synovia. An occasional patient may complain of increasing difficulty with "palpitations." These can be caused by arrhythmias, which may be immunological in origin, as suggested by the presence of Bracht-Wächter bodies in the myocardium, or may be the result of spread of infection from the valve to the conducting system in the interventricular septum. That the initial presentation of subacute endocarditis may be related to the development of immunological reactions is supported by the observation that the Osler node and probably the Roth spot may be, in part, due to vasculitis (see below).

LUMBAR PAIN. Persistent pain in the lumbar area has become an increasingly common early complaint of patients with subacute endocarditis.[186] This is not due to vertebral osteomyelitis, as evidenced by failure to demonstrate any changes in the vertebral bodies over months of radiographic examination, and by the rapid disappearance of the pain after effective antimicrobial therapy is initiated.

PROSTHETIC VALVULAR INFECTIONS. The onset of infection involving prosthetic valves is often difficult to recognize because there may be no signs or symptoms, with the exception of fever, that clearly indicate the presence of this disease.

DRUG USERS. The mode of onset of infective endocarditis in persons who use illicit drugs intravenously is not sufficiently suggestive to permit a diagnosis; however, two features may indicate the presence of valvular infection in such patients. In those in whom the tricuspid valve is involved, the appearance of repeated episodes of pulmonary embolism, sometimes accompanied by infarction, is suggestive of the diagnosis. In persons with fungal infection of the mitral or aortic valve, the first manifestation may be embolic occlusion of a major artery, most often in one of the legs, because of the large size of the vegetations characteristic of this type of disease. In such cases diagnosis is often established by embolectomy and isolation of the organism from the clot.

Acute Endocarditis

The mode of onset of acute infective endocarditis is distinctly different from that of the subacute form. Patients are usually previously well and become ill rapidly, with manifestations of severe infection. Normally there are no signs indicating the presence of valvular disease in the early stage. Unlike subacute endocarditis, complications related directly to the rapidly advancing destructive process occur commonly within a week or less after infection and are often reflected by the rapid development of heart failure, especially when the aortic valve is involved. Because the thrombi on the affected valve are moderately large and soft, embolization is often the first manifestation of the disease, and patients may first be seen by a physician because of multiple petechiae or purpuric lesions of the skin, acute onset of neurological signs, or, if the infection involves the right side of the heart, "pneumonia" or single or multiple abscesses of the lung.

SIGNS AND SYMPTOMS

Fever is by far the most common sign of infective endocarditis. The type and course of the fever are variable; normal or subnormal temperatures may be present in from 3 to 15 per cent of cases.[187] Absence of fever is not uncommon in elderly persons with the subacute form of infection. This may be so because, with increasing age, basal (96.7°F or 36°C) and maximal (98.6°F or 37°C) daily temperatures tend to become lower than in young persons. It is probably for this reason that older patients with subacute infective endocarditis have "normal" temperatures. The author has seen a number of patients with this disease in their 70's who have been thought to be free of fever. However, when the course of the daily temperatures is charted over a period, variations ranging from 96.8°F (36°C) in the early morning to 98.6°F (37°C) in the late afternoon are noted, representing fever in such persons. Absence of an elevated temperature should not preclude obtaining blood cultures when other signs and symptoms suggest endocarditis.

Other conditions in which fever may be absent in the face of subacute endocarditis are massive intracerebral or subarachnoid hemorrhage, cardiac failure, uremia, and administration of antimicrobial drugs in doses sufficient to decrease elevated temperatures but inadequate to eradicate the valvular infection. Repeated short courses of antimicrobial therapy, interspersed with periods during which treatment is withheld in patients with undiagnosed endocarditis, produce a characteristic pattern of repetitive episodes of remission and relapse of fever; this course should alert physicians to the possibility of the disease in any patient in whom a murmur is audible. With few exceptions the maximal daily temperature of patients with acute infective endocarditis is higher (102 to 104°F or 39 to 40°C) than when the disease is subacute. Shaking chills are strikingly infrequent in the subacute infection unless salicylates are administered at inappropriate intervals; rigor will usually appear as the antipyretic activity disappears and the temperature begins to increase. In sharp contrast, patients with the acute form of infective endocarditis frequently experience high-grade fever in the range of 102 to 104°F (39 to 40°C) or higher early in the disease; shaking chills are common even when salicylates are not given.

CARDIAC MURMURS

It was accepted dogma for many years that absence of a murmur ruled out the possibility of infective endocarditis, especially the subacute form of the disease. However, it is now apparent that up to 10 per cent of patients with subacute endocarditis do not have a detectable murmur when they first come to medical attention. In most instances a murmur appears at some time during the period of treatment; less frequently, a murmur may not be detected until 2 to 3 months after therapy has been discontinued; in a rare patient a murmur may never appear, even many years after cure of the infection.

One of 167 patients with subacute and 7 of 54 patients with acute endocarditis were reported by Pankey to be free of murmurs.[188] He noted that *changes* in the character of the murmur occurred in 16.7 per cent of the subacute cases. This has not been the experience of this author, who, in studies of more than 900 patients with *subacute* valvular infections, has found changing murmurs to be uncommon. A change in a murmur occurs much more frequently in patients with *acute* valvular infections. One-third of cases of endocarditis of the right side of the heart, especially the tricuspid valve, and all with infection of the mural endocardium are free of murmurs. Basal systolic murmurs, caused either by the flow of blood from the left ventricle into a widened tortuous aorta or by atherosclerotic changes in the aortic valve, often pose a problem in the diagnosis of infective endocarditis, especially the subacute form, since the physician detects no change in the character of the murmur, the presence of which he may have been aware of for a long time. It must be stressed that, in older patients with unexplained fever who are known to have had a murmur for many years, the possibility of bacterial endocarditis must always be entertained, even in the occasional instance in which blood cultures are negative (p. 1113). With respect to infective endocarditis, *no murmur can be considered "innocent."* Personal experience has taught that the discovery of a so-called "flow" or systolic "ejection" murmur that remains unchanged over long periods of observation has resulted in failure to consider the possibility of valvular infection.

Anemia is a universal feature of both acute and subacute infective endocarditis; *pallor* of the skin and mucous membranes is common. Libman and Friedberg called attention to rare patients who exhibited erythema of the nose and surrounding skin, especially the cheeks, bearing a slight resemblance to the facial lesion in systemic lupus erythematosus.[184]

CHARACTERISTIC DIAGNOSTIC LESIONS ("PERIPHERAL STIGMATA")

Five lesions involving the skin and its appendages and the eye have, for many years, been considered the classic peripheral manifestations of subacute bacterial endocarditis: *petechiae, subungual hemorrhages, Osler nodes, Janeway lesions*, and *Roth spots*. Because of the long course of the active disease in the pre-antibiotic era, these peripheral lesions were much more common than now, when effective antibiotic therapy usually rapidly brings the disease under control.[187] There has been a decrease in the incidence of *petechiae*, especially in the subacute form of the disease, from about 85 per cent before antimicrobial agents were available to 19 to 40 per cent at present.[1, 4, 185, 189, 190] Libman and Friedberg pointed out that petechiae with pale centers are of greater diagnostic importance than those with yellow centers.[184] These lesions are often present in the conjunctivae and are detectable, in some cases, only when the upper eyelids are everted. They also tend to occur most prominently on the skin on the dorsa of the hands and feet but are also commonly seen over the anterior chest and abdominal wall, oral and pharyngeal mucosa, and soft palate. Purpuric lesions develop occasionally and are seldom associated with thrombocytopenia. The presence of petechiae is not always diagnostic of infective endocarditis, since these lesions develop in patients with various types of hematological disorders (especially when the number of circulating platelets is markedly reduced), systemic lupus erythematosus, scurvy, renal insufficiency, bacteremia without endocarditis (staphylococcal, streptococcal, meningococcal, and gonococcal), atrial myxoma, and verrucous endocardiosis ("marantic endocarditis"). Over 50 per cent of patients who undergo cardiopulmonary bypass develop conjunctival petechiae in the immediate postoperative period, in the absence of infection, presumably owing to fat microemboli.[191] Because these persons are especially susceptible to valvular infection, physicians must be aware of this "false-positive" sign.

Subungual ("splinter") hemorrhages are uncommon in patients with bacterial endocarditis. At present they are observed more frequently in general hospital populations than in persons with valvular infections[192] and are often related to advanced age and trauma. The characteristic features of a splinter hemorrhage are its linear form and the fact that its distal end does not reach the anterior edge of the nail bed; the latter distinguishes this lesion from a true splinter. The number of fingers involved is variable and ranges from a single nail bed with only one hemorrhage to several fingers, each of which contains several "splinters." In some cases the toes may be involved, either alone or together with the fingers. In trichinosis, subungual hemorrhages are common and each nail bed contains large numbers of these lesions.

Osler nodes are small, raised, nodular, red to purple, painful, tender lesions that are present most often in the pulp spaces of the terminal phalanges of the fingers. They may also be present on the back of the toes, the soles, and the thenar and hypothenar eminences. They are less common on the sides of the fingers, the forearms, and the ears and seldom occur on the trunk. The most characteristic feature of these lesions is their tenderness. At times, patients can anticipate the development of Osler nodes because of an antecedent peculiar, local "sensation" or pain at a site in which the lesion later appears. They may be fleeting in some cases and disappear within a few hours after they have developed; however, they usually persist for 4 to 5 days but remain tender for only 2 to 3 days and seldom become necrotic. Although almost completely restricted to the subacute type of endocarditis, Osler nodes are rarely present in the acute form of valvular infection. There has been a striking decrease in the incidence of Osler nodes over the past 30 years.

Janeway lesions are small (1 to 4 mm in diameter),

irregular, flat, erythematous, nontender, painless macules present most often on the thenar and hypothenar eminences of the hands and the soles of patients with subacute infective endocarditis. They appear less often on the tips of the fingers and plantar surfaces of the toes; rarely they take the form of a diffuse macular erythematous rash over the extremities and trunk. The lesions on the hands and feet blanch with pressure and with elevation of the extremities. When present in cases of acute valvular infection, the lesions tend to be purple and hemorrhagic.

Clubbing of fingers and/or toes was present in virtually all patients with subacute bacterial endocarditis 25 to 30 years ago but is now quite uncommon.

Ocular signs are occasionally present in patients with infective endocarditis, especially the subacute type. In addition to the conjunctival petechiae, these lesions may appear in the sclera and the retiina, where they are circular or flame-shaped. The *Roth spot*, as first described, is located in the retina and has the appearance of a "cotton-wool" exudate; it consists of aggregations of cytoid bodies.[193] Histological study of these lesions has shown them to be perivascular collections of lymphocytes in the nerve layer of the retina that may or may not be surrounded by edema and hemorrhage. Because the association of these lesions with infective endocarditis was first recognized by Litten,[194] they are referred to as "Litten's sign" in the French literature. The boat-shaped hemorrhage in the retina, erroneously called a Roth spot, was first described by Doherty and Trubek, who attributed it to recurrent crops of petechiae.[195] They noted that these lesions often appeared over a period of only a few hours. Both the cytoid bodies and hemorrhagic spots have decreased in incidence over the years and are now present in less than 5 per cent of cases. Round white spots are occasionally present in the retina; they are noted more often in the acute than in the subacute form of the disease. Optic neuritis occasionally occurs.

Splenomegaly is still a relatively frequent sign in patients with endocarditis, but it is not as common as in the preantibiotic era, when it occurred in 80 to 90 per cent of cases. The spleen may be only slightly enlarged and barely palpable; in the acute form of the disease it may be large, soft, painful, and tender.

A number of other signs and symptoms, some of which are uncommon or rare, may be present in infective endocarditis. Among these are pericardial friction rub, manifestations of congestive heart failure, cardiac arrhythmias of various types, hematuria (in the absence of renal infarction), cough that may occur early and be distressing, hoarseness, arthritis, and pain and tenderness of the long bones and of the sternum (especially when anemia is severe).

BACTERIA-FREE STAGE

The "bacteria-free stage" of endocarditis, first described by Libman in 1913,[196] is now rare as a result of early diagnosis and treatment of the disease. However, this syndrome is still seen, albeit uncommonly, in patients in whom the disease remains unsuspected and untreated for months. The outstanding features of this form of valvular infection include congestive heart failure, diaphoresis, joint pains, leg swelling, and thigh pain. Fever is absent in most cases but develops if and when embolism occurs. The emboli are often sterile. New murmurs are rare. The kidney is usually involved; macroscopic hematuria is common, even in the absence of infarction. Renal failure is frequent, as is anemia. The white blood count is usually low, and granulocytopenia may develop. The spleen may be markedly enlarged. Petechiae are much less common than in the active stage of the disease, but purpuric lesions are frequent. Osler nodes are uncommon. Two of the most frequent signs of the bacteria-free stage of endocarditis are marked tenderness of the sternum and a striking brown pigmentation of the face and back of the hands.

The criteria for the diagnosis of this syndrome are absence of manifestations indicating active valvular infection, during which bacteremia may have been present; negative blood cultures but organisms still present in the vegetations; renal insufficiency; severe progressive anemia; embolic phenomena; striking splenomegaly; brown pigmentation of the face; and absence of fever. Patients with this syndrome have survived for as long as 3 years and usually die of renal insufficiency or congestive heart failure.

COMPLICATIONS OF ENDOCARDITIS

(Table 34–3)

CARDIAC COMPLICATIONS

HEART FAILURE. Congestive heart failure resulting from acute aortic regurgitation is currently the leading cause of death from infective endocarditis. This may occur over a varying period of time in untreated cases of the subacute form of the disease. In contrast, cardiac failure may appear with startling rapidity in acute endocarditis when the aortic valve is infected and may become so severe within a week after the onset of infection that replacement of the valve becomes an emergency procedure. In a review of 144 cases of infective endocarditis, Mills et al. noted congestive failure in 55 per cent.[198] Eighty per cent of those with heart failure had regurgitant aortic valves and/or enterococcal infection. Cardiac decompensation occurred in about 50 per cent of patients with mitral valve regurgitation and in less than 20 per cent of those with congenital heart disease or infection of the tricuspid valve. Nearly 95 per cent of patients who experienced cardiac failure within 6 months after the onset of endocarditis had premonitory manifestations within 1 month after infection. The organisms involved were (in order of frequency) enterococcus, *Strep. pneumoniae*, *Staph. aureus*, and *Strep. viridans*. Review of collected studies of congestive heart failure complicating infective endocarditis indicates an incidence ranging from 15 to 65 per cent. Aortic or mitral valve regurgitation may develop as early as 1 month after infection and nearly always within 6 months; in some instances it may not occur until as long as 1 year after the appearance of endocarditis. Although it had been suggested that myocarditis is the basis of cardiac failure, it now seems clear that the primary cause is valvular destruction.

Another complication responsible for heart failure, said

TABLE 34–3 LIFE-THREATENING COMPLICATIONS OF INFECTIVE ENDOCARDITIS[197]

Intracardiac Complications	Extracardiac Complications
Intractable cardiac failure	Embolization of coronary arteries
Myocardial (or septal) abscess	Stroke
Rupture of papillary muscles	Embolus to spinal cord
Annular abscess	Abscess of spleen
Destruction of valvular leaflets	Mycotic aneurysm in brain
Mycotic aneurysm of sinus of Valsalva	Recurrence of endocarditis
Aortocardiac and other fistulas	Cerebral abscess(es)
Suppurative pericarditis	Multiple embolic episodes
Obstruction of outlet of Starr-Edwards valve	
Separation of prosthetic valve from annulus	
Infection of intracardiac patches	

to be common in patients with severe aortic regurgitation, is the impact of the jet stream created by the regurgitant aortic valve on the mitral valve, leading to the development of a secondary lesion that varies in character from erosion to perforation of a cusp; the regurgitant stream may occasionally cause rupture of the chordae tendineae.[199] Severe involvement of the mitral valve accentuates the left ventricular overload imposed by the aortic regurgitation and markedly exaggerates the heart failure.

Hemodynamically important valvular stenosis may result from infective endocarditis when the vegetations are unusually large, as in fungal infection, and obstruct the flow of blood to and from the left ventricle.[200, 201] One of the reasons for the development of congestive heart failure in patients with the Starr-Edwards prosthesis is progressive obstruction of the valvular outlet during the course of infection; this is most common when the invading organism is *Candida* or *Aspergillus* because of the characteristically large vegetations. The hemodynamic changes in aortic regurgitation produced by infective endocarditis have been evaluated by Mann and his colleagues.[202] They noted that the mean pulse pressure, left ventricular end-diastolic volume, and stroke volume were significantly smaller in patients who developed aortic regurgitation acutely than in those with the chronic condition.

Other Cardiac Complications

A number of intracardiac complications directly related to the valvular involvement may develop in the course of infective endocarditis and are much more common in the acute than in the subacute form of the disease.[183, 185] Some, but not all, are associated with rapid or progressive congestive heart failure, a change in the character of an existing murmur, or the appearance of a murmur not previously detected. Some of the complications result from disruption of the valves and their supporting structures. Among these are fenestration or tears of a leaflet, detachment of one or more areas of a valve from its annulus, and rupture of the chordae tendineae or papillary muscles. Another group of intracardiac complications includes the formation of fistulas, aneurysms (particularly of the sinus of Valsalva) that often involve the fibrous atrioventricular body, perforation of valve cusps, septal and other abscesses, and acute pericarditis with cardiac tamponade. In studies correlating anatomical and electrocardiographic abnormalities in 24 patients with aortic valve endocarditis. Roberts and Somerville found prolonged P-R intervals unrelated to digitalis therapy in 18 patients and atrioventricular dissociation in 4 patients.[203] In four of six patients with prolonged P-R intervals and in three of four with normal conduction and left bundle branch block, abscesses had invaded the interventricular septum; four out of six patients with prolonged conduction died suddenly.

MYOCARDIAL ABSCESSES. One of the most serious intracardiac complications of bacterial endocarditis is the development of myocardial abscesses (Fig. 34–8) that are thought to be present in about 20 per cent of patients who succumb to valvular infections.[204, 205] Abscesses occur most often when *Staph. aureus* and enterococci are involved and are rare when infection is caused by *Strep. viridans*. Multiple myocardial abscesses may be present, especially when coagulase-positive staphylococci cause the disease and when antimicrobial therapy is not instituted until relatively late in the course of infection. A single large abscess may be present and rupture into the pericardial sac, causing rapid death from the resulting pyohemopericardium (Fig. 34–2). Septal abscesses are not uncommon in patients with acute staphylococcal endocarditis. In some instances these completely destroy the involved area and produce a left-to-right shunt.

Abscesses of the interventricular septum secondary to infection of the mitral valve are usually located in the lower part of the septum. The presence of this complication may be suspected on the basis of serial changes in the electrocardiogram, consisting of a gradual increase in atrioventricular conduction time and eventually left bundle branch block; the right bundle is much less frequently involved. Recognition of this entity during life is of great importance because surgical removal of the abscess and its replacement by a patch may be life-saving. A much more serious threat because it is less often manageable surgically and is usually not suspected clinically is an abscess involving the upper portion of the interventricular septum that develops as a result of contiguous spread from an acutely

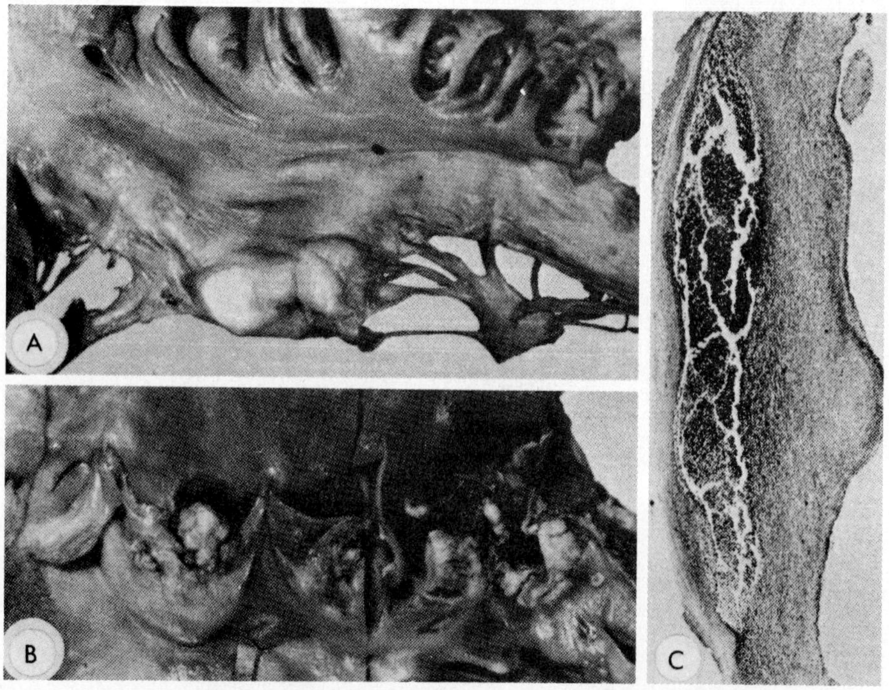

FIGURE 34–8. Pneumococcal endocarditis involving tricuspid (*A*) and aortic (*B*) valves. The vegetation on the tricuspid valve is small, whereas the vegetations on the aortic valve are large and cause extensive destruction of the cusps. *C*, Histological section of a portion of the tricuspid leaflet showing abscess formation. (From Roberts, W. C., and Buchbinder, N. A.: Right-sided valvular infective endocarditis. Am. J Med. *53*:7, 1972.)

infected aortic valve. In such cases the electrocardiographic changes are not as characteristic as in the lower septal lesions; the diagnosis is usually overlooked. However, the appearance of various types of arrhythmias, including varying degrees of heart block, especially complete block, should alert the physician to the possibility of this type of abscess. Surgical removal is required for cure. Septal abscess is a rare complication of subacute endocarditis, especially when caused by viridans streptococci.

A specific type of *intracardiac abscess* involving the valvular ring has been described by Arnett and Roberts in 27 patients who succumbed to infective endocarditis.[206] The aortic annulus was involved most often, and abscess of the atrioventricular ring was observed in a few instances. The following criteria were found to be of value in the diagnosis of abscesses of valvular rings: (a) infection of the aortic valve, (b) recent appearance of regurgitation, (c) the presence of pericarditis, (d) a high degree of atrioventricular block (complete in five cases and Mobitz type II in one case), and (e) short duration of symptoms, followed by the rapid development of severe disability and death. Abscess of the mitral and/or tricuspid and pulmonic valves may also complicate the course of endocarditis.

PERICARDITIS. This rare complication of the subacute type of infective endocarditis is not the result of bacterial invasion of the pericardial space in the vast majority of cases. It probably represents an immunological reaction, possibly deposition of immune complexes, in most instances. In contrast, the pericarditis that occasionally complicates the acute type of valvular infection is usually purulent and results from hematogenous deposition of organisms in the pericardial space or from rupture of a myocardial abscess into the sac (Fig. 34–2). Other causes of pericarditis in patients with infective endocarditis include erosion of a mycotic aneurysm of the sinus of Valsalva, extension of infection from the aortic valve into the pericardial wedge between the root of the aorta and the pulmonary artery, uremia, and reactivation of rheumatic fever during the course of endocarditis (Table 34–3).

MYOCARDITIS. Although its pathogenesis is unclear, many observers consider myocarditis one of the important complications of infective endocarditis.[207, 208] A recent study[209] has indicated that an immunological phenomenon may be involved. Antibodies to endocardium and sarcolemma are present in all patients with chronic infective endocarditis. The detection of such antibodies may indicate the presence of myocardial involvement before it is identified clinically or electrocardiographically. Only low levels of these antibodies are present in cases of acute endocarditis. The typical lesions associated with the myocarditis are the so-called Bracht-Wächter bodies (see earlier). Diffuse collections of lymphocytes or aggregations of polymorphonuclear leukocytes, with or without myocardial necrosis or miliary abscesses, are occasionally present. The myocardium may show areas of degeneration. Proliferation of the cells of capillaries and arterioles, arteriolitis or necrosis of the media or adventitia, and perivascular cellular infiltrations are detectable in some cases.

EMBOLIZATION. Although its incidence has decreased over the past 30 years, next to complications involving the heart itself, arterial embolization is the most common potentially serious complication of infective endocarditis. Emboli were clinically detected in 70 to 97 per cent of patients in the preantibiotic era but are now found in only 15 to 35 per cent.[1, 4, 189, 210, 211] The most common sites are the spleen, kidneys, coronary vessels, and brain, although almost every tissue and organ may be involved. Splenic emboli have been discovered at autopsy in 44 per cent of cases but are suspected only rarely during life. Renal infarcts have been detected in as many as 56 per cent of patients studied at necropsy but are recognized clinically less often.[212] Bell has reported embolic glomerular lesions in the kidneys of 52 per cent of patients with subacute and in 7 per cent of patients with acute bacterial endocarditis.[213] Myocardial infarction, often undetected by electrocardiography, has been found in 40 to 60 per cent of autopsied patients with valvular infections and is due to embolization of the coronary arterial bed. When the aortic valve is infected, infarction of the myocardium often leads to the development of congestive heart failure.[210, 214–216] Major cerebral emboli have been observed in almost one-third of patients with endocarditis at autopsy.[183] *Paradoxical embolization* may occur in the course of endocarditis, involving the tricuspid valve in patients with a patent foramen ovale.[217]

The middle cerebral artery and its branches are most frequently involved, and hemiplegia is the most frequent consequence.[183, 218] Jochman's dictum, "in hemiplegia in young adults or children always think of subacute bacterial endocarditis," is as applicable today as when it was first stated, in 1914.[219] Three per cent of all emboli to the brain arise from infections of the cardiac valves.[220] Embolic occlusion of cerebral vessels may be the presenting sign of endocarditis. The clinical manifestations resulting from this are discussed below. Embolization of the vascular supply of the spinal cord is rare; it usually produces girdle pain and paraplegia.[221] Weakness, peripheral neuropathy, nerve tenderness, sensory disturbances, and localized pain may develop when emboli invade supplying peripheral nerves.[222–224] Unilateral blindness resulting from embolization of the retinal artery, infarction of the retina with formation of a hole, and mononeuropathy may complicate valvular infections.[225]

Embolic occlusion of large arteries (e.g., the femoral) is rare in bacterial endocarditis; the most likely cause is fungal valvular disease or atrial myxoma. Large vegetations may also be present in an occasional case caused by *Staph. aureus*. The larger the vegetation, the higher the risk of embolization and vascular occlusion.[226] It is well known that embolic phenomena may occur weeks to months after the infectious process on the valve has been eradicated. This is probably because as long as 6 months may be required before the vegetations on the affected valve become covered by endothelium.

METASTATIC INFECTIONS

In the acute infection, especially that due to *Staph. aureus*, an abscess develops at every site at which an embolus is deposited. In most patients who succumb to staphylococcal endocarditis, abscesses are present in almost every organ and tissue. If such lesions are not present at other sites, they are practically always detected in the kidneys and myocardium; the abscesses are usually small. The clinical course of staphylococcal endocarditis complicated by multiple diffuse abscesses may often be sufficiently characteristic to be diagnostic. The distinguishing features are (a) defervescence early during antimicrobial therapy; (b) return of fever either during treatment or after it has been discontinued; (c) failure to respond to the drug given initially or to the administration of another "effective" agent; and (d) negative blood cultures. If organisms are recovered from the blood, they are frequently still sensitive to the drug used at the beginning of treatment.

In contrast, metastatic infection after deposition of emboli in the course of subacute endocarditis, particularly that caused by *Strep. viridans*, is distinctly rare, probably because the number of organisms in the embolus is small, the bacteria have a low invasive capability, and most patients with this type of infection have high titers of specific bactericidal antibody that, in the presence of normal serum levels of complement, rapidly kills the few streptococci that are deposited. Thus, although infarctions of the myocardium, brain, kidneys, and spleen develop in patients with subacute endocarditis, abscesses in these organs—suppurative myocarditis, pyogenic meningitis, splenic abscess, or pyelonephritis—are rare. However, a sterile meningitis, with the biochemical and cellular characteristics of so-called aseptic meningitis, or a syndrome consistent with diffuse encephalitis with an abnormal or normal cerebrospinal fluid, may occur in the subacute type of valvular infection and provide the first clue to the diagnosis, especially in cases where an audible murmur is not present.

MYCOTIC ANEURYSMS. Mycotic aneurysms are a major complication of infective endocarditis. Although they have probably not decreased in incidence over the years, as indicated by the results of studies of autopsied cases, they are now detected clinically less often and are not as frequently fatal as they were in the past. They have been reported to occur in about 2.5 per cent of patients with valvular infections[227] and constitute 2.5 to 6.2 per cent of *all* aneurysms involving the brain. These lesions usually develop during the active phase of the infectious process but may not become manifest for months to years after it has been eradicated. They are most common when relatively noninvasive organisms, such as *Strep. viridans*, are involved and are less frequent when *Staph. aureus* is the causative agent. Several mechanisms may be involved in their pathogenesis. Among these are injury produced by deposition of immune complexes in the arterial wall, embolic occlusion of the vasa vasorum and sterile infarction of a blood vessel (usually in subacute endocarditis), and direct invasion by organisms or deposition of bacteria-laden emboli, followed by infarction and the formation of an abscess in the vascular wall (common in acute infections). When mycotic aneurysms develop in the course of endocarditis owing to *Staph. aureus*, there is a high incidence of rupture at the area of involvement of the blood vessel. Although any artery may be the site of an aneurysm, the vessels most often involved are those in the brain; the sinuses of Valsalva; ligated ductus arteriosus; the abdominal aorta and its branches; and the coronary and pulmonary arteries.[212, 228] Among other areas in which mycotic aneurysms may develop in the course of infective endocarditis are the peripheral pulmonary[229] and intrapulmonary arteries,[230] primarily in drug addicts, the vessels of the lower extremities,[231] the small bowel,[232] the mitral valve leaflets,[233] and the mitral annulus.[234] The development of aneurysms is usually silent; clinical manifestations appear usually after the lesions have started to leak slowly or rupture and produce gross hemorrhages. When present in the brain, their pressure effects may produce headache or cranial nerve palsies. Areas in which mycotic aneurysms pose the greatest threat to life are the brain, abdominal aorta, the superior mesenteric, splenic and coronary arteries, and ligated ductus arteriosus.

NEUROLOGICAL COMPLICATIONS

Neurological complications occur in about 30 per cent of cases of infective endocarditis and are a major cause of death.[235] Embolization of the brain is the most common problem. The development of cerebral mycotic aneurysms, meningitis, meningoencephalitis, or abscesses of the brain is related to the deposition of infected emboli. Embolization occurs more frequently when the mitral valve is involved, especially when the infection is caused by a highly invasive organism (e.g., *Staph. aureus*). Mycotic aneurysms of the brain are more common and appear earlier in acute infective endocarditis and later in the subacute disease. The presence of hemorrhage in a patient with a cerebral mycotic aneurysm dictates the need for surgery. However, healing may occur in some instances in which the disease is produced by relatively nonvirulent bacteria, such as viridans streptococci. In such instances emboli produce sterile lesions in the brain and, for this reason, rupture much less frequently than when highly invasive bacteria are involved. The meningitis associated with acute endocarditis is usually purulent but most often aseptic when viridans streptococci are the causative agents. It is important to be aware that seizures in patients with endocarditis receiving penicillin may be caused by the drug, especially when it is administered in large doses to persons with normal renal function and in the usual quantities to those with an important degree of renal insufficiency.

Ziment[236] grouped the neurological manifestations of endocarditis on the basis of their cause as follows:

Toxic—headache, impaired concentration, drowsiness, insomnia, vertigo, and irritability

Psychiatric—neurosis, psychosis, confusion, disorientation, emotional instability, delirium, auditory and visual disturbances, apathy, and altered personality

Cerebrovascular—hemi-, di,- para-, or quadriplegia, sensory and motor aphasia, aphonia, stupor, and coma

Meningoencephalitis—acute brain syndrome

Cranial nerves—visual disturbances, palsies of various cranial nerves, pseudobulbar palsy, and sensory impairment

Dyskinesia—tremor, ataxia, parkinsonism, seizures, chorea, hemifacial dyskinesia, hiccupping, and myoclonus

Spinal cord or peripheral nerves—girdle pain, weakness, paraplegia, paresis, sensory disturbances, myalgia, and peripheral neuropathy

The brain may be the site of embolic abscesses in about 1 per cent of patients with subacute and in about 25 per cent of patients with acute infective endocarditis. Subdural empyema has also occurred. Ziment noted that encephalomalacia and endarteritis due to vasculitis of the cerebral arteries may be present. Petechiae and purpuric lesions may develop in the brain; they appear mostly in white matter adjacent to the lateral ventricles but also in the gray matter along the aqueduct and the corpus callosum. Meningeal or cerebral edema is present in some cases but usually produces no signs or symptoms. In addition to embolic retinal arterial occlusion, multiple retinal and conjunctival hemorrhages may develop. Other ocular complications of infective endocarditis are papilledema, iridocyclitis, panophthalmitis (usually in acute endocarditis), nystagmus, conjugate deviation of the eyes, and paresis of the third cranial nerve.

A study of the neurological complications observed in 281 cases of infective endocarditis admitted to the Massachusetts General Hospital has been reported by Pruitt et al.[237] Eighty-four patients (39 per cent) experienced neurological dysfunction during the course of the disease. The sex distribution of the cases was even; ages ranged from 3 months to 89 years, with most patients older than 50 years. The fatality rate was 58 per cent in those with manifestations of nervous system disorders, compared with 20 per cent in patients without neurological abnormalities. Neurological complications were most common with valvular infections caused by *Staph. aureus,* followed by streptococci, *Strep. pneumoniae*, and *Enterobacter.* Disturbances in function of the nervous system were noted in 79 of 84 patients with underlying cardiac valvular disease but in none with nonvalvular congenital heart disease.

Embolic cerebral infarction. This is the most common neurological complication of infective endocarditis. It occurs in 6 to 31 per cent of patients with this disease and is associated more often with infection of the mitral valve than that of the aortic valve. The infarctions are both macroscopic and microscopic. Emboli are present in other organs simultaneously with those in the brain in about half of cases. Cerebral infarction tends to occur within 2 weeks after the onset of valvular infection when highly invasive organisms, such as *Staph. aureus,* enterococci, and *E. coli*, are involved. When other bacteria, principally streptococci, produce the disease, cerebral infarctions develop in a biphasic manner and occur either 2 to 4 weeks or 1 to 3 months after the onset of the endocarditis. The fatality rate of cerebral infarction complicating infective endocarditis ranges from 17 to 81 per cent in patients who experience embolic strokes; approximately three-fourths die within 1 year after onset of their valvular infection.[237]

Mycotic aneurysms of cerebral arteries. These are present in 2 to 10 per cent of patients with infective endocarditis and account for 2.5 to 6.2 per cent of all intracranial aneurysms.[237] A study of 85 cases of endocarditis in which the presence of cerebral mycotic aneurysms was demonstrated by angiography indicated a fatality rate of 80 per cent in cases in which the lesions ruptured and 30 per cent in those in which it remained intact; the overall death rate was 46 per cent.[238] Multiple aneurysms were present in 15 patients (17.6 per cent). Sixty-five per cent of the aneurysms ruptured spontaneously.

Cerebral abscesses. These were noted at necropsy in 9 of the 218 patients (4.1 per cent); these lesions were not detected during life. In eight cases the abscesses were microscopic (< 1 cm^3). In six cases multiple microabscesses in the brain were associated with similar lesions in other organs.

MUSCULOSKELETAL SYSTEM

Involvement of the musculoskeletal system occurs in 44 per cent of patients with infective endocarditis.[239] In 27 per cent, symptoms and signs of dysfunction of the muscles or joints were the first, or among the first complaints. The most common manifestation was arthralgia. The shoulder joint was most often involved, followed, in descending order of frequency, by the knees, hips, wrists, ankles, and metatarsophalangeal and metacarpophalangeal joints. Multiple joints were affected in some cases. Objective evidence of arthritis was present in about one third of the cases. The ankle was most often involved, followed by the knees and wrists. Migrating polyarthritis was present in some instances. Pain in the lumbar area of the back, diffuse myalgias, and synovitis were also noted. Acute arthritis or arthralgia is present in 33 per cent of cases of gonococcal and 50 per cent of meningococcal endocarditis.

RENAL INVOLVEMENT

An excellent review of the gross and histological lesions of the kidneys in patients with infective endocarditis has been published by Feinstein and his associates.[240] Listed in Table 34–4 are the types of renal abnormalities present in association with valvular infection.

TABLE 34–4 RENAL COMPLICATIONS OF ENDOCARDITIS

Renal infarction.	Most common lesion; present in ⅔ of untreated cases. Occurs in 10 to 15% of right-sided endocarditis.
Focal glomerulonephritis.	Second most common lesion. Occurs in 50% of untreated cases and 15% of treated ones. May be associated with renal failure and nephrotic syndrome.
Diffuse glomerulonephritis.	30 to 60% of untreated cases and 10% in treated cases.
"Flea-bitten" kidney.	Multiple emboli and hemorrhages.
Renal abscess(es).	Usually with highly invasive organisms, e.g., *Staph. aureus.*
Cortical necrosis.	In patients with disseminated intravascular coagulation.
Renal lesions related to antimicrobial therapy.	Interstitial nephritis, toxic nephropathy, acute tubular necrosis. Renal failure may occur in the course of subacute endocarditis.[240]

IMMUNOLOGICAL PHENOMENA

IMMUNOGLOBULINS. Specific agglutinating, complement-fixing, and bactericidal antibodies and cryoglobulins are present in the serum of patients with infective endocarditis, especially the subacute form. *Hypergammaglobulinemia* has been demonstrated by Cordeiro et al.,[241] who noted an early increase in 19S and 7S globulins, followed by a rise in alpha$_2$-globulin. Immunoglobulins with specific affinities for the renal glomerular basement membrane, vascular walls, and myocardium of normal persons were present. In patients with subacute endocarditis, gamma globulin was fixed in the sarcolemma and myofibrils of the myocardium; in the walls of blood vessels, especially in the intima and subintima; in the cardiac valves and vegetations (Fig. 34–9), and in the basal layer of the glomeruli of the kidney.

Williams and Kunkel[242] described the presence of *rheumatoid factor* in the blood of patients with subacute infective endocarditis. They demonstrated positive latex fixation reactions in about 50 per cent of cases of the subacute type of endocardial infection, with high titers in most instances. The reactive factor was 19S globulin. With successful treatment, titers of circulating rheumatoid factor fell rapidly. The latex fixation test is positive in about 50 per cent of patients with valvular infections present for 6 or more weeks. Other immunological abnormalities detected in some patients with infective endocarditis are antinuclear antibody and depression of total hemolytic complement as well as both C_3 and C_4.[243] The presence of *circulating immune complexes* has been demonstrated by Bayer and his colleagues in 97 per cent of patients with infective endocarditis.[244] Blood levels of the complexes were greater than 12 μg/ml in all instances and were significantly higher than in patients with sepsis without endocarditis.

McKenzie and his colleagues[245] detected circulating immune complexes (IC) in 75 per cent of patients with valvular infections. This correlated with a subacute course and associated cutaneous vasculitis, glomerulonephritis, involvement of joints, and tissue deposits of immunoglobulins and complement. Serial determinations of IC were found to be useful in monitoring the activity of the disease in patients whose blood cultures were negative, and in those with continued extravalvular manifestations of activity of the disease. Levels of circulating immune complexes are low in patients with acute endocarditis.[246] Immune complexes have been detected in 45 per cent of cases of endocarditis in which cultures of the blood were negative.[247]

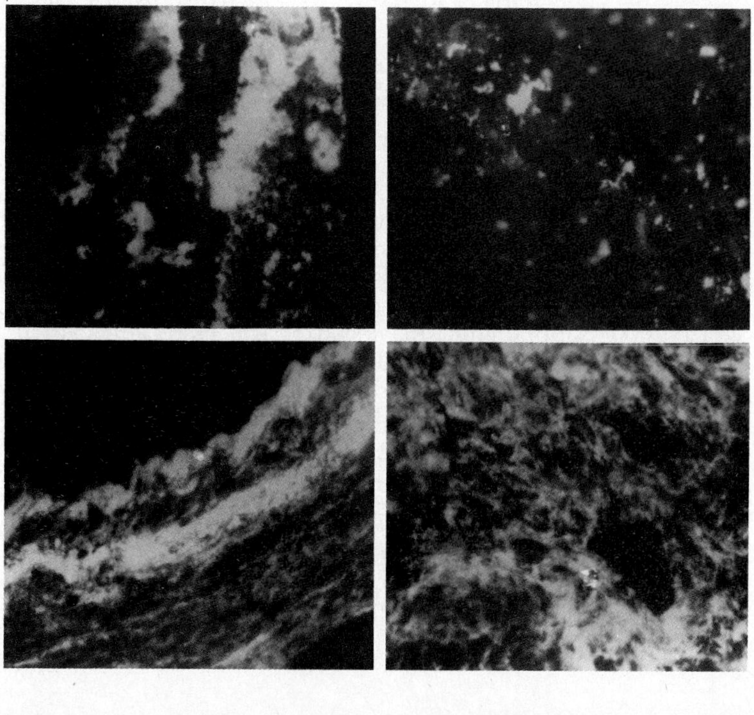

FIGURE 34–9. ***Top left,*** **Mitral valve vegetation from patient with infective endocarditis stained for human IgG. Extensive intravalvular and surface IgG is present (× 160).** ***Top right,*** **Infective endocarditis heart valve stained for IgM. Focal collections of IgM in areas of cellular inflammation are present (× 350).** ***Bottom left,*** **Valvular tissue from patient with infective endocarditis stained for C5b-C9 activated complement neoantigen, showing diffuse deposition on endocardium and subendocardial layer in area of intense chronic inflammatory cellular infiltrate (× 160).** ***Bottom right,*** **Infective endocarditis valvular vegetation stained with fluorescein-conjugated aggregates of IgG, showing diffuse interstitial deposition of rheumatoid factor in tissue (× 350). (From Williams, R. C., and Kilpatrick, K.: Immunofluorescence studies of cardiac valves in infective endocarditis. Arch. Intern. Med. *145*:297, 1985.)**

Immunofluorescence of valves removed at surgery from patients with infective endocarditis caused by viridans streptococcus has disclosed heavy intravalvular deposits of IgG and bacterial antigen in the vegetations and substance of the valve, much more focal interstitial IgM and C_3 in some areas, and diffuse endocardial and subendocardial deposits of C_3 and C_3 complement as well as neoantigens and large quantities of rheumatoid factor in the interstitium of the valve[248] (Fig. 34–9).

Immunological phenomena play a critical role throughout the course of subacute infective endocarditis. A prime factor involved in the pathogenesis of this syndrome is the gradual development of *specific agglutinating antibody* as a result of repeated episodes of transient bacteremia over a period of years. It has been suggested that this finally stimulates development of a sufficient level of agglutinin to cause conglutination of the small number of organisms present in a transient bacteremia and leads to deposition of a bacterial inoculum of sufficient size to initiate infection in the sterile platelet-fibrin clot. Until a high concentration of this antibody develops in the circulation over a period of years, usually as a result of multiple intrusions of organisms (most often *Strep. viridans*) infection does not occur because the bacteria are few in number, have low invasive capability, remain in the bloodstream for a short time (usually no longer than 5 to 10 minutes), and are rapidly eliminated by effective humoral and cellular clearing mechanisms.

CLINICAL MANIFESTATIONS OF IMMUNOLOGICAL ORIGIN. Several of the manifestations present during the early stage of subacute bacterial endocarditis are probably immunological in origin. *Roth spots* resemble the cytoid bodies that may appear in systemic lupus erythematosus and other vasculitides. *Janeway lesions* may represent an immunological reaction.[243] It has also been postulated that the pathology of *Osler nodes* is strongly suggestive of an Arthus reaction. Howard has demonstrated a perivasculitis in many tiny vessels in the malpighian layers, without evidence of emboli or bacteria in these lesions.[249] Alpert et al.[250] have isolated *Staph. aureus* and *Candida* from these lesions and have suggested, as did Kerr,[4, 212] that Osler nodes "are in all probability caused by minute emboli." The arthralgias of infective endocarditis are now also thought to be caused by deposition of immune complexes in the synovia; however, this has not been proved.

Sterile pericarditis, dermal vasculitis, deposition of immunoglobulin in blood vessels of normal skin, and leukocytoclastic angiitis of skin (purpuric lesions) may be related to disposition of immune complexes.[251, 252] The best-proved example of the operation of immunological reactions in the pathogenesis of complications of both acute and subacute valvular infection is acute, subacute, and chronic proliferative glomerulonephritis. These have been demonstrated in endocarditis caused by viridans streptococci as well as *Staph. aureus.*[253, 254] Gutman and his associates noted discrete deposits of fibrin containing IgG and complement in the basement membrane and/or in the mesangial region of the glomeruli. Antibody eluted from the kidney of a patient with subacute endocarditis who died of renal failure was shown by Levy and Hong to combine specifically with the bacteria cultured from the blood.[255] The elute also contained antiglomerular antibody and activated complement in the destroyed basement membrane. Lumpy-bumpy glomerular fluorescence, when stained for IgG and β_1C, has been demonstrated in patients with subacute endocarditis.[256]

ENDOCARDITIS INVOLVING THE RIGHT SIDE OF THE HEART

Infective endocarditis involving the right side of the heart is increasing in frequency, probably as a result of the widespread use of intravenous illicit drugs; it now accounts for about 5 to 10 per cent of all instances of valvular infections.[257] The tricuspid valve is infected most often. Isolated pulmonary valvular endocarditis, although occurring most often in the presence of congenital abnormalities of the heart, may occur in the absence of any congenital lesions. Both right-sided valves are infected in some cases. The clinical picture is dominated by extracardiac manifestations. Pneumonia or pulmonary emboli occur in 60 to 100 per cent of patients with involvement of the tricuspid valve, while splenomegaly, hematuria, renal failure, and peripheral stigmata are uncommon. Combined tricuspid and mitral endocarditis in a patient with a ventricular septal defect has been described.[258]

Two-thirds of the cases of right-sided endocarditis studied at the Mayo Clinic were acute, with prominent pulmonary manifestations; murmurs, splenomegaly, or multiple cutaneous and renal abscesses were present in about one-third of cases.[258a] Blood cultures were usually positive. *Staph. aureus* was isolated in half the cases; *Strep. pneumoniae, N. gonorrhoeae*, streptococci (*viridans, faecalis,* and *pyogenes*), and gram-negative bacilli have also been recovered. Hearts with congenital malformations or normal ones are most often involved. Infections of skin wounds, respiratory tract (*Strep. pneumoniae*), and urethra; prostatic massage; dental sepsis; normal parturition; septic abortion; and narcotic addiction are among the reported pathogenetic factors.[258a, 259] In 80 per cent of the cases with tricuspid valve involvement a murmur was not heard, and the diagnosis was not suspected during life.[258a] Renal involvement, most commonly abscesses or diffuse pyelonephritis, was present in 65 per cent of patients. Glomerular and tubular hemorrhage and focal embolic glomerulonephritis have also been noted. In congenita lesions with exclusive or predominant left-to-right shunts, defects of the interventricular septum, or patent ductus arteriosus complicated by endocarditis, emboli are deposited almost exclusively in the lungs early in the course of the disease and may produce hemoptysis, pleurisy, or pneumonia[260]; systemic embolization may occur later.

Myocarditis is one of the complications of endocarditis involving the right side of the heart. Histologically, this consists of small foci of perivascular collections of polymorphonuclear leukocytes or diffuse infiltrates with the same type of cell or miliary abscesses. The lungs are the primary site for the deposition of emboli, resulting in the development of single or multiple *pulmonary infarcts*. If the infecting organisms are relatively avirulent (e.g., *Strep. viridans*), the infarcted areas will only rarely be infected. In contrast, when a highly invasive bacterium, such as *Staph. aureus*, is the causative agent, the infarcts are almost always infected and are rapidly converted to abscesses. Other pulmonary complications include pneumonia, thrombosis, and septic arteritis of the branches of the pulmonary artery. Among the *renal complications* of endocarditis involving the right side of the heart are suppurative nephritis, focal or diffuse proliferative glomerular nephritis, and tubular hemorrhages.

The sequential appearance of repeated episodes of "pneumonia" (infarcts of the lung), followed by hepatomegaly, often associated with a mild degree of jaundice, and finally the development of progressive renal failure in patients with persistent fever, should raise the possibility of infection of the right heart, even in the absence of a murmur. Blood cultures are frequently negative when relatively noninvasive organisms are involved. However, when infectious process is caused by *Staph. aureus*, blood culture is often positive *after* the development of infected pulmonary infarcts, which become the source of bacteria entering the systemic circulation. Causes of death in untreated persons with involvement of the right side of the heart, and even in some who receive appropriate therapy, are multiple pulmonary infarcts and abscesses and cardiac failure.

INFECTIVE ENDOCARDITIS IN CHILDREN

(See also p. 906)

An analysis by Zakrzewski and Keith of 50 cases of infective endocarditis in children has indicated that underlying rheumatic heart disease is an uncommon predisposing factor[261]; the most common one appears to be the tetralogy of Fallot, followed in order of frequency by congenital aortic stenosis, patent ductus arteriosus, and pulmonic stenosis. There is a striking difference in the factors that predispose to valvular infection in children and adults. In children, these include severe burns, osteomyelitis, asthma, bronchitis, infection of the urinary tract, otitis media, thrombophlebitis, pneumonia, pansinusitis, diarrhea, dermatitis, circumcision, and acute rheumatic fever.

A difference in the frequency of specific organisms responsible for endocarditis in children was noted by Zakrzewski and Keith in a comparison of cases studied from 1952 to 1961 and those observed between 1958 and 1962.[261] *Staph. aureus* was responsible for 37 per cent and *Strep. viridans* for 32 per cent in the first period; in the latter one *Staph. aureus* and *epidermidis* caused 72 per cent, whereas *Strep. viridans* was involved in about 20 per cent; the marked increase in staphylococcal valvular disease is undoubtedly related to the greater frequency of cardiac surgery.

Infective endocarditis in infants younger than 2 years of age, most of whom were only a few weeks or months old, was characterized by a number of features that distinguish it from that involving older children[148]; all cases were of the acute type and involved more than one valve. Congenital heart disease was present in only 8 per cent. About 60 per cent had infection of the mitral valve; the tricuspid valve was affected in 32 per cent, the aortic valve in 17 per cent, and the pulmonic valve in 6.5 per cent. Embolic phenomena were present in only 18 per cent. In every instance there was evidence of disease at extracardiac sites. Among these were infections of the skin, enteritis, empyema, osteomyelitis, and tuberculosis. Diagnosis of endocarditis in these infants was usually made post mortem.

An extensive review of 149 instances of bacterial endocarditis in 141 children studied at the Children's Hospital Medical Center in Boston has been presented by Johnson and coworkers.[262] Six of the patients had two and one had three episodes of the disease. Predisposing factors, in order of frequency, included infected extracardiac foci (urinary tract infection, meningitis, and osteomyelitis), dental manipulation, cardiac surgery, catheterization, and orthopedic and otolaryngological surgical procedures. The most common underlying types of heart disease were congenital (118 cases) and rheumatic (14 cases). There were no significant disorders of the heart in 17 patients. The most frequent underlying lesion was the tetralogy of Fallot; the others, in order of incidence, were ventricular septal defect, aortic stenosis, rheumatic heart disease, patent ductus arteriosus, and transposition of the great arteries. Blood cultures were sterile in 19 children. Presenting clinical manifestations consisted of fever (87 per cent), splenomegaly (65 per cent), petechiae (42 per cent), and heart failure (34 per cent). In 21 per cent heart murmurs were present and underwent changes during the course of the disease. The most frequent complication was congestive heart failure; others included central nervous system disorders, pulmonary emboli, and aortic regurgitation.

Stanton et al.[263] have pointed out that there has been a change in the spectrum of infective endocarditis in children. Any analysis of the syndrome as it appeared before the 1970's and was reported during the next 10 years disclosed a number of important differences. A large proportion of the more recently reported patients developed endocarditis postoperatively, and a number of children developed valvular infections after they underwent cardiac catheterization. All instances of endocarditis in children with normal hearts were associated with the presence of intravenous catheters. The organisms most commonly responsible for the disease were viridans streptococci and staphylococci. Complications developed in 58 per cent of the children.

A recent report from the Mayo Clinic[264] noted that the fatality rate in infective endocarditis was particularly high in children younger than 10 years; the poor prognosis of endocarditis in neonates has been reemphasized.[265] Mycotic aneurysms continue to be strikingly uncommon in children with this infection.[266]

PROSTHETIC VALVE ENDOCARDITIS

The clinical features of infection of prosthetic valves are, for the major part, the same as those that characterize endocarditis involving natural valves. Infection of the surgical wound in the sternum, or sternal osteomyelitis, is a common predisposing factor for early prosthetic valve endocarditis. Variations in the period of time elapsing between operation and the onset of prosthetic infection were discussed earlier (p. 1095). The development of fever associated with or following detection of a new heart murmur suggestive of a paravalvular leak suggests the presence of endocarditis.

Several complications are peculiar to prosthetic valvular endocarditis. One is associated primarily with the presence of a ball-type prosthesis, especially the Starr-Edwards valve (Fig. 34–3), and consists of the gradual development of congestive heart failure owing to progressive obstruction of the outlet of the valve by growth of bacteria or, more commonly, yeasts or fungi. Paravalvular leak caused by a valve ring abscess in patients with mechanical prostheses may lead to heart failure subsequent to progressive valvular regurgitation. In patients with bioprostheses, destruction of the valve leaflets themselves may cause regurgitation. Another complication of endocarditis of prosthetic valves, which is shared by patients addicted to intravenously administered drugs, is an increased incidence of embolization of large arteries owing to the greater frequency of fungal colonization and infection. Persistent elevation of temperature in patients with valvular prostheses, in the absence of another cause and either a change in an existing murmur or the development of a new one, together with sterile cultures of blood, is highly suggestive of an abscess in the annulus, frequently at the site of one or more of the sutures anchoring the prosthesis, leading to severe valvular regurgitation. Synthetic materials used to close septal defects may also become infected.

Endocarditis During Pregnancy and the Puerperium

Endocarditis is an uncommon complication of pregnancy; however, Libman and Friedberg pointed out that bacterial endocarditis may occur during pregnancy or shortly after childbirth.[184] They suggested that, in the presence of pelvic inflammatory disease, a transient bacteremia occurring during labor and delivery might be followed by subacute endocarditis in women with underlying cardiac disease. Although the organisms most often involved are viridans streptococci and *Staph. aureus*, *Listeria monocytogenes* and *Chlamydia* may also be responsible. Blood cultures may be sterile. If the uterus becomes infected during the puerperium (puerperal sepsis), especially when the infection is exogenous in origin, the endocarditis may be of the acute type because of the high frequency with which *Strep. pyogenes* is the responsible organism.

Among unusual organisms reported as causes of endocarditis during pregnancy are *Haemophilus aphrophilus, Listeria monocytogenes, Salmonella entertidis,* group B streptococcus, *Strep. anaerobius,* and *Chlamydia trachomatis.*[266a]

Diabetics and Elderly Patients

Endocarditis is more common in patients with diabetes mellitus than in those free of this disease,[266b] and a primary extracardiac focus of infection plays an important role in the pathogenesis of endocarditis in diabetics. Diabetics with staphylococcal bacteremia are more likely to develop endocarditis than are nondiabetics.

The organisms most often responsible for infective endocarditis in elderly patients are streptococci.[266c] *Strep. bovis is the most common cause of the disease* in the elderly. This is of great clinical importance because of the association of endocardial infection by this organism with colonic cancer. *Staph. aureus* and *Staph. epidermidis* are involved in 20 to 30 per cent of community-acquired cases; gram-negative organisms are common when the disease develops nosocomially (hospital or nursing home).

RELAPSE AND RECURRENCE OF INFECTIVE ENDOCARDITIS

Early or intercurrent relapses are defined as the development of manifestations of infection together with positive blood cultures that appear within 3 months of completion of treatment with antimicrobial agents. Among the factors responsible are (a) superinfection (by an organism different from the one initially present) often associated with the use of "broad-spectrum" antibiotics; (b) spread, by way of the circulation, of a drug-resistant bacterium or fungus from an extracardiac site such as a colonized intravenous catheter, suppurative thrombophlebitis, or infection of the urinary tract; (c) the development of resistance of the organism initially responsible for the disease; and (d) the appearance of "cell wall–deficient" organisms ("persisters"), especially when drugs that inhibit the synthesis of the bacterial cell wall (penicillins, cephalosporins) are administered. This last factor has been suggested, but its importance in intercurrent relapses remains to be proved.

A syndrome that appears to be an early relapse but is actually due to an intracardiac or extracardiac complication occasionally occurs in patients with endocarditis caused by *Staph. aureus.* As pointed out above (p. 1107), the development of abscesses in one or more other organs is usually accompanied by a return of fever and bacteremia after a period of what appears to be a satisfactory therapeutic response; however, this is not due to relapse of infection in the affected valve.

Late relapse is defined as return of all the features of active endocarditis 3 to 6 months or longer after antimicrobial treatment has led to apparent "cure" of the infection. The causative agent of the relapse may be different from or the same as the one initially responsible for the valvular disease. Late relapse is relatively common in patients with endocarditis caused by yeasts or fungi. The reasons for this are (a) relative insensitivity of the organism to the drug used for treatment, (b) failure of the antifungal agent to penetrate the valvular lesion to a depth great enough to eradicate all the organisms, and (c) spread of the infection to sites in the heart contiguous to the affected valve. Late relapses are also quite common when endocarditis involves prosthetic valves, and the causative agent is often the one initially involved. However, in some instances the initial bacterial infection may be followed, either during treatment or within 6 months, by invasion of the prosthesis by a fungus or yeast, especially when combined broad-spectrum antimicrobial therapy is given.

RECURRENT ENDOCARDITIS. This is defined as the reappearance of all the cardinal manifestations of infective endocarditis and positive blood cultures later than 6 months after cure of the initial episode. It may be caused by the same organism that produced the first episode but is often due to a different bacterium or fungus. A mechanism that may be responsible for recurrent endocarditis has been suggested by Welton and his colleagues.[267] They noted that bacteria frequently persist in healed valvular lesions for longer than 10 months after a clinical "cure" had been accomplished by means of appropriate chemotherapy and compared this situation with "inactive" tuberculosis. The incidence of recurrent endocarditis has been reported to range from 2 to 8 per cent. Patients with prosthetic valves may experience recurrent infections over a period of months or years. The author has studied one patient who experienced a mixture of five relapses and recurrences. The first involved a natural valve; the others were infections of various types of valvular prostheses, each of which was removed. A different organism was responsible for each of the episodes.

LABORATORY FINDINGS

Elevation of the erythrocyte sedimentation rate is the most common and almost universal abnormal laboratory finding in infective endocarditis. It may be as high as 100 mm/hr. or more (Westergren method) in a few cases. *Anemia* is present in from 50 to 80 per cent of patients with this disease when they first come to medical attention and may be severe. The characteristics of the anemia are those observed in all types of infection.

In subacute infective endocarditis the *white blood count,* in most instances, does not exceed 7000 to 8000 mm^3. However, in almost all cases there is a shift to the left, and a small percentage of "band" forms is the rule. In contrast, leukocytosis, with white blood counts ranging from 15,000 to 20,000/mm^3 or higher, with a shift to the left when the acute disease is present. However, a normal white blood count and even leukopenia may be present in the acute infection.

Hyperstimulation of the reticuloendothelial system, as evidenced by an *increase in the number of plasma cells in the bone marrow,* is common in subacute endocarditis. Large lymphocytic cells, histiocytes, are detectable in the capillary blood in 15 to 25 per cent of the subacute cases. These are usually not present in the peripheral blood but are demonstrable in blood obtained from a fingertip or earlobe.

Although *thrombocytopenia* due to disseminated intravascular coagulation occurs as a rare complication of acute bacterial endocarditis, this may be an infrequent, isolated finding in both the subacute and acute types of valvular infection.

The *urine* is normal in uncomplicated cases of infective endocarditis. In some instances *proteinuria* may be the only abnormality and is often related to the presence of fever. Red blood cells in the urine usually indicate renal infarction. *Hematuria, red blood cell casts,* and *proteinuria* suggest acute proliferative glomerulonephritis.

DIAGNOSIS

CLINICAL FEATURES. The characteristic features, especially of the subacute form of infective endocarditis, have undergone such remarkable changes since the introduction of antibiotics more than 40 years ago that if present day physicians relied on the clinical diagnostic criteria established in the years preceding 1950, the disease would not be suspected in 90 per cent or more of the cases.[1, 190, 268] Thus, as already pointed out, Osler nodes, Janeway lesions, and Roth spots have become quite uncommon. Even subungual hemorrhages and petechiae are seen only occasionally now.

The most striking feature of infective endocarditis in the antibiotic era is the increasing frequency with which *cardiac murmurs are absent* in both acute and subacute forms of the disease. Forty years ago the absence of a murmur was considered to rule out subacute endocarditis. Now an increasing number of patients with this type of infection have no detectable murmur when first seen; the diagnosis is usually suspected on the basis of multiple positive blood cultures, the absence of any other source of infection and, quite often, the development of an embolic complication. In most of these patients a murmur develops during the course of treatment; in a few it does not become detectable until 2 to 3 months after cure is accomplished and is not related to recurrence of the infection; in a rare instance a murmur may never develop. The increased number of patients who do not have murmurs when they first come to medical attention is due, in part, to the higher frequency of acute endocarditis involving the left side of the heart and acute or subacute infection of the tricuspid valve. These forms of endocarditis are characterized by absence of a murmur in about one-third of cases early in the course of the disease.

Most physicians are still under the impression that a change in the character of the murmur is common in infective endocarditis and that this is a diagnostic feature of the disease. This is rarely the case in subacute valvular infection. It is, however, common in patients in whom the process is acute. The cause of the change is practically always destruction of the valve and its supporting structures. Common in patients with staphylococcal endocarditis involving the aortic valve is the sudden appearance of a loud diastolic blowing murmur related to the development of aortic regurgitation. Less common, but also responsible for a change in murmur in the acute disease, is rupture of the chordae tendineae or papillary muscles or separation of a leaflet of the valve from the annulus. In patients with prosthetic valves the appearance of a murmur or a change in one already present is often associated with a paravalvular leak that may or may not be induced by infection.

One of the most difficult diagnostic problems is presented by the older patient known to have had a grade 2/6 or 3/6 basal systolic murmur for years, who develops fever, whose blood culture may or may not be positive, and who presents with none of the peripheral manifestations of infective endocarditis. This type of murmur is usually caused by calcific, degenerative changes in the aortic valve (p. 1055), or it may be due only to the widening and tortuosity of the aorta associated with aging. Often the diagnosis of valvular infection is not seriously considered in such persons, especially when blood cultures are negative. A similar problem is encountered with younger patients in whom a grade 2 "ejection" or "flow" murmur is considered "innocent," whereas, in fact, it represents a valvular abnormality on which either acute or subacute infection may become superimposed.

The availability of effective antimicrobial agents has resulted in an important diagnostic problem, which, if not appreciated, may lead to potentially life-threatening complications of subacute infective endocarditis. Typically, the patient seeks medical attention because of fever. Despite detection of a murmur, blood cultures are not carried out, but oral therapy with an antibiotic is initiated. In the person with valvular infection caused by an organism susceptible to the drug administered, defervescence often occurs within 4 to 5 days. However, when the fever is the only manifestation of endocarditis, it usually returns about 7 to 10 days after treatment has been discontinued. This usually leads to another visit to the physician, who often makes a diagnosis of "viral infection" and reinstitutes treatment with the antibiotic that had previously reduced the elevated temperature. Such short periods of exposure to one or more antimicrobial agents may be repeated several times before it becomes apparent that the patient is becoming increasingly ill, or until an embolic episode, heart failure, or some other complication develops, when the patient is finally hospitalized, blood samples are cultured, and the diagnosis is established. This course of events in a patient with fever and cardiac murmur is so highly suggestive of infective endocarditis that a full course of antimicrobial therapy with bactericidal agents should be instituted even when multiple blood cultures prove to be sterile. Each recurrence of fever, because it represents the recrudescence of the valvular infection, adds to the valvular damage.

BLOOD CULTURES. The sine qua non for the diagnosis of infective endocarditis is recovery of the causative organism from the blood.

Whether or not bacteria or other infectious agents are grown depends on a number of factors, some of which are technical and some of which involve specific clinical and immunological phenomena.[269] It is now clear that the bacteremia of endocarditis is qualitatively continuous but quantitatively discontinuous (i.e., organisms are probably always present but their numbers vary considerably). This is illustrated by the study of Beeson et al.,[270] who showed that only about 3 per cent of blood cultures of patients with subacute valvular infections contained more than 100 organisms per milliliter. The incidence of positive blood cultures, as recorded by various observers, has varied considerably. Werner and his colleagues obtained positive cultures in 95 per cent of 789 cultures in 206 patients.[271] The first culture of the blood of persons with streptococcal endocarditis was positive in 95 per cent of the cases; one of the first two cultures yielded the causative agent in 98 per cent. When infection was caused by organisms other than streptococcus, positive cultures were obtained in only 82 per cent. The bacteremia was commonly of "low magnitude"; only 17 per cent of the blood samples contained more than 100 organisms per milliliter. Others have reported an incidence of positive blood cultures ranging from 53 to 74 per cent.[271, 272] Belli and Waisbren noted that the organism responsible for the valvular infection could be isolated from one of the three initial blood cultures in only 82 per cent of their patients.[273] Differences in the colony counts in blood collected from different arterial and venous sites were noted by Beeson and his coworkers.[270] In general, mixed venous blood entering the heart contained about 35 per cent fewer colonies than did arterial blood. Despite this finding, a number of other observers have noted no advantage in culture of arterial over venous blood in establishing the presence of clinically significant bacteremia in cases of infective endocarditis.

Recovery of *Staph. aureus* from the bloodstream always raises the problem of distinguishing endocarditis from uncomplicated bacteremia, especially in the absence of a murmur, a situation present in about one-third of patients early in the course of endocardial infection.[274] In patients with fungal endocarditis, especially when the causative agent is *Aspergillus*, blood cultures are frequently negative. However, the fungus responsible for the valvular infection may often be recovered from an embolus that lodges in a large artery—a relatively frequent occurrence in this type of disease.

NEGATIVE CULTURES. A number of factors responsible for failure to recover bacteria from the peripheral circulation of patients with infective endocarditis has been identified by Van Scoy[275] and others.[276] These are presented in

TABLE 34–5 CATEGORIES OF APPARENT CULTURE-NEGATIVE ENDOCARDITIS

1. Noninfective endocarditis
2. Prior antimicrobial treatment
3. "Fastidious" bacteria
4. Q fever
5. Fungi
6. Acid-fast bacteria
7. *Chlamydia*
8. ? L forms of bacteria
9. ? Virus
10. Right-sided endocarditis
11. Uremia

Adapted from Van Scoy, R. E.: Culture-negative endocarditis. Mayo Clin. Proc. 57:149–154, 1982.

Table 34–5. An increasingly important reason for the greater frequency of negative blood cultures is treatment with one or more antimicrobial agents before the diagnosis is established.[277, 278] As short a period of exposure to an antibiotic as 2 days may make it impossible to retrieve organisms from the blood, despite the fact that they are still present on the vegetations.

It is impossible to state categorically, in any patient, how long it would take for blood rendered sterile by an antimicrobial agent to yield organisms after cessation of treatment. In some instances, especially when the period of treatment has been only 2 to 3 days, cultures may become positive 48 hours after the drug has been withdrawn. In contrast, when an antiinfective compound has been administered for longer periods, cultures may not become positive until a week or more after its use has been discontinued. Because of this, patients who are suspected on clinical grounds of having infective endocarditis and who have been treated must no longer receive the drug. Culturing of the blood should be initiated 24 to 48 hours after therapy has been withdrawn. If results are negative, cultures should not be repeated until 7 to 10 days have elapsed. If the blood is still sterile at that time, a factor other than the antimicrobial therapy, the presence of an unusual organism, or a diagnosis other than infective endocarditis should be considered. When subacute bacterial endocarditis is present, there is no real danger in delaying therapy for as long as a week, since (1) if, as in the bulk of instances, fever is absent, the patient has already been partially treated, and (2) early death is not related to the infectious process, but to a potentially lethal embolic episode—an unpredictable event that is not prevented by the most effective antimicrobial therapy. This is not true in acute endocarditis, in which a delay of 24 to 48 hours in initiating treatment may be seriously life-threatening.

In a number of cases, technical factors, including the use of inadequate quantities of blood or medium, improper timing of the culture, too small a number of specimens, and inappropriate incubation, are responsible for failure to recover the causative agent from patients with infective endocarditis. Because the number of organisms in the blood is small and variable, the optimal quantity drawn should be no less than 10 ml, in order to furnish an inoculum adequate to initiate bacterial growth. Many patients, especially those who have had the subacute form of the disease, have moderate concentrations of bactericidal antibody or have received treatment with minimal doses of an orally administered antibiotic; therefore, the quantity of medium into which a single specimen of blood is inoculated should be 100 ml. The optimal ratio of blood to medium is about 1:10. This may sufficiently dilute the quantity of circulating antibody or antibiotic to inhibit antibacterial activity. Clearly the quantity of blood drawn cannot always be 10 ml, particularly since several cultures are required to establish the diagnosis; this presents the greatest problem in young children. In such cases the ratio of blood to medium should still be at least 1:10. It must be stressed, however, that the quantity of blood obtained should be maximum for a given clinical situation.

TECHNIQUES. There has been considerable discussion concerning the optimal time for drawing blood and the number of cultures required to establish the presence of endocarditis. A single positive culture is of no diagnostic value because, regardless of the nature of the organism recovered, it may represent contamination. The minimal number of cultures of the blood required to establish the presence of infective endocarditis has been reported by Belli and Waisbren to be five.[273] Probably the best time for obtaining a blood culture is 2 hours before the temperature begins to rise. This is based on the well-established observation that this is the period required for bacterial endotoxin to stimulate the production of endogenous pyrogen by neutrophilic leukocytes and macrophages. However, this is not always practical. The author uses the following approach to timing and number of blood cultures. Temperature is monitored, from a normal level, every hour until about 1° F of fever is present. At this point a specimen is drawn every 5 to 10 minutes until six samples have been obtained. In most instances three or more of these will be positive; a similar approach the next day usually yields the same results. If the first six cultures are all negative, all succeeding sets of the same number are usually also sterile.

All blood obtained must be cultured aerobically and anaerobically. Because about 10 per cent of cases of infective endocarditis are caused by microaerophilic streptococci and a small number are caused by strict anaerobes such as *Peptostreptococcus, Peptococcus,* or *Bacteroides,* it is imperative that the blood also be incubated anaerobically. Some organisms (e.g., *N. gonorrhoeae, N. meningitidis,* and *Brucella abortus*) grow best in an atmosphere of 5 to 10 per cent carbon dioxide. "Nutritionally deficient" streptococci require pyridoxine for growth. The presence of *H. influenzae* in the blood will be overlooked unless Levinthal liquid medium or chocolate agar is used for culture. If cell wall–deficient organisms are suspected, culture of the blood in an osmotically stable medium is required; on repeated subculture these bacteria may revert to the parent cell wall–containing form.

Inappropriate periods of incubation may be responsible for "negative" blood cultures when some organisms are involved. Although most bacteria grow in cultures of blood within a few days to a week, some require a considerably longer period. Cultures for *Brucella* may not become positive until after 4 to 6 weeks of incubation. Growth of many common organisms, including most of the fungi involved in endocarditis, may be delayed for a week or longer in cases in which antibiotics have been administered.

SEROLOGICAL TESTS. A positive serological test may be of value in establishing the diagnosis of infective endocarditis. Examples of this are *Coxiella burnetii, Chlamydia, Brucella, Cryptococcus,* and *Candida.*

The importance of serological tests for teichoic acid in establishing the diagnosis of valvular infection caused by *Staph. aureus* has been demonstrated.[279]

Concomitant elevation of IgG and IgM antibody levels has been demonstrated by Wheat et al.[280] in 50 per cent of patients with endocarditis or complicated bacteremia. These antibodies were detected in only about 5 per cent of cases of other types of staphylococcal infections and in about 3 per cent of normal persons. Antibody to the peptidoglycan of *Staph. aureus* has been detected in 50 to 100 per cent of patients with endocarditis caused by this organism.[281, 282] Shanson et al. have reported that detection of elevated titers of fluorescent antibody for viridans streptococci distinguishes endocarditis from bacteremia without cardiac involvement.[283] Serological studies in patients with candidal endocarditis have indicated that persisting or rising levels of precipitating or agglutinating antibodies, or both, whether or not associated with candidemia, signal invasion of prosthetic valves by the organism.[284]

SCINTILLATION SCANNING. Scanning of the heart with gallium-67 appears to be of diagnostic value in some instances of infective endocarditis. Scintillation scanning of the precordial region 2 to 7 days after the intravenous administration of 3 mc of the radionuclide has been reported to yield positive results in seven persons, three of which were confirmed by postmortem imaging at autopsy.[285] The scans were negative at 48 hours and positive from 3 to 8 days after injection. Fifteen patients without endocarditis, who served as controls, showed no uptake of the isotope in the region of the myocardium 48 or more hours after it was injected. A ventricular abscess in a patient was first suspected on the basis of a positive gallium-67 scan[286]; the disadvantages of this approach to the diagnosis of infective endocarditis are an insufficient degree of resolution to indicate the site of infection, the length of time (48 hours) required for localization of the radionuclide, and a 40 per cent incidence of false-negative results.[287]

ELECTROCARDIOGRAPHY. Changes in the electrocardiogram are not diagnostic in uncomplicated infective endocarditis. However, as pointed out earlier (p. 1107), this approach is helpful in that incomplete or complete heart block, bundle branch block, and premature ventricular contractions are associated with septal abscesses or myocarditis.[287] The author recommends serial electrocardiography every 48 hours in all cases of acute endocarditis, especially when caused by *Staph. aureus.* This permits early identification of septal abscess and the need for surgical removal of the lesion. The anatomical relation of the noncoronary cusp of the aortic valve and the mitral annulus to the conduction apparatus has been considered responsible for the development of abnormalities of conduction and is of some value in localizing the site of the lesion.

RADIOGRAPHY. Radiological findings in patients with endocarditis involving the left side of the heart are usually not impressive until destruction of the affected valve is so far advanced that congestive failure develops.[288] There are no diagnostic radiographic abnormalities in cases in which the right side of the heart is involved until pulmonary infarction, with or without infection, develops.

ECHOCARDIOGRAPHY (See also p. 111)

Echocardiography provides another approach to the diagnosis of infective endocarditis and some of its intracardiac complications (Figs. 5–53, p. 107; 5–63, p. 111; and 5–64, p. 112). An increasing number of studies have pointed out the limitations of this technique, the features that permit recognition of the specific valve involved, as well as the characteristics of specific complications.[289]

An evaluation of the diagnostic effectiveness of echocardiography by Amsterdam[290] indicated that two-dimensional echocardiography detects 50 to 80 per cent of cases of infective endocarditis. The factors important for the detection of valvular vegetations are the size of the lesion (3 mm or larger), its intracardiac location, duration of the disease for at least 2 weeks (vegetations are usually not seen before this), the presence of abscess of the myocardium or valvular ring, and aneurysm of the sinus of Valsalva. Echocardiography is also valuable in identifying flutter of the ventricular septum and flail leaflets. Doppler echocardiography may be of value in detecting early valvular regurgitation and in assessing the severity of regurgitation; patients may be followed serially and the decision in favor of surgical treatment may be made if valvular regurgitation is progressive.

The limitation of echocardiography is its nonspecificity; the presence of vegetations is associated with abnormalities similar to those observed with rupture of the chordae tendineae, flail valvular leaflets, nodular thickening of the leaflets, and the presence of valvular tumors.

The value of echocardiography in staphylococcal infection of the aortic valve has been reported by Fox and his colleagues.[291] "Shaggy" echoes were recorded from the aortic leaflets in diastole as well as irregular diastolic densities in the left ventricular outflow tract, suggesting that the infection caused flailing of the aortic leaflets. Echocardiographic detection of flail aortic leaflets and premature closure of the mitral valve indicated the need for immediate replacement of the aortic valve.

Of 14 patients with endocarditis involving the aortic valve studied by Berger et al.,[292] 12 had vegetations demonstrated by two-dimensional echocardiography; in the others the presence of the disease was identified anatomically. This technique was found to be superior to the M-mode in determining the size, shape, and movement of the vegetations. The authors summarized their findings as follows: "In those patients with negative two-dimensional echocardiograms, the vegetations were 3 mm in diameter or less at surgery or autopsy. Vegetations that were visualized on two-dimensional echocardiography (Fig. 34–10) were found to be at least 5 mm in diameter at the time of operation."

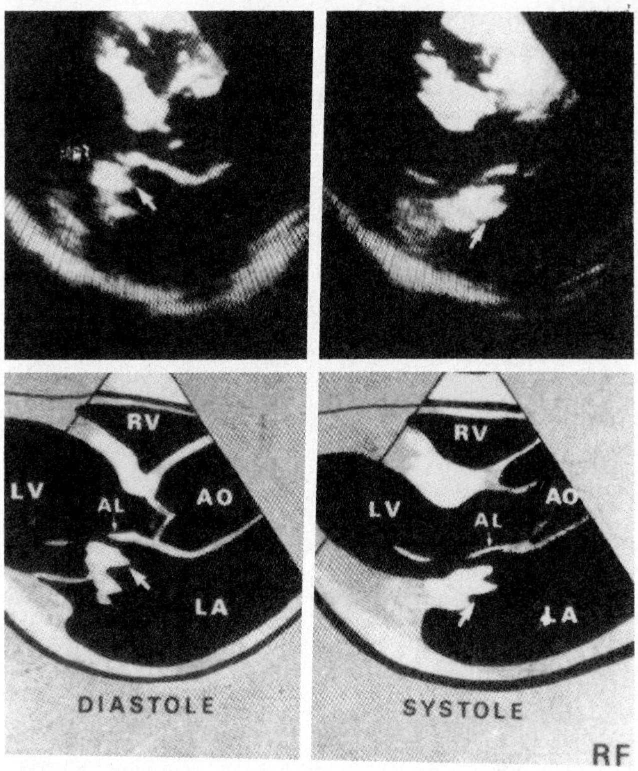

FIGURE 34–10. Long-axis echocardiograms in diastole (*left*) and systole (*right*) from a patient who had a native mitral valve vegetation. A large mass of echoes involving the posterior mitral leaflet (arrows) is seen in the left ventricle (LV) during diastole and in the left atrium (LA) during systole. Note the thin and delicate appearance of the normal anterior mitral leaflet (AL). RV = right ventricle, Ao = aorta. (From Rubenson, D. S., et al.: The use of echocardiography in diagnosing culture-negative endocarditis. Circulation *64*:641, 1981, by permission of the American Heart Association, Inc.)

Echocardiography has also been found to be of value in identification of myocardial and valvular ring abscesses[293] (Fig. 5–64, p. 112). Echocardiography of an aortic perivalvular abscess in patients with prosthetic valve endocarditis may disclose rocking of the prosthesis, the presence of an aneurysm of the sinus of Valsalva, thickening of the posterior area of the aortic root, and perivalvular density in the ventricular septum.[294]

An extensive study by Andy and his colleagues of the efficacy of echocardiography in the detection of infective endocarditis and its complications, especially in relation to involvement of specific valves, indicated that vegetations on the tricuspid valve, as visualized by echocardiography (Fig. 5–63, p. 111; Fig. 34–11), were always larger than those on the mitral valve.[295] No patients with tricuspid regurgitation demonstrated torn cusps. Two-dimensional echocardiograms were found by Berger and his colleagues[296] to be superior to the M-mode technique in identifying endocarditis involving the tricuspid and pulmonic valves.

Two-dimensional echocardiography has also been noted to be useful in establishing the diagnosis of isolated pulmonic valve endocarditis[297, 298] (Fig. 34–12) and in demonstrating infection in cases of interventricular septal defect.

Because size is critical to detection of the valvular vegetations in patients with infective endocarditis, echocardiography might be expected to give positive results more often when infections are caused by fungi because of the characteristically large valvular lesions. The features of aortic valvular disease caused by *C. parapsilosis* have been described by Gomes and his associates[299] and include clusters of abnormal echoes visible intermittently in the aortic root; thickening of the valve leaflets, with abnormal

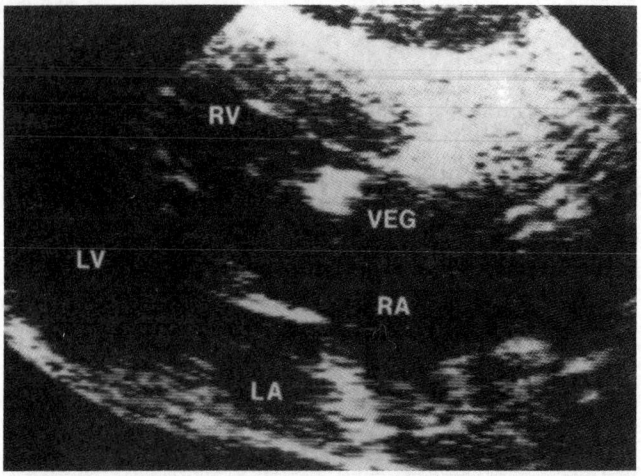

FIGURE 34–11. Two-dimensional echocardiographic study (parasternal long-axis view) demonstrating large echo-dense object attached to the tricuspid valve suggesting a tricuspid vegetation. LA = left atrium; LV = left ventricle; RA = right atrium; RV = right ventricle; VEG = tricuspid valve vegetation. (From Fernandez, G. C., et al.: Gonococcal endocarditis: A case series demonstrating modern presentation of an old disease. Am. Heart J. *108*:1326, 1984.)

"shaggy" echoes in both systole and diastole; and normal excursion of the leaflets except when damage is extensive.

Eighty-seven patients with clinical evidence of infective endocarditis studied by Stewart et al.[300] were divided into two groups on the basis of positive and negative echocardiography (M-mode and two-dimensional). The individuals in whom one or more vegetations were demonstrated by the noninvasive technique were found to be at a higher risk of developing complications (emboli, congestive cardiac failure, and need for surgery) than those in whom echocardiography demonstrated no vegetations. The authors stressed the point that "although the detection of vegetations by echocardiography in patients with the clinical syndrome of endocarditis clearly identifies a subgroup at risk of complications, decisions regarding clinical management made solely on the basis of the presence or absence of vegetative lesions are hazardous. Management of such patients must continue to be based on the clinical integration of multiple factors."

An interesting study of the value of echocardiography in the diagnosis of endocarditis in 11 patients with negative blood cultures in whom the presence of the disease was established during cardiac surgery was carried out by Rubenson et al.[301] Both natural (five cases) and prosthetic valves (six cases) were involved. Valvular masses were identified by echocardiography in eight cases. The other three had prosthetic aortic valves that showed the diastolic mitral valve vibration characteristic of aortic regurgitation. In three instances the illness was poorly defined clinically. The authors emphasize the point that, in these persons, echocardiography was a prime factor in identifying the presence of endocarditis.

Dillon et al.[302] have suggested that initial and serial echocardiographic studies carried out over the course of treatment not only play an important role in diagnosis, but are also of value in assessing the size of vegetations and the state of valvular function while antimicrobial therapy is being administered. Vik-Mo[303] has pointed out that the results of echocardiography may identify premature mitral closure and high left ventricular filling pressure in patients with aortic valvular endocarditis. Echocardiography during the first 2 weeks of an episode of endocarditis may fail to disclose vegetations. When they appear they may be massive and disappear without embolization, increase in size, or remain unchanged despite therapy.[304]

As discussed above, one of the important points to remember about the use of echocardiography in the diagnosis of infective endocarditis is related to the size of the vegetations on the affected valve. Clearly the larger the lesions, the more likely their presence is to be detected by echocardiography. Thus, this technique produces positive results in fungal valvular infections because, as a rule, the vegetations are large. The technique is of less value, but still useful, in acute endocarditis caused by *Staph. aureus*, in which endocardial lesions are often of moderate size, but may be quite large. The primary difficulty of echocardiographic diagnosis arises in patients with the subacute form of the disease because of the small size of the vegetations associated with infection by viridans streptococci and other relatively avirulent organisms.

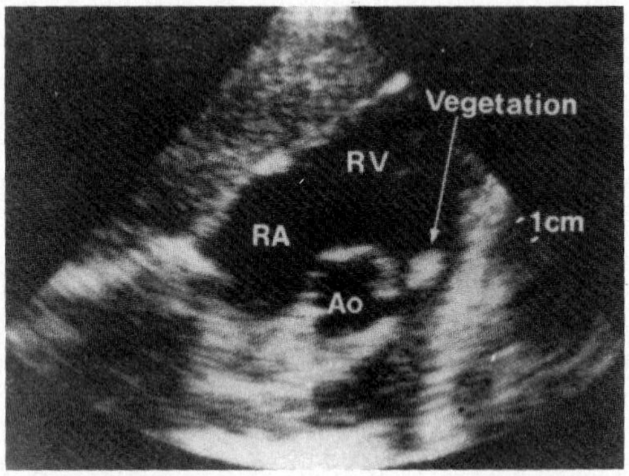

FIGURE 34–12. Cross-sectional echocardiogram of the right side of the heart from the subxiphoid region. A 2 cm mass attached to the pulmonary valve is clearly evident. RA = right atrium, RV = right ventricle, Ao = aortic root. (From Rosoff, M. H., Cohen, M. V., and Jacquette, G.: Pulmonary valve gonococcal endocarditis—A forgotten disease. Br. Heart J. *50*:290, 1983.)

MANAGEMENT OF INFECTIVE ENDOCARDITIS

Before the antibiotic era, attempts to treat infective endocarditis were relatively unsuccessful. For the most part physicians were limited to observation and study of the "natural history" of this almost invariably fatal disease. The development of highly potent antimicrobial agents, followed by refinements of and advances in the techniques of cardiac surgery, have so altered this heretofore "hopeless" situation that today young physicians are often perplexed when defervescence fails to occur within 24 to 48 hours after initiation of treatment, and older physicians are upset by a fatal outcome when, previously, they were amazed if their patients recovered.

ANTIMICROBIAL THERAPY

Although penicillin—the first antibiotic effective in the management of infective endocarditis—is still the agent of choice in most cases, the increasing involvement of uncommon bacterial species and fungi in the pathogenesis of the disease has posed difficult and, at times, insurmountable therapeutic problems and underscores the need for careful application of sensitive microbiological techniques not only to isolate all organisms involved, but also to identify them and evaluate their susceptibility to a wide range of antimicrobial agents.

SELECTION OF DRUGS. The choice of specific antimicrobial therapy for infective endocarditis depends strictly on the nature of the organism recovered from the blood and its susceptibility to various drugs. Treatment should be begun promptly but usually need not be immediate in the subacute form of infection, since most of these patients have been ill for several weeks to as long as 3 or more months before the diagnosis is established. Therefore, a delay in instituting treatment of 2 or 3 days until definitive microbiological data become available is of little or no prognostic importance. If death occurs before therapy is begun in such cases, it is most often due, not to the infectious process, but to one of its sequelae, such as rupture of a mycotic aneurysm or embolic occlusion of a coronary artery—complications not prevented by chemotherapy.

In contrast, it is imperative that there be no delay in treatment in acute bacterial endocarditis, especially when it involves a highly destructive organism, such as *Staph. aureus*, because of the rapidity with which valve leaflets, papillary muscles, or chordae tendineae may rupture or myocardial and/or septal abscesses may develop. In the absence of bacteriological evidence, the etiology of acute endocarditis may, at times, be suspected on the basis of the circumstances in which it developed. For example, a staphylococcal skin infection in a patient with endocarditis should implicate this organism as the cause of the valvular infection. Examination of stained smears of petechial lesions or of the "buffy coat" of the peripheral blood may reveal the causative organism 1 or 2 days before results of blood cultures are available. Despite the urgent need for treatment in such cases, administration of antimicrobial agents should be withheld until sufficient blood cultures have been obtained, a procedure that usually involves a delay of no more than 1 hour. Antibiotic therapy should be begun, with the drugs chosen empirically, before the organism has been identified and before sensitivity tests have become available; if these tests indicate that a drug other than the one being given is preferable, the appropriate agent should be substituted.

ANTIBACTERIAL EFFECTIVENESS. It is important that, in addition to its antimicrobial activity, the agent selected pose minimal risk of untoward effects, be administered by a route acceptable to the patient, and present no problems with respect to the physiological, biochemical, and anatomical characteristics of the host.[305] In general, bactericidal drugs appear to be more effective than bacteriostatic ones not only in eradicating the valvular infection, but also in reducing the risk of relapse after therapy has been completed.

Although it has been generally accepted that the effectiveness of treatment of endocarditis could be evaluated by determination of the antibacterial activity of the blood against the responsible organism,[306] this has recently been brought into question. A multicenter collaborative study of the value of the serum in vitro bactericidal test (SBT) as a determinant of the effectiveness of the treatment of infective endocarditis has shown that the test can predict bacteriological success accurately but not bacteriological failure or clinical outcome.[307] A peak SBT level of 1/64 and trough level of 1/32 are considered to represent optimal therapy. However, Mellors et al.[308] have concluded, from a review of the literature, that the results of these determinations do not furnish useful information about most patients with endocarditis and did not warrant their use routinely in patients with this disease. This recommendation is supported by a report of a lack of correlation between the level of antibacterial activity in the blood and the clinical outcome.[309] The lack of clinical importance of the test is underscored by experimental observations indicating that the concentration of an antibiotic in a fibrin clot, a model for the vegetation, is directly related to the peak serum concentration and degree of protein-binding of the drug. Evidence also exists that antibacterial activity persists in the mass of fibrin for long periods after the antibiotic is no longer detectable in the circulation.[310, 311]

DOSAGE CONSIDERATIONS. Despite the fact that antimicrobial agents have been used for more than 40 years in the treatment of infective endocarditis, no firm data are available concerning the proper daily dose of any of these drugs. Regimens vary greatly and depend on the experience of the physician. Thus, doses of penicillin ranging from as low as 4 to 6 million units to as high as 20 to 30 million units per day have been administered to patients with subacute disease when the responsible agent has been a highly susceptible strain of viridans streptococcus or other organism. Unfortunately there is no proof that either of these extremes of dosage is necessary or ideal. For this reason the doses of antibiotics recommended below for the management of valvular infections are necessarily based on published experiences and are perforce empirical.

In terms of generating the highest levels and longest duration of antimicrobial activity, Barza et al. have shown that the bolus injection of an antibiotic is more effective than a constant intravenous infusion.[312] Although the question of what constitutes an optimal interval between doses in the management of infective endocarditis remains unsettled, experimental data obtained from studies of the penetration and persistence of antimicrobial activity in fibrin, combined with 40 years of experience treating both acute and subacute infective endocarditis, have convinced this author that an interval of 6 hours between doses of a parenterally administered drug is effective in most adults. This might be extended in older persons because of decreased renal tubular secretory function. In children, however, a shorter interval (3 to 4 hours) between doses may be required to maintain effective concentrations of drug in the infected platelet-fibrin thrombus because of the high level of tubular secretory function that leads to rapid urinary excretion of penicillins and cephalosporins.

DURATION OF THERAPY. The duration of therapy required to cure infective endocarditis is, like the dosage, for the most part, also empirical and therefore often controversial. Although many physicians continue treatment for only 4 weeks, there is an increasing tendency to extend this to 6 weeks, despite the lack of statistically significant evidence that this leads to a higher percentage of cures or reduces the incidence of relapse in most cases, especially when the organisms are highly susceptible to the antibiotic used. It remains to be proved whether 6 weeks of exposure to an antibiotic is required when the infection is caused by uncommon bacterial species, by strains less sensitive to antimicrobial agents, or by fungi. The observation that the risk of superinfection is directly related to the length of time over which an antibiotic is administered, especially when the drug used has a broad spectrum of activity,[313] suggests that there may actually be some danger in prolonging therapy beyond 4 weeks. Attempts have also been made to limit the duration of treatment to 2 weeks in patients with subacute bacterial endocarditis caused by such noninvasive organisms as *Strep. viridans*.[314] Although cure has been reported in some instances, this approach cannot yet be recommended until considerably more data regarding rate of cure and risk of relapse become available.

ROUTES OF ADMINISTRATION. Most physicians experienced in the treatment of subacute infective endocarditis recommend parenteral administration of antibiotics, usually by the intravenous route. However, in a number of cases, successful treatment of this disease with oral penicillin has been reported. The stimulus for this approach has been the desire to avoid the pain of intramuscular or intravenous injection, to eliminate such complications as thrombophlebitis and sterile or infected abscesses in muscle, and the desire to shorten hospitalization. Antimicrobial agents that have been administered orally include buffered penicillin G and phenoxymethylpenicillin (penicillin V).[314–317] In many instances oral treatment with one of the penicillins has been combined with the intramuscular injection of streptomycin. Therapy with this regimen has also been continued for only 2 weeks in a number of cases.[314] While high rates of cure have been reported by several investigators,[314–317] relapses have occurred in a relatively small number of cases. This type of therapy must be restricted to patients with *subacute* bacterial endocarditis caused by organisms that are highly susceptible to the antibiotic used; it has no place and is extremely dangerous in treatment of the acute type of valvular infections. Although Burman et al.[318] have recently reported a cure of refractory staphylococcal endocarditis with rifampin and erythromycin, it must be pointed out that this approach is potentially dangerous and should not be used except in the most unusual circumstances.

A review by Phillips and Watson of oral therapy for infective endocarditis points out that "despite much discussion, no final conclusion has been reached about the optimum duration of oral treatment."[319] Short courses (2 weeks) have been reported to be effective, while some investigators have recommended therapy for as long as 6 or more weeks. Despite the reports of success with oral antibiotics, many physicians prefer to treat this disease parenterally. The following objections to oral administration have been raised.[320]

1. Large groups of patients treated with parenteral antibiotics have experienced no relapses, an important consideration, since each recrudescence of valvular infection not only adds an increment of permanent damage to an already functionally poor valve, but also presents a risk of death.
2. Orally administered antibiotics may be irregularly absorbed, especially in patients who are quite ill; this necessitates constant monitoring of blood levels of the antibiotic, a technique not available in most "routine" diagnostic microbiological laboratories.
3. Patients may fail to take each dose of drug unless under the continuous watchful eye of the physician or nurse.
4. Gastrointestinal irritation leading to nausea, vomiting, and diarrhea is associated with the oral use of antibiotics in some persons.
5. The risk of superinfections, even rapidly fatal ones, is not eliminated when antibiotics are taken orally.

Although 4 weeks of intravenous or intramuscular injection of an antimicrobial agent causes discomfort in most persons, vast clinical experience has indicated that, with proper attention and encouragement from the physician, almost all patients accept this form of treatment with minimal complaint.

PROBLEMS OF THERAPY. A fairly common therapeutic problem arises when the clinical picture is highly suggestive of subacute bacterial endocarditis but the blood cultures are repeatedly sterile. Because of the high fatality rate when the disease is not treated, therapy is usually based on experience and clinical judgment. Initially therapy should be directed at possible enterococcal infection, as discussed below (p. 2540). Cannady and Sandford[310] have made the following suggestions regarding therapy of patients with suspected endocarditis when blood cultures have failed to yield an organism: If there is no satisfactory response after 2 weeks of empirical treatment, administration should be continued for an additional 14 days, during which cultures and serological tests may indicate the presence of infection caused by fungi, *Chlamydia, Rickettsia,* or *Brucella*. If all these studies are negative, treatment should be discontinued and the patient reevaluated. These investigators also point out that the most difficult problem involves the compromised host who has received many antibiotic regimens or the patient with a prosthetic heart valve. The latter may have fungal endocarditis and may well be a candidate for empirical therapy with amphotericin B, but surgical removal of the infected valve may be necessary to cure the disease.

Negative cultures of the blood are seldom, if ever, a problem in acute infections involving the left side of the heart. In endocarditis involving the right side of the heart, organisms may not be recovered from the peripheral circulation until pulmonary infarction and infection occur, after which cultures of the blood become positive. However, if embolization to the lungs does not occur and the blood remains sterile, therapy must be undertaken as soon as possible and should be directed against organisms known to be most often responsible for this kind of disease, especially coagulase-positive staphylococcus. When the enterococcus may be the causative agent, the use of a penicillinase-resistant penicillin or ampicillin plus an aminoglycoside or vancomycin is recommended; an optimal choice is nafcillin or oxacillin (12 gm/day, in divided doses) plus gentamicin or tobramycin (80 mg every 8 hours).

Anticoagulants

The use of anticoagulants in patients with infective endocarditis has been and remains controversial.[321] It is clear that anticoagulants are of no benefit in the management of valvular infections because these drugs do not prevent separation of small fragments from the valvular thrombus and the vegetations do not increase in size if antimicrobial therapy is effective. Anticoagulation may cause bleeding at the site of deposition of an embolus. It is this author's view that when a condition such as phlebothrombosis of the extremities or pelvis results in pulmonary embolism, with or without infarction, and requires anticoagulation with heparin or coumadin, the presence of infective endocarditis does not absolutely contraindicate the use of these drugs. When embolization from the infected valve occurs, the situation must be reevaluated relative to the risks of hemorrhage at the sites where emboli have been deposited, on the one hand, and of a fatal pulmonary infarct, on the other; anticoagulation is likely to be of no value in this situation. When the phlebothrombosis involves the extremities or pelvis, the issue can be resolved by insertion of an umbrella into the inferior vena cava (p. 1590). Wilson et al.[322] have reported that the morbidity and mortality in patients with prosthetic valve endocarditis did not increase when an anticoagulant was given. However, when it was discontinued, the incidence of major complications involving the central nervous system increased. The fatality rate was 47 per cent with adequate anticoagulation and 57 per cent when it was inadequate; this difference may not be statistically significant.

TREATMENT OF ENDOCARDITIS CAUSED BY SPECIFIC ORGANISMS

(Tables 34–6 and 34–7)

GRAM-POSITIVE COCCI

STAPHYLOCOCCI. Despite the use of antimicrobial agents effective against *Staph. aureus* in vitro, the clinical results of therapy of endocarditis caused by this organism are relatively poor, when compared with subacute disease produced by alpha-streptococci. In patients not sensitized to penicillins, this group of agents is first choice. About 15 per cent of infections caused by *Staph. aureus* that occur outside hospitals and more than 90 per cent that develop during hospitalization are caused by penicillin-resistant strains. Nafcillin, oxacillin, or cephalothin are the choices in such cases.

The most recently recommended regimens for the treatment of both methicillin-sensitive and -resistant strains of *Staph. aureus* and *Staph. epidermidis*[333] are presented in Table 34–6.

The following program for the treatment of staphylococcal endocarditis involving native and prosthetic valves, using one of the recently developed antimicrobial agents has been recommended by the Working Party of the British Society for Antimicrobial Therapy[334]; flucloxacillin, 2 gm intravenously every 4 hours plus fusidic acid, 500 mg orally every 8 hours plus gentamicin, 120 mg for the first dose, followed by 80 mg intravenously every 8 hours. Vancomycin is recommended for patients who are sensitized to

TABLE 34–6 ANTIBIOTIC THERAPY FOR STAPHYLOCOCCAL ENDOCARDITIS IN ADULTS*

ORGANISM/SETTING	DRUG OF CHOICE	ALTERNATE THERAPY**	DURATION (WEEKS)	COMMENTS
Staphylococcus aureus				
Methicillin-susceptible				
Non-addicts	Oxacillin or nafcillin 1.5–2.0 gm intravenously every 4 hours	Cephalothin 1.5–2.0 gm intravenously every 4 hours Cefazolin 1.5–2.0 gm intravenously every 6 hours Vancomycin 500 mg (7.5 mg/kg) intravenously every 6 hours	4–6	For prosthetic valve endocarditis, possibly native valve endocarditis: add gentamicin 1 mg/kg intravenously every 8 hours to nafcillin first 5 days Poor response at 7 days: continue and add gentamicin or rifampin 300 mg orally every 8 hours
Addicts	As above	As above	4	For complicated native valve endocarditis: treat 6 weeks
Methicillin-resistant				
Non-addicts	Vancomycin 500 mg (7.5 mg/kg) intravenously every 6 hours	Select based on susceptibility data	4–6	Role of combined therapy not clear: aminoglycoside resistance common
Addicts	Vancomycin, as above	Trimethoprim/sulfamethoxazole 240/1,200 mg intravenously every 12 hours	4	Trimethoprim/sulfamethoxazole limited to right-sided native valve endocarditis
Staphylococcus epidermidis				
Methicillin-susceptible				
Prosthetic valve endocarditis	Oxacillin or nafcillin 1.5–2.0 gm intravenously every 4 hours, plus rifampin 300 mg orally every 8 hours; gentamicin 1 mg/kg intravenously every 8 hours for initial 2 weeks	A cephalosporin or vancomycin at above doses plus gentamicin and rifampin	6	
Native valve endocarditis	Oxacillin or nafcillin for *S. aureus*	Cephalothin, cefazolin, or vancomycin per *S. aureus*	4	
Methicillin-resistant				
Prosthetic valve endocarditis	Vancomycin 500 mg (7.5 mg/kg) intravenously every 6 hours, plus rifampin 300 mg orally every 8 hours; gentamicin 1 mg/kg intravenously every 8 hours for initial 2 weeks	Select based on susceptibility data	6	Test isolates recovered after therapy for rifampin resistance
Native valve endocarditis	Vancomycin for methicillin-resistant *S. aureus*	Select based on susceptibility data	4	

*Adjust doses of vancomycin, gentamicin, and trimethoprim/sulfamethoxazole for renal insufficiency.
**If patient cannot tolerate drug of choice: cephalosporins used in mild penicillin allergy, vancomycin used if penicillins cause anaphylaxis or hives.

penicillin or who are infected by an organism resistant to the above program.

A therapeutic approach to the problem presented by patients strongly suspected of having infective endocarditis on clinical grounds but when blood cultures are persistently negative has been recommended by Bayer[335] (Table 34–9).

The fatality rate from staphylococcal endocarditis in 25 patients treated with a single antibiotic (penicillin G, methicillin, nafcillin, cephalothin, or vancomycin) was noted to be 40 per cent. It was identical in 15 patients who received combined therapy (nafcillin plus gentamicin, penicillin plus gentamicin, or methicillin plus gentamicin).[336] A recent study has indicated that treatment with a single effective antibiotic (a penicillinase-resistant penicillin or a cephalosporin) is curative, and that adding an aminoglycoside does not increase the rate of cure.[337]

In the author's experience even large dosages of the most active antimicrobial drugs fail to cure the infection in patients in whom a large number of abscesses develop either before or after therapy has been initiated. An important determinant of the eventual outcome of this disease is failure to institute treatment early in the course of the disease; a delay as short as 4 to 5 days may increase the risk of a fatal outcome.

Despite the low invasive capacity of *Staph. epidermidis*. the prognosis for recovery from endocarditis produced by this organism is generally poor, even when patients are treated with an antibiotic that is considered to be sensitive to it on the basis of in vitro study. A common course of events in this type of valvular infection is relapse after discontinuation of treatment. This may occur several times, despite repeated administration of an effective drug, and may finally lead to congestive failure. At this point, replacement of the affected valve with a prosthesis is indicated.

STREPTOCOCCI. Of the organisms responsible for subacute infective endocarditis, *Streptococcus viridans* is the most common. Although most of these bacteria are highly sensitive to penicillin G, it must be emphasized that all strains in this group do not constitute a single species, and all are not susceptible to this antibiotic.

Treatment of streptococcal (viridans) endocarditis with a combination of penicillin and streptomycin or gentamicin has been recommended on the basis of in vitro synergy of the drugs.[323] However, this author's experience with more than 900 cases given penicillin alone does not support this recommendation; all the patients survived, and none relapsed over the 6 months after discontinuation of treatment. Two reports have confirmed this experience.[324, 324a]

For patients sensitized to penicillin, several approaches

TABLE 34–7 TREATMENT OF ENDOCARDITIS

Microorganism	Antimicrobial Therapy	Duration of Treatment (weeks)	Alternative Therapy	Duration of Treatment (weeks)
Streptococcal Endocarditis				
Penicillin-sensitive streptococci (MIC less than 0.2 μg/ml); nonenterococcal group D	Aqueous penicillin G (20 mill. units/day IV)	4	Cephalothin (1.5 gm IV every 4 hr)	4
	or		**or**	
	Aqueous penicillin G (20 mill. units/day IV)	2	Vancomycin (7.5 mg/kg every 6 hr)	4
	plus			
	Gentamicin (1 mg/kg IV every 8 hr)	2		
	or			
	Aqueous penicillin G (20 mill. units/day IV)	4		
	plus			
	Gentamicin (1 mg/kg IV every 8 hr)	2		
Relative penicillin-resistance (MIC greater than 0.2 μg/ml); nutritionally variant viridans streptococci	Aqueous penicillin G (20 mill. units/day IV) **plus** Gentamicin (1 mg/kg IV every 8 hr)	4	Vancomycin (7.5 mg/kg IV every 6 hr)	4
Enterococcal endocarditis	Aqueous penicillin G (20–40 mill. units/day IV)	4–6	Vancomycin (7.5 mg/kg IV every 6 hr)	4–6
	or			
	Ampicillin (12 gm/day IV)	4–6		
	plus		**plus**	
	Gentamicin (1 mg/kg IV every 8 hr)		Gentamicin (1 mg/kg IV every 8 hr)	
Staphylococcal Endocarditis	See Table 34–6			
Enterobacteriaceae				
E. coli, Klebsiella, Proteus, etc.	Ampicillin (12 gm/day IV)	4–6	Cephalothin (8–12 gm/day IV)	4–6
	or		**or**	
	Gentamicin (1.7 mg/kg IV every 8 hr)		Cefotaxime (2 gm IV every 8 hr)	4–6
	can add			
	Ticarcillin (3 gm IV every 4 hr)			
	or			
	Piperacillin (4 gm IV every 6 hr)			

Adapted from Wilson, W. R., and Geraci, J. E.: Antibiotic treatment of infective endocarditis. Ann. Rev. Med. *34*:413–427, 1983.

Table continued on opposite page

are available: one involves desensitization to this drug—a simple and minimally dangerous procedure that is often not necessary because of the availability of other effective antimicrobial agents. An adequate substitute for penicillin G in these cases is intravenous cephalothin, 2 gm every 4 hours. (The risk of cross-reactivity between these agents has been less than 1 per cent in the experience of this author.) Another cephalosporin, cefazolin, has been reported by Quinn et al. to be effective in the treatment of staphylococcal endocarditis.[325] However, relapses have been noted when this antibiotic has been used.[326] Vancomycin (2 gm/day) has been reported to be effective in some instances of this type of endocarditis.[327] Most strains of *Strep. viridans* susceptible to penicillin are sensitive to erythromycin, 1 gm given intravenously every 6 hours. In endocarditis caused by alpha-streptococci, clindamycin is thought to be a "third-line" drug for use in patients who have previously had a serious reaction to both penicillins and cephalosporins[328] because relapse has occurred after therapy was discontinued.

It is now clear that optimal therapy for enterococcal endocarditis requires combined therapy with a beta-lactam antibiotic (a penicillin, but *not* cephalothin) plus an aminoglycoside (streptomycin, gentamicin, tobramycin, amikacin, netilmicin).[329–331] Failure to achieve synergism against the organism is related to its resistance to the aminoglycoside being administered and is corrected by substitution of an active drug in the same class.[332] In vitro resistance to 2000 mg/ml of streptomycin mitigates against the use of this antibiotic.

A number of regimens have been found to be of value in the management of endocarditis caused by enterococci. Among these are penicillin G (25 million units intravenously every 6 hours) plus streptomycin (0.5 gm intramuscularly every 12 hours) or gentamicin or tobramycin (3 to 5 mg/kg in three equally divided doses at 8-hour intervals). A combination that has proved to be more effective than penicillin plus an aminoglycoside in vitro is nafcillin plus gentamicin or tobramycin; the intravenous dose of nafcillin is 1 gm every 3 hours or 2 gm every 4 hours. Some strains of enterococci are quite sensitive to ampicillin; the dose of this drug for subacute endocarditis is 8 to 12 gm/day, in three or four equally divided and spaced intravenous injections, together with gentamicin or tobramycin. In patients sensitized to penicillins, the administration of 4 gm/day of erythromycin (1 gm intravenously every 6 hours) has proved to be highly effective when the organism is sensitive to this drug.

TABLE 34–7 TREATMENT OF ENDOCARDITIS *Continued*

Microorganism	Antimicrobial Therapy	Duration of Treatment (weeks)	Alternative Therapy	Duration of Treatment (weeks)
P. aeruginosa	Tobramycin (1.7 mg/kg IV every 8 hr) **plus** Ticarcillin (3 gm IV every 4 hr) **or** Piperacillin (4 gm IV every 6 hr)	6		
HACEK Organisms				
Haemophilus, Actinobacillus, Cardiobacterium, Eikenella, Kingella	Ampicillin (12 gm/day IV) **can add** Gentamicin (1.7 mg/kg IV every 8 hr)	3	Desensitize patient and treat with ampicillin	
***Corynebacterium* spp.**				
Penicillin-sensitive	Aqueous penicillin G (20 mill. units/day IV) **plus** Gentamicin (1 mg/kg IV every 8 hr)	4–6	Vancomycin (7.5 mg/kg IV every 6 hr)	4–6
Penicillin-resistant	Vancomycin (7.5 mg/kg IV every 6 hr)	4–6		
Fungi				
Candida spp.	Amphotericin B (1–1.5 mg/kg/day IV) **plus** 5-fluorocytosine (150 mg/kg/day by mouth in divided doses)	6–8	None	
Culture-negative Endocarditis				
Normal valve	Penicillin G (20–40 mill. units/day IV) **plus** Gentamicin (1.7 mg/kg IV every 8 hr)	4–6	Vancomycin (7.5 mg/kg IV every 6 hr) **plus** Gentamicin (1.7 mg/kg IV every 8 hr)	
Prosthetic valve (See also Table 34–9)	Vancomycin (7.5 mg/kg IV every 6 hr) **plus** Gentamicin (1.7 mg/kg IV every 8 hr)	4–6		

YEASTS AND FUNGI

More than a decade of use has demonstrated the effectiveness of amphotericin B in the management of infections caused by a wide variety of yeasts and fungi. Therapy with this agent has been beneficial in histoplasmosis, cryptococcosis, and candidiasis. Experience indicates, however, that the treatment of fungal infections of the heart presents a number of problems that are unique to this organ and that are quite different from those encountered when this kind of disease involves other organs. Although sporadic reports have suggested that candidal endocarditis has been eradicated by administration of amphotericin B alone, the diagnosis in such cases has been largely based on the demonstration of candidemia, a finding not always diagnostic of cardiac or systemic disease.[338, 339]

The relatively poor results of chemotherapy of fungal infections of cardiac valves has prompted consideration of adjunct therapy (i.e., surgical removal of the infected site). In 1961 Kay and his colleagues reported an instance of candidal endocarditis resistant to amphotericin B that was ultimately cured by debridement of an infected tricuspid valve.[340] Experience since then has emphasized the intolerably high frequency of primary drug failure and underscores the need for surgical intervention in infections not only of natural valves, but especially of prosthetic valves.[341] It must be pointed out, however, that not even this combined therapeutic approach results in an acceptable cure rate. When the diagnosis of fungal endocarditis is established, treatment with amphotericin B must be promptly initiated. After about a week of administration of the antibiotic, it is best to remove the infected valve, replace it with a prosthesis, and continue chemotherapy for at least 6 to 8 weeks. When this fails it has been the practice, in some instances, to replace the prosthetic valve with a new one. However, even this has failed to eradicate the disease in many cases.

Another approach to this problem has been suggested. In patients in whom endocarditis is limited to the tricuspid valve, total valvulectomy without prosthetic replacement has been carried out.[342] Unless pulmonary hypertension is present, patients apparently get along fairly well after operation. Administration of amphotericin B was continued for a number of weeks until there was a clinical impression of eradication of the infectious process. A prosthesis is then inserted, and treatment continued. It must be emphasized that of all types of endocarditis, the prognosis for recovery is poorest in those caused by yeasts and fungi.

Several regimens have been recommended for intravenous therapy with amphotericin B.[343, 344] One involves administration of 0.25 mg/kg the first day, followed by an increase of 0.25 mg/kg each day until a dose of 1 mg/kg/day is reached. This is continued until the completion of therapy. In severe infections, such as is the case in fungal endocarditis, the daily dose may be increased to 1.5 mg/kg/day. Another approach involves the administration of 1 mg the first day and 5 mg the second day, followed by daily increases of 5 to 10 mg until 1 mg/kg/day is being administered.

Treatment is commonly continued for 6 to 8 weeks. If relapse follows discontinuation of therapy, it may be necessary to administer a second, or even third, course of the antibiotic.

A compound of potential value in the management of fungal diseases is 5-fluorocytosine, a drug that can be administered orally. In most instances this agent is being used, together with amphotericin B, for the treatment of fungal endocarditis when the responsible organism is susceptible to both drugs. In some instances in which the organism is susceptible, 5-fluorocytosine has been given alone for varying periods of time, often many months, after "cure" has been accomplished by combined therapy.

When given orally, 5-fluorocytosine is well absorbed from the gastrointestinal tract and reaches clinically effective concentrations.[345–347] Blood levels may be bactericidal for some strains of *Candida* but only bacteristatic for others.[347] The dosage is 50 to 150 mg/kg given at 6-hour intervals; this must be reduced in the presence of renal insufficiency. The most frequent side effects are hepatotoxicity and depression of the bone marrow, which are usually reversible when the drug is discontinued. Nausea and vomiting are fairly common.

Assessment of cure of fungal endocarditis should be made with caution because symptoms of the disease may remain suppressed for long periods.[348] A more accurate view of this situation is that it is "stabilized." Patients should be followed from the time chemotherapy is discontinued because relapse may occur as long as 2 years after completing treatment. Blood cultures are usually negative. Antibodies to *Candida* may be absent in the presence of infection, and their detection does not identify an active infectious process because precipitins to *Candida* are present in 40 per cent of patients who undergo cardiac surgery and are not infected, as well as in those in whom there has been an apparent cure.[349]

PROSTHETIC VALVE ENDOCARDITIS

In Table 34–8 are presented the recommendations of Wilson and Geraci[350] for the treatment of infective endocarditis in prosthetic valve endocarditis. It must be emphasized that monitoring of blood levels and renal, auditory, and labryinthine function is mandatory in patients receiving any of the aminoglycosides and vancomycin. Van Scoy[275] has suggested the use of specific antimicrobial agents for the management of both native and prosthetic valve infections with negative blood cultures (Table 34–9).

SURGICAL THERAPY

Despite the emphasis on the medical management of infective endocarditis over the past 40 years, it must be pointed out that the first spontaneous cure of an infection of the cardiovascular system was accomplished by Touroff and Vessell in 1940, when they ligated an infected patent ductus arteriosus.[350a] After a hiatus of many years, during which the prognosis of endocarditis changed from almost complete hopelessness to a high expectancy of recovery as more and more highly effective antimicrobial agents be-

TABLE 34–8 ANTIMICROBIAL THERAPY FOR PATIENTS WITH PROSTHETIC VALVE ENDOCARDITIS†

ORGANISM	ROUTINE ANTIMICROBIAL THERAPY	THERAPY FOR PATIENTS ALLERGIC TO PENICILLIN
S. aureus or *S. epidermidis*		
Penicillin-sensitive (MIC* ≤ 0.1 μg/ml)	Penicillin G, 20 million units IV/24 hr by continuous drip or in 6 equally divided doses for 4–6 weeks	Vancomycin, ‡ 7.5 mg/kg IV every 6 hr for 4–6 weeks, or cefazolin,§ 2 gm IV every 8 hr, or cephalothin, 2 gm IV every 4 hr, for 4–6 weeks
Penicillin-resistant (MIC >0.1 μg/ml)	Nafcillin, oxacillin, or methicillin, 2 gm IV every 4 hr for 4–6 weeks	Same as above
Methicillin-resistant	Vancomycin,‡ 7.5 mg/kg IV every 6 hr, plus rifampin, 300 mg orally every 12 hr for 4–6 weeks	Cefazolin, 2 gm IV every 8 hr, or cephalothin, 2 gm IV every 4 hr plus rifampin, 300 mg orally every 12 hr for 4–6 weeks
Streptococci		
Penicillin-sensitive viridans and non-enterococcal Group D (MIC ≤0.2 μg/ml)	Penicillin G, 20 million units IV/24 hr by continuous drip or in 6 equally divided doses for 4 weeks, plus streptomycin,‡ 7.5 mg/kg IM every 12 hr for first 14 days of treatment	Same as for penicillin-sensitive staphylococci above
Enterococci and penicillin-resistant (MIC >0.2 μg/ml)	Penicillin G, 20 million units IV/24 hr by continuous drip or in 6 equally divided doses, plus streptomycin,‡ 7.5 mg/kg IM every 12 hr, or gentamicin, 1 mg/kg IV every 8 hr for 4–6 weeks	Vancomycin,‡ 7.5 mg/kg IV every 6 hr plus streptomycin,‡ 7.5 mg/kg IM every 12 hr, or gentamicin, 1 mg/kg IV every 8 hr for 4–6 weeks or desensitize to penicillin
Diphtheroids	Penicillin G, 20 million units IV/24 hr by continuous drip or in 6 equally divided doses, plus gentamicin, 1 mg/kg IV every 8 hr, for 4–6 weeks	Vancomycin,‡ 7.5 mg/kg IV every 6 hr for 4–6 weeks
Gram-negative bacilli	Most effective and least toxic agent, given IV for 4–6 weeks. Selection of single- or combination-drug therapy should be based on results of in vitro MIC, MBC,* and synergy tests	
Fungi	Amphotericin B plus 5-fluorocytosine plus cardiac valve replacement	

*MBC, minimal bactericidal concentration; MIC, minimal inhibitory concentration.
†Dosages suggested are for adults with normal renal and hepatic function.
‡Vancomycin and streptomycin should not exceed 500 mg/dose.
§Other cephalosporins may be used in equivalent dosage, depending on results of in vitro susceptibility studies.
Adapted from Wilson, W. R., Danielson, G. K., Giuliani, E. R., and Geraci, J. E.: Prosthetic valve endocarditis. Mayo Clin. Proc. 57:155–161, 1982.

came available, surgical approaches have again become the ultimate therapeutic modality in patients in whom all other forms of treatment have been successful. However, as is often the case with progress in medicine, the development of new methods of management, while solving one set of problems, has frequently created new ones that are often more difficult to solve than the ones they replace. This is unquestionably the case in the surgical treatment of infective endocarditis. On the one hand, successful surgical manipulation of the uninfected heart has been responsible for an appreciable increment in the incidence of cardiovascular infections. On the other hand, although it is often the final successful approach to the eradication of valvular infections, surgical intervention raises difficult questions in relation not only to its advisability and indications, but also, once such a course has been accepted as necessary, to the time when it should be undertaken.[351]

One of the most critical and unquestioned indications for surgical intervention in cases of infective endocarditis is the development of intractable cardiac failure due to disruption of valve leaflets or their supporting structures. The role of intractable congestive failure in death from infective endocarditis is emphasized by the fact that this is the most common cause of fatality in this disease. Involvement of the aortic valve is most often the cause of this problem,[352–354] but severe mitral regurgitation, although less common, has also required replacement of the damaged valve with a prosthesis.[355, 356] It has become increasingly clear that the *presence of active infection is not a contraindication to cardiac surgery* in patients whose valves and their supporting structures have been severely injured or destroyed by infection.[357, 358]

The fatality rate in *emergency* aortic valve replacement has been reported to be about 33 per cent, but it is declining[352–354]; it is far less when it is carried out electively.[352] The necessity of surgical intervention in patients with perforation of the aortic valve leading to regurgitation during the course of endocarditis is emphasized by a report of eight patients in whom operation was not carried out and all of whom died; of seven patients with the same lesion who underwent repair of the perforation or replacement of the valve, only three succumbed.[359] Griffin et al. have stressed the need for immediate insertion of a prosthesis when severe cardiac failure complicates valvular infections.[360] They also suggested that this procedure be performed early in patients with mild decompensation of the heart because of a significant risk of sudden death from embolic myocardial infarction or the development of potentially lethal arrhythmias.

INDICATIONS. The following are the important indications for cardiac surgery in patients with infective endocarditis: (1) *Congestive heart failure* that does not respond to intensive medical management. Active infection is not a contraindication. (2) *No response of the infectious process* on the involved valve despite appropriate, intensive antimicrobial therapy for about 1 week. (3) *Repeated embolic occlusions*, especially when vital areas such as brain, eyes, coronary arteries, and kidneys are involved. In this situation the problem that arises involves a decision as to when surgery should be performed. Should this be after the first, second, third, or more embolic episode? There are no data that indicate the answer to this question. (4) *Presence of a septal abscess*. (5) *Relapse of infection* (3 months or less after "cure"). It is the author's practice to treat the first relapse over the same length of time as the original infection. A second relapse should prompt serious consideration of removal of the affected valve. (6) *Recurrence of endocarditis* (>6 months after "cure") involving the valve initially affected or a different one. If it is the same valve, management involves the same approach as that used for the first *relapse*. If the recurrence involves a different valve, treatment is the same as for an initial episode. (7) *Endocarditis involving aneurysms of sinus of Valsalva or atrioventricular junctional tissues*. (8) *Fungal endocarditis*; treatment is replacement by a prosthesis after 7 to 10 days of antifungal therapy. In addition, Alsip et al.[361] have suggested the following indications for surgery in patients with endocarditis: Hemodynamic compromise, valvular obstruction, unstable prosthesis, rupture chordae tendineae or papillary muscles, mitral valve preclosure in aortic regurgitation, early prosthetic infection, periprosthetic leak, and intracardiac extension of infection.

The indications for surgery in patients who develop heart block in the course of endocarditis have been defined by Dinubile[362] as follows: The observed appearance of progression of established heart block, involvement of the aortic valve, persistence of block for at least 1 week of optimal antimicrobial therapy, and elimination of other potential causes of abnormalities in conduction. Robbins et al.[363] recommend operation when fever persists for 3 weeks and the vegetation is 1 cm in diameter, provided that all cardiac causes for the elevated temperature have been ruled out. Kay et al.[364] have suggested that the demonstration by echocardiography of premature closure of the mitral valve, signifying severe aortic regurgitation, is an indication for surgery, even in the absence of cardiac failure.

Wilson et al. have indicated that replacement of the cardiac valve may be successfully carried out in patients with active infective endocarditis, even when blood cultures are positive.[365] They believe that hemodynamic status of such patients is the factor that determines the time when the valve should be replaced. The activity of the infection or the duration of antimicrobial therapy before surgery is of little or no importance in the decision to insert a prosthesis. In patients with myocardial or aortic abscesses in whom conventional aortic valve replacement is not possible, a radical surgical procedure may be necessary. Richardson and his colleagues have reported that heart failure and annular and myocardial abscesses—present most often with staphylococcal and fungal endocarditis—were the primary cause of death in infection involving natural as well as prosthetic valves.[366] Operation significantly improved survival in cases with moderate or severe cardiac decompensation, in infection of natural valves when moderate or severe heart failure was present, and in patients with staphylococcal infection of prosthetic valves. Rappaport[367] has pointed out that the conclusions reached by Richardson and associates[366] do not apply to endocarditis involving the tricuspid valve because the prognosis for cure by medical therapy alone is very good.

If this fails, and especially if hemodynamic difficulties develop, surgical removal of the affected valve is indicated.

RIGHT-SIDED ENDOCARDITIS. This often presents a special problem with respect to the need for surgical treatment. It has been suggested that excision of the tricuspid valve may be the treatment of choice when there is failure to respond to antimicrobial agents. It is now clear that the prognosis for cure of infection involving this valve, when it is caused by *Pseudomonas* and other gram-negative bacteria, fungi, and other organisms, is dramatically improved by surgical removal of the valve and not replacing it with a prosthesis.[368, 369] With normal pulmonary artery pressure, cardiac output can be maintained for at least limited periods in the absence of the tricuspid valve.

There is general agreement that tricuspid valvular endocarditis caused by these organisms, especially when they are only moderately sensitive or resistant to available

TABLE 34–9 ANTIMICROBIAL THERAPY OF APPARENT CULTURE-NEGATIVE ENDOCARDITIS

Type of Infection	Antimicrobial Therapy		Alternative Therapy
	WITHOUT PRIOR TREATMENT*		
Acute, natural valve	Oxacillin or nafcillin 2 gm IV every 4 hr plus penicillin G or ampicillin 20 to 40 million units IV per 24 hr or 2 gm IV every 4 hr, respectively, plus streptomycin 7.5 mg/kg IM every 12 hr		Vancomycin 7.5 mg/kg IV every 6 hr plus cephalothin† 2 g IV every 4 hr plus streptomycin 7.5 mg/kg IM every 12 hr
Subacute, natural valve	Penicillin G or ampicillin 20 to 40 million units IV per 24 hr or 2 gm IV every 4 hr, respectively, plus streptomycin 7.5 mg/kg IM every 12 hr		Vancomycin 7.5 mg/kg IV every 6 hr plus streptomycin 7.5 mg/kg IM every 12 hr
Prosthetic valve	Vancomycin 7.5 mg/kg IV every 6 hr plus an aminoglycoside, for example, gentamicin 1.5 mg/kg IV every 8 hr with or without rifampin 600 mg orally every 12 hr		
	WITH PRIOR ANTIMICROBIAL THERAPY*		
Natural valve in nonaddict	Same as treatment of acute, natural valve endocarditis patient without prior antimicrobial therapy		
Prosthetic valve	Vancomycin 7.5 mg/kg IV every 6 hr plus gentamicin or tobramycin 1.5 mg/kg IV every 8 hr plus ticarcillin 5 gm IV every 6 hr with or without rifampin 600 mg orally every 12 hr	or	Vancomycin 7.5 mg/kg IV every 6 hr plus gentamicin or tobramycin 1.5 mg/kg IV every 8 hr plus third-generation cephamycin,† for example, moxalactam 20 mg/kg IV every 6 to 8 hr, with or without rifampin 600 mg orally every 12 hr

*Doses should be adjusted according to renal and hepatic function.
†Another cephalosporin or cephamycin may be considered.
Adapted from Van Scoy, R. E.: Culture-negative endocarditis. Mayo Clin. Proc. 57:149–154, 1982.

antimicrobial agents, is best treated by valvulectomy without replacement by a prosthesis, followed by the administration of antibiotics for 6 weeks.[368–370] This approach is supported by the experience of Arbulu and Asfaw,[371] who restudied a small number of patients who had undergone this procedure 10 years earlier and compared their clinical status with a group of patients who had had valvulectomy with placement of a prosthesis at about the same time as the other patients. No significant differences were identified.

Silverman et al.[372] noted that cardiac failure was the most frequent indication for surgery with replacement of any infected valve by a prosthesis. Twenty-one per cent of the patients undergoing this procedure developed endocarditis and required reoperation 3 to 18 months later; the fatality rate was 38 per cent. They concluded that surgery was not precluded by infection of multiple valves. The fatality rate of the disease was high, despite treatment with potentially effective antimicrobial agents. Reyes and Lerner[373] have recommended therapy with azlocillin plus an aminoglycoside, but different approaches, based on which side of the heart was involved. In patients with right-sided endocarditis in whom bacteremia persists after 2 weeks of therapy with a beta-lactam antibiotic (ticarcillin) plus a high dose of a potent aminoglycoside, or if the organism is still present in the blood after 6 weeks of appropriate antimicrobial therapy, the tricuspid valve needs to be removed and *not replaced.* Immediate replacement of the infected valve by a prosthesis plus 6 weeks of treatment with appropriate antimicrobial therapy was recommended when the valves on the right side of the heart were infected.

SURGICAL COMPLICATIONS. Complications resulting from the insertion of prosthetic valves in patients with endocarditis include paravalvular leaks, congestive heart failure, complete heart block, systemic arterial emboli, and valvular obstruction; these are often associated with the preoperative presence of annular and myocardial abscesses. Infective endocarditis may recur after insertion of a cardiac prosthesis; the incidence ranges from 1 to 4 per cent.[374] It often becomes apparent within 2 months of the original operation and seems to be related to inadequate debridement, occult sources of infection from preoperative septic emboli, and the characteristics of the original organism.[374] Retained local infection, preexisting peripheral abscesses, and virulent bacteria limit the effectiveness of valve replacement in such patients. It is well known that endocarditis involving a prosthetic valve may appear months to years after operation.

PROSTHETIC VALVE INFECTION (Table 34–10). Infection superimposed on prosthetic valves or on "patches" inserted into previously uninfected hearts poses difficult problems in management.[101] Although chemotherapy based on the sensitivity of the responsible organism is effective in a small number of cases, especially those in which the diagnosis is made and treatment is instituted early, medical management alone often fails to eradicate the disease.[375–378] The development of bacteremia after insertion of a prosthetic valve poses a dilemma difficult to resolve because its source may be extracardiac as well as intracardiac. A study has suggested criteria that may be helpful in indicating the site of the infectious process from which organisms have invaded the bloodstream: (a) if the interval between operation and the detection of organisms in the circulation is less than 25 days, it is more likely that the infection is extracardiac; (b) a longer period is suggestive of an intracardiac infection; (c) the appearance of new murmurs suggests the possibility that bacteria have colonized the prosthesis; and (d) detectable extracardiac sources of bacteremia (e.g., sternal infection, the presence of indwelling venous or urinary tract catheters, suppurative phlebitis, or pneumonia) suggest, but do not prove, that the prosthetic valve is not the source of the organisms.[165] It must be emphasized, however, that none of these criteria, singly or together, always distinguishes extracardiac from intracardiac infections.[166] The author recommends no more than one attempt at eradication of the infection by medical means. Treatment should involve two drugs with a bactericidal effect on the organism, and if the patient appears to respond, therapy should be continued for 6 to 8 weeks. Late streptococcal valve endocarditis involving a bioprosthesis is most often amenable to intensive antibiotic therapy. Early prosthetic valve endocarditis, particularly involving a mechanical prosthesis, is rarely responsive to medical therapy.[101a] If medical therapy fails, the infected valve is removed and replaced by a prosthesis,

TABLE 34–10 FEATURES OF PROSTHETIC VALVE ENDOCARDITIS

MICROBIOLOGY			
Early PVE	**Percent**	**Late PVE**	**Percent**
Staphylococci	45	Streptococci	40
Staph. epidermidis	25	*Strep. viridans*	30
Staph. aureus	20	Group D, *Strep. pneumoniae*	10
Gram-negative	20		
Fungi	10	Staphylococci	35
Diphtheroids	10	*Staph. epidermidis*	25
Streptococci	10	*Staph. aureus*	10
Other	5	Gram-negative	10
		Fungi	5
		Other	5
CLINICAL MANIFESTATIONS			
Fever	97		
Murmur (new/changing)	56		
Petechiae	33		
Splenomegaly	33		
Emboli	33		
Roth spots	5		
Osler's nodes	5		
Janeway lesions	5		
INDICATIONS FOR SURGERY			
Absolute			
Congestive heart failure			
Ongoing sepsis			
Fungal etiology			
Valve obstruction			
Unstable prosthesis by fluoroscopy			
New-onset heart block			
Relative			
Mild congestive heart failure			
Nonstreptococcal organism			
Early PVE			
Embolism			
Paravalvular leak			
Vegetations by echocardiography			
Relapse			
Culture-negative without response			

PVE, prosthetic valve endocarditis.

Modified from Cowgill, L. D., Addonizio, V. P., Hopeman, A. R., and Harken, A. H.: Prosthetic valve endocarditis. Curr. Probl. Cardiol. *11*:626, 628, 635, 646, 1986.

and treatment is continued for 3 to 4 weeks after surgery. One study of the natural history of infective endocarditis after insertion of prostheses into the heart has indicated that antibiotic therapy alone may be effective in eradicating disease that develops 6 or more months after operation.[379] When infection of the prosthesis appeared within 2 months of its insertion, 40 per cent of the patients died before chemotherapy was instituted; the others survived after replacement of the prosthesis and treatment with vancomycin. It was suggested that the prognosis of prosthetic valvular infection that occurs later than 6 months after operation is the same as that for endocarditis involving a natural valve. These conclusions differ from the experience of Sande et al., who noted a 100 per cent fatality rate in patients treated with antibiotics for infectious processes involving cardiac prostheses.[165] The management of infection of prosthetic valves recommended by Wilson et al.[167] is presented in Table 34–8.

The absolute and relative indications for surgery in prosthetic valve endocarditis are shown in Table 34–10. Valve replacement is necessary in all patients with heart failure and/or fungal infections, since mortality with medical therapy alone approaches 100 per cent in these patients. Mortality in patients with heart failure with combined medical and surgical treatment is approximately 50 per cent.[101a] At operation all infected material and tissue and sources of emboli should be excised and major hemodynamic abnormalities corrected. Often the surgical procedures are quite formidable, as in the example shown in Figure 34–13. Combining major series, the overall mortality of patients with prosthetic valve endocarditis managed with antibiotics was 61.4 per cent, whereas those treated surgically (generally a sicker group of patients) was 38.5 per cent.[101a]

PROGNOSIS

Despite the availability of effective antibiotics and the increasing effectiveness of surgical treatment, the mortality and morbidity of infective endocarditis are still significant. The overall 5-year survival has been reported to range from 47 to 90 per cent; of the patients who live, about 15 to 24 per cent are incapacitated by heart failure or the sequelae of embolization.[380–382] Prominent factors in determining the ultimate outcome are age, type of organism, duration of illness before institution of therapy, site and extent of valvular involvement, presence of renal insuffi-

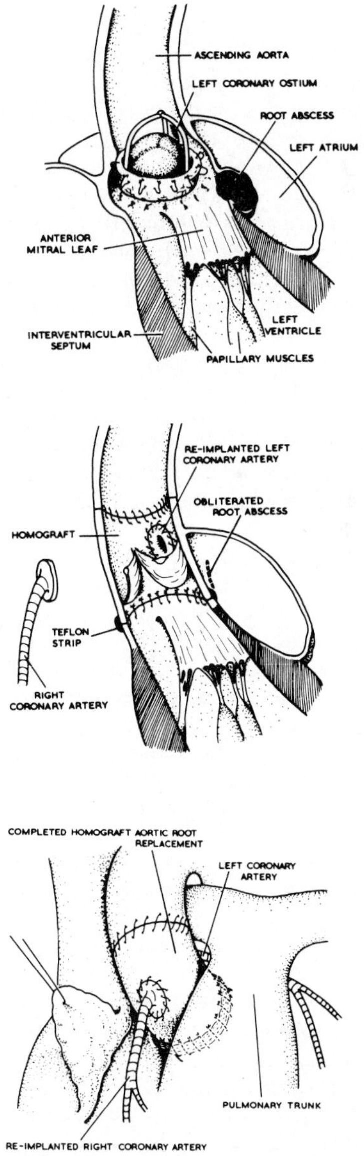

FIGURE 34–13. *Top*, Prosthetic endocarditis. Valve dehiscence and aortic root abscess formation are pictured. *Center*, Aortic root replacement with a homograft showing the reimplanted left coronary artery. *Bottom*, Completed aortic root replacement also showing the reimplanted right coronary artery. (From Lau, J. K. H., Robles, A., Cherian, A., and Ross, D. N.: Surgical treatment of prosthetic endocarditis. J. Thorac. Cardiovasc. Surg. *87*:714, 1984.)

ciency, congestive heart failure, and complications such as embolization, mycotic aneurysms, superinfections, myocarditis, and myocardial abscess. Pearce and Guze suggested that all electrocardiographic abnormalities (except left ventricular hypertrophy and P mitrale) as well as severe alcoholism and/or portal cirrhosis are associated with a poor prognosis for recovery from infective endocarditis.[383]

Age of 60 or older, preexisting cardiovascular disease, prior hospitalization within 30 days of onset of illness, and the development of neurological complications have been identified by Julander[384] and others[384a] as poor prognostic factors in addicted and nonaddicted patients with endocarditis. A history of congestive cardiac failure before the onset of the valvular infection, the presence of diabetes mellitus, cancer, or cirrhosis, a vegetation demonstrated by echocardiography, and involvement of the aortic valve also augur a poor outcome.

Endocarditis caused by *Staph. aureus*, enterococci, gram-negative bacteria, and fungi is associated with an appreciably higher death rate than when it is caused by alpha-streptococci. The prognosis for survival is best when *Strep. viridans* is involved and is worst when *Staph. epidermidis* and *Staph. aureus*, yeasts, and fungi cause the disease. The fatality rate of endocarditis caused by *Candida* is about 80 per cent when patients are treated by either medical or surgical methods alone. However, when these therapeutic modalities are combined, the risk of death is reduced to 20 per cent, especially when the involved valve is replaced by a prosthesis within a few days after the diagnosis of candidal endocarditis is established.

Delay in diagnosis with late initiation of therapy worsens the prognosis in subacute endocarditis. Lerner and Weinstein observed that, of the patients with the subacute disease treated within 2 weeks after the onset of symptoms, 90 per cent survived; only 74 per cent were cured when therapy was withheld for longer than 8 weeks.[1] The survival rate falls appreciably when therapy is delayed longer than 8 weeks and when complications (embolic phenomena, heart failure, and central nervous system involvement) develop.

Perforated valves, torn cusps, or ruptured chordae tendineae—lesions heralded by the appearance of new murmurs, aortic regurgitation, or rapidly developing heart failure—often precede a fatal issue. Although these complications are relatively common in acute infective endocarditis, they have also been observed occasionally in patients with the subacute type of disease.[1]

Cardiac decompensation increases the incidence of failure of antimicrobial therapy and of early and late death. Lerner and Weinstein reported that 6 months after completion of treatment, the survival rate was four times greater in patients with normal than in those with abnormal cardiac function.[1] This has also been observed by others.[382, 384]

Several observers have noted that *myocarditis* is common and is probably an important factor in determining the prognosis of endocarditis.[208, 385, 386] The presence of myocardial abscesses involving either the septum or walls of the ventricles increases the risk of death. However, if these are recognized early and are surgically removed, the prognosis improves.

Although the presence of *myocardial infarction* is seldom detected during life, it is a relatively common finding at autopsy in patients with infective endocarditis.[387–389] Coronary occlusions, even those of minor degree, but especially when multiple, threaten prognosis. Jackson and Allison have presented strong evidence in support of the role of myocardial infarction in the congestive heart failure that occurs in infective endocarditis.[390]

The development of *renal dysfunction* during or after recovery from infective endocarditis is also an ominous prognostic sign, especially if heart failure is also present. About 5 to 10 per cent of the deaths in treated endocarditis are associated with renal failure.[380] However, many observers have documented that even severe uremia may be reversed by intensive antimicrobial therapy.

When *embolic phenomena* supervene, the prognosis for survival depends greatly on the site at which the emboli are deposited, the time in the course of the disease when they develop, and whether or not they produce suppuration.[185, 380] Thus embolization of the coronary arteries or vital areas of the brain and lung (if cardiac failure is present) is a considerably greater threat to survival than involvement of other organs. Systemic emboli have been found in 60 and 45 per cent, respectively, of fatal cases of acute and subacute endocarditis studied at the Massachusetts General Hospital.[380] Cerebral vessels were involved in more than 60 per cent. Embolization may occur longer than 6 months after successful treatment of the cardiac infection but is seldom fatal at that time.[382, 386, 391, 392]

Mycotic aneurysms often begin to develop in the early stages of infective endocarditis but may not rupture until many weeks or months after apparent recovery.[1] The degree of danger with which they are associated depends on their location; tears do not mean inevitable death. Pearce and Guze noted that when cerebral emboli and mycotic aneurysms are not immediately fatal, the prognosis for recovery is good.[383] Of 20 patients with mycotic aneurysms studied by Cates and Christie,[392a] 17 died; the cerebral vessels were involved in all but one of the fatal cases. In addition to the cerebral arteries, which are the most common and most dangerous sites, aneurysms have been found in the abdominal aorta, superior mesenteric artery, sinus of Valsalva, mitral valve, splenic artery, ligated ductus arteriosus, and coronary arteries.[150, 393–396]

PROSTHETIC VALVULAR INFECTIONS. The prognosis in infection of prosthetic valves is determined, in general, by the same factors that influence the outcome in patients with endocarditis involving natural valves. In addition, it depends on whether complications develop, such as obstruction of the valve, paravalvular leaks, or separation of the prosthesis to a degree that causes congestive heart failure. The fatality rate in infections that developed when a previously infected natural valve was replaced with a prosthesis was found to be 28 per cent by Boyd et al.[397] and was 90 per cent in patients treated for 4 to 6 weeks without control of the infection or surgical intervention. In those with uncontrolled disease who were operated on within 10 days, the survival rate was 83 per cent. A review of the literature indicated that the average fatality rate in patients with infected intracardiac prostheses was about 70 per cent.[398]

The overall case-fatality rate in patients with prosthetic valve endocarditis between 1960 and 1980 has been reported to be 58 per cent by Mayer and Schoenbaum.[169] It was appreciably higher when the infection developed "early" ($<$60 days postoperatively); this may be related to infection by staphylococci, gram-negative bacteria, and fungi, as indicated by the fact that the fatality rate was lower when streptococci were involved. The factors that played a role in a poor outcome were congestive heart failure, systemic emboli, "early" prosthetic valve endocarditis, infection by bacteria other than streptococci, infection in a heterograft, and fever persisting for longer than 10 days.

PREVENTION

An approach to the prevention of infective endocarditis involves three considerations:[399]

1. Identification of Patients at Risk. These are all patients (with exceptions noted) with congenital heart disease, both before and after operation, including patients with mitral valve prolapse who have mitral regurgitation; patients with rheumatic valvular heart disease, other acquired forms of valvular disease (both preoperative and postoperative), and hypertrophic obstructive cardiomyopathy; patients with a history of infective endocarditis; patients with indwelling transvenous pacemakers; renal dialysis patients with shunts; and patients with ventriculoatrial shunts for hydrocephalus. Patients particularly at *high risk* are those with prosthetic valves, conduits, patches, and surgically created shunts. Patients who do *not* ordinarily require prophylaxis are those with isolated ostium secundum atrial septal defect, patients more than 6 months after repair of such a defect without a patch, patients more than 6 months after ligation of a patent ductus arteriosus, and postcoronary bypass patients.

2. Identification of Procedures for Which Chemoprophylaxis is Indicated. These include all procedures which potentially produce substantial bacteremia, such as dental and oral surgical procedures, open heart surgery, tonsilloadenoidectomy, gastrointestinal and genitourinary operations, instrumentation and biopsies, nasal intubation, rigid bronchoscopy, as well as incision and drainage of an abscess. Except for the patients at high risk mentioned above, prophylaxis is not *ordinarily* required for percutaneous liver biopsy, gastrointestinal endoscopy without biopsy, barium enema, uncomplicated vaginal delivery, brief bladder catheterization with sterile urine, and diagnostic cardiac catheterization.

3. Selection of a Specific Prophylactic Program. A number of different approaches to this have been recommended, all of which have the same purpose but vary with respect to the choice of specific drugs, their dosage, and the time over which they are applied. They are summarized in Tables 30–4 (p. 907) and 34–11.

Selection of appropriate prophylactic antibiotics requires knowing not only the organisms most likely to be involved in transient bacteremias but also knowing when these are most likely to be responsible for infection of cardiac valves. For example, the bacteria present in the blood after dental manipulation or operations on the upper respiratory tract are, for the most part, viridans streptococci, but enterococci or staphylococci may also invade the circulation after these procedures. Transient bacteremia associated with procedures involving the urinary, gastrointestinal, and genital tracts is usually characterized by the presence of various species of streptococci, gram-negative bacteria, and, occasionally, *Bacteroides. Staph. aureus* is a common culprit in cardiac surgery involving extracorporeal circulation because this decreases the activity of phagocytic cells. When incision and drainage of an abscess or debridement of contaminated tissue is carried out, the choice of prophylactic agent is based on the type or organism recovered from the infected site and its sensitivity to various antimicrobial agents.

A number of programs for the prevention of endocarditis in patients at risk has been proposed by various groups and individual investigators. Among these are the American Heart Association,[400] the Canadian Pediatric Society,[401] the Working Party of the British Society for Antimicrobial Therapy,[402] the European Society of Cardiology,[403] the Medical Letter,[404] and Shanson.[405] These differ to varying degrees, not only in the choice of specific antimicrobial agents but also in dosage and the time and duration of their administration.

TABLE 34–11 RECOMMENDATIONS FOR PROPHYLAXIS

Category	Antibiotic Regimen
DENTAL PROCEDURES	
Local anesthesia	
Not allergic to penicillin	A. Amoxicillin 3 gm orally 1 hr before
Allergic to penicillin or had penicillin recently	B. Erythromycin 1.5 gm orally 1 hr before; 0.5 gm 6 hr later
General anesthesia	
No special risk	C. Amoxicillin 1 gm IM or IV; 0.5 gm orally or IM 6 hr later
Patients at special risk*	
Not allergic to penicillin	D. Amoxicillin 1 gm IM or IV plus gentamicin 120 mg IM or IV: amoxicillin 0.5 gm orally or IM 7 hr later
Allergic to penicillin	E. Vancomycin 1 gm IV plus gentamicin 120 mg IM or IV
SURGERY OR INSTRUMENTATION OF THE UPPER RESPIRATORY TRACT	
Category	**Antibiotic Regimen**
No special risk	Recommendation C
Special risk	Recommendation D or E
GENITOURINARY SURGERY OR INSTRUMENTATION	
Category	**Antibiotic Regimen**
Not allergic to penicillin	Recommendation D
Allergic to penicillin	Recommendation E
Patient with infected urine	Regimen to cover organisms isolated

OBSTETRICAL AND GYNECOLOGICAL PROCEDURES

Endocarditis is very uncommon after these procedures; however, patients at special risk of infection should receive antibiotic cover as for genitourinary surgery.

PEDIATRIC DOSES

Amoxicillin: Children under 10 years—one-half the adult dose
Erythromycin: Children under 5 years—one-quarter the adult dose
Gentamicin: 2 mg/kg
Vancomycin: 20 mg/kg

*Patients at special risk include those with prosthetic valves, those who have a past history of endocarditis, or those who require general anesthesia and are allergic to penicillin. The latter group requires vancomycin, which must be administered IV over a 30-minute period. IM administration of 1 gm of amoxicillin may be painful. It is recommended that it be given in 2.5 mg of 1% lidocaine. Patients at special risk should always undergo procedures within the hospital.

Adapted from Working Party of the British Society for Antimicrobial Chemotherapy: The antibiotic prophylaxis of infective endocarditis. Lancet 2:1323–1326, 1982.

The following statement by the American Heart Association[400] places the prophylaxis of infective endocarditis in perspective: "The American Heart Association Committee on Rheumatic Fever and Endocarditis recognizes that it is not possible to make recommendations for all possible situations. Practitioners must exercise their clinical judgment in determining the duration and choice of antibiotic when special circumstances apply. . . . Because there are not controlled clinical trials, the choice of antibiotic regimens for prevention of endocarditis in humans must be based on indirect information."

OPEN HEART AND OTHER SURGICAL PROCEDURES. The purpose of prophylaxis in patients undergoing open heart or other types of surgery is not only the prevention of endocarditis, which may not be a threat in some cases, but also to decrease the risk of other infections, such as those involving the sternal wound and lungs, and to prevent episodes of bacteremia that may occur during surgery and lead to metastatic infections. Infections that develop early in the postoperative period are often caused by *Staph. aureus* or *Staph. epidermidis.* Bacteria less frequently responsible are streptococci, gram-negative bacteria, and fungi. Because there is no chemoprophylactic program that will protect against invasion by all organisms, prudence suggests that in surgical patients it be directed primarily against the staphylococcus. For this reason the antibiotics most frequently used have been oxacillin, nafcillin, or cephalothin, the latter protecting against invasion not only by staphylococci, but also by common gram-negative bacilli, such as *E. coli, Proteus mirabilis,* and *K. pneumoniae.* An acceptable regimen for these antibiotics is 2 gm intravenously 2 hours before operation, 1 gm intraoperatively, and 1 gm every 4 hours for no longer than 2 days, in order to minimize the risk of superinfection. The author prefers cephalothin because of its activity against most staphylococci and streptococci as well as against the common gram-negative bacteria. Vancomycin, 1 gm intravenously 2 hours before surgery, followed by the same dose every 12 hours for 2 days may be first choice in some cases or used in persons sensitized to the penicillins or cephalosporins. Although penicillinase-resistant penicillins and first-generation cephalosporin are usually administered, the eventual choice rests on information concerning a hospital's experiences with the antimicrobial activities of various drugs. If it is known that methicillin-resistant staphylococcus are present, vancomycin is the optimal choice for prophylaxis.

UNDERLYING CARDIAC DISEASE. Patients with underlying cardiac disease, especially abnormal valves, who undergo surgical or other manipulations of the gastrointestinal and genitourinary tracts or dental procedures should be given chemoprophylaxis. The programs included here are the ones recommended by the American Heart Association (Table 30–4, p. 907) and the Working Party of the British Society for Antimicrobial Chemotherapy (Table 34–11). For information furnished in the other programs, the reader is directed to the specific reference.

The American Heart Assocation[400] has recommended prophylaxis of endocarditis in patients undergoing surgery involving infected tissue or incision and drainage of abscesses, and for surgical and dental procedures in persons who have had a documented episode of endocarditis in the past. Prophylaxis should be considered for patients with arteriovenous shunts for renal dialysis, or those with ventriculoatrial shunts who are subjected to surgical or dental manipulation.

SPECIAL SITUATIONS. Prophylaxis of infective endocarditis in persons with mitral valve prolapse (MVP) is not indicated unless the murmur of mitral regurgitation is present.[406] Clemens and Ransohoff[407] have pointed out that the risk of endocardial infections with MVP is "so very small" that it is outweighed by the greater danger of fatal reactions associated with the parenteral (15 deaths per 10 million courses) or oral (0.9 deaths per 10 million courses) administration of penicillin. Murphy et al.[408] have recommended that prophylaxis for transurethral surgery be initiated more than 24 hours before the procedure is carried out.

It must be emphasized that the chemoprophylactic programs currently in use for the prevention of recurrences of rheumatic fever may not eliminate the risk of the development of infective endocarditis. For this reason all patients on such programs who are subjected to manipulations of the oral cavity or the upper respiratory, urinary, or gastrointestinal tract must receive additional prophylaxis.

DENTAL HYGIENE. Several reports have stressed the role of good dental hygiene in the prevention of infective endocarditis in patients at risk who are subjected to various kinds of dental manipulation. This approach has been encouraged by Shanson's statement that "direct evidence that any antibiotic prophylaxis is effective for preventing endocarditis in dental patients is completely lacking." Microbiological sampling of dental plaque is of little value in selecting appropriate prophylaxis for dental procedures in patients who have recently received antibiotics but may be important in those who have been exposed to these agents over an extended period.[409]

It has been suggested that meticulous dental hygiene may be more important than antimicrobial prophylaxis in preventing infective endocarditis in patients undergoing various dental procedures.[410] In commenting about chemoprophylaxis in susceptible patients, Oakley and Somerville[411] noted that a rise in the standard of oral hygiene would probably help more than any other measure to reduce the incidence of streptococcal infective endocarditis. Seldin[412] urged that all patients at risk of valvular infection be maintained as free of any type of dental disease as possible.

REFERENCES

PATHOGENESIS

1. Lerner, P. I., and Weinstein, L.: Infective endocarditis in the antibiotic era. N. Engl. J. Med. *274*:199, 259, 323, 387, 1966.
2. Kelson, S. R., and White, P. D.: Notes on 250 cases of subacute bacterial streptococcal endocarditis studied and treated between 1927 and 1939. Ann. Intern. Med. 22:40, 1940.
3. Kaye, D.: Changing pattern of infective endocarditis. Am. J. Med. 78:157, 1985.
4. Kerr, A., Jr.: Subacute bacterial endocarditis. *In* Pullen, R. L. (ed.): Springfield, Ill, Charles C Thomas, 1955. (No. 274, Am. Lecture Series, Monograph of Bannerstone Division of Am. Lectures in Internal Medicine.)
5. Weinstein, L., and Rubin, R. H.: Infective endocarditis—1973. Prog. Cardiovasc. Dis. *16*:239, 1973.
6. Levandowski, R. A.: *Streptococcus milleri* endocarditis complicated by myocardial abscess. South. Med. J. *78*:892, 1985.
7. Coto, H., and Berk, S. L.: Endocarditis caused by *Streptococcus morbillorum.* Am. J. Med. Sci. *287*:54, 1984.
8. Bayliss, R., Clarke, C., Oakley, C. M., Somerville, W., Whitfield, A. G. W., and Young, S. E. J.: The microbiology and pathogenesis of infective endocarditis. Br. Heart J. *50*:513, 1983.
9. Levin, R. M., Pulliam, L., Mondry, C., Levy, D., Hadley, K., and Grossman, M.: Penicillin-resistant *Streptococcus constellatus* as a cause of endocarditis. Am. J. Dis. Child. *136*:42, 1982.
10. Harder, E. J., Wilkowske, C. J., Washington, J. A., III, and Geraci, J. E.: *Streptococcus mutans* endocarditis. Ann. Intern. Med. *80*:364, 1974.
11. Roberts, K. B., and Sidlak, M. E.: Satellite streptococci: A major cause of "negative" blood cultures in bacterial endocarditis? JAMA *241*:2293, 1979.
12. Eisenberg, F. P., Lorber, B., Suh, B., and McDonough, M. T.: Case Report: Prosthetic valve endocarditis due to a nutritionally variant streptococcus. Am. J. Med. Sci. *289*:249, 1985.
13. Ramirez, C. A., Naraqi, S., and McCulley, D. J.: Group A beta-hemolytic streptococcus endocarditis. Am. Heart J. *108*:1383, 1984.
14. Gallagher, P. C., and Watankunakorn, C.: Group B streptococcal endocarditis: Report of seven cases and review of the literature, 1962–1985. Rev. Infect. Dis. *8*:175, 1986.
15. Stein, D. S., and Panwalker, A. P.: Group C streptococcal endocarditis: Case report and review of literature. Infection *13*:282, 1985.
16. Rolston, K. V. I., Chandrasekar, P. H., and LeFrock, J. H.: Clinical features and anti-microbial therapy of infections caused by Group G streptococci. Infection *13*:203, 1985.
17. Bevanger, L., and Stames, T. I.: Group L streptococci as the cause of bacteraemia and endocarditis. Acta Pathol. Microbiol. Scand. *87*:301, 1979.
18. Missri, J. C., and Rohatgi, P.: Pneumococcal endocarditis following splenectomy for trauma. Am. Heart J. *108*:622, 1984.
19. Prag, J., Kjoller, E., and Espersen, F.: Stomatococcus mucilaginosus endocarditis. Eur. J. Clin. Microbiol. *4*:422, 1985.
20. Pein, E. D., Wilson, W. R., Kunz, K., and Washington, J. A., II: *Aerococcus viridans* endocarditis. Mayo Clin. Proc. *59*:47, 1984.
21. Wilkowske, C. J.: Enterococcal endocarditis. Mayo Clin. Proc. *57*:101, 1982.
22. Klein, R. S., Recco, R. A., Catalano, M. T., Edberg, C. S., Casey, J. I., and Steigbigel, N. H.: Association of *Streptoccus bovis* with carcinoma of the colon. N. Engl. J. Med. *297*:800, 1977.
23. Bayer, A. S.: Staphylococcal bacteremia and endocarditis. State of the art. Arch. Intern. Med. *142*:1169, 1982.
24. Karchmer, A. W., Archer, G. L., and Dismukes, W. E.: *Staphylococcus epidermidis* causing prosthetic valve endocarditis: Microbiologic and clinical observations as guides to therapy. Ann. Intern. Med. *98*:447, 1983.
25. Baddour, I. M., Phillips, T. N., and Bisno, A. L.: Coagulase-negative staphylococcal endocarditis. Occurrence in patients with mitral valve prolapse. Arch. Intern. Med. *146*:119, 1986.
26. Conrad, S. A., and West, B. C.: Endocarditis caused by *Staphylococcus xylosus* associated with intravenous drug abuse. J. Infect. Dis. *149*:826, 1984.
27. Dan, M., Marien, G. I., and Goldsand, G.: Endocarditis caused by *Staphylococcus warneri* on a normal aortic valve following vasectomy. Can. Med. Assoc. J. *131*:211, 1984.
28. Trepeta, R. W., and Edberg, S. C.: *Corynebacterium diphtheriae* endocarditis: Sustained potential of a classical pathogen. Am. J. Clin. Pathol. *81*:679, 1984.
29. Adoue, D., LeFèvre, J. C., Chamontin, B., Couret, B., Arlet-Suau, E., and Fédou, R.: *Corynebacterium* (JK group) endocarditis. Apropos of a case. Sem. Hop. Paris *60*:1075, 1984.
30. Austin, G. E., and Hill, E. O.: Endocarditis due to *Corynebacterium* CDC Group G2. J. Infect. Dis. *147*:1106, 1983.
31. Murray, B. E., Karchmer, A. W., and Moellering, R. C., Jr.: Diphtheroid prosthetic valve endocarditis. A study of clinical features and infecting organisms. Am. J. Med. *69*:838, 1980.
32. Worthington, M. G., Daly, B. D. I., and Smith, F. E.: *Corynebacterium hemolyticum* endocarditis on a native valve. South. Med. J. *78*:1261, 1985.
33. Davis, A. J., James, P. A., and Hawkey, P. M.: *Lactobacillus* endocarditis. J. Infect. *12*:169, 1986.
34. Gallagher, P. G., Amedia, C. A., and Watanakunakorn, C.: *Listeria monocytogenes* endocarditis in a patient on chronic hemodialysis, successfully treated with vancomycin-gentamicin. Infection *14*:125, 1986.
35. Vlachakin, N. D., Gazes, P. C., and Hairston, P.: Nocardial endocarditis following mitral valve replacement. Chest *63*:276, 1975.
36. Waters, E. W, Romansky, M. J., Johnson, A. C., and Conway, S. J.: *Actinomyces bovis* endocarditis: An uncommon and complex problem. *In* Sylvester, J. C. (ed.): Antimicrobial Agents and Chemotherapy—1962. American Society of Microbiology, Washington, DC, 1963, p. 517.
37. McCabe, R. S., Baldwin, J. C., McGregor, C. A., Miller, D. C., and Vosti, K. L.: Prosthetic valve endocarditis by *Legionella pneumophilia.* Ann. Intern. Med. *100*:525, 1984.
38. Broeren, S. A., and Peel, M. M.: Endocarditis caused by *Rothia dentocariosa.* J. Clin. Pathol. *37*:1298, 1984.
39. Fliegelman, R. M., Cohen, R. S., and Zakhireh, B.: *Erysipelothrix rhusiopathiae* endocarditis. Report of a case and review of literature. J. Am. Osteopathic Assoc. *85*:39, 1985.
40. McCormack, R. C., Kaye, D., and Hook, E. W.: Endocarditis due to *Streptobacillus moniliformis.* A report of two cases and review of the literature. *200*:183, 1967.

41. Reller, L. B.: Endocarditis caused by *Bacillus subtilis*. Am. J. Clin. Pathol. *60*:714, 1973.
42. Block, C. S., Levy, M. L., and Fritz, V. U.: *Bacillus cereus* endocarditis. A case report. S. Afr. Med. J. *53*:556, 1978.
43. Alvarez-Elcoro, S., and Sifuentes-Osorio, J.: *Clostridium perfringens* bacteremia in prosthetic valve endocarditis. Diagnosis by peripheral blood smear. Arch. Intern. Med. *144*:849, 1984.
44. Cohen, P. S., Maguire, J. H., and Weinstein, L.: Infective endocarditis caused by gram-negative bacteria. Prog. Cardiovasc. Dis. *22*:205, 1980.
45. Wieland, M., Lederman, M. M., Klein-King, C., et al.: Left-sided endocarditis due to *Pseudomonas aeruginosa*. A report of 10 cases and review of the literature. Medicine *65*:180, 1986.
46. Noriega, E. R., Rubinstein, E., Simberkoff, M. S., and Rahal, J. J., Jr.: Subacute and acute endocarditis due to *Pseudomonas cepacia* in heroin addicts. Am. J. Med. *59*:29, 1975.
47. Yu, V. L., Rumans, L. W., Wing, E. J., McLeod, R., Sattler, F.N., Horvey, R.M., and Beresinski, S.C.: *Pseudomonas multophilia* causing heroin-associated infective endocarditis. Arch. Intern. Med. *138*:1667, 1978.
48. Valenstein, P., Bardy, G. H., Cox, C. C., and Zwadyk, P.: *Pseudomonas alcaligenes* endocarditis. Am. J. Clin. Pathol. *79*:245, 1983.
49. Cooper, R. and Mills, J.: *Serratia* endocarditis: A follow-up report. Arch. Intern. Med. *140*:199, 1980.
50. Chowdhury, M. N. H., Al-Nozha, M., Husain, I. S., and Akhtar, J.: Endocarditis due to *Actinobacillus actinomycetemcomitans*. J. Infect. *10*:158, 1985.
51. Blair, T. P., and Baker, W. P.: *Haemophilus influenzae* endocarditis. South. Med. J. *78*:759, 1985.
52. Graninger, W., Pirich, K., Kronik, G., Hirschl, M., and Gossinger, H.: *Haemophilus parainfluenzae* endocarditis on tricuspid valve. Cardiology *71*:215, 1984.
53. Root, T. E., Silva, E. A., Edwards, L. D., and Topp, J. H.: *Hemophilus aphrophilus* endocarditis with a probable dental focus of infection. Chest *80*:109, 1981.
54. Lane, T., MacGregor, R. R., Wright, D., and Hollander, J.: *Cardiobacterium hominis*: An elusive cause of endocarditis. J. Infect. Dis. 675, 1983.
55. Appelbaum, J. S., Wilding, G., and Morse, L. J.: *Yersinia enterocolitica* endocarditis. Arch. Intern. Med. *143*:2150, 1983.
56. Schmidt, U., Chmel, H., Kaminski, Z., and Sen, P.: The clinical spectrum of *Campylobacter* fetus infections: Report of five cases and review of the literature. Q. J. Med. *49*:431, 1980.
57. Almer, L-O.: A case of brucellosis complicated by endocarditis and disseminated intravascular coagulation. Acta Med. Scand. *217*:139, 1985.
58. McCullough, D., Menzies, R., and Corthere, B. M.: Endocarditis due to *Citrobacter diversus* developing resistance to cephalothin. N.Z. Med. J. *85*:182, 1977.
59. LeFrock, L. J., Klainer, A. S., and Zuckerman, K.: *Edwardsiella tarda* bacteremia. South. Med. J. *69*:188, 1976.
60. O'Leary, T., and Fong, I. W.: Prosthetic valve endocarditis caused by Group Ve-1 bacteria (*Chromobacterium typhiflavus*). J. Clin. Microbiol. *20*:995, 1984.
61. Claesson, B., Falsen, E., and Kjellman, B.: *Kingella kingae* infections: A review and a presentatiaon of data from 10 Swedish cases. Scand. J. Infect. Dis. *17*:233, 1985.
62. Elansary, E. H., and Earis, J. E.: *Pasteurella multocida* endocarditis. Br. Med. J. *286*:1862, 1983.
63. Alvarez-Elcoro, S., Soto-Ramirez, L., and Mateos-Mora, M.: *Salmonella* bacteremia in patients with prosthetic heart valves. Am. J. Med. *77*:61, 1984.
64. Landis, S. J., and Korver, J.: *Eikenella corrodens* endocarditis: Case report and review of the literature. Can. Med. Assoc. J. *128*:822, 1983.
65. Fredericka, D. N.: Endocarditis and brain abscess due to *Bacteroides oralis*. *J. Infect. Dis. 145*:918, 1982.
66. Duperval, R., Beland, S., and Marcoux, J. A.: Infective endocarditis due to *Leptotrichia buccalis*: A case report. Can. Med. Assoc. J. *130*:422, 1984.
67. Porath, A., Wanderman, K., Simu, A., Vinde, B., and Alkan, M.: Case Report. Endocarditis caused by *Haemophilus aegyptius*. Am. J. Med. Sci. *282*:110, 1986.
68. Fernandez, G. C., Chapman, A. J., Jr., Bolli, R., Rose, S. D., O'Meara, M. E., Luck, J. C., Pratt, C. M., and Young, J. B.: Gonococcal endocarditis: A case series demonstrating modern presentation of an old disease. Am. Heart J. *108*:1326, 1984.
69. Weetman, A. P., Matthews, N., O'Hara, S. P., Amos, N., Williams, B. D., and Thomas, J. P.: Meningococcal endocarditis with profound acquired hypocomplementaemia. J. Infect. *10*:51, 1985.
70. Pollack, S., Mogtader, A., and Lange, M.: *Neisseria subflava* endocarditis. Case report and review of the literature. Am. J. Med. *76*:752, 1984.
71. Davis, C. L., Towns, M., Henrich, W. L., and Melby, K.: *Neisseria mucosus* endocarditis following drug abuse. Case report and review of the literature. Arch. Intern. Med. *143*:583, 1983.
72. Thornhill-Jones, M. L., Canwati, H. N., Ibrahim, M. Z., and Sapico, F. L.: *Neisseria sicca* endocarditis in intravenous drug abusers. West. J. Med. *142*:255, 1985.
73. Simor, A. E., and Salit, I. E.: Endocarditis caused by M6. J. Clin. Microbiol. *17*:931, 1983.
74. Kannangara, D. W., Salem, F. A., Rao, B. S., and Thadepalli, H.: Cardiac tuberculosis: TB of endocardium. Am. J. Med. Sci. *287*:45, 1984.
75. Rumisek, J. D., Albus, R. A., and Clarke, J. S.: Late *Mycobacterium chelonei* bioprosthetic valve endocarditis: Activation of implanted contaminant? Ann. Thorac. Surg. *39*:277, 1985.
76. Lohr, D. C., Goeken, J. A., Doty, D. B., and Donta, S.: *Mycobacterium gordonae* infection of a prosthetic valve. J.A.M.A. *239*:1528, 1978.
77. Kuritsky, J. N., Bullen, C., Broome, C. V., Silcox, V. A., Good, R. C., and Wallace, R. J., Jr.: Sternal wound infections and endocarditis due to organisms of the *Mycobacterium fortuitum* complex. Ann. Intern. Med. *98*:938, 1983.
78. Editorial: Chronic Q fever. J. Infect. *8*:1, 1984.
79. Van der Bel-Kahn, J. M., Watanakunakorn, C., Menefee, N. G., Long, H. D., and Dicter, R.: *Chlamydia trachomatis* endocarditis. Am. Heart J. *95*:627, 1978.
80. Jones, R. B., Priest, J. B., and Kuo, C-C: Subacute chlamydial endocarditis. J.A.M.A. *247*:655, 1982.
81. Seelig, M. S., Goldberg, P., Kozinn, P. J., and Berger, A. R.: Fungal endocarditis: Patients at risk and their treatment. Postgrad. Med. J. *55*:632, 1979.
82. Herling, I. M., Kotler, M. N., Segal, B. L.: *Candida parapsilosis* endocarditis without predisposing cause. Int. J. Cardiol. *5*:753, 1984.
83. Holliday, H. D., Keipper, V., and Kaiser, A. B.: *Torulopsis glabrata* endocarditis. J.A.M.A. *244*:2088, 1980.
84. Wilkowske, C. J., and Hermans, P. E.: General principles of antimicrobial therapy. Mayo Clin. Proc. *58*:6, 1983.
85. Svirbely, J. R. Ayers, L. W., and Buesching, W. J.: Filamentous *Histoplasma capsulatum* endocarditis involving mitral and aortic valve porcine bioprostheses. Arch. Pathol. Lab. Med. *109*:273, 1985.
86. Merchant, R. K., Louria, D. B., Gersher, P. H., Edycomb, J. H., and Utz, J. P.: Fungal endocarditis: Review of the literature and report of three cases. Ann. Intern. Med. *48*:242, 1958.
87. Barst, R. I., Prince, A. S., and Neu, H. C.: *Aspergillus* endocarditis in children: Case report and review of the literature. Pediatrics *68*:73, 1981.
88. Erdos, M. S., Butt, K., and Weinstein, L.: Mucomycotic endocarditis of the pulmonary valve. J.A.M.A. *222*:951, 1972.
89. Reyes, C. V., Stanley, M. M., and Rippon, J. W.: *Trichosporon beigelii* endocarditis as a complication of peritoneovenous shunt. Hum. Pathol. *16*:857, 1985.
90. DelRossi, A. J., Morse, D., Spagna, P. M., and Lemole, C. M.: Successful management of *Penicillium* endocarditis. J. Thorac. Cardiovasc. Surg. *80*:945, 1980.
91. Davis, W. A., Isner, J. M., Bracey, A. W., Roberts, W. C., and Garagusi, V. E.: Disseminated *Petriellidium boydii* and pacemaker endocarditis. Am. J. Med. *69*:929, 1980.
92. Kalish, S. B., Goldschmidt, R., Li, C., Knop, R., Cook, F. V., Wilner, G., and Victor, T. A.: Infective endocarditis caused by *Paecilomyces varioti*. Am. J. Clin. Pathol. *78*:249, 1982.
93. Varitian, C. V., Shlaes, D. M., Padye, A. A., and Ajello, L.: *Wangiella dermatitidis* endocarditis in an intravenous drug user. Am. J. Med. *78*:703, 1984.
94. Toshinowal, R., Goodman, S., Ally, S., Ray, V., Bodino, C., and Kullick, C. A.: Endocarditis due to *Chromosporium* species. A disease of medical progress. J. Infect. Dis. *153*:638, 1986.
95. Sklaver, A. R., Hoffman, T. A., and Greenman, R. I.: Staphylococcal endocarditis in addicts. South. Med. J. *71*:638, 1978.
96. Dreyer, N. P., and Fields, B. N.: Heroin-associated infective endocarditis. Ann. Intern. Med. *78*:699, 1973.
97. Bailey, I. K., and Richards, J. G.: Infective endocarditis in a Sydney teaching hospital—1962–1971. Aust. N.Z. Med. *5*:413, 1975.
98. Pankey, G. A.: The prevention and treatment of bacterial endocarditis. Am. Heart J. *98*:102, 1979.
99. Buchbinder, N. A., and Roberts, W. C.: Left-sided valvular active endocarditis. Am. J. Med. *53*:20, 1972.
100. Roberts, W. C., and Buchbinder, N. A.: Healed left-sided infective endocarditis. A clinicopathological study of 59 patients. Am. J. Cardiol. *40*:876, 1976.
101. Roberts. W. C., and Buchbinder, N. A.: Right-sided valvular infective endocarditis. Am. J. Med. *53*:7, 1972.
101a. Cowgill, L. D., Addonizio, V. P., Hopewau, A. R., and Harken, A. H.: Prosthetic valve endocarditis. Curr. Probl. Cardiol. *11*:620, 1986.
102. Arnett, E. N., and Roberts, W. C.: Prosthetic valve endocarditis. Clinicopathological analysis of 22 necropsy patients with comparison of observations in 74 necropsy patients with active infective endocarditis involving natural left-sided cardiac valves. Am. J. Cardiol. *38*:281, 1976.
103. Anderson, D. J., Buckley, B. H., and Hutchins, G. M.: A clinicopathologic study of prosthetic valve endocarditis in 22 patients: Morphologic basis for diagnosis and therapy. Am. Heart J. *94*:325, 1977.
104. Bartolotti, U., Thiene, G., Milano, A. Panizzon G., Valente, M., and Gallucci, V.: Pathological study of infective endocarditis on Hancock porcine bioprostheses. J. Thorac. Cardiovasc. Surg. *81*:934, 1981.
105. Ferrans, V. J., Boyce, S. W., Billingham, M. E., Spray, T. L., and Roberts, W. C.: Infection of glutaraldehyde-preserved porcine valve heterografts. Am. J. Cardiol. *43*:1123, 1979.
106. Schoen, F. J., Titus, J. L., and Lawrie, G. M.: Autopsy determined causes of death after cardiac valve replacement. J.A.M.A. *249*:899, 1983.
107. Schoen, F. J., Levy, R. J.: Bioprosthetic heart valve failure. Pathology and pathogenesis. Cardiol. Clin. *2*:717, 1984.
108. Schoen, F. J.: Pathology of cardiac valve replacement. *In* Steiner, M. D., and Fernandez, R. M. (eds.): Guide to Prosthetic Cardiac Valves. New York, Springer-Verlag, 1985, p. 209.
109. Peterson, L. J., and Peacock, R.: The incidence of bacteremia in pediatric patients following tooth extraction. Circulation *53*:676, 1976.
110. Goodman, J. S., Kolhouse, J. F., and Koenig, M. G.: Recurrent endocarditis due to *Streptococcus viridans* in an edentulous man. South. Med. J. *66*:352, 1973.
111. Bayliss, R., Clarke, C., Oakley, C., Somerville, W., and Whitfield, A. G. W.: The teeth and infective endocarditis. Br. Heart J. *50*:506, 1983.
112. LeFrock, J. L., Ellis, C. A., Klainer, A., and Weinstein, L.: Transient bacteremia associated with barium enema. Arch. Intern. Med. *135*:835, 1975.

113. LeFrock, J. L., Ellis, C. A., Turchik, J. B., and Weinstein, L.: Transient bacteremia associated with sigmoidoscopy. N. Engl. J. Med. *289*:469, 1973.
114. Rigilano, J., Mahapatra, R., Barnhill, J., and Gutierrez, J.: Enterococcal endocarditis following sigmoidoscopy and mitral valve prolapse. Arch. Intern. Med. *144*:850, 1984.
115. Shull, H. J., Green, B. M., Allen, S. R., Dunn, G. D., and Schenker, S.: Bacteremia with upper gastrointestinal endoscopy. Ann. Intern. Med. *212*, 1975.
116. Rafoth, A. J., Sorenson, R. M., and Bond, J. H.: Bacteremia following colonoscopy. Gastrointest. Endosc. *22*:32, 1975.
117. LeFrock, J. L., Ellis, C. A., Turchik, J. B., Zawacki, J. K., and Weinstein, L.: Transient bacteremia associated with percutaneous liver biopsy. J. Infect. Dis. *131*(Suppl.):104, 1975.
118. Sullivan, N. M., Sutter, V. L., Mims, M. M., Marsh, V. H., and Finegold, S. M.: Clinical aspects of bacteremia after manipulation of the genitourinary tract. J. Infect. Dis. *127*:49, 1973.
119. Ritvo, R., Monroe, P., and Andriole, V. T.: Transient bacteremia due to suction abortion. Implications for SBE prophylaxis. Yale J. Biol. Med. *50*:471, 1977.
120. McShane, A. L., and Hone, R.: Prevention of bacterial endocarditis: *Does nasal intubation* warrant prophylaxis? Br. Med. J. *292*:26, 1986.
121. Low, D. E., Shoenut, J. P., Kennedy, J. K., Harding, G. K. M., Den Boer, B., and Micflikies, A. B.: Infectious complications of endoscopic injection sclerotherapy. Arch. Intern. Med. *146*:569, 1986.
122. Niv, Y., Bat, L., and Motro, M.: Bacterial endocarditis after Hurst bouginage in a patient with a benign esophageal stricture and mitral valve prolapse. Gastrointest. Endosc. *31*:265, 1985.
123. Goldman, G., Ziberman, M., and Werbin, N.: Bacteremia in anal dilatation. Dis. Colon Rectum *29*:304, 1986.
124. Iwamura, K., Ueno, F., Itakura, M., and Sugimoto, E.: Evaluation of blood cultures following laparoscopy. Tokai J. Exp. Clin. Med. *5*:323, 1980.
125. Valla, D., Pariente, E-A., Degott, C.,. Fabiani-Saloff, B., Bernuau, J., Rueff, B., and Benhamou, J-P.: Right-sided endocarditis complicating peritoneovenous shunting for ascites. Arch. Intern. Med. *143*:1801, 1983.
126. Connors, A. F., Castele, R. J., Farhat, N. Z., and Tomashefski, J. F.: Complications of right heart catheterization—a prospective autopsy study. Chest *88*:567, 1985.
127. Tsao, M. M. P., and Katz, D.: Central venous catheter-induced endocarditis: Human correlate of the animal experimental model of endocarditis. Rev. Infect. Dis. *6*:783, 1984.
128. Rowley, K. M., Clubb, K. S., Smith, G. J. W., and Cabin, H. S.: Right-sided infective endocarditis as a consequence of flow-directed pulmonary artery catheterization. A clinicopathological study of 55 autopsied patients. N. Engl. J. Med. *311*:1152, 1984.
129. Parker, F. B., Greiner-Hayes, C., Tomar, R. H., Markowitz, A. H., Bove, E. L., and Marvasti, M. A.: Bacteremia following prosthetic valve replacement. Ann. Surg. *197*:147, 1983.
130. Cookson, W. O., and Harris, A. R. C.: Diphtheroid endocarditis after electrolysis. Br. Med. J. *282*:1513, 1981.
131. Lee, R. J. E., and McIlwain, J. C.: Subacute bacterial endocarditis following ear acupuncture. Int. J. Cardiol. *7*:62, 1985.
132. Dan, M., Marien, G. J. R., and Goldsand, G.: Endocarditis caused by *Staphylococcus warneri* on a normal aortic valve following vasectomy. Can. Med. Assoc. J. *131*:211, 1984.
133. Snyder, N., Atterbury, C. E., Correia, J. P., and Conn, H. F.: Increased concurrence of cirrhosis and bacterial endocarditis. Gastroenterology *73*:1107, 1977
134. Baskin, T. W., Rosenthal, A., and Pruitt, B. A., Jr.: Acute bacterial endocarditis: A silent source of sepsis in the burn patient. Ann. Surg. *184*:618, 1976.
135. Lemire, G. G., Morin, J. E., and Dobell, A. R. C.: Pacemaker infections: A 12-year review. Can. J. Surg. *18*:181–184, 1975.
136. Garvey, G. J., and Neu, H. C.: Infective endocarditis—an evolving disease. A review of endocarditis at the Columbia-Presbyterian Medical Center, 1968–1973. Medicine *57*:105, 1978.
137. Whitby, M., Fraser, S., Gemmell, C. G., Wright, P. A.: Toxic shock syndrome and endocarditis. Br. Med. J. *286*:1613, 1983.
138. Rosen, P., and Armstrong, D.: Infective endocarditis in patients treated for malignant neoplastic disease. Am. J. Clin. Pathol. *60*:241, 1973.
139. Tornos, M. P., Galve, E., and Pahissa, A.: Clinical considerations regarding infective Libman-Sacks endocarditis. Int. J. Cardiol. *7*:409, 1985.
140. Cross, A. S., and Steigbigel, R. T.: Infective endocarditis and access site infections in patients on hemodialysis. Medicine *55*:453, 1976.
141. Markowitz, S. M., Szentpetery, S., Lower, R. R., and Duma, R. J.: Endocarditis due to accidental penetrating foreign bodies. Am. J. Med. *60*:571, 1976.
142. Shevchenko, Iu. L.: Infectious intracardiac complications of gunshot wounds of the heart. Vestn. Khir. *131*:86, 1983.
143. Dehan, M., Vermont, P., and Casasoprana, G.: Endocarditis bacteriennes sur cardiopathies congenitales. Arch. Mal. Coeur *75*:1049, 1982.
144. Gelfman, R., and Levine, S. A.: The incidence of acute and subacute bacterial endocarditis in congenital heart disease. Am. J. Med. Sci. *204*:324, 1942.
145. Johnson, C. M., and Rhodes, H. K.: Pediatric endocarditis. Mayo Clin. Proc. *57*:86, 1982.
146. McGuinness, G. A., Schieken, R. M., and Maguire, G. F.: Endocarditis in the newborn. Am. J. Dis. Child. *134*:577, 1980.
147. Shah, P., Singh, W. S. A., Rose V., and Keith, J. D.: Incidence of bacterial endocarditis in ventricular septal defects. Circulation *34*:127, 1966.
148. Hallidie-Smith, K. A., Olsen, E. G. J., Oakley, C. M., Goodwin, J. F., and Cleland, W. P.: Ventricular septal defect and aortic regurgitation. Thorax *24*:257, 1969.
149. Rodbard, S.: Blood velocity and endocarditis. Circulation *27*:18, 1963.
150. Glenn, F., Stewart, H. J., Engle, M. A., Lukas, D. S., Artusio, J., Steinberg, I. S., and Holswade, G. R.: Coarctation of aorta complicated by bacterial endocarditis and an aneurysm of the sinus of Valsalva. Circulation *17*:432, 1958.
151. Blumenthal, S., Griffiths, S. P., and Morgan, B. C.: Bacterial endocarditis in children with heart disease. Pediatrics *26*:933, 1960.
152. Bove, E. L., Kavey, R-E. W., Sondheimer, H. M., and Parker, F. B., Jr.: Subacute bacterial endocarditis and complete endocardial cushion defect. Ann. Thorac. Surg. *34*:466, 1982.
153. Vosa, C., Arciprete, P., Bellitti, R., Agozzino, L., and Cotrufo, M.: Bacterial endocarditis of the aortic valve associated with diaphragmatic subaortic stenosis—account of two operated cases. Int. J. Cardiol. *6*:84, 1984.
154. Korn, D., DeSanctis, R. W., and Sell, S.: Massive calcification of the mitral annulus: A clinicopathologic study of fourteen cases. N. Engl. J. Med. *267*:900, 1962.
155. Watanakunakorn, C.: *Staphylococcus aureus* endocarditis on the calcified mitral annulus fibrosus. Am. J. Med. Sci. *266*:219, 1973.
156. Chagnac, A., Rudniki, C., and Loebel, H.: Infectious endocarditis in idiopathic hypertrophic subaortic stenosis. Report of three cases and review of the literature. Chest *81*:346, 1982.
157. Wang, K., Gobel, F. L., and Gleason, D. F.: Bacterial endocarditis in idiopathic hypertrophic subacute stenosis. Am. Heart J. *89*:359, 1975.
158. Lachman, A. S., Branwell-Jones, D. M., Lakier, J. B., Pocock, W. A., and Barlow, J. B.: Infective endocarditis in the billowing mitral leaflet syndrome. Br. Heart J. *37*:326, 1975.
159. Clemens, J. D., Horwitz, R. J., Jaffe, C. C., Feinstein, A. K., and Stanton, B. F.: A controlled evaluation of the risk of bacterial endocarditis in persons with mitral valve prolapse. N. Engl. J. Med. *307*:776, 1982.
160. Retchin, S. M., Fletcher, R. H., and Waugh, R. A.: Endocarditis and mitral valve prolapse: What is "risk"? Int. J. Cardiol. *5*:653, 1984.
161. Hickey, S. W., and Wilcken, D. E. L.: Mitral valve prolapse and bacterial endocarditis: When is antibiotic prophylaxis necessary? Am. Heart J. *109*:431, 1985.
162. Soman, V. R., Breton, G., Hershkowitz, M., and Mark, H.: Bacterial endocarditis of mitral valve in Marfan's syndrome. Br. Heart J. *36*:1247, 1974.
163. Starkebaum, M., Durack, D., and Beeson, P.: The "incubation period" of subacute bacterial endocarditis. Yale J. Biol. Med. *50*:49–58, 1977.
164. Kaplan, E., Helmsworth, J. A., Ahearn, E. N., Benzing, G., III, Daoud, G., and Schwartz, D. C.: Results of palliative procedures for tetralogy of Fallot in infants and young children. Ann. Thorac. Surg. *5*:489, 1968.
165. Sande, M. A., Johnson, W. D., Jr., Hook, E. W., and Kaye, D.: Sustained bacteremia in patients with prosthetic valves. N. Engl. J. Med. *286*:1067,1972.
166. Weinstein, L.: Infected prosthetic valves: A diagnostic and therapeutic dilemma. N. Engl. J. Med. *286*:1108, 1972.
167. Wilson, W. R., Danielson, G. K., Giuliani, E. R., and Geraci, J. E.: Prosthetic valve endocarditis. Mayo Clin. Proc. *57*:155, 1982.
168. Karchmer, A. W., Archer, G. L., and Dismukes, W. E.: *Staphylococcus epidermidis* causing prosthetic valve endocarditis. Microbiologic and clinical observations as guides to therapy. Ann. Intern. Med. *98*:447, 1983.
169. Mayer, K. H., and Schoenbaum, S. C.: Evaluation and management of prosthetic valve endocarditis. Prog. Cardiovasc. Dis. *25*:43, 1982.
170. Calderwood, S. B., Swinski, L. A., Waternaux, C. M., Karchmer, A. W., and Buckley, M. J.: Risk factors for the development of prosthetic valve endocarditis. Circulation *72*:31, 1985.
171. Rutledge, R., Kim, B. J., and Applebaum, R. E.: Actuarial analysis of the risk of prosthetic valve endocarditis in 1598 patients with mechanical and bioprosthetic valves. Arch. Surg. *120*:469, 1985.
172. Ivert, T. S. A., Dismukes, W. E., Cobbs, C. G., Blackstone, E. H., Kirklin, J. W., and Bergdahl, L. A. L.: Prosthetic valve endocarditis. Circulation *69*:223, 1984.
173. Dismukes, W. E., Karchmer, A. W., Buckley, M. J., Austen, W. G., and Swartz, M. N.: Prosthetic valve endocarditis. Circulation *48*:365, 1973.
174. Persaud, V.: Two unusual cases of mural endocarditis with a review of the literature. Am. J. Clin. Pathol. *53*:832, 1970.
175. Graham, H. V., von Hartitzch, B., Medina, J. R.: Infected atrial myxoma. Am. J. Cardiol. *38*:658, 1976.
176. Rogers, E. W., Weyman, A. E., Nobel, R. J., and Burns, S. C.: Left atrial myxoma infected with *Histoplasma capsulatum*. Am. J. Med. *64*:683, 1978.
177. Osler, W.: Malignant endocarditis. Gulstonian Lectures. Lancet *1*:459, 1885.
178. Lepeschkin, E.: On the relation between the site of valvular involvement in endocarditis and the blood pressure resting on the valve. Am. J. Med. Sci. *224*:318, 1952.
179. Allen, A. C.: Mechanism of localization of vegetations of bacterial endocarditis. Arch. Pathol. *27*:399, 1939.
180. Wadsworth, A. B.: A study of the endocardial lesions developing during pneumococcus infection in horses. J. Med. Res. *34*:279, 1919.
181. Gould, K., Ramirez-Ronda, C. H., Holmes, R. K., and Sanford, J. P.: Adherence of bacteria to heart valves *in vitro*. J. Clin. Invest. *56*:1364, 1975.
182. Holmes, R. K., and Ramirez-Ronda, C. H.: Adherence of bacteria to the endothelium of heart valves. Infective Endocarditis, an American Heart Association Monograph. No. 52, 1977, pp. 382, 12–13.

CLINICAL MANIFESTATIONS

183. Weinstein, L., and Schlesinger, J. J.: Pathoanatomic, pathophysiologic and clinical correlations in endocarditis. N. Engl. J. Med. *291*:832, 1122, 1974.

184. Libman, E., and Friedberg, C. K.: Subacute Bacterial Endocarditis. 2nd ed. New York, Oxford University Press, 1948.
185. Weinstein, L., and Rubin, R. H.: Infective endocarditis—1973. Prog. Cardiovasc. Dis. *16*:239, 1973.
186. Harkonen, M., Olin, P. E., et al.: Severe backache as a presenting sign of bacterial endocarditis. Acta Med. Scand. *210*:329, 1981.
187. Weinstein, L: Infective endocarditis: Past, present and future. J. R. Coll. Physicians Lond. 6:161, 1972.
188. Pankey, G. A.: Acute bacterial endocarditis at University of Minnesota Hospitals, 1939–1959. Am. Heart J. *64*:583, 1962.
189. Wedgewood, J.: Early diagnosis of subacute bacterial endocarditis. Lancet 2:1058, 1955.
190. Weinstein, L.: Modern infective endocarditis. JAMA *233*:260, 1975.
191. Willerson, J. T., Moellering, R. C., Jr., Buckley, M. J., and Austen, W. G.: Conjunctival petechiae after open-heart surgery. N. Engl. J. Med. *284*:539, 1971.
192. Kilpatrick, Z. M., Greenberg, P. A., and Sanford, J. P.: Splinter hemorrhages—their clinical significance. Arch. Intern. Med. *115*:730, 1965.
193. Roth, M.: Ueber Netzhautaffectionen bei Wundfiebern. Dtsch. Z. Chir. *1*:471, 1872.
194. Litten, M.: Ueber akute maligne Endocarditis und die dabei vorkommender Retinalveränderungen. Charit. Ann. *3*:137, 1878.
195. Doherty, W. B., and Trubek, M.: Significant hemorrhagic retinal lesions in bacterial endocarditis (Roth's spots). JAMA *97*:308, 1931.
196. Libman, E.: The clinical features of cases of subacute bacterial endocarditis that have spontaneously become bacteria-free. Am. J. Med. Sci. *146*:625, 1913.
197. Weinstein, L.: Life-threatening complications of infective endocarditis and their management. Arch. Intern. Med. *146*:953, 1986.
198. Mills, J., Utley, J., and Abbott, J.: Heart failure in infective endocarditis: Predisposing factors, course and treatment. Chest *66*:151, 1974.
199. Gonzalez-Lavin, L., Lise, M., and Ross, D.: The importance of the "jet lesion" in bacterial endocarditis involving the left heart: Surgical considerations. J. Thorac. Cardiovasc. Surg. *59*:185, 1970.
200. Roberts, W. C., Ewy, G. A., Glancy, D. L., and Marcus, F. I.: Valvular stenosis produced by active infective endocarditis. Circulation *36*:449, 1967.
201. Sacks, P. V., Lakier, J. B., and Barlow, J. B.: Severe aortic stenosis produced by bacterial endocarditis. Br. Med. J. *3*:97, 1969.
202. Mann, T., McLaurin, L., Grossman, W., and Craige, E. E.: Assessing the hemodynamic severity of acute regurgitation due to infective endocarditis. N. Engl. J. Med. *293*:108, 1975.
203. Roberts, N. K., and Somerville, J.: Pathological significance of electrocardiographic changes in aortic valve endocarditis. Br. Heart J. *31*:395, 1969.
204. Gopalakrishna, K. V., Kwan, K., and Shah, A.: Metastatic myocardial abscess due to group F streptococci. Am. J. Med. Sci. *274*:329, 1977.
205. Kin, H-S., Weilbacher, D. G., Lie, J. T., and Titus, J. L.: Myocardial abscesses. Am. J. Clin. Pathol. *70*:18, 1978.
206. Arnett, E. N., and Roberts, W. C.: Valve ring abscess in active infective endocarditis. Frequency, location and clues to clinical diagnosis from the study of 95 necropsy patients. Circulation *54*:140, 1976.
207. Perry, E. L., Fleming, R. G., and Edwards, J. E.: Myocardial lesions in subacute bacterial endocarditis. Ann. Intern. Med. *36*:126, 1952.
208. Blankenhorn, M. A., and Gall, E. A.: Myocarditis and myocardiosis: Clinicopathologic appraisal. Circulation *13*:217, 1956.
209. Maisch, B., Eichstadt, H., and Kochsiek, K.: Immune reactions in infective endocarditis: I. Clinical data and diagnostic relevance of antimyocardial antibodies. Am. Heart J. *106*:329, 1983.
210. Cates, J. E., and Christie, R. V.: Subacute bacterial endocarditis. A review of 442 patients treated in 14 centers appointed by the Penicillin Trials Committee of the Medical Research Council. Q. J. Med. *20*:93, 1951.
211. Vogler, W. R., and Dorney, E. R.: Bacterial endocarditis in congenital heart disease. Am. Heart J. *64*:198, 1962.
212. Kerr, A., Jr.: Bacterial endocarditis—revisited. Mod. Con. Cardiovasc. Dis. *33*:831, 1964.
213. Bell, E. T.: Glomerular lesions associated with endocarditis. Am. J. Pathol. *8*:639, 1932.
214. Pfeifer, J. F., Lipton, M. J., Oury, J. H., Angell, W. W., and Hulgren, H. N.: Acute coronary embolism complicating bacterial endocarditis: Operative treatment. Am. J. Cardiol. *37*:920, 1976.
215. Menzies, C. J. G.: Coronary embolism with infarction in bacterial endocarditis. Br. Heart J. *23*:464, 1961.
216. Brunson, J. G.: Coronary embolism in bacterial endocarditis. Am. J. Pathol. *29*:689, 1953.
217. Shenoy, M. M., Grief, E., Friedman, S. A., and Leibowitz, I.: Paradoxical embolism secondary to tricuspid valve endocarditis. Am. J. Cardiol. *54*:1374, 1984.
218. Horder, T. J.: Infective endocarditis: With an analysis of 150 cases and with special reference to the chronic form of the disease. Q. J. Med. *2*:289, 1909.
219. Jochman, G.: Lehrbuch der Infektionskrankheiten für Artze und Studierende. Berlin, Julius Springer, 1914, pp. 144–148.
220. McDevitt, E.: Treatment of cerebral embolism. Mod. Treat. *2*:52, 1965.
221. Harrington, A. W.: Embolism of the spinal cord. Glasgow Med. J. *103*:28, 1925.
222. Harrison, M. J. G., and Hampton, J. R.: Neurological presentation of bacterial endocarditis. Br. Med. J. *2*:148, 1967.
223. Kernohan, J. W., Woltman, H. W., and Barnes, A. R.: Involvement of the nervous system associated with endocarditis: Neuropsychiatric and neuropathological observations in forty-two cases of fatal outcome. Arch. Neurol. Psychol. *42*:789, 1939.
224. Jones, H. R., Jr., and Siekert, R. G.: Embolic mononeuropathy and bacterial endocarditis. Arch. Neurol. *19*:535, 1968.
225. Schocket, S., and Braver, D.: Cilioretinal artery occlusion in a patient with suspected bacterial endocarditis. South. Med. J. *63*:1, 1970.
226. Wong, D., Chandraratna, P. A. N., Wishnow, R. M., Dusitanond, V., and Nimalasuriya, A.: Clinical implications of large vegetations in infectious endocarditis. Arch. Intern. Med. *143*:1874, 1983.
227. Roach, M. R., and Drake, C. G.: Ruptured cerebral aneurysms caused by microorganisms. N. Engl. J. Med. *273*:240, 1963.
228. Kauffman, S. L., Lynfield, J., and Henningar, G. R.: Mycotic aneurysms of the intrapulmonary arteries. Circulation *35*:90, 1967.
229. Navarro, C., Dickinson, P. C. T., Kondlapoodi, P., and Hagstrom, J. W. C.: Mycotic aneurysms of the pulmonary arteries in intravenous drug addicts. Report of three cases and review of the literature. Am. J. Med. *76*:1124, 1984.
230. Godin, N., Pinget, L., and Waldvogel, F.: Mycotic aneurysms of the intrapulmonary arteries: Unusual manifestation of right-sided endocarditis. Rev. Fr. Mal. Respir. *11*:907, 1983.
231. Escudier, B., Becquemin, J. P., Alexandre, J. B., Piquois, A., Larde, D., and Jacotot, B.: Aneurysmes jambiers compliquant les endocardites bacteriennes. Deux observations. La Presse Med. *12*:1595, 1983.
232. Wilson, J. W., Ellis, D., Leyden, M. J., Thomas, R., and Sullivan, J. R.: Mycotic aneurysm of the small bowel presenting as gastrointestinal hemorrhage. Med. J. Aust. *141*:114, 1984.
233. Enia, F., Celona, G., and Filippone, V.: Echocardiographic detection of mitral valve aneurysm in patient with infective endocarditis. Br. Heart J. *49*:98, 1983.
234. Fein, S. A., Daudiss, K., McIlduff, J. B., Sanders, W., and Wolff, M. L.: Ruptured aneurysm of mitral annulus in bacterial endocarditis. Am. Heart J. *108*:171, 1984.
235. Lerner, P. I.: Neurologic complications of infective endocarditis. Med. Clin. North Am. *69*:385, 1985.
236. Ziment, I.: Nervous system complications in bacterial endocarditis. Am. J. Med. *47*:593, 1969.
237. Pruitt, A. A., Rubin, R. H., Karchmer, A. W., and Duncan, G. W.: Neurologic complications of bacterial endocarditis. Medicine *57*:329, 1978.
238. Bohmfalk, G. L., Story, J. L., Wissinger, J. P., and Brown, W. E.: Bacterial intracranial aneurysm. J. Neurosurg. *48*:369, 1978.
239. Churchill, M. A., Geraci, J. E., and Hunder, G. G.: Musculoskeletal manifestations of bacterial endocarditis. Ann. Intern. Med. *87*:754, 1977.
240. Feinstein, E. I., Eknoyan, G., Lister, B. J., Kim, H. F., and Greenberg, S. D.: Renal complications of bacterial endocarditis. Am. J. Nephrol. *5*:457, 1985.
241. Cordeiro, A., Costa, H., and Lagenha, F.: Editorial. Immunologic phase of subacute bacterial endocarditis. A new concept and general considerations. Am. J. Cardiol. *16*:477, 1965.
242. Williams, R. C., and Kunkel, H. G.: Rheumatoid factor, complement and conglutinin aberrations in patients with subacute bacterial endocarditis. J. Clin. Invest. *41*:666, 1962.
243. Williams, R. C.: Bacterial endocarditis—an analysis of immunopathology of infective endocarditis. An American Heart Association Symposium (No. 52) 1977, pp. 20–23.
244. Bayer, A. S., Theofilopoulos, A. N., Eisenberg, R., Dixon, F. J., and Guze, J. B.: Circulating immune complexes in infective endocarditis. N. Engl. J. Med. *295*:1500, 1976.
244a. Hooper, D. C., Bayer, A. S., Karchmer, A. W., Theofilopoulos, A. N., and Swartz, M. N.: Circulating immune complexes in prosthetic valve endocarditis. Arch. Intern. Med. *143*:2081, 1983.
245. McKenzie, P. E., Hawke, D., Woodroffe A. J., Thompson, A. J., Seymour, A. E., and Clarkson, A. R.: Serum and tissue immune complexes in infective endocarditis. J. Clin. Lab. Immunol. *4*:125, 1980.
246. Kauffman, R. H., Thompson, J., Valentijn, R. M., Daha, M. R., and Van Es, L. A.: The clinical implications and the pathogenetic significance of circulating immune complexes in infective endocarditis. Am. J. Med. *71*:17, 1981.
247. Maisch, B., Mayer, E., Schubert, U., Bert, P. A., and Kochsiek, K.: Immune reactions in infective endocarditis. II. Relevance of circulating immune complexes, serum inhibition factors, lymphocytoxic reactions, and antibody-dependent cellular cytotoxicity against cardiac target cells. Am. Heart J. *106*:338, 1983.
248. Williams, R. C., Jr., and Kilpatrick, K.: Immunofluorescence studies of cardiac valves in infective endocarditis. Arch. Intern. Med. *145*:297, 1985.
249. Howard, E. J.: Osler's nodes. Am. Heart J. *59*:633, 1960.
250. Alpert, J. S., Krous, H. F., Dalen, J. E., O'Rourke, R. A., and Bloor, C. M.: Pathogenesis of Osler's nodes. Ann. Intern. Med. *85*:471, 1976.
251. Davis, J. A., Weisman, M. H., and Dail, D. H.: Vascular disease in infective endocarditis: Report of immune-mediated events in skin and brain. Arch. Intern. Med. *138*:480, 1978.
252. Rubenfeld, S., and Kyung-Whan, M.: Leucocytoclastic angiitis in subacute bacterial endocarditis. Arch. Dermatol. *113*:1073, 1977.
253. Tu, W. H., Shearn, M. A., and Lee, J. C.: Acute diffuse glomerulonephritis in acute staphylococcal endocarditis. Ann. Intern. Med. *71*:335, 1969.
254. Gutman, R. A., Striker, G. E., Gilliland, B. C., and Cutler, R. E.: The immune complex glomerulonephritis of bacterial endocarditis. Medicine *51*:1, 1972.
255. Levy, R. L., and Hong, R.: The immune nature of subacute bacterial endocarditis (SBE) nephritis. Am. J. Med. *64*:645, 1973.
256. Keslin, M. H., Messner, R. P., and Williams, R. C., Jr.: Glomerulonephritis with subacute bacterial endocarditis. Arch. Intern. Med. *132*:578, 1973.
257. Panidis, I. P., Kotler, M. N., Mintz, G. S., Segal, B. L., and Ross, J. J.: Right heart endocarditis: Clinical and echocardiographic features. Am. Heart J. *107*:759, 1984.
258. Itoh, N., Shigematu, H., Itoh, M., and Yamada, H.: Right-sided infective endocarditis combined with mitral involvement in a patient with ventricular septal defect. Acta Pathol. Jpn. *35*:459, 1985.

258a. Bain, R. C., Edwards, J. E., Scheiffey, C. H., and Geraci, J. E.: Right-sided bacterial endocarditis and endarteritis: Clinical and pathologic study. Am. J. Med. *24*:98, 1958.
259. Bashour, F. A., and Winchell, C. P.: Right-sided bacterial endocarditis. Am. J. Med. Sci. *240*:411, 1960.
260. Altschule, M. D.: Subacute bacterial endocarditis of the right heart. Med. Sci. *15*:50, 1964.
261. Zakrzewski, T., and Keith, J.: Bacterial endocarditis in infants and children. J. Pediatr. *67*:1179, 1965.
262. Johnson, D. H., Rosenthal, A., and Nadas, A. S.: A forty-year review of bacterial endocarditis in infancy and childhood. Circulation *51*:581, 1975.
263. Stanton, B. F., Baltimore, R. S., and Clemens, J. D.: Changing spectrum of infective endocarditis in children. Am. J. Dis. Child. *138*:720, 1984.
264. Johnson, C. M., and Rhodes, K. H.: Pediatric endocarditis. Mayo Clin. Proc. 57:86, 19182.
265. Eliaou, J. F., Montoya, F., Sibille, G., Adda, M., Grolleau, R., and Bonnet, H.: Infectious endocarditis in the neonatal period. Pediatric 38:561, 1983.
266. Bergsland, J., Kawaguchi, A., Roland, M., Pieroni, D. R., and Subramanian, S.: Mycotic aortic aneurysms in children. Ann. Thorac. Surg. 37:314, 1984.
266a. Payne, D. G., Fishburne, J. I., Jr., Rufty, A. J., and Johnston, F. R.: Bacterial endocarditis in pregnancy. Obstet. Gynecol. *60*:247, 1982.
266b. Cooper, G., and Platt, R.: *Staphylococcus aureus* bacteremia in diabetic patients. Endocarditis and mortality. Am. J. Med. *73*:658, 1982.
266c. Cantrell, M., and Yoshikawa, T. T.: Infective endocarditis in the aging patient. Gerontology *30*:316, 1984.
267. Welton, D. E., Young, J. B., Gentry, W. O., Raizner, A. E., Alexander, J. K., Chahine, R. A., and Miller, R. R.: Recurrent infective endocarditis. Am. J. Med. *66*:932, 1979.
268. Uwaydah, M. M., and Weinberg, A. N.: Bacterial endocarditis—a changing pattern. N. Engl. J. Med. *273*:1231, 1965.
269. Pankey, G. A.: The prevention and treatment of bacterial endocarditis. Am. Heart J. *98*:102, 1979.
270. Beeson, P. B., Brannon, E. S., and Warren, J. V.: Observations on the sites of removal of bacteria from the blood in patients with bacterial endocarditis. J. Exp. Med. *81*:9, 1945.
271. Werner, A. S., Cobbs, C. G., Kaye, D., and Hook, E. W.: Studies on the bacteremia of bacterial endocarditis. J.A.M.A. *202*:127, 1967.
272. Kelson, S. E., and White, P. D.: Notes on 250 cases of subacute bacterial (streptococcal) endocarditis studied and treated between 1927 and 1929. Ann. Intern. Med. *22*:40, 1945.
273. Belli, J., and Waisbren, B. A.: The number of blood cultures necessary to diagnose most cases of bacterial endocarditis. Am. J. Med. Sci. *232*:284, 1956.
274. Thompson, R. L.: Staphylococcal infective endocarditis. Mayo Clin. Proc. 57:106, 1982.
275. Van Scoy, R. E.: Culture-negative endocarditis. Mayo Clin. Proc. *57*:149, 1982.
276. Cannady, P. B., Jr., and Sandford, J. P.: Negative blood cultures in infective endocarditis: A review. South. Med. J. *69*:1420, 1976.
277. Pesanti, E. L., and Smith, I. M.: Infective endocarditis with negative blood cultures. An analysis of 52 cases. Am. J. Med. *66*:43, 1979.
278. Pazin, G. J., Saul, S., and Thompson, M. E.: Blood culture positivity. Suppression by outpatient antibiotic therapy in patients with bacterial endocarditis. Arch. Intern. Med. *142*:263, 1982.
279. Nagel, J. G., Tuazon, C. U., Cardella, T. A., and Sheagren, J. N.: Teichoic acid serologic diagnosis of staphylococcal endocarditis. Use of gel diffusion and counterimmunoelectrophoretic methods. Ann. Intern. Med. *82*:13, 1975.
280. Wheat, L. J., Kohler, R. B., Tabarah, Z. A., and White, A.: IgM antibody response to staphylococcal infection. J. Infect. Dis. *144*:307, 1981.
281. Christensson, B., Hedström, S. A., and Kronvall, G.: The clinical significance of serological methods in the diagnosis of staphylococcal septicaemia and endocarditis. Scand. J. Infect. Dis. *41*(Suppl.):140, 1983.
282. Wheat, L. J., Wilkinson, B. J., Kohler, R. B., and White, A. C.: Antibody response to peptidoglycan during staphylococcal infections. J. Infect. Dis. *147*:16, 1983.
283. Shanson, D. C., Kirk, N., and Humphrey, R.: Clinical evaluation of a fluorescent antibody test for the serological diagnosis of streptococcal endocarditis. J. Clin. Pathol. *38*:92, 1985.
284. Seelig, M. S., Speth, C. P., Kozinn, P. J., Taschdjian, C. L., Toni, E. F., and Goldberg, P.: Patterns of *Candida* endocarditis following cardiac surgery: Importance of early diagnosis and therapy (an analysis of 91 cases). Prog. Cardiovasc. Dis. *17*:125, 1974.
285. Wiseman, J., Rouleau, J., Rigo, P., Strauss, H. W., and Pitt, B.: Gallium-67 myocardial imaging for the detection of bacterial endocarditis. Radiology *120*:135, 1976.
286. Spies, S. M., Myers, S. M., Barresi, V., Grais, I. M., and DeBoer, A.: A case of myocardial abscess evaluated by radionuclide techniques: A case report. J. Nucl. Med. *18*:1089, 1977.
287. Miller, M. H., and Casey, J. I.: Infective endocarditis: New diagnostic techniques. Am. Heart J. *96*:123, 1978.
288. Ellis, K., Jaffe, C., Malm, J. R., and Bowman, F. O., Jr.: Infective endocarditis: Roentgenographic considerations. Radiol. Clin. North Am. *11*:415, 1973.
289. Stewart, J. A., Silimperi, D., Harris, P., Wise, N. K., Fraker, T. D., Jr., and Kisslo, J. A.: Echocardiographic documentation of vegetative lesions in infective endocarditis: Clinical implications. Circulation *61*:374, 1980.
290. Amsterdam, E. A.: Value and limitations of echocardiography in endocarditis. Cardiology *71*:229, 1984.
291. Fox, S., Kotler, M. N., Segal, B. L., and Parry, W.: Echocardiographic diagnosis of acute aortic value endocarditis. Arch. Intern. Med. *137*:85, 1977.
292. Berger, M., Gallerstein, P. E., Benhuri, P., Balla, R., and Goldberg, E.: Evaluation of aortic valve endocarditis by two-dimensional echocardiography. Chest *80*:61, 1981.
293. Scanlan, J. G., Seward, J. B., and Tajik, A. J.: Valve ring abscess in infective endocarditis: Visualization with wide-angle two-dimensional echocardiography. Am. J. Cardiol. *49*:1794, 1982.
294. Ellis, S. G., Goldstein, J., and Popp, R. H.: Detection of endocarditis-associated perivalvular abscesses by two-dimensional echocardiography. J. Am. Coll. Cardiol. *5*:647, 1985.
295. Andy, J. J., Sheikh, M. U., Nayab, A., Barores, B. O., Fox, L. M., Curry, C. L., and Roberts, W. C.: Echocardiographic observations in opiate addicts with infective endocarditis. Am. J. Cardiol. *40*:17, 1977.
296. Berger, M., Delfin, L. A., Helveh, M., and Goldberg, E.: Two-dimensional echocardiographic findings in right-sided infective endocarditis. Circulation *61*:855, 1980.
297. Dander, B., Richetti, B., and Poppi, B.: Echocardiographic diagnosis of isolated pulmonary valve endocarditis. Br. Heart J. *47*:298, 1982.
298. Berger, M., Wilkes, H. S., Gallerstein, P. E., Berdoff, R. L., and Goldberg, E.: M-mode and two-dimensional echocardiographic findings in pulmonic valve endocarditis. Am. Heart J. *107*:391, 1984.
299. Gomes, J. A., Calderon, J., Lajam, F., Sakurai, H., Friedman, H. S., and Tatz, J. S.: Echocardiographic detection of fungal vegetations in *Candida parapsilosis* endocarditis. Am. J. Med. *61*:273, 1976.
300. Stewart, J. A., Silimperi, D., Harris, P., Wise, N. K., Fraker, T. D., and Kisslo, J. A.: Echocardiographic documentation of vegetative lesions in infective endocarditis: Clinical implications. Circulation *61*:374, 1980.
301. Rubenson, D. A., Tucker, C. R., Stinson, E. B., London, E. J., Oyer, P., Moreno-Cabral, R., and Popp, R. L.: The use of echocardiography in diagnosing culture-negative endocarditis. Circulation *64*:641, 1981.
302. Dillon, T., Meyer, R. A., Korfhagen, J. C., Kaplan, S., and Chung, K. J.: Management of infective endocarditis using endocardiography. J. Pediatr. *96*:552, 1980.
303. Vik-Mo, H.: Left ventricular function in aortic valve endocarditis. Echocardiographic evaluation and comparison with findings in chronic aortic regurgitation. Acta Med. Scand *219*:3, 1986.
304. Neimann, J. L., Fischer, M., Kownator, S., and Faivre, G.: Echocardiographic follow-up of vegetations in infectious endocarditis. Arch. Mal. Coeur. *75*:1329, 1982.

MANAGEMENT OF INFECTIVE CARDITIS

305. Weinstein, L., and Dalton, A. C.: Host determinants of response to antimicrobial agents. N. Engl. J. Med. *279*:467, 524, 580, 1968.
306. Schlichter, J. G., MacLean, H., and Milzer, A.: Effective penicillin therapy in subacute bacterial endocarditis and other chronic infections. Am. J. Med. Sci. *217*:600, 1949.
307. Weinstein, M. P., Stratton, C. W., Ackley, A., Hawley, H. B., Robinson, P. A., Fisher, B. C., Alcid, D. V., Stephens, D. S., and Reller, L. B.: Multicenter collaborative evaluation of a standardized serum bactericidal test as a prognostic indicator in infective endocarditis. Am. J. Med. *78*:262, 1985.
308. Mellors, J. W., Coleman, D. L., and Andriole, V. T.: Value of the serum bactericidal test in management of patients with bacterial endocarditis. Eur. J. Clin. Microbiol. *5*:67, 1986.
309. Cooper, R., and Mills, J.: Serratia endocarditis. A follow-up report. Arch. Intern. Med. *140*:199, 1980.
310. Cannady, P. B., Jr., and Sandford, J. P.: Negative blood cultures in infective endocarditis: A review. South. Med. J. *69*:1420, 1976.
311. Barza, M., Samuelson, T., and Weinstein, L.: Penetration of antibiotics into fibrin loci *in vivo*. II. Comparison of nine antibiotics: Effect of dose and degree of protein binding. J. Infect. Dis. *129*:66, 1974.
312. Barza, M., Brusch, J., Bergeron, M. G., and Weinstein, L.: Penetration of antibiotics into fibrin loci *in vivo*. III. Intermittent versus continuous infusion and effect of probenecid. J. Infect. Dis. *129*:73, 1974.
313. Weinstein, L., Goldfield, M., and Chang, T-W.: Infections occurring during chemotherapy: A study of their frequency, type and predisposing factors. N. Engl. J. Med. *251*:247, 1954.
314. Tan, J. S., Kaplan, S., Terhune, C. A., Jr., and Hamburger, M.: Successful two-week treatment schedule for penicillin-susceptible *Streptococcus viridans* endocarditis. Lancet 2:1340, 1971.
315. Walker, W. F., and Hamburger, M.: Penicillin-sensitive streptococcal endocarditis. Arch. Intern. Med. *100*:359, 1957.
316. Goodman, S., Berry, R. H., Benjamin, J. E., Schiro, H. S., and Hamburger, M.: Subacute bacterial endocarditis treated with oral penicillin. Arch. Intern. Med. *104*:625, 1959.
317. Hamburger, M., Kaplan, S., and Walker, W. F.: Subacute bacterial endocarditis caused by penicillin-sensitive streptococi. JAMA *175*:554, 1961.
318. Burman, N. D., Joffe, H. S., and Watson, C.: Oral antibiotic cure of staphylococcal endocarditis. Postgrad. Med. J. *49*:920, 1973.
319. Phillips, B., and Watson, G. H.: Oral treatment of subacute bacterial endocarditis in children. Arch. Dis. Child. *52*:235, 1977.
320. Weinstein, L., and Schlesinger, J.: Treatment of infective endocarditis—1973. Prog. Cardiovasc. Dis. *6*:275, 1973.
321. Kanis, J. A.: The use of anticoagulants in bacterial endocarditis. Postgrad. Med. J. *50*:312, 1974.
322. Wilson, W. R., Geraci, J. E., Danielson, G. K., Thompson, R. L., Spittell, J. A., Jr., Washington, J. A., II, and Giuliani, E. R.: Anticoagulant therapy

and central nervous system complications in patients with prosthetic valve endocarditis. Circulation 57:1004, 1978.

323. Wolfe, J. C., and Johnson, W. D.: Penicillin-sensitive streptococcal endocarditis. *In vitro* and clinical observations on penicillin-streptomycin therapy. Ann. Intern. Med. *81*:178, 1974.
324. Karchmer, A. W., Moellering, R. C., Jr., Maki, D. G., and Swartz, M. N.: Single-antibiotic therapy for streptococcal endocarditis. JAMA *241*:1801, 1979.
324a. Malacoff, R. F., Frank, E., and Andriole, V. T.: Streptococcal endocarditis (nonenterococcal, non-group A). J.A.M.A. *241*:1807, 1979.
325. Quinn, E. L., Pohlod, D., Madhaven, T., Burch, K., Fisher, E., and Cox, F.: Clinical experience with cefazolin and other cephalosporins in bacterial endocarditis. J. Infect. Dis. *128*(Suppl.):S386, 1973.
326. Bryant, R. E., and Alford, R. H.: Unsuccessful treatment of staphylococcal endocarditis with cefazolin. J.A.M.A. *237*:569, 1977.
327. Geraci, J. E., and Wilson, W. R.: Vancomycin therapy for infective endocarditis. Rev. Infect. Dis. *3*:S250, 1981.
328. Hinthom, D. R., Baker, L. H., Romig, D. A., Voth, D. W., and Liu, C.: Endocarditis treated with clindamycin: Relapse and liver dysfunction. South. Med. J. *70*:823, 1977.
329. Hunter, T. H.: Use of streptomycin in the treatment of bacterial endocarditis. Am. J. Med. *2*:436, 1974.
330. Moellering, R. C., Jr., and Weinberg, A. N.: Studies on antibiotic synergism against enterococci. J. Clin. Invest. *50*:2580, 1971.
331. Standiford, H. D., de Maine, J. B., and Kirby, W. M. M.: Antibiotic synergism of enterococci. Arch. Intern. Med. *126*:255, 1970.
332. Moellering, R. C., Jr., Wennersten, C., and Weinberg, A. N.: Synergy of penicillin and gentamicin against enterococci. J. Infect. Dis. *124*(Suppl.):207, 1971.
333. Karchmer, A. W.: Staphylococcal endocarditis. Laboratory and clinical basis for antibiotic therapy. Am. J. Med. *78*:116, 1985.
334. Working Party of the British Society for Antimicrobial Chemotherapy: Antibiotic treatment of streptococcal and staphylococcal endocarditis. Lancet *2*:815, 1985.
335. Bayer, A. S.: Staphylococcal bacteremia and endocarditis. State of the art. Arch. Intern. Med. *142*:1169, 1982.
336. Watanakunakorn, C., and Baird, I. M.: Prognostic factors in *Staphylococcus aureus* endocarditis and results of therapy with penicillin and gentamicin. Am. J. Med. Sci. *273*:133, 1977.
337. Abrams, B., Sklaver, A.,. Hoffman, T., and Greenman, R.: Single or combination therapy of staphylococcal endocarditis in intravenous drug abusers. Ann. Intern. Med. *90*:789, 1979.
338. Menda, K. B., and Gorbach, S. L.: Favorable experience with bacterial endocarditis in heroin addicts. Ann. Intern. Med. *78*:25, 1973.
339. Mayrer, A. R., Brown, A., Weintraub, R. A., Ragni, M., and Postic, B.: Successful medical therapy for endocarditis due to *Candida parapsilosis*. Chest *73*:546, 1978.
340. Kay, J. H., Bernstein, S., Feinstein, D., and Biddle, M.: Surgical cure of *Candida albicans* endocarditis with open heart surgery. N. Engl. J. Med. *364*:907, 1961.
341. Kay, J. H., Bernstein, S., Tsuji, H. K., Redington, J. V., Milgram, M., and Brem, T.: Surgical treatment of *Candida endocarditis*. J.A.M.A. *203*:621, 1968.
342. Arbulu, A., Thomas, N. W., and Wilson, R. F.: Valvulectomy without prosthetic replacement. A life-saving operation for tricuspid *Pseudomonas* endocarditis. J. Thorac. Cardiovasc. Surg. *64*:103, 1972.
343. Bindschadler, D. D., and Bennett, J. E.: A pharmacologic guide to the clinical use of amphotericin. Br. J. Infect. Dis. *120*:427, 1969.
344. Drutz, D. J., Spickard, A., Rogers, D. E., and Koenig, M. G.: Treatment of disseminated mycotic infections: A new approach to amphotericin B therapy. Am. J. Med. *45*:405, 1968.
345. Fass, R. J., and Perkins, R. L.: 5-Fluorocytosine in the treatment of cryptococcal and *Candida* mycoses. Ann. Intern. Med. *74*:535, 1971.
346. Vandevelde, A. G., Mauceri, A. A., and Johnson, J. E., III: 5-Fluorocytosine in the treatment of mycotic infections. Ann. Intern. Med. *77*:43, 1972.
347. Record, C. O., Skinner, J. M., Sleight, P., and Speller, D. C. E.: *Candida* endocarditis treated with 5-fluorocytosine. Br. Med. J. *1*:262, 1971.
348. Galgiani, J. N., and Stevens, D. A.: Fungal endocarditis: Need for guidelines in evaluating therapy. J. Thorac. Cardiovasc. Surg. *73*:293, 1977.
349. Parsons, E. R., and Nassau, E.: *Candida* serology in open-heart surgery. J. Med. Microbiol. *7*:415, 1974.
350. Wilson, W. E., and Geraci, J. E.: Antibiotic treatment of infective endocarditis. Ann. Rev. Med. *34*:413, 1983.
350a. Touroff, A. S. W., and Vessell, H.: Subacute *Streptococcus viridans* endarteritis complicating patent ductus arteriosus. J.A.M.A. *115*:1270, 1940.
351. Croft, C. H., Woodward, W., Elliott, A., Commerford, P. J., Barnard, C. N., and Beck, W.: Analysis of surgical versus medical therapy in active complicated native valve infective endocarditis. Am. J. Cardiol. *51*:1650, 1983.
352. Hancock, E. W., Shumway, N. E., and Remington, J. S.: Valve replacement in active bacterial endocarditis. J. Infect. Dis. *123*:106, 1971.
353. Kaiser, G. C., Williams, V. L., Thurmann, M., and Hanlon, C. R.: Valve replacement in cases of aortic insufficiency due to active endocarditis. J. Thorac. Cardiovasc. Surg. *54*:491, 1967.
354. Wise, J. R., Jr., Cleland, W. P., Halldie-Smith, K. A., Bentall, H. H., Goodwin, J. F., and Oakley, C. M.: Urgent aortic-valve replacement for acute aortic regurgitation due to infective endocarditis. Lancet *2*:115, 1971.
355. Robicsek, F., Payne, R. B., Daugherty, H. K., and Sanger, P. W.: Bacterial endocarditis of the mitral valve treated by excision and replacement. Ann. Surg. *166*:854, 1967.
356. Khonsari, S., Bahabozurgui, S., Cook, W. A., and Frater, R. W. M.: Urgent open-heart surgery for endocarditis of mitral valve. N.Y. State J. Med. *71*:2650, 1971.
357. Jung, J. Y., Saab, S. B., and Almond, C. H.: The case for early surgical treatment of left-sided primary infective endocarditis. A collective review. Thorac. Cardiovasc. Surg. *70*:509, 1975.
358. Stinson, E. B., Griepp, R. B., Vosti, K., Copeland, J. G., and Shumway, N. E.: Operation treatment of active endocarditis. J. Thorac. Cardiovasc. Surg. *71*:659, 1976.
359. Fowler, N. O., Hamburger, M. H., and Bove, K. E.: Aortic valve perforation. Am. J. Med. *42*:539, 1967.
360. Griffin, F. M., Jr., Jones, G., and Cobbs, C. G.: Aortic insufficiency in bacterial endocarditis. Ann. Intern. Med. *76*:23, 1972.
361. Alsip, S. G., Blackstone, E. H., Kirklin, J. W., and Cobbs, C. G.: Indications for cardiac surgery in patients with active infective endocarditis. Am. J. Med. *78*:138, 1985.
362. Dinubile, M. J.: Heart block during bacterial endocarditis: A review of the literature and guidelines for surgical intervention. Am. J. Med. Sci. *287*:30, 1984.
363. Robbins, M. J., Frater, R. W. N., Soeiro, R., Fishman, W. H., and Strom, J. A.: Influence of vegetation size on clinical outcome of right-sided infective endocarditis. Am. J. Med. *80*:165, 1986.
364. Kay, P. H., Oldershaw, P. J., Dawkins, K., Lennox, S. C., and Paneth, M.: The results of surgery for active endocarditis of the native aortic valve. J. Cardiovasc. Surg. *25*:321, 1984.
365. Wilson, W. R., Danielson, G. K., Givliani, E. R., Washington, J. A., III, Jaumin, P. M., and Geraci, J. E.: Valve replacement in patients with active infective endocarditis. Circulation *58*:585, 1978.
366. Richardson, J. V., Karp, R. B., Kirklin, J. W., and Dismukes, W. E.: Treatment of infective endocarditis: A 10-year comparative analysis. Circulation *58*:589, 1978.
367. Rapaport E.: Editorial. The changing role of surgery in the management of infective endocarditis. Circulation *58*:598, 1978.
368. Simberkoff, M. S., Isom, W., Smithivast, T., Noriega, E. R., and Rahal, J. J., Jr.: Two-stage tricuspid valve replacement for mixed bacterial endocarditis. Arch. Intern. Med. *133*:212, 1974.
369. Sethia, B., and Williams, B. T.: Tricuspid valve excision without replacement in a case of endocarditis secondary to drug abuse. Br. Heart J. *40*:579, 1978.
370. Robin, E., Thoms, N. W., Arbulu, A., Ganguly, S. N., and Magnisalis, K.: Hemodynamic consequences of total removal of the tricuspid valve without prosthetic replacement. Am. J. Cardiol. *35*:481, 1975.
371. Arbulu, A., and Asfaw, I.: Tricuspid valvulectomy with prosthetic replacement. J. Thorac. Cardiovasc. Surg. *82*:684, 1981.
372. Silverman, N. A., Levitsky, S., and Mammana, R.: Acute endocarditis in drug addicts: Surgical treatment for multiple valve infection. Am. Coll. Cardiol. *4*:680, 1984.
373. Reyes, M. P., and Lerner, A. M.: Current problems in the treatment of infective endocarditis due to *Pseudomonas aeruginosa*. Rev. Infect. Dis. *5*:314, 1983.
374. Bogart, D. B., Hodges, G. R., Lewis, H. D., Jr., and Fixley, M. S.: Prosthetic valve endocarditis: Reviewing the problem. Postgrad. Med. *62*:119, 1977.
375. Robinson, M. J., Greenberg, J. J., Korn, M., and Rywlin, A. M.: Infective endocarditis at autopsy: 1965–1969. Am. J. Med. *52*:492, 1972.
376. Walker, S. R., Shumway, N. E., and Merigan, T. C.: Management of infected cardiac valve prostheses. J.A.M.A. *208*:531, 1969.
377. Watanakunakorn, C., and Hamburger, M.: *Staphylococcus epidermidis* endocarditis complicating a Starr-Edwards prosthesis: A therapeutic dilemma. Arch. Intern. Med. *126*:1014, 1970.
378. Okies, J. E., Viroslav, J., and Williams, T. W., Jr.: Endocarditis after cardiac valve replacement. Chest *59*:198, 1971.
379. Dorney, E. R., and King, S. R.: Bacterial endocarditis following prosthetic valve surgery: Early and late occurrence. Circulation *41*(Suppl. 3):150, 1970.
380. Morgan, W. L., and Bland, E. F.: Bacterial endocarditis in antibiotic era. Circulation *19*:753, 1959.
381. Wallach, J. B., Glass, M., Lakash, L., and Angrist, A. A.: Bacterial endocarditis in aged. Ann. Intern. Med. *42*:1206, 1955.
382. Bunn, P., and Lunn, J.: Late follow up of 64 patients with subacute bacterial endocarditis treated with penicillin. Am. J. Med. Sci. *243*:549, 1962.
383. Pearce, M. L., and Guze, L. B.: Some factors affecting prognosis in bacterial endocarditis. Ann. Intern. Med. *55*:270, 1961.
384. Julanger, I.: Unfavourable prognostic factors in *Staphylococcus aureus* septicemia and endocarditis. Scand. J. Infect. Dis. *17*:179, 1985.
384a. Wedgewood, J.: Prognosis in subacute bacterial endocarditis. Lancet *2*:922, 1957.
385. Guze, L. B., and Pearce, M. L.: Hospital-acquired bacterial endocarditis. Arch. Intern. Med. *112*:56, 1963.
386. Zeman, F. D.: Subacute bacterial endocarditis in aged. Am. Heart J. *29*:661, 1945.
387. Menzies, C. J.: Coronary embolism with infarction in bacterial endocarditis. Br. Heart J. *23*:464, 1961.
388. Marietta, J. S.: Acute bacterial endocarditis and coronary embolism. Tex. State J. Med. *56*:426, 1960.
389. Brunson, J. G.: Coronary embolism in bacterial endocarditis. Am. J. Pathol. *29*:689, 1953.
390. Jackson, J.F., and Allison, F., Jr.: Bacterial endocarditis. South Med. J. *54*:1331, 1961.
391. Priest, W. S., and Smith, J. M.: Effect of healed subacute bacterial endocarditis on cardiac dynamics. Arch. Intern. Med. *95*:646, 1955.
392. Mendelson, C. E., Cahue, A., Katz, L. N., and Brams, W. A.: Long-term outlook for healed subacute bacterial endocarditis. J.A.M.A. *160*:437, 1956.

392a. Cates, J. E., and Christie, R. V.: Subacute bacterial endocarditis: A review of 442 patients treated in 14 centers appointed by the Penicillin Trials Committee of the Medical Research Council. Q. J. Med. *20*:93, 1951.
393. Hoffman, F. G., and Robinson, J. J.: Aneurysm of mitral valve associated with bacterial endocarditis. Am. Heart J. *63*:826, 1962.
394. Blum, L.: Development of current concept of mycotic aneurysm. N.Y. State J. Med. *64*:1317, 1964.
395. Poblacion, D., McKenty, J., and Campbell, M.: Mycotic aneurysm of the superior mesenteric artery complicating subacute bacterial endocarditis: Successful resection. Can. Med. Assoc. J. *90*:744, 1964.
396. Case Records of the Massachusetts General Hospital (Case 43371). N. Engl. J. Med. 257:515, 1957.
397. Boyd, A. A., Spencer, F. C., Isom, O. W., Cunningham, J. N., Reed, G. E., Acinapura, A. J., and Tice, D. A.: Infective endocarditis: An analysis of 54 surgically treated patients. J. Thorac. Cardiovasc. Surg. *73*:23, 1977.
398. Sandza, J. G., Clark, R. E., Ferguson, T. B., and Connors, J. P., and Weldon, C. S.: Replacement of prosthetic heart valves. J. Thorac. Cardiovasc. Surg. *74*:864, 1977.
399. Kaplan, E. L., Anthony, B. F., et al.: Prevention of bacterial endocarditis. Circulation *56*:139A, 1977.
400. Shulman, S. T., Amren, D. P., Bisno, A. L., et al.: Prevention of bacterial endocarditis: A statement for health professionals by the committee on rheumatic fever and infective endocarditis of the council on cardiovascular disease in the young. Circulation *70*:1123A, 1984.
401. Infectious Diseases and Immunization Committee, Canadian Paediatric Society: Bacterial endocarditis. Can. Med. Assoc. J. *134*:28, 1986.
402. Working Party of the British Society for Antimicrobial Chemotherapy: The antibiotic prophylaxis of infective endocarditis. Lancet 2:1323, 1982.
403. Delaye, J., Etienne, J., et al.: Prophylaxis of infective endocarditis for dental procedures. Report of a Working Party of the European Society of Cardiology. Eur. Heart J. *6*:826, 1985.
404. Prevention of bacterial endocarditis. Med. Lett. *23*:91, 1981.
405. Shanson, D. C.: Prophylaxis and treatment of infective endocarditis. Drugs 25:433, 1983.
406. Bor, D. H., and Himmelstein, D. U.: Endocarditis prophylaxis for patients with mitral valve prolapse. A quantitative analysis. Am. J. Med. *76*:711, 1984.
407. Clemens, J. D., and Ransohoff, D. E.: A quantitative assessment of pre-dental antibiotic prophylaxis for patients with mitral-valve prolapse. J. Chronic Dis. 37:531, 1984.
408. Murphy, D. M., Stassen, L., Carr, M. E., Gillespie, W. A., Caffertey, M. T., and Falkner, F. R.: Bacteraemia during prostatectomy and other transurethral operations: Influence of timing of antibiotic administration. J. Clin. Pathol. *37*:673, 1984.
409. MacFarlane, T. W., McGowan, D. A., Hunter, K., et al.: Prophylaxis for infective endocarditis: Antibiotic sensitivity of dental plaque. J. Clin. Pathol. *36*:459, 1982.
410. Bayliss, R., Clarke, C., Oakley, W., Somerville, W., and Whitfield, A. G. W.: The teeth and endocarditis. Br. Heart J. *50*:506, 1983.
411. Oakley, C., and Somerville, W.: Prevention of infective endocarditis. Br. Heart J. *45*:233, 1981.
412. Seldin, E. B.: Dental factors in infective endocarditis. Circulation *71*:1093, 1985.

35 THE PATHOGENESIS OF ATHEROSCLEROSIS

by RUSSELL ROSS, Ph.D., D.D.S.

Atherosclerosis, the principal cause of death in Western civilization,[1] is a progressive disease process that generally begins in childhood and has clinical manifestations in middle to late adulthood. Two decades ago, atherosclerosis was considered to be a degenerative process because of the accumulation of lipid and necrotic debris in the advanced lesions. We now recognize that it is a multifactorial process which, if it leads to clinical sequelae, requires extensive proliferation of smooth muscle cells within the intima of the affected artery. The form and content of the advanced lesions of atherosclerosis demonstrate the results of three fundamental biological processes. These are: (1) proliferation of intimal smooth muscle cells together with variable numbers of accumulated macrophages; (2) formation by the proliferated smooth muscle cells of large amounts of connective tissue matrix, including collagen, elastic fibers, and proteoglycans; and (3) accumulation of lipid, principally in the form of cholesteryl esters and free cholesterol within the cells as well as in the surrounding connective tissues.[2–5] Despite the fact that the term "atherosclerosis" is derived from the Greek "athero" (gruel or porridge) and "sclerosis" (hardening), it is important to note that there may be great variability in the relative amounts of tissue formed by each of these processes in the lesions. Consequently, many lesions of atherosclerosis are dense and fibrous, whereas others may contain large amounts of lipid and necrotic debris, with most demonstrating combinations and variations of each of these characteristics.

RISK FACTORS

(See also Chapter 36)

The development of the concept of "risk factors" and their relationships to the incidence of coronary artery disease evolved from prospective epidemiological studies in the United States and Europe.[6–9] These studies demonstrated a consistent association among characteristics observed at one point in time in apparently healthy individuals with the subsequent incidence of coronary artery disease in these individuals. These associations include that between an increase in the concentration of plasma cholesterol and the rate of occurrence of new events of coronary artery disease, and among the incidence of cigarette smoking, hypertension, clinical diabetes, obesity, age, or male sex, and the occurrence of coronary artery disease.[10–12] As a result of these associations, each characteristic has been termed a risk factor for coronary artery disease, and this terminology has been generally accepted and has become part of the scientific literature associated with this problem.

It is important to remember, however, that the presence of a risk factor does not necessarily imply a direct causal relationship. In most instances, a risk factor is the trait that predicts the risk of development of clinically significant disease within a population. In some cases, it may be involved in the causation of the disease; however, to achieve the latter requires a proved epidemiological association that is statistically valid. The risk factor concept has been extremely useful because it permits one to assess the importance not only of the aforementioned risk factors but also of genetic traits in given individuals, such as a family history of premature coronary artery disease. Using such information, it has become possible to determine whether modification of a given risk factor will result in modification of the risk of a particular disease.

Thus, a risk factor may be defined broadly as "any habit or trait that can be used to predict an individual's probability of developing that disease."[1] A risk factor so defined may be a causative agent but is not necessarily one. A more limited and specific definition is that a risk factor is a causative agent or condition that can be used to predict an individual's probability of developing disease. Used in this fashion, there are at least three independent predictors of risk for individuals within a population of the incidence of atherosclerosis. These are: plasma cholesterol concentration,[13–17] cigarette smoking,[18, 19] and elevated blood pressure.[19–21]

THE NORMAL ARTERY

The normal artery (Fig. 35–1) consists of an intima lined by endothelium on the inner (luminal) aspect of the vessel and bounded by the internal elastic lamina on its outer

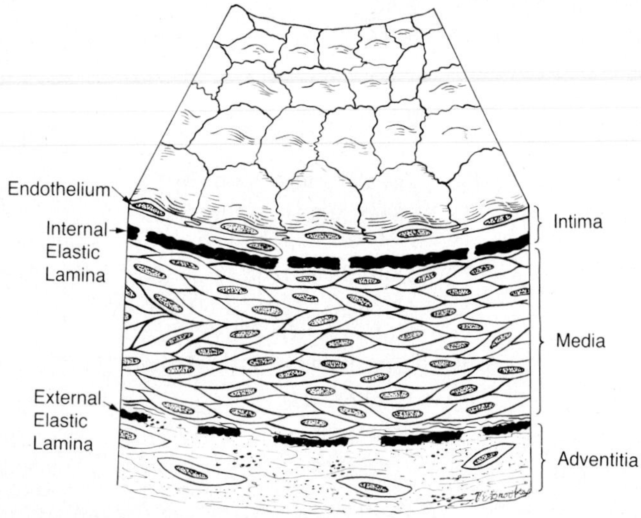

FIGURE 35–1. Structure of a normal muscular artery. (Reprinted by permission from Ross, R., and Glomset J.: The pathogenesis of atherosclerosis. N. Engl. J. Med. *295*:369, 1976.)

aspect. The media is bounded by the internal elastic lamina and, in well-developed muscular and elastic arteries, by an external elastic lamina. The adventitia is bounded by the external elastic lamina and the exterior of the vessel itself.

The Intima

At birth, the intima consists of a relatively thin layer of connective tissue which contains occasional solitary smooth muscle cells. Most of the connective tissue at birth consists of basement membrane. With increasing age, the amount of connective tissue increases, principally as a result of thickening of the basement membrane and formation of collagen fibrils and new elastic fibers. With increasing age, there appears to be a concentric increase in the numbers of intimal smooth muscle cells.

The intima is the site at which the lesions of atherosclerosis form. The lesions of atherosclerosis appear to be able to form in two ways in different individuals. In those who develop clinical sequelae, the lesions form by a generally asymmetrical thickening of the intima which continually encroaches upon the lumen, resulting in a decrease in the flow of blood. The second form of intimal thickening is one in which the increase in the intima may be associated with a continued dilation of the artery so that the actual lumen changes little, if at all, in diameter. In the latter case, although lesions of atherosclerosis may form, they are generally more symmetrical and concentric; few if any clinical sequelae appear to result.

The Media

The media is the muscular wall of the artery, bounded by the internal and external elastic laminae (Fig. 35–1). These laminae consist of fenestrated sheets of elastic fibers with numerous openings large enough to permit both substances and cells to pass in either direction. The media of muscular arteries consists of spiraling layers of smooth muscle cells attached to one another, each cell surrounded by a discontinuous basement membrane and by interspersed collagen fibrils and proteoglycan. Elastic arteries contain multiple lamellae of smooth muscle cells, each equivalent to a single media in a small muscular artery, or arteriole. Each lamella is bounded by an elastic lamina on its inner and outer aspects. The number of lamellar units present in elastic arteries has been shown to be highly predictable in relation to the size of the animal and to other factors, such as the anatomical position of the artery. Twenty-nine lamellar units have been suggested to represent the thickest amount of artery wall capable of transporting oxygenated metabolites from the lumen of the aorta to the outermost lamella. When more than 29 lamellar units are present, vasa vasorum that are derived from the adventitia appear to be necessary. These can provide nutrients to the remaining outer lamellar units.[22, 23]

The Adventitia

The adventitia consists of a dense collagenous structure containing numerous bundles of collagen fibrils, elastic fibers, and many fibroblasts together with some smooth muscle cells (Fig. 35–1). It is a highly vascular tissue. As indicated earlier, the adventitia provides the outermost portion of the media of large elastic arteries with much of their nutrition via vasa vasorum, as well as with lymphatic channels and innervation. Wolinsky and Glagov[23] have observed that the abdominal aorta in humans lacks vasa vasorum in its outermost aspects and have suggested that this may be one of the reasons why the abdominal aorta is particularly vulnerable to atherogenesis.

CELLS OF THE ARTERY AND FROM THE BLOOD POTENTIALLY INVOLVED IN ATHEROGENESIS

Endothelium

The endothelial cells probably represent the largest and most extensive tissue in the body since they line the entire vascular tree. In the arterial system, the endothelial cells form a continuous smooth, uninterrupted surface and represent the principal barrier between the elements of the blood and the artery wall (Fig. 35–2). In adulthood, the turnover of endothelial cells in those arteries that have been studied is relatively low; however, Schwartz and Benditt[24, 25] have observed that there are "hot spots" where turnover of endothelium is high in the aorta, even in adults. These hot spots do not appear to be necessarily located at particular anatomical sites. The endothelium forms a highly selective permeability barrier,[26–28] is usually thought to be a nonthrombogenic surface,[29] is a highly active metabolic tissue,[30] and is capable of forming several vasoactive substances[29, 31, 32] and connective tissue macromolecules.[33] Endothelial cells examined in culture also have procoagulant properties[34]; however, it is probable that these procoagulant properties are manifested at times of "injury" to the endothelium and are probably not present in situ in the normal artery.

Although the endothelial cells, as seen *en face* by light and scanning electron microscopy (Fig. 35–3) and in cross section by light and transmission electron microscopy (Fig. 35–4), appear to be highly similar morphologically in different parts of the arterial tree, there may be functional differences in these lining cells in arteries in different anatomical sites. If this were so, one might anticipate that there might be differences in the way in which endothelial cells respond to injury after exposure to various injurious agents in different parts of the arterial tree. Endothelial cells are normally attached to each other by tight junctions and by gap junctions. They transport substances in both directions via the process of bulk-phase endocytosis, some-

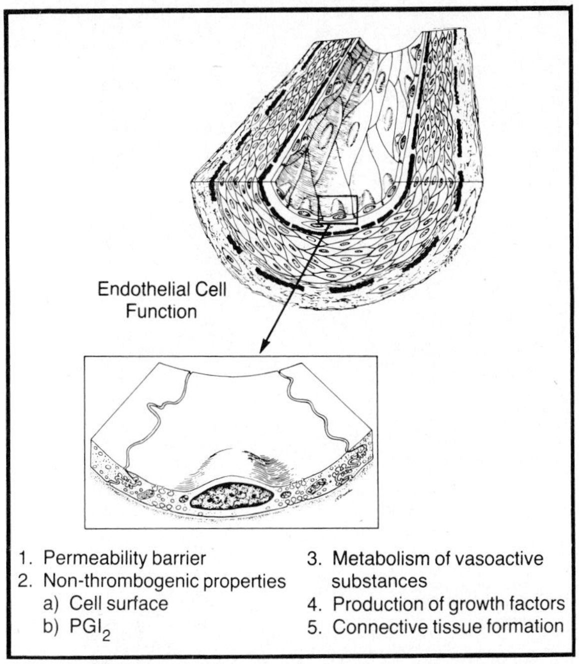
Endothelial Cell
Function
1. Permeability barrier
2. Non-thrombogenic properties
a) Cell surface
b) PGI_2
3. Metabolism of vasoactive substances
4. Production of growth factors
5. Connective tissue formation

FIGURE 35–2. Diagram showing the endothelial barrier present in the normal artery wall. In the higher magnification insert, the borders between the endothelial cells are irregular, allowing the cells to interdigitate. Vesicles and infoldings at either cell surface permit the cells to transport materials from the lumen of the artery to the tissue by pinocytosis. Transport also occurs below the cell junctions, demonstrated by vesicles that fuse in these regions. In the artery, the cell rests on a connective-tissue matrix that consists of a basement membrane intermixed with collagen fibrils. (Reprinted by permission from Ross, R., and Glomset, J.: The pathogenesis of atherosclerosis. N. Engl. J. Med. *295*:371, 1976.)

times called *transcytosis*. Transendothelial channels have been observed in capillary endothelium; however, it is not clear whether they play a role in macromolecular transport in arterial tissue. It has also been suggested that the junctions between endothelial cells may serve as potential sites of increased endothelial transport, particularly when the endothelium has been injured.

Endothelial cells rest on a basement membrane that consists of a particular form of collagen (type IV collagen) intermixed with particular types of proteoglycan molecules. The endothelial cells are undoubtedly responsible for the synthesis of these connective tissue molecules.[33] The basement membrane probably also serves as a crude form of filter.

Endothelial cells have receptors for many different molecules on their surface, including receptors for low-density lipoprotein,[35] for growth factors, and probably for a number of pharmacological agents. The endothelium theoretically provides a nonthrombogenic surface because of its capacity to form prostaglandin derivatives, particularly prostacyclin (PGI_2) (Chap. 56), a potent vasodilator that is an effective inhibitor of platelet aggregation,[29, 32] and because of its surface coat of heparan sulfate. Endothelial cells can also secrete agents that are effective in lysing fibrin clots, including plasminogen, as well as procoagulant materials such as von Willebrand factor.[34] They also secrete a number of vasoactive agents, such as angiotensin-converting enzyme and platelet-derived growth factor, which may be important in vasoconstriction.

A particular characteristic of the endothelium that may be of great importance is the fact that endothelial cells grow in an obligate monolayer. Such growth is representative of cells that line most body surfaces, including epithelial surfaces, and is characterized by the fact that the endothelial cells cannot crawl over one another at sites of injury to facilitate repair of a surface that has been deendothelialized. In other words, only the cells at the margin of an injury can participate in the regenerative response. Thus if a particular anatomical site is repeatedly injured over a prolonged period of time, and if the endothelial cells that regenerate lose their replication capacity, cells distal to the site, capable of replicating, may not be able to participate simply because they cannot reach the site to do so.

Arterial endothelial cells are capable of synthesizing and secreting at least two mitogens, one of which is a form of platelet-derived growth factor (PDGF).[36–38] PDGF is a growth factor for mesenchymally derived, connective tissue–forming cells such as fibroblasts and smooth muscle, but not for endothelial cells. The capacity of endothelium, when it has been appropriately "activated," to form such growth factors may be important in atherogenesis. This will be discussed further in the section concerning the response-to-injury hypothesis of atherosclerosis (see p. 1142).

Thus, the endothelium forms an obligate monolayer that lines the entire arterial tree, is metabolically active, produces vasoactive substances, has a nonthrombogenic surface, and can form procoagulant materials. It also serves as the permeability barrier that controls the passage of molecules into the artery. All of these activities demonstrate the dynamic nature of the endothelial lining and how potentially important this cell layer is in the maintenance of arterial homeostasis.

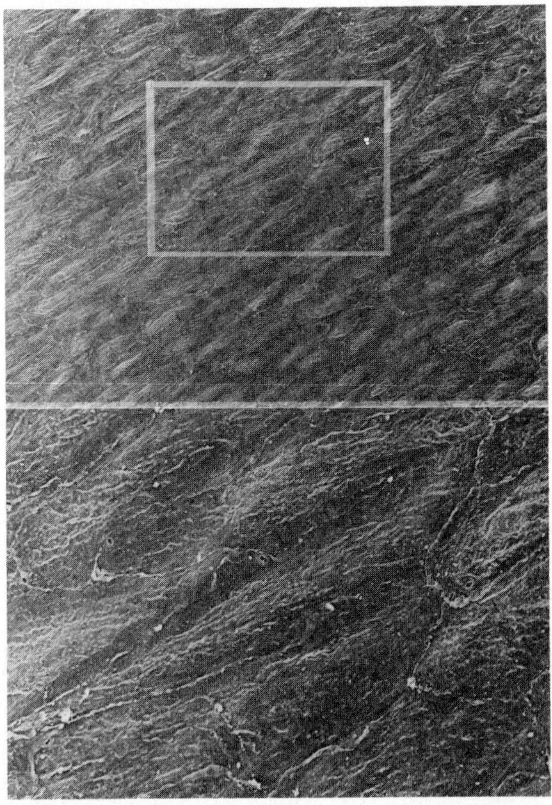

FIGURE 35–3. Scanning electron micrographs of the thoracic aorta endothelium from normal monkey (Macacca nemestrina). × 540. At somewhat higher magnification, the overlapping folds of the endothelial cells can be clearly visualized. The elongated and elliptical appearance of the endothelium can also be seen. The long axes of the cells appear to be diagonal and are oriented in the main direction of the flow of blood in the artery. × 2100. (From Ross, R.: Atherosclerosis: A problem of the biology of arterial wall cells and their interactions with blood components. Arteriosclerosis *1*:297, 1981, by permission of the American Heart Association.)

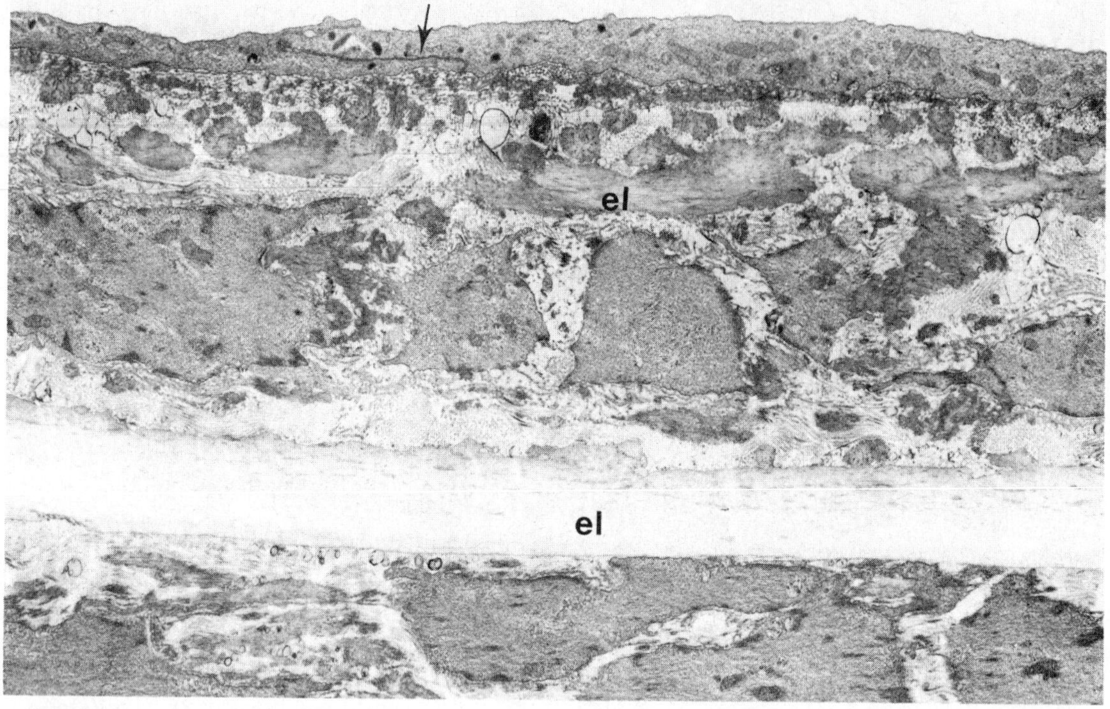

FIGURE 35–4. Transmission electron micrograph of a developing monkey aorta. Two endothelial cells can be seen at the lumen with a junction between them (arrow). Beneath the endothelial cells are newly forming elastic fibers (el) that are separated from the endothelium by basement membrane and collagen fibrils. Beneath the newly forming elastic fibers is a layer of smooth muscle cells separated from another layer by a well-formed elastica (el). No nuclei are apparent in the endothelial cells in this particular thin section.

Smooth Muscle

The cell that proliferates in the arterial intima to form the advanced lesions of atherosclerosis, the smooth muscle cell, is originally derived from the media. In his early work, Wissler[39] described this cell as a "multifunctional medial mesenchymal cell." It is now widely accepted that proliferation of smooth muscle cells in the intima represents the sine qua non of the lesions of advanced atherosclerosis (Fig. 35–5).

Less than 20 years ago, the only functional capacity attributed to the smooth muscle cell was its ability to contract. In 1971, it became possible to maintain and propagate pure populations of smooth muscle cells in culture and to demonstrate that this cell, like the fibroblast, is one of the principal connective tissue–forming cells in the body.[40] It is capable of synthesizing and secreting several forms of collagen, both elastic fiber proteins and several different types of proteoglycans.[41] The principal role of the smooth muscle cell in the fully formed adult artery is presumably to maintain the tone of the arterial wall by its capacity to maintain the slow contractions peculiar to smooth muscle. The smooth muscle cell responds to numerous vasoactive agents, such as epinephrine and angiotensin, which induce contraction and vasoconstriction, and prostacyclin, which can induce relaxation and vasodilation. Smooth muscle cells, like fibroblasts, contain specific high-affinity receptors for a number of ligands. These ligands include low-density lipoprotein[42] (see p. 1161) (which is the principal cholesterol-carrying plasma lipoprotein that participates in regulation of cholesterol metabolism), insulin (which is involved in glucose metabolism), and growth factors such as PDGF[43] (which help to regulate cell multiplication). Arterial smooth muscle cells of the newborn rat have been shown to be capable of synthesizing and secreting PDGF in contrast to adult rat smooth muscle.[44] These observations suggest possible roles for smooth muscle in growth and development and possibly in atherosclerosis as well (to be discussed below). It is not clear whether this capacity to form PDGF is the same in smooth muscle from man or other species.

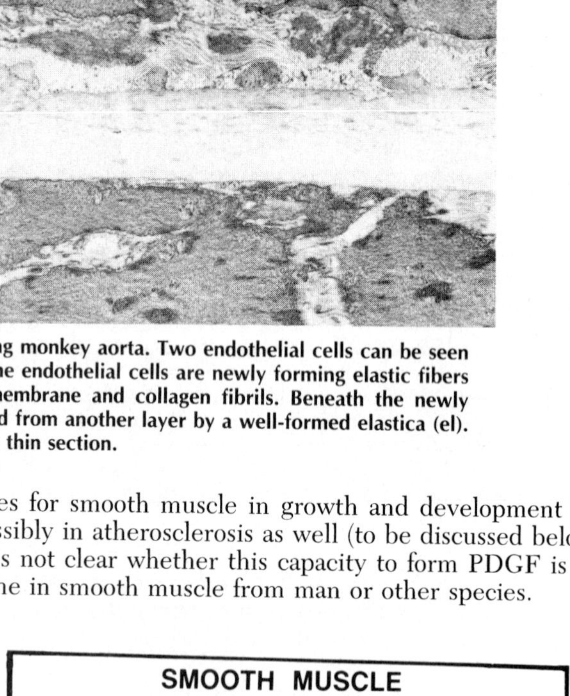

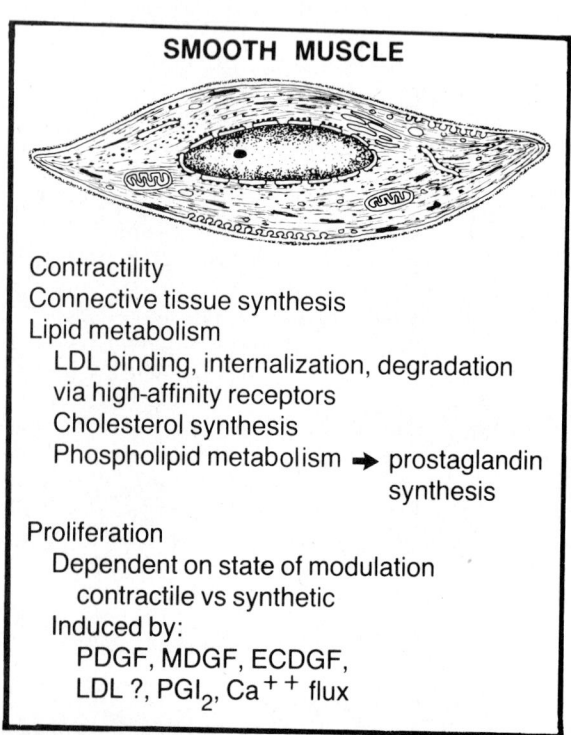

FIGURE 35–5. Diagram of a smooth muscle cell showing many of the phenotypic characteristics of normal smooth muscle, as well as factors that can induce smooth muscle proliferation. (From Ross, R.: Atherosclerosis: A problem of the biology of arterial wall cells and their interactions with blood components. Arteriosclerosis *1*:304, 1981, by permission of the American Heart Association.)

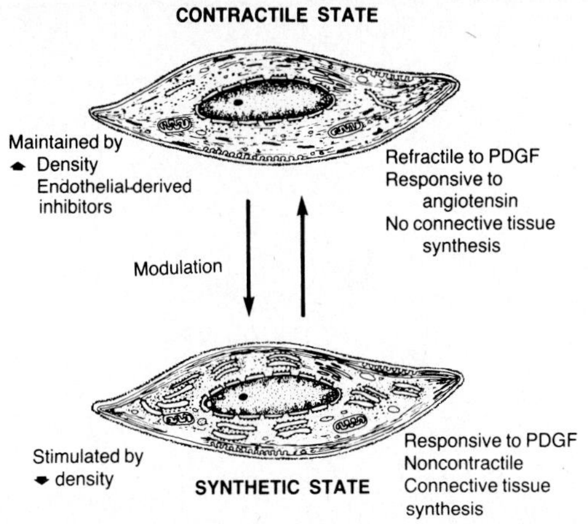

FIGURE 35–6. Diagram illustrating the state of modulation of smooth muscle cells in which the contractile versus the synthetic state are maintained by different sets of factors. (From Ross, R.: Atherosclerosis: A problem of the biology of arterial wall cells and their interactions with blood components. Arteriosclerosis *1*:305, 1981, by permission of the American Heart Association.)

Smooth muscle cells appear to be capable of presenting two different phenotypes in culture.[45, 46] The first of these, the *contractile phenotype*, is generally thought to be associated with cell contractility because the cells contain extensive myofibrils throughout their cytoplasm consisting of actin and myosin filaments. These contractile filaments bind to one another and to the subplasmalemmal surface of the cell by dense bodies. Such cells do *not* appear to be capable of responding to mitogens such as PDGF. When a smooth muscle cell becomes appropriately stimulated, it loses its contractile phenotype and changes to a cell that has decreased content of myofilaments and that contains an extensively developed rough endoplasmic reticulum and Golgi complex. Such a cell has been described as being in a *synthetic phenotype*. Smooth muscle cells in the synthetic phenotype appear to be involved in the formation of numerous secretory proteins, including connective tissue matrix macromolecules. These two different smooth muscle phenotypes have been described in cell culture as well as in the artery wall.

It has been suggested that the phenotypic differentiation of the smooth muscle cell may be important in terms of its capacity to respond to mitogens such as PDGF, and thus to form the lesions of atherosclerosis. Smooth muscle cells in the contractile phenotype have been described as nonresponsive to mitogens, whereas those in the synthetic phenotype have been described as responsive.[45, 46] For the lesions of atherosclerosis to form, the smooth muscle cells must, in most cases, migrate from the media into the intima, where they can respond mitogenically. Consequently, control of the phenotypic state of smooth muscle cells could be important in understanding and preventing atherogenesis (Fig. 35–6).

One characteristic feature of the smooth muscle cells found in the lesions of atherosclerosis is the accumulation of lipid that results in formation of vacuolated cells, or foam cells. Most of the lipids that are deposited in these cells are in the form of cholesteryl esters that result from increase in cholesterol synthesis and esterification, and also a decrease in degradation of cholesteryl esters in the lysosomes of the cell.

Finally, it has recently been shown that under special circumstances some smooth muscle cells may be capable of releasing a form of PDGF to which they and their neighbors could respond. It is well known that a marked intimal smooth muscle proliferative lesion can be induced by passing an intraarterial balloon embolectomy catheter through an artery sufficient to strip off the lining endothelium. The exposed subendothelial connective tissue attracts platelets to adhere and degranulate. This is followed by migration of smooth muscle cells from the media into the intima, where they proliferate and form a myointimal, hyperplastic, fibrotic lesion. If the smooth muscle cells are cultured from such a lesion induced in the rat carotid artery, and are compared with smooth muscle cells cultured from a contralateral uninjured artery, those from the proliferative lesion secrete a form of PDGF (see section on Growth Factors) and thus may participate in further lesion enlargement by an autocrine form of stimulation. There is no evidence as yet that smooth muscle cells from human lesions are capable of similar activity. In fact, there are data to suggest that smooth muscle cells derived from occlusive fibrous plaques in the superficial femoral arteries of a series of patients who had bypass surgery cannot divide. When placed in culture, these cells respond less well to mitogens and act like senescent cells that have undergone numerous cell doublings.[47]

Macrophages

Macrophages in all tissues, whether they are resident macrophages or cells that have entered the tissue during an inflammatory response, are derived at some point in their life span from circulating blood monocytes.[48] When the monocyte enters a tissue, it appears to take on characteristics peculiar to the host tissue. In most inflammatory sites, the macrophage acts as a scavenger cell to remove foreign substances by phagocytosis and intracellular hydrolysis, and as a second line of defense after the neutrophil against microbial organisms.[49]

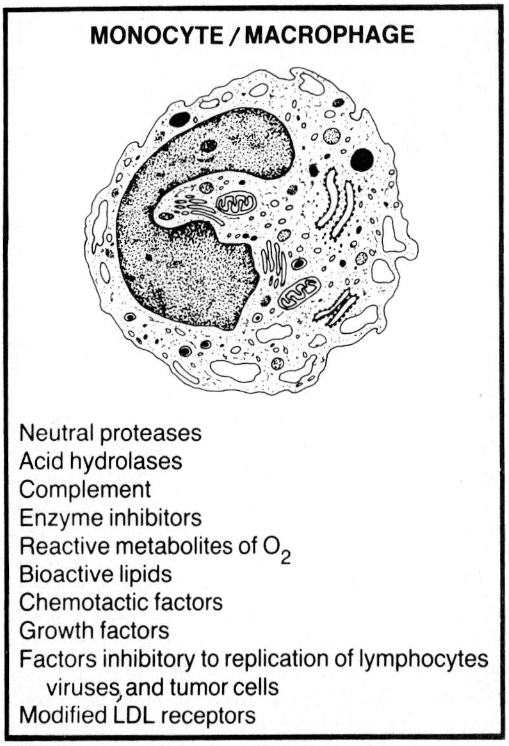

MONOCYTE / MACROPHAGE
Neutral proteases
Acid hydrolases
Complement
Enzyme inhibitors
Reactive metabolites of O_2
Bioactive lipids
Chemotactic factors
Growth factors
Factors inhibitory to replication of lymphocytes viruses, and tumor cells
Modified LDL receptors

FIGURE 35–7. Diagram of a monocyte/macrophage cell containing a large number of substances, many of which are not present in the circulating monocyte but are formed after the monocyte leaves the blood and enters a specific tissue. A few of the components that can be found in macrophages are listed beneath the diagram. (From Ross, R.: Atherosclerosis: A problem of the biology of arterial wall cells and their interactions with blood components. Arteriosclerosis *1*:302, 1981, by permission of the American Heart Association.)

Macrophages are capable of secreting a large number of biologically important substances, including chemotactic agents such as leukotriene B4[50] and interleukin 1,[51] and oxygen metabolites such as superoxide anion,[52] which can be toxic to other cells. Macrophages have recently been shown to be capable of synthesizing and secreting at least five different growth factors.[53] These include (1) PDGF,[54] a growth factor for mesenchymal cells such as smooth muscle and fibroblasts; (2) interleukin 1, which is also somewhat mitogenic for fibroblasts;[51] (3) fibroblast growth factor (FGF),[55] a mitogen for endothelial cells and thus a potentially important angiogenic agent; (4) epidermal growth factor (EGF) and EGF-like molecules (e.g., transforming growth factor alpha [TGF α]), both of which bind to the same receptor and are capable of stimulating the growth of epithelial cells; (5) transforming growth factor beta (TGF β), a substance that participates in a synergistic way with some of the aforementioned growth factors in aiding the proliferation of many cells in different tissues, and in some instances in inhibiting cell growth (Fig. 35–7).

As a result of its scavenging capacity and its ability to form and secrete growth factors, the macrophage is probably the key cell responsible for the promotion of connective tissue proliferation so commonly associated with chronic inflammatory responses. Macrophages, like smooth muscle, are a major source of foam cells in the lesions of atherosclerosis. In fact, they are the principal cells in the fatty streak, the initial lesion of atherosclerosis. They accumulate large amounts of lipid in the form of droplets that contain large amounts of cholesteryl ester. The role of the macrophage in atherogenesis will be discussed below.

Platelets (See also Chap. 56)

Although they are probably uninvolved in the generation of many lesions, platelets are clearly implicated in the genesis of some of the lesions of atherosclerosis. (This will be discussed in greater detail below.) However, platelets are also important because they are regularly involved in one of the principal sequelae of atherosclerosis, thrombosis. It is usually a mural or occlusive thrombus or both that leads to infarction.

Platelets are amazing cells in that, although they are capable of little to no protein synthesis, they contain, sequestered in their granules, numerous prepacked extraordinarily potent molecules (Fig. 35–8).[56, 57] Among these are a number of factors that participate in the coagulation cascade and, in addition, at least four extremely potent growth factors or mitogens. These are the same growth factors that can be formed by the activated macrophage; namely, PDGF,[58] FGF, EGF[59] or TGF α, and TGF β.[60] It appears that each of these growth factors is present in a class of granules, the alpha granules, which were originally thought to represent a single class on the basis of cell fractionation studies. They may, however, represent several different granules that are similar in morphological and flotation characteristics. Thus when they are separated by cell fractionation and density gradient centrifugation, they appear to sequester into a single population.

When the platelet is exposed to substrates that induce platelet adherence, aggregation, and degranulation, each of these growth factors is potentially released and thus is capable of eliciting a proliferative response by essentially all of the resident cells in a particular tissue. In other words, platelets contain growth factors potentially stimulatory for each of the cell types present in any tissue in which platelet aggregation and release may occur. Thus, at sites of injury in which collagen exposure, thrombin and fibrin formation, or adenosine diphosphate release occur, platelet aggregation and thrombosis can occur, leading to release of the numerous vasoactive, stimulatory, and proliferative agents carried by the platelets. Each of these agents may play an important role in stimulating an early vasoconstrictive and proliferative response.[61] This early reparative response to injury may be important in the initiation of the lesions of atherosclerosis as well.

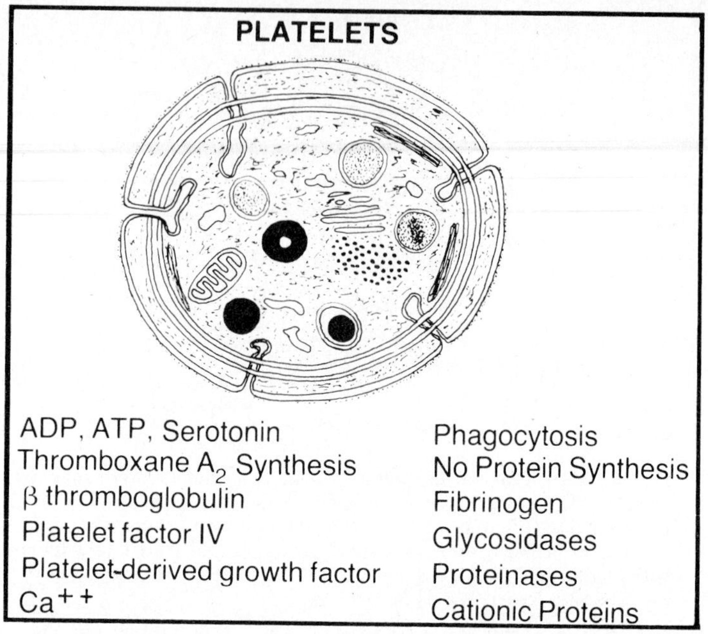

PLATELETS
ADP, ATP, Serotonin
Thromboxane A_2 Synthesis
β thromboglobulin
Platelet factor IV
Platelet-derived growth factor
Ca++
Phagocytosis
No Protein Synthesis
Fibrinogen
Glycosidases
Proteinases
Cationic Proteins

FIGURE 35–8. Diagram of a platelet demonstrating the principal constituents of the platelet, which are listed beneath the figure. (From Ross, R.: Atherosclerosis: A problem of the biology of arterial wall cells and their interactions with blood components. Arteriosclerosis *1*:301, 1981, by permission of the American Heart Association.)

THE LESIONS OF ATHEROSCLEROSIS

Although atherosclerosis has been known for many centuries, its clinical effects are manifested principally in medium-sized muscular arteries, including the coronary, carotid, basilar, and vertebral arteries, as well as several arteries affecting the lower extremities, particularly the iliac and superficial femoral arteries. Larger arteries, such as the aorta and the iliac arteries, can also be involved, and the principal clinical sequelae in these large arteries is usually aneurysmal dilatation and its related effects.[62]

The earliest lesions of atherosclerosis can usually be found in young children and infants in the form of a lesion called the *fatty streak*, whereas the advanced lesion, the fibrous plaque, generally appears during early adulthood and progresses with age.[63–66] Until recently, most tissues that had been prepared for examination were derived from autopsy specimens and were sufficiently poorly preserved so that when the cells became laden with lipid and appeared as foam cells, it was virtually impossible to determine the origin of the cell. Recent advances in tissue fixation and embedding have permitted new modes of preservation. Furthermore, monoclonal antibodies have been developed that are specific for smooth muscle cells, for macrophages, and for lymphocytes. With the use of these antibodies and with improved preservation techniques, it has been possible to identify specifically the origin of the cells in the different lesions of atherosclerosis.

The Fatty Streak

Fatty streaks were observed by Stary[66] in his studies of a series of children and young adults. He demonstrated that by the age of 10 years, the fatty streaks consisted principally of lipid-laden macrophages, together with varying (but usually small) numbers of lipid-filled smooth muscle cells that accumulated beneath them as the lesions increased in size. Grossly, the fatty streak appears as an area of yellow discoloration due to the large amount of lipid deposited in the foam cells. The bulk of this lipid is in the form of cholesterol and cholesteryl ester, which probably enters the fatty streak by transport of lipoproteins from the plasma via the endothelial cells, after which it is taken up by macrophages and smooth muscle cells. The plasma lipids present in the intima are ingested by macrophages and are hydrolyzed and re-esterified once they have been taken up by these cells.

Stary also studied fatty streaks in the coronary arteries of a series of children and young adults and observed that they were localized at anatomical sites that were the same as the sites in other older individuals that were occupied by advanced fibromuscular lesions, or fibrous plaques. His data and that of others suggested that over a period of time, fatty streaks at particular sites are converted by a series of changes into the more advanced fibroproliferative lesions of atherosclerosis, whereas fatty streaks at other anatomical sites either remain the same or regress and disappear. McGill[67] has gone on to review data to demonstrate that with time, fatty streaks occupy increasing surface areas of the coronary arteries and that these sites also precede the formation of advanced lesions. Thus, although it is difficult to derive firm conclusions from these types of data, such observations suggest that the fatty streak in many instances, if not the large majority, is the precursor lesion that becomes converted into the advanced occlusive form of atherosclerosis.

Once foam cells have formed in fatty streaks and in advanced lesions, it may become extremely difficult to define the cell of origin. The cells become filled with lipid droplets that appear as empty vacuoles in paraffin-embedded tissues which are often surrounded by a very thin rim of cytoplasm (Fig. 35–9). Electron microscopic examination may permit identification of some of these cells; however, large numbers remain difficult if not impossible to identify using standard techniques of tissue staining.

Several monoclonal antibodies have been developed, at least two of which appear to be specific for cell type. Tsukada et al.[68] have developed monoclonal antibodies against smooth muscle–alpha actin and against a cytoplasmic antigen present in macrophages. Fortunately, these antigens resist some modes of fixation and embedding in paraffin. With these monoclonal antibodies, it has been possible to identify positively both macrophages and smooth muscle cells in lesions of atherosclerosis. Thus it can be said definitively that the fatty streak consists principally of lipid-laden macrophages together with small and variable numbers of smooth muscle cells (Fig. 35–9).

Diffuse Intimal Thickening

One form of lesion, described as a diffuse intimal thickening, consists of increased numbers of intimal smooth muscle cells surrounded by variable amounts of connective tissue. It is not entirely clear whether these sites of thickened intima represent developmental thickenings or whether such multilayered cushions of intimal smooth muscle cells are sites that formed because of increased stress on the artery wall, but which do not progress to advanced lesions of atherosclerosis. This is a somewhat poorly understood and controversial subject.

The Fibrous Plaque

The advanced lesion of atherosclerosis is generally called a fibrous plaque. When the fibrous plaque becomes involved with thrombosis, hemorrhage, and/or calcification, it is often called a *complicated lesion*.

Fibrous plaques are grossly white in appearance and are usually elevated. In many cases they protrude into the lumen of the artery and, if sufficiently large, compromise the flow of blood. These lesions consist of large numbers of intimal smooth muscle cells, together with numerous macrophages. When these cells contain lipid, the lipid is

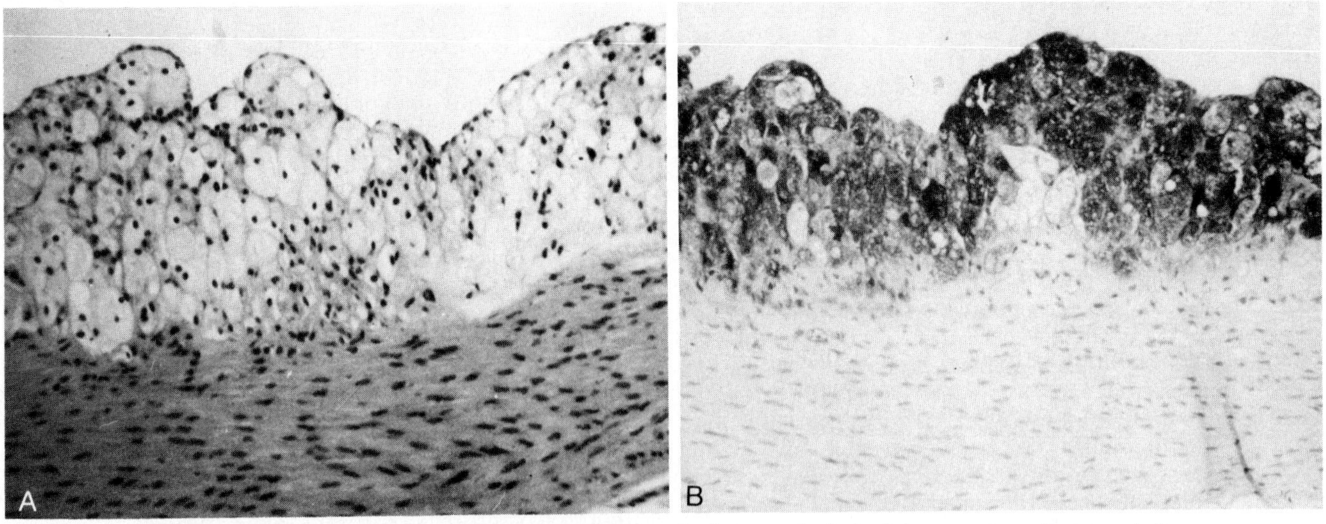

FIGURE 35–9. Light micrographs demonstrating portions of a fatty streak obtained from an aorta of a hypercholesterolemic monkey. This particular fatty streak contains several layers of macrophages. *A* is a routinely fixed and embedded paraffin section that has been stained with hematoxylin and eosin. The macrophage-rich areas are seen as clear, since they are lipid-containing and the lipid has been extracted during the process of dehydration and embedding. *B* demonstrates an adjacent section that has been stained with immunoperoxidase coupled to an antibody specific for a cytoplasmic antigen present within the macrophage. The macrophages stain densely black in this micrograph, demonstrating that the large majority of the lipid-rich cells in the fatty streak are macrophages. Such antibodies make it possible to recognize cell type, even after the cells have become distorted by inclusions.

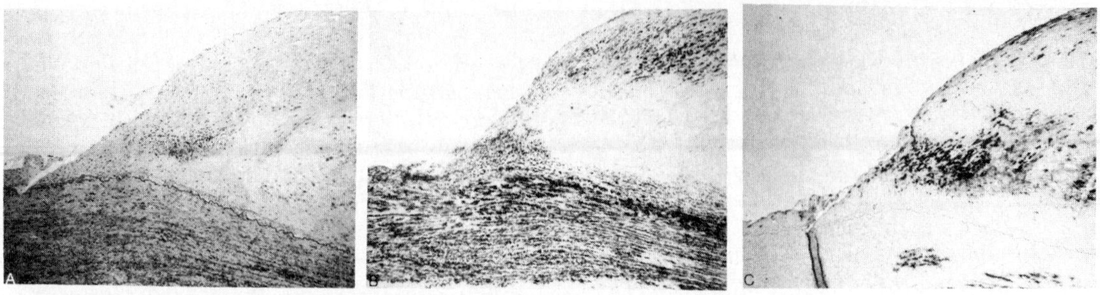

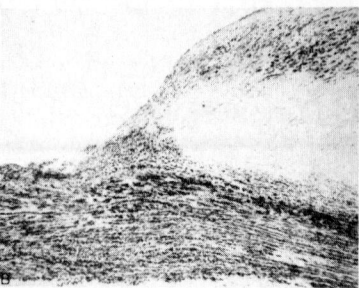

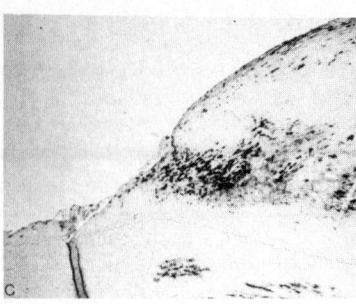

FIGURE 35–10. Three light micrographs demonstrating adjacent sections of a human fibrous plaque from a carotid endarterectomy specimen. *A* was stained with hematoxylin and eosin. In the elevated portion of the lesion, the area adjacent to the lumen consists of a fibrous cap of parallel layers of smooth muscle cells covering a mixture of cells. With H & E it is impossible to determine cell type. *B* is an adjacent section that has been stained using immunoperoxidase coupled to an anti-smooth muscle actin antibody. The smooth muscle cells in the fibrous cap, in the media underlying the lesion, and in patches and individual cells located throughout the lesion, are stained black. *C* is an adjacent section stained with immunoperoxidase coupled to an anti-macrophage antibody. Individual macrophages can be seen dispersed among the smooth muscle cells in the fibrous cap, but are found principally in the area deep to the fibrous cap between the fibrous cap and the media, where most of the lipid-containing cells in this particular lesion can be found.

primarily in the form of cholesterol and cholesteryl ester. The proliferated smooth muscle cells are surrounded by collagen and elastic fibers, by large amounts of proteoglycan, and, in individuals who are hypercholesterolemic, by varying amounts of lipid deposited in the cells and in the connective tissue. Fibrous plaques characteristically are covered by a fibrous cap.

In a study of a large series of male patients who had advanced occlusive lesions of the superficial femoral artery, we observed that the fibrous cap of each lesion consisted largely of a particular form of smooth muscle cell that is thin and pancake-shaped and that is surrounded by numerous lamellae of basement membrane, proteoglycan, and large numbers of collagen fibrils. The connective tissue in the fibrous cap is exceedingly dense. Beneath the fibrous cap lies a mixture of smooth muscle cells, macrophages, and numerous lymphocytes, including both B cells and T cells. Using the monoclonal antibodies already described, as well as antibodies to lymphocytes, it has been possible to identify definitively each of these cell types in the advanced lesions of atherosclerosis. In this highly cellular portion of the fibrous plaque, there are also large amounts of connective tissue. Beneath the cell-rich region, there is often a zone of necrotic tissue and debris which may contain cholesterol crystals and regions of calcification as well as numerous enlarged foam cells (Fig. 35–10).

Some fibrous plaques are densely fibrous and contain relatively little lipid, whereas others are rich in lipid deposits. Such differences can be found in different arteries within a given individual but are often associated with different risk factors. For example, it is common that the fibrous plaques observed in the superficial femoral arteries of those who are heavy cigarette smokers are extremely fibrous and contain relatively little lipid. On the other hand, individuals who are hypercholesterolemic and have advanced lesions in the coronary arteries often have large amounts of lipid within the lesions.[47]

There appears to be a general pattern in the distribution of advanced lesions of atherosclerosis in humans. Generally, the abdominal aorta is more extensively involved than the thoracic aorta.[22] Lesions in the aorta are usually most prominent near the ostia of major branches that leave the aorta. Some arteries such as the renal arteries appear to be spared from atherosclerosis, except at their ostia.[69] The coronary arteries generally demonstrate the most intense involvement, with lesions of atherosclerosis located within the first 6 cm of the artery.[70] It has been suggested that the severity of lesion formation in a given artery may be related in part to the particular nature of the characteristics of the blood flow in the artery, and that rheological forces play a major role in determining the localization, extent, and severity of lesions in susceptible individuals.[71, 72]

The principal clinical results of advanced lesions of atherosclerosis are derived either from the fact that they partially or totally occlude the lumen of the affected artery or because cracks and fissures develop in the lesions, leading to thrombosis and embolism, or to aneurysmal dilatation (which usually occurs in large arteries such as the aorta).

HYPOTHESES OF ATHEROGENESIS

Current theories of the pathogenesis of the lesions of atherosclerosis relate back to early proposals made by Virchow,[73] Rokitansky,[74] and Duguid.[75] Virchow believed that a form of low-grade injury to the artery wall resulted in a type of inflammatory insudate, which in turn caused increased passage and accumulation of plasma constituents in the intima of the artery.[73] Rokitansky's belief, subsequently elaborated upon by Duguid, was that an encrustation of small mural thrombi existed at sites of arterial injury, that these thrombi went on to organize by the growth of smooth muscle cells into them, and they would become incorporated into the lesions and thus serve as sites where the lesions would progress.[74, 75]

In 1973, these two notions about atherogenesis were combined with new knowledge of the cellular and molecular biology of the artery wall in a hypothesis termed the *response-to-injury hypothesis of atherosclerosis.*[2] This hypothesis has been modified as new data have come forth. It now takes into account many aspects of the behavior of arterial and blood cells described above, as well as the numerous risk factors that have been associated with atherogenesis, including hyperlipidemia, hormone dysfunction, altered rheological forces as may occur in hypertension, and alteration of the endothelial barrier by factors associated with cigarette smoking, diabetes, and so on.[3, 6, 76]

A second hypothesis that was also formulated in 1973, the *monoclonal hypothesis*, suggests that the lesions of atherosclerosis may represent some form of neoplasia.[14] Both of these are discussed below.

The Response-to-Injury Hypothesis

The response-to-injury hypothesis of atherosclerosis states that some form of "injury" may occur to the lining endothelial cells at particular anatomical sites in the artery wall. "Injury" to the endothelium is a key event in this hypothesis, and defining and understanding the subtleties of the nature of the various possible forms of injury is paramount in both testing the hypothesis and, if it is found to be correct, in developing means of prevention and intervention.

Endothelial injury may be manifested as a number of forms of endothelial dysfunction. For example, interference with the permeability barrier role of the endothelium, alterations in the nonthrombogenic properties of the endothelial surface, and promotion of the procoagulant properties of the endothelium would all represent forms of dysfunction and injury that could result in some of the changes to be discussed below. Furthermore, maintenance of the continuity of the endothelial surface and maintenance of the normal low rates of turnover of the endothelial cells at most sites in the arterial tree are important in maintaining homeostasis. When turnover of the endothelium increases, it is possible that such turnover may be related to a series of changes in the endothelium, including the synthesis and secretion of vasoactive substances, of lipolytic enzymes, and of growth factors by the endothelial cells. Thus, endothelial injury could potentially lead to a host of changes in the lining of endothelial cells which could then lead to a critical sequence of cellular interactions, culminating in formation of lesions of atherosclerosis (Fig. 35–11).

In the case of chronic hyperlipidemia, the response-to-injury hypothesis proposes that an increase in plasma lipoproteins, principally low-density lipoproteins and thus cholesterol, would result in changes in the surface characteristics of both the endothelial cells and in the circulating leukocytes, particularly circulating monocytes and possibly platelets as well. Hypercholesterolemia somehow leads to increased adhesion of monocytes to endothelium at sites throughout the arterial tree.[77] When these monocytes adhere, they probe and are chemotactically attracted to migrate between endothelial cells and localize subendothelially, where they can become active as scavenger cells and are converted to macrophages. When they become macrophages, these cells take up lipid. The lipid may enter the subendothelium in large quantities in the hypercholesterolemic state, resulting in the formation of foam cells and in the development of fatty streaks. The accumulation of macrophages in the intimal space would then establish conditions that could lead to further alterations in the endothelium. Macrophages are well known to be capable of synthesizing and secreting numerous injurious agents

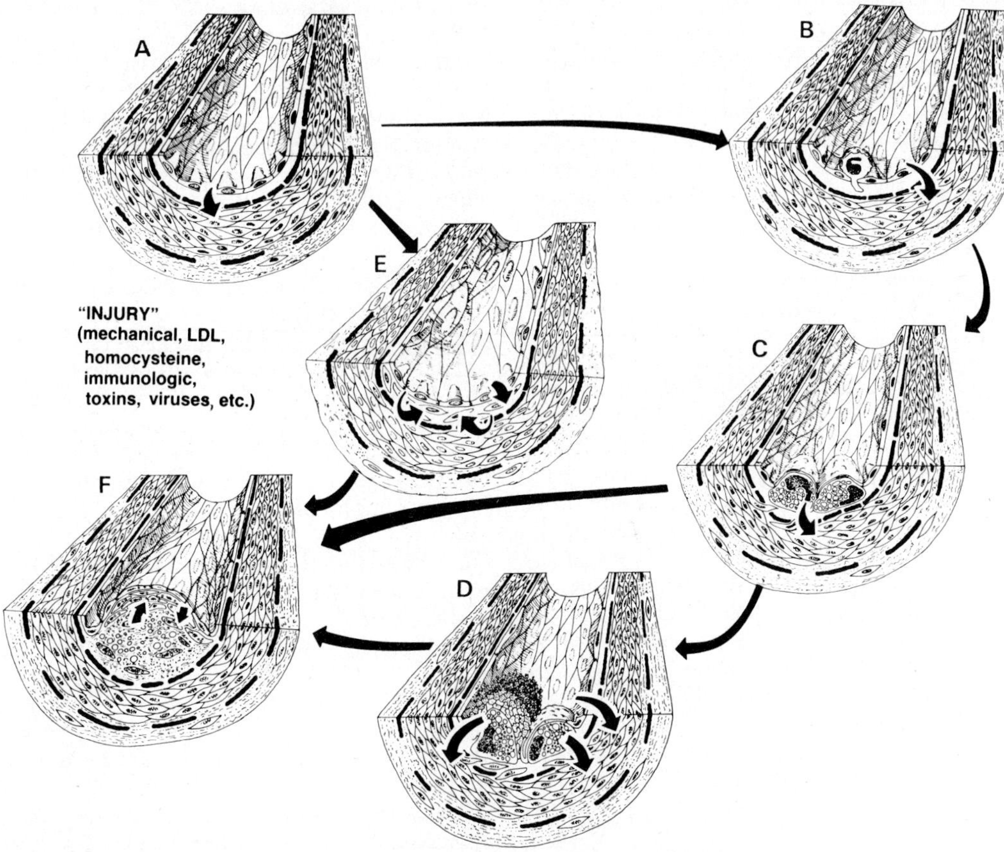

FIGURE 35–11. The response-to-injury hypothesis. Advanced intimal proliferative lesions of atherosclerosis may develop by at least two pathways. The pathway demonstrated by the clockwise (long) arrows to the right has been observed in experimentally induced hypercholesterolemia. Injury to the endothelium (*A*) may induce growth factor secretion (short arrow). Monocytes attach to endothelium (*B*), which may continue to secrete growth factors (short arrow). Subendothelial migration of monocytes (*C*) may lead to fatty streak formation and release of growth factors such as PDGF (short arrow). Fatty streaks may become directly converted to fibrous plaques (long arrow from *C* to *F*) through release of growth factors from macrophages or endothelial cells or both. Macrophages may also stimulate or injure the overlying endothelium. In some cases, macrophages may lose their endothelial cover and platelet attachment may occur (D), providing three possible sources of growth factors—platelets, macrophages, and endothelium (short arrows). An alternative pathway for development of advanced lesions of atherosclerosis is shown by the arrows from *A* to *E* to *F*. In this case, the endothelium may be injured but remain intact. Increased endothelial turnover may result in growth factor formation by endothelial cells (*A*). This may stimulate migration of smooth muscle cells from the media into the intima, accompanied by endogenous production of PDGF by smooth muscle as well as growth factor secretion from the "injured" endothelial cells (*E*). These interactions could then lead to fibrous plaque formation and further lesion progression (*F*). (Reprinted by permission from Ross, R.: The pathogenesis of atherosclerosis—an update. N. Engl. J. Med. *314*:496, 1986.)

that normally could play a role in killing ingested microorganisms or in nullifying toxic substances.[49] In this instance, the macrophages could potentially secrete oxidative metabolites such as superoxide anion, which could further injure the overlying endothelial cells. It has been demonstrated that lipid-laden macrophages are capable of forming peroxide and superoxide anion in vitro,[52] suggesting that this may occur in vivo as well.

A further and potentially important reaction of the macrophage is related to its capacity to form growth factors. Activated macrophages can, as already noted, synthesize and secrete at least four potent growth factors: PDGF, FGF, an EGF-like factor, and TGF β. PDGF is a potent mitogen for smooth muscle cells, as is FGF under some circumstances. The combination of these growth factors, together with TGF β, has been shown in vivo to be extremely potent in stimulating the migration and proliferation of fibroblasts and potentially of smooth muscle cells, and in stimulating formation of new connective tissue by these cells.[78] Thus, if the macrophage-derived foam cells are appropriately activated in the subendothelial space, they could potentially be involved in the secretion of growth factors that could chemotactically attract smooth muscle cells to migrate from the media into the intima, to proliferate within the intima, and to set up a series of conditions that could lead to the formation of an intimal, fibromuscular, proliferative lesion. The stage would thus have been set by these circumstances for the development of an advanced lesion of atherosclerosis. If the cycle of "endothelial injury" and macrophage accumulation and stimulation is repeated, at least two cells capable of releasing growth factors into the intima—the activated endothelial cell and the activated macrophage—may continue to contribute to progression of the lesions.

The response-to-injury hypothesis also provides an opportunity for the interaction of a third cell, the platelet. The hypothesis suggests that if the flow properties of the blood at particular anatomical sites are such that these properties participate in the endothelial injury, endothelial cell-cell attachment may be affected and cell disjunction may occur, leading to retraction of endothelial cells and exposure of the underlying foam cells or connective tissue or both. In either case, this would permit opportunities for platelets to interact, adhere, aggregate, and form mural thrombi.[79–83] Should this occur, the platelet could provide a third potent source of growth factors, including the same four factors that can be released by the activated macrophage. Thus, there are numerous opportunities for mitogens to be deposited in the artery wall, which, under proper circumstances, could play critical roles in the genesis of proliferative smooth muscle lesions of atherosclerosis (Fig. 35–11).

It is important to point out that injury to the endothelium need not result in denudation of the endothelial cells. Endothelial injury may simply be manifested by relatively rapid replacement of individual endothelial cells that are lost, or it may simply be reflected in alterations in endothelial permeability or by release of growth factors.

Finally, it has been shown in some special cases, such as in the rat, that arterial smooth muscle cells that have been induced to proliferate in vivo also may be stimulated to secrete a form of PDGF when they are grown in cell culture. If this were to occur in vivo, then as smooth muscle cells proliferate in developing lesions, they might be able to induce further progression of the lesions by release of growth factors. Whether this will be shown to occur in species other than the rat remains to be determined.

The Monoclonal Hypothesis

The monoclonal hypothesis suggests that each lesion of atherosclerosis is derived from a single smooth muscle cell that serves as a source of all of the cells within the lesion. This hypothesis is based upon the Lyon, or inactive X chromosome, hypothesis, which states that each tissue is made of a small "patch" of related cells that have either an active maternal or an active paternal X chromosome, but not both. Such a fact would make little to no metabolic difference, since each X chromosome codes for similar enzymes. However, there is a special case that permits analysis of lesions by utilizing this fact. This is the case of some black females who are heterozygous for the enzyme glucose-6-phosphate dehydrogenase (G-6-PD). This enzyme is coded for by the X chromosome and occurs in two isozymic forms that can be separated by electrophoresis. When an individual is heterozygous for these two isozymes, one X chromosome codes for one and the second X chromosome for the other isoenzyme. Progenitor cells that have been committed to one or the other of the two X chromosomes therefore can replicate and form patches that will contain either one or the other isoenzyme.

This principle was taken advantage of by Lindner and Gartler,[84] who demonstrated that multiple samples of uterine leiomyomas are composed of cells that contain the same active X chromosome as denoted by G-6-PD, whereas when they examined samples of adjacent normal myometrium, they found both isozymes. More recently, studies of some tumors have also demonstrated similar phenomena, suggesting that in some tumors the tumor cells arose from a single cell; that is, they are monoclonal.

These observations were utilized in the proposal that some atherosclerotic plaques, which frequently appear as isolated nodules surrounded by areas of normal tissue, might be monoclonal. Benditt and Benditt[14] examined a series of plaques from a small number of black females that were obtained at autopsy. They dissected very small samples of each plaque and examined the isozyme content of each sample and determined the number of lesions that contained one or the other isozyme, or both isozymes. They interpreted their data to signify that each lesion of atherosclerosis represents a clone derived from a single smooth muscle cell, which they have recently termed monotypic rather than monoclonal. They have gone on to suggest, therefore, that each lesion of atherosclerosis is a benign neoplasm derived from a cell that has been transformed by viruses, by chemicals, or by other mutagens. More recently, investigators have looked for the presence of particular viruses, such as the herpes virus.[85] It is possible that some virally induced lesions could result in monoclonal lesions. It should be pointed out that contradictory data both supporting and refuting the monoclonal hypothesis have been published.

There are other possible interpretations of the data supporting the monoclonal hypothesis. Fialkow[86] has pointed out that the presence of a single-enzyme phenotype in a lesion does not necessarily mean that the lesion is clonal in origin. A single lesion could arise by the participation of more than one cell. If each cell that participated contained the same isozyme, and if some cells had a replicative advantage over others, it is possible that cells with a given isozyme type would replicate in preference to cells with the second isozyme type. The probability of such an origin would depend on the smooth muscle cell mosaic composition or patch size and distribution in the normal intima, which unfortunately is not known. If there were repeated cycles of cell death and cell proliferation in which a particular cell type had a selective advantage in proliferating, then repetitive sampling of these cells could lead to a single-enzyme phenotype, despite the fact that the lesions were multicellular in origin. In addition, clonal selection with evolution toward a single-enzyme phenotype has been shown to occur in several forms of focal hyperplasia. This makes it difficult if not impossible to determine whether the single-enzyme phenotype that has been observed is caused by monoclonality or by polyclonality based on selection as noted earlier.

LIPIDS AND LIPOPROTEINS IN ATHEROSCLEROSIS

Since hypercholesterolemia is the major risk factor associated with the increased incidence of atherosclerosis in the United States and Western Europe, it is important to understand the role that lipids play in this process. Although many lesions of atherosclerosis are fibrous and contain relatively little lipid, the effects of lipid on endothelium, monocytes, and smooth muscle, and the accumulation of lipid in the lesions of hypercholesterolemic individuals, are critical components of the process of atherogenesis. Consequently, it is important to understand specifically how elevated levels of cholesterol-bearing lipoproteins are related to the process of atherogenesis. These subjects are discussed in detail elsewhere in this book (pp. 1154 to 1167 and 1637 to 1645).

The Lipid Research Clinic Trials have provided data suggesting that it would be beneficial to lower plasma low-density lipoprotein (LDL) levels.[16, 17] Those studies showed that the decrease in plasma cholesterol can be correlated with a reduction in the incidence of myocardial infarction, and presumably atherosclerosis. The genetic basis for the increase in plasma LDL is not known for most individuals in the population who are hypercholesterolemic, although some may be heterozygous for the familial hypercholesterolemia (FH) trait. Nevertheless, our understanding of the LDL receptor control of HMG CoA reductase, and thus cholesterol synthesis, has been critical in permitting us to understand how cholesterol metabolism is regulated. As important as these studies are, however, they do not provide data that permit us to understand how the lesions of atherosclerosis form. In other words, although the LDL receptor pathway provides an understanding of the control of cholesterol metabolism, it yields no information concerning the basis of the cellular changes and interactions that occur when elevated plasma cholesterol leads to atherosclerosis.

To answer this question, it has been necessary to devise experiments using appropriate animal models and appropriate cell culture systems. These tests provide opportunities to determine how smooth muscle cells proliferate and under what circumstances, what cellular interactions occur during the pathogenesis of this disease process, and what factors are elaborated by the cells that control not only smooth muscle multiplication but also connective tissue formation and lipid accumulation.

The response-to-injury hypothesis of atherosclerosis already discussed can be taken one step further in terms of asking how chronic hypercholesterolemia may "injure" endothelium. Jackson and Gotto[87] have suggested that one form of endothelial injury which may occur upon exposure to chronically elevated levels of LDL may result from the effects of an increase in the number of cholesterol molecules in the plasma membranes of cells, including the endothelial cells. When the cholesterol/phospholipid ratio of endothelial plasma membranes is elevated, this could theoretically lead to an increase in the viscosity of the membranes. Changes such as these would decrease the malleability of the endothelial cell surface and, should this occur, could have critical effects at particular anatomical sites such as branches or bifurcations in the arterial tree, where the endothelial cells are exposed to changes in the flow of blood. Such rheological changes could cause an otherwise normally malleable endothelial surface, if it becomes more viscous and thus more rigid, to be incapable of dealing with the stresses caused by these changes in the flow characteristics. This could lead to endothelial cell-cell separation and endothelial retraction, particularly at sites where the blood flow has already been modified owing to the formation of fatty streaks, as has been found to occur in hypercholesterolemic monkeys, swine, and man. As already discussed, hypercholesterolemia also leads to changes in monocyte-endothelial adhesion properties and to the development of fatty streaks themselves. It is also possible that hypercholesterolemia may alter the endothelial cells so that they are stimulated to produce increased amounts of growth factor. All or any of these responses could lead to important changes that, step by step, lead to atherogenesis.

GROWTH FACTORS

As discussed earlier, growth factors can be elaborated by all four cells potentially involved in the lesions of atherosclerosis: endothelium, monocyte/macrophages, platelets, and smooth muscle. Although the first three of these cells can produce more than one growth factor, platelet-derived growth factor (PDGF) could play a critical role in the genesis of atherosclerosis because of its chemotactic and mitogenic effects on smooth muscle cells.

PDGF is a two-chain molecule of approximately 30,000 molecular weight that is highly cationic and highly disulfide bonded.[88–91] It is an extraordinarily potent mitogen that binds with very high affinity to responsive cells[92, 93] and is chemotactic for the same cells for which it is mitogenic.[94, 95] When it binds to its high-affinity cell-surface receptor, it induces a series of biological events, some of which are probably related to induction of DNA synthesis and cell division. These cellular responses include phosphorylation of the PDGF receptor through the activation of a tyrosine kinase on the receptor, and the activation of C-kinase in the subplasmalemmal cytoplasm resulting from phospholipase activation at the cell surface. C-kinase activation could ultimately lead to calcium transfer from intracellular compartments, which in itself may possibly be important in induction of the mitogenic signal.[53]

PDGF also induces increased binding of LDL to cells by increasing the numbers of LDL receptors,[42, 96] increased cholesterol synthesis, increased endocytosis, increased flux of ions into the cell, reorganization of actin cables within the cells, and change in cell shape. It also has recently been found to be a potent vasoactive agent, even more potent than angiotensin II.[53] Thus, if PDGF is released from platelets when they adhere to the artery wall at sites of injury, from activated macrophages after they enter the artery wall (particularly during fatty streak formation), from activated endothelial cells if they are appropriately stimulated, and perhaps in some special instances from appropriately activated smooth muscle cells, then such responses would enhance lesion formation.

PDGF has an extremely short half-life when it is injected into the circulation.[97] This short half-life suggests that

PDGF that is not bound locally to tissue would be cleared rapidly and thus would be unavailable at sites distant from its release. Furthermore, PDGF binds to a number of proteins in the plasma, including alpha$_2$-macroglobulin. These binding proteins could serve to increase further the capacity of PDGF to act as a tissue mitogen at local sites where PDGF has been released and is bound to the tissue.[98]

There is a striking homology between the amino acid sequence of purified PDGF and that of a transforming protein derived from an oncogene of the simian sarcoma virus. This homology is not only striking but also suggests that PDGF may be important in proliferation of cells transformed by the simian sarcoma virus.[99, 100] Furthermore, numerous lines of transformed cells secrete a form of PDGF and have downregulated receptors for PDGF, suggesting that a form of PDGF may play a role in the proliferation of cells that are neoplastically transformed in other ways.[101] Both chains of PDGF have been cloned, and cDNA probes are available for each of them. This will make it possible to explore the PDGF molecule in great detail and to probe the controls of genetic expression at the molecular level in each of the different cells capable of secreting PDGF. Such studies should permit us to understand more about how PDGF participates in disease processes such as atherosclerosis, as well as its potential role in other tissue responses, including wound repair and perhaps even embryogenesis and development.

CELLULAR EVENTS THAT OCCUR DURING ATHEROGENESIS

Several animals form lesions of atherosclerosis similar to humans when they develop hypercholesterolemia from eating a fatty diet. This has made it possible to study the effects of hypercholesterolemia in terms of understanding the cellular interactions that occur that lead to the lesions of atherosclerosis. Such studies have been performed by Faggiotto et al. on nonhuman primates,[102, 103] by Gerrity[104–106] and his colleagues on swine, and by Rosenfeld et al.[107] on fat-fed rabbits and the Watanabe heritable hyperlipemic rabbit (WHHL rabbit). The latter studies have provided highly detailed observations concerning the sequence of cellular events that occur in endogenous hypercholesterolemia (the WHHL rabbit, a model of familial homozygous hypercholesterolemia) as compared with those that take place during diet-induced hypercholesterolemia.

The data of Faggiotto et al.[102, 103] show that the first and most striking event occurs after 7 to 14 days of diet-induced hypercholesterolemia. This consists of the attachment of larger numbers of leukocytes, principally monocytes, to the surface of the arterial endothelium (Fig. 35–12). The monocytes attach to the endothelial cells in clusters that appear to be randomly located throughout the arterial tree in all large and medium-sized arteries. The attached monocytes then migrate over the surface of the endothelium, where they probe, find a junction between the endothelial cells and use this junctional site to slip between the cells and localize in the subendothelial space (Fig. 35–13). This process, as viewed in cell culture, appears to occur very rapidly and presumably does so in vivo as well. After finding their way into the subendothelial intimal space, the monocytes become converted into macrophages, so that within less than one month large numbers of foam cells, or lipid-filled macrophages, are found beneath an intact endothelium. These cells continue to enlarge as they fill with lipid. Such accumulations of foam cells represent the establishment of the first and ubiquitous lesion of atherosclerosis, the fatty streak (Fig. 35–14). The fatty streaks continue to expand over a period of 4 to 5

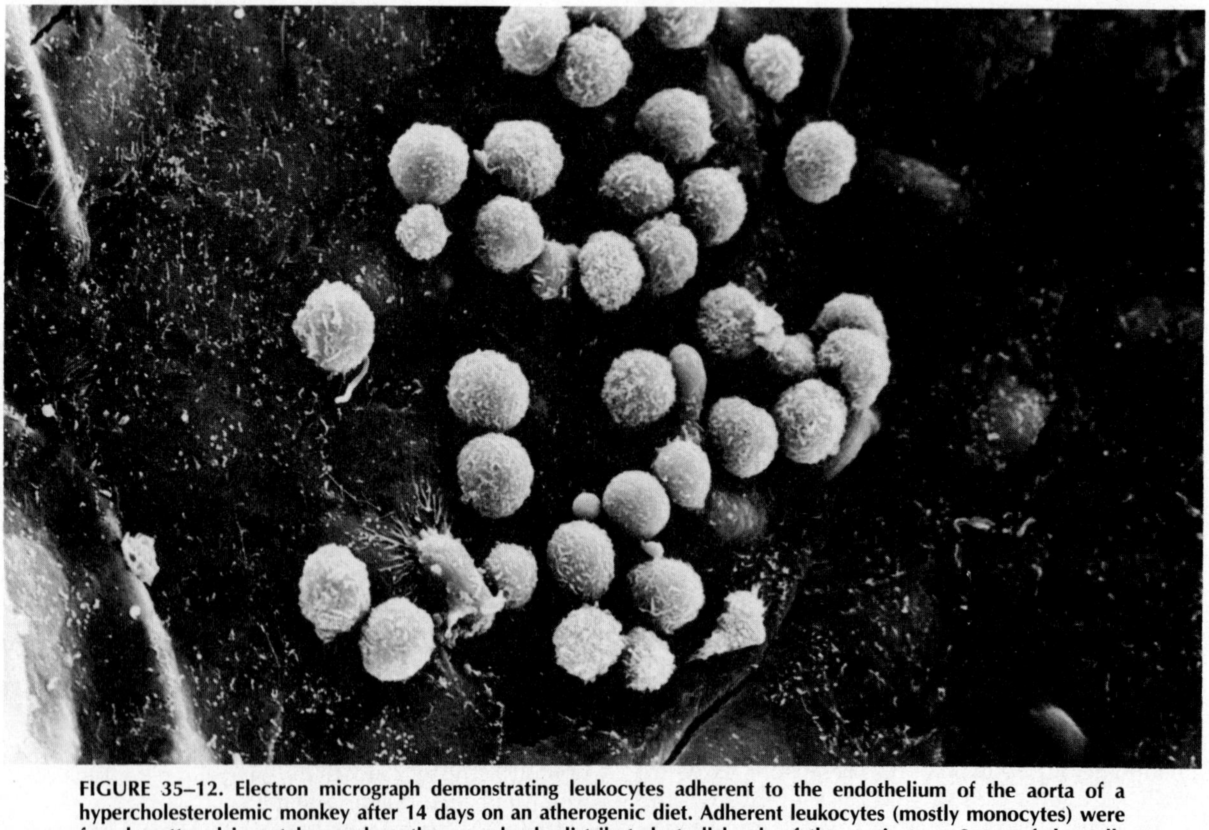

FIGURE 35–12. Electron micrograph demonstrating leukocytes adherent to the endothelium of the aorta of a hypercholesterolemic monkey after 14 days on an atherogenic diet. Adherent leukocytes (mostly monocytes) were found scattered in patches such as these randomly distributed at all levels of the aortic tree. Some of the cells appear spread on the surface, whereas others are rounded in appearance.

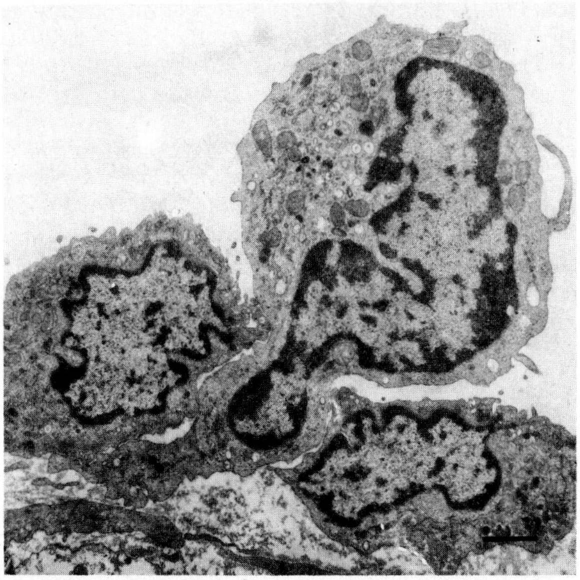

FIGURE 35–13. Electron micrograph showing a monocyte which has come between two endothelial cells as it was apparently in the process of entering the intimal space. This was easily observed at 14 days of hypercholesterolemia in fat-fed nonhuman primates. Bar = 1 μ. (From Faggiotto, A., Ross, R., and Harker, L.: Studies of hypercholesterolemia in the nonhuman primate. I. Changes that lead to fatty streak formation. Arteriosclerosis *4*:330, 1984, by permission of the American Heart Association.)

months in the hypercholesterolemic monkeys by continuing the process of monocyte adherence, subendothelial migration and localization, and lipid accumulation. As the fatty streaks expand, the surface of the artery becomes highly irregular and convoluted (Fig. 35–15). With increasing time, small numbers of smooth muscle cells begin to appear beneath the accumulated macrophages within the intima and also begin to accumulate deposits of lipid and take on the appearance of foam cells. As discussed earlier, monoclonal antibodies specific for smooth muscle and macrophages have made it possible to show that both types of cell become foam cells as the lesions expand. The cholesterol levels in the plasma of the fat-fed monkeys ranged between 500 to 1000 mg/dl, which are not dissimilar from the levels of plasma cholesterol found in humans with FH disease.

After approximately 5 to 6 months at these very high cholesterol and LDL levels, a second series of changes occurred in the monkeys, initially at branches and bifurcations in the iliac arteries and subsequently at higher regions in the arterial tree. The changes that were found at branches and bifurcations suggest that they may be associated with the flow characteristics at these particular sites in the vessel. They consisted of retraction of the endothelial cells covering some of the fatty streaks caused by endothelial cell-cell detachment. Endothelial retraction exposed the numerous lipid-filled macrophages to the circulation (Fig. 35–16). In some instances, these macro-

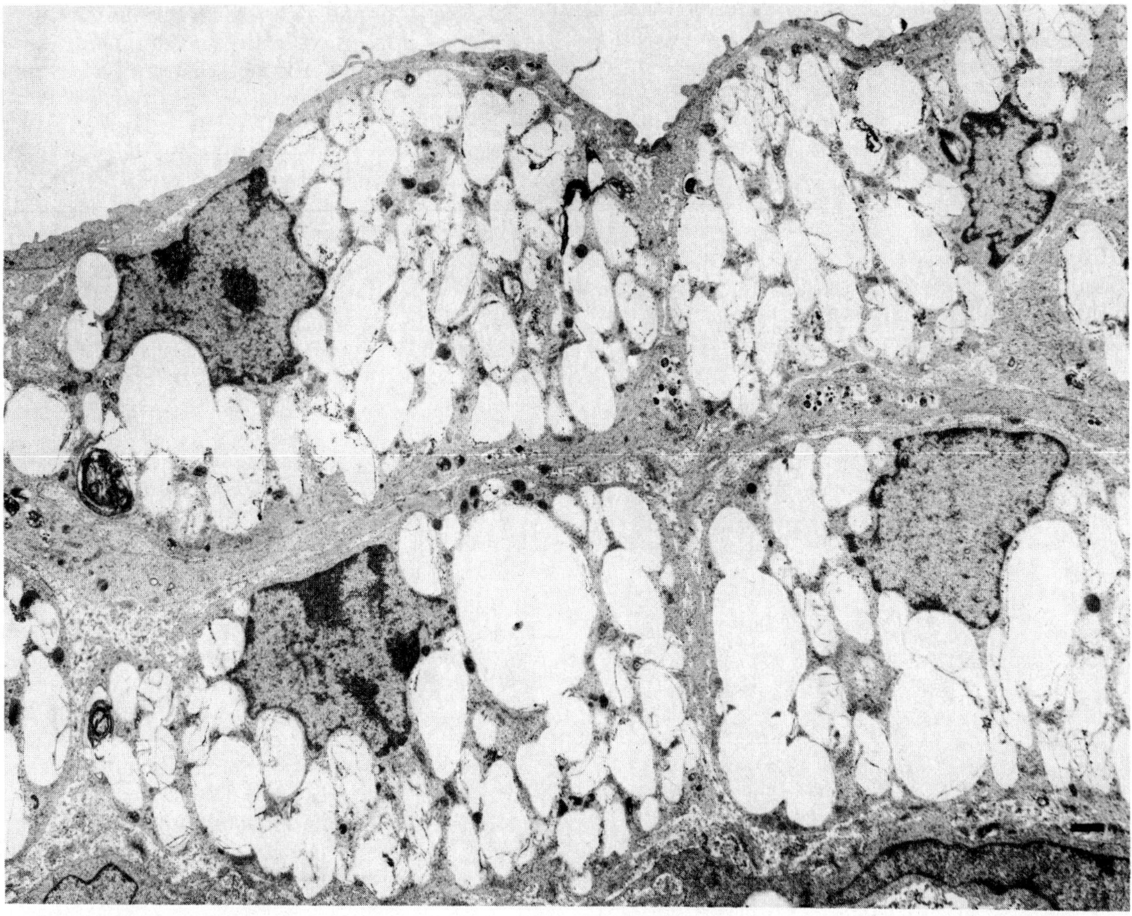

FIGURE 35–14. Transmission electron micrograpn snowing a fatty streak containing two layers of subendothelial foam cells after 2 months of hypercholesterolemia in a fat-fed nonhuman primate. The large lipid-filled macrophages are distributed focally in multilayers. The cells are four- to six-fold larger than lipid-laden macrophages observed in control animals. There is a small amount of intercellular matrix and some lipid debris. The macrophages maintain a close relationship to the intact endothelium. The endothelium is markedly stretched so that the endothelial cells have become very thin. (From Faggiotto, A., Ross, R., and Harker, L.: Studies of hypercholesterolemia in the nonhuman primate. I. Changes that lead to fatty streak formation. Arteriosclerosis *4*:332, 1984, by permission of the American Heart Association.)

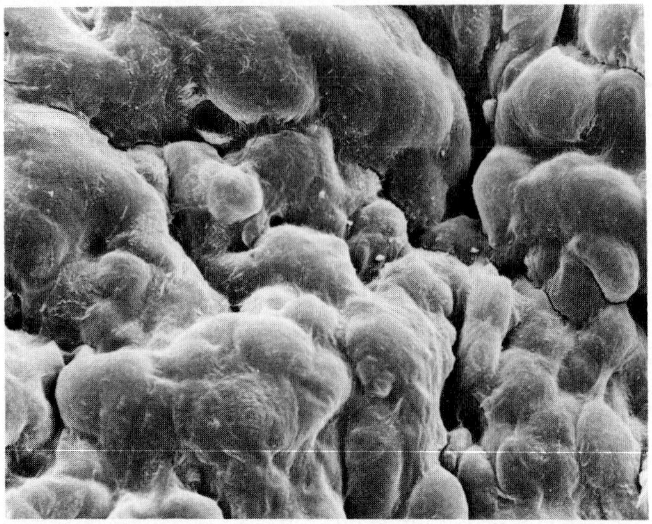

FIGURE 35–15. Scanning electron micrograph providing a surface view of a fatty streak from a fat-fed monkey after 2 months of hypercholesterolemia. The surface of the fatty streak has become highly irregular and has a striking nodular pattern with deep crevices between the nodules. Such a pattern forms by continuing adherence of monocytes to the endothelial cells that probe and migrate subendothelially between cells to continually expand the fatty streak.

phages appear to be swept into the circulation, leading to the presence of foam cells in the blood. When this occurred, the exposed connective tissue upon which these macrophages resided served as sites for platelet adherence and for microthrombi to form. In other areas, some of the exposed macrophages also served as a nidus for platelets to adhere, and thrombi formed on the surfaces of the macrophages, demonstrating that the macrophages may represent a potent site for platelet interactions (Fig. 35–17). In either of these cases where platelet interactions such as those just described occurred, similar anatomical sites were observed 1 to 2 months later to be occupied by space-filling lesions of advanced atherosclerosis, or fibrous

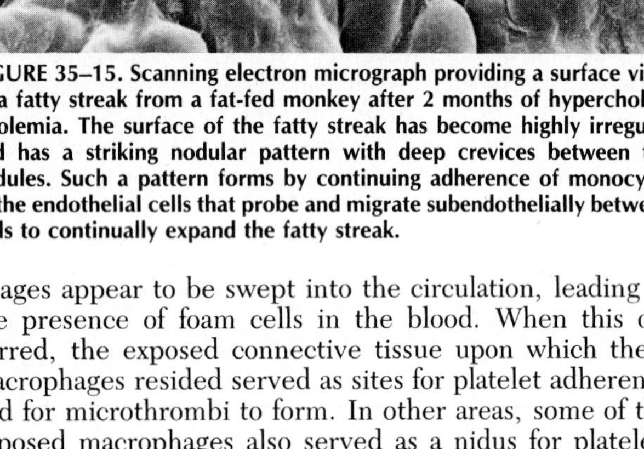

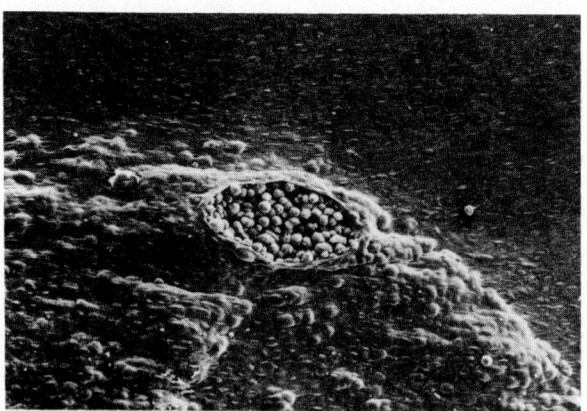

FIGURE 35–16. Low-power scanning electron micrograph demonstrating a fatty streak in a hypercholesterolemic monkey that had been on the high-fat, high-cholesterol diet for 5 months. The center of the fatty streak has lost its endothelial cover, exposing the underlying macrophages. This has occurred by detachment of endothelial cells and retraction of these endothelial cells, exposing the underlying macrophages to the flowing blood. The fatty streak can be seen to cover the bottom half of the micrograph in a crescentic pattern, and the area of endothelial retraction can be observed in the center of the micrograph. (From Faggiotto, A., and Ross, R.: Studies of hypercholesterolemia in the nonhuman primate. II. Fatty streak conversion to fibrous plaque. Arteriosclerosis *4*:347, 1984, by permission of the American Heart Association.)

plaques. These fibrous plaques had all of the characteristic appearances of fibrous plaques in humans, including a dense fibrous cap that overlay areas of extensive proliferation of smooth muscle cells intermixed with lipid-filled macrophages, beneath which were found areas of cell debris, lipid accumulation, and sometimes calcification (Fig. 35–18). The same changes occurred at the iliac bifurcation after approximately 7 months, in the abdominal aorta after 9 months, in the thoracic aorta by 11 months, and in the coronary arteries after a year to 13 months. By analyzing the distribution of these changes and correlating this distribution with the levels of cholesterol in the animals with time, Faggiotto et al.[102, 103] were able to demonstrate that there was a correlation among three factors: the level of plasma cholesterol, the duration of the maintenance of this increased level of cholesterol, and the changes that occur at particular anatomical sites with time.

Another important observation was that there were many advanced lesions of atherosclerosis that also occurred at sites where fatty streaks were present but where there was no clear evidence of endothelial cell-cell separation and exposure of the subendothelium.[103] Thus, one has to conclude that proliferative lesions of atherosclerosis can occur at sites where the endothelium remains intact over preexisting lesions such as fatty streaks. This can undoubtedly be explained by the fact that both activated macrophages and endothelium can serve as sources of growth factors so that platelet interactions are not required for smooth muscle proliferation to occur.

This leads to the need to determine what constitutes endothelial injury. It also suggests that there can be nondenuding forms of injury that are just as important as denuding forms described already. Reidy and Schwartz[108, 109] have indicated that one of the most common results of endothelial injury may be detachment of individual endothelial cells, which are rapidly replaced by neighboring cells so that endothelial continuity is maintained. Several markers have been developed that can be used to identify sites of endothelial injury. Hansson et al.[110] demonstrated that injured endothelial cells take up IgG whereas normal endothelium will not, and that such IgG uptake can be correlated with increased replication of the endothelium. Furthermore, Reidy and Schwartz[111] showed that a linear correlation exists between the extent of endothelial injury (the number of denuded cells) and the localization of indium-111–labeled platelets at these sites. Platelets would adhere because injured endothelium appears to have lost its nonthrombogenic properties. Thus there may be several different forms of endothelial injury and more subtle techniques may be necessary to uncover them. This raises the interesting question, as suggested earlier, of whether one subtle form of endothelial injury may be the stimulation of these cells to synthesize and secrete growth factors, including PDGF, that could then play a critical role in the genesis of the events previously described. If this were the case, then endothelial disjunction, retraction, and subendothelial exposure are clearly not necessary for lesions of atherosclerosis to develop, since both activated endothelium and macrophages could be sufficient in themselves to provide a mitogenic stimulus for smooth muscle cells to form lesions of atherosclerosis.

REGRESSION OF ATHEROSCLEROSIS

A number of studies have demonstrated that lesions of experimentally induced atherosclerosis can in fact regress. When hypercholesterolemic swine and nonhuman primates that have developed severe lesions are placed on a

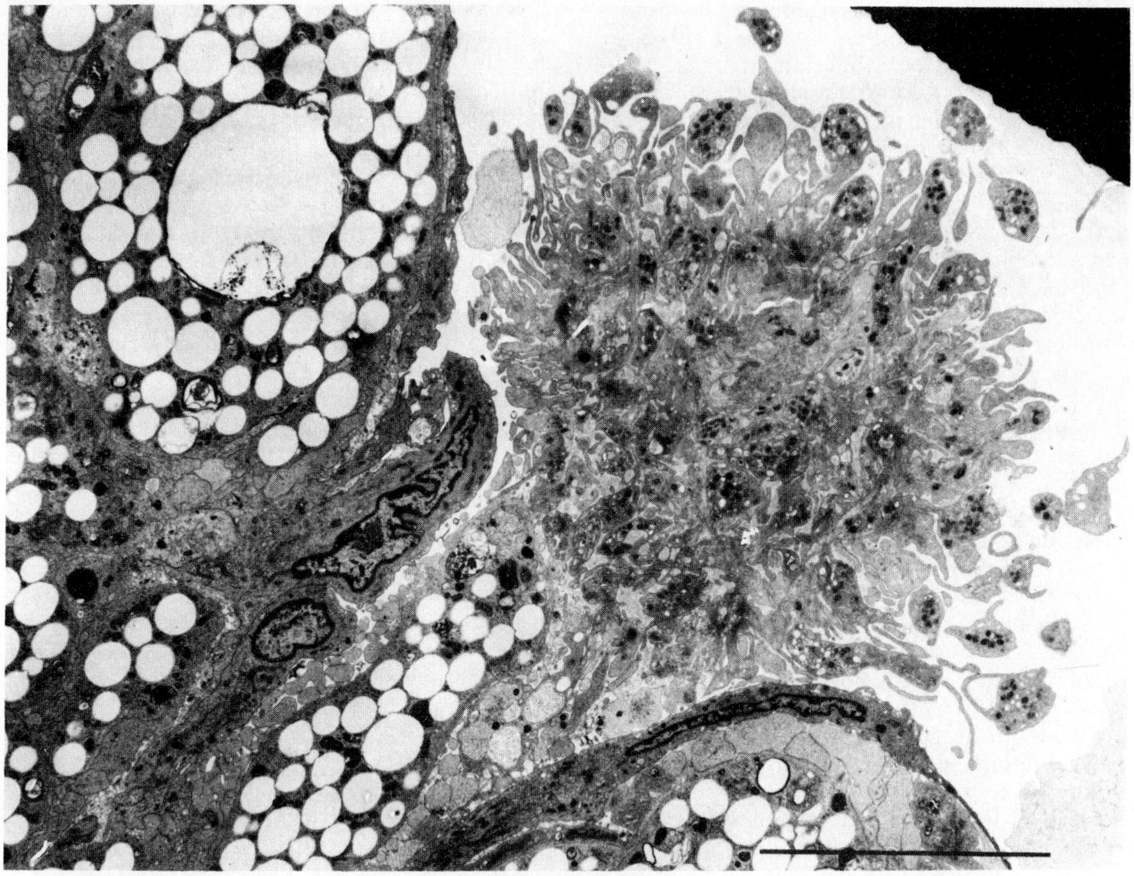

FIGURE 35–17. Transmission electron micrograph of platelets adherent to an exposed macrophage from a fatty streak in a fat-fed monkey that had been hypercholesterolemic for 6 months. The platelets in this thrombus are generally adherent to exposed foam cells and penetrate into the depth of a crevice in the fatty streak. Many of the platelets have undergone degranulation and have released their contents. Bar = 10 μ. (From Faggiotto, A., and Ross, R.: Studies of hypercholesterolemia in the nonhuman primate. II. Fatty streak conversion to fibrous plaque. Arteriosclerosis *4*:349, 1984, by permission of the American Heart Association.)

normocholesterolemic diet, these lesions can regress. Fatty streaks formed in the monkeys studied on the high-fat, high-cholesterol diet of Faggiotto et al.[102] were found to regress completely within one month after the animals were placed on a normal diet. Most of the studies of regression of the advanced lesions of atherosclerosis have been performed in nonhuman primates, principally in different strains of macaques and in squirrel monkeys. The studies were performed by providing the monkeys with atherogenic diets that took them through stages of fatty streak development and on to fibrous plaque formation. When cholesterol was removed from the diet and plasma cholesterol concentrations returned to normal, Faggiotto et al.[102] observed that reasonably rapid regression of fatty streaks occurred. Of greater potential interest, significant reduction in the size of the smooth muscle proliferative

FIGURE 35–18. Light micrograph demonstrating an advanced fibrous plaque that formed in the internal iliac artery of a monkey that was hypercholesterolemic for 7 months. The lesion has occluded approximately 70 per cent of the arterial lumen and consists of numerous layers of smooth muscle cells surrounded by fibrous connective tissue. An area of lipid and necrotic tissue occupies the left side and upper portion of this lesion. (From Faggiotto, A., and Ross, R.: Studies of hypercholesterolemia in the nonhuman primate. II. Fatty streak conversion to fibrous plaque. Arteriosclerosis *4*:345, 1984, by permission of the American Heart Association.)

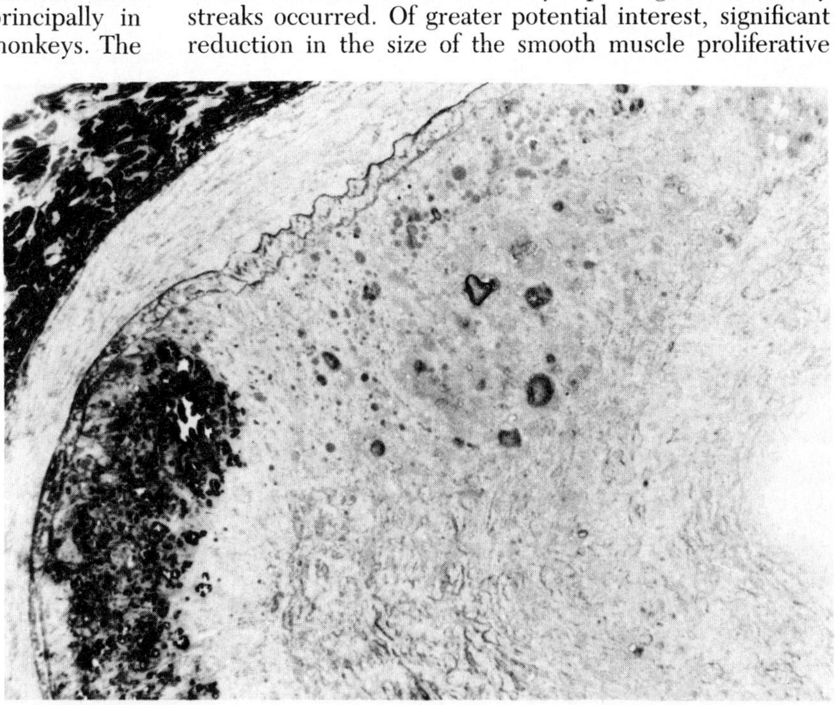

lesions has been observed by several different investigators. Some of the earliest studies were performed by Armstrong et al.,[102a] who demonstrated that coronary atherosclerosis could regress. These studies were subsequently confirmed by Wissler and Vesselinovitch.[102b] Perhaps the largest number of studies have been performed by Clarkson and his colleagues.[102c] They demonstrated the clear therapeutic benefit of lowering plasma cholesterol concentrations after having induced fibrous plaques in animals on hypercholesterolemic regimens for periods of 12 months and longer. Regression occurred principally in lesions in the abdominal aorta and in the coronary arteries, in contrast to those that formed at the carotid bifurcation, which appeared, on some occasions, to develop lesions relatively independently of plasma lipid concentrations. When regression occurs and plasma-cholesterol levels return to baseline, the lesions of atherosclerosis become smaller, contain less lipid, and demonstrate marked decreases in their content of cholesterol and cholesteryl esters. Remodeling of connective tissue proteins also appears to take place, as shown by decreases in both collagen and elastic fiber proteins in these lesions. Thus it seems that, over a sufficiently long period of time, advanced lesions can in some cases also regress.

Recently, a number of investigators have been probing the capacity of fish oils, which contain large amounts of omega-3 fatty acids, to decrease plasma-cholesterol levels and potentially to induce lesion regression when added to the diet of hypercholesterolemic individuals.[112] Not only do these diets lead to decrease in plasma-cholesterol levels, but they also change the balance of prostaglandins that are formed by the cells. It is well known that platelets have the capacity to use arachidonic acid to form the prostaglandin derivative thromboxane A_2, a proaggregating factor for platelets. On the other hand, endothelial cells and smooth muscle use the same fatty acid to form, via cyclooxygenase, the prostaglandin metabolite prostacyclin (PGI_2), an extraordinarily potent antiaggregant and vasodilator. When the omega-3 fatty acids are fed to animals (and if they are particularly rich in eicosapentaenoic acid), they shift the balance because thromboxane A_3 derived from this fatty acid is inactive as a platelet aggregant, whereas PGI_3 is as active as PGI_2, thus favoring antiaggregant, vasodilator effects over effects that might lead to platelet aggregation and thrombosis.

THROMBOSIS (See also Chapter 56)

As described at the beginning of this chapter, thrombosis was originally considered to be an important component in the initiation and progression of the lesions of atherosclerosis. It now appears that thrombosis may play several roles. One prominent and potentially important clinical role is that of thrombi which become incorporated into existing advanced lesions of atherosclerosis, rapidly resulting in lumen narrowing and increase in lesion dimensions. Perhaps one of the most persistent and common complications of atherosclerosis is the formation of cracks and fissures in the advanced lesions of atherosclerosis that can act as sites for platelet attachment and formation of mural and potentially occlusive thrombi, which could lead to unstable angina or myocardial infarction.

As discussed earlier, there is good evidence in nonhuman primates and in rabbits that mural thrombi can contribute to the initiation and development of lesions of atherosclerosis.[79–83] This has also been demonstrated in humans at the perianastomotic site of coronary bypass surgery, where new lesions of atherosclerosis form in approximately 30 per cent of all bypass grafts.[113] In monkeys or rabbits on a hyperlipemic diet, intraarterial balloon catheter deendothelialization can lead to intimal smooth muscle proliferative lesions that appear very much like those found in hypercholesterolemic patients.

Thrombi have been observed in the coronary arteries of the vast majority of individuals who die from transmural myocardial infarction. However, thrombi are much less common in individuals who die from subendocardial infarction. Thrombosis is even less common in individuals who die of sudden cardiac death, although both thrombosis and embolism are well recognized as complications of cerebrovascular disease as well as peripheral vascular disease.

The role of the endothelium in the process of thrombosis is not entirely clear since, as discussed earlier, endothelial cells have both nonthrombogenic and procoagulant activities. Endothelial cells produce von Willebrand factor as well as plasminogen activator and prostacyclin. The development of agents that can alter thromboxane formation and thus prevent platelet interaction, or alter prostacyclin formation and thus promote platelet interactions, should make it possible to obtain a clearer idea of the role of these agents as compared with others that can be produced by the endothelial cells in the process of thrombosis in general.

CONCLUSIONS

It is clear that knowledge in the field of atherosclerosis has exploded and is changing rapidly. The opportunity to use the tools of cell and molecular biology, as well as new noninvasive methods for examining individuals at the clinical level, has broadened our understanding of the roles of the cells in atherogenesis. Cell and molecular biology have rapidly increased our understanding of the principal cells involved in atherosclerosis: endothelium, smooth muscle, platelets, and monocyte/macrophages. How the risk factors that are commonly associated with an increased incidence of atherosclerosis are related to these cellular interactions is beginning to be understood, particularly in relation to hypercholesterolemia. Unfortunately, there are no good animal models that permit us to study the questions related to cigarette smoking, hypertension, diabetes, or some of the other risk factors that are epidemiologically associated with atherosclerosis. Without these, it is difficult to know the nature of the cellular interactions that occur during the genesis of the disease process as it is associated with each of these important risk factors.

Perhaps the most critical aspect of this problem is the need to understand the basis of the genetic susceptibility of individuals to these risk factors and thus to circumstances that can lead to these increased cellular interactions. Once the genetic loci for the various apoproteins are identified, and once it is possible to demonstrate altered genetic loci for these and other factors important in atherogenesis in individuals who are at increased risk for heart attack and/or stroke, it should be possible to begin to probe this question using these new tools.

Acknowledgments

This work was supported in part by grants from U.S. Public Health Service Grant HL-18645, a grant from RJR Nabisco, Inc., and NIH grant RR-00166 to the Northwest Regional Primate Center. The author is particularly indebted to Elaine Raines, Agostino Faggiotto, Michael Rosenfeld, Toyohiro Tsukada, Allen Gown, and to Daniel Bowen-Pope, with whom work reported from his laboratory was performed.

REFERENCES

RISK FACTORS

1. Report of the Working Group on Arteriosclerosis of the National Heart, Lung, and Blood Institute, Vol. 2. DHEW Publication No. (NIH) 82–2035, Washington D.C., U.S. Government Printing Office, 1981.
2. Ross, R., and Glomset, J.: Atherosclerosis and the arterial smooth muscle cell. Science *180*:1332, 1973.
3. Ross, R., and Glomset, J. A.: The pathogenesis of atherosclerosis. N. Engl. J. Med. *295*:369, 1976.
4. Ross, R., and Harker, L.: Hyperlipidemia and atherosclerosis. Science *193*:1094, 1976.
5. Wissler, R. W., Vesselinovitch, D., and Getz, G. J.: Abnormalities of the arterial wall and its metabolism in atherogenesis. Prog. Cardiovasc. Dis. *18*:341, 1976.
6. Dawber, T. R., Moore, F. E., and Mann, G. V.: Measuring the risk of coronary heart disease in adult population groups. II. Coronary heart disease in the Framingham study. Am. J. Public Health *47*:4, 1957.
7. Chapman, J. M., Goerke, L. S., Dixon, W., Loveland, D. B., and Phillips, E.: Measuring the risk of coronary heart disease in adult population groups. IV. The clinical status of a population group in Los Angeles under observation for two or three years. Am. J. Public Health *47*:33, 1957.
8. Doyle, J. T., Heslin, A. S., Hillboe, H. E., Formel, P. F., and Korns, R. F.: Measuring the risk of coronary heart disease in adult population groups. III. A prospective study of degenerative cardiovascular disease in Albany: Report of three years' experience. I. Ischemic heart disease. Am. J. Public Health *47*:25, 1957.
9. Drake, R. M., Buechley, R. W., and Breslow, L.: Measuring the risk of coronary heart disease in adult population groups. V. An epidemiological investigation of coronary heart disease in the California health survey population. Am. J. Public Health *47*:43, 1957.
10. Report of Inter-Society Commission for Heart Disease Resources. Primary prevention of the atherosclerotic disease. Circulation *42*:55, 1970.
11. Stamler, J., Berkson, D. M., and Lindberg, H. A.: Risk factors: Their role in the etiology and pathogenesis of the atherosclerotic diseases. *In* Wissler, R. W., Geer, J. C., and Kaufman, N. (eds.): The Pathogenesis of Atherosclerosis. Baltimore, Williams and Wilkins, 1962, p. 41.
12. Kuller, L. H.: Epidemiology of cardiovascular disease: Current perspectives. Am. J. Epidemiol. *104*:425, 1976.
13. Ross, R.: The pathogenesis of atherosclerosis—an update. N. Engl. J. Med. *314*:488, 1986.
14. Benditt, E. P., and Benditt, J. M.: Evidence for a monoclonal origin of human atherosclerotic plaques. Proc. Natl. Acad. Sci. USA *70*:1753, 1973.
15. Inkeles, S., and Eisenberg, D.: Hyperlipidemia and coronary atherosclerosis: a review. Medicine (Baltimore) *70*:110, 1981.
16. Lipid Research Clinics Program. The Lipid Research Clinics Coronary Primary Prevention Trial Results. I. Reduction in incidence of coronary heart disease. J.A.M.A. *251*:351, 1984.
17. Lipid Research Clinics Program. The Lipid Research Clinics Coronary Primary Prevention Trial Results. II. The relationship of reduction in incidence of coronary heart disease to cholesterol lowering. J.A.M.A. *251*:365, 1984.
18. Smoking and Health. Chapt. 3. Criteria for Judgment. DHEW Publication No. (NIH) 1103, Washington, D.C., U.S. Government Printing Office, 1964.
19. The Pooling Project Research Group: Relationship of blood pressure, serum cholesterol, smoking habit, relative weight, and ECG abnormalities to incidence of major coronary events: final report of the pooling project. J. Chronic Dis. *31*:201, 1978.
20. Oberman, A., Harlan, W. R., Smith, M., and Graybiel, A.: The cardiovascular risk associated with different levels and types of elevated blood pressure. Minn. Med. 52:1283, 1969.

THE NORMAL ARTERY

21. Report of the Hypertension Task Force, Vol. 1. DHEW Publication No. (NIH) 79–1623, Washington, D.C., U.S. Government Printing Office, 1964.
22. Glagov, S.: Hemodynamic risk factors: mechanical stress, mural architecture, medial nutrition and the vulnerability of arteries to atherosclerosis. *In* Wissler, R. W., and Geer, J. C. (eds.): The Pathogenesis of Atherosclerosis. Baltimore, Williams and Wilkins, 1972, p. 164.
23. Wolinsky, H., and Glagov, S.: Comparison of abdominal and thoracic aortic medial structure in mammals. Deviation of man from the usual pattern. Circ. Res. 25:677, 1969.

CELLS OF THE ARTERY AND FROM THE BLOOD POTENTIALLY INVOLVED IN ATHEROGENESIS

24. Schwartz, S. M., and Benditt, E. P.: Clustering of replicating cells in aortic endothelium. Proc. Natl. Acad. Sci. USA *73*:651, 1976.
25. Schwartz, S. M., and Benditt, E. P.: Aortic endothelial cell replication. Effects of age and hypertension in the rat. Circ. Res. *41*:248, 1977.
26. Simionescu, N., Simionescu, M., and Palade, G. E.: Permeability of muscle capillaries to small heme-peptides. Evidence for the existence of patent transendothelial channels. J. Cell Biol. *64*:586, 1975.
27. Huttner, I., Boutet, M., and More, R. H.: Studies on protein passage through arterial endothelium. I. Structural correlates of permeability in rat arterial endothelium. Lab. Invest. *28*:672, 1973.
28. Renkin, E. M.: Multiple pathways of capillary permeability. Circ. Res. *41*:735, 1977.
29. Moncada, S., Herman, A. G., Higgs, E. A., and Vane, J. R.: Differential formation of prostacyclin (PGX or PGI_2) by layers of the arterial wall. An explanation for the antithrombotic properties of vascular endothelium. Thromb. Res. *11*:323, 1977.
30. Fielding, C. J.: Metabolism of cholesterol-rich chylomicrons. Mechanism of binding and uptake of cholesteryl esters by the vascular bed of the perfused rat heart. J. Clin. Invest. *62*:141, 1978.
31. Furchgott, R. F.: Role of endothelium in responses of vascular smooth muscle. Circ. Res. *53*:557, 1983.
32. Gimbrone, M. A. Jr., and Alexander, R. W.: Angiotensin II stimulation of prostaglandin production in cultured human vascular endothelium. Science *189*:219, 1975.
33. Jaffe, E. A., Minick, C. R., Adelman, B., Becker, C. G., and Nachman, R.: Synthesis of basement membrane by cultured human endothelial cells. J. Exp. Med. *144*:209, 1976.
34. Jaffe, E. A., Hoyer, L. W., and Nachman, R. L.: Synthesis of antihemophilic factor antigen by cultured human endothelial cells. J. Clin. Invest. *52*:2757, 1973.
35. Steinberg, D.: Lipoproteins and atherosclerosis. A look back and a look ahead. Arteriosclerosis *3*:283, 1983.
36. Gajdusek, C. M., DiCorleto, P. E., Ross, R., and Schwartz, S. M.: An endothelial cell-derived growth factor. J. Cell Biol. *85*:467, 1980.
37. DiCorleto, P. E.,Gajdusek, C. M., Schwartz, S. M., and Ross, R.: Biochemical properties of the endothelium-derived growth factor: Comparison to other growth factors. J. Cell. Physiol. *114*:339, 1983.
38. DiCorleto, P. E., and Bowen-Pope, D. F.: Cultured endothelial cells produce a platelet-derived growth factor-like protein. Proc. Natl. Acad. Sci. USA *80*:1919, 1983.
39. Wissler, R. W.: The arterial medial cell, smooth muscle, or multifunctional mesenchyme? J. Atheroscl. Res. *8*:201, 1968.
40. Ross, R.: The smooth muscle cell. II. Growth of smooth muscle in culture and formation of elastic fibers. J. Cell Biol. *50*:172, 1971.
41. Burke, J. M., and Ross, R.: Synthesis of connective tissue macromolecules by smooth muscle. Int. Rev. Connect. Tissue Res. *8*:119, 1979.
42. Chait, A., Ross, R., Albers, J. J., and Bierman, E. L.: Platelet-derived growth factor stimulates activity of low density lipoprotein receptors. Proc. Natl. Acad. Sci. USA *77*:4084, 1980.
43. Bowen-Pope, D. F., Seifert, R. A., and Ross, R.: The platelet-derived growth factor receptor. *In* Boynton, A. L., and Leffert, H. L. (eds.): Control of Animal Cell Proliferation: Recent Advances. Vol. 1. New York, Academic Press, 1985, p. 281.
44. Seifert, R. A., Schwartz, S. M., and Bowen-Pope, D. F.: Developmentally regulated production of platelet-derived growth factor–like molecules. Nature *311*:669, 1984.
45. Chamley-Campbell, J., Campbell, G., and Ross, R.: Phenotype-dependent response of cultured aortic smooth muscle to serum mitogens. J. Cell Biol. *89*:379, 1981.
46. Thyberg, J., Palmberg, L., Nilsson, J., Ksiazek, T., and Sjolund, M.: Phenotype modulations in primary cultures of arterial smooth muscle cells. On the role of platelet-derived growth factor. Differentiation *25*:156, 1983.
47. Ross, R., Wight, T. N., Strandness, E., and Thiele, B.: Human atherosclerosis: I. Cell constitution and characteristics of advanced lesions of the superficial femoral artery. Am. J. Pathol. *114*:79, 1984.
48. Van Furth, R.: Current view on the mononuclear phagocyte system. Immunobiology *161*:178, 1982.
49. Nathan, C. F., Murray, H. W., and Cohn, Z. A.: Current concepts: The macrophage as an effector cell. N. Engl. J. Med. *303*:622, 1980.
50. Martin, T. R., Altman, L. C., Albert, R. K., and Henderson, W. R.: Leukotriene B4 production by human alveolar macrophage: A potential mechanism for amplifying inflammation in the lung. Am. Rev. Respir. Dis. *129*:106, 1984.
51. Bevilacqua, M. P., Pober, J. S., Cotran, R. S., and Gimbrone, M. A. Jr.: Interleukin 1 (IL1) acts upon vascular endothelium to stimulate procoagulant activity and leukocyte adhesion. J. Cell. Biochem. Suppl. *9A*:148, 1985.
52. Cathcart, M. K., Morel, D. W., and Chisolm, G. III.: Monocytes and neutrophils oxidize low-density lipoprotein making it cytotoxic. J. Leuk. Biol. *38*:341, 1985.
53. Ross, R., Raines, E. W., and Bowen-Pope, D. F.: The biology of platelet-derived growth factor. Cell *46*:155, 1986.
54. Shimokado, K., Raines, E. W., Madtes, D. K., Barrett, T. B., Benditt, E. P., and Ross, R.: A significant part of macrophage-derived growth factor consists of at least two forms of PDGF. Cell *43*:277, 1985.
55. Baird, A., Mormede, P., and Bohlen, P.: Immunoreactive fibroblast growth factor in cells of peritoneal exudate suggests its identity with macrophage-derived growth factor. Biochem. Biophys. Res. Commun. *126*:358, 1985.
56. Holmsen, H., and Weiss, H. J.: Secretable storage pools in platelets. Annu. Rev. Med. *30*:119, 1979.
57. Pepper, D. S.: Macromolecules released from platelet storage organelles. Thrombos. Haemost. (Stuttg.) *42*:1667, 1980.
58. Ross, R., Glomset, J., Kariya, B., and Harker, L.: A platelet-dependent serum factor that stimulates the proliferation of arterial smooth muscle cells in vitro. Proc. Natl. Acad. Sci. USA *71*:1207, 1974.
59. Oka, Y., and Orth, D. N.: Human plasma epidermal growth factor/beta-urogastrone is associated with blood platelets. J. Clin. Invest. *72*:249, 1983.
60. Assoian, R. K., Komoriya, A., Meyers, C. A., Miller, D. M., and Sporn, M. B.: Transforming growth factor-β in human platelets. Identification of a major storage site, purification, and characterization. J. Biol. Chem. 258:7155, 1983.
61. Baumgartner, H. R.: Platelet-interaction with vascular structures. Thromb. Diath. Haemorrh. *51*(Suppl.):161, 1972.

THE LESIONS OF ATHEROSCLEROSIS

62. McGill, H. C. Jr. (ed.): The Geographic Pathology of Atherosclerosis. Baltimore, Williams and Wilkins, 1968.
63. Geer, J. C., McGill, H. C. Jr., and Strong, J. P.: The fine structure of human atherosclerotic lesions. Am. J. Pathol. 38:263, 1961.
64. Geer, J.C.: Fine structure of human aortic intimal thickening and fatty streaks. Lab. Invest. *14*:1764, 1965.
65. Ghidoni, J. J., and O'Neal, R. M.: Recent advances in molecular pathology. A review: Ultrastructure of human atheroma. Exp. Mol. Pathol. 7:378, 1967.
66. Stary, H. C.: Evolution of atherosclerotic plaques in the coronary arteries of young adults. Arteriosclerosis 3:471a, 1983.
67. McGill, H. C. Jr.: Persistent problems in the pathogenesis of atherosclerosis. Arteriosclerosis *4*:443, 1984.
68. Tsukada, T., Rosenfeld, M., Ross, R., and Gown, A. M.: Immunocytochemical analysis of cellular components in lesions of atherosclerosis in the Watanabe and fat-fed rabbit using monoclonal antibodies. Arteriosclerosis (*in press*).
69. Glagov, S., and Oxoa, A.: Significance of the relatively low incidence of atherosclerosis in the pulmonary, renal and mesenteric arteries. Ann. N.Y. Acad. Sci. *149*:940, 1968.
70. Strong, J. P., Eggen, D. A., and Oalmann, M. C.: The natural history, geographic pathology, and epidemiology of atherosclerosis. *In* Wissler, R. W, and Geer, J. C. (eds.): The Pathogenesis of Atherosclerosis. Baltimore, Williams and Wilkins, 1972, p. 20.
71. Glagov, S., Rowley, D. A., Cramer, D. B., and Page, R. G.: Heart rate during 24 hours of usual activity 100 normal men. J. Appl. Physiol. *29*:799, 1970.
72. Wissler, R. W., and Vesselinovitch, D.: Atherosclerosis—relationship to coronary blood flow. Am. J. Cardiol. *52*(2):2A, 1983.

THE HYPOTHESES OF ATHEROGENESIS

73. Virchow, R.: Phlogose und thrombose im gefassystem, gesammelte abhandlungen zur wissenschaftlichen medicin. Frankfurt-am-Main, Meidinger Sohn and Co., 1856, p. 458.
74. Rokitansky, C. von: A Manual of Pathological Anatomy, translated by Day, G. E. Vol. 4. London, The Sydenham Society, 1852.
75. Duguid, J. B.: Thrombosis as a factor in the pathogenesis of coronary atherosclerosis. J. Pathol. Bacteriol. *58*:207, 1946.
76. Ross, R.: Atherosclerosis—a problem of the biology of arterial wall cells and their interaction with blood components. Arteriosclerosis *1*:293, 1981.
77. Leary, T.: The genesis of atherosclerosis. Arch. Pathol. *32*:507, 1941.
78. Assoian, R. K., Grotendorst, G. R., Miller, D. M., and Sporn, M. B.: Cellular transformation by coordinated action of three peptide growth factors from human platelets. Nature *309*:804, 1984.
79. Stemerman, M. B., and Ross, R.: Experimental arteriosclerosis. I. Fibrous plaque formation in primates, an electron microscope study. J. Exp. Med. *136*:769, 1972.
80. Sheppard, B. L., and French, J. E.: Platelet adhesion in the rabbit abdominal aorta following the removal of the endothelium: A scanning and transmission electron microscopical study. Proc. R. Soc. Lond. (Biol.) *176*:427, 1971.
81. More, S.: Thromboatherosclerosis in normolipemic rabbits: A result of continued endothelial damage. Lab. Invest. *29*:478, 1973.
82. Friedman, R. J., Moore, S., and Singal, D. P.: Repeated endothelial injury and induction of atherosclerosis in normolipemic rabbits by human serum. Lab. Invest. *32*:404, 1975.
83. Harker, L. A., Ross, R., Slichter, S. J., and Scott, C. R.: Homocystine-induced arteriosclerosis: The role of endothelial cell injury and platelet response in genesis. J. Clin. Invest. *58*:731, 1976.
84. Lindner, D., and Gartler, S. M.: Glucose-6-phosphate dehydrogenase mosaicism: Utilization as a cell marker in the study of leiomyomas. Science *150*:67, 1965.
85. Hajjar, D. P., Fabricant, C. G., Minick, C. R., and Fabricant, J.: Virus-induced artherosclerosis: Herpesvirus infection alters aortic cholesterol metabolism and accumulation. Am. J. Pathol. *122*:62, 1986.
86. Fialkow, P. J.: Use of genetic markers to study cellular origin and development of tumor in human females. Adv. Cancer Res. *15*:191, 1972.

LIPIDS AND LIPOPROTEINS IN ATHEROSCLEROSIS

87. Jackson, R. L., and Gotto, A. M. Jr.: Hypothesis concerning membrane structure, cholesterol, and atherosclerosis. *In* Paoletti, R., and Gotto, A. M., Jr. (eds.): Atherosclerosis Reviews. Vol. 1. New York, Raven Press, 1976, p. 1.

GROWTH FACTORS

88. Heldin, C.-H., Westermark, B., and Wasteson, A.: Platelet-derived growth factor: Purification and partial characterization. Proc. Natl. Acad. Sci. USA 76:3722, 1979.
89. Antoniades, H. N.: Human platelet-derived growth factor (PDGF): Purification of PDGF-I and PDGF-II and separation of their reduced subunits. Proc. Natl. Acad. Sci. USA 78:7314, 1981.
90. Raines, E. W., and Ross, R.: Platelet-derived growth factor. I. High yield purification and evidence for multiple forms. J. Biol. Chem. *257*:5154, 1982.
91. Huang, J. S., Huang, S. S., Kennedy, B., and Deuel, T. F.: Platelet-derived growth factor: Specific binding to target cells. J. Biol. Chem. *257*:8130, 1982.
92. Heldin, C.-H., Westermark, B., and Wasteson, A.: Specific receptors for platelet-derived growth factors on cells derived from connective tissue and glia. Proc. Natl. Acad. Sci. USA *78*:3664, 1981.
93. Bowen-Pope, D. F., and Ross, R.: Platelet-derived growth factor. II. Specific binding to cultured cells. J. Biol. Chem. *257*:5161, 1982.
94. Grotendorst, G., Seppa, H. E. J., Kleinman, H. K., and Martin, G.: Attachment of smooth muscle cells to collagen and their migration toward platelet-derived growth factor. Proc. Natl. Acad. Sci. USA *78*:3669, 1981.
95. Grotendorst, G. R., Chang, T., Seppa, H. E. J., Kleinman, H. K., and Martin, G. R.: Platelet-derived growth factor is a chemoattractant for vascular smooth muscle cells. J. Cell. Physiol. *113*:261, 1982.
96. Witte, L. D., and Cornicelli, J. A.: Platelet-derived growth factor stimulates low density lipoprotein receptor activity in cultured human fibroblasts. Proc. Natl. Acad. Sci. USA *77*:5962, 1980.
97. Bowen-Pope, D. F., Malpass, T. W., Foster, D. M., and Ross, R.: Platelet-derived growth factor in vivo: Levels, activity, and rate of clearance. Blood *46*:458, 1984.
98. Raines, E. W., Bowen-Pope, D. F., and Ross, R.: Plasma binding proteins for platelet-derived growth factor that inhibit its binding to cell-surface receptors. Proc. Natl. Acad. Sci. USA *81*:3424, 1984.
99. Doolittle, R. F., Hunkapiller, M. W., Hood, L. E., Devare, S. G., Robbins, K. C., Aaronson, S. A., and Antoniades, H. N.: Simian sarcoma virus onc gene, v-sis, is derived from the gene (or genes) encoding a platelet-derived growth factor. Science *221*:275, 1983.
100. Waterfield, M. D., Scrace, G. T., Whittle, N., Stroobant, P., Johnsson, A., Wasteson, A., Westermark, B., Heldin, C.-H., Huang, J. S., and Deuel, T. F.: Platelet-derived growth factor is structurally related to the putative transforming protein p^{28sis} of simian sarcoma virus. Nature *304*:35, 1983.
101. Bowen-Pope, D. F., Vogel, A., and Ross, R.: Production of platelet-derived growth factor-like molecules and reduced expression of platelet-derived growth factor receptors accompany transformation by a wide spectrum of agents. Proc. Natl. Acad. Sci. USA *81*:2396, 1984.

CELLULAR EVENTS THAT OCCUR DURING ATHEROSCLEROSIS

102. Faggiotto, A., Ross, R., and Harker, L.: Studies of hypercholesterolemia in the nonhuman primate. I. Changes that lead to fatty streak formation. Arteriosclerosis *4*:323, 1984.
102a. Armstrong, M. L., Warner, E. D., and Conner, W. E.: Regression of coronary atheromatosis in rhesus monkeys. Circ. Res. *27*:59, 1970.
102b. Wissler, R. W., and Vesselinovitch, D.: Studies of regression of advanced atherosclerosis in experimental animals and man. Ann. N.Y. Acad. Sci. *275*:363, 1976.
102c. Clarkson, T. B., Bond, M. G., Bullock, B. C., McLaughlin, K. J., and Sawyer, J. K.: A study of atherosclerosis regression in Macaca mulatta. V. Changes in abdominal aorta and carotid and coronary arteries from animals with atherosclerosis induced for 38 months and then regressed for 24 or 48 months at plasma cholesterol concentrations of 300 or 200 mg/dl. Exp. Mol. Pathol. *41*:96, 1984.
103. Faggiotto, A., and Ross, R.: Studies of hypercholesterolemia in the nonhuman primate. II. Fatty streak conversion to fibrous plaque. Arteriosclerosis *4*:341, 1984.
104. Gerrity, R. G., Naito, H. K., Richardson, M., and Schwartz, C. J.: Dietary induced atherogenesis in swine: Morphology of the intima in prelesion stages. Am. J. Pathol. *95*:775, 1979.
105. Gerrity, R. G.: The role of the monocyte in atherogenesis. I. Transition of blood-borne monocytes into foam cells in fatty lesions. Am. J. Pathol. *103*:181, 1981.
106. Gerrity, R. G., Goss, J. A., and Soby, L.: Control of monocyte recruitment by chemotactic factor(s) in lesion-prone areas of swine aorta. Arteriosclerosis *5*:55, 1985.
107. Rosenfeld, M. E., Faggiotto, A., and Ross, R.: The role of the mononuclear phagocyte in primate and rabbit models of atherosclerosis. *In* Van Furth, R. (ed.): Mononuclear Phagocytes: Characteristics, Physiology, and Function. The Hague, Netherlands, Martinus Nijhoff, 1985, p. 795.
108. Reidy, M. A., and Schwartz, S. M.: Endothelial regeneration. III. Time course of intimal changes after small defined injury to rat aortic endothelium. Lab. Invest. *44*:301, 1981.
109. Reidy, M.A., and Schwartz, S. M.: Endothelial injury and regeneration. IV. Endotoxin: a nondenuding injury to aortic endothelium. Lab. Invest. *48*:25, 1983.
110. Hansson, G. K., Bondjers, G., Bylock, A., and Hjalmarsson, L.: Ultrastructural studies on nonatherosclerotic rabbits. Exp. Mol. Pathol. *33*:301, 1980.

REGRESSION OF ATHEROSCLEROSIS

111. Reidy, M. A., and Schwartz, S. M.: Recent advances in molecular pathology: arterial endothelium—assessment of in vivo injury. Exp. Mol. Pathol. *41*:419, 1984.
112. Cannon, P. J.: Eicosanoids and the blood vessel wall. Circulation 70:00, 1984.
113. Chesebro, J. H., Clements, L. P., Fuster, V., Elveback, L.R., Smith, H. C., Bardsley, W. T., Frye, R. L., Holmes, D. H. Jr., Vliestra, R. E., Pluth, J. R., Wallace, R. B., Puga, F. J., Orszulak, T. A., Piehler, J. M., Schaff, H. V., and Danielson, G. K.: A platelet-inhibitor-drug trial in coronary-artery bypass operations. Benefit of perioperative dipyridamole and aspirin therapy on early postoperative vein-graft patency. N. Engl. J. Med. *307*:73, 1982.

36 RISK FACTORS FOR CORONARY ARTERY DISEASE

by ANTONIO M. GOTTO, Jr., M.D., D.Phil., and
JOHN A. FARMER, M.D.

EPIDEMIOLOGY AND THE DECLINING DEATH RATE

Coronary artery disease (CAD) remains the major cause of death in the United States despite the decline noted over the past several years. Every year 5.4 million individuals are diagnosed as having CAD, and over 550,000 deaths per year are attributable to coronary atherosclerosis. A significant proportion of deaths occur in relatively young patients. The National Center for Health Statistics estimates that there are over 5,000,000 myocardial infarction survivors, half of whom are physically limited by their disease. CAD is associated with $8 billion annually in direct health costs and $60 billion in economic costs.

In the United States a dramatic decline in the death rate from CAD has occurred over the past 25 years. Many hypotheses have been put forward, none of which can fully explain the decline. Kuller[1] has suggested that the declining death rate from coronary disease in this country can be accounted for primarily by changes in attitudes toward the habit of tobacco smoking, particularly on the part of middle-aged men. In the authors' opinion, treatment programs designed to alter and prevent the modifiable risk factors have probably contributed to the decline in death rates from CAD.

The Haynes Survey[2] has confirmed a decrease in serum cholesterol levels, and there has certainly been an improvement in detection and treatment of hypertension. Also, cigarette smoking in middle-aged men has declined, and there has been an enormous increase in participation in leisure-time physical activity. Dietary habits have changed substantially; there has been a decrease in consumption of saturated fat, of certain red meats (particularly beef), of eggs, butter, and cream, and an increase in consumption of polyunsaturated or vegetable fats and low-fat milk.

Hypertension control has shown a steady improvement over the past two decades (Chap. 28). The proportion of persons of both sexes and all racial groups whose hypertension has been treated and controlled has risen. This possibly has contributed to the decline in coronary mortality, especially among blacks and women. However, none of the commonly involved epidemiological correlates of CAD totally explains the decline in mortality in the United States; other unknown mechanisms apparently exist.[2]

Other factors such as prehospital care, the availability of coronary care units, improved medical therapy, and newer surgical techniques have also emerged to play a role in the management of CAD and the secondary prevention of mortality. Although their contributions to the decline in cardiovascular mortality are unknown, it should be noted that the downward trend in mortality preceded the widespread introduction of coronary care units and the advent of bypass surgery.

The decline in incidence of CAD is seen in both sexes, although the incidence remains lower in women, especially in the younger age groups. It has declined more in blacks than in whites since 1968. Currently, mortality from coronary heart disease is similar in black and white males but higher in black than in white females. Hispanics also have demonstrated a decline in mortality and may have a lower incidence of CAD than do whites.

DEFINITION OF RISK FACTORS

Large-scale epidemiological studies have demonstrated that CAD and its complications are associated with a variety of risk factors. Some of these studies have identified significant risk factors for CAD within a given population while others have compared relative risk between different populations. The Framingham Study in the United States was one of the first to describe the primary and secondary risk factors for CAD.[4]

Coronary risk factors refer to conditions which have been demonstrated by statistical procedures to increase the susceptibility of an individual to the morbidity and mortality of coronary atherosclerosis. Some factors may be statistically significant in a univariate analysis but not in a multivariate analysis—that is, when multiple risk factors are considered. Potential benefit may be derived by identifying a risk factor which may be altered through intervention, thus possibly preventing the formation of an atherosclerotic plaque, retarding its growth, or reducing its size. Direct evidence in humans for reversal of atherosclerosis by risk factor intervention is in its early stages. Several recent secondary intervention studies have shown that lowering levels of cholesterol and low density lipoprotein (LDL) cholesterol will slow the progression of either femoral or coronary artery plaques. The primary alterable risk factors for CAD are hypercholesterolemia, hypertension, and tobacco smoking. Diabetes mellitus and low levels of high density lipoprotein (HDL) cholesterol are also well established as risk factors for CAD. Other alterable risk factors whose relative importance is still being established include serum triglyceride concentration, personality type, level of physical activity, and obesity.

Multiple Risk Factors

The Honolulu Heart Program[5] related 14 biological and life style characteristics in Japanese men living in Hawaii, Japanese men living in Japan, and U.S. white men. The study showed very inconsistent relationships with the different factors used to measure coronary disease. The incidence of nonfatal and fatal myocardial infarction of Japanese men living in Hawaii was about half that of U.S. white men and approximately twice that of Japanese men living in Japan. For example, systolic blood pressure was the most powerful and consistent risk factor for all manifestations of CAD except angina pectoris. A similar association was shown for cigarette smoking. Although serum cholesterol had a significant association with fatal coronary disease and nonfatal myocardial infarction, its contribution was less than that of either systolic blood pressure or cigarette smoking. Glucose intolerance was strongly associated with fatal coronary disease, but not with other manifestations. Alcohol consumption had a strong deterrent effect on fatal coronary disease and nonfatal myocardial infarction. Umcomplicated angina pectoris, in contrast to the other manifestations of CAD, had no association with blood pressure, serum cholesterol, or cigarette smoking. As of this writing, it is not possible to determine whether the consumption of carbohydrates and alcohol in a normal, nonrestricted population, which was observed in the Honolulu Heart Program, protected against CAD or whether the association reflected a decrease in the percentage of dietary calories from fat.[6]

One of the problems in such correlations is in measuring the different endpoints in CAD. For example, correlations with angina pectoris may be different from those with nonfatal myocardial infarction, with acute coronary insufficiency, and with death from coronary disease. Therefore, a number of problems arise in classification. The weakest associations are usually with angina pectoris because this is the softest endpoint and the most difficult to define. Furthermore, there may well be differences in etiology of coronary heart disease death in different individuals. Thrombosis may play an important role in myocardial infarction and may be more important in some individuals than in others. Some individuals may have an increased susceptibility of the myocardium to fail or of the specialized conduction system to become unstable, leading to fatal arrhythmias.

HYPERCHOLESTEROLEMIA

Hypercholesterolemia has been one of the most extensively studied risk factors for the development of CAD. Studies from the 19th century demonstrated that arteriosclerotic plaques were laden with cholesterol. In the early part of this century Anitschkow and his colleagues in the U.S.S.R. produced atherosclerosis in rabbits by cholesterol feeding and, in fact, Anitschkow[7] stated that cholesterol was an essential ingredient for atherosclerosis.

In comparisons between countries, such as the Seven Countries Study, the 5 and 10 year rates of CAD were much lower in Japan and the Mediterranean countries as compared with the United States, Finland, and the Netherlands. The percentage of calories consumed from saturated fats, and consequently the concentrations of serum cholesterol, were significantly lower in Japan and in the Mediterranean countries.[8] Similarly, in the International Atherosclerosis Project, Holman and McGill[9] described the extent of atherosclerosis in the aorta and coronary arteries in about 3100 individuals. They also established a correlation between the proportion of calories derived from saturated fat, and level of serum cholesterol, and the severity of coronary atherosclerosis.

The World Health Organization is currently gathering data on cardiovascular disease mortality from 27 industrialized countries. Simons[10] reported on partially complete information from 19 of the countries and found that in men, 45 per cent of the interpopulation variation in CAD mortality was related to a variation in serum cholesterol levels; 32 per cent was related to variation in HDL cholesterol, and 55 per cent to variation in the ratio of total serum cholesterol:HDL cholesterol. Figure 36–1 shows CAD mortality rates compared with serum cholesterol levels for men in the 19 nations.

Every major epidemiologic study performed to date has shown a significant correlation between the level of serum cholesterol at the time of entry and the risk of coronary heart disease. Hypercholesterolemia was defined as one of the three primary risk factors in the Framingham Study; the earlier the age at which hypercholesterolemia was detected, the greater the risk of developing coronary disease during the period of observation. The relationship between the level of cholesterol and risk of coronary heart disease appears to be a continuous one, as shown in Figure 36–2. In a recent review of new prospective epidemiological studies, Peto was unable to identify any threshold in the range of cholesterol values classed as "normal" in the U.S. and United Kingdom.[10a] Thus, in these two popula-

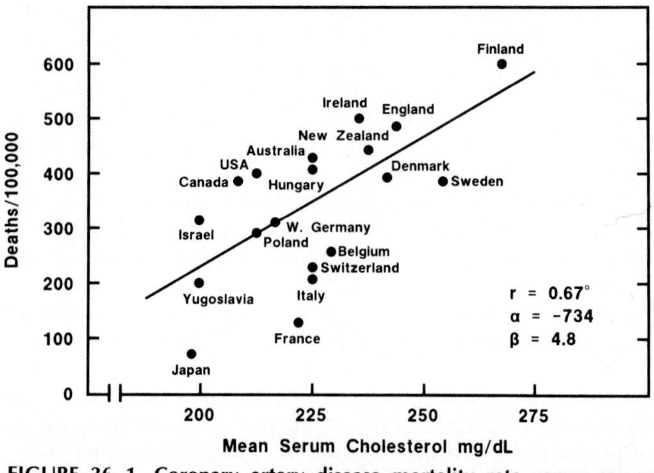

FIGURE 36–1. Coronary artery disease mortality rate versus serum cholesterol. (From Simons, L. A.: Interrelations of lipids and lipoproteins with coronary artery disease mortality in 19 countries. Am. J. Cardiol. 57:5G, 1986.)

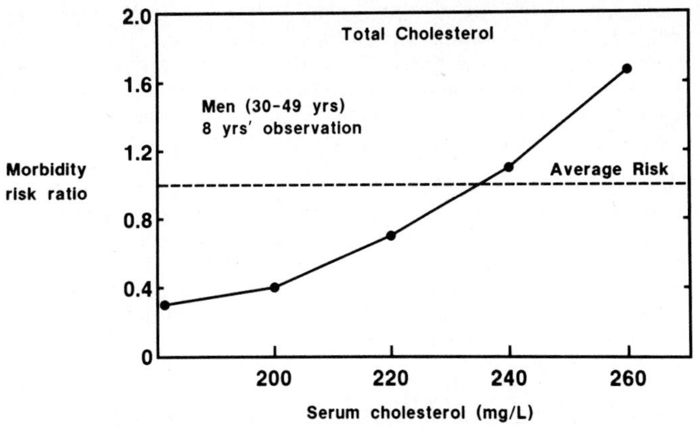

FIGURE 36–2. Various cholesterol fractions as related to coronary artery disease risk. Men in Framingham aged 39 to 49 with cholesterol values over 240 mg/dl were found to have significantly higher risk than those whose total cholesterol levels were below the mean values of approximately 25 mg/dl.

tions, there was no threshold for coronary heart disease avoidance. While it is difficult to define a safe base level of cholesterol, we know that in those societies where the level is under about 150 mg/dl and where levels of LDL cholesterol are quite low, atherosclerosis and coronary heart disease are extremely rare. Over the years an enormous body of data has been generated linking the level of serum cholesterol to the development of occlusive CAD. This evidence comes from metabolic, epidemiological, genetic, and animal studies, and from studies of plaque and experimental evidence in man.

SECONDARY PREVENTION STUDIES.* Establishing a statistical correlation between level of serum cholesterol and risk of CAD does not prove that reducing cholesterol levels will actually decrease this risk. The testing of this theory has been referred to as the cholesterol hypothesis (or lipid or LDL hypothesis) because, as will be discussed later, LDL is the primary atherogenic lipoprotein. A number of studies have provided supportive evidence that reducing cholesterol will reduce risk. One of these, a study at the Wadsworth Veterans Administration Hospital in Los Angeles,[11] used a randomized control involving 846 hospitalized veterans. This trial included patients both with and without clinical evidence of CAD at time of entry. The average age at entry was 65 years. The difference between the two groups was in the proportion of calories fed as saturated fat versus the polyunsaturated type. After an 8-year follow-up, the combined endpoints of nonfatal and fatal atherosclerotic events were decreased by 31 per cent in the group receiving the polyunsaturated fat diet. Mortality was not significantly different. In another secondary study on post-myocardial infarction patients, carried out to study the use of nicotinic acid,[12] a 9 per cent decrease in cholesterol over 5 years was reported. This translated to a significant reduction in incidence of nonfatal myocardial infarctions.

In a Finnish cross-over study of men and women in two mental hospitals performed by Turpeinen et al.[13] diet was used to lower cholesterol. The CAD mortality rate for those on the fat-modified diet was 53 per cent lower in men and 34 per cent lower in women; mortality differences from all causes were small and not statistically significant. Another complicating factor of this study was that, because patient turnover was relatively high, the same group of patients was not followed for the entire period of the study.

*Secondary prevention refers to prevention or postponement of appearance or recurrence of manifestations of CAD.

PRIMARY PREVENTION STUDIES.* Several *primary* prevention studies (on subjects without any clinical history or manifestations of CAD) have also been conducted. In the World Health Organization trial[14] a large group of European men with mild to moderate hypercholesterolemia were randomized and treated with placebo or with clofibrate. In moderately hypercholesterolemic men, clofibrate reduced cholesterol by about 10 per cent and the incidence of nonfatal myocardial infarction by about 20 per cent. However, an increased mortality was observed in the group receiving clofibrate; this led to the recommendation that this drug not be used routinely for community studies. An increased incidence of cholelithiasis had previously been noted with this drug in the Coronary Drug Project.

The Oslo study[15] was a primary prevention trial in which intervention consisted of reducing cholesterol with diet. In this study of 1232 men aged 40 to 49 who had marked hypercholesterolemia but normal blood pressures, 25 per cent in the special intervention group and 17 per cent in the control group reported that they had stopped smoking. There was a 13 per cent greater reduction in the cholesterol level in the special intervention group. The incidence of nonfatal and fatal myocardial infarctions was reduced by 42 per cent in the special intervention group compared with the usual care group. In the special group the death rate from all forms of coronary heart disease was decreased by 56 per cent, although this difference did not reach statistical significance because of the relatively small size of the sample. A significant decrease in coronary heart disease, measured as the sum of nonfatal and fatal myocardial infarctions, was observed in this study, but it was difficult to fractionate the effects of cholesterol and smoking.

Another large primary prevention trial was carried out in the U.S., called the Multiple-Risk Factor Intervention Trial (MRFIT).[16] High-risk men were either referred to their own physician for standard, usual care or were enrolled in an intensive treatment program consisting of dietary treatment for lowering plasma cholesterol, advice against cigarette smoking, and treatment of elevated blood pressure with diet and medication. No significant differences were observed between the two overall groups with respect to coronary disease at the end of the study. As it turned out, the two groups received similar treatment. As an after-the-fact observation, it was noted that for 2087 men in the trial who resembled those in the Oslo study (meaning that their blood pressures were normal and they had hypercholesterolemia and smoked cigarettes), mortality from coronary heart disease was 49 per cent lower in the special intervention group compared with the usual care group. This type of subgroup analysis may not be valid. However, data from over 300,000 subjects screened for the MRFIT study showed a continuous relationship between the concentration of serum cholesterol and coronary heart disease mortality.

THE CORONARY PRIMARY PREVENTION TRIAL. Yet, with all of this preexisting evidence, it remained for the Coronary Primary Prevention Trial (CPPT)[17] to provide the most definitive proof of the cholesterol, low-density lipoprotein (LDL), or lipid hypothesis. The study was carried out in 12 lipid research clinics across North America. For this purpose, over 300,000 men were screened to identify 3806 who met strictly defined criteria. At time of entry, the men were free of clinical manifestations of coronary disease, were between ages 35 and 59, had Type II hyperlipoproteinemia with cholesterol levels over 265 mg/dl, and had an LDL cholesterol over 170 mg/dl. The average cholesterol readings were 291 to 292 mg/dl in the two groups. The men were followed for a period of 7 to 10 years. The "hard endpoints" were nonfatal myocardial

*Primary prevention refers to prevention or postponement of CAD.

infarction and coronary heart disease death. Men with severe hypertriglyceridemia, diabetes, and a number of other preexisting conditions were excluded from the study.

The men were randomized on the basis of cigarette smoking and various other factors and assigned either to a treatment or a placebo group. Each group was placed on a diet which lowered cholesterol by about 4 per cent. The control group received a placebo and the treatment group the bile acid sequestrant cholestyramine. The recommended dosage was up to 24 gm per day; however, only a minority of the participants were able to take this level of the drug. Use of the drug resulted in a lowering of cholesterol of approximately 9 per cent in the treatment versus the control group and a reduction of LDL cholesterol of about 12 per cent.

Results. The reduction in cholesterol of approximately 9 per cent was associated with a decrease in hard endpoints of coronary heart disease by 19 per cent. A graded effect was observed; that is, in those individuals who did not take the medication and had no reduction in cholesterol, there was no reduction in coronary risk. In those individuals who were able to take the full dose of medication, a 19 per cent reduction in cholesterol was observed, and a decrease in coronary disease of 39 per cent occurred (Fig. 36–3). As a rough rule of thumb in this study, a 1 per cent reduction in cholesterol reduced the risk of developing coronary disease by 2 per cent. Actually, the reduction of coronary heart disease observed in the CPPT is very close to that predicted by the Framingham study data. Results of the study were internally consistent in that there was a graded effect between degree of cholesterol and LDL lowering and reduction of coronary heart disease. Furthermore, "secondary endpoints" such as the development of angina pectoris, appearance of positive exercise electrocardiograms, and number of coronary bypass operations performed were also reduced in the treatment groups.

A few instances of oral or pharyngeal cancer were noted in the group receiving cholestyramine, but no particular significance can be attached to this. While the treatment group exhibited a decrease in cardiovascular-related deaths, it also exhibited an increase in noncardiovascular-related deaths. This increase is unexplained, but does not appear to be related to taking the drug or lowering cholesterol; some of the deaths were related to traffic accidents. Because of the relatively small number of participants in the study, it was unlikely that the trial would show a significant decrease in overall mortality, although the CPPT has been criticized on this point as well as others.

Within the limitations defined by the investigators at the beginning of the trial, which are both acceptable and proper in clinical trial practice, the difference in the hard endpoints of myocardial infarction and/or coronary heart disease death was reduced significantly by 19 per cent through lowering cholesterol with a p value of less than 0.05. Possibly, greater differences would have been observed if the cholesterol lowering had been greater. Adherence to the regimen involving the bile acid sequestrant required a great deal of dedication on the part of the physician and the patient. In the authors' opinion, this study fulfilled the requirements for establishing the cholesterol hypothesis.

Relationship to Other Trials. The data from the MRFIT trial have been analyzed with respect to cholesterol levels and CAD mortality as referred to above. A significant and continuous relationship was shown between the level of cholesterol and CAD mortality during the study. Peto et al. have provided a new analysis of all "unconfounded" randomized lipid trials.[10a] They concluded that no significant adverse effect could be shown with cholesterol lowering, and that the curve relating cholesterol lowering to CAD is steeper than previously recognized. In the trials analyzed, an average cholesterol reduction of 10 per cent for 2 years reduced CAD by 16 per cent. However, a prolonged 10 per cent reduction of cholesterol lowered CAD by 33 per cent, a greater degree of reduction than was seen in the CPPT over 7 years. Similarly, for between-population comparisons such as the Seven Countries studies, Peto and colleagues report that a lifetime reduction of cholesterol by 10 per cent is associated with one-third fewer instances of CAD. They point out the pitfalls in interpreting both randomized trials and epidemiological studies; one of the most serious problems is interpretation of the "timescale" question, as will be illustrated below in connection with the Framingham study.

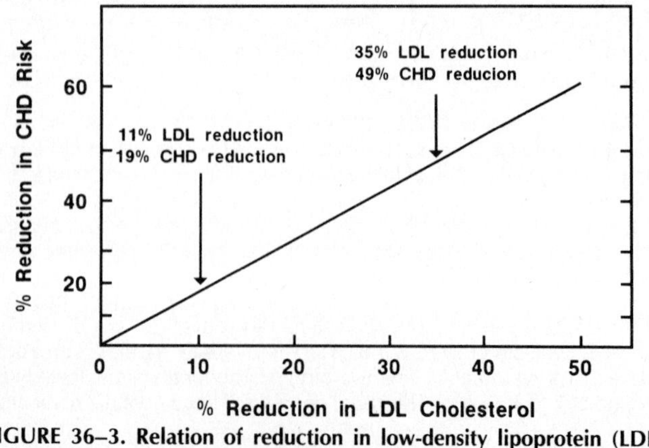

FIGURE 36–3. Relation of reduction in low-density lipoprotein (LDL) cholesterol to reduction in coronary heart disease (CHD) risk (Cox Proportional Hazards Model) in the Coronary Primary Prevention Trial.

The problem of all-cause mortality and serum cholesterol has recently been addressed by Castelli,[18] who emphasized the importance of longitudinal observations rather than cross-sectional measurements. In a follow-up of Framingham subjects, in which all-cause mortality was compared with quartile values of cholesterol, no differences were observed during the first 10 years. Thereafter and up to 30 years there were significant differences, with lower cholesterol groups enjoying a significant reduction in all-cause mortality. As of this writing, there is no convincing evidence that lowering cholesterol or LDL to the extent carried out in the trials or to the extent recommended by the American Heart Association or the National Institutes of Health produces adverse effects including colon cancer.

HYPERTRIGLYCERIDEMIA

Whether hypertriglyceridemia is an independent risk factor for coronary disease has been controversial. Various statistical analyses have not, in many cases, found serum triglyceride values to be an independent predictor of coronary disease. However, analysis of the Framingham data[19] does indicate that the concentration of serum triglycerides is an independent risk factor in females. Carlson and Bottiger carried out a follow-up study of deaths in 321 men and 55 women from myocardial infarction over a 19-year period. Fasting triglyceride concentration was an independent risk factor for cause of death or myocardial infarction in both sexes. Other independent risk factors include age, systolic blood pressure, smoking (for men), cholesterol, hemoglobin, and erythrocyte sedimentation rate.[20]

The Triglyceride Consensus Conference sponsored by the NIH defined a fasting triglyceride value in excess of 500 mg/dl as definitely abnormal and from 250 to 500 mg/dl as the borderline range. The authors believe these values are too high and would consider less than 200 to 250 mg/dl to be a more desirable triglyceride level. In some individuals with hypertriglyceridemia, there is an associated elevation of LDL. A strong statistical association exists between hypertriglyceridemia and low levels of HDL. Herein may lie part of the explanation for the association between triglyceride levels and coronary disease in studies of individuals who were symptomatic and were studied by coronary arteriography.

Hypertriglyceridemia is also a hallmark of Type III hyperlipoproteinemia or dysbetalipoproteinemia, and is also associated with hyperuricemia. Severe hypertriglyceridemia exists in the hyperchylomicronemic syndromes, namely Types I and V hyperlipoproteinemia. In these circumstances, the chylomicronemia and the hypertriglyceridemia are causes of abdominal pain and potentially fatal attacks of pancreatitis. Medical indications for treating hypertriglyceridemia exist; however, perhaps the most important concept about this condition is that it signals the presence of other metabolic disorders.

CAN THE PROGRESSION OF ATHEROSCLEROSIS BE HALTED?

Data from the Bogalusa Heart Study (Fig. 36–4) show a direct stepwise correlation between LDL concentrations and the percentage of total involvement of the aorta by fatty streak in young persons. The aortic fatty streaks were strongly correlated with antemortem levels of LDL and total serum cholesterol and were inversely related to the ratio of HDL cholesterol to LDL cholesterol.[21]

Cabin and Roberts[22] studied the relationship between serum cholesterol and triglyceride levels and the amount and extent of coronary narrowing by atherosclerotic plaques at necropsy. They performed a quantitative analysis of 2037 5-mm segments of 160 major epicardial coronary arteries in 40 patients. They found a positive correlation between the total cholesterol concentration and the number of severely narrowed coronary arteries per subject. The total serum cholesterol did not correlate with the amount of severe narrowing; however, there was a significant correlation between serum triglyceride levels and the percentage of severely narrowed 5-mm segments. This study suggests that in patients with fatal coronary heart disease, triglyceride levels correlate more strongly with the amount of severe coronary narrowing than do total cholesterol levels. In other studies utilizing coronary angiography, triglycerides were found to correlate with coronary obstruction. One cannot draw definitive conclusions from such studies about the relative significance of cholesterol and triglyceride as risk factors for coronary disease.

Data from several studies have shown that lowering cholesterol and LDL reduces the rate of progression of atherosclerosis. The first such controlled trial was a small study performed in the United Kingdom[23] in patients with femoral artery disease. Total cholesterol reductions of 25 per cent and LDL-cholesterol reductions of 28 per cent were achieved by diet combined with several lipid-lowering drugs and resulted in a significant decline in the rate of progression of femoral atherosclerosis, as noted by arteriography.

In the Type II hyperlipidemia trial[24] performed at the National Heart, Lung, and Blood Institute (NHLBI), patients with CAD were treated with cholestyramine. Reducing LDL or improving the ratio of HDL to total cholesterol was associated with a decrease in the rate of progression of coronary blockage in patients who had at least 50 per cent blockage in one or more major coronary arteries (Fig. 36–5). In a nonrandomized study in Leiden in the Netherlands, Arntzenius[25] and his colleagues used diet alone to lower cholesterol. They also observed a decrease in the rate of progression of coronary disease based on the ratio of plasma cholesterol to HDL cholesterol.

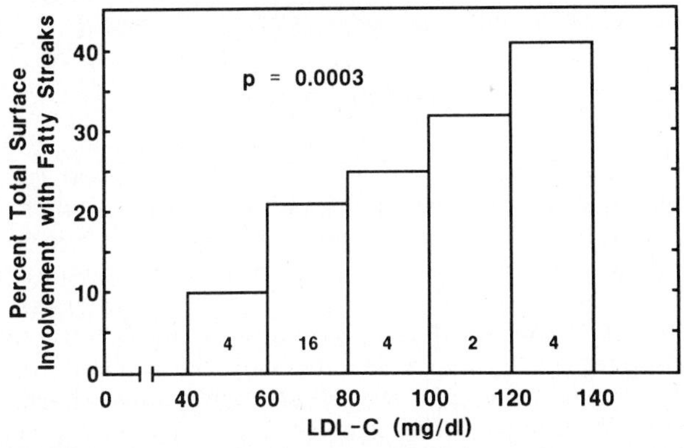

FIGURE 36–4. Atherosclerotic fatty streak involvement of the aorta related to levels of low-density lipoprotein cholesterol (LDL-C) in 30 young persons. Increasing LDL-C levels are significantly related to increasing amounts of aortic fatty streaks. (To convert values for cholesterol to millimoles per liter, multiply by 0.026.) (Reprinted by permission from Newman, W. P., Freedman, D. S., and Voors, A. W.: Relation of serum lipoprotein levels and systolic blood pressure to early atherosclerosis. The Bogalusa Heart Study. N. Engl. J. Med. *314*:138, 1986.)

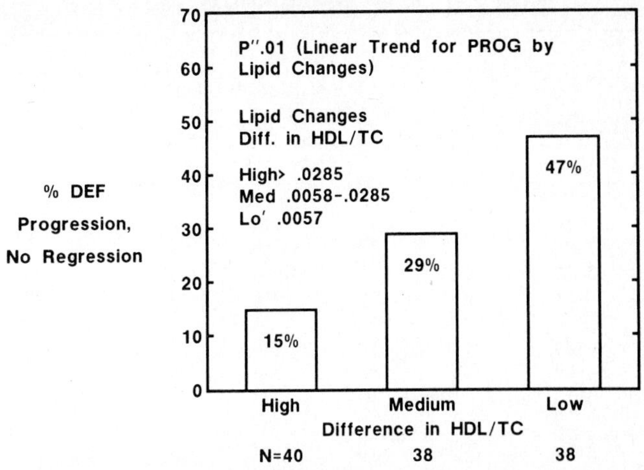

FIGURE 36–5. Results of the NHLBI Type II coronary intervention trial: A plot of the percentage of patients with either definite progression or no regression of coronary obstruction versus the ratio of HDL cholesterol to total cholesterol. The lower the ratio, the greater the percentage of subjects with progression or absence of regression.

THE CHOLESTEROL CONSENSUS CONFERENCE

The traditional way of defining hyperlipoproteinemia has been based on plasma cholesterol or triglyceride levels exceeding the 95th percentile value for age and sex, in comparison with measurements in a comparable nonrestricted population. The Lipid Research Clinic data provide the most complete sets available (Table 36–1). However, on the basis of metabolic, epidemiological, pathological, and genetic animal experimental studies, and primary and secondary intervention trials, a cholesterol consensus conference was held at the National Institutes of Health in 1984 to review the data and to establish new guidelines for defining hyperlipoproteinemia.[26] The panel concluded that the available evidence "established beyond a reasonable doubt that lowering definitely elevated blood cholesterol (specifically, blood levels of low-density lipoprotein [LDL] cholesterol) will reduce the risk of heart attacks caused by coronary heart disease. After careful review of genetic, experimental, epidemiologic, and clinical trial evidence, we recommend treatment of individuals with blood cholesterol levels above the 75th percentile (upper 25 per cent of values) (Table 36–2). . . . Furthermore, we are persuaded that the blood cholesterol levels of most Americans are undesirably high, in large part because of a high dietary intake of calories, saturated fat, and cholesterol."

The cholesterol values for selecting adults at moderate risk for CAD are between the 75th and 90th percentiles. For ages 20 to 29, these values fall between 200 and 220 mg/dl or between 5.17 and 5.69 mM; for ages 30 to 39, the values are between 220 and 240 mg/dl or between 5.69 and 6.21 mM. Over age 40, the values are between 240 and 260 mg/dl or between 6.21 and 6.72 mM. The high-risk group contains those whose values exceed the 90th percentile, namely over 220 for ages 20 to 29, over 240 for ages 30 to 39, and over 260 for those 40 and over. The panel made further recommendations on the desirability for the cholesterol readings of individuals over age 30 to

TABLE 36–1 REFERENCE VALUES FOR PLASMA CHOLESTEROL AND LIPOPROTEIN CHOLESTEROL*

	mg/dl												
	PLASMA CHOLESTEROL					LDL CHOLESTEROL				HDL CHOLESTEROL			
PERCENTILE	5	50	75	90	95	5	50	75	95	5	10	50	95
AGE (YR)													
						Men							
5–19	115	155	170	185	200	65	95	105	130	35†	40†	55†	75†
20–24	125	165	185	205	220	65	105	120	145	30	30	45	65
25–29	135	180	200	225	245	70	115	140	165	30	30	45	65
30–34	140	190	215	240	255	80	125	145	185	30	30	45	60
35–39	145	200	225	250	270	80	135	155	190	30	30	45	60
40–44	150	205	230	250	270	85	135	155	185	25	30	45	65
45–69	160	215	235	260	275	90	145	165	205	30	30	50	70
70+	150	205	230	250	270	90	145	165	185	30	35	50	75
						Women							
5–19	120	160	175	190	200	65	100	110	140	35	40	55	70
20–24	125	170	190	215	230	55	105	120	160	35	35	55	80
25–34	130	175	195	220	235	70	110	125	160	35	40	55	80
35–39	140	185	205	230	245	75	120	140	170	35	40	55	80
40–44	145	195	215	235	255	75	125	145	175	35	40	60	90
45–49	150	205	225	250	270	80	130	150	185	35	40	60	85
50–54	165	220	240	265	285	90	140	160	200	35	40	60	90
55+	170	230	250	295	295	95	150	170	215	35	40	60	95

*From the Lipid Research Clinics program–North American Prevalence Study.
†For HDL values for men aged 15–19 yr use values for age group 20–24 yr.
LDL = low-density lipoprotein; HDL = high-density lipoprotein.

be under 200 mg/dl and for those under age 30, a value under 180 mg/dl.

Two basic approaches are recommended for reducing the risk of cholesterol in the population. One, which may be called the high-risk strategy, aims at identifying those above the 75th percentile through testing carried out by screening in physicians' offices, in the workplace, and at health care facilities. New automated methods for measuring cholesterol rapidly from a drop of blood or a small quantity of serum make mass screening technically feasible. Those individuals with results above the 75th percentile would be singled out for intensive treatment, initially with diet. Most of those individuals with readings between the 75th and 90th percentiles could be treated with diet alone; those with levels above the 90th percentile would be treated initially with diet, and if necessary a drug could be added.

The mass-strategy approach is aimed at changing the dietary habits of the general population in an attempt to achieve a universal lowering of cholesterol. The mass-strategy approach involves educational activities such as those used over the last 25 years by the American Heart Association. Through this and other efforts U.S. eating habits have already changed: the U.S. diet of today contains fewer eggs, less butter, cream, and whole milk, less animal fat, beef, and other red meat, and more vegetable and polyunsaturated fats than it once did. A high-risk strategy and a mass population strategy are not mutually exclusive but could be promoted at the same time.

The basic strategy for measuring cholesterol is testing of all adults when they visit their physicians; on average, U.S. citizens see their physicians once a year. If measurements were made then, it would be theoretically possible for patients to know their cholesterol value within a relatively short period of time. If the cholesterol value for individuals over age 30 is less than 200 mg/dl, the authors recommend retesting in 1 to 2 years or, at the most, in 5 years. If the value is over 200 mg/dl, the test should be repeated; if the second result is over 200 mg/dl, the individual should be referred to a physician for evaluation of lipoproteins as discussed below.

In the mass-strategy approach, a national effort would be required to educate adults and children to make informed dietary choices. The question of changing the diet of children remains controversial. The American Heart Association recommends that the basic Phase I (the AHA's Prudent Diet) should be adopted by families and for all individuals over age 2. Furthermore, children of high-risk families, such as those with histories of early "heart attack," hypertension, diabetes, or hyperlipidemia, should be screened at an early age for elevated cholesterol.

TABLE 36–2 BLOOD CHOLESTEROL VALUES FOR SELECTING MEN AND WOMEN WHO REQUIRE TREATMENT

AGE	MODERATE RISK (75TH PERCENTILE)	HIGH RISK (90TH PERCENTILE)
20–29	200–220 mg/dl	220–240 mg/dl
30–39	220–240 mg/dl	240–260 mg/dl
≥40	240–260 mg/dl	>260 mg/dl

From the NIH Consensus Conference on Lowering Blood Cholesterol to Prevent Coronary Heart Disease, 1984.

LIPOPROTEINS

The major plasma lipids include cholesterol, cholesteryl ester, triglyceride, and phospholipid. None of these is water soluble and they do not circulate in a free form in the blood. Instead, they are complexed and bound to a specific group of protein carriers called *apolipoproteins*, which are found on the surface of the lipoproteins. Lipids and apolipoproteins circulate through the bloodstream in macromolecular complexes called *lipoproteins*. There are five major groups of lipoproteins which may be separated by ultracentrifugation: the chylomicrons, very low-density lipoproteins (VLDL), low-density lipoproteins (LDL), intermediate-density lipoproteins (IDL), and high-density lipoproteins (HDL) (Table 36–3). A thorough knowledge of lipoproteins and their functions is essential to an understanding of hypercholesterolemia.

Figure 36–6 represents a schematic representation of a lipoprotein particle (see also Fig. 49–5, p. 1638). The

TABLE 36–3 COMPOSITION AND PROPERTIES OF HUMAN PLASMA LIPOPROTEINS

Properties	Chylomicrons	VLDL*	IDL†	LDL‡	HDL§
Density	0.95	0.95–1.006	1.006–1.019	1.019–1.063	1.061–1.210
Electrophoretic mobility	Origin	Pre-β	β	β	α
Major lipid constituents	Triglyceride ("exogenous")	Triglyceride ("enogenous"), phospholipid	Esterified cholesterol, phospholipid	Triglyceride, esterified cholesterol	Phospholipid cholesterol
Apoprotein constituents	ApoA-I ApoII ApoIV ApoB-48	ApoB-100 ApoC-I ApoC-II ApoC-III ApoE	ApoB-100 ApoE	ApoB-100	ApoA-I ApoA-II ApoC-II ApoE

*Very low-density lipoproteins. †Intermediate-density lipoproteins. ‡Low-density lipoproteins. §High-density lipoproteins.
From Beigel, Y., and Gotto, A.: Lipoproteins in Health and Disease: Diagnosis and Management. The Baylor College of Medicine Cardiology Series 9:6, No. 1, 1986.

typical structure of a plasma lipoprotein is a spherical particle in which the water-insoluble nonpolar lipids (in particular the triglyceride and the cholesteryl ester) are protected by a surface monolayer consisting of phospholipids and apolipoproteins. Unesterified cholesterol occupies an intermediate position between the surface layer of apolipoproteins and phospholipid and the core of neutral lipid. Chylomicrons are the largest of the lipoprotein particles, their core consisting mainly of triglyceride. In moving from the larger chylomicron particles to VLDL to LDL, the lipid core shifts from a triglyceride to cholesteryl ester. The core of VLDL is predominantly triglyceride made endogenously in the liver while the core of LDL is largely cholesteryl ester. The HDL are very small particles and are relatively rich in protein, cholesteryl ester, and phospholipid.

APOLIPOPROTEINS

A great deal of research has been conducted in the use of apolipoproteins as markers for CAD (Table 36–4). The apolipoproteins exhibit the type of polymorphism and heterogeneity seen with other plasma proteins. One can almost certainly predict that a group of apolipoproteinopathies will be identified that is comparable to the hemoglobinopathies which have been so extensively described. As far as clinical utility is concerned, some investigators have found that either apolipoprotein A-1 (apoA-I) or the concentration of apolipoprotein B-100 (apoB-100) in LDL and VLDL are better predictors of CAD than are total plasma lipids or lipoproteins. It has been reported that apoA-I was the best predictor of the likelihood of finding significant arteriosclerosis in patients undergoing coronary arteriography.[27] In this study, an inverse relationship existed; the higher the concentration of apoA-I, the lower the likelihood of finding significant coronary obstruction. ApoA-I was a better predictor than total cholesterol or HDL in this particular study.

ApoA-I is a major protein in HDL, has a molecular weight of 28,000, is synthesized in the gut and in the liver, and is also present in chylomicrons. The apolipoproteins contain specific regions, *amphipathic helices*. These regions are relatively rich in charged amino acids but have the property of binding phospholipid and forming an outer face of polar amino acids and an inner face of hydrophobic amino acids. ApoA-I is the prototype of the apoproteins containing such structures and it appears that this structure has been maintained through evolution by the process of gene duplication. ApoA-I has several stretches of this structure; typically an amphipathic region contains approximately 33 amino acids divided into thirds by a proline. In addition to its function of binding lipids, apoA-I is an activator of the enzyme lecithin cholesterol acyl transferase (LCAT).

ApoA-II is a minor constituent of HDL and does not

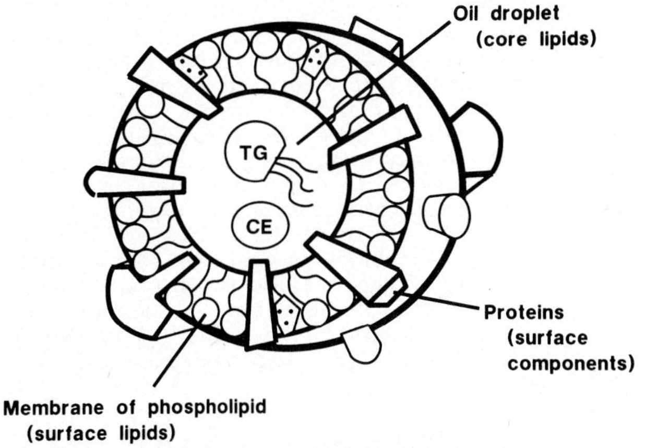

FIGURE 36–6. General structure of a lipoprotein particle, consisting of an inner droplet of neutral (or water-insoluble) core lipids, primarily triglyceride and cholesteryl ester, and a solubilizing surface layer of phospholipid and lesser amounts of free cholesterol. Specific protein components, the apolipoproteins, are bound to the outer membrane of the molecule through their specific lipophilic regions. These proteins are the primary determinants of the class and of the metabolic behavior of the lipoprotein molecules. (From Cholesterol and coronary disease . . . reducing the risk. Lecture Guide. New York, Science and Medicine, 1986.)

TABLE 36–4 SUMMARY OF APOLIPOPROTEINS

The Plasma Apolipoproteins

Name	Lipoprotein	Molecular Weight	Function
apo-AI	HDL, chylomicrons*	28,000	Structural; activator of LCAT enzyme
apo-AII	HDL, chylomicrons	16,000	Structural
apo-AIV	HDL, chylomicrons,* VLDL	46,000	Unknown
apo-B-100	LDL, VLDL	550,000	Structural; synthesis and secretion of VLDL; binds to LDL receptor (BE)
apo-B-48	Chylomicrons	250,000	Structural; synthesis and secretion from intestine
apo-CI	HDL, chylomicrons, VLDL	6,000	Activator of LCAT
apo-CII	HDL, chylomicrons, VLDL	7,000	Activator of lipoprotein lipase
apo-CIII	HDL, chylomicrons, VLDL	7,000	Stabilizes surface; provides negative charge
apo-D	HDL, chylomicrons*	21,000	Cholesteryl ester exchange
apo-E	HDL, VLDL, chylomicrons*	34,000	Binds to receptor on cell membrane of liver (E and BE) and macrophage

*Only in nascent chylomicrons.
From Cholesterol & Coronary Disease . . . Reducing the Risk. Lecture Guide. New York, Science & Medicine, 1986.

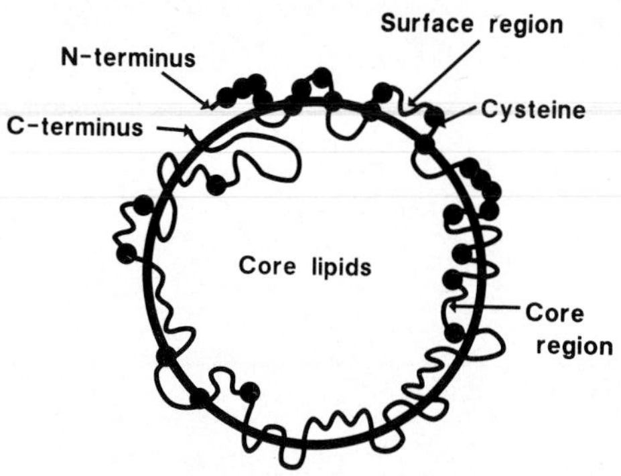

FIGURE 36–7. Hypothetical model of apoB-100 structure on LDL. For simplicity, the trypsin-accessible regions are shown on the surface, and the trypsin-inaccessible regions inside the core of the LDL particle (not to scale). The surface-core orientation is presented to allow easy visualization of trypsin-accessibility. It does not imply that the different parts of apoB-100 are physically on the surface or buried inside the lipoprotein particle. (From Yang, C.-Y., Chen, S.-H., Gianturco, S. H., Bradley, W. A., Sparrow, J. T., Tanimura, M., Li, W.-H., Sparrow, D. A., DeLoof, H., Rosseneu, M., Lee, F.-S., Gu, Z.-W., Gotto, A. M., Jr., and Chan, L.: Sequence, structure, receptor-binding domains and internal repeats of human apolipoprotein B-100. Nature *323*:738, 1986.)

appear to be present in all species. In man, apoA-II consists of two identical chains connected by single disulfide linkage; in other species, it consists of a single chain. It has been reported to be an activator of hepatic triglyceride lipase, which also hydrolyzes triglyceride and phospholipid, HDL_2 being a preferred substrate. ApoA-IV is synthesized in the gut, is present in HDL, chylomicrons, and VLDL, has a molecular weight of 46,000, and is a highly helical structure. Although its function is unknown, it has been reported to be an activator of LCAT.

ApoB occurs in two forms; ApoB-100 is secreted by the liver while apoB-48 is synthesized by the small intestine. ApoB-48 is present on the surface of chylomicrons and chylomicron remnants and is probably required for the synthesis of chylomicrons. ApoB-100 is found in VLDL, IDL, and LDL and accounts for approximately 25 per cent of the protein by weight in LDL. ApoB-100 represents the recognition site for the LDL or ApoB,E receptor on cell surfaces (Fig. 36–7). Genetic variations of apoB have been noted, and their effect on atherogenesis has been described recently.[27a] However, the polymorphism associated with CAD was not associated with increased levels of LDL, cholesterol, or apoB.

Until recently, the structure of apoB-100 was unknown. One problem in determining the structure was its size; another was the fact that once the lipid is removed, the protein is highly insoluble. This property is due in part to the relatively high content of beta structure or pleated sheet structure in apoB-100. The cDNA structure of apoB has been recently defined: it contains 14.1 kilobases and codes for the 4563 amino acids, which includes a 27-amino acid signal protein. The mature protein contains 4536 residues. The sequence was deduced by the cloning and sequencing of overlapping DNA's from human liver specimen libraries. A dot matrix analysis of the amino acid sequence was performed and showed the presence of several long internal repetitions in apoB-100, a property in common with other apolipoproteins. With the use of synthetic peptides, it was possible to determine lipid-binding regions. ApoB-100 contains two types, the amphipathic helical binding region sites present in other apolipoproteins as well as the highly hydrophobic beta structure or pleated sheet regions. It is postulated that the amphipathic helical regions are localized at the surface of the LDL particle while the beta or pleated sheet regions may be buried within the neutral lipid core of cholesteryl ester.[28, 29]

In an earlier publication describing the partial sequence of the cDNA by Knott et al.,[30] a region of apoB was identified that showed a significant homology to residues 140 to 150 of apoE, the putative binding site to the apoB/E receptor. These presumed binding sites, which enable the LDL or apoB/E receptor to recognize the lipoprotein, contain clusters of positively charged amino acids, lysine, and arginine, which could bind to a negatively charged region of the LDL receptor.[31] Yang et al.[29] have prepared a synthetic fragment of apoB-100 consisting of amino acid residues 3345 to 3381, which has homology to residues 140 to 150 of apoE. Indeed, it was found that this synthetic peptide from apoB-100 was able to bind to the LDL receptor, which supports the concept that this region is recognized by the B/E receptor and provides the opportunity of pinpointing the precise structural determinants for recognition by the B/E receptor. Mutations within this region could alter the receptor-binding properties of LDL.

ApoC-I, C-II, and C-III are synthesized in the liver and are found in VLDL and HDL. HDL's appear to serve as a reservoir for these apoproteins, which may be transferred to the triglyceride-rich lipoproteins following a meal and participate in the clearance of dietary fat. ApoC-II is an obligatory activator of lipoprotein lipase. ApoC-I is an LCAT activator while the function of apoC-III is unclear. ApoC-III has been reported to decrease the uptake of triglyceride-rich lipoprotein remnants by the liver.

ApoD. This apoprotein is a relatively minor constituent found in HDL and chylomicrons. Its molecular weight is 21,000. It has been reported to be involved in cholesteryl ester exchange but does not appear to be the exchange enzyme itself.

ApoE. This apoprotein is synthesized in the liver; however, other tissues that have the ability to synthesize apoE include the small bowel, kidney, adrenal gland, and the cells of the reticuloendothelial system. ApoE makes up about 15 per cent of the protein of VLDL, 7 per cent of the protein of chylomicron remnants, and 1 to 2 per cent of the protein of HDL. It can be recognized both by the apoB,E receptor and by a specific receptor in the liver whose function appears to be the removal of chylomicron remnants. As noted above, the ability of apoE to interact with the LDL receptor is thought to be a result of a ligand recognition site between residues 140 and 150.

ApoE contains three major alleles: apoE-II, apoE-III, and apoE-IV. ApoE-II contains cysteines at residues 112 and 158; apoE-III cys and arg, respectively, and E-IV arg, arg. In experiments with fibroblasts, E-II exhibits diminished binding to the B,E receptor (the LDL receptor) compared with E-III and E-IV. Substitution for the arg at 158 is presumed to alter the conformation of the positively charged amino acids between residues 140 and 150 which bind to the receptor. Other alleles are present but are less common. The E-III allele has a frequency of about 76 per cent in white populations, E-IV about 13 per cent, and E-II 10 per cent. The various combinations of these alleles are homozygotes for E-II/E-II, E-III/E-III, E-IV/E-IV, and heterozygotes for E-II/E-III, E-II/E-IV, and E-III/E-IV. The ApoE-II allele has been found to be associated with lower levels of cholesterol and the E-IV allele with higher levels in population studies. The delayed clearance of apoE-containing chylomicron remnants by the hepatic apoE receptor theoretically could lead to an up-regulation of the B,E (LDL) receptor and an enhanced clearance of LDL. ApoE-IV–containing remnants, on the other hand, would have the opposite effect, i.e., an enhanced uptake, down-regulation of B,E receptor, decreased LDL clearance, and higher cholesterol levels.[31a]

Over 90 per cent of patients with dysbetalipoproteinemia or Type III hyperlipoproteinemia are homozygous for the E-II/E-II phenotype. This disorder is characterized by hypercholesterolemia, hypertriglyceridemia, and abnormal IDL or VLDL particles that are cholesterol enriched. The particles have beta electrophoretic mobility and are termed beta-VLDL. Premature coronary and peripheral vascular disease is characteristically associated with Type III hyperlipoproteinemia. Whereas in a normal individual the chylomicron remnants have a half-life in the blood of less than 10 minutes, in Type III hyperlipoproteinemia they may persist for hours. Although apoE-II does not bind to lipoprotein receptors or isolated cells as well as E-III and E-IV, a second abnormality must be superimposed in order to produce the relatively uncommon type III hyperlipoproteinemia, since the E-II/E-II phenotype occurs in 1 per cent of the population.

LIPOPROTEIN METABOLISM

(See also Fig. 49–6, p. 1638)

CHYLOMICRONS. The largest of the lipoproteins, the chylomicrons originate from the gut, are mainly composed of triglycerides, and transport dietary triglyceride and cholesterol. The predominant function of chylomicrons is the transfer of the exogenously derived triglyceride and cholesterol from the intestinal lumen to sites of metabolism or storage. Dietary fat is broken down to free fatty acids and monoglycerides in the intestinal lumen. The lipid components, cholesterol, and partially digested triglycerides enter the intestinal villi especially in the jejunum, where they are reconstituted into triglycerides. In the cells of the intestinal wall, cholesterol is esterified to cholesteryl ester, mainly cholesterol oleate, through the enzymatic reaction catalyzed by acyl cholesterol acyl transferase (ACAT). The triglyceride particles are then complexed with apoB-48, apoA-I, and probably apoA-II and A-IV within the intestinal wall. The chylomicrons enter the systemic circulation via the lymphatic circulation. ApoE and apoC proteins are added in the lymph or blood; these proteins are made in the liver but not the intestine. The chylomicron particles are rapidly cleared from the blood.

The clearing of the chylomicrons is modulated by lipoprotein lipase and results in the formation of remnant particles which are rich in cholesterol and apoE, apoC, and apoB-48.[32] Partially degraded chylomicron particles are called *remnants* and are cleared very rapidly from the circulation by a receptor that is present on the surface of liver cells. This receptor is called the *apoE* or *chylomicron remnant receptor*. It recognizes apoE and, unlike the LDL apoB/E receptor in the liver, does not appear to be down-regulated as remnant particles are taken up. Dietary cholesterol presumably would be taken up by the liver through the apoE receptor–mediated endocytosis.

The presence of chylomicrons in fasting plasma is abnormal. Chylomicronemia represents part of the criteria for the diagnosis of Type I and Type V hyperlipoproteinemia. Also, in uncontrolled Type III hyperlipoproteinemia, or dysbetalipoproteinemia, fasting chylomicronemia may be present. While chylomicronemia per se is not thought to result in premature coronary disease, the accumulation of remnant particles is thought to be atherogenic. It has been postulated that a prolonged clearance of the dietary remnant particles could be damaging to the vascular endothelium and could predispose to atherosclerosis.

VERY LOW-DENSITY LIPOPROTEINS (VLDL). These lipoproteins are endogenously produced by the liver and contain apoB-100. Although triglyceride is the predominant lipid, cholesterol, cholesteryl ester, and phospholipid are also present. The synthesis of VLDL is increased in obesity, alcohol use, and diabetes. The function of VLDL is the transport of cholesterol and endogenously produced triglyceride from the liver to their sites of utilization.

INTERMEDIATE-DENSITY LIPOPROTEINS (IDL). These lipoproteins are formed from metabolism of VLDL. HDL acts as a reservoir for apoE and apoC, which are added to VLDL prior to its breakdown. After their formation from VLDL, IDL's are transported to the liver where roughly one-half is metabolized in man. The remainder is converted to LDL. The IDL's have a high cholesterol content and migrate in the beta region on electrophoresis.[33] Elevations of IDL are thought to predispose to premature coronary and peripheral vascular disease.[34]

The metabolism of VLDL requires lipoprotein lipase. Normal individuals maintain the apoB-100 associated with VLDL during metabolism to IDL and subsequently LDL. During hydrolysis of triglyceride, apoE and apoC's are transferred to HDL. The role of elevated VLDL in atherogenesis is controversial and is discussed on page 1166.

LOW-DENSITY LIPOPROTEINS (LDL). These are the major cholesterol-carrying components of plasma. ApoB-100 is virtually the exclusive protein present in LDL and comprises 25 per cent of LDL mass. LDL's are mainly formed from VLDL breakdown but may be synthesized directly.[35] After formation and transport they are bound by specific B,E or LDL receptors on hepatic and a variety of extrahepatic tissues.[36] About one-third to three-fourths of LDL are removed by hepatic B,E receptors. (For detailed discussion see page 1641.) After binding, the LDL is removed and metabolized. The LDL receptor also can bind IDL prior to its peripheral conversion to LDL. If the number of LDL receptors is decreased, the plasma concentration of LDL rises.[37] In familial hypercholesterolemia, heterozygotes have one-half of the LDL receptors of normal persons, while homozygotes have little or no receptor activity (p. 1640). Over 80 per cent of patients with elevated cholesterol, however, do not have monogenically determined hypercholesterolemia but rather have polygenic hypercholesterolemia (p. 1637). Therefore, elevations of LDL due to a primary receptor defect are relatively uncommon.

HIGH-DENSITY LIPOPROTEINS (HDL). These lipoproteins are produced by the liver and the gut, and by peripheral catabolism of chylomicrons and VLDL. They contain by weight approximately 30 per cent cholesterol, 45 per cent protein, 25 per cent phospholipid (predominantly phosphatidyl choline), and a small amount of triglyceride. HDL's serve as a reservoir for apolipoproteins that may be exchanged between this family of lipoproteins and VLDL and chylomicrons. At least one of these apolipoproteins, apoC-II, is an obligatory activator of lipoprotein lipase. HDL plays a role in the transport of cholesterol, removing it from peripheral tissue. There is evidence for the existence of an HDL receptor which may facilitate cholesterol removal from cells by this lipoprotein. ApoA-I or apoA-II has been reported to interact with this receptor.[38]

Some investigators have proposed that a phenomenon exists in which HDL facilitates cholesterol removal from cells, particularly the cells of the reticuloendothelial system.[39] This process has been viewed as the reverse or opposite of the one in which LDL-cholesterol is delivered to the cell by receptor-mediated endocytosis. Therefore, it has been called "reverse endocytosis." Deficiency of this function could theoretically account for the accumulation of cholesteryl ester in cells—for example, as in Tangier disease. Once cholesterol is removed from cells by HDL, the cholesterol can be converted to cholesteryl ester through a step mediated by the enzyme LCAT. The cholesteryl ester can then be transferred from HDL to VLDL, IDL, and LDL via an enzyme or enzymes which catalyze the transfer of cholesteryl ester between different lipoprotein families. Eventually the choleserol removed from peripheral tissues by HDL would reach the liver (Fig. 36–8). Another function of HDL is to serve as a source of cholesterol for endocrine tissues such as the adrenal cortex, the ovary, and the testes.

HDL_2 and HDL_3. HDL may be subdivided into several fractions; the two most thoroughly studied ones are HDL_2 and HDL_3. HDL_2 consists of larger particles that are more lipid-rich and of lower density, while HDL_3 particles are smaller and more protein rich, lipid poor, and denser. Little epidemiological data exist as to the relative protective effects of HDL_2 versus HDL_3 with respect to CAD. Patsch and colleagues carried out extensive studies on the metabolism of HDL, its subfractions, and its relationship to dietary lipemia. They used zonal ultracentrifuge to separate and isolate the HDL subfractions and showed that an inverse relationship exists between the degree of postprandial lipemia and the concentration of HDL, apoA-I, and HDL_2.[40]

Concentrations of HDL_2 are higher in women than in men and are increased by estrogen or physical exercise. The condition known as *familial hyperalphalipoproteinemia* is one in which the HDL_2 fraction primarily is in-

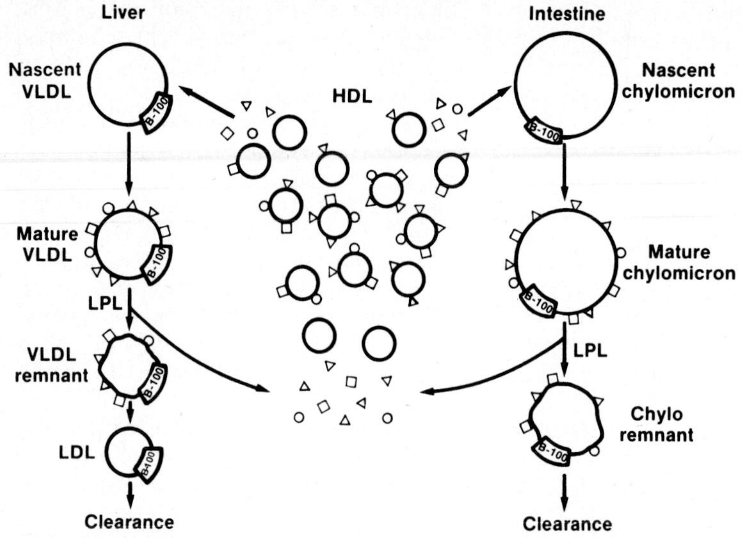

FIGURE 36–8. Function of HDL. An additional source of HDL lipid and protein is derived from the peripheral hydrolysis of chylomicrons and VLDL by the lipoprotein lipase. During hydrolysis of the triglyceride component, the surface coat components, phospholipid and apolipoprotein, are released into the plasma and are incorporated into HDL. This contribution from VLDL provides a significant source of HDL apolipoproteins C-I, C-II, C-III, and E. HDL apolipoproteins A-I and A-IV can also come from nascent chylomicrons. The net result is a heterogeneous population of HDL particles containing various quantities of different apolipoproteins and maintaining in equilibrium a rapid exchange of many of these components. (From Cholesterol and coronary disease . . . reducing the risk. Lecture Guide. New York, Science and Medicine, 1986.)

creased. Persons with this condition are said to live frequently into their 80's and 90's. Thus, all of the factors which would be expected to be associated with protection against CAD are associated with HDL influence, primarily with HDL_2. It is interesting that alcohol, which is known to raise levels of HDL, has been found to increase the levels of both HDL_3 and HDL_2. The clinical significance of this observation remains to be determined.

Concentrations of HDL show a strong inverse relationship with coronary disease, and HDL levels may be altered by many factors, including exercise, alcohol consumption, and hormones.[41, 42] A number of factors are associated with low levels of HDL: one is hypertriglyceridemia; another is cigarette smoking. While the concentration of lipoprotein lipase is positively correlated with the concentration of HDL, that of hepatic triglyceride lipase is inversely related to HDL, as one might expect since HDL_2 is a substrate for hepatic triglyceride lipase.

Pocock et al.[43] recently reported results from the British Regional Heart Study, which they interpreted as showing that HDL cholesterol is not a major risk factor in the etiology of ischemic heart disease. However, these investigators used samples from nonfasting subjects and combined VLDL-cholesterol and LDL-cholesterol as nonHDL cholesterol. This was a large prospective study of men aged 40 to 59, patients of general practitioners in 24 British towns. After an average follow-up of over 4 years, 193 cases of major coronary events were recorded in 7415 men. It is possible that the results reflected the statistical approach the investigators used, and the fact that they did not distinguish between LDL and VLDL cholesterol. The non-HDL cholesterol remained significant after all multivariate analyses. In the Framingham study, in older individuals, HDL cholesterol became a more important predictor of coronary heart disease than did either total or LDL cholesterol. The British group was a somewhat younger group than the Framingham one, which showed the strongest correlation of coronary disease with HDL.

LP (a). This is a unique lipoprotein found mainly in the density range of HDL. It is a relatively minor lipoprotein, containing less than 15 per cent of the plasma cholesterol. Although it resembles LDL in that it contains apoB, it also contains apolipoprotein (a) to which it is linked by disulfide bonds. While relatively little is known about it in comparison with the other lipoproteins, a recent study has implicated it in coronary disease and atherosclerosis. In a study of 307 patients undergoing coronary angiography, LP (a) was associated with CAD in women of all ages and in men 55 years or older.[44]

GENETIC VARIATION OF APOLIPOPROTEINS

Restriction fragment length polymorphism (RFLP) is a powerful tool for studying genetic variation. This term describes an altered pattern of gene fragments which are produced when the genomic DNA molecules from different individuals are digested with enzymes called *restriction endonucleases.* Each restriction nuclease is specific for a defined sequence of recognition of DNA. A change in the pattern of polymorphism could represent simply a point mutation or could be due to a deletion, insertion, or rearrangement of the DNA. Such analysis was initially used with the enzyme EcoR1 to detect the abnormality in the DNA of patients with the familial deficiency of apoA-I and apoC-III.

The genes for apoA-I, apoC-III, and apoA-IV have been shown to be localized on chromosome 11. That a genetic effect involving the apoA-I gene can produce atherosclerosis was established in a careful clinical investigation of two sisters[45] who developed coronary disease in their 20's. ApoA-I and apoC-III were absent from the blood of both patients, and HDL levels were very low. The apoA-I gene and apoC-III gene are located on opposite strands of the DNA. The two sisters, in addition to coronary disease, had xanthomas on the skin and tendons, corneal clouding, and their first-degree relatives had one-half the normal levels of apoA-I and apoC-III. It was found that the two sisters had a gene rearrangement due to an inversion of a DNA segment that contained a displacement which affected the functioning of both the genes for apoA-I and apoC-III. It is thought that a part of the apoC-III gene is inserted into the apoA-I gene, and that this is the basis of the combined apoprotein deficiency.

Extensive population screening has shown at least 11 different variants of the apoA-I, mainly with the use of electrophoresis and isoelectric focusing. These have appeared in individuals who are heterozygotes for one normal apoA-I allele and for one abnormal one. The abnormal gene produces mutants which contain either one additional acid unit or two additional basic amino acids. Two such mutants, apoA-I Milano and apoA-I Marburg, were associated with reduced levels of HDL.[46, 47] Each of these had an additional acidic amino acid. Three of the mutants, apoA-I Giessen, apoA-I Marburg, and apoA-I Muenster 2a, have been reported to be defective in the ability to activate LCAT.

RFLP studies with apoA-II[48] suggest that there are alleles for the apoA-II gene. These alleles are produced by

RFLP using the restrictive endonuclease MspI. One allele with a frequency of 15 to 20 per cent is associated with an increase in the plasma concentration of apoA-II in the homozygous state. In this allele, the composition of HDL is altered. This could have physiological importance since apoA-II has been reported to be an activator of hepatic triglyceride lipase. Patsch et al.[40] have suggested that the fraction of HDL containing apoA-II would represent a substrate for this enzyme and might be converted to HDL_3.

RFLPs have been used to study the cluster of genes for apoA-I, apoC-III, and apoA-IV on chromosome 11.[49] Two different alleles have been identified in the apoC-III region, one called S-1 and the other S-2. These vary in different racial groups; furthermore, the S-2 allele has been reported to be increased in individuals with hypertriglyceridemia, with Type V hyperlipoproteinemia, with low levels of HDL, and in survivors of myocardial infarction. The DNA polymorphism lies in the 3′ untranslated region of the apoC-III gene, and the associated clinical abnormalities in lipoproteins have been described in whites. Whether the base changes cause the lipoprotein abnormalities has not been established. These studies were done with a restriction enzyme called Sst1.

In another clinical study examining the polymorphism of apoA-I, a minor allele, X2, detected with the restrictive endonuclease XmnI, was associated with Type IIb, Type III, and Type V hyperlipoproteinemia but not with Type IIa or Type IV.[50] The X2 allele was associated with the highest levels of triglyceride. Ordovas et al.[51] described apoA-I polymorphism associated with premature coronary artery disease and familial hyperalphalipoproteinemia. This study used another restriction endonuclease, Pst1. In one clinical study, the P-2 allele, which is missing the Pst1 site and is a 3.3-kilobase fragment, showed no association with a lipoprotein abnormality. However, Ordovas et al. used the Pst1 polymorphism to define an association with premature CAD. The 3.3-kb band, called the P-2 allele, was found in 4 per cent of 123 randomly selected controlled subjects and in 3 per cent of 30 subjects without angiographic evidence of CAD. By contrast, this allele was found in 32 per cent of 88 patients who had angiographically documented CAD before the age of 60. It was also found in 8 of 12 index cases of kindreds with familial hypoalphalipoproteinemia.[52–55] This latter disorder has been described as a dominant one, and affected individuals have HDL cholesterol values below the 10th percentile for their age and sex.

CAD is associated with low levels of HDL. An earlier study had shown that 60 per cent of 224 consecutive patients under age 60 with angiographically documented coronary obstruction had HDL levels below the 10th percentile; this represented the most common lipid abnormality in these subjects. Within kindreds with familial hypoalphalipoproteinemia and in first-degree relatives of patients with CAD, the P-2 allele was associated with decreased levels of HDL cholesterol. Of those patients with CAD examined by Ordovas et al.,[51] 58 per cent had HDL cholesterol levels below the 10th percentile of normal values. The authors interpreted the findings to indicate that polymorphism in the region between apoA-I and apoC-III may be a useful marker of both familial hypoalphalipoproteinemia and premature CAD. It should be noted, however, that such observations do not establish causality.

FAMILIAL apoC-II DEFICIENCY. This condition was first described by Breckenridge et al.,[56] and a number of families have been reported in different parts of the world.[57] No abnormality in the gene or the DNA of this apoprotein has been discovered as of this writing, although there are reports of DNA polymorphism. The deficiency of apoC-II produces a hyperchylomicronemic syndrome with either a Type I or Type V hyperlipoproteinemia pattern, usually the Type I variety. In individuals and in kindreds in whom apoC-II is deficient, severe hypertriglyceridemia occurs due to a lipoprotein lipase which is functionally inactive. So far, genetic polymorphism has not been described in individuals who are missing apoC-II.

Genetic variability detected by RFLP in the apoC-III region has been described in association with hypertriglyceridemia as noted above. The exact significance of the polymorphic variance of apoC-III in this condition remains to be established. Further studies to clone the alleles of patients affected with the polymorphism might clarify the nature of the abnormality, and linkage studies should also be performed by examining a phenotype found in a family. The RFLP technique, which potentially is a powerful one, can be applied by isolating DNA from white blood cells and analyzing it.

On the basis of polymorphism of apoB observed in case-control studies in whites with and without CAD, it has been postulated that there may be changes in the apoB structure that could influence CAD—for example, affecting the interaction with monocytes, endothelial cells, or smooth muscle cells without influencing the interaction with the LDL receptor.[27a] The apoB gene is located on chromosome 2. The polymorphism was not associated with either an increase or a decrease in the concentration of LDL on apoB, although the X1 allele with endonuclease XbaI, the BI allele with EcoRI, and the ID1 with MspI all occurred with increased frequency in those patients with CHD.

Earlier studies on patients who had received multiple blood transfusions had led to the recognition of various alleles referred to as Ag. Some of the Ag alleles had small effects on risk of CHD and on the concentrations of plasma cholesterol. Genetic polymorphism in the protein structure of apoB-100 and apoB-48 has been described by Young et al.,[58, 58a] especially with the use of the monoclonal antibody MB19. These changes did not appear to affect the composition of LDL or its binding to the B,E receptor.

DEFECTS IN THE SYNTHESIS OF APOLIPOPROTEIN B. Two different genetic diseases have been described in which a deficiency exists in the synthesis of apoB.[58a] One is *abetalipoproteinemia*, in which no circulating LDL is present; VLDL and chylomicrons are also absent and only HDL's are present. This appears to be an autosomal recessive disorder and is associated with acanthocytosis, an atypical form of retinitis pigmentosa, spinocerebellar dysfunction, kyphosis of the spine, and fat malabsorption. ApoB-100 and B-48 appear to be absent and the normal transport of lipid from both the intestine and liver is severely impaired. Heterozygotes do not show any clinical or physiological abnormalities. In the second disorder involving the synthesis of apoB, called *homozygous hypobetalipoproteinemia,* the clinical manifestations are much the same as those in abetalipoproteinemia. However, unlike abetalipoproteinemia, in which the parents of subjects have normal concentrations of apoB, in homozygous hypobetalipoproteinemia the parents have one-half the normal level of apoB. They are free, however, of clinical symptoms. CAD has not been associated with abetalipoproteinemia or hypobetalipoproteinemia, although the number of subjects studied thus far has been relatively small.

In another genetic disorder involving apoB in which apoB-48 appears to be synthesized, chylomicron particles can be formed from fat; however, apoB-100 is not synthesized by the liver and is absent from the circulation.

A group of families has been studied with premature coronary disease but with normal levels of total cholesterol and LDL cholesterol and an increased proportion of apoB in LDL and VLDL, a condition termed *hyperapolipoproteinemia B.*[59] The VLDL particles are smaller, denser, and more protein-enriched. A group of individuals was also observed with coronary disease who had apoB levels in the same range as patients with familial hypercholesterolemia, but who had much lower concentrations of total cholesterol and LDL cholesterol than did individuals with familial hypercholesterolemia. Whether the hyperapoB as it was defined is an independent risk factor and whether apoB itself is in some way atherogenic remains to be determined.

DIAGNOSIS OF HYPERLIPOPROTEINEMIA

The first step in the approach to the patient with suspected hyperlipoproteinemia is an accurate determination of plasma lipoprotein concentrations. Cholesterol screening may be done on nonfasting subjects. If the cholesterol value is over 200 mg/dl, the test should be repeated. If the results again are over 200 mg/dl, lipoprotein testing should be done after an overnight fast. Patients should be on their usual diet, and at a stable weight. If possible, they should not be taking antihyperlipidemic medications and should not be acutely ill. From the fasting sample, cholesterol, HDL, and triglyceride should be measured. LDL cholesterol can be calculated by a formula, unless the patient has severe hypertriglyceridemia (triglyceride over 400 mg/dl) or has Type III hyperlipoproteinemia.

HDL is determined by measuring the cholesterol that is in solution after precipitating the apoB-containing lipoproteins, VLDL, IDL, and LDL. (IDL is included with the VLDL.) The LDL cholesterol is calculated by the following formula:

$$\text{LDL} = \text{Total cholesterol} - \text{HDL} - \frac{\text{Triglyceride}}{5}$$

The latter ratio is used as an estimate of VLDL and IDL cholesterol concentrations.

As a general guideline to relate risk to level of LDL, the high-risk group is considered to include individuals with LDL cholesterol over 170 mg/dl, although some clinicians would use a value as low as 140 or 150 mg/dl. The low-risk group is those with LDL cholesterols under 100 mg/dl, while an intermediate-risk group would be individuals with LDL cholesterol levels of 100 to 170 mg/dl. Recently, ratios of LDL to HDL cholesterol have been used as another indicator of risk, especially for individuals in the intermediate-risk group. A patient with ratio greater than 5 would be considered at high risk, 3 to 5 at significant risk, 3 at average risk, 2 to 3 at modest risk, and less than 2, low risk. Thus, the high-risk category would include individuals with total LDL cholesterol values over 170 mg/dl, or who had an HDL/LDL cholesterol value greater than 5. The treatment goal for the high-risk group is to lower the LDL cholesterol below 140 to 150 mg/dl and to reduce the LDL/HDL cholesterol value to less than 3. Although these are rough guidelines and should be considered only as approximations, they may be of use in interpreting the HDL/LDL ratios.

TYPING OF HYPERLIPOPROTEINEMIA

As of this writing, the classification of hyperlipoproteinemias proposed by Fredrickson and Lees[59a] remains a practical approach for the physician. The system is based on laboratory definitions and does not define genetic abnormalities, underlying pathophysiology, or take into account HDL. The various forms or the genetic hyperlipoproteinemias, their characteristics, and the lipoprotein types they may produce are summarized in Table 36–5.

TYPE I HYPERLIPOPROTEINEMIA AND EXOGENOUS HYPERTRIGLYCERIDEMIA. The accumulation of chylomicrons in the fasting plasma result in a creamy supernatant above a clear infranatant and is characteristic of Type I hyperlipoproteinemia. Clinically, Type I hyperlipoproteinemia may be associated with poorly controlled diabetes mellitus, pancreatitis, or dysglobulinemia as secondary conditions. The primary form is not associated with the complications of premature atherosclerosis. The primary familial forms are quite rare and have two underlying causes: one is the absence or inactivity of the enzyme lipoprotein lipase and the other is the lack of its activator, apoC-II. Familial lipoprotein lipase deficiency is indicated clinically by lipemia retinalis, eruptive xanthomas, and hepatosplenomegaly in the presence of massive hypertriglyceridemia and normal cholesterol. Abdominal pain and pancreatitis are frequent complications. The genetic absence of lipoprotein lipase is rare and occurs only with a frequency of 1 per million. The disease may be suspected from plasma samples in a patient with the aforementioned clinical manifestations, and with fasting chylomicronemia plus normal or only slightly elevated cholesterol and VLDL. Specific assays for lipoprotein lipase and apoC-II are available if necessary.

TYPE II HYPERLIPOPROTEINEMIA. This type of hyperli-

TABLE 36–5 HYPERLIPOPROTEINEMIA PHENOTYPE DEFINITIONS AND THEIR ASSOCIATION WITH GENETIC AND OTHER DISORDERS

Phenotype	Laboratory Definition	Associated with Genetic Disorders	Conditions Associated with Secondary Hyperlipoproteinemia
Type I	Hyperchylomicronemia and absolute deficiency of LPL Cholesterol normal Triglycerides greatly increased	Familial LPL* deficiency ApoC-II deficiency	Dysglobulinemia, pancreatitis, poorly controlled diabetes mellitus
Type IIa	LDL† increased Cholesterol increased Triglycerides normal	Familial hypercholesterolemia LDL receptor abnormal Familial combined hyperlipidemia Polygenic hypercholesterolemia	Hypothyroidism, acute intermittent porphyria, nephrosis, idiopathic hypercalcemia, dysglobulinemia, anorexia nervosa
Type IIb	LDL increased VLDL‡ increased Cholesterol increased Triglycerides increased	Familial hypercholesterolemia Familial combined hyperlipidemia	
Type III	Floating β lipoproteins VLDL cholesterol/VLDL triglyceride >0.35 ApoE-II homozygote on isoelectric focusing Cholesterol increased Triglycerides increased	Familial dysbetalipoproteinemia	Diabetes mellitus, hypothyroidism, dysglobulinemia (monoclonal gammopathy)
Type IV	VLDL increased Cholesterol normal or increased Triglycerides increased	Familial hypertriglyceridemia Familial combined hyperlipidemia	Glycogen storage disease, hypothyroidism, disseminated lupus erythematosus, diabetes mellitus, nephrotic syndrome, renal failure, ethanol abuse
Type V	Chylomicrons and VLDL increased LDL present but reduced Cholesterol increased Triglycerides greatly increased	Familial hypertriglyceridemia Familial multiple lipoprotein type hyperlipidemia	Poorly controlled diabetes mellitus, glycogen storage disease, hypothyroidism, nephrotic syndrome, dysglobulinemia, pregnancy, estrogen administration (either contraceptive or therapeutic) in women with familial hypertriglyceridemia

From Gotto, A. M.: Practical approach to phenotyping hyperlipoproteinemia. *In* Kligfield, P. D. (ed.): Cardiology Reference Book. New York, Co-Medica, Inc., 1984.
*Lipoprotein lipase.
†Low-density lipoproteins.
‡Very low-density lipoproteins.

poproteinemia is defined as an elevation of total plasma cholesterol and, predominantly, LDL cholesterol. In Type IIa hyperlipoproteinemia, triglycerides and VLDL are normal and in Type IIb, they are elevated. Type IIa, or isolated elevation of LDL, may be genetic or secondary to underlying diseases such as hypothyroidism, nephrosis, and dysglobulinemia.

The most common cause of an isolated elevation of cholesterol and LDL-cholesterol is *polygenic hypercholesterolemia* (p. 1637). This may account for as many as 85 per cent of individuals detected to have hypercholesterolemia by routine screening, although the exact incidence of polygenic hypercholesterolemia in patients with Type II phenotype is unknown. Polygenic hypercholesterolemia is not well understood from a genetic standpoint; it is a disease state in which LDL is elevated without a definite single-gene disorder being implicated. Presumably, exogenous factors interact with poorly understood genetic factors. Increased LDL synthesis, defective LDL catabolism, or both are implicated. Dietary treatment alone significantly reduces cholesterol levels in most of these patients.

Primary Type II hyperlipoproteinemia may be due to familial hypercholesterolemia, which is inherited as an autosomal dominant; the gene frequency is 1 in 500 for the heterozygote and 1 in 1 million for the homozygote (p. 1639). Familial hypercholesterolemia has a strong association with premature atherosclerosis and may be expressed in childhood in the homozygous form. While levels of LDL are elevated, the HDL levels are reduced.[60] Deficiency of the cell-surface receptor for LDL is the biochemical hallmark of familial hypercholesterolemia: heterozygotes have approximately 50 per cent fewer LDL receptors.

Patients with familial hypercholesterolemia frequently have dermatological manifestations of elevated LDL such as tendinous xanthomas (Figs. 2–2, p. 17, and Fig. 49–6, p. 1638) which are relatively specific for Type II. These lesions appear on extensor tendons such as the Achilles and forearm tendons and may result in exercise-associated tendinitis.[61] Additionally, these patients have corneal arcus and xanthomas in other areas. Premature development of arcus is an indication for lipid evaluation but may occur in normal persons and may be absent in patients with marked elevation of cholesterol.[62] Xanthomas are a common clinical finding in patients with Type II hyperlipoproteinemia but are not specific or sensitive for diagnostic purposes.

Cholesterol concentrations in the heterozygote range from 300 to 500 mg/dl, with an average of 350 mg/dl; *homozygotes* have levels of 600 to 1200 mg/dl. The vascular complications for familial hypercholesterolemia are well described and may occur in infancy or early childhood in the homozygote. Homozygous Type II patients have relentless coronary and peripheral atherosclerosis, with the disease generally becoming clinically evident by adolescence. Valvular structures may also be involved and aortic stenosis is well documented.[63] Heterozygotes are also affected and early myocardial infarction is the rule. There is an increased severity of disease manifestations in males; in one study, the mean age at onset of an acute ischemic myocardial event was 43 in heterozygous males and 53 in females.[64]

In addition to familial hypercholesterolemia and polygenic hypercholesterolemia, *familial combined hyperlipoproteinemia* (p. 1643) may present as a Type II phenotype.[65, 66] This disease is associated with premature atherosclerosis. Gene frequency of the autosomal dominant disorder is estimated at 1 in 200.[67] It may be manifested phenotypically as Type IIa, IIb, or IV. The metabolic abnormality is thought to be an overproduction of hepatic apoB which is found in LDL and VLDL.[68] The actual clinical manifestations are a function of fat intake, obesity, and other unknown factors. The diagnosis is difficult to establish and may require family studies. Tendon xanthomas are rare.[69]

A number of *secondary* causes of Type II hyperlipoproteinemia have been recognized. The nephrotic syndrome and hypothyroidism may produce Type IIa or IIb HLP. Hepatic VLDL synthesis is increased in the nephrotic syndrome. Biliary obstruction is unique in that an abnormal lipoprotein (LpX) accumulates and accounts for a significant fraction of the resultant hypercholesterolemia. This lipoprotein is similar in electrophoretic mobility to LDL but contains an increased proportion of unesterified cholesterol and phospholipid. Acute intermittent porphyria is a rare cause of Type II hyperlipoproteinemia.

Pe'er et al.[70] examined the relationship between corneal arcus and coronary artery disease in 150 adults aged 55 in Israel. The corneal arcus (Fig. 36–9) occurs commonly with aging and has also long been known to be associated with hypercholesterolemia, particularly Type II hyperlipoproteinemia, and familial hypercholesterolemia. The histological characteristic is an accumulation of lipids at the periphery of the cornea and the peripheral corneal stroma, Bowman's membrane, and Descemet's membrane. This forms a ringlike opacity. The central part of the cornea is not involved in the arcus. The association of corneal arcus with Type II and Type III hyperlipoproteinemia is of interest. In the Israeli study, it was found that the corneal arcus occurred with more frequency in males and that the frequency and size of corneal arcus correlated positively with age. There was also a positive correlation between the levels of cholesterol and LDL levels in males and the size of the arcus. Of interest is the fact that diastolic blood pressure was negatively correlated with corneal arcus. Other coronary risk factors including concentrations of plasma triglyceride, HDL, and VLDL, weight, glucose, smoking, and obesity did not correlate with corneal arcus.

TYPE III HYPERLIPOPROTEINEMIA. This form of hyperlipoproteinemia (also called broad beta disease or dysbetalipoproteinemia) is an uncommon disorder which is usually diagnosed after the patient reaches age 20 and is associated with premature atherosclerosis.[71] Patients with Type III hyperlipoproteinemia have markedly elevated cholesterol (from 300 to 1000 mg/dl) and triglyceride levels which are derived from incomplete catabolism of chylomicrons and VLDL. Lipoprotein electrophoresis reveals an increase in VLDL (pre-beta) and a second band which encompasses both VLDL and LDL fractions. This broad band contains remnant intermediates called beta-VLDL's. The normal ratio of VLDL cholesterol to total triglycerides is less than 0.2. In Type III, this ratio is higher than 0.3.[72]

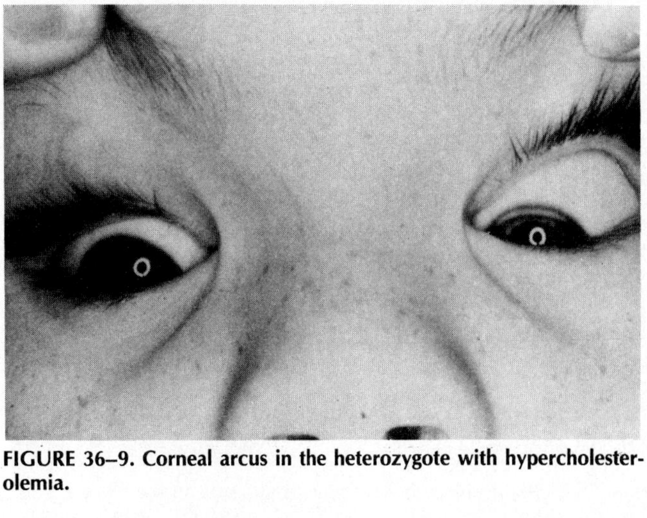

FIGURE 36–9. Corneal arcus in the heterozygote with hypercholesterolemia.

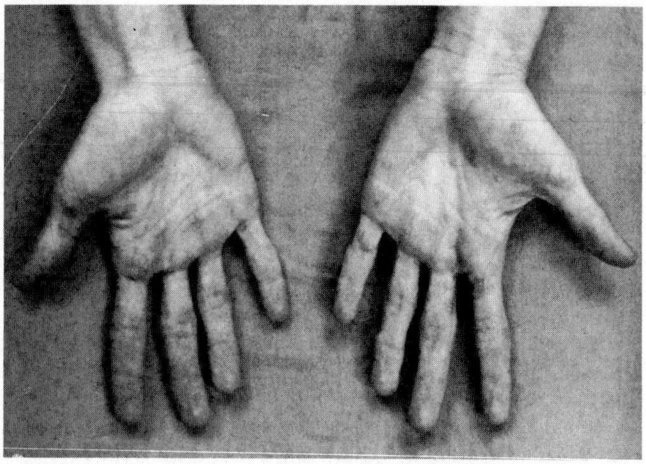

FIGURE 36–10. Palmar xanthomas.

The beta-VLDL contains the apoE-II isomorph described above.[73] ApoE normally facilitates the uptake by the liver of chylomicron remnants which accumulate in Type III.[74] In addition to the apoE-II homozygotes, some patients may rarely manifest a Type III pattern in association with a deficiency of hepatic triglyceride lipase.[75] Delineation of apoE subtypes is a very useful diagnostic tool for Type III but is not readily available.[76] Type III is associated with premature vascular disease and may be unmasked by excessive alcohol intake or hypothyroidism. The physical examination may be normal in Type III. However, a characteristic palmar lesion, xanthoma stria palmaris, which consists of yellow streaks in the palmar creases, is frequently present (Fig. 36–10). Xanthomas called *tuberoeruptive xanthomas* may also be present over the tibial tuberosities and elbows (Fig 36–11). *Tendon xanthomas* which are common in Type II are rare in Type III.[77]

TYPE IV HYPERLIPOPROTEINEMIA. This form is caused by an accumulation of VLDL, which results in a cloudy appearance of fasting plasma. Type IV may be genetic in origin or may occur secondary to another disease. Two main genetic patterns are recognized. Familial or primary endogenous hypertriglyceridemia is transmitted as an autosomal dominant disorder. The disorder is relatively common and the incidence of the heterozygote form is 1 per cent of the general population. VLDL production is increased in this condition[78] and HDL concentrations are often low. The metabolic defect appears to be an oversynthesis of triglyceride and VLDL by the liver in which large, triglyceride-rich particles are produced. Triglyceride levels are generally in the 200 to 500 mg/dl range. Familial combined hyperlipoproteinemia, discussed above, is a disorder with variable expression and may also present as Type IV. Triglyceride, cholesterol, or both may be elevated and the variable phenotypes in a given family are common in the familial combined type. Regardless of the phenotypic pattern in individual patients, there is a tendency for the premature development of vascular disease in the familial combined hyperlipidemias. The risk for patients with familial hypertriglyceridemia is less clearly delineated since their ratio of LDL to total cholesterol is frequently normal.[79]

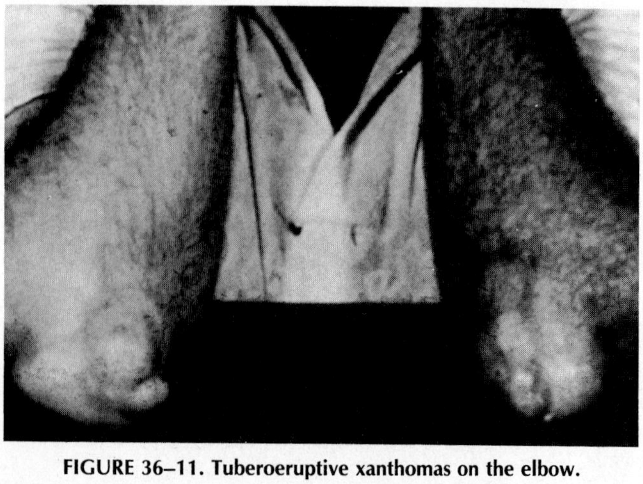

FIGURE 36–11. Tuberoeruptive xanthomas on the elbow.

Secondary causes of a Type IV pattern are common and should be actively sought; a few include excess dietary calories or alcohol, renal failure, diabetes mellitus, hepatocellular disease (glycogen or lipid storage), and dysproteinemias. Diabetes is frequently associated with elevated triglycerides. Multiple mechanisms are probably involved in the elevated triglyceride in diabetes. Obese diabetics who are insensitive to the action of insulin require elevated levels of insulin to maintain a given level of glucose. VLDL synthesis is increased secondary to the elevated insulin levels. In diabetics who lack insulin, the mechanism is more complex and relates to the level of lipoprotein lipase activity. The antilipolytic action of insulin lowers substrate availability for hepatic free fatty acid incorporation into triglycerides by diminishing free fatty acid release from adipocytes. Additionally, insulin is required to maintain adequate activity of lipoprotein lipase. With insulin deficiency, the enzyme activity required for breakdown of triglycerides and chylomicrons is diminished and these substances may accumulate in the blood. Exogenous insulin restores lipoprotein lipase and prevents marked elevations of VLDL and chylomicrons. Reduced lipoprotein lipase activity also occurs in myxedema and renal failure, and this may account for the elevated triglyceride levels in these conditions, although hypercholesterolemia is usually present as well as hyperthyroidism.

TYPE V HYPERLIPOPROTEINEMIA. This unusual form of hyperlipoproteinemia, or mixed hypertriglyceridemia, is characterized by marked elevations of VLDL and chylomicrons and normal to low levels of LDL. The diagnosis is generally made in the adult age group. Type V plasma has a creamy supernatant overlying a turbid, VLDL-rich serum. The underlying causes are complex and include genetic and secondary factors. The mode of inheritance and expression are not well delineated because of the rarity of the condition and its variable expression. Although elevations of chylomicrons are generally associated with a decreased level of lipoprotein lipase, some activity is present, unlike the situation in Type I. However, in Type V there appear to be both an overproduction of VLDL and a diminished clearance of VLDL and chylomicrons.

The familial forms of Type V are frequently associated with glucose intolerance and hyperuricemia. Obesity, especially when associated with rapid weight gain, also predisposes to a Type V pattern. The Type V pattern may also be seen in patients with the genetic forms of hypertriglyceridemia; effective treatment will remove chylomicrons and revert the phenotype to Type IV or in some instances to Type IIb. Other secondary factors involved in Type V hyperlipoproteinemia are excessive alcohol consumption and exogenous estrogens.[80] Marked elevations of triglyceride may result in pancreatitis, which may be fatal. Triglyceride levels over approximately 2000 mg/dl are associated with eruptive xanthoma, lipemia retinalis, and hepatosplenomegaly. A polyneuropathy associated with numbness and tingling in the extremities may be noted, although, on a clinical basis, it may be difficult to separate the hyperlipidemic-associated neuropathy from that caused by associated diabetes.[81] The involvement of other risk factors for premature atherosclerosis such as diabetes, hypertension, and obesity cloud the evaluation of the primary risk with Type V per se.[82, 83]

TREATMENT OF HYPERLIPOPROTEINEMIA

Before treatment is initiated, a careful medical examination should be performed to determine if the hyperlipoproteinemia is secondary to an underlying disease or is primary or genetic. A careful dietary history should be taken to obtain information about the relative proportions of cholesterol and total and saturated fat in the diet. Underlying diseases such as diabetes mellitus, renal insufficiency, hypothyroidism, biliary obstruction, nephrotic liver disease, and dysproteinemia should be optimally treated and separated from the primary hyperlipoproteinemias, which are presumably genetic and for which no underlying disease is present. Lipid values should be repeated sequentially both to assess efficacy of therapy and to determine whether the phenotypic pattern has changed.

The use of medications that can affect lipids should be documented and the need for continuation determined. Commonly used medications which elevate cholesterol, LDL, triglyceride, and VLDL include the thiazide diuretics and beta blockers. Estrogens tend to raise HDL cholesterol and VLDL-triglyceride levels, although their effect on cardiac risk, especially in postmenopausal females, is the subject of current debate.[84–86] Users of oral contraceptives tend to have increased levels of serum cholesterol[87, 88]; however, the effect on blood lipids is a function of the relative amounts of estrogen and progesterone in the different preparations.[89, 90] Progesterone analogs decrease elevated levels of triglyceride but also decrease HDL. The effect of antihypertensive agents on blood lipids is complex. Beta blockers, except those with intrinsic sympathomimetic activity, have been shown to lower the HDL fraction of total cholesterol.[91] This effect on HDL was verified in the BHAT study, although propranolol had been shown to improve survival after a myocardial infarction.[92] Alpha-adrenoceptor blockers such as prazosin do not adversely affect plasma lipids and lipoproteins, but whether or not this will translate into a protective effect on survival has not been demonstrated.[93, 94] The calcium antagonists, the angiotensin-converting enzyme inhibitors, and drugs affecting the central nervous system, such as clonidine and guanabenz have generally been found to have neutral effects on plasma lipids. Diuretics also adversely affect plasma lipoproteins and lipids, mainly by increasing LDL, VLDL, cholesterol, and triglyceride rather than by lowering HDL.

DIET THERAPY

Since it has been shown that lowering of serum cholesterol translates to a lower risk, all patients with hyperlipoproteinemia should have a careful dietary assessment. Diet therapy should be the initial mode of therapy and should be continued even if pharmacological treatment is instituted. Weight loss and moderate exercise may aid in lowering serum cholesterol and should be encouraged. Lipid levels may be altered by the total caloric and cholesterol intake, the percentage of fat ingested relative to other nutrients, and the type of fat ingested. Dietary cholesterol may indirectly affect the plasma cholesterol by increasing the level of intrahepatic cholesterol, thereby decreasing the number or activity of LDL receptors. This results in a secondary risk in plasma levels due to diminished hepatic LDL uptake. Dietary cholesterol should be limited to less than 300 mg/day.

TABLE 36–6 DIETARY GOALS OF PHASES 1, 2, AND 3 IN PREVENTION AND TREATMENT OF CAD

PHASE	1	2	3
Fat (% calories)	30	25	20
Carbohydrate (% calories)	55	60	65
Protein (% calories)	15	15	15
Cholesterol (mg)	300	200–250	100–150
P/S*	1	1	1–2

Adapted from American Heart Association Special Report: Recommendations for treatment by hyperlipidemia in adults. Circulation 69:1065A, 1984, by permission of the American Heart Association, Inc.

*Ratio of polyunsaturated fat to saturated fat.

The American Heart Association has developed a progressive diet approach for patients with hyperlipidemia, and for persons who want to prevent CAD (Table 36–6). Levels of fat, carbohydrate, protein, and cholesterol are given in three phases and are graded according to the person's total caloric needs. The patient can progress to a more restrictive level if necessary. Phase I is the diet recommended to the general population for prevention of CAD.[95] The quantity of calories is based on achieving and maintaining ideal body weight. The total percentage of calories from fat should not exceed 30, and the absolute quantity of fat calories is proportionately scaled down for weight reduction, i.e., saturated, mono-, and polyunsaturated fats are proportionately reduced if the caloric intake decreases. Daily cholesterol intake is also based on total calories consumed but should not exceed 100 mg/1000 kcal of energy and would average 250 to 300 mg/day for a 2500- to 3000-calorie diet.

Polyunsaturated fats of the n-6 family lower serum cholesterol to the extent that they are used to replace saturated fat. Recent studies with monounsaturates suggest that they also lower LDL and cholesterol when substituted for saturated fat.[96] The diet recommended by the American Heart Association reduces total dietary fat to 30 per cent of calories, to be equally distributed between polyunsaturated, saturated, and monounsaturated fat. Carbohydrate intake affects triglyceride levels. Transient hypertriglyceridemia may occur in patients who begin a high carbohydrate diet after being on a high fat diet. However, kinetic studies have demonstrated that lower sustained levels of triglycerides will occur with a high carbohydrate diet. Alcohol should be restricted to 2 oz per day in persons with hypertriglyceridemia.

Omega-3 Unsaturated Fatty Acids

The value of consuming oil from cold-water fish for protection against coronary disease has been debated. Greenland Eskimos have been reported to have a relatively low incidence of atherosclerotic heart disease,[97] although this assumption is not backed by extensive data. In research on this effect, several metabolic changes were noted in subjects consuming the fish. These fish oils are rich in eicosopentaenoic acid, an omega-3 unsaturated fat, which replaces arachidonic acid in the membrane of platelets. A prolonged bleeding time has been described with a reduction in platelet aggregation, as has a decrease in thrombotic tendency. Eicosopentaenoic acid and docosahexaenoic acid appear to be the most important omega-3 fatty acids in the cold-water fish.[98, 99] Fish that contain omega-3 fatty acids include salmon (Chinook, sockeye, coho, pink, and Atlantic), mackerel, rainbow trout, sardines, lake whitefish, sablefish, bluefin, and albacore tuna.

The exact mechanism by which omega-3 fats affect the bleeding time has not been elucidated. The change in bleeding time may not necessarily be explained in terms of ratio of prostacyclin to thromboxane A_2 or to PGI_3 formation (p. 1760). The most striking effect of the omega-3 fatty acids on plasma lipids is a reduction in the concentration of triglycerides and VLDL. At high concentrations of omega-3 fatty acids, LDL and cholesterol concentrations may also be suppressed, but this is quantitatively less significant than the reduction of VLDL. There appears to be a suppression of VLDL synthesis by the liver.[100]

Simons et al.[101] fed an encapsulated preparation of fish oil called Maxepa to hyperlipidemic patients in a dosage of 6 to 16 gm per day over a 3-month period. In Types IIa and IIb hyperlipoproteinemia, there was no substantial decrease in cholesterol concentrations. However, triglycerides were significantly reduced in Types IIb and IV, by 28 and 41 per cent, respectively. In patients with Type V, 16 gm of fish oil per day reduced triglycerides by 58 per cent. In Type V, while VLDL cholesterol was reduced by 42 per cent, LDL cholesterol rose by 7 per cent and HDL cholesterol by 6 per cent. These investigators observed no significant change in bleeding time, platelet count, and blood viscosity during their studies.

Thorngren et al.[102] fed healthy male volunteers a fish diet for 6 weeks. The fatty acid composition of the platelet membranes changed within a week of the beginning of the fish diet, with the composition of the omega-6 fatty acids decreasing and that of omega-3 increasing. There was also a decrease in the ability of adenosine diphosphate and collagen to aggregate the platelets, but the bleeding time was not changed. The bleeding time increased after 6 weeks on the diet, by 37 per cent. The bleeding time was still increased 3 weeks after the diet was terminated when the fatty acid composition of the platelets had returned to normal.

There was no correlation between the decrease in the aggregability of the platelets and their fatty acid composition and in the bleeding time. The platelets were less sensitive to aggregation by ADP and collagen, even several weeks after the fatty acid composition had reverted to the predietary level and after the bleeding time became normal. No change in thromboxane A_2 occurred in vivo as a consequence of the diet. There were changes in the in vitro formation of thromboxane A_2 in clotting venous blood. These observations illustrate the complexities of the effects of fish diet on thrombostasis and show that their effects on hemostasis cannot be explained simply by a decrease in the formation of thromboxane A_2 locally, by a decrease in the aggregability of platelets, or by a change in the fatty acid composition of the membranes.

The authors suggest that the discrepancy between the effects of the fish diet on thromboxane A_2 formation in vitro and in vivo might be based on the fact that all of the platelets in clotting venous blood are maximally activated and produce all the thromboxane that can be formed from available arachidonic acid. The rest of the explanation would be that in vivo only a small part of the platelets are activated, and only a part of the total thromboxane A_2 forming capacity is used. Thus, in bleeding time blood (that is, the blood used in determining a bleeding time), much less thromboxane A_2 would be required and formed, and no difference would be observed between those on the diet and controls. The fact that the effects of diet continue after the diet is stopped and after the platelet fatty acid composition reverts indicates that some other unknown factor or factors must be involved. Since hemostasis depends on the platelets, the reactivity of injured vessels, and plasma coagulation, dietary changes might also influence bleeding by altering the coagulation mechanism or the properties of the endothelial cells.

Brox et al.[103] fed cod liver oil to patients with familial hypercholesterolemia, or Type IIa hyperlipoproteinemia. After 30 ml of cod liver oil was ingested as a dietary supplement for 6 weeks, the bleeding times were not significantly prolonged, unlike in the study of Thorngren et al. However, these authors did find a decrease in thromboxane generation in vitro and a decrease in collagen-induced platelet aggregation. Neither of these changes correlated with any changes in platelet behavior similar to the results of Thorngren et al. These investigators did not note any change in HDL, cholesterol, or triglyceride during the trial. One cautionary note in the feeding of cod liver oil is that toxic levels of vitamin A may be obtained if too high a dose is taken.

In a study[104] in which Western diet was supplemented with 40 ml of cod liver oil per day, providing approximately 10 gm of omega-3 fatty acids (about one-third more than what was provided in the study by Brox et al.), bleeding time increased while platelet aggregation decreased. The in vitro changes in thromboxane B_2 formation as noted above were observed. Both the blood pressure and the blood pressure response to norepinepherine and angiotensin II decreased in these subjects. It is important to note that the in vitro observations do not necessarily correspond to what occurs in vivo, as described in the article by Thorngren et al.

As of this writing, omega-3 fatty acid agents are being advertised for the prevention of CAD. At relatively low doses, 3 to 5 mg/day, the effect is primarily on the blood platelets and eicosanoid metabolism. At much higher doses, the synthesis of VLDL and triglycerides is inhibited. In the absence of any controlled clinical trial, the authors favor a cautious approach of increasing the dietary consumption of cold-water fish such as salmon, which are rich in omega-3 fatty acids. Incorporation of such fish into the diet a minimum of twice a week seems prudent, pending further information. The authors do not recommend the routine use of omega-3 supplements as of this writing.

DRUG TREATMENT

Drug therapy of lipid disorders should not be employed until a diagnosis is firmly established and a maximal dietary effort has been sustained. Diet therapy is the mainstay of treatment; a strenuous effort must be made to lower elevated lipid values by nonpharmacological means. Secondary causes of hyperlipidemia should also be identified and treated. If these measures fail, drug therapy should be initiated, with diet therapy continued even after pharmacological therapy is begun.

One can find various approaches and algorithms to treating hyperlipoproteinemia. Hoeg et al.[105] recommend that individuals with LDL cholesterol above the 75th percentile be treated with diet and that those whose cholesterol levels are not reduced below 200 mg/dl by diet alone be treated with diet and drugs. They recommend treating with diet those patients with triglyceride levels between 200 and 500 mg/dl. If the triglyceride level stays above 500 and the patient is at high risk for pancreatitis or has a strong personal or family history of coronary disease, drugs along with diet are recommended. For those with triglyceride levels over 1000 mg/dl, Hoeg et al. recommend dietary modification and referral to a specialized center for evaluation and treatment if levels are not adequately controlled. If the LDL cholesterol remains over 200 mg/dl after 3 to 6 months on a diet, they recommend nicotinic acid as the drug of choice, unless diabetes mellitus, peptic ulcer disease, or symptomatic gout is present.

The authors' approach[106, 107] is as follows: For individuals with cholesterol values above the 75th percentile due to a primary elevation of LDL, the diet is begun, with 4 to 6 weeks allowed for each progressive phase. Cholesterol and lipoprotein levels are retested before the next phase of the diet is undertaken. For most individuals, in the 75th to 90th percentile range, diet alone will be sufficient. If cholesterol and LDL levels remain above the 75th percentile after 3 to 6 months of maximal dietary therapy, the patient is evaluated for possible drug therapy. An LDL cholesterol level of over 170 mg/dl after a dietary trial is an indication for drug therapy. Individuals with LDL cholesterol values under 100 mg/dl are at relatively low risk. Depending on the age and individual circumstance, a question may be raised about the use of a cholesterol-lowering drug for LDL cholesterol levels between 140 and 170 mg/dl. Each case must be individualized, taking into account age, family history, and clinical status. A ratio of LDL cholesterol to HDL cholesterol of greater than 3 or total cholesterol to HDL cholesterol of greater than 4.5 place the patient at additional risk, since HDL and LDL are independent risk factors for CAD. One of the bile acid sequestrants, cholestyramine or colestipol, is the authors' choice for lowering cholesterol. Nicotinic acid should be added if this drug fails or if a second drug is added, such as gemfibrozil, clofibrate, probucol, or neomycin. If neomycin is used, the patient should be followed closely with audiograms for ototoxicity.

BILE ACID SEQUESTRANTS. Cholestyramine and colestipol are quarternary ammonium salts that act as anion exchange resins which bind bile salts in the intestine. This binding results in an interruption of the enterohepatic circulation of bile salts with resultant loss in the stool. The increased loss of cholesterol will lower the level within the liver, augment LDL receptor activity, and increase the uptake via the receptor. Cholestyramine and colestipol are effective in Type II hyperlipoproteinemia,[108] particularly if the cholesterol is moderately elevated as in the sporadic or polygenic forms. They are usually not sufficient as single agents if the cholesterol is severely elevated in cases of heterozygotes with Type II. No single-drug therapy is usually effective in the rare homozygous Type II, although combination drug therapy with a bile acid sequestrant and HMG CoA reductase inhibitor may be beneficial in patients with some residual LDL receptor activity. Probucol has been reported to be useful in some homozygotes in South Africa.[108a]

The bile acid sequestrants are difficult to administer due to frequent and often severe side effects and problems with drug interactions. Major side effects are gastrointestinal; systemic effects are uncommon due to lack of absorption. However, the resins may bind concomitantly administered medications such as digitalis, phenobarbital, thiazide, warfarin, thyroxine, tetracycline, and phenylbutazone, and decrease their absorption.

If possible, blood levels or the effects of the drugs should be monitored. The resins come in a granulated preparation in 4 or 5 gm packets, and should be mixed with fluids and taken with meals. They should not be taken with drugs that may be bound. The initial dose for both should be low (e.g., one packet per day before a meal) and should be increased by 1 packet per day after a week or more. For patients who tolerate the drug, the average dosage is 3 to 6 packets per day, usually given in divided doses with meals. Although the maximum dosage is difficult to attain due to poor patient compliance, it will produce an LDL lowering of 25 to 30 per cent. However, a 20 per cent reduction is considered a good response. Only a 9 per cent reduction of cholesterol was achieved in the CPPT despite the extensive use of counseling by adherence counselors as well as physicians. The degree of cholesterol lowering is proportional to the dosage of drug taken; continued use of these drugs will result in a lowering of LDL cholesterol which translates into a decreased risk from atherosclerosis.

NICOTINIC ACID. This is a B vitamin which is used in dosages that far exceed the levels required for its action as a vitamin; at a daily dose of 3 to 5 gm per day, it is effective in all types of hyperlipoproteinemia except Type I. It decreases LDL by about 25 per cent and VLDL by approximately 75 per cent by blocking hepatic VLDL synthesis with a subsequent reduction in LDL formation.[109] Nicotinic acid also inhibits the release of fatty acids from adipose tissue and thus decreases the substrate available to the liver for triglyceride synthesis. Nicotinic acid increases HDL levels by 20 to 40 per cent, probably as a result of decreased VLDL production.[110] Side effects common with nicotinic acid are cutaneous flushing and gastrointestinal symptoms. Flushing and pruritus usually occur within an hour of administration and can best be minimized by taking the drug with meals plus aspirin. The flushing tends to decrease with time; its basis is a prostaglandin-mediated capillary dilation. The gastrointestinal side effects relate to elevations of liver enzymes and gastritis, which may be severe. The drug should be avoided in patients with a propensity for peptic ulcer disease. Increased pigmentation of the skin may occur, especially in the axilla and groin. Because elevations of hepatic enzymes may occur, liver function tests should be monitored. Other problems caused by the drug are impaired glucose tolerance and hyperuricemia; however, this is rarely a problem except in patients with gout or hyperuricemia. The dose should initially be low (e.g., 50 mg with each meal) and gradually advanced to 1 gram 3 times a day. A major benefit of nicotinic acid is the lowering of LDL when it is given in combination with colestipol or cholestyramine.

PROBUCOL. This drug lowers both HDL and LDL fractions.[111] LDL cholesterol reductions of an average of 20 per cent can be expected. The lowering of HDL is of concern; however, an intervention study with probucol and colestipol using angiographic endpoints[111a] was interpreted as showing stabilization of established coronary lesions and prevention of new ones despite a concomitant reduction of both HDL and LDL. In some patients, the level of LDL might overshadow the significance of changes in HDL, which might be of importance in individuals with lower levels of LDL. For example, the most consistent finding in patients with myocardial infarction is a low level of HDL. Intervention in these patients may require a different strategy from that in patients with severe Type II hyperlipoproteinemia. The mechanism of action is unknown, but cholesterol synthesis has been reported to decrease in combination with decreased absorption of cholesterol and increased excretion.[112] The drug is lipophilic and may be incorporated into LDL. In Watanabe rabbits lacking the LDL receptor, probucol enhances LDL clearance, presumably by the macrophage or scavenger pathway, with no apparent effect on VLDL. Hence, probucol is most efficacious in the treatment of patients with Type II hyperlipoproteinemia. Probucol may be combined with a bile acid sequestering agent for an additional effect on LDL lowering. The effect of HDL lowering on CAD risk is unknown. The major side effects of probucol are gastrointestinal in nature and are generally mild when the drug is used as a single agent. The usual dosage is 500 mg twice a day with meals.

GEMFIBROZIL. This is a fibric acid derivative which is effective in lowering VLDL, IDL, and triglycerides.[113] Although the exact mechanism of action is unknown, one apparent effect is to increase lipoprotein lipase activity, thus increasing clearance of VLDL and VLDL remnants on IDL. Cholesterol excretion into bile is also increased. The drug is quite effective in lowering triglycerides; decreases of 50 per cent can be seen without significant toxicity. Additionally, HDL levels have been increased by as much as 20 per cent.[114] LDL levels may increase, particularly in the face of severe hypertriglyceridemia. While the most common side effects are nausea and gastrointestinal discomfort, myositis and impaired glucose tolerance have been noted. It is important to be aware that all fibric acid derivatives may potentiate the effect of Coumadin anticoagulants. The usual dose is 600 mg twice a day.

CLOFIBRATE. This drug decreases LDL and VLDL cholesterol and is mainly used to treat Type III and IV hyperlipoproteinemias. In the World Health Organization's primary intervention trial, clofibrate use was associated with a decline in nonfatal myocardial infarction. However, an increase in noncardiac death and in overall mortality was reported.[115] Also, clofibrate use has been associated with lithogenic bile and an increased frequency of gallstones. Other side effects are nausea, abdominal discomfort, and, uncommonly, ventricular arrhythmia, changes in liver function, and a syndrome of muscle tenderness and increase in muscle enzymes. Clofibrate acts to increase lipoprotein lipase and the biliary excretion of sterols, with a resultant decrease in triglyceride level of about 40 per cent. If the triglycerides are elevated, clofibrate may increase the conversion of VLDL to LDL with an untoward elevation of LDL. In general, with Type II hyperlipoproteinemia, the reduction in cholesterol is modest and is approximately 10 per cent. The IDL fraction which is increased in Type III hyperlipoproteinemia is markedly reduced and clofibrate is a mainstay of therapy. However, until the effects of clofibrate on noncardiac mortality are more clearly defined from a cause-and-effect standpoint, its use should be restricted to patients in whom other medications have failed and in those with Type III hyperlipoproteinemia.

DEXTROTHYROXINE. This drug, the dextroisomer of the naturally occurring thyroid hormone levothyroxine, is used as a secondary drug in the treatment of Type II hyperlipoproteinemia. Although its effects are unknown, it appears to increase the activity of LDL receptors in hypothyroid animals. This drug should not be used in patients with hypertension, arrhythmias, or suspected significan' underlying coronary atherosclerosis.

HMG CoA REDUCTASE INHIBITORS. Compactin, lovastatin (formerly known as mevinolin), synvinolin,* and eptastatin* are agents that inhibit 3-hydroxy-3-methylglutaryl coenzyme A reductase (HMG CoA), an enzyme in the cholesterol biosynthetic pathway.[116, 117] They can be used in combination with the bile acid sequestrants because they inhibit the resultant increase in the enzyme system induced by these agents. The HMG CoA reductase inhibitors are competitive inhibitors of the rate-limiting enzyme in cholesterol biosynthesis; their side chain resembles the structure of HMG CoA. Compactin and lovastatin are quite similar in structure, differing only in a methyl group on lovastatin in a site where compactin contains a proton. For unexplained reasons, the development of compactin was dropped in Japan because of presumed toxicity in animal experiments. Since these agents do not block the synthesis of HMG CoA reductase but rather inhibit its action competitively, their use actually results in an increased synthesis of the enzyme as the cell attempts to overcome the effects of the competitive inhibition. The main indication for the use of HMG CoA reductase inhibitors is an elevation of LDL cholesterol. In a dosage of 20 to 80 mg/day, lovastatin has been reported to reduce LDL cholesterol by 30 to 40 per cent in heterozygotes for familial hypercholesterolemia. The HMG CoA reductase results in a decrease in cholesterol synthesis and a secondary increase in the level of hepatic LDL receptors. This new class of drugs is very promising.

*Not approved by the FDA at the time of this writing.

OXYSTEROLS. Another type of drug currently being tested is inhibitors of oxysterols. A drug discovered by Schroepfer,[118] 15-ketosterol, has been tested. This drug, the mechanism of which is unknown, shows great promise in primates, in which it has been reported to double the level of HDL, while decreasing LDL concentrations by approximately 50 per cent.

MISCELLANEOUS AND EXPERIMENTAL DRUGS

Neomycin Sulfate. This is an amino glycosite antibiotic which is reported to decrease LDL and LDL cholesterol at a usual dosage of 2 gm/day in divided doses. The drug is not well absorbed in the gastrointestinal tract and has potential nephrotoxicity and ototoxicity. Hoeg et al., who have experience using the drug, have reported decreases in LDL cholesterol of up to 20 to 25 per cent.[105]

Beta Sitosterol. This is another structural analog of cholesterol that contains plant sterols and that acts to decrease cholesterol absorption.[119] It has a relatively mild effect on serum lipids and produces approximately 10 per cent reduction in the concentration of cholesterol and LDL.

Another new class of drug under development is the *inhibitors of acyl cholesterol acyl transferase (ACAT)*. Inhibition of this enzyme in the gut might interfere with the esterification of cholesterol and its subsequent incorporation into chylomicrons, although this has not been established. The binding of LDL to the B,E receptor triggers a set of events that leads to an activation of ACAT and to the intracellular esterification of cholesterol to cholesteryl oleate. By blocking ACAT and increasing the proportion of unesterifed cholesterol in the cell, the ability of the cell to remove cholesterol might be enhanced.

Some potential mechanisms being considered to treat hypercholesterolemia are listed in Table 36–7.

Although probably all of the drugs have multiple actions, a summary of the established mechanisms of drug action on lipoprotein metabolism follows: (1) Nicotinic acid works at the level of the liver, suppressing VLDL synthesis. (2) The fibric acid derivatives gemfibrozil and clofibrate increase the catabolism of VLDL and IDL by enhancing the activity of lipoprotein lipase. (3) The bile acid sequestrants (cholestyramine and colestipol), the HMG CoA reductase inhibitors, and dextrothyroxine increase the activity of hepatic LDL receptors. (4) Probucol may increase clearance via the scavenger or macrophage pathway.

Combination drug therapy, as mentioned above, holds great promise for the future. The bile acid sequestrants have been used in conjunction with nicotinic acid in treating heterozygotes for familial hypercholesterolemia. The bile acid sequestrants have also been used in conjunction with fibric acid derivatives, with HMG CoA reductase

TABLE 36–7 HYPOTHETICAL MECHANISMS OF DRUGS AFFECTING LIPOPROTEIN REGULATION

Scavenger pathway
Lipoprotein lipase (LPL)
Hepatic lipase
Increase hepatic clearance or metabolism
Increase HDL (nicotinic acid, gemfibrozil)
HDL peptide analogs

inhibitors (in which case they reduce LDL cholesterol by over 50 per cent in heterozygotes for familial hypercholesterolemia), and in conjunction with probucol. A combination of nicotinic acid, which decreases the secretion of VLDL, and neomycin sulfate, which decreases cholesterol absorption, reduces LDL cholesterol by about 40 per cent.

TREATMENT SPECIFIC FOR THE HYPERLIPOPROTEINEMIA TYPES

TREATMENT OF TYPE I. Type I is generally diagnosed in the pediatric age group. The treatment for primary Type I is quite difficult—drug therapy is ineffective for lipoprotein lipase–deficient patients and has no role in the treatment plan. With a fat-restricted diet as the cornerstone of therapy, the aim is to lower triglycerides to levels that minimize the risk of recurrent pancreatitis (generally less than 1000 mg/dl). Dietary fat is limited to 10 to 25 gm per day. Medium-chain triglycerides may be used to enhance dietary compliance and provide calories, because they are directly absorbed while being transported from the lacteal via chylomicrons.

The clinical presentation is different for hyperchylomicronemia due to ApoC-II deficiency, and possibly the treatment should be different also. This disease is generally manifested in somewhat older patients; hepatosplenomegaly is not prominent. Although drug therapy is ineffective, ApoC-II may be supplied by plasma infusions in life-threatening situations. While lipoprotein lipase may be absent or lack activation, its biochemical activity may be limited by specific inactivators.[120] Heparin activates lipoprotein lipase and if it is inactivated by high levels of gamma globulin, as in systematic lupus erythematosus, a secondary form of Type I hyperlipidemia may result.

TREATMENT OF TYPE II. Aggressive therapy is mandatory for all patients with the Type II hyperlipoproteinemia because of the high incidence of premature coronary atherosclerosis and vascular disease. Therapy should be based on a proper diagnosis, and secondary causes of elevated cholesterol should be excluded. The common secondary causes are generally clinically evident and include use of some medications, biliary obstruction, nephrotic syndrome, and myxedema. The patient should scrupulously follow a diet beginning with phase I and progressing to phases II and III of the AHA dietary plan for the stepwise treatment of hyperlipoproteinemia. The majority of patients with mild Type II hyperlipoproteinemia have polygenic hypercholesterolemia and may be treated with diet alone. For those with more severe cases, particularly those with familial hypercholesterolemia, treatment will require diet as well as medication. The drug of choice is a bile acid sequestrant, cholestyramine, in doses of 4 to 8 gm three times a day or Colestipol, in doses of 5 to 10 gm three times a day. Added to this may be nicotinic acid in doses of 1 to 1.5 gm three times daily with meals. Another alternative is the HMG CoA reductase inhibitor in conjunction with the bile acid sequestrant; however, as noted above, the HMG CoA reductase inhibitor does not have FDA approval at the time of this writing. Probucol may also be used either alone in mild cases or in conjunction with a bile acid sequestrant. Hoeg and colleagues[105] have used niacin in conjunction with neomycin sulfate, but this latter drug also is not approved. In mild cases in which triglycerides are normal, and when other drugs cannot be tolerated, gemfibrozil might be used to reduce cholesterol and LDL by approximately 10 per cent.

Plasma exchange and ileal bypass may be used for heterozygotes for familial hypercholesterolemia. LDL pheresis or various types of extracorporeal procedures may be used to remove LDL from the circulation. In rare cases in homozygotes for familial hypercholesterolemia, liver transplant may be required. The authors believe that this has been done in two cases to date.[121]

TREATMENT OF TYPE III. Type III patients respond to correction of secondary causes such as excessive alcohol or caloric intake, thyroid deficiency, and hyperglycemia. Drug therapy is also effective when other corrective measures fail. Clofibrate is generally effective in correcting the elevated cholesterol and triglyceride levels[122]; however, nicotinic acid may be equally effective and has fewer side effects. Although estrogens paradoxically have also been reported to have a therapeutic effect, they should only be used when other measures have been ineffective.[123]

TREATMENT OF TYPE IV. The treatment of Type IV hyperlipoproteinemia involves dietary management and weight control. Alcohol consumption should be minimized and diabetes, if present, should be controlled. A phase I diet may be used. If drug therapy is necessary for patients at risk of pancreatitis or other complications of hypertriglyceridemia, it should be individualized according to the etiology of the elevated VLDL. The most commonly used medication is gemfibrozil, although nicotinic acid is quite effective. These drugs should be used when triglyceride levels exceed 500 mg/dl after secondary causes are treated and after diet therapy has been utilized. Estrogen replacement therapy should be used with great caution in the presence of hypertriglyceridemia.

TREATMENT OF TYPE V. Treatment of Type V hyperlipoproteinemia centers on the underlying causes, especially alcohol use and diabetes. Estrogen use should be avoided if possible. Dietary therapy should be directed toward the achievement of ideal body weight. Fats (preferably polyunsaturated) should not exceed 30 per cent of caloric intake and cholesterol should be less than 500 mg per day. If drug therapy is required, nicotinic acid or gemfibrozil is usually employed; however, nicotinic acid may cause worsening of glucose tolerance and this may limit its use in patients with Type V. Norethindrone acetate has been used in women and oxandralone in men, although these drugs are not approved by the FDA for the treatment of hyperlipoproteinemia.

OTHER TYPES OF THERAPY FOR HYPERLIPOPROTEINEMIA

If diet and hypolipidemic agents are ineffective in lowering cholesterol to acceptable levels, other more aggressive therapies are available. Bypassing the terminal 200 cm of the ileum may be utilized to interrupt the intrahepatic circulation for reabsorption of bile salts.[124] Portocaval shunt appears to decrease LDL synthesis in familial hypercholesterolemia and will result in significant reductions in cholesterol; however, this treatment is no longer recommended because of long-term side effects.[125, 126] Additionally, liver transplantation may be used in patients with total absence of LDL receptors[121] as mentioned above. All of the surgical techniques are fraught with obvious serious problems and should be considered only when diet and medications have failed to lower LDL cholesterol to acceptable levels.

Plasma exchange columns for LDL pheresis and anti-LDL are available, but their use currently is limited by expense and inconvenience.[127] Thompson et al.[128] reported an improved survival of patients with homozygous familial hypercholesterolemia who were treated with plasma exchange. The interval of treatment was an average of 2 weeks over a mean of 8.4 years. The patients treated with plasma exchange had an average decrease in serum cholesterol concentration of 37 per cent and an average increase in survival of 5.5 years.

OTHER RISK FACTORS

TOBACCO SMOKING

The surgeon general has named smoking the most preventable risk factor for cardiovascular disease.[129] The potential of developing coronary heart disease in male cigarette smokers is approximately 2.14 times greater than in nonsmokers.[130] The risk taken by cigar and pipe smokers may be less than that of cigarette smokers, but at least in one study their risk was still greater than for that of nonsmokers (Table 36–8).

Some facts about smoking are (1) about 50 million Americans smoke on a regular basis, (2) the number of adult smokers and the per capita cigarette consumption has declined over the past ten years, and (3) the number of teenage girls who begin smoking has increased.[131] Major effects of smoking on the cardiovascular system are the stimulation of the sympathetic nervous system by nicotine and the displacement of oxygen from hemoglobin by carbon monoxide. Other postulated mechanisms include an induced immunological reaction of the vessel wall related to some constituent of smoke, and potentially some increase in adhesiveness of platelets.[132] The incidence in myocardial infarction and mortality from heart disease increases progressively with the number of cigarettes smoked,[133] and the incidence of sudden death is higher in smokers than in nonsmokers. Individuals who stop smoking have a lower incidence of both myocardial infarction and coronary heart disease than those who continue to smoke.[134] Studies by Auerback have shown a correlation between cigarette smoking and the presence of coronary atherosclerosis, even in asymptomatic individuals.[135] Peripheral vascular disease appears to be especially aggravated by cigarette smoking, possibly due to a decrease in the supply of oxygen delivered to tissues, resulting from the desaturation of hemoglobin by carbon monoxide. Cigarette smoking lowers HDL and increases the risk of myocardial infarction and coronary heart disease in women taking oral contraceptives. The risk for cerebral vascular disease is increased about 1 1/2 times in smokers.

Without question, the most important factor in the initiation of smoking by teenagers is peer pressure. The studies of Schachter indicate that nicotine is addicting to smokers.[136] Recently, a form of nicotine-containing chewing gum has been approved by the FDA to help smokers satisfy their craving for nicotine, but its efficacy remains to be established in long-term studies. On the average, 50 to 150 μg of nicotine are absorbed through the lungs and oral mucosa with each puff of tobacco, or about 1 to 2 mg per cigarette. A habitual smoker requires a boost of nicotine approximately every 20 to 30 minutes while awake to prevent the occurrence of withdrawal symptoms. Various forms of behavioral modification and psychological approaches have been tested to determine their efficacy in stopping smoking. Various techniques were employed in the MRFIT study, some involving individuals, others involving group sessions with spouses, and all involving educational techniques and behavior modification. In the MRFIT study, 36 per cent of individuals who initially smoked over 40 cigarettes per day remained off cigarettes at a 4-year follow-up study.[137]

TABLE 36–8 INCIDENCE OF CHD MORBIDITY RELATED TO CIGARETTE SMOKING*

Smoking Pattern	Incidence Ratio
Nonsmokers	58
Cigar and pipe smokers only	71
Cigarette smokers	
About 0.5 pack/day	104
About 1 pack/day	120
More than 1 pack/day	183

From Aronow, W. S., and Kaplan, N. M.: Smoking. *In* Kaplan, N. M., and Stamler, J. (eds.): Prevention of Coronary Heart Disease: Practical Management of the Risk Factors. Philadelphia, W. B. Saunders Company, 1983, p. 55.

*Data from the Pooling Project Research Group: Relationship of blood pressure, serum cholesterol, smoking habit, relative weight and ECG abnormalities to incidence of major coronary events: final report of the Pooling Project. J. Chron. Dis. *31*:201, 1978.

Among Framingham Study participants,[138] within 2 years of stopping smoking, a decrease in incidence of myocardial infarction was demonstrated. Men aged 45 to 54 who quit smoking had one-half the risk of coronary events as compared with those who smoked over an 18-year period.[139] In a study of British physicians by Doll and Peto,[140] the mortality rate was decreased by 5 years after smoking was stopped, although the mortality rate of ex-smokers was never as favorable as that of individuals who had never smoked.

Individuals who smoke more than 25 cigarettes a day have lower levels of HDL and higher levels of VLDL cholesterol and triglyceride than nonsmokers, ex-smokers, and those who smoke less than 25 per day. No differences were observed in those who smoked less than 15 cigarettes per day.[141] Additionally, patients who suffer a myocardial infarction and have normal arteriograms frequently have smoking as their sole major risk factor. However, in populations following a diet low in saturated fat and cholesterol, the evidence for increased independent risk from tobacco is poor.[142] The level of risk of CAD to smokers is related to the presence of other major risk factors and to the number of cigarettes smoked.

Kelly et al. studied a group of 2955 patients who had had myocardial infarction and followed them for 1 year or until death. While the investigators reported a decreased mortality rate in smokers compared with nonsmokers at 1 month, 6 months, and 1 year, the fact was that the smokers were on the average 10 years younger than the nonsmokers. Adjusting for age eliminated the differences in mortality rates at 6 and 12 months.[143] Jugdutt et al., in observations in young women, speculated that cigarette smoking may have precipitated spasm by a nicotine-induced release of norepinephrine and a decrease in the ratio of prostacyclin to thromboxane A_2.[144] Infarction was actually observed in one patient in whom a noncritical lesion was already present. This patient also used oral contraceptives, which along with norepinephrine and thromboxane A_2 increases platelet aggregation and platelet clumping, both of which may induce spasm. It was suggested that the combination of cigarette smoking and estrogens could have induced a sequence of platelet aggregation, vasoconstriction, and thrombosis leading to myocardial infarction in one young woman with normal coronary arteries.

Kaufman et al. evaluated the components of cigarette smoke in relationship to risk of myocardial infarction in young men. These investigators compared 502 cases with 835 hospital controls between ages 30 and 54.[145] The risk of myocardial infarction increased by 2.8 with the number of cigarettes smoked. Risk, however, did not vary with the quantity of nicotine or carbon monoxide in the cigarette. Kaufman et al. interpreted these results as showing that men who smoked cigarettes containing less tar and nicotine and less carbon monoxide do not have a corresponding decrease in risk of myocardial infarction. The risk in these individuals was just as high in those smoking cigarettes containing larger amounts of nicotine and carbon monoxide. Thus, the newer cigarettes do not appear to offer any protection against coronary disease.[145]

The authors do not believe that cigarettes with less nicotine and tar and more effective filters are safer than regular cigarettes. In the Framingham Study, smokers who used filtered cigarettes possibly had an even higher incidence of coronary heart disease than did smokers of nonfiltered cigarettes.[146] The authors believe that those smokers who switched to lower nicotine cigarettes very likely inhaled more deeply, took larger puffs, and perhaps smoked the cigarette longer in order to compensate for a lower level of nicotine. Also, studies by Wald did not show that the delivery of carbon monoxide was reduced by the use of filtered cigarettes.[147] Therefore, the authors do not advocate the use of low tar, low nicotine cigarettes.

Smoking cessation has been demonstrated to be associated with a decline in cardiovascular death. Despite an encouraging decline in the percentage of people who smoke, a large number of U.S. citizens continue to smoke and represent a sizable pool of patients whose cardiac risk could be dramatically lowered by intervention. The incidence of myocardial infarction has been definitely diminished in patients who discontinue tobacco use. The risk reduction occurs quite early and may approach 50 per cent 12 months after cessation of smoking.[148] Major public health measures have been enacted to protect the nonsmoker from passive inhalation and to discourage consumption by reducing cigarette advertising and by increasing excise taxes.

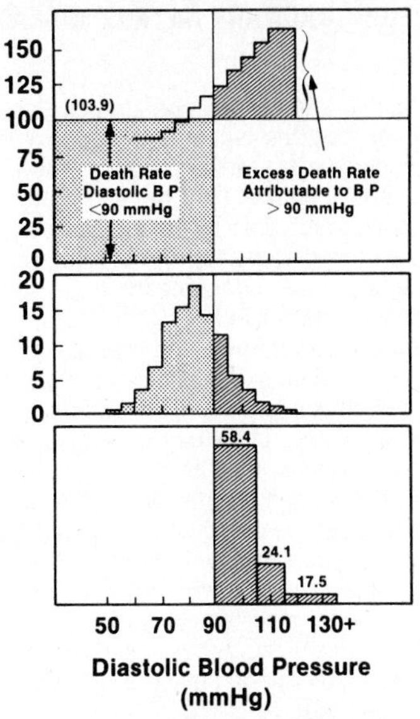

FIGURE 36–12. An estimate of the percentage of excess deaths attributable to hypertension by varying levels of diastolic blood pressure (DBP) (*bottom*), derived by multiplying the death rate per 10,000 person years at different levels of DBP in the Framingham study (*top*) by the distribution of DBP in the population (*center*). When the large number of people with diastolic blood pressure (DBP) from 90 to 104 mm Hg is multiplied by the excess risk associated with this range of blood pressure, the percentage of excess deaths attributable to DBP of 90 to 104 mm Hg is shown to be 58.4 per cent of the total excess mortality associated with hypertension. (From Hypertension Detection and Follow-up Program Cooperative Group: The hypertension detection and follow-up program; a progress report. Circ. Res. *40*(Suppl I):106, 1977, by permission of the American Heart Association, Inc.)

HYPERTENSION

(See also p. 824)

Hypertension has been well established as a major risk factor for the development of coronary atherosclerosis.[149] This has been demonstrated in both sexes and among various age groups and racial groups; the prevalence of hypertension ranges from 9 to 20 per cent of the population. Risk increases if hypertension is present along with the other established risks of hypercholesterolemia and smoking. Risk for the development of CAD due to hypertension is continuous and graded.[149] Hence, there is no threshold below which a given level of blood pressure is definitely safe; this renders definitions of hypertension that are based on statistical population and distributions inappropriate. It is more reasonable clinically to define hypertension as the level of blood pressure elevation which adds significantly to the risk of developing complications.

The Hypertension Detection and Follow-up Program obviously has had an enormous impact on the detection and control of hypertension in the U.S. and on the decrease in mortality from cardiovascular disease, particularly cerebrovascular disease.[150] In the early 1960's it was estimated that the condition in only one out of eight hypertensives in this country was under good control.[151] This increased to as many as three out of four by the early 1980's.[152] If 90 mm Hg is used as a cutoff point for defining diastolic hypertension, approximately one-fourth of the U.S. population would be classified as hypertensive.

Figure 27–2 (p. 820) shows data from 160,000 people aged 30 to 69. The blood pressure readings were obtained in their homes. This population contained a higher proportion of low-income blacks than is representative of the U.S. population; also, the readings are higher than would be obtained when testing is repeated. In a clinical setting, when the blood pressure is rechecked with a second reading, in about 35 per cent of those with an initial diastolic blood pressure reading of over 95 mm/Hg, there is a fall below 90 mm Hg.[153]

CONTROL OF HYPERTENSION. For otherwise healthy adults with borderline readings between 90 to 95 mm Hg, the physician should provide general guidelines for blood pressure control. Figure 36–12, from the Hypertension, Detection, and Follow-up Cooperative Group, gives the percentage of excess deaths attributable to hypertension at various degrees of diastolic blood pressure. When a diastolic blood pressure from 90 to 104 mm Hg is multiplied by the excess risk associated with this range of blood pressure, the percentage of excess deaths attributable to the high blood pressure is 58.4 per cent of the total excess mortality associated with hypertension. Therefore, those having such a diastolic reading constitute a large group who might benefit most from treatment. While the importance of diastolic blood pressure is emphasized, systolic blood pressure appears, in epidemiological studies, to have a close correlation with cardiovascular mortality and morbidity. Environmental factors predisposing to hypertension include obesity, high sodium intake, heavy alcohol consumption, and stress. Less than 5 per cent of hypertension is secondary to renal, endocrine, or adrenal disorders.

HYPERTENSION IN CHILDREN. The data of Berenson and associates from the Bogalusa Heart Study suggest that the tendency toward high blood pressure can be traced to childhood (pp. 852 and 1016). A tendency exists for hypertension to run in families.[154] Several risk markers have been identified in children of hypertensive patients who themselves may have blood pressures in the high normal range; Zinner[155] identified the urinary excretion of kallikrein as a marker.

ELECTROLYTE FLUX IN HYPERTENSION. Berenson and associates have also studied renal processing of sodium as a marker, mainly in blacks. Another defect, described by Edmonson et al.,[156] is in the transport of sodium and potassium across the cell membrane of leukocytes (p. 833). Garay et al.[157] reported abnormalities in hypertensives in the rate of sodium and potassium flux in and out of erythrocytes. In about one-half of normotensive children of hypertensive patients, the net flux of sodium to potassium was lower in members of families with "hypertension." These investigators thus use a laboratory test to distinguish between essential and secondary hypertension on the basis of cation fluxes across erythrocytes. Haddy et al. described an etiology of hypertension involving a defect in sodium transport, possibly across the renal tubule.[158] This defect in combination with excess sodium intake and sodium retention by the kidney is compounded by a circulating natriuretic hormone which hypothetically might cause an increased contractility of smooth muscle cells in blood vessels in arterioles by altering the calcium influx.

RELATION OF DIET TO HYPERTENSION. While the causal relationship between high sodium intake and hypertension has not been proved, an enormous body of evidence is available on this point. The average U.S. consumption of salt of about 10 to 15 gm per day, or 150 to 200 mEq of sodium, is much more than the body needs. About two-thirds of this is obtained in processed foods, and the other third is added in cooking or at the table. The more processed and precooked foods consumed and the lower the consumption of fresh vegetables, fruits, and protein sources, the higher is the sodium intake.

In populations in which hypertension is uncommon or absent, sodium intake is very low, usually below 70 mEq/day. A rough correlation exists between the prevalence of hypertension and the level of sodium intake. Early in the course of hypertension, cardiac output tends to be high. Extreme salt restriction will undoubtedly lower an elevated blood pressure. In various animal experiments in which a genetically determined hypertension is a factor, the blood pressure becomes even more elevated by salt intake. Obesity is positively correlated with high blood pressure, but the correlation is primarily with body mass. Consumption of two or more ounces of alcohol per day is associated with an increased prevalence of hypertension as well as cardiovascular mortality.[159, 160]

McCarron[161] and associates have claimed that a reduced intake of calcium is more significant than salt intake as a determinant of blood pressure. The role of dietary calcium intake in hypertension needs to be clarified. A few studies have been carried out involving the feeding of calcium supplements to hypertensive subjects.[162] The results reportedly were variable; in some instances, calcium supplementation was credited with decreasing the blood pressure, while in others an increase in blood pressure was noted (p. 834).

EFFECTS OF TREATING HYPERTENSION. In five randomized controlled trials of treating mild hypertension (diastolic blood pressure 90 to 104 mm Hg) (Table 36–9), antihypertensive drugs were used. In three of the studies, the drugs were compared with placebo, while in the other two, the comparison group was a "less intensively treated group designated as referred care." The VA Cooperative Study[163] provided firm evidence for the benefit of decreasing diastolic blood pressure exceeding 104 mm Hg, but morbidity and mortality were not decreased in the group with pressures between 90 and 104 mm Hg. The numbers in this group were relatively small.

The Hypertension Detection and Follow-up Program (HDFP). Over 7800 patients in the group with diastolic pressures between 90 to 104 mm Hg were enrolled in the Hypertension Detection and Follow-up Program.[164] One-half of the patients were referred to their usual medical care, designated referred care, while the other half received more intensive treatment under the so-called stepped care program. In the stepped care program, one drug at a time was added sequentially to bring the blood pressure below a given goal. The initial drug used was a diuretic, followed by an adrenergic inhibitor, followed by hydralazine. After 5 years, the group given the more intensive treatment had a mean diastolic blood pressure of 83 mm Hg, while the referred care group had an average of 88. There was a decrease in mortality of 20 per cent in the stepped care group, this difference in mortality being highly significant in establishing the benefit in lowering blood pressure to between 90 and 104 mm Hg. The stepped care group also had a significant decrease in both noncardiovascular and cardiovascular mortality, primarily cerebrovascular mortality. On the basis of these findings, the second Joint National Committee on Hypertension (1980) recommended that the initial goal of antihypertensive therapy is to achieve and maintain diastolic pressure under 90 mm Hg.[165]

The Australian Therapeutic Trial. In this trial,[166] patients with diastolic blood pressures between 95 and 109 mm Hg who were free of evidence of cardiovascular disease were enrolled. Patients were randomly assigned to placebo or to stepped care drug therapy similar to the therapeutic regimen used in the Hypertension Detection and Follow-up Program. The trial was stopped after a statistically significant difference in mortality between the two groups of 30 per cent was reached, after 3 years. The average decrease in diastolic blood pressure of the stepped care group was 12.2 mm Hg, compared with 6.6 mm Hg in the placebo group. Therefore, both the Australian trial and the Hypertension Detection Follow-up showed a significant protection against cardiovascular, mainly cerebrovascular, complications by a decrease in diastolic blood pressure of 5 to 6 mm Hg. In neither study was any protection shown for patients under age 50, but there were relatively few of them. Nor was any protection shown for women in the Australian trial.

Multiple-Risk Factor Intervention Trial (MRFIT). This was a very large trial carried out under the auspices of the NHLBI in the United States and described above[167] (p. 1155). The 12,866 men selected were between the ages of 35 and 57, had no clinical evidence of cardiovascular disease, and were chosen on the basis of their serum cholesterol levels, cigarette smoking, and blood pressure. At the beginning of the trial, 8011 had hypertension, defined as a diastolic blood pressure of over 90 mm Hg, the majority falling between 90 and 104 mm Hg. After 7 years of follow-up of the hypertensive subjects, the more intensively treated group had a reduction in coronary heart disease of 23.7 per cent, and of all-cause mortality of 17.3 per cent. For the 70 per cent of the total group in whom the resting ECG was normal at the time of entry, the results were quite consistent with the Hypertension Detection Follow-up and Australian trials. However, for the 30 per cent of hypertensive individuals who had abnormal ECG at time of entry, the mortality rates from heart disease and all-cause mortality were actually higher in the stepped care group than in the usual care group. A reason for these findings is not immediately clear. The increased mortality in the stepped care group with abnormal ECG's has been thought to be a result of the high-dose diuretic regimen used, but this has not been proved. Hypokalemia also has not been established as a cause for these findings.

The Medical Research Council (MRC) Trial. This was a very large trial of drug treatment of mild hypertension carried out in the United Kingdom.[168] In the previous trials, diuretics were used invariably as the first step of treatment after nonpharmacological means were employed. In the MRC Trial, benefit in terms of decreased mortality was limited to a reduction in mortality from cerebrovascular disease. Note that this was the only trial in which a direct comparison was made between a diuretic and a beta blocker. Some differences were observed in the relative effect between these two agents; the reductions in blood pressure were slightly greater for those treated with diuretics than for those receiving beta blockers. Of course, differences exist between all of the trials. For example, there were fewer blacks in the MRC Trial as compared with the Hypertension Detection Follow-up Trial in the United States.

In none of the trials with hypertensive agents was a reduction in coronary heart disease observed in the range of what had been predicted from the Framingham Study. Only about one-fourth of the reduction in heart disease predicted in the Framingham study was observed. A number of theories have been proposed to account for this, none of which has been established. The side effects of diuretics, such as elevations of cholesterol and triglyceride and production of hypokalemia, may be operative here. It could be argued that the benefits of antihypertensive therapy to patients with existing coronary artery disease come too late. It also might be argued that some unknown effect of antihypertensive therapy interfered with the expected reduction in coronary disease.

The physician must consider the risk-to-benefit ratio in treating patients with mild hypertension, particularly those with diastolic pressures between 90 and 95 mm Hg. If diuretics are used, the authors recommend that the initial dose be no more than the equivalent of 25 mg of hydrochlorothiazide. An effort should be made to avoid hypokalemia, and if the patient has an abnormal resting ECG or hyperlipidemia, then consideration might be given to using an initial drug other than a diuretic. There may well be heterogeneous effects of lowering blood pressure in different racial groups. In conclusion, the question of whether or not lowering blood pressure below 104 mm Hg in those with mild to moderate hypertension will reduce mortality from myocardial infarction and coronary heart disease remains to be established.

TABLE 36–9 CONTROLLED TRIALS OF THERAPY FOR MILD HYPERTENSION

Study	Number of Patients	DBP (mm Hg)	Design: Control	Design: Active	Reductions of Complications (per cent)
VA, 1970	170	90–104	Placebo	Stepped Care	35
USPHS, 1977	389	90–114	Placebo	Stepped Care	44
HDFP, 1979	7,825	90–104	Referred Care	Stepped Care	20
Australian, 1980	3,427	95–109	Placebo	Stepped Care	30
MRFIT, 1982	8,011	≥90	Referred Care	Stepped Care	See text

From Kaplan, N. M.: Hypertension. *In* Kaplan, N. M., and Stamler, J. (eds.): Prevention of Coronary Heart Disease: Practical Management of the Risk Factors. Philadelphia, W. B. Saunders Company, 1983, p. 68.

PHYSICAL ACTIVITY

EPIDEMIOLOGICAL CONSIDERATIONS

The role of physical activity in preventing coronary disease and in decreasing mortality after myocardial infarction remains controversial. Long-term physical activity is known to be important in maintaining body weight and muscle tissue, in lowering blood pressure and triglycerides, and in raising the level of HDL cholesterol, particularly the HDL_2 fraction. Persons who exercise regularly have been reported to have a lower incidence of sudden death, but some increase in likelihood of sudden cardiac death occurs in sedentary individuals when an exercise program is initiated. Because of this, for patients over age 35, the authors strongly recommend consulting with a physician and taking an exercise test before undertaking a new program of vigorous physical activity.

Epidemiological studies in several countries have shown a consistent inverse relationship between caloric intake per kilogram of body mass and coronary heart disease. This is presumed to be related to a protective effect of increased physical activity. In a study by Siltanen et al.,[169] vigorous physical conditioning of at least 4 hours per week appeared to decrease mortality after an initial myocardial infarction and possibly during the subsequent 2 years.

LaRosa et al.,[170] in a study termed the National Exercise and Heart Disease Project, tested total cholesterol, HDL, LDL, and triglyceride and did not find that long-term moderate physical exercise affected lipoprotein levels. Most likely, the level of exercise in this study was not sufficient to alter the concentrations of the plasma lipoproteins, since these changes have been well documented in many cross-sectional studies. In the Ontario Exercise-Heart Collaborative Study,[171] Rechnitzer et al. failed to find that a high-intensity exercise program prevented recurrent myocardial infarction in men. The 4-year recurrence rate in 379 patients on a high-intensity program did not differ from that among 354 patients on a program of light exercise.

Hartung et al.,[172] studied the relationship between exercise and alcohol consumption on HDL in runners and inactive men. They found that exercise was a more significant determinant of HDL levels than alcohol. Individuals who ran 12 or more miles a week had leaner body mass, lower levels of lipids, and higher levels of HDL cholesterol than did sedentary individuals. Consuming as much as 3 (12-oz) beers (38.88 gm ethanol) a day raised the HDL levels in sedentary men but not in exercising men. Hartung et al.[173] also studied the relationship between exercise, alcohol consumption, and lipoproteins in women, and found that exercise appeared to be a more significant determinant of HDL levels than was alcohol consumption in premenopausal women. Women who ran had higher levels of HDL_2 than inactive women. Consuming 35 gm/day of alcohol did not significantly change lipoprotein levels in either active or inactive groups of women.

Rigorous testing of the concept that physical inactivity is a risk factor for the development of coronary artery disease has been limited by methodological problems. There are obvious problems in large-scale epidemiological studies that attempt to correlate such factors as occupation, leisure activity, and historical documentation of activity with cardiovascular mortality. These studies are often not well controlled as to other risk or genetic factors. Experimental evidence in primates[174] indicates that aerobic exercise reduces the severity of atherosclerosis despite an atherogenic diet. These conditioned primates also had lower pulse rates, elevated HDL, low VLDL, and loss of body fat. While these studies may not be directly applicable to humans, it is well documented that similar changes in lipid levels occur in humans who exercise,[175] even though direct pathological or angiographic correlations have not been made in a systematic manner. However, indirect studies using the double product at which ischemia occurred on treadmill testing after intense physical training and extent of ST depression at the same double product show a favorable response to training.[176] The indirect treadmill data have been supported in a longitudinal study which showed that men who are less physically fit are twice as likely to suffer a subsequent myocardial infarction when bicycle ergotomy was used as the standard for fitness.[177]

MECHANISMS OF POSSIBLE BENEFIT. If the extensive suggestive epidemiological data which supports reduced risk from coronary atherosclerosis are correct, the exact mechanism which provides protection is probably multifactorial. Regular aerobic exercise lowers both systolic and diastolic blood pressures, albeit not markedly[178] (p. 1165). This has been demonstrated in longitudinal studies that revealed an inverse relationship between physical activity and hypertension. Hence, continued dynamic exercise at a level that would maintain lean body mass and blood pressure at normal levels would be expected to lower long-term cardiac risk.

The effect of exercise on blood lipids has been extensively studied. Of special interest is the effect of physical exertion on HDL levels, which in turn is inversely correlated with the incidence of CAD.[179] Regular exercise raises HDL.[180] An inverse relationship between HDL and obesity has been documented.[181] Hence, the rise in HDL may be a consequence of loss of body fat rather than exercise per se, although the precise mechanisms would not alter the presumed statistical decrease in risk from elevated HDL.

Another benefit from regular exercise is improved glucose tolerance, although it is not clear that reduction of elevated blood glucose levels lowers cardiovascular mortality.[182] The resultant alterations of physical activity on clotting activity have uncertain clinical implications. However, physically active individuals have increased fibrinolytic activity when venous clots are formed.[183]

EXERCISE LEVELS. The exercise level required to improve a patient's risk factor profile has not been established; however, if basically sedentary patients undertake a moderate exercise program, a considerable reduction in cardiovascular risk may be attained. Whether or not an increased benefit is attained with more sustained exercise has not been documented. An excess energy expenditure of approximately 2000 kilocalories per week apparently provides the same protection as that seen in runners preparing for a marathon.[184]

A practical exercise prescription is a function of the clinical status of the patient and the presence or absence of coronary artery disease. Patients at increased risk of CAD—for example, hypertensives, hypercholesterolemics, smokers, diabetics, and those with suspected CAD—should undergo a monitored exercise treadmill test in addition to having a clinical history and physical. Treadmill testing should generally be done in patients over the age of 35 who plan to begin an exercise program. If the patient has no evidence or history of ischemic heart disease, exercise programs may not need close monitoring due to the low risk involved. Adherence to an exercise program is a major problem, and half of those who begin a regular program may drop out. Unfortunately, high-risk groups such as smokers who might be expected to benefit most tend to have higher dropout rates than nonsmokers.[185] For patients with documented ischemic disease, more precautions are needed because of the risk of exercise-induced arrhythmias, lack of training, and the possibility of inducing a myocardial infarction secondary to unfavorable oxygen supply and demand relationships. All patients with known ischemic disease should undergo treadmill testing prior to the institution of a progressive exercise program. If a myocardial infarction has occurred, the patient may undergo a submaximal treadmill test prior to discharge from the hospital[186] (Chap. 41). Prognosis may be estimated by ST shifts, exercise time, ectopy, and inappropriate blood pressure response.

While exercise may alter the sense of well-being and physical capacity and favorably alter modifiable risk factors, its quantitative effect on mortality and morbidity is less definite as a secondary preventive measure.[187] Studies have been performed which addressed the use of exercise as a secondary preventive measure for reducing cardiac morbidity and mortality.[188] Statistically significant reductions in mortality could not be documented, although trends which favor exercise have been noted. Continued adherence to the recommended exercise level was a problem, and the dropout rate tended to decrease the intended differences in control and exercise groups. Also, the controlled studies have had relatively small numbers of subjects.

Most of the epidemiological studies reported to date are consistent with the theory that the risk of coronary heart disease may be reduced with vigorous physical activity. However, the results contain a number of inconsistencies and the studies have limitations based on self-selection, physical status of the subjects at the time of initial study, complications from other health problems, and difficulties in quantifying physical activity. As discussed above, physical activity is expected to have beneficial effects on blood pressure, on plasma triglycerides and HDL, on glucose tolerance, and on control of obesity. Also, so-called aerobic exercise is expected to improve cardiovascular function and possibly to reduce thrombosis and the reactivity of the cardiovascular system to stress. It must be emphasized that firm evidence establishing that physical conditioning will decrease coronary heart disease and cardiovascular mortality is lacking, and experiments to establish such may never be possible.

RECOMMENDATIONS. Nonetheless, the physician often has to base judgment on the best evidence available, and the authors agree with the recommendations of the American Heart Association, the U.S. Department of HHS, and the report of the British Joint Working Party.[189–191] Regular physical activity is part of an overall life style aimed at decreasing the risk factors for CAD and of maintaining an improved state of metabolic function of the cardiovascular system. There appears to be a relatively low risk involved in a careful exercise program, and it seems to be a relatively inexpensive way to improve the general state of health and well-being of the population.

In order to bring about a significant improvement in aerobic capacity or the $\dot{V}O_{2max}$, a minimum of three sessions per week are required, each lasting between 20 and 30 min. Five sessions produce a maximal result, which is achieved after 4 to 6 weeks of training. For sedentary individuals contemplating initiating a program of physical activity, the importance of a medical evaluation before beginning must be emphasized.

The role of the physician is pivotal in helping the patient to establish attainable goals for an exercise program. A regular routine should be advocated with flexibility as to the type of calorie expenditure allowed. The physician should encourage and support the patient to maximize benefits and minimize dropout.

OBESITY

As with so many other risk factors, the precise role of obesity as a risk factor in CAD is uncertain. In a reexamination of the incidence of CAD in the data from the Framingham cohort involving 5209 of the men and women originally in the study, Hubert et al.[192] reported that obesity was a significant independent risk predictor for CAD, especially among females. The observations were made over a 26-year period on the basis of the Metropolitan Relative Weight. While the statistical correlation was weaker in men, CAD and congestive heart failure in men was related to percentage of desirable weight at the time of initial observation. This correlation was independent of age, cholesterol level, systolic blood pressure, cigarette smoking, left ventricular hypertrophy, and glucose intolerance. In women, weight was positively and independently associated with CAD, stroke, congestive heart failure, and coronary and cardiovascular death. The investigators interpret these data as showing that weight gain after the early adult years carries an increased risk of cardiovascular disease that is not related either to initial weight or to the levels of other risk factors which may have resulted from the weight gain, such as hypertension, diabetes, hypercholesterolemia, and hypertriglyceridemia.

The definition of obesity is somewhat arbitrary and differs from definition of body fatness. The most commonly used tables for determining obesity are those developed by the Metropolitan Life Insurance Company. In these tables, a desirable weight is defined as that weight at which the lowest mortality rates occur in individuals who are applying for life insurance. Bray[193] expresses guidelines for body weight as a median rate with a range of acceptable body weights for each height. Bray has recommended the use of body mass index (BMI) of weight/height^2 as the best approach at estimating obesity. The prevalence of obesity in the U. S. averages approximately 20 per cent for men aged 45 to 54 and 15 per cent for women. Approximately 16 per cent of men are 20 per cent or more overweight, and 28 per cent of women are 20 per cent or more overweight.

An NIH consensus conference panel on obesity reached the conclusion that obesity has adverse effects on both health and longevity. Obesity has a direct relationship with all of the major coronary risk factors other than smoking. The strongest correlations with obesity exist with blood pressure, hypertriglyceridemia, hyperinsulinemia and very inversely with the concentration of HDL cholesterol. No threshold of obesity could be detected at which this relationship occurred.

MECHANISM OF THE ADVERSE EFFECTS OF OBESITY. Knuiman et al.[194] measured serum cholesterol, HDL, and body mass index in adult men from 13 countries. Body mass index showed a positive correlation with total cholesterol and was negatively related to HDL cholesterol and the ratio of HDL cholesterol to total cholesterol.

Obese patients have a higher incidence of hypertension, although the exact mechanism involved in the genesis of the elevated blood pressure is not definite and may differ from that in nonobese patients with essential hypertension. A correlation exists between the extent of obesity and blood pressure elevation, although the relationship is not linear.[195] Elevation in blood pressure is the major risk factor which is definitely correlated with excess weight and may explain the excess risk for CAD associated with obesity. Lipid abnormalities are well documented in obesity, but their epidemiological significance has yet to be determined. Although hypertriglyceridemia is the most common abnormality seen in obese patients, its causal role in the production of coronary atherosclerosis is unclear.

Recent epidemiological studies have determined that obese patients tend to have increased serum cholesterol levels.[196] However, the elevation in total cholesterol is small and the excess mortality due to this elevation is not clear. HDL cholesterol is generally low in obese patients and the ratio of total cholesterol to HDL is increased. In addition, in individual obese patients who continue to gain more weight, the HDL levels will continue to decline. While it is well documented that low HDL levels are associated with excess cardiac risk,[41] it remains to be determined if primarily elevating the HDL will decrease risk.[197] Obese patients who lose weight do not show an increase in HDL,[198] so the exact role that HDL plays in cardiac risk related to obesity is unknown.

Patients whose weight is greater than 30 per cent of the established norms have higher levels of serum glucose secondary to insulin resistance which is imparted by obesity. This level of increased weight is compatible with the level associated with increased cardiac risk due to ischemic heart disease. However, patients with glucose intolerance tend to have higher blood pressure and altered lipid levels: this makes an independent risk assessment involving glucose intolerance difficult to prove. In patients with established diabetes, the rise in mortality occurs again only in those patients with markedly excessive weight. The exact role that hyperinsulinemia per se plays in obesity is unclear. It has been demonstrated that an elevated level of insulin is an independent risk,[199] although the exact role that the factor of high insulin levels plays has not been evaluated in obesity.

DISTRIBUTION OF FAT

Studies now carried out in different countries have shown the importance of the distribution of fat as a coronary risk factor. In a 13-year study of 54-year-old Swedish men, the waist-to-hip circumference ratio showed a linear relationship with CAD risk, while body mass index and skinfold thicknesses were not correlated.

In a 12-year follow-up study of females from Gothenburg, Sweden, Lapidus et al.[200] showed a positive association in 1462 women between the incidence of myocardial infarction, angina pectoris, and stroke and/or death and waist-to-hip circumference ratio. The association with myocardial infarction was independent of age, smoking, serum cholesterol, triglyceride, systolic blood pressure, and body mass index. In another report[201] a high ratio of waist-to-hip circumference was associated with an increase of CAD in men. Measures of total obesity had no predictive power. The waist-to-hip ratio appears to be more significant as a predictor of CAD than the total degree of obesity. Thus, a masculine distribution of adipose tissue increases the risk of coronary disease in both males and females on the basis of the Gothenburg data (Fig. 36–13). In females, the risk ratio between the highest quintile and the lowest quintile was 8.2 for myocardial infarction, 3.8 for strokes, and 2.0 for death of any cause.

The Seven Countries Study was a prospective one consisting of 15 cohorts of southern European men between ages 40 to 59. No statistically significant relationship could be shown between coronary death and obesity.[202] In the Pooling Project, 12,381 white men aged 40 to 64 from eight different U.S. populations were followed from 4.9 to 9.6 years. The data were plotted on the basis of ideal weight in

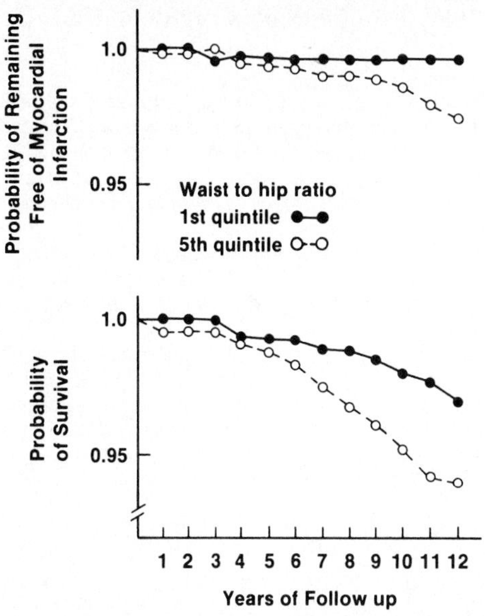

FIGURE 36–13. Probability of remaining free of myocardial infarction and dying of any cause for every year of a 12-year follow-up by highest and lowest quintiles of ratio of waist-to-hip circumference at entry. (From Lapidus, L., et al: Distribution of adipose tissue and risk of cardiovascular disease and death: A 12-year follow-up of participants in the population study of women in Gothenburg, Sweden. Br. Med. J. *289*:1257, 1984.)

quintiles. The pooled data from six cohorts had a statistically significant linear relationship with coronary death (Fig. 36–14). One of the six did not show such a relationship; the Chicago People's Gas Study showed a U-shaped relationship. A stepwise increase was seen only in Framingham, about which the observations of Hubert et al. have already been mentioned. In the prospective studies on obesity and cardiovascular disease and mortality, data from the Framingham study showed a U-shaped curve with highest mortality at the lower and upper end of the body mass index. However, other epidemiological studies have not found obesity to be an independent predictor of CAD. When other risk factors such as blood pressure and cholesterol level were taken into account, obesity appeared to be less significant. On the basis of the foregoing, the analysis of Barrett-Conner and Khaw is somewhat surprising.[203] In studies composed predominantly of white men, these investigators found inconsistency in the relationship between coronary mortality and obesity, and they believe that a misclassification of obesity may account for some of these discrepancies. They analyzed in detail the Seven Countries Study of 15 cohorts and the Pooling Project Study of 8 cohorts.[204] The strongest evidence for the relationship between obesity and atherosclerosis came from patients who were extremely obese—for example, more than 30 per cent above the ideal body weight.

The NIH Obesity Consensus Conference suggested that the apparent contradiction between higher levels of CAD risk factors in association with obesity but with an inconsistent correlation of coronary death might

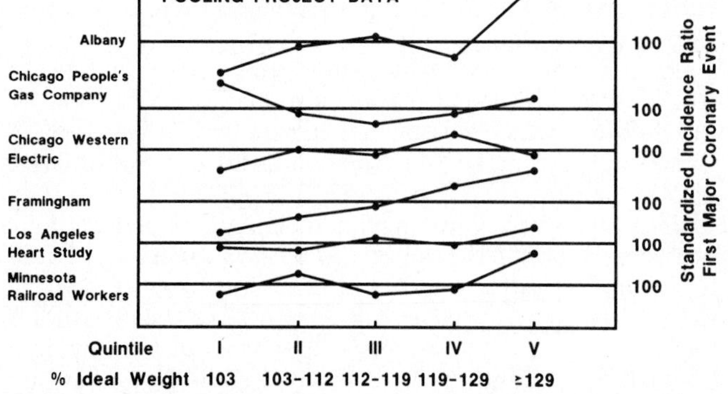

FIGURE 36–14. Coronary disease by relative weight quintile. Pooling Project. (From Barrett-Connor, E., and Khaw, K-T.: Is obesity a risk factor for coronary artery disease? Perspect. Lipid Dis. *3*:18, 1986.)

be due to differences in duration of follow-up, or a self-selection bias of healthy workers that may have existed in some of the cohorts.

Barrett-Connor and Khaw reject these suggestions and instead they favor a misclassification based on the differences used to define obesity, such as relative body weight, body mass index, and skinfold thickness. For example, in patients who are not in exercise programs, the percentage of body fat increases with age, even though total body weight may remain constant. Barrett-Connor and Khaw suggest that the duration or location of body fat may be more important than the overall measure of degree of obesity.

The explanation for the paradox of the inconsistency of obesity as a predictive factor of CAD risk in white men remains, and there is no adequate explanation as of this writing. In summary, obesity is associated with other cardiac risk factors and may add to the total risk in these patients. Hence, weight reduction should be encouraged in patients who have these additional risks.

Diet therapy should aim at weight reduction to approach ideal body weight and to maintain the weight loss and should also aim at controlling hyperlipidemia if necessary. Since eating is a behavior, changing of behavioral habits of eating is a key element in the control of obesity. Exercise and physical activity are obviously important adjuncts to weight control.

DIET

When a nutrient analysis was done in over 8000 men on the island of Oahu,[205] those who developed coronary disease had a lower consumption of calories. This finding is consistent with the other studies from Puerto Rico and Framingham. The men with CAD also had a lower consumption of carbohydrates, starch, and vegetable protein. While the percentage of calories from polyunsaturated fat and saturated fat loses its significance in multivariate analysis, men who developed CAD had a higher mean intake of percentage of calories from saturated fatty acids, polyunsaturated fatty acids, fat protein, and a higher cholesterol intake per thousand calories than those who were free of CAD. The lower mean intake of calories was not due to a decrease in the total consumption of fat, because this was roughly the same in the coronary and noncoronary groups. The main difference was that those with coronary disease had a lower mean intake of carbohydrate and alcohol. Previous studies from Puerto Rico and Framingham had shown that men with CAD had a lower consumption of carbohydrate and starch, but the means were not significantly different in Framingham.

The Zutphen Study reported by Kromhout and Coulander,[206] as well as several previous ones,[207–209] showed that men who developed CAD consumed fewer calories per day than men who did not. The difference in consumption varied from 170 to 270 kcal per day. This inverse relationship between energy intake and heart disease shows an even stronger relationship when the energy intake is related to body weight. The most likely explanation for this finding, which has been suggested by Marr et al.,[210] is that energy intake shows a significant correlation with physical activity.

These data therefore suggest that physical activity may protect against CAD. Energy intake was inversely related to serum cholesterol and was also inversely related to skinfold thickness.[211] The conclusions from such studies appear to be that energy intake per mass of body weight is not independently related to CAD, but Kromhout and Coulander conclude that energy intake is important in regulating body fat and serum cholesterol, which were major risk factors for coronary disease in their study. Dietary cholesterol was related to coronary risk in a univariate regression analysis, but in a multivariate analysis, dietary cholesterol intake per 100 kcal was not independently related to CAD. This contrasted with the results of the Western Electric Study,[212] which reported that cholesterol intake per 100 kg had a positive relationship with CAD independent of age, systolic blood pressure, cigarette smoking, Quetelet index,* and alcohol consumption, and surprisingly, serum cholesterol levels. Kromhout and Coulander concluded that in an unrestricted population of middle-aged men, energy intake in relationship to body weight is a stronger determinant of CAD than is the consumption of various individual nutrients. Kushi et al. performed a large prospective epidemiological study of 1001 middle-aged men in whom they found that diet was related to CAD but that the relationship was a relatively weak one.[213] In general, therefore, a high intake of dietary saturated fat and cholesterol, a low intake of polyunsaturated fat, and a low intake of fiber increased the risk for coronary disease in this study.

Riemersma[214] et al. measured the linoleic acid content in adipose tissue in apparently healthy men age 40 to 49 from four European regions which had different rates of CAD. The proportion of linoleic acid in adipose tissue was lowest in men from Northern Karelia in Finland, who had the highest mortality rates from coronary heart disease. The highest content was in Italy, where this mortality was lowest; intermediate contents were found in men in Scotland and southwest Finland, which also had intermediate mortality rates from heart disease. It is assumed that in these relations differences occur in the content of linoleic acid in the diet.

Also in the Riemersma study, the desaturation and elongation product dihomo-γ-linolenic acid was highest in Italy and lowest in Northern Karelia, and the concentration of arachidonic acid in adipose tissue was also highest in Italy. Furthermore, Italian men had the highest adipose tissue content of oleate, most likely reflecting the high concentration of this monounsaturated fat in the Italian or Mediterranean diet containing olive oil. Blood pressures were higher in Finland and there was a greater degree of obesity. There was a gradient of serum cholesterol concentration with the highest values being in Northern Karelia and Southwest Finland and the lowest in Italy. HDL cholesterol concentrations were related to the serum cholesterol levels, and were highest in Finland and lowest in Italy, although the ratio of HDL cholesterol to total cholesterol was not significantly different. The regional differences in the linoleic acid content of adipose tissue were of high statistical significance when other risk factors for heart disease were taken into account in multivariate analysis.

In one study in Finland[215, 216] a low linoleic content in serum phospholipids was suggested as a possible independent predictor of CHD. A previous study of Scottish men had also found low linoleic acid content in adipose tissue associated with heart disease.[217] The saturation-elongation product of linoleic acid, dihomo-γ-linolenic acid (20:3n-6), in the Scottish study was even more powerful an independent predictor of CHD. Thus, a diet rich in linoleic acid and/or relatively poor in saturated fatty acids appears to be associated with protection against CAD. The higher tissue content of linoleic acid and its elongation product would reflect lower concentrations of serum cholesterol, lower blood pressure, and possible changes in platelet aggregation, all of which could contribute to a lower incidence of CAD.

PLATELETS

(See also p. 1759)

The exact role of platelets in coronary disease remains to be defined. Platelets produce the platelet-derived growth factor (PDGF), which promotes the growth and proliferation of smooth muscle cells. A similar factor can be formed also by endothelial cells, macrophages, and smooth muscle cells under certain conditions. Platelets also produce a substance which inhibits endothelial cell regeneration.[218] Platelets most likely play a role in coronary artery spasm and, along with the endothelial cell, may contribute to changes in the vessel wall after angioplasty or fibrinolytic therapy.

The platelet itself is involved in intrinsic coagulation at several steps,

*Body mass index (BMI) height/cube root of weight $h/\sqrt[3]{w}$, also known as the Ponderal index.

including the activation of factor VIII and of prothrombin. Rao et al.[219] studied 23 patients with chest pain, 7 with normal arteriograms and 16 with proved coronary disease. These investigators believe that what they define as platelet coagulant activity is an important determinant of hemostasis. Measuring this activity involves the activation of platelets with various agents which are then used to activate the coagulation system. These investigators reported a higher platelet coagulant activity in the patients with CAD as compared with the control group. Obviously, further studies of this phenomenon and a more precise definition of the platelet coagulant activity would be desirable.

FAMILY HISTORY AND FAMILY AGGREGATION

Both case control and prospective studies point to the familial aggregation of CAD. The aggregation of risk factors is well known and includes cholesterol, lipoproteins, blood pressure, diabetes, and obesity. As Feinleib[220] has pointed out, it is a mistake to conclude that genetic and environmental factors operate in a simple additive manner—rather, they are often interconnected. For example, a genetic predisposition to high blood pressure or hypercholesterolemia may be determined by the salt, saturated fat, or caloric consumption of the overall population. The homogeneity or heterogeneity of a given population may also greatly confound an attempt to distinguish between genetic and environmental factors. Obviously, as far as the physician is concerned, the important point is to identify those risk factors which are modifiable and to concentrate on their control.

It is unusual for coronary heart disease to be the manifestation of a single-gene disorder, as in familial hypercholesterolemia or in the A-I/C-III deficiency discussed above (p. 1160). Another familial disorder associated with vascular disease is homocystinuria. Heterozygotes in this disorder do not appear to have an increased risk for coronary heart disease. In Chapter 49 the genetic basis for heart disease, including hyperlipidemia and CAD, is reviewed.

Studies have indicated a familial aggregation of coronary heart disease, but this aggregation cannot be completely explained by the familial clustering of currently known risk factors for coronary disease.[221] Thus, there may be other genetic or environmental factors which remain to be defined. The question also arises as to when a possible family history is in itself an independent predictor of CAD, apart from known risk factors.

Shea and Nichols addressed the issue of the importance of family history in CAD.[222] They took the position that family history identifying the clustering or aggregation of risk factors in a family (called familial clustering or aggregation) is extremely important in populations with very high rates of cardiovascular disease. On the other hand, they believe that family history per se is more likely to be an independent predictor of CAD in families with a more moderate level of cardiovascular risk and in populations with a lower rate of CAD mortality. A positive family history could be explained on the basis of known risk factors. Conroy et al.[223] suggested that there may be familial aggregation of individuals with a high susceptibility to the effects of cigarette smoking, hypertension, and hyperlipoproteinemia, as in high-risk populations. Friedlander and associates, in an Israeli study, also confirmed the importance of a family history of myocardial infarction. However, this group also found that a positive family history was a predictor of myocardial infarction independent of other variables.[224] It is quite possible that differences in the genetic and environmental characteristics of the different populations studied could influence the extent to which a positive family history can be considered an independent variable for CAD.

Neufeld and Goldbourt emphasized the importance of genetics as determinants of the degree, time, course, and severity of atherosclerosis and symptomatic coronary disease. They suggested that the genetic component is very relevant to any intervention strategy, and they appear to favor the high-risk strategy, i.e., identifying high-risk individuals for special care.[225]

With respect to aggregation of coronary heart disease, Jorde et al. found no familial aggregation for earlobe creases.[226]

PSYCHOSOCIAL AND BEHAVIORAL FACTORS

The authors believe that psychosocial factors have played an important role in the incidence of CAD in Western society in this century. The mechanism of many psychosocial factors such as stress are not so well known. There have been six prospective studies[227] and many case control reports which have analyzed the relationships between depression, anxiety, and neuroticism and the conditions of CAD, angina pectoris, and angiographic findings of coronary artery blockage (Table 36–10). The most convincing evidence from these prospective studies come from those carried out in the United States, Israel, and Sweden; they provide strong evidence that emotional distress precedes the development of symptoms of CAD. If one attempts to relate the same measurements to myocardial infarction, the results are quite different, and in most cases there is a failure to show a statistical association between these

TABLE 36–10 SUMMARY OF STUDIES RELATING ANXIETY, DEPRESSION, AND NEUROTICISM TO CORONARY HEART DISEASE

Study	Place	Study Design*	Type of CHD†	Anxiety‡	Depression	Neuroticism
Medalie et al. (Am. J. Med. *55*:583, 1973)	Israel	P	AP	+		
Ostfeld et al. (J. Chron. Dis. *17*:265, 1964)	Chicago	P	AP		+/−	+
Lebovits et al. (Psychosom. Med. *29*:265, 1967)	Chicago	P	D	+	+	+
Floderus et al. (Nord. Hyg. Tid. Supp 6, 1974)	Sweden	P	AP-D			+
Bengtsson et al. (Acta Med. Scand. Supp 82, 1973)	Sweden	RC	AP-D	+		
Bruhn et al. (J. Psychosom. Res. *18*:187, 1974)	Oklahoma	P	D		+	
Paffenbarger et al. (Am. J. Epidemiol. *83*:314, 1966)	Pennsylvania/ Massachusetts	P	D	+		
Zyzanski et al. (Arch. Intern. Med. *136*:1234, 1976)	Boston	RC	Angio	+	+	

*P = Prospective study, RC = Retrospective study with control group.
†AP = Angina pectoris, D = Coronary death, Angio = Coronary angiography.
‡+ = A finding of a positive association, +/− = An equivocal association or different findings in different subgroups, O = A finding of no association.
From Jenkins, C. D.: Psychosocial and behavioral factors. *In* Kaplan, N. M., and Stamler, J. (eds.): Prevention of Coronary Heart Disease: Practical Management of the Risk Factors. Philadelphia, W. B. Saunders Company, 1983, p. 99.

various factors and myocardial infarction. The largest prospective study, reported in 1975, involved Swedish construction workers and showed a relationship between emotional factors and fatal and nonfatal myocardial infarctions. Mechanisms for accelerating CAD by chronic emotional disturbances have not been established but would include an overbalance of sympathetic versus parasympathetic activity, release of epinephrine and norepinephrine, and acute increases in blood pressure.

Liu et al.[228] analyzed educational background in relation to risk factors and long-term mortality from coronary disease, cardiovascular disease, and all-cause mortality for middle-aged men in the Chicago Heart Association Detection Project in Industry, from the People's Gas Company Study, and from the Western Electric Study. For all three cohorts, a graded inverse association was noted at baseline between educational level and blood pressure and between educational level and cigarette use at entry. No clear pattern was observed with cholesterol levels at time of entry. There was a statistically significant graded, inverse relationship between educational level and age-adjusted mortality rates from CAD, cardiovascular disease, and all causes. These investigators believed that the inverse relationship between educational level and mortality is explained at least in part by changes in the established known risk factors for coronary disease.

This interpretation is consistent with a study of DuPont Company employees.[229] A decline in myocardial infarction and in risk-factor modification did not occur uniformly across all socioeconomic groups; the higher the level of education and socioeconomic status, the greater the modification in life style and the greater the decline in incidence of coronary heart disease. Such observations do not establish causality, but it is obvious that the more affluent and highly educated individuals were more likely to follow a low-fat diet, control their weight, exercise regularly, and avoid tobacco. The great challenge presented to the U.S. health care delivery system is to insure that such changes are introduced and occur across all levels of society.

STRESS AND OCCUPATION

Davidson[230] has described the effects of physiological and psychological factors associated with occupation on the incidence of cardiovascular disease. Psychosocial factors which appear to influence the induction or exacerbation of cardiovascular disease include perceived job stress, role ambiguity or conflict, job autonomy, job-person fit, job change, unemployment, and retirement. Of course, actual physical factors can also be related to occupational mortality from heart disease, as has been established for carbon disulfide exposure and CAD, which has recently been reported by Wilcosky and Tyroler[231] in rubber industry–related jobs. These investigators observed an increase in cardiovascular mortality among workers exposed to carbon disulfide. Although others had previously observed this relationship, Wilcosky and Tyroler also raised the question of a possible relationship between ethanol and phenol and CAD.

STRESS AND TYPE A PERSONALITY

(See also p. 1883)

In addition to a type of stress called chronic disturbing emotion, a second type of psychosocial factor related to CAD is the so-called Type A behavior, or intense behavioral activation. Type A behavior has been extensively described by Friedman[232] and Rosenman and Chesney[233] and also supported by the investigations of Jenkins.[234] Available evidence led an expert panel at the NHLBI[235] to accept as valid an association between Type A behavior and CAD.

Type A persons, characterized as highly competitive, ambitious, and impatient, are in constant struggle with their environment. The Type B personality, on the other hand, is considered to be more passive and less disturbed by environmental stress. The relationship of Type A personality to CAD has been evaluated in several large studies, including the Framingham Study.[236] Type A personality traits seem to predispose a person to the complications of CAD even when studies were controlled for the more traditional risk factors such as hypertension, hypercholesterolemia, and smoking. Furthermore, the association between CAD and Type A personality has been correlated anatomically by angiography and physiologically by thallium-perfusion studies.[237, 238] A significant proportion of the population is at risk when as many as 50 per cent of men may be classed as Type A[236]; the incidence of this type of behavior may be increasing.

The Western Collaborative Study[239] showed that Type A men had 2.2 times the prevalence of CAD compared with Type B men. According to Rosenman et al., the risk ratio for developing CAD for Type A versus Type B varies with the length of follow-up from approximately 2:1 to 3:1.[240] Jenkins[241, 242] found a dose-response gradient between the Type A score and risk of first or recurrent myocardial infarction. In a prospective study of two separate cohorts by de Baker et al.,[243] a Jenkins Activity Survey Type A score and Speed and Impatience score showed a positive correlation with predictability for CAD. A retrospective analysis of the Framingham data reveals a relative risk of 1.6/1 for Type A men between ages 45 to 55 but an insignificant risk for those over age 55. The association of Type A with CAD was stronger with females, ranging from 8:1 in women aged 45 to 64 and 2:1 in women aged 65 to 74. The relationship was stronger between Type A behavior and angina, a weaker endpoint, than with Type A and myocardial infarction. One point of interest from the 8-year incidence data for CAD from Framingham was that the relationship of Type A behavior to CAD was much stronger in white-collar than in blue-collar workers. Jenkins has concluded from available evidence that Type A behavior is an independent contributor to CAD and has approximately the same strength as a risk factor such as cigarette smoking, elevated blood pressure, or serum cholesterol.

However, there are recent negative findings concerning Type A behavior and CAD. In the Aspirin Myocardial Infarction Study, Type A behavior did not correlate with the risk of reinfarction or coronary death.[244] Likewise, in the MRFIT study of men randomized to the usual care group, there was no relationship between the personality typing A or B (as determined by the so-called structured interview, or Jenkins Activity Survey score) and the 7-year mortality for CAD.[245]* Thus, some of the more recent studies have raised questions about the interpretation of earlier studies relating Type A personality to CAD. The

*The Jenkins Activity Survey is a questionnaire of self-reported multiple choices. The answers are scored by a computer on the basis of algorithms based on cross-validation against the structured interview ratings. The structured interview, developed by Rosenman et al., consists of 25 to 30 questions and observations of the study subjects. A four-point scale is used to rate behavior, more on the manner in which the recipient responds than on the content of the responses.

inconsistency between these more recent results and the earlier ones requires further analysis or studies for clarification.

Ruberman et al.[246] have described the psychosocial effects after myocardial infarction and their relation to mortality and noted the adverse effects of social isolation and a high degree of life stress on mortality after myocardial infarction. These investigators, in contrast, found that Type A behavior had no such independent influence. Thus, it may be very difficult to evaluate the effects of the separate concepts of stress and personality type on coronary mortality. Moser et al.[247] also analyzed psychosocial stress, in particular unemployment, and found that mortality from all causes was increased among the unemployed. Although Appels and Mulder in a recent study found no association between Type A behavior and incidence of myocardial infarction in 243 men in Rotterdam, a weak association existed between fatal coronary events and Type A personality ($p = .04$). This 9.5 year study led the investigators to conclude that the relationship between Type A behavior and fatal coronary disease also occurs in Europe, but the effect was a relatively weak one.[248] Friedman et al.[249] found that altering Type A behavior in post-myocardial infarction patients reduced their rate of recurrence and death from CAD when compared with controls. The 4.5 year cardiac recurrence rate was 12.9 per cent for those who received cardiac counseling and Type A counseling compared with a recurrence rate of 21.2 per cent in the comparison group, who received no special counseling. After a year, a significant difference occurred between the number of cardiac deaths in the Type A treated group and the control group and continued throughout the remaining 3.5 years of the study.

The precise way in which stress and Type A behavior patterns are manifested in ischemic heart disease is unclear and cannot be explained by a single mechanism. Stress may increase the risk imparted to a person by traditional factors and this may be modulated by the personal response. A rise in blood pressure might be anticipated to result from excess adrenergic response. However, there are little data to support the relationship of Type A personality and hypertension. Although some studies have shown a correlation between psychological factors and elevated blood pressure, the relationship is not definite.[250] Whether persons with Type A personality tend to be more likely to use tobacco has not been clearly established. There are slight changes in lipid values in patients under stress, but this has not been conclusively shown to add to total cardiac risk.[251] Type A patients may also react differently to nonstressful situations. Hence, while stress may play a role in the modification of traditional risk factors, this effect of stress appears to be a relatively minor one and apparently would not explain the epidemiologically documented increased risk.

Stress management has been advocated for primary and secondary prevention of coronary heart disease and has been shown prospectively to decrease the reaction to anxiety-provoking situations. Whether this type of intervention translates into reduced mortality from coronary artery disease has not been demonstrated. While stress management has also been utilized in the secondary treatment of post-myocardial infarction patients, the results are not conclusive for analysis of long-term survival data. Hence, while stress reduction and behavior modification have attractive features, they have not been evaluated to the point where they can be routinely recommended.[252] As Wilcox points out, personality scores and stress scores do not measure the same thing, although individuals' personalities influence their reaction to the external environment.[253] Better means of defining what is being measured and how to measure it are needed in order to explore further this difficult area.

GLUCOSE INTOLERANCE

Frank diabetes mellitus is a well-known risk factor for coronary artery disease.[254] However, problems have arisen in defining standardized criteria for the diagnosis of diabetes and in comparing the risk inherent in diabetics with that of patients who have glucose intolerance without overt diabetes. The definition of diabetes mellitus of the National Diabetes Data Group is given in Table 36–11. The mechanism of coronary effects is multifactorial for patients with overt diabetes and may relate to altered platelet function[255] or to increased red blood cell adhesion[256] in addition to the frequent association of hypertension, obesity, and lipid abnormalities. The Framingham Study found diabetes to be a major risk factor for CAD on the basis of the criteria of a fasting glucose of over 120 mg/dl, on the presence of glucosuria, and on oral glucose tolerance test showing a blood glucose greater than 160 mg/dl at one hour and more than 110 at 2 hours. This rather liberal definition of glucose intolerance was most likely responsible for inconsistencies of findings on various international studies relating hyperglycemia and CAD.

Frank diabetes occurs in 2 to 6 per cent of the general population, and impaired glucose tolerance may occur in up to 20 per cent, depending on the levels of glucose employed for the diagnosis.[255] However, overt diabetes will develop in only a small (<5%) percentage of patients with moderate glucose intolerance (2-hour plasma glucose of 140 to 200 mg/dl). Hence, the use of more conservative criteria to diagnose impaired glucose tolerance may alter the epidemiological findings.

The risk of ischemic heart disease in patients who have asymptomatic elevations of blood glucose is not clear. In a multivariate analysis of 15 different studies, the International Collaborative Group raised the issue of the absolute risk of asymptomatic hyperglycemia, especially when other risk factors such as hypertension, smoking, and hypercholesterolemia are present.[257] A critical analysis of a number of studies does not support a strong correlation between ischemic heart disease and asymptomatic hyperglycemia. In a review of more than a dozen studies, only data from the Chicago People's Gas Study showed a positive correlation between the 1-hour postprandial glucose level and death rate from CAD after correction of other risk factors[258]

TABLE 36–11 CRITERIA FOR DIABETES AND GLUCOSE INTOLERANCE IN NONPREGNANT ADULTS*

Diabetes Mellitus
(Type I = Insulin dependent; Type 2 = Noninsulin dependent)
Fasting plasma glucose ≥ 140 mg/dl
Sustained elevated plasma glucose levels during the OGTT†
Two hour ≥ 200 mg/dl
One other value between 0 and 2 hours ≥ 200 mg/dl
Classic symptoms of diabetes with unequivocal elevation of plasma glucose
Impaired Glucose Tolerance (OGTT)
Fasting plasma glucose <140 mg/dl
One value between 0 and 2 hours ≥ 200 mg/dl
Two hour = 140–199 mg/dl

*Reproduced from the National Diabetes Data Group: Classification and diagnosis of diabetes mellitus and other categories of glucose intolerance. Diabetes 28:1039, 1979.

†OGTT = Oral glucose tolerance test.

From Kaplan, N. M.: Diabetes and glucose intolerance. *In* Kaplan, N. M., and Stamler, J. (eds.): Prevention of Coronary Heart Disease: Practical Management of the Risk Factors. Philadelphia, W. B. Saunders Company, 1983, p. 114.

TABLE 36–12 CORONARY HEART DISEASE (CHD) AND CARDIOVASCULAR DISEASE (CVD) MORTALITY RATES FOR MIDDLE-AGED MEN IN THE HIGHEST PERCENTILES OF POSTLOAD BLOOD GLUCOSE

Series	Number of Men in Series	Percentile Chosen as Threshold	Number of Men above Threshold	CHD Mortality Rate per 1,000*		CVD Mortality Rate per 1,000*	
				Above Threshold†	Below Threshold	Above Threshold	Below Threshold
Stamler et al, 1979	6,596	97.5	164	10.5 (2)	11.2 (67)	15.8 (3)	13.5 (80)
Fuller et al, 1980	15,344	98.0	320	24.7 (10)	10.9 (171)	24.7 (10)	13.6 (213)
Reunanen et al, 1979	3,267	95.0	161	4.5 (1)	12.8 (38)	16.0 (3)	21.5 (64)
Ducimetiere et al, 1979	6,589	97.5	115	2.2 (1)‡	1.0 (35)‡	2.2 (1)‡	1.2 (42)‡

*Rates for follow-up periods of 4 to 5 years, except as specified.
†Number of deaths in parentheses.
‡Mean annual rates.
From Kaplan, N. M.: Diabetes and glucose intolerance. *In* Kaplan, N. M., and Stamler, J. (eds.): Prevention of Coronary Heart Disease: Practical Management of the Risk Factors. Philadelphia, W. B. Saunders Company, 1983, p. 115.

(Table 36–12). However, there is no question that established diabetes increases the risk of CAD. The same risk factors for CAD that apply to nondiabetics appear also to apply to diabetics, and diabetics are susceptible to both macro- and microvascular disease. The protective mechanism against CAD existing in premenopausal women is inoperative in Type I diabetes. Positive associations exist between diabetes and the following disorders: hypertension, hypertriglyceridemia, and low levels of HDL.

Control of hypertension appears to be particularly important in protection against microvascular diabetic complications in the eye and the kidney. Formation of glycosylated LDL has been suggested as a possible predisposing factor to macrovascular disease or atherosclerosis in diabetics. Evidence does not exist at this time as to whether or not maintaining normal glucose levels will reduce the risk of macrovascular or atheroscerotic complications in diabetics.

The approach to risk reduction in diabetes should be multifaceted. Weight control improves glucose control, and lipid abnormalities should be corrected by diet or drugs. Smoking should be discontinued and hypertension controlled, although alternatives to drugs which adversely alter glucose control or lipid levels should be sought. The benefits of tight control of blood glucose on the long-term vascular complications of diabetes has been controversial; however, the consensus is that the small vessel microangiopathies affecting the retina and kidney are reduced by maintaining more normal levels of plasma glucose. Normalization of fasting glucose may also improve lipid abnormalities.[259]

ESTROGENS AND SEX

It is well established that females have a lower incidence of CAD than males. In Western society, women have a life span averaging 8 years longer than men. It has been estimated that 40 per cent of the excess of male mortality is caused by CAD. In U.S. whites under age 45, males are 10 times more likely to develop myocardial infarction than are females. Wingard[260] published a 9-year follow-up of 6928 adults. Sixteen demographic and behavioral risk factors were analyzed, yet none could adequately account for the sex difference in CAD. In the Framingham data, differences in coronary risk could be accounted for by risk factor levels in individuals between ages 45 and 55 but not in individuals over age 55. Females have higher levels of HDL cholesterol and lower levels of LDL cholesterol and total cholesterol than do males under age 50. A striking increase in CAD occurs after menopause.

The question remains open as to the benefit of estrogen to postmenopausal women in protection against coronary disease. Rosenberg et al.[261] reported no association, as did Pfeffer et al.[262] The Harvard School of Public Health Study reported a significant decrease in coronary mortality in postmenopausal women receiving estrogens, particularly in smokers.[263] Postmenopausal women have a substantial increase in the incidence of coronary events.[264] The marked difference in coronary risk in men and women narrows with age.

EFFECT OF ESTROGENS IN FEMALES. Two conflicting reports have appeared concerning the question of whether estrogen will prevent heart attack in women. One of these studies, from the Harvard Medical School,[265] was a survey of more than 120,000 registered nurses. The investigators examined results from 33,317 postmenopausal females who were initially free of coronary disease. In 1976, 53 per cent had used estrogens at some time and 35 per cent were current users. The great majority were using Premarin or conjugated estrogen in a dosage of 1.2 or 0.6 mg per day. Of the women who had used estrogen, the risk of heart attack, either fatal or nonfatal, was approximately one-half of that in those who had never used them. Of the current users, the risk was about one-third of that in those who had never used estrogen. These results were not changed by correcting for age, cigarette smoking, past use of oral contraceptives, hypertension, diabetes, serum cholesterol, obesity, or family history.

A report based on the Framingham Study presented conflicting results.[266] The effect of estrogen use on morbidity from CAD was studied in 1234 postmenopausal women aged 50 to 83 years. Postmenopausal women who had taken estrogen had over a 50 per cent elevated risk of cardiovascular morbidity and more than a twofold risk for cerebrovascular disease compared with women who had not taken estrogen. Those who smoked while taking estrogen were at increased risk for myocardial infarction. Among nonsmokers, estrogen use was associated with only an increased incidence of stroke. Mortality from CAD and from all causes did not differ for either those who had taken estrogen or those who had not. Therefore, in postmenopausal women, little evidence exists beyond that of the Framingham Study that use of moderate doses of noncontraceptive estrogens are harmful to the cardiovascular system and, in fact, some evidence exists that such use might protect against CAD.

ESTROGEN IN MEN. The use of estrogen in men appears, if anything, to increase cardiovascular complications. In the Coronary Drug Project, mortality and complications due to thrombophlebitis and pulmonary embolism were increased by administration of estrogen in men who had already had one or more myocardial infarctions.[267] The effects of estrogens include an increase in serum HDL cholesterol, in VLDL, and in triglycerides, and a decrease in LDL cholesterol. In individuals who begin with a fasting plasma triglyceride level of over 500 mg/dl, the use of Premarin or other forms of estrogen or, for example, diethylstilbestrol in men with prostatic cancer, may exacerbate hypertriglyceridemia to the point of causing pancreatitis. Estrogen is not contraindicated in such patients, but it must be used with great caution and attention to its effects on the plasma triglyceride level. Some investigators have reported an association of estrogen and an impairment of glucose tolerance, an increased tendency toward thrombosis, an increase in blood pressure in susceptible individuals, and an increase in the tone of the smooth muscles of the coronary arteries possibly leading to spasm.

ORAL CONTRACEPTIVES. The use of these agents is more complicated than that of estrogens alone because most contain both estrogen and progesterone in varying quantities. Progesterone analogs decrease both triglyceride and HDL levels. The study of Mann et al.[268] was one of the first to demonstrate an increased risk of acute myocardial infarction associated with the use of oral contraceptives. The relative risk in oral contraceptive users was estimated at 4.5 compared with that in healthy nonusers. Other case-controlled studies also showed an association between the use of oral contraceptives and nonfatal myocardial infarctions in young women.[269, 270] Two large prospective studies in the United Kingdom also confirmed an increase of nonfatal myocardial infarction in users of oral contraceptives.[271, 272] The occurrence of the myocardial infarction was predominantly in cigarette smokers over age 35, and the risk was very slight in otherwise healthy women under age 40.

Linquist observed in a population of women in Gothenburg, Sweden,[273] that premature menopause was associated with an increased incidence of CAD; premature menopause per se might be a predisposing factor. It is also known that cigarette smokers have a higher incidence of premature menopause, so the effect could have been secondary to other risk factors. In women both in Scandinavia and in Framingham, serum triglyceride levels appeared to be an important predictor of coronary disease while myocardial infarction, hypertension, and smoking were also important indicators. Salonen[274] studied the use of oral contraceptives and smoking habits in samples of women from Eastern Finland, and observed an excessive risk of acute myocardial infarction in oral contraceptive users who also smoked. Engle et al.[275] studied the role of oral contraceptives in atherosclerosis and myocardial infarction in young women. In 34 patients who had myocardial infarctions without atherosclerosis, 27 had used oral contraceptives at the time of infarction; however, cigarette smoking was also common in this group. In the group with myocardial infarction with typical atherosclerosis, the usual atherogenic risk factors were present. Oral contraceptives were used by 15 of 42 of these patients. Thus, in the patients who had a myocardial infarction while taking oral contraceptive medication, 64 per cent did not have angiographically determined coronary atherosclerosis, which raises the possibility of an effect of the drug on coronary artery spasm. Oral contraceptives, particularly in association with cigarette smoking, might increase the risk of myocardial infarction in some women. On the basis of a study by the Royal College of General Practitioners,[271] the incidence of hypertension was increased 2.6 times in 23,000 women taking oral contraceptives as compared with a similar group who did not use them. A Scottish Study[276] also showed higher blood pressure readings in women on oral contraceptives; thus, hypertension may also contribute to myocardial infarction in women as a complication of oral contraceptives.

When comparing myocardial infarction in young men and young women, Wei and Bulkley found atherosclerosis to be more common in the men, while the women had a greater preponderance of nonatherosclerotic myocardial infarction. This suggests the greater importance of coronary spasm or thrombosis in young women with myocardial infarction.[277] Uhl studied 165 patients under age 40 with myocardial infarction and compared them with 100 patients over age 40.[278] The group under age 40 had more risk factors—in particular, smoking, hyperlipoproteinemia, hypertension, diabetes, and family history of CAD and obesity. It was of interest that physical exertion at the time of the infarction was more common in the younger patients. Mortality rate was lower in the younger patients as might be expected.

ALCOHOL

There is universal agreement that a high consumption of alcohol is an important preventable cause of death. It is also well established that consumption of more than approximately two alcoholic drinks per day is associated with higher levels of blood pressure (p. 837). While heavy drinking has been shown in at least seven different studies to increase mortality, including CAD mortality, other studies raise the possibility that moderate alcohol consumption might be beneficial. As described above (p. 1162), alcohol increases the level of HDL. Some studies have reported increases only in the HDL_3 fraction while another[279] found that both HDL_2 and HDL_3 were raised.

A study by St. Leger et al. of subjects ages 55 to 64 from 18 countries provided evidence for an inverse relationship between alcohol consumption and cardiac mortality.[280] The alcohol consumed was mainly wine. LaPorte et al.[281] also reported an inverse relationship between alcohol consumption and CAD in men aged 55 to 64 from 20 countries. The results of five case-controlled studies (Table 36–13) also show an inverse relationship between the daily consumption of small to moderate amounts of ethanol and CAD. Of five prospective studies, four also showed generally an inverse relationship of coronary heart disease in light-to-moderate drinkers.

TABLE 36–13 CASE-CONTROL STUDIES OF ALCOHOL CONSUMPTION AND CORONARY HEART DISEASE

Study	Size of Population	Level of Consumption	Relative Risk Drinkers: Nondrinkers
Klatsky et al., 1974	661 cases* 661 controls	≤2 drinks/day	0.7
		3–5 drinks/day	0.7
		6 + drinks/day	0.4
Stason et al., 1976	399 cases† 2486 controls	<6 drinks/day	1.0
		6 + drinks/day	0.6
Hennekens et al., 1978	568 cases‡	≤2 oz alcohol/day	0.4
		>2 oz alcohol/day	0.7
Petitti et al., 1979	not given†	Any	0.3
Rosenberg et al., 1981	513 cases† 918 controls	Any	0.7

*Both fatal and nonfatal.
†Nonfatal.
‡Fatal.
From Hennekens, C. H.: Alcohol. *In* Kaplan, N. M., and Stamler, J. (eds.): Prevention of Coronary Heart Disease: Practical Management of the Risk Factors. Philadelphia, W. B. Saunders Company, 1983, p. 132.

Stason[282] analyzed the Framingham Study cohort and arrived at a figure of 0.7 as the relative risk of those drinking 30 or more oz of ethanol per month, compared to those drinking less than this. Marmot et al.[283] in a 10-year study of male civil servants reported finding a lower total mortality among moderate drinkers than for nondrinkers or those consuming less than 34 gm of alcohol per day. The Chicago Western Electric Study,[284] by contrast, showed an insignificant relationship between moderate use of alcohol and CAD mortality. This study also showed a direct significant relationship between coronary mortality and heavy drinking. In a study on nonhuman primates fed a high cholesterol diet, it was found that those given alcohol had atherosclerotic blockage in 8 per cent of arteries as opposed to 48 per cent blockage in the same animals given a placebo.[285]

It is of interest that St. Leger et al. found that the inverse relationship between alcohol drinking and CAD mortality could be accounted for solely on the basis of the intake of wine by patients. The results may have been skewed by the data from France. A great deal of variability exists in the reporting of alcohol consumption, and in accounting for other cardiovascular risk factors. Although moderate drinking is associated with less coronary disease, there are many unanswered questions in this area. Several autopsy studies[286–288] have shown an inverse relationship between the level of alcohol consumption and extent of atherosclerosis. Barboriak[288] also found an inverse relationship between extent of CAD and levels of HDL, which is consistent with the hypothesis that inverse relationships between alcohol and CAD are mediated by HDL levels. Furthermore, because alcohol has such complex clinical and metabolic effects, and because of the social and medical implications of excess alcohol consumption, the authors do not advise patients to drink alcohol as a preventive measure.

MINOR RISK FACTORS

Because CAD is a multifactorial disease, several minor risk factors have been implicated in its genesis whose effects are not fully documented or understood. Some of these associated factors which we have not yet discussed include trace elements, water hardness, hypercalcemia, fibrinogen, vasectomy, coffee consumption, and hyperuricemia.

TRACE MINERALS. In the zinc-copper hypothesis, Klevay proposes that a relative deficiency of copper or an excess of zinc predisposes to hypercholesterolemia and CAD.[289, 290]

WATER HARDNESS. Leoni et al. studied the pattern of cardiovascular mortality in Abruzzo, Italy, between 1969 and 1978. They found an inverse relationship between water hardness and mortality due to cardiovascular disease similar to that reported previously from other countries.[291] Crawford et al.[292] extensively reviewed the subject of hardness of water compared with cardiovascular mortality from different regions and described an inverse relationship between cardiovascular mortality and water hardness. Unfortunately, an identification linking protection or risk to specific components has not yielded any definite results. Magnesium, selenium, and zinc have been noted in some studies as conferring protection, while manganese, lead, and cadmium have been reported to carry increased risk. The inconsistency of the findings makes it difficult to draw any definite conclusions or make recommendations concerning hardness of water as of this writing. Luoma et al.[293] reported a low concentration of fluoride and a low magnesium intake in Finnish men age 30 to 64 who were discharged after a first myocardial infarction in comparison with the control population.

HYPERCALCEMIA. Roberts and Waller[294] described chronic hypercalcemia as a risk factor for coronary atherosclerosis, noting that chronic hypercalcemia was associated with an accelerated deposition of calcium in the cardiac anuli and valvular cusps, in the media and intima of coronary arteries, and in myocardial fibers. These workers suggest that chronic hypercalcemia might be viewed as a risk factor for accelerated coronary atherosclerosis. This condition exists in a variety of metabolic situations, including primary hyperparathyroidism.

FIBRINOGEN. A stong association between fibrinogen concentration and CAD has been noted. As a risk factor, concentrations of fibrinogen have been reported to carry as much weight as any other risk factor that has been studied. This has been confirmed not only in the Framingham Study but in two others. Also, Meade et al. have shown that the concentration of factor VII is predictive of CAD up to 5 years.[295] Fibrinogen is positively correlated with concentrations of cholesterol and triglyceride and therefore is associated with hyperlipidemia. It is also correlated with smoking, obesity, and socioeconomic stress. Factor VII is also positively correlated with hyperlipoproteinemia, especially with Type IV. Miller et al. have reported that sudden administration of a fat load has no effect on the concentration of fibrinogen.[296]

Since over 90 per cent of patients with myocardial infarction exhibit a coronary thrombosis, one might expect high concentrations of fibrinogen to predispose to thrombotic events. Whether or not levels of fibrinogen and factor VII relate exclusively to the thrombotic aspect of CAD or whether they might play some role in atherogenesis is not known. In clinical trials in which atherosclerosis is studied, or in primary prevention trials, the endpoints measured are myocardial infarction, and/or death due to CAD. Therefore, there is a strong thrombotic contribution to the primary endpoints apart from any effect on atherosclerosis. The build-up of the atherosclerotic plaque is thought to be most closely related to levels of LDL, of other atherogenic lipoproteins, and inversely to levels of HDL. On the other hand, the events actually used to measure the effect on the atherosclerotic process are themselves dependent on thrombosis. Hence, fibrinogen and clotting factors have a strong potential effect on the way that the atherosclerotic process is assessed in primary prevention trials.

The concept that fibrin and the thrombotic process is related to atherogenesis is an old one; early researchers had postulated that fibrin contributes to the growth of atherosclerotic plaques. This might occur by the incorporation of a mural thrombus into the intima of an artery. Smith and Ashall have shown that fibrin is present in the normal arterial intima.[297] Fibrin may be diffusely or discretely deposited within an atherosclerotic plaque. Thus, it is arguable that the early proliferative plaque may arise from a mural fibrin thrombus. All of the clotting factors are present in the intima. Prothrombin is present in the gelatinous atherosclerotic lesion, but the ratio of the antithrombin III inhibitor to prothrombin is about 3:1. In patients dying of a myocardial infarction, Smith and Ashall did not find plasminogen to be present within the intima.[298] Therefore, it can be concluded that the intima has a high potential for formation of fibrin and a low potential for fibrinolysis.

Split fibrin products are present within the intima and exert potentially toxic effects including chemotaxis, increase of vascular permeability, and stimulation of fibroblast proliferation causing angiogenesis. Fibrin deposition might also be associated with the trapping of LDL. Smith et al. have shown that the intima contains not only extractable soluble LDL but also an insoluble apoB-containing substance which remains in the tissues.[299] This latter substance can be released by treatment with proteolytic enzymes, including plasminogen.

In summary, fibrin may be deposited in situ, and, as part of a mural thrombus, may initiate lesion formation or contribute to its development. Regardless of its relation to the atherogenic process per se, high concentrations of fibrinogen and factor VII, in conjunction with a high activity of prothrombin, a low activity of antithrombin III, and a low activity of plasminogen, would appear to enhance fibrin deposition and thrombus formation.

VASECTOMY. The subject of vasectomy and nonfatal myocardial infarction has been fraught with controversy. In animal studies, vasectomy increased the severity in diet-induced atherosclerosis in the Macaca fascicularis and in rhesus monkeys.[300, 301] Different investigators observed no excess risk for myocardial infarction in vasectomized men, nor was there an increase in the prevalence of hypertension or of hypercholesterolemia.[302] In a more recent study of 4733 vasectomized men,[303] the incidence of nonfatal myocardial infarction was 1.3 cases per 1000 man-years. This was virtually identical with a much larger series of comparable nonvasectomized men. Thus, at the present time, there is no established association between vasectomy and myocardial infarction up to 10 years after vasectomy.

COFFEE. The Tromso Heart Study has raised the interesting question of coffee consumption and serum cholesterol concentrations.[304] In persons consuming more than 9 cups of coffee a day compared to those consuming less than 1 cup, total cholesterol levels were significantly higher—6.23 versus 5.56 mmol in men and 5.92 versus 5.32 mmol in women. (One mmol is approximately 40 mg/dl.) In another report from the Tromso Heart Study,[305] the rise in cholesterol appeared to be related to consuming boiled rather than filtered coffee. Recently, LaCroix et al.[306] found an independent dose-responsive association between coffee consumption and clinically evident CAD. Over a period of 19 to 35 years, 1130 male medical students were followed and examined for clinically significant evidence of CAD, and changes in coffee consumption and cigarette smoking were documented. Heavy coffee drinkers were found to be at a twofold to threefold greater risk for CAD as compared with noncoffee drinkers.

CARDIAC TRANSPLANTATION. Accelerated atherosclerosis is an important problem affecting long-term survival after cardiac transplantation (p. 530). Hess et al.[307] have postulated that a mechanism of chronic immune injury due to cytotoxic B-cell antibodies and/or hypercholesterolemia led to accelerated atherosclerosis in transplanted hearts. These investigators followed 14 long-term survivors of cardiac transplantation and measured cytotoxic B-cell antibodies and hyperlipidemia and observed them for the development of CAD. Three patients in whom the underlying cardiac disease leading to the transplantation was cardiomyopathy developed no antibodies, had normal serum lipids, and were free of CAD for up to 6 months. Ten patients whose cardiac transplantations were necessitated by ischemic cardiomyopathy, and one who had idiopathic cardiomyopathy, developed severe hypercholesterolemia. Six of these 11 had cytotoxic B-cell antibodies; all 6 of these developed diffuse atherosclerosis and died between 8 and 30 months. The investigators postulated that the combination of hypercholesterolemia with cytotoxic B-cell antibodies is a predictor of accelerated atherosclerosis, myocardial infarction, and sudden death in transplant patients. The atherosclerotic lesions contained lymphocytic and monocytic infiltrates. In the five hypercholesterolemic patients without cytotoxic antibodies, atherosclerosis developed after 3 years with more proximal and discrete lesions. These investigators believed that hypercholesterolemia, due to an increase in LDL, in association with low levels of HDL and the presence of cytotoxic B-cell antibodies distinguish the patients who are most susceptible to accelerated atherosclerosis, death, and early myocardial infarction. Hypercholesterolemia and an absence of the B-cell antibodies predisposes to atherosclerosis but at a less accelerated rate than in those with the antibodies.

HYPERURICEMIA. This has long been of interest because of its association with CAD. A statistical association exists between hyperuricemia and hypertriglyceridemia. The Framingham Study[308] found that the concentration of serum uric acid was correlated with both the systolic and diastolic blood pressure. Uric acid was a predictor of myocardial infarction, but in multivariate analyses (including age, systolic blood pressure, relative weight, cigarette smoking, and serum cholesterol) serum uric acid was not an independent predictor of coronary disease. Rather, hyperuricemia is viewed as an indication of a metabolic disturbance or of disturbances which themselves may predispose to coronary disease.

Acknowledgment

We wish to acknowledge the excellent assistance of Mrs. Beth Flinn in the preparation of this chapter.

REFERENCES

EPIDEMIOLOGY AND THE DECLINING DEATH RATE

1. Kuller, L. H.: Controlling coronary heart disease: Where we will stand by the end of this decade. Presp. Lipid Dis. (*In press.*)
2. Goor, R., Hosking, J. D., Dennis, B. H., Graves, K. L., Waldman, G. T., and Haynes, S. G.: Nutrient intakes among selected North American populations in the Lipid Research Clinics Prevalence Study: Composition of fat intake. Am. J. Clin. Nutr. *41*:299, 1985.
3. Stallones, R. E.: Mortality due to ischemic heart disease: Observations and explanations. *In* Gotto, A. M. Jr., and Paoletti, R. (eds.): Atherosclerosis Reviews 9:43, 1982.

DEFINITION OF RISK FACTORS

4. Kannel, W. B., and Gordon, T.: The Framingham Study: An epidemiological investigation of cardiovascular disease, Section 30. Some characteristics related to the incidence of cardiovascular disease and death: the Framingham Study. 18-year follow-up. Washington, D.C., Dept. of Health, Education, and Welfare, Publication No. (NIH) 74–599, 1974.
5. Yano, K., Reed, S. M., and McGee, D. L.: Ten-year incidence of coronary heart disease in the Honolulu heart program. Relationship to biologic and lifestyle characteristics. Am. J. Epidemiol. *119*:653, 1984.
6. Carter, C., McGee, D., Reed, D., Yano, K., and Stemmerman, G.: Hematocrit and the risk of coronary heart disease: The Honolulu Heart Program. Am. Heart J. *105*:674, 1983.

HYPERCHOLESTEROLEMIA

7. Anitschkow, N., and Chalatow, S.: Uber experimentelle Cholesterinsteatose. Centralbl. Allg. Pathol. Anat. *24*:1, 1913.
8. Keyes, A. (ed.): Coronary heart disease in seven countries. Circulation *41*, Suppl. 1, 1970.
9. Holman, R. L., McGill, H. C., Jr., Strong J. P., and Greer, J. C.: The natural history of atherosclerosis. Am. J. Pathol. *34*:209, 1958.
10. Simons, L. A.: Interrelations of lipids and lipoproteins with coronary artery disease mortality in 19 countries. Am. J. Cardiol. *57*:5G, 1986.
10a. Peto, R.: Personal communication, 1986.
11. Dayton, S., and Pearce, M. L.: Diet high in unsaturated fat. A controlled clinical trial. Minn. Med. *52*:1237, 1969.
12. Coronary Drug Project Research Group: Clofibrate and niacin in coronary heart disease. J.A.M.A. *231*:360, 1975.
13. Turpeinen, O., Karvonen, M. J., Pekkarinen, M., Miettinen, M., Elosuo, R., and Paavilainen, E.: Dietary prevention of coronary heart disease: The Finnish mental hospital study. Int. J. Epidemiol. *8*:99, 1979.
14. Committee of Principal Investigators: WHO Clofibrate Trial. WHO cooperative trial on primary prevention of ischemic heart disease using clofibrate to lower serum cholesterol: Mortality follow-up report. Lancet 2:379, 1980.
15. Hjermann, I., Holme, I. Byre, K., and Leren, P.: Effect of diet and smoking on the incidence of coronary heart disease: Report from the Oslo study group of a randomized trial in healthy men. Lancet 2:1303, 1981.
16. Multiple-Risk Factor Intervention Trial Research Group: Multiple-Risk Factor Intervention Trial: Risk factor changes in mortality results. J.A.M.A. *248*:1465, 1982.
17. Lipid Research Clinics' Program: The Lipid Research Clinics' coronary primary prevention trial results. I. Reduction in incidence of coronary heart disease. II. The relationships of reduction in incidence of coronary heart disease to cholesterol lowering. J.A.M.A. *251*:351, 1984.
18. Castelli, W. P.: Personal communication, 1986.
19. Castelli, P.: Framingham heart study update: Cholesterol, triglycerides, lipoproteins, and the risk of coronary heart disease. Perspect. Lipid Dis. *3*:20, 1986.
20. Carlson, L. A., and Bottiger, L. E.: Risk factors for ischemic heart disease in men and women. Acta. Med. Scand. *218*:207, 1985.
21. Newman, W. P., Freedman, D. S., Voors, A. W., Gard, P. D., Srinivasen, S. R., Cresanta, J. L., Williamson, G. D., Webber, L. S., and Berenson, G. S.: Relation of serum lipoprotein levels and systolic blood pressure to early atherosclerosis—The Bogalusa Heart Study. N. Engl. J. Med. *314*:138, 1986.
22. Cabin, H. S., and Roberts, W. C.: Relation of serum total cholesterol and triglyceride levels to the amount and extent of coronary arterial narrowing by atherosclerotic plaque in coronary heart disease. Am. J. Med. *73*:227, 1982.
23. Duffield, R. G. M., Lewis, B., Miller, N. E., Jamieson, C. W., Brunt, J. N. H., and Colchester, A. C. F.: Treatment of HLP retards progression of symptomatic femoral atherosclerosis: A randomized controlled trial. Lancet 2:639, 1985.
24. Levy, R. I., Brensike, J. F., Epstein, S. E., Kelsey, S. F., Passamani, E. R., Richardson, J. M., Loh, I. K., Stone, N. J., Aldrich, R. F., and Battaglini, J. W.: The influence of changes in lipid values induced by cholestyramine and diet on progression of coronary artery disease: Results of the NHLBI Type II coronary intervention study. Circulation *69*:325, 1984.
25. Arntzenius, A. C., Kromhout, D., Barth, J. D., Reiber, J. H. C., Bruschke, A. V., Buis, B., van Gent, C. M., Kempen-Voogd, N., and Strikwerda, S.: Diet, lipoproteins, and the progression of coronary atherosclerosis. N. Engl. J. Med. *312*:805, 1985.
26. Consensus Conference Statement: Lowering blood cholesterol to prevent heart disease. J.A.M.A. *253*:2080, 1985.

LIPOPROTEINS

27. Kottke, B. A., Zinmeister, A. R., Holmes, D. R. Jr., Kneller, R. W., Hallaway, B. J., and Mao S. J.: Apolipoproteins and coronary artery disease. Mayo Clin. Proc. *61*:313, 1986.
27a. Hegele, R. A., Huang, L.-S., Herbert, P. N., Blum, C. B., Buring, J. E., Hennekens, C. H., and Breslow, J. L.: Apolipoprotein B—Gene DNA polymorphism associated with myocardial infarction. N. Engl. J. Med. *315*:1509, 1986.
28. Chen, S.-H., Yang, C.-Y., Chen, P.-F., Setzer, D., Tanimura, M., Li, W.-H., Gotto, A. M., Jr., and Chan, L.: The complete cDNA and amino acid sequence of human apolipoprotein B-100. J. Biol. Chem. *261*:12918, 1986.
29. Yang, C.-Y., Chen, S.-H., Gianturco, S. H., Bradley, W. A., Sparrow, J. T., Tanimura, M., Li, W.-H., Sparrow, D. A., DeLoof, H., Rosseneu, M., Lee, F.-S., Gu, Z.-W., Gotto, A. M., Jr., and Chan, L.: Sequence, structure, receptor-binding domains and internal repeats of human apolipoprotein B-100. Nature *323*:738, 1986.
30. Knott, T. J., Rall, S. C., Innerarity, T. L., Jacobson, S. F., Urdea, M. S., Levy-Wilson, B., Powell, L. M., Pease, R. J., and Nakai, H.: Human apolipoprotein B: Structure of carboxyl-terminal domains, sites of gene expression, and chromosomal localization. Science *230*:37–43, 1985.
31. Goldstein, J. L., and Brown, M. S.: Familial hypercholesterolemia. *In* Stanbury, J. B., Wyngaarden, J. B., Fredrickson, D. S., Goldstein, J. L., and Brown, M. S. (eds.): The Metabolic Basis of Inherited Disease. 5th ed. New York, McGraw-Hill Book Co., 1985, pp. 672–712.
31a. Lenzen, H. J., Assmann, G., Buchwalsky, R., and Schulte, H.: Association of apolipoprotein E polymorphism, low-density lipoprotein cholesterol, and coronary artery disease. Clin. Chem. *32*:778, 1986.
32. Sherril, B. C., Innerarity, T. L., and Mahley, R. W.: Rapid hepatic clearance of the canine lipoproteins containing only the E apoprotein by a high affinity receptor. J. Biol. Chem. *255*:1804, 1980.
33. Havel, R. J.: Familial dysbetalipoproteinemia: New aspects of pathogenesis and diagnosis. Med. Clin. N. Am. *66*:441, 1982.
34. Hazzard, W. R.: Primary Type III hyperlipidemia. *In* Rifkind, B. M., and Levy, R. I. (eds.): Hyperlipidemia: Diagnosis and Therapy. New York, Grune and Stratton, 1977, p. 137.
35. Schaefer, E. J., and Levy, R. I.: Pathogenesis and management of lipoprotein disorders. N. Engl. J. Med. *312*:1300, 1985.
36. Goldstein, J. L., and Brown, M. S.: Atherosclerosis: The low-density lipoprotein receptor hypothesis. Metabolism *26*:1257, 1977.
37. Witztum, J. L.: The role of lipoprotein receptor in the regulation of plasma low density lipoprotein levels. *In* Haft, J., and Karliner, J. S. (eds.): Receptor Science in Cardiology. Mt. Kisco, N. Y., Futura Publishing Co. 1983, pp. 227–258.
38. Oram, J. F., Brinton, E. A., and Bierman, E. L.: Regulation of high density lipoprotein in cultured human skin fibroblasts and human arterial smooth muscle cells. J. Clin. Invest. *72*:1611, 1983.
39. Schmitz, G., Robenek, H., Lohmann, U., and Assmann, G.: Interaction of high-density lipoproteins with cholesteryl ester–laden macrophages: Biochemical and morphological characterization of cell surface receptor binding, endocytosis, and resecretion of high-density lipoproteins by macrophages. E.M.B.O.J., *4*:613, 1985.
40. Patsch, W., Schonfeld, G., Gotto, A. M., Jr., and Patsch, J. R.: Characterization of human high-density lipoproteins by zonal ultracentrifugation. J. Biol. Chem. *255*:3178, 1980.
41. Gordon, T., Castelli, W. P., Hjortland, M. C., Kannel, W. B., and Dawber, T. R.: High density lipoprotein as a protective factor against coronary heart disease. The Framingham Study. Am. J. Med. *62*:707, 1977.
42. Fraser, G. E., Anderson, J. T., Foster, N., Goldberg, R., Jacobs, D., and Blackburn, H.: The effect of alcohol on serum high density lipoproteins. Atherosclerosis *46*:275, 1983.
43. Pocock, S. J., Shaper, A. G., Phillips, A. N., Walker, M., and Whitehead, T.

P.: High-density lipoprotein cholesterol is not a major risk factor for ischaemic heart disease in British men. Br. Med. J. *292*:515, 1986.
44. Dahlen, G. H., Guyton, J. R., Attar, M., Farmer, J. A., Kautz, J. A., and Gotto, A. M., Jr.: Association of levels of lipoprotein Lp (a), plasma lipids and other lipoproteins with coronary artery disease documented by angiography. Circulation *74*:758, 1986.
45. Karathanasis, S. K., Norum, R. A., Zannis, V. I., and Breslow, J. L.: An inherited polymorphism in the human apolipoproteinA-I gene locus related to the development of atherosclerosis. Nature *301*:1718, 1983.
46. Franceschini, G., Sirtori, C. R., Capurso, A., Weisgraber, K. H., and Mahley, R. W.: A-I Milano apoprotein. Decreased high-density lipoprotein cholesterol levels with significant lipoprotein modifications and without clinical atherosclerosis in an Italian family. J. Clin. Invest. *66*:892, 1980.
47. Utermann, G., Steinmetz, A., Paetzold, R., Wilk, J., Feussner, G., Kaffarnik, H., Mueller-Eckhardt, C., Seidel, D., Vogelberg, K. H., and Zimmer, F.: Apolipoprotein A-I Marburg: Studies on two kindreds with a mutant of human apolipoprotein A-I. Hum. Genet. *61*:329, 1982.
48. Breslow, J. L.: Apolipoprotein defects. Hosp. Pract. *20*:43, 1985.
49. Seilhamer, J. J., Protter, A. A., Frossard, P., and Levy-Wilson, B.: Isolation and DNA sequence of full-length cDNA and of the entire gene for human apolipoprotein AI—discovery of a new genetic polymorphism in the apo AI gene. DNA *3*:309, 1984.
50. Protter, A. A., Levy-Wilson, B., Miller, J., Bencen, G., White, T., and Seilhamer, J. J.: Isolation and sequence analysis of the human apolipoprotein CIII gene and the intergenic region between the apo AI and apo CIII genes. DNA *3*:449, 1984.
51. Ordovas, J. M., Schaefer, E. J., Salem, D., Ward, R. H., Glueck, C. J., Vergani, C., Wilson, P. W., and Karathanasis, S. K.: Apolipoprotein A-I gene polymorphism associated with premature coronary artery disease and familial hyperalphalipoproteinemia. N. Engl. J. Med. *314*:671, 1986.
52. Vergani, C., and Bettale, G.: Familial hypoalphalipoproteinemia. Clin. Chim. Acta. *114*:45–52, 1981.
53. Third, J. L. H. C., Montag, J., Flynn, M., Freidel, J., Laskarzewski, P., and Glueck, C. J.: Primary and familial hypoalphalipoproteinemia. Metabolism *33*:136, 1984.
54. Glueck, C. J., Daniels, S. R., Bates, S., Benton, C., Tracy, T., and Third, J. L. C. H.: Pediatric victims of unexplained stroke and their families: Familial lipid and lipoprotein abnormalities. Pediatrics *69*:308, 1982.
55. Daniels, S. R., Bates, S., Lukin, R. R., Benton, C., Third, J., and Glueck, C. J.: Cerebrovascular arteriopathy (arteriosclerosis) and ischemic childhood stroke. Stroke *13*:360, 1982.
56. Breckenridge, W. C., Little, J. A., Steiner, G., Chow, A., and Poapst, M.: Hypertriglyceridemia associated with deficiency of apolipoprotein C-II. N. Engl. J. Med. *298*:1265, 1978.
57. Gotto, A. M., Jr.: ApoC-II deficiency revisited. N. Engl. J. Med. *310*:1664, 1984.
58. Herbert, P. N., Assmann, G., Gotto, A. M., Jr., and Frederickson, D. S.: Familial lipoprotein deficiency: Abetalipoproteinemia, hypobetalipoproteinemia, and Tangier disease. *In* Stanbury, J. B., et al.: The Metabolic Basis of Inherited Disease. New York, McGraw-Hill Book Co., 1983, p. 589.
58a. Young, S. G., Bertics, S. J., Curtiss, L. K., Casal, D. C., and Witztum, J. L.: Monoclonal antibody MB19 detects genetic polymorphism in human apolipoprotein B. Proc. Natl. Acad. Sci. USA *8*:1101, 1986.
59. Teng, B., Sniderman, A. D., Soutar, A. K., and Thompson, G. R.: Metabolic basis of hyperapobetalipoproteinemia. Turnover of apolipoprotein B in low density lipoprotein and its precursors and subfractions compared with normal and familial hypercholesterolemia. J. Clin. Invest. *77*:663, 1986.
59a. Fredrickson, D. S., and Lees, R. S.: System for phenotyping hyperlipoproteinemia. Circulation *31*:321, 1965.
60. Streja, D., Steiner, G., and Kwitterovick, P. O.: Plasma high density lipoproteins and ischemic heart disease. Studies in a large kindred with familial hypercholesterolemia. Ann. Intern. Med. *89*:871, 1978.
61. Shapiro, J. R., Fallet, R. W., Tsang, R. C., and Glueck, C. J.: Achilles tendinitis and tenosynovitis. A diagnostic manifestation of familial Type II hyperlipoproteinemia in children. Am. J. Dis. Child. *128*:486, 1974.
62. Gagne, C., Moorjani, S., Brun, D., Toussaint, M., and Lupien, P. J.: Heterozygous familial hypercholesterolemia: Relationship between plasma lipids, lipoproteins, clinical manifestations and ischemic heart disease in men and women. Atherosclerosis *34*:13, 1979.
63. Goldstein, J. L.: The cardiac manifestations of homozygous and heterozygous forms of Type II hyperbetalipoproteinemia. Birth Defects *8*:202, 1972.
64. Slack, J.: Risks of ischemic heart disease in familial hyperlipoproteinemic states. Lancet *2*:1380, 1969.
65. Goldstein, J. L., Schratt, H. G., Hazzard, W. R., Bierman, E. L., and Motulsky, A. G.: Hyperlipidemia in coronary heart disease. II. Genetic analysis of lipid levels in 176 families and delineation of a new inherited disorder, combined hyperlipidemia. J. Clin. Invest. *52*:1544, 1973.
66. Rose, H. G., Kranz, P., Weinstock, M., Juliano, J., and Haft, J. I.: Inheritance of combined hyperlipoproteinemia. Evidence for a new lipoprotein phenotype. Am. J. Med. *54*:148, 1973.
67. Goldstein, J. L.: Hyperlipidemia in coronary heart disease: I. Lipid levels in 500 survivors of myocardial infarction. J. Clin. Invest. *52*:1533, 1973.
68. Brunzell, J. D., Albers, J. J., Chait, A., Grundy, S. M., Groszek, E., and McDonald, G. B.: Plasma lipoproteins in familial combined hyperlipidemia and monogenic familial hypertriglyceridemia. J. Lipid Res. *24*:147, 1983.
69. Vega, G. L., Illingworth, R. P., and Grundy, S. M.: Normocholesterolemic tendon xanthomatosis with overproduction of apolipoprotein B. Metabolism *32*:118, 1963.
70. Pe'er, J., Vidaurri, J., Halfon, S.-T., Eisenberg, S., and Zauberman, H.: Association between corneal arcus and some of the risk factors for coronary artery disease. Br. J. Ophthalmol. *67*:795, 1983.
71. Tatomi, R., Mabuchi, H., and Veda, K.: Intermediate density lipoprotein and cholesterol rich VLDL in angiographically determined coronary artery disease. Circulation *64*:1174, 1981.
72. Fredrickson, D. S., Morganroth, J., and Levy, R. I.: Type III hyperlipoproteinemia. Ann. Intern. Med. *82*:150, 1975.
73. Utermann, G., Jaeschke, M., and Menz, J.: Familial hyperlipoproteinemia. Type III: Deficiency of apoE-III in VLDL. F.E.B.S. Lett. *56*:352, 1975.
74. Schaeffer, E. J., and Levy, R. I.: Pathogenesis and management of lipoprotein disorders. N. Engl. J. Med. *312*:1300, 1985.
75. Breckenridge, W. C., Little, J. A., Alaupovic, P., Wang, C. S., Kuksis, A., Kakis, G., Lindgren, F., and Gardiner, G.: Type III hyperlipoproteinemia associated with a familial deficiency of hepatic lipase. Atherosclerosis *45*:161, 1982.
76. Havel, R. J.: Familial dysbetalipoproteinemia: New aspects of pathogenesis and diagnosis. Med. Clin. N. Am. *66*:441, 1982.
77. Morganroth, J., Levy, R. I., and Fredrickson, D. S.: The biochemical, clinical, and genetic features of Type III hyperlipoproteinemia. Ann. Intern. Med. *82*:158, 1977.
78. Janus, E. D., Nicoll, A. M., Turner, P. R., Magill, P., and Lewis, B.: Kinetic basis of the primary hyperlipoproteinemia. Eur. J. Clin. Invest. *10*:161, 1980.
79. Sniderman, A. D., Wolfson, C., Teng, B., Franklin, F. A., Bachorik, P. S., and Kwiterovich, P. O. J.: Association of hyperapobetalipoproteinemia with endogenous hypertriglyceridemia and atherosclerosis. Ann. Intern. Med. *97*:833, 1982.
80. Chait, A., Mancini, M., February, A. W., and Lewis, B.: Clinical and metabolic study of alcoholic hyperlipidemia. Lancet *2*:62, 1972.
81. Sadbank, V., Bechan, M., and Bonnstein, B.: Hyperlipidemia neuropathy. Acta Neuropathol. *19*:290, 1971.
82. Fallat, R. W., and Glueck, C. J.: Familial and acquired type V hyperlipoproteinemia. Atherosclerosis *23*:41, 1976.
83. Zilversmit, D. B.: Atherogenesis: A postprandial phenomenon. Circulation *60*:473, 1979.

TREATMENT OF HYPERLIPOPROTEINEMIA

84. Rosenberg, L., Armstrong, B., and Jick, H.: Myocardial infarction and estrogen therapy in postmenopausal women. N. Engl. J. Med. *294*:1256, 1976.
85. Pfeffer, R. I., Whipple, G. H., Kurosaki, T. T., and Chapman, J. M.: Coronary risk and estrogen use in post menopausal women. Am. J. Epidemiol. *107*:479, 1978.
86. Barrett-Conner, E., Brown, W. V., Turner, J., Austin, M., and Criqui, M. H.: Heart disease risk factors and hormone use in postmenopausal women. J.A.M.A. *241*:2167, 1979.
87. Wynn, V., Adams, P. W., Godsland, I., Melrose, J., Mithyananthen, R., Oakley, N. W., and Seed, M.: Comparison of the effects of different combined oral contraceptive formulations on carbohydrate and lipid metabolism. Lancet *1*:1045, 1979.
88. Lipid Research Clinics Program Epidemiology Committee: Plasma lipid distribution in selected North American populations. The LRC Program Prevalence Study. Circulation *60*:427, 1979.
89. Wahl, P., Walden, C., Knopp, R., Hoover, J., Wallace, R., Neiss, G., and Rifkind, B.: Effect of estrogen/progestin potency on lipid/lipoprotein cholesterol. N. Engl. J. Med. *308*:862, 1983.
90. Bradley, D. D., Wingerd, J., Petitt, D. B., Krauss, R. M., and Ramcharan, S.: Serum high density lipoprotein cholesterol in women using oral contraceptives, estrogen, and progestin. N. Engl. J. Med. *299*:17, 1978.
91. Leren, P., Foss, P. O., Helgeland, A., Hjermann, I., Holme, I., and Lund-Larsen, P. G.: Effect of propranolol and prazosin on blood lipids. The Oslo Study. Lancet *2*:4, 1980.
92. Shulman, R. S., Herbert, P. N., Capone, R., et al.: Effects of propranolol on blood lipids and lipoproteins in myocardial infarction. Circulation 67(suppl I): 19, 1983.
93. Velasco, M., Silva, H., Morillo, J., Pellicer, R., Urbana-Quintana, A., and Hernandez-Pieretti, O.: Effect of prazosin on blood lipids and on thyroid function in hypertensive patients. J. Cardiovasc. Pharmacol. 4(Suppl 2):S 225, 1982.
94. Zanchetti, A.: Summary of prozosin lipid studies. Am. J. Med. *76*(2A):122, 1984.
95. AHA Special Report: Recommendations for treatment of hyperlipidemia in adults. Circulation *69*:1065, 1984.
96. Mattson, F. H., and Grundy, S. M.: Comparison of effects of dietary saturated, monounsaturated, and polyunsaturated fatty acids on plasma lipids and lipoproteins in man. J. Lipid Res. *26*:194, 1985.
97. Bang, H. O., Dyerberg, J., and Hjrne, N.: The composition of food consumed by Greenland Eskimos. Acta. Med. Scand. *69*:200, 1976.
98. Dyerberg, J., and Bang, H. O.: Haemostatic function and platelet polyunsaturated fatty acids in Eskimos. Lancet *2*:433, 1979.
99. Bang, H. O., Dyerberg, J., and Sinclair, H. M.: The composition of the Eskimo food in northwestern Greenland. Am. J. Clin. Nutr. *33*:2657, 1980.
100. Philipson, B. E., Rothrode, D. W., Connor, W. E., Harris, W. S., and Illingworth, D. R.: Reduction of plasma lipids, lipoproteins, and apoproteins

by dietary fish oils in patients with hypertriglyceridemia. N. Engl. J. Med. *312*:1210, 1216, 1985.

101. Simons, L. A., Hickie, J. B., and Balasubramaniam, S.: On the effects of dietary n-3 fatty acids (Maxepa) on plasma lipids and lipoproteins in patients with hyperlipidemia. Atherosclerosis *54*:75, 1985.
102. Thorngren, M., Shafi, S., and Born, G. V. R.: Delay in primary haemostasis produced by a fish diet without change in local thromboxane A_2. Br. J. Haematol *58*:567, 1984.
103. Brox, J. H., Killie, J. E., Osterud, B., Holme, S., and Nordy, A.: Effects of cod liver oil on platelets and coagulation in familial hypercholesterolemia (Type IIa). Acta Med. Scand. *213*:137, 1983.
104. Lorenz, R., Spengler, U., Fishcer, S. Duhm, J., and Weber, P. C.: Platelet function, thromboxane formation and blood pressure control during supplementation of the Western diet with cod liver oil. Circulation *67*:504, 1983.
105. Hoeg, J. M., Gregg, R. E., and Brewer, H. B.: An approach to the management of hyperlipoproteinemia. J.A.M.A. *255*:512, 1986.
106. Gotto, A. M., Jr., Jones, P. H., and Scott, L. W.: The diagnosis and management of hyperlipidemia. Disease-A-Month *321*:245, 1986.
107. Jones, P. H., and Gotto, A. M., Jr.: Drug treatment of hyperlipidemia. Mod. Concepts Cardiovasc. Dis. *53*:53, 1984.
108. Levy, R. I.: Drugs used in the treatment of hyperlipoproteinemia. *In* Goodman, A. S., Gilman, L. S., Gilman, A. (eds.): The Pharmacologic Basis of Therapeutics. New York, Macmillan, 1980, pp. 834–877.
108a. Baker, S. G., Joffe, B. I., Mendelsohn, D., and Seftel, H. C.: Treatment of homozygous familial hypercholesterolemia with probucol. S. Afr. Med. J. *62*:7, 1982.
109. Grundy, S. M., Mok, H. Y. I., Zech, L., and Berman, M.: Influence of nicotinic acid on metabolism of cholesterol and triglycerides in man. J. Lipid Res. *22*:24, 1981.
110. Shepherd, J., Packard, C. J., Patsch, J. R., Gotto, A. M., Jr., and Taunton, O. D.: Effects of nicotinic acid therapy on plasma high density lipoprotein subfraction distribution and composition on apolipoprotein A metabolism. J. Clin. Invest. *63*:858, 1979.
111. Mellies, M. J., Gartside, P. S., Glatfelter, L., Vink, P. Guy, G., Schonfeld, G., and Glueck, C. J.: Effects of probucol on plasma cholesterol, high- and low-density lipoprotein cholesterol and apolipoprotein A-I and A-II in adults with primary familial hypercholesterolemia. Metabolism *29*:956, 1980.
111a. Kuo, P. T., Wilson, A. C., Kostis, J. B., and Moreyra, A. E.: Effects of combined probucol-colestipol treatment for familial hypercholesterolemia and coronary artery disease. Am. J. Med. 57:43H, 1986.
112. Nestel, P. J., and Billington, T.: Effects of probucol on low density lipoprotein removal and high-density lipoprotein synthesis. Atherosclerosis 38:203, 1981.
113. Samuel, P.: Effects of gemfibrozil on serum lipids. Am. J. Med. *74*:23, 1983.
114. Lewis, J. E.: Long-term use of gemfibrozil in the treatment of dyslipidemia. Angiology *33*:603, 1982.
115. WHO cooperative trial on primary prevention of ischaemic heart disease using clofibrate to lower serum cholesterol: Mortality follow-up. Lancet *2*:379, 1980.
116. Mabuchi, H., Sakai, T., and Sakai, Y.: Reduction of serum cholesterol in heterozygous patients with familial hypercholesterolemia. Additive effects of compactin and cholestyramine. N. Engl. J. Med. *308*:609, 1983.
117. Bilheimer, D. W., Grundy, S. M., Brown, M. S., and Goldstein, J. L.: Mevinolin and colestipol stimulate receptor mediated clearance of low density lipoproteins from plasma in familial hypercholesterolemic heterozygotes. Proc. Natl. Acad. Sci. USA *80*:4124, 1983.
118. Schroepfer, G. J., Jr., Sherill, B. C., Wang, K.-S., Wilson, W. K., Kisic, A., and Clarkson, T. B.: 5α-cholest-8(14)-en-3 β-01-15-one lowers serum cholesterol and induces profound changes in levels of lipoprotein cholesterol and apoproteins in monkeys fed a diet of moderate cholesterol content. Proc. Natl. Acad. Sci. USA *81*:6861, 1984.
119. Tilvis, R. S., and Miettinen, T. A.: Serum plant sterols and their relation to cholesterol absorption. Am. J. Clin. Nutr. *43*:92, 1986.
120. Brunzell, J. D., Miller, N. E., Alaupovic, P., St. Hilaire, R. J., Wang, C. S., Sarson, P. L., Bloom, S. R., and Lewis, B.: Familial chylomicronemia due to a circulating inhibitor of lipoprotein lipase activity. J. Lipid Res. *24*:12, 1983.
121. Bilheimer, D. W., Goldstein, J. L., Grundy, S. M., Starzl, T. E., and Brown, M. S.: Liver transplantation to provide low density lipoprotein receptors and lower plasma cholesterol in a child with homozygous familial hypercholesterolemia. N. Engl. J. Med. *311*:1658, 1984.
122. Schaefer, E. J.: Dietary and Drug Treatment. *In* Brewer, H. B. (moderator): Type III Hyperlipoproteinemia: Diagnosis, molecular effects, pathology, and treatment. Ann. Intern. Med. 98:623, 1983.
123. Kushwaha, R. S., Hazzard, W. R., Gagne, C., Chait, A., and Albers, J.: Type III hyperlipoproteinemia: Paradoxical hypolipidemic response to estrogen. Ann. Intern. Med. 87:517, 1977.
124. Miettinen, T. A., and Lempinen, M.: Cholestyramine and ileal bypass in the treatment of familial hypercholesterolemia. Eur. J. Clin. Invest. 7:509, 1977.
125. Starzl, T. E., Putnam, C. W., Chase, H. P., and Porter, K. A., Portacaval shunt in hyperlipoproteinemia. Lancet *2*:940, 1972.
126. Forman, M. B., Baker, S. G., and Meny, C. J.: Treatment of homozygous familial hypercholesterolemia with portacaval shunt. Atherosclerosis *41*:349, 1982.
127. Lupien, P. J., Moorjani, S., Lou, M., Brun, D., and Gagne, C.: Removal of cholesterol from blood by affinity binding to heparin-agarose: Evaluation and treatment in homozygous familial hypercholesterolemia. Pediatr. Res. *14*:113, 1980.
128. Thompson, G. R., Myant, N. B., Kilpatrick, D., Oakley, C. M., Raphael, M. J., and Steiner, R. E.: Assessment of long term plasma exchange for familial hypercholesterolemia. Br. Heart J. *43*:680, 1980.

OTHER RISK FACTORS

129. Report of the Surgeon General: Smoking and Health. Washington, D.C., U.S. Department of Health, Education, and Welfare, Public Health Service Publication No. 79–50066, 1979.
130. Shapiro, S., Weinblatt, E., Frank, C. W., and Sager, R. V.: Incidence of coronary heart disease in a population insured for medical care (HIP): Myocardial infarction, angina pectoris, and possible myocardial infarction. Am. J. Publ. Health *59*(Suppl):*1*, 1969.
131. Aronow, W. S., and Kaplan, N. M.: Smoking. *In* Kaplan, N. M., and Stamler, J. S., (eds.): Prevention of Coronary Heart Disease. Practical management of the risk factors. Philadelphia, WB Saunders Company, 1983, p. 51.
132. Levine, P. H.: An acute effect of cigarette smoking on platelet function: A possible link between smoking and arterial thrombosis. Circulation *48*:619, 1973.
133. Kannel, W. B.: Update on the role of cigarette smoking in coronary artery disease. Am. Heart J. *101*:319, 1981.
134. Friedman, G. D., Dales, L. G., and Ury, H. K.: Mortality in middle-aged smokers and nonsmokers. N. Engl. J. Med. *300*:213, 1979.
135. Auerback, O., Carter, H. W., Garfinkel, L., and Hammond, E. C.: Cigarette smoking and coronary artery disease: A macroscopic and microscopic study. Chest *70*:697, 1976.
136. Schachter, S.: Urinary pH in the psychology of nicotine addiction. *In* Davidson, P. O., and Davidson, S. M. (eds.): Behavioral Medicine: Changing Health Lifestyles. New York, Brunner Mazel, 1979, pp. 70–93.
137. Hughes, G. H., Hymowitz, N., Ockene, J. K., Simon, N., and Vogt, T. M.: The multiple-risk factor intervention trial (MRFIT). Prev. Med. *10*:476, 1981.
138. Kannel, W. B.: Hypertension, blood lipids, and cigarette smoking as co-risk factors for coronary heart disease. N.Y. Acad. Sci. *304*:128, 1978.
139. Gordon, T., Kannel, W. B., and McGee, D.: Death and coronary attacks in men after giving up cigarette smoking. Lancet *2*:1345, 1974.
140. Doll, R., and Peto, R.: Mortality in relation to smoking: 20 years observations on male British doctors. Br. Med. J. *2*:1525, 1976.
141. Brischetto, C. S., Connor, W. E., and Connor, S. L.: Plasma lipid and lipoprotein profiles of cigarette smokers from randomly selected families: Enhancement of hyperlipidemia and depression of high density lipoprotein. Am. J. Cardiol. *52*:675, 1983.
142. Keys, A. (ed.): Smoking habits in seven countries. A multivariate analysis of death and coronary heart disease. Vol. 9. Cambridge, Harvard University Press, 1980, pp. 136–160.
143. Kelly, T. L., Gilpin, E., Ahnve, S., Henning, H., and Ross, J., Jr.: Smoking status at the time of acute myocardial infarction and subsequent prognosis. Am. Heart J. *110*:535, 1985.
144. Jugdutt, B. I., Stevens, G. F., Zacks, D. J., Lee, S. J., and Taylor, R. F.: Myocardial infarction, oral contraception, cigarette smoking, and coronary artery spasm in young women. Am. Heart J. *106*:757, 1983.
145. Kaufman, D. W., Helmrich, S. P., Rosenberg, L., Miettinen, O. S., and Shapiro, S.: Nicotine and carbon monoxide content of cigarette smoke and the risk of myocardial infarction in young men. N. Eng. J. Med. *308*:409, 1983.
146. Castelli, W. P., Garrison, R. J., Dawber, T. R., McNamara, P. M., Feinleib, M., and Kannel, W. B.: The filter cigarette and CHD: The Framingham study. Lancet *2*:109, 1981.
147. Wald, N. J.: Mortality from lung cancer and coronary heart disease in relation to changes in smoking habits. Lancet *1*:136, 1976.
148. Hammond, E. C.: Smoking in relation to mortality and morbidity. Findings in the first 34 months of follow-up in a prospective study started in 1959. JNCI 32:1161, 1969.
149. Stamler, J., Stamler, R., and Liu, K. J.: High blood pressure. *In* Connor, W. E., and Bristow J. D. (eds.): Coronary Heart Disease. Prevention, Complications and Treatment. Philadelphia, J.B. Lippincott, 1985.
150. Hypertension Detection and Follow-up Program Cooperative Group: Five-year findings of the hypertension detection and follow-up program: I. Reduction in mortality of persons with high blood pressure, including mild hypertension. J.A.M.A. *242*:2562, 1979.
151. The Joint National Committee on Detection, Evaluation, and Treatment of High Blood Pressure: The 1980 report of the Joint National Committee on Detection, Evaluation, and Treatment of High Blood Pressure. Arch. Intern. Med. *140*:1280, 1980.
152. Kaplan, N. M.: Clinical Hypertension. 3rd ed. Baltimore, Williams and Wilkins, 1982.
153. Hypertension Detection and Follow-up Program Cooperative Group: Patient participation in a hypertension control program. J.A.M.A. 239:1507, 1978.
154. Newman, W. P., Freedman, D. S., Voors, A. W., Gard, P. D., Srinirasan, S. R., Cresanta, J. L., Williamson, G. D., Webber, L. S., and Berenson, G. S.: Relation of serum lipoprotein levels and systolic blood pressure to early atherosclerosis. N. Engl. J. Med. *314*:138, 1986.
155. Zinner, S. H., Margolius, H. S., Rosner, B., and Kass, E. H.: Stability of blood pressure rank and urinary kallikrein concentration in childhood: An eight-year follow-up. Circulation 58:908, 1978.
156. Edmondson, R. P., Thomas, R. D., Hilton, P. J., Patrick, J., and Jones, N. F.: Abnormal leukocyte composition and sodium transport in essential hypertension. Lancet *1*:1003, 1975.
157. Garay, R. P., Elghozi, J. L., Dagher, G., and Meyer, P.: Laboratory distinction between essential and secondary hypertension by measurement of erythrocyte cation fluxes. N. Engl. J. Med. *302*:769, 1980.
158. Haddy, F. J.: Mechanism, prevention and therapy of sodium-dependent hypertension. Am. J. Med. *69*:746, 1980.

159. Kannel, W. B., and Sorlie, P.: Hypertension in Framingham. *In* Paul, O. (ed.): Epidemiology and Control of Hypertension. Miami, Symposia Specialists, 1975, pp. 553–592.
160. Dyer, A. R., Stamler, J., Paul, O., Berkson, D. M., Lepper, M. H., McKean, H., Shekelle, R. B., Lindberg, H. A., and Garside, D.: Alcohol consumption, cardiovascular risk factors, and mortality in two Chicago epidemiologic studies. Circulation *56*:1067, 1977.
161. Carron, D. A., Morris, C. D., and Cole, C.: Dietary calcium in human hypertension. Science *217*:267, 1982.
162. Kaplan, N.: Personal communication, 1986.
163. Veteran's Administration Cooperative Study Group on antihypertensive agents: Effects of treatment on morbidity in hypertension. J.A.M.A. *213*:1143, 1970.
164. Hypertension Detection and Follow-up Program Cooperative Group: Five-year findings of the hypertension detection and follow-up program. I. Reduction in mortality of persons with high blood pressure, including mild hypertension. J.A.M.A. *242*:2562, 1979.
165. The Joint National Committee on Detection, Evaluation, and Treatment of High Blood Pressure: The 1980 report of the Joint National Committee on Detection, Evaluation, and Treatment of High Blood Pressure. Arch. Intern. Med. *140*:1280, 1980.
166. Management Committee: The Australian therapeutic trial in mild hypertension. Lancet 1:1261, 1980.
167. Multiple-Risk Factor Intervention Trial Research Group: Multiple-Risk Factor Intervention Trial. J.A.M.A. *248*:1465, 1982.
168. Paul, O.: The Medical Research Council Trial. Hypertension *8*:733, 1986.
169. Siltanen, P., Romo, M., and Haapakoske, J.: The influence of previous physical activity on survival and reinfarction after first myocardial infarction. Acta Med. Scand. *668*:34, 1982.
170. LaRosa, J. C., Cleary, P., and Muesing, R. A.: Effect of long-term moderate physical exercise on plasma lipoproteins. The National Exercise and Heart Disease Project. Arch. Intern. Med. *142*:2269, 1982.
171. Rechnitzer, P. A., Cunningham, D. A., and Andrew, G. M.: Relation of exercise to the recurrence rate of myocardial infarction in men. Ontario Exercise-Heart Collaborative Study. Am. J. Cardiol. *51*:65, 1983.
172. Hartung, G. H., Foreyt, J. P., Mitchell, J. G., Reeves, R. S., and Gotto, A. M., Jr.: Effect of alcohol intake on high-density lipoprotein cholesterol levels in runners and inactive men. J.A.M.A. *249*:747, 1983.
173. Hartung, G. H., Reeves, R. S., Foreyt, J. P., Patsch, W., and Gotto, A. M., Jr.: Effect of alcohol intake and exercise on plasma high density lipoprotein cholesterol subfractions and apolipoprotein A-I in women. Am. J. Cardiol. 58:148, 1986.
174. Kramsch, D. M., Aspen, A. J., Abramowitz, B. M., Kreimendahl, T., and Hood, W. B., Jr.: Reduction of coronary atherosclerosis by moderate conditioning in monkeys on an atherogenic diet. N. Engl. J. Med. *305*:1483, 1981.
175. Ehsani, A. A., Martin, W. H., Heath, G. W., and Coyle, E. F.: Cardiac effects of prolonged and intense exercise training in patients with coronary artery disease. Am. J. Cardiol. *50*:246, 1982.
176. Ehsani, A. A., Heath, G. W., and Hagberg, J. M.: Effects of 12 months of intense exercise training on ischemic ST segment depression in patients with coronary artery disease. Circulation *64*:1116, 1981.
177. Peters, P. K., Cady, L. D., and Bischoff, D. B.: Physical fitness and subsequent myocardial infarction in healthy workers. J.A.M.A. *249*:3052, 1983.
178. Wilcox, R. G., Bennett, T., Brown, A. M., and Macdonald, I. A.: Is exercise good for high blood pressure? Br. Med. J. *285*:767, 1982.
179. Miller, N. E.: Coronary atherosclerosis and plasma lipoproteins. J. Cardiovasc. Pharmacol. (Suppl. 2) *4*:190, 1982.
180. Wood, P. D., Haskell, W. L., and Blair, S. M.: Increased exercise level and plasma lipoproteins. Metabolism *32*:31, 1983.
181. Gordon, T., Castelli, W. P., Hjortland, M. C., Kannel, W. B., and Dawber, T. R.: High-density lipoprotein as a protective factor against coronary heart disease. The Framingham Study. Am. J Med. *62*:707, 1977.
182. Garcia, M. J., McNamara, P. M., and Gordon, T.: Morbidity and mortality of diabetics in the Framingham population. Diabetes *23*:103, 1974.
183. Williams, R. S., Lague, E. E., and Lewis, J. L.: Physical conditioning augments the fibrinolytic response to venous occlusion in healthy adults. N. Engl. J. Med. *302*:987, 1980.
184. Milvy, P., and Siegel, A. J.: Physical activity levels and altered mortalities from CHD with emphasis on marathon running: A critical review. Cardiovasc. Rev. Res. 2:233, 1981.
185. Oldridge, N. B., Donner, A. P., and Duck, C. W.: Predictors of dropout from cardiac exercise rehabilitation. Am. J. Cardiol. *51*:701, 1983.
186. Theroux, P., Waters, D. D., Halphen, C., Debaisieu, J. C., and Mizgala, H. F.: Prognostic value of exercise testing soon after myocardial infarction. N. Engl. J. Med. *301*:341, 1979.
187. Mayou, R. A.: A controlled trial of early rehabilitation after myocardial infarction. J. Cardiac Rehab. *3*:397, 1983.
188. Shaw, L. W.: Effects of a prescribed supervised exercise program on mortality and cardiovascular morbidity in patients after a myocardial infarction. Am. J. Cardiol. *48*:39, 1981.
189. American Heart Association: The Committee on Exercise. Exercise and Training Apparently Healthy Individuals. A Handbook for Physicians, AHA, 1972.
190. Department of Health and Human Services (PHS): Promoting health, preventing disease: Objectives for the nation. Washington, D.C., U.S. Government Printing Office, 1980, pp. 155–162.
191. Report of Joint Working Party of the Royal College of Physicians and the British Cardiac Society: Prevention of coronary heart disease. J. R. Coll. Physicians (Lond.) *10*:213, 1976.
192. Hubert, H. B., Feinleib, M., McNamara, P. M., and Castelli, W. P.: Obesity as an independent risk factor for cardiovascular disease: A 26-year follow-up of participants in the Framingham Heart Study. Circulation *67*:968, 1983.
193. Bray, GA: Obesity in America. Washington, D.C., U.S. Dept. of Health, Education and Welfare, Publication No. (NIH) 79–359, 1979.
194. Knuiman, J. T., West, C. E., and Burema, J.: Serum total and high density lipoprotein cholesterol concentrations and body mass index in adult men from 13 countries. Am. J. Epidemiol. *116*:631, 1982.
195. Johnson, A. L., Cornoni, J. C., and Cassel, J. C.: Influence of race, sex, and weight on blood pressure behavior in young adults. Am. J. Cardiol. *35*:523, 1975.
196. Thelle, D. S., Shaper, A. G., and Whitehead, T. P.: Blood lipids in middle aged British men. Br. Heart J. *49*:205, 1983.
197. Havel, R. J.: Treatment of hyperlipidemia: Where do we stand? Am. J. Med. *73*:301, 1982.
198. Rossner, S., and Hallurg, D.: Long-term follow-up of serum lipoproteins after jejunoileal bypass surgery for marked obesity. Int. J. Obes. *4*:197, 1980.
199. Pell, S., and D'Alonso, C.: Factors associated with long-term survival of diabetes. J.A.M.A. *214*:1833, 1970.
200. Lapidus, L., Bengtsson, C., Larsson, B., Pennert, K., Rybo, E., and Sjostrom, L.: Distribution of adipose tissue and risk of cardiovascular disease and death: A 12 year follow-up of participants in the population study of women in Gothenburg, Sweden. Br. Med. J. *289*:1257, 1984.
201. Larsson, B., Svardsudd, K., Welin, L., Wilhelmsen, L., Bjorntorp, P., and Tibblin, G.: Abdominal adipose tissue distribution, obesity, and risk of cardiovascular disease and death: A 13-year follow-up of participants in the study of men born in 1913. Br. Med. J. *288*:1401, 1984.
202. Keys, A., Menotti, A, Arvanis, C., Blackburn, H., Djordevic, B. S., Buzina, R., Dontas, A. S., Fidanza, F., Karvonen, M. J., and Kimura, N.: The Seven Countries Study: 2289 deaths in 15 years. Prev. Med. *13*:141, 1984.
203. Barrett-Conner, E., and Khaw, K-T.: Is obesity a risk factor for coronary artery disease? Persp. Lipid Dis. *3*:18, 1986.
204. Blackburn, H., Djordevic, B. S., Buzina, R., Dortas, A. S., Fidanza, F., Karvonen, M. J., and Kimura, N.: The Pooling Research Group. Relationship of blood pressure, serum cholesterol, smoking habit, relative weight and ECG abnormalities to incidence of major coronary events: Final report of the pooling project. J. Chron. Dis. *31*:201, 1978.
205. McGee, D. L., Reed, D. M., Yano, J., Kagan, A., and Tillotson, J.: Ten-year incidence of coronary heart disease in the Honolulu heart program. Am. J. Epidemiol. *119*:667, 1984.
206. Kromhout, D., and Coulander, C.: Diet, prevalence, and 10-year mortality from coronary heart disease in 871 middle-aged men. The Zutphen Study. Am. J. Epidemiol. *119*:733, 1984.
207. Morris, J. N., Marr, J. W., and Clayton, D. G.: Diet and heart: A postscript. Br. Med. J. *2*:1307, 1977.
208. Yano, K., Rhoads, G. G., Kagan, A., and Tillotson, J.: Dietary intake and the risk of coronary heart disease in Japanese men living in Hawaii. Am. J. Clin. Nutr. *31*:1270, 1978.
209. Garcia-Palmieri, M. R., Sorlie, P., Tillotson, J., Costas, R., Jr., Cordero, E., and Rodriguez, M.: Relationship of dietary intake to subsequent coronary heart disease incidence: The Puerto Rico Heart Health Program. Am. J. Clin. Nutr. *33*:1818, 1980.
210. Marr, J. W., and Morris, J. N.: Re: Dietary intake and the risk of coronary heart disease in Japanese men living in Hawaii. Letter to the editor. Am. J. Clin. Nutr. *34*:1156, 1981.
211. Kromhout, D.: Energy and macronutrient intake in lean and obese middle-aged men during 10-year follow-up (The Zutphen study). Am. J. Clin. Nutr. *38*:591, 1983.
212. Shekelle, R. B., Schryrock, A., Paul O., Lepper, M., Stamler, J., Liu, S., and Raynor, W. J., Jr.: Diet, serum cholesterol, and death from coronary heart disease: The Western Electric Study. N. Engl. J. Med. *304*:65, 1981.
213. Kushi, L. H., Lew, R. A., Stare, F. J., Ellison, C. R., el Lozy, M., Bourke, G., Daly, L., Graham, I., Hickey, N., and Mulcahy, R.: Diet and 20-year mortality from coronary heart disease: The Ireland-Boston Diet-heart study. N. Engl. J. Med. *312*:811, 1985.
214. Riemersma, R. A., Wood, D. A., Butler, S., Elton, R. A., Oliver, M., Salo, M., Nikkari, T., Vartiainen, E., Puska, P., and Gey, F.: Linoleic acid content in adipose tissue in coronary heart disease. Br. Med. J. *292*:1423, 1986.
215. Nikkari, T., Salo, M., Mastela, J., and Aromas, A.: Serum fatty acids in Finnish men. Atherosclerosis *49*:139, 1983.
216. Nikkari, T., and Salo, M.: Serum fatty acids in Finnish population groups. *In* Marcuse, R. (ed.): Proceedings of the 12th Scandinavia Symposium on Lipids. 1983. Góteborg: Lipid forum c/o Slk, 1984, pp 80–86.
217. Keys, A.: Coronary heart disease in seven countries. Circulation *41*(Suppl. 1)1, 1970.
218. Heimark, R. L., Twardzik, D. R., and Schwartz, S. M.: Inhibition of endothelial regeneration by type-beta transforming growth factor from platelets. Science *233*:1078, 1986.
219. Rao, A. K., Mintz, P. D., and Lavine, S. J.: Coagulant activities of platelets in coronary artery disease. Circulation *69*:15, 1984.
220. Feinleib, M.: Genetics. *In* Kaplan, N. M., and Stamler, J. (eds.): Prevention of Coronary Heart Disease. Practical Management of the Risk Factors. Philadelphia, W. B. Saunders Company, 1983.
221. ten Kate, L. P., Boman, H., Daiger, S. P., and Motulsky, A. G.: Familial aggregation of coronary heart disease and its relation to known genetic risk factors. Am. J. Cardiol. *50*:945, 1982.

222. Shea, S., and Nichols, A.: The clinical importance of family history of ischemic heart disease. Cardiovasc. Rev. Rep. *4*:1343, 1983.
223. Conroy, R. M., Mulcahy, R., Hickey, N., and Daly, L.: Is a family history of coronary heart disease an independent coronary risk factor? Br. Heart J. *53*:378, 1985.
224. Friedlander, Y., Kark, J. D., and Stein, Y.: Family history of myocardial infarction as an independent risk factor for coronary heart disease. Br. Heart J. *53*:382, 1985.
225. Neufeld, H. N., and Goldbourt, U.: Coronary heart disease: Genetic aspects. Circulation *67*:943, 1983.
226. Jorde, L. B., Williams, R. R., and Hunt, S. C.: Lack of association of diagonal earlobe crease with other cardiovascular risk factors. West. J. Med. *140*:220, 1984.
227. Jenkins, C. D.: Psychosocial and behavioral factors. *In* Kaplan, N. M., and Stamler, J. (eds.): Prevention of Coronary Heart Disease. Philadelphia, W. B. Saunders Company, 1983, p. 99.
228. Liu, K., Cedres, L. B., and Stamler, J.: Relationship of education to major risk factors and death from coronary heart disease, cardiovascular diseases and all causes. Findings of three Chicago epidemiologic studies. Circulation *66*:1308, 1982.
229. Colbourn, A. W.: The decline in coronary heart disease mortality: The DuPont experience. Del. Med. J. *58*:351, 1986.
230. Davidson, D. M.: Cardiovascular disease and occupation. Cardiovasc. Rev. Rep. *5*:503, 1984.
231. Wilcosky, T. C., and Tyroler, H. A.: Mortality from heart disease among workers exposed to solvents. J. Occup. Med. *25*:879, 1983.
232. Friedman, M.: Pathogenesis of Coronary Artery Disease. New York, McGraw-Hill Book Co., 1969.
233. Rosenman, R. H., and Chesney, M. A.: The relationship of Type A behavior pattern. J. Psychosom. Res. *21*:323, 1977.
234. Jenkins, C. D.: The Coronary Prone Personality. *In* Gentry, W. D., and Williams, R. B. (eds.): Psychological Aspects of Myocardial Infarction and Coronary Care. 2nd ed. St. Louis, C. V. Mosby, 1979.
235. Review Panel on Coronary-Prone Behavior and Coronary Heart Disease: Coronary-prone behavior and coronary heart disease. A critical review. Circulation *63*:1199, 1981.
236. Haynes, S. A., Feinleib, M., and Kannel, W.: The relationship of psychosocial factors to coronary heart disease in the Framingham Study. Am. J. Publ. Health 3:37, 1980.
237. Frank, K. A., Heller, S. S., Kornfeld, D. S., Sporn, A. A., and Weiss, W. B.: Type A behavior pattern and coronary angiographic findings. J.A.M.A. *240*:761, 1978.
238. Kahn, J. P., Kornfeld, D. S., Blood, D. K., Lynn, R. B., Heller, S. S., and Frank, K. A.: Type A behavior and the thallium stress test. Pychosom. Med. *44*:431, 1982.
239. Rosenman, R. H., Friedman, M., Straus, R., Wurm, M., Kositchek, R., Hahn, W., Werthessem, N. T.: A predictive study of coronary heart disease. The Western Collaborative Group Study. J.A.M.A. *189*:15, 1964.
240. Rosenman, R. H., Brand, R. J., Jenkins, D., Friedman, M., Straus, R., and Wurm, M.: Coronary heart disease in the Western Collaborative Group Study: Final follow-up experience of 8½ years. J.A.M.A. 233:872, 1975.
241. Jenkins, C. D., Rosenman, R. H., and Zyzanski, S. J.: Prediction of clinical coronary heart disease by a test for coronary-prone behavior pattern. N. Engl. J. Med. *290*:1271, 1974.
242. Jenkins, C. D., Zyzanski, S. J., and Rosenman, R. H.: Risk of new myocardial infarction in middle-aged men with manifest coronary heart disease. Circulation *53*:342, 1976.
243. de Baker, G., Kornitzer, M., Kittel, F., and Dramaix, M.: Behavior, stress and psychosocial traits as risk factors. Prev. Med. *12*:32, 1983.
244. Shekelle, R. B., Gale, M., and Norusis, M.: Type A score (Jenkins Activity Survey) and risk of recurrent coronary heart disease in the aspirin–myocardial infarction study. Am. J. Cardiol *56*:221, 1985.
245. Shekelle, R. B., Hulley, S., Neaton, J., Billings, J. H., Borhani, N. O., Gerace, T. A., Jacobs, D. R., Lasser, N. L., Mittlemark, M. B., and Stamler, J.: Type A behavior and risk of coronary death in MRFIT. Proceedings of the Council on Epidemiology, American Heart Association, San Diego, California, March 3, 1983.
246. Ruberman, W., Weinblatt, E., Goldberg, J. D., and Chaudhary, B. S.: Psychosocial influences on mortality after myocardial infarction. N. Engl. J. Med. *311*:552, 1974.
247. Moser, K. A., Fox, A. J., and Jones, D. R.: Unemployment and mortality in the POCS longitudinal study. Lancet *2*:1324, 1984.
248. Appels, A., and Mulder, P.: Type A behavior and myocardial infarction. A 9.5 year follow-up of a small cohort. Int. J. Cardiol. *8*:465, 1985.
249. Friedman, M., Thoresen, C. E., Gill, J. J., Ulmer, D., Powell, L. H., Price, V. A., Brown, B., Thompson, L., Rabin, D. D., Breall, W. S., Bourg, E., Levy, R., and Dixon, T.: Alteration of Type A behavior and its effects on cardiac recurrences in post myocardial infarction patients: Summary results of the recurrent coronary prevention project. Am. Heart J. *112*:653, 1986.
250. Harrel, J. P.: Psychological factors and hypertension: Status report. Psychol. Bull. *87*: 482, 1980.
251. Friedman, M., Rossenman, R. H., and Carrol, V.: Changes in serum cholesterol and blood clotting time in men subjects to cycle variations of occupational stress. Circulation *17*:852, 1980.
252. The Review Panel on Coronary-Prone Behavior and Coronary Heart Disease: Coronary-prone behavior and coronary heart disease: A critical review. Circulation *63*:1199, 1981.
253. Wilcox, R. G.: Ischaemic heart disease: Behavior type A equals American type behaviour? Int. J. Cardiol. *8*:471, 1985.
254. Garcia, M. I., McNamara, P. M., and Gordon, T.: Morbidity and mortality in diabetics in the Framingham population. Diabetes *23*:105, 1976.
255. West, K. M.: Epidemiology of diabetes and its vascular lesions. New York, Elsevier, 1978.
256. Silberhaus, K., Schernthaner, G., and Sinzinger, H.: Decreased vascular prostacycline in juvenile onset diabetes. N. Engl. J. Med. *300*:366, 1979.
257. Joint Discussion: The International Collaborative Group. J. Chron. Dis. *32*:829, 1979.
258. Stamler, R., Stamler, J., Lindberg, H. A., Marquard, J., Berkson, D. M., Paul, O., Lepper, M., Dyer, A., and Stevens, E.: Asymptomatic hyperglycemia and coronary heart disease in middle-aged men in two employed populations in Chicago, J. Chron. Dis. *32*:805, 1979.
259. Glasgow, A. M., August, G. P., and King, W.: Relationship between control and serum lipids in juvenile onset diabetes. Diabetes Care *4*:76, 1981.
260. Wingard, D. L.: The sex differential in mortality rates. Demographic and behavioral factors. Am. J. Epidemiol. *115*:205, 1982.
261. Rosenberg, L., Armstrong, B., and Jick, H.: Myocardial infarction and estrogen therapy in postmenopausal women. N. Engl. J. Med. *294*:1256, 1976.
262. Pfeffer, R. I., Whipple, G. H., Kurosaki, T. T., and Chapman, J. M.: Coronary risk and estrogen use in postmenopausal women. Am. J. Epidemiol. *107*:479, 1978.
263. Haynes, S. G., and Feinleib, M.: Women, work and coronary heart disease: Prospective findings from the Framingham Heart Study. Am. J. Public Health *70*:133, 1980.
264. Kannel, W. B., Hjortland, M. C., McNamara, P. M., and Gordon, T.: Menopause and the risk of cardiovascular disease. Ann. Intern. Med. *85*:447, 1976.
265. Stampfer, M. J., Willett, W. C., Colditz, G. A., Rosner, B., Speizer, F. E., and Hennekens, C. H.: A prospective study of postmenopausal estrogen therapy and coronary heart disease. N. Engl. J. Med. *313*:1044, 1985.
266. Wilson, P. W. F., Garrison, R. J., and Castelli, W. P.: Original article: Postmenopausal estrogen use, cigarette smoking, and cardiovascular morbidity in women over 50: The Framingham Study. N. Engl. J. Med. *313*:1038, 1985.
267. Coronary Drug Project Research Group: The Coronary Drug Project. Findings leading to discontinuation of the 2.5 mg/day estrogen group. J.A.M.A. *226*:652, 1973.
268. Mann, J. I., Vessey, M. P., Thorogood, M., and Doll, R.: Myocardial infarction in young women with special reference to oral contraceptive practice. Br. Med. J. *2*:241, 1975.
269. Jick, H., Dinan, B., and Rothman, K. J.: Oral contraceptives and nonfatal myocardial infarction. J.A.M.A. *239*:1403, 1978.
270. Shapiro, S., Slone, D., Rosenberg, L., Kaufman, D. W., Stolley, P. D., and Miettinen, O. S.: Oral-contraceptive use in relation to myocardial infarction. Lancet *1*:743, 1979.
271. Royal College of General Practitioners: Oral Contraceptives and Health. London, Pitman Medical Publishing Company, 1974.
272. Vessey, M., Doll, R., Peto, R., Johnson, B., and Wiggins, P.: A long-term follow-up study of women using different methods of contraception: An interim report. J. Biosoc. Sci. *8*:373, 1976.
273. Lindquist, O.: Influence of the menopause of ischaemic heart disease and its risk factors and on bone mineral content. Acta Obstet. Gynecol. Scand. Suppl. 110, p. 1–32, 1982.
274. Salonen, J. T.: Oral contraceptives, smoking and risk of myocardial infarction in young women. Acta Med. Scand. *212*:141, 1982.
275. Engle, H.-J., Engel, E., and Lichtlen, P. R.: Coronary atherosclerosis and myocardial infarction in young women—role of oral contraceptives. Eur. Heart J. *4*:1, 1983.
276. Weir, R. J.: Effect on blood pressure or changing from high to low dose steroid preparations in women with oral contraceptive induced hypertension. South. Med. J. *27*:212, 1982.
277. Wei, J. Y., and Bulkley, B. H.: Myocardial infarction before age 36 years in women: Predominance of apparent nonatherosclerotic events. Am. Heart. J. *104*:561, 1982.
278. Uhl, G. S., and Farrell, P. W.: Myocardial infarction in young adults: Risk factors and natural history. Am. Heart J. *105*:548, 1985.
279. Hartung, G. H., Reeves, R. S., Krock, L. P., Foreyt, J. P., and Patsch, W.: Effect of alcohol and exercise on plasma HDL cholesterol subfractions and apolipoprotein A-I (APOA-I) in middle-aged men. Circulation *72*:(Suppl. III):452, 1985.
280. St. Leger, A. S., Cochrane, A. L., and Moore, F.: Factors associated with cardiac mortality in developed countries with particular reference to the consumption of wine. Lancet *1*:1017, 1979.
281. LaPorte, R. E., Cresanta, J. L., and Kuller, L. H.: The relationship of alcohol consumption to atherosclerotic heart disease. Prev. Med. *9*:22, 1980.
282. Stason, W. B., Neff, R. K., Miettinen, D. S., and Jick, H.: Alcohol consumption and nonfatal myocardial infarction. Am. J. Epidemiol. *104*:603, 1976.
283. Marmot, M. G., Rose, G., Shipley, M. J., and Thomas B. J.: Alcohol and mortality: A U-shaped curve. Lancet *1*:580, 1981.
284. Dyer, A. R., Stamler, J., Paul, O., Lepper, M., Shekelle, R. B., McKean, H., and Garside, D.: Alcohol consumption and 17-year mortality in the Chicago Western Electric Company study. Prev. Med. *9*:78, 1980.
285. Clarkson, T.: Alcohol, atherosclerosis, and lipoproteins in primate studies. Presented at the American Heart Association Symposium on Alcohol and Cardiovascular Diseases, San Diego, 1980.
286. Anderson, A. J., Barboriak, J. J., and Rimm, A. A.: Risk factors and angiographically determined coronary occlusion. Am. J. Epidemiol. *107*:8, 1978.
287. Barboriak, J. J., Rimm, A. A., and Anderson, A. J.: Coronary artery occlusion and alcohol intake. Br. Heart. J. *39*:289, 1977.

288. Barboriak, J. J., Anderson, A. J., and Hoffmann, R. G.: Interrelationships between coronary artery occlusion, high-density lipoprotein cholesterol, and alcohol intake. J. Lab. Clin. Med. *94*:348, 1979.
289. Klevay, L. M.: The role of copper, zinc, and other chemical elements in ischemic heart disease. *In* Rennert, O. W., and Chan, W.-Y. (eds.): Metabolism of Trace Metals in Man. Vol. I. Boca Raton, CRC Press, 1984.
290. Klevay, L. M.: Copper and ischemic heart disease. Bio. Trace Element Res. *5*:245, 1983.
291. Leoni, V., Fabiani, L., and Ticchiarelli, L.: Water hardness and cardiovascular mortality rate in Abruzzo, Italy. Arch. Environ. Health *40*:274, 1985.
292. Crawford, M. D., Clayton, D. G., Stanley, F., and Shaper, A. G.: An epidemiological study of sudden death in hard and soft water areas. J. Chron. Dis. *30*:69, 1977.
293. Luoma, H., Aromaa, A., and Helminen, S.: Risk of myocardial infarction in Finnish men in relation to fluoride, magnesium and calcium concentration in drinking water. Acta Med. Scand. *213*:171, 1983.
294. Roberts, W., and Waller, B. F.: Chronic hypercalcemia as a risk factor for coronary atherosclerosis. Cardiovasc. Res. Rep. *4*:1275, 1983.
295. Meade, T. W., Mellows, S., Brozovic, M., Miller, G. J., Cakrabarti, R. R., North, W. R., et al.: Haemostatic function and ischemic heart disease: Principal results of the Northwick Park Heart Study. Lancet *2*:533, 1986.
296. Miller, G. J., Martin, J. C., Webster, J., Wilkes, H., Miller, N. E., Wilkinson, W. H., and Meade, T. W.: Association between dietary fat intake and plasma factor VII coagulant activity—a predictor of cardiovascular mortality. Atherosclerosis *60*:269, 1986.
297. Smith, E. B., and Ashall, C.: Fibronectin distribution in human aortic intima and atherosclerotic lesions: Concentration of soluble and collagenase-releasable fractions. Biochem. Biophys. Acta *880*:10, 1986.
298. Smith, E. B., and Ashall, C.: Fibrinolysis and plasminogen concentration in aortic intima in relation to death following myocardial infarction. Atherosclerosis *55*:171, 1985.
299. Smith, E. B., Massie, I. B, and Alexander, K. M.: The release of an immobilized lipoprotein fraction from atherosclerotic lesions by incubation with plasmin. Atherosclerosis *25*:71, 1976.
300. Alexander, N. J., and Clark, T. B.: Vasectomy increases the severity of diet-induced atherosclerosis in Macaca fascicularis. Science *201*:538, 1978.
301. Clarkson, T. B., and Alexander, N. J.: Long-term vasectomy: Affects on the occurrence and extent of atherosclerosis in rhesus monkeys. J. Clin. Invest. *65*:15, 1980.
302. Walker, A. M., Jick, H., Hunter, J. R., Danford, A., Watkins, R. N., Alhedeff, L., and Rothman, K. J.: Vasectomy and non-fatal myocardial infarction. Lancet *1*:13, 1981.
303. Walker, A. M., Jick, H., Hunter, J. R., and McEvoy, J.: Vasectomy and nonfatal myocardial infarction: Continued observations indicates no elevation of risk. J. Urol. *130*:936, 1983.
304. Thelle, D. S., Arnesen, E., and Forde, O. H.: The Tromso heart study. Does coffee raise serum cholesterol? N. Engl. J. Med. *308*:1454, 1983.
305. Forde, O. H., Knutsen, S. F., Arnesen, E., and Thelle, D. S.: The Tromso heart study: Coffee consumption and serum lipid concentrations in men with hypercholesterolemia: A randomised intervention study. Br. Med. J. *290*:893, 1985.
306. LaCroix, A. Z., Mead, L. A., Liang, K.-Y., Thomas, C. B., and Pearson, T. A.: Coffee consumption and the incidence of coronary heart disease. N. Engl. J. Med. *315*:977, 1986.
307. Hess, M. L., Hastillo, A., Mohanakumar, T., Cowley, M. J., Vetrovac, G., Szentpetery, S., Wolfgang, T. C., and Lower, R. R.: Accelerated atherosclerosis in cardiac transplantation: Role of cytotoxic B-cell antibodies and hyperlipidemia. Circulation *69*:(suppl. II),94, 1983.
308. Brand, F. N., McGee, D. L., Kannel, W. B., Stokes, J., and Castelli, W. P.: Hyperuricemia as a risk factor of coronary heart disease: The Framingham Study. Am. J. Epidemiol. *121*:11, 1985.

37 CORONARY BLOOD FLOW AND MYOCARDIAL ISCHEMIA

by EUGENE BRAUNWALD, M.D., and
BURTON E. SOBEL, M.D.

Hypoxia, or *hypoxemia*, is a state of reduced oxygen supply to tissue despite adequate perfusion; *anoxia* is the absence of oxygen supply despite adequate perfusion; *ischemia* is the condition of oxygen deprivation accompanied by inadequate removal of metabolites consequent to reduced perfusion. Although clinical manifestations of coronary insufficiency generally reflect the effects of ischemia, under selected experimental and clinical conditions, deprivation of oxygen can be separated from reduced washout of metabolites.[1] For example, in isolated hearts perfused at high flow rates with media equilibrated with a gas mixture poor in oxygen, anoxia without ischemia results, since washout of metabolites is not hindered. An analogous situation occurs in patients with cyanotic congenital heart disease, as well as in those with cor pulmonale, severe anemia, asphyxiation, and carbon monoxide poisoning.

Neither ischemia nor hypoxia can be defined in absolute terms, since the blood flow and quantity of oxygen required to support myocardium under one set of conditions will not necessarily pertain under another. In man, blood flow of 60 to 90 ml/min per 100 gm of myocardium is generally required under basal physiological conditions. On the other hand, when the mechanical activity of the heart and its metabolic requirements are markedly reduced, myocardial viability may be maintained by perfusion at much lower rates, approximately 10 to 20 ml/min per 100 gm, or even with complete interruption of perfusion for periods of up to 100 minutes. Examples of conditions that reduce oxygen needs markedly include hypothermia with ventricular fibrillation and asystole, techniques widely used in cardiovascular surgery. Another example of lowered cardiac oxygen needs occurs following the administration of nitroglycerin and other nitrates, which reduce the preload and afterload, and of beta-adrenoceptor blockers, which lower heart rate and contractility. This reduction of oxygen needs is perhaps the *principal* mechanism by which these agents relieve anginal pain (p. 1330).

The importance of defining ischemia in *relative* rather than absolute terms is underscored by the use of a variety of stress tests to detect or assess the severity of coronary artery disease. During relative ischemia an imbalance between myocardial oxygen demands and supply occurs, as a consequence of increased demands with a fixed supply or as a consequence of reduced supply. Whether the ischemia manifests as anginal discomfort, deviation of the ST-segment on the electrocardiogram (Chap. 8), relative diminution of accumulation of ^{201}Tl in myocardial "perfusion images," regional wall motion disorders, or diminution of ejection fraction detectable with gated blood pool images (Chap. 11), the underlying principle is the same. Induction of stress by exercise, atrial pacing, handgrip, or any other means leads to a transitory disparity in the balance between oxygen supply and demand. Although this balance may be adequate under conditions of rest, the disparity becomes manifest when the increased oxygen demands cannot be satisfied by an adequate augmentation of myocardial delivery.

DETERMINANTS OF MYOCARDIAL OXYGEN CONSUMPTION

The heart is an aerobic organ; that is, it relies almost exclusively on the oxidation of substrates for the generation of energy, and it can develop only a small oxygen debt. Therefore, in a steady state, determination of the rate of myocardial oxygen consumption ($M\dot{V}O_2$) provides an accurate measure of its total metabolism.

It has been known for many years that the total metabolism of the arrested, quiescent heart is only a small fraction of that of the working organ. The $M\dot{V}O_2$ of the beating canine heart ranges from 8 to 15 ml/min per 100 gm, while the oxygen of the noncontracting heart is approximately 1.5 ml/min per 100 gm.[2-4] This quantity of oxygen is required for those physiological metabolic processes not directly associated with contraction. Increases in the frequency of depolarization of the noncontracting heart are accompanied by only very small increases of $M\dot{V}O_2$. Indeed, the quantity of oxygen required for electrical activation of the heart is approximately only 0.5 per cent of the $M\dot{V}O_2$ of the normal working heart; thus, the oxygen cost of electrical depolarization is trivial in relation to the cost of contractile activity.[5]

MYOCARDIAL TENSION. In 1915 Evans and Matsuoka concluded from studies on the Starling heart-lung preparation that "there is a relation between the tension set up on contraction and the metabolism of the contractile tissue."[6] Subsequently, experimental techniques for regulating the external performance of the heart improved enormously. In 1955, in a systematic investigation of the relative effects of aortic pressure, stroke volume, and heart rate on $M\dot{V}O_2$, it became apparent that it is not possible to estimate the energy needs of the myocardium simply from the external work produced by the heart when work is calculated in the classic manner as the product of developed pressure and stroke volume. As a corollary, it was shown that myocardial efficiency, i.e., the ratio of the work performed to the oxygen consumed, varies widely depending on the hemodynamic conditions.[7, 8] These investigations suggested that the tension-time index, i.e., the area under the left ventricular pressure curve, is an important determinant of the $M\dot{V}O_2$. Subsequently, it was emphasized that the tension in the wall of the ventricle is a direct function of the radius and the intraventricular pressure and is inversely related to ventricular wall thickness. Also, myocardial wall tension and the force-time integrals were shown to be more definitive determinants of myocardial energy utilization than was developed pressure.[9, 10] Later studies demonstrated that velocity of myocardial contraction—a reflection of the heart's contractile state—is an additional, important determinant of $M\dot{V}O_2$ (Fig. 37–1).[11]

Recent reexamination of the determinants of $M\dot{V}O_2$ has emphasized that it correlates closely with the left ventricular systolic pressure-volume area, which consists of the sum of the area within the systolic pressure-volume loop, i.e., the external mechanical work, and the end-systolic elastic potential energy in the ventricular wall[4, 12, 13] (Fig. 37–2). Rooke and Feigl have provided impressive evidence that $M\dot{V}O_2$ is influenced by stroke volume, although less so than by pressure development.[3] They have also provided an experimental basis for the use of the systolic pressure-rate product (plus an estimate of the oxygen requirements of the noncontracting heart) as a clinically useful index of $M\dot{V}O_2$. These observations are consistent with Fenn's classic observations on skeletal muscle, which showed that the energy release (a variable related to oxygen consumption) is proportional to the sum of tension development and external work of the muscle.[14, 15] Thus, both skeletal muscle and myocardium have the capacity to adjust their energy costs to external conditions imposed *after* stimulation.[10]

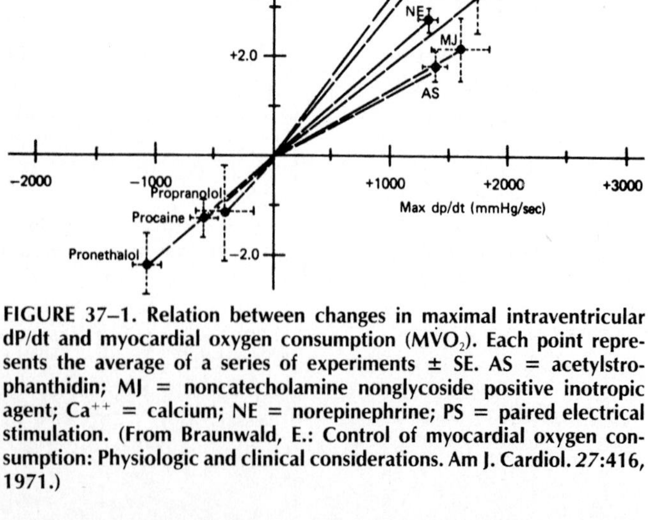

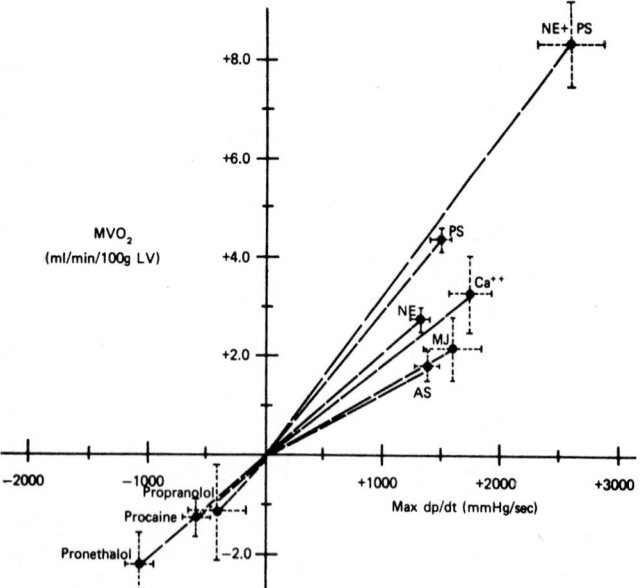

FIGURE 37–1. Relation between changes in maximal intraventricular dP/dt and myocardial oxygen consumption ($M\dot{V}O_2$). Each point represents the average of a series of experiments ± SE. AS = acetylstrophanthidin; MJ = noncatecholamine nonglycoside positive inotropic agent; Ca^{++} = calcium; NE = norepinephrine; PS = paired electrical stimulation. (From Braunwald, E.: Control of myocardial oxygen consumption: Physiologic and clinical considerations. Am J. Cardiol. *27*:416, 1971.)

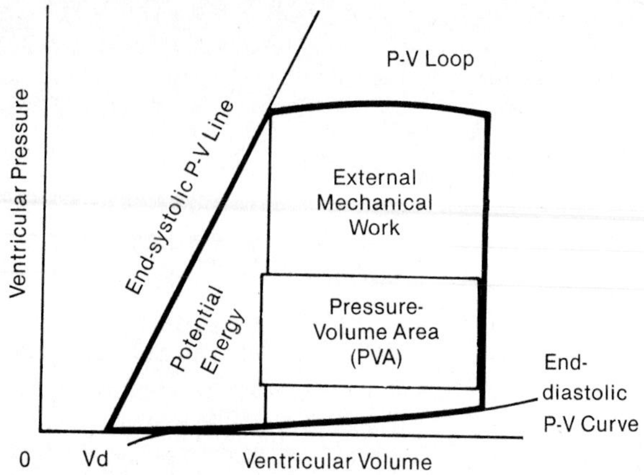

FIGURE 37–2. Schematic illustration of systolic pressure-volume area and its two components, external mechanical work (the P-V loop) and potential energy. End-systole is the time at which the P-V loop touches the end-systolic P-V relation line. The systolic segment of the P-V loop consists of the segments for the isovolumic contraction phase and the ejection phase. The diastolic segment of the P-V loop consists of the segments for the isovolumic relaxation phase and the filling phase. (From Suga, H., Goto, Y., Yamada, O., and Igarashi, Y.: Independence of myocardial oxygen consumption from pressure-volume trajectory during diastole in canine left ventricle. Circ. Res. *55*:735, 1984, by permission of the American Heart Association, Inc.)

MYOCARDIAL CONTRACTILITY. The effect on $M\dot{V}O_2$ of positive inotropic stimuli, such as Ca^{++}, cardiac glycosides, and catecholamines, is the end result of their influence on two major determinants of $M\dot{V}O_2$ that change in opposite directions in the intact heart. These are tension, which declines as a consequence of a reduction in heart size, and myocardial contractility, which, by definition, is augmented. In the failing, dilated ventricle, the increased contractility reduces the left ventricular end-diastolic pressure and volume. On the basis of the Laplace relation (p. 405), this reduction in ventricular volume leads to a decline in intramyocardial tension, which tends to reduce $M\dot{V}O_2$. However, the decrease in $M\dot{V}O_2$ that might be expected to result from falling tension in the ventricular wall is offset by the increase in contractility, which tends to augment $M\dot{V}O_2$. The net result of these opposing effects is to produce no change, a small increase, or a small decrease in $M\dot{V}O_2$. Thus, the change in $M\dot{V}O_2$ that follows the stimulation of contractility depends on the extent to which intramyocardial tension is reduced in relation to the extent to which contractility is augmented.[16] In the absence of heart failure, drugs that stimulate myocardial contractility elevate $M\dot{V}O_2$, since heart size and therefore wall tension are not reduced and do not offset the effect on metabolism of the stimulation of contractility.

The conclusion that myocardial contractility is an important determinant of $M\dot{V}O_2$ is supported by observations on the effects of reducing contractility. Thus, in animal experiments reductions in contractility and in the velocity of contraction produced by cardiac depressant drugs, including propranolol, and procainamide, were shown to reduce $M\dot{V}O_2$ when wall tension was held constant, or almost so.[17]

The results of experiments in which the relative effects on $M\dot{V}O_2$ of changes in tension development and in myocardial contractility were assessed in the same heart, and it was concluded that the quantitative effects on $M\dot{V}O_2$ of changes in contractility and tension development are both substantial and of the same order of magnitude.[17] In these experiments heart rate was purposely held constant, since heart rate itself is an important determinant of $M\dot{V}O_2$. An augmentation of rate elevates the level of $M\dot{V}O_2$ by increasing the frequency of tension development per unit of time, as well as by increasing contractility.[7, 18]

Although the precise energy costs of maintenance of the active state of the myocardium have not yet been clearly defined, they are likely to be relatively low. In studies of isolated papillary muscles, $M\dot{V}O_2$ was found to be a function of the tension that is developed and the velocity of shortening of the unloaded muscle. Shortening against a load requires oxygen above and beyond that required for the development of tension. It has been suggested by Suga et al. that almost the entire increase in $M\dot{V}O_2$ produced by the administration of positive inotropic agents such as Ca^{++} and epinephrine results from energy costs of enhanced excitation-contraction coupling, specifically the energy cost of greater and more rapid Ca^{++} uptake by the SR,[12] the increased contractile activity produced, rather than from a direct stimulating effect of the catecholamines on basal myocardial metabolism. It has been suggested that increased severe valvular regurgitation does not increase $M\dot{V}O_2$ significantly when myocardial tension is held constant because of the relatively low oxygen cost of the additional muscle shortening associated with valvular regurgitation[7, 19] (Table 37–1). $M\dot{V}O_2$ is influenced also by the substrate utilized. Specifically, it varies directly with the fraction of energy derived from the metabolism of fatty acids, which in turn varies directly with the arterial concentration of fatty acids and inversely with that of glucose and insulin.[20]

TABLE 37–1 DETERMINANTS OF MYOCARDIAL OXYGEN CONSUMPTION

1.	Tension development
2.	Contractile state
3.	Heart rate
4.	Shortening against a load (Fenn effect)
5.	Maintenance of cell viability in basal state
6.	Depolarization
7.	Activation
8.	Maintenance of active state
9.	Direct metabolic effect of catecholamines
10.	Fatty acid uptake

REGULATION OF CORONARY BLOOD FLOW

ANATOMIC FACTORS. Coronary blood flow is influenced by anatomic, hydraulic, mechanical, and metabolic factors.[8, 21–23] During diastole, when the aortic valve is closed, aortic diastolic pressure is transmitted without impediment through the dilated sinuses of Valsalva to the ostia. The aortic arch and sinuses then act as a miniature reservoir, facilitating maintenance of relatively uniform coronary inflow through diastole. Both the left and right coronary arteries course across the epicardial surface of the heart (Chap. 10). The major vessels and their principal branches serve as conductance vessels and normally offer little resistance to coronary blood flow. The epicardial conductance vessels can alter their tone by vasoconstricting to alpha-adrenergic stimuli and vasodilating to nitroglycerin.[24] These vessels give rise to smaller penetrating vessels approximately at right angles (Fig. 37–3). A large pressure drop occurs in these intramural vessels and in the coronary arterioles, hence their designation as "resistance vessels." The dense capillary network of about 4000 capillaries/sq mm cross-section of the heart is not uniformly patent, since precapillary sphincters appear to serve a regulatory function,[25] depending on the flow needs of the myocardium.

Collaterals. Anastomotic connections without an intervening capillary bed exist between portions of the same coronary artery and between different coronary arteries. The distribution and extent of these collateral vessels differ markedly between species, as well as among different individuals of the same species. In canine hearts, an extensive epicardial network of collateral vessels is common, but epicardial collateral vessels are not prominent in porcine or primate hearts. In human hearts, the distribution and extent of collateral vessels are quite variable. Under physiological conditions, such vessels are generally less than 40 μm in diameter and appear to have little or no functional role. However, when myocardial perfusion is compromised by obstructions affecting major vessels, these collateral vessels enlarge over several weeks and blood flow through them increases.[26] Exercise,[27, 28] severe anemia,[29] and gradual (rather than abrupt) coronary occlusion[30] appear to enhance the development of collat-

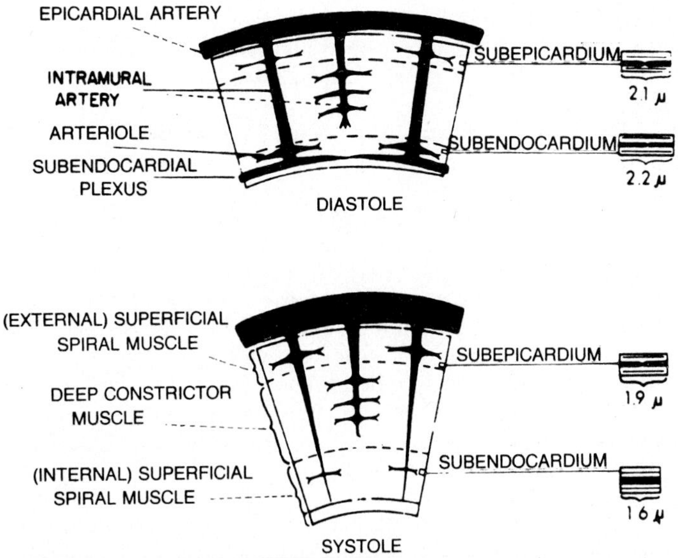

FIGURE 37–3. Cross-section of the left ventricular wall in systole and diastole. Factors involved in the susceptibility of the subendocardium to the development of ischemia include the greater dependence of this region on diastolic perfusion and the greater degree of shortening, and therefore of energy expenditure, of this region during systole. (From Bell, J. R., and Fox, A. C.: Pathogenesis of subendocardial ischemia. Am. J. Med. Sci. *268*:2, 1974.)

erals, although in experimental animals exercise does not reduce mortality resulting from coronary occlusion.[31] Perfusion via collaterals in the presence of total coronary occlusion may equal perfusion via a vessel with 90 per cent obstruction of the luminal diameter.[32]

Although debate continues concerning the functional significance of collaterals, two facts are clear: (1) collaterals become visible angiographically only when coronary occlusion is complete or virtually so, and (2) the presence of collaterals occasionally can prevent the development of a myocardial infarction in the presence of a total coronary occlusion. However, even when collaterals prevent myocardial infarction in the presence of coronary occlusion, they provide perfusion just sufficient to maintain myocardial viability; an increase in $M\dot{V}O_2$ induced by electrical pacing results in a deterioration of myocardial function.[33] Some studies have shown that the presence of collaterals appears to reduce the frequency of wall motion disorders in the face of coronary obstruction,[32] while others have not confirmed this.[32a] Therefore, when cardiac muscle is supplied entirely or largely by collateral vessels, it often becomes ischemic if its oxygen demands increase above basal levels.

PERFUSION PRESSURE. As in any vascular bed, blood flow in the coronary bed depends on the driving pressure and the resistance offered by this bed. However, the coronary circulation differs from other circulations in that the resistance offered by the bed is influenced considerably by phasic systolic compression of the coronary vessels coursing through the myocardium. The effective driving or perfusion pressure is the pressure gradient between the coronary arteries and the pressure either in the right atrium or the left ventricle in diastole, since coronary flow drains into both of these chambers. However, effective perfusion pressure is not constant throughout the cardiac cycle. When the aortic valve is open and ejected blood flows rapidly past the coronary ostia, perfusion pressure is reduced slightly below aortic pressure because of the Venturi effect. In addition, phasic changes in right atrial pressure occurring during the cardiac cycle and in the left ventricle during diastole modify the effective perfusion pressure gradient, albeit only slightly, except in the presence of a tall right atrial v wave, as in tricuspid regurgitation.

FACTORS EXTRINSIC TO THE VASCULAR BED. Coronary vascular resistance is influenced both by factors *extrinsic* to the bed, particularly compressive forces within the myocardium (intramyocardial pressure acting on the intramyocardial vessels), and by metabolic, neural, and humoral factors *intrinsic* to the bed causing changes in the cross-sectional area of coronary resistance vessels. Intramyocardial pressure is determined primarily by the ventricular pressure throughout the cardiac cycle.[33, 34] Because ventricular pressure is so much higher in systole than it is in diastole, myocardial compressive forces acting on intramyocardial vessels are much greater during this phase of the cardiac cycle. Accordingly, most of the coronary blood flow to the left ventricle occurs during diastole. Indeed, there may even be some backflow in the major coronary arteries during systole. Since an increase in heart rate diminishes the total amount of diastolic time per minute while increasing myocardial oxygen demands, tachycardia may compromise coronary perfusion. This "throttling" effect of systole on myocardial perfusion[21] is particularly important when systolic intraventricular pressure is elevated but coronary perfusion pressure is not, as in the case of obstruction to left ventricular outflow by valvular or subvalvular aortic stenosis, or in severe aortic regurgitation.

Extravascular Compressive Forces. The dramatic impact of left ventricular compression on coronary blood flow can be demonstrated experimentally with a beating heart perfused at constant pressure in which asystole is induced transiently by vagal stimulation. At this time, coronary blood flow suddenly increases by approximately 50 per cent because of relief of the compressive effect.[22] Since compressive forces exerted by the right ventricle are ordinarily far less than those of the left ventricle, perfusion of the right ventricle is not interrupted during systole.

The calculation of coronary vascular resistance is complicated by the observation that under normal conditions coronary blood flow ceases when coronary driving pressure reaches levels of approximately 40 mm Hg, the so-called P_{zf} or pressure at zero flow (Fig. 37–4). Although there is no question concerning the existence of a P_{zf} substantially above coronary venous pressure, considerable debate continues about the mechanism responsible for it.[35, 36]

The Greater Susceptibility of the Subendocardium. Extravascular compressive forces during systole are greater in subendocardial zones of the heart compared with subepicardial ones (Fig. 37–3). Therefore, systolic flow is greatly reduced in this region.

Under physiological conditions, marked transitory disparities exist between endocardial and epicardial wall stresses and, correspondingly, between endocardial and epicardial flow throughout the cardiac cycle. Nevertheless, under physiological conditions, in conscious dogs the ratio of endocardial to epicardial flow averaged throughout the cardiac cycle is approximately 1.25:1 as a consequence of preferential dilatation of the subendocardial vessels.[37] Total flow is greater in the subendocardium because calculated wall stress and oxygen consumption are greater in this region than in the subepicardium. Interventions that re-

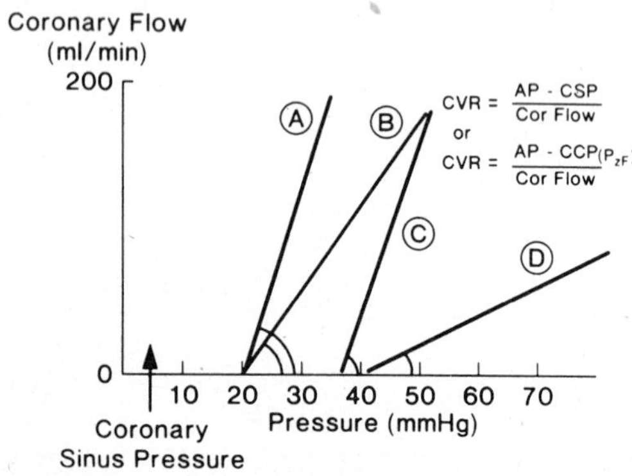

FIGURE 37–4. Diagram illustrating the potential importance of critical closing pressure (CCP) or the pressure at zero flow (P_{zF}) on the calculation of coronary vascular resistance (CVR). The slopes of the lines reflect coronary conductance, the inverse of coronary resistance: the pressure at zero flow is closely related to critical closing pressure, or : P_{zF}. Line D depicts the normal situation. The coronary bed is not dilated because the pressure-flow relationship has a relatively shallow slope. Also, in line D, P_{zF} is almost 40 mm Hg. Line A shows a theoretical pressure-flow relationship obtained in a maximally dilated coronary bed. The slope of line A is much steeper than that of line D, and P_{zF} is much lower in line A than in line D (approximately 20 mm Hg). Lines B and C illustrate that either P_{zF} or conductance can be responsible for major changes in the pressure-flow relationships. This implies that without knowledge of P_{zF} calculations of resistance or conductance in the coronary bed may be seriously in error. In addition, it is obvious that coronary vascular resistance will be much different if coronary driving pressure is aortic pressure (AP)—critical closing pressure P_{zF} instead of AP—coronary sinus pressure (CSP). Cor Flow = coronary flow. (From Marcus, M. L.: Autoregulation in the coronary circulation. *In* The Coronary Circulation in Health and Disease. New York, McGraw-Hill Book Company, 1983, p. 105.)

duce the perfusion pressure gradient during diastole (as occurs with coronary obstruction, elevation of ventricular diastolic pressure, and tachycardia) lower the ratio of subendocardial to subepicardial flow and may cause the subendocardium to become ischemic.

The combination of a greater wall stress, and hence greater resistance to flow, and higher metabolic demands results in lower coronary vascular tone in the subendocardium than in the subepicardium. As a consequence, the reserve for vasodilatation is also less in the subendocardium than in the subepicardium, and as perfusion is reduced the deeper layers of myocardium become ischemic before the more superficial ones. This phenomenon is manifested by reduced intracellular oxygen tension and contractility and increased production of lactate in the inner layers of the ventricular wall as the heart becomes ischemic[38] (see Fig. 37–21, p. 1206).

The susceptibility of the subendocardium to ischemia by the combination of limited reserve for vasodilation, extrinsic compression from the higher wall stress to which it is subjected,[39] and the resultant high metabolic demands accounts for ST-segment depression on the electrocardiogram characteristically associated with episodes of transient ischemia (Fig. 7–35, p. 204). Injury currents from the subendocardium, resulting in ST-segment depression, accompany the maldistribution of transmural flow and metabolic impairment of subendocardial tissue under these circumstances, even though net transmural flow may remain near normal[40] (Fig. 37–5). These considerations provide the basis for the recognition of myocardial ischemia by ST-segment depression during exercise stress testing (Chap. 8). When coronary flow is restricted, the adaptive changes of the subendocardial zone include its greater potential for glycolytic metabolism[41] due to higher glycolytic enzyme activity and, consequently, higher lactate production rates.[42] However, even though the glycogen content of subendocardium is higher than that of the subepicardium under aerobic conditions, concentrations of high-energy phosphate compounds are generally lower

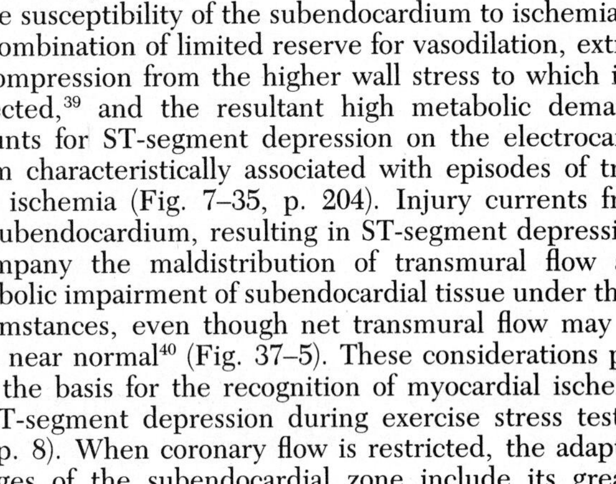

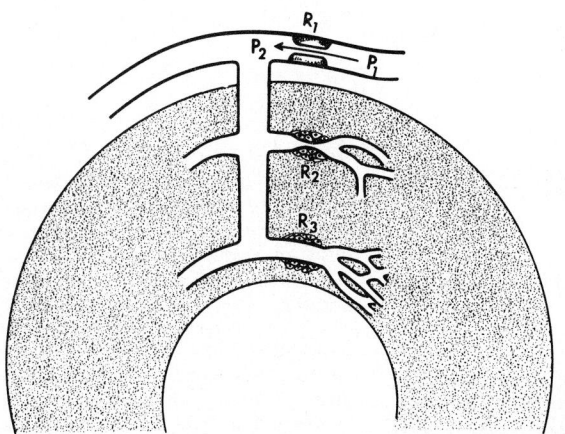

FIGURE 37–5. Effects of a stenosis in an epicardial vessel (R_1) on endocardial and epicardial flow. Endocardial vessels (R_3) are maximally dilated, whereas epicardial vessels (R_2) are not. A vasodilator stimulus resulting (for example, from an increase in heart rate) will augment transmural flow owing to dilation of subepicardial vessels. Increase in flow will cause a greater pressure drop across the stenosis (P_1-P_2) and the coronary driving pressure (P_2) will drop. As long as the fall in resistance in subepicardial vessels (R_2) is greater than the resulting fall in driving pressure, flow will increase in the subepicardial region. However, because subendocardial vessels are already maximally dilated, the fall in coronary driving pressure will not be accompanied by a fall in resistance. Hence, flow to subendocardial vessels will fall. (From Epstein, S. E., Cannon, R. O., III, and Talbot, T. L.: Hemodynamic principles in the control of coronary blood flow. Am. J. Cardiol. *56*:8E, 1985.)

than those in the midepicardium and subepicardium when coronary flow is restricted (Fig. 37–2, p. 1192), because of the inability of anaerobic metabolism to fulfill energy requirements completely.

Prediction of Subendocardial Ischemia. Griggs, Hoffman, Buckberg, Brazier and their collaborators have developed indexes for the evaluation of transmural blood flow and the prediction of subendocardial ischemia in the absence of coronary artery obstruction.[37, 40–43] They reasoned that the delivery of oxygen to the subendocardium represents the product of arterial oxygen content and the driving force for subendocardial blood flow, which in turn depend on the integrated pressure difference between the aorta and left ventricle during diastole, termed the *diastolic pressure–time index* (DPTI). The demand for blood flow, i.e., $M\dot{V}O_2$, is closely related to the area beneath the systolic portion of the ventricular pressure curve, i.e., the *systolic pressure–time index* (SPTI). The ratio DPTI × oxygen content/SPTI has been used as an index of the relation between subendocardial oxygen supply and demand. This ratio can be reduced by (1) opening an arteriovenous fistula or patent ductus arteriosus or inducing aortic regurgitation to diminish aortic diastolic pressure and thereby reducing DPTI; (2) increasing preload or afterload, causing left ventricular dysfunction, or reducing left ventricular compliance; these maneuvers all raise left ventricular diastolic pressure and also reduce DPTI; (3) inducing tachycardia to shorten diastole[44]; and (4) causing severe anemia or hypoxemia to reduce arterial oxygen content. With reduction of the DPTI × oxygen content/SPTI below a critical value of approximately 10, the endocardial/epicardial blood flow ratio also decreased.

Although it is recognized that this index provides only an approximation of the oxygen supply-to-demand relationship,[33] it can explain a number of clinical findings, such as the development of angina and the electrocardiographic and biochemical evidence of ischemia caused by tachycardia in patients with aortic stenosis; in this situation DPTI falls and SPTI rises. Myocardial lactate production has been observed to occur during beta-adrenoceptor stimulation with isoproterenol in patients with aortic stenosis,[45] when left ventricular systolic pressure, contractility, heart rate, and therefore, $M\dot{V}O_2$ rise. When adrenergic stimulation was carried out in dogs with experimentally produced aortic stenosis, the myocardial lactate concentration and the lactate-pyruvate ratio rose while the reduction of ATP stores was more prominent in the inner than the outer half of the ventricle.[38] This indicates that the subendocardium is more vulnerable to ischemia and therefore becomes dependent on anaerobic metabolism more readily than does the subepicardium. In experimentally produced aortic regurgitation, diastolic coronary blood flow falls but systolic flow rises, so that total coronary flow does not change.[46] However, with severe reductions in aortic diastolic pressure, DPTI declines and the subendocardial region exhibits biochemical evidence of anaerobic metabolism. As the DPTI × oxygen content/SPTI declines, the subendocardial lactate-pyruvate ratio rises, evidence of anaerobic metabolism in this region of myocardium. These observations are clinically relevant considering that angina pectoris occurs in a significant number of patients with severe aortic stenosis and/or regurgitation in the absence of coronary artery disease (Chap. 33). Other conditions in which subendocardial ischemia occurs include marked systemic hypotension, regardless of etiology (Chap. 19), and pulmonary embolism, particularly when complicated by fever, tachycardia, and anemia. In these conditions the ischemia results from a combination of lowered coronary perfusion pressure, tachycardia, and increased subendo-

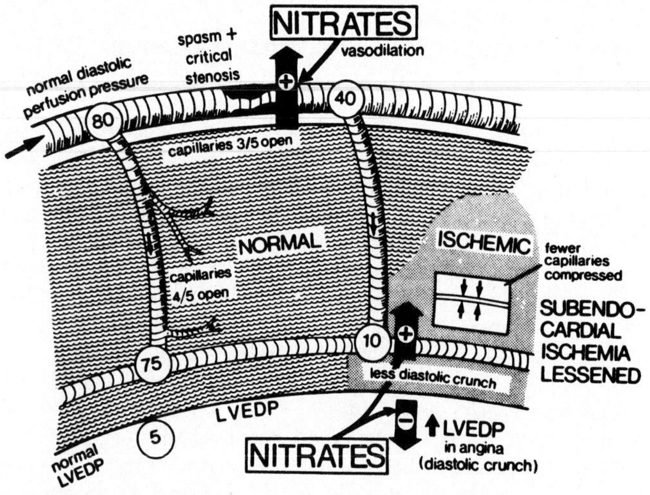

FIGURE 37–6. Effects of a critical stenosis in an epicardial vessel and of nitrates on myocardial perfusion and function. When a patient with a critical stenosis exercises, subendocardial ischemia and an increase in left ventricular end-diastolic pressure (LVEDP) occur; this is accompanied by compression ("crunch") of subendocardial vessels. Alternatively, angina at rest can develop if there is superimposed coronary spasm. Nitrates bring relief by increasing the diameter of large coronary arteries, by relaxing spasm, by reducing LVEDP, and by decreasing diastolic compression. (Adapted from Parratt, J. R., Marshall, R. J., and Ledingham, M. C. A.: J. Physiol. [Paris] *76*:791, 1980.)

cardial tension secondary to sympathetic stimulation of myocardial contractility. Since coronary blood flow ceases at a pressure higher than ventricular diastolic pressure (see discussion of P_{zf} above), as arterial pressure declines with systemic hypotension or aortic regurgitation, the coronary perfusion pressure declines to quite low levels.

In the presence of coronary obstruction the *effective* pressure perfusing the subendocardial region is determined by the gradient between the diastolic coronary pressure *distal* to the obstruction and the left ventricular end-diastolic pressure; hence the DPTI no longer reflects or even approximates the driving force for subendocardial blood flow. When left ventricular diastolic pressure is elevated in the ischemic ventricle, the endocardial/epicardial flow ratio declines, further reducing subendocardial blood flow.[47] Intensification of subendocardial ischemia can raise ventricular diastolic pressure further, causing a vicious circle. Since maldistribution of transmural blood flow compromises the subendocardial tissue, antianginal drugs may be effective if they improve the ratio of subendocardial to subepicardial flow even if they do not augment net transmural perfusion. Analysis of the washout of ^{86}Rb and fractional uptake of radioactive-labeled microspheres has shown that both nitroglycerin and beta-adrenoceptor blockers redistribute blood flow to the subendocardium.[48, 49] This phenomenon may, in the case of nitroglycerin, reflect in part the direct effects of the drugs on the coronary vascular bed as well as the reduction of extravascular compressive forces induced by a lowering of ventricular diastolic pressure resulting from a reduction of preload (Fig. 37–6). Beta blockers reduce $M\dot{V}O_2$ and thereby ischemia; the relief of ischemia in turn abolishes the reduction of subendocardial blood flow and tends to restore to normal the ratio of subendocardial to subepicardial blood flow.

CONTROL OF CORONARY VASCULAR RESISTANCE

Resistance is influenced markedly by changes in the tone of the vascular bed, changes that are mediated by neural, metabolic, pharmacological, and myogenic factors, as well as substances released by the endothelium.

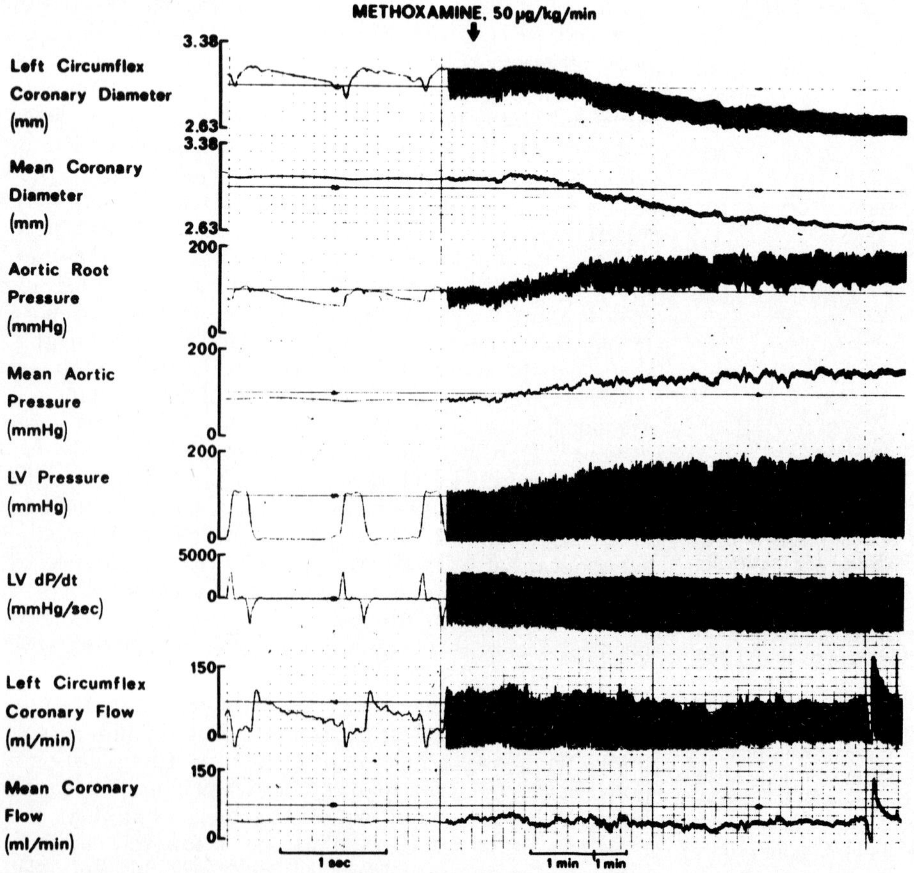

FIGURE 37–7. The effects of a 10-minute infusion of methoxamine, 50 µg/kg/min, in a conscious dog are depicted on simultaneous and continuous measurements of phasic and mean left circumflex coronary artery diameter, aortic root pressure, left ventricular pressure, left ventricular dP/dt, and phasic and mean left circumflex coronary blood flow. Methoxamine increases coronary diameters only initially and transiently and then induces striking sustained reductions in coronary diameters at a markedly elevated aortic pressure. At the end of the response, the vessel was transiently occluded to obtain a zero blood flow reference. (From Vatner, S. F., Pagani, M., Manders, W. T., and Pasipoularides, A. D.: Alpha-adrenergic vasoconstriction and nitroglycerin vasodilation of large coronary arteries in the conscious dog. J. Clin. Invest. *65*:5, 1980.)

NEURAL FACTORS. The coronary arteries are richly innervated by sympathetic and parasympathetic nerves.[22, 24] Both $alpha_1$ and $alpha_2$ receptors are present in the coronary arteries,[50a] and when activated by neuronally released or circulating norepinephrine both cause coronary vasoconstriction[50] (Fig. 37–7), which appears to be mediated largely by an increased concentration of calcium in coronary vascular smooth muscle.[50b, 50c, 50d] Stimulation of cardiac sympathetic nerves causes coronary vasoconstriction when inotropic and chronotropic effects are blocked.[51] The activation of $alpha_1$ receptors induced by the infusion of methoxamine has been demonstrated to reduce the diameter of coronary arteries while increasing intraluminal pressure.[24, 52] The carotid chemoreceptor reflex causes marked coronary vasoconstriction, which can be blocked by surgical denervation or by the alpha blocker phentolamine.[52] $Beta_1$ and $beta_2$ receptors in the large and small coronary arteries mediate vasodilation.[24, 53] Beta-adrenoceptor blockade induces coronary constriction, but this effect appears *not* to be a direct action on the coronary arteries but rather results from blockade of $beta_1$-mediated increases in $M\dot{V}O_2$.[54] The extent of cholinergic regulation of large coronary arteries is controversial,[55] although parasympathetic stimulation appears to dilate small coronary arteries.[24]

Intravenous administration of norepinephrine induces a brief fall, followed by a sustained rise, in coronary vascular resistance, accompanied by a decline in coronary sinus pO_2 (Fig. 37–8).[56] The early vasodilatation can be eliminated by beta-adrenoceptor blockade and presumably results from the augmented myocardial oxygen needs consequent to stimulation of myocardial beta receptors; the later increase in coronary vascular resistance can be prevented by alpha-adrenoceptor blockade and presumably results from stimulation of alpha receptors in the coronary vascular bed. Blockade of $alpha_1$ receptors in patients with coronary artery disease attenuates the coronary vasoconstrictor response to the cold pressor test[57] and cigarette smoking,[58, 58a] indicating that both responses are mediated by stimulation of alpha receptors.

Baroreceptor activity affects coronary vascular resistance reflexly. In the dog with sectioned vagal nerves, occlusion of the carotid arteries to produce baroreceptor hypotension induces an increase in heart rate and blood pressure, accompanied by a reduction in coronary vascular resistance.[59] When the reflex tachycardia and myocardial contractility (which would be expected to increase $M\dot{V}O_2$ and thereby lower coronary vascular resistance) are blocked with propranolol, an increase in coronary vascular resistance is observed, which can be prevented by cardiac sympathectomy. It may be concluded that with intact sympathetic nerves and beta receptors, the coronary dilatation consequent to carotid occlusion is due to heightened cardiac metabolic activity induced reflexly by baroreceptor hypotension. When this augmentation of myocardial beta-receptor-mediated activity is prevented with beta blockade, reflex coronary *vasoconstriction* secondary to carotid hypotension is unmasked.[60] Stimulation of the distal ends of the vagi produces coronary vasodilatation,[60, 61] an effect that is mediated by the release of acetylcholine from vagal nerve endings and that can be blocked by atropine.[22]

There is also evidence for some *tonic* coronary constriction mediated by the sympathetic nerves.[62] Acute surgical denervation of the heart produces a fall in coronary vascular resistance with a decrease in arteriovenous oxygen extraction.[63] Coronary vascular resistance in patients as well as in dogs[64] with innervated hearts declines by almost 25 per cent in response to alpha-adrenoceptor blockade, suggesting that basal coronary constrictor tone mediated by alpha receptors is released. Coronary vascular resistance does not diminish when patients with cardiac transplants receive alpha-adrenoceptor blockade, suggesting that cardiac denervation had previously released the coronary constrictor tone. However, in the unanesthetized dog, cardiac denervation does not protect the myocardium that has been rendered ischemic by coronary occlusion.[65]

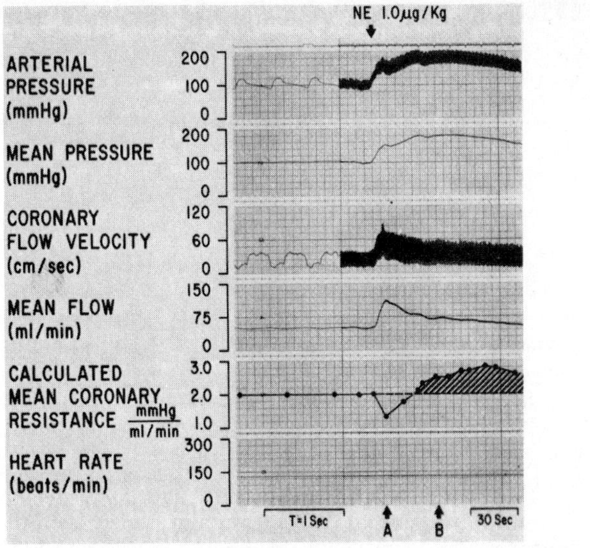

FIGURE 37–8. Effects of intravenously administered norepinephrine (NE) in the intact unanesthetized dog with heart rate held constant. Coronary vascular resistance fell initially (*A*) and then showed a sustained increase (*B*). (From Vatner, S. F., Higgins, C. B., and Braunwald, E.: Effects of norepinephrine on coronary circulation and left ventricular dynamics in the conscious dog. Circ. Res. *34*:812, 1974, by permission of the American Heart Association, Inc.)

In the conscious dog, stimulation of the carotid sinus nerves results in a substantial reduction in coronary vascular resistance.[62] This effect can be prevented by alpha-receptor blockade, suggesting that sympathetic coronary constrictor tone is present in the resting conscious dog and that coronary vasodilatation attendant upon electrical stimulation of the carotid sinus nerves results from a reduction in this resting vasoconstrictor tone. Coronary vasodilatation resulting from stimulation of the carotid sinus nerves occurs also during exercise, suggesting that alpha-receptor–mediated constrictor tone persists in the coronary vascular bed during exercise, despite the coexisting metabolic vasodilatation. This conclusion is supported by studies using alpha-adrenoceptor blocking drugs. These studies have shown that the increase in coronary blood flow and oxygen delivery to the myocardium during normal exercise is limited by alpha-adrenergic vasoconstriction.[66]

Efferent neural influences on the coronary vascular bed may also be activated reflexly by cardiopulmonary parasympathetic receptors. Stimulation of parasympathetic receptors leads to reflex systemic and coronary vasodilatation.[67] Chemoreceptor activation initially causes coronary dilatation, a reflex that is mediated by the vagi and can be abolished by atropine.[22] As already noted, the late response is coronary vasoconstriction.[52] Intracoronary injection of veratrum alkaloids, as well as other metabolically active substances, induces reflex bradycardia and hypotension (the Bezold-Jarisch reflex),[68] the afferent limb of which involves the vagus nerves. The effects of efferent vagus nerve activity causing *coronary* vasodilatation[69] have been documented, indicating that the Bezold-Jarisch reflex involves coronary efferent as well as afferent parasympathetic components.[67] Reflex constriction of stenotic lesions of the coronary vascular bed in humans has been demonstrated by studying the effects of handgrip by means of coronary arteriography.[70] However, an increase in sympathetic outflow does *not* appear to be responsible for episodes of coronary spasm in patients with Prinzmetal's (variant) angina.[71]

AUTOREGULATION OF CORONARY BLOOD FLOW

When sudden alterations in perfusion pressure in many vascular beds are imposed, the abrupt changes in blood flow are only transitory, with flow promptly returning toward the previous steady-state level.[72] This phenomenon, termed autoregulation (Fig. 37–9), applies also to the coronary vascular bed and tends to maintain myocardial perfusion within a relatively narrow range, regardless of transitory changes in perfusion pressure between upper limits of 120 to 140 mm Hg and lower levels of 50 to 70 mm Hg.[34] Demonstration of autoregulation in intact animals is difficult because modification of coronary perfusion pressure also changes both $M\dot{V}O_2$ and extrinsic compression of the coronary vessels. However, under experimental conditions in which perfusion pressure is altered but ventricular pressure, cardiac contractility, and heart rate—the principal determinants of $M\dot{V}O_2$—are maintained constant, autoregulation is clearly evident. Autoregulation is more prominent in the subepicardial than in the subendocardial layers of the left ventricle. Drugs that cause relaxation of coronary vascular smooth muscle diminish autoregulation.[33] It has been observed that when coronary perfusion pressure falls to below the critical levels of 60 to 70 mm Hg, the coronary vessels become maximally dilated and flow becomes pressure-dependent, i.e., autoregulation is lost (Fig. 37–9). This observation explains the importance of maintaining coronary perfusion pressure in patients with hypotension of any cause, including acute myocardial infarction. When obstructive coronary artery disease is present, coronary perfusion pressure is lower than aortic pressure. A small reduction of the latter could lower perfusion pressure below the critical levels, thereby depressing myocardial perfusion, intensifying myocardial ischemia, and increasing left ventricular filling pressure, which decreases the perfusion pressure gradient further. In patients with cardiogenic shock, the reduction of perfusion pressure below this critical level at which autoregulation is lost lowers coronary blood flow even through nonobstructed vessels and may reduce collateral blood flow to the periinfarction zone, thereby enlarging the infarct (Fig. 38–9, p. 1231).

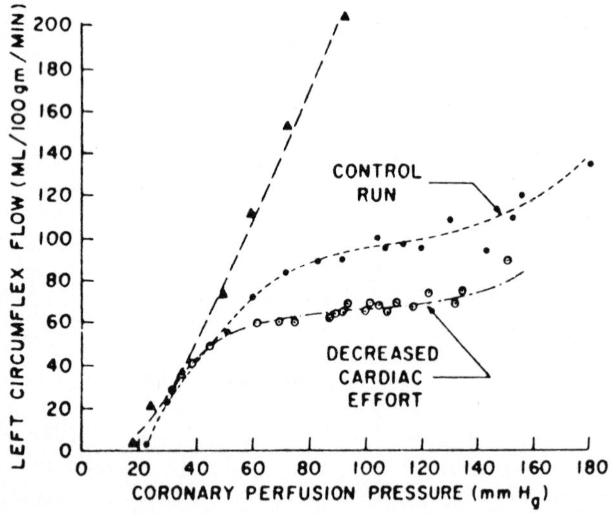

FIGURE 37–9. Relation between left circumflex coronary flow and coronary perfusion pressure. Coronary perfusion pressure has been altered independently of aortic pressure, which is maintained essentially constant. Triangles represent the immediate change in flow with various sudden increases in perfusion pressure from a pressure of 40 mm Hg. Closed circles along the middle curve represent the readjusted steady-state flow levels over a range of perfusion pressures after autoregulation has occurred. Note the relative independence of flow from coronary perfusion pressure between approximately 70 and 130 mm Hg. When cardiac effort was reduced by lowering aortic pressure (open circles), the steady-state level of left circumflex flow was also reduced but again remained relatively independent of coronary perfusion pressure over a broad range of perfusion pressure changes. (From Mosher, P., et al.: Control of coronary blood flow by an autoregulatory mechanism. Circ. Res. *14*:250, 1964, by permission of the American Heart Association, Inc.)

Several mechanisms have been implicated, including myogenic and metabolic factors as well as extravascular compressive forces, i.e., interstitial pressure.[21, 22]

MYOGENIC FACTORS. Stretch of vascular smooth muscle resulting from an increase in perfusion pressure stimulates the muscle to contract.[73] The consequent augmentation of resistance tends to return blood flow toward normal despite the higher perfusion pressure. Although the myogenic mechanism, sometimes called the Bayliss effect, appears to be a general characteristic of vascular smooth muscle,[74] its role in the regulation of coronary blood flow has not been explicitly defined and is probably a modest one.[22]

METABOLIC CONTROL OF CORONARY BLOOD FLOW (Fig. 37–10). It is likely that changes in regional myocardial metabolism are important determinants of autoregulation (and therefore coronary blood flow). Several mediators have been implicated, including oxygen, carbon dioxide, and vasodilator metabolites, such as adenosine, that accumulate in hypoperfused regions of myocardium. There is a tight coupling between $M\dot{V}O_2$ and coronary blood flow.[8, 34] It has been suggested that with increased energy expenditure by the heart there is a proportionally increased production of vasodilator metabolites, which in turn reduce coronary vascular resistance and raise coronary blood flow so that only small changes in myocardial oxygen extraction occur. Insofar as the role of metabolic factors in mediating acute regulation of coronary blood flow is concerned, it has been suggested that a marked reduction in coronary arterial perfusion pressure (while $M\dot{V}O_2$ is held constant) causes an immediate decrease in coronary flow. This would be expected to cause an increased myocardial oxygen extraction and a reduced myocardial oxygen tension; the resultant hypoxia and accompanying accumulation of vasodilator metabolites then would cause coronary vasodilatation.[75] It is possible that oxygen acts on vascular smooth muscle directly, possibly by altering the electrochemical potential of the muscle cells. Direct vasodilating effects of diminished oxygen tension have been demonstrated in the coronary, femoral, and other vessels.[76] Molecular oxygen diffusing across the walls of the vessels appears to be a primary determinant of constrictor tone of precapillary sphincters under physiological conditions.[77] Thus, diminution of oxygen tension increases the number of capillaries perfused within a predefined region of myocardium, presumably by relaxation of these sphincters.[78] In this manner coronary blood flow would be expected to remain constant despite a reduction of coronary perfusion pressure. Transitory augmentation of the concentration of potassium in extracellular fluid, an early consequence of myocardial ischemia, may also modify the transmembrane potential of vascular smooth muscle cells and result in vasodilatation.

Role of Adenosine (Fig. 37–11). Degradation of adenine nucleotides under conditions in which ATP utilization exceeds the capacity of myocardial cells to resynthesize high-energy phosphate compounds (a process dependent on oxidative phosphorylation in mitochondria) results in the production of adenosine monophosphate (AMP). The

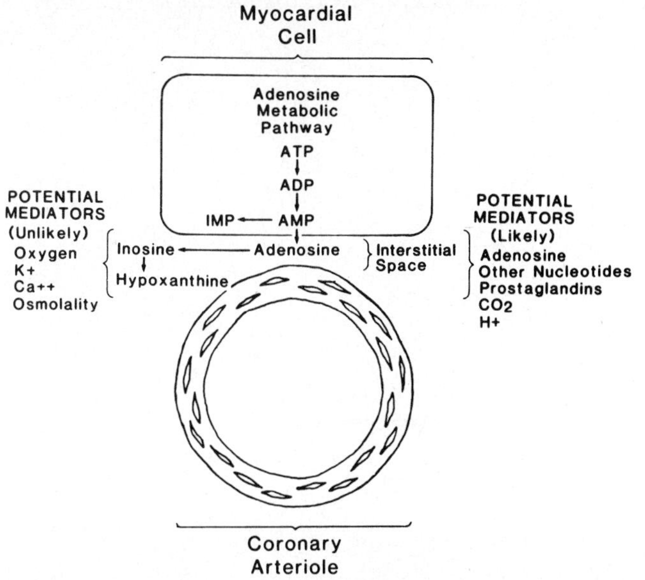

FIGURE 37–10. Diagram illustrating potential mediators that may couple myocardial cellular metabolism and coronary vascular resistance. These potential mediators are divided into unlikely and likely categories on the basis of presently available evidence. The metabolic pathway of the most likely mediator (adenosine) is also illustrated. ATP = adenosine triphosphate; ADP = adenosine diphosphate; IMP = inosine monophosphate; AMP = adenosine monophosphate; K^+ = potassium ions; CA^{++} = calcium; CO_2 = carbon dioxide; H^+ = hydrogen ion. (From Marcus, M. L.: Metabolic regulation of coronary blood flow. *In* The Coronary Circulation in Health and Disease. New York, McGraw-Hill Book Company, 1983, p. 85.)

enzyme 5′-nucleotidase is responsible for the formation of adenosine.[79] Accordingly, adenosine and its metabolites, inosine and hypoxanthine, appear in interstitial fluid and in the coronary sinus venous effluent. *Adenosine* is a powerful vasodilator[80] that is considered to be an important, perhaps *the critical, mediator* linking metabolically induced vasodilatation to diminished coronary perfusion (Fig. 37–11). There is substantial evidence that an imbalance (a reduction) in the supply-to-demand ratio for oxygen is the primary determinant of adenosine formation.[79, 81]

Concentrations of adenosine in the venous effluent are much lower than those in interstitial fluid, in part because capillary endothelium rapidly converts adenosine to inosine and hypoxanthine.[82] However, when the enzyme responsible for this conversion, adenosine deaminase, is inhibited by administration of 8-azaguanine, prominent increases occur in the concentration of adenosine in the effluent.[83] If, at a constant level of myocardial metabolism, adenosine were being released at a constant rate, an elevation of coronary perfusion pressure and the resultant increase in coronary blood flow would augment the washout of adenosine, reduce its concentration, and thus increase coronary vascular resistance. Such a mechanism could provide a feedback to account for autoregulation of coronary blood flow. More important, it could also explain the close correlation between the energy expenditure of the heart and the level of coronary blood flow.[83, 83a] According to this concept, as the former rises, the ratio of oxygen supply to demand declines, and more ATP is degraded to AMP, which becomes available for and enhances adenosine formation. The latter causes coronary relaxation, thereby increasing coronary blood flow to a level appropriate to the $M\dot{V}O_2$.

It appears that adenosine acts on the surface of vascular smooth muscle cells, apparently at a receptor site on the cell membrane; presumably adenosine blocks entry of Ca^{++} into these cells and thereby causes vasodilatation.[22] In addition to its potent vasodilating action, adenosine exerts a generally depressant activity on cardiac automaticity and atrioventricular conduction and attenuates the effects of adrenergic influences on myocardial contractility.[84]

Despite its importance, adenosine is almost certainly not the only metabolic factor involved. It is possible that adenosine does not act alone but interacts with other agents in response to hypoxia in causing coronary relaxation.[85] Prostaglandins, kinins, acetate, potassium, and a number of metabolites alter coronary vascular resistance profoundly and may play a role in mediating vasodilatation in response to hypoxia. The infusion of at least two prostaglandins synthesized in the heart (PGI_2 and PGE_2) can cause coronary vasodilatation,[85a] and the inhibition of prostaglandin synthesis with indomethacin causes an increase in coronary vascular resistance in humans.[86]

Autoregulation in the bed distal to the obstruction may be compromised because the bed is already maximally dilated in the basal state. As a consequence, perfusion of this distal bed becomes dependent entirely on perfusion pressure (Fig. 37–5). Under these circumstances, augmentation of cardiac oxygen requirements, as occurs during exercise, *without* an increase in perfusion pressure results in or intensifies ischemia. Since blood flow to regions supplied by normal vessels can be increased (because regional vasodilatation in these regions is possible), while blood flow to the compromised zone cannot (because its

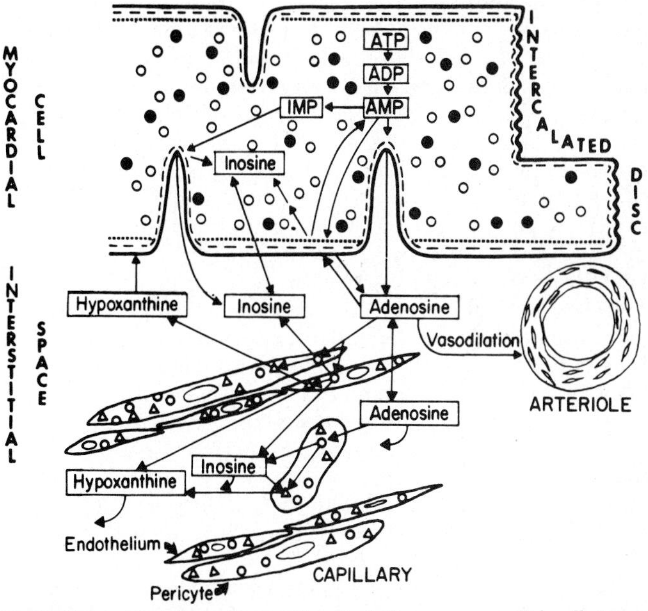

FIGURE 37–11. Schematic drawing depicting a myocardial cell, interstitial space, an arteriole, and a capillary with the localization of enzymes involved in the formation and fate of adenosine. Adenosine formed by 5′-nucleotidase from AMP (which in turn arises from ATP) can enter the interstitial space. There it can induce arteriolar dilation and reenter the myocardial cell, where it is either phosphorylated to AMP by adenosine kinase or deaminated to inosine by adenosine deaminase, or it can enter the capillaries and leave the tissue. A large fraction of adenosine that crosses the capillary wall is deaminated to inosine, which in turn is split to hypoxanthine and ribose-1-PO_4 by nucleoside phosphorylase located in the endothelial cells, pericytes, and erythrocytes. Most of the adenosine is taken up by the myocardial cells, and that escaping into the circulation is largely in the form of inosine and hypoxanthine. Since adenylic acid deaminase (which deaminates AMP to IMP) is in low concentration in heart muscle, the major degradative pathway from AMP is via dephosphorylation to adenosine. ○ = Adenosine deaminase; ● = adenylic acid deaminase; △ = nucleoside phosphorylase; (---) = 5′-nucleotidase; (·····) = adenosine kinase. (From Berne, R. M., and Rubio, R.: Coronary circulation. *In* Berne, R. M., Sperelakis, N., and Geiger, S. R. [eds.]: Handbook of Physiology, Section 2. The Cardiovascular System. Bethesda, Md., American Physiological Society, 1979, p. 924.)

vessels are already maximally dilated), disparities in regional perfusion can become intensified. This explains the exercise-induced disparity in uptake of ^{201}Thallium in ischemic heart disease (p. 331), as well as the exercise-induced regional dysfunction in the presence of subcritical coronary stenosis.[87] In addition, vasodilatation in the normal zones may reduce perfusion pressure to the ischemic zones and deprive them further of blood flow, a phenomenon sometimes termed "coronary steal."

ENDOTHELIAL-MEDIATED CORONARY VASODILATATION. Furchgott and associates[88, 89] and other investigators[90, 90a] have observed that an intact endothelium is required for a large number of compounds, such as acetylcholine, ADP, ATP, bradykinin, and histamine, to elicit a vasodilator response in muscular arteries, including the coronary arteries. These vasodilators thus do not act directly on vascular smooth muscle. In the absence of endothelium, several of these substances—particularly acetylcholine—cause constriction of the coronary (and other) arteries. The endothelium of muscular arteries appears to have receptors for these vasodilators. When they are bound to the receptors, these vasodilators cause release from endothelial cells of a substance that produces relaxation of adjacent vascular smooth muscle, a substance termed *endothelial-derived relaxant factor* (EDRF). EDRF is a labile compound that has not yet been characterized; it does not appear to be a prostaglandin, but it may be a lipoxygenase metabolite of arachidonic acid or other unsaturated fatty acid released by activation of phospholipase. It activates guanylate cyclase in vascular smooth muscle, resulting in an increase in intracellular cyclic guanosine monophosphate (cyclic GMP), which presumably is responsible for the vascular relaxation. Nitroglycerin and sodium nitroprusside, agents with vasodilator action that is not dependent on endothelial cells, produce a direct increase in smooth muscle cyclic GMP without requiring EDRF.

Experimentally produced atherosclerosis in primates impairs the endothelial-dependent vascular relaxation to acetylcholine.[91] Acetylcholine infused into normal coronary arteries of patients undergoing coronary arteriography causes a dose-dependent dilatation; in contrast, when infused into severely stenotic coronary vessels, it causes marked constriction[92] (Fig. 37–12). Thus, coronary atherosclerosis may be associated with a defect in endothelial vasodilator function that may play a role in the pathogenesis of coronary vasospasm.

An increase in coronary blood flow, however it is induced, causes vasodilation, a phenomenon termed *blood-flow mediated vasodilation* or *reactive dilation*. The mechanism responsible for this phenomenon is not clear. One possibility is that the increase in blood flow augments the shear stress on the endothelium, which in turn releases EDRF.[93]

PHARMACOLOGICAL AGENTS. As already pointed out, alpha-adrenoceptor agonists can cause constriction of both coronary conduction vessels, i.e., the large epicardial arteries, as well as coronary resistance vessels, i.e., the small intramural arteries and arterioles[24] (Figs. 37–7 and 37–8). This effect is counteracted by the passive distention of these vessels consequent to an elevation of intravascular pressure as well as by the metabolically induced coronary vasodilatation resulting from the increase in $M\dot{V}O_2$ accompanying the arterial hypertension induced by these drugs. Directly acting coronary vasodilators, such as nitroglycerin and isosorbide dinitrate,[93a, 94, 94a] augment perfusion of ischemic zones, as reflected by increased clearance of ^{133}Xe

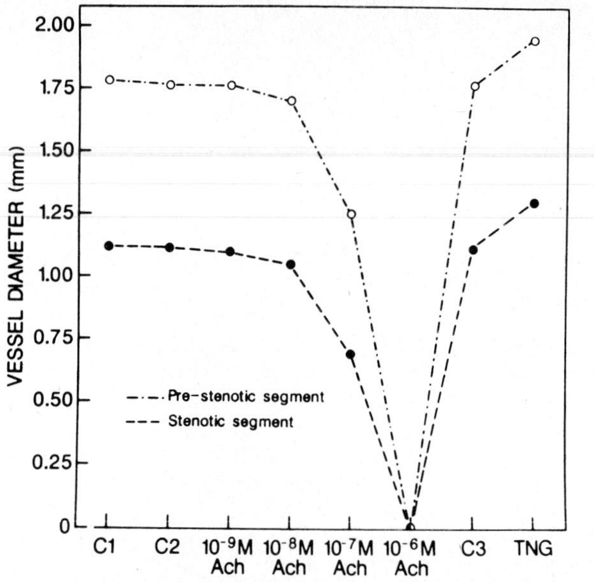

FIGURE 37–12. Response of one patient with an atherosclerotic coronary artery to intracoronary administration of an endothelium-dependent vasodilator (acetylcholine) and a direct smooth-muscle vasodilator (nitroglycerin). C1 = control, C2 = vehicle control, Ach = acetylcholine, C3 = repeated control, and TNG = nitroglycerin. (From Ludmer, P. L., Selwyn, A. P., Shook, T. L., Wayne, R. R., Mudge, G. H., Alexander, R. W., and Ganz, P.: Paradoxical vasoconstriction induced by acetylcholine in atherosclerotic coronary arteries. N. Engl. J. Med. *315*:1049, 1986.)

in patients with coronary artery disease[95]; these drugs have been shown to dilate coronary conductance vessels, coronary collaterals, and even atherosclerotic stenoses[96–98] (Fig. 39–4, p. 1327) as well as to reduce the ventricular diastolic tension which tends to limit flow to the subendocardium; they have a lesser effect on resistance vessels[92] (Fig. 37–6).

Papaverine and calcium antagonists exert a direct action on the large epicardial conductance vessels as well as on the resistance vessels.[98] These agents increase blood flow to normal as well as ischemic myocardium.[99] Dipyridamole dilates the distal (resistance) vessels.[93a, 93b] Because these are acted upon also by the endogenous vasodilator (adenosine), this agent is of little if any value in the treatment of acute myocardial ischemia. Prostaglandin I_2, which inhibits platelet aggregation, also is a potent coronary vasodilator,[85] whereas thromboxane A_2, which is produced by and aggregates platelets, is also a potent coronary vasoconstrictor. Dazoxiben, a thromboxane A_2 synthetase inhibitor, can prevent cyclic increases in coronary vascular resistance in stenotic coronary arteries.[100] Serotonin is an extremely potent coronary vasoconstrictor acting on serotonergic receptors.[24, 100a] It can be blocked by the serotonergic antagonists methysergide and ketanserin. Ergonovine and related ergot alkaloids are used diagnostically to provoke coronary spasm in patients suspected of having Prinzmetal's (variant) angina (p. 1360); these compounds cause coronary constriction by acting both on alpha-adrenergic and serotonergic receptors.[24]

REACTIVE HYPEREMIA AND CORONARY FLOW RESERVE. Transient ischemia in the zone of supply of any vascular bed, including the coronary vascular bed, is followed by an increase in blood flow above control levels, a response called *reactive hyperemia*. The flow debt (although not the oxygen debt) is overpaid by marked vasodilation during reactive hyperemia, a process that is probably related to the accumulation of vasodilator metabolites.[33] The difference between resting coronary blood flow and peak flow during reactive hyperemia represents the *coronary flow* *reserve*, which has been measured not only in experimental animals[100b] but also in patients at the time of cardiac surgery.[101] As anticipated, the coronary reserve has been found to be reduced, even absent, in patients with severe obstructive coronary disease, and can be restored to normal by bypass grafting. It is also reduced in the left ventricle of patients with severe left ventricular hypertrophy secondary to aortic stenosis.[102, 102a] Perhaps this reduction is caused by failure of growth of the coronary circulation to keep pace with the increase in ventricular mass.[102]

There has been considerable interest in estimating coronary flow reserve in patients who have not undergone surgery. A reduction of the coronary blood flow response to the vasodilating actions of dipyridamole has been demonstrated in patients with hypertension.[103] Using electrical pacing of the heart to evoke a vasodilator response, Cannon and associates described an abnormally reduced reserve in patients with hypertrophic cardiomyopathy, in whom elevation of left ventricular filling pressure, probably related to an ischemia-induced reduction in ventricular compliance during tachycardia, was associated with a decline in coronary blood flow.[104] Similar reductions in vasodilator reserve were demonstrated in patients with angina pectoris and angiographically normal epicardial coronary arteries.[105, 106]

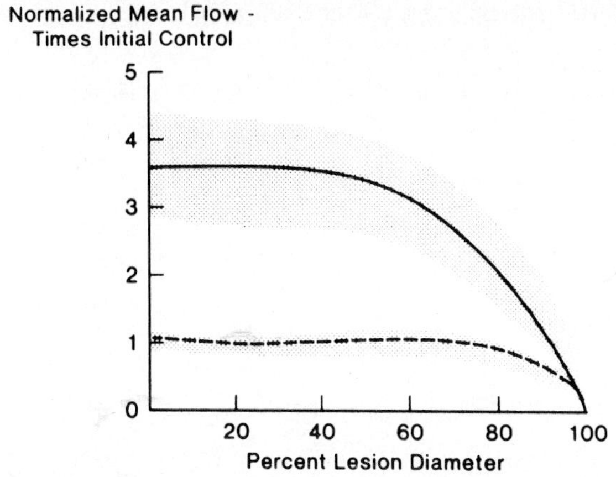

FIGURE 37–13. Relationship between resting (*dashed line*) and maximal coronary blood flow (*solid line*) and percentage of diameter stenosis in a dog. Progressive coronary stenosis was achieved by progressively narrowing a short segment of a proximal coronary artery. Resting coronary blood flow did not change until coronary diameter stenosis exceeded 80 percent. Maximal coronary blood flow began to decrease when percent diameter stenosis exceeded 50 percent. (From Marcus, M. L.: The Coronary Circulation in Health and Disease. New York, McGraw-Hill, 1983, and modified from Gould, K. L., Lipscomb, K.: Effects of coronary stenoses on coronary flow reserve and resistance. Am. J. Cardiol. *34*:50, 1974.)

FACTORS LIMITING CORONARY PERFUSION

The normal coronary vascular bed has the capacity to reduce its resistance to approximately 20 per cent of basal levels during the stress of maximal exercise; i.e., a five- to sixfold increase in coronary blood flow can occur during maximal exercise, which is generally accompanied by an increase in arterial pressure and a marked tachycardia. It is then not surprising that, in the basal state, the diameter of a proximal coronary artery can be reduced by up to approximately 80 per cent of normal, and dilatation of the coronary resistance vessels distal to the obstruction can maintain blood flow without the development of ischemia at rest. In other words, the dilatation of the intramural resistance is sufficient to offset the obstruction in the epicardial conductance vessel so that total coronary resistance in the resting state, and therefore coronary blood flow, remains constant (Fig. 37–13). However, since coronary blood flow cannot rise with this degree of obstruction in the proximal coronary bed, any stimulus that increases $M\dot{V}O_2$, such as exercise- or pacing-induced tachycardia, will elicit ischemia. With lesser degrees of obstruction, the distal bed is not maximally dilated in the basal state and, although the capacity for further dilatation exists, when the diameter is reduced by between about 40 and 80 per cent, this capacity is subnormal and ischemia may develop, depending on the extent to which myocardial oxygen demands are augmented. With less than 40 per cent diameter stenosis maximum flow during exercise is usually normal (Fig. 37–13). When obstruction of a proximal coronary artery reduces the lumen by more than approximately 80 to 85 per cent of normal, ischemia will be present even in the basal state, despite maximal dilatation of the resistance vessels (unless the myocardium distal to the obstructed vessel is perfused by collateral vessels). Transient severe obstruction, as may occur with coronary spasm, will result in brief periods of ischemia, chest pain, electrocardiographic changes, and myocardial dysfunction. When severe ischemia persists, myocardial necrosis ensues.

Basic considerations of fluid mechanics indicate that the pressure drop across a stenosis varies directly with the length of the stenosis and inversely with the fourth power of the radius (Bernoulli's theorem), emphasizing the greater importance of changes in the latter compared with the former[107, 108] (Fig. 37–14). Stenosis resistance changes relatively little with mild degrees of vascular narrowing but rises progressively and precipitously with severe obstruction; indeed, resistance almost triples as stenosis severity increases from 80 to 90 per cent.[109] As a consequence, with even a slight change in the severity of stenosis—as might occur when the resistance of the distal bed and therefore the pressure distending the narrowed coronary artery declines, as during exercise or following dipyridamole—the perfusion pressure distal to the obstruction may become reduced and subendocardial perfusion impaired.[107] Even in the presence of an "organic" athero-

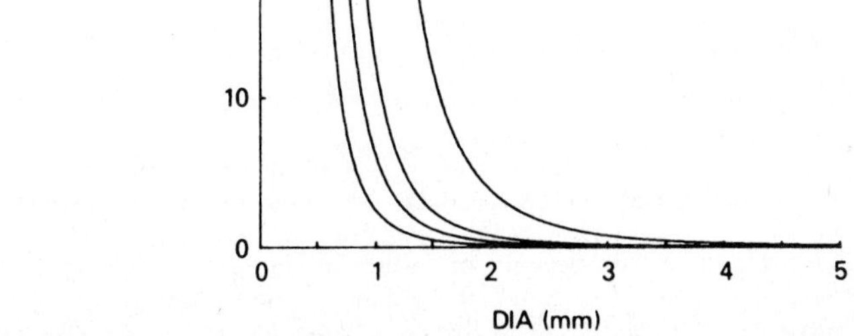

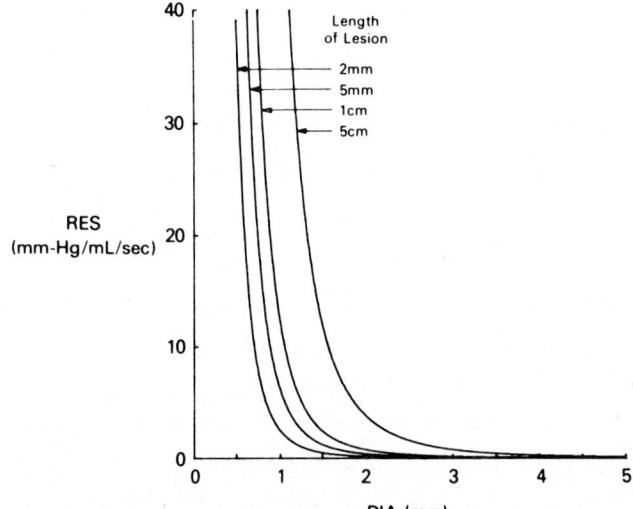

FIGURE 37–14. Relationship between coronary artery diameter (DIA) and resistance (RES) to flow. Obstructive lesions of different lengths are depicted by the four different curves; as length of the lesion increases, the resistance to flow increases at any given vessel diameter. However, because resistance is proportional to the fourth power of vessel diameter, vessel diameter is the preponderant influence on resistance to flow. (From Epstein, S. E., and Talbot, T. L.: Dynamic coronary tone in precipitation, exacerbation, and relief of angina pectoris. Am. J. Cardiol. *48*:797, 1981.)

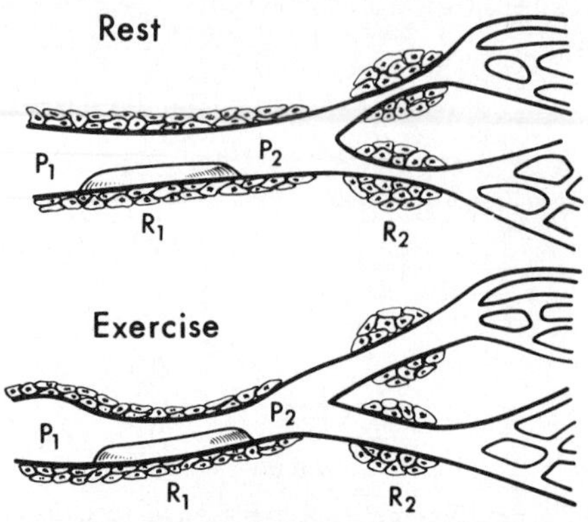

FIGURE 37–15. Diagrammatic representation of vessel collapse when myocardial flow increases. Under baseline conditions (Rest, *top*), flow across the stenosis (R_1) is modest and a large pressure gradient (P_1-P_2) does not develop. With a vasodilator intervention such as exercise, (*bottom*) the pressure gradient across the stenosis (P_1-P_2) increases. The resulting fall in intraluminal pressure may lead to collapse of the vessel at the level of the obstruction, thereby increasing the degree of stenosis. This leads to dilatation of the distal vessels (R_2). (From Epstein, S. E., Cannon, R. O., III, and Talbot, T. L.: Hemodynamic principles in the control of coronary blood flow. Am. J. Cardiol. *56*:9E, 1985.)

sclerotic lesion, resistance is not fixed. As flow across such a lesion rises, substantial energy losses due to turbulence occur; these are proportional to the flow squared. As a result, as flow rises, there is an exponential rise in the pressure gradient across the stenosis. At any flow rate the gradient rises with the degree of stenosis. As the trans-stenotic pressure drop increases, so does the pressure distending the artery. This may result in passive collapse[110] (Fig. 37–15).

FIXED AND DYNAMIC OBSTRUCTION. Myocardial ischemia and its consequences may occur as a result of fixed atherosclerotic lesions or may be secondary to transitory reduction of myocardial blood flow caused by coronary spasm or platelet aggregation.[111, 111a] The clinical sequelae of myocardial ischemia, whether produced by an increase in MVO_2 in the face of fixed obstruction or by a reduction in myocardial oxygen supply resulting from coronary spasm or transient aggregation of platelets, may be manifested clinically as angina pectoris, electrical instability, characteristic electrocardiographic changes, or depression of myocardial function, alone or in combination.

Maseri has clarified the interrelation between fixed and dynamic (variable) obstruction to blood flow. Normal subjects can carry out maximal exercise, develop a fifteen- to twentyfold increase in body $\dot{V}O_2$ above resting levels, yet

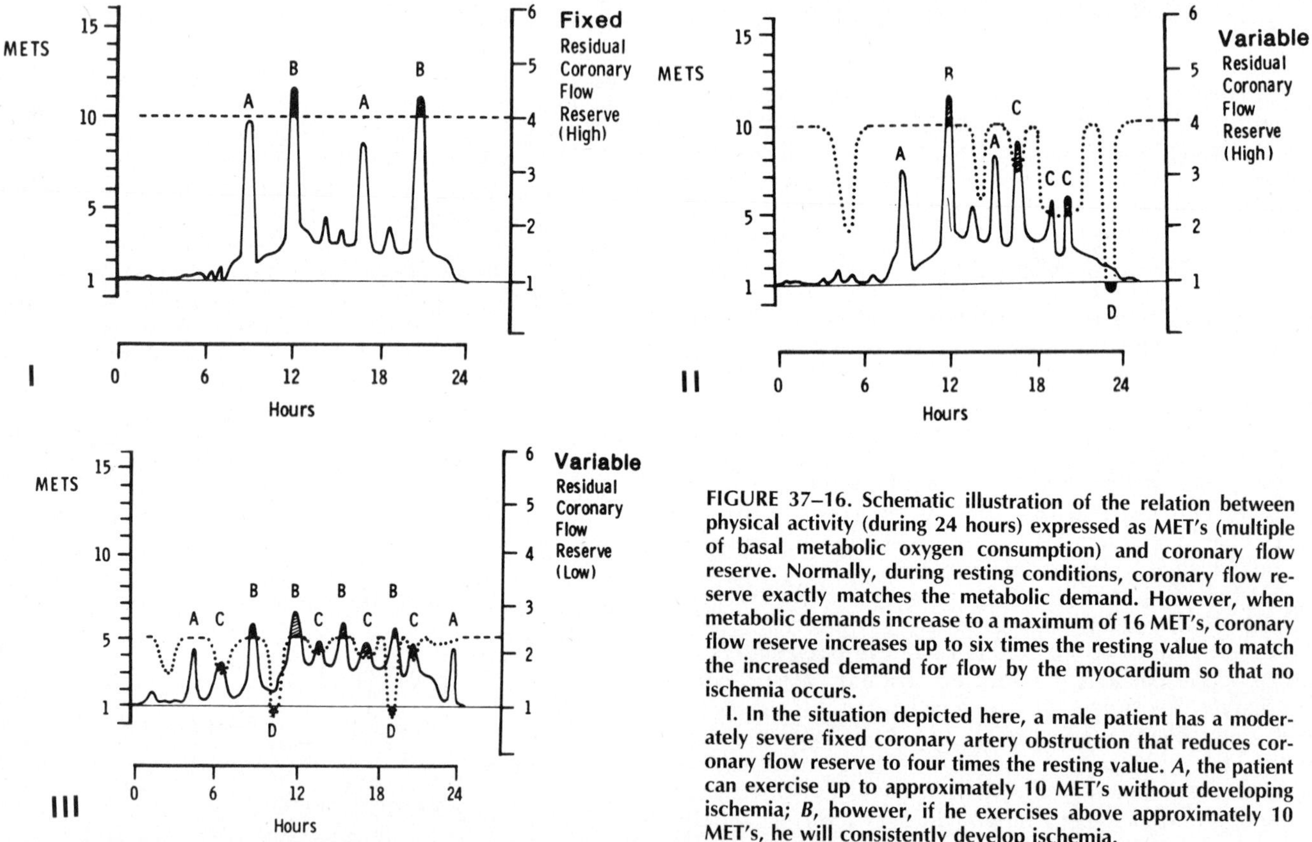

FIGURE 37–16. Schematic illustration of the relation between physical activity (during 24 hours) expressed as MET's (multiple of basal metabolic oxygen consumption) and coronary flow reserve. Normally, during resting conditions, coronary flow reserve exactly matches the metabolic demand. However, when metabolic demands increase to a maximum of 16 MET's, coronary flow reserve increases up to six times the resting value to match the increased demand for flow by the myocardium so that no ischemia occurs.

I. In the situation depicted here, a male patient has a moderately severe fixed coronary artery obstruction that reduces coronary flow reserve to four times the resting value. *A*, the patient can exercise up to approximately 10 MET's without developing ischemia; *B*, however, if he exercises above approximately 10 MET's, he will consistently develop ischemia.

II. In the situation depicted here, the patient has a moderately severe stenosis which fixes the coronary reserve at four times resting levels as in I. In addition, he has a variable stenosis. Therefore, residual coronary flow reserve has an upper limit that is fixed but that can decrease because of the presence of the mechanisms that transiently interfere with coronary blood flow. Thus, the residual coronary flow reserve can vary throughout the day. Under these conditions, if the patient exercises beyond the maximal residual coronary flow reserve, he will always develop ischemia (*B*). However, he may also develop ischemia on other occasions after smaller degrees of exercise, when residual coronary flow reserve is decreased by these functional factors (*C*). Occasionally, coronary flow reserve decreases so that resting flow is impaired and ischemia occurs at rest (*D*). At other times of the day, this patient can exercise below the level of his maximal residual coronary flow reserve without experiencing ischemia (*A*).

III. In the situation depicted here, the patient has a very severe fixed stenosis and also variable stenosis. Maximal residual coronary flow reserve is reduced to little more than two times the resting value of coronary flow, thus allowing the patient to exercise up to a level of about 5 MET's in the absence of any transient impairment of coronary flow. The combination of markedly reduced coronary flow reserve and of transient impairment of coronary flow results in frequent occurrences of ischemic episodes caused by excessive increase of demand above the maximal residual coronary flow (*B*) or by transient impairment of flow during exertion (*C*) or at rest (*D*). However, in the absence of transient impairment of flow, the patient can tolerate activities below 5 MET's (*A*). (Modified from Maseri, A., Chierchia, S., and Kaski, J. C.: Mixed angina pectoris. Am. J. Cardiol., *56*:31E and 32E, 1985.)

not develop myocardial ischemia because they operate within their normal coronary reserve. Figure 37–16 I shows the effects of fixed coronary obstruction that allows a fourfold increase in coronary blood flow. Ischemia occurs whenever $M\dot{V}O_2$ rises to a level that cannot be met by this coronary flow reserve. It is clear that transient reductions of coronary reserve below this level will occur in many patients with coronary atherosclerosis. In these patients, the anginal threshold will be quite variable (Fig. 37–16 II), a condition referred to as mixed angina.[112]

MYOCARDIAL ISCHEMIA AND ISCHEMIC INJURY

EFFECTS OF ISCHEMIA ON MYOCARDIAL FUNCTION

EFFECTS ON VENTRICULAR CONTRACTION. In 1935 Tennant and Wiggers demonstrated that after ligation of a coronary artery the contraction of cardiac muscle supplied by this vessel ceases, and the affected area appears cyanotic, dilated, and bulging.[113] In the basal state there is no reserve in blood flow; any reduction in flow, even one as small as 10 to 20 per cent, results in an approximately similar percentage reduction of myocardial segment shortening.[114] Myocardial ischemia is generally associated with elimination of the normal contractile performance in a *localized area* of myocardium, resulting in an asynergic contraction.[115] Figure 37–17 shows the immediate regional myocardial functional responses to acute coronary occlusion: there is paradoxical motion in the central ischemic zone, reduced contraction in the adjacent area, and compensatory hyperfunction of the uninvolved normal myocardium, the latter mediated in part by vasodilation and the Frank-Starling mechanism.[116, 117] A reduction of blood flow of 80 per cent results in akinesis, while a 95 per cent reduction causes systolic bulging (dyskinesis).[118] Animals and patients with coronary artery disease and a previous myocardial infarction exhibit impaired regional left ventricular function; although, if the damage is limited, hyperfunction of the residual myocardium will maintain global left ventricular function (Fig. 15–7, p. 456). In the isolated heart, global ischemia causes a depression of myocardial contractility reflected as a decrease in the slope of the end-systolic pressure-volume relation (E_{max}) (p. 459).[119] On the other hand, regional ischemia shifts the relationship rightward without affecting the slope (E_{max}). The shift reflects the behavior of the noncontractile is-

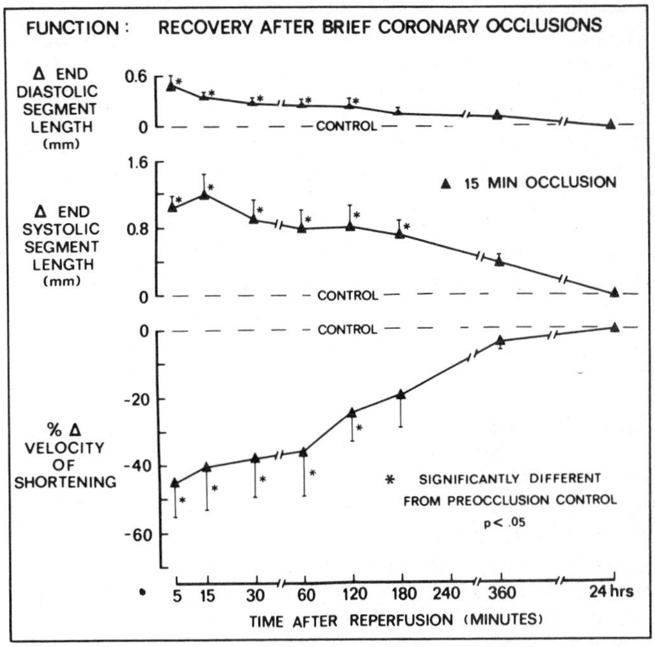

FIGURE 37–18. Prolonged recovery of regional function expressed as changes in end-diastolic segment length, end-systolic segment length, and velocity of shortening after 15 minutes of coronary artery occlusion. Recovery times from 5 minutes to 24 hours after reperfusion are shown. Values that are significantly different from control are shown by the asterisks ($p < 0.05$). (From Vatner, S. F., Heyndrickx, G. R., and Fallon, J. T.: Effects of brief periods of myocardial ischemia on regional myocardial function and creatine kinase release in conscious dogs and baboons. Can. J. Cardiol. Suppl. *A* (July):22A, 1986.)

chemic segment of the ventricle, while the normal slope results from the compensatory hyperfunction of the nonischemic segment.[120] Transient episodes of myocardial ischemia cause left ventricular systolic and diastolic dysfunction. The duration of impaired function may be quite prolonged, and post-ischemic depression ("stunning") of the myocardium, with impaired mechanical performance, reduced high-energy phosphate stores, and abnormal ultrastructure may persist for several days following a brief—15-minute—period of coronary occlusion, which is not enough to cause myocardial necrosis[121, 121a] (Fig. 37–18). The mechanism of stunning has not been defined. The contractility of stunned but viable myocardium can be stimulated by infused sympathomimetics.[122–124] However, it does not respond to sympathetic nerve stimulation[125]; accumulation of oxygen-derived free radicals may also play a role in its dysfunction (p. 1212).

Regional loss of myocardial contractile activity, whether sustained or transient, if sufficiently widespread, depresses overall left ventricular function, producing reductions of stroke volume, stroke work, cardiac output, and ejection fraction and elevation of end-diastolic volume and pressure. Clinical evidence of heart failure occurs when regional asynergy is so severe and extensive that the uninvolved myocardium cannot sustain the excess load. Hemodynamic evidence of left ventricular failure develops when contrac-

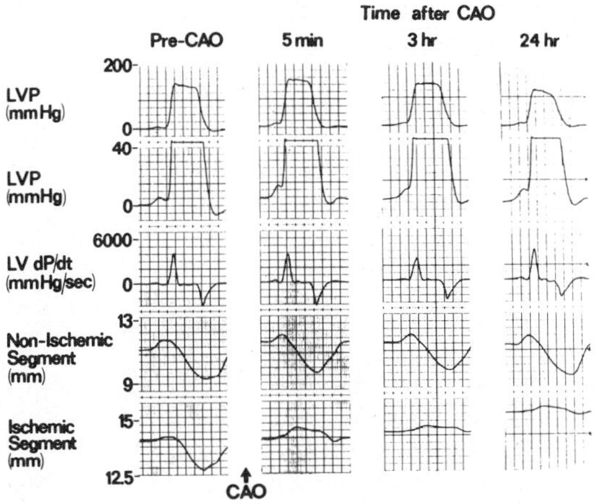

FIGURE 37–17. Phasic recordings are shown for left ventricular (LV) systolic (1st trace) and end-diastolic (2nd trace) pressures, LV dP/dt, and segment shortening in nonischemic and ischemic zones in a normal dog, before coronary artery occlusion (CAO), at 5 minutes and 3 and 24 hours after CAO. (From Amano, J., Thomas J. X., Jr., Lavallee, M., Mirsky, I., Glover, D., Manders, W. T., Randall, W. C., and Vatner, S. F.: Effects of myocardial ischemia on regional function and stiffness in conscious dogs. Am. J. Physiol. *252*:H113, 1987.)

tion ceases in 20 to 25 per cent of the left ventricle; with loss of 40 per cent or more of left ventricular myocardium, severe pump failure ensues and, if this loss is acute, fatal or near-fatal cardiogenic shock usually develops.

Since the heart has virtually no stores of oxygen, its high rate of energy expenditure results in a sudden, striking decline of myocardial oxygen tension within seconds of coronary occlusion, coincident with the loss of contractility. The marginal zone contracts weakly, whereas the nonischemic myocardium exhibits a compensatory increase in its force of contraction. The rapid decline in contractility induced by ischemia cannot be attributed to alterations in excitability. Although ischemia does not produce major changes in the amplitude and upstroke velocity of the action potential,[126] the duration of the plateau phase of the action potential is shortened, which may signify a reduction in the slow inward current, carried largely by Ca^{++}.

Mechanisms. The precise mechanism by which ischemia impairs left ventricular systolic function has not been defined.[127] It is possible that ischemia reduces the release of Ca^{++} from the sarcolemma, the sarcoplasmic reticulum (SR), or both, and thereby interferes with the interaction of Ca^{++} with the contractile proteins.[128, 129] As outlined in Chapter 13, contraction is normally initiated by the rapid release of Ca^{++} from the SR, and this release is triggered by a rise in the local concentration of Ca^{++} in the vicinity of the SR. According to this concept, when the Ca^{++} concentration in the cytoplasm reaches a critical level, a massive release of Ca^{++} from the SR occurs, leading to muscle contraction. Changes in intracellular pH may influence this Ca^{++} trigger mechanism—i.e., a fall in intracellular pH, as occurs in ischemia, may reduce the sensitivity of the SR to the local concentration of Ca^{++}. As discussed on page 389, once Ca^{++} is released from the SR, it combines with specific receptor sites on the regulator protein, troponin, which ultimately leads to muscle tension and shortening. One theory for the depression of systolic function during systole says that the high intracellular $[H^+]$ induced by ischemia may compete with Ca^{++} for the receptors on the troponin molecules. Thus, the actin-myosin interaction is impaired and it has been postulated that as a result of these two processes, i.e., reduction of the sensitivity of the SR to any given concentration of Ca^{++} and competition between H^+ and Ca^{++} for the troponin receptor sites, contractility is reduced.[127, 128, 130] This idea is supported by the observations that the functional changes induced by primary acidosis in the face of adequate myocardial oxygenation are similar to those produced by ischemia,[131] and that the reversal of acidosis by the administration of alkali improves contractile performance.[132] In addition to the role played by intracellular $[H^+]$, minor reductions of ATP may be important. It is possible that the concentrations of high-energy phosphate compounds in critical locations—such as the SR, a locus of Ca^{++} binding and release, or the sarcolemma (where ion fluxes and cell volume may be affected)—are reduced by ischemia,[127] even when the overall intracellular concentration of these compounds is still normal or near normal.

In summary, it is likely that the abnormalities of contraction caused by ischemia result from the reduced release of Ca^{++} by the SR, ultimately making less Ca^{++} available to the contractile sites, and/or from the accumulation of intracellular H^+ and its interference with the interaction of Ca^{++} and the contractile proteins. Further exploration is needed of the roles of reduced transsarcolemmal passage of Ca^{++} during the plateau of the action potential and of lowered intracellular oxygen tension on stores of high-energy phosphate compounds in critical locations within the myocardial cell.

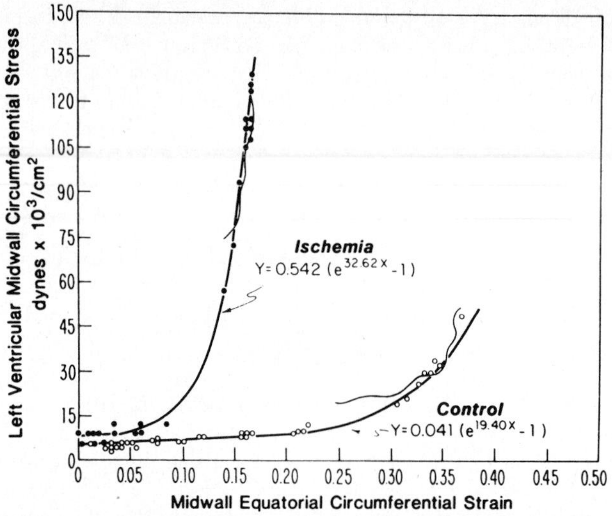

FIGURE 37–19. Diastolic pressure-strain and stress-strain relationships constructed from observations during control period and during ischemia. (From Visner, M. S., Arentzen, C. E., Parrish, D. G., Larson, E. V., O'Connor, M. J., Crumbley, A. J., III, Bache, R. J., and Anderson, R. W.: Effects of global ischemia on the diastolic properties of the left ventricle in the conscious dog. Circulation *71*:616, 1985, by permission of the American Heart Association, Inc.)

EFFECTS ON VENTRICULAR DIASTOLIC PROPERTIES. Myocardial ischemia and infarction alter not only the contractile properties of the heart but also the diastolic pressure-volume relations of the left ventricle. Myocardial ischemia impairs ventricular relaxation[132a–136] as evidenced by a decreased rate of left ventricular pressure decline (negative dP/dt) and ventricular wall thinning and prolongs the isovolumetric relaxation period.[136–139] The globally ischemic ventricle is less compliant than normal[135, 136] (Fig. 37–19). In the presence of regional ischemia, the reduction of compliance involves the ischemic region,[140, 141] while the behavior of the nonischemic region conforms to that described by a higher and steeper portion of the pressure-volume curve. In turn, the ischemia induced changes in diastolic properties increase the resistance to ventricular filling and together with the reduced systolic properties of the ventricle contribute to the elevation of left ventricular diastolic pressure during ischemia. The mechanism responsible for the ischemia-induced impairment of myocardial relaxation has not been fully elucidated, but it has been proposed that reductions of myocardial high-energy stores impair the rate of uptake of Ca^{++} from the vicinity of the myofilaments into the SR, thus prolonging contraction.[142] Ca^{++} channel blockade will antagonize this process and by diminishing Ca^{++} influx into the cell will lower cytosolic $[Ca^{++}]$, restoring rapid relaxation. On the other hand, caffeine, an agent known to prolong Ca^{++} availability, potentiates the ischemia-induced impairment of ventricular relaxation.[143]

Ischemia thus causes impairment of cardiac contraction and incomplete ventricular emptying (systolic failure). In addition, it impairs ventricular relaxation and shifts the diastolic pressure-volume curve upward (diastolic failure). The combination of systolic and diastolic failure leads to elevated ventricular filling pressures, ultimately causing symptoms of pulmonary congestion.

ELECTROPHYSIOLOGICAL CONSEQUENCES OF ISCHEMIA

ST-SEGMENT CHANGES IN THE DETECTION OF ISCHEMIA. It has been known for more than a half century that ST-segment elevation is an electrocardiographic sign of coronary artery occlusion. Within 30 to 60 seconds after occlusion in dogs with open chests, epicardial leads from within the area of cyanosis show ST-segment elevation, reaching a maximum 5 to 7 minutes after occlusion. ST-segment elevation in the central area of cyanosis is usually more marked than at the periphery. With the use of small intracavitary electrodes, simultaneous ST-segment elevation is noted on the endocardial surface, although it is less marked than that recorded on the epicardium.[144]

The electrophysiological basis of ST-segment changes in myocardial ischemia is discussed on page 204; an altered ion transport across the myocardial cell membrane apparently is the underlying cause. In the nonischemic myocardium, cell volume is regulated within narrow limits by the sarcolemmal "sodium pump" (p. 491). This active, metabolically dependent pump maintains a high extracellular [Na^+] as well as high intracellular [K^+] and colloids, thus stabilizing cell volume.[145] It has been postulated that with ischemia, the availability of energy necessary for this pumping is reduced. According to this concept, Na^+, accompanied by $C1^+$ and H_2O, accumulates intracellularly and K^+ begins to leak into the extracellular space.[146] The reduction in intracellular [K^+] or the accumulation of extracellular K^+ or both are critical in the generation of the elevated ST segment, since small changes in the ratio of intracellular to extracellular [K^+] have a marked effect on the polarity of cellular membranes.[126, 147]

Interpretation of ST-Segment Elevations. The magnitude of epicardial ST-segment elevation generally correlates with the decrease in blood flow, lactate accumulation, and depletion of high-energy phosphate compounds in the underlying myocardium.[148] In addition, ST-segment elevation is associated with a reduction in oxygen tension in the affected tissue below 65 per cent of control,[149] and the magnitude of the elevation correlates with intramyocardial oxygen tension.[150] Measurements with a mass spectrometer have shown that intramyocardial ST-segment elevations are correlated with changes in myocardial gas tensions.[151] Also, epicardial ST-segment elevations shortly after coronary artery occlusion correlate closely with subsequent depletion of myocardial creatine phosphokinase (CK) activity and with histological evidence of necrosis in the subjacent myocardium.[152–154] It is now clear that the distribution of *epicardial* ST-segment elevation provides a reasonably useful index of the extent of myocardial ischemia, but that the *intramyocardial* ST segment is a more sensitive index than the epicardial. However, it must be appreciated that ST-segment elevation, wherever measured, is not specific for myocardial ischemia, since the ST segment is also affected by changes in temperature, by drugs (including the digitalis glycosides and quinidine), by sympathetic stimulation of the heart,[155] by epicardial injury due to pericarditis, and by localized intraventricular conduction defects.[156]

ALTERATIONS IN CELLULAR ELECTROPHYSIOLOGY INDUCED BY ISCHEMIA. The effects of ischemia on the electrophysiological properties of cardiac muscle are numerous and complex.[157] Ischemia-induced ventricular tachyarrhythmias can be caused by increased automaticity (p. 596), triggered activity (p. 597), and reentry (p. 600). However, knowledge of the effects of acute ischemia on the electrophysiology of the human heart is limited. Although studies in animal models provide major insights, these models may not mirror the clinical condition in several aspects, including the nature of the occlusive coronary artery lesion, the presence of multiple lesions, and differences in collateral blood flow. After acute coronary artery ligation *in the dog*, ventricular arrhythmias occur in three phases.[158, 159]

The Early Period. An early phase begins almost immediately after coronary ligation, frequently culminates in ventricular fibrillation within 3 to 6 minutes, and usually lasts less than 30 minutes. Within minutes after coronary occlusion, marked alterations occur in the electrophysiological properties of ventricular myocardial cells, with shortening of action potential duration and refractoriness, decreased amplitude, upstroke velocity, and resting potential.[126] Extracellular recordings from the epicardial surface of the ischemic zone show marked loss of amplitude and delay and fractionation of recorded electrograms, suggesting that activation in myocardium is irregular and that the effects of ischemia are heterogeneous.[160] Conduction velocity initially increases after coronary occlusion, presumably related to the increase in extracellular K^+ (which may also contribute to the abbreviation of the action potential). Subsequently, conduction velocity slows.[157] Available evidence suggests that inhomogeneities in the conduction velocity and in the shortening of the refractory period create the conditions necessary for reentry, which in turn is responsible for ventricular tachycardia and ventricular fibrillation early during ischemia. The cause of ventricular premature beats is less clear but may be related to the triggering of automatic activity by the current of injury.[161] This early arrhythmic phase observed in experimental animals could be related to the "prehospital" phase of arrhythmias observed in patients, which is also marked by a high incidence of ventricular fibrillation and sudden death. The arrhythmias of the early phase are intimately rate-related.[158, 160, 162] Thus, vagally induced cardiac slowing can avert or abort ectopic ventricular rhythms.[160, 162] Conversely, ectopic ventricular rhythm can be induced by cardiac pacing.[158]

There is evidence that regional myocardial sympathetic stimulation contributes to the early malignant phase of ventricular arrhythmia after the onset of ischemia. During ischemia, beta-adrenoceptors are redistributed from intracellular vesicles to the sarcolemma. This may enhance the response of the ischemic myocardium to sympathomimetics, causing arrhythmia, increase of $M\dot{V}O_2$, and extension of the ischemic zone.[163] In patients with coronary artery disease, recovery of metabolic function as reflected in uptake of labeled deoxyglucose following exercise-induced ischemia suggests a possible metabolic basis.[163a] Sympathectomy and beta-adrenoceptor blockade mitigate both the regional augmentation of cyclic AMP and the frequency and severity of the early phase of ventricular arrhythmias.[164] On the other hand, the effectiveness of antiarrhythmic drugs such as quinidine and lidocaine during the early phase is controversial.[165]

The Intermediate Period. After a period of quiescence, a delayed arrhythmic phase begins at about 6 to 9 hours following coronary occlusion in the dog and lasts for 24 to 72 hours. During this period spontaneous polymorphic ventricular rhythms occur, but ventricular fibrillation is uncommon. Multiple electrophysiological mechanisms are probably involved in the delayed arrhythmic phase, particularly abnormal automaticity of subendocardial Purkinje fibers.[166] This phase may correspond to ventricular tachycardia and "accelerated idioventricular rhythms" (p. 698) commonly seen on the second and third days following infarction in humans. Antiarrhythmic drugs such as quinidine, procainamide, lidocaine, and disopyramide suppress these arrhythmias by reducing automaticity.

The Late Phase. By 72 hours after coronary ligation in the dog, the spontaneous polymorphic ventricular rhythms have nearly subsided, but the heart is still prone to ventricular tachyarrhythmias and, occasionally, ventricular fibrillation.[166a] These arrhythmias may be easily induced by rapid cardiac pacing or programmed premature stimulation[167] and may be the result of reentrant circuits in the subepicardial layer of the infarction, including the boundary zone between the infarction and surrounding viable myocardium. This late phase of ventricular vulnerability may correspond to the "post-coronary care unit" ventricular arrhythmias and late in-hospital ventricular fibrillation. Antiarrhythmic drugs, such as lidocaine or procainamide, seem to abolish these late reentrant arrhythmias by further depression or block of the already slowed conduction in the reentrant circuit.[168] Electrophysiological abnormalities persist for long periods after myocardial infarction. These may be responsible, in part, for the prolonged increased risk of sudden death in such patients.

REPERFUSION ARRHYTHMIAS. There has been considerable interest in the mechanism of ventricular arrhythmias that occur with release of coronary occlusion and reperfusion (whether induced or spontaneous)[169] as opposed to occlusion arrhythmias. Ventricular fibrillation is likely to occur abruptly without warning following reperfusion, whereas it is often heralded by ventricular ectopic beats with increasing frequency after occlusion. Chemical and electrical gradients caused by washout of metabolites and electrolytes that have accumulated in the ischemic zone are probably responsible for the electrophysiological derangement responsible for reperfusion arrhythmias.[170, 171] Reperfusion is accompanied by changes in regional concentrations of K^+, Ca^{++}, H^+, catecholamines, and lysophosphoglycerides; the last are derived from degradation of membrane phospholipids in cells undergoing infarction.[172] Reperfusion arrhythmias are more common in experimental animals such as the dog and pig. However, while they are less common in patients, the occasional abrupt onset of ventricular fibrillation in those with coronary occlusion and myocardial infarction who are undergoing thrombolytic, mechanical, or spontaneous reperfusion and in those with Prinzmetal's angina at the termination of an episode of coronary spasm is a clinical example of reocclusion arrhythmia.

Biochemical Mechanisms of Ischemia. The biochemical correlates of ischemia-induced electrophysiological changes have not been identified with certainty. Ischemia depresses the energy-dependent sarcolemmal Na pump, which leads to a gain in intracellular Na and loss of intracellular K with consequent elevation of extracellular K concentration in the vicinity of the sarcolemma.[173, 174] As a result of anaerobic metabolism, intracellular pH declines. Ischemia also results in release of norepinephrine from adrenergic nerve endings and an increase of tissue levels of cyclic AMP.[175] It has been postulated that in the ischemic zone, high concentrations of extracellular K^+ may depolarize the cells to the extent that the rapid Na^+ channel is inactivated, and high concentrations of catecholamines may stimulate the slow current carried principally by Ca^{++}, resulting in slow response action potentials. The latter could explain the slowed conduction and reentrant ventricular arrhythmias associated with ischemia. Although this hypothesis is attractive, its validity has not been established, and indeed has been questioned.[165, 170, 176]

It is less likely that slow response action potentials are responsible for ischemia-induced electrophysiological disturbances in the later stage of myocardial infarction. The extracellular K^+ concentration is probably not as high as in the early stage of ischemia. Besides, total catecholamines in the ischemic region decline to a very low level on the day after coronary occlusion.[177] However, ischemic myocardium still shows markedly depressed action potentials, slow conduction, and a high propensity for reentrant rhythms.[178] In the later stage of ischemia, ischemic myocardial cells have been found to be exquisitely sensitive to the depressant effect of tetrodotoxin, a specific blocker of the fast Na^+ channel, and not to verapamil and D600, which are blockers of the slow Ca^{++} channel.[178] These observations suggest that poor membrane responses of ischemic myocardial cells are related to depression of the fast Na^+ channel. The clinical relevance of studies of ischemia-induced ionic conductance changes relates to the choice of ideal antiarrhythmic therapy following ischemia. Thus, the antiarrhythmic effect of lidocaine on ischemia-induced reentrant ventricular arrhythmias (pp. 625 and 694) may be due to selective depression of ischemic myocardial cells forming part of the reentrant pathway. The finding that the effect of lidocaine on depressed ischemic cells is similar to that of tetrodotoxin suggests that lidocaine acts by further depressing the tenuous Na^+ channel in ischemic cells.[168]

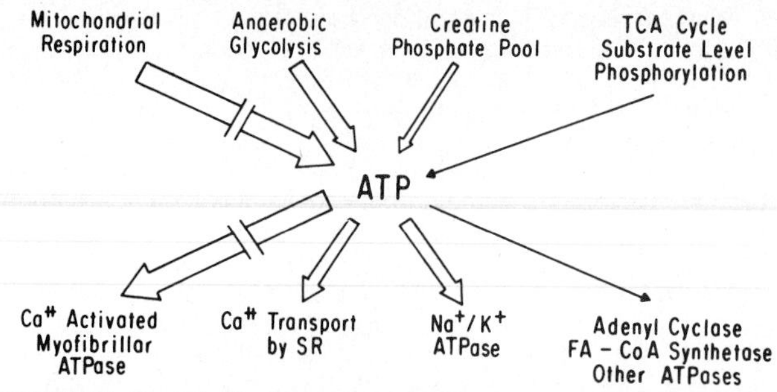

FIGURE 37–20. Principal reactions producing and utilizing high energy phosphates (HEP) in ischemic tissue. The width of the arrows indicates the estimated quantitative importance of the various reactions. In severe ischemia, aerobic respiration is abolished. The preexisting stores of HEP, in the form of creatine phosphate (CP) or ATP, are relatively small. Thus, anaerobic glycolysis becomes the principal source of energy, producing 80 to 90 per cent of the HEP bonds that can be utilized by severely ischemic tissue. Substrate-level phosphorylation of α-ketoglutarate in the mitochondria does not require oxygen, but the tissue content of substrates that can be shuttled to α-ketoglutarate is small. Energy utilized also is markedly reduced during ischemia. Cardiac contraction, which is mediated by Ca^{++}-activated myofibrillar ATPase, consumes much of the ATP produced in aerobic myocardium. However, contraction is abolished or severely depressed in areas of severe ischemia. Nevertheless, ATP continues to be required to remove NA^+ from the cell, to keep Ca^{++} sequestered in the sarcoplasmic reticulum, and for a variety of other cellular processes that may continue to compete for the remaining ATP. (From Jennings, R. B., and Reimer, K. A.: Lethal myocardial ischemic injury. Am. J. Pathol. *102*:241, 1981.)

EFFECTS OF ISCHEMIA ON MYOCARDIAL METABOLISM

HIGH-ENERGY PHOSPHATE METABOLISM. During the first minutes of severe ischemia, the production of high-energy phosphates (the sum of ATP and creatine phosphate [CP]) declines and is greatly exceeded by the utilization (Figs. 37–20 and 37–21). Therefore, tissue stores decline progressively, with CP stores falling more rapidly than ATP stores. CP is depleted by transferring its high-energy phosphate to ADP in an attempt to maintain ATP stores.[178a] In the presence of normal aerobic mitochondrial function, ADP is converted to ATP (through the myokinase reaction). In the absence of normal oxidative phosphorylation it is converted to AMP (Fig. 37–22), which in turn is broken down to adenosine and ultimately to inosine, hypoxanthine, and xanthine (Fig. 37–11).[179] Reimer and Jennings have shown that when ATP was reduced below 20 per cent of control values the ability to regenerate high-energy phosphate, preserve cell volume, and maintain ionic regulation is lost.[180] The combination of reduced myocardial high-energy phosphate concentration and cell swelling results in damage to the sarcolemma, which may play a key role in cell death during ischemia or reperfusion (Fig. 37–23).[180, 181] When tissue is *reversibly* injured by ischemia (i.e., its viability can be maintained by reperfusion), ATP stores are usually greater than 60 per cent of control and electronmicroscopy may reveal only glycogen loss, nuclear

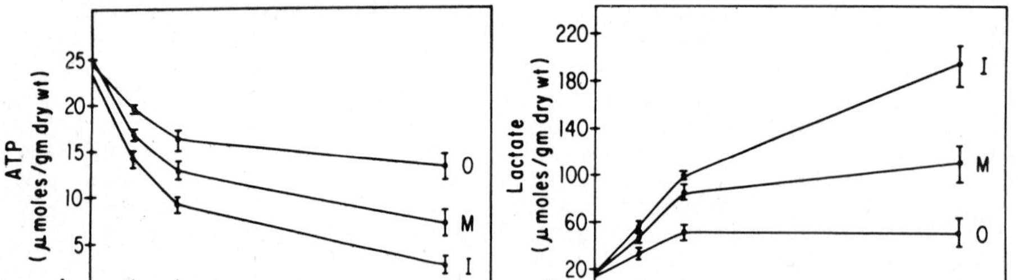

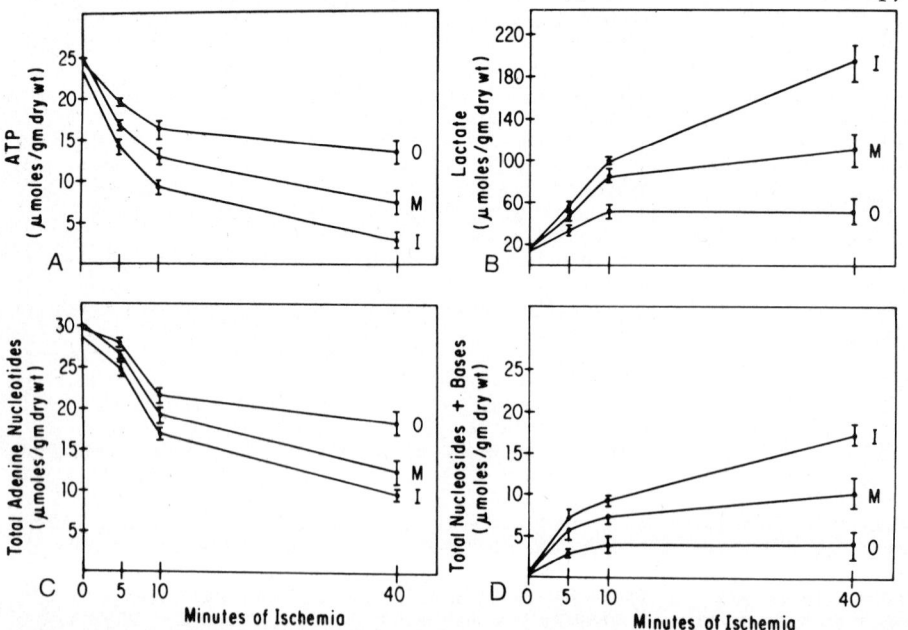

FIGURE 37–21. Time course of metabolic changes during myocardial ischemia plotted by transmural layer (I = inner, subendocardial; M = middle; O = outer subepicardial). Ischemia was induced by circumflex occlusion in anesthetized dogs. Data for different times are based on different groups of dogs; N = 4 to 6; brackets indicate plus or minus one standard error of the mean. *A*, More rapid depletion of ATP in the inner layer, highly significant after 5 min of ischemia ($p < 0.01$). *B*, Tissue lactate accumulation, with the most rapid accumulation in the subendocardium. For all layers there was a progressive increase in lactate content during the first 10 min of ischemia. Between 10 and 40 min there was continued lactate accumulation in the inner and middle layers, but not in the outer layer. *C*, Total adenine nucleotide content (ATP + ADP + AMP). Adenine nucleotide degradation was most rapid in the subendocardium. Note the time lag between ATP depletion (graph A) and adenine nucleotide breakdown. *D*, Total nucleosides and bases, which are the products of adenine nucleotide degradation. Accumulation was fastest in the subendocardium. As with lactate (graph B), nucleoside and base content in the outer layer was maximal by 10 minutes and was not further increased at 40 minutes, even though adenine nucleotide breakdown in this layer continued (graph C). (From Reimer, K. A., and Jennings, R. B.: Myocardial ischemia, hypoxia and infarction. *In* Fozzard, H. A., Jennings, R. B., Haber, E., Katz, A. M., and Morgan, H. E. [eds.]: The Heart and Cardiovascular System. New York, Raven Press, 1986, p. 1144. From the studies of Murry, C. E. et al.: Collateral blood flow and transmural location: Independent determinants of ATP in ischemic canine myocardium. Fed. Proc. *44*:823, 1985.)

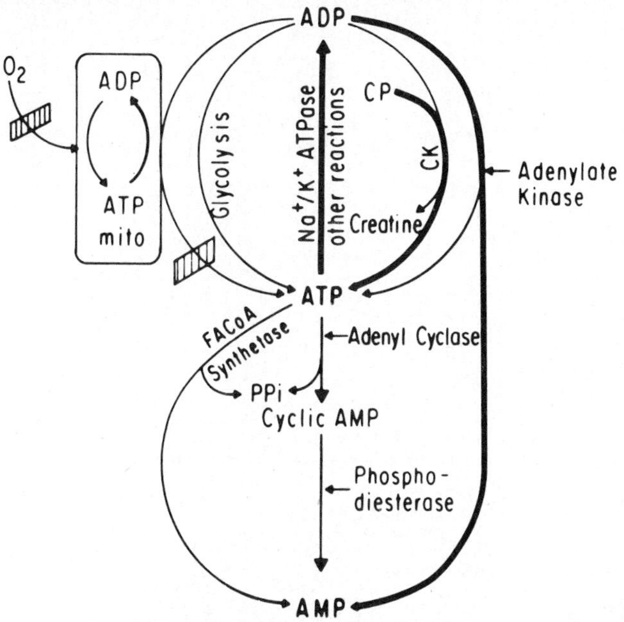

FIGURE 37–22. The major metabolic pathways of adenine nucleotide degradation during myocardial ischemia. The quantitatively most important pathways are indicated by the solid arrows. (From Jennings, R. B., Reimer, K. A., Hill, M. L., and Mayer, S. E.: Total ischemia in dog hearts, in vitro. 1. Comparison of high energy phosphate production, utilization, and depletion, and of adenine nucleotide catabolism in total ischemia in vitro vs. severe ischemia in vivo. Circ. Res. *49*:892, 1981, by permission of the American Heart Association, Inc.)

chromatin clumping, intermyofibrillar edema, and mitochondrial swelling but no sarcolemmal damage or accumulation of amorphous dense bodies in the mitochondria. Reduction of ATP below 30 per cent is usually associated with visible sarcolemmal damage and irreversible injury (i.e., the tissue is not viable despite reperfusion)[182, 183] (Fig. 37–24).

The technique of phosphorus-31 nuclear magnetic resonance (NMR) spectroscopy is providing important new information concerning high-energy phosphate stores and intracellular pH in ischemic myocardium. Multiple sequential measurements can be made on the same tissue and correlated with mechanical activity.[169, 183a] This technique has demonstrated that the magnitude of intracellular acidosis and associated increase in inorganic phosphate correlate inversely with post-ischemic structure and recovery of function. ATP but not CP content correlates with return of contractile function after reperfusion.[184, 185]

CARBOHYDRATE METABOLISM IN ISCHEMIA. Under normal aerobic conditions, myocardium derives its energy primarily from oxidative phosphorylation, a process localized to the mitochondria.[186] Although many types of substrate can be utilized, oxidation of fatty acids predominates. Oxidative phosphorylation is regulated to a large extent by the phosphate potential: (ATP)/(ADP) × (P_i). When oxygen availability is limited, the rate of ATP synthesis declines and high-energy phosphate stores decline. Depletion of purine nucleotide pools is prompt. It persists for hours to days after even brief intervals of ischemia, in part because of the limited capacity of myocardium for de novo purine synthesis. The reduction in the phosphate potential and the prevailing concentrations of intermediates such as glucose-6-phosphate alter the activity of enzymes involved in intermediary metabolism. During hypoxia, glycolytic flux increases because of enhanced uptake of glucose and also phosphorylation, reflecting (1) decline of glucose-6-phosphate and release of inhibition of hexokinase; (2) release of inhibition of phosphofructokinase (PFK) by citrate and ATP; and (3) activation of PFK by inorganic phosphate. Glycogenolysis accelerates because of transformation of phosphorylase b, an inactive form of the enzyme under physiological conditions, to the active, phosphorylated form, phosphorylase a. Later, glycogenolysis is potentiated by activation of phosphorylase b itself, by accumulating metabolites such as adenosine monophosphate, and by release of inhibition by glucose-6-phosphate (Fig. 37–25). There is evidence for functional compartmentalization of glycolytic versus oxidative metabolism in that energy from glycolysis preferentially supports sarcolemmal function, while oxidative phosphorylation preferentially supports contractile function.[187]

The augmentation of glycolytic flux so characteristic of hypoxia and of the initial response to ischemia may contribute to maintenance of viability of the heart by providing ATP. The importance of glycolysis in the generation of energy is reflected in the observation that inhibition of glycolysis with iodoacetate results in cessation of beating of the anoxic heart even though the agent does not influence the apparent function of the well-oxygenated heart. Augmentation of glycolytic flux by provision of glucose or prior augmentation of glycogen stores confers some resistance to the deterioration of function induced by anoxia or ischemia. Nevertheless, even with insulin present in the perfusion medium, anaerobic metabolism can supply less than half the energy requirement for maintenance of viability of the nonworking, isolated, perfused, anoxic heart. Thus, anaerobic metabolism alone cannot maintain myocardial ATP stores indefinitely in the nonworking heart, let alone in myocardium with markedly great energy requirements associated with contractile function.

Anaerobic Glycolysis. Under aerobic conditions, carbohydrate metabolism proceeds via oxidation through the tricarboxylic acid (Krebs) cycle. However, when anoxia supervenes, the lack of oxygen inhibits the activity of this cycle and the metabolism of glucose can proceed only via anaerobic glycolysis. When the cause of anoxia is ischemia, lactate accumulates, since oxidation of pyruvate is precluded by the inhibition of the tricarboxylic acid cycle, and washout of metabolites is reduced because of the limited perfusion. The initial burst of glycolytic activity accompanying hypoxia with or without ischemia appears to depend on allosteric effects of adenine nucleotides and other regulators of enzymes such as phosphorylase b, hexokinase, and phosphofructokinase.[188] However, under conditions of limited perfusion sufficient to induce hypoxia, the rapidly increasing concentration of lactic acid within the cell, the decline of pH, and the accumulation of other metabolites inhibit glycolytic flux at the phosphofructokinase and glyceraldehyde-3-phosphate dehydrogenase[188, 189] steps, among others (Fig. 37–25).

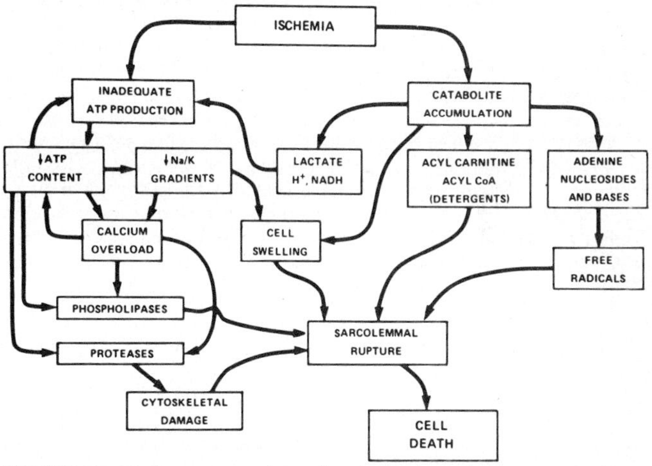

FIGURE 37–23. Some potential pathways leading to sarcolemmal damage, which form the basis for various hypotheses of events leading to irreversible ischemic cell injury. In general terms, two major facets of ischemia are the inadequate production of ATP and the accumulation of potentially noxious catabolites. Declining ATP content could have many adverse consequences including loss of sodium and potassium gradients, calcium overload, and activation of endogenous phospholipases or proteases. The latter could damage the sarcolemma and/or its cytoskeletal supports. Accumulation of catabolites such as lactate, H^+, and NADH inhibit anaerobic glycolysis and thereby inhibit ATP production in ischemia. Products of lipid degradation may act as detergents and damage cell membranes. Adenine nucleosides and bases accumulate and might be a major source of free radicals via the xanthine oxidase reaction. In addition, accumulating catabolites are an intracellular osmotic load that may accentuate cell swelling and facilitate the rupture of already weakened membranes. The relative importance of these various pathways in the pathogenesis of ischemic cell death has not been established. Moreover, many reactions occur in ischemic myocardium which have been less well studied and are not included on this diagram; it is not even certain that the most important assays are illustrated. (From Reimer, K. A., and Jennings, R. B.: Myocardial ischemia, hypoxia and infarction. *In* Fozzard, H. A., Jennings, R. B., Haber, E., Katz, A. M., and Morgan, H. E. [eds.]: The Heart and Cardiovascular System. New York, Raven Press, 1986, p. 1163.)

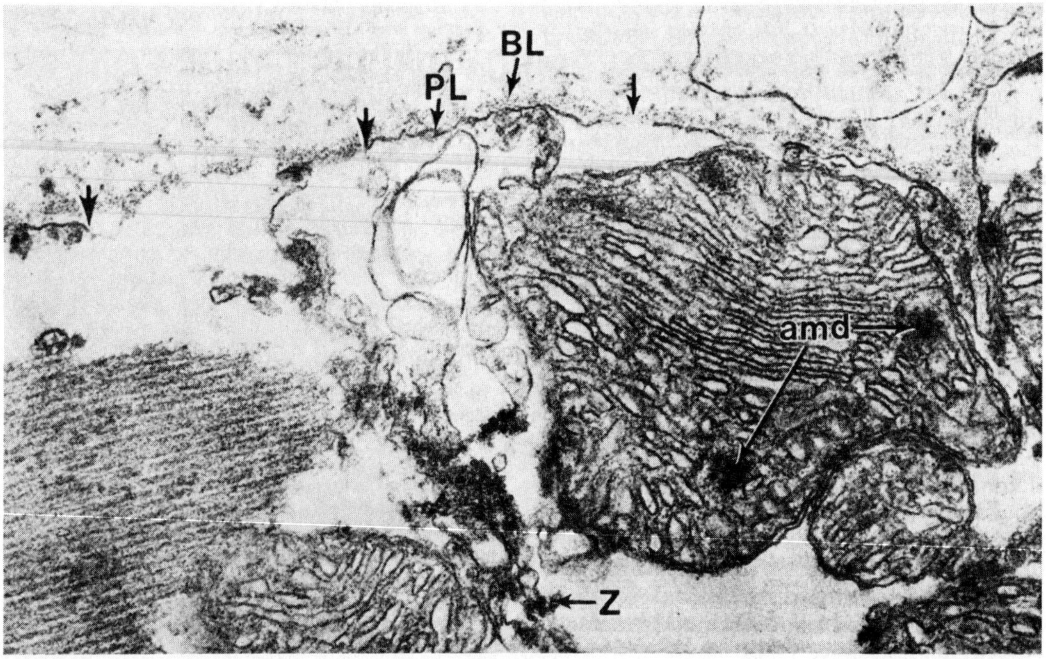

FIGURE 37–24. Characteristic changes in the sarcolemma of severely ischemic left ventricular myocytes that were irreversibly injured by 40 minutes of in vivo ischemia. There is a relatively small gap in the plasmalemma (thin arrow) and another much larger gap (between the two thick arrows). Note that the attachment between the plasmalemma and the underlying myofibril at the level of the Z line (Z) is broken. (Perfusion fixation with glutaraldehyde and paraformaldehyde followed by postosmication × 62,500.) (From Jennings, R. B., and Hawkins, H. K.: Ultrastructural changes of acute myocardial ischemia. *In* Wildenthal, K. [ed.]: Degradative Processes in Heart and Skeletal Muscle. New York, Elsevier/North Holland, 1980, pp. 295–346.)

The Role of Lactate. In isolated perfused hearts, lactate exerts a deleterious effect on glycolytic flux independent of pH[190] by inhibiting the glyceraldehyde-phosphate dehydrogenase reaction, which is responsible for conversion of glyceraldehyde-3-phosphate to 1,3-diphosphoglyceric acid. On the other hand, acidosis itself inhibits glycolytic flux and the malate-aspartate cycle.[190] This and other similar cycles provide a shuttle via intermediates to which the mitochondrial membranes are permeable, permitting transport of reducing equivalents formed in the cytosol across the mitochondrial membranes and thereby allowing their oxidation by the respiratory chain. Persistent or prolonged ischemia results in inhibition of the shuttle reactions because of accumulation of reducing equivalents in the mitochondria (due to the lack of oxygen as a terminal electron and hydrogen receptor), with consequent accumulation of reducing equivalents and hydrogen ions in the cytosol as well. The acidosis and accumulation of metabolites contribute directly to inhibition of glycolytic flux.[191] Thus, because glycolytic flux in ischemic tissue becomes limited relatively soon after the initial burst of activity, it is capable of meeting only a significantly smaller proportion of energy requirements than in anoxic tissue.

The above-described changes in carbohydrate metabolism induced by myocardial ischemia account for the relationship between lactate production and the severity of impaired perfusion; this relationship may be exploited diagnostically. Under normal aerobic conditions, myocardium extracts lactate from the arterial blood with extraction fractions in

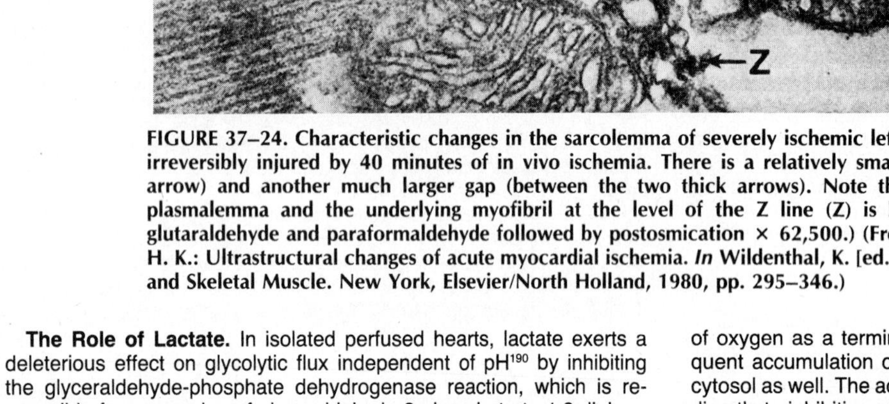

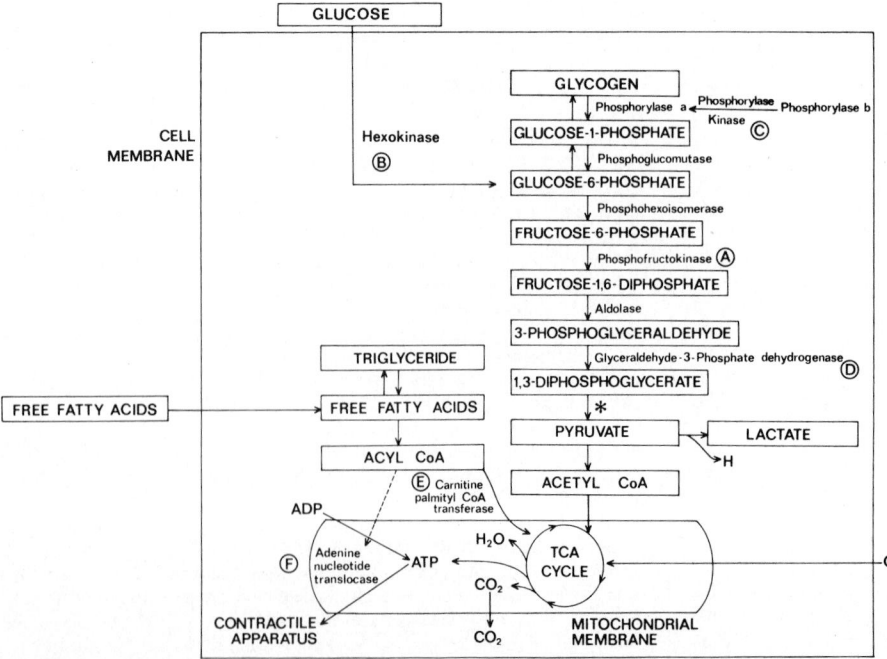

FIGURE 37–25. Effects of ischemia on glycolysis and free fatty acid metabolism. Ischemia increases intracellular lactate concentration; this accumulation inhibits several enzymes in the glycolytic pathway: Phosphofructokinase (*A*); hexokinase (*B*); and phosphorylase kinase (*C*), which prevents activation of phosphorylase b to phosphorylase a and therefore suppresses conversion of glycogen to glucose-1-phosphate. Glyceraldehyde-3-phosphate dehydrogenase (*D*) is suppressed by an elevation of intracellular lactate. (* denotes that the glycolytic pathway has been condensed at this point.) Ischemia increases the intracellular concentration of acyl CoA esters, in part because the intracellular accumulation of lactate inhibits carnitine palmityl coenzyme A transferase (*E*), the enzyme that catalyzes the transfer of acyl CoA from the cell cytoplasm to the mitochondria. Acyl CoA esters inhibit the effective exchange of ADP and ATP between the cytoplasm of the cell and the mitochondria by suppressing the activity of adenine nucleotide translocase (*F*). The antilipolytic agents are effective because they prevent a build-up of acyl CoA esters within the cytoplasm, and 1-carnitine exerts a salutary effect on ischemic myocardium by reversing the inhibition of adenine nucleotide translocase, thus allowing continued movement of ADP and ATP between the cell cytoplasm and the mitochondria. (TCA = tricarboxylic acid.) (Reproduced with permission from Hillis, L. D., and Braunwald, E.: Myocardial ischemia. N. Engl. J. Med. *296*:971, 1034, and 1093; 1977.)

the range of 20 per cent. In normal subjects extraction persists despite acceleration of ventricular rate by pacing.[192] However, when myocardial ischemia is present at rest or develops in response to stress induced by pacing or other physiological stimuli, lactate extraction declines or is replaced by net lactate production.[193] Dual carbon-labeled isotopic experiments have demonstrated that in patients with coronary artery disease simultaneous lactate production and extraction can occur. During a pacing stress test, significant lactate release occurs even in the presence of *net* lactate extraction.[194] In general, both decreased lactate extraction and an increase in lactate production are accompanied by an increase in coronary venous lactate/pyruvate ratios, compared with values in arterial blood. Unfortunately, relationships between the concentrations of lactate in coronary sinus blood and in extracellular fluid, cytosol, and mitochondrial compartments are complex and are influenced by nonspecific factors such as acid-base balance, adrenergic stimulation of the heart, substrate availability, permeability of cell membranes to lactate and pyruvate, concomitant disorders such as diabetes mellitus, and prevailing levels of plasma free fatty acids. Furthermore, net lactate extraction is a relatively insensitive index of changes occurring in localized regions of the heart. Accordingly, the diagnostic sensitivity and specificity of altered lactate extraction for the detection or assessment of severity of ischemia are somewhat limited.

DIFFERENCES BETWEEN ISCHEMIA AND ANOXIA. A number of important differences exist between anoxia and ischemia.[1] Not only is oxidative metabolism reduced during ischemia, as it is in anoxia, but the anaerobic production of ATP also proceeds at less than maximal capacity. In the ischemic working heart the concentration of lactic acid rises and the intracellular pH falls rapidly as the acid products of glycolysis accumulate (Fig. 37–21). In contrast, in the anoxic heart perfusion results in the washout of the acid products of glycolysis, thereby retarding the rate of development of intracellular acidosis. The increased lactate production is not sustained by the ischemic heart, which has a glycolytic rate about one-fourth that of the anoxic heart in a steady state. This is unrelated to a reduction of substrate availability. Thus, the addition of insulin and glucose to the perfusion medium fails to stimulate glycolysis to the extent observed in anoxia or under normal aerobic conditions. While insulin and elevated glucose in the perfusate are able to increase glucose transport and augment the intracellular glucose concentration, they do not prevent ischemia from inhibiting glucose utilization.

The lower glycolytic flux in the ischemic as compared to the anoxic heart probably results in part from the inhibition by intracellular acidosis of PFK (Fig. 37–25), a key enzyme in the glycolytic chain. The reduction of glycolytic flux through the inhibition of PFK results in the accumulation of glucose-6-phosphate, and this inhibits hexokinase, further decreasing the phosphorylation of glucose. As a consequence, glycolysis provides less energy to the ischemic than to the anoxic heart. The importance of intracellular pH is further supported by the observation that pretreatment of rat myocardium to an alkaline pH of 7.9 maintains tension during a subsequent period of hypoxia.[194a]

FATTY ACID METABOLISM IN ISCHEMIA. Under normal aerobic conditions, 60 to 90 per cent of myocardial energy requirements is met by oxidation of free fatty acids (FFA),[195, 196] which are trapped in cells in the form of fatty (acyl) esters containing coenzyme A (acyl-CoA). The preferential utilization of FFA by myocardium appears to depend on the high activity of several enzyme systems, including the acyl-CoA-carnitine transferase systems that facilitate continuing transport of acyl-CoA from the cytosol to the mitochondria in a series of steps in which acyl-CoA and acyl-carnitine are interconverted.

After fatty acids are taken up by myocardial cells and undergo esterification with CoA, the acyl-CoA intermediates generally remain trapped in the cell. Acyl-CoA may be incorporated into triglycerides in the cytosol or oxidized after transport through the mitochondrial membrane. Under aerobic conditions, oxidation predominates since the products formed (two carbon moieties called acetyl groups) are readily incorporated as intermediates into the citric acid cycle and oxidized to carbon dioxide and water. Oxidation of fatty acids inhibits glucose uptake, glycolytic flux, and glycogenolysis. The increased production of acetyl-CoA accompanying fatty acid oxidation inhibits pyruvate dehydrogenase,[197] thereby limiting the flow of carbohydrate metabolism through the citric acid cycle. Accumulation of glucose-6-phosphate inhibits hexokinase, decreasing phosphorylation of glucose. The decreased phosphorylation, coupled with direct inhibition of membrane transport of glucose mediated by fatty acids, contributes to the overall reduction of carbohydrate metabolism when fatty acid availability is high and oxygenation adequate.[198]

Striking changes in fatty acid metabolism result from myocardial ischemia. The limited supply of oxygen inhibits beta-oxidation—as does the increased ratio of NADH/NAD and the reduced concentration of flavoproteins.[188] With more prolonged ischemia, oxidation of fatty acids is inhibited by another mechanism: inhibition or loss of long-chain acyl-carnitine transferase enzyme activity, necessary for transport of cytosolic acyl-CoA to the mitochondria before oxidation.[199] Accordingly, intracellular concentrations of acyl-CoA increase and acetyl-CoA content declines.[200] The increased acyl-CoA accompanied by increased production of glycerol, a byproduct of the enhanced glycolytic flux induced by ischemia, leads to increased synthesis of triglycerides, which accumulate in the ischemic myocardium.

Intramyocardial Accumulation of Acyl-CoA in Ischemia. Accumulation of acyl-CoA may be deleterious because it inhibits further formation of CoA esters of fatty acids. Thus, fatty acids entering the cell cannot be esterified and trapped and are therefore prone to egress promptly. Furthermore, oxidation of fatty acids entering the cell cannot proceed without initial esterification with CoA. Accordingly, accumulation of fatty acid labeled with carbon-11, which can be monitored externally in vivo by positron tomography (p. 338) (Fig. 37–26), is diminished in ischemic or hypoxic zones.[201, 202] Restored metabolism accompanying reperfusion implemented promptly enough to maintain cell viability is reflected by a return of myocardial accumulation of fatty acid toward normal,[203, 204] although the return of recovery may sometimes be prolonged.[163a, 204a]

Accumulation of acyl-CoA esters also inhibits activity of an enzyme in the inner mitochondrial membrane, adenine nucleotide translocase—important in myocardial energy metabolism[205] and required for transport of ATP synthesized in the mitochondria to the cytosol. Although definitive information is not yet available, inhibition of the translocase and consequent failure of repletion of cytosolic ATP may be one factor accounting for the prompt decline of creatine phosphate in ischemic myocardium. Creatine kinase facilitates phosphorylation of ADP to form ATP, with concomitant conversion of creatine phosphate to creatine when cytosolic ATP concentrations decline. Thus, cytosolic creatine phosphate content declines as the cell compensates for diminished transport of ATP from mitochondria to cytosol. Accordingly, the effects of limited oxygen availability in ischemic myocardium on fatty acid metabolism may result in impaired energy production not only by direct limitation of oxidation of fatty acids, but also because of deleterious effects of the accumulating acyl-CoA intermediates on cellular function.

Ischemia-Induced Defects in Fatty-Acid Metabolism. Detection of altered fatty acid metabolism is the basis for recognition of ischemic myocardium in experimental animals and patients after intravenous administration of cyclotron-produced, positron-emitting, ^{11}C-labeled fatty acids. In isolated perfused hearts, transitory diminution of perfusion leads to a reversible reduction of ^{11}C-palmitate accumulation, reflecting decreased uptake and oxidation of fatty acids in the perfusate.[202, 206] The uptake of tracer is independent of flow per se, as long as metabolic activity of the myocardium remains constant. In patients with myocardial infarction, diminished accumulation of ^{11}C-palmitate is evident in computer-reconstructed images obtained by positron-emission, transaxial tomography[201] (Fig. 37–26). Because this technique permits quantitative delineation of the distribution of the tracer in a cross-section of the heart after intravenous administration, the diminution of ^{11}C-palmitate uptake detectable tomographically corresponds quantitatively to biochemical and morphometric criteria of infarction.[207]

Reduced flow alone does not diminish uptake of a substrate if intermediary metabolism is not altered, since the extraction fraction increases. Thus, transitory ischemia without reduction of either myocardial oxygen consumption or fatty acid utilization would not be manifested tomographically by decreased ^{11}C-palmitate uptake.[208] However, prolonged ischemia, with impairment of oxidative metabolism but without necrosis, would give rise to a zone of decreased accumulation of the tracer evident by tomography. The two conditions (prolonged ischemia without necrosis and infarction per se) can be readily differentiated with the use of serial studies. Prolonged and persistent diminution of oxidative metabolism and hence persistently impaired regional uptake of ^{11}C-palmitate detectable tomographically are tantamount to necrosis in view of the well-established irreversibility of injury sustained by myocardium rendered ischemic for 2 hours or more.

PROTEIN METABOLISM IN ISCHEMIA. Characteristic changes in

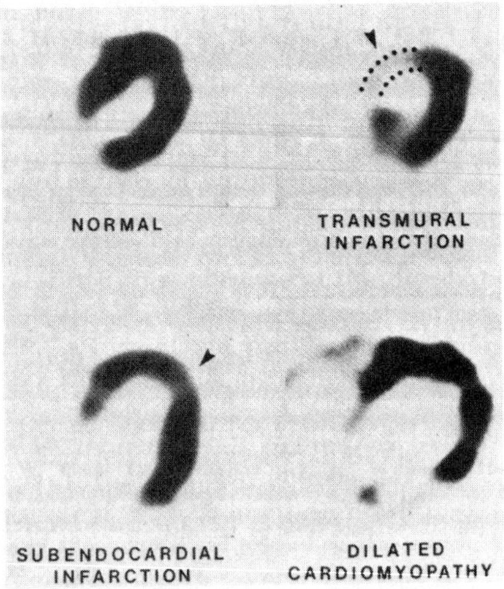

FIGURE 37–26. Myocardial uptake of ^{11}C-palmitate in a patient with dilated cardiomyopathy (*bottom right*) compared with uptake in a normal volunteer (*upper left*), a patient with nontransmural infarction (*upper right*), and a patient with transmural myocardial infarction (*lower left*). Note the heterogeneous uptake of tracer in the patient with dilated cardiomyopathy as compared with the discrete defects in tracer uptake in the patients with myocardial infarctions and the homogeneous uptake in the normal volunteer. (From Schelbert, H. R.: Positron-emission tomography: Assessment of myocardial blood flow and metabolism. Circulation *72* (Suppl. IV):129, 1985, by permission of the American Heart Association, Inc.)

synthesis and degradation of myocardial proteins accompany ischemia.[209] Synthesis decreases because of inhibition of peptide chain initiation and elongation.[210] Efflux of alanine reflects not only its diminished utilization in protein synthesis but also augmented synthesis by transamination of pyruvate, a precursor accumulating because of impaired carbohydrate exudation.[211] Thus, alanine release from the ischemic heart is analogous to lactate production.

Release of another amino acid, phenylalanine, has been employed in experimental preparations in which reincorporation into protein is prevented by pretreatment with cycloheximide (an inhibitor of protein synthesis) to provide an index of protein degradation under a variety of conditions, including normal oxygenation, anoxia, and simulated ischemia. The process of protein degradation requires energy derived from oxidative metabolism under physiological conditions based on observations with such preparations, since the rate of protein degradation declines by as much as 80 per cent in isolated hearts subjected to severe ischemia.[212] Although proteolysis mediated by lysosomal hydrolases has been implicated as a factor leading to irreversible injury in myocardium undergoing ischemic injury, increases in free and total lysosomal hydrolase activity do not occur until several hours after the onset of ischemia.[213] Accordingly, it appears likely that the early loss of functional sarcolemmal integrity accompanied by electrophysiological manifestations, subsequent impairment of cell volume regulation, and leakage of cytoplasmic constituents reflects primary damage to the cell membrane itself. Only later during the evolution of ischemic injury do activation and liberation of lysosomal enzymes or activation of proteases appear to be prominent. It has been postulated that a Ca^{++}-activated neutral protease degrades subunits of troponin within the first few hours of severe ischemia.[214] These and related observations suggest that the irreversible nature of injury sustained by ischemic myocardium is not due to proteolysis, even though activation of these enzymes may account for the release of relatively late markers of cell death and result in protein degradation late in the evolution of necrosis.

Under physiological conditions, the myocardium extracts glutamic acid from arterial blood and produces ammonia and glutamine, which appear in the coronary venous effluent. When ischemia supervenes, ammonia derived from amino acids that cannot be incorporated into protein under these conditions is incorporated into alanine and glutamine with a consequent increase in their concentrations in the coronary sinus effluent. The increased production of alanine has been viewed as analogous to the increased production of lactate. Both are markers of ischemia. In the case of alanine, transamination of pyruvate serves as a sink for ammonia that would otherwise accumulate. In the case of lactate, the pyruvate serves as a sink for hydrogen ions.

OXIDATIVE PHOSPHORYLATION. The importance of oxidative phosphorylation, i.e., the coupling of ATP synthesis to aerobic respiration, for the metabolic integrity of myocardium is underscored by some simple quantitative considerations. Complete oxidation of one mole of glucose gives rise to the net production of 36 moles of ATP. In contrast, only 2 moles of ATP are produced from complete anaerobic metabolism of 1 mole of glucose. Thus, even if the profound derangements in intermediary metabolism associated with increased production of reducing equivalents accompanying anaerobic glycolysis could be corrected, an 18-fold increase in glycolytic flux would be required for myocardium to synthesize comparable quantities of ATP via anaerobic compared to aerobic metabolism. The failure of energy production to keep pace with demand in ischemic cells is manifested by a prompt decline in the concentration of creatine phosphate, a major constituent of myocardial high-energy phosphate stores.[215]

The dependence of myocardial viability on the availability of oxygen has stimulated careful assessment of the gradients of oxygen present within ischemic zones of the heart, based on analysis of the oxidation-reduction state of specific components of the electron transport chain and different spectra reflecting changes in the oxygenation of myoglobin.[216, 217] Results obtained with optical techniques applied to the infarcted heart in vitro suggest that individual cells, and possibly individual mitochondria, are either fully aerobic or fully anaerobic in regions of myocardium subjected to ischemia. Thus, at any given instant, borders between anoxic and oxygenated tissue are very sharp. This phenomenon is in part a reflection of the very high affinity of mitochondria for oxygen. In response to ischemia, the mitochondria remain oxidized, despite very low levels of tissue oxygen tension, and become reduced only when virtually the last remaining oxygen has been utilized within a region. Thus, there appears to be a sharp, anatomically definable border between regions in which mitochondria are aerobic and anaerobic. However, this border is not static. As ischemia persists, there is expansion of the mass of severely ischemic tissue judging from morphological observations in canine hearts subjected to coronary occlusion. Early in the course of severe ischemia there is a potentially large mass of jeopardized but not yet irreversibly injured ischemic myocardium, susceptible to favorable influence by selected interventions.

The percentage of transmural necrosis ultimately developing within a zone of myocardium rendered ischemic by coronary occlusion maintained for 40 minutes, 3 hours, 6 hours, and 24 hours, followed by reperfusion for 2 to 4 days, varies from 38 to 85 per cent with a "wavefront" of necrosis progressing from subendocardial to epicardial tissue,[1, 217a] presumably because the subendocardium has a greater oxygen demand and smaller oxygen supply than the epicardium (Fig. 37–27). Metabolic studies have shown greater and more rapid reductions of ATP and total adenosine nucleotides and a greater and more rapid accumulation of lactate and nucleotides and bases, i.e., the products of degradation of adenine nucleotides in the subendocardium (Fig. 37–21). A cell in the subendocardium may be able to tolerate severe ischemia for a brief interval although it will become necrotic after 20 minutes. A cell with similar energy requirements in the subepicardium will be able to tolerate the milder degree of ischemia to which it is exposed following coronary occlusion for a longer period before becoming necrotic. As a consequence, when ischemic myocardium is reperfused 20 min to 5 hours after coronary occlusion, a progressively smaller epicardial zone of myocardium survives.[217b]

ACTIVATION OF LYSOSOMAL ENZYMES. Most tissues

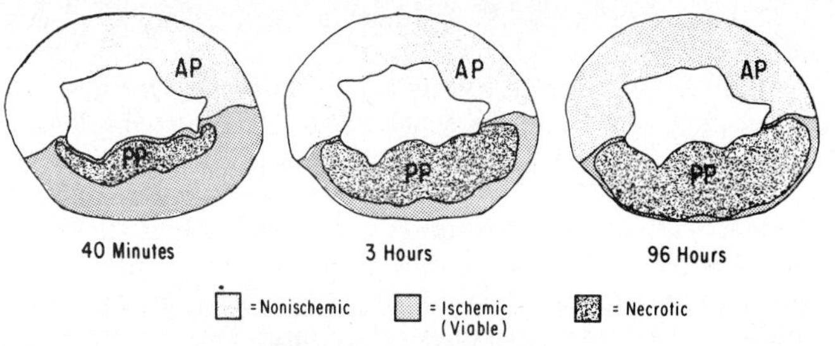

FIGURE 37–27. Progression of cell death versus time after circumflex coronary occlusion in dogs. Necrosis occurs first in the subendocardial myocardium. With longer occlusions, a wavefront of cell death moves from the subendocardial zone across the wall to involve progressively more of the transmural thickness of the ischemic zone. In contrast, the lateral margins in the subendocardial region of the infarct are established as early as 40 minutes after occlusion and are sharply defined by the anatomic boundaries of the ischemic bed. AP = anterior papillary muscle; PP = posterior papillary muscle. (From Reimer, K. A., Hill, M. L., and Jennings, R. B.: Prolonged depletion of ATP and of the adenine nucleotide pool due to delayed resynthesis of adenine nucleotides following reversible myocardial ischemic injury in dogs. J. Mol. Cell. Cardiol. *13*:229, 1981.)

contain latent lysosomal hydrolases capable of mediating proteolysis under certain conditions. Lysosomal hydrolases are activated by an acid pH, although mammalian cells contain neutral proteases as well. Relatively late reparative processes in myocardium undergoing infarction are accompanied by consistent increases in lysosomal hydrolase activity in tissue extracts as well as in the circulation, suggesting that activation of proteases with dissolution of cellular debris is a component to the response to irreversible injury. However, the extent to which activation of lysosomal hydrolase contributes to early manifestations of ischemia or irreversibility remains controversial. What is clear is that much of the lysosomal activity in the heart undergoing infarction comes from cells participating in the response to inflammation, such as polymorphonuclear leukocytes rather than myocardial cells per se.

ROLE OF CALCIUM IN ISCHEMIC INJURY. Myocardial injury induced by ischemia is associated with complexes of calcium in the tissue detectable by electron microscopy.[1, 218, 219] The interaction between myocardial ischemia and myoplasmic [Ca^{++}] is complex, as illustrated in Figure 37–28. Ischemia, however produced, is characterized by a reduction of myocardial ATP stores, which interferes with the transsarcolemmal $Na^{+}-K^{+}$ exchange, which in turn elevates intracellular [Na^{+}], raising intracellular [Ca^{++}] through an enhanced $Na^{+}-Ca^{++}$ exchange. Lowered ATP stores also reduce Ca^{++} uptake by the sarcoplasmic reticulum and reduce extrusion of Ca^{++} from cells. The resultant augmented intracellular [Ca^{++}] causes mitochondrial Ca^{++} overload, which depresses ATP production further. Activation of intracellular Ca^{++} ATPases augments ATP usage and activates sarcolemmal phospholipases, which release membrane phospholipid degradation products whose detergent properties impair the integrity of the cell membrane.[220, 221] Calcium antagonists interfere with Ca^{++} influx through voltage-dependent channels. Beta-adrenoceptor agonists recruit additional receptor-operated channels, and beta-adrenoceptor blockers reduce Ca^{++} influx by interfering with this recruitment of receptor-operated channels. Thus, one would expect beta blockers and Ca^{++} antagonists to have similar effects in the treatment of ischemia. Indeed, both groups of compounds delay ischemia-induced necrosis and, particularly when combined with reperfusion, reduce the extent of myocardial necrosis.[222–227]

The hypothesis that the entry of Ca^{++} into ischemic cells may be harmful is based on the observation that after a period of myocardial ischemia and subsequent reperfusion the accumulation of excess Ca^{++} in the mitochondria may interfere with their capacity to generate ATP. The destructive chain of metabolic events provoked by increased intracellular [Ca^{++}] appears to be responsible, at least in part, for the death of cells in the ischemic myocardium. Henry and associates[227a] found that during one hour of severe ischemia, the left ventricle undergoes progressive ischemic contracture, with the development of an elevated ventricular diastolic pressure and a fourfold increase in mitochondrial Ca^{++}. With subsequent reperfusion, both myocardial systolic function and relaxation remain abnormal, and a further marked increase in Ca^{++} accumulation occurs. Administration of nifedipine prevents ischemic contracture and permits recovery of systolic contractile function and of myocardial relaxation. These favorable hemodynamic changes are accompanied by a marked reduction in the accumulation of Ca^{++} in the mitochondria. Ca^{++} antagonists have also been shown to reduce ATP depletion and myocardial damage during coronary occlusion, and particularly during reperfusion,[227–230] and nifedi-

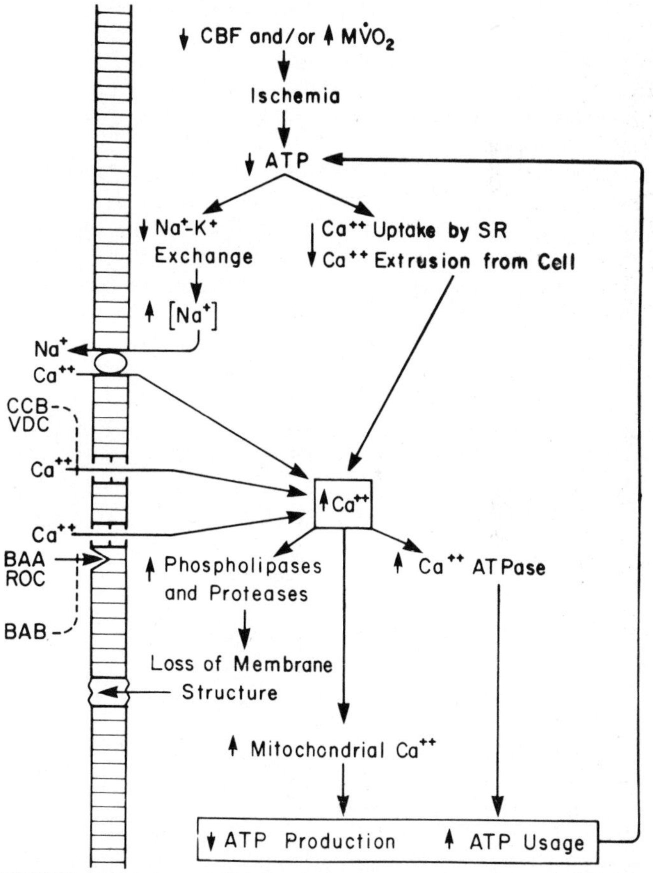

FIGURE 37–28. Interactions between myocardial ischemia and [Ca^{++}]. A reduction of coronary blood flow (CBF), sometimes accompanied by an increase in myocardial oxygen requirements ($M\dot{V}O_2$), causes myocardial ischemia, which in turn reduces cellular ATP stores. This reduction interferes with the transsarcolemmal NA^{+}-K^{+} exchange, which elevates intracellular [NA^{+}], raising intracellular [Ca^{++}] through an enhanced Na^{+}-Ca^{++} exchange. Lowered ATP stores also reduce Ca^{++} uptake by the sarcoplasmic reticulum (SR) and reduce extrusion of Ca^{++} from cells. The resultant augmented intracellular [Ca^{++}] causes mitochondrial Ca^{++} overload, which depresses ATP production further; activation of intracellular Ca^{++} ATPases, which augment ATP usage; and activation of sarcolemmal phospholipases and proteases, which impair the integrity of the cell membrane. Calcium-channel blockers (CCB) interfere with Ca^{++} influx through voltage-dependent channels (VDA). Beta-adrenoceptor agonists (BAA) recruit additional receptor-operated channels (ROC). Beta-adrenoceptor blockers (BAB) reduce Ca^{++} influx by interfering with the recruitment of ROC. (Reproduced with permission from Braunwald, E.: Mechanism of action of calcium channel blocking agents. N. Engl. J. Med. *307*:1618, 1982.)

pine preserved left ventricular function in dogs with cardiopulmonary bypass that were subjected to prolonged total ischemia.[231] These experiments demonstrate that in a setting analogous to the clinical practice of cardiac surgery, Ca^{++} antagonists protect myocardium, which is at first ischemic and is then reperfused. Thus, Ca^{++} antagonists may be valuable in protecting the myocardium from the Ca^{++}-associated ischemic injury occurring during open heart surgery. However, Ca^{++} antagonists do *not* appear to inhibit Ca^{++} influx into irreversibly injured myocardium. Instead, their protective action depends on an antiischemic effect resulting from a reduction of $M\dot{V}O_2$ (p. 1214).

The accumulation of Ca^{++} in myocardium undergoing ischemic injury has important diagnostic implications. Myocardial infarct scintigraphy with agents such as ^{99m}Tc-stannous pyrophosphate permits detection and localization of infarction after intravenous injection of tracer. The tissue's avidity for the tracer appears to depend on the accumulation of Ca^{++} (p. 342).

OXYGEN-DERIVED FREE RADICALS IN ISCHEMIC TISSUE INJURY. There is substantial evidence that ischemic tissue generates oxygen-derived free radicals (oxygen radicals), i.e., oxygen molecules containing an odd number of electrons, making them chemically reactive, and often leading to chain reactions.[232, 233, 233a] There are three principal oxygen radicals: the superoxide anion ($\cdot O_2^-$), hydrogen peroxide (H_2O_2), and the hydroxyl radical ($\cdot OH$) (Fig. 37–29). Acute, severe ischemia appears to increase the production of oxygen radicals by several mechanisms: (1) dissociation of intramitochondrial electron transport; (2) ischemia-induced Ca^{++} influx activates phospholipase which enhances arachidonic acid metabolism, which in turn may produce oxygen radicals; (3) ischemia converts the normal myocardial enzyme xanthine dehydrogenase to xanthine oxidase in some species, which in the presence of xanthine produces oxygen radicals; (4) complement is activated in ischemic tissue and this enhances the accumulation of neutrophils which in turn release oxygen radicals.[233a]

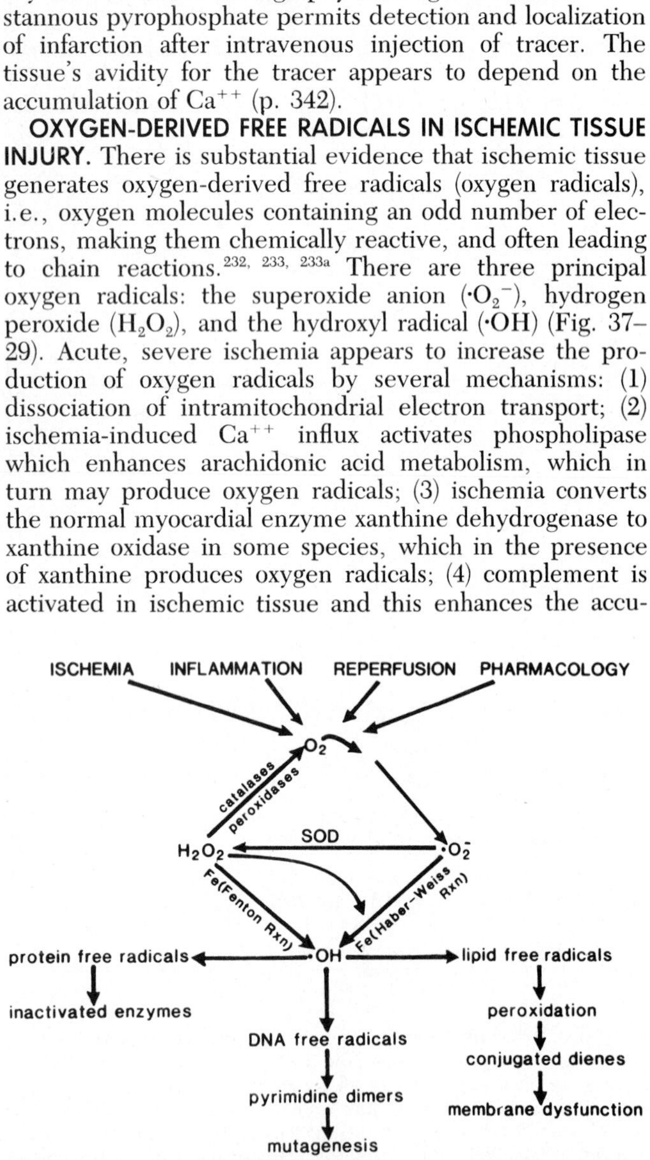

FIGURE 37–29. The proposed cellular and subcellular effects of the oxygen free radical system as a result of ischemia or reperfusion. These entities result in the univalent reduction of molecular oxygen to the superoxide anion ($\cdot O_2^-$). The superoxide anion can then be dismutated to hydrogen peroxide by the superoxide dismutase enzymes (SOD, MnSOD and CuZnSOD) and then either by a Fenton reaction (Rxn) or a Haber-Weiss reaction produce the hydroxyl radical, which is a potent oxidizing species. The hydroxyl radical in turn can produce protein free radicals, DNA free radicals, and lipid free radicals, which can have profound effects on the cell. (From Hammond, B., and Hess, M. L.: The oxygen-free radical system: Potential mediator of myocardial injury. Reprinted by permission of the American College of Cardiology. J. Am. Coll. Cardiol. 6:216, 1985.)

The oxygen radicals, in turn, can contribute to ischemic damage. These moieties react with almost any biological molecule in their vicinity. It has been proposed[232] that by causing perioxidation of cell membranes, oxygen radicals damage cell membranes and contribute to cell death. It has also been postulated that they can contribute to the development of irreversible injury by acting on the mitochondria and sarcoplasmic reticulum. This postulate is based largely on the observation that free radical scavengers such as superoxide dismutase and catalase prevent the ischemia-induced loss of Ca^{++} sequestration by the SR[234] and preserve mitochondrial function.[235]

The observation that scavengers of oxygen radicals enhance the rate of recovery of myocardial function after a brief period of ischemia suggests that these substances also play a significant role in the genesis of postischemic depression of myocardial function (myocardial stunning).[236, 236a] When oxygen is reintroduced into ischemic tissue, there is a burst of production of oxygen radicals. This may cause substantial injury and limit the immediate benefit of reperfusion.

RELEASE OF MYOCARDIAL ENZYMES IN DETECTION OF ACUTE MYOCARDIAL INFARCTION. Since biochemical markers of ischemic injury have become important clinical tools, some considerations required for their proper interpretation merit particular attention. Loss of functional integrity of the sarcolemma is a primary common denominator underlying liberation of cytoplasmic constituents into the circulation, such as transaminase (SGOT, AST), lactic dehydrogenase (LDH), and creatine kinase (CK)[237] (see p. 1239). Species of lower molecular weight, such as myoglobin, are liberated, but elevated concentrations persist in the circulation only briefly because of rapid renal clearance. Furthermore, myoglobin released from hypoperfused skeletal muscle may cloud interpretation of elevated values in plasma.[238]

Accurate assessment of myocardial infarction based on analysis of plasma enzyme time-activity curves has been facilitated by the demonstration that one isoenzyme of creatine kinase, CK-MB, is localized primarily in the heart in humans.[237–239] Under carefully defined conditions in experimental animals, depletion of myocardial CK activity correlates with infarct size estimated independently by morphometric techniques or with the use of radioactively labeled microspheres.[240] The corollary of these observations, namely, that increases in plasma enzyme activity reflect infarct size, has been recognized for many years.

On the basis of many clinical studies and observations in conscious experimental animals,[237, 241] it has become clear that release of myocardial cytosolic enzymes into the circulation is tantamount to cell death when the cause of enzyme release is myocardial ischemia. Accordingly, infarct size has been estimated from analysis of plasma enzyme CK time-activity curves,[242–244] and from curves obtained by quantitative assay of plasma samples for CK-MB activity.[245] Despite obvious imperfections, enzymatic estimates of infarct size have correlated with biochemical and morphological analyses of infarction in hearts of experimental animals, morbidity and mortality in patients, histochemical assessment of necrosis among patients who succumb to acute myocardial infarction,[246, 247] early and late ventricular arrhythmia, and impairment of ventricular function.[248, 249] Time-activity curves are influenced by regional myocardial perfusion, local degradation of enzyme in the heart, the ratio of enzyme released compared to that destroyed,[250] inactivation of enzyme in lymph,[251] exchange of enzyme between vascular and extravascular compartments,[243] and potential variation in the rate of inactivation and removal of enzyme once it has reached the circulation.[251] Thus, the pattern of enzyme release and its overall magnitude may be influenced by interventions resulting in early reperfusion and accelerated washout. Nevertheless, analysis of plasma time-activity curves of CK-MB and other biochemical markers of ischemic injury has proved useful in quantitative assessment of the progress and extent of myocardial infarction in the clinical setting.

Creatine Kinase Isoforms. Subforms of individual isoenzymes of CK-MM (isoforms), which may be distinguished by differences in isoelectric points (PI), exist in the plasma soon after myocardial infarction. When CK-MM is released into the bloodstream it is in the MM_3 isoform; this evolves in the plasma sequentially and in a time-dependent fashion into two other isoforms, MM_2 and MM_1, having lower isoelectric points. Both in experimental animals and in patients with coronary occlusion, within one hour after occlusion the percentage of total circulating MM comprised by the MM_3 isoform rises, with a reciprocal reduction of MM_2. No conversion of isoforms appears to occur in normal, ischemic, or necrotic myocardium.[252] It appears possible to use a single blood sample in which relative distribution of CK-MM isoforms is estimated both to diagnose and to time the onset of myocardial infarction. The isoform profile may be distinctly abnormal in the face of normal total CK or CK-MB.[253] However, since the MM_3 isoform is present in tissues other than the heart, the isoform profile in plasma is less specific for myocardial damage than is the CK-MB. The isoform profile (the percentage of concentrations of total CK activity in plasma comprised by MM_3) changes rapidly following myocardial reperfusion and appears to provide a prompt, reliable, and noninvasive index of the presence of myocardial reperfusion.[254]

MODIFICATION OF ISCHEMIC INJURY

A variety of interventions have been shown in animal experiments to modify the severity of ischemic injury, and in some instances parallel changes in infarct size have been observed. The theoretical basis for these interventions and the experimental results are discussed below. The clinical application of these observations is discussed on page 1258. The potency of any intervention designed to limit ischemic injury is inversely related to the interval between the onset of the ischemic stimulus and the time the intervention is applied.[255] In the normothermic working dog heart no intervention can be expected to exert a significant beneficial effect if it is initiated more than 4 to 6 hours after the onset of severe ischemia, because by this time all tissue in the distribution of the occluded vessel is likely to have become irreversibly injured.

INTERVENTIONS THAT INCREASE MYOCARDIAL INJURY AFTER CORONARY ARTERY OCCLUSION (Table 37–2)

The extent and severity of myocardial ischemic injury, and ultimately of myocardial infarction after coronary occlusion, depend on the balance between oxygen supply and demand in the jeopardized myocardium. Certain interventions known to increase $M\dot{V}O_2$ also increase the severity and extent of myocardial injury in the presence of residual, albeit restricted coronary blood flow. In the dog without heart failure, isoproterenol, digitalis (in the absence of heart failure), and amrinone[256, 257] have a deleterious effect on ischemic myocardium. Exercise can precipitate ischemia in the presence of obstruction not severe enough to cause ischemia at rest. Also, pacing-induced tachycardia increases ischemic damage,[257, 258] and a similar observation in patients has been reported.[259] Hypoxemia,[260] anemia,[261] and hypotension, regardless of how produced,[262] increase myocardial ischemic injury after coronary occlusion, since in all of these conditions the delivery of oxygen to the ischemic tissue is reduced; similarly, hypoglycemia augments ischemic injury.[263] Hyperthermia impairs mechanical performance of the ischemic myocardium[264]; through its direct stimulation of $M\dot{V}O_2$ and heart rate, it exerts an adverse effect on myocardial oxygen balance.

TABLE 37–2 INTERVENTIONS THAT INCREASE MYOCARDIAL INJURY AFTER CORONARY ARTERY OCCLUSION

Increase Myocardial Oxygen Requirements
Isoproterenol
Digitalis and amrinone (in the absence of heart failure)
Tachycardia
Hyperthermia
Decrease Myocardial Oxygen Supply
Directly
Hypoxemia
Anemia
Through collateral vessels, reducing coronary perfusion pressure
Hemorrhage
Sodium nitroprusside
Other vasodilators (including isoproterenol)
Coronary vasoconstriction (indomethacin)
Decrease substrate availability
Hypoglycemia

The positive inotropic and chronotropic effects of isoproterenol improve the function of normal myocardium and elevate $M\dot{V}O_2$. When isoproterenol is administered in the presence of global myocardial ischemia, however, myocardial function deteriorates rapidly because of the intensification of ischemia.[265–267] The effects of isoproterenol on myocardial function in the presence of regional ischemia are more complex. In the conscious dog with regional myocardial ischemia, isoproterenol elicits a spectrum of reactions in areas with different degrees of ischemia.[268] Severely ischemic sites exhibit no increase in blood flow and a deterioration of function occurs during infusion of isoproterenol, as a result of an increase in $M\dot{V}O_2$, whereas normal or moderately ischemic areas show an improvement of both myocardial function and regional blood flow. The positive chronotropic and inotropic actions of isoproterenol cause an increase in infarct size in anesthetized dogs and myocardial lactate production increases when isoproterenol is administered to patients with acute myocardial infarction.[269]

An increase in the concentration of circulating fatty acids also aggravates ischemia following coronary occlusion.[270] They augment $M\dot{V}O_2$[271] in the presence of limited oxygen supply; this intensifies ischemia, depresses myocardial contractility, and probably precipitates arrhythmias.[272]

As discussed on page 1212, release of oxygen-derived free radicals also increases myocardial ischemic injury.

INTERVENTIONS THAT REDUCE MYOCARDIAL INJURY AFTER CORONARY ARTERY OCCLUSION (Table 37–3)

The balance between myocardial oxygen supply and demand in the ischemic myocardium can be improved by augmenting the supply and/or reducing the demand. Restoration of perfusion is by far the most effective means of salvaging ischemic myocardium. Several studies in animals have shown that early reperfusion results in smaller infarction than if the occlusion is sustained. As might be expected, the extent of salvage depends on the duration of occlusion.[1, 217, 273, 274] Reperfusion after less than 15 to 20 minutes of coronary occlusion salvages essentially all of the ischemic tissue.[1] With longer periods of ischemia, a wavefront of necrosis beginning in the subendocardium and

TABLE 37–3 INTERVENTIONS THAT REDUCE EXPERIMENTAL MYOCARDIAL INJURY FOLLOWING CORONARY OCCLUSION

- Increasing myocardial oxygen supply
  - Directly
    - Coronary artery reperfusion (surgery, PTCA, thrombolysis)
    - Elevating arterial pO_2, hyperbaric oxygenation
    - Fluorocarbons
  - Through collateral vessels
    - Elevation of coronary perfusion pressure (e.g., methoxamine, neosynephrine)
    - Intraaortic balloon counterpulsation
  - Coronary vasodilatation (calcium antagonists, nitroglycerin, prostacyclin)
  - Coronary venous retroperfusion
- Decreasing myocardial O_2 demand
  - Beta-adrenoceptor blockers
  - Cardiac glycoside in the failing heart
  - Intraaortic balloon in counterpulsation
  - Decreasing afterload in hypertensive individuals
  - Decreasing preload (nitroglycerin)
  - Inhibiting calcium influx (Ca^{++} antagonists)
  - Hypothermia
- Preventing myocardial edema
  - Increasing plasma osmolality (mannitol, hypertonic glucose)
- Augmenting anaerobic metabolism
  - Glucose-insulin-potassium, fructose diphosphate, ribose
  - hypertonic glucose
- Enhancing transport to the ischemic zone of substrate utilized in energy production (presumed)
  - Hyaluronidase
- Prevention of injury by oxygen-free radicals (e.g., superoxide dismutase, allopurinol)
- Reduction of catabolism
  - Inhibition of adenine nucleotide catabolism (allopurinol)
  - Inhibition of lipolysis (β-pyridilcarbinol)
- Prevention of cell swelling
  - Osmotic agents (mannitol), Ca^{++} antagonists
- Reduction of inflammatory response
  - Glucocorticosteroids
  - Nonsteroidal inflammatory drugs (e.g., ibuprofen)
- Reduction of microvascular damage
  - Prevention of injury of vessels by free radicals
  - Prevention of platelet aggregation
  - Prevention of endothelial swelling (hypertonic agents)

moving progressively outward, i.e., to the epicardium and laterally, occurs[275] (Fig. 37–27). When reperfusion is carried out after 6 hours of coronary occlusion, most of the jeopardized myocardium becomes necrotic and no tissue is salvaged. The inhalation of an *oxygen-rich gas mixture* exerts a slight beneficial effect on the ischemic myocardium, also presumably by enhancing delivery of oxygen to ischemic tissue through collaterals.[276] This may be greatly enhanced by combining inhalation of 100 per cent oxygen with fluorocarbon mixtures, i.e., so-called artificial blood, which greatly augments delivery.[277, 277a]

Intraaortic balloon counterpulsation (p. 573) reduces the severity of ischemic injury, presumably by reducing $M\dot{V}O_2$, as a consequence of lowering systolic wall tension, while simultaneously augmenting oxygen delivery by increasing aortic diastolic (coronary perfusion) pressure. In experimental animals, *beta-adrenoceptor blockers* appear to prolong the survival of severely ischemic tissue, judging from changes in ST segments, QRS complexes, myocardial creatine kinase activity, and electronmicroscopic, histochemical, and histological criteria.[278] In addition, these drugs appear to improve the ratio of subendocardial to subepicardial blood flow in both ischemic and normal areas of myocardium in dogs with coronary occlusion. Beta-adrenoceptor blockade appears to be more useful in *delaying* than preventing cell death and is especially effective in limiting infarct size in animals subjected to coronary occlusion and reperfusion.[224, 225, 279] As discussed above (p. 1211), an influx of Ca^{++} into the myocardial cell is associated with and may play a role in cell necrosis. It has been observed that the Ca^{++} antagonists[279a, 279b] verapamil,[219, 222, 228] nifedipine,[280] and diltiazem[281] reduce the severity of ischemic injury as well as infarct size. The best available evidence suggests that the reduction of infarct size observed with Ca^{++} antagonists in experimental animals results from the ability of these compounds to exert an antiischemic effect, presumably by blocking Ca^{++} entry into ischemic cells, thereby lowering their $M\dot{V}O_2$ and reducing the ischemia-induced reduction of high-energy phosphates. An effect on Ca^{++} entry into irreversibly injured cells is probably not involved in the cardiac protection offered by these agents. Ca^{++} antagonists are particularly helpful when they are administered prophylactically, i.e., before the development of ischemia or early in the course of ischemia.[226, 227, 229, 230]

A number of *metabolic interventions* may also improve the energy balance of ischemic myocardium. As fatty acid oxidation is impaired by ischemia, glucose becomes the principal source of energy.[282] In the ischemic dog heart, oxidative phosphorylation and cardiac function are enhanced by the infusion of glucose-insulin-potassium (GIK).[283] In the anoxic, isolated heart, both electrical and mechanical function improve and recovery occurs more rapidly when glucose is added to the perfusate.[284] Other beneficial effects that have been attributed either to glucose alone or to glucose-insulin-potassium include (1) an increase in contractility due to the hyperosmolar action of glucose,[285] (2) a reduction in the concentration and myocardial uptake of circulating free fatty acids (which reduces $M\dot{V}O_2$), (3) a restoration of the intracellular K^+ concentration, and (4) reducing the frequency of serious ventricular dysrhythmias. In the open-chest dog, administration of GIK begun 30 minutes after coronary occlusion and maintained for 24 hours reduces the extent of myocardial necrosis that eventually develops.[286] Hypertonic glucose without insulin and potassium also reduces myocardial necrosis, but its salutary effect is not as great as that of GIK. In the baboon, GIK infusion after acute coronary occlusion preserves myocardial energy stores, with greater amounts of ATP, creatine phosphate, and glycogen in the ischemic zones of treated than in those of untreated animals.[287]

In the dog with experimentally produced coronary occlusion, myocardial ischemic injury is reduced by other agents that inhibit myocardial extraction of free fatty acids (i.e., antilipolytic agents, such as beta-pyridyl carbinol, and lipid-free albumin infusion), thus indirectly favoring glucose metabolism.[288] Injury is also reduced by sodium dichloroacetate,[289] which enhances the utilization of glucose relative to that of free fatty acids and by l-carnitine, which, by reversing the inhibition of adenine nucleotide translocase, prevents the depletion of cytoplasmic high-energy phosphate stores (Fig. 37–25).[290]

A number of agents that limit the inflammatory response reduce myocardial ischemic injury in the laboratory animal, and some have been used in limited numbers of patients (Chap. 38). Ischemia is characterized by the release of leukotactic factors and increased capillary permeability, leading to interstitial edema. As a result of the edema, the microvasculature is compressed, further diminishing blood flow to the ischemic area.[291] *Cobra venom factor*, a protein that enzymatically cleaves C3 and prevents the effects of the complement system, reduces myocardial injury.[292] Similarly, the kallikrein system enhances leukotactic activity, capillary permeability, interstitial edema, and proteolytic activity, and *aprotinin*, an inhibitor of this system, diminishes ischemic injury.[293] Large doses of a *glucocorticoster-*

oid also reduces myocardial infarct size in the dog with coronary occlusion.[294, 295] These compounds limit myocardial necrosis through mechanisms that are not clearly defined. They may also increase blood flow to the ischemic myocardium. Regardless of the effect of corticosteroids on the extent of myocardial ischemic injury, there is also evidence that when multiple doses are employed they may inhibit healing of the infarct, increasing the risk of ventricular rupture or aneurysm formation.[296] *Ibuprofen*, a nonsteroidal antiinflammatory compound, has also been shown to reduce infarct size in experimental animals,[297] but, like corticosteroids, interferes with infarct healing and scar formation.[298]

Mannitol reduces the extent of ischemic injury and improves the function of the ischemic myocardium. This hyperosmotic agent reduces cell swelling and also presumably improves collateral blood flow to the ischemic myocardium.[299]

Hyaluronidase has also been shown to reduce myocardial necrosis[300] in the dog and rabbit.[301] The depolymerization of mucopolysaccharides caused by hyaluronidase may increase the supply of nutrients to the myocardium or increase the washout of damaging metabolites. This agent decreases ST-segment elevations in dogs with coronary occlusion and decreases the ultimate extent of damage, estimated electrocardiographically, biochemically, and morphologically.

For decades *nitroglycerin* was avoided in patients with acute myocardial infarction because nitroglycerin-induced reductions in systemic arterial pressure and concomitant reflex increases in heart rate were believed to intensify ischemic injury. However, it has been shown in the dog that intravenous nitroglycerin, administered at a rate sufficient to cause a mild diminution in systemic arterial pressure, reduces the magnitude and extent of ischemic injury,[302] and that this injury can be further lessened if the blood pressure decrease and reflex tachycardia induced by nitroglycerin are abolished by the simultaneous infusion of methoxamine and phenylephrine. In addition, the administration of nitroglycerin shortly after coronary artery occlusion partially reverses the ventricular fibrillation threshold, whereas nitroglycerin and phenylephrine in combination restore this threshold to normal.[303] Nitroglycerin is presumed to act by augmenting perfusion of the border of the ischemic zone[304] by dilating collaterals and by reducing myocardial demands by lowering preload and afterload (Fig. 37–6).

The idea that oxygen-derived free radicals play a role in myocardial injury due to ischemia and reperfusion is discussed on page 1212. A variety of scavengers of oxygen radicals have been shown to reduce the size of myocardial infarction in some[233a] but certainly not all experiments.[304a, 304b] These agents include superoxide dismutase, catalase,[236, 236a] their combination,[305] *N*-2-mercaptopropionyl glycine,[306] and allopurinol, an inhibitor of xanthine oxidase.[307, 308] Neutrophils accumulate rapidly in ischemic tissue and the injury they cause is mediated in large part through release of oxygen radicals. Neutrophil depletion also limits infarct size[310]; however, free radical scavengers are effective in this respect even in animals depleted of neutrophils.[306] With increasing evidence for the effectiveness of thrombolytic therapy of acute myocardial infarction (p. 1253), the combination of administering free radical scavengers and carrying out reperfusion therapy appears to be an attractive one in limiting infarct size. However, for the scavengers to be effective in the setting of reperfusion, it will be necessary to deliver them to the infarct before or certainly no later than at the time of reperfusion.

REPERFUSION INJURY. As already indicated, it is generally agreed that the establishment of reperfusion represents by far the most effective technique for limiting cell death in the presence of severe ischemia. At the same time reperfusion elicits a number of adverse reactions that at the most can negate and at the least may limit the beneficial actions.

Acceleration of Myocyte Necrosis. Reperfusion obviously is necessary to supply the oxygen and substrates vital for the recovery of severely ischemic cells and to remove noxious metabolites. However, after reperfusion such cells often suddenly develop ultrastructural changes of irreversible cell death, including "explosive cell swelling" and widespread architectural disruption. Nevertheless, it is likely that most—and perhaps all—of the myocytes in which necrosis is accelerated by reperfusion were already irreversibly injured by the time reperfusion occurred and that reperfusion merely hastened the death of cells already destined not to recover. If reperfusion does cause necrosis of *reversibly* injured myocardium, the quantity of tissue so affected is likely to be small.

Ischemic Cell Swelling. This causes compression of myocardial capillaries interfering further with myocardial perfusion. During reperfusion this process is greatly intensified; it is possible that reperfusion-induced cell swelling

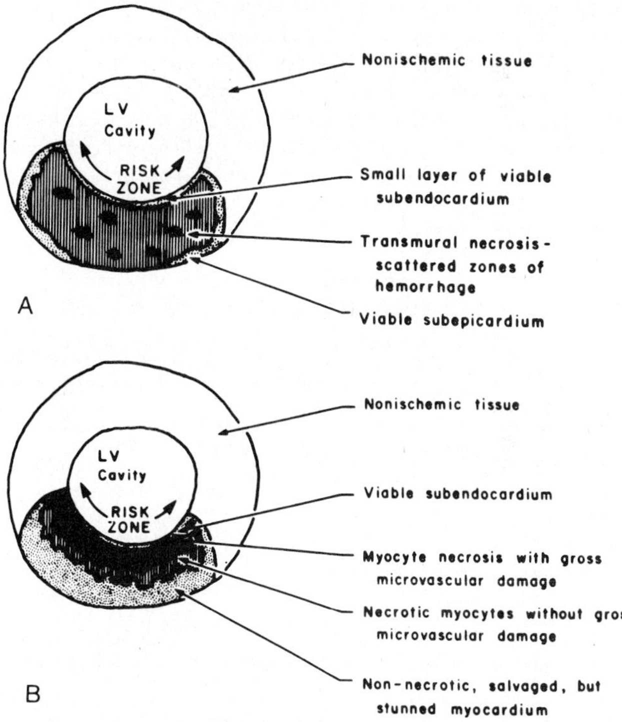

FIGURE 37–30. *A*, Schematic diagram showing a transverse section through a canine left ventricle subjected to a permanent coronary occlusion without reperfusion. The white area represents nonischemic myocardium supplied by the nonoccluded vessel. The infarct (hatched area) is transmural or near-transmural. There are scattered zones of hemorrhage (solid black). A small layer of viable subendocardium is present, which derives its oxygen directly from the ventricular cavity. Where collateral flow is high, there may be a small rim of surviving subepicardium (stippled areas). *B*, Schematic diagram showing a transverse section through a canine left ventricle subjected to coronary occlusion followed within 1 or 2 hours by coronary reperfusion. The hatched and solid black areas represent the infarct that is confined to the inner half of the myocardium. The solid black area represents the zone of gross microvascular damage including the zones of no-reflow and hemorrhage. It is smaller than and contained within the total infarct. The remainder of the infarct without severe microvascular damage is represented by the hatched area and is located in the midmyocardium. The epicardial portion of the ischemic zone (stippled area) has been salvaged by coronary reperfusion. It is nonnecrotic but stunned (postischemic ventricular dysfunction) for hours to days following coronary reperfusion. (From Braunwald, E., and Kloner, R. A.: Myocardial reperfusion: A double-edge sword? J. Clin. Invest. *76*:1715, 1985.)

and vascular compression can be responsible for the necrosis of reversibly injured cells.[311]

The "No-Reflow" Phenomenon. This refers to the failure of achieving sustained reperfusion after a prolonged period of ischemia. The areas of reduced or absent reflow often show and appear to result from ischemia-induced microvascular damage and myocardial contracture. The no-reflow phenomenon does *not* appear to augment myocyte death, because the zone of reflow is contained within areas in which myocytes were already necrotic at the time of the onset of reperfusion (Fig. 37–30).

Reperfusion-Induced Hemorrhage. Reperfused infarcts frequently contain hemorrhagic areas.[312] Reperfusion-induced hemorrhage, like the "no-reflow" phenomenon, is caused largely by microvascular damage. This is generally contained within areas of myocardium already necrotic at the time of reperfusion.[313]

The Calcium Paradox and the Oxygen Paradox. The reintroduction of Ca^{++} and/or of oxygen to hearts previously perfused with Ca^{++}-free hypoxic media causes marked damage to the sarcolemma and entry of large quantities of Ca^{++} into the ischemic cells. These phenomena have been termed the *calcium paradox*[314] and the *oxygen paradox*, respectively.[315] Perfusion of ischemic cells with Ca^{++}-free solution occurs clinically only in the special circumstances when cardioplegia is produced during cardiac surgery by means of a Ca^{++}-free solution. However, the oxygen paradox does appear to have widespread clinical relevance in that it may be mediated by oxygen-derived free radicals and potentially can be limited by scavengers of these substances.

REFERENCES

CONTROL OF MYOCARDIAL OXYGEN CONSUMPTION

1. Reimer, K. A., and Jennings, R. B.: Myocardial ischemia, hypoxia and infarction. *In* Fozzard, H. A., Jennings, R. B., Haber, E., Katz, A. M., and Morgan, H. E. (eds.): The Heart and Cardiovascular System. New York, Raven Press, 1986, pp. 1133–1202.
2. McKeever, W. P., Gregg, D. E., and Canney, P. C.: Oxygen uptake of the nonworking left ventricle. Circ. Res. 6:612, 1958.
3. Rooke, G. A., and Feigl, E. O.: Work as a correlate of canine left ventricular oxygen consumption, and the problem of catecholamine oxygen wasting. Circ. Res. *50*:273, 1982.
4. Suga, H., Goto, Y., Yamada, O., and Igarashi, Y.: Independence of myocardial oxygen consumption from pressure-volume trajectory during diastole in canine left ventricle. Circ. Res. *55*:734, 1984.
5. Klocke, F. J., Braunwald, E., and Ross, J., Jr.: Oxygen cost of electrical activation of the heart. Circ. Res. *18*:357, 1966.
6. Evans, C. L., and Matsuoka, Y.: The effect of various mechanical conditions on the gaseous metabolism and efficiency of the mammalian heart. J. Physiol. *49*:378, 1915.
7. Sarnoff, S. J., Braunwald, E., Welch, G. H., Jr., Case, R. B., Stainsby, W. N., and Macruz, R.: Hemodynamic determinants of oxygen consumption of the heart with special reference to the tension-time index. Am. J. Physiol. *192*:148, 1958.
8. Braunwald, E., Sarnoff, S. J., Case, R. B., Stainsby, W. N., and Welch, G. H., Jr.: Hemodynamic determinants of coronary flow: Effect of changes in aortic pressure and cardiac output on the relationship between myocardial oxygen consumption and coronary flow. Am. J. Physiol. *192*:157, 1958.
9. Rodbard, S., Williams, C. B., and Rodbard, D.: Myocardial tension and oxygen uptake. Circ. Res. *14*:139, 1964.
10. Teplick, R., Haas, G. S., Trautman, E., Titus, J., Geffin, G., and Daggett, W. M.: Time dependence of the oxygen cost of force development during systole in the canine left ventricle. Circ. Res. *59*:27, 1986.
11. Sonnenblick, E. H., Ross, J., Jr., Covell, J. W., and Braunwald, E.: Velocity of contraction as a determinant of myocardial oxygen consumption. Am. J. Physiol. *209*:919, 1965.
12. Suga, H., Hisano, R., Goto, Y., Yamada, O., and Igarashi, Y.: Effect of positive inotropic agents on the relation between oxygen consumption and systolic pressure volume area in canine left ventricle. Circ. Res. *53*:306, 1983.
13. Suga, H., Yamada, O., Goto, Y., and Igarashi, Y.: Oxygen consumption and pressure-volume area of abnormal contractions in canine heart. Am. J. Physiol. *246*:H154, 1984.
14. Fenn, W. O.: A quantitative comparison between the energy liberated and the work performed by the isolated sartorius muscle of the frog. J. Physiol. (Lond.) *58*:175, 1923.
15. Rall, J. A.: Sense and nonsense about the Fenn effect. Am. J. Physiol. *242*(Heart Circ. Physiol. 11):H1, 1982.
16. Covell, J. W., Braunwald, E., Ross, J., Jr., and Sonnenblick, E. H.: Studies on digitalis. XVI. Effects on myocardial oxygen consumption. J. Clin. Invest. *45*:1535, 1966.
17. Graham, T. P., Jr., Covell, J. W., Sonnenblick, E. H., Ross, J., Jr., and Braunwald, E.: Control of myocardial oxygen consumption: Relative influence of contractile state and tension development. J. Clin. Invest. *47*:375, 1968.
18. Boerth, R. C., Covell, J. W., Pool, P. E., and Ross, J., Jr.: Increased myocardial oxygen consumption and contractile state associated with increased heart rate in dogs. Circ. Res. *24*:725, 1969.
19. Urschel, C. W., Covell, J. W., Graham, T. P., Clancy, R. L., Ross, J., Jr., Sonnenblick, E. H., and Braunwald, E.: Effects of acute valvular regurgitation on the oxygen consumption of the canine heart. Circ. Res. *23*:33, 1968.

REGULATION OF CORONARY BLOOD FLOW

20. Vik-Mo, H., and Mjos, O. E.: Influence of free fatty acids on myocardial oxygen consumption and ischemic injury. Am. J. Cardiol. *48*:361, 1981.
21. Braunwald, E., Ross, J., Jr., and Sonnenblick, E. H.: Regulation of coronary blood flow. *In* Mechanisms of Contraction of the Normal and Failing Heart. 2nd ed. Boston, Little, Brown, 1976, p. 200.
22. Berne, R. M., and Rubio, R.: Coronary circulation. *In* Berne, R. M., Sperelakis, N., and Geiger, S. R. (eds.): Handbook of Physiology; Section 2, The Cardiovascular System. Bethesda, American Physiological Society, 1979, p. 897.
23. Feigl, E. O.: Coronary physiology. Physiol. Rev. *63*:1, 1983.
24. Young, M. A., and Vatner, S. F.: Regulation of large coronary arteries. Circ. Res. *59*:579, 1986.
25. Provenza, D. V., and Scherlis, S.: Coronary circulation in dog's heart: Demonstration of muscle sphincters in capillaries. Circ. Res. *7*:318, 1959.
26. Schaper, W.: The physiology of the collateral circulation in the normal and hypoxic myocardium. Rev. Physiol. Biochem. Pharmacol. *63*:102, 1971.
27. Cohen, M. V., Yipintsoi, T., and Scheuer, J.: Coronary collateral stimulation by exercise in dogs with stenotic coronary arteries. J. Appl. Physiol. *52*:664, 1982.
28. Bloor, C. M., White, F. C., and Sanders, M.: Effects of exercise on collateral development in myocardial ischemia in pigs. J. Appl. Physiol. *56*:656, 1984.
29. Scheel, K. W., and Williams, S. E.: Hypertrophy and coronary and collateral vascularity in dogs with severe chronic anemia. Am. J. Physiol. *249*:H1031, 1985.
30. Patterson, R. E., Jones-Collins, B. A., Aamodt, R., and Ro, Y. M.: Differences in collateral myocardial blood flow following gradual vs. abrupt coronary occlusion. Cardiovasc. Res. *17*:207, 1983.
31. Schaper, W.: Influence of physical exercise on coronary collateral blood flow in chronic experimental two-vessel occlusion. Circulation *65*:905, 1982.
32. Verani, M. S.: The functional significance of coronary collateral vessels: Anecdote confronts science. Cathet. Cardiovasc. Diagn. *9*:333, 1983.
32a. Elayda, M. A., Mathur, V. S., Hall, R. J., Massumi, G. A., Garcia, E., and deCastro, C. M.: Collateral circulation in coronary artery disease. Am. J. Cardiol. *55*:58, 1985.
33. Marcus, M. L.: The Coronary Circulation in Health and Disease. New York, McGraw-Hill and Company, 1983, 465 pp.
34. Olsson, R. A., and Bugni, W. J.: Coronary circulation. *In* Fozzard, H. A., et al. (eds.): The Heart and Cardiovascular System. New York, Raven Press, 1986, pp. 987–1038.
35. Klocke, F. J., Mates, R. E., Canty, J. M., Jr., and Ellis, A. K.: Coronary pressure-flow relationships. Controversial issues and probable implications. Circ. Res. *56*:311, 1985.
36. Spaan, J. A. E.: Coronary diastolic pressure-flow relation and zero flow pressure explained on the basis of intramyocardial compliance. Circ. Res. *56*:293, 1985.
37. Klocke, F. J.: Coronary blood flow in man. Prog. Cardiovasc. Dis. *19*:117, 1976.
38. Griggs, D. M., Jr., Chen, C. C., and Tchokoev, V. V.: Subendocardial metabolism in experimental aortic stenosis. Am. J. Physiol. *224*:607, 1973.
39. Sabbah, H. N., and Stein, P. D.: Effect of acute regional ischemia on pressure in the subepicardium and subendocardium. Am. J. Physiol. *242*(Heart Circ. Physiol. 11):H240, 1982.
40. Brazier, J., Cooper, N., and Buckberg, G.: The adequacy of subendocardial oxygen delivery: The interaction of determinants of flow, arterial oxygen content and myocardial oxygen need. Circulation *49*:968, 1974.
41. Lundsgaard-Hansen, P., Meyer, C., and Riedwyl, H.: Transmural gradients of glycolytic enzyme activities in left ventricular myocardium. I. The normal state. Pfluegers Arch. *297*:89, 1967.
42. Buckberg, G. D., Fixler, D. E., Archie, J. P., and Hoffman, J. I. E.: Experimental subendocardial ischemia in dogs with normal coronary arteries. Circ. Res. *30*:67, 1972.
43. Hoffman, J. I. E.: Determinants of prediction of transmural myocardial perfusion. Circulation *58*:381, 1978.
44. Neill, W. A., Oxendine, J., Phelps, N., and Anderson, R. P.: Subendocardial ischemia provoked by tachycardia in conscious dogs with coronary stenosis. Am. J. Cardiol. *35*:30, 1975.
45. Fallen, E. L., Elliott, W. C., and Gorlin, R.: Mechanisms of angina in aortic stenosis. Circulation *36*:480, 1967.
46. Griggs, D. M., Jr., and Chen, C. C.: Coronary hemodynamics and regional myocardial metabolism in experimental aortic insufficiency. J. Clin. Invest. *53*:1599, 1974.
47. Dunn, R. B., and Griggs, D. M., Jr.: Ventricular filling pressure as a determinant of coronary blood flow during ischemia. Am. J. Physiol. *244*:H429, 1983.
48. Becker, L. C., Fortuin, N. J., and Pitt, B.: Effect of ischemia and antianginal

drugs on the distribution of radioactive microspheres in the canine left ventricle. Circ. Res. *28*:263, 1971.

49. Mathes, P., and Rival, J.: Effect of nitroglycerin on total and regional coronary blood flow in the normal and ischaemic canine myocardium. Cardiovasc. Res. 5:54, 1971.
50. Woodman, O. L., and Vatner, S. F.: Coronary vasoconstriction mediated by $alpha_1$ and $alpha_2$ adrenoceptors in the conscious dog. Am. J. Physiol. (*in press*).

50a. Vatner, S. F.: Alpha-adrenergic tone in the coronary circulation of the conscious dog. Fed. Proc. *43*:2867, 1984.

50b. Morgan, K. G.: Role of calcium ion in maintenance of vascular smooth muscle tone. Am. J. Cardiol. *59*:24A, 1987.

50c. Johns, A., Leijten, P., Yamamoto, H., Hwang, K., and van Breemen, C.: Calcium regulation in vascular smooth muscle contractility. Am. J. Cardiol. *59*:18A, 1987.

50d. Adelstein, R. S., and Sellers, J. R.: Effects of calcium on vascular smooth muscle contraction. Am. J. Cardiol. *59*:4B, 1987.

51. Rinkema, L. E., Thomas, J. X., Jr., and Randall, W. C.: Regional coronary vasoconstriction in response to stimulation of stellate ganglia. Am. J. Physiol. *243*:H410, 1982.
52. Murray, P. A., Lavallee, M., and Vatner, S. F.: Alpha-adrenergic–mediated reduction in coronary blood flow secondary to carotid chemoreceptor reflex activation in conscious dogs. Circ. Res. *54*:96, 1984.
53. Vatner, D. E., Knight, D. R., Homcy, C. J., Vatner, S. F., and Young, M. A.: Subtypes of beta-adrenergic receptors in bovine coronary arteries. Circ. Res. *59*:463, 1986.

53a. Pitt, B., Elliot, E. C., and Gregg, D. E.: Adrenergic receptor activity in the coronary arteries of the unanesthetized dog. Circ. Res. *21*:75, 1967.

54. Vatner, S. F., and Hintze, T. H.: Mechanism of constriction of large coronary arteries by beta-adrenergic receptor blockade. Circ. Res. *53*:389, 1983.
55. Cox, D. A., Hintze, T. H., and Vatner, S. F.: Effects of acetylcholine on large and small coronary arteries in conscious dogs. J. Pharmacol. Exp. Ther. *225*:764, 1983.
56. Vatner, S. F., Higgins, C. B., and Braunwald, E.: Effects of norepinephrine on coronary circulation and left ventricular dynamics in the conscious dog. Circ. Res. *34*:812, 1974.
57. Kern, M. J., Horowitz, J. D., Ganz, P., Gaspar, J., Colucci, W. S., Lorell, B. H., Barry, W. H., and Mudge, G. H., Jr.: Attenuation of coronary vascular resistance by selective $alpha_1$-adrenergic blockade in patients with coronary artery disease. J. Am. Coll. Cardiol. *5*:840, 1985.
58. Winniford, M. D., Wheelan, K. R., Kremers, M. S., Ugolini, V., van den Berg, E., Jr., Niggemann, E. H., Jansen, D. E., and Hillis, L. D.: Smoking-induced coronary vasoconstriction in patients with atherosclerotic coronary artery disease: Evidence for adrenergically mediated alterations in coronary artery tone. Circulation *74*:662, 1986.

58a. Winniford, M. D., Jansen, D. E., Reynolds, G. A., Apprill, P., Black, W. H., and Hillis, L. D.: Cigarette smoking-induced coronary vasoconstriction in atherosclerotic coronary artery disease and prevention by calcium antagonists and nitroglycerin. Am. J. Cardiol. *59*:203, 1987.

59. Szentivanyi, M., and Juhasz-Nagy, N.: Physiological role of the coronary constrictor fibers. Q. J. Exp. Physiol. *48*:93, 1963.
60. Hackett, J. G., Abboud, F. M., Mark, A. L., Schmid, P. G., and Heistad, D. D.: Coronary vascular responses to stimulation of chemoreceptors and baroreceptors. Circ. Res. *21*:8, 1972.
61. Higgins, C. B., Vatner, S. F., and Braunwald, E.: Parasympathetic control of the heart. Pharmacol. Rev. *25*:119, 1973.
62. Vatner, S. F., Franklin, D., VanCitters, R. L., and Braunwald, E.: Effects of carotid sinus nerve stimulation on the coronary circulation of the conscious dog. Circ. Res. *27*:11, 1970.
63. Brachfeld, N., Monroe, R. G., and Gorlin, R.: Effects of pericoronary denervation on coronary hemodynamics. Am. J. Physiol. *199*:174, 1960.
64. Macho, P., and Vatner, S. F.: Effects of prazosin on coronary and left ventricular dynamics in conscious dogs. Circulation *65*:1186, 1982.
65. Lavallee, M., Amano, J., Vatner, S. F., Manders, W. T., Randall, W. C., and Thomas, J. X., Jr.: Adverse effects of chronic cardiac denervation in conscious dogs with myocardial ischemia. Circ. Res. *57*:383, 1985.
66. Heyndrickx, G. R., Muylaert, P., and Pannier, J. L.: Alpha-adrenergic control of oxygen delivery to myocardium during exercise in conscious dog. Am. J. Physiol. *242*(Heart Circ. Physiol. 11):H805, 1982.
67. Feigl, E. O.: Reflex parasympathetic coronary vasodilation elicited from cardiac receptors in the dog. Circ. Res. *37*:175, 1975.
68. Jarisch, A., and Zotterman, Y.: Depressor reflexes from the heart. Acta Physiol. Scand. *16*:31, 1948.
69. Feigl, E. O.: Parasympathetic control of coronary blood flow in dogs. Circ. Res. *25*:509, 1969.
70. Brown, B. G., Lee, A. B., Bolson, E. L., and Dodge, H. T.: Reflex constriction of significant coronary stenosis as a mechanism contributing to ischemic left ventricular dysfunction during isometric exercise. Circulation *70*:18, 1984.
71. Chierchia, S., Davies, G., Berkenboom, B., Crea, F., Crean, P., and Maseri, A.: Alpha-adrenergic receptors and coronary spasm: An elusive link. Circulation *69*:8, 1984.
72. Driscol, T. E., Moir, T. W., and Eckstein, R. W.: Vascular effects of changes in perfusion pressure in the nonischemic and ischemic heart. Circ. Res. *15*(Suppl. I):94, 1964.
73. Oien, A. H., and Aukland, K.: A mathematical analysis of the myogenic hypothesis with special reference to autoregulation of renal blood flow. Circ. Res. *52*:241, 1983.
74. Bayliss, W. M.: On the local reaction of the arterial wall to changes in arterial pressure. J. Physiol. (Lond.) *28*:220, 1902.
75. Coffman, J. D., and Gregg, D. E.: Oxygen metabolism and oxygen debt repayment after myocardial ischemia. Am. J. Physiol. *201*:881, 1961.
76. Detar, R., and Bohr, D. F.: Oxygen and vascular smooth muscle contraction. Am. J. Physiol. *214*:241, 1968.
77. Duling, B. R.: Microvascular responses to alterations in oxygen tension. Circ. Res. *31*:481, 1972.

77a. Duling, B. R.: Changes in microvascular diameter and oxygen tension induced by carbon dioxide. Circ. Res. *32*:370, 1973.

78. Martini, J., and Honig, C. R.: Direct measurement of intercapillary distance in beating rat heart in situ under various conditions of O_2 supply. Microvasc. Res. *1*:244, 1969.
79. Sparks, H. V., Jr., and Bardenheuer, H.: Regulation of adenosine formation by the heart. Circ. Res. *58*:193, 1986.
80. Rubio, R., and Berne, R. M.: Release of adenosine by the normal myocardium and its relationship to the regulation of coronary resistance. Circ. Res. *25*:407, 1969.
81. Bardenheuer, H., and Schrader, J.: Supply-to-demand ratio for oxygen determines formation of adenosine by the heart. Am. J. Physiol. *250*:H-173, 1986.
82. Rubio, R., Berne, R. M., and Dobson, J. G., Jr.: Sites of adenosine production in cardiac and skeletal muscle. Am. J. Physiol. *225*:938, 1973.
83. Rubio, R., Berne, R. M., and Katori, M.: Release of adenosine in reactive hyperemia of the dog heart. Am. J. Physiol. *216*:56, 1969.

83a. McKenzie, J. E., Steffen, R. P., and Haddy, F. J.: Relations between adenosine and coronary resistance in conscious exercising dogs. Am. J. Physiol. *242*:H24, 1982.

84. Belardinelli, L., Vogel, S., Linden, J., and Berne, R. M.: Anti-adrenergic action of adenosine on ventricular myocardium in embryonic chick hearts. J. Mol. Cell. Cardiol. *14*:291, 1982.
85. Gellai, M., Norton, J. M., and Detar, R.: Evidence for direct control of coronary vascular tone by oxygen. Circ. Res. *32*:279, 1973.

85a. Bergman, G., Atkinson, L., Richardson, P. J., Daly, K., Rothman, M., Jackson, G., and Jewitt, D. E.: Prostacyclin: Haemodynamic and metabolic effects in patients with coronary artery disease. Lancet *1*:569, 1981.

86. Friedman, P. L., Brugada, P., Kuck, K. H., Bar, F. W. H. M., and Wellens, H. J. J.: Coronary vasoconstrictor effect of indomethacin in patients with coronary artery disease. N. Engl. J. Med. *305*:1171, 1981.
87. Lee, J.-D., Tajimi, T., Guth, B., Seitelberger, R., Miller, M., and Ross, J., Jr.: Exercise-induced regional dysfunction with subcritical coronary stenosis. Circulation *73*:596, 1986.
88. Furchgott, R. F., and Zawadski, J. V.: The obligatory role of endothelial cells in the relaxation of arterial smooth muscle by acetylcholine. Nature *288*:373, 1980.
89. DeBoer, L. W. V., Rude, R. E., Davis, R. F., Maroko, P. R., and Braunwald, E.: Extension of myocardial necrosis into normal epicardium following hypotension during experimental coronary occlusion. Cardiovasc. Res. *16*:423, 1982.

89a. Furchgott, R. F.: Role of endothelium in responses of vascular smooth muscle. Circ. Res. *53*:557, 1983.

90. Peach, M. J., Loeb, A. L., Singer, H. A., and Saye, J. A.: Endothelium-derived vascular relaxing factor. Hypertension *7*(Suppl. 1):94, 1985.

90a. Peach, M. J., Singer, H. A., Izzo, N. J., Jr., and Loeb, A. L.: Role of calcium in endothelium-dependent relaxation of arterial smooth muscle. Am. J. Cardiol. *59*:35A, 1987.

91. Freiman, P. C., Mitchell, G. G., Heistad, D. D., Armstrong, M. L., and Harrison, D. G.: Atherosclerosis impairs endothelium-dependent vascular relaxation to acetylcholine and thrombin in primates. Circ. Res. *58*:783, 1986.
92. Ludmer, P. L., Selwyn, A. P., Shook, T. L., Wayne, R. R., Mudge, G. H., Alexander, R. W., and Ganz, P.: Paradoxical vasoconstriction induced by acetylcholine in atherosclerotic coronary arteries. N. Engl. J. Med. *315*:1046, 1986.
93. Hintze, T. H., and Vatner, S. F.: Reactive dilation of large coronary arteries in conscious dogs. Circ. Res. *54*:50, 1984.

93a. Fam, W. M., and McGregor, M.: Effect of coronary vasodilator drugs on retrograde flow in areas of chronic myocardial ischemia. Circ. Res. *15*:355, 1964.

93b. Cannon, R. O., III, Schenke, W. H., Leon, M. B., Rosing, D. R., Urquhart, J., and Epstein, S. E.: Limited coronary flow reserve after dipyridamole in patients with ergonovine-induced coronary vasoconstriction. Circulation *75*:163, 1987.

94. Cohen, M. V., Downey, J. M., Sonnenblick, E. H., and Kirk, E. S.: The effects of nitroglycerin on coronary collaterals and myocardial contractility. J. Clin. Invest. *52*:2836, 1973.

94a. Schwartz, J. S., and Bache, R. J.: Pharmacologic vasodilators in the coronary circulation. Circulation *75*:I–162, 1987.

95. Vatner, S. F., Pagani, M., Manders, T., and Pasipoularides, A. D.: Alpha-adrenergic vasoconstriction and nitroglycerin vasodilation of large coronary arteries in the conscious dog. J. Clin. Invest. *65*:5, 1980.
96. Feldman, R. L., Marx, J. D., Pepine, C. J., and Conti, C. R.: Analysis of coronary responses to various doses of intracoronary nitroglycerin. Circulation *66*:321, 1982.
97. Macho, P., and Vatner, S. F.: Effects of nitroglycerin and nitroprusside on large and small coronary vessels in conscious dogs. Circulation *64*:1101, 1981.
98. Hinte, T. H., and Vatner, S. F.: Comparison of effects of nifedipine and nitroglycerin on large and small coronary arteries and cardiac function in conscious dogs. Circ. Res. *52*(Suppl. I):139, 1983.
99. Engle, H.-J., and Lichten, P. R.: Beneficial enhancement of coronary blood flow by nifedipine: Comparison with nitroglycerin and beta blocking agents. Am. J. Med. *71*:658, 1981.
100. Bush, L. R., Campbell, W. B., Buja, L. M., Tilton, G. D., and Willerson, J. T.: Effects of the selective thromboxane synthetase inhibitor dazoxiben on variations in cyclic blood flow in stenosed canine coronary arteries. Circulation *69*:1161, 1984.

100a. Bush, L. R., Campbell, W. B., Kern, K., Tilton, G. D., Apprill, P., Ashton,

J., Schmitz, J., Buja, L. M., and Willerson, J. T.: The effects of alpha$_2$-adrenergic and serotonergic receptor antagonists on cyclic blood flow alterations in stenosed canine coronary arteries. Circ. Res. *55*:642, 1984.

100b. Hoffman, J. I. E.: A critical review of coronary reserve. Circulation 75:I–6, 1987.

101. Marcus, M. L., Harrison, D. G., White, C. W., and Hiratzka, L. F.: Assessing the physiological significance of coronary obstruction in man. Can. J. Cardiol. Suppl. A:195A, 1986.

102. Marcus, M. L., Dotty, D. B., Hiratzka, L. F., Wright, C. B., and Eastham, C. L.: Decreased coronary reserve. A mechanism for angina pectoris in patients with aortic stenosis and normal coronary arteries. N. Engl. J. Med. *307*:1362, 1982.

102a. Marcus, M. L., Harrison, D. G., Chilian, W. M., Koyanagi, S., Inou, T., Tomanek, R. J., Martins, J. B., Eastham, C. L., and Hiratzka, L. F.: Alterations in the coronary circulation in hypertrophied ventricles. Circulation *75*:I–19, 1987.

103. Opherk, D., Mall, G., Zebe, H., Schwarz, F., Weihe, E., Manthey, J., and Kubler, W.: Reduction of coronary reserve: A mechanism for angina pectoris in patients with arterial hypertension and normal coronary arteries. Circulation *69*:1, 1984.

104. Cannon, R. O., III, Rosing, D. R., Maron, B. J., Leon, M. B., Bonow, R. O., Watson, R. M., and Epstein, S. E.: Myocardial ischemia in patients with hypertrophic cardiomyopathy: contribution of inadequate vasodilator reserve and elevated left ventricular filling pressures. Circulation *71*:234, 1985.

105. Cannon, R. O., III, Bonow, R. O., Bacharach, S. L., Green, M. V., Rosing, D. R., Leon, M. B., Watson, R. M., and Epstein, S. E.: Left ventricular dysfunction in patients with angina pectoris, normal epicardial coronary arteries, and abnormal vasodilator reserve. Circulation *71*:218, 1985.

106. Cannon, R. O., III, Leon, M. B., Watson, R. M., Rosing, D. R., and Epstein, S. E.: Chest pain and "normal" coronary arteries—Role of small coronary arteries. Am. J. Cardiol. *55*:50B, 1985.

107. Gould, K. L.: Assessing coronary stenosis severity: A recurrent clinical need. J. Am. Coll. Cardiol. *8*:91, 1986.

108. Epstein, S. E., and Talbot, T. L.: Dynamic coronary tone in precipitation, exacerbation, and relief of angina pectoris. Am. J. Cardiol. *48*:797, 1981.

109. Klocke, F. J.: Measurements of coronary blood flow and degree of stenosis: Current clinical implications and continuing uncertainties. J. Am. Coll. Cardiol. *1*:31, 1983.

110. Epstein, S. E., Cannon, R. O., III, and Talbot, T. L.: Hemodynamic principles in the control of coronary blood flow. Am. J. Cardiol. *56*:4E, 1985.

111. Maseri, A.: Myocardial ischemia in man: Current concepts, changing views and future investigation. Can. J. Cardiol. Suppl. A:225A, 1986.

111a. Ganz, P., Abben, R. P., and Barry, W. H.: Dynamic variations in resistance of coronary arterial narrowings in angina pectoris at rest. Am. J. Cardiol. *59*:66, 1987.

MYOCARDIAL ISCHEMIA AND ISCHEMIC INJURY

112. Maseri, A., Chierchia, S., and Kaski, J. C.: Mixed angina pectoris. Am. J. Cardiol. *56*:30E, 1985.

113. Tennant, R., and Wiggers, C. J.: The effect of coronary occlusion on myocardial contractions. Am. J. Physiol. *112*:351, 1935.

114. Ross, J., Jr., Gallagher, K., Matzusaki, M., Lee, J. D., Guth, B., and Goldfarb, R.: Regional myocardial blood flow and function in experimental myocardial ischemia. Can. J. Cardiol. Suppl. A:9A, 1986.

115. Osakada, G., Hess, O. M., Gallather, K. P., Kemper, W. S., and Ross, J., Jr.: End-systolic dimension-wall thickness relations during myocardial ischemia in conscious dogs. Am. J. Cardiol. *51*:1750, 1983.

116. Amano, J., Thomas, J. X., Jr., Lavallee, M., Mirsky, I., Glover, D., Manders, W. T., Randall, W. C., and Vatner, S. F.: Effects of myocardial ischemia on regional function and stiffness in conscious dogs. Am. J. Physiol. 252:H110, 1987.

117. Lew, W. Y. W., Chen, Z., Guth, B., and Covell, J. W.: Mechanisms of augmented segment shortening in nonischemic areas during acute ischemia of the canine left ventricle. Circ. Res. *56*:351, 1985.

118. Vatner, S. F.: Correlation between acute reductions in myocardial blood flow and function in conscious dogs. Circ. Res. *47*:201, 1980.

119. Sunagawa, K., Maughan, W. L., Friesinger, G., Guzman, P., Chang, M., and Sagawa, K.: Effect of coronary arterial pressure on left ventricular end-systolic pressure-volume relation of isolated canine heart. Circ. Res. *50*:727, 1982.

120. Sunagawa, K., Maughan, W. L., and Sagawa, K.: Effect of regional ischemia on the left ventricular end-systolic pressure-volume relationship of isolated canine hearts. Circ. Res. *52*:170, 1983.

121. Braunwald, E., and Kloner, R. A.: The stunned myocardium: Prolonged, post-ischemic ventricular dysfunction. Circulation *66*:1146, 1982.

122. Vatner, S. F., Heyndrickx, G. R., and Fallon, J. T.: Effects of brief periods of myocardial ischemia on regional myocardial function and creatine kinase release in conscious dogs and baboons. Can. J. Cardiol. (Suppl. A):19A, 1986.

123. Ellis, S. G., Wynne, J., Braunwald, E., Henschke, C. I., Sandor, T., and Kloner, R. A.: Response of reperfusion-salvaged stunned myocardium to inotropic stimulation. Am. Heart J. *107*:13, 1984.

124. Arnold, J. M. O., Braunwald, E., Sandor, T., and Kloner, R. A.: Inotropic stimulation of reperfused myocardium with dopamine: Effects on infarct size and myocardial function. J. Am. Coll. Cardiol. *6*:1026, 1985.

125. Ekmekci, A., Toyoshima, H., Dowczynski, J. K., Nagaya, T., and Prinzmetal, M.: Angina pectoris. IV. Clinical and experimental difference between ischemia with S-T elevation and ischemia with S-T depression. Am. J. Cardiol. 7:412, 1961.

125a. Ciuffo, A. A., Ouyang, P., Becker, L. C., Levin, L., and Weisfeldt, M. L.: Reduction of sympathetic inotropic response after ischemia in dogs. J. Clin. Invest. 75:1504, 1985.

126. Janse, M. J.: Electrophysiology and electrocardiology of acute myocardial ischemia. Can. J. Cardiol. Suppl. *A*:46A, 1986.

127. Carmeliet, E.: Myocardial ischemia: Reversible and irreversible changes. Circulation *70*:149, 1984.

128. Katz, A. M.: Effects of ischemia on the contractile processes of heart muscle. Am. J. Cardiol. *32*:456, 1973.

129. Chesnais, J. M., Coraboeuf, E., Sauviat, M. P., and Vassas, J. M.: Sensitivity of H, Li and Mg ions of the slow inward sodium current in frog atrial fibres. J. Mol. Cell. Cardiol. *7*:627, 1975.

130. Braunwald, E., Ross, J., Jr., and Sonnenblick, E. H.: Mechanisms of Contractions in the Normal and Failing Heart. 2nd Ed. Boston, Little, Brown and Company, 1976, p. 357.

131. Williamson, J. R., Schaffer, S. W., Ford, C., and Safer, B.: Contribution of tissue acidosis to ischemic injury in the perfused rat heart. Circulation *53*(Suppl I):3, 1976.

132. Regan, T. J., Effros, R. M., Haider, B., Oldewurtel, H.A., Ettinger, P. O., and Ahmed, S. S.: Myocardial ischemia and cell acidosis: Modification by alkali and the effects on ventricular function and cation composition. Am. J. Cardiol. *37*:501, 1976.

133. Gewirtz, H., Ohley, W., Walsh, J., Shearer, D., Sullivan, M. J., and Most, A. S.: Ischemia-induced impairment of left ventricular relaxation: Relation to reduced diastolic filling rates of the left ventricle. Am. Heart J. *105*:72, 1983.

134. Carroll, J. D., Hess, O. M., Hirzel, H. O., and Krayenbuehl, H. P.: Exercise-induced ischemia: The influence of altered relaxation on early diastolic pressures. Circulation *67*:521, 1983.

135. Momomura, S-I., Ingwall, J. S., Parker, J. A., Sahagian, P., Ferguson, J. J., and Grossman, W.: The relationships of high energy phosphates, tissue pH, and regional blood flow to diastolic distensibility in the ischemic dog myocardium. Circ. Res. *57*:822, 1985.

136. Visner, M. S., Arentzen, C. E., Parrish, G. D., Larson, E. V., O'Connor, M. J., Crumbley, A. J., III, Bache, R. J., and Anderson, R. W.: Effects of global ischemia on the diastolic properties of the left ventricle in the conscious dog. Circulation *71*:610, 1985.

137. Grossman, W., and McLaurin, L. P.: Diastolic properties of the left ventricle. Ann. Intern. Med. *84*:316, 1976.

138. Bourdillon, P. D., Lorell, B. H., Mirsky, I., Paulus, W. J., Wynne, J., and Grossman, W.: Increased regional myocardial stiffness of the left ventricle during pacing-induced angina in man. Circulation *67*:316, 1983.

139. Carroll, J. D., Hess, O. M., Hirzel, H. O., and Krayenbuehl, H. P.: Exercise-induced ischemia: The influence of altered relaxation on early diastolic pressures. Circulation *67*:521, 1983.

140. Sasayama, S., Nonogi, H., Miyazaki, S., Sakurai, T., Kawai, C., Eiho, S., and Kuwahara, M.: Changes in diastolic properties of the regional myocardium during pacing-induced ischemia in human subjects. J. Am. Coll. Cardiol. *5*:599, 1985.

141. Grossman, W.: Why is left ventricular diastolic pressure increased during angina pectoris? J. Am. Coll. Cardiol. *5*:607, 1985.

142. Imai, K., Wang, T., Millard, R. W., Ashraf, M., Kranias, E. G., Asano, G., Grassi di Gende, A. O., Nagao, T., Solaro, R. J., and Schwartz, A.: Ischaemia-induced changes in canine cardiac sarcoplasmic reticulum. Cardiovasc. Res. *17*:696, 1983.

143. Paulus, W. J., Serizawa, T., and Grossman, W.: Altered left ventricular diastolic properties during pacing-induced ischemia in dogs with coronary stenoses. Potentiation by caffeine. Circ. Res. *50*:218, 1982.

144. Rakita, L., Borduas, J. L., Rothman, S., and Prinzmetal, M.: Studies on the mechanism of ventricular activity. XII. Early changes in the RS-T segment and QRS complex following acute coronary artery occlusion: Experimental study and clinical applications. Am. Heart J. *48*:351, 1954.

145. Leaf, A.: Cell swelling: A factor in ischemic tissue injury. Circulation *48*:455, 1973.

146. Opie, L. H., Owen, P., Thomas, M., and Samson, R.: Coronary sinus lactate measurements in assessment of myocardial ischemia: Comparison with changes in lactate/pyruvate and beta-hydroxybutyrate/acetoacetate ratios and with release of hydrogen, phosphate and potassium ions from the heart. Am. J. Cardiol. *32*:295, 1973.

147. Surawicz, B.: ST-segment, T-wave, and U-wave changes during myocardial ischemia and after myocardial infarction. Can. J. Cardiol. (Suppl.) *A*:71, 1986.

148. Karlsson, J., Templeton, G. H., and Willerson, J. T.: Relationship between epicardial S-T segment changes and myocardial metabolism during acute coronary insufficiency. Circ. Res. *32*:725, 1973.

149. Sayen, J. J., Peirce, G., Katcher, A. H., and Sheldon, W. F.: Correlation of intramyocardial electrocardiograms with polarographic oxygen and contractility in the nonischemic and regional ischemic left ventricle. Circ. Res. *9*:1268, 1961.

150. Angell, C. S., Lakatta, E. G., Weisfeldt, M. L., and Shock, N. W.: Relationship of intramyocardial oxygen tension and epicardial ST segment changes following acute coronary artery ligation: Effects of coronary perfusion pressure. Cardiovasc. Res. *9*:12, 1975.

151. Khuri, S. F., Flaherty, J. T., O'Riordan, J. B., Pitt, B., Brawley, R. K., Donahoo, J. S., and Gott, V. L.: Changes in intramyocardial ST segment voltage and gas tensions with regional myocardial ischemia in the dog. Circ. Res. *37*:455, 1975.

152. Braunwald, E., and Maroko, P. R.: ST-segment mapping: Realistic and unrealistic expectations. Circulation *54*:529, 1976.

153. Maroko, P. R., Kjekshus, J. K., Sobel, B. E., Covell, J. W., Ross, J., Jr., and Braunwald, E.: Factors influencing infarct size following experimental coronary artery occlusions. Circulation *43*:67, 1971.

154. Hillis, L. D., Askenazi, J., Braunwald, E., Radvany, P., Muller, J. E., Fishbein, M. C., and Maroko, P. R.: Use of changes in epicardial QRS complex to assess interventions which modify the extent of myocardial necrosis following coronary artery occlusion. Circulation *54*:591, 1976.

155. Kralios, F. A., Martin, L., Burgess, M. J., and Millar, K.: Local ventricular repolarization changes due to sympathetic nerve-branch stimulation. Am. J. Physiol. *228*:1621, 1975.
156. Muller, J. E., Maroko, P. R., and Braunwald, E.: Evaluation of precordial electrocardiographic mapping as a means of assessing changes in myocardial ischemic injury. Circulation *52*:16, 1975.
157. Gettes, L. S.: Effect of ischemia on cardiac electrophysiology. *In* Fozzard, H. A., Jennings, R. B., Haber, E., Katz, A. M., and Morgan, H. E. (eds.): The Heart and Cardiovascular System. New York, Raven Press, 1986, pp. 1317–1342.
158. Elharrar, V., and Zipes, D. P.: Cardiac electrophysiological alterations during myocardial ischemia. *In* Levy, M. N., and Vassalle, M. (eds.): Excitation and Neural Control of the Heart. Baltimore, Williams and Wilkins, 1982, pp. 149–180.
159. Mehra, R., Zeiler, R. H., Gough, W. B., and El-Sherif, N.: Reentrant ventricular arrhythmias in the late myocardial infarction period. 9. Electrophysiologic-anatomic correlation of reentrant circuits. Circulation *67*:11, 1983.
160. El-Sherif, N., Scherlag, B. J., and Lazzara, R.: Electrode catheter recording during malignant ventricular arrhythmias following experimental acute myocardial ischemia. Evidence for reentry due to conduction delay and block in ischemic myocardium. Circulation *51*:1003, 1975.
161. Janse, M. J., and Kleber, A. G.: Electrophysiological changes and ventricular arrhythmias in the early phase of regional myocardial ischemia. Circ. Res. *49*:1069, 1981.
162. Kent, F. K., Smith, E. R., Redwood, D. R., and Epstein, S. E.: Electrical stability of acutely ischemic myocardium. Influence of heart rate and vagal stimulation. Circulation *47*:291, 1973.
163. Maisel, A. S., Motulsky, H. J., and Insel, P. A.: Externalization of beta-adrenergic receptors promoted by myocardial ischemia. Science *230*:183, 1985.
163a. Camici, P., Araujo, L., Spinks, T., Lammertsma, A. L., Sohanpal, S. K., Jones, T., and Maseri, A.: Prolonged metabolic recovery allows late identification of ischemia in the absence of electrocardiographic and perfusion changes in patients with exertional angina. Can. J. Cardiol. (Suppl. A):131A, July, 1986.
164. Corr, P. B., Witkowski, F. X., and Sobel, B. E.: Mechanisms contributing to malignant dysrhythmias induced by ischemia in the cat. J. Clin. Invest. *61*:109, 1978.
165. Elharrar, J., Gaum, W. E., and Zipes, D. P.: Effect of drugs on conduction delay and incidence of ventricular arrhythmias induced by acute coronary occlusion in dogs. Am. J. Cardiol. *39*:544, 1977.
166. Horowitz, L. N., Spear, J. F., and Moore, E. N.: Subendocardial origin of ventricular arrhythmias in 24-hour-old experimental myocardial infarction. Circulation *53*:56, 1976.
166a. Kimura, S., Basset, A. L., Kohya, T., Kozlovskis, P. L., and Myerburg, R. J.: Automaticity, triggered activity, and responses to adrenergic stimulation in cat subendocardial Purkinje fibers after healing of myocardial infarction. Circulation *75*:651, 1987.
167. El-Sherif, N., Hope, R. R., Scherlag, B. J., and Lazzara, R.: Re-entrant ventricular arrhythmias in the late myocardial infarction period. 2. Patterns of initiation and termination of reentry. Circulation *55*:702, 1977.
168. Lazzara, R., Hope, R. R., El-Sherif, N., and Scherlag, B. J.: Effects of lidocaine on hypoxic and ischemic cardiac cells. Am. J. Cardiol. *41*:872, 1978.
169. Murdock, D. K., Loeb, J. M., Euler, D. E., and Randall, W. C.: Electrophysiology of coronary reperfusion. A mechanism for reperfusion arrhythmias. Circulation *61*:175, 1980.
170. Downar, E., Janse, M.S., and Durrer, D.: The effect of "ischemic" blood on transmembrane potentials of normal porcine ventricular myocardium. Circulation *55*:455, 1977.
171. Sobel, B. E., Corr, P. B., Robinson, A. K., Goldstein, R. A., Witkowski, F. X., and Klein, M. S.: Accumulation of lysophosphoglycerides with arrhythmogenic properties in ischemic myocardium. J. Clin. Invest. *61*:109, 1978.
172. Corr, P. B., Cain, M. E., Witkowski, F. X., Price, D. A., and Sobel, B. E.: Potential arrhythmogenic electrophysiological derangements in canine Purkinje fibers induced by lysophosphoglycerides. Circ. Res. *44*:822, 1979.
173. Schwartz, A., Wood, J. M., Allen, J. C., Barret, E., Entman, M. L., Goldstein, M. A., Sordahl, L. Z., Suzuki, M., and Lewis, R. M.: Biochemical and morphologic correlates of cardiac ischemia. 1. Membrane systems. Am. J. Cardiol. *32*:46, 1973.
174. Cherry, G., and Myers, M. B.: The relationship to ventricular fibrillation of early tissue sodium and potassium shifts and coronary vein potassium levels in experimental myocardial infarction. J. Thorac. Cardiovasc. Surg. *61*:587, 1971.
175. Podzuweit, T., Dalby, A. J., Cherry, G. W., and Opie, L. H.: Tissue levels of cyclic AMP in ischemic and non-ischemic myocardium following coronary artery ligation. J. Mol. Cell. Cardiol. *10*:81, 1978.
176. Kuppersmith, J., Shaing, H., Litwak, R. S., and Harman, M. V.: Electrophysiologic effects of verapamil in canine myocardial ischemia. Am. J. Cardiol. *37*:149, 1976.
177. Griffith, J., and Leung, F.: The sequential estimation of plasma catecholamines and whole blood histamine in myocardial infarction. Am. Heart J. *82*:171, 1971.
178. El-Sherif, N., and Lazzara, K.: Reentrant ventricular arrhythmias in the late myocardial infarction period. 7. Effect of verapamil and D-600 and role of the "slow channel." Circulation *60*:3, 1979.
178a. Ugurbil, K.: Magnetization transfer measurements of creatine kinase and ATPase rates in intact hearts. Circulation *72*(Suppl. IV):94, 1985.
179. Jennings, R. B., Reimer, K. A., Hill, M. L., and Mayer, S. E.: Total ischemia in dog hearts in vitro. I. Comparison of high energy phosphate production, utilization and depletion, and of adenine nucleotide catabolism in total ischemia in vitro vs. severe ischemia in vivo. Circ. Res. *49*:892, 1981.
180. Steenberger, C., Hill, M. L., and Jennings, R. B.: Volume regulation and plasma membrane injury in aerobic, anaerobic, and ischemic myocardium in vitro. Circ. Res. *57*:864, 1985.
181. Reimer, K. A., Jennings, R. B., and Hill, M. L.: Total ischemia in dog hearts, in vitro. 2. High energy phosphate depletion and associated defects in energy metabolism, cell volume regulation, and sarcolemmal integrity. Circ. Res. *49*:901, 1981.
182. Rude, R. E., DeBoer, L. W. V., Ingwall, J. S., Kloner, R. A., Hale, S. L., Davis, M., Maroko, P. R., and Braunwald, E.: Prediction of biochemical derangement in ischemic myocardium following experimental coronary artery occlusion. Am. J. Cardiol. *45*:415, 1980.
183. Ingwall, J. S.: Phosphorus nuclear magnetic resonance spectroscopy of cardiac and skeletal muscles. Am. J. Physiol. *242*(Heart Circ. Physiol. 11):H729, 1982.
183a. Barrett, E. J., Alger, J. R., and Zaret, B. L.: Nuclear magnetic resonance spectroscopy: Its evolving role in the study of myocardial metabolism. J. Am. Coll. Cardiol. *6*:497, 1985.
184. Flaherty, J. T., Weisfeldt, M. L., Bulkley, B. H., Gardner, T. J., Gott, V. L., and Jacobus, W. E.: Mechanisms of ischemic myocardial cell damage assessed by phosphorus-31 nuclear magnetic resonance. Circulation *65*:561, 1982.
185. Pernot, A.-C., Ingwall, J. S., Menasche, P., Grousset, C., Bercot, M., Pinwnica, A., and Fossel, E. T.: Evaluation of high-energy phosphate metabolism during cardioplegic arrest and reperfusion: A phosphorus-31 nuclear magnetic resonance study. Circulation *67*:1296, 1983.
186. Taegtmeyer, H.: Carbohydrate interconversions and energy production. Circulation *72*(Suppl. IV):1, 1985.
187. Weiss, J., and Hiltbrand, B.: Functional compartmentation of glycolytic versus oxidative metabolism in isolated rabbit heart. J. Clin. Invest. *75*:436, 1985.
188. Rovetto, M. J., Lamberton, W. F., and Neely, J. R.: Mechanisms of glycolytic inhibition in ischemic rat hearts. Circ. Res. *37*:742, 1975.
189. Sobel, B. E., and Mayer, S. E.: Cyclic adenosine monophosphate and cardiac contractility. Circ. Res. *32*:407, 1973.
190. Williamson, J. R., Schaffer, S. W., Ford, C., and Safer, B.: Contribution of tissue acidosis to ischemic injury in the perfused rat heart. Circulation *53*(Suppl. I):3, 1976.
191. LaNoue, K. F., and Williamson, J. R.: Interrelationships between malate-aspartate shuttle and critic acid cycle in rat heart mitochondria. Metabolism *20*:119, 1971.
192. Most, A. S., Gorlin, R., and Soeldner, J. S.: Glucose extraction by the human myocardium during pacing stress. Circulation *45*:92, 1972.
193. Opie, L. H., Owen, P., Thomas, M., and Samson, R.: Coronary sinus lactate measurements in assessment of myocardial ischemia: Comparison with changes in lactate/pyruvate and beta-hydroxybutyrate/acetoacetate ratios and with release of hydrogen, phosphate and potassium ions from the heart. Am. J. Cardiol. *32*:295, 1973.
194. Wisneski, J. A., Gertz, E. W., Neese, R. A., Gruenke, L. D., and Craig, J. C.: Dual carbon-labeled isotope experiments using D-[6-^{14}C] glucose and L-[1, 2, 3^{-13} C_3] lactate: A new approach for investigating human myocardial metabolism during ischemia. J. Am. Coll. Cardiol. *5*:1138, 1985.
194a. Regan, T. J., Effros, R. M., Haider, R., Oldewurtel, H. A., Ettinger, P. O., and Ahmed, S. S.: Myocardial ischemia and cell acidosis: Modification by alkali and the effects on ventricular function and cation composition. Am. J. Cardiol. *27*:501, 1976.
195. Hansen, C. A., Fellenius, E., and Neely, J. R.: Metabolic rates in normal and infarcted myocardium. Can. J. Cardiol. Suppl. A:1A, 1986.
196. Bieber, L. L., and Fiol, C. J.: Fatty acid and ketone metabolism. Circulation *72*(Suppl IV):9, 1985.
197. Crass, M. F., III, McCaskill, E. S., and Shipp, J. C.: Glucose-free fatty acid interactions in the working heart. J. Appl. Physiol. *29*:87, 1970.
198. Neely, J. R., and Morgan, H. E.: Relationship between carbohydrate and lipid metabolism and the energy balance of heart muscle. Annu. Rev. Physiol. *36*:413, 1974.
199. Wood, J. M., Sordahl, L. A., Lewis, R. M., and Schwartz, A.: Effect of chronic myocardial ischemia on the activity of carnitine palmityl-coenzyme A transferase of isolate canine heart mitochondria. Circ. Res. *32*:340, 1973.
200. Neely, J. R., Rovetto, M. J., Whitmer, J. T., and Morgan, H. E.: Effects of ischemia on ventricular function and metabolism in the isolated working rat heart. Am. J. Physiol. *225*:651, 1973.
201. Sobel, B. E.: Positron tomography and myocardial metabolism: An overview. Circulation *72*(Suppl. IV):22, 1985.
202. Schelbert, H. R.: Positron-emission tomography: Assessment of myocardial blood flow and metabolism. Circulation *72*(Suppl. IV):122, 1985.
203. Bergmann, S. R., Lerch, R. A., Fox, K. A. A., Ludbrook, P. A., Welch, M. J., Ter-Pogossian, M. M., and Sobel, B. E.: Temporal dependence of beneficial effects of coronary thrombolysis characterized by positron tomography. Am. J. Med. *73*:573, 1982.
204. Sobel, B. E., and Bergmann, S. R.: Coronary thrombolysis: Some unresolved issues. Am. J. Med. *72*:1, 1982.
204a. Schelbert, H. R.: Evaluation of "metabolic fingerprints" of myocardial ischemia. Can. J. Cardiol.(Suppl. A):121A, 1986.
205. Shrago, E., Shug, A., and Elson, C.: Regulation of cell metabolism by mitochondrial transport systems. *In* Hanson, R. W., and Mehlman, M. A. (eds.): Gluconeogenesis: Its Regulation in Mammalian Species. New York, John Wiley and Sons, 1976, p. 221.
206. Geltman, E. M., and Sobel, B. E.: Cardiac positron tomography. Chest *83*:553, 1983.
207. Weiss, E. S., Ahmed, S. A., Welch, M. J., Williamson, J. R., Ter-Pogossian, M. M., and Sobel, B. E.: Quantification of infarction in cross sections of canine myocardium in vivo with positron emission transaxial tomography and ^{11}C-palmitate. Circulation *55*:66, 1977.

208. Fox, K. A. A., Nomura, H., Sobel, B. E., and Bergmann, S. R.: Consistent substrate utilization despite reduced flow in hearts with maintained work. Am. J. Physiol. *244*:H799, 1983.
209. Zak, R.: Nitrogen metabolism and mechanisms of protein synthesis and degradation. Circulation 72(Suppl. IV):13, 1985.
210. Kao, R., Rannels, E., and Morgan, H. E.: Effects of anoxia and ischemia on protein synthesis in perfused rat hearts. Circ. Res. *38*(Suppl. I):124, 1976.
211. Taegtmeyer, H., Peterson, M. B., Ragavan, V. V., Ferguson, A. G., and Lesch, M.: De novo alanine synthesis in isolated oxygen-deprived rabbit myocardium. J. Biol. Chem. *252*:5010, 1977.
212. Rannels, D. E., McKee, E. E., and Morgan, H. E.: Regulation of protein synthesis and degradation in heart and skeletal muscle. *In* Litwack, G. (ed.): Biochemical Actions of Hormones. New York, Academic Press, 1976.
213. Weissman, G., Hoffstein, S., Gennaro, D., and Fox, A. C.: Lysosomes in ischemic myocardium, with observations on the effects of methyl-prednisolone. *In* Lefer, A. M., Kelliher, G. J., and Rovetto, M. J. (eds.): Pathophysiology and Therapeutics of Myocardial Ischemia. New York, Spectrum Publications, Inc., 1977, p. 367.
214. Toyo-Oka, T., and Masaki, T.: Calcium-activated neutral protease from bovine ventricular muscle. J. Mol. Cell. Cardiol. *11*:769, 1979.
215. Williamson, J. R., Steenbergen, C., Rich, T., Deleeuw, G., Barlow, C., and Chance, B.: The nature of ischemic injury in cardiac tissue. *In* Lefer, A. M., Kelliher, G. J., and Rovetto, M. J. (eds.): Pathophysiology and Therapeutics of Myocardial Ischemia. New York, Spectrum Publications, Inc., 1977, p. 193.
216. Chance, B.: Discussion. Circ. Res. 38(Suppl. I):69, 1976.
217. Reimer, K. A., Lowe, J. E., Rasmussen, M. M., and Jennings, R. B.: The wavefront phenomenon of ischemic cell death. I. Myocardial infarct size vs duration of coronary occlusion in dogs. Circulation *56*:786, 1977.
217a. Chance, B., Clark, B. J., Nioka, S., Subramanian, H., Maris, J. M., and Bode, H.: Phosphorus nuclear magnetic resonance spectroscopy in vivo. Circulation 72(Suppl. IV):103, 1985.
217b. Lavallee, M., Cox, D., Patrick, T. A., and Vatner, S. F.: Salvage of myocardial function by coronary artery reperfusion 1, 2, and 3 hours after occlusion in conscious dogs. Circ. Res. *53*:235, 1983.
218. Fleckenstein, A.: Calcium Antagonism in Heart and Smooth Muscle. New York, John Wiley and Sons, 1983.
219. Braunwald, E.: Mechanism of action of calcium channel blocking agents. N. Engl. J. Med. *307*:1618, 1982.
220. Corr, P. B., Gross, R. W., and Sobel, B. E.: Arrhythmogenic amphiphilic lipids and the myocardial cell membrane. J. Mol. Cell. Cardiol. *14*:619, 1982.
221. Sedlis, S. P., Corr, P. B., Sobel, B. E., and Ahumada, G. G.: Lysophosphatidyl choline potentiates Ca^{++} accumulation in rat cardiac myocytes. Am. J. Physiol. *13*:H32, 1983.
222. Kloner, R. A., DeBoer, L. W. V., Carlson, N., and Braunwald, E.: The effect of verapamil on myocardial ultrastructure during and following release of coronary artery occlusion. Exp. Mol. Pathol. *36*:277, 1982.
223. Braunwald, E., Muller, J. E., Kloner, R. A., and Maroko, P. R.: Role of beta-adrenergic blockade in the therapy of patients with myocardial infarction. Am. J. Med. *784*:113, 1983.
224. Hammerman, H., Kloner, R. A., Briggs, L. L., and Braunwald, E.: Enhancement of salvage of reperfused myocardium by early beta-adrenergic blockade. J. Am. Coll. Cardiol. *3*:1438, 1984.
225. Miyazawa, K., Fukuyama, H., Komatsu, E., and Yamaguchi, I.: Effects of propranolol on myocardial damage resulting from coronary artery occlusion followed by reperfusion. Am. Heart J. *111*:519, 1986.
226. Lo, H.-M., Kloner, R. A., and Braunwald, K.: Effect of intracoronary verapamil on infarct size in the ischemic, reperfused canine heart: Critical importance of the timing of treatment. Am. J. Cardiol. *56*:672, 1985.
227. Campbell, C. A., Kloner, R. A., Alker, K. J., and Braunwald, E.: Effect of verapamil on infarct size in dogs subjected to coronary artery occlusion with transient reperfusion. J. Am. Coll. Cardiol. *8*:1169, 1986.
227a. Henry, P. D., Shuchleib, R., Davis, J., Weiss, E. S., and Sobel, B. E.: Myocardial contracture and accumulation of mitochondrial calcium in ischemic rabbit heart. Am. J. Physiol. (Heart Circ. Physiol.) *2*:H677, 1977.
228. DeBoer, L. W. V., Strauss, H. W., Kloner, R. A., Rude, R. E., David, R. F., Maroko, P. R., and Braunwald, E.: Autoradiographic method for measuring the ischemic myocardium at risk: Effects of verapamil on infarct size after experimental coronary artery occlusion. Proc. Natl. Acad. Sci. *77*:6119, 1980.
229. Nayler, W. G., Panagiotopoulos, S., Elz, J. S., and Sturrock, W. J.: Fundamental mechanisms of action of calcium antagonist in myocardial ischemia. Am. J. Cardiol. *59*:75B, 1987.
230. Kloner, R. A., and Braunwald, E.: Effects of calcium antagonists on infarcting myocardium. Am. J. Cardiol. *59*:84B, 1987.
231. Clark, R. E., Christlieb, I. Y., and Ferguson, T. B.: Laboratory and initial clinical studies of nifedipine, a calcium antagonist for improved myocardial preservation. Ann. Surg. *193*:719, 1981.
232. Hammond, B., and Hess, M. L.: The oxygen-free radical system: Potential mediator of myocardial injury. J. Am. Coll. Cardiol. *6*:215, 1985.
233. McCord, J. M.: Oxygen-derived free radicals in postischemic tissue injury. N. Engl. J. Med. *312*:159, 1985.
233a. Ambrosio, G., Weisfeldt, M. L., Jacobus, W. E., and Flaherty, J. T.: Evidence for a reversible oxygen radical-mediated component of reperfusion injury: reduction by recombinant human superoxide dismutase administered at the time of reflow. Circulation *75*:282, 1987.
233b. Rossen, R. D., Swain, J. L., Michael, L. H., Weakley, S., Giannini, E., and Entman, M. L.: Selective accumulation of the first component of complement and leukocytes in ischemic canine heart muscle. Circ. Res. *57*:119, 1985.
234. Krause, S. M., and Hess, M. L.: Characterization of canine, cardiac sarcoplasmic reticulum function during short term, normothermic global ischemia. Circ. Res. *55*:176, 1984.
235. Shlafer, M., Kane, P. E., and Kirsh, M. M.: Superoxide dismutase plus catalase enhances the efficacy of hypothermic cardioplegia to protect the globally ischemic reperfused heart. J. Thorac. Cardiovasc. Surg. *83*:830, 1982.
236. Myers, M. L., Bolli, R., Lekich, R. F., Hartley, C. J., and Roberts, R.: Enhancement of recovery of myocardial function by oxygen free-radical scavengers after reversible regional ischemia. Circulation *72*:915, 1985.
236a. Przyklenk, K., and Kloner, R. A.: Superoxide dismutase plus catalase improve contractile function in the canine model of the "stunned myocardium." Circ. Res. *58*:148, 1986.
237. Ahumada, G., Roberts, R., and Sobel, B. E.: Evaluation of myocardial infarction with enzymatic indices. Prog. Cardiovasc. Dis. *18*:405, 1976.
238. Stone, M. J., Willerson, J. T., Gomez-Sanchez, C. E., and Waterman, M. R.: Radioimmunoassay of myoglobin in human serum: Results in patients with acute myocardial infarction. J. Clin. Invest. *56*:1334, 1975.
239. Wagner, G. S., Roe, C. R., Limbird, L. E., Rosati, R. A., and Wallace, A. G.: The importance of identification of the myocardial specific isoenzyme of creatine phosphokinase (MB form) in the diagnosis of acute myocardial infarction. Circulation *47*:263, 1973.
240. Braunwald, E., and Maroko, P. R.: Limitation of infarct size. Curr. Probl. Cardiol. *3*:51, 1978.
241. Ahmed, S. A., Williamson, J. R., Roberts, R., Clark, R. E., and Sobel, B. E.: The association of increased plasma MB CPK activity and irreversible ischemic myocardial injury in the dog. Circulation *54*:187, 1976.
242. Shell, W. E., Kjekshus, J. K., and Sobel, B. E.: Quantitative assessment of the extent of myocardial infarction in the conscious dog by means of analysis of serial changes in serum creatine phosphokinase activity. J. Clin. Invest. *50*:2614, 1971.
243. Sobel, B. E., Markam, J., Karlsberg, R. P., and Roberts, R.: The nature of disappearance of creatine kinase from the circulation and its influence on enzymatic estimation of infarct size. Circ. Res. *41*:836, 1977.
244. Geltman, E. M., Ehsani, A. A., Campbell, M. K., Schechtman, K., Roberts, R., and Sobel, B. E.: The influence of location and extent of myocardial infarction on long-term ventricular dysrhythmia and mortality. Circulation *60*:805, 1979.
245. Roberts, R., Gowda, K. S., Ludbrook, P. A., and Sobel, B. E.: Specificity of elevated serum MB creatine phosphokinase activity in the diagnosis of acute myocardial infarction. Am. J. Cardiol. *36*:433, 1975.
246. Bleifeld, W., Mathey, D., Hanrath, P., Buss, H., and Effert, S.: Infarct size estimated from serial serum creatine phosphokinase in relation to left ventricular hemodynamics. Circulation *55*:303, 1977.
247. Hackel, D. B., Reimer, K. A., Ideker, R. E., Mikat, E. M., Hartwell, T. D., Parker, C. B., Braunwald, E., Buja, M., Gold, H. K., Jaffe, A. S., Muller, J. E., Raabe, D. S., Rude, R. E., Sobel, B. E., Stone, P.H., Roberts, R., and the MILIS Study Group: Comparison of enzymatic and anatomic estimates of myocardial infarct size in man. Circulation *70*:824, 1984.
248. Mathey, D., Bleifeld, W., Hanrath, P., and Effert, S.: Attempt to quantitate relation between cardiac function and infarct size in acute myocardial infarction. Br. Heart J. *36*:271, 1974.
249. Norris, R. M., Whitlock, R. M. L., Barratt-Boyes, C., and Small, C. W.: Clinical measurement of myocardial infarct size. Modification of a method for the estimation of total creatine phosphokinase release after myocardial infarction. Circulation *51*:614, 1975.
250. Vatner, S. F., Baig, H., Manders, W. T., and Maroko, P. R.: Effects of coronary artery reperfusion on myocardial infarct size calculated from creatine kinase. J. Clin. Invest. *61*:1048, 1978.
251. Clark, G. L., Robison, A. K., Gnepp, D. R., Roberts, R., and Sobel, B. E.: Effects of lymphatic transport of enzyme on plasma CK time-activity curves after myocardial infarction. Circ. Res. *43*:162, 1978.
252. Hashimoto, H., Abendschein, D. R., Strauss, A. W., and Sobel, B. E.: Early detection of myocardial infarction in conscious dogs by analysis of plasma MM creatine kinase isoforms. Circulation *71*:363, 1985.
253. Jaffe, A. S., Serota, H, Grace, A., and Sobel, B. E.: Diagnostic changes in plasma creatine kinase isoforms early after the onset of acute myocardial infarction. Circulation *74*:105, 1986.
254. Devries, S. R., Sobel, B. E., and Abendschein, D. R.: Early detection of myocardial reperfusion by assay of plasma MM-creatine kinase isoforms in dogs. Circulation *74*:567, 1986.
255. Rude, R. E., Muller, J. E., and Braunwald, E.: Efforts to limit the size of myocardial infarcts. Ann. Intern. Med. *95*:736, 1981.
256. Maroko, P. R., Kjekshus, J. K., Sobel, B. E., Watanabe, T., Covell, J. W., Ross, J., Jr., and Braunwald, E.: Factors influencing infarct size following experimental coronary artery occlusion. Circulation *43*:67, 1971.
257. Kloner, R. A., and Braunwald, E.: Review—Observations on experimental myocardial ischemia. Cardiovasc. Res. *14*:371, 1980.
258. Shell, W. E., and Sobel, B. E.: Deleterious effects of increased heart rate on infarct size in the conscious dog. Am. J. Cardiol. *31*:474, 1973.
259. Richman, S.: Adverse effect of atropine during myocardial infarction: Enhancement of ischemia following intravenously administered atropine. J.A.M.A. *228*:1414, 1974.
260. Radvany, P., Maroko, P. R., and Braunwald, E.: Effect of hypoxemia on the extent of myocardial necrosis after experimental coronary occlusion. Am. J. Cardiol. *35*:795, 1975.
261. Yoshikawa, H., Powell, W. J., Jr., Bland, J. H. L., and Lowenstein, E.: Effect of acute anemia on experimental myocardial ischemia. Am. J. Cardiol. *32*:670, 1973.
262. DeBoer, L. W. V., Rude, R. E., Davis, R. F., Maroko, P. R., and Braunwald, E.: Extension of myocardial necrosis into normal epicardium following hypotension during experimental coronary occlusion. Cardiovasc. Res. *16*:423, 1982.
263. Libby, P., Maroko, P. R., and Braunwald, E.: The effect of hypoglycemia on myocardial ischemic injury during acute experiment coronary artery occlusion. Circulation *51*:621, 1975.

264. Leidtke, A. J., and Hughes, H. C.: Hyperthermic insult to ischemic myocardium: Implications of fever as an energy draining process in myocardial infarct. Clin. Res. *24*:227A, 1976.
265. Vatner, S. F., McRitchie, R. J., Maroko, P. R., Patrick, T. A., and Braunwald, E.: Effects of catecholamines, exercise, and nitroglycerin on the normal and ischemic myocardium in conscious dogs. J. Clin. Invest. *54*:563, 1974.
266. Maroko, P. R., Libby, P., and Braunwald, E.: Effect of pharmacologic agents on the function of the ischemic heart. Am. J. Cardiol. *32*:930, 1973.
267. Davidson, S., Maroko, P. R., and Braunwald, E.: Effects of isoproterenol on contractile function of the ischemic and anoxic heart. Am. J. Physiol. *227*:439, 1974.
268. Vatner, S. F., Millard, R. W., Patrick, T. A., and Heyndrickx, G. R.: Effects of isoproterenol on regional myocardial function, electrogram, and blood flow in conscious dogs with myocardial ischemia. J. Clin. Invest. *57*:1261, 1976.
269. Mueller, H., Ayres, S. M., Gregory, J. J., Giannelli, S., Jr., and Grace, W. J.: Hemodynamics, coronary blood flow, and myocardial metabolism in coronary shock: Response to 1-norepinephrine and isoproterenol. J. Clin. Invest. *49*:1885, 1970.
270. Shug, A., and Shrago, E.: A proposed mechanism for fatty acid effects on energy metabolism of the heart. J. Lab. Clin. Med. *81*:214, 1973.
271. Mjøs, O. D., Kjekshus, J. K., and Lekven, J.: Importance of free fatty acids as a determinant of myocardial oxygen consumption and myocardial ischemic injury during norepinephrine infusion in dogs. J. Clin. Invest. *53*:1290, 1974.
272. Kjekshus, J. K., and Mjøs, O. D.: Effect of free fatty acids on myocardial function and metabolism in the ischemic dog heart. J. Clin. Invest. *51*:1767, 1972.
273. Schaper, J., and Schaper, W.: Reperfusion of ischemic myocardium: Ultrastructural and histochemical aspects. J. Am. Coll. Cardiol. *1*:1037, 1983.
274. Ellis, S. G., Henschke, C. I., Sandor, T., Wynne, J., Braunwald, E., and Kloner, R. A.: Time course of functional and biochemical recovery of myocardium salvaged by reperfusion. J. Am. Coll. Cardiol. *1*:1047, 1983.
275. Lavallee, M., Cox, D. A., and Vatner, S. F.: Effects of coronary artery reperfusion on recovery of regional myocardial function in conscious dogs. Eur. Heart J. *6*:109, 1985.
276. Maroko, P. R., Radvany, P., Braunwald, E., and Hale, S. L.: Reduction of infarct size by oxygen inhalation following acute coronary occlusion. Circulation *52*:360, 1975.
277. Glogar, D. H., Kloner, R. A., Muller, J., DeBoer, L. W. V., and Braunwald, E.: Fluorocarbons reduce myocardial ischemic damage after coronary occlusion. Science *211*:1439, 1981.
277a. Tokioka, H., Miyazaki, A., Fung, P., Rajagopalan, R. A., Kar, S., Meerbaum, S., Corday, E., and Drury, J. K.: Effects of intracoronary infusion of arterial blood or Fluosol-DA 20% on regional myocardial metabolism and function during brief coronary artery occlusions. Circulation *75*:473, 1987.
278. Braunwald, E., Muller, J. E., Kloner, R. A., and Maroko, P. R.: Role of beta-adrenergic blockade in the therapy of patients with myocardial infarction. Am. J. Med. *74*:113, 1983.
279. Lange, R., Kloner, R. A., and Braunwald, E.: First ultrashort-acting-beta-adrenergic blocking agent: Its effect on size and segmental wall dynamics of reperfused myocardial infarcts in dogs. Am. J. Cardiol. *51*:1759, 1983.
279a. Nayler, W. G., Panagiotopoulos, S., Elz, J. S., and Sturrock, W. J.: Fundamental mechanisms of action of calcium antagonists in myocardial ischemia. Am. J. Cardiol. *59*:75B, 1987.
279b. Kloner, R. A., and Braunwald, E.: Effects of calcium antagonists on infarcting myocardium. Am. J. Cardiol. *59*:84B, 1987.
280. Henry, P. R., Shuchleib, R., Borda, L. J., Roberts, R., Williamson, J. R., and Sobel, B. E.: Effects of nifedipine on myocardial perfusion and ischemic injury in dogs. Circ. Res. *43*:372, 1978.
281. Drury, J. K., Haendchen, R. V., Meerbaum, S., Fishbein, M C., Y-Rit, J., and Corday, E.: Diltiazem improves function and reduces infarct size after acute coronary occlusion. J. Am. Coll. Cardiol. *1*:692, 1983.
282. Opie, L. H.: Metabolism of free fatty acids, glucose and catecholamines in acute myocardial infarction: Relation to myocardial ischemia and infarct size. Am. J. Cardiol. *36*:938, 1975.
283. Calva, E., Mujica, A., Bisteni, A., and Sodi-Pallares, D.: Oxidative phosphorylation in cardiac infarct: Effect of glucose-KCl-insulin solution. Am. J. Physiol. *209*:371, 1965.
284. Henry, P. D., Sobel, B. E., and Braunwald, E.: Protection of hypoxic guinea pig hearts with glucose and insulin. Am. J. Physiol. *226*:390, 1974.
285. Wildenthal, K., Mierzwiak, D. S., and Mitchell, J. H.: Acute effects of increased serum osmolality on left ventricular performance. Am. J. Physiol. *216*:898, 1969.
286. Maroko, P. R., Libby, Sobel, B. E., Bloor, C. M., Sybers, H. D., Shell, W. E., Covell, J. W., and Braunwald, E.: Effect of glucose-insulin-potassium infusion on myocardial infarction following experimental coronary artery occlusion. Circulation 45:1160, 1972.
287. Opie, L. H., Bruyneel, K., and Owen, P.: Effects of glucose, insulin, and potassium infusion on tissue metabolic changes within the first hour of myocardial infarction in the baboon. Circulation *52*:49, 975.
288. Kjekshus, J. K.: Effect of lipolytic and inotropic stimulation on myocardialischemic injury. *In* Hjalmarson, A., and Werko, L. (eds.): Experimental and Clinical Aspects on Preservation of the Ischemic Myocardium. Sweden, Molndal, 1976, p. 35.
289. Mjøs, O. D.: Effect of reduction of myocardial free fatty acid metabolism relative to that of glucose on the ischemic injury during experimental coronary artery occlusion in dogs. *In* Hjalmarson, A., and Werko, L. (eds.): Experimental and Clinical Aspects on Preservation of the Ischemic Myocardium. Sweden, Molndal, 1976, p. 29.
290. Folts, J. D., Shug, A. S., Koke, J. R., and Bittar, N.: Protection of the ischemic dog myocardium with L-carnitine. Clin. Res. *24*:217A, 1976.
291. Flores, J., DiBona, D. R., Beck, C. H., and Leaf, A.: The role of cell swelling in ischemic renal damage and the protective effect of hypertonic solute. J. Clin. Invest. *51*:118, 1972.
292. Maroko, P. R., Carpenter, C. B., Chiariello, M., Fishbein, M. C., Radvany, P., Knostman, J. B., and Hale, S. L.: Reduction by cobra venom factor of myocardial necrosis following coronary artrery occlusion. J. Clin. Invest. *61*:661, 1978.
293. Diaz, P. E., Fishbein, M. C., Davis, M. A., Askenazi, J., and Maroko, P. R.: Effect of kallikrein inhibitor aprotinin on myocardial ischemic injury following coronary artery occlusion in the dog. Am. J. Cardiol. *40*:541, 1977.
294. Libby, P., Maroko, P. R., Bloor, C. M., Sobel, B. E., and Braunwald, E.: Reduction of experimental myocardial infarct size by corticosteroid administration. J. Clin. Invest. *52*:599, 1973.
295. Masters, T. N., Harbold, N. B., Jr., Hall, D. G., Jackson, R. D., Mullen, D. C., Daugherty, H. K., and Robicsek, F.: Beneficial metabolic effects of methylprednisolone sodium succinate in acute myocardial ischemia. Am. J. Cardiol. *37*:557, 1976.
296. Hammerman, H., Kloner, R. A., Hale, S., Schoen, F. J., and Braunwald, E.: Dose-dependent effects of short-term methylprednisolone on myocardial infarct extent, scar formation, and ventricular function. Circulation *68*:446,1983.
297. Jugdutt, B. I., Hutchins, G. M., Bulkley, B. H., and Becker, L .C.: Salvage of ischemic myocardium by ibuprofen during infarction in the conscious dog. Am. J. Cardiol. *46*:74, 1980.
298. Brown, E. J., Kloner, R. A., Schoen, F. J., Hammerman, H., Hale, S., and Braunwald, E.: Scar thinning due to ibuprofen administration following experimental myocardial infarction. Am. J. Cardiol. *51*:877, 1983.
299. Willerson, J. T., Watson, J. T., and Platt, M. R.: Effect of hypertonic mannitol and intraaortic counterpulsation on regional myocardial blood flow and ventricular performance in dogs during myocardial ischemia. Am. J. Cardiol. *37*:514, 1976.
300. Maroko, P. R., Libby, P., Bloor, C. M., Sobel, B. E., and Braunwald, E.: Reduction by hyaluronidase of myocardial necrosis following coronary artery occlusion. Circulation *46*:430, 1972.
301. Wetstein, L., Simson, M. B., Haselgrove, J., Barlow, C. H., and Harken, A. H.: Mechanism of action of hyaluronidase in decreasing myocardial ischemia post coronary occlusion in the isolated perfused rabbit heart. Am. Heart J. *104*:529, 1982.
302. Myers, R. W., Scherer, J. L., Goldstein, R. A., Goldstein, R. E., Kent, K. M., and Epstein, S. E.: Effects of nitroglycerin and nitroglycerin-methoxamine during acute myocardial ischemia in dogs with preexisting multivessel coronary occlusive disease. Circulation *51*:632, 1975.
303. Kent, K. M., Smith, E. R., Redwood, D. R., and Epstein, S. E.: Beneficial electrophysiologic effects of nitroglycerin during acute myocardial infarction. Am. J. Cardiol. *33*:513, 1974.
304. Forman, R., Eng, C., and Kirk, E. S.: Comparative effect of verapamil and nitroglycerin on collateral blood flow. Circulation *67*:1200, 1983.
304a. Gallagher, K. P., Buda, A. J., Pace, D., Gerreu, R. A., and Shlafer, M.: Failure of superoxide dismutase and catalase to alter size of infarction in conscious dogs after three hours of occlusion followed by reperfusion. Circulation 73:1065, 1986.
304b. Uraizee, A., Reiner, K. A., Murry, C. E., and Jennings, R. B.: Failure of superoxide dismutase to limit size of myocardial infarction after 40 minutes of ischemia and four days of reperfusion in dogs. Circulation *75*:1237, 1987.
305. Jolly, S. R., Kane, W. J., Bailie, M. B., Abrams, G. D., and Lucchesi, B. R.: Canine myocardial reperfusion injury: Its reduction by the combined administration of superoxide dismutase and catalase. Circ. Res. *54*:277, 1984.
306. Mitsos, S. E., Askew, T. E., Fantone, J. C., Kunkel, S. L., Abrams, G. D., Schork, A., and Lucchesi, B. R.: Protective effects of N-2-mercaptopropionyl glycine against myocardial reperfusion injury after neutrophil depletion in the dog: Evidence for the role of intracellular-derived free radicals. Circulation *73*:1077, 1986.
307. Akizuki, S., Yoshida, S., Chambers, D. E., Eddy, L.J., Parmley, L. F., Yellon, D. M., and Downey, J. M.: Infarct size limitation by the xanthine oxidase inhibitor, allopurinol, in closed-chest dogs with small infarcts. Cardiovasc. Res. *19*:686, 1985.
308. Werns, S. W., Shea, M. J., Mitsos, S. E., Dysko, R. C., Fantone, J. C., Schork, M. A., Abrams, G. D., Pitt, B., and Lucchesi, B. R.: Reduction of the size of infarction by allopurinol in the ischemic-reperfused canine heart. Circulation *73*:518, 1986.
309. Romson, J. L., Hook, B. G., Kunkel, S. L., Abrams, G. D., Schork, M. A., and Lucchesi, B. R.: Reduction of the extent of ischemic myocardial injury by neutrophil depletion in the dog. Circulation *67*:1016, 1983.
310. Braunwald, E., and Kloner, R. A.: Myocardial reperfusion: A double-edged sword? J. Clin. Invest. *76*:1713, 1985.
311. Jennings, R. B., Schaper, J., Hill, M. L., Steenbergen, C., Jr., and Reimer, K. A.: Effect of reperfusion late in the phase of reversible ischemic injury: Changes in cell volume, electrolytes, metabolites, and ultrastructure. Circ. Res. *56*:262, 1985.
312. Kloner, R. A., Ellis, S. G., Lange, R., and Braunwald, E.: Studies of experimental coronary artery reperfusion: Effects on infarct size, myocardial function, biochemistry, ultrastructure, and microvascular damage. Circulation *68*(Suppl. I):8, 1983.
313. Kloner, R. A., Ellis, S.G., Carlson, N. V., and Braunwald, E.: Coronary reperfusion for the treatment of acute myocardial infarction. Postischemic ventricular dysfunction. Cardiology *70*:233, 1983.
314. Hearse, D. J.: Reperfusion of the ischemic myocardium. J. Mol. Cell. Cardiol. *9*:605, 1977.
315. Hess, M. L., and Manson, N. H.: Molecular oxygen: Friend and foe. The role of the oxygen free radical system in the calcium paradox, the oxygen paradox and ischemia/reperfusion injury. J. Mol. Cell. Cardiol. *16*:969, 1984.

38 ACUTE MYOCARDIAL INFARCTION

by RICHARD C. PASTERNAK, M.D., EUGENE BRAUNWALD, M.D., and BURTON E. SOBEL, M.D.

INTRODUCTION

Nearly 1,500,000 patients suffer from acute myocardial infarction (AMI) annually and approximately one-fourth of all deaths in the United States are due to AMI.[1] More than 60 per cent of the deaths associated with AMI occur within one hour of the event and are attributable to arrhythmias, most often ventricular fibrillation (Chap. 24). About 500,000 patients with confirmed AMI are hospitalized yearly in the U.S. and at least as many additional patients are admitted because of suspected AMI. The mortality rates during hospitalization and the year following infarction are approximately 10 per cent each. However, there is considerable variation in prognosis depending on a wide variety of clinical factors, as discussed later. In the U.S., the yearly economic burden of coronary artery disease is in excess of $100 billion.[2] Perhaps as much as half of this cost is related to myocardial infarction (MI) and its prevention and treatment.

DIMINISHING MORTALITY IN MYOCARDIAL INFARCTION. The decline in death rate from coronary artery disease (p. 1153) has been accompanied by diminished mortality from AMI. This fall in the mortality appears to be caused by two factors: a fall in the incidence of AMI by 25 per cent or more[3] and a similarly marked fall in the case fatality rate once a myocardial infarction has occurred.[3-6] The reasons for this decline in mortality have been extensively debated[7, 8]; undoubtedly they are multifactorial. According to recent estimates,[9, 10] about 40 per cent of the fall in mortality is caused by such medical interventions as coronary care units, prehospital resuscitation, and newer mechanical and medical treatments of coronary artery disease.

There is no doubt that careful monitoring of cardiac rhythm and prompt treatment of primary arrhythmias have reduced sharply the incidence of in-hospital deaths from AMI.[11] Accordingly, most deaths among patients with this condition who reach the hospital are now attributable to left ventricular failure and shock, and occur within the 3 or 4 days after the onset of infarction.[12, 13] Only a minority of in-hospital deaths now result from primary arrhythmias and most of these occur in settings in which monitoring and/or treatment is inadequate. However, arrhythmias occurring in the setting of extensive infarction and left ventricular failure (secondary arrhythmias) still represent a common cause of death.[11, 14, 15]

Before the advent of coronary care units, treatment of AMI was directed almost exclusively toward allowing healing of the infarct, preventing cardiac rupture and other complications such as pulmonary and systemic embolism, and sustaining arterial pressure and urine output. Subsequently, the major emphasis was on the prevention and aggressive treatment of arrhythmias. The concept that infarct size is an important determinant of prognosis and that its ultimate extent might be modified favorably by early implementation of selected physiological and pharmacological interventions has directed attention to the protection of jeopardized myocardium by attempts to decrease myocardial oxygen demand as well as by restoration of perfusion to ischemic tissue.[15–17] There have been recent dramatic strides, particularly in the area of thrombolytic therapy for AMI.[17–19] We are now in an era in which the management of AMI may be characterized as "aggressive,"[20] in which there is wide recognition of the dynamic nature of the infarction process, and in which technological advances are occurring rapidly. This chapter addresses the underlying pathophysiology of AMI and the resulting clinical manifestations. Rapidly evolving management strategies are discussed in this pathophysiological context.

PATHOLOGY OF ACUTE MYOCARDIAL INFARCTION

Almost all myocardial infarctions result from atherosclerosis of the coronary arteries, generally with superimposed coronary thrombosis. The genesis of the coronary atherosclerotic lesion is a complex and controversial issue (see Chap. 35), and a number of risk factors have been associated with the development of atherosclerosis (see Chap. 36). However, regardless of the etiology and pathogenesis of the atherosclerotic process, the end result is plaques that cause luminal narrowing of the coronary arterial tree and thus reduce the blood supply to the myocardium and, in many instances, a thrombus that causes further narrowing and often total occlusion. Below a certain critical level of blood flow, myocardial cells develop ischemic injury, a process described in detail in Chapter 37. When severe ischemia is prolonged, irreversible damage, i.e., MI, occurs.

Since the coronary luminal narrowing affects the major coronary arteries and their various branches to a different extent, MI usually occurs focally in specific regions of the heart. The location and size of a particular infarction depend on a number of different factors: (1) the location and severity of the atherosclerotic narrowings in the coronary arterial tree; (2) the size of the vascular bed perfused by the narrowed vessel(s); (3) the oxygen needs of the poorly perfused myocardium; (4) the extent of development of collateral blood vessels; (5) the presence, site, and severity of coronary arterial spasm; and (6) the presence of tissue factors capable of modifying the necrotic process.

GROSS PATHOLOGICAL CHANGES

Myocardial infarction may be divided into two major types: *transmural infarcts*, in which myocardial necrosis involves the full thickness of the ventricular wall, and *subendocardial (nontransmural) infarcts*, in which the necrosis involves the subendocardium, the intramural myocardium, or both without extending all the way through the ventricular wall to the epicardium (Fig. 38–1).

Acute coronary thrombosis appears to be far more common when the infarction is transmural.[21, 22] Furthermore, the histological pattern of necrosis may differ, with contraction band injury (see below) seen almost twice as often in nontransmural as in transmural infarction.[21] Transmural infarcts are more frequently localized to the zone of distribution of a single coronary artery. Nontransmural infarctions, however, frequently occur in the setting of severely narrowed but still patent coronary arteries, often in patients with pulmonary embolism, hypertension, hypotension, anemia, aortic stenosis, operative procedures, or cerebrovascular accidents. In the presence of severe atherosclerotic narrowing of the coronary arteries, these and other conditions associated with increased myocardial metabolic demands or decreased myocardial oxygen delivery or both are capable of producing patchy nontransmural myocardial necrosis, which tends to involve the subendocardium. In other instances, nontransmural infarcts appear to result from a total thrombotic occlusion that undergoes early spontaneous thrombolysis.

Myocardial infarction most commonly involves the left ventricle and interventricular septum; however, depending upon the criteria used, approximately one-third to two-thirds of patients with inferior infarction have some involvement of the right ventricle.[23–26] Among these patients, right ventricular infarction occurs exclusively in those with transmural infarction of the inferior posterior wall and the posterior portion of the septum. Although right ventricular infarction almost invariably develops in association with infarction of the adjacent septum and left ventricular myocardium, *isolated* infarction of the right ventricle is seen in 3 to 5 per cent of autopsy-proven cases of myocardial infarction, usually in patients with chronic lung disease and right ventricular hypertrophy.[27]

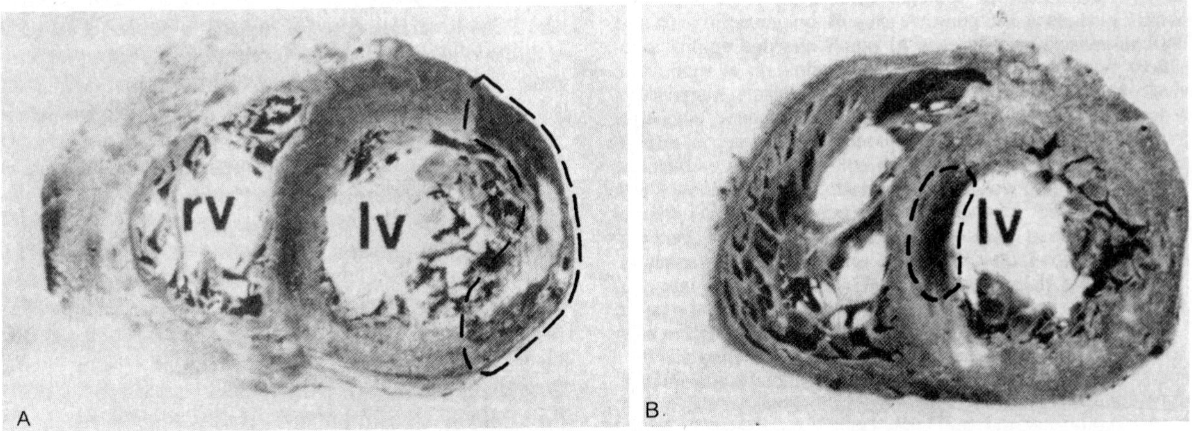

FIGURE 38–1. Transverse slices through right (rv) and left (lv) ventricle showing a transmural lateral wall infarction (*A*) and recent septal subendocardial infarction in *B*. (Infarcts outlined by ---.) (From Friedfeld, A. G., et al.: Nontransmural versus transmural myocardial infarction. A morphologic study. Am. J. Med. *75*:425, 1983.)

ATRIAL INFARCTION. This occurs in 7 to 17 per cent of autopsy-proven cases of MI,[28-31] is often seen in conjunction with left ventricular infarction, and can result in rupture of the atrial wall. This type of infarct is more common on the right than the left side[31] and occurs more frequently in the atrial appendages than in the lateral or posterior walls of the atrium. These differences in incidence might be explained by the considerably higher oxygen content of left atrial blood, which may nourish the thin atrial wall despite obstructive disease involving the coronary arterial system perfusing it. Since right atrial infarction is usually asociated with obstructive disease of the sinus node artery, it is accompanied frequently by atrial arrhythmias.

Gross changes do not appear in the myocardium until 6 hours after the onset of MI.[32, 33] Initially, the myocardium in the affected region appears pale, bluish, and slightly swollen. Eighteen to 36 hours after the onset of the infarct, the myocardium appears tan or reddish-purple, with a serofibrinous exudate evident on the epicardium in transmural infarcts. These changes persist for approximately 48 hours; the infarct then turns gray, and fine yellow lines, secondary to neutrophilic infiltration, appear at its periphery. This zone gradually widens and during the next few days extends throughout the infarct.

Eight to 10 days following infarction, the thickness of the cardiac wall in the area of the infarct is reduced as necrotic muscle is removed by mononuclear cells. The cut surface of an infarct of this age is yellow, surrounded by a reddish-purple band of granulation tissue (Fig. 38–2) that extends through the necrotic tissue by 3 to 4 weeks. Commencing at this time and extending over the next 2 to 3 months, the infarcted area gradually acquires a gelatinous, ground-glass, gray appearance, eventually converting into a shrunken, thin, firm scar, which whitens and firms progressively with time[34-36]; this process begins at the periphery of the infarct and gradually moves centrally. The endocardium below the infarct increases in thickness and becomes gray and opaque.

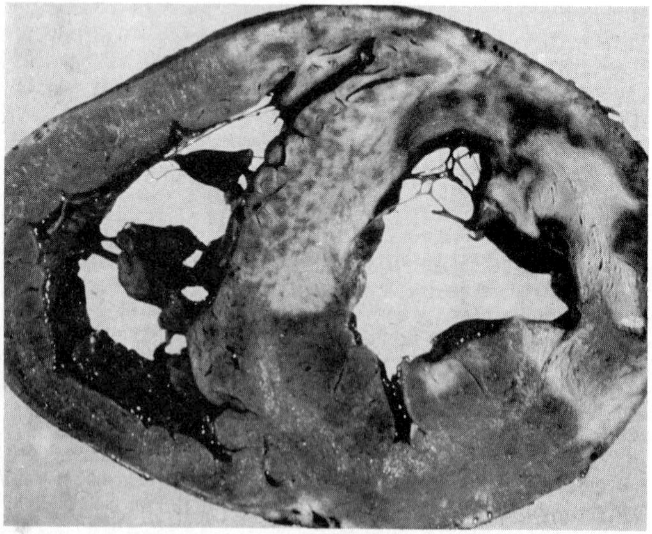

FIGURE 38–2. Acute myocardial infarct. Cross section of the heart shows myocardial infarct about a week old, involving the posterior half of the interventricular septum and the posterior lateral left ventricular walls. This infarct is secondary to occlusion of the left circumflex coronary artery. The myocardium has a mottled appearance, and the margins of the infarct are well demarcated. In the central portion of the infarct involving the posterior papillary muscle, there is evidence of hemorrhage. (From Bloor, C. M.: Cardiac Pathology. Philadelphia, J. B. Lippincott Co., 1978.)

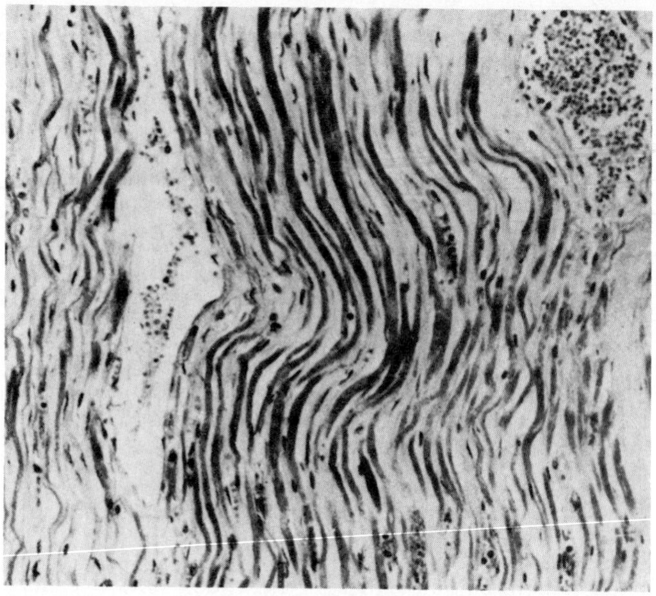

FIGURE 38–3. Wavy and stretched appearance of necrotic muscle cells in an acute myocardial infarct. The wavy myocardial fibers have pyknotic nuclei and hypereosinophilic cytoplasm. (Hematoxylin and eosin × 128). (From Willerson J. T., Hillis, L. D., and Buja, L. M. [eds.]: Pathogenesis and pathology of ischemic heart disease. *In* Ischemic Heart Disease. Clinical and Pathophysiologic Aspects. New York, Raven Press, 1982, p. 46.)

HISTOLOGICAL AND ULTRASTRUCTURAL CHANGES

LIGHT MICROSCOPY. Severe ischemia, which is potentially reversible, causes cloudy swelling, as well as hydropic, vascular, and fatty degeneration.[37] For many years it was believed that no light microscopic changes could be seen in infarcted myocardium until 8 hours after interruption of blood flow. Bouchardy and Majno, however, have called attention to a wavy pattern of myocardial cells that occurs shortly after the onset of infarction (Fig. 38–3), a pattern that is probably the result of agonal contraction of myocardial cells.[38, 39] With careful light microscopy, contraction bands and small spaces between myocardial cells are also revealed. After 8 hours, edema of the interstitium becomes evident, as do increased fatty deposits in the muscle fibers, along with infiltration of neutrophilic polymorphonuclear leukocytes and red blood cells. Muscle cell nuclei become pyknotic and then undergo karyolysis, and small blood vessels undergo necrosis.

By 24 hours there is clumping of the cytoplasm and loss of cross striations, with appearance of focal hyalinization and irregular cross bands in the involved myocardial fibers. The nuclei become pyknotic and sometimes even disappear. The myocardial capillaries in the involved region dilate, and polymorphonuclear leukocytes accumulate, first at the periphery and then in the center of the infarct.[39a] During the first 3 days, the interstitial tissue becomes edematous and red blood cells may extravasate. Generally, on about the fourth day after infarction, removal of necrotic fibers begins, again commencing at the periphery. Later, lymphocytes, macrophages, and fibroblasts infiltrate between myocytes, which become fragmented. At 8 days the necrotic muscle fibers have become dissolved; by about 10 days the number of polymorphonuclear leukocytes is reduced, and granulation tissue first appears at the periphery. Ingrowth of blood vessels and fibroblasts continues, along with removal of necrotic muscle cells, until the fourth to sixth week following infarction, by which time much of the necrotic myocardium has been removed. This process continues along with increasing collagenization of the infarcted area. By the sixth week, the infarcted area has usually been converted into a firm connective tissue scar with interspersed intact muscle fibers.[35]

HISTOCHEMISTRY. A variety of *histochemical* approaches have been used to detect myocardial changes compatible with infarction before routine microscopic changes become evident at 6 hours. These include estimation of glycogen, using a periodic acid-Schiff stain (PAS) and succinic dehydrogenase activity. Glycogen stores may become depleted within 3 to 4 hours after the onset of severe myocardial ischemia. However, the reliability of these procedures diminishes with lengthening of the interval between death and the examination of the myocardium.[33]

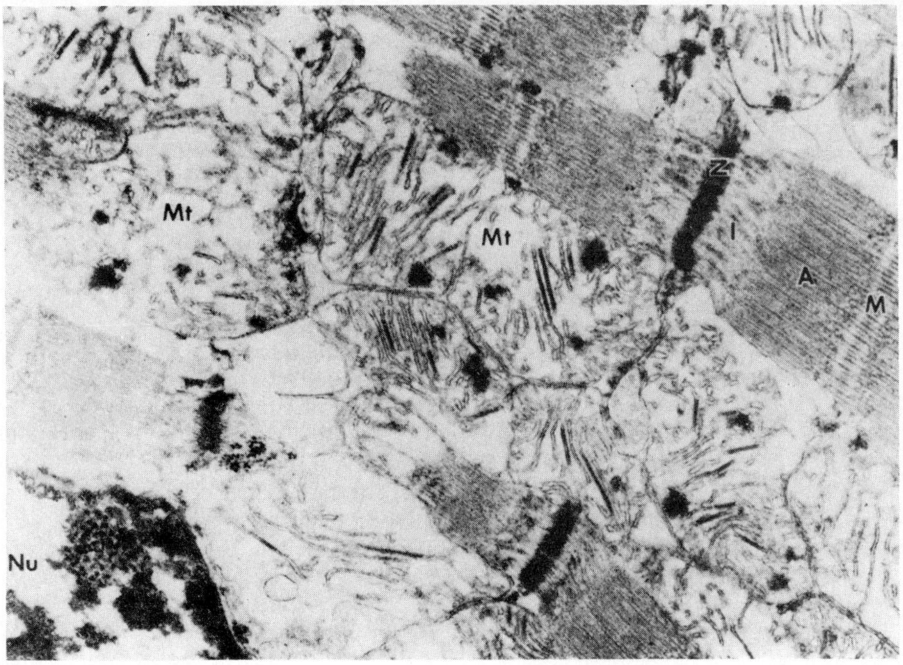

FIGURE 38–4. Electron micrograph of a muscle cell from the center of an infarct produced by permanent coronary occlusion in the dog. The myofibrils are fixed in a relaxed state and exhibit I, A, M, and Z bands. There is slight edema and no glycogen. (The clusters of granules resembling glycogen probably are ribosomes.) The mitochondria (Mt) are swollen and have linear densities and amorphous matrix (flocculent) densities. The nucleus (Nu) has clumped chromatin along the nuclear membrane and large lucent areas. (Tissue fixed with glutaraldehyde and osmium. Epoxy section stained with uranyl acetate and lead citrate, × 19,500.) (From Willerson, J. T., Hillis, L. D., and Buja, L. M. [eds.]: Pathogenesis and pathology of ischemic heart disease. *In* Ischemic Heart Disease. Clinical and Pathophysiological Aspects. New York, Raven Press, 1982, p. 47.)

One of the most useful histochemical methods is the nitro–blue tetrazolium staining technique; the heart is sliced transversely into several sections. These sections are washed and incubated in buffered tetrazolium solution, which is reduced to a dark blue compound, formazan, in viable zones of myocardium. Reduction of tetrazolium is accomplished by endogenous substrates, coenzymes, and dehydrogenases; these are absent or deficient in necrotic areas of myocardium, which therefore remain uncolored and hence identifiable. This reaction can distinguish infarcted myocardium 6 to 8 hours after the start of infarction.[40]

ELECTRONMICROSCOPY. Although the *alterations in cardiac ultrastructure* to be described are based on animal experiments and are not directly applicable to clinical diagnosis, they provide important information concerning the process of myocardial infarction. The earliest ultrastructural changes in cardiac muscle following ligation of a coronary artery, noted within 20 minutes, consist of reduction in the size and number of glycogen granules, development of intracellular edema, and swelling and distortion of the transverse tubular system, the sarcoplasmic reticulum, and the mitochondria (Fig. 38–4).[41–44] When these changes are relatively mild, they are compatible with reversible ischemic injury. Changes after 60 minutes of occlusion include myocardial cell swelling, mitochondrial abnormalities such as swelling and internal disruption, aggregation and margination of nuclear chromatin, and relaxation of myofibrils. After 20 minutes to 2 hours of ischemia, changes in some cells become irreversible, and there is progression of these alterations; additional changes include indistinct, tight junctions at the intercalated discs, swollen sacs of the sarcoplasmic reticulum at the level of the A band, greatly enlarged mitochondria with few cristae, thinning and fractionation of myofilaments, disappearance of the heterochromatin, rarefaction of the euchromatin and peripheral aggregation of chromatin in the nucleus, disorientation of myofibrils, and clumping of mitochondria. Cells irreversibly damaged by ischemia are usually swollen, with an enlarged sarcoplasmic space; the sarcolemma may peel off the cells, defects in the plasma membrane may appear, and the mitochondria are fragmented.

The swollen mitochondria obtained from ischemic myocardium contain deposits of calcium phosphate and amorphous matrix densities[45]; many of these changes become more intense when blood flow is restored.[46] However, it appears unlikely that the structural and functional deterioration of mitochondria—the hallmark of ischemic injury—is the primary mediator of myocardial cell death. In experimental infarction, reflow into an area rendered ischemic for 40 to 60 minutes results in violent cell swelling with vacuolization of myocardial cell cytoplasm and marked swelling of mitochondria. Cell membranes are lifted off the myofibrils, and subsarcolemmal blebs appear. The speed with which these morphological changes occur early after ischemic reflow suggests that ischemia produces a defect of volume regulation in myocardial cells.

PATTERNS OF MYOCARDIAL NECROSIS. Coagulation Necrosis.[47, 47a] This results from severe, persistent ischemia and is usually present in the central region of infarcts, which results in the arrest of muscle cells in the relaxed state and the passive stretching of ischemic muscle cells. On light microscopy the myofibrils are stretched, many with unclear pyknosis, with vascular congestion and healing by phagocytosis of necrotic muscle cells. There is evidence of mitochondrial damage with prominent amorphous (flocculent) densities but no calcification.

Coagulative Myocytolysis.[38, 48, 49] This form of myocardial necrosis, also termed contraction band necrosis,[50] results primarily from severe ischemia followed by reflow.[41] It is caused by increased Ca^{++} influx into dying cells, resulting in the arrest of cells in the contracted state. It is seen in the periphery of large infarcts and is present to a greater extent in nontransmural infarcts than in transmural ones.[21] The entire infarct may show this form of necrosis when reperfusion occurs experimentally[51] or by surgery[50] or thrombolysis. Its presence in a large segment of some infarcts suggests that reperfusion through spontaneous thrombolysis or the release of spasm or both have occurred. It is characterized by hypercontracted myofibrils with contraction bands and mitochondrial damage, frequently with calcification, marked vascular congestion, and healing by lysis of muscle cells.

Myocytolysis. This results from prolonged moderate ischemia and, like coagulative myocytolysis, is also frequently seen at the borders of an infarct as well as in patchy areas of infarction in patients with chronic ischemic heart disease. It is characterized by edema and cell swelling, early lysis of myofibrils, late lysis of nuclei, no neutrophilic response, and healing by lysis and phagocytosis of necrotic myocytes.[36, 48]

CORONARY ANATOMY AND PATHOLOGICAL ANATOMY

The importance of coronary artery obstruction has been the subject of much controversy since 1912 when Herrick proposed that AMI was due to occlusion of an epicardial coronary artery.[52] In the 3 decades following Herrick's description of the condition, the clinical manifestations of myocardial infarction were believed to stem from sudden coronary arterial occlusion, usually due to thrombosis; hence the terms *coronary thrombosis* and *acute myocardial infarction* became almost synonymous. One weakness of this concept was shown by Blumgart and colleagues, who demonstrated that *coronary occlusion could occur in the absence of infarction*, when the collateral circulation was adequate to maintain myocardial nutrition.[53] Equally important, Friedberg and Horn observed that *infarction could occur in the absence of coronary occlusion*.[54] The patients whom they described had severe coronary arterial narrowing. The areas of patchy, subendocardial infarction which occurred were thought to have developed secondary to relative insufficiency of coronary blood flow. Miller et al. then expanded on these observations, demonstrating that predominantly subendocardial infarcts were rarely associated with coronary occlusion, whereas transmural infarctions were frequently so.[55]

Coronary arteriographic studies have clarified the usual pathological anatomy associated with AMI. Generally, in patients with MI who come to necropsy, more than one coronary artery is severely narrowed.[36, 56] One-third to two-thirds of patients with AMI have critical obstruction (to less than 25 per cent of luminal area) of all three coronary arteries, whereas the remainder are equally divided between those having one-vessel disease and those having two-vessel disease.[57, 58] Most transmural infarcts occur distal to a totally occluded coronary artery. However, the converse is not the case, in that total occlusion of a coronary artery is not always associated with myocardial infarction. Collateral blood flow and other factors—such as the level of myocardial metabolism, the presence and location of stenoses in other coronary arteries, the rate of development of the obstruction, and the quantity of myocardium supplied by the obstructed vessel—all influence the viability of myocardial cells distal to the occlusion. In many series of patients studied at necropsy or by coronary arteriography, a small number (< 5 per cent) of patients with MI are found to have normal coronary vessels.[36, 56–58] In these patients, an embolus that has lysed or a prolonged episode of severe coronary spasm may have been responsible for the reduction in coronary flow.

Obstruction of the left anterior descending coronary artery usually causes infarction or threatens the viability of the anterior and apical regions of the left ventricle; portions of the septum, anterolateral wall, papillary muscles, and inferoapical wall of the left ventricle may also be involved. Obstruction of the left circumflex artery can cause infarction of the lateral or inferoposterior wall of the left ventricle, whereas occlusion of the right coronary artery usually results in infarction of the inferoposterior wall of the left ventricle, the inferior portions of the septum, and posteromedial papillary muscle, and portions of the right ventricle. The size of the infarction and its location depend on the distribution of the obstructed coronary vessels. Thus, with occlusion of a dominant right coronary artery which supplies the posterior descending artery and posterior left ventricular wall, the inferoposterior wall of the left ventricle becomes infarcted, whereas the same region of the myocardium becomes involved with occlusion of the left circumflex coronary artery in the presence of a dominant left coronary artery.

RIGHT VENTRICULAR INFARCTION. Regardless of whether or not it is combined with involvement of the left ventricle, right ventricular infarction is generally associated with obstructive lesions of the right coronary artery. However, right ventricular infarction occurs less commonly than would be anticipated from the frequency of atherosclerotic lesions involving the right coronary artery.[59] This discrepancy probably can be explained by the lower oxygen demands of the right ventricle, since right ventricular infarcts occur more commonly in conditions such as pulmonary hypertension associated with increased right ventricular needs.[29] Moreover, the intercoronary collateral system of the right ventricle is richer than that of the left, and the thinness of the right ventricular wall allows the chamber to derive some nutrition from the blood within the right ventricular cavity.

Rather frequently, when an area of the ventricle is perfused by collateral vessels, an infarct occurs at a distance from a coronary occlusion. For example, following the gradual obliteration of the lumen of the right coronary artery, the inferior wall of the left ventricle may be maintained viable by collateral vessels arising from the left anterior descending coronary artery. In this circumstance, an occlusion of the left anterior descending artery may cause an infarct of the diaphragmatic wall.

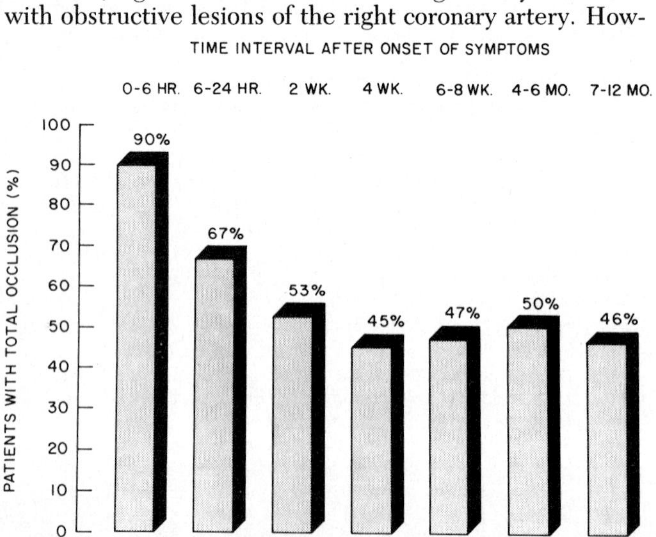

FIGURE 38–5. Percentage of patients with total coronary occlusion at different time intervals after the onset of symptoms of AMI. (Adapted from deFeyter, P. J., van den Brand, M., Serruys, P. W., and Wijns, W.: Early angiography after myocardial infarction: What have we learned? Am. Heart J. *109*:194, 1985.)

CORONARY THROMBOSIS

Conclusions drawn from autopsy studies of the coronary arteries following AMI are limited by both the selection bias (obviously only patients who die can be studied), and by postmorten events, including lysis of clots that were present premortem. For many years coronary angiography was avoided in the acute phases of MI because of potential complications.[60, 61] Experience of the last decade, however, has shown that angiography is safe even during the acute phase of MI.[62] Angiographic studies performed in the earliest hours of transmural MI have revealed an approximate 90 per cent incidence of total occlusion in the infarct-related vessel.[62–64] Recanalization from spontaneous thrombolysis[65–67] as well as attrition due to some mortality among those patients with total occlusion results in a diminishing incidence of totally occluded vessels found in the period following myocardial infarction (Fig. 38–5).[57, 62, 65, 68]

Occlusion of a coronary artery leading to MI appears to be the final common pathway resulting from a complex and dynamic interaction among coronary atherosclerosis, vasospasm, and platelet activation, ultimately leading to coronary artery thrombosis.[36, 69–71a]

CORONARY ATHEROSCLEROSIS IN MYOCARDIAL INFARCTION. Roberts has quantified the extent and severity of atherosclerosis in autopsied patients with a history of MI.[56, 72, 73] The entire length of the epicardial coronary tree was examined by dividing each coronary artery into 5-mm segments and assessing a cross-sectional area of each segment. The extent of severe narrowing (76 to 100 per cent) was largely unpredictable from clinical factors and varied between roughly 20 and 45 per cent of all coronary artery segments. Of the remaining segments without severe stenosis, approximately two-thirds showed moderate stenoses (51 to 75 per cent) and one-third, mild stenoses (26 to 50 per cent). Less than 6 per cent of segments examined were 25 per cent narrowed or less. Thus, the atherosclerotic processes were virtually ubiquitous in most patients with MI. However, as in all studies carried out at necropsy, the results apply only to patients who have died. Less advanced atherosclerosis may be present in survivors.

The atherosclerotic plaques that are associated with thrombosis and a total occlusion, located in infarct-related vessels, are generally more complex and irregular than those in vessels not associated with MI.[74] Histological studies of these lesions often reveal plaque rupture or fissuring (Fig. 38–6).[75, 76] Angiographic morphology suggestive of plaque rupture has been identified in the majority of stenoses associated with AMI or abrupt onset of unstable angina.[77, 78] This finding is rare in the noninfarct-related vessels of AMI patients and in the vessels of patients with chronic stable angina pectoris.[78] While controversy exists regarding the exact role that plaque rupture plays in the sequence of events leading to coronary artery occlusion, it is probable that hemorrhage into

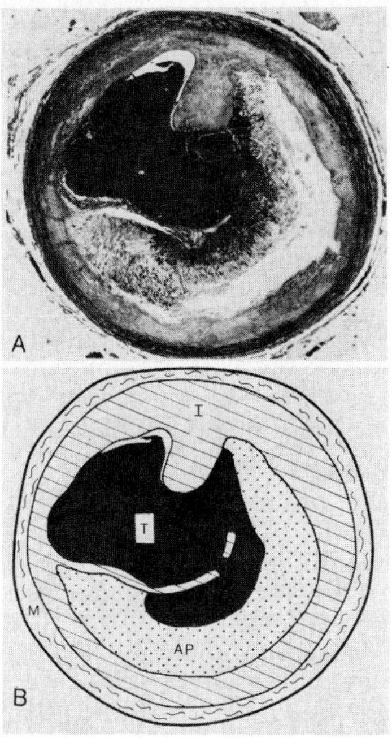

FIGURE 38–6. Histological cross section of a major plaque rupture (*a*) and accompanying diagram (*b*). The plaque (AP) has a large defect in the fibrous cap, through which a dumb bell mass of thrombus has formed, part being within the plaque and part virtually occluding the lumen. (From Davies, M. J., and Thomas, A. C.: Plaque fissuring—the cause of acute myocardial infarction, sudden ischemic death, and crescendo angina. Br. Heart J. *53*:363, 1985.)

an atherosclerotic plaque can initiate a chain of events leading to coronary artery thrombus in MI.[71, 76]

Roberts has pointed out that (1) in patients with *fatal* ischemic heart disease, the lumina of at least two of the three major coronary arteries are usually narrowed by more than 75 per cent by atherosclerotic plaques; (2) the atherosclerotic process is limited to the epicardial arteries and spares the intramural vessels; and (3) the degree of luminal narrowing by atherosclerotic plaques is similar irrespective of the type of fatal coronary event.[79]

While it is now clear that transmural MI usually is caused by coronary thrombosis, the precise pathophysiological sequence leading from coronary atherosclerosis to MI is not precisely understood.[69–71] The incidence of coronary thrombosis in subendocardial infarction is less clear, because angiographic studies provide only indirect evidence of thrombosis. The results of postmortem studies are difficult to interpret because thrombi can undergo organization or recanalization that makes their pathological characteristics indistinguishable from nonocclusive atherosclerotic plaques.[79, 80] Angiographic studies have suggested a wide variability in the frequency of coronary thrombosis with nontransmural infarction ranging from 20 to nearly 90 per cent.[17, 22, 81] The increasingly persuasive evidence that thrombosis plays a major role in patients with unstable ischemic syndromes[77, 78, 81] suggests that previous estimates of the incidence of thrombosis in nontransmural MI may have been less than the true frequency.

Rarely, coronary thrombosis may cause multifocal or circumferential infarction. However, the latter is more often the consequence of a severe imbalance between myocardial oxygen supply and demand when multiple high-grade fixed atherosclerotic lesions exist and myocardial oxygen demand is increased by such causes as tachycardia, increased ventricular wall tension, and increased myocardial contractility.

The rapidity with which thrombosis develops and the extent of coronary collaterals can determine whether acute coronary occlusion causes a transmural infarct, a subendocardial infarct, or no infarct.[41]

COMPOSITION OF THROMBI. At necropsy, coronary arterial thrombi, which are approximately 1 cm in length in most cases,[55] adhere to the luminal surface of an artery and are composed of platelets, fibrin, erythrocytes, and leukocytes. The composition of the thrombus may vary at different levels: A white thrombus is composed of platelets, fibrin, or both distally, and a red thrombus is composed of erythrocytes, fibrin, platelets, and leukocytes proximally. Early thrombi are usually small and nonocclusive and are composed almost exclusively of platelets.

In patients with MI, coronary thrombi are usually superimposed on or adjacent to atherosclerotic plaques. It has been suggested that degenerative changes in the atherosclerotic intima damage supportive perivascular tissue with resultant rupture of a plaque, sometimes accompanied by intramural hemorrhage.[41] This process may enlarge the volume of the plaque so that it occludes the arterial lumen without the occurrence of thrombosis, or the fissuring may disrupt the intima covering the plaque, thereby exposing collagen to flowing blood, a strong stimulus for thrombus formation.[75, 76, 82] Thus a possible mechanism for coronary thrombosis is ulceration or erosion of an atherosclerotic plaque with resultant exposure of collagen and other thrombogenic materials to the bloodstream.[69–71]

THE UNSTABLE PLAQUE. Angiographic studies have suggested that ulceration and plaque fissuring can be radiographically characterized as stenoses showing irregular borders and intraluminal lucencies. (The latter may be due to thrombus associated with the atherosclerotic lesion.) It has also been theorized that an angiographic pattern suggesting disruption of the atherosclerotic plaque is associated with histopathological evidence of coronary thrombosis as well as being associated with the clinical syndromes of unstable angina (p. 1353) and AMI.[71a, 74, 76–78, 83]

ROLE OF PLATELETS AND COAGULATION FACTORS. While it is increasingly clear that platelets play an important role in the pathogenesis of atherosclerosis (Chap. 35), their precise *causal* role in MI remains controversial (p. 2759). It is quite likely that they are involved in the pathogenesis of coronary thrombosis.[69, 70, 84] Radiolabeled platelets incorporated into coronary thrombi have been identified scintigraphically in patients with AMI.[85, 86] When atherosclerotic plaques undergo the changes noted above, exposed collagen leads to prompt platelet adhesion followed by formation of platelet aggregates, release of platelet granular constituents, and possible microembolization. The platelet in AMI has been characterized as hyperaggregable; this phenomenon is probably related to the production, by aggregating platelets, of increased amounts of thromboxane A_2 (a potent platelet-aggregating prostaglandin that is also a powerful vasoconstrictor).[69, 87, 88]

An imbalance in the clotting system between prothrombotic activity and the fibrinolytic system may also be related to the development of AMI. A hypercoagulable state may lead to MI in some patients who do not have atherosclerotic lesions (see below). A reduced fibrinolytic capacity due to the presence of a plasma inhibitor of tissue plasminogen activator may be important in the pathogenesis of AMI in certain patients.[89]

TEMPORAL CORRELATIONS. In order to define the precise relationship between coronary thrombosis and AMI, it is important to know the time course of thrombus formation in relation to the onset of infarction. Unfortunately, estimates of the age of coronary thrombi and myocardial infarction by histological criteria may be quite imprecise,[79, 90, 91] but several lines of evidence suggest that a thrombus is present acutely. As already noted, studies in which coronary arteriography performed on patients within the first few hours after the onset of AMI have demonstrated that the coronary artery supplying the area of evolving infarction is totally occluded in the majority of these individuals.[62, 63, 92–95] If fibrinolytic agents are infused into the occluded artery, patency is achieved in a high percentage of cases. Angiography performed after fibrinolytic therapy usually demonstrates residual high-grade stenotic lesions at the site where coronary arterial occlusion had existed. Fresh thrombi have been recovered from the majority of patients with acute myocardial infarction undergoing emergency coronary bypass surgery,[62] and have been directly visualized through coronary angioscopy in the setting of unstable angina, a condition that frequently precedes the development of AMI.[77, 96]

CORONARY ARTERY SPASM

In addition to causing AMI in rare patients with normal coronary arteries (see below), coronary artery spasm may also play a broader role in patients with atherosclerotic coronary artery disease[71a, 97] (p. 294). It has been postulated that spasm may cause intimal damage that can initiate formation of an atherosclerotic plaque.[98–100] Epicardial coronary artery spasm has been identified in patients with fixed atherosclerotic coronary artery stenosis before, during, and after AMI.[101–103] An association between coronary artery spasm and coronary artery thrombosis has also been documented clinically.[104, 105]

In the setting of AMI, there is evidence of increased production of vasodilating and vasoconstricting prostaglandins,[86, 106] but it appears that the vasoconstricting activity of thromboxane A_2 predominates.[69, 87] Thus, the presence of thromboxane A_2 or other vasoconstricting substances released by the aggregating platelets at the site of a coronary artery stenosis has the potential to initiate or maintain coronary artery constriction. It may be responsible for some observed cases of coronary artery spasm occurring with and perhaps contributing to the pathogenesis of AMI. Postulated interactions of spasm with platelet aggregation and coronary artery thrombosis are outlined in Figure 38–7.

COLLATERAL CIRCULATION

Normal hearts contain an extensive network of interarterial anastomotic blood vessels, greater than 60 μm in diameter, involving epicardial, intramyocardial, and subendocardial connections. This collateral circulation exists

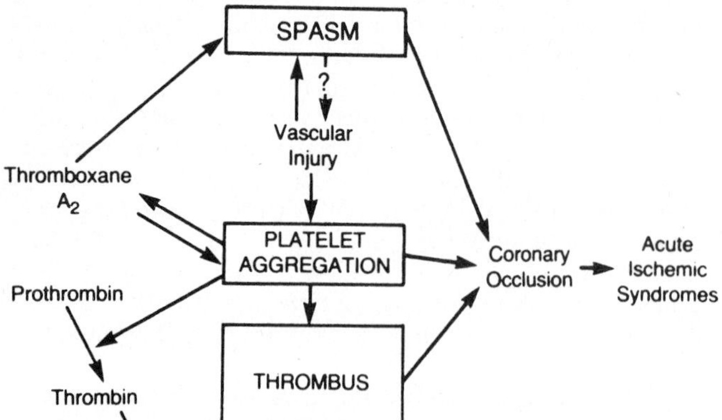

FIGURE 38–7. The interrelationship of dynamic mechanisms that may cause or contribute to the clinical presentation of acute ischemic syndromes. (From Epstein, S. E., and Palmeri, S. T.: Mechanisms contributing to precipitation of unstable angina and myocardial infarction: Implications regarding therapy. Am. J. Cardiol. *54*:1245, 1984.)

at birth and apparently grows in size along with the rest of the coronary circulation but is beyond the limit of resolution of coronary arteriographic techniques and is not seen in living subjects without disease. In patients with coronary artery disease, these preexisting channels progressively enlarge, presumably as a consequence of the release of local vasodilators; flow through the collaterals will occur when pressure differences exist across these channels.[107] The coronary collateral circulation is particularly well developed in patients with (1) coronary occlusive disease, especially when it is severe, with the reduction of the luminal cross-sectional area by more than 75 per cent in one or more major vessels; (2) chronic hypoxia, as occurs in severe anemia, chronic obstructive pulmonary disease, and cyanotic congenital heart disease; and (3) left ventricular hypertrophy, which intensifies coronary collaterals.

There is considerable variability in the development of collateral channels that exists among patients with comparable degrees of coronary artery disease. Although the increases in the collateral circulation in patients with ischemic heart disease are due primarily to enlargement of already existing anastomoses, the possibility exists that new anastomotic channels are formed during the reparative phase following AMI.

CORONARY COLLATERALS IN ACUTE MYOCARDIAL INFARCTION. Early angiography in patients with AMI and the performance of serial catheterizations for trials on the effects of reperfusion in these patients have allowed for more careful study of the angiographic appearance of collaterals. Although well-developed collaterals are not the rule at the time of infarction, some collaterals are seen in nearly 40 per cent of patients with an acute total occlusion,[108] and more begin to appear soon after the total occlusion occurs.[22, 109, 110] The incidence of collaterals 1 to 2 weeks following AMI varies considerably and may be as high as 85 to 100 per cent in patients with persistent total occlusions of the infarct vessel, or as low as 17 to 42 per cent in patients with subtotal occlusions.[22, 109–111]

That the appearance of collaterals is closely related to the presence of a totally occluded vessel has been shown by studies at the time of coronary angioplasty. These studies have allowed for the demonstration that filling of collaterals improves within 1 to 2 minutes of a sudden temporary coronary artery occlusion induced by an angioplasty balloon.[112, 113] Likewise, a total occlusion induced by transient coronary artery spasm may allow for the visualization of collaterals not seen before the spasm.[114] It is likely that the presence of a high-grade stenosis (> 90 per cent), possibly with periods of intermittent total occlusion, permits the development of collaterals that remain only as *potential* conduits until a total occlusion occurs or recurs. The latter event then brings these channels into full operation.

Supporting the argument in favor of a functional role for coronary collateral vessels is the finding that in patients with coronary occlusion and collaterals the area of myocardial necrosis is frequently smaller than the area supplied by an occluded coronary artery when collaterals are not present.[111, 115] Indeed, it is rather common for patients with abundant collaterals to have totally occluded coronary arteries without evidence of infarction in the distribution of that coronary vessel; thus, the survival of the myocardium distal to such occlusions must be dependent on collateral blood flow.

In conclusion, collateral coronary vessels, present from birth, frequently enlarge and may become functional in the presence of severe myocardial hypoxia or ischemia and following acute coronary occlusion and MI. Although blood flow through collaterals may be capable of contributing importantly to the maintenance of the resting energy requirements of the heart, and although the collaterals may limit infarct size in the face of total coronary occlusion and thereby contribute to patient survival, blood flow through collaterals is not sufficient to meet the needs of the myocardium when the latter are augmented by stress or to prevent myocardial necrosis in the majority of instances.[107, 111, 116]

NONATHEROSCLEROTIC CAUSES OF ACUTE MYOCARDIAL INFARCTION

Numerous pathological processes other than atherosclerosis can, on occasion, involve the coronary arteries and

TABLE 38–1 CAUSES OF MYOCARDIAL INFARCTION WITHOUT CORONARY ATHEROSCLEROSIS

Coronary Artery Disease Other Than Atherosclerosis
Arteritis
Luetic
Granulomatous (Takayasu's disease)
Polyarteritis nodosa
Mucocutaneous lymph node (Kawasaki's) syndrome
Disseminated lupus erythematosus
Rheumatoid arthritis
Ankylosing spondylitis
Trauma to coronary arteries
Laceration
Thrombosis
Iatrogenic
Coronary mural thickening with metabolic diseases or intimal proliferative disease
Mucopolysaccharidoses (Hurler's disease)
Homocystinuria
Fabry's disease
Amyloidosis
Juvenile intimal sclerosis (idiopathic arterial calcification of infancy)
Intimal hyperplasia associated with contraceptive steroids or with the postpartum period
Pseudoxanthoma elasticum
Coronary fibrosis caused by radiation therapy
Luminal narrowing by other mechanisms
Spasm of coronary arteries (Prinzmetal's angina with normal coronary arteries)
Spasm after nitroglycerin withdrawal
Dissection of the aorta
Dissection of the coronary artery
Mucocutaneous lymph node syndrome (Kawasaki's disease)
Emboli to Coronary Arteries
Infective endocarditis
Prolapse of mitral valve
Mural thrombus from left atrium, left ventricle
Prosthetic valve emboli
Cardiac myxoma
Associated with cardiopulmonary bypass surgery and coronary arteriography
Paradoxical emboli
Papillary fibroelastoma of the aortic valve ("fixed embolus")
Congenital Coronary Artery Anomalies
Anomalous origin of left coronary from pulmonary artery
Left coronary artery from anterior sinus of Valsalva
Coronary arteriovenous and arteriocameral fistulas
Coronary artery aneurysms
Myocardial Oxygen Demand-Supply Disproportion
Aortic stenosis, all forms
Incomplete differentiation of the aortic valve
Aortic insufficiency
Carbon monoxide poisoning
Thyrotoxicosis
Prolonged hypotension
Hematological (in situ Thrombosis)
Polycythemia vera
Thrombocytosis
Disseminated intravascular coagulation
Hypercoagulability
Hypercoagulability, thrombosis, thrombocytopenic purpura
Miscellaneous
Cocaine abuse
Myocardial contusion
Myocardial infarction with normal coronary arteries

Modified from Cheitlin, M., et al.: Myocardial infarction without atherosclerosis. J.A.M.A. *231*:951, 1975. Copyright 1975, American Medical Association.

result in myocardial infarction (Table 38–1).[117] For example, coronary arterial occlusions can be the result of embolization of a coronary artery. Emboli most frequently lodge in the distribution of the left anterior descending coronary artery, commonly in the distal epicardial and intramural branches.[55] The causes of coronary embolism are numerous: infective and marantic endocarditis (Chap. 34), mural thrombi, prosthetic valves, and calcium deposits from manipulation of calcified valves at operation (Chap. 33). In situ thrombosis of coronary arteries can occur secondary to chest-wall trauma (Chap. 45). Oral contraceptive use probably is associated with AMI in healthy women,[118, 119] although this point remains controversial.[120] The mechanism of this association may operate through an increased tendency for thrombosis.

A variety of inflammatory processes can be responsible for coronary artery abnormalities, some of which mimic atherosclerotic disease and may predispose to true atherosclerosis.[121] There is suggestive epidemiological evidence that viral infections, particularly with coxsackie B, may be an uncommon cause of MI.[122] Viral illnesses precede AMI occasionally in young persons who are later shown to have normal coronary arteries.[122–124]

Syphilitic aortitis may produce marked narrowing or occlusion of one or both coronary ostia,[125] whereas Takayasu's arteritis may result in obstruction of the coronary arteries (Chap. 46).[126] Necrotizing arteries, polyarteritis nodosa,[127] mucocutaneous lymph node syndrome (Kawasaki's disease) (p. 1014),[128] systemic lupus erythematosus,[129] and syphilis can cause coronary occlusion. Therapeutic levels of mediastinal radiation can cause thickening and hyalinization of the walls of coronary arteries, with subsequent infarction.[130] MI may also be the result of coronary arterial involvement in amyloidosis (p. 1431), Hurler syndrome, pseudoxanthoma elasticum, and homocystinuria (Chap 54).[131]

Involvement of the small coronary arteries (0.1 to 1.0 mm in diameter) by a number of disease processes may produce intimal and medial hyperplasia, necrosis, dissection, and thrombosis,[132] resulting in occlusions that produce *focal* areas of infarction and ultimately of fibrosis. Depending on the location and extent of the fibrotic reaction, arrhythmias, conduction defects, heart block, and heart failure can occur.

As *cocaine abuse* has become more common, reports of AMI following the use of cocaine have appeared with increasing frequency. Cocaine may cause AMI in patients with normal coronary arteries,[133, 134, 134a] preexisting MI,[135] documented coronary artery disease,[136–138] or known coronary artery spasm.[139] Recurrent MI after further cocaine abuse has been reported as well.[133, 138] Cocaine may cause MI by two mechanisms: (1) increasing myocardial oxygen demand via increases in heart rate and blood pressure, and (2) diminishing coronary artery flow resulting from either coronary vasospasms and/or thrombosis.[134] In very high doses, cocaine appears to have a direct toxic effect on heart muscle that may produce cardiac failure and sudden death.[140, 141]

MYOCARDIAL INFARCTION WITH ANGIOGRAPHICALLY NORMAL CORONARY VESSELS

Approximately 6 per cent of all patients with AMI and perhaps four times that percentage of patients with this diagnosis under the age of 35 years do not have coronary atherosclerosis demonstrated by coronary arteriography or at autopsy.[57, 67] Perhaps half the patients of this group, in turn, have a variety of other lesions involving the coronary vessels or myocardium (Table 38–1), whereas the others have no detectable coronary obstructive lesions.[142–144] Patients with AMI and normal coronary arteries tend to be young and to have relatively few coronary risk factors, except that they often have a history of cigarette smoking.[145–147] Usually they have no history of angina pectoris prior to the infarction.[148] The infarction in these patients is usually not preceded by any prodrome, but the clinical, laboratory, and electrocardiographic features of AMI are otherwise indistinguishable from those present in the overwhelming majority of patients with AMI who have classic obstructive atherosclerotic coronary artery disease. In patients without coronary obstruction, the prognosis for survival of the acute event is usually excellent, but a few fatalities have occurred; therefore it has been possible to document the presence of this syndrome at autopsy.[144, 149] In 10 such patients, infarcts ranged from 5 to 33 per cent (mean of 18 per cent) of the left ventricle.[149] No thromboembolic material was seen in the coronary arterial tree despite the fact that the infarcts were only 2 days old in five patients and 3 or 4 days old in three others.

In patients who recover, areas of localized dyskinesis and hypokinesis can often be demonstrated by left ventricular angiography. One patient having angiographically normal coronary arteries after thrombolytic therapy for AMI was found to have a 75 per cent atherosclerotic narrowing of the infarct-related artery at autopsy 4 months later.[150] At least nine patients have been described as having both occlusion of the infarct-related artery during the acute phase of MI and normal coronary arteries during the convalescent phase.[146] In most cases, the initial total occlusion appears to have been due to thrombosis as thrombolytic therapy was used to produce complete recanalization. In several cases, a component of spasm was probably present because the process was partially reversed by nitroglycerin.

POSSIBLE MECHANISMS. Coronary Spasm. Numerous theories have been proposed to explain the occurrence of AMI in patients with normal coronary arteriograms. Patients with vasospastic angina are clearly at risk for MI: coronary spasm has been shown to cause MI in some patients with normal coronary arteries.[101, 103, 105, 151] The administration of agents that provoke coronary artery spasm has been reported to cause MI in patients with normal coronary arteries,[152] and withdrawal of chronic nitrate vasodilation is presumably responsible for MI in others.[153] However, spasm may be induced in only a minority of patients with MI and normal coronary arteries.[145–147, 154] Intracoronary vasodilators often have no effect when administered acutely in MI, even when patients are later (after thrombolysis) shown to have normal coronary arteries. It is attractive to hypothesize that many of these cases are caused by combined coronary artery spasm and thrombosis, perhaps with underlying endothelial irregularities or small plaques that are not apparent on coronary angiography.[105, 146, 155]

Other Causes. Additional suggested causes include (1) coronary emboli (perhaps from a small mural thrombus, a prolapsed mitral valve,[156] or a myxoma); (2) coronary artery disease in vessels too small to be visualized by coronary arteriography or coronary arterial thrombosis with subsequent recanalization (Table 38–1); (3) a variety of hematological disorders causing in situ thrombosis in the presence of normal coronary arteries[144] (polycythemia vera, cyanotic heart disease with polycythemia,[157] sickle cell anemia,[158] disseminated intravascular coagulation, thrombocytosis, and thrombotic thrombocytopenic purpura); (4) augmented oxygen needs; and (5) hypotension secondary to sepsis, blood loss, or pharmacological agents and anatomical variations such as anomalous origin of a coronary artery (p. 927) and coronary arteriovenous fistula (p. 927).

PROGNOSIS. The long-term outlook for patients who have survived an AMI with normal coronary vessels on arteriography appears to be substantially better than for patients with MI and obstructive coronary artery disease.[142–145, 149, 159] Following recovery from the initial infarct, recurrent infarction, heart failure, and death are unusual in patients with normal coronary arteries. Indeed, most of these individuals have normal exercise electrocardiograms[160] and only a minority develop angina pectoris.

PATHOPHYSIOLOGY OF ACUTE MYOCARDIAL INFARCTION

SYSTOLIC FUNCTION

The fundamental pathological alteration underlying left ventricular dysfunction in AMI is loss of functioning segments of myocardium. Depression of cardiac function in myocardial infarction is directly related to the extent of left ventricular damage.[161] Cessation of blood flow to a region of myocardium produces four sequential abnormal contraction patterns[162]: (1) *dyssynchrony*, dissociation in the time course of contraction of adjacent segments of myocardial segments; (2) *hypokinesis*, reduction in the extent of shortening; (3) *akinesis*, cessation of shortening; and (4) *dyskinesis*, paradoxical expansion, systolic bulging.[163, 164] Accompanying dysfunction of the infarcting segment is initial *hyperkinesis* of the remaining normal myocardium in the intact ventricle.[165] This increased motion of the noninfarcted region subsides within 2 weeks of infarction. It is thought to be the result of acute compensatory mechanisms including the Frank-Starling mechanism and increased levels of circulating catecholamines (p. 1233).[165] If a sufficient amount of myocardium undergoes ischemic injury, left ventricular pump function becomes depressed, and cardiac output, stroke volume, blood pressure, and peak dP/dt are reduced.[161, 164] The paradoxical systolic expansion of an area of ventricular myocardium decreases the stroke output of the left ventricle. With the passage of time, edema and cellular infiltration and ultimately fibrosis increase the stiffness of the infarcted myocardium back to and beyond control values.[166] Increasing stiffness in the infarcted zone of myocardium improves left ventricular function, since it prevents systolic paradoxical wall motion.

Areas with reduced and absent wall motion are universally seen in patients with transmural AMI. Rackley and collaborators have demonstrated a linear relationship between specific parameters of left ventricular function and clinical symptoms.[167] The earliest abnormality is a reduction in diastolic distensibility, which can be observed with infarcts that involve only 8 per cent of the total left ventricle on angiographic examination. When the abnormally contracting segment exceeds 10 per cent, the ejection fraction is reduced; with 15 per cent involvement, elevations of left ventricular end-diastolic pressure and volume occur. Clinical heart failure accompanies areas of abnormal contraction exceeding 25 per cent, and cardiogenic shock, often fatal, accompanies loss of more than 40 per cent of the left ventricular myocardium.[167]

Unless extension of the infarct occurs, some improvement in abnormal wall motion takes place during the healing phase, as recovery of function occurs in initially reversibly injured myocardium. Regardless of the age of the infarct, patients who continue to demonstrate abnormal wall motion of 20 to 25 per cent of the left ventricle manifest hemodynamic signs of left ventricular failure.[168] Physical signs and symptoms of left ventricular failure also increase proportional to increasing areas of abnormal left ventricular wall motion.[164] The findings are of interest in view of the experimental work of Pfeffer et al., who produced infarcts of varying sizes and studied left ventricular performance 3 weeks later.[161] Rats with relatively small infarcts (< 30 per cent of the left ventricle) had no detectable impairment of function; those with moderate-sized infarcts (31 to 46 per cent) exhibited normal baseline measurements but inadequate responses to hemodynamic stresses; rats with large infarcts (> 46 per cent) uniformly exhibited left ventricular failure.

Patients with AMI often also show reduced myocardial contractile function in noninfarcted zones of myocardium.[169] This may result from obstruction of the coronary artery supplying this region of the ventricle, which is perfused by collaterals from the vessel that becomes occluded, a condition that has been termed *ischemia at a distance*.[170] Conversely, the presence of collaterals developing before MI may allow for greater preservation of regional systolic function in an area of distribution of the occluded artery[111, 171] and improvement in left ventricular ejection fraction early after infarction.[110]

DIASTOLIC FUNCTION

As pointed out on page 1204, myocardial ischemia alters not only the systolic performance but also the diastolic characteristics of the left ventricle, ultimately raising its diastolic pressure at any given volume.[166, 172–174] Left ventricular diastolic properties are altered in infarcted and ischemic myocardium, leading initially to an increase but later to a reduction in left ventricular compliance. These changes are associated with an initial rise in left ventricular end-diastolic pressure. Over a period of 2 weeks, this pressure begins to fall toward normal, as there is a compensatory increase in end-diastolic volume.[175] As with impairment of systolic function, the magnitude of diastolic abnormality appears to be related to the size of the initial infarct. Patients who have recovered from AMI frequently continue to manifest decreased left ventricular compliance secondary to the fibrous scar that remains in the left ventricle.

CIRCULATORY REGULATION IN ACUTE MYOCARDIAL INFARCTION

The abnormality in circulatory regulation that is present in AMI is diagrammed in Figure 38–8. The process begins with an anatomical or functional obstruction in the coronary vascular bed, which results in regional myocardial ischemia and, if the ischemia persists, in infarction. If the infarct is of sufficient size, it depresses overall left ventricular function so that left ventricular stroke volume falls and filling pressures rise. The hemodynamic deterioration is more severe if an atrioventricular conduction disturbance develops or if a mechanical complication such as mitral regurgitation or ventricular septal rupture occurs. A marked depression of left ventricular stroke volume ultimately lowers aortic pressure and reduces coronary perfusion pressure; this condition may intensify myocardial ischemia and thereby initiate a vicious circle (Fig. 38–9). The inability of the left ventricle to empty also leads to an increased preload—that is, it dilates the well-perfused, normally functioning portion of the left ventricle. This compensatory mechanism tends to restore stroke volume to normal levels. However, the dilatation of the left ventricle also elevates ventricular afterload, because Laplace's law (p. 405) dictates that at any given arterial pressure the dilated ventricle must develop a higher wall tension. The increased afterload not only depresses left ventricular stroke volume but also elevates myocardial oxygen consumption, which in turn intensifies regional myocardial ischemia. When regional myocardial dysfunction is limited

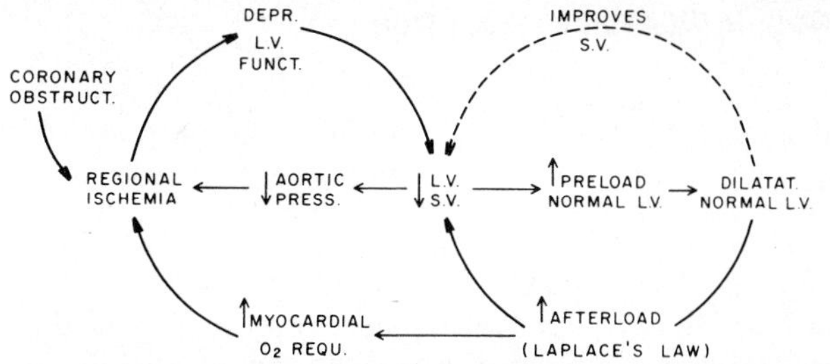

FIGURE 38–8. Changes in circulatory regulation in ischemic heart disease. DEPR. L.V. FUNCT., depressed left ventricular function; S.V., stroke volume; DILATAT., dilatation; O_2 REQU., oxygen requirements. Solid lines indicate that the effect is produced or intensified; broken lines indicate that it is diminished. (From Braunwald, E.: Regulation of the circulation. N. Engl. J. Med. *290*:1420, 1974.)

and the function of the remainder of the left ventricle is normal, compensatory mechanisms will sustain overall left ventricular function. If a large portion of the left ventricle becomes necrotic, pump failure occurs, i.e., overall left ventricular function becomes so depressed that the circulation cannot be sustained despite the dilatation of the remaining viable portion of the ventricle.

EFFECTS OF TREATMENT. Some of the consequences of treating pump failure, discussed on pages 1276–1280, should be considered. The favorable effect of raising a depressed arterial pressure results from the increased coronary perfusion pressure and the subsequent augmented blood flow across the stenotic areas and through the collateral vessels. This improvement of coronary blood flow may limit the size of the infarction by improving oxygen delivery to the periinfarction zone. In this manner, myocardial fiber shortening may be augmented, thereby increasing stroke volume and cardiac output and elevating arterial pressure.

However, there are also some unfavorable effects of increasing arterial pressure because this intervention usually necessitates an elevation of left ventricular intracavitary pressure (unless it is achieved by a circulatory assist device, such as an intraaortic balloon). The increased afterload causes cardiac dilatation; intramyocardial tension rises, not

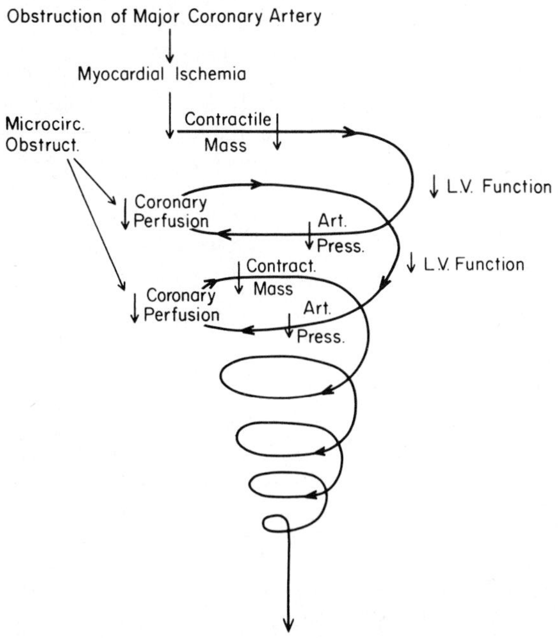

FIGURE 38–9. The sequence of events in the vicious cycle in which coronary artery obstruction leads to cardiogenic shock and progressive circulatory deterioration. (From Pasternak, R. C., Braunwald, E., and Alpert, J. S. Acute myocardial infarction. *In* Braunwald, E., et al. [eds.]: Harrison's Principles of Internal Medicine. New York, McGraw-Hill Book Co., 1987.)

only because of the higher intraventricular pressure but also because of the cardiac dilatation (p. 405). The increased wall tension augments myocardial oxygen needs and reduces myocardial fiber shortening (p. 396). These changes can cause further ischemia of the marginally viable myocardium adjacent to that supplied exclusively by the occluded vessel, and the area of infarction may be enlarged. Thus, cardiac function may deteriorate further.

It is obvious that the circulation is delicately balanced in patients with AMI. Unless the loss of viable myocardium is so extensive that it precludes survival, or is so small that the patient's survival is not threatened, the outcome may well depend on the clinician's appreciation of the interaction of the many factors that influence circulatory performance and their judicious manipulation.

VENTRICULAR REMODELING

INFARCT EXPANSION. For decades clinicians have been aware that left ventricular dilatation occurs as a consequence of MI,[176] which leads to changes in both the infarcted and the noninfarcted segments of the ventricle. These changes alter left ventricular size, shape, and wall thickness. Increases in the size of the infarct segment, known as infarct expansion, appear to be due to disruption of the normal myocardial cells and tissue loss within the necrotic zone leading to localized thinning and dilatation of the infarct.[177–180] At autopsy following MI, 50 per cent of hearts show no infarct expansion, but more than one-fourth have severe infarct expansion and wall thinning while the remainder have lesser degrees of infarct dilatation.[181] Infarct extension occurs almost exclusively in transmural infarcts. It is far more common with anterior than with inferior infarction, and it correlates directly with the size of the infarct.[178, 181] Additionally, the degree of infarct expansion appears to be related to the preinfarction wall thickness, with existing hypertrophy possibly protecting against infarct thinning.[181] Marked infarct expansion can be associated with rupture of the infarct segment.[181, 182]

While infarct expansion plays an important role in the ventricular dilatation that occurs in the early weeks following myocardial infarction,[183] ventricular remodeling is also caused by changes in the noninfarcted segment.[169, 175, 183] Wynne et al. reported that regional ejection fraction in the noninfarcted segment was abnormal in about two-thirds of patients with anterior wall myocardial infarction and in about one-third of patients with inferior myocardial infarction.[169]

VENTRICULAR DILATATION. Segmental lengthening of the endocardial perimeter occurs even in normally contracting ventricular walls early after MI,[175] and in some patients this process continues for many months.[183, 184] Lengthening of the noninfarcted segment appears to occur *without* regional wall thinning; therefore, the mass of the noninfarcted segment can actually increase. An increase in myocardial mass without disproportionate wall thickening has been termed "volume load hypertrophy" by Grossman[185] (p. 432); this concept may be applied to regional myocardium as well as the entire left ventricle.[175] Following MI, an extra burden is placed on the residual functioning myocardium of the noninfarcted segment,[162, 168] which presumably is responsible for the hypertrophy. The adaptive hypertrophy could help compensate for the functional impairment induced by the infarct itself and may be responsible for some of the initial hemodynamic improvement seen in the weeks after infarction in some patients. However, as illustrated in Figure 38–10, adaptive hypertrophy may undergo a transition with ultimate impairment of contractile function in the presence of a large infarction, leading to further cardiac dilatation, loss of global function, and ultimately heart failure.[175]

In conclusion, remodeling is a complex process that is not limited to areas of infarction and occurs to an increasing extent with larger infarcts. It begins at the time of AMI and, while limited in patients with small infarction, it probably continues for months to years after the infarct until either a stable hemodynamic state is achieved or progressively severe cardiac decompensation occurs leading to death from congestive heart failure. The process may, of course, be accelerated by ischemia of the noninfarcted myocardium and by additional infarcts.

PATHOPHYSIOLOGY OF OTHER ORGAN SYSTEMS IN ACUTE MYOCARDIAL INFARCTION

Alterations in Pulmonary Function (see also p. 1874)

Significant changes in the pulmonary function and arterial blood gases of patients with AMI are described in Chapter 61. Changes in pulmonary gas exchange, ventilation, and distribution of perfusion all occur with AMI. Hypoxemia is a frequent consequence, with its severity, in general, proportional to that of left ventricular failure. Thus, there is an inverse relation between arterial oxygen tension and pulmonary artery diastolic pressure in patients with AMI suggesting that increased pulmonary capillary hydrostatic pressure leads to interstitial edema, which results in arteriolar and bronchiolar compression that ultimately causes perfusion of poorly ventilated alveoli with resultant hypoxemia.[186] In addition to hypoxemia, there is a fall in diffusing capacity of carbon monoxide.[187] Hyperventilation often occurs in patients with AMI and

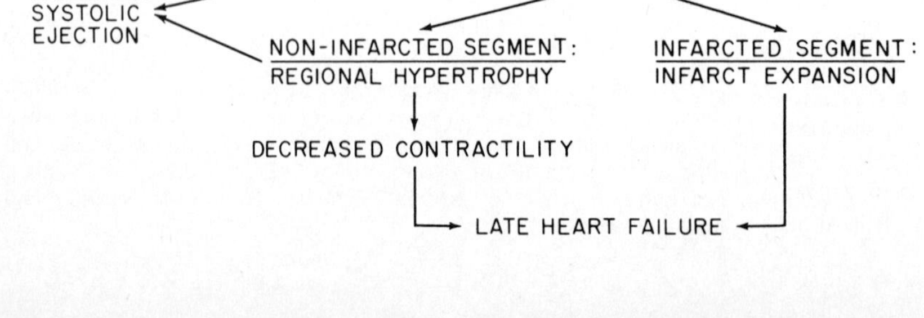

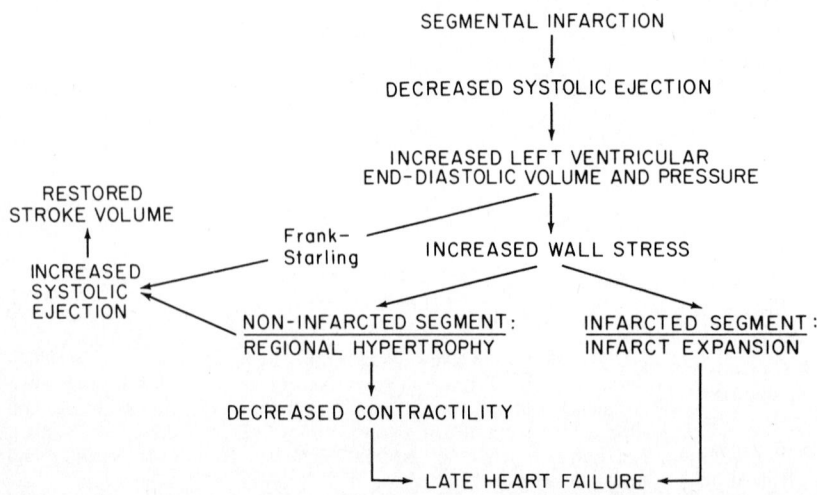

FIGURE 38–10. Hypothesis proposed to account for the mechanisms of left ventricular remodeling. (From McKay, R. G., et al.: Left ventricular remodeling after myocardial infarction: A corollary to infarct expansion. Circulation *74*:693, 1986, by permission of the American Heart Association.)

may cause hypocapnia and respiratory alkalosis, particularly in restless, anxious patients with pain. Intrapulmonary shunting of blood has been noted in patients in whom left ventricular failure complicates AMI. With improvement in heart failure, hypoxemia and intrapulmonary shunting diminish.

INCREASE IN INTERSTITIAL WATER. With a double radioisotope indicator dilution technique, a positive correlation has been demonstrated between pulmonary extravascular (interstitial) water content, left ventricular filling pressure, and the clinical signs and symptoms of left ventricular failure.[186] Over a period of 2 to 4 days following AMI, both the pulmonary extravascular water content and the wedge pressure decline. Presumably the increased pulmonary extravascular water represents a transudate secondary to increased pulmonary capillary pressure.

The increase in pulmonary extravascular water may also be responsible for the alterations in pulmonary mechanics observed in patients with AMI, i.e., reduction of airway conductance, pulmonary compliance, forced expiratory volume and midexpiratory flow rate, and an increase in closing volume—the last presumably related to the widespread closure of small, dependent airways during the first 3 days following AMI.[188] Recovery of left ventricular function or diuresis reduces abnormally elevated values for closing volumes to normal. Presumably, competition for space between arteries and small airways in the bronchovascular sheath accounts for some of the elevation in airway resistance, particularly at left atrial pressures under 15 mm Hg. Higher left atrial pressures produce increases in airway resistance secondary to interstitial, alveolar, and peribronchial edema.

REDUCTION OF VITAL CAPACITY. For over 70 years it has been recognized that a fall in vital capacity is related to shortened life expectancy for the cardiac patient.[189] It is now clear that virtually all indices of lung volume—total lung capacity, functional residual capacity, residual volume, as well as vital capacity—fall in the setting of AMI.[190] These reductions correlate with the elevations of left-sided filling pressure and are most probably due to increases in pulmonary extravascular water. Lung volumes, oxygenation, and airway resistance all return toward normal by the time of discharge for most patients.[190]

Increased pulmonary venous pressure also results in redistribution of pulmonary blood flow from the bases to the apices of the lung in patients with AMI,[191] altering the relationship between ventilation and perfusion. However, at follow-up examination 3 to 25 weeks after MI, the ventilation/perfusion relationship has usually returned to normal or almost so.

REDUCTION OF AFFINITY OF HEMOGLOBIN FOR OXYGEN. In patients with MI, particularly when complicated by left ventricular failure or cardiogenic shock, the affinity of hemoglobin for oxygen is reduced, i.e., the P_{50} is increased.[192] The increase in P_{50} results from increased levels of erythrocyte 2,3-diphosphoglycerate (2,3-DPG), is maximal after 24 hours, and constitutes an important compensatory mechanism, responsible for an estimated 18 per cent increase in oxygen release from oxyhemoglobin in patients with cardiogenic shock.[192]

Alterations in Endocrine Function (Fig. 38–11)

PANCREAS. Hyperglycemia and impaired glucose tolerance are common in patients with AMI. Although the absolute levels of blood insulin are often in the normal range in patients with uncomplicated AMI, they are usually inappropriately low for the level of blood sugar elevation, and there may be relative insulin resistance as well.[193] Patients with cardiogenic shock often demonstrate marked hyperglycemia and depressed levels of circulating insulin, often with complete suppression of insulin secretion in response to tolbutamide.[194] These abnormalities in insulin secretion and the resultant impaired glucose tolerance appear to be secondary to a reduction in pancreatic blood flow as a consequence of splanchnic vasoconstriction, which accompanies severe left ventricular failure. In addition, increased activity of the sympathetic nervous system with augmented circulating catecholamines[195] inhibits insulin secretion[196, 197] and augments glycogenolysis, also contributing to the elevation of blood sugar.[198]

Since hypoxic heart muscle derives a considerable portion of its energy from the metabolism of glucose (Chap. 37), and since insulin is essential for the uptake of glucose by the myocardium as well as for myocardial protein synthesis and inhibition of lysosomal activity, the deleterious effects of insulin deficiency are clear.[199]

ADRENAL MEDULLA. Excessive secretion of catecholamines produces many of the characteristic signs and symptoms of AMI. The plasma and urinary catecholamine levels are highest during the first 24 hours after the onset of chest pain,[198] with the greatest rise in plasma catecholamine secretion occurring during the first hour after the onset of MI,[200] when it may be in the range observed in racing car drivers immediately upon completion of a race.[201] These high levels of circulating catecholamines in patients with AMI correlate with the occurrence of serious arrhythmias[197, 202] and result in the stimulation of myocardial oxygen consumption, both directly and indirectly, as a consequence of catecholamine-induced elevation of circulating free fatty acids.[200] As might be anticipated, the concentration of circulating catecholamines correlates with extent of myocardial damage, incidence of cardiogenic shock, as well as both early and late mortality rates.[197, 203]

It is not clear, however, whether the elevation in plasma catecholamines plays some role in determining the amount of myocardium that becomes necrotic or whether this elevation is a consequence of the myocardial damage, i.e., whether it is cause or effect or both. The time course of sympathetic activation, which begins extremely early before extensive myocardial necrosis is present, suggests at least a potential role for these circulating hormones in extending myocardial damage and certainly in the genesis of arrhythmias.[203] Circulating catecholamines enhance platelet aggregation; when this occurs in the coronary microcirculation, the release of the potent vasoconstrictor thromboxane A_2 may further impair cardiac perfusion.[198]

ADRENAL CORTEX. Plasma and urinary 17-hydroxycorticosteroids and ketosteroids, as well as aldosterone, are also markedly elevated in patients with AMI.[198] Their concentrations correlate directly with the

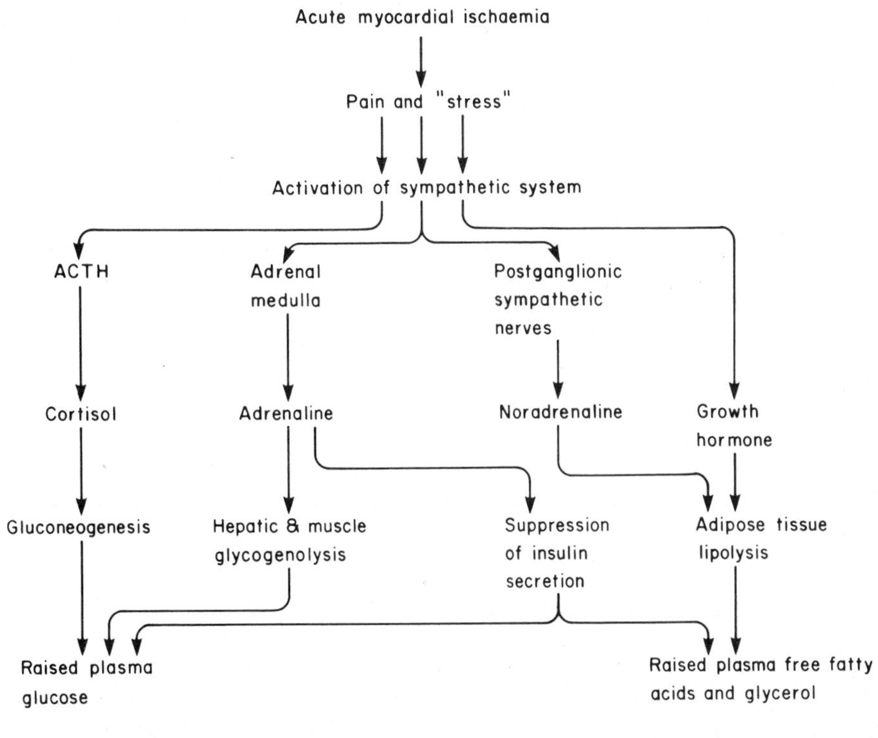

FIGURE 38–11. Principal hormonal and metabolic effects of myocardial infarction. (From Oliver, M. F.: Metabolic response during impending myocardial infarction. II. Clinical implications. Circulation *45*:491, 1972 by permission of the American Heart Association, Inc.)

peak level of serum glutamic oxaloacetic transaminase[204] and serum creatine kinase,[203] implying that the stress imposed by larger infarcts is associated with greater secretion of adrenal steroids. Glucocorticosteroids also contribute to the impairment of glucose tolerance. Although it has been suggested that the secretion of glucocorticoids is increased, it is inadequate to meet the demands for the stress imposed by a massive AMI, particularly if it is accompanied by cardiogenic shock.[198]

THYROID GLAND. Although patients with AMI are generally euthyroid, there is evidence for a significant transient decrease in serum T_3 levels, a fall that is most marked on about the third day after the infarct.[205–207] This fall in T_3 is usually accompanied by a rise in reverse T_3 with variable changes or no change in T_4 and TSH levels. The alteration in peripheral thyroxin metabolism appears to correlate with infarct size[206] and may be mediated by the rise in endogenous levels of cortisol that accompanies AMI.[205, 207]

HEMATOLOGICAL FUNCTION. Platelets. AMI generally occurs in the presence of extensive coronary and systemic atherosclerotic plaques, which may serve as the site for the formation of platelet aggregates, a sequence that has been suggested as the initial step in the process of coronary thrombosis, coronary occlusion, and subsequent MI. Circulating platelets are hyperaggregable in patients with AMI.[88] Approximately one-third of these patients demonstrate shortened platelet survival times.[208] Types III and IV hyperlipoproteinemia, frequently present in patients with AMI, can also be responsible for shortening platelet survival. Findings suggestive of a hypercoagulable state as a risk factor for AMI are discussed on page 1770.

Coagulation Tests. Elevated levels of serum fibrinogen degradation products, an end product of thrombosis[209]—as well as release of distinctive proteins when platelets are activated, i.e., platelet factor 4[210] and beta thromboglobulin[211]— have been reported in some patients with AMI. Fibrinopeptide A, a protein released from fibrin by thrombin, is a marker of ongoing thrombosis and is elevated during the early hours of AMI.[212] The interpretation of the coagulation tests in patients with AMI may be complicated by elevated blood levels of catecholamines, concomitant shock, and/or pulmonary embolism, conditions which are all capable of altering various tests of platelet and coagulation function.[213, 214] Thus, it is not yet clear whether the above-mentioned changes are the causes or consequences of AMI.

Leukocytes. AMI is usually accompanied by leukocytosis that is thought to be related both to the necrotic process and its magnitude, in which leukocytes play an active role, and to their stimulation by elevated glucocorticoids that occur with infarction. It is now recognized that leukocytes also participate in the thrombotic process.[215] Activation of neutrophils may serve to produce important intermediates, such as leukotriene B_4 and oxygen-free radicals,[216, 217] that exert important microcirculatory effects.[215]

Blood Viscosity. An elevation of blood viscosity also occurs in patients with AMI.[218] During the first few days after infarction, this is mainly attributable to hemoconcentration, but later the increases in plasma viscosity and red cell aggregation correlate with elevated serum concentrations of $alpha_2$ globulin and fibrinogen, which are nonspecific reactions to tissue necrosis and which are also responsible for the elevated sedimentation rate characteristic of AMI.[219] The high values of blood viscosity are observed most frequently in patients with complications, such as left ventricular failure, cardiogenic shock, and thromboembolism.

ALTERATIONS IN RENAL FUNCTION. Both prerenal azotemia and acute renal failure can complicate the marked reduction of cardiac output that occurs in cardiogenic shock. These conditions are discussed on page 566.

CLINICAL FEATURES OF ACUTE MYOCARDIAL INFARCTION

PRECIPITATING FACTORS

In most patients with AMI, no precipitating factor can be identified. An early study noted the following patient activities at the onset of AMI: heavy physical exertion, 13 per cent; modest or usual exertion, 18 per cent; surgical procedure, 6 per cent; rest, 51 per cent; and sleep, 8 per cent.[220] Another study showed similar results except that only 2 per cent of patients experienced MI during heavy physical exertion.[221] Others, however, have reported that a significant number of AMI's occur within a few hours of severe physical exertion.[222, 223] It has been pointed out that the *severe exertion* which preceded an infarction was often performed at times when the patient was unduly fatigued or emotionally stressed.[224] Exertion before infarction is somewhat more common among patients without preexisting angina than in patients who have had a history of angina.[225] Thus, although adequate control studies have not been carried out, there is *suggestive* evidence that heavy exercise may play a precipitating role in some patients. Such infarctions are presumably the result of marked increases in myocardial oxygen consumption in the presence of severe coronary arterial narrowing. Supporting this hypothesis is the finding that fatal MI occurring during heavy exertion is often associated with severe coronary arterial narrowing but no occlusion.[223]

Surgical procedures associated with acute blood loss have also been noted as frequent precursors of AMI (p. 1696). Reduced myocardial perfusion secondary to hypotension and increased myocardial oxygen demands secondary to fever, tachycardia, and agitation are presumably responsible for the myocardial necrosis. Other factors reported as predisposing to AMI include respiratory infections, hypoxemia of any cause, pulmonary embolism, hypoglycemia, administration of ergot preparations, serum sickness, allergy, and wasp stings.[226–229] In patients with Prinzmetal's angina (p. 1360), AMI may develop in the territory of the coronary artery, which repeatedly undergoes spasm. Rarely, munition workers exposed to high concentrations of nitroglycerin may develop myocardial infarction when they are withdrawn from this exposure, suggesting that it is caused by vasospasm.[153] Accelerating angina and rest angina, two forms of unstable angina, may culminate as infarction of the myocardium, again in the distribution of the affected vessel.[230]

Considerable evidence has accumulated that *emotional stresses* may be a precipitating factor in the initiation of AMI.[231] A number of reports have documented that upsetting life events occur commonly in patients who subsequently suffer an MI (p. 1885).[232] Such events have been quantified and scored as *Life Change Units.* Rahe and coworkers noted, on retrospective analysis, a significant buildup of Life Change Units in patients who subsequently suffered myocardial infarction or died suddenly.[232]

Trauma may precipitate an AMI in one of two ways. Myocardial contusion and hemorrhage into the myocardium may actually cause cell necrosis, or the injury may involve a coronary artery, causing occlusion of that vessel with resultant MI (Chap. 45). *Neurological disturbances* (transient ischemic attacks or strokes) may also precipitate AMI.[11, 233]

CIRCADIAN PERIODICITY. An analysis of a large number of patients hospitalized with myocardial infarction, studied as part of the Multicenter Investigation of Limitation of Infarct Size (MILIS), has revealed a pronounced circadian periodicity for the time of onset of AMI.[234] In this retrospective review, a peak incidence of onset at about 9 AM was found when timing was estimated from either the occurrence of symptoms or from the first elevation of plasma creatine kinase MB (Fig. 38–12). Other studies, including a large World Health Organization report[235] and a study of sudden death,[236] have also found this morning peak incidence of AMI, but this phenomenon has escaped clinical attention until recently. Mitler and Kripke have

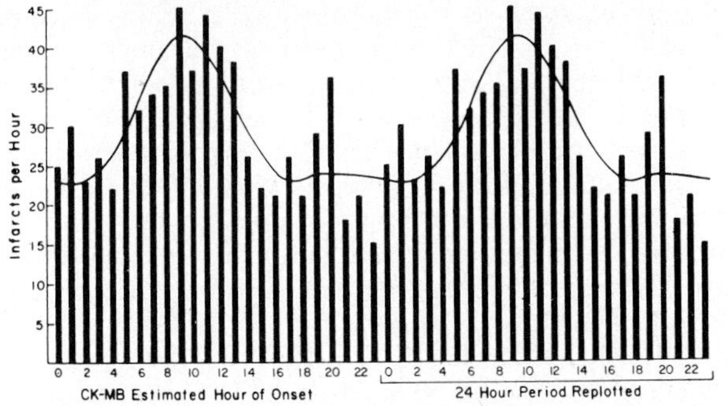

FIGURE 38–12. The hourly frequency of onset of myocardial infarction as determined by the CK-MB method in 703 patients. The number of infarctions beginning during each of the 24 hours of the day is plotted on the left. On the right, the identical data are plotted again to show the relation between the end and the beginning of the day. A two-harmonic-regression equation for the frequency of onset of myocardial infarction has been fitted to the data (curved line). A prominent circadian rhythm is present, with primary peak incidence of infarction at 9 AM and a secondary peak at 8 PM. (Reprinted by permission from Muller, J. E., et al.: Circadian variation in the frequency of onset of acute myocardial infarction. N. Engl. J. Med. *313*:1315, 1985.)

pointed out that the early-morning peak in MI parallels the peak incidence of death from ischemic heart disease occurring at 8 AM.[237] Circadian rhythms affect many physiological and biochemical parameters; the early morning hours are associated with rises in plasma catecholamines and cortisol and increases in platelet aggregability. Interestingly, the characteristic circadian peak was absent in patients receiving beta-blocker therapy before their presentation with AMI.[234] A study of ambulatory ST-segment monitoring in patients with coronary artery disease has found that ST shifts occur most commonly in the morning hours.[238] Thus, it is possible that some cyclical aspects of combined vasospastic and prothrombotic factors, in the setting of preexisting atherosclerosis, lead to AMI. The apparent relationship between a patient's biological rhythm and the onset of AMI appears to be of both pathophysiological and clinical importance.

CLINICAL HISTORY

PRODROMAL SYMPTOMS. Despite recent advances in the laboratory detection of AMI, the history remains of substantial value in establishing a diagnosis. A prodromal history can be elicited in 20 to 60 per cent of patients with AMI.[233, 239] The prodrome is usually characterized by chest discomfort, resembling classic angina pectoris (described on pp. 4 and 1316), but it occurs at rest or with less activity than usual and can therefore be classified as unstable angina. However, the latter is often not disturbing enough to induce patients to seek medical attention, and if they do, they are not usually hospitalized. Among patients who are hospitalized for unstable angina, fewer than 15 per cent develop AMI (p. 1359). Of the patients with AMI presenting with prodromal symptoms of unstable angina, approximately one-third have had symptoms from 1 to 4 weeks before hospitalization; in the remaining two-thirds, symptoms predated admission by a week or less, with one-third of these patients (20 per cent of all with prodromes) having had symptoms for 24 hours or less.[240]

NATURE OF THE PAIN. The pain of AMI is variable in intensity; in most patients it is severe and, in some instances, intolerable. The pain is prolonged, usually lasting for more than 30 minutes and frequently for a number of hours. The discomfort is described as constricting, crushing, oppressing, or compressing; often the patient complains of something sitting on or squeezing the chest. Although usually described as a squeezing, choking, vise-like, or heavy pain, it may also be characterized as a stabbing, knifelike, boring, or burning discomfort. The pain is usually retrosternal in location, spreading frequently to both sides of the anterior chest, with predilection for the left side. Often the pain radiates down the ulnar aspect of the left arm, producing a tingling sensation in the left wrist, hand, and even fingers. Some patients note only a dull ache or numbness of the wrists in association with severe substernal or precordial discomfort. In some instances, the pain of AMI may begin in the epigastrium and simulate a variety of abdominal disorders, a fact which often causes MI to be misdiagnosed as "indigestion." In other patients the discomfort of AMI radiates to the shoulders, upper extremities, neck, jaw, and interscapular region, again usually favoring the left side. In patients with preexisting angina pectoris, the pain of infarction usually resembles that of angina with respect to quality and location. However, it is generally much more severe, lasts longer, and is not relieved by rest and nitroglycerin.

What follows is a lucid, personal, published description of the pain of AMI, provided by a distinguished, experienced physician:

> During the first 15 to 20 minutes when the pain was waxing and waning, I was pretending it was esophageal and popping a few Tums and drinking a glass of milk. After this, the pain certainly told me just what it seems to have told other patients. I felt I must sit down very, very quietly. Although I did so, the pain became a steadily expanding, deep, penetrating ache spreading from beneath mid-breast bone, around the sides of my chest, up my neck into my lower jaw, and down the inner aspect of my left arm into my fourth and fifth fingers. It cycled a bit. Sometimes it seemed most dreadful in my chest—then in my jaw and lower teeth—then in my left arm. But it conveyed one clear message. What I thought from the outset and continued to think through about 2 hours of what seemed absolutely intolerable pain was that if I remained *absolutely* immobile, not moving even an eyelash, perhaps it would let go of me. I would guess it took about 10 to 12 minutes to build to maximal intensity and there it stayed. During the entire period I sat absolutely still with my eyes closed, conscious of the fact that I was sweating profusely and that I probably looked very pale and lousy. Although my wife was bustling cheerfully about in the kitchen not 15 feet away, I said absolutely nothing, feeling that even moving my tongue or vocal chords was simply too much. There was no inclination to groan or cry out.
>
> There was another aspect of the pain frequently alluded to by others. There was absolutely no doubt in my mind that I was about to die. As the pain remained, I simply wished exodus would go ahead and happen. . . . The quality of the pain is as difficult for me to describe as it seems to have been for other observers over the last 70 plus years. It was not the bright or burning or well-localized pain one feels with a cut, a puncture, or a burn, from which one instinctively and swiftly retreats. A very different set of nerve endings is involved. It was a dreadful, deep, nauseating ache. If you would try multiplying a hundredfold the kind of ache you experience after working too long trying to screw a recalcitrant light bulb into a ceiling socket that's a little too high over your head to reach decently, you would be close. . . .
>
> As to intensity, I keep wanting to use the word *unbearable*. Obviously, this word is not really appropriate, as I did manage somehow to bear the pain. But it was an absolutely monstrous, awful sensation, and it was totally untouched by 20 or 30 or 40 milligrams of morphine administered to me over the next 2 hours. That morphine gave so little relief has made me empathize deeply with the hundreds of patients with the same disease I've treated with this drug over the years.[241]

In some patients, particularly the elderly, AMI is manifested clinically not by chest pain but rather by symptoms of acute left ventricular failure and chest tightness or by overwhelming weakness, accompanied by diaphoresis, nausea, vomiting, and diarrhea.[11] The pain of AMI may have disappeared by the time the physician first encounters the patient (or the patient reaches the hospital), or it may persist for many hours. Opiates—in particular, morphine—usually relieve the pain, although a persistent soreness, pressure, or dull ache may remain for several hours or more despite intensive treatment with analgesics. The longer a patient requires analgesic administration after hospital admission for ischemic pain, the more likely that MI will be confirmed in that patient.[242] Both angina pectoris and the pain of AMI are thought to arise from nerve endings in ischemic or injured, but not necrotic, myocardium.[243] Thus, in MI, stimulation of nerve fibers in an ischemic zone of myocardium surrounding the necrotic central area of infarction probably gives rise to the pain.

It has been suggested that the phenomenon of referred pain is modulated by the spatial and temporal patterns of excitation of these afferent sympathetic fibers as well as a variable contribution of vagal afferent fibers.[244] Experience with patients undergoing procedures to reperfuse myocardium in the setting of AMI suggests that pain often disappears suddenly and completely once blood flow to the infarct territory is restored.[245] In patients in whom reocclusion occurs after thrombolysis, pain recurs if the initial reperfusion has left viable myocardium. Thus, what has previously been thought of as "the pain of infarction," sometimes lasting for many hours, probably represents pain caused by ongoing ischemia. The recognition that pain implies ischemia and not inevitable infarction has important clinical implications and heightens the importance of seeking ways to improve the ischemia, for which the pain is a marker. This finding suggests that the clinician should not be complacent about ongoing cardiac pain under any circumstances.

Differential Diagnosis. The pain of AMI may simulate the pain of *acute pericarditis* (p. 1388), which is usually associated with some pleuritic features, i.e., it is aggravated by respiratory movements and coughing and often involves the shoulder, ridge of the trapezius, and neck. *Pleural pain* is usually sharp, knifelike, and aggravated by each breath, which distinguishes it from the deep, dull, steady pain of AMI. *Pulmonary embolism* (Chap. 47) generally produces pain laterally in the chest, is often pleuritic in nature, and may be associated with hemoptysis. The pain due to *acute dissection of the aorta* (p. 1554) is usually localized in the center of the chest, is extremely severe, persists for many hours, and often radiates to the lower back and sometimes into the legs. Often one or more major arterial pulses are absent. Pain arising from the *costochondral and chondrosternal articulations* may be associated with localized swelling and redness; it is usually sharp and "darting" and is characterized by marked localized tenderness.

OTHER SYMPTOMS. Nausea and vomiting occur in more than 50 per cent of patients with transmural MI and severe chest pain,[246] presumably owing to activation of vagal reflex or to stimulation of left ventricular receptors as part of the Bezold-Jarisch reflex (p. 1555).[247] These occur more commonly in patients with inferior MI than in those with anterior MI. Occasionally a patient complains of diarrhea or a violent urge to evacuate the bowels during the acute phase of MI. Moreover, nausea and vomiting are common side effects of opiates. When the pain of AMI is epigastric in location and is associated with nausea and vomiting, the clinical picture may easily be confused with that of acute cholecystitis, gastritis, or peptic ulcer. Other symptoms include feelings of profound weakness, dizziness, palpitations, cold perspiration, and a sense of impending doom. On occasion, symptoms arising from an episode of cerebral embolism or other systemic arterial embolism are the first signs of an AMI. Rarely, patients with inferior infarction report intractable hiccupping, a finding which has been attributed to diaphragmatic irritation by the infarct. The aforementioned symptoms may or may not be accompanied by chest pain.[248]

SILENT MI AND ATYPICAL PRESENTATION. Population studies suggest that between 20 and 60 per cent of nonfatal MI's are unrecognized by the patient and are discovered only on subsequent routine electrocardiographic[249–252] or postmortem examinations. Of these unrecognized infarctions, approximately half are truly silent, with the patients unable to recall any symptoms whatsoever referable to the infarction. The other half of patients with so-called silent infarction can recall an event characterized by symptoms compatible with acute infarction when leading questions are posed after the abnormal electrocardiogram is discovered. Unrecognized or silent infarction occurs more commonly in patients without antecendant angina pectoris, and is more common in patients with diabetes and hypertension,[250] although the association with diabetes is controversial.[253]

In an analysis of atypical presentations of AMI, Bean[254] lists the following: (1) congestive heart failure—beginning de novo or worsening of established failure; (2) classic angina pectoris without a particularly severe or prolonged attack; (3) atypical location of the pain; (4) central nervous system manifestations, resembling those of stroke, secondary to a sharp reduction in cardiac output in a patient with cerebral arteriosclerosis; (5) apprehension and nervousness; (6) sudden mania or psychosis; (7) syncope; (8) overwhelming weakness; (9) acute indigestion; and (10) peripheral embolism.

PHYSICAL EXAMINATION

GENERAL APPEARANCE. Patients suffering an AMI usually appear anxious and in considerable distress. An anguished facial expression is common, and—in contrast to patients with angina pectoris, who often lie, sit, or stand quite still, realizing that all forms of activity increase the discomfort—patients suffering an AMI may be restless and move about in an effort to find a comfortable position. Others, like the physician who described his own symptoms, prefer to sit still. They often massage or clutch their chests and frequently describe their pain with a clenched fist held against the sternum (a sign of ischemic pain popularized by Dr. Samuel A. Levine). In patients with left ventricular failure and sympathetic stimulation, cold perspiration and skin pallor may be evident; they usually sit or are propped up in bed, gasping for breath. Between breaths, they may complain of chest discomfort or a feeling of suffocation. Cough productive of frothy, pink, or blood-streaked sputum is common.

Patients in cardiogenic shock often lie listlessly, making few if any spontaneous movements. The skin is cool and clammy, with a bluish or mottled color over the extremities, and there is marked facial pallor with severe cyanosis of the lips and nailbeds. Depending on the degree of cerebral perfusion, the patient in shock may converse normally or may evidence confusion and disorientation. The patient is often anxious and frightened but may profess interest in only minimal communication.

VITAL SIGNS. The heart rate may vary from a marked bradycardia to rapid regular or irregular tachycardia, depending on the underlying rhythm and the degree of left ventricular failure. Most commonly, the pulse is rapid and regular initially (sinus tachycardia at 100 to 110 beats/min), slowing as the patient's pain and anxiety are relieved; premature ventricular beats are common, occurring in more than 95 per cent of patients evaluated early after the onset of symptoms.

Blood Pressure. The majority of patients with uncomplicated AMI are normotensive, although the reduced stroke volume accompanying the tachycardia may cause a small decline in systolic pressure and an elevation of diastolic pressure. Among previously normotensive patients, a hypertensive response frequently occurs, with the arterial pressure exceeding 160/90 mm Hg, presumably as a consequence of adrenergic discharge secondary to pain and agitation. The arterial pressure rarely exceeds 200/110 mm Hg. It is rather common for previously hypertensive patients to become normotensive without treatment following AMI, although approximately two-thirds of these previously hypertensive patients eventually regain their elevated levels of blood pressure, generally 3 to 6 months after infarction. In patients with massive infarcts, arterial pressure falls acutely, owing to left ventricular dysfunction and venous pooling secondary to administration of morphine or nitrates or both; as recovery occurs, the arterial pressure tends to return to preinfarction levels. Patients in cardiogenic shock (p. 572), by definition, have systolic pressures below 90 mm Hg. However, hypotension does not necessarily signify cardiogenic shock, since some patients with inferior infarction, in whom the Bezold-Jarisch reflex is activated, may also have systolic blood pressure below 90 mm Hg.[255] These patients do not demonstrate peripheral manifestations of hypoperfusion; their prognosis is generally good and their hypotension eventually resolves spontaneously, although this resolution can be accelerated by atropine and assumption of the Trendelenburg position. Other patients who are initially only slightly hypotensive may demonstrate gradually falling blood pressures with progressive reduction in cardiac output over several hours or days as they gradually develop cardiogenic shock as a consequence of increasing ischemia and extension of infarction (Fig. 38–9). Evidence of autonomic hyperactivity is common, varying in type with the location of the infarction. At some time in their initial presentation, more than half of patients with inferior MI have evidence of excess parasympathetic stimulation, with hypotension, bradycardia, or both, while about half of patients with anterior MI show signs of sympathetic excess, having hypertension, tachycardia, or both.[256]

Temperature and Respiration. Most patients with AMI develop *fever*, a nonspecific response to tissue necrosis, within 24 to 48 hours of the onset of infarction. Body temperature often begins to rise within 4 to 8 hours after the onset of infarction, and rectal temperature often reaches 101 to 102° F. Fever usually resolves by the seventh or eighth day following infarction.

The *respiratory rate* may be slightly elevated soon after the development of an AMI; in patients without heart failure, it results from anxiety and pain, since it returns to normal with treatment of physical and psychological discomfort. In patients with left ventricular failure, the respiratory rate correlates with the severity of failure; patients with pulmonary edema may have respiratory rates exceeding 40 per minute. However, the respiratory rate is not necessarily elevated in patients with cardiogenic shock. Cheyne-Stokes (periodic) respiration (p. 481) may occur in elderly individuals with cardiogenic shock and heart failure, particularly after opiate therapy and in the presence of cerebrovascular disease.

JUGULAR VENOUS PULSE. The height and contour of the jugular venous pulse reflect right atrial and right ventricular diastolic pressures (p. 19). Since these pressures are usually normal or only slightly elevated in patients with AMI (even in the presence of mild to moderate left ventricular failure), it is not surprising that the jugular venous pulse does not appear to be abnormal. The *a* wave may be prominent in patients with pulmonary hypertension secondary to left ventricular failure or reduced compliance.[257] In contrast, right ventricular infarction (whether or not it accompanies left ventricular infarction) often results in marked jugular venous distention and, when it is complicated by necrosis of right ventricular papillary muscles, tall *v* waves of tricuspid regurgitation are evident. In patients with AMI and cardiogenic shock, the jugular venous pressure is usually elevated. In patients with AMI, hypotension, and hypoperfusion, whose signs may specifically resemble those of patients with cardiogenic shock but who have flat neck veins, it is likely that the depression of left ventricular performance may be related, at least in part, to hypovolemia, but the differentiation can be made only by assessing left ventricular performance.

CAROTID PULSE. Palpation of the carotid arterial pulse provides a clue to the left ventricular stroke volume; a small pulse suggests a reduced stroke volume, whereas a sharp, brief upstroke is often observed in patients with mitral regurgitation or ruptured ventricular septum with a left-to-right shunt. Pulsus alternans reflects severe left ventricular dysfunction.

THE CHEST. Moist rales are audible in patients who develop left ventricular failure and/or a reduction of left ventricular compliance with AMI. An early assessment of prognosis may be made in relation to the fraction of the lung field over which rales are heard (Table 38–2). Diffuse wheezing may be present in patients with severe left ventricular failure. Cough with hemoptysis, suggesting pulmonary embolism with infarction, may also occur.

CARDIAC EXAMINATION. Despite severe symptoms and extensive myocardial damage, the findings on examination of the heart may be surprisingly unremarkable in patients with AMI. Palpation of the precordium may yield normal findings but more commonly reveals (in patients with sinus rhythm) a presystolic pulsation, synchronous with an audible fourth heart sound, reflecting a vigorous left atrial

TABLE 38–2 KILLIP CLASSIFICATION OF PATIENTS WITH ACUTE MYOCARDIAL INFARCTION

	Definition	Patients with Acute Myocardial Infarction Admitted to CCU in This Category (%)	Approximate Mortality (%)†
Class I	Absence of rales over the lung fields and absence of S3	30–40	8
Class II	Rales over 50 per cent or less of the lung fields or the presence of an S3	30–50	30
Class III	Rales over more than 50 per cent of the lung fields (frequently pulmonary edema)	5–10	44
Class IV	Shock	10	80–100

Adapted from Killip, T., and Kimball, J. T.: Treatment of myocardial infarction in a coronary care unit. A two year experience with 250 patients. Am. J. Cardiol. *20*:457, 1967.

†Estimated mortality in the 1960's. Mortality still rises with increased class, although the values in each class are lower today than in the 1960's.

contraction filling a ventricle with reduced compliance. In the presence of left ventricular systolic dysfunction, an outward movement of the left ventricle may be palpated in early diastole, coincident with a third heart sound. When the anterior or lateral portion of the ventricle is dyskinetic, an abnormal systolic pulsation is present in the third, fourth, or fifth interspaces to the left of the sternum. In some patients, this abnormal paradoxical precordial impulse is clearly separable from the point of maximal impulse, which is more lateral and to the left. In other patients, the abnormal impulse is a diffuse, rippling, precordial movement, approximately 5 to 10 cm in diameter, not clearly separable from the point of maximal impulse. Patients with longstanding hypertension or previous infarction with left ventricular hypertrophy often demonstrate a laterally displaced, sustained apical impulse.

Auscultation. The heart sounds, particularly the first sound, are frequently muffled[258] and occasionally inaudible immediately after the infarct, and their intensity increases as healing occurs.[259] A soft first sound may also reflect prolongation of the P-R interval. Patients with marked ventricular dysfunction and/or left bundle branch block may have paradoxical splitting of the second heart sound (p. 47). Individuals with postinfarction angina also may develop transient, paradoxically split second heart sounds during anginal episodes because of prolongation of the left ventricular preejection period.

A *fourth heart sound* is almost universally present in patients in sinus rhythm with AMI and is usually best heard between the left sternal border and the apex. This sound reflects atrial contraction and a reduction in left ventricular compliance (p. 50) and is associated with an elevation of left ventricular end-diastolic pressure, even in the absence of left ventricular systolic dysfunction. It is of little diagnostic value, since it is commonly audible in most patients with chronic ischemic heart disease and is recordable, although not often audible, in many normal subjects older than 45 years.

A *third heart sound* in AMI usually reflects extensive left ventricular dysfunction. It is usually heard in patients with large infarctions. This sound is heard best at the apex, with the patient in the left lateral recumbent position, and is more common in patients with transmural anterior infarctions than in those with inferior or nontransmural infarctions.[260] Patients with a third heart sound often have elevated left ventricular filling pressure. The mortality of patients who manifest a third heart sound during the acute phase of MI is higher than that of patients without such a sound.[260] A third sound may be caused not only by left ventricular failure but also by increased inflow into the left ventricle, as occurs when mitral regurgitation or ventricular septal defect complicate AMI. Third and fourth heart sounds emanating from the left ventricle are heard best at the apex; in patients with right ventricular infarcts, these sounds may be heard along the left sternal border and are intensified by inspiration.

Systolic murmurs, transient or persistent, are commonly audible in patients with AMI and generally result from mitral regurgitation secondary to papillary muscle dysfunction or left ventricular dilatation. A new, prominent holosystolic murmur at the apex, accompanied by a thrill, may represent rupture of a head of a papillary muscle (p. 1037). The findings in rupture of the interventricular septum are similar, although the murmur and thrill are usually most prominent along the left sternal border while being audible at the right sternal border as well. The systolic murmur of tricuspid regurgitation (caused by right ventricular failure due to pulmonary hypertension and/or right ventricular infarction or by infarction of a right ventricular papillary muscle) is also heard along the left sternal border but is characteristically intensified by inspiration and is accompanied by a prominent *v* wave in the jugular venous pulse. In evaluating systolic murmurs in patients with chest pain, it is important to note that aortic stenosis is a common cause of ischemic pain (p. 1055) and that it occurs, like coronary artery disease, most commonly in middle-aged and elderly men. Therefore, the diagnosis of aortic stenosis should be considered in patients suspected of having suffered an MI who have a systolic murmur at the base of the heart. Rarely, *diastolic murmurs* are produced by blood flowing through a severe coronary arterial stenosis. A *continuous murmur* is an unusual finding that may occur as a result of a variety of congenital abnormalities including a coronary artery arteriovenous fistula, a very rare cause of myocardial ischemia or infarction.[261]

Pericardial friction rubs are audible in 7 to 20 per cent of all patients with AMI and in a higher percentage of patients with transmural infarcts.[262, 263] Rubs are notorious for their evanescence and, hence, are probably even more common than reported; frequent auscultation in patients with transmural infarction often results in the discovery of a rub which might otherwise have gone unnoticed. Although friction rubs may be heard by 24 hours or as late as 2 weeks after the onset of infarction, most commonly they are noted on the second or third day.[263] Occasionally, in patients with extensive infarction, a loud rub may be heard for many days. About 40 per cent of patients with a friction rub in the setting of AMI have a pericardial effusion on echocardiographic study[264] but only rarely are the classic electrocardiographic changes of pericarditis (p. 1489) seen.[263] Delayed onset of the rub and the associated discomfort of pericarditis (as late as 3 months postinfarction) are characteristic of the postmyocardial infarction (Dressler) syndrome (p. 1287).[264–268]

Pericardial rubs are most readily audible along the left sternal border or just inside the point of maximal impulse and occur after either anterior or inferoposterior transmural infarction. Loud rubs may be audible over the entire precordium and even over the back. Occasionally, only the systolic portion of a rub is heard; it may be confused with a systolic murmur, and the diagnosis of rupture of the ventricular septum or mitral regurgitation may be considered. The presence of a pericardial friction rub does not exclude the presence of a significant pericardial effusion.

THE FUNDI. Hypertension, diabetes, and generalized atherosclerosis commonly accompany AMI, and since these conditions may produce characteristic changes in the fundus, a careful funduscopic examination may provide information concerning the underlying vascular status; this is particularly useful in patients unable to provide a detailed history.

THE ABDOMEN. As noted above, in patients with AMI (particularly inferior infarcts) with diaphragmatic irritation, the pain may localize in the epigastrium or the right upper quadrant. Pain in the abdomen associated with nausea, vomiting, restlessness, and even abdominal distention is often interpreted by patients as a sign of "indigestion,"[254] resulting in self-medication with antacids, and it may suggest an acute abdominal process to the physician. A normal abdominal examination aids in ruling this out and in pointing to the correct diagnosis. Right heart failure, characterized by hepatomegaly and a positive abdominojugular reflux, is unusual in patients with acute left ventricular infarction but does occur in patients with severe and usually prolonged left ventricular failure or right ventricular infarction.

THE EXTREMITIES. Coronary atherosclerosis is often associated with systemic atherosclerosis, and it is therefore common for patients with AMI to have a history of intermittent claudication and to demonstrate physical findings of peripheral vascular disease. Thus, diminished peripheral arterial pulses, loss of hair, and atrophic skin in the lower extremities are noted frequently in patients with coronary artery disease. Peripheral edema is a manifestation of right ventricular failure and, like congestive hepatomegaly, is unusual in patients with acute left ventricular infarction. Cyanosis of the nailbeds is common in patients with severe left ventricular failure and is particularly striking in patients with cardiogenic shock.

NEUROPSYCHIATRIC FINDINGS. Except for the altered mental status that occurs in patients with AMI who have a markedly reduced cardiac output and cerebral hypoperfusion, the neurological examination is normal unless the patient has suffered cerebral embolism secondary to a mural thrombus. Indeed, an underlying MI is common in patients with cerebral embolic stroke. There is an increased coincidence of cerebrovascular accidents and AMI. In a prospective study of patients with cerebrovascular accidents admitted to the hospital within 72 hours of the onset, 12.7 per cent have an associated AMI; in contrast, in a series of patients with AMI, only 1.7 per cent suffered a stroke. The coincidence was confined to patients with large myocardial infarcts as reflected in markedly elevated serum creatine kinase concentrations.[269] The coincidence between these two conditions may be explained by systemic hypotension due to MI precipitating a cerebral infarction and the converse, as well as by mural emboli from the heart causing cerebral emboli.

As discussed in Chapter 62, patients with AMI often exhibit alterations of the emotional state, including intense anxiety, denial, and depression.

LABORATORY EXAMINATIONS

ENZYMES

Irreversibly injured myocardial cells release a number of enzymes into the circulation, where they can be measured by specific chemical reactions (p. 1212).[270] Increased activities of many enzymes have been found in the serum or plasma of patients with AMI.[271, 272] Following experimental MI, a small but significant myocardial venoarterial difference of enzyme activity can be measured,[273] and elevated plasma levels of enzymes correlate with corresponding depletion of these same eyzymes from infarcted tissue.[274] Determinations of serum activity of creatine kinase (CK), glutamic oxaloacetic transferase (GOT), and lactic dehydrogenase (LDH) are frequently used in the laboratory diagnosis of AMI.

Serum glutamic oxaloacetic transferase (SGOT) activity usually exceeds the normal range within 8 to 12 hours following the onset of chest pain; peak SGOT levels occur 18 to 36 hours after infarction and fall to normal within 3 to 4 days (Fig. 38–13). False-positive elevations of this enzyme occur in patients with primary liver disease, hepatic congestion, and skeletal muscle disease and following intramuscular injections, pulmonary embolism, and various forms of shock.[270] Elevated levels of SGOT have also been noted in patients with pericarditis and epicardial involvement. Since the time course of elevation and fall of SGOT is intermediate between that of CK and LDH, and since SGOT elevation is nonspecific, its incremental benefit for

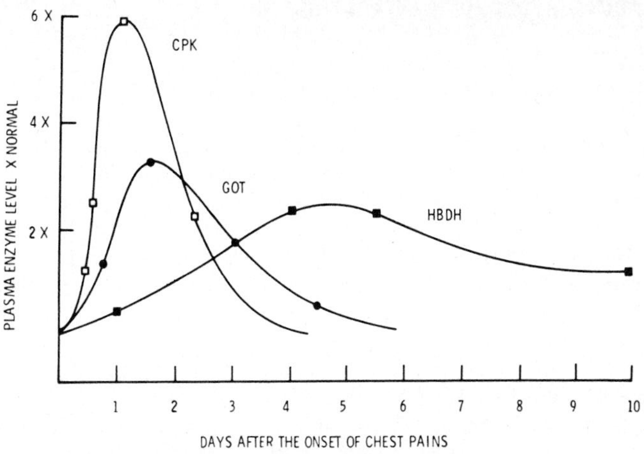

FIGURE 38–13. Typical plasma profiles for creatine kinase (CPK), glutamate oxalocetate transaminase (GOT), and hydroxybutyrate dehydrogenase (HBDH, LDH) activities following the onset of acute myocardial infarction. (From Hearse, D. J.: Myocardial enzyme leakage. J. Molec. Med. *2*:185, 1977.)

the diagnosis of AMI when the other two enzymes are tested is negligible.[271, 275]

LDH activity rises and falls more slowly than SGOT and exceeds the normal range by 24 to 48 hours after the onset of AMI, reaches a peak 3 to 6 days after the onset of pain, and returns to normal levels 8 to 14 days after the infarction. Like SGOT, the total LDH, while sensitive, is not specific; false-positive elevations occur in patients with hemolysis, megaloblastic anemia, leukemia, liver disease, hepatic congestion, renal disease, a variety of neoplasms, pulmonary embolism, myocarditis, skeletal muscle disease, and shock.[270, 271]

LDH has five isoenzymes, which are numbered in the order of the rapidity of their migration toward the anode of an electrophoretic field. LDH_1 moves most rapidly, whereas LDH_5 is the slowest. Fractionation of serum LDH into its five isoenzymes increases diagnostic accuracy, since the heart contains principally LDH_1, whereas liver and skeletal muscle contain primarily LDH_4 and LDH_5. Thus, LDH_5 is commonly elevated in patients with congestive hepatomegaly. Most conditions causing elevated serum total LDH activity, such as liver or skeletal muscle disease or injury, are readily distinguished from AMI by analysis of LDH isoenzymes. Increased serum LDH_1 activity precedes elevation of serum total LDH and usually occurs within 8 to 24 hours after infarction.[276] Elevations of LDH and in the ratio of LDH_1 to total LDH occur in more than 95 per cent of patients with AMI.[270, 277] Since hemolysis also raises serum LDH_1 activity, particular care must be taken in the withdrawal and handling of the blood specimens.

Many laboratories report the ratio of LDH_1 to LDH_2, which is elevated in MI. An LDH_1/LDH_2 ratio greater than 1.0 is commonly used as a cutoff defining abnormality in most series[271]; however, even a ratio as low as 0.76 has been reported to be more than 90 per cent sensitive and specific for the diagnosis of AMI.[276] LDH or LDH isoenzyme analysis for the diagnosis of AMI should be reserved for cases in which the CK has already fallen to normal—that is, when infarction is suspected to have occurred 2 to 4 days earlier. Although LDH isoenzyme testing may be useful, as indicated above, like SGOT, the *routine* use of LDH and LDH isoenzyme determination is not justified and accounts for a considerable waste of resources.[278, 279]

CREATINE KINASE (CK) (See also p. 2632). Serum CK activity exceeds the normal range within 4 to 8 hours following the onset of AMI and declines to normal within

3 to 4 days after the onset of chest pain (Fig. 38–13).[270] The time of peak serum CK activity varies considerably, occurring as early as 8 hours after the onset of pain to as long as 58 hours later.[280] While the mean peak CK for AMI occurs at about 24 hours, peak levels occur earlier in patients who have had reperfusion as a result of the administration of thrombolytic therapy or mechanical recanalization (as well as in patients with early spontaneous thrombolysis), with peak CK occurring at about 12 hours after infarction in such cases.[271, 281] With reperfusion, enzyme is released into the circulation more rapidly than for an infarct of comparable size without reperfusion.[282] Thus, reperfusion renders estimation of infarct size by enzyme analysis less accurate. Because the time-activity curve of serum CK is influenced by reperfusion, and because reperfusion itself influences infarct size, it has been suggested that the time to peak CK activity should be incorporated into estimates of infarct size.[283]

Although elevation of the serum CK is the most sensitive enzymatic detector of AMI that can be used routinely,[270, 276, 277, 284, 285] 15 per cent false-positive results will occur in patients with muscle disease, alcohol intoxication, diabetes mellitus, skeletal muscle trauma, vigorous exercise, convulsions, intramuscular injections, thoracic outlet syndrome, and pulmonary embolism.[270, 275, 286] However, serum CK activity is normal in patients with heart failure and hepatic disease. CK values in women are normally about two-thirds of those in men.

TABLE 38–3 RECOMMENDATIONS ON THE USE OF SERUM ENZYME ASSAYS IN THE DIAGNOSIS OF ACUTE MYOCARDIAL INFARCTION

1. A single set of cardiac enzyme values in the emergency room is not sufficiently sensitive to exclude myocardial infarction. Although a single, markedly positive CK-MB value will greatly increase the probability of acute infarction, data are insufficient to support or reject a policy whereby low-risk patients, who otherwise would be sent home, would be observed until one or more CK-MB values are obtained.
2. If myocardial infarction is suspected, then samples of total CK and CK-MB levels should be measured on admission and about 12 and 24 hours later, although condensed versions of this strategy may ultimately prove to be equally efficacious and more cost effective. If myocardial infarction may have occurred more than 24 hours before admission, and if CK and CK-MB levels are not diagnostic, a total LDH level should be ordered. If the total LDH level is elevated, an assay of LDH isoenzymes should be obtained. If the first LDH1/LDH2 ratio is only slightly less than 1.0, a second assay is probably indicated.
3. If chest pain recurs after admission, CK and CK-MB assays should be done at 0, 12, and 24 hours. "Surveillance" enzyme assays are not recommended in asymptomatic patients without electrocardiographic changes.
4. Routine use of enzyme assays other than those for CK, CK-MB, and LDH isoenzymes is not recommended.
5. If more than 2 hours may pass before CK isoenzymes will be assayed, the serum sample should be preserved on ice.
6. Strategies including CK-MB assays can be used to diagnose myocardial infarction in the setting of noncardiac surgery and cardiac catheterization and after electrical countershock.
7. In the setting of cardiac surgery, myocardial infarction should be diagnosed if any two of the following are present: CK-MB elevation persisting more than 12 hours; new Q waves on an electrocardiogram; or regional defect on technetium pyrophosphate scintigraphy.
8. False-positive elevations of CK-MB can be minimized by diluting samples with marked elevations of total CK; detecting isoenzyme variants that masquerade as CK-MB on column chromatography assays by retesting the sample on an electrophoretic assay if the clinical presentation is atypical for myocardial infarction; or consideration of other sources of CK-MB (for example, myocarditis, renal failure, neuromuscular diseases, trauma) if a true elevation of CK-MB levels is found in the absence of a typical rise and fall of CK and CK-MB levels and other evidence for myocardial infarction.

From Lee, T., and Goldman, L.: Serum enzyme assays in the diagnosis of acute myocardial infarction. Recommendations based on a quantitative analysis. Ann. Intern. Med. *102*:221, 1986.

CK ISOENZYMES. Three isoenzymes of CK (MM, BB, and MB) have been identified by electrophoresis. Extracts of brain and kidney contain predominantly the BB isoenzyme, skeletal muscle contains principally MM, and both MM and MB isoenzymes are present in cardiac muscle. The MB isoenzymes of CK may also be present in minor quantities in the small intestine, tongue, diaphragm, uterus, and prostate.[285, 287] Strenuous exercise, particularly in trained long-distance runners or professional athletes, may cause elevation of both total CK and CK-MB.[288, 289] For some athletes, both the percentage of MB released and the characteristic rise and fall of CK-MB may be similar to the changes seen after MI. Recent evidence raises the possibility that isoenzyme production is at least partially dynamic, with the relative portion of MB isoenzyme in cardiac muscle perhaps depending on maturation, preexisting coronary artery disease, or left ventricular hypertrophy.[290] Despite these issues and the fact that small amounts of CK-MB isoenzyme are found in tissues other than heart, elevated serum activity of CK-MB may be considered, for practical purposes, to be the result of AMI (except in the case of trauma or surgery on the above-mentioned organs, which contain small quantities of the enzyme).

Three isoforms of the MM isoenzyme have been identified.[291, 292] One of these isoforms is released into the blood quite rapidly—perhaps as soon as one hour—after the onset of infarction. An assay of this MM isoform may permit early identification of patients with AMI (see p. 2633). Nevertheless, measurement of serum CK-MB isoenzyme continues to be a most useful and widely available test for myocardial necrosis.[271, 287, 293, 294] The development of radioimmunoassay for the measurement of serum CK-MB has been helpful in increasing the accuracy, sensitivity, and specificity of this test.[295] In addition to AMI secondary to coronary obstruction, other forms of injury to cardiac muscle—such as those resulting from myocarditis, trauma, cardiac catheterization, shock,[296] and cardiac surgery—may also produce elevated serum CK-MB activity.[297–299] These latter causes of elevations of serum CK-MB values can usually be readily distinguished from AMI by the clinical setting. In approximately 15 per cent of patients with apparent AMI, the CK-MB may be elevated despite a normal total CK.[300–301] The importance of this finding is unclear. In an animal model, it has been shown that CK-MB may be released into the blood by transient severe ischemia without myocardial necrosis[302]; thus, minor elevation of CK-MB may not be diagnostic of AMI. Patients with minimally elevated CK-MB and normal CK, however, do have a prognosis that is generally worse than patients with suspected MI and no CK-MB elevation.[301, 303, 303a] Thus, whether or not such elevations represent true "microinfarctions" may be less important than the prognostic connotations of this isolated elevation. Therefore, total CK is not a sensitive adequate screening test. On the basis of a careful analysis of factors affecting serum enzyme assays and a rational approach to minimizing resource consumption without adversely affecting diagnostic accuracy, Lee and Goldman[271] have proposed the series of recommendations on the use of serum enzyme assays for the diagnosis of AMI, shown in Table 38–3. Serial measurement of CK-MB and application of the methods devised by Sobel and Shell (p. 1212)[270] allow prediction of infarct size determined at necropsy[304]; infarct size estimated by this method varies inversely with ejection fraction[305] and with survival.[306] Coronary artery reperfusion influences infarct size estimates by CK-MB as it does for total CK-derived estimates. Thus, further refinements in the estimation of infarct size from CK-MB will depend on the incorporation of the effect of acute reperfusion into such estimates.[307]

OTHER LABORATORY MEASUREMENTS

Numerous nonspecific manifestations may be recognized in patients with AMI. Although they are not generally employed in establishing the diagnosis, awareness of their coexistence with infarction is important in order to avoid misinterpretation or erroneous diagnosis of other disorders.

HYPERGLYCEMIA. This occurs frequently following AMI, not only in diabetic patients, in whom ketoacidosis may be precipitated, but also (with a lower frequency) in nondiabetics, in whom several weeks may elapse before carbohydrate tolerance returns to normal[308] (p. 1233). The plasma urea and creatinine concentrations are normal, except in patients with severe left ventricular failure, in whom reduced renal perfusion and glomerular filtration may result in azotemia.

Hypokalemic alkalosis may be present in patients who develop an AMI while receiving thiazide or loop diruetics for antecedent hypertension or heart failure.

SERUM LIPIDS. These are often determined in patients with AMI. However, the results may be misleading, since numerous factors that can alter the values are operating at the time of the patient's admission to the hospital; for example, stress increases serum cholesterol, whereas recumbency decreases it.[309] Serum triglycerides are affected by caloric intake, intravenous glucose, and recumbency.[309]

During the first 24 to 48 hours after admission, total cholesterol and HDL cholesterol remain at or near baseline values but generally fall precipitously after that.[310, 311] The fall in HDL cholesterol after AMI is greater than the total cholesterol; thus, the ratio of total cholesterol to HDL cholesterol is no longer useful for risk assessment early after MI.[312] Therefore, unless values are obtained very early in patients admitted for AMI, it is best to defer determinations of serum lipid levels until at least 8 weeks after the infarction has occurred.

MYOGLOBIN. This protein is released into the circulation from injured myocardial cells and can be demonstrated within a few hours after the onset of infarction; myoglobinemia is common in patients with AMI. Peak levels of serum myoglobin are reached considerably earlier (3 to 20 hours, mean = 11.4 hours after onset of infarction) than peak values of serum CK.[313] However, the time of earlier appearance of myoglobin in the serum, its peak level, and the duration of detectable myoglobin release do *not* correlate well with these same parameters for serum CK and with clinical estimates of the severity of infarction. Myoglobin appears in the serum in multiple short bursts which last for only an hour or two; in contrast to CK, myoglobin (which has a molecular weight of only 17,000) is readily excreted into the urine. This pattern of myoglobin release suggests that MI may be occurring in a series of short bursts rather than as a single episode.[313] The clinical value of serial determinations of myoglobin in AMI is limited because of the brief duration of its elevation and the lack of specificity resulting from the fact that myoglobin is a constituent of skeletal muscle and is readily detected in the serum following damage to skeletal muscle.

TRACE METALS. Alterations in serum concentrations of various *trace metals* have been noted during AMI. Elevations in serum concentration of copper and nickel have been observed that seem to parallel elevations in the sedimentation rate.[314, 315] Significant decreases in serum zinc,[316] iron,[317] and magnesium[318] concentration occur within a day after infarction. The significance of alterations in serum concentrations of trace metals after infarction is currently unknown.

HEMATOLOGICAL MANIFESTATIONS. An increase in the *white blood count* occurs frequently following AMI; it may be a response to tissue necrosis or increased secretion of adrenal glucocorticoids or both. The elevation of the white count usually develops within 2 hours after the onset of chest pain, reaches a peak 2 to 4 days following infarction, and returns to normal in 1 week; the peak white blood cell count usually ranges between 12 and 15 $\times$ 10^3 per cubic millimeter but occasionally rises to as high as 20 $\times$ 10^3 per cubic millimeter. Often there is an increase in the percentage of polymorphonuclear leukocytes and a shift of the differential count to band forms. The *erythrocyte sedimentation rate* (ESR) is usually normal during the first day or two after infarction, even though fever and leukocytosis may be present. It then rises to a peak on the fourth or fifth day and may remain elevated for several weeks. The increase in the ESR is secondary to elevated plasma alpha$_2$ globulin and fibrinogen,[319] but the peak does not correlate well with the size of the infarction or with the prognosis. The *hematocrit* often increases during the first few days following infarction as a consequence of hemoconcentration.[218]

ELECTROCARDIOGRAPHIC FINDINGS

(See also p. 203)

In the majority of patients with AMI, some change can be documented when serial electrocardiograms are compared. However, many factors limit the ability of the ECG to diagnose and localize MI: the extent of myocardial injury, the age of the infarct, its location, the presence of conduction defects, the presence of previous infarcts or acute pericarditis, changes in electrolyte concentrations, and the administration of cardioactive drugs. Nevertheless, serial standard 12-lead ECG's remain a clinically useful method for the detection and localization of MI.[294, 320]

Although there is general agreement of ECG and vectorcardiographic criteria for the recognition of infarction of the anterior and inferior myocardial walls (Table 7–5, p. 211), there is less agreement on criteria for lateral and posterior infarcts[321]; here even the terminology may be confusing.[322] Although most patients continue to demonstrate the ECG changes from an infarction, particularly if they evolve Q waves for the rest of their lives, in a substantial minority the typical changes disappear and the electrocardiogram returns to normal after a number of months or, more commonly, years.[323] Under many circumstances Q wave patterns may simulate MI.[324] Conditions that may mimic the electrocardiographic features of MI by producing a pattern of "pseudoinfarction" are listed in Table 38–4.

Q WAVE AND NON-Q-WAVE INFARCTION. In the past an AMI (by enzyme or other clinical criteria) in which Q waves fail to develop on the electrocardiogram was referred to as a "subendocardial" or "nontransmural" MI. However, the presence or absence of Q waves on the surface ECG does not predict reliably the distinction between transmural and nontransmural or subendocardial MI.[325, 326] True pathological subendocardial MI, as recognized at autopsy, is seen with ST-segment depression and/or T wave changes only about 50 per cent of the time.[327] Nevertheless, for the prognostic importance of identifying two different populations, a distinction should be made between AMI's with or without Q waves.[328, 329] Changes in the ST segment and T wave are quite nonspecific and may occur in a variety of conditions, including stable and unstable angina pectoris, ventricular hypertrophy, acute and chronic pericarditis, myocarditis, early repolarization, electrolyte imbalance,

TABLE 38–4 CONDITIONS SIMULATING INFARCTION ON ECG

Ventricular hypertrophy
Right ventricular (cor pulmonale)
Left ventricular
Conduction disturbances
Left bundle branch block
Left anterior fascicular block
Wolff-Parkinson-White syndrome
Primary myocardial disease
Myocarditis
Dilated cardiomyopathy
Hypertrophic cardiomyopathy (both obstructive and nonobstructive)
Friedreich's ataxia
Muscular dystrophy
Pneumothorax
Pulmonary embolus
Amyloid heart disease
Primary and metastatic tumors to the heart
Traumatic heart disease
Intracranial hemorrhage
Hyperkalemia
Pericarditis
Early repolarization
Sarcoidosis involving the heart

From Taussig, A. S., et al.: Misleading ECGs: Patterns of infarction. J. Cardiovasc. Med. 9:1147, 1983.

shock, metabolic disorders, and following the administration of digitalis (Ch. 7).[321] Serial electrocardiograms may be of considerable aid in differentiating these conditions from non-Q-wave infarction.[329a] Transient changes favor angina or electrolyte disturbances, whereas persistent changes argue for infarction if other causes such as shock, administration of glycoside, and persistent metabolic disorders can be eliminated. In the final analysis, the diagnosis of nontransmural infarction rests more on the combination of clinical findings and the elevation of serum enzymes than on the electrocardiogram.

ISCHEMIA AT A DISTANCE. Patients with new Q waves and ST segment elevation diagnostic for MI in one territory often have ST-segment depression in other territories. These additional ST-segment changes may be caused by ischemia in a territory other than the area of infarction, termed "ischemia at a distance,"[330] or by reciprocal electrical phenomena.[331] A good deal of attention has been directed to associated ST-segment depression in the anterior leads, which occurs in the majority of patients with acute interior MI.[332] However, despite the clinical importance of differentiation among causes of anterior ST-segment depression in such patients—including anterior ischemia, posterior wall infarction, and true reciprocal changes—such a differentiation cannot be made reliably by electrocardiographic or even vectorcardiographic[332] techniques. Although precordial ST-segment depression is more commonly associated with extensive infarction of the posterior, lateral, or inferior septal segments—rather than anterior wall subendocardial ischemia[333–335]—ancillary scintigraphic or angiographic techniques are necessary to document this. Regardless of whether the anterior ST-segment changes reflect anterior wall ischemia or are reciprocal to changes elsewhere, this finding, as with ischemia at a distance, implies a poorer prognosis than is the case if such changes are not present.[330, 333]

RIGHT VENTRICULAR INFARCTION. This is difficult to diagnose by the electrocardiogram, presumably because the right ventricular myocardial mass is small in comparison with the left. However, ST-segment elevation in right precordial leads (V_1, V_3R–V_6R) has been noted to be a relatively sensitive and specific sign of right ventricular infarction[336–340] (Fig. 38–14). Occasionally ST-segment elevation in the usual precordial leads (particularly V_2 and V_3) may be due to acute right ventricular infarction; this appears to occur only when the injury to the left ventricular inferior wall is minimal.[341] Usually, the concurrent inferior wall injury suppresses this anterior ST-segment elevation resulting from right ventricular injury. Likewise, right ventricular infarction itself appears to reduce the anterior ST-segment depression often seen with inferior wall myocardial infarction.[342]

ATRIAL INFARCTION. This can be suspected occasionally from the electrocardiogram[343, 344]; the most common electrocardiographic patterns are depression or elevation of the PQ segment, alterations in the contour of the P wave and abnormal atrial rhythms, including atrial flutter, atrial fibrillation, wandering atrial pacemaker, and AV nodal rhythm.[321]

While the relative values of vectorcardiography and conventional scalar electrocardiography in the recognition of MI can be debated,[345–347] vectorcardiography is used only rarely in the diagnosis of AMI today.

IMAGING IN ACUTE MYOCARDIAL INFARCTION

Roentgenography (See also p. 156)

The initial chest roentgenogram in patients with AMI is almost invariably a portable film obtained in the emergency room or the coronary care unit. Two findings are common: signs of left ventricular failure and cardiomegaly. Although the pulmonary vascular markings on the roentgenogram generally reflect the left ventricular end-diastolic pressure, significant discrepancies may occur because of what have been termed *diagnostic lags* and *post-therapeutic lags*. In the former, patients may have elevated left ventricular filling pressure and normal chest roentgenogram, and, because of the time required for pulmonary edema to accumulate after left ventricular filling pressure has become elevated, 12 hours may elapse before the radiographic findings reflect the hemodynamic status. The post-therapeutic phase lag represents the longer time interval, generally 1 or 2 days, required for pulmonary edema to resorb and the radiographic signs of pulmonary congestion to clear after left ventricular filling pressure has returned toward normal.[348]

Cardiomegaly in a patient with AMI usually signifies prior infarction or another form of antecedent cardiovascular disease such as chronic hypertension with subsequent left ventricular dilatation, and it is usually associated with impaired left ventricular function.[349] Since the chest film (especially the portable film in the A-P projection) is not a sensitive indicator of ventricular size, the converse is not true, in that patients may have increased end-diastolic volume and still demonstrate a normal-sized heart on roentgenographic examination. The degree of congestion and the size of the left side of the heart on the chest film are highly useful predictors for defining groups of patients with AMI who are at increased risk of dying after the acute event.[350]

Radioisotopic Studies

All major forms of nuclear cardiac imaging—radionuclide angiography, perfusion scintigraphy, infarct avid scintigraphy, and positive-emission tomography—are useful in detecting AMI, in assessing infarct size and jeopardized myocardium, in determining the effects of the infarct on ventricular function, and in establishing prognosis. The application of these techniques is discussed in Chapter 11.[294, 351–355]

Magnetic Resonance Imaging

(See Figs. 12–27, 12–28, and 12–29, p. 372)

Cardiac imaging with magnetic resonance imaging (MRI) has been employed in experimental and clinical studies of AMI.[356, 357] In addition to localizing and sizing the area of infarction, it has been suggested that MRI techniques may be capable of early recognition of MI[358] and of providing an assessment of the severity of the ischemic insult.[359] By electrocardiographically gating MR images, it has been possible to differentiate infarcted from noninfarcted myocardium in humans.[357, 360] While imaging with this technique presents practical problems for routine studies in coronary care unit patients because patients must be transported to the MRI facility, this safe, noninvasive modality holds much promise. Potential capabilities of MR imaging are likely to include not only the ability to detect, localize, and size AMI but also to assess perfusion of infarcted and noninfarcted tissue; to identify areas of jeopardized but not infarcted myocardium; to identify myocardial edema, fibrosis, wall thinning, and hypertrophy; to assess ventricular chamber size and segmental wall motion; and to identify the temporal transition between ischemia and infarction.

With the great potential of this new technique, increasing attention is being directed to its use as reflected in the literature, and extensive resources are being consumed for the installation of clinical units. Nevertheless, the role of MRI must be carefully evaluated in comparison to other less costly and complex alternatives.[361]

Echocardiography (See also p. 121)

As major technical improvements have been made, echocardiography has emerged as an extremely important imaging modality in all cardiac patients. The relative portability of echocardiographic equipment makes this technique ideal for the assessment of patients with AMI hospitalized in the critical care setting.[361a]

M-MODE ECHOCARDIOGRAPHY. This is a sensitive technique for examining regional left ventricular wall motion.[362] It is limited to the imaging of small segments of the interventricular septum and posterior left ventricular wall; rarely, small segments of the anterior wall can be imaged as well. Therefore, abnormalities of regional wall motion and even left ventricular aneurysms, particularly those involving the anterior wall, may be missed completely.[363] Despite this obvious shortcoming, some useful information can be obtained from patients with acute or old MI, particularly in the diagnosis of complications of MI (Table 38–5). Abnormalities of left ventricular wall motion, usually corresponding to the electrocardiographic site of infarction, may be recognized in the majority of patients with transmural infarction, and hyperkinetic motion can be found in noninfarcted areas in approximately one-third of patients.[364] An increased internal diameter of the left ventricle, determined by echocardiography, correlates closely with clinical, hemodynamic, and angiographic signs of heart failure.[365]

M-mode echocardiography is also useful in detecting small pericardial effusions in patients with postinfarction pericarditis.[366] A number of changes—including increased amplitude of upper septal wall motion; dilatation of the right ventricle; and abnormal mitral valve motion in diastole, suggesting increased mitral valve flow—have been noted in the echocardiograms of patients with rupture of the ventricular septum after MI. Although not specific, this combination of echocardiographic findings provides a useful clue to the diagnosis of septal rupture.[367, 368] M-mode echocardiography can also be employed in the noninvasive diagnosis of right ventricular infarction. Findings include an increased right ventricular end-diastolic diameter and an increased ratio of right ventricular to left ventricular end-diastolic diameter.[369]

TWO-DIMENSIONAL ECHOCARDIOGRAPHY (See Figs. 5–90 to 5–94, pp. 121 to 123). This technique can provide both longitudinal and transverse views of the left ventricle, and a much larger fraction of the ventricular wall—including significant portions of the left ventricular apical, anterior, septal, inferior, and posterior walls—can be imaged[370] by this method than by the M-mode technique. Areas of abnormal regional wall motion are observed almost universally in patients with AMI.[371, 372] Abnormal wall motion is less often noted echocardiographically when the infarction is nontransmural; however, abnormalities are still present in more than two-thirds of patients.[373] Left ventricular function, estimated from two-dimensional echocardiograms,[373] correlates well with estimates for angiographic studies[374] and sometimes predicts the clinical course.[375]

In addition to the abnormal wall motion seen following AMI, myocardium in the area of infarction is usually much thinner than noninfarcted myocardium. Ultrasonic tissue characterization techniques, which take advantage of the known increase in echo intensity from myocardial scar, appear to aid in the differentiation between ischemic and infarcted myocardium.[376] The extent of abnormal wall motion generally does not change in serial two-dimensional echocardiographic studies unless infarct expansion occurs—a poor prognostic sign.[183] However, motion within the originally defined area of dyssynergy may improve during the recovery phase of AMI. Computer-aided contour systems have improved the accuracy of two-dimensional wall motion assessment and may be useful for quantitative studies of MI patients, particularly when analysis of regional wall thickening, radial length changes, and regional segment lengths are of interest.[377] While reliably detecting and localizing an AMI, two-dimensional echocardiography has been less useful for quantifying the area of infarction because of difficulties in distinguishing between ischemic and infarcted tissue. Both fail to contract normally; in such assessments the area of actual tissue necrosis usually is overestimated.[378]

Two-dimensional echocardiography is extremely useful for the detection of most mechanical complications of AMI. Left ventricular aneurysms[379] and pseudoaneurysms[380] usually are easily and reliably identified. In addition, in patients with AMI who develop a loud systolic murmur, this type of echocardiography can be used to detect and localize a ventricular septal defect, as well as detect mitral

TABLE 38–5 COMPLICATIONS OF ACUTE MYOCARDIAL INFARCTION DETECTED BY ECHOCARDIOGRAPHY

Complication	Echocardiographic Manifestations
Early	
Arrhythmias	Not applicable
Heart block and/or marked bradycardia	Not applicable
Shock	Large areas of noncontractile LV myocardium
	Right ventricular infarction: impaired RV wall motion; increased RV size with or without abnormal septal motion; absence of pericardial fluid
Pulmonary edema (congestive heart failure)	Large areas of noncontractile LV myocardium and/or anatomical complications (e.g., ventricular septal defect)
Subacute	
Infarct extension/expansion	Expansion demonstrated by disproportionate transmural diastolic thinning and associated regional ventricular dilation on two-dimensional echocardiography (2DE)
Severe mitral regurgitation secondary to papillary muscle dysfunction or rupture	Rupture demonstrated by visualization of untethered mitral valve leaflet on 2DE
Acute ventricular septal defect	2DE visualization of septal rent; negative contrast effect after IV fluid injection
Subacute to late	
Ventricular aneurysm	Localized interruption in the diastolic configuration of LV wall; orifice to aneurysm is wide
Ventricular pseudoaneurysm	Demonstration of narrow neck leading into the false aneurysm cavity
Thromboembolism	Visualization of LV thrombus

From Strauss, W. E., and Parisi, A. F.: Echocardiography. *In* Morganroth. J., Parisi, A., and Pohost, G. M. (eds.): Noninvasive Cardiac Imaging. Copyright © 1983 by Year Book Medical Publishers. Inc., Chicago.

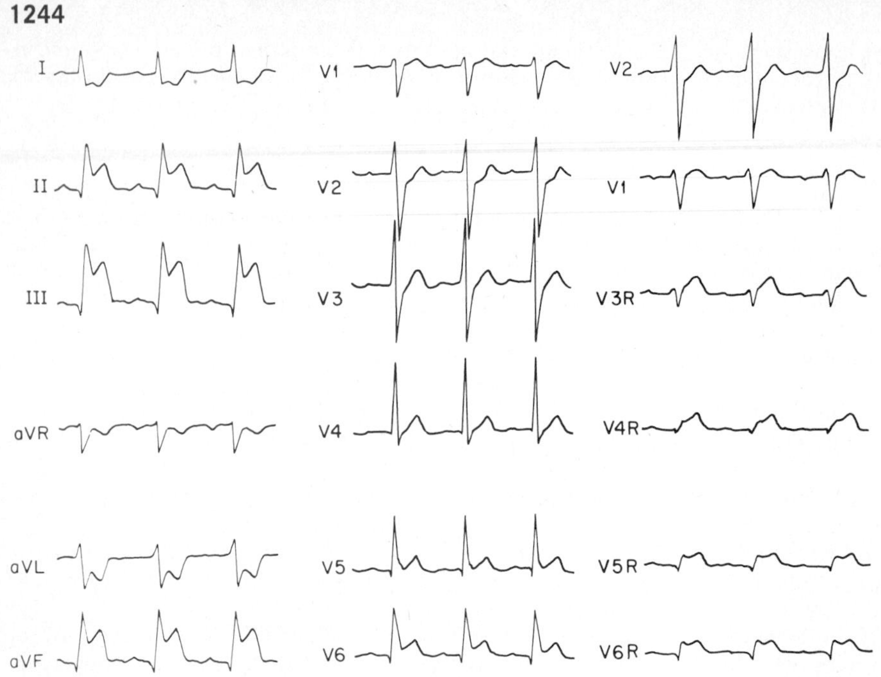

FIGURE 38–14. Leads I, II, III, aVr, AVl, aVf, leads V_1, V_2, V_3, V_4, V_5, V_6, and right precordial leads V_2, V_1, V_3R, V_4R, V_5R, and V_6R are recorded simultaneously. The ECG shows an acute inferoposterior wall myocardial infarction. The right precordial leads show ST-segment elevation in leads V_3R, V_4R, V_5R, and V_6R indicating right ventricular infarction as well. (From Brant, S. H.: Value of electrocardiogram in diagnosing right ventricular involvement in patients with an acute inferior wall myocardial infarction. Br. Heart J. *49*:368, 1983.)

regurgitation, and elucidate its cause.[381–383] Myocardial rupture, pericardial effusion,[377] and left ventricular thrombus formation,[384] all of which occur with AMI, may also be detected by this method.

DOPPLER ECHOCARDIOGRAPHY. This technique (p. 87) allows for assessment of blood flow in the cardiac chambers and across cardiac valves.[385] Used in conjunction with two-dimensional echocardiography, it is of benefit in detecting and assessing the severity of mitral or tricuspid regurgitation following AMI. Identification of the site of acute ventricular septal rupture, as well as quantification of shunt flow across the resulting defect, is also possible. Reliable estimation of cardiac output has been made by combining Doppler echocardiographic measurements of flow with two-dimensional echocardiographic measurements of ascending aortic cross-sectional area through which blood flows.[386]

SYSTOLIC TIME INTERVALS. The preejection period (PEP) and left ventricular ejection time (LVET) (p. 54) have been employed to estimate the state of left ventricular function in patients with AMI, but considerable disagreement exists concerning the value of these measurements in this condition.[387, 388] Because of the adrenergic hyperactivity commonly present in patients with AMI, comparison of systolic time intervals in patients with AMI with those obtained from patients with chronic, stable, left ventricular dysfunction is not valid. In general, patients with AMI demonstrate an abnormally short LVET, reflecting a reduction of stroke volume and a normal or only slightly prolonged PEP. The normal or nearly normal PEP should, in reality, be considered to be abnormally prolonged, since a markedly shortened PEP is normally obtained in the presence of excess adrenergic activity. Patients with AMI and normal PEP/LVET ratios demonstrate fewer clinical signs of left ventricular failure than do patients with abnormally elevated ratios. The PEP/LVET ratio becomes progressively increased with greater degrees of left ventricular failure, and patients who succumb to pump failure usually have the most abnormally elevated ratios.

Serial measurements of systolic time intervals usually reflect the changes in left ventricular function that frequently occur during the course of an acute myocardial infarction. Thus, the PEP/LVET ratio rises in patients with infarct extension.

APEXCARDIOGRAPHY. This technique can be employed to gain information about left ventricular systolic and diastolic function (p. 57). Abnormalities of the *a* wave and systolic wave of the apexcardiogram correlate with measurements of left ventricular function obtained at the time of cardiac catheterization.[389] Moreover, paradoxical motion of the left ventricle secondary to an aneurysm can be identified by apexcardiography. Increased amplitude of the *a* wave and an abnormal morphology of the systolic wave (presence of an abnormally shaped systolic wave or a secondary systolic bulge) of the apexcardiogram correlates well with akinesia or dyskinesia (or both) identified angiographically.[389]

ESTIMATION OF MYOCARDIAL INFARCT SIZE

ELECTROCARDIOGRAPHY. Interest in limiting infarct size, in large part because of the recognition that the quantity of myocardium infarcted has important prognostic implications, has focused attention on the accurate determination of MI size. The ECG initially received greatest attention. Early studies by Maroko and others demonstrated that measurement of the sum of ST-segment elevation from many precordial leads was useful for assessing the extent of myocardial injury in patients with anterior MI.[390, 391] While this technique is practical and easily utilized, it is applicable only to anterior infarctions. It is limited by the inability to distinguish between reversibly and irreversibly ischemic tissue, and it depends on the influence of myocardial geometry.[392] QRS scoring systems with planar[393–395] or vectorcardiographic[396, 397] techniques to estimate infarct size have been developed. While demonstrating good correlations with infarct size at autopsy and with enzymatic estimates, these ECG techniques are also subject to major limitations. These include the effects of ventricular geometry[392] as well as the inability to size infarcts in patients with conduction defects, nontransmural MI, and multiple infarctions.[398]

ENZYMATIC METHODS. Serial measurements of enzymes released by necrotic myocardium, particularly creatine kinase (CK) and the MB isoenzyme, are helpful in determining AMI size. Clinically, the peak CK or CK-MB is useful for a rough estimate of infarct size and is widely used prognostically. However, coronary artery recanalization—spontaneous or pharmacologically or mechanically achieved—dramatically changes the wash-out kinetics of CK from myocardium, resulting in early and exaggerated peak enzyme levels.[281, 282] Quantification of the cumulative release of CK[396, 399] or CK-MB[304, 400, 401] has been closely correlated with other techniques for estimating infarct size and with the area of necrosis at autopsy. This quantitative approach has proved useful for determining, in clinical trials on groups of patients, the effects (if any) of different forms of therapy for AMI and for prognostic assessment. However, accurate quantitation by this method is not available early enough to be useful for the clinician caring for patients with AMI.

NONINVASIVE IMAGING TECHNIQUES. Echocardiography (Chap. 5; p. 121), radionuclide scintigraphy (Chap. 11; p. 341), CT scanning (Chap. 12), and magnetic resonance imaging (Chap. 12; p. 368) have all been utilized for the clinical and experimental assessment of infarct size. Contrast enhancement[402] may improve upon the tendency of two-dimensional echocardiography to overestimate infarct size.[403, 404] Infarct-avid scintigraphy and the myocardial perfusion and wall motion types all have been used experimentally to quantify infarct size, but are limited by the inability to detect small infarcts, by ventricular geometry, and again by difficulty in distinguishing ischemic from infarcted myocardium. Tomography has improved on techniques employing technetium-99m pyrophosphate to image AMI.[405, 406] Imaging of radiolabeled myosin-specific antibodies, which bind to myosin exposed by the loss of plasma membrane in early myocardial necrosis, is the newest scintigraphic technique and holds promise for highly accurate quantification of infarct size.[355]

MANAGEMENT OF ACUTE MYOCARDIAL INFARCTION

Many options are available for the treatment of AMI. Newer approaches include the use of pharmacological agents to dissolve occluding thrombi and to delay necrosis of jeopardized myocardium and mechanical procedures to recanalize occluded coronary arteries. While such approaches have been termed "aggressive,"[20] they are clearly warranted in increasing numbers of patients. Nevertheless, the sound management of patients with AMI still depends on a variety of conventional management measures that have come into use in the decades since Herrick's original description of the condition at the beginning of this century. These measures, which consist of bed rest, oxygen, treatment of arrhythmias, and prevention of complications will be considered in this section before the more invasive therapies are discussed.

Physician practices have changed dramatically as newer approaches to the care of the AMI patient have become available.[407] Virtually all physicians in the U.S. have intensive care facilities available for their patients with AMI. In 1970, such facilities were *unavailable* to almost 20 per cent of family physicians and general practitioners. The routine use of antiarrhythmic agents has increased markedly, while the regular prescription of long-term anticoagulant therapy has fallen by 50 per cent or more. Nitrates and/or beta blockers, rarely prescribed in 1970, are now given to the majority of patients. Average hospital stay is probably one-half of what it was in 1970, or even shorter. Finally, invasive and/or noninvasive procedures to evaluate prognosis and the need for further therapy are now used in most post-MI patients, whereas only a small percentage of patients had such procedures performed in 1970.

PREHOSPITAL CARE

It is now well established that most deaths associated with AMI occur within the first hour after its onset and that death usually is due to ventricular fibrillation (Chap. 24).[408, 409] Accordingly, the importance of the immediate implementation of definitive resuscitative efforts and of rapidly transporting the patient to a hospital cannot be overemphasized. First and foremost, patients must be educated to seek immediate medical attention should they develop manifestations of MI. In patients with previous infarcts or in those with chronic stable angina, these manifestations are not difficult to describe—severe chest pain resembling that with the first infarct or more severe and prolonged than with ordinary angina. The task is more difficult in patients in whom the AMI is the first clinical manifestation of coronary artery disease.

Public campaigns must inform the susceptible population (most adults) about the clinical manifestations of AMI. People must be educated concerning the benefits of seeking immediate medical help if they are suffering an AMI, both in terms of prevention and treatment of potentially fatal arrhythmias as well as salvage of jeopardized myocardium by reperfusion. Well-equipped ambulances and helicopters staffed by personnel trained in the care of the infarct victim allow definitive therapy to commence while the patient is being transported to the hospital.[410] These specially equipped and staffed ambulances have been termed *mobile coronary care units*; to be used effectively, they must be placed strategically within a community and excellent radio communication systems must be available. They should be equipped with battery-operated monitoring equipment and direct writing electrocardiograph, a battery-operated DC defibrillator, oxygen, endotracheal tubes and suction apparatus, and commonly used cardiovascular drugs. A radiotelemetry system that allows transmission of the electrocardiogram to the hospital is desirable but not essential. The effectiveness of such a system depends upon the competency of paramedics, transmission distances, and the availability of expert consultation on the receiving end.[411]

The effectiveness of these systems in Belfast, Ireland,[410] Seattle, Washington,[412] and Columbus, Ohio[413] has been amply documented. The rapid initiation of prehospital cardiopulmonary resuscitation facilitated by mobile coronary care units and trained paramedical personnel results in initially successful resuscitation in approximately two-thirds of patients. It has been demonstrated that the frequency of death *during* transportation can be diminished from 22 to 9 per cent when defibrillation equipment and trained paramedical personnel are available.[414] In addition to prompt defibrillation, the efficacy of prehospital care appears to depend on several factors, including early relief of pain with its deleterious physiological sequelae, reduction of excessive activity of the autonomic nervous system, and abolition of prelethal arrhythmias, such as ventricular tachycardia.

Communication systems capable of transmitting the electrocardiogram over regular telephone lines are now available for the home. The prehospital use of such a system has been shown to reduce morbidity and mortality in a high-risk subset of patients supplied with the device.[415] Mobile intensive care and prehospital monitoring systems have also facilitated the acquisition of data about the earliest signs and symptoms of AMI, both for the understanding of early complications of AMI and for identifying patient subgroups with differing risks.[416] Observations of simple variables such as heart rate and blood pressure permit initial classification to high- or low-risk subgroups because patients initially presenting with hypotension have a mortality in excess of 50 per cent, whereas patients with isolated sinus bradycardia (and a normal or elevated blood pressure) appear to have a mortality that approaches zero.[416]

CORONARY CARE UNITS

During the past two and a half decades the mortality of patients with AMI treated in coronary care units has declined significantly from what it had been before the introduction of these units.[3, 5, 6] Reduction in mortality has resulted in large part from the elimination of *primary* arrhythmias as a cause of death.[11] Actually, most instances of primary arrhythmias occur *before* the patient reaches the hospital, and only about 5 per cent of patients develop a primary ventricular arrhythmia *after* they reach the hospital, an average of 5 to 6 hours after the onset of the attack in most series. Deaths from primary ventricular fibrillation have been prevented because the coronary care unit allows continuous monitoring of cardiac rhythm by highly trained nurses with the authority to administer immediate treatment and prophylaxis of arrhythmias in the absence of physicians, and because of the specialized equipment (defibrillators, pacemakers) and drugs available for instantaneous use.[417] Although all these benefits can certainly be achieved for patients scattered throughout the hospital, the clustering of patients with AMI has greatly improved the efficient use of the trained personnel, facilities, and equipment. In recent years, with increasing emphasis on hemodynamic monitoring and treatment of the serious complications of AMI with such modalities as afterload reduction and intra-aortic balloon counter pulsation, the coronary care unit has assumed even greater importance. As interventional strategies including thrombolytic therapy and acute coronary angioplasty become used more routinely in AMI patients, facilities in which patients may undergo diagnostic and therapeutic angiographic procedures are being integrated into the coronary care unit structure.

At the same time, the value of coronary care units for patients with *uncomplicated AMI* has been questioned and restudied.[418] In one widely publicized randomized trial, patients with suspected infarction were evaluated initially at home; after a 2-hour observation interval they were divided at random into home-management and hospital-management groups.[419] Although the 6-week mortality rate among patients with infarction in the two groups was similar (13 per cent and 11 per cent, respectively), such low overall mortality rates make detection of small although real differences difficult. Furthermore, approximately one-fourth of the patients with significant electrophysiological or hemodynamic complications were excluded. Thus, hospital care was provided for all high-risk patients. Furthermore, under the general conditions of medical practice in the United States, it is difficult to provide the same immediate intensive care at home for all patients with suspected infarction that was made available in this study. Since prediction of the occurrence of early complications is imperfect, it appears that the observation and prompt treatment possible in a well-staffed coronary care unit continue to justify the reliance placed upon this setting as the primary one for early management of patients with suspected or confirmed AMI. Patient delay in seeking medical attention and the medical system's delay in responding reduce the potential impact of the coronary care unit because the patients do not reach the unit until the maximum danger has passed. Therefore, education of the public, of patients at high risk of AMI, and those members of the medical profession involved in responding to the initial complaints of these patients is likely to be rewarded by further reductions of mortality.[418]

SELECTION OF PATIENTS FOR THE CCU. With increasing attention directed to the limitation of resources and to the economic impact of intensive care, there have been efforts to identify patients for whom hospitalization in a coronary care unit would likely be of benefit (p. 1687). A single set of cardiac enzyme measurements obtained in the emergency room is not of sufficient sensitivity to rule out an AMI.[271] On the other hand, the ECG, particularly in conjunction with a general clinical assessment, can be useful both for predicting which patients will have the diagnosis of AMI confirmed and identifying low-risk patients who may require less intensive care. Of patients with a classic history of chest pain but with a normal ECG in the emergency room, less than 20 per cent will ultimately have an AMI on that admission, and less than 1 per cent will develop any significant complication (Fig. 38–15).[420] Thus, a patient with a normal ECG may not require admission to a full-fledged coronary care unit. Careful analysis of the quality of pain may help identify such low-risk patients as well. Patients without a history of angina pectoris or MI presenting with pain that is sharp or stabbing and pleuritic, positional, or reproduced by palpation of the chest wall are extremely unlikely to have an AMI.[421]

More complex decision protocols, which have been utilized with the aid of simple computer programs accessible to the emergency room staff, have been successfully tested and found capable of accurately predicting which patients with acute chest pain are having an MI[422] and which have acute ischemic heart disease (including unstable angina).[423] These instruments, which incorporate clinical variables including ECG changes, the quality of pain and other symptoms, and the patient's age, have not yet achieved widespread use. As pressures increase to eliminate inappropriate coronary care unit admissions, clinicians in the emergency room may find it important to take advantage of such tools.

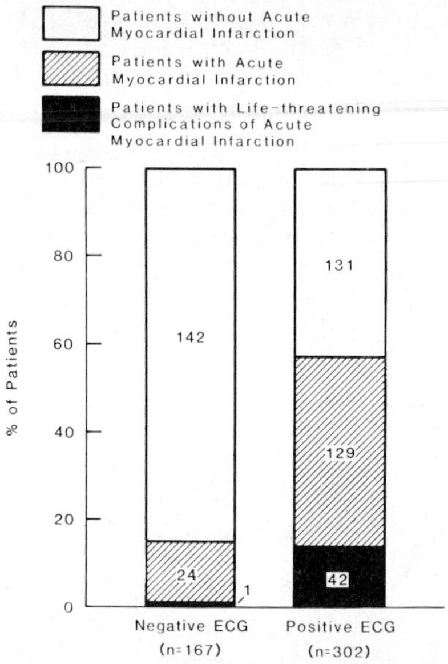

FIGURE 38–15. The initial emergency room electrocardiogram predicts percentages of patients with acute myocardial infarction and immediately life-threatening complications (ventricular fibrillation, sustained ventricular tachycardia, or heart block). Numbers of patients are shown within the bars. The differences in the rate of myocardial infarction and in the rates of complications between the two ECG groups are both statistically significant ($P < 0.01$). A positive ECG includes any of the following: repolarization changes, new Q waves, left ventricular hypertrophy, left bundle branch block, or a paced rhythm. (From Brush, J. E., et al.: Use of the initial electrocardiogram to predict in-hospital complications of acute myocardial infarction. N. Engl. J. Med. *312*:1137, 1985.)

For patients with a low probability of MI, the clinician should consider admission to an intermediate care facility equipped with simple ECG monitoring and resuscitation equipment. This strategy has been shown to be cost-effective.[424] It may be preferable for many such patients who stand to gain little benefit from the high staffing, intense activity, and elaborate technology available to current coronary care units (with their attendant high costs) and who may be disturbed by that activity and equipment. Use of a nonintensive care facility for low-risk patients may reduce coronary care unit utilization by one-third, shorten hospital stays, and have no deleterious effect on patients' recovery.

RECOMMENDATIONS. While it is true that there is both a lack of direct evidence for the value of coronary care units and a lack of consensus concerning general admission policies and therapeutic strategies for these units,[425] several common principles and guidelines may be proposed: (1) Most patients with clear-cut AMI should be admitted to an intensive (coronary) care unit. Patients with hemodynamic instability, other serious medical problems, or continuing symptoms also should be admitted, even if the diagnosis of AMI is uncertain. Most patients with unstable angina (p. 1353), particularly if episodes of chest pain are occurring at rest, should also be admitted to the coronary care unit. (2) Once an AMI is ruled out, which may be as early as 24 hours after admission,[425a] and symptoms are controlled with oral or topical pharmacological agents, discharge from the coronary care unit should be considered. (3) In AMI patients with uncomplicated status, stays in the unit need be no longer than 2 days. (4) In patients with complicated AMI, the duration of the coronary care unit stay should depend on the need for "intensive" care—that is, hemodynamic monitoring, close nursing supervision, intravenous vasoactive drugs, and frequent changes in the medical regimen.

GENERAL MEASURES

General care measures should include (1) a liquid diet for 24 hours, because of the risk of nausea and vomiting or cardiac arrest early after infarction and the need to reduce the risk of aspiration. This should be followed by a 1500 calorie soft diet, with no added salt, divided into multiple small feedings for several days. Then, in the absence of heart failure, a regular diet, low in cholesterol and saturated fats, is appropriate. Caffeine-rich beverages should be avoided because of their possible arrhythmogenic effects. (2) Dioctyl sodium sulfosuccinate, 100 mg daily, or another stool softener should be used to prevent constipation and straining. (3) The emotional impact of an AMI and of hospitalization in a coronary care unit (Ch. 62) should be offset by thoughtful explanations of the nature of the illness, the function of the equipment, and the purpose of the procedures. A deliberate effort should be made to maintain the atmosphere in the coronary care unit as quiet and restful as possible. Diazepam, 2 to 5 mg orally four times a day, is useful to allay the anxiety that is so common in this setting. Flurazepam, 15 to 30 mg, or an equivalent may be given for sleep. (4) Derangements potentially contributing to arrhythmias, such as hypoxemia, hypovolemia, disturbances of acid-base balance or of electrolytes, and drug toxicity should be identified and corrected.

CONTROL OF CARDIAC PAIN

The alleviation or reduction of pain is a critical factor in the care of patients with AMI. Since the pain associated with MI is related to ongoing ischemia (p. 1236), many interventions that act to improve the oxygen supply-demand relationship (either by increasing supply or decreasing demand) may lessen the pain associated with AMI.

NITRATES. As long as hypotension is not present, careful administration of nitrates may lessen pain. Once it is ascertained that hypotension is not present, a sublingual nitroglycerin tablet should be administered and the patient observed carefully for improvement in symptoms or change in hemodynamics. If an initial dose is well tolerated and appears to be of benefit, further nitrates should be administered, with careful monitoring of the vital signs. However, long-acting nitrate preparations should be avoided in the very early course of AMI. In patients with a prolonged period of waxing and waning chest pain, intravenous nitroglycerin may be of benefit in controlling symptoms and improving ischemia, but careful monitoring of blood pressure is required.[426] Nitrates should be used cautiously in patients with inferior wall infarction because even small doses may produce sudden hypotension and bradycardia; a reaction that can be life-threatening can usually be easily reversed with intravenous atropine if it is recognized quickly.[427] In patients with suspected right ventricular myocardial infarction, nitrates should be used with *extreme caution*, if at all, since these patients may be particularly sensitive to the venodilating effects of the drug, with sudden hypotension resulting from inadequate right ventricular filling.[428]

NIFEDIPINE. Sublingual nifedipine may alleviate the pain or improve ischemia in some patients with AMI, but this drug should be administered with caution as hypotension may result. In the setting of ischemia and infarction, hypotension of any cause may increase pain if the fall in blood pressure lowers coronary filling, thereby intensifying ischemia. Thus, correction of hypotension itself may lessen pain in some patients.

ANALGESICS. Although a wide variety of analgesic agents has been used to treat the pain associated with MI, including meperidine, pentazocine, and morphine, the latter agent remains the drug of choice except in patients with well-documented morphine hypersensitivity. Four to 8 mg should be administered intravenously and doses of 2 to 8 mg repeated at intervals of 5 to 15 minutes until the pain is relieved or evident toxicity—i.e., hypotension, depression of respiration, or severe vomiting—precludes further administration of the drug. In some patients, remarkably large cumulative doses of morphine (2 to 3 mg/kg) may be required and are usually tolerated.

The reduction of anxiety resulting from morphine diminishes the patient's restlessness and the activity of the autonomic nervous system, with a consequent reduction of the heart's metabolic demands. The beneficial effect of morphine in patients with pulmonary edema is unequivocal (p. 555) and may relate to several factors, including peripheral arterial and venous dilatation (particularly among patients with excessive sympathoadrenal activity), reduction of the work of breathing, and slowing of heart rate secondary to combined withdrawal of sympathetic tone and augmentation of vagal tone.[429]

Hypotension following the administration of morphine can be minimized by maintaining the patient in a supine position and elevating the lower extremities if systolic arterial pressure declines below 100 mm Hg. Obviously, such positioning is undesirable in the presence of pulmonary edema, but morphine rarely produces hypotension under these circumstances. The concomitant administration of atropine in doses of 0.5 to 1.5 mg intravenously may be helpful in reducing the excessive vagomimetic effects of morphine, particularly when hypotension and bradycardia are present before it is administered. Respiratory depression is an unusual complication of morphine in the presence of severe pain or pulmonary edema, but as the patient's cardiovascular status improves, impairment of ventilation may supervene and should be watched for. It can be treated with Naloxone, in doses of 0.1 to 0.2 mg intravenously initially, repeated after 15 minutes if necessary. Nausea and vomiting may be troublesome side effects of large doses of morphine and may be treated with a phenothiazine in order to avoid the marked stress on the circulation resulting from emesis.

Other analgesics such as meperidine are less effective than is morphine but equally likely to produce side effects and prone to augment ventricular rate. Inhalation of *nitrous oxide*, in concentrations of from 20 to 50 per cent, combined with oxygen, is utilized widely in Europe and to a lesser extent in the United States. It frequently provides effective analgesia, particularly in patients with relatively mild pain,[430, 431] and in those having recurrent prolonged episodes of pain. Nitrous oxide appears to influence myocardial oxygen demands favorably, since its sedative action diminishes the patient's total metabolic needs. It does not depress left ventricular function or produce significant hemodynamic changes or adverse reactions.

OXYGENATION. Hypoxemia is common in patients with AMI and is usually secondary to ventilation-perfusion abnormalities[432] that are sequelae of left ventricular failure; pneumonia and intrinsic pulmonary disease are additional causes of hypoxemia. It is common practice to treat all patients hospitalized with AMI with oxygen for 24 to 48 hours, based on the very common occurrence of arterial hypoxemia and both experimental[433] and clinical[434] evidence that increased oxygen in the inspired air may protect ischemic myocardium. However, augmentation of the fraction of oxygen in the inspired air does not elevate oxygen delivery significantly in patients who are not hypoxemic. Furthermore, it may increase systemic vascular resistance and arterial pressure and thereby lower cardiac output slightly.

In view of these considerations, arterial oxygen tension

should be measured at the time of the patient's admission to the coronary care unit; oxygen therapy may be omitted if it is normal. On the other hand, oxygen should be administered to patients with AMI when arterial hypoxemia is clinically evident or can be documented by measurement.[435] In these patients, serial arterial blood gas measurements may be employed to follow the efficacy of oxygen therapy. Although patients with AMI may exhibit a reduction in precordial ST-segment elevation during 100 per cent oxygen breathing, no long-term effect on survival or on the development of complications has been documented.[434]

In general, the delivery of 2 to 4 liters/min of 100 per cent oxygen by mask or nasal prongs for 2 to 3 days is satisfactory for most patients with mild hypoxemia. If arterial oxygenation is still depressed on this regimen, the flow rate may have to be increased. In patients with pulmonary edema, endotracheal intubation and controlled ventilation at a positive pressure may be necessary.

BETA-ADRENOCEPTOR BLOCKERS. Beta blocking agents have been used in the early hours of AMI in attempts to limit the size of infarction (p. 1258). In the course of these studies, it has been recognized that beta blockers improve pain and reduce the need for analgesics in many patients, presumably by reducing ischemia.[436, 437] Patients most suited for the use of beta blockers early in the course of AMI are those who also have sinus tachycardia and hypertension, since beta blockers will improve the heart rate and blood pressure, thereby lowering myocardial oxygen demand. A popular and relatively safe protocol for the use of a beta blocker in this situation is as follows: (1) Patients with heart failure, hypotension, bradycardia, or heart block are first excluded. (2) Metoprolol is given in three 5-mg boluses. (3) Patients are observed for *2 to 5 minutes* after each bolus and if heart rate falls below 60 beats per minute, or systolic blood pressure falls below 100 mm Hg, no further drug is given; a total of three intravenous doses (15 mg) are administered. (4) If hemodynamic stability continues, 6 to 8 hours later the patient is begun on oral metoprolol 50 mg for one day, then advanced to 100 mg twice daily if the lower dose is well tolerated. A new, extremely short-acting beta blocker, esmolol, may prove useful and even safer than currently available drugs.[437a]

PHYSICAL ACTIVITY. In the absence of all complications, patients with AMI need not be confined to bed for more than 24 to 36 hours and, unless they are hemodynamically compromised, they may use a bedside commode from the time of admission. Progression of activity regimens should be individualized depending upon patients' clinical status, age, and physical capacity. A typical patient may sit in a chair for two half-hour periods on the second and for two one-hour periods on the third day. If arrhythmia, heart failure, and other significant complications have not occurred or if they are controlled, the patient may be transferred out of the coronary care unit after 3 days. Monitoring for at least an additional two days in an intermediate care unit is desirable.

In patients without hemodynamic compromise, early ambulation—including dangling feet on the side of the bed, sitting in a chair, standing, and walking around the bed—does not cause important changes in heart rate, blood pressure, or pulmonary wedge pressure.[438] While heart rate increases slightly (usually by less than 10 per cent), pulmonary wedge pressures fall slightly as the patient assumes the upright posture for activities. Early ambulatory activities are only rarely associated with any symptoms, and when symptoms do occur, they generally are related to hypotension.[438] Thus, when Levine and Lown proposed the "armchair" treatment of AMI 25 years ago, they were undoubtedly correct that stress to the myocardium is less in the upright position.[439] As long as blood pressure and heart rate are monitored carefully, early ambulation offers considerable psychological and physical benefit without any clear medical risk.

HEMODYNAMIC ASSESSMENT

Major advances in the management of AMI have resulted from hemodynamic monitoring that has become widespread in coronary care units in recent years.[440–443] This often consists of both an intraarterial catheter and a pulmonary artery catheter. The former is usually inserted into the radial artery for continuous monitoring of systemic pressure and for sampling for blood gas determination. Pulmonary artery catheterization is accomplished with a balloon-tipped flotation catheter, often advanced, with fluoroscopic guidance, from a peripheral vein through the right heart and into the pulmonary artery. Judicious positioning of the catheter allows recording of the pulmonary arterial pressure when the balloon is inflated.[440] Blood may be sampled from the tip of the catheter in the pulmonary artery and, in certain catheters, from a second lumen opening into the right atrium. Pulmonary artery balloon catheters with a thermistor near the tip for recording thermodilution cardiac output are used frequently.[444] Thus, a single catheter in the right heart can yield the following information: saturation of blood in the pulmonary artery and right atrium, pressures in the pulmonary artery, pulmonary wedge position, and right atrium and cardiac output. A good correlation has been found between pulmonary artery wedge pressure (which is equal to pulmonary capillary pressure) and left ventricular diastolic pressure in patients with AMI.[445]

Balloon-tipped catheters are now available with a fiberoptic bundle for transmission of light. By connecting this catheter to an oximeter, continuous pulmonary artery venous blood oxygen saturation can be monitored.[446] This interesting technique is not yet widely used, as it has not been demonstrated to be of a major benefit in the coronary care unit setting.

In the past, central venous or right atrial pressure was used to gauge the degree of *left* ventricular failure in patients with AMI. However, this technique is fraught with error, since central venous pressure actually reflects *right* rather than left ventricular function. Right ventricular function, and therefore systemic venous pressure, may be normal or nearly so in patients with significant left ventricular failure.[443] Conversely, patients with right ventricular failure due to right ventricular infarction or pulmonary embolism may exhibit elevated right atrial and central venous pressures despite normal left ventricular function.[447] Low values for right atrial and central venous pressures imply hypovolemia, whereas elevated right atrial pressures usually result from right ventricular failure secondary to left ventricular failure, pulmonary hypertension, or right ventricular infarction, or less commonly from tricuspid regurgitation or pericardial tamponade.

The prognosis and the clinical status are related to both the cardiac output and pulmonary artery wedge pressure. Patients with normal cardiac output after AMI have an extremely low expected mortality; prognosis worsens as cardiac output declines. Patients with cardiac indices in the range of 2.7 to 4.3 liters/min/sq meter usually have no clinical signs of impaired perfusion, whereas patients with cardiac indices ranging from 1.8 to 2.2 liters/min/sq meter

TABLE 38–6 CONTROLLED TRIALS OF EARLY DISCHARGE FOLLOWING AMI

Authors	No. of Patients	Eligible for Early Discharge (%)	Discharge Day		Follow-up Months	Mortality After Discharge (%)	
			Early	Late		Early	Late
Harpur et al	262	76	15	28	8.0	5.0	8.0
Hutter et al	925	15	14	21	6.0	4.0	7.0
Hayes et al	268	70	9	16	1.5	6.7	7.3
McNeer et al	158	42	7	11	6.0	0	0
Ahlmark et al	383	66	8	15	3.0	4.7	2.0

From: Madsen, E. B.: Time of discharge for patients with acute myocardial infarction. Cardiovasc. Rev. Reports *4*:1301, 1983.
See reference for further information about these studies.

demonstrate early signs of hypoperfusion (cool skin and decreasing urine output and mental acuity). Patients whose cardiac index is less than 1.8 liters/min/sq meter are usually in shock. The pulmonary artery wedge pressure reflects the state of left ventricular filling, its compliance, and its ability to empty. As pulmonary pressure rises, progressive increases in pulmonary congestion occur. Mortality is greater for patients with elevated pulmonary wedge pressures.[448]

Patients with intraventricular conduction defects or AV block or both after *anterior* infarction have lower cardiac indices and higher pulmonary capillary wedge pressures than do patients without these conduction disturbances. On the other hand, patients with these conduction defects and *inferior* myocardial infarction usually do not demonstrate such hemodynamic abnormalities. The difference in hemodynamic measurements between these two groups is the result of the more extensive myocardial necrosis in patients with anterior infarction.[449]

PULMONARY ARTERY CATHETERIZATION. Before inserting a pulmonary artery catheter into a patient with an AMI, the physician must decide that the potential benefit of the information to be obtained outweighs any potential risks. Complications from pulmonary artery catheters are relatively rare, but severe problems can occur, including sepsis, pulmonary infarction, and pulmonary artery rupture. By minimization of the duration of catheterization and by adherence to careful sterile techniques, risk may be diminished.[450, 451] Accurate determination of hemodynamics by clinical assessment is difficult in critically ill patients. The use of a pulmonary artery catheter often leads to important changes in therapy that would not have occurred if the hemodynamic information had not been available.[452, 453] Some believe, however, that the pulmonary artery catheter is often overused. It has been suggested that until a clinical trial assessing its benefit is performed, the use of this technique should be curbed.[454] This view emphasizes the importance of careful patient selection, meticulous technique, and correct interpretation of the data obtained.

Patients most likely to benefit from pulmonary artery catheter monitoring include those whose AMI is complicated by: (1) hypotension that is not easily corrected by volume administration; (2) hypotension in the presence of congestive heart failure; (3) hemodynamic compromise severe enough to require intravenous vasopressors or vasodilators or intraaortic balloon counterpulsation; (4) mechanical lesions (or suspected ones) such as cardiac tamponade, severe mitral regurgitation, and a ruptured ventricular septum.[451]

THE INTERMEDIATE CORONARY CARE UNIT

Since the hazard of *primary* ventricular fibrillation is essentially over in 24 to 36 hours, there is little need for patients with entirely *uncomplicated* infarcts to remain in a coronary care unit for more than 2 days. Obviously, patients with complicated infarcts, particularly those with arrhythmias, pump failure, and recurrent ischemia, require continued care in such a unit. Patients who have undergone reperfusion and may be at risk of recurrent infarction also may require an extra day or so in the intensive cardiac care unit. There is an increased risk of ventricular tachycardia and ventricular fibrillation in the late MI period, particularly among patients with impaired left ventricular function or anterior infarction, accounting for between 10 and 30 per cent of total hospital deaths.[455] Recurrent ischemia or infarction also places such patients at increased risk.[456] In view of this significant in-hospital mortality after discharge from the coronary care unit, continued surveillance in intermediate coronary care units (also called step-down units) is justifiable. In fact, patients at an extremely low risk for complications should be considered as candidates for initial direct admission to such a facility.

Risk factors for mortality in the hospital *after* discharge from the coronary care unit include intraventricular conduction defects,[457] sinus tachycardia persisting for more than 2 days, and extensive anterior infarction, as well as episodes of ventricular fibrillation and of atrial flutter or fibrillation occurring while the patient is in the coronary care unit, and, possibly, marked electrocardiographic ST-segment abnormalities induced by low levels of activity.[458] It is possible that a reduction in late hospital mortality can be achieved with the use of intermediate coronary care units, which permit prolonged continuous monitoring of the electrocardiogram and prompt, effective treatment of ventricular fibrillation and other serious arrhythmias. The availability of these units may be useful also in helping to identify those patients who remain free from complications for a minimum of one week, since early discharge from the hospital appears to be feasible for this subset.[459]

The timing of hospital discharge is discussed on page 1287 (see also Table 38–6).

EARLY REHABILITATION (See p. 1287 and Ch. 41). Following myocardial infarction, patients are often eager for information, in need of reassurance, confused by misinformation and prior impressions, capable of counterproductive denial, and simply frightened. Cardiac rehabilitation should be carefully structured and often requires a considerable period of time, optimally beginning as early as possible once the patient is no longer in extreme danger. Intermediate care facilities provide ideal settings and ample opportunities to begin the rehabilitation process. Although intermediate care units were introduced for the purpose of decreasing mortality after coronary care unit discharge, studies have not shown any conclusive benefit in that regard.[460–462] Nevertheless, the capacity for the early detection of problems following AMI and the social and educational benefits of grouping such patients together strongly argue for continued utilization of the concept of intermediate coronary care. Furthermore, the economic advantage of grouping such patients together for sharing of resources, in terms of improving utilization of coronary care units and possibly for facilitating early discharge, outweighs any questions raised by the lack of a clear consensus regarding reduced mortality. An additional potential advantage that should not be underestimated is facilitation of patient education in a group setting with formal lectures and various types of audiovisual programs.

LIMITATION OF INFARCT SIZE

Infarct size is an important determinant of prognosis in patients with AMI. Patients who succumb from cardiogenic shock exhibit massive infarcts.[463, 464] Early impairment of ventricular function, presaging a poor prognosis, is correlated with extensive infarcts.[464, 465] Survivors with large infarcts frequently exhibit late impairment of ventricular function, and the long-term mortality rate is higher than that for survivors with small infarcts (Fig. 38–16), who tend not to develop cardiac decompensation.[465–469] The influence of infarct size on mortality is most apparent during the patient's hospital course and in the first few months after infarction. The hospital mortality in patients with large infarcts, as estimated by technetium pyrophosphate scanning, is several times greater than it is in patients with small infarcts.[468] However, the importance of infarct size declines somewhat with time after the initial episode[469]; after recovery from an AMI it is the quantity of remaining myocardium whose viability is threatened because it is perfused by obstructed coronary vessels that becomes critical to the prognosis.

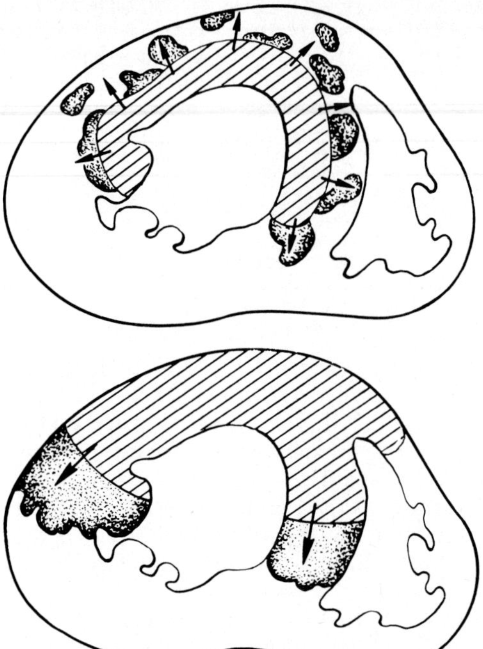

FIGURE 38–17. Two types of extension of myocardial infarction. Type A (top) was observed at the edges of an infarct, usually subepicardially. Type B (bottom) occurred at the lateral margins. (From Alonso, D. R., et al.: Pathophysiology of cardiogenic shock: Quantification of myocardial necrosis, clinical, pathological and electrocardiographic correlation. Circulation *48*:588, 1973, by permission of the American Heart Association, Inc.)

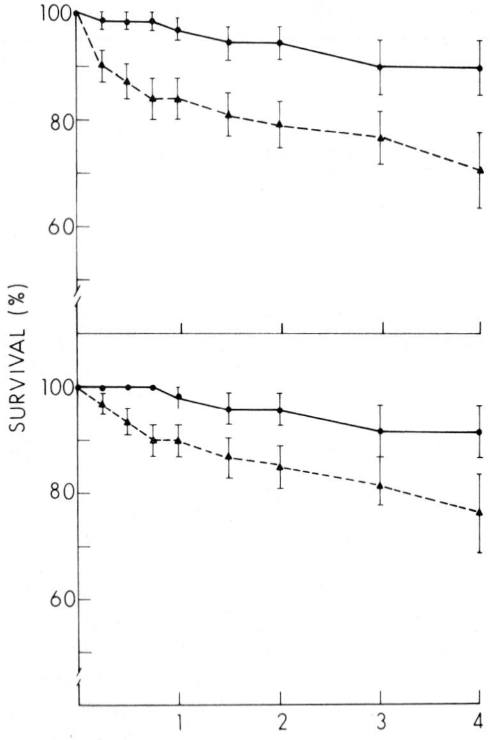

FIGURE 38–16. The influence of the extent of initial myocardial infarction on survival. Survival is shown after initial myocardial infarction in a total of 173 patients with infarct size index (expressed in terms of CK-gram-equivalents/m^2) of <15 (solid line) vs. ≥ 15 (interrupted line). Brackets indicate standard errors. The upper panel depicts survival curves for all patients who survived for at least 24 hours after the onset of an initial myocardial infarction. The lower panel depicts curves for those patients who survived at least 21 days after infarction. In both groups, survival was significantly greater for patients with small compared to large infarcts ($p < 0.05$). (From Geltman, E. M., et al.: The influence of location and extent of myocardial infarction on long-term ventricular dysrhythmia and mortality. Circulation *60*:805, 1979, by permission of the American Heart Association, Inc.)

In view of the prognostic importance of infarct size, the concept that modification of infarct size is possible has attracted a great deal of experimental and clinical attention over the past 2 decades.[15, 16, 470, 471] Efforts to limit the size of infarction have been divided among three different (sometimes overlapping) approaches: early reperfusion, reduction of myocardial energy demands, and stimulation of anaerobic energy production.[472] Before these areas are considered in more detail, issues concerning the infarction process and general clinical measures are discussed.

THE DYNAMIC NATURE OF INFARCTION. AMI is a dynamic process that often does not occur instantaneously but sometimes evolves relatively slowly (Fig. 38–17). As has been pointed out (p. 1213), in experimental animals the fate of jeopardized, ischemic tissue may be affected favorably by interventions that restore perfusion, reduce myocardial oxygen requirements, inhibit accumulation or facilitate washout of noxious metabolites, augment the availability of substrate for anaerobic metabolism,[15, 16, 470–473] or blunt the effects of mediators of injury such as calcium or free oxygen radicals,[474, 475] metabolites, and constituents of cell membranes.[476, 477]

The perfusion of the myocardium associated with AMI appears to be reduced maximally immediately following coronary occlusion. In experimental animals, increases in blood flow to the peripheral portions of the ischemic zones become evident within 24 hours of acute coronary occlusion,[478] suggesting that dynamic factors contribute to the early limitation of perfusion. These may include the efflux of potassium from injured myocardial cells[479] as well as the release of catecholamines as a consequence of ischemia of adrenergic neurons (and the resultant vasospasm). Spasm of coronary vessels has been implicated not only in Prinzmetal's variant angina (p. 1360) but also in association with MI induced by atherosclerosis,[101, 480–482] as well as in patients experiencing postinfarction angina at rest.[483, 484] While it may play a contributory role, other than in patients with Prinzmetal's angina it is unlikely to be the principal cause. While coronary spasm might play a role at the inception of coronary occlusion, by the time an angiogram is performed intracoronary nitroglycerin very rarely results in reperfusion.

Relatively prompt, *partial* restoration of reduced blood flow to the ischemic zone may result from spontaneous thrombolysis, from relief of coronary spasm (see above), or from improved systemic hemodynamics; the latter includes augmented coronary perfusion pressure and reduced left ventricular end-diastolic pressure. Subsequently, perfusion may be enhanced by the development of collateral circulation.[485] The prompt implementation of measures designed to protect ischemic myocardium and support myocardial perfusion may provide sufficient time for the development of anatomical and physiological compensatory mechanisms that limit the ultimate extent of infarction.

AMI in hospitalized patients may be complicated by extension of infarction or early reinfarction (p. 1286). Depending on the criteria utilized for detection, the incidence of these complications ranges from 8 to 30 per cent.[486–488] It is possible that interventions designed to protect ischemic myocardium during the initial event may also reduce the incidence of extension of infarction or early reinfarction. On the other hand, it has been suggested that preservation of ischemic myocardium could lead to persistent survival of cells in regions subjected to repetitive episodes of severe ischemia, leading to the development of arrhythmias. The relatively poor *late* prognosis of patients with non-Q-wave infarction[489, 490] is consistent with this possibility. However, despite these hazards, there is no evidence that the implementation of interventions designed to protect ischemic myocardium results in any late deleterious effects. Furthermore, it has been reported that preservation of ischemic myocardium by trimethaphan in hypertensive patients with evolving infarction,[491] by intravenous nitroglycerin in normotensive patients,[492] and by the early administration of beta-adrenoceptor blocking agents[493–496] is actually associated with a reduced rather than an increased mortality.

Proof of the clinical efficacy of specific interventions has been difficult to acquire, in part because of the wide variations in the size of infarcts and their rate of evolution, in part because of the difficulties involved in measuring infarct size, and in part because it is difficult to predict what the size any given infarction would have been had the intervention under study not taken place. In addition, since many patients usually reach the hospital 5 hours or even later after the onset of ischemia, it may be too late in these patients to salvage substantial quantities of ischemic myocardium in the first place.

ROUTINE MEASURES FOR INFARCT SIZE LIMITATION

Recognition that the ultimate size of an MI does not depend solely on the pathological anatomy of the coronary vascular bed, but also on a variety of physiological variables, suggests emphasis on a number of principles in the management of AMI. These principles can and should be applied in routine care. It is mandatory to maintain an optimal balance between myocardial oxygen supply and demand so that as much of the jeopardized zone of the myocardium surrounding the most profoundly ischemic zones of the infarct can be salvaged. During the period before irreversible injury has occurred, myocardial oxygen consumption should be minimized by maintaining the patient at rest, physically and emotionally, and by utilizing mild sedation and a quiet atmosphere that may lower heart rate, a major determinant of myocardial oxygen consumption. If the patient was receiving a beta-adrenoceptor blocking agent at the time the clinical manifestations of the infarct commenced, the drug should not be discontinued unless a specific contraindication develops, such as left ventricular systolic failure or bradyarrhythmia. Marked sinus bradycardia (heart rate less than approximately 50 beats/min) and the frequently coexisting hypotension should be treated with postural maneuvers (the reverse Trendelenburg position) to increase central blood volume and atropine or electrical pacing, but *not* with isoproterenol. On the other hand, the *routine* administration of atropine, with the resultant increase in heart rate, to patients without serious bradycardia is contraindicated. All forms of tachyarrhythmias require prompt and direct treatment, since they increase myocardial oxygen needs.

Diuretics are the first line of drugs indicated in the treatment of congestive heart failure. If they prove insufficient, vasodilators should be added,[497] unless the patient is already hypotensive. Inotropic agents such as the digitalis glycosides and cardioactive sympathomimetics should be added only if there is evidence of persistent and severe ventricular failure despite diuretics and vasodilators; these agents should *not* be given prophylactically. Of the various sympathomimetic amines available, isoproterenol with its chronotropic and vasodilator effects is the most hazardous. *Dobutamine* (or small doses of dopamine), which has less effect on heart rate and systemic vascular resistance than do norepinephrine, epinephrine or isoproterenol is the drug of choice when cardiac contractility *must* be augmented.

Particular attention must be paid to preserving arterial oxygenation in patients with hypoxemia, such as occurs in patients with chronic pulmonary disease, pneumonia, or left ventricular failure. Oxygen-enriched air should be administered to patients with hypoxemia, and bronchodilators and expectorants should be used when indicated. Severe anemia, which can also extend the area of ischemic injury, should be corrected by the cautious administration of packed red cells, accompanied by a diuretic if there is any evidence of left ventricular failure. Associated conditions, particularly infections and the accompanying tachycardia, fever, and elevated myocardial oxygen needs, require immediate attention.

Systolic arterial pressure should not be allowed to deviate by more than approximately 25 to 30 mm Hg from the patient's usual level, unless marked hypertension had been present before the AMI. In regard to the effect of changes in arterial pressure on myocardial injury, it is likely that each patient has an optimum level of arterial pressure. As coronary perfusion pressure deviates from this level, the unfavorable balance between oxygen supply (which is related to coronary perfusion pressure) and myocardial oxygen demand (which is related to ventricular wall tension) that ensues will increase the extent of ischemic injury.

Rather than simply maintaining the patient's vital signs, the physician's attention should be directed toward controlling ischemia and preserving the myocardium as well as maintaining perfusion of peripheral organs. However,

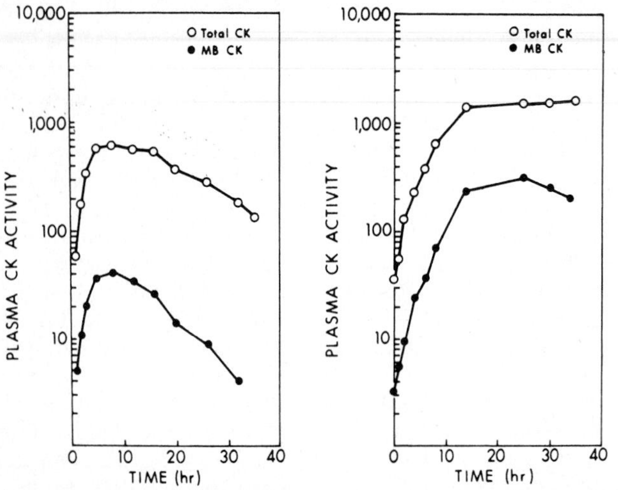

FIGURE 38–18. Plasma CK time-activity curves in a patient with uncomplicated acute myocardial infarction (*left*) and one with acute myocardial infarction associated with cardiogenic shock (*right*). As shown on the left, hemodynamically uncomplicated acute myocardial infarction is characterized by a relatively early occurrence of peak total and MB-CK activity, with a gradual subsequent smooth decline. On the other hand, as shown on the right, myocardial infarction associated with cardiogenic shock is characterized by a more prolonged interval prior to occurrence of peak enzyme activity in blood, indicative of persistent release of enzyme reflecting progressive damage of myocardium. Total CK activity may remain elevated in patients with myocardial infarction because of extracardiac release of enzyme, but the sustained elevation of MB-CK activity accompanying cardiogenic shock, as evident in the example shown on the right, is attributable to continuing cardiac damage. (From Gutovitz, A. L., et al.: The progressive nature of myocardial injury in selected patients with cardiogenic shock. Am. J. Cardiol. *41*:469, 1978.)

these two objects may sometimes conflict. In the first 4 to 6 hours after the onset of the clinical event, when the ultimate size of the infarct has not yet been established, myocardial preservation should ordinarily be given the highest priority. This may mean foregoing the stimulation of cardiac contractility by inotropic agents. Later, once the size of the infarct is fixed and if heart failure supervenes, it may be appropriate to stimulate the heart with positive inotropic agents, i.e., to employ an intervention that might have increased infarct size if given at an earlier time.

In some patients, particularly those with cardiogenic shock, tissue damage occurs in a "stuttering" manner with persistent release of CK into the bloodstream (Fig. 38–18) rather than abruptly, a condition that might more properly be termed *subacute infarction*.[464, 469] This concept of the dynamic nature of the infarct process as well as the observation that the incidence of ventricular ectopic activity in both the early and late post-infarct period is a function of infarct size[469] greatly expands the horizon for what can *potentially* be accomplished by techniques to limit myocardial necrosis.

REPERFUSION OF MYOCARDIAL INFARCTION

One of the two most important developments in the treatment of patients with AMI since Herrick's description of the syndrome more than 75 years ago[52] consists of establishing reperfusion of ischemic heart muscle in the early hours of myocardial infarction. (The second is the prevention and treatment of life-threatening arrhythmias.) While reperfusion occurs spontaneously in some patients,[281] this may not occur early enough to salvage ischemic myocardium, and in any event it is now well recognized that a persistent thrombotic occlusion is present in the majority of patients with AMI while the myocardium is undergoing necrosis.[62] Efforts to recanalize an occluded coronary artery by pharmacological and/or mechanical means have been increasingly successful. When carried out within the first several hours after coronary occlusion, in several species of experimental animals reperfusion improves hemodynamics and decreases infarct size, as assessed by epicardial ST-segment recordings, precordial QRS maps, myocardial CK depletion, positron-emission tomography, and morphology.[498–503] The extent of protection appears to be directly related to the rapidity with which reperfusion is implemented after the onset of coronary occlusion.[504]

While surgical reperfusion by coronary artery bypass grafting has been undertaken with variable success since the early 1970's,[505] the current era was launched by the pioneering efforts of Chazov[506] and Rentrop[507] and their collaborators. The investigators demonstrated successful reperfusion of an occluded coronary artery by the intracoronary infusion of a thrombolytic agent, sometimes in conjunction with recanalization by means of a guidewire. Many different therapeutic approaches are now available

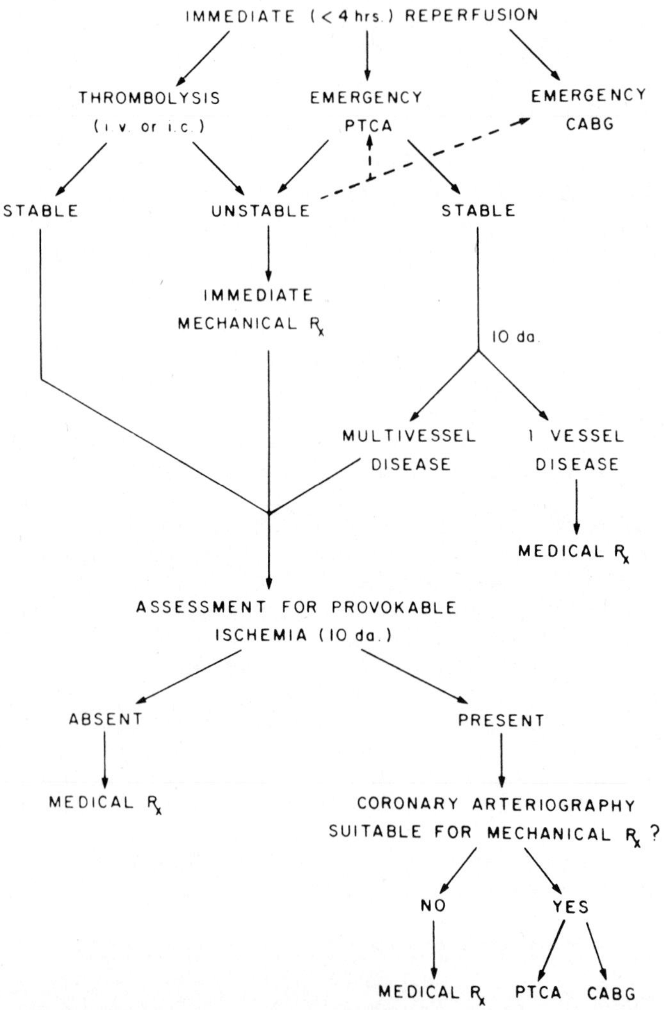

FIGURE 38–19. Approaches to the treatment of AMI. Rx = treatment, PTCA = percutaneous transluminal coronary angioplasty, CABG = coronary artery bypass grafting, i.v. = intravenous, i.c. = intracoronary. (From Braunwald, E.: The aggressive treatment of acute myocardial infarction. Circulation *71*:1087, 1985, by permission of the American Heart Association, Inc.)

to the clinician.[20] Much clinical research is currently directed at deciding on optimal reperfusion strategies and at understanding ancillary clinical issues such as patient selection, follow-up noninvasive testing, and the need for additional secondary preventive measures. One approach, based on current clinical evidence and on different availability of resources, is outlined in Figure 38–19.

PATHOPHYSIOLOGY OF MYOCARDIAL REPERFUSION

By delivering oxygen to ischemic muscle, reperfusion has the potential to relieve ischemia. Prevention of cell death by the restoration of blood flow depends on the severity and duration of preexisting ischemia. Substantial experimental evidence for this concept[508, 509] is supported by clinical studies showing that both recovery of ventricular function[510, 511, 511a] and overall mortality[19] are improved the earlier that blood flow is restored. Collateral coronary vessels also appear to play a role in the successful restoration of left ventricular function following reperfusion.[511a, 512] Collaterals are probably of greater importance in patients having reperfusion later than with reperfusion 1 to 2 hours after coronary artery occlusion; they provide sufficient perfusion of the myocardium to retard cell death.

A specific form of "reperfusion injury" has been described as cell death that occurs following reperfusion in tissue that previously had been ischemic but not necessarily irreversibly damaged.[475, 513] The possibility that reperfusion is a "double-edged sword" has been raised.[514] On the one hand, blood flow must be restored to salvage ischemic myocardium, but it is possible, although not yet unequivocally established, that the process of restoring flow may damage cells not yet irreversibly injured. Reperfusion does increase the cell swelling that occurs with ischemia,[475, 515] and this alone or with the condition known as the "no-reflow" phenomenon (when swollen cells impinge on the restoring of flow at the microvascular level[515]), could potentially lead to cellular injury. Available evidence indicates that, while reperfusion may accelerate necrosis of irreversibly injured myocytes, it does not add to the area of myocardium ultimately damaged, for such cells are already destined to die.[17] Reperfusion of myocardium in which the microvasculature is damaged leads to the creation of a hemorrhagic infarct.[508, 516] Reperfusion by means of thrombolytic therapy appears more likely to produce a hemorrhagic infarction than reperfusion by mechanical means.[516] While concern has been raised that this hemorrhage may lead to extension of the infarct,[517] this apparently is not the case.[514, 518] Histological study of patients not surviving in spite of successful reperfusion has revealed hemorrhagic infarcts, but this hemorrhage usually does *not* extend beyond the area of necrosis.[516, 519] Necrosis in the reperfused myocardium generally is of the contraction band type rather than the coagulation necrosis type seen after AMI (Fig. 38–20).[519]

The sudden exposure to both calcium and oxygen with the restoration of flow and anaerobic metabolism has been observed to affect the severity of ischemic damage.[513, 514] Toxicity from oxygen-derived free radicals, mediated at least in part by stimulated leukocytes, has attracted considerable attention[475, 514, 520] for its possible role in extending myocardial injury. Although unsupported by clinical evidence as of this writing, future therapy, likely to be carried out with reperfusion, may well include administration of agents that reduce leukocyte activation and scavenge oxygen-free radicals.[475, 514] In addition, drugs such as beta-adrenoceptor blockers and verapamil, which *delay* the death of ischemic cells, may, if administered prophylactically to patients at high risk of occlusion (or reocclusion) or in the earliest phases of the development of an AMI, enhance the quantity of myocardium salvaged by early reperfusion.

Reperfusion frequently causes changes in the cardiac rhythm. Transient sinus bradycardia occurs in many patients with inferior infarcts at the time of acute reperfusion; it is most often accompanied by some degree of hypotension. This combination of hypotension and bradycardia with a sudden increase in coronary flow has been ascribed to the Bezold-Jarisch reflex.[521] Premature ventricular contractions are the most common arrhythmia noted at the time of reperfusion, but these are frequent in all patients with AMI and it is not clear whether or not reperfusion actually increases their incidence. An accelerated idioventricular rhythm and ventricular tachycardia are more common acutely after successful reperfusion than after failed therapy.[522] When present, these rhythm disturbances may actually be a marker of successful restoration of coronary flow.[523] The need for treatment of these arrhythmias should be anticipated in any patient receiving therapy designed to recanalize a totally occluded coronary artery in the setting of AMI. Occasionally, reperfusion may actually improve ventricular arrhythmias due to ongoing ischemia or may improve heart block associated with an AMI.[524]

CORONARY THROMBOLYSIS

The knowledge that coronary thrombosis is often responsible for the initiation and/or the perpetuation of infarction (p. 1226) and the discovery that administration

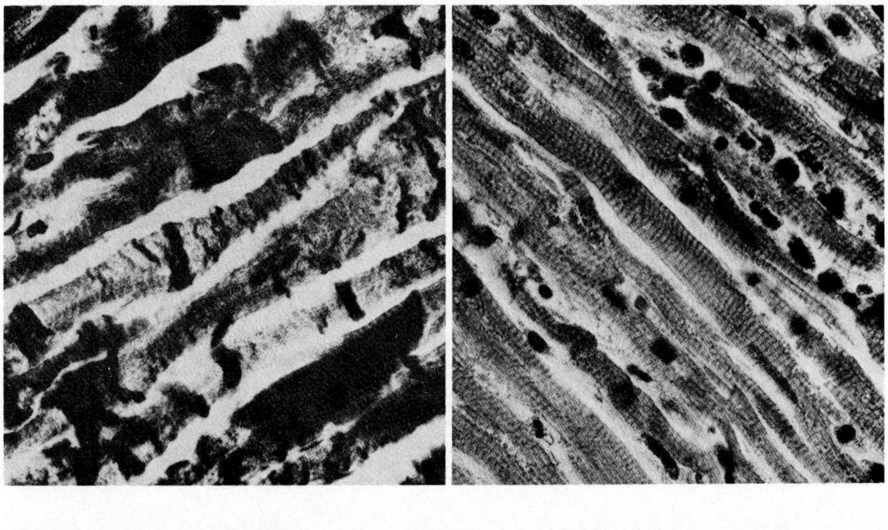

FIGURE 38–20. ***Left,*** **Contraction band necrosis of muscle fibers after successful thrombolysis.** ***Right,*** **Coagulation necrosis after unsuccessful thrombolysis: sarcomeres remain in register. (Masson-Goldner trichrome stain; final magnification 500:1, reduced 30%.) (From Mattefeldt, T., et al.: Necropsy evaluation in seven patients with evolving acute myocardial infarction treated with thrombolytic therapy. Am. J. Cardiol.** ***54*****:530, 1984.)**

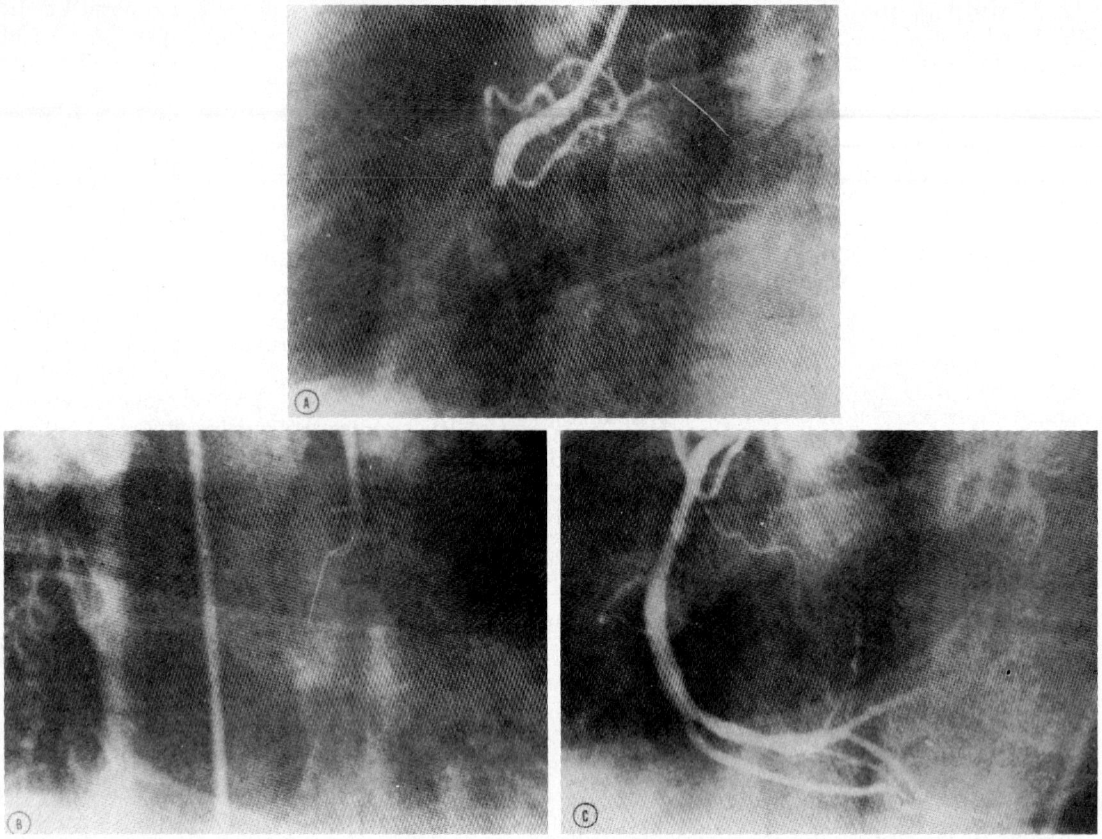

FIGURE 38–21. *A*, Complete occlusion of the right coronary artery in a 38-year-old male patient with evolving inferoposterolateral myocardial infarction. *B*, Infusion catheter advanced to site of occlusion. *C*, The artery was patent after 20 minutes of thrombolysin infusion rate of 4,000 IU/min. The arteriogram was taken after an additional infusion of thrombolysin, 120,000 IU in 60 minutes, which further improved patency. (From Ganz, W., Buchbinder, N., Marcus H., Mondkar, A., Maddahi, J., Charuzi, Y., O'Connor, L., Shell, W., Fishbein, M. C., Kass, R., Miyamoto, A., and Swan, H. J. C.: Intracoronary thrombolysis in evolving myocardial infarction. Am. Heart J. *101*:4, 1981.)

of thrombolytic agents restores angiographic patency to coronary vessels in a majority of cases[63, 94, 525, 526] have sparked interest in the potential value of clot lysis in salvaging jeopardized tissue and limiting the extent of injury sustained in patients with evolving MI.

Clinical investigation in this area initially focused on the use of *intracoronary* thrombolysis in the early hours of AMI.[63, 94, 527] Viability will be maintained in a portion of the successfully reperfused myocardium, as reflected in the restoration of contractile activity.[165, 528] On the basis of results of several successful trials, the Food and Drug Administration approved the use of *intracoronary* streptokinase and urokinase for the treatment of myocardial infarction.[17] Many factors affect the usefulness of this technique, which is dependent on the availability of a skilled catheterization team and well-equipped catheterization facility. Most reported experience with intracoronary thrombolysis has not been in both randomized and controlled trials, largely because it has been thought difficult to withhold thrombolytic therapy once a thrombotic coronary artery occlusion has been visualized angiographically, and it has not been considered ethical to catheterize patients if randomization to no thrombolytic therapy were possible for a portion of the patients. A review of a series of the most carefully performed trials has failed to show significant improvement in mortality even when the data are pooled.[18, 528a] Because of the delay involved in catheterizing patients with AMI and because of the greater potency and, theoretically, the greater safety of the newer clot-specific thrombolytic agents such as tissue plasminogen activator (t-PA) (p. 1758), there is a growing consensus that intracoronary administration of thrombolytic therapy should be reserved for patients who develop coronary thrombosis during the course of an angiographic procedure and in whom a coronary catheter is either already in place or such placement is easily and rapidly achieved.

INTRAVENOUS THROMBOLYSIS. This form of thrombolytic therapy has several important advantages over intracoronary use.[528a] Since only the placement of a peripheral intravenous line is required, therapy may be initiated early, in a variety of locations (emergency room, ambulance, helicopter, or even at home[529]) and at relatively low cost. While treatment with intravenous streptokinase seems less effective in achieving recanalization than intracoronary streptokinase, and reocclusion appears to be more frequent with intravenous therapy,[17] newer, apparently more effective thrombolytic agents appear to make up for this difference.[530, 531] Intravenous streptokinase has been used in the treatment of AMI for decades, preceding our recent definitive knowledge that thrombosis is the focal event in initiating AMI. The impact of this treatment on mortality in the most carefully performed studies is shown in Figure 38–22. Although only a minority of these trials were statistically significant when considered alone, overall results were highly significant for an improvement in mortality.[18]

One exceptionally important study has had a great impact in demonstrating the therapeutic benefit of intravenous thrombolytic treatment. The GISSI trial[19] randomized a total of 11,806 patients at 176 participating centers into two groups: conventional treatment without a thrombolytic agent and conventional therapy plus 1.5 million units of intravenous streptokinase given over 60 minutes as soon as possible after randomization. Eligible patients

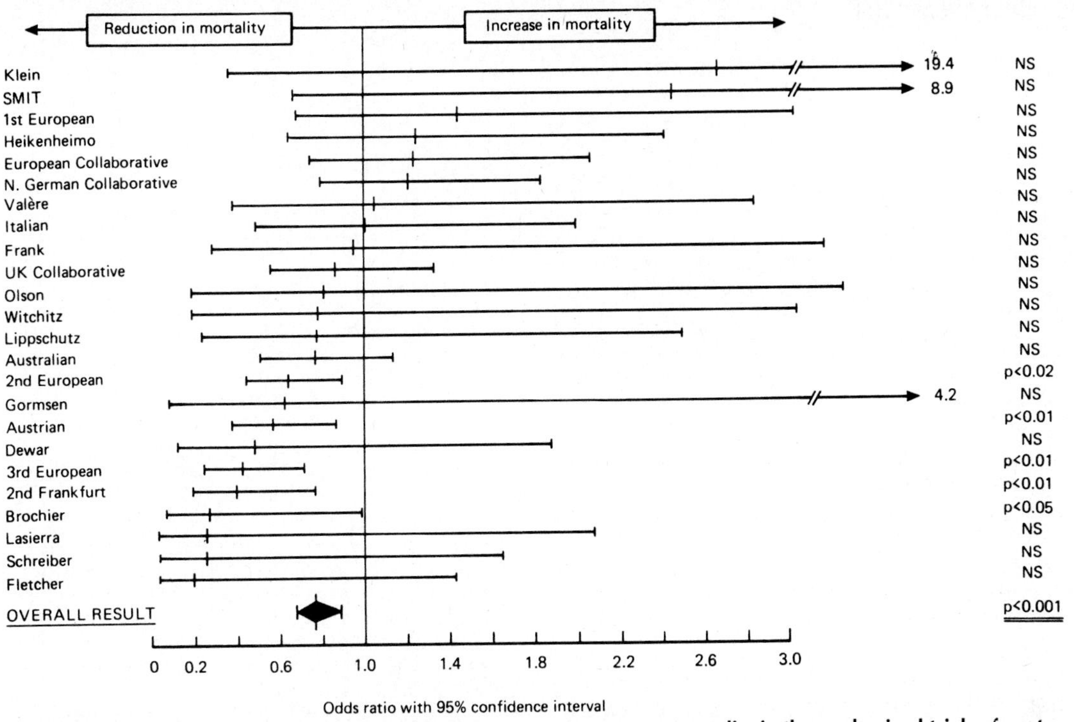

FIGURE 38–22. Apparent effects of intravenous fibrinolytic treatment on mortality in the randomized trials of acute myocardial infarction. (From: Yusuf, S., et al.: Intravenous and intracoronary fibrinolytic therapy in acute myocardial infarction: Overview of results on mortality, reinfarction, and side effects from 33 randomized controlled trials. Eur. Heart J. 6:556, 1985.)

included (1) those who had chest pain and ST-segment elevation *or* depression of 1 mm or less in any limb lead and/or of 2 mm or less in any precordial lead, *and* (2) those who were admitted to the coronary care unit within 12 hours of the onset of symptoms. Patients with recent bleeding problems, a cerebrovascular accident within 2 months, a surgical or invasive procedure or trauma in the previous 10 days, uncontrolled hypertension, previous treatment with streptokinase, or other life-threatening conditions were excluded. Complete data were available in over 99 per cent of the randomized patients. In-hospital mortality was 10.7 per cent in the streptokinase-treated group and 13.0 per cent in the control group, a highly significant difference. Mortality in subgroups stratified according to elapsed time between the onset of symptoms and randomization is shown in Table 38–7. The most profound treatment effect was seen among patients randomized early, with patients treated within one hour showing a nearly 50 per cent reduction in mortality by streptokinase.

Streptokinase treatment appeared to be most beneficial in patients 65 years of age or younger, patients with anterior infarction, patients without previous infarction, and patients at low risk as determined by Killip scale.[19] Streptokinase-treated patients experienced twice as many in-hospital reinfarctions as control patients (4 per cent vs. 2 per cent, respectively). The increase in the reinfarction rate after streptokinase has recently been confirmed.[532] The incidence of other complications in both studies was relatively low and did not differ importantly between groups. Adverse reactions to streptokinase occurred in less than 12 per cent of patients, but most were minor. Only 0.3 per cent of patients suffered a major bleeding complication, and the incidence of cerebrovascular accidents was similar in both treated and untreated groups at 0.2 per cent. The improvement in survival in the streptokinase-treated patients noted at the time of hospital discharge was sustained at one year.[531a]

In the absence of contraindications such as those applied in the GISSI trial, thrombolytic therapy is acceptable and recommended treatment for patients seen within 4 to 6 hours of onset of the clinical manifestations of AMI. Such therapy should be confined to patients younger than 75 years.[532a] Tissue plasminogen activator is a more effective lytic agent with a less pronounced systemic lytic effect than streptokinase.[530, 531, 533] As such agents become available after careful study, they are likely to be superior to intravenous streptokinase (or urokinase).

REOCCLUSION. There is evidence that patients with severe residual stenosis following thrombolysis are at higher risk for reocclusion than those without such obstruction, but whether percutaneous transluminal coronary an-

TABLE 38–7 MORTALITY BY HOURS FROM ONSET OF SYMPTOMS IN GISSI INTRAVENOUS STREPTOKINASE TRIAL

Hours After Symptoms' Onset	Deaths: Total (%)	SK patients (%)	C patients (%)	P Value
< 1	11.8	8.2	15.4	0.0001
≤ 3	10.6	9.2	12.0	0.0005
> 3–6	12.9	11.7	14.1	0.03
> 6–9	13.3	12.6	14.1	NS
> 9–12	14.6	15.8	13.6	NS

SK = streptokinase, C = control, NS = not significant.
Adapted from Gruppo Italiano Per Lo Studio Della Streptochinasi Nell'Infarto Miocardico (GISSI): Effectiveness of intravenous thrombolytic treatment in acute myocardial infarction. Lancet *1*:397, 1986.

gioplasty (PTCA) can prevent this and improve global ventricular function is not yet clear. If PTCA is useful, the most appropriate timing needs to be established. In one series 42 per cent of patients who after successful thrombolysis were left with a coronary luminal diameter less than 0.6 mm suffered reocclusion, whereas no reocclusion occurred in those with a larger lumen.[534] Most patients are now treated with heparin[18, 540] and aspirin following thrombolytic therapy in an effort to minimize the risk of reocclusion, but the effectiveness of these drugs and of other pharmacological therapy such as beta blockers is not clear. A number of strategies are currently under consideration: (1) Immediate (less than 2 hours after onset of thrombolytic therapy), or early (18 to 48 hours) follow-up coronary angiography performed in an attempt to identify patients at high risk for reocclusion or reinfarction so that mechanical revascularization might be carried out (percutaneous transluminal coronary angioplasty [PTCA] or coronary artery bypass grafting).[535–538] (2) Intracoronary thrombolysis following emergency intravenous therapy. (3) Longer-term maintenance infusion of the thrombolytic agent to reduce reocclusion.[541] (4) Use of thrombolytic agents with a prolonged rather than short half-life.[542] The relative benefits and risks of these strategies in various subgroups of patients are being studied.

INFARCT SIZE AND VENTRICULAR FUNCTION. Keeping in mind that infarct size is difficult to measure in patients, evidence suggests that myocardial infarcts are smaller in those receiving thrombolytic therapy than in those not receiving such therapy.[17, 543, 543a] This reduction in infarct size is greatest in patients treated earliest,[544, 545] particularly if treatment is begun within 2 hours of symptom onset.[528] While the effect of thrombolysis on left ventricular function has not always been shown to be beneficial,[546, 547] preservation of or improvement in left ventricular ejection fraction is often observed if patients are treated within 4 or especially 2 hours of the onset of the event.[17, 165, 511a, 523, 543, 544, 548] The improvement in ventricular function is probably greatest in patients with initially reduced left ventricular ejection fraction.[527, 549, 550] When a coronary artery occlusion causes right ventricular infarction, successful thrombolysis usually results in restoration of normal right ventricular function,[551] although this may occur without thrombolysis as well.[552] Postinfarction ischemia, as determined by clinical observation at the time of subsequent coronary arteriography[553] or on follow-up exercise stress testing or stress thallium scintigraphy,[554] is more common in patients with successful recanalization by thrombolysis, reflecting the presence of preserved but jeopardized myocardium. Sustained ventricular arrhythmias may be less inducible by programmed electrical stimulation (Chap. 21) after successful early reperfusion than after unsuccessful thrombolytic therapy.[555]

CORONARY ANGIOPLASTY

(See also Chap. 41)

Reperfusion can be achieved by emergency percutaneous transluminal coronary angioplasty (PTCA).[535, 556–559] Using a guidewire and balloon catheter, it is technically easier to cross a total occlusion consisting of a fresh thrombus than to cross a longstanding occlusion of a coronary artery. Thus, wire-guided balloon angioplasty can be useful to achieve prompt reperfusion in three situations: (1) in lieu of thrombolytic therapy, (2) when thrombolysis has failed, or (3) after successful thrombolysis when a severe residual stenosis remains. Successful angioplasty can be anticipated in the majority of patients in whom thrombolysis has failed.[535] However, in such cases angioplasty is probably of clinical benefit only when the duration of ischemia is short enough so that successful reperfusion is able to reverse a portion of the ischemic injury.[537] (It is not yet clear that it is beneficial to open an occluded vessel in the absence of reversibly injured myocardium). In addition to the need for ready availability of an experienced catheterization team and complete catheterization facilities, there are other problems and potential disadvantages of PTCA in AMI. These include the potential for propagation of a thrombus as a consequence of trauma to the vessel wall, trauma induced by angioplasty, and occlusion of the vessel by dissection, spasm, or subintimal hematoma.[516, 535] One small prospective trial comparing PTCA with thrombolysis by streptokinase has shown that the two forms of therapy appear to be equally effective at inducing early reperfusion,[560] with PTCA producing significantly less severe residual coronary artery stenosis (Fig. 38–23) and less exercise-induced post-MI ischemia.[561] In fact, all patients who develop ischemia (as assessed by thallium-201 imaging during submaximal exercise) had 50 per cent or more residual stenosis of the infarct-related vessel.[561] The strategy of using coronary angioplasty *after* thrombolysis has also been tested in small prospective trials[537, 538, 562] and is the subject of ongoing investigation as part of the multicenter thrombolysis in myocardial infarction (TIMI) study.[530] Angioplasty after thrombolysis can improve the recanalization rate[558, 559] and might diminish the incidence of in-hospital reocclusion, but this has not been proved.[538, 563]

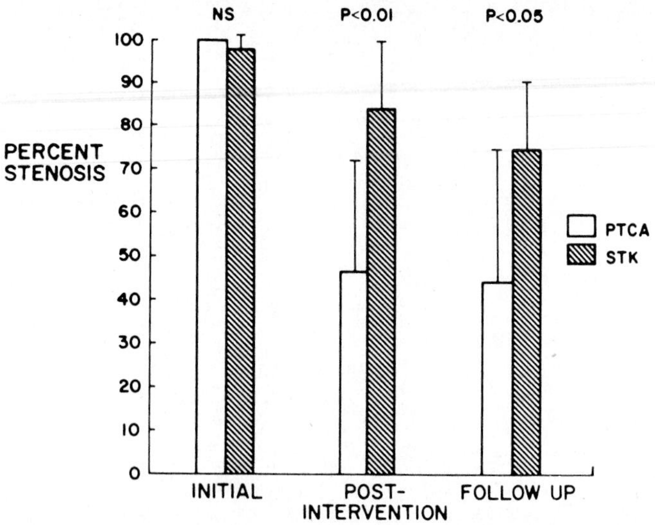

FIGURE 38–23. Severity of stenosis of infarct-related coronary artery before intervention, immediately after intervention, and at recatheterization 10 days after intervention. NS = not significant, PTCA = percutaneous transluminal coronary angioplasty, STK = intracoronary streptokinase. (From Fung, A. Y., et al.: Prevention of subsequent exercise-induced peri-infarct ischemia by emergency coronary angioplasty in acute myocardial infarction: Comparison with intracoronary streptokinase. By permission of The American College of Cardiology. J. Am. Coll. Cardiol. *8*:496, 1986.)

Although PTCA can be performed quickly and relatively safely after the onset of ischemia,[559] the majority of patients with AMI do not have rapid access to facilities in which this procedure can be performed. Therefore, the most important role of PTCA in AMI probably is as an adjunct to early, more readily available thrombolysis, with angioplasty being utilized to prevent infarct extension or reinfarction. While it is likely that coronary angioplasty will not play a major role in reducing infarct size initially (probably this will be accomplished by pharmacological therapy), it is the hope that angioplasty will be most important in keeping the infarct small once such therapy is used.

Newer catheterization techniques (Chap. 41) including the use of laser angioplasty,[564, 565] rotational thrombectomy catheters,[566] or mechanical atherectomy devices[567] may improve on current balloon angioplasty techniques, but all these will continue to be limited in their application by the requirements for trained personnel and accessible facilities.

RECOMMENDATIONS

On the basis of the above considerations and information from existing studies, as well as our own experience in the NIH-sponsored TIMI trial, and recognizing fully that this field is in rapid evolution, we recommend the following reperfusion strategy as of this writing:

1. Tissue plasminogen activator (t-PA)* should be given intravenously (a 6 mg bolus, a total of 60 mg during the first hour, 20 mg during the second hour, and 5 mg per hour during each of the next 4 hours for a total of 100 mg) to all patients with impending or evolving transmural infarction (characteristic ischemic pain for ≥ 30 min, clear-cut new ST segment elevation), if the drug can be administered within 4 hours of the onset of symptoms and if contraindications to the administration of this drug are not present (see below). If tPA is not available, 1.5 million units of intravenous streptokinase, administered over one hour, should be substituted.

2. If symptoms have been present for more than 4 hours, thrombolytic therapy should be employed only if there is clinical evidence of ongoing ischemia, including continuing or recurrent chest pain and/or continuing elevation of electrocardiographic ST segments.

3. Absolute contraindications to thrombolytic therapy include major surgery within one month, a history of significant gastrointestinal bleeding, a history of cerebrovascular disease (an intracerebral hemorrhage, stroke, or transient ischemic attack), a major bleeding diathesis, prolonged cardiopulmonary resuscitation within the past 2 weeks, severe uncontrolled hypertension (systolic BP > 180 or diastolic BP > 110), or severe trauma in the past 6 weeks. Relative contraindications include advanced age (greater than 75 years), any history of peptic ulcer disease, agitation, lethargy, or confusion.

4. Prior to the institution of thrombolytic therapy, consideration should be given to the patient's need for intravascular catheterization, as would be required for the placement of an arterial pressure monitoring line, a pulmonary artery catheter for hemodynamic monitoring, or a temporary transvenous pacemaker. If any of these are required, ideally they should be placed, as expeditiously as possible, before the thrombolytic agent is begun. If such procedures would require an additional delay of more than 30 minutes, they should be deferred for as long as possible after thrombolytic therapy is begun. In the early hours *after* institution of thrombolytic therapy, such catheterization should be performed only if of critical importance, and then sites where excessive bleeding can be controlled should be chosen (e.g., subclavian vein catheterization should be avoided).

5. With infusion of t-PA, intravenous heparin should be employed initially given as a bolus of 5000 units intravenously, followed by a continuous infusion. It should be begun at the rate of 1000 units/hr and adjusted to keep the partial thromboplastin time at 1½ to 2 times control value.

6. If a skilled cardiac catheterization team that is highly experienced in the performance of coronary angioplasty is readily available, and if myocardial salvage appears to have occurred after thrombolysis (symptoms resolved rapidly, ST-segment changes improved, and/or an early peak in the serum creatine kinase was seen), coronary angiography should be performed within 18 to 48 hours after the patient's initial presentation. If the infarct-related vessel is suitable for angioplasty, that procedure should be carried out during the catheterization. If angioplasty is unsuccessful, if the infarct-related vessel is unsuitable for that procedure, or if severe multivessel disease is present, consideration should be given to coronary artery bypass surgery. The timing of surgery should depend upon both the patient's clinical status (that is, *early* if ischemia recurs and *deferred* in the patient who remains pain-free and hemodynamically stable), and upon the precariousness of the coronary anatomy (e.g., early surgery should be considered for patients with high-grade stenosis of the left main coronary artery).

7. If ischemia recurs prior to catheterization, or if such a procedure cannot readily be performed, consideration should be given to retreatment with t-PA, particularly if thrombolytic therapy initially had been successful.

8. If, following thrombolytic therapy, a qualified catheterization team and well-equipped laboratory are not available in the facility in which the patient is located, it is reasonable to keep the patient in that facility while watchfully waiting for signs of recurrent ischemia. In the event of recurrent ischemia, the patient should be transferred promptly to a tertiary care center. On the other hand, if the patient's condition remains stable, cardiac catheterization and coronary arteriography may be deferred, and the decision whether to proceed with these procedures can be based upon the results of predischarge noninvasive testing, just as for patients not having undergone thrombolytic therapy (p. 1294).

9. Additional medical therapy with nitrates, calcium antagonists, beta blockers, and/or antiplatelet agents should be routinely employed, as required, just as they are for other patients with AMI or for coronary angioplasty.

SURGICAL REPERFUSION IN ACUTE MYOCARDIAL INFARCTION

There have been extensive improvements in intraoperative myocardial preservation with cardioplegia and hypothermia and of surgical techniques that have allowed surgical reperfusion in patients with AMI to be carried out at a quite low mortality—approximately 2 per cent in selected centers. This has kept alive the concept of emergency coronary revascularization as a possible measure to protect jeopardized myocardium in patients suffering AMI.[568–570] As appears to be the case for all methods designed to limit infarct size, this therapy can be successful only if it is applied within the first 4 to 6 hours (preferably the first 2 hours) of the onset of the acute event. In the usual patient who develops an AMI outside of the hospital, it is logistically difficult to bring the patient to the hospital, carry out a clinical evaluation, outline the coronary anatomy by arteriography, assemble the surgical team, commence operation, and place the patient on cardiopulmonary bypass in less than 4 hours after the onset of the event. It is therefore unlikely that surgical reperfusion can or will be widely applied on a regular basis in the routine treatment of AMI. Indeed, operation is contraindicated in patients with uncomplicated transmural infarcts more than

---

*At the time of this writing, t-PA has not been approved by the U.S. Food and Drug Administration.

6 hours after the onset of the event. When carried out at this time, surgical reperfusion appears to produce marked hemorrhage into the area of infarction.[571]

However, in some patients with AMI, including some with cardiogenic shock, infarction appears to occur in a stuttering fashion over an interval of several days.[572] Theoretically, revascularization carried out more than 6 hours after the onset of the event might be of benefit in this group, but this has yet to be established. Also, coronary bypass surgery can be carried out promptly in patients who develop coronary occlusion in the course of cardiac catheterization, coronary arteriography, and PTCA,[573–575] as well as in patients whose coronary anatomy has been assessed recently by coronary arteriography and who develop an infarction in the hospital while awaiting operation.

Patients undergoing successful thrombolysis but with important residual stenoses, who on anatomic grounds are more suitable for surgical revascularization than for PTCA, have undergone coronary artery bypass surgery with quite low mortality and morbidity.[576–578] Although postoperative chest tube drainage with relatively minor bleeding occurs more commonly than after elective bypass surgery, this problem is not of major concern.[577] PTCA is preferable in patients suitable for this procedure, whereas surgery should be reserved for those in whom PTCA has not been successful or could not be performed, or for patients with left main or extensive multivessel coronary artery disease for whom coronary artery bypass graft surgery would be recommended even in the absence of AMI. Thus, it is in this group of patients with AMI, i.e., those who have undergone or who are undergoing thrombolytic therapy, that a small subgroup can be identified who are likely to benefit from emergency revascularization. In this group, coronary artery bypass surgery is likely to be effective in limiting myocardial infarct size, since it can be carried out before irreversible myocardial damage has occurred. At the same time, bypass of noninfarct-related coronary obstructions can be expected to produce additional benefit.

PHARMACOLOGICAL THERAPY OF ACUTE MYOCARDIAL INFARCTION

BETA-ADRENOCEPTOR BLOCKADE

Beta blockers decrease cardiac index, stroke index, heart rate, blood pressure, and tension-time index (Fig. 38–24). The net effect of these drugs is a reduction in myocardial oxygen consumption per minute and per beat. Favorable effects of beta-adrenoceptor blockade on the balance of myocardial oxygen supply and demand are reflected in the reduction of myocardial lactate production[579] and diminution of ventricular arrhythmias.[580] Since beta-adrenoceptor blockade diminishes circulating levels of free fatty acids by antagonizing the lipolytic effects of catecholamines, and since elevated levels of fatty acids augment myocardial oxygen consumption and probably increase the incidence of arrhythmias, these metabolic actions of beta-blocking agents may be beneficial to the ischemic heart.[579]

Objective evidence of beneficial effects of beta blockers in acute myocardial ischemia has been reported by several investigators using various modifications of the precordial ST-segment mapping technique (Fig. 38–25).[581–583] For example, Gold et al.[581] found that the likelihood of a beneficial clinical and electrocardiographic response increased in the presence of residual antegrade or collateral blood flow to the infarct zone, as determined by coronary arteriography.

However, just as is the case in the experimental situations, not all clinical trials of beta blockers in AMI have reported salutary effects. Thus, practolol (oral or intravenous followed by oral) begun early during the course of AMI did not result in major differences in the clinical course, although there was a lower mortality in the subgroup of practolol-treated patients who had tachycardia at the time of entry into the study.[584]

Until recently studies of the effect of beta blockade on indexes of infarct size in patients were limited. Peter et al.[585] found that patients treated *within 4 hours of onset of symptoms* of uncomplicated MI had significantly lower peak serum creatine kinase levels and less cumulative creatine kinase release into plasma than did patients without specific therapy. The same group[586] also found that patients with suspected MI, treated with propranolol within 4 hours of the onset of

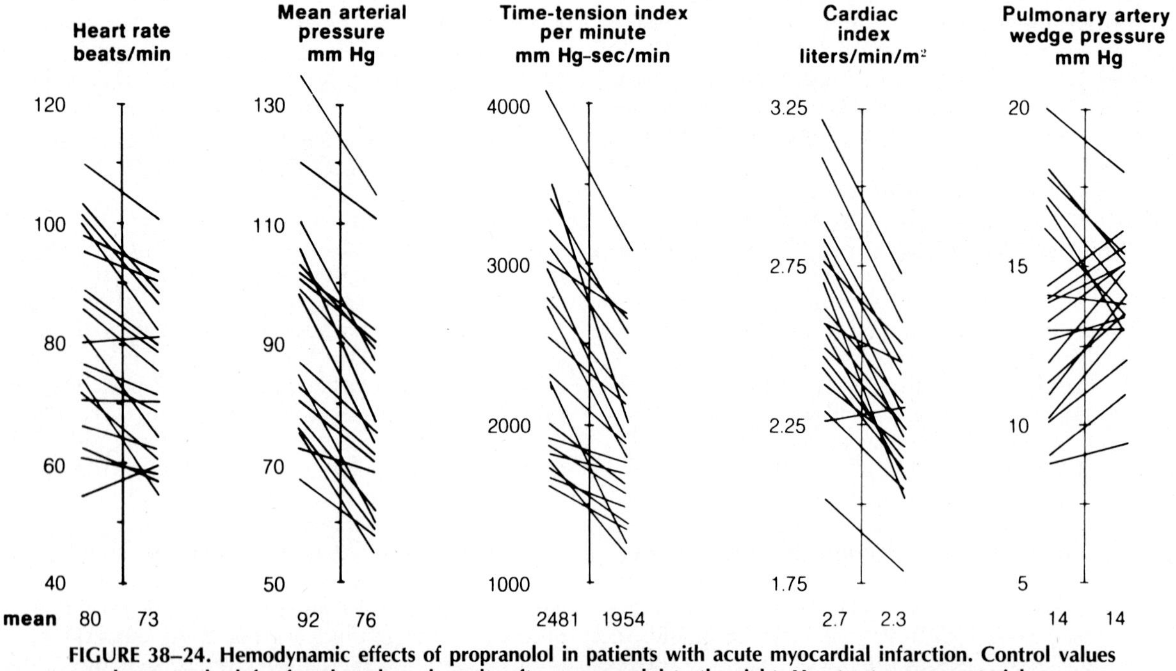

FIGURE 38–24. Hemodynamic effects of propranolol in patients with acute myocardial infarction. Control values are shown to the left of each scale and results after propranolol to the right. Heart rate, mean arterial pressure, and time-tension index are uniformly decreased after propranolol, and cardiac index is decreased in all but one patient. The response of pulmonary artery wedge pressure, however, is variable; in 6 patients with pressures above 15 mm Hg before treatment, propranolol produced a substantial reduction, whereas in the remaining patients, pressure was slightly increased. (From Mueller, H. S., et al.: How, when and why to use propranolol in acute MI. Cardiovasc. Med. *2*:321, 1977.)

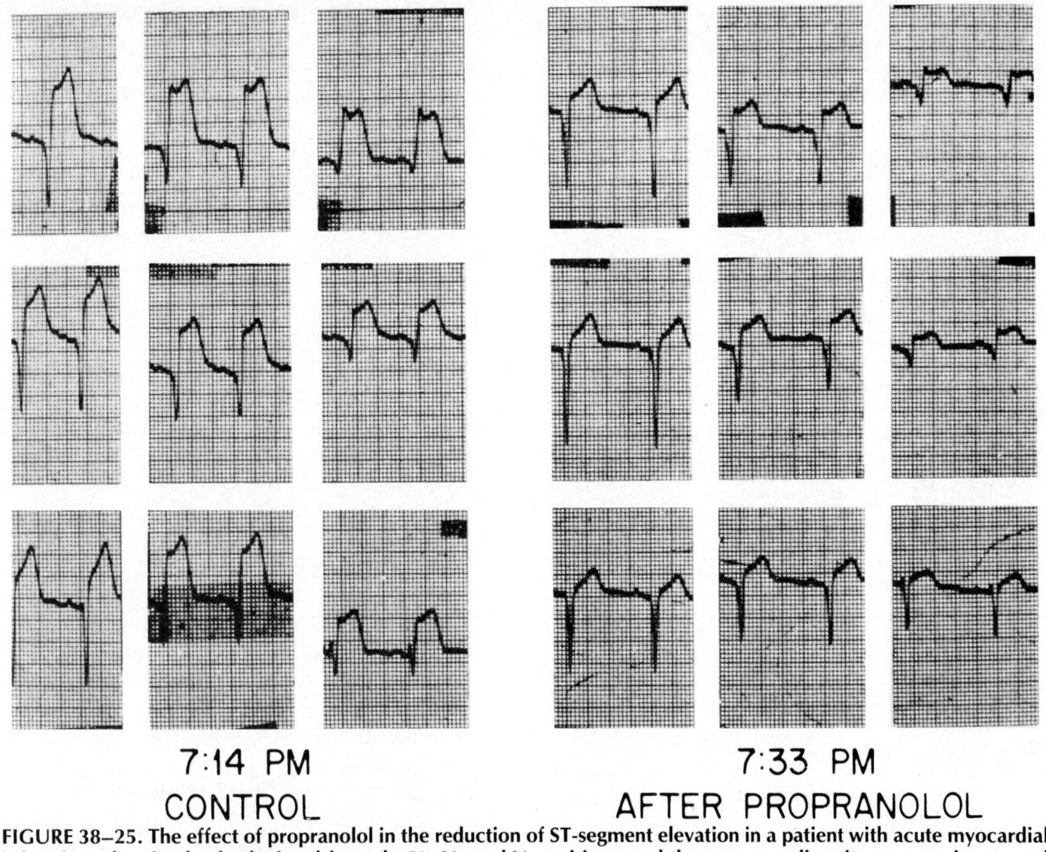

FIGURE 38–25. The effect of propranolol in the reduction of ST-segment elevation in a patient with acute myocardial infarction. The nine leads, depicted from the V_1, V_3, and V_5 positions, and the corresponding sites are one intercostal space above and below the standard positions. Note the marked reduction in ST-segment elevations after propranolol administration. (From Gold, H. K., et al.: Propranolol-induced reduction of signs of ischemic injury during acute myocardial infarction. Am. J. Cardiol. *38*:689, 1976.)

symptoms, had a significantly lower incidence of infarction. This suggests that threatened infarction might actually be prevented by early beta blockade. Similarly, Yusuf et al. have reported that intravenous atenolol, given a median of 4 hours following symptoms of AMI, decreased the incidence of AMI and of CK-MB release, the electrocardiographic evolution of infarction,[587, 588] and the severity of ischemic pain.[589] Alprenolol[590] and metoprolol[591] begun early in the course of infarction and then maintained have been shown to limit enzymatically estimated infarct size.

RESULTS OF MULTICENTER TRIALS. The results of four large trials designed to test the effects of early beta blockade in myocardial infarction are available. In the *Multicenter Investigation for the Limitation of Infarct Size* (MILIS) study, propranolol administered an average of 8.5 hours after the onset of symptoms, when compared to control, failed to reduce infarct size. More favorable results were reported by the *International Collaborative Study Group*, which reported on the use of intravenous timolol in the early phase of AMI.[592] In this study, patients were treated a mean of 3.4 hours after the onset of symptoms, and infarct size was smaller in timolol-treated patients as assessed by cumulative release of CK (Fig. 38–26), and by electrocardiographic indices.

In a large randomized trial using intravenous metoprolol (*the MIAMI Trial*[593]), infarct size was found to be smaller by enzymatic criteria (maximum serum activity of aspartate amino transferase) in the metoprolol group but only in patients treated within 7 hours.[593] All these studies are consistent with experimental and other clinical evidence that ischemic myocardium can be spared from irreversible injury only if treated early enough in the infarction process. For most patients, the outside time limit for salvaging viable myocardium is probably in the range of 4 to 6 hours. Benefit is highly variable if treatment is begun between 6 and 12 hours.

In an additional large multicenter trial (*ISIS 1*) involving over 16,000 patients, investigators reported a significant reduction in mortality among the patients randomized to intravenous atenolol when compared to placebo-treated patients (Fig. 38–27).[594] Patients were treated at a mean of 5 hours after the onset of suspected AMI. Mortality was reduced by 15 per cent by one week and this difference was maintained for the first year of follow-up. The study further suggests that treatment of approximately 200 patients would result in avoidance of one reinfarction, one cardiac arrest, and one death in the first week of an AMI.[594]

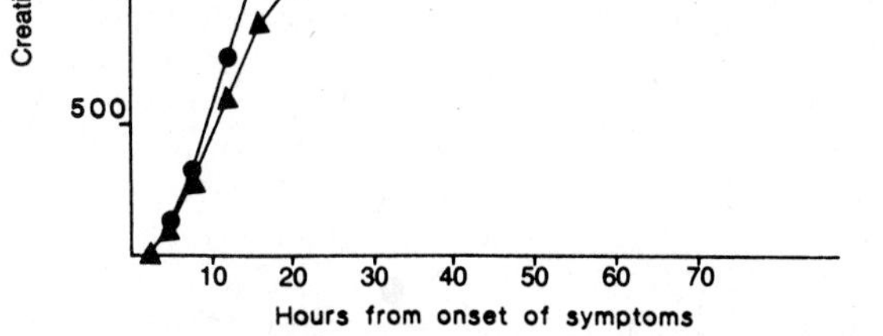

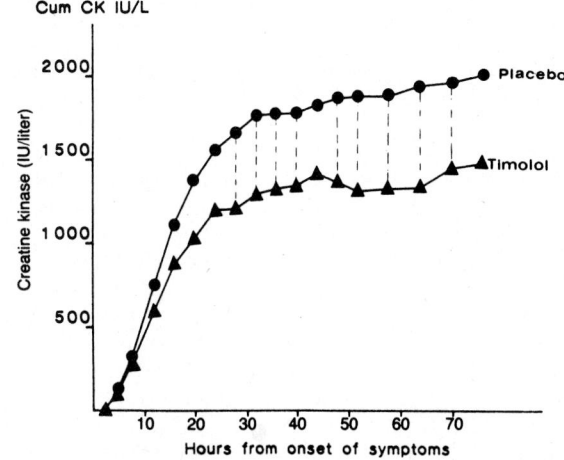

FIGURE 38–26. Mean cumulative release of creatine kinase during the evolution of acute myocardial infarction. Time zero denotes onset of symptoms. Significant differences between the two groups are indicated by vertical dashed lines. (From The International Collaborative Study Group: Reduction of infarct size with the early use of timolol in acute myocardial infarction. N. Engl. J. Med. *310*:9, 1984.)

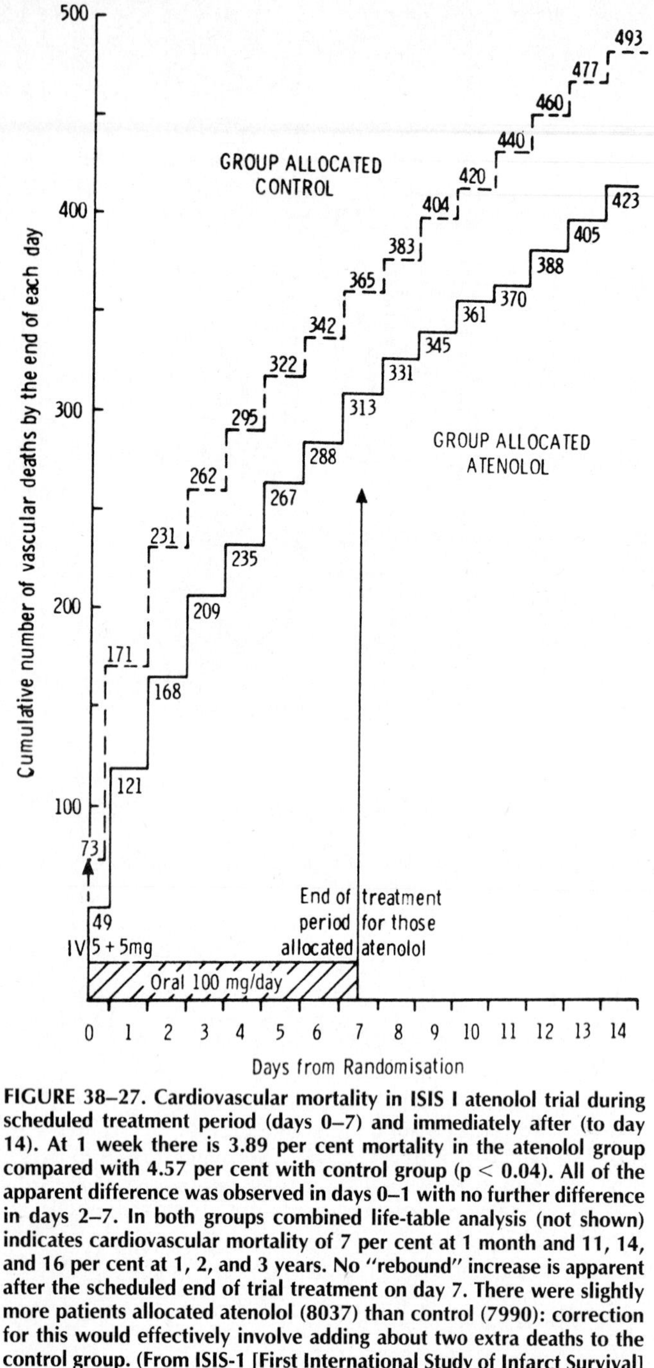

FIGURE 38–27. Cardiovascular mortality in ISIS I atenolol trial during scheduled treatment period (days 0–7) and immediately after (to day 14). At 1 week there is 3.89 per cent mortality in the atenolol group compared with 4.57 per cent with control group ($p < 0.04$). All of the apparent difference was observed in days 0–1 with no further difference in days 2–7. In both groups combined life-table analysis (not shown) indicates cardiovascular mortality of 7 per cent at 1 month and 11, 14, and 16 per cent at 1, 2, and 3 years. No "rebound" increase is apparent after the scheduled end of trial treatment on day 7. There were slightly more patients allocated atenolol (8037) than control (7990): correction for this would effectively involve adding about two extra deaths to the control group. (From ISIS-1 [First International Study of Infarct Survival] Collaboration Group: Randomized trial of intravenous atenolol among 16,027 cases of suspected acute myocardial infarction: ISIS-1. Lancet *2*:57, 1986.)

Given the favorable effects of beta blockade in the aforementioned clinical trials, as well as the observation in experimental animals that beta blockade enhances the quantity of myocardium salvaged by reperfusion (p. 1214), addition of a beta-adrenoceptor blocking agent to thrombolytic therapy may prove useful in patients without contraindications. Also, patients in a hyperdynamic state (sinus tachycardia, hypertension, no evidence of heart failure) as well as patients seen in the first 4 hours would appear to be good candidates for this therapy, regardless of whether thrombolytic therapy is employed. Unless there are contraindications, beta blockade probably should be continued in patients who develop AMI while receiving one of these agents. In addition, beta blockers are indicated in patients in whom infarction is complicated by persistent or recurrent ischemic pain, progressive or repetitive serum enzyme elevations suggestive of infarct extension, or tachyarrhythmias refractory to lidocaine and procainamide early after the onset of infarction. If adverse effects of beta blockers develop, or if patients present with complications of infarction that are contraindications to beta blockade such as heart failure or heart block, the beta blocker should be withheld or can be discontinued safely.[595]

RECOMMENDATIONS. In patients with AMI who have not received beta blockers in the preceding 24 hours, this therapy may be administered as metoprolol 15 mg intravenously, divided into three equal doses given at 2- to 5-minute intervals. During this period, heart rate and arterial pressure should be determined, and an electrocardiographic strip should be recorded after each injection. Intravenous beta blockade should not be administered in patients with a history of bronchial asthma, and its administration should be halted if any of the following events are present or develop:

1. Second- or third-degree AV block or lengthening of the P-R interval beyond 0.24 sec.
2. Rales extending more than one-third of the way up the lung fields, or wheezes detected on auscultation.
3. Ventricular rate below 50 per minute.
4. Systolic arterial pressure below 90 to 95 mm Hg.
5. Pulmonary artery wedge pressure above 20 to 24 mm Hg. (While it is useful to monitor this pressure in patients in whom a beta blocker will be administered, it is by no means essential.)

The intravenous administration of metoprolol is followed 6 to 8 hours later by oral metoprolol given first as 50 mg twice daily for the first day and then advanced to 100 mg twice daily, if the lower dose is tolerated. Ideally, the dose should keep the heart rate between 50 and 65 beats/min and the systolic pressure above 95 mm Hg in the absence of heart failure, wheezing, or advanced AV block.

Selection of Beta Blocker. At the time of this writing, the selection of the particular beta blocker is difficult; only metoprolol has been approved for intravenous use in AMI by the Food and Drug Administration. However, favorable effects have also been reported with atenolol, timolol, and alprenolol.

In the absence of any favorable evidence supporting the benefit of agents with intrinsic sympathomimetic activity (ISA) such as pindolol and oxprenolol, and with some unfavorable evidence for their role in secondary prevention,[596, 597] beta blockers with ISA probably should not be chosen for treatment of AMI. Occasionally the clinician may wish to proceed with beta blocker therapy even in the presence of relative contraindications, such as a history of mild asthma, mild bradycardia, mild heart failure, or first-degree heart block. In this situation, a trial of the very short-acting beta blocker esmolol may help determine whether the patient can tolerate beta blockade.[598, 599] Since the hemodynamic effects of this drug are reversed in less than 30 minutes, it offers considerable advantage over longer-acting agents when the risk of a beta blocker complication is relatively high.

Although antagonism of sympathetic stimulation to the heart might be expected to exacerbate pulmonary edema in patients with occult heart failure, usually only small changes in pulmonary capillary wedge pressure occur when the drug is used in patients with AMI.[579]

NITRATES

(See also p. 1327)

Intravenous nitroglycerin has been reported to affect infarct size in patients. Derrida and associates[600] have reported that this drug causes a greater reduction in ST-segment elevations and less R-wave fall at initially ischemic sites. Furthermore, in patients with heart failure, mortality and serious ventricular arrhythmias appeared to be reduced in the nitroglycerin-treated group. Bussmann and associates[601, 602] found significantly lower values of peak serum CK, lower rates of CK release, and smaller calculated infarct sizes in nitroglycerin-treated patients. Becker and colleagues[603, 604] have shown in a prospective, randomized trial that treatment with intravenous nitroglycerin for 48 hours followed by nitroglycerin ointment therapy for 72 hours enhanced postinfarction improvement of myocardial perfusion measured with ^{201}Tl scintigraphy.

As with other interventions to spare ischemic myocardium in AMI, the benefit of intravenous nitroglycerin appears to be confined to patients treated earliest.[604] Patients with inferior wall infarction are particularly sensitive to an excessive fall in preload, particularly if concurrent right ventricular infarction is present.[428] In such cases nitrate-induced venodilatation could impair cardiac output and reduce coronary blood flow, thus worsening myocardial oxygenation rather than improving it.[605]

In patients with AMI, the administration of nitroglycerin and other nitrates such as isosorbide dinitrate diminishes pulmonary capillary wedge pressure and systemic arterial pressure as well as left ventricular end-systolic and end-diastolic volumes. It also reduces ventricular asynergy, to the extent that the local impairment of the left ventricular function is due to reversibly injured, depressed myocardium rather than to zones of completed infarction or scar.[606]

As is true in experimental animals, the administration of nitroglycerin to patients with AMI depends on the existing hemodynamics. When systemic arterial and pulmonary capillary wedge pressures are normal or low prior to the administration of nitroglycerin, reflex tachycardia may result from the further reduction of ventricular filling and arterial pressures.

Intravenous nitroglycerin can be administered safely to patients with evolving MI as long as the dose is titrated carefully to avoid induction of reflex tachycardia or systemic arterial hypotension (systolic blood pressure $\leq$ 95 mm Hg).[497] One useful regimen employs an initial infusion rate of 10 μg/min with stepwise increases of 10 μg/min. Alternatively, it may be administered sublingually at doses of 0.3 to 0.6 mg. This route may be more hazardous, since the rate of absorption is difficult to control and arterial pressure may decline precipitously. Nitroglycerin is often useful for the relief of persistent pain and as a vasodilator in patients with infarction associated with left ventricular failure.

When continuous infusion of intravenous nitroglycerin is used, two important potential complications must be considered. First, most commercially available nitroglycerin for intravenous use is prepared in a solution with ethanolol as a diluent. When high infusion rates are continued for several days, signs and symptoms of alcohol intoxication may occur.[607] Second, clinically significant methemoglobinemia has been reported to occur during administration of intravenous nitroglycerin.[608] Although uncommon, this problem is seen when unusually large doses of nitrates are administered. It is important not only for its potential to cause symptoms of lethargy and headache but also because elevated methemoglobin levels can impair the oxygen-carrying capacity of blood, potentially exacerbating ischemia.

According to all of the available evidence, nitroglycerin very rarely opens previously occluded coronary arteries. Nevertheless, one or two 0.3 mg tablets of nitroglycerin should be given when a patient presents with acute chest pain, particularly if the diagnosis of AMI is not clear. Patients in whom the pain is caused by unstable angina may respond. Despite the evidence of a favorable effect of nitroglycerin on infarct size reviewed above, *routine* use of this drug is not recommended in patients with established AMI. However, in patients with pump failure, pulmonary edema, or continuing ischemia, intravenous nitroglycerin may be useful for lowering preload and afterload, and for improving flow to ischemic myocardium. It is contraindicated in the presence of hypotension.

OTHER POTENTIALLY USEFUL APPROACHES TO PROTECTION OF ISCHEMIC MYOCARDIUM

The experimental observations indicating the potential usefulness of the interventions described below are summarized on pages 1213 to 1215.

CALCIUM ANTAGONISTS. Two multicenter prospective, randomized trials in evolving MI have failed to show any reduction in infarct size by the early administration of nifedipine.[609, 610] Both trials used enzymatic estimates of infarct size, and nifedipine may alter the release of CK in a complex manner which could obscure the possible benefit of the drug.[611] Both diltiazem[612, 613] and verapamil[614, 615] have been administered safely to patients with AMI, but data on infarct size are unavailable. Promising evidence from animal models of AMI with diltiazem[616] and with experimental calcium channel blockers such as nisoldipine[617] as of this writing have yet to be replicated in patients.[617a]

GLUCOSE-INSULIN-POTASSIUM. Administration of a solution of glucose-insulin-potassium (300 gm of glucose, 50 units of insulin, and 80 mEq of KCl in 1000 ml of water administered at a rate of 1.5 ml/kg/hr) lowers the concentration of plasma free fatty acids and improves ventricular performance, as reflected in systolic arterial pressure, cardiac output, and stroke work at any level of left ventricular filling pressure[618]; also the frequency of ventricular premature beats decreases.[619] In a nonrandomized study, mortality appeared to be reduced,[620] hemodynamics improved, global ejection fraction increased, and asynergy in the ischemic zone and pulmonary artery diastolic pressure reduced.[621] However, no definitive effect on enzymatically estimated infarct size or long-term mortality has been described in a prospective, controlled, randomized trial.

CORTICOSTEROIDS AND NONSTEROIDAL ANTIINFLAMMATORY AGENTS. Administration of a single large dose of methylprednisolone has been reported to decrease infarct size, estimated enzymatically.[622] However, the control and treated groups were not strictly comparable with respect to the apparent extent of infarction prior to the administration of the drug. In contrast to these favorable effects, in another study infarct size estimated enzymatically appeared to be *increased* by multiple doses of methylprednisolone.[623] Administration of the drug has led to persistent elevation of plasma CK-MB and the suspicion of an excessively high incidence of ventricular rupture, as well as an increase in mortality, perhaps because administration of corticosteroids inhibits healing of the infarct.[624] High doses of steroids compared with low doses (30 mg/kg) appear to impair healing and cause scar thinning.[625] Accordingly, administration of multiple high doses of corticosteroids beginning several hours after the onset of ischemic injury appears to be deleterious rather than beneficial.

The nonsteroidal antiinflammatory compounds ibuprofen and indomethacin also result in marked scar thinning when given after experimental MI.[626, 627] Therefore, such agents should be avoided in early AMI, both because of these findings and because of the possibility that indomethacin and similar drugs may impair coronary blood flow by increasing coronary vascular resistance.[628] However, aspirin does not produce similar scar thinning,[627] and in addition to its potentially favorable antiplatelet effect (p. 1767), aspirin may improve blood flow at the margins of an infarction.[629] Thus, the clinical caution raised for steroids and other nonsteroidal antiinflammatory agents need not be extended to aspirin.

INTRAAORTIC BALLOON COUNTERPULSATION. From a theoretical standpoint, intraaortic balloon counterpulsation might be expected to limit infarct size for several reasons. In experimental animals, intraaortic balloon counterpulsation decreases afterload and myocardial oxygen consumption,[630] decreases preload, increases coronary blood flow, and improves cardiac performance.[631] When intraaortic balloon counterpulsation is carried out in experimental animals immediately after coronary occlusion, ischemic myocardium appears to be protected.[632] No definitive information is available indicating that intraaortic balloon counterpulsation alters the prognosis in patients with relatively uncomplicated infarction. Leinbach et al., however, have reported an immediate, persistent fall in ST-segment elevation. This occurred in patients with anterior MI who had preservation of precordial R waves and good ventricular function,[633] in whom the left anterior descending coronary artery was not totally occluded and who underwent intraaortic balloon pumping within 6 hours.

In a relatively small prospective trial intraaortic balloon pumping with intravenous nitroglycerin appeared to preserve function only in noninfarcted segments.[634] Given the relatively frequent rate of complications[635] following intraaortic balloon insertion and the absence of convincing data for infarct size reduction, intraaortic balloon pumping should be reserved for hemodynamically compromised patients and for those with refractory ischemia, for whom the benefit of this approach has been demonstrated.

MISCELLANEOUS AGENTS. Oxygen-derived free radicals are abundant in ischemic tissue and may contribute to myocardial injury, particularly following reperfusion (p. 1212). Evidence from studies in animals suggests that the extent of myocardial necrosis can be affected favorably by treatment with oxygen-free radical scavengers such as superoxide dismutase.[636, 637] Additionally, myocardial function is improved by the enhanced recovery induced by oxygen-free radical scavengers after severe ischemia.[638] Studies in humans are under way to test the efficacy of this type of therapy for sparing injured myocardium.

The genesis and diagnosis of arrhythmias are presented in Chapters 20 and 22 and their treatment in Chapter 21. The role of arrhythmias in complicating the course of patients with AMI and the prevention and treatment of these arrhythmias in this setting are discussed here (Table 38–8).

Some abnormality of cardiac rhythm has been noted in 72 to 96 per cent of patients with acute myocardial infarction treated in coronary care units (Table 38–9).[233, 639] The incidence of arrhythmias is higher in those patients seen earlier after the onset of symptoms (Fig. 38–28).[640] Moreover, many arrhythmias occur prior to hospitalization, before the patient is monitored.[641] Thus, the overall incidence of rhythm disturbance in AMI may actually be as high as 100 per cent. However, these data are difficult to interpret, since ambulatory electrocardiographic monitoring has also disclosed arrhythmias in a high percentage of asymptomatic, apparently healthy middle-aged men.[642]

Arrhythmias occurring in patients with AMI require vigorous treatment when they impair hemodynamics, compromise myocardial viability by augmenting myocardial oxygen requirements, or predispose to malignant ventricular arrhythmias, i.e., ventricular tachycardia, ventricular fibrillation, or asystole.[643] There is evidence that both the diminished threshold to ventricular fibrillation[644] and the incidence of malignant ventricular arrhythmias associated with infarction[469, 645] are affected by the extent of the underlying infarction.

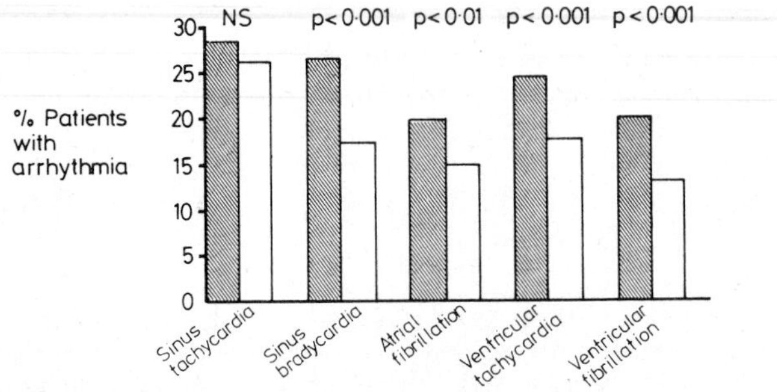

FIGURE 38–28. Comparison of incidence and major disorders of cardiac rhythm in patients with acute myocardial infarction observed in less than one hour after onset of symptoms (shaded bars) and those first observed after longer delay (open bars). (From O'Doherty, M., et al.: Five hundred patients with myocardial infarction monitored within one hour of symptoms. Br. Med. J. *286*:1405, 1983.)

When patients are seen very early during the course of MI they almost invariably exhibit evidence of increased activity of the autonomic nervous system. Thus sinus bradycardia, sometimes associated with AV block, and hypotension reflect the augmented vagal activity. Hypotension, regardless of cause, is hazardous in patients with AMI, since it impairs perfusion of marginally ischemic zones, intensifies ischemia, and may initiate or perpetuate the vicious circle illustrated in Figure 38–9 (p. 1231).

Activation of receptors within atrial and ventricular

TABLE 38–8 CARDIAC ARRHYTHMIAS AND THEIR MANAGEMENT DURING ACUTE MYOCARDIAL INFARCTION

Category	Arrhythmia	Objective of Treatment	Therapeutic Options
I. *Electrical instability*	Ventricular premature beats	Prophylaxis against ventricular fibrillation	Antiarrhythmic agents (lidocaine, procainamide)
	Ventricular tachycardia	Prophylaxis against ventricular fibrillation; restoration of hemodynamic stability	Antiarrhythmic agents; cardioversion/defibrillation
	Ventricular fibrillation	Urgent reversion to sinus rhythm	Defibrillation; bretylium tosylate
	Accelerated idioventricular rhythm	Observation unless hemodynamic function is compromised	Increase sinus rate (atropine, atrial pacing); antiarrhythmic agents
	Nonparoxysmal AV junctional tachycardia	Search for precipitating causes (e.g., digitalis intoxication); suppress arrhythmia only if hemodynamic function is compromised	Atrial overdrive pacing; antiarrhythmic agents; cardioversion relatively contraindicated if digitalis intoxication present
II. *Pump failure/ Excessive sympathetic stimulation*	Sinus tachycardia	Reduce heart rate to diminish myocardial oxygen demands	Antipyretics; analgesics; evaluate level of PCW pressure and treat accordingly
	Atrial fibrillation and/or atrial flutter	Reduce ventricular rate; restore sinus rhythm	Verapamil, digitalis glycosides; anticongestive measures (diuretics, afterload reduction); cardioversion; rapid atrial pacing (for atrial flutter)
	Paroxysmal supraventricular tachycardia	Reduce ventricular rate; restore sinus rhythm	Vagal maneuvers; verapamil, cardiac glycosides, beta-adrenergic blockers; cardioversion; rapid atrial pacing
III. *Bradyarrhythmias and conduction disturbances*	Sinus bradycardia	Acceleration of heart rate only if hemodynamic function is compromised	Atropine; atrial pacing
	Junctional escape rhythm	Acceleration of sinus rate only if loss of atrial "kick" causes hemodynamic compromise	Atropine; atrial pacing
	Atrioventricular block and intraventricular block	(See p. 1266)	Insertion of pacemaker

Modified from Antman, E. M., and Rutherford, J. D. (eds.): Coronary Care Medicine: A Practical Approach. Boston, Martinus Nijhoff Publishing, 1986, p. 78.

TABLE 38–9 ARRHYTHMIAS DETECTED BY ECG MONITORING IN A CORONARY CARE UNIT IN 1000 CONSECUTIVE PATIENTS WITH INFARCTION 1967–71

ARRHYTHMIA	INCIDENCE (%)	MORTALITY (%)	ASSOCIATION WITH VENTRICULAR FIBRILLATION (%)
All ventricular ectopics	57	19	14
i. Salvos (runs)	17	35	26
ii. Bigemini	7	36	22
iii. R on T	6	41	40
iv. VPBs not i, ii or iii	36	15	8
Ventricular tachycardia	10	55	52
Ventricular fibrillation	8	61	
Accelerated idioventricular rhythm	9	19	12
Atrial fibrillation	11	28	
Atrial flutter	3	24	
Paroxysmal supraventricular tachycardia	3	37	
Sinus tachycardia	41	26	11
Sinus bradycardia	25	9	8
All cases		18	8

From Norris, R. M., and Singh, B. N.: Arrhythmias in acute myocardial infarction. *In* Norris, R. M. (ed.): Myocardial Infarction. Its Presentation, Pathogenesis and Treatment. Edinburgh, Churchill Livingstone, 1982, p. 55.

myocardium by necrotic tissue may cause enhanced efferent sympathetic activity, increased concentrations of circulating catecholamines, and local release of catecholamines from nerve endings within the heart.[646] The latter may also result from direct ischemic damage of adrenergic neurons. In addition, ischemic myocardium may be hyperreactive to the arrhythmogenic effects of norepinephrine,[647] which may vary strikingly in concentration in different portions of the ischemic heart.[648] Sympathetic stimulation of the heart may also enhance the automaticity of ischemic Purkinje fibers. Furthermore, catecholamines facilitate propagation of slow current responses mediated by calcium (p. 599), and stimulation of ischemic myocardium by catecholamines may exacerbate arrhythmias dependent on such currents.[647] Finally, it has been demonstrated that transmural infarction can interrupt both afferent and efferent limbs of the sympathetic nervous system innervating myocardium distal (but still viable) to

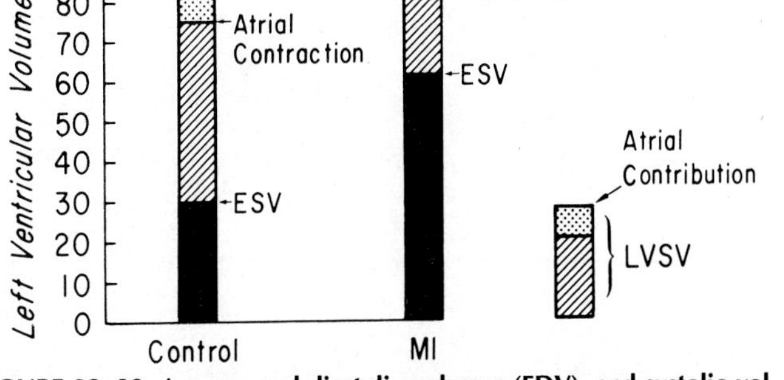

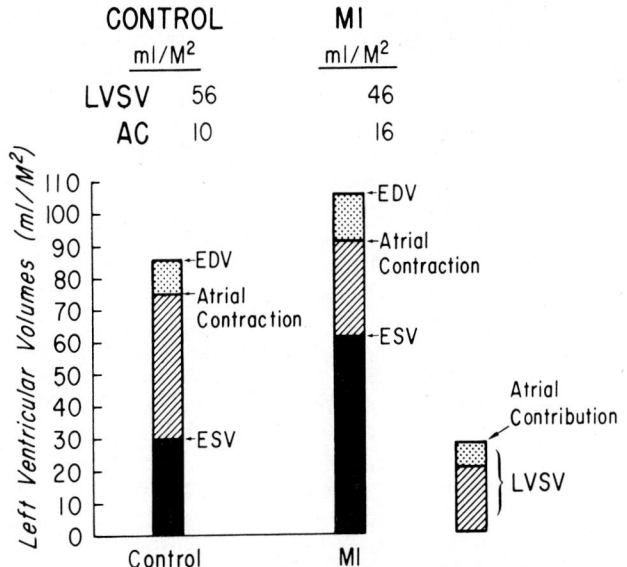

FIGURE 38–29. Average end-diastolic volumes (EDV), end-systolic volumes (ESV), left ventricular stroke volumes (LVSV), and atrial contribution (AC) in a control group of patients and in patients after myocardial infarction (MI). (From Rahimtoola, S. H., et al.: Left atrial transport function in myocardial infarction. Am. J. Med. *59*:686, 1975.)

the area of infarction.[648] In addition to the potential for modifying a variety of cardiovascular reflexes, this creation of autonomic imbalance may promote the development of arrhythmias.[648] Cardiac catecholamine depletion induced by mediastinal ablation[649] or reduction of adrenergic stimulation by pharmacological means[14] protects against ventricular arrhythmias in experimental animals. This explains why beta-adrenoceptor blocking agents may also be helpful in the treatment of ventricular arrhythmias, particularly when the latter are associated with other signs of heightened adrenergic activity.

The treatment of tachyarrhythmias involves not only the use of antiarrhythmic drugs but also correction of abnormalities of plasma electrolyte concentrations, acid-base balance disturbances, hypoxemia, anemia, and digitalis intoxication. In addition, it is essential to treat pericarditis, pulmonary emboli, and pneumonia or other infections, which may give rise to sinus tachycardia or other supraventricular tachyarrhythmias.

HEMODYNAMIC CONSEQUENCES OF CARDIAC ARRHYTHMIAS. Patients with significant left ventricular dysfunction have a relatively fixed stroke volume and depend on changes in heart rate to alter cardiac output. However, there is a narrow range over which the cardiac output is maximal, with significant reductions occurring at faster and lower rates.[650] Thus, all forms of bradycardia and tachycardia may depress the cardiac output in patients with AMI. Although the optimal rate insofar as cardiac output is concerned may exceed 100 per minute, it is important to consider that heart rate is one of the major determinants of myocardial oxygen consumption (p. 1193) and that at more rapid heart rates myocardial energy needs can be elevated to levels that adversely affect ischemic myocardium. Therefore, in patients with AMI, the optimal rate is usually somewhat lower, in the range of 80 beats/min.

A second factor to consider in assessing the hemodynamic consequences of a particular arrhythmia is the loss of atrial transport function, i.e., the atrial "kick."[651] Studies in patients without AMI have demonstrated that loss of atrial transport decreases left ventricular output by 15 to 20 per cent.[652] However, in patients with reduced diastolic left ventricular compliance of any cause (including AMI), atrial systole is of greater importance for left ventricular filling. In patients with AMI, atrial systole boosts end-diastolic volume by 15 per cent, end-diastolic pressure by 29 per cent, and stroke volume by 35 per cent (Fig. 38–29).[653]

BRADYARRHYTHMIAS

SINUS BRADYCARDIA

(See also p. 664)

Sinus bradycardia is the most common arrhythmia occurring during the early phases of AMI, and it is particularly frequent in patients with inferior and posterior infarction.[654–656] Observations in mobile coronary care units indicate that 25 to 40 per cent of patients with AMI have electrocardiographic evidence of sinus bradycardia within the first hour after the onset of symptoms; however, 4 hours after infarction commences, the incidence of sinus bradycardia has declined to 15 to 20 per cent.[640, 641] The cause of the vagotonia and resultant bradycardia and hypotension accompanying AMI is not entirely clear. One factor appears to be stimulation of cardiac vago-afferent receptors[657] (which are more common in the inferoposterior than the anterior or lateral portions of the left ventricle) with resulting efferent cholinergic stimulation of the heart.

The phenomenon is a manifestation of the Bezold-Jarisch reflex.[658] This reflex is mediated by the vagi and occurs during thrombolytic reperfusion, particularly of the right coronary artery.[521] Often sinus bradycardia is a component of a vasovagal or vasodepressor response, which may be intensified by severe pain as well as by morphine, and may be related to vasovagal syncope (p. 889).

The clinical significance of sinus bradycardia is debated. There is evidence, on the one hand, that this arrhythmia is an important risk factor during the very early phase of AMI and predisposes the patient to the development of repetitive ventricular arrhythmias and hypotension.[656] On the other hand, it has been suggested on the basis of data obtained in experimental infarction and from some clinical observations that the increased vagal tone that produces sinus bradycardia during the early phase of AMI may actually be protective, perhaps because it reduces myocardial oxygen demands.[655] Thus the acute mortality rate appears to be as low in patients with sinus bradycardia as in patients without this arrhythmia (Table 38–9).

MANAGEMENT. This depends upon the timing and severity, and on other clinical manifestations. Isolated sinus bradycardia, unaccompanied by hypotension or ventricular ectopy, should be observed rather than treated initially. In the first 4 to 6 hours following infarction, if the sinus rate is extremely slow (under 40/min), administration of intravenous atropine in aliquots of 0.3 to 0.6 mg every 3 to 10 minutes (with a total dose not exceeding 2 mg) to bring heart rate up to approximately 60/min often abolishes the premature ventricular beats commonly associated with this degree of sinus bradycardia.[659, 660] Atropine often contributes to restoration of arterial pressure[408] and hence coronary perfusion, and should be employed if hypotension accompanying any degree of sinus bradycardia is present.

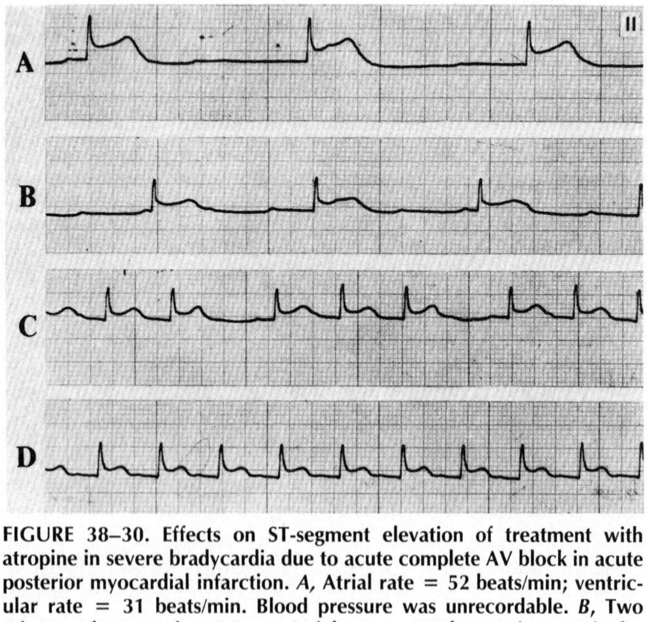

FIGURE 38–30. Effects on ST-segment elevation of treatment with atropine in severe bradycardia due to acute complete AV block in acute posterior myocardial infarction. *A,* Atrial rate = 52 beats/min; ventricular rate = 31 beats/min. Blood pressure was unrecordable. *B,* Two minutes after atropine, 0.6 mg: Atrial rate = 105 beats/min; ventricular rate = 40 beats/min. Systolic blood pressure = 75 mm Hg. A reduction in ST segment is seen when compared with *A. C,* Three minutes after atropine, 1.2 mg: Second-degree AV block. Atrial rate = 115 beats/min; ventricular rate = 88 beats/min. D, Four and a half minutes after atropine, 1.2 mg: normal AV conduction. P-R interval = 0.2 sec. Ventricular rate = 110 beats/min. Blood pressure = 170/110 mm Hg. (From Adgey, A. A. J., et al.: Acute phase of myocardial infarction. Prehospital management of the coronary patient. Minnesota Med. 59:347, 1976.)

The favorable effects of atropine are frequently accompanied by regression of ST-segment elevation (Fig. 38–30). Elevation of the lower extremities will also often elevate arterial pressure by redistributing blood from the systemic venous bed to the thorax, thereby augmenting ventricular preload, cardiac output, and arterial pressure.

Sinus bradycardia occurring more than 6 hours after the onset of the AMI is often transitory, is caused by sinus node dysfunction or atrial ischemia rather than vagal hyperactivity, is usually not accompanied by hypotension, and does not usually predispose to ventricular arrhythmias. Treatment is not required unless ventricular performance is compromised or administration of a beta-adrenoceptor blocker or high doses of antiarrhythmic drugs, which may slow the sinus rate further, is planned. When atropine is ineffective and the patient is symptomatic and/or hypotensive, electrical pacing is indicated. In patients with depressed ventricular performance, who require the "atrial kick," atrial pacing or atrioventricular sequential pacing is superior to simple ventricular pacing.[661]

CONDUCTION DISTURBANCES: ATRIOVENTRICULAR AND INTRAVENTRICULAR BLOCK

Ischemic injury can produce blocks at any level of the atrioventricular or intraventricular conduction system. Such blocks may occur in the atrioventricular node, producing various grades of AV block; in either main bundle branch, producing various grades of AV block; in either main bundle branch, producing right or left bundle branch block; and in the anterior and posterior divisions of the left bundle, producing left anterior or left posterior (fascicular) divisional blocks (Table 38–10). Disturbances of conduction can, of course, occur in various combinations. The mechanisms and recognition of intraventricular conduction disturbances are discussed in Chapter 7 and of atrioventricular conduction disturbances in Chapter 22.

FIRST-DEGREE AV BLOCK. First-degree AV block (Fig. 22–40, p. 702) occurs in 4 to 14 per cent of patients with AMI admitted to coronary care units. His bundle electrocardiographic studies have shown that almost all patients with first-degree AV block have disturbances in conduction *above* the bundle of His, i.e., intranodal. The localization of the site of block is of considerable importance, since the development of complete heart block and ventricular asystole is restricted almost exclusively to those patients with first-degree block in whom the conduction disturbance is *below* the bundle of His,[662] and this occurs more commonly in patients with anterior infarction and in those with associated bifascicular block.[663, 664]

First-degree AV block generally does not require specific treatment. However, if digitalis intoxication is suspected as the cause, this drug should be discontinued. Beta blockers and calcium antagonists (other than nifedipine) prolong AV conduction and may be responsible for first-degree AV block as well. However, discontinuation of these drugs in the setting of AMI has the potential of increasing ischemia and ischemic injury. Therefore, in the presence of first-degree block alone, the clinician may consider decreasing the dosage of these drugs but for this reason alone should not discontinue them. Only if higher degree block or hemodynamic impairment occurs should these agents be stopped. If the block is a manifestation of excessive vagotonia and is associated with sinus bradycardia and hypotension, administration of atropine, as outlined above, may be helpful. In all circumstances, careful surveillance is important in view of the possibility of progression to higher degrees of block.[665]

TABLE 38–10 INCIDENCE AND PROGNOSES OF CONDUCTION BLOCKS IN ACUTE MYOCARDIAL INFARCTION

Type of Conduction Block	Incidence of Conduction Block (%)	Patients with Conduction Block Who Develop Complete AV Block (%)	Mortality (%)
None		6	15
LAH	5	3	27
LPH	1	0	42
RBBB ± LAH	5	46	45
RBBB + LPH	1	43	57
RBBB	2	43	46
LBBB	5	20	44

Adapted from Mullins, C. B., and Atkins, J. M.: Prognoses and management of ventricular conduction blocks in acute myocardial infarction. Mod. Concepts Cardiovasc. Dis. *45*:129, 1976, by permission of the American Heart Association, Inc.

SECOND-DEGREE AV BLOCK. Mobitz Type I, or Wenckebach. Mobitz type I block (Fig. 22–43, p. 703) occurs in 4 to 10 per cent of patients with AMI admitted to coronary care units[663] and accounts for about 90 per cent of all patients with AMI and second-degree AV block. This type of block (1) generally occurs within the AV node, (2) is usually associated with narrow QRS complexes, (3) is presumably secondary to ischemic injury, (4) occurs more commonly in patients with inferior than anterior myocardial infarction, (5) is usually transient and does not persist for more than 72 hours after infarction, (6) may be intermittent, and (7) rarely progresses to complete AV block. First-degree and type I second-degree AV block do not appear to affect survival, are most commonly associated with occlusion of the right coronary artery, and are caused by ischemia of the AV node.

Mobitz Type II. This is a rare conduction defect (Fig. 22–44, p. 704) following AMI, occurring in only 10 per cent of all cases of second-degree block[639]; thus, the overall incidence of Mobitz type II block after infarction is less than 1 per cent. In contrast to Mobitz type I block, type II second-degree block (1) usually originates from a lesion in the conduction system below the bundle of His,[663] (2) is associated with a wide QRS complex, (3) often but not invariably reflects trifascicular block with impaired conduction distal to the bundle of His, (4) often progresses suddenly to complete AV block, and (5) is almost always associated with anterior rather than inferior infarction.

Specific therapy also is not required in patients with second-degree AV block of the Mobitz type I variety when the average ventricular rate is adequate and ventricular irritability, heart failure, and bundle branch block are absent. However, if these complications develop or if the ventricular rate falls below approximately 50/min, immediate treatment with a temporary pacemaker is indicated. Because of its potential for progression to complete heart block, Mobitz type II second-degree AV block should be treated with a temporary demand pacemaker with the rate set at approximately 60/min.[666]

COMPLETE (THIRD-DEGREE) AV BLOCK. The atrioventricular conduction system has a dual blood supply, the AV branch of the right coronary artery and the septal perforating branch from the left anterior descending coronary artery.[667] Therefore, complete AV block can occur in patients with either anterior or inferior infarction. Complete AV block develops in 5 to 8 per cent of patients with AMI. As with other forms of AV block, the prognosis depends on the anatomical location of the block in the conduction system and the size of the infarction.

In general, complete heart block in patients with inferior infarction results from an intranodal or prenodal lesion[667a] and develops gradually, often progressing from first-degree and type I second-degree block. The escape rhythm is usually stable without asystole and often junctional, with a rate exceeding 40/min and a narrow QRS complex in 70 per cent of cases and a slower rate and wide QRS in the others. This form of complete AV block is often transient and resolves in a week.[664, 668] The mortality is approximately 15 per cent.

In patients with anterior infarction, third-degree AV block often occurs suddenly, 12 to 24 hours after the onset of the infarct, although it is usually preceded by intraventricular block and often a Mobitz type II pattern (not first-degree or Mobitz type I) AV block. Such patients have unstable escape rhythms with wide QRS complexes and rates less than 40 beats/min; ventricular asystole may occur quite suddenly. The mortality in this group of patients is extremely high, approximately 70 to 80 per cent.[669–671]

Prognosis. The prognosis for patients with AV block complicating AMI depends on the extent and secondarily on the anatomical site of the myocardial injury.[667] Thus, patients with inferior infarction often have concomitant ischemia or infarction of the AV node secondary to hypoperfusion of the AV node artery. However, the His-Purkinje system usually escapes injury in such individuals. Patients with inferior MI who develop AV block usually have lesions in both the right and left anterior descending arteries.[672] Likewise, patients with inferior MI and AV block have larger infarcts and more depressed right ventricular and left ventricular function than do patients with inferior infarct and no AV block.[673] As noted above, junctional escape rhythms with narrow QRS complexes occur commonly in this setting. Hemodynamic derangements are often mild in these patients, and mortality is only slightly increased.[449] In patients with anterior infarction, AV block usually develops as a result of extensive septal necrosis that involves the bundle branches. The high mortality in this group of patients with slow idioventricular rhythm and wide QRS complexes is the consequence of extensive myocardial necrosis resulting in severe left ventricular failure and often shock.[449]

Definitive data are not available concerning the importance of *complete AV block* as an *independent* risk factor for mortality and whether temporary transvenous pacing per se improves survival of patients with AMI. Some investigators contend that ventricular pacing is useless when employed to correct complete AV block in patients with *anterior* infarction in view of the poor prognosis in this group regardless of therapy. We agree with others,[667, 674, 675] however, that ventricular or atrioventricular sequential pacing is indicated in essentially *all* patients with AMI with complete AV block. Pacing is likely to protect against transient hypotension with its attendant risks of extending infarction and precipitating malignant ventricular arrhythmias. Also, pacing protects against asystole, a particular hazard in patients with anterior infarction and infranodal block. Improved survival with pacing probably occurs in only a small fraction of patients with complete AV block and anterior wall infarcts, since the extensive destruction of the myocardium that almost invariably accompanies this condition results in a very high mortality rate, even in paced patients. Therefore, a large series of patients would be required to demonstrate the small reduction of mortality that might be achieved by pacing. The absence of data supporting such an effect, however, by no means excludes the possibility that it may be present. While it is generally agreed that pacing is indicated in patients with *inferior* wall infarction and complete AV block, it is of particular importance if the ventricular rate is very slow (<45 beats/min), if ventricular irritability or hypotension is present, or if pump failure develops; atropine is only rarely of value in these patients. Only when complete heart block develops in less than 6 hours after the onset of symptoms is atropine likely to abolish the AV block or cause acceleration of the escape rhythm.[676] In such cases the AV block is more likely to be transient and related to increases in vagal tone rather than the more persistent block seen later in the course of MI, which generally requires cardiac pacing.

INTRAVENTRICULAR BLOCK. Intraventricular conduction disturbances, i.e., block within one or more of the three subdivisions (fascicles) of the His-Purkinje system (the anterior and posterior divisions of the left bundle and the right bundle, p. 198) occur in 10 to 20 per cent of patients with AMI (Table 38–10). The right bundle branch and the left posterior division have a dual blood supply from the left anterior descending and right coronary artery, whereas the left anterior division is supplied by septal perforators originating from the left anterior descending coronary artery. Not all conduction blocks observed in patients with AMI can be considered to be complications of infarcts, since almost half are already present at the time the first electrocardiogram is recorded, and they may represent antecedent disease of the conduction system.

Isolated Left Anterior Divisional Block (Fig. 7–22, p. 196). This occurs in 3 to 5 per cent of patients with AMI,[677, 678] and in an additional 5 per cent of patients with associated right bundle branch block and AMI.[677] As noted in Table 38–10, mortality is increased in these patients, although not as much as in patients with other forms of conduction block.

Left Posterior Divisional Block. This occurs in only 1 to 2 per cent of patients with AMI admitted to coronary care units. The posterior fascicle is larger than the anterior fascicle, and, in general, a larger infarct is required to block it. As a consequence, mortality is markedly increased (Table 38–10).[677] Complete AV block is not a frequent complication of *either* form of isolated divisional block.

Right Bundle Branch Block. This defect alone occurs in approximately 2 per cent of patients with AMI and frequently leads to AV block because it is often a new lesion, associated with anteroseptal infarction. The mortality is high even if complete AV block does not occur (Table 38–10).[639, 674, 677–679]

Bifascicular Block. The combination of right bundle branch block with either left anterior or posterior divisional block or the combination of left anterior and posterior divisional blocks (i.e., left bundle branch block) is known as bidivisional or bifascicular block (p. 200). If new block occurs in two of the three divisions of the conduction system, the risk of developing complete AV block is quite high.[639, 677] Mortality is also high because of the occurrence of severe pump failure secondary to the extensive myocardial necrosis required to produce such an extensive intraventricular block.[680] Left bundle branch block occurs in approximately 5 per cent of patients with AMI (Table 38–10). Although the latter defect progresses to complete AV block only half as frequently as does right bundle branch block, it is associated with as high a mortality as right bundle branch block and the other two forms of bifascicular block,[639, 677, 679] and with a high late mortality.[233] Patients with intraventricular conduction defects, particularly right bundle branch block, account for the majority of patients who develop ventricular fibrillation late in their hospital stay. However, the high mortality in these patients occurs even in the absence of AV block and appears to be related to cardiac failure and massive infarction rather than to the conduction disturbance. Preexisting bundle branch block or divisional block is less often associated with the development of complete heart block in patients with AMI than are conduction defects acquired during the course of the infarct.[679] Bidivisional block in the presence of prolongation of the P-R interval (first-degree AV block) may indicate disease of the third subdivision[681] rather than disease of the AV node. In such cases, termed trifascicular block, nearly 40 per cent will progress to complete heart block, a risk that is considerably greater than the risk of complete heart block without first-degree AV block.[675, 682]

Complete bundle branch block (either left or right), the combination of right bundle branch block and left anterior divisional (fascicular) block, or any of the various forms of trifascicular block are all more often associated with anterior than inferoposterior infarction.

Use of Pacemakers in Acute Myocardial Infarction

TEMPORARY PACING. Just as is the case for complete AV block, transvenous ventricular pacing has not resulted in statistically demonstrable improvement in prognosis among patients with AMI who develop intraventricular conduction defects. However, temporary pacing is advisable in certain of these patients because of the high risk of developing complete AV block. This includes patients with *new* bilateral (bifascicular) bundle branch block, i.e., right bundle branch block with left anterior or posterior divisional block and alternating right and left bundle branch block; first-degree AV block adds to this risk. Isolated new block in only one of the three fascicles even with P-R prolongation and preexisting bifascicular block and normal P-R interval poses somewhat less risk; these patients should be monitored closely with insertion of a temporary pacemaker deferred unless higher degree AV block occurs.

The risk of developing complete heart block following AMI can be predicted on the basis of results of an analysis of several large series of well-characterized patients with AMI.[683] The presence (new or preexisting) of any of the following conduction disturbances was considered a risk factor: first-degree AV block, Mobitz type I second-degree AV block, Mobitz type II second-degree AV block, left anterior hemiblock, left posterior hemiblock, right bundle branch block, and left bundle branch block. Each risk factor was assigned a score of 1, and the risk score was calculated as the sum of these electrocardiographic risk factors. The incidence of *complete heart block* occurred as follows: Risk score *0*, 1.2 to 6.8 per cent incidence, risk score *1*, 7.8 to 10.4 per cent incidence, risk score *2*, 25.0 to 30.1 per cent incidence, and risk score *3* to 36 or greater per cent incidence.[683]

We believe that failure to demonstrate improved prognosis statistically does not belie the potential value of pacemaker therapy; it probably reflects the overriding impact on mortality of the extensive infarction responsible for the development of the conduction abnormality and the large number of patients required to permit statistical documentation of reduction of mortality.

Temporary pacing in AMI (p. 717) has been successfully employed for the last 2 decades. In assessing the need for temporary pacing (Table 38–11), the clinician must keep in mind that between 10 and 20 per cent of patients develop pacemaker-related complications.[684, 685] A pericardial friction rub is heard in approximately 5 per cent of patients but does not necessarily indicate cardiac perforation, nor is such a finding an indication for withdrawal of

TABLE 38–11 SUGGESTED USE OF TEMPORARY PACING WITH AMI

	Strength of Indication (−, +, ++)
Rate Disturbances	
Sinus bradycardia without hypotension, VEA, angina, left ventricular failure, or syncope	−
Sinus bradycardia with any of the above despite atropine	+
Accelerated idioventricular rhythm	−
Idioventricular rhythm with bradycardia, and hypotension or rate <45	+
Recurrent sick sinus syndrome, prolonged sinus pauses	+
Ventricular tachycardia (especially overdrive pacing for torsades de pointes)	+
Conduction Disturbances	
First-degree AV block	−
Second-degree AV block	
Mobitz I without bradycardia or hypotension	−
Mobitz I with bradycardia and hypotension	+
Mobitz II	++
Complete (third-degree) AV block	++
Isolated new or preexisting LAH, LPH *or* RBBB	−
New LBBB	+
New Bifascicular block*	++
Pre-existing Bifascicular block	−†

Indications are graded as −, Temporary pacing not indicated; +, Temporary pacing should be considered, particularly if other therapeutic maneuvers have failed or if emergency pacer insertion would be difficult or logistically impossible at some other time (e.g., skilled personnel not always available); ++, Temporary pacing should be instituted.

VEA = Ventricular ectopic activity, AV = atrioventricular, LAH = Left anterior hemiblock, LPH = Left posterior hemiblock, RBBB = Right bundle branch block, LBBB = Left bundle branch block.

*Bifascicular block includes alternating right and left bundle branch block, right bundle branch block with left axis deviation, right bundle branch block with right axis deviation, and left bundle branch block with P-R interval prolongation.

†If duration of block is uncertain or if preexisting block occurs with new first-degree AV block, stronger consideration should be given.

the pacemaker electrode. Arrhythmias requiring cardioversion, right ventricular perforation, and local infectious complications occur in 1 to 3 per cent of cases.[684] Pacemaker malfunction also occurs rather frequently and is, in part, related to the experience of the clinical team in managing the device and its insertion.

Although external temporary cardiac pacing was introduced in 1952,[686] its widespread clinical use has not occurred until recently, due to technical refinements making the technique safe, quickly applicable, and relatively well tolerated.[687] Noninvasive external temporary cardiac pacing is now possible routinely in conscious patients and is acceptable to many but not all patients because of the discomfort[688] (Fig. 38–31). Used in a standby mode, it is virtually free of complications and contraindications and provides an important alternative to transvenous endocardial pacing. However, until its effectiveness has been more clearly documented, its routine use should be reserved for patients with moderate (or less) risk of complete heart block. Furthermore, once continuous pacing is required, external pacing is generally not well tolerated for more than minutes to hours. In such situations, it should be replaced by a temporary transvenous pacemaker.

PERMANENT PACING. The question of permanent pacing in survivors of AMI associated with conduction defects is still controversial[679, 689–691] (Table 38–12). Patients with inferior infarction with *transient* type II second-degree block or complete AV block without an associated intraventricular conduction defect do not appear to require

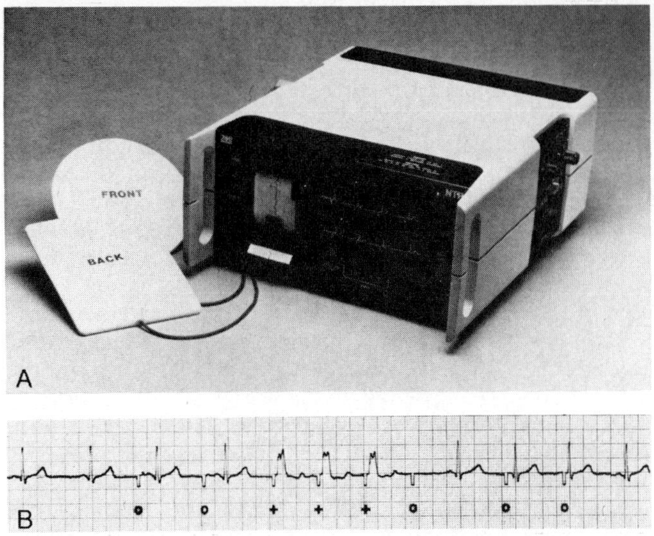

FIGURE 38–31. *A*, Noninvasive temporary pacing device shown with patient electrodes. The electrodes are self-adhering and applied to the left precordium (front) and posteriorly (back). The pacemaker includes an oscilloscopic monitor and strip recorder. Sensitivity, output, and rate adjustments can be made from the controls on the side of the device. *B*, Electrocardiographic strip during pacing with capture (+); also shown is the pacing artifact (0) when output of the pacer is lowered so as not to capture. The pacer rate is approximately 80 beats/min; the patient's intrinsic rate is approximately 60 beats/min. (Courtesy of P. Zoll, M.D.)

permanent pacing. Some contend that prophylactic pacing makes little difference in the long-term survival of patients with AMI and bundle branch block complicated by transient high-degree block.[690] On the other hand, in a retrospective multicenter study, survivors of AMI and bundle branch block who experienced transient high-degree (Mobitz type II second-degree, or third-degree) block had a high incidence of recurrent high-degree AV block and sudden death, and this incidence was reduced by insertion of a permanent demand pacemaker.[675, 679] Thus, these findings suggest a role for prophylactic permanent pacing in patients with AMI and bundle branch block with transient high-degree atrioventricular block.

The question of the advisability of permanent pacemaker insertions is complicated by the fact that not all sudden deaths in this population are due to recurrent high-degree block. A high incidence of late in-hospital ventricular fibrillation occurs in coronary care unit survivors with anteroseptal myocardial infarction complicated by either right or left bundle branch block.[692] If the propensity for this arrhythmia continued, ventricular fibrillation rather than asystole due to failure of atrioventricular conduction

TABLE 38–12 SUGGESTED USE OF PERMANENT PACING FOLLOWING AMI

	Strength of Indication (−, +, ++)
Transient AV conduction disturbances in the absence of intraventricular conduction defects	−
Transient advanced* AV block and associated bundle branch block	+
Persistent first degree AV block with new bundle branch block	+
Persistent advanced* AV block	++

Indications are graded as −, Permanent pacing not indicated; +, Permanent pacing frequently used but opinion is divided (certain patients in this category warrant further testing (such as Holter monitoring or measurement of H-V conduction time before decision can be made); ++, Permanent pacing indicated (insertion of pacemaker should take place before hospital discharge).

*Advanced heart block is defined as Mobitz II second-degree AV block *or* third-degree (complete) AV block.

and of the infranodal pacemaker could be responsible for late sudden death.

ASYSTOLE. This arrhythmia has been reported to occur in 1 to 14 per cent of patients with AMI admitted to coronary care units.[693] This wide variation in incidence reflects differences in the definition of this event. The lower incidence rates include only patients who develop asystole either as a primary event or following abnormalities of atrioventricular or intraventricular conduction, whereas the higher rates include patients who develop asystole as a terminal complication. In either event, the mortality is very high, ranging upward from 90 per cent.[639]

Appearance of apparent ventricular asystole on monitor displays of continuously recorded electrocardiograms may be misleading, since the mechanism may in fact be fine ventricular fibrillation. Because of the predominance of ventricular fibrillation as the cause of cardiac arrest in this setting, initial therapy should include electrical countershock, even if definitive electrocardiographic documentation of this arrhythmia is not available. In the rare instance in which asystole can be documented to be the responsible electrophysiological disturbance, immediate transthoracic pacing (or stimulation with a transvenous pacemaker if one is already in place) is indicated. In this situation temporary noninvasive pacing with an external stimulating device may be life-saving.[688]

SUPRAVENTRICULAR TACHYARRHYTHMIAS

SINUS TACHYCARDIA. Almost one-third of patients with an AMI will develop sinus tachycardia (p. 663) at some time during the first few days after the infarction,[639] an arrhythmia that may be associated with transient hypertension or hypotension and augmented sympathetic activity.[646, 694] The most common causes of sinus tachycardia are anxiety, persistent pain, and left ventricular failure. Other causes include fever, pericarditis, hypovolemia, atrial infarction, pulmonary embolism, and the administration of cardioaccelerator drugs such as atropine, epinephrine, or isoproterenol. Sinus tachycardia is particularly common in patients with anterior infarction. It is an undesirable rhythm in patients with AMI, since it results in an augmentation of myocardial oxygen consumption, as well as a reduction in the time available for coronary perfusion. Persistent sinus tachycardia may signify persistent heart failure and under these circumstances is a poor prognostic sign associated with an excess mortality. An underlying cause should be sought and appropriate treatment instituted, e.g., analgesics for pain, diuretics for heart failure, oxygen, beta blockers and nitroglycerin for ischemia, and aspirin for fever or pericarditis.[695]

Administration of beta-adrenoceptor blocking agents, in the dosage and manner described on page 634, may be helpful in the treatment of sinus tachycardia, particularly when this arrhythmia is a manifestation of a hyperdynamic circulation, which is seen particularly in young patients with an initial MI without extensive cardiac damage (p. 1274). However, beta blockade is contraindicated in patients in whom the sinus tachycardia is a manifestation of hypovolemia or pump failure, the latter reflected by a systolic arterial pressure below 100 mm Hg, rales involving more than one-third of the lung fields, a pulmonary capillary wedge pressure exceeding 20 to 25 mm Hg, or a cardiac index below approximately 2.3 liters/min/m^2.

ATRIAL PREMATURE CONTRACTIONS. Atrial premature contractions (p. 669) are relatively common after MI, occurring in up to half of all patients.[639, 696] Atrial premature contractions, and the atrial tachyarrhythmias (paroxysmal supraventricular tachycardia, atrial flutter, and atrial fibrillation) which they often herald, may be caused by atrial distention secondary to increases in left ventricular diastolic pressure, by pericarditis with its associated atrial epicarditis, or, less commonly, by ischemic injury to the atria[697] and sinus node. Atrial premature beats per se are not associated with an increase in mortality, and cardiac output is unaffected.[698] Occasionally an atrial premature beat may initiate ventricular tachycardia[699] or even ventricular fibrillation[700] in the presence of AMI.

Premature atrial contractions require no specific therapy and may indicate atrial dilatation, excessive autonomic stimulation, or the presence of overt or occult heart failure. If they are related to heart failure, they often respond to treatment of this condition.

PAROXYSMAL SUPRAVENTRICULAR TACHYCARDIA (See also pp. 603 and 680). This arrhythmia occurs in 2 to 5 per cent of patients with AMI.[701] It tends to be both transient and recurrent.[696] Its deleterious effects result from the elevation of myocardial oxygen consumption and the impairment of ventricular performance consequent to the rapid ventricular rate; it is associated with an increase in mortality.

Aggressive management is indicated for paroxysmal supraventricular tachycardia because of the rapid rate. Augmentation of vagal tone by manual carotid sinus stimulation or intravenous administration of 10 mg of edrophonium (Tensilon) may restore sinus rhythm. Alpha-adrenoceptor agonists to increase arterial pressure and activate carotid sinus baroreceptors, an acceptable form of therapy for paroxysmal supraventricular tachycardia under other circumstances, are hazardous in patients with AMI, and intravenous verapamil is preferable.[702, 703] Although digitalis glycosides may be useful in augmenting vagal tone, thereby terminating the arrhythmia, their effect is often delayed. Accordingly, low-energy DC countershock or rapid atrial stimulation via a transvenous intra-atrial electrode should be utilized if hemodynamic decompensation occurs or if the rhythm is refractory to conventional measures. *Paroxysmal atrial tachycardia with AV block* (p. 674) may be a manifestation of digitalis intoxication and should be treated by withholding this drug and instituting potassium therapy, when it is accompanied by hypokalemia.

ATRIAL FLUTTER AND FIBRILLATION (See also pp. 671 and 672). Atrial flutter is the least common atrial arrhythmia associated with AMI, occurring in only 1 to 3 per cent of all patients. As in patients who develop this arrhythmia in the absence of infarction, atrial flutter is usually associated with 2:1 atrioventricular block. Since the atrial rate ranges from 250 to 350 beats/min, the ventricular rate is usually 125 to 175 beats/min. Atrial flutter is usually transient and is a consequence of augmented sympathetic stimulation of the atria, often occurring in patients with left ventricular failure or pulmonary emboli. Atrial flutter often intensifies hemodynamic deterioration.[633, 647, 698]

Atrial fibrillation is far more common than flutter, occurring in 10 to 15 per cent of patients with AMI.[641, 693, 696, 698, 701] As with atrial premature contractions and atrial flutter, fibrillation is usually transient and tends to occur in patients with left ventricular failure but is also observed in patients with pericarditis and ischemic injury to the atria; it occurs more frequently following anterior than inferior infarction and appears to be a consequence of left atrial ischemia in the majority of cases.[704] The increased ventricular rate and the loss of the atrial contribution to left ventricular filling—i.e., the atrial kick—result in a significant reduction in cardiac output. Both atrial flutter and fibrillation are more common during the first 24 hours after infarction than later and are associated with increased mortality, particularly in patients with anterior wall infarction. However, because they are more common in patients with clinical and hemodynamic manifestations of extensive infarction and a poor prognosis, their *independent* contributions to increased mortality are not clear. Unfortunately, their management is complicated by frequent recurrence, particularly when they result from left atrial dilatation secondary to left ventricular failure.

Management. Atrial flutter and fibrillation in patients with AMI are treated in a manner similar to that in other settings (pp. 672 and 673). However, because of the possibility that a rapid ventricular rate can increase infarct size and because of the important role played by atrial contraction in the support of cardiac output in patients with AMI (Fig. 38–29), treatment must be prompt, especially when the ventricular rate exceeds 100/min. *Digitalis glycosides* are the principal agents used to slow the ventricular response. Digitalis may be supplemented by small intravenous doses of a beta blocker which also prolongs the AV nodal refractory period: 1 to 4 mg of propranolol in divided doses is often quite effective in reducing the ventricular rate and is well tolerated even in patients with mild heart failure and a rapid ventricular rate. Reduction of the rate of ventricular response to atrial fibrillation may be achieved also with verapamil administered intravenously[702] via bolus injections of 60 to 120 μg/kg, followed by a continuous infusion of 2.5 to 5.0 μg/kg/min, although caution must be exercised to avoid systemic arterial hypotension. On the other hand, when hemodynamic decompensation is prominent, electrical cardioversion is indicated with anterior and laterally placed paddles,[705] beginning with 25 watt-seconds for atrial flutter and 50 watt-seconds for atrial fibrillation with gradual increase if the initial shock is not successful.

An additional important option for the treatment of atrial flutter is the use of rapid atrial stimulation via a transvenous intraatrial electrode (p. 672); in contrast to DC cardioversion, this technique can be employed in the presence of possible digitalis intoxication, is less prone than DC countershock to elicit bradycardia after conversion to sinus rhythm, provides control of ventricular rate via atrial or ventricular pacing should this be necessary, and can be reapplied with less difficulty than cardioversion, should the patient experience recurrent atrial flutter. Following restoration of sinus rhythm, attention should be directed to the management of the underlying cause, usually heart failure, and to the prevention of recurrences, with antiarrhythmic agents such as quinidine. Patients with recurrent episodes should be treated with oral anticoagulants.

JUNCTIONAL RHYTHMS (See also p. 676). Sustained junctional rhythms fall into three categories:

1. *AV junctional rhythm* at a rate of 35 to 60 beats/min in which the AV junctional tissue simply assumes the role of the dominant pacemaker when the sinus node is depressed.

2. *Accelerated junctional rhythm* in which increased rhythmicity of the junctional tissue usurps the role of pacemaker, usually at a rate of 70 to 130 beats/min.

These two arrhythmias are often transient, occur during the first 48 hours of the infarction, usually develop and terminate gradually, and are characterized by QRS complexes that resemble those of normally conducted beats. Retrograde P waves may be evident, or atrioventricular dissociation may occur, with the junctional rate slightly in excess of the underlying sinus rate. Disagreement exists concerning the prognostic implications of these arrhythmias; some observers attach a poor prognosis to these arrhythmias, whereas others believe that they are benign.[633, 696, 706] However, in patients with relatively slow junctional rhythm, the process is generally a benign protective escape rhythm and is commonly seen among patients with a slow sinus rate in the presence of inferior myocardial infarction.

3. *Paroxysmal junctional tachycardia* usually produces rates between 160 and 220 beats/min.[633, 696] This arrhythmia is uncommon in AMI, occurring in only 1 to 2 per cent of patients. In contrast to accelerated junctional rhythms, episodes of paroxysmal junctional tachycardia commence and terminate abruptly, thereby resembling other forms of paroxysmal supraventricular tachycardia, and they often occur in the presence of left ventricular failure, ischemia of the conduction system, or digitalis excess.[698] When intraventricular conduction defects are present, it may be difficult to distinguish paroxysmal atrial or junctional tachycardia from ventricular tachycardia. The hemodynamic and prognostic significance of paroxysmal junctional tachycardia is similar to that for paroxysmal atrial tachycardia except that the atrial kick is lost with the junctional rhythm. As indicated above, the loss of atrial transport function may be tolerated poorly. When a junctional rhythm is present and there is hemodynamic impairment, transvenous sequential atrioventricular pacing may be required to facilitate ventricular performance and maintain adequate peripheral perfusion.

VENTRICULAR ARRHYTHMIAS

VENTRICULAR PREMATURE BEATS (VPB's) (See also p. 692). Although VPB's are very frequent, indeed almost universal[707, 708] in the presence of AMI, the value of the so-called warning arrhythmias in the prediction of ventricular fibrillation is not clear. It was believed that warning arrhythmias—defined as frequent VPB's (more than five per minute), VPB's with multiform configuration, early coupling (the "R-on-T" phenomenon), and repetitive patterns in the form of couplets or salvos—presage ventricular fibrillation. However, it is now clear that they are present in as many patients who develop fibrillation as who do not.[11] Several reports have shown that primary ventricular fibrillation (see below) occurs without antecedent warning arrhythmias in 40 to 83 per cent of cases.[709–711] On the other hand, frequent and complex VPB's are commonly observed in patients with AMI who never develop ventricular fibrillation.[709, 710]

Prognosis. The significance of early coupling ("R-on-T" phenomenon) has been reassessed in experimental[712] and clinical[710] studies. These have shown that ventricular tachyarrhythmias in patients with AMI are often initiated by a VPB that does *not* fall on an antecedent T wave. In fact, a majority of ventricular tachycardias in patients with AMI appear to be initiated by a *late*-coupled VPB.[713, 714] In two clinical reports on electrocardiographic antecedents of primary ventricular fibrillation, 45 per cent[709] and 41 per cent [710] of episodes of ventricular fibrillation, respectively, were initiated by a late-coupled VPB. However, in one study[715] frequent VPB's showing the R-on-T phenomenon did appear to herald the development of ventricular fibrillation but not of ventricular tachycardia. Thus, the prognostic value, if any, of various forms of VPB's in AMI remains unclear.

Management. A large number of randomized trials have compared the routine (including prehospital[716]) administration of several potent antiarrhythmic drugs—lidocaine, quinidine, procainamide, and disopyramide, as well as beta-adrenoceptor blocking agents—against placebo.[715a] All of these agents reduced the frequency of ventricular premature contractions, and in the case of lidocaine, routine administration lowered the incidence of ventricular fibrillation in some studies,[716–719] but not in all.[720] None of the agents administered in this fashion, however, reduced mortality.[721, 722]

Despite the results of these large trials and despite the complexity of the relationship between ventricular premature contractions and ventricular fibrillation, we favor the prophylactic administration of antiarrhythmic drugs in *selected* patients. This position is based partly on the concept that the abolition or reduction of ventricular premature contractions serves as a useful endpoint that reflects an adequate overall pharmacological effect. Thus, when an appropriately selected agent is administered in sufficiently high doses, it can reduce the incidence of ventricular fibrillation even though its antifibrillatory activity can be monitored only indirectly, i.e., by reducing the incidence of ventricular premature contractions. It seems eminently desirable to reduce the incidence of ventricular fibrillation; although primary ventricular fibrillation (not preceded by pump failure) may be treated effectively in centers where clinical trials on patients with AMI are being carried out, which usually have well-staffed and equipped coronary care units, this does not guarantee similar results in different settings.

Frequent ventricular premature contractions occurring very soon after the onset of MI, particularly during the first hour, may depend primarily on reentry rather than on increased automaticity.[723] At this time, lidocaine, which impairs conduction in ventricular myocardium and diminishes automaticity, may be somewhat less effective than it is later.[721] When, at the very inception of an infarction, ventricular premature contractions are encountered in the presence of sinus tachycardia, augmented sympathoadrenal stimulation is often a contributing factor, and may be improved by beta-adrenoceptor blockade. In fact, early administration of an intravenous beta blocker is effective in reducing the incidence of ventricular fibrillation in evolving MI.[724] The effectiveness of beta-adrenoceptor blocking drugs under these circumstances may, in fact, play a role in the reduction in sudden deaths reported in patients who have recovered from AMI and are at high risk of recurrence.[594, 597] The dosages and modes of administration as well as the contraindications to beta blockade are discussed on page 633.

Lidocaine. In the absence of specific, correctable factors, such as sympathoadrenal hyperactivity with tachycardia, lidocaine should be administered to patients with AMI and frequent ventricular premature contractions (> 6/min), multiform premature contractions, extrasystoles occurring in pairs or salvos, and early premature contractions (R on T), even though it is acknowledged that it may not be appropriate to consider these to be "warning arrhythmias." We favor the prophylactic administration of lidocaine, as described below, particularly in patients with AMI at high risk of developing ventricular fibrillation. This includes younger patients (< 50 years) without a prior history of heart failure or AMI and who present within the first 6 hours of infarction. Older patients (> 70 years) who are seen more than 6 hours after the onset of the MI are less likely to develop ventricular fibrillation and are at high risk of developing lidocaine toxicity and should probably not receive prophylaxis routinely. The management of other patients must be individualized. The setting in which the patient is treated must also be considered. Obviously, the risk to life of ventricular fibrillation is greater at home or on a general hospital floor than in an expertly and fully staffed and equipped coronary care unit.

The pharmacology and pharmacokinetics of lidocaine are discussed on page 625. With regimens depending on continuous infusion alone, therapeutic blood levels (1.5 to 5 μg/ml) are reached only after several hours because of the short half-life of the drug. Therefore, a loading dose of 100 mg or 1.5 mg/kg should be given intravenously as a bolus injection at the time of admission or during the patient's transportation to the hospital, followed in 5 to 10 minutes by an injection of 0.5 mg/kg. An intravenous infusion should be started concomitantly; a dose of 50 μg/kg/min in patients without heart failure, hypotension, or primary hepatic dysfunction and of 20 μg/kg/min in patients with any of these problems is advised.[725] Intramuscular injections into the deltoid or gluteal muscles with conventional syringes and needles do not achieve therapeutic concentrations as promptly as those following intravenous injection.

The maintenance dose of lidocaine should be adjusted within the range of 1 to 4 mg/min to reduce sharply or abolish premature ventricular contractions. It should be recognized that the metabolism of lidocaine is slowed not only in patients with heart failure or hypotension[726] but also in those with diminution of hepatic blood flow due to effects of pharmacological agents such as propranolol.[727] The rate of infusion should be lower in patients on cimetidine and in patients with renal failure. Therefore, careful titration is needed to avoid toxicity, manifested primarily by central nervous system hyperactivity, as well as by depression of intraventricular and atrioventricular conduction and cardiac contractility. Saturation of an extravascular pool normally occurs after a continuous infusion of approximately three hours, at which time blood levels will increase despite maintenance of a constant infusion rate.[728] At this time, it may be desirable to reduce the rate of administration by about 25 per cent.

This regimen is effective in suppressing ventricular premature contractions in approximately 75 per cent of patients seen within the first hour after the onset of ischemia[408]; it is effective in an even higher percentage—80 to 90 per cent—of patients seen later after the onset of ischemia, perhaps because enhanced automaticity becomes a progressively more important factor in the etiology of ventricular premature contractions with the passage of time from the onset of infarction and because of the particular effectiveness of the drug for arrhythmias on this basis.[729–731] Lidocaine has been shown to abolish reentrant ventricular arrhythmias in the late myocardial infarction phase by further depression and block of conduction in the reentrant pathway.[732]

Procainamide. When ventricular premature contractions compromise hemodynamics and persist despite administration of lidocaine, or when lidocaine is contraindicated for other reasons (e.g., allergy), administration of procainamide intravenously in bolus doses of approximately 1 to 2 mg/kg intravenously over intervals of 5 minutes to a cumulative dose of approximately 1000 mg, followed by maintenance therapy with an intravenous infusion (20 to 80 μg/kg/min), may be effective. In patients with AMI, suppression of premature ventricular beats occurs at lower plasma concentrations of procainamide than is required in patients with chronic heart disease. This difference appears to reflect an electrophysiological difference, with the myocardium being more sensitive to the drug, rather than a change in procainamide pharmacokinetics, which is apparently normal in patients with AMI.[733]

Other Drugs. Other drugs such as tocainide[734] and the experimental agent propafenone,[735] appear to be as effective as lidocaine for suppressing premature ventricular beats. Ventricular premature contractions that are unresponsive to lidocaine, procainamide, or tocainide in approximately the first 6 hours following AMI, particularly in the presence of sinus tachycardia, may be responsive to beta-adrenoceptor blocking agents.

Although phenytoin (Dilantin) (p. 632) (50 to 100 mg intravenously at 5 to 10 minute intervals to a total of 1000 mg) may diminish ventricular arrhythmia by decreasing the rate of phase IV depolarization, suppressing efferent cardiac sympathetic stimulation,[736] and further depressing and blocking conduction in ischemia-induced reentrant pathways,[737] it does not confer protection against ventricular fibrillation either in the first few hours[738] or later in the course of AMI. On the other hand, this drug may be effective when ventricular arrhythmias are initiated or potentiated by digitalis intoxication.

If ventricular premature contractions recur following initial intravenous treatment, oral administration of conventional antiarrhythmic agents is justified, including quinidine, procainamide, flecainide, tocainide, mexiletine, disopyramide, phenytoin, and propranolol, selected on the basis of the criteria outlined above and described in Chapter 21.

In the post-myocardial infarction period, the prognostic significance of VPB's, particularly frequent ones, appears to be less controversial. Although there is little correlation between ventricular arrhythmias occurring in the early hours or days of AMI and those observed in the late post infarction period,[739, 740] frequent VPB's or ventricular tachycardia *following* hospital discharge do appear to be an independent risk factor for sudden death (p. 1294).[741, 742]

ACCELERATED IDIOVENTRICULAR RHYTHM (Fig. 22–35, p. 698). Commonly defined as a ventricular rhythm with a rate of 60 to 110 (or 125) beats/min,[743, 744] and frequently called "slow ventricular tachycardia," this arrhythmia is seen in 8 to 20 per cent of patients with AMI, usually in the first 2 days, and seems to be equally common in anterior and inferior infarctions. About half of all episodes of accelerated idioventricular rhythm are manifested as an escape rhythm occurring during slowing of the sinus rhythm or gradual speeding of the ventricular pacemaker; the other half of accelerated idioventricular rhythms is initiated by a premature beat.[745] Most episodes are of short duration, and the arrhythmia may terminate abruptly, slow gradually before termination, or be overdriven by acceleration of the basic cardiac rhythm. Variation of the rate is common. Accelerated idioventricular rhythms in patients with AMI probably result from enhanced automaticity of Purkinje fibers. In contrast to rapid ventricular tachycardia, accelerated idioventricular rhythms are thought not to affect prognosis.[11, 744, 745] However, accelerated idioventricular rhythms are frequently associated with episodes of rapid ventricular tachycardia, and in many patients increased automaticity is manifested at times as accelerated idioventricular rhythms and at other times as ventricular tachycardia.

The need for treatment of this arrhythmia is controversial. Since these rhythms may deteriorate into ventricular tachycardia and since they may compromise cardiac function because of impairment of the physiological sequential relationship between atrial and ventricular contraction, it may be prudent to treat them by accelerating the sinus rate with atropine or atrial pacing or by suppressing the ventricular pacemaker with the administration of lidocaine intravenously. However, there is no definitive evidence that this arrhythmia, when left untreated, increases the incidence of either ventricular fibrillation or mortality.[746]

VENTRICULAR TACHYCARDIA (See also p. 694). This arrhythmia is generally defined as three or more consecutive ventricular ectopic beats occurring at a frequency exceeding 120 beats/min. The reported incidence of ventricular tachycardia in AMI is in the range of 10 to 40 per cent.[11, 639] When this arrhythmia occurs within the first 24 hours, it is often precipitated by a late VPB and is transient and benign. Ventricular tachycardia occurring late in the course of AMI is more common in patients with transmural infarction and left ventricular dysfunction, is sustained, usually induces marked hemodynamic deterioration, and is associated with a relatively high hospital mortality rate—40 to 50 per cent[639] (Table 38–8). However, the relative contribution to the high mortality rate of this arrhythmia per se, compared with that of the underlying impairment of left ventricular performance due to large infarction, is not clear. In addition, the long-term mortality in patients who exhibit ventricular tachycardia in the late hospital phase of AMI is greatly increased.[747]

Hypokalemia increases the risk of all ventricular tachycardia[748, 749] (Fig. 38–32). Low serum potassium should be identified quickly after a patient's admission for AMI and should be treated promptly. During the course of the patient's hospitalization, care should be taken to insure that the serum potassium level remains consistently above 4.0 mEq/liter. Rapid abolition of ventricular tachycardia in patients with AMI is mandatory because of its deleterious effect on pump function and because it frequently deteriorates into ventricular fibrillation. When the ventricular rate is rapid (> 150/min) and/or there is a decline in arterial pressure, a single attempt at "thumpversion," i.e., striking a sharp blow to the precordium, is indicated (p. 697). If this maneuver is unsuccessful, it should be followed immediately by synchronized DC countershock, beginning with relatively low energies, i.e., 10 watt-seconds. When the ventricular rate is very rapid and synchronization is not possible, a defibrillatory impulse of 100 to 200 watt-seconds should be delivered. When the ventricular rate is slower than approximately 150/min and

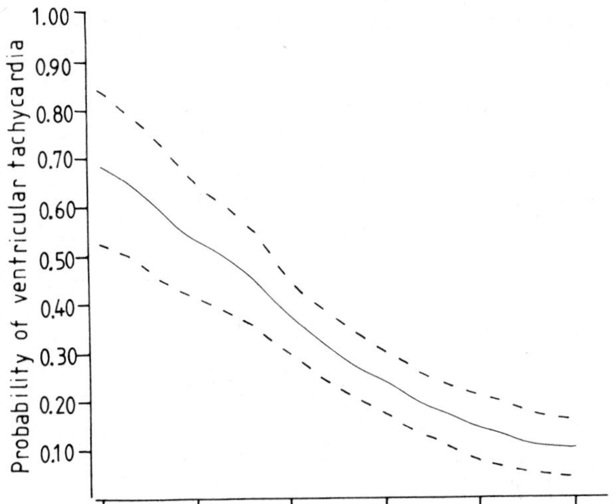

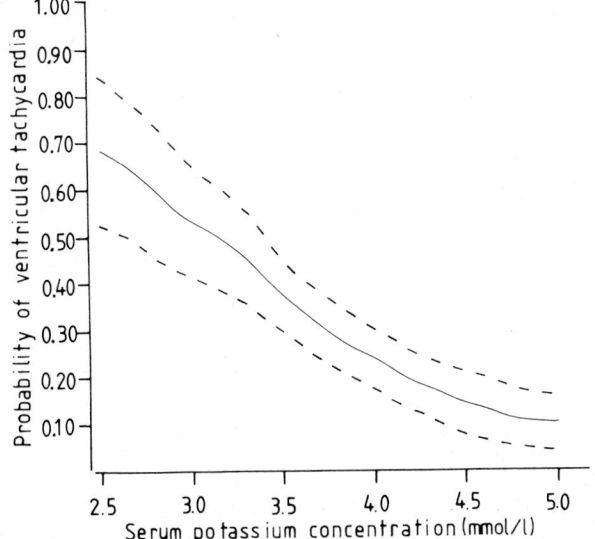

FIGURE 38–32. Probability of ventricular tachycardia in relation to serum potassium concentration. Dotted lines denote standard deviation. (From Nordrehany, J. E., et al.: Serum potassium concentration as a risk factor of ventricular arrhythmias early in acute myocardial infarction. Circulation *71*:645, 1985, by permission of the American Heart Association, Inc.)

the arrhythmia is well tolerated hemodynamically, a brief (15 to 20 min) trial of treatment with lidocaine or procainamide, using the loading doses described on pages 627 and 630, is in order. If these measures are unsuccessful, an infusion of bretylium tosylate (1 to 2 mg/min) may be tried. After reversion to sinus rhythm, every effort should be made to correct underlying abnormalities such as hypoxia, hypotension, acid-base or electrolyte disturbances, and digitalis excess. Recurrent or refractory ventricular tachycardia may respond to aneurysm resection, encircling endocardial ventriculotomy, or endocardial resection with or without coronary artery bypass grafting; these surgical procedures are generally reserved for use until after the acute phase.[750–752]

VENTRICULAR FIBRILLATION (See also p. 701). This arrhythmia occurs in 4 to 18 per cent of patients with AMI treated in coronary care units.[709–711] It occurs with equal incidence in patients with anterior and with inferior Q-wave infarctions[693] and is rare in patients with non-Q-wave infarction. This arrhythmia may occur in three settings in hospitalized patients with AMI. Its occurrence as a mechanism of sudden death is discussed in Chapter 24. *Primary* ventricular fibrillation, responsible for more than 80 per cent of all instances of this arrhythmia,[711] occurs suddenly and unexpectedly in patients with no or few signs or symptoms of left ventricular failure. Approximately 60 per cent of episodes occur within 4 hours and 80 per cent within 12 hours of the onset of symptoms.[711] *Secondary* ventricular fibrillation, on the other hand, is the final phase of a progressive downhill course with left ventricular failure and cardiogenic shock.[693] So-called *late* ventricular fibrillation usually occurs 1 to 6 weeks following AMI. Patients with intraventricular conduction defects and anterior wall infarction, patients with persistent sinus tachycardia, atrial flutter, or fibrillation early in their course, and those with right ventricular infarction who require ventricular pacing[753] all are at higher risk for suffering late *in-hospital* ventricular fibrillation than patients without these features.

Coronary care unit survivors with anteroseptal infarction complicated by right or left bundle branch block are particularly vulnerable to this late complication.[754] Those patients discharged alive with an anterior MI complicated by ventricular fibrillation face a much worse prognosis than those with inferior MI and ventricular fibrillation. In a case-controlled study, cumulative mortality at 5-year follow-up for the anterior MI group (54 per cent) was twice that for the inferior MI group (26 per cent).[755]

The effect of *primary* ventricular fibrillation on prognosis continues to be debated.[753, 756, 757] The MILIS study showed that it does not have an adverse effect.[756] On the other hand, secondary ventricular fibrillation occurring in association with marked left ventricular failure or hypotension clearly entails a dire prognosis, with only 20 to 25 per cent of patients surviving hospitalization.[746] The prognosis is intermediate in so-called late in-hospital ventricular fibrillation.[11] In the latter two forms it is the impairment of cardiac function consequent to the loss of contracting myocardium rather than the arrhythmia per se that is responsible for the poor prognosis.

Procainamide, lidocaine,[716, 717] and the beta-adrenoceptor blockers propranolol[724] and metoprolol[758] administered prophylactically have all been reported to reduce the incidence of primary ventricular fibrillation in hospitalized patients.[729, 759] However, they may not reduce overall mortality substantially because treatment of this arrhythmia is so successful in an efficient coronary care unit.

Management. The treatment of ventricular fibrillation, described in detail on pages 701 and 702, is *electrical countershock*, implemented as rapidly as possible. The likelihood of successful restoration of an effective cardiac rhythm declines rapidly with time after the onset of uncorrected ventricular fibrillation. Irreversible brain damage may occur within 1 to 2 minutes, particularly in elderly patients. Despite the superficial appeal of "thump version," which may sometimes terminate ventricular tachycardia (as opposed to fibrillation), no time should be lost before treating patients with ventricular fibrillation with electrical countershock.

Prompt electrical countershock generally interrupts fibrillation and restores an effective cardiac rhythm in patients under direct medical observation in the coronary care unit. When ventricular fibrillation occurs outside of an intensive care unit, resuscitative efforts are much less likely to be successful, primarily because the time interval between the onset of the episode and institution of definitive therapy tends to be prolonged. Since closed-chest cardiopulmonary resuscitation with external cardiac compression provides only a marginal cardiac output even under optimal circumstances, countershock should be implemented as soon as possible after the detection of ventricular fibrillation rather than deferred under the mistaken impression that adequate circulatory and respiratory support can be maintained in the interim. Failure of electrical countershock to restore an effective cardiac rhythm is due almost always to rapidly recurrent ventricular tachycardia or ventricular fibrillation, to electromechanical dissociation, or, very rarely, to electrical asystole.

Ventricular fibrillation often recurs rapidly and repeatedly when the metabolic milieu of the heart has been compromised by severe or prolonged hypoxemia, acidosis, electrolyte abnormalities, or digitalis intoxication. Under these conditions, continued cardiopulmonary resuscitation, prompt implementation of pharmacological and ventilatory maneuvers designed to correct these abnormalities, treatment with antiarrhythmic agents such as lidocaine, and rapidly repeated attempts with electrical countershock may be effective. Even though repeated shocks with excessive energy may damage the myocardium[760, 761] and elicit arrhythmias,[762] speed is essential and prompt efforts with high-intensity shocks (generally 300 to 400 watt-seconds initially) are justified. When ventricular fibrillation persists without documented interruption by electrical countershock, the intracardiac administration of epinephrine (up to 10 ml of a 1:10, 000 concentration) or calcium gluconate (up to 15 ml of 10 per cent calcium gluconate) may facilitate success in a subsequent attempt. Conversion of fine to coarse ventricular fibrillation by either or both of these drugs may augur well for subsequent successful defibrillation.

Successful interruption of ventricular fibrillation or prevention of refractory recurrent episodes may be facilitated by administration of *bretylium tosylate*, 5 mg/kg intravenously, repeated 20 minutes later if necessary (p. 635).[763] When synchronous cardiac electrical activity is restored by countershock, but contraction is ineffective, i.e., during electromechanical dissociation—the usual underlying cause is very extensive myocardial ischemia, or necrosis, or rupture of the ventricular free wall or septum. If rupture has not occurred, intracardiac administration of calcium gluconate or epinephrine may facilitate restoration of an effective heartbeat. Another antifibrillatory agent is amiodarone (p. 637). It has a slow onset of action; therefore, its principal role may prove to be in the *prevention* rather than treatment of ventricular fibrillation.

HEMODYNAMIC DISTURBANCES IN ACUTE MYOCARDIAL INFARCTION

Swan, Forrester, and their associates have examined the cardiac output and wedge pressure together and have identified four major hemodynamic subsets of patients with AMI (Table 38–13): patients with normal perfusion and without pulmonary congestion (normal cardiac output and normal wedge pressure), patients with normal perfusion and pulmonary congestion (normal cardiac output and elevated wedge pressure), patients with decreased perfusion but without pulmonary congestion (reduced cardiac output and normal wedge pressure), and patients with decreased perfusion and pulmonary congestion (reduced cardiac output and elevated wedge pressure).[764] Although this classification is useful, it must be appreciated that patients frequently pass from one category to another with therapy and, sometimes, even apparently spontaneously.

HEMODYNAMIC SUBSETS. These usually reflect the clinical status of the patients.[443] Hypoperfusion usually becomes evident clinically when the cardiac index falls below approximately 2.2 liters/min/sq meter, whereas pulmonary congestion is noted when the wedge pressure exceeds approximately 20 mm Hg. However, approximately 25 per cent of patients with cardiac indices less than 2.2 liters/min/sq meter and 15 per cent of patients with elevated pulmonary capillary wedge pressures are not recognized clinically. Discrepancies in hemodynamic and clinical classification of patients with AMI arise for a variety of reasons. Patients may exhibit "phase lags" as clinical pulmonary congestion develops or resolves, symptoms secondary to chronic obstructive pulmonary disease may be confused with those resulting from pulmonary congestion, or long-standing left ventricular dysfunction may mask signs of hypoperfusion secondary to compensatory vasoconstriction.[764]

The hemodynamic subsets shown in Table 38–13 may be further divided and characterized by means of hemodynamic monitoring. Such a classification system allows for rational approaches to therapy as indicated in Table 38–14. The goals of hemodynamic therapy are to maintain ventricular performance, support blood pressure, and protect jeopardized myocardium. Since these goals occasionally may be at cross purposes, careful recognition of the hemodynamic profile, as assessed clinically or as available from hemodynamic monitoring, is required before optimal therapeutic interventions can be chosen.

INVASIVE HEMODYNAMIC MONITORING (See also p. 611). Hemodynamic assessment becomes possible once the patient reaches the hospital. An estimation of the presence or absence of gross abnormalities in cardiac index and left ventricular filling pressure can be made on the basis of clinical examination in approximately 80 per cent of patients. However, as noted above, severe depression of cardiac index and/or elevation of left ventricular filling

TABLE 38–13 HEMODYNAMIC SUBSETS IN ACUTE MYOCARDIAL INFARCTION

Clinical Subset	Cardiac Index (liter/min/sq meter)	Pulmonary Capillary Wedge Pressure (mm Hg)	Mortality (%)
I. No pulmonary congestion or peripheral hypoperfusion	2.7 ± 0.5	12 ± 7	2.2
II. Isolated pulmonary congestion	2.3 ± 0.4	23 ± 5	10.1
III. Isolated peripheral hypoperfusion	1.9 ± 0.4	12 ± 5	22.4
IV. Both pulmonary congestion and hypoperfusion	1.6 ± 0.6	27 ± 8	55.5

From Forrester, J. S., et al.: Medical therapy of acute myocardial infarction by application of hemodynamic subsets. N. Engl. J. Med. 295:1404, 1976.

TABLE 38–14 POTENTIALLY USEFUL THERAPEUTIC INTERVENTIONS IN HEMODYNAMIC CATEGORIES OF PATIENTS WITH ACUTE MYOCARDIAL INFARCTION

Hemodynamic Category	P_a*	$\overline{PA}_0$†	CI‡	Suggested Intervention	Remarks
Normal	≤15	≤12	2.7–3.5‡	None	β-blockade may be beneficial
Hyperdynamic state	≤15	≤12	≥3.0	β-adrenoceptor blockage	Tachycardia is a hallmark of subset
Hypotension or shock secondary to hypovolemia	≤15	≤9	≤2.7	Repletion of vascular volume	Reclassification may be necessary after PA_0 is increased to range of 14 to 18 mm Hg
LV failure					
Mild	≥22	≥18–≤22	≤2.5	Diuretics	Dyspnea, hypoxemia, or mild pulmonary vascular congestion
Severe	≥25	≥22	≤1.8	Vasodilators + diuretics	Pulmonary vascular congestion and pulmonary edema; cardiac glycosides; positive pressure ventilation and/or circulatory assist may be useful
Cardiogenic hypotension or shock	≥22	≥18	≤1.8	Circulatory assist	Sympathomimetic agents with positive inotropic effects such as dopamine or dobutamine may be useful

*P_a mean pulmonary artery pressure in mm Hg.
†$\overline{PA}_0$, mean pulmonary artery occlusive pressure in mm Hg.
‡CI, cardiac index in liters/minute/m^2.

pressure may be unsuspected in as many as 15 per cent of patients when estimates are based exclusively on clinical criteria.[443]

In patients with *clinically uncomplicated AMI,* invasive hemodynamic monitoring is generally not necessary, since the status of the circulation can be assessed by careful clinical evaluation. This ordinarily consists of monitoring of heart rate and rhythm, measurement of systemic arterial pressure by cuff, obtaining chest roentgenograms to detect heart failure, careful and repeated auscultation of the lung fields for pulmonary congestion, measurement of urine flow, examination of the skin and mucous membranes for evidence of the adequacy of perfusion, and arterial sampling for pO_2, pCO_2, and pH when hypoxemia or metabolic acidosis is suspected.

Invasive monitoring ordinarily consists of inserting an arterial line for the continuous measurement of arterial pressure and a balloon flotation catheter for measurement of pulmonary artery, pulmonary artery occlusive (equivalent to pulmonary wedge), and right atrial pressures, and cardiac output by thermodilution. In patients with hypotension, a Foley catheter provides accurate and continuous measurement of urine output.

The importance of invasive hemodynamic monitoring[443] is based on the following principal factors:

1. Difficulty of interpreting clinical and radiographic findings of pulmonary congestion because of phase lags, such as those occurring after diuretic therapy.
2. Need for identifying noncardiac causes of arterial hypotension, particularly hypovolemia.
3. Possible contributions of reduced ventricular compliance to impaired hemodynamics, requiring judicious adjustment of intravascular volume to optimize left ventricular filling pressure.
4. Difficulty in assessing the severity and sometimes even determining the presence of lesions such as mitral regurgitation and ventricular septal defect when the cardiac output or the systemic pressures are depressed.
5. Establishing a baseline of hemodynamic measurements and guiding therapy in patients with clinically apparent pulmonary edema or cardiogenic shock.
6. Underestimation of systemic arterial pressure by the cuff method in patients with intense vasoconstriction (Fig. 19–2, p. 562).

HYPOTENSION IN THE PREHOSPITAL PHASE

During the *prehospital phase of AMI,* invasive hemodynamic monitoring is usually not practical, and during this period, therapy should be guided by frequent clinical assessment and measurement of arterial pressure by the cuff method, with the recognition that intense vasoconstriction can provide a falsely low pressure measured by this method. Hypotension associated with bradycardia often reflects excessive vagotonia, which may be responsive to atropine and elevation of the lower extremities. Relative or absolute hypovolemia is often present when hypotension occurs with a normal or rapid heart rate, particularly among patients receiving diuretics just prior to the occurrence of infarction. Marked diaphoresis, reduction of fluid intake, or vomiting during the period preceding and accompanying the onset of AMI may all contribute to the development of hypovolemia. Even if the effective vascular volume is normal, *relative* hypovolemia may be present, since ventricular compliance is reduced in AMI (p. 1204) and a left ventricular filling pressure as high as 20 mm Hg may be needed to provide an optimal preload.

MANAGEMENT. In the absence of rales involving more than one-third of the lung fields, the patient should be put in the reverse Trendelenburg position and in those with sinus bradycardia and hypotension, atropine should be administered (0.5 mg intravenously repeated at 5-min intervals up to 2.0 mg). If these measures do not correct the hypotension, crystalloid solutions should be administered intravenously, beginning with a bolus of 100 ml followed by 50-ml increments every 5 minutes. The patient should be carefully observed and the infusion stopped when the systolic pressure returns to approximately 100 mm Hg, if the patient becomes dyspneic, or if pulmonary rales develop or increase. Because of the poor correlation between left ventricular filling pressure and mean right atrial pressure, assessment of systemic (even central) venous pressure is of limited value as a guide to fluid therapy.

Administration of cardiotonic agents (see below) is indicated during the prehospital phase if systemic arterial hypotension persists and is refractory to correction of hypovolemia and excessive vagotonia. In the absence of invasive hemodynamic monitoring, assessment of peripheral vascular resistance must be based on clinical observations. If cutaneous vasoconstriction is present, therapy with dobutamine, which stimulates cardiac contractility without unduly accelerating heart rate and which does not increase the impedance to ventricular outflow, may be helpful (p. 525). In hypotensive patients with AMI, when there is clinical evidence of vasodilatation, an uncommon circumstance, neosynephrine is preferable.

HYPOVOLEMIC HYPOTENSION

Recognition of hypovolemia is of particular importance in hypotensive patients with AMI, because improvement in circulatory dynamics is so readily and safely achieved by augmentation of vascular volume. Since hypovolemia is often occult, it is frequently overlooked in the absence of invasive hemodynamic monitoring. It may be absolute, with low left ventricular filling pressure ($<$ 8 mm Hg), or relative, with normal (8 to 12 mm Hg) or even modestly increased (13 to 18 mm Hg) left ventricular filling pressures. Because of the reduction of left ventricular compliance that occurs with acute ischemia and infarction (p. 1204), left ventricular filling pressures between 13 and 18 mm Hg, while above the upper limits of normal, may be suboptimal.

Exclusion of hypovolemia as the cause of hypotension requires documentation of a reduced cardiac output despite left ventricular filling pressure exceeding 18 mm Hg. If, in a hypotensive patient, the pulmonary capillary wedge pressure (ordinarily measured as the pulmonary artery occlusive pressure) is below this level, fluid challenge should be carried out with sequential 50-ml intravenous bolus infusions[765] and serial assessments should be made of pulmonary capillary wedge pressure and cardiac output. Elevation of pulmonary capillary wedge pressure to between 18 and 24 mm Hg reflects the achievement of a left ventricular filling pressure associated with an optimal cardiac output. If hypovolemia is documented or suspected, the fluid replaced should resemble the fluid lost. Thus, when a low hematocrit complicates AMI, infusion of whole blood is the treatment of choice. On the other hand, crystalloid or colloid solutions should be administered when the hematocrit is normal or elevated.

Hypotension caused by *right ventricular infarction* may be confused with that caused by hypovolemia, because both are associated with a low, normal, or minimally elevated left ventricular filling pressure. The findings and management in right ventricular infarction are discussed on page 1280.

THE HYPERDYNAMIC STATE

When infarction is not complicated by hemodynamic impairment, no therapy other than general supportive measures and treatment of arrhythmias is necessary. However, if the hemodynamic profile is of the hyperdynamic state, i.e., elevation of sinus rate, arterial pressure, and cardiac index, occurring singly or together in the presence of a normal or low left ventricular filling pressure, and if other causes of tachycardia such as fever, infection, and pericarditis can be excluded, treatment with beta-adrenergic blocking agents is indicated. The rationale, dose, and mode of administration are discussed on page 633. Presumably, the increased heart rate and blood pressure are the result of inappropriate activation of the sympathetic nervous system, possibly secondary to augmented release of catecholamines or anxiety or both.

LEFT VENTRICULAR FAILURE AND CARDIOGENIC SHOCK

In patients with AMI, heart failure is characterized by either diastolic dysfunction alone or by both systolic and diastolic dysfunction. Left ventricular diastolic dysfunction leads to pulmonary venous hypertension and pulmonary congestion, often associated with a depression of cardiac output. Clinical manifestations of left ventricular failure become more common as the extent of the injury to the left ventricle increases.

Clinical application of the Frank-Starling principle is useful for characterizing myocardial function in the AMI patient. If the cardiac index is plotted as a function of the pulmonary capillary wedge pressure (a modified Starling relationship) in patients with AMI, a wide range of left ventricular performances is apparent (Fig. 38–33). It is clear from this figure that mortality in AMI increases in association with the severity of the hemodynamic deficit. In addition, one-third of patients with AMI have normal resting left ventricular hemodynamics.[764]

Physiological assessment of left ventricular function refines the information obtained by clinical means.[443] Among patients with AMI who are clinically uncomplicated (Killip Class I, p. 1237), approximately 50 per cent have a reduced cardiac output and 75 per cent have an elevated ventricular filling pressure. Patients with one or both of these hemodynamic abnormalities have a worse prognosis than those without any hemodynamic disturbance, even though they may be clinically uncomplicated.[443] Similarly, the prognosis of patients in Killip Class IV (cardiogenic shock) is a function of the hemodynamic status. Rackley et al. reported that in such patients a filling pressure greater than 29 mm Hg was associated with a mortality of 100 per cent, a filling pressure greater than 15 mm Hg and a cardiac index less than 2 liters/min/sq meter with a mortality of 93 per cent, and a filling pressure less than 15 mm Hg and a cardiac index less than 2 liters/min/sq meter with a mortality of 63 per cent.[443] Thus, it is clear that hemodynamics vary widely among patients with AMI with similar clinical presentations. Therefore, measurement of pertinent hemodynamic variables may be of great value in patients with complications.[766]

THERAPEUTIC IMPLICATIONS. Classification of patients with AMI by hemodynamic subsets has therapeutic relevance. As already noted, patients with normal wedge pressures and hypoperfusion often benefit from infusion of fluids, since the peak value of stroke volume is usually not attained until left ventricular filling pressure reaches 20 to 24 mm Hg.[443] However, a low level of left ventricular filling pressure does not imply that left ventricular damage is necessarily slight. Such patients may be relatively hypovolemic and/or may have suffered a right ventricular infarct with or without severe left ventricular damage.[767]

The relation between ventricular filling pressure and cardiac index when preload is increased by an infusion of saline or dextran can provide valuable hemodynamic information, in addition to that obtained from baseline measurements. For example, the ventricular function curve rises steeply (marked increase in cardiac index, small increase in filling pressure) in patients with normal left ventricular function and hypovolemia, whereas the curve rises gradually or remains flat in those patients with a combination of hypovolemia and depressed cardiac function. The slope of the ventricular function curve, obtained 2 or 3 days following the infarction, correlates well with the ejection fraction determined 4 to 6 weeks later.[443]

Cardiogenic Shock (See also p. 572)

PATHOLOGICAL FINDINGS. The severest clinical expression of left ventricular failure, cardiogenic shock, is associated with extensive damage to the left ventricular myocardium.[768–770] Page et al., who studied 20 such patients at autopsy, found that all exhibited necrosis of at least 40 per cent of the left ventricle. In contrast, 35 per cent or less of the left ventricle had been destroyed in all but 1 of 14 patients who succumbed without having been in cardiogenic shock.[768] Similar findings were reported by Alonso

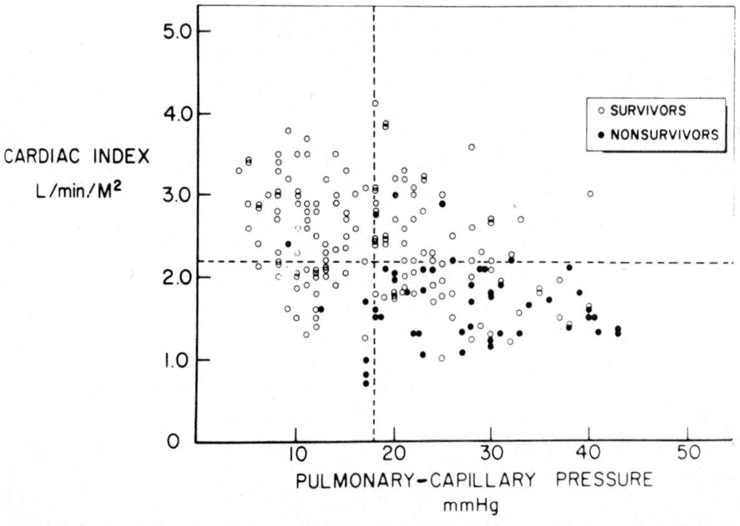

FIGURE 38–33. Relation between pulmonary-capillary pressure and cardiac index in 200 patients with acute myocardial infarction. The dotted lines are placed at the levels of 18 mm Hg for pulmonary-capillary pressure and 2.1 liters per minute per square meter for cardiac index. There is a wide degree of variability in left ventricular performance in patients with acute myocardial infarction, and mortality rate increases as cardiac performance deteriorates. (From Forrester, J. S., et al.: Medical therapy of acute myocardial infarction by application of hemodynamic subsets. N. Engl. J. Med. *295*:1356, 1976.)

et al.: Patients with cardiogenic shock had lost an average of 51 per cent of the left ventricular myocardium (range: 35 to 68 per cent), whereas in a group of infarcted patients who died suddenly from arrhythmias and who had never been in cardiogenic shock, necrosis averaged 23 per cent (range: 14 to 31 per cent) of the left ventricle.[769] Patients who die as a consequence of cardiogenic shock usually develop this complication while in the hospital. These individuals often have "piecemeal" necrosis, progressive myocardial necrosis from marginal extension of their infarct in an ischemic zone bordering on the infarction. This is associated with persistent elevation of CK-MB.[771] Early deterioration in left ventricular function secondary to apparent extension of infarction may, in some cases, result from *expansion* of the necrotic zone of myocardium without actual *extension* of the necrotic process. Shearing forces that develop during ventricular systole can disrupt necrotic myocardial muscle bundles, with resultant expansion and thinning of the akinetic zone of myocardium, which in turn results in deterioration of overall left ventricular function.[183]

At autopsy, patients with cardiogenic shock consistently demonstrate marginal extension of recent areas of infarction (Fig. 38–17).[768–770, 772] Additionally, focal areas of necrosis are frequently found in regions of the left and right ventricles that are not adjacent to the major area of recent infarction.[768] Such extensions and focal lesions are probably in part the result of the shock state itself, since they can also be found in the hearts of patients dying of noncardiogenic shock. Infarction of the ischemic periinfarction zone can be precipitated by a number of factors that adversely affect the supply of oxygen or the metabolic demand in the zone of myocardium, including a reduction of coronary perfusion pressure and an augmentation of myocardial oxygen demand resulting from the local release of catecholamines from ischemic adrenergic nerve endings in the heart as well as from circulating endogenous or infused catecholamines. Patients with rupture of the ventricular septum or of a papillary muscle can also manifest with cardiogenic shock. These patients often have smaller infarcts than do those with cardiogenic shock secondary to ventricular failure without a mechanical lesion. The prognosis is better in such patients, since the smaller infarct allows their left ventricle to support the circulation once the mechanical defect has been corrected surgically.

PATHOPHYSIOLOGY. The shock state in patients with AMI appears to be the result of a vicious circle, demonstrated in Figure 38–9, p. 1231. According to this formulation, coronary obstruction leads to myocardial ischemia that impairs myocardial contractility and ventricular performance. This, in turn, reduces arterial pressure and therefore coronary perfusion pressure, leading to further ischemia and extension of necrosis until the left ventricle has insufficient contracting myocardium to sustain life. Stasis in the smaller arteries and arterioles distal to a major proximal occlusion may result in secondary microvascular obstruction, further impairing myocardial perfusion. The progressive nature of the myocardial insult in this syndrome is reflected in the stuttering and progressive evolution of elevations in the plasma enzyme–time activity curves of markers specific for myocardial injury.[772]

At autopsy, more than two-thirds of patients with cardiogenic shock demonstrate stenosis of 75 per cent or more of the luminal diameter of all three major coronary vessels, usually including the left anterior descending coronary artery.[773] Almost all patients with cardiogenic shock are found to have thrombosis of the artery supplying the major region of recent infarction.[768, 769]

MANAGEMENT OF LEFT VENTRICULAR FAILURE

Invasive hemodynamic monitoring is essential to guide therapy of patients with moderate to severe left ventricular failure.

AVOIDANCE OF HYPOXEMIA. The treatment of left ventricular failure with AMI requires meticulous attention to ventilation, since hypoxemia can impair the function of ischemic tissue at the margin of the infarct and thereby contribute to establishing or perpetuating the vicious circle (Fig. 38–9, p. 1231). The combination of pulmonary vascular congestion (or when it is severe, pulmonary edema), reduced pulmonary compliance, and the respiratory depression that may be associated with excessive doses of analgesics conspires to impair ventilatory function and arterial oxygenation (p. 1874). When in patients with left ventricular failure secondary to AMI arterial oxygen tension cannot be maintained above 60 mm Hg despite inhalation of 100 per cent oxygen delivered at 8 liters/min by mask and the adequate use of bronchodilators, endotracheal intubation, assisted ventilation, and positive pressure should be considered. The improvement of arterial oxygenation and hence myocardial oxygen supply may help to restore ventricular performance. Positive end-expiratory pressure may diminish systemic venous return and reduce effective left ventricular filling pressure. Once a patient is intubated and mechanically ventilated, withdrawal of the support during the recovery phase must be undertaken extremely carefully. Since myocardial ischemia frequently occurs during the return to unsupported spontaneous breathing,[774] the weaning process should be accompanied by careful observation for signs of ischemia and is potentially facilitated by a period of intermittent mandatory ventilation before extubation. Continuous ST-segment monitoring has been recommended for these patients.[774]

When wheezing complicates pulmonary congestion, bronchodilators that act primarily on $beta_2$-adrenoceptors, such as isoetharine or metaproterenol, given as aerosols, or terbutaline, which can be administered subcutaneously or orally, are more desirable than conventional bronchodilators, such as isoproterenol or epinephrine, whose primary effects are on $beta_1$-receptors.

Although positive inotropic agents may be useful, they do *not* represent the *initial* therapy of choice in patients with AMI. Instead, heart failure in this setting is managed most effectively first by reduction of blood volume and ventricular preload, and, if possible, by lowering afterload. Arrhythmias may contribute to hemodynamic compromise as discussed on page 1263 and should be treated promptly in patients with left ventricular failure.

DIURETICS (See also p. 507). Mild heart failure in patients with AMI frequently responds well to diuretics such as furosemide, administered intravenously in doses of 10 to 40 mg, repeated at 3- to 4-hour intervals if necessary. The resultant reduction of pulmonary capillary pressure reduces dyspnea, and the lowering of left ventricular wall tension that accompanies the reduction of left ventricular diastolic volume diminishes myocardial oxygen requirements and may lead to improvement of contractility and augmentation of the ejection fraction, stroke volume, and cardiac output. The reduction of elevated left ventricular filling pressure may also enhance myocardial oxygen delivery by diminishing the impedance to coronary perfusion attributable to elevated ventricular wall tension (p. 519). It may also improve arterial oxygenation by reducing pulmonary vascular congestion.

The intravenous administration of furosemide reduces

pulmonary vascular congestion and pulmonary venous pressure within 15 minutes, before renal excretion of sodium and water have occurred; presumably this action results from a direct dilating effect of this drug on the systemic arterial bed (p. 513). It is important not to "overshoot" the mark by reducing left ventricular filling pressure much below 18 mm Hg, the lower range associated with optimal left ventricular performance, since this may reduce cardiac output further and cause arterial hypotension. Excessive diuresis may also result in hypokalemia, with its attendant risk of digitalis intoxication.

VASODILATORS (See also p. 515). Myocardial oxygen requirements depend on left ventricular wall stress, which in turn is proportional to the product of peak developed left ventricular pressure, volume, and wall thickness (p. 518). Vasodilator therapy is not currently recommended in patients with uncomplicated AMI, but is useful in patients whose MI is complicated by: (1) heart failure unresponsive to treatment with diuretics, (2) hypertension, (3) mitral regurgitation, or (4) ventricular septal defect. In these patients, treatment with vasodilator agents increases stroke volume and may reduce myocardial oxygen requirements and thereby lessen ischemia. The necessity for hemodynamic monitoring of systemic arterial and pulmonary capillary wedge (or at least pulmonary artery) pressure and cardiac output in patients treated with these agents must be emphasized, since improvement of cardiac performance and energetics requires three simultaneous effects: (1) reduction of left ventricular afterload, (2) avoidance of excessive systemic arterial hypotension in order to maintain effective coronary perfusion pressure, and (3) avoidance of excessive reduction of ventricular filling pressure with consequent diminution of cardiac output. In general, pulmonary capillary wedge pressure should be maintained at approximately 20 mm Hg and arterial diastolic blood pressure above 60 mm Hg in patients who were normotensive before developing the AMI.

Appropriate doses of vasodilators generally enhance stroke volume and cardiac output, reduce left ventricular filling pressure and volume and calculated systemic vascular resistance, without causing serious reflex tachycardia. While available data are not conclusive and do not apply to all subsets of patients with AMI, at least one vasodilator, nitroglycerin, when given early in the course of AMI, has been reported also to protect ischemic myocardium and limit infarct size (p. 1215). Excessive doses of vasodilators may decrease cardiac output by reducing preload and left ventricular filling pressure below optimal levels or may decrease coronary perfusion by excessive depression of systemic arterial pressure. Compromise of coronary perfusion, in turn, may impair ventricular performance further, extend infarction, and give rise to lethal arrhythmias.

Vasodilator therapy is particularly useful when AMI is complicated by mitral regurgitation or rupture of the ventricular septum. In such patients, vasodilators alone or in combination with intraaortic balloon counterpulsation can sometimes serve as a "holding maneuver" and provide hemodynamic stabilization to permit definitive catheterization and angiographic studies to be carried out and to prepare the patient for early surgical intervention. Because of the precarious state of patients with complicated infarcts and the need for meticulous adjustment of dosage, therapy is best initiated with agents that can be administered intravenously and that have a short duration of action, such as nitroprusside,[775–778] nitroglycerin,[779–781] or isosorbide dinitrate.[782] After initial stabilization, medications that may be useful are long-acting nitrates given by mouth, sublingually, or by ointment[783, 784]; calcium antagonists such as

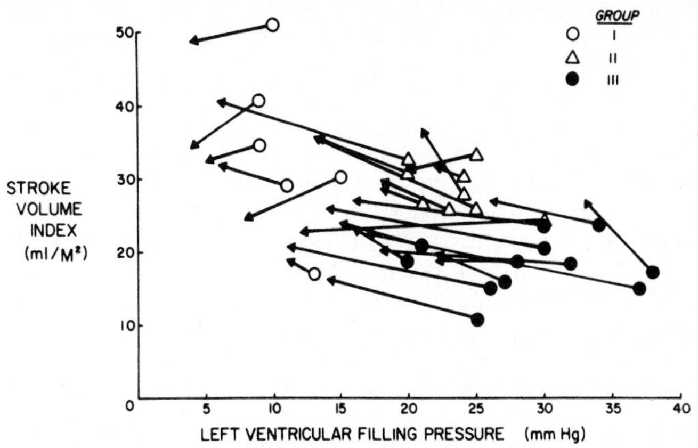

FIGURE 38–34. Hemodynamic responses to nitroprusside infusion in patients with acute myocardial infarction. Patients in Groups II and III with elevated left ventricular filling pressures (20 mm Hg or more) tend to respond to the vasodilator with an increase in the stroke volume and a marked drop in the filling pressure, whereas patients with left ventricular filling pressures below 15 mm Hg (Group I) show a reduction in the stroke volume and tend to have less marked decreases in filling pressures during nitroprusside infusion. Group III patients had stroke work indices below 20 g-m/m². (From Chatterjee, K., and Parmley, W. W.: The role of vasodilator therapy in heart failure. Prog. Cardiovasc. Dis. *19*:301, 1977.)

nifedipine[785]; and angiotensin-converting enzyme inhibitors such as captopril.[786]

Nitroprusside. There has been more experience with the intravenous infusion of sodium nitroprusside in patients with AMI than with other vasodilators. It is generally given initially in doses of 0.5 μg/kg/min[787] and may be gradually and progressively increased up to 50 μg/kg/min. While increasing stroke volume and cardiac output in patients with AMI and left ventricular failure (Fig. 38–34), nitroprusside diminishes arteriolar resistance and impedance to left ventricular ejection, pulmonary capillary wedge pressure, myocardial oxygen requirements, and sometimes the frequency of ventricular premature contractions. With optimization of dose, improved segmental ventricular function of zones of apparent infarction has been observed.[775] Nitroprusside may augment cardiac output even in patients with cardiogenic shock, if arterial diastolic and coronary perfusion pressure are maintained by concomitant intraaortic balloon counterpulsation.

Nitroglycerin. This drug has been shown in animal experiments to be less likely than nitroprusside to produce a "coronary steal," i.e., to divert blood flow from the ischemic to the nonischemic zone.[780] Therefore, used intravenously, it (or isosorbide dinitrate, which has a similar action[782]) may be a particularly useful vasodilator in patients with AMI.[781] Ten to 15 μg/min is infused and the dose is increased by 10 μg/min every 5 minutes until the desired effect (improvement of hemodynamics or relief of ischemic chest pain) or a decline in systolic arterial pressure to 90 mm Hg, or by more than 15 mm Hg, has occurred. Although both nitroglycerin and nitroprusside lower systemic arterial pressure, systemic vascular resistance, and the heart rate–systolic blood pressure product, the reduction of left ventricular filling pressure is more prominent with nitroglycerin because of its relatively greater effect than nitroprusside on venous capacitance vessels. Nevertheless, in patients with severe left ventricular failure, cardiac output often increases despite the reduction in left ventricular filling pressure produced by nitroglycerin.

Oral Vasodilators. The use of oral vasodilators in the treatment of chronic congestive heart failure is discussed on page 516. In patients who have persistent heart failure, long-term treatment with a converting-enzyme inhibitor should be carried out. Studies are under way to determine the efficacy of these agents in patients with left ventricular dysfunction without heart failure. It is hoped that this reduced ventricular load will decrease the remodeling of the left ventricle that occurs commonly in the period after MI and thereby defer the development of heart failure and death therefrom[788] (Fig. 38–10, p. 1232).

DIGITALIS (See also p. 489). Although digitalis increases contractility and the oxygen consumption of normal hearts, when heart failure is present the diminution of heart size and wall tension frequently results in a net reduction of myocardial oxygen requirements.[789] In animal experiments it fails to improve ventricular performance immediately following experimental coronary occlusion, but salutary effects are elicited when it is administered several days later.[790] The absence of early beneficial effects may be due to the inability of ischemic tissue to respond to digitalis, the already maximal stimulation of contractility of the normal heart by circulating and neuronally released catecholamines, or the dissipation of the force of contraction of normal myocardium into dyskinetic areas. In experimental animals without congestive heart failure who are subjected to coronary occlusion, digitalis increases the severity of ischemia, presumably by stimulating oxygen requirements.[473] Digitalis reduces the severity of ischemia occurring in the presence of experimentally induced congestive heart failure,[791] presumably because of the reduction in myocardial oxygen requirements.

Although the issue is still controversial, arrhythmias may be increased by digitalis glycosides when they are given to patients in the first few hours after the onset of MI, particularly in the presence of hypokalemia. Also, undesirable peripheral systemic and coronary vasoconstriction may result from the rapid intravenous administration of rapidly acting glycosides such as ouabain.[792]

Administration of digitalis to patients hospitalized with AMI should generally be reserved for the management of supraventricular tachyarrhythmias such as atrial flutter and fibrillation and of heart failure that persists despite treatment with diuretics and vasodilators. Digitalis causes modest improvement of cardiac performance in patients with mild heart failure (Killip Class II).[793, 794] There is no indication for its use as an inotropic agent in patients without clinical evidence of left ventricular dysfunction (Killip Class I), and it is too weak an inotropic agent to be relied upon as the principal cardiac stimulant in patients in overt pulmonary edema or cardiogenic shock (Classes III or IV). It may, however, be useful as a supplement to vasodilator agents and in the treatment of persistent or recurrent left ventricular failure.[795] Cardiac glycosides appear to become progressively more effective in the treatment of heart failure as the interval from the acute events lengthens; i.e., they are more effective in the treatment of chronic than of acute heart failure secondary to ischemic heart disease. However, the possibility that continued administration of digitalis might contribute to late mortality in the two years following AMI has been raised[796] and debated.[797] While it is clear that mortality is greater in patients treated with digoxin after AMI, it is not clear that this increase in mortality is due to digoxin itself or to confounding variables that correlate with use of digoxin.[798] The possible long-term hazards of digitalis administration must be clarified before a definitive recommendation about its use in the convalescent phase can be made. At this time, it would appear to be indicated only if there is overt heart failure and/or supraventricular tachyarrhythmias.

BETA-ADRENOCEPTOR AGONISTS (See also p. 524). When left ventricular failure is severe, as manifested by marked reduction of cardiac index (< 2 liters/min/square meter), and pulmonary capillary wedge pressure is at optimal (18 to 24 mm Hg) or excessive (> 24 mm Hg) levels despite therapy with diuretics, beta-adrenoceptor agonists are indicated. Although isoproterenol is a potent cardiac stimulant and improves ventricular performance, it should be avoided in the MI patient. It also causes tachycardia and augments myocardial oxygen consumption and lactate production[799]; in addition, it reduces coronary perfusion pressure by causing systemic vasodilation and in animal experiments increases the extent of experimentally induced infarction.[473, 800] Norepinephrine and metaraminol also increase myocardial oxygen consumption because of their peripheral vasoconstrictor as well as positive inotropic actions.

Dopamine (p. 524) and *dobutamine* (p. 525), which are relatively cardio-selective and stimulate $beta_1$ receptors, exert predominantly positive inotropic effects and may be particularly useful in patients with AMI and reduced cardiac output, increased left ventricular filling pressure, pulmonary vascular congestion, and hypotension.[801] Fortunately, the potentially deleterious alpha-adrenergic vasoconstrictor effects exerted by *dopamine* occur only at higher doses than those required to increase contractility. Its vasodilating actions on renal and splanchnic vessels and its positive inotropic effects generally improve hemodynamics and renal function.[802] In patients with AMI and left ventricular failure, this drug should be administered at a dose of 3 μg/kg/min, while monitoring pulmonary capillary wedge and systemic arterial pressures as well as cardiac output. The dose may be increased stepwise to 20 μg/kg/min, in order to reduce pulmonary capillary wedge pressure to approximately 20 mm Hg and elevate cardiac index to exceed 2 liters/min/square meter. However, it must be recognized that doses exceeding 5 μg/kg/min activate peripheral alpha receptors and cause vasoconstriction. While concern has been raised that the positive inotropic effect of even low-dose dopamine could extend infarct size, experimental evidence suggests that the enhancement in contractility by dopamine does not increase infarct size or lead to late deterioration of cardiac function even when the drug is administered to acutely reperfused, severely ischemic myocardium.[803] Presumably, the absence of a powerful chronotropic effect and maintenance of arterial pressure distinguish it from isoproterenol.

Dobutamine has a positive inotropic effect comparable to that of dopamine but a slightly less positive chronotropic effect,[804] with less vasoconstrictor activity at higher doses. In patients with AMI dobutamine improves left ventricular performance without augmenting enzymatically estimated infarct size.[805, 806] It may be administered in a starting dose of 2.5 μg/kg/min and increased stepwise to a maximum of 30 μg/kg/min. Both dopamine and dobutamine must be given carefully and with constant monitoring of the electrocardiogram, systemic arterial pressure, pulmonary artery or pulmonary artery occlusive pressure, and, if possible, frequent measurements of cardiac output. The dose must be reduced if systolic pressure exceeds 130 to 140 mm Hg, heart rate exceeds 100 to 110 beats/min, supraventricular or ventricular tachyarrhythmias are precipitated, or if ST-segment changes increase.

AMRINONE (p. 527). This is a noncatecholamine, nonglycoside, inotropic, and vasodilating agent that has recently been approved for clinical use parenterally.[807] Experience with it in the setting of AMI is relatively limited, but it appears to be an ideal agent for selected patients with heart failure despite treatment with diuretics, who are not hypotensive and who are likely to benefit from both an enhancement in contractility and afterload reduction.

An increase in infarct size has been reported in dogs given amrinone after experimental AMI.[808] However, studies in patients with a similar experimental compound, milrinone, suggest that in the failing heart this class of agent does not increase myocardial oxygen consumption.[809] In patients with left ventricular failure following AMI amrinone increases cardiac output while reducing pulmonary wedge pressure and systemic vascular resistance.[810, 811] Heart rate increases only at relatively high doses.[811] In MI patients studied, no exacerbation of angina or increased incidence of arrhythmias has been reported.[810] The initial intravenous dosage of amrinone is 0.75 mg/kg infused slowly over several minutes. This is then followed by a continued maintenance infusion started at 5 to 10 μg/kg/min and titrated to the patient's hemodynamic response. The total daily dose should not be greater than 10 mg/kg.[812]

TREATMENT OF CARDIOGENIC SHOCK

(See also p. 569)

When a massive AMI produces profound global impairment of left ventricular function, cardiogenic shock supervenes. This condition is characterized by marked hypotension with systolic arterial pressure less than 80 mm Hg and a marked reduction of cardiac index (generally < 1.8 liters/mm/sq meter) in the face of elevated left ventricular filling pressure (pulmonary capillary wedge pressure > 18 mm Hg.[770] Spurious estimates of left ventricular filling pressure based on measurements of the pulmonary artery occlusive pressure can occur in the presence of marked mitral regurgitation, in which the tall *v* wave in the left atrial (and pulmonary artery occlusive) pressure tracing elevates the mean pressure above left ventricular end-diastolic pressure. Accordingly, mitral regurgitation and other mechanical lesions such as ventricular septal defect, ventricular aneurysm, and pseudoaneurysm must be excluded before the diagnosis of cardiogenic shock due to global impairment of left ventricular function can be established. These potentially catastrophic mechanical complications should be suspected in any patient with AMI in whom circulatory collapse occurs. Immediate hemodynamic and angiographic evaluations are necessary in these patients with cardiogenic shock. It is important to exclude these complications because primary therapy of such lesions usually requires immediate operative treatment with intervening support of the circulation by intra-aortic balloon counterpulsation.

When these mechanical complications are not present, cardiogenic shock is due to global impairment of left ventricular function.[813] While dopamine and dobutamine usually improve hemodynamics in these patients, unfortunately they do not appear to improve hospital survival significantly. Similarly, vasodilators have been utilized in an effort to elevate cardiac output and to reduce left ventricular filling pressure. However, by lowering the already markedly reduced coronary perfusion pressure, myocardial perfusion can be compromised further, accelerating the vicious circle illustrated in Figure 38–9, page 1231. Vasodilators may nonetheless be employed in conjunction with intra-aortic balloon counterpulsation and inotropic agents in an effort to increase cardiac output while sustaining or elevating coronary perfusion pressure.

The systemic vascular resistance is usually elevated in patients with cardiogenic shock, but occasionally resistance is normal, and in a few cases vasodilation actually predominates. When systemic vascular resistance is *not* elevated in patients with cardiogenic shock, norepinephrine (in doses ranging from 2 to 10 μg/min), which has both alpha- and beta-adrenoceptor agonist properties, may be employed to increase diastolic arterial pressure, maintain coronary perfusion, and improve contractility, but, again, there is no definitive evidence that ultimate outcome is affected by this drug.[719, 814] Norepinephrine should be used only when other means, including balloon counterpulsation, fail to maintain arterial diastolic pressure above 50 to 60 mm Hg in a previously normotensive patient. The use of alpha-adrenoceptor agents such as phenylephrine or methoxamine is contraindicated in most patients with cardiogenic shock (unless systemic vascular resistance is inordinately low).

REPERFUSION. Reversal of cardiogenic shock by acute reperfusion has been reported, usually with thrombolytic therapy, emergency PTCA, or a combination of these measures.[17, 535, 556, 558, 559, 815] In several reported cases, cardiogenic shock due to total occlusion of the left main coronary artery was reversed by intravenous thrombolysis with streptokinase.[816, 817] While these techniques may occasionally be useful, since myocardial salvage may only be accomplished in the earliest hours of AMI, reperfusion is likely to be of benefit only in patients seen within 4 to 6 hours of the onset of symptoms. Most patients, however, do not develop cardiogenic shock until 24 to 48 hours following the onset of AMI and by that time sufficient myocardial necrosis has occurred so that successful reperfusion is unlikely to improve left ventricular performance substantially.

INTRAAORTIC BALLOON COUNTERPULSATION (See also p. 563). Cardiogenic shock due to mechanical defects following AMI (pp. 1283 to 1285) or to severe left ventricular dysfunction may be stabilized by means of the appropriate use of intraaortic balloon counterpulsation (IABP) when other medical measures fail.[818–821] In present practice, the balloon is inserted percutaneously[822] or, rarely, via an arterial cutdown in the femoral artery and advanced into the thoracic aorta via the femoral artery. Phased pulsations, electrocardiographically synchronized, allow for inflation at the time of closure of the aortic valve and deflation just before the onset of systole. The augmented coronary perfusion pressure during diastole enhances coronary blood flow because coronary vascular resistance is minimal during this portion of the cardiac cycle (Fig. 38–35). Since the balloon is deflated throughout systole, the left ventricle ejects against a lower impedance. Hemodynamic changes generally include a 10 to 20 per cent increase in cardiac output, a reduction in systolic and increase in diastolic arterial pressure with little change in mean pressure, a diminution of heart rate, and an increase in urine output.[818, 820, 823] The reduction in left ventricular afterload reduces myocardial oxygen consumption,[823] and, as a consequence, anaerobic metabolism and myocardial ischemia are diminished.[824] Favorable effects are sometimes reflected in prompt resolution of electrocardiographic signs of ischemia.

Indications. Intraaortic balloon counterpulsation is utilized in the treatment of AMI in three groups of patients: (1) those whose condition is hemodynamically unstable and in whom support of the circulation is required for the performance of diagnostic studies which are carried out to assess lesions that are potentially correctable surgically, (2) in cardiogenic shock that is unresponsive to medical management, and (3) rarely in the unusual presence of persistent ischemic pain that is unresponsive to treatment with inhalation of 100 per cent oxygen, beta-adrenoceptor block-

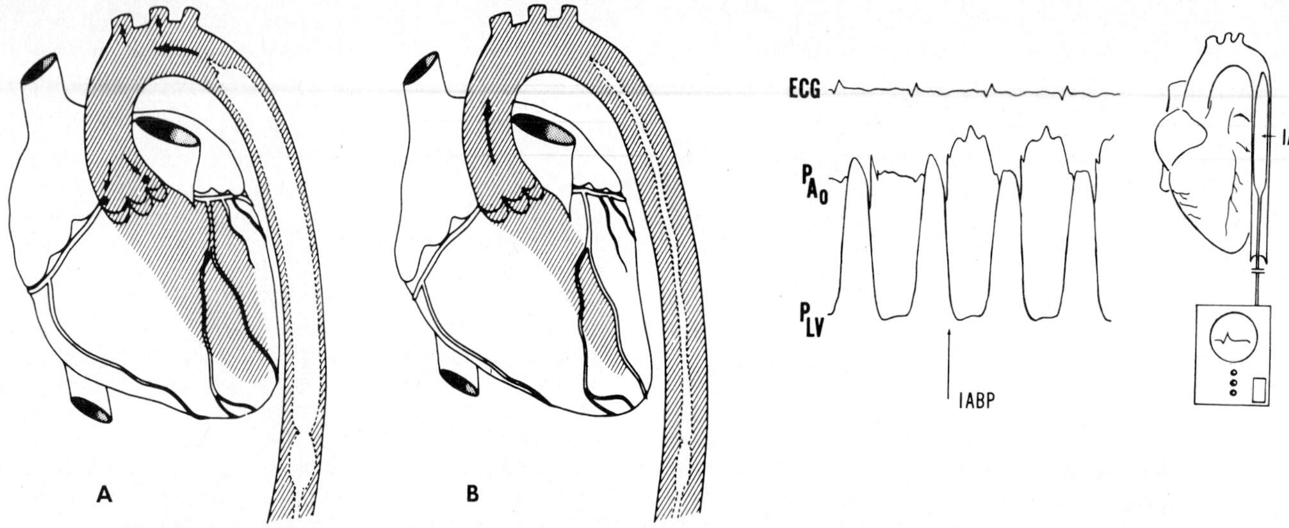

FIGURE 38–35. The relationship between the cardiac cycle and balloon inflation when intraaortic balloon counterpulsation is being utilized. During diastole (panel A) the balloon is inflated, augmenting the prevailing pressure in the proximal aorta and hence coronary arterial perfusion pressure. During systole (panel B) the left ventricular chamber dimension decreases with antegrade ejection of blood into the proximal aorta. During this portion of the cardiac cycle the balloon is deflated, facilitating ejection of blood into the periphery where systemic arterial resistance vessels are dilated maximally because of the preceding inhibition of perfusion by the inflated balloon during diastole. As shown in the inset on the right, utilization of intraaortic balloon counterpulsation (IABP) results in augmentation of diastolic arterial blood pressure (P_{Ao}) with a modest reduction in systolic left ventricular pressure (P_{LV}). (From Bolooki, H.: Clinical Application of Intra-aortic Balloon Pump. Mt. Kisco, NY, Futura Publishing Co., 1977.)

ade, nitrates, and calcium channel blocking agents during the postinfarction state. Unfortunately, among patients with cardiogenic shock, improvement is often only temporary, and "balloon dependence" is common.[821, 826, 827] Patients with cardiogenic shock treated with this modality can be successfully weaned from the supporting system only occasionally. Counterpulsation alone does not improve overall mortality, either in patients with or those without a surgically remediable mechanical lesion.[819, 828, 829] However, it may be life-saving in allowing the patient to tolerate catheterization and coronary arteriography and to be brought to the operating room for definitive treatment without irreversible organ damage. Surgical treatment in cardiogenic shock (aside from correcting mechanical abnormalities) may involve bypassing severely obstructed nonoccluded vessels. Occlusion of one major vessel may cause left ventricular dysfunction and hypotension, which can then lead to hypoperfusion and ischemia of myocardium subserved by the other diseased vessels. Left ventricular function may be improved by relief of this ischemia with revascularization. It is possible that left ventricular bypass (p. 532), a technique that reduces left ventricular oxygen demands more drastically, may ultimately prove to be more effective in improving survival in patients with cardiogenic shock than intraaortic balloon counterpulsation[830]; however, it is still experimental.

Noninvasive approaches to circulatory assistance have been developed such as external devices that apply pressure to the lower extremities during diastole, thereby promoting increased runoff during systole. However, this form of therapy likewise does not alter outcome decisively; its hemodynamic effects are, in fact, less than those of intraaortic counterpulsation.[831]

Complications. These are infrequent but include damage to or perforation of the aortic wall, ischemia distal to the site of insertion of the balloon in the femoral artery, thrombocytopenia, hemolysis, renal emboli, and mechanical failure such as rupture of the balloon.[635, 825] Although left ventricular rupture has been observed with increased frequency in patients undergoing balloon pumping,[819] this phenomenon appears to be a manifestation of the underlying extensive transmural infarction rather than a complication of IABP itself.

Right Ventricular Infarction

A characteristic hemodynamic pattern (Table 38–15) has been observed in patients with right ventricular infarction,[25, 832, 832a] which frequently accompanies inferior left ventricular infarction,[833] or rarely occurs in isolated form.[834, 835] Right-heart filling pressures (central venous, right atrial, and right ventricular end-diastolic pressures) are elevated while left ventricular filling pressure is normal or only slightly raised[767]; right ventricular systolic and pulse pressures are decreased, and cardiac output is often markedly depressed. Rarely, this disproportionate elevation of right-sided filling pressure causes right-to-left shunting through a patent foramen ovale.[836] This possibility should be considered in patients with right ventricular infarction who have unexplained systemic hypoxemia.

DIAGNOSIS. Many patients with the combination of normal left ventricular filling pressure and depressed cardiac index in fact have right ventricular infarcts (with accompanying inferior left ventricular infarcts). The hemodynamic picture may superficially resemble that seen in patients with pericardial disease (Chap. 44).[767] In it are seen elevated right ventricular filling pressure; well-preserved, steep, right atrial *v* descent; and an early diastolic dip and plateau (square root sign) in the right ventricular pressure tracing. Moreover, Kussmaul's sign (inspiratory fall > 10 mm Hg in systolic arterial blood pressure) may be present in patients with right ventricular infarction. In fact, Kussmaul's sign in the setting of inferior wall AMI is highly predictive of right ventricular involvement.[25] The ECG may provide the first clue that right ventricular involvement is present in the patient with inferior wall MI (Fig. 38–14, p. 1244). Most patients with right ventricular infarction have ST-segment elevation in lead V_4R (right precordial lead in V_4 position).[837] Transient elevation of the ST segment in any of the right precordial leads may occur with right ventricular MI[838] and the presence of 0.1 mV or

TABLE 38–15 FEATURES OF RIGHT VENTRICULAR INFARCTION

1. Inferior-posterior myocardial infarction
2. Clinical findings may include:
   A. Normal or depressed right ventricular function
   B. Shock
   C. Tricuspid regurgitation
   D. Ruptured ventricular septum
3. Hemodynamic measurements
   A. Abnormally elevated right atrial pressure
   B. Normal right ventricular and pulmonary artery systolic pressures
   C. Increased ratio of right ventricular to left ventricular filling pressure
   D. Depressed right ventricular function curve
4. Scintigraphy
   A. Uptake in right ventricular free wall
   B. Increased right ventricular dimensions and decreased wall motion
5. Echocardiography
   A. Increased right ventricular dimension
   B. Absence of pericardial effusion
6. Cardiac enzymes
   A. Increased magnitude of enzyme values to left ventricular dysfunction
7. Cardiac catheterization
   A. Involvement of right or left circumflex coronary arteries
   B. Right ventricular akinesis
8. Differential diagnosis
   A. Hypotension with acute myocardial infarction
   B. Pericardial tamponade
   C. Constrictive pericarditis
   D. Pulmonary embolus

From Rackley, C. E., Russell, R. O., Jr., Mantle, J. A., Rogers, W. J., Papapietro, S. E., and Schwartz, K. M.: Right ventricular infarction and function. Am. Heart J. *101*:215, 1981.

more ST-segment elevation in any one or combination of leads V_4R, V_5R, or V_6R in patients with the clinical picture of acute MI is highly sensitive and specific for the diagnosis of right ventricular MI.[839]

Echocardiography. This technique is helpful in the differential diagnosis[840] because in right ventricular infarction—in contrast to pericardial tamponade—no significant quantities of pericardial fluid are seen. On two-dimensional echocardiography, abnormal wall motion of the right ventricle as well as dilatation and depression of the right ventricular ejection fraction can be noted.[25, 841, 842] Gated equilibrium radionuclide angiography also is useful for recognizing right ventricular MI.[25, 843] Serial scintigraphic studies have shown that some degree of recovery of an initially depressed right ventricular ejection fraction is the rule with right ventricular myocardial infarction,[26, 844] whereas this is not necessarily true for left ventricular ejection fraction (Fig. 38–36).

Hemodynamics. Loss of atrial transport in patients with right ventricular infarction can result in marked reductions in stroke volume and arterial blood pressure.[845] Likewise, ventricular pacing, when required, may fail to increase cardiac output.[846] The hemodynamic importance of right ventricular infarction in patients with inferior infarction is reflected in the observations of Marmor et al. They noted that although infarct size (reflected in CK release curves) was similar in patients with anterior and inferior infarcts, the former had more severe depression of the left ventricular ejection fraction and the latter had more severe depression of the right ventricular ejection fraction.[847]

TREATMENT. In patients with hypotension due to right ventricular MI, hemodynamics may be improved by a combination of expanding plasma volume to augment right ventricular preload and cardiac output, and, when left ventricular failure is present, by adding arterial vasodilators. These drugs reduce the impedance to left ventricular outflow and in turn left ventricular diastolic, left atrial, and pulmonary (arterial) pressures, thereby lowering the impedance to right ventricular outflow and enhancing right ventricular output. A remarkably high survival rate of 60 per cent, albeit in a small series, emphasizes the importance of recognition and vigorous medical therapy of this cause of serious hypotension in MI.[848] Right ventricular infarction is common among patients with inferior left ventricular infarction. Therefore, otherwise unexplained systemic arterial hypotension or diminished cardiac output, or marked hypotension in response to small doses of nitroglycerin,[428] should lead to the prompt consideration of this diagnosis. In view of the importance of atrial transport, as noted above, patients requiring pacing should have atrial or atrioventricular sequential pacing.[845, 846] Replacement of the tricuspid valve has been carried out in the treatment of severe tricuspid regurgitation secondary to right ventricular infarction.[849]

MECHANICAL CAUSES OF HEART FAILURE AND SHOCK FOLLOWING ACUTE MYOCARDIAL INFARCTION

Myocardial Rupture

The most dramatic complications of AMI are those that involve tearing or rupture of acutely infarcted tissue. The clinical characteristics of these events vary considerably and depend largely on the site of rupture, which may involve the papillary muscles, the interventricular septum, or the free wall of either ventricle. The overall incidence of these complications is hard to assess because clinical and autopsy series differ considerably. However, as a group

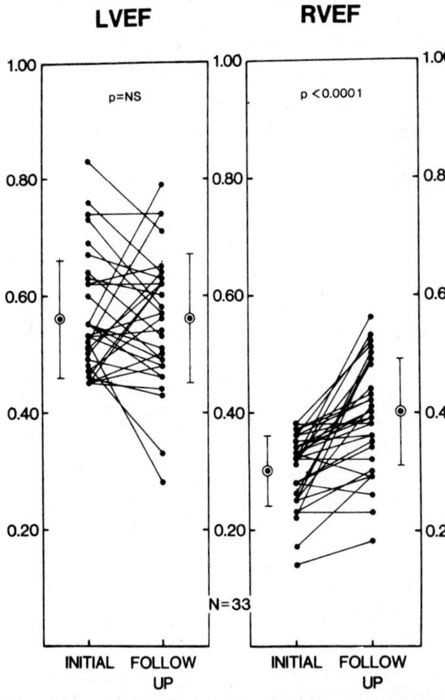

FIGURE 38–36. Sequential changes in global ventricular function in 33 patients with inferior myocardial infarction and predominant right ventricular dysfunction. LVEF = left ventricular ejection fraction, RVEF = right ventricular ejection fraction, closed circles within rings = mean ± SD. Note that left ventricular function was normal or almost so and did not change between initial and follow-up examinations. The latter was carried out at an average of 9.6 days after AMI. In contrast, right ventricular ejection fraction is markedly depressed and rises strikingly, albeit not to normal levels. (From Shah, P. K., et al.: Scintigraphically detected predominant right ventricular dysfunction in acute myocardial infarction: Clinical and hemodynamic correlates and implications for therapy and prognosis. J. Am. Coll. Cardiol. 6:1264, 1985. By permission of the American College of Cardiology.)

TABLE 38–16 CLINICAL PROFILE OF MECHANICAL COMPLICATIONS OF MYOCARDIAL INFARCTION

Variable	VSD	Free Wall Rupture	Papillary Muscle Rupture
Age (mean, years)	63	69	65
Days post-MI	3–5	3–6	3–5
Anterior MI	66%	50%	25%
New murmur	90%	25%	50%
Palpable thrill	Yes	No	Rare
Previous MI	25%	25%	30%
Incidence	2%–4%	Up to 10%	1%
Mortality			
Medical	90%	90%	90%
Surgical	50%	Case reports 40%–90%	

MI = myocardial infarction; VSD = ventricular septal defect.
From Labovitz, A. J., et al.: Mechanical complications of acute myocardial infarction. Cardiovasc. Rev. Rep. 5:948, 1984.

they are probably responsible for about 15 per cent of all deaths from AMI. The comparative clinical profile of these complications, as gathered from different studies, is shown in Table 38–16.

Rupture of the Free Wall

Rupture of the free wall of the infarcted ventricle occurs in up to 10 per cent of patients dying in the hospital of AMI. Thinness of the apical wall, marked intensity of necrosis at the terminal end of the blood supply, poor collateral flow, the shearing effect of muscular contraction against an inert and stiffened necrotic area, and aging of the myocardium with laceration of the myocardial microstructure have all been proposed as the local factors that lead to rupture.[850–852]

The following are some features that characterize this serious complication of AMI. Rupture of the free wall:

1. Occurs more frequently in women than in men with infarction and more frequently in the elderly;
2. Is more common in hypertensive than normotensive patients[853];
3. Occurs approximately seven times more frequently in the left than the right ventricle and seldom occurs in the atria;
4. Usually involves the anterior or lateral walls of the ventricle in the area of the terminal distribution of the left anterior descending coronary artery;
5. Is usually associated with transmural infarction involving at least 20 per cent of the left ventricle;
6. Occurs between 1 day and 3 weeks, but most commonly 3 to 6 days, following the infarct;
7. Is usually preceded by infarct expansion, i.e., thinning and a disproportionate dilatation within the softened necrotic zone[182];
8. Most commonly results from a distinct tear in the myocardial wall or a dissecting hematoma that perforates a necrotic area of myocardium (Fig. 38–37);
9. Usually occurs near the junction of the infarct and the normal muscle;
10. Occurs less frequently in the center of the infarct, but when rupture occurs here, it is usually during the second rather than the first week following the infarct;
11. Rarely occurs in a hypertrophied ventricle or in an area of excellent collateral vessels.[850]

Rupture of the free wall of the left ventricle usually leads to hemopericardium and death from cardiac tamponade. Occasionally, rupture of the free wall of the ventricle occurs as the first clinical manifestation in patients with undetected or silent myocardial infarction, and then it may be considered a form of "sudden cardiac death" (Chap. 24).

The course of rupture varies from catastrophic, with an acute tear leading to immediate death, to slow and incomplete, leading to late rupture or formation of a false aneurysm.[854] In either case, survival depends on the recognition of this complication, hemodynamic stabilization of the patient—usually with inotropic agents and/or intraaortic balloon pump—and most importantly on immediate surgical repair.[855–857] Survival has occasionally been reported even in the most dire of circumstances, i.e., when the diagnosis is correctly made within moments of rupture, and through a well-coordinated operating room effort, the patients were placed on cardiopulmonary bypass within one hour and the defects then successfully repaired.[858–860]

Incomplete rupture of the heart may occur when organizing thrombus and hematoma, together with pericardium, seal a rupture of the left ventricle and thus prevent the development of hemopericardium (Figs. 38–38 and 38–39). With time, this area of organized thrombus and pericardium can become a small, left ventricular diverticulum or a large pseudoaneurysm which maintains communication with the cavity of the left ventricle.[861] In contrast to true aneurysms, which always contain some myocardial elements in their walls, the walls of false aneurysms are composed of organized hematoma and pericardium and lack any elements of the original myocardial wall. False aneurysms can become quite large, even equaling the true ventricular cavity in size, and they communicate with the left ventricular cavity through a narrow neck. Frequently, false aneurysms contain significant quantities of old and recent thrombus, superficial portions of which can cause arterial emboli. False aneurysms can drain off a portion of

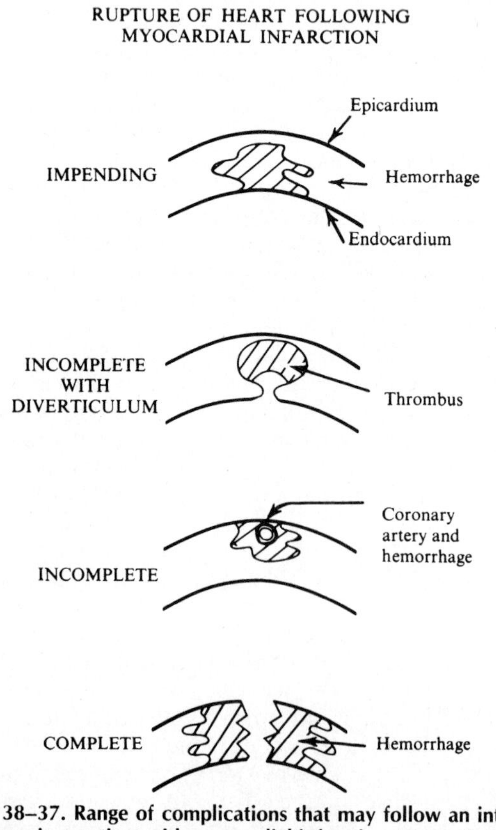

FIGURE 38–37. Range of complications that may follow an intramural hemorrhage in a patient with myocardial infarction. (From Datta, B. N., et al.: Incomplete rupture of the heart with diverticulum formation. Pathology 7:179, 1975.)

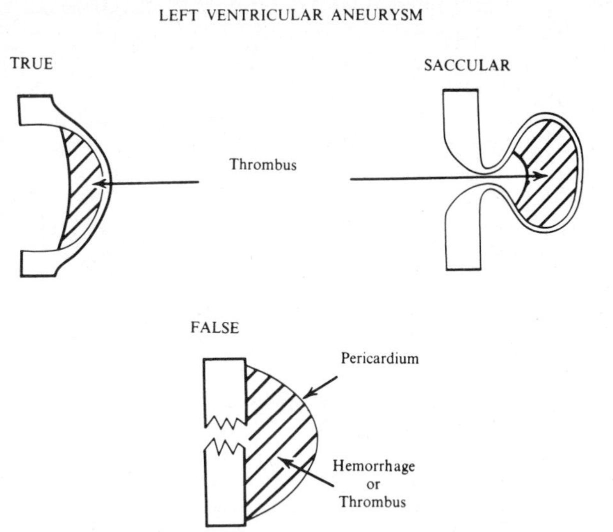

FIGURE 38–38. Appearance of aneurysms that may develop following myocardial infarction. (From Datta, B. N., et al.: Incomplete rupture of the heart with diverticulum formation. Pathology 7:179, 1975.)

each ventricular stroke volume exactly as do true aneurysms. The diagnosis of pseudoaneurysm can be made by two-dimensional echocardiography (Fig. 5–91, p. 122) and contrast angiography.

DIAGNOSIS. The recognition of rupture usually is first suggested by the development of sudden profound right heart failure associated with shock, often rapidly leading to electromechanical dissociation. Immediate pericardiocentesis will confirm the diagnosis and relieve the pericardial tamponade, at least momentarily.[862] If the patient's condition is relatively stable, echocardiography may help in establishing the diagnosis of tamponade. Under the most favorable conditions, cardiac catheterization can be carried out, not necessarily to confirm the diagnosis of rupture but to delineate the coronary anatomy. This is so that, in addition to ventricular repair, coronary artery bypass surgery can be performed in patients in whom high-grade lesions are seen. In situations in which hemodynamics are critically compromised, establishment of the diagnosis should be followed immediately by surgery for resection of the necrotic and ruptured myocardium with primary reconstruction. In the absence of previous coronary angiography, it has been suggested that "blind" bypass should be done if proximal coronary artery lesions are palpable at the time of surgery.[862] When rupture is subacute and a pseudoaneurysm is suspected or present, elective surgery is indicated because rupture of the pseudoaneurysm occurs relatively frequently.[861, 863]

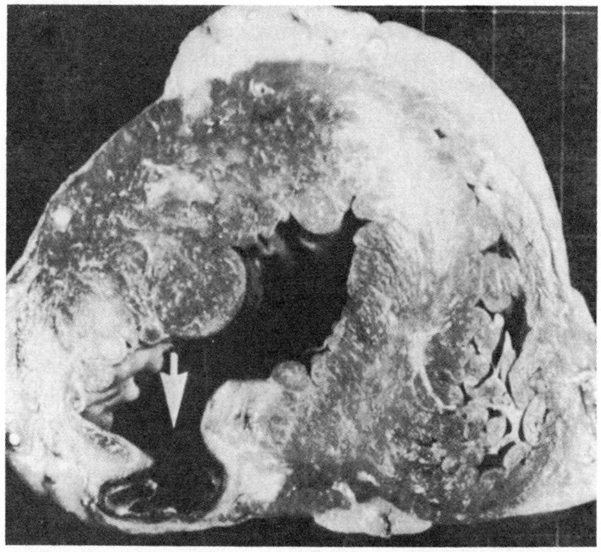

FIGURE 38–39. Heart slice showing incomplete rupture with diverticulum formation in the posterior wall of the left ventricle (arrow). Its lumen contains thrombus. Note scarring of the walls of the left ventricle. Coronary arteries have barium in their lumens. (From Datta, B. N., et al.: Incomplete rupture of the heart with diverticulum formation. Pathology 7:179, 1975.)

Rupture of the Interventricular Septum

Although rupture of the interventricular septum is said to be less common than rupture of the free wall at autopsy,[850, 853, 864–866] our clinical experience has been otherwise, perhaps because death usually is not immediate, and patients can reach a referral center where this complication is treated frequently. The perforation usually is single and ranges in length from one to several centimeters. It may be a direct through-and-through hole or may be more irregular and serpiginous.[867] The size of the defect determines the magnitude of the left-to-right shunt and the extent of hemodynamic deterioration, which in turn affects the likelihood of survival. The development of shock and the likelihood of survival appear to depend critically on impairment of right ventricular function.[865] As in rupture of the free wall of the ventricle, transmural infarction underlies rupture of the ventricular septum. Anterior and anterolateral MI's are somewhat more common than inferior or inferolateral infarcts in patients with ventricular septal rupture.[864] Rupture of the septum with an anterior infarction tends to be apical in location, whereas inferior infarctions are associated with perforation of the basal septum. Virtually all patients have multivessel coronary artery disease, with the majority exhibiting lesions in all of their major vessels.[865]

The diagnosis of a ruptured interventricular septum is usually heralded by the appearance of a new harsh, loud holosystolic murmur that is heard best at the lower left and usually right sternal borders. A thrill may occur with the murmur. Biventricular failure generally ensues within hours to days. Confirmation of the diagnosis usually requires insertion of a pulmonary artery balloon catheter to document the left-to-right shunt. The defect can also be recognized by two-dimensional echocardiography.

Recently, catheter placement of an umbrella-shaped device within the ruptured septum has been reported to stabilize the conditions of critically ill patients with acute septal rupture following AMI.[867a]

Rupture of a Papillary Muscle

Partial or total rupture of a papillary muscle is a rare but often fatal complication of transmural MI [868] Inferior wall infarction can lead to rupture of the posteromedial papillary muscle, which occurs more commonly than rupture of the anterolateral muscle, a consequence of anterolateral MI.[869] Rupture of a right ventricular papillary muscle is rare but can cause massive tricuspid regurgitation and right ventricular failure. Complete transection of a left ventricular papillary muscle is incompatible with life because the sudden massive mitral regurgitation that develops cannot be tolerated.[870, 871] Rupture of a portion of a papillary muscle resulting in severe, although not necessarily overwhelming, mitral regurgitation is much more frequent (Fig. 33–13, p. 1037). Unlike rupture of the ventricular septum, which occurs with large infarcts, papillary muscle rupture occurs with a relatively small infarction in approximately one-half of the cases seen.[868] The extent of coronary artery disease in these patients may be relatively modest as well.[869]

In a small number of patients, rupture of more than one cardiac structure is noted clinically[872, 873] or at postmortem examination; all possible combinations of rupture of the free left ventricular wall, the interventricular septum, and papillary muscles have been described.[864, 867]

As with patients who have a ruptured ventricular septal defect, those with papillary muscle rupture manifest a new holosystolic murmur followed by the development of increasingly severe heart failure. In both situations the murmur may disappear as arterial pressure falls. Partial or complete rupture of a papillary muscle may be promptly recognized echocardiographically;[874] therefore, an echocardiogram should be obtained immediately on any patient in whom the diagnosis is suspected, because hemodynamic deterioration can ensue rapidly. Echocardiography also allows for differentiation of papillary muscle rupture from other generally less severe forms of mitral regurgitation that occur with AMI.[875]

Hemodynamic Findings and Management in Ventricular Septal Rupture and Mitral Regurgitation

It may be difficult, on clinical grounds, to distinguish between acute mitral regurgitation and rupture of the ventricular septum in patients with AMI who suddenly develop a loud systolic murmur.[876] This differentiation can be made by two-dimensional and Doppler echocardiography as well as first-pass radionuclide ventriculography. In addition, a right-heart catheterization with a balloon-tipped catheter can readily distinguish between these two complications. As noted above, patients with ventricular septal rupture demonstrate a "step-up" in oxygen saturation in blood samples from the right ventricle and pulmonary artery compared with those from the right atrium. Patients with acute mitral regurgitation lack this step-up; they may demonstrate tall *v* waves in both the pulmonary capillary and the pulmonary arterial pressure tracings (Fig. 38–40). However, patients with septal rupture may also develop large *v* waves and thus, the presence of this finding is not necessarily useful in an individual patient. Cardiac output is usually significantly decreased in both conditions.

Invasive monitoring, which is essential in these patients, also allows for the critically important assessment of right ventricular function. Right and left ventricular filling pressures (right atrial pressure and pulmonary capillary wedge pressure) dictate fluid administration and the use of diuretics, while measurements of cardiac output and mean arterial pressure are obtained for calculation of systemic vascular resistance as a guide for vasodilator therapy. The latter, generally using nitroprusside, should be instituted as early as possible once hemodynamic monitoring is available. This may be critically important for stabilizing the patient's condition in preparation for further diagnostic studies and surgical repair. If vasodilator therapy is not tolerated or if it fails to achieve hemodynamic stability, intraaortic balloon counterpulsation should be rapidly instituted.

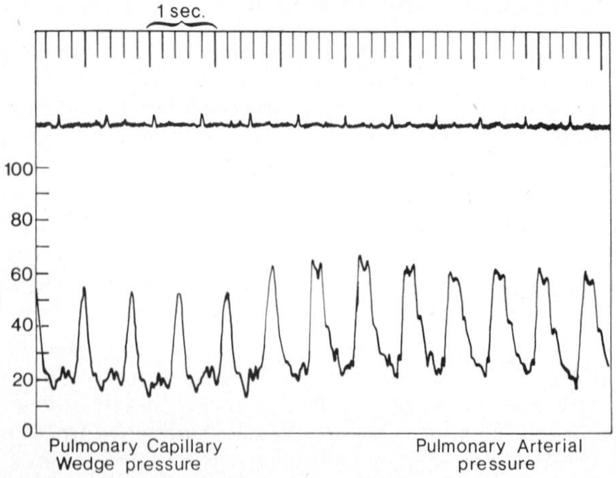

FIGURE 38–40. Acute mitral regurgitation secondary to ruptured chord from infarcted papillary muscle in a 45-year-old man. Tracing shows mitral regurgitation, tall *v* waves in pulmonary capillary wedge and pulmonary artery tracings. (Courtesy of Ira S. Ockene, M.D.)

Surgical Treatment of Hemodynamic Impairment

Operative intervention is most successful in patients with AMI and circulatory collapse when a surgically correctable mechanical lesion can be identified and repaired, such as ventricular septal defect.[877, 878] In such patients the circulation should at first be supported by intraaortic balloon pulsation and a positive inotropic agent such as dopamine or dobutamine in combination with a vasodilator unless the patient is hypotensive. Operation should not be delayed in patients with a correctable lesion who require pharmacological and/or mechanical (counterpulsation) support (Fig. 38–41).[856, 862, 877, 879–881] Such patients frequently develop a serious complication—infection, adult respiratory distress syndrome, extension of the infarct, or renal failure—if operation is delayed. On the other hand, when the hemodynamic status of a patient with one of these mechanical lesions complicating an AMI remains stable *after* the patient has been weaned off pharmacological and/or mechanical support, it may be desirable to postpone operation for 2 to 4 weeks to allow some healing of the infarct to occur. Surgical repair may involve either repair of a ventricular septal defect or insertion of a prosthetic mitral valve usually accompanied by coronary revascularization.

Left Ventricular Aneurysm

A ventricular aneurysm, which is a circumscribed, noncontractile outpouching of the left ventricle, develops in 12 to 15 per cent of patients who survive a myocardial infarction.[882] The wall of the aneurysm is thin in comparison with the rest of the left ventricle (Fig. 38–38), and it is usually composed of fibrous tissue as well as necrotic muscle, occasionally mixed with viable myocardium.[883] Aneurysm formation presumably occurs when intraventricular tension stretches the noncontracting infarcted heart muscle, thus producing infarct expansion,[182, 884] a relatively weak, thin layer of necrotic muscle, and fibrous tissue that bulges with each cardiac contraction. With the passage of time, the wall of the aneurysm becomes more densely fibrotic, but it continues to bulge with systole, thus "stealing" some of the left ventricular stroke volume during each systole.[163]

When an aneurysm is present after anterior MI, there is generally a total occlusion of a poorly collateralized left anterior descending coronary artery.[885] An aneurysm is rarely seen with multivessel disease when there are either extensive collaterals or a nonoccluded left anterior descending artery.[885] Aneurysms usually range from 1 to 8 cm in diameter.[882] They occur approximately four times more often at the apex and in the anterior wall than in the inferoposterior wall.[882] The overlying pericardium is usually densely adherent to the wall of the aneurysm, which may

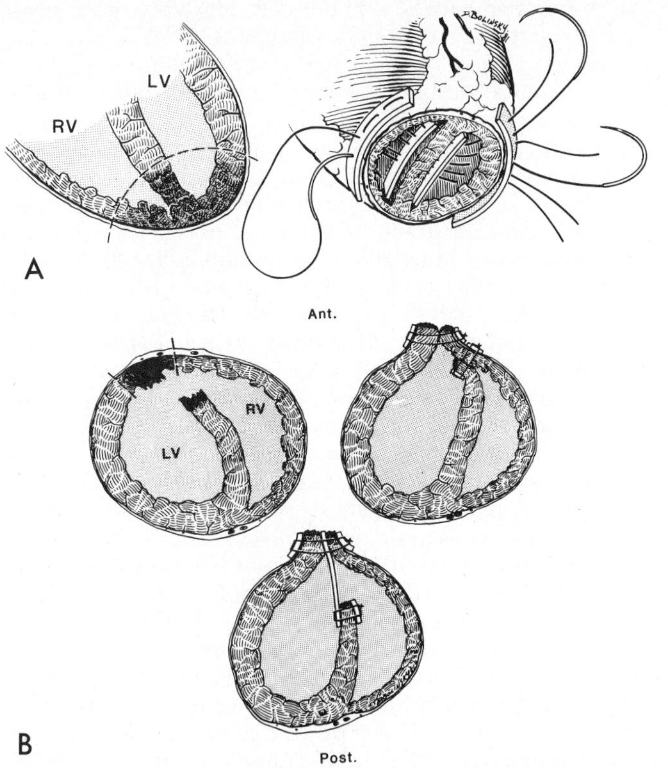

FIGURE 38–41. *A*, **Closure of apical ventricular septal rupture. The infarcted apex is resected, and the remaining viable myocardium of the septum and the left and right ventricular free walls are buttressed together using Telfon felt inside and outside the ventricle. LV = left ventricle; RV = right ventricle.** *B*, **Closure of a ventricular septal rupture with an extensive anterior infarct. The septum is reconstructed with a heavy Dacron patch that is sewn to the base of remaining septum using Teflon bolsters on both sides. The free edge of the patch is then brought out and the left and right ventricular free walls are attached to it, as shown in C. Ant. = anterior; LV = left ventricle; Post = posterior; RV = right ventricle. (Reproduced with permission from Kopf, G. S., Meshkov, A., Laks, H., Hammond, G. L., and Geha, A. S.: Changing patterns in the surgical management of ventricular septal rupture after myocardial infarction. Am. J. Surg.** ***143*****:465, 1982.)**

even become partially calcified after several years. Rarely, a true left ventricular aneurysm ruptures soon after its development. In isolated cases this has been attributed to a degree of early myocardial rupture interrupted by subepicardial aneurysm formation, susceptible to later complete rupture.[886] Ordinarily, late rupture, when the aneurysm has become stabilized by the formation of dense fibrous tissue in its wall, almost never occurs.[861, 882]

Mortality in patients with a left ventricular aneurysm is up to six times higher than among patients without aneurysms, even when compared to that in patients with comparable left ventricular ejection fraction.[887] Death in these patients is often sudden and presumably related to the high incidence of ventricular tachyarrhythmias that occur with aneurysms.

The presence of persistent ST-segment elevation in an electrocardiographic area of infarction, classically thought to suggest aneurysm formation, actually indicates a large infarct but does not necessarily imply an aneurysm.[888] The diagnosis of aneurysm is best made noninvasively by an echocardiographic study (Figs. 5–87, p. 120, and 5–90, p. 121), by radionuclide ventriculography, or at the time of cardiac catheterization by left ventriculography. With the loss of shortening from the area of the aneurysm, the remainder of the ventricle is required to compensate. With relatively large aneurysms, complete compensation is impossible. The stroke volume falls, or if maintained, it is at the expense of an increase in end-diastolic volume, which in turn leads to increased wall tension and myocardial oxygen demand. Heart failure may ensue, and angina may appear or worsen.

TREATMENT. Surgical aneurysmectomy generally is successful only if there is relative preservation of contractile performance in the nonaneurysmal portion of the left ventricle.[862] In such circumstances, when the operation is performed for worsening heart failure or angina, operative mortality is relatively low and clinical improvement can be expected.[862, 889] Aneurysmectomy and special procedures carried out to control ventricular tachyarrhythmias occurring with left ventricular aneurysms are described on page 647.

OTHER COMPLICATIONS OF ACUTE MYOCARDIAL INFARCTION

LEFT VENTRICULAR THROMBUS AND ARTERIAL EMBOLISM

Mural thrombi are common in patients succumbing to AMI.[890] In one report, 44 per cent of 924 patients dying of AMI were found to have mural thrombi attached to the endocardium overlying the infarct[891]; thrombi are more common in patients with large than small infarcts and therefore are probably more frequently found in nonsurvivors than in survivors. They are almost universally located in the left ventricle, particularly at its apex. With extensive transmural infarction of the septum, however, mural thrombi may overlie infarcted myocardium in both ventricles. As noted earlier, mural thrombus is rather common in a ventricular aneurysm or pseudoaneurysm. Mural thrombi can be recognized premortem by two-dimensional echocardiography in approximately one-third of all patients with acute transmural anterior or apical infarctions (Fig. 5–94, p. 123); they are rare in patients with inferior-posterior infarcts.[892] Mural thrombi may be more frequent in patients treated with beta-adrenoceptor blockade after AMI.[892a]

Although a mural thrombus adheres to the endocardium overlying the infarcted myocardium, superficial portions of it can become detached and produce systemic arterial emboli. Approximately half the patients with mural thrombi at autopsy also have evidence of systemic emboli.[882, 892, 893] In one study, systemic emboli were noted at autopsy in 10 per cent of 500 patients who died of acute myocardial infarction; half of the emboli were cerebral.[894] The other half usually lodged in the kidney or spleen or at the bifurcation of the aorta or iliac or femoral arteries; rarely, intestinal infarction results from embolization of the superior mesenteric artery. Occasionally, embolism from a mural thrombus is the presenting symptom, with the underlying myocardial infarction either silent or overlooked.

Most echocardiographic studies of this condition are either retrospective or highly selective, and thus the premortem incidence of thrombosis and its clinical importance remain unclear. One recent study shed some light on this problem; Spirito et al. prospectively evaluated 58 patients daily for the first 5 days of infarction, every other day until day 15, and then monthly for a mean of 7 months following infarction.[384] Left ventricular thrombi were identified in 41 per cent of the patients, nearly half within 48 hours of infarction. Over 90 per cent of the patients developing a thrombus within 48 hours died, all of causes related to their large infarction (shock, reinfarction, rupture, and ventricular tachyarrhythmia), while none had clinical evidence of emboli from their left ventricular thrombus.[384] Only 1 of the 24 patients with thrombus had a clinically apparent embolic episode. (None of the patients were receiving anticoagulation therapy.) Other studies have shown a higher incidence of embolization, with as many as 27 per cent of patients with left ventricular thrombus suffering cerebrovascular accidents.[895] However, this often occurs despite adequate anticoagulant therapy.

MANAGEMENT. It is not clear whether heparinization or therapy with streptokinase plus heparin affects the development of left ventricular thrombus.[896–899] Therefore, it is not our practice to recommend routine anticoagulation, even if a left ventricular thrombus is present, unless: (1) an embolic event has already occurred or (2) the thrombus appears highly mobile and/or markedly protuberant and shaggy on the echocardiogram.[900]

Antiplatelet therapy, while probably not capable of affecting thrombus size in most patients, has been shown to prevent further platelet deposition on existing thrombi.[901] For this benefit, and because it is generally so benign, antiplatelet therapy is recommended for most patients with left ventricular thrombi in whom systemic anticoagulation is not undertaken. Independent of therapy, spontaneous regression of a thrombus occurs in 20 per cent or more of patients,[384] while systemic thrombolytic therapy causes echocardiographic regression or disappearance of the thrombus in most patients so treated.[902]

VENOUS THROMBOSIS AND EMBOLISM

Almost all pulmonary emboli originate from thrombi in the veins of the lower extremities (Chap. 47); much less commonly, they originate from mural thrombi overlying an area of infarction in the right ventricle. Bed rest and heart failure predispose to venous thrombosis and subsequent pulmonary embolism, and both of these factors occur commonly in patients with AMI, particularly those with large infarctions. In one autopsy study, major pulmonary emboli were present (though not always responsible for a fatal outcome) in 11 per cent of patients dying of AMI.[894]

Several decades ago, at a time when patients with AMI were subjected to prolonged periods of bed rest, significant pulmonary embolism was found in more than 20 per cent of patients with MI at autopsy,[903] and massive pulmonary embolism accounted for 10 per cent of deaths from AMI.[891] In recent years, with early mobilization and the widespread use of low-dose anticoagulant prophylaxis, pulmonary embolism has become an uncommon cause of death in this condition.

POSTINFARCTION ISCHEMIA AND EXTENSION

Angina developing within the first 10 days following AMI is disconcerting to patients and physicians alike. In many patients, it responds to rest, nitroglycerin, beta-adrenoceptor blockade, and calcium channel antagonists,[904] just as does classic angina. In a minority of patients, postinfarction angina may be refractory to treatment and is provoked by minimal activity, meals, or emotional upset. When accompanied by ST-T–wave changes in the same area where Q waves have appeared, it may be due to coronary spasm,[905, 906] to occlusion of an initially patent vessel, or to reocclusion of a recanalized one.

Regardless of whether postinfarction angina is persistent or limited, its presence is important, for both short and long-term mortality is higher among such patients.[330, 907] For this reason we concur with the recommendation of others[908] that most patients who develop spontaneous angina early after AMI should undergo cardiac catheterization and coronary arteriography to assess their suitability for a revascularization procedure. While the patient's age and general medical condition should be considered in the decision, the availability of coronary angioplasty has made this relatively broad recommendation more reasonable than when the only alternative was coronary artery bypass graft surgery. Even in the most experienced hands, this latter operation carries a 20 per cent mortality when done for recurrent angina within a week of AMI.[909]

Exercise stress testing, particularly when used with stress-thallium scintigraphy may be helpful in discerning whether chest pain following an AMI is due to ischemia. However, such tests should be avoided if symptoms have been persistent, accompanied by ECG changes, or have occurred at rest or with minimal activity. Recently, positron-emission tomography has proved useful for recognizing hypoperfused but viable myocardium following AMI.[910]

Infarct extension occurs in approximately 10 per cent of patients with AMI during the first 10 days.[911, 912] It is frequently difficult to distinguish post-infarction angina from infarct extension. The latter is usually associated with more severe and prolonged discomfort, and *persistent* electrocardiographic changes (ST-T changes or QRS changes or both) may occur. It is generally defined as reelevation or reappearance of CK-MB in the serum after the initial peak. Neither chest pain nor the electrocardiogram provides accurate markers for recognizing infarct extension, as both occur in only about half of patients with extension. The majority of patients with cardiogenic shock have developed infarct extension.[769] In a prospective study of patients, it was found that mortality in those experiencing extension is more than double that noted in patients in whom extension did not occur.[913] Marmor reported that infarct extension occurred most frequently in obese females and was most common in patients with nontransmural infarction.[914] It is apparently more common in patients with diabetes mellitus, a previous MI, and in those with an early peaking CK-MB curve (< 15 hours).[912] Presumably, the higher mortality associated with infarct extension is related to the larger mass of myocardium whose function becomes compromised.

PERICARDIAL EFFUSION AND PERICARDITIS (See also p. 1514)

PERICARDIAL EFFUSIONS. These are common after AMI. Generally detected echocardiographically, their incidence varies with technique, criteria, and laboratory expertise. They occur in approximately 25 per cent of patients after MI.[377, 915] This finding cannot be viewed as a complication because it does not necessarily lead to clinical problems. (When tamponade occurs, it is usually due to ventricular rupture or hemorrhagic pericarditis.) Effusions are more common with anterior MI's, larger infarcts, and when congestive failure is present.[377, 915, 916]

The reabsorption rate of a post-infarction pericardial effusion is slow, often taking several months to resolve.[377] The presence of an effusion does not indicate that pericarditis is present. Although they may occur together, the majority of effusions occur without other evidence of pericarditis.

PERICARDITIS. When secondary to transmural AMI, pericarditis may produce pain as early as the first day and as late as 6 weeks after MI. This may be confused with pain resulting from persistent ischemia or extension of the infarct or both. Transmural myocardial infarction, by definition, extends to the epicardial surface and is responsible for producing local pericardial inflammation. Although transitory pericardial friction rubs are relatively common among patients with transmural infarction within the first 48 hours, the pain or electrocardiographic changes occur much less often. In one recent study of 423 consecutive patients with AMI, 31 (7.3 per cent) developed a pericardial friction rub, but only one patient had electrocardiographic changes diagnostic of acute pericarditis[263] (p. 1489). Pericarditis is more common in males, among patients with Q-wave infarction, and in those in whom congestive heart failure is present.[263, 917] Although fibrinous or serofibrinous pericarditis may be seen in up to 15 per cent of patients with AMI at autopsy, clinical studies rarely suggest the presence of active pericarditis in more than 10 per cent of patients,[917] whereas pericardial effusion without evidence of pericarditis is far more common.[377, 915] The discomfort of pericarditis usually becomes worse during a deep inspiration, but it may be somewhat relieved when the patient sits up and leans forward (Chap. 44).

Pericarditis generally occurs between the second and fourth days after the infarction. In some patients with diffuse pericarditis, an accompanying pericardial effusion may be large, but tamponade is rare, and as noted above no effusion is present in the majority of patients. Occasionally, hemorrhagic effusion with cardiac tamponade develops after myocardial infarction in patients who have been treated with anticoagulants.[918] A case of late pericardial constriction due to anticoagulant-induced hemopericardium has been reported.[919] While anticoagulation clearly increases the risk for hemorrhagic pericarditis early after MI, this complication has not been reported with sufficient frequency during heparinization or following thrombolytic therapy to warrant *absolute* prohibition of such agents when a rub is present. In cases in which continuation or initiation of anticoagulant therapy is *strongly* indicated (such as during cardiac catheterization or following coronary angioplasty), particularly careful attention is warranted to the clotting parameters and the duration of anticoagulation, and in observation for clinical signs of possible tamponade.

DRESSLER SYNDROME. Also known as the *post-myocardial infarction syndrome,*[265, 268] this usually occurs 2 to 10 weeks after infarction. Its incidence is difficult to define because it often blends imperceptibly with the more common early post-myocardial infarction pericarditis. This incidence has decreased dramatically since the use of chronic anticoagulation has fallen out of favor and since antiinflammatory agents are used more vigorously. However, it has probably not disappeared completely as some have contended.[920, 921] At autopsy, patients with this syndrome usually demonstrate localized fibrinous pericarditis[917] containing polymorphonuclear leukocytes.[265] The post-myocardial infarction syndrome is probably the result of an autoimmune antibody response against certain pericardial and myocardial antigens exposed to the immune system at the time of infarction.[267] It is treated with aspirin 650 mg, as often as every 4 hours. Other nonsteroidal antiinflammatory agents are best avoided in the AMI patient because of their potential to impair infarct healing,[626] to cause ventricular rupture,[627a] and to increase coronary vascular resistance.[628] In occasional patients full-dose steroids are necessary to control what may be very severe symptoms.

CONVALESCENCE, DISCHARGE, AND POST-MYOCARDIAL INFARCTION CARE (See also Chaps. 41 and 62)

The patient with uncomplicated AMI should be washed by an attendant during the first 3 to 5 days. If the convalescence continues uneventfully, limited ambulation within the room can be begun on the third or fourth day. Once early ambulatory activities are begun, advancement in the activity should depend on the patient's condition. Activity can then increase progressively, and a shower may be allowed some time after the seventh day.

Prolonged hospitalization and enforced bed rest for any illness may lead to complications (particularly in elderly patients), such as constipation, decubitus ulcers, excessive resorption of bone with formation of renal calculi, atelectasis, thrombophlebitis, pulmonary emboli, urinary retention, mild anemia due to repetitive blood sampling for diagnostic tests, impaired oral intake of fluids, bleeding from the gastrointestinal tract due to stress ulcers, and deconditioning of cardiovascular reflex responses to postural changes. Because of the precarious status of the heart recovering from AMI, avoidance of such complications is of primary importance. For example, constipation may lead to straining, transitory reduction of venous return and diminution of cardiac output, impaired coronary perfusion, and ventricular arrhythmias, occasionally culminating in ventricular fibrillation. Early implementation of a bed-chair regimen appears to be useful in avoiding many of the difficulties encountered previously among patients confined to bed for several weeks.

TIMING OF HOSPITAL DISCHARGE

The time of discharge from the hospital is variable. It may be as early as 6 or 7 days after admission for patients who experience no complications, who can be followed readily at home, and for whom the family setting is conducive to convalescence.[922, 923] Most complications that would preclude early discharge occur within the first day or so of admission and therefore, patients suitable for early discharge can be identified early during the hospitalization.[923] Ordinarily, discharge of patients without complications is deferred until approximately 10 days following infarction, at a time when the patient has become fully ambulatory. For patients who have experienced a complication, discharge is deferred until their condition has been stable for several days and it is clear that they are responding appropriately to necessary medications such as antiarrhythmic agents, vasodilators, or positive inotropic agents.

There have been several controlled trials (Table 38–6, p. 1249) and many uncontrolled trials of early discharge after AMI.[924] None have shown any increase in risk with early discharge, and some have actually shown significantly worse mortality and morbidity in the group discharged later,[925] although this may have been due to confounding variables. When considered together, the studies of early discharge are quite encouraging. Results involving 892 patients in 8 different trials of discharge between 7 and 14 days after admission for AMI suggest that there is no unfavorable effect on mortality and morbidity.[924] A multivariant statistical technique to determine risk of discharge for individual patients has been proposed.[926] Using 19 clinical variables, this technique was developed with the following assumption: discharge would take place when the risk of a serious complication occurring in the 2 weeks following discharge was below 5 per cent, and the risk of death in the first 30 days after admission for AMI was also less than 5 per cent. Tested retrospectively in over 1000 patients and prospectively in almost 200 patients, this statistical system confirmed that about 50 per cent of patients could be discharged safely after 5 days, and that up to a 20 per cent saving in hospitalization days could be obtained.[926] Use of this model requires a small programmable calculator.

While early discharge certainly is feasible for the majority of patients with uncomplicated MI, there are two caveats. The first is that it is often useful and convenient, before hospital discharge, to attempt to identify patients at considerable risk of reinfarction or cardiac death. This usually involves noninvasive testing, which may lead to cardiac catheterization and coronary arteriography and, if indicated, to coronary revascularization. Much can be said for accomplishing all of this, if it is necessary, before hospital discharge. Second, we do not yet know of the potential adverse effects on scar formation or ventricular remodeling of early increased physical activity: thinning of myocardial scars has been demonstrated in animals that are exercised early after coronary ligation[927] and in which arterial pressure is elevated.[928] The latter concern can be minimized by strict instructions to the patient and family concerning the gradual resumption of activity following discharge.

Before discharge from the hospital, the patient should receive detailed instruction concerning physical activity. Initially, this should consist of being ambulatory at home but avoiding isometric activity such as lifting; several rest periods should be taken daily. In addition, the patient should be given fresh nitroglycerin tablets and instructed in their use and should receive careful instructions about the use of any other medication prescribed. As convalescence progresses, graded resumption of activity should be encouraged. Many approaches have been utilized, ranging from formal rigid guidelines to general advice advocating moderation and avoidance of any activity that evokes symptoms. Sexual counseling is often overlooked during recovery from MI[929, 930] and should also be included as part of the educational process. There is some evidence that behavior alteration is possible after recovery from MI and that this may improve prognosis.[931, 932] The physical and psychological rehabilitation of patients convalescing from AMI are discussed in Chapters 41 and 62.

SECONDARY PREVENTION OF MYOCARDIAL INFARCTION

The concept of secondary prevention of reinfarction and death after recovery from an AMI has been investigated actively during the past 2 decades. Until quite recently, however, nearly all efforts at demonstrating secondary prevention had failed. Problems in proving the efficacy of various interventions have been related both to the ineffectiveness of certain strategies and to the difficulty in proving a benefit as mortality and morbidity have improved following AMI. Nevertheless, patients who survive the initial course of AMI are at increased risk due to coronary artery disease and its complications; therefore, it is imperative that efforts be made to reduce this risk in each patient. While secondary prevention drug trials generally have tested one form of therapy against placebo in an attempt to demonstrate a benefit of that therapy, the physician must remember that disciplined clinical care of the individual patient is far more important than rote use of an agent found beneficial in the latest drug trial.[933]

In reviewing the results of any secondary prevention trial, the clinician must consider several issues before deciding on its relevance to a particular patient: (1) Was the intervention begun immediately (once AMI was identified) or was it applied later, and what is the relationship of its expected effectiveness to this timing? (2) Were patients in the trial similar to the patient for whom the intervention is contemplated, or would the specific patient under consideration have been excluded from the trial, thus rendering the trial's conclusion less meaningful for that particular patient? (3) Is there some reason to anticipate that the intervention being considered might be unusually risky in certain patients for whom it may be used (e.g., beta-adrenoceptor blockers in a patient with a history of obstructive lung disease)? (4) Once the intervention is started, how long should it be continued, or is this information unavailable because studies have not been ongoing for a sufficient time? (5) What is the underlying risk that the individual patient faces? As detailed on pages 1291 to 1295, patients with low risk can be separated from those with higher risk. In interventional strategies, the level of risk should be taken into consideration when any therapy, particularly if it is to be long term, is contemplated.

It is likely that secondary prevention efforts are, in fact, responsible in part for the remarkable decline in mortality and morbidity[9] in patients with coronary artery disease, although the magnitude of the impact is not clear. Efforts to improve survival and the quality of survival after MI that relate to modification of known risk factors are considered in Chapter 36. Of the risk factors considered, cessation of smoking and control of hypertension are probably most important. It has been shown that within 2 years of quitting smoking, the risk of a nonfatal MI in these former smokers falls to a level compatible with that in never-smokers.[934] Being hospitalized for an AMI is a powerful motivation for patients to cease cigarette smoking, and this is an ideal time to encourage that clearly beneficial change. It is also an ideal time to begin to treat hypertension, to counsel patients to achieve optimal body weight, and to consider various strategies to improve the patient's lipid profile. Unfortunately, unless prior values of total cholesterol and HDL cholesterol are known, or unless measurements are obtained within the first 24 to 48 hours,[310–312] reliable values, necessary to guide therapy, will not be available until approximately 2 to 3 months after the MI. As discussed in Chapter 41, cardiac rehabilitation efforts that include exercise programs and the teaching of stress reduction techniques are also likely to have an impact on secondary prevention. However, despite the general desirability of these measures, for many patients with AMI, particularly the elderly, it is unlikely that much change in the underlying coronary atherosclerosis will take place with their institution.

Beta-Adrenoceptor Blockers

These drugs have been the most intensively investigated group of drugs for secondary prevention following AMI. Numerous studies have now shown that beta blocker administration improves survival after AMI, and as a result, prescribing patterns for these agents have changed dramatically.[935] The first beta blocker trial was reported by Snow in 1965,[936] arousing a great deal of interest. Of the many beta blocking agents tested since then, propranolol,[937, 938] metoprolol,[493, 939] timolol,[940, 941] and oxprenolol[596, 942] have been tried in the greatest number of patients. Large trials with timolol, propranolol, and metoprolol have demonstrated that these drugs improve survival in a wide spectrum of postinfarction patients and also reduce the incidence of sudden death and reinfarction. Results with oxprenolol, a beta blocker with intrinsic sympathomimetic activity (ISA), are far less encouraging, with at least one trial of this agent appearing to show a slight adverse effect on mortality.[596] The structure of the various trials have varied considerably, making comparisons exceedingly difficult.[597] While increasingly rigorous trial design and analysis have allowed for more definitive conclusions, considerable controversy continues regarding optimal selection of patients, variety of beta blocker, initial route (intravenous followed by oral vs. oral vs. intravenous), and timing of administration.

Although differences in trials have made it statistically unsound to pool data from studies, one useful strategy has been to compare by graphs estimates of the mortality benefit (or lack of benefit) and the trial's 95 per cent confidence limits.[597, 943]

Of the individual trials displayed in Figure 38–42*A*,[597] 11 of 13 showed improved mortality with beta blockade, and in three of these the benefits were statistically significant. This form of analysis has been applied to beta blocker trials to demonstrate both the mode of benefit (Fig. 38–42*B*), and the effect of ancillary properties of the beta blocker (Fig. 38–42*C*). It appears that improved mortality is related primarily to the prevention of sudden death and that, while there is no difference between cardioselective and noncardioselective beta blockers, agents with ISA are markedly less beneficial than those without ISA.[597]

ADVERSE EFFECTS. While adverse effects have required withdrawal of the beta blocker in approximately 10 per cent of patients, most of these effects can be ameliorated by varying the choice of beta blocker, reducing the dosage, or discontinuing the medication if necessary. There has been natural concern that, because of the beta blockers'

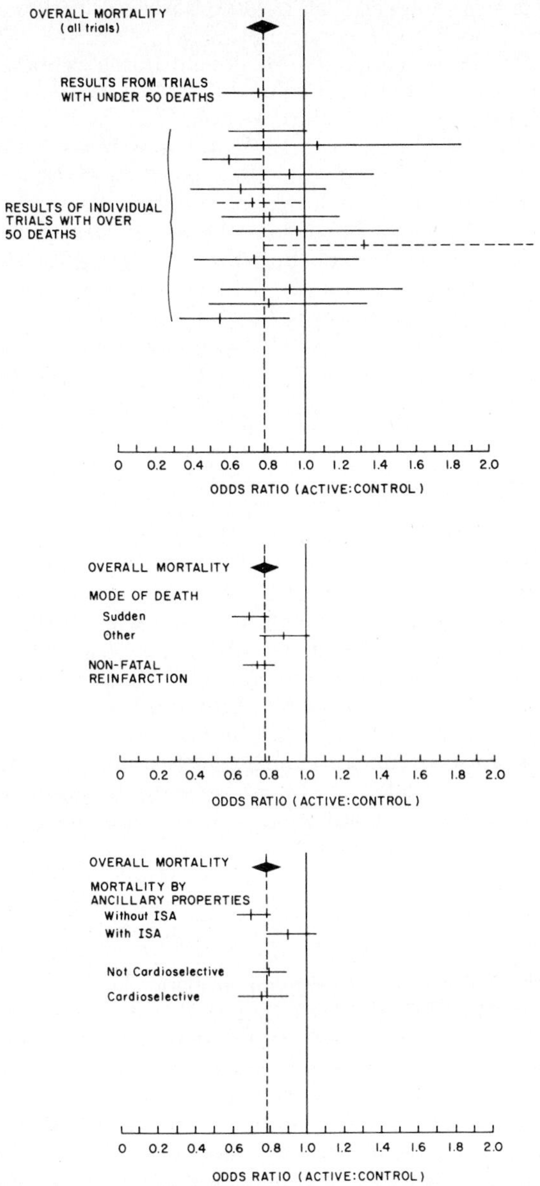

FIGURE 38–42. ***Top,*** **Mortality by allocated treatment in randomized trials of long-term beta blockade following myocardial infarction: odds ratios (active:control), together with approximately 95 or 99 per cent confidence ranges are shown —+— 95 per cent confidence range for trials that ran to scheduled finish, – –+– – 99 per cent confidence range for trials stopped early due to good/bad trend. Pooled data from ten trials with under 50 deaths are shown, individual results of thirteen trials are displayed, while pooled data from all twenty-three trials is shown at top (◆). *Center,* Mode of death (pooled data from 14 trials), and nonfatal reinfarction (pooled data from 20 trials) in long-term beta blocker trials that reported these end points separately (95 per cent confidence ranges). *Bottom,* Mortality in long-term beta blocker trials, by ancillary properties of agent tested. Pooled data from 14 beta blocker trials without intrinsic sympathomimetic activity (ISA) are compared to data from 11 trials of those with ISA; pooled data from 8 trials utilizing a cardioselective beta blocker are compared to data from 17 trials of drugs without cardioselectivity. (Adapted from Yusuf, S., et al.: Beta blockade during and after myocardial infarction: An overview of the randomized trials. Prog. Cardiovasc. Dis. *27*:335, 1985, by permission of Grune and Stratton.)**

negative inotropic effect, heart failure would complicate the administration of these agents to patients after AMI. Although a slight excess of clinical heart failure has been reported in some trials,[597] this difference appears to be at most trivial. Most studies have excluded patients with heart failure at entry, but even those including patients with mild failure do not show any increase in either death or subsequent heart failure.[597] Subgroup analysis of patients from the Norwegian timolol study showed a more marked ability to prevent sudden death in patients with cardiac enlargement than in patients with normal heart size.[944] In the BHAT trial propranolol decreased the incidence of sudden death by 13 per cent in patients without heart failure and by 47 per cent in patients who had prior failure.[945] Early administration of beta blockers may reduce the incidence of heart failure by improving ischemia and by preventing reinfarction. At least one of the large trials suggests that this concept may be accurate. In the Göteborg metoprolol trial, a similar percentage of patients developed heart failure after AMI (27 per cent in the metoprolol group and 30 per cent in the control group), but significantly less diuretic was required among metoprolol-treated patients than among controls.[946]

The mechanism by which beta blockers improve survival is not completely clear. It is likely that many factors are important, including control of hypertension and ischemia, an antiarrhythmic effect, perhaps an antiplatelet effect, an improvement in scar size, and possibly vascularity of the myocardium.[597] Blockade of the direct toxic effect of adrenergic stimulation on the myocardium may also be important. Since neither cardioselectivity or membrane-stabilizing activity appears to be requisite, the mechanism of beneficial effect appears to be due to a "class effect," i.e., it is secondary to beta blockade itself. The reduction in mortality is seen in all age groups for all types of infarction, and in all risk groups.

RECOMMENDATIONS. On the basis of currently available evidence, patients without a contraindication to beta blockade (asthma, moderate congestive heart failure, bradyarrhythmias) should have prophylactic treatment with beta blockers initiated after AMI. The dosage should be sufficient to blunt the heart rate response through stress or exercise. Since, in different trials, therapy has been initiated over a wide range of starting times (from hours to weeks) it is impossible to know which time is best from the available data. However, since the safety of early administration of beta blockers has been well documented,[936, 939] it is reasonable to suggest that beta blocker administration should begin as early as possible, certainly before hospital discharge, as long as contraindications are not present. A convenient time is *after* the patient has had any noninvasive stress test but before hospital discharge. Since much of the impact in preventing mortality occurs in the first few weeks, an excess degree of caution is not only unwarranted, but delay may lead to failure to prevent a proportion of early deaths.[597] It is unclear how long patients should be treated. While it is reasonable to conclude that treatment need not extend beyond the period when mortality curves no longer diverge, this rationale is problematic: Will discontinuation of therapy lead to increasing mortality in some patients? Do mortality curves actually continue to diverge? Will continuing the drug lead to some degree of continued protection? In the absence of answers to such questions, it is reasonable to suggest that therapy be continued for at least 2 years. At that time, if the beta blocker is well tolerated and if there is no reason to discontinue therapy, such therapy probably should be continued in most patients.

The 1 to 2 per cent overall reduction in patients after MI mortality that would come from long-term use of beta blockers and secondary prevention may seem small, but it is comparable to the reduction in mortality achieved by long-term antihypertensive therapy, and would result in the saving of approximately 6000 lives per year in the United States.[597] While it should not be considered "ethically imperative" to treat all post-infarction patients, the fact that over 35,000 patients have been randomized into placebo-controlled beta blocker trials does make it important that the clinician be aware of the results of these trials, and at least consider beta blocker therapy in AMI patients, including the elderly, who survive MI.[597, 947] Beta blockade should not be given to patients who have clear contraindications, and *probably* need not be given to patients with an *extremely* good prognosis (first AMI, good ventricular function, no angina, negative stress test, and no complex ventricular ectopy) in whom a mortality rate of less than 1 per cent per year can be anticipated.[948, 949]

Anticoagulants

There are at least three theoretical reasons for anticipating that anticoagulants might be beneficial in the management of AMI: (1) Since the coronary occlusion responsible for the AMI is often a thrombus (p. 1226), anticoagulants might be expected to halt or slow progression and to prevent the development of new thrombi elsewhere in the coronary arterial tree. (2) Anticoagulants might be expected to diminish the formation of mural thrombi and resultant systemic embolization. (3) Anticoagulants might be expected to reduce the incidence of venous thrombosis and pulmonary embolization.

Despite several decades of evaluation, the results of the treatment of AMI with anticoagulants are inconclusive. However, sporadic reports continue to appear of the favorable effects of anticoagulants on mortality among patients hospitalized with AMI.[950–953] Salutary effects on the underlying coronary disease, progression, or recurrence of infarction have not been clearly demonstrated with conventional anticoagulant drugs, yet it is probable that they decrease the incidence of cerebral emboli resulting from mural thrombi.[954] In addition, the administration of heparin in doses sufficient to influence activation of factor X without affecting conventional laboratory tests of the coagulation system substantially diminishes the incidence of deep vein thrombosis[955] and thereby reduces the incidence of pulmonary emboli. It appears advisable, therefore, to administer minidose heparin (5000 units subcutaneously) every 8 to 12 hours in the absence of specific contraindications.[956–958] The drug should be continued until 2 to 3 days before hospital discharge, although it is recognized that in patients with uncomplicated AMI's, there is no evidence that it reduces mortality.

In patients at high risk of embolism (e.g., those with ventricular aneurysm, marked obesity, cardiogenic shock, low output state, present or past thrombophlebitis, arterial or pulmonary embolism), in the absence of contraindications, anticoagulant treatment does exert a favorable effect on survival, and full-dose anticoagulation with heparin is indicated (e.g., intravenous administration of 10,000 units, followed by continuous infusion of 1000 units per hour) to maintain the clotting time and partial thromboplastin time at 1.5 to 2.0 times normal. After 5 to 7 days of therapy, warfarin or continued administration of subcutaneous, adjusted doses of heparin may be employed if conditions exist that suggest that venous thrombosis and embolism are likely to recur. These include continued or worsening heart failure, persistent thrombophlebitis, or the need for prolonged bed rest.

The long-term benefit of anticoagulants *following hospital discharge* is especially controversial. In one well-designed clinical trial on survivors of AMI exceeding 60 years of age, intensive and stable anticoagulant therapy reduced the risk of recurrent infarction and of cardiac death.[959] Among patients with demonstrated protuberant left ventricular thrombi following AMI, anticoagulation may reduce the risk of embolization.[900] However, review of well-designed acute phase[960] and long-term[961] anticoagulation trials have failed to show conclusively that anticoagulant administration lowers mortality in the phase after discharge. Anticoagulation does, however, clearly reduce the occurrence of thromboembolic complications. Therefore, it is reasonable to limit the use of chronic anticoagulants to patients in the post-hospital phase to those with specific indications, including thrombophlebitis, a history of pulmonary or systemic embolism, evidence of a mural thrombus in the left ventricle on two-dimensional echocardiography (Fig. 5–94, p. 123), and severe heart failure.[962]

Antiplatelet Agents

Secondary prevention trials with antiplatelet agents are based on the suggestion that platelets play a role in MI and sudden death by the participation of thrombi composed of platelet aggregates at the site of an atherosclerotic coronary artery narrowing, by aggregates obstructing microcoronary vessels, by the induction of coronary vasospasm, via the vasoconstrictor thromboxane A_2 produced by platelets, by their role in atherogenesis, and by their potential for causing arrhythmias. In two different careful reviews of the major secondary prevention aspirin trials performed over the last 15 years, opposite conclusions were reached about the efficacy of aspirin after AMI.[963, 964] Although seven of the eight trials reviewed showed a lower mean mortality with aspirin, the difference was statistically significant in only one (Table 56–3, p. 1776). Pooling of the data suggests that aspirin prophylaxis could result in at least a 10 per cent reduction in total deaths and a 20 per cent reduction in reinfarction.[963] The statistical validity of such pooling is questionable; therefore, the role of aspirin in secondary prevention is still unsettled. However, in the absence of contraindications to aspirin administration, particularly the history of peptic ulcer disease or gastrointestinal bleeding, we recommend 80 to 325 mg aspirin daily; this can be administered as an enteric-coated tablet. This dosage should minimize the risk of accompanying gastrointestinal side effects; the cost is low and inconvenience trivial. Although it is possible that sulfinpyrazone may also reduce the risk of sudden death and reinfarction after AMI,[965] there is no reason to anticipate that its antiplatelet effect is different from, or superior to, aspirin. Therefore, use of sulfinpyrazone in place of aspirin is not recommended.[966] The addition of dipyridamole to aspirin for possible potentiation of antiplatelet effect has not convincingly improved on the effect of aspirin alone[967, 968]; therefore, coadministration of dipyridamole is also not recommended as of this writing.

Other Measures

The effectiveness of secondary prevention with other agents, including calcium antagonists, antiarrhythmics, lipid-lowering drugs, prostacyclin analogs, and thromboxane synthetase inhibitors, requires further investigation.

CALCIUM ANTAGONISTS. Studies of verapamil[614] and nifedipine[609] have failed to show any benefit with the early administration of these agents. In fact, one study[610] has actually shown a higher early mortality (at 2 weeks) when nifedipine was given early to patients with threatened or acute MI. One trial in patients with non-Q-wave infarction showed a 50 per cent reduction in reinfarction in patients taking diltiazem compared with a randomized placebo-controlled group (Fig. 38–43).[612] In some patients at high risk for reinfarction, such therapy is warranted, but these patients generally undergo further investigation (p. 1292).

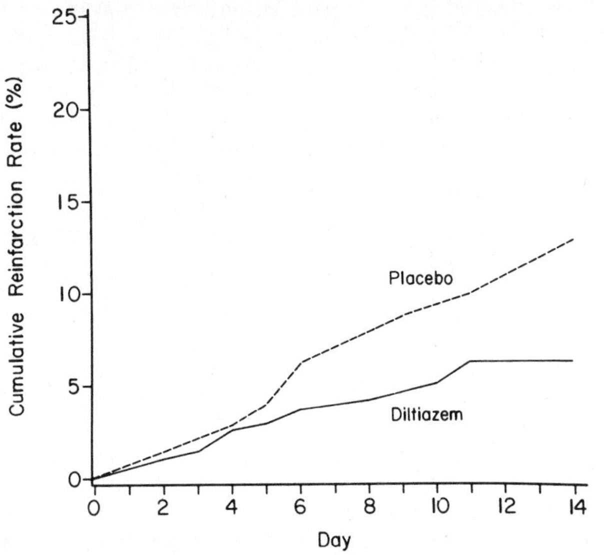

FIGURE 38–43. Life-table cumulative reinfarction rate, according to treatment group, from randomized study of 576 patients with non-Q-wave myocardial infarction. (From Gibson R. S., et al.: Diltiazem and reinfarction in patients with non-Q-wave myocardial infarction. N. Engl. J. Med. *315*:423, 1986.)

NITRATES. These agents are widely prescribed to patients following AMI, usually for prevention of recurrent ischemia. However, controlled trials to test the efficacy of this strategy have not been carried out, and such an approach cannot be recommended. In one retrospective study, patients treated with long-acting nitrates had a significantly lower mortality (10 per cent vs. 26 per cent) than those not receiving this therapy.[969] This observational study cannot be used as justification for applying such therapy to all patients unless a specific indication, such as continuing angina, is present.

ANTIARRHYTHMICS. While it has been recognized for decades that antiarrhythmic therapy can control atrial and ventricular arrhythmias effectively in many patients, such agents have never been shown conclusively to effect long-term mortality following AMI. Careful reviews of clinical trials have failed to suggest that routine use of these agents would be of any benefit.[960, 961] Even the newest agents do not appear to be of substantial benefit.[969a] Whether subgroups with complex arrhythmias should be treated remains unanswered by such studies, yet treatment of such patients with antiarrhythmic agents does seem reasonable in the absence of contraindications or newer data to the contrary.

RISK FACTOR MODIFICATION. This strategy applied following AMI also has not been shown convincingly to effect long-term mortality and morbidity by controlled studies. However, two trials are worthy of note. In the first, late follow-up (at a mean of 15 years) from the Coronary Drug Project, begun in 1966, has revealed lower mortality among patients treated with niacin for its favorable effect on serum lipids.[970] Remarkably, this benefit was seen nearly 9 years after termination of the study, when patients were no longer taking niacin. Second, it is known that type A behavior (an excessive sense of time urgency and easily aroused hostility, p. 1884) can be improved by training techniques, and it has been reported, although not yet confirmed, that the use of such techniques following AMI may reduce significantly the risk of recurrent AMI and sudden death.[971] It is clearly prudent to follow strategies known to improve long-term cardiac risks such as encouraging smoking cessation, control of diabetes and hypertension if present, and treatment of elevated serum cholesterol or other prognostically unfavorable lipid profiles.

ASSESSMENT OF PROGNOSIS

Both short-term and long-term survival after AMI depend on a number of factors,[972, 973] the most important of which is the state of left ventricular function. Additional importance is ascribed to the severity and extent of the obstructive lesions in the coronary vascular bed perfusing residual viable myocardium.[974, 975] In other words, survival relates to the quantity of myocardium that has become necrotic and the quantity at risk of becoming necrotic. At one extreme, the prognosis is best for the patient with normal intrinsic coronary vessels whose completed infarction constitutes a small area (less than 5 per cent) of the left ventricle as a consequence of a coronary embolus and who has no jeopardized myocardium. At the other extreme is the patient with a massive infarct who is in cardiogenic shock and whose residual myocardium is perfused by markedly obstructed vessels; obviously, progression of atherosclerosis or lowering of perfusion pressure in these vessels will impair the function and viability of the residual myocardium on which left ventricular function depends. The situation may not be hopeless even in such a patient, however, since revascularization may abolish the threat to the jeopardized myocardium.

CLINICAL FACTORS. Soon after coronary care units were instituted, it became apparent that left ventricular function is an important early determinant of survival. Thus, Killip studied patients divided into four groups on the basis of the clinical severity of left ventricular failure as assessed by physical examination at the time of admission to the coronary care unit. As noted in Tables 38–2 and 38–13, hospital mortality from AMI depends directly on the severity of left ventricular dysfunction present at the time of admission.[976] Similarly, Peel[977] and Norris[978] and their collaborators developed clinical prognostic indices for patients with AMI. Although they used historical, electrocardiographic, and radiological data to predict hospital mortality, evidence of left ventricular failure heavily weigh these indices in the direction of poor prognosis.

Certain demographic and historical factors are associated with a poor prognosis after infarction, including female sex,[978a] age greater than 65 years, a history of diabetes mellitus, hypertension, prior angina pectoris, and previous myocardial infarction.[979, 980] *Diabetes mellitus*, in particular, appears to confer a three- to fourfold increase in risk[981]; whether this is due to accelerated atherosclerosis or some other characteristic induced by the diabetic state (such as a larger infarct size[982]) remains unclear.[983] Isolated elevation of systolic blood pressure and combined systolic and diastolic hypertension are also unfavorable prognostic factors.[984] Interestingly, however, patients whose blood pressure falls after AMI seem to have a worse prognosis than those whose blood pressure increases or remains unchanged.[984] There is also greater mortality after anterior wall MI than after inferior MI, even when corrected for infarct size.[985, 986] As has already been discussed, infarct extension (p. 1286) influences prognosis adversely. Poor prognosis comes from the loss of viable myocardium with the resulting larger area of infarction creating a greater compromise in overall ventricular function. Postinfarction angina generally connotes a less favorable prognosis because it indicates the presence of jeopardized myocardium[986a]; however, if it is due to coronary artery spasm rather than critical organic obstruction, prognosis may be relatively good.[987]

Although the incidence of unrecognized MI is less than that of clinically apparent MI,[252] the long-term prognosis from unrecognized infarction appears to be similar to, and as serious as, that following recognized infarction.[988] Although the risk of angina recurring after an unrecognized MI is less than after a clinically apparent MI, the incidence of late stroke and heart failure may be even greater among patients with unrecognized MI.[988]

Increasingly sophisticated statistical techniques have been applied to risk assessment following AMI. Madsen et al. have developed a discriminate function analysis score based on the presence or absence of four factors: heart failure, ventricular tachycardia, AV block, and previous infarction or extension of infarction.[989] The accuracy of this score has been tested in several different populations and is useful for predicting both the risk of reinfarction and that of death following AMI.[989] This group has also shown that reliable long-term prediction of outcome is possible using data from the first 24 hours of hospitalization,[990] without a substantial increase in accuracy when further data from the rest of the hospitalization are added.[991]

HEMODYNAMICS AND VENTRICULAR FUNCTION. Physiological evidence of compromised left ventricular function also correlates with hospital mortality in AMI,[992] as already discussed (Table 38–2). Thus, patients with hemodynamic (elevated pulmonary capillary wedge pressure and/or depressed cardiac index) or ventriculographic (depressed ejection fraction and elevated end-systolic volume by radionuclide angiography) evidence of left ventricular failure have a worse prognosis than patients without these findings.[993–996] Acute pulmonary edema with AMI, even if due to diastolic dysfunction and associated with a normal ejection fraction, can be used to identify a high-risk group.[997] However, the presence or absence of concomitant right ventricular dysfunction with AMI (usually with inferior MI) does *not* appear to influence long-term outcome.[998] The *chest roentgenogram* is also of prognostic value because patients with cardiomegaly after infarction do not fare as well as individuals without this feature.

Because impaired ventricular function generally is a manifestation of the cumulative extent of myocardial damage sustained, one important determinant of prognosis is *infarct size*. This may be determined from an analysis of CK (or CK-MB) samples obtained at frequent intervals[271] or less accurately from analysis of the peak enzyme level. Thus, patients with markedly elevated plasma enzyme levels (CK > 2000 IU) often manifest left ventricular failure with concomitant poor prognosis. Furthermore, prognosis for as long as 4 years after an initial infarction is related to infarct size estimated from plasma CK time-activity curves at the time of the acute episode[306] (Fig. 38–16, p. 1250). A large defect or multiple defects on a thallium-201 perfusion scintigram obtained early in the course of AMI, also presumably related to infarct size, is associated with a high incidence of mortality or subsequent cardiac events.[995, 998] Similarly, patients with large infarcts on technetium-99m scintigrams have an adverse prognosis.[352, 999]

Experimental evidence suggests that an intervention aimed at improving ventricular function and ventricular remodeling after AMI (p. 1232), such as vasodilator therapy with captopril, may lessen ventricular dilatation and improve survival in the chronic phase of infarction.[1000] A trial is now under way to assess the possible benefit of this strategy in patients. Thus, in the future, ways may be found to improve upon the altered prognosis associated with large infarcts and compromised ventricular function.

Q-WAVE VERSUS NON-Q-WAVE INFARCTION. Myocardial infarction occurring without the development of new Q waves has been called subendocardial, nontransmural, and non-Q-wave infarction. However, the correlation between the electrocardiographic findings of transmural or subendocardial myocardial infarction and the pathological counterparts is not good.[326] Indeed, many patients with pathological transmural infarctions have no Q waves or have loss of R waves and vice versa. Consequently, it has been suggested that the description of MI based on electrocardiographic findings be confined to what is actually observed on the electrocardiogram—that is, "Q-wave" and "non-Q-wave" infarctions.

The acute mortality in patients with non-Q-wave infarcts is approximately half of that in patients with Q-wave infarcts,[456, 1001, 1002] unless early recurrent infarction or infarct extension occurs, in which case mortality is similar to that for Q-wave infarction.[456] Patients with non-Q-wave infarction tend to have smaller infarctions initially and only infrequently have total occlusions of the infarct-related vessel when compared with patients with Q-wave infarction.[22, 1002] Consistent with this finding are a lower incidence of heart failure early after infarction (as a consequence of a lesser degree of ventricular function impairment), and more frequent angina (related to the presence of preserved myocardium with marginal blood supply).[1002–1004] However, it is now clear that uncomplicated non-Q-wave infarctions are not benign conditions.[329, 1003–1006] Thus, 60 per cent of these patients have critical obstruction in two or three of the major coronary arteries, and approximately 20 per cent go on to develop an acute Q-wave infarction within 3 months of the non-Q-wave infarct.[1007] In one series almost half of the patients with non-Q-wave infarction developed unstable angina during a follow-up period averaging 11 months.[1008] In another, the incidence of infarct extension or early recurrent infarction was high.[1007] Hutter et al. have reported high early and late reinfarction rates in patients with "subendocardial" infarctions and comparable late mortalities in patients with both types of infarctions.[1001] In-hospital extension of a non-Q-wave infarction appears to increase long-term risk, with a doubling of one-year mortality in one study.[1009]

Thus, it is clear that patients with non-Q-wave infarctions have a natural history different from that in patients with Q-wave infarction. The former may be considered relatively unstable conditions associated with a low initial mortality rate, a high risk of later infarction, and a high late mortality rate. The recognition of differences between the natural histories of these two forms of infarction suggests the need for a more aggressive diagnostic approach, including coronary arteriography perhaps followed by early coronary angioplasty[1009a] or surgical treatment even in selected asymptomatic patients who have sustained an acute non-Q-wave infarction.

Despite the logic inherent in this approach, there is no firm evidence that this strategy influences the course favorably, although it has been shown that the calcium antagonist diltiazem may be effective in preventing early recurrent MI and angina following non-Q-wave infarction. A multicenter study of this intervention in over 500 randomized patients showed a 50 per cent reduction in the cumulative incidence of such events 2 weeks after infarction (Fig. 38–43).[612]

All patients with evidence of recurrent ischemia after infarction (regardless of location or ECG configuration) should receive medical therapy (bedrest, oxygen, nitrates, beta blockers, and calcium antagonists as tolerated) and should be considered for revascularization if this is appropriate (Chap. 39). However, it is particularly important to carefully follow symptomatic patients with non-Q-wave infarction because of the frequent presence of jeopardized but viable myocardium in such patients. Symptoms of recurrent angina or findings on noninvasive testing compatible with ischemia should be pursued vigorously and treated appropriately.[1010]

ELECTROCARDIOGRAM. Patients whose electrocardiogram demonstrates persistent advanced heart block (e.g., Mobitz type II, second-degree, or third-degree atrioventricular block) or new intraventricular conduction abnormalities (bifascicular or trifascicular) in the course of an AMI have a worse prognosis than do patients without these abnormalities (Table 38–10). Other electrocardiographic findings that augur poorly for the postinfarction patient are repetitive ventricular ectopic activity (Table 38–9) (couplets, runs), persistent horizontal or downsloping ST-segment depression and Q waves in multiple leads, atrial arrhythmias (especially atrial fibrillation), voltage criteria for left ventricular hypertrophy, and an abnormal signal-averaged electrocardiogram (on a specially filtered and processed QRS complex).[1010a, 1010b, 1010c]

ST-segment depressions in leads other than those with acute Q waves are also a poor prognostic sign; for example, patients with acute inferior wall infarcts who demonstrate ST-segment depressions in precordial leads have a worse prognosis than do patients without this finding. There is controversy concerning whether these ST-segment depressions reflect reciprocal electrical changes, associated disease of the left anterior descending coronary artery, or, most likely, a larger inferior infarct.[331–335, 1011] Similarly, patients who develop angina during the first 10 days following infarction, with new electrocardiographic changes distant from the acute infarct, i.e., angina "at a distance," have a distinctly worse prognosis than do patients having postinfarct angina with ischemia in the infarct zone.[330]

LATE POSTINFARCT ASSESSMENT OF PROGNOSIS

Following recovery from AMI—i.e., by 10 days to 6 weeks after the event—long-term prognosis can be evaluated by ambulatory electrocardiographic monitoring and exercise testing.[972, 1012] The development of ST-segment abnormalities, typical angina or exercise limitation by dyspnea at low levels of exercise (heart rate < 120 beats/min or exercise duration < 6 minutes on the Bruce protocol [p. 229]), and a major (> 2 mm) ST-segment depression and a stress-induced fall in blood pressure at any level of exercise signify a poor prognosis.[1013–1018] A predischarge submaximal exercise test is useful for early screening and can detect ischemia and arrhythmias among patients in whom these clinical features were not necessarily apparent during their hospital stay.[1019–1021] However, maximal stress tests performed 4 to 6 weeks later identify a significantly greater number of patients with residual myocardial ischemia.[1022, 1023] Radionuclide angiography,[1024, 1025] echocardiography,[374, 377] thallium scintigraphy,[1019] as well as coronary arteriography and left ventriculography, can provide additional important prognostic information. However, the invasive tests are ordinarily carried out only if the patient is symptomatic or if the noninvasive tests suggest a poor prognosis and if the results of these examinations would alter the management (Chap. 39).[1007, 1026] A progressive increase in one-year mortality is seen as ejection fraction, as measured by radionuclide angiography during hospitalization, falls below 0.40 (Fig. 38–44).[1027] Evidence indicates that electrical instability, as reflected in frequent, multiple, or complex ventricular extrasystoles, and left ventricular dysfunction, as reflected in a depressed left ventricular ejection fraction (< 40 per cent) 10 days after the occurrence of an AMI, are independent risk factors[1028]; the presence of both risk factors was associated with an increased 15-month mortality.[972, 1029, 1030]

Despite the clear prognostic importance of severe ventricular ectopy when detected during in-patient bedside or ambulatory monitoring, studies utilizing invasive programmed ventricular stimulation have provided conflicting evidence that ventricular arrhythmias provoked by this technique have any prognostic significance.[1017, 1031, 1032] Patients who develop sustained ventricular tachycardia or fibrillation spontaneously in the early recovery period are

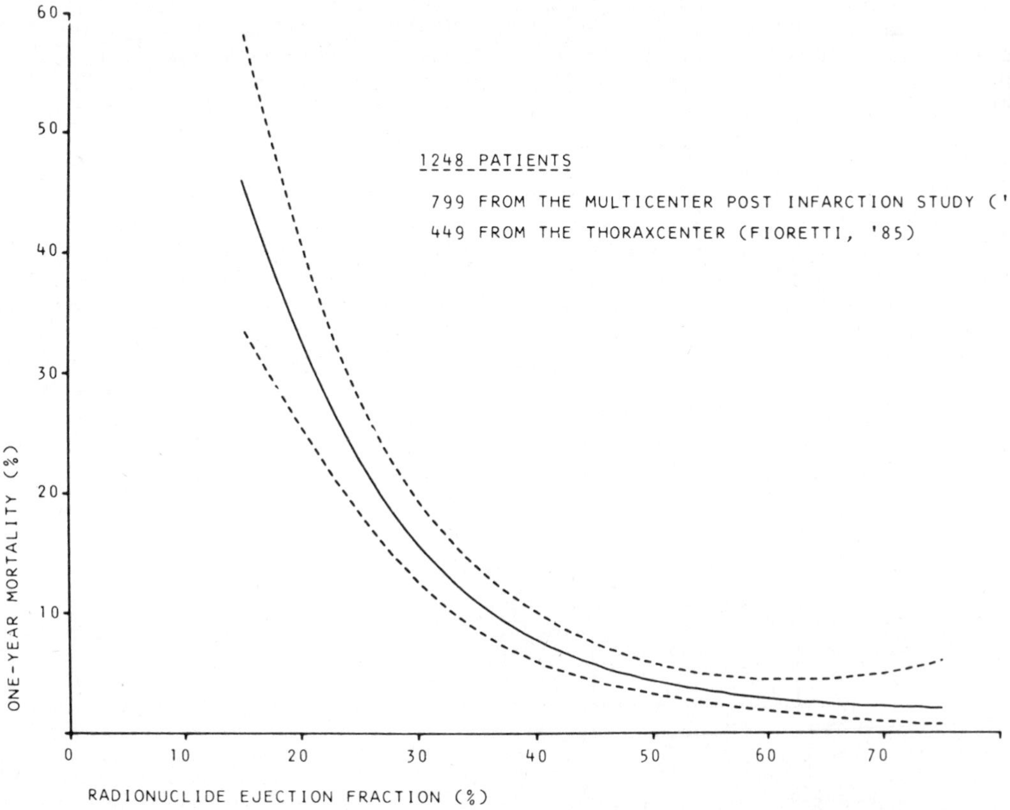

FIGURE 38–44. One-year mortality as a function of radionuclide ejection fraction (per cent) measured at hospital discharge after acute myocardial infarction. The solid line between the *dashed lines* indicates the corresponding 95 per cent confidence interval. The calculations are based on pooled data from the Multicenter Postinfarction Study and the Thoraxcenter. (From Serray, P. W., et al.: Preservation of global and regional left ventricular function after early thrombolysis in acute myocardial infarction. J. Am. Coll. Cardiol. *7*:729, 1986. By permission of the American College of Cardiology.)

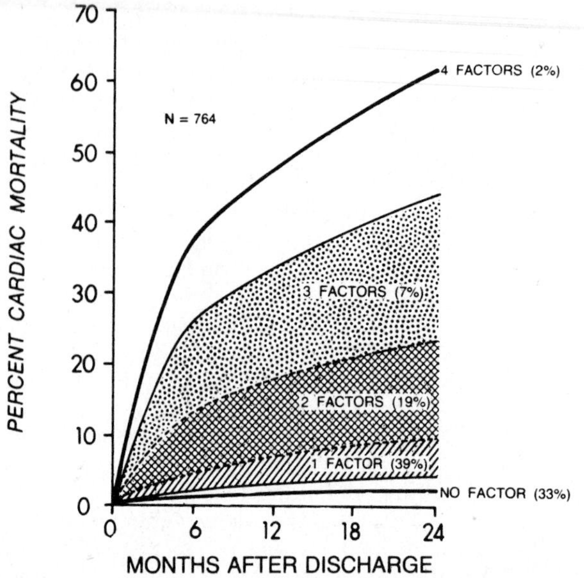

FIGURE 38–45. Mortality curves and zones of risk, according to number of risk factors. Individual risk factors included New York Heart Association functional classes II through IV (not class I) before admission, pulmonary rales, occurrence of 10 or more ventricular ectopic depolarizations per hour, and a radionuclide ejection fraction below 0.40. The variation of risk within each zone reflects the spectrum of relative risk for individual factors as well as the range of multiplicative risks for combinations of two and three factors. The numbers in the parentheses denote the percentage of the population with the specified number of factors. (From The Multicenter Post-infarction Research Group: Risk stratification and survival after myocardial infarction. N. Engl. J. Med. *309*:331, 1983.)

at increased risk of sudden cardiac death following hospital discharge. Control of ventricular arrhythmias in such patients, by medical and (if necessary) surgical therapy, may improve long-term mortality but has not been shown definitely to do this.[1033] When considered together, the combination of clinical factors, radionuclide ejection fraction, and frequent ventricular extrasystoles as detected from ambulatory monitoring can provide an accurate assessment of prognosis—not surprisingly, the more risk factors present, the greater mortality at any time following AMI (Fig. 38–45).[12, 1027]

Use of readily available clinical variables and exercise electrocardiography is probably sufficient for risk stratification in most patients following AMI. The additional techniques of echocardiography, radionuclide angiography, thallium-201 scintigraphy (if necessary with dipyridamole), and ambulatory electrocardiography should probably be reserved for (1) patients who cannot undergo exercise electrocardiography, (2) those in whom it is not diagnostic, e.g. patients with left bundle branch block, and (3) those who are already thought to be at relatively high risk and in whom a search for specific risks (e.g. ventricular arrhythmia, myocardial dysfunction, or left ventricular thrombus) is appropriate and might lead to specific forms of therapy.[1034]

While there are many different strategies for the overall assessment of prognosis following AMI, a consensus approach has been formulated and is presented in Figure 38–46. This approach is based on the recognition that an increase in cardiac risk results from left ventricular dysfunction, reflecting damaged myocardium as well as provokable ischemia, and reflecting myocardium at risk.[1035] The strategy outlined is directed at identifying patients at more than low risk who can expect some benefit from anticipated interventions. Unfortunately, in patients at greatest risk—those with very severe left ventricular dysfunction—most currently available medical and surgical therapies are of little long-term benefit.

RECOMMENDATIONS. On the basis of the above information, and in particular on the prognostic stratification shown in Figure 38–46, the following general approach to the post-MI patient is proposed. In the first 5 days of hospitalization invasive or noninvasive testing generally is not necessary for patients with uncomplicated AMI. However, if ischemia recurs after the first 24 hours, at any time before discharge, and is not readily controlled by medical therapy, and if the patient is a suitable candidate for revascularization, consideration should be given to proceeding with early cardiac catheterization and coronary arteriography to define the coronary anatomy and assess left ventricular function. Following AMI symptoms secondary to left ventricular dysfunction should be treated medically unless accompanied by evidence of reversible ischemia (angina, electrocardiographic changes, and/or reversible thallium-201 defects on imaging following an exercise stress test).

Before hospital discharge, patients without evidence of overt pump failure or ischemia and whose overall medical condition permits (e.g., excluding the very elderly or those with serious associated systemic diseases), should undergo noninvasive testing. For most patients this means limited exercise stress (treadmill or bicycle) electrocardiography combined with thallium imaging for those with marked resting ECG abnormalities, or radionuclide ventriculography for those in whom an assessment of left ventricular function has not been obtained already (by echocardiography, for example). Patients at high risk of recurrent MI or death should have cardiac catheterization and coronary

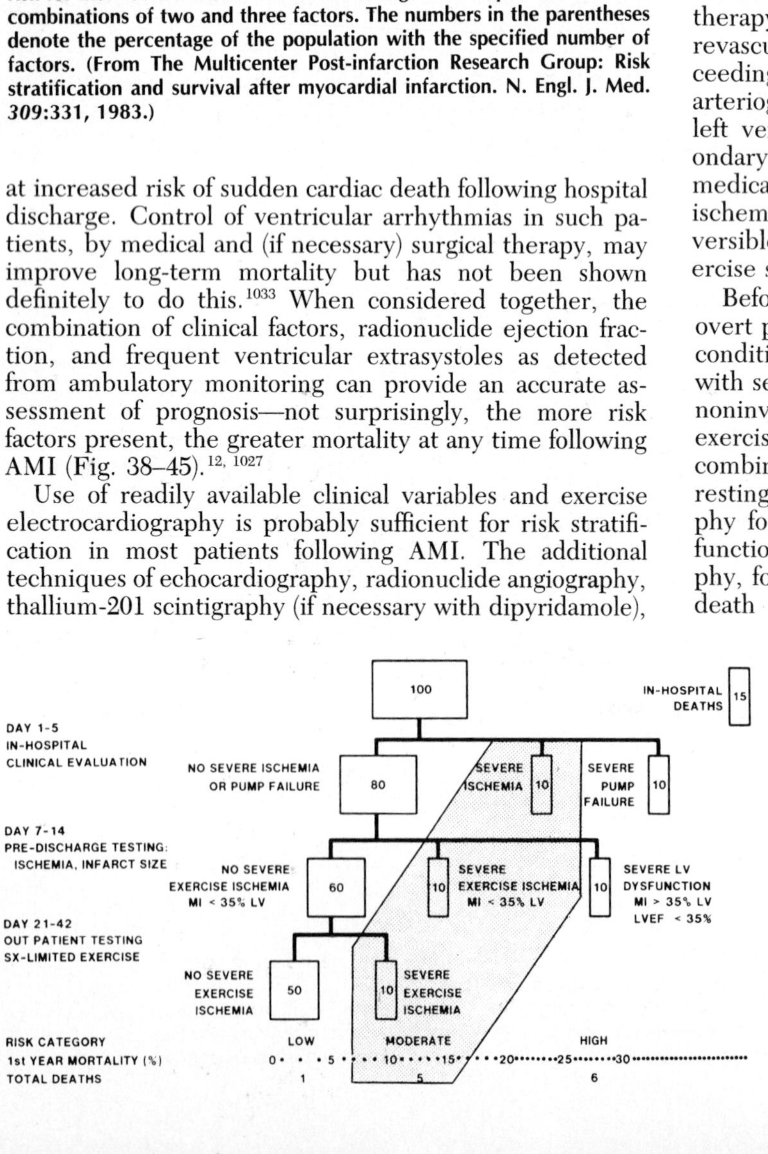

FIGURE 38–46. Prognostic stratification after acute myocardial infarction. The size of each patient subset (numbers in boxes) in the algorithm is approximate and will vary according to the patient population. Stratification of patients into the three main risk categories (low, moderate, and high) is based on the extent of myocardial ischemia (MI) and left ventricular (LV) dysfunction. A variety of clinical observations and tests may be used to detect these abnormalities at various times after acute myocardial infarction. Patients in the shaded area are those most likely to experience a reduction in mortality from coronary revascularization. LVEF = left ventricular ejection fraction, SX = symptom. (From DeBusk, R. F., et al.: Identification and treatment of low-risk patients after acute myocardial infarction and coronary-artery bypass graft surgery. N. Engl. J. Med. *314*:161, 1986.)

arteriography. This includes patients with angina induced at a low level of exercise, particularly if associated with marked ECG changes (ST depressions >0.2 mV or serious electrical instability). Others in this category are those with a large reversible defect on thallium-201 imaging and those with an exercise-induced fall in left ventricular ejection fraction (more than 5 to 10 per cent) on radionuclide ventriculography. If exercise testing is negative or only mildly positive (in which case antianginal agents should be administered), the patient may be discharged.

The predischarge exercise test is useful not only for the detection of ischemia, arrhythmias, or symptoms of left ventricular dysfunction, but it also serves the patient and physician as a useful guide in developing activity recommendations and limitations for the early post-MI period. Patients with ventricular ectopy during hospitalization and those with severe left ventricular dysfunction should generally undergo ambulatory electrocardiographic monitoring before discharge as well. If malignant ventricular arrhythmias (frequent VPB's, couplets, or bouts of ventricular tachycardia) are detected, we recommend treatment with antiarrhythmic agents, recognizing that the value of this approach has not been established definitively.

Four to six weeks after hospital discharge, further noninvasive testing, including maximal (symptom-limited) exercise stress testing, is appropriate for patients who are suitable candidates for revascularization (and have not already undergone such therapy). This would include those patients not already selected for invasive work-up by prior testing, those not suffering from associated debilitating diseases and those not very elderly—in other words, all patients for whom the results of noninvasive testing might lead to a change in the treatment program and for whom that change could affect the prognosis favorably. Catheterization and arteriography should be performed in patients whose noninvasive work-up suggests the presence of remaining jeopardized myocardium following AMI. Proceeding with an invasive work-up is therefore a consideration in any patient with a positive exercise stress test in the post-MI period. However angiography is most strongly indicated in patients who have an exercise-induced fall in blood pressure, signs or symptoms of ischemia at a low workload, more than 0.2 mV of ST-segment depression on exercise electrocardiography, large (or multiple) reversible defects on thallium-201 imaging, or a marked fall in left ventricular ejection fraction with exercise radionuclide ventriculography.

REFERENCES

INTRODUCTION

1. American Heart Association: 1987 Heart Facts. Dallas, American Heart Association National Center.
2. Weinstein, M. C., and Stason, W. B.: Cost-effectiveness of interventions to prevent or treat coronary heart disease. Ann. Rev. Public Health 6:41, 1985.
3. Peli, S., and Fayerweather, W. E.: Trends in the incidence of myocardial infarction and in associated mortality and morbidity in a large employed population, 1957–1983. N. Engl. J. Med. *312*:1005, 1985.
4. Pryor, D. B., Harrell, F. E., Jr., Lee, K. L., Califf, R. M., and Rosati, R. A.: An improving prognosis over time in medically treated patients with coronary artery disease. Am. J. Cardiol. 52:444, 1983.
5. Gillum, R. F., Folsom, A., Luepker, R. V., Jacobs, D. R., Jr., Kottke, T. E., Gomez-Marin, O., Prineas, R. J., Taylor, H. L., and Blackburn, H.: Sudden death and acute myocardial infarction in a metropolitan area, 1970–1980. N. Engl. J. Med. *309*:1353, 1983.
6. Elveback, L. R., and Connolly, D. C.: Coronary heart disease in residents of Rochester, Minnesota. V. Prognosis of patients with coronary heart disease based on initial manifestation. Mayo Clin. Proc. *60*:305, 1985.
7. Stern, M. P.: The recent decline in ischemic heart disease mortality. Ann. Intern. Med. *91*:630, 1979.
8. Kannel, W. B.: Meaning of the downward trend in cardiovascular mortality. J.A.M.A. *247*:877, 1982.
9. Goldman, L., and Cook, E. F.: The decline in ischemic heart disease mortality rates. An analysis of the comparative effects of medical interventions and changes in lifestyle. Ann. Intern. Med. *101*:825, 1984.
10. Beaglehole, R.: Medical management and the decline in mortality from coronary heart disease. Br. Med. J. *292*:33, 1986.
11. Norris, R. M.: Myocardial Infarction. New York, Churchill Livingstone, 1982, 322 pp.
12. Ong, L., Green, S., Reiser, P., and Morrison, J.: Early prediction of mortality in patients with acute myocardial infarction: A prospective study of clinical and radionuclide risk factors. Am. J. Cardiol. *57*:33, 1986.
13. Gillespie, T. A., and Sobel, B. E.: A rationale for therapy of acute myocardial infarction: Limitation of infarct size. Adv. Intern. Med. *22*:319, 1976.
14. Spann, J. F.: Changing concepts of pathophysiology, prognosis, and therapy in acute myocardial infarction. Am. J. Med. *74*:877, 1983.
15. Rude, R. E., Muller, J. E., and Braunwald, E.: Efforts to limit the size of myocardial infarcts. Ann. Intern. Med. *95*:736, 1981.
16. Lange, L. G., and Sobel, B. E.: Pharmacological salvage of myocardium. Ann. Rev. Pharmacol. Toxicol. *22*:115, 1982.
17. Laffel, G. L., and Braunwald, E.: Thrombolytic therapy. A new strategy for treatment of acute myocardial infarction. N. Engl. J. Med. *311*:710, 770, 1984.
18. Yusuf, S., Collins, R., Peto, R., Furberg, C., Stampfer, M. J., Goldhaber, S. Z., and Hennekens, C. H.: Intravenous and intracoronary fibrinolytic therapy in acute myocardial infarction: Overview of results on mortality, reinfarction, and side effects from 33 randomized control trials. Eur. Heart J. *6*:556, 1985.
19. Gruppo Italiano Per Lo Studio Della Streptochinasi Nell'Infarcto Miocardico (GISSI): Effectiveness of Intravenous thrombolytic treatment in acute myocardial infarction. Lancet *1*:397, 1986.
20. Braunwald, E.: The aggressive treatment of acute myocardial infarction. Circulation *71*:1087, 1985.

PATHOLOGY OF ACUTE MYOCARDIAL INFARCTION

21. Freifeld, A. G., Schuster, E. H., and Bulkley, B. H.: Nontransmural versus transmural myocardial infarction. Am. J. Med. *75*:423, 1983.
22. DeWood, M. A., Stifter, W. F., Simpson, C. S., Spores, J., Eugster, G. S., Judge, T. P., and Hinnen, M. L.: Coronary arteriographic findings soon after non-Q wave myocardial infarction. N. Engl. J. Med. *315*:417, 1986.
23. Nixon, J. V.. Right ventricular myocardial infarction. Arch. Intern. Med. *142*:945, 1982.
24. Haupt, H. M., Hutchins, G. M., and Moore, G. W.: Right ventricular infarction: Role of the moderator band artery in determining infarct size. Circulation *67*:1268, 1983.
25. Baigrie, R. S., Haq, A., Morgan, C. D., Rakowski, H., Drobac, M., and McLaughlin, P.: The spectrum of right ventricular involvement in inferior wall myocardial infarction: A clinical hemodynamic and noninvasive study. J. Am. Coll. Cardiol. *1*:1396, 1983.
26. Shah, P. K., Maddahi, J., Berman, D. S., Pichler, M., and Swan, H. J. C.: Scintigraphically detected predominant right ventricular dysfunction in acute myocardial infarction: Clinical and hemodynamic correlates and implications for therapy and prognosis. J. Am. Coll. Cardiol. *6*:1264, 1985.
27. Kopelman, H. A., Forman, M. B., Wilson, B. H., Kolodgie, F. D., Smith, R. F., Friesinger, G. C., and Virmani, R.: Right ventricular myocardial infarction in patients with chronic lung disease: Possible role of right ventricular hypertrophy. J. Am. Coll. Cardiol. *5*:1302, 1985.
28. Laurie, W., and Woods, J. D.: Infarction (ischemic fibrosis) in the right ventricle of the heart. Acta Cardiol. *18*:399, 1963.
29. Wade, W. G.: The pathogenesis of infarction of the right ventricle. Br. Heart J. *21*:545, 1957.
30. Cushing, E. H., Feil, H. S., Stanton, E. J., and Wartman, W. B.: Infarction of the cardiac auricles (atria): Clinical, pathological and experimental studies. Br. Heart J. *4*:17, 1942.
31. Lowe, T. E., and Wartman, W. B.: Myocardial infarction. Br. Heart J. *6*:115, 183, 1944.
32. Gould, S. E., and Ioannides, G.: Ischemic heart disease. *In* Gould, S. E. (ed.): Pathology of the Heart and Blood Vessels. 3rd ed. Springfield, Charles C Thomas, 1968, p. 613.
33. Bloor, C. M.: Cardiac Pathology. Philadelphia, J. B. Lippincott Co., 1978, p. 176.
34. Mallory, G. K., White, P. D., and Salcedo-Salger, J.: The speed of healing of myocardial infarction: A study of the pathological anatomy in 72 cases. Am. Heart J. *18*:647, 1939.
35. Fishbein, M. C., Maclean, D., and Maroko, P. R.: The histopathological evolution of myocardial infarction. Chest *73*:843, 1978.
36. Buja, L. M., and Willerson, J. T.: Clinicopathologic correlates of acute ischemic heart disease syndromes. Am. J. Cardiol. *47*:343, 1981.
37. Schlesinger, M. J., and Reiner, L.: Focal myocytolysis of the heart. Am. J. Pathol. *31*:443, 1955.
38. Bouchardy, B., and Majno, G.: Histopathology of early myocardial infarcts. Am. J. Physiol. *74*:301, 1974.
39. Derias, N. W., and Adams, C. W. M.: The nonspecific nature of the myocardial wave fiber. Histopathology *3*:241, 1979.
39a. Chatelain, P., Latour, J. G., Tran, D., de Lorgeril, M., Dupras, G., and Bourassa, M.: Neutrophil accumulation in experimental myocardial infarcts: Relation with extent of injury and effect of reperfusion. Circulation *75*:1083, 1987.
40. Kloner, R. A., Ganote, C. E., Whalen, D. A., Jr., and Jennings, R. B.: Effect of a transient period of ischemia on myocardial cells: Fine structure during the first few minutes of reflow. Am. J. Pathol. *74*:399, 1974.
41. Willerson, J. T., Hillis, L. D., and Buja, L. M.: Ischemic Heart Disease. New York, Raven Press, 1982, 374 pp.

42. Kloner, R. A., Rude, R. E., Carlson, N., Maroko, P. R., Karaffa, S., DeBoer, L. W. V., and Braunwald, E.: Ultrastructural evidence of microvascular damage and myocardial cell injury after coronary artery occlusion: Which comes first? Circulation *62*:945, 1980.
43. Kloner, R. A., and Braunwald, E.: Review—Observations on experimental myocardial ischemia. Cardiovasc. Res. *14*:371, 1980.
44. Kloner, R. A., DeBoer, L. W. V., Carlson, N., and Braunwald, E.: The effect of verapamil on myocardial ultrastructure during and following release of coronary artery occlusion. Exp. Mol. Pathol. *36*:277, 1982.
45. Caulfield, J., and Klionsky, B.: Myocardial ischemia and early infarction. An electron microscopic study. Am. J. Pathol. *35*:489, 1959.
46. Jennings, R. B., and Ganote, C. E.: Structural change in myocardium during acute ischemia. Circ. Res. *35*(Suppl. 3):156, 1974.
47. Kloner, R. A., Fishbein, M. C., Hare, C. M., and Maroko, P. R.: Early ischemic ultrastructural and histochemical alterations in the myocardium of the rat following coronary artery occlusion. Exp. Mol. Pathol. *30*:129, 1979.
47a. Miyazaki, S., Fujiwara, H., Onodera, T., Kihara, Y., Matsuda, M., Wu, D. J., Nakamura, Y., Kumada, T., Sasayama, S., Kawai, C., and Hamashima, Y.: Quantitative analysis of contraction band and coagulation necrosis after ischemia and reperfusion in the porcine heart. Circulation *75*:1074, 1987.
48. Baroldi, G.: Different types of myocardial necrosis in coronary heart disease: A pathophysiologic review of their functional significance. Am. Heart J. *89*:742, 1875.
49. Hagler, H. K., Sherwin, L., and Buja, L. M.: Effect of different methods of tissue preparation on mitochondrial inclusions of ischemic and infarcted canine myocardium: Transmission and analytical electron microscopic study. Lab. Invest. *40*:529, 1979.
50. Hutchins, G. M., and Bulkley, B. H.: Correlation of myocardial contraction band necrosis and vascular patency: A study of coronary artery bypass graft anastomoses at branch points. Lab. Invest. *36*:642, 1977.
51. Kloner, R. A., Ellis, S. G., Lange, R., and Braunwald, E.: Studies of experimental coronary artery reperfusion: Effects on infarct size, myocardial function, biochemistry, ultrastructure, and microvascular damage. Circulation *68*:(Suppl I):I–8, 1983.
52. Herrick, J. B.: Clinical features of sudden obstruction of the coronary arteries. J.A.M.A. *59*:2015, 1912.
53. Blumgart, H. L., Schlesinger, M. J., and Davis, D.: Studies on the relation of the clinical manifestations of angina pectoris, coronary thrombosis, and myocardial infarction to the pathologic findings with particular reference to the significance of the collateral circulation. Am. Heart J. *19*:1, 1940.
54. Friedberg, C. K., and Horn, H.: Acute myocardial infarction not due to coronary artery occlusion. J.A.M.A. *112*:1675, 1939.
55. Miller, R. D., Burchell, H. B., and Edwards, J. E.: Myocardial infarction with and without acute coronary occlusion; a pathologic study. Arch. Intern. Med. *88*:597, 1951.
56. Roberts. W. C., and Jones, A. A.: Quantification of coronary arterial narrowing at necropsy in acute transmural myocardial infarction. Analysis and comparison of findings in 27 patients and 22 controls. Circulation *61*:786, 1980.
57. Betriu, A., Castaner, A., Sanz, G. A., Pare, J. C., Roig, E., Coll, S., Magrina, J., and Navarro-Lopez, F.: Angiographic finding 1 month after myocardial infarction: A prospective study of 259 survivors. Circulation *65*:1099, 1982.
58. Silver, M. D., Baroldi, G., and Mariani, F.: The relationship between acute occlusive coronary thrombi and myocardial infarction studied in 100 consecutive patients. Circulation *61*:219, 1980.
59. Rackley, C. E., Russell, R. O., Jr., Mantle, J. A., Rogers, W. J., Papapietro, S. E., and Schwartz, K. M.: Right ventricular infarction and function. Am. Heart J. *101*:215, 1981.
60. deFeyter, P. J., van den Brand, M., Serruys, P. W., and Wijns, W.: Early angiography after myocardial infarction: What have we learned? Am. Heart J. *109*:194, 1985.
61. Bristow, J. D., Burchell, H. B., Campbell, R. W., Ebert, P. A., Hall, R. J., Leonard, J. J., and Reeves, T.: Report of the Ad Hoc Committee on the indications for coronary arteriography. Circulation *55*:969A, 1977.
62. DeWood, M. A., Spores, J., Notske, R., Mouser, L. T., Burroughs, R., Golden, M. S., and Lang, H. T.: Prevalence of total coronary occlusion during the early hours of transmural myocardial infarction. N. Engl. J. Med. *303*:897, 1980.
63. Ganz, W., Buchbinder, N., Marcus, H., Mondkar, A., Madahi, J., Charuzi, Y., O'Connor, L., Shell, W., Fishbein, M. C., Kass, R., Miyamoto, A., and Swan, H. J. C.: Intracoronary thrombolysis in evolving myocardial infarction. Am. Heart J. *101*:4, 1981.
64. Timmis, G. C., Gangadharan, V., Hauser, A. M., Ramos, R. C., Westveer, D. C., and Gordon, S.: Intracoronary streptokinase in clinical practice. Am. Heart J. *104*:925, 1982.
65. deFeyter, P. J., van Eenige, M. J., van der Wall, E. E., Bezemer, P. D., van Engelen, C. L. J., Funke-Kupper, A. J., Kerkkamp, H. J. J., Visser, F. C., and Roos, J. P.: Effects of spontaneous and streptokinase-induced recanalization on left ventricular function after myocardial infarction. Circulation *67*:1039, 1983.
66. Ong, L., Reiser, P., Coromilas, J., Scherr, L., and Morrison, J.: Left ventricular function and rapid release of creatine kinase MB in acute myocardial infarction: Evidence for spontaneous reperfusion. N. Engl. J. Med. *309*:1, 1983.
67. DeWood, M. A., Notske, R. N., Simpson, C. S., Stifter, W. F., and Shields, J. P.: Prevalence and significance of spontaneous thrombolysis in transmural myocardial infarction. Eur. Heart J. *6*:33, 1985.
68. Pichard, A. D., Ziff, C., Rentrop, P., Holt, J., Blanke, H., and Smith, H.: Angiographic study of infarct-related coronary artery in the chronic stage of acute myocardial infarction. Am. Heart J. *106*:687, 1983.
69. Willerson, J. T., Campbell, W. B., Winniford, M. D., Schmitz, J., Apprill, P., Firth, B. G., Ashton, J., Smitherman, T., Bush, L., and Buja, L. M.: Conversion from chronic to acute coronary artery disease: Speculation regarding mechanisms. Am. J. Cardiol. *54*:1349, 1984.
70. Epstein, S. E., and Palmeri, S. T.: Mechanisms contributing to precipitation of unstable angina and acute myocardial infarction: Implications regarding therapy. Am. J. Cardiol. *54*:1245, 1984.
71. Alpert, J. S.: Coronary vasomotion, coronary thrombosis, myocardial infarction, and the camel's back. J. Am. Col. Cardiol. *5*:617, 1985.
71a. Feldman, R. L.: Editorial. Coronary thrombosis, coronary spasm and coronary atherosclerosis and speculation on the link between unstable angina and acute myocardial infarction. Am. J. Cardiol. *59*:1187, 1987.
72. Brosius, F. C., and Roberts, W. C.: Comparison of degree of and extent of coronary narrowing by atherosclerotic plaque in anterior and posterior transmural acute myocardial infarction. Circulation *64*:715, 1981.
73. Cabin, H. S., and Roberts, W. C.: Comparison of amount and extent of coronary narrowing by atherosclerotic plaque and of myocardial scarring at necropsy in anterior and posterior healed transmural myocardial infarction. Circulation *66*:93, 1982.
74. Levin, D. C., and Fallon, J. T.: Significance of the angiographic morphology of localized coronary stenoses: Histopathologic correlations. Circulation *66*:316, 1982.
75. Falk, E.: Plaque rupture with severe pre-existing stenosis precipitating thrombosis: Characteristics of coronary atherosclerotic plaque underlying fatal occlusion thrombi. Br. Heart J. *50*:127, 1983.
76. Davies, M. J., and Thomas, A. C.: Plaque fissuring—the cause of acute myocardial infarction, sudden ischemic death, and crescendo angina. Br. Heart J. *53*:363, 1985.
77. Forrester, J. S., Litvack, F., Grundfest, W., and Hickey, A.: A perspective of coronary disease seen through the arteries of a living man. Circulation *75*:505, 1987.
78. Wilson, R. F., Holida, M. D., and White, C. W.: Quantitative angiographic morphology of coronary stenoses leading to myocardial infarction or unstable angina. Circulation *73*:286, 1986.
79. Roberts, W. C.: The coronary arteries in fatal coronary events. *In* Chung, E. K. (ed.): Controversies in Cardiology. New York, Springer-Verlag, 1976, p. 1.
80. Ridolfi, R. L., and Hutchins, G. M.: Relationship between coronary artery lesions and myocardial infarcts: Ulceration of atherosclerotic plaques precipitating coronary thrombosis. Am. Heart J. *93*:468, 1977.
81. Mandelkorn, J. B., Wolf, N. M., Singh, S., Shechter, J. A., Kersh, R. I., Rodgers, D. M., Workman, M. B., Bentivoglio, L. G., LaPorte, S. M., and Meister, S. G.: Intracoronary thrombus in nontransmural myocardial infarction and in unstable angina pectoris. Am. J. Cardiol. *52*:1, 1983.
82. Davies, M. J., and Thomas, A.: Thrombosis and acute coronary-artery lesions in sudden cardiac ischemic death. N. Engl. J. Med. *310*:1137, 1984.
83. Falk, E.: Unstable angina with fatal outcome: Dynamic coronary thrombosis leading to infarction and/or sudden death. Circulation *71*:699, 1985.
84. Harker, L. A., and Ritchie, J. L.: The role of platelets in acute vascular events: Circulation *62*:(Suppl V):13, 1980.
85. Bergmann, S. R., Lerch, R. A., Mathias, C. J., Sobel, B. E., and Welch, M. J.: Noninvasive detection of coronary thrombi with In-111 platelets: Concise communication. J. Nucl. Med. *24*:130, 1983.
86. Fox, K. A. A., Bergmann, S. R., Mathias, C. J., Powers, W. J., Siegel, B. A., Welch, M. J., and Sobel, B. E.: Scintigraphic detection of coronary artery thrombi in patients with acute myocardial infarction. J. Am. Coll. Cardiol. *4*:975, 1984.
87. Hirsh, P., Campbell, W. B., Willerson, J. D., and Hillis, L. D.: Prostaglandins and ischemic heart disease. Am. J. Med. *71*:1009, 1981.
88. Mueller, H. S., Rao, P. S., Greenberg, M. A., Buttrick, P. M., Sussman, I. I., Levite, H. A., Grose, R. M., Perez-Davila, V., Strain, J. E., and Spaet, T. H.: Systemic and transcardiac platelet activity in acute myocardial infarction in man: Resistance to prostacyclin. Circulation *72*:1336, 1985.
89. Hamstein, A., Wiman, B., De Faire, U., Blomback, M.: Increased plasma levels of a rapid inhibitor of tissue plasminogen activator in young survivors of myocardial infarction. N. Engl. J. Med. *313*:1557, 1985.
90. Chandler, A. B.: Relationship of coronary thrombosis to myocardial infarction. Mod. Concepts Cardiovasc. Dis. *44*:1, 1975.
91. Barold, G.: Pathological anatomy of myocardial infarction. *In* Wilhelmsen, L., and Hjalmarson, A. (eds.): Acute and Long-Term Medical Management of Myocardial Ischemia. Sweden, Mölndal, 1978, p. 41.
92. Mathey, D. G., Kuck, K. H., Tilsner, V., Krebber, H. J., and Bleifeld, W.: Nonsurgical coronary artery recanalization in acute myocardial infarction. Circulation *63*:489, 1981.
93. Rentrop, P., Blanke, H., Karsch, K. R., Kaiser, H., Kostering, H., and Leitz, K.: Selective intracoronary thrombolysis in acute myocardial infarction and unstable angina pectoris. Circulation *63*:307, 1981.
94. Markis, J. E., Malagold, M., Parker, J. A., Silverman, K. J., Barry, W. H., Als, A. V., Paulin, S., Grossman, W., and Braunwald, E.: Myocardial salvage after intracoronary thrombolysis with streptokinase in acute myocardial infarction. N. Engl. J. Med. *305*:777, 1981.
95. Gagnon, R. M., Morissette, M., Bensimon, H., Beaudet, R., Poirier, N., Noel, C., Presant, S., and Lemire, J.: The role of coronary thrombosis in myocardial infarction: Further evidence shown by intracoronary thrombolysis with streptokinase. Cathet. Cardiovasc. Diagn. 8:393, 1982.

96. Sherman, C. T., Litvack, F., Grundfest, W., Lee, M., Hickey, A., Chaux, A., Kass, R., Blanche, C., Matloff, J., Morgenstern, L., Ganz, W., Swan, H. J. C., and Forrester, J.: Coronary angioscopy in patients with unstable angina pectoris. N. Engl. J. Med. *315*:913, 1986.
97. Conti, C. R.: Myocardial infarction: Thoughts about pathogenesis and the role of coronary artery spasm. Am. Heart J. *110*:187, 1985.
98. Gertz, S. D., Merin, G., Pasternak, R. C., Gotsman, M. S., Blaumanis, O. R., and Nelson, E.: Endothelial damage and thrombosis following partial coronary artery constriction: Relevance to the pathogenesis of myocardial infarction. Israel J. Med. Sci. *14*:384, 1978.
99. Maseri, A., L'Abbate, A., Chierchia, S., Parodi, O., Severi, S., Biagini, A., Distante, A., Marzilli, M., and Ballerstra, A. M.: Significance of spasm in the pathogenesis of ischemic heart disease. Am. J. Cardiol. *44*:788, 1979.
100. Marzilli, M., Goldstein, S., Trivella, M. G., Palumbo, C., and Maseri, A.: Some clinical considerations regarding the relation of coronary vasospasm to coronary atherosclerosis: A hypothetical pathogenesis. Am. J. Cardiol. *45*:882, 1980.
101. Oliva, P. B., and Breckenridge, J. C.: Arteriographic evidence of coronary arterial spasm in acute myocardial infarction. Circulation *56*:366, 1977.
102. Cipriano, P. R., Koch, F. H., Rosenthal, S. M. K., Baim, D. S., Ginsburg, R., and Schroeder, J. S.: Myocardial infarction in patients with coronary artery spasm demonstrated by angiography. Am. Heart J. *105*:542, 1983.
103. Bertrand, M. E., Leblanche, J. M., Tilmant, P. Y., Thieuleux, F. A., Delforge, M. G., and Chahine, R. A.: The provocation of coronary arterial spasm in patients with recent transmural myocardial infarction. Eur. Heart J. *4*:532, 1983.
104. Benacerraf, A., Scholl, J. M., Achard, F., Tonnelier, M., and Lavergne, G.: Coronary spasm and thrombosis associated with myocardial infarction in a patient with nearly normal coronary arteries. Circulation *67*:1147, 1983.
105. Vincent, G. M., Anderson, J. L., and Marshall, H. W.: Coronary spasm producing coronary thrombosis and myocardial infarction. N. Engl. J. Med. *309*:220, 1983.
106. Friedrich, T., Lichey, J., Nigam, S., Priesnitz, M., and Wegscheider, K.: Follow-up of prostaglandin plasma levels after an acute myocardial infarction. Am. Heart J. *109*:222, 1985.
107. Gorlin, R.: Coronary collaterals. *In* Coronary Artery Disease. Philadelphia, W. B. Saunders Company, 1976, p. 59.
108. Markis, J. E., Brewer, C. C., Alderman, J., McKay, R. G., Forman, S., Braunwald, E., and TIMI Investigators: Myocardial infarction without early coronary angiographic evidence of occlusion: The NHLBI thrombolysis in myocardial infarction trial (TIMI). Circulation 72(Suppl. III):56, 1985.
109. Schwartz, H., Leiboff, R. H., Bren, G. B., Wasserman, A. G., Katz, R. J., Varghese, P. J., Sokil, A. B., and Ross, A. M.: Temporal evolution of the human coronary collateral circulation after myocardial infarction. J. Am. Coll. Cardiol. *4*:1088, 1984.
110. Nitzberg, W. D., Nath, H. P., Rogers, W. J., Hood, W. P., Whitlow, P. L., Reeves, R., and Baxley, W. A.: Collateral flow in patients with acute myocardial infarction. Am. J. Cardiol. *56*:729, 1985.
111. Freedman, S. B., Dunn, R. F., Bernstein, L., Morris, J., and Kelly, D. T.: Influence of coronary collateral blood flow on the development of exertional ischemia and Q wave infarction in patients with severe single-vessel disease. Circulation *71*:681, 1985.
112. Rentrop, K. P., Cohen, M., Blanke, H., and Phillips, R. A.: Changes in collateral channel filling immediately after controlled coronary artery occlusion by an angioplasty balloon in human subjects. J. Am. Coll. Cardiol. *5*:587, 1985.
113. Meier, B., and Luethy, P.: Coronary wedge pressure as predictor of recruitable collateral arteries. Circulation *70*(Suppl. II): 266, 1984.
114. Tada, M., Yamagishi, M., Kodama, K., Kuzuya, T., Nanto, S., Inoue, M., and Abe, H.: Transient collateral augmentation during coronary arterial spasm associated with ST-segment depression. Circulation *67*:693, 1983.
115. Newman, P. E.: The coronary collateral circulation: Determinants and functional significance in ischemic heart disease. Am. Heart J. *102*:431, 1981.
116. Horwitz, L. D., Groves, B. M., Walsh, R. A., Sorensen, S. M., and Latson, T. W.: Functional significance of coronary collateral vessels in patients with coronary artery disease. Am. Heart J. *104*:221, 1982.
117. Cheitlin, M. D., McAllister, H. A., and deCastro, C. M.: Myocardial infarction without atherosclerosis. J.A.M.A. *231*:951, 1975.
118. Mann, J. D., Vessey, M. P., Thorogood, M., and Doll, R.: Myocardial infarction in young women with special reference to oral contraceptive practice. Br. Med. J. *2*:214, 1975.
119. Wei, J. Y., and Bulkley, B. H.: Myocardial infarction before age 36 years in women: Predominance of apparent nonatherosclerotic events. Am. Heart J. *104*:561, 1982.
120. Porter, J. B., Hunter, J. R., Jick, H., and Stergachis, A.: Oral contraceptives and nonfatal vascular disease. J. Am. Coll. Obstet. Gynecol. *66*:1, 1985.
121. Parrillo, J. E., and Fauci, A. S.: Necrotizing vasculitis, coronary angiitis, and the cardiologist. Am. Heart J. *99*:547, 1980.
122. Spodick, D. H.: Inflammation and the onset of myocardial infarction. Ann. Intern. Med. *102*:699, 1985.
123. Miklozek, C. L., and Abelmann, W. H.: Viral myopericarditis presenting as acute myocardial infarction. Circulation *64*(Suppl. IV):25, 1982.
124. Kron, J., Lucas, L., Lee, T. D., and McAnulty, J.: Myocardial infarction following an acute viral illness. Arch. Intern. Med. *143*:1466, 1983.
125. Connolley, J. E., Eldridge, F. L., Calvin, J. W., and Stemmer, E. A.: Proximal coronary artery obstruction. N. Engl. J. Med. *271*:213, 1964.
126. Roberts, W. C., MacGregor, R. R., DeBlanc, H. J., Beiser, G. D., and Wolff, S. M.: The prepulseless phase of pulseless disease, or pulseless disease with pulses. Am. J. Med. *46*:313, 1969.
127. Pick, R. A., Glover, M. U., and Vieweg, W. V. R.: Myocardial infarction in a young woman with isolated coronary arteritis. Chest *82*:378, 1982.
128. Kegel, S. M., Dorsey, T. J., Rowen, M., and Taylor, W. F.: Cardiac death in mucocutaneous lymph node syndrome. Am. J. Cardiol. *40*:282, 1977.
129. Homcy, C. J., Liberthson, R. R., Fallon, J. T., Gross, S., and Miller, L. M.: Ischemic heart disease in systemic lupus erythematosus in the young patient: Report of six cases. Am. J. Cardiol. *49*:481, 1982.
130. Taymor-Luria, H., Cohn, K., and Pasternak, R. C.: How to identify radiation heart disease. J. Cardiovasc. Med. *8*:113, 1983.
131. Huang, S., Kumar, G., Steele, H. D., and Parker, J. O.: Cardiac involvement in pseudoxanthoma elasticum. Am. Heart J. *74*:680, 1967.
132. James, T. N.: Small arteries of the heart. Circulation *56*:2, 1977.
133. Cregler, L. L., and Mark, H.: Relation of acute myocardial infarction to cocaine abuse. Am. J. Cardiol. *56*:793, 1985.
134. Zimmerman, F. H., Gustafson, G. M., and Kemp, H. G.: Recurrent myocardial infarction associated with cocaine abuse in a young man with normal coronary arteries: Evidence for coronary artery spasm culminating in thrombosis. J. Am. Coll. Cardiol. *9*:964, 1987.
134a. Rod, J. L., and Zucker, R. P.: Acute myocardial infarction shortly after cocaine inhalation. Am. J. Cardiology *59*:161, 1987.
135. Coleman, D. L., Ross, T. F., and Naughton, J. L.: Myocardial ischemia and infarction related to recreational cocaine use. West. J. Med. *136*:445, 1982.
136. Kossowsky, W. A., and Lyon, A. F.: Cocaine and acute myocardial infarction. A probable connection. Chest *86*:729, 1984.
137. Pasternack, P. F., Colvin, S. B., and Baumann, F. G.: Cocaine-induced angina pectoris and acute myocardial infarction in patients younger than 40 years. Am. J. Cardiol. *55*:847, 1985.
138. Weiss, R. J.: Recurrent myocardial infarction caused by cocaine abuse. Am. Heart J. *111*:793, 1986.
139. Schachne, J. S., Roberts, B. H., and Thompson, P. D.: Coronary artery spasm and myocardial infarction associated with cocaine use. N. Engl. J. Med. *310*:1665, 1984.
140. Ritchie, J. M., and Greene, N. M.: Local anesthetics. *In* Goodman, L. S., and Gilman, A. G. (eds.): The Pharmacologic Basis of Therapeutics. 6th ed. New York, Macmillan, 1980, p. 307.
141. Benchimo, A., Bartall, J., and Desser, K. B.: Accelerated ventricular rhythm and cocaine abuse. Ann. Intern. Med. *88*:518, 1978.
142. Glover, M. V., Kuber, M. T., Warren, S. E., and Vieweg, W. V. R.: Myocardial infarction before age 36: Risk factor and arteriographic analysis. Am. J. Cardiol. *49*:1600, 1982.
143. Ciraulo, D. A., Bresnahan, G. F., Frankel, P. S., Isely, P. E., Zimmerman, W. R., and Chesne, R. B.: Transmural myocardial infarction with normal coronary angiograms and with single-vessel coronary obstruction. Clinical-angiographic features and five-year follow-up. Chest *83*:196, 1983.
144. Achuff, S. C., Bell, W. R., and Bulkley, B. H.: Thromboses in previously normal coronary arteries. Primary Cardiol. *8*:137, 1982.
145. Pasternak, R. C., Thibault, G. E., Savola, M., DeSanctis, R. W., and Hutter, A. M., Jr.: Chest pain with angiographically insignificant coronary arterial obstruction. Clinical presentation and long term follow-up. Am. J. Med. *68*:813, 1980.
146. Lindsay, J., and Pichard, A.: Acute myocardial infarction with normal coronary arteries. Am. J. Cardiol. *54*:902, 1984.
147. Salem, B. I., Haikal, M., Zambrano, A., Bollis, A., and Gowda, S.: Acute myocardial infarction with "normal" coronary arteries: Clinical and angiographic profiles, with ergonovine testing. Tex. Heart Inst. J. *12*:1, 1985.
148. Rosenblatt, A., and Selzer, A.: The nature and clinical features of myocardial infarction with normal coronary arteriograms. Circulation *55*:578, 1977.
149. Eliot, R. S., Baroldi, G., and Leone, A.: Necropsy studies in myocardial infarction with minimal or no coronary luminal reduction due to atherosclerosis. Circulation *49*:1127, 1974.
150. Lindsay, J., Dwyer, S., and Punja, U.: Angiographic demonstration of coronary occlusion during spontaneous acute myocardial infarction and subsequent angiographically normal coronary arteries. Am. J. Cardiol. *51*:1227, 1982.
151. Heulpler, F. A.: Syndrome of symptomatic coronary arterial spasm with nearly normal coronary arteriograms. Am. J. Cardiol. *45*:833, 1981.
152. Klein, L. S., Simpson, R. J., Stern, R., Hayward, J. C., and Foster, J. R.: Myocardial infarction following administration of sublingual ergotamine. Chest *82*:375, 1982.
153. Lange, R. L., Reid, M. S., Tresch, D. D., Keelan, M. H., Bernard, V. M., and Coolidge, G.: Nonatheromatous ischemic heart disease following withdrawal from chronic industrial nitroglycerin exposure. Circulation *46*:666, 1972.
154. Heulpler, F. A , Proudfit, W. L., Razavi, M., Shirey, E. R., Greenstreet, R., and Sheldon, W. C.: Ergonovine maleate provocative test for coronary arterial spasm. Am. J. Cardiol. *41*:631, 1978.
155. Braunwald, E.: Coronary spasm and acute myocardial infarction—New possibility for treatment and prevention (Editorial). N. Engl. J. Med. *299*:1301, 1978.
156. Makino, H., and Al-Sadir, J.: Myocardial infarction in patients with mitral valve prolapse and normal coronary arteries. J. Am. Coll. Cardiol. *1*:661, 1983.
157. Yeager, S. B., and Freed, M. D.: Myocardial infarction as a manifestation of polycythemia in cyanotic heart disease. Am. J. Cardiol. *53*:952, 1984.
158. Martin, C. R., Cobb, C., Tatter, D., Johnson, C., and Haywood, J.: Acute myocardial infarction in sickle cell anemia. Arch. Intern. Med. *143*:830, 1983.
159. Eslami, B., Russell, R. O., Jr., Bailey, M. T., Oberman, A., Tieszen, R. L., and Rackley, C. E.: Acute myocardial infarction in the absence of coronary arterial insufficiency. Ala. J. Med. Sci. *12*:322, 1975.
160. Arnett, E. N., and Roberts, W. C.: Acute myocardial infarction and angiographically normal coronary arteries: An unproved combination. Circulation *53*:395, 1976.
161. Pfeffer, M. A., Pfeffer, J. M., Fishbein, M. C., Fletcher, P. J., Spadaro, J.,

Kloner, R. A., and Braunwald, E.: Myocardial infarct size and ventricular function in rats. Circ. Res. 44:503, 1979.

PATHOPHYSIOLOGY OF ACUTE MYOCARDIAL INFARCTION

162. Herman, M. V., Heinle, R. A., Klein, M. D., and Gorlin, R.: Localized disorders in myocardial contraction. N. Engl. J. Med. 227:222, 1967.
163. Swan, H. J. C., Forrester, J. S., Diamond, G., Chatterjee, K., and Parmley, W. W.: Hemodynamic spectrum of myocardial infarction and cardiogenic shock. Circulation 45:1097, 1972.
164. Forrester, J. S., Wyatt, H. L., Daluz, P. L., Tyberg, J. V., Diamond, G. A., and Swan, H. J. C.: Functional significance of regional ischemic contraction abnormalities. Circulation 54:64, 1976.
165. Serruys, P. W., Simoons, M. L., Suryapranata, H., Vermeer, F., Wijns, W., van den Brand, M., Bar, F., Zwann, C., Krauss, X. H., Remme, W. J., Res, J., Verheugt, F. W. A., van Domburg, R., Lubsen, J., and Hugenholtz, P. G.: Preservation of global and regional left ventricular function after early thrombolysis in acute myocardial infarction. J. Am. Coll. Cardiol. 7:729, 1986.
166. Diamond, G., and Forrester, J. S.: Effect of coronary artery disease and acute myocardial infarction on left ventricular compliance in man. Circulation 45:11, 1972.
167. Rackley, C. E., Russell, R. O., Jr., Mantle, J. A., and Rogers, W. J.: Modern approach to the patient with acute myocardial infarction. Curr. Prob. Cardiol. 1:49, 1977.
168. Klein, M. D., Herman, M. V., and Gorlin, R. G.: A hemodynamic study of left ventricular aneurysm. Circulation 35:614, 1967.
169. Wynne, J., Sayres, M., Maddox, D. E., Idoine, J., Alpert, J. S., Neill, J., and Holman, B. L.: Regional left ventricular function in acute myocardial infarction: Evaluation with quantitative radionuclide ventriculography. Am. J. Cardiol. 45:203, 1980.
170. Schuster, E. H., and Bulkley, B. H.: Ischemia at a distance after acute myocardial infarction: A cause of early postinfarction angina. Circulation 62:509, 1980.
171. Cortina, A., Ambrose, J. A., Prieto-Granada, J., Moris, C., Simarro, E., Holt, J., and Fuster, V.: Left ventricular function after myocardial infarction: Clinical and angiographic correlations. J. Am. Coll. Cardiol. 5:619, 1985.
172. Pirzada, F. A., Ekong, E. A., Vokonas, P. S., Apstein, C. S., and Hood, W. B., Jr.: Experimental myocardial infarction. XIII. Sequential changes in left ventricular pressure-length relationships in the acute phase. Circulation 53:970, 1976.
173. Paulus, W. J., Grossman, W., Serizawa, T., Bourdillon, P. D., Pasipoularides, A., and Mirsky, I.: Different effects of two types of ischemia on myocardial systolic and diastolic function. Am. J. Physiol. 248:H719, 1985.
174. Aroesty, J. M., McKay, R. G., Heller, G. V., Royal, H. D., Als, A. V., and Grossman, W.: Simultaneous assessment of left ventricular systolic and diastolic function during pacing-induced ischemia. Circulation 71:889, 1985.
175. McKay, R. G., Pfeffer, M. A., Pasternak, R. C., Markis, J. E., Come, P. C., Nakao, S., Alderman, J. D., Ferguson, J. J., Safian, R. D., and Grossman, W.: Left ventricular remodeling following myocardial infarction: A corollary to infarct expansion. Circulation 74:693, 1986.
176. White, P. D.: Heart Disease. 2nd ed. New York, Macmillan, 1937, p. 357.
177. Stewart, D. K., Hamilton, G. W., Murray, J. A., and Kennedy, J. W.: Left ventricular function and coronary artery anatomy before and after myocardial infarction: A study of six cases. Circulation 49:47, 1974.
178. Hutchins, G. M., and Bulkley, B. H.: Infarct expansion versus extension: Two different complications of acute myocardial infarction. Am. J. Cardiol. 41:1127, 1978.
179. Eaton, L. W., Weiss, J. L., Bulkley, B. H., Carrison, J. B., and Weisfeldt, M. L.: Regional cardiac dilatation after acute myocardial infarction. N. Engl. J. Med. 300:57, 1979.
180. Roberts, C. S., Maclean, D., Maroko, P. R., and Kloner, R. A.: Early and late remodeling of the left ventricle after acute myocardial infarction. Am. J. Cardiol. 54:407, 1984.
181. Pirolo, J. S., Hutchins, G. M., and Moore, G. W.: Infarct expansion: Pathologic analysis of 204 patients with a single myocardial infarct. J. Am. Coll. Cardiol. 7:349, 1986.
182. Schuster, E. H., and Bulkley, B. H.: Expansion of transmural myocardial infarction: A pathophysiologic factor in cardiac rupture. Circulation 60:1532, 1979.
183. Erlebacher, J. A., Weiss, J. L., Eaton, L. W., Kallman, C., Weisfeldt, M. L., and Bulkley, B. H.: Late effects of acute infarct dilation on heart size: A two-dimensional echocardiographic study. Am. J. Cardiol. 49:1120, 1982.
184. Warren, S. E., McKay, R. G., Royal, H. D., Parker, J. A., Ransil, B. J., Markis, J. E., and Grossman, W.: Time course of left ventricular dilatation following acute myocardial infarction. Circulation. 72(Suppl. III): 439, 1985.
185. Grossman, W.: Cardiac hypertrophy: Useful adaptations or pathologic process? Am. J. Med. 69:576, 1980.
186. Biddle, T. L., Yu, P. N., Hodges, M., Chance, J. R., Ehrlich, D. A., Kronenberg, M. W., and Roberts, D. L.: Hypoxemia and lung water in acute myocardial infarction. Am. Heart J. 92:692, 1976.
187. Hales, C. A., and Kazemi, H.: Clinical significance of pulmonary function tests. Pulmonary function after uncomplicated myocardial infarction. Chest 72:350, 1977.
188. Hales, C. A., and Kazemi, H.: Small-airways function in myocardial infarction. N. Engl. J. Med. 290:761, 1974.
189. Peabody, F. W., and Wentworth, J. A.: Clinical studies of the respiration. IV. The vital capacity of the lungs and its relation to dyspnea. Arch. Intern. Med. 20:443, 1917.
190. Gray, B. A., Hyde, R. W., Hodges, M., and Yu, P. N.: Alterations in lung volume and pulmonary function in relation to hemodynamic changes in acute myocardial infarction. Circulation 59:551, 1979.
191. Kazemi, H., Parsons, E. F., Valenca, L. M., and Strieder, D. J.: Distribution of pulmonary blood flow after myocardial ischemia and infarction. Circulation 41:1025, 1970.
192. DaLuz, P. L., Cavanilles, J. M., Michaels, S., Weill, M. H., and Shubin, H.: Oxygen delivery, anoxic metabolism and hemoglobin-oxygen affinity (P_{50}) in patients with acute myocardial infarction and shock. Am. J. Cardiol. 36:148, 1975.
193. Datey, K. K., and Nanda, N. C.: Hyperglycemia after acute myocardial infarction. N. Engl. J. Med. 276:262, 1976.
194. Vetter, N. J., Adams, W., Strange, R. C., and Oliver, M. F.: Initial metabolic and hormonal response to acute myocardial infarction. Lancet 1:284, 1974.
195. Bertel, O., Buhler, F. R., Baitsch, G., Ritz, R., and Burkart, F.: Plasma adrenaline and noradrenaline in patients with acute myocardial infarction. Relationship to ventricular arrhythmias in varying severity. Chest 82:64, 1982.
196. Taylor, S. H., Saxton, C., Majid, P. A., Dykes, J. R. W., Ghosh, P., and Stoker, J. B.: Insulin secretion following myocardial infarction with particular respect to pathogenesis of cardiogenic shock. Lancet 2:1373, 1969.
197. Taylor, S. H., Majid, P. A., Saxton, C., and Sharma, B.: Insulin secretion in heart failure. Am. Heart J. 83:281, 1972.
198. Ceremuzynski, L.: Hormonal and metabolic reactions evoked by acute myocardial infarction. Circ. Res. 48:767, 1981.
199. Jefferson, L. S., Rannels, D. E., Munger, B. L., and Morgan, H. E.: Insulin in the regulation of protein turnover in heart and skeletal muscle. Fed. Proc. 33:1098, 1974.
200. Opie, L. H.: Metabolism of free fatty acids, glucose, and catecholamines in acute myocardial infarction: Relation to myocardial ischemia and infarct size. Am. J. Cardiol. 36:938, 1975.
201. Taggart, P., and Carruthers, M.: Endogenous hyperlipidemia induced by emotional stress of racing driving. Lancet 1:363, 1971.
202. Jequier, E., and Perret, C.: Urinary excretion of catecholamines and their main metabolites after myocardial infarction: Relationship to the clinical syndrome. Eur. J. Clin. Invest. 1:77, 1970.
203. Karlsberg, R. P., Cryer, P. E., and Roberts, R.: Serial plasma catecholamine response early in the course of clinical acute myocardial infarction: Relationship to infarct extent and mortality. Am. Heart J. 102:24, 1981.
204. Logan, R. W., and Murdoch, W. R.: Blood levels of hydrocortisone, transaminases, and cholesterol after myocardial infarction. Lancet 2:521, 1966.
205. Ljunggren, J. G., Falkenberg, C., and Savidge, G.: The influence of endogenous cortisol on the peripheral conversion of thyroxine in patients with acute myocardial infarction. Acta Med. Scand. 205:267, 1979.
206. Wiersinga, W. M., Lie, K. I., and Touber, J. L.: Thyroid hormones in acute myocardial infarction. Clin. Endocrinol. 14:367, 1981.
207. Kahana, L., Keidar, S., Sheinfeld, M., and Palant, A.: Endogenous cortisol and thyroid hormone levels in patients with acute myocardial infarction. Clin. Endocrinol. 19:131, 1983.
208. Steele, P., Rainwater, J., and Vogel, R.: Abnormal platelet survival time in men with myocardial infarction and normal coronary arteriogram. Am. J. Cardiol. 41:60, 1978.
209. Laursen, B., and Gormsen, J.: Spontaneous fibrinolysis demonstrated by immunological technique. Thromb. Diath. Haemorrh. 17:42, 1967.
210. Handin, R. I., McDonough, M., and Lesch, M.: Elevation of platelet factor IV in acute myocardial infarction: Measurement by radioimmunoassay. J. Lab. Clin. Med. 91:340, 1978.
211. Smitherman, T. C., Milam, M., Woo, J., Willerson, J. T., and Frenkel, E. P.: Elevated beta thromboglobulin in peripheral venous blood of patients with acute myocardial ischemia: Direct evidence for enhanced platelet reactivity in vivo. Am. J. Cardiol. 48:395, 1981.
212. Eisenberg, P., Sherman, L. A., Schechtman, K., Perez, J., Sobel, B. E., and Jaffe, A. S.: Fibrinopeptide A: A marker for acute coronary thrombosis. Circulation 71:912, 1985.
213. Rickman, F. D., Handin, R., Howe, J. P., Alpert, J. S., Dexter, L., and Dalen, J. E.: Fibrin split products in acute pulmonary embolism. Ann. Intern. Med. 79:664, 1973.
214. Cowan, D. H.: Acquired disorders of platelet function. *In* Colman, R. W., Hirsch, J., Marker, V. J., and Salzman, E. W. (eds.): Hemostasis and Thrombosis: Basic Principles and Clinical Practice. Philadelphia, J. B. Lippincott Co., 1982, pp. 516–524.
215. Marcus, A. J., Safier, L. B., Ullman, H. L., Broekman, M. J., Islam, N., Oglesby, T. D., Gorman, R. R., and Ward, J. W.: Inhibition of platelet function in thrombosis. Circulation 72:698, 1985.
216. Fantone, J. C., and Ward, P. A.: Role of oxygen-derived free radicals and metabolites in leukocyte-dependent inflammatory reactions. Am. J. Physiol. 107:397, 1982.
217. Engler, R. L., Dahlgren, M. D., Morris, D. D., Peterson, M. A., and Schmid-Schonbein, G. W.: Role of leukocytes in response to acute myocardial ischemia and reflow in dogs. Am. J. Physiol 251:H314, 1986.
218. Jan, K. M., Chien, S., and Bigger, J. T., Jr.: Observation on blood viscosity changes after acute myocardial infarction. Circulation 51:1079, 1972.
219. Hershberg, P. I., Wells, R. E., and McGandy, R. B.: Hematocrit and prognosis in patients with acute myocardial infarction. J.A.M.A. 219:855, 1972.

220. Phipps, C.: Contributory causes of coronary thrombosis. J.A.M.A. *106*:761, 1936.
221. Master, A. M., Dack, S., and Jaffe, H. L.: Factors and events associated with onset of coronary artery thrombosis. J.A.M.A. *109*:546, 1937.
222. Smith, C., Sauls, H. C., and Ballew, J.: Coronary occlusion: A clinical study of 100 patients. Ann. Intern. Med. *17*:681, 1942.
223. French, A. J., and Dock, W.: Fatal coronary arteriosclerosis in young soldiers. J.A.M.A. *124*:1233, 1944.
224. Fitzhugh, G., and Hamilton, B. E.: Coronary occlusion and fatal angina pectoris: Study of the immediate causes and their prevention. J.A.M.A. *100*:475, 1933.
225. Matsuda, M., Matsuda, Y., Ogawa, H., Moritani, K., and Kusukawa, R.: Angina pectoris before and during acute myocardial infarction: Relation to degree of physical activity. Am. J. Cardiol. *55*:1255, 1985.
226. Knapp, R. B., Topkins, M. J., and Artusio, J. F., Jr.: The cerebrovascular accident and coronary occlusion in anesthesia. J.A.M.A. *182*:332, 1962.
227. Goldfischer, J. D.: Acute myocardial infarction secondary to ergot therapy. N. Engl. J. Med. *262*:860, 1960.
228. Roussak, N. J.: Myocardial infarction during serum sickness. Br. Heart J. *16*:218, 1954.
229. Levine, H. D.: Acute myocardial infarction following wasp sting. Report of two cases and critical survey of the literature. Am. Heart J. *91*:365, 1976.
230. Maseri, A., L'Abbate, A., Baroldi, G., Chierchia, S., Marzilli, M., Ballestra, A. M., Severi, S., Parodi, W., Biagini, A., Distante, A., and Pesola, A.: Coronary vasospasm as a possible cause of myocardial infarction. A conclusion derived from the study of "preinfarction" angina. N. Engl. J. Med. *299*:1271, 1978.
231. Jenkins, C. D.: Recent evidence supporting psychologic and social risk factors for coronary disease. N. Engl. J. Med. *294*:987, 1033, 1976.
232. Rahe, R. H., Romo, M., Bennett, L., and Siltanen, P.: Recent life changes, myocardial infarction, and abrupt coronary death. Arch. Intern. Med. *133*:221, 1974.
233. vonArbin, M., Britton, M., deFaire, U., Helmers, C., Miah, K., and Murray, V.: Myocardial infarction in patients with acute cerebrovascular disease. Eur. Heart J. *3*:136, 1982.
234. Muller, J. E., Stone, P. H., Turi, Z. G., Rutherford, J. D., Czeisler, C. A., Parker, C., Poole, W. K., Passamani, E., Roberts, R., Robertson, T., Sobel, B. E., Willerson, J. T., and Braunwald, E.: Circadian variation in the frequency of onset of acute myocardial infarction. N. Engl. J. Med. *313*:1315, 1985.
235. Myocardial infarction community registers: Results of a WHO international collaborative study coordinated by the regional office for Europe. *In*: Public Health in Europe, No. 5. Copenhagen, Regional Office for Europe (World Health Organization), 1976, pp. 1–230.
236. Muller, J., Ludmer, P. L., Willich, S. N., Tofler, G. H., Aylmer, G., Klangos, I., and Stone, P. H.: Circadian variation in the frequency of sudden cardiac death. Circulation *75*:131, 1987.
237. Mitler, M. M., and Kripke, D. F.: Circadian variation in myocardial infarction. N. Engl. J. Med. *314*:1187, 1986.
238. Quyyumi, A. A., Mockus, L., Wright, C., and Fox, K. M.: Morphology of ambulatory ST-segment changes in patients with varying severity of coronary artery disease: Investigation of the frequency of nocturnal ischemia and coronary spasm. Br. Heart J. *53*:186, 1985.
239. Alonzo, A. M., Simon, A. B., and Feinleib, M.: Prodromata of myocardial infarction and sudden death. Circulation *52*:1056, 1975.
240. Harper, R. W., Kennedy, G., DeSanctis, R. W., and Hutter, A. M., Jr.: The incidence and pattern of angina prior to acute myocardial infarction: A study of 577 cases. Am. Heart J. *97*:178, 1979.
241. Rogers, D. E.: Some observations on having a coronary. The Pharos of Alpha Omega Alpha *49*:12, 1986.
242. Baker, P.: Suspected myocardial infarction: Early diagnostic value of analgesic requirements. Br. Med. J. *290*:27, 1985.
243. Malliani, A., and Lombardi, F.: Consideration of the fundamental mechanisms eliciting cardiac pain. Am. Heart J. *103*:575, 1982.
244. Malliani, A.: The elusive link between transient myocardial ischemia and pain. Circulation *73*:201, 1986.
245. Ganz, W., Geft, I., Shah, P. K., Lew, A. S., Rodriguez, L., Weiss, T., Maddahi, J., Berman, D. S., Charuzi, Y., and Swan, H. J. C.: Intravenous streptokinase in evolving acute myocardial infarction. Am. J. Cardiol. *53*:1209, 1984.
246. Ingram, D. A., Fulton, R. A., Portal, R. W., and Aber, C. P.: Vomiting as a diagnostic aid in acute ischemic cardiac pain. Br. Med. J. *281*:636, 1980.
247. Sleight, P.: Cardiac vomiting. Br. Heart J. *46*:5, 1981.
248. Uretsky, B. F., Farquhar, D. S., Borezin, A., and Hood, W. B.: Symptomatic myocardial infarction without chest pain: Prevalence and clinical course. Am. J. Cardiol. *40*:498, 1977.
249. Roseman, M. D.: Painless myocardial infarction: A review of the literature and analysis of 220 cases. Ann. Intern. Med. *41*:1, 1954.
250. Margolis, J. R., Kannel, W. B., Feinleib, M., Dawber, T. R., and McNamara, P. M.: Clinical features of unrecognized myocardial infarction—silent and symptomatic. Eighteen-year follow-up: The Framingham Study. Am. J. Cardiol. *32*:1, 1973.
251. Sullivan, W., Vlodaver, Z., Tuna, N., Long, L., and Edward, J. E.: Correlation of electrocardiographic and pathologic findings in healed myocardial infarction. Am. J. Cardiol. *42*:724, 1978.
252. Aronow, W., Starling, L., Etienne, F., D'Alba, P., Edwards, M., Lee, N. H., and Parungao, R. F.: Unrecognized Q-wave myocardial infarction in patients older than 64 years in a long-term health-care facility. Am. J. Cardiol. *56*:483, 1985.
253. Medalie, J. H., and Goldbourt, U.: Unrecognized myocardial infarction: Five-year incidence, mortality, and risk factors. Ann. Intern. Med. *84*:526, 1976.
254. Bean, W. B.: Masquerade of myocardial infarction. Lancet *1*:1044, 1977.
255. Chadda, K. D., Lichstein, E., Gupta, P. K., and Choy, R.: Bradycardia-hypotension syndrome in acute myocardial infarction. Reappraisal of the overdrive effects of atropine. Am. J. Med. *59*:158, 1975.
256. Webb, S. W., Adgey, A. A., and Pantridge, J. F.: Autonomic disturbance at onset of acute myocardial infarction. Br. Med. J. *818*:89, 1982.
257. Chizner, M. A.: Bedside diagnosis of the acute myocardial infarction and its complications. Curr. Probl. Cardiol. *7*:1, 1982.
258. Renner, W. F., and Renner, G. W.: The quality of resonance of the first sound after myocardial infarction: Clinical significance. Circulation *59*:1144, 1979.
259. Stein, P. D., Sabbah, H. N., and Barr, I.: Intensity of heart sounds in the evaluation of patients following myocardial infarction. Chest *75*:679, 1979.
260. Riley, C. P., Russell, R. O., Jr., and Rackley, C. E.: Left ventricular gallop sound and acute myocardial infarction. Am. Heart J. *86*:598, 1973.
261. Case Records of the Massachusetts General Hospital (Case 49-1986). N. Engl. J. Med. *315*:1533, 1986.
262. Sawaya, J. I., Mujais, S. K., and Armenian, H. K.: Early diagnosis of pericarditis in acute myocardial infarction. Am. Heart J. *100*:144, 1980.
263. Krainin, F. M., Flessas, A. P., and Spodick, D. H.: Infarction-associated pericarditis. Rarity of diagnostic electrocardiogram. N. Engl. J. Med. *311*:1211, 1984.
264. Galve, E., Garcia-Del-Castillo, H., Evangelista, A., Battle, J., Permanyer-Miralda, G., and Soler-Soler, J.: Pericardial effusion in the course of myocardial infarction: Incidence, natural history, and clinical relevance. Circulation *73*:294, 1986.
265. Dressler, W.: The post-myocardial infarction syndrome: A report of 44 cases. Arch. Intern. Med. *103*:28, 1959.
266. Soloff, L. A.: Pericardial cellular response during the postmyocardial infarction syndrome. Am. Heart J. *82*:812, 1971.
267. McCabe, J. C., Ebert, P. A., Engle, M. A., and Zabriskie, J. B.: Circulating heart-reactive antibodies in the postpericardial syndrome. J. Surg. Res. *14*:158, 1973.
268. Lichstein, E., Arsura, E., Hollander, G., Greengart, A., and Sanders, M.: Current incidence of postmyocardial infarction (Dressler's) syndrome. Am. J. Cardiol. *50*:1269, 1982.
269. Thompson, P. L., and Robinson, J. S.: Stroke after acute myocardial infarction: Relation to infarct size. Br. Med. J. *2*:457, 1978.
270. Sobel, B. E., and Shell, W. E.: Serum enzyme determinations in the diagnosis and assessment of myocardial infarction. Circulation *45*:471, 1972.
271. Lee, T. H., and Goldman, L.: Serum enzyme assays in the diagnosis of acute myocardial infarction. Ann. Intern. Med. *105*:221, 1986.
272. Hearse, D. J.: Myocardial enzyme leakage. J. Mol. Med. *2*:185, 1977.
273. Pasyk, S., Bloor, C. M., Khouri, E. M., and Gress, D. E.: Systemic and coronary effects of coronary artery occlusion in the unanesthetized dog. Am. J. Physiol. *220*:646, 1971.
274. Shell, W. E., Kjekshus, J. K., and Sobel, B. E.: Quantitative assessment of the extent of myocardial infarction in the conscious dog by means of analysis of serial changes in serum creatine phosphokinase activity. J. Clin. Invest. *50*:2614, 1971.
275. Lott, J. A.: Serum enzyme determinations in the diagnosis of acute myocardial infarction: An update. Hum. Pathol. *15*:706, 1984.
276. Vasudevan, G., Mercer, D. W., and Varat, M. A.: Lactic dehydrogenase isoenzyme determination in the diagnosis of acute myocardial infarction. Circulation *57*:1055, 1978.
277. Weidner, N.: Laboratory diagnosis of acute myocardial infarct. Usefulness of determination of lactate dehydrogenase (LDH)-1 level and the ratio of LDH-1 to total LDH. Arch. Pathol. Lab. Med. *106*:375, 1982.
278. Fisher, M. L., Kelemen, M. H., Collins, D., Morris, F., Moran, G. W., Carliner, N. H., and Plotnick, G. D.: Routine serum enzyme tests in the diagnosis of acute myocardial infarction. Arch. Intern. Med. *143*:1541, 1983.
279. Reis, G. J., Kaufman, H. W., Horowitz, G. L., and Pasternak, R. C.: Marginal benefits of LDH and LDH isoenzymes in diagnosis of myocardial infarction: Are they worth it? J. Am. Coll. Cardiol. *9*:22A, 1987.
280. Herlitz, J.: Time lapse from estimated onset of acute myocardial infarction to peak serum enzyme activity. Clin. Cardiol. *7*:433, 1984.
281. Ong, L., Reiser, P., Coromilas, J., Scherr, L., and Morrison, J.: Left ventricular function and rapid release of creatine kinase MB in acute myocardial infarction: Evidence for spontaneous reperfusion. N. Engl. J. Med. *309*:1, 1983.
282. Blanke, H., von Hardenberg, D., Cohen, M., Kaiser, H., Karsch, K. R., Holt, J., Smith, H., Jr., and Rentrop, P.: Patterns of creatine kinase release during acute myocardial infarction after nonsurgical reperfusion: Comparison with conventional treatment and correlation with infarct size. J. Am. Coll. Cardiol. *3*:675, 1984.
283. Horie, M., Yasue, H., Omote, S., Takizawa, A., Nagao, M., Nishida, S., and Kubota, J.: A new approach for the enzymatic estimation of infarct size: Serum peak creatine kinase and time to peak creatine kinase activity. Am. J. Cardiol. *57*:76, 1986.
284. Goldberg, D. M., and Windfield, D. A.: Diagnostic accuracy of serum enzyme assays for myocardial infarction in a general hospital population. Br. Heart J. *34*:597, 1972.
285. Roberts, R., and Sobel, B. E.: Isoenzymes of creatine phosphokinase and diagnosis of myocardial infarction. Ann. Intern. Med. *79*:741, 1973.

286. Godfrey, N. F., Halter, D. G., Minna, D. A., Weiss, M., and Lorber, A.: Thoracic outlet syndrome mimicking angina pectoris with elevated creatine phosphokinase values. Chest 83:461, 1983.
287. Tsung, S. H.: Several conditions causing elevation of serum CK-BB. Am. J. Clin. Pathol. 75:711, 1981.
288. Apple, F. S., Rogers, M. A., Sherman, W. M., and Ivy, J. L.: Comparison of serum creatine kinase and creatine kinase MB activities post-marathon race versus post myocardial infarction. Clin. Chim. Acta *138*:111, 1984.
289. Jaffe, A. S., Garfinkel, B. T., Ritter, C. S., and Sobel, B. E.: Plasma MB creatine kinase after vigorous exercise in professional athletes. Am. J. Cardiol. 53:856, 1984.
290. Ingwall, J. S., Kramer, M. F., Fifer, M. A., Lorell, B. H., Shemin, R., Grossman, W., and Allen, P. D.: The creatine kinase system in normal and diseased human myocardium. N. Engl. J. Med. *313*:1050, 1985.
291. Morelli, R. L., Carlson, D. J., Emilson, B., Abendschein, D. R., and Rapaport, E.: Serum creatine kinase MM isoenzyme sub-bands after acute myocardial infarction in man. Circulation 67:1283, 1983.
292. Hashimoto, H., Abendschein, D. R., Strauss, A. W., and Sobel, B. E.: Early detection of myocardial infarction in conscious dogs by analysis of plasma MM creatine kinase isoforms. Circulation *71*:363, 1985.
293. Roberts, R., Gowda, K. S., Ludbrook, P. A., and Sobel, B. E.: Specificity of elevated serum MB creatine phosphokinase activity in the diagnosis of acute myocardial infarction. Am. J. Cardiol. *36*:433, 1975.
294. Turi, Z. G., and cooperating investigators from the MILIS study group: Electrocardiographic, enzymatic and scintigraphic criteria of acute myocardial infarction as determined from study of 726 patients. Am. J. Cardiol. 55:1463–1465, 1985.
295. Roberts, R., Sobel, B. E., and Parker, C. W.: Radioimmunoassay for creatine kinase isoenzymes. Science *194*:855, 1976.
296. McGrath, R. B., and Revtyak, G.: Secondary myocardial injuries. Crit. Care Med. *12*:1024, 1984.
297. Alderman, E. L., Matlof, H. J., Shumway, N. E., and Harrison, D. C.: Evaluation of enzyme testing for the detection of myocardial infarction following direct coronary surgery. Circulation *48*:135, 1973.
298. Klein, M. S., Coleman, R. E., Weldon, C. S., Sobel, B. E., and Robert, R.: Concordance of electrocardiographic and scintigraphic criteria of myocardial injury after cardiac surgery. J. Thorac. Cardiovasc. Surg. *71*:934, 1976.
299. Roberts, R., Sobel, B. E., and Ludbrook, P. A.: Determination of the origin of elevated plasma CPK after cardiac catheterization. Cathet. Cardiovasc. Diagn. *2*:239, 1976.
300. Smith, J. L., Ambos, D., Gold, H. K., Muller, J. E., Poole, W. K., Raabe, D. S., Jr., Rude, R. E., Passamani, E., Braunwald, E., Sobel, B. E., Roberts, R., and the MILIS Study Group: Enzymatic estimation of myocardial infarct size when early creatine kinase values are not available. Am. J. Cardiol. *51*:1294, 1983.
301. Hong, R. A., Licht, J. D., Wei, J. Y., Heller, G. V., Blaustein, A. S., and Pasternak, R. C.: Elevated CK-MB with normal total creatine kinase in suspected myocardial infarction: Associated clinical findings and early prognosis. Am. Heart J. *111*:1041, 1986.
302. Heyndrickx, G. R., Amano, J., Kenna, T., Fallon, J. T., Patrick, T. A., Manders, T., Rogers, G. G., Rosendorff, C., and Vatner, S. F.: Creatine kinase release not associated with myocardial necrosis after short periods of coronary artery occlusion in conscious baboons. J. Am. Coll. Cardiol. *6*:1299, 1985.
303. White, R. D., Grande, P., Califf, L., Palmeri, S. T., Califf, R. M., and Wagner, G. S.: Diagnostic and prognostic significance of minimally elevated creatine kinase-MB in suspected acute myocardial infarction. Am. J. Cardiol. 55:1478, 1985.
303a. Yusuf, S., Collins, R., Lin, L., Sterry, H., Pearson, M., and Sleight, P.: Significance of elevated MB isoenzyme with normal creatine kinase in acute myocardial infarction. Am J. Cardiol. 59:245, 1987.
304. Grande, P., Hansen, B. F., Christiansen, C., and Naestoft, J.: Estimation of acute myocardial infarct size in man by serum CK-MB measurements. Circulation *65*:756, 1982.
305. Hori, M., Inoue, M., Fukui, S., Shimazu, T., Mishima, M., Ohgitani, N., Minamino, T., and Abe, H.: Correlation of ejection fraction and infarct size estimated from the total CK released in patients with acute myocardial infarction. Br. Heart J. *41*:433, 1979.
306. Geltman, E. M., Ehsani, A. A., Campbell, M. K., Schechtman, K., Roberts, R., and Sobel, B. E.: The influence of location and extent of myocardial infarction on long-term ventricular dysrhythmia and mortality. Circulation *60*:805, 1979.
307. Tamaki, S., Murakami, T., Kadota, K., Kambara, H., Yui, Y., Nakajima, H., Suzuki, Y., Nohara, R., Takatsu, Y., Kawai, C., Tamaki, N., Mukai, T., and Torizuka, K.: Effects of coronary artery reperfusion on relation between creatine kinase-MB release and infarct size estimated by myocardial emission tomography with thallium-201 in man. J. Am. Coll. Cardiol. 2:1031, 1983.
308. Goldberger, E., Alesio, J., and Woll, F.: The significance of hyperglycemia in myocardial infarction. N.Y. State Med. J. *45*:391, 1945.
309. Tan, M. H., Wilmshurst, E. G., Gleason, R. E., and Soeldner, J. S.: Effect of posture on serum lipids. N. Engl. J. Med. *289*:416, 1973.
310. Gore, J. M., Goldberg, R. J., Matsumoto, A. S., Castelli, W. P., McNamara, P. M., and Dalen, J. E.: Validity of serum total cholesterol level obtained within 24 hours of acute myocardial infarction. Am. J. Cardiol. *54*:722, 1984.
311. Ryder, R. E. J., Hayes, T. M., Mulligan, I. P., Kingswood, J. C., Williams, S., and Owens, D. R.: How soon after myocardial infarction should plasma lipid values be assessed? Br. Med. J. *289*:1651, 1984.
312. Ronnemaa, T., Viikari, J., Irjala, K., and Peltola, O.: Marked decrease in serum HDL cholesterol level during acute myocardial infarction. Acta Med. Scand. *207*:161, 1980.
313. Kagen, L., Scheidt, S., and Butt, A.: Serum myoglobin in myocardial infarction: The "staccato phenomenon." Is acute myocardial infarction in man an intermittent event? Am. J. Med. *62*:86, 1977.
314. Vallee, B. L.: The time course of serum copper concentrations of patients with myocardial infarction. Metabolism *1*:420, 1952.
315. Sunderman, F. W., Jr., Nomoto, S., Pradhan, A. M., Levine, H., Bernstein, S. H., and Hirsch, R.: Increased concentration of serum nickel after acute myocardial infarction. N. Engl. J. Med. *283*:896, 1970.
316. Wacker, W. E. C., Ulmer, D. D., and Vallee, B. L.: Metalloenzymes and myocardial infarction. II. Malic and lactic dehydrogenase activities and zinc concentrations in serum. N. Engl. J. Med. *255*:449, 1956.
317. Fitzsimons, E. J., and Kaplan, K.: Rapid drop in serum iron concentration in myocardial infarction. Am. J. Clin. Pathol. *73*:552, 1980.
318. Rector, W. G., Jr., DeWood, M. A., Williams, R. V., and Sullivan, J. F.: Serum magnesium and copper levels in myocardial infarction. Am. J. Med. Sci. *281*:25, 1981.
319. Eastham, R. D., and Morgan, E. H.: Plasma-fibrinogen levels in coronary-artery disease. Lancet *2*:1196, 1963.
320. Savage, R. M., Wagner, G. S., Ideker, R. E., Podolsky, S. A., and Hackel, D. B.: Correlation of postmortem anatomic findings with electrocardiographic changes in patients with myocardial infarction. Circulation *55*:279, 1977.
321. Cooksey, J. D., Dunn, M., and Massie, E.: Clinical Vectorcardiography and Electrocardiography. 2nd ed. Chicago, Year Book Medical Publishers, Inc., 1977, p. 361.
322. Seyal, M. S., and Swiryn, S.: True posterior myocardial infarction. Arch. Intern. Med. *143*:983, 1983.
323. Haiat, R., Worthington, F. X., Castellanos, A., and Lemberg, L.: Unusual normalization of the electrocardiogram on the 6th day of myocardial infarction. J. Electrocardiol. *4*:363, 1971.
324. Goldberger, A. L.: Myocardial infarction. St. Louis, C. V. Mosby, 1984, pp. 29–146.
325. Pipberger, H. V., and Lopez, E. A.: "Silent" subendocardial infarcts: Fact or fiction? Am. Heart J. *100*:597, 1980.
326. Phibbs, B.: "Transmural" versus "Subendocardial" myocardial infarction: An electrocardiographic myth. J. Am. Coll. Cardiol. *1*:561, 1983.
327. Levine, H. D.: Subendocardial infarction in retrospect: Pathologic, cardiographic, and ancillary features. Circulation *72*:790, 1985.
328. Spodick, D. H.: Q-wave infarction versus S-T infarction: Nonspecificity of electrocardiographic criteria for differentiating transmural and nontransmural lesions. Am. J. Cardiol. *51*:913, 1983.
329. Zema, M. J.: Q-wave, S-T segment, and T-wave myocardial infarction. Am. J. Med. *78*:391, 1985.
329a. Goldberg, R. J., Gore, J. M., Alpert, J. S., and Dalen, J. E.: Non-Q wave myocardial infarction: Recent changes in occurrence and prognosis—a community-wide perspective. Am. Heart J. *113*:273, 1987.
330. Schuster, E. H., and Bulkley, B. H.: Early postinfarction angina. Ischemia at a distance and ischemia in the infarct zone. N. Engl. J. Med. *305*:1101, 1981.
331. Ferguson, D. W., Pandian, N., Kioschos, J. M., Marcus, M. L., and White, C. W.: Angiographic evidence that reciprocal ST-segment depression during acute myocardial infarction does not indicate remote ischemia: Analysis of 23 patients. Am. J. Cardiol. *53*:55, 1984.
332. Mukharji, J., Murray, S., Lewis, S. E., Croft, C. H., Corbett, J. R., Willerson, J. T., and Rude, R. E.: Is anterior ST-depression with acute transmural inferior infarction due to posterior infarction? J. Am. Coll. Cardiol. *4*:28, 1984.
333. Gibson, R. S., Crampton, R. S., Watson, D. D., Taylor, G. J., Carabello, B. A., Holt, N. D., and Beller, G. A.: Precordial ST-segment depression during acute inferior myocardial infarction: Clinical, scintigraphic and angiographic correlations. Circulation *66*:742, 1982.
334. Little, W. C., Rogers, E. W., and Sodums, M. T.: Mechanism of anterior ST-segment depression during acute inferior myocardial infarction. Ann. Intern. Med. *100*:26, 1984.
335. Lew, A. S., Weiss, A. T., Shah, P. K., Maddahi, J., Peter, T., Ganz, W., Swan, H. J. C., and Berman, D. S.: Precordial ST-segment depression during acute inferior myocardial infarction: Early thallium-201 scintigraphic evidence of adjacent posterolateral or inferoseptal involvement. J. Am. Coll. Cardiol. *5*:203, 1985.
336. Candell-Riera, J., Figueras, J., Valle, V., Alvarez, A., Gutierrez, L., Cortadellas, J., Cinca, J., Salas, A., and Rius, J.: Right ventricular infarction: Relationships between ST-segment elevation in V_4R and hemodynamic, scintigraphic, and echocardiographic findings in patients with acute inferior myocardial infarction. Am. Heart J. *101*:281, 1981.
337. Chou, T., Van Der Bel-Kahn, J., Allen, J., Brockmeier, L., and Fowler, N. O.: Electrocardiographic diagnosis of right ventricular infarction. Am. J. Med. *70*:1175, 1981.
338. Klein, H. O., Tordiman, T., Ninio, R., Sareli, P., Oren, V., Lang, R., Gefen, J., Pauzner, C., DiSegni, E., David, D., and Kaplinsky, E.: The early recognition of right ventricular infarction: Diagnostic accuracy of the electrocardiogram V_4R lead. Circulation *67*:558, 1983.
339. Braat, S. H., Brugada, P., DeZwaan, C., Coenegracht, J. M., and Wellens, H. J. J.: Value of electrocardiogram in diagnosing right ventricular involvement in patients with an acute inferior wall myocardial infarction. Br. Heart J. *49*:368, 1983.
340. Lopez-Sendon, J., Coma-Canella, I., Alcasena, S., Seoane, J., and Gamallo, C.: Electrocardiographic findings in acute right ventricular infarction: Sensitivity and specificity of electrocardiographic alterations in right precordial leads V_4R, V_3R, V_1, V_2, and V_3. J. Am. Coll. Cardiol. *6*:1273, 1985.

341. Geft, I. L., Shah, P. K., Rodriguez, L., Hulse, S., Maddahi, J., Berman, D. S., and Ganz, W.: ST elevations in leads V_1 to V_5 may be caused by right coronary artery occlusion and acute right ventricular infarction. Am. J. Cardiol. *53*:991, 1984.
342. Lew, A. S., Maddahi, J., Shah, P. K., Weiss, A. T., Peter, T., Berman, D. S., and Ganz, W.: Factors that determine the direction and magnitude of precordial ST-segment deviations during inferior wall acute myocardial infarction. Am. J. Cardiol. *55*:883, 1985.
343. Lieu, C. K., Greenspan, G., and Piccirillo, R. T.: Atrial infarction of the heart. Circulation *23*:331, 1961.
344. Silvertssen, E., Hoel, B., Bay, G., and Jorgensen, L.: Electrocardiographic atrial complex and acute atrial myocardial infarction. Am. J. Cardiol. *31*:450, 1973.
345. Stein, P. D., and Simon, A. P.: Vectorcardiographic diagnosis of diaphragmatic myocardial infarction. Am. J. Cardiol. *38*:568, 1976.
346. Howard, P. F., Benchimol, A., Desser, K. B., Reich, F. D., and Graves, C.: Correlation of electrocardiogram and vectorcardiogram with coronary occlusion and myocardial contraction abnormality. Am. J. Cardiol. *38*:582, 1976.
347. Levine, H. D., Young, E., and Williams, R. A.: Electrocardiogram and vectorcardiogram in myocardial infarction. Circulation *45*:457, 1972.
348. Timmis, A. D., Fowler, M. B., Burwood, R. J., Gishen, P., Vincent, R., and Chamberlain, D. A.: Pulmonary oedema without critical increase in left atrial pressure in acute myocardial infarction. Br. Med. J. *283*:636, 1981.
349. Field, B. J., Russell, R. O., Jr., Moraski, R. E., Soto, B., Hood, W. P., Jr., Burdenshaw, J. A., Smith, M., Maurer, B. J., and Rackley, C. E.: Left ventricular size and function and heart size in the year following myocardial infarction. Circulation *50*:331, 1974.
350. Waris, E. K., Siitonen, L., and Himanka, E.: Heart size and prognosis in myocardial infarction. Am. Heart J. *71*:187, 1966.
351. Gibson, R. S., Taylor, G. J., Watson, D. D., Stebbins, P. T., Martin, R. P., Crampton, R. S., and Beller, G. A.: Predicting the extent and location of coronary artery disease during the early postinfarction period by quantitative thallium-201 scintigraphy. Am. J. Cardiol. *47*:1010, 1981.
352. Willerson, J. T., Parkey, R. W., Lewis, S. E., Bonte, F. J., and Buja, L. M.: Hot-spot imaging for patients with acute myocardial infarction. J. Cardiovasc. Med. *7*:291, 1982.
353. Geltman, E. M., Biello, D., Welch, M. J., Ter-Pogossian, M. M., Roberts, R., and Sobel, B. E.: Characterization of nontransmural myocardial infarction by positron-emission tomography. Circulation *65*:747, 1982.
354. Leppo, J. A., O'Brien, J. O., Rothendler, J. A., Getchell, J. D., and Lee, V. W.: Dipyridamole-thallium-201 scintigraphy in the prediction of future cardiac events after acute myocardial infarction. N. Engl. J. Med. *310*:1014, 1984.
355. Khaw, B. A., Gold, H. K., Yasuda, T., Leinbach, R. C., Kanke, M., Fallon, J. T., Barlai-Kovach, M., Strauss, H. W., Sheehan, F., and Haber, E.: Scintigraphic quantification of myocardial necrosis in patients after intravenous injection of myosin-specific antibody. Circulation *74*:501, 1986.
356. Wesbey, G., Higgins, C. B., Lanzer, P., Botvinick, E., and Lipton, M. J.: Imaging and characterization of acute myocardial infarction in vivo by gated nuclear magnetic resonance. Circulation *69*:125, 1984.
357. Johnston, D. L., Thompson, R. C., Liu, P., Dinsmore, R. E., Wismer, G. L., Saini, S., Kaul, S., Rosen, B. R., Brady, T. J., and Okada, R. D.: Magnetic resonance imaging during acute myocardial infarction. Am. J. Cardiol. *57*:1059, 1986.
358. Pflugfelder, P. W., Wisenberg, G., Prato, F. S., Carroll, S. E., and Turner, K. L.: Early detection of canine myocardial infarction by magnetic resonance imaging in vivo. Circulation *71*:587, 1985.
359. Ratner, A. V., Okada, R. D., Newell, J. B., and Pohost, G. M.: The relationship between proton nuclear magnetic resonance relaxation parameters and myocardial perfusion with acute coronary arterial occlusion and reperfusion. Circulation *71*:823, 1985.
360. McNamara, M. T., Higgins, C. B., Schechtmann, N., Botvinick, E., Lipton, M. J., Chatterjee, K., and Ampara, E. G.: Detection and characterization of acute myocardial infarction in man with use of gated magnetic resonance. Circulation *71*:717, 1985.
361. Reeves, R. C., Evanochko, W. T., and Pohost, G. M.: Potential approaches to evaluating the cardiovascular system using NMR. Prog. Cardiovasc. Dis. *29*:53, 1986.
361a. Kloner, R. A., and Parisi, A. F.: Acute myocardial infarction: diagnostic and prognostic applications of two-dimensional echocardiography. Circulation *75*:521, 1987.
362. Lindvall, K., Erhardt, L., and Sjogren, A.: Serial M-mode echocardiographic mapping in myocardial infarction: A quantitative evaluation of left ventricular wall motion abnormalities. Clin. Cardiol. *6*:220, 1983.
363. Teichholz, L. E., Kreulen, T., Herman, M. V., and Gorlin, R.: Problems in echocardiographic volume determinations; echocardiographic-angiographic correlations in the presence or absence of asynergy. Am. J. Cardiol. *37*:7, 1976.
364. Corya, B. C., Rasmussen, S., Knoebel, S. B., and Feigenbaum, H.: Echocardiography in acute myocardial infarction. Am. J. Cardiol. *36*:1, 1975.
365. Nieminen, M., and Heikkila, J.: Echoventriculography in acute myocardial infarction. II. Monitoring of left ventricular performance. Br. Heart J. *38*:271, 1976.
366. Feigenbaum, H., Corya, B. C., Dillon, J. C., Weyman, A. E., Rasmussen, S., Black, M. J., and Chang, S.: Role of echocardiography in patients with coronary artery disease. Am. J. Cardiol. *37*:775, 1976.
367. Chandraratna, P. A. N., Balachandran, P. K., Shah, P. M., and Hodges, M.: Echocardiographic observation on ventricular septal rupture complicating acute myocardial infarction. Circulation *51*:506, 1975.
368. DeJoseph, R. L., Seides, S. F., Lindner, A., and Damato, A. N.: Echocardiographic findings of ventricular septal rupture in acute myocardial infarction. Am. J. Cardiol. *36*:346, 1975.
369. Sharpe, D. N., Botvinick, E. H., Shames, D. M., Schiller, N. B., Massie, B. M., Chatterjee, D., and Parmley, W. W.: The noninvasive diagnosis of right ventricular infarction. Circulation *57*:483, 1978.
370. Heger, J. J., Weyman, A. E., Wann, L. S., Dillon, J. C., and Feigenbaum, H.: Cross-sectional echocardiography in acute myocardial infarction: Detection and localization of regional left ventricular asynergy. Circulation *60*:531, 1979.
371. Visser, C. A., Lie, K. I., Becker, A. E., and Durrer, D.: Apex two-dimensional echocardiography. Alternative approach to quantification of acute myocardial infarction. Br. Heart J. *47*:461, 1982.
372. Gibson, R. S., Bishop, H. L., Stamm, R. B., Crampton, R. S., Beller, G. A., and Martin, R. P.: Value of early two-dimensional echocardiography in patients with acute myocardial infarction. Am. J. Cardiol. *49*:1110, 1982.
373. Mann, D. L., Gillam, L. D., and Weyman, A. E.: Cross-sectional echocardiographic assessment of regional left ventricular performance and myocardial perfusion. Prog. Cardiovasc. Dis. *23*:1, 1986.
374. Parisi, A. F., Moynihan, P. F., Folland, E. D., and Feldman, C. L.: Quantitative detection of regional left ventricular contraction abnormalities by two-dimensional echocardiography. II. Accuracy in coronary artery disease. Circulation *63*:761, 1981.
375. Oh, J. K., Miller, F. A., Shub, C., Reeder, G. S., and Tajik, A. J.: Evaluation of acute chest pain syndromes by two-dimensional echocardiography: Its potential application in the selection of patients for acute reperfusion therapy. Mayo Clin. Proc. *62*:59, 1987.
376. Parisi, A. F., Nieminen, M., O'Boyle, J. E., Moynihan, P. F., Khuri, S. F., Kloner, R. A., Folland, E. D., and Schoen, F. J.: Enhanced detection of the evolution of tissue changes after acute myocardial infarction using color-coded two-dimensional echocardiography. Circulation *66*:764, 1982.
377. Weiss, J. L.: Echocardiographic evaluation of coronary artery disease. *In* Come, P. C. (ed.): Diagnostic Cardiology. Noninvasive Imaging Techniques. Philadelphia, J. B. Lippincott Co., 1985, pp. 343–363.
378. Weiss, J. L., Bulkley, B. H., Hutchins, G. M., and Mason, S. J.: Two-dimensional echocardiographic recognition of myocardial injury in man: Comparison with postmortem studies. Circulation *63*:401, 1981.
379. Barrett, J. J., Charuzi, Y., and Corday, E.: Ventricular aneurysm: Cross-sectional echocardiographic approach. Am. J. Cardiol. *46*:1133, 1980.
380. Catherwood, E., Mintz, G. S., Kotler, M. N., Parry, W. R., and Segal, B. L.: Two-dimensional echocardiographic recognition of left ventricular pseudoaneurysm. Circulation *62*:294, 1980.
381. Richards, K. L., Hoekenga, D. E., Leach, J. K., and Blaustein, J. C.: Dopplercardiographic diagnosis of interventricular septal rupture. Chest *76*:101, 1979.
382. Bishop, H. L., Gibson, R. S., Stamm, R. B., Beller, G. A., and Martin, R. P.: Role of two-dimensional echocardiography in the evaluation of patients with ventricular septal rupture postmyocardial infarction. Am. Heart J. *102*:965, 1981.
383. Donaldson, R. M., and Ballester, M.: Echocardiographic visualization of the anatomic causes of mitral regurgitation resulting from myocardial infarction. Postgrad. Med. J. *58*:257, 1982.
384. Spirito, P., Bellotti, P., Chiarella, F., Domenicucci, S., Sementa, A., and Vecchio, C.: Prognostic significance and natural history of left ventricular thrombi in patients with acute anterior myocardial infarction: A two-dimensional echocardiographic study. Circulation *72*:774, 1985.
385. Nishimura, R. A., Miller, F. A., Callahan, M. J., Benassi, R. C., Seward, J. B., and Tajik, A. J.: Doppler echocardiography: Theory, instrumentation, technique, and application. Mayo Clinic Proc. *60*:321, 1985.
386. Chandraratna, P. A., Nanna, M., McKay, C., Nimalasuriya, A., Swinney, R., Elkayam, U., and Rahimtoola, S. H.: Determination of cardiac output by transcutaneous continuous-wave ultrasonic Doppler computer. Am. J. Cardiol. *53*:234, 1984.
387. Parker, M. E., and Just, H. G.: Systolic time intervals in coronary artery disease as indices of left ventricular function: Fact or fancy? Br. Heart J. *36*:368, 1974.
388. Brubakk, O., and Overskeid, K.: Systolic time intervals in acute myocardial infarction. Acta Med. Scand. *199*:33, 1976.
389. Khan, A. H., and Haywood, L. J.: Value of serial apexcardiograms during and after myocardial infarction. Chest *70*:367, 1976.
390. Maroko, P. R., Libby, P., Covell, J. W., Sobel, B. E., Ross, J., and Braunwald, E.: Precordial ST-T segment elevation mapping: An atraumatic method for assessing alterations in the extent of myocardial ischemic injury. Am. J. Cardiol. *29*:227, 1972.
391. Reid, P. R., Taylor, D. R., Kelly, D. T., Weisfeldt, M. L., Humphries, J. O., Ross, R. S., and Pitt, B.: Myocardial-infarct extension detected by precordial ST-segment mapping. N. Engl. J. Med. *290*:123, 1974.
392. Lekven, J., Chatterjee, K., Tyberg, J. V., and Parmley, W. W.: Influence of left ventricular dimensions on endocardial and epicardial QRS amplitude and ST segment elevations during acute myocardial ischemia. Circulation *61*:679, 1980.
393. Hillis, L. D., Askenazi, J., Braunwald, E., Radvany, P., Muller, J. E., Fischbein, M. C., and Maroko, P. R.: Use of changes in the epicardial QRS complex to assess interventions which modify the extent of myocardial necrosis following coronary artery occlusion. Circulation *54*:591, 1976.
394. Ideker, R. E., Wagner, G. S., Ruth, W. K., Alonso, D. R., Bishop, S. P., Bloor, C. M., Fallon, J. T., Gottlieb, G. J., Hackel, D. B., Phillips, H. R., Reimer, K. A., Roark, S. F., Rogers, W. J., Savage, R. M., White, R. D., and Selvester, R. H.: Evaluation of a QRS scoring system for estimating myocardial infarct size. II. Correlation with quantitative anatomic findings for anterior infarcts. Am. J. Cardiol. *49*:1604, 1982.

395. Roark, S. F., Ideker, R. E., Wagner, G. S., Alonso, D. R., Bishop, S. P., Bloor, C. M., Bramlet, D. A., Edwards, J. E., Fallon, J. T., Gottlieb, G. J., Hackel, D. B., Phillips, H. R., Reimer, K. A., Rogers, W. J., Ruth, W. K., Savage, R. M., White, R. D., and Selvester, R. H.: Evaluation of a QRS scoring system for estimating myocardial infarct size. III. Correlation with quantitative anatomic findings for inferior infarcts. Am. J. Cardiol. *51*:382, 1983.
396. Sederholm, M., Grottum, P., Erhardt, L., and Kjekshus, J.: Quantitative assessment of myocardial ischemia and necrosis by continuous vector-cardiography and measurements of creatine kinase release in patients. Circulation *68*:1006, 1983.
397. Cowan, M. J., Bruce, R. A., and Reichenbach, D. D.: Validation of a computerized QRS criterion for estimating myocardial infarction size and correlation with quantitative morphologic measurements. Am. J. Cardiol. *57*:60, 1986.
398. Hinohara, T., Hindman, N. B., White, R. D., Ideker, R. E., and Wagner, G. S.: Quantitative QRS criteria for diagnosing and sizing myocardial infarcts. Am. J. Cardiol. *53*:875, 1984.
399. Witteveen, S. A. G. J., Hemker, H. C., Hollaar, L., and Hermens, W. T.: Quantitation of infarct size in man by means of plasma enzyme levels. Br. Heart J. *37*:795, 1975.
400. Morrison, J., Coromilas, J., Munsey, D., Robbins, M., Zema, M., Chiaramida, S., Reiser, P., and Scherr, L.: Correlation of radionuclide estimates of myocardial infarction size and release of creatine kinase-MB in man. Circulation *62*:277, 1980.
401. Hackel, D. B., Reimer, K. A., Ideker, R. E., Mikat, E. M., Hartwell, T. D., Parker, C. B., Braunwald, E. B., Buja, M., Gold, H. K., Jaffe, A. S., Muller, J. E., Raabe, D. S., Rude, R. E., Sobel, S. E., Stone, P. H., Roberts, R., and the MILIS Study Group: Comparison of enzymatic and anatomic estimates of myocardial infarct size in man. Circulation *70*:824, 1984.
402. Armstrong, W. F., West, S. R., Dillon, J. C., and Feigenbaum, H.: Assessment of location and size of myocardial infarction with contrast-enhanced echocardiography. II. Application of digital imaging techniques. J. Am. Coll. Cardiol. *4*:141, 1984.
403. Weiss, J. L., Bulkley, B. H., Hutchins, G. M., and Mason, S. J.: Two-dimensional echocardiographic recognition of myocardial injury in man: Comparison with postmortem studies. Circulation *63*:401, 1981.
404. Force, T., Kemper, A., Perkins, L., Gilfoil, M., Cohen, C., and Parisi, A. F.: Overestimation of infarct size by quantitative two-dimensional echocardiography: The role of tethering and of analytic procedures. Circulation *63*:1360, 1986.
405. Holman, B. L., Goldhaber, S. Z., Kirsch, C. M., Polak, J. F., Friedman, B. J., English, R. J., and Wynne, J.: Measurement of infarct size using single photon emission computed tomography and technetium-99m pyrophosphate: A description of the method and comparison with patient prognosis. Am. J. Cardiol. *50*:503, 1982.
406. Corbett, J. R., Lewis, S. E., Wolfe, C. L., Jansen, D. E., Lewis, M., Rellas, J. S., Parkey, R. W., Rude, R. E., Buja, M., and Willerson, J. T.: Measurement of myocardial infarct size by technetium pyrophosphate single-photon tomography. Am. J. Cardiol. *54*:1231, 1984.

MANAGEMENT OF ACUTE MYOCARDIAL INFARCTION

407. Wenger, N. K., Hellerstein, H. K., Blackburn, H., and Castranova. S. J.: Physician practice in the management of patients with uncomplicated myocardial infarction: Changes in the past decade. Circulation *65*:421, 1982.
408. Pantridge, J. F., Webb, S. W., Adgey, A. A. J., and Geddes, J. S.: The first hour after the onset of acute myocardial infarction. *In* Yu, P. N., and Goodwin, J. F. (eds.): Progress in Cardiology. Philadelphia, Lea and Febiger, 1974, p. 173.
409. Antman, E. M., and Rutherford, J. D.: Coronary Care Medicine. Martinus Nijhoff, Boston, 1986, p. 20.
410. Pantridge, J. R., and Geddes, J. S.: Diseases of the cardiovascular system. Management of acute myocardial infarction. Br. Med. J. *2*:168, 1976.
411. Dillon, J. C., Vasu, C. M., Berman, D. S., DeMaria, A. N., Goldstein, S. Y., Mandell, W. J., and Warren, J. V.: Thirteenth Bethesda Conference—Task Force III: Diagnostic procedures. Am. J. Cardiol. *50*:377, 1982.
412. Cobb, L. A., Baum, R. S., Alverez, H., III, and Schaffer, W. A.: Resuscitation from out-of-hospital ventricular fibrillation: 4 years' follow-up. Circulation *51-52*(Suppl. III):223, 1975.
413. Lewis, R. P., Lanese, R. R., Stang, J. M., Chirikos, T. N., Keller, M. D., and Warren, J. V.: Reduction of mortality from prehospital myocardial infarction by prudent patient activation of mobile coronary care system. Am. Heart J. *103*:123, 1982.
414. Crampton, R. S., Aldrich, F. R., Gascho, J. A., Miles, J. R., Jr., and Stillerman, R.: Reduction of prehospital, ambulance and community coronary death rates by the community-wide emergency cardiac care system. Am. J. Med. *58*:151, 1975.
415. Capone, R. J., Visco, J., Curwen, E., and VanEvery, S.: The effect of early prehospital transtelephonic coronary intervention on morbidity and mortality: Experience with 284 postmyocardial infarction patients in a pilot program. Am. Heart J. *107*:1153, 1984.
416. Pressley, J. C., Wilson, B. H., Severance, H. W., Raney, M. P., KcKinnis, R. A., Smith, M. W., Hindman, M. C., and Wagner, G. S.: Basic emergency medical care of patients with acute myocardial infarction: Initial prehospital characteristics and in-hospital complications. J. Am. Coll. Cardiol. *4*:487, 1984.
417. Goldman, L.: Coronary care units: A perspective on their epidemiologic impact. Int. J. Cardiol. *2*:284, 1982.
418. Morris, A. L., Nernberg, V., Roos, N. P., Henteleff, P., and Ross, L., Jr.: Acute myocardial infarction: Survey of urban and rural hospital mortality. Am. Heart J. *105*:44, 1983.
419. Hill, J. D., Hampton, J. R., and Mitchell, J. R. A.: A randomized trial of home-versus-hospital management for patients with suspected myocardial infarction. Lancet *1*:837, 1978.
420. Brush, J. E., Brand, D. A., Acampora, D., Chalmer, B., and Wackers, F. J.: Use of the initial electrocardiogram to predict in-hospital complications of acute myocardial infarction. N. Engl. J. Med. *312*:1137, 1985.
421. Lee, T. L., Cook, E. F., Weisberg, M., Sargent, R. K., Wilson, C., and Goldman, L.: Acute chest pain in the emergency ward: Identification and evaluation of low-risk patients, Arch. Intern. Med. *145*:65, 1985.
422. Goldman, L., Weinberg, M., Weisberg, M., Olshen, R., Cook, E. F., Sargent, R. K., Lamas, G. A., Dennis, C., Wilson, C., Deckelbaum, L., Fineberg, H., and Stiratelli, R.: A computer-derived protocol to aid in the diagnosis of emergency room patients with acute chest pain. N. Engl. J. Med. *307*:588, 1982.
423. Pozen, M. W., D'Agostino, R. B., Mitchell, J. B., Rosenfeld, D. M., Gugliemino, J. T., Schwartz, M. L., Teebagy, N., Valentine, M., and Hood, W. B.: The usefulness of a predictive instrument to reduce inappropriate admissions to the coronary care unit. Ann. Intern. Med. *92*:238, 1980.
424. Fineberg, H., Scadden, D., and Goldman, L.: Management of patients with a low probability of acute myocardial infarction: Cost-effectiveness of alternatives to coronary care unit admission. N. Engl. J. Med. *310*:1301, 1984.
425. McGregor, M.: The coronary care unit. A lack of consensus. Am. J. Med. *78*:378, 1985.
425a. Lee, T. H., Rouan, G. W., Weisberg, M. C., Brand, D. A., Cook, F., Acampora, D., Goldman, L., and the Chest Pain Study Group: Sensitivity of routine clinical criteria for diagnosing myocardial infarction within 24 hours of hospitalization. Ann. Intern. Med. *106*:181, 1987.
426. Mikolich, J. R., Nicoloff, N. B., Robinson, P. H., and Logue, H. B.: Relief of refractory angina with continuous intravenous infusion of nitroglycerin. Chest *77*:375, 1980.
427. Come, P. C., and Pitt, B.: Nitroglycerin-induced severe hypotension and bradycardia in patients with acute myocardial infarction. Circulation *54*:624, 1976.
428. Ferguson, J. J., Diver, D. J., Boldt, M., and Pasternak, R. C.: Nitroglycerin induced hypotension with acute myocardial infarction: A marker of right ventricular involvement? Circulation *72*(Suppl III):460, 1985.
429. Zelis, R., Mansour, E. J., Capone, R. J., and Mason, D. T.: The cardiovascular effects of morphine: The peripheral capacitance and resistance vessels in human subjects. J. Clin. Invest. *54*:1247, 1974.
430. Wynne, J., Mann, T., Alpert, J. S., and Grossman, W.: Beneficial effects of nitrous oxide in patients with ischemic heart disease. Circulation *55-56*(Suppl. III):18, 1977.
431. Thompson, P. L., and Lown, B.: Nitrous oxide as an analgesic in acute myocardial infarction. J.A.M.A. *235*:924, 1976.
432. Fillmore, S. J., Shapiro, M., and Killip, T.: Arterial oxygen tension in acute myocardial infarction. Serial analysis of clinical state and blood gas changes. Am. Heart J. *79*:620, 1970.
433. Maroko, P. R., Radvany, P., Braunwald, E., and Hale, S. L.: Reduction of infarct size by oxygen inhalation following acute coronary occlusion. Circulation *52*:360, 1975.
434. Madias, J. E., and Hood, W. B., Jr.: Reduction of precordial ST-segment elevation in patients with anterior myocardial infarction by oxygen breathing. Circulation *53* (Suppl. I):198, 1976.
435. Singer, M. M., Wright, F., Stanley, L. K., Roe, B. B., and Hamilton, W. K.: Oxygen toxicity in man: A prospective study in patients after open-heart surgery. N. Engl. J. Med. *283*:1473, 1970.
436. Ramsdale, D. R., Faragher, E. B., Bennett, D. H., Bray, C. L., Ward, C., Cruickshank, J. M., Yusuf, S., and Sleight, P.: Ischemic pain relief in patients with acute myocardial infarction by intravenous atenolol. Am. Heart J. *203*:459, 1982.
437. Richterova, A., Herlitz, J., Holmesberg, S., Swedberg, K., Waagstein, F., Waldenström, A., Vedin, A., Wennerblom, B., Wilhelmsson, C., and Hjalmarson, A.: Göteborg metoprolol trial: Effects on chest pain. J. Cardiol. *53*:32D, 1984.
437a. Kirshenbaum, J. M., Antman, E., McGowan, N., and Kloner, R. A.: Use of esmolol in patients with acute myocardial ischemia and contraindications to beta blockade. J. Am. Coll. Cardiol. *9*:24A, 1987.
438. Magder, S.: Assessment of myocardial stress from early ambulatory activities following myocardial infarction. Chest *87*:442, 1985.
439. Levine, S. A., and Lown, B.: "Armchair" treatment of acute coronary thrombosis. J.A.M.A. *148*:1365, 1952.
440. Swan, H. J. C.: Ganz, W., Forrester, J. S., Marcus, H., Diamond, G., and Chonette, D.: Catheterization of the heart in man with use of a flow-directed balloon-tipped catheter. N. Engl. J. Med. *283*:447, 1970.
441. Crexells, C., Chatterjee, K., Forrester, J. S., Dikshit, K., and Swan, H. J. C.: Optimal level of filling pressure in the left side of the heart in acute myocardial infarction. N. Engl. J. Med. *289*:1263, 1973.
442. Raphael, L. D., Mantle, J. A., Moraski, R. E., Rogers, W. J., Russell, R. O., Jr., and Rackley, C. E.: Quantitative assessment of ventricular performance in unstable ischemic heart disease by dextran function curves. Circulation *55*:858, 1977.
443. Rackley, C. E., Satler, L. F., Pearle, D. L., Del Negro, A. A., Pallas, R. S., and Kent, K. E.: Use of hemodynamic measurements for management of

acute myocardial infarction. *In* Rackley, C. E. (ed.): Advances in Critical Care Cardiology. Philadelphia, F. A. Davis Co., 1986, pp. 3-16.

444. Weisel, R. D., Berger, R. L., and Hechtman, H. B.: Measurement of cardiac output by thermodilution. N. Engl. J. Med. *292*:682, 1975.
445. Rahimtoola, S. H., Loeb, H. S., Ehsani, A., Sinno, Z., Chuquimia, R., Lal, R., Rosen, K. M., and Gunnar, R. M.: Relationship of pulmonary artery to left ventricular diastolic pressures in acute myocardial infarction. Circulation *46*:283, 1972.
446. McMichan, J. C., Baele, P. L., and Wignes, M. W.: Insertion of pulmonary artery catheters—a comparison of fiberoptic and nonfiberoptic catheters. Crit. Care Med. *12*:517, 1984.
447. Gewirtz, H., Gold, H. K., Fallon, J. T., Pasternak, R. C., and Leinbach, R. C.: Role of right ventricular infarction in cardiogenic shock associated with inferior myocardial infarction. Br. Heart J. *42*:719, 1979.
448. Shell, W. E., DeWood, M. A., Peter, T., Mickle, D., Prause, J., Forrester, J. S., and Swan, H. J. C.: Comparison of clinical signs and hemodynamic state in the early hours of transmural myocardial infarction. Am. Heart J. *104*:521, 1982.
449. Biddle, T. L., Ehrich, D. A., Hu, P. N., and Hodges, M.: Relation of heart block and left ventricular dysfunction in acute myocardial infarction. Am. J. Cardiol. *39*:961, 1977.
450. Applefield, J. J., Caruthers, T. E., Reno, D. J., and Civetta, J. M.: Assessment of the sterility of long-term cardiac catheterization using the thermodilution Swan-Ganz catheter. Chest *74*:377, 1978.
451. Goldenheim, P. D., and Kazemi, H.: Cardiopulmonary monitoring of critically ill patients. N. Engl. J. Med. *311*:776, 1984.
452. Eisenberg, P. R., Jaffe, A. S., and Schuster, D. P.: Clinical evaluation compared to pulmonary artery catheterization in the hemodynamic assessment of critically ill patients. Crit. Care Med. *12*:549, 1984.
453. Breisblatt, W., Harvey, M. R., Levy, W., Mirto, G., Cohen, L. S., and Feinstein, A. R.: Monitoring the use of Swan-Ganz catheters. Circulation *68*(Suppl. III):410, 1983.
454. Robin, E. D.: The cult of the Swan-Ganz catheter. Ann. Intern. Med. *103*:445, 1985.
455. Graboys, T. B.: In-hospital sudden death after coronary care unit discharge: A high-risk profile. Arch. Intern. Med. *135*:512, 1975.
456. Marmor, A., Geltman, E. M., Schechtman, K., Sobel, B. E., and Roberts, R.: Recurrent myocardial infarction: Clinical predictors and prognostic implications. Circulation *66*:415, 1982.
457. Lie, K. I., Liem, K. L., Schuilenburg, R. M., David, G. K., and Durrer, D.: Early identification of patients developing late in-hospital ventricular fibrillation after discharge from the Coronary Care Unit. Am. J. Cardiol. *41*:674, 1978.
458. Starling, M. R., Crawford, M. H., Kennedy, G. T., and O'Rourke, R. A.: Treadmill exercise tests predischarge and six week post-myocardial infarction to detect abnormalities of known prognostic value. Ann. Intern. Med. *94*:721, 1981.
459. Severance, H. W., Jr., Morris, K. G., and Wagner, G. S.: Criteria for early discharge after acute myocardial infarction. Validation in a community hospital. Arch. Intern. Med. *142*:39, 1982.
460. Resnekov, L.: The intermediate care unit—a stage in continued coronary care. Br. Heart J. *39*:357, 1977.
461. Weinberg, S. L.: Intermediate coronary care—observations on the validity of the concept. Chest *73*:154, 1978.
462. Leak, D., and Eydt, J. E.: An assessment of intermediate coronary care. Arch. Intern. Med. *138*:1780, 1978.
463. Page, D. L., Caulfield, J. B., Kastor, J. A., DeSanctis, R. W., and Sanders, C. A.: Myocardial changes associated with cardiogenic shock. N. Engl. J. Med. 285:133, 1971.
464. Gutovitz, A. L., Sobel, B. E., and Roberts, R.: Progressive nature of myocardial injury in selected patients with cardiogenic shock. Am. J. Cardiol. *41*:469, 1978.
465. Rogers, W. J., McDaniel, H. G., Smith, L. R., Mantle, J. A., Russell, R. O., Jr., and Rackley, C. E.: Correlation of angiographic estimates of myocardial infarct size and accumulated release of creatine kinase MB isoenzyme in man. Circulation *56*:199, 1977.
466. Sobel, B. E., Bresnahan, G. F., Shell, W. E., and Yoder, R. D.: Estimation of infarct size in man and its relation to prognosis. Circulation *46*:640, 1972.
467. Bleifield, W., Mathey, D., Hanrath, P., Buss, H., and Effert, S.: Infarct size estimated from serial serum creatine phosphokinase in relation to left ventricular hemodynamics. Circulation *55*:303, 1977.
468. Holman, B. L., Chisholm, R. J., and Braunwald, E.: The prognostic implications of acute myocardial infarct scintigraphy with ^{99m}Tc-pyrophosphate. Circulation *57*:320, 1978.
469. Geltman, E. M., Ehsani, A. A., Campbell, M. K., Schechtman, K., Roberts, R., and Sobel, B. E.: The influence of location and extent of myocardial infarction on long-term ventricular dysrhythmia and mortality. Circulation *60*:805, 1979.
470. Sobel, B. E., and Shell, W. E.: Jeopardized, blighted, and necrotic myocardium. Circulation *47*:215, 1973.
471. Braunwald, E., and Maroko, P. R.: The reduction of infarct size—an idea whose time (for testing) has come. Circulation *50*:206, 1974.
472. Kubler, W., and Doorey, A.: Reduction of infarct size. An attractive concept: Useful or possible in human? Br. Heart J. *53*:5, 1985.
473. Maroko, P. R., Kjekshus, J. K., Sobel, B. E., Watanabe, T., Covell, J. W., Ross, J., Jr., and Braunwald, E.: Factors influencing infarct size following experimental coronary artery occlusions. Circulation *43*:67, 1971.
474. Christlieb, I. Y., Clark, R. E., and Sobel, B. E.: Three-hour preservation of the hypothermic globally ischemic heart with nifedipine. Surgery *90*:947, 1981.
475. Weisfeldt, M. L.: Reperfusion and reperfusion injury. Clin. Res. *35*:13, 1987.
476. Corr, P. B., Snyder, D. W., Lee, B. I., Gross, R. W., Keim, C. R., and Sobel, B. E.: Pathophysiological concentrations of lysophosphatides and the slow response. Am. J. Physiol. *12*:187, 1982.
477. Gross, R. W., Corr, P. B., Lee, B. I., Saffitz, J. E., Crafford, W. A., Jr., and Sobel, B. E.: Incorporation of radiolabeled lysophosphatidylcholine into canine Purkinje fibers and ventricular muscle: Electrophysiological, biochemical and autoradiographic correlations. Circ. Res. *51*:27, 1982.
478. Schaper, W., and Pasyk, S.: Influence of collateral flow on the ischemic tolerance of the heart following acute and subacute coronary occlusion. Circulation *53*(Suppl. I):I-57, 1976.
479. Borda, L., Shuchleib, R., and Henry, P. D.: Effects of potassium on isolated canine arteries. Circ. Res. *41*:778, 1977.
480. Braunwald, E.: Coronary artery spasm as a cause of myocardial ischemia. J. Lab. Clin. Med. *97*:299, 1981.
481. Maseri, A., L'Abbate, A., Baroldi, G., Chierchia, S., Marzilli, M., Ballestra, A. M., Severi, S., Parodi, O., Biagini, A., Distante, A., and Pesola, A.: Coronary vasospasm as a possible cause of myocardial infarction. N. Engl. J. Med. *299*:1271, 1978.
482. Henry, P. D., and Yokoyama, M.: Supersensitivity of atherosclerotic rabbit aorta to ergonovine: Mediation by aserotonergic mechanism. J. Clin. Invest. *66*:306, 1980.
483. Morgan, T. J., French, W. J., Abrams, H. F., and Criley, J. M.: Post-myocardial infarction angina and coronary spasm. Am. J. Cardiol. *50*:192, 1982.
484. Koiwaya, Y., Torii, S., Takeshita, A., Nakagaki, O., and Nakamura, M.: Postinfarction angina caused by coronary arterial spasm. Circulation *65*:275, 1982.
485. Williams, D. O., Amsterdam, E. A., Miller, R. R., and Mason, D. T.: Functional significance of coronary collateral vessels in patients with acute myocardial infarction: Relation to pump performance, cardiogenic shock, and survival. Am. J. Cardiol. *37*:345, 1976.
486. Strauss, H. D.: Myocardial infarction extension: Clinical significance. Primary Cardiol. *8*:14, 1982.
487. Baker, J. T., Bramlet, D. A., Lester, R. M., Harrison, D. C., Roe, C. R., and Cobb, F. R.: Myocardial infarction extension: Incidence and relationship to survival. Circulation *65*:918, 1982.
488. Marmor, A., Sobel, B. E., and Roberts, R.: Factors presaging early recurrent myocardial infarction ("extension"). Am. J. Cardiol. *48*:603, 1981.
489. Cannom, D. S., Levy, W., and Cohen, L. S.: The short- and long-term prognosis of patients with transmural and nontransmural myocardial infarction. Am. J. Med. *61*:452, 1976.
490. Hutter, A. M., Jr., DeSanctis, R. W., Flynn, T., and Yeatman, L. A.: Nontransmural myocardial infarction. A comparison of hospital and late clinical course of patients with that of matched patients with transmural anterior and transmural inferior myocardial infarction. Am. J. Cardiol. *48*:595, 1981.
491. Shell, W. E., and Sobel, B. E.: Protection of jeopardized ischemic myocardium by reduction of ventricular afterload. N. Engl. J. Med. *291*:481, 1974.
492. Derrida, J. P., Sal, R., and Chiche, P.: Nitroglycerin infusion in acute myocardial infarction. N. Engl. J. Med. *297*:336, 1977.
493. Hjalmarson, A., Herlitz, J., Malek, I., Ryden, L., Vedin, A., Waldenstroj, A., Wedel, H., Elmfeldt, D., Holmberg, S., Nyberg, G., Swedberg, K., Waagstein, F., Waldenstrom, J., Wilhemsen, L., and Wilhelmsson, C.: Effect on mortality of metoprolol in acute myocardial infarction. Lancet *2*:823, 1981.
494. Yusuf, S., Ramsdale, E., Peto, R., Furse, L., Bennet, D., Bray, C., and Sleight, P.: Early intravenous atenolol treatment in suspected acute myocardial infarction. Preliminary report of a randomized trial. Lancet *2*:73, 1980.
495. Lange, R., Kloner, R. A., and Braunwald, E.: First ultrashort-acting beta-adrenergic blocking agent: Its effect on size and segmental wall dynamics of reperfused myocardial infarcts in dogs. Am. J. Cardiol. *51*:1759, 1983.
496. Braunwald, E., Muller, J. E., Kloner, R. A., and Maroko, P. R.: Role of beta-adrenergic blockade in the therapy of patients with myocardial infarction. Am. J. Med. *74*:113, 1983.
497. Chatterjee, K., and Parmley, W. W.: Vasodilator therapy for acute myocardial infarction and chronic congestive heart failure. J. Am. Coll. Cardiol. *1*:133, 1983.
498. Ginks, W. R., Sybers, H. D., Maroko, P. R., Covell, J. W., Sobel, B. E., and Ross, J., Jr.: Coronary artery reperfusion: II. Reduction of myocardial infarct size at 1 week after the coronary occlusion. *51*:2717, 1972.
499. Lang, T., Corday, E., Gold, H., Meerbaum, S., Rubins, S., Costantini, C., Hirose, S., Osher, J., and Rosen, V.: Consequences of reperfusion after coronary occlusion: Effects on hemodynamic and regional myocardial metabolic function. Am. J. Cardiol. *33*:69, 1974.
500. Smith, G. T., Soeter, J. R., Haston, H. H., and McNamara, J. J.: Coronary reperfusion in primates: Serial electrocardiographic and histologic assessment. J. Clin. Invest. *54*:1420, 1974.
501. Kloner, R. A., Fishbein, M. C., Cotran, R. S., Braunwald, E., and Maroko, P. R.: The effect of propranolol on microvascular injury in acute myocardial ischemia. Circulation *55*:872, 1977.
502. Deloche, A., Fabiaini, J. N., Camilleri, J. P., Relland, J., Joseph, D., Carpentier, A., and Dubost, C.: The effect of coronary artery reperfusion on the extent of myocardial infarction. Am. Heart J. *93*:358, 1977.
503. Bergmann, S. R., Lerch, R. A., Fox, K. A. A., Ludbrook, P. A., Welch, M. J., Ter-Pogossian, M. M., and Sobel, B. E.: The temporal dependence of beneficial effects of coronary thrombolysis characterized by positron tomography. Am. J Med. *73*:573, 1982.
504. Reimer, K. A., and Jennings, R. B.: The wavefront phenomenon of myocardial ischemic cell death. II. Transmural progression of necrosis within the

framework of ischemic bed size (myocardium at risk) and collateral flow. Lab. Invest. *40*:633, 1979.
505. Cheauvechai, C., Effler, D. B., Loop, F. D., Groves, L. K., Sheldon, W. C., Razavi, M., and Sones, F. M., Jr.: Emergency myocardial revascularization. Am. J. Cardiol. 32:901, 1973.
506. Chazov, E. I., Mateeva, L. S., Mazaev, A. V., Sargin, K. E., and Sadovskaia, G. V.: Intracoronary administration of fibrinolysin in acute myocardial infarction. Ter. Arkh. *48*:8, 1976.
507. Rentrop, P., DeVivie, E. R., Karsch, K. R., and Kreuzer, H.: Acute coronary occlusion with impending infarction as an angiographic complication relieved by a guide-wire recanalization. Clin. Cardiol. *1*:101, 1978.
508. Kloner, R. A., Ellis, S. G., Lange, R., and Braunwald, E.: Studies of experimental coronary artery reperfusion: Effects on infarct size, myocardial function, biochemistry, ultastructure, and microvascular damage. Circulation *68* (Suppl. I):8, 1983.
509. Reimer, K. A., Lower, J. E., Rasmussen, M. M., and Jennings, R. B.: The wavefront phenomenon of ischemic cell death. I. Myocardial infarct size vs. duration of coronary occlusion in dogs. Circulation *56*:786, 1977.
510. Schwartz, F., Schuler, G., Katus, H., Hofmann, M., Manthy, J., Tillmanns, H., Mehmel, H. C., and Kubler, W.: Intracoronary thrombolysis in acute myocardial infarction: Duration of ischemia as a major determinant of late results after recanalization. Am. J. Cardiol. *50*:933, 1982.
511. Sheehan, F. H., Mathey, D. G., Schofer, J., Dodge, H. T., and Bolson, E. L.: Factors that determine recovery of left ventricular function after thrombolysis in patients with acute myocardial infarction. Circulation *71*:1121, 1985.
511a. Sheehan, F. H., Braunwald, E., Canner, P., Dodge, H. T., Gore, J., Van Natta, P., Passamani, E. R., Williams, D. O., Zaret, B., and Co-investigators: The effect of intravenous thrombolytic therapy on left ventricular function: a report on tissue-type plasminogen activator and streptokinase from the thrombolysis in myocardial infarction (TIMI Phase I) trial. Circulation *75*:817, 1987.
512. Saito, Y., Yasuno, M., Ishida, M., Suzuki, K., Matoba, Y., Emura, M., and Takahashi, M.: Importance of coronary collaterals for restoration of left ventricular function after intracoronary thrombolysis. Am. J. Cardiol. *55*:1259, 1985.
513. Nayler, W. G., and Elz, J. S.: Reperfusion injury: Laboratory artifact or clinical dilemma? Circulation *74*:215, 1986.
514. Braunwald, E., and Kloner, R. A.: Myocardial reperfusion: A double-edged sword? J. Clin. Invest. *76*:1713, 1985.
515. Kloner, R. A., Ganote, C. E., and Jennings, R. B.: The "no-reflow" phenomenon after temporary coronary occlusion in the dog. J. Clin. Invest. *54*:1496, 1974.
516. Waller, B. F., Rothbaum, D. A., Pinkerton, C. A., Cowley, M. J., Linnemeier, T. J., Orr, C., Irons, M., Helmuth, R. A., Wills, E. R., and Aust, C.: Status of the myocardium and infarct-related coronary artery in 19 necropsy patients with acute recanalization using pharmacologic (streptokinase, r-tissue plasminogen activator), mechanical (percutaneous transluminal coronary angioplasty) or combined types of reperfusion therapy. J. Am. Coll. Cardiol. *9*:785, 1987.
517. Bresnahan, G. F., Roberts, R., Shell, W. E., Ross, J., Jr., and Sobel, B. E.: Deleterious effects due to hemorrhage after myocardial reperfusion. Am. J. Cardiol. *32*:82, 1974.
518. Fujiwara, H., Onodera, T., Tanaka, M., Fujiwara, T., Wu, D. J., Kawai, C., and Hamashima, Y.: A clinicopathologic study of patients with hemorrhagic myocardial infarction treated with selective coronary thrombolysis with urokinase. Circulation *73*:749, 1986.
519. Mattfeldt, T., Schwarz, F., Schuler, G., Hofmann, M., and Kubler, W.: Necropsy evaluation in seven patients with evolving acute myocardial infarction treated with thrombolytic therapy. Am. J. Cardiol. *54*:530, 1984.
520. Werns, S. W., Shea, M. J., and Lucchesi, B. R.: Free radicals and myocardial injury: Pharmacologic implications. Circulation *74*:1, 1986.
521. Wei, J. Y., Markis, J. E., Malagold, M., and Braunwald, E.: Cardiovascular reflexes stimulated by reperfusion of ischemic myocardium in acute myocardial infarction. Circulation *67*:796, 1983.
522. Cercek, B., and Horvat, M.: Arrhythmias with brief, high-dose intravenous streptokinase infusion in acute myocardial infarction. Eur. Heart J. *6*:109, 1985.
523. Goldberg, S., Greenspon, A. J., Urban, P. L., Muza, B., Berger, B., Walinsky, P., and Maroko, P. R.: Reperfusion arrhythmia: A marker of restoration of antegrade flow during intracoronary thrombolysis for acute myocardial infarction. Am. Heart J. *105*:26, 1983.
524. Wilber, D., Walton, J., O'Neill, W., Laufer, N., and Pitt, B.: Effects of reperfusion on complete heart block complicating anterior myocardial infarction. J. Am. Coll. Cardiol. *4*:1315, 1984.
525. Rentrop, P., Blanke, H., Marsch, K. R., Kaiser, H., Kostering, H., and Leitz, K.: Selective intracoronary thrombolysis in acute myocardial infarction and unstable angina pectoris. Circulation *63*:307, 1981.
526. Khaja, F., Walton, J. A., Brymer, J. F., Lo, E., Osterburger, L. E., O'Neill, W. W., Colfer, H. T., Weiss, R., Lee, T., Kurian, T., Goldberg, D., Pitt, B., and Goldstein, S.: Intracoronary fibrinolytic therapy in acute myocardial infarction, report of a prospective randomized trial. N. Engl. J. Med. *308*:1305, 1983.
527. Smalling, R. W., Fuentes, F., Matthews, M. W., Kuhn, J., Nishikawa, A., Walker, W. E., Adams, P. R., and Gould, K. L.: Factors affecting outcome of coronary reperfusion with intracoronary streptokinase in acute myocardial infarction. Am. J. Cardiol. *59*:505, 1987.
528. Mathey, D. G., Sheehan, F. H., Schofer, J., and Dodge, H. T.: Time from onset of symptoms to thrombolytic therapy: A major determinant of myocardial salvage in patients with acute transmural infarction. J. Am. Coll. Cardiol. *6*:581, 1985.
528a. Patel, B., and Kloner, R. A.: Analysis of reported randomized trials of streptokinase therapy for acute myocardial infarction in the 1980s. Am. J. Cardiol. *59*:501, 1987.
529. Koren, G., Weiss, A. T., Hasin, Y., Applebaum, D., Welber, S., Rozenman, Y., Lotan, C., Mosseri, M., Sapoznikov, D., Luria, M. H., and Gotsman, M. S.: Prevention of myocardial damage in acute myocardial ischemia by early treatment with intraveneous streptokinase. N. Engl. J. Med. *313*:1384, 1985.
530. The TIMI Study Group: The thrombolysis in myocardial infarction (TIMI) trial. Phase I Findings. N. Engl. J. Med. *312*:932, 1985.
531. Verstraete, M., Bory, M., Collen, D. Erbel, R., Lennane, R. J., Mathey, D., Michels, H. R., Schartl, M., Uebis, R., Bernard, R., Brower, R. W., DeBono, D. P., Huhmann, W., Lursen, J., Meyer, J., Rutsch, W., Schmidt, W., and Von Essen, R.: Randomised trial of intravenous recombinant tissue-type plasminogen activator versus intravenous streptokinase in acute myocardial infarction. Lancet *1*:842, 1985.
531a. Piccolo, E., and co-investigators: In-hospital results and one-year follow-up of the G.I.S.S.I. trial. G. Ital. Cardiol. *17*:20, 1987.
532. Schroder, R., Karl-Ludwig, N., Leizorovicz, A., Linderer, T., and Tebbe, U.: A prospective placebo-controlled double-blind multicenter trial of intravenous streptokinase in acute myocardial infarction (ISAM): Long-term mortality and morbidity. J. Am. Coll. Cardiol. *9*:197, 1987.
532a. Lew, A. S., Hod, H., Cercek, B., Shah, P. K., and Ganz, W.: Mortality and morbidity rates of patients older and younger than 75 years with acute myocardial infarction treated with intravenous streptokinase. Am. J. Cardiol. *59*:1, 1987.
533. Sherry, S.: Tissue plasminogen activator (t-PA). Will it fulfull its promise? N. Engl. J. Med. *313*:1014, 1985.
534. Badger, R. S., Brown, B. G., Kennedy, J. W., Mathey, D., Gallery, C. A., Bolson, E. L., and Dodge, H. T.: Usefulness of recanalization to luminal diameter of 0.6 millimeter or more with intracoronary streptokinase during acute myocardial infarction in predicting "normal" perfusion status, continued arterial patency and survival at one year. Am. J. Cardiol. *59*:519, 1987.
535. Holmes, D. R., Smith, H. C., Vliestra, R. D., Nishimura, R. A., Reeder, G. S., Bove, A. A., Breshahan, J. F., Chesbro, J. H., and Piehler, J. M.: Percutaneous transluminal coronary angioplasty alone or in combination with streptokinase therapy, during acute myocardial infarction. Mayo Clin. Proc. *60*:449, 1985.
536. Schroder, R., Vohringer, H., Linderer, T., Giamino, G., Bruggeman, T., and Leitner, E. V.: Follow-up after coronary arterial reperfusion with intravenous streptokinase in relation to residual myocardial infarct artery narrowings. Am. J. Cardiol. *55*:313, 1985.
537. Miller, H. I., Almagor, Y., Keren, G., Chernilas, J., Roth, A., Eschar, Y., Shapira, I., Shargorodsky, B., Berenfeld, D., and Laniado, S.: Early intervention in acute myocardial infarction: Significance for myocardial salvage of immediate intravenous streptokinase therapy followed by coronary angioplasty. J. Am. Coll. Cardiol. *9*:608, 1987.
538. Meyer, J., Erbel, R., Pop, T., Von Olshausen, K., Schuster, C. J., Treese, N., Rupprecht, H. J., Heinrichs, K. J., Diefenbach, C., Eissner, D., and Hohn, K.: Balloon coronary angioplasty in patients with acute myocardial infarction. Tex. Heart Inst. J. *13*:393, 1986.
539. Simoons, M. L., Brands, M., De Zwaan, C., Verheugt, F. W. A., Remme, W. J., Serruys, P. W., Bar, F., Res, J., Krauss, X. H., Vermeer, F., and Lubsen, J.: Improved survival after early thrombolysis in acute myocardial infarction. Lancet 2:578, 1985.
540. Kaplan, K., Davison, R., Parker, M., Mayberry, B., Feiereisel, P., and Salinger, M.: Role of heparin after intravenous thrombolytic therapy for acute myocardial infarction. Am. J. Cardiol. *59*:241, 1987.
541. Gold, H. K., Leinbach, R. C., Garabedian, H. D., Yasuda, T., Johns, J. A., Grossbard, E. B., Palacios, I., and Collen, D.: Acute coronary reocclusion after thrombosis with recombinant human tissue-type plasminogen activator: Prevention by a maintenance infusion. Circulation *73*:347, 1986.
542. Marder, V. J., Rothbard, R. L., Fitzpatrick, P. G., and Francis, C. W.: Rapid lysis of coronary artery thrombi with anisoylated plasminogen: Streptokinase activator complex. Ann. Intern. Med. *104*:304, 1986.
543. The I.S.A.M. Study Group: A prospective trial of intravenous streptokinase in acute myocardial infarction. Mortality, morbidity, and infarct size at 21 days. N. Engl. J. Med. *314*:1465, 1986.
543a. Schroder, R., Neuhaus, K.-L., Leizorovicz, A., Linderer, T., Tebbe, U. for the ISAM Study Group: A prospective placebo-controlled double-blind multicenter trial of intravenous streptokinase in acute myocardial infarction (ISAM): Long-term mortality and morbidity. J. Am. Coll. Cardiol. *9*:197, 1987.
544. Schwartz, F., Schuler, G., Katus, H. Hofmann, M., Manthey, J., Tillmanns, H., Mehmel, H. C., and Kubler, W.: Intracoronary thrombolysis in acute myocardial infarction: Duration of ischemia as a major determinant of late results after recanalization. Am. J. Cardiol. *50*:933, 1982.
545. Simoons, M. L., Serruys, P. W., van den Brand, M., Res, J., Verheugt, F. W. A., Krauss, X. H., Remme, W. J., Bar, F., deZwaan, C., van der Laarse, A., Vermeer, F., and Lubsen, J.: Early thrombolysis in acute myocardial infarction: Limitation of infarct size and improved survival. J. Am. Coll. Cardiol. *7*:717, 1986.
546. Lolley, D. M., Fulton, R., Hamman, J., Reader, G. S., Johnson, J. L., Clarke, J. A., Sheth, M. K., and Hearne, M. J.: Early coronary artery surgery after intracoronary streptokinase thrombolytic therapy. J. Am. Coll. Cardiol. *1*:632, 1983.

547. Ritchie, J. L., Davis, K. B., Williams, D., Caldwell, J., and Kennedy, J. W.: Global and regional left ventricular function and tomographic radionuclide perfusion: The Western Washington Intracoronary Streptokinase in Myocardial Infarction Trial. Circulation *70*:867, 1984.
548. Spann, J. F., Sherry, S., Carabello, B. A., Denenberg, B. S., Mann, R. M., McCann, W. D., Gault, J. H, Gentzler, R. D., Belber, A. D., Maurer, A. H., and Cooper, E. M.: Coronary thrombolysis by intravenous streptokinase in acute myocardial infarction: Acute and follow-up studies. Am. J. Cardiol. *53*:655, 1984.
549. Ferguson, D. W., White, C. W., Schwartz, J. L., Brayden, G. P., Kelly, K. J., Kioschos, J. M., Kirchner, P. T., and Marcus, M. L.: Influence of baseline ejection fraction and success of thrombolysis on mortality and ventricular function after acute myocardial infarction. Am. J. Cardiol. *54*:705, 1984.
550. Raizner, A. E., Tortoledo, F. A., Verani, M. S., VanReet, R. E., Young, J. B., Rickman, F. D., Cashion, R., Samuels, D. A., Pratt, C. M., Attar, M., Rubin, H. S., Lewis, J. M., Klein, M. S., and Roberts, R.: Intracoronary thrombolytic therapy in acute myocardial infarction: A prospective, randomized, controlled trial. Am. J. Cardiol. *55*:301, 1985.
551. Schuler, G., Hofmann, M., Schwartz, F., Mehmel, H., Manthey, J., Tillmanns, H., Harathmann, S., and Kubler, W.: Effect of successful thrombolytic therapy on right ventricular function in acute inferior wall myocardial infarction. Am. J. Cardiol. *54*:951, 1984.
552. Verani, M., Tortoledo, F. E., Batty, J. W., and Raizner, A. E.: Effect of coronary artery recanalization on right ventricular function in patients with acute myocardial infarction. J. Am. Coll. Cardiol. *5*:1029, 1985.
553. Satler, L. F., Rackley, C. E., Green, C. E., Pallas, R. S., Pearle, D. L., Del Negro, A. A., and Kent, K. M.: Ischemia during angioplasty after streptokinase: A marker of myocardial salvage. Am. J. Cardiol. *56*:749, 1985.
554. Melin, J. A., De Coster, P. M., Renkin, J., Detry, J. R., Beckers, C., and Col, J.: Effect of intracoronary thrombolytic therapy on exercise-induced ischemia after acute myocardial infarction. Am. J. Cardiol. *56*:705, 1985.
555. Kersschot, I. E., Brugada, P., Ramentol, M., Zehender, M., Waldecker, B., Stevenson, W. G., Geibel, A., DeZwaan, C., and Wellens, H. J. J.: Effects of early reperfusion in acute myocardial infarction on arrhythmias induced by programmed stimulation: A prospective, randomized study. J. Am. Coll. Cardiol. *7*:1234, 1986.
556. Meyer, J., Merx, W., Dorr, R., Lambertz, H., Bethge, C., and Effert, S.: Successful treatment of acute myocardial infarction shock by combined percutaneous transluminal coronary recanalization (PTCR) and percutaneous transluminal coronary angioplasty (PTCA). Am. Heart J. *103*:132, 1982.
557. Papapietro, S. E., MacLean, W. A. H., Stanley, A. W. H., Jr., Cooper, T. B., Hess, R. G., Siler, W., and Geer, D. A.: Percutaneous transluminal coronary angioplasty in acute myocardial infarction. J. Am. Coll. Cardiol. *1*:580, 1983.
558. Hartzler, G. O., Rutherford, B. D., and McConahay, D. R.: Percutaneous transluminal coronary angioplasty: Application for acute myocardial infarction. Am. J. Cardiol. *53*:1176, 1984.
559. Sriram, R., Mullen, G. M., Foschi, A., and Bicoff, J. P.: Percutaneous transluminal coronary angioplasty in acute myocardial infarction without prior thrombolytic therapy. Am. J. Cardiol. *55*:842, 1985.
560. O'Neill, W., Timmis, G. C., Bourdillon, P. D., Lai, P., Ganghadarhan, V., Walton, J., Ramos, R., Laufer, N., Gordon, S., Shork, M. A., and Pitt, B.: A prospective randomized clinical trial of intracoronary streptokinase versus coronary angioplasty for acute myocardial infarction. N. Engl. J. Med. *314*:812, 1986.
561. Fung, A. Y., Lai, P., Juni, J. E., Bourdillon, P. D. V., Walton, J. A., Laufer, N., Buda, A. J., Pitt, B., and O'Neill, W. W.: Prevention of subsequent exercise-induced periinfarct ischemia by emergency coronary angioplasty in acute myocardial infarction: Comparison with intracoronary streptokinase. J. Am. Coll. Cardiol. *8*:496, 1986.
562. Erbel, R., Pop, T., Meinertz, T., Kasper, W., Schreiner, G., Henkel, B., Henricks, K. J., Pfeiffer, C., Rupprecht, H. J., and Meyer, J.: Combined medial and mechanical recanalization in acute myocardial infarction. Cathet. Cardiovasc. Diagn. *11*:361, 1985.
563. Erbel, R., Pop, T., Jurgen-Henricks, K., vonOlshausen, K., Schuster, C. J., Rupprecht, H. J., Steuernagel, C., and Meyer, J.: Percutaneous transluminal coronary angioplasty after thrombolytic therapy: A prospective controlled randomized trial. J. Am. Coll. Cardiol. *8*:485, 1986.
564. Abela, G. S., Normann, S. J., Cohen, D. M., Frauzini, D., Feldman, R. L., Crea, F., French, A., Pepia, C. J., and Conti, C. R.: Laser recanalization of occluded atherosclerotic arteries in vivo and in vitro. Circulation *71*:403, 1985.
565. Cumberland, D. C., Sanborn, T. A., Tayler, D. I., Moore, D. J., Welsch, C. L., Greenfield, A. J., Gruben, J. K., and Ryan, T. J.: Percutaneous laser thermal angioplasty: Initial clinical results with a laser probe in total peripheral artery occlusion. Lancet *1*:1457, 1986.
566. Ritchie, J. L., Hansen, D., Vracko, R., and Auth, D. C.: Mechanical thrombolysis: A new rotational catheter approach for acute thrombi. Circulation *73*:1006, 1986.
567. Simpson, J. B., Johnson, D. E., Thapliyal, H. V., Marks, D. S., and Broden, L. J.: Transluminal atherectomy: A new approach to the treatment of atherosclerotic vascular disease. Circulation *72*(Suppl. III):146, 1985.
568. DeWood, M. A., Heit, J., Spores, J., Berg, R., Jr., Selinger, S. L., Rudy, L. W., Hensley, G. R., and Shields, J. P.: Anterior transmural myocardial infarction: Effects of surgical coronary reperfusion on global and regional left ventricular function. J. Am. Coll. Cardiol. *1*:1223, 1983.
569. DeWood, M. A., Spores, J., Berg, R., Kendall, R. W., Graunwald, R. P., Selinger, S. L., Hensley, G. R., Sutherland, K. I., and Shields, J. P.: Acute myocardial infarction: A decade of experience with surgical reperfusion in 701 patients. Circulation *68*(Suppl. II):8, 1983.
570. Phillips, S. J., Zeff, R. H., Skinner, J. R., Toon, R. S., Gryonon, A., and Kouptakworu, C.: Reperfusion protocol and results in 738 patients with evolving myocardial infarction. Ann. Thor. Surg. *41*:119, 1986.
571. Montoya, A., Mulet, J., Pifarre, R., Brynjolfsson, G., Moran, J. M., Sullivan, H. J., and Gunnar, R. M.: Hemorrhagic infarct following myocardial revascularization. J. Thorac. Cardiovasc. Surg. *75*:206, 1978.
572. Kagen, L., Scheidt, S., and Butt, A.: Serum myoglobin in myocardial infarction: The "staccato phenomenon": Is acute myocardial infarction in man an intermittent event? Am. J. Med. *62*:86, 1977.
573. Loop, F. D., Cheanvechai, C., Sheldon, W. C., Taylor, P. C., and Effler, D. B.: Early myocardial revascularization during acute myocardial infarction. Chest *66*:478, 1974.
574. Gruntzig, A. R., Senning, A., and Siegenthaler, W. E.: Non-operative dilatation of coronary artery stenosis. N. Engl. J. Med. *301*:61, 1979.
575. Kent, K. M., Bonow, R. O., Rosing, D. R., Ewels, C. J., Lipson, L. C., McIntosh, C. L., Bacharach, S., Green, M., and Epstein, S. E.: Improved myocardial function during exercise after successful percutaneous transluminal coronary angioplasty. N. Engl. J. Med. *306*:441, 1982.
576. Wellons, H. A., Schnieder, J. A., Mikell, F. L., Moses, H., Dove, J. T., Batchelder, J. E., and Taylor, G. T.: Early operative intervention after thrombolytic therapy for acute myocardial infarction. J. Vasc. Surg. *2*:186, 1985.
577. Kay, P., Ahmad, A., Floten, S., and Starr, A.: Emergency coronary artery bypass surgery after intracoronary thrombolysis for evolving myocardial infarction. Int. J. Cardiol. *7*:281, 1985.
578. Meyer, J., Merx, W., Dorr, R., Erbel, R., vonEssen, R., Lambertz, H., Bethge, C., Josef-Schmitz, H., Bardos, P., Minale, C., Josef-Messmer, B., and Effert, S.: Sequential intervention procedures after intracoronary thrombolysis; balloon dilatation, bypass surgery, and medical treatment. Int. J. Cardiol. *7*:281, 1985.
579. Mueller, H. S., and Ayres, S. M.: The role of propranolol in the treatment of acute myocardial infarction. Prog. Cardiovasc. Dis. *19*:405, 1977.
580. Ahumada, G. G., Karlsberg, R. P., Jaffe, A. S., Ambos, H. D., Sobel, B. E., and Roberts, R.: Reduction of early ventricular arrhythmia by acebutolol in patients with acute myocardial infarction. Br. Heart J. *41*:654, 1979.
581. Gold, H. K., Leinbach, C., and Maroko, P. R.: Propranolol-induced reduction of signs of ischemic injury during acute myocardial infarction. Am. J. Cardiol. *38*:689, 1976.
582. Libby, P., Maroko, P. R., Covell, J. W., Malloch, C. I., Ross, J., Jr., and Braunwald, E.: Effect of practolol on the extent of myocardial ischemic injury after experimental coronary occlusion and its effect on ventricular function in the normal and ischemic heart. Cardiovasc. Res. *7*:167, 1973.
583. Pelides, L. J., Reid, D. S., Thomas, M., and Shillingford, J. P.: Inhibition by beta-blockade of the ST-segment elevation after acute myocardial infarction in man. Cardiovasc. Res. *2*:295, 1972.
584. Barber, J. M., Boyle, D. M., Chaturvedi, N. C., Singh, N., and Walsh, M. J.: Practolol in acute myocardial infarction. Acta Med. Scand. *587*(Suppl.):213, 1976.
585. Peter, T., Norris, R. M., and Clarke, E. D.: Reduction of enzyme levels by propranolol after acute myocardial infarction. Circulation *57*:1091, 1978.
586. Norris, R. M., Clarke, E. D., Sammel, N. L., Smith, W. M., and Williams, B.: Protective effect of propranolol in threatened myocardial infarction. Lancet *2*:907, 1978.
587. Yusuf, S., Sleight, P., Rossi, P., Ramsdale, D., Peto, R., Furze, L., Sterry, H., Pearson, M., Motwani, R., Parish, S., Gray, R., Bennett, D., and Bray, C.: Reduction in infarct size, arrhythmias and chest pain by early intravenous beta blockade in suspected acute myocardial infarction. Circulation *67*:12, 1983.
588. Yusuf, S., Ramsdale, D., Rossi, P., Peto, R., Pearson, M., Sterry, H., Furse, L., Motwani, R., Parish, S., Gray, R., Bennett, D., Bray, C., and Sleight, P.: Reduction in infarct size, morbidity and short-term mortality by early intravenous beta blockade. J. Am. Coll. Cardiol. *1*:676, 1983.
589. Ramsdale, D. R., Faragher, E. G., Bennett, D. H., Bray, C. L., Ward, C., Cruickshank, J. M., Yusuf, S., and Sleight, P.: Ischemic pain relief in patients with acute myocardial infarction by intravenous atenolol. Am. Heart J. *103*:459, 1982.
590. Jurgensen, H. J., Frederiksen, J., Hansen, D. A., and Pedersen-Bjorgaard, D.: Limitation of myocardial infarct size in patients less than 66 years treated with alprenolol. Br. Heart J. *45*:583, 1981.
591. Hjalmarson, A., Herlitz, J., Holmberg, S., Ryden, L., Swedberg. K., Vedin, A., Waagstein, F., Waldenstrom, A., Waldenstrom, J., Wedel, H., Wilhelmsen, L., and Wilhelmsson, C.: The Göteborg metoprolol trial. Effects on mortality and morbidity in acute myocardial infarction. Circulation *67*:26, 1983.
592. The International Collaborative Study Group: Reduction of infarct size with the early use of timolol in acute myocardial infarction. N. Engl. J. Med. *310*:9, 1984.
593. The MIAMI Trial Research Group: Metoprolol In Acute Myocardial Infarction (MIAMI). A randomized placebo-controlled international trial. Eur. Heart J. *6*:199, 1985.
594. ISIS-1 (First International Study of Infarct Survival) Collaborative Group: Randomized trial of intravenous atenolol among 16,027 cases of suspected acute myocardial infarction: ISIS-I. Lancet *2*:57, 1986.
595. Croft, C. H., Rude, R. E., Gustafson, N., Stone, P. H., Poole, K., Roberts, R., Strauss, H. W., Raabe, D. S., Thomas, L. J., Jaffe, A. S., Muller, J., Hoagland, P., Sobel, B., Passamini, E. R., Braunwald, E., Willerson, J. T., and the MILIS Study Group: Abrupt withdrawal of β-blockade therapy in patients with myocardial infarction: Effects on infarct size, left ventricular function, and hospital course. Circulation *73*:1281, 1986.
596. European Infarction Study Group: European Infarction Study (E.I.S.). A

secondary prevention study with slow-release oxprenolol after myocardial infarction: Morbidity and mortality. Eur. Heart J. *5*:189, 1984.
597. Yusuf, S., Peto, R., Lewis, J., Collins, R., and Sleight, P.: Beta blockade during and after myocardial infarction: An overview of the randomized trials. Prog. Cardiovasc. Dis. *27*:335, 1985.
598. Kirschenbaum, J. M., Kloner, R. A., Antman, E. M., and Braunwald, E.: Use of an ultra short-acting β-blocker in patients with acute myocardial ischaemia. Circulation *72*:873, 1985.
599. Sung, R. J., Blanski, L., Kirschenbaum, J., MacCosbe, P., Turlapaty, P., and Laddu, A. R.: Clinical experience with esmolol, a short-acting beta-adrenergic blocker in cardiac arrhythmias and myocardial ischaemia. J. Clin. Pharmacol. *26*(Suppl. A):A-15, 1986.
600. Derrida, J. P., Sal, R., and Chiche, P.: Favorable effects of prolonged nitroglycerin infusion in patients with acute myocardial infarction. Am. Heart J. *96*:833, 1978.
601. Bussmann, W. D., Passek, D., Seidel, W., and Kaltenbach, M.: Reduction of CK and CK-MB indexes of infarct size by intravenous nitroglycerin. Circulation *63*:615, 1981.
602. Bussmann, W. D., Barthe, G., Klepzig, H., and Kaltenbach, M.: Controlled study of intravenous nitroglycerin treatment for two days in patients with recent myocardial infarction. Clin. Cardiol. *3*:399, 1980.
603. Becker, L. C., Bulkley, B. H., and Pitt, B.: Enhanced reduction of thallium-201 defects in acute myocardial infarction by nitroglycerin treatment: Initial results of a prospective randomized trial. Clin. Res. *26*:219A, 1978.
604. Flaherty, J. T., Becker, L. C., Bulkley, B. H., Weiss, J. L., Gerstenblith, G., Kallman, C. H., Silverman, K. J., Wei, J. Y., Pitt, B., and Weisfeldt, M. L.: A randomized prospective trial of intravenous nitroglycerin in patients with acute myocardial infarction. Circulation *68*:576, 1983.
605. Osuna, P. B., Moreno, M. G., Jimenez, A. A., Sanchez-Castillo, S., Luengo, 1 C. M., Hernandez, J. S., Bazo, L. C., Bueno, M. C., Dominguez, M. D., and Garcia, C. L.: Isosorbide dinitrate sublingual therapy for inferior myocardial infarction: Randomized trial to assess infarct size limitation. Am. J. Cardiol. *55*:330, 1985.
606. Shah, R., Bodenheimer, M. M., Banka, V. S., and Helfant, R. H.: Nitroglycerin and ventricular performance: Differential effect in the presence of reversible and irreversible asynergy. Chest *70*:473, 1976.
607. Shook, T. L., Kirschenbaum, J. M., Hundley, R. F., Shorey, J. M., and Lamas, G. A.: Ethanol intoxication complicating intravenous nitroglycerin therapy. Ann. Intern. Med. *101*:498, 1984.
608. Kaplan, K. J., Taber, M., Teagarden, J. R., Parker, M., and Davison, R.: Association of methemoglobinemia and intravenous nitroglycerin adminstration. Am. J. Cardiol. *55*:181, 1985.
609. Sirnes, P. A., Overskeid, K., Pederson, T. R., Bathen, J., Drivenes, A., Froland, G. S., Kiekshus, J. K., Landmark, K., Rokseth, R., Sirnes, K. E., Sundoy, A., Torgussen, B. R., Westlund, K. M., and Wik, B. J.: Evolution of infarct size during the early use of nifedipine in patients with acute myocardial infarction: The Norwegian nifedipine multicenter trial. Circulation *70*:738, 1984.
610. Muller, J. E., Morrison, J., Stone, P. H., Rude, R. E., Rossner, B., Roberts, R., Pearle, D. L., Turi, Z. G., Schneider, J. F., Serfas, D. H., Tate, C., Schneider, E., Sobel, B. E., Hennekens, C. H., and Braunwald, E.: Nifedipine therapy for patients with threatened and acute myocardial infarction: A randomized, double-blind, placebo-controlled comparison. Circulation *69*:740, 1984.
611. Loogna, E., Sylven, C., Groth, T., and Mogensen, L.: Complexity of enzyme release during acute myocardial infarction in a controlled study with early nifedipine treatment. Eur. Heart J. *6*:114, 1985.
612. Gibson, R. S., Boden, W. E., Theroux, P., Strauss, H. D., Pratt, C. M., Gheorghiade, M., Capone, R. J., Crawford, M. H., Schlant, R. C., Kleiger, R. E., Young, P. M., Schechtman, K., Perryman, M. B., Roberts, R., and the Diltiazem Reinfarction Study Group: Diltiazem and reinfarction in patients with non-Q-wave myocardial infarction. N. Engl. J. Med. *315*:423, 1986.
613. Gibelin, P., Benoit, P., Camous, J. P., Baudouy, M., and Monrand, P.: Tolerance clinique et hemodynamique du diltiazem intraveineux a la phase aigue de l'infarctus du myocarde. Ann. Cardiol. Angeiol. *34*:263, 1985.
614. The Danish Study Group on Verapamil in Myocardial Infarction: Verapamil in acute myocardial infarction. Eur. Heart J. *5*:515, 1984.
615. Crea, F., Deanfield, J., Crean, P., Sharom, M., Davies, G., and Maseri, A.: Effects of verapamil in preventing early postinfarction angina and reinfarction. Am. J. Cardiol. *55*:900, 1985.
616. Klein, H. H., Schubothe, M., Nebeudahl, K., and Kreuzer, H.: The effect of two different diltiazem treatments on infarct size in ischemic, reperfused porcine hearts. Circulation *69*:1000, 1984.
617. Tumas, J., Deth, R., and Kloner, R. A.: Effects of nisoldipine, a new calcium antagonist, on myocardial infarct size and cardiac dynamics following acute myocardial infarction. J. Cardiovasc. Pharmacol. *7*:361, 1985.
617a. Kloner, R. A., and Braunwald, E.: Effects of calcium antagonists on infarcting myocardium. Am. J. Cardiol. *59*:84B, 1987.
618. Mantle, J. A., Rogers, W. J., McDaniel, H. G., Holmes, R. A., Russell, R. O., Jr., and Rackley, C. E.: Metabolic support of mechanical performance in myocardial infarction in man—a ramdomized clinical trial of glucose-insulin-potassium. Am. J. Cardiol. *43*:395, 1979.
619. Rogers, W. J., Segall, P. H., McDaniel, H. G., Mantle, J. A., Russell, R. O., Jr., and Rackley, C. E.: Prospective randomized trial of glucose-insulin-potassium in acute myocardial infarction. Am. J. Cardiol. *43*:801, 1979.
620. Heng, M. K., Norris, R. M., Singh, B. N., and Barratt-Boyes, C.: Effects of glucose and glucose-insulin-potassium on haemodynamics and enzyme release after acute myocardial infarction. Br. Heart J. *39*:748, 1977.
621. Rogers, W. J., McDaniel, H. G., Mantle, J. A., and Rackley, C. E.: Prospective randomized trial of glucose-insulin-potassium in acute myocardial infarction: Effects on hemodynamics, short- and long-term survival. J. Am. Coll. Cardiol. *1*:628, 1983.
622. Morrison, J., Reduto, L., Pizzarello, R., Geller, K., Maley, T., and Gulotta, S.: Modification of myocardial injury in man by corticosteroid administration. Circulation *53*(Suppl. I):200, 1976.
623. Roberts, R., DeMello, V., and Sobel, B. E.: Deleterious effects of methylprednisolone in patients with myocardial infarction. Circulation *53*(Suppl. I):204, 1976.
624. Bulkley, B. H., and Roberts, W. C.: Steroid therapy during acute myocardial infarction: A cause of delayed healing and of ventricular aneurysm. Am. J. Med. *56*:244, 1974.
625. Hammerman, H., Kloner, R. A., Hale, S., Schoen, F. J., and Braunwald, E.: Dose-dependent effects of short-term methylprednisolone on myocardial infarct extent, scar formation, and ventricular function. Circulation *68*:446, 1983.
626. Brown, E. J., Jr., Kloner, R. A., Schoen, F. J., Hammerman, H., Hale, S., and Braunwald, E.: Scar thinning due to ibuprofen administration following experimental myocardial infarction. Am. J. Cardiol. *51*:877, 1983.
627. Hammerman, H., Kloner, R. A., Schoen, F. J., Brown, E. J., Jr., Hale, S., and Braunwald, E.: Indomethacin-induced scar thinning after experimental myocardial infarction. Circulation *67*:1290, 1983.
627a. Silverman, H. W., and Pfeifer, M. P.: Relation between use of anti-inflammatory agents and left ventricular free wall rupture during acute myocardial infarction. Am. J. Cardiol. *59*:363, 1987.
628. Friedman, P. L., Brown, E. J., Jr., Gunther, S., Alexander, R. W., Barry, W. H., Mudge, G. H., and Grossman, W.: Coronary vasoconstrictor effect of indomethacin in patients with coronary artery disease. N. Engl. J. Med. *305*:1171, 1981.
629. Ruf, W., Suehiro, G. T., Suehiro, A., and McNamara, J. J.: Regional myocardial blood flow in experimental myocardial infarction after pretreatment with aspirin. J. Am. Coll. Cardiol. *7*:1057, 1986.
630. Powell, W. J., Jr., Daggett, W. M., Magro, A. E., Bianco, J. A., Buckley, M. J., Sanders, C. A., Kantrowitz, A. R., and Austen, W. G.: Effects of intra-aortic balloon counterpulsation on cardiac performance, oxygen consumption, and coronary blood flow in dogs. Circ. Res. *26*:753, 1970.
631. Saini, V. K., Hood, W. B., Jr., Hechtman, H. G., and Berger, R. L.: Nutrient myocardial blood flow in experimental myocardial ischemia. Circulation *52*:1086, 1975.
632. Maroko, P. R., Bernstein, E. F., Libby, P., DeLaria, G. A., Covell, J. W., Ross, J., Jr., and Braunwald, E.: Effects of intra-aortic balloon counterpulsation on the severity of myocardial ischemic injury following acute coronary occlusion. Circulation *45*:1150, 1972.
633. Leinbach, R. C., Gold, H. K., Harper, R. W., Buckley, M. J., and Austen, W. G.: Early intra-aortic balloon pumping for anterior myocardial infarction without shock. Circulation *58*:204, 1978.
634. Flaherty, J. T., Becker, L. C., Weiss, J. L., Brinker, J. A., Bulkley, B. H., Gerstenblish, G., Kallman, C. H., and Weisfeldt, M. L.: Results of a randomized prospective trial of intra-aortic balloon counterpulsation and intravenous nitroglycerin in patients with acute myocardial infarction. J. Am. Coll. Cardiol. *6*:434, 1985.
635. Alderman, J. D., Gabliani, G. I., McCabe, C. H., Brewer, C. C., Lorell, B. H., Pasternak, R. C., Skillman, J. J., Steer, M. L., and Baim, D.: Incidence and management of limb ischemia with percutaneous wire-guided intra-aortic balloon catheters. J. Am. Coll. Cardiol. (*In press*).
636. Jolly, S. R., Kane, W. J., Bathe, M. B., Abrams, G. D., and Lucchesi, B. R.: Canine myocardial reperfusion injury. Its reduction by the combined administration of superoxide dismutase and catalase. Circ. Res. *54*:277, 1984.
637. Werns, S. W., Shea, M. J., Driscoll, E. M., Cohen, C., Abrams, G. D., Pitt, B., and Lucchesi, B. R.: The independent effects of oxygen radial scavengers on canine infarct size reduction by superoxide dismutase but not catalase. Circ. Res. *56*:895, 1985.
638. Myers, M. L., Bolli, R., Lekich, R. F., Hartley, C., and Roberts, R.: Enhancement of recovery of myocardial function by oxygen free-radical scavengers after reversible regional ischemia. Circulation *72*:915, 1985.

ARRHYTHMIAS IN ACUTE MYOCARDIAL INFARCTION

639. Meltzer, L. E., and Cohen, H. E.: The incidence of arrhythmias associated with acute myocardial infarction. *In* Meltzer, L. E., and Dunning, A. J. (eds.): Textbook of Coronary Care. Philadelphia, Charles Press, 1972.
640. O'Doherty, M., Tayler, D. I., Quinn, E., Vincent, R., and Chamberlain, D. A.: Five hundred patients with myocardial infarction monitored within one hour of symptoms. Br. Med. J. *286*:1405, 1983.
641. Pantridge, J. F., and Adgey, A. A. J.: Pre-hospital coronary care. The mobile coronary care unit. Am. J. Cardiol. *24*:666, 1969.
642. Hinkel, L. E., Jr., Carver, S. T., and Steven, M.: The frequency of asymptomatic disturbances of cardiac rhythm and conduction in middle-aged men. Am. J. Cardiol. *24*:629, 1969.
643. Corday, E., and Corday, S. R.: Advances in clinical management of acute myocardial infarction in the past 25 years. J. Am. Coll. Cardiol. *1*:126, 1983.
644. Bloor, C. M., Ehsani, A., White, F. C., and Sobel, B. E.: Ventricular fibrillation threshold in acute myocardial infarction and its relation to myocardial infarct size. Cardiovasc. Res. *9*:468, 1975.
645. Cox, J. R., Jr., Roberts, R., Ambos, H. D., Oliver G. C., and Sobel, B. E.: Relations between enzymatically estimated myocardial infarct size and early ventricular dysrhythmia. Circulation *53*(Suppl. I):150, 1976.
646. Malliani, A., Schwartz, P. J., and Zanchetti, A.: A sympathetic reflex elicited by experimental coronary occlusion. Am. J. Physiol. *217*:703, 1969.
647. Corr, P. B., and Gillis, R. A.: Autonomic neural influences on the dysrhythmias resulting from myocardial infarction. Circ. Res. *43*:1, 1978.

648. Barber, M. J., Mueller, T. M., Davies, B. G., Gill, R. M., and Zipes, D. P.: Interruption of sympathetic and vagal-mediated afferent responses by transmural myocardial infarction. Circulation *72*:623, 1985.
649. Ebert, P. A., Venderbeek, R. B., Allgood, R. J., and Sabiston, D. C., Jr.: Effect of chronic cardiac denervation on arrhythmias after coronary artery ligation. Cardiovasc. Res. *4*:141, 1970.
650. Shillingford, J., and Thomas, M.: Hemodynamic effects of acute myocardial infarction in man. Prog. Cardiovasc. Dis. *9*:571, 1967.
651. Lassers, B. E., Anderton, J. L., George, M., Muir, A. L., and Julian, D. G.: Hemodynamic effects of artificial pacing in complete heart block complicating acute myocardial infarction. Circulation *38*:308, 1968.
652. Ruskin, J., McHale, P. A., Harley, A., and Greenfield, J. C., Jr.: Pressure-flow studies in man; effects of atrial systole on left ventricular function. J. Clin. Invest. *49*:472, 1970.
653. Rahimtoola, S. H., Ehsani, A., Sinno, M. Z., Loeb, H. S., Rosen, K. M., and Gunnar, R. M.: Left atrial transport function in myocardial infarction: Importance of its booster function. Am. J. Med. *59*:686, 1975.
654. Adgey, A. A. J., Alley, J. D., Geddes, J. S., James, R. G. G., Webb, S. W., and Zaidi, S. A.: Acute phase of myocardial infarction. Lancet *2*:501, 1971.
655. Graner, L. E., Gershen, B. J., Orlando, M. M., and Epstein, S. E.: Bradycardia and its complications in the pre-hospital phase of acute myocardial infarction. Am. J. Cardiol. *32*:607, 1973.
656. Zipes, D. P.: The clinical significance of bradycardic rhythms in acute myocardial infarction. Am. J. Cardiol. *24*:814, 1969.
657. Thorén, P. N.: Activation of left ventricular receptors with nonmedullated vagal afferent fibers during occlusion of a coronary artery in the cat. Am. J. Cardiol. *37*:1046, 1976.
658. Mark, A. L.: The Bezold-Jarisch reflex revisited: Clinical implications of inhibitory reflexes originating in the heart. J. Am. Coll. Cardiol. *1*:90, 1983.
659. Chadda, K. D., Lichstein, E., Gupta, P. K., and Choy, R.: Bradycardia-hypotension syndrome in acute myocardial infarction: Reappraisal of the overdrive effects of atropine. Am. J. Med. *59*:158, 1975.
660. Warren, J. V., and Lewis, R. P.: Beneficial effects of atropine in the pre-hospital phase of coronary care. Am. J. Cardiol. *37*:68, 1976.
661. Topol, E. J., Goldschlager, N., Ports, T. A., DiCarlo, L. A., Jr., Schiller, N. B., Botvinick, E. H., and Chatterjee, K.: Hemodynamic benefit of atrial pacing in right ventricular myocardial infarction. Ann. Intern. Med. *96*:594, 1982.
662. Damato, A. N., and Lau, S. H.: Clinical value of the electrogram of the conduction system. Prog. Cardiovasc. Dis. *13*:119, 1970.
663. Johansson, B. W.: Atrioventricular and bundle branch block in acute myocardial infarction. Natural history and prognosis. *In* Meltzer, L. E., and Dunning, A. J. (eds.): Textbook of Coronary Care. Philadelphia, Charles Press, 1972, p. 328.
664. Rotman, M., Wagner, G. S., and Wallace, A. G. P.: Bradyarrhythmias in acute myocardial infarction. Circulation *45*:703, 1972.
665. Norris, R. M., and Mercer, C. J.: Significance of idioventricular rhythms in acute myocardial infarction. Prog. Cardiovasc. Dis. *16*:455, 1974.
666. Haft, J. I.: Clinical implications of atrioventricular and intraventricular conduction abnormalities. II. Acute myocardial infarction. *In* Rios, J. C. (ed.): Clinical-Electrocardiographic Correlations. Philadelphia, F. A. Davis Co., 1977, p. 65.
667. Fisch, G. R., Zipes, D. P., and Fisch, C.: Bundle branch block and sudden death. Prog. Cardiovasc. Dis. *23*:187, 1980.
667a. Bilbao, F. J., Zabalza, I. E., Vilanova, J. R., and Froupe, J.: Atrioventricular block in posterior acute myocardial infarction: A clinicopathologic correlation. Circulation *75*:733, 1987.
668. Friedberg, C. K., Cohen, H., and Donoso, E.: Advanced heart block as a complication of acute myocardial infarction. Role of pacemaker therapy. Prog. Cardiovasc. Dis. *10*:466, 1968.
669. Bergovich, J., Fenig, S., and Lassers, J.: Management of acute myocardial infarction complicated by advanced atrioventricular block: Role of artificial pacing. Am. J. Cardiol. *23*:54, 1969.
670. Chatterjee, K., Harris, A., and Leatham, A.: The risk of pacing after infarction, and current recommendation. Lancet *2*:1061, 1969.
671. Kostuk, W. J., and Beanland, D. S.: Complete heart block associated with acute myocardial infarction. Am. J. Cardiol. *26*:380, 1970.
672. Bassan, R., Maia, I. G., Bozza, A., Amino, J. G. C., and Santos, M.: Atrioventricular block in acute inferior wall myocardial infarction: Harbinger of associated obstruction of the left anterior descending coronary artery. J. Am. Coll. Cardiol. *8*:773, 1986.
673. Strasberg, B., Pinchas, A., Arditti, A., Lewin, R. F., Sclarovsky, S., Hellman, C., Zafrir, N., and Agmon, J.: Left and right ventricular function in inferior acute myocardial infarction and significance of advanced atrioventricular block. Am. J. Cardiol. *54*:985, 1984.
674. Atkins, J. M., Leshin, S. J., Blomquist, G., and Mullins, C. B.: Ventricular conduction blocks and sudden death in acute myocardial infarction. N. Engl. J. Med. *288*:281, 1973.
675. Hindman, M. C., Wagner, G. S., JaRo, M., Atkins, J. M., Scheinman, M. M., DeSanctis, R. W., Hutter, A. H., Jr., Yeatman, L., Rubenfire, M., Pujura, C., Rubin, M., and Morris, J. J.: The clinical significance of bundle branch block complicating acute myocardial infarction. 2. Indications for temporary and permanent pacemaker insertion. Circulation *58*:689, 1978.
676. Feigl, D., Ashkenazy, J., and Kishon, Y.: Early and late atrioventricular block in acute inferior myocardial infarction. J. Am. Coll. Cardiol. *4*:35, 1984.
677. Mullins, C. B., and Atkins, J. M.: Prognoses and management of ventricular conduction blocks in acute myocardial infarction. Mod. Concepts Cardiovasc. Dis. *45*:129, 1976.
678. Scheinman, M. M., and Gonzalez, R. P.: Fascicular block and acute myocardial infarction. J.A.M.A. *244*:2646, 1980.
679. Hindman, M. C., Wagner, G. S., JaRo, M., Atkins, J. M., Scheinman, M. M., DeSanctis, R. W., Hutter, A. H., Yeatman, L., Rubenfire, M., Pujure, C., Rubin, M., and Morris, J. J.: The clinical significance of bundle branch block complicating acute myocardial infarction. I. Clinical characteristics, hospital mortality, and one-year follow-up. Circulation *58*:679, 1978.
680. Godman, M. J., Lassers, B. W., and Julian, D. G.: Complete bundle branch block complicating acute myocardial infarction. N. Engl. J. Med. *282*:237, 1970.
681. Rosen, K. M., Rahimtoola, H., Chuquimia, R., Loeb, H. S., and Gunnar, R. M.: Electrophysiological significance of first-degree atrioventricular conduction disturbance. Circulation *43*:491, 1971.
682. Lie, K. I., Wellens, H. J., and Schuilenburg, R. M.: Bundle branch block and acute myocardial infarction. *In* Wellens, H. J. J., Lie, K. I., and Janse, M. J. (eds.): The Conduction System of the Heart: Structure, Function and Clinical Implications. Philadelphia, Lea and Febiger, 1976, pp. 662–672.
683. Lamas, G. A., Muller, J. E., Turi, Z. G., Stone, P. H., Rutherford, J. D., Jaffe, A. S., Raabe, D. S., Rude, R. E., Mark, D. B., Califf, R. M., Gold, H. K., Robertson, T., Passamani, E. R., Braunwald, E., and the MILIS Study Group: A simplified method to predict occurrence of complete heart block during acute myocardial infarction. Am. J. Cardiol. *57*:1213, 1986.
684. Hynes, J. K., Holmes, D. R., Jr., and Harrison, C. E.: Five-year experience with temporary pacemaker therapy in the coronary care unit. Mayo Clin. Proc. *58*:122, 1983.
685. Austin, J. L., Preis, L. K., Crampton, R. S., Beller, G. A., and Martin, R. P.: Analysis of pacemaker malfunction and complications of temporary pacing in the coronary care unit. Am. J. Cardiol. *49*:301, 1982.
686. Zoll, P.: Resuscitation of the heart in ventricular standstill by external electrical stimulation. N. Engl. J. Med. *247*:768, 1952.
687. Falk, R. H., Zoll, P. M., and Zoll, R.H.: Safety and efficacy of noninvasive cardiac pacing. N. Engl. J. Med. *309*:1166, 1983.
688. Zoll, P. M., Zoll, R. H., Falk, R. H., Clinton, J. E., Eitel, D. R., and Antman, E. M.: External noninvasive temporary cardiac pacing: Clinical trials. Circulation *71*:937, 1985.
689. Ritter, W. S., Atkins, J.M., Blomqvist, C. G., and Mullins, C. B.: Permanent pacing in patient with transient trifascicular block during acute myocardial infarction. Am. J. Cardiol. *38*:205, 1976.
690. Ginks, W. R., Sutton, R., Oh, W., and Leatham, A.: Long-term prognosis after acute inferior infarction with atrioventricular block. Br. Heart J. *39*:186, 1977.
691. Frye, R. L., Collins, J. J., DeSanctis, R. W., Dodge, H. T., Dreifus, L. S., Fisch, C., Gettes, L., Gillette, P. C., Parsonnet, V., Reeves, T. J., and Weinberg, S. L.: Guidelines for permanent cardiac pacemaker implantation, May 1984. J. Am. Coll. Cardiol. *4*:434, 1984.
692. Wilson, C., and Adgey, A. A. J.: Survival of patients with late ventricular fibrillation after acute myocardial infarction. Lancet *2*:214, 1974.
693. Meltzer, L. E., and Kitchell, J. B.: The incidence of arrhythmias associated with acute myocardial infarction. Prog. Cardiovasc. Dis. *9*:50, 1966.
694. Peterson, D. F., and Brown, A. M.: Pressor reflexes produced by stimulation of afferent fibers in the cardiac sympathetic nerves of the cat. Circ. Res. *28*:605, 1971.
695. Berman, J., Haffajee, C. I., and Alpert, J. S.: Therapy of symptomatic pericarditis after myocardial infarction: Retrospective and prospective studies of aspirin, indomethacin, prednisone, and spontaneous resolution. Am. Heart J. *101*:750, 1981.
696. DeSanctis, R. W., Block, P., and Hutter, A. M.: Tachyarrhythmias in myocardial infarction. Circulation *45*:681, 1972.
697. Gordon, S., Finck, D. R., Perera, R. D., Levine, J., and Barnes, S. J.: Atrial infarction complicating an acute inferior myocardial infarction. Arch. Intern. Med. *144*:193, 1984.
698. Jewitt, D. E., Balcon, R., Raftery, E. B., and Oram, S.: Incidence and management of supraventricular arrhythmias after acute myocardial infarction. Lancet *2*:734, 1967.
699. Rothfeld, E. L., Parsonnet, J., McGorman, W., and Linden, S.: Harbingers of paroxysmal ventricular tachycardia in acute myocardial infarction. Chest *71*:142, 1977.
700. El-Sherif, N., Gann, D., and Sung, R. J.: Initiation of ventricular fibrillation by supraventricular beats in patients with acute myocardial infarcton. (Abstr.) Circulation *58*(Suppl. II):195, 1978.
701. James, T. N.: Myocardial infarction and atrial arrhythmias. Circulation *24*:761, 1961.
702. Krikler, D. M., and Rowland, E.: The role of calcium-ion antagonists in cardiac arrhythmias. *In* Fleckenstein, A., and Roskamm, G. (eds.): Calcium Antagonists. New York, Springer-Verlag, 1980, p. 55.
703. Zipes, D. P., and Troup, P. J.: New antiarrhythmic agents: Amiodarone, aprindine, disopyramide, ethmozin, mexiletine, tocainide, verapamil. Am. J. Cardiol. *41*:1005, 1978.
704. Hod, H., Lew, A. S., Keltai, M., Cercek, B., Geft, I. O., Shah, P., and Ganz, W.: Early atrial fibrillation during evolving myocardial infarction: A consequence of impaired left atrial perfusion. Circulation *75*:146, 1987.
705. Kerber, R. E., Jensen, S. R., Grayzel, J., Kennedy, J., and Hoyt, R.: Elective cardioversion: Influence of paddle-electrode location and size on success rates and energy requirements. N. Engl. J. Med. *305*:658, 1981.
706. Konecke, L. L., and Knoebel, S. B.: Nonparoxysmal junctional tachycardia complicating acute myocardial infarction. Circulation *45*:367, 1972.
707. Lown, B., Fakhro, A., Hood, W. B., and Thorn, G. W.: The coronary care unit—new perspectives and directions. J.A.M.A. *199*:188, 1967.
708. Julian, D. T., Valentine, P. Z., and Miller, G. G.: Disturbances of rate, rhythm, and conduction in acute myocardial infarction. A prospective study of 100 unselected patients with the aid of electrocardiographic monitoring. Am. J. Med. *37*:915, 1964.

709. Lie, K. J., Wellens, H. J. J., Dorsnar, E., and Durrer, D.: Observations on patients with primary ventricular fibrillation complicating acute myocardial infarction. Circulation *52*:755, 1975.
710. El-Sherif, N., Myerburg, R. J., Scherlag, B. J., Befeler, B., Aranda, J. M., Castellanos, A., and Lazzara, R.: Electrocardiographic antecedents of primary ventricular fibrillation. Value of the R-on-T phenomenon in myocardial infarction. Br. Heart J. *38*:415, 1976.
711. Lawrie, D. M., Higgins, M. R., Godman, M. J., Julian, D. G, and Donald, K. W.: Ventricular fibrillation complicating acute myocardial infarction. Lancet 2:523, 1968.
712. El-Sherif, N., Scherlag, B. J., and Lazzara, R.: Electrode catheter recordings during malignant ventricular arrhythmias following experimental acute myocardial ischemia. Evidence for reentry due to conduction delay and block in ischemic myocardium. Circulation *51*:1003, 1975.
713. Roberts, R., Ambos, H. D., Loh, C. W., and Sobel, B. E.: Initiation of repetitive ventricular depolarizations by relatively late premature complexes in patients with acute myocardial infarction. Am. J. Cardiol. *41*:678, 1978.
714. DeSoyza, N., Meacham, D., Murphy, M. L., Kane, J. J., Doherty, J. E., and Bissett, J. K.: Evaluation of warning arrhythmias before paroxysmal ventricular tachycardia during acute myocardial infarction in man. Circulation *60*:814, 1979.
715. Campbell, R. W. F., Murray, A., and Julian, D. G.: Relation of ventricular arrhythmias to ventricular fibrillation. Br. Heart J. *43*:109, 1980.
715a. Josephson, M. E.: Treatment of ventricular arrhythmias after myocardial infarction. Circulation *74*:653, 1986.
716. Koster, R. W., and Dunning, J.: Intramuscular lidocaine for prevention of lethal arrhythmias in the prehospitalization phase of acute myocardial infarction. N. Engl. J. Med. *313*:1105, 1985.
717. Lie, K. I., Wellens, H. J., and Van Capelli, F. J.: Lidocaine in the prevention of primary ventricular fibrillation. A double-blind randomized study of 212 consecutive patients. N. Engl. J. Med. *291*:1324, 1974.
718. Routledge, P. A., Stargel, W. W., Barchowsky, A., Wagner, G. S., and Shand, D. G.: Control of lidocaine therapy: New perspectives. Therap. Drug Monitoring *4*:265, 1982.
719. DeSilva, R. E., Hennekens, C. H., Lown, B., and Casscells, S. W.: Lidocaine prophylaxis in acute myocardial infarction: An evaluation of methodology. Lancet *1*:855, 1981.
720. Dunn, H. M., McComb, J. M., Kinney, C. D., Campbell, N. P. S., Shanks, R. G., MacKenzie, G., and Adgey, A. A. J.: Prophylactic lidocaine in the early phase of suspected myocardial infarction. Am. Heart J. *110*:353, 1985.
721. May, G. S., Furberg, C. D., Eberlein, K. A., and Geraci, B. J.: Secondary prevention after myocardial infarction. A review of short-term acute phase trials. Prog. Cardiovasc. Dis. *25*:335, 1983.
722. Lie, K. J.: Lidocaine and prevention of ventricular fibrillation complicating acute myocardial infarction. Int. J. Cardiol. *7*:321, 1985.
723. Mehra, R., Zeiler, R. H., Gough, W. B., and El-Sherif, N.: Re-entrant ventricular arrhythmias in the later myocardial infarction period. 9. Electrophysiologic-anatomic correlation of re-entrant circuits. Circulation *67*:11, 1983.
724. Norris, R. M., Brown, M. A., Clarke, E. D., Barnaby, P. F., Geary, G. G., Logan, R. L., and Sharpe, D. N.: Prevention of ventricular fibrillation during acute myocardial infarction by intravenous propranolol. Lancet 2:883, 1984.
725. Lopez, L. M., Mehta, J. L., Robinson, J. D., and Roberts, R. J.: Optimal lidocaine dosing in patients with myocardial infarction. Ther. Drug Monit. *4*:271, 1982.
726. Feely, J., Wade, D., McAllister, C. B., Wilkinson, G. R., and Robertson, D.: Effect of hypotension on liver blood flow and lidocaine disposition. N. Engl. J. Med. *307*:866, 1982.
727. Prescott, L. F., Adjepon-Yamoah, K.K., and Talbot, R. G.: Impaired lignocaine metabolism in patients with myocardial infarction and cardiac failure. Br. Med. J. *1*:939, 1976.
728. LeLorier, J., Grenon, D., Latour, Y., Caille, G., Dumont, G., Brosseau, A., and Solignac, A.: Pharmacokinetics of lidocaine after prolonged intravenous infusions in uncomplicated myocardial infarction. Ann. Intern. Med. *87*:700, 1977.
729. Corr, P. B., and Sobel, B. E.: Mechanisms contributing to dysrhythmias induced by ischemia and their therapeutic implications. Adv. Cardiol. *22*:110, 1978.
730. Lown, B., and Vassaux, C.: Lidocaine in acute myocardial infarction. Am. Heart J. *76*:586, 1968.
731. Fehmers, M. C. O., and Dunning, A. J.: Intramuscularly and orally administered lidocaine in the treatment of ventricular arrhythmias in acute myocardial infarction. Am. J. Cardiol. *29*:514, 1972.
732. El-Sherif, N., Scherlag, B. J., Lazzara, R., and Hope, R. R.: Re-entrant ventricular arrhythmias in the late myocardial infarction period. 4. Mechanism of action of lidocaine. Circulation *56*:395, 1977.
733. Kessler, K. M., Kayden, D. S., Estes, D. M., Koslovskis, P. L., Sequeira, R., Trohman, R. G., Palomo, A. R., and Myerburg, R. J.: Procainamide pharmacokinetics in patients with acute myocardial infarction or congestive heart failure. J. Am. Coll. Cardiol. *7*:1131, 1986.
734. Keefe, D. L., Williams, S., Torres, V., Flowers, D., and Somberg, J. C.: Prophylactic tocainide or lidocaine in acute myocardial infarction. Am. J. Cardiol. *57*:527, 1986.
735. Rehnqvist, N., Ericsson, G. G., Ericsson, S., Olsson, G., and Svensson, G.: Comparative investigation of the antiarrhythmic effect of propafenone and lidocaine in patients with ventricular arrhythmias during acute myocardial infarction. Acta Med. Scand. *216*:525, 1984.
736. Gillis, R. A., McClellan,J. R., Sauer, T. S., and Standaert, F. G.: Depression of cardiac sympathetic nerve activity by diphenylhydantoin. J. Pharmacol. Exp. Ther. *179*:599, 1971.
737. El-Sherif, N., and Lazzara, R.: Re-entrant ventricular arrhythmnias in the late myocardial infarction period. 5. Mechanism of action of diphenylhydantoin. Circulation *57*:405, 1978.
738. Lown, B., and Wolf;, M.: Approaches to sudden death from coronary heart disease. Circulation *44*:130, 1971.
739. Wenger, T. L., Bigger, J. T., Jr., and Merrill, G. S.: Ventricular arrhythmias in the late hospital phase of acute myocardial infarction. Circulation *59*:110, 1975.
740. Schulze, R. A., Rouleau, J., Rigo, P., Bowers, S., Strauss, H. W., and Pitt, B.: Ventricular arrhythmias in the late phase of acute myocardial infarction: Relation to left ventricular function detected by gated cardiac blood pool scanning. Circulation *52*:1006, 1975.
741. Moss, A. J., De Camilla, J. J., Davis, H. P., and Bayer, L.: Clinical significance of ventricular ectopic beats in the early posthospital phase of myocardial infarction. Am. J. Cardiol. *39*:635, 1977.
742. Mukharji, J., and MILIS Study Group: Risk factors for sudden death after acute myocardial infarction. Am. J. Cardiol. *54*::31, 1984.
743. Doherty, J. E.: AssociatIon of accelerated idioventricular rhythm and paroxysmal ventricular tachycardia in acute myocardial infarction. Am. J. Cardiol. *34*:667, 1974.
744. Sclarovsky, S., Strasberg, B., Martonovich, G., and Agmon, J.: Ventricular rhythms with intermediate rates in acute myocardial infarction. Chest *74*:180, 1978.
745. Lichstein, E., Ribas-Meneclier, C., Gupta, P. K., and Chadda, K. D.: Incidence and description of accelerated idioventricular rhythm complicating acute myocardial infarction. Am. J. Med. *58*:192, 1975.
746. Bigger, J. T., Jr., Dresdale, R. J., and Heissenbuttel, R. H., Weld, F. M., and Wit, A. L.: Ventricular arrhythmias in ischemic heart disease: Mechanism, prevalence, significance, and management. Prog. Cardiovasc. Dis. *19*:255, 1977.
747. Bigger, J. T., Jr., Weld, F. M., and Rolnitzky, L. M.: Prevalence, characteristics and significance of ventricular tachycardia (three or more complexes) detected with ambulatory electrocardiographic recording in the late hospital phase of acute myocardial infarction. Am. J. Cardiol. *48*:815, 1981.
748. Solomon, R. J., and Cole, A. G.: Importance of potassium in patients with acute myocardial infarction. Acta Med. Scand. *647*(Suppl):87, 1981.
749. Nordehaug, J. E., Johannessen, K. A., and von der Lippe, G.: Serum potassium concentration as a risk factor of ventricular arrhythmias early in acute myocardial infarction. Circulation *71*:645, 1985.
750. Wald, R. W., Waxman, M. B., Corey, P, N., Gunstensen, J., and Goldman, B. S.: Management of intractable ventricular trachyarrhythmias after myocardial infarction. Am. J. Cardiol. *44*:329, 1979.
751. Guiraudon, G., Fontaine, G., Frank, R., Escande, G., Etievent, P., and Cabrol, C.: Encircling endocardial ventriculotomy: A new surgical treatment for life-threatening tachycardias resistant to medical treatment following myocardial infarction. Ann. Thorac. Surg. *26*:438, 1978.
752. Josephson, M. E., Harken, A. H., and Horowitz, L. N.: Endocardial excision: A new surgical technique for the treatment of recurrent ventricular tachycardia. Circulation *60*:1430, 1979.
753. Schwartz, P. J., Zaza, A., Grazi, S., Lombardo, M., Lotto, A., Sbressa, C., and Zappa, P.: Effect of ventricular fibrillation complicating acute myocardial infarction on long-term prognosis: Importance of the site of infarction. Am. J. Cardiol. *56*:384, 1985.
754. Lie, K. I., Liem, K. L., Schuilenburg, R. M., David, G. K., and Durrer, D.: Early identification of patients developing late in-hospital ventricular fibrillation after discharge from the coronary care unit. Am. J. Cardiol. *41*:674, 1978.
755. Sclarovsky, S., Zafrir, N., Strasberg, B., Kracoff, O., Lewin, R. F., Arditi, A., Rosen, K. M., and Agmon, J.: Ventricular fibrillation complicating temporary ventricular pacing in acute myocardial infarction: Significance of right ventricular infarction. Am. J. Cardiol. *48*:1160, 1981.
756. Toffler, G. H., Stone, P. H., Muller, J. E., Rutherford, J., Willitck, S. N., Gustafson, N. K., Pool, K., Robertston, T., and Braunwald, E.: Prognosis after myocardial infarction complicated by ventricular fibrillation. Circulation *74*(Suppl. II):304, 1986.
757. Conley, M. J., McNeer, J. F., Lee, K. L., Wagner, G. S., and Rosati, R. A.: Cardiac arrest complicating acute myocardial infarction. Predictability and prognosis. Am. J. Cardiol. *39*:7, 1977.
758. Ryden, L., Ariniego, R., Arnman, K., Herlitz, J., Hjalmarson, A., Holmberg, S., Reyes, C., Smedgard, P., Svedberg, K., Vedin, A., Waagstein, F., Waldenstrom, A., Wilhelmsson, C., Wedel, H., and Yamamoto, M.: A double-blind trial of metoprolol in acute myocardial infarction. Effects on ventricular tachyarrhythmias. N. Engl. J. Med. 308:614, 1983.
759. Engler, R. L., and LeWinter, M. M.: Ventricular arrhythmias: Diagnosis, treatment and prognosis. *In* Karliner, J. (ed.): Coronary Care. New York, Churchill Livingstone, 1981, pp. 367–390.
760. Van Vleet, J. F., Tacker, W. A., Jr., Geddes, L. A., and Ferrans, V. J.: Acute cardiac damage in dogs given multiple transthoracic shocks with a trapezoidal wave-form defibrillator. Am. J. Vet. Res. *38*:617, 1977.
761. Ehsani, A., Ewy, G. A., and Sobel, B. E.: Effects of electrical countershock on serum creatine phosphokinase (CPK) isoenzyme activity. Am. J. Cardiol. *37*:12, 1976.
762. Abboud, F. M., Pansegrau, D. G., and Mark, A. L.: Automatic responses to ventricular defibrillation. In Proceedings, Cardiac Defibrillation Conference, Purdue University, West Lafayette, Indiana, 1975.
763. Heissenbuttel, R. H., and Bigger, J. T., Jr.: Bretylium tosylate, a newly available antiarrhythmic drug for ventricular arrhythmias. Ann. Intern. Med. *91*:229, 1979.

HEMODYNAMIC DISTURBANCES IN ACUTE MYOCARDIAL INFARCTION

764. Forrester, J. S., Diamond, G., Chatterjee, K., and Swan, H. J. C.: Medical therapy of acute myocardial infarction by application of hemodynamic subsets. N. Engl. J. Med. 295:1356, 1404, 1976.
765. Russell, R. O., Jr., Rackley, C. E., Pambo, J., Hunt, D., Potanin, C., and Dodge, H. T.: Effects of increasing left ventricular filling pressure in patients with acute myocardial infarction. J. Clin. Invest. 49:1539, 1970.
766. Carabello, B., Cohn, P. F., and Alpert, J. S.: Hemodynamic monitoring in patients with hypotension after myocardial infarction. Chest 74:5, 1978.
767. Coma-Canella, I., Lopez-Sendon, J., and Gamallo, C.: Low output syndrome in right ventricular infarction. Am. Heart J. 98:613, 1979.
768. Page, D. L., Caulfield, J. B., Kastor, J. A., DeSanctis, R. W., and Sanders, C. A.: Myocardial changes associated with cardiogenic shock. N. Engl. J. Med. 285:133, 1971.
769. Alonso, D. R., Scheidt, S., Post, M., and Killip, T.: Pathophysiology of cardiogenic shock; quantification of myocardial necrosis, clinical, pathologic and electrocardiographic correlation. Circulation 48:588, 1973.
770. Resnekov, L.: Cardiogenic shock. Chest 83:893, 1983.
771. Ratshin, R. A., Rackley, C. E., and Russell, R. O., Jr.: Hemodynamic evaluation of left ventricular function in shock complicating myocardial infarction. Circulation 45:127, 1972.
772. Gutovitz, A. L., Sobel, B. E., and Roberts, R.: Progressive nature of myocardial injury in selected patients with cardiogenic shock. Am. J. Cardiol. 41:469, 1978.
773. Wackers, F. J., Lie, K. I., Becker, A. E., Durrer, D., and Wellens, H. J. J.: Coronary artery disease in patients dying from cardiogenic shock or congestive heart failure in the setting of acute myocardial infarction. Br. Heart J. 38:906, 1976.
774. Rasanen, J., Nikki, O. P., and Heikkila, J.: Acute myocardial infarction complicated by respiratory failure. The effects of mechanical ventilation. Chest 85:21, 1984.
775. Bodenheimer, M. M., Ramanathan, K., Banka, V. S., and Helfant, R. H.: Effect of progressive pressure reduction with nitroprusside on acute myocardial infarction in humans. Determination of optimal afterload. Ann. Intern. Med. 94:435, 1981.
776. Durrer, J. D., Lie, K. I., Van Capelle, F. J. L., and Durrer, D.: Effect of sodium nitroprusside on mortality in acute myocardial infarction. N. Engl. J. Med. 306:1121, 1982.
777. Cohn, J. N., Franciosa, J. A., Francis, G. S., Archibald, D., Tristani, F., Fletcher, R., Montero, A., Cintron, G., Clarke, J., Hager, D., Saunders, R., Cobb, F., Smith, R., Hoeb, H., and Settle, H.: Effect of short-term infusion on sodium nitroprusside on mortality rate in acute myocardial infarction complicated by left ventricular failure. Results of a Veterans Administration Cooperative Study. N. Engl. J. Med. 306:1129, 1982.
778. Passamani, E. R.: Nitroprusside in myocardial infarction. N. Engl. J. Med. 306:1168, 1982.
779. Borer, J. S., Redwood, D. R., Levitt, B., Cagin, N., Bianchi, C., Vallin, H., and Epstein, S. E.: Reduction in myocardial ischemia with nitroglycerin or nitroglycerin plus phenylephrine administered during acute myocardial infarction. N. Engl. J. Med. 293:1008, 1975.
780. Chiariello, M., Gold, H. K., Leinbach, R. C., Davis, M. A., and Maroko, P. R.: Comparison between the effects of nitroprusside and nitroglycerin on ischemic injury during acute myocardial infarction. Circulation 54:766, 1976.
781. Flaherty, J. T.: Intravenous nitroglycerin. Johns Hopkions Med. J. 151:36, 1982.
782. Rabinowitz, B., Tamari, I., Elazar, E., and Neufeld, H. N.: Intravenous isosorbide dinitrate in patients with refractory pump failure and acute myocardial infarction. Circulation 65:771, 1982.
783. Gold, H. K., Leinbach, R. C., and Sanders, C. A.: Use of sublingual nitroglycerin in congestive failure following acute myocardial infarction. Circulation 46:839, 1972.
784. Franciosa, J. A., Mikulic, E., Cohn, J. N., Jose, E., and Fabie, A.: Hemodynamic effects of orally administered isosorbide dinitrate in patients with congestive heart failure. Circulation 50:1020, 1974.
785. Cohen, R., A., Shepherd, J. T., and Vanhoutte, P. M.: Prejunctional and postjunctional actions of endogenous norepinephrine at the sympathetic neuroeffector junction in canine coronary arteries. Circ. Res. 52:16, 1983.
786. Cohn, J. N.: Editorial—Progress in vasodilator therapy for heart failure. N. Engl. J. Med. 302:1414, 1980.
787. Franciosa, J. A., Guiha, N. H., Limas, C. J., Rodriguera, E., and Cohn, J. N.: Improved left ventricular function during nitroprusside infusion in acute myocardial infarction. Lancet 1:650, 1972.
788. Pfeffer, J. M., Pfeffer, M. A., and Braunwald, E.: Hemodynamic benefits and prolonged survival with long-term captopril therapy in rats with myocardial infarction and heart failure. Circulation 75(Suppl. I):149, 1987.
789. Covell, J. W., Braunwald, E., Ross, J., Jr., and Sonnenblick, E. H.: Studies on digitalis XVI. Effects on myocardial oxygen consumption. J. Clin. Invest. 45:1535, 1966.
790. Kumar, R., Hood, W. B., Jr., Joison, J., Gilmour, D. P., Norman, J. C., and Abelmann, W. H.: Experimental myocardial infarction. VI. Efficacy and toxicity of digitalis in acute and healing phase in intact conscious dog. J. Clin. Invest. 49:358, 1970.
791. Watanabe, T., Covell, J. W., Maroko, P. R., Braunwald, E., and Ross, J.: The effects of increased arterial pressure and positive inotropic agents on the severity of myocardial ischemia in the acutely depressed heart. Am. J. Cardiol. 30:371, 1972.
792. Ross, J., Jr., Waldhausen, J. S., and Braunwald, E.: Studies on digitalis. I. Direct effects on peripheral vascular resistance. J. Clin. Invest. 39:930, 1960.
793. Morrison, J., Coromilas, J., Robbins, M., Ong, L., Eisenberg, S., Stechel, R., Zema, M., Reiser, P., and Scherr, L.: Digitalis and myocardial infarction in man. Circulation 62:8, 1980.
794. Marcus, F. I.: Use of digitalis in acute myocardial infarction (Editorial). Circulation 62:17, 1980.
795. Marchionni, N., Pini, R., Vannucci, A., Conti, A., DeAlfieri, W., Calamandrei, M., Di Bari, M., Ferrucci, L., Moschi, G., Lombardi, A., and Greppi, B.: Hemodynamic effects of digoxin in acute myocardial infarction in man: A randomized controlled trial. Am. Heart J. 109:63, 1985.
796. Moss, A. J., Davis, H. T., Conrad, D. L., Decamilla, J. J., and Odoroff, C. L.: Digitalis-associated cardiac mortality after myocardial infarction. Circulation 64:1150, 1981.
797. Muller, J. E., Turi, Z. G., Stone, P. H., Rude, R. E., Raabe, D. S., Jaffe, A. S., Gold, H. K., Gustafson, N., Poole, W. R., Passamani, E., Smith, T. W., Bruanwald, E., and the MILIS Study Group: Digoxin therapy and mortality after myocardial infarction. Experience in the MILIS Study. N. Engl. J. Med. 314:265, 1986.
798. Bigger, J. T., Jr., Fleiss, J. L., Rolnitzky, L. M., Merab, J. P., and Ferrick, K. J.: Effects of digitalis treatment on survival after acute myocardial infarction. Am. J. Cardiol. 55:623, 1985.
799. Mueller, H., Ayres, S. M., Giannelli, S., Jr., Conklin, E. F., Mazzara, J. T., and Grace, W. J.: Effect of isoproterenol, 1-norepinephrine, and intra-aortic counterpulsation on hemodynamics and myocardial metabolism in shock following acute myocardial infarction. Circulation 45:335, 1972.
800. Shell, W. E., and Sobel, B. E.: Deleterious effects of increased heart rate on infarct size in the conscious dog. Am. J. Cardiol. 31:474, 1973.
801. Ichard, C., Ricome, J. L., Rimailho, A., Bottineau, G., and Auzepy, P.: Combined hemodynamic effects of dopamine and dobutamine in cardiogenic shock. Circulation 67:620, 1983.
802. Holzer, J., Karliner, J. S., O'Rourke, R. A., Pitt, W., and Ross, J., Jr.: Effectiveness of dopamine in patients with cardiogenic shock. Am. J. Cardiol. 32:79, 1973.
803. Arnold, J. M. O., Braunwald, E., Sandor, T., and Kloner, R. A.: Inotropic stimulation of reperfused myocardium with dopamine: Effects on infarct size and myocardial function. J. Am. Coll. Cardiol. 6:1026, 1985.
804. Tuttle, R. R., and Mills, J.: Development of a new catecholamine to selectively increase cardiac contractility. Circ. Res. 36:185, 1975.
805. Goldstein, R. A., Passamani, E. R., and Roberts, E.: Comparison of digoxin and dobutamine in patients with acute infarction and cardiac failure. N. Engl. J. Med. 303:846, 1980.
806. Maekawa, K., Liang, C-S., and Hood, W. B., Jr.: Comparison of dobutamine and dopamine in acute myocardial infarction. Effects of systemic hemodynamics, plasma catecholamines, blood flows, and infarct size. Circulation 67:750, 1983.
807. Mancini, D., LeJemtel, T., and Sonnenblick, E.: Intravenous use of amrinone for the treatment of the failing heart. Am. J. Cardiol. 56:8B, 1985.
808. Rude, R. E., Kloner, R. A., Maroko, P. R., Khuyri, S., Karoffa, S., DeBoer, L. W., and Braunwald, E.: Effects of amrinone on experimental acute myocardial ischemic injury. Cardiovasc. Res. 14:419, 1980.
809. Monrad, E. S., Baim, D. S., Smith, J. S., Lanoue, A., Braunwald, E., and Grossman, W.: Effects of milrinone on coronary hemodynamics and myocardial energetics in patients with congestive heart failure. Circulation 71:972, 1985.
810. Taylor, S. H., Verma, S. P., Hussain, M., Reynolds, G., Jackson, N. C., Hafizullah, M., Richmond, A., and Silke, B.: Intravenous amrinone in left ventricular failure complicated by acute myocardial infarction. Am. J. Cardiol. 56:29B, 1985.
811. Verma, S. P., Silke, B., and Taylor, S. H.: Hemodynamic dose-response effects of amrinone in left ventricular failure complicating myocardial infarction. Br. J. Clin. Pharmacol. 19:540P, 1985.
812. Colucci, W. S., Wright, R. F., and Braunwald, E.: New positive inotropic agents in the treatment of congestive heart failure. N. Engl. J. Med. 314:349, 1986.
813. Gunnar, R. M., and Loeb, H. S.: Shock in acute myocardial infarction: Evolution of physiologic therapy. J. Am. Coll. Cardiol. 1:154, 1983.
814. Mueller, H., Ayres, S. M., Gregory, J. J., Gianelli, S., Jr., and Grace, W. J.: Hemodynamics, coronary blood flow, and myocardial metabolism in coronary shock: Response to L-norepinephrine and isoproterenol. J. Clin. Invest. 49:1885, 1970.
815. Mathey, D., Kuck, K. H., Remmecke, J., Tilsner, V., and Bleifeld, W.: Transluminal recanalization of coronary artery thrombosis: A preliminary report of its application in cardiogenic shock. Eur. Heart J. 1:207, 1980.
816. Lew, A., Weiss, A. T., Shah, P. K., Fishbein, M. C., Berman, D. S., Maddahi, J.: Extensive myocardial salvage and reversal of cardiogenic shock after reperfusion of the left main coronary artery by intravenous streptokinase. Am. J. Cardiol. 54:450, 1984.
817. Alosilla, C. E., Bell, W. W., Ferree, J., and De La Torre, A.: Thrombolytic therapy during acute myocardial infarction due to sudden occlusion of the left main coronary artery. J. Am. Coll. Cardiol. 5:1253, 1985.
818. Kantrowitz, A., Krakauer, J. S., Rosenbaum, A., Butner, A. M., Freed, P. S., and Jaron, D.: Phase-shift balloon pumping medically refractory cardiogenic shock: Results in 27 patients. Arch. Surg. 99:739, 1969.
819. Scheidt, S., Wilner, G., Mueller, H., Summers, D., Lesch, M., Wolff, G., Krakauer, J., Rubenfire, M., Felming, P., Noon, G., Oldham, N., Killip, T., and Kantrowitz, A.: Intra-aortic balloon counterpulsation in cardiogenic shock: Report of a co-operative clinical trial. N. Engl. J. Med. 288:979, 1973.
820. Mundth, E. D., Buckley, M. J., Daggatt, W. M., McEnany, M. T., Leinbach, R. C., Gold, H. K., and Austen, W. B.: Intra-aortic balloon pump assistance and early surgery in cardiogenic shock. Adv. Cardiol. 15:159, 1975.
821. Corral, C. H., and Vaughn, C. C.: Intra-aortic balloon counterpulsation: An eleven-year review and analysis of determinants of survival. Tex. Heart Inst. J. 13:39, 1986.

822. Goldberg, M. J., Rubenfire, M., Kantrowitz, A., Goodman, G., Freed, P. S., Hallen, L., and Reimann, P.: Intraaortic balloon pump insertion: A randomized study comparing percutaneous and surgical techniques. J. Am. Coll. Cardiol. *9*:515, 1987.
823. Mueller, H., Ayres, S. M., Conklin, E. F., Giamelli, S., Jr., Mazzara, J. T., Grace, W. T., and Nealon, T. F., Jr.: The effects of intra-aortic counterpulsation on cardiac performance and metabolism in shock associated with acute myocardial infarction. J. Clin. Invest. *50*:1885, 1971.
824. Gold, H. K., Leinbach, R. C., Mundth, E. D., Sanders, C. A., and Buckley, M. J.: Reversal of myocardial ischemia complicating acute infarction by intra-aorta balloon pumping. Circulation *45-46*(Suppl. II):22, 1972.
825. Isner, J. M., Cohen, S. J., Viruari, R., Lawrikson, W., and Roberts, W. C.: Complications of the intra-aortic balloon counterpulsation device: Clinical and morphologic observations in 45 necropsy patients. Am. J. Cardiol. *45*:250, 1980.
826. DeLaria, G. A., Johansen, K. H., Sobel, B. E., Sybers, H. D., and Bernstein, E. F.: Delayed evolution of myocardial ischemic injury after intra-aortic balloon counterpulsation. Circulation *50*(Suppl. II):242, 1974.
827. Johnson, S. A., Scanlon, P. J., Loeb, H. S., Moran, J. M., Pifarre, R., and Gunnar, R. M.: Treatment of cardiogenic shock in myocardial infarction by intra-aortic balloon counterpulsation and surgery. Am. J. Med. *62*:687, 1977.
828. O'Rourke, M. F., Norris, R. M., Campbell, T. J., Chang, V. P., and Sammel, N. L.: Randomized controlled trial of intra-aortic balloon counterpulsation in early myocardial infarction with acute heart failure. Am. J. Cardiol., *47*:815, 1981.
829. Bitran, D., Hasin, Y., Weiss, A., Shefer, A., Freiman, I., Shimon, D., and Gotsman, M. S.: Intra-aortic balloon counterpulsation in acute myocardial infarction. Israel J. Med. Sci.*18*:215, 1982.
830. Pae, W. E., Jr., and Pierce, W. S.: Temporary left ventricular assistance in acute myocardial infarction and cardiogenic shock. Rationale and criteria for utilization. Chest *79*:692, 1981.
831. Gowda, S. K., Gillespie, T. A., Byrne, J. D., Ambos, H. D., Sobel, B. E., and Roberts, R.: Effects of external counterpulsation on enzymatically estimated infarct size and ventricular arrhythmia. Br. Heart J. *40*:308, 1978.
832. Chou, T-C., Fowler, N. O., Gabel, M., van der Bel-Kahn, J., and Feltner, E. J.: Electrocardiographic and hemodynamic changes in experimental right ventricular infarction. Circulation *67*:1258, 1983.
832a. Dell'Italia, L. J., Lembo, N. J., Starling, M. R., Crawford, M. H., Simmons, R. S., Lasher, J. C., Blumhardt, R., Lancaster, J. M., and O'Rourke, R. A.: Hemodynamically important right ventricular infarction: Follow-up evaluation of right ventricular systolic function at rest and during exercise with radionuclide ventriculography and respiratory gas exchange. Circulation *75*:996, 1987.
833. Lloyd, E. A., Gersh, B. J., and Kennelly, B. M.: Hemodynamic spectrum of dominant right ventricular infarction. Am. J. Cardiol. *48*:1016, 1981.
834. Roberts, N., Harrision, D. G., Reimer, K. A., Crain, B. S., and Wagner, M. D.: Right ventricular infarction with shock but without significant left ventricular infarction: A new clinical syndrome. Am. Heart J. *110*:1047, 1985.
835. Forman, M. B., Goodin, J., Phelan, B., Kopelman, H., and Virmani, R.: Electrocardiographic changes associated with isolated right ventricular infarction. J. Am. Coll. Cardiol. *4*:640, 1984.
836. Bansal, R. C., Marsa, R. J., Holland, D., Beehler, C., and Gold, P. M.: Severe hypoxemia due to shunting through a patent foramen ovale: A correctable complication of right ventricular infarction. J. Am. Coll. Cardiol. *5*:188, 1985.
837. Braat, S. H., Brugada, P., DeZwaan, C., DenDulk, K., and Wellens, H. J. J.: Right and left ventricular ejection fraction in acute inferior wall infarction with or without ST-segment elevation in lead V_4R. J. Am. Coll. Cardiol. *4*:940, 1984.
838. Chou, T., Van Der Bel-Kahn, J., Allen, J., Brockmeier, L., and Fowler, N. O.: Electrocardiographic diagnosis of right ventricular function. Am. J. Med. *70*:1175, 1981.
839. Croft, C. H., Nicod, P., Corbett, J. R., Lewis, S. E., Huxley, R., Mukharji, J., Willerson, J. T., and Rude, R. E.: Detection of acute right ventricular infarction by right precordial electrocardiography. Am. J. Cardiol. *50*:421, 1982.
840. Lopez-Sendon, J., Garcia-Fernandez, M. A., Coma-Canella, I., Yanguela, M. M., and Banuelos, F.: Segmental right ventricular function after acute myocardial infarction: Two-dimensional echocardiographic study in 63 patients. Am. J. Cardiol. *51*:390, 1983.
841. Jugdutt, B. I., Sussex, B. A., Sivaram, C. A., and Rossall, R. E.: Right ventricular infarction: Two-dimensional echocardiographic evaluation. Am. Heart J. *107*:505, 1984.
842. Arditti, A., Lewin, R. F., Hellman, C., Sclarovsky, S., Strasberg, B., and Agmon, J.: Right ventricular dysfunction in acute inferoposterior myocardial infarction. An echocardiographic isotopic study. Chest *87*:307, 1985.
843. Starling, M. R., Dell'italia, L. J., Chaudhuri, T. K., Boros, B. L., and O'Rourke, R. A.: First transit and equilibrium radionuclide angiography in patients with inferior transmural myocardial infarction: Criteria for the diagnosis of associated hemodynamically significant right ventricular infarction. J. Am. Coll. Cardiol. *4*:923, 1984.
844. Dell'italia, L. J., Starling, M. R., Crawford, M. H., Boros, B. L., Chaudhuri, T. K., and O'Rourke, R. A.: Right ventricular infarction: Identification by hemodynamic measurements before and after volume loading and correlation with noninvasive techniques. J. Am. Coll. Cardiol. *4*:931, 1984.
845. Haffajee, C. I., Love, J., Gore, J. M., and Alpert, J. S.: Reversibility of shock by atrial or atrioventricular sequential pacing in right ventricular infarction. Am. J. Cardiol. *49*:1025, 1982.
846. Topol, E. J ., Goldschlager, N., Ports, T. A., Dicarlo, L. A., Schiller, N. B., Botvinick, E. H., and Chatterjee, K.: Hemodynamic benefit of atrial pacing in right ventricular myocardial infarction. Ann. Intern. Med. *96*:594, 1982.
847. Marmor, A., Geltman, E. M., Biello, D. R., Sobel, B. E., Siegel, B. S., and Roberts, R.: Functional response to the right ventricle to myocardial infarction: Dependence on the site of left ventricular infarction. Circulation *64*:1005, 1981.
848. Lorell, B., Leinbach, R. C., Pohost, G. M., Gold, H. K., Dinsmore, R. E., Hutter, A. M., Jr., Pastore, J. O., and DeSanctis, R. W.: Right ventricular infarction. Clinical diagnosis and differentiation from cardiac tamponade and pericardial constriction. Am. J. Cardiol. *43*:465, 1979.
849. Korr, K. S., Lewvinson, H., Bough, E. W., Gheorghiade, M., Stone, J., McEnany, T., and Shulman, R. S.: Tricuspid valve replacement for cardiogenic shock after acute right ventricular infarction. J.A.M.A. *244*:1958, 1980.
850. London, R. E., and London, S. B.: Rupture of the heart. A critical analysis of 47 consecutive autopsy cases. Circulation *31*:202, 1965.
851. Björck, G., Mogensen, L., Nyquist, O., Orinius, E., and Sjogren, A.: Studies of myocardial rupture with cardiac tamponade in acute myocardial infarction. Chest *61*:4, 1972.
852. Kassis, E., Vogelsang, M., and Lyngoborg, K.: Cardiac rupture complicating myocardial infarction. A study concerning early diagnosis and possible management. Dan. Med. Bull. *48*:164, 1981.
853. Edmondson, H. A., and Hozie, H. J.: Hypertension and cardiac rupture: Clinical and pathological study of 72 cases, in 13 of which rupture of the interventricular septum occurred. Am. Heart J. *24*:719, 1942.
854. Balakumaran, K., Verbaan, C. J., Essed;, C. E., Nauta, J., Bos, E., Haalebos, M. M. P., Penn, O., Simoons, M. L., and Hugenholtz, P. G.: Ventricular free wall rupture: Sudden, subacute, slow, sealed and stabilized varieties. Eur. Heart J. *5*:282, 1984.
855. Coma-Canella, I., Lopez-Sendon, J., Gonzalez, L. N., and Ferrufino, O.: Subacute left ventricular free wall rupture following acute myocardial infarction: Bedside hemodynamics, differential diagnosis, and treatment. Am. Heart J. *106*:278, 1983.
856. Feneley, M. P., Chang, V. P., and O'Rourke, M.: Myocardial rupture after acute myocardial infarction. Br. Heart J. *49*:550, 1983.
857. Pifarre, R., Sullivan, H. J., Grieco, J., Montoya, A., Bakhos, M., Scanlon, P. J., and Gunnar, R. M.: Management of left ventricular rupture complicating myocardial infarction. J. Thorac. Cardiovasc. Surg. *86*:441, 1983.
858. Eisenmann, B., Bareiss, P., Pacifico, A. D., Jeanblanc, B., Kretz, J. G., Baehret, B., Warter, J., and Kieny, R.: Anatomic, clinical and therapeutic features of acute cardiac rupture. J. Thorac. Cardiovasc. Surg. *76*:78, 1978.
859. Russell, R. O., Jr., Turner, J. D., Rogers, W. J., Mantle, J. A., and Rackley, C. E.: Mortality reduction after acute myocardial infarction in a myocardial infarction research unit. Clin. Res. *26*:752A, 1978.
860. McMullan, M. H., Kilgore, T. L., Dear, H. D., and Hindman, S. H.: Sudden blowout rupture of the myocardium after infarction: Urgent management. J. Thorac. Cardiovasc. Surg. *89*:259, 1985.
861. Vlodaver, Z., Coe, J. L., and Edwards, J. E.: True and false left ventricular aneurysms. Circulation *51*:567, 1975.
862. Cohn, L. H.: Surgical management of acute and chronic cardiac mechanical complications due to myocardial infarction. Am. Heart J. *102*:1049, 1981.
863. Shabbo, F. P., Dymond, D. S., Rees, G. M., and Hill, I. M.: Surgical treatment of false aneurysm of the left ventricle after myocardial infarction. Thorax *38*:25, 1983.
864. Vlodaver, Z., and Edwards, J. E.: Rupture of ventricular septum or papillary muscle complicating myocardial infarction. Circulation *55*:815, 1977.
865. Radford, M. J., Johnson, R. A., Daggett, W. M., Fallon, J. T., Buckley, M. J., Gold, H. K., and Leinbach, R. C.: Ventricular septal rupture: A review of clinical and physiologic features and an analysis of survival. Circulation *64*:545, 1981.
866. Matsui, K., Kay, J. H., Mendez, M., Zubiate, P., Vanstrom, N., and Yokoyama, T.: Ventricular septal rupture secondary to myocardial infarction. Clinical approach and surgical results. J.A.M.A. *245*:1537, 1981.
867. Edwards, B. S., Edwards, W. D., and Edwards, J. E.: Ventricular septal rupture complicating acute myocardial infarction: Identification of simple and complex types in 53 autopsied hearts. Am. J. Cardiol. *54*:1201, 1984.
867a. Lock, J. E., Block, P. C., McKay, R. G., Baim, D. S., and Keane, J. F.: Catheter closure of post infarction-postoperative ventricular defects: Initial experience. Circulation (*in press*).
868. Nishimura, R. A., Schaff, H. V., Shub, C., Gersh, B. J., Edwards, W. D., and Tajik, A.: Papillary muscle rupture complicating acute myocardial infarction: Analysis of 17 patients. Am. J. Cardiol. *51*:373, 1983.
869. Barbour, D. J., and Roberts, W. C.: Rupture of a left ventricular papillary muscle during acute myocardial infarction: Analysis of 22 necropsy patients. J. Am. Coll. Cardiol. *8*:588, 1986.
870. Roberts, W. C., and Perloff, J. K.: Mitral valvular disease—A clinicopathologic survey of the conditions causing the mitral valve to function abnormally. Ann. Intern. Med. *77*:939, 1972.
871. Wei, J. Y., Hutchins, G. M., and Bulkley, B. H.: Papillary muscle rupture in fatal acute myocardial infarction. Ann. Intern. Med. *90*:149, 1979.
872. Lader, E., Colvin, S., and Tunick, P.: Myocardial infarction complicated by rupture of both ventricular septum and right ventricular papillary muscle. Am. J. Cardiol. *52*:424, 1983.
873. Gonzalez-Lavin, L., and Friedman, J. P.: Surgical treatment of ventricular septal rupture and mitral regurgitation complicating acute myocardial infarction: Report of a case and review of the literature. Clin. Cardiol. *6*:603, 1983.
874. Come, P. C., Riley, M. F., Weintraub, R., Morgan, J. P., and Nakao, S.: Echocardiographic detection of complete and partial papillary muscle rupture during acute myocardial infarction. Am. J. Cardiol. *56*:787, 1985.
875. Ballester, M., Tasca, R., Marin, L., Rees, S., Richard, A., and McDonald, L.: Different mechanisms of mitral regurgitation in acute and chronic forms of coronary heart disease. Eur. Heart J. *4*:557, 1983.

876. Meister, S. G., and Helfant, R. H.: Rapid bedside differentiation of ruptured interventricular septum from acute mitral insufficiency. N. Engl. J. Med. *287*:1024, 1972.
877. Kopf, G. S., Meshkov, A., Laks, H., Hammond, G. L., and Beha, A. S.: Changing patterns in the surgical management of ventricular septal rupture after myocardial infarction. Am. J. Surg. *143*:465, 1982.
878. Montoya, A., McKeever, L., Scanlon, P., Sullivan, H. J., Gunnar, R. M., and Pifarre, R.: Early repair of ventricular septal rupture after infarction. Am. J. Cardiol. *45*:345, 1980.
879. Miller, D. C., and Stinson, E. B.: Surgical management of acute mechanical defects secondary to myocardial infarction. Am. J. Surg. *141*:677, 1981.
880. Thomas, C. S., Jr., Alford, W. C., Jr., Burrus, G. R., Glassford, D. M., Jr., and Stoney, W. S.: Urgent operation for acquired ventricular septal defect. Ann. Surg. *195*:706, 1982.
881. Daggett, W. M., Buckley, M. J., Akins, C. W., Leinbach, R. C., Gold, H. K., Block, P. C., and Susten, W. G.: Improved results of surgical management of postinfarction ventricular septal rupture. Ann. Surg. *196*:269, 1982.
882. Abrams, D. L., Edelist, A., Luria, M. H., and Miller, A. J.: Ventricular aneurysm: A reappraisal based on a study in 65 consecutive autopsied cases. Circulation *27*:164, 1963.
883. Schlicter, J., Hellerstein, H. K., and Katz, L. N.: Aneurysm of the heart: A correlative study of 102 proved cases. Medicine *33*:43, 1954.
884. Eaton, L. W., and Bulkley, B. H.: Expansion of acute myocardial infarction: Its relationship to infarct morphology in canine model. Circ. Res. *49*:80, 1981.
885. Forman, M. D., Collins, H. W., Kipelman, H. A., Vaughn, W. K., Perry, J. M., Virmani, R., and Friesinger, G. C.: Determinants of left ventricular aneurysm formation after anterior myocardial infarction: A clinical and angiographic study. J. Am. Coll. Cardiol. *8*:1256, 1986.
886. Epstein, J. I., and Hutchins, G. M.: Subepicardial aneurysm: A rare complication of myocardial infarction. Am. J. Med. *75*:639, 1983.
887. Meizlish, J. L., Berger, H. J., Plankey, M., Errico, D., Levy, W., and Zaret, B. L.: Functional left ventricular aneurysm formation after acute anterior transmural myocardial infarction: Incidence, natural history, and prognostic implications. N. Engl. J. Med. *311*:1001, 1984.
888. Lindsay, J., Jr., Dewey, R. C., Talesnick, B. S., and Nolan, N. G.: Relation of ST-segment elevation after healing of acute myocardial infarction to the presence of left ventricular aneurysm. Am. J. Cardiol. *54*:84, 1984.
889. Brawley, R. K., Magovern, G. J., Jr., Gott, V. L., Donahoo, J. S., Gardner, T. J., and Watkins, L., Jr.: Left ventricular aneurysmectomy. Factors influencing postoperative results. J. Thorac. Cardiovasc. Surg. *85*:712, 1983.
890. Visser, C. A., Kan, G., Lie, K. I., and Durrer, D.: Incidence and one-year follow-up of left ventricular thrombus following acute myocardial infarction: An echocardiographic study of 96 patients. J. Am. Coll. Cardiol. *1*:648, 1983.
891. Hellerstein, H. K., and Martin, J. W.: Incidence of thromboembolic lesions accompanying myocardial infarction. Am. Heart J. *33*:443, 1947.
892. Asinger, R. W., Mikell, F. L., Elsperger, J., and Hodges, M.: Incidence of left ventricular thrombosis after acute transmural myocardial infarction. Serial evaluation of two-dimensional echocardiography. N. Engl. J. Med. *305*:297, 1981.
892a. Johannessen, K. A., Nordrehaug, J. E., and von der Lippe, G.: Increased occurrence of left ventricular thrombi during early treatment with timolol in patients with acute myocardial infarction. Circulation *75*:151, 1987.
893. Graber, J. D., Oakley, C. M., Pickering, J. F., Goodwin, J. F., Raphael, M. J., and Steiner, R. E.: Ventricular aneurysm and appraisal of diagnosis and surgical therapy. Br. Heart J. *34*:830, 1972.
894. Davies, M. J., Woolf, N., and Robertson, W. B.: Pathology of acute myocardial infarction with particular reference to occlusive coronary thrombi. Br. Heart J. *38*:659, 1976.
895. Johannessen, K. A., Nordrehaug, J. E., and von der Lippe, G.: Left ventricular thrombosis and cerebrovascular accident in acute myocardial infarction. Br. Heart J. *51*:553, 1984.
896. Gueret, P., Dubourg, O., Ferrier, A., Farcot, J. C., Riguad, M., and Bourdarias, J. P.: Effects of full-dose heparin anticoagulation on the development of left ventricular thrombosis in acute transmural myocardial infarction. J. Am. Coll. Cardiol. *8*:419, 1986.
897. Sharma, B., Carvalho, A., Wyeth, R., and Franciosa, J. A.: Left ventricular thrombi diagnosed by echocardiography in patients with acute myocardial infarction treated with intracoronary streptokinase followed by intravenous heparin. Am. J. Cardiol. *56*:422, 1985.
898. Eigler, N., Maurer, G., and Shah, P. K.: Effect of early systemic thrombolytic therapy on left ventricular mural thrombus formation in acute anterior myocardial infarction. Am. J. Cardiol. *54*:261, 1984.
899. Nordrehaug, J. E., Johannessen, K. A., and von der Lippe, G.: Usefulness of high-dose anticoagulants in preventing left ventricular thrombus in acute myocardial infarction. Am. J. Cardiol. *55*:1941, 1985.
900. Visser, C. A., Kan, G., Meltzer, R. S., Dunning, A. J., and Roelandt, J.: Embolic potential of left ventricular thrombus after myocardial infarction: A two-dimensional echocardiographic study of 119 patients. J. Am. Coll. Cardiol. *5*:1276, 1985.
901. Stratton, J. R., and Ritchie, J. L.: The effects of antithrombotic drugs in patients with left ventricular thrombi: Assessment with indium-111 platelet imaging and two-dimensional echocardiography. Circulation *69*:561, 1984.
902. Kremer, P., Fiebig, R., Tilsner, V., Bleifeld, W., and Mathey D. G.: Lysis of left ventricular thrombi with urokinase. Circulation *72*:112, 1985.
903. Eppinger, E. C., and Kennedy, J. A.: The cause of death in coronary thrombosis, with special reference to pulmonary embolism. Am. J. Med. Sci. *195*:104, 1938.
904. Stone, P., and Muller, J. E.: Nifedipine therapy for recurrent ischemic pain following myocardial infarction. Clin. Cardiol. *5*:223, 1982.
905. Moran, T. J., French, W. J., Abrams, H. F., and Criley, J. M.: Post-myocardial infarction angina and coronary spasm. Am J. Cardiol. *50*:197, 1982.
906. Koiwaya, Y., Torii, S., Takeshita, A., Nakagaki, O., and Nakamura, M.: Postinfarction angina caused by coronary arterial spasm. Circulation *65*:275, 1982.
907. Chaturvedi, N. C., Walsh, M. J., Evans, A., Munro, P., Boyle, D. M., and Barber, J. M.: Selection of patients for early discharge after acute myocardial infarction. Br. Heart J. *36*:533, 1974.
908. Epstein, S. E., Palmeri, S. T., and Patterson, R. E.: Evaluation of patients after acute myocardial infarction. Indications for cardiac catheterization and surgical intervention. N. Engl. J. Med. *307*:1467, 1982.
909. Disesa, V. J., O'Neil, A. C., Bitran, D., Cohn, L. H., Shemin, R. J., and Collins, J. J.: Aggressive surgical management of post-infarction angina: Results of myocardial revascularization early after transmural infarction. Tex. Heart J. *12*:333, 1985.
910. Brunken, R., Tillisch, J., Schwaiger, M., Child, J. S., Marshall, R., Mandelkern, M., Phelphs, M. E., and Schelbert, H. R.: Regional perfusion, glucose metabolism, and wall motion in patients with chronic electrocardiographic Q wave infarctions: Evidence for persistence of viable tissue in some infarct regions by positron emission tomography. Circulation *73*:951, 1986.
911. Buda, A. J., Macdonald, I. L., Dubbin, J. D., Orr, S. A., and Strauss, H. D. Myocardial infarct extension: Prevalence, clinical significance, and problems in diagnosis. Am. Heart J. *105*:744, 1983.
912. Rude, R. E., and the MILIS Study Group: Myocardial infarct extension: Incidence and clinical significance in MILIS. Circulation (Suppl. III) *72*:55, 1985.
913. Baker, J. T., Bramlet, D. A., Lester, R. M., Harrison, D. G., Roe, C. R., and Cobb, F. R.: Myocardial infarct extension: Incidence and relationship to survival. Circulation *65*:918, 1982.
914. Marmor, A., Sobel, B. E., and Roberts, E.: Factors presaging early recurrent myocardial infarction ("extension"). Am. J. Cardiol. *48*:603, 1981.
915. Pierard, L. A., Albert, A., Henrard, L., Lempereur, P., Sprynger, M., Carlier, J., and Kulbertus, H. E.: Incidence and significance of pericardial effusion in acute myocardial infarction as determined by two-dimensional echocardiography. J. Am. Coll. Cardiol. *8*:517, 1986.
916. Wunderink, R. G.: Incidence of pericardial effusions in acute myocardial infarctions. Chest *85*:492, 1985.
917. Lichstein, E., Liu, H.-M., and Gupta, P.: Pericarditis complicating acute myocardial infarction: Incidence of complications and significance of electrocardiogram on admission. Am. Heart J. *87*:246, 1974.
918. Blau, N., Shen, B. A., Pittman, D. E., and Joyner, C. E.: Massive hemopericardium in a patient with post-myocardial infarction syndrome. Chest *71*:549, 1977.
919. Karim, A. H., and Salomon, J.: Constrictive pericarditis after myocardial infarction. Sequelae of anticoagulant-induced hyperpericardium. Am. J. Med. *79*:389, 1985.
920. Lichstein, E., Arsura, E., Hollander, G., Greengart, A., and Sanders, M.: Current incidence of postmyocardial infarction (Dressler's) syndrome. Am. J. Cardiol. *50*:1269, 1982.
921. Northocte, R. J., Hutchinson, S. J., and McGuinness, J. B.: Evidence of the continued existence of the postmyocardial infarction (Dressler's Syndrome). Am. J. Cardiol. *53*:1201, 1984.

CONVALESCENCE, DISCHARGE, AND POST-MYOCARDIAL INFARCTION CARE

922. Madsen, E. B.: Time of discharge for patients with acute myocardial infarction. Cardiovasc. Rev. Reports *4*:1301, 1983.
923. Lau, Y. K., Smigh, J., Morrison, S. L., and Chamberlain, D. A.: Policy for early discharge after acute myocardial infarction. Br. Med. J. *281*:1489, 1980.
924. Pryor, D. B., Hindman, M. C., Wagner, G. S., Califf, R. M., Rhoads, M. K., and Rosati, R. A.: Early discharge after acute myocardial infarction. Ann. Intern. Med. *99*:528, 1983.
925. Abraham, A. S., Sever, Y., Weinstein, M., Dollberg, M., and Menczel, J.: Value of early ambulation in patients with and without complications after acute myocardial infarction. N. Engl. J. Med. *292*:719, 1975.
926. Madsen, E. B., Hougaard, P., Gilpin, E., and Pedersen, S.: The length of hospitalization after acute myocardial infarction determined by risk calculation. Circulation *68*:9, 1983.
927. Kloner, R. A., and Kloner, J. A.: The effect of early exercise on myocardial infarct scar formation. Am. Heart J. *106*:1009, 1983.
928. Hammerman, H., Kloner, R. A., Alker, K. U., Schoen, F. J., and Braunwald, E.: Effects of transient increased afterload during experimentally induced acute myocardial infarction in dogs. Am. J. Cardiol. *55*:566, 1985.
929. Papadopoulos, C.: A survey of sexual activity after myocardial infarction. Cardiovasc. Med. *3*:821, 1978.
930. Papadopoulos, C., Beaumont, C., Shelley, S. I., and Larrimore, P.: Myocardial infarction and sexual activity of the female patient. Arch. Intern. Med. *143*:1528, 1983.
931. Friedman, M., Thoresen, C. E., Gill, J. J., Ulmer, D., Thompson, L., Powell, L., Price, V., Elek, S. R., Rabin, D. D., Breall, W. S., Piaget, G., Dixon, T., Bourg, E., Levy, R. A., and Tasto, D. L.: Feasibility of altering type A behavior pattern after myocardial infarction. Recurrent coronary prevention project study: Methods, baseline results and preliminary findings. Circulation *66*:83, 1982.
932. Ewart, C. K., Taylor, C. B., Reese, L., and DeBusk, R. F.: Effects of early postinfarction exercise testing on self perception and subsequent physical activity. J. Am. Coll. Cardiol. *1*:662, 1983.
933. Taylor, S. H.: Secondary prevention after myocardial infarction: Facts and fallacies. J. Cardiovasc. Pharmacol. *6*:5914, 1984.

934. Rosenberg, L., Kaufman, D. W., Helmrich, S. P., and Shapiro, S.: The risk of myocardial infarction after quitting smoking in men under 55 years of age. N. Engl. J. Med. *313*:1511, 1985.
935. Myers, M. G.: Changing patterns in drug therapy for ischemic heart disease. Can. Med. Assoc. J. *312*:644, 1984.
936. Snow, P. J. D.: Effect of propranolol in myocardial infarction. Lancet *2*:735, 1965.
937. Roberts, R., Croft, C., Gold, H. K., Hartwell, T. D., Jaffe, A. S., Muller, J. E., Mullin, S. M., Parker, C., Passamani, E. R., Poole, W. K., Raabe, D. S., Rude, R. E., Stone, P. H., Turi, Z. G., Sobel, B. E., Willerson, J. T., Braunwald, E., and the MILIS Study Group: Effect of propranolol on myocardial infarct size in a randomized, blinded, multicenter trial. N. Engl. J. Med. *311*:218, 1984.
938. Beta Blocker Heart Attack Study Group: The Beta-Blocker Heart Attack Trial. J.A.M.A. *246*:2073, 1981.
939. Herlitz, J., Elmfeldt, D., Holmberg, S., Malek, I., Nyberg, G., Pennert, K., Ryden, L., Swedberg, K., Vedin, A., Waagstein, F., Waldenstrom, A., Waldenstrom, J., Wedel, H., Wilhelmsen, C., and Hjalmarson, A.: Göteborg metoprolol trial: Mortality and causes of death. Am. J. Cardiol. *53*:9D, 1984.
940. The Norwegian Multicenter Study Group: Timolol-induced reduction in mortality and reinfarction in patients surviving acute myocardial infarction, N. Engl. J. Med. *304*:801, 1981.
941. Pedersen, T. R., and the Norwegian Multicenter Study Group: Six-year follow-up of the Norwegian multicenter study on timolol after acute myocardial infarction. N. Engl. J. Med. *313*:1055, 1985.
942. Taylor, S. H., Silke, B., Ebbutt, A., Sutton, G. C., Prout, B. J., and Burley, D. M.: A long-term prevention study with oxprenolol in coronary heart disease. N. Engl. J. Med. *307*:1293, 1982.
943. May, G. S.: A review of acute-phase beta-blocker trials in patients with myocardial infarction. Circulation *67*(Suppl. I):21, 1983.
944. Gundersen, T.: Seconary prevention after myocardial infarction: Subgroup analysis of patients at risk in the Norwegian timolol multicenter study. Clin. Cardiol. *8*:253, 1985.
945. Chadda, K., Goldstein, S., Byington, R., and Curb, J. D.: Effect of propranolol after acute myocardial infarction in patients with congestive heart failure. Circulation *73*:503, 1986.
946. Herlitz, J., Hjalmarson, A., Holmberg, S., Sedberg, K., Vedin, A., Waagstein, F., Waldenstrom, A., Wedel, H., Wilhemsen, L., and Wilhelmsson, C.: Development of congestive heart failure after treatment with metoprolol in acute myocardial infarction. Br. Heart J. *51*:539, 1984.
947. Gundersen, T., Abrahamsen, A. M., Kjekshus, J., and Ronnevik, P. K.: Timolol-related reduction in mortality and reinfarction in patients ages 65–77 years surviving acute myocardial infarction. Circulation *66*:1179, 1982.
948. Griggs, T. R., Wagner, G. S., and Gettes, L. S.: Beta-adrenergic blocking agents after myocardial infarction: An undocumented need in patients at lowest risk. J. Am. Coll. Cardiol. *6*:1530, 1983.
949. Ahumada, G. G.: Identification of patients who do not require beta antagonists after myocardial infarction. Am. J. Med. *76*:900, 1984.
950. Modan, B., Shani, M., Schor, S., and Modan, M.: Reduction of hospital mortality from acute myocardial infarction by anticoagulant therapy. N. Engl. J. Med. *292*:1359, 1975.
951. Wessler, S.: Antithrombotic agents are indicated in the therapy of acute myocardial infarction. Cardiovasc. Clin. *8*:131, 1977.
952. Tonaschia, J., Gordis, L., and Schmerler, H.: Retrospective evidence favoring use of anticoagulants for myocardial infarctions. N. Engl. J. Med. *292*:1362, 1975.
953. Horwitz, R. I., and Feinstein, A. R.: The application of therapeutic trial principles to improve the design of epidemiologic research: A case-control study suggesting that anticoagulants reduce mortality in patients with myocardial infarction. J. Chronic Dis. *34*:575, 1981.
954. Anticoagulants in acute myocardial infarction: Results of a cooperative clinical trial. J.A.M.A. *225*:724, 1973.
955. Wray, R., Maurer, B., and Shillingford, J.: Prophylactic anticoagulant therapy in the prevention of calf-vein thrombosis after myocardial infarction. N. Engl. J. Med. *288*:815, 1973.
956. Rosenberg, R. D.: Actions and interactions of antithrombin and heparin. N. Engl. J. Med. *292*:146, 1975.
957. Hull, R., Delmore, T., Carter, C., Hirsh, J., Genton, E., Gent, M., Turpie, G., and McLaughlin, D.: Adjusted subcutaneous heparin versus warfarin sodium in the long-term treatment of venous thrombosis. N. Engl. J. Med. *306*:198, 1982.
958. Pitt, A., Anderson, S. T., Habersberger, P. G., and Rosengarten, D. S.: Low-dose heparin in the prevention of deep thromboses in patients with acute myocardial infarction. Am. Heart J. *99*:574, 1980.
959. A double-blind trial to asses long-term oral anticoagulant therapy in elderly patients with myocardial infarction. Report of the Sixty-plus Reinfarction Study Research group. Lancet *2*:989, 1980.
960. May, G. S., Furberg, C. D., Eberlein, K. A., and Geraci, B. J.: Secondary prevention after myocardial infarction: A review of short-term acute phase trials. Prog. Cardiovasc. Dis. *25*:335, 1983.
961. May, G. S., Eberlein, K. A., Furberg, C. D., Passamani, E. R., and DeMets, D. L.: Secondary prevention after myocardial infarction: A review of long-term trials. Prog. Cardiovasc. Dis. *25*:331, 1982.
962. Goldberg, R. J., Gore, J. J., Dalen, J. E., and Alpert, J. S.: Long-term anticoagulant therapy after acute myocardial infarction. Am. Heart J. *109*:616, 1985.
963. Elwood, P. C.: Aspirin in the prevention of myocardial infarction: Current status. Drugs *28*:1, 1984.
964. Friedewald, W. T., Furberg, C. D., and May, G. S.: Aspirin and myocardial infarction. Cardiovasc. Rev. Rep. *5*:1285, 1984.
965. Anturane Reinfarction Trial Research Group: Sulfinpyrazone in the prevention of sudden death after myocardial infarction. N. Engl. J. Med. *302*:250, 1980.
966. Davies, J. A.: Secondary prevention of myocardial infarction. Int. J. Clin. Pharmacol. Res. *5*:303, 1985.
967. Persantine-Aspirin Reinfarction Study Research Group: Persantine and aspirin in coronary heart disease. Circulation *62*:449, 1980.
968. Klimt, C. R., Knatterud, G. L., Stamler, J., and Meier, P.: Persantine-aspirin reinfarction study. Part II. Secondary coronary prevention with persantine and aspirin. J. Am. Coll. Cardiol. *7*:251, 1986.
969. Rapport, E.: Influence of long-acting nitrate therapy on the risk of reinfarction, sudden death, and total mortality in survivors of acute myocardial infarction. Am. Heart J. *110*:276, 1985.
969a. Gottlieb, S. H., Achuff, S. C., Mellits, E. D., Gerstenblith, G., Baughman, K. L., Becker, L., Chandra, N. C., Henley, S., Humphries, J. O., Heck, C., Kennedy, M. M., Weisfeldt, M. L., and Reid, P. R.: Prophylactic antiarrhythmic therapy of high-risk survivors of myocardial infarction: Lower mortality at 1 month but not at 1 year. Circulation *75*:792, 1987.
970. Canner, P. L., Berge, K. G., Weuger, N. K., Stamler, J., Friedman, L., Prineas, R. J., and Friedewald, W.: Fifteen-year mortality in Coronary Drug Project patients: Long-term benefits with niacin, J. Am. Coll. Cardiol. *8*:1245, 1986.
971. Friedman, M., Thoresen, C. E., Gill, J. J., Ulmer, D., Powell, L. H., Price, V. A., Brown, B., Thompson, L., Rabin, D. D., Breall, W. S., Bourg, E., Levy, R., and Dixon, T.: Alteration of type A behavior and its effect on cardiac recurrences in post-myocardial infarction patients: Summary results of the recurrent coronary prevention project. Am. Heart J. *112*:653, 1986.
972. Rapaport, E., and Remedios, P.: The high-risk patient after recovery from myocardial infarction: Recognition and management. J. Am. Coll. Cardiol. *1*:391, 1983.
973. Madsen, E. B., Hougaard, P., and Gilpin, E.: Dynamic evaluation of prognosis from time-dependent variables in acute myocardial infarction. Am. J. Cardiol. *51*:1579, 1983.
974. Taylor, G. J., Humphries, J. O., Mellits, E. D., Pitt, B., Schulze, R. A., Griffith, L. S. C., and Achuff, S. C.: Predictors of clinical course, coronary anatomy, and left ventricular function after recovery from acute myocardial infarction. Circulation *62*:960, 1980.
975. Norris, R. M., Barnaby, P. F., Brandt, P. W. T., Geary, G. G., Whitlock, R. M. L., Wild, C. J., and Barratt-Boyes, B. G.: Prognosis after recovery from first acute myocardial infarction: Determinants of reinfarction and sudden death. Am. J. Cardiol. *53*:408, 1984.
976. Killip, T., and Kimball, J. I.: Treatment of myocardial infarction in a coronary care unit. A two-year experience with 250 patients. Am. J. Cardiol. *20*:457, 1967.
977. Peel, A. A. F., Semple, T. Wang, I., Lancaster, W. M., and Dall, J. L. G.: A coronary prognostic index for grading the severity of infarction. Br. Heart J. *24*:745, 1962.
978. Norris, R. M., Brandt, P. W. T., Caughey, D. E., Lee, A. J., and Scott, P. J.: A new coronary prognostic index. Lancet *1*:274, 1969.
978a. Tofler, G. H., Stone, P. H., Muller, J. E., Willich, S. N., Davis, V. G., Poole, W. K., Strauss, H. W., Willerson, J. T., Jaffe, A. S., Robertson, T., Passamani, E., Braunwald, E., and the MILIS Study Group: Effects of gender and race on prognosis after myocardial infarction: Adverse prognosis for women, particularly black women. J. Am. Coll. Cardiol. 9:473, 1987.
979. DeBusk, R. F., Kraemer, H. C., and Nash, E.: Stepwise risk stratification soon after acute myocardial infarction. Am. J. Cardiol. *52*:1161, 1983.
980. Merrilees, M. A., Scott, P. J., and Norris, R. M.: Prognosis after myocardial infarction: Results of 15-year follow-up. Br. Med. J. *288*:356, 1984.
981. Smith, J. W., Marcus, F. I., and Serokman, R., with the Multicenter Postinfarction Research Group: Prognosis of patients with diabetes mellitus after acute myocardial infarction. Am. J. Cardiol. *54*:718, 1984.
982. Rennert, G., Saltz-Rennerts, H., Wanderman, K., and Weitzman, S.: Size of acute myocardial infarcts in patients with diabetes mellitus. Am. J. Cardiol. *55*:1629, 1985.
983. Gwilt, D. J. G., Petri, M., Lewis, P. W., Nattrass, M., and Pentecost, B. L.: Myocardial infarct size and mortality in diabetic patients. Br. Heart J. *54*:466, 1985.
984. The Coronary Drug Project Research Group: Blood pressure in survivors of myocardial infarction. J. Am. Coll. Cardiol. *4*:1134, 1984.
985. Maisel, A. S., Gilpin, E., Holt, B., LeWinter, M., Ahnve, S., Henning, H., Collins, D., and Ross, J.: Survival after hospital discharge in matched populations with inferior or anterior myocardial infarction. J. Am. Coll. Cardiol. *6*:731, 1985.
986. Hands, M. E., Lloyd, B. L., Robinson, J. S., DeKlerk, N., and Thompson, P. L.: Prognostic significance of electrocardiographic site of infarction after correction for enzymatic size of infarction. Circulation 73:885, 1986.
986a. Bosch, X., Theroux, P., Waters, D. D., Pelletier, G. B., and Roy, D.: Early postinfarction ischemia: Clinical, angiographic, and prognostic significance. Circulation 75:988, 1987.
987. Koiwaya, Y., Nakagaki, O., Takeshita, A., and Nakamura, M.: Clinical characteristics and prognosis of patients with postinfarction angina caused by coronary artery spasm. Clin. Cardiol. 7:68, 1984.
988. Kannell, W. B., and Abbott, R. D.: Incidence and prognosis of unrecognized myocardial infarction. N. Engl. J. Med. *311*:1144, 1984.
989. Madsen, E. B., Gilpin, E., and Henning, H.: Evaluation and prognosis one year after myocardial infarction. J. Am. Coll. Cardiol. *4*:985, 1983.
990. Henning, H., Gilpin, E., Covell, J. W., Swan, E. A., O'Rourke, R. A., and Ross, J., Jr.: Prognosis after acute myocardial infarction: A multivariate analysis of mortality and survival. Circulation 59:1124, 1979.
991. Madsen, E. B., Gilpin, E., Henning, H., Ahnve, S., LeWinter, M., Ceretto, W., Joswig, W., Collins, D., Pitt, W., and Ross, J.: Prediction of late

mortality after myocardial infarction from variables measured at different times during hospitalization. Am. J. Cardiol. *53*:47, 1984.

992. Verdouw, P. D., Hagemeijer, F., van Dorp, W. G., van der Vorm, A., and Hugenholtz, P. G.: Short-term survival after acute myocardial infarction predicted by hemodynamic parameters. Circulation 52:413, 1975.
993. Sanford, C. F., Corbett, J., Nicod, P., Curry, G. L., Lewis, S. E., Dehmer, G. J., Anderson, A., Moses, B., and Willerson, J. T.: Value of radionuclide ventriculography in the immediate characterization of patients with acute myocardial infarction. Am. J. Cardiol. *49*:637, 1982.
994. Shell, W. E., DeWood, M. A., Peter, T., Mickle, D., Prause, J. A., Forrester, J. S., and Swan, H. J. C.: Comparison of clinical signs and hemodynamic state in the early hours of transmural myocardial infarction. Am. Heart J. *103*:521, 1982.
995. Becker, L. C., Silverman, K. J., Bulkley, B. H., Kallman, C. H., Mellits, E. D., and Weisfeldt, M.: Comparison of early thallium-201 scintigraphy and gated blood pool imaging for predicting mortality in patients with acute myocardial infarction. Circulation *67*:1272, 1983.
996. Shiina, A., Tajik, A. J., Smith, H C., Lengyel, M., and Seward, J. B.: Prognostic significance of regional wall motion abnormality in patients with prior myocardial infarction: A prospective correlative study of two-dimensional echocardiography and angiography. Mayo Clin. Proc. *61*:254, 1986.
997. Warnowicz, M. A., Parker, H., and Cheitlin, M. D.: Prognosis of patients with acute pulmonary edema and normal ejection fraction after acute myocardial infarction. Circulation *67*:330, 1983.
998. Haines, D. E., Beller, G. A., Watson, D. D., Nygaard, T. W., Craddock, G. B., Cooper, A. A., and Gibson, R. S.: A prospective clinical, scintigraphic, angiographic and functional evaluation of patient after inferior myocardial infarction with and without right ventricular dysfunction. J. Am. Coll. Cardiol. *6*:995, 1985.
999. Holman, B. L., Chisholm, R. J., and Braunwald, E.: The prognostic implications of acute myocardial infarct scintigraphy with ^{99m}Tc-pyrophosphate. Circulation *57*:320, 1978.
1000. Pfeffer, M. A., Pfeffer, J. M., Steinberg, C., and Finn, P.: Survival after an experimental myocardial infarction: Beneficial effects of long-term therapy with captopril. Circulation *72*:406, 1985.
1001. Hutter, A. M., Jr., DeSanctis, R. W.: Flynn, T., and Yeatman, L. A.: Nontransmural myocardial infarction: A comparison of hospital and late clinical course of patients with that of matched patients with transmural anterior and transmural inferior myocardial infarction. Am. J. Cardiol. *48*:595, 1981.
1002. Nicholson, M. R., Roubin, G. S., Bernstein, L., Harris, P. J., and Kelly, D. T.: Prognosis after an initial non-Q-wave myocardial infarction related to coronary arterial anatomy. Am. J. Cardiol. *52*:462, 1983.
1003. Gibson, R. S., Beller, G. A., Gheorghiade, M., Nygaard, T. W., Watson, D. D., Huey, B. L., Sayre, S. L., and Kaiser, D. L.: The prevalence and clinical significance of residual myocardial ischemia 2 weeks after uncomplicated non-Q wave infarction: A prospective natural history study. Circulation *73*:1186, 1986.
1004. Connolly, D. C., and Elveback, L. R.: Coronary heart disease in residents of Rochester, Minnesota. VI. Hospital and posthospital course of patients with transmural and subendocardial myocardial infarction. Mayo Clin. Proc. *60*:375, 1985.
1005. Rigo, R., Murray, M., Taylor, D. R., Weisfeldt, M. L., Strauss, H. W., and Pitts, B.: Hemodynamic and prognostic findings in patients with transmural and nontransmural infarction. Circulation *51*:1064, 1975.
1006. Madias, J. E., and Gorlin, R.: The myth of "mild" myocardial infarction. Ann. Intern. Med. *86*:347, 1977.
1007. Madias, J. E., Chahine, R. A., Gorlin, R., and Blacklow, D. J.: A comparison of transmural and nontransmural acute myocardial infarction. Circulation *49*:498, 1974.
1008. Madigan, N. P., Rutherford, B. D., and Frye, R. L.: The clinical course, early prognosis and coronary anatomy of subendocardial infarction. Am. J. Med. *60*:634, 1976.
1009. Maisel, A. S., Ahnve, S., Gilpin, E., Henning, H., Goldberger, A. L., Collins, D., LeWinter, M., and Ross, J., Jr.: Prognosis after extension of myocardial infarct: The role of Q-wave or non-Q-wave infarction. Circulation *71*:211, 1985.
1009a. Safian, R. D., Snyder, L. D., Snyder, B. A., McKay, R. G., Lorell, B. H., Aroesty, J. M., Pasternak, R. C., Bradley, A. B., Monrad, E. S., and Baim, D. S.: Usefulness of percutaneous transluminal coronary angioplasty for unstable angina pectoris after non-Q-wave acute myocardial infarction. Am. J. Cardiol. *59*:263, 1987.
1010. Kennedy, J. W.: Non-Q-wave myocardial infarction. N. Engl. J. Med. *315*:451, 1986.
1010a. Kuchar, D. L., Thorburn, C. W., and Sammel, N. L.: Prediction of serious arrhythmic events after myocardial infarction: signal-averaged electrocardiogram, Holter monitoring and radionuclide ventriculography. J. Am. Coll. Cardiol. *9*:531, 1987.
1010b. Gomes, J. A., Horowitz, S. F., Millner, M., Machac, J., Winters, S. L., and Barreca, P.: Relation of late potentials to ejection fraction and wall motion abnormalities in acute myocardial infarction. Am. J. Cardiol. *59*:1071, 1987.
1010c. Denniss, A. R., Richards, D. A., Cody, D. V., Russell, P. A., Young, A. A., Cooper, M. J., Ross, D. L., and Uther, J. B.: Prognostic significance of ventricular tachycardia and fibrillation induced at programmed stimulation and delayed potentials detected on the signal-averaged electrocardiograms of survivors of acute myocardial infarction. Circulation *74*:731, 1986.
1011. Ong, L., Valdellon, B., Coromilas, J., Brody, R., Reiser, P., and Morrison, J.: Precordial ST-T segment depression in inferior myocardial infarction. Evaluation by quantitative thallium-201 scintigraphy and technetium-99m ventriculography. Am. J. Cardiol. *51*:734, 1983.
1012. DeFeyter, P. J., van Eenige, M. J., Dighton, D. H., and Roos, J. P.: Exercise testing early after myocardial infarction. Chest *83*:853, 1983.
1013. Fuller, C. M., Raizner, A. E., Verani, M., Nahormek, P. A., Chahine, R. A., McEntee, C. W., and Miller, R. R.: Early postmyocardial infarction treadmill stress testing. Ann. Intern. Med. *94*:734, 1981.
1014. Nair, R., Allan, K., Reg, N., Baird, M. G., Beanlands, D. A., and Higginson, L. A.: A comparison of clinical treadmill predictors of prognosis following acute myocardial infarction. J. Am. Coll. Cardiol. *1*:717, 1983.
1015. Waters, D. W., Bosch, X., Bouchard, A., Moise, A., Roy, D., Pelletier, G., and Therous, P.: Comparison of clinical variables and variables derived from a limited predischarge exercise test: A predictory of early and later mortality after myocardial infarction. J. Am. Coll. Cardiol. *5*:1, 1985.
1016. Fioretti, P., Brower, R. W., Simoons, M. L., Bos, R. J., Baardman, T., Beelen, A., and Hugenholtz, P. G.: Prediction of mortality during the first year after acute myocardial infarction with clinical variables and stress test at hospital discharge. Am. J. Cardiol. *55*:1313, 1985.
1017. Denniss, A. R., Baaijens, H., Cody, D. V., Richards, D. A., Russell, P. A., Young, A. A., Ross, D. L., and Uther, J. B.: Value of programmed stimulation and exercise testing in predicting one-year mortality after acute myocardial infarction. Am. J. Cardiol. *56*:213, 1985.
1018. Madsen, E. B., Gilpin, E., Ahnve, S., Henning, H., and Ross, J., Jr.: Prediction of functional capacity and use of exercise testing for predicting risk after acute myocardial infarction. Am. J. Cardiol. *56*:839, 1985.
1019. Gibson, R. S., Watson, D. D., Crampton, R. S., and Beller, G. A.: Prospective comparison of submaximal exercise TL-201 scintigraphy 2 weeks after symptom-limited maximal testing 3 months after myocardial infarction. J. Am. Coll. Cardiol. *1*:654, 1983.
1020. Krone, R. J., Gillespie, J. A., Weld, F. M., Miller, J. P., Moss, A. J.: Low-level exercise testing after myocardial infarction: Usefulness in enhancing clinical risk stratification. Circulation *71*:80, 1985.
1021. Starling, M. R., Crawford, M. H., Henry R. L., Lembo, N. J., Kennedy, G. T., and O'Rourke, R. A.: Prognostic value of electrocardiographic exercise testing and noninvasive assessment of left ventricular ejection fraction soon after acute myocardial infarction. Am. J. Cardiol. *57*:532, 1986.
1022. Handler, C. E., and Sowton, E.: Stress testing predischarge and six weeks after myocardial infarction to compare submaximal and maximal exercise predischarge and to assess the reproducibility of induced abnormalities. Int. J. Cardiol. *9*:173, 1985.
1023. Starling, M. R., Crawford, M. H., Kennedy, D. T., and O'Rourke, R. A.: Treadmill exercise tests predischarge and six weeks post-myocardial infarction to detect abnormalities of known prognostic value. Ann. Intern. Med. *94*:721, 1981.
1024. Hung, J., Goris, M. L., Nash, E., Kraemer, H. C., and DeBusk, R. F.: The comparative prognostic value of standard treadmill testing, rest and exercise thallium myocardial perfusion scintigraphy and radionuclide ventriculography 3 weeks after myocardial infarction. J. Am. Coll. Cardiol. *1*:654, 1983.
1025. Morris, K. G., Palmeri, S. T., Califf, R. M., McKinnis, R. A., Higginbotham, M. B., Coleman, R. E., and Cobb, F. R.: Value of radionuclide angiography for predicting specific cardiac events after acute myocardial infarction. Am. J. Cardiol. *55*:318, 1985.
1026. Borer, J. S., Rosing, D. R., Miller, R. H., Stark, R. M., Kent, K. M., Bacharach, S. L., Green, M. V., Lake, C. R., Cohen, H., Holmes, D., Donohue, D., Baker, W., and Epstein, S. E.: Natural history of left ventricular function during 1 year after acute myocardial infarction: Comparison with clinical electrocardiographic and biochemical determinations. Am. J. Cardiol. *46*:1, 1980.
1027. The Multicenter Postinfarction Research Group: Risk Stratification and survival after myocardial infarction. N. Engl. J. Med. *309*:331, 1983.
1028. Bigger, J. T., Jr., Fleiss, J. L., Kleiger, R., Miller, J. P., Rolnitzky, L. M., and the Multicenter Post-infarction Research Group: The relationships among ventricular arrhythmias, left ventricular dysfunction, and mortality in the 2 years after myocardial infarction. Circulation *69*:250, 1984.
1029. Mukharji, J., Rude, R., Gustafson, N., Poole, K., Passamani, E., Thomas, L. J., Jr., Strauss, H. W., Muller, J. E., Roberts, R., Raabe, D. S., Jr., Braunwald, E., Willerson, J. T., and cooperating investigators, MILIS: Late sudden death following myocardial infarction: Interdependence of risk factors. J. Am. Coll. Cardiol. *1*:585, 1983.
1030. Moss, A. J., Bigger, J. T., Case, R. B., Gillespie, J., Goldstein, R., Greenberg, H., Krone, R., Marcus, F. I., Odoroff, C. L., and Oliver, G. C.: Risk stratification and prognostication after myocardial infarction. J. Am. Coll. Cardiol. *1*:716, 1983.
1031. Richards, D. A., Cody, D. V., Denniss, A. R., Russell, P. A., Young, A. A., and Uther, J. B.: Ventricular electrical instability: A predictor of death after myocardial infarction. Am. J. Cardiol. *51*:75, 1983.
1032. Roy, D., Marchangd, E., Theroux, P., Waters, D. D., Pelletier, G. B., Cartier, R., and Bourassa, M. G.: Long-term reproducibility and significance of provokable ventricular arrhythmias after myocardial infarction. J. Am. Coll. Cardiol. *8*:32, 1986.
1033. DiMarco, J. P., Lerman, B. B., Kron, I. L., and Sellers, T. D.: Sustained ventricular tachyarrhythmias within 2 months of acute myocardial infarction: Results of medical and surgical therapy in patients resuscitated from the initial episode. J. Am. Coll. Cardiol. *6*:759, 1985.
1034. Fioretti, P., Brower, R. W., Simoons, M. L., tenKaten, H., Beelan, A., Baardman, T., Lubsen, J., and Hugenholtz, P. G.: Relative value of clinical variables, biycle ergometry, rest radionuclide ventriculography and 24-hour ambulatory electrocardiographic monitoring at discharge to predict 1-year survival after myocardial infarction. J. Am. Coll. Cardiol. *8*:40, 1986.
1035. DeBusk, R. F., Blomqvist, G., Kouchoukos, N. T., Luepker, R. V., Miller, H. S., Moss, A. J., Pollock, M. L., Reeves, T. J., Selvester, R. H., Stason, W. B., Wagner, G. S., and Willman, V. L.: Identification and treatment of low-risk patients after acute myocardial infarction and coronary-artery bypass graft surgery. N. Engl. J. Med. *314*:161, 1986.

39 CHRONIC ISCHEMIC HEART DISEASE

by JOHN D. RUTHERFORD, M. B.,
EUGENE BRAUNWALD, M. D., and
PETER F. COHN, M.D.

INTRODUCTION

Chronic ischemic heart disease is most commonly due to obstruction of the coronary arteries, which in turn usually results from atherosclerosis, the pathogenesis of which is described in Chapter 35. The importance of ischemic heart disease in contemporary society is attested to by the almost epidemic number of persons afflicted—especially when this number is compared with the anecdotal reports of its occurrence in the medical literature prior to this century. Coronary artery disease causes more deaths, disability, and economic loss in industrialized nations than any other group of diseases. In the United States arteriosclerosis is responsible for nearly half of all deaths. Each year, at least 200,000 Americans under the age of 65 die with what has been called *premature* ischemic heart disease and another five million people are afflicted with it. In addition to enormous personal and family suffering, it has been estimated that in 1987 the economic costs of cardiovascular diseases, with ischemic heart disease being a major contributor, will be more than eighty-five billion dollars in health expenditures and lost productivity.

In this century a dramatic increase in coronary heart disease mortality has occurred, with a peak being reached in the late 1960's in most industrialized countries. Since then a continuing downward trend in coronary heart disease mortality has been noted in North America, Belgium, Finland, Israel, Japan, Australia, and New Zealand.[1] In contrast, in most Eastern European countries and in the U.S.S.R. and Sweden, death rates from coronary heart disease are still increasing.

Of great interest are community-based studies carried out in Rochester, Minnesota, which showed that the incidence of coronary heart disease had been increasing up until 1959, fell to the level recorded in 1954 over the next 5 years, and thereafter slowly declined until 1969 with no change from 1969 to 1975.[2, 3] These observations applied to angina pectoris, myocardial infarction, and sudden unexpected death, with the greatest decline being noted in the incidence of sudden death. This fall in coronary heart disease incidence was followed a decade later by lowering of the overall annual mortality rate and probably was a contributing factor. The 5-year survival of patients with angina pectoris improved from 75 per cent in the years 1950 to 1970 to 87 per cent during 1970 to 1975.

It remains to be seen whether the decline in coronary heart disease mortality (in the countries in which it has been observed) is due to a reduction in incidence, a change in case fatality rates, or both of these factors. Whereas changing incidence might suggest that preventive programs are having an impact, changing case fatality rates would suggest improvements in medical and surgical management of patients known to have coronary heart disease. As we assess such data, it is important to consider carefully the composition of the population under study with respect to the natural history of coronary artery disease (Fig. 39–1).

The widespread decline in mortality secondary to coronary artery disease noted in different countries with differ-

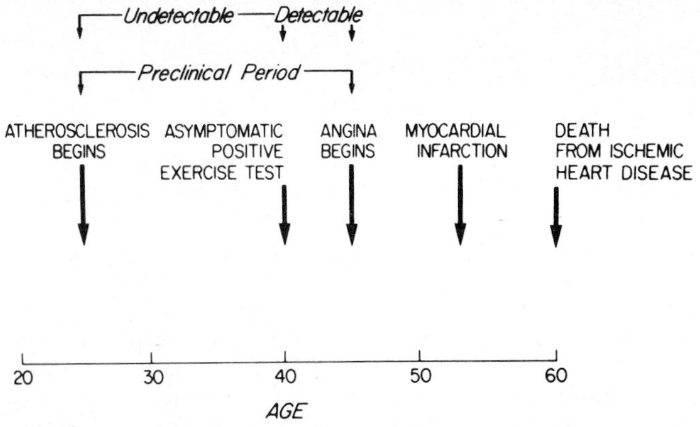

FIGURE 39–1. The natural history of a prototypical patient with coronary artery disease. Atherosclerosis begins as an asymptomatic, undetectable pathological process that usually, but not always, proceeds through an asymptomatic period in which it is undetectable, then detectable. This is often followed by a symptomatic period with a duration and expression that vary from patient to patient. The reported natural history of a group of symptomatic patients differs, depending on the rate of progression. For many patients, however, the first clinical manifestation of their disease is infarction or sudden death. (From Goldman, L. et al.: The changing "natural history" of symptomatic coronary artery disease: Basis versus bias. Am. J. Cardiol. *51*:449, 1983.)

ent health systems and in all age groups appears to be real rather than the result of changes in methods of classifying patients. Studies in Rochester mentioned above[2, 3] suggest that both the incidence and the case fatality rates may be falling. The fact that the population rates of coronary heart disease can change substantially over the course of several years provides a strong argument that efforts to prevent and/or treat the disease have the potential for success.[4]

There is no uniform presenting syndrome for chronic ischemic heart disease. Although chest discomfort is usually the predominant symptom in chronic (stable), unstable, or variant angina and acute myocardial infarction, syndromes of ischemic heart disease also occur in which ischemic chest discomfort is absent or not prominent. These include asymptomatic (silent) myocardial ischemia, cardiac arrhythmias, and congestive heart failure. Myocardial ischemia may also occur in the absence of coronary atherosclerosis (as in aortic valve disease, hypertrophic cardiomyopathy, and syphilitic aortitis), and coronary artery disease may occur together with these other forms of heart disease. Finally, the various syndromes characteristic of ischemic heart disease may complicate noncardiac disease, e.g., coronary artery disease may occur in patients with chronic renal failure requiring dialysis.

HISTORICAL PERSPECTIVES

To appreciate this disease entity, some historical perspective is useful. Angina pectoris serves as a good example, since it is the most common clinical presentation of chronic ischemic heart disease. The term was first used by Dr. William Heberden in a report published in 1772.[5] Unlike the word "dolor," which means grief or pain, the word "angina" was intended to indicate a sense of *strangling*. Heberden noted that fear of death ("angor animi") often accompanies this sensation in the chest (or rather, observed with this symptom complex, episodes of discomfort in the "breast"). Heberden's description of angina is as accurate today as it was more than 2 centuries ago:

> "There is a disorder of the breast, marked with strong and peculiar symptoms considerable for the kind of danger belonging to it, and not extremely rare, of which I do not recollect any mention among medical authors. The seat of it, and sense of strangling and anxiety, with which it is attended, may make it not improperly be called angina pectoris. Those, who are afflicted with it, are seized while they are walking and most particularly when they walk soon after eating, with a painful and most disagreeable sensation in the breast, which seems as if it would take their life away, if it were to increase or to continue; the moment they stand still, all this uneasiness vanishes."

The pathophysiological mechanism of angina pectoris as being related to an imbalance between myocardial oxygen supply and demand was first described in 1799 by C.H. Parry:

> "The rigidity of the coronary arteries may act, proportionately to the extent of the ossification, as a mechanical impediment to the free motion of the heart; and though a quantity of blood may circulate through these arteries, sufficient to nourish the heart, yet there may probably be less than what is requisite for ready and vigorous action. Hence, though a heart so diseased may be fit for the purposes of common circulation, during a state of bodily and mental tranquility, and of health otherwise good, yet when any unusual exertion is required, its powers may fail, under the new and extraordinary demand."[6]

An indirect commentary on the incidence of recognized coronary atherosclerosis is provided by the medical literature dealing with angina. Following Heberden's original account of angina pectoris, few reports dealt with this syndrome before the beginning of the 20th century. For example, in a textbook of medicine by Austin Flint published in 1866,[7] only two pages were devoted to angina pectoris. There appears to have been far less coronary artery disease 100 years ago than now, for it seems hard to believe that it could have escaped attention if acute myocardial infarction and sudden death occurred with any frequency in young and middle-aged men. In the mid-19th century, renewed interest in angina pectoris was stimulated by Brunton's report on the use of amyl nitrate for the treatment of angina pectoris,[8] yet when William Osler published his textbook of medicine in 1892,[9] he still referred to angina as a rare condition. Osler believed that complete obliteration of a coronary artery, if produced suddenly, was usually fatal. Although he recognized different gradations of anginal pain, nonfatal acute myocardial infarction as a separate entity was recognized for the first time with the reports of Obraztov and Strazhesko in Russia in 1910[10] and of Herrick in the United States in 1912.[11]

P. D. White became interested in coronary artery disease early in the 20th century, stating that while a student at Harvard Medical School he received no instruction or experience that helped him recognize this condition. In 1968, he reviewed the hospital records of 800 patients who had been under his care as an intern at the Massachusetts General Hospital in 1912–1913.[12] Of 700 men, mainly between the ages of 20 and 60 years, only eight were diagnosed as having angina pectoris; three had syphilitic aortitis as the cause of their pain, and one had rheumatic aortic regurgitation. Thus, it appears that symptomatic ischemic heart disease was quite uncommon (or rarely recognized) at the Massachusetts General Hospital at the beginning of the 20th century. In the early 1920's, ischemic heart disease aroused more interest, and there were increasing reports of its occurrence. Wearn, at the Peter Bent Brigham Hospital, described a premonitory chest pain syndrome before the actual myocardial infarction occurred—the syndrome currently named unstable angina.[13]

With the development of cardiology as a speciality, interest in coronary artery disease grew rapidly. The diagnostic value of the electrocardiogram became recognized, especially during exercise. Perhaps the most important next step in understanding the pathophysiology of chronic ischemic heart disease was the clinical-pathological correlation described by Blumgart, Schlesinger, and Zoll at Boston's Beth Israel Hospital.[14] Their studies were particularly important because they demonstrated the different histopathological findings in patients with angina pectoris and myocardial infarction, and they stressed the importance of the collateral circulation. Two decades after the work of Blumgart and associates the modern era of study of coronary artery disease began with the introduction of coronary arteriography by Sones in 1959,[15] allowing the evaluation of coronary anatomy in vivo.

CHRONIC STABLE ANGINA PECTORIS

CLINICAL MANIFESTATIONS

CHARACTERISTICS OF ANGINA (See also p. 3). Angina pectoris is a discomfort in the chest or adjacent areas, which is caused by myocardial ischemia and is associated with a disturbance of myocardial function but without myocardial necrosis.[16] Heberden's initial description of the chest discomfort as conveying a sense of "strangling and anxiety" is still remarkably pertinent today, although adjectives used to describe this distress now include "vise-like," "constricting," "suffocating," "crushing," "heavy," and "squeezing." In other patients, the quality of the sensation is even more vague and may be described as a mild pressure-like discomfort or an uncomfortable numb sensation. The site of the discomfort is usually retrosternal, but radiation is common and usually occurs down the ulnar surface of the left arm; commonly, the right arm and the outer surfaces of both arms are also involved[17] (Fig. 1–1, p. 5). Sampson and Cheitlin have documented the large number of regions that can be sites of radiation, with neck, jaw, and throat pain observed most commonly.[18] Headache is uncommon, and discomfort below the epigastrium due to angina is rare. Anginal "equivalents" (i.e., symptoms of myocardial ischemia other than angina) such as breathlessness, faintness, fatigue, and belching have also been reported.

The symptom complex leading to the diagnosis of angina is invariably important even if the intensity of the discomfort described by the patient appears slight. Pain seldom occurs only in the left pectoral area and a discomfort lasting all day is unlikely to be cardiac ischemia unless it is caused by myocardial infarction or an uncorrected cardiac rhythm disturbance. It is characteristic that patients with angina will usually prefer to rest, sit, or stop walking during attacks.[16]

ETIOLOGY. The etiology of angina pectoris is complex and not fully understood.[19] For example, the specific substance that actually stimulates sympathetic afferents and begins the series of interactions that culminate in chest discomfort has not been identified. Some evidence favors agents that are released from cells as a result of transient ischemia, such as adenosine,[20] bradykinin, histamine, or serotonin.[21] Acidosis or elevated potassium concentration in the involved tissues may trigger release of these substances to which the sensory end-plates of the intracardiac sympathetic nerves appear to be particularly sensitive. The end-plates are the receptors of a network of unmyelinated nerves that lie between cardiac muscle fibers and that are also found around coronary vessels, travel to the cardiac plexus, and then ascend to the sympathetic ganglia (C7-T4). Impulses are transmitted to corresponding spinal ganglia, then via the spinal cord to the thalamus, and finally to the cerebral cortex.

The discomfort of myocardial ischemia is perceived in various regions of the chest because it is "referred" to the corresponding peripheral dermatomes that supply afferent nerves to the same segment of the spinal cord as the heart. A plausible explanation is that a common pool of secondary neurons can be stimulated by somatic and visceral afferent impulses.[22] If visceral stimuli are excessive, the nearby intermediate neurons that are receptors for somatic impulses may be excited, and the discomfort will then be perceived as being cutaneous in origin. Thus, pain impulses can be referred to the medial aspects of the arm via common connections to the brachial plexus and can be referred to the neck via connections with the cervical roots.

It is not clear why some patients with clear-cut evidence of ischemic heart disease experience no chest discomfort; diabetics appear to have a higher frequency of "silent" ischemia, perhaps because of autonomic denervation. In some patients chest pain disappears after a myocardial infarction, even though other evidence of paroxysmal ischemia, such as ST-segment depression, may persist. It is postulated that in these patients the nerve endings may have been damaged as a result of the infarction. Finally, patients with reproducible evidence of myocardial ischemia may or may not experience chest pain with each of the various episodes. Ambulatory electrocardiography has revealed that the majority of patients with angina also experience numerous episodes of silent ischemia, i.e., ST-segment and T-wave changes identical to those occurring during typical angina but unaccompanied by chest discomfort. These episodes are accompanied by reductions of myocardial perfusion, as measured by uptake of radioactive rubidium.[23] The frequency is reduced by treatment with nitrates, beta blockers, and calcium antagonists, supporting the contention that they represent instances of myocardial ischemia. (See p. 1362 for further discussion of silent ischemia).

Features of Anginal Discomfort. The fact that the discomfort of angina is not uniform and that other entities can mimic it often makes the differential diagnosis of chest pain difficult[16, 17, 24] (Table 1–1, p. 3). Constant[25] has suggested that physicians should ask specific questions to differentiate "nonanginal chest pain" from angina. He notes that some of the characteristics of nonanginal pain are a pain lasting less than 5 seconds or greater than 20 to 30 minutes (provided infarction is excluded); a pain aggravated or precipitated by one deep breath; pain precipitated by a single movement of the trunk or arm; pain relieved within a few seconds of lying horizontally (patients with angina rarely lie down to get relief); pain relieved within a few seconds of one or two swallows of food or water; pain localized to a very small area, e.g., an area the size of the tip of a finger; pain associated with tenderness of chest wall (unless the anginal pain is referred to a site of previous chest wall trauma). Differentiating the discomfort resulting from these noncardiac disorders from angina pectoris is usually possible when the *quality* of the pain and its *duration*, *precipitating factors*, and *associated symptoms* are taken into consideration (Table 1–3, p. 4).[18] Thus, the *typical* anginal episode usually begins gradually and reaches maximum intensity over a period of minutes before dissipating—usually as a result of cessation of the activity that precipitated it. *Noncoronary* causes should be considered in patients with sharp, stabbing, or burning chest pain that comes and goes in a matter of seconds or with a dull, continuous ache in the chest. Similarly, changes in posture do not usually affect the discomfort of myocardial ischemia, and this maneuver helps to distinguish angina from pericardial disease or hiatus hernia.

Angina Due to Increased Oxygen Demand. In typical angina, the pain is related to an increase in myocardial oxygen demands, most commonly brought about by physical activity; the *rate* at which a task is carried out is important. Hurrying is particularly likely to precipitate angina, as are efforts involving motion of the hands over the head. Emotion or eating, particularly when combined with physical activity, commonly causes angina, as do a variety of other factors, including the excessive metabolic demands imposed by chills and fever, thyrotoxicosis, tachycardia from any cause, severe anemia, and hypoglycemia. In all these conditions, underlying fixed coronary artery obstruction in the form of atheromatous disease is usually present, and the other factors (e.g., exercise, fever) in-

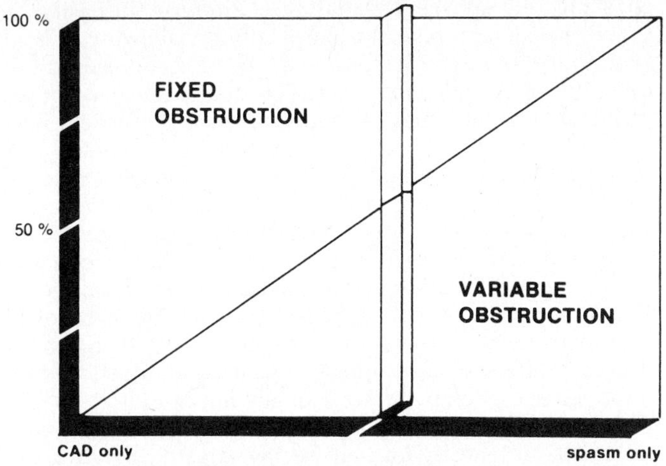

FIGURE 39–2. Different mixtures of fixed and variable obstruction may produce myocardial ischemia. The vertical bar represents a patient in whom both spasm (variable obstruction) and fixed obstruction play significant roles in occluding a coronary artery. This variable mixture of spasm and fixed obstruction may be present not only in Prinzmetal's angina but in classic angina and acute myocardial infarction as well. (From Muller, J. E.: Prinzmetal's angina: A model for the role of spasm in ischemic heart disease. J. Cardiovasc. Med. 5:19, 1980.)

crease the activity of the heart, stimulate myocardial oxygen needs in the presence of a fixed and limited oxygen supply, and thus precipitate ischemia and chest discomfort.

Angina Due to Transient Decreased Oxygen Supply. There is increasing evidence, however, that angina may also be caused by transient reductions of oxygen supply as a consequence of *coronary vasoconstriction.*[26–28] As pointed out on page 1193, the coronary arterial bed is well innervated and a variety of stimuli alter coronary tone. There is a reciprocal relationship between the severity of dynamic and organic obstruction required to cause myocardial ischemia (Fig. 37–16, p. 1202). Thus, in the occasional patient with no organic lesions, only severe dynamic obstruction can cause myocardial ischemia and resultant angina. On the other hand, in patients with severe, although subcritical, fixed obstruction to coronary flow, only a minor increase in dynamic obstruction is necessary to cause blood flow to fall below a critical level and cause myocardial ischemia (Fig. 39–2).

FIXED- VS. VARIABLE-THRESHOLD ANGINA. The variability of the threshold for angina differs among patients. In patients with *fixed-threshold angina* due largely to increased oxygen demands, with few if any dynamic (vasoconstrictive) components, the level of physical activity—a reflection of myocardial oxygen consumption—required to precipitate angina is relatively constant. Characteristically, these patients can predict with precision the amount of physical activity that causes angina, e.g., walking up exactly two and a half flights of stairs. When these patients are tested on a treadmill or bicycle, the pressure-rate product that elicits angina and/or electrocardiographic evidence of ischemia is fixed or almost so. Patients with *variable-threshold angina*, the majority of whom have a fixed obstructive lesion but in whom dynamic obstruction caused by vasoconstriction plays an important role in causing myocardial ischemia, typically have "good days," when they are capable of substantial physical activity, and "bad days," when even minimal activity can cause clinical and/or electrocardiographic evidence of myocardial ischemia or when angina occurs at rest. Often, even in the course of a single day, they may be capable of substantial physical activity at one time, while at another time minimal activity will result in angina. Patients with variable-threshold angina often complain of angina precipitated by cold temperatures, emotion, and meals and occasionally of angina occurring at rest or nocturnally. It is presumed that coronary vasoconstriction contributes to the development of angina under these circumstances. The anginal threshold tends to be lower in the morning than in the afternoon, correlating with the angiographic finding of smaller coronary arterial lumina at that time of day.[29] However, even in patients with angina at rest and nocturnal angina, an increase in myocardial oxygen demand may play a role.[30] In the many patients who fall between these two extremes (Fig. 39–2), the anginal threshold is *moderately variable*; the term *mixed angina* has been suggested to describe this large group.[31]

Changes in the blood pressure–heart rate product (the double product) provide a rough approximation of myocardial oxygen requirements (p. 1193). In patients with effort-induced fixed-threshold angina, the threshold at which ischemia develops (as reflected in angina and ST-segment depression) is a function of myocardial oxygen requirement. In patients with (relatively) fixed-threshold angina, the time and effort required for the development of angina during treadmill exercise is relatively predictable and reproducible; it is probable that as the performance of the ventricle (and therefore its oxygen consumption) increases, a point is reached at which myocardial perfusion distal to a major coronary arterial obstruction can no longer increase, and ischemia ensues as oxygen consumption rises.

Observations in patients experiencing angina under circumstances other than exercise help to explain the pathophysiological bases of angina. For example, some patients with ischemic heart disease characteristically experience angina on exposure to *cold weather* or *during or after meals.* A cold environment has been shown to increase peripheral resistance at rest and during exercise.[32] The rise in arterial pressure, by augmenting myocardial oxygen requirements, lowers the threshold for the development of angina. An alternative, or additional, explanation is the development of cold-induced coronary vasoconstriction.[33, 34] The reduction in exercise capacity during or after meals has been explained by a more rapid rise in heart rate and blood pressure compared to preprandial values,[35] but the postprandial increase in myocardial oxygen needs may not be sufficient to explain the development of ischemia, and a dynamic component, i.e., coronary vasoconstriction, may also be involved.[36] Similarly, during angina induced by *emotional stress*, heart rate and blood pressure and therefore myocardial oxygen needs rise but usually not to the level required to produce angina during exercise. Therefore, a dynamic component probably plays a role here as well.[37]

Relief of anginal discomfort is usually afforded by rest (not by "walking through") and by sublingual nitroglycerin; indeed, the response to the drug is often a useful diagnostic tool.[38] A long delay before relief is obtained, i.e., more than 5 to 10 minutes, suggests that the pain is not ischemic in origin. As described by Levine, carotid sinus pressure can also often bring about rapid alleviation of discomfort.[39]

In *atypical angina* the precipitating factors may be similar, but the quality of the discomfort is different (sharp and stabbing, for example); or, if the quality of the discomfort is angina-like, the precipitating causes are unusual, such as varying body positions; or the discomfort may be typical in quality and occur only at rest but may not be accompanied by characteristic ST-segment changes. *Nonanginal chest pain* has neither the quality of typical angina nor its usual precipitating causes.

GRADING OF ANGINA PECTORIS. A system of grading effort angina proposed by the Canadian Cardiovascular Society in 1972 has gained widespread acceptance and was used in the Coronary Artery Surgery Study.[40] This grading system is the New York Heart Association (NYHA) functional classification, which is modified to allow independent observers to categorize patients in more precise terms. The Specific Activity Scale described by Goldman et al.[41] is also useful in estimating symptomatic severity. These systems are described on pages 11 and 12 and in Table 1–5.

CLINICAL-PATHOLOGICAL CORRELATIONS. The prevalence of coronary artery disease in subsets of patients with typical angina, atypical angina, and nonanginal chest pain has been estimated by Diamond and Forrester to be about 90 per cent, 50 per cent, and 16 per cent, respectively, while the prevalence of coronary artery disease in asymptomatic adults of comparable age is estimated to be 3 to 4 per cent.[42] Pasternak et al. reported that among 3242 patients in whom coronary angiograms were obtained for chest pain, 175 (5.4 per cent) had essentially normal coronary vessels. Of the latter, about one-third had chest pain typical of angina and in two-thirds it was atypical.[43] Several reports[44–46] suggest that the clinical manifestations of ischemia may be more severe in patients with multivessel than single-vessel disease, but in any individual patient the nature of the underlying disease cannot be predicted from the severity, nature, duration, or quality of the discomfort. Perhaps the best examples of this lack of clinical-pathological correlation are two groups of patients who have been well characterized: those with advanced obstructive disease and so-called "silent ischemia)"[47–49] (p. 1362) and those with Prinzmetal's angina (p. 1360). For comparable degrees of obstructive coronary artery disease, as defined arteriographically, asymptomatic or minimally symptomatic patients have a better prognosis than do those with severe angina.[50] When infarction (without angina) is the first manifestation of ischemic heart disease, it is often associated with single-vessel disease; when angina occurs before infarction, two- or three-vessel disease is usually present.[51] Gender also appears to influence the clinical expression of coronary artery disease. Among women, angina pectoris is by far the most frequent clinical expression, as compared with men, in whom fatal and nonfatal myocardial infarction proportionately are more common than in women.[52] While a natural menopause does not appear to increase the risk of coronary heart disease, bilateral oophorectomy does; however, this latter risk may be prevented by estrogen replacement.[52a]

DIFFERENTIAL DIAGNOSIS OF CHEST PAIN

(Table 1–1, p. 3)

The differentiation of various disorders from coronary artery disease is challenging because, as has already been noted, the severity of the chest pain and the seriousness of the underlying disorder are not necessarily related. Compounding the difficulty in differential diagnosis is the common myth that pain in the left arm or left side of the chest is an ominous sign signifying the presence of coronary artery disease. A host of disorders can cause these types of discomfort.

ESOPHAGEAL DISORDERS. These may produce symptoms that can mimic myocardial ischemia.[52b, 52c] Abnormal regurgitation of acid from the stomach to the esophagus—esophageal reflux—is relatively common. This can cause inflammation of the esophageal mucosa and is often associated with a retrosternal burning—"heartburn," indigestion, and/or belching. Spasm of the esophagus may cause constant retrosternal discomfort of uniform intensity or severe spasmodic pain during or after swallowing. These symptoms are intermittent and often accompanied by difficulty in swallowing, although the pain may occur spontaneously at times. While esophageal disorders may produce substernal "burning," features more suggestive of esophageal than anginal pain include a background of continuous aching, a discomfort confined to the retrosternal area that does not radiate laterally, a pain that is not associated with exercise, and a pain disturbing sleep and occurring in association with some esophageal symptoms.[53] Discomfort caused by esophageal spasm is often relieved by nitroglycerin (although not usually in less than 3 minutes). Unlike angina, esophageal pain is often relieved by milk, antacids, foods, or occasionally hot liquids.[25]

Acid regurgitation, or acid-induced esophageal spasm, as a cause of chest pain may be investigated by alternate infusions of dilute acid and normal saline via a nasogastric catheter with the tip at the level of the mid-esophagus (Bernstein test). In patients with subjective and objective evidence of gastroesophageal acid reflux, acid infusion will readily produce pain within 2 to 4 minutes; however, pain may continue for over 20 minutes in patients after the acid infusion is stopped despite the fact that the esophageal pH returns to normal much earlier.[54] Acid reflux into the esophagus can also be recognized by recording pH from an electrode at the tip of a catheter inserted into the distal esophagus.[55]

Gastric reflux is often associated with *hiatus hernia*, which can be diagnosed radiographically. In patients with hiatus hernia, postprandial distress is most marked in the recumbent position, a feature that helps to differentiate it from angina pectoris. The differentiation between esophageal pain and angina is complicated by the observation that infusion of acid into the esophagus of patients with coronary artery disease can increase the rate pressure product, can cause angina as well as ECG evidence of ischemia, and can also cause pain indistinguishable from angina in patients with infrequent or absent reflux symptoms.[56] Also, esophageal stimulation with acid will lower the threshold for exertional angina pectoris, especially in patients who have concurrent, regular esophageal symptoms.[57]

In patients with retrosternal chest pain of unclear cause, esophageal motility disorders are not uncommon[58–60] and should be specifically excluded or confirmed. In addition to chest pain, the majority of such patients have dysphagia.[58, 59] While barium studies may reveal motility problems, esophageal manometry may reveal diffuse esophageal spasm, increased pressure at the lower esophageal sphincter, and other disorders.[58–60] Provocative pharmacological agents such as ergonovine[61] and metacholine[60] may provoke esophageal pain and manometric signs of spasm (in patients with normal coronary arteries). Surgical or medical therapy of esophageal reflux will improve symptoms in patients with normal coronary arteries whose experience of chest pain coincides with documented episodes of reflux (using 24-hour esophageal pH monitoring).[55]

BILIARY COLIC. This symptom is sometimes confused with angina pectoris. It is usually caused by a rapid rise in biliary pressure due to obstruction of the cystic or bile duct. Accordingly, the pain is usually abrupt in onset and steady in nature, subsiding slowly over minutes or hours. It is usually most intense in the right upper abdomen but may also be felt in the epigastrium, left abdomen, or precordium. This discomfort is often referred to the scapula, may radiate around the costal margin to the back, or rarely may be felt in the shoulder, suggesting diaphragmatic irritation. Although nausea and vomiting are common, the relationship of the pain to meals is variable. While a history of dyspepsia, flatulence, fatty food intolerance, and indigestion may be associated with cholelithiasis, these symptoms are also commonly experienced by the general normal population. Ultrasonic scanning will often help to confirm the diagnosis. Usually oral cholecystography will show if stones are present in the gallbladder; failure to opacify the gallbladder may indicate nonfunction due to disease. Cholangiography performed after episodes of acute cholangitis may demonstrate cholelithiasis; if these are radiopaque, they may be seen on a plain x-ray.

Distention of the splenic flexure of the colon can also mimic anginal pain, but, unlike angina, relief of symptoms often follows a bowel movement.

COSTOSTERNAL SYNDROME. In 1921, Tietze first described a syndrome of local pain and tenderness, usually limited to the anterior chest wall, associated with swelling of the costal cartilages. This condition causes pain that can resemble angina pectoris. The full-blown Tietze syndrome, i.e., pain associated with tender swelling of the costochondral junctions, is uncommon, whereas costochondritis causing tenderness of the costochondral junctions (without swelling) is relatively common.[62, 63] Pain on palpation of these joints is a useful clinical sign. Local pressure should be applied routinely to the anterior chest wall during the examination of the patient being evaluated for angina pectoris. Treatment usually consists of reassurance, antiinflammatory agents, and occasionally local steroids.[64]

CERVICAL RADICULITIS. This may occur as a constant ache, often resulting in a sensory deficit. The pain may be related to motion of the neck, just as motion of the shoulder triggers attacks of pain due to bursitis. A hyperalgesic area of skin noted by running the finger down the back and exerting pressure may lead to the suspicion of thoracic root pain.[25] Occasionally, pain mimicking angina can be due to compression of the brachial plexus via *cervical ribs*. Physical examination may also detect pain brought about by movement of an arthritic shoulder, a calcified shoulder tendon, and the like. The musculoskeletal disorders that can mimic angina include subacromial bursitis and costochondritis.

OTHER CAUSES OF ANGINA-LIKE PAIN. *Pulmonary hypertension* of severe degree may be associated with exertional chest pain with the characteristics of angina pectoris. Other associated symptoms include dyspnea on exertion and faintness, dizziness, or syncope associated with exertion. Associated findings on physical examination, such as a parasternal lift, palpable and loud pulmonary component of the second sound, and right ventricular hypertrophy on the electrocardiogram usually are readily recognized (p. 810). *Pulmonary embolism* (Chap. 47) causes chest pain that is usually associated with dyspnea.[65] Associated pleuritic pain suggests pulmonary infarction, and a history of exacerbation of the pain with inspiration with findings of a pleural friction rub usually readily distinguish this from angina pectoris.

The pain of *acute pericarditis* (p. 1488) at times may be difficult to distinguish from angina pectoris. Pericarditis tends to occur in a younger age group and the diagnosis depends on chest pain, a pericardial friction rub, and ECG changes. The chest pain usually is fairly sudden in onset, severe and persistent, and is intensified by coughing, swallowing, and inspiration. Relief may be obtained by sitting up and leaning forward. Palpation of the trapezius ridge often causes discomfort. A pericardial friction rub can be detected in most patients if listened for carefully, at different times, with the patient in different positions. Early widespread ST-segment elevation may be seen in leads in which the positive electrode faces the ventricular cavity rather than the epicardial surface (that is, leads aV_r, III, and/or V_1).

Acute myocardial infarction (Chap. 38) is usually associated with prolonged (> 30 minutes), severe pain that apart from duration and intensity may be similar to a patient's previous episodes of angina pectoris. It is associated with characteristic electrocardiographic and enzyme findings.

In many of the disorders just mentioned, angina pectoris can usually be excluded by a careful history and physical examination. It must be stressed, however, that ischemic heart disease can and frequently does *coexist* with any of these other disorders and that occasionally noncardiac disease can trigger a true anginal attack in a patient with coronary artery disease.

CHEST PAIN WITH NORMAL CORONARY ARTERIOGRAM

The syndrome of angina or angina-like chest pain with a normal coronary arteriogram is an important clinical entity to be differentiated from classic ischemic heart disease caused by coronary atherosclerosis.[43, 66, 67] In this condition, sometimes referred to as *Syndrome X*, the prognosis is usually excellent[68, 69]—contrasted with that in patients with coronary atherosclerosis—and its recognition is of clinical importance. Patients with chest pain who have normal coronary arteriograms may constitute as many as 10 to 20 per cent of those undergoing coronary arteriography because of the strong suspicion of angina. The cause of the syndrome is unknown. True myocardial ischemia, reflected in the production of lactate by the myocardium during exercise or pacing, is present in only a small fraction of these patients.[70]

INADEQUATE VASODILATOR RESERVE. Several studies suggest that many patients with chest pain with angiographically normal coronary arteries and no evidence of large vessel spasm, even after an ergonovine challenge, demonstrate an abnormally reduced capacity to decrease coronary resistance and increase coronary flow in response to atrial pacing.[71] This abnormality appears to affect the smaller resistance vessels that are not visible angiographically, while the large proximal conductance vessels appear to be normal. This "abnormal vasodilator reserve" may be associated with exercise-induced regional wall motion abnormalities and abnormalities of resting diastolic function.[72] Such patients, with low coronary flow reserve, may exhibit abnormal thallium-201 perfusion scintigrams during exercise that are indicative of true blood flow or perfusion abnormalities.[73] Interestingly, in patients with hypertension and secondary left ventricular hypertrophy with angina pectoris and a normal coronary arteriogram, a reduced coronary blood flow response to dipyridamole has been observed, suggesting a similar pathogenic mechanism.[74] Other patients with angina and normal coronary arteries are found on extensive investigation to have a cardiomyopathy—either hypertrophic[75] or congestive—and in these cases reduced perfusion, especially of the subendocardium, may be responsible for myocardial ischemia and resultant angina. This finding correlates well with the autopsy observation of thickening of the walls of the coronary arterioles in hypertrophic obstructive cardiomyopathy.[76]

OTHER CAUSES. Patients with psychogenic chest pain, neurocirculatory asthenia, and DaCosta syndrome may also manifest chest pain and have normal coronary arteries. Recently, platelet hyperaggregability in vitro has been demonstrated in some patients with chest pain and normal coronary arteries.[77] The role that this finding may play in the pathogenesis of this syndrome is unknown.

CLINICAL FEATURES. The syndrome of angina or angina-like chest pain with normal large coronary arteries occurs more frequently in women, while obstructive coronary artery disease is found more commonly in men. Fewer than half of the patients with chest pain and normal coronary arteriograms have typical angina; the majority have a variety of forms of atypical chest pain. In some patients with minimal or no coronary disease, an exaggerated preoccupation with personal health is prospectively associated with continued chest pain.[78]

PHYSICAL AND LABORATORY FINDINGS. Abnormal physical findings indicative of ischemia, such as precordial bulges, gallop sounds, and murmurs of mitral regurgitation, are uncommon. The resting electrocardiogram may be normal, but nonspecific ST-T abnormalities are often observed. Commonly, perusal of serial electrocardiograms during multiple episodes of chest pain reveals no significant change from baseline. A minority, approximately 20 per cent of patients with chest pain and normal coronary arteriograms, have positive exercise tests. However, many patients with this chest pain syndrome fail to complete the exercise test, discontinuing because of fatigue or mild chest discomfort. Left ventricular function is usually normal at rest and after pacing,[70, 79] unlike the situation in obstructive coronary artery disease in which function often becomes impaired during stress. However, a small percentage of these patients exhibit lactate production and ST-segment depression during exercise (signifying ischemia), for as yet unexplained reasons. Some patients show abnormal myocardial perfusion,[73] but there is no consistent pattern of abnormal myocardial blood flow,[80, 81] although coronary vasodilator reserve may be impaired.[71–74]

In patients with a persistent chest pain syndrome and normal coronary arteries, esophageal abnormalities should be considered.[55] Such patients may show either motility disorders of the esophagus or abnormal reflux. In patients whose experience of chest pain coincides with documented reflux, either surgical or medical therapy may give gratifying relief of symptoms.[55]

Important prognostic information on patients with either normal or near-normal coronary arteriograms has been obtained from the CASS Registry.[69] In patients with an ejection fraction of at least 50 per cent, the 7-year survival rate was 96 per cent for patients with a normal arteriogram and 92 per cent with those whose arteriographic study revealed mild disease (less than 50 per cent luminal stenosis). In such patients, an ischemic response to exercise was not associated with increased mortality although a history of smoking or hypertension was. Bass and Wade found that two-thirds of patients with chest pain and normal coronary arteries had predominantly psychiatric disorders.[82] Others have found that the incidence of coronary artery disease is extremely low in patients with atypical chest pain who are anxious and/or depressed.[83]

In *summary*, there are a number of possible explanations in patients having chest pain and normal coronary arteriograms. Sometimes review of angiography will reveal that significant coronary artery disease exists (i.e., incorrect interpretation of angiograms with a false-negative result). When there is no evidence of coronary artery narrowing, other causes of pain may be defined (e.g., esophageal disease, mitral valve prolapse syndrome), although often other causes cannot be found after exhaustive tests. It should be remembered that there may be "abnormal vasodilator reserve" of smaller coronary resistance vessels with, or without, associated cardiac hypertrophy.

MANAGEMENT. This should focus on the explanation of the relatively benign nature of the condition to the patient, psychological counseling, and analgesics to provide pain relief. Calcium antagonists appear to be effective in reducing the frequency and severity of angina and improving exercise tolerance in most patients with chest pain resulting from abnormal vasodilator reserve.[84] However, some patients continue to remain disabled with long-term chest discomfort. This can lead to multiple medical consultations and be responsible for a great deal of anxiety. Behavioral therapy may teach the patient with pain how to function more effectively,[85, 86] although unfortunately chronic symptoms may persist.

PHYSICAL EXAMINATION OF THE PATIENT WITH CHRONIC STABLE ANGINA

GENERAL EXAMINATION. In the patient with chronic ischemic heart disease and angina pectoris, the general examination may be entirely normal or may reveal the presence of risk factors for the development of coronary atherosclerosis. Inspection of the eyes may reveal a *corneal arcus* and examination of the skin may reveal xanthomas. A corneal arcus is found more frequently in middle-aged men than women.[87] In families with hypercholesterolemia it is present in proportion to the duration of the hypercholesterolemia rather than with the pattern of the particular disorder.[88] In men, the size of the corneal arcus appears to correlate positively with age and levels of cholesterol and low-density lipoproteins. The corneal arcus is not known to regress in humans and is unaffected by a reduction in the level of lipids.[88] *Xanthelasma*, in which lipid deposits are intracellular, appears to be promoted by increased levels of triglycerides and a relative deficiency of high-density lipoproteins. In the Lipid Research Clinic's study,[89] the prevalence of both xanthelasma and corneal arcus increased with age and was highest in persons with Type II dyslipoproteinemia and usually low in those with the Type IV phenotype. Both were associated with increased levels of total and low-density lipoprotein cholesterol, especially in young men. In young people, both xanthelasma and corneal arcus were highly associated with each other, and seemed to identify persons with plasma lipoprotein abnormalities. Neither showed a consistent association with manifestations of peripheral arterial disease.[89] Adjusted odds ratios for the presence of ischemic heart disease in individuals with xanthelasma and corneal arcus generally were increased.

There appears to be a correlation between coronary artery disease and *diagonal earlobe crease*, except in native American Indians, Orientals, and children with Beckwith-Wiedemann syndrome (exomphalos, macroglossia, giantism).[90] The diagonal earlobe crease is often unilateral in younger persons with coronary artery disease, becoming bilateral with advancing age. It is not believed to be inherited but rather develops along with coronary heart disease.[91] Some have suggested that associated ear canal hair may also be associated with coronary artery disease.[92]

The *blood pressure* may be chronically elevated or may rise acutely (along with the heart rate) during an anginal attack. These changes may precede (and precipitate) or follow (and be caused by) the ongoing episode. *Retinal arteriolar changes* are common in patients with coronary artery disease, even those without diabetes mellitus or hypertension. An abnormal light reflex is the most sensitive sign, while abnormal vessel tortuosity and decreased caliber are less sensitive but more specific signs. Other features of the general physical examination that are important to seek are abnormalities of the arterial pulses and of the venous system. Major abnormalities of the carotid artery pulse, or bruits, associated with cerebral symptoms usually will lead to echocardiography and perhaps carotid arteriography. Abnormality to palpation of the peripheral arterial pulses (femoral and popliteal) or the presence of bruit is not as accurate as are actual measurements of limb perfusion.[93] However, correlation of coronary artery disease with carotid and peripheral arterial disease makes physical examination of these vessels an important part of the investigation of these patients.

Evaluation of the patient's venous system, particularly in the legs, may have an important bearing on the type of grafting procedure employed in subsequent coronary artery surgery.

CARDIAC EXAMINATION. This may supply useful clues to both the diagnosis of ischemic heart disease and the functional state of the myocardium. First, the presence of murmurs of hypertrophic obstructive cardiomyopathy or aortic valve disease suggests that the ischemic chest pain may be due to conditions other than, or in addition to, coronary artery disease. Second, certain findings such as a third or loud fourth heart sound and early diastolic or presystolic filling waves on the apex cardiogram suggest ischemia as the basis for chest pain if other obvious cardiac diseases are absent. These are common findings in patients with angina at rest and their frequency is increased during handgrip exercise,[94] even if the latter does not precipitate angina pectoris. These sounds and pulsations are related to the functional state of the left ventricle, particularly its pressure and compliance during diastole (p. 402). In patients with moderate to severe left ventricular dysfunction, a sustained apical cardiac impulse is common. The presence of a palpable presystolic impulse may be more indicative of moderate than severe left ventricular dysfunction.[95] While a fourth heart sound may be recorded phonocardiographically in many apparently normal subjects over the age of 45, we agree with Tavel[96] that a clear, loud fourth heart sound accompanied by a palpable presystolic wave is an abnormal finding. It is not specific for ischemic heart disease but may be elicited in other conditions associated with left ventricular hypertrophy such as aortic stenosis, hypertrophic cardiomyopathy, and hypertension, in which left ventricular compliance is reduced (p. 51). Paradoxical splitting of the second heart sound (p. 47) may occur transiently during an anginal attack and appears to be related to asynergy and prolongation of left ventricular contraction.

When patients with ischemic heart disease lie in the left lateral recumbent position, dyskinetic bulges at the apex may be palpated or recorded by means of apexcardiography (p. 58); the bulges correspond to dyskinetic areas and often complement the auscultatory findings of diastolic filling sounds. Transient or persistent apical systolic murmurs are quite common and have been attributed to reversible papillary muscle dysfunction secondary to transient myocardial ischemia or to fibrosis, a manifestation of subendocardial infarction. They are more prevalent in patients with extensive coronary artery disease, especially those with prior myocardial infarction and left ventricular dysfunction. The systolic murmur may assume a variety of configurations (early, late, or holosystolic) and may be accentuated by exertion or during angina. A midsystolic click, often followed by a late systolic murmur characteristic of mitral regurgitation produced by papillary muscle dysfunction (Fig. 33–12, p. 1036), also occurs in patients with coronary artery disease. A diastolic murmur or a continuous murmur is an uncommon finding and has been attributed to turbulent flow across a proximal coronary artery stenosis.[97]

Abnormal left ventricular function during myocardial ischemia may be documented by abnormalities in systolic time intervals, i.e., prolongation of the preejection period (PEP), shortening of the systolic ejection period (SEP), and an increase in the PEP/SEP ratio (p. 54).

LABORATORY TESTS IN CHRONIC STABLE ANGINA

ELECTROCARDIOGRAM

The resting electrocardiogram is normal in one-fourth to one-half of patients with chronic stable angina pectoris, depending on the incidence of previous myocardial infarction in the particular series of patients.[98] Patients with normal tracings may have severe angina, but they usually have not previously suffered extensive infarctions. When the electrocardiogram is abnormal, the most common findings are nonspecific ST-T changes with or without evidence of prior transmural infarction; however, a variety of conduction disturbances, most frequently left bundle branch block and left anterior divisional block, have also been reported.

When left bundle branch block is found with coronary artery disease, it is often associated with marked impairment in left ventricular function,[99] presumably reflecting extensive coronary artery disease. The finding of incomplete right bundle branch block does not appear to be associated with an increased risk of death from coronary heart disease or cardiovascular disease.[100] A variety of arrhythmias, especially ventricular premature beats, may be present, but they are not specific for identifying coronary artery disease. Abnormal Q waves are relatively specific but insensitive indicators of myocardial necrosis. Correlation between the electrocardiographic pattern of myocardial infarction and total obstruction of the coronary artery perfusing that segment of the ventricle is excellent.[101]

Interval electrocardiograms may reveal the development of Q-wave infarction that are unrecognized clinically either by patients or their physicians. Such electrocardiographic abnormalities have as serious a prognosis as recognized infarction.[102] The increasing use of ambulatory electrocardiographic monitoring has shown that many patients with symptomatic myocardial ischemia also have episodes of silent ischemia which would otherwise go unrecognized during normal daily activities (p. 1363).

Exercise Electrocardiography (See Chap. 8)

For appropriate application of noninvasive tests, it is important to consider Bayes' theorem (pp. 235 and 1683), which states that while the reliability of any test is defined by its sensitivity and specificity,* its predictability depends on the prevalence of the disease in the population under study (Table 52–2, p. 1683).

Exercise electrocardiography is of limited value in predicting the *presence or absence* of coronary artery disease after other easily obtainable clinical data have been taken into account, e.g., the presence or absence of typical anginal symptoms, the presence or absence of Q waves, a clinical history of acute myocardial infarction, a history of cigarette smoking, elevated cholesterol, and the age of the patient.[103] However, the recording of an electrocardiogram during and after exercise—especially if angina is precipitated—is valuable in assessing the severity and prognosis of patients suspected of having ischemic heart disease.[104, 105, 105a] Indeed, simple clinical parameters are valuable in assessing the results of exercise testing.

*For definitions of these terms, see p. 235.

ASSESSMENT OF SEVERITY AND PROGNOSIS. The occurrence of *chest pain*, in addition to ST-segment depression, at a light level of activity during an exercise test (< 4 METS) signifies that the likelihood of subsequent coronary events (myocardial infarction, progression of angina or coronary death) is substantially greater than in patients who exhibit ST-segment depression alone or the combination of pain and ST depression at a heavier workload (8 to 9 METS).[106] Failure to achieve a normal *heart rate* response to exercise (chronotropic incompetence) is also frequently observed in patients with extensive coronary artery disease.[107, 108] A low maximal heart rate along with ST-segment depression increases the sensitivity of exercise electrocardiography, but the specificity declines progressively as maximal heart rate increases.[107]

Exercise-induced *hypotension* is an independent predictor of the outcome in patients with chest pain.[109, 110] It has been reported to occur in 10 to 20 per cent of patients with either three-vessel or left main coronary artery disease[111–113] or in patients with abnormal left ventricular function.[114] These findings apply to patients whose blood pressure increases by 20 mm Hg or less or decreases during exercise.

In patients with symptom-limited exercise tests who have 2 mm or more of ST-segment depression, i.e., a strongly positive exercise test, *the duration of exercise* alone (which reflects the functional state of the left ventricle) is an important indicator of subsequent prognosis.[104] The degree of ST-segment depression, the time of onset, and the configuration and the persistence of abnormalities combine to increase the sensitivity and specificity of the test.[115] Early onset of ST-segment depression, its long persistence following exercise, and most importantly its shape (Fig. 39–3) are all strongly associated with the extent of coronary artery disease.

The appearance of *conduction abnormalities*[116, 117] or *ectopic activity* may be exposed by exercise testing. The development of a transient intraventricular conduction abnormality is uncommon in patients with exercise-induced angina but may suggest significant coronary artery disease,[116] particularly when it occurs at a low heart rate.[117] While the exercise test is useful for exposing ventricular ectopic activity, and while patients with more severe forms

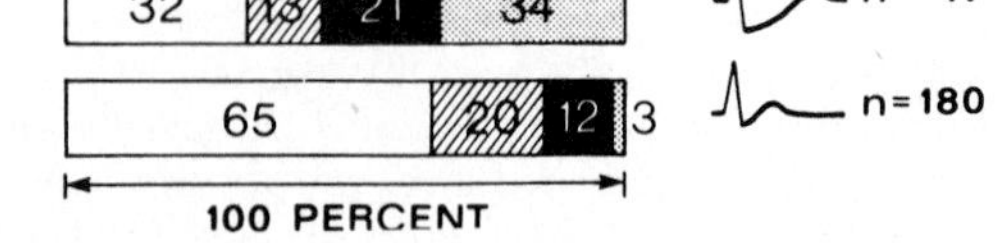

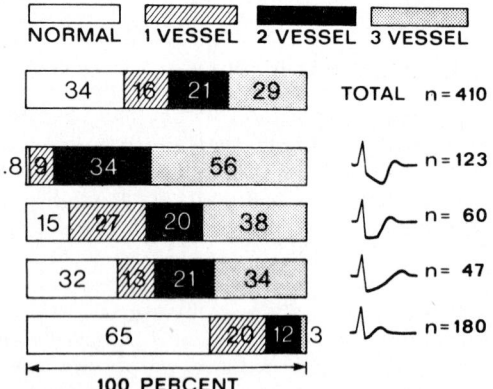

FIGURE 39–3. Relation between the type of ST-segment response in an exercise test and the extent of coronary artery disease. All numbers represent percentages. The total study population is represented at the top. Downsloping ST segments are highly specific for coronary disease, with only one false-positive response (0.8 per cent) encountered; most patients with this response (90 per cent) have double- and triple-vessel involvement. Neither the horizontal nor the slowly upsloping ST segments aid in identifying severe disease. A small percentage (15 per cent) of patients with entirely normal treadmill tests have double- and triple-vessel disease. (From Goldschlager, N., et al.: Treadmill stress tests as indicators of presence and severity of coronary artery disease. Ann. Intern. Med. *85*:277, 1976.)

of coronary artery disease and abnormal left ventricular function have been shown to have a greater prevalence of exercise-induced arrhythmias,[118, 119] this approach is less sensitive than 24-hour ambulatory electrocardiographic monitoring.

INFLUENCE OF ANTIANGINAL THERAPY. It is important to recognize that antianginal pharmacological therapy reduces the sensitivity of exercise testing as a screening tool for left main coronary disease or three-vessel disease[120] and that beta blockade will increase the exercise duration and either suppress or delay the appearance of ST-segment depression and thus obscure the diagnostic interpretation of exercise testing.[121] Even in patients receiving antianginal medications a positive exercise test will have the usual implications for management. A negative exercise test in patients on antianginal drugs does not exclude significant and possibly threatening myocardial ischemia. Therefore, if the purpose of the exercise test is to diagnose ischemia, it should be performed in the absence of antianginal medications. The advisability of withdrawing medications in an individual patient before exercise testing is a matter of judgment. Unless the patient has severe angina, sublingual nitroglycerin for 1 or 2 days will be sufficient to control symptoms if other therapy is withdrawn. For long-acting nitrates, calcium antagonists, and short-acting beta blockers, stopping the medications the day before testing usually will suffice. Two or three days are required for patients on long-acting beta blockers. If the purpose of the exercise test is to identify safe levels of daily activity, the test should be done while the patient is on medications.

INCONCLUSIVE TESTS. In patients with vascular, orthopedic, or neurological conditions who cannot perform leg exercise, arm exercise is a reasonable but not equivalent alternative.[122] A negative test using arm exercise may be inconclusive.

In view of the relatively low sensitivity (70 to 85 per cent) of exercise stress electrocardiography (p. 1683), a negative result does not rule out ischemic heart disease; however, it makes three-vessel or left main disease much less likely. Conversely, an adequate maximum exercise test—one achieving more than 85 per cent of predicted maximal heart rate—is unlikely to miss three-vessel or left main coronary artery disease. A major limitation of the sensitivity of the exercise electrocardiogram is that it cannot be interpreted in many patients. This includes patients who are incapable of reaching the level of exercise required for near-maximal effort (85 per cent or more of maximal predicted heart rate), particularly those on beta-adrenoceptor blockers or those who develop fatigue, leg cramps, or dyspnea, and patients with abnormalities in the baseline electrocardiogram, including those on digitalis. In such patients radionuclide imaging may be very helpful.

RADIONUCLIDE IMAGING

STRESS THALLIUM-201 MYOCARDIAL PERFUSION IMAGING. In this technique, the details of which are described on pp. 329 to 334, the radionuclide is injected at peak exercise and the image is obtained several minutes later when the patient is at rest[122a]; it demonstrates the regional perfusion pattern that existed during the stress of exercise. Defects represent either areas of stress-induced impairment of blood flow or infarction. If a delayed image is obtained 2 to 3 hours later and the initial defect persists, it is probably due to an infarction. On the other hand, if it exhibits delayed uptake (i.e., redistribution), it represents an area of ischemic, transiently hypoperfused but viable myocardium.

In a summary of 22 published studies involving more

than 2000 patients, the stress thallium-201 scintigram was usually superior to the exercise electrocardiogram, with a sensitivity of 83 per cent (compared with 73 per cent for the electrocardiogram) and a specificity of 90 per cent (compared with 82 per cent).[123]

Stress thallium-201 scintigraphy is useful in a number of clinical situations in the assessment of patients with known or suspected chronic stable angina:

1. Patients with chest pain and normal findings during exercise scintigraphy have an excellent prognosis,[124, 124a] even if angiography has demonstrated underlying coronary artery disease.[125]
2. In patients with single-vessel coronary artery disease (a situation in which the sensitivity of the electrocardiographic exercise test is particularly low), exercise thallium-201 perfusion imaging is often much more sensitive.[126]
3. In patients who cannot perform routine exercise tests, dipyridamole-induced maximal coronary vasodilation (p. 331), when used in conjunction with thallium myocardial imaging, has been shown to have a sensitivity and specificity for the detection of coronary artery disease comparable to that of exercise thallium imaging. Imaging 45 minutes after administration of oral dipyridamole is effective in unmasking regions of underperfused but viable myocardium.[127]
4. If multiple thallium-201 redistribution defects are observed with exercise (or following dipyridamole administration), especially if associated with abnormal lung uptake (reflecting a sudden rise in left ventricular diastolic pressure), multivessel coronary artery disease causing significant ischemia is usually present.[128] The finding of a larger left ventricle on the immediate post-stress image than on the delayed image, i.e., transient ischemic dilatation of the ventricle, is a highly specific marker of multivessel critical stenosis.[129]

Limitations of thallium scintigraphy include relatively high cost, difficulties with interpretation, and difficulties with imaging markedly obese patients.

EXERCISE RADIONUCLIDE ANGIOGRAPHY. In this test, described in detail on pp. 323 to 324, measurements of ejection fraction and of regional wall motion are obtained both at rest and at increasing workloads.[128a] In a summary of 12 published studies comprising 771 patients, Gibson and Beller reported that the radionuclide angiogram had both sensitivity and specificity of approximately 90 per cent when both failure of a rise in ejection fraction and presence of a new regional wall motion abnormality were required for the test to be deemed positive.[123] It is important to include exercise-induced regional wall motion abnormalities in order to define a positive exercise radionuclide angiogram, since the ejection fraction may fail to rise in patients with conditions other than ischemic heart disease, including cardiomyopathies, valvular heart disease, or hypertension, and in normal individuals receiving a beta-adrenoceptor blocker. Furthermore, radionuclide imaging at the peak of exercise is necessary to achieve maximal sensitivity for the detection of coronary artery disease.[130]

The greater sensitivity of the two radionuclide techniques, i.e., radionuclide angiography and stress thallium perfusion scintigraphy, compared to exercise electrocardiography, is probably related to the fact that abnormalities of perfusion and left ventricular contraction occur at a lower ischemic threshold than does exercise-induced ST-segment depression. Both radionuclide techniques are superior to exercise electrocardiography primarily because they allow evaluation of patients with electrocardiographic abnormalities at rest and of those who are unable to achieve adequate levels of exercise.

The sensitivity and specificity of both radionuclide techniques have been found to be similar in seven studies, comprising a total of 391 patients.[123] There is no consensus as to which of the two tests should be carried out first. We prefer to obtain the stress thallium-201 scintigram initially, since exercise radionuclide angiography can usually be performed on the same day after myocardial perfusion scintigraphy if the need arises, whereas the converse is not possible.

Clinical Application of Noninvasive Tests (See also p. 232)

In asymptomatic persons or in those with nonanginal chest pain who are being screened or evaluated for coronary artery disease, i.e., patients in whom the pretest likelihood of coronary disease is low (less than 15 per cent), a negative exercise electrocardiogram generally provides sufficient information to confirm the absence of ischemic heart disease; a positive test result should be followed by a thallium perfusion scan. When both of these tests are abnormal, the likelihood of significant coronary artery disease exceeds 80 per cent; however, if there is a discrepancy in the results of the two tests, either coronary arteriography or radionuclide angiography (and arteriography if the result is positive) is in order.

In patients with *atypical angina*, if two noninvasive tests are abnormal, the likelihood of coronary artery disease exceeds 95 per cent; if both tests are normal, this likelihood falls below 5 per cent. Results of noninvasive stress tests are independent of each other, and whenever they are discordant, a third noninvasive test will often be helpful. Also, when test results are discordant, they should be evaluated in the light of the level of exercise achieved as well as the degree of positivity (e.g., the presence of accompanying symptoms, the depth of the ST-segment response, the heart rate at which it occurred, and the persistence of the ST-segment response on the stress electrocardiogram; the size and number of perfusion defects on the stress perfusion scintigram; and the magnitude of the exercise-induced change in ejection fraction and regional wall motion disorder on the exercise radionuclide angiogram). Thus, a patient with a normal exercise electrocardiogram who develops multiple large perfusion defects on a thallium-201 scintigram (accompanied by chest pain at a heart rate of 160 beats/min) has a much greater likelihood of having ischemic heart disease than one who has a normal exercise electrocardiogram and develops a single small perfusion defect without chest pain at a heart rate of 195 beats/mm.

In patients with *typical angina* (i.e., those with a high pretest likelihood of disease) noninvasive testing is most valuable for estimating the extent and severity of coronary artery disease, and thereby the prognosis. The development of exertional hypotension, marked or prolonged ST-segment depression at low work levels and/or heart rate, striking decreases in ejection fraction and wall motion, and large or multiple defects on the exercise thallium scintigram all point to severe multivessel disease in patients at high risk of subsequent coronary events, including sudden death.[131]

OTHER LABORATORY TESTS IN PATIENTS WITH KNOWN CORONARY DISEASE

ECHOCARDIOGRAPHY (See also p. 119). The areas of the ventricle that can be imaged by M-mode echocardiography are limited; the apex and inferior and lateral walls of the left ventricle are usually missed. Larger sections of the ventricle can be visualized by two-dimensional echocardiography. Serial tracings often reveal disorders of wall motion as ischemia waxes or wanes.

Echocardiography performed immediately after exercise (p. 120) is useful in the detection of wall motion abnormalities and may enhance the diagnostic yield of a treadmill exercise test[132] (Fig. 5–89, p. 121). The sensitivity of postexercise two-dimensional echocardiography for detecting coronary artery disease (based on an abnormal ejection fraction response and/or regional wall motion abnormalities evaluated by slow motion, bidirectional, and stop-frame video playback) is 91 per cent and the specificity 88 per cent with sensitivities for one-, two-, and three-vessel disease being 64, 95, and 100 per cent, respectively.[133] Recently, a transducer has been developed so that wall motion abnormalities may be detected during exercise with a sensitivity of 100 per cent and specificity of 93 per cent.[134] Despite new transducer design, two-dimensional echocardiography during or immediately after bicycle or treadmill exercise has not been used widely because of technical difficulties. An alternative approach may be to use isometric handgrip or to pace patients with a transesophageal atrial technique during two-dimensional echocardiography, which yields results similar to studies using isotonic exercise.[135] Two-dimensional echocardiography has also been used for defining obstructive lesions of the left main coronary artery.[136]

BIOCHEMICAL TESTS. Serum levels of cardiac enzymes (p. 1239) are normal in angina pectoris and serve to differentiate these patients from those with acute myocardial infarction. One of the striking features of chronic ischemic heart disease in *relatively young persons* is the frequency with which certain metabolic abnormalities are detected. Since *hypercholesterolemia* and *carbohydrate intolerance* are recognized as risk factors for the development of ischemic heart disease, this finding is not unexpected, and the prevalence of these abnormalities, particularly in patients under the age of 50 years, is impressive (Chap. 36). Over 90 per cent of patients under the age of 50 with angiographically proven ischemic heart disease can have either carbohydrate intolerance of Type II or IV hyperlipoproteinemia.[137, 138]

Chest Roentgenogram. This is usually within normal limits in patients with chronic ischemic heart disease. However, coronary artery calcification detected fluoroscopically may be more diagnostic of coronary artery disease than was once thought, especially in young people. More than 90 per cent of patients with coronary artery calcification were found to have critical coronary artery obstruction; however, coronary calcification on fluoroscopy is not a very sensitive test, since it is found in only 40 per cent of patients with angiographically documented coronary artery disease.[139] When fluoroscopic evidence of coronary calcification is present in combination with a positive exercise test, the probability of finding coronary artery disease on subsequent coronary angiography is very high.[140]

CATHETERIZATION, ANGIOGRAPHY, AND CORONARY ARTERIOGRAPHY

Although the clinical examination and noninvasive techniques described above are valuable, the definitive diagnosis of coronary artery disease and a precise assessment of its anatomical severity and its effects on cardiac performance and myocardial metabolism require cardiac catheterization (Chap. 9), coronary arteriography (Chap. 10), and left ventricular angiography (Chap. 6). Among patients with chronic stable angina pectoris, coronary arteriography usually reveals relatively equal distribution (approximately 25 per cent each) of critical (> 70 per cent luminal diameter) narrowing of one, two, and three of the major coronary arteries. About 5 to 10 per cent of patients have obstruction of the left main coronary artery, and in approximately 15 per cent no critical obstruction is detectable (Chap. 10). Total occlusion of at least one major coronary artery is more common in patients with chronic angina who have had prior infarctions than in those without infarction. The risk of complications of cardiac catheterization is increased in patients with left main coronary artery disease and is highest in patients with unstable angina and very proximal stenoses.[51]

Coronary artery ectasia, i.e., aneurysmal dilatation, is present in approximately 2 per cent of patients with ischemic heart disease. This angiographic lesion does not appear to affect symptoms, survival, or the incidence of myocardial infarction; it is considered to be a variant of coronary atherosclerosis rather than a distinct clinical entity.[141] *Coronary collaterals* are observed only when there is 50 to 75 per cent stenosis* of a coronary artery, but in up to 20 per cent of patients with this degree of stenosis, no collaterals are visible. The functional significance of collateral vessels is unclear. When they are well developed, coronary collaterals may be adequate to protect against resting ischemia even in the presence of total occlusion, but they fail to meet the increased needs of exercise and therefore may not reduce the frequency or severity of angina. Also, patients with abundant collaterals appear to suffer smaller myocardial infarctions.[142, 143] On the basis of canine experiments, it is not clear whether or not exercise alters the development of collaterals.[144, 145]

Diastolic ventricular performance, as reflected in the early diastolic ventricular filling rate, is impaired at rest as a consequence of scarring (and/or ischemia) in many patients with chronic stable angina, even when systolic performance, as reflected in the ejection fraction, is normal. Diastolic filling becomes even more abnormal (slowed) during exercise, when ischemia intensifies.

The frequency of abnormal elevations of left ventricular end-diastolic pressure and of reduced cardiac output increases with the number of vessels exhibiting critical narrowing and with the number of prior infarctions,[146] but there is a great deal of overlap among individual patients so that the severity of coronary arterial disease cannot be predicted from these two measurements. The left ventricular end-diastolic pressure may be elevated because of reduced ventricular compliance, left ventricular systolic failure, or a combination of these two processes[147]; both impaired diastolic and systolic failure may occur as a consequence of acute ischemia and chronic scar formation. The elevation of left ventricular diastolic pressure has its clinical correlate in the presence of diastolic (third and fourth) heart sounds. In many patients with normal hemodynamics in the basal state, abnormalities of left ventricular function can be elicited by dynamic or static exercise. Elevations of left ventricular end-diastolic pressure usually occur *before* the patient complains of chest discomfort and before there is electrocardiographic ST-segment depression.

Pacing-induced and post-pacing angina and/or ST-segment depression can also be observed in the catheterization laboratory. This form of stress testing is especially useful for combined hemodynamic-metabolic-ventriculographic studies[148] because quantitative left ventricular angiography

*Unless otherwise noted, "per cent stenosis" refers to reduction of luminal diameter.

and myocardial lactate metabolism can be studied during or immediately after pacing, uncomplicated by an elevation of systemic arterial lactate levels, as occurs in dynamic exercise. When atrial pacing to induce ischemia is carried out in patients with chronic angina secondary to chronic obstructive coronary artery disease, elevations in ventricular end-diastolic presure occur frequently and usually in association with the development of angina and at a reproducible heart rate–blood pressure product.[148] Impaired ventricular relaxation and increased regional myocardial stiffness have also been demonstrated during pacing-induced ischemia[149] and represent one component of the altered diastolic properties of the ischemic ventricle (p. 1204).

LEFT VENTRICULAR FUNCTION. Ischemia-induced left ventricular dysfunction can be detected with greatest accuracy by means of biplane contrast ventriculography. *Global* abnormalities of left ventricular function are expressed in elevations of left ventricular end-diastolic and end-systolic volumes and depression of the ejection fraction (p. 454). However, abnormalities of *regional* wall motion (hypokinesia, akinesia, or dyskinesia, Fig. 10–56, p. 306, and Figs. 15-6 and 7, p. 456) are more sensitive, specific, and characteristic of coronary artery disease, since the latter is usually regional in distribution. Also, hyperkinetic contraction of normal myocardium may compensate for hypokinetic or akinetic ischemic or necrotic myocardium, thereby maintaining normal or almost-normal global left ventricular function, despite marked depression of function in one region of the ventricle.

Left ventricular function (global or regional) may be normal at rest in patients with chronic coronary artery disease without previous myocardial infarction but becomes abnormal during or after stress (exercise, pacing). However, the converse is not necessarily the case. While in most instances resting abnormalities signify irreversible damage, i.e., prior infarction, chronic ischemia sufficient to maintain the viability of the myocardium can result in persistent ventricular dysfunction, a condition termed "hibernating myocardium."[150, 151] This form of reversible left ventricular dysfunction may or may not be accompanied by angina pectoris or electrocardiographic changes of ischemia. The reversibility of this form of left ventricular function is reflected in long-term improvement after revascularization (by surgery or percutaneous transluminal coronary angioplasty) or transiently after an inotropic stimulus (postextrasystolic) potentiation[152] or the infusion of a sympathomimetic amine.[153]

Histopathological studies performed on myocardial biopsy specimens obtained at the time of coronary artery bypass operations have demonstrated that those segments which exhibit reversible asynergy at angiography are made up predominantly of histologically normal myocardium, while the nonresponsive segments exhibit marked muscle loss and replacement by fibrous tissue.[154] The more responsive areas are usually better perfused, either by the native coronary artery or by collateral vessels, and are associated with a lower frequency of Q waves on the electrocardiogram.[155] The most severe aspect of left ventricular asynergy is the well-demarcated aneurysm, which not only exhibits contractile failure but also is unable to resist expansion during ventricular systole; in other words, it exhibits dyskinesis (paradoxical pulsation).

In addition to demonstrating areas of asynergy, left ventriculography may also show mitral valve prolapse (Fig. 33–22, p. 1051), which occurs in 20 to 25 per cent of patients with obstructive coronary artery disease[156] and probably results from impaired contractility of the ventricular myocardium and papillary muscles.

Abnormal myocardial metabolism has also been documented by means of cardiac catheterization in patients with chronic stable angina. With a catheter in place in the coronary sinus, coronary arteriovenous lactate measurements are obtained at rest and after suitable stresses, such as the infusion of isoproterenol[157] or pacing.[158] Since lactate is a byproduct of anaerobic glycolysis, its production by the heart and subsequent appearance in coronary sinus blood is a sign of myocardial ischemia. When combined with coronary arteriography, this technique may be helpful in localizing significant coronary obstructive lesions and myocardial ischemia.[157]

MYOCARDIAL PERFUSION STUDIES. Several techniques based on wash-out of radioactive inert gases from the myocardium following injection into the coronary arteries can be used to measure regional myocardial blood flow, as described on page 339. Using these techniques, reductions in the perfusion of areas of myocardium subserved by totally obstructed coronary arteries compared with areas that are normally perfused have been demonstrated. Less striking differences were observed with lesions compromising the lumen by 50 to 90 per cent.[159] Coronary blood flow measured by the regional xenon-133 technique has also been shown to be diminished in areas of abnormal ventricular wall motion, both at sites of previous infarction[160] and in noninfarcted regions.[161]

MANAGEMENT

The management of ischemic heart disease involves four aspects: (1) correction of specific coronary risk factors, discussed in Chap. 36; (2) general and nonpharmacological methods, with particular attention toward adjustment of the patient's life style; (3) various specific medications used to treat angina; and (4) revascularization by percutaneous transluminal angioplasty and coronary bypass surgery.

GENERAL MEASURES

General measures include the treatment of hypertension (Chap. 28), which not only is a risk factor for the development and progression of atherosclerosis but also causes cardiac hypertrophy, augments myocardial oxygen requirements and thereby intensifies myocardial ischemia in patients with obstructive coronary disease. Attainment of an ideal weight is particularly important in the obese patient, in whom weight reduction raises the threshold for the development of angina pectoris.

It is imperative for patients with chronic coronary artery disease who are *cigarette smokers* to discontinue this practice. Among patients with angiographically documented coronary artery disease, cigarette smokers have a higher 5-year mortality and relative risk of infarction or sudden death than those who have quit smoking.[162] Habitual smokers who survive out-of-hospital cardiac arrest have a lower incidence of recurrent arrest at 3 years if they stop smoking then do patients who continue to smoke.[163] There appears to be a strong association between the risk of myocardial infarction and smoking,[164, 165] and this risk appears related more to the number of cigarettes smoked per day rather than the duration of smoking. This risk of infarction returns to a level similar to that in men who have never smoked within a few years of stopping smoking.[166] These observations suggest that cigarette smoking may be responsible for hemodynamic events other than progression of atherosclerosis. Indeed, while cigarette smoking may increase myocardial oxygen demand and 24-hour energy expenditure (by approximately 10 per cent),[167] it can also induce decreases in coronary blood flow[168] due to an alpha-adrenergically mediated increase in coronary artery tone.[169, 169a] In addition, cigarette smoking appears to interfere with the efficacy of antianginal drugs. Improvement in exercise tolerance and a reduction in angina pectoris were noted when cigarette smokers stopped smoking while on therapy with beta blockers and nifedipine.[170] Both active and passive cigarette smoking,[171] the inhalation of smog, and ascent to high altitude all lower the threshold for angina, and their avoidance represents an important aspect of therapy.

In addition, fever, anemia, thyrotoxicosis, infection, tachycardia, hypoxemia as occurs in acute and chronic pulmonary disease, and certain drugs used to treat noncardiac diseases (such as amphetamines and isoproterenol mists) all increase myocardial oxygen needs and may precipitate or intensify angina; cocaine can cause coronary spasm. These conditions and drugs should be eliminated. Congestive heart failure (by causing cardiac dilatation) and cardiac tachyarrhythmias can increase myocardial oxygen needs. Their treatment, as outlined in Chapters 17 and 22, will frequently diminish the frequency and severity of angina.

COUNSELING AND CHANGES IN LIFE STYLE. Effective communication with both the patient and the family is essential. The psychosocial issues faced by the patient who develops chronic stable angina are similar to, although usually less intense than, those experienced by the patient with an acute myocardial infarction, discussed on page 1887. Many patients have an unrealistically gloomy perception of their prognosis; they should be offered a realistic appraisal, together with an understandable explanation of the pertinent clinical features of the disease.

An important aspect of the physician's role is to counsel patients in the kind of work they can do, in their leisure activities, eating habits, vacation plans, and the like. It is desirable, if possible, to consult with the closest member(s) of the family, both to insure an accurate and full assessment of the patient's activities and to inform the family of what can be expected in the course of the patient's disease.

Certain changes in life style may be helpful, such as modifying strenuous activities if they constantly and repeatedly produce angina. These changes may be minor in many instances. For example, golfing could be modified to include use of a golfcart instead of walking. Many activities, such as shopping or climbing stairs, need not be discontinued. Often, it is merely necessary to perform them more slowly or to pause for brief periods of rest. The patient with chronic stable angina should avoid excessive fatigue and exhaustion; one or two regular rest periods during each day are often helpful. While it is desirable to minimize the number of bouts of angina, an occasional episode is not to be feared. The vast majority of patients with chronic stable angina should not be treated like invalids. Often, the propensity for angina actually declines, perhaps as a result of the development of collaterals or because of training effects, discussed later; indeed, unless patients occasionally reach their anginal threshold, they may not appreciate the extent of their exercise capacity.

Eliminating or reducing the factors that precipitate anginal episodes is of obvious importance. Patients learn their usual threshold by trial and error. Since many anginal episodes are precipitated by increases in the mechanical activity of the heart (due to increases in myocardial oxygen consumption), the patient should avoid *sudden* bursts of activity, particularly after long periods of rest. There is a circadian rhythm characterized by a lower anginal threshold shortly after arising.[172] Therefore, morning activities such as showering, shaving, and dressing should be done at a slower pace, and if necessary with use of prophylactic nitroglycerin. The stress of sexual intercourse is ordinarily approximately equal to that of climbing one flight of stairs at a normal pace or of any activity that induces a heart rate of approximately 120 beats/min. With proper precautions, i.e., commencing more than 2 hours postprandially and taking an additional dose of a short-acting beta blocker one hour before and nitroglycerin 15 minutes before, the majority of patients with chronic stable angina are able to continue a satisfactory sexual life.

Just as there is a role for exercise in the management of coronary artery disease, so is there a role for rest, especially in situations in which angina has become frequent or severe. Marked restriction of activity or even complete bed rest, in addition to drug therapy, may be necessary to control symptoms. In less critical situations, merely reducing the amount of time spent working or increasing the rest periods will have a beneficial effect. For example, a long lunch break including a short nap may be beneficial. It may be helpful for the patient to use a face mask or scarf to cover the mouth or nose in cold weather. A hot, humid environment may also precipitate angina, and air conditioning may be a necessity rather than a luxury for patients with ischemic heart disease. Large meals can have a similar effect if they are followed by exertion. An effort should be made to minimize emotional outbursts, since they too increase myocardial oxygen requirements and sometimes induce coronary vasoconstriction. Occasionally antianxiety drugs or sedation may be useful.

PREVENTION OF MYOCARDIAL (RE)INFARCTION. A variety of measures are used widely in the secondary prevention of acute myocardial infarction (p. 1288). These include discontinuation of smoking, treatment of abnormally elevated low-density lipoproteins and hypertension, modification of Type A personality, and administration of antiplatelet agents, anticoagulants, and beta blockers. Several of these (discontinuing smoking and using beta blockers) have been shown to improve survival and to reduce the incidence of reinfarction. The data in support of the other measures are more controversial, and in many trials, their effectiveness is limited to the early postinfarction period.

Many patients with chronic stable angina have never experienced an infarction, and others have not reached the time frame in which the interventions have been found to be helpful. One must be cautious about applying to patients with chronic stable angina, without a recent myocardial infarction, the result of studies carried out in patients with recent infarction. While we await additional information, it seems sensible for patients with chronic stable angina to cease smoking, to assume an ideal body weight, and to control blood pressure. The administration of low-dose aspirin (80 mg/day or 325 mg every other day) is probably not hazardous and may be beneficial in reducing the incidence of myocardial infarction, although this is not proved. Whether beta blockers in this population have any value is not clear. Since the beneficial effects observed in the post-myocardial infarction population (p. 1288) also possibly occur in the chronic stable angina group, it seems sensible to administer these drugs when angina and/or hypertension are present in these patients and when these drugs are well tolerated. Perhaps the antiarrhythmic and antiischemic effects exhibited in patients with recent myocardial infarction treated with beta blockers are also beneficial in patients with chronic stable angina. There is no evidence that chronic anticoagulants are indicated except in patients with other indications. While sensible efforts should be made to lower elevated cholesterol, *intense* dietary and pharmacological measures need not be undertaken in the elderly (> 65 years) or in those in whom serum cholesterol is not elevated unless the LDL/HDL ratio is especially unfavorable.

EXERCISE (See also Chap. 41). The *conditioning effect of exercise* on skeletal muscle allows the patient to expend a greater workload at any level of total body oxygen consumption, and the conditioning effect of exercise on the heart, by decreasing the heart rate at any level of exercise, allows a higher cardiac output to be achieved at any level of myocardial oxygen consumption. The combination of these two effects of exercise permits the patient with chronic stable angina to increase physical performance substantially following institution of a continuing exercise program. The reduced pressure-rate product reduces myocardial requirements during exertion and enables the patient with coronary artery disease to perform at higher workloads before reaching the ischemic threshold.[173] Therefore, physical conditioning reduces the amount of oxygen needed by the heart for any given amount of total body work. An example of this effect is seen in the study of Redwood et al., who noted that a 6-week training program improved exercise performance by reducing the responses of heart rate and arterial pressure to bicycle exercise and by prolonging the duration of exercise before angina occurred.[174] There is also some evidence that in patients with chronic ischemic heart disease after training, a greater ejection fraction was achieved at equivalent workloads.[175] The psychological benefits of exercise are difficult to evaluate. However, exercise may be very helpful in increasing the confidence of patients recovering from myocardial infarction, although the question of whether or not exercise accelerates the development of collateral vessels is unsettled in patients with chronic coronary artery disease.[144, 145]

For all of the aforementioned reasons, patients are urged to participate in regular exercise programs—usually walking (see below)—in conjunction with their drug therapy. Patients who are involved in exercise programs usually are also more likely to be health-conscious, to pay attention to diet and weight, and to discontinue cigarette smoking. Thus, in addition to a conditioning effect on skeletal and cardiac muscle, regular dynamic exercise provides the individual with a feeling of well-being, an important consideration in the management of any chronic disease. The rationale and specific details for establishing an exercise program in patients with coronary artery disease are outlined in Chapter 41. Despite the many favorable effects of regular physical exercise in patients with coronary artery disease and chronic stable angina enumerated above, it must be acknowledged that there is no hard evidence that such programs affect survival or the need for surgery in these patients.

NITRATES (See also p. 520)

MECHANISM OF ACTION. Although the clinical effectiveness of amyl nitrite was first described in 1867 by Brunton,[8] organic nitrates are still the most common medications physicians employ to treat patients with angina pectoris. The action of these agents is to relax vascular smooth muscle. The vasodilator effects of nitrates are evident in both systemic (including coronary) arteries and veins in normal subjects and in patients with ischemic heart disease, but they appear to be predominant in the venous circulation.[176] The decrease in venous tone reduces the return of blood to the heart and reduces preload and ventricular dimensions,[177] which in turn reduces wall tension and afterload. The actions of nitrates to reduce preload and afterload also make them useful in the treatment of heart failure as well as angina pectoris.

Posture is important in evaluating the hemodynamic effects of nitrates. In the supine position, venous return is normally greater while exercise tolerance and the anginal threshold are lower than in the upright position. The hemodynamic and angina-relieving effects of nitrates are most marked when patients are sitting or standing, i.e., when these drugs can reduce preload, and these effects resemble those of phlebotomy. By reducing the heart's mechanical activity, volume, and oxygen consumption, nitrates increase exercise capacity in patients with ischemic heart disease, i.e., a greater total body workload can be achieved before the anginal threshold is reached.

A vasodilating effect of the nitrates on the larger (conductance) coronary arteries can also be readily demonstrated, and there is evidence, obtained from quantitative, computer-assisted measurements of coronary arterial diameter, that nitroglycerin causes vasodilatation of epicardial stenoses. Presumably, these are eccentric lesions, and nitroglycerin causes relaxation of smooth muscle in the wall of the coronary artery not encompassed by the plaque. Even a small increase in the narrowed arterial lumen can produce a significant reduction in resistance to blood flow across the narrowed lesion (Fig. 39–4).[178]

Studies in experimental animals with coronary obstruction have shown that nitroglycerin causes redistribution of blood flow to ischemic areas, particularly in the subendocardium,[179] perhaps mediated in part by an increase in collateral blood flow[180] and in part by a lowering of ventricular diastolic pressure, reducing subendocardial compression. Results of studies of nitroglycerin on coronary

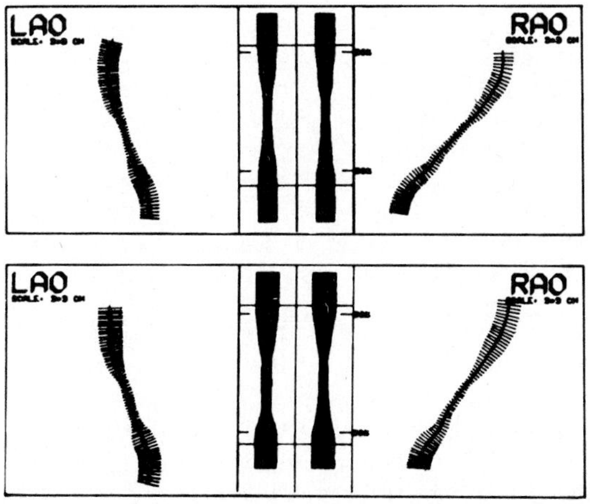

	NORMAL AREA [mm²]	MINIMUM DIAMETER [mm]	MINIMUM AREA [mm²]	FLOW RESISTANCE [mm Hg/cm³/sec]
CONTROL				
ABSOLUTE	5.2	1.03	0.87	10.3
% STENOSIS		60%	83%	
NITROGLYCERIN				
ABSOLUTE	7.6	1.18	1.12	6.5
% STENOSIS		59%	83%	
CHANGE with NITROGLYCERIN	2.4 (46%)	0.15 (15%)	0.25 (29%)	-3.8 (37%)

FIGURE 39–4. Representative computer printout of segmental stenosis images and dimensional data for pre- and post-nitroglycerin (0.4 mg, sublingual) angiograms of this 60 per cent mid-right coronary artery stenosis. Each value is averaged from eight estimates. LAO = left anterior oblique, RAO = right anterior oblique. (From Brown, B. G., et al.: The mechanisms of nitroglycerin action: Stenosis vasodilation as a major component of the drug response. Circulation *64*:1089, 1981, by permission of the American Heart Association, Inc.)

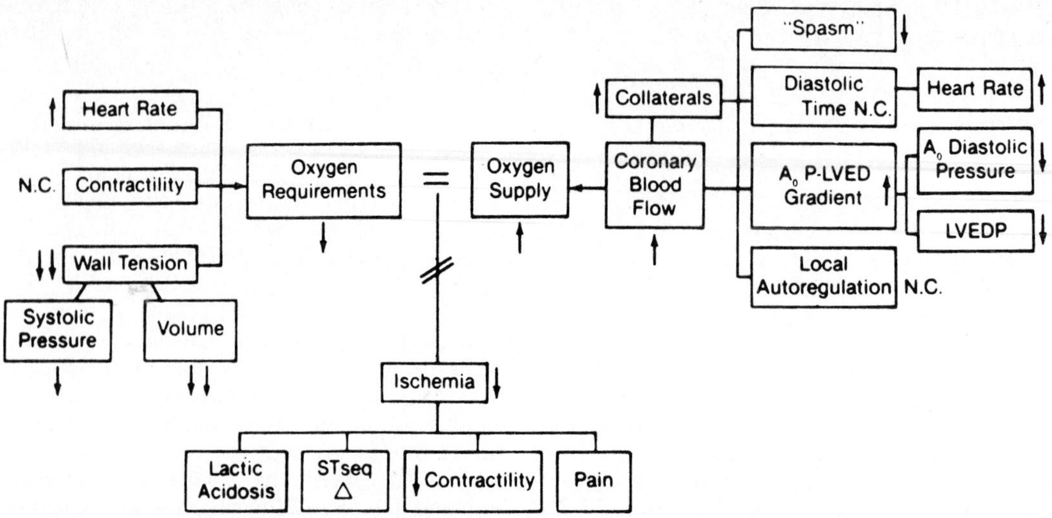

FIGURE 39–5. Factors influencing balance between myocardial oxygen requirements (*left*) and supply (*right*). Arrows indicate effects of nitrates. In relieving angina pectoris, nitrates exert favorable effects on the balance between oxygen requirements and supply. Although a reflex increase in heart rate would tend to reduce the time for coronary flow, dilation of collaterals and enhancement of the pressure gradient for flow to occur as the LVEDP falls tends to increase coronary flow. AoP = aortic pressure, LVEDP = left ventricular end-diastolic pressure, NC = no change. (From Frishman, W. H.: Pharmacology of the nitrates in angina pectoris. Am. J. Cardiol. *56*:81, 1985.)

blood flow have been conflicting. Some studies in patients have reported increased blood flow after sublingual or intravenous nitroglycerin,[181] but most report no change or reduced flow.[182–184] However, as myocardial oxygen demands fell, the net effect on oxygen balance became favorable. In studies employing intracoronary injection of xenon-133[185] (as well as in retrograde perfusion studies performed during coronary bypass surgery[186]), regional myocardial blood flow in areas perfused by stenotic coronary arteries rose after nitroglycerin when well-developed collaterals supplying those regions were present. Atrial pacing studies indicate that after nitroglycerin the heart can be paced to higher rates before angina occurs.[187] The nitrates have also been shown to improve ventricular wall motion in patients with ischemic heart disease, as demonstrated by contrast ventriculography,[188] echocardiography, and radionuclide ventriculography, at rest and during exercise.[189]

The mechanism of the nitrates' antianginal actions is complex (Fig. 39–5). Nitrates are not considered to exert a *direct* effect on the contractile state of the heart, although heart rate may rise reflexly as a consequence of the decline in blood pressure. When beta blockers are administered concurrently, the reflex tachycardia accompanying the nitrate-induced hypotension is eliminated.[190] Apparently, one action is to reduce the mechanical activity of the heart through the previously noted systemic effects, with subsequent reduction in development of the left ventricular wall tension (which results from reduction of arterial pressure and ventricular volume) and of myocardial oxygen consumption.[191] Reduced left ventricular end-diastolic pressure may also decrease the resistance to coronary blood flow. It is probable that the cardiac actions of the nitrates—dilating epicardial stenoses, dilating coronary collateral vessels, and reducing ventricular diastolic pressure and thereby lowering extravascular resistance to endocardial perfusion—all act to increase oxygen delivery to ischemic myocardium. In the final analysis, some combination of a reduction of myocardial oxygen requirements and increased oxygen delivery to the ischemic area relieves or prevents the development of myocardial ischemia in patients with chronic stable angina.

An assessment of the relative importance of these two actions of nitroglycerin (reducing oxygen demand and increasing oxygen supply) has been complicated by the differing results of studies on the effects of intracoronary nitroglycerin. Any effect of the drug administered by this route must derive from its direct action on the coronary vascular bed, i.e., by improving myocardial oxygen supply; some studies have demonstrated a beneficial effect of intracoronary nitroglycerin,[178] while others have not. It is of interest that smoking-induced coronary vasoconstriction is prevented by nitroglycerin and calcium antagonists.[192] Perhaps the principal action of nitrates differs in different patients; in patients with a strong vasoconstrictive component their principal action may be to increase oxygen delivery to ischemic myocardium, and in patients with relatively fixed lesions and constant-threshold angina their principal action may be to reduce myocardial oxygen demands.

Cellular Mechanism of Action. It has been postulated that vascular smooth muscle cells have nitrate receptors, with sulfhydryl groups, which become oxidized by nitrates, initiating the process of vascular relaxation.[193] Nitroglycerin-induced vasodilation can be enhanced by previous administration of *N*-acetylcysteine, an agent that increases the availability of sulfhydryl groups.[194] This action has been demonstrated to potentiate peripheral hemodynamic responses[194] and the coronary vasodilator effect of nitroglycerin.[195] Nitrates also enter smooth muscle and are converted into S-nitrosothiols; these activate intracellular guanylate cyclase and cause an increase in cyclic guanosine monophosphate, which triggers smooth muscle relaxation.[196] Nitrates may also act through the prostaglandin system.[197, 198] In both in vivo and in vitro experiments, nitroglycerin has been shown to induce prostacyclin synthesis, although a clear role for the prostaglandin system as a modulator of nitroglycerin action has yet to be demonstrated.[199, 200]

Types of Preparations and Routes of Administration

Nitroglycerin administered sublingually remains the drug of choice for treatment of an acute anginal episode. A transient but effective concentration of the drug rapidly appears in the circulation because sublingual administra-

TABLE 39–1 DOSAGE AND KINETICS OF NITROGLYCERIN AND LONG-ACTING NITRATES

Medication	Usual Dosage	Onset of Action	Duration of Action
Sublingual NTG	0.3–0.6 mg	2–5 min	10–30 min
Aerosol NTG	0.4 mg	2–5 min	10–30 min
Sublingual and chewable ISDN	2.5–10 mg	3–15 min	1–2 hr
Sublingual and chewable ET	5–15 mg, 10 mg	3–15 min	2 hr
Transmucosal NTG	1–3 mg	2–5 min	3–5 hr*
Oral NTG (SR)	2.5–9 mg	30–45 min	2–8 hr*
Oral ISDN	5–30 mg	15–30 min	3–6 hr
Oral ISDN (SR)	40 mg	30–60 min	6–10 hr
Oral ET	10 mg	30 min	Variable
Oral PET	10–40 mg	30 min	3–6 hr
Oral PET (SR)	30–80 mg	Slow	6–10 hr
NTG ointment (2%)	½–2 inches	20–60 min	3–8 hr
Transdermal NTG	5–10 mg	30–60 min	Up to 24 hr

*Duration of action lengthens with increasing dosage.

ET = erythrityl tetranitrate, ISDN = isosorbide dinitrate, NTG = nitroglycerin, PET = penaerythrityl tetranitrate, SR = sustained release.

Modified from Frishman, W. H.: Pharmacology of the nitrates in angina pectoris. Am. J. Cardiol. 56:81, 1985.

tion avoids first-pass hepatic metabolism. The half-life of nitroglycerin itself is brief and it is rapidly converted to two inactive metabolites, both of which are found in the urine after nitroglycerin administration. The liver possesses large amounts of hepatic glutathione organic nitrate reductase, but there is also evidence that blood vessels (veins and arteries) may metabolize nitrates directly.[200] Thus, within 30 to 60 minutes hepatic breakdown has abolished the hemodynamic and clinical effects. Nitroglycerin is also available in oral, ointment, and transdermal forms (Table 39–1). The usual sublingual dosage is 0.3 to 0.6 mg, and most patients respond within 5 minutes to one or two 0.3 mg tablets. If symptoms are not relieved by a single dose, additional doses of 0.3 mg may be taken at 5-minute intervals, but no more than 1.2 mg should be used within a 15-minute period. The development of tolerance is rarely a problem with intermittent usage. Sublingual nitroglycerin is especially useful when it is taken prophylactically shortly before activities are begun that are likely to cause angina. Used for this purpose, it may prevent anginal attacks for up to 30 to 40 minutes.

ADVERSE REACTIONS. These are common and include headache, flushing, and hypotension. The last is only rarely severe but can be potentially dangerous if the chest pain is due to a myocardial infarction rather than angina and arterial pressure has already declined because of pump failure and/or vagal reaction or hypovolemia. In addition, the partial pressure of oxygen in arterial blood may fall after large doses of nitroglycerin because of a ventilation-perfusion imbalance owing to inability of the pulmonary vascular bed to vasoconstrict in areas of alveolar hypoxia and thereby redirect perfusion to less hypoxic tissues.[201] Methemoglobinemia is a rare complication of very large doses of nitrates (p. 519). Commonly used doses of nitrates cause small elevations of methemoglobin that probably are not of clinical significance.

PREPARATIONS. Nitroglycerin tablets tend to lose their potency, especially if exposed to light, and should be kept in dark containers. Other nitrate preparations are available in sublingual, buccal, oral, spray, and ointment form (Table 39–1). Isosorbide dinitrate and other long-acting preparations are available in 2.5 and 5.0 mg sublingual tablets, and 10-mg buccal (chewable) form, and 5-, 10-, and 20-mg tablets for oral use as well as in 40-mg (sustained-release) capsules. An oral nitroglycerin spray that dispenses metered, aerosolized doses of 0.4 mg may be better absorbed in patients with dry mucosal membranes. It can also be quickly sprayed onto, or under, the tongue with one hand and has a 3-year shelf-life. For prophylaxis, the spray should be used 5 to 10 minutes before attack-provoking activities.[202]

Intermittent nitrate therapy appears to be preferable to the administration schedules that are designed to produce steady-state nitrate levels. Since orally administered nitrates undergo rapid hepatic metabolism,[203] large doses (5 mg nitroglycerin and 20 mg isosorbide dinitrate or pentaerythritol tetranitrate) may be required. Oral nitrates are not very potent agents, but they can raise the threshold of activity required for the development of angina and reduce the incidence of anginal attacks and the need for sublingual nitroglycerin.[204] They do not appear to cause tolerance to sublingual nitroglycerin.[205]

ISOSORBIDE DINITRATE. This long-acting nitrate has two metabolites (one of which has a potent vasodilatory action) which are cleared less rapidly than the parent drug and are excreted unchanged in the urine. Some investigators believe that the clinical effects of this agent relate to the actions of isosorbide dinitrate itself, as well as its metabolites.[199] The more protracted actions are believed to be the result of the metabolite 5-isosorbide mononitrate. Isosorbide dinitrate, like nitroglycerin, has been shown to dilate directly both atherosclerotic lesions and normal coronary segments and was shown to be particularly effective in dilating diseased segments in small and medium-sized arteries, with peak dilatation occurring at 30 minutes.[206] Oral isosorbide (5 to 30 mg) has been shown to augment the exercise response to beta-adrenoceptor blockers.[207]

TOLERANCE. In patients with stable angina pectoris, tolerance appears to develop during four-times-daily therapy with oral isosorbide dinitrate, but not when it is given two or three times daily.[207a] After 2 weeks of therapy, no diminished efficacy has been seen with buccal nitroglycerin administered three times daily.[208] Isosorbide dinitrate, continually administered in doses of 30, 60, and 120 mg four times daily, is less effective in sustaining a reduction in systolic pressure and increased exercise duration until the onset of angina than when it is administered as a single dose. During sustained therapy, exercise tolerance increased to the same magnitude after a dosage of 15 mg four times daily as with much higher dosages. Sustained therapy with isosorbide dinitrate, even in high dosage, results in tolerance to the antianginal and circulatory effects.[209]

TOPICAL NITROGLYCERIN. Nitroglycerin ointment (15 mg per inch) is efficacious when applied (most commonly to the chest) in strips of 0.5 to 2.0 inches. Delay in the onset of action is approximately 30 minutes.[176] However, this form of the drug is particularly useful in patients with severe angina who are confined to bed and chair since it is effective for 4 to 6 hours. It may also be used prophylactically after retiring by patients with nocturnal angina. Skin permeability increases with increased hydration and thus absorption is enhanced if paste is covered with plastic and the edges taped.

TRANSDERMAL NITROGLYCERIN DISCS. A silicone gel or polymer matrix is impregnated with nitroglycerin and absorption is then maintained for 24 to 48 hours at a rate determined by various methods of preparation, including a semipermeable membrane placed between the drug reservoir and the skin.[210] The dose depends on the size of the unit (5 to 30 cm), which releases 25 to 144 mg nitroglycerin over a 24-hour period. Most investigators believe that a minimal therapeutic level of nitroglycerin is at least 1 ng/ml.[211] Relatively low doses of the disc (5 to 10 mg/24 hours) probably do not produce sufficient plasma and tissue concentrations to sustain consistent, effective antianginal effects.[212]

Continuous delivery of organic nitrates over a 24-hour period appears to induce the rapid onset of partial or complete tolerance, with loss of clinical and hemodynamic effects of nitroglycerin within 18 to 24 hours after initial (acute) dosing. Long-acting formulations of higher doses, or schedules using frequent dosing, appear to produce greater evidence of nitrate tolerance than regimens using smaller doses, shorter-acting compounds, or less frequent dosing intervals. Once a state of tolerance has been induced, a nitrate-free interval will restore responsiveness. The minimal duration of this interval is unclear. Some data suggest that once tolerance has been established, responsiveness returns within 24 hours after the last dose, although a shorter interval may suffice.[213]

Transdermal nitroglycerin in a dose of 100 mg is effective for 8 hours during acute therapy. However, during sustained therapy, after only 7 to 10 days of 100 mg of transdermal isosorbide dinitrate per day, walking treadmill time at 4, 8, and 24 hours after drug application was similar to that seen during therapy with placebo.[213]

WITHDRAWAL OF NITRATES. Regardless of the route of administration and specific preparation used, the lowest effective dosage of long-acting nitrates should be employed, since tolerance to large doses may develop.[214] Because of the possibility of nitrate dependence, nitrate therapy should be withdrawn carefully. Indeed, in individuals exposed to industrial doses of nitroglycerin, nitrate tolerance, nitrate dependence, and withdrawal symptoms may cause serious problems. During the manufacturing of dynamite, substantial levels of nitrates are often present in the surrounding atmosphere and can be absorbed from the skin and lungs. After an acute response of headache, hypertension, palpitations, and gastrointestinal disturbance, adaptation ocurs. Withdrawal from this environment may result in angina unrelated to exertion or emotion usually within 1 to 3 days of nonexposure. In fact, spontaneous coronary vasospasm and acute myocardial infarction have been documented during a period of withdrawal.[215]

BETA-ADRENOCEPTOR BLOCKING AGENTS (See also pp. 874 and 1333)

These drugs constitute a cornerstone of therapy for effort-induced chronic stable angina.[216, 217] A number of studies have shown that beta-adrenoceptor blockers, in doses that are generally well tolerated, reduce the frequency of anginal episodes and raise the anginal threshold when given alone[218–220] and in combination with other antianginal agents. The salutatory action of these drugs, which have a chemical structure resembling that of isoproterenol and other beta-adrenoceptor agonists,[221] depends on their ability to cause competitive inhibition of the effects of neuronally released and circulating catecholamines on beta-adrenoceptors.[222] In this manner, these drugs attenuate the cardiac responses to adrenergic stimulation (chiefly increases in heart rate and contractility). Thus, beta blockers reduce myocardial oxygen demands primarily during activity or excitement when surges of increased sympathetic activity occur. Effects on heart rate and myocardial contractility at rest, while significant, are less profound because of the lower adrenergic drive to the heart in the basal state. Beta-adrenoceptor blockers also lower myocardial oxygen needs by reducing arterial pressure, and they are extremely useful antihypertensive agents (p. 874).

CHARACTERISTICS OF DIFFERENT BETA BLOCKERS. The differing pharmacological properties of these agents affect their relative actions (Table 39–2).

Selectivity. Two major subtypes of beta receptors, designated $beta_1$ and $beta_2$,[223] are present in different proportions in different tissues. $Beta_1$ receptors predominate in the heart and their stimulation leads to an increase in heart rate and A-V conduction and contractility, whereas elsewhere stimulation of these receptors leads to the release of renin in juxtaglomerular cells and lipolysis in adipocytes. $Beta_2$ stimulation results in bronchodilation, vasodilatation, and glycogenolysis. The beta blockers have been classified according to their relative cardioselectivity: nonselective beta-blocking drugs (propranolol, timolol, pindolol, and nadolol) block both $beta_1$ and $beta_2$ receptors, whereas cardioselective beta blockers (atenolol, metoprolol, and acebutolol) produce selective blockade of $beta_1$ receptors, while having lesser effects on $beta_2$ receptors. Thus, cardioselective beta blockers will reduce myocardial oxygen demands while tending not to block bronchodilation, vasodilatation, or glycogenolysis. As the dosages administered are increased, this cardioselectivity diminishes.[224] Since cardioselectivity is only relative, the use of such drugs in doses sufficient to prevent angina may still cause bronchoconstriction in some susceptible patients.

Membrane-Stabilizing Activity. Membrane-stabilizing activity refers to the "quinidine-like" effect of certain beta blockers that reduce the rate of rise of the cardiac action potential (p. 628). The clinical relevance of this effect is questionable because it is observed only at concentrations far exceeding therapeutic levels of the beta blockers that exhibit this action at all (propranolol, metoprolol, pindolol).

Intrinsic Sympathomimetic Activity. Beta blockers with intrinsic sympathomimetic activity (pindolol and acebutolol) are "partial agonists" and produce blockade by shielding beta receptors from more potent beta agonists. Pindolol and acebutolol produce low-grade beta stimulation when sympathetic activity is low (at rest), while under conditions of stress and exercise, when sympathetic activity is high, partial agonists behave more like conventional beta blockers.

Pindolol causes little if any lowering of heart rate, depression or atrioventricular (A-V) conduction, or depression of contractility at rest but still blocks the effects of exercise on these parameters. Its partial agonist activity also induces bronchodilation.[225–227] The clinical value of these actions remains to be established.[219, 228] In patients with severe symptoms and nocturnal angina, agents with partial agonist activity may not be as effective at reducing heart rate, reducing the frequency, duration, and magnitude of ambulatory ST-segment changes (monitored over 48 hours), or increasing the duration of exercise.[229]

Potency. This is the ability of beta blockers to inhibit the tachycardia produced by isoproterenol. All drugs are considered in reference to propranolol, which is given a value of 1.0 (see Table 39–5). Timolol and pindolol are the most potent agents, while acebutolol and labetalol are the least.

Lipid Solubility. The lipid solubility or hydrophylicity of beta blockers is a major determinant of their absorption and metabolism. The lipid-soluble beta blockers, propranolol, metoprolol, and pindolol (see Table 39–5), are readily absorbed from the gastrointestinal tract. They are metabolized predominantly by the liver, have a relatively short half-life, and usually require administration twice or more daily in order to achieve continuing pharmacological ef-

TABLE 39–2 PHARMACOKINETICS AND PHARMACOLOGY OF SOME BETA-ADRENOCEPTOR BLOCKERS

	Drug									
	Atenolol	Metoprolol	Nadolol	Pindolol	Propranolol	Timolol	Propranolol HCl	Propranolol LA	Acebutolol	Labetalol
Extent of absorption (%)	≃50	>95	≃30	>90	90	>90	>90	>90	≃70	>90
Extent of bioavailability (% of dose)	≃40	≃50	≃30	≃90	≃30	75	≃30	≃20	≃50	≃25
Beta-blocking plasma concentration	0.2 to 0.5 μg/ml	50 to 100 ng/ml	50 to 100 ng/ml	50 to 100 ng/ml	50 to 100 ng/ml	5 to 10 ng/ml	50–100 ng/ml	20–100 ng/ml	0.2–2.0 μg/ml	0.7–3.0 μg/ml
Protein binding (%)	<5	12	≃30	57	93	≃10	93	93	30–40	≃50
Lipophilicity*	Low	Moderate	Low	Moderate	High	Low	High	High	Low	Low
Elimination half-life (hr)	6 to 9	3 to 4	14 to 25	3 to 4	3.5 to 6.0	3 to 4	3–4	10	3–4‡	≃6
Urinary recovery of unchanged drug (% of dose)	≃40	≃3	70	≃40	<1	≃20	<1	<1	≃40	<1
Total urinary recovery (% of dose)	>95	>95	70	>90	>90	65	>90	>90	>90	>90
Drug accumulation in renal disease	Yes	No	Yes	No	No	No	No	No	Yes§	No
Predominant route of elimination†	RE (mostly unchanged)	HM	RE	RE (≃40% unchanged) and HM	HM	RE (≃20% unchanged) and HM	HM	HM	HM§	HM
Active metabolites	No	No	No	No	Yes	No	Yes	Yes	Yes	No
β_1-blocker potency ratio (propranolol = 1)	1.0	1.0	1.0	6.0	1.0	6.0	1.0	1.0	0.3	0.3
Relative β_1 sensitivity	+	+	0	0	0	0	0	0	Yes	0
Intrinsic sympathetic activity	0	0	0	+	0	0	0	0	+	0
Membrane-stabilizing activity	0	0	0	+	+ +	0	+ +	+ +	+	0
Usual maintenance dose	50 to 100 mg/qd	50 to 100 mg/qid	40 to 80 mg/qd	5 to 20 mg/tid	60 mg/qid	20 mg/bid	60 mg/qid	80 to 160 mg/qd	200 to 600 mg/bid	100 to 600 mg/bid

*Determined by the distribution ratio between octanol and water.
†RE = renal excretion, HM = hepatic metabolism.
‡Half-life of the active metabolite, diacetolol, is 12 to 15 hours.
§Acebutolol is mainly eliminated by the liver but its major metabolite, diacetolol, is excreted by the kidney.
Modified from Frishman, W. H., Kaftka, K. R., and Meltzer, A. H.: Antianginal Agents, Part 2: β-Blockers. Hosp. Formul. *21*:62, 1986.

fects. The water-soluble beta blockers (hydrophylic), atenolol and nadolol, are not as readily absorbed from the gastrointestinal tract, are not as extensively metabolized, have relatively long plasma half-lives, and can be administered once daily. In addition, they are less likely to cross the blood-brain barrier and cause central nervous system side effects such as mental depression, sleep disturbances, nightmares, fatigue, and weakness. Indeed, controlled trials have shown that atenolol causes less frequent nightmares and hallucinations than does metoprolol or propranolol.[229–232]

Alpha-Adrenoceptor Blocking Activity. The only available beta blocker that also possessses alpha-adrenoceptor blocking activity is labetalol.[233] The alpha blocking potency of this agent is four to six times less than its beta blocking potency and it is one of the weaker beta blockers compared with propranolol (see Table 39–2). Its combined alpha and beta blocking effects make it a particularly useful antihypertensive agent (p. 875).

Oxidation Phenotype. A possible explanation for the widely varying differences in plasma concentrations in patients taking the same dose of a beta blocker may be due to differences in oxidation phenotypes. Metoprolol is one of several beta blockers that undergo oxidative metabolism in human beings. It has been found that the metabolism of metoprolol exhibits the debrisoquine type of genetic polymorphism and that poor hydroxylators have a threefold prolongation of the elimination half-life of metoprolol as compared with extensive hydroxylators.[234] Thus, angina might be controlled by a single daily dose of metoprolol in poor hydroxylators, whereas extensive hydroxylators would need the same dose two or three times a day. Such observations might also apply to propranolol, timolol, and alprenolol, which have all been reported to produce high plasma concentrations or symptoms of excessive beta blockade in poor hydroxylators of debrisoquine.[235]

First-Pass Effects. Certain beta blockers, e.g., propranolol, metoprolol, and timolol, are extensively metabolized by the liver. Following absorption via the gastrointestinal tract, metabolism occurs in the liver before the agents reach the systemic circulation. This effect is most significant for propranolol, which is transformed into inactive metabolites by the liver following oral administration so that only a relatively small amount of drug reaches the bloodstream. If propranolol is administered intravenously, however, a much higher concentration reaches the bloodstream and thus the intravenous dose has greater potency than an orally administered one.

DOSAGE. For optimal results, the dosage of beta blocker should be carefully titrated. In the case of propranolol, it is useful to start with 80 mg of propranolol daily (20 mg four times a day) or comparable doses of other blockers. It should be realized that with such a dosage regimen 24 to 48 hours will be required for the drug to reach levels of 100 ng/ml needed to reduce resting heart rates to 50 to 60 beats/min and to cause less than a 20 beat/min increase with modest exercise (e.g., climbing one flight of stairs) and to produce 70 to 80 per cent reduction in the tachycardia induced by strenuous exercise on a treadmill.[236] The usual dosage of propranolol ranges from 80 to 320 mg per day, but some patients require (and tolerate) doses as high as 1000 mg daily.

ADVERSE EFFECTS. Most of the adverse reactions to beta blockers are a consequence of their beta-blocking properties and include myocardial effects (severe sinus bradycardia, sinus arrest, AV block, reduced left ventricular contractility), bronchoconstriction, fatigue, mental depression, nightmares, gastrointestinal upset, sexual dysfunction, intensification of insulin-induced hypoglycemia, cutaneous reactions, and withdrawal syndrome.[235, 237] Lethargy, weakness, and fatigue may be caused by reduced cardiac output or may arise from a direct effect on the central nervous system. Nightmares, depression, and even psychoses may occur. Agents with a lower lipid solubility, e.g., atenolol, nadolol, and acebutolol, may not penetrate into the central nervous system as much and may benefit the patient. Bronchoconstriction results from a blockade of $beta_2$ receptors in the tracheobronchial tree. As a consequence, asthma and chronic obstructive lung disease are contraindications to the use of such agents. Cardioselectivity of beta blockers such as metoprolol and atenolol is only relative, and the use of such drugs in dosages sufficient to prevent angina may still cause bronchoconstriction in susceptible patients. In general, we believe that [illegible]tory of asthma or wheezing probably constitutes an absolute contraindication to the use of beta blockers. Finally, other side effects include skin rash, fever, GI symptoms (nausea, diarrhea, or constipation), and pharyngitis. In patients who already have impaired left ventricular function, congestive heart failure may be intensified, an effect that can be counteracted by the use of digitalis or diuretics. Beta blockers should not be used in patients with bradyarrhythmias of any kind unless a pacemaker is in place. In patients with partial AV block, they may further impair conduction. Blockade of noncardiac $beta_2$ receptors inhibits catecholamine-induced glycogenolysis so that noncardioselective beta blockers may impair the defense to insulin-induced hypoglycemia. Blockade of noncardiac $beta_2$ receptors also inhibits the vasodilating effects of catecholamines in peripheral blood vessels and leaves the constrictive (alpha-adrenergic) receptors unopposed and enhances vasoconstriction. Noncardioselective beta blockers may precipitate episodes of Raynaud's phenomenon and may cause uncomfortable coldness of the distal extremities. In patients with peripheral vascular disease, reduced flow to the limbs may occur.[238]

Sudden withdrawal of beta blockers in ambulatory patients has been reported to result in acute ischemic episodes.[237] This rebound is much less marked in hospitalized patients, suggesting that increased physical activity combined with a reduction of beta blockade results in the clinical worsening. Other possible mechanisms involve unmasking of the underlying coronary obstruction that has progressed during the course of drug administration, a sudden elevation of arterial pressure, and an increase in the number of adrenergic beta receptors ("up-regulation").[239] Chronic beta-adrenoceptor blockade in vivo has been shown to increase myocardial sensitivity to catecholamine action upon its withdrawal by more effective coupling of the activated receptor to cyclic AMP generation rather than by up-regulation.[240]

Drug interactions involving beta blockers also occur. Most of the available information relates to propranolol, but detailed information regarding other beta blockers is available[241] (Table 39–3).

TABLE 39–3 INTERACTIONS OF BETA-ADRENOCEPTOR BLOCKING AGENTS AND OTHER DRUGS

PHARMACOKINETIC INTERACTIONS

1. Cimetidine:	Reduces hepatic metabolism of beta blockers; increased plasma levels of beta-blockers and serum half-life prolonged. Bradycardia may be excessive. *Management:* Monitor heart rate and reduce dose of one or both drugs.
2. Aluminum hydroxide gel:	Delay or reduction in GI absorption with reduced plasma levels of beta blocker. *Management:* Take drugs at different times or increase beta-blocker dose.
3. Barbiturates:	Induction of hepatic enzymes enhances metabolism of beta blockers and reduces plasma levels. *Management:* Avoid barbiturates or increase beta-blocker dosage.
4. Lidocaine:	Propranolol therapy reduces hepatic clearance of lidocaine; serum lidocaine levels may increase and toxicity may ensue. *Management:* Monitor plasma lidocaine concentration and reduce dosage if appropriate.

PHARMACODYNAMIC INTERACTIONS

1. Verapamil: Hypotension, bradycardia, negative inotropic responses and abnormal AV conduction are all additive with beta blockers. Avoid concurrent use (especially in patients with depressed left ventricular function). Monitor patients carefully if concurrent use unavoidable.
2. Epinephrine: Hypertension (and reflex bradycardia) result from unopposed alpha-vasoconstrictive effects of epinephrine.
3. Aminophylline: By phosphodiesterase inhibition, aminophylline increases cyclic AMP. Antagonism results from concurrent use with beta blockers.
4. Antidiabetic agents: Propranolol may induce hypoglycemia (reduced glycogenolysis), hyperglycemia (inhibition of insulin release); hypertension (release of endogenous epinephrine with hypoglycemia and unopposed alpha-vasoconstrictor effects ensue), absence of tachycardia with hypoglycemia. Avoid beta blockers in diabetics if possible. Cardioselective agents preferable.
5. Clonidine: Sudden withdrawal (and norepinephrine release) may result in severe hypertension if unopposed alpha-adrenergic tone exists due to beta-adrenergic blockade.
   Management: Withdraw beta blockers before clonidine.
6. Cyclopropane: Combined effects of cyclopropane and beta blockade may result in depression of LV function.

OTHER INTERACTIONS

1. Indomethacin: May reduce antihypertensive effect of beta blockers.
2. Ergot alkaloids: With beta blockers may cause excessive vasoconstriction.
3. Tricyclic antidepressants: May inhibit the bradycardia and negative inotropic effects of beta blockers.
4. Monoamine oxidase inhibitors: Enhance hypotensive effect of beta blockers.
5. Tubocurarine, succinylcholine, and pancuronium: Potentiate muscle relaxation when used with beta blockers.

CALCIUM ANTAGONISTS

The critical role played by calcium ions in the normal contraction of cardiac and vascular smooth muscle is discussed on page 389 and in myocardial ischemia on page 1211. Calcium antagonists block the entry of calcium into cardiac and vascular smooth muscle cells. Despite their chemical heterogeneity,[242, 243] calcium antagonists' major action is to interfere with the entry of calcium into cells through voltage-sensitive channels, whereas processes that involve the release of intracellular stores of calcium are relatively insensitive to these drugs. They are effective in the treatment of chronic stable angina, either alone or in combination with beta-adrenoceptor blockers and nitrates.[244–246] Calcium-channel antagonists appear to be beneficial in controlling angina and improving exercise tolerance in patients with chronic stable angina pectoris due to coronary atherosclerosis as well as in those with Prinzmetal's variant angina (p. 1360) and angina resulting from abnormally small coronary arteries with limited vasodilator reserve.[84]

Three calcium antagonists—nifedipine, verapamil, and diltiazem—are available in the United States (Table 39–4). All three agents are effective in causing relaxation of vascular smooth muscle in both the systemic arterial and coronary arterial beds. There has also been interest in the observations that calcium antagonists appear to have antiatherogenic effects in rabbits and monkeys.[247]

NIFEDIPINE. Nifedipine is a dihydropyridine that is particularly effective in reducing the contractility of smooth muscle, especially vascular smooth muscle. Ninety per cent of the administered drug is absorbed following oral or buccal administration and is detectable in the serum after 20 and 3 minutes, respectively. Its peak concentration occurs between 1 and 2 hours following oral use. The drug is highly protein-bound and is metabolized to inert products, most of which are eliminated by the kidney and some through the gastrointestinal tract.[244] The plasma half-life is 4 to 5 hours. The dose of nifedipine is 10 mg orally every 8 (or 6) hours increased to 20 mg every 8 (or 6) hours, guided by blood pressure response. The dosage of 160 mg daily is considered to be maximal.

Nifedipine is a more potent vasodilator than diltiazem

TABLE 39–4 CLINICAL PHARMACOKINETICS OF MAJOR CALCIUM ANTAGONISTS

Agent	Usual Adult Dose	Absorption	Onset of Action	Peak Effect	Plasma Half-Life
Verapamil	IV: 0.075 to 0.15 mg/kg	—	≈2 min	3 to 5 min	<½ hr
	Oral: 80 to 120 mg tid or qid	90%	2 hr	3 to 4 hr	3 to 7 hr*
Nifedipine	SL: 10 to 30 mg tid or qid	90%	<3 min	Not available	
	Oral: 10 to 30 mg tid or qid	90%	<20 min	1 to 2 hr	4 hr
Diltiazem	IV: 0.075 to 0.15 mg/kg	—		Not available	
	Oral: 30 to 90 mg tid or qid	90%	<15 min	30 min	4 hr

IV = intravenous, SL = sublingual.
*Single dose; may be lengthened to 4.5 to 12 hours after 6 to 10 consecutive oral doses.
From Singh, B. N.: Clinical pharmacology of calcium antagonist drugs. Cornell Postgraduate Course on Calcium Antagonists. New York, Medcom, Inc., 1982, p. 5.

and verapamil. Although its in vitro actions on myocardium and specialized cardiac tissue, i.e., the sinoatrial and AV nodes, are similar to those of the other agents, the concentration required to reproduce effects on these tissues is not reached in vivo because of the early appearance of its powerful vasodilating effects. Thus in clinical practice the potential negative chronotropic, inotropic, and dromotropic (on A-V conduction) effects of nifedipine are seldom a problem.

The beneficial effects of nifedipine in the treatment of angina result from its capacity to reduce myocardial oxygen needs consequent to afterload reduction, and to increase myocardial oxygen delivery consequent to its dilating action on the coronary vascular bed. In conscious animals, nifedipine has been shown to dilate both large coronary arteries and coronary resistance vessels.[248] Nifedipine decreases left ventricular afterload, while ejection fraction, velocity of circumferential fiber shortening, heart rate, and cardiac index all show slight reflex increases; these increases can be blocked by simultaneous administration of beta-adrenoceptor blockers. In patients with elevated left ventricular end-diastolic volumes and pressures, nifedipine reduces ventricular end-diastolic pressure and left ventricular end-diastolic and end-systolic volumes and enhances ejection fraction more than it does in patients with normal baseline left ventricular function[249] (Fig. 39–6 and Table 39–5).

Adverse Effects. These occur in 15 to 20 per cent of patients; they lead to discontinuation of medication in 5 per cent[250] (Table 39–6). Many are related to the systemic vasodilation and include headache, dizziness, flushing, hypotension, and troublesome leg edema (not related to heart failure). Gastrointestinal side effects, including nausea, epigastric pressure, and vomiting, are noted in approximately 5 per cent of patients. Occasionally, nifedipine aggravates angina, presumably by lowering arterial pressure excessively with subsequent reflex tachycardia in patients with extremely severe, fixed obstructions. For this reason, combined therapy of nifedipine with a beta blocker is particularly effective in the treatment of chronic stable angina and is superior to single-drug therapy.[251, 252]

A comparison of the side effects of nifedipine with those of other calcium antagonists is shown in Table 39–6. Because of its potent vasodilator effects, nifedipine is contraindicated in patients who are already hypotensive.[253] In patients with mild left ventricular dysfunction, sinus bradycardia, sick sinus syndrome, and AV block (particularly if a beta-adrenoceptor blocking agent is concurrently administered and additional drug therapy of angina is indicated), nifedipine is the calcium antagonist of choice.[254]

TABLE 39–5 COMPARISON OF DRUG EFFECTS ON GLOBAL AND REGIONAL LEFT VENTRICULAR FUNCTION DURING EXERCISE (VS. CONTROL)

	Global LV Function								Regional LV Function		
	HR	SBP	DPB	PAPD	CI	TVR	EF	EDVI	NL	ISCH	SCAR
Nitroglycerin	(↑)	—	(↓)	↓	—	—	(↑)	(↓)	—	↑	—
Nifedipine	↑	↓	↓	↓	↑	↓	(↑)	—	—	↑	—
Metoprolol	↓	↓	—	↑	(↓)	↑	—	—	↓	(↑)	—

Significant group differences are represented by different symbols: arrows indicate changes vs. control; arrows in parentheses indicate changes that are significant by single comparison but not by multiple group comparison.

Abbreviations: LV = left ventricular, HR = heart rate, SBP = systolic blood pressure, DBP = diastolic blood pressure, PAPD = pulmonary artery diastolic pressure, CI = cardiac index, TVR = total vascular resistance, EF = ejection fraction, EDVI = end-diastolic volume index, NL = normal segment, ISCH = ischemic segment, SCAR = scar segment, ↑ = increase, ↓ = decrease, — = no significant change vs. control.

From Pfisterer, M., et al.: Comparative effects of nitroglycerin, nifedipine and metoprolol on regional left ventricular function in patients with one-vessel coronary disease. Circulation 67:291, 1983.

TABLE 39–6 SIDE EFFECTS OF ANTIANGINAL DRUGS*

	Hypotension Flushing, Headache	Left Ventricular Dysfunction	Decreased Heart Rate Atrioventricular Block†	Gastrointestinal Symptoms	Broncho-constriction‡
Beta blockers	0	+ +	+ + +	+	+ + +
Nitrates	+ + +	0	0	0	0
Diltiazem	+	+	+	0	0
Nifedipine	+ + +	0	0	0	0
Verapamil	+	+	+ +	+ +	0

*0 = absent, + = mild, + + = moderate, + + + = sometimes severe.
†In patients with sick sinus node syndrome or conduction system disease.
‡In patients with obstructive lung disease.
From Braunwald, E.: Mechanism of action of calcium channel blocking agents. N. Engl. J. Med. *307*:1618, 1982.

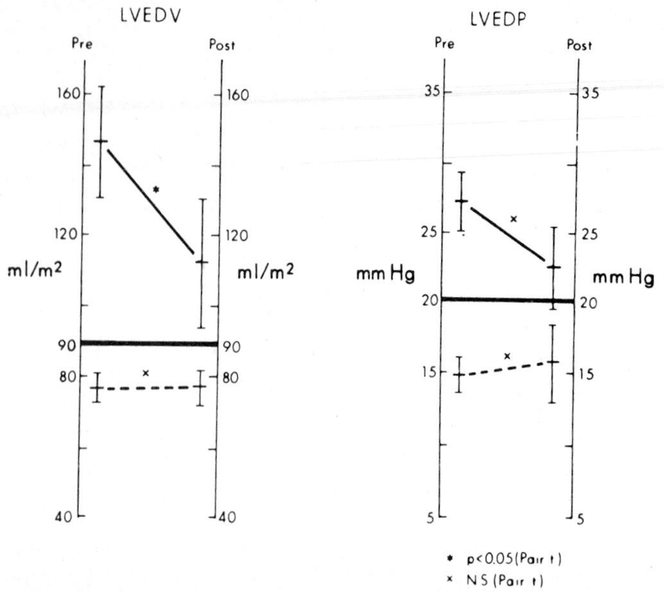

FIGURE 39–6. Left ventricular end-diastolic volume (LVEDV) and end-diastolic pressure (LVEDP) before and after nifedipine. Average EDV declined significantly in group 2 patients, in whom baseline LVEDV exceeded 90 ml/m², but was unchanged in group 1 patients, in whom initial LVEDV was normal. Average LVEDP declined in group 2 patients but did not change significantly in those in group 1. (From Ludbrook, P. A., et al.: Acute hemodynamic responses to sublingual nifedipine: Dependence on left ventricular function. Circulation 65:489, 1982, by permission of the American Heart Association, Inc.)

This is because in the clinical dosage range tolerated it has fewer negative effects on myocardial contractility or on the specialized automatic or conduction system than does verapamil or diltiazem. In patients already receiving maximal doses of nitrates and beta-blocker therapy, the addition of nifedipine (80 to 100 mg per day) has been shown to improve diastolic function of the left ventricle at rest and during exercise.[255] However, in patients with severe left ventricular dysfunction, the addition of nifedipine may precipitate left ventricular failure.

VERAPAMIL (See also p. 636). The drug is well absorbed after oral administration, although 85 per cent is eliminated by the liver as a first-pass effect. Ninety per cent of verapamil is bound to protein and plasma levels of its metabolites may be much higher than those of the parent drug. The usual starting dose of verapamil for oral administration is 40 to 80 mg three times daily. It may later be increased to 80 to 120 mg three or four times daily to a maximum dose of 480 mg/day (Table 39–4).

Parenteral verapamil dilates the systemic and coronary small-vessel resistance beds without clearly increasing myocardial metabolic demands. In addition, it has been shown to dilate large conductance vessels in both normal and diseased arterial segments, although this effect is not as potent as that of nitroglycerin.[256] Verapamil appears to decrease myocardial oxygen demand without any change in the anginal threshold, i.e., in the rate-pressure product at the onset of angina.[256, 257] Trials comparing verapamil with beta blockade (usually propranolol) in the treatment of effort-related angina[258] have shown that the drugs are comparable in producing dose-dependent reductions in frequency of anginal attacks. In a comparison of propranolol (480 mg per day) and verapamil (320 mg per day), verapamil was found to be a more effective antianginal agent than propranolol, although the combination of both drugs resulted in better exercise capacity than did either drug alone.[254, 259]

Verapamil enhances left ventricular diastolic filling at rest and during exercise in patients with chronic stable angina, whereas beta blockade does not have this effect.[259] Despite marked negative inotropic effects of verapamil in isolated cardiac muscle preparations, changes in contractility are modest in patients with normal cardiac function.[250] In patients with cardiac dysfunction, verapamil, like beta blockade, may reduce cardiac output and elevate left ventricular filling pressure.

In clinical doses, verapamil also inhibits calcium influx into specialized cardiac cells, sometimes causing slowing of heart rate and A-V conduction. It may cause slight P-R prolongation. Although the drug depresses the sinus node automaticity, the systemic vasodilator effects of the drug activate reflexes that counteract or minimize this effect. Verapamil is therefore contraindicated in patients with sick sinus syndrome, A-V conduction abnormalities, and in suspected digitalis toxicity. In treatment of angina pectoris, intravenous verapamil should not be used together with an orally administered beta blocker nor should a beta blocker be administered intravenously in patients receiving oral verapamil, and certainly intravenous verapamil and a beta blocker should not be used together.[254]

Adverse effects of verapamil are noted in approximately 10 per cent of patients and relate to systemic dilation (hypotension and facial flushing), gastrointestinal symptoms (constipation and nausea), and central nervous system reactions such as headache and dizziness.

DILTIAZEM. This calcium antagonist is absorbed rapidly and almost completely, with peak concentrations occurring after 30 minutes and a half-life of approximately 4 hours. Eighty per cent of the drug is bound to plasma proteins, 60 per cent is metabolized by the liver, and the remainder is excreted by the kidneys.

The dosage of diltiazem is 30 to 60 mg four times daily,[260] although higher doses are sometimes more effective.[261, 262]

Diltiazem's actions are intermediate between those of nifedipine and verapamil. In clinically useful doses its vasodilator effects are somewhat less profound than nifedipine's while its cardiac depressant action (on the sinoatrial and A-V nodes and myocardium) may be less than those of verapamil. Thus, the remarkably low incidence of adverse effects of this drug may be explained. Diltiazem is a systemic vasodilator, lowering arterial pressure at rest and during exertion and increasing the workload required to produce myocardial ischemia, but there is some evidence that the drug may also increase myocardial oxygen delivery.[263] In patients with coronary artery disease, diltiazem reduces afterload and depresses myocardial systolic function, although it improves left ventricular relaxation, which may contribute in part to enhancement of early diastolic filling.[264] Studies in patients during tachycardia-induced angina pectoris suggest that the major benefit of diltiazem is related to reduction of myocardial oxygen demand rather than to enhancing myocardial oxygen delivery.[265]

Diltiazem is a highly efficacious antianginal agent with minimal side effects when given to patients with medically refractory stable angina who are already taking nitrates and beta blockers.[266, 266a] High doses of diltiazem (mean dose 340 mg) have been shown to be a safe addition to maximally tolerated doses of isosorbide dinitrate and a beta blocker, causing increases in exercise tolerance and resting and exercise left ventricular ejection fraction without increasing side effects.[261] The combination of high doses of diltiazem with beta blockers is more effective in reducing symptoms and improving exercise capacity without increasing adverse effects than is the use of diltiazem alone.[262, 267] Like verapamil, diltiazem should be used only with caution in patients with sick sinus syndrome and advanced degrees of AV block and left ventricular function.

SELECTION OF DRUGS FOR THE TREATMENT OF CHRONIC STABLE ANGINA

Verapamil (360 mg/day) and diltiazem (360 mg/day) appear to be equipotent antianginal agents and similar in efficacy to propranolol (320 mg/day). Nifedipine 60 mg/day appears to be equivalent to propranolol 160 to 240 mg/day. Diltiazem and verapamil, which reduce resting heart rate, appear to be more effective as single drugs for angina than is nifedipine, which causes reflex sympathetic stimulation; the latter is most effective when combined with a beta blocker.[254]

RELATIVE ADVANTAGES OF BETA BLOCKERS AND CALCIUM ANTAGONISTS. There is some controversy about whether a calcium antagonist or a beta blocker should be employed first in the treatment of chronic stable angina in patients in whom more than an occasional sublingual nitroglycerin tablet is required. As indicated in the foregoing discussion, both classes of agents appear to be about equally effective. Chronic administration of beta-adrenoceptor blockers has been found to prolong life in patients after acute myocardial infarction, but this has not yet been demonstrated for calcium antagonists. However, diltiazem is effective in preventing severe angina and early reinfarction after non-Q-wave infarction.[268] On the other hand, a number of conditions, such as moderate to severe left ventricular failure, sinus bradycardia, sick sinus syndrome, and advanced AV block as well as obstructive lung disease, are contraindications to beta blockade, and in such patients nifedipine is preferable. Hypertensive patients do well with both beta blockers and calcium antagonists, since both agents have antihypertensive effects.

One logical way to make a choice between a calcium antagonist and a beta blocker in patients who have no contraindications to either class of agents and who tolerate them well is to take a detailed history and determine whether the patient's anginal threshold is fixed or variable, as discussed on page 1317. When it is relatively fixed, it may be presumed that myocardial ischemia is caused primarily by an increase in myocardial oxygen needs during exercise in the face of a fixed supply, and a beta blocker would be considered the agent of choice; conversely, in patients with variable-threshold angina, in whom a reduction of myocardial blood supply caused by coronary vasospasm plays a role in the development of ischemia and angina, a calcium antagonist may be preferable to a beta blocker.

COMBINATION THERAPY. In patients with more severe angina, a combination of a beta-adrenoceptor blocker, a calcium antagonist, and a long-acting nitrate may be employed. The hemodynamic spectrum of action of nitroglycerin, calcium antagonists, and beta blockers is sufficiently different to suggest that combination therapy might be useful (Tables 39–5 and 39–7). Indeed, a number of studies[254] have shown that the combination of a beta blocker and a calcium antagonist is superior to either drug alone. While combined treatment is usually well tolerated,[266a] this combination should be approached with caution, since it can occasionally produce severe left ventricular dysfunction.[269, 270] It is often possible to use low doses of each agent, so that the adverse effects of each drug are diminished.

In patients with angina severe enough to require combination therapy but without specific contraindications to any antianginal agents, the combination of a beta blocker and nifedipine or of verapamil or diltiazem with a long-acting nitrate is appropriate. As already stated, since beta blockers and both verapamil and diltiazem exert negative inotropic effects and depress cardiac automaticity and conduction, this combination may be hazardous in patients who already have left ventricular dysfunction and in those with impaired function of the sinoatrial or AV nodes. The combination of nifedipine and nitrates may also be less than ideal, since both agents are potent vasodilators. Triple-drug therapy (long-acting nitrates, a beta blocker, and a calcium antagonist) is used widely and effectively in many patients with severe angina. In practice, antianginal drugs are begun in low doses and are gradually raised to tolerance. If the patient's life style is limited by persistent angina despite all the aforementioned measures, and if there are no contraindications, mechanical revascularization should be considered.

In decisions about the management of individual patients with angina, the effects of the antianginal agents on indices of myocardial oxygen supply and demand should be con-

TABLE 39–7 EFFECTS OF ANTIANGINAL AGENTS ON INDICES OF MYOCARDIAL OXYGEN SUPPLY AND DEMAND*

		Beta-Adrenoceptor Blockers				Calcium Antagonists		
		ISA†		Cardioselective				
Index	Nitrates	No	Yes	No	Yes	Nifedipine	Verapamil	Diltiazem
Supply								
Coronary resistance								
Vascular tone	↓ ↓	↑	0	↑	0 ↑	↓ ↓ ↓	↓ ↓ ↓	↓ ↓ ↓
Intramyocardial diastolic tension	↓ ↓ ↓	↑	0	↑	↑	↓ ↓	0 ↑	0
Coronary collateral circulation	↑	0	0	0	0	↑	0	↑
Duration of diastole	0 (↓)	↑ ↑ ↑	0 ↓	↑ ↑ ↑	↑ ↑ ↑	0 ↑ (↓ ↓)	↑ ↑ ↑ (↓)	↑ ↑ (↓)
Demand								
Intramyocardial systolic tension								
Preload	↓ ↓ ↓	↑	0	↑	↑	↓ 0	↑ 0 ↓	0 ↓
Afterload (peripheral vascular resistance)	↓	↑	↑	↑ ↑	↑	↓ ↓	↓	↓
Contractility	0 (↑)	↓ ↓ ↓	↓	↓ ↓ ↓	↓ ↓ ↓	↓ (↑ ↑)‡	↓ ↓ (↑)‡	↓ (↑)‡
Heart rate	0 (↑)	↓ ↓ ↓	0 ↓	↓ ↓ ↓	↓ ↓ ↓	0 (↑ ↑)	↓ ↓ (↑)	↓ ↓ (↑)

*↑ = increase, ↓ = decrease, 0 = little or no definite effect. Number of arrows represents relative intensity of effect. Symbols in parentheses indicate reflex-mediated effects.

†ISA = intrinsic sympathomimetic activity.

‡Effect of calcium entry blockers on left ventricular *contractility*, as assessed in the intact animal model. The net effect on *left ventricular performance* is variable, being influenced by alterations in afterload, reflex cardiac stimulation, and the underlying state of the myocardium.

From Shub, C., Vlietstra, R. E., and McGoon, M. D.: Selection of optimal drug therapy for the patient with angina pectoris. Mayo Clin. Proc. *60*:539, 1985.

TABLE 39–8 RECOMMENDED DRUG THERAPY (CALCIUM ANTAGONIST VERSUS BETA BLOCKER) IN PATIENTS WHO HAVE ANGINA IN CONJUNCTION WITH OTHER MEDICAL CONDITIONS*

CLINICAL CONDITION	RECOMMENDED DRUG (ALTERNATIVE DRUG)
Cardiac arrhythmias and conduction abnormalities	
Sinus bradycardia	Nifedipine
Sinus tachycardia (not due to cardiac failure)	Beta blocker
Supraventricular tachycardia	Verapamil or beta blocker
Atrioventricular block	Nifedipine
Rapid atrial fibrillation (with digitalis)	Verapamil or beta blocker
Ventricular arrhythmias	Beta blocker (± group 1 antiarrhythmic agent)
Left ventricular dysfunction	
Congestive heart failure	
Mild (LVEF ≥40%)	Nifedipine (verapamil, diltiazem, or beta blockers cautiously)
Moderate to severe (LVEF <40%)	Nifedipine (cautiously, in combination with other therapy)
Left-sided valvular heart disease†	
Aortic stenosis (mild)‡	Beta blocker
Aortic insufficiency	Nifedipine
Mitral regurgitation	Nifedipine
Mitral stenosis§	Beta blocker
Miscellaneous medical conditions	
Systemic hypertension	Beta blocker (calcium antagonists)
Severe preexisting headaches	Beta blockers (verapamil or diltiazem)
COPD with bronchospasm or asthma	Nifedipine, verapamil, or diltiazem
Hyperthyroidism	Beta blocker
Raynaud's syndrome	Nifedipine
Claudication	Nifedipine, verapamil, or diltiazem (low-dose $beta_1$ blocker or beta-ISA)
Depression	Nifedipine, verapamil, or diltiazem
Neurasthenia or fatigue states	Nifedipine, verapamil, or diltiazem
Insulin-dependent diabetes mellitus	Nifedipine, verapamil, or diltiazem (low-dose $beta_1$ or beta-ISA)

*Beta-ISA = beta blocker with intrinsic sympathomimetic activity such as pindolol or acebutolol, COPD = chronic obstructive pulmonary disease, LVEF = left ventricular ejection fraction.

†Surgical therapy should be considered for patients with severe valvular heart disease; beta blockers are not routinely used in patients with valvular heart disease and left ventricular failure.

‡Vasodilators may increase aortic valve gradient, and beta blockers can cause left ventricular failure. Any of these drugs should be used with extreme caution in patients with severe aortic stenosis.

§If congestive heart failure (associated with normal left ventricular function) occurs in a patient with angina, severe mitral stenosis, and rapid atrial fibrillation, a beta blocker (in combination with digitalis) may be used to decrease the heart rate.

From Shub, C., Vlietstra, R. E., and McGoon, M. D.: Selection of optimal drug therapy for the patient with angina pectoris. Mayo Clin. Proc. *60*:539, 1985.

sidered.[271] When angina pectoris exists with other conditions, such as asthma and diabetes mellitus, which can complicate drug therapy, the choice of therapy should be made carefully (Table 39–8).

PERCUTANEOUS TRANSLUMINAL CORONARY ANGIOPLASTY (PTCA)

(See also Chap. 40)

The use of PTCA in the treatment of chronic coronary artery disease occupies an intermediate position in the spectrum between medical therapy and coronary artery surgery. With improved equipment and increasing numbers of experienced operators, the primary success rate of PTCA has improved over the last 10 years[272, 272a] so that the number of procedures performed has risen rapidly. Although there has been a liberalization of the indications for PTCA, some general guidelines for selecting suitable candidates have evolved in this rapidly changing field.[272b]

PATIENT SELECTION. Patients for PTCA should, in general, have symptoms, objective evidence of more than trivial myocardial ischemia, and an optimal, significant coronary lesion (or lesions) with the potential for complete revascularization. Ideally, such patients should also be suitable surgical candidates; however, selected patients who are not suitable (e.g., with severe pulmonary or renal disease, and advanced age with infirmity) may be considered. In such patients PTCA may be undertaken as a palliative procedure and may be useful even in those with multivessel disease in whom all lesions are not suitable for dilatation.

The optimal lesion for PTCA in a patient with stable angina pectoris involves a single coronary artery and is easily accessible. It is concentric, smooth, noncalcified, short (less than 0.5 cm), subtotal, and occupies a straight portion of the artery that has no side branches and that supplies an area of myocardium "protected" by distal collateral vessels.[273] PTCA of such lesions has a primary success rate of greater than 85 to 90 per cent.[272, 274, 275] If at the end of the PTCA procedure there is evidence of intimal dissection and a residual diameter of less than 30 per cent narrowing (or a pressure gradient of less than 15 mm Hg) at the site of the coronary lesion, the risk of restenosis is low[276] and there is a high chance of symptomatic relief.[275] However, PTCA is being carried out with increasing frequency in lesions that are eccentric, calcified, less accessible and totally occluded.[276a] Each of these factors reduces the chance of primary success and adds risk to the procedure.

RISKS. Careful documentation of the risks of elective PTCA performed by experienced operators has shown that almost 90 per cent of procedures will be uneventful. However, "minor" complications (side-branch closure, blood loss requiring transfusion, and need for emergency recatheterization or femoral artery repair) will occur in approximately 7 per cent of cases and "major" complications (need for emergency surgery, myocardial infarction, and death) in approximately 4 per cent.[274] In one series the overall myocardial infarction rate was 2.6 per cent and total mortality was 0.1 per cent. The risk of complications is increased in females, in patients with multivessel disease, and those with eccentric or calcified lesions. Of particular importance is the observation that the presence of angiographic intimal dissection after PTCA substantially increases the immediate risk of a major complication[274, 274a] but also favors long-term patency of the vessel.[276]

Consideration of *multivessel PTCA* must take into account the experience of several groups. This research strongly suggests that incomplete revascularization following multivessel PTCA may be associated with an increased restenosis rate and recurrence of angina,[277–279] morbid events, and the need for coronary artery surgery. The risk of restenosis of a lesion is approximately 30 per cent[276] within the first 6 months of the procedure with angina recurring in the majority of patients with significant restenoses. Accordingly, the rate of restenosis is greater following multivessel angioplasty. However, the success rate of reangioplasty procedures is at least equivalent to initial procedures.

An essential requirement for any institution performing PTCA is the availability of prompt surgical revascularization. Emergency surgery will be required in approximately 5 per cent[274, 275] of patients undergoing elective PTCA (for severe coronary artery dissection, occlusion, or intractable angina) and is usually associated with a higher morbidity and mortality.[280]

Left main coronary artery lesions are usually associated with significant disease elsewhere in the coronary arteries and thus present major potential risks, both at the time of PTCA and later if restenosis occurs. In our view, attempts at PTCA in this situation are almost always contraindicated unless some protection is provided by a patent graft to the circumflex or anterior descending coronary arteries.

If left ventricular function is impaired, successful reperfusion by PTCA can improve both systolic[281] and diastolic[282] function, even though the risks of the procedure are increased. Indeed, significant long-term improvement in coronary artery hemodynamics (equivalent to results of coronary artery surgery) is seen following successful PTCA.[283] This improvement is reflected in improved myocardial function during exercise[284, 284a] and long-term improvements in symptoms[275] and reduction in morbid events.[277–279, 285]

PTCA of the native coronary circulation or grafts is feasible after previous coronary artery bypass surgery to improve symptomatic status and avoid the need for reoperation.[286] Better long-term results are achieved with dilatation of distal graft lesions than of those located proximally or in the graft body.[279] Even totally occluded coronary arteries can be dilated,[287–289] especially if there is a short nonvisualized segment of occluded artery of known short duration.[288]

Invariably, a number of issues should be considered as the risks and benefits of PTCA are balanced against those of coronary artery surgery in individual patients. There are no absolute rules, but the following questions should be considered:

1. How experienced is the angioplasty team and is there adequate surgical backup?
2. How "favorable" is the lesion?
3. What are the potential consequences of abrupt total occlusion of the vessel to be dilated?
4. What are the chances of achieving complete revascularization?

These factors involve judgment and discussion among cardiologists, surgeons, patients, and their families.

Laser Angioplasty

Successful vaporization of atherosclerotic plaques and intracoronary thrombi using an argon laser passed through a fiberoptic catheter (i.e., transluminal laser coronary angioplasty) has been reported in a variety of animal and human necropsy models.[290–292] Laser-generated light eliminates plaque by converting it from solid-phase matter to a soluble gas. However, perforation of the vessel wall under the target lesion remains a major obstacle to widespread clinical use. The development of pulsed lasers[290] and excimer systems (which operate in the near-ultraviolet range)[291] may minimize adjacent thermal injury, and in conjunction with adequate visual control could be widely applicable. In addition to reperfusion, it is possible that laser-induced thermal fusion of separated layers of atheromatous arterial wall may eventually be useful in the treatment of arterial dissections.[293]

GUIDELINES FOR MEDICAL TREATMENT OF CHRONIC STABLE ANGINA

Risk factor modification is most important in younger patients with chronic stable angina (under the age of approximately 50 to 55). This is most easily accomplished by cessation of cigarette smoking and treatment of hypertension. What effect reduction of serum cholesterol levels will have on the regression of atheromas is unclear, but it is unlikely to be significant unless a markedly elevated serum cholesterol is radically reduced. Perhaps currently available methods of diet and drug therapy may slow the progression of the disease. Similarly, the relationship between maintenance of blood sugar within the normal range in diabetics and preventing vascular disease is far from settled.

In mild chronic stable angina, drug therapy may be limited to sublingual nitroglycerin on an "as necessary" basis if pain episodes are relatively infrequent (once or twice a week). It should also be used prophylactically in situations known to precipitate angina. If nitroglycerin is required on a daily basis, either long-acting nitrate preparations or moderate doses of a beta blocker (e.g., atenolol 25 to 50 mg/day) or both may also be employed. The doses of the drugs will depend on how well they are tolerated and on the clinical response. Resting heart rate should be lowered to 50 to 60 beats/min and heart rate during ordinary activity should be below 100 beats/min to assure adequate beta blockade. The clinical response can often be estimated by an improvement in exercise tolerance or the degree of ST-segment depression during a standard treadmill test. If the patient is still symptomatic at high doses of a beta blocker (> 320 to 400 mg/day propranolol or the equivalent) and long-acting nitrates (e.g., isosorbide dinitrate, 40 to 80 mg/day), a calcium antagonist should be added. The relative advantages and disadvantages of the three available agents have been discussed. Whichever is selected, a relatively low dose is given to begin and dosage is increased gradually.

There is no unanimity concerning when a patient with chronic angina pectoris should undergo cardiac catheterization, coronary arteriography, and left ventriculography. Some physicians take a more aggressive posture with patients under 50 years of age, with the hope of finding a lesion that demands revascularization; others prefer to wait for development of refractoriness to medical therapy, regardless of the patient's age. We believe that the use of noninvasive tests, as outlined on page 1321, can be extremely helpful in identifying patients with chronic stable angina at high risk of coronary events or early death; if there are no contraindications to coronary revascularization in such patients, they should be subjected to coronary arteriography. Similarly, patients for whom medical therapy fails should undergo coronary arteriography.

CORONARY ARTERY SURGERY

OPERATIVE PROCEDURE (See also Chap. 51)

Beta-adrenoceptor blockers, nitrates, and calcium antagonists are continued until surgery. Most surgeons perform coronary artery surgery using cardiopulmonary bypass at moderate hypothermia (24° to 32°C) with hemodilution. A motionless heart is achieved by continuous aortic cross-clamping with profound cardiac hypothermia and cardioplegia induced with cold potassium solution.[294] Simultaneous topical and core myocardial hypothermia (such as achieved by direct injection of cold solutions into the coronary arteries) have been recommended to provide uniform myocardial cooling. Rapid diastolic cardiac arrest is the aim and in the U.S. the most commonly used agent to achieve this is a high-concentration potassium chloride solution. Both crystalloid and blood cardioplegic solutions have been used with success.[295]

VENOUS CONDUITS. When vein grafts are used, the autologous saphenous vein remains the first choice. Arm vein grafts do not appear as effective as either saphenous

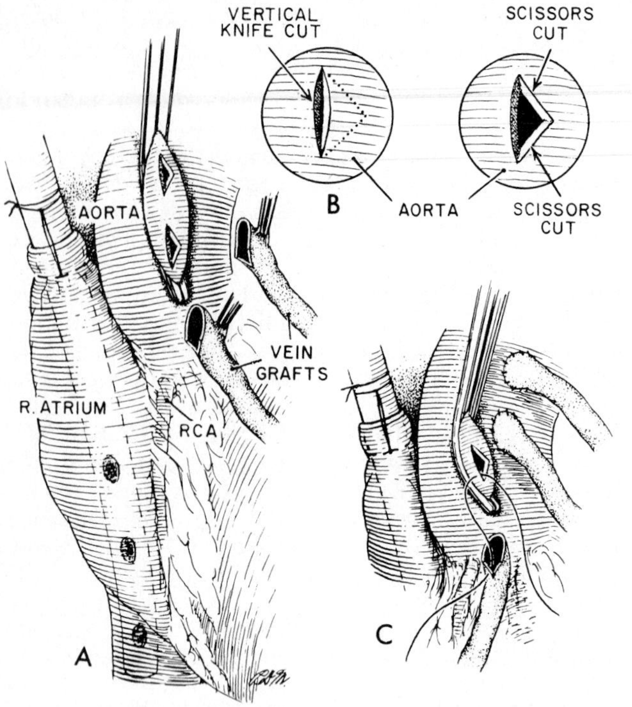

FIGURE 39–7. The aorticovenous anastomosis. *A* shows the direction of the anastomotic site for left-sided grafts; *B* shows details of aortic orifices; *C* shows the direction of right coronary artery (RCA) grafts. (From Cohn, L. H.: Surgical techniques of emergency coronary revascularization. *In* Cohn, L. H. [ed.]: The Treatment of Acute Myocardial Ischemia: An Integrated Medical-Surgical Approach. Mt. Kisco, N.Y., Futura Publishing Co., 1979, p. 87.)

veins or internal mammary artery grafts.[296, 297] Care in harvesting and handling veins before insertion may have a major influence on structural postoperative changes in vein grafts.

The vein grafts are inverted so that the distal end of the vein is placed proximally as an end-to-side anastomosis on the aorta (Fig. 39–7). The distal end of the vein is then placed as an end-to-side anastomosis on the coronary artery (Fig. 39–8); side-to-side anastomoses permit revascularization of several coronary artery branches with a single saphenous vein graft. In order to avoid obstruction of the graft by thrombotic occlusion, care must be exercised in the physical handling as well as in the positioning and arching of the vessels. Revascularization should include bypass of all major arterial segments with more than 50 per cent stenoses of the luminal diameter.[298]

INTERNAL MAMMARY ARTERY BYPASS GRAFTS. In patients under the age of 65 years, the internal mammary artery usually is remarkably free of atheroma. When it is grafted to a coronary artery, it appears to be immune to the development of intimal hyperplasia, which is almost universally seen in aortocoronary vein grafts, and atherosclerotic changes develop in only a small percentage of patients after coronary artery surgery.[299] The internal mammary artery is delicate and great care has to be taken to mobilize the vessel satisfactorily without traumatizing it (Fig. 39–9). This prolongs the operative time and often involves entry into the pleural space. The internal mammary is therefore not usually used for emergency surgery or in patients with left main coronary artery disease. Some investigators believe that the reason for better results obtained with internal mammary grafting in virtually all studies is patient selection bias, i.e., fewer patients with

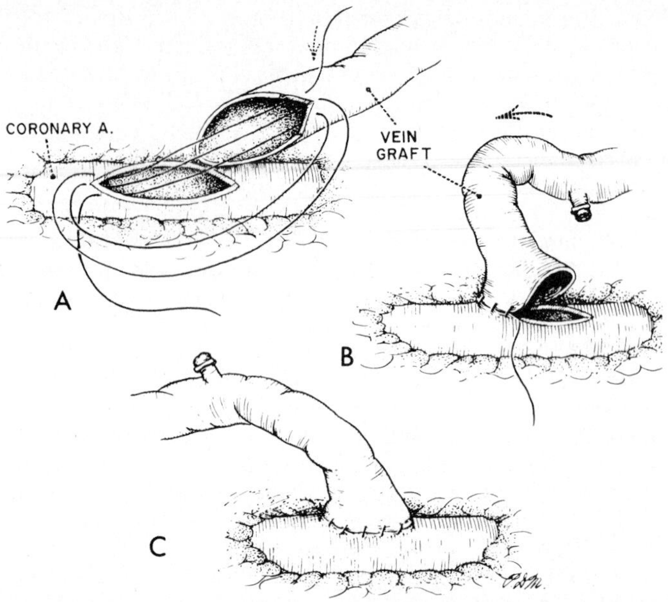

FIGURE 39–8. The venocoronary anastomosis to the proximal portion of the arteriotomy. (From Cohn, L. H.: Surgical techniques of emergency coronary revascularization. *In* Cohn, L. H. [ed.]: The Treatment of Acute Myocardial Ischemia: An Integrated Medical-Surgical Approach. Mt. Kisco, N.Y., Futura Publishing Co., 1979, p. 87.)

poor left ventricular function, clinical instability, left main coronary artery disease, and unstable angina receive internal mammary grafts. With rare exceptions, numerous studies have demonstrated patency of the internal mammary artery grafts of about 95 per cent at one year. After 7 to 10 years the patency of internal mammary artery grafts is 85 to 95 per cent.[300, 301] Loop et al.[302] have compared results in patients who received an internal mammary artery graft to the anterior descending coronary artery alone or combined with one or more saphenous grafts with those in patients who had only saphenous vein bypass grafts. The patency of the internal mammary artery was

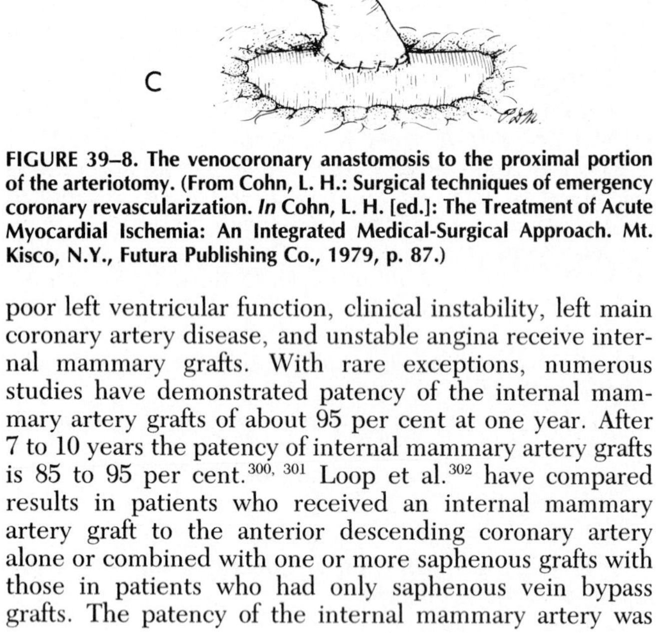

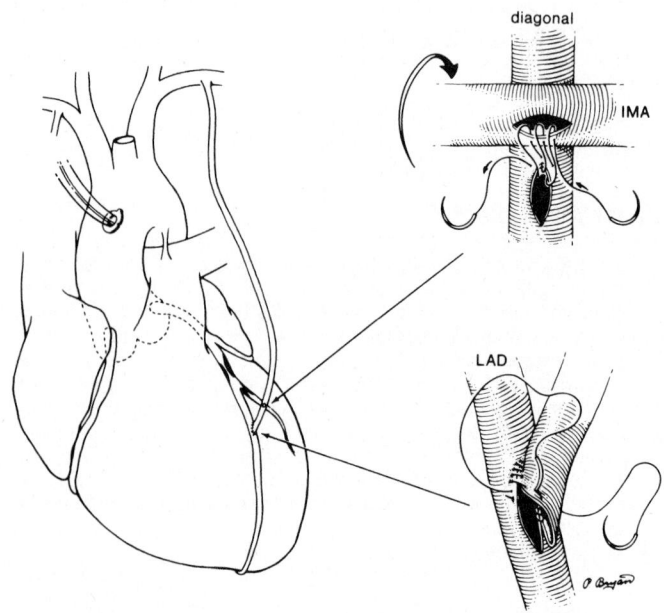

FIGURE 39–9. Internal mammary grafting: Schematic representation of in situ left internal mammary artery (IMA) graft to the left anterior descending (end-to-side) and diagonal branch (side-to-side) employing the diamond anastomotic technique to the latter. The details show the IMA pedicle rolled up over the diagonal coronary artery to facilitate exposure and use of continuous suture. (From Jones, E. L.: Extended use of the internal mammary coronary artery bypass. J. Cardiac Surg. 1:13, 1986.)

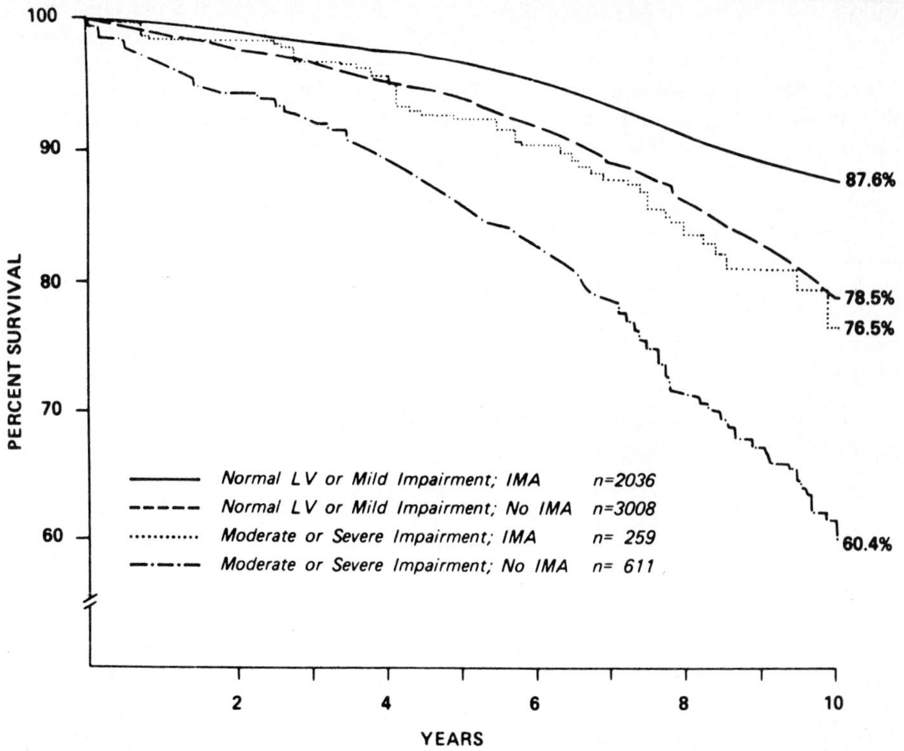

FIGURE 39–10. Influence of the internal mammary artery graft on ten-year survival. Patients who received an internal mammary artery graft to the anterior descending coronary artery alone or combined with one or more saphenous vein grafts were compared with patients who had only saphenous vein bypass grafts. The internal mammary artery (IMA) group had significantly higher survival rates for all categories of left ventricular performance, as compared with the vein-graft-only group. (Reprinted with permission from Loop, F. D., et al.: Influence of the internal mammary artery graft on 10-year survival and other cardiac events. N. Engl. J. Med. *314*:1, 1986.)

higher than that of the saphenous vein grafts. The 10-year actuarial survival was better among the patients receiving internal mammary grafts for patients with one-, two-, and three-vessel disease (Fig. 39–10).

The use of internal mammary artery grafting is safe and not associated with increased surgical morbidity or mortality.[303] Recently, reports have shown that multiple internal mammary artery grafts can be used[304] as well as sequential[305, 306] and other types of grafts[307] (Fig. 39–11). The diameter of the internal mammary artery graft more nearly matches that of the recipient coronary artery than does the saphenous vein. Whereas total flow through an internal mammary graft is less, the velocity of flow may be greater than a vein graft because of the smaller diameter of the artery.[308] Many surgeons now believe that whenever indicated and if technically feasible, internal mammary artery grafting (at least for lesions of the anterior descending coronary artery) is the preferable treatment. Except in emergency situations, they use internal mammary grafts.[309–311]

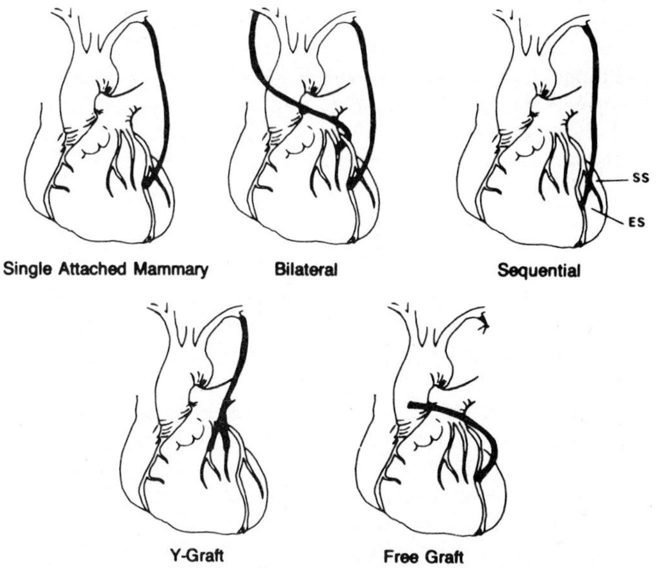

FIGURE 39–11. Different types of internal mammary artery grafts. A single attached internal mammary artery graft (either the right or left) remains attached proximally to the subclavian artery and is connected to the coronary arteries. Bilateral internal mammary artery grafts (right and left) are joined end-to-side to coronary arteries. Sequential internal mammary artery grafts consist of an attached or free internal mammary artery with one or more side-to-side anastomoses and one end-to-side anastomosis. The internal mammary artery Y graft has two terminal branches of either the attached or free internal mammary artery sutured to two coronary arteries. A free internal mammary graft is placed by transsecting the right or left internal mammary artery near its origin in the subclavian artery, and the proximal artery is anastomosed to the aorta with the distal end to the coronary artery. (From Tector, A. J., et al.: Expanding the use of the internal mammary artery to improve patency in coronary artery bypass grafting. J. Thorac. Cardiovasc. Surg. *97*:9, 1986.)

Mild Obstruction. Intraoperative studies have shown that arteries with less than 50 per cent obstruction of the luminal diameter often have minimal, if any, pressure gradients across the lesions and little difference in blood flow through the artery, as measured by clearance of xenon-133, when the bypass graft is opened.[312] Patients with higher-grade obstructions usually have greater pressure gradients across the lesions, and flow through the artery may increase significantly when the bypass graft is opened.

The Distal Vasculature. The state of the distal coronary arterial vasculature is also important. Late patency of grafts is related to coronary arterial runoff, as determined by the diameter of the coronary artery into which the graft is inserted, the size of the distal vascular bed, and to a lesser degree the severity of coronary atherosclerosis distal to the site of insertion of the graft.[313] The highest graft patency rates are found when the lumina of the vessels distal to the graft insertion are greater than 1.5 mm in diameter, perfuse a large peripheral vascular bed, and are free of atheroma occluding more than 25 per cent of the vessel lumen. Vessel diameters measured at coronary arteriography correlate satisfactorily with those obtained at operation.[314] Whenever there is any question about the ability of a vessel to accept a graft, the surgeon should attempt the anastomosis (consistent with patient safety, of course), because subjective improvement clearly depends on the completeness of revascularization.[315]

Flow Rates. When measured at the time of operation, flow rates through saphenous vein grafts average nearly 70 ml/min. Those in which the flow is less than 45 ml/min—and especially less than 25 ml/min—are frequently associated with graft closure, whereas closure is less common at flow rates exceeding 45 ml/min.[316, 317] The possible causes for reduced flow include subcritical obstruction of a proximal coronary artery; a technically poor anastomosis, with narrowing of the lumen due to kinking of the vessel or pinching at the site of the anastomosis; and a small myocardial mass perfused by the graft, which may in turn be due to diseased distal vasculature.

OTHER SURGICAL PROCEDURES FOR ISCHEMIC HEART DISEASE. Replacement of the aortic or mitral valve or both (Chap. 33) and left ventricular aneurysmectomy (p. 1365) may be performed with or without associated bypass grafting in patients with ischemic heart disease. When valve replacement or aneurysmectomy is carried out as the sole procedure, it is usually because of the presence of heart failure refractory to medical management. In most instances, these procedures are performed along with coronary revascularization; the fact that these procedures may add to the operative risk of simple bypass grafting may be related to the prolongation and greater complexity of the procedure, as well as to the fact that they are carried out on patients with left ventricular failure who are poor operative risks.

RESULTS OF SURGERY

OPERATIVE MORTALITY. Operative mortality for the treatment of stable and unstable angina pectoris has been declining steadily despite the fact that the median age of patients being operated on has increased by 15 years since the operation was developed in the late 1960's.[318] During the last 5 years excellent operative results have been obtained in patients with coronary artery disease and impaired ventricular function.[319-324] It is noteworthy that in patients of small stature (which probably correlates with small cardiac size and small coronary arteries), operative mortality is significantly increased and relief of angina is not as complete (see p. 1352). In the CASS, the overall mortality for patients operated on between 1975 and 1978 was 2.3 per cent. With increasing left ventricular dysfunction, operative mortality increased and operative mortality was also affected by age: 0 in patients under 30 years to 7.9 per cent in those over 70 years. As expected, operative mortality was 1.7 per cent for elective surgery, 3.5 per cent for urgent surgery, and 10.8 per cent for emergency surgery.[325] The risk was 8 per cent in patients undergoing resectional plication of aneurysm; it rose to 24 per cent in patients undergoing mitral valve replacement.

There were 8991 patients in the CASS Registry who underwent nonrandomized primary isolated coronary artery bypass grafting; 8971 had follow-up of more than 30 days.[326] The operative mortality was 2.4 per cent and the 5-year survival, 90 per cent. Patients with left main coronary artery disease had an operative mortality of 3.8 per cent and a five-year survival of 85 per cent, while patients with three-vessel disease had an operative mortality of 2.6 per cent and a 5-year survival of 88 per cent. In the CASS, operative mortality among the 15 participating centers ranged from 0.3 to 6.4 per cent; this emphasizes that the experience and skill of the team (surgeons, anesthesiologists, and cardiologists) play decisive roles in determining the outcome. In more recent series, mortalities as low as 0.8 per cent are reported for elective surgery.[327] The major areas of management that have been responsible for the currently low operative mortality of coronary artery surgery involve measures in both the intraoperative and perioperative periods. Improved anesthetic techniques, intraoperative protection of myocardium, conduit selection and preservation, blood conservation, perioperative hemodynamic monitoring, pharmacological left ventricular unloading, intraaortic balloon assistance, and arrhythmia control have all contributed.[295] In patients with active ischemia or extremely poor left ventricular function, operative mortality may be reduced when the intraaortic balloon is used to support the circulation during the perioperative period. There is still considerable variability among surgical groups, and the physician considering the referral of a particular patient for surgical treatment must be aware of the recent results obtained by the surgical group selected.

PERIOPERATIVE COMPLICATIONS

Perioperative Myocardial Infarction. This complication occurs in approximately 5 per cent of elective coronary revascularization.[328-331] In the CASS patients operated on between 1975 and 1979 the perioperative infarction rate, defined as the appearance of Q waves in the perioperative period, was reported as 6.4 per cent.[328] The incidence of perioperative infarction is usually related to the obstruction of a graft and correlates with the number of bypass grafts. Therefore, meticulous attention to anastomosis of the graft to the coronary artery is vital.[329] Although the loss of any viable myocardium obviously is undesirable, in most patients the perioperative infarcts are small. Patients experiencing a perioperative myocardial infarction have a higher perioperative mortality but no difference in 5-year survival than do patients without this complication.[330, 331]

Intellectual Dysfunction. It is common for patients to show impaired cognitive function early following coronary artery bypass surgery. This occurs in the absence of overt evidence of a perioperative stroke.[332] It is important that the physician reassure the patient and family that this is usually a temporary phenomenon which resolves in time.[333]

Hypertension. This complication can occur in up to one-third of all patients after coronary artery surgery.[334] The mechanism is unclear, but it may be related to increased levels of circulating catecholamines and renin. With the use of afterload-reducing agents such as intravenous sodium nitroprusside in the perioperative period, it rarely presents a problem. However, it is important that hypertension be adequately controlled to prevent cardiac failure and excessive perioperative bleeding.

Intraventricular Conduction Disturbances. In general, patients with coronary artery disease who develop fascicular conduction disturbances have diffuse myocardial disease and an unfavorable prognosis. A study of patients operated on in the mid 1970's indicated that patients with preoperative or surgically related left bundle branch block or intraventricular conduction defects had a higher mortality rate following bypass surgery than those without these findings.[335] The predominant causes of death were ventricular arrhythmias and cardiac failure. However, in patients operated on between 1976 and 1981 the development of new perioperative ventricular conduction disturbances did not worsen survival rate in patients followed up to 3 years.[335a] It is uncertain whether or not prophylactic pacemaker insertion would be of benefit.

Complications in the Obese. Physicians, nurses, and physiotherapists involved in the perioperative care of obese patients are well aware of the need for aggressive chest physiotherapy, the importance of mobilizing the patient rapidly, and potential problems with persistent immobilization in bed. One study compared patients who were markedly obese (33 per cent over ideal body weight) with a group of patients who were up to 8 per cent over ideal body weight. Although the markedly obese patients had a higher incidence of preoperative hypertension and hyperlipidemia, their operative mortality was not significantly higher. The markedly obese patients were more likely to have postoperative hypertension and wound infection and required more bronchodilator therapy.[336]

SYMPTOMATIC RESULTS. Major relief of angina pectoris occurs in most patients after coronary artery surgery[337–343]; however, return to full employment is disappointing in many series.[344] Factors that adversely affect the prospects of patients returning to work include increasing age,[345–348] postoperative angina,[345, 347–349] and either unemployment or a disability period before surgery.[345, 347, 348] Approximately half of patients will return to presurgery levels of household activity[350] and most will experience improved physical and sexual functional status.[351] By 10 years after coronary vein graft surgery the relief of symptoms and improved exercise performance noted at 5 years have decreased to levels seen in medically treated patients.[351a]

GRAFT PATENCY RATE AND CHANGES IN NATIVE CIRCULATION. Experimental studies and observations in humans suggest that there are several consecutive phases of disease development in venous aortocoronary artery bypass grafts[352–354] (Fig. 39–12).

Early Occlusion. Risk factors for early occlusion of venous grafts (which is reported to be 18 per cent in the month after operation[353] and is usually due to platelet thrombotic occlusion at the distal anastomotic site) include a small luminal size of the artery grafted, low vein graft blood flow, and kinking of the grafts. Bypass to the circumflex or right coronary artery is associated with a higher incidence of occlusion than the left anterior descending coronary artery. In addition, atheroma at the arteriotomy site or extension of the arteriotomy into a branch vessel may predispose to early occlusion. Perioperative platelet inhibitor therapy with aspirin and persantin appears to diminish the rate of early occlusion.

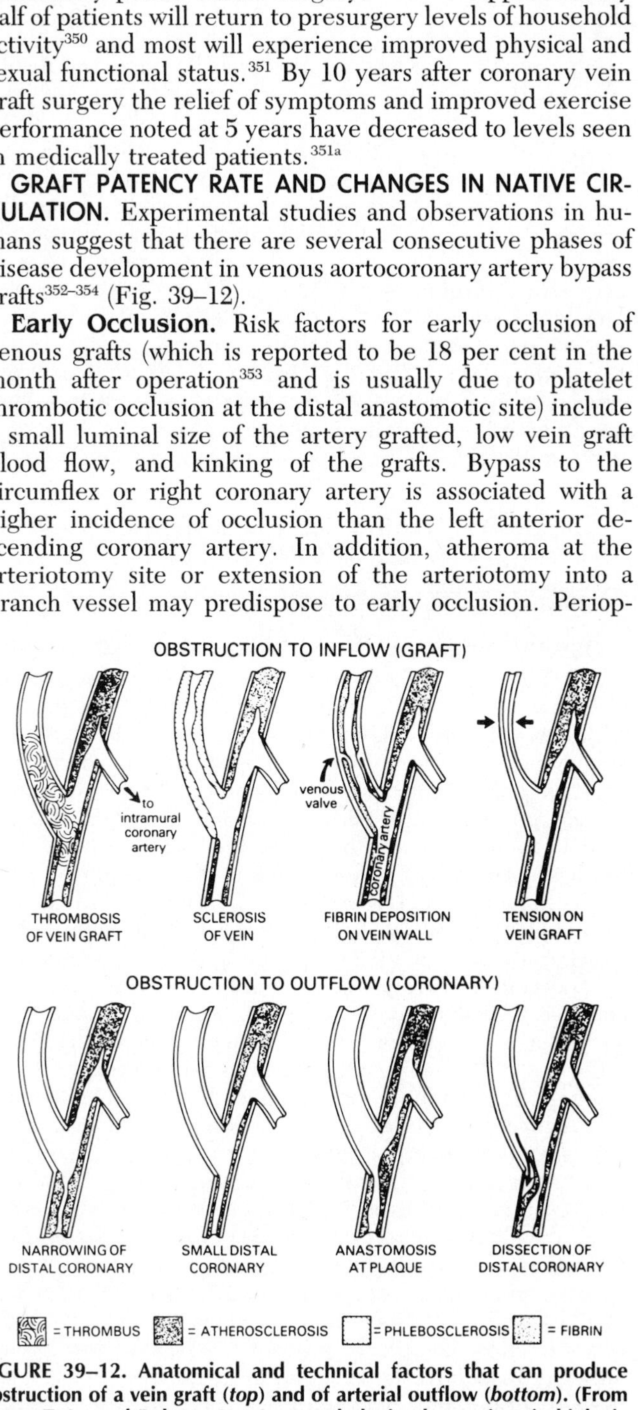

FIGURE 39–12. Anatomical and technical factors that can produce obstruction of a vein graft (*top*) and of arterial outflow (*bottom*). (From Spray, T. L., and Roberts, W. C.: Morphologic observations in biologic conduits between aorta and coronary artery. *In* Rahimtoola, S. [ed.]: Coronary Bypass Surgery. Philadelphia, F. A. Davis, 1977, p. 11.)

Intermediate Phase of Platelet-Related Intimal Hyperplasia. Intimal hyperplasia and smooth muscle cell proliferation of the vein graft are apparent within one month of operation and progress during the first postoperative year. This accelerated process of intimal hyperplasia is an early stage of atherosclerotic plaque formation and is believed to occur because of an interaction between platelets and chronic mild endothelial damage. If proliferation is severe and localized (as occurs at the site of the anastomosis between the graft and the recipient artery), total occlusion can occur within a year. However, if the proliferation is less severe and diffuse, the overall caliber of the vein graft can decrease by 25 to 30 per cent in diameter during this period. This phase of platelet deposition leading to smooth muscle cell proliferation and intimal hyperplasia is not prevented by platelet-inhibitor therapy.[353]

Late Occlusion. By the end of the first year, the overall occlusion rate per distal anastomosis is between 16 and 26 per cent and the chance of one or more distal anastomoses being occluded in an individual patient with multiple venous grafts are 41 to 47 per cent.[355–357] Both platelet thrombi and intimal hyperplasia contribute to this occlusion, and platelet inhibitor therapy is of benefit in preventing it. Eicosapentaenoic acid (found in high concentrations in salt water fish and synthetically refined cod liver oil) inhibits platelet-mediated intimal hyperplasia. Studies suggest that cod liver oil might be used to prevent intimal hyperplasia in vein grafts used for myocardial revascularization.[358]

In a prospective, randomized, double-blind trial, dipyridamole (started 48 hours before operation) plus aspirin (started 7 hours after operation) was compared with placebo treatment (Fig. 56-16, p. 1777). The daily maintenance therapy was dipyridamole 75 mg and aspirin 325 mg orally three times a day. Within one month of operation 3 per cent of vein graft distal anastomoses were occluded in the treated patients and 10 per cent in the placebo group. The proportion of patients with one or more distal anastomoses occluded was 8 per cent in the treated group and 21 per cent in the placebo group.[356] At angiography performed one year after operation, 11 per cent of 478 vein-graft distal anastomoses were occluded in the treated group and 25 per cent of 486 were occluded in the placebo group. The proportion of patients with one or more distal anastomoses occluded was 22 per cent of 171 patients in the treated group and 47 per cent of 172 in the placebo group.[357] This regimen of aspirin and dipyridamole was not associated with excess bleeding; its use appears reasonable in patients undergoing venous bypass grafting in the doses employed by the original investigators. It is possible, however, that dipyridamole is not essential[358a] and that much lower doses of aspirin (40 to 80 mg/day) may be sufficient.

Atherosclerosis in Venous Bypass Grafts. Beyond the first year, a histological picture indistinguishable from that of arterial atherosclerotic disease occurs[359] (Fig. 39–13). Some investigators think that, as in arteries, the development of atherosclerosis in vein grafts is a continuum starting from platelet deposition to smooth muscle cell proliferation, and finally to lipid incorporation into the plaque. The overall occlusion rate per distal anastomosis is 25 to 35 per cent at 5 to 7 years and 40 to 50 per cent at 10 years. At 11-year follow-up by the Montreal Heart Institute, only 60 per cent of grafts were patent and of these 46 per cent showed relatively severe atherosclerosis.[360]

Thus, the attrition rate of saphenous vein grafts and the

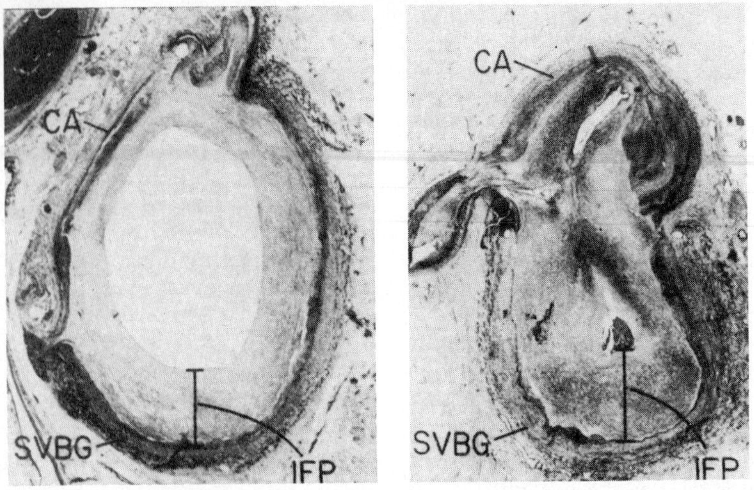

FIGURE 39–13. Postmortem histological sections through coronary artery (CA) anastomosis sites of saphenous vein bypass grafts (SVBG) show extensive fibrous tissue proliferation in the grafts' intimal layers. In the graft at left, the circumferential intimal fibrous plaque (IFP) developed in 5 months. In the graft at right, the process resulted in greater than 90 per cent stenosis 8 months after implantation. With time, such fibrous plaques may become infiltrated with lipids and calcium and increasingly resemble atherosclerotic plaques. (From Bulkley, B. H.: Why coronary bypass grafts fail: Early and late pathologic changes. J. Cardiovasc. Med. 5:1025, 1980.)

processes involved are fairly well known. There is a 15 to 20 per cent loss of patent grafts during the first year after operation, due to early thrombosis or intimal hyperplasia, or a combination of both. For the next 5 years the attrition rate is approximately 2 per cent per year; however, between 6 and 11 years after operation the mean attrition rate increases to 4 per cent per year.[355]

Nongrafted Coronary Arteries. Progression of disease in nongrafted diseased coronary arteries occurs at a rate of approximately 4 to 5 per cent per year during the first 11 years after operation.[359, 361] While determination of graft patency usually involves postoperative angiography, radionuclide techniques assessing myocardial perfusion may also indicate graft patency.[362, 363] Serial imaging after coronary surgery may identify patients with a greater or lesser likelihood of graft occlusion. In patients who have no or atypical chest pain, the absence of new thallium perfusion defects correlates well with patency of all grafts. In contrast, the development of new perfusion defects in addition to the return of typical or atypical chest pain indicates a high probability of graft occlusion.[363] Contrast-enhanced computer tomography also may be used to assess patency of saphenous vein grafts (Fig. 12–10, p. 363).

Effects of Hypercholesterolemia. It has been observed that LDL and LDL-B cholesterol levels are higher and that HDL cholesterol levels are lower 11 years after operation in patients with atherosclerotic grafts than in patients with normal grafts.[364] Seventy-nine per cent of patients without new atherosclerotic lesions had normal lipid and normal plasma LDL apoprotein levels compared with only 8 per cent of patients whose grafts showed new atherosclerotic lesions. These observations suggest strongly (but do not prove) that efforts should be made to establish as normal as possible a lipid profile, i.e., LDL and HDL concentrations, postoperatively, utilizing dietary and pharmacological methods described on page 1167. In addition, body weight should be at an ideal level and cessation of smoking in the postoperative period should be mandatory.

LATE SURVIVAL. The large randomized trials of coronary artery surgery have provided detailed information of late survival (p. 1347). The important influence of left ventricular function on both operative mortality and long-term survival has been described (p. 1348). Other factors that may influence long-term postoperative survival adversely include NYHA functional class III or IV,[365] ST-segment depression on the resting baseline electrocardiogram,[365, 366] a history of hypertension and myocardial infarction,[365] evidence of peripheral arterial disease,[366] advanced age, continued cigarette smoking, and hypercholesterolemia.[367] Progressive atherosclerosis in both grafts and native vessels following coronary artery surgery may be adversely affected by abnormal plasma lipoprotein levels.[364] When the results of coronary artery surgery were compared in patients with and without diabetes mellitus at a mean follow-up of 3.8 years, there was no significant difference with respect to relief of symptoms or survival in the two groups[368] despite the fact that associated hypertension, peripheral vascular disease, and prior myocardial infarction were twice as common in diabetic patients. The 10-year results of coronary artery surgery in patients age 35 or younger showed excellent actuarial survival rates of 94 per cent at 5 years and 85 per cent at 10 years despite the severity of the underlying disease and the rapidity of the atherosclerotic process in these patients.[369] However, during longer follow-up, atherosclerosis of the venous grafts becomes an increasingly important problem.[369a]

MEDICAL VERSUS SURGICAL THERAPY OF (STABLE) ANGINA PECTORIS

Prognostic Considerations

OBSERVATIONS WITHOUT ANGIOGRAPHIC ASSESSMENT. The Framingham Study revealed over a long period of follow-up that the average annual mortality of patients with chronic stable angina was 4 per cent.[370] Remission of angina may occur in up to one-third of patients with angina of recent onset. However, if the condition has been present for several years, remission is unusual. Survivors of myocardial infarction had a 5 per cent annual mortality after the first postinfarction year.[370] Others have reported similar,[371] higher,[372] and lower mortality rates.[373] In a long-term follow-up study of 586 men who had survived an attack of unstable angina or acute infarction and who were treated conservatively, the survival at 5 years was 80 per cent, at 10 years was 61 per cent, and at 15 years it was 43 per cent.[373] The severity of angina pectoris has some influence on the survival of patients with coronary artery disease. In a patient population with normal ventricular function and a similar extent of coronary disease, those with severe angina (perhaps reflecting albeit indirectly the severity of ischemia) have a worse prognosis.[374] Data from the Veterans Administration Study have shown that clinical factors such as the severity of symptoms, the presence of an abnormal resting electrocardiogram (ST-segment depression), and a history of either myocardial infarction or hypertension all adversely affect outcome, particularly if two or more factors are present.[375] The European Coronary Study Group showed that an abnormal resting electrocardiogram and peripheral vascular disease also adversely affect survival in medically managed patients with chronic coronary artery disease.[338] Others have reported the adverse influence of hypertension on prognosis in patients with established coronary artery disease, and cigarette smoking appears to increase the incidence of sudden death. Cardiomegaly on a routine chest x-ray and the presence of a third sound on physical examination have adverse effects on prognosis because they reflect more extensive myocardial damage.[376]

In patients presenting with acute myocardial infarction, there are four easily measurable clinical factors that contribute to prognosis as long as 6 to 15 years after infarction.[377] These are (1) the patient's age, (2) the presence or absence of cardiac enlargement on the first chest x-ray after admission, (3) the presence or absence of pulmonary congestion or edema on the first chest x-ray, and (4) the presence or absence of a previous infarction at the time of the index infarction. A number of studies have confirmed the adverse prognostic significance of myocardial dysfunction and cardiac arrhythmias in survivors of infarction.[378–383] It is widely accepted that a low left ventricular ejection fraction and significant ventricular ectopy after infarction are important independent determinants of poor long-term prognosis, the former being more important than the latter.[384] Not surprisingly, electrocardiographic abnormalities, particularly Q waves in multiple leads, intraventricular conduction defects, and left ventricular hypertrophy (three signs common in patients with significant left ventricular dysfunction), are associated with a poor prognosis in coronary artery disease.[385, 386]

PROGNOSIS BASED ON ANGIOGRAPHIC CRITERIA. In angiographic criteria for prognostic evaluation, the two important variables are (1) left ventricular function and (2) the severity and extent of coronary artery disease. In general, the extent of left ventricular dysfunction is a more important determinant of prognosis than the extent and severity of coronary artery disease.[387] The follow-up of patients in the CASS Registry has allowed the accurate study of survival of medically treated patients with angiographically assessed coronary artery disease. Both the number of major coronary arteries with severe obstruction and the degree of depression of left ventricular ejection fraction were independent adverse risk factors, the latter again exerting the dominant influence.[388] These two risk factors are synergistic in that the adverse effects on prognosis of impaired ventricular function are more pronounced as the number of stenotic vessels increases (Fig. 39–14).

Studies in *symptomatic* patients have revealed that if only one of the three major coronary arteries has more than 50 per cent stenosis, the annual mortality rate will be approximately 2 per cent.[389, 390] The importance of the quantity of myocardium that is jeopardized is reflected in the observation that an obstructive lesion proximal to the first septal perforator of the left anterior descending coronary artery was associated with a 5-year survival of 90 per cent, compared with one of 98 per cent in patients with more distal lesions.[390] Proximal lesions of the right coronary artery or left circumflex coronary artery were not associated with decreased survival compared with distal lesions. The survival rate of patients with right coronary artery disease at 5 years appeared to be higher (96 per cent) than in patients with disease of the left anterior descending coro-

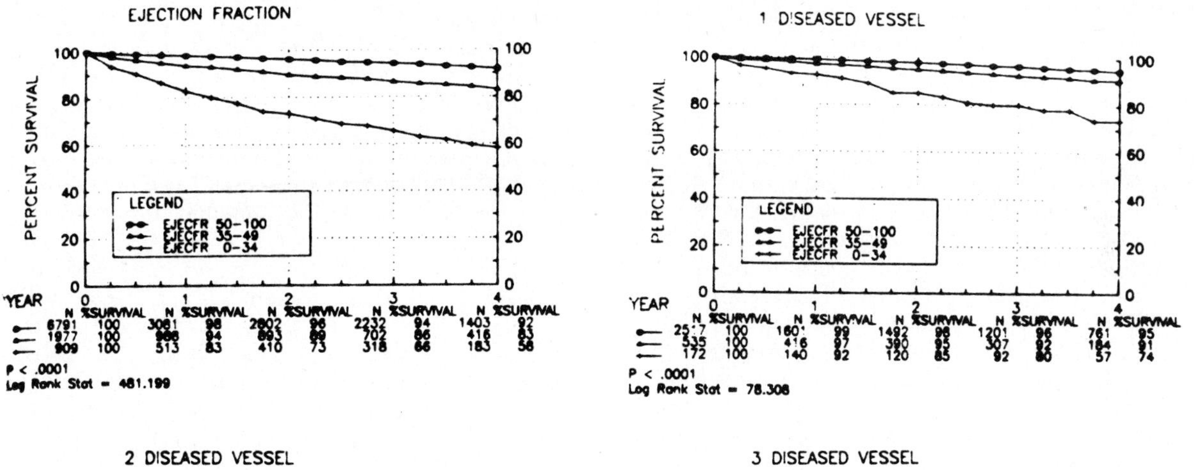

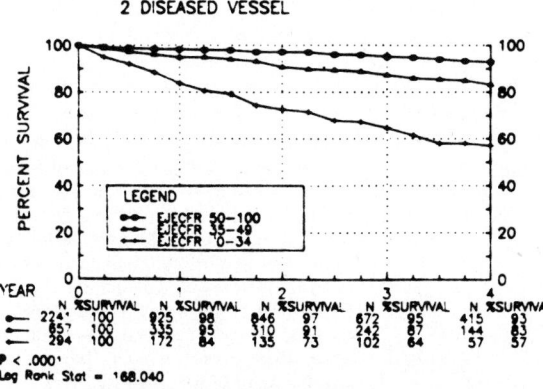

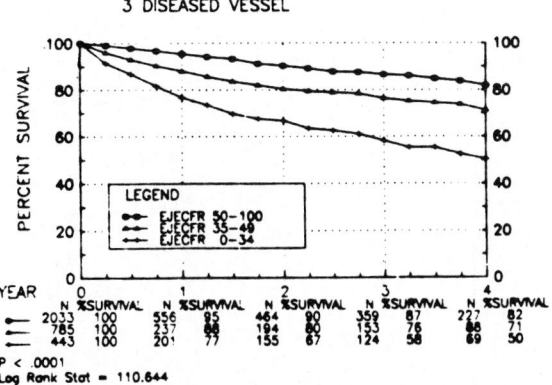

FIGURE 39–14. Effect of the anatomical extent of obstructive coronary artery disease and left ventricular function on survival in medically treated patients in CASS Registry. Survival of medically treated patients with no significant obstructive disease was 97 per cent in contrast to 92 per cent, 84 per cent and 68 per cent of patients with one-, two-, and three-vessel disease, respectively. In patients with less than 50 per cent left main coronary artery obstruction and measured ejection fraction (EJEC FR), the effect of decreasing ejection fraction on survival is evident, even when the probability of survival is already high, such as in patients with one or two obstructed arteries. As the severity of arterial disease increases, the impact of left ventricular dysfunction is even greater upon survival. (From Mock, M. B., et al.: Survival of medically treated patients in the Coronary Artery Surgery (CASS) Registry. Circulation 66:562, 1982, by permission of the American Heart Association, Inc.)

nary artery (92 per cent). The overall survival of nonsurgically treated patients with left anterior descending and left circumflex coronary artery disease was not significantly different, but both were less than the survival of patients with isolated right coronary artery disease.[390] The risk of cardiac events does not appear to be related to the presence or absence of collateral vessels in patients with one-vessel coronary disease[391]; however, even in patients with single-vessel disease, left ventricular ejection fraction was the baseline descriptor most strongly associated with survival.

In symptomatic patients, if two of the three major arteries exhibit severe (>75 per cent) stenosis, the annual mortality is approximately 7 per cent and if all three vessels are stenotic it rises to approximately 11 per cent.[392–394] In an observational study of patients with obstructive coronary disease who initially were treated medically, 15-year survival rates were 48, 28, 18, and 9 per cent for patients with single-, double-, triple-, and left main vessel disease, respectively.[395] Sixty of the original 598 patients had operations for coronary disease during the period of the study. In addition to the number of vessels involved, the severity of obstruction is also important. Prognosis for patients with 50 to 75 per cent narrowing is better than for those with more than 75 per cent narrowing.[396]

High-grade lesions of the *left main coronary artery* are particularly life-threatening. Mortality among medically treated patients has been reported as 29 per cent at 18 months,[397] 39 per cent at 2 years,[398] 48 per cent at 2 years,[399] and 50 per cent at 3 years.[400] Survival is better for patients having a 50 to 70 per cent stenosis (1- and 3-year survivals of 91 per cent and 66 per cent, respectively) than for patients with a greater than 70 per cent left main stenosis (1- and 3-year survivals of 72 and 41 per cent)[400] (Fig. 39–15). Furthermore, a number of noninvasive and catheterization characteristics are predictors of an adverse prognosis in patients with 70 per cent or greater left main stenosis; these include chest pain at rest, ST-T wave changes on the resting electrocardiogram, cardiomegaly on the chest roentgenogram, a history of congestive heart failure, findings of left ventricular dysfunction at catheterization, and elevation of the arterial-mixed venous oxygen difference.[400] Characterization of patients with left main coronary artery stenosis with a lesser degree of risk adds flexibility to their management.

The *severity of symptoms* is a useful prognostic factor in conjunction with arteriographic findings. In asymptomatic or mildly symptomatic patients with one- or two-vessel disease, the prognosis is excellent and annual mortality is approximately 1.5 per cent. In patients with three-vessel disease with good exercise capacity (achievement of 85 per cent predicted heart rate or workload of 100 watts or more), the annual mortality rate is also only 4 per cent, but in those with poor exercise capacity it is much higher.[401] During exercise testing in the CASS randomized study (a group of patients with mild angina or history of infarction and a left ventricular ejection fraction of greater than 35 per cent), the presence of exercise-induced angina identified patients who had a survival advantage over 7 years if assigned to surgical therapy (94 per cent survival), compared with medical therapy (87 per cent survival).[402]

The assessment of *ventricular function* and extent and severity of coronary artery disease have been major influences in determining our understanding of the natural history of coronary artery disease and have been of help in determining which patients should be selected for surgical therapy (p. 1348). Taken together, the available information suggests that the volume of myocardium perfused by critically narrowed vessels (and therefore at risk of necrosis) and the rate of progression of coronary atherosclerosis are the principal determinants of prognosis in patients with coronary artery disease. In some patients, the conversion of a stable atherosclerotic plaque into an ulcerated plaque and the proclivity for development of coronary thrombosis (p. 1227) as well as the development of electrical instability may also affect prognosis.

EXERCISE ELECTROCARDIOGRAPHY AND OTHER NONINVASIVE TESTS FOR PROGNOSTIC EVALUATION. The aims of exercise electrocardiographic testing, thallium scintigraphy, and exercise radionuclide ventriculography are to provide data about ventricular function and the quantity of myocardium becoming ischemic during stress. In this manner, an assessment of the patient's functional status and the quantity of "jeopardized" myocardium can be assessed. In patients in whom left ventricular function and coronary anatomy have also been defined, exercise stress testing can provide important additional prognostic information. In patients with known coronary anatomy undergo-

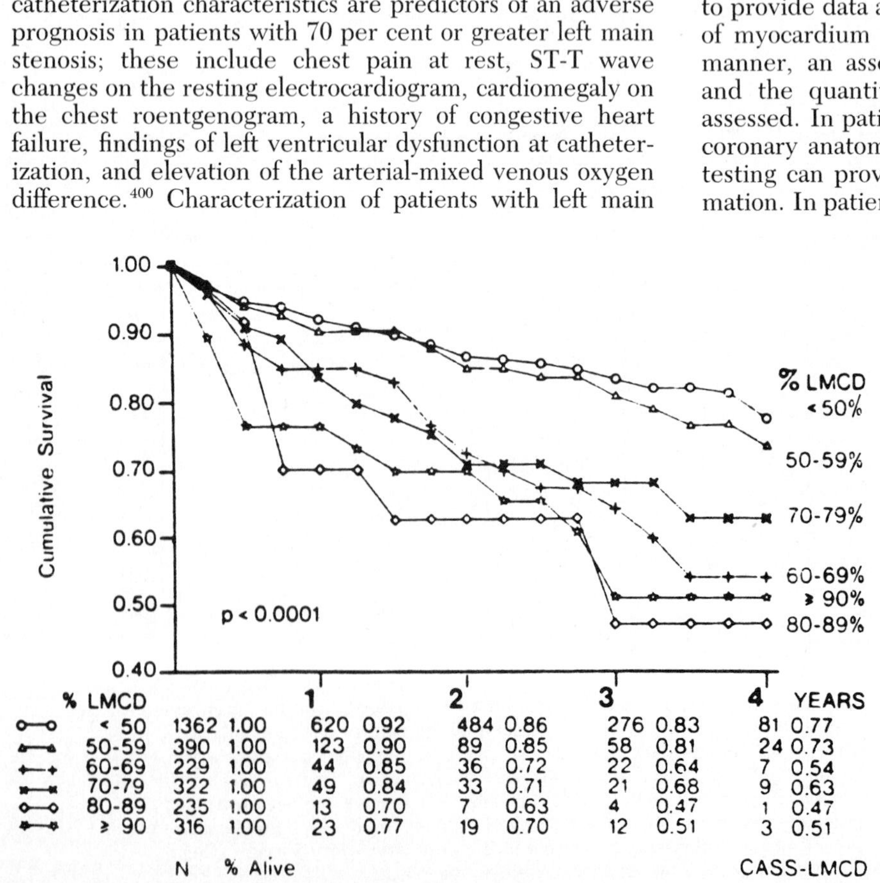

FIGURE 39–15. Survival curves for medically treated patients with left main coronary disease. The cumulative survival rates of nonsurgically treated patients with left main coronary disease (LMCD) in the CASS Registry analyzed according to per cent intraluminal narrowing are demonstrated. The survival curves separate when the degree of angiographically assessed stenosis exceeds 60 per cent, so that patients with a lesser degree of narrowing have relatively favorable long-term prognosis. (From Chaitman, B. R., et al.: Effect of coronary bypass surgery on survival patterns in subsets of patients with left main coronary artery disease. Am. J. Cardiol. *48*:765, 1981.)

TABLE 39–9 RISK STRATIFICATION BY EXERCISE TESTING

Study	Patients (N)	Risk Classification: Low	Intermediate	High
McNeer et al Circulation 57:64, 1978	1,472	<1 mm ST ↓ FS ≥ IV Peak HR ≥ 160 beats/min		≥1 mm ST ↓ FS I or II
Bruce et al (Seattle Heart Watch) Circulation 60:638, 1979	2,001	<1 mm ST ↓ No LV dysfunction	≥1 mm ST ↓ No LV dysfunction	FS ≤ I Peak SBP <130 mm Hg Cardiomegaly
Dagenais et al Circulation 65:452, 1982	107	≤2 mm ST ↓ FS ≥ IV	≤2 mm ST ↓ FS ≥ III	≥2 mm ST ↓ FS ≤ I
Schneider et al Am. J. Cardiol. 50:682, 1982	80			>1 mm ST ↓ FS I or II
Weiner et al Am. Heart J. 105:749, 1983	292	≤2 mm ST ↓ No LV dysfunction		LV dysfunction or ≥ 2 mm ST ↓ beginning in stage I
Weiner et al (CASS) J. Am. Coll. Cardiol. 3:772, 1984	4,083	<1 mm ST ↓ FS ≥ III	≥1 mm ST ↓ FS ≥ III	≥1 mm ST ↓ FS ≤ I

N = number, FS = final exercise stage (Bruce protocol), LV = left ventricular, SBP = systolic blood pressure, HR = heart rate, CASS = Coronary Artery Surgery Study.

From Deering, T. F., and Weiner, D. A.: Prognosis of patients with coronary artery disease. J. Cardiopulmon. Rehabil. 5:325, 1985.

ing graded, multistage exercise testing which is terminated for symptoms or marked ST-segment changes, the duration of exercise (exercise stage entered) and the presence or absence of ST-segment change during exercise (greater than 0.1 mV of ST-segment change) identifies subgroups at high and low risk (Table 39–9). Patients able to exercise into or beyond stage IV of the Bruce protocol (or its equivalent) or able to achieve a maximum heart rate of greater than or equal to 160 beats/min and/or with a negative ST-segment response have a one-year survival of greater than 98 per cent even if significant coronary artery disease is present. Patients stopping exercise in the early stages (Bruce stages I or II) at a low heart rate with a positive ST-segment response have a survival of only 80 to 85 per cent at 12 months.[104, 403]

Using the CASS Registry, 30 clinical and exercise variables were analyzed in 4083 patients with defined ventricular function and coronary anatomy to assess factors of prognostic importance.[404] The duration of exercise and the ST-segment response emerged as the most important exercise test variables. In a subgroup of 570 patients with three-vessel coronary disease and preserved left ventricular function, the probability of survival at 4 years ranged from 53 per cent for patients only able to achieve stage 1 of exercise to 100 per cent for patients able to exercise into stage V of the standard or modified Bruce protocol. Patients showing less than 0.1 mV of ST-segment depression who could exercise into stage III of the Bruce protocol or higher had an annual mortality of 1 per cent or less, while those with at least 0.1 mV ST-segment depression who could not complete stage I had an annual mortality of 5 per cent or more. In patients with two-vessel disease and good ventricular function, noninvasive exercise test parameters also distinguished between high- and low-risk subsets.[405]

STRESS THALLIUM-201 MYOCARDIAL PERFUSION IMAGING (see also p. 335). Exercise thallium scintigraphy may be helpful in identifying areas of myocardium in which ischemia may be induced and that may benefit from revascularization. It is known that in patients with chest pain, a normal exercise scintigram confers an excellent prognosis even if underlying coronary artery disease has been demonstrated angiographically.[406, 407] Predictors of adverse prognosis following thallium-201 scintigraphy performed during exercise, or after administration of dipyridamole, include a delayed tracer redistribution, multiple large perfusion defects, and abnormal lung uptake.[334] The limitations of 201-thallium scintigraphy include the high cost, the long imaging time, interpretation difficulties by nonexperts, and poor imaging in markedly obese individuals. Furthermore, the patient has to be able to attain a sufficient level of exercise before a normal perfusion pattern can be assumed confidently to indicate no significant underlying coronary artery disease. However, dipyridamole can be employed in patients with severe exercise limitations.

EXERCISE RADIONUCLIDE ANGIOGRAPHY (see also p. 314). A number of studies suggest that the exercise left ventricular ejection fraction is one of the best prognostic predictors of major future cardiac events or of high-risk coronary artery disease.[408] In patients with known coronary artery disease, if the exercise left ventricular ejection fraction does not rise appropriately or if it falls, this suggests that there is sufficient ischemia to prevent the normal decrease in end-systolic volume observed with exercise. A fall of left ventricular ejection fraction in patients whose initial resting left ventricular ejection fraction is 30 per cent or higher may be associated with left main coronary disease or severe three-vessel disease and may indicate a high mortality over the next 1 to 2 years.[408] Jones et al. found that during preoperative evaluation patients who had the most profound exercise-induced left ventricular dysfunction prior to myocardial revascularization had an improved survival,[409, 410] while those with a normal ejection fraction response to exercise did not.

In patients whose left ventricular function and coronary anatomy have been defined, the demonstration of ischemia or jeopardized myocardium may have a profound bearing on management. In a study of minimally symptomatic patients with preserved resting left ventricular function and three-vessel disease, evidence of impaired exercise capacity combined with the demonstration of inducible myocardial ischemia identified those at high risk of death during medical therapy.[411] Patients who did not manifest ischemia during exercise by radionuclide angiography or exercise electrocardiography had an excellent prognosis compared with those with impaired exercise capacity, especially if it occurred at a low workload (Fig. 39–16).

EFFECT OF SURGICAL THERAPY ON RELIEF OF ANGINA, LONG-TERM SURVIVAL, AND OCCURRENCE OF MYOCARDIAL INFARCTION

RELIEF OF ANGINA PECTORIS. As early as 1972, a committee of the American Heart Association indicated that the most widely accepted indication for surgical re-

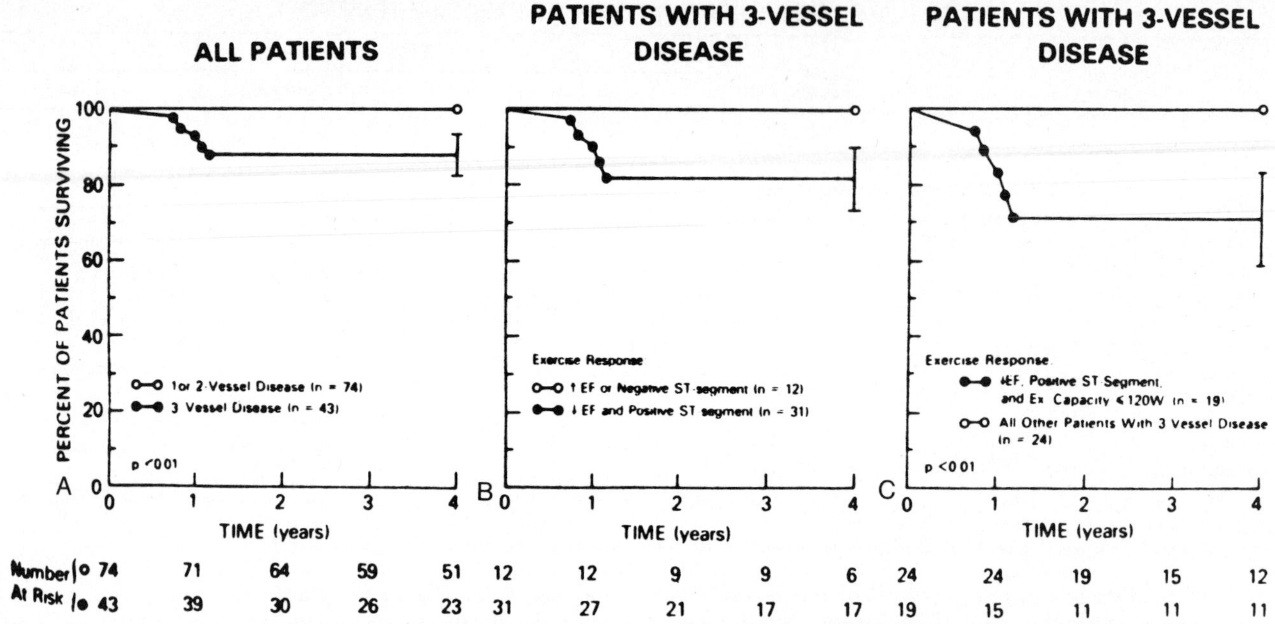

FIGURE 39–16. Influence of anatomical severity of coronary artery disease, reversible ischemia, and exercise capacity on survival in mildly symptomatic patients with coronary artery disease and left ventricular ejection fractions greater than 40 per cent. Survival curves are shown for patients with three-vessel disease as compared with those with one- or two-vessel disease (*A*), patients with three-vessel disease and an increase in ejection fraction (EF) or a negative ST-segment response to exercise as compared with those with three-vessel disease and both a decreased ejection fraction and a positive ST-segment response with exercise (*B*), and patients with three-vessel disease and a decrease in ejection fraction during exercise, a positive ST-segment response, and exercise capacity of 120 watts or less as compared with all other patients with three-vessel disease (*C*). The number of patients with potential follow-up at each time is shown for each group. Evidence of impaired exercise capacity associated with evidence of reversible myocardial ischemia defines a group of patients with three-vessel disease with an adverse prognosis long term. (Reprinted with permission from Bonow, R. O., et al.: Exercise-induced ischemia in mildly symptomatic patients with coronary artery disease and preserved left ventricular function. N. Engl. J. Med. *311*:1339, 1984.)

vascularization was "significant disability from moderate to severe angina pectoris, unresponsive to optimal medical care."[412] This remains the principal indication; however, myocardial revascularization is now being carried out in increasing numbers of patients with unstable angina unresponsive to medical therapy (p. 1358) and in patients with postmyocardial infarction angina.[413]

Relief of angina pectoris occurs in up to 95 per cent of patients with chronic stable angina following coronary artery surgery. Over half the patients become totally asymptomatic, at least initially. Most of the others exhibit substantial although not total symptomatic relief.[337] Five years after coronary artery surgery, the major randomized trials have all demonstrated greater relief of angina, better exercise performance, and a lower requirement for cardiac medications for these patients as compared with medically treated patients.[338–340] Follow-up studies show a reoperation rate of 5 per cent per year for recurrence of symptoms.[414] By 5 years after operation the percentage of surgical patients who retain marked symptomatic improvement has decreased to 40 to 50 per cent and the use of beta blockers has increased progressively[337, 340] (Fig. 39–17). Improvement is maintained best in those with the most complete revascularization.[341]

Prospective assessment of progression of coronary artery disease in randomized medical and surgical patients over a 5-year angiographic period of follow-up shows that two-thirds of patients in each group will show progression of coronary artery disease. This is most likely to occur at the site of a previously documented lesion.[361] In surgically treated patients, the rate of progression in ungrafted arteries and in the portions of the arteries distal to grafts occurs at the same rate as in medically treated patients. However, progression of disease in both obstructed and normal segments of coronary artery proximal to a graft occurs at a higher and faster rate than in corresponding segments in a medically treated group.[361]

For patients with persistent angina despite adequate medical therapy and for those who cannot tolerate the usual antianginal medications and who are not ideal candidates for PTCA, coronary artery surgery provides excellent symptomatic relief. It is likely that with increasing use of internal mammary artery grafts long-term relief of angina and freedom from subsequent cardiac events will improve compared with previous patient populations who have received coronary artery vein grafts alone (p. 1338).

Long-Term Survival

LEFT MAIN CORONARY ARTERY STENOSIS. There is general agreement that surgical treatment improves survival in patients with left main coronary artery obstruction[415, 416] (Fig. 39–15). As already pointed out (p. 1344), the presence of left main coronary artery stenosis does not define a homogeneous population.[400, 415, 416] Coronary bypass surgery appears to confer the most benefit on patients with severe degrees of left main coronary artery disease and/or those patients with impaired left ventricular function. However, it is still beneficial in all patients with stenoses greater than 50 per cent and for patients with normal left ventricular function.[416]

There is continuing debate about whether there is "a left main equivalent," which has a natural history similar to that of left main coronary disease. The condition in question may consist of disease in the proximal portions of both the left anterior descending and left circumflex coronary arteries. We believe that the ominous nature of significant left main coronary disease exists because a single

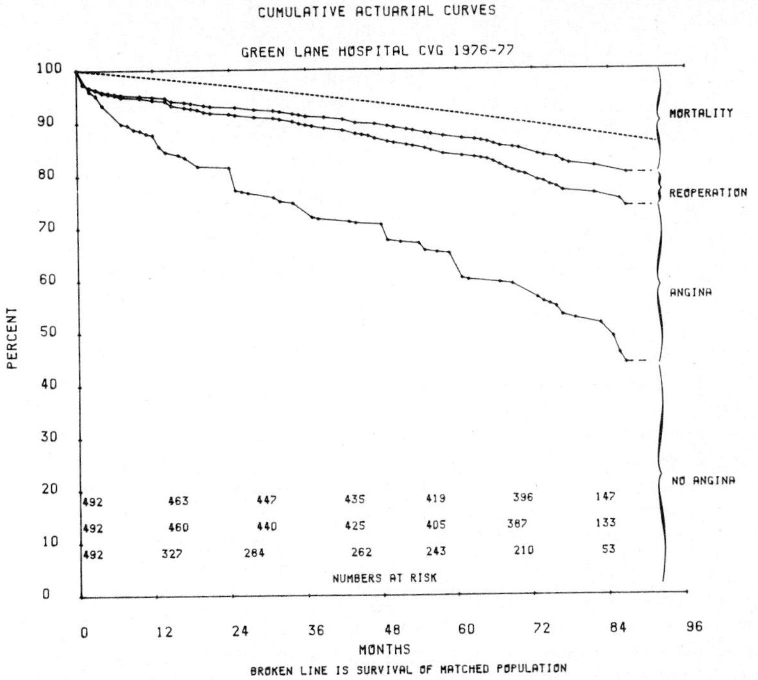

FIGURE 39–17. Cumulative actuarial morbidity and mortality curves for patients following coronary artery surgery. The results of 492 consecutive coronary artery bypass grafting operations performed for angina (1976–1977) were evaluated 77 months after surgery during a 2-month period. Cumulative actuarial curves (Kaplan-Meier) for patients were constructed for the variables of death, reoperation for recurrence of angina, and presence or absence of postoperative angina. Numbers of patients at risk at different time intervals for each of the three variables are shown at base of graph (numbers at risk). The mortality of an age-matched population for the years 1976 and 1977 is shown by the broken line. Six years after coronary artery surgery, 84 per cent of the population was alive, 5 per cent had undergone reoperation for angina, and 57 per cent of the population was alive and free of angina after initial operation. (From Rutherford, J. D., et al.: Multivariate analysis of the long-term results of coronary artery bypass grafting performed during 1976 and 1977. Am. J. Cardiol. *57*:1264, 1986.)

pathophysiological event can cause infarction of a large quantity of myocardium. While combined disease of the proximal left anterior descending and circumflex coronary arteries does identify a subgroup of high-risk patients, their prognosis is not as poor as those with left main coronary disease.[417]

ONE-VESSEL, TWO-VESSEL, OR THREE-VESSEL CORONARY ARTERY DISEASE WITH OR WITHOUT IMPAIRED VENTRICULAR FUNCTION. There has been considerable interest in and debate of the question of whether coronary artery surgery will prolong life or prevent myocardial infarction in patients who do not have severe symptoms and who have obstructive coronary artery disease other than left main coronary artery disease. Three major randomized clinical trials enrolling patients at different time periods and with different entry criteria have provided data that help answer these questions.

THE VETERANS ADMINISTRATION COOPERATIVE STUDY. This study prospectively examined the effects of coronary artery surgery as opposed to medical treatment in 686 adult males, randomly allocated to surgical or medical management in 1972 to 1974.[365, 375, 418–420] The patients were males who had stable angina pectoris of at least 6 months' duration, electrocardiographic evidence of either prior infarction or ischemia at rest or during exercise, significant coronary disease of at least one major coronary artery with a graftable distal segment, and a left ventricular ejection fraction greater than 25 to 30 per cent.

By 7 years after randomization survival rates were 70 per cent with medical treatment and 77 per cent with surgical treatment ($p = 0.043$), but by 11 years the rates were 57 and 58 per cent, respectively, presumably because of late occlusion of the venous grafts.[419] *Retrospective* analyses have revealed that coronary artery surgery appears to confer an advantage over medical therapy in patients at high *clinical* risk (having two or more of the following: NYHA class III or IV, a history of hypertension, previous myocardial infarction, and ST depression on the resting electrocardiogram). It also conferred an advantage in a high *angiographic* risk group (impaired left ventricular function and three-vessel coronary artery disease).

The Veterans Administration Study participants have summarized their long-term survival results as follows: coronary artery surgery did not significantly improve *overall* survival in patients without left main disease, while a significant survival benefit was seen with surgery at 5 to 7 years in subgroups of patients with multiple clinical and angiographic risk factors. This benefit diminished gradually when follow-up was extended to 11 years. The majority of patients who did not belong to high-risk subgroups derived no benefit from surgical treatment at any time.[420]

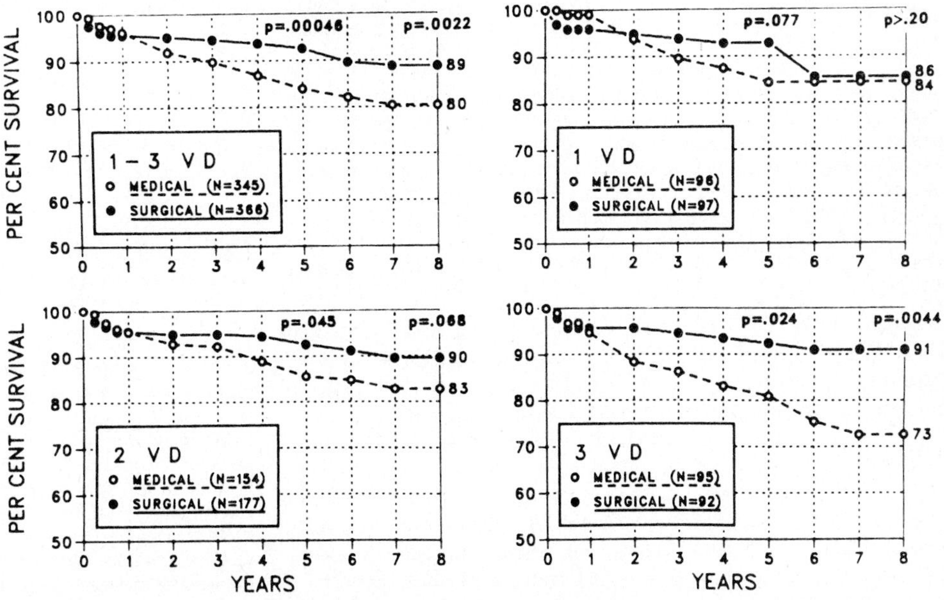

FIGURE 39–18. Cumulative survival curves for patients in the European Coronary Surgery Study. In order to compare the European prospective randomized coronary surgery study with other studies a cohort of 711 patients were identified as having greater than 75 per cent obstruction in one, two, or three vessels. A significant improvement in survival with surgery was found in the total cohort and in the subgroup with three-vessel disease; however, there was no significant difference in survival between the two treatments in patients with one-vessel disease and those with two-vessel disease without proximal left anterior descending stenosis. (From Varnauskas, E., and the European Coronary Surgery Study Group: Survival, myocardial infarction, and employment status in a prospective, randomized study of coronary bypass surgery. Circulation *72*[Suppl. V]:90, 1985, by permission of the American Heart Association, Inc.)

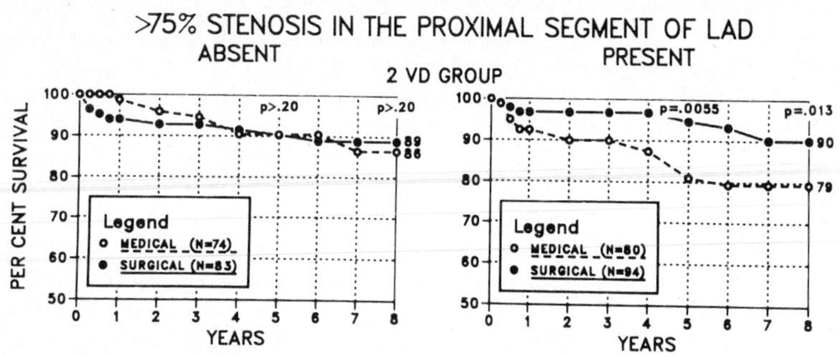

FIGURE 39–19. Cumulative survival for the subgroup of patients with double-vessel disease (2 VD group) in the European Coronary Study Group when disease is defined as 75 per cent or greater narrowing and is subdivided by the presence or absence of disease in the proximal segment of the left anterior descending coronary artery (LAD). This retrospective analysis suggests that surgery may confer an advantage over medical therapy in patients with two-vessel disease in whom both narrowings are greater than 75 per cent of luminal diameter and one of them is the proximal segment of the left anterior descending coronary artery. (From Varnauskas, E., and European Coronary Surgery Study Group: Survival, myocardial infarction, and employment status in a prospective, randomized study of coronary bypass surgery. Circulation *72*[Suppl. V]:90, 1985, by permission of the American Heart Association, Inc.)

THE EUROPEAN CORONARY SURGERY STUDY GROUP. Men under the age of 65 with mild to moderate chronic stable angina (57 per cent were in classes I or II Canadian Cardiovascular Society and 42 per cent were in class III), significant stenoses in at least two major coronary arteries, and good left ventricular function (ejection fraction greater than 50 per cent) were randomized to medical or surgical treatment between 1973 and 1976.[338, 366, 421–423] At 8 years of follow-up the policy of early surgery improved survival significantly compared with medical treatment in the total population (89 vs. 80 per cent) and in the subgroup with three-vessel disease (92 vs. 77 per cent) (Fig. 39–18) and in the patients with two-vessel disease in which one of the diseased vessels was the proximal segment of the left anterior descending coronary artery (90 vs. 79 per cent) (Fig. 39–19). There was no significant difference in survival between medical and surgical treatment in patients with one-vessel disease and in those with two-vessel disease without stenosis of the proximal left anterior descending coronary artery. Other variables that signified a better survival with surgery included an abnormal electrocardiogram at rest, ST-segment depression greater than 1.5 mm during exercise, peripheral arterial disease, and age over 50 years (Table 39–10).

The study participants believed that in "high-risk" patients with mild-to-moderate chronic angina pectoris and good left ventricular function, coronary arteriography should be performed if two or more of the above-mentioned noninvasive high-risk predictors exist. Subsequently, they would advise surgery for patients who show stenoses of at least three major coronary arteries or those who have greater than 75 per cent stenoses in two major vessels, one of which is the proximal segment of the left anterior descending coronary artery, as well as in patients with a 50 per cent or greater stenosis of the left main coronary artery.[366]

CORONARY ARTERY SURGERY STUDY (CASS). In this, the most recent prospective randomized trial of coronary artery surgery,[319, 320, 328] patients age 65 or younger with mild angina or with a myocardial infarction more than 3 weeks previously were randomized to medical or surgical therapy between 1975 and 1979 if they had significant operable coronary artery disease. After 7 years, cumulative survival in patients with one-, two-, and three-vessel disease assigned to surgical and medical treatment were 92 and 90 per cent for one-vessel disease, 88 per cent in each group for two-vessel disease, and 88 and 83 per cent respectively for patients with three-vessel disease.[320] A significant advantage favoring surgical assignment was observed in patients with three-vessel disease and ejection fractions between 35 per cent (Fig. 39–20) and 50 per cent. Eighty-eight per cent of patients in the surgical group and 65 per cent of those in the medical group were alive (p = 0.009). An important CASS Registry study has demonstrated that in patients with *severe* angina, surgery improves survival in those with three-vessel disease regardless of whether ventricular function is normal or depressed.[374] Other studies have also suggested that patients who demonstrate the most severe ischemia-induced ventricular dysfunction during exercise are most likely to benefit subsequently with respect to survival, relief of pain, and improvement in exercise capacity.[409, 410, 424]

TREATMENT OF PATIENTS WITH SEVERELY DEPRESSED LEFT VENTRICULAR FUNCTION.

A number of studies have examined the outcome of medical as opposed to surgical therapy in patients with coronary artery disease and severely depressed left ventricular function.[321–324, 324a] In a CASS Registry study[322] surgical treatment was shown to prolong survival, particularly in patients with ejection fractions below 0.26 per cent. A 43 per cent 5-year survival was noted with medical treatment compared with 63 per cent 5-year survival with surgical treatment (Fig. 39–21). In a more recent study examining the late results of surgical and medical therapy for patients with coronary artery disease and resting ejection fractions of less than 36 per cent, 7-year survival and freedom from nonfatal infarction were greater in the surgically treated patients than in the medically treated ones. Surgical treatment also was associated with improved survival in the patients with an ejection fraction of 25 per cent or less.[324] These studies suggest that if operative mortality is lower than approximately 7 per cent, surgery is likely to offer an advantage over medical therapy in terms of survival and relief of anginal symptoms in patients with ischemic jeopardized myocardium and severely depressed left ventricular function. There is no evidence that surgery improves survival in asymptomatic survivors of two or three myocardial infarctions with multivessel disease.[425]

The relationship between poor surgical outcome and clinical evidence of congestive heart failure, hemodynamic evidence of left ventricular dysfunction, and extensive wall motion disorders on left ventricular angiography is well recognized. Clinical descriptors such as a history of heart failure (particularly if such a history predominates over a history of angina pectoris), pulmonary rales, previous need of a diuretic or digitalis, and a cardiothoracic ratio of 0.50 or more are all associated with a significantly higher operative risk. In the Coronary Artery Surgery Study (CASS)[325] and the CASS Registry,[326] there was increasing operative mortality with increasing evidence of left ventricular dysfunction; 5-year survival was also adversely affected. Patients with normal or near-normal left ventricular function had an operative mortality rate of 2 per cent and a 5-year survival of 92 cent. Patients with moderate impairment had an operative mortality of 4.2 per cent and a 5-year

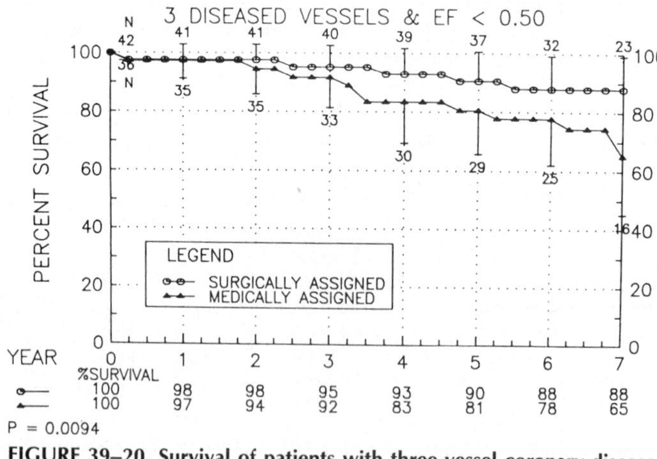

FIGURE 39–20. Survival of patients with three-vessel coronary disease and left ventricular dysfunction. In the CASS trial, the survival of patients with three diseased vessels and left ventricular ejection fractions less than 0.50 after 7 years of follow-up was 88 per cent in patients assigned to surgical treatment and 65 per cent in patients assigned to medical treatment. The numbers of patients at risk each year, for each treatment, are shown on the graphs. (From Killip, T., et al.: Coronary artery surgery study [CASS]: a randomized trial of coronary bypass surgery. Eight years follow-up and survival in patients with reduced ejection fraction. Circulation *72*(Suppl. V):102, 1985, by permission of the American Heart Association, Inc.)

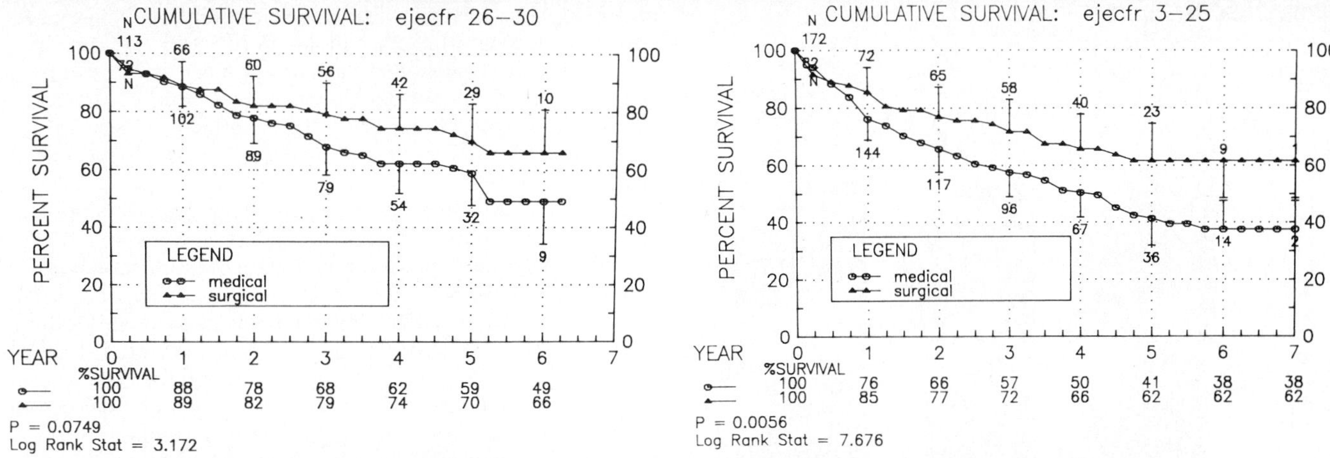

FIGURE 39–21. Life table cumulative survival curves for patients with severe left ventricular dysfunction. A CASS Registry study identified 420 medically treated and 231 surgically treated patients (coronary graft plus myocardial surgery in 30 per cent) who had severe left ventricular dysfunction manifested by an ejection fraction below 0.36 and markedly abnormal wall motion. Life table cumulative survival for patients with an ejection fraction of 0.26 to 0.30 (*left panel*), and for patients with ejection fractions of 0.03 to 0.25 (*right panel*) are shown. The survival curves are adjusted for all other significant prognostic variables. The P values associated with each analysis are shown in the bottom left corner of the figures. Surgical benefit was most apparent for patients with ejection fractions below 0.26 who had a 43 per cent 5-year survival with medical treatment versus a 63 per cent 5-year survival with surgery. Surgically treated patients experienced substantial symptomatic benefit compared with medically treated patients if their presenting symptoms were predominantly angina; however, there was no relief of symptoms caused primarily by heart failure. The operative mortality in this high-risk subset was 6.9 per cent. (From Alderman, E. L., et al.: Results of coronary artery surgery in patients with poor left ventricular function [CASS]. Circulation *68*:785, 1983, by permission of the American Heart Association, Inc.)

survival of 80 per cent, and in those with poor ventricular function the operative mortality was 6.2 per cent and 5-year survival was 65 per cent.

ASSESSMENT OF CONTRACTILE RESERVE. In patients with impaired left ventricular function it may be useful to estimate ejection fraction and left ventricular wall motion in the basal state as well as after inotropic stimulation or afterload reduction in order to show enhancement of otherwise depressed wall motion.[152–153] The term *contractile reserve* is used to describe the ability of ventricular wall segments that contract abnormally in the basal state to exhibit augmented contractility, often with an increase in overall ejection fraction in response to a suitable stimulus. Zones of the myocardium responding to inotropic stimulation or to a decrease in afterload may improve functionally after revascularization (Fig. 39–22).[152] Nesto et al. have reported that survival following revascularization is better among patients whose ejection fraction rose by more than 10 per cent when stimulated by either epinephrine or postextrasystolic potentiation than in those in whom this failed to occur.[153] The demonstration of augmentation of contractility acutely, and similar improvement after revascularization, is related to the finding that many hypokinetic (and even akinetic) areas of ventricular wall are composed either of ischemic, although viable, muscle or of a mixture of the latter and fibrous scar. The viable muscle is capable of responding to the inotropic stimulation and its contraction may respond to improved perfusion after operation.[154] In contrast, necrotic tissue obviously cannot be stimulated to contract by any pharmacological or hemodynamic intervention nor by improved perfusion.

In patients with poor left ventricular function and poor contractile reserve (less than 10 per cent increase in ejection fraction with inotropic stimulation), perioperative mortality is high and long-term survival is poorer than in patients with equally depressed left ventricular function but with normal contractile reserve.[152–154]

Myocardial Stunning and Hibernation. Two related pathophysiologic conditions termed *myocardial stunning* (prolonged but temporary postischemic ventricular dysfunction without myocardial necrosis) and *myocardial hibernation* (persistent left ventricular dysfunction when myocardial perfusion is chronically reduced but is still sufficient to maintain the viability of tissue) have been defined (p. 1203). Hibernating myocardium results from months or years of ischemia, and ventricular dysfunction persists until blood flow is restored (p. 1325). In these patients the predominant clinical feature of myocardial ischemia may be elevation of left ventricular pressure and dyspnea secondary to ventricular systolic and/or diastolic dysfunction. Symptoms resulting from chronic left ventricular dysfunction may be inappropriately ascribed to myocardial necrosis and scarring when they may, in fact, be reversed when the chronic ischemia is relieved by coronary revascularization.[426–429]

Surgical Results in Patients With Left-Ventricular Dysfunction. While the risk of operation is higher in patients with depressed left ventricular function, it has been found that patients with moderately impaired[319] and

TABLE 39–10 FIVE-YEAR SURVIVAL IN MEDICALLY MANAGED PATIENTS WITH TWO- OR THREE-VESSEL CORONARY ARTERY DISEASE

Risk Factors				5-Year Survival (%)	
Proximal LAD stenosis	ST depression > 1.5 mm with exercise	Peripheral vascular disease	Abnormal resting ECG	2-Vessel disease	3-Vessel disease
−	−	−	−	98	96
+	−	−	−	94	92
+	+	−	−	88	83
+	+	+	−	69	60
+	+	+	+	−	40

LAD = Left anterior descending coronary artery.

From Rutherford, J. D.: Coronary artery surgery, 1984. N. Z. Med. J. 97:813, 1984. Adapted from European Surgery Study Group: Long-term results of prospective, randomized study of coronary artery bypass surgery in stable angina pectoris. Lancet 2:1173, 1982.

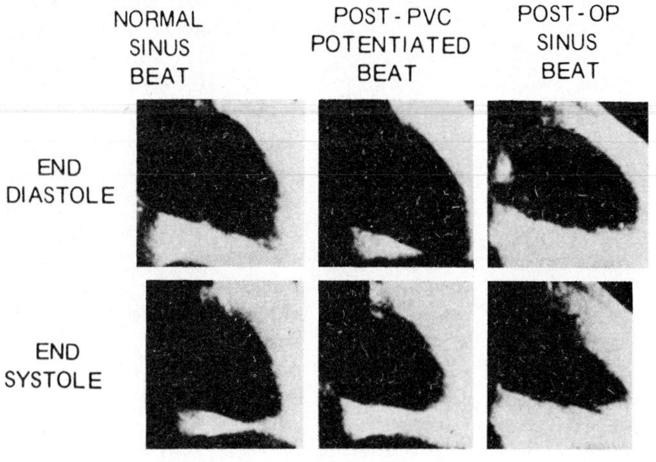

	PRE-OP NSB	PRE-OP pPVC	POST-OP
EDVI	138	151	156
ESVI	88	83	55
SVI	50	68	101
EF	36%	45%	65%

FIGURE 39–22. Examples of the ventriculographic analysis performed to evaluate the effects of an inotropic stimulus, including some of the calculations made. PVC = premature ventricular contraction, PRE-OP = preoperative, POST-OP = postoperative, NSB = normal sinus beat, pPVC = after premature ventricular contraction, EDVI = end-diastolic volume index (ml/m^2), ESVI = end-systolic volume index (ml/m^2), SVI = stroke volume index (ml/m^2), EF = ejection fraction. (From Popio, K. A., et al.: Post extrasystolic potentiation as a predictor of potential myocardial viability. Am. J. Cardiol. 39:944, 1977.)

even severely impaired left ventricular function[321–324] may have improved long-term survival as compared with similar patients with coronary artery disease treated medically. Indeed, patients with the worst ventricular function may show the most striking symptomatic and functional response to revascularization.[323] Furthermore, in patients with a history of heart failure and 3-vessel disease, coronary artery surgery may reduce the incidence of sudden death compared with those having medical therapy.[323a] Therefore, it is important to evaluate patients with heart failure secondary to coronary artery disease to determine whether their myocardium exhibits contractile reserve. If it does and the anatomy is appropriate we recommend surgical treatment, recognizing that higher than usual risks are involved.

CONCLUSIONS. In considering which groups of patients are likely to achieve a greater survival benefit from coronary artery surgery rather than medical therapy, the large randomized trials and CASS Registry studies all contribute important information. Clearly, coronary artery surgery is a procedure which prolongs survival in patients with significant left main coronary artery disease and is likely to confer even greater benefits to patients with severe stenoses with clinical or catheterization evidence of impaired ventricular function. In patients with moderately severe, stable angina pectoris and normal left ventricular function, the European study suggests that if several factors such as age greater than 50 years, an abnormal ECG at rest, ST-segment depression greater than 1.5 mm during exercise, and peripheral arterial disease are present (Table 39–10), coronary angiography should be performed. In such patients with three-vessel disease or coronary artery stenoses of greater than 75 per cent reduction in luminal diameter in the proximal left anterior descending coronary artery and one other major vessel, surgery appears superior to medical therapy.

Surgery also appears to have an advantage over medical therapy in patients with no or mild symptoms and three-vessel disease and moderately impaired ventricular function (ejection fraction 35 to 50 per cent). Other clinical risk factors in patients with three-vessel disease and either normal or impaired ventricular function that might lead to surgical rather than medical therapy include severe angina pectoris (class III or IV NYHA), a history of myocardial infarction or hypertension, and resting ST-segment depression on the electrocardiogram. There is no evidence that surgical therapy confers any advantage over medical therapy in patients with two-vessel disease (which does not include severe proximal involvement of the left anterior descending coronary artery) and single-vessel disease. Patients in this latter category are being treated with increasing frequency, whether or not they have symptoms or jeopardized myocardium, by PTCA. As yet there is no evidence to suggest that the benefits of successful dilatation outweigh the risks of the procedure or whether any survival advantage is conferred upon such patients.

The randomized trials have also suggested that both medical and surgical treatments have improved over time. In patients with angiographically confirmed three-vessel coronary artery disease treated medically, the annual mortality in the later 1960's was 11.4 per cent. Fifteen years later in the CASS it was only 2.1 per cent. (It is not clear how similar these two patient groups are.) For patients who have less than severe angina or who are free of angina after a recent infarction, if ventricular function is normal, surgical therapy does not appear to confer any benefits over medical therapy in terms of long-term survival for patients with one-, two-, or three-vessel coronary disease. If moderate angina pectoris exists, if the left ventricular ejection fraction decreases during exercise,[424] or if there is a positive symptom-limited exercise test in stages I or II of a standard Bruce protocol (or its equivalent) associated with 1.5 mm or greater ST-segment electrocardiographic depression, surgical therapy may confer some survival advantage to patients with three-vessel and with two-vessel disease involving the proximal left anterior descending coronary artery (Table 39–11).

For patients with coronary artery disease whose dominant symptom is angina pectoris and who have severely depressed left ventricular function (ejection fraction 35 per cent or less), surgery appears to offer survival advantages if critically narrowed vessels perfuse viable myocardium. In patients whose dominant symptoms are heart failure without angina and diffuse poor contraction of the left ventricle *without contractile reserve*, revascularization is unlikely to be beneficial.

OCCURRENCE OF MYOCARDIAL INFARCTION. In patients with chronic stable angina who do not satisfy the indications for operation shown in Table 39–11, there is no evidence that survival is improved. Bypass grafting is associated with some small risk (1 per cent mortality, 5 per cent incidence of infarction), and a progressive attrition of venous grafts occurs, particularly after 5 years.[355] Therefore, it is suggested that, in patients with normal ventricular function and mild to moderate symptoms on medical therapy, bypass surgery be postponed until the symptoms warrant consideration of this intervention.

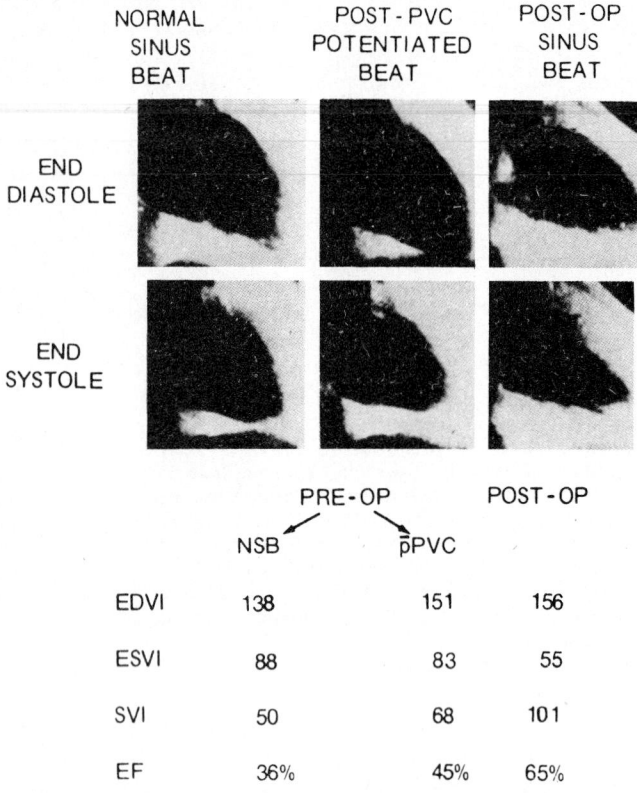

The major randomized trials do not suggest that coronary

TABLE 39–11 INDICATIONS FOR CORONARY ARTERY SURGERY IN PATIENTS WITH CHRONIC STABLE ANGINA

1. Angina pectoris that is severe, disabling, or interfering with life style on maximally tolerated medical therapy.
2. Results of noninvasive stress testing indicate extensive inducible ischemia, poor functional capacity, associated with critical (> 70%) obstruction in one or more vessels.
3. Left main coronary artery stenosis (> 60%).
4. Critical obstruction (> 70%) in three major coronary arteries with:
   a. Resting left ventricular dysfunction
   b. Normal resting left ventricular function + evidence of inducible ischemia or a poor exercise tolerance.
5. Critical obstruction of proximal left anterior descending artery with significant obstruction of one other major vessel + moderate angina pectoris and/or inducible ischemia.

artery surgery reduces the likelihood of myocardial infarction.[365, 430, 431] In the European Coronary Surgery study, separation of perioperative from late postoperative infarctions is not possible; however, after 5-year follow-up the incidence in the medical group (11 per cent) was not significantly different from that in the surgical group (15 per cent). In the CASS, in which the perioperative myocardial infarction rate was 6.4 per cent, surgery did not appear to prevent the occurrence of subsequent infarction.[431] In the Veterans Administration study there also was no significant difference in the incidence of nonfatal myocardial infarction between medically and surgically treated patients during the first 5 years of follow-up.

Although operative mortality and myocardial preservation techniques have improved greatly during the 15 years since the Veterans Administration study, there is still no evidence that surgical therapy is superior to medical therapy in reducing the incidence of myocardial infarction. The CASS reported an annual risk of nonfatal myocardial infarction (Q-wave positive) of 2.2 per cent per year with medical treatment compared with 2.8 per cent per year for surgical treatment. However, a recent study suggests that patients who have undergone previous coronary artery surgery are likely to have smaller myocardial infarctions and better residual left ventricular function after infarction because of the presence of less jeopardized myocardium distal to the infarct-producing lesion.[432]

PATIENT SELECTION FOR CORONARY ARTERY SURGERY

To undergo coronary artery bypass grafting, patients with chronic stable angina must usually meet certain clinical criteria. A plan for work-up and management of patients with mild to moderate angina is shown in Figure 39–23.

The most widely accepted indication for coronary artery bypass surgery in stable angina pectoris is significant disability from symptoms despite optimal medical care. Although this disability usually results from the coronary artery disease itself, it may be related to the side effects of the medication required to control the discomfort of myocardial ischemia, or patients may find taking large amounts of medication intolerable. Lastly, if the level of angina pectoris on a medical regimen clearly interferes with a patient's work or recreational activity or expecta-

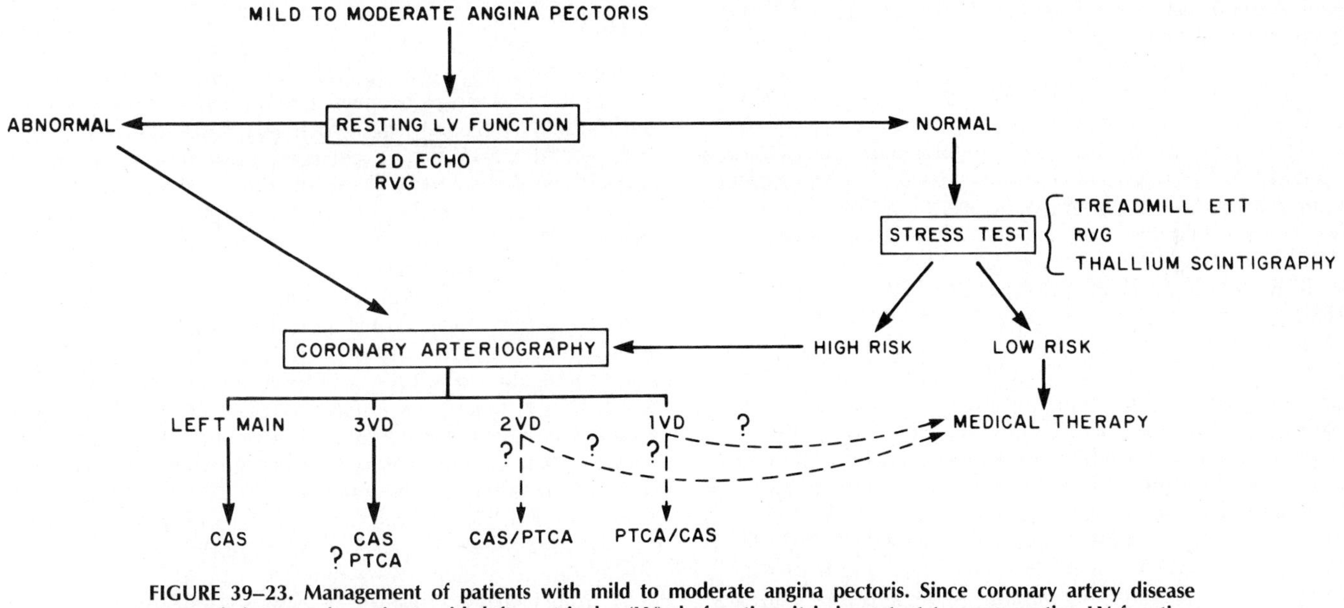

FIGURE 39–23. Management of patients with mild to moderate angina pectoris. Since coronary artery disease prognosis is worse in patients with left ventricular (LV) dysfunction, it is important to assess resting LV function (most readily accomplished noninvasively by either two-dimensional echocardiography [2D-echo] or radionuclide ventriculography [RVG].) If LV function is abnormal at rest, coronary angiography should be performed; if normal, some form of stress testing should be performed, e.g., treadmill exercise testing, radionuclide ventriculography at rest and during exercise, and thallium scintigraphy (with exercise or dipyridamole). If there is evidence of significant exercise-induced ischemia or LV dysfunction, coronary arteriography should be performed. If stress is accomplished that is equivalent to or greater than completion of stage III of a Bruce protocol treadmill test without evidence of significant exercise-induced ischemia or LV dysfunction, a trial of medical therapy is reasonable. Using this approach, the results of coronary arteriography will lead to logical management choices. For all patients with significant (>60%) left main coronary artery disease and for most with significant (>70%) three-vessel coronary artery disease (3VD), coronary surgery (CAS) is advised. With significant two- (2VD) and one-vessel disease (1VD) the options of CAS, percutaneous transluminal angioplasty (PTCA), or medical therapy will be considered. In patients with critical obstruction of the proximal left anterior descending artery with significant obstruction of one other major vessel and moderate angina pectoris and/or inducible ischemia, either CAS or PTCA is usually advised. In patients with significant one-vessel coronary artery disease, the decision for CAS, PTCA, or medical therapy is made individually. Either PTCA or CAS is favored in those with results of noninvasive testing indicating extensive inducible ischemia, poor functional capacity, and a critical (>70%) obstruction present. (Adapted from Corne, R. A.: Risk stratification in stable angina pectoris. [Editorial] Am. J. Cardiol. *59*:695, 1987.)

tions, a recommendation for coronary artery surgery may be entirely appropriate.

Optimal medical care, as described earlier (p. 1325), involves achievement of satisfactory body weight, control of medical conditions such as thyrotoxicosis or anemia that might intensify myocardial ischemia, maintenance of normal blood pressure, assessment and control of arrhythmias (particularly in patients with impaired ventricular function), and treatment of metabolic abnormalities such as carbohydrate intolerance and hyperlipidemia. Abstinence from smoking is encouraged and a range of medications including beta blockers, short- and long-acting nitrates, and calcium antagonists are used to control symptoms.

The average age of operation has risen from 50 years in the mid-60's to 64 years in the mid-80's, and many patients have had previous myocardial infarction. This trend has continued because of excellent results achieved in the elderly.[433] In the early 1970's most patients selected for operation were in functional classes III and IV but now patients with three-vessel disease and left ventricular dysfunction at rest or inducible for exercise, regardless of the presence or severity of symptoms, are appropriately undergoing coronary artery surgery.

WOMEN AS SURGICAL CANDIDATES. In the CASS study, 15 institutions carried out isolated coronary artery bypass grafting on 6258 men and 1153 women from 1975 to 1980. The operative mortality in men was 1.9 per cent, while the operative mortality for women undergoing coronary artery bypass grafting at the same institutions, during the same period, was 4.5 per cent. When matched for age, severity of angina, and the extent of coronary atherosclerosis, women appear to have twice the operative mortality of men.[434] After 2 years of follow-up, women were shown to have lower overall graft patency rates and at 5 to 10 years postoperatively they had a higher incidence of angina than men.[434] Women's smaller physical size and the smaller diameter of grafted coronary arteries may be responsible for this poorer response[435]; operative mortality increases in both men and women as physical size decreases.

CORONARY ARTERY BYPASS GRAFTING IN THE ELDERLY. During the past decade the hospital mortality of coronary artery surgery in the elderly (65 or older) has declined to between 2.7 and 7.7 per cent.[433, 436–442] In general, mortality is greater in patients over 75,[437, 440] and women in this age group seem to be at higher risk of hospital death.[437] Variables predictive of perioperative mortality are the same as in younger patients and include the presence of 70 per cent or more severe stenosis of the left main coronary artery, severe left ventricular dysfunction,[433, 438, 440] and the presence of one or more associated medical disease.[438, 440] Compared with younger patients, the elderly spend more time in the hospital[438, 441] and are more prone to complications.[441] These in turn are associated with a higher perioperative mortality.[440, 442] However, angina is relieved or diminished in approximately 90 per cent of patients[438, 439] and the 5-year survival of patients older than 65 is generally excellent.[433] Thus, advanced age per se is not a contraindication to surgery.

REOPERATION. Approximately 5 per cent of all coronary artery surgery procedures now are reoperations.[414] Recurrent severe angina pectoris occurs at rates of 4 to 7 per cent per year in patients who have had prior coronary artery surgery; angiographic changes in these patients include primary bypass graft obstruction, progressive coronary arteriosclerosis, or a combination of these factors. Campeau et al. have reported that 10 years after initial operation 40 per cent of saphenous vein grafts had occluded and 50 per cent of the remainder were significantly narrowed.[355] Operative mortality rates for repeat coronary artery surgery are about two to three times those of the initial procedure and range from 2 to 5.3 per cent.[414] The CASS Registry reported that patients requiring reoperation tended to be young females with less extensive coronary artery disease, less ventricular impairment, and fewer coronary vessels bypassed at the initial operation.[443] After reoperation, symptomatic relief of angina pectoris is not as frequent as with primary revascularization[444] but freedom from serious cardiac events and substantial relief of severe angina are noted in more than 60 per cent of patients 5 years later.[444] Long-term patency of internal mammary artery grafts is better than for vein grafts; if it is technically feasible, this is the preferred graft for both initial and repeat coronary artery surgery procedures.[318]

PATIENTS WITH ASSOCIATED CAROTID, ABDOMINAL AORTIC, AND PERIPHERAL VASCULAR DISEASE. The incidence of carotid arterial disease in patients undergoing coronary artery surgery varies from 2 to 12 per cent in most series. Postoperative strokes occur in approximately 2 to 3 per cent of all patients following coronary revascularization, but in selected patients with known carotid disease it may occur in approximately 20 per cent.[445] Conversely, myocardial infarction is responsible for a substantial number of late deaths following carotid endarterectomy. The risk factors for the development of stroke after coronary bypass grafting are increasing age, preexisting cerebrovascular disease, severe atheroma of the ascending aorta, prolonged cardiopulmonary bypass, and severe perioperative hypotension.[446]

Simultaneous carotid-coronary operations should be considered in patients with symptomatic carotid disease with bilateral carotid arterial obstructions and concurrent unstable angina, left main coronary artery obstruction, or diffuse multivessel coronary artery disease. Combined coronary and carotid arterial[447] and coronary arterial and abdominal aortic[448] procedures can be performed with mortality and morbidity similar to that of isolated surgery on the carotid artery and abdominal aorta. Most patients with asymptomatic cervical bruits or mild to moderate carotid artery obstruction can undergo coronary artery surgery alone with a low incidence of perioperative stroke.[449] In patients with unstable angina and a prior stroke the perioperative risk of neurological injury may be increased, and decisions need to be made on a case-by-case basis. Usually, if patients have symptoms suggestive of carotid disease or a cervical bruit, noninvasive carotid testing will identify reliably which patients have significant carotid lesions. Asymptomatic, unilateral, internal carotid artery stenosis or occlusion does not appear to increase the stroke risk during coronary artery surgery.[450]

Coronary artery disease is commonly associated with peripheral vascular disease and is the leading cause of mortality and morbidity in the perioperative period of patients undergoing peripheral vascular surgery.[451] Commonly, these patients have major exercise limitations because of peripheral vascular insufficiency and they may have significant coronary artery disease. However, their angina is masked by the limitation in their physical activities. Routine exercise testing may be impossible. In patients admitted for nonemergency surgery on the abdominal aorta or vessels of the lower extremities, preoperative thallium imaging after administration of dipyridamole may identify ischemic myocardium. With this technique, one half of patients with thallium redistribution had cardiac events, whereas there were no such events in patients whose thallium scan was either normal or showed only persistent defects.[452] These findings suggest that patients with redistribution following dipyridamole-thallium imaging should be considered for preoperative coronary angiography and possible myocardial revascularization in order to avoid postoperative myocardial ischemia and possibly improve survival.

HEART FAILURE AND MYOCARDIAL INFARCTION. As discussed elsewhere (p. 1366), in the absence of severe angina, patients with overt heart failure secondary to multiple myocardial infarctions are not good candidates for coronary revascularization. However, in patients in whom left ventricular dysfunction is due to chronically ischemic but not irreversibly damaged tissue, surgical revascularization can improve left ventricular function.[426–429] The most striking clinical improvement may be observed in patients with the most severe dysfunction.[323] Survival may be improved as well.[323, 324] Patients with overt heart failure should be studied carefully to exclude a mechanical lesion such as mitral regurgitation or a ventricular aneurysm, which is usually amenable to surgical treatment.

Indications for coronary revascularization in patients with acute myocardial infarction or cardiogenic shock and intractable ventricular arrhythmias are discussed elsewhere (p. 1257).

UNSTABLE ANGINA

Unstable angina (previously also known as preinfarction angina, crescendo angina, [acute] coronary insufficiency, and intermediate coronary syndrome) is clinically important because of its frightening and disabling nature and the possibility that it heralds acute myocardial infarction. Pathological studies of patients with this syndrome who do *not* develop an acute fatal myocardial infarction are rare, but those that are available usually reveal multivessel disease but a low incidence of recent *occlusive* thrombi. These findings suggest that coronary vasospasm, transient platelet aggregation, and/or nonocclusive thrombi may play a role in the development of the acute ischemic episodes occurring in the presence of severe organic obstructive disease. Thus, ischemic heart disease may really represent a spectrum of severity of myocardial necrosis, with transmural infarction at one end of the spectrum, ranging through acute subendocardial infarction, to unstable angina, to chronic stable angina at the other end of the spectrum.[453]

DEFINITION. In addition to the absence of clear-cut electrocardiographic and cardiac enzyme changes diagnostic of a myocardial infarction, the currently used definition of unstable angina pectoris depends on the presence of *one* or more of the following three historical features, accompanied by electrocardiographic changes: (1) crescendo angina (more severe, prolonged, or frequent) superimposed on a preexisting pattern of relatively stable, exertion-related angina pectoris; (2) angina pectoris at rest as well as with minimal exertion; or (3) angina pectoris of new onset (usually within one month), which is brought on by minimal exertion. The ischemic episodes of unstable angina pectoris are *not* related to obvious precipitating factors, such as anemia, infection, thyrotoxicosis, or cardiac arrhythmias. Prinzmetal's ("variant") angina is a different entity and is discussed on page 1360.

CLINICAL AND LABORATORY FINDINGS

SYMPTOMS. The chest discomfort in this syndrome is similar in quality to that of classic effort-induced angina, although it is usually more intense, is usually described as pain, may persist for as long as 30 minutes, and occasionally awakens the patient from sleep. Longer episodes of ischemic pain are usually associated with acute myocardial infarction. The usual therapeutic regimen of nitroglycerin administration and physical rest often provides only temporary or incomplete relief. Several clues should alert the physician to a changing anginal pattern and the development of unstable angina; these include an abrupt and persistent reduction in the threshold of physical activity that provokes angina; an increase in the frequency, severity, and duration of angina; radiation of the discomfort to a new site; and onset of new features associated with the pain, such as diaphoresis, nausea, or palpitation.

The proportion of patients with unstable angina who have angina of new onset, a crescendo pattern superimposed on stable angina, or rest angina varies among different series and depends on how the observers defined the syndrome. Patients in whom unstable angina is superimposed on longstanding, stable angina almost always have multivessel disease, while patients with new onset of severe angina may have a strong dynamic (vasoconstrictive) component superimposed on fixed obstructive disease, involving only a single coronary artery.[454]

PHYSICAL EXAMINATION. This may reveal transient diastolic (third and fourth) heart sounds and dyskinetic apical impulses, suggesting left ventricular dysfunction, or a transient murmur of mitral regurgitation during or immediately after an ischemic episode.[455] These findings are nonspecific, since they may also be present in patients with chronic angina pectoris or acute myocardial infarction.

ELECTROCARDIOGRAM. Transient deviations of the ST-segment (depression or elevation) and/or T-wave inversions occur commonly in unstable angina. Usually, these clear completely or partially with the relief of pain. Persistence of electrocardiographic changes for more than 6 to 12 hours may suggest that a non-Q-wave infarction has occurred.

If patients have a typical history of chronic stable angina pectoris or established coronary artery disease (previous myocardial infarction, abnormal coronary arteriograms, or a history of a positive noninvasive stress test) before the development of symptoms of unstable angina, the diagnosis of unstable angina may be made with reasonable reliability if typical symptoms exist, even in the absence of electrocardiographic changes. It is in the subgroup of patients without evidence of previous coronary artery disease and no electrocardiographic changes from baseline associated with pain that the diagnosis may be inaccurate. Also, in these patients no underlying coronary artery disease may be found at coronary arteriography.

Ischemic chest pain is not a reliable or sensitive marker of transient acute myocardial ischemia. Episodes of primary reduction in coronary flow may be associated with variable and minor electrocardiographic changes that precede symptoms of pain or discomfort.[456] In continuously monitored patients who demonstrated large falls in coronary sinus oxygen saturation, reflecting changes in myocardial blood flow, the ischemic episodes were associated with pseudonormalization of previously inverted or flat T waves in the majority of instances of ischemia (77 per cent), ST-segment elevation in some (20 per cent), and ST-segment depression in a few (2 per cent). In those instances of transient myocardial ischemia associated with chest pain

(10 of 37), the pain always occurred 50 to 120 seconds *after* the onset of the ST-T changes.[456] It is now widely recognized that patients with either stable or unstable angina have a high incidence of ischemic electrocardiographic changes without accompanying symptoms when continuous electrocardiographic monitoring is performed.[23, 47–49, 457–464] Transient abnormalities in myocardial perfusion and function have been associated with these electrocardiographic changes.[23, 456, 462, 463]

STANDARD LABORATORY TESTS. Findings on chest roentgenogram, serum cholesterol level, and carbohydrate tolerance are similar to those observed in patients with chronic stable angina. Unlike acute myocardial infarction, nonspecific indicators of gross tissue necrosis, such as leukocytosis and fever, are usually absent. Cardiac enzymes are not abnormally elevated; when cardiac-specific enzymes are elevated, by definition the diagnosis is acute myocardial infarction and not unstable angina.

CARDIAC CATHETERIZATION AND CORONARY ARTERIOGRAPHY

Coronary arteriographic findings in patients with unstable angina have generally shown the same distribution of no disease and one-, two-, and three-vessel disease found in patients with chronic angina pectoris and in patients who have suffered a myocardial infarction; the incidence of left main coronary artery disease may be somewhat higher.[465] The left anterior descending coronary artery is the most commonly affected vessel in patients with unstable (as well as chronic stable) angina.[466] The collateral circulation appears less well developed in patients with unstable angina than in those with stable angina pectoris, an arteriographic impression that is supported by findings at operation in which retrograde flow, measured directly by cannulation of the opened artery, was less in patients with unstable angina than in those with chronic stable angina.[467] The incidence of normal coronary arteriograms among patients with unstable angina varies among different series and averages 5 per cent. No obvious explanation other than coronary spasm exists for this finding.

Correlation of coronary angiographic morphology and histology of coronary artery stenotic lesions has suggested that significant stenoses (50 to 99 per cent reduction of luminal diameter on postmortem angiograms) which have smooth borders, an hourglass shape, and no intraluminal lucencies are more likely to have fatty or fibrous plaques with intact intimal surfaces and no superimposed thrombus. In contrast, lesions causing similar degrees of obstruction, which have irregular borders or intraluminal lucencies, are more likely to show plaque rupture, plaque hemorrhage, superimposed partially occlusive thrombus, or recanalized thrombus.[468] Postmortem studies have also shown that about 70 per cent of specimens of diseased arterial segments with significant narrowings (greater than or equal to 50 per cent diameter loss) have an eccentric, residual arterial lumen that is partially circumscribed by an arc of at least 60 degrees of normal arterial wall.[469] The presence of this pliable, muscular elastic arc of normal wall provides a mechanism whereby variations in intraluminal pressure and/or vasomotor tone may alter lumen caliber and thus flow resistance. The mean disease-free wall arc length is approximately 20 per cent of the total vessel circumference in eccentric coronary artery lesions that obstruct 50 to 90 per cent of the cross-sectional area irrespective of the lesion's location within the vessel or the size of the vessel.[470]

CORONARY MORPHOLOGY. Recently, Ambrose and colleagues examined coronary artery morphology at cardiac catheterization in patients with either stable or unstable angina.[471, 472] All had coronary lesions that obstructed the luminal diameter by 50 per cent or more. They found that coronary artery lesions seen on angiograms as asymmetrical lesions with a narrow neck, irregular borders, or both, are more likely to be found in patients with unstable angina. In contrast, lesions with concentric, symmetrical narrowing, or asymmetrical narrowing with smooth borders and a broad neck are more common in patients with stable angina (Fig. 10–44, p. 296). In patients with known coronary artery anatomy and stable angina pectoris who were restudied after an acute episode of unstable angina, it appeared that acute progression had evolved from a previously insignificant lesion in most instances and that the eccentric lesion (type II lesion, that is, eccentrically placed convex stenosis with a narrow neck due to one or more overhanging edges or irregular, scalloped borders, or both) is the most common morphological feature of disease progression and may represent either a disrupted atherosclerotic plaque or a partially lysed thrombus, or both. This lesion appears to be a major cause of unstable angina.[472] Others have confirmed a similar morphology in patients with the abrupt onset of stable angina.[473]

Intracoronary filling defects with appearances consistent with thrombus have also been found more commonly in patients with recent rest pain and unstable angina pectoris. Coronary angioscopy frequently reveals complex plaques or thrombi not detected by coronary angiography in such patients.[474]

The notion that eccentric coronary artery lesions may be seen frequently in patients with either new-onset or unstable angina is an interesting one. It is not difficult to conceive that alterations in coronary artery tone at the site of irregular plaques may initiate and/or be exacerbated by local formation of subtotally occlusive platelet thrombi, with resulting intensification of angina. Unstable angina is also associated with progression in the extent and severity of coronary obstructive lesions.[475]

Findings on left ventriculography are similar to those in patients with chronic stable angina and generally show good wall motion *between* episodes of acute ischemia, except of course in patients who have had prior myocardial infarctions. During episodes of acute ischemia, localized areas of asynergy are present and stroke volume and ejection fraction decline, while left ventricular end-systolic

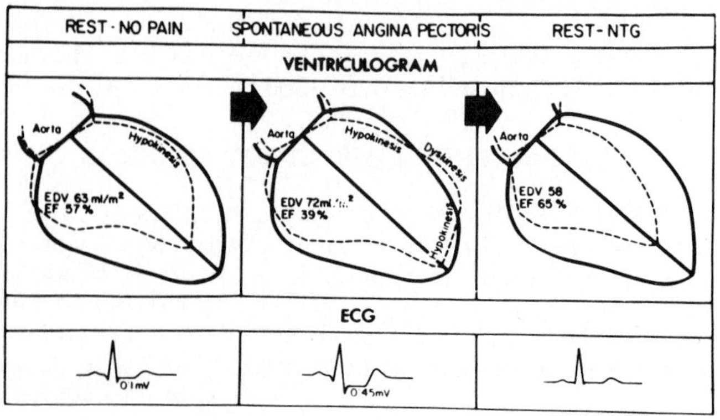

FIGURE 39–24. Diagrammatic representation of left ventricular end-systolic and end-diastolic frames. Note that during spontaneous angina pectoris, when ST-segment depression of 0.45 mV develops, there is an increase in end-diastolic volume (EDV) with a decrease in ejection fraction (EF); regional wall motion abnormality also develops. These values revert to normal after nitroglycerin (NTG) therapy. (From Sharma, B., et al.: Left ventricular function during spontaneous angina pectoris: Effect of sublingual nitroglycerin. Am. J. Cardiol. *46*:34, 1980.)

and end-diastolic volumes rise, as does left ventricular filling pressure[476]; nitroglycerin restores both global and regional left ventricular function (Fig. 39–24).

PATHOPHYSIOLOGY

Most patients with unstable angina have severe obstructive coronary artery disease; episodes of myocardial ischemia can be precipitated by either an increase in myocardial oxygen demand and/or a reduction in supply. Episodes of spontaneous (rest) angina can be preceded by arterial hypertension and/or tachycardia, which lead to increases in myocardial oxygen requirements, as is the case for exertion-related fixed-threshold angina pectoris. It has also been demonstrated that in patients with fixed atherosclerotic obstructive lesions, a primary reduction of myocardial oxygen supply (due to either coronary vasoconstriction, i.e., a further reduction in lumen diameter consequent to normal vasoconstrictor influences or perhaps to platelet aggregation) may be responsible for many cases of angina at rest and not merely those associated with Prinzmetal's angina in which there is abnormal severe spasm of a proximal coronary artery[31] (p. 1360).

In patients with unstable angina who are continuously monitored, an interesting sequence of events is characteristic (Fig. 39–25). First, there is usually a reduction of coronary sinus oxygen saturation (which, in the presence of constant oxygen needs, signifies a reduction of coronary blood flow). This is followed in turn by characteristic electrocardiographic changes discussed above, and then chest discomfort appears. Secondary to the latter, blood pressure and/or heart rate may rise.[456] Thus, in many patients with angina at rest, ischemia appears to be precipitated by a reduction in oxygen supply rather than an increase in demand. It is also possible that in some instances an increase in myocardial oxygen demand and a reduction in supply occur simultaneously. Thus, in patients with angina, coronary vasoconstriction has been observed during exercise.[477] This is an example of simultaneous augmentation of myocardial oxygen needs with concurrent reduced availability. Occasionally, a similar mechanism may be operative in patients with unstable angina.

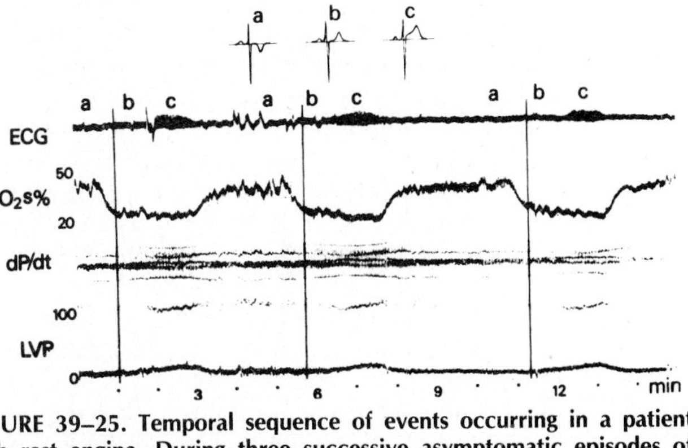

FIGURE 39–25. Temporal sequence of events occurring in a patient with rest angina. During three successive asymptomatic episodes of primary reductions in coronary blood flow (as indicated by a fall in the great cardiac vein oxygen saturation, CSO_2S), over a 15-minute period, recordings were made of electrocardiogram (lead V_2), left ventricular pressure (LVP), and dP/dt. Electrocardiographic patterns are recorded in resting conditions (a), at the onset of the ischemic episode (b), and at the peak of the ischemic episode (c). Vertical lines correspond to the onset of the ST-T changes. A sharp drop in CSO_2S (indicating a fall in coronary blood flow) consistently precedes the onset of hemodynamic changes (a fall in LVP and LVdP/dt) and electrocardiographic changes. If angina occurs, the electrocardiographic events are consistently shown to precede the onset of symptoms. (From Chierchia, S., et al.: Sequence of events in angina at rest: Primary reduction in coronary flow. Circulation *61*:759, 1980, by permission of the American Heart Association, Inc.)

Mechanisms contributing to the reduction of oxygen supply, and therefore to the precipitation of ischemic episodes in patients with unstable angina pectoris who have severe underlying obstructive coronary artery disease, include progression of atherosclerosis, platelet aggregation, thrombosis, and coronary spasm.[478]

PROGRESSION OF ATHEROSCLEROSIS. Evidence exists that the development of unstable angina may be associated with marked recent progression in extent and severity of coronary artery disease greater than that seen in patients with chronic stable angina.[475]

PLATELET AGGREGATION. There is substantial evidence to support the role of platelet aggregates in the precipitation of ischemic episodes. Thus, animal models have shown that spontaneous decreases in coronary blood flow distal to coronary artery stenoses may be due to episodes of platelet aggregation[479–481] (which may occlude a partially constricted coronary artery) and that cyclic reductions in coronary blood flow can be prevented by aspirin.[481] This suggests that platelet aggregation rather than fibrin deposition may cause the observed cyclic reductions of coronary flow.[482] Platelets and the coronary vascular endothelium interact in a complex manner; platelets produce the proaggregatory and vasoconstrictive thromboxane A_2, while the endothelium produces antiaggregatory prostacyclin (prostaglandin I_2). It is likely that other factors such as change in sympathetic vascular tone[483] and the activation of platelet receptors (alpha$_2$ adrenergic and serotonergic)[484] may promote platelet aggregation.

In patients with unstable angina who have had pain within 24 hours, the finding of elevated metabolites of thromboxane A_2 in plasma and urine suggests that local thromboxane release may be associated with episodes of unstable angina pectoris.[485] The reductions in coronary blood flow in canine experiments appear to be abolished by platelet inhibitors including aspirin, sulfinpyrazone, prostacyclin, ibuprofen, and indomethacin but not by heparin, nitroglycerin, or papaverine.[482, 486] Again this suggests that they are mediated by platelet aggregation rather than by vasospasm or fibrin deposition. Furthermore, two large-scale clinical trials indicate that aspirin can protect against death and nonfatal acute myocardial infarction in patients with unstable angina.[487, 488] Finally, in patients with unstable angina who suffer sudden ischemic cardiac death, platelet aggregates have been found in small intramyocardial vessels. These occur in segments of myocardium immediately downstream of a major epicardial coronary artery containing an atheromatous plaque that has undergone fissuring and on which mural thrombus had developed.[489]

THROMBOSIS. Several clinical studies have shown that when coronary angiography is performed in patients with unstable angina or rest angina, intracoronary filling defects having the appearance of thrombus are found and coronary angioscopy has confirmed this interpretation.[474] Furthermore, when thrombolytic therapy (streptokinase) is given to patients with unstable angina and recent pain, a decrease in the severity of coronary stenosis, dissolution of intracoronary filling defects, and opening of an occluded artery have all been observed.[490] Finally, pathological observations in patients with unstable angina who died have suggested an ongoing thrombotic process in a major coronary artery during the period of unstable angina. This process culminates in total vascular occlusion, which causes infarction and/or sudden death.[491]

CORONARY SPASM OR ALTERATIONS IN VASOMOTOR TONE. Quantitative angiography in patients with unstable angina has shown vasomotor hyperreactivity localized to regions of preexisting coronary atheroma.[492] Also, clinical studies have reported large-vessel coronary spasm as a cause of ST-segment elevation in patients with rest angina.[493] Postmortem studies have shown that in the majority of significantly diseased coronary arteries a portion of the circumference is circumscribed by normal arterial walls. Because of this and because unstable angina pectoris is obviously a dynamic, multifactorial process, it is likely that a normal pliable muscular elastic arc of vessel wall provides a mechanism whereby normal (vasoconstriction) or abnormally intense (vasospasm) increases in vasomotor tone may affect lumen caliber and thus flow resistance. Therefore, alterations in coronary artery tone at the site of plaques may initiate and/or be exacerbated by local formation of platelet thrombi with resulting angina.

It is likely that progression of atherosclerosis, platelet aggregation, thrombus formation, and changes in vasomotor tone (or spasm) may operate either alone or together at different times in individual patients. The pathophysiology of the unstable angina pectoris syndrome is a complex, dynamic process that may be interrupted by a variety of measures aimed at modifying these processes. Furthermore, unstable angina is often a precursor of myocardial infarction and both conditions may occur acutely and suddenly and may share a common pathological link.[494]

NONINVASIVE TESTS

Most patients who are hospitalized with unstable angina, after initial therapy of bed rest, oxygen, analgesics, nitrates, beta-adrenoceptor blocking drugs and/or calcium antagonists, will be stabilized quite quickly, will become asymptomatic, and their electrocardiographic signs of continuing ischemia will disappear. During this period, serial electrocardiographic and enzyme evaluations will confirm that no infarction has taken place. Noninvasive tests may help determine whether or not angiography should be performed promptly.

POSITIVE TECHNETIUM-99m STANNOUS PYROPHOSPHATE SCINTIGRAMS (p. 341). These scintigrams, suggesting diffuse subendocardial necrosis, are positive in approximately 30 per cent of patients with unstable angina without electrocardiographic or enzyme changes diagnostic of acute myocardial infarction. Such findings suggest that these patients have either sustained minor degrees of otherwise unrecognized subendocardial necrosis or infarction has occurred in the recent past. Continuing angina during hospital treatment, ischemic electrocardiographic changes, and positive technetium pyrophosphate scintigrams identify a subgroup of patients at high risk of cardiac death and nonfatal myocardial infarctions.[495]

THALLIUM SCINTIGRAPHY. This may reveal a transient defect of myocardial perfusion in patients developing angina at rest, accompanied by ST-segment alterations, supporting the concept that a reduction of blood flow is responsible.[496]

TWO-DIMENSIONAL ECHOCARDIOGRAPHY. This examination may reveal transient abnormalities of ventricular wall motion. Persistent abnormalities of wall motion are associated with an adverse prognosis.[497]

SILENT ISCHEMIA IN UNSTABLE ANGINA. Ischemic electrocardiographic changes without accompanying symptoms, i.e., episodes of silent myocardial ischemia, occur frequently in patients with unstable angina. Such changes correlate with transient reductions in myocardial perfusion and abnormalities of ventricular function.[463] In one study, silent ischemia detected by continuous electrocardiographic monitoring occurred in more than half of the patients with unstable angina while they were receiving intensive medical therapy. Patients with such ST-segment changes during the first 48 hours after admission to a coronary care unit were more likely to suffer a myocardial infarction, require bypass surgery or angioplasty, or develop recurrent symptomatic angina during the next month. Multivariate analyses showed that silent ischemia was the best predictor of these various adverse outcomes[498] (Fig. 39–26). While this latter approach may not be applicable to all patients, it may prove helpful as a particularly sensitive way of detecting continuing ischemia in hospitalized patients.

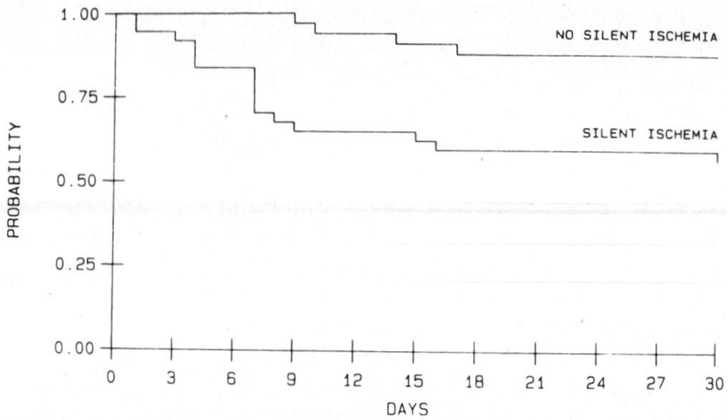

FIGURE 39–26. Influence of presence or absence of silent ischemia on morbid events in patients with unstable angina. Seventy patients with unstable angina had continuous electrocardiographic monitoring. Thirty-seven patients had at least one episode of silent ischemia and 33 patients had no silent ischemia. Those patients *with no silent ischemia* had a higher probability of *not* experiencing myocardial infarction or requiring revascularization for recurrent angina during the next 30 days as shown in the Kaplan-Meier curves comparing the cumulative probabilities of these events. (Reprinted by permission from Gottlieb, S. O., et al.: Silent ischemia as a marker for early unfavorable outcomes in patients with unstable angina. N. Engl. J. Med. *314*:1214, 1986.)

INDICATIONS FOR CATHETERIZATION AND ANGIOGRAPHY. As is the case in patients with chronic stable angina, several questions need to be resolved: How will these tests aid in further management of the syndrome? In what patients should they be performed? What are the risks involved? Are any special precautions necessary? Although there is no unanimity of opinion regarding the answers to these questions, we believe that in most instances coronary arteriography is very helpful in the management of patients with unstable angina. For patients in whom medical therapy fails, coronary arteriography should be carried out immediately, i.e., as soon as their hemodynamic condition has been stabilized, unless there are obvious contraindications to possible angioplasty or coronary bypass surgery. On the other hand, in patients who respond to medical therapy, we recommend catheterization and arteriography several days after symptoms have stabilized. These procedures are helpful in that they identify several subgroups of patients with unstable angina pectoris and can thus be used to dictate therapy: (1) Patients with left main coronary artery disease—the most life-threatening form of the disease—in whom there is now general agreement that urgent surgery is indicated. (2) Patients with multivessel obstructive disease without a clear "culprit" lesion and who are not suitable for angioplasty. Unless there are contraindications, we recommend that operation be planned on a semiurgent basis (within 10 days) after the patient's condition has stabilized. (3) A small number of patients (about 5 per cent of all patients with unstable angina) with no demonstrable coronary artery disease, in whom the prognosis appears excellent and in whom no further surgical consideration is necessary. In some of these patients coronary spasm is responsible for the angina, and this can be established by an ergonovine test at the time of coronary arteriography (p. 1361); intensification of therapy with nitrates and calcium antagonists would then be indicated. (4) Patients with single-vessel or double-vessel disease with a discrete narrow proximal lesion (i.e., "culprit lesion") amenable to percutaneous transluminal angioplasty (p. 295). (5) Patients with diffuse distal coronary artery disease unsuitable for angioplasty bypass grafting.

Which patients are unsuitable for study? Obviously, patients who are suffering from another serious life-threatening illness with a poor prognosis do not require study. Advanced age is not considered to be a contraindication. The risks of coronary arteriography may be somewhat greater in patients with unstable angina than in those with chronic stable angina, but the addition of intraaortic balloon counterpulsation has reduced mortality to near zero.[499, 500] Maximal medical therapy, as described below, should be maintained up to and continued through the time of cardiac catheterization and arteriography.

MANAGEMENT

Unstable angina pectoris is a serious, potentially dangerous condition, and its management must be approached with this in mind. The patient should be admitted to the hospital and immediately placed at bed rest. Removal from an emotionally taxing situation, a quiet atmosphere, physical and emotional rest, the physician's reassurance, mild sedation, and antianxiety drugs are all helpful and will diminish or relieve episodes of rest pain in perhaps half of all patients. A vigorous effort must be undertaken immediately to diagnose and treat conditions that may be responsible for transient increases in myocardial oxygen demands, such as infection, fever, thyrotoxicosis, anemia, exacerbation of preexisting heart failure, concurrent illnesses (particularly of the pulmonary tract, leading to coughing and hypoxemia, and acute gastrointestinal disturbances, causing vomiting, retching, or severe diarrhea), tachyarrhythmias (that increase myocardial oxygen demand), and severe bradyarrhythmias that reduce myocardial perfusion. Control of these aggravating factors will be helpful in 10 to 15 per cent of patients. Placing the bed into the reverse Trendelenburg position (feet down) is a simple measure that may be helpful[501] as may the inhalation of 100 per cent oxygen during periods of pain.

The electrocardiogram should be monitored continuously; diagnostic tests to rule out a myocardial infarction should include serial CK-MB enzymes. Invasive monitoring is usually not necessary unless a serious hemodynamic disturbance is suspected. Frequent radionuclide angiograms, thallium perfusion scans, and two-dimensional echocardiograms, although useful in elucidating the mechanism and consequences of unstable angina, are not very helpful in acute patient management and may actually be harmful in that they disturb the patient's rest.

NITRATES. These are a mainstay of therapy. In addition to frequently relieving and preventing the pain of unstable angina, they have been shown to improve global and regional left ventricular function, as indicated above (Fig. 39–24). Nitrates may be given sublingually, orally, topically, or intravenously, and they may be of the short- or long-acting variety. *Intravenous nitroglycerin* offers the advantage of more consistent control of ischemic episodes during the first 24 hours of treatment.[502] An additional advantage of intravenous nitroglycerin in patients already receiving standard therapy of oral or topical nitrates and beta-blocking drugs is that it will reduce the number of anginal episodes, reduce the need for sublingual nitroglycerin use, and also reduce the amount of analgesia required.[503] A dosage schedule designed to reduce mean arterial pressure by 10 per cent is a safe and effective way of treating unstable angina unresponsive to standard medical therapy.[504] Nitroglycerin is relatively stable when stored in glass containers; however, plastic bags should be avoided because the drug is absorbed by the plastic. Polyvinyl chloride tubing also has a great affinity for nitroglycerin.[505] Therefore, the quantity of nitroglycerin delivered to the patient may be much less than that ordered. Several companies offer a nonpolyvinyl chloride infusion set with preparations of intravenous nitroglycerin. Also, commercial preparations of intravenous nitroglycerin contain alcohol in quantities of 0.01 to 0.14 ml/mg of nitroglycerin, so that when large doses of the agent are administered the quantity of alcohol delivered may be substantial.

BETA-ADRENOCEPTOR BLOCKERS. The role of beta-adrenoceptor blockade in the treatment of unstable angina pectoris is being reexamined because many episodes of myocardial ischemia in these patients are not preceded by increases in heart rate or blood pressure, which are the major determinants of myocardial oxygen consumption. However, immediately after the onset of ischemia, increases in heart rate and blood pressure commonly occur and may perpetuate the ischemia.[506] In patients with chronic stable angina pectoris, potentiation of coronary vasoconstriction has been demonstrated after beta-adrenoceptor blockade presumably mediated by unopposed alpha-adrenoceptor vasomotor tone.[507] However, despite their extensive clinical use, beta blockers do not appear to aggravate myocardial ischemia except in patients with normal coronary vessels and vasotonic angina pectoris.[508]

Several randomized trials have placed the role of beta blockers in the treatment of unstable angina pectoris in better perspective. In one study, patients who were not receiving beta blockers at the time of entry into the hospital responded more rapidly when they received the combination of beta blockers and nitrates than nifedipine alone.[509] In another trial the addition of propranolol to therapy with nitrates and nifedipine reduced the frequency and duration of both symptomatic and silent ischemic episodes.[510] Propranolol and diltiazem have been shown to be equally effective in reducing both episodes of chest pain during hospitalization and the symptoms present one month after initiation of therapy. After 5 months, myocardial infarction rate, death rate, and number of patients undergoing coronary artery surgery were similar.[511] Patients with rest angina randomized to single-drug therapy with propranolol or verapamil had similar, significant reductions in the number of episodes of angina and nitroglycerin tablets consumed.[512] However, verapamil reduced the average number of ischemic ST-segment deviations, while propranolol did not. In conclusion, beta blockers continue to play an important role in the management of patients with unstable angina pectoris.[512a]

In patients who are already taking beta blockers at the time when unstable angina develops, the drug should be continued unless contraindications are present. The dosage of beta blockers should be adjusted so that the resting heart rate is between 50 and 60 beats/min. This usually requires 240 to 320 mg of propranolol per day (or the equivalent for other beta blockers). Beta blockade may improve pulmonary congestion if the elevated pulmonary venous pressure is due to an ischemia-induced reduction of left ventricular compliance or left ventricular systolic failure. Rarely, heart failure may be precipitated by beta blockade in patients with previous infarction. In this situation the drug should be discontinued or the dose reduced and treatment with diuretics instituted.

CALCIUM ANTAGONISTS. When administered as initial therapy or along with nitrates, calcium antagonists appear to be about as effective as beta-adrenoceptor blockers.[513] However, it is common for patients to be receiving nitrates, or a combination of nitrates and beta blockers, before initiation of therapy with calcium antagonists. Two major double-blind, randomized trials have more clearly defined the role of calcium antagonists. In patients with unstable angina receiving conventional medical therapy of propranolol and long-acting nitrates, the addition of nifedipine improved outcome significantly. After 4 months, failure of medical treatment (defined as sudden death, myocardial infarction, or coronary artery surgery) occurred in 44 per cent of patients given nifedipine compared with 61 per cent of patients given placebo (Fig. 39–27). In those patients with ST-segment elevation during pain, in whom vasomotor tone changes were presumably playing a major role, the combined regimen of nifedipine plus nitrates and propranolol failed in 36 per cent, whereas nitrates and propranolol failed in 66 per cent.[514] In a second study, nifedipine alone was compared to the combination of propranolol and isosorbide dinitrate. For the study population as a whole, therapy with nifedipine alone was equivalent to the combination.[509] In patients who developed unstable angina while on beta blockers, nifedipine relieved pain more rapidly than did additional propranolol and/or nitrates. This latter study supports the use of nifedipine in patients with unstable angina who are already receiving beta blockade as does a multicenter Dutch study.[512a]

ANTICOAGULANTS. The benefits of the use of anticoagulants in patients with unstable angina have not been fully established by rigorous trials. An early study was stopped prematurely.[515] Also, a randomized study showed a marked reduction in mortality and frequency of infarction in patients assigned to either heparin or heparin and atenolol (compared with those assigned to placebo or atenolol alone). However, this study is difficult to interpret because, of 400 patients entered, 186 were withdrawn subsequently because of incorrect recruitment.[516] More recently, 102 patients were prospectively randomized to

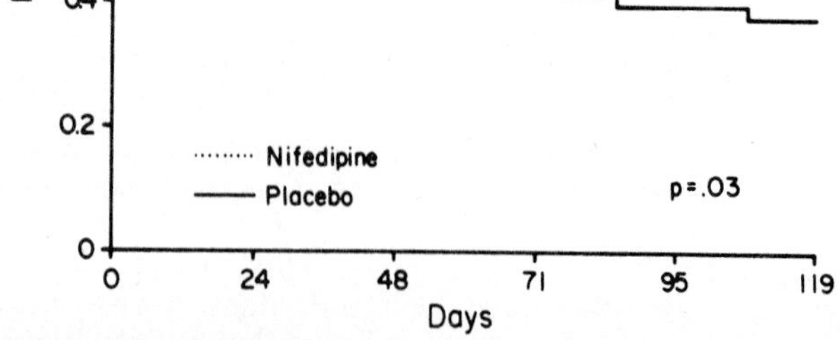

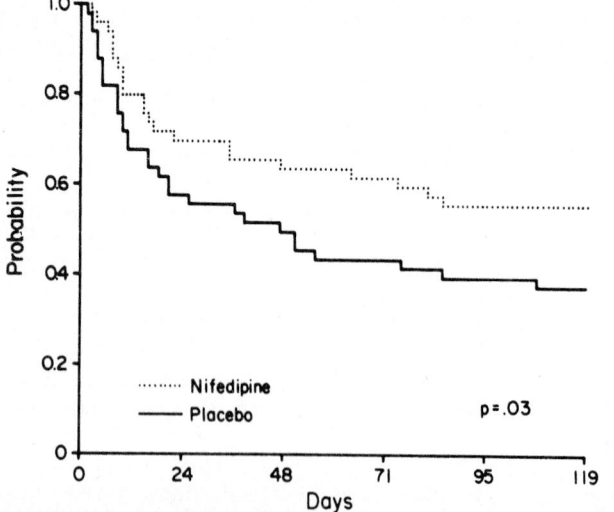

FIGURE 39–27. Effect of nifedipine on the cumulative probability of no failure of medical therapy in all patients. (Reprinted with permission from Gerstenblith, G., et al.: Nifedipine in unstable angina. A double-blind, randomized trial. N. Engl. J. Med. *306*:885, 1982.)

anticoagulants (heparin 10,000 units every 6 hours for 2 days and warfarin for 6 months); death, recurrent unstable angina, and myocardial infarction occurred in 17 of the control group and only 6 of the treated group ($p < 0.05$).[517]

We believe that heparin therapy may reduce morbid events in patients with unstable angina, and use it as a constant intravenous infusion, recognizing that its routine use cannot be recommended on the available evidence.

INTRAAORTIC BALLOON COUNTERPULSATION. This mode of therapy is considered when others have failed and is usually effective in stabilization of the patient's condition, both symptomatically and hemodynamically. Intraaortic balloon counterpulsation is usually initiated either before or during coronary arteriography with a view to continuing it through revascularization. This technique is useful primarily because it allows the safe performance of coronary arteriography and insures that the patient goes to coronary artery surgery or PTCA under optimal conditions.

REVASCULARIZATION. In the last 5 years as PTCA has become commonly used in patients with chronic stable angina, it has also been used with increasing frequency in patients with unstable angina. The patient with severe proximal lesions of one major vessel can undergo coronary angioplasty safely. Successful dilatation will relieve unstable angina, increase the patient's functional capacity, and relieve ischemia as reflected in exercise electrocardiograms and thallium scintigraphy.[518, 519] Comparable results with PTCA have been demonstrated in patients with single-vessel coronary disease whether they have stable or unstable angina.[520, 521] Indeed, observational studies suggest that coronary angioplasty compares favorably with coronary artery surgery in patients with unstable angina because the procedure is associated with a low mortality and morbidity. Marked improvement in symptoms can be expected initially in over 90 per cent of patients.[521, 522] In one report emergency PTCA was performed safely and successfully (93 per cent initial success rate) in 60 patients with mostly single-vessel coronary disease and unstable angina pectoris refractory to maximal medical therapy.[523] The restenosis rate was 28 per cent at 6 months. Improved functional status after sustained, successful coronary angioplasty was seen with an almost-normal capacity on bicycle exercise testing and absence of ischemia during thallium isotope studies in 80 per cent of patients. In patients with multivessel disease dilatation of the "culprit" vessel is effective acutely but there is a high recurrence rate of angina pectoris because of only partial revascularization.[524]

SURGICAL THERAPY. Surgical revascularization remains a mainstay of therapy for unstable angina. One large series showed that the operative mortality in patients with unstable angina operated on between 1974 and 1982 was 1.7 per cent; the survival rates and reoperation rates at 5 years were 92 and 6 per cent, and at 10 years the respective values were 83 and 17 per cent. No differences were observed in long-term survival for any of the clinical subgroups of patients whether they had angina at rest, angina after recovery from acute myocardial infarction, or progressive angina of recent onset at the time of presentation.[525] No difference in 2-year mortality was seen in a recent study of patients randomized to medical and surgical therapy, although in patients with lower ejection fractions surgical therapy conferred a survival advantage.[525a] Patients in the CASS registry who underwent surgical therapy for unstable angina showed a 7-year cumulative survival rate of 79 per cent. Features predictive of an adverse long-term outcome were clinical and angiographic markers of left ventricular dysfunction, the extent of coronary disease, and the presence of other illnesses such as hypertension, diabetes, peripheral vascular disease, and stroke.[526]

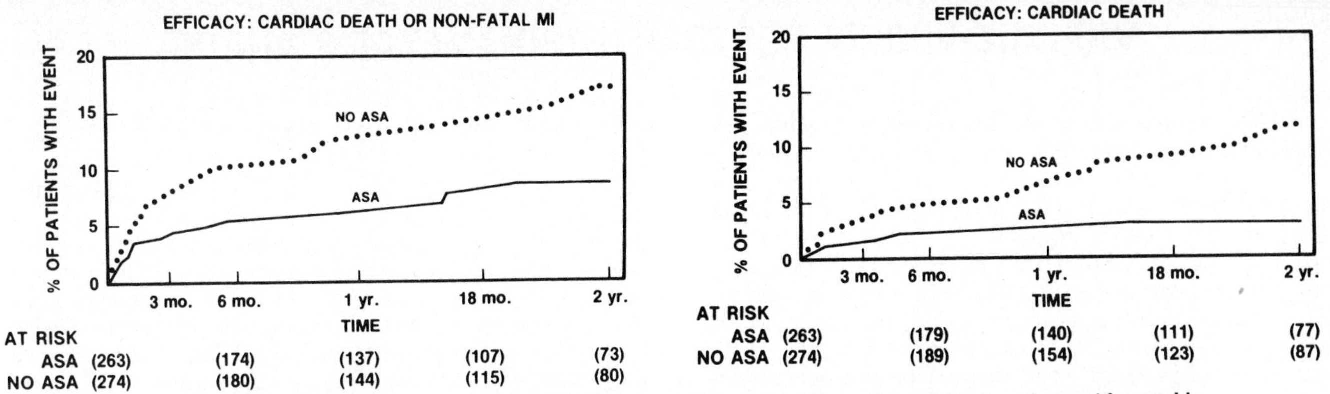

FIGURE 39–28. Influence of aspirin and sulfinpyrazone therapy on mortality and morbidity in patients with unstable angina. Buffered aspirin (324 mg per day) was administered to patients with unstable angina for a 3-month period. *Left panel*: The occurrence of cardiac death or nonfatal myocardial infarction (MI) in the aspirin (ASA) and no aspirin groups are shown. The graph is a life table depiction of the cumulative risk and time of the first occurrence of an outcome event, according to aspirin allocation. The numbers of patients at risk are noted below the graph. Patients were entered into the trial within 8 days of hospitalization and were treated and followed for up to 2 years. The incidence of cardiac death and nonfatal myocardial infarction was 8.6 per cent in the groups given aspirin and 17 per cent in other groups, representing a risk reduction with aspirin. *Right panel*: Curves demonstrating the occurrence of cardiac death in the aspirin (ASA) and no aspirin groups are shown. The incidence of cardiac death alone or from any cause was 3 per cent in the groups given aspirin and 11.7 per cent in the other groups, representing a risk reduction in the aspirin treated group. (Reprinted with permission from Cairns, J. A., et al.: Aspirin, sulfinpyrazone, or both in unstable angina. N. Engl. J. Med. *313*:1369, 1985.)

The role of coronary arteriography and reperfusion and the timing of such therapy remain controversial. The choice of reperfusion technique depends on the findings in an individual patient, the local expertise, and experience. If a patient has received intensive medical therapy for a 48-hour period and there is persistent evidence of continuing ischemia, it is our policy to proceed with catheterization and coronary arteriography. Intraaortic balloon counterpulsation is often instituted either before or during cardiac catheterization if the patient exhibits any hemodynamic instability. If the patient has single-vessel disease and well-maintained left ventricular function, then commonly coronary angioplasty is performed, if technically feasible. On the other hand, in patients in whom there is evidence of left main coronary disease or multivessel disease and the anatomy is suitable for bypass grafting, operation is performed immediately.

Patients who respond to intensive medical therapy are gradually ambulated. If angina on mild effort recurs despite maximal medical therapy, coronary arteriography is performed and PTCA or bypass grafting is carried out as in patients who did not respond to medical therapy initially. Patients who improve on medical management without recurrence of pain may be discharged from the hospital. The decision for further therapy can be made on the basis of clinical response and electrocardiographic or scintigraphic response to exercise just as for patients with chronic stable angina. Such patients undergo exercise stress testing before hospital discharge. In many patients, the results of these tests will be positive and angiography will be performed.[526a]

LONG-TERM ASPIRIN THERAPY. Two large, well-designed studies have demonstrated the beneficial effects of aspirin in patients with unstable angina. The Veterans Administration study[487] showed that buffered aspirin (324 mg per day) administered to patients with unstable angina for a 3-month period reduced mortality as well as the occurrence of fatal or nonfatal acute myocardial infarctions. A multicenter trial in Canada provided similar results with a larger dose of aspirin (325 mg four times daily)[488] (Fig. 39–28).

PROGNOSIS

Unstable angina and acute myocardial infarction are closely related pathogenetically (p. 1227) and clinically. While it has been pointed out that the majority of patients with acute myocardial infarction reported a prodrome of more intense or longer periods of angina, i.e., unstable angina, shortly before infarction,[527] the opposite is not the case, i.e., only a minority of patients with unstable angina pectoris develop early infarction. While patients with unstable angina may present difficult management problems, it is generally recognized that most do not in fact develop myocardial infarction over the short term.

Hospital death occurs in approximately 1 per cent of patients; 3-month mortality ranges from 2 to 10 per cent, and one-year mortality from 8 to 18 per cent.[528, 529] Nonfatal myocardial infarction occurs in 7 to 9 per cent of hospitalized patients, between 16 and 21 per cent at 3 months[529] and between 14 and 22 per cent at one year.[530]

There are two situations in which unstable angina appears to have a worse prognosis. The first involves patients whose pain does not respond to intensive medical therapy within 48 hours of therapy.[454, 530] In one study, those patients who had persistent rest pain after 48 hours of therapy had a one-year survival of 57 per cent compared with 96 per cent in those patients whose pain was quickly relieved.[529] The second situation involves patients who have either persistent ECG changes with angina pectoris or who have episodes of silent ischemia detected by continuous electrocardiographic monitoring.[498]

VARIANT ANGINA PECTORIS (PRINZMETAL'S ANGINA)

In 1959, Prinzmetal et al. described an unusual syndrome of cardiac pain that occurs almost exclusively at rest, usually is not precipitated by physical exertion or emotional stress, and is associated with ST-segment elevations on the electrocardiogram.[531] This syndrome, now known as *Prinzmetal's* or *variant angina*, may be associated with acute myocardial infarction, severe cardiac arrhythmias, including ventricular tachycardia, and fibrillation, as well as sudden death. Its incidence relative to that of the other forms of ischemic heart disease has not been established.

MECHANISM

Variant angina pectoris has been demonstrated convincingly to be due to coronary artery spasm.[493] It is defined as a transient, abrupt, marked reduction in the diameter of an epicardial (or large septal) coronary artery resulting in myocardial ischemia in the absence of any preceding increases in myocardial oxygen demand reflected in elevations of heart rate or blood pressure. This reduction in diameter can be reversed by nitroglycerin and can occur in either normal or diseased coronary arteries.[532] The striking reduction in luminal diameter is focal, usually involving one or occasionally more than one site. It should not be confused with vasoconstriction of the small coronary resistance vessels, a normal response to stimuli such as exercise and cold exposure. This response is much less intense and occurs diffusely throughout the coronary vascular bed. Sites of spasm in Prinzmetal's are often adjacent to atheromatous plaques. It has been suggested that in these patients the basic abnormality of coronary artery spasm may be hypercontractility of the arterial wall associated with the atherosclerotic process itself.[533] Other mechanisms suggested include endothelial injury (which reverses the dilator response to a variety of stimuli to a vasoconstrictor response[534]), and hypercontractility of vascular smooth muscle due to vasoconstrictor mitogens and leukotrienes and higher local concentrations of blood-borne vasoconstrictors in areas of neovascularized atherosclerotic plaques.[533] Vasospasm is unlikely to be initiated by platelet-derived thromboxane A_2.[535] In keeping with this is the finding that aspirin and thromboxane A_2 blockade *fail* to prevent attacks of vasospastic angina.[536] In support of the possibility that vasoactive substances may have an important role in the pathogenesis of coronary spasm is the observation that an excessive number of mast cells have been seen in the adventitia of a vasospastic artery of a young patient succumbing to coronary artery spasm.[537] Another indication that vasoactive amines may be important in this condition is the occurrence of coronary artery spasm in carcinoid heart disease.[538]

CLINICAL MANIFESTATIONS

The history differs from that of typical angina: the principal finding is angina *at rest*.[539] In contrast to unstable angina, the rest pain does not usually represent an "evolution" from an earlier period in which pain occurred with decreasing levels of effort. Although exercise capacity is usually well preserved, some patients experience typical pain and ST-segment elevations not only at rest but during or after exertion as well.[477] The anginal discomfort may be extremely severe and accompanied by syncope, the latter presumably caused by arrhythmias. Attacks of variant angina tend to be clustered between midnight and 8 A.M.[540] Patients studied with 48-hour Holter electrocardiograms show more frequent abnormalities in the morning than in the afternoon, even patients without clinically apparent angina pectoris.[541] Clinical features do not reliably differentiate patients with Prinzmetal's angina with normal or mildly abnormal coronary arteriograms from those with fixed severe coronary obstruction.[542] A large percentage of the former are heavy smokers.[543] This supports the observations that cigarette smoking may influence vasomotor tone. These patients often have a combination of fixed-threshold exertion-induced angina with ST-segment depression and variant angina (rest angina with ST-segment elevation). Rarely, variant angina develops following coronary artery bypass grafting[544] and coronary artery spasm has also been observed intraoperatively after the application of coronary vein grafts. In a subset of patients, variant angina appears to be a manifestation of a generalized vasospastic disorder associated with attacks of migraine and Raynaud's phenomenon.[545] Patients with Prinzmetal's angina tend to be younger than those patients with classic exertion-induced angina, and the male preponderance in the latter group is not evident.[546] In some patients there appears to be a distinct relationship between emotional distress and episodes of coronary vasospasm.[547]

Although patients with Prinzmetal's angina are often heavy cigarette smokers, on physical examination they do not usually exhibit the risk factors for coronary atherosclerosis (p. 1320). Cardiac examination is usually normal in the absence of ischemia (unless the patient has suffered a previous myocardial infarction) but often reveals signs of dyskinesis and impaired left ventricular function during episodes of myocardial ischemia.

ELECTROCARDIOGRAM. The electrocardiogram is the key to the diagnosis of variant angina. ST segments, usually normal at rest, develop characteristic elevations with pain (Fig. 39–29). In some patients episodes of ST-segment elevation alternate with episodes of ST-segment depression accompanied by pseudonormalization of the T waves. Many patients exhibit multiple attacks of asymptomatic ST-segment deviation (silent ischemia). The ST-segment deviations may be present in any leads but are particularly frequent in inferior leads, reflecting the frequency of involvement of the right coronary artery, and disappear as pain subsides. Arrhythmias and conduction disturbances occur during episodes of ischemia.[548] Experimental work and clinical observations suggest that the incidence of arrhythmias depends on the severity of the ischemia. The risk of ventricular fibrillation during release of coronary spasm may be greater when there are no flow-limiting stenoses and the initial reduction in coronary blood flow is greater.[549] Myocardial cell damage, as reflected in the release of small quantities of myoglobin or CK-MB, may occur in the absence of persistent electrocardiographic changes in patients with prolonged attacks.[550] Transient Q waves have been observed.[551]

Exercise testing in patients with variant angina is of limited value since there is such a variable response of patients to exercise. Equal numbers of patients will show ST-segment elevation, ST-segment depression, or no change in ST segments during exercise, reflecting the variability of the underlying fixed coronary artery disease in some patients and the absence of significant lesions in others.

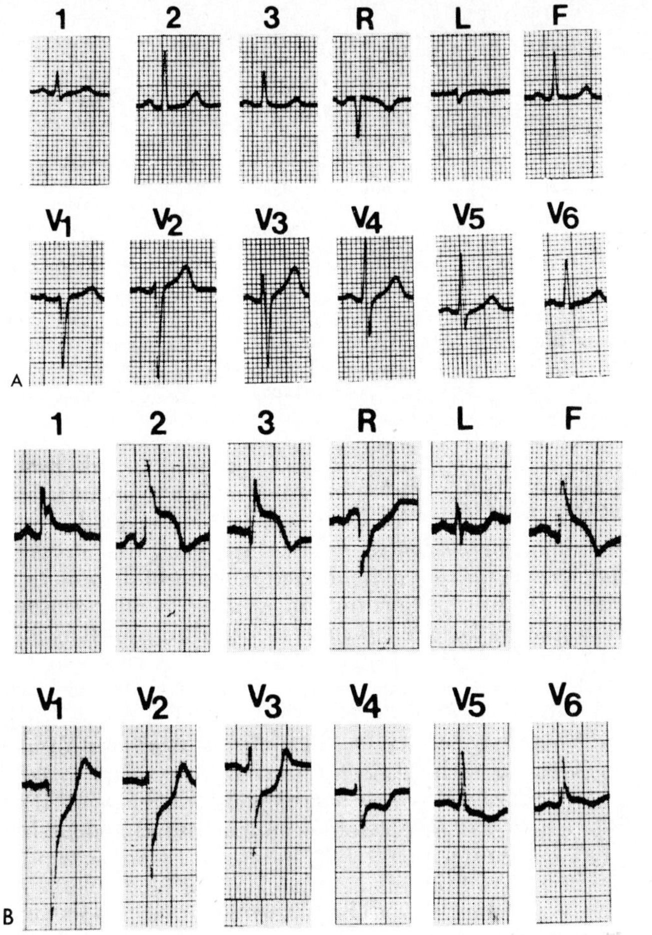

FIGURE 39–29. Electrocardiogram (*A*) prior to an episode of Prinzmetal's angina and (*B*) during an episode of Prinzmetal's angina. ST segments are now markedly elevated in the inferior leads, with reciprocal depression in the anterior leads. After nitroglycerin was given, the ECG returned to baseline. (From Berman, N. D., et al.: Prinzmetal's angina with coronary artery spasm. Angiographic, pharmacologic, metabolic and radionuclide perfusion studies. Am. J. Med. *60*:727, 1976.)

HEMODYNAMIC AND ARTERIOGRAPHIC STUDIES

Hemodynamic data obtained during episodes of spontaneous pain[552, 553] have provided information about patients with variant angina. In contrast to the finding in patients with chronic stable (effort-induced) angina, episodes of Prinzmetal's angina often occur at rest or during mild exertion and are not preceded by increases in heart rate, arterial pressure, or myocardial contractility—all of which increase cardiac work or oxygen consumption. Spasm of a proximal coronary artery with resultant transmural ischemia, first postulated as the cause of variant angina, has been convincingly documented arteriographically (p. 295). Exercise-induced ST-segment elevation can be associated with partial or total obstruction of large epicardial arteries in a manner similar to episodes observed during spontaneous or ergonovine-induced angina.[554, 555] This suggests that coronary spasm may have a common mechanism despite being initiated by different stimuli.

The coronary anatomy of Prinzmetal's angina has been defined both at autopsy and during coronary arteriography (Fig. 10–42, p. 295). Severe proximal coronary atherosclerosis of at least one major vessel occurs in approximately two-thirds of patients and in them spasm usually occurs within 1 cm of the organic obstruction. The remainder have normal coronary arteries in the absence of ischemia.[556] Spasm may occur at one or multiple sites in one artery or occur in multiple arteries simultaneously, and is more common in the right coronary artery than in the others. Patients with variant angina with normal coronary arteriograms are more likely to have purely nonexertional angina and ST-segment elevations involving inferior leads, while patients with variant angina who have organic obstructive lesions with superimposed coronary artery spasm often have associated effort angina and ischemia in anterolateral leads.[556] Patients with no or mild fixed coronary obstruction tend to experience a more benign course than do patients with associated severe obstructive lesions.[557]

THE ERGONOVINE TEST. A number of provocative tests for coronary spasm have been developed. Of these, the ergonovine test is the most sensitive and useful. Ergonovine maleate, an ergot alkaloid that stimulates both alpha-adrenergic and serotonergic receptors and therefore exerts a direct constrictive effect on vascular smooth muscle, has been used to induce coronary artery spasm in patients with Prinzmetal's angina. Coronary arteries that constrict spontaneously appear to be abnormally sensitive to this agent. When administered intravenously in doses ranging from 0.05 to 0.40 mg, ergonovine provides a sensitive and specific test for provoking coronary artery spasm.[558] There is some correlation between the dose of ergonovine required to induce a positive test and the frequency of spontaneous attacks.[559] In low doses and in carefully controlled clinical situations, ergonovine is a relatively safe drug, but prolonged coronary artery spasm precipitated by ergonovine may cause myocardial infarction. Because of this hazard, it is recommended that ergonovine be administered only to patients in whom coronary arteriography has demonstrated normal or nearly normal coronary arteries and in gradually increasing doses, beginning with a very low dose. The test should be carried out only in a setting where appropriate resuscitative equipment, drugs, and personnel are readily available, usually in the cardiac catheterization laboratory, so that the angiographic diagnosis of spasm can be made and intracoronary nitroglycerin can be administered to abolish the spasm. Some investigators have also found that the ergonovine test can be carried out safely in the coronary care unit, with a positive test being reflected in the development of chest pain and ST-segment depression[560]; however, the safety of the test in this setting has not been firmly established.[561] The normal response of the coronary arterial bed to larger doses (0.40 mg) of ergonovine is a diffuse reduction in arterial caliber by approximately 30 per cent. This dose-dependent phenomenon differs from the abnormal response in Prinzmetal's angina, which is characterized by severe *focal* spasm, usually to much lower doses of the agent.

Methacholine,[562] a parasympathomimetic drug, *dopamine*,[562a] and *histamine*[563] can also induce coronary artery spasm. Like ergonovine, these agents are capable of producing marked coronary artery spasm both in patients with variant angina who have severe underlying arteriosclerotic coronary artery narrowing and in those without such fixed stenoses. Exercise, the cold pressor test, and induced alkalosis can all cause coronary spasm in patients with variant angina, but none of these tests is as sensitive as ergonovine.[564] Catheter-induced coronary ostial spasm is nonspecific and not helpful in the diagnosis of Prinzmetal's angina.

MYOCARDIAL PERFUSION STUDIES. Localization of the myocardial perfusion defect to an area perfused by a coronary artery in which spasm can be demonstrated by arteriography has been reported using intravenous thallium-201,[565, 566] and a reduction in coronary sinus flow during episodes of spasm has also been noted.[567] These studies support the relationship between coronary spasm and the resultant myocardial perfusion and ischemia.

MANAGEMENT

Although the management of Prinzmetal's variant angina is similar in some respects to that of chronic stable angina pectoris, there are important differences:

1. Patients with both forms of angina respond promptly to nitrates; sublingual or intravenous nitroglycerin can often abolish attacks of variant angina promptly, and long-acting nitrates are useful in preventing attacks.[568] However, the mechanism of action of the drugs may differ in the two types of angina. As already discussed (p. 1328), in chronic (effort-induced) stable angina, one important action of the nitrates appears to involve reducing myocardial oxygen needs. In Prinzmetal's angina, the nitrates abolish or prevent myocardial ischemia only by exerting a direct vasodilating effect on the spastic coronary arteries.
2. In patients with chronic stable angina pectoris, beta-adrenoceptor blockade is usually beneficial, but the response of patients with Prinzmetal's angina is variable. Some of the latter, particularly those with associated fixed lesions, exhibit a reduction in the frequency of exertion-induced angina caused primarily by an augmentation of myocardial oxygen requirements. In others, however, propranolol or any nonselective beta-adrenoceptor blocker may actually be detrimental, since blockade of the $beta_2$ receptors, which subserve coronary dilation, allows unopposed alpha-receptor–mediated coronary artery vasoconstriction to occur; the duration of episodes of vasotonic angina has been reported to be prolonged by propranolol.[569]
3. In contrast to beta blockers, the calcium antagonists have been found to be extremely effective in preventing the coronary artery spasm of variant angina.[546, 570] These drugs, along with long- and short-acting nitrates, are the mainstay of therapy in Prinzmetal's angina. Similar efficacy rates have been noted for nifedipine, diltiazem, and verapamil.[571] Rarely, a patient will respond to only one of these three agents, and even less commonly simultaneous administration of two or even three antagonists is required.[571a] A multicenter trial with nifedipine showed dramatic reductions in the frequency of episodes and in the need for nitroglycerin (Fig. 39–30). Because calcium antagonists act through a different mechanism, the vasodilatory actions of these drugs may be additive to those of the nitrates. There have been reports suggesting a rebound of symptoms when nifedipine or verapamil is abruptly discontinued, but not diltiazem.[572] Calcium antagonists ordinarily should be used in maximally tolerated doses.

The natural history of Prinzmetal's angina is cyclic periods of frequent spasm that alternate with asymptomatic periods. After 6 to 12 months of therapy, gradual tapering of the drug with careful observation may be considered.

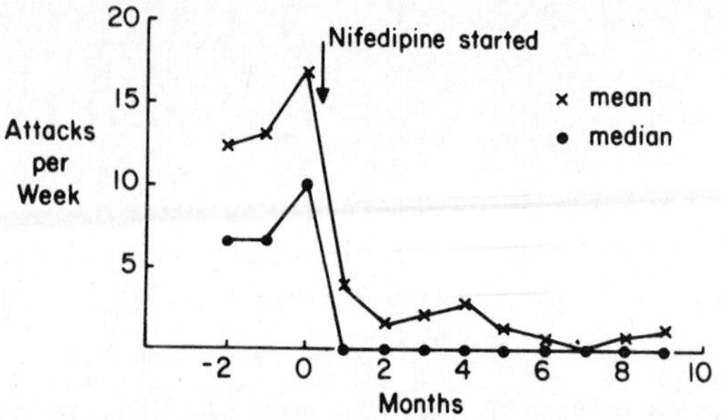

FIGURE 39–30. Mean and median weekly attack rates at various times before and during nifedipine therapy in 127 patients with Prinzmetal's angina. (Reprinted with permission from Antman, E., et al.: Nifedipine therapy for coronary artery spasm: Experience in 127 patients. N. Engl. J. Med. *302*:1269, 1980.)

4. *Prazosin*, a selective alpha-adrenoceptor blocker (p. 873), has also been found to be of value in patients with Prinzmetal's angina.[573] Aspirin, helpful in unstable angina (p. 1359), may actually increase the severity of ischemic episodes in patients with Prinzmetal's angina, because in high dosage aspirin inhibits biosynthesis of the naturally occurring coronary vasodilator prostaglandin I_2.[574]
5. Recent work has suggested that PTCA may be helpful in patients with variant angina[575] who have discrete proximal noncalcified obstructive lesions in a single major coronary artery. Calcium antagonists should be continued for at least 6 months. In patients with isolated coronary artery spasm without accompanying obstructive disease, PTCA and coronary artery bypass surgery are not indicated.

PROGNOSIS

Many patients with variant angina appear to go through an acute, active phase, with frequent episodes of angina and cardiac events during the first 6 months after their presentation. Over this period of time, nonfatal myocardial infarction occurs in up to 20 per cent of patients and death in up to 10 per cent.[576–580] Patients with variant angina who develop serious arrhythmias, ventricular tachycardia, ventricular fibrillation, high-degree atrioventricular block, or asystole during spontaneous episodes of pain have higher maximal ST-segment elevation and are at a higher risk for sudden death.[581] Patients with severe obstructive coronary artery lesions are at greater risk for persistent anginal symptoms, acute myocardial infarction, and death.[577–580] In most patients who survive an infarction or the initial 3- to 6-month period, the condition stabilizes and there is a tendency for symptoms and cardiac events to diminish with time.[580] In time, variant angina may go into remission, with the results of ergonovine testing becoming negative,[559] especially in patients showing a favorable initial response to calcium antagonist treatment.[581a] Then it is possible to attempt cautious tapering of dosage and ultimate withdrawal of calcium antagonists.

ISCHEMIC HEART DISEASE IN WHICH DISCOMFORT IS NOT THE DOMINANT SYMPTOM

"SILENT" MYOCARDIAL ISCHEMIA

There appear to be two forms of "silent" myocardial ischemia. The first and less common form, which we have designated Type I silent ischemia, occurs in patients with severe coronary artery disease who never experience angina; indeed, some do not even experience pain in the course of myocardial infarction. The second and much more frequent form, designated Type II silent ischemia, occurs in patients with the usual forms of chronic stable angina, unstable angina, or Prinzmetal's angina. When carefully monitored, patients with Type II are shown to have some episodes of ischemia that are associated with chest discomfort and other episodes that are not—i.e., episodes of "silent ischemia." Epidemiological studies of sudden death (p. 745), clinical and postmortem studies of patients with "silent" myocardial infarction, and studies of patients with chronic angina pectoris suggest that many individuals with extensive coronary artery obstruction do not have angina pectoris in any of its recognized forms (stable, unstable, or variant).[47–49a, 581b, 581c] These individuals, representative of Type I silent ischemia, have a defective anginal "warning system." Both the patient and physician may be unaware of the presence of ischemic heart disease until a fatal event ensues or an old infarction is detected on a routine electrocardiogram.

During long-term follow-up in the Framingham Study, one-quarter of patients had "unrecognized" myocardial infarction detected only by pathological Q waves on routine 2-yearly electrocardiogram, and of these approximately half of the episodes were truly "silent."[102] In other patients, a myocardial infarction is the first clinical manifestation of ischemic heart disease, although postmortem or angiographic studies indicate that the coronary atherosclerosis must have existed for many years. Such patients may be identified prior to such an event because of cardiac arrhythmias, abnormal electrocardiograms (occasionally at rest, more commonly during exercise), or by means of coronary arteriography performed as a result of a positive exercise test.

AMBULATORY ELECTROCARDIOGRAPHY. The extensive use of ambulatory electrocardiographic monitoring has led to a greater appreciation of "silent" ischemia: It has become apparent that anginal pain is a poor indicator of and underestimator of the frequency of significant cardiac ischemia.[47] Hemodynamic changes indicative of myocardial ischemia (increasing left ventricular end-diastolic pressure and decreasing left ventricular ejection fraction with exercise) occur in patients with coronary artery disease irrespective of the occurrence of angina pectoris.[582] Ambulatory studies in patients with chronic stable angina have also emphasized that, while increases in myocardial oxygen demand lead to ischemia, in many episodes of ischemia, both symptomatic and silent, heart rate is not accelerated and arterial pressure does not rise, suggesting that reductions in myocardial supply make an important contribution to the initiation of ischemia in such patients.[583] Using frequency-modulated ambulatory electrocardiographic recordings, it has been found that transient ST-segment depression of 0.1 mV or greater, which lasts for more than 30 seconds, is a very rare finding in normal subjects.[584] However, in patients known to have coronary artery disease there is a strong correlation between such transient ST-segment depression and independent measurements of regional myocardial perfusion and ischemia using rubidium-82 uptake measured by positron-emission tomography.[23] Perfusion defects occurred in the same myocardial segment during painful and silent episodes of ST-segment depression. These responses were significantly different from those observed in normal subjects studied similarly[23] (Fig. 39–31).

Analyses of ambulatory electrocardiographic recordings in patients with angina (exertion induced, and occurring at rest) suggest that the majority of ischemic episodes occurring during normal daily activities are asymptomatic[459–461, 584–586b] (Fig. 39–32) (Type II silent ischemia). Episodes of ST-segment depression, both symptomatic and silent, are more common in the morning.[172] Nocturnal ST-segment changes are almost invariably an indicator of two- or three-vessel coronary artery disease or left main stem stenosis.[587]

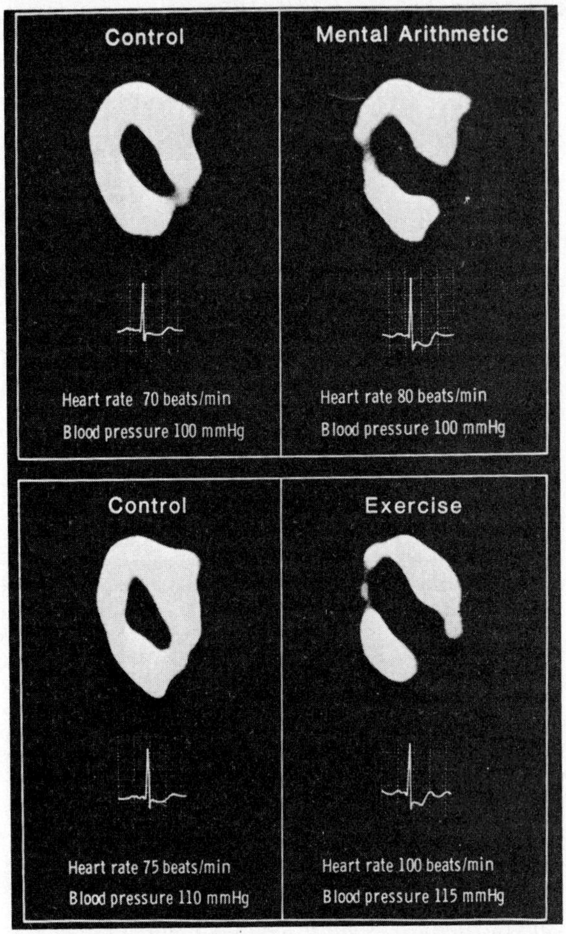

FIGURE 39–31. These images are tomographic slices of the myocardium recorded using positron-emission tomography in a patient with chronic stable angina, a positive exercise test, and proven coronary artery disease. The information from the heart is obtained from the short-lived tracer rubidium-82, which provides a measure of the distribution and changes in regional myocardial perfusion. The first image (control, *top left*) shows uniform perfusion to the posterior wall, free wall, anterior wall, and septum of the left ventricle. Regional myocardial perfusion during mental arithmetic (*top right*) shows a regional decrease in myocardial perfusion to the left ventricular free wall accompanied by ST-segment depression but not associated with chest pain. The second control image (*bottom left*) shows a return of myocardial perfusion to normal. During exercise (*bottom right*) there is a recurrence of ischemia in the same area of the myocardium in which a perfusion abnormality occurred during the stress of mental arithmetic. With exercise, there was both ST-segment depression and symptoms of angina pectoris. Thus, in this patient the ischemia provoked by mental arithmetic (asymptomatic) and exercise (symptomatic) showed similar ST-segment depression and myocardial perfusion abnormalities. (From Deanfield, J. E., et al.: Silent myocardial ischemia due to mental stress. Lancet *2*:1001, 1984.)

MECHANISM OF SILENT ISCHEMIA. It is unclear why some episodes of myocardial ischemia are silent while others are symptomatic. It has been theorized that patients who have no episodes of symptomatic ischemia have a higher pain threshold.[588] Some studies suggest that silent episodes may reflect less severe ischemia[460] with less evidence of left ventricular dysfunction.[463] Among patients who experience both symptomatic and asymptomatic ischemia, the ST segment changes recorded by ambulatory ECG monitoring are similar, although there is a tendency for symptomatic episodes to be accompanied by longer periods of ST segment deviation and more marked ST depressions.[587] In keeping with the increased incidence of silent myocardial infarction in patients with diabetes mel-

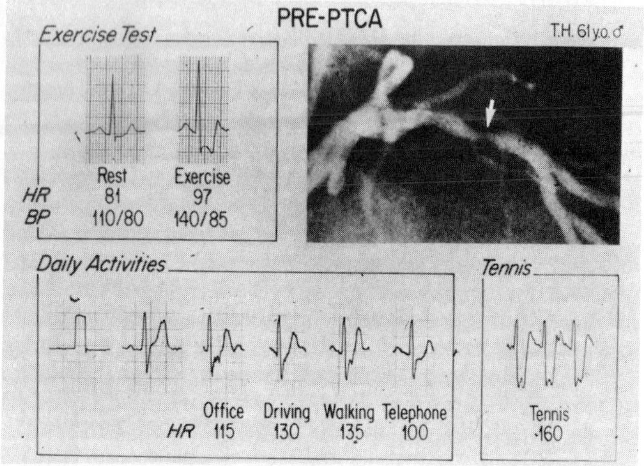

FIGURE 39–32. The ambulant electrocardiograms and coronary angiograms of a severe left anterior descending stenosis of a patient who presented with fatigue (but not angina) during a singles tennis match are shown. In stage II of a treadmill exercise test (Bruce protocol), 4 mm of ST-segment depression was seen in lead V5. Ambulatory Holter monitoring of lead V_5 demonstrates ischemic ST-segment depressions during a number of ordinary activities, e.g., walking, telephoning. During a game of tennis, marked ST-segment depression was recorded when the patient was asymptomatic. (From Nabel, E. G., et al.: Characteristics and significance of ischemia detected by ambulatory electrocardiographic monitoring. Circulation *75*[Suppl. II]74, 1987, by permission of the American Heart Association, Inc.)

litus, there is an increased incidence of asymptomatic ischemia in patients with coronary artery disease and type II diabetes mellitus than in nondiabetic patients.[589] Smokers with coronary artery disease may have profound silent disturbances of regional myocardial perfusion and ST-segment depressions during smoking.[590] It is not yet clear whether frequent episodes of silent ischemia, i.e., asymptomatic episodes of ST-segment depression, occurring in patients who also experience exercise-induced angina indicate a worse prognosis in these patients. Pharmacological agents which reduce or abolish episodes of symptomatic ischemia, i.e., nitrates, beta blockers and calcium antagonists, also reduce or abolish episodes of silent ischemia.[590a] It is also not clear whether abolition of silent ischemia should be the endpoint of therapy and whether this will influence prognosis favorably. It should be noted that monitoring of patients with unstable angina pectoris identifies a subset of patients with a worse long-term prognosis.[498]

DETECTION. At the present time, the detection of patients with coronary artery disease without angina (Type I silent ischemia) is largely fortuitous. It is likely that screening of populations on a mass basis for silent ischemia would be extraordinarily costly.[591] Many false-positive tests occur in normal individuals.[592, 593] In Norway, an effort to detect such patients was carried out using a combination of screening techniques (questionnaires, resting and exercise electrocardiograms) in over 2000 asymptomatic and presumably healthy men aged 40 to 50 years.[594] Patients known to have heart disease, hypertension, or diabetes mellitus were excluded. As a result of the screening, more than 105 men were referred for coronary angiography: only 20 on the basis of a suspicious history and the rest because of electrocardiographic abnormality. Two-thirds were found to have coronary artery disease. Overall, less than 4 per cent of this population had silent myocardial ischemia, i.e., more than 75 per cent luminal stenosis of one or more coronary arteries. This figure is close to the 4 to 5 per cent of the population estimated by others to be the size of this subgroup.[42]

However, many patients with Type I asymptomatic ischemia are identified because of an asymptomatic positive exercise electrocardiogram performed following myocardial infarction.[593a] In those patients with a defective anginal warning system it would appear to be useful to obtain coronary arteriograms. Consideration should be given to treating critically obstructive lesions by revascularization so that severe asymptomatic ischemia is not induced repeatedly during normal life.

HEART FAILURE

Manifestations of congestive heart failure are common in patients with coronary artery disease but may be predominant in some, especially those who have sustained prior myocardial infarctions and in whom the ischemic focus may have become replaced by fibrous scar, with disappearance or reduction of the angina. The three most common causes of congestive heart failure are (1) left ventricular aneurysm, (2) mitral regurgitation due to papillary muscle dysfunction, and (3) an inadequate quantity of normally contracting myocardium. The latter may be secondary to extensive myocardial infarction, a large quantity of viable but "hibernating" myocardium, or a combination of these.

LEFT VENTRICULAR ANEURYSM

This is usually defined as paradoxical (dyskinetic) systolic expansion of a portion of the ventricular wall, most commonly the anterior or apical segment. In vitro length-tension studies of tissue taken from human ventricular aneurysms have demonstrated that chronic fibrous aneurysms interfere with ventricular performance principally through loss of contractile tissue but that the extent of expansion and "lost work" by the normal left ventricle is minor.[595] These might be considered to be anatomical but not functional aneurysms (Fig. 39–33). In contrast, aneurysms made up largely of a mixture of scar tissue and viable myocardium or of thin scar tissue produce a mechanical disadvantage by a combination of paradoxical expansion and loss of effective contraction[596]; these might be considered to be functional aneurysms. *False aneurysms* (pseudoaneurysms), which represent localized myocardial rupture, in which the hemorrhage is limited by pericardial adhesions (Figs. 5–91, p. 122, and 39–33) have a mouth that is considerably smaller than the maximal diameter.

The frequency of the development of ventricular aneurysms after myocardial infarction depends on the incidence of transmural myocardial infarction and congestive heart failure in the population studied. Left ventricular aneurysm in the absence of coronary artery disease but with prior infarction has been reported, but it is a rare occurrence. Anterior aneurysms are often associated with total occlusion of the left anterior descending coronary artery, and a poor collateral blood supply, but are unusual in the presence of multivessel disease with a good collateral circulation or a patent anterior descending coronary artery.[596a]

Over 80 per cent of left ventricular aneurysms are located anterolaterally near the apex, with approximately 5 to 10 per cent located posteriorly. Most anterior aneurysms are true aneurysms, whereas nearly half of the posterior aneurysms are false aneurysms.[597] Three-quarters of patients with aneurysms have multivessel coronary artery disease.[598] Almost half of patients with moderate or large aneurysms present with symptoms of heart failure,

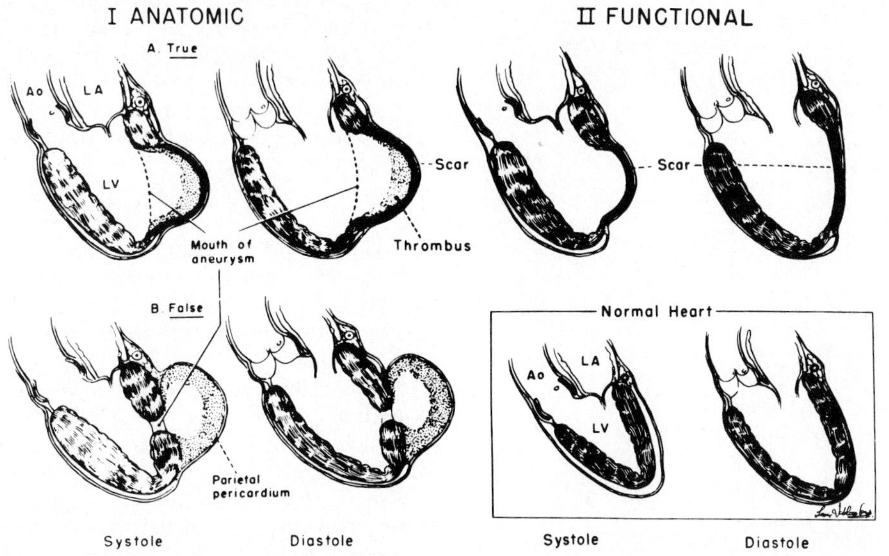

FIGURE 39–33. Diagrams of hearts in systole and diastole with true and false anatomical and functional left ventricular aneurysms and healed myocardial infarction. A diagram of a normal heart in systole and diastole is shown for comparison. The *true anatomical left ventricular aneurysm* protrudes during both systole and diastole, has a mouth that is as wide as or wider than the maximal diameter, has a wall that was formerly the wall of the left ventricle, and is composed of fibrous tissue with or without residual myocardial fibers. A true aneurysm may or may not contain thrombus and almost never ruptures once the wall is healed. The *false anatomical left ventricular aneurysm* protrudes during both systole and diastole, has a mouth that is considerably smaller than the maximal diameter of the aneurysm and represents a myocardial rupture site, has a wall made up of parietal pericardium, virtually always contains thrombus, and often ruptures. The *functional left ventricular aneurysm* protrudes during ventricular systole but not during diastole and consists of fibrous tissue with or without myocardial fibers. (From Cabin, H. S., and Roberts, W. C.: Left ventricular aneurysm, intraaneurysmal thrombus and systemic embolus in coronary heart disease. Chest *77*:586, 1980.)

with or without associated angina. One-third present with severe angina alone, and approximately 15 per cent have symptoms related to ventricular arrhythmias. Thrombosis is found in almost half of patients with left ventricular aneurysms.[599] Embolic events in patients with left ventricular thrombi occur infrequently, tend to occur within the initial 4 to 6 months after infarction, and can be devastating. Thrombi within the left ventricle can be detected by angiography, two-dimensional echocardiography (Fig. 5–94, p. 123), or indium-111-labeled autologous platelets.[600] Beyond the first 6 months after infarction the data are insufficient to suggest that long-term anticoagulant treatment is routinely indicated.[601] Some patients with ventricular aneurysms have a high incidence of arrhythmias, and some have intractable life-threatening ventricular arrhythmia requiring surgery (p. 645).

DETECTION. Diagnostic clues to the presence of aneurysm include persistent ST-segment elevations on the electrocardiogram and a characteristic contour (bulge) of cardiac silhouette of the left ventricle on a chest roentgenogram (Fig. 6–23, p. 154). These findings, when clear-cut, are relatively specific but they have limited sensitivity. Radionuclide ventriculography (Fig. 11–13, p. 327) and two-dimensional echocardiography (Fig. 5–87, p. 120) can demonstrate ventricular aneurysm. Two-dimensional echocardiography has also been used to evaluate the function and size of the nonaneurysmal or residual myocardium[602] and shortening of minor axis dimensions at the base of the heart,[603] which both provide prognostic information. As expected, those patients with the best function of residual myocardium have a better outcome after surgery. Computer tomography may be a relatively reliable noninvasive technique for the identification of left ventricular aneurysms and screening for resectability (Fig. 12–8, p. 362).[604] However, biplane left ventriculography remains the most precise method available for outlining a left ventricular aneurysm, assessing septal motion, and determining the quantity of functioning residual myocardium.

The motion of the interventricular septum, as assessed by radionuclide[605, 606] or contrast angiography[607] or echocardiography, is also of importance in evaluating the function of residual myocardium. Patients with akinesis of the interventricular septum tend to have less favorable outcomes following surgery compared with patients who exhibit septal motion.[607] On the other hand, patients who exhibit the most paradoxical systolic movement of the aneurysm tend to do better after operation than those showing akinesis.[605, 606]

LEFT VENTRICULAR ANEURYSMECTOMY. Indications for this procedure include congestive heart failure, refractory ventricular tachycardia, recurrent thromboembolism, and refractory angina. A large left ventricular aneurysm in a patient with symptoms of heart failure, particularly if angina pectoris is also present, is an indication for operation. Among patients with advanced chronic congestive heart failure, operation carries a particularly high risk in those with symptoms of severe heart failure or a low output state, a requirement for more than 80 mg of furosemide daily, and akinesis of the interventricular septum. Akinesia or dyskinesia of the posterior basal segment of the left ventricle and significant right coronary artery stenoses are additional risk factors.[598] The presence of angina pectoris appears to be a more benign symptom preoperatively than heart failure and is associated with a better prognosis following operation.[597, 598]

Hospital mortality for left ventricular aneurysmectomy is under 10 per cent,[597] with acute cardiac failure and intractable ventricular arrhythmias identifying patients at highest risk. Risk factors for poor late survival include incomplete revascularization, impaired systolic function of the basal segments of the ventricle and of the septum, and the presence of dominant symptoms of cardiac failure

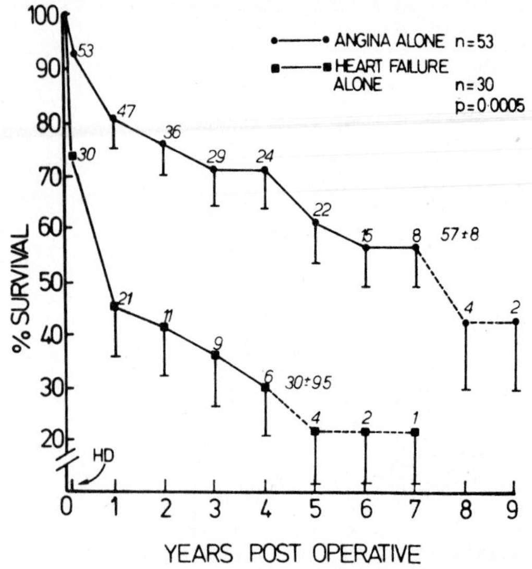

FIGURE 39–34. Survival curves for surgically treated patients with left ventricular aneurysm. Those patients complaining of angina rather than heart failure before operation have a more favorable long-term survival. The numbers of patients at risk are noted. (From Barratt-Boyes, B. G., et al: The results of surgical treatment of left ventricular aneurysms: An assessment of risk factors affecting early and late mortality. J. Thorac. Cardiovasc. Surg. *87*:87, 1984.)

rather than angina pectoris[597, 598] (Fig. 39–34). Long-term follow-up in survivors usually shows impressive clinical improvement. After 5 years, 70 to 80 per cent of survivors are in NYHA class I or II,[608, 609] with a 10-year actuarial survival of 69 per cent in patients undergoing left ventricular aneurysmectomy and revascularization compared with 57 per cent in those undergoing left ventricular aneurysmectomy alone.[608] Ejection fraction during exercise has been shown to improve up to one year after operation.[610]

True ventricular aneurysms do not rupture, and operative excision is carried out in order to improve the clinical manifestations (most often heart failure but sometimes also angina and life-threatening tachyarrhythmias). Pseudoaneurysms do rupture, on the other hand, and they should be resected on an urgent basis as soon as the diagnosis is established.

MITRAL REGURGITATION

Rupture of a papillary muscle, or of the head of a papillary muscle, usually causes severe acute mitral regurgitation in the course of an acute myocardial infarction (Fig. 33–13, p. 1037). Chronic mitral regurgitation in patients with ischemic heart disease is caused, most commonly, by papillary muscle dysfunction due to ischemia or fibrosis (Fig. 33–11, p. 1036) and/or by dilatation of the mitral annulus; many of the latter patients have ventricular aneurysms (p. 1037). Most patients with chronic coronary artery disease and mitral regurgitation suffered prior myocardial infarction, but the frequency of this syndrome (as with aneurysm) varies depending on the population studied. Clinical features that help to identify mitral regurgitation due to papillary muscle dysfunction as the cause of acute pulmonary edema or of milder symptoms of left-sided failure include a typical heart murmur and demonstration of a flail mitral valve leaflet on echocardiography. The latter is the preferred diagnostic technique, since the timing and duration of the murmur are variable. Instead of being only mid- to late systolic, as was originally thought, murmurs may be holosystolic or early systolic. Doppler echocardiography is helpful in assessing the severity of the regurgitation. The left atrium is usually not greatly enlarged unless severe mitral regurgitation has been present for almost a year. The electrocardiogram is nonspecific, and most patients have angiographic evidence of multivessel coronary artery disease. Mitral valve replacement alone is rarely indicated but may be undertaken in combination with coronary artery bypass grafting.

ISCHEMIC CARDIOMYOPATHY

Burch and colleagues used the term *ischemic cardiomyopathy* to describe the condition in which coronary artery disease results in severe myocardial dysfunction, often indistinguishable from manifestations of primary cardiomyopathy.[611] The fact that manifestations of cardiac dysfunction such as dyspnea or heart failure rather than anginal pain may be the predominant feature of ischemic myocardium is well known. Recent observations have confirmed that in ambulatory patients with coronary artery disease the occurrence or frequency of angina pectoris is an insensitive indicator of significant cardiac ischemia[587] and of ventricular dysfunction occurring during exertion.[582] Thus, symptoms of heart failure (caused by ischemic myocardial dysfunction, diffuse fibrosis, and multiple infarctions, alone or in combination) rather than a single discrete ventricular aneurysm may dominate the clinical picture. In some patients with chronic coronary artery disease angina may be the principal clinical manifestation at one time but later diminishes or even disappears as heart failure becomes more prominent. Other patients have no history of angina or myocardial infarction (Type I silent ischemia, p. 1363) and it is in this subgroup that ischemic cardiomyopathy may be confused with dilated cardiomyopathy (p. 1414).

The electrocardiogram may also be misleading. Myocardium with apparent electrocardiographic evidence of infarction, namely pathological Q waves and diminished R wave height, can be successfully reperfused with improvement in myocardial function.[612] Further evidence that electrocardiographic Q waves may overlie ischemic, rather than necrotic, myocardium is provided by the observation that Q waves may be induced by exercise and subsequently disappear with rest.[613]

When considering ischemic myopathy, it is important to recognize that chronic reduction of myocardial perfusion may cause persistent left ventricular dysfunction without tissue necrosis occurring so that as long as myocardial flow is inadequate, function remains impaired ("hibernating myocardium," pp. 1325 and 1349).[150] Thus, hibernating myocardium can result from months or years of ischemia and ventricular dysfunction will persist until blood flow is restored. Stunned myocardium, on the other hand, results from a brief period of ischemia which is followed by impaired contractile performance, persisting much longer. The concept of "myocardial hibernation" is a useful one because symptoms resulting from chronic left ventricular dysfunction may be incorrectly thought to result from necrotic and scarred myocardium rather than from a reversible ischemic process.

It is for this reason that attempts have been made to decide whether cardiac dysfunction is irreversible (due to necrosis) or potentially reversible (due to ischemia). If myocardial contractility can be improved by an inotropic stimulus such as postextrasystolic potentiation or the infusion of a sympathomimetic amine, it is said to exhibit contractile reserve. Hibernating myocardium may be present in patients with known or suspected coronary artery disease with a degree of cardiac dysfunction or heart failure not readily accounted for by other possible causes, e.g., cardiomyopathy of other etiology, longstanding hypertension, and prior myocardial infarctions. In patients in whom this condition is suspected, cardiac catheterization and coronary arteriography should be carried out to assess hemodynamic parameters, ventricular function, and coronary anatomy. If myocardium exhibiting a contractile defect is supplied by stenotic or collateral vessels, efforts are made to see whether it exhibits contractile reserve. If improvement in ventricular function occurs with inotropic stimulation it is possible that revascularization carried out by surgery or coronary angioplasty may result in improved survival (p. 1349).[324, 614, 615] The outlook for patients with ischemic cardiomyopathy treated medically is very poor.[616] Associated ventricular arrhythmias occurring in such patients with poor ventricular function usually are an ominous sign. Patients with diffuse disease have the worst outlook, with a slightly better clinical course being observed in patients with isolated wall motion disorders.

CARDIAC ARRHYTHMIAS

Many patients with ischemic heart disease with serious cardiac arrhythmias have other manifestations of active myocardial ischemia, such as acute myocardial infarction. Various degrees of ventricular ectopic activity are the most common arrhythmias. The frequency and severity of ventricular arrhythmias induced during exercise tests and ambulatory monitoring correlate with the degree of arteriographically documented coronary artery disease. Patients with severe left ventricular dysfunction associated with multivessel disease have more high-grade ectopic activity than do those with normal ventricular function and single-vessel disease.[617] In some patients with coronary artery disease cardiac arrhythmias are the *predominant* manifestation of their disease. That there is a substantial subgroup of patients with coronary artery disease and occult arrhythmias is suggested by the frequency with which sudden death is the first manifestation of ischemic heart disease (Chap. 24). When arrhythmias are the predominant clinical manifestation, they are also the main focus of therapeutic interventions. This ordinarily involves pharmacological therapy, but in cases of drug failure, electrical (p. 642) and surgical (p. 645) therapy may be useful.

NONATHEROMATOUS CORONARY ARTERY DISEASE

Nonatheromatous ischemic heart disease may result from congenital abnormalities in the origin or distribution of the coronary arteries (pp. 288 and 927). The most important of these are anomalous origin of a coronary artery (usually the left) from the pulmonary artery, origin of both coronary arteries from either the right or left sinus of Valsalva, and coronary arteriovenous fistula.

A number of inherited connective tissue disorders are associated with myocardial ischemia.[618] These include the Marfan syndrome (aortic dissection) (p. 1725), Hurler syndrome (coronary obstruction) (p. 1726), homocystinuria (coronary artery thrombosis) (p. 1726), Ehlers-Danlos syndrome (coronary arterial dissection) (p. 1727), and pseudoxanthoma elasticum (accelerated coronary artery disease) (p. 1726). Kawasaki disease, the mucocutaneous lymph node syndrome, may cause coronary artery aneurysms and ischemic heart disease in children (p. 1014).

Perhaps the most common cause of nonatheromatous coronary disease resulting in myocardial ischemia is the syndrome of angina-like pain despite normal coronary arteriograms. Myocardial ischemia *not* caused by coronary atherosclerosis can also result from embolism, as in infective endocarditis (Chap. 34); prosthetic valve thrombi (Chap. 33); primary tumors of the heart (Chap. 43); calcific emboli from calcified aortic valves, especially from mural thrombi. Luetic aortitis may also produce myocardial ischemia by causing obstruction of coronary ostia.

An interesting nonatherosclerotic ischemic syndrome has been described in workers in the nitrate industry who apparently experience nitrate withdrawal symptoms on weekends, presumed to be secondary to coronary spasm when there is no counterstimulation to the vasoconstriction that they undergo as an adaptation to the vasodilating actions of the high concentrations of nitrates to which they are exposed.[619]

Acknowledgment

The authors gratefully acknowledge the secretarial help of Lisa J. McHale.

REFERENCES

INTRODUCTION

1. Marmot, M. G.: Interpretation of trends in coronary heart disease mortality. Acta Med. Scand (Suppl.) *701*:58, 1985.
2. Connolly, D. C., Oxman, A. J., Nobrega, F. T., Kurland, L. T., Kennedy, M. A., and Elveback, L. R.: Coronary heart disease in residents of Rochester, Minnesota, 1950–1975. I. Background in study design. Mayo Clinic Proc. *56*:661, 1981.
3. Elveback, L. R., Connolly, D. C., and Kurland, L. T.: Coronary heart disease in residents of Rochester, Minnesota, 1950–1975. II. Mortality, incidence, and survival. Mayo Clin. Proc. *56*:665, 1981.
4. WHO Expert Committee: Prevention of coronary heart disease. Tech. Rep. Ser. WHO 1982; No. 678.
5. Heberden, W.: Some account of a disorder of the breast. Med. Trans. Coll. Physicians (Lond.) *2*:59, 1772.
6. Parry, C. H.: An inquiry into the symptoms and causes of the syncope anginosa, commonly called angina pectoris. Vols. 3 and 4. Bath, England, K. Cuttwell, 1799, p. 113.
7. Flint, A.: Diseases affecting the circulatory system. *In* A Treatise on the Principles and Practice of Medicine. Philadelphia, Henry C. Lea, 1866.
8. Brunton, T. L.: On the use of nitrite of amyl in angina pectoris. Lancet *2*:97, 1867.
9. Osler, W.: The Principles and Practice of Medicine. New York, Appleton, 1892.
10. Muller, J. E.: Diagnosis of myocardial infarction: Historical notes from the Soviet Union and the United States. Am. J. Cardiol. *40*:269, 1977.
11. Herrick, J. B.: Clinical features of sudden obstruction of the coronary arteries. J.A.M.A. *59*:2015, 1912.
12. White, P. D.: The prevalence of coronary heart disease. *In* Blumgart, H. I. (ed.): Symposium on Coronary Heart Disease. New York, American Heart Association, 1968.
13. Wearn, J. T.: Thrombosis of the coronary arteries, with infarction of the heart. Am. J. Med. Sci. *165*:250, 1923.
14. Blumgart, H. L., Schlesinger, M. J., and Zoll, P. M.: Angina pectoris, coronary failure and acute myocardial infarction: The role of coronary occlusions and collateral circulation. J.A.M.A. *116*:91, 1941.
15. Sones, F. M., Jr.: Acquired heart disease: Symposium on the Present and Future of Cineangiography. Am. J. Cardiol. 3:710, 1959.

CHRONIC (STABLE) ANGINA PECTORIS

16. Matthews, M. B., and Julian, D. G.: Angina pectoris: Definition and description. *In* Julian, D. G. (ed.): Angina Pectoris. 2nd ed. New York, Churchill Livingstone, 1985, p. 2.
17. Christie, L. G., Jr., and Conti, C. R.: Systematic approach to evaluation of angina-like chest pain: Pathophysiology and clinical testing with emphasis on objective documentation of myocardial ischemia. Am. Heart J. *102*:897, 1981.
18. Sampson, J. J., and Cheitlin, M. D.: Pathophysiology and differential diagnosis of cardiac pain. Prog. Cardiovasc. Dis. *13*:507, 1971.
19. Malliani, A.: The elusive link between transient myocardial ischemia and pain. Circulation *73*:201, 1986.
20. Sylven, C., Beermann, B., Jonzon, B., and Brandt, R.: Angina pectoris-like pain provoked by intravenous adenosine in healthy volunteers. Br. Med. J. *293*:227, 1986.
21. Del Banco, P. L., Del Bene, E., and Sicuteri, F.: Heart pain. *In* Bonica, J. J. (ed.): Advances in Neurology. Vol. 4. New York, Raven Press, 1974, p. 375.
22. Mountcastle, V. B.: Pain and temperature sensibilities. *In* Mountcastle, V. B. (ed.): Medical Physiology. 13th ed. St. Louis. C. V. Mosby Co., 1974.
23. Deanfield, J., Shea, M., Ribeiro, P., de Landsheere, C. M., Wilson, R. A., Horlock, P., and Selwyn, A. P.: Transient ST-segment depression as a marker of myocardial ischemia during daily life. Am. J. Cardiol. *54*:1195, 1984.
24. Branch, W. T., Jr.: Severe chest pain: Noncardiac emergencies. J. Cardiovasc. Med. *8*:159, 1983.
25. Constant, J.: The clinical diagnosis of nonanginal chest pain: The differentiation of angina from nonanginal chest pain by history. Clin. Cardiol. *6*:11, 1983.
26. Hillis, L. D., and Braunwald, E.: Coronary artery spasm. N. Engl. J. Med. *299*:695, 1978.
27. Epstein, S. E., and Talbot, T. L.: Dynamic coronary tone in precipitation, exacerbation and relief of angina pectoris. Am. J. Cardiol., *48*:797, 1981.
28. Ganz, P., Abben, R. P., and Barry, W. H.: Dynamic variations in resistance of coronary arterial narrowings in angina pectoris at rest. Am. J. Cardiol. *59*:66, 1987.
29. Yasue, H.: Pathophysiology and treatment of coronary arterial spasm. Chest *78*:216, 1980.
30. Quyyumi, A. A., Mockus, L. J., Wright, C. A., and Fox, K. M.: Mechanisms of nocturnal angina pectoris: Importance of increased myocardial oxygen demand in patients with severe coronary artery disease. Lancet *1*:1207, 1984.
31. Maseri, A.: Mixed angina pectoris. Am. J. Cardiol. *56*:30E, 1985.
32. Epstein, S. E., Stampfer, M., Beiser, G. D., Goldstein, R. E., and Braunwald, E.: Effect of a reduction in environmental temperature on the circulatory response to exercise in man. Implications concerning angina pectoris. N. Engl. J. Med. *280*:7, 1969.
33. Mudge, G. H., Jr., Grossman, W., Mills, R. M., Jr., Lesch, M., and Braunwald, E.: Reflex increase in coronary vascular resistance in patients with ischemic heart disease. N. Engl. J. Med. 295:1333, 1976.
34. Mudge, G. H., Jr., Goldberg, S., Gunther, S., Mann, T., and Grossman, W.: Comparison of metabolic and vasoconstrictor stimuli on coronary vascular resistance in man. Circulation *59*:544, 1979.

35. Goldstein, R. E., Redwood, D. R., Beiser, G. D., and Epstein, S. E.: Alterations in the circulatory response to exercise following a meal and their relationship in postprandial angina pectoris. Circulation *44*:90, 1971.
36. Figueras, J., Singh, B. N., Ganz, W., and Swan, H. J. C.: Hemodynamic and electrocardiographic accompaniments of resting postprandial angina. Br. Heart J. *42*:402, 1979.
37. Schiffer, F., Hartley, L. H., Schulman, C. L., and Abelmann, W. H.: Evidence for emotionally induced coronary arterial spasm in patients with angina pectoris. Br. Heart J. *44*:62, 1980.
38. Horowitz, L. D., Herman, M. V., and Gorlin, R.: Clinical response to nitroglycerin as a diagnostic test for coronary artery disease. Am. J. Cardiol. *29*:149, 1972.
39. Levine, S. A.: Carotid sinus massage: A new diagnostic test for angina pectoris. J.A.M.A. *182*:1332, 1962.
40. Campeau, L.: Grading of angina pectoris. Circulation *54*:522, 1976.
41. Goldman, L., Hashimoto, B., and Cook, E. F.: Comparative reproducibility and validity of systems for assessing cardiovascular functional class: Advantages of a new specific activity scale. Circulation *64*:1227, 1981.
42. Diamond, G. A., and Forrester, J. S.: Analysis of probability as an aid in the clinical diagnosis of coronary artery disease. N. Engl. J. Med. *300*:1350, 1979.
43. Pasternak, R. C., Thibault, G. E., Savoia, M., DeSanctis, R. W., and Hutter, A. M., Jr.: Chest pain with angiographically insignificant coronary arterial obstruction. Clinical presentation and long-term follow-up. Am. J. Med. *68*:813, 1980.
44. Proudfit, W. L., Shirey, E. K., Sheldon, W. C., and Sones, F. M., Jr.: Certain clinical characteristics correlated with extent of obstructive lesions demonstrated by selective cine coronary arteriography. Circulation *38*:947, 1968.
45. Hamby, R. I., Gupta, M. P., and Young, M. W.: Clinical and hemodynamic aspects of single-vessel coronary artery disease. Am. Heart J. *85*:458, 1973.
46. Welch, C. C., Proudfit, W. L., and Sheldon, W. C.: Coronary arteriographic findings in 1000 women under age 50. Am. J. Cardiol. *35*:211, 1975.
47. Quyyumi, A. A., Wright, C. M., Mockus, L. J., and Fox, K. M.: How important is a history of chest pain in determining the degree of ischemia in patients with angina pectoris? Br. Heart J. *54*:22, 1985.
48. Singh, B. N., Nademanee, K., Figueras, J., and Josephson, M. A.: Hemodynamic and electrocardiographic correlates of symptomatic and silent myocardial ischemia: Pathophysiologic and therapeutic implications. Am. J. Cardiol. *58*:3B–10B, 1986.
49. Selwyn, A. P., Shea, M., Deanfield, J. E., Wilson, R., Horlock, P., and O'Brien, H. A.: Character of transient ischemia in angina pectoris. Am. J. Cardiol. *58*:21B–25B, 1986.
49a. Coy, K. M., Imperi, G. A., Lambert, C. R., and Pepine, C. J.: Silent myocardial ischemia during daily activities in asymptomatic men with positive exercise test responses. Am. J. Cardiol. *59*:45, 1987.
50. Cohn, P. F., Harris, P., Barry, W. H., Rosati, R. A., Rosenbaum, P., and Waternaux, C.: Prognostic importance of anginal symptoms in angiographically defined coronary artery disease. Am. J. Cardiol. *47*:233, 1981.
51. Gordon, P. R., Abrams, C., Gash, A. K., and Carabello, B. A.: Pericatheterization risk factors in left main coronary artery stenosis. Am. J. Cardiol. *59*:1080, 1987.
52. Reunanen, A., Suhonen, O., Aromaa, A., Knekt, P., and Pyorala, K.: Incidence of different manifestations of coronary heart disease in middle-aged Finnish men and women. Acta Med. Scand. *218*:19, 1985.
52a. Colditz, G. A., Willett, W. C., Stampfer, M. J., Rosner, B., Speizer, F. E., and Hennekens, C. H.: Menopause and the risk of coronary heart disease in women. N. Engl. J. Med. *316*:1105, 1987.
52b. Vantrappen, G., and Janssens, J.: Angina and oesophageal pain—a gastroenterologist's point of view. Eur. Heart J. *7*:828, 1986.
52c. Rapaport, E.: Angina and oesophageal pain. Eur. Heart J. *7*:824, 1986.
53. Davies, H. A., Jones, D. B., Rhodes, J., and Newcombe, R. G.: Anginal-like esophageal pain: differentiation from cardiac pain by history. J. Clin. Gastroenterol. *7*:477, 1985.
54. Winnan, G. R., Meyer, C. T., and McCallum, R. W.: Interpretation of the Bernstein Test: A reappraisal of criteria. Ann. Intern. Med. *96*:320, 1982.
55. DeMeester, T. R., O'Sullivan, G. C., Bermudez, G., Midell, A. I., Cimochowski, G. E., O'Drobinak, J.: Esophageal function in patients with angina-type chest pain and normal coronary angiograms. Ann. Surg. *196*:488, 1982.
56. Mellow, M. H., Simpson, A. G., Watt, L., Schoolmeester, L., and Haye, O. L.: Esophageal acid perfusion in coronary artery disease. Gastroenterology *85*:306, 1983.
57. Davies, H. A., Rush, E. M., Lewis, M. J., Page, Z., Brown, A. L., and Petch, M. C.: Oesophageal stimulation lowers exertional angina threshold. Lancet *1*:1011, 1985.
58. Patterson, D. R.: Diffuse esophageal spasm in patients with undiagnosed chest pain. J. Clin. Gastroenterol. *4*:415, 1982.
59. Traube, M., Albibi, R., and McCallum, R. W.: High-amplitude peristaltic esophageal contractions associated with chest pain. J.A.M.A. *250*:2655, 1983.
60. Lee, M. G., Sullivan, S. N., Watson, W. C., and Melendez, L. J.: Chest pain—esophageal, cardiac, or both? Am. J. Gastroenterol. *80*:320, 1985.
61. Eastwood, G. L., Weiner, B. H., Dickerson, W. J., White, E. M., Ockene, I. S., Haffajee, C. I., and Alpert, J. S.: Use of ergonovine to identify esophageal spasm in patients with chest pain. Ann. Intern. Med. *94*:768, 1981.
62. Wolf, E., and Stern, S.: Costosternal syndrome. Its frequency and importance in differential diagnosis of coronary heart disease. Arch. Intern. Med. *136*:189, 1976.
63. Peyton, F. W.: Unexpected frequency of idiopathic costochondral pain. Obstet. Gynecol. *62*:605, 1983.
64. Epstein, S. E., Gerber, L. H., and Borer, J. S.: Chest wall syndrome. A common cause of unexpected cardiac pain. J.A.M.A. *241*:2793, 1979.
65. Bettmann, M. A., and Salzman, E. W.: Current concepts in the diagnosis of pulmonary embolism. Mod. Concepts Cardiovasc. Dis. *53*:1, 1984.
66. Cohn, P. F., Gorlin, R., Vokonas, P., Williams, R. A., and Herman, M. V.: A quantitative clinical index for the diagnosis of symptomatic coronary artery disease. N. Engl. J. Med. *286*:901, 1972.
67. Ockene, I. S., Shay, M. J., Alpert, J. S., Weiner, B. H., and Dalen, J. E.: Unexplained chest pain in patients with normal coronary arteriograms. N. Engl. J. Med. *303*:1249, 1980.
68. Papanicolaou, M. N., Califf, R. M., Hlatky, M. A., McKinnis, R. A., Harrell, F. E., Jr., Mark, D. B., McCants, B., Rosati, R. A., Lee, K. L., and Pryor, D. B.: Prognostic implications of angiographically normal and insignificantly narrowed coronary arteries. Am. J. Cardiol. *58*:1181, 1986.
69. Kemp, H. G., Kronmal, R. A., Vlietstra, R. E., Frye, R. L., and participants in the Coronary Artery Surgery Study: Seven-year survival of patients with normal or near normal coronary arteriograms: A CASS Registry study. J. Am. Coll. Cardiol. *7*:479, 1986.
70. Greenberg, M. A., Grose, R. M., Neuburger, N., Silverman, R., Strain, J. E., and Cohen, M. V.: Impaired coronary vasodilator responsiveness as a cause of lactate production during pacing-induced ischemia in patients with angina pectoris and normal coronary arteries. J. Am. Coll. Cardiol. *9*:743, 1987.
71. Cannon, R. O., Leon, M. B., Watson, R. M., Rosing, D. R., and Epstein, S. E.: Chest pain and "normal" coronary arteries—role of small coronary arteries. Am. J. Cardiol. *55*:50B, 1985.
72. Cannon, R. O., Bonow, R. O., Bacharach, S. L., Green, M. V., Rosing, D. R., Leon, M. B., Watson, R. M., and Epstein, S. E.: Left ventricular dysfunction in patients with angina pectoris, normal epicardial coronary arteries, and abnormal vasodilator reserve. Circulation *71*:218, 1985.
73. Legrand, V., Hodgson, J. McB., Bates, E. R., Aueron, F. M., Mancini, J., Smith, J. S., Gross, M. D., and Vogel, R. A.: Abnormal coronary flow reserve and abnormal radionuclide exercise test results in patients with normal coronary angiograms. J. Am. Coll. Cardiol. *6*:1245, 1985.
74. Opherk, D., Zebe, H., Weihe, E., Mall, G., Durr, C., Gravert, B., Nehmel, H. C., Schwarz, F., and Kubler, W.: Reduced coronary dilatory capacity and ultrastructural changes of the myocardium in patients with angina pectoris but normal coronary arteriograms. Circulation *63*:817, 1981.
75. Pasternac, A., Noble, J., Streulens, Y., Elie, R., Henschke, C., and Bourassa, M. G.: Pathophysiology of chest pain in patients with cardiomyopathies and normal coronary arteries. Circulation *65*:778, 1982.
76. Spray, T. L., Maron, B. J., Morrow, A. G., Epstein, S. E., and Roberts, W. C.: Clinical pathologic conference. A discussion on hypertrophic cardiomyopathy. Am. Heart J. *95*:511, 1978.
77. Rubenfire, M., Blevins, R. D., Barnhart, M., Housholder, S., Selik, N., and Mammen, E. F.: Platelet hyperaggregability in patients with chest pain and angiographically normal coronary arteries. Am. J. Cardiol. *57*:657, 1986.
78. Wielgosz, A. T., Fletcher, R. H., McCants, C. B., McKinnis, R. A., Haney, T. L., and Williams, R. B.: Unimproved chest pain in patients with minimal or no coronary disease: A behavioral phenomenon. Am. Heart J. *108*:67, 1984.
79. Mammohansingh, P., and Parker, J. O.: Angina pectoris with normal coronary arteriograms: Hemodynamic and metabolic response to pacing. Am. Heart J. *90*:555, 1975.
80. Meller, J., Goldsmith, S. J., Rudin, A., Pichard, A. D., Gorlin, R., Teichholz, L. E., and Herman, M. V.: Spectrum of exercise thallium-201 myocardial perfusion imaging in patients with chest pain and normal coronary angiograms. Am. J. Cardiol. *43*:717, 1979.
81. Green, L. H., Cohn, P. F., Holman, B. L., Adams, D. F., and Markis, J. E.: Regional myocardial blood flow in patients with chest pain syndromes and normal coronary arteriograms. Br. Heart J. *40*:242, 1978.
82. Bass, C., and Wade, C.: Chest pain with normal coronary arteries. A comparative study of psychiatric and social morbidity. Psychol. Med. *14*:51, 1984.
83. Channer, K. S., James, M. A., Papouchado, M., and Rees, J. R.: Anxiety and depression in patients with chest pain referred for exercise testing. Lancet *2*:820, 1985.
84. Cannon, R. O., Watson, R. M., Rosing, D. R., and Epstein, S. E.: Efficacy of calcium channel blocker therapy for angina pectoris resulting from small-vessel coronary artery disease and abnormal vasodilator reserve. Am. J. Cardiol. *56*:242, 1985.
85. Ockene, I. S., and Ockene, J. K.: Chest pain in the patient with normal coronary arteries. Primary Cardiol. pp. 83, Feb., 1983.
86. Levenkron, J. C., Goldstein, M. G., Adamides, O., Jr., and Greenland, P.: Chronic chest pain with normal coronary arteries: A behavioral approach to rehabilitation. J. Cardiopulmon. Rehabil. *5*:475, 1985.
87. Pe'er J., Vidaurri, J., Halfon, S.-T., Eisenberg, S., and Zauberman, H.: Association between corneal arcus and some of the risk factors for coronary artery disease. Br. J. Ophthal. *67*:795, 1983.
88. Winder, A. F.: Relationship between corneal arcus and hyperlipidaemia is clarified by studies in familial hypercholesterolaemia. Br. J. Ophthal. *67*:789, 1983.
89. Segal, P., Insull, W., Chambless, L. E., Stinnett, S., LaRosa, J. C., Weissfeld, L., Halfon, S., Kwiterovitch, P. O., and Little, J. A.: The association of dyslipoproteinemia with corneal arcus and xanthelasma. The Lipid Research Clinic's Program Prevalence Study. Circulation *73*:108, 1986.
90. Elliot, W. J.: Ear lobe crease and coronary artery disease. 1,000 patients and review of the literature. Am. J. Med. *75*:1024, 1983.
91. Kaukola, S.: The diagonal ear-lobe crease, heredity and coronary heart disease. Acta Med. Scand. (Suppl.) *668*:60, 1982.
92. Wagner, R. F., Reinfeld, H. B., Wagner, K. D., Gambino, A. T., Falco, T. A., Sokol, J. A., Katz, S., and Zeldis, S. M.: Ear-canal hair and the ear-lobe crease as predictors for coronary-artery disease (letter). N. Engl. J. Med. *311*:1317, 1984.

93. Criqui, M. H., Coughlin, S. S., and Fronek, A.: Noninvasively diagnosed peripheral arterial disease as a predictor of mortality: Results from a prospective study. Circulation *72*:768, 1985.
94. Cohn, P. F., Thompson, S., Strauss, W., Todd, J., and Gorlin, R.: Diastolic heart sounds during static (handgrip) exercise in patients with chest pain. Circulation *47*:1217, 1973.
95. Ranganathan, N., Juma, Z., and Sivaciyan, V.: The apical impulse in coronary heart disease. Clin. Cardiol. *8*:20, 1985.
96. Tavel, M. E.: The fourth heart sound—a premature requiem? Circulation *49*:4, 1974.
97. Sangster, J. F., and Oakley, C. M.: Diastolic murmur of coronary artery stenosis. Br. Heart J. *35*:840, 1973.
98. Gorlin, R.: Evaluation of the patient with coronary heart disease. *In* Gorlin, R. (ed.): Coronary Artery Disease. Philadelphia, W. B. Saunders Company, 1976, p. 178.
99. Hamby, R. I., Weissman, R. H., Prakash, M. N., and Hoffman, I.: Left bundle branch block: A predictor of poor left ventricular function in coronary artery disease. Am. Heart J. *106*:471, 1983.
100. Liao, Y., Emidy, L. A., Dyer, A., Hewitt, J. S., Shekelle, R. B., Paul, O., Prineas, R., and Stamler, J.: Characteristics and prognosis of incomplete right bundle branch block: An epidemiologic study. J. Am. Coll. Cardiol. *7*:492, 1986.
101. McQueen, M. J., Holder, D., and El-Maraghi, N. R. H.: Assessment of the accuracy of serial electrocardiograms in the diagnosis of myocardial infarction. Am. Heart J. *105*:258, 1983.
102. Kannel, W. B., and Abbott, R. D.: Incidence and prognosis of unrecognized myocardial infarction. N. Engl. J. Med. *311*:1144, 1984.
103. Goldman, L., Cook, E. F., Mitchell, N., Flatley, M., Sherman, H., Rosati, R., Harrell, F., Lee, K., and Cohn, P. F.: Incremental value of the exercise test for diagnosing the presence or absence of coronary artery disease. Circulation *66*:945, 1982.
104. Dagenais, G. R., Rouleau, J. R., Christen, A., and Fabia, J.: Survival of patients with a strongly positive exercise electrocardiogram. Circulation *65*:452, 1982.
105. Deering, T. F., and Weiner, D. A.: Prognosis of patients with coronary artery disease. J. Cardiopulmon. Rehabil. *5*:325, 1985.
105a. Gordon, D. J., Ekelund, L.-G., Karon, J. M., Probstfield, J. L., Rubenstein, C., Sheffield, L. T., and Weissfeld, L.: Predictive value of the exercise tolerance test for mortality in North American men: The Lipid Research Clinics Mortality Follow-up Study. Circulation *74*:252, 1986.
106. Cole, J. R., and Ellestad, M. H.: Significance of chest pain during treadmill exercise: Correlation with coronary events. Am. J. Cardiol. *41*:227, 1978.
107. Hlatky, M. A., Pryor, D. B., Harrell, F. E., Jr., Califf, R. M., Mark, D. B., and Rosati, R. A.: Factors affecting sensitivity and specificity of exercise electrocardiography. Am. J. Med. *77*:64, 1984.
108. Weins, R. D., Lafia, P., Marder, C. M., Evans, R. G., Kennedy, H. L.: Chronotropic incompetence in clinical exercise testing. Am. J. Cardiol. *54*:74, 1984.
109. Thompson, P. D., and Kelemer, M. H.: Hypotension accompanying the onset of exertional angina. A sign of severe compromise of left ventricular blood supply. Circulation *52*:28, 1975.
110. Irving, J. B., Bruce, R. A., and DeRouen, T. A.: Variations in and significance of systolic pressure during maximal exercise (treadmill) testing. Relation to severity of coronary artery disease and cardiac mortality. Am. J. Cardiol. *39*:841, 1977.
111. Stone, P. H., LaFolette, E. L., and Cohn, K.: Patterns of exercise treadmill test performance in patients with left main coronary artery disease: Detection dependent on left coronary dominance or coexistent dominant right coronary disease. Am. Heart J. *104*:13, 1982.
112. Nygaard, T. W., Gibson, R. S., Ryan, J. M., Gascho, J. A., Watson, D. D., and Beller, G. A.: Prevalence of high-risk thallium-201 scintigraphic findings in left main coronary artery stenosis: Comparison of patients with multiple- and single-vessel coronary artery disease. Am. J. Cardiol. *53*:462, 1984.
113. Weiner, D. A., McCabe, C. H., Cutler, S. S., and Ryan, T. J.: Decrease in systolic blood pressure during exercise testing: Reproducibility, response to coronary artery bypass surgery, and prognostic significance. Am. J. Cardiol. *49*:1627, 1982.
114. Hakki, A. -H., Munley, B. M., Hadjimiltiades, S., Meissner, M. D., and Iskandrian, A. S.: Determinants of abnormal blood pressure response to exercise in coronary artery disease. Am. J. Cardiol. *57*:71, 1986.
115. Goldschlager, N., Selzer, A., and Cohn, K.: Treadmill stress tests and indicators of presence and severity of coronary artery disease. Ann. Intern. Med. *85*:277, 1976.
116. Boran, K. G., Oliveros, R. A., Boucher, C. A., Beckmann, C. H., and Seaworth, J. F.: Ischemia-associated intraventricular conduction disturbances during exercise testing as a predictor of proximal left anterior descending coronary artery disease. Am. J. Cardiol. *51*:1098, 1983.
117. Vasey, C., O'Donnell, J., Morris, S., and McHenry, P.: Exercise-induced left bundle branch block and its relation to coronary artery disease. Am. J. Cardiol. *56*:892, 1985.
118. Helfant, R. H., Pine, R., Kabde, V., and Banka, V. S.: Exercise-related ventricular premature complexes in coronary heart disease. Correlations with ischemia and angiographic severity. Ann. Intern. Med. *80*:589, 1974.
119. McHenry, P. L., Morris, S. N., Kavalier, M., and Jordan, J. W.: Comparative study of exercise-induced ventricular arrhythmias in normal subjects and patients with documented coronary artery disease. Am. J. Cardiol. *37*:609, 1976.
120. Mukharji, J., Kremers, M., Lipscomb, K., and Blomqvist, C. G.: Early positive exericse test and extensive coronary disease: Effect of antianginal therapy. Am. J. Cardiol. *55*:267, 1985.
121. Ho, S. W. -C., McComish, M. J., and Taylor, R. R.: Effect of beta-adrenergic blockade on the results of exercise testing related to the extent of coronary artery disease. Am. J. Cardiol. *55*:258, 1985.
122. Balady, G. J., Weiner, D. A., McCabe, C. H., and Ryan, T. J.: Value of arm exercise testing in detecting coronary artery disease. Am. J. Cardiol. *55*:37, 1985.
122a. Koss, J. H., Kobren, S. M., Grunwald, A. M., and Bodenheimer, M. M.: Role of exercise thallium-201 myocardial perfusion scintigraphy in predicting prognosis in suspected coronary artery disease. Am. J. Cardiol. *59*:531, 1987.
123. Gibson, R. S., and Beller, G. A.: Should exercise electrocardiography testing be replaced by radioisotope methods? *In* Rahimtoola, S. H. (ed.): Controversies in Coronary Artery Disease. Philadelphia, F. A. Davis Co., 1983, pp. 1–31.
124. Wackers, F. J. T., Russo, D. J., Russo, D., and Clements, J. P.: Prognostic significance of normal quantitative planar thallium-201 stress scintigraphy in patients with chest pain. J. Am. Coll. Cardiol. *6*:27, 1985.
124a. Koss, J. H., Kobren, S. M., Grunwald, A. M., and Bodenheimer, M. M.: Role of exercise thallium-201 myocardial perfusion scintigraphy in predicting prognosis in suspected coronary artery disease. Am. J. Cardiol. *59*:531, 1987.
125. Pamelia, F. X., Gibson, R. S., Watson, D. D., Craddock, G. B., Sirowatka, J., and Beller, G. A.: Prognosis with chest pain and normal thallium-201 exercise scintigrams. Am. J. Cardiol. *55*:920, 1985.
126. Port, S. C., Oshima, M., Ray, G., McNamee, P., and Schmidt, D. H.: Assessment of single-vessel coronary artery disease: Results of exercise electrocardiography, thallium-201 myocardial perfusion imaging and radionuclide angiography. J. Am. Coll. Cardiol. *6*:75, 1985.
127. Kaul, S., Kiess, M., Liu, P., Guiney, T. E., Pohost, G. M., Okada, R. D., and Boucher, C. A.: Comparison of exercise electrocardiography and quantitative thallium imaging for one-vessel coronary artery disease. Am. J. Cardiol. *56*:257, 1985.
128. Gibson, R. S., Watson, D. D., Carabello, B. A., Holt, N. D., and Beller, G. A.: Clinical implications of increased lung uptake of thallium-201 during exercise scintigraphy 2 weeks after myocardial infarction. Am. J. Cardiol. *49*:1586, 1982.
128a. Bonow, R. O.: Exercise testing and radionuclide procedures in high-risk populations. Circulation *75*(Suppl. II):18, 1987.
129. Weiss, A. T., Berman, D. S., Lew, A. S., Nielsen, J., Potkin, B., Swan, H. J. C., Waxman, A., and Maddahi, J.: Transient ischemic dilation of the left ventricle on stress thallium-201 scintigraphy: A marker of severe and extensive coronary artery disease. J. Am. Coll. Cardiol. *9*:752, 1987.
130. Dymond, D. S., Foster, C., Grenier, R. P., Carpenter, J., and Schmidt, D. H.: Peak exercise and immediate postexercise imaging for the detection of left ventricular functional abnormalities in coronary artery disease. Am. J. Cardiol. *53*:1532, 1984.
131. Patterson, R. E., Horowitz, S. F., Eng, C., Meller, J., Goldsmith, S. J., Pichard, A. D., Halgash, D. A., Herman, M. V., and Gorlin, R.: Can noninvasive exercise test criteria identify patients with left main or 3-vessel coronary disease after a first myocardial infarction? Am. J. Cardiol. *51*:361, 1983.
132. Robertson, W. S., Feigenbaum, H., Armstrong, W. F., Dillon, J. C., O'Donnell, J., and McHenry, P. W.: Exercise echocardiography: A clinically practical addition in the evaluation of coronary artery disease. J. Am. Coll. Cardiol. *2*:1085, 1983.
133. Limacher, M. C., Quinones, M. A., Poliner, L. R., Nelson, J. G., Winters, W. L., and Waggoner, A. D.: Detection of coronary artery disease with exercise two-dimensional echocardiography. Circulation *67*:1211, 1983.
134. Heng, M. K., Simard, M., Lake, R., and Udhoji, V. H.: Exercise two-dimensional echocardiography for diagnosis of coronary artery disease. Am. J. Cardiol. *54*:502, 1984.
135. Iliceto, S., D'Ambrosio, G., Sorino, M., Papa, A., Amico, A., Ricci, A., and Rizzon, P.: Comparison of postexercise and transesophageal atrial pacing two-dimensional echocardiography for detection of coronary artery disease. Am. J. Cardiol. *57*:547, 1986.
136. Rink, L. D., Fiegenbaum, H., Godley, R. W., Weyman, A. E., Dillon, J. C., Phillips, J. F., and Marshall, J. E.: Echocardiographic detection of left main coronary artery obstruction. Circulation *65*:719, 1982.
137. Neinle, R. A., Levy, R. I., Frederickson, D. S., and Gorlin, R.: Lipid and carbohydrate abnormalities in patients with angiographically documented coronary artery disease. Am. J. Cardiol. *24*:178, 1969.
138. Falsetti, H. L., Schnatz, J. D., Greene, D. G., and Bunelli, I. L.: Lipid and carbohydrate studies in coronary artery disease. Circulation *37*:184, 1968.
139. Margolis, J. R., Chan, J. T. T., Kong, Y., Peter, R. H., Behar, V. S., and Kisslo, J. A.: The diagnostic and prognostic significance of coronary artery calcification. A report of 800 cases. Radiology *127*:609, 1980.
140. Detrano, R., Salcedo, E. E., Hobbs, R. E., and Yiannikas, J.: Cardiac cinefluoroscopy as an inexpensive aid in the diagnosis of coronary artery disease. Am. J. Cardiol. *57*:1041, 1986.
141. Hartnell, G. G., Parnell, B. M., and Pridie, R. B.: Coronary artery ectasia: Its prevalence and clinical significance in 4993 patients. Br. Heart J. *54*:392, 1985.
142. Newman, P. E.: The coronary collateral circulation: Determinants and functional significance in ischemic heart disease. Am. Heart J. *102*:431, 1981.
143. Gregg, D. E., and Patterson, R. E.: Functional importance of the coronary collaterals. N. Engl. J. Med. *303*:1404, 1980.
144. Schaper, W.: Influence of physical exercise on coronary collateral blood flow in chronic experimental two-vessel occlusion. Circulation *65*:905, 1982.
145. Cohen, M. V., Yipintsol, T., and Scheuer, J.: Coronary collateral stimulation by exercise in dogs with stenotic coronary arteries. J. Appl. Physiol. Resp. Environ. Exercise Physiol. *52*:664, 1982.
146. Moraski, R. E., Russell, R. O., Jr., Smith, M., and Rackley, C. E.: Left ventricular function in patients with and without myocardial infarction and one, two or three vessel coronary artery disease. Am. J. Cardiol. *35*:1, 1975.

147. Mann, T., Brodie, B. R., Grossman, W., and McLaurin, L. P.: Effect of angina on the left ventricular diastolic pressure-volume relationship. Circulation *35*:761, 1977.
148. Helfant, R. H., Forrester, J. S., Hampton, J. R., Haft, J. I., Kemp, H. G., and Gorlin, R.: Coronary heart disease. Differential hemodynamic, metabolic, and electrocardiographic effects in subjects with and without angina pectoris during atrial pacing. Circulation *42*:601, 1970.
149. Bourdillon, P. D., Lorell, B. H., Mirsky, I., Paulus, W. J., Wynne, J., and Grossman, W.: Increased regional myocardial stiffness of the left ventricle during pacing-induced angina in man. Circulation *67*:316, 1983.
150. Rahimtoola, S. H.: A perspective on the three large multicenter randomized clinical trials of coronary bypass surgery for chronic stable angina. Circulation *72*(Suppl. V):123, 1985.
151. Braunwald, E., and Rutherford, J. D.: Reversible ischemic left ventricular dysfunction: Evidence for the "hibernating myocardium." J. Am. Coll. Cardiol. *8*:1467, 1986.
152. Popio, K. A., Gorlin, R., Bechtel, D., and Levine, J. A.: Postextrasystolic potentiation as a predictor of potential myocardial viability: Preoperative analyses compared with studies after coronary bypass surgery. Am. J. Cardiol. *39*:944, 1977.
153. Nesto, R. W., Cohn, L. H., Collins, J. J., Jr., Wynne, J., Holman, L., and Cohn, P. F.: Inotropic contractile reserve: a useful predictor of increased 5-year survival and improved postoperative left ventricular function in patients with coronary artery disease and reduced ejection fraction. Am. J. Cardiol. *50*:39, 1982.
154. Bodenheimer, M. M., Banka, V. S., Hermann, G. A., Trout, R. G., Pasdar, H., and Helfant, R. H.: Reversible asynergy: Histopathologic and electrographic correlations in patients with coronary artery disease. Circulation *53*:792, 1976.
155. Banka, V. S., Bodenheimer, M. M., and Helfant, R. H.: Determinants of reversible asynergy: The native coronary circulation. Circulation *52*:810, 1975.
156. Verani, M. S., Carroll, R. J., and Falsetti, H. L.: Mitral valve prolapse in coronary artery disease. Am. J. Cardiol. *37*:1, 1976.
157. Herman, M. V., Elliott, W. C., and Gorlin, R.: An electrocardiographic, anatomic, and metabolic study of zonal myocardial ischemia in coronary heart disease. Circulation *35*:834, 1967.
158. Gertz, E. W., Wisneski, J. A., Neese, R., Bristow, J. D., Searle, G. L., and Hanlon, J. T.: Myocardial lactate metabolism: Evidence of lactate release during net chemical extraction in man. Circulation *63*:1273, 1981.
159. Cannon, P. J., Weiss, M. B., and Sciacca, R. R.: Myocardial blood flow in coronary artery disease: Studies at rest and during stress with inert gas washout techniques. Prog. Cardiovasc. Dis. *20*:95, 1977.
160. Dwyer, E. M., Jr., Dell, R. B., and Cannon, P. J.: Regional myocardial flow in transmural myocardial infarction. Circulation *48*:924, 1973.
161. See, J. R., Cohn, P. F., Holman, B. L., Roberts, B. H., and Adams, D. F.: Angiographic abnormalities associated with alterations in regional myocardial blood flow in coronary artery disease. Br. Heart J. *38*:1278, 1976.
162. Kronmal, R. A., Oberman, A., Frye, R. L., and Killip, T., III: Effect of cigarette smoking on survival of patients with angiographically documented coronary artery disease. Report from CASS Registry. J.A.M.A. *255*:1023, 1986.
163. Hallstrom, A. P., Cobb, L. A., and Ray, R.: Smoking as a risk factor for recurrence of sudden cardiac arrest. N. Engl. J. Med. *314*:271, 1986.
164. Rogot, E., and Murray, J. L.: Smoking and causes of death among U.S. veterans: 16 years of observation. Public Health Rep. *95*:213, 1980.
165. Kannel, W. B., Castelli, W. P., and McNamara, P. M.: Cigarette smoking and risk of CHD: Epidemiologic clues to pathogenesis: The Framingham Study. N.C.I. Monogr. *28*:9, 1968.
166. Kaufman, D. W., Helmich, S. P., and Shapiro, S.: The risk of myocardial infarction after quitting smoking in men under 55 years of age. N. Engl. J. Med. *313*:1511, 1985.
167. Hofstetter, A., Schutz, Y., Jequier, E., and Wahren, J.: Increased 24-hour energy expenditure in cigarette smokers. N. Engl. J. Med. *314*:79, 1986.
168. Nicod, P., Rehr, R., Winniford, M. D., Campbell, W. B., Firth, B. G., and Hillis, L. D.: Acute systemic and coronary hemodynamic and serologic responses to cigarette smoking in long-term smokers with atherosclerotic coronary artery disease. J. Am. Coll. Cardiol. *4*:964, 1984.
169. Winniford, M. D., Wheelan, K. R., Kremers, M. S., Ugolini, V., van den Berg, E., Jr., Niggemann, E. H., Jansen, D. E., and Hillis, L. D.: Smoking-induced coronary vasoconstriction in patients with atherosclerotic coronary artery disease: Evidence for adrenergically mediated alterations in coronary artery tone. Circulation *73*:662, 1986.
169a. Winniford, M. D., Jansen, D. E., Reynolds, G. A., Apprill, P., Black, W. H., and Hillis, L. D.: Cigarette smoking-induced coronary vasoconstriction in atherosclerotic coronary artery disease and prevention by calcium antagonists and nitroglycerin. Am. J. Cardiol. *59*:203, 1987.
170. Deanfield, J., Wright, C., Kirkler, S., Ribeiro, P., and Fox, K.: Cigarette smoking and the treatment of angina with propranolol, atenolol, and nifedipine. N. Engl. J. Med. *310*:951, 1984.
171. Aronow, W. S.: Effect of passive smoking on angina pectoris. N. Engl. J. Med. *299*:21, 1978.
172. Rocco, M. B., Barry, J., Campbell, S., Nabel, E., Cook, E. F., Goldman, L., and Selwyn, A. P.: Circadian variation of transient myocardial ischemia in patients with coronary artery disease. Circulation *75*:395, 1987.
173. Ferguson, R. J., Taylor, A. W., Cote, P., Charlebois, J., Dinelle, Y., Peronnet, F., de Champlain, J., and Bourassa, M. G.: Skeletal muscle and cardiac changes with training in patients with angina pectoris. Am. J. Physiol. *243*:H830, 1982.
174. Redwood, D. R., Rosing, D. R., and Epstein, S. E.: Circulatory and symptomatic effects of physical training in patients with coronary artery disease and angina pectoris. N. Engl. J. Med. *286*:959, 1972.
175. Jensen, D., Atwood, J. E., Froelicher, V., McKirnan, M. D., Battler, A., Ashburn, W., and Ross, J., Jr.: Improvement in ventricular function during exercise studied with radionuclide ventriculography after cardiac rehabilitation. Am. J. Cardiol. *46*:770, 1980.
176. Frishman, W. H.: Pharmacology of the nitrates in angina pectoris. Am. J. Cardiol. *56*:81, 1985.
177. Williams, J. F., Jr., Glick, G., and Braunwald, E.: Studies on cardiac dimensions in intact unanesthetized man. V. Effects of nitroglycerin. Circulation *32*:76, 1965.
178. Brown, B. G., Bolson, E., Petersen, R. B., Pierce, C. D., and Dodge, H. T.: The mechanisms of nitroglycerin action: Stenosis vasodilation as a major component of the drug response. Circulation *64*:1089, 1981.
179. Bache, R. J., Ball, R. M., Cobb, F. R., Rembert, J. C., and Greenfield, J. C., Jr.: Effects of nitroglycerin on transmural myocardial blood flow in the unanesthetized dog. J. Clin. Invest. *55*:1219, 1975.
180. Cohen, M. V., Downey, J. M., Sonnenblick, E. H., and Kirk, E. S.: The effects of nitroglycerin on coronary collaterals and myocardial contractility. J. Clin. Invest. *52*:2836, 1973.
181. Cowan, C., Duran, P. V. M., Corsini, G., Goldschlager, N., and Bing, R. J.: The effects of nitroglycerin on myocardial blood flow in man. Measured by coincidence counting and bolus injections of 84-rubidium. Am. J. Cardiol. *24*:154, 1969.
182. Parker, J. O., West, R. O., and DiGiorgi, S.: The effect of nitroglycerin on coronary blood flow and the hemodynamic response to exercise in coronary artery disease. Am. J. Cardiol. *27*:59, 1971.
183. Ganz, W., and Marcus, H. S.: Failure of intracoronary nitroglycerin to alleviate pacing-induced angina. Circulation *46*:880, 1972.
184. Bernstein, L., Friesinger, G. C., Lichtlen, P. R., and Ross, R. S.: The effect of nitroglycerin on the systemic circulation in man and dog. Circulation *33*:107, 1966.
185. Cohn, P. F., Maddox, D. E., Holman, B. L., Markis, J. E., Adams, D. F., and See, J. R.: Effect of sublingually administered nitroglycerin on regional myocardial blood flow in patients with coronary artery disease. Am. J. Cardiol. *39*:672, 1977.
186. Goldstein, R. E., Stinson, E. B., Scherer, J. L., Seningen, R. P., Grehl, T. M., and Epstein, S. E.: Intraoperative coronary collateral function in patients with coronary occlusive disease. Nitroglycerin responsiveness and angiographic correlations. Circulation *49*:298, 1974.
187. Chiong, M. A., West, R. O., and Parker, J. O.: Influence of nitroglycerin on myocardial metabolism and hemodynamics during angina induced by atrial pacing. Circulation *45*:1044, 1972.
188. Dove, J. T., Shah, P. M., and Schreiner, B. F.: Effects of nitroglycerin on left ventricular wall motion in coronary artery disease. Circulation *49*:682, 1974.
189. Borer, J. S., Bacharach, S. L., Green, M. V., Kent, K. M., Johnston, G. S., and Epstein, S. E.: Effect of nitroglycerin on exercise-induced abnormalities of left ventricular regional function and ejection fraction in coronary artery disease. Assessment by radionuclide cineangiography in symptomatic and asymptomatic patients. Circulation *57*:314, 1978.
190. Epstein, S. E., and Braunwald, E.: Inhibition of the adrenergic nervous system in the treatment of angina pectoris. Med. Clin. North Am. *52*:1031, 1968.
191. Lee, S. J. K., Sung, Y. K., and Zaragoza, A. J.: Effects of nitroglycerin on left ventricular volumes and wall tension in patients with ischemic heart disease. Br. Heart J. *32*:790, 1970.
192. Winniford, M. D., Jansen, D. E., Reynolds, G. A., Apprill, P., Black, W. H., and Hillis, L. D.: Cigarette smoking-induced coronary vasoconstriction in atherosclerotic coronary artery disease and prevention by calcium antagonists and nitroglycerin. Am. J. Cardiol. *59*:203, 1987.
193. Needleman, P., and Johnson, E. M.: Pharmacological, biological, and biochemical interaction of organic nitrates with sulfhydryls: Possible correlations with a mechanism for tolerance development, vasodilation, and mitochondrial and acetyline reaction. *In* Needleman, P. (ed.): Organic Nitrates: Handbook of Experimental Pharmacology. Vol. 40. New York, Springer-Verlag, 1975, pp. 97–114.
194. Horowitz, J. D., Antman, E. M., Lorell, B. H., Barry, W. H., and Smith, T. W.: Potentiation of the cardiovascular effects of nitroglycerin by *N*-acetylcysteine. Circulation *68*:1247, 1983.
195. Winniford, M. D., Kennedy, P. L., Wells, P. J., and Hillis, L. D.: Potentiation of nitroglycerin-induced coronary dilatation by *N*-acetylcysteine. Circulation *73*:138, 1986.
196. Ignarro, L. J., Lippton, H., Edwards, J. C., Barocos, W. H., Hyman, A. L., Kadowitz, P. J., and Gruelter, C. A.: Mechanism of vascular smooth muscle relaxation by organic nitrates, nitrites, nitroprusside, and nitric oxide: Evidence for the involvement of S-nitrosothiols as active intermediates. J. Pharmacol. Exp. Ther. *218*:739, 1981.
197. Levin, R. I., Jaffe, E. A., Weksler, B. B., and Tack-Goldman, K.: Nitroglycerin stimulates synthesis of prostacyclin by cultured human endothelial cells. J. Clin. Invest. *67*:762, 1981.
198. Mehta, J., Mehta, P., and Ostrowksi, N.: Effects of nitroglycerin on human vascular prostacyclin and thromboxane A_2 generation. J. Lab. Clin. Med. *102*:116, 1983.
199. Abrams, J.: Pharmacology of nitroglycerin and long-acting nitrates. Am. J. Cardiol. *56*:12A, 1985.
200. Fung, H. -L.: Pharmacokinetics of nitroglycerin and long-acting nitrate esters. Am. J. Med. *74*:13, 1983.
201. Hales, C. A., and Westphal, D.: Hypoxemia following the administration of sublingual nitroglycerin. Am. J. Med. *65*:911, 1978.
202. Parker, J. O., Vankoughnett, K. A., and Farrell, B.: Nitroglycerin lingual spray: Clinical efficacy and dose response relation. Am. J. Cardiol. 57:1, 1986.

203. Needleman, P., Lang, S., and Johnson, E. M., Jr.: Organic nitrates: Relationship between biotransformation and rational angina pectoris therapy. J. Pharmacol. Exp. Ther. *181*:489, 1972.
204. Markis, J. E., Gorlin, R., Mills, R. M., Williams, R. A., Schweitzer, P., and Ransil, B. J.: Sustained effect of orally administered isosorbide dinitrate on exercise performance of patients with angina pectoris. Am. J. Cardiol. *43*:265, 1979.
205. Lee, G., Mason, D. T., and DeMaria, A. N.: Effects of long-term oral administration of isosorbide dinitrate on the antianginal response to nitroglycerin. Am. J. Cardiol. *41*:82, 1978.
206. Badger, R. S., Brown, B. G., Gallery, C. A., Bolson, E. L., and Dodge, H. T.: Coronary artery dilation and hemodynamic responses after isosorbide dinitrate therapy in patients with coronary artery disease. Am. J. Cardiol. *56*:390, 1985.
207. Bassan, M. M., and Weiler-Ravell, D.: The additive antianginal action of oral isosorbide dinitrate in patients receiving propranolol. Magnitude and duration of effect. Chest *83*:233, 1983.
207a. Parker, J. O., Farrell, B., Lahey, K. A., and Moe, G.: Effect of intervals between doses on the development of tolerance to isosorbide dinitrate. N. Engl. J. Med. *316*:1440, 1987.
208. Parker, J. O., Vankoughnett, K. A., and Farrell, B.: Comparison of buccal nitroglycerin and oral isosorbide dinitrate for nitrate tolerance in stable angina pectoris. Am. J. Cardiol. *56*:724, 1985.
209. Thadani, U., Fung, H. L., Darke, A. C., and Parker, J. O.: Oral isosorbide dinitrate in angina pectoris: Comparison of duration of action and dose-response relation during acute and sustained therapy. Am. J. Cardiol. *49*:411, 1982.
210. Transdermal delivery systems for nitroglycerin. Med. Lett. *24*:35, 1982.
211. Armstrong, P. W., Armstrong, J. A., and Marks, G. S.: Blood levels after sublingual nitroglycerin. Circulation *59*:585, 1979.
212. Abrams, J.: The brief saga of transdermal nitroglycerin discs: Paradise lost? Am. J. Cardiol. *54*:220, 1984.
213. Parker, J. O., Vankoughnett, K. A., and Fung, F. -L.: Transdermal isosorbide dinitrate in patients receiving propranolol. Magnitude and duration of effect. Chest *83*:233, 1983.
214. Abrams, J.: Transdermal nitroglycerin and nitrate tolerance. Ann. Intern. Med. *104*:424, 1986.
215. Przybojewski, J. Z., and Heyns, M. H.: Acute coronary vasospasm secondary to industrial nitroglycerin withdrawal. S. Afr. Med. J. *63*:158, 1983.
216. Braunwald, E. (ed.): Beta-Adrenergic Blockade—A New Era in Cardiovascular Medicine. New York, Exerpta Medica, 1978, 309 pp.
217. Rogers, W. J.: Use of beta blockers in the treatment of ischemic heart disease: A comparison of the available agents. Cardiovasc. Rev. Rep. *5*:31, 1984.
218. Miller, R. R., Olson, H. G., and Pratt, C. M.: Efficacy of beta-adrenergic blockade in coronary heart disease: Propranolol in angina pectoris. Clin. Pharmacol. Ther. *18*:598, 1975.
219. Manyari, D. E., Kostuk, W. J., Carruthers, G., Johnston, D. J., and Purves, P.: Pindolol and propranolol in patients with angina pectoris and normal or near-normal ventricular function. Lack of influence of intrinsic sympathomimetic activity on global and segmental left ventricular function assessed by radionuclide ventriculography. Am. J. Cardiol. *51*:427, 1983.
220. Harris, F. J., Low, R. I., Palmer, L., Amsterdam, E. A., and Mason, D. T.: Antianginal efficacy and improved exercise performance with timolol. Twice-daily beta blockade in ischemic heart disease. Am. J. Cardiol. *51*:13, 1983.
221. Clark, B. J.: Beta-adrenoceptor-blocking agents: Are pharmacologic differences relevant? Am. Heart J. *104*:334, 1982.
222. Watanabe, A. G.: Recent advances in knowledge about beta-adrenergic receptors: Application to clinical cardiology. J. Am. Coll. Cardiol. *1*:82, 1983.
223. Lands, A. M., Arnold, A., McAuliff, J. P., Luduena, F. P., and Brown, T. G.: Differentiation of receptor systems activated by sympathomimetic amines. Nature *214*:597, 1967.
224. Conolly, M. E., Kersting, F., and Dollery, C. T.: The clinical pharmacology of beta-adrenoreceptor blocking drugs. Prog. Cardiovasc. Dis. *19*:203, 1976.
225. Frishman, W. H., and Kostis, J.: The significance of intrinsic sympathomimetic activity in beta-adrenoceptor blocking drugs. Cardiovasc. Rev. Rep. *3*:503, 1982.
226. Kostis, J. B., Frishman, W., Hosler, M. H., Thorsen, N. L., Gonasun, L., and Weinstein, J.: Treatment of angina pectoris with pindolol: The significance of intrinsic sympathomimetic activity of beta blockers. Am. Heart J. *104*:496, 1982.
227. Cannon, R. E., Slavin, R. G., and Gonasun, L. M.: The effect on asthma of a new beta blocker, pindolol. Am. Heart J. *104*:438, 1982.
228. Gebhardt, V. A., and Wisenberg, E.: The role of beta blockade, with and without intrinsic sympathomimetic activity in preserving compromised left ventricular function in patients with ischemic heart disease. Am. Heart J. *109*:1013, 1985.
229. Quyyumi, A. A., Wright, C., Mockus, L., and Fox, K. M.: Effect of partial agonist activity in beta blockers in severe angina pectoris: A double-blind comparison of pindolol and atenolol. Br. Med. J. *289*:951, 1984.
230. Betts, T. A., and Alford, C.: Beta blocking drugs and sleep. A controlled trial. Drugs 25 (Suppl. 2):268, 1983.
231. Greminger, P., Vetter, H., Boerlin, H. J., Havelka, J., Baumgart, P., Walger, P., Luscher, T., Siegenthaler, W., and Vetter, W.: A comparative study between 100 mg atenolol and 20 mg pindolol slow-release in essential hypertension. Drugs 25 (Suppl. 2):37, 1983.
232. Westerlund, A.: Central nervous system side effects with hydrophilic and lipophilic beta blockers. Eur. J. Clin. Pharmacol. 28(Suppl. 2): 73, 1985.
233. Frishman, W., and Halprin, S.: Clinical pharmacology of the new beta-adrenergic blocking drugs. VII. New horizons in beta-adrenoceptor blocking therapy—labetalol. Am. Heart J. 98:660, 1979.
234. Lennard, M. S., Silas, J. H., Freestone, S., Ramsay, L. E., Tucker, G. T., and Woods, H. F.: Oxidation phenotype—a major determinant of metoprolol metabolism and response. N. Engl. J. Med. *307*:1558, 1982.
235. Koch-Wesler, J.: Beta-adrenoceptor antagonists: New drugs and new indications. N. Engl. J. Med. *305*:500, 1981.
236. Rutherford, J. D., Singh, B. N., Ambler, P. K., and Norris, R. M.: Plasma propranolol concentration in patients with angina and acute myocardial infarction. Clin. Exp. Pharmacol. Physiol. *3*:297, 1976.
237. Miller, R. R., Olson, H. G., Amsterdam, E. A., and Mason, D. T.: Propranolol withdrawal rebound phenomenon. Exacerbation of coronary events after abrupt cessation of antianginal therapy. N. Engl. J. Med. *293*:416, 1975.
238. Hiatt, W. R., Stoll, S., and Nies, A. S.: Effect of beta-adrenergic blockers on the peripheral circulation in patients with peripheral vascular disease. Circulation *72*:1226, 1985.
239. Aarons, R. D., and Molinoff, P. B.: Changes in the density of beta adrenergic receptors in rat lymphocytes, heart, and lung after chronic treatment with propranolol. J. Pharmacol. Exp. Ther. *221*:439, 1982.
240. Cooper, G., Kent, R. L., McGonigle, P., and Watanabe, A.: Beta adrenergic receptor blockade of feline myocardium. Cardiac mechanics, energetics, and beta adrenoceptor regulation. J. Clin. Invest. *77*:441, 1986.
241. McDevitt, D. G.: Drug interactions involving beta-adrenoceptor blocking drugs. *In* Petri, J. C. (ed.): Cardiovascular and Respiratory Disease Therapy. Elsevier/North Holland, 1980, pp. 21–41.
242. Vaghy, P. L., Williams, J. S., and Schwartz, A.: Receptor pharmacology of calcium entry blocking agents. Am. J. Cardiol. *59*:9A, 1987.
243. Godfraind, T.: Classification of calcium antagonists. Am. J. Cardiol. *59*:11B, 1987.
244. Stone, P. H., Antman, E. M., Muller, J. E., and Braunwald, E.: Calcium channel blocking agents in the treatment of cardiovascular disorders. Part II. Hemodynamic effects and clinical applications. Ann. Intern. Med. *93*:886, 1980.
245. Krikler, D. M.: Calcium antagonists for chronic stable angina pectoris. Am. J. Cardiol. *59*:95B, 1987.
246. Stone, P. H., Turi, Z., Muller, J. E., Geltman, E., Jaffe, A., and Braunwald, E.: Experience with nifedipine in 845 patients with refractory angina pectoris. J. Am. Coll. Cardiol. *1*:596, 1983.
247. Henry, P. D.: Atherosclerosis, calcium, and calcium antagonists. Circulation *72*:456, 1985.
248. Vatner, S. F., and Hintze, T. H.: Effects of a calcium-channel antagonist on large and small coronary arteries in conscious dogs. Circulation *66*:579, 1982.
249. Ludbrook, P. A., Tiefenbrunn, A. J., Reed, F. R., and Sobel, B. E.: Acute hemodynamic responses to sublingual nifedipine: Dependence on left ventricular function. Circulation *65*:489, 1982.
250. Flaim, S. F., and Zelis, R.: Clinical use of calcium entry blockers. Fed. Proc. *40*:2877, 1981.
251. Morse, J. R., and Nesto, R. W.: Double-blind crossover comparison of the antianginal effects of nifedipine and isosorbide dinitrate in patients with exertional angina receiving propranolol. J. Am. Coll. Cardiol. *6*:1395, 1985.
252. Uusitalo, A., Arstila, M., Bae, E. A., Harkonen, R., Keyrilainen, O., Rytkonen, U., Schjelderup-Mathiesen, P. M., and Wendelin, H.: Metoprolol, nifedipine, and the combination in stable effort angina pectoris. Am. J. Cardiol. *57*:733, 1986.
253. Marra, S., Paolillo, V., Baduini, G., Spadaccini, F., and Angelino, P. F.: Acute effects of chewable nifedipine on hemodynamic responses to upright exercise in patients with prior myocardial infarction and effort angina. Chest *83*:50, 1983.
254. Subramanian, V. B.: Combined therapy with calcium-channel and beta blockers: Facts, fiction, and practical aspects. Cardiovasc. Rev. Rep. *7*:259, 1986.
255. White, H. D., Polak, J. F., Wynne, J., Holman, B. L., Antman, E. M., and Nesto, R. W.: Addition of nifedipine to maximal nitrate and beta-adrenoreceptor blocker therapy in coronary artery disease. Am. J. Cardiol. *55*:1303, 1985.
256. Chew, C. Y. C., Brown, B. G., Singh, B. N., Wong, M. M., Pierce, C., and Petersen, R.: Effects of verapamil on coronary hemodynamic function and vasomobility relative to its mechanism of antianginal action. Am. J. Cardiol. *51*:699, 1983.
257. Rouleau, J., Chatterjee, K., Ports, T. A., Doyle, M. B., Hiramatsu, B., and Parmley, W. W.: Mechanism of relief of pacing-induced angina with oral verapamil: Reduced oxygen demand. Circulation *67*:94, 1983.
258. Charlap, S., and Frishman, W. H.: Comparative effects of verapamil and beta blockers in the therapy for patients with stable angina pectoris. Cardiovasc. Rev. Rep. *4*:66, 1983.
259. Leon, M. B., Rosing, D. R., Bonow, R. O., Lipson, L. C., and Epstein, S. E.: Clinical efficacy of verapamil alone and combined with propranolol in treating patients with chronic stable angina pectoris. Am. J. Cardiol. *48*:131, 1981.
260. Smith, M. S., Verghese, C. P., Shand, D. G., and Pritchett, E. L. C.: Pharmacokinetic and pharmacodynamic effects of diltiazem. Am. J. Cardiol. *51*:1369, 1983.
261. Boden, W. E., Bough, E. W., Reichman, M. J., Rich, V. B., Young, P. M., Korr, K. S., and Shulman, R. S.: Beneficial effects of high-dose diltiazem in patients with persistent effort angina on beta blockers and nitrates: A randomized, double-blind, placebo-controlled cross-over study. Circulation *71*:1197, 1985.
262. Humen, D. P., O'Brien, P., Purves, P., Johnson, D., and Kostuk, W. J.: Effort angina with adequate beta-receptor blockade: Comparison with diltiazem alone and in combination. J. Am. Coll. Cardiol. *7*:329, 1986.
263. Wagniart, P., Ferguson, R. J., Chaitman, B. R., Achard, F., Benacerraf, A., Delanguenhagen, B., Morin, B., Pasternac, A., and Bourassa, M. G.: Increased exercise tolerance and reduced electrocardiographic ischemia with diltiazem in patients with stable angina pectoris. Circulation *66*:23, 1982.

264. Murakami, T., Hess, O. M., and Krayenbuehl, H. P.: Left ventricular function before and after diltiazem in patients with coronary artery disease. J. Am. Coll. Cardiol. 5:723, 1985.
265. DeServi, S., Ferrario, M., Ghio, S., Bartoli, A., Mussini, A., Poma, E., Angoli, L., Bramucci, E., Aimè, E., Rondanelli, R., and Specchia, G.: Effects of diltiazem on regional coronary hemodynamics during atrial pacing in patients with stable exertional angina: Implications for mechanism of action. Circulation 73:1248, 1986.
266. Schroeder, J. S., Beier-Scott, L., Ginsburg, R., Bristow, M. R., and McAuley, B. J.: Efficacy of diltiazem for medically refractory stable angina: Long-term follow-up. Clin. Cardiol. 8:480, 1985.
266a. O'Hara, M. J., Khurmi, N. S., Bowles, M. J., and Raftery, E. B.: Diltiazem and propranolol combination for the treatment of chronic stable angina pectoris. Clin. Cardiol. 10:115, 1987.
267. Strauss, W. E., and Parisi, A. F.: Superiority of combined diltiazem and propranolol therapy for angina pectoris. Circulation 71:951, 1985.
268. Gibson, R. S., Boden, W. E., Theroux, P., Strauss, H. D., Pratt, C. M., Gheorghiade, M., Capone, R. J., Crawford, M. H., Schlant, R. C., Kleiger, R. E., Young, P. M., Schechtman, K., Perryman, B., Roberts, R., and the Diltiazem Reinfarction Study Group: Diltiazem and reinfarction in patients with non-Q-wave myocardial infarction. Results of a double-blind, randomized, multicenter trial. N. Engl. J. Med. 315:423, 1986.
269. Packer, M., Meller, J., Medina, N., Yushak, M., Smith, H., Holt, J., Guerrera, J., Todd, G. D., McAllister, R. G., Jr., and Gorlin, R.: Hemodynamic consequences of combined beta-adrenergic and slow calcium channel blockade in man. Circulation 65:660, 1982.
270. Kieval, J., Kirsten, E. B., Kessler, K. M., Mallon, S. M., and Myerburg, R. J.: The effects of intravenous verapamil on hemodynamic status of patients with coronary artery disease receiving propranolol. Circulation 65:653, 1982.
271. Shub, C., Vlietstra, R. E., and McGoon, M. D.: Selection of optional drug therapy for the patient with angina pectoris. Mayo Clin. Proc. 60:539, 1985.
272. Anderson, H. V., Roubin, G. S., Leimgruber, P. P., Douglas, J. S., Jr., King, S. B., and Gruentzig, A. R.: Primary angiographic success rates of percutaneous transluminal coronary angioplasty. Am. J. Cardiol. 56:712, 1985.
272a. Ernst, S. M. P. G., van der Feltz, T. A., Bal, E. T., Bogerijen, L. V., van den Berg, E., Ascoop, C. A. P. L., and Plokker, H. W. T.: Long-term angiographic followup, cardiac events, and survival in patients undergoing percutaneous transluminal coronary angioplasty. Brit. Heart J. 57:220, 1987.
273. Vlietstra, R. E., and Holmes, D. R. (eds.): PTCA Percutaneous Transluminal Coronary Angioplasty 1987. Philadelphia, F. A. Davis Co.
274. Bredlau, C. E., Roubin, G. S., Leimgruber, P. P., Douglas J. S., Jr., King, S. B., and Gruentzig, A. R.: In-hospital morbidity and mortality in patients undergoing elective coronary angioplasty. Circulation 72:1044, 1985.
274a. Simpfendorfer, C., Belardi, J., Bellamy, G., Galan, K., Franco, I., and Hollman, J.: Frequency, management and follow-up of patients with acute coronary occlusions after percutaneous transluminal coronary angioplasty. Am. J. Cardiol. 59:267, 1987.
275. Cowley, M. J., Vetrovec, G. W., DiSciascio, G., Lewis, S. A., Hirsch, P. D., and Wolfgang, T. C.: Coronary angioplasty of multiple vessels: Short-term outcome and long-term results. Circulation 72:1314, 1985.
276. Leimgruber, P. P., Roubin, G. S., Hollman, J., Cotsonis, G. A., Meier, B., Douglas, J. S., King, S. B., and Gruentzig, A. R.: Restenosis after successful coronary angioplasty in patients with single-vessel disease. Circulation 73:710, 1986.
276a. Melchior, J. P., Meier, B., Urban, P., Finci, L., Steffenino, G., Noble, J., and Rutishauser, W.: Percutaneous transluminal coronary angioplasty for chronic total coronary arterial occlusion. Am. J. Cardiol. 59:535, 1987.
277. Mabin, T. A., Holmes, D. R., Jr., Smith, H. C., Vlietstra, R. E., Reeder, G. S., Bresnahan, J. F., Bove, A. A., Hammes, L. N., Elveback, L. R., and Orszulak, T. A.: Follow-up clinical results in patients undergoing percutaneous transluminal coronary angioplasty. Circulation 71:754, 1985.
278. Vandormael, M. G., Chaitman, B. R., Ischinger, T., Aker, U. T., Harper, M., Hernandez, J., Deligonul, U., and Kennedy, H. L.: Immediate and short-term benefit of multilesion coronary angioplasty: Influence of degree of revascularization. J. Am. Coll. Cardiol. 6:983, 1985.
279. Reeder, G. S., Vlietstra, R. E., Mock, M. B., Holmes, D. R., Smith, H. C., and Piehler, J. M.: Comparison of angioplasty and bypass surgery in multivessel coronary artery disease. Int. J. Cardiol. 10:213, 1986.
280. Brahos, G. J., Baker, N. H., Ewy, G., Moore, P. J., Thomas, J. W., Sanfelippo, P. M., McVicker, R. F., and Fankhauser, D. J.: Aortocoronary bypass following unsuccessful PTCA: Experience in 100 consecutive patients. Ann. Thor. Surg. 40:7, 1985.
281. Bentivoglio, L. G., Van Raden, M. J., Kelsey, S. F., and Detre, K. M.: Percutaneous transluminal coronary angioplasty (PTCA) in patients with relative contraindications: Results of the National Heart, Lung, and Blood Institute PTCA Registry. Am. J. Cardiol. 53 (Suppl. 1):82C, 1984.
282. Bonow, R. O., Kent, K. M., Rosing, D. R., Lipson, L. C., Bacharach, S. L., Green, M. V., and Epstein, S. E.: Improved left ventricular diastolic filling in patients with coronary artery disease after percutaneous transluminal coronary angioplasty. Circulation 66:1159, 1982.
283. Bates, E. R., Aueron, F. M., Legrand, V., LeFree, M. T., Mancini, G. B. J., Hodgson, J. M., and Vogel, R. A.: Comparative long-term effects of coronary artery bypass graft surgery and percutaneous transluminal coronary angioplasty on regional coronary flow reserve. Circulation 72:833, 1985.
284. Kent, K. M., Bonow, R. O., Rosing, D. R., Ewels, C. J., Lipson, L. C., McIntosh, C. L., Bacharach, S., Green, M., and Epstein, S. E.: Improved myocardial function during exercise after successful percutaneous transluminal coronary angioplasty. N. Engl. J. Med. 306:441, 1982.
284a. Gruentzig, A. R., King, S. B., Schlumpf, M., and Siegenthaler, W.: Long-term follow-up after percutaneous transluminal coronary angioplasty. The early Zurich experience. N. Engl. J. Med. 316:1127, 1987.
285. Berger, E., Williams, D. O., Reinert, S., and Most, A. S.: Sustained efficacy of percutaneous transluminal coronary angioplasty. Am. Heart J. 111:233, 1986.
286. Cote, G., Myler, R. K., Stertzer, S. H., Clark, D. A., Fishman-Rosen, J., Murphy, M., and Shaw, R. E.: Percutaneous transluminal angioplasty of stenotic coronary artery bypass grafts: 5 years' experience. J. Am. Coll. Cardiol. 9:8, 1987.
287. Serruys, P. W., Umans, V., Heyndrickx, G. R., Brand, M. V. D., de Feyter, P. J., Wijns, W., Jaski, B., and Hugenholtz, P. G.: Elective PTCA of totally occluded coronary arteries not associated with acute myocardial infarction; short-term and long-term results. Eur. Heart J. 6:2, 1985.
288. Kereiakes, D. J., Selmon, M. R., McAuley, B. J., McAuley, D. B., Sheehan, D. J., and Simpson, J. B.: Angioplasty in total coronary artery occlusion: Experience in 76 consecutive patients. J. Am. Coll. Cardiol. 6:526, 1985.
289. DiSciascio, G., Vetrovec, G. W., Cowley, M. J., and Wolfgang, T. C.: Early and late outcome of percutaneous transluminal coronary angioplasty for subacute and chronic total coronary occlusion. Am. Heart J. 111:833, 1986.
290. Isner, J. M., and Clarke, R. H.: Laser angioplasty: Unraveling the Gordian knot. J. Am. Coll. Cardiol. 7:705, 1986.
291. Forrester, J. S., Litvack, F., and Grundfest, W. S.: Laser angioplasty and cardiovascular disease. Am. J. Cardiol. 57:990, 1986.
292. Choy, D. S., Stertzer, H., Quilici, P., Wallsh, E., Bruno, M. S., Loubeau, J. -M., Kaminow, I., and Rotterdam, H.: Argon laser angioplasty in cadaver and animal models. J. Am. Coll. Cardiol. 1:690, 1983.
293. Hiehle, J. F., Jr., Bourgelais, D. B. C., Shapshay, S., Schoen, F. J., Kim, D., and Spears, R.: Nd-YAG laser fusion of human atheromatous plaque-arterial wall separations in vitro. Am. J. Cardiol. 56:953, 1985.

CORONARY ARTERY SURGERY

294. Loop, F. D., Sheldon, W. C., Lytle, B. W., Cosgrove, D. M., III, and Proudfit, W. L.: The efficacy of coronary artery surgery. Am. Heart J. 101:86, 1981.
295. Kaiser, G. C.: CABG 1984: technical aspects of bypass surgery. Circulation 72(Suppl. V):46, 1985.
296. Preito, I., Basil, E. F., and Abdulnou, R. E.: Upper extremity vein graft for aortocoronary bypass. Ann. Thorac. Surg. 37:218, 1984.
297. Stoney, W. S., Alford, W. C., Burrus, G. R., Glassford, D. M., Petracek, M. R., and Thomas, C. S.: The fate of arm vein grafts used for coronary artery bypass grafts. J. Thorac. Cardiovasc. Surg. 88:522, 1984.
298. Jones, E. L., Carver, J. M., Guyton, R. P., Bone, D. K., Hatcher, C. R., Jr., and Riechwalt, N.: Importance of complete revascularization in performance of the coronary bypass operation. Am. J. Cardiol. 51:7, 1983.
299. Frazier, B. L., Flemma, R. J., Tector, A. J., and Korns, M. E.: Atherosclerosis involving the internal mammary artery. Ann. Thorac. Surg. 18:305, 1974.
300. Grondin, C. M., Campeau, L., Lesperance, J., Enjalber, T. M., and Bourassa, M. G.: Comparison of late changes in internal mammary artery in saphenous vein grafts in two consecutive series of patients ten years after operation. Circulation 70(I):I-208, 1984.
301. Lytle, B. W., Loop, F. D., Cosgrove, D. W., Ratliff, N. B., Easley, K., and Taylor, P. C.: Long-term (5 to 12 years) serial studies of internal mammary artery and saphenous vein coronary bypass grafts. J. Thorac. Cardiovasc. Surg. 89:248, 1985.
302. Loop, F. D., Lytle, B. W., Cosgrove, D. M., Stewart, R. W., Goormastic, M., Williams, G. W., Golding, L. A. R., Gill, C. C., Taylor, P. C., Sheldon, W. C., and Proudfit, W. L.: Influence of the internal mammary artery graft on 10-year survival and other cardiac events. N. Engl. J. Med. 314:1, 1986.
303. Cosgrove, D. M., Loop, F. D., Lytle, B. W, Goormastic, M., Stewart, R. W., Gill, C. C., and Golding, L. R.: Does mammary artery grafting increase surgical risk? Circulation 72(Suppl. II): 170, 1985.
304. Tector, A. J., and Schmahl, T. M.: Techniques for multiple internal mammary artery bypass grafts. Ann. Thorac. Surg. 38:281, 1984.
305. Kamath, M. L., Matyski, L. S., Schmidt, D. H., and Smith, L. L.: Sequential internal mammary artery grafts. Expanded utilization of an ideal conduit. J. Thorac. Cardiovasc. Surg. 89:163, 1985.
306. Hodgson, J. M., Singh, A. K., Drew, T. M., Riley, R. S., and Williams, D. O.: Coronary flow reserve provided by sequential internal mammary artery grafts. J. Am. Coll. Cardiol. 7:32, 1986.
307. Tector, A. J., Schmahl, T. M., and Canino, V. R.: Expanding the use of the internal mammary artery to improve patency in coronary artery bypass grafting. J. Thorac. Cardiovasc. Surg. 91:9, 1986.
308. Dobrin, P., Canfield, T., Moran, J., Sullivan, H., and Pifarre, R.: Coronary artery bypass. The physiological basis for differences in flow with internal mammary artery and saphenous vein grafts. J. Thorac. Cardiovasc. Surg. 74:445, 1977.
309. Lewis, M. R., and Dehmer, G. J.: Coronary bypass using the internal mammary artery. Am. J. Cardiol. 56:480, 1985.
310. Spencer, F. C.: The internal mammary artery: The ideal coronary bypass graft? N. Engl. J. Med. 314:50, 1986.
311. Barnes, H. B., Standevan, J. W., and Reese, J.: Twelve year experience with internal mammary artery for coronary artery grafts. J. Thorac. Cardiovasc. Surg. 90:668, 1985.
312. Smith, S. C., Jr., Gorlin, R., Herman, M. V., Taylor, W. J., and Collins, J. J., Jr.: Myocardial blood flow in man. Effect of coronary collateral circulation and coronary artery bypass surgery. J. Clin. Invest. 51:2556, 1972.

313. Lesperance, J., Bourassa, M. G., Biron, P., Campeau, L., and Saltiel, J.: Aorta to coronary artery saphenous vein grafts. Preoperative angiographic criteria for successful surgery. Am. J. Cardiol. *30*:459, 1972.
314. Rosch, J., Dotter, C. T., Antonovic, R., Bonchek, L., and Starr, A.: Angiographic appraisal of distal vessel suitability for aortocoronary bypass graft surgery. Circulation *48*:202, 1973.
315. Cukingnan, R. A., Carey, J. S., Wittig, J. H., and Brown, B. G.: Influence of complete coronary revascularization on relief of angina. J. Thorac. Cardiovasc. Surg. *79*:188, 1980.
316. Walker, J. A., Friedberg, H. D., Flemma, R. J., and Johnson, W. D.: Determinants of angiographic patency of aortocoronary vein bypass grafts. Circulation *45, 46* (Suppl. I):86, 1972.
317. Grondin, C. M., Lapage, G., Castoguay, Y. R., Meere, C., and Grondin, P.: Aortocoronary bypass graft. Initial blood flow through the graft, and early postoperative patency. Circulation *44*:815, 1971.
318. Loop, F. D.: CASS continued. Circulation 72(Suppl. II):1, 1985.
319. Passamani, E., Davis, K. B., Gillespie, M. J., Killip, T., and the CASS principal investigators and their associates: A randomized trial of coronary artery bypass surgery. Survival of patients with a low ejection fraction. N. Engl. J. Med. *312*:1665, 1985.
320. Killip, T., Passamani, E., Davis, K., and the CASS Principal Investigators and their Associates: Coronary artery surgery study (CASS): A randomized trial of coronary bypass surgery. Eight-year follow-up and survival in patients with reduced ejection fraction. Circulation *72*(Suppl. V):102, 1985.
321. Zubiate, P., Kay, J. H., and Dunne, E.F.: Myocardial revascularization for patients with an ejection fraction of 0.2 or less. 12 years' results. West. J. Med. *140*:745, 1984.
322. Freeman, A. P., Walsh, W. F., Giles, R. W., Choy, D., Newman, D. C., Horton, D. A., Wright, J. S., and Murray, I. P.: Early and long-term results of coronary artery bypass grafting with severely depressed left ventricular performance. Am. J. Cardiol. *54*:749, 1984.
323. Alderman, E. L., Fisher, L. D., Litwin, P., Kaiser, G. C., Myers, W. O., Maynard, C., Levine, F., and Schloss, M.: Results of coronary artery surgery in patients with poor left ventricular function (CASS). Circulation *68*:785, 1983.
323a. Holmes, D. R., Davis, K. B., Mock, M. B., Fisher, L. D., Gersh, B. J., Killip, T., Pettinger, M., and Participants in the Coronary Artery Surgery Study: The effect of medical and surgical treatment on subsequent sudden cardiac death in patients with coronary artery disease: A report from the Coronary Artery Surgery Study. Circulation *73*:1254, 1986.
324. Pigott, J. D., Kouchoukos, N. T., Oberman, A., and Cutter, G. R.: Late results of surgical and medical therapy for patients with coronary artery disease and depressed left ventricular function. J. Am. Coll. Cardiol. *5*:1036, 1985.
324a. Vigilante, G. J., Weintraub, W. S., Klein, L. W., Schneider, R. M., Seelaus, P. A., Parr, G. V. S., Lemole, G., Agarwal, J. B., and Helfant, R. H.: Improved survival with coronary bypass surgery in patients with three-vessel coronary disease and abnormal left ventricular function. Matched case-control study in patient with potentially operable disease. Am. J. Med. *82*:697, 1987.
325. Kennedy, J. W., Kaiser, G. C., Fisher, L. D., Fritz, J. K., Myers, W., Mudd, J. G., and Ryan, T. J.: Clinical and angiographic predictors of operative mortality from the collaborative study in coronary artery surgery (CASS). Circulation *63*:793, 1981.
326. Myers, W. O., Davis, K., Foster, E. D., Maynard, C., and Kaiser, G. C.: Surgical survival in the Coronary Artery Surgery Study (CASS) Registry. Ann. Thorac. Surg. *40*:245, 1985.
327. Adler, D. S., Goldman, L., O'Neil, A., Cook, E. F., Mudge, G. H., Shemin, R. J., DiSesa, V., Cohn, L. H., and Collins, J. J.: Long-term survival of more than 2,000 patients after coronary artery bypass grafting. Am. J. Cardiol. *58*:195, 1986.
328. CASS Principal Investigators and their Associates: Coronary Artery Surgery Study (CASS): A randomized trial of coronary artery bypass surgery. Survival data. Circulation *68*:939, 1983.
329. Burton, J. R., Fitzgibbon, G. H., Keon, W. J., and Leach, A. J.: Perioperative myocardial infarction complicating coronary bypass. Clinical and angiographic correlations and prognosis. J. Thorac. Cardiovasc. Surg. *82*:758, 1981.
330. Gray, R. J., Matloff, J. M., Conklin, C. M., Ganz, W., Charuzi, Y., Wolfstein, R., and Swan, H. J. C.: Perioperative myocardial infarction: Late clinical course after coronary artery bypass surgery. Circulation *66*:1185, 1982.
331. Chaitman, B. R., Alderman, E. L., Sheffield, L. T., Tong, T., Fisher, L., Mock, M. B., Weins, R. D., Kaiser, G. C., Roitman, D., Berger, R., Gersh, B., Schaff, H., Bourassa, M. G., and Killip, T.: Use of survival analysis to determine the clinical significance of new Q waves after coronary bypass surgery. Circulation *67*:302, 1983.
332. Shaw, P. J., Bates, D., Cartlidge, N. E. F., French, J. M., Heaviside, D., Julian, D. G., and Shaw, D. A.: Early intellectual dysfunction following coronary bypass surgery. Q. J. Med. *58*:59, 1986.
333. Raymond, M., Conklin, C., Schaeffer, J., Newstadt, G., Matloff, J. M., and Gray, R. J.: Coping with transient intellectual dysfunction after coronary bypass surgery. Heart Lung *13*:531, 1984.
334. Roberts, A. J., Subramanian, V. A., Herman, S. D., Case, D. B., Johnson, G. A., Jr., and Gay, W. A., Jr.: Systemic hypertension associated with coronary artery bypass surgery. J. Thorac. Cardiovasc. Surg. *74*:846, 1977.
335. Bateman, T. M., Weiss, M. H., Czer, L. S. C., Conklin, C. M., Kass, R. M., Steward, M. E., Matloff, J. M., and Gray, R. J.: Fascicular conduction disturbances and ischemic heart disease: Adverse prognosis despite coronary revascularization. J. Am. Coll. Cardiol. *5*:632, 1985.
335a. Chu, A., Califf, R. M., Pryor, D. B., McKinnis, R. A., Harrell, F. E., Jr., Lee, K. L., Curtis, S. E., Oldham, H. N., and Wagner, G. S.: Prognostic effect of bundle branch block related to coronary artery bypass grafting. Am. J. Cardiol. *59*:798, 1987.
336. Koshal, A., Hendry, P., Roman, S. V., and Keon, W. J.: Should obese patients not undergo coronary artery surgery? Can. J. Surg. *28*:331, 1985.
337. Rutherford, J. D., Whitlock, R. M. L., McDonald, B. W., Barratt-Boyes, B. G., and Kerr, A. R.: Multivariate analysis of the long-term results of coronary artery bypass grafting performed during 1976 and 1977. Am. J. Cardiol. *57*:1264, 1986.
338. European Coronary Surgery Study Group: Long-term results of prospective randomised study of coronary artery bypass surgery in stable angina pectoris. Lancet *2*:1173, 1982.
339. CASS Principal Investigators and their Associates: Coronary Artery Surgery Study (CASS): A randomized trial of coronary artery bypass surgery. Quality of life in patients randomly assigned to treatment groups. Circulation *68*:951, 1983.
340. Hultgren, H. M., Peduzzi, P., Detre, K., Takaro, T., and the study participants: The 5-year effect of bypass surgery on relief of angina and exercise performance. Circulation 72(Suppl. V):79, 1985.
341. Frick, M. H., Harjola, P.-T., and Valle, M.: Persistent improvement after coronary bypass surgery: Ergometric and angiographic correlations at 5 years. Circulation *67*:491, 1983.
342. Lawrie, G. M., Morris, G. C., Calhoon, J. H., Safi, H., Zamore, J. L., Beltengady, M., Baron, A., Silbers, A., and Chapman, P. W.: Clinical results of coronary bypass in 500 patients at least 10 years after operation. Circulation *66*(Suppl. I):1, 1982.
343. Johnson, W. D., Kayser, K. L., and Pedraza, P. M.: Angina pectoris and coronary bypass surgery: Patterns of prevalence and recurrence in 3105 consecutive patients followed up to 11 years. Am. Heart J. *108*:1190, 1984.
344. Wenger, N. K.: Rehabilitation of the coronary patient: status 1986. Prog. Cardiovasc. Dis. *29*:181, 1986.
345. Hammermeister, K. E., DeRoden, T. A., English, M. T., and Dodge, H. T.: Effect of surgical versus medical therapy on return to work in patients with coronary artery disease. Am. J. Cardiol. *44*:105, 1978.
346. David, P.: Contributing factors preventing return to work of cardiac surgery patients. Cleve. Clin. Q. *45*:177, 1978.
347. Hymowitz, Z., Freiman, I., Borman, J., Applebaum, A., and Gotsman, M. S.: Work status before and after coronary artery bypass surgery. Publ. Health (Lond.) *99*:367, 1985.
348. Misra, K. K., Kazanchi, B. N., Davies, G. J., Westaby, S., Sapsford, R. N.,and Bentall, H. H.: Determinants of work capability and employment after coronary artery surgery. Eur. Heart J. *6*:176, 1985.
349. Sergeant, P., Lesaffre, E., Flameng, W., and Suy, R.: How predictable is the postoperative work resumption after aortocoronary bypass surgery? Acta Cardiologica *41*:41, 1986.
350. Hall, R.: Coronary artery bypass long-term follow-up on 22,284 consecutive patients. Circulation *68*(Suppl. II):20, 1983.
351. Stanton, B., Jenkins, C. D., Savageau, J. A., and Thurer, R. L.: Functional benefits following coronary artery bypass graft surgery. Ann. Thorac. Surg. *37*:286, 1984.
351a. Peduzzi, P., Hultgren, H., Thomsen, J., and Detre, K.: Ten-year effect of medical and surgical therapy on quality of life: Veterans Administration Cooperative Study of Coronary Artery Surgery. Am. J. Cardiol. *59*:1017, 1987.
352. Fuster, V., and Chesebro, J. J.: Aortocoronary artery vein-graft disease: Experimental and clinical approach for the understanding of the role of platelets and platelet inhibitors. Circulation 72(Suppl. V):65, 1985.
353. Fuster, V., and Chesebro, J. H.: Role of platelets and platelet inhibitors in aortocoronary artery vein-graft disease. Circulation *73*:227, 1986.
354. Smith, S. H., and Geer, J. C.: Morphology of saphenous vein-coronary artery bypass grafts. Seven to 116 months after surgery. Arch. Pathol. Lab. Med. *107*:13, 1983.
355. Campeau, L., Enjalbert, M., Lesperance, J., Vaislic, C., Grondin, C. M., and Bourassa, M. G.: Atherosclerosis and late closure of aortocoronary saphenous vein grafts: Sequential angiographic studies at 2 weeks, 1 year, 5 to 7 years, and 10 to 12 years after surgery. Circulation *68*(Suppl. II):1, 1983.
356. Chesebro, J. H., Clements, I. P., Fuster, V., Elveback, L. R., Smith, H. C., Bardsley, W. T., Frye, R. L., Holmes, D. R., Jr., Vlietstra, R. E., Pluth, J. R., Wallace, R. B., Puga, F. J., Orszulak, T. A., Piehler, J. M., Schaff, H. V., and Danielson, G. K.: A platelet-inhibitor drug trial in coronary-artery bypass operations. Benefit of perioperative dipyridamole and aspirin therapy on early postoperative vein-graft patency. N. Engl. J. Med. *307*:73, 1982.
357. Chesebro, J. H., Fuster, V., Elveback, L. R., Clements, I. P., Smith, H. C., Holmes, D. R., Jr., Bardsley, W. T., Pluth, J. R., Wallace, R. B., Puga, F. J., Orszulak, T. A. Piehler, J. M., Danielson, G. K., Schaff, H. V., and Frye, R. L.: Effect of dipyridamole and aspirin on late vein-graft patency after coronary bypass operations. N. Engl. J. Med. *310*:209, 1984.
358. Landymore, R. W., MacAulay, M., Sheridan, B., and Cameron, C.: Comparison of cod-liver oil and aspirin-dipyridamole for the prevention of intimal hyperplasia in autogenous vein grafts. Ann. Thorac. Surg. *41*:54, 1986.
358a. Fitzgerald, G. A.: Dipyridamole. N. Engl. J. Med. *316*:1247, 1987.
359. Lie, J. T., Lawrie, G. M., and Morris, G. C.: Aortocoronary bypass saphenous vein graft atherosclerosis. Am. J. Cardiol. *40*:906, 1977.
360. Bourassa, M. G., Fisher, L. D., Campeau, L., Gillespie, M. J., McConney, M., and Lesperance, J.: Long-term fate of bypass grafts. The coronary artery surgery study (CASS) and Montreal Heart Institute experiences. Circulation 72(Suppl. V):71, 1985.
361. Frick, M. H., Valle, M., and Harjola, P.-T.: Progression of coronary artery disease in randomized medical and surgical patients over a 5-year angiographic follow-up. Am. J. Cardiol. *52*:681, 1983.
362. Pfisterer, M., Emmenegger, H., Schmitt, H. E., Muller-Brand, J., Hasse, J., Gradel, E., Laver, M. B., Burckhardt, D., and Burkart, F.: Accuracy of serial myocardial perfusion scintigraphy with Thallium-201 for prediction of graft patency early and late after coronary artery bypass surgery. A controlled prospective study. Circulation *66*:1017, 1982.

363. Rasmussen, S. L., Nielsen, S. L., Amtorp, O., Folke, K., and Fritz-Hansen, P.: 201-Thallium imaging as an indicator of graft patency after coronary artery bypass surgery. Eur. Heart J. 5:494, 1984.
364. Campeau, L., Enjalbert, M., Lesperance, J., Bourassa, M. G., Kwiterovich, P., Jr., Wacholder, S., and Sniderman, A.: The relation of risk factors to the development of atherosclerosis in saphenous-vein bypass grafts and the progression of disease in the native circulation. A study 10 years after aortocoronary bypass surgery. N. Engl. J. Med. *311*:1329, 1984.
365. Detre, K. M., Takaro, T. Hultgren, H., Peduzzi, P., and the Study Participants: Long-term mortality and morbidity results of the Veterans Administration randomized trial of coronary artery bypass surgery. Circulation 72(Suppl. V): 84, 1985.
366. Varnauskas, E., and the European Coronary Surgery Study Group: Survival, myocardial infarction, and employment status in a prospective randomized study of coronary bypass surgery. Circulation 72(Suppl. V):90, 1985.
367. Barboriak, J. J., Rimm, A. A., and Anderson, A. J.: Risk factors and mortality in patients with aortocoronary vein bypass operations. Cardiology *63*:237, 1978.
368. Devineni, R., and McKenzie, F. N.: Surgery for coronary artery disease in patients with diabetes mellitus. Can. J. Surg. *28*:367, 1985.
369. Lytle, B. W., Kramer, J. R., Golding, L. R., Cosgrove, D. M., Borsh, J. A., Goormastic, M., and Loop, F.D.: Young adults with coronary atherosclerosis: 10-year results of surgical myocardial revascularization. J. Am. Coll. Cardiol. *4*:445, 1984.
369a. Fitzgibbon, G. M., Hamilton, M. G., Leach, A. J., Kafka, H. P., Markle, H. V., and Keon, W. J.: Coronary artery disease and coronary bypass grafting in young men: Experience with 138 subjects 39 years of age and younger. J. Am. Coll. Cardiol. *9*:977, 1987.
370. Kannel, W. B., and Feinlieb, M.: Natural history of angina pectoris in the Framingham study: Progress and survival. Am. J. Cardiol. *29*:154, 1972.
371. Frank, C. W., Weinblatt, W., and Shapiro, S.: Angina pectoris in men: Prognostic significance of related medical factors. Circulation *47*:509, 1973.
372. Vedin, A., Wilhelmsson, C., Elmfeldt, D., Save-Soderbergh, J., Tibblin, G., and Wilhelmsen, L.: Death and non-fatal reinfarctions during two years' follow-up after myocardial infarction. Acta Med. Scand. *198*:353, 1975.
373. Graham, I., Mulcahy, R., Hickey, N., O'Neill, W., and Daly, L.: Natural history of coronary heart disease: A study of 586 men surviving an initial acute attack. Am. Heart J. *105*:249, 1983.
374. Kaiser, G. C., Davis, K. B., Fisher, L. D., Myers, W. O., Foster, E. D., Passamani, E. R., and Gillespie, M. J.: Survival following coronary artery bypass grafting in patients with severe angina pectoris (CASS). J. Thorac. Cardiovasc. Surg. *89*:513, 1985.
375. Detre, K., Peduzzi, P., Murphy, M., Hultgren, H., Thomsen, J., Oberman, A., and Takaro, T.: Effect of bypass surgery on survival in patients with low- and high-risk groups delineated by the use of simple clinical variables. Circulation *63*:1329, 1981.
376. Harlan, W. R., Oberman, A., Grimm, R., and Rosati, R. A.: Chronic congestive heart failure in coronary artery disease: Clinical criteria. Ann. Intern. Med. *86*:133, 1977.
377. Merrilees, M. A., Scott, P. J., and Norris, R. M.: Prognosis after myocardial infarction. Results of 15-year follow-up. Br. Med. J. *288*:356, 1984.
378. Peel, A. A. F., Semple, T., Wang, I., Lancaster, W. M., and Dall, J. L. G.: A coronary prognostic index for grading the severity of infarction. Br. Heart J. *24*:745, 1962.
379. Killip, T., and Kimball, J. T.: Treatment of myocardial infarction in a coronary care unit. A two-year experience with 250 patients. Am. J. Cardiol. *20*:457, 1967.
380. Luria, M. H., Knoke, J. D., Wach, J. S., and Luria, M. A.: Survival after recovery from acute myocardial infarction. Two- and five-year prognostic indices. Am. J. Med. 67:7, 1979.
381. Bigger, J. T., Haller, C. A., Wenger, T. L., and Weld, F. M.: Risk stratification after acute myocardial infarction. Am. J. Cardiol. *42*:202, 1979.
382. Moss, A. J., DeCamilla, J., Davis, H., and Baker, L.: The early post-hospital phase of myocardial infarction. Prognostic stratification. Circulation *54*:58, 1976.
383. Kitchin, A. H., and Pocock, S. J.: Prognosis of patients with acute myocardial infarction admitted to a coronary care unit. II. Survival after hospital discharge. Br. Heart J. 39:1167, 1977.
384. The Multicenter Postinfarction Research Group: Risk stratification and survival after myocardial infarction. N. Engl. J. Med. *309*:331, 1983.
385. Blackburn, H: The prognostic importance of the electrocardiogram after myocardial infarction: Experience in the Coronary Drug Project. Ann. Intern. Med. 77:677, 1972.
386. Kannel, W. B., Boyle, J. T., McNamara, P., Quickenton, P., and Gordon, T.: Precursors of sudden coronary death: Factors related to the incidence of sudden death. Circulation *51*:606, 1975.
387. Sanz, G., Castaner, A., Betriu, A., Magrina, J., Roig, E., Coll, S., Pare, J. C., and Navarro-Lopez, F.: Determinants of prognosis in survivors of myocardial infarction. A prospective clinical angiographic study. N. Engl. J. Med. *306*:1065, 1982.
388. Mock, M. B., Ringqvist, I., Fisher, L. D., Davis, K. B., Chaitman, B. R., Kouchoukos, N. T., Kaiser, G. C., Alderman, E., Ryan, T. J., Russell, R. O., Jr., Mullin, S., Fray, D., Killip, T., III, and participants in the Coronary Artery Surgery Study: Survival of medically treated patients in the Coronary Artery Surgery Study (CASS) Registry. Circulation *66*:562, 1982.
389. Reeves, T. J., Oberman, A., Jones, W. B., and Sheffield, L. T.: Natural history of angina pectoris. Am. J. Cardiol. 33:423, 1974.
390. Califf, R. M., Tomabechi, Y., Lee, K. L., Phillips, H., Pryor, D. B., Harrell, F. E., Jr., Harris, P. J., Peter, R. H., Behar, V. S., Kong, Y., and Rosati, R. A.: Outcome in one-vessel coronary artery disease. Circulation 67:283, 1983.
391. Nestico, P. F., Hakki, A.-H., Meissner, M. D., and Bemis, C. E., Kimbiris, D., Mintz, G. S., Segal, B. L., and Iskandrian, A. S.: Effect of collateral vessels on prognosis in patients with one-vessel coronary artery disease. J. Am. Coll. Cardiol. *6*:1257, 1985.
392. Burggraf, G. W., and Parker, J. O.: Prognosis in coronary artery disease—angiographic, hemodynamic and clinical factors. Circulation *51*:146, 1975.
393. Humphries, J. O., Kuller, L., Ross, R. S., Friesinger, G. C., and Page, E. E.: Natural history of ischemic heart disease in relation to angiographic findings. Circulation *49*:489, 1974.
394. Oberman, A., Jones, W. B., and Riley, C. P.: Natural history of coronary artery disease. Bull. N.Y. Acad. Med. *48*:1109, 1972.
395. Proudfit, W. J., Bruschke, A. V. G., MacMillan, J. P., Williams, G. W., and Sones, F. M., Jr.: Fifteen-year survival study of patients with obstructive coronary artery disease. Circulation *68*:986, 1983.
396. Harris, P. J., Behar, V. S., Conley, M. J., Harrell, F. E., Jr., Lee, K. L., Peter, R. H., Kong, Y., and Rosati, R. A.: The prognostic significance of 50 per cent coronary stenosis in medically treated patients with coronary artery disease. Circulation *62*:240, 1980.
397. Conti, C. R., Selby, J. H., and Christie, L. G.: Left main coronary artery stenosis: Clinical spectrum, pathophysiology and management. Prog. Cardiovasc. Dis. *22*:73, 1979.
398. Talano, J., Scanlon, P., Meadows, W., Kahn, M., Pifarre, R., and Gunnar, R.: Influence of surgery on survival in 145 patients with left main coronary artery disease. Circulation *51*, *52*(Suppl. I):105, 1975.
399. Demots, H., Boncheck, L., Roesch, J., Anderson, R., Starr, A., and Rahimtoola, S.: Left main coronary artery disease. Am. J. Cardiol. *36*:136, 1975.
400. Conley, M. J., Ely, R. L., Kisslo, J., Lee, K. L., McNeer, J. F., and Rosati, R. A.: The prognostic spectrum of left main stenosis. Circulation *57*:947, 1978.
401. Kent, K. M., Rosing, D. R., Ewels, C. J., Lipson, L., Bonow, R., and Epstein, S. E.: Prognosis of asymptomatic or mildly symptomatic patients with coronary artery disease. Am. J. Cardiol. *49*:1823, 1982.
402. Ryan, T. J., Weiner, D. A., McCabe, C. H., Davis, K. B., Sheffield, L. T., Chaitman, B. R., Tristani, F. E., and Fisher, L. D.: Exercise testing in the Coronary Artery Surgery Study randomized population. Circulation 72(Suppl. V):31, 1985.
403. McNeer, J. F., et al.: The role of the exercise test in the evaluation of patients with ischemic heart disease. Circulation *57*:64, 1978.
404. Weiner, D. A., Ryan, T. J., McCabe, C. H., Chaitman, B. R., Sheffield, L. T., Ferguson, J. C., Fisher, L. D., and Tristani, F.: Prognostic importance of a clinical profile and exercise test in medically treated patients with coronary artery disease. J. Am. Coll. Cardiol. *3*:772, 1984.
405. Gohlke, H., Samek, L., Betz, P., and Roskamm, H.: Exercise testing provides additional prognostic information in angiographically defined subgroups of patients with coronary artery disease. Circulation *68*:979, 1983.
406. Wahl, J., Hakki, A. H., and Iskadrian, A. S.: Prognostic implications of normal exercise thallium-201 images. Arch. Intern. Med. *145*:253, 1985.
407. Damelia, F. X., Gibson, R. S., Watson, D. D., Craddock, G. B., Sirowatka, J., and Beller, G. A.: Prognosis with chest pain and normal thallium-201 exercise scintigrams. Am. J. Cardiol. *55*:920, 1985.
408. Beller, G. A., Gibson, R. S., and Watson, D. D.: Radionuclide methods of identifying patients who may require coronary artery bypass surgery. Circulation 72(Suppl. V):9, 1985.
409. Jones, R. H., Floyd, R. D., Austin, E. H., and Sabiston, D. C.: The role of radionuclide angiography in the preoperative prediction of pain relief and prolonged survival following coronary artery bypass grafting. Ann. Surg. *197*:743, 1983.
410. Kronenberg, M. W., Pederson, R. W., Harston, W. E., Born, M. L., Bender, H. W., and Friesinger, G. C.: Left ventricular performance after coronary artery bypass surgery. Ann. Intern. Med. *99*:305, 1983.
411. Bonow, R. O., Kent, K. M., Rosing, D. R., Lan, K. K. G., Lakatos, E., Borer, J. S., Bacharach, S. L., Green, M. V., and Epstein, S. E.: Exercise-induced ischemia in mildly symptomatic patients with coronary artery disease and preserved left ventricular function. N. Engl. J. Med. *311*:1339, 1984.
412. Report of Inter-Society Commission for Heart Disease Resources: Optimal resources for coronary artery surgery. Circulation *46*:A-325, 1972.
413. Breyer, H., Engelman, R. M., Rousou, J. A., and Lemeshow, W. S.: Postinfarction angina: An expanding subset of patients undergoing coronary artery bypass. J. Thorac. Cardiovasc. Surg. *90*:532, 1985.
414. Foster, E. D.: Re-operation for coronary artery disease. Circulation 72(Suppl. V):59, 1985.
415. Takaro, T., Pifarre, R., and Fish, R.: Left main coronary artery disease. Prog. Cardiovasc. Dis. 28:229, 1985.
416. Chaitman, B. P., Fisher, L. D., and Bourassa, M. G.: Effect of coronary bypass surgery on survival patterns in subsets of patients with left main coronary artery disease. Report of the Collaborative Study in Coronary Artery Surgery (CASS). Am. J. Cardiol. *48*:765, 1981.
417. Califf, R. M., Conley, M. J., Behar, V. S., Harrell, F. E., Jr., Lee, K. L., Pryor, D. B., McKinnis, R. A., and Rosati, R. A.: "Left main equivalent" coronary artery disease: Its clinical presentation and prognostic significance with nonsurgical therapy. Am. J. Cardiol. *53*:1489, 1984.
418. Takaro, T., Hultgren, H. N., Detre, K. M., and Peduzzi, P.: The Veterans Administration Cooperative Study of Stable Angina: Current status. Circulation *65* (Part II):60, 1982.
419. The Veterans Administration Coronary Artery Bypass Surgery Cooperative Study Group: Eleven-year survival in the Veterans Administration randomized trial of coronary bypass surgery for stable angina. N. Engl. J. Med. *311*:1333, 1984.
420. Detre, K., Peduzzi, P., Scott, S. M., and Davies, B.: Long-term survival results in medically and surgically randomized patients. Prog. Cardiovasc. Dis. 28:235, 1985.

421. European Coronary Surgery Study Group: Coronary-artery bypass surgery in stable angina pectoris: Survival at two years. Lancet *1*:889, 1979.
422. European Coronary Surgery Study Group: Prospective randomised study of coronary artery bypass surgery in stable angina pectoris. Lancet *2*:491, 1980.
423. European Coronary Surgery Study Group: Prospective randomized study of coronary artery bypass surgery in stable angina pectoris: A progress report on survival. Circulation *65*(Suppl. II):67, 1982.
424. Iskandrian, A. S., Hakki, A.-H., Goel, I. P., Mundth, E.D., Kane-Marsch, S. A., and Schenk, C. L.: The use of rest and exercise radionuclide ventriculography in risk stratification in patients with suspected coronary artery disease. Am. Heart J. *110*:864, 1985.
425. Norris, R. M., Agnew, T. N., Brandt, P. W.T., et al.: Coronary surgery after recurrent myocardial infarction: Progress of a trial comparing surgical with nonsurgical management for asymptomatic patients with advanced coronary disease. Circulation *63*:785, 1981.
426. Rozanski, A., Berman, D., Gray, R., Diamond, G., Raymond, J., Prause, J., Maddahi, J., Swan, H. J. C., and Matloff, J.: Preoperative prediction of reversible myocardial asynergy to postexercise radionuclide ventriculography. N. Engl. J. Med. *307*:212, 1982.
427. Brundage, B. H., Massie, B. M., and Borvinick, E. H.: Improved regional ventricular function after successful surgical revascularization. J. Am. Coll. Cardiol. *3*:902, 1984.
428. Akins, C. W., Pohost, G. M., DeSanctis, R. W., and Block, P. C.: Selection of angina-free patients with severe left ventricular dysfunction for myocardial revascularization. Am. J. Cardiol. *46*:695, 1980.
429. Shanes, J. G., Kondos, G. T., Levitsky, S., Pavel, D., Subramanian, R., and Brundage, B. H.: Coronary artery obstruction: A potentially reversible cause of dilated cardiomyopathy. Am. Heart J. *110*:173, 1985.
430. Murphy, M. L., Meadows, W. R., Thomsen, J., Hultgren, H. N., Takaro, T., Fish, R., and Read, R.: The effect of coronary artery bypass surgery on the incidence of myocardial infarction and hospitalization. Prog. Cardiovasc. Dis. *28*:309, 1986.
431. CASS principal investigators and their associates: Myocardial infarction and mortality in the Coronary Artery Surgery Study (CASS) randomized trial. N. Engl. J. Med. *310*:750, 1984.
432. Crean, P. A., Waters, D. D., Bosch, X., Pelletier, G. B., Roy, D., and Theroux, P.: Angiographic findings after myocardial infarction in patients with previous bypass surgery: Explanations for smaller infarcts in this group compared with control patients. Circulation *71*:693, 1985.
433. Gersh, B. J., Kronmal, R. A., Schaff, H. V., Frye, R. L., Ryan, T. J., Mock, M. B., Myers, W. O., Athearn, M. W., Gosselin, A. J., Kaiser, G. C., Bourassa, M. G., Killip, T., III, and the Participants in the Coronary Artery Surgery Study: Comparison of coronary artery bypass surgery and medical therapy in patients 65 years of age or older. N. Engl. J. Med. *313*:217, 1985.
434. Loop, F. D., Golding, L. R., Macmillan, J. P., Cosgrove, D. M., Lytle, B. W., and Sheldon, W. C.: Coronary artery surgery in women compared with men: Analyses of risks and long-term results. J. Am. Coll. Cardiol. *1*:383, 1983.
435. Fisher, L. D., Kennedy, J. W., Davis, K. B., Maynard, C., Fritz, J. K., Kaiser, G., Myers, W. O., and the participating CASS clinics: Association of sex, physical size, and operative mortality after coronary artery bypass in the Coronary Artery Surgery Study (CASS). J. Thorac. Cardiovasc. Surg. *84*:334, 1982.
436. Janusz, M. T., Jamieson, W. R. E., Causton, N., Burr, L. H., Allen, P., and Munro, A. I.: Coronary artery bypass in patients over 65 years of age. Can. J. Surg. *26*:186, 1983.
437. Faro, R. S., Golden, M. D., Javid, H., Serry, C., DeLaria, G. A., Monson, D., Weinberg, M., Hunter, J. A., and Najafi, H.: Coronary revascularization in septuagenarians. J. Thorac. Cardiovasc. Surg. *86*:616, 1983.
438. Gersh, B. J., Kronmal, R. A., Frye, R. L., Schaff, H. V., Ryan, T. J., Gosselin, A. J., Kaiser, G. C., Killip, T., III, and participants in the Coronary Artery Surgery Study: Coronary arteriography and coronary artery bypass surgery: Morbidity and mortality in patients aged 65 years or older. A report from the Coronary Artery Surgery Study. Circulation *67*:483, 1983.
439. Elayda, M. A., Hall, R. J., Gray, A. G., Mathur, V. S., and Cooley, D. A.: Coronary revascularization in the elderly patient. J. Am. Coll. Cardiol. *3*:1398, 1984.
440. Montague, N. T., Kouchoukos, N. T., Wilson, T. A. S., Bennett, A. L., Knott, H. W., Lochridge, S. K., Erath, H. G., Jr., and Clayton, O. W.: Morbidity and mortality of coronary bypass grafting in patients 70 years of age and older. Ann. Thorac. Surg. *39*:552, 1985.
441. Roberts, A. J., Woodhall, D. D., Conti, C. R., Ellison, D. W., Fisher, R., Richards, C., Marks, R. G., Knauf, D. G., and Alexander, J. A.: Mortality, morbidity, and cost-accounting related to coronary artery bypass graft surgery in the elderly. Ann. Thorac. Surg. *39*:426, 1985.
442. Rose, D. M., Gelbfish, J., Jacobowitz, I. J., Kramer, M., Zisbrod, Z., Acinapura, A., Cappabiana, P., and Cunningham, J. N.: Analysis of morbidity and mortality in patients 70 years of age and over undergoing isolated coronary artery bypass surgery. Am. Heart J. *110*:361, 1985.
443. Foster, E. D., Fisher, L. D., Kaiser, G. C., Myers, W. O., and CASS principal investigators and their associates: Comparison of operative mortality and morbidity results for initial and repeat coronary artery bypass grafting: The Coronary Artery Surgery Study (CASS) Registry experience. Ann. Thorac. Surg. *38*:563, 1984.
444. Schaff, H. V., Orzulak, T. A., Gersh, B. J., Piehler, J. M., Puga, F. J., Danielson, G. K. and Pluth, J. R.: The morbidity and mortality of reoperation for coronary artery disease and analysis of late results with use of actuarial estimate of event-free interval. J. Thorac. Cardiovasc. Surg. *85*:508, 1983.
445. Brener, B. J., Brief, D. K., Alpert, J., et al.: A four-year experience with preoperative noninvasive carotid evaluation of 2,026 patients undergoing cardiac surgery. J. Vasc. Surg. *1*:326, 1984.
446. Gardner, T. J., Horneffer, P. J., Manolio, T. A., Pearson, T. A., Gott, V. L., Baumgartner, W. A., Borkon, A. M., Watkins, L., and Reitz, B. A.: Stroke following coronary artery bypass grafting: A ten-year study. Ann. Thorac. Surg. *40*:574, 1985.
447. Babu, S. C., Shah, P. M., Singh, B. M., Semel, L., Clauss, R. H., and Reed, G. E.: Coexisting carotid stenosis in patients undergoing cardiac surgery: Indications and guidelines for simultaneous operations. Am. J. Surg. *150*:207, 1985.
448. David, T. E.: Combined cardiac and abdominal aortic surgery. Circulation *72*(Suppl. II):18, 1985.
449. Jones, E. L., Craver, J. M., Michalik, R. A., Murphy, D. A., Guyton, R. A., Bone, D. K., Hatcher, C. R., and Reichwald, N. A.: Combined carotid and coronary operations: When are they necessary? J. Thorac. Cardiovasc. Surg. *87*:7, 1984.
450. Furlan, A. J., and Craciun, A. R.: Risk of stroke during coronary artery bypass graft surgery in patients with internal carotid artery disease documented by angiography. Stroke *16*:797, 1985.
451. Debakey, M. E., and Lawrie, G. M.: Combined coronary artery and peripheral vascular disease: Recognition and treatment. J. Vasc. Surg. *1*:605, 1984.
452. Boucher, C. A., Brewster, D. C., Darling, R. C., Okada, R. D., Strauss, H. W., and Pohost, G. M.: Determination of cardiac risk by dipyridamole-thallium imaging before peripheral vascular surgery. N. Engl. J. Med. *312*:389, 1985.

UNSTABLE ANGINA

453. Gorlin, R., Fuster, V., and Ambrose, J. A.: Anatomic-physiologic links between acute coronary syndromes. (Editorial) Circulation *74*:6, 1986.
454. Victor, M. F., Likoff, M. J., Mintz, G. S., and Likoff, W.: Unstable angina pectoris of new onset: A prospective clinical and arteriographic study of 75 patients. Am. J. Cardiol. *47*:228, 1981.
455. Fischl, S., Gorlin, R., and Herman, M. V.: The intermediate coronary syndrome. Clinical, angiographic, and therapeutic aspects. N. Engl. J. Med. *228*:1193, 1973.
456. Chierchia, S., Brunelli, C., Simonetti, I., Lazzari, M., and Maseri, A.: Sequence of events in angina at rest: Primary reduction in coronary blood flow. Circulation *61*:759, 1980.
457. Biagini, A., Mazzei, M. G., Carpeggiani, C., Testa, R., Antonelli, R., Michelassi, C., L'Abbate, A., and Maseri, A.: Vasospastic ischemic mechanism of frequent asymptomatic transient ST-T changes during continuous electrocardiographic monitoring in selected unstable patients. Am. Heart J. *103*:13, 1982.
458. Johnson, S. M., Mauritson, D. R., Winniford, M. D., Willerson, J. T., Firth, B. G., Cary, J. R., and Hillis, L. D.: Continuous electrocardiographic monitoring in patients with unstable angina pectoris: Identification of high-risk subgroup with severe coronary disease, variant angina, and/or impaired early prognosis. Am. Heart J. *103*:4, 1982.
459. Stern, S., and Tzivoni, D.: Early detection of silent ischemic heart disease by 24-hour electrocardiographic monitoring of active subjects. Br. Heart J. *36*:481, 1976.
460. Cecchi, A. C., Dovellini, E. V., Marchi, F., Pucci, P., Santoro, G. M., and Fazzini, P. F.: Silent myocardial ischemia during ambulatory electrocardiographic monitoring in patients with effort angina. J. Am. Coll. Cardiol. *1*:934, 1983.
461. Deanfield, J. E., Maseri, A., Selwyn, A. P., Ribeiro, P., Chierchia, S., Krikler, S., and Morgan, M.: Myocardial ischaemia during daily life in patients with stable angina: its relation to symptoms and heart rate changes. Lancet *2*:753, 1983.
462. Cohn, P. F., Brown, A. J., Jr., Wynne, J., Holman, B. L., and Atkins, H. L.: Global and regional left ventricular ejection fraction abnormalities during exercise in patients with silent myocardial ischemia. J. Am. Coll. Cardiol. *1*:931, 1983.
463. Chierchia, S., Lazzari, M., Freedman, B., Brunelli, C., and Maseri, A.: Impairment of myocardial perfusion and function during painless myocardial ischemia. J. Am. Coll. Cardiol. *1*:924, 1983.
464. Campbell, S., Barry, J., Rocco, M. B., Nabel, E. G., Mead-Walters, K., Rebecca, G. S., and Selwyn, A. P.: Features of the exercise test that reflect the activity of ischemic heart disease out of hospital. Circulation *74*:72, 1986.
465. Alison, H. W., Russell, R. O., Jr., Mantle, J. A., Kouchoukos, N. T., and Rackley, C. E.: Coronary anatomy and arteriography in patients with unstable angina pectoris. Am. J. Cardiol. *41*:204, 1978.
466. Roberts, W. C., and Virmani, Z.: Quantitation of coronary arterial narrowing in clinically isolated unstable angina pectoris: An analysis of 22 necropsy patients. Am. J. Med. *67*:792, 1979.
467. Parker, F. B., Jr., Neville, J. F., Jr., Hanson, E. C., and Webb, W. R.: Retrograde and antegrade pressures and flows in preinfarction syndrome. Circulation *50*(Suppl. 11):122, 1974.
468. Levin, D. C., and Fallon, J. T.: Significance of the angiographic morphology of localized coronary stenoses: Histopathologic correlations. Circulation *66*:316, 1984.
469. Freudenberg, H., and Lichtlen, P. R.: The normal segment in coronary stenosis—a postmortem study. Z. Cardiol. *70*:863, 1981.
470. Saner, G. E., Gobel, F. L., Salomonowitz, E., Erien, D. A., and Edwards, J. E.: The disease-free wall in coronary atherosclerosis: Its relation to degree of obstruction. J. Am. Coll. Cardiol. *6*:1096, 1985.
471. Ambrose, J. A., Winters, S. L., Stern, A., Eng, A., Teichholz, L. E., Gorlin, R., and Fuster, F.: Angiographic morphology and the pathogenesis of unstable angina pectoris. J. Am. Coll. Cardiol. *5*:609, 1985.
472. Ambrose, J. A., Winters, S. L., Arora, R. R., Eng, A., Riccio, A., Gorlin, R.,

and Fuster, V.: Angiographic evolution of coronary artery morphology in unstable angina. J. Am. Coll. Cardiol. 7:472, 1986.
473. Wilson, R. F., Holida, M. D., and White, C. W.: Quantitative angiographic morphology of coronary stenoses leading to myocardial infarction or unstable angina. Circulation 73:286, 1986.
474. Sherman, C. T., Litvack, F., Grundfest, W., Lee, M., Hickey, A., Chaux, A., Kass, R., Blanche, C., Matloff, J., Morgenstern, L., Ganz, W., Swan, H. J. C., and Forrester, J.: Coronary angioscopy in patients with unstable angina pectoris. N. Engl. J. Med. 315:913, 1986.
475. Moise, A., Theroux, P., Taeymans, Y., Descoings, B., Lesperance, J., Waters, D. D., Pelletier, G. B., and Bourassa, M. G.: Unstable angina and progression of coronary atherosclerosis. N. Engl. J. Med. 309:685, 1983.
476. Sharma, B., Hodges, M., Asinger, R. W., Goodwin, J. F., and Francis, G. S.: Left ventricular function during spontaneous angina pectoris: Effect of sublingual nitroglycerin. Am. J. Cardiol. 46:34, 1980.
477. Specchia, G., De Servi, S., Falcon, C., Bramucci, E., Angoli, L., Mussini, A., Marioni, G. P., Montemartini, C., and Bobba, P.: Coronary arterial spasm as a cause of exercise-induced ST-segment elevation in patients with variant angina. Circulation 59:948, 1979.
478. Epstein, S. E., and Palmeri, S. T.: Mechanisms contributing to precipitation of unstable angina and acute myocardial infarction: Implications regarding therapy. Am. J. Cardiol. 54:1245, 1984.
479. Aiken, J. W., Gorman, R. R., and Shebuski, R. J.: Prevention of blockage of partially obstructed coronary arteries with prostacyclin correlates with inhibition of platelet aggregation. Prostaglandins 17:483, 1979.
480. Uchida, Y., Yoshimoto, N., and Murao, S.: Cyclic fluctuations in coronary blood pressure and flow induced by coronary artery constriction. Jpn. Heart J. 16:454, 1975.
481. Folts, J. D., Crowell, E. B., and Rowe, G. G.: Platelet aggregation in partially obstructed vessels and its elimination with aspirin. Circulation 54:365, 1976.
482. Bolli, R., Ware, J. A., Brandon, T. A., Weilbaecher, D. G., Mace, M. L., Jr.: Platelet-mediated thrombosis in stenosed canine coronary arteries: Inhibition by nicergoline, a platelet-active alpha-adrenergic antagonist. J. Am. Coll. Cardiol. 3:1417, 1984.
483. Raeder, E. A., Verrier, R. L., and Lown, B.: Influence of the autonomic nervous system on coronary blood flow during partial stenosis. Am. Heart J. 104:249, 1982.
484. Bush, L. R., Campbell, W. B., Kern, K., Tilton, G. D., Apprill, P., Ashton, J., Schmitz, J., Buja, L. J., and Willerson, J. T.: The effects of α-2 adrenergic and serotonergic receptor antagonists in cyclic blood flow alterations in stenosed canine coronary arteries. Circ. Res. 55:642, 1984.
485. Fitzgerald, D. J., Roy, L., Catella, F., and Fitzgerald, G. A.: Platelet activation in unstable coronary disease. N. Engl. J. Med. 315:983, 1986.
486. Folts, J. D., Gallagher, K., and Rowe, G. G.: Blood flow reductions in stenosed canine coronary arteries: Vasospasm or platelet aggregation. Circulation 65:248, 1982.
487. Lewis, H. D., Davis, J. W., Archibald, D. G., Steinke, W. E., Smitherman, T. C., Doherty, J. E., III, Schnaper, H. W., LeWinter, M. M., Linares, E., Pouget, J. M., Sabharwal, S. C., Chesler, E., and DeMots, H.: Protective effects of aspirin against acute myocardial infarction and death in men with unstable angina. N. Engl. J. Med. 309:396, 1983.
488. Cairns, J. A., Gent, M., Singer, J., Finnie, K. J., Froggatt, G. M., Holder, D. A., Jablonsky, G., Kostuk, W. J., Melendez, L. J., Myers, M. G., Sackett, D. L., Sealey, B. J., and Tanser, P. H.: Aspirin, sulfinpyrazone, or both in unstable angina. Results of a Canadian multicenter trial. N. Engl. J. Med. 313:1369, 1985.
489. Davies, M. J., Thomas, A. C., Knapman, P. A., and Hangartner, J. R.: Intramyocardial platelet aggregation in patients with unstable angina suffering sudden ischemic cardiac death. Circulation 73:418, 1986.
490. Mandelkorn, J. B., Wolf, N. M., Singh, S., Shechter, J. A., Kersh, R. I., Rodgers, D. M., Workman, M. B., Bentivoglio, L. G., LaPorte, S. M., and Meister, S. G.: Intracoronary thrombus in nontransmural myocardial infarction and in unstable angina pectoris. Am. J. Cardiol. 52:1, 1983.
491. Falk, E.: Unstable angina with fatal outcome: Dynamic coronary thrombosis leading to infarction and/or sudden death. Circulation 71:699, 1985.
492. Brown, B. G., Bolson, E. L., and Dodge, H. T.: Dynamic mechanisms in human coronary stenosis. Circulation 70:917, 1984.
493. Oliva, P. B., Potts, D. E., and Pluss, R. G.: Coronary arterial spasm in Prinzmetal angina. Documentation by coronary arteriography. N. Engl. J. Med. 288:745, 1973.
494. Ambrose, J. A., Winters, S. L., Arora, R. R., Haft, J. I., Goldstein, J., Rentrop, K. P., Gorlin, R., and Fuster, V.: Coronary angiographic morphology in myocardial infarction: A link between the pathogenesis of unstable angina and myocardial infarction. J. Am. Coll. Cardiol. 6:1233, 1985.
495. Olson, H. G., Lyons, K. P., Aronow, W. S., Stinson, P. J., Kuperus, J., and Waters, H. J.: The high-risk angina patient. Circulation 64:674, 1981.
496. Uthurralt, N., Davies, G. J., Parodi, O., Bencivelli, W., and Maseri, A.: Comparative study of myocardial ischemia during angina at rest and on exertion using thallium-201 scintigraphy. Am. J. Cardiol. 48:410, 1981.
497. Nixon, J. V., Brown, C. N., and Smitherman, T. C.: Identification of transient and persistent segmental wall motion abnormalities in patients with unstable angina by two-dimensional echocardiography. Circulation 65:1497, 1982.
498. Gottlieb, S. O., Weisfeldt, M. L., Ouyang, P., Mellits, E. D., and Gerstenblith, G.: Silent ischemia as a marker for early unfavorable outcomes in patients with unstable angina. N. Engl. J. Med. 314:1214, 1986.
499. Weintraub, R. M., Aroesty, J. M., Paulin, S., Levine, F. H., Markis, J. E., LaRaia, P. J., Cohen, S. I., and Kurland, G. S.: Medically refractory unstable angina pectoris. I. Long-term follow-up of patients undergoing intra-aortic balloon counterpulsation and operation. Am. J. Cardiol. 43:877, 1979.
500. Levine, F. H., Gold, H. K., Leinbach, R. C., Daggett, W. M., Austen, W. G., and Buckley, M. J.: Management of acute myocardial ischemia with intra-aortic balloon pumping and coronary bypass surgery. Circulation 58(Suppl. I):69, 1978.
501. Mohr, R., Smolinsky, A., and Goor, D. A.: Treatment of nocturnal angina with 10 degree Trendelenburg bed position. Lancet 1:1325, 1982.
502. Curfman, G. D., Heinsimer, J. A., Lozner, E. C., and Fung, H.: Intravenous nitroglycerin in the treatment of spontaneous angina pectoris: A prospective, randomized trial. Circulation 67:276, 1983.
503. Kaplan, K., Davison, R., Parker, M., Przybylek, J., Teagarden, J. R., and Lesch, M.: Intravenous nitroglycerin for the treatment of angina at rest unresponsive to standard nitrate therapy. Am. J. Cardiol. 51:694, 1983.
504. Lin, S.-G. and Flaherty, J. T.: Crossover from intravenous to transdermal nitroglycerin therapy in unstable angina pectoris. Am. J. Cardiol. 56:742, 1985.
505. Baaske, D. M., Amann, A. H., Wagenknecht, D. M., Mooers, M., Carter, J. E., Hoyt, H. F., and Stoll, R. G.: Nitroglycerin compatibility with intravenous fluid filters, containers, and administration sets. Am. J. Hosp. Pharm. 37:201, 1980.
506. Figueras, J., Singh, B. N., Ganz, W., Charuzi, Y., and Swan, H. J. C.: Mechanism of rest and nocturnal angina: Observations during continuous hemodynamic and electrocardiographic monitoring. Circulation 59:955, 1979.
507. Kern, M. J., Petru, M. A., Ferry, D. R., Eilen, S. P., Barr, W. K., Porter, C. B., and O'Rourke, R. A.: Regional coronary vasoconstriction after combined beta-adrenergic and calcium channel blockade in patients with coronary artery disease. J. Am. Coll. Cardiol. 5:1438, 1985.
508. Tilmant, P. Y., Lablanche, J. M., Thieuleux, F. A., Depuis, B. A., and Bertrand, M. E.: Detrimental effect of propranolol in patients with coronary arterial spasm countered by combination with diltiazem. Am. J. Cardiol. 52:230, 1983.
509. Muller, J. E., Turi, Z. G., Pearle, D. L., Schneider, J. F., Serfas, D. H., Morrison, J., Stone, P. J., Rude, R. E., Rosner, B., Sobel, B. E., Tate, C., Scheiner, E., Roberts, R., Hennekens, C. H., and Braunwald, E.: Nifedipine and conventional therapy for unstable angina pectoris: A randomized, double-blind comparison. Circulation 69:728, 1984.
510. Gottlieb, S. O., Weisfeldt, M. L., Ouyang, P., Achuff, S. C., Baughman, K. L., Traill, T. A., Brinker, J. A., Shapiro, E. P., Chandra, N. C., Mellits, E. D., Townsend, S. N., and Gerstenblith, G.: Effect of the addition of propranolol therapy with nifedipine for unstable angina pectoris: A randomized, double-blind, placebo-controlled trial. Circulation 73:331, 1986.
511. Theroux, P., Taeymans, Y., Morissette, D., Bosch, X., Pelletier, G. B., and Waters, D. D.: A randomized study comparing propranolol and diltiazem in the treatment of unstable angina. J. Am. Coll. Cardiol. 5:717, 1985.
512. Parodi, O., Simonetti, I., Michelassi, C., Carpeggiani, C., Biagini, A., L'Abbate, A., and Maseri, A.: Comparison of verapamil and propranolol therapy for angina pectoris at rest: A randomized, multiple-crossover, controlled trial in the coronary care unit. Am. J. Cardiol. 57:899, 1986.
512a. Holland Interuniversity Nifedipine/Metoprolol Trial (HINT) Research Group: Early treatment of unstable angina in the coronary care unit: A randomised, double-blind, placebo-controlled comparison of recurrent ischaemia in patients treated with nifedipine or metoprolol or both. Br. Heart J. 56:400, 1986.
513. Mehta, J., Pepine, C. J., Day, M., Guerrero, J. R., and Conti, C. R.: Short-term efficacy of oral verapamil in rest angina. A double-blind placebo-controlled trial in CCU patients. Am. J. Med. 71:977, 1981.
514. Gerstenblith, G., Ouyang, P., Achuff, S. C., Bulkley, B. H., Becker, L. C., Mellits, E. D., Baughman, K. L., Weiss, J. L., Flaherty, J. T., Kallman, C. H., Llewellyn, M., and Weisfeldt, M. L.: Nifedipine in unstable angina: A double-blind, randomized trial. N. Engl. J. Med. 306:885, 1982.
515. Wood, P.: Acute and subacute coronary insufficiency. Br. Med. J. 1:1779, 1961.
516. Telford, A. M., and Wilson, C.: Trial of heparin versus atenolol in prevention of myocardial infarction in intermediate coronary syndrome. Lancet 1:1225, 1981.
517. Williams, D. O., Kirby, M. G., McPherson, K., and Phear, D. N.: Anticoagulant treatment in unstable angina. Br. J. Clin. Pract. 40:114, 1986.
518. Williams, D. O., Riley, R. S., Singh, A. K., Gewirtz, H., and Most, A. S.: Evaluation of the role of coronary angioplasty in patients with unstable angina pectoris. Am. Heart J. 102:1, 1981.
519. Meyer, J., Schmidt, H., Erbel, R., Kiesslich, T., Bocker-Josephs, B., Krebs, W., Braun, P. C., Bardos, P., Minale, C., Messmer, B. J., and Effert, S.: Treatment of unstable angina pectoris with percutaneous transluminal coronary angioplasty (PTCA). Cathet. Cardiovasc. Diagn. 7:361, 1981.
520. Meyer, J., Schmitz, H.-J., Kiesslich, T., Erbel, R., Krebs, W., Schulz, W., Bardos, P., Minale, C., Messmer, B. J., and Effert, S.: Percutaneous transluminal coronary angioplasty in patients with stable and unstable angina pectoris: Analysis of early and late results. Am. Heart J. 106:973, 1983.
521. Faxon, D. P., Detre, K. M., McCabe, C. H., Fisher, L., Holmes, D. R., Cowley, M. J., Bourassa, M. G., Van Raden, M., and Ryan, T. J.: Role of percutaneous transluminal coronary angioplasty in the treatment of unstable angina. Am. J. Cardiol. 53:131C, 1983.
522. Quigley, P. J., Erwin, J., Maurer, B. J., Walsh, M. J., and Gearty, G. F.: Percutaneous transluminal coronary angioplasty in unstable angina: Comparison with stable angina. Br. Heart J. 55:227, 1986.
523. de Feyter, P. J., Serruys, P. W., van den Brand, M., Balakumaran, K., Mochtar, B., Soward, A. L., Arnold, A. E. R., and Hugenholtz, P. G.: Emergency coronary angioplasty in refractory unstable angina. N. Engl. J. Med. 313:342, 1985.

524. DeFeyter, P. J., Serruys, P. W., Arnold, A., Simoons, M. L., Wijns, W., Geuskens, R., Soward, A., van den Brand, M., and Hugenholtz, P. G.: Coronary angioplasty of the unstable angina-related vessel in patients with multivessel disease. Eur. Heart J. 7:460, 1986.
525. Rahimtoola, S. H., Nunley, D., Grunkemeier, G., Tepley, J., Lambert, L., and Starr, A.: Ten-year survival after coronary bypass surgery for unstable angina. N. Engl. J. Med. *308*:676, 1983.
525a. Luchi, R. J., Scott, S. M., Deupree, R. H., and the principal investigators and their associates of Veterans Administration Cooperative Study No. 28: Comparison of medical and surgical treatment for unstable angina pectoris. N. Engl. J. Med. *316*:977, 1987.
526. McCormick, J. R., Schick, E. C., Jr., McCabe, C. H., Kronmal, R. A., and Ryan, T. J.: Determinants of operative mortality and long-term survival in patients with unstable angina. The CASS experience. J. Thorac. Cardiovasc. Surg. *89*:683, 1985.
526a. Swahn, E., Areskog, M., Berglund, U., Walfridsson, H., and Wallentin, L.: Predictive importance of clinical findings and a predischarge exercise test in patients with suspected unstable coronary artery disease. Am. J. Cardiol. *59*:208, 1987.
527. Solomon, H. A., Edwards, A. L., and Killip, T.: Prodromata in acute myocardial infarction. Circulation *40*:463, 1969.
528. Roberts, K. B., Califf, R. M., Harrell, F. E., Jr., Lee, K. L., Pryor, D. B., and Rosati, R. A.: The prognosis for patients with new-onset angina who have undergone cardiac catheterization. Circulation *68*:970–978, 1983.
529. Gazes, P. C., Mobley, E. M., Jr., Faris, H. M., Jr., Duncan, R. C., and Humphries, G. B.: Preinfarction (stable) angina—a prospective study: Ten-year follow-up. Prognostic significance of electrocardiographic changes. Circulation *48*:331, 1973.
530. Mulcahy, R., Awadhi, A. H. A., deBuitleor, M., Tobin, G., Johnson, H., and Contoy, R.: Natural history and prognosis of unstable angina. Am. Heart J. *109*:753, 1985.

VARIANT ANGINA PECTORIS (PRINZMETAL'S ANGINA)

531. Prinzmetal, M., Kennamer, R., Merliss, R., Wada, T., and Bor, N.: A variant form of angina pectoris. Am. J. Med. *27*:375, 1959.
532. Conti, C. R.: Coronary Artery Spasm: Pathophysiology, Diagnosis, and Treatment. New York, Marcel Dekker, 1986, p. 1.
533. Ganz, P., and Alexander, R. W.: New insights into the cellular mechanisms of vasospasm. Am. J. Cardiol. *56*:11E, 1985.
534. Ludmer, P. L., Selwyn, A. P., Shook, T. L., Wayne, R. R., Mudge, G. H., Jr., Alexander, R. W., and Ganz, P.: Paradoxical vasoconstriction induced by acetylcholine in atherosclerotic coronary arteries. N. Engl. J. Med. *315*:1046, 1986.
535. Yui, Y., Hattori, R., Takatsu, Y., and Kawai, C.: Selective thromboxane A_2 synthetase inhibition in vasospastic angina pectoris. J. Am. Coll. Cardiol. 7:25, 1986.
536. Chierchia, S., de Caterina, R., Crea, F., Patrono, C., and Maseri, A.: Failure of thromboxane A_2 blockade to prevent attacks of vasospastic angina. Circulation *66*:702, 1982.
537. Forman, M. B., Oates, J. A., Robertson, D., Robertson, R. M., Roberts, L. J., and Virmani, R.: Increased adventitial mast cells in a patient with coronary spasm. N. Engl. J. Med. *313*:1138, 1985.
538. Topol, E. J., and Fortuin, N. J.: Coronary artery spasm and cardiac arrest in carcinoid heart disease. Am. J. Med. 77:950, 1984.
539. Stein, J. H., Ambrose, J. A., King, B. D., and Herman, M. V.: An integrated approach to the recognition and treatment of variant angina. Cardiovasc. Rev. Rep. *3*:1297, 1982.
540. Yasue, H., Omote, S., Takizawa, A., Nagao, M., Miwa, K., and Tanaka, S.: Cardiac variations of exercise-induced coronary arterial spasm. Circulation *59*:938, 1979.
541. Waters, D. D., Miller, D., Bouchard, A., Bosch, X., and Theroux, P.: Circadian variation in variant angina. Am. J. Cardiol. *54*:61, 1984.
542. Bott-Silverman, C., Heupler, F. A., and Yiannikas, J.: Variant angina: Comparison of patients with and without fixed severe coronary artery disease. Am. J. Cardiol. *54*:1173, 1984.
543. Scholl, J.-M., Benacerraf, A., Ducimetiere, P., Chabas, D., Brau, J., Chappelle, J., and Thery, J. L.: Comparison of risk factors in vasospastic angina without significant fixed coronary narrowing to significant fixed coronary narrowing and no vasospastic angina. Am. J. Cardiol. *57*:199, 1986.
544. Waters, D. D., Theroux, P., Crittin, J., Dauwe, F., and Mizgala, H. F.: Previously undiagnosed variant angina as a cause of chest pain after coronary artery bypass surgery. Circulation *61*:1159, 1980.
545. Miller, D., Waters, D. D., Warnica, W., Szlachcic, J., Kreeft, J., and Theroux, P.: Is variant angina the coronary manifestation of a generalized vasospastic disorder? N. Engl. J. Med. *304*:763, 1981.
546. Antman, E., Muller, J., Goldberg, S., MacAlpin, R., Rubenfire, M., Tabatznik, B., Liang, C., Heupler, F., Achuff, S., Reichek, N., Geltman, E., Kerin, N. Z., Neff, R. K., and Braunwald, E.: Nifedipine therapy for coronary-artery spasm. Experience in 127 patients. N. Engl. J. Med. *302*:12, 1980.
547. Bashour, T. T., Hakim, O., and Cheng, T. O.: Coronary spastic angina in middle-aged women: A psychosomatic disorder? Am. Heart J. *106*:609, 1983.
548. Gabliani, G. I., Winniford, M. D., Fulton, K. L., Johnson, S. M., Mauritson, D. R., and Hillis, L. D.: Ventricular ectopic activity with spontaneous variant angina: Frequency and relation to transient ST-segment deviation. Am. Heart J. *110*:40, 1985.
549. Sheehan, F. H., and Epstein, S. E.: Determinants of arrhythmic death due to coronary spasm: Effect of preexisting coronary artery stenosis on the incidence of reperfusion arrhythmia. Circulation *65*:259, 1982.
550. Biagini, A., Mazzei, M. G., Carpeggiani, C., Buzzigoli, G., Zucchelli, G., Parodi, O., L'Abbate, A., and Maseri, A.: Myocardial cell damage during attacks of vasospastic angina in the absence of persistent electrocardiographic changes. Clin. Cardiol. *4*:315, 1981.
551. Meller, J., Conde, C. A., Donoso, E., and Dack, S.: Transient Q waves in Prinzmetal's angina. Am. J. Cardiol. *35*:691, 1975.
552. Guazzi, M., Polese, A., Fiorentini, C., Magrini, F., and Bartorelli, C.: Left ventricular performance and related hemodynamic changes in Prinzmetal's variant angina pectoris. Br. Heart J. *33*:84, 1971.
553. Gaasch, W. H., Adyantha, A. V., Wang, V. H., Pickering, E., Quinons, M. A., and Alexander, J. K.: Prinzmetal's variant angina: Hemodynamic and angiographic observations during pain. Am. J. Cardiol. *35*:683, 1977.
554. Matsuda, Y., Ozaki, M., Ogawa, H., Naito, H., Yoshino, F., Katayama, F., Fujii, T., Matsuazaki, M., and Kusukawa, R.: Coronary arteriography and left ventriculography during spontaneous and exercise-induced ST-segment elevation in patients with variant angina. Am. Heart J. *106*:509, 1983.
555. Crea, F., Davies, G., Romeo, F., Chierchia, S., Bugiardini, R., Kaski, J. C., Freedman, B., and Maseri, A.: Myocardial ischemia during ergonovine testing: Different susceptibility to coronary vasoconstriction in patients with exertional and variant angina. Circulation *69*:690, 1984.
556. Selzer, A., Langston, M., Ruggeroli, C., and Cohn, K.: Clinical syndrome of variant angina with normal coronary arteriogram. N. Engl. J. Med. *295*:1343, 1976.
557. Cipriano, P. R., Koch, F. H., Rosenthal, S. J., and Schroeder, J. S.: Clinical course of patients following the demonstration of coronary artery spasm by angiography. Am. Heart J. *101*:127, 1981.
558. Winniford, M. D., Johnson, S. M., Mauritson, D. R., and Hillis, L. D.: Ergonovine provocation to assess efficacy of long-term therapy with calcium antagonists in Prinzmetal's variant angina. Am. J. Cardiol. *51*:684, 1983.
559. Waters, D. D., Szlachcic, J., Theroux, P., Dauwe, F., and Mizgala, H. F.: Ergonovine testing to detect spontaneous remissions of variant angina during long-term treatment with calcium antagonist drugs. Am. J. Cardiol. *47*:179, 1981.
560. Waters, D. D., Theroux, P., Szlachcic, J., Dauwe, F., Crittin, J., Bonan, R., and Mizgala, H. F.: Ergonovine testing in a coronary care unit. Am. J. Cardiol. *46*:922, 1980.
561. Heupler, F. A., Jr.: Provocative testing for coronary arterial spasm: Risk, method, and rationale. Am. J. Cardiol. *46*:335, 1980.
562. Yasue, H., Touyama, M., Shimamoto, M., Kato, H., Tanaka, S., and Akiyama, F.: Role of autonomic nervous system in the pathogenesis of Prinzmetal's variant angina. Circulation *50*:534, 1974.
562a. Crea, F., Chierchia, S., Kaski, J. C., Davies, G. J., Margonato, A., Miran, D. O., and Maseri, A.: Provocation of coronary spasm by dopamine in patients with active variant angina pectoris. Circulation *74*:262, 1986.
563. Ginsburg, R., Bristow, M. R., Kantrowitz, N., Baim, D. S., and Harrison, D. C.: Histamine provocation of clinical coronary artery spasm: Implications concerning pathogenesis of variant angina pectoris. Am. Heart J. *102*:819, 1981.
564. Waters, D. D., Szlachcic, J., Bonan, R., Miller, D. D., Dauwe, F., and Theroux, P.: Comparative sensitivity of exercise, cold pressor and ergonovine testing in provoking attacks of variant angina in patients with active disease. Circulation *67*:310, 1983.
565. Maseri, A., Parodi, O., Severi, S., and Pesola, A.: Transient transmural reduction of myocardial blood flow, demonstrated by thallium-201 scintigraphy, as a cause of variant angina. Circulation *54*:280, 1976.
566. McLaughlin, P. R., Doherty, P. W., Martin, P. R., Goris, M. L., and Harrison, D. L: Myocardial imaging in a patient with reproducible variant angina. Am. J. Cardiol. *39*:129, 1977.
567. Ricci, D. R., Orlick, A. E., Doherty, P. W., Cipriano, P. R., and Harrison, D. R.: Reduction of coronary blood flow during coronary artery spasm occurring spontaneously and after provocation by ergonovine maleate. Circulation *57*:392, 1978.
568. Ginsburg, R., Lamb, I. H., Schroeder J. S., Hu, M., and Harrison, D. C.: Randomized double-blind comparison of nifedipine and isosorbide dinitrate therapy in variant angina pectoris due to coronary artery spasm. Am. Heart J. *103*:44, 1982.
569. Robertson, R. M., Wood, A. J. J., Vaughn, W. K., and Robertson, D.: Exacerbation of vasotonic angina pectoris by propranolol. Circulation *65*:281, 1982.
570. Schroeder, J. S., Lamb, I. H., Bristow, M. R., Ginsburg, R., Hung, J., and McAuley, B. J.: Prevention of cardiovascular events in variant angina by long-term diltiazem therapy. J. Am. Coll. Cardiol. *1*:1507, 1983.
571. Kimura, E., and Kishida, H.: Treatment of variant angina with drugs: A survey of 11 cardiology institutes in Japan. Circulation *63*:844, 1981.
571a. Prida, Z. E., Gelman, J. S., Feldman, R. L., Hill, J. A., Pepine, C. J., and Scott, E.: Comparison of diltiazem and nifedipine alone and in combination in patients with coronary artery spasm. J. Am. Coll. Cardiol. *9*:412, 1987.
572. Schroeder, J. S., Walker, S. D., Skalland, L., and Hemberger, J. A.: Absence of rebound from diltiazem therapy in Prinzmetal's variant angina. J. Am. Coll. Cardiol. *6*:174, 1985.
573. Tzivoni, D., Keren, A., Benhorin, J., Gottlieb, S., Atlas, D., and Stern, S.: Prazosin therapy for refractory variant angina. Am. Heart J. *105*:262, 1983.
574. Miwa, K., Kambara, H., and Kawai, C.: Effect of aspirin in large doses on attacks of variant angina. Am. Heart J. *105*:351, 1983.
575. Corcos, T., David, P. R., Bourassa, M. G., Guiteras Val., P., Robert, J., Mata, L. A., and Waters, D. D.: Percutaneous transluminal coronary angioplasty for the treatment of variant angina. J. Am. Coll. Cardiol. *5*:1046, 1985.
576. Waters, D. D., Szlachcic, J., Miller, D., and Theroux, P.: Clinical characteristics of patients with variant angina complicated by myocardial infarction or death within 1 month. Am. J. Cardiol. *49*:658, 1982.

577. Severi, S., Davies, G., Maseri, A., Marzullo, P., and L'Abbate, A.: Long-term prognosis of "variant" angina with medical treatment. Am. J. Cardiol. *46*:226, 1980.
578. Waters, D. D., Miller, D., Szlachcic, J., Bouchard, A., Methe, M., Kreeft, J., and Theroux, P.: Factors influencing the long-term prognosis of treated patients with variant angina. Circulation *68*:258, 1983.
579. Mark, D. B., Califf, R. M., Morris, K. G., Harrell, F. E., Jr., Pryor, D. B., Hlatky, M. A., Lee, K. L., and Rosati, R. A.: Clinical characteristics and long-term survival of patients with variant angina. Circulation *69*:880, 1984.
580. Mark, D. B., and Califf, R. M.: Variant angina: Prognosis and therapy. Primary Cardiol. pp. 25, June, 1986.
581. Miller, D. D., Waters, D. D., Szlachcic, J., and Theroux, P.: Clinical characteristics associated with sudden death in patients with variant angina. Circulation *66*:588, 1982.
581a. Previtali, M., Panciroli, C., Ardissino, D., Chimienti, M., Angoli, L., and Salerno, J. A.: Spontaneous remission of variant angina documented by Holter monitoring and ergonovine testing in patients treated with calcium antagonists. Am. J. Cardiol. *59*:235, 1987.

ISCHEMIC HEART DISEASE IN WHICH DISCOMFORT IS NOT THE DOMINANT SYMPTOM

581b. Cohn, P. F., and Kannel, W. B.: Recognition, pathogenesis, and management options in silent coronary artery disease. Circulation *75*(Suppl. II):54 pp, 1987.
581c. Cohn, P. F.: The concept and pathogenesis of active but asymptomatic coronary artery disease. Circulation 75(Suppl II):2, 1987.
582. Hirzel, H. O., Leutwyler, R., and Krayenbuehl, H. P.: Silent myocardial ischemia: Hemodynamic changes during dynamic exercise in patients with proven coronary artery disease despite absence of angina pectoris. J. Am. Coll. Cardiol. *6*:275, 1985.
583. Chierchia, S., Smith, G., Morgan, M., Gallino, A., Deanfield, J., Croom, M., and Maseri, A.: Role of heart rate in pathophysiology of chronic stable angina. Lancet 2:1353, 1984.
584. Deanfield, J. E., Ribiero, P., Oakley, K., Krikler, S., and Selwyn, A. P.: Analysis of ST-segment changes in normal subjects: Implications for ambulatory monitoring in angina pectoris. Am. J. Cardiol. *54*:1321, 1984.
585. Schang, S. J., Jr., and Pepine, C. J.: Transient asymptomatic S-T depression during daily activity. Am. J. Cardiol. *39*:396, 1977.
586. Selwyn, A. P., Fox, K., Eves, M., Oakley, D., Dargie, H., and Shillingford, J.: Myocardial ischaemia in patients with frequent angina pectoris. Br. Med. J. 2:1594, 1978.
586a. Gibson, R. S., Beller, G. A., and Kaiser, D. L.: Prevalence and clinical significance of painless ST segment depression during early postinfarction exercise testing. Circulation 75(Suppl. II):36, 1987.
586b. Singh, B. N., Nademanee, K.: Prevalence and prognostic significance of silent myocardial ischemia in patients with unstable angina. Circulation 75(Suppl II):40, 1987.
587. Quyyumi, A. A., Mockus, L., Wright, C., and Fox, K. M.: Morphology of ambulatory ST-segment changes in patients with varying severity of coronary artery disease. Investigation of the frequency of nocturnal ischaemia and coronary spasm. Br. Heart J. *53*:186, 1985.
588. Droste, C., and Roskamm, H.: Experimental pain measurement in patients with asymptomatic myocardial ischemia. J. Am. Coll. Cardiol. *1*:940, 1983.
589. Chiariello, M., Indolfi, C., Cotecchia, M. R., Sifola, C., Romano, M., and Condorelli, M.: Asymptomatic transient ST changes during ambulatory ECG monitoring in diabetic patients. Am. Heart J. *110*:529, 1985.
590. Deanfield, J. E., Shea, M. J., Wilson, R. A., Horlock, P., de Landsheere, C. M., and Selwyn, A. P.: Direct effects of smoking on the heart: Silent ischemic disturbances of coronary flow. Am. J. Cardiol. *57*:1005, 1986.
590a. Stone, P. H.: Calcium antagonists for Prinzmetal's variant angina, unstable angina and silent myocardial ischemia: Therapeutic tool and probe for identification of pathophysiologic mechanisms. Am. J. Cardiol. 59:101B, 1987.
591. Epstein, S. E., Kent, K. M., Goldstein, R. E., Borer, J. S., and Rosing, D. R.: Strategy for evaluation and surgical treatment of the asymptomatic or mildly symptomatic patient with coronary artery disease. Am. J. Cardiol. *43*:1015, 1979.
592. Froelicher, V. F., Yanowitz, F. G., Thompson, A. J., and Lancaster, M. C.: The correlation of coronary angiography and the electrocardiographic response to maximal treadmill testing in 76 asymptomatic men. Circulation *48*:597, 1973.
593. Borer, J. S., Brensike, J. D., Redwood, D. R., Itscoitz, S. B., Passamanin, E. R., Stone, N. J., Richardson, J. M., Levy, R. I., and Epstein, S. E.: Limitations of electrocardiographic response to exercise in predicting coronary artery disease. N. Engl. J. Med. *293*:367, 1975.
593a. Weiner, D. A.: The diagnostic and prognostic significance of an asymptomatic positive exercise test. Circulation 75(Suppl. II):20, 1987.
594. Erikssen, J., Enge, I., Forfang, K., and Storstein, O.: False-positive diagnostic tests and coronary angiographic findings in 105 presumably healthy males. Circulation *54*:371, 1976.
595. Parmley, W. W., Chuck, L., Kivowitz, C., Matloff, J. M., and Swan, H. J. C.: In vitro length-tension relations of human ventricular aneurysms. Relation of stiffness to mechanical disadvantage. Am. J. Cardiol. *32*:889, 1973.
596. Erikson, U., Hallen, A., Helmius, G., and Sawada, S.: On the pathophysiology of left ventricular aneurysm. An analysis by cineangiography and videodensitometry. Fortschr. Röntgenstr. *137*:85, 1982.
596a. Forman, M. B., Collins, H. W., Kopelman, H. A., Vaughn, W. K., Perry, J. M., Virmani, R., and Friesinger, G. C.: Determinants of left ventricular aneurysm formation after anterior myocardial infarction: A clinical and angiographic study. J. Am. Coll. Cardiol. 8:1256, 1986.
597. Kirklin, J. W., Barratt-Boyes, B. G.: Left ventricular aneurysmectomy *In* Cardiac Surgery. New York, John Wiley and Sons, Inc., 1986, p. 279.
598. Barratt-Boyes, B. G., White, H. D., Agnew, T. M., Pemberton, J. R., and Wild, C. J.: The results of surgical treatment of left ventricular aneurysms: An assessment of the risk factors affecting early and late mortality. J. Thorac. Cardiovasc. Surg. *87*:87, 1984.
599. Cabin, H. S., and Roberts, W. C.: Left ventricular aneurysm, intra-aneurysmal thrombus and systemic embolus in coronary heart disease. Chest 77:586, 1980.
600. Ezekowitz, M. D., Wilson, D. A., Smith, E. O., Burow, R. D., Harrison, L. H., Parker, D. E., Elkins, R. C., Peyton, M., and Taylor, F. B.: Comparison of indium-111 platelet scintigraphy and two-dimensional echocardiography in the diagnosis of left ventricular thrombi. N. Engl. J. Med. *306*:1409, 1982.
601. Meltzer, R. S., Visser, C. A., and Fuster, V.: Intracardiac thrombi and systemic embolization. Ann. Intern. Med. *104*:689, 1986.
602. Visser, C. A., Kan, G., Meltzer, R. S., Moulijn, A. C., David, G. D., and Dunning, A. J.: Assessment of left ventricular aneurysm resectability by two-dimensional echocardiography. Am. J. Cardiol. *56*:857, 1985.
603. Ryan, T., Petrovic, O., Armstrong, W. F., Dillon, J. C., and Feigenbaum, H.: Quantitative two-dimensional echocardiographic assessment of patients undergoing left ventricular aneurysmectomy. Am. Heart J. *111*:714, 1986.
604. Foster, C. J., Sekiya, T., Brownlee, W. C., Griffin, J. F., and Isherwood, I.: Computed tomographic assessment of left ventricular aneurysms. Br. Heart J. *52*:332, 1984.
605. Yiannikas, J., MacIntyre, W. J., Underwood, D. A., Takatani, S., Cook, S. A., Go, R. T., and Loop, F. D.: Prediction of improvement of left ventricular function after ventricular aneurysmectomy using Fourier phase and amplitude analysis of radionuclide cardiac blood pool scans. Am. J. Cardiol. *55*:1308, 1985.
606. Ormerod, O. J., Barber, R. W., Stone, D. L., Taylor, N. C., Wraight, E. P., and Petch, M. C.: Improved selection of patients for aneurysmectomy by combined phase and amplitude analysis of gated cardiac scintigraphy. Eur. Heart J. *6*:921, 1985.
607. Mullen, D. C., Posey, L., Gabriel, R., Singh, H. M., Flemma, R. J., and Lepley, D., Jr.: Prognostic considerations in the management of left ventricular aneurysms. Ann. Thorac. Surg. *23*:455, 1977.
608. Olearchyk, A. S., Lemole, G. M., and Spagna, P. M.: Left ventricular aneurysm. Ten years' experience in surgical treatment of 244 cases. Improved clinical status, hemodynamics, and long-term longevity. J. Thorac. Cardiovasc. Surg. *88*:544, 1984.
609. Keenan, D. J., Monro, J. L., Ross, J. K., Manners, J. M., Conway, N., and Johnson, A. M.: Left ventricular aneurysm. The Wessex experience. Br. Heart J. *54*:269, 1985.
610. Yabe, Y., Yamashita, T., Komatsu, H., Koyama, N., Ito, N., and Kamegai, T.: Study of left ventricular function and myocardial viability in patients with left ventricular aneurysm developed after myocardial infarction. A comparative study of medical and surgical therapy. Jpn. Heart J. *26*:53, 1985.
611. Burch, G. E., Giles, T. D., and Colcolough, H. L.: Ischemic cardiomyopathy. Am. Heart J. *79*:291, 1970.
612. Kolibash, A. J., Goodenow, J. S., Bush, C. A., Tetalman, M. R., and Lewis, R. P.: Improvement of myocardial perfusion and left ventricular function after coronary artery bypass grafting patients with unstable angina. Circulation *59*:66, 1979.
613. Bateman, T. M., Czer, L. S. C., Gray, R. J., Maddahi, J., Raymond, M. J., Geft, I. L., Ganz, W., Shah, P. K., and Berman, D. S.: Transient pathologic Q waves during acute ischemic events: An electrocardiographic correlate of stunned but viable myocardium. Am. Heart J. *106*:1421, 1983.
614. Manley, J. C., King, J. F., and Zeft, H. F.: The "bad" left ventricle. Results of coronary surgery and effect on late survival. J. Thorac. Cardiovasc. Surg. *72*:841, 1976.
615. Shearn, D. L., and Brent, B. N.: Coronary artery bypass surgery in patients with left ventricular dysfunction. Am. J. Med. *80*:405, 1986.
616. Yatteau, R. F., Peter, R. H., Behar, V. S., Bartel, A. G., Rosati, R. A., and Kong, Y.: Ischemic cardiomyopathy: The myopathy of coronary artery disease. Natural history and results of medical versus surgical treatment. Am. J. Cardiol. *34*:520, 1974.
617. Calvert, A., Lown, B., and Gorlin, R.: Ventricular premature beats and anatomically defined coronary heart disease. Am. J. Cardiol. *39*:4, 1977.
618. Oakley, C. M.: Nonatheromatous ischemic heart disease. Postgrad. Med. J. *52*:438, 1976.
619. Lange, R. L., Reid, M. S., Tresch, D. D., Keelan, M. H., Bernhard, J. M., and Coolidge, G.: Nonatheromatous ischemic heart disease following withdrawal from chronic industrial nitroglycerin exposure. Circulation *46*:666, 1972.

40 INTERVENTIONAL CATHETERIZATION TECHNIQUES: Percutaneous Transluminal Balloon Angioplasty, Valvuloplasty, and Related Procedures

by DONALD S. BAIM, M.D.

From 1950 through the late 1970's essentially all cardiac catheterizations were performed to evaluate individual disease states, to guide medical therapy, or to provide a plan for cardiac surgical techniques (see Chaps. 9 and 10). Beginning in the 1980's, however, cardiac catheterization has begun to play an increasingly important role in *treating* as well as *diagnosing* cardiovascular lesions. This new application of catheterization-based treatment has become known as "interventional" cardiology and may involve delivery of mechanical, thermal, microsurgical, or light energy to cardiovascular lesions by means of specialized percutaneously inserted catheters. The end result may be to open stenotic blood vessels or cardiac valves, or to close undesired channels for blood flow, in an effort to achieve a physiological correction of the underlying cardiac pathology comparable to that obtained by traditional surgical techniques. If such a correction is possible, it may be obtained frequently at a fraction of the expense, disability, and discomfort of surgery. The explosive growth of this area has already had a major impact on health care delivery and is likely to increase as these interventional techniques continue to mature. The delivery of electric currents to the heart and specialized conduction tissue through catheters for therapeutic purposes is another application of interventional catheterization and is described on pages 644 and 645.

TREATMENT OF VASCULAR STENOSIS

The development of vascular angiography made it possible to visualize atherosclerotic and fibromuscular stenoses in various arterial beds. In the course of such angiographic procedures, Dotter and Judkins noted that it was frequently possible to pass first a guidewire and then a catheter or rigid dilator through an area of stenosis in the iliac-femoral system, thereby enlarging the lumen and improving antegrade blood blow (Fig. 40–1).[1–3] While the so-called *Dotter technique* was used to some extent in Europe between 1964 and 1974,[4] its application was limited by the trauma to the artery which resulted from exertion of axial force on the stenosis, and the local complications which were related to the percutaneous introduction of the large-caliber rigid dilators. In 1974 Gruentzig and Kumpe modified the technique by substituting a balloon-tipped catheter for the rigid dilator.[5] This nonelastomeric balloon catheter could be introduced and passed across the stenosis in its smaller collapsed state and then inflated to a predetermined size with liquid contrast material in order to achieve the desired enlargement in luminal caliber (Fig. 40–2). The so-called *Gruentzig technique* was applied first to peripheral[5] and then to renal arterial stenoses.[6] In 1977, after cadaver and intraoperative studies during bypass surgery, percutaneous balloon angioplasty was extended

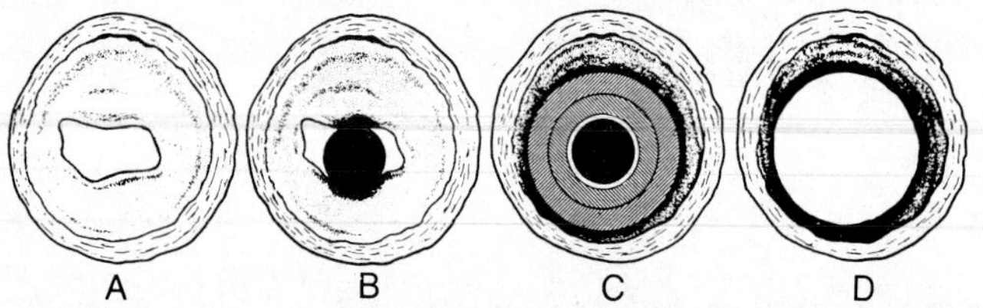

FIGURE 40–1. The Dotter technique. Cross sections of a stenotic arterial lumen are shown at baseline, during the passage of the initial catheter, during the passage of the coaxial dilators, and after the procedure. Note the improvement in lumenal diameter without enlargement of the outer vessel caliber, suggesting compaction of the atheroma as the mechanism of dilatation. (From Dotter, C. T., Rosch, J., and Judkins, M. P.: Transluminal dilatation of atherosclerotic stenosis. Surg. Gynecol. Obstet. *127*:794, 1968.)

to stenoses of the epicardial coronary arteries.[7] Balloon anioplasty—albeit with some technical refinements—still constitutes the core of interventional cardiology and has provided major encouragement for the subsequent development of a variety of other interventional techniques for application in the heart and extracardiac vasculature.

PERCUTANEOUS TRANSLUMINAL CORONARY ANGIOPLASTY (PTCA)

EARLY EXPERIENCE. Between 1977 and 1980 coronary angioplasty used the original Gruentzig catheter,[7] a two-lumen device in which one lumen was used to inflate and deflate the polyvinylchloride (PVC) balloon, while the second lumen was used to monitor pressure or inject radiographic contrast through a port near the catheter tip. A short segment of flexible guidewire was attached to the tip of the dilatation catheter. Although this guidewire reduced the chance of intimal dissection and subintimal passage, it could not be reshaped or manipulated once introduced into the patient, sharply limiting the ability to advance the dilatation catheter beyond all but the most proximal coronary stenoses. Moreover, the large diameter of these early balloon catheters in their deflated state (0.060 inch, or 1.5 mm) made it difficult to cross severe or inelastic stenoses, since the diameter of the deflated balloon was frequently larger than that of the stenotic lumen (i.e., 0.6 mm for an 80 per cent stenosis of a typical 3-mm diameter coronary artery). To deal with this problem, the dilatation catheter had to be advanced through a large (No. 8 or 9 French, 2.7 or 3.0 mm outer diameter), stiff "guiding catheter" positioned in the coronary ostium. The third limitation of the original Gruentzig catheter was its comparatively low balloon rupture pressure (6 atm, or 90 psi), which made it difficult to dilate rigid lesions adequately. In an effort to mitigate these problems, early angioplasty operators attempted to select patients considered to have "soft" rather than rigid lesions (as reflected by recent onset of anginal symptoms and absence of calcification of the lesion on fluoroscopy), and particularly those patients whose lesions were located in the proximal coronary segments.

To define better the results, complications, and long-term efficacy of this new technique, the National Heart, Lung, and Blood Institute (NHLBI) established a PTCA Registry in 1979.[8, 9] Candidates for PTCA were selected to have severe enough angina to warrant consideration of bypass surgery, objective evidence of myocardial ischemia, and coronary anatomy (proximal, subtotal, discrete, concentric, noncalcified stenosis of a single coronary artery) thought to be approachable with the limited equipment then available. Although such patients were believed to represent fewer than 5 to 10 per cent of the symptomatic coronary artery disease population, more than 3000 patients underwent PTCA before the Registry was closed in late 1981. Despite the careful selection of ideal candidates, the primary success rate of PTCA in the Registry was less than 60 per cent, with failure to cross the stenosis with the dilatation system in 29 per cent and failure to dilate the stenosis in 12 per cent of patients attempted. Two other important problems were identified: (1) approximately 6 per cent of patients required emergency bypass to correct acute, severe myocardial ischemia which resulted from abrupt reclosure of the dilated artery, and (2) between 20 and 30 per cent of patients with an initially successful procedure experienced return of angina owing to angiographically evident renarrowing ("restenosis") of the dilated segment within 6 months after the procedure.

TECHNICAL IMPROVEMENTS. Shortly after the NHLBI

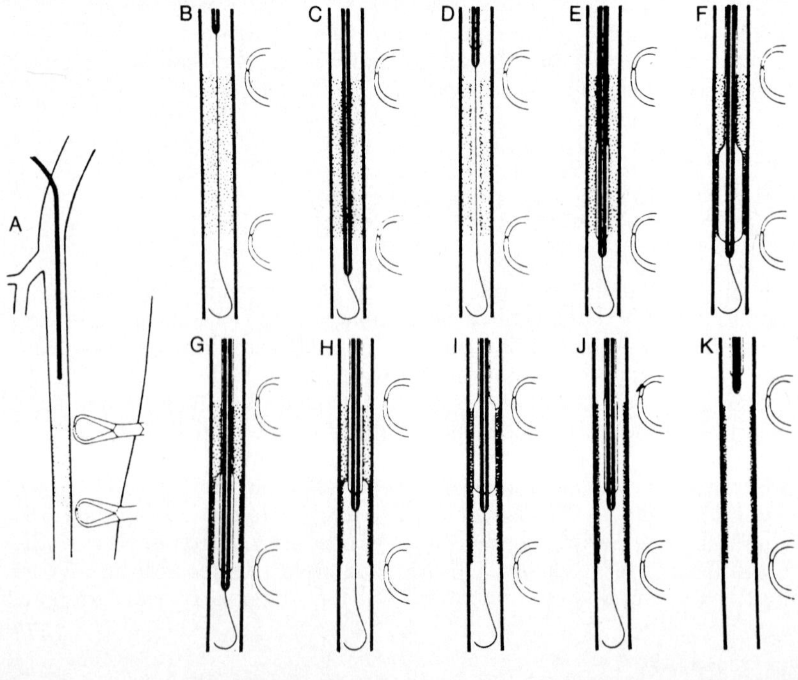

FIGURE 40–2. The Gruentzig technique. This series of diagrams depicts the application of balloon angioplasty to the treatment of a totally occluded peripheral artery (*A*). After diagnostic angiography a guidewire (*B*) and an angiographic catheter (*C*) are passed through the area of total occlusion. This creates a lumen for passage of the deflated dilatation catheter (*D, E*). The dilatation balloon is then inflated at several points throughout the stenotic lumen (*F* to *I*), resulting in improvement in vessel patency. Again note the absence of enlargement in the outer diameter, suggesting compaction of atherosclerotic material as the mechanism for lumenal enhancement. (From Gruentzig, A., and Kumpe, D. A.: Technique of percutaneous transluminal angioplasty with the Gruentzig balloon catheter. Am. J. Radiol. *132*:547, 1979.)

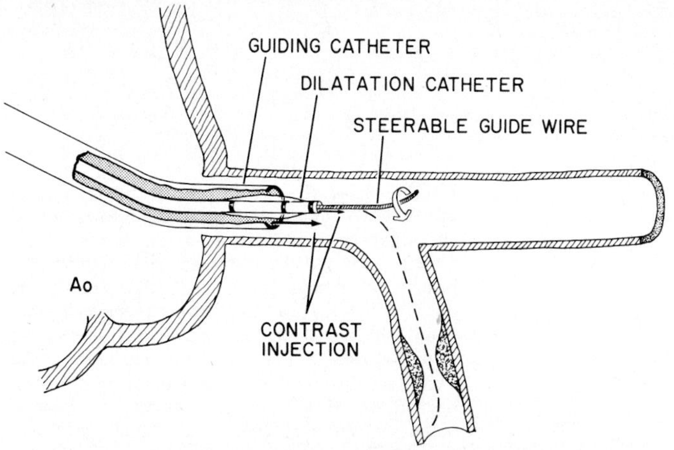

FIGURE 40–3. Movable guidewire dilatation system. The dilatation catheter is shown here at the end of a large (No. 8 or 9 French, 2.7- or 3.0-mm) guiding catheter, which is positioned at the ostium of the involved vessel. The soft, yet steerable guidewire is then advanced through the central lumen of the dilatation catheter and directed through and beyond the target lesion. The position of this guidewire relative to coronary branches and lesions can be revealed by contrast injection through the guiding catheter or through the central lumen of the dilatation catheter. Once the guidewire has been successfully positioned, it serves as a "track" over which the dilatation catheter itself can be advanced. (From Baim, D. S., and Faxon, D. P.: Coronary angioplasty. *In* Grossman, W. [ed.]: Cardiac Catheterization and Angiography. 3rd ed. Philadelphia, Lea and Febiger, 1986.)

Registry was closed, a variety of technical improvements in PTCA equipment, coupled with the availability of more experienced operators, facilitated major improvements in the overall success of PTCA.[10, 11] The original dilatation catheter was redesigned so that the guidewire now extended the entire length of the dilatation catheter, allowing the wire to be advanced, withdrawn, reshaped, or steered during the procedure (Fig. 40–3).[12, 13] Although these specialized guidewires are only 0.014 to 0.018 inch (0.3 to 0.5 mm) in diameter, sophisticated engineering has allowed the fabrication of devices with soft atraumatic tips, excellent torque control, and superb radiographic visibility. Current guidewires can be manipulated across stenoses located virtually anywhere in the coronary tree, and then serve as a "railroad track" over which advancement of the dilatation catheter can be performed. Special "exchange-length" guidewires (300 cm long) are also available which can be left positioned in the distal coronary artery as one balloon catheter is withdrawn and a second is inserted, or as contrast injection is performed through the guiding catheter to assess adequacy of dilatation.[14] Improvements in the design of dilatation catheters[10, 11, 13, 15] have led to the development of devices with deflated diameters as small as 0.030 inch (0.75 mm), inflated diameters between 2.0 and 4.0 mm, and the ability to tolerate inflation pressures as high as 20 atm (300 psi). These devices can be used to cross and dilate even the severest and most rigid stenoses.

CURRENT TECHNIQUES

Patients undergoing coronary angioplasty are usually admitted to the hospital the day before the procedure. Prior catheterization and exercise test data are reviewed, and a dilatation strategy is developed detailing the specific lesions, the sequence, and the equipment to be used for dilatation. The procedure—including the likelihood of successful dilatation, abrupt reclosure with emergency surgery, and late restenosis—is discussed with the patient and the family. Consent forms for both PTCA and possible emergency coronary artery bypass surgery are signed. Patients are proscribed from oral intake after midnight and asked to bathe with an antiseptic scrub. Aspirin (325 mg/day), dipyridamole (200 mg/day), and a calcium channel blocker are added to existing medical therapy.

At the time of PTCA appropriate vascular access (by way of either brachial artery cutdown or femoral artery puncture) is obtained (Fig. 9–2, p. 245), and a guiding catheter is positioned at the ostium of the involved coronary artery. A venous catheter for monitoring right heart pressure and/or temporary ventricular pacing is usually placed, and full systemic heparinization is achieved using 10,000 units of intravenous heparin. Baseline angiography is performed to clarify any uncertainties (e.g., location of side branches relative to the target stenosis) and to document continued suitability of the lesion for dilatation. The guidewire is then passed across the target lesion and positioned in the distal segment of the involved vessel. A dilatation catheter comparable to the size of the adjacent normal artery is advanced into the lesion and adequately pressurized to expand the balloon to its full diameter. Adequate dilatation is confirmed by repeat angiography and/or measurement of the translesional pressure gradient, after which the dilated segment is observed over 5 to 10 minutes to document stability of the result. Additional lesions may then be dilated according to the predetermined dilatation strategy. The effect of heparin is allowed to wear off before removal of the vascular sheaths, although intravenous heparin infusion may be resumed for 24 to 48 hours if significant intimal dissection is present at the dilatation site. After 8 to 24 hours of bed rest, the patient is ambulated and discharged.

INDICATIONS

The indication for PTCA is myocardial ischemia owing to coronary stenosis(es) deemed suitable for this procedure.[8, 9] With the advantage of improved guidewires, dilatation catheters, and guiding catheters, successful crossing and dilatation is now achieved in well over 90 per cent of lesions in which it is attempted, compared with only 60 per cent in the original NHLBI Registry. This improvement in success is reflected in new NHLBI Registry of 723 patients treated at 15 centers during 1985[16] and in the data reported by a number of individual centers.[17–19] Moreover, this higher success rate has occurred despite the inclusion of patients with progressively more challenging anatomical and clinical disease. Whereas PTCA was originally limited to proximal stenoses, more distal, eccentric, and calcified lesions are now approached on a routine basis.[10] Lesions involving *coronary bifurcations*—previously avoided because of the 14 per cent incidence of "snowplow" occlusion of the side branch (Fig. 40–4)[20]—can now be dilated using the "kissing balloon"[21] or double wire (Fig. 40–5)[22] techniques to preserve both the main and the side branch lumens. *Totally occluded coronary arteries* are also approachable by PTCA,[21a] in order to revascularize areas of viable myocardium supplied by inadequate collateral flow (Fig. 40–6) or to provide collateral flow to other stenotic vessels undergoing dilatation (Fig. 40–7).[23–28] Although the primary success rate in dilatation of chronic total occlusions remains lower than that for other stenotic lesions (75 per cent for occlusions less than 3 months old and below 50 per cent for older occlusions), dilatation of total occlusions now accounts for 10 to 20 per cent of PTCA volume in large centers.[27, 28]

MULTIVESSEL CORONARY ARTERY DISEASE. An increasing number of patients with multivessel coronary artery

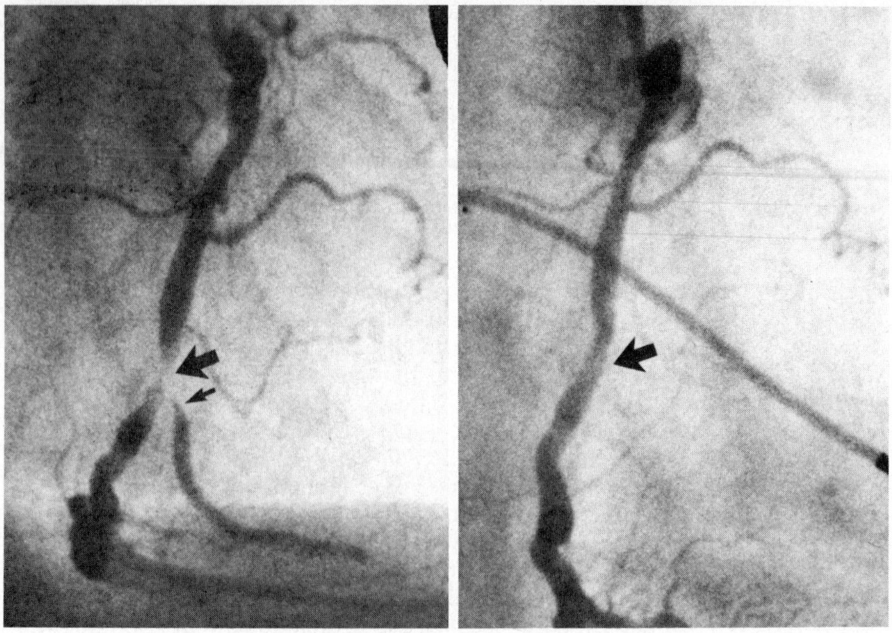

FIGURE 40–4. The "snowplow" effect. The left panel shows severe stenosis of the midportion of the right coronary artery (large arrow), from which a proximally diseased right ventricular branch (small arrow) originates. After PTCA (*right panel*), dilatation of the right coronary lesion has been achieved at the expense of occlusion of the right ventricular side branch. (From Baim, D. S.: Percutaneous transluminal angioplasty. *In* Petersdorf, R. G., et al. [eds.]: Harrison's Principles of Internal Medicine, Update VI. New York, McGraw-Hill Book Co., 1985.)

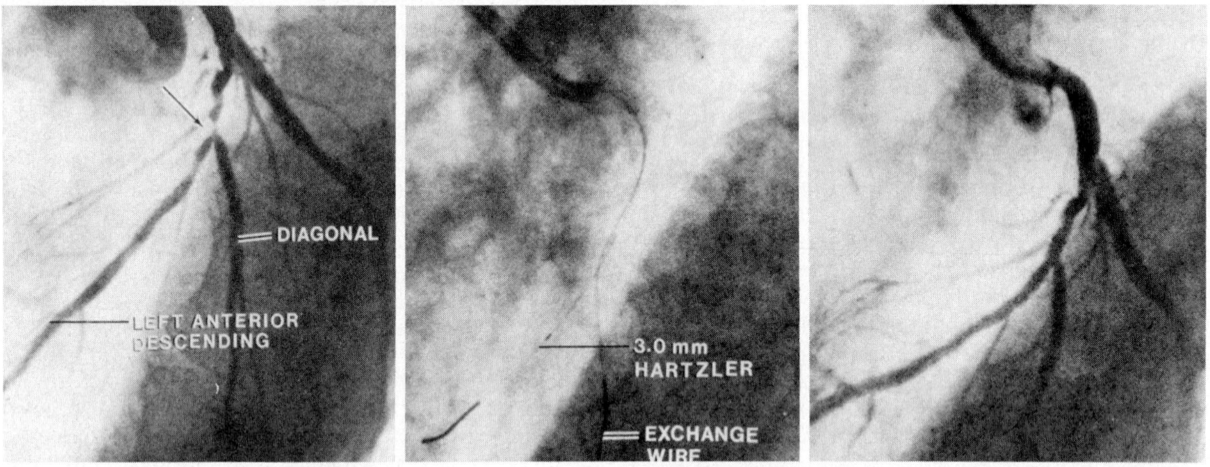

FIGURE 40–5. "Double wire" technique. To avoid occlusion of major branches involved in bifurcation lesions, two separate dilatation systems can be positioned—one in the main vessel and one in the involved branch vessel—through a single guiding catheter. *Alternate* inflation of these two dilatation systems can then be performed. In contrast, the "kissing balloon" technique would require *simultaneous* inflations of two dilatation systems, each passing through its own guiding catheter. (From Oesterle, S. N., McAuley, B. J., Buchbinder, M., and Simpson, J. B.: Angioplasty at coronary bifurcations: Single guide, two-wire technique. Cathet. Cardiovasc. Diagn. *12*:57, 1986.)

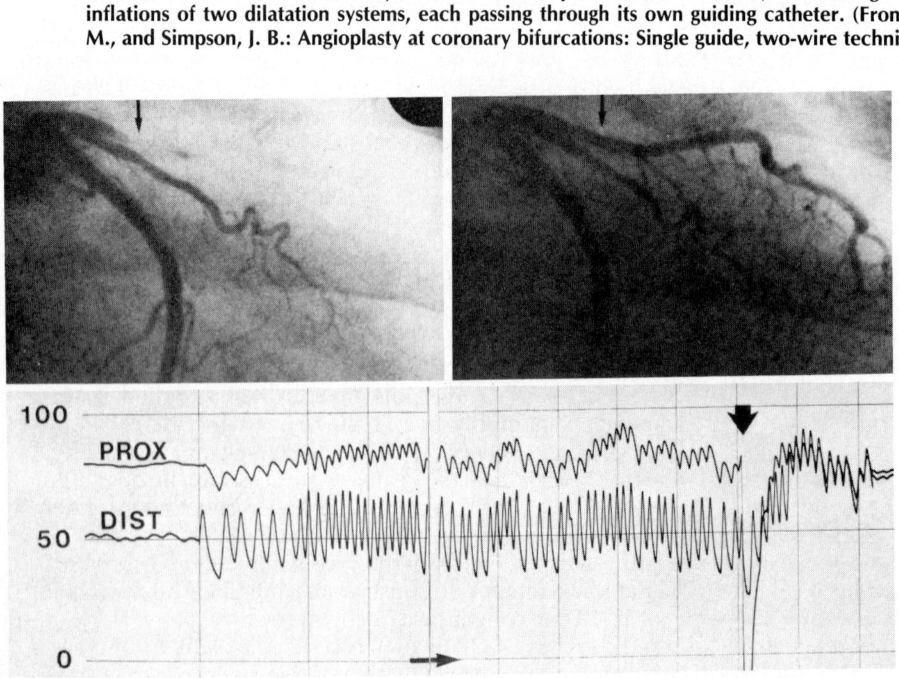

FIGURE 40–6. Angioplasty of a totally occluded coronary artery. Baseline angiography (*upper left*) shows total occlusion of the proximal left anterior descending. Prominent collateral filling of the distal vessel was evident during right coronary injection (not shown). Despite the presence of total occlusion of the involved vessel, this lesion was successfully crossed and dilated, with the result shown in the upper right. The bottom panel shows measurement of the "proximal" aortic and "distal" intracoronary pressure during inflation, and after deflation (bold arrow) of the dilatation catheter. Note the presence of a high distal occluded coronary artery pressure (50 mm Hg) consistent with good collateral function, and the resolution of the pressure difference between the proximal and distal sampling sites after balloon deflation (residual transstenotic gradient 5 mm Hg). (From Dervan, J. P., Baim, D. S., Cherniles, J., and Grossman, W.: Transluminal angioplasty of occluded coronary arteries: Use of a movable guidewire system. Circulation *68*:776, 1983, by permission of the American Heart Association, Inc.)

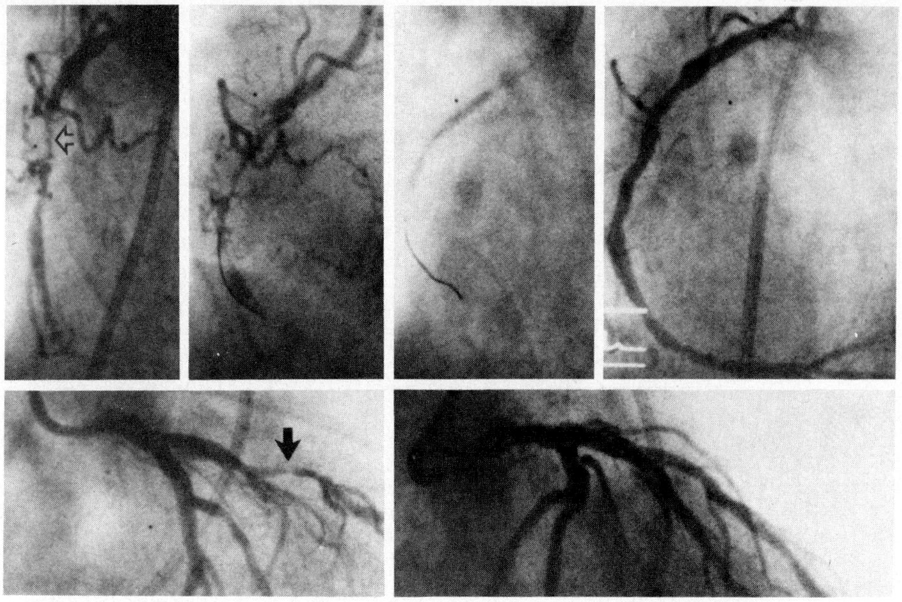

FIGURE 40–7. "Boot strap" two-vessel dilatation. Upper panel shows functionally occluded mid-right coronary artery, with filling of the distal vessel by way of bridging (right-to-right) and left-to-right collaterals. Successful dilatation of this lesion (*upper right*) restored antegrade flow in the right coronary artery and allowed reversal of the left-to-right collaterals to support the left anterior descending territory during dilatation of that vessel (bold arrow). (From Baim, D. S., and Faxon, D. P.: Coronary angioplasty. *In* Grossman, W. [ed.]: Cardiac Catheterization and Angiography. 3rd ed. Philadelphia, Lea and Febiger, 1986.)

disease are being subjected to PTCA as an alternative to bypass surgery (Figs. 40–7 and 40–8).[29–31] These patients account for more than half of those entered into the 1985 Registry, although fewer than two-thirds of patients identified as having multivessel *disease* actually underwent multivessel *dilatation*.[16] Although preliminary data suggest that many patients with multivessel coronary artery disease may derive substantial clinical benefit from successful PTCA, multivessel disease clearly imposes several additional difficulties compared with single-vessel disease. These include (1) longer duration of the procedure and greater usage of radiographic contrast material, (2) more diffuse myocardial ischemia if abrupt reclosure should occur, (3) a greater chance that not all significant coronary lesions will be successfully dilated (incomplete revascularization), and (4) a greater chance that recurrent angina will develop owing to restenosis of a dilated segment or progression of disease in one or more undilated segments (Fig. 40–9).[32–35] These difficulties affect both the selection of patients for and the performance of the actual PTCA procedure. The operator must decide which lesions are responsible for the patient's symptoms (the "culprit" lesions[36]) and therefore must be dilated, which lesions are mild enough to be left alone, what the sequence of dilatations should be, and whether a suboptimal result in one lesion necessitates deferral of other dilatations to a separate sitting (a "staged" multivessel PTCA procedure). These issues must be addressed on a case-by-case basis, but the general goal of PTCA in a patient with multivessel disease is to dilate all lesions which narrow the diameter of major coronary segments by more than 70 per cent. While milder lesions can be dilated easily, dilatation is not usually required to control symptoms and still entails some risk of abrupt reclosure or accelerated restenosis.[37] If natural progression of these mild lesions leads to recurrent ischemic symptoms, they can be addressed in a subsequent procedure. Given these uncertainties about PTCA in multivessel disease, an adequately controlled

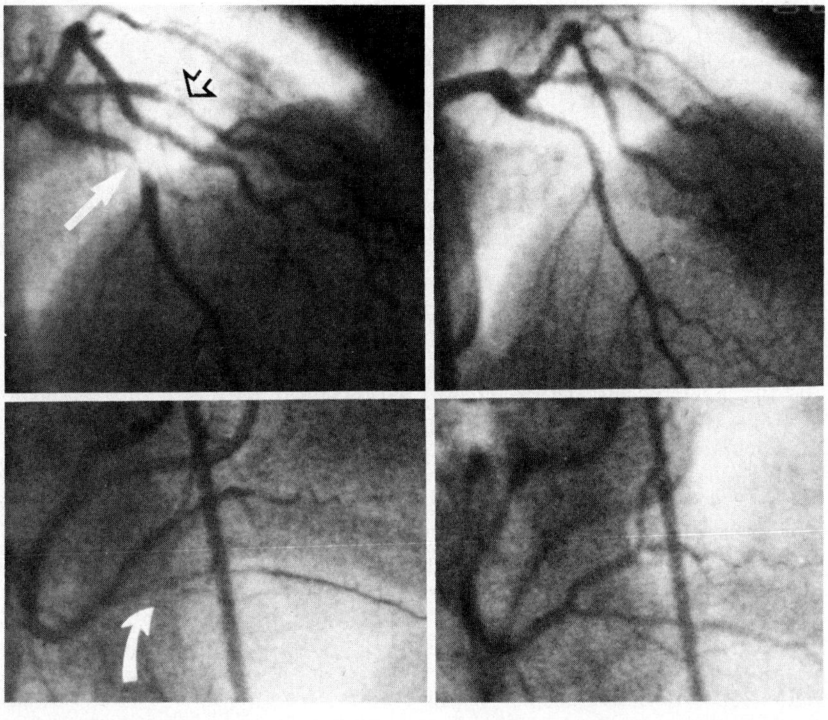

FIGURE 40–8. Multivessel dilatation. Upper panel shows severe stenosis of the proximal left anterior descending (bold arrow) and moderate stenosis of the large diagonal branch (open arrow) as seen before and after dilatation. Severe stenosis in the midportion of the posterior descending branch of the right coronary artery (curved arrow) was also dilated using a prototype 1.5-mm low-profile dilatation catheter.

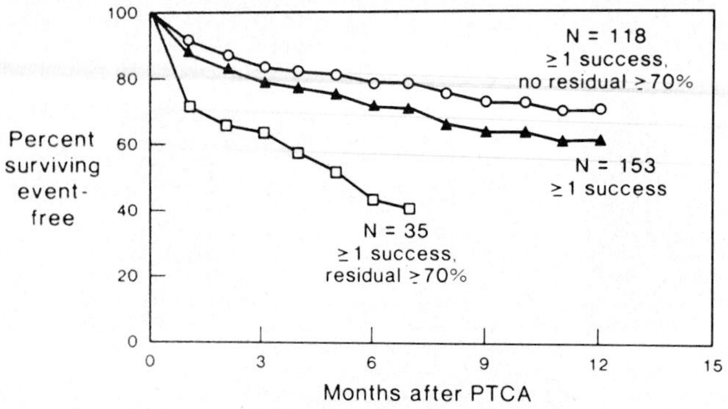

FIGURE 40–9. Recurrent angina in multivessel disease. Life table analysis shows the cumulative incidence of recurrent angina in patients undergoing successful angioplasty for coronary artery disease. Note the more rapid development of symptomatic failure in the subgroup (open squares) in which one or more lesions greater than or equal to 70 per cent diameter reduction remained owing to incomplete revascularization by PTCA, compared with the subgroup (open circles) in which no lesions greater than 70 per cent remained, or the overall group of 153 patients (closed triangles). (From Mabin, T. A., Holmes, D. R., Smith, H. C., Vlietstra, R. E., Reeder, G. S., Bresnehan, J. F., Bove, A. A., Hammes, L. N., Elveback, L. R., and Orszulak, T. A.: Follow-up clinical results in patients undergoing percutaneous transluminal coronary angioplasty. Circulation *71*:754, 1985, by permission of the American Heart Association, Inc.)

comparison of PTCA with bypass surgery—as proposed in the Bypass Angioplasty Revascularization Intervention (BARI) Trial currently being designed under the sponsorship of the NHLBI—will be required to establish the optimal application of PTCA in this important patient population.[38]

UNSTABLE ANGINA. At the same time as PTCA has been applied to progressively more difficult *anatomical* situations, it has also been applied to a broader spectrum of *clinical* disease states. Whereas PTCA was initially used largely in patients with chronic, stable angina, it is now used increasingly in patients with more unstable patterns, i.e., new onset, rest, or preinfarction angina (p. 1353).[19, 36, 39] Between one-half and three-quarters of such patients are anatomically suitable for PTCA, particularly if revascularization can be limited to dilatation of one or more severe "culprit" lesions responsible for the unstable clinical picture[36] without attempting revascularization of other milder lesions, small branches, or chronic total occlusions. In many instances PTCA can be performed in patients with unstable angina as an extension of the initial diagnostic catheterization procedure.[40]

ACUTE MYOCARDIAL INFARCTION. The majority of patients with acute myocardial infarction have the anatomical features making them suitable for PTCA, after (or instead of) thrombolytic therapy (p. 1253).[41–43] Prompt PTCA of the infarct-related occlusion or stenosis appears to improve the probability of opening the involved vessel and reduce the incidence of subsequent vessel reocclusion or postinfarction ischemia, and leads to better recovery of left ventricular function than thrombolytic therapy alone.[44, 45] Preliminary studies have suggested that prompt PTCA may also reduce the mortality in patients with cardiogenic shock associated with acute myocardial infarction.[46] These issues, as well as the optimal timing of PTCA after the administration of thrombolytic therapy, are currently being investigated in the Thrombolysis in Myocardial Infarction (TIMI) Trial conducted by the NHLBI, as well as in a number of smaller trials. Given the large number of patients presenting to hospital within the first several hours of myocardial infarction, and the major commitment of human and physical resources which would be required to make PTCA available to patients with acute myocardial infarction on a timely basis,[19, 41] sound demonstration of major long-term clinical benefit will be required before broad adoption of this management strategy can be recommended.

OTHER INDICATIONS. Another rapidly growing indication for PTCA consists of patients with *recurrent angina after bypass surgery*, who may undergo dilatation of either a bypass graft stenosis, or a lesion in a previously grafted or ungrafted native coronary artery (Fig. 40–10).[47–49] Patients with other factors *increasing the risk of surgery* (advanced age,[50] poor left ventricular function, or severe pulmonary disease) may also be favored for PTCA if suitable anatomy is found at the diagnostic catheterization. Such high-risk patients may even be offered PTCA of lesions (left main stenosis, left main equivalent, or diffuse three-vessel coronary disease) who would otherwise be rejected for angioplasty in favor of bypass surgery. At the other end of the spectrum, some patients with *milder anginal symptoms* (Canadian Heart Class I or II) may be subjected to catheterization followed by dilatation of one or more severe underlying lesions, rather than remaining on medical antianginal therapy. Although such patients constitute less than 20 per cent of those currently subjected to PTCA,[19] it should be pointed out that there is no evidence that PTCA is superior to medical therapy for this patient group in terms of longevity, freedom from subsequent myocardial infarction, or reduced long-term health costs.

ECONOMIC AND REGULATORY IMPLICATIONS

The rapidly growing role of PTCA is reflected in current (1986) statistics. An estimated 110,000 PTCA procedures

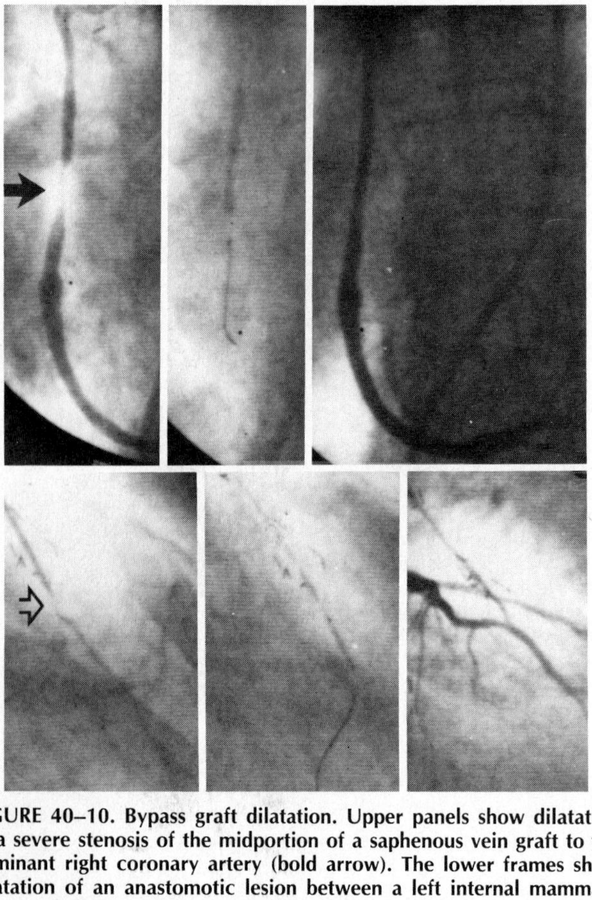

FIGURE 40–10. Bypass graft dilatation. Upper panels show dilatation of a severe stenosis of the midportion of a saphenous vein graft to the dominant right coronary artery (bold arrow). The lower frames show dilatation of an anastomotic lesion between a left internal mammary artery and the distal left anterior descending (open arrow).

are being performed annually, compared with approximately 240,000 coronary artery bypass operations. From another perspective, the current utilization of PTCA is reflected in the revascularization outcome of patients undergoing first-time diagnostic catheterizations for coronary artery disease. In the author's institution approximately 60 per cent of such patients are referred for revascularization, which consists of nearly equal numbers of PTCA and surgical bypass procedures.[19] Because PTCA can be performed for approximately one-half to one-third the in-hospital cost of bypass surgery, with a shorter length of stay and convalescent period, it is being increasingly favored by third-party payers.[19, 51] Most cost studies, however, do not factor in the hidden expenses of standby bypass surgery[52] or the late expenses associated with treatment of restenosis, so that the magnitude of this cost savings is difficult to quantitate accurately. Finally, both the success rate of PTCA and the resultant cost savings depend heavily on the experience and track record of the individual operator.[53] Standards for training in PTCA as a specialized part of fellowship are being developed,[54] but no precise guidelines are available for training or maintaining the PTCA skills of individuals who have already entered practice.[55–57] It is clear, however, that not all invasive cardiologists can or should perform PTCA.[57] Moreover, because of the requirement for high-quality radiographic imaging and in-house cardiac surgical backup to deal promptly with abrupt vessel reclosure, PTCA is likely to continue to be restricted to a fraction of the hospitals which currently perform diagnostic cardiac catheterization.

COMPLICATIONS

Beyond continued refinement of angioplasty catheters and concomitant improvement in the primary success rate, it is likely that the next several years will see additional advances in our understanding of the factors influencing the initial dilatation and subsequent vessel healing. While angioplasty was initially thought to rely on compression of the atherosclerotic plaque (Figs. 40–1 and 40–2),[1, 2, 5] experimental studies disclose neither significant compression nor embolization of plaque elements. Instead, the majority of improvement in vessel lumen appears to result from "cracking" and outward displacement of the plaque, associated with local plastic stretching of the media and adventitia (Fig. 40–11).[58–61] The use of a nonelastomeric balloon with an inflated diameter comparable to the diameter of the normal lumen adjacent to the stenotic segment is usually sufficient to achieve adequate dilatation, while minimizing the likelihood of excessive vessel trauma or vessel rupture precipitated by overdilatation.[62] Particularly rigid lesions may require inflation of the balloon to high pressure (10 to 20 atm, 150 to 300 psi) to achieve this result, while eccentric lesions (Fig. 40–12) may require use of a slightly oversized balloon catheter, repeated inflations, or prolonged (1 minute) inflations to overcome the intrinsic elasticity of the normal arterial wall opposite the atherosclerotic plaque.[63, 64] Fortunately, these repeated transient coronary occlusions are usually well tolerated hemodynamically and do not cause serious arrhythmias,[65] although angina may develop during balloon inflation in those patients who do not have good collateral flow to the dilated vessels.

In the process of achieving adequate dilatation, neither too little nor too much "controlled injury" should be inflicted on the vessel wall. It is therefore important to monitor the adequacy of dilatation closely during the procedure, either by repeated angiographic examination of the dilated segment[66] or by ongoing estimation of the residual translesional gradient,[67] i.e., the difference between mean aortic pressure and the mean coronary pressure distal to the dilated segment measured through the central lumen of the deflated balloon catheter (Fig. 40–6). Residual stenoses less than 50 per cent and residual translesional gradients below 15 mm Hg are indicative of a successful procedure, although better results are commonly achieved.

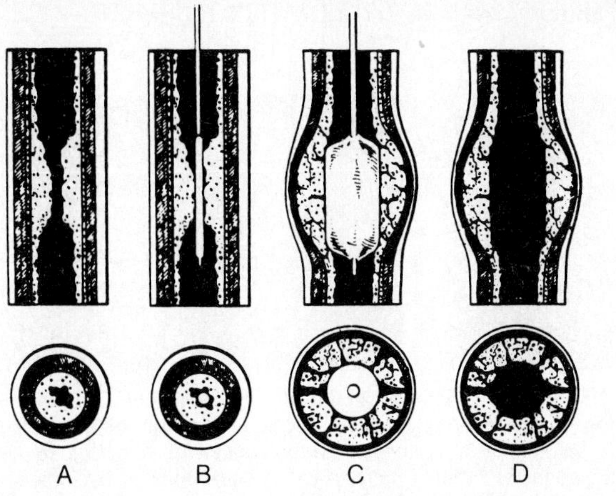

FIGURE 40–11. Current concept of the mechanism of balloon dilatation. Serial panels show the baseline stenosis, passage of the deflated balloon catheter, balloon inflation, and the post dilatation appearance, as drawn in longitudinal and transverse cross-sectional views. Balloon inflation (panel C) is associated with fracture and outward displacement of the atherosclerotic plaque, as well as plastic stretching of the media and adventitia. The result (panel D) is enlargement of the lumen owing to expansion of the entire vessel wall, rather than compaction of atherosclerotic material. (From Castaneda-Zuniga, W. R., Formanek, A., Tadavarthy, M., Vlodaver, Z., Edwards, J. E., Zollikofer, C., and Amplatz, K.: The mechanism of balloon angioplasty. Radiology *135*:565, 1980.)

Even when the dilatation procedure has been successful, evidence of the vascular injury associated with PTCA is often evident in the radiographic appearance of intimal dissection at the dilatation site (Fig. 40–13).[68] Although patients with moderately large dissections may have some chest discomfort owing to local vessel trauma,[69] limited dissection does not usually interfere with antegrade flow and goes on to heal by reendothelialization within 6 weeks of the dilatation procedure.

ABRUPT RECLOSURE. In approximately 4 per cent of patients—particularly those undergoing dilatation of long (more than 2 cm), eccentric, or curved stenotic seg-

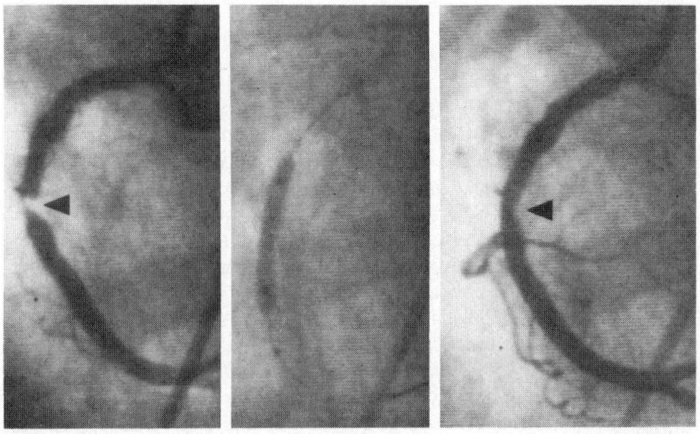

FIGURE 40–12. Dilatation of an eccentric lesion. Baseline angiography (*left panel*) shows a profoundly eccentric stenosis of the midportion of the right coronary artery, with essentially no involvement of the opposite wall. Repeated, prolonged dilatations using a 3.5-mm balloon catheter (*center panel*) were required to overcome the elasticity of this vessel. Although a satisfactory result has been obtained (*right panel*), some residual narrowing is evident.

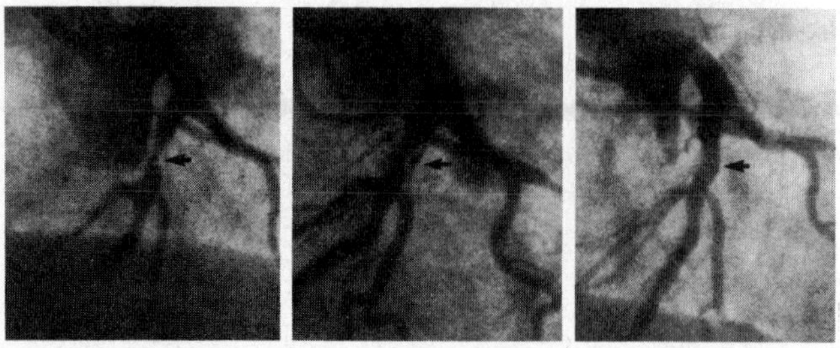

FIGURE 40–13. Intimal dissection during successful dilatation. Examination of the mid-left anterior descending (arrow) before (*left panel*) and immediately after (*center panel*) successful dilatation shows both enlargement of luminal caliber and the presence of two linear filling defects within the vessel lumen. This localized dissection did not impede antegrade flow and healed to leave an essentially normal vessel at 3-month restudy (*right panel*). (From Baim, D. S.: Percutaneous transluminal angioplasty. *In* Petersdorf, R. G., et al. [eds.]: Harrison's Principles of Internal Medicine, Update VI. New York, McGraw-Hill Book Co., 1985.)

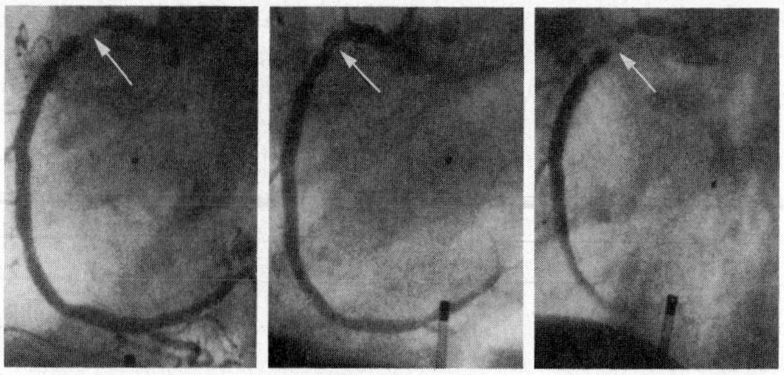

FIGURE 40–14. Dissection leading to abrupt reclosure. Baseline angiography (*left panel*) shows severe stenosis of the proximal right coronary artery. Immediately after dilatation (*center panel*) overall luminal caliber was improved, but a moderate dissection was evident. Within 15 minutes this dissection progressed to abrupt vessel reclosure with delayed antegrade perfusion, chest pain, and ST-segment elevation in the inferior leads. At the time this procedure was performed (1980) the value of repeat dilatation had not yet been recognized and no devices to restore antegrade flow were available. Accordingly, this patient underwent uncomplicated emergency saphenous vein bypass grafting of the dominant right coronary artery. (From Baim, D. S.: Percutaneous transluminal coronary angioplasty: Analysis of unsuccessful procedures as a guide toward improved results. Cardiovasc. Intervent. Radiol. *5*:186, 1982.)

ments—local injury produces more extensive dissection. This may (in conjunction with local vasospasm or thrombus formation) progress to abrupt vessel closure within 30 minutes of dilatation (Fig. 40–14).[70, 71] Half the vessels which manifest abrupt reclosure can be reopened by redilatation,[72] but the other half (or approximately 2.5 per cent of the total PTCA attempts) currently require emergency surgery if vessel closure recurs and is associated with clinical and electrocardiographic evidence of myocardial ischema.[52, 73, 74] Management of this complication necessitates prompt availability of an experienced cardiac surgical team and highlights the need for close cooperation between interventional cardiologists and their surgical colleagues. Despite prompt revascularization, most patients requiring emergency surgery still sustain some degree of

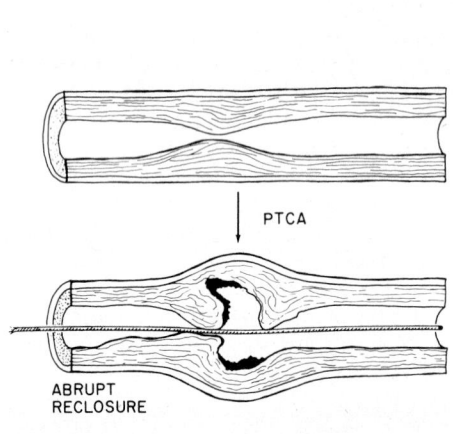

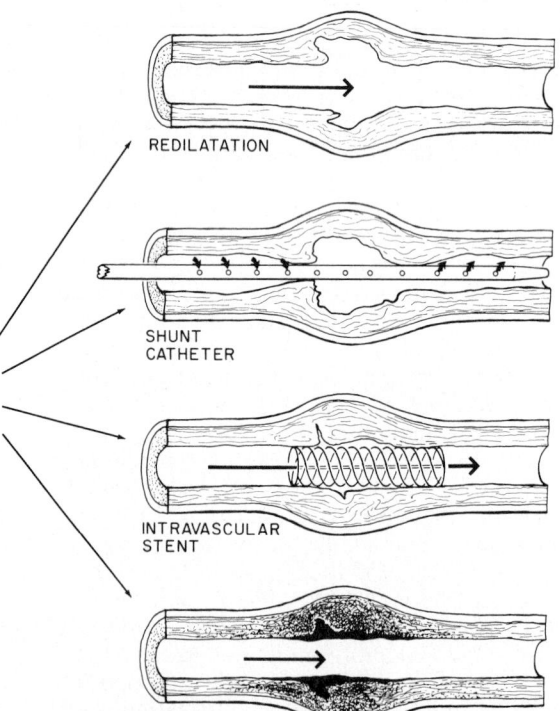

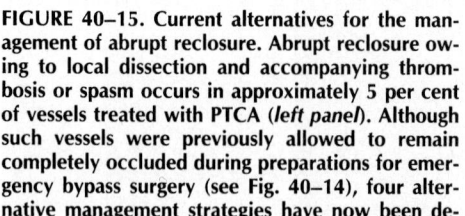

FIGURE 40–15. Current alternatives for the management of abrupt reclosure. Abrupt reclosure owing to local dissection and accompanying thrombosis or spasm occurs in approximately 5 per cent of vessels treated with PTCA (*left panel*). Although such vessels were previously allowed to remain completely occluded during preparations for emergency bypass surgery (see Fig. 40–14), four alternative management strategies have now been developed: *Redilatation* using multiple, prolonged inflations of the balloon catheter is successful in remolding the dissected vessel into a stable patent configuration in approximately one-half of the cases of abrupt reclosure. In the remaining cases a *shunt catheter* can be positioned within the occluded segment, over an exchange-length guidewire. Arterial blood can enter this catheter through side holes located proximal to the point of occlusion and exit through side holes located distally, to maintain perfusion of the distal vessel as the patient is transported to the operating room. The catheter is then removed after the local delivery of cardioplegic solution and before placement of the aortic cross clamp. Two investigational approaches to abrupt reclosure include placement of an *intravascular stent* which can be delivered into the affected segment over a dilatation catheter and expanded to the caliber of the adjacent normal vessel by balloon inflation. This prevents the dissection flaps from acutely compromising lumen caliber and permits long-term patency and reendothelialization in the presence of anticoagulant drugs. *Thermal welding* uses a laser-heated balloon catheter to coagulate and seal the local dissection and maintain vessel patency without placement of a prosthetic material.

a myocardial infarction and contribute heavily to the 0.4 per cent mortality associated with elective PTCA.[71, 75] Management of abrupt reclosure has been improved recently with the advent of special perfusion or "shunt" catheters (Fig. 40–15),[76] which can be placed across the occluded segment, to permit perfusion of the distal bed to continue while surgical control of the situation is being achieved. While better understanding of the dilatation process may allow more predictable responses and lower the incidence of significant dissection,[77] newer adjunctive techniques, i.e., the use of even more prolonged balloon inflations, thermal welding of the dissection plane,[78] or placement of an intraluminal vascular stent (Fig. 40–15),[79] may allow more consistent reversal of the reclosure phenomenon. These advances may reduce further the incidence of emergency coronary bypass grafting and might even obviate the need for in-house surgical standby during PTCA procedures.

RESTENOSIS. The second area in which enhanced understanding of the biology of angioplasty is required is in the prevention of restenosis of the dilated segment. After successful PTCA there should be no clinical, electrocardiographic, and thallium perfusion evidence of myocardial ischemia.[80–85] In approximately 20 per cent of patients, however, evidence of myocardial ischemia reappears within 6 months of the dilatation, coupled with angiographic evidence of restenosis of the dilated segment (Fig. 40–16).[86] An additional 5 to 10 per cent of patients may remain free of recurrent symptoms but demonstrate partial angiographic renarrowing of the dilated segment. Some clinical parameters—severe baseline stenosis, incomplete dilatation, unstable angina with a brief duration of symptoms, male gender, stenosis of the left anterior descending coronary artery, ostial stenosis, uncontrolled vasospasm at the dilatation site,[87–89] or a soft lesion which dilates without visible dissection—are associated with a higher incidence of late restenosis.

Animal studies suggest that post-PTCA restenosis results from platelet adhesion to the area of endothelial damage at the dilatation site, with subsequent release of potent smooth muscle vasoconstrictors and mitogens, such as platelet-derived growth factor (PDGF).[90] According to this hypothesis, restenosis may represent a human correlate of the arterial injury technique used to create atherosclerotic plaques in experimental animals. In support of this, postmortem studies show that areas of restenosis tend to have a different, more proliferative histological appearance compared with the underlying primary plaque (Fig. 40–17).[66, 91] On the other hand, adjunctive therapy with currently available antiplatelet agents (aspirin and dipyridamole) has thus far failed to decrease the incidence of restenosis in PTCA patients, despite a favorable effect in some animal models. Clinical trials with other antiplatelet agents (prostacyclin analogs, omega-3-fatty acids), pharmacological blockers of PDGF,[92] or techniques to leave behind a smoother and less platelet-attractive surface (thermal "smoothing" or mechanical plaque resection) are now in progress in an effort to decrease the restenosis rate. In the meantime, patients who have undergone successful PTCA should have their clinical symptoms and exercise test performance monitored closely over the 6 months following the procedure.

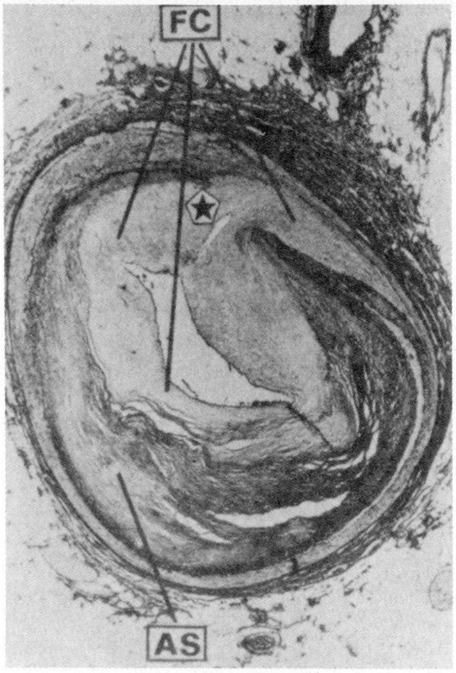

FIGURE 40–17. Histological appearance of restenosis. Cross-sectional view of the left anterior descending coronary artery of a patient with restenosis after successful dilatation. The original atherosclerotic plaque (and associated fracture) are evident as the darker staining material (AS). The proliferative fibrocellular material (FC) responsible for restenosis is evident by its differential staining characteristics. (From Serruys, P. W., Reiber, J. H. C., Wijns, W., van den Brand, M., Kooijman, C. J., tenKaten, H. J., and Hugenholtz, P. G.: Assessment of percutaneous transluminal coronary angioplasty by quantitative coronary angiography: Diameter versus videodensitometric area measurements. Am. J. Cardiol. *54*:482, 1984.)

If clinical evidence of restenosis develops, repeat catheterization, including repeat PTCA, is the best management (Fig. 40–16). Repeat PTCA is almost always successful[93] and is preferable to relying on intensified medical therapy alone, since the restenotic lesion may progress rapidly and produce escalating symptoms. Re-restenosis may develop in 20 to 30 per cent of patients after re-PTCA, necessitating a third (or even a fourth) dilatation before long-term patency is secured. If symptoms and signs of restenosis do not develop within 6 months of the dilatation procedure, they are unlikely to do so in future years, although anginal symptoms may develop due to progression of disease at other sites, and require additional dilatation procedures.[17, 84, 85] Routine follow-up angiography is not clinically justified after PTCA, except in special situations (high-risk patients, commercial pilots). With the use of repeat PTCA for management of restenosis and progressive disease at other sites, fewer than 12 per cent of patients undergoing initially successful dilatation will require bypass surgery during the next several years.[9]

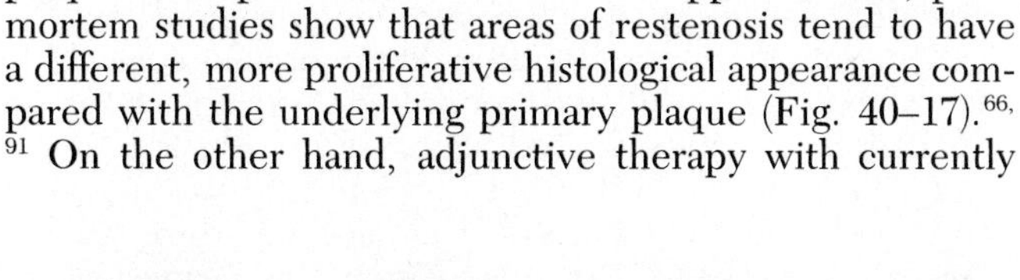

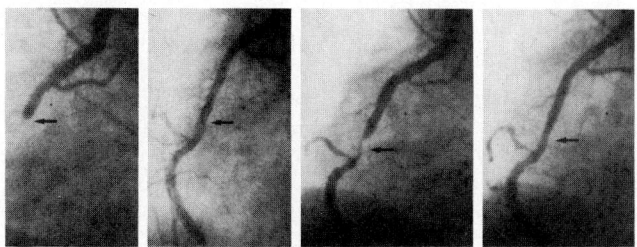

FIGURE 40–16. Restenosis of a dilated segment. The left panels show the appearance of a totally occluded mid-right coronary artery before and immediately after successful dilatation. Despite the absence of residual stenosis, this patient experienced recurrent symptoms 6 weeks after the procedure. Repeat catheterization (*right panels*) showed severe recurrence of the original lesion, which was successfully redilated. Restenosis developed again 6 weeks later (not shown), but this patient has now remained entirely asymptomatic for more than 4 years after a successful third dilatation.

NEWER TECHNIQUES FOR TREATING VASCULAR STENOSIS

While essentially all experience in the treatment of coronary stenoses has involved the use of balloon dilatation, a number of other methods are under investigation. Given the advanced state and evident success of balloon dilatation, these methods must strive for the following goals: (1) to improve the crossing rate for difficult (i.e., totally occluded) lesions; (2) to minimize or correct local injury responsible for abrupt vessel reclosure; or (3) to remove physically plaque and/or leave behind a smoother luminal surface in an effort to reduce the incidence of late restenosis. *Mechanical devices* include "cut-and-retrieve" systems to remove the plaque from the vessel lumen (Fig. 40–18),[94, 95] miniature drills or rotating wires to penetrate or fragment the plaque, and permanent vascular stents which can be positioned within the stenotic lumen.[79]

LASER ANGIOPLASTY. Lasers emitting any of several wavelengths from the infrared to the ultraviolet bands can be used to deliver energy to the stenotic vessel by means of 0.3- to 0.4-mm-diameter fiberoptic catheter guides. The original goal of laser angioplasty was direct ablation of plaque material,[96, 97] but this usually produces prothrombotic thermal charring and surrounding acoustic ("blast") injury of the adjacent vessel wall. In contrast with the comparatively long wavelength lasers used in other medical applications (CO_2 = 10.6 μ, Nd:YAG = 1.06 μ, argon = 0.5 μ), there is some evidence that the shorter wavelength excimer laser (less than 0.3 μ) achieves ablation of plaques with less surrounding thermal and acoustic injury.[98] Similar effects may be obtained by rapid-pulsing, high-energy lasers of longer wavelengths. In addition to the uncertainties regarding optimal laser wavelength, all studies of direct laser energy have been plagued by a high incidence of vessel perforation, owing either to ablation of the vessel wall by the laser or to mechanical effects of the stiff laser fibers.[99–101] Efforts are being made to improve the sensitivity of plaque over normal wall (using tetracycline[102] or hematoporphyrin[103] staining) and to improve the delivery of laser energy along the vessel lumen (using wire guides, centralizing balloons, or angioscopic visualization of the laser fiber). Lasers can also be used to deliver controlled thermal energy to the diseased vessel using a specially designed balloon catheter with a light-diffusing fiber, or a laser-heated metallic tip to "melt" the plaque.[104, 105] Both direct and indirect (thermal) laser techniques have been evaluated in peripheral arterial disease and are now undergoing early clinical trials in the coronary circulation.[106]

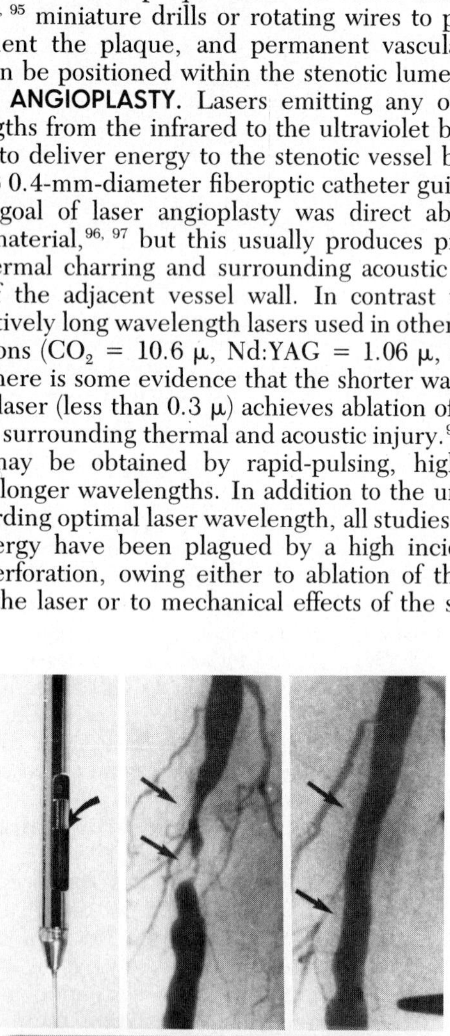

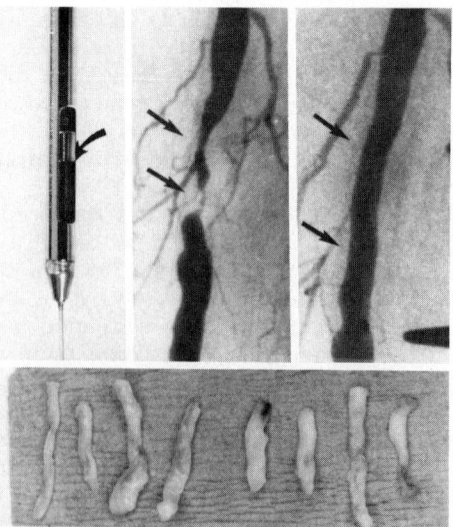

FIGURE 40–18. Mechanical "cut-and-retrieve" system. The upper left panel shows this specialized device which uses a cutting blade (curved arrow) spun at 2000 rpm as it is advanced downward through the device's cutting zone after placement within the stenotic segment. This technique was used to treat a severe superficial femoral arterial stenosis (double arrows, *center panel*) with the result shown (*upper right panel*). The strips of atheroma removed during the process are shown in the lower panel. (Courtesy of John B. Simpson, M.D., Devices for Vascular Intervention, Redwood City, Calif.).

ANGIOPLASTY OF OTHER (NONCORONARY) ARTERIES

Although most interventional techniques have been developed and tested in peripheral vessels (femoral or iliac arteries), the number of peripheral angioplasty procedures remains much smaller than the number of coronary angioplasties. In general, the results of peripheral angioplasty are similar to those described for PTCA. Primary success rates for peripheral arterial balloon dilatation exceed 95 per cent for the iliac and 87 per cent for the femoral arteries, with a 5-year restenosis rate which varies from 10 per cent for iliac vessels up to 40 per cent for smaller popliteal vessels.[107–110] Peripheral lesions, however, are more likely to be long (up to 10 cm) or totally occluded, in comparison to coronary arterial lesions. These technical challenges, coupled with better end-organ tolerance of ischemia and the absence of cardiac tamponade as a complication of vessel perforation or rupture, have fostered more aggressive trials of mechanical, thermal, or laser techniques in the peripheral circulation.

As in coronary angioplasty, peripheral angioplasty of technically suitable lesions may offer significant clinical and economic benefits over surgical repair, particularly since patients with peripheral vascular disease frequently have other cardiac or pulmonary disease which increase the risk of general anesthesia.[111] Because peripheral angiography is viewed as a preparation for vascular surgery, however, only a small fraction of patients with mildly or moderately symptomatic peripheral vascular disease are currently offered the option of peripheral angioplasty.[112]

Dilatation of atherosclerotic or fibromuscular stenoses in the *renal arteries* followed peripheral angioplasty as an application of balloon angioplasty (Fig. 40–19).[6] Renal artery angioplasty continues to be applied with excellent short- and long-term success as an alternative to vascular surgery in patients with renovascular hypertension (p. 844) or renal insufficiency as the result of anatomically suitable stenoses in the main artery or its principal branch.[113, 114]

In their original paper,[1] Dotter and Judkins predicted that interventional techniques would ultimately be applied to a variety of other vascular territories, including the *brachiocephalic and cerebral circulation.* Although the underlying disease processes (atherosclerosis and fibromuscular disease) are similar to those treated by balloon angioplasty in other vascular beds, carotid lesions are more likely to exhibit ulceration and adherent thrombus. At the same time, the brain is less tolerant of microembolic debris than any other end organ. Although obvious distal embolization has not been a frequent occurrence during balloon dilatation at other sites, this problem should be carefully evaluated in the cerebral circulation to decide whether adjunctive measures (e.g., distal particle filters) will be required. Until that time, balloon angioplasty continues to be used in inoperable lesions of the posterior circulation and in small numbers of patients with stenosis of the extracranial carotid artery (Fig. 40–20).[115–117] Use of these applications is likely to increase rapidly over the next decade, however, since surgical correction of cerebrovascular disease is performed in approximately 100,000 patients per year in the United States and continues to be associated with significant morbidity.

Balloon dilatation of other stenotic vessels has also been used. This includes dilatation of stenoses in pulmonary arteries or veins, and vascular shunts.[118–120] A conventional catheter is generally used to cross the target stenosis and place an exchange-length guidewire. The conventional catheter is then removed, and replaced by a balloon dilatation catheter of appropriate diameter. Because of the elasticity of most congenital stenoses, balloon diameters of 10 to 12 mm (two to three times that of the stenotic segment) may be required to produce significant dilatation. Balloon dilatation has also been used to maintain patency of the *ductus arteriosus* in children with cyanotic congenital heart disease, and to treat *coarctation of the aorta*. The site of coarctation is crossed with a guidewire, which permits advancement of a diagnostic catheter for performance of baseline angiography and calculation of the aortic diameter adjacent to the area of narrowing. A balloon catheter with a diameter 1 or 2 mm less than that of the normal segment is then advanced over the guidewire, positioned within the stenotic segment, and inflated with dilute contrast material. Successful procedures are marked by at least a 30 per cent increase in the diameter of the treated segment and at least a 50 per cent reduction in the associated pressure gradient. Because primary dilatation of coarctation is associated with a significant incidence of late aneurysm formation, it may be appropriate to reserve balloon dilatation for recurrent stenoses which develop after primary surgical repair (p. 931).[121, 122]

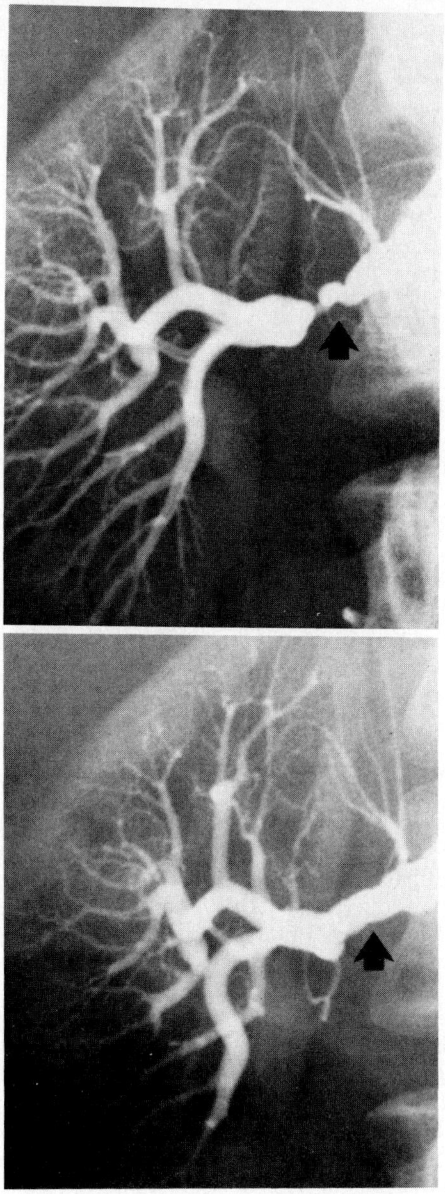

FIGURE 40–19. Renal artery angioplasty. *Top,* Severe stenosis of the right renal artery (arrow) owing to fibromuscular disease in a patient with refractory hypertension. *Bottom,* Luminal caliber improved after successful dilatation. (Courtesy of Ducksoo Kim, M.D.)

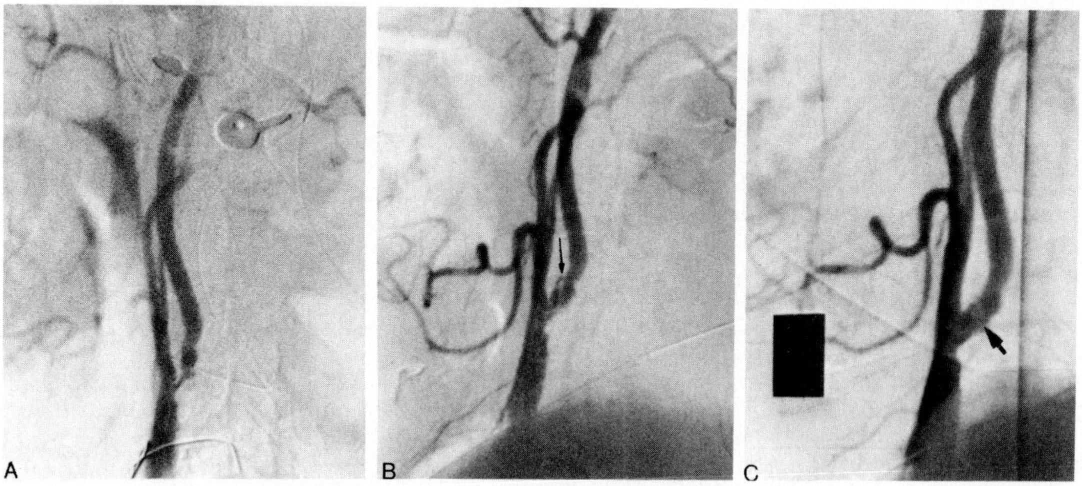

FIGURE 40–20. Carotid angioplasty. The left panels show severe stenosis at the origin of the right internal carotid artery before and immediately after balloon dilatation. Note the appearance of intimal dissection (*center panel*). At restudy 6 months later, luminal caliber was preserved, with resolution of intimal dissection. (From Tsai, F. Y., Matovich, V., Hieshima, G., Shah, D. C., Mehringer, C. M., Tiu, G., Higashida, R., and Pribam, H. F. W.: Percutaneous transluminal angioplasty of the carotid artery. Am. J. Neurol. Radiol. *7*:349, 1986.)

TREATMENT OF VALVULAR STENOSIS

PULMONARY VALVULOPLASTY

Pulmonary valvular stenosis (p. 942), a relatively common congenital cardiac lesion, was traditionally corrected by surgical "valvuloplasty," i.e., incision of fused commissures under direct vision. Beginning in 1982 pediatric cardiologists began using balloon dilatation catheters with inflated diameters 1 to 2 mm larger than the annulus size (20 to 25 mm) to produce similar commissural splitting by way of a closed transluminal approach.[123–125] This procedure has been quite successful, with a reduction of the pulmonic valve gradient to approximately one-third of its baseline valve. Given the high success rate and low incidence of complication, balloon valvuloplasty has essentially replaced open surgical repair for valvular pulmonic stenosis (p. 944). Application of balloon valvuloplasty for the treatment of *congenital* aortic stenosis has also been reported (p. 981), with a 70 per cent reduction in valve gradient and no significant increase in aortic regurgitation.[125, 126]

MITRAL VALVULOPLASTY

In contrast to congenital pulmonic stenosis, it was believed until recently that adult *acquired* rheumatic and/or calcific stenosis of the mitral or aortic valves would *not* be amenable to balloon valvuloplasty because of (1) the more rigid structure of such lesions, (2) the potential for systemic embolization of valve debris, and (3) the potential for creating severe regurgitation. In 1985, however, balloon valvuloplasty was first applied to young adult patients with acquired (rheumatic) mitral stenosis, using a transseptal approach.[127]

TECHNIQUE. After puncture of the intraatrial septum with a needle and long sheath, a small balloon flotation catheter is advanced from the left atrium to the left ventricle and then across the aortic valve into the descending aorta (Fig. 40–21). An exchange-length (260 cm) guidewire is then positioned through this catheter to allow removal of the balloon flotation catheter and advancement of a small (8 mm) dilatation catheter for enlargement of the opening made in the intraatrial septum. This step is required to facilitate passage of the larger (23 to 25-mm diameter) valvuloplasty balloon through the intraatrial septum and across the stenotic mitral valve. Inflation of this larger balloon results in separation of the fused commissures analogous to the earlier surgical technique of closed or open mitral commissurotomy. Subsequent variations of the technique have included the use of two smaller (12 to 18 mm) balloon catheters, which can be advanced individually across the atrial septum and then inflated simultaneously within the mitral orifice.[128]

After these encouraging results in young adults with rheumatic mitral stenosis, similar procedures were attempted in adult patients with more rigid calcific lesions (p. 1034).[129, 130] Using this technique, it has been possible to achieve physiologically adequate enlargement of the mitral orifice area (from 0.9 to 1.5 cm^2).[131, 131a] There has been no significant overall increase in the degree of mitral regurgitation, and no evidence of systemic emboli in patients preselected for absence of left atrial thrombus. Approximately one-third of patients show evidence of a persistent small left-to-right shunt at the atrial level, owing to dilatation of the atrial septal puncture during passage of the valvuloplasty balloon. This minor complication should become less prevalent as improved technology permits the production of valvuloplasty balloons with smaller collapsed profiles. Similarly, balloon catheters capable of more rapid inflation and deflation will be of value in minimizing the period of systemic arterial hypotension which invariably results from transient occlusion of left ventricular inflow during balloon inflation. Early (6- to 12-month) follow-up studies have demonstrated preservation of the improved mitral orifice and similar physiological improvements (fall in filling pressures and pulmonary vascular resistance) to those seen after surgical correction of mitral stenosis. At this time, however, it is difficult to predict whether late (5 to 10-year) restenosis will be as evident after valvuloplasty as it is after surgical commissurotomy.

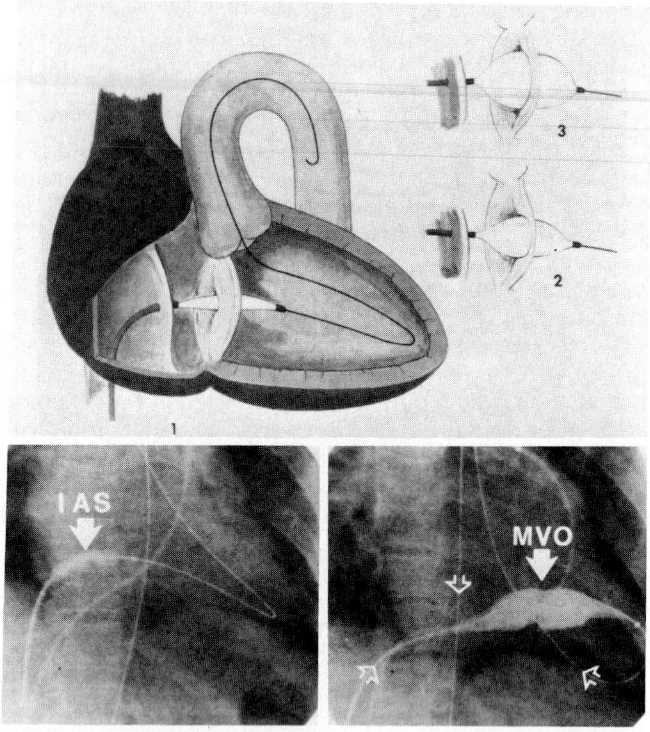

FIGURE 40–21. Mitral valvuloplasty. The top panel shows a schematic diagram of the transseptal approach to mitral valvuloplasty, while the bottom panel shows radiographic frames obtained during an actual procedure. After dilatation of the intraatrial septum by an 8-mm balloon catheter, a 25-mm dilatation catheter is advanced into the mitral valve orifice (MVO) and inflated. Note the appearance of a "waist" corresponding to the impression of the stenotic mitral orifice on the partially inflated dilatation catheter. This waist resolved with full inflation of the balloon, associated with an increase in mitral valve area from 0.9 to 1.6 cm^2. The path of the guidewire from right atrium to left atrium, to left ventricle, to descending aorta is shown by the open arrows.

AORTIC VALVULOPLASTY

With evident success of balloon valvuloplasty in the treatment of acquired mitral stenosis, attention has now been turned to dilatation of calcific aortic stenosis in the adult. This disorder is the principal indication for most of the approximately 20,000 aortic valve replacements performed each year in the United States. Narrowing of the valve orifice is due to a combination of an underlying congenital structural abnormality (i.e., a bicuspid aortic valve), commissural fusion, and stiffening of the leaflets by extensive calcium deposition.[132] Postmortem and intraoperative balloon dilatations have demonstrated both separation of fused commissures and increased leaflet pliability owing to microfractures and macrofractures through the calcium deposits. These findings suggested that percutaneous aortic valvuloplasty might be possible in advanced aortic stenosis. By the end of 1986 this procedure had been performed in several hundred patients, using principally the retrograde approach (Fig. 40–22).[132, 133]

TECHNIQUE. A conventional catheter is advanced retrogradely across the stenotic valve and into the left ventricle. Through this catheter an exchange-length guidewire is then positioned in the left ventricular apex and used to advance a series of balloon dilatation catheters (12, 15, 18, 20, and, occasionally, 23 mm in diameter) across the stenotic valve. Each balloon is inflated several times using dilute liquid radiographic contrast material. Maintenance of the balloon within the aortic orifice during inflation is difficult because of a tendency for the balloon to be ejected by the force of left ventricular contraction but is facilitated by the use of catheters with longer (i.e., 6-cm rather than 3-cm) balloon segments. A small number of aortic balloon valvuloplasty procedures have also been performed using the antegrade (transseptal) approach, similar to that used for mitral valvuloplasty.

RESULTS. The magnitude of orifice improvement during aortic valvuloplasty (0.6 to 1.0 cm^2) appears to be less than seen with mitral valvuloplasty, but this is usually adequate to produce marked improvement in clinical status, filling pressures, and left ventricular performance in patients with severe resting symptoms caused by critical aortic stenosis.[134, 134a] There have been no significant problems with systemic emboli or worsened aortic regurgitation, and balloon inflation seems to cause less hemodynamic compromise than it does during mitral dilatation because some left ventricular ejection can occur between the inflated balloon and the aortic commissures. While aortic balloon valvuloplasty is likely to play an increasing role in the treatment of patients whose advanced age or other medical problems place them at high risk for surgical aortic valve replacement, improvement in the orifice area seems to be less than that usually obtained with a valve replacement. Unless changes in technique achieve greater dilatation, valve replacement will probably still be preferred in young active patients with severe aortic stenosis.

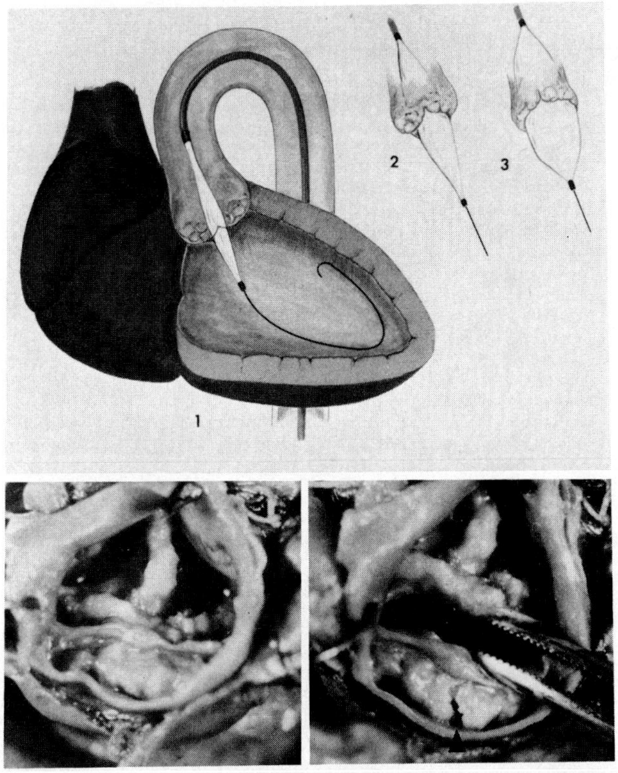

FIGURE 40–22. Aortic valvuloplasty. The top panel shows a schematic diagram of the retrograde approach to aortic valvuloplasty, while the bottom panels show the gross appearance of a stenotic aortic valve before (*left*) and after (*right*) postmortem balloon valvuloplasty. Note the fracture through the large calcified nodule (arrow) and the overall improvement in leaflet compliance.

OTHER INTERVENTIONAL CATHETERIZATION TECHNIQUES

Some of the earliest applications of interventional cardiology were in patients with congenital heart disease. In 1966 Rashkind described passage of a balloon catheter through a preexisting patent foramen ovale, followed by withdrawal of the inflated balloon to create a functional atrial septal defect in patients with transposition of the great arteries (p. 953), tricuspid atresia, pulmonic atresia, mitral atresia, total anomalous pulmonary venous return, or single ventricle.[135] Sixteen years later Park and coworkers modified this technique by use of a catheter with a surgical blade, which can be deployed in the left atrium after transseptal puncture and then used to incise the atrial septum during withdrawal.[136] The resulting atrial septal defect can then be enlarged using a balloon catheter as described by Rashkind. More recently, animal experimentation has suggested the potential use of laser ablation to create similar atrial septal defects.[137]

In addition to the creation or enlargement of vascular channels, pediatric cardiologists have also developed devices for closing aberrant vascular channels. Rashkind developed a "double disc" prosthesis which can be passed across an unwanted atrial septal defect or patent ductus arteriosis (Fig. 40–23).[135, 138] The first disc is deployed on the far side of the defect and then held in place by three spring struts, as the remaining disc and struts are pulled back across the defect and deployed on its near side. The result is sealing of the defect between two layers of prosthetic material.

Methods have also been developed for preoperative closure of unwanted systemic-pulmonary collateral vessels in patients undergoing correction of tetralogy of Fallot, using preformed steel coils embolized into the unwanted vessel through a catheter delivery system. This approach—similar to that used by vascular radiologists to treat arteriovenous malformations or actively bleeding vessels in other beds—leads to occlusion of the target vessel by local thrombosis.

SUMMARY

After the first tentative exploration of mechanical dilatation in the peripheral arterial circulation, the past decade has seen the explosive growth of interventional techniques for the treatment of a number of common cardiovascular diseases. Of these techniques, balloon dilatation is the most highly developed. It provides a safe and effective alternative to bypass surgery in up to one-half of patients requiring revascularization of coronary, renal, or peripheral artery lesions. Extension of this technique to the cerebral circulation and to valvular stenosis is in its infancy but promises to make inroads into current surgical practice. Other interventional techniques, such as the use of mechanical cut-and-retrieve, thermal, or direct laser devices,

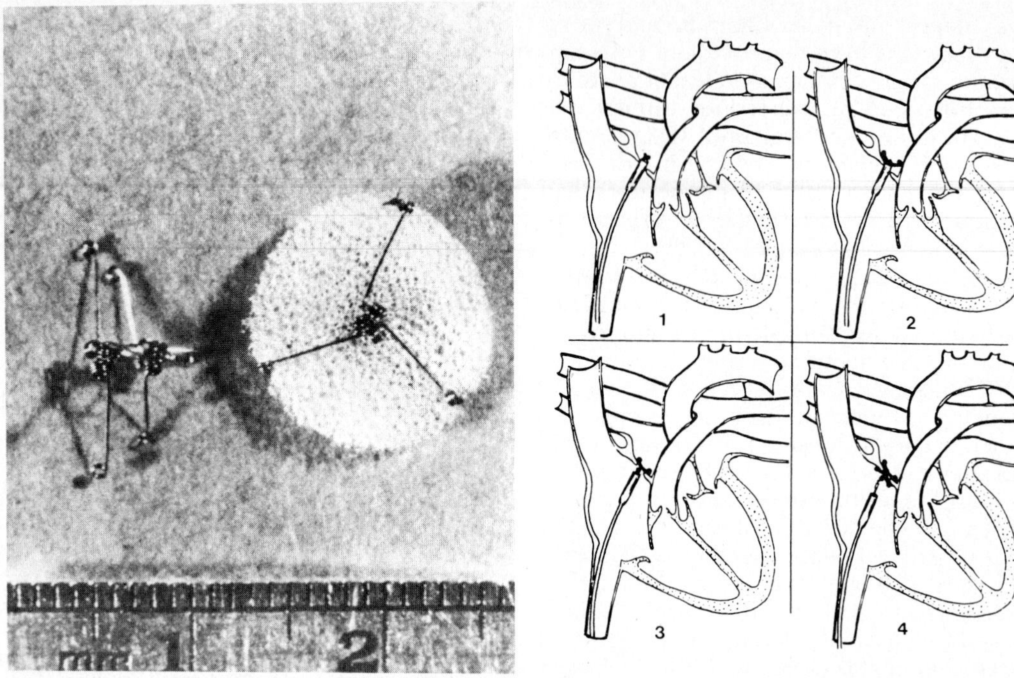

FIGURE 40–23. Closure of an atrial septal defect using a double-disc prosthesis. The left panel shows the spring skeleton of the prosthesis, as well as an enface view of the spring struts covered with prosthetic material. The diagram at right shows the placement of this device: the device is loaded into a delivery catheter in a collapsed configuration. The catheter is passed across the atrial septal defect (*panel 1*) and the distal struts are deployed (*panel 2*). The delivery catheter is withdrawn slightly, so that the second set of struts can be deployed on the right atrial side of the defect (*panel 3*). The double-disc prosthesis is then detached from the delivery system (*panel 4*) and left in place as the delivery catheter is withdrawn. (From Rashkind, W. J.: Transcatheter treatment of congenital heart disease. Circulation 67:711, 1983, by permission of the American Heart Association, Inc.)

have undergone only preliminary testing but may enhance one or more existing applications or create entirely new applications for interventional cardiology.

At a time of rising health care costs and an aging population, these interventional techniques offer the chance of equivalent symptomatic improvement with less discomfort, disability, and expense than conventional surgery. As with all new techniques, however, careful validation of their utility in comparison with existing medical and surgical techniques will be necessary in order to insure their optimal use in patient care.

REFERENCES

TREATMENT OF VASCULAR STENOSIS

1. Dotter, C. T., and Judkins, M. P.: Transluminal treatment of arteriosclerotic obstruction: Description of a new technique and a preliminary report of its application. Circulation *30*:654, 1964.
2. Dotter, C. T., Rosch, J., and Judkins, M. P.: Transluminal dilatation of atherosclerotic stenosis. Surg. Gynecol. Obstet. *127*:794, 1968.
3. Dotter, C. T.: Transluminal angioplasty: A long view. Radiology *135*:561, 1980.
4. Zeitler, E., Schoop, W., and Zahnow, W.: The treatment of occlusive arterial disease by transluminal catheter angioplasty. Radiology *99*:19, 1971.
5. Gruentzig, A., and Kumpe, D. A.: Technique of percutaneous transluminal angioplasty with the Gruentzig balloon catheter. Am. J. Radiol. *132*:547, 1979.
6. Gruentzig, A., Kuhlmann, U., Vetter, W., Luetof, U., Meier, B. and Siegenthaler, W.: Treatment of renovascular hypertension with percutaneous transluminal dilatation of a renal-artery stenosis. Lancet *1*:801, 1978.
7. Gruentzig, A. R., Senning, A., and Siegenthaler, W. E.: Non-operative dilatation of coronary artery stenosis—percutaneous transluminal coronary angioplasty. N. Engl. J. Med. *301*:61, 1979.
8. Kent, K. M., Bentivoglio, L. G., Block, P. C., et al.: Percutaneous transluminal coronary angioplasty: Report from the registry of the National Heart, Lung, and Blood Institute. Am. J. Cardiol. *49*:2011, 1982.
9. Kent, K. M., Mullin, S. M., and Passamani, E. R. (eds.): Proceedings of the National Heart, Lung, and Blood Institute workshop on the outcome of percutaneous transluminal angioplasty (June 7-8, 1983). Am. J. Cardiol. *53*:1C, 1984.
10. Baim, D. S., and Faxon, D. P.: Coronary angioplasty. *In* Grossman, W. (ed.): Cardiac Catheterization and Angiography. 3rd ed. Philadelphia, Lea and Febiger, 1986.
11. Topol, E. J., Myler, R. K., and Stertzer, S. H.: Selection of dilatation hardware for PTCA—1985. Cathet. Cardiovasc. Diagn. *11*:629, 1985.
12. Simpson, J. B., Baim, D. S., Robert, E. W., and Harrison, D. C.: A new catheter system for coronary angioplasty. Am. J. Cardiol. *49*:1216, 1982.
13. Anderson, H. V., Roubin, G. S., Leimgruber, P. P., Douglas, J. S., King, S. B., and Gruentzig, A. R.: Primary angiographic success rates of percutaneous transluminal coronary angioplasty. Am. J. Cardiol. *56*:712, 1985.
14. Dervan, J. P., McKay, R. G., and Baim, D. S.: The use of an exchange wire in coronary angioplasty. Cathet. Cardiovasc. Diagn. *11*:207, 1985.
15. Abele, J.: Balloon catheters and transluminal dilatation: Technical considerations. Am. J. Radiol. *135*:901, 1980.
16. Detre, K., Costigan, T., Kelsey, S., et al.: PTCA in 1985: The NHLBI Resistry. (Abs.) J. Am. Coll. Cardiol. *9*:19A, 1987.
17. Hirzel, H. O., Eichhorn, P., Kappenberger, L., Gander, M. P., Schlumpf, M., and Gruentzig, A. R.: Percutaneous transluminal coronary angioplasty: Late results at 5 years following intervention. Am. Heart J. *109*:575, 1985.
18. Libow, M., Gruentzig, A. R., and Greene, L.: Percutaneous transluminal coronary angioplasty. Curr. Prob. Cardiol. *1*:3, 1985.
19. Barbash, G. I., Rabkin, M. T., Kane, N. M., and Baim, D. S.: Coronary angioplasty under the prospective payment system: The need for a severity-adjusted payment scheme. J. Am. Coll. Cardiol. *8*:784, 1986.
20. Meier, B., Gruentzig, A. R., King, S. B., Douglas, J. S., Hollman, J., Ischinger, T., Aueron, F., and Galan, K.: Risk of side branch occlusion during coronary angioplasty. Am. J. Cardiol. *53*:10, 1984.
21. Meier, B.: Kissing balloon coronary angioplasty. Am. J. Cardiol. *54*:918, 1984.
21a. Melchior, J-P., Meier, B., Urban, P., Finci, L., Steffenino, G., Noble, J., and Rutishauser, W.: Percutaneous transluminal coronary angioplasty for chronic total coronary arterial occlusion. Am. J. Cardiol. *59*:535, 1987.
22. Oesterle, S. N., McAuley, B. J., Buchbinder, M., and Simpson, J. B.: Angioplasty at coronary bifurcations: Single guide, two-wire technique. Cathet. Cardiovasc. Diagn. *12*:57, 1986.
23. Dervan, J. P., Baim, D. S., Cherniles, J., and Grossman, W.: Transluminal angioplasty of occluded coronary arteries: Use of a movable guide wire system. Circulation *68*:776, 1983.
24. Holmes, D. R., Vlietstra, R. E., Reeder, G. S., Bresnahan, J. F., Smith, H. C., Bove, A. A., and Schaff, H. V.: Angioplasty in total coronary artery occlusion. J. Am. Coll. Cardiol. *3*:845, 1984.
25. Kimbiris, D., Iskandrian, A., Saras, H., Goel, I., Bemis, C., Segal, B. L., and Mundth, E.: Rapid progression of coronary stenosis in patients with unstable angina pectoris selected for coronary angioplasty. Cathet. Cardiovasc. Diagn. *10*:101, 1984.
26. Serruys, P. W., Umans, V., Hendrickx, G. R., Van Brand, M. V., DeFeyter, P. J., Wijns, W., Jaski, B., and Hugenholtz, P.G.: Elective PTCA of totally occluded coronary arteries not associated with acute myocardial infarction; short-term and long-term results. Eur. Heart J. *6*:2, 1985.
27. Kereiakes, D. J., Selmon, M. R., McAuley, B. J., McAuley, D. B., Sheehan, D. J., and Simpson, J. B.: Angioplasty of total coronary occlusion: Experience in 76 consecutive patients. J. Am. Coll. Cardiol. *6*:526, 1985.
28. Safian, R. D., Snyder, L. D., Snyder, B. A., McKay, R. G., Lorell, B. H., Aroesty, J. M., Bradley, A. B., Monrad, E. S., and Baim, D. S.: Long-term results and follow-up of coronary angioplasty of totally occluded coronary arteries. Circulation 72:(Suppl III)141, 1985.

29. Hartzler, G. O.: Percutaneous transluminal coronary angioplasty in multivessel disease. Cathet. Cardiovasc. Diagn. *9*:537, 1983.
30. Vlietstra, R. E., Holmes, D. R., Reeder, G. S., Mock, M. B., Smith, H. C., Bove, A. A., Bresnahan, J. F., and Piehler, J. M.: Balloon angioplasty in multivessel coronary artery disease. Mayo Clin. Proc. *58*:563, 1983.
31. Cowley, M. J., Vetrovec, G. W., DiSciascio, G., Lewis, S. A., Hirsh, P. D., and Wolfgang, T. C.: Coronary angioplasty in multiple vessels: Short-term outcome and long-term results. Circulation *72*:1314, 1985.
32. Jones, E. L., Craver, J. M., Guyton, R. A., Bone, D. K., Hatcher, C. R., and Riechwald, N.: Importance of complete revascularization in performance of the coronary bypass operation. Am. J. Cardiol. *51*:7, 1983.
33. Mabin, T. A., Holmes, D. R., Smith, H. C., Vlietstra, R. E., Reeder, G. S., Bresnehan, J. F., Bove, A. A., Hammes, L. N., Elveback, L. R., and Orszulak, T. A.: Follow-up clinical results in patients undergoing percutaneous transluminal coronary angioplasty. Circulation *71*:754, 1985.
34. Vandormael, M. G., Chaitman, B. R., Ischinger, T., Aker, U. T., Harper, M., Hernandez, J., Deligonul, U., and Kennedy, H. L.: Immediate and short-term benefit of multilesion coronary angioplasty: Influence of degree of revascularization. J. Am. Coll. Cardiol. *6*:983, 1985.
35. Mata, L. A., Bosch, X., David, P. R., Rapold, H. J., Corcos, T. and Bourassa, M. G.: Clinical and angiographic assessment 6 months after double vessel percutaneous coronary angioplasty. J. Am. Coll. Cardiol. *6*:1239, 1985.
36. Wohlgelernter, D., Cleman, M., Highman, H. A., and Zaret, B. L.: Percutaneous transluminal coronary angioplasty of the "culprit lesion" for the management of unstable angina pectoris in patients with multivessel coronary artery disease. Am. J. Cardiol. *58*:460, 1986.
37. Ischinger, T., Gruentzig, A. R., Hollman, J., King, S., Douglas, J., Meier, B., Bradford, J., and Tankersley, R.: Should coronary arteries with less than 60% diameter stenosis be treated by angioplasty? Circulation *68*:148, 1983.
38. Mock, M. B., Reeder, G. S., Schaff, H. V., Holmes, D. R., Vlietstra, R. E., Smith, H. C., and Gersh, B. J.: Percutaneous transluminal coronary angioplasty versus coronary artery bypass. Isn't it time for a randomized trial? N. Engl. J. Med. *312*:916, 1985.
39. DeFeyter, P. J., Serruys, P. W., Van den Brand, M., Balakumaran, K., Mochtar, B., Soward, A. L., Arnold, A.E.R., and Hugenholtz, P. G.: Emergency coronary angioplasty in refractory unstable angina. N. Engl. J. Med. *313*:342, 1985.
40. Feldman, R. L., Macdonald, R. G., Hill, J. A., Conti, R., Pepine, C. J., Carmichael, M. G., Knauff, D. G., and Alexander, J. A.: Coronary angioplasty at the time of initial cardiac catheterization. Cathet. Cardiovasc. Diagn. *12*:219, 1986.
41. Braunwald, E.: The aggressive treatment of acute myocardial infarction. Circulation *71*:1087, 1985.
42. Meyer, J., Merx, W., Schmitz, H., Erbel, R., Kiesslich, T., Dorr, R., Lambertz, H., Bethge, C., Krebs, W., Bardos, P., Minale, C., Messmer, B. J., and Effert, S.: Percutaneous transluminal coronary angioplasty immediately after intracoronary streptolysis of transmural myocardial infarction. Circulation *66*:905, 1982.
43. Hartzler, G. O., Rutherford, B. D., McConahay, D. R., Johnson, W. L., McCallister, B. D., Gura, G. A., Conn, R. C., and Crockett, J. E.: Percutaneous transluminal coronary angioplasty with and without thrombolytic therapy for treatment of acute myocardial infarction. Am. Heart J. *106*:965, 1983.
44. O'Neill, W., Timmis, G. C., Bourdillon, P. D., Lai, P., Ganghadarhan, V., Walton, J., Ramos, R., Laufer, N., Gordon, S., Schork, A., and Pitt, B.: A prospective randomized clinical trial of intracoronary streptokinase versus coronary angioplasty for acute myocardial infarction. N. Engl. J. Med. *314*:812, 1986.
45. Fung, A. Y., Lai, P., Juni, J. E., Bourdillon, P. D., Walton, J. A., Laufer, N., Buda, A. J., Pitt, B., and O'Neill, W.: Prevention of subsequent exercise-induced periinfarct ischemia by emergency coronary angioplasty in acute myocardial infarction: Comparison with intracoronary streptokinase. J. Am. Coll. Cardiol. 8:496, 1986.
46. O'Neill, W., Erbel, R., Laufer, N., Walton, J., Bates, E., Topol, E., Bourdillon, P. D., Meyer, J., and Pitt, B.: Coronary angioplasty therapy of cardiogenic shock complicating acute myocardial infarction. Circulation 72(Suppl III):309, 1985.
47. Douglas, J. S., Gruentzig, A. R., King, S. B., Hollman, J., Ischinger, T., Meier, B., Craver, J. M., Jones, E. L., Waller, J. L., Bone, D. K., and Guyton, R.: Percutaneous transluminal coronary angioplasty in patients with prior coronary bypass surgery. J. Am. Coll. Cardiol. 2:745, 1983.
48. Block, P. C., Cowley, M., Kaltenbach, M., Kent, K. M., and Simpson, J.: Percutaneous angioplasty of stenoses of bypass grafts or of bypass graft anastomotic sites. Am. J. Cardiol. *53*:666, 1984.
49. Waller, B. F., Rothbaum, D. A., Gorfinkel, H. J., Ulbright, T. M., Linnemeir, T. J., and Berger, S. M.: Morphologic observations after percutaneous transluminal balloon angioplasty of early and late aortocoronary saphenous vein bypass grafts. J. Am. Coll. Cardiol. *4*:784, 1984.
50. Dorros, G., and Janke, L.: Percutaneous transluminal coronary angioplasty in patients over the age of 70 years. Cathet. Cardiovasc. Diagn. *12*:223, 1986.
51. Reeder, G. S., Krishan, I., Nobrega, F. T., Naessens, J., Kelly, M., Christianson, J. B., and McAfee, M. K.: Is percutaneous coronary angioplasty less expensive than bypass surgery? N. Engl. J. Med. *311*:1157, 1984.
52. Wilson, J. M., Dunn, E. J., Wright, C. B., Bailey, W. W., Callard, G. M., Melvin, D. B., Mitts, D. L., Will, R. J., and Flege, J. B.: The cost of simultaneous surgical standby for percutaneous transluminal coronary angioplasty. J. Thorac. Cardiovasc. Surg. *91*:362, 1986.
53. Roubin, G. S., Douglas, J. S., and King, S. B.: Percutaneous coronary angioplasty: Influence of operator experience on results. Am. J. Cardiol. *57*:873, 1986.
54. Weaver, W., Myler, R. K., Sheldon, W. E., Huston, J. T., Judkins, M. P., and the Laboratory Standard Committee: Guidelines for physician performance of percutaneous transluminal coronary angioplasty. Cathet. Cardiovasc. Diagn. *11*:109, 1985.
55. Scanlon, P. J.: The training for and practice of percutaneous transluminal coronary angioplasty: Results of two surveys. Cathet. Cardiovasc. Diagn. *11*:561, 1985.
56. Harston, W. E., Tilley, S., Rodeheffer, R., Forman, M. B., and Perry, J. M.: Safety and success of the beginning percutaneous transluminal coronary angioplasty program using the steerable guidewire system. Am. J. Cardiol. *57*:717, 1986.
57. Hartzler, G. O.: Percutaneous transluminal coronary angioplasty: View of a single relatively high frequency operator. Am. J. Cardiol. *57*:869, 1986.
58. Sanborn, T. A., Faxon, D. P., Haudenschild, C., Gottsman, S. B., and Ryan, T. J.: The mechanism of transluminal angioplasty: Evidence for formation of aneurysms in experimental atherosclerosis. Circulation *68*:1136, 1983.
59. Block, P. C., Baughman, K. L., Pasternak, R. C., and Fallon, J. T.: Transluminal angioplasty: Correlation of morphologic and angiographic findings in an experimental model. Circulation *61*:778, 1980.
60. Castaneda-Zuniga, W. R., Formanek, A., Tadavarthy, M., Vlodaver, Z., Edwards, J. E., Zollikofer, C., and Amplatz, K.: The mechanism of balloon angioplasty. Radiology *135*:565, 1980.
61. Sanborn, T. A., Faxon, D. P., Waugh, D., Small, D. M., Haudenschild, C., Gottsman, S. B., and Ryan, T. J.: Transluminal angioplasty in experimental atherosclerosis: Analysis for embolization using an in vivo perfusion system. Circulation *66*:917, 1982.
62. Saffitz, J. E., Rose, T. E., Oaks, J. B., and Roberts, W. C.: Coronary artery rupture during coronary angioplasty. Am. J. Cardiol. *51*:902, 1983.
63. Saner, H. E., Gobel, F. L., Salomonowitz, E., Erlein, D. A., and Edwards, J. E.: The disease-free wall in coronary atherosclerosis: Its relation to degree of obstruction. J. Am. Coll. Cardiol. *6*:1096, 1985.
64. Kaltenbach, M., Beyer, J., Walter, S., Klepzig, H., and Schmidts, L.: Prolonged application of pressure in transluminal angioplasty. Cathet. Cardiovasc. Diagn. *10*:213, 1984.
65. Serruys, P. W., Wijns, W., van den Brand, M., Meij, S., Slager, C., Schuurbiers, J.C.H., Hugenholtz, P. G., and Brower, R. W.: Left ventricular performance, regional blood flow and lactate metabolism during transluminal angioplasty. Circulation *70*:25, 1984.
66. Serruys, P. W., Reiber, J. H. C., Wijns, W., van den Brand, M., Kooijman, C. J., tenKaten, H. J., and Hugenholtz, P. G.: Assessment of percutaneous transluminal coronary angioplasty by quantitative coronary angiography: Diameter versus videodensitometric area measurements. Am. J. Cardiol. *54*:482, 1984.
67. Anderson, H. V., Roubin, G. S., Leimgruber, P. P., Cox, W. R., Douglas, J. S., King, S. B., and Gruentzig, A. R.: Measurement of transstenotic pressure gradient during percutaneous transluminal coronary angioplasty. Circulation *73*:1223, 1986.
68. Holmes, D. R., Vlietstra, R. E., Mock, M. B., Reeder, G. S., Smith, H. C., Bove, A. A., Bresnahan, J. F., Piehler, S. M., Schaff, H., and Orszulak, T. A.: Angiographic changes produced by percutaneous transluminal coronary angioplasty. Am. J. Cardiol. *51*:676, 1983.
69. Aueron, F., and Gruentzig, A.: Significance of chest pain during percutaneous transluminal coronary angioplasty. Am. Heart J. *107*:578, 1984.
70. Meier, B., Gruentzig, A. R., Hollman, J., Ischinger, T., and Bradford, J. M.: Does length or eccentricity of coronary stenoses influence the outcome of transluminal dilatation? Circulation *67*:497, 1983.
71. Dorros, G., Cowley, M. J., Simpson, J., et al.: Percutaneous transluminal coronary angioplasty: Report of complications from the National Heart, Lung, and Blood Institute PTCA Registry. Circulation *67*:723, 1983.
72. Hollman, J., Gruentzig, A. R., Douglas, J. S., King, S. B., Ischinger, T., and Meier, B.: Acute occlusion after percutaneous transluminal angioplasty—new approach. Circulation *68*:725, 1983.
73. Murphy, D. A., Craver, J. M., Jones, E. L., Gruentzig, A. R., King, S. B., and Hatcher, C. R.: Surgical revascularization following unsuccessful percutaneous transluminal coronary angioplasty. J. Thorac. Cardiovasc. Surg. *84*:342, 1982.
74. Kabbani, S. S., Bashour, T. T., Jones, R., Myler, R. K., Hanna, E. S., Ellerston, D. G., Bronstein, M., and McBride, P.: Surgical experience following transluminal coronary angioplasty. Tex. Heart Inst. J. *11*:112, 1984.
75. Bredlau, C. E., Roubin, G. S., Leimgruber, P. P., Douglas, J. S., King, S. B., and Gruentzig, A. R.: In-hospital morbidity and mortality in elective coronary angioplasty. Circulation *72*:1044, 1985.
76. Hinohara, T., Simpson, J. B., Phillips, H. R., Behar, V. S., Peter, R. H., Kong, Y., Carlson, E. B., and Stack, R. S.: Transluminal catheter reperfusion: A new technique to reestablish blood flow after coronary occlusion during percutaneous transluminal coronary angioplasty. Am. J. Cardiol. *57*:684, 1986.
77. Demer, L. L., Jain, A., Hartley, C. J., Raizner, A. E., Lewis, J. M., and Roberts, R.: Quantitative assessment of lesion dilatation during coronary angioplasty in man. J. Am. Coll. Cardiol. *7*(Abs.):64A, 1986.
78. Hiehle, J. F., Bourgelais, D.B.C., Shapshay, S., Schoen, F. S., Kim, D., and Spears, R.: Nd-YAF laser fusion of human atherosclerotic plaque—arterial wall separations in vitro. Am. J. Cardiol. *56*:953, 1985.
79. Sigwart, U., Puel, J., Mirkovitch, V., Joffre, F., and Kappenberger, L.: Intravascular stents to prevent occlusion and restenosis after transluminal angioplasty. N. Engl. J. Med. *316*:701, 1987.
80. Williams, D. O., Riley, R. S., Singh, A. K., and Most, A. S.: Restoration of normal coronary hemodynamics and myocardial metabolism after percutaneous transluminal coronary angioplasty. Circulation *62*:653, 1980.
81. Hirzel, H. O., Neusch, K., Gruentzig, A. R., and Luetolf, U. M.: Short- and long-term changes in myocardial perfusion after percutaneous transluminal coronary angioplasty assessed by thallium-201 exercise scintigraphy. Circulation *63*:1001, 1981.

82. Kent, K. M., Bonow, R. O., Rosing, D. R., Ewels, C. J., Lipson, L. C., McIntosh, C. L., Bacharach, S., Green, M., and Epstein, S. E.: Improved myocardial function during exercise after successful percutaneous transluminal coronary angioplasty. N. Engl J. Med. *306*:441, 1982.
83. O'Neill, W. W., Walton, J. A., Bates, E. R., Colfer, H. T., Aueron, F. M., LeFree, M. T., Pitt, B., and Vogel, R. A.: Criteria for successful coronary angioplasty as assessed by alterations in coronary vasodilatory reserve. J. Am. Coll. Cardiol. *3*:1382, 1984.
84. Meier, B., Gruentzig, A. R., Siegenthaler, W. E., and Schlumpf, M.: Long-term exercise performance after percutaneous transluminal coronary angioplasty and coronary artery bypass grafting. Circulation *68*:796, 1983.
85. Gruentzig, A. R., King, S. B., III, Schlumpf, M., and Siegenthaler, W.: Long-term follow-up after percutaneous transluminal coronary angioplasty. N. Engl. J. Med. *316*:1127, 1987.
86. Leimgruber, P. P., Roubin, G. S., Hollman, J., Cotsonis, G. A., Meier, B., Douglas, J. S., King, S. B., and Gruentzig, A. R.: Restenosis after successful coronary angioplasty in patients with single vessel disease. Circulation *73*:710, 1986.
87. Hollman, J., Austin, G. E., Gruentzig, A. R., Douglas, J. S., and King, S. B.: Coronary artery spasm at the site of angioplasty in the first two months after successful percutaneous transluminal coronary angioplasty. J. Am. Coll. Cardiol. *2*:1039, 1983.
88. Corcos, T., David, P. R., Bourassa, M. G., Val, P. G., Robert, J., Mata, L. A., and Waters, D. D.: Percutaneous transluminal coronary angioplasty for the treatment of variant angina. J. Am. Coll. Cardiol. *5*:1046, 1985.
89. Bertrand, M. E., LaBlanche, J. M., Thieuleux, F. A., Fourrier, J. L., Trainsel, G., and Asseman, P.: Comparative results of percutaneous transluminal coronary angioplasty in patients with dynamic versus fixed coronary stenosis. J. Am. Coll. Cardiol. *8*:504, 1986.
90. Faxon, D. P., and Sanborn, T. A.: Restenosis following transluminal angioplasty in experimental atherosclerosis. Arteriosclerosis *4*:189, 1984.
91. Essed, C. E., van den Brand, M., and Becker, A. E.: Transluminal coronary angioplasty and early restenosis: Fibrocellular occlusion after wall laceration. Br. Heart J. *49*:393, 1983.
92. Castellot, J. J., Favreau, L. V., Karnovsky, M. J, and Rosenberg, R. D.: Inhibition of vascular smooth muscle cell growth by endothelial cell-derived heparin. J. Biol. Chem. 257:11256, 1982.
93. Meier, B., King, S. B., Gruentzig, A. R., Douglas, J. S., Hollman, J., Ischinger, T., Galan, K., and Tankersly, R.: Repeat coronary angioplasty. J. Am. Coll. Cardiol. *4*:463, 1984.
94. Simpson, J. B., Johnson, D. E., Tapliyal, H. V., Marks, D. S., and Braden, L. J.: Transluminal atherectomy: A new approach to the treatment of atherosclerotic vascular disease. Circulation 72(Suppl III):146, 1985.
95. Leyser, L. J., Bundy, M. A., Abreo, F., Hanley, H. G., Fadely, D., and Walker, J. M.: Evaluation of a coronary lysing system: Results of a preclinical safety and efficacy study. Cathet. Cardiovasc. Diagn. *12*:246, 1986.
96. Abela, G. S., Normann, S. J., Cohen, D. M., Franzini, D., Feldman, R. L., Crea, F., French, A., Pepine, C. J., and Conti, C. R.: Laser recanalization of occluded atherosclerotic arteries in vivo and in vitro. Circulation *71*:403, 1985.
97. Eldar, M., Battler, A., Neufeld, H. N., Gaton, E., Arieli, R., Akselrod, S., Levite, A., and Katzir, A.: Transluminal carbon dioxide-laser catheter angioplasty for dissolution of atherosclerotic plaques. J. Am. Coll. Cardiol. *3*:135, 1984.
98. Isner, J. M., Donaldson, R. F., Deckelbaum, L. I., Clarke, R. H., Laliberte, S. M., Ucci, A. A., Salem, D. N., and Konstam, M. A.: The excimer laser: Gross, light microscopic and ultrastructural analysis of potential advantages for use in laser therapy of cardiovascular disease. J. Am. Coll. Cardiol. *6*:1102, 1985.
99. Lee, G., Ikeda, R. M., Chan, M. C., Lee, M. H., Rink, J. L., Reis, R. L., Theis, J. H., Low, R., Bommer, W. J., Kung, A. H., Hanna, E. S., and Mason, D. T.: Limitations, risks and complications of laser recanalization: A cautious approach warranted. Am. J. Cardiol. *56*:181, 1985.
100. Choy, D.S.J., Stertzer, S. H., Myler, R. K., Marco, J. and Fournial, G.: Human coronary laser recanalization. Clin. Cardiol. 7:377, 1984.
101. Ginsburg, R., Wexler, L., Mitchell, R. S., and Profitt, D.: Percutaneous transluminal laser angioplasty for treatment of peripheral vascular disease. Clinical experience with 16 patients. Radiology *156*:619, 1985.
102. Murphy-Chutorian, D., Kosek, J., Mok, W., Quay, S., Huestis, W., Mehigan, J., Profitt, D., and Ginsburg, R.: Selective absorption of ultraviolet laser energy by human atherosclerotic plaque treated with tetracycline. Am. J. Cardiol. *55*:1293, 1985.
103. Spears, J. R., Shropshire, D., and Paulin, S.: Fluorescence of experimental atheromatous plaques with hematoporphyrin derivatives. J. Clin. Invest. *71*:395, 1983.
104. Sanborn, T. A., Faxon, D. P., Haudenschild, C. C., and Ryan, T. J.: Experimental angioplasty: Circumferential distribution of laser energy with a laser probe. J. Am. Coll. Cardiol. *5*:934, 1985.
105. Cumberland, D. C., Sanborn, T. A., Tayler, D. I., Moore, D. J., Welsh, C. L., Greenfield, A. J., Guben, J. K., and Ryan, T. J.: Percutaneous laser thermal angioplasty: Initial clinical results with a laser probe in total peripheral artery occlusions. Lancet 1:1457, 1986.
106. Sanborn, T. A., Faxon, D. P., Kellett, M. A., and Ryan, T. J.: Percutaneous coronary laser thermal angioplasty. J. Am. Coll. Cardiol. *8*:1437, 1986.
107. Spence, R. K., Freiman, D. B., Gatenby, R., Hobbs, C. L., Barker, C. F., Berkowitz, H. D., Roberts, B., McClean, G., Oleaga, J., and Ring, E. J.: Long-term results of transluminal angioplasty of the iliac and femoral arteries. Arch. Surg. *116*:1377, 1981.
108. Kadir, S., White, R. I., Kaufman, S. L., Barth, K. H., Williams, G. M., Burdick, J. F., O'Mara, C. S., Smith, G. W., Stonesifer, G. L., Ernst, C. B., and Minken, S. L.: Long-term results of aortoiliac angioplasty. Surgery *94*:10, 1983.
109. Gallino, A., Mahler, F., Probst, P., and Nachbur, B.: Percutaneous transluminal angioplasty of the arteries of the lower limbs: A 5-year follow-up. Circulation *70*:619, 1984.
110. Hewes, R. C., White, R. I., Murray, R. R., Kaufman, S. L., Chang, R., Kadir, S., Kinnison, M. L., Mitchell, S. E., and Auster, M.: Long-term results of superficial femoral artery angioplasty. Am. J. Radiol. *146*:1025, 1986.
111. Kinnison, M. L., White, R. I., Bowers, W. P., and Dunlap, E. D.: Cost incentives for peripheral angioplasty. Am. J. Radiol. *145*:1241, 1985.
112. Doubilet, P., and Abrams, H. L.: The cost of underutilization—percutaneous transluminal angioplasty for peripheral vascular disease. N. Engl. J. Med. *310*:95, 1984.
113. Sos, T. A., Pickering, T. G., Sniderman, K., Saddenki, S., Case, D. B., Silane, M. F., Vaughan, E. D., and Laragh, J. H.: Percutaneous transluminal renal angioplasty in renovascular hypertension due to atheroma or fibromuscular dysplasia. N. Engl. J. Med. *309*:274, 1983.
114. Miller, G. A., Ford, K. K., Braun, S. D., Newman, G. E., Moore, A. V., Malone, R., and Dunnick. N. R.: Percutaneous transluminal angioplasty vs. surgery for renovascular hypertension. Am. J. Radiol. *144*:447, 1985.
115. Motarjeme, A., Keifer, J. W., and Zuska, A. J.: Percutaneous transluminal angioplasty of the brachiocephalic arteries. Am. J. Neurol. Radiol. *3*:169, 1982.
116. Motarjeme, A., Keifer, J. W., and Zuska, A. J.: Percutaneous transluminal angioplasty of the vertebral arteries. Radiology *139*:715, 1981.
117. Tsai, F. Y., Matovich, V., Hieshima, G., Shah, D. C., Mehringer, C. M., Tiu, G., Higashida, R. and Pribam, H.F.W.: Percutaneous transluminal angioplasty of the carotid artery. Am. J. Neurol. Radiol. *7*:349, 1986.
118. Lock, J. E., Bass, J. L., Castaneda-Zuniga, W., Fuhrman, B. P., Rashkind, W. J., and Lucas, R. V.: Dilatation angioplasty of congenital or operative narrowings of venous channels. Circulation *70*:457, 1984.
119. Driscoll, D. J., Hesslein, P. S., and Mullins, C. E.: Congenital stenosis of individual pulmonary veins: Clinical spectrum and unsuccessful treatment by transvenous balloon dilation. Am. J. Cardiol. *49*:1767, 1982.
120. Lock, J. E., Castaneda-Zuniga, W. R., Fuhrman, B. P., and Bass, J. L.: Balloon dilatation of hypoplastic and stenotic pulmonary arteries. Circulation *67*:962, 1983.
121. Kan, J. S., White, R. I., Mitchell, S. E., Farmlett, E. J., Donahoo, J. S., and Gardner, T. J.: Treatment of restenosis of coarctation by percutaneous transluminal angioplasty. Circulation *68*:1087, 1983.
122. Lock, J. E., Bass, J. L., Amplatz, K., Fuhrman, B. P., and Castaneda-Zuniga, W.: Balloon angioplasty of aortic coarctations in infants and children. Circulation *68*:109, 1983.
123. Kan, J. S., White, R. I., Mitchell, S. E., and Gardner, T. J.: Percutaneous balloon valvuloplasty: A new method for treating congenital pulmonary valve stenosis. N. Engl. J. Med. *307*:540, 1982.
124. Kan, J. S., White, R. I., Mitchell, S. E., Anderson, J. H., and Gardner, T. J.: Percutaneous transluminal balloon valvuloplasty for pulmonary valve stenosis. Circulation *69*:554, 1984.
125. Walls, J. T., Lababidi, Z., Curtis, J. J., and Silver, D.: Assessment of percutaneous balloon pulmonary and aortic valvuloplasty. J. Thorac. Cardiovasc. Surg. *88*:352, 1984.
126. Lababidi, Z., Wu, J., and Walls, J. T.: Percutaneous balloon aortic valvuloplasty: Results in 23 patients. Am. J. Cardiol. 53:194, 1984.
127. Lock, J. E., Khalilullah, M., Shrivastava, S., Bahl, V., and Keane, J. F.: Percutaneous catheter commissurotomy in rheumatic mitral stenosis. N. Engl. J. Med. *313*:1515, 1985.
128. Zaibag, M. A., Kasab, S. A., Ribeiro, P. A., and Al Fagih, M. R.: Percutaneous double-balloon mitral valvotomy for rheumatic mitral stenosis. Lancet 1:757, 1986.
129. McKay, R. G., Lock, J. E., Keane, J. F., Safian, R. D., Aroesty, J. M., and Grossman, W.: Percutaneous mitral valvuloplasty in an adult patient with calcific rheumatic mitral stenosis. J. Am. Coll. Cardiol. *7*:1410, 1986.
130. Block, P. C., Palacios, I. F., Jacobs, M. L., and Fallon, J. T.: Mechanism of percutaneous mitral valvotomy. Am. J. Cardiol. *59*:178, 1987.
131. McKay, R. G., Lock, J. E., Safian, R. D., Come, P. C., Diver, D. J., Baim, D. S., Berman, A. D., Warren, S. E., Mandell, V. E., Royal, H. D., and Grossman, W.: Balloon dilatation of mitral stenosis in adult patients: Postmortem and percutaneous mitral valvuloplasty studies. J. Am. Coll. Cardiol. *9*:723, 1987.
132. Rahimtoola, S. H.: Catheter balloon valvuloplasty of aortic and mitral valve stenosis in adults. Circulation *75*:895, 1987.
133. Cribier, A., Savin, T., Berland, J., Rocha, P., Mechmeche, R., Saoudi, N., Behar, P., and Letac, B.: Percutaneous transluminal balloon valvuloplasty of adult aortic stenosis: Report of 92 cases. J. Am. Coll. Cardiol. *9*:381, 1987.
134. McKay, R. G., Safian, R. D., Lock, J. E., Diver, D. J., Berman, A. D., Warren, S. E., Come, P. C., Baim, D. S., Mandell, V. E., Royal, H. D., and Grossman, W.: Assessment of left ventricular and aortic valve function after aortic balloon valvuloplasty in adult patients with critical aortic stenosis. Circulation 75:192, 1987.
135. Rashkind, W. J.: Transcatheter treatment of congenital heart disease. Circulation *67*:711, 1983.
136. Park, S. C., Neches, W. H., Mullins, C. E., Girod, D. A., Olley, P. M., Falkowski, G., Garibjan, V. A., Mathews, R. A., Fricker, F. J., Beerman, L. B., Lenox, C. C., and Zuberbuhler, J. R.: Blade atrial septostomy: Collaborative study. Circulation *66*:258, 1982.
137. Bommer, W. J., Lee, G., Riemenschneider, T. A., Ikeda, R. M., Rebeck, K., Stobe, D., Ogata, C., Theis, J. H., Reis, R. L., and Mason, D. T.: Laser atrial septostomy. Am. Heart J. *106*:1152, 1983.
138. Lock, J. E., Cockerham, J. T., Keane, J. F., Finley, J. P., Wakely, P. E., Jr., and Fellows, K. E.: Transcatheter umbrella closure of congenital heart defects. Circulation *75*:593, 1987.

41 REHABILITATION OF PATIENTS WITH CORONARY ARTERY DISEASE

by ALBERT OBERMAN, M.D.

Through a series of transitional stages, cardiac rehabilitation enables patients to attain the highest level of performance compatible with the extent of their disease. A comprehensive program involves physical fitness, secondary prevention, psychosocial adaptations, and vocational counseling. The ultimate goal of these activities is to allow the patient with coronary artery disease to regain or even exceed former physical capabilities and general level of well-being. Techniques for cardiac rehabilitation evolved from the work evaluation units of the 1950's.[1, 2] Since then the scope of rehabilitation has been expanded to encompass most aspects of quality of life, and the domain has been broadened to include nearly all patients with cardiovascular disease, especially those who have had therapeutic procedures—coronary artery bypass grafting,[3–5] heart valve replacement,[6, 7] coronary angioplasty,[7] aneurysmectomy,[8] and cardiac transplantation.[9, 10]

The greatest losses to society, both direct and indirect, can be attributed to diseases of the circulatory system.[11] Coronary artery disease, the most prominent cause of premature disability and death, accounts for 19 per cent of the disability allowances paid by the Social Security Administration.[12] Despite therapeutic advances, return-to-work rates have diminished since 1970 for patients with uncomplicated myocardial infarction.[13] In 1970, 85 to 89 per cent of previously employed patients less than 55 years of age returned to work, but only 79 to 84 per cent did so in 1979. Referral to special work evaluation units can return even those with complex medical, psychological, and vocational problems to nearly normal levels of work and leisure activities.[14] The progressive aging of the population accompanied by rising costs of social services will accelerate the need for comprehensive rehabilitation services to maintain the work force.[15]

However, return to work is but one of several potential benefits arising from rehabilitative efforts. Equally important outcomes expected from a successful program include capability of attaining near maximal performance, favorable physiological adaptations, relief of symptoms, a sense of well-being, and the preservation of the patient's role in the family and society. Less certain is whether the exercise component in combination with other elements of a rehabilitation program can retard atherosclerosis, protect against further cardiac complications, and prolong life.

COMPONENTS OF A REHABILITATION PROGRAM

EXERCISE TRAINING

INDICATIONS. Exercise, a key element in the rehabilitative process, can produce improved musculoskeletal fitness, multiple training adaptations, and salutary psychological and attitudinal changes.

Musculoskeletal Disability. Reduced physical activity and prolonged bed rest lead to reduction in skeletal muscle mass, strength, and joint flexibility. Patients who have had surgical procedures are especially vulnerable to musculoskeletal problems because of operative manipulation of the sternum and chest wall. Musculoskeletal problems affect the morale of the patient and, if not managed properly, lead to chronic disability. Appropriate exercise in combination with early mobilization counters these adverse influences by restoring strength, flexibility, and joint mobility.

Improved Functional Capacity. Most importantly, exercise training leads to improved functional work capacity. Properly designed physical training programs increase maximal oxygen uptake (VO_{2max}) from 9 to 56 per cent, depending upon the extent of the training program and patient characteristics.[16–18] Exercise involving large muscle groups at sufficient intensity and duration enhances oxygen transport within the circulatory system and oxidative metabolic capacity of skeletal muscles, resulting in greater exercise tolerance.[16, 19, 20] Those patients with initially low capacity but without left ventricular dysfunction tend to show the greatest improvement.

Because $\dot{V}O_{2max}$ is greater after training, the fraction of $\dot{V}O_{2max}$ required for a given submaximal task is reduced. Because of this decreased relative workload, the metabolic and circulatory demands are reduced for trained patients, even those with impaired left ventricular function.[19, 21, 22] However, patients with compromised ventricular function have already realized much of their adaptive capacity, by widening of the A-$\dot{V}O_2$ difference and shunting of blood to working tissues.[16] Ordinarily, the threshold for symptoms becomes manifest at about 75 per cent of functional aerobic capacity so that exertion below this threshold should not cause severe dyspnea.[23] Therefore, even a modest increment in physical capacity may permit a marked improvement in the quality of life by allowing stair climbing, shopping, and other daily activities.

From mild efforts such as walking, training may result because of improved work efficiency or habituation rather than increased aerobic capacity alone (Fig. 41–1).[24] Another explanation for training benefits relates to the anaerobic threshold, also termed the *lactate*[25] or *ventilatory*[26] *threshold.* Sustained physical performance results in lactate accumulation and fatigue in working muscles associated with breathlessness whenever oxygen utilization exceeds oxygen availability. There is some evidence that patients adapt to training by increasing the lactate threshold so that they are able to maintain sustained physical activity close to their maximal oxygen uptake.[25] This could explain the ability of patients with coronary artery disease to maintain a pace greater than anticipated from their $\dot{V}O_{2max}$. But other investigators believe that the lactate threshold cannot be altered by training.[26] Not infrequently, patients are limited by leg fatigue, claudication, or angina pectoris rather than by aerobic capacity.[27, 28] Although data are sparse, training over a period of 3 or more months, when conducted to the point of leg intolerance, appears to increase the ability to extend walking distance.[28, 29]

Psychosocial Adaptations. Low-level exercise appears sufficient to stimulate positive psychosocial changes among men who have had myocardial infarctions.[30] Physical conditioning provides a means for allaying anxiety and preventing depression, conditions not infrequently encountered in such patients. Exercise offers a positive and constructive approach by helping to encourage participation in new activities and dispelling fears associated with physical exertion.[31–33] Such improvement in physical capacity allows patients to see themselves in the context of health rather than as cardiac cripples, strengthening feelings of well-being, self-esteem, and self-confidence. These psychological benefits derived from exercise training can result in an enhanced quality of life.[33]

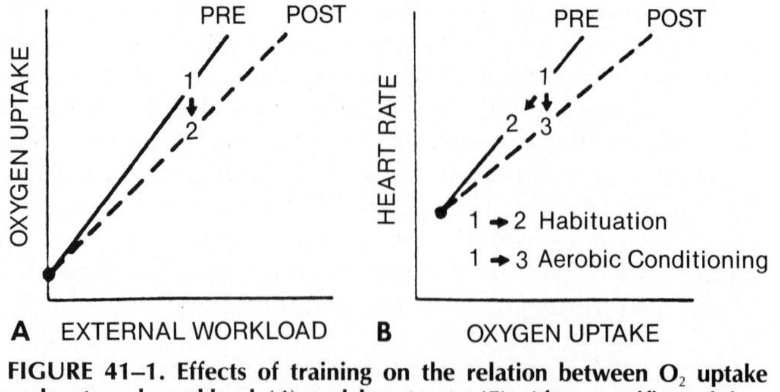

FIGURE 41–1. Effects of training on the relation between O_2 uptake and external workload (*A*) and heart rate (*B*). After specific training, patients become more efficient in performing a given task. This improved work efficiency (*A*) results in a decreased oxygen requirement for exercise at a constant external workload as shown (point 1 to point 2). A decreased submaximal exercise heart rate (*B*) at the same external workload may be due either to improved work efficiency (point 1 to point 2) or to aerobic conditioning (point 1 to point 3). The term "habituation" may be used to distinguish increased work efficiency from aerobic conditioning in which the heart rate becomes lower, but at the same oxygen consumption. (Adapted from Dressendorfer, R. H., Smith, J. L., Amsterdam, E. A., and Mason, D. T.: Reduction of submaximal exercise myocardial oxygen demand post-walk training program in coronary patients due to improved physical work efficiency. Am. Heart J. *103*:358, 1982.)

ASSESSMENT FOR EXERCISE. Aside from the prognostic implications, clinical evaluation and exercise testing provide a baseline standard from which to evaluate potential benefits from training programs, progression of disease, and other conditions that might preclude vigorous activities. However, it is difficult to predict training effects in men with coronary artery disease, even with extensive clinical, treadmill, and radionuclide data.[22] Because of the many possible gains from physical activity enumerated above, excluding patients without definite contraindications seems inappropriate. Even after initial evaluation, further observation of patients at monitored exercise sessions allows more precise recommendations for long-term exercise.[34, 35]

Clinical Evaluation. Although few absolute contraindications to physical activity exist, the presence of any acute illness, poorly controlled systemic disease, or unstable condition carries an unacceptable risk with exertional activities. Cardiovascular contraindications to exercise include: (1) acute myocardial infarction, (2) unstable angina pectoris, (3) resting blood pressure greater than 200/110 mm Hg, (4) arrhythmias (ventricular tachycardia or any rhythm significantly compromising cardiac function), (5) unpaced third-degree heart block, (6) uncompensated congestive heart failure, (7) severe aortic stenosis or left ventricular outflow tract obstruction, (8) aortic dissection, (9) cardiomyopathy, (10) active myocarditis within the past year, (11) recent thrombophlebitis, and (12) recent systemic or pulmonary embolism. Possible contraindications and precautions for exercise are reviewed in recent publications.[5, 36–39] Patients with diabetes, obstructive lung disease, renal disease, hernia, anemia, orthopedic disabilities, or other chronic illnesses require special attention, but such disorders rarely proscribe physical activity. Patients who exhibit sternal instability after coronary artery bypass grafting should not perform exercise involving the upper extremity or trunk.[5] While pacemakers do not preclude exercise training, they do raise the need for certain precautions,[37, 38, 40] especially an inadequate heart rate response to exercise. Recently introduced activity-sensitive pacemakers permit a wide range of physical activity.[41]

Drugs may influence the exercise response as well as generate associated symptoms, signs, and metabolic changes.[37, 42, 43, 43a] Although a consistent drug regimen does not influence serial exercise responses, variation in drugs used, dosage, or patient adherence may alter the response. Even though drugs may change the exercise response, they do not necessarily vitiate training effects.[37, 42–44] "Cold" remedies and "mood elevators" exaggerate the sympathetic response to exercise and may predispose to dysrhythmias. Individuals on anticoagulants must be observed carefully so that local trauma and possible bleeding can be avoided. Insulin requirements for diabetics decrease with exercise, while drug-induced hypokalemia can reduce exercise tolerance. Digitalis, diuretics, tranquilizers, and antihypertensives may augment ST-segment depression. Beta blockers, calcium channel antagonists, and vasodilators may modify heart rate, blood pressure, and angina threshold. Even though beta blockers alter the heart rate at given exercise intensities, the training effect will be preserved, as will the heart rate–exercise relationship.[42, 43] In fact, such agents often increase exercise capacity in patients with angina or exercise-induced ventricular dysfunction by permitting a greater intensity and therefore a greater likelihood of achieving a training effect.

Exercise Testing. Although a variety of protocols can be used for exercise testing,[43a, 44] the routine selected should be conducted in a standard fashion in order to compare data in the same patient longitudinally and pemit comparison among patients. Submaximal exercise tests can be used, but it must be realized that age-predicted heart rates from available tables do not always apply to coronary artery disease patients. Maximal heart rate can be highly variable among individuals of the same sex and age. Moreover, cardiac diseases and drugs commonly used for treatment may attenuate the heart rate response to exercise.

An exercise test determining functional aerobic capacity is considered maximal when peak exertional effort is reached or the test is terminated because of electrocardiographic or clinical endpoints. The peak value of maximal oxygen uptake during symptom-limited treadmill exercise appears to be a valid measure of maximal cardiovascular capacity, irrespective of the limiting symptoms or pattern of oxygen consumption in the final 90 seconds.[45] Workloads achieved can also be expressed through the metabolic equivalent system (METS). A MET is a unit of energy that approximates 3.5 ml O_2/kg-min, the amount of oxygen required under basal conditions.

Generally, ischemic symptoms and signs occur at the same heart rate or at the same double product (heart rate times systolic pressure), regardless of environmental conditions or the mix of dynamic-static exercise.[14] With the increasing concern for silent ischemia (p. 1362),[46] the ECG abnormalities induced with exercise assume new importance, even in the absence of exercise-induced ischemia. Opinions vary regarding the significance of exercise-induced premature ventricular contractions (PVC's) compared with those occurring at rest but decreasing with exercise.[47, 48] Neither exercise testing nor prolonged ambulatory monitoring for PVC's has yet clarified the significance of such dysrhythmias for patients entering an exercise program.[47–49] However, a characteristic and reproducible relationship between PVC frequency and heart rate over the range of heart rates encountered during routine activities is demonstrable.[50]

The test situation can be used to advantage in observing the patient during exercise for symptoms, signs, and general appearance, and for teaching him how to judge his own performance. The Borg scale, a technique for rating perceived exertion (RPE) which is used by having the patient rate the workload on a scale from 6 to 20, should be employed.[51] Each odd number is characterized by appropriate descriptors, ranging from very, very light (7 rating) to very, very hard (19 rating). Such ratings can be used for assessing the patient's work tolerance and as a means for estimating training level independent of heart rate measurement.[52] Those who overestimate their ability to jog tend to exceed heart rate targets while those who overestimate their heart rate during exercise tend to maintain heart rate levels that are less than optimal.[53] The use of RPE can be especially valuable in unsupervised situations and for those instances in which the patient's heart rate is an unreliable measure of external workload such as with a change in drug regimens.

Arm exercise testing protocols are available for patients who are unable to exercise because of lower extremity difficulties or whose occupational or recreational activities are predominantly arm work. Descriptions of ergometer exercise testing protocols and implications of such findings for training programs have been reviewed recently by Franklin.[54]

Types of Exercise

DYNAMIC VS. STATIC EXERCISE. Muscular contractions can generally be classified as dynamic (isotonic) or static (isometric). *Dynamic* activities initiate muscle tension resulting in movement through a range of motion. *Static* exercise characterizes muscle tension without appreciable movement. Actually, most dynamic activities contain static elements but static exercise does not necessarily have a dynamic component. Dynamic exercise involving large muscle groups and designed to overload the oxygen transport system of the body may also improve left ventricular responses to static exercise and should be the primary emphasis in a training program. Because adaptive training responses are specific to the muscle group involved, the patient's occupational and leisure time activities should be considered in establishing an appropriate exercise routine.[16, 55, 56]

Ideally, training programs should simulate the daily activities and exercise patterns of the patient to insure training of the proper muscle groups. Commonly used dynamic exercises include walking, jogging, swimming, bicycling, rope skipping, calisthenics, aerobics, and long-distance running. Swimming, an ideal exercise from the standpoint of involving large muscle groups in both arms and legs, also provides relief for weight-bearing joints. However, swimming has relatively high energy costs and can mask ischemic symptoms.[57, 58] Despite the many advantages to be derived from water activities, several limitations must be taken into account: accessibility of a swimming pool, the need for careful monitoring, and special requirements for cardiopulmonary resuscitation. The bicycle is also weight supporting, and bicycling is relatively low in energy cost per unit.[55] Although rope skipping is a convenient way to exercise, even low levels of skipping may result in excessive oxygen requirements for many patients. Only a small percentage of cardiac patients, estimated at about 2 to 5 per cent, can participate in long-distance running.[59] The training program to prepare for such activities requires an intensity of activity well above that needed for cardiovascular fitness. Yet participation in marathons has been demonstrated to be feasible and safe for selected patients,[59] even those who have had a cardiac transplant.[59a]

Since patients must invariably perform some types of static exercise, such as lifting or carrying heavy objects, the inclusion of such activities in training routine enables the cardiac patient to improve daily activities. Recent studies suggest no difference between combined dynamic-static exercise compared with dynamic exercise alone at peak loads in provoking ischemia, left ventricular dysfunction, or ventricular arrhythmias.[60–62] However, patients with inadequate left ventricular function cannot increase cardiac output at the higher afterload conditions imposed by isometric work.[63] As a result, static activities by such individuals can lead to abnormalities or left ventricular function and ectopy.[16, 18, 60] Although static exercise can lead to an exaggerated blood pressure response,[18] ischemic changes are less frequent at the same rate pressure product required to evoke changes with dynamic exercise, possibly because of increased aortic blood pressure and enhanced coronary perfusion.[60] Static activity may be prescribed for a patient if his tolerance and hemodynamic responses at various intensities with differing muscle mass are evaluated.

Many cardiac patients require upper body strength for daily activities. Contrary to previous beliefs, weight training has now been demonstrated to be feasible and safe in selected patients after a myocardial infarction.[56, 60] Weight training, when added to a dynamic endurance program, provides a well-rounded conditioning program. Typical routines employ dumbbells from 2 to 10 pounds with 5 to 10 repetitions for each muscle group exercised. More comprehensive routines have incorporated weights initially set at 40 per cent of one-repetition maximum.[56] If desired, patients should be instructed on proper techniques for weight training and monitored.

INTERMITTENT VS. CONTINUOUS EXERCISE. Most rehabilitation programs incorporate interval training techniques, a series of repeated bouts of exercise followed by recovery periods of low-level activity (Fig. 41–2). Intermittent exercise offers several advantages over continuous training techniques: (1) the low-level activity recovery period allows subsequent higher intensity levels with less fatigue; (2) intermittent activity lends itself to changing modes of exercise; (3) diverse activities permit different muscle groups to be stressed; (4) development of ischemia is less likely; and (5) patients can be monitored during the recovery period intervals. However, even with intermittent exercise, complete recovery may not take place after exercise bouts as reflected by the increasing heart rate and fatigue levels for comparable workloads later in the sequence.

Exercise Prescriptions

For most training adaptations, exercise must tax the cardiorespiratory system. Beginning with supervised exercise is essential to insure the greatest benefit with minimal risk. The primary determinants of the magnitude

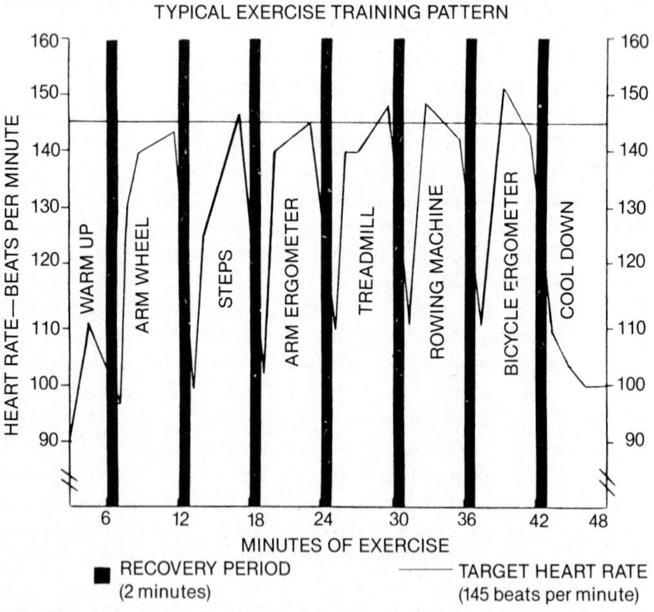

FIGURE 41–2. Exercise during a monitored group training session. This is best carried out on a series of training devices after a warm-up period of 5 to 10 minutes. The patient alternates between arm and leg devices with a 2-minute recovery period between the devices, which allows the attaining of a greater work load with less fatigue and the use of intermittent monitoring. On each device, the patient attains target heart rate within a minute or two and maintains this heart rate for the remainder of the 4-minute exercise period. There does tend to be a sequential increase in aerobic requirements due to incomplete recovery between exercise periods. The heart rate for most patients is easily maintained within 5 per cent of the target heart rate.

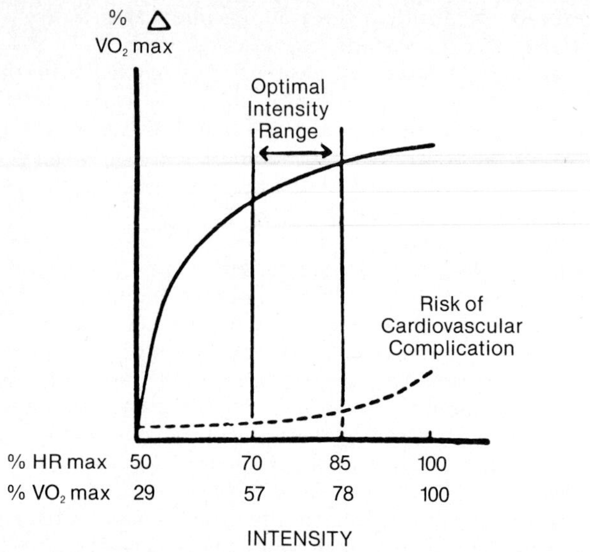

FIGURE 41–3. Relationship between per cent gain in aerobic capacity ($\dot{V}O_{2max}$) and intensity of exercise expressed as per cent of maximal heart rate (HR max) or per cent of $\dot{V}O_{2max}$. The optimal intensity range is 70 to 85 per cent of HR max equivalent to 57 to 78 per cent $\dot{V}O_{2max}$. As the intensity of exercise exceeds 85 per cent HR max, the relative risks of arrhythmias, angina pectoris, and other ischemic manifestations increase abruptly, whereas the improvement in aerobic capacity levels off. (Adapted from Hellerstein, H. K., and Franklin, B. A.: Exercise testing and prescription. *In* Wenger, N. K., and Hellerstein, H.K. (eds.): Rehabilitation of the Coronary Patient. New York, John Wiley and Sons, 1978, pp. 149–202.)

of the adaptive response to various types of exercise involve the intensity, frequency, and duration of the exercise sessions.

INTENSITY OF EXERCISE. Intensity appears to be the single most important determinant in achieving the desired training effects. Patients should have a target exercise intensity that takes into consideration symptoms, signs, and perceived exertion. Training intensity should never exceed the point at which ischemia occurs. By actually testing the patient, the monitoring physician can take into account aberrant exercise responses due to intrinsic cardiac disease, other disorders, metabolic changes, or medications.[63a] The cardiac patient should train at about 50 to 75 per cent of maximal oxygen uptake, although a relative load of 40 per cent has sufficed in some instances (Fig. 41–3).[19, 37, 38, 55]

Ample data indicate that a heart rate at 70 to 85 per cent of maximal capacity corresponds to the 50 to 75 per cent levels of maximal oxygen uptake required for training.[5, 37, 38, 55] This relationship of heart rate to oxygen uptake remains consistent for persons of all ages in the presence or absence of coronary artery disease and at all levels of training under usual environmental circumstances.[64] Because of the high linear correlation between oxygen uptake and heart rate at submaximal workloads, the heart rate may be substituted for the more difficult measurement of oxygen consumption.

The submaximal workload or the heart rate at a given workload for training can be taken directly from the exercise test results. In practice, several methods are generally used for estimating a "target" heart rate (THR) range to regulate the physical activity intensity during training sessions:

Method 1: The simplest technique is to compute the target heart rate zone using 70 to 85 per cent of the maximal heart rate (MHR) achieved on prior exercise testing. The calculation for an MHR of 160 is as follows: $0.85 \times 160 = 136$ (upper limit); $0.70 \times 160 = 112$ (lower limit). The THR ranges from 112 to 126 beats per minute.

Method 2: This approach takes the variability of the resting heart rate into account and gives a slightly higher range for target heart rate. In this method, 70 to 85 per cent of the difference between resting heart rate (RHR) and MHR is added to the RHR: 0.85 × (160–60) + 60 = 145 (upper limit); 0.70 × (160–60) + 60 = 130 (lower limit). The THR ranges from 130 to 145 beats per minute.

A more complicated technique, the *sliding scale method*, uses a relative training intensity that takes into consideration both resting heart rate and the symptom-limited functional aerobic capacity.[37] The prescription can also be given in METS taken as a direct percentage of maximal capacity. In published tables (Table 41–4) METS are transformed into energy requirements for common activities at work and home. METS provide only an approximate index because individual differences in energy expenditure vary according to environmental factors, physical condition, skills, and motivation.

In practice, a person rarely maintains an exact target heart rate but varies about 5 per cent above and below THR. Because of this variability in heart rate during exercise, the simpler techniques for estimating exercise intensity may be preferred to more complex methods. Upper limits of prescribed training heart rates during early rehabilitation generally correspond to an RPE of 12 to 15. The RPE is especially useful when heart rate responses are difficult to determine, are calculated incorrectly, or are unreliable because of a change in clinical status.

DURATION OF EXERCISE. Duration can be tailored to exercise intensity; the greater the intensity, the less the duration need be. Although training adaptations can occur with brief high-intensity sessions, this is certainly not advisable from the standpoint of safety. Besides, the logistics of getting to and from exercise sessions make longer, less frequent exercise meetings more practical. Generally, exercise sessions should range from 30 to 45 minutes in duration. Longer training periods are associated with an increased incidence of orthopedic injuries.[65, 66] Training effects may be noted as soon as 2 weeks or as late as 6 weeks after starting but can be highly variable among individuals, depending upon initial functional capacity, health status, and response to specific activities.[64]

FREQUENCY OF EXERCISE. To improve cardiorespiratory fitness, the exercise program should be performed at least 3 days a week, preferably nonconsecutively to minimize musculoskeletal stress. Frequent low-level brief sessions may be valuable for patients unable to tolerate 30 minutes of moderate-intensity exercise. Maintenance programs of 2 to 3 days per week generally suffice to retain exercise adaptations. Frequency of training appears to be less important than either intensity or duration but probably plays a role for those interested in attaining higher levels of fitness.

HAZARDS OF EXERCISE. Not to be ignored are the possible risks from exercise. Foremost are those injuries related to the musculoskeletal system, especially the lower extremities.[66] A variety of other disorders have been reported. Extremes of temperature may predispose to heat exhaustion, heat stroke, or even frostbite of exposed parts of the body in cold climates.[67–69] More unusual problems associated with vigorous exertion are hypersensitivity reactions ranging from pruritus and urticaria to generalized anaphylactic reactions.[70] Although relatively rare, such episodes during or after exercising can be life threatening. Cardiac patients attempting long-distance running may also encounter complications associated with extremely strenuous exertion, such as hematuria, myoglobinuria, diarrhea, gastrointestinal bleeding, and rhabdomyolysis.[71, 72]

Serious complications result from an increased susceptibility to cardiovascular events during exertion and immediately afterward (Fig. 41–3). Haskell[73] surveyed major supervised cardiac rehabilitation programs and calculated the occurrence of major cardiovascular complications during exercise training as one fatal event per 34,673 exercise hours and one nonfatal event per 116,402 hours. Others have reported similar or lower rates of cardiac events[74, 74a] and called attention to the risk of "primary" arrhythmic events.[75] Many complications occur during warm-up or

TABLE 41–1 APPROXIMATE ENERGY REQUIREMENTS FOR SELECTED ACTIVITIES

Energy Category	Self-Care or Home	Occupational	Recreational	Physical Conditioning
Very light < 3 METS < 11 ml/kg/min < 4 kcal	Washing, shaving, dressing Desk work, writing Washing dishes Driving car	Sitting (clerical, assembling) Standing (store clerk, bartender) Driving truck Janitorial work	Playing cards Horseshoes Bait casting Billiards Sewing, knitting Golf (cart)	Walking (level @ 2 mph) Stationary bicycle (very low resistance) Very light calisthenics
Light 3–5 METS 11–18 ml/kg/min 4–6 kcal	Cleaning windows Raking leaves Weeding Power lawn mowing Waxing floors (slowly) Painting Carrying objects (15–30 lbs)	Stocking shelves (light objects) Light welding Light carpentry Machine assembly Auto repair Paperhanging	Dancing (social and square) Golf (walking) Sailing Horseback riding Volleyball (6 man) Tennis (doubles)	Walking (3–4 mph) Level bicycling (6–8 mph) Light calisthenics
Moderate 5–7 METS 18–25 ml/kg/min 6–8 kcal	Easy digging in garden Climbing stairs (slowly) Carrying objects (30–60 lb)	Carpentry (exterior home building) Shoveling dirt Using pneumatic tools	Light backpacking Tennis (singles) Water skiing Skating (ice & roller) Horseback riding (gallop)	Walking (4.5–5 mph) Bicycling (9–10 mph) Swimming (breast stroke)
Heavy 7–9 METS 25–32 ml/kg/min 8–10 kcal	Sawing wood Heavy shoveling Climbing stairs (moderate speed) Carrying objects (60–90 lb)	Tending furnace Digging ditches Using pick and shovel	Canoeing Mountain climbing Touch football Paddleball	Jog (5 mph) Swim (crawl stroke) Rowing machine Bicycling (12 mph) Heavy calisthenics)
Very Heavy > 9 METS > 32 ml/kg/min > 10 kcal	Carrying loads upstairs Carrying objects (> 90 lb) Climbing stairs (quickly) Shoveling heavy snow	Lumberjacking Heavy labor	Handball Squash Cross country skiing	Running (≥ 6 mph) Bicycle (≥ 13 mph or up steep hill) Rope jumping

Adapted from Haskell WL: Design and implementation of cardiac conditioning programs. *In* Wenger, N. K., and Hellerstein, H. (eds.): Rehabilitation of the Coronary Patient. New York, John Wiley and Sons, 1978, pp. 203–241.

cool-down; this suggests the need for adequate supervision during rest breaks and a minimum of 15 minutes of postexercise surveillance.[36] Because of the established risk during the immediate postexertional period, surveillance of locker rooms, showers, and rest rooms must be maintained. There generally appears to be no effective way to identify individuals at greater risk for exertional-related cardiac arrest, although increased risk may result from exceeding target heart rates.[74]

SECONDARY PREVENTION

Recent studies document the importance of drugs,[76–78] invasive treatment,[79] and life style intervention programs[80–82] in reducing the sequelae of coronary disease, prolonging life, and positively influencing daily activities (Chap. 36). Such findings emphasize the importance of selectively combining therapeutic modalities with rehabilitation measures for optimal clinical management.

RETARDATION OF ATHEROSCLEROSIS. Accumulating evidence suggests that modification of factors predisposing to coronary artery disease influence the atherosclerotic process.[80–83, 83a] The data indicate that an elevated serum cholesterol level, especially with a low proportion of high-density lipoprotein cholesterol and possibly disordered apoprotein moieties, accelerates the progression of atherosclerosis and its complications.[81, 82] For those patients undergoing coronary artery bypass grafting, the prevention of atherosclerosis in the vein grafts themselves constitutes a serious long-term concern. More importantly, lowering lipids by means of diet and drugs introduces the possibility of not only preventing or delaying progression of coronary artery lesions but of causing their actual regression.[81, 82] Data from the controlled trials justifying reduction of plasma lipids by means of drugs are mixed,[84, 85] but long-term follow-up data in the Coronary Drug Project indicate significantly greater survival in those treated with nicotinic acid.[77] Even small reductions in the progression or induction of regression in coronary artery lesions should diminish subsequent morbidity and mortality.[81]

Patients should be advised to discontinue smoking as early in the course of the disease as possible, since cigarettes can cause profound impairment of regional myocardial perfusion.[86, 87] Repeated insults may provide a mechanism linking smoking to coronary events.[86] In the Coronary Artery Surgery Study (CASS) registry, 5-year survival was significantly lower among those who continued to smoke.[88] Lowering elevated arterial pressure in patients with coronary artery disease should diminish symptoms, enhance left ventricular function, and retard progression of disease. However, no documentation from controlled trials among such populations is available. To justify treatment, one must extrapolate from the studies on the efficacy of antihypertensive treatment for the general population,[89] and the anticipated greater myocardial oxygen costs in hypertension.

Through multiple mechanisms, exercise induces the following physiological benefits: (1) reduction of weight and an associated increase in lean body mass when caloric intake is constant,[90] and (2) a modified lipoprotein profile, including lower levels of serum triglycerides and a greater amount of cholesterol carried by high-density lipoproteins, particularly HDL_2.[82, 91, 91a] In addition, exercise-induced weight loss appears to produce elevation of HDL cholesterol more readily than weight loss by diet alone.[92] However, to bring about higher HDL levels, several reports suggest that a threshold of about 10 miles run per week for a period of months is needed.[82, 93] No clear consensus exists on the relationship of total cholesterol concentration to habitual exercise independent of weight changes. Other benefits include: (3) improved carbohydrate metabolism resulting in improved glucose tolerance and consequently reduced serum insulin values,[94] (4) probably a lowered resting diastolic blood pressure with a decrease in mean blood pressure during submaximal exercise,[16, 95, 96, 96a] (5) impetus for development of desirable health habits including modification of behavior,[31] (6) decreased platelet adhesiveness and enhanced fibrinolysis,[91] and (7) lessened adrenergic response to stress.[16, 97] However, coronary patients in exercise-only programs demonstrate minimal improvement in major risk factors.[98] The lack of more striking changes may be attributed to an inability to attain the necessary levels of exertion,[82] or inadequate counseling. Yet, exercise might aid in secondary prevention indirectly by blocking the effects of major risk factors by lowering heart rate, accelerating carbon monoxide metabolism, or diminishing platelet aggregation. Any or all of these metabolic changes might counter the adverse effect of smoking.

PROTECTION AGAINST CLINICAL MANIFESTATIONS. Through properly executed training programs, coronary artery disease patients can increase their exercise tolerance and, consequently, the ability to sustain higher work loads without myocardial ischemia.[16, 20, 99] In some instances coronary patients can reach a degree of fitness seldom attained even by healthy individuals—that demanded for marathon races.[59] Such clinical improvement results from a more favorable ratio between myocardial and total body work resulting from peripheral and regulatory adaptations.[16, 19] The increased maximal oxygen uptake realized with training depends chiefly upon enhanced peripheral extraction of oxygen by redistribution of blood to working skeletal muscles and local adaptive changes in the skeletal muscle's capacity for aerobic metabolism.[16, 20] As a result there is a lessened myocardial oxygen demand due to a reduction in heart rate, and to a lesser extent, systolic blood pressure at a given workload during exercise. Heart rate and rate pressure product (RPP) correlate well with myocardial oxygen demand during large-muscle dynamic exercise and have been demonstrated to be a good index for demand in patients with coronary artery disease.[16] The RPP of cardiac patients at a similar workload or oxygen uptake after training decreases from 8 to 22 per cent.[16]

Some clinical studies found that training actually improves myocardial oxygen delivery or utilization, leading to not only an increased exercise tolerance but also to a possible increase in the absolute threshold for myocardial ischemia.[100–102] Ehsani and colleagues[102] found that patients able to exercise at 65 to 85 per cent of $\dot{V}O_{2max}$ for 1 hour per day, 4 or 5 days per week, achieved a 38 per cent increase in $\dot{V}O_{2max}$. The extent of ST-segment displacement at the maximal workload was less after training, even though the RPP increased by 20 per cent. These findings were interpreted as indicative of a reduction in myocardial ischemia. Indirect evidence for a more favorable oxygen supply-demand relationship includes reversion of aberrant ballistocardiographic waveforms,[103] decrease in the number of electrocardiographic abnormalities,[104] and diminishing of ventricular ectopic activity.[16]

Experimental data suggest that physical training has direct effects on the coronary vascular bed,[105] on myocardial perfusion and myocardial performance, and even on proximal coronary vasomotor reactivity.[106, 107] Nevertheless, studies of physical activity in patients with coronary artery disease have not yet demonstrated expanded collateral circulation.[108]

Several preliminary studies have suggested that lack of improvement in cardiac function results from an inadequate training stimulus.[16, 109–111] These data indicate that more prolonged and intense training can effect desirable cardiac adaptations in patients with coronary artery disease. Exercise intensity appears to be an important factor in determining the volume load associated with exercise and consequently the changes that take place in physically trained individuals.[112] It is possible that several months of moderate exercise training in coronary artery disease patients produces adaptations primarily in the autonomic nervous system and skeletal muscles, and that more prolonged and higher intensity exercise leads to cardiovascular adaptations. Improvement in exercise performance has been attributed to enhanced left ventricular function and increased stroke volume.[113–115] Using perfusion scintigraphy and radionuclide ventriculography, Froelicher and associates[116] demonstrated changes in myocardial perfusion and function in men with coronary artery disease who exercised for a year, but the changes were relatively modest and were observed only in subgroups of patients. Williams and coworkers[110] found a small but apparently real increase in left ventricular ejection fraction after 6 to 12 months of conditioning. The extent of training bradycardia correlated with the increment in ejection fraction at the pretraining maximum workload. Thus, exercise-induced cardiac adaptations in addition to the favorable metabolic changes already noted in trained muscles remain a distinct possibility.

Clinical Trials of Secondary Prevention

Over the last decade a growing series of randomized trials with a single exception[117–124] have demonstrated a lower mortality among survivors of myocardial infarction randomized to an exercise training group than those in a "control" group (Table 41–2). Typically, the studies were based on supervised training programs consisting of two to four sessions per week lasting 20 to 60 minutes each. Such trials were inadequate to test rigorously the hypothesis that exercise reduces overall mortality because of deficiencies in their design and small numbers of participants. Yet all the studies but one showed reductions in mortality ranging from 20.6 to 42.9 per cent in the exercise group. Little effect on the incidence of reinfarction was noted. In this country, the National Exercise and Heart Disease Project showed substantially fewer deaths from recurrent myocardial infarction, associated with a 37 per cent reduction in total mortality.[125] The benefits of exercise were most striking in those patients whose physical capacity exceeded 7 METS and in whom the systolic blood pressure response to exercise testing exceeded 140 mm Hg, presumably reflecting better left ventricular function. Pooling of the results from five of the earlier studies with comparable methodology is consistent with a 19 per cent reduction ($p<0.05$) in total mortality for an exercise intervention group.[85] From recent selected trials, Collins and coworkers[126] calculated a 20 per cent reduction in mortality, more marked if exercise rehabilitation started early after myocardial infarction.

COMPREHENSIVE PROGRAMS. More comprehensive rehabilitation intervention programs have emphasized health education, risk factor modification, and pharmacological management in addition to exercise. In a controlled but nonrandomized study, functional, economic, and psychosocial benefits persisted for as long as 58 months after coronary artery bypass grafting.[127] In the North Karelia Study[128, 129] participants experienced a reduction in the incidence of recurrent infarction and new vocational invalidity pensions. Two Finnish centers collaborated to assess the effects of comprehensive rehabilitation on morbidity and mortality in addition to other outcomes.[130] Beginning 2 weeks after hospital discharge, the cumulative coronary mortality was 18.6 per cent in the intervention group and 29.4 per cent in the control group at 3-year follow-up, with differences mainly related to reduced numbers of sudden deaths after infarction. At a special clinic in Göteborg a reduction in cardiovascular events was noted in patients after 2 years of attendance[131]; a reduction was also observed in a group in the Netherlands.[132] However, total mortality was not changed significantly in either program.

On the basis of available data, substantial opportunities exist for secondary prevention among patients with coronary artery disease. Further refinement in identifying those patients most likely to benefit from such intervention and advances in other therapeutic modalities should further reduce morbidity and mortality for those participating in rehabilitation programs.

APPROACH TO PSYCHOSOCIAL SEQUELAE OF HEART DISEASE. The patient and family are forced to make a number of social, emotional, and psychological adjustments to heart disease (Chap. 62).[133–135] Realizing the sources of these emotional reactions may aid in ameliorating unnecessary emotional arousal. Fear of death, reinfarction, or inability to resume formal living patterns is commonly amenable to counseling. Postmyocardial infarction depres-

TABLE 41–2 SECONDARY PREVENTION WITH PHYSICAL TRAINING PREVIOUS RANDOMIZED CONTROLLED TRIALS

TRIAL (Reference)	N	INTERVENTION	FOLLOW-UP (MONTHS)	TOTAL MORTALITY (%) Control	Intervention	EFFECTIVENESS (%)*
Sweden (117) (1968–72)	315	Supervised exercise, 3×/week	48	22.3	17.7	20.6
Finland (118) (1969–72)	298	Supervised exercise, 2–3×/week	12	21.9	17.1	21.9
Finland (119) (1969–72)	380	Daily home exercise	29	14.0	10.0	28.6
Canada (120) (1972–78)	733	Partially supervised exercise, 2–4×/week	48	7.3	9.5	−30.0
U.S. (122) (1974–79)	651	Supervised exercise, 3×/week	36	7.3	4.6	37.0
Chile (123) (1973–82)	193	Supervised exercise, 3×/week	108	27.0†	17.2†	36.3
England (124) (unknown)	303	Supervised exercise, 2×/week	25	14.0	8.0	42.9

$$\text{*Effectiveness} = \frac{\text{control mortality} - \text{intervention mortality}}{\text{control mortality}} \times 100$$

†Personal communication

sion and anxiety are very common and can lead to permanent psychological problems, unless they are counteracted by appropriate counseling. Since few patients express their fears to their physician spontaneously, prompting patients to ask questions about discomfort and prognosis will aid some patients in talking and seeking help.[136]

Patients who undergo coronary artery bypass grafting experience psychological difficulty in several spheres. Patients who are asymptomatic after operation are uncertain about their limitations and are fearful of precipitating pain, whereas those with continued symptoms become discouraged and depressed. Impairment of psychological functioning has been observed after coronary artery bypass procedures.[137] Heller and coworkers[138] reported that despite physical improvement after surgery, psychological problems remained a major barrier to rehabilitation in approximately one-third of their patients. Patients may experience anxiety, depression, increased somatic preoccupation, loss of self-esteem, and impaired sexual functioning. Patients' perception of their health status is probably as important as their actual functional capacity in determining the extent of disability after operation.[139]

Relaxation and stress management training have met with some success in improving psychological and morbidity measures.[140] Cay[141] has summarized the methods of treatment as informing the patient of the natural history of the disease, explaining the rationale of treatment, supplying reassurance and encouragement, giving practical help with concrete problems, providing nondirective guidance, prescribing drug therapy, and gradually increasing physical exercise. In addition, patients and their families should be informed about community resources including counseling services, home care agencies and services, vocational rehabilitation facilities, and coronary clubs. Group sessions allow patients to exchange information, gain social group support, express their feelings, and share solutions to common problems.[142]

Information given patients early in the course of myocardial infarction has differential effects depending on how an individual patient copes.[143] *Denial* is a common defense reaction effectively used by many patients[136, 144] during early phases that frequently results in compliance problems during later phases of rehabilitation. Patients who use *repression* as a defense respond poorly when a great deal of information is provided.[144] Anxiety, fatigue, and the need for complicated care in the hospital setting often limit educational opportunities. After the patient has left the hospital, a more detailed educational program is possible. At this time further explanation of the illness, natural history of the disease, and possibilities for long-term management should be addressed.

Although some patients profit from formal support and intervention, it is best that patients and their families assume responsibility for rehabilitation and deal with the emotional aspects of the illness. Social support systems are of great value in the rehabilitation process and should be fostered.[145] Involving patients in planning for recovery by teaching them to self-monitor physical activities and identify areas in which they can make decisions for their own care helps to encourage adherence to the medical regimen. Family counseling should include discussion of life style adjustments to be anticipated during convalescence and the harm of voluntary unnecessary restriction of activity.

The spouse often finds it difficult to provide care while allowing the patient to be independent and resume activities. The spouse's anxiety and uncertainty may be as great as those of the patient.[134] As a result of these conflicts and the stress from major changes in roles, marital tensions tend to increase. Resumption of sexual activity is a potential source of difficulty in the marital relationship during these stressful readjustment periods. A common misconception is that sexual intercourse may be too strenuous for patients with coronary disease. Yet the average heart rate during peak sexual activity is less than 120 beats/min, and the exertional requirements correspond to walking up one or two flights of stairs or taking a brisk walk for several blocks.[146, 147, 147a]

Social isolation combined with a high degree of life stress increased the risk of death fourfold in the Beta-Blocker Heart Attack Trial.[147a] Data from recent studies indicate that behavioral management alone or in combination with other interventions may influence prognosis.[148, 149] The Recurrent Coronary Prevention Project reported that patients receiving a combined Type A and cardiac counseling intervention had a lower infarction and cardiovascular mortality rate than patients who received only medical advice.[150, 151] Long-term compliance with life style recommendations, which has been notoriously poor, is an important area for behavioral intervention.[152]

Patients' perceptions of their own physical handicaps are greatly influenced by emotional state; not surprisingly, disability varies markedly at comparable levels of disease. Marked psychological improvements may be the most striking aspect of a comprehensive rehabilitation program and may do much to restore an active life style for those impaired.

VOCATIONAL REHABILITATION. Work outcomes can be viewed from several perspectives: time required for resumption of usual work activities, number of hours worked per week, work capabilities, or job compared with usual occupation. The anticipated loss to the work force in the general male population of age similar to that of patients with coronary artery disease is about 4 per cent per year.[153] Over 80 per cent of patients with an uncomplicated posthospitalization course return to their former jobs within 3 months of infarction compared with about 65 per cent of patients after coronary artery bypass grafting.[13] Relief of symptoms and physiological improvements suffice in many instances to bring patients back to gainful employment. Others require additional motivation and reassurance from their physician and families. Activity limitations play a role, but the presence or absence of angina pectoris has a somewhat limited impact on the percentage of patients resuming work after infarction.[154, 155] Severe infarctions may delay the return to work and lessen the proportion of patients returning to work.[155] However, neither severity of disease nor mode of treatment greatly influence subsequent employability after coronary artery bypass grafting.[139, 156]

What does seem to be important in determining whether individuals will return to work is their work history before infarction or surgery. Individuals previously not working rarely seek employment after medical treatment and cite "doctor's advice" as a major reason for not doing so.[15, 153] The likelihood of the patient returning to work one year after catheterization for coronary artery disease depends on functional class, work history, occupation, and age.[156] Other factors found useful in determining whether a patient will return to work include presence of a non-work income, availability of the previous job, perception of health, educational level, family and social stability, and psychological factors.[139, 157]

Barriers to work rehabilitation include noncardiac disabilities, unsatisfactory work records, low occupational skills, unavailability of jobs, availability of worker's compensation, legal concerns, and other related factors. Anticipated higher than average health care and retirement costs further influence rehiring practices for coronary artery disease patients. Also, the misconception that myocardial infarction patients are not capable of physical labor has led firms to reject them from industrial positions even though only 5 per cent of patients now perform occupational duties that could be classified as heavy.[14] For those jobs involving peak exertional loads, such activity tends to be in short bursts so that myocardial work is less than required for prolonged steady-state efforts. If the strenuous activity is brief with the usual rest periods interspersed, even patients with relatively low physical work capacity can reach surprisingly high exertional levels before developing symptoms or signs of ischemia. The totality of peak loads, average work requirements, and environmental conditions must be weighed in estimating work limitations. Useful publications for disability evaluation are available.[158–160]

Historically, determination of fitness to work has been established by work evaluation units. If patients exhibit no limitations under the physical stress of symptom-limited treadmill exercise testing, the probability is high that they will not encounter difficulties during ordinary working conditions. The heart rate and workload at which ischemic abnormalities appear during dynamic effort signify the likelihood of encountering problems during daily activities.[161] The absence of symptoms and signs at low to moderate workloads indicates capabilities for physical activity without special restrictions.[14] Ambulatory electrocardiograms or special monitoring may be useful in special circumstances but is unnecessary for most typical jobs.

In order to advise patients on return to gainful employment, physicians must understand patients' occupational requirements. Medical practitioners can work with employers to establish a satisfactory work environment perceived by the patient as nonthreatening to health by recommending temporary limited-duty jobs, modified work routines, alternative job assignments, or job transfers that do not involve severe physiological or psychological stress. As the supply of younger workers becomes less and that of older workers continues to increase, the cost of the failure of cardiac patients capable of productive employment to return to work will escalate.[15]

PHASES OF REHABILITATION

Typically, a cardiac rehabilitation program consists of three successive phases: Phase one, in-hospital, early convalescence during hospitalization; phase two, intermediate, a highly structured routine for the transition period between hospitalization and resumption of ordinary activities; and phase three, a long-term, supervised program for further development of fitness and maintenance of gains. For selected patients who meet eligibility requirements, an individualized maintenance program can begin anywhere from 6 months to several years after indoctrination into the long-term program (Table 41–3). Although the general guidelines remain the same throughout these program phases, the objectives and methods differ somewhat in each.

PHASE ONE: IN-HOSPITAL. As early as the 1940's, Tinsley Harrison questioned the wisdom of 6 to 8 weeks of absolute bed rest after a myocardial infarction.[162] Controversy surrounded early mobilization after infarction until a series of investigations, progressing from an "armchair regimen"[163] to rapid mobilization and early exercise testing, demonstrated the safety and efficacy of such activities for some patients.[164–167] Coronary artery bypass grafting creates a situation not unlike that after myocardial infarction, in which carefully supervised activity programs result in shortened hospital stays, with no greater immediate risk than prolonged bed rest.[168]

Mobilization early during convalescence has become an integral part of the rehabilitation of patients who are free of continued ischemia, cardiac failure, and electrical instability or acute problems. The presence and the extent of silent ischemia also provides an important measure of high risk for early unfavorable outcomes.[46] The value of early physical activity is primarily to avert or limit the harmful effect of prolonged bed rest rather than to promote training adaptations.[169] Sivarajan and colleagues[170] could not detect any beneficial or detrimental effects on performance at 3 months after an early in-hospital exercise program. Another report indicated significant functional improvement from early low-intensity exercises months after hospitalization but only in a small subgroup of patients who were able to exercise without evidence of ischemia.[171] Not to be neglected is patient education,[172] an integral part of the in-hospital rehabilitation program. The immediate convalescent period is an appropriate time to introduce behavioral changes; however, such intervention must be followed by continuous support after hospital discharge for sustained effect.

As early as the first few days after infarction or coronary artery bypass grafting, patients without complications can be started on self-care activities limited to several METS (Fig. 41–4). This modest exertional level rarely increases the heart rate more than 10 beats/min and permits patients

TABLE 41–3 TIME SEQUENCE AND SCOPE OF ACTIVITIES IN VARIOUS PHASES OF A CARDIAC REHABILITATION PROGRAM

TIME SEQUENCE (MO)	1	2	4	10
PHASE	I In-Hospital	II Intermediate Convalescence	III Long-Term Program	IV Individualized Programs
DURATION (WEEKS)	1–3	3–12	24+	Indefinite
FREQUENCY	2–3×/day	3×/week	3–4×/week	3–5×/week
ACTIVITIES				
Range of motion, self-care	X			
Slow walking	X	X	X	X
Calisthenics	X	X	X	X
Dynamic exercise		X	X	X
Exercise devices		X	X	X
Weight training:				
Light dumbbells		X	X	X
Circuit wt. training			X	X
Recreational sports			X	X

Step	Education and Activities Following Myocardial Infarction
1 CCU	**Orient and answer questions;** bed rest; partial self-care; bedpan/bedside commode; dangle legs; passive ROM to major joints as tolerated; ankle plantar and dorsiflexion 5 reps 5 x /day; supine deep breathing 5 reps 2 x /day.
2 CCU	**Orient to rehabilitation and plan transfer from CCU;** up in chair 15 min 2–3 x /day; bed bath; bedside commode; active ROM as tolerated; ankle exercises 5 x /day; sitting: deep breathing 2 x /day.
3 Ward	**Cardiac anatomy and physiology, atherosclerosis and MI;** sit in chair ad lib; walk in room; self-care; active exercises 5 reps 1 x /day sitting: [2]shoulder flexion and [3]abduction, [4]knee extension, [5]elbow flexion; standing: [6]toe raises, [7]hip flexion.
4 Ward	**Risk factors and management of CAD;** walk in hall with supervision 75 ft 3 x /day; active exercises: increase to include [8]arm circles and [9]hip abduction 5 reps 2 x /day.
5 Ward	**Management of CAD: meds, exercise and pulse taking, diet, CABG, and percutaneous transluminal coronary angioplasty;** walk 100 ft 4 x /day with supervision, if needed; active exercises: increase to include [10]trunk forward flexion and [11]side stretching 5 reps 2 x /day.
6 Ward	**Behavioral counseling; patient and family adjustments;** walk in hall, ad lib, 3 x /day; stair climbing 2–4 steps with supervision and pulse taking; treadmill/bike testing; active exercises 7–10 reps 2 x /day.
7 Ward	**Discharge planning: meds; return appointments; diet; home activities and exercise; community resources; return to work, sexual activity and driving car;** walk in hall, ab lib, 4 x /day; stair climbing 6–8 steps with supervision and pulse taking; active exercises 7–10 reps 3 x /day.

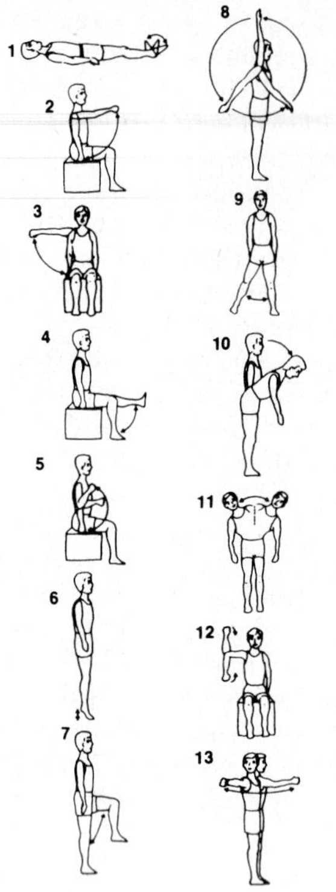

Step	Education and Activities Following Coronary Artery Bypass Grafting
1 SICU	**Orient and answer questions;** up in chair when stable 3–5 x /day 15 min; partial self-care; bedside commode; deep breathing and coughing each hour while awake; walk 50–100 ft with supervision when stable; ankle plantar and dorsiflexion 5 x / day.
2 SICU	**Orient to rehabilitation and plan transfer from SICU;** partial self-care; in chair, ad lib; deep breathing and coughing; walk 100 ft with supervision 3 x /day; ankle exercises 5 x /day.
3 Ward	**Cardiac anatomy and physiology: atherosclerosis and MI;** [12]self-care; active exercises: shoulder flexion, abduction, and rotation, backward circumduction; elbow flexion; knee extension: 5–10 reps 2 x /day; increase walking to 200–300 ft 3 x /day.
4 Ward	**Risk factors and management of CAD;** active exercises 10–15 reps 2 x /day to include [13]shoulder horizontal flexion; walk 400 ft 3 x /day.
5 Ward	**Behavioral counseling: patient and family adjustments;** walk in hall, ad lib, 4 x /day; stair climbing 8–12 steps with supervision and pulse taking; treadmill/bike testing; active exercises 10–15 reps 3 x /day.
6 Ward	**Discharge planning: meds; return appointments; diet; home activities and exercise; community resources; incision care; return to work, sexual activity and driving car;** walking in hall ad lib 4 x / day; stair climbing up to 16 steps with supervision and pulse taking; active exercises 15 reps 3 x /day.

FIGURE 41–4. Inpatient activity schedule. Exercise instructions: (1) Supine exercises should be used for range of motion (ROM) activities while patient remains in bed; (2) sitting exercises may be performed when patient has become comfortable sitting in chair, with progression to (3) standing exercises as tolerated by the patient.

1. *Ankle exercise* (1,2)–With leg fully extended and parallel to the floor, point toes up and down. Follow by rotating feet in a circle, with motion occurring at ankle; relax and repeat with other leg.

2. *Shoulder flexion* (1,2,3)–With arm at side and elbow straight, lift arm toward front and over head and return to side; relax and repeat with opposite arm.

3. *Shoulder abduction* (1,2,3)–With arm at side and elbow straight, lift arm to side away from body and then return to side; relax and repeat with opposite arm.

4. *Knee extension* (1,2)–Raise leg parallel to bed (floor) by fully extending it and return to starting position; relax and repeat with opposite leg.

5. *Elbow flexion* (1,2,3)–With arm at side, bend elbow and touch shoulder with fingertips; relax and repeat with opposite arm.

6. *Toe raises* (3)–Raise heels as high as possible with toes touching floor.

7. *Hip flexion* (1,3)–With knee bent, raise knee toward chest and then return to starting position; relax and repeat with opposite leg.

8. *Arm circles* (2,3)–With elbow relaxed, make large backward arm circles similar to the back stroke for swimming; relax and repeat with opposite arm.

9. *Hip abduction* (1,3)–With legs straight, move leg out to side of body and return to starting position (may use support for balance); relax and repeat with opposite leg.

10. *Trunk forward flexion* (2,3)–With knees relaxed, bow forward from the waist.

11. *Side stretching* (2,3)–With arms hanging loosely at sides and with knees relaxed, bend trunk to the side; relax and repeat to the opposite side.

12. *Shoulder rotation* (1,2,3)–Lift arm straight out to the side so that arm is parallel to the floor and at shoulder level. Bend elbow to a 90-degree angle so that forearm is pointing upward with palm facing forward. With arm in the fixed position, lower forearm and palm toward the floor so that palm faces downward; relax and repeat with opposite arm.

13. *Shoulder horizontal flexion* (1,2,3)–Lift arm straight out to the side so that arm is parallel to the floor and at shoulder level. In the same plane, move arm forward and backward in a sweeping motion; relax and repeat with opposite arm.

(Adapted from Metier, C. P. et al.: J. Cardiol. Rehabil. 6:89, 1986.)

to feed themselves, wash their hands and face, shave, and use the bedside commode with assistance. Progressive self-care activities allow patients to maintain the expectation of an independent life style. Sitting in a chair several times daily as suggested years ago[163] prevents orthostatic intolerance from bed rest. Intermittent exposure to gravitational stress usually suffices to protect against the increased cardiovascular stress induced by physical activity after bed rest.[173] Exercise involves a gradual approach that begins with an active range of motion as tolerated, progressing to more active exercises in conjunction with a walking program. Specific upper extremity and trunk exercises have been developed for postoperative patients without evidence of sternal instability.[3–5] Isometric exercises are avoided because of the presumed excessive myocardial oxygen consumption and dysrhythmias imposed by the predominantly "pressure" workload, especially in patients with compromised left ventricular function.[63] Physical activity should be carried out under the supervision of the nursing staff with frequent reassessment of symptoms and signs during the early physical activity sessions.

Early Postmyocardial Infarction Exercise Testing.

This technique is useful in formulating discharge planning and rehabilitation guidelines in low-risk patients.[39, 174] A low-level testing protocol provides additional data to detect the threshold for adverse symptoms or signs, to judge whether a patient can tolerate self-care activities at home, and to indicate the need for additional diagnostic studies and prognostic information. The safety of early exercise testing appears to be more related to the severity of disease than to the length of the interval following infarction or to the details of the test protocol. In patients without interference from medication, the standing heart rate of approximately 20 to 30 beats/min or an RPE of 12 to 13 can be used as guides for an appropriate intensity.[42] Patients with estimated or tested capacity at 3 or more METS should be able to follow the progressive exercise routine without difficulty. Before activities are increased to greater than 5 METS, an exercise evaluation should be conducted for guidance. If problems occur, the level of activity should be either reduced or discontinued temporarily until the patient can resume the physical activity routine safely. Criteria for termination of inpatient exercise sessions have been detailed[37] and generally involve undue fatigue, onset of angina, ST segment displacement of 3 mm or more, dysrhythmias, excessively high heart rates or blood pressure, an inappropriate drop in systolic blood pressure, or bradycardia.

PHASE TWO: INTERMEDIATE CONVALESCENCE. This phase of the program has as its objective the reversal of deconditioning and the initiation of a structured conditioning program. At the time of discharge from the hospital, the patient should be able to perform activities at peak levels of 3.5 to 4.0 METS, long enough to allow customary sedentary activities at home. Women may encounter special difficulties by attempting to resume total household tasks immediately upon discharge from the hospital.[175] During initial days at home, patients should continue the activities started at the hospital as warm-up exercises followed by walking at a graduated distance and pace. After the initial posthospitalization examination, further advice about exercise can be given to those ready to increase their physical activity. During this period, the patient is asked first to walk at least a quarter mile on level ground in 5 to 10 minutes for a period of 7 days, then a half mile in 10 to 15 minutes for another 7 days. Provided that there are no contraindications, the walking program is accelerated first in distance and then in pace. Generally, if the distance can be doubled at a given intensity without producing symptoms or excessive heart rate response, the next higher level of intensity may be undertaken.[176] The walk is gradually lengthened to achievable goals, such as a full mile at a 20 to 30 minute pace for a period of 7 to 14 days followed by further lengthening of the distance so that the total time approximates 30 to 45 minutes.

Approximately 6 weeks after hospitalization, a *symptom-limited maximal exercise test* should be conducted in order to determine limitations of activity. After evaluation the emphasis shifts toward dynamic exercises at greater intensity to improve cardiopulmonary function. At this point patients must be carefully reevaluated to detect possible abnormal responses to more vigorous exertion or conditions requiring special precautions. Some examples include inappropriate blood pressure or heart rate responses, ST-segment depression or elevation; angina, unusual fatigue, severe dyspnea, and a need for prolonged recovery. Any changes in the medication regimen must be taken into account. An inappropriately high intensity of exercise can lead to ischemia, orthopedic problems, and poor compliance, whereas homeopathic levels nullify any likely improvement and discourage patients from resuming ordinary activities.

A progressive individualized approach can prevent early unwarranted disability. Patients able to perform at levels of 5 METS or more should exercise at least three times per week, preferably on alternate days to avoid excessive bone and joint stress. During the first few weeks the duration of the exercise should range from 20 to 30 minutes and then increase to as much as 45 minutes.

For those patients with functional capacities below 5 METS the duration can be set empirically and adjusted according to the individual response to exercise. The frequency of exercise should be prescribed for three to five periods per week. Daily sessions for persons with capacities between 3 and 5 METS may be advisable, and for patients with functional capacities less than 3 METS, sessions of 5 minutes or so several times daily.[37] Within these guidelines, the exercise prescription for most patients will result in training adaptations without undue fatigue or hazard.

Monitored Group Program. An exercise facility offers the substantial advantages of trained personnel, monitoring capabilities for validating exercise prescriptions, established emergency routines, educational programs, and social reinforcements by other participants. The first week or so of the program should be used as a transition period toward a structured endurance training routine.[34] Patients should receive proper exercise instruction and be observed for new symptoms and signs not apparent on previous exercise testing. In addition, this initial period is used to adjust proposed work loads to attain target heart rates.

A training session may proceed as depicted in Figure 41–2. After an initial clinical evaluation, blood pressure, heart rate, and a single-lead ECG are evaluated. Warm-up activities should be employed to facilitate transition from rest to dynamic exercise by stretching muscles and increasing blood flow.[55] Sudden strenuous exertion has been found to provoke ischemic changes even in healthy men with normal ECG responses to exercise testing. Abnormal left ventricular ejection fractions and wall motion changes also have been observed among healthy men subjected to sudden strenuous activities.[55] Such abnormalities can be attenuated when the exercise is preceded by a low-level warm-up.[177] Slow walking and stretching exercises comprise the warm-up during the initial 10 minutes of the session. The patient then exercises at the target rate set initially at about 60 per cent of maximal capacity or 70 to 75 per cent of the maximal heart rate achieved on the prior exercise test. Continuous or intermittent monitoring can be used.

Useful training devices include the treadmill, stationary bicycle, steps, rowing machine, arm ergometer, and arm wheel. On each device, the patient reaches the target rate within a minute or so and maintains this heart rate for the remainder of a 4-minute exercise period. The prescribed heart rate is maintained by adjusting work loads and monitoring for heart rates outside the training range. After the 4th minute there is a 2-minute recovery or light activity period before the patient moves to the next exercise station. The patient alternates between arm and leg devices. In this way the patient achieves a larger overall work load before the onset of fatigue or symptoms and enjoys the other advantages of an intermittent program. However, there does tend to be a sequential increase in aerobic requirements, presumably because of incomplete recovery between exercise periods. After completion of these stages, a session of calisthenics or weight training can provide additional activities before a final cool-down period.

The cool-down period provides an interval for circulatory adjustments thus reducing the likelihood of postexertional hypotension, facilitating dissipation of body heat, promoting more rapid removal of lactic acid,[55] and reducing the potential adverse effects of the postexercise rise in plasma catecholamines.[178] Afterward, a brief evaluation consisting of pertinent questions and evaluation of heart rate, blood pressure, and ECG is appropriate. Most patients are ready to begin their own long-term program after 6 to 12 weeks of phase two.

Home Program. Medically directed rehabilitation at home provides an alternative to group training programs for selected patients. Some patients prefer not to participate in group programs for various reasons: inaccessibility of the exercise facility, financial difficulties, inconvenience, and personal preference. Several prototypes for training at home have been established.[179, 180] In the training program described by Miller and coworkers,[181] low-risk patients receive detailed written instructions for exercises and monitoring, including anticipated changes in clinical status that obviate continuation of exercise. Special self-monitoring devices are worn and the ECG is transmitted over the telephone to a special unit for external monitoring at prearranged times twice weekly. Training results apparently compare favorably with group sessions conducted at a medical facility.

PHASE THREE: LONG-TERM PROGRAM. After a suitable period of instruction and monitoring, usually no longer than 12 weeks, transfer to a long-term program is desirable. Criteria for entry into a community program include an understanding of the rationale for physical activity, an exercise capacity of at least 5 METS, stable medical status, a basic knowledge of the disease process and medications, and an awareness of possible abnormal symptoms and signs.[37] As with the first two phases, preliminary evaluation and exercise testing are necessary for determining exercise activities. This phase is designed to retain training adaptations made and stimulate further progress. The need for supervision is critical during the transition to more vigorous exertion with less structured routines. Except for those patients benefiting from low-level activities such as walking, it is best to delay a less structured long-term program until patients can meet the entry criteria. Recreational activities equivalent to the peak energy requirements of the previous exercise test can be introduced in the absence of known contraindications. Sports and games vary in the need for the basic elements of fitness—endurance, strength, and flexibility—and should be selected accordingly.

A typical long-term exercise session would consist of the following segments: (1) warm-up with slow walking and stretching exercise for 5 to 10 minutes; (2) endurance training consisting of 30 minutes of walking, jogging, cycling, or swimming at the target exertional level; (3) a 5-minute transitional period of light activity followed by (4) a 20- to 30-minute recreational period; and (5) a final cool-down 5-minute walk. The allotted time for structured endurance and recreational activities depends on individual preference, capabilities, and facilities. The introduction of a weight training circuit as part of the recreational activities offers several advantages:[56] development of increased upper body strength, improved physical appearance, and variation in the exercise routine. Initial data indicate that weight training improves compliance and contributes to endurance as well.

Heart rate estimates are more difficult to make during recreational activities, and the patient's subjective feeling of exertion (RPE) becomes more important. Recreational activities can be modified to decrease the peak levels of intensity and to provide continuous involvement of players throughout the game period so that the heart rate remains within the target zone. As the patient adapts to the training routine, the heart rate for a given workload will decrease, allowing progressive increments in external work. Clinical wisdom dictates the importance of the cool-down period as it is well recognized that many cardiac events occur immediately after exercise. Periodic evaluation aids in adjusting the exercise prescription and in assessing progress.

INDIVIDUALIZED PROGRAMS. Individual preferences, economic concerns, and other factors necessitate the use of individual exercise programs for patients who qualify. Patients may proceed to an individualized maintenance program after a period of at least 3 months in a supervised program. Evaluations should confirm: (1) a stable health status, (2) relatively low risk for subsequent cardiac events, (3) functional performance of at least 5 METS, (4) an understanding of the principles of exercise training, (5) knowledge of the disease process and treatment including medication, and (6) mechanisms for follow-up. Provisions for periodic assessment and training with others in a group should be made for enhancing safety and long-term adherence. Physicians can maintain surveillance through exercise diaries and telephone monitoring, among other means.

Within such constraints, cardiac patients can undertake rehabilitation programs at the least risk and greatest benefit. Major modifications in cardiac rehabilitation programs are taking place to allow maximum participation by the greatest number of individuals possible. At the same time, emphasis is shifting away from morbidity and mortality outcomes toward those factors benefiting work and leisure activities. Cardiac rehabilitation should allow patients to attain the best possible physical, mental, and social conditions so that they may lead active and productive lives in the community.[182] With an increasing number of participants in programs of larger scope, cardiac rehabilitation will play a growing role in the long-term clinical management of patients with coronary artery disease.

REFERENCES

COMPONENTS OF A REHABILITATION PROGRAM

1. Hellerstein, H.K.: Cardiac rehabilitation: A retrospective view. *In* Pollock, M.L., and Schmidt, D.H. (ed.): Heart Disease and Rehabilitation. New York, John Wiley and Sons, 1986, pp. 701–711.
2. Kellerman, J.: Rehabilitation of patients with coronary heart disease. Prog. Cardiovasc. Dis. *17*:303, 1975.
3. Oberman, A., and Kouchoukos, N.T.: Role of exercise after coronary artery surgery. *In* Wenger, N.K. (ed.): Exercise and the Heart. Philadelphia, F. A. Davis Co.., 1978, pp. 155–172.
4. Robinson, G., Froelicher, V.F., and Utley, J.R.: Rehabilitation of the coronary artery bypass graft surgery patient. J. Cardiac Rehabil. *4*:74, 1984.
5. Metier, C.P., Pollock, M.L., and Graves, J.E.: Exercise prescription for the coronary artery bypass graft surgery patient. J. Cardiac Rehabil. *6*:85, 1986.
6. Newell, J.P., Kappagoda, C.T., Stoker, J.B., Deverall, P.B., Watson, D.A., and Linden, R.J.: Physical training after heart valve replacement. Br. Heart J. *44*:638, 1980.
7. Cantwell, J.D.: Cardiac rehabilitation in the mid-1980s. Phys. Sports Med. *14*:89, 1986.
8. Lampman, R.M., Stewart, J.R., Collins, J.A., and Thrall, J.H.: Exercise training soon after left ventricular aneurysmectomy and endocardial resection. J. Cardiac Rehabil. 2:134, 1982.
9. Hassell, L.A., Fowles, R.E., and Stinson, E.B.: Patients with congestive cardiomyopathy as cardiac transplant recipients. Am. J. Cardiol. *47*:1205, 1981.
10. Squires, R.W., Arthur, P.R., Gau, G.T., Muri, A., and Lambert, W.B.: Exercise after cardiac transplantation: A report of two cases. J. Cardiac Rehabil. *3*:570, 1983.
11. Rice, D.P., Hodgson, T.A., and Kopstein, A.N.: The economic cost of illness: A replication and update. Health Care Financing, Winter 1985.
12. Momentum Toward Health: U.S. Department of Health and Human Services, NIH Pub. No. 85–2353, November 1985.

13. Wenger, N.K., Hellerstein, H.K., and Blackburn, H.: Physician practice in the management of patients with uncomplicated myocardial infarction: Changes in the past decade. Circulation *65*:421, 1982.
14. DeBusk, R.F., and Dennis, C.A.: Occupational work evaluation of patients with cardiac disease: A guide for physicians. West. J. Med. *137*:515, 1982.
15. Oberman, A., and Finklea, J.F.: Return to work after coronary artery bypass grafting. Ann. Thorac. Surg. *34*:353, 1982.

EXERCISE

16. Haskell, W.L.: Mechanisms by which physical activity may enhance the clinical status of cardiac patients. *In* Pollock, M.L., and Schmidt, D.H. (eds.): Heart Disease and Rehabilitation. New York, John Wiley and Sons, 1986, pp. 303–324.
17. Hartung, G.H., and Rangel, R.: Exercise training in postmyocardial infarction patients: Comparison of results with high risk coronary and post-bypass patients. Arch. Phys. Med. Rehabil. *62*:147, 1981.
18. Schlant, R.C.: Physiology of exercise. *In* Fletcher, G.F.: Exercise in the Practice of Medicine. Mt. Kisco, N.Y., Futura Publishing Co., 1982, pp. 1–43.
19. Blomquist, C.G., and Lewis, S.F.: Physiological effects of training: Geneal circulatory adjustments. *In* Cohen, L.S., Mock, M.B., and Ringqvist, I. (eds.): Physical Conditioning and Cardiovascular Rehabilitation. New York, John Wiley and Sons, 1981, pp. 57–76.
20. Scheuer, J., and Tipton, C.M.: Cardiovascular adaptations to physical training. Ann. Rev. Physiol. *39*:221, 1977.
21. Conn, E.H., Williams, R.S., and Wallace, A.G.: Exercise responses before and after physical conditioning in patients with severely depressed left ventricular function. Am. J. Cardiol. *49*:296, 1982.
22. Hammond, H.K., Kelly, T.L., Froelicher, V.F., and Pewen, W.: Use of clinical data in predicting improvement in exercise capacity after cardiac rehabilitation. J. Am. Coll. Cardiol. *6*:19, 1985.
23. Report of the Task Force on Cardiovascular Rehabilitation of the National Heart and Lung Institute: Needs and Opportunities for Rehabilitating the Coronary Heart Disease Patient. DHEW Publication No. (NIH) 75–750, Washington, D.C., U.S. Government Printing Office, 1974.
24. Dressendorfer, R.H., Smith, J.L., Amsterdam, E.A., and Mason, D.T.: Reduction of submaximal exercise myocardial oxygen demand post-walk training program in coronary patients due to improved physical work efficiency. Am. Heart J. *103*:258, 1982.
25. Coyle, E.F., Martin, W.H., Ehsani, A.A., Hagberg, S.A., Bloomfield, D.R., Sinacore, D.R., and Holloszy, J.O.: Blood lactate threshold in some well-trained ischemic heart disease patients. J. Appl. Physiol. *54*:18, 1983.
26. Sullivan, M., Ahnve, S., Froelicher, V.F., and Meyers, J.: The influence of exercise training on the ventilatory threshold of patients with coronary heart disease. Am. Heart J. *109*:458, 1985.
27. Wilson, J.R., Martin, J.L., Schwartz, D., and Ferraro, N.: Exercise intolerance in patients with chronic heart failure: Role of impaired nutritive flow to skeletal muscle. Circulation *69*:1079, 1984.
28. Jonason, A., Jonzon, B., Ringqvist, I., and Omar-Rydbert, A.: Effects of physical training on different categories of patients with intermittent claudication. Acta Med. Scand. *206*:253, 1979.
29. Saltin, B.: Physical training in patients with intermittent claudication. *In* Cohen, L.S., Mock, M.B., and Ringqvist, I. (eds.): Physical Conditioning and Cardiovascular Rehabilitation. New York, John Wiley and Sons, 1981, pp. 181–196.
30. Stern, M.J., and Cleary, P.: National Exercise and Heart Disease Project: Psychosocial changes observed during a low-level exercise program. Arch. Intern. Med. *141*:1463, 1981.
31. Prosser, G., Carson, P., and Phillips, R.: Exercise after myocardial infarction: Long-term rehabilitation effects. J. Psychosom. Res. *29*:535, 1985.
32. Fontana, A.F., Kerns, R.D., Rosenberg, R.L., Marcus, J.L., and Colonese, K.D.: Exercise training for cardiac patients: Adherence, fitness, and benefits. J. Cardiopul. Rehabil. *6*:4, 1986.
33. Ott, C., and Bergner, M.: The effect of rehabilitation after myocardial infarction on quality of life. Quality of Life and Cardiovascular Care *1*:176, 1985.
34. Fletcher, B.J., Thiel, J., and Fletcher, G.F.: Phase II intensive monitored cardiac rehabilitation for coronary artery disease and coronary risk factors—a six-session protocol. Am. J. Cardiol. *57*:751, 1986.
35. Williams, M.A., Esterbrooks, D.J., Aronow, W.S., and Sketch, M.H.: Limitations of exercise testing to screen cardiac patients for early nonmonitored rehabilitation exercise programs. J. Cardiac Rehabil. *4*:396, 1984.
36. Pollock, M.L., Wilmore, J.H., and Fox, S.M.: Prescribing exercise for rehabilitation of the cardiac patient. *In* Exercise in Health and Disease: Evaluation and prescription for prevention and rehabilitation. Philadelphia, W. B. Saunders Company, 1984, pp. 298–373.
37. Exercise prescription for cardiac patients. *In* Blair, S.N., Gibbons, L.W., Painter, P., Pate, R.R., Taylor, C.B., and Will, J. (eds.): American College of Sports Medicine. Guidelines for Exercise Testing and Prescriptions, 3rd Ed. Philadelphia, Lea and Febiger, 1986, pp. 53–71.
38. Council on Scientific Affairs: Physician-supervised exercise programs in rehabilitation of patients with coronary heart disease. J.A.M.A. *245*:1463, 1981.
39. DeBusk, R.F., Blomqvist, C.G., Kouchoukos, N.T., Luepker, R.V., Miller, H.S., Moss, A.J., Pollock, M.L., Reeves, T.J., Selvester, R.H., Staston, W.B., Wagner, G.S., and Willman, V.L.: Identification and treatment of low-risk patients after acute myocardial infarction and coronary-artery bypass graft surgery. N. Engl. J. Med. *314*:161, 1986.
40. Superko, H.R.: The effects of cardiac rehabilitation in permanently paced patients with third degree heart block. J. Cardiac Rehabil. *3*:561, 1983.
41. Humen, D.P., Kostuk, W.J., and Klein, G.: Activity-sensing, rate-responsive pacing: Improvement in myocardial performance with exercise. PACE *8*:52, 1985.
42. Beta Blockers and Exercise: A Symposium. *In* Harrison, D.C. (ed.): Am. J. Cardiol. *55*:167D–171D, 1985.
43. Lowenthal, D.T., Stein, D.T., Hare, T.W., Yarnoff, A., Lowenthall, P.J., Saris, S., Falkner, B., and Affrime, M.B.: The clinical pharmacology of cardiovascular drugs during exercise. J. Cardiac Rehabil. *3*:829, 1983.
43a. Guidelines for Exercise Testing: A report of the Joint American College of Cardiology/American Heart Association Task Force on Assessment of Cardiovascular Procedures. Circulation *74*:653A, 1986.
44. Guidelines for exercise test administration: *In* Blair, S.N., Gibbons, L.W., Painter, P., Pate, R.R., Taylor, C.B., and Will, J. (eds.): American College of Sports Medicine. Guidelines for Exercise Testing and Prescription, 3d Ed. Philadelphia, Lea and Febiger, 1986, pp. 9–30.
45. Eldridge, J.E., Ramsey-Green, C.L., and Hossack, K.F.: Effects of the limiting symptom on the achievement of maximal oxygen consumption in patients with coronary artery disease. Am. J. Cardiol. *57*:513, 1986.
46. Gottlieb, S.O., Weisfeldt, M.L., Ouyang, P., Mellits, D.E., and Gerstenblith, G.: Silent ischemia as a marker for early unfavorable outcomes in patients with unstable angina. N. Engl. J. Med. *314*:1214, 1986.
47. Viitasalo, M.T., Kala, R., Eisalo, A., and Halonen, A.: Ventricular arrhythmias during exercise testing, jogging, and sedentary life. Chest *76*:21, 1979.
48. McKinnis, R.A., Burks, H., Lee, K.L., Harrell, F.E., Behar, V.S., Pryor, V.S., Pryor, D.B., Wagner, G.S., and Rosati, R.A.: Prognostic implications of ventricular arrhythmias during 24-hour ambulatory monitoring in patients undergoing cardiac catheterization for coronary artery disease. Am. J. Cardiol. *50*:23, 1982.
49. Simoons, M., Lap, C., and Pool, J.: Heart rate levels and ventricular ectopic activity during cardiac rehabilitation. Am. Heart J. *100*:9, 1980.
50. Winkle, R.A.: The relationship between ventricular ectopic beat frequency and heart rate. Circulation *66*:439, 1982.
51. Borg, G.A.: Psychophysical bases of perceived exertion. Med. Sci. Sports Exercise *14*:377, 1982.
52. Chow, R.J., and Wilmore, J.H.: The regulation of exercise intensity by ratings of perceived exertion. J. Cardiac Rehabil. *4*:382, 1984.
53. Ewart, C.K., Stewart, K.J., Gillilan, R.E., Kelemen, M.H., Valenti, S.A., Manley, J.D., and Kelemen, M.D.: Usefulness of self-efficacy in predicting overexertion during programmed exercise in coronary artery disease. Am. J. Cardiol. *57*:557, 1986.
54. Franklin, B.A.: Exercise testing, training and arm ergometry. Sports Med. *2*:100, 1985.
55. Franklin, B.A., Hellerstein, H.K., Gordon, S., and Timmis, G.C.: Exercise prescription for the myocardial infarction patient. J. Cardiopul. Rehabil. *6*:62, 1986
56. Keleman, M.H., Stewart, K.J., Gillilan, R.E., Ewart, C.K., Valenti, S.A., and Manley, J.D.: Circuit weight training in cardiac patients. J. Am. Coll. Cardiol. *7*:38, 1986.
57. Madger, S., Linnarsson, D., and Gullstrand, L.: The effect of swimming on patients with ischemic heart disease. Circulation *63*:979, 1981.
58. Thompson, D.L., Boone, T.W., and Miller, H.S.: Comparison of treadmill exercise and tethered swimming to determine validity of exercise prescription. J. Cardiac Rehabil. *2*:363, 1982.
59. Shephard, R.J., Kavanagh, T., Tuck, J., and Kennedy, J.: Marathon jogging in postmyocardial infarction patients. J. Cardiac Rehabil. *3*:321, 1983.
59a. Kavanagh, T., Yacoub, M., Campbell, R., and Mertens, D.: Marathon running after cardiac transplantation: A case history. J. Cardiopulmonary Rehabil. *6*:16, 1986.
60. Painter, P., and Hanson, P.: Isometric exercise: Implications for the cardiac patient. Cardiac Rev. Rep. *5*:261, 1984.
61. DeBusk, R.F., and Davidson, D.M.: The work evaluation of the cardiac patient. J. Occup. Med. *22*:715, 1980.
62. Ferguson, R.J., Cote, P., Bourassa, M.G., and Corbara, F.: Coronary blood flow during isometric and dynamic exercise in angina pectoris patients. J. Cardiac Rehabil. *1*:21, 1981.
63. Mitchell, J.H., and Blomqvist, C.G.: Response of patients with heart disease to dynamic and static exercise. *In* Pollock, M.L., and Schmidt, D.H. (eds.): Heart Disease and Rehabilitation. New York, John Wiley and Sons, 1986, pp. 85–96.
63a. Coplan, N.L., Gleim G.W., and Nicholas, J.A.: Principles of exercise prescription for patients with coronary artery disease. Am. Heart J. *122*:145, 1986.
64. Wilson, P.K., Fardy, P.S., and Froelicher, V.F.: Cardiac Rehabilitation, Adult Fitness and Exercise Testing. Philadelphia, Lea and Febiger, 1981, pp. 333–351.
65. Pollock, M.L., Gettman, L.R., Milesis, C.A., Bah, M.D., Durstine, L., and Johnson, R.B.: Effects of frequency and duration of training on attrition and incidence of injury. Med. Sci. Sports *9*:31, 1977.
66. Powell, K.E., Kohl, H.W., Caspersen, C.J., and Blair, S.N.: An epidemiological perspective on the causes of running injuries. Phys. Sports Med. *14*(6):100, 1986.
67. Balke, B.: Altitude and cold: The cardiac patient. *In* Pollock, M.L., and Schmidt, D.H. (eds.): Heart Disease and Rehabilitation. New York, John Wiley and Sons, 1986, pp. 537–547.
68. Raven, P.B.: Heat and air pollution: The cardiac patient. *In* Pollock, M.L., and Schmidt, D.H. (eds.): Heart Disease and Rehabilitation. New York, John Wiley and Sons, 1986, pp. 549–574.
69. Fletcher, G.F.: Influence of environmental factors on exercise activities in patient care. *In* Fletcher, G.F. (ed.): Exercise in the Practice of Medicine. Mt. Kisco, N.Y., Futura Publishing Co., 1982, pp. 347–358.

70. Casale, T.B., Keahey, T.M., Kaliner, M.: Exercise-induced anaphylactic syndromes: Insights into diagnostic and pathophysiologic features. J.A.M.A. *255*:2049, 1986.
71. Fletcher, G.F.: Influence of environmental factors on exercise activities in patient care. *In* Exercise in the Practice of Medicine. Mt. Kisco, N.Y., Futura Publishing Co., 1982, pp. 347–358.
72. Oberman, A.: Healthy exercise. *In* Personal health maintenance (Special Issue). West. J. Med. *141*:864, 1984.
73. Haskell, W.L.: Cardiovascular complications during medically supervised exercise training. *In* Cohen, L .S., Mock, M.B., and Ringqvist, I. (eds.): Physical Conditioning and Cardiac Rehabilitation. New York, John Wiley and Sons, 1981, pp. 159–167.
74. Hossack, K.F., and Hartwig, R.: Cardiac arrest associated with supervised cardiac rehabilitation. J. Cardiac Rehabil. *2*:402, 1982.
74a. Van Camp, S.P., and Peterson, R.A.: Cardiovascular complications of outpatient cardiac rehabilitation programs. J.A.M.A. *256*:1160, 1986.
75. Cobb, L.A., and Weaver, W.D.: Exercise: A risk for sudden death in patients with coronary heart disease. J. Am. Coll. Cardiol. *7*:215, 1986.

SECONDARY PREVENTION

76. Turi, Z.G., and Braunwald, E.: The use of beta-blockers after myocardial infarction. J.A.M.A. *249*:2512, 1983.
77. Canner, P.L.: Mortality in coronary drug project patients during a nine-year post-treatment period. J. Am. Coll. Cardiol. *5*:442, 1985.
78. Harker, L.A.: Clinical trials evaluating platelet-modifying drugs in patients with atherosclerotic cardiovascular disease and thrombosis. Circulation *73*:206, 1986.
79. Kirklin, J.W., Blackstone, E.H., and Rogers, W.J.: The plights of the invasive treatment of ischemic heart disease. J. Am. Coll. Cardiol. *5*:158, 1985.
80. Kannel, W.B., Doyle, J.T., Ostfeld, A.M., Jenkins, C.D., Kuller, L., Podell, R.N., and Stamler, J.: Optimal resources for primary prevention of atherosclerotic diseases: Atherosclerosis study group. Circulation *70*:153A, 1984.
81. Glueck, C.J.: Role of risk factor management in progression and regression of coronary and femoral artery atherosclerosis. Am. J. Cardiol. *57*:35G, 1986.
82. Superko, H.R., Wood, P.D., and Haskell, W.L.: Coronary heart disease and risk factor modification: Is there a threshold? Am. J. Med. *78*:826, 1985.
83. Raichlen, J.S., Healy, B., Achuff, S.C., and Pearson, T. A.: Importance of risk factors in the angiographic progression of coronary artery disease. Am. J. Cardiol. *57*:66, 1986.
83a. Mahley, R.W.: Atherogenic lipoproteins and coronary artery disease: Concepts derived from recent advances in cellular and molecular biology. Circulation *72*:943, 1985.
84. Oliver, M.F.: Prevention of coronary heart disease—propaganda, promises, problems, and prospects. Circulation *73*:1, 1986.
85. May, G.S., Eberlein, K.A., Furberg, C.D., Passamani, E.R., and DeMets, D.L.: Secondary prevention after myocardial infarction: A view of long-term trials. Prog. Cardiovasc. Dis. *24*:331, 1982.
86. Deanfield, J.E., Shea, M.J., Wilson, R.A., Horlock, P., deLandsheere, C.M., and Selwyn, A.P.: Direct effects of smoking on the heart: Silent ischemic disturbances of coronary flow. Am. J. Cardiol. *57*:1005, 1986.
87. Klein, L.W., Ambrose, J., Pichard, A., Holt, J., Gorlin, R., and Teichholz, L.E.: Acute coronary hemodynamic response to cigarette smoking in patients with coronary artery disease. J. Am. Coll. Cardiol. *3*:879, 1984.
88. Vliesstra, R.E., Kronmal, R.A., Oberman, A., Frye, R.L., and Killip, T.: Effect of cigarette smoking on survival of patients with angiographically documented coronary artery disease. J.A.M.A. *255*:1023, 1986.
89. The 1984 Report of the Joint National Committee on Detection, Evaluation, and Treatment of High Blood Pressure. Arch. Intern. Med. *144*:1045, 1984.
90. American College of Sports Medicine: Position statement on proper and improper weight loss programs, 1983.
91. Oberman, A.: Exercise and the primary prevention of cardiovascular disease. Am. J. Cardiol. *55*:10-D, 1985.
91a. Goldberg, L., and Elliot, D.L.: The effect of physical activity on lipid and lipoprotein levels. Med. Clin. North Am. *69*:41, 1985.
92. Wood, P.D., Haskell, W.L., and Fortmann, S.P.: Effects on lipoproteins of weight loss by dieting versus exercise in a controlled trial. CVD Epidemiology Newsletter *39*:50, 1986.
93. Williams, P.T., Wood, P.D., Haskell, W.L., and Vranizan, K.: The effects of running mileage and duration on plasma lipoprotein levels. J.A.M.A. *247*:2674, 1982.
94. Heath, G.W., Gavin, J.R., III, Hinderliter, J.M., et al.: Effects of exercise and lack of exercise on glucose tolerance and insulin sensitivity. J. Appl. Physiol. *55*:512, 1983.
95. Tipton, C.M.: Exercise training and hypertension. Exercise Sports Sciences Rev. *12*:245, 1984.
96. Martin, J.E., and Dubbert, P.M.: Exercise in hypertension. Ann. Behavioral Med. *7*:1, 13, 1985.
96a. Nelson, L., Jennings, G.L., Esler, M.D., and Korner, P.L.: Effect of changing levels of physical activity on blood-pressure and hemodynamics in essential hypertension. Lancet *2*:473, 1986.
97. Ehsani, A.A., Heath, G.W., Martin, W.H., III, Hagberg, J.M., and Holloszy, J.O.: Effects of intense exercise training on plasma catecholamines in coronary patients. J. Appl. Physiol. *57*:155, 1984.
98. Oberman, A., Cleary, P., LaRosa, J.C., Hellerstein, H.K., and Naughton, J.: Changes in risk factors among long-term exercise rehabilitation program participants. Adv. Cardiol. *31*:168, 1982.
99. Foster, C., Pollock, M.L., Anholm, J.D., Squires, R.W., Ward, A., Dymond, D.S., Rod, J.L., Saichek, R.P., and Schmidt, D.H.: Work capacity and left ventricular function during rehabilitation after myocardial revascularization surgery. Circulation *69*:748, 1984.
100. Laslett, L.J., Paumer, L., and Amsterdam, E.A.: Increase in myocardial oxygen consumption indexes by exercise training at onset of ischemia inpatients with coronary artery disease. Circulation *71*:958, 1985.
101. Redwood, D.R., Rosing, D.R., and Epstein, S.E.: Circulatory and symptomatic effects of physical training in patients with coronary-artery disease and angina pectoris. N. Engl. J. Med. *286*:959, 1972.
102. Ehsani, A.A., Heath, G.W., Hagberg, J.M., Sobel, B.E., and Holloszy, J.O.: Effects of 12 months of intense exercise training on ischemic ST-segment depression in patients with coronary artery disease. Circulation *57*:549, 1978.
103. Holloszy, J.O., Skinner, J.S., Barry, A.J., et al.: Effect of physical conditioning on cardiovascular function—a ballistocardiographic study. Am. J. Cardiol. *14*:761, 1964.
104. Epstein, L., Miller, G.J., Stitt, F.W., and Morris, J.N.: Vigorous exercise in leisure time, coronary risk factors, and resting electrocardiogram in middle-aged male civil servants. Br. Heart J. *38*:403, 1976.
105. Kramsch, D.M., Aspen, A.J., Abramowitz, B.M., Kreimendahl, T., and Hood, W.B.: Reduction of coronary atherosclerosis by moderate conditioning exercise in monkeys on an atherogenic diet. N. Engl. J. Med. *305*:1483, 1981.
106. Froelicher, V.F.: The Cardiovascular Effects of Chronic Exercise. *In* Exercise Testing and Training. Chicago, Year Book Medical Publishers, Inc., 1984, pp. 179–235.
107. Bove, A.A., and Dewey, J.D.: Proximal coronary vasomotor reactivity after exercise training in dogs. Circulation *71*:620, 1985.
108. Scheuer, J.: Effects of physical training on myocardial vascularity and perfusion. Circulation *66*:491, 1982.
109. Hagberg, J.M., Ehsani, A.A., and Holloszy, J.O.: Effect of 12 months of intense exercise training on stroke volume in patients with coronary artery disease. Circulation *67*:1194, 1983.
109a. Ehsani, A.A., Biello, D.R., Schultz, J., Sobel, B.E., and Holloszy, J.O.: Improvement of left ventricular contractile function by exercise training in patients with coronary artery disease. Circulation *74*:350, 1986.
110. Williams, R.S., McKinnis, R.A., Cobb, F.R., Higginbotham, M.B., Wallace, A.G., Coleman, R.E., and Califf, R.M.: Effects of physical conditioning on left ventricular ejection fraction in patients with coronary artery disease. Circulation *70*:69, 1984.
111. Paterson, D.H., Shephard, R.J., Cunningham, D., Jones, N.L., and Andrew, G.: Effects of physical training on cardiovascular function following myocardial infarction. J. Appl. Physiol. *47*:482, 1979.
112. Schaible, T.F., and Scheuer, J.: Cardiac adaptations to chronic exercise. Prog. Cardiovasc. Dis. *27*(5):297, 1985.
113. Cobb, F.R., Williams, R.S., McEwan, P., Jones, R.H., Coleman, R.E., and Wallace, A.G.: Effects of exercise training on ventricular function in patients with recent myocardial infarction. Circulation *66*:100, 1982.
114. DeMaria, A.N., Neumann, A., Lee, G., Fowler, W., and Mason, D.T.: Alterations in ventricular mass and performance induced by exercise training in men evaluated by echocardiography. Circulation *57*:237, 1978.
115. Jensen, D., Atwood, J.E., Froelicher, V., McKirnam, M.D., Battler, A., Ashburn, W., and Ross, J.: Improvement in ventricular function during exercise studied with radionuclide ventriculography after cardiac rehabilitation. Am. J. Cardiol. *46*:770, 1980.
116. Froelicher, V., Jensen, D., Genter, F., Sullivan, M., McKirnan, M.D., Witztum, K., Scharf, J., Strong, M.L., and Ashburn, W.: A randomized trial of exercise training in patients with coronary heart disease. J.A.M.A., *252*:1291, 1984.
117. Wilhelmsen, L., Sanne, H., Elmfeldt, D., Grimby, G., Tibblin, G., and Wedel, H.: A controlled trial of physical training after myocardial infarction. Prev. Med. *4*:491, 1975.
118. Kentala, E.: Physical fitness and feasibility of physical rehabilitation after myocardial infarction in men of working age. Ann. Clin. Res. *4*:1, 1972.
119. Palatsi, I.: Feasibility of physical training after myocardial infarction and its effect on return to work, morbidity and mortality. Acta Med. Scand. *599*(Suppl):7, 1976.
120. Shephard, R.J.: Evaluation of earlier studies: Canada. *In* Cohen, L.S., Mock, M.B., and Ringqvist, I. (eds.): Physical Conditioning and Cardiovascular Rehabilitation. New York, John Wiley and Sons, 1981, pp. 271–288.
121. Rechnitzer, P.A., Cunningham, D.A., Andrew, G.M., Buck, C.W., Jones, N.L., Kavanagh, T., Oldridge, N.B., Parker, J.O., Shephard, R.J., Sutton, J.R., and Donner, A.P.: Relation of exercise to the recurrence rate of myocardial infarction in men: Ontario exercise-heart collaborative study. Am. J. Cardiol. *51*:65, 1983.
122. Shaw, L.W.: Effects of a prescribed supervised exercise program on mortality and cardiovascular morbidity in patients after a myocardial infarction. Am. J. Cardiol. *48*:39, 1981.
123. Roman, O., Guitierrez, M., Luksic, I., Chavez, E., Camuzzi, A.L., Villalon, E., Klenner, C., and Cumsille, F.: Cardiac rehabilitation after myocardial infarction: 9-year controlled follow-up study. Cardiology *70*:223, 1983.
124. Carson, P., Philips, R., Lloyd, M., Tucker, H., Neophytou, M., Buch, N.J., Gelson, A., Lawton, A., and Simpson, T.: Exercise after a myocardial infarction: A controlled trial. J. R. Coll. Physicians Lond. *16*:147, 1982.

125. Oberman, A., and Naughton, J.: The national exercise and heart disease project. *In* Pollock, M.L., and Schmidt, D.H., (eds.): Heart Disease and Rehabilitation. New York, John Wiley and Sons, 1986, pp. 369–385.
126. Collins, R., Yusuf, S., and Peto, R.: Exercise after myocardial infarction reduces mortality: Evidence from randomized controlled trials (RCTs). J. Am. Coll. Cardiol. 3(Abs):622, 1984.
127. Ben-Ari, E., Kellermann, J.J., Fisman, E., Pines, A., Peled, B., and Drory, Y.: Benefits of long-term physical training in patients after coronary artery bypass grafting—A 58-month follow-up and comparison with a nontrained group. J. Cardiopul. Rehabil. *6*:165, 1986.
128. Salonen, J.T., and Puska, P.: A community programme for rehabilitation and secondary prevention of patients with acute myocardial infarction as part of a comprehensive community programme for control of cardiovascular disease (North Karelia Project). Scand. J. Rehabil. Med. *12*:33, 1980.
129. Puska, P., Tuomilehto, J., Salonen, J.T., et al.: Community control of cardiovascular disease: Evaluation of a comprehensive community programme for control of cardiovascular diseases in 1972–1977 in North Karelia, Finland. Geneva, WHO Monograph Series, 1981.
130. Kallio, V., Hamalainen, H., Kakkila, J., and Luurila, O.J.: Reduction in sudden deaths by a multifactorial intervention programme after acute myocardial infarction. Lancet 2:1091, 1979.
131. Vedin, A., Wilhemsson, C., Tibblin, G., and Wilhemsen, L.: The postinfarction clinic in Göteborg, Sweden. A controlled trial of therapeutic organization. Acta Med. Scand. *200*:453, 1976.
132. Vermueulen, A., Lie, K.I., and Durrer, D.: Effects of cardiac rehabilitation after myocardial infarction: Changes in coronary risk factors and long-term prognosis. Am. Heart J. *105*:798, 1983.

PSYCHOSOCIAL REHABILITATION

133. Eliot, R.S.: Stress and the Major Cardiovascular Disorders. Mt. Kisco, N.Y., Futura Publishing Co., 1979.
134. Croog, S.H., and Levine, S.: The Heart Patient Recovers. New York, Human Sciences Press, 1977.
135. Blumenthal, J.A.: Psychologic assessment in cardiac rehabilitation. J. Cardiopul. Rehabil. *5*:208, 1985.
136. Tesar, G.E., and Hackett, T.P.: Psychiatric management of the hospitalized cardiac patient. J. Cardiopul. Rehabil. *5*:219, 1985.
137. Kinchla, J., and Weiss, T.: Psychologic and social outcomes following coronary artery bypass surgery. J. Cardiopul. Rehabil. *5*:274, 1985.
138. Heller, S.S., Frank, K.A., Kornfeld, D.S., et al.: Psychological outcome following open heart surgery. Arch. Intern. Med. *5*:67, 1974.
139. Oberman, A., Wayne, J.B., Kouchoukos, N.T., Charles, E.D., Russell, R.O., and Rogers, W.J.: Employment status after coronary artery bypass surgery. Circulation *65*(Suppl.II):115, 1982.
140. Baer, P.E., Cleveland, S.E., Montero, A.C., Revel, K.F., Clancy, C., and Bowen, R.: Improving post-myocardial infarction recovery status by stress management training during hospitalization. J. Cardiac Rehabil. *5*:191, 1985.
141. Cay, E.L.: Psychological approach in patient after a myocardial infarction. Adv. Cardiol. *24*:120, 1978.
142. Hackett, T.P.: The use of groups in the rehabilitation of the postcoronary patient. Adv. Cardiol. *24*:127, 1978.
143. Rejeski, W.J., Morley, D., and Sotile, W.: Cardiac rehabilitation: A conceptual framework for psychologic assessment. J. Cardiac Rehabil. *5*:172, 1985.
144. Shaw, R.E., Cohen, F., Doyle, B., and Palesky, J.: The impact of denial and repressive style on information gain and rehabilitation outcomes in myocardial infarction patients. Psychosom. Med. *47*:262, 1985.
145. Friis, R., and Armstrong, T.: Social support and social networks, and coronary heart disease and rehabilitation. J. Cardiopul. Rehabil. *6*:132, 1986.
146. Hellerstein, H.K., and Friedman, E.H.: Sexual activity and the postcoronary patient. Med. Aspects Hum. Sex. *3*:70, 1973.
147. McLane, M., Krop, H., and Mehta, J.: Psychosexual adjustment and counseling after myocardial infarction. Ann. Intern. Med. *92*:514, 1980.
147a. Ruberman, W., Weinblatt, E., Goldberg, J.D., and Chaudhary, B.S.: Psychosocial influences on mortality after myocardial infarction. N. Engl. J. Med. *311*:552, 1984.
148. Oldenberg, B., Perkins, R.J., and Andrews, G.: Controlled trial of psychological intervention in myocardial infarction. J. Consult. Clin. Psychol. *53*:852, 1985.
149. Ornish, D., Scherwitz, L.W., Doody, R.S., et al.: Effects of stress management training and dietary changes in treating ischemic heart disease. J.A.M.A. *249*:54, 1983.
150. Friedman, M., Thoresen, C.E., Gill, J.J., Powell, L.H., Ulmer, D., Thompson, L., Price, V.A., Rabin, D.D., Breall, W.S., Dixon, T., Levy, R., and Bourg, E.: Alteration of Type A behavior and reduction in cardiac recurrences in postmyocardial infarction patients. Am. Heart J. *108*:237, 1984.
151. Thoresen, C.E., Friedman, M., Powell, L.H., Fill, J.J., and Ulmer, D.: Altering the Type A behavior pattern in postinfarction patients. J. Cardiopul. Rehabil. *5*:258, 1985.
152. Martin, J.E., and Dubbert, P.M.: Behavioral management strategies for improving health and fitness. J. Cardiac Rehabil. *4*:200, 1984.

VOCATIONAL REHABILITATION

153. Johnson, W.D., Kayser, K.L., Pedraza, P.M., and Shore, R.T.: Employment patterns in males before and after myocardial revascularization surgery. A study of 229 consecutive male patients followed for as long as 10 years. Circulation *65*:1086, 1982.
154. Guvendik, L., Rahan, M., and Yacoub, M.: Symptomatic status and pattern of employment during a five-year period following myocardial revascularization for angina. Ann. Thorac. Surg. *34*:383, 1982.
155. Wiklund, I., Sanne, H., Vedin, A., and Wilhelmsson, C.: Determinants of return to work one year after a first myocardial infarction. J. Cardiac Rehabil. *5*:62, 1985.
156. Oberman, A., Fisher, C., Maynard, L., Mullin, S.M., Charles, E.D., and Tristani, F.: Long-term changes in work status among patients in the Coronary Artery Surgery Study (CASS) Registry. *In* Walter, P.J.F. (ed.): Return to Work After Coronary Artery Bypass Surgery. New York, Springer-Verlag, 1985, pp. 137–147.
157. Return to Work After Coronary Artery Bypass Surgery: Incidence and Main Factors. *In* Walter, P.J.F. (ed.): Return to Work After Coronary Artery Bypass Surgery. New York, Springer-Verlag, 1985, pp. 1–121.
158. American Medical Association: Guides to the evaluation of permanent impairment, 2nd Ed. Chicago, 1984.
159. Disability Evaluation Under Social Security: U.S. Department of Health and Human Services, Social Security Administration, SSA Pub. No. 05–10089, February, 1986, pp. 34–44.
160. Carey, T.S., and Hadler, N.: The role of the primary physician in disability determination for social security insurance and workers' compensation. Ann. Intern. Med. *104*:706, 1986.
161. Sheldahl, L.M., Wilke, N.A., Tristani, F.E., and Hughes, C.V.: Heart rate responses during home activities soon after myocardial infarction. J. Cardiac Rehabil. *4*:327, 1984.

PHASES OF REHABILITATION

162. Harrison, T.R.: Abuse of rest as a therapeutic measure for patients with cardiovascular disease. J.A.M.A. *125*:1075, 1944.
163. Levine, S.A., and Lown, B.: "Armchair" treatment of acute coronary thrombosis. J.A.M.A. *148*:1365, 1952.
164. Pryor, D.B., Hindman, M.C., Wagner, G.S., Califf, R.M., Rhoads, M.K., and Rosati, R.A.: Early discharge after acute myocardial infarction. Ann. Intern. Med. *99*:528, 1983.
165. Lindvall, K., Erhardt, L.R., Lundman, T., Rehnqvist, N., and Sjogren, A.: Early mobilization and discharge of patients with acute myocardial infarction. A prospective study using risk indicators and early exercist test. Acta Med. Scand. *206*:169, 1979.
166. Theroux, P., Waters, D.D., Halphen, C., Debaisieux, J.-C., and Mizgala, H.F.: Prognostic value of exercise testing soon after myocardial infarction. N. Engl. J. Med. *301*:341, 1979.
167. Waters, D.D., Bosch, X., Bouchard, A., Moise, A., Roy, D., Pelletier, G., and Theroux, P.: Comparison of clinical variables and variables derived from a limited predischarge exercise test as predictors of early and late mortality after myocardial infarction. J. Am. Coll. Cardiol. 5(1):1, 1985.
168. Silvidi, G.E., Squires, R.W., Pollock, M.L., and Foster, C.: Hemodynamic responses and medical problems associated with early exercise and ambulation in coronary artery bypass graft surgery patients. J. Cardiac Rehabil. *2*:355, 1982.
169. Wenger, N.K.: Early ambulation after myocardial infarction: Rationale, program components, and results. *In* Wenger, N.K., and Hellerstein, H.K. (eds.): Rehabilitation of the Coronary Patient, 2nd Ed. New York, John Wiley and Sons, Inc., 1984, p. 97.
170. Sivarajan, E.S., Bruce, R.A., Almes, M.J., Green, B., Belanger, L., Lindskog, B.D., Newton, K.M., and Mansfield, L.W.: In-hospital exercise after myocardial infarction does not improve treadmill performance. N. Engl. J. Med. *305*:358, 1981.
171. DeBusk, R.F., Houston, N., Haskell, W., Fry, G., and Parker, M.: Exercise training soon after myocardial infarction. Am. J. Cardiol. *44*:1225, 1979.
172. Wenger, N.K.: The Education of the Patient with Cardiac Disease in the Twenty-first Century. New York, Le Jacq Publishing Co., 1986.
173. Convertino, V.A.: Effect of orthostatic stress on exercise performance after bed rest: Relation to inhospital rehabilitation. J. Cardiac Rehabil. *3*:660, 1983.
174. Weld, F.M.: Exercise testing early after myocardial infarction. J. Cardiac Rehabil. *5*:20, 1985.
175. Boogaard, M.A.K., and Briody, M.E.: Comparison of the rehabilitation of men and women post-myocardial infarction. J. Cardiopul. Rehabil. *5*:379, 1985.
176. The Committee on Exercise: Exercise testing and training of individuals with heart disease or at high risk for its development: A handbook for physicians. Dallas, American Heart Association, 1975.
177. Williams, D.O., Bass, T.A., Gewirtz, H., and Most, A.A.: Adaptation to the stress of tachycardia in patients with coronary artery disease: Insight into the mechanism of the warm-up phenomenon. Circulation *71*:687, 1985.
178. Dimsdale, J.E., Hartley, L.H., Guiney, T., Ruskin, J.N., and Greenblatt, D.: Postexercise peril: Plasma catecholamines and exercise. J.A.M.A. *251*:630, 1984.
179. DeBusk, R.F., Haskell, W.L., Miller, N.H., Berra, K., and Taylor, C.B., in cooperation with Berger, W.E., and Lew, H.: Medically directed at-home rehabilitation soon after clinically uncomplicated acute myocardial infarction: A new model for patient care. Am. J. Cardiol. *55*:251, 1985.
180. Fletcher, G.F., Chiaramida, A.J., LeMay, M.R., Johnston, B.L., Thiel, J.E., and Spratlin, M.C.: Telephonically monitored home exercise early after coronary artery bypass surgery. Chest *86*:198, 1984.
181. Miller, N.H., Haskell, W.L., Berra, K., and DeBusk, R.F.: Home versus group exercise training for increasing functional capacity after myocardial infarction. Circulation *70*:645, 1984.
182. Oldridge, N.B.: Cardiac rehabilitation, self-responsibility, and quality of life. J. Cardiopul. Rehabil. *6*:153, 1986.

42 THE CARDIOMYOPATHIES AND MYOCARDITIDES

by JOSHUA WYNNE, M. D., and
EUGENE BRAUNWALD, M. D.

CLASSIFICATION

The cardiomyopathies constitute a group of diseases, often of unknown etiology, in which the dominant feature is involvement of the heart muscle itself.[1–3] They are unique in that they are not the result of ischemic,[4]* hypertensive, congenital, valvular, or pericardial diseases (Table 42–1). While the diagnosis of cardiomyopathy requires the exclusion of these etiological factors, the features of cardiomyopathy are often sufficiently distinctive—both clinically and hemodynamically—to allow a positive diagnosis to be made.[4a] With increasing awareness of this condition by clinicians, along with improvements in diagnostic techniques, cardiomyopathy is being recognized as a significant cause of morbidity and mortality.[5]

A variety of schemes have been proposed for classifying the cardiomyopathies.[2, 3, 6] Most useful from a clinical standpoint is a *functional* classification that emphasizes common pathophysiological abnormalities. Three basic categories of functional impairment have been described (Table 42–2 and Fig. 42–1): (1) *dilated* (formerly called congestive), characterized by ventricular dilatation, contractile dysfunction, and often symptoms of congestive heart failure; (2) *hypertrophic*, recognized by inappropriate left ventricular hypertrophy, often with asymmetrical involvement of the septum, with preserved or enhanced contractile function; and (3) *restrictive*, marked by endocardial scarring of the ventricle, with impairment of diastolic filling. The distinctions between these three functional categories are not absolute, and there is often overlap; in particular, patients with hypertrophic cardiomyopathy also have increased wall stiffness (as a consequence of the myocardial hypertrophy) and thus present some of the features of a restrictive cardiomyopathy. Table 42–3 shows the echocardiographic characteristics of the three types of cardiomyopathies.

A second approach to classification is to divide the cardiomyopathies into primary and secondary forms.[6] *Primary cardiomyopathies* are conditions in which: (1) the basic pathological process involves the myocardium rather than the valves or other cardiac structures, and (2) the cause of the heart disease is unknown and not part of a disorder affecting other organs. *Secondary cardiomyopathies* are conditions in which the cause of the myocardial abnormality is known or in which the cardiomyopathy is one manifestation of a systemic disease process, such as sarcoid. The secondary cardiomyopathies are further subdivided into the etiologies listed in Table 42–1. The functional and etiological approaches can be combined as in *dilated cardiomyopathy secondary to alcohol*, or *primary hypertrophic cardiomyopathy* (etiology unknown).

ENDOMYOCARDIAL BIOPSY. Evaluation of the patient suspected of suffering from a cardiomyopathy has been facilitated by the use of endomyocardial biopsy (p. 262).[7] Using a flexible bioptome, the clinician may obtain a tissue

*The term *ischemic cardiomyopathy* refers to the condition in which ischemic heart disease causes diffuse fibrosis or multiple infarctions and leads to heart failure with left ventricular dilatation; it may or may not be associated with angina pectoris[4] (p. 1362).

sample with surprising ease and safety from the right or left ventricle via a transvenous or transarterial approach (Fig. 42–2).[8–10] Two-dimensional echocardiography may help guide the placement of the bioptome and reduce radiation exposure.[11, 12] Endomyocardial biopsy results in a small tissue sample (average size 1–4 mm), and five or

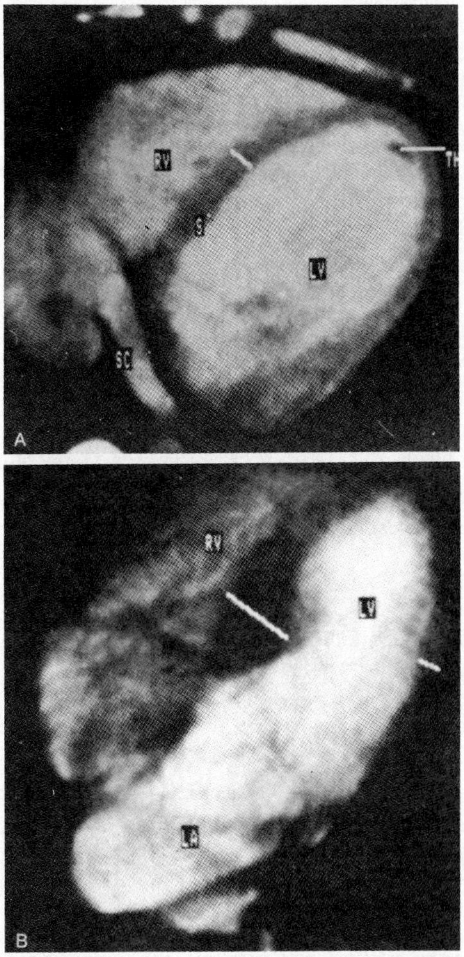

FIGURE 42–1. Computed tomographic four-chamber images in cardiomyopathy. *A*, Dilated cardiomyopathy, with marked left ventricular (LV) and right ventricular (RV) dilatation. There is an apical thrombus (TH). *B*, Hypertrophic cardiomyopathy, with asymmetric septal hypertrophy. White line shows marked septal (left) thickening compared with posterolateral wall (right). LA = left atrium; S = septum; SC = coronary sinus. (From Wojtowicz, J., et al.: Cardiac chambers and their walls in cardiomyopathies as evaluated with CT. Eur. J. Radiol. *4*:93, 1984.)

TABLE 42–1 IMPORTANT CAUSES OF CARDIOMYOPATHY AND MYOCARDITIS

1. Inflammatory
   - a. Infective
     - Viral
     - Rickettsial
     - Bacterial
     - Mycobacterial
     - Spirochetal
     - Fungal
     - Parasitic
   - b. Noninfective
     - Collagen diseases
     - Granulomatous
2. Metabolic
   - a. Nutritional
     - Thiamine
     - Kwashiorkor
     - Pellagra
     - Scurvy
     - Hypervitaminosis D
     - Obesity
     - Selenium deficiency
   - b. Endocrine
     - Acromegaly
     - Thyrotoxicosis
     - Myxedema
     - Uremia
     - Cushing's disease
     - Pheochromocytoma
     - Diabetes mellitus
   - c. Altered metabolism
     - Gout
     - Oxalosis
     - Porphyria
   - d. Electrolyte imbalance
3. Toxic
   - a. Cobalt
   - b. Alcohol
   - c. Bleomycin
   - d. Adriamycin
   - e. Phenothiazines and antidepressants
   - f. Antimony compounds
   - g. Carbon monoxide
   - h. Lead
   - i. Emetine and dehydroemetine
   - j. Chloroquine
   - k. Lithium
   - l. Cyclophosphamide
   - m. Hydrocarbons
   - n. Catecholamines
   - o. Phosphorus
   - p. Mercury
   - q. Insect stings
   - r. Snake bites
   - s. Paracetamol
   - t. Reserpine
   - u. Corticosteroids
   - v. Cocaine
   - w. Methylsergide
4. Infiltrative
   - a. Amyloidosis
   - b. Hemochromatosis
   - c. Neoplastic
   - d. Glycogen storage disorders
   - e. Sarcoidosis
   - f. Mucopolysaccharidosis
   - g. Fabry's disease
   - h. Whipple's disease
   - i. Gaucher's disease
   - j. Sphingolipidoses
5. Fibroplastic
   - a. Endomyocardial fibrosis
   - b. Endocardial fibroelastosis
   - c. Löffler's fibroplastic endocarditis
   - d. Becker's disease
   - e. Carcinoid
6. Hematological
   - a. Sickle cell anemia
   - b. Polycythemia vera
   - c. Thrombotic thrombocytopenic purpura
   - d. Leukemia
7. Hypersensitivity
   - a. Methyldopa
   - b. Penicillin
   - c. Sulfonamides
   - d. Tetracycline
   - e. Phenindione
   - f. Phenylbutazone
   - g. Antituberculous drugs
   - h. Giant cell myocarditis
   - i. Cardiac transplant rejection
8. Genetic
   - a. Hypertrophic cardiomyopathy
     - With gradient
     - Without gradient
   - b. Neuromuscular
     - Duchenne muscular dystrophy
     - Facioscapulohumeral muscular dystrophy
     - Limb-girdle dystrophy of Erb
     - Myotonia dystrophica
     - Friedreich's ataxia
9. Miscellaneous acquired
   - a. Postpartum cardiomyopathy
   - b. Obesity
10. Idiopathic
    - a. Idiopathic dilated cardiomyopathy
    - b. Idiopathic restrictive cardiomyopathy
    - c. Idiopathic hypertrophic cardiomyopathy
11. Physical agents
    - a. Heat stroke
    - b. Hypothermia
    - c. Radiation

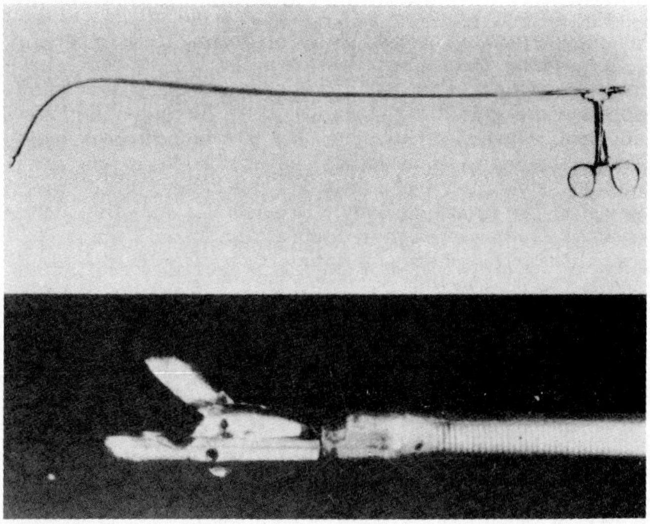

FIGURE 42–2. *Top*, The Stanford bioptome for performing endomyocardial biopsy. *Bottom*, Close-up of the cutting jaws in the open position. (From O'Connell, J. B., et al.: Dilated cardiomyopathy: Emerging role of endomyocardial biopsy. Curr. Probl. Cardiol. *11*:450, 1986.)

TABLE 42–2 FUNCTIONAL CLASSIFICATION OF THE CARDIOMYOPATHIES

	DILATED	RESTRICTIVE	HYPERTROPHIC
Symptoms	Congestive heart failure, particularly left-sided	Dyspnea, fatigue	Dyspnea, angina pectoris
	Fatigue and weakness	Right-sided congestive heart failure	Fatigue, syncope, palpitations
	Systemic or pulmonary emboli	Signs and symptoms of systemic disease: amyloidosis, iron storage disease, etc.	
Physical Examination	Moderate to severe cardiomegaly; S_3 and S_4	Mild to moderate cardiomegaly; S_3 or S_4	Mild cardiomegaly Apical systolic thrill and heave; brisk carotid upstroke
	Atrioventricular valve regurgitation, especially mitral	Atrioventricular valve regurgitation; inspiratory increase in venous pressure (Kussmaul's sign)	S_4 common Systolic murmur that increases with Valsalva maneuver
Chest Roentgenogram	Moderate to marked cardiac enlargement, especially left ventricular	Mild cardiac enlargement	Mild to moderate cardiac enlargment
	Pulmonary venous hypertension	Pulmonary venous hypertension	Left atrial enlargement
Electrocardiogram	Sinus tachycardia	Low voltage	Left ventricular hypertrophy
	Atrial and ventricular arrhythmias	Intraventricular conduction defects	ST-segment and T-wave abnormalities
	ST-segment and T-wave abnormalities	AV conduction defects	Abnormal Q waves
	Intraventricular conduction defects		Atrial and ventricular arrhythmias
Echocardiogram	Left ventricular dilatation and dysfunction	Increased left ventricular wall thickness and mass	Asymmetrical septal hypertrophy (ASH)
	Abnormal diastolic mitral valve motion secondary to abnormal compliance and filling pressures	Small or normal-sized left ventricular cavity	Narrow left ventricular outflow tract
		Normal systolic function	Systolic anterior motion (SAM) of the mitral valve
		Pericardial effusion	Small or normal-sized left ventricle
Radionuclide Studies	Left ventricular dilatation and dysfunction (RVG)	Infiltration of myocardium (^{201}Tl)	Small or normal-sized left ventricle (RVG)
		Small or normal-sized left ventricle (RVG)	Vigorous systolic function (RVG)
		Normal systolic function (RVG)	Asymmetrical septal hypertrophy (RVG or ^{201}Tl)
Cardiac Catheterization	Left ventricular enlargement and dysfunction	Diminished left ventricular compliance	Diminished left ventricular compliance
	Mitral and/or tricuspid regurgitation	"Square root sign" in ventricular pressure recordings	Mitral regurgitation
	Elevated left- and often right-sided filling pressures	Preserved systolic function	Vigorous systolic function
	Diminished cardiac output	Elevated left- and right-sided filling pressures	Dynamic left ventricular outflow gradient

RVG = Radionuclide ventriculogram; ^{201} Tl = thallium-201

more biopsies are often required to be certain of a given histological finding, since pronounced topographic variations may be found within the myocardium.[13] It remains controversial as to which patients with cardiomyopathy should be subjected to biopsy, but there is general agreement that biopsy may be of benefit in certain specific situations (Table 42–4).[14, 15] Although on occasion endomyocardial biopsy may identify a specific etiological agent in an individual patient with cardiac disease of uncertain cause (Table 42–5 and Fig. 42–3), the clinical utility of routine biopsy in cardiomyopathy remains uncertain, particularly since no definitive pattern has been found in dilated cardiomyopathy. Interpretation of biopsy specimens has been facilitated by the recent adaptation of a universally accepted set of histological definitions, the *Dallas criteria.*[16]

TABLE 42–3 ECHOCARDIOGRAPHIC FINDINGS IN THREE TYPES OF CARDIOMYOPATHY

	DILATED	HYPERTROPHIC	RESTRICTIVE
LV cavity	+ +	− or N	N
LV wall thickness	N	+	+
LV contractility	−	+ or N	N or −

LV = left ventricular; − = decreased; N = normal; + = increased.
From DeMaria, A. N., Bommer, W., Lee, G., and Mason, D. T.: Value and limitations of two dimensional echocardiography in assessment of cardiomyopathy. Am. J. Cardiol. *46*:1225, 1980.

TABLE 42–4 COMMON INDICATIONS FOR ENDOMYOCARDIAL BIOPSY

1. To differentiate restrictive from constrictive disease.
2. To evaluate cardiac involvement in systemic disease.
3. To evaluate myocarditis.
4. To detect cardiotoxicity due to cardiotoxic agents.
5. To evaluate cardiac transplant rejection.
6. To evaluate cardiac tumors.

TABLE 42–5 SPECIFIC PATHOLOGICAL ENTITIES DETECTED BY ENDOMYOCARDIAL BIOPSY

1. Cardiac transplant rejection	7. Endocardial fibroelastosis
2. Myocarditis	8. Endomyocardial fibrosis
3. Adriamycin cardiotoxicity	9. Carcinoid
4. Amyloidosis	10. Glycogen storage disease
5. Sarcoidosis	11. Cardiac tumor
6. Hemochromatosis	12. Fabry's disease

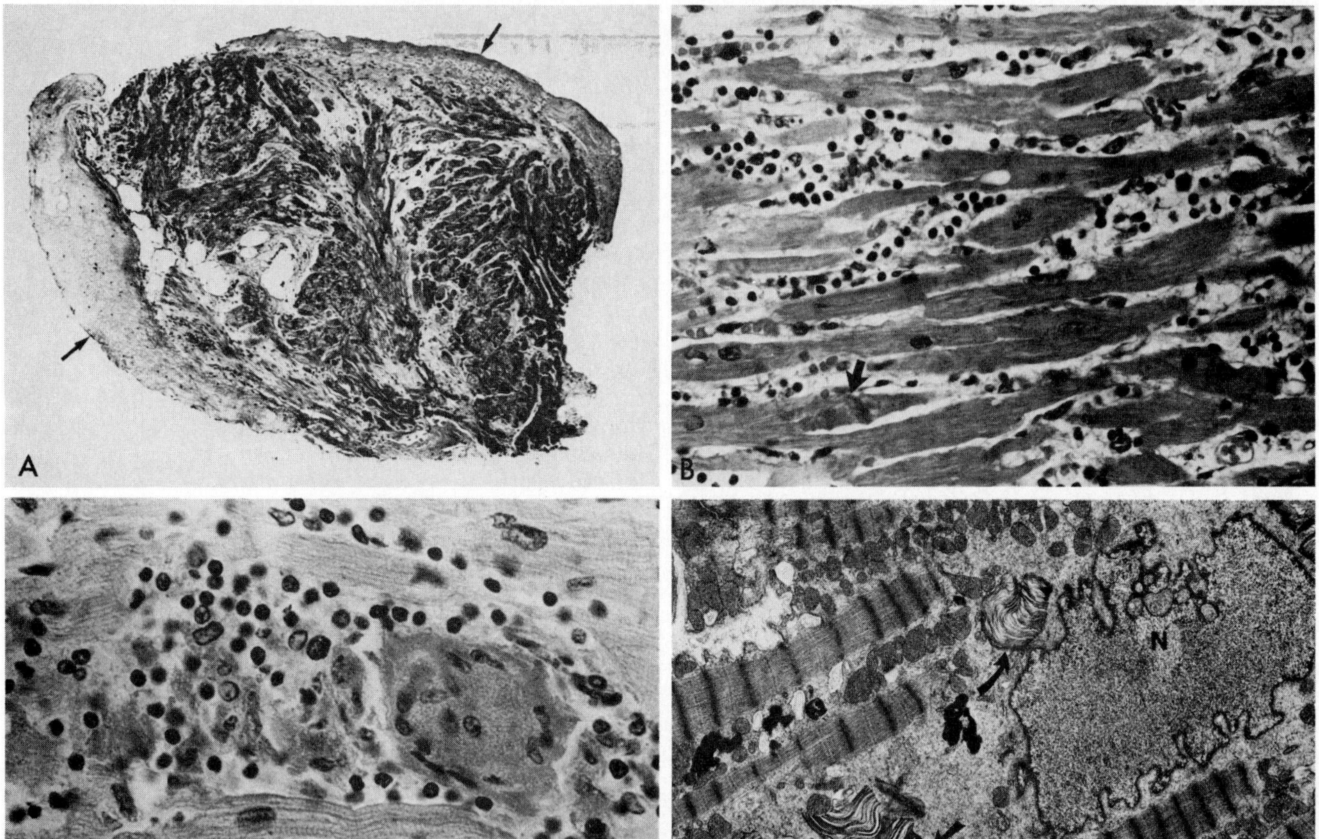

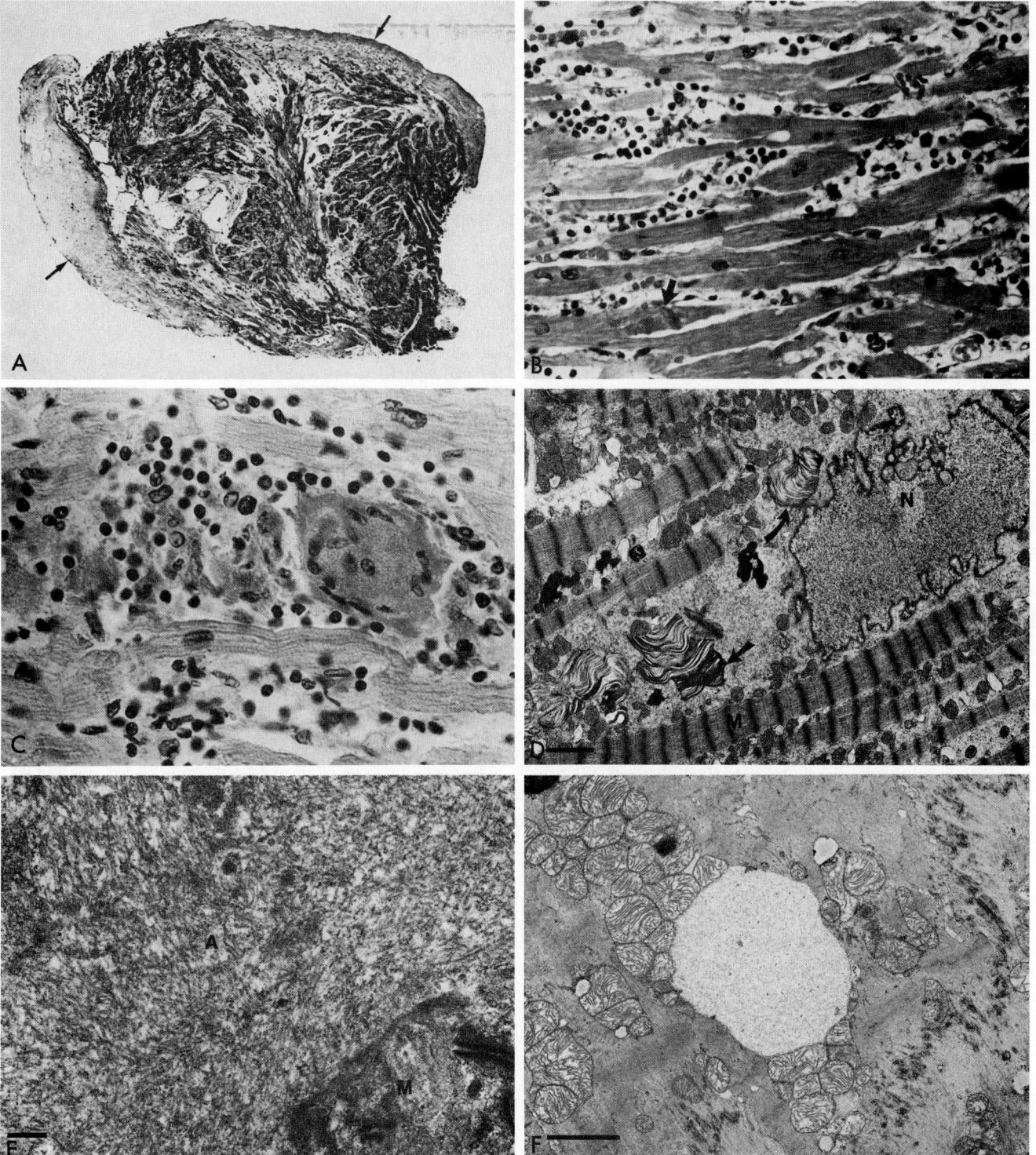

FIGURE 42–3. Representative examples of findings by endomyocardial biopsy. *A*, Low-power view of an entire transvenous right ventricular endomyocardial biopsy specimen. The endocardial surface is indicated by arrows. (Hematoxylin and eosin stain; original magnification × 90.) *B*, Inflammatory myocarditis with moderate, predominantly lymphocytic interstitial infiltrate throughout the myocardium. Focal myocardial cell necrosis is indicated by the arrow. (Hematoxylin and eosin stain; original magnification × 550.) *C*, Typical myocardial lesion in giant cell myocarditis with foci of mixed inflammatory infiltrate and multinucleated giant cells. (Hematoxylin and eosin stain; original magnification × 550.) *D*, Endomyocardial biopsy in patient with Fabry's disease. Transmission electron micrograph of cardiac muscle cell showing nucleus (N), myofibrils (M), and cytoplasmic inclusions (arrows) characteristic of Fabry's disease. (Original magnification × 3000. Bar at lower left-hand corner = 2 μm.) *E*, Cardiac amyloidosis revealed by endomyocardial biopsy. A very high magnification transmission electron photomicrograph (× 50,000) shows finely fibrillar amyloid material (A) in the interstitium surrounding individual myocytes. A portion of one myocyte is seen (M). (Bar at lower left = 0.1 μm.) *F*, Electron micrograph of endomyocardial biopsy specimen from a patient with Adriamycin cardiotoxicity. The myocyte shown demonstrates swelling of the sarcoplasmic reticulum and diffuse myofibrillar loss. (Original magnification × 4500. Bar at lower left = 2 μm.) (Courtesy of Frederick J. Schoen, M.D., Department of Pathology, Brigham and Women's Hospital.)

DILATED CARDIOMYOPATHY

IDIOPATHIC DILATED CARDIOMYOPATHY

Dilated cardiomyopathy is a syndrome, probably pluricausal, characterized by cardiac enlargement, and ultimately by symptoms resulting from left ventricular dysfunction, often by the development of congestive heart failure. Formerly called congestive cardiomyopathy, the term *dilated cardiomyopathy* is now preferred, since the earliest abnormality is ventricular enlargement and systolic contractile dysfunction, with congestive heart failure often (but not invariably) developing later. In an occasional patient, the predominant finding is that of contractile dysfunction with only a mildly dilated left ventricle.[17]

Although the etiology is not definable in many cases, the dilated cardiomyopathies probably represent a final common pathway that is the end result of myocardial damage produced by a variety of toxic, metabolic, or infectious agents.[18] Alcohol, for example, may lead to severe cardiac dysfunction and congestive heart failure and present clinical, hemodynamic, and pathological findings identical to those present in idiopathic dilated cardiomyopathy. The course of idiopathic dilated cardiomyopathy is usually one of progressive deterioration, with three-fourths of patients dying within 5 years after the onset of symptoms, although a minority improve, with a reduction in cardiac size and longer survival.[17, 19] Factors that are associated with high mortality include left ventricular conduction delay, marked elevation of right and/or left ventricular filling pressure, absence of left ventricular thickening, age greater than 55 years, a cardiothoracic ratio greater than 0.55, and a cardiac index less than 2.6 liters/min/m^2.[19–22] Surprisingly, there is not a good correlation between the extent of impairment of ventricular function and mortality.[23] Specific endomyocardial biopsy morphological findings may offer some predictive information regarding prognosis.[24] Children with dilated cardiomyopathy have a particularly grave prognosis, although a minority may show unexpected clinical improvement.[25, 26]

PATHOLOGY

POSTMORTEM EXAMINATION. This reveals enlargement and dilatation of all four chambers; the ventricles are more dilated than the atria. While the thickness of the ventricular wall is increased in some cases, the degree of hypertrophy is often inadequate for the severe dilatation present.[27] The development of left ventricular hypertrophy appears to have a protective or beneficial role in dilated cardiomyopathy, since it may serve to reduce systolic wall stress and protect against further cavity dilatation[27–29] (p. 433). The cardiac valves are intrinsically normal, and intracavitary thrombi, particularly in the ventricular apex, are common. The coronary arteries are usually normal.[30] The right ventricle is preferentially involved in some cases of dilated cardiomyopathy, sometimes on a familial basis.[31, 32]

HISTOLOGICAL EXAMINATION. Microscopic study reveals extensive areas of interstitial and perivascular fibrosis, particularly involving the left ventricular subendocardium.[33, 34] Small areas of necrosis and cellular infiltrate are seen on occasion, but these typically are not prominent features.[35, 36] Quantitative analysis of myocardial samples has shown a reduction in the number of nerve cells in dilated cardiomyopathy, but the significance of this finding is unclear at present.[37] Cardiac biopsy specimens obtained during life by a transvenous or transthoracic approach demonstrate a variety of abnormalities, including interstitial fibrosis, cellular infiltrates, cellular hypertrophy, and myocardial cell degeneration.[38] Both left and right ventricular tissues possess reduced activities of mitochondrial enzymes, with elevated levels of lactate dehydrogenase.[39] These abnormalities of mitochondrial function are not unexpected in view of the known ultrastructural abnormalities of the mitochondria, and it is thought that the elevated levels of lactate dehydrogenase result from enhanced anaerobic glycolysis due to mitochondrial dysfunction.[39] No viruses or other etiological agents have been identified with any regularity in tissue from patients with dilated cardiomyopathy. Particularly disappointing has been the failure to identify any immunological, histochemical, morphological, ultrastructural, or microbiological markers that might be used to establish the diagnosis of idiopathic dilated cardiomyopathy or to clarify its cause.

ETIOLOGY

It is likely that primary dilated cardiomyopathy is a common expression of myocardial damage that has been produced by a variety of myocardial insults. While the cause or causes remain unclear, at least four conditions, if not etiologically linked, appear to lower the threshold for the development of cardiomyopathy, and it is possible that in some cases a combination of factors results in severe myocardial damage. Chronic ingestion of excessive alcohol, pregnancy (see Chap. 60), systemic hypertension (see Chap. 27), and a variety of infections (pp. 1440 to 1449) may each be associated with myocardial dysfunction and congestive failure and are important causes of secondary dilated cardiomyopathy. Cigarette smoking has also been found to be associated with dilated cardiomyopathy,[40] independently of its important role as a risk factor in the development of ischemic heart disease (p. 1172).

The possible progression of viral myocarditis to cardiomyopathy as a consequence of an autoimmune reaction, has engendered the greatest speculation as a possible cause of "idiopathic" dilated cardiomyopathy.[41] While this hypothesis is inviting, it remains largely unsupported; there have been few observations of a transition from myocarditis to dilated cardiomyopathy[42] and little evidence to suggest prior viral infections in most patients with unequivocal cardiomyopathy.[41] However, there are patients who manifest the clinical features of a dilated cardiomyopathy in whom endomyocardial biopsy reveals evidence of an inflammatory myocarditis. The frequency of finding evidence of an inflammatory infiltrate in dilated cardiomyopathy varies widely and undoubtedly depends largely on criteria used for diagnosis.[43–50] Other evidence favoring the concept that dilated cardiomyopathy is a post-viral disorder includes the presence of high antibody viral titers,[51] viral-specific RNA sequences,[52] and apparent viral particles[54] in patients with "idiopathic" dilated cardiomyopathy. What remains lacking is the demonstration of an etiological role of the lymphocytic infiltrate, since the presence of round cells in the myocardium of patients with dilated cardiomyopathy does not necessarily imply the presence of active myocarditis.[35] Myocardial uptake of the radionuclide gallium-67 may provide a noninvasive means of identifying patients likely to have a prominent lymphocytic infiltrate, and it may thus help select patients for biopsy.[54–58]

Although the findings have not been completely reproducible, abnormalities of both humoral and cellular immunity have been found in patients with dilated cardiomyopathy.[59, 60] Circulating antimyocardial antibodies[60–64] and abnormalities of various T cells, particularly suppressor T cells,[60, 65–69] have been found in some, but not all, studies. It has been suggested that these putative immunological abnormalities may be the consequence of prior viral myocarditis.[70] Viral components may be incorporated into the cardiac sarcolemma, only to serve as an antigenic source that directs the heart responses to attack the myocardium.[71]

A variety of other possible causes has been proposed although none is accepted as *the* cause of dilated cardiomyopathy. Thus, endocrine abnormalities as well as the effects of chemical or toxins, notably doxorubicin (p. 1748), have been suggested as possible etiological factors.[71a] It has been suggested that microvascular hyperreactivity (spasm) may lead to myocellular necrosis and scarring, with resultant heart failure, although this remains speculative.[72]

In contrast to hypertrophic cardiomyopathy, in which familial transmission is quite common, in dilated cardiomyopathy it is rare. Occasional instances have been reported[73–77, 77a]; one intriguing familial metabolic deficiency is that of carnitine, with improvement occurring in the myopathy with carnitine repletion.[78, 79]

CLINICAL MANIFESTATIONS

HISTORY. Symptoms usually develop gradually in patients with dilated cardiomyopathy. Some patients may be asymptomatic yet have left ventricular dilatation for months or even years.[80] An unrecognized illness may result in left ventricular dilatation, which is clinically recognized only years later when symptoms develop or when routine chest roentgenography demonstrates cardiomegaly. Other patients, after recovery from what appears to be a systemic viral infection, develop symptoms of heart failure for the first time. In still others, severe heart failure develops acutely during an episode of myocarditis; while some recovery occurs, chronic manifestations of diminished cardiac reserve persist and heart failure reappears months or years later. Although patients of any age may be affected, the disease is most common in middle age and is more frequent in men than in women.[81]

The most striking symptoms are those of left ventricular failure. Fatigue and weakness due to diminished cardiac output are common. Right heart failure is a late and ominous sign and is associated with a particularly poor prognosis (p. 473). Chest pain occurs in one-fourth to one-half of patients and may suggest concomitant ischemic heart disease.[80, 82] In some patients there appears to be a reduction in myocardial perfusion despite normal coronary arteries, suggesting that subendocardial ischemia may play a role in the genesis of chest pain.[83–85] Chest pain secondary to pulmonary embolism and abdominal pain secondary to congestive hepatomegaly are frequent in the late stages of the illness.

PHYSICAL EXAMINATION. This usually reveals variable degrees of cardiac enlargement and findings of congestive heart failure. The systolic blood pressure is usually normal or low, and the pulse pressure is narrow, reflecting a diminished stroke volume. Pulsus alternans (p. 23) is common when severe left ventricular failure is present. The jugular veins are frequently distended. Prominent *a* and *v* waves are visible—the latter a late manifestation of the presence of tricuspid valvular regurgitation. The liver may be engorged and pulsatile. Peripheral edema and ascites may be present.

The precordium usually reveals left and, occasionally, right ventricular impulses, but the heaves are not sustained, as they are in patients with considerable ventricular hypertrophy. The apical impulse is usually displaced laterally, reflecting left ventricular dilatation. A presystolic *a* wave may be palpable. The second heart sound is usually normally split, although paradoxical splitting (p. 47) may be detected in the presence of left bundle branch block, an electrocardiographic finding which is not unusual in dilated cardiomyopathy. If pulmonary hypertension is present the pulmonary component of the second heart sound may be accentuated, and the splitting may be narrow. Presystolic gallop sounds (S_4) often precede the development of overt congestive heart failure. Ventricular gallops (S_3) are the rule once cardiac decompensation occurs, and a summation gallop is often heard when there is tachycardia. Systolic murmurs are common and are usually due to mitral or, less commonly, tricuspid valvular regurgitation. Atrioventricular valvular regurgitation results from enlargement of the circumference of the mitral or tricuspid annulus; ventricular dilatation with resultant distortion of the geometry of the subvalvar apparatus ("papillary muscle dysfunction") plays a lesser role.[86] Gallop sounds and regurgitant murmurs can often be elicited or intensified by isometric handgrip exercise with its attendant enhancement of systemic vascular resistance and impedance to left ventricular outflow (p. 37). Systemic emboli resulting from dislodgment of intracardiac thrombi from the left atrium and ventricle and pulmonary emboli that originate in the venous system of the legs are common late complications.

NONINVASIVE EXAMINATION. To identify potentially reversible secondary causes of dilated cardiomyopathy, several basic screening biochemical *tests* are often indicated, including determination of serum phosphorus (hypophosphatemia), serum calcium (hypocalcemia), serum creatinine and urea nitrogen (uremia), and serum iron (hemochromatosis)[18] (Table 42–6). The *chest roentgenogram* usually reveals left ventricular enlargement, although

TABLE 42–6 SCREENING PROCEDURE FOR DISTINGUISHING IDIOPATHIC DILATED CARDIOMYOPATHY FROM REVERSIBLE CAUSES

Possible Diagnosis	Tests	Treatment
In all cases:		
Alcoholic CM	Repeated questioning of the patient and family members	Complete abstinence from alcohol
Uremic CM	BUN, serum creatinine	Renal dialysis
Hypophosphatemia	Serum phosphorus	Phosphate repletion
Hypocalcemia	Serum calcium	Calcium repletion
Iron overload	Serum iron studies; endomyocardial or liver biopsy in some cases	Treatment for hemochromatosis
Pheochromocytoma	Urinary screening tests	Operative removal of tumor
If there is recurrent VT, BBB, or CHB in a young person:		
Sarcoid heart disease	Thallium scan, tissue biopsy, angiotensin I converting enzyme (serum)	Corticosteroids*
If course is < 6 weeks to 6 months, especially with febrile illness at onset:		
Acute inflammatory myopericarditis	Serum antibody titers for enteroviruses, toxoplasma, cold agglutinins, ANA, rheumatoid factor, ASLO	Antibiotics for toxoplasma or myocoplasmal infection
	Endomyocardial biopsy; gallium scan (?)	Immunosuppressive treatment* for post-viral or noninfectious cases (see text)

CM = cardiomyopathy; VT = ventricular tachycardia; BBB = bilateral bundle branch block; CHB = advanced atrioventricular block; BUN = blood urea nitrogen; ANA = antinuclear antibody; ASLO = antistreptolysin-O.

*Treatment not yet proved to be beneficial; referral for entry in an investigative protocol may be advisable.

From Johnson, R. A., and Palacios, I.: Dilated cardiomyopathies of the adult. N. Engl. J. Med. 307:1119, 1982.

generalized cardiomegaly is often seen. Left ventricular failure may result in signs of pulmonary venous hypertension (i.e., pulmonary vascular redistribution) as well as interstitial and even alveolar edema (p. 164). Pleural effusions may be present, and the azygos vein and superior vena cava may be dilated when right heart failure supervenes. The *electrocardiogram* often shows sinus tachycardia when heart failure is present. The entire spectrum of atrial and ventricular tachyarrhythmias and atrioventricular conduction disturbances may be seen. Indeed, arrhythmias are second in frequency only to heart failure as clinical manifestations of congestive cardiomyopathy.[87] Although ventricular arrhythmias are common, there is no unequivocal relationship between the severity of arrhythmias and clinical features nor with the risk of sudden death,[88–92] although those dying suddenly tend to have worse left ventricular function.[93] In rare cases, recurrent and/or incessant supraventricular tachyarrhythmias may actually be the *cause* (rather than the result) of ventricular dysfunction, particularly in children.[94–97] In these cases, restoration of sinus rhythm or slowing of the heart rate may be therapeutic. A variety of intraventricular conduction defects is common, and Q waves may be present when there is extensive left ventricular fibrosis without discrete myocardial infarction. ST-segment and T-wave abnormalities are common.

M-mode, two-dimensional and Doppler *echocardiography* are useful in assessing the degree of impairment of left ventricular function and for excluding concomitant valvular or pericardial disease (Chap. 5).[98, 99] In addition to examining all four cardiac valves for evidence of structural or functional abnormalities, echocardiography permits the size of the ventricular cavity to be assessed, the thickness of the left and right ventricular walls to be evaluated, and an estimate to be made of ventricular function.[100] Although some degree of right ventricular contractile dysfunction is common,[101] marked right ventricular enlargement is noted late in the illness. A pericardial effusion may sometimes be demonstrated. *Thallium-201 imaging* at rest and with exercise is of limited value in distinguishing left ventricular enlargement due to dilated cardiomyopathy from that due to coronary artery disease unless a large defect indicative of a myocardial infarction is seen.[102, 103]

Radionuclide ventriculography, like echocardiography, reveals increased end-diastolic and end-systolic left ventricular volumes, reduced ejection fractions in both ventricles and wall-motion abnormalities.[104] This technique is helpful both in the assessment of ventricular function and in evaluating the response to therapy.[105] In many cases, however, it is not necessary to carry out serial *batteries* of noninvasive tests in order to follow patients with dilated cardiomyopathy and evaluate their response to treatment. This is true particularly when the studies are performed only with the patient at rest, since clinical symptoms correlate best with exercise capacity, which in turn bears only a general relationship to resting ventricular performance.[106]

CARDIAC CATHETERIZATION AND ANGIOCARDIOGRAPHY. The left ventricular end-diastolic, left atrial, and pulmonary artery wedge pressures are usually elevated. Modest degrees of pulmonary arterial hypertension are common.[18] Advanced cases may demonstrate right ventricular dilatation and failure as well, with resultant elevation of the right ventricular end-diastolic, right atrial, and central venous pressures.

Left ventriculography demonstrates enlargement of this chamber, typically with diffuse reduction in wall motion. Segmental wall motion abnormalities are not uncommon, and may simulate the angiographic findings in coronary artery disease.[18, 107, 107a] However, prominent localized wall disorders are more characteristic of coronary artery disease, while diffuse, global dysfunction is more typical of dilated cardiomyopathy. The ejection fraction is reduced and the end-systolic volume is increased as a result of the impairment of left ventricular contractility. Sometimes left ventricular thrombi may be visualized within the left ventricle as intracavitary filling defects. Mild mitral regurgitation is often present. On occasion, it may be difficult to distinguish left ventricular dilatation secondary to severe mitral regurgitation from a dilated cardiomyopathy with secondary mitral regurgitation.

Coronary arteriography usually reveals normal vessels,[18] although coronary dilatory capacity may be impaired.[108] This technique may be of particular value in patients with abnormal Q waves on the electrocardiogram or regional left ventricular wall motion abnormalities on noninvasive testing, since such findings may be due to myocardial infarction as a result of obstructive coronary artery disease or, alternatively, extensive localized myocardial fibrosis secondary to severe dilated cardiomyopathy in the absence of coronary artery obstruction.

TREATMENT

Since the cause of idiopathic dilated cardiomyopathy is unknown, specific therapy is not possible. Treatment, therefore, is on the same basis as that for heart failure, discussed in detail in Chapter 17. Physical, dietary, pharmacological, mechanical, and surgical interventions may help to control symptoms; only cardiac transplantation and specific vasodilator therapy (hydralazine plus nitrates) have been shown to prolong life.[109, 110]

Patients with moderately severe left ventricular failure may be comfortable at rest but develop severe symptoms with exercise, when they are unable to increase their cardiac output commensurately. It is reasonable to restrict activity for these patients to avoid precipitation of unwanted and poorly tolerated symptoms (Fig. 17–1, p. 486). Because of recent evidence that activation of the sympathetic nervous system may have deleterious cardiac effects (rather than being an important compensatory mechanism as traditionally thought), beta-adrenoceptor blockade has been suggested as a means to prolong survival.[111, 112] Results to date have been inconsistent, but improvement in symptoms (sometimes dramatic) and survival have been suggested.[113–120] Beta-adrenoceptor blockade has been surprisingly well tolerated, with infrequent aggravation of heart failure (which, on occasion, may be profound).[114] The mechanism of beneficial action of beta blockers may relate to five factors: (1) negative chronotropic effect with reduced myocardial oxygen demand; (2) reduced myocardial damage due to catecholamines; (3) improved diastolic relaxation; (4) inhibition of sympathetically mediated vasoconstriction; and (5) increase in myocardial beta-adrenoceptor density.[121, 122]

While there is no evidence that antiarrhythmic agents prolong life or prevent sudden death in dilated cardiomyopathy, it is appropriate to use them in the treatment of symptomatic or serious arrhythmias.[23] Because of the adverse effects of most available agents, many of which depress myocardial contractility (Chap. 21), treatment should be individualized, with both efficacy and toxicity carefully monitored.[123] Unfortunately, even improved arrhythmia control documented by electrophysiological testing may not translate into prevention of sudden death or the recurrence of arrhythmias; implantation of the automatic internal defibrillator (p. 768) should be considered in appropriate candidates.[124] Because of the frequency and hazards of embolization,[125] patients with dilated cardiomyopathy and heart failure should be treated with anticoagulants, even without direct evidence of thrombus formation if there are no specific contraindications to these agents.[19, 126–128] In those patients with chronic heart failure secondary to a dilated cardiomyopathy and a lymphocytic infiltrate on myocardial biopsy, treatment with corticosteroids and immunosuppressive agents has been advocated. The appropriateness and results of such therapy are controversial and the subject of ongoing investigation.[43, 47–49, 55, 129, 130]

Surgical replacement of regurgitant valves has been attempted in some patients with progressive atrioventricular valvular regurgitation (almost always mitral) that appeared to result in progressive cardiac enlargement and failure. The results of operation are usually less than satisfactory because of the degree of preexisting cardiac dysfunction and damage. In appropriate patients, cardiac transplantation may be an alternative (p. 1664), with a 1-year survival rate of over 80 per cent compared with less than 5 per cent in nontransplanted patients[131, 132] and a 3-year survival of 70 per cent.[133]

ALCOHOLIC CARDIOMYOPATHY

Chronic excessive consumption of alcohol may be associated with congestive heart failure, hypertension, arrhythmias, and sudden death; it is the major cause of secondary, non-ischemic dilated cardiomyopathy in the Western world.[134, 135] It is estimated that two-thirds of the adult population use alcohol to some extent, and more than 10 per cent are heavy users. Therefore, it is not surprising that alcoholic cardiomyopathy is a major problem.[136] Ceasing alcohol consumption may halt the progression or even reverse alcoholic cardiomyopathy, which, unlike primary dilated cardiomyopathy, is otherwise usually marked by progressive deterioration.[124, 137]

The consumption of alcohol may result in myocardial damage by three basic mechanisms: (1) a presumed direct toxic effect of alcohol or of its metabolites; (2) nutritional effects, most commonly in association with thiamine deficiency which leads to beriberi heart disease (p. 786); and (3) rarely, toxic effects due to additives in the alcoholic beverage (cobalt)[138, 139] (p. 1418). There had been speculation that alcohol caused myocardial damage only through dietary deficiencies, but it is now clear that alcoholic cardiomyopathy occurs in the absence of nutritional deficiencies.[139]

Typical Oriental beriberi (p. 786) may coexist with alcoholic cardiomyopathy more commonly than has been suspected. The distinguishing features of each include peripheral vasodilatation and high output failure, often right-sided, in the former and reduced contractility with typically left-sided low output failure in the latter.[140, 141] Beriberi responds to thiamine administration, often dramatically.[141]

Alcohol results in acute as well as chronic depression of myocardial contractility and may produce demonstrable cardiac dysfunction even when ingested by normal individuals in quantities consumed in social drinking.[142-145] The acute hemodynamic effects of alcohol appear to depend on its blood levels, since ventricular dysfunction following acute ethanol ingestion may be reversed within 15 to 30 minutes of hemodialysis.[146] Prior exposure to alcohol appears to modulate the hemodynamic response to acute challenge with alcohol. Larger doses of alcohol are required to produce cardiac dysfunction in chronic alcoholic patients without obvious heart disease than in normal subjects. On the other hand, the alcoholic person with clinically evident cardiac dysfunction appears to be more susceptible to the deleterious effects of alcohol than normal.[146]

The mechanism of the cardiac depression produced by alcohol remains unclear, and a direct causal relationship between alcohol and the development of cardiomyopathy has not been proved. In acute studies, alcohol and its metabolite acetaldehyde have been shown to interfere with a number of cellular functions that involve the transport and binding of calcium, mitochondrial respiration, myocardial lipid metabolism, myocardial protein synthesis, and myofibrillar ATPase.[136, 147-149] The accumulation of metabolites of ethanol in the myocardium may interfere with normal myocardial lipid metabolism and may play a role in the pathogenesis of alcohol-induced myocardial damage.[139] Alcohol results in loss of potassium ions from myocardial cells, along with diminished uptake of free fatty acids but enhanced myocardial extraction of triglyceride.[150] The roles that other associated electrolyte imbalances (hypokalemia, hypophosphatemia, hypomagnesemia) may play in alcohol-mediated damage have not been clarified.[136] The major unanswered question is precisely how these metabolic effects result in persistent myocardial injury.

PATHOLOGY. The gross and microscopic pathological findings are nonspecific and similar to those observed in idiopathic dilated cardiomyopathy, although certain ultrastructural details suggest alcoholic cardiomyopathy.[151] Edema of the vascular wall and perivascular fibrosis of the intramyocardial coronary arteries has been observed,[152, 153] and it has been suggested that the myocardial damage in alcoholic cardiomyopathy may be the result of ischemia produced by disease of the small intramural coronary arteries.[153] Alcohol, even in small amounts, may result in alterations of mitochondrial structure and function.[154, 155]

Clinical Manifestations

Alcoholic cardiomyopathy most commonly occurs in males 30 to 55 years of age who have been heavy consumers of whiskey, wine, or beer, usually for more than 10 years.[146, 156] The male predominance appears to be largely the result of the higher frequency of alcoholism in this sex, although noninvasive testing of cardiac function in male and female alcoholic patients suggests that cardiac dysfunction is more prevalent in men than in women.[157] While alcoholic cardiomyopathy may be observed in the homeless, malnourished, "skid row" alcoholic man who is a candidate for and may often suffer from alcoholic cirrhosis, many patients are well-nourished individuals of middle and even upper socioeconomic status without liver disease or peripheral neuropathy.[146] Therefore, unless a high index of suspicion is maintained, it may be easy to miss a history of alcohol abuse. Persistent questioning of the patient and particularly the relatives of patients with unexplained cardiomegaly or cardiomyopathy is often required to elicit a history of alcoholism.

It is frequently possible to demonstrate mild depression of cardiac function in chronic alcoholics even before cardiac dysfunction becomes clinically manifested.[158] Abnormalities of both systolic function (reduced ejection fraction) and diastolic function (increased myocardial wall stiffness) have been demonstrated in alcoholic patients without cardiac symptoms by a variety of invasive and noninvasive techniques.[158-161] Two basic patterns have been observed: (1) left ventricular dilatation with impaired systolic function and (2) left ventricular hypertrophy with diminished compliance and normal or increased contractile performance;

left ventricular size is most substantially increased.[161-163] While overt alcoholic liver disease and cardiac involvement often do not occur together, even cirrhotic patients without signs or symptoms of heart disease have inducible evidence of asymptomatic myocardial disease.[158-160]

The development of symptoms may be insidious, although some patients have acute and florid left-sided congestive heart failure. A paroxysm of atrial fibrillation is a relatively frequent initial presenting finding.[136] More advanced cases involve findings of biventricular failure, with left ventricular dysfunction usually dominating. Dyspnea, orthopnea, and paroxysmal nocturnal dyspnea are frequently observed. Palpitations and syncope due to tachyarrhythmias, usually supraventricular, are occasionally present. Angina pectoris does not occur unless there is concomitant coronary artery disease or aortic stenosis.

PHYSICAL EXAMINATION. This usually reveals a narrow pulse pressure, often with an elevated diastolic pressure secondary to excessive peripheral vasoconstriction. There is cardiomegaly, and protodiastolic (S_3) and presystolic (S_4) gallop sounds are common. An apical systolic murmur of mitral regurgitation due to papillary muscle dysfunction is often found. The severity of right heart failure varies, but jugular venous distention and peripheral edema are common.

LABORATORY EXAMINATION. The *chest roentgenogram* in the advanced case demonstrates cardiac enlargement, pulmonary congestion, and pulmonary venous hypertension (p. 163). Pleural effusions are often seen. *Electrocardiographic abnormalities* are common and are frequently the only indication of alcoholic heart disease during the preclinical phase. Alcoholic patients without other evidence of heart disease often are seen after developing palpitations, chest discomfort, or syncope typically following a binge of alcohol consumption on a weekend, particularly during the year-end holiday season.[164] This is dubbed the "holiday heart syndrome." The most common arrhythmia observed is atrial fibrillation, followed by atrial flutter and frequent ventricular premature contractions.[164, 165] Alcohol consumption may even predispose to atrial fibrillation or flutter in nonalcoholics.[166] Hypokalemia may play a role in the genesis of some of these arrhythmias. Supraventricular arrhythmias are also frequently observed in patients with overt alcoholic cardiomyopathy. Sudden, unexpected death is not uncommon in young adult alcoholics, and it is likely that ventricular fibrillation is responsible.[146, 167]

Atrioventricular conduction disturbances (most commonly first-degree heart block), bundle branch block, and left ventricular hypertrophy are common electrocardiographic findings.[168] Prolongation of the Q-T interval is noted frequently.[163] ST-segment and T-wave changes are often restored to normal within several days after cessation of alcohol consumption.[169]

The hemodynamic findings observed at cardiac catheterization and the assessment of left ventricular function by noninvasive methods (echocardiography, isotope angiography, and systolic time intervals) resemble those found in idiopathic dilated cardiomyopathy.

The *natural history* of alcoholic cardiomyopathy depends on the drinking habits of the patient. Total abstinence in the earlier stages of the disease frequently leads to resolution of the manifestation of congestive heart failure and a return of heart size to normal.[156, 170] Continued alcohol consumption leads to further myocardial damage and fibrosis, with the development of refractory congestive heart failure. Death may also be due to arrhythmia, heart block, and systemic or pulmonary embolism.

TREATMENT. The key to the long-term treatment of alcoholic cardiomyopathy is *immediate and complete abstinence*, as early in the course of the disease as possible. The prognosis in patients who continue to drink, particularly if they have been symptomatic for a long period, is poor. In one study, 80 per cent of such patients died within a 3-year period.[156] In the overall population of patients with alcoholic cardiomyopathy, between 40 and 50 per cent succumb within a 3- to 6-year period.[156, 170] Prolonged bed rest is also thought to result in functional improvement,[170] although its major benefit may simply be the decreased alcohol consumption.

The management of acute episodes of congestive heart failure is similar to that of idiopathic dilated cardiomyopathy. For patients with severe congestive heart failure, it is prudent to administer thiamine on the chance that beriberi may be contributing to the heart failure.

COBALT CARDIOMYOPATHY

A previously unrecognized syndrome of fulminating congestive heart failure appeared in 1966, first in Quebec City, Canada, and subsequently in Omaha, Nebraska; Minneapolis, Minnesota; and Belgium.[138] The disease was found in people who drank a particular brand of beer to which cobalt sulfate had been added as a foam stabilizer. After cobalt had been removed from the process, no more cases of the disease were reported. Rare cases of cobalt cardiomyopathy have been found after industrial exposure to cobalt[171] and after the therapeutic ingestion of cobalt salts in the treatment of anemia.[172]

Pathological findings are those of a dilated, hypertrophied heart, often surrounded by a sizable pericardial effusion. Mural thrombi are present in over one-third of patients.[173] Microscopic examination reveals myofibrillar hyaline necrosis as well as myocardial vacuolization and degeneration. The mechanism responsible for the development of cobalt cardiotoxicity remains unclear.

CLINICAL MANIFESTATIONS. The typical patient who developed cobalt-beer cardiomyopathy was a middle-aged man who had consumed large quantities of the contaminated beer.[138] The disease was characterized by severe heart failure, with death occurring in more than 40 per cent of patients, often within 3 days of hospital admission.[138] The typical presentation was that of the abrupt onset of left followed by right heart failure. Hemodynamic findings were those of biventricular failure with depressed cardiac output.[138]

HYPERTROPHIC CARDIOMYOPATHY

DEFINITIONS

The gross pathological features of hypertrophic cardiomyopathy (HCM) were first systematically described in 1958.[174] The characteristic finding is inappropriate myocardial hypertrophy, often involving the interventricular septum of a nondilated left ventricle. A distinctive clinical feature was soon recognized in many patients with HCM: a dynamic pressure gradient in the subaortic area, evanescent in some patients, which divides the left ventricle into a high-pressure apical region and a lower-pressure subaortic region. Hence the terms *idiopathic hypertrophic subaortic stenosis (IHSS)* and muscular subaortic stenosis were suggested, although subsequent findings have indicated that many patients do not, in fact, ever have obstruction to left ventricular outflow, and thus HCM is a more appropriate and inclusive way to describe the disease. Since hypertrophy often occurs in the absence of a pressure gradient, the characteristic feature of HCM is myocardial hypertrophy that is out of proportion to the hemodynamic load.

The most characteristic pathophysiological abnormality in HCM is not systolic but rather *diastolic* dysfunction.[5, 174a] Thus, HCM is characterized by abnormal stiffness of the left ventricle during diastole, with resultant impaired ventricular filling. This abnormality in diastolic relaxation results in elevation of the left ventricular end-diastolic pressure. The elevated left ventricular filling pressure is associated with elevated left atrial, pulmonary venous, and pulmonary capillary pressures, causing dyspnea—the most common symptom in HCM, despite typically *hypercontractile* left ventricular function. The disease appears to be genetically transmitted as an autosomal dominant trait with a high degree of penetrance in somewhat more than half the patients, although sporadic cases occur, some of which may represent new mutations.[176, 177] Evidence of the disease is found in about one-fourth the first-degree relatives of a patient with HCM; in many of the relatives the disease is milder than in the propositus, the degree of hypertrophy is less and more localized, and outflow gradients are usually lacking.[177] Symptoms are often absent, and the disease is detected only by echocardiography.[176]

PATHOLOGY

MACROSCOPIC EXAMINATION. This typically discloses a marked increase in myocardial mass, and the ventricular cavities are small (Fig. 42–4). The left ventricle is usually more involved with the hypertrophic process than is the right.[178] The atria are dilated and often hypertrophied,[179] reflecting the high resistance to filling of the ventricles and the effects of atrioventricular valve regurgitation (Table 42–7). The pattern of hypertrophy of the left ventricle typically is distinctive and differs from that seen with secondary hypertrophy (as in systemic hypertension or discrete obstruction to left ventricular outflow, i.e., subaortic, valvular, or supravalvular aortic stenosis) in that it is commonly associated with disproportionate involvement of the interventricular septum compared with the free wall of the left ventricle (Fig. 42–4). Both in normal subjects as well as in patients with left ventricular hypertrophy without HCM, the ratio of the thickness of the interventricular septum to that of the left ventricular free wall has been shown at autopsy and by echocardiography to be approximately 1.0 and nearly always less than 1.3. However, this ratio usually exceeds 1.3 to 1.5 in HCM. Asymmetrical septal hypertrophy (ASH) was at one time believed to be pathognomonic of HCM, but modifications of this concept have been required.[180-191] Thus, it is now recognized that concentric left ventricular hypertrophy, with symmetrical thickening of the left ventricle, involving the septum and free wall equally, may occasionally be seen in patients with the genetically transmitted as well as the sporadic forms of hypertrophic cardiomyopathy.[181, 182] Even in the majority of patients who manifest ASH the hypertrophy often extends beyond the septum to involve portions of the anterolateral left ventricular wall.[192] In some patients with HCM there is substantial hypertrophy in unusual locations, such as the posterior portion of the septum, the posterobasal free wall, and the midventricular level; this may result in diagnostic confusion, since the hypertrophy may not be detectable by M-mode echocardiography but only by two-dimensional echocardiography.[193-196]

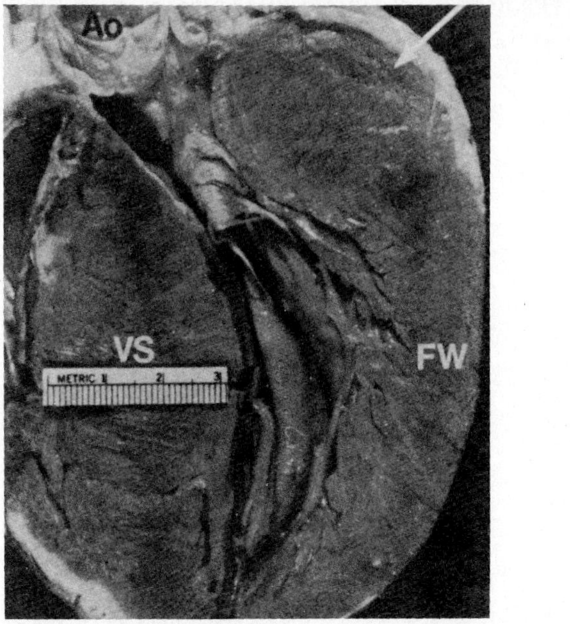

FIGURE 42–4. Hypertrophic cardiomyopathy with massive hypertrophy of interventricular septum (VS). The VS is disproportionately hypertrophied compared with the left ventricular free wall (FW), but the hypertrophy of the FW is not uniform. The posterobasal left ventricular free wall behind the posterior mitral leaflet (arrow) is much thicker than the portion of the free wall located closer to the apex. (From Ciro, E., et al.: Coexistence of asymmetric and symmetric left ventricular hypertrophy in a family with hypertrophic cardiomyopathy. Am. Heart J. *104*:643, 1982.)

TABLE 42–7 PATHOLOGICAL FINDINGS IN HYPERTROPHIC CARDIOMYOPATHY

Finding	Frequency (%)
Asymmetrical septal hypertrophy	95
Small or normal-sized ventricular cavities	95
Mural plaque in left ventricular outflow tract	75
Thickened mitral valve	75
Dilated atria	100
Abnormal intramural coronary arteries	50
Disarray of ventricular septal myocardial fibers	95

Data from Roberts, W. C., and Ferrans, V. J.: Pathologic anatomy of the cardiomyopathies. Idiopathic dilated and hypertrophic types, infiltrative types and endomyocardial disease with and without eosinophilia. Hum. Pathol. 6:287, 1975.

Apical HCM. Two types of an unusual form of HCM localized to the *apical* portion of the left ventricle have been noted. One form, originally described in Japanese patients, imparts a characteristic spadelike configuration to the left ventricular chamber on two dimensional echocardiographic or contrast ventriculographic study[197-204] (Fig. 42–5). Patients with apical hypertrophy of this type may demonstrate giant negative T waves in the precordial electrocardiographic leads, but they typically do not demonstrate pressure gradients.[205] The other form involves a small, poorly contractile apical segment that communicates with the subaortic area through a markedly narrowed midventricular channel. In this form of apical HCM the T waves are not deeply inverted, and an intraventricular pressure gradient may be found.[206] Another variant of HCM, frequently seen in elderly patients, demonstrates severe concentric left ventricular hypertrophy, small left ventricular cavity size, and is associated with hypertension; this syndrome has been termed hypertensive hypertrophic cardiomyopathy of the elderly.[207] Disproportionate septal hypertrophy (ASH) may be found in patients with a variety of acquired or congenital lesions in the absence of HCM.[183, 190]

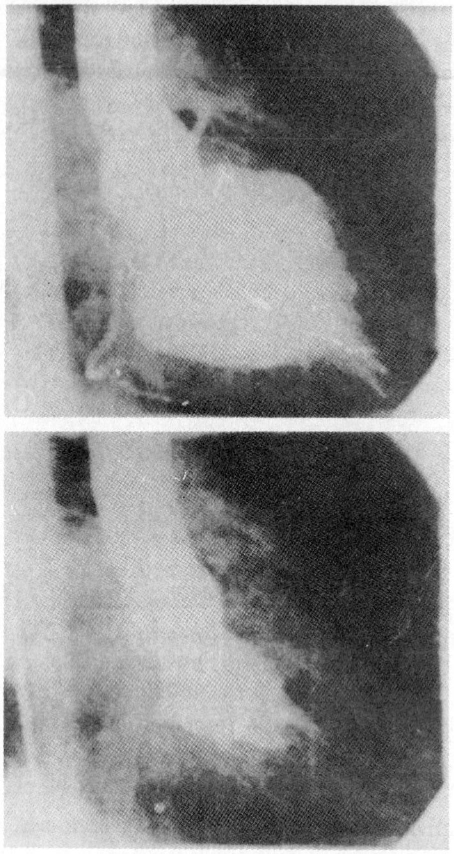

FIGURE 42–5. Left ventriculogram in the right anterior oblique view in apical hypertrophic cardiomyopathy, shown in end-diastole (*top*) and end-systole (*bottom*). The ventricle demonstrates an "ace of spades" configuration with marked hypertrophy of the apex and papillary muscles. (From Vacek, J. L., et al.: Apical hypertrophic cardiomyopathy in American patients. Am. Heart J. *108*:1501, 1984.)

Thus, ASH is a normal finding during fetal life, in neonates, and in infants but normally disappears by the age of 1 or 2 years.[189, 208] Conditions resulting in right ventricular pressure overload and thus right ventricular hypertrophy, such as pulmonic stenosis or primary pulmonary hypertension, often result in thickening of the interventricular septum, without affecting the free wall of the left ventricle.[188, 189] Abnormal thickness of the septum relative to that of the free wall may also occur in coronary artery disease, presumably when infarction leads to fibrosis and thinning of the free wall of the left ventricle, while the noninfarcted septum exhibits compensatory hypertrophy.[209, 210] Other conditions that may present similar patterns of disproportionate septal hypertrophy include lentiginosis, Turner syndrome, acromegaly, hyper- and hypothyroidism, hyperparathyroidism, and Friedreich's ataxia (p. 1789).[211-214] A discrete localized muscular bulge may be seen in the septum of patients with aortic stenosis, and the bulge may become more prominent after aortic valve replacement.[215, 216] Athletes, weight lifters, and infants of diabetic mothers (p. 1012) may demonstrate similar patterns. Rarely, apparent left ventricular hypertrophy is due to infiltration of the septum by tumor,[217, 218] Pompe's disease[219] (p. 1013), amyloid[220] or Fabry's disease.[221]

To differentiate the various causes of septal–free wall disproportion, the term *disproportionate septal thickening* has been used to indicate the secondary form, while ASH is often reserved for the primary form found in HCM. In the latter, the degree of thickening of the interventricular septum appears to be unrelated to the presence or absence of a pressure gradient. However, patients who have had a left ventricular outflow pressure gradient during life demonstrate secondary hypertrophy of the posterobasal wall, including the area immediately behind the posterior leaflet of the mitral valve and below the mitral annulus.[222]

A "contact lesion" in the form of a mural plaque on the endocardium of the left ventricular outflow tract is frequently found in patients with marked intraventricular pressure gradients at rest[30] (Table 42–7). This fibrous thickening appears to result from the trauma of the anterior mitral valve leaflet apposing the septum during systole. The thickening of the mitral valve that is often seen probably has a similar basis.[30]

HISTOLOGY. Microscopic findings in HCM are distinctive, with gross disorganization of the muscle bundles resulting in a characteristic whorled pattern; abnormalities are found in the cell-to-cell arrangement (disarray), and disorganization of the myofibrillar architecture within a given cell[223] (Fig. 42–6). Fibrosis is usually prominent.[224, 224a] The myocardial cells are wider and shorter than in other conditions, and they often have bizarre shapes.[222] Foci of disorganized cells are often interspersed between areas of hypertrophied but otherwise normal-appearing muscle cells.[222] Similar cellular disorganization is found in a spontaneously occurring primary myocardial disease of dogs and cats.[225] While initially considered specific for HCM, it is now recognized that abnormally arranged cardiac muscle cells may be found not only in a variety of disease states, including concentric left ventricular hypertrophy secondary to pressure overload, coronary artery disease, congenital heart disease, and cor pulmonale, but in normal hearts as well.[226-229] Although disarray itself is not a specific indication of HCM, there appears to be a *quantitative* relationship between the extent of cellular disarray and HCM, since the disorganization of myocardial

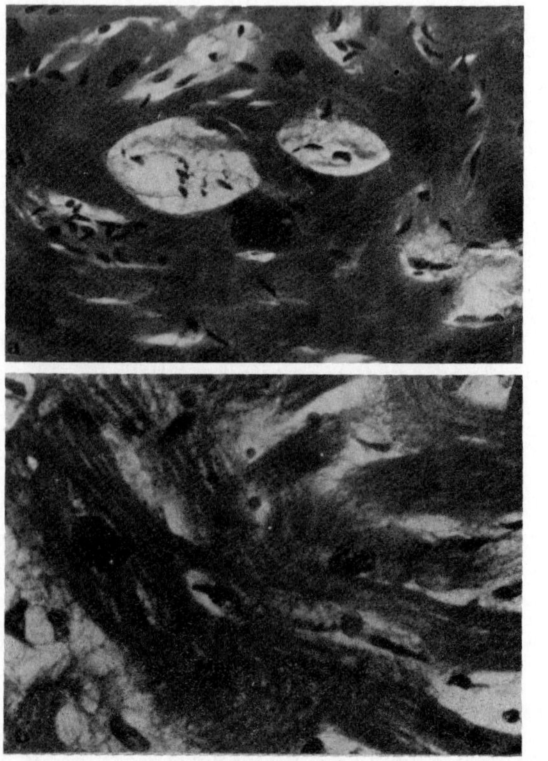

FIGURE 42–6. Histological specimen from a patient with hypertrophic cardiomyopathy, showing marked disarray and whorls of muscle fibers (*top*) and myofibrils (*bottom*). (Original magnification × 773.) (From Davis, M. J.: The cardiomyopathies: A review of terminology, pathology and pathogenesis. Histopathology *8*:363, 1984.)

fibers is far greater in HCM than in other disorders.[230] There is a suggestion that the greater the extent of cellular disorganization, the worse the clinical outcome. However, a somewhat surprising finding is that there is little correlation between the extent of cellular disorganization in surgically excised septectomy samples in patients with HCM and the amount observed at subsequent necropsy.[231]

The *distribution* of cellular disarray differs in patients with and without pressure gradients. While both forms have interventricular septal cellular disarray, patients without gradients tend to have disarray in the left ventricular free wall as well, suggesting a diffuse myopathic process.[222, 232, 233] Conversely, patients with gradients have less abnormalities in the free wall,[233] although these findings are controversial. The changes in the free wall resemble those seen in valvular aortic stenosis. This indicates that they are secondary to the high intraventricular pressure caused by the gradient.

Abnormal intramural coronary arteries, with a reduction in the size of the lumen and thickening of the vessel wall, is common in HCM.[233a] This abnormality occurs most frequently in the ventricular septum; it also has been observed in infants who died of this condition and could represent a congenital component of the condition. The prominence of abnormal intramural coronary arteries in areas of extensive myocardial fibrosis is consistent with the hypothesis that these abnormalities may be responsible for the development of myocardial ischemia.[233a]

ETIOLOGY

The cause of the myocardial hypertrophy in HCM remains unknown. While there are persuasive data that in many patients the disease is inherited,[194] and in at least some instances linked to the HLA system,[234-238] the basic defect is unknown. It has been proposed that it is the *susceptibility* to development of HCM that is inherited.[239] The disorganized myocardial fibers may be the result of mechanical stresses placed on the fibers within the septum, since myocardial disarray is also seen frequently in other conditions characterized by excessive systolic pressure.[228] Pressure overload has been shown to alter myocardial myosin isoenzyme composition, establishing the linkage of mechanical stress and muscle biochemistry.[240] It has been suggested that the genetic defect in HCM results in a catenoid shape and configuration of the septum that is concave to the left in the transverse plane but concave to the right in the apex-to-base plane. This abnormal configuration of the septum leads to prominent isometric contraction which might result in fiber disarray.[241] The reverse argument has also been made that the isometric contraction inherent in malaligned cells itself stimulates hypertrophy.[242]

Other suggested etiologies of HCM include (1) abnormal sympathetic stimulation because of excessive production of or heightened responsiveness of the heart to circulating catecholamines[5, 242-247]; (2) abnormally thickened intramural coronary arteries that do not dilate normally and lead to myocardial ischemia, with resultant fibrosis and abnormal compensatory hypertrophy[248]; (3) a primary abnormality of collagen that may lead to an abnormal and disorganized fibrous skeleton which, with the development of hypertrophy, leads to myocardial cellular disorganization and disarray[248]; (4) subendocardial ischemia,[249] possibly related to abnormalities of the microcirculation,[250] that depletes the energy stores essential for the sequestration of calcium during diastole, resulting in persistent interaction of the contractile elements during diastole and attendant increased diastolic stiffness[251]; and (5) abnormal handling of calcium ion by the myocardium.[252, 253, 253a]

PATHOPHYSIOLOGY

Since the initial descriptions of hypertrophic cardiomyopathy, the feature that has attracted the greatest attention and has been the source of considerable controversy is the dynamic pressure gradient (Fig. 42–7).[251] While this pressure gradient was initially thought to be due to a muscular sphincter action in the subaortic region, it appears to be related to further narrowing of an already small outflow tract (narrowed by the prominent septal hypertrophy and possibly abnormal location of the mitral valve) by systolic anterior motion (SAM) of the mitral valve against the septum. There is a strong temporal and quantitative relationship between SAM and the outflow gradient[254-256, 256a] (Fig. 42–8). Yet even the view that the pressure gradient in HCM is the result of mechanical obstruction as a consequence of SAM may require modification. The generation of a pressure gradient due to subaortic obstruction would imply that left ventricular ejection is slowed or impeded at some point during systole. Yet characteristic features of HCM are rapid ventricular emptying and high ejection fractions. Hemodynamic studies have shown that the majority of flow (at least 80 per cent) is unusually rapid in patients with HCM and is completed earlier in systole than normal, regardless of whether gradients are absent, provocable, or present.[257-259] In patients with intraventricular pressure gradients, a portion of the stroke volume is, in fact, expelled before obstruction commences. However, evidence exists that later in systole "true obstruction" is present. Since the total duration of systole is prolonged only in patients with intraventricular pressure gradients,[257] it is likely that a certain amount of blood is in fact impeded in its ejection from the left ventricle as a consequence of dynamic obstruction, even though most of the blood flow is not "obstructed" in a true fluid dynamic sense.[258-260]

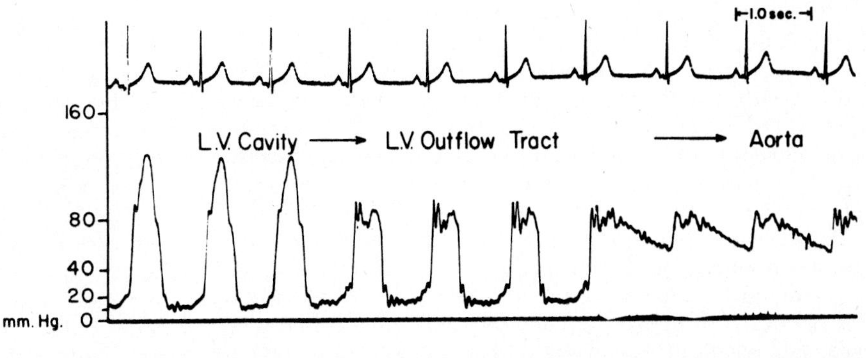

FIGURE 42–7. Pressure tracing recorded as retrograde aortic catheter was withdrawn from the left ventricular (LV) cavity through the left ventricular outflow tract and into the ascending aorta. Note that the pressure gradient occurs within the left ventricle. There is a notch on the left ventricular pressure pulse at approximately 100 mm Hg, the value of the peak systolic pressure distal to the obstruction. In the left ventricular outflow tract the pressure pulse exhibits a midsystolic dip and a secondary elevation late in systole. A similar contour is present during systole in the aortic pressure pulse. (From Braunwald, E., et al.: Idiopathic hypertrophic subaortic stenosis. Circulation *30*(Suppl. IV):67, 1964, by permission of the American Heart Association, Inc.)

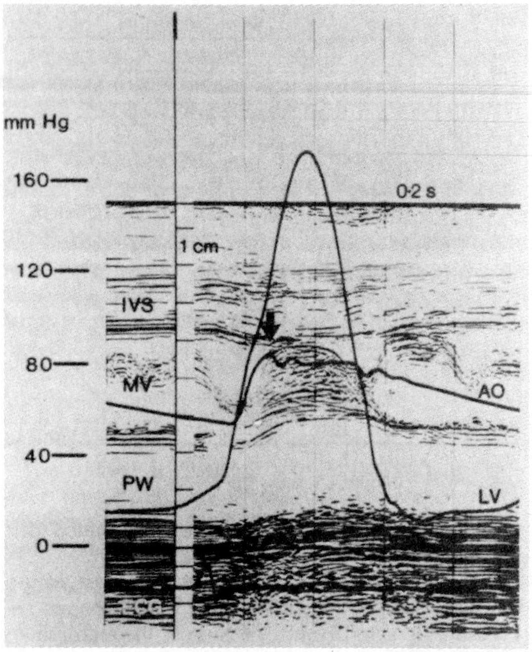

FIGURE 42–8. Simultaneous hemodynamic and echocardiographic recordings in a patient with HCM with 86 mm Hg outflow gradient. The arrow indicates the onset of systolic anterior motion–septal contact and the onset of the pressure gradient, which are simultaneous. IVS = interventricular septum; MV = mitral valve; PW = posterior wall; AO = central aortic pressure; LV = left ventricular pressure. (From Pollick, C., et al.: Muscular subaortic stenosis: The temporal relationship between systolic anterior motion of the anterior mitral leaflet and the pressure gradient. Circulation 66:1087, 1982, by permission of the American Heart Association, Inc.)

CLINICAL MANIFESTATIONS

SYMPTOMS. Although symptomatic HCM is most commonly a disease of young adulthood (the average age of presentation is 26 years),[261] it occurs more commonly than often suspected in elderly patients.[262] The condition has been observed at necropsy in stillborns and both clinically and pathologically in octogenarians. The importance of recognizing this disorder in children at the earliest possible time is highlighted by the high mortality rate; death is often sudden and unexpected.[5] Since syncope and sudden death have been associated with competitive sports and severe exertion in patients with HCM it is important to diagnose this condition so that these activities may be proscribed. A particularly high index of suspicion of this condition must be maintained to make the clinical diagnosis in the elderly, since their symptoms may easily be confused with those of coronary artery or aortic valve disease.[262] No sex predilection is apparent, although females are more likely to be severely disabled and may initially present at a younger age than males.[263]

The clinical picture varies considerably, ranging from the asymptomatic relative of a patient with recognized HCM who has ASH on echocardiogram but no other manifestation of the illness to the patient with incapacitating symptoms.[261] Most patients with HCM are asymptomatic and are the relatives of patients with known disease. Unfortunately, the first clinical manifestation of the disease in asymptomatic individuals may be sudden death.[264]

The most common symptom is *dyspnea*, occurring in up to 90 per cent of symptomatic patients, which is largely a consequence of the elevated left ventricular diastolic (and therefore left atrial and pulmonary venous) pressure, which results largely from impaired ventricular filling and increased wall stiffness secondary to ventricular hypertrophy.[179, 261] Angina pectoris (found in about three-fourths of symptomatic patients), fatigue, and syncope are also common.[179, 261] Palpitations, paroxysmal nocturnal dyspnea, overt congestive heart failure, and dizziness are found less frequently,[261] although marked congestive heart failure culminating in death may be seen in infants with hypertrophic cardiomyopathy.[265] Exertion tends to exacerbate many of the symptoms. A variety of mechanisms may contribute to the production of angina pectoris. It is at least in part the result of an imbalance between oxygen supply and demand as a consequence of the greatly increased myocardial mass.[266] Transmural infarction may occur in the absence of narrowing in the extramural coronary arteries.[267] Narrowing of the small coronary arteries may contribute to myocardial ischemia,[248] particularly during exertion, and older patients with hypertrophic cardiomyopathy may have concurrent atheromatous obstructive coronary artery disease. Impaired diastolic relaxation may produce subendocardial ischemia as a result of prolonged maintenance of wall tension with a concomitant slower-than-normal decrease in the impedance to coronary blood flow. As in patients with valvular aortic stenosis, syncope may result from inadequate cardiac output with exertion or from cardiac arrhythmias.[268, 269] Near-syncopal ("graying out") spells that occur in the erect posture and that can be relieved by immediately lying down are common, occurring in about half of symptomatic patients.[179] However, in contrast to valvular aortic stenosis, syncope or near-syncope may not be an ominous finding in HCM; some patients have a history of such episodes dating back many years without deterioration.[261]

PHYSICAL EXAMINATION. This may be normal in asymptomatic patients without gradients, particularly those with the apical variant of HCM, save for a left ventricular lift and a loud fourth heart sound, but there are usually prominent findings in patients with a pressure gradient in the left ventricular outflow tract. The apical precordial impulse is often displaced laterally and is usually abnormally forceful and enlarged.[179, 261] Because of decreased left ventricular compliance, a prominent presystolic apical impulse which results from forceful atrial systole is often present. This may result in a double apical impulse as a result of the prominent *a* wave. A more characteristic but less frequently recognized abnormality is a triple apical beat, the third impulse being a late systolic bulge that occurs when the heart is nearly empty and is performing near-isometric contraction. These findings may be readily recorded by apexcardiography (Fig. 3–30, p. 59).

A systolic thrill is commonly present, is most frequently palpable at the apex or along the lower left sternal border,[263] and bears only a rough relationship to the severity of the pressure gradient.[261, 263] The jugular venous pulse may demonstrate a prominent *a* wave, reflecting diminished right ventricular compliance secondary to the massive hypertrophy of the ventricular septum. The carotid pulse typically rises briskly and then declines in midsystole as the gradient develops, followed by a secondary rise. This may be well appreciated on physical examination and can be demonstrated more clearly by means of indirect pulse tracings (Figs. 42–9 and 3–23, p. 56).

The first heart sound is normal and is often preceded by a fourth heart sound that corresponds to the apical presystolic impulse.[261, 263] The second heart sound is usually normally split. In some patients, however, it is narrowly split and in others, particularly those with severe outflow gradients, paradoxical splitting may be noted.[261, 263] A third

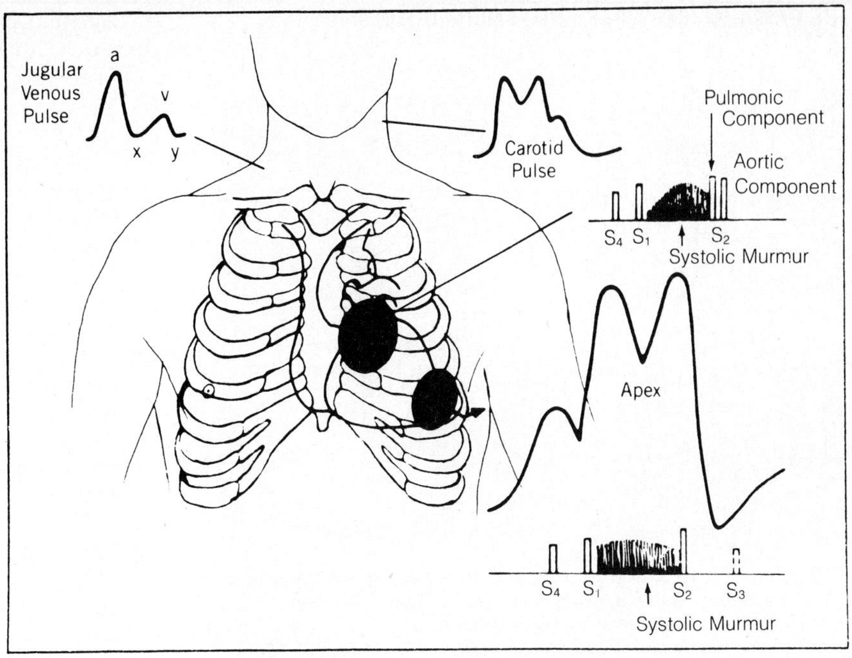

FIGURE 42–9. Salient physical signs of hypertrophic obstructive cardiomyopathy. Jugular venous pulse shows prominent *a* wave. Carotid pulse shows rapid rise and bifid pulse. Left ventricular apex shows prominent *a* wave and bifid systolic impulse. Auscultatory features are schematized. S_4 = fourth heart sound; S_1 = first heart sound; S_3 = third heart sound. (From Shah, P. M.: Newer concepts in hypertrophic obstructive cardiomyopathy II. J.A.M.A. *242*:1771, 1979. Copyright 1979, American Medical Association.)

heart sound is common but does not have the same ominous significance as in patients with valvular aortic stenosis. Systolic ejection sounds relating to rapid acceleration of blood flow, may be found on occasion.[270] The auscultatory hallmark of HCM is a systolic murmur which is typically harsh and crescendo-decrescendo in configuration; it usually commences well after the first heart sound and is best heard between the apex and the left sternal border. It often radiates well to the lower sternal border, the axillae, and base of the heart but not into the neck vessels.[261] In patients with prominent SAM, the murmur usually reflects both outflow tract turbulence and concomitant mitral regurgitation, while in patients without SAM, turbulence in the outflow tract is the only cause.[271, 272] Accordingly, the murmur is often more holosystolic and blowing at the apex and in the axillae (probably due to mitral regurgitation) and midsystolic and harsher along the lower sternal border (due to flow across the outflow tract).[263]

The murmur is labile in intensity and duration, and a variety of maneuvers may be utilized to augment or suppress it (Table 42–8; see also Tables 2–6, p. 35 and 2–7, p. 37). A diastolic rumbling murmur, reflecting increased transmitral flow, may occur in patients with marked mitral regurgitation. The murmur of aortic regurgitation is observed only rarely in patients with HCM, although it may develop after operation to correct the outflow gradient[261, 263] or following infective endocarditis.[273]

It is important to emphasize the features of physical examination that permit differentiation of HCM from fixed orifice obstruction, most commonly due to valvular aortic stenosis (Table 33–12, p. 1056). The character of the carotid pulse is the most useful feature in this regard.[274] Because there is obstruction to left ventricular emptying from the beginning of systole with fixed valvular stenosis, the carotid upstroke is slowed and of low amplitude (pulsus parvus et tardus) (Figs. 3–23, p. 56, and 4–4, p. 67). With HCM, as already pointed out, initial ejection of blood from the left ventricle is unimpeded, and therefore the arterial upstroke is brisk. Other features that may be helpful but are of considerably less significance are the location of the murmur (it radiates along the carotid arteries in valvular aortic stenosis but not in HCM), and the location of the systolic thrill (most prominent in the second right intercostal space in valvular aortic stenosis and in the fourth interspace along the left sternal border in HCM).

ELECTROCARDIOGRAM. This is usually abnormal in HCM and invariably so in symptomatic patients with left ventricular outflow gradients[275] (Fig. 42–10). Normal electrocardiograms are seen in only one-fourth of asymptomatic patients without gradients,[261] and usually are found in the presence of only localized left ventricular hypertrophy.[274] The most common abnormalities are ST-segment and T-wave abnormalities, followed by evidence of left ventricular hypertrophy, with QRS complexes that are tallest in the midprecordial leads.[274, 276] There may be progressive electrocardiographic evidence of hypertrophy over time.[277] Giant negative T-waves in the midprecordial leads are characteristic of HCM involving the apex[205] (Fig. 42–11). Prominent, abnormal Q waves are relatively common, occurring in 20 to 50 per cent of patients.[263] The Q-wave abnormalities often involve the inferior (II, III, aV_1) and/or lateral (V_4–V_6) leads (Fig. 42–10). They appear to be due to depolarization of myopathic cells in the septum that have abnormal electrophysiological properties.[278] A variety

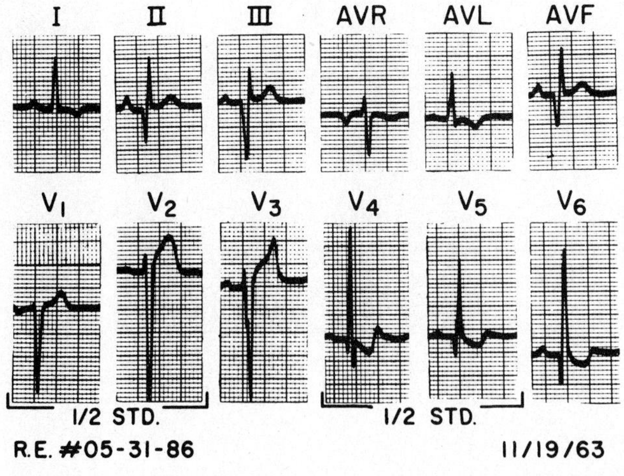

FIGURE 42–10. Electrocardiogram showing abnormal Q waves in leads II, III, aV_F, V_5, and V_6 in a patient with HCM. Precordial leads exhibit the voltage criteria for left ventricular hypertrophy. (From Braunwald, E., et al.: Idiopathic hypertrophic subaortic stenosis. Circulation *30*(Suppl. IV):26, 1964, by permission of the American Heart Association, Inc.)

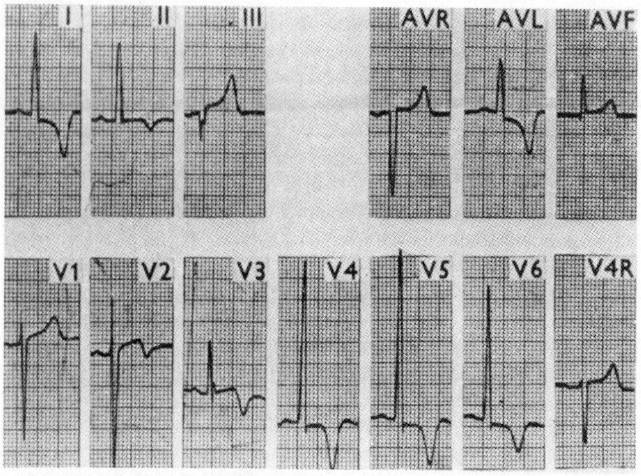

FIGURE 42–11. Electrocardiogram in patient with apical hypertrophic cardiomyopathy. There is prominent QRS voltage with deep T wave inversion across the precordial leads. (From Steingo, L., et al.: Apical hypertrophic nonobstructive cardiomyopathy. Am. Heart J. *104*:635, 1982.)

of other electrocardiographic abnormalities may occur, including abnormal electrical axis (usually left-axis deviation) and P-wave abnormalities (usually left atrial enlargement). Accessory atrioventricular pathways have been found in hypertrophic cardiomyopathy, although they appear to be rare.[279] A short P-R interval followed by slurring of a tall R wave with normal QRS duration is a relatively frequent finding[261]; in many cases this appears to be unassociated with evidence of preexcitation.[280] Clinically significant abnormalities of AV conduction are uncommon but may cause syncope.[281]

Although a hemodynamic mechanism may play a role in the death of patients with HCM, many and perhaps most deaths, particularly those that are known to have been sudden, are probably due to an arrhythmia. Because of the systolic and diastolic abnormalities in this disorder rhythm disturbances are less well tolerated.

Ventricular arrhythmias are common in patients with HCM, occurring in over three-fourths of patients undergoing continuous ambulatory electrocardiographic monitoring.[282] Ventricular tachycardia is found in about one-fourth of the patients studied, and in some it is a harbinger of subsequent sudden death.[282-284] A similar spectrum of arrhythmias may be detected in those asymptomatic relatives of patients with HCM who themselves have the disease (often undiagnosed).[285] Treadmill testing may expose arrhythmias that are not present at rest, although continuous ambulatory monitoring is superior in detecting repetitive ventricular tachyarrhythmias.[286] Supraventricular tachycardia may be found in one-fourth to one-half of patients.[284, 287] Atrial fibrillation occurs in 5 to 10 per cent of patients, and the resultant loss of the atrial contribution to the filling of a hypertrophied, stiff ventricle may result in marked clinical deterioration—as a consequence of a reduction in cardiac output or elevation of the left atrial pressure or both.[263, 288] *Electrophysiological testing* may induce sustained symptomatic supraventricular or ventricular tachyarrhythmias not detectable by continuous ambulatory monitoring.[289]

CHEST ROENTGENOGRAM. The findings on radiographic examination are variable; heart size, principally the left ventricle, may range from normal to markedly enlarged, but there is little correlation between heart size and the severity of the outflow tract gradient. Left atrial enlargement is frequently observed, especially when significant mitral regurgitation is present.[261] Aortic root enlargement and valvular calcification are not seen unless associated diseases are present, although calcification of the mitral annulus is common in HCM.[290]

ECHOCARDIOGRAPHY (See also p. 124). Because echocardiography combines the attributes of high resolution and no known risk, it has been widely utilized in the evaluation of hypertrophic cardiomyopathy[180, 291, 292] (Fig. 42–12, Figs. 5–97 to 5–100, p. 124 to 126). It is useful in the study of patients with suspected HCM and also in the screening of relatives of patients in whom this condition

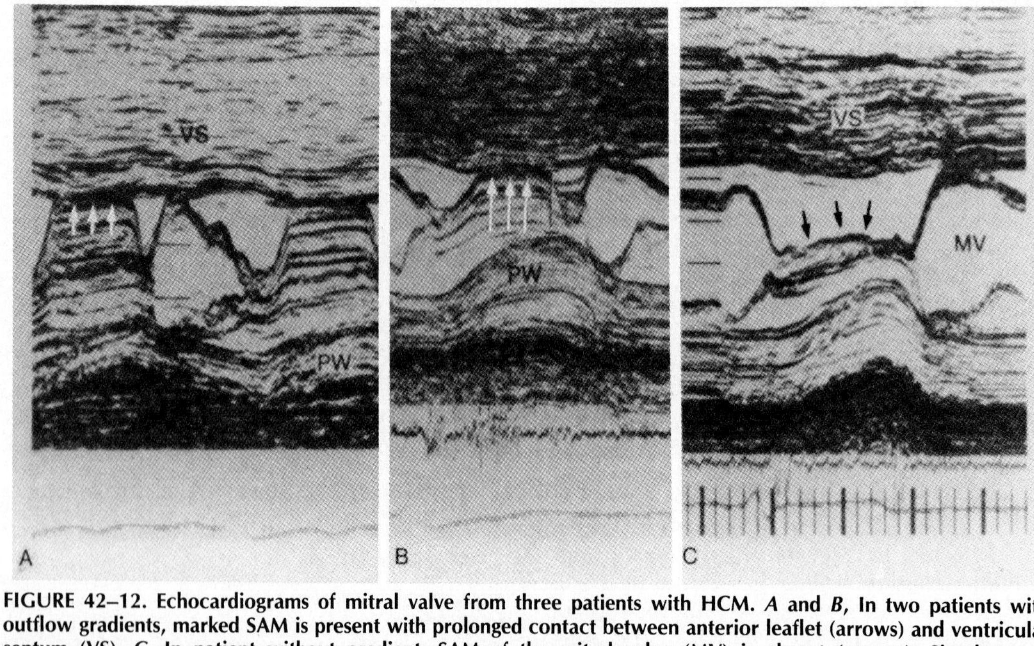

FIGURE 42–12. Echocardiograms of mitral valve from three patients with HCM. *A* and *B*, In two patients with outflow gradients, marked SAM is present with prolonged contact between anterior leaflet (arrows) and ventricular septum (VS). *C*, In patient without gradient, SAM of the mitral valve (MV) is absent (arrows). Simultaneous phonocardiograms and lead II electrocardiograms are shown below. PW = posterior left ventricular wall. (From Maron, B. J., et al.: Dynamic subaortic obstruction in hypertrophic cardiomyopathy: Analysis by pulsed Doppler echocardiography. J. Am. Coll. Cardiol. 6:1, 1985. Reprinted with permission of the American College of Cardiology.)

has been documented. The echocardiogram is of value in identifying and quantifying morphological (i.e., distribution of septal hypertrophy) as well as functional features (e.g., hypercontractile left ventricle).

The cardinal echocardiographic feature of HCM myopathy is left ventricular hypertrophy. Although the characteristic feature is hypertrophy of the septum and anterolateral free wall, other left ventricular locations may be involved, including portions of the free wall and the apex; on occasion concentric involvement is seen.[291, 293-295] Although controversial, it has been suggested that apical involvement accounts for 10 per cent of HCM cases, and concentric, more than one-third.[292] Maximal hypertrophy of the septum often occurs midway between the base and apex of the left ventricle. The finding of a thickened septum that is at least 1.3 to 1.5 times the thickness of the posterior wall when measured in diastole just prior to atrial systole has been the time-honored criterion for the diagnosis of asymmetrical septal hypertrophy (ASH).[179, 180] The septum not only is relatively thicker than the posterior wall but is typically at least 15 mm in thickness (normal ≦ 11 mm). Approximately half the first-degree relatives of patients with HCM will have such an abnormal septal/free wall ratio, despite the fact that they are often asymptomatic, have normal physical examinations, and are often unaware of any cardiac disease.[175] There is usually substantial heterogeneity in the distribution of hypertrophy when the patterns of involvement of relatives are compared.[194, 296] In patients with concentric left ventricular hypertrophy (due to systemic hypertension or aortic valve disease, for example), the septal/free wall ratio will often be close to 1:1, although occasional patients with hypertension will manifest ASH.[297-300] The use of a septal/free wall ratio of 1.5:1 may be more specific for HCM, although some patients with HCM will not be identified.

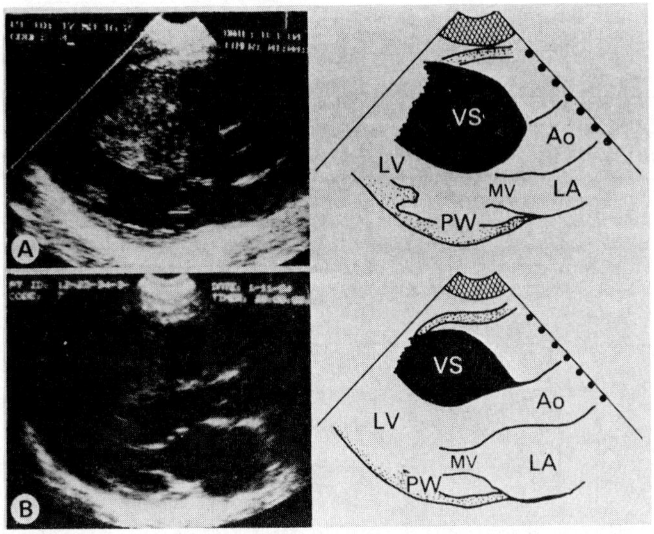

FIGURE 42–13. Two-dimensional echocardiograms obtained in end-diastole in the parasternal long-axis view. Accompanying schematic illustrations are on the right. These two patients with HCM and massive left ventricular hypertrophy illustrate variations in the distribution of ventricular septal hypertrophy in the basal to apical cross-sectional plane. *A*, Massive hypertrophy of the ventricular septum (VS) with similar magnitude of wall thickening in the basal and apical segments, resulting in the appearance of a "lemon drop" protruding into both ventricles. The left ventricular (LV) outflow tract appears narrowed. *B*, Septal thickening is most substantial distal to the mitral valve (MV) and the basal septum is less markedly thickened. The left ventricular (LV) outflow tract appears normal in size and the septum does not bulge into the outflow tract. Ao = aorta; LA = left atrium; PW = posterior free wall. (From Louie, E. K. and Maron, B. J.: Hypertrophic cardiomyopathy with extreme increase in left ventricular wall thickness: functional and morphologic features and clinical significance. J. Am. Coll. Cardiol. *8*:57, 1986. Reprinted with permission of the American College of Cardiology.)

M-mode echocardiography will not always provide accurate measurements of true septal thickness, however. In many cases in which the M-mode echocardiogram falsely suggests ASH, the finding is due to oblique imaging of an acutely anteriorly angled interventricular septum.[301] Two-dimensional echocardiography is therefore preferred in the evaluation of HCM patients, and should be used to clarify septal orientation and thickness in questionable or equivocal cases (Fig. 42–13). Two-dimensional echocardiography is also useful for identifying patients with localized hypertrophy in unusual locations not accessible to the M-mode beam, such as the posterior or apical septum, the anterior or lateral left ventricular free wall,[193] and the apex.[205, 206] An unusual echocardiographic pattern consisting of a ground-glass appearance has been noted in portions of the hypertrophied myocardium in HCM.[302] It has been speculated that this pattern may be related to the abnormal cellular architecture and myocardial fibrosis that has been noted in pathological studies. Two-dimensional echocardiograms in HCM have suggested, in concordance with autopsy specimens, that the interventricular septum is configured in the shape of a catenoid, i.e., a curved surface with net zero curvature at all points.[303]

A second echocardiographic feature often found in hypertrophic cardiomyopathy in addition to ASH is narrowing of the left ventricular outflow tract, which is formed by the interventricular septum anteriorly and the anterior leaflet of the mitral valve posteriorly.[304] The mitral valve apparatus is positioned abnormally close to the septum, possibly the result of the posterior bulging of the septum. When HCM is associated with a pressure gradient, there is abnormal systolic anterior motion (SAM) of the anterior leaflet, and occasionally the posterior leaflet of the mitral valve (Fig. 42–12).[305, 306] Although the role of SAM in *producing* the gradient is controversial, there is a close relationship between the degree of SAM and the size of the outflow gradient.[305] Prolonged interventricular septal contact of the mitral apparatus is limited to HCM with resting pressure gradients,[307] and there is a close temporal relationship between the onset of the pressure gradient and the onset of septal apposition of the mitral apparatus.[308]

Three explanations have been offered for SAM: (1) the mitral valve is *pulled* against the septum by contraction of the papillary muscles, because of the abnormal location and orientation of these muscles resulting from septal hypertrophy; (2) the mitral valve is *pushed* against the septum because of its abnormal position in the outflow tract; (3) the mitral valve is drawn toward the septum because of the lower pressure that occurs as blood is ejected at a high velocity through a narrowed outflow tract (Venturi effect). However, contrary to initial reports, SAM of the mitral valve and dynamic left ventricular gradients are not pathognomonic of HCM but may be found in a variety of other conditions, including hypercontractile states, left ventricular hypertrophy, transposition of the great arteries, and infiltration of the septum.[181, 182, 309, 310] Even mild degrees of left ventricular hypertrophy may be associated with SAM and outflow gradients, particularly under conditions of enhanced sympathetic tone.[311] In many cases in conditions other than HCM, SAM is due to buckling of the chordae tendineae rather than to movement of the anterior mitral valve leaflet as occurs in HCM (although the chordae tendineae and papillary muscles may contribute to SAM in HCM).[312-314]

Several other echocardiographic findings may be present: (1) a small left ventricular cavity; (2) reduced septal motion and thickening during systole, particularly of the upper septum[315] (presumably because of the disarray of the myofibrillar architecture and abnormal contractile function); (3) normal or increased motion of the posterior wall; (4) a reduced rate of closure of the mitral valve in mid-diastole secondary to a decrease in left ventricular compliance or abnormal transmitral flow during diastole;[316] (5) mitral valve prolapse; and (6) partial systolic closure or, more commonly, coarse systolic fluttering of the aortic valve related to turbulent blood flow in the outflow tract.[317] The echocardiographic findings that accompany a left ventricular outflow tract gradient (SAM and aortic valve partial closure) may be quite labile, and provocative measures such as the Valsalva maneuver or pharmacologically induced vasodilatation with amyl nitrite (Fig. 3–23, p. 56), stimulation of contractility with isoproterenol, or an induced premature ventricular contraction may be required to precipitate the findings.

Abnormalities of diastolic function may be demonstrated by echocardiography in many patients with HCM, independent of the presence or absence of a systolic pressure gradient. The isovolumetric relaxation time, measured from aortic valve closure to mitral valve opening, is frequently prolonged and the peak velocity of left ventricular filling is reduced.[318] Because the septum is typically hypokinetic, the rate of left ventricular filling is determined primarily by the rate of free wall thinning. While there is a general relationship between the extent of hypertrophy and the severity of abnormalities of diastolic function, even nonhypertrophied regions of the HCM ventricle appear to contribute to the impairment of diastolic function seen in HCM.[319]

Doppler ultrasound has confirmed the virtual ubiquity of mitral regurgitation when an outflow gradient is present,[320, 321] and a marked deceleration of aortic blood flow that occurs coincident with SAM.[305] Doppler color flow imaging reveals mitral regurgitation, most prominent in late systole, with the appearance of turbulent flow in the left ventricular outflow tract; in one study, the velocity of the latter was correlated with the degree of SAM, supporting the concept of left ventricular outflow tract obstruction.[317a]

RADIONUCLIDE SCANNING. These techniques are gaining popularity in the detection of HCM. Thallium-201 myocardial imaging, particularly when tomographic imaging is performed, permits direct determination of the relative thicknesses of the septum and free wall and may be of particular value when technical constraints limit the reliability of echocardiographic evaluation in a given patient with presumed HCM.[322] The utility of rest and exercise thallium-201 scintigraphy in identifying patients with HCM whose angina pectoris is due to obstructive epicardial coronary artery disease is controversial; at least in some patients, thallium-201 defects suggestive of regional myocardial ischemia are found despite angiographically normal coronary arteries.[323, 324] Gated radionuclide ventriculography with blood pool labeling permits the evaluation of not only the size but also the motion of the septum and left ventricle. Disproportionate thickening of the upper septum is a distinctive scintigraphic feature that may be seen in the steep left anterior oblique view. As with the echocardiogram, abnormal diastolic filling of the ventricle has been observed in patients with HCM (both with and without gradients) by computer analysis of the blood pool scan.[325, 326]

HEMODYNAMICS

Cardiac catheterization discloses diminished diastolic left ventricular compliance and a pressure gradient, when present, within the body of the left ventricle, which is separated from a subaortic chamber by the thickened septum and the anterior leaflet of the mitral valve that abuts the septum (Figs. 42–7 and 42–14).[256a] The pressure gradient may be quite labile and may vary between 0 and 175 mm Hg. There is often a notch on the ascending limb of the left ventricular pressure curve, occurring at the onset of left ventricular ejection[261] and the pressure tracing may, on occasion, demonstrate a pattern of pulsus alternans.[327] The arterial pressure tracing may demonstrate a "spike and dome" configuration similar to the carotid pulse recording. As a consequence of diminished left ventricular compliance, the mean and particularly the *a* wave in the left atrial pressure pulse and the left ventricular end-diastolic pressures are usually elevated.[261] Artifactual outflow gradients may occur if the left ventricular catheter becomes entrapped in the trabeculae of a markedly hypertrophied left ventricle. Proper technique and choice of catheters with side holes should clarify the mechanism of such gradients. Cardiac output may be depressed in patients with longstanding severe gradients. In the majority of patients it is normal; occasionally it is elevated.

Hemodynamic abnormalities in HCM are not limited to the left heart. Approximately one-fourth of patients demonstrate pulmonary hypertension, which is usually mild but occasionally may be moderate to severe. This may be due to elevated mean left atrial pressures. A pressure gradient in the right ventricular outflow tract occurs in approximately 15 per cent of patients who have obstruction to left ventricular outflow[261, 263] and appears to result from muscular contraction of the infundibulum. Right atrial and right ventricular end-diastolic pressures may be slightly elevated.

ANGIOCARDIOGRAPHY. Left ventriculography shows a hypertrophied ventricle in which the anterior leaflet of the mitral valve moves anteriorly during systole and encroaches upon the outflow tract (Fig. 42–15). Associated with this motion of the leaflet is mitral regurgitation, which appears to be a constant finding in patients with gradients. The left ventricular cavity is often small, and systolic ejection is typically vigorous, resulting in virtual oblitera-

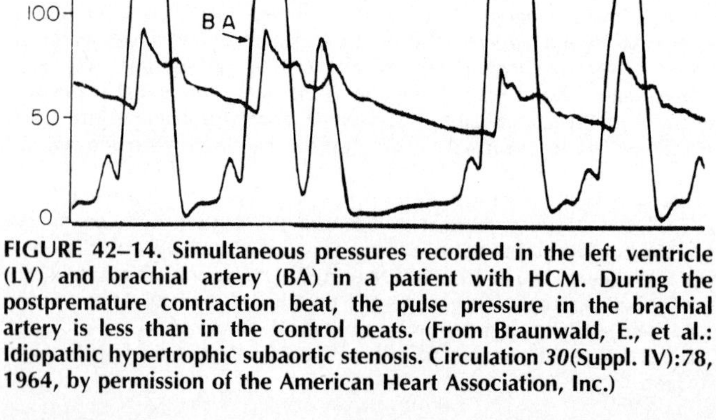

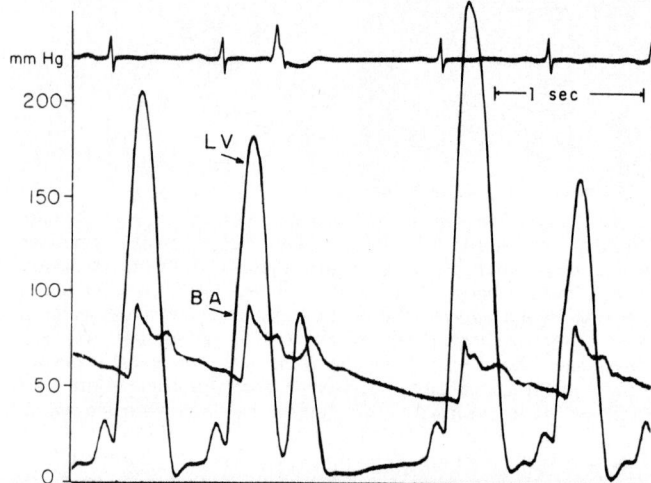

FIGURE 42–14. Simultaneous pressures recorded in the left ventricle (LV) and brachial artery (BA) in a patient with HCM. During the postpremature contraction beat, the pulse pressure in the brachial artery is less than in the control beats. (From Braunwald, E., et al.: Idiopathic hypertrophic subaortic stenosis. Circulation *30*(Suppl. IV):78, 1964, by permission of the American Heart Association, Inc.)

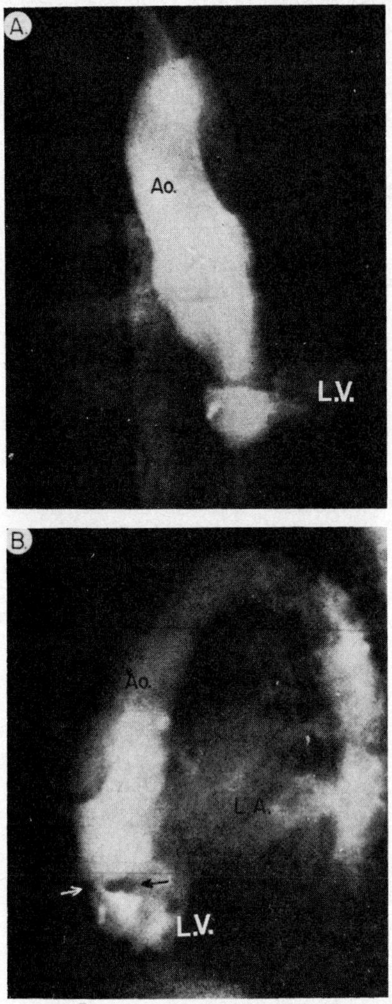

FIGURE 42–15. Angiograms showing obstruction in a patient with familial HCM. Films were obtained during selective left ventricular angiography, in the frontal (*A*) and lateral (*B*) projections during systole. A linear area of narrowing is apparent (arrows), which lies at the point where the hypertrophied septum impinges on the closed anterior leaflet of the mitral valve. Ao. = aorta, L.A. = left atrium, L.V. = left ventricle. (From Ross, J., Jr., Braunwald, E., Gault, J. H., Mason, D. T., and Morrow, A. G.: The mechanism of the intraventricular pressure gradient in idiopathic hypertrophic subaortic stenosis. Circulation *34*:558, 1966, by permission of the American Heart Association, Inc.)

tion of the cavity at end systole, although the apparent hypercontractile state may relate more to reduced afterload (end-systolic wall stress) than enhanced inotropy.[328, 329] The papillary muscles are often prominent and may fill the left ventricular cavity in late systole. In some cases, the hypertrophy of the papillary muscles and midventricular myocardium may result in true muscular stenosis owing to a sphincter mechanism.[330] In patients with apical involvement, the extensive hypertrophy may convey a spade-like configuration to the left ventricular angiogram[197] (Fig. 42–5).

It is often helpful to supplement angiographic evaluation of the left ventricle with simultaneous right ventriculography in a cranially angulated LAO projection in order to obtain optimal visualization of the size, shape, and configuration of the interventricular septum.[331] The left septal surface either is flat or bulges into the left ventricular cavity at its mid or lower portion, in contrast to the normal findings of the septum curving toward the right ventricle.

In patients over 45 years of age, coronary artery obstructive disease is rather common, although the symptoms of ischemic pain are indistinguishable from those of patients with normal coronary angiograms and hypertrophic cardiomyopathy.[332] The left anterior descending[333] and septal perforator coronary arteries may demonstrate phasic narrowing during systole in the absence of fixed obstructive lesions.[334]

LABILITY OF GRADIENT. A feature characteristic of HCM already referred to is the variability and lability of the left ventricular outflow gradient. A given patient may demonstrate a large outflow gradient on one occasion but have none at another time. In some patients without a resting gradient, it may be temporarily provoked.[335] Three basic mechanisms are involved in the production of dynamic gradients, all of which act by reducing ventricular volume and presumably accentuate the apposition of the anterior mitral leaflet against the septum: (1) increased contractility, (2) decreased preload, and (3) decreased afterload.[261, 335] In a minority of patients with HCM, the gradient is midventricular[330] and may be intensified by increased contractility, which exerts a direct muscular sphincteric action. The stimuli that provoke or intensify left ventricular outflow tract gradients in HCM generally improve myocardial performance in normal subjects and in patients with most other forms of heart disease. Conversely, reductions in contractility or increases in preload or afterload, which increase left ventricular dimensions, reduce or abolish the left ventricular outflow gradient.

Alterations in the magnitude of the gradient are reflected by changes in the findings on physical examination, noninvasive tests, and catheterization findings (Table 42–8). An increase in the gradient results in a louder murmur, a longer ejection period with a more characteristic spike and dome configuration in the carotid pulse, and more flagrant echocardiographic evidence of SAM of the anterior mitral leaflet. *It is this dynamic characteristic of HCM that distinguishes it from the discrete forms of obstruction to ventricular outflow.*

A number of bedside procedures may be useful in the evaluation of suspected hypertrophic cardiomyopathy.[336] Perhaps the most helpful is sudden standing from a squatting position. Squatting results in an increase in venous return and an increase in aortic pressure, which increases ventricular volume, diminishing the gradient and decreasing the intensity of the murmur. Sudden standing has the

TABLE 42–8 EFFECTS OF INTERVENTIONS ON OUTFLOW GRADIENT AND SYSTOLIC MURMUR IN HCM

	CONTRACTILITY	PRELOAD	AFTERLOAD
Increase in Gradient and Murmur			
Valsalva maneuver (during strain)	—	↓	↓
Standing	—	↓	—
Postextrasystole	↑	↑	—
Isoproterenol	↑	↓	↓
Digitalis	↑	↓	—
Amyl nitrite	— then ↑	↓ then ↑	↓
Nitroglycerin	—	↓	↓
Exercise	↑	↑	↑
Tachycardia	↑	↓	—
Hypovolemia	↑	↓	↓
Decrease in Gradient and Murmur			
Mueller maneuver	—	↑	↑
Valsalva overshoot	—	↑	↑
Squatting	—	↑	↑
Alpha-adrenoceptor stimulation (phenylephrine)	—	—	↑
Beta-adrenoceptor blockade	↓	↑	—
General anesthesia	↓	—	—
Isometric handgrip	—	—	↑

↑ = increase; ↓ = decrease; — = no major change.

opposite effects and results in accentuation of the gradient and the murmur. The Valsalva maneuver is another useful bedside technique for eliciting or exacerbating the gradient (Table 42–8). Following a transient increase in arterial pressure that usually lasts for four or five cardiac cycles after the onset of the strain coincident with an increase in heart rate, the arterial systolic and pulse pressures and ventricular volume decline, and the gradient (and murmur) increase. Following release of the strain, there is a compensatory overshoot of arterial pressure and venous return and cardiac slowing, all of which increase ventricular volume and reduce the magnitude of the gradient and the murmur.[336] In occasional patients, there may be paradoxical attenuation of the systolic murmur despite an increase in the pressure gradient, presumably related to a critical reduction in stroke volume. The characteristic finding in this setting is striking attenuation of the arterial pulses.[337] The Mueller maneuver, i.e., deep inspiration against a closed glottis (the opposite of the Valsalva maneuver), results in the *lessening* of dynamic obstruction to left ventricular outflow.[338] Inhalation of amyl nitrite also intensifies the murmur and the abnormality of the arterial pulse (Fig. 3–23, p. 56).

One of the most potent stimuli for enhancing the gradient is *postextrasystolic potentiation* (p. 412), which may occur following a spontaneous premature contraction or be induced by mechanical stimulation with a catheter or an external precordial mechanical stimulator.[339] The resultant increase in contractility in the beat following the extrasystole is so marked that it outweighs the otherwise salutary effect of increased ventricular filling caused by the compensatory pause and produces an increase in the gradient and often of the murmur as well. A characteristic change often occurs in the directly recorded arterial pressure tracing, which, in addition to displaying a more marked spike and dome configuration, exhibits a pulse pressure that fails to increase as expected or actually decreases (Fig. 42–14). This is one of the most reliable signs of dynamic obstruction of the left ventricular outflow tract.[340] In some patients, the postextrasystolic murmur is attenuated despite an increase in the outflow gradient, apparently because in this setting the murmur (a hybrid of outflow tract turbulence and mitral regurgitation) is mirroring to a greater degree changes in the degree of mitral regurgitation rather than changes in the outflow tract gradient.[272]

Digitalis glycosides and the beta-adrenoceptor agonist isoproterenol augment the gradient, since they increase myocardial contractility, while nitroglycerin and amyl nitrite exaggerate the gradient by decreasing arterial pressure and ventricular volume.[261] Hypovolemia (as a result of hemorrhage or overly aggressive diuresis) may also provoke overt obstruction to left ventricular outflow. The intensity of the murmur and the left ventricular outflow gradient may be decreased by beta-adrenoceptor blockade, although the effect of the latter is often not dramatic and is of most hemodynamic benefit in protecting against the *increase* in the gradient that may be provoked by exercise.[239] In most patients the severity of mitral regurgitation and the intensity of the apical blowing regurgitant murmur vary with the degree of obstruction of left ventricular outflow.[336]

MANAGEMENT

Interventions that decrease ventricular contractility or increase ventricular volume, systemic arterial pressure, the dimensions of the outflow tract, or ventricular compliance usually exert a salutary effect on the symptoms and vice versa. Since digitalis glycosides increase contractility and thus the obstruction; these drugs are generally proscribed unless atrial fibrillation with a very rapid ventricular rate and/or left ventricular dilatation and dysfunction without a gradient (see below) are present. Similarly, nitrates and beta-adrenoceptor stimulants are best avoided. Dyspnea is a prominent symptom in patients with HCM but is not usually due to systolic dysfunction. Diuretics should be used sparingly, if at all, since reduction of intravascular volume may reduce ventricular size and increase the systolic pressure gradient, as well as causing a reduction in cardiac output or blood pressure. This is of particular concern in patients with small left ventricular cavities and limited stroke volume, especially the variant of HCM termed the hypertensive hypertrophic cardiomyopathy of the elderly.[207]

Beta-Adrenoceptor Blockers. These drugs are the mainstay of medical therapy. Most of the experience to date has been with propranolol. Beta blockade may prevent the increase in outflow obstruction that accompanies exercise, although resting gradients are largely unchanged.[5, 342] It decreases the determinants of myocardial oxygen consumption and thus angina pectoris, and perhaps exerts an antiarrhythmic action.[5] Angina pectoris generally responds more favorably to treatment with a beta blocker than does dyspnea.[343] It has also been suggested that beta blockade may prevent sudden death, but its efficacy for this purpose has not been established.[5] Beta blockade also blunts the chronotropic response, thus limiting the demand for increased myocardial oxygen delivery.[344] Beta-adrenoceptor blockade may also have a beneficial effect on diastolic ventricular filling possibly by improving the distensibility of the left ventricle.[341, 345] The overall clinical response to beta blockade is variable, however, since only about one-third to two-thirds of patients experience symptomatic improvement[346, 347]; a blinded, properly controlled test of this therapy has not been reported. It is reasonable to try large doses of propranolol (greater than 320 mg per day) in patients without contraindications who have not experienced adequate symptomatic improvement with conventional doses[348]; some patients so treated experience symptomatic improvement and improved exercise capacity.[349]

Calcium Antagonists. These are an increasingly popular alternative to beta-adrenoceptor blockade in the management of HCM[359a]; exercise performance in particular may be improved when patients are changed from a beta-adrenoceptor blocker to verapamil.[350] Both the hypercontractile systolic function and the abnormalities of diastolic filling may be related to abnormal calcium kinetics, and drugs that block the inward transport of calcium across the myocardial cell membrane may be able to rectify both abnormalities.

Verapamil has been the most widely studied calcium-channel blocking agent in this condition (Fig. 42–16). Its use was suggested, at least in part, by the observation that it produces a protective and beneficial effect in the hereditary cardiomyopathy of the Syrian hamster, a condition marked by intracellular calcium overload, in which propranolol is ineffective.[351] Although the vasodilator effects of verapamil should not be helpful in HCM, it appears that by depressing myocardial contractility, verapamil can decrease the left ventricular outflow gradient when given intravenously or orally.[352-355] Perhaps more important from a symptomatic point of view, verapamil improves diastolic filling in HCM.[325, 356-359] Verapamil appears to improve diastolic filling by improved relaxation rather than by

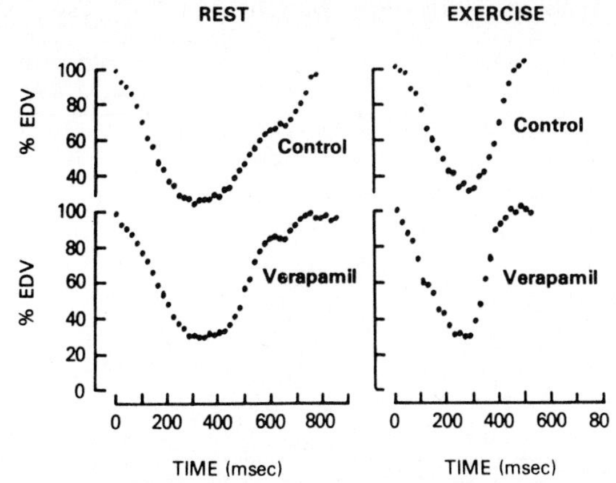

FIGURE 42–16. Relative left ventricular volume, determined by radionuclide ventriculography, plotted against time, showing ejection and filling of the left ventricle in HCM before and after verapamil. The left ventricular volume curves were obtained at rest (*left*) and during exercise (*right*). Verapamil increased left ventricular filling at rest and during exercise. (From Bonow, R. O., et al.: Verapamil-induced improvement in left ventricular diastolic filling and increased exercise tolerance in patients with hypertrophic cardiomyopathy: Short- and long-term effects. Circulation *72*:853, 1985, by permission of the American Heart Association, Inc.)

changes in left ventricular diastolic stiffness[360]; at any given diastolic volume, filling pressure is reduced.[361, 362] While variable clinical responses have been reported with verapamil, about two-thirds of patients show increased exercise capacity and an improved symptomatic status.[363-369] Sustained symptomatic improvement has been noted with the long-term administration of verapamil in ambulatory patients,[356, 370] although important adverse effects, including sudden death, have been observed in a small fraction of patients so treated.[371] Complications with verapamil include suppression of sinus node automaticity and inhibition of atrioventricular conduction, vasodilatation, and negative inotropic effects.[372, 373] These side effects may culminate in hypotension, pulmonary edema, and death; there is a suggestion that antiarrhythmic agents, especially quinidine, may exacerbate the deleterious hemodynamic effects of verapamil.[371] Because of these adverse effects, it has been suggested that verapamil should not be used, or be used only with extreme caution, in patients with high left ventricular filling pressure or symptoms of paroxysmal nocturnal dyspnea or orthopnea.[371] Unfortunately, these are usually the patients who are in greatest need of therapy. In addition, patients with abnormalities of electrical impulse generation or conduction should not receive verapamil unless a pacemaker is in place.

Nifedipine has also been used in HCM, and it may have advantages over verapamil, since it causes less depression of atrioventricular conduction, although it is a more potent vasodilator.[251] It improves diastolic function in HCM without depressing systolic function, apparently by increasing left ventricular compliance.[251, 374] Nifedipine may also improve the chest pain in these patients.[375] Combined administration of nifedipine and propranolol may be of benefit in some patients, particularly those with outflow gradients.[376] However, it should be recognized that the potent vasodilator effects of nifedipine may lead to systemic hypotension and an increase in the outflow gradient.[377, 378]

Diltiazem has also shown beneficial effects in HCM, producing improved diastolic function.[379, 380] Although the data are not conclusive, there are suggestive findings that calcium-channel blocker therapy may promote regression of left ventricular hypertrophy with a reduction in muscle mass.[381, 382]

Disopyramide, an antiarrhythmic drug that alters calcium kinetics, has produced symptomatic improvement and abolition of the pressure gradient in a small number of patients with HCM, presumably as a consequence of depression of left ventricular systolic performance.[383]

Beta-adrenoceptor blockers, calcium antagonists, and the conventional antiarrhythmic agents do not appear to suppress serious ventricular arrhythmias or reduce the frequency of supraventricular arrhythmias.[284] However, *amiodarone* is effective in the treatment of both supraventricular and ventricular tachyarrhythmias in HCM without significantly affecting left ventricular function.[384, 385]

Strenuous exercise should be avoided because of the risk of sudden death; it is the major cause of a fatal outcome in HCM cardiomyopathy.[346] Even though there are many individuals with subclinical HCM who exercise vigorously,[386] the risk of sudden death is sufficiently real that competitive sports are proscribed in patients with marked hypertrophy or other factors believed to be associated with increased risk[387] (Table 42–9). Atrial fibrillation should usually be electrically converted to sinus rhythm without delay because of the often catastrophic hemodynamic consequences of the loss of the atrial contribution to ventricular filling in this disorder. Infective endocarditis may occur in about 5 per cent of patients, and antibiotic prophylaxis is indicated.[263, 388] The infection usually occurs on the aortic valve or mitral apparatus, on the endocardium, or at the site of the contact lesion on the septum; thus, chronic endocardial trauma may provide a nidus foı subsequent infection. Anticoagulants should be given to patients with chronic atrial fibrillation when no contraindication exists.

SURGICAL TREATMENT. A variety of surgical procedures aimed at reducing the outflow gradient have been developed and are most commonly utilized in the markedly symptomatic patient who has not responded well to medical management (Table 42–10).[388a] The most popular operation for HCM consists of excising a portion of the hypertrophied septum. A transaortic approach with septal myotomy-myectomy[399] is probably the most widely utilized procedure, although left transventricular as well as combined transaortic and left ventricular approaches have also been employed successfully.[388a] Operation often relieves the obstruction as well as the mitral regurgitation, although even when performed by surgeons experienced with this procedure, operative mortality is in the range of 5 to 10 per cent.[5, 390-393] Patients over the age of 65 years have undergone successful operations with benefits and risks comparable to those of younger adults.[394] Since symptoms in HCM are not closely correlated with the presence or magnitude of the pressure gradient, it is possible that the operation produces beneficial effects aside from the reduction in outflow gradient that is routinely produced.[395] Although replacement of the mitral valve has been advo-

TABLE 42–9 RECOMMENDATIONS FOR PARTICIPATION IN SPORTS FOR PATIENTS WITH HYPERTROPHIC CARDIOMYOPATHY

1. Competitive sports *not* allowed if any of the following are present:
   a. Marked left ventricular hypertrophy
   b. Evidence of significant outflow gradient (by echocardiography or catheterization)
   c. Important supraventricular or ventricular arrhythmias
   d. History of sudden death in relatives with hypertrophic cardiomyopathy
2. Low-intensity competitive sports allowed if none of above conditions present

Adapted from Maron, B. J., et al.: Task force III: Hypertrophic cardiomyopathy, other myopericardial diseases and mitral valve prolapse. J. Am. Coll. Cardiol. 6:1215, 1985. Reprinted with permission from the American College of Cardiology.

TABLE 42–10 OPERATIONS FOR HYPERTROPHIC CARDIOMYOPATHY

Operation	Indications	How it works	Results	Effects on prognosis
Septal resection	Severe symptoms; fixed gradient > 50 mm Hg; localized hypertrophy; huge papillary muscles	Increases ventricular volume; decreases systolic force; ? other effects	Relieves symptoms; lowers LVEDP	0
Mitral valve replacement	Severe mitral regurgitation; pulmonary edema	Lowers left atrial pressure; improves ventricular volume by removing papillary muscles	Dramatic	?
CABG-septal resection	Intractable angina; "dangerous" proximal CAD	Improves myocardial blood supply	To be assessed	?

CABG = Coronary artery bypass grafting; CAD = Coronary artery disease; LVEDP = Left ventricular end diastolic pressure.
From Goodwin, J. F. and Oakley, C. M.: Medical and surgical treatment of hypertrophic cardiomyopathy. Eur. Heart J. *4*(Suppl. F): 209, 1983.

cated, myotomy-myectomy alone is usually adequate and remains the surgical procedure of choice.[390] Surgery results in improvement in symptoms and exercise capacity and an increase in the peak exercise cardiac output.[391, 396] Furthermore, septal myotomy-myectomy does not produce important impairment of global left ventricular function at rest or during exercise.[397] Myotomy-myectomy may be combined with other necessary operative procedures (particularly coronary artery bypass grafting and mitral valve replacement) without a substantial increase in risk and with generally favorable postoperative outcome.[398, 399] An innovative approach is to perform the myotomy-myectomy with a laser, with similar morphological results as are obtained with the conventional blade approach.[400]

NATURAL HISTORY

The clinical course in HCM is varied, although in most patients symptoms remain stable and in some instances even improve over a period of 5 to 10 years.[263, 346] The annual attrition is about 4 per cent a year, and clinical deterioration (aside from sudden death) is usually slow. Although symptoms are unrelated to the severity or even the presence of a gradient, the percentage of severely symptomatic patients does increase with age.[5, 263, 346] The onset of atrial fibrillation usually leads to a striking increase in symptoms, and prompt cardioversion is usually indicated.[5] Pregnancy is generally well tolerated, although maternal death has been reported.[401, 402]

Progression of HCM to left ventricular dilatation and dysfunction without a gradient, i.e., dilated cardiomyopathy, is an interesting, serious, but unusual occurrence.[346, 403-407] Sometimes it occurs after prior surgical resection of the septum or as a consequence of myocardial infarction.[266, 408] In patients with infarction, the extramural coronary arteries may be normal. Extensive areas of the myocardium may be scarred, resulting in left ventricular dilatation.[266] The extent of left ventricular hypertrophy usually remains stable over time, although a minority of patients may develop increasing degrees of hypertrophy.[409] Substantial changes in the magnitude of the gradient occur in a small proportion of patients; both the appearance (or intensification) of a gradient are usually accompanied by an increase in symptoms.[410]

Death is usually sudden in HCM and may occur in previously asymptomatic patients, in individuals who were unaware they had the disease, or in patients with an otherwise stable course.[5, 263, 346, 411] Paradoxically, younger patients, those without functional limitation, and those with mild or no gradients appear to be at particular risk of sudden death.[264, 412] There is a subgroup of patients with HCM in whose families premature death is unusually frequent.[411] Even individuals without such "malignant" family histories are at risk of sudden death. No specific clinical feature (other than a family history of sudden death due to HCM cardiomyopathy and young age) appears to identify patients at risk of sudden death,[412] although it has been suggested that a history of syncope, severe dyspnea, and ventricular tachycardia may be more common in patients at risk of sudden death.[413-415] Sudden death often occurs during exercise, and strenuous exertion should probably be proscribed in all patients with HCM whether or not symptoms are prominent, although the risk of sudden death appears to decrease above the age of 40 years.[264, 412] Unsuspected HCM is the most common abnormality found at autopsy in young competitive athletes who die suddenly.[416] The development of atrial fibrillation also may be a poor prognostic sign.[417] The degree of left ventricular hypertrophy does not appear to correlate well with prognosis, since patients with massive hypertrophy are often no more than minimally symptomatic and appear to have no more malignant courses than do patients with moderate hypertrophy.[418]

It is presumed, but not established, that sudden death is due to a ventricular arrhythmia, although atrial arrhythmias may play a role in sensitizing the heart so that ventricular arrhythmias appear subsequently.[264] The protective effect of beta-adrenoceptor blockade or calcium-antagonists in preventing sudden death has still not been established. However, amiodarone is effective in suppressing repetitive ventricular tachyarrhythmias in hypertrophic cardiomyopathy, and there are data suggesting that it may prevent sudden death.[419, 420]

RESTRICTIVE AND INFILTRATIVE CARDIOMYOPATHIES

Of the three major functional categories of the cardiomyopathies (dilated, hypertrophic, and restrictive), the restrictive are the least common in Western countries. The hallmark of the restrictive cardiomyopathies is abnormal diastolic function; the ventricular walls are excessively rigid and impede ventricular filling. Contractile function, on the other hand, is often relatively unimpaired. Thus, restrictive cardiomyopathy bears some functional resemblance to constrictive pericarditis, which is also characterized by normal or near-normal systolic function but abnormal ventricular filling.[421-424, 424a] Differentiation of the two conditions is mandatory because of the potential for surgical intervention in the latter.

A variety of specific pathological processes may result in restrictive cardiomyopathy, although the cause often remains unknown.[421] Myocardial fibrosis, hypertrophy, or infiltration is usually responsible for the abnormal diastolic behavior. Myocardial involvement with amyloid is a common cause of secondary restrictive cardiomyopathy, although restriction is also seen in hemochromatosis, glycogen deposition, endomyocardial fibrosis, and, less commonly, fibroelastosis, the eosinophilias, neoplastic infiltration, pseudoxanthoma elasticum, collagen-vascular diseases, and myocardial fibrosis of diverse etiologies.[425-427]

Some patients may manifest all the features of a restrictive cardiomyopathy and exhibit the pathological findings of left ventricular hypertrophy and fibrosis[425]; certainly ventricular hypertrophy can cause diminished ventricular compliance. Other pathological findings include biatrial dilatation, often with thrombi in the atrial appendages, and normal left ventricular cavity size.[425] It has been suggested that myocardial fibrosis of any cause may result in restrictive physiology when it is sufficiently severe.[426] Rare patients may present with findings of restrictive physiology but without fibrosis, infiltration, or other pathological findings demonstrable in the heart. It has been suggested that a defect in myocardial relaxation is present in these patients.[426]

HEMODYNAMICS. The clinical and hemodynamic features of restrictive heart disease simulate those of chronic constrictive pericarditis[5, 425, 428]; endomyocardial biopsy, CT scanning (Fig. 12–11, p. 364), and MR imaging (Fig. 12–32, p. 373) may be particularly useful in differentiating the two diseases. Exploratory thoracotomy may be required on rare occasions. The characteristic hemodynamic feature in both conditions is a deep and rapid early decline in ventricular pressure at the onset of diastole, with a rapid rise to a plateau in early diastole.[425] This dip and plateau has been termed the "square root" sign (Fig. 44–14, p. 1501) and is manifested in the atrial pressure tracing as a prominent *y* descent followed by a rapid rise and plateau. The *x* descent may also be rapid, and the combination results in the characteristic M or W waveform in the atrial pressure tracing. The *a* wave is prominent and often is of the same amplitude as the *v* wave.[5, 429] Both systemic and pulmonary venous pressures are elevated, although patients with restrictive heart disease typically have left ventricular filling pressures which exceed right ventricular filling pressure by more than 5 mm Hg, and this difference is accentuated by exercise. In this respect they differ from patients with constrictive pericarditis, in whom diastolic pressures are similar in both ventricles, usually differing by not more than 5 mm Hg. The pulmonary artery systolic pressure is often greater than 45 mm Hg in patients with restrictive cardiomyopathy but is lower in constrictive pericarditis.[429] Furthermore, the plateau of the right ventricular diastolic pressure is usually at least one-third of the peak right ventricular systolic pressure in patients with constrictive pericarditis, while it is frequently less in restrictive cardiomyopathy.

CLINICAL MANIFESTATIONS. Exercise intolerance is frequent because of the inability of patients with restrictive cardiomyopathy to increase their cardiac output by tachycardia without further compromising ventricular filling. Weakness and dyspnea are often prominent.[425] Chest pain may be prominent in a small fraction of patients but is usually absent. Particularly in advanced cases, an elevated central venous pressure, with peripheral edema, enlarged liver, ascites, and anasarca may be present.[425] *Physical examination* may reveal jugular venous distention; and an S_3, S_4, or both. An inspiratory increase in venous pressure (Kussmaul sign) may be seen.[5] However, in contrast to constrictive pericarditis, the apex impulse is usually palpable, and the apexcardiogram demonstrates a prominent rapid filling wave in restrictive cardiomyopathy.

Various ancillary laboratory findings in addition to endomyocardial biopsy may be useful in distinguishing between constrictive and restrictive disease. While pericardial calcification is neither absolutely sensitive nor specific for constrictive pericarditis[425] (p. 1501), its presence in a patient in whom the differential diagnosis rests between restrictive cardiomyopathy and constrictive pericarditis lends strong support to the latter diagnosis. The echocardiogram may demonstrate thickening of the left ventricular wall and an increase of left ventricular mass in patients with infiltrative disease causing restrictive cardiomyopathy,[430] and the pattern of filling of the left ventricle as shown on echocardiography differs in the two conditions.[428] The accuracy of distinguishing between pericardial and myocardial thickening by CT scanning and magnetic resonance imaging is extremely helpful in the differential diagnosis (Chap. 12).

AMYLOIDOSIS

ETIOLOGY AND TYPES. Amyloidosis is a disease complex that results from deposition of unique twisted β-pleated sheet fibrils formed from various proteins by several different pathogenic mechanisms.[431] Amyloid may be found in almost any organ, but clinically evident disease does not appear unless there is extensive infiltration. Several different types of amyloid fibrils have been described; the two most common are those composed of immunoglobulin light chains (designated AL) and those composed of a nonimmunoglobulin protein (designated AA).[431]

Amyloidosis presents in one of three clinicopathological forms: (1) acquired systemic amyloidosis, (2) organ-limited amyloidosis, and (3) localized deposition. Three forms of acquired systemic amyloidosis are seen: (a) associated with an immunocyte dyscrasia (e.g., multiple myeloma), (b) reactive (e.g., due to chronic infectious or inflammatory conditions), and (c) heredofamilial. Three different forms of familial involvement are recognized, depending upon the principal organ system involved: nephropathic, neuropathic, and cardiopathic.[432] Organ-limited amyloidosis may involve several organ systems, including the heart, and is more common with aging, thus the designation *senile* amyloidosis.

Senile amyloidosis is becoming increasingly common as the average age of the population increases. Scattered deposits of amyloid localized to the aorta or atria are virtually ubiquitous in individuals over the age of 80; one-fourth have diffuse cardiac involvement with a specific fibrillar protein (termed ASc) that is unlike that found in other forms of amyloidosis.[433, 434] Small deposits of amyloid may often be found in the pulmonary vessels or the vessels of other organs as well.

CARDIAC AMYLOIDOSIS

Involvement of the heart is a common finding and is the most frequent cause of death in amyloidosis associated with an immunocyte dyscrasia.[433] In reactive amyloidosis, on the other hand, clinically significant cardiac involvement is uncommon[431]; the myocardial deposits are typically small and perivascular and usually do not result in significant myocardial dysfunction. Familial amyloidosis is only occasionally associated with overt cardiac involvement and then usually only late in the course of the disease.[435] The clinical course is usually dominated by neurological or renal dysfunction. Cardiac involvement in senile amyloidosis varies from small atrial deposits that do not result in functional impairment to extensive ventricular involvement with resultant cardiac failure.[436]

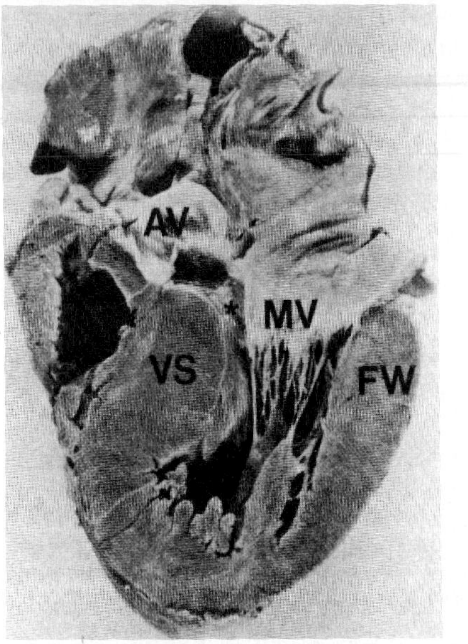

FIGURE 42–17. Massive cardiac enlargement due to amyloidosis, simulating HCM. The atrial endocardium contains grossly evident amyloid deposits. The ventricular septum (VS) is disproportionately thickened compared with the posterior free wall (FW) and narrows the left ventricular outflow tract. An endocardial fibrous plaque is present under the aortic valve (AV) and is the result of contact due to SAM of the mitral valve (MV). (From Sedlis, S. P., et al.: Cardiac amyloidosis simulating hypertrophic cardiomyopathy. Am. J. Cardiol. *53*:969, 1984.)

Cardiac amyloidosis occurs more commonly in men than in women, and it is rare before the age of 30 years.[436, 437] Even in the familial form, the onset of clinical cardiac disease usually does not occur before the age of 35 years and generally occurs much later in life.

PATHOLOGY. The pathological findings often include mild atrial enlargement, usually without significant ventricular dilatation (Fig. 42–17). The walls of both ventricles are typically firm, rubbery, noncompliant, and thickened.[437] Thrombi are often found in the atrial appendages.[437] Amyloid is present between the myocardial fibers,

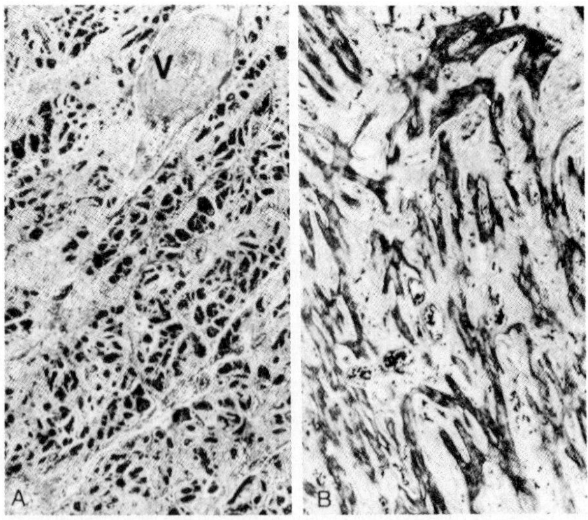

FIGURE 42–18. Photomicrographs of myocardium from the left ventricular free wall (*A*) and ventricular septum (*B*) illustrating extensive accumulation of amyloid filling the interstitial spaces, focally replacing cardiac myocytes and infiltrating the walls of small blood vessels (V). (Original magnification × 38 (A) and × 80 (B).) (From Sedlis, S. P., et al.: Cardiac amyloidosis simulating hypertrophic cardiomyopathy. Am. J. Cardiol. *53*:969, 1984.)

with extensive deposition in the papillary muscles occurring commonly.[438] Serial sections of the sinoatrial and atrioventricular nodes and the bundle branches may disclose amyloid deposits,[439] particularly in the familial forms,[440] although fibrosis of these structures is perhaps more common. In addition, endocardial involvement of the atria and ventricles is frequent (Fig. 42–18), sometimes associated with overlying thrombi. The pericardium may contain focal deposits of amyloid as well. Amyloidosis often results in focal thickening or deposits on the cardiac valves, but whether these abnormalities interfere with valvular function, other than the production of murmurs, is not clear.[433, 442] The intramural coronary arteries and veins frequently contain amyloid deposits in the media and adventitia, occasionally compromising the lumina of the vessels,[443] with attendant localized areas of ischemic necrosis that may produce intractable congestive heart failure.[444]

CLINICAL MANIFESTATIONS. Involvement of the cardiovascular system by amyloidosis occurs in one of four general forms. Many patients exhibit some combination of these forms.

1. The most common is congestive heart failure due to *systolic dysfunction*, which occurs in the majority of patients.[433] Hemodynamic evidence of restriction of ventricular filling may not be prominent in these patients. The course of this form of the disease is often one of relentless progression, usually poorly responsive to treatment. The progress is usually rapid, with death due to cardiac failure generally occurring within 2 years after the onset of symptoms[433]; the majority succumb within 1 year. Cardiomegaly is often demonstrated on chest roentgenography, although massive cardiac enlargement is uncommon. Angina pectoris is not a common finding unless there is concomitant atherosclerotic disease.[437]

2. A second presentation of cardiac amyloidosis is that of a *restrictive cardiomyopathy*.[445] Right-sided findings dominate the clinical presentation, with peripheral edema a prominent finding while paroxysmal nocturnal dyspnea and orthopnea are absent. Amyloid infiltration of the myocardium results in increased stiffness of the myocardium, producing the characteristic diastolic dip and plateau (square root sign) in the ventricular pressure pulse that may simulate constrictive pericarditis.[446] In contrast to the accelerated early left ventricular diastolic filling found in constrictive pericarditis, cardiac amyloidosis is marked by an impaired rate of early diastolic filling, as a consequence of the stiffness of the ventricle.[447]

3. *Orthostatic hypotension* is the third mode of presentation, occurring in about 10 per cent of cases.[443] Although most likely due to amyloid infiltration of the autonomic nervous system or of blood vessels (p. 1634), amyloid deposition in the heart and adrenals may contribute to this manifestation. Hypovolemia as a result of the nephrotic syndrome secondary to renal amyloidosis may aggravate the postural hypotension.

4. An *abnormality of cardiac impulse formation and conduction* is the fourth and least common mode of presentation and may result in arrhythmias and conduction disturbances. Sudden death, presumably arrhythmic in origin, is relatively common.[445]

Physical examination often reveals findings of congestive heart failure; a systolic murmur due to atrioventricular valvular regurgitation may be present. Particularly in patients with restrictive cardiomyopathy, jugular venous distention, a protodiastolic gallop, hepatomegaly, peripheral edema, and a narrow pulse pressure are found.[448] Patients typically are normotensive or hypotensive; even previously hypertensive individuals usually have a fall in blood pressure as the disease progresses.[437]

TABLE 42–11 ELECTROCARDIOGRAPHIC ABNORMALITIES IN CARDIAC AMYLOIDOSIS

Low-voltage potentials	50%
QRS-axis shifts	66%
Myocardial necrosis	64%
AV block	35%
Bundle branch block	16%
Atrial fibrillation	19%
Junctional rhythm	7%
Paroxysmal atrial tachycardia	1%

AV = atrioventricular.

Modified from Buja, L. M., et al.: Clinically significant cardiac amyloidosis. Am. J. Cardiol. *26*:394, 1970.

The *chest roentgenogram* usually shows cardiomegaly in patients with systolic dysfunction, although heart size may be normal in patients with the restrictive form. Pulmonary congestion may be prominent in patients with congestive heart failure. Pleural effusions are common. *The electrocardiogram* is usually abnormal; the most characteristic feature is diffusely diminished voltage, occurring in approximately half the patients[433] (Table 42–11). Myocardial infarction is often simulated because of small or absent R waves in right precordial leads or, less frequently, by Q waves in the inferior leads. Left-axis deviation is seen in more than half the patients. Arrhythmias are common,[449] particularly atrial fibrillation, which has been reported in 20 per cent of the patients.[432] Complex ventricular arrhythmias are found in 50 per cent of the patients with cardiac amyloidosis, and in some may be a harbinger of sudden death. Various forms of AV conduction defects are often seen and have been found in one-third of patients with cardiac amyloidosis. Abnormalities of AV conduction appear to be particularly common in familial amyloidosis with polyneuropathy.[451] Sinus node involvement is common, and the clinical and electrocardiographic features of the sick sinus syndrome may be present (p. 667).[452, 453]

Echocardiography (Figs. 42–19 and 5–101, p. 126) in advanced cases most commonly reveals increased thickness of the walls of the ventricles, small ventricular chambers, dilated atria, and impaired left ventricular function.[454, 454a] Early preclinical unsuspected cardiac involvement may be detectable only by echocardiography.[455] Although the cardiac valves may be thickened, they usually move normally.[456, 457] A pericardial effusion is common, but rarely results in tamponade.[458] The appearance of the thickened cardiac walls is often distinctive on two-dimensional echocardiography, demonstrating a granular sparkling texture, presumably due to the amyloid deposit.[454, 459, 460] The echocardiographic appearance probably results from the presence of nodules containing amyloid and collagen.[461] In some cases the pattern of increased wall thickness is nonuniform and may resemble HCM with ASH.[462, 463] Echocardiographic demonstration of thick left ventricular walls with concomitant low voltage on the electrocardiogram appears to distinguish cardiac amyloidosis from pericardial disease or left ventricular hypertrophy, and this distinctive voltage/mass ratio is characteristic of myocardial infiltration by the amyloid fibrils.[464, 465] Computer-assisted analysis of echocardiograms in amyloidosis has shown reduced ventricular distensibility and impaired diastolic filling.[466]

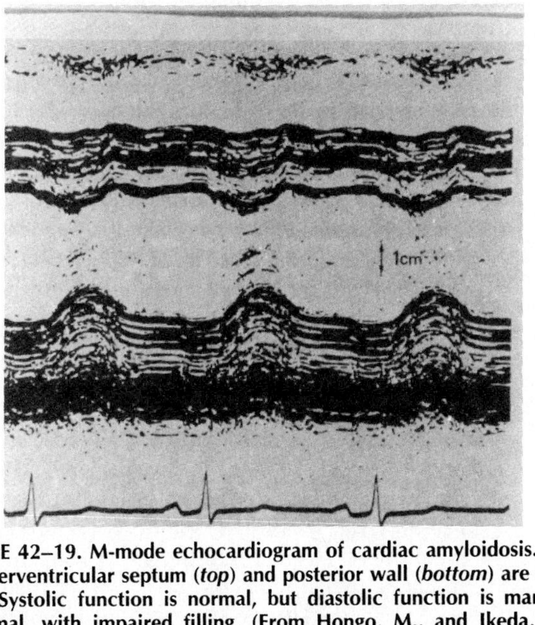

FIGURE 42–19. M-mode echocardiogram of cardiac amyloidosis. Both the interventricular septum (*top*) and posterior wall (*bottom*) are thickened. Systolic function is normal, but diastolic function is markedly abnormal, with impaired filling. (From Hongo, M., and Ikeda, S.-I.: Echocardiographic assessment of the evolution of amyloid heart disease: A study with familial amyloid polyneuropathy. Circulation *73*:249, 1986, by permission of the American Heart Association, Inc.)

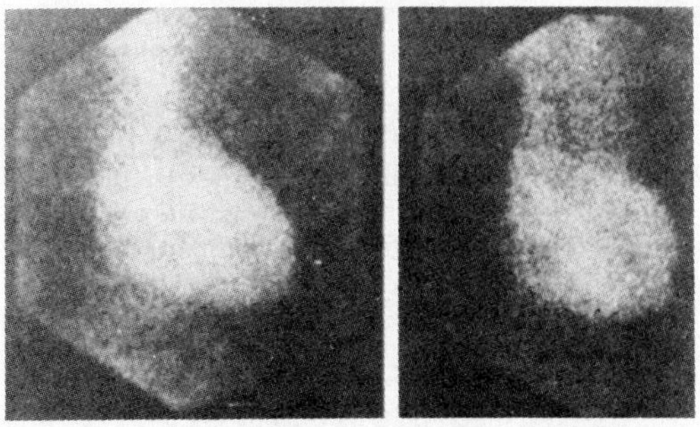

FIGURE 42–20. Technetium-99m-pyrophosphate myocardial scan in a patient with cardiac amyloidosis. There is intense uptake in all myocardial segments, including the right ventricle. ANT = anterior view; LAO 30° = 30-degree left anterior oblique view. (From Schiff, S., et al.: Diagnostic considerations in cardiomyopathy: Unique scintigraphic pattern of diffuse biventricular technetium-99m-pyrophosphate uptake in amyloid heart disease. Am. Heart J. *103*:562, 1982.)

Scintigraphy with technetium-99m-pyrophosphate is often strongly positive with prominent cardiac involvement, although in a minority of cases it is inexplicably falsely negative[467-472] (Fig. 42–20). Positive scans tend to correlate with extensive cardiac involvement; scans are usually negative when the echocardiogram does not demonstrate abnormalities.[467]

Computed tomography may suggest the presence of myocardial amyloid when diffuse ventricular thickening is associated with a radiographic myocardial density lower than seen when myocardial hypertrophy exists alone.[468]

DIAGNOSIS. Whereas 2 or 3 decades ago the clinical diagnosis of systemic amyloidosis was made correctly antemortem only 25 per cent of the time, with more recent clinical awareness of the disease and the utilization of *biopsy techniques* the diagnosis is now made antemortem in the majority of cases. Rectal biopsy has been the single most useful diagnostic procedure, combining the attributes of relative ease of performance, sensitivity, and safety.[473] Biopsy of gingiva, bone marrow, liver, kidney, and various other tissues has also been employed. Endomyocardial biopsy of the right or left ventricles may be helpful in establishing the diagnosis of cardiac amyloidosis.

TREATMENT. The treatment of cardiac amyloidosis is generally unsatisfactory and ineffective, since there is no known way to halt the progression of the underlying disease, although several experimental trials are under way.[474] Digitalis glycosides should be used with caution because patients with cardiac amyloidosis appear to be particularly sensitive to digitalis preparations, and the use of ordinary doses may lead to serious arrhythmias; this may relate to selective binding of digoxin to amyloid fibrils in the myocardium.[475] Similarly, nifedipine binds to amyloid fibrils[476]; its use may lead to exacerbation of congestive heart failure symptoms due to an enhanced negative inotropic effect.[477, 478] Insertion of a permanent pacemaker may be beneficial in patients with symptomatic conducting system disease.[479]

INHERITED INFILTRATIVE DISORDERS CAUSING CARDIOMYOPATHY

The intramyocardial accumulation of an abnormal metabolic product may result in abnormal systolic contractile performance. However, it may also impair the filling of the ventricles, thereby adding a restrictive component. A variety of infiltrative diseases, often inherited, may result in this hemodynamic picture, including the glycogenoses (p. 1013), the mucopolysaccharidoses (p. 1728), Fabry's disease, and Gaucher's disease.[480]

FABRY'S DISEASE

Fabry's disease (angiokeratoma corporis diffusum universale) is an X-linked disorder of glycosphingolipid metabolism due to a deficiency of the enzyme ceramide trihexosidase. It is characterized by an intracellular accumulation of a neutral glycolipid, with prominent involvement of the skin and kidneys as well as the myocardium. *Histological examination* often reveals widespread involvement of the myocardium, vascular endothelium, conducting tissues, and valves—particularly the mitral valve.[481, 482] The major clinical manifestations of the disease result from the accumulation of the glycolipid substrate in endothelial cells, with eventual occlusion of small arterioles.[483] The accumulation of the glycolipid occurs in the lysosomes of the cardiac tissues and is responsible for the multiple cardiovascular manifestations of Fabry's disease.[481] Symptomatic cardiovascular involvement occurs eventually in most affected males, while female carriers are usually asymptomatic or only minimally symptomatic.[481] Systemic hypertension, renovascular hypertension, mitral valve prolapse, and congestive heart failure are common clinical manifestations.[481] Altered vasomotor activity is found in Fabry's disease, resulting in a Raynaud-like picture.[484] Electrocardiographic abnormalities include left ventricular hypertrophy, P-wave abnormalities, conduction defects, and arrhythmias.[485, 485a] The echocardiogram usually reveals increased left ventricular wall thickness, presumably the result of glycolipid deposition, which may simulate hypertrophic cardiomyopathy[221] and mitral valve prolapse. Differentiation from other restrictive processes (such as cardiac amyloidosis) may not be possible on echocardiographic grounds.[486] Endomyocardial biopsy may be of considerable value in differentiating the two conditions[221, 487, 488] and a low alpha-galactosidase activity in leukocytes is also helpful diagnostically.

Whether renal transplantation prevents progressive cardiac involvement in Fabry's disease is not clear.[489]

GAUCHER'S DISEASE. Gaucher's disease is an uncommon, inherited disorder of glycosyl ceramide metabolism. It is secondary to a deficiency of the enzyme beta-glucosidase and results in accumulation of cerebrosides in the spleen, liver, bone marrow, lymph nodes, brain, and myocardium. Diffuse interstitial infiltration of the left ventricle by cells laden with cerebroside occurs in Gaucher's disease, associated with reduced left ventricular compliance and cardiac output. Clinical evidence of cardiac involvement is uncommon, but when present it is characterized by left ventricular dysfunction, hemorrhagic pericardial effusion, increase in left ventricular wall mass, and calcification of the left-sided valves.[490-492]

HEMOCHROMATOSIS AND HEMOSIDEROSIS

(See also p. 1739)

Hemochromatosis is characterized by excessive deposition of iron in a variety of parenchymal tissues (heart, liver, gonads, and pancreas). It may occur (1) as a familial or idiopathic disorder, (2) in association with a defect in hemoglobin synthesis resulting in ineffective erythropoiesis, (3) in chronic liver disease, and (4) with excessive oral intake of iron over many years. While patients who have iron deposits in the myocardium almost always have deposits in other organs (e.g., liver, spleen, pancreas, bone marrow), the severity of myocardial involvement varies widely and parallels only roughly that in other organs.[493]

The *pathological findings* (Fig. 55–8, p. 1740) are a dilated heart with thickened ventricular walls. Myocardial iron deposits, often grossly visible, are most common in the subepicardial region, followed by the subendocardial region and papillary muscles, and are least common in the midmyocardial wall. They are more extensive in ventricular than atrial myocardium.[493] Iron deposits in myocardial cells are typically perinuclear in location initially but eventually occupy much of the fiber. Involvement of the cardiac conducting system is limited, compared with the relatively heavy infiltration of contracting cells.[494] Myocardial degeneration and fibrosis may also occur.

The severity of myocardial dysfunction is proportional to the amount of iron present in the myocardium.[494] Extensive deposits of cardiac iron (particularly those grossly visible at postmortem examination) are invariably associated with cardiac dysfunction—usually chronic congestive heart failure, which is often the cause of death. Extensive cardiac deposits usually occur in patients who receive more than 100 blood transfusions (unless there is associated iron loss due to bleeding).[493]

The *clinical manifestations* vary widely, depending on the extent of myocardial involvement. Some patients remain asymptomatic despite echocardiographic evidence of myocardial infiltration, which is expressed as an increase in left ventricular wall thickness.[430, 494] In such cases, a variety of noninvasive techniques, including exercise radionuclide ventriculography, may demonstrate early subclinical myocardial involvement in which treatment is most effective.[495-498] Symptomatic cardiac involvement is usually associated with electrocardiographic abnormalities, including ST-segment and T-wave changes, as well as supraventricular arrhythmias; these electrocardiographic changes correlate with the degree of iron deposits in the heart.[493] Atrioventricular conduction disturbances and ventricular arrhythmias are uncommon.

Advanced iron storage disease involving the heart usually produces a dilated or a restrictive cardiomyopathy, characterized by exertional dyspnea, orthopnea, peripheral edema, and protodiastolic gallop sounds. The diagnosis is aided by finding elevated plasma iron levels (180 to 300 μg/dl; normal = 50 to 150), a normal or low total iron-binding capacity (200 to 300 μg/dl; normal = 250 to 370), and markedly elevated values for saturation of transferrin (80 to 100 per cent; normal = 22 to 46 per cent), serum ferritin (900 to 6000 ng/ml; normal = 3 to 180), urinary iron (9 to 23 mg/24 hr; normal = 0 to 2), and liver iron (600 to 1800 μg/100 mg dry wt; normal = 30 to 140).[499] Cardiac failure is usually progressive and largely refractory to therapy,[493] although repeated phlebotomies or the use of the chelating agent desferrioxamine may be beneficial.[500, 501] (For further discussion of the treatment of iron storage disease see p. 1741.)

SARCOIDOSIS

Sarcoidosis is a granulomatous disorder of unknown etiology, characterized by multisystem involvement. Infiltration of the lungs, reticuloendothelial system, and skin usually dominates the clinical picture, but virtually any tissue may be affected. The most important manifestation results from pulmonary involvement. This often leads to diffuse fibrosis which may result in fatal right heart failure.[502, 503] Primary cardiac involvement is not often recognized clinically, although it may be demonstrated at autopsy in 20 to 30 per cent of cases of sarcoid, most of which demonstrate generalized sarcoidosis.[504, 505] Clinical manifestations of sarcoid heart disease are present in less than 5 per cent of patients, although myocardial involvement may result in heart block, congestive heart failure, ventricular arrhythmias, and sudden death, particularly in youngsters.[504, 506, 507, 507a] Myocardial sarcoidosis may have restrictive as well as congestive features, since cardiac infiltration by sarcoid granulomas results not only in increased stiffness of the ventricular wall but diminished systolic contractile function as well. Myocardial sarcoidosis typically affects young or middle-aged adults (mean age, 40 years) of either sex; there is usually evidence of generalized sarcoidosis.[502, 506]

PATHOLOGY. The typical pathological feature of sarcoidosis is the presence of noncaseating granulomas, which occur in many organs. They infiltrate the myocardium and may eventually become fibrotic scars. The granulomas may involve any region of the heart, although the left ventricular free wall and the interventricular septum are the most common sites, and extensive granulomas and scar tissue in the cephalad portion of the interventricular septum is a constant finding in patients with abnormalities of the conduction system.[506] Cardiac effects may range from a few scattered lesions to extensive involvement.[508] Because of the variable cardiac involvement, myocardial biopsy may be positive in only about half of the patients, and therefore a negative biopsy by no means excludes the diagnosis.[509, 510] Transmural involvement is common,[506] and large portions of the ventricular wall may be replaced by sarcoid tissue, which may lead to aneurysm formation. While involvement of small coronary artery branches may be found in sarcoidosis, the pathophysiological importance of this observation remains unclear.[511]

CLINICAL MANIFESTATIONS. Death was sudden in two-thirds of the patients in a large autopsy study of sarcoidosis of the heart; indeed, sudden death is the most common manifestation of cardiac sarcoidosis.[506] Many of the patients experienced antecedent arrhythmias or complete AV block.[506, 511, 512] Conduction disturbance is the most frequent clinical indication of myocardial sarcoid in nonfatal cases. Syncope is common and may reflect paroxysmal arrhythmias or conduction disturbances.[513] Atrial and ventricular arrhythmias, especially ventricular tachycardia, are observed frequently.[506, 514, 515] Congestive heart failure is the other major manifestation of myocardial involvement. While cor pulmonale as a consequence of pulmonary sarcoidosis accounts for some of the symptoms of heart failure, many symptoms are caused by direct myocardial involvement by granulomas and scar tissue, and the patients show the clinical features of restrictive or dilated cardiomyopathy.[503, 506, 512, 516, 517] Symptoms of myocardial sarcoid may be present for variable lengths of time; however, the disease may progress rapidly to death, and in some patients the interval from the onset of the cardiac symptoms to death is less than 2 years.[506] Survival may be as long as 10 to 20 years, however.[509, 518]

Cardiac dysfunction is often severe and progressive. Occasionally, patients with extensive involvement develop overt left ventricular aneurysms.[506, 519] Pericardial effusions are found in about 10 to 15 per cent of patients with sarcoidosis, and only rarely progress to tamponade.[504, 520]

The *physical examination* may reveal findings of extracardiac sarcoid or may be totally normal. A systolic murmur reflecting mitral regurgitation is common.[506] This appears to be more the result of left ventricular dilatation or infiltration than of direct sarcoid involvement of the papillary muscles.[506]

The *electrocardiogram* is frequently abnormal in patients with known sarcoid and most commonly demonstrates T-wave abnormalities.[521] Sarcoidosis appears to have an affinity for involvement of the AV junction and bundle of His, and thus varying degrees of AV block are common.[506, 511, 521] With extensive myocardial involvement, pathological Q waves may appear and simulate myocardial infarction.

DIAGNOSIS. In many cases the diagnosis may be suspected in patients with bilateral hilar lymphadenopathy on chest roentgenogram in whom there is clinical or electrocardiographic evidence of myocardial disease. Percutaneous endomyocardial biopsy may be particularly useful in establishing the diagnosis.[522, 523] Myocardial imaging with thallium-201 may also be helpful in demonstrating segmental filling defects representing areas of infiltration of the myocardium and may indicate myocardial involvement in more than one-third of patients with sarcoid but without clinical evidence of cardiac involvement.[524] Imaging may also indicate the presence of right ventricular hypertrophy in patients with right ventricular overload due to pulmonary fibrosis and pulmonary hypertension. Myocardial uptake of technetium pyrophosphate and gallium in myocardial sarcoidosis has also been reported.[525]

TREATMENT. The treatment of myocardial sarcoidosis is difficult. Arrhythmias are often refractory to antiarrhythmic drugs,[526] although quinidine with or without propranolol is sometimes efficacious.[527] Permanent pacing may be helpful,[511] and since sudden death is so common in sarcoid, it should be applied in patients with advanced heart block. While the matter is not settled, it appears that corticosteroids may be of some benefit in treating the conduction disturbances, arrhythmias, and myocardial dysfunction of sarcoidosis.[528] Since the risk of sudden death appears to be greatest in patients with extensive myocardial involvement, it is reasonable to attempt to halt the progression of the disease with steroids before irreversible fibrosis occurs.[505] Some evidence suggests that steroids may result in the healing of granulomas, although formation of a ventricular aneurysm may be a possible side effect.[506]

BECKER'S DISEASE

Becker's disease (also called African cardiomyopathy) is an uncommon condition of obscure etiology that occurs most commonly in South Africa. It is characterized by cardiac dilatation without hypertrophy and by fibrosis of the papillary muscles, subendocardium, and endocardium; it is associated with pericardial effusion, myocardial necrosis, and mural thrombosis.[529, 530] The disease appears to progress from an acute edematous serous myocarditis marked by fibrinoid necrosis to a chronic stage with endocardial necrosis and fibrosis, mural thrombosis, and organization leading to endocardial sclerosis.

The disease occurs in all ages and in all races in South Africa. It may present as congestive heart failure, which may be acute and rapidly progressive, with death occurring within 6 months, or may be chronic, with survival for up to 3 years.[530] Patients may show an acute illness marked by fever; leukocytosis (without eosinophilia); multiple emboli with infarction of the lungs, spleen, kidneys, or brain; and progressive congestive heart failure.[529, 530] Dyspnea is almost a ubiquitous symptom, often associated with cough, peripheral edema, chest pain, and hemoptysis.[529]

ENDOMYOCARDIAL DISEASE

Endomyocardial disease (EMD) is a common form of restrictive cardiomyopathy in equatorial Africa and is encountered with less frequency in South America, Asia, and nontropical countries, including the United States.[531-534] It is marked by intense endocardial fibrotic thickening of the apex and subvalvular regions of one or both ventricles that results in obstruction to inflow of blood into the respective ventricle, thus producing restrictive physiology. Two variants of the disease have been described, one occurring principally in tropical countries (termed endomyocardial fibrosis, EMF), and the other in temperate countries (Löffler's endocarditis parietalis fibroplastica).

Although long considered separate entities, if only because Löffler's endocarditis is marked by intense tissue and often peripheral eosinophilia, there is now general agreement that EMF and Löffler's endocarditis are different manifestations of the same disease, since the pathological findings in advanced cases are identical.[343, 535, 536] Despite the pathological similarities, there are differences in clinical presentation (Fig. 42–21). In addition to the geographic differences, the temperate form of the disease (Löffler's endocarditis) acts as a more aggressive and rapidly progressive disorder, affecting principally males, and is associated with hypereosinophilia, thromboembolic phenomena, and a generalized arteritis. EMF, conversely, shows no sex predilection, occurs in younger patients, and usually is not associated with an intense eosinophilia or thromboembolic phenomena.[536]

It has been postulated that Löffler's endocarditis and EMF are different phases in a progressive disease that results from the toxic effect of eosinophils on the heart.[535, 537] Under this formulation, an initial hypereosinophilia of whatever course results in damage to the myocardium that produces the first phase of EMD: a necrotic phase, marked by an intense myocarditis, rich in eosinophils, and with an associated arteritis (i.e., Löffler's endocarditis). This initial phase occurs within the first few months of illness. It appears to be followed by a thrombotic stage, occurring about a year after initial presentation, during which the myocarditis has receded, nonspecific thickening of the myocardium is beginning, and there is a variable degree of superimposed thrombus formation. The last stage is one of fibrosis, presenting all of the features of EMF.[535] The three stages—necrotic, thrombotic, and fibrotic—have been defined on the basis of postmortem material, and it is not suggested that each patient with advanced disease (manifested by EMF) has necessarily passed through the earlier phases.

The possible role of *eosinophils* in the production of the cardiac abnormalities has intrigued investigators for years.[537, 538] Eosinophils may damage tissues by direct invasion or the release of toxic substances.[539] The presence of degranulated peripheral eosinophils in patients with Löffler's endocarditis suggests that the protein constituents of the eosinophil's granule may be cardiotoxic,[536-538, 540, 541] producing first the necrotic phase of EMD, followed by the thrombotic and fibrotic phases after the disappearance of the initial eosinophilia.[539]

Since the clinical manifestations of EMD demonstrate geographical and clinical differences, Löffler's endocarditis and EMF will be discussed separately, even though they appear to be part of the same disease continuum.

LÖFFLER'S ENDOCARDITIS

Hypereosinophilic Syndrome

Marked eosinophilia of any cause may be associated with endomyocardial disease. The typical patient who presents with Löffler's endocarditis is a male in his fourth decade who lives in a temperate climate and has the hypereosinophilic syndrome (i.e., persistent eosinophilia with ≧ 1500 eosinophils/mm^3 for at least 6 months or until death, with evidence of organ involvement).[538] Cardiac involvement in the hypereosinophilic syndrome is the rule, occurring in more than three-fourths of patients.[542] Hypereosinophilia and cardiac involvement is also seen in the Churg-Strauss syndrome, which is differentiated by asthma, nasal polyposis, and a necrotizing vasculitis.[543] The cause of the eosinophilia in most patients with Löffler's endocarditis is unknown, although in some it may be the result of leukemia, or it may be reactive (that is, secondary to various parasitic, allergic, granulomatous, hypersensitivity, or neoplastic disorders[538]). The relationship of the eosinophilia to possible parasitic infestation is unclear.[544]

PATHOLOGY. In the hypereosinophilic syndrome, a variety of organs are usually involved besides the heart, including the lungs, bone marrow, and brain.[539, 542] Renal, gastrointestinal, dermatological and hepatic involvement is observed less frequently.[545] Cardiac involvement is often biventricular, with mural endocardial thickening of the inflow portions and apex of the ventricles (Fig. 42–22). Histological findings include variable degrees of: (1) an acute inflammatory eosinophilic myocarditis involving the myo- and endocardium; (2) thrombosis, fibrinoid change, and inflammatory reaction involving small intramural coronary vessels; (3) mural thrombosis, often containing eosinophils; and (4) fibrotic thickening of up to several millimeters.[538, 539] In some patients without manifest cardiac involvement, abnormalities in endomyocardial biopsy spec-

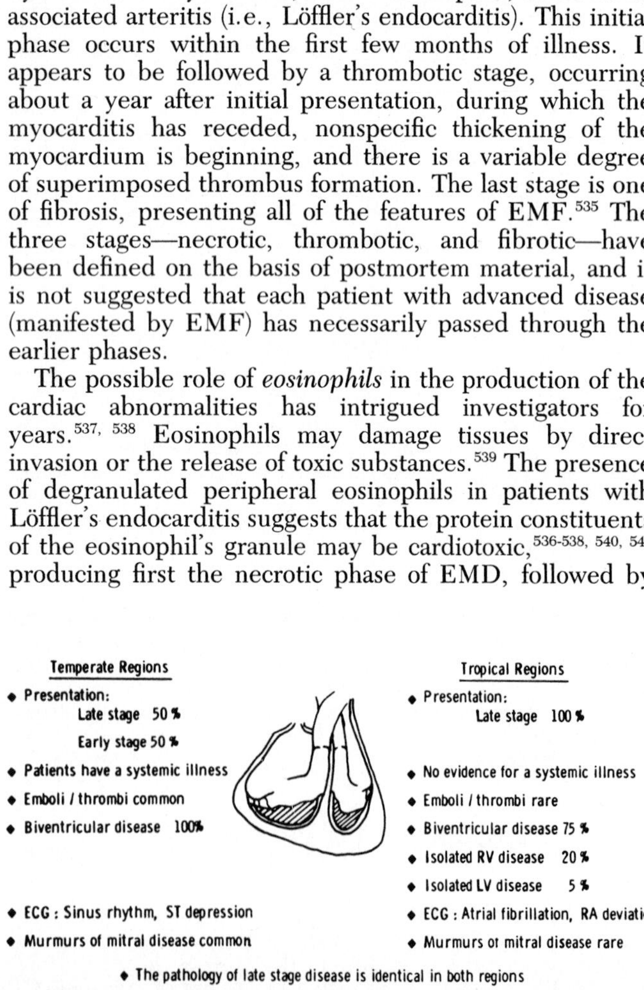
Temperate Regions
Presentation:
Late stage 50 %
Early stage 50 %
Patients have a systemic illness
Emboli / thrombi common
Biventricular disease 100%
ECG : Sinus rhythm, ST depression
Murmurs of mitral disease common
Tropical Regions
Presentation:
Late stage 100 %
No evidence for a systemic illness
Emboli / thrombi rare
Biventricular disease 75 %
Isolated RV disease 20 %
Isolated LV disease 5 %
ECG : Atrial fibrillation, RA deviation
Murmurs of mitral disease rare
The pathology of late stage disease is identical in both regions

FIGURE 42–21. Comparison of the differences between tropical and temperate endomyocardial disease: ECG = electrocardiogram. (From Olsen, E. G. J., and Spry, C. J. F.: Relation between eosinophilia and endomyocardial disease. Prog. Cardiovasc. Dis. *27*:241, 1985.)

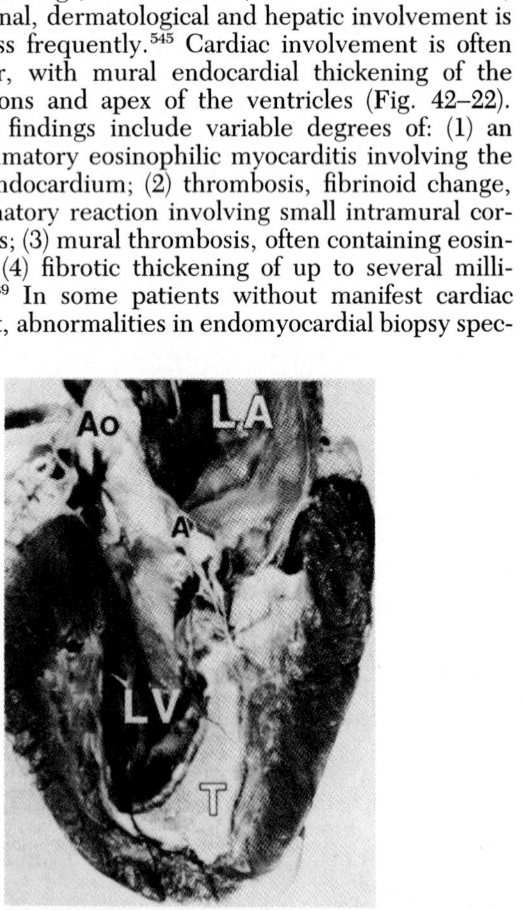

FIGURE 42–22. Longitudinal section of the left ventricle (LV) in a patient with Löffler's endocarditis showing a large thrombus (T) in the inflow portion of the ventricle. A = anterior mitral leaflet; Ao = aorta; LA = left atrium. (From Fauci, A. S., et al.: The idiopathic hypereosinophilic syndrome. Ann. Intern. Med. *97*:78, 1982.)

imens may be limited to changes in endothelial cells in the endocardium and changes of the microvasculature without other myopathic abnormalities.[539] Whether these early changes result simply from the eosinophilia remains unclear.

CLINICAL MANIFESTATIONS. The principal clinical features include weight loss, fever, cough, skin rash, and congestive heart failure. Although early cardiac involvement may be asymptomatic, overt cardiac dysfunction occurs in more than half the patients and may be right- and/or left-sided.[538, 539] Cardiomegaly, often without overt symptoms of congestive heart failure, may be present, and the murmur of mitral regurgitation is common. Progressive mitral regurgitation is seen in one-third of patients.[539] Systemic embolism is frequent and may lead to neurological and renal dysfunction. Death is usually due to congestive heart failure, often with associated renal, hepatic, or respiratory dysfunction.

LABORATORY EXAMINATION. A variety of abnormalities of the blood may be seen in addition to the eosinophilia. The erythrocyte sedimentation rate is frequently elevated, and occasionally patients have abnormal or depressed leukocyte alkaline phosphatase levels and chromosomal abnormalities (including the Philadelphia [Ph^1] chromosome).[542]

The *chest roentgenogram* may reveal cardiomegaly and pulmonary congestion or, less commonly, pulmonary infiltrates. The *electrocardiogram* most commonly shows nonspecific ST-segment and T-wave abnormalities. Arrhythmias, especially atrial fibrillation, and conduction defects, particularly right bundle branch block, may also be present.[531, 538]

The *echocardiogram* commonly demonstrates localized thickening of the posterobasal left ventricular wall, with absent or markedly limited motion of the posterior leaflet of the mitral valve.[538, 546, 547] There may be obliteration of the apex by thrombus material.[546, 548] Enlargement of the atria may be seen,[548] along with Doppler ultrasound evidence of AV valve regurgitation. The endocardium may be unusually echo-reflective as a consequence of fibrosis,[548] even in the absence of other apparent structural abnormalities.[549]

The *hemodynamic consequences* of the dense endocardial scarring seen in Löffler's endocarditis are those of a restrictive cardiomyopathy as described above (p. 1431) with abnormal diastolic filling due to increased stiffness of the ventricles and a reduction in the size of the ventricular cavity by organized thrombus. Systolic performance is also impaired and atrioventricular valvular regurgitation may occur because of involvement of the supporting apparatus of the mitral or tricuspid valves.[538] *Cardiac catheterization* reveals markedly elevated ventricular filling pressures, and there may be evidence of tricuspid or mitral regurgitation. A characteristic feature on angiocardiography is largely preserved systolic function with obliteration of the apex of the ventricles.[531] The diagnosis is often confirmed by percutaneous endomyocardial biopsy.[531, 538]

TREATMENT. Medical therapy during the course of early Löffler's endocarditis, and surgical therapy during the later phases of fibrosis, appear to have had a positive effect on symptoms and survival.[343, 538, 539] Corticosteroids appear to have a beneficial effect on acute myocarditis,[538, 539, 550, 551] and together with cytotoxic drugs (hydroxyurea in particular), appear to have improved survival substantially.[343, 538, 539] Routine cardiac therapy with digitalis, diuretics, afterload reduction, and anticoagulation as indicated are adjuncts in the management of these patients. Surgical therapy appears to offer significant palliation of symptoms once the fibrotic stage has been reached.[343, 552, 553]

ENDOMYOCARDIAL FIBROSIS

Endomyocardial fibrosis occurs most commonly in tropical and subtropical Africa, particularly Uganda and Nigeria. It is typified by fibrous endocardial lesions of the inflow portion of the right or left ventricle or both and often involves the atrioventricular valves, resulting in regurgitation. It is a relatively frequent cause of heart failure and death in equatorial Africa, accounting for 10 to 20 per cent of deaths due to heart disease.[343, 530]

While most prominent in Africa, it is also found in tropical and subtropical regions in the rest of the world, including India, Brazil, Colombia, and Sri Lanka.[554] It is most common in specific ethnic groups, notably the Rwanda tribe in Uganda and in people of low socioeconomic status.[554] The disease is equally frequent in both sexes, and, although most common in children and young adults, its reported age range is from 4 to 70 years of age.[343] It is most common in blacks, but cases have been reported occasionally in whites in temperate climates who previously resided in tropical areas.

PATHOLOGY. A pericardial effusion, which may be quite large, may be present. The heart is normal in size or slightly enlarged, but massive cardiomegaly does not occur. The right atrium is often dilated, and in patients with severe right ventricular involvement there may be massive enlargement of this chamber. Indentation of the right border of the heart above the apex as a result of apical scarring may occur.

Combined right and left ventricular disease occurs in about half the cases, with pure left ventricular involvement occurring in 40 per cent and pure right ventricular involvement in the remaining 10 per cent of patients who are examined post mortem.[343] When affected, the right ventricle exhibits extensive, dense, fibrous thickening of the inflow tract and apex, with involvement of the papillary muscles and chordae tendineae. Involvement of the right ventricle may lead to obliteration of the apex, with a mass of thrombus and fibrous tissue filling the cavity.[530] The tricuspid valve is often pulled down and distorted by the fibrous process involving the supporting structures.[530] Right atrial thrombi occur commonly. Left ventricular involvement is similar, with fibrosis extending from the apex up the inflow portion of the left ventricle to the posterior mitral valve leaflet. The anterior leaflet of the mitral valve and the outflow portion of the left ventricle are usually spared. Thrombi often overlie the endocardial lesions, and widely distributed endocardial calcific deposits may occur.[555] The coronary arteries are uninvolved, as is the remainder of the body.[343, 535]

Microscopically, the involved endocardium demonstrates a thick layer of collagen tissue on top of a layer of loosely arranged connective tissue[556] (Fig. 42–23). Septa composed of fibrous and granulation tissue extend for variable distances into the myocardium.[343, 530] Interstitial edema is often present, but there is no cellular infiltration.[530] Small patches of fibroelastosis may occur in both ventricular outflow tracts beneath the semilunar valves but are thought to be a secondary phenomenon due to local trauma rather than a result of the basic pathological process.[530]

CLINICAL MANIFESTATIONS. Endomyocardial fibrosis may involve both ventricles or either ventricle selectively; left-sided involvement results in symptoms of pulmonary congestion, while predominant right-sided disease may present features of a restrictive cardiomyopathy and therefore simulate constrictive pericarditis. There is often regurgitation of one or both atrioventricular valves. The onset of the disease is usually insidious, but it is sometimes

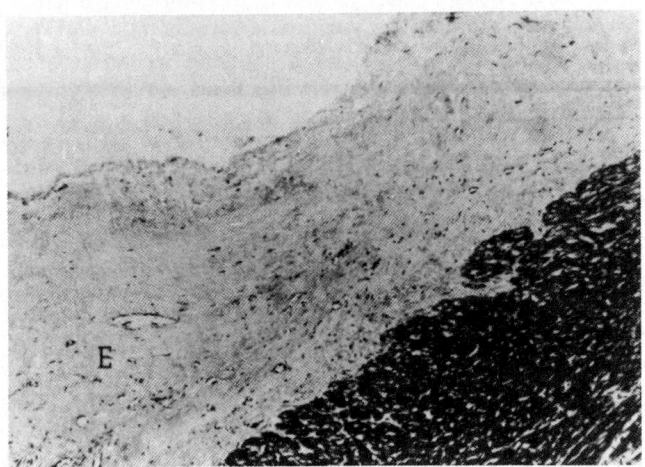

FIGURE 42–23. Photomicrograph of endomyocardial biopsy specimen in endomyocardial fibrosis showing marked fibrotic thickening of the endocardium (E). (Original magnification × 250.) (From Fawzy, M. E., et al.: Endomyocardial fibrosis: Report of eight cases. J. Am. Coll. Cardiol. *5*:983, 1985. Reprinted with permission from the American College of Cardiology.)

ushered in by an acute febrile illness.[530] Rarely, the disease appears to stabilize, and survival for up to 12 years has been observed, but it is usually relentlessly progressive.[530] In contrast to Becker's disease (p. 1435), pulmonary or systemic embolization is uncommon.[530] Death is due to progressive myocardial failure, often associated with pulmonary congestion, infection, or infarction. The most important immediate cause of death is sudden, unexpected cardiovascular collapse, presumably arrhythmic in origin.[343] Patients with prominent involvement of the right side of the heart appear to survive longer than those with principally left-sided involvement.

RIGHT VENTRICULAR ENDOMYOCARDIAL FIBROSIS. Pure or predominant right ventricular involvement is characterized by fibrous obliteration of the right ventricular apex that diminishes the capacity of this chamber. The fibrosis often extends to the supporting apparatus of the tricuspid valve, resulting in tricuspid regurgitation. Therefore, clinical manifestations in patients with right-sided involvement include an elevated jugular venous pressure, a prominent *v* wave, and a rapid *y* descent. A protodiastolic gallop sound may be heard along the lower sternal border, reflecting right ventricular dysfunction. The liver is usually large and pulsatile, and ascites, splenomegaly, and peripheral edema are common. Pulmonary congestion is not present in the absence of left-sided involvement, and the pulmonary artery and pulmonary capillary wedge pressures are normal. A pericardial effusion, which is sometimes quite large, may be present. The right atrium is often enlarged, sometimes massively so.

The *electrocardiogram* is usually abnormal, with diminished QRS voltage (probably resulting from the presence of a pericardial effusion), ST-segment and T-wave abnormalities, and findings of right atrial enlargement.[557] Occasionally, atrial fibrillation occurs.[343] The *chest roentgenogram* demonstrates cardiac enlargement, usually with gross prominence of the right atrium and a pericardial effusion. Calcification in the region of the right ventricular apex may be found. *Echocardiography* may demonstrate right ventricular thickening, obliteration of the apex, dilated atrium, strong echoes emanating from the endocardial surface, and abnormal septal motion in patients with tricuspid regurgitation.[533, 548, 558, 559] At *angiography* the right ventricular apex is characteristically not visualized because of obliteration by the fibrous endocardium, but tricuspid regurgitation, right atrial enlargement, and filling defects in the right atrium due to intraatrial thrombi are sometimes seen.[343] Early angiographic changes that may be present before advanced disease develops include a change in the endocardial appearance, small apical filling defects, and mild tricuspid regurgitation.[560]

LEFT VENTRICULAR ENDOMYOCARDIAL FIBROSIS. Predominant *left-sided* involvement results in a different clinical picture. The endomyocardial fibrosis involves the apex of the ventricle and usually the chordae tendineae or the posterior mitral valve leaflet as well, leading to mitral regurgitation.[535] The murmur may be confined to late systole, as is characteristic of the papillary muscle dysfunction type of murmur, or it may be pansystolic. Findings of pulmonary hypertension may be prominent. A protodiastolic gallop is commonly heard.

The *electrocardiogram* usually shows T-wave abnormalities and diminished QRS voltage in the presence of a pericardial effusion, although left ventricular hypertrophy may be present.[343, 557] There may be findings of left atrial abnormality. Occasionally, atrial fibrillation is present. *Echocardiographic* features include thickening and reduced motion of the posterobasal wall and posterior mitral leaflet, increased echo-reflectivity of the endocardium, preserved systolic wall motion in the presence of apical obliteration, dilated atrium, and Doppler ultrasound evidence of mitral regurgitation.[533, 548, 558, 559] *Cardiac catheterization* usually reveals pulmonary hypertension, with elevated left ventricular filling pressures and a reduced cardiac index. The left ventriculogram usually shows mitral regurgitation, and a filling defect due to an intracavitary thrombus within the ventricle may be seen on occasion.[343, 531] Although coronary arteriography does not reveal obstructive disease, a peculiar vascular blush may be seen in about 50 per cent of patients, presumably related to vascular changes in the endocardium.[561]

BIVENTRICULAR ENDOMYOCARDIAL FIBROSIS. This form of endomyocardial fibrosis occurs more frequently than either isolated right- or left-sided disease. If there is more than minimal right ventricular involvement, severe pulmonary hypertension does not occur, and the right-sided findings dominate the clinical presentation. The typical patient with biventricular involvement may have the features of right ventricular endomyocardial fibrosis, as described above, with only a mitral regurgitant murmur to suggest left ventricular involvement. Systemic embolization may occur in up to 15 per cent of patients; infective endocarditis is even less frequent and is found in less than 2 per cent.

DIAGNOSIS. This is based on the presence of the typical clinical and laboratory features, particularly angiography,[531, 534, 559, 562] in an individual from the appropriate geographical area. Eosinophilia is usually not a prominent feature and when present may reflect associated parasitic infestation. *Endomyocardial biopsy* may occasionally be helpful in establishing the diagnosis[559] (Fig. 42–23). However, this risks dislodging a mural thrombus, with resultant embolization, and left-sided biopsy is *not* recommended.[531] In addition, because the disease is often focal, the biopsy may miss the pathological process, particularly if a right ventricular biopsy is performed in a patient with isolated left-sided disease.[559]

TREATMENT. The medical treatment of endomyocardial fibrosis is often difficult and not particularly effective. Digitalis glycosides may be helpful in controlling the ventricular rate in patients with atrial fibrillation, but the response of congestive symptoms is disappointing. Diuret-

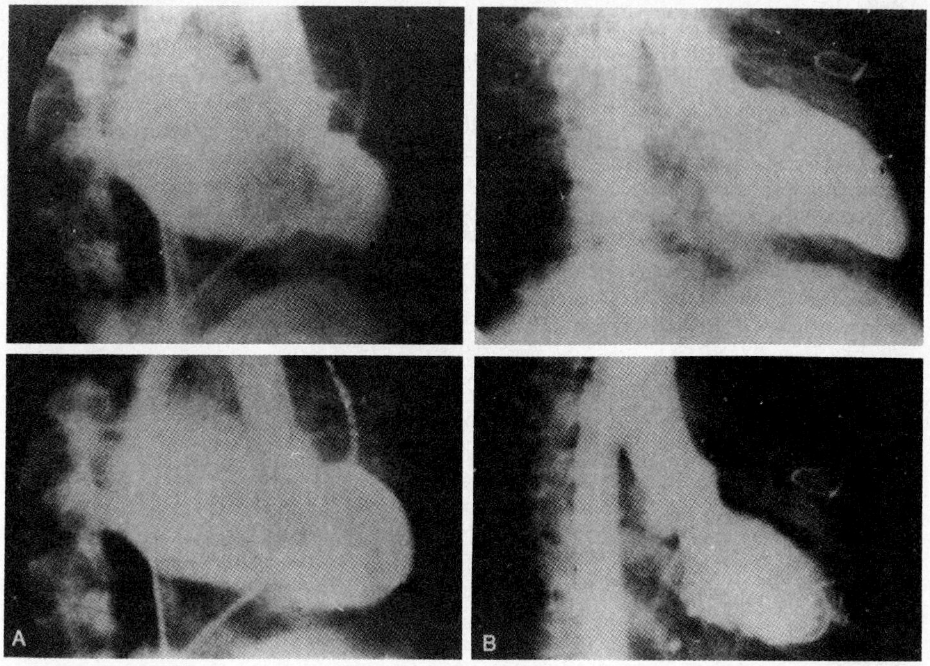

FIGURE 42–24. Right anterior oblique left ventriculogram in a patient with extensive EMF (*top*, systole; *bottom*, diastole). *A*, Preoperatively, there is amputation of the apex and mitral regurgitation. *B*, After extensive endocardiectomy and mitral valvuloplasty, the angiographic appearance is virtually normal. (From Metras, D., et al.: The surgical treatment of endomyocardial fibrosis: results in 55 patients. Circulation *72*:II-274, 1985, by permission of the American Heart Association, Inc.)

ics are not particularly helpful in the treatment of ascites. Once endomyocardial disease has reached the fibrotic stage, surgery offers the possibility of symptomatic improvement and is the treatment of choice.[343] Operative excision of the fibrotic endocardium and replacement of the mitral and/or tricuspid valves has led to substantial symptomatic improvement.[532, 534, 563-570] Mitral valve repair, rather than replacement, can be accomplished in some patients.[565, 571] Postoperative catheterization has also provided objective evidence of hemodynamic improvement with a reduction in ventricular filling pressures, an increase in cardiac output, and normalization of the angiographic appearance[565] (Fig. 42–24). Operative mortality has been high, running between 15 and 25 per cent in the larger series.[532, 564, 565]

ENDOCARDIAL FIBROELASTOSIS

(See p. 1011)

CARCINOID HEART DISEASE

ETIOLOGY AND PATHOLOGY. The carcinoid syndrome is caused by a metastasizing carcinoid tumor and is characterized by cutaneous flushing, diarrhea, bronchoconstriction, and endocardial plaques composed of a unique type of fibrous tissue.[572] The vasomotor, bronchoconstrictor, and cardiac manifestations are undoubtedly related to circulating humoral substances secreted by the tumor.[573] The diarrhea is probably caused by serotonin, which is secreted in large amounts by carcinoid tumors, while the dermal flushes and bronchospasm appear to be related to the release of kinin peptides. Virtually all patients develop diarrhea and flushing, while cardiac abnormalities occur in over one-half the patients and bronchospasm in one-third.[572, 574] Unusually, patients may demonstrate coronary artery spasm.[575]

Sixty to 90 per cent of tumors arise in the appendix, while the rest originate in the ileum, stomach, duodenum, other areas of the gastrointestinal tract, and bronchus.[573, 576] Carcinoid tumors of the ileum are the most likely to metastasize, with involvement of the regional lymph nodes and liver. Also, it is usual that only carcinoid tumors that invade the liver result in carcinoid heart disease.[577] The cardiac lesions may be related to large circulating quantities of serotonin (5-hydroxytryptamine), bradykinin, or other substances secreted by the tumor, which are usually inactivated by the liver, lungs, and brain.[576, 578] Hepatic metastases apparently allow large quantities of tumor products to reach the heart without being inactivated by the liver.[576] Left-sided cardiac involvement occurs in about one-third of patients with fatal cardiac carcinoid; when it occurs, it typically is of little hemodynamic significance, in contrast to right-sided involvement.[573] The preferential right-sided involvement presumably is related to inactivation of the offending humoral substance(s) by the lungs.

The characteristic *pathological* findings are fibrous plaques that involve the "downstream" aspect of the tricuspid and pulmonic valves, the endocardium of the cardiac chambers, and the intima of the venae cavae, pulmonary artery, and coronary sinus.[572, 573] The fibrous tissue in the plaques results in distortion of the valves, leading to pulmonic stenosis and tricuspid regurgitation,[573] sometimes with some degree of stenosis.[573] Histologically, the plaques consist of deposits of fibrous tissue located superficially on the endocardium with little or no extension into the underlying layers.[573] Ultrastructural studies have demonstrated that the plaques are composed of smooth muscle cells embedded in a stroma rich in acid mucopolysaccharides and collagen.[572] The plaques may form as a result of healing of a superficial endocardial injury, which is produced by a compound secreted by or derived from the tumor.[572]

CLINICAL MANIFESTATIONS. *Physical examination* usually reveals a systolic murmur along the left sternal border, produced by pulmonic stenosis, tricuspid regurgitation, or both. A murmur of pulmonary regurgitation may be found as well.[573, 578-584]

The *chest roentgenogram* may reveal enlargement of the heart; the pulmonary artery trunk is typically of normal size, without evidence of poststenotic dilatation as occurs in congenital pulmonic stenosis.[578] No specific *electrocardiographic pattern* is diagnostic of carcinoid heart disease, although low voltage is often present. Evidence of right atrial enlargement may be seen on occasion, but electrocardiographic evidence of right ventricular hypertrophy is usually lacking. Nonspecific ST-segment and T-wave abnormalities and right bundle branch block have also been reported.[578] *Echocardiography* may reveal evidence of tricuspid and/or pulmonary valve thickening, along with right atrial and right ventricular dilatation.[585]

The *hemodynamic findings* most commonly encountered are those of tricuspid regurgitation and pulmonic stenosis. Some patients with the carcinoid syndrome appear to be in a hyperkinetic state, which may lead to high-output heart failure[586] (Chap. 25).

TREATMENT. Treatment of patients with mild congestive heart failure consists of digitalis and diuretics. Some of the vasomotor symptoms may be controlled with alpha-adrenoceptor blockers and serotonin antagonists. Surgical replacement of the tricuspid valve and pulmonic valvotomy may be beneficial in severely symptomatic patients with serious valvular dysfunction.[576, 587, 588]

OBESITY HEART DISEASE

(See p. 1819)

DIABETIC CARDIOMYOPATHY

(See p. 1816)

MYOCARDITIS

When the heart is involved in an inflammatory process, often caused by an infectious agent, myocarditis is said to be present. The inflammation may involve the myocytes, interstitium, vascular elements, and/or pericardium; involvement of the latter structure is discussed in Chapter 44.

Myocarditis has been described during and following a wide variety of viral, rickettsial, bacterial, protozoal, and metazoal diseases; indeed, virtually any infectious agent may produce cardiac inflammation. Infectious agents cause myocardial damage by three basic mechanisms: (1) invasion of the myocardium[589]; (2) production of a myocardial toxin, e.g., diphtheria; and (3) immunologically mediated myocardial damage.[589] Although often mistakenly limited to inflammation due to an infective agent, myocarditis may also be caused by radiation and other physical agents, chemicals (e.g., lead), pharmacological agents (e.g., Adriamycin, p. 1748), and metabolic disorders (e.g., uremia, Chap. 59), as is discussed later in this chapter.[590]

Myocarditis may be an acute or a chronic process. In North America, viruses are the most common agents producing myocarditis, while in South America, Chagas' disease (produced by *Trypanosoma cruzi*) is far more common. The identification of the specific etiological agent responsible for infectious myocarditis usually rests on the associated extracardiac findings, since the cardiovascular signs and symptoms are often nonspecific. The histological findings vary, depending on the stage of the disease, the mechanism of myocardial damage, and the specific etiological agent. Myocardial involvement may be focal or diffuse, but the myocardial lesions are generally randomly distributed in the heart, and thus the clinical consequences depend to a large extent on the size and number of the lesions. However, a single small lesion may have profound consequences if it is located within the cardiac conducting system.[591] The histological findings are usually nonspecific (except for some parasitic and granulomatous forms of myocarditis), and, with the exception of Adriamycin cardiotoxicity, myocardial biopsy is usually not rewarding in elucidating the specific etiological agent.

INFECTIOUS MYOCARDITIS

CLINICAL MANIFESTATIONS

The clinical expression of myocarditis ranges from the asymptomatic state secondary to focal inflammation to fulminant fatal congestive heart failure due to diffuse myocarditis. An initial episode of viral myocarditis, perhaps unrecognized and forgotten, may be the initial event that eventually culminates in an "idiopathic" dilated cardiomyopathy.[589] In experimental animals, the structural and functional myocardial alterations that follow viral myocarditis may persist well beyond the stage of viral replication and myocardial inflammatory response,[589] and the late changes resemble those of dilated cardiomyopathy.[592, 593]

The outcome after viral myocarditis is quite variable. In most patients, the event is entirely self-limited and often unrecognized (Fig. 42–25). More overt myocarditis results in acute congestive heart failure.[589] In others, unrecognized myocarditis may be the cause of arrhythmias in what appears to be a structurally normal heart.[130] Some patients with chest pain and angiographically normal coronary arteries may have had subclinical myocarditis at some point in the past.[594] Most intriguing is the real possibility that viral myocarditis may culminate in dilated cardiomyopathy, presumably as a consequence of viral-mediated immunological cardiac damage.[343, 595, 596]

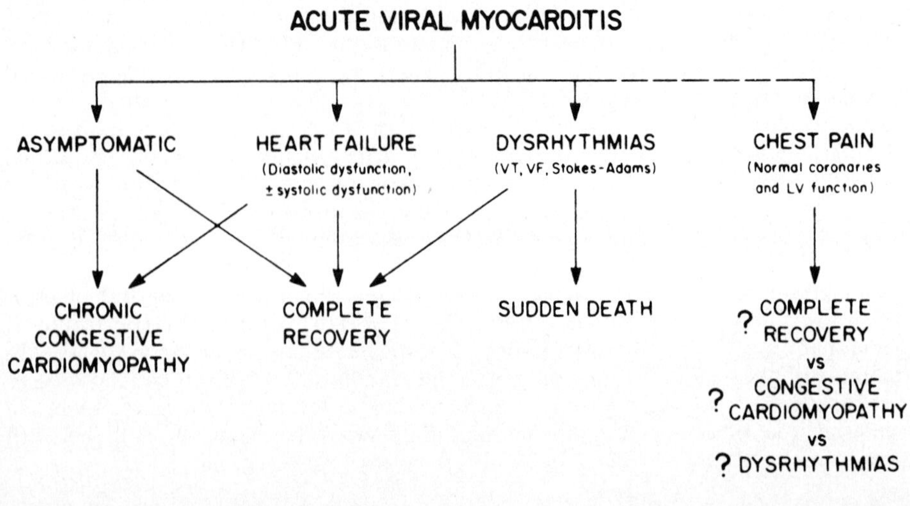

FIGURE 42–25. Schematic representation of the diversity of clinical presentation and outcome following acute viral myocarditis. VT = ventricular tachycardia; VF = ventricular fibrillation; LV = left ventricular. (From Kereiakes, D. J., and Parmley, W. W.: Myocarditis and cardiomyopathy. Am. Heart J. *108*:1318, 1984.)

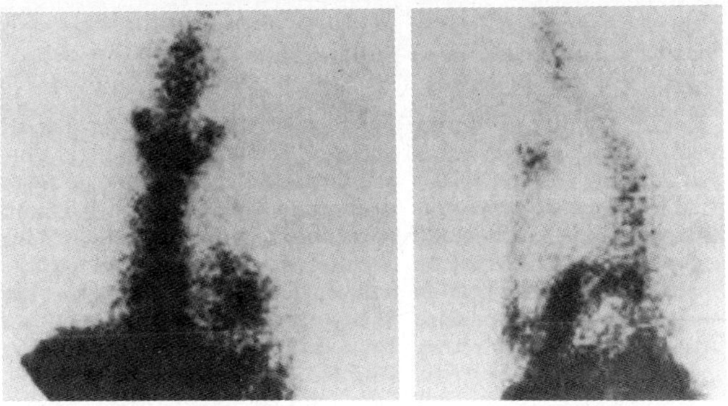

FIGURE 42–26. Gallium-67 images in a patient with active myocarditis in the setting of apparent dilated cardiomyopathy. Left = anterior, Right = 60-degree, left anterior oblique projections. (From O'Connell, J. B., and Gunnar, R. M.: Dilated-congestive cardiomyopathy: Prognostic features and therapy. J. Heart Transplant *2*:7, 1982.)

While transient electrocardiographic abnormalities suggesting myocardial involvement are noted in many patients with infectious diseases, most patients do not have other clinical manifestations of myocarditis. It is postulated that these electrocardiographic changes reflect subclinical myocardial involvement. That frequent but unrecognized myocardial involvement occurs with systemic infections is supported by histological evidence of myocarditis in 4 to 10 per cent of routine postmortem examinations.[597-599] Some degree of myocardial involvement, often subepicardial in location, also frequently occurs in patients with acute pericarditis.[600]

Since myocardial involvement is subclinical in most acute infectious diseases, the majority of patients have no specific complaints referable to the cardiovascular system; the presence of myocarditis is often inferred from the ST-segment and T-wave changes on the electrocardiogram.[589] From a clinical viewpoint, myocardial involvement is associated with nonspecific symptoms, including fatigue, dyspnea, palpitations, and precordial discomfort. Chest pain usually reflects associated pericarditis, but precordial discomfort suggestive of myocardial ischemia is occasionally observed.[601]

On *physical examination*, tachycardia is usual and may be out of proportion to the temperature elevation.[589, 597] The first heart sound is often muffled, and a protodiastolic gallop may be present. A transient apical systolic murmur may appear, but diastolic murmurs are rare.[602] Clinical evidence of congestive heart failure occurs only in the more severe cases.[589, 597, 602] The heart is usually normal in size in the clinically silent cases, but it may be dilated in patients with congestive heart failure. Pulmonary and systemic emboli may occur.

Electrocardiographic abnormalities are usually transient and occur far more frequently than does clinical myocardial involvement.[589] The most common changes are abnormalities of the ST segment and T wave, but atrial and in particular ventricular arrhythmias, atrioventricular (AV) and intraventricular conduction defects, and, rarely, Q waves may be seen.[589] Complete AV block is usually transient and resolves without sequelae, but it is occasionally a cause of sudden death in patients with myocarditis.[603] On *radiological examination*, heart size may range from normal to markedly enlarged, and pulmonary congestion may be present in patients with fulminant disease. *Radionuclide scanning* after the administration of gallium-67 or technetium-99m pyrophosphate may identify inflammatory and necrotic changes characteristic of myocarditis[604, 605] (Fig. 42–26).

The *diagnosis* is often predicated on the identification of the associated systemic illness and its characteristic features. The diagnosis of viral myocarditis is supported by the identification of the virus in stool, throat washings, blood, myocardium, feces, or pericardial fluid, or by a distinct (usually fourfold) increase in virus neutralizing antibody, complement-fixation, or hemagglutination inhibition titers.[589] Even in fatal cases, isolation of virus from the myocardium at necropsy is difficult and is accomplished with regularity only with the Coxsackie, echo-, and poliomyelitis viruses.[606] cDNA clones representing various regions of the Coxsackie B virus-specific RNA sequences have been used to detect and quantify virus-specific sequences in tissue.[606a]

PATHOLOGY. Patients dying of or with myocarditis demonstrate a wide spectrum of gross and histological pathological changes, reflecting the range of disease seen clinically (Fig. 42–27). Grossly, the hearts may be normal, dilated, hypertrophied, or flabby. An interstitial inflammatory reaction is usually observed and myocytolysis and necrosis may be seen. Routine histological examination of the heart rarely provides a specific diagnosis, although in

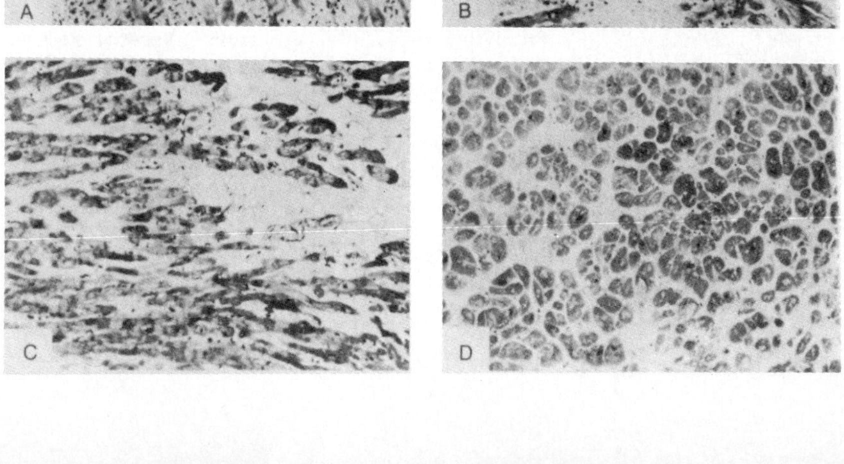

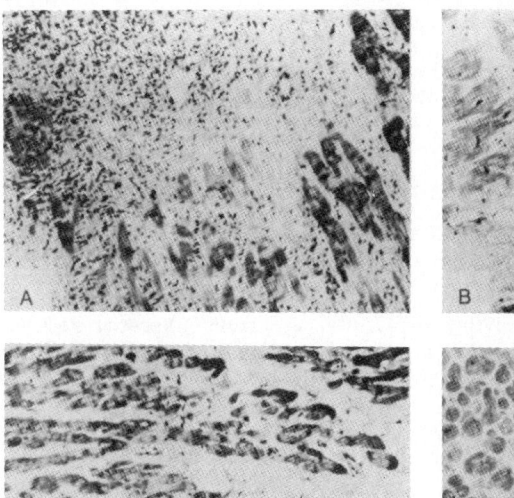

FIGURE 42–27. Representative endomyocardial biopsy specimens in myocarditis showing spectrum of infiltrative, fibrotic, and necrotic features. *A*, Diffuse mononuclear cell infiltrate, myocyte necrosis, marked interstitial edema and loose interstitial fibrosis. *B*, Single focus of mononuclear cells adjacent to a necrotic myocyte (arrow) with diffuse widening of interstitial spaces containing increased numbers of mononuclear cells. *C*, Widened interstitial spaces containing occasional mononuclear cells without evidence of myocyte necrosis or degeneration. *D*, Irregular hypertrophy of myocytes and dense interstitial fibrosis without evidence of an inflammatory-cell infiltrate. (Original magnification × 160.) (From Dec, G. W. Jr., et al.: Active myocarditis in the spectrum of acute dilated cardiomyopathies. Clinical features, histologic correlates, and clinical outcome. N. Engl. J. Med *312*:885, 1985.)

some instances electron microscopic and immunofluorescent techniques may allow elucidation of a specific etiology.

TREATMENT. Therapy is often supportive and is usually directed at the more prominent systemic manifestations of the disease. The demonstration of a particular predilection for involvement of the AV conducting system in some forms of myocarditis[589] suggests that patients with suspected myocarditis should be observed closely for any evidence of conduction abnormality. Since hypoxia and exercise intensify the damage from myocarditis in experimental animals, adequate oxygenation and rest are indicated.[607] Congestive heart failure responds to routine management, including digitalization and diuresis, although patients with myocarditis appear to be particularly sensitive to digitalis, and toxicity should be watched for. Significant arrhythmias should be treated with antiarrhythmic agents, although beta-adrenoceptor blockers are probably best avoided in view of their negative inotropic action. The use of corticosteroids is controversial, but they are proscribed in acute viral myocarditis, since increased tissue necrosis and viral replication have been demonstrated following their use.[589] In some patients with rapidly progressive congestive heart failure of no identifiable cause, an inflammatory myocarditis may be demonstrable by right ventricular endomyocardial biopsy. A small number of patients have responded favorably to treatment with immunosuppressive agents, usually prednisone and azathioprine.[129, 130, 606, 608] Serial endomyocardial biopsies have confirmed the resolution of the inflammatory infiltrate with treatment.[609] However, the value of antiinflammatory therapy for immune suppression has not been established unequivocally. Given the variability in the course of myocarditis and of the cardiomyopathy to which it may lead, the results of the ongoing blinded, controlled, randomized trial with this therapy will be crucial. Nonsteroidal antiinflammatory agents—indomethacin, salicylates, and ibuprofen,[610, 611] along with cyclosporine[612, 613]—are contraindicated during the acute phase of viral myocarditis, since they increase myocardial damage.

It is hoped that effective antiviral agents for treating viral myocarditis will be developed.[614] It may also be possible, in the future, to treat patients with myocarditis with agents that stimulate production of interferon, since this substance affords protection against the effects of viral myocarditis, at least in experimental animals.[615] Antibiotics may also be employed with benefit in infections caused by atypical pneumonia and psittacosis.

VIRAL MYOCARDITIS*

Systemic infection with numerous viruses may be associated with clinical evidence of myocarditis[616] (Table 42–12). The myocarditis characteristically develops after a lag period of several weeks following the initial systemic infection, suggesting involvement of an immunological mechanism. In animals, a variety of factors appears to enhance susceptibility to myocardial damage, including radiation, malnutrition, steroids, exercise, and previous myocardial injury. Viral myocarditis may be particularly virulent in infants and in pregnant women.[589]

COXSACKIE VIRUS. Both Coxsackie A and B viruses may produce myocarditis, although infection with Coxsackie B is more common, and this agent is the most frequent cause of viral myocarditis.[589] The myocardium appears to be particularly susceptible to the effects of this virus because of the apparent affinity of myocardial membrane receptors for the viral particles.[589] Necropsy often demonstrates a pericardial effusion, pericarditis, cardiac enlargement, and a predominantly mononuclear inflammatory infiltrate, with necrosis of the atrial and ventricular myocardium.[617] In some cases, focal myocardial necrosis simulating myocardial infarction is seen, despite normal coronary arteries.[618-622]

TABLE 42–12 PRINCIPAL VIRAL CAUSES OF MYOCARDITIS

Coxsackie (Groups A and B)
Echovirus
Adenovirus
Influenza
Varicella
Poliomyelitis
Mumps
Rabies
Viral hepatitis
Rubella
Rubeola
Infectious mononucleosis
Cytomegalovirus
Arbovirus (Groups A and B)
Variola and vaccinia
Viral encephalitis
Yellow fever
Herpes simplex

Although most infections are probably benign, self-limited, and subclinical,[589] Coxsackie myocarditis appears to be particularly virulent in the neonate.[623] In most infections in adults, the other clinical manifestations of viral involvement, such as pleurodynia, myalgia, upper respiratory tract symptoms, and arthralgias, predominate. Severe cases in the adult are characterized by myopericardial involvement with pleuritic or pericarditic chest pain, palpitations, and fever. Many patients with overt myocardial involvement develop congestive heart failure with cardiomegaly and pulmonary edema.

The *electrocardiogram* is virtually always abnormal, with ST-segment and T-wave changes and arrhythmias, often ventricular in origin; AV conduction disturbances are common.[624] Blood levels of myocardial enzymes (serum glutamic oxaloacetic transaminase, creatine kinase) may be normal or elevated, reflecting the absence or presence of variable degrees of myocardial necrosis.[625] *Echocardiography* may reveal diffuse and regional left ventricular wall motion abnormalities which usually improve or disappear over time.[626, 627]

Most patients recover completely within weeks, although it may require months for the electrocardiogram and ventricular function to return to normal.[628, 629] Rarely, Coxsackie myocarditis is fatal in adults.[630] Some patients become symptomatic following resolution of the infection, and they may present years later with dilated cardiomyopathy.[624] Occasionally, patients appear to recover completely only to develop symptoms subsequently.[631]

Treatment is symptomatic, and despite occasional postmortem evidence of intracardiac thrombi, anticoagulation should probably be avoided because of the risk of a hemorrhagic pericardial effusion.[624] Bed rest is indicated during the acute course of myocarditis, but there is no convincing evidence that a period of prolonged rest after apparent resolution of the acute process is useful.[632] Heart failure and cardiac arrhythmias are treated in the usual fashion.

ECHOVIRUS. Closely akin to the Coxsackie virus, the echoviruses may also be associated with myopericarditis, often during the course of an acute, pleurodynia-like illness,[633, 634] although clinically apparent myocardial involvement during the course of an echovirus infection is rare. Ventricular arrhythmias, complete AV block, and transient, nonspecific electrocardiographic changes have been reported.[635]

ADENOVIRUS. Myocarditis is rare in adenovirus infection. Postmortem findings include dilated right and left ventricles, with a mononuclear infiltrate with fragmentation of the myocardial fibers.[636]

INFLUENZA. Cardiovascular involvement may play an important role in patients with influenza, since one-third of fatal cases have evidence of active myocarditis.[637] Postmortem findings in fatal cases include biventricular dilatation, with evidence of subendocardial and subepicardial petechiae and hemorrhage. A mononuclear inflammation is prominent, especially in perivascular areas. Occasional fibrinoid necroses of the myocardial arterioles may be seen. The earliest histological abnormalities include petechial hemorrhages and loss of myofibrillar striations. Subsequently, fragmentation of the myocardial fibers becomes marked, and there is interstitial edema and hemorrhage.[637]

Cardiac involvement typically occurs within 1 to 2 weeks of the onset

*Myocarditis secondary to psittacosis and *Mycoplasma pneumoniae* is described later in this chapter.

of the illness and may be severe, sometimes contributing to mortality.[638] The *clinical manifestations* include dyspnea, palpitations, anginal chest pain, arrhythmia, and heart failure[639]; there is often concomitant involvement of the pericardium. Sinus tachycardia or, less commonly, sinus bradycardia may be seen. The *electrocardiogram* may show transient ST-segment and T-wave abnormalities, conduction defects, and even complete AV block.[637] Sudden death is common and may be associated with massive hemorrhagic pulmonary edema due to viral involvement of the lungs.[637]

VARICELLA. Clinical myocarditis is a rare finding in varicella, although unsuspected myocarditis is common in fatal varicella.[640] Occasionally a patient may develop overt evidence of myocarditis with congestive heart failure.[640, 641] Histological findings include rare but characteristic intranuclear inclusion bodies within the myocardial cells, along with interstitial edema, cellular infiltrates, and myonecrosis.[642] The electrocardiogram may show conduction abnormalities, and sudden death occurs rarely.[641]

POLIOMYELITIS. Myocarditis is a frequent finding in fatal cases of poliomyelitis, particularly during epidemics,[643] occurring in half or more of all patients dying with this disease; death may be sudden.[644] While myocardial involvement is usually focal and minimal in extent, some patients with bulbar disease succumb early in the course of the illness, often with cardiovascular collapse.[643, 645] These patients all have viral infection of the medulla and severe systemic vasoconstriction that leads to pulmonary edema. Myocarditis appears to contribute to the heart failure.[643] The *electrocardiogram* is frequently abnormal, with ST-segment and T-wave abnormalities, prolongation of the P-R and Q-T intervals,[646] extrasystoles, tachycardia, and atrial fibrillation. *Treatment* is symptomatic, with aggressive support of pulmonary function; tracheostomy and prolonged mechanical ventilatory support may be required. Fortunately, this disease has been largely eliminated by immunization.

MUMPS. Myocardial involvement during the course of mumps is a rare phenomenon, occurring in less than 10 per cent of adults infected with this virus, and even less frequently in children.[647] The hearts of only a few patients with mumps have come to postmortem examination and they have been found to be both dilated and hypertrophied. Histologically, there is diffuse interstitial fibrosis, with infiltration of mononuclear cells and areas of focal necrosis.[648]

Cardiac involvement is usually unrecognized clinically, and the diagnosis of myocarditis is based on nonspecific electrocardiographic changes.[649] Transient ST-segment and T-wave abnormalities are most common, but extrasystoles and AV conduction block may occur; in a rare case, persistent complete heart block requires insertion of a permanent pacemaker.[650] Myocarditis generally occurs in the first week of illness and is transient, in most cases resolving within several weeks.[649] A few patients develop precordial chest pain, dyspnea, palpitations, and fatigue; cardiomegaly and congestive heart failure occur on occasion.[648] Tachycardia, a transient apical systolic murmur, and protodiastolic gallop may be present.[649]

VIRAL HEPATITIS. The characteristic *pathological changes* in the myocardium associated with viral hepatitis are minute foci of necrosis of isolated muscle bundles, often surrounded by lymphocytes, and a diffuse serous inflammation.[651] The ventricles may be dilated, with petechial hemorrhages.[652] Hemorrhage into the interventricular septum involving the area of the conduction system is a conspicuous finding,[651, 652] and electrocardiographic surveillance for evidence of conduction defects may be warranted in patients with clinical evidence of myocarditis during the course of viral hepatitis. Myocardial damage may be produced indirectly through an immune-mediated mechanism, or directly by viral invasion of the heart.[653]

Symptomatic myocarditis is generally observed in the first to third week of illness.[654] Patients may have dyspnea, palpitations and anginal chest pain; fatalities have been reported.[653, 655] *Electrocardiographic changes*, including bradycardia, ventricular premature beats, and ST-segment and T-wave changes, may be seen during the course of hepatitis.[651] These abnormalities are usually transient and asymptomatic, although congestive heart failure, cardiomegaly, and sudden death have been reported.[652]

HUMAN IMMUNODEFICIENCY VIRUS. Cardiac involvement in the acquired immunodeficiency syndrome (AIDS) is common but usually clinically silent. Pericardial effusion, right-sided marantic endocarditis, right ventricular dilatation, left ventricular dysfunction, and mitral regurgitation may be found by echocardiography in many AIDS patients.[656] Pathological findings include metastatic Kaposi's sarcoma involving the epicardium or myocardium, thrombotic endocarditis with embolization, fibrinous pericarditis, and myocarditis, particularly caused by toxoplasmosis and cryptococcosis.[657-660]

INFECTIOUS MONONUCLEOSIS. Examination of the hearts of patients with the myocarditis associated with infectious mononucleosis may reveal atypical lymphocytes within the myocardium, along with focal myocardial infiltrates and necrosis.[661] *Electrocardiographic changes* associated with infectious mononucleosis are common, although symptomatic cardiac involvement is only rarely observed.[661-663] ST-segment and T-wave changes may be observed, along with varying degrees of AV block. Ventricular arrhythmias occur rarely but may be fatal. Symptomatic patients may demonstrate a pericardial friction rub, an apical systolic murmur,and evidence of congestive heart failure.[661] Most patients follow an uncomplicated and nonfatal clinical course.[664]

RUBELLA AND RUBEOLA. Congenital cardiovascular lesions may develop in the offspring when *rubella* is contracted by the mother during the first trimester of pregnancy, with persistent ductus arteriosus and pulmonary artery maldevelopment as prominent anomalies (Chap. 30). Abnormalities of the conduction system have been reported in postnatal rubella[665] and myocarditis occurs on rare occasions.[666]

In *rubeola*, transient electrocardiographic abnormalities,[667, 668] including prolongation of the P-R interval, ST-segment and T-wave changes, AV conduction abnormalities, and ventricular tachycardia, have been reported.[602, 667, 668] The electrocardiographic changes are usually transient. Congestive heart failure occurs on rare occasions, and its appearance is a poor prognostic sign, often indicating a fatal outcome.[669] Histological examination of the heart in fatal cases has revealed evidence of myocarditis characterized predominantly by a perivascular lymphocytic infiltrate.[668]

CYTOMEGALOVIRUS. Unrecognized infection with cytomegalovirus (CMV) is extremely common in childhood, and the majority of the adult population have antibodies to CMV.[670, 671] Primary infection after the age of 35 years is uncommon, and generalized infection usually occurs only in immunosuppressed patients with neoplastic disease. The cardiovascular manifestations in adults are generally limited to asymptomatic and transient electrocardiographic changes. Symptomatic cardiac involvement is rare, although a hemorrhagic pericardial effusion may occur.[672] While fatalities are unusual, when they do occur histological examination of the heart may reveal focal lymphocytic infiltration and fibrosis.[672]

ARBOVIRUS. Infections due to group A arbovirus (e.g., chikungunya) and group B arbovirus (e.g., dengue) often result in symptomatic cardiac involvement.[673] In addition to symptoms due to systemic involvement (fever, headache, sweating), chest pain, dyspnea, palpitations, fatigue, dizziness, and paroxysmal nocturnal dyspnea are often prominent features. A protodiastolic gallop, apical systolic murmur, and cardiomegaly are common.[674-676] The latter often persists after the acute illness has resolved. The *electrocardiogram* is virtually always abnormal in patients with myocardial involvement, and ST segment and T wave abnormalities, sinus tachycardia, sinus bradycardia, conduction disturbances, and arrhythmias are found.[676] Atrial fibrillation, atrial premature depolarizations, and ventricular premature depolarizations are also seen. Sudden death may occur, most often due to ventricular arrhythmias or embolization.[674] Complete recovery is unusual, and most patients have persistent cardiomegaly and abnormalities of the electrocardiogram.[674, 676]

VARIOLA AND VACCINIA. Cardiac involvement following smallpox is rare, although several cases of myocarditis associated with acute cardiac failure and death have been reported.[677] Myocarditis with pericardial effusion and congestive heart failure has also been observed as a complication of smallpox vaccination[678]; an immunological mechanism has been suggested and dramatic responses to steroids have been reported. The histological changes include a mixed mononuclear infiltrate, with interstitial edema and occasional degenerating or necrotic muscle bundles.[679]

YELLOW FEVER. Myocardial changes are occasionally seen in fatal cases of yellow fever, with petechial hemorrhages of the endocardial and epicardial surfaces, foci of myocardial necrosis, and cellular infiltration.[680]

RESPIRATORY SYNCYTIAL VIRUS. Although respiratory syncytial virus is an important cause of respiratory disease, particularly in children, it rarely results in cardiac involvement.[681] Several patients have developed clinical congestive heart failure after an infection with this virus, with symptoms appearing several days after the initial respiratory manifestations.[681, 682] Complete heart block is a prominent feature,[683] although cardiomegaly, ventricular arrhythmias, and cardiac decompensation may also be noted.

MYCOPLASMA PNEUMONIAE. Electrocardiographic abnormalities are common during the course of atypical pneumonia, occurring in up to one-third of patients.[684] Nonspecific ST-segment and T-wave abnormalities are most common, particularly involving the right-sided precordial leads, but first-degree AV block is occasionally seen.[669, 684] The electrocardiographic findings usually resolve within 1 to 2 weeks. A cell-mediated myocarditis has been postulated as the cause of the changes.[685] Pericarditis may be a prominent finding, and congestive heart failure is occasionally seen.[686, 687] A protodiastolic gallop and pericardial friction rub may be noted in occasional cases.[669] No specific treatment for the cardiovascular involvement is usually indicated. Complete recovery is the rule in most patients.[686]

PSITTACOSIS. Myocarditis complicating psittacosis is a relatively common occurrence and is characterized by congestive heart failure and acute pericarditis.[688, 689] *Pathological changes* include a fibrinous pericarditis, subendocardial hemorrhages, and interstitial edema, with lymphocytic and plasma cell infiltrates. Fatty degeneration or cloudy swelling of the muscle fibers may be seen. Fever, chest pain, electrocardiographic changes, cardiomegaly, systemic emboli, tachycardia, and hypotension may occur. While most patients recover completely, fatalities have been reported in a small fraction.[688] The systemic infection may be treated effectively with tetracycline, but the effect of the antibiotic on the myocardium is unknown.

RICKETTSIAL MYOCARDITIS

The rickettsial diseases are frequently associated with evidence of myocardial involvement. Transient ST-segment and T-wave alterations in particular are observed commonly. The circulatory collapse that may accompany these diseases is largely a manifestation of abnormalities of the peripheral vascular bed, but a myocardial component may also be present. The basic histopathological process is a vasculitis, with a periarterial interstitial infiltrate.

SCRUB TYPHUS. Myocarditis is common during the course of scrub typhus (tsutsugamushi disease, caused by *R. tsutsugamushi*). The histological findings are those of a focal panvasculitis involving the small blood vessels. Myocardial necrosis is unusual, but hemorrhage into the heart and subepicardial petechiae may occur. Clinical evidence of myocardial involvement typically is not severe and is usually not associated with residual cardiac damage.[690, 691] The electrocardiogram may show nonspecific ST-segment and T-wave abnormalities, as well as first-degree AV block. A protodiastolic gallop and apical systolic murmur suggestive of mitral regurgitation are occasionally found.

ROCKY MOUNTAIN SPOTTED FEVER. Clinical evidence of myocarditis is more common than often recognized in Rocky Mountain spotted fever (caused by *R. rickettsii*), and the heart is often involved in the multisystem damage that occurs as the result of a widespread vasculitis.[692-694] Unsuspected left ventricular dysfunction is common, and echocardiographic evidence of dysfunction may persist in some patients.[692]

Q FEVER. Endocarditis is the most common cardiac manifestation of infection with *R. burnettii* (Q fever). Myocarditis is not a prominent feature, although dyspnea and chest pain, perhaps reflecting associated pericarditis, occur frequently.[695] The electrocardiogram may demonstrate transient ST-segment and T-wave changes as well as paroxysmal ventricular arrhythmias.[695, 696] Abnormalities of the immune system have been implicated in the pathogenesis of the disease.[697, 698]

BACTERIAL MYOCARDITIS

DIPHTHERIA. Myocardial involvement is one of the most serious complications of diphtheria[699] and occurs in at least one-fourth of cases. Indeed, myocardial involvement is the most common cause of death in this infection.[700] Cardiac damage is due to the liberation by the diphtheria bacillus of a toxin that inhibits protein synthesis by interfering with the transfer of amino acids from soluble RNA to polypeptide chains under construction.[701]

Pathological findings include a flabby and dilated heart with a myocardium that has a "streaky" appearance. Microscopic examination reveals characteristic fatty infiltration of the myocytes, often with an interstitial inflammatory infiltrate, myocytolysis, and hyaline necrosis of muscle fibers.[669] With time, fibrosis and hypertrophy of the remaining myocardial cells develop. The conduction system is often involved.

Typically, *clinical* signs of cardiac dysfunction appear at the end of the first week of the illness.[699] Cardiomegaly and severe congestive heart failure are often present.[699] A protodiastolic gallop and pulmonary congestion may be prominent features. Elevation of the serum transaminase levels may be seen; a high level is associated with a poor prognosis.[699] Sudden circulatory failure and death may occur.[669] Many patients develop ST-segment and T-wave abnormalities, but atrial and ventricular arrhythmias may also occur.[702] Persistently abnormal electrocardiograms are common following diphtheritic myocarditis, as are cardiomegaly and symptoms of reduced cardiac reserve.[669] Some patients recover fully.[699]

Because of the serious effects of the toxin on the myocardium, antitoxin should be administered as rapidly as possible. Antibiotic therapy is of less urgency. General supportive measures are indicated. Overt congestive heart failure may be resistant to therapy with cardiac glycosides. The development of complete AV block is a serious complication, but it may be amenable to treatment with a transvenous pacemaker.[703] Corticosteroids do not appear to have any place in the treatment of the cardiac abnormalities[704]; treatment with carnitine seems to reduce the incidence of heart failure and the need for pacemaker, and to lower mortality.[705]

SALMONELLA. Symptomatic myocardial involvement during salmonella infections is rare, although electrocardiographic abnormalities are often seen, suggesting subclinical myocarditis. *Postmortem findings* in salmonella myocarditis may reveal a shaggy, fibrinous pericarditis and, in some cases, evidence of endocarditis.[706, 707] Myocardial petechiae and hemorrhagic necrosis may occur, with evidence of biventricular dilatation. A polymorphonuclear leukocytic infiltrate with evidence of coronary arteritis may be found.[708] The arteritis may lead to thrombosis, infarction, and death. Other cardiovascular complications include infected mural thrombi, occasionally resulting in pulmonary and systemic emboli, and mycotic aneurysms.[706] Myocardial abscesses often develop and may rupture, producing fatal cardiac tamponade.[706] Myocarditis with congestive heart failure occurs most commonly in children who are severely ill with salmonellosis, and it is associated with a high mortality.[709] When myocarditis occurs, it often develops rapidly, with evidence of biventricular failure, tachycardia, a protodiastolic gallop, an apical systolic murmur of mitral regurgitation, and peripheral edema.[710]

Electrocardiographic abnormalities include ST-segment and T-wave changes, and prolonged P-R or Q-T intervals. These electrocardiographic changes typically appear in the second week of illness and usually resolve completely within a week.[710]

TUBERCULOSIS. Tuberculous involvement of the myocardium is extremely rare, particularly since the introduction of drugs effective against tuberculosis.[711, 712] Children are more susceptible than adults to myocardial involvement.[713] Cardiac involvement may occur by direct extension from tuberculous hilar lymph nodes (probably the most common); lymphatic spread; and hematogenous spread.[714, 715]

Most cases of myocardial tuberculosis are clinically silent and are diagnosed only at postmortem examination.[711] On rare occasions, tuberculosis involvement of the myocardium may lead to arrhythmias, including atrial fibrillation and ventricular tachycardia, complete AV block, congestive heart failure, and sudden death.[711]

STREPTOCOCCUS. The most common detected cardiac finding following beta-hemolytic streptococcal infection is acute rheumatic fever, which is discussed in detail in Chapter 54.

Direct infection of the heart by the streptococcus produces a myocarditis that is distinct from acute rheumatic carditis. It is characterized by an interstitial infiltrate composed of mononuclear cells with occasional polymorphonuclear leukocytes; the infiltrate may be focal or diffuse and may be localized to the subendocardial or perivascular region. There may be small areas of myocardial necrosis,[716] and direct bacterial invasion of the myocardium can sometimes be detected. *Electrocardiographic abnormalities*, including prolongation of the P-R and Q-T intervals, occur frequently.[669] While these abnormalities are rarely associated with other clinical manifestations of myocardial involvement, sudden death, conduction disturbances, and arrhythmias may occur.[717]

MENINGOCOCCUS. Myocardial involvement is common during the course of meningococcal infections, particularly in men with fatal meningococcal infections.[718] *Pathological findings* include hemorrhagic myocardial lesions, occasionally associated with intracellular organisms. An interstitial myocarditis composed of lymphocytes, plasma cells, and polymorphonuclear leukocytes is often observed, occasionally with muscle necrosis.[718] Fulminating meningococcemia associated with the Waterhouse-Friderichsen syndrome may exhibit focal muscle necrosis, severe fatty change, and cloudy swelling of the myocytes.[719]

Meningococcal myocarditis may result in congestive heart failure, which may be fatal, as well as in pericardial effusion.[720] Death may also occur suddenly and be associated with involvement of the AV node. It is advisable to monitor the heart rhythm of patients with meningococcemia. In milder cases, transient electrocardiographic abnormalities, principally ST-segment and T-wave changes, are often seen and may resolve completely with time.[720]

CLOSTRIDIA. Cardiac involvement is common in patients with clostridial infections with multiple organ involvement[721]; the myocardial damage results from the toxin elaborated by the bacteria. The *pathological findings* are distinctive, with gas bubbles usually present in the myocardium. Areas of degenerated muscle fibers are apparent, but an inflammatory infiltrate is usually absent.[721] *C. perfringens* may cause myocardial abscess formation with myocardial perforation and resultant purulent pericarditis.[722]

INFECTIVE ENDOCARDITIS. Myocardial infection is frequently observed as a consequence of infective endocarditis (Chap. 34).

LEGIONNAIRE'S DISEASE. Although pneumonia, rhabdomyolysis, renal failure, and hepatic as well as central nervous system involvement are common with *Legionella pneumophila*, overt cardiac involvement is not. Occasional electrocardiographic changes may be noted, consisting primarily of ST-segment and T-wave abnormalities; ventricular arrhythmias may be seen.[723] Rarely, pericardial effusion or myocarditis with evidence of myocardial necrosis and congestive heart failure may be seen.[724, 725]

BRUCELLOSIS. Cardiac involvement in the course of brucellosis is uncommon, usually consisting of endocarditis.[726, 727] Myocardial involvement, when it occurs, is manifested by T-wave changes and prolongation of AV conduction.[726] An occasional patient develops fulminant myocarditis, with a lymphocytic and polymorphonuclear infiltrate.[726]

WHIPPLE'S DISEASE

Intestinal lipodystrophy, or Whipple's disease, may be associated with myocardial involvement, and PAS-positive macrophages may be found in the myocardium, pericardium, and heart valves of patients with this disorder.[728] Coronary artery lesions, with smooth muscle necrosis, panarteritis, and medial scarring, are not rare.[729] Unusually, patients may develop pulmonary hypertension.[730] Electron microscopy has demonstrated rod-shaped structures in the myocardium similar to those found in the small intestine, and it has been suggested that they are the causative agent of the myocardial abnormalities. There is often an associated inflammatory infiltrate and foci of fibrosis. The valvular fibrosis may be severe enough to result in aortic regurgitation and mitral stenosis.[729] While asymptomatic, nonspecific electrocardiographic changes are most common, systolic murmurs, pericarditis, and even overt congestive heart failure may occur.[728] Antibiotic therapy appears to be effective in treating the basic disease; however, relapses can occur, often more than 2 years after initial diagnosis.[731, 732]

SPIROCHETAL INFECTIONS

SYPHILIS. Aortitis is the most common manifestation of luetic involvement of the cardiovascular system. Aortic regurgitation and coronary ostial narrowing are associated findings (p. 1566). Syphilitic involvement of the myocardium itself in the form of gumma formation is rare and is usually unsuspected clinically. Involvement of the interventricular septum may result in damage to the conducting system and AV block.[733] Gummae may also impinge on the heart valves and interfere with their function.[734] While congenital syphilis may lead to a diffuse myocarditis,[735] the existence of this in adults is disputed.[736]

LEPTOSPIROSIS (WEIL'S DISEASE). Cardiac involvement is common in leptospirosis. The *pathological findings* include petechiae or larger foci of hemorrhage, often located in the epicardium.[737] An interstitial myocardial infiltration, often subendocardial in location, may occur, with involvement of the papillary muscles.[737] Involvement of the AV conduction system may be a prominent feature. The most common manifestations of cardiac involvement are ST-segment and T-wave changes; atrial and ventricular arrhythmias, sinus bradycardia, and conduction defects may occur.[738-741] Cardiomegaly, pulmonary congestion, a protodiastolic gallop, pericarditis, and symptoms of congestive heart failure occur rarely.[738]

RELAPSING FEVER. Many infections are currently observed in Ethiopia. During pandemics, mortality may be particularly high, reaching 70 per cent, although sporadic cases are often more benign.[742] Cardiac involvement is a common complication and is often implicated as a cause of death. AV conduction defects occur frequently and may be responsible for sudden death, although tachyarrhythmias have also been implicated.[742] Numerous petechiae are observed with a diffuse histiocytic interstitial infiltrate, particularly around small arterioles in the left ventricle.

FUNGAL INFECTIONS

Cardiac fungal infections occur most frequently in patients with malignant disease and/or those receiving chemotherapy, steroids, radiation, or immunosuppressive therapy. Cardiac surgery, intravenous drug abuse, and infection with HIV are also predisposing factors for fungal cardiac involvement.[743]

ASPERGILLOSIS. Myocardial involvement is not uncommon in generalized aspergillosis. On *pathological examination*, myocardial necrosis and infarction caused by thrombosis of vessels that contain fungal mycelia are commonly seen. The fungus often extends beyond the vessel walls and invades the surrounding necrotic myocardium.[744] The electrocardiogram may be normal in the face of significant myocardial damage but T-wave changes may be present.[745] The *diagnosis* of aspergillus infection is often difficult. Identification of aspergillus through open lung biopsy, aspiration lung biopsy, transtracheal aspiration, or bronchial brush technique is usually successful. Early institution of prolonged therapy with amphotericin B may result in significant improvement.[744]

ACTINOMYCOSIS. Myocarditis is a rare complication of actinomycotic infection, occurring in less than 2 per cent of patients.[746] However, cardiac involvement is quite serious when it does occur. Involvement of the heart most commonly is the result of direct extension of disease within the thorax.[746] Initially the pericardium is invaded, with eventual obliteration of the pericardial space.[747] The myocardium is commonly involved by extension of the pericardial process. Myocardial seeding is less common. The myocardial lesion is a suppurative, necrotizing abscess containing the organism, surrounded by granulation tissue.[747] Both right- and left-sided failure are common manifestations.[747] A pericardial rub may be heard, sometimes associated with clinical evidence of a pericardial effusion. Arrhythmias occur infrequently.[746]

BLASTOMYCOSIS. Blastomycosis involves the myocardium by spread from mediastinal lymph nodes, by hematogenous miliary seeding,[748, 749] and most frequently by direct extension from the pericardium. *Pathological findings* include cardiac dilatation without hypertrophy but with caseation and tubercle formation. Thrombi may form above the endocardial lesions. Dyspnea, cyanosis, and peripheral edema may be prominent. Tachycardia and a systolic murmur are often present.[749]

CRYPTOCOCCOSIS. Cryptococcal infection of the myocardium occurs most commonly in patients with disseminated malignancy.[750] *Pathological examination* may show cardiac dilatation, with epithelial granulomas and giant cells and variable degrees of fibrosis.[751] Congestive heart failure occurs[751]; pulmonary congestion and muffled heart sounds may be found on physical examination, and cardiomegaly on the chest roentgenogram. The *electrocardiogram* may show first-degree AV block and T-wave inversions; ventricular arrhythmias have been observed.

CANDIDIASIS. Disseminated monilial infections are common opportunistic infections, particularly in the compromised host.[752] Endocarditis is the most frequent manifestation of cardiac involvement (p. 1121), occurring most commonly in cardiac surgical patients or drug addicts, although abscesses of the myocardium may occur as associated or independent findings. Complete heart block may be caused by microabscesses of the conduction system. A myocarditic pattern may be seen in immunosuppressed patients,[753] with pseudohyphae and yeast forms, and multiple foci in the myocardium.

COCCIDIOIDOMYCOSIS. Involvement of the heart is seen on occasion in patients with generalized coccidioidomycosis. The hearts may be grossly normal, although epicardial lesions with resultant pericarditis are frequent,[754] and progression to constrictive pericarditis may occur[755] (p. 1501). A nonspecific, focal, interstitial, and perivascular cellular infiltrate with associated muscle fiber degeneration and interstitial edema is commonly found, although granulomas containing fungi are also seen sometimes.

HISTOPLASMOSIS. Cardiac involvement in histoplasmosis is rare and usually is in the form of endocarditis (Chap. 34).[756] Pericarditis with effusion may also occur (p. 1513) and superior vena caval obstruction has been observed.[757] Myocardial involvement occurs less frequently, although atrial arrhythmias and T-wave abnormalities have been reported.[757]

PROTOZOAL MYOCARDITIS

Trypanosomiasis (Chagas' Disease)

Chagas' disease is caused by the protozoan *Trypanosoma cruzi*. The major cardiovascular manifestation is an extensive myocarditis that typically becomes evident years after the initial infection. The disease is prevalent in Central and South America, particularly in Brazil, Argentina, and Chile, where it is a major public health problem. Between 10 and 20 million people in South America may be infected with the parasite.[758]

The natural history of Chagas' disease is characterized by three phases: acute, latent, and chronic. During the *acute phase*, the disease is transmitted to humans through the bite of a reduviid bug (subfamily *Triatominae*), which harbors the parasite in its gastrointestinal tract. This insect acquires the disease from feeding on infected animals, including the armadillo, raccoon, opossum, and skunk as well as domestic dogs and cats. The reduviid bug, popularly known in Argentina as "vinchuca," meaning "to let oneself drop," lives in the walls and roofs of houses and, during nocturnal feeding, drops from the ceiling onto the sleeping person below.[759] The bug then often bites the person around the eyes, and infection of the human host occurs when the trypanosomes in the animal's feces gain entry through abraded skin or through the conjunctivae. Occasionally, this results in unilateral periorbital edema and swelling of the eyelid, termed *Romaña's sign*,[760] while entry through the skin may result in a lesion called a *chagoma*. Transmission may also occur through blood transfusions as well as congenitally.

ACUTE TRYPANOSOMIASIS. Following inoculation, the protozoa multiply and then migrate widely throughout the body. In a minority of cases an acute illness occurs, although inapparent acute infections are more common.[759]

Pathological examination during the acute phase often reveals parasites in the cardiac fibers with a marked cellular infiltrate, particularly around cardiac cells that have ruptured and released the parasites. Involvement may extend into the endocardium, resulting in thrombus formation, and into the epicardium resulting in pericardial effusion. The pathogenesis of the myocardial lesions of acute Chagas' disease appears to relate in large part to immune lysis by antibody and cell-mediated immunity directed against antigens released from *T. cruzi*–infected cells, which become adsorbed onto the surface of infected and noninfected host cells.[761-763]

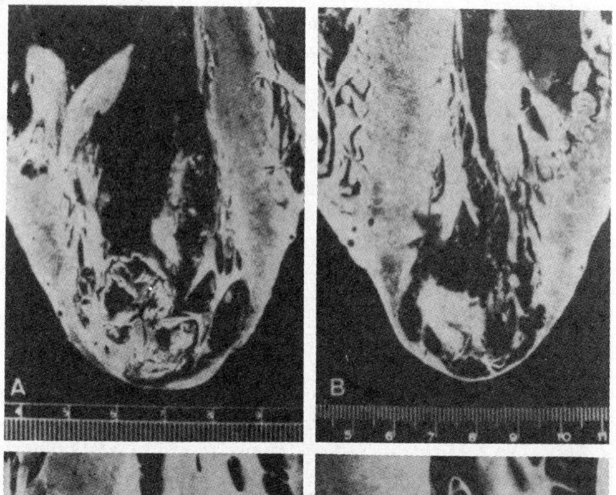

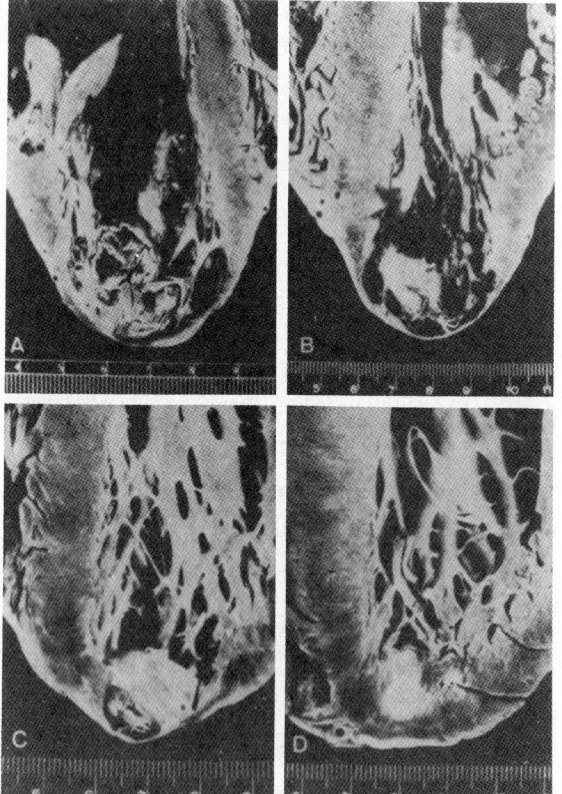

FIGURE 42–28. Four examples of gross pathological findings in Chagas' disease with apical thrombosis, demonstrating apical puriform softening (*A*), different phases of organization (*B* and *C*), and complete hyalinization (*D*). (From Oliveria, J. S. M., et al.: Cardiac thrombosis and thromboembolism in chronic Chagas' heart disease. Am. J. Cardiol. *52*:147, 1983.)

Clinical Manifestations. These include fever, muscle pains, sweating, hepatosplenomegaly, myocarditis with congestive heart failure, and, occasionally, meningoencephalitis.[759] Most patients recover, and their symptoms resolve over several months. Young children most commonly develop clinical acute disease and generally are more seriously ill, than adults.

CHRONIC TRYPANOSOMIASIS. The disease then enters a *latent phase*, not to reappear for 10 to 30 years. At an average of 20 years after the initial (and usually unrecognized) infestation, approximately 30 per cent of infected individuals develop findings of *chronic Chagas' disease*, the manifestations of which cover a wide spectrum from asymptomatic but seropositive patients through those with electrocardiographic abnormalities to those with advanced disease characterized by cardiomegaly, congestive heart failure, arrhythmias, thromboembolic phenomenon, right bundle branch block, and sudden death. In the advanced stage, cardiac dilatation typically involves all the cardiac chambers, although right-sided enlargement may predominate.[764] Even those individuals whose only clinical evidence of the disease is seropositivity often have subclinical cardiac involvement that may be demonstrated by endomyocardial biopsy.[765, 766]

The central paradox in the pathogenesis of this disorder is the negative correlation between the severity of disease and the level of parasitemia.[762] It is not unusual to be unable to detect parasites in patients dying of Chagas' disease.[767] An autoimmune mechanism is thus suggested. It appears (at least in an animal model) that self-reactive cytotoxic T lymphocytes develop following the initial infection, and these lymphocytes are able to lyse normal host cells, perhaps related to cross-reacting antigens of *T. cruzi* and striated muscle.[761, 768, 769] Stimulation of polyclonal B cells also has been suggested as a possible mediator of damage in this disease.[770] It is thought that the acute phase results in the release from parasite-modified host cells of self components that are immunogenic.

Pathology. Nerves and autonomic ganglia are frequently abnormal; megaesophagus and megacolon may occur; less commonly, there is dilatation of the stomach, duodenum, ureter, and bronchi.[771] Different strains of *T. cruzi* may account for the geographic differences in the expression of Chagas' disease; in Brazil, megaesophagus and megacolon are uncommon, but these conditions are usual in Venezuela.[772] Lesions of the cardiac nerves are routinely found in patients with chronic Chagas' disease, with evidence of cardiac parasympathetic denervation.[764, 773] Pathological cardiac findings include cardiac enlargement with dilatation and hypertrophy of all cardiac chambers.[759, 764, 771] The left ventricular apex is often thin and bulging, resembling an aneurysm[774] (Fig. 42–28). Thrombus formation is frequent and may fill much of the apex; the right atrium also frequently contains thrombus.[771] It has been suggested that this characteristic apical aneurysm may be the result of intravascular platelet aggregation leading to focal myocardial necrosis.[775]

The microscopic findings are principally those of extensive fibrosis, particularly of the left ventricle. A chronic cellular infiltrate composed of lymphocytes, plasma cells, and macrophages is often present.[771] Preferential involvement of the right bundle branch and the anterior fascicle of the left bundle branch by inflammatory and fibrotic changes explains the frequent occurrence of right bundle branch and left anterior fascicular block.[776] Parasites may be identified in one-fourth of patients[764]; the frequency with which they are found depends upon the diligence of the search for them.

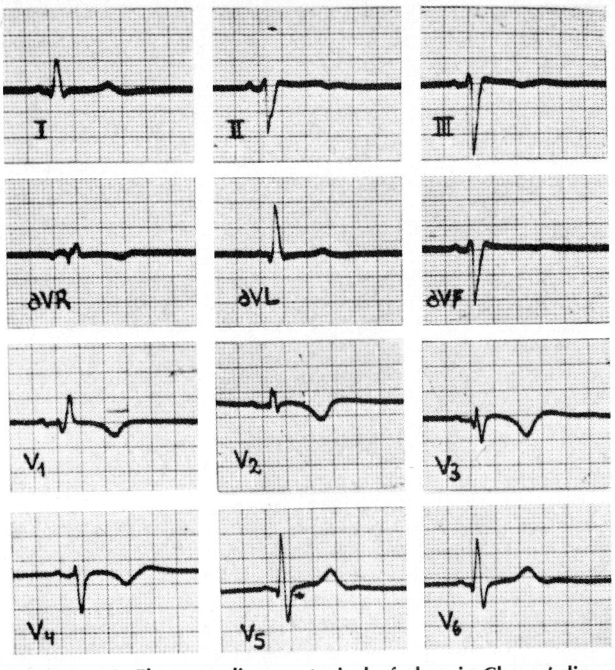

FIGURE 42–29. Electrocardiogram typical of chronic Chagas' disease, demonstrating left anterior hemiblock, right bundle branch block, and T-wave changes. (From Rosenbaum, M. B.: Chagasic myocardiopathy. Progr. Cardiovasc. Dis. *7*:199, 1964, by permission of Grune and Stratton.)

Clinical Manifestations. Chronic progressive heart failure, often predominantly right-sided, is the rule in advanced cases. Thus, while pulmonary congestion is occasionally noted, the usual findings generally include fatigue due to diminished cardiac output, peripheral edema, ascites, and hepatic congestion.[759] Tricuspid regurgitation is often present, particularly in patients with severe right-sided heart failure, although mitral regurgitation is frequently present as well.[771] The second heart sound is widely split, often with an accentuated pulmonic component,[759] reflecting the combined effects of right bundle branch block and pulmonary hypertension. Autonomic dysfunction is common, with marked abnormalities in the expected reflex changes in heart rate produced by various maneuvers.[777-779]

The *chest roentgenogram* often demonstrates severe cardiomegaly, with or without pulmonary venous hypertension.[771] *Electrocardiographic abnormalities* are the rule, particularly in patients who are seroreactive to *T. cruzi* antigen, with right bundle branch block and left anterior hemiblock being the most common changes in patients with chronic Chagas' disease[759, 771, 780, 781] (Fig. 42–29). ST-segment and T-wave abnormalities are common,[759] while Q waves involving the inferior leads,[771] P-wave abnormalities, and AV block are occasionally seen. Early in the disease, the electrocardiogram may be normal or nearly so. Administration of the antiarrhythmic agent ajmaline may precipitate the appearance of electrocardiographic abnormalities and thus identify patients with as yet clinically silent cardiac involvement.[782] Furthermore, electrophysiological testing of asymptomatic patients, even those with normal electrocardiograms, may demonstrate abnormalities of the conducting system in the majority.[783]

Ventricular arrhythmias are a prominent feature of chronic Chagas' disease. Frequent ventricular premature depolarizations, often with multiple morphologies, are seen frequently, and bouts of ventricular tachycardia may occur. Ventricular arrhythmias are particularly common during and following exercise, occurring in the majority of patients subjected to stress electrocardiographic testing (including some without any clinical evidence of cardiac involvement).[771, 784] Syncope and sudden death due to ventricular fibrillation are a constant threat and may develop even before cardiomegaly or heart failure.[759] Sinus bradycardia may also be seen, even in patients with severe heart failure when a tachycardia would be expected, presumably related to cardiac autonomic dysfunction.[759, 764] Atrial arrhythmias, including atrial fibrillation, may also occur. Thromboembolic phenomena are a frequent complication,[771] occurring in more than 50 per cent of the patients.[785]

The *echocardiographic findings* in some are those of a dilated cardiomyopathy, with dilatation, increased end-diastolic and end-systolic volumes, reduced fractional systolic shortening of the left ventricle, and ejection fraction, often with enlargement of the left atrium and right ventricle.[771] Diastolic filling of the left ventricle is frequently abnormal, even in those without other clinical or echocardiographic evidence of cardiac involvement.[786, 787] In the majority of advanced cases, the echocardiographic appearance is distinctive, with left ventricular posterior wall hypokinesis and relatively preserved interventricular septal motion; an apical aneurysm is often seen on two-dimensional echocardiography.

Radionuclide ventriculography may, like echocardiography, demonstrate regional left ventricular wall motion abnormalities in the absence of an overall depression of global ventricular function.[788]

Left ventricular cineangiography in advanced cases shows a dilated, hypokinetic left ventricle with a large apical aneurysm containing intracavitary thrombus, often with evidence of mitral regurgitation (Fig. 42–30).[789] Mild asynergy in the anteroapical region, often associated with right ventricular enlargement and dysfunction, may be seen in some patients despite the absence of clinical, radiological, or electrocardiographic evidence of cardiac involvement.[790-792] *Coronary angiography* is usually normal, although abnormalities of the coronary microcirculation have been suggested as the cause of the clinical manifestations of Chagas' disease.[793]

The *complement-fixation* test (Machado-Guerreiro test) is useful in diagnosis; it has a sensitivity of greater than 90 per cent, with a specificity of 99 per cent[759] for the identification of chronic Chagas' disease. Also used in diagnosis are the indirect immunofluorescent antibody, the enzyme-linked immunosorbent assay (ELISA), and the hemagglutination tests.[794, 795] Another test that is occasionally useful is the detection of parasites in the blood of

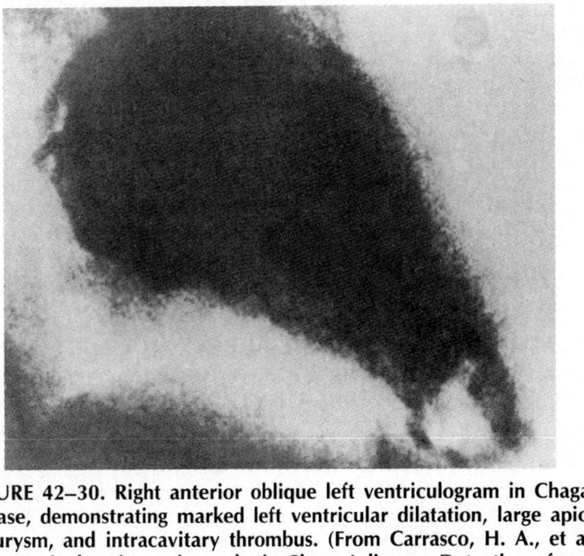

FIGURE 42–30. Right anterior oblique left ventriculogram in Chagas' disease, demonstrating marked left ventricular dilatation, large apical aneurysm, and intracavitary thrombus. (From Carrasco, H. A., et al.: Left ventricular cineangiography in Chagas' disease: Detection of early myocardial damage. Am. Heart J. *104*:595, 1982.)

patients with chronic Chagas' disease (which occurs in 30 to 40 per cent of cases) by means of *xenodiagnosis*. The patient is bitten by reduviid bugs bred in the laboratory; the subsequent identification of parasites in the intestine of the insect is proof of infection in the human host.[759]

TREATMENT. The management of Chagas' disease remains difficult; although slowly progressive at first, once cardiac decompensation develops, there is usually a rapid and inexorable progression to death, which is usually due to arrhythmia, congestive failure, and systemic thromboembolism.[796, 797] Prevention of the disease by control of transmission to humans is logical but expensive,[798] and has not been uniformly successful thus far.[781, 799] Amiodarone appears to be particularly effective in controlling the ubiquitous ventricular arrhythmias seen in Chagas' disease, although whether this translates into improved survival remains unestablished; intravenous amiodarone may result in myocardial depression.[758, 800-804] Anticoagulation may be of some benefit in preventing recurrent thromboembolic episodes.[785] While antiparasitic agents such as nifurtimox and benzimidazole are effective in reducing parasitemia, there is no evidence that they are efficacious in curing the disease.[799] A more promising avenue of approach appears to be immunoprophylaxis, although a clinically useful vaccine is not yet available.[760, 762]

AFRICAN TRYPANOSOMIASIS. African sleeping sickness, due to *Trypanosoma gambiense* or *T. rhodesiense*, may be associated with myocardial abnormalities, although they are usually of less functional significance than in so-called American trypanosomiasis (Chagas' disease).[805] *T. rhodesiense*, in particular, may lead to cardiac failure, although the central nervous system findings (excessive somnolence) usually dominate the clinical picture.

Pathological examination uniformly reveals pericardial fluid. The heart is not as greatly dilated and hypertrophied as it is in Chagas' disease and may appear grossly to be normal. There is often epicardial thickening with a cellular exudate composed of lymphocytes, plasma cells, and histiocytes.[806] The myocardium typically displays a diffuse interstitial infiltrate, often with zones of patchy fibrosis and interstitial edema.[806, 807]

Nonspecific *electrocardiographic* changes, usually T-wave abnormalities and prolongation of the Q-T interval,[805] are often observed. Unlike Chagas' disease, arrhythmias and conduction disturbances are usually not prominent features and the arterial pressure is usually normal. Some of the patients have asymptomatic cardiomegaly, although both pulmonary congestion and peripheral edema have been reported.

TOXOPLASMOSIS. *Toxoplasma* infections are caused by an obligate intracellular parasite (*T. gondii*); both congenital and acquired forms may occur. Symptomatic, acquired, toxoplasmic infections occur most commonly in immunosuppressed patients with malignant diseases, and occasionally in patients with acquired immune deficiency syndrome.[659, 808] *Pathological findings* include cardiac enlargement and hypertrophy, with occasional endocardial thrombi.[809] Petechial hemorrhages, an inflammatory infiltrate with variable degrees of edema and degeneration of the muscle bundles, and pericardial effusion are often present.

Most adult cases are asymptomatic, but *Toxoplasma* infections may produce a severe, fatal disease with multisystem involvement.[808] Toxoplasmic myocarditis, often with pericarditis, may occur as an isolated disease process or as part of a multisystem disseminated disease.[810] Manifestations may include arrhythmia (atrial and ventricular), AV block, pericarditis, and heart failure.[811] Large pericardial effusions may be seen on occasion.[812] Palpitations, tachycardia, chest discomfort, fatigue, pulmonary congestion, and peripheral edema may be prominent symptoms. *Physical examination* usually reveals cardiomegaly, congestive heart failure, gallop rhythm, systolic murmurs, and hypotension. The *electrocardiogram* may show a variety of abnormalities, including atrial and ventricular arrhythmias, bundle branch block or hypertrophy patterns, or AV conduction defects.[809, 813] When the myocardial involvement is one manifestation of disseminated disease, the antibody titers are typically quite high or rise rapidly. On the other hand, isolated myocarditis may be associated with low and nondiagnostic titers.

Treatment is with a combination of pyrimethamine and triple sulfonamides, but the response to therapy is variable.[813, 814] Corticosteroids may be helpful in treating arrhythmias or conduction defects.

MALARIA. While myocardial changes may be demonstrated during the course of malaria, particularly with *Plasmodium falciparum*, clinical findings to indicate cardiac involvement are rare. The heart generally demonstrates few gross abnormalities. The principal findings are histological. The capillaries are often filled and even distended with an accumulation of parasites, sometimes totally occluding the lumen of the vessels. Thrombosis of the capillaries and ischemic myocardial changes may be seen.[815, 816] Focal myocardial damage may be present, along with an interstitial infiltrate composed of lymphocytes, plasma cells, and macrophages. In rare cases, cardiac failure may contribute to or even cause death,[817] although it has not been demonstrated that chronic heart disease results from malaria. Slight ST-segment and T-wave changes on the electrocardiogram may be the only clinical indications of myocarditis.[818]

METAZOAL MYOCARDIAL DISEASE

SCHISTOSOMIASIS. Schistosomiasis is a major public health problem, with an infection rate as high as 85 per cent in heavily endemic areas, such as the Nile River basin in Africa and the Yangtze River basin in the Orient. Its principal cardiac effect is right heart overload secondary to pulmonary hypertension. Embolization of the schistosomal ova to the pulmonary vasculature results in an allergic pulmonary arteritis and a paravascular granulomatous reaction, which results in pulmonary hypertension. Right ventricular hypertrophy and right heart failure with chronic cor pulmonale occur typically in young adults.[819, 820]

Direct myocardial involvement, on the other hand, is quite infrequent.[821] Myocardial invasion by the ova may result in an inflammatory myocarditis, with a perivasculitis composed principally of mononuclear cells and eosinophils.[821] It has also been proposed that a myocarditis may occur in the absence of direct invasion by the parasite, and a toxic or allergic etiology has been postulated.[822]

HETEROPHYIASIS. This condition results from infestation by several intestinal flukes and is common, particularly in the Far East. The heart may become involved, presumably by hematogenous spread. The heart may be slightly dilated, particularly the right side, with prominent subepicardial hemorrhages. Chronic congestive heart failure is present for some time and may eventually culminate in the patient's death.[822, 823]

CYSTICERCOSIS. Cardiac involvement with *Cysticercus cellulosae*, the larval form of *Taenia solium*, is occasionally seen following a disseminated systemic infection. While electrocardiographic changes, including P- and T-wave abnormalities, as well as congestive heart failure have been reported, most cases of cardiac involvement are not apparent clinically.[824–826]

ECHINOCOCCUS (HYDATID CYST). *Echinococcus* is endemic in many sheep-raising areas of the world, particularly Argentina, Uruguay, New Zealand, Greece, North Africa, and Iceland, but cardiac involvement in hydatid disease is uncommon, occurring in less than 2 per cent of cases.[827] The usual host of *Echinococcus granulosus* is the dog, but human beings may serve as intermediate hosts (rather than the sheep, the usual intermediate host) if they accidentally ingest ova from contaminated dog feces.

The left ventricle is the most common site of cardiac involvement, presumably because of its richer coronary circulation.[828] Involvement of the interventricular septum and right ventricle may also occur.[828] A myocardial cyst may degenerate and calcify, develop daughter cysts, or rupture. Rupture of the cyst is the most dreaded complication; rupture into the pericardium may result in acute pericarditis, which may progress to chronic constrictive pericarditis. Rupture into the cardiac chambers may result in systemic or pulmonary emboli.[829] The liberation of hydatid fluid into the circulation may produce profound, fatal circulatory collapse due to an anaphylactic reaction to the protein constituents of the fluid.

Most patients with intact cysts are minimally symptomatic or asymptomatic.[830, 831] The *electrocardiogram* often reflects the location of the cyst; T-wave changes and loss of QRS voltage may occur with left ventricular involvement, while AV conduction defects or right bundle branch block may be seen with involvement of the interventricular septum. Chest pain is usually due to rupture of the cyst into the pericardial space with resultant pericarditis. Protrusion of a cyst from the interventricular septum into the right ventricular outflow tract may result in partial obstruction.[828]

Diagnosis. Recognition of an echinococcal cyst of the heart is a relatively simple matter if there is evidence of cysts in other organs, particularly the liver and lung. Unfortunately, the cardiac cyst is often an isolated, solitary finding. The *chest roentgenogram* frequently shows an abnormal cardiac silhouette or a calcified lobular mass adjacent to

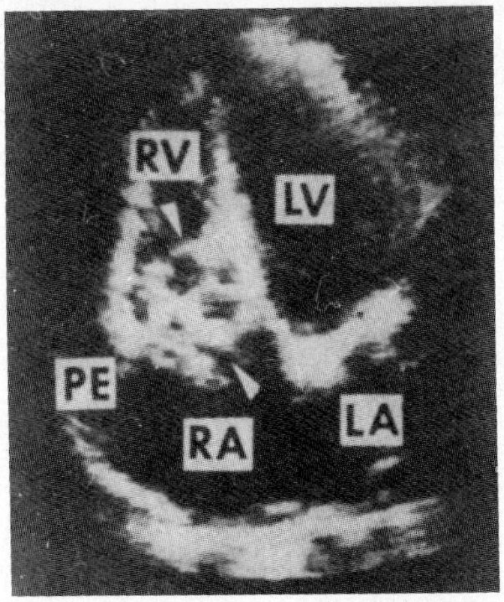

FIGURE 42–31. Two-dimensional echocardiogram in the apical four-chamber view in a patient with a large hydatid cyst (arrows) at the level of the tricuspid valve. The cyst was attached to the upper portion of the interventricular septum, just under the septal leaflet of the tricuspid valve. LA = left atrium; LV = left ventricle; PE = pericardial effusion; RA = right atrium; RV = right ventricle. (From Erol, C., et al.: Cardiac hydatid cyst simulating tricuspid stenosis. Am. J. Cardiol. 56:833, 1985.)

the left ventricle.[828] Two-dimensional echocardiography and computed tomography may prove useful in the early detection of cardiac involvement[827, 828, 832, 833] (Fig. 42–31). Definitive diagnosis is provided by cardiac catheterization and angiography. Hemodynamic measurements may demonstrate a gradient between the right ventricle and pulmonary artery in patients with obstruction to right ventricular outflow. *Eosinophilia*, present in some patients, is a useful adjunctive finding. The *Casoni skin test* is not very helpful because both false-positive and false-negative results occur. Serological tests, including hemagglutination and complement-fixation, are more useful.[830]

Management. Until recently treatment for hydatid disease was limited to surgical excision. Recent experience suggests that the benzimidazole derivative mebendazole may be an effective agent in the medical management of this disease.[834] Because of the significant risk of rupture of the cyst and its attendant serious and sometimes fatal consequences, surgical excision is generally recommended, even for asymptomatic patients.[827] The surgical results have been generally favorable, with complete recovery in many cases.[828]

VISCERAL LARVA MIGRANS. People are occasional accidental hosts of the roundworm infestations of dogs due to *Toxocara canis*. Most cases occur in children 1 to 3 years of age.[835] Myocarditis may occur in association with invasion of the myocardium by larvae. The myocardial lesions include granulomas or extensive inflammatory infiltrates with foci of muscle necrosis.[836] Congestive failure and death may occur, although complete recovery following the use of corticosteroids has been reported.[835, 836]

TRICHINOSIS. Infestation with *Trichinella spiralis* is the most common human helminthic disease, and evidence of involvement may be found in almost 1 per cent of routine autopsies.[837] Unlike some parasitic diseases with cardiac involvement, myocarditis plays a prominent role in trichinosis and is in fact responsible for the majority of fatalities.[838] The mortality of acute trichinosis is reported to be approximately 5 per cent. Less frequently, death is due to pulmonary embolism secondary to venous thrombosis as well as encephalitis.[838]

Although the parasite frequently invades the heart, it does not usually encyst there, and it is rare to find larvae or larval fragments in the myocardium. Nonetheless, *pathological findings* at postmortem examination may be impressive. The heart may be dilated and flabby and a pericardial effusion may be present. A prominent focal infiltrate composed of lymphocytes and eosinophils, with interstitial edema, hyperemia, and scattered hemorrhages, is commonly found.[822, 837, 838] Areas of muscle degeneration and necrosis are present. The lesions may be due to toxic effects of the products produced in the course of the host reaction.

Clinical Manifestations. These consist of congestive heart failure and chest pain, usually appearing around the third week of the disease, when the general constitutional symptoms are abating.[837, 839] Often, the cardiac symptoms are mild or absent or are overshadowed by other symptoms. Physical examination may be normal, or there may be gross cardiomegaly with severe congestive heart failure.[840] Sudden death may occur, usually in the fourth to eighth week of the illness.[822, 839]

Electrocardiographic abnormalities may be detected in one-fourth of patients with trichinosis and parallel the time course of clinical cardiac involvement, initially appearing in the second or third week and usually resolving by the seventh week of the illness.[837, 840] The most common electrocardiographic abnormalities are T-wave changes, followed by prolongation of the QRS complex, diminished QRS voltage, first-degree AV block,[840] and ventricular arrhythmias. The electrocardiographic changes usually resolve completely.

The definitive *diagnosis* is based on the demonstration of larval forms in tissue biopsy samples, usually of the gastrocnemius muscle. Eosinophilia, when present, is a supportive finding.[822] The skin test is usually but not invariably positive. Treatment is with corticosteroids; dramatic improvement in cardiac function has been reported following their use.[837, 838] Recovery from myocarditis may occur without residual cardiac damage.

NONINFECTIOUS MYOCARDIAL DAMAGE

A wide variety of stimuli other than those produced by infection may act on the heart and damage the myocardium.[841, 842] In some cases, the damage is acute, transient, and associated with evidence of myocardial inflammation (myocarditis). Other agents that damage the myocardium may lead to chronic changes with resulting histological evidence of fibrosis and a clinical picture of a dilated cardiomyopathy. Furthermore, many offending stimuli may be associated with both acute and chronic phases (e.g., alcohol, Adriamycin). The response often is related to the dose and rate of exposure.

Numerous chemicals and drugs (both industrial and therapeutic) may lead to cardiac damage and dysfunction. Several physical agents (e.g., radiation and excessive heat) may also result in myocardial damage. Furthermore, myocardial involvement may be evident in a variety of systemic diseases, which are described in Part IV of this book.

TOXIC, CHEMICAL, AND DRUG EFFECTS

COCAINE. Although the precise mechanism is as yet unestablished, a variety of cardiovascular complications are associated with cocaine abuse, including myocardial infarction (Chap. 38), ventricular arrhythmia, rupture of the ascending aorta, myocarditis, and sudden death.[843-849] Proposed mechanisms include peripheral and coronary vasoconstriction as a result of cocaine-mediated inhibition of reuptake of catecholamines by adrenergic nerve endings, increased myocardial oxygen demand, coronary spasm, or nonatherosclerotic obstructive coronary lesions.[850-853] The cardiovascular effects of cocaine are often countered with beta-adrenoceptor blockers; more recently, calcium channel blockers have been suggested as antagonists to the toxic cardiac effects of cocaine.[854]

TRICYCLIC ANTIDEPRESSANTS (See also p. 1894). Although sudden death, disturbances in rhythm, and abnormalities of AV conduction may be seen with the tricyclic antidepressants, particularly when taken as an overdose, important depression of left ventricular function is usually not seen, even in patients with preexisting heart disease.[855, 856] It is not clear if there is a synergistic depression of ventricular function when a tricyclic antidepressant is given with another drug (such as an antiarrhythmic) that also has negative inotropic effects.[857] Postural hypotension may be exacerbated, however, and heart block precipitated in patients with preexisting conducting system disease.[858, 859]

PHENOTHIAZINES (See also p. 1896). The phenothiazines may be associated with a variety of cardiac disturbances, including electrocardiographic changes, atrial and ventricular arrhythmias, and sudden death.[860, 861] Postural hypotension may also be seen.[857] The cardiac effects are largely dose-dependent. Electrocardiographic abnormalities may be seen with as little as 200 mg of thioridazine per day and consist of lengthening of the Q-T interval and T-wave changes. Prolongation of the Q-T interval may set the stage for the emergence of ventricular arrhythmias, particularly torsades de pointes (p. 698).[862, 863] Higher doses may lead to frank T-wave inversion and increase in the amplitude of the U wave.[860] Changes in the P wave, QRS complex, and ST segment are usually absent. The electrocardiographic abnormalities and arrhythmias resolve with discontinuation of the drug, usually within 48 hours.[864]

Pathological changes in the hearts of patients who have received psychotropic drugs and who have died suddenly include the deposition of acid mucopolysaccharide between muscle bundles in periarteriolar regions as well as the conduction system, with myofibrillar degeneration, and endothelial proliferation in the smaller blood vessels, although a direct causal relationship between drug administration and cardiomyopathic changes is only inferential.[857] A variety of explanations have been invoked for apparent cardiac damage, including direct toxic effects of the phenothiazines on the myocardium, stimulation of higher autonomic centers, and changes in circulating or myocardial levels of catecholamines.[865]

EMETINE. Cardiovascular changes are common with the use of emetine, a drug often employed in the treatment of amebiasis and schistosomiasis, presumably because of its prolonged duration of action and consequent potential for accumulation with resultant toxicity.[857] Myocardial lesions may be observed in some but not all patients at autopsy, and similar cardiac damage is noted in experimental animals given emetine.[860] The myocardial lesions consist of myofibrillar degeneration and necrosis, with an interstitial infiltrate of mononuclear cells and histiocytes. Emetine appears to inhibit oxidative phosphorylation and results in reversible damage to the mitochondria.[866] However, the observation that potassium administration often results in normalization of the T waves suggests that the electrocardiographic changes are due to transient intracellular ionic shifts.[867]

The *electrocardiogram,* which may be abnormal in 50 per cent of treated patients, most commonly shows reduced T-wave amplitude or inversion. Prolongation of the Q-T interval and ST-segment shifts may also be seen, although abnormalities of the P wave, P-R segment, and QRS complex are infrequent. The electrocardiographic changes usually resolve within weeks or months after cessation of treatment. Sinus tachycardia and hypotension may also be seen, although clinical evidence of myocardial toxicity is usually lacking. Only rare fatalities have been reported. *Dehydroemetine* results in electrocardiographic abnormalities similar to those of emetine, but they are less prominent and of shorter duration.

Emetine and dehydroemetine therapy should be discontinued upon appearance of clinical evidence of cardiac toxicity, but treatment may be continued cautiously if electrocardiographic changes are the only manifestation. Potassium supplementation may be employed so long as the serum potassium level is closely monitored.

METHYSERGIDE. The widespread fibrotic reactions seen with this drug can also involve the heart. Up to 1 per cent of patients treated long-term may develop typically left-sided valvular lesions resulting in stenosis and regurgitation.[857] Fibrotic endocardial and pericardial lesions are also seen on occasion, producing a hemodynamic picture of restrictive and constrictive disease.[868]

CHLOROQUINE. This drug has been widely used in the prophylaxis and treatment of a variety of parasitic diseases and has potent toxic cardiac effects, which appear to be related to its ability to inhibit cellular respiration by blocking the Krebs cycle.[869] It is a myocardial depressant in large doses, although routine doses are not usually associated with clinical evidence of cardiac dysfunction.[867, 869, 869a] Electrocardiographic changes may be seen and are similar to those seen with emetine, although they are less pronounced and of shorter duration. In toxic doses, chloroquine may result in depressed cardiac output, bradycardia, arrhythmias, heart block, and death.[869]

ANTIMONY COMPOUNDS. Various antimony compounds, such as stibophen and tartar emetic, have been widely used in the treatment of schistosomiasis; less toxic agents are now becoming available. The antimony compounds are associated with electrocardiographic changes in almost all patients.[870] Typical *electrocardiographic changes* include prolongation of the Q-T interval with flattening or inversion of T waves. ST-segment shifts and P-wave changes may be seen, although the QRS complex usually demonstrates no abnormality.[860] Most patients do not demonstrate cardiac findings, although chest pain, bradycardia, hypotension, ventricular arrhythmias (including paroxysmal ventricular tachycardia), and sudden death may occur.[871]

LITHIUM (See also p. 1897). Lithium carbonate, used in the treatment of manic-depressive disorders, is associated with T-wave changes in one-fourth or more of patients who receive the drug.[859, 872] Clinical evidence of myocardial involvement is usually lacking, although intoxication with lithium may be associated with ventricular arrhythmias, symptomatic sinus node abnormalities, atrioventricular conduction disturbances, congestive heart failure, and death.[872-875] In fatal lithium toxicity, the heart is dilated and there is evidence of myofibrillar degeneration associated with a lymphocytic interstitial infiltrate and fibrosis.[872] The risk of lithium toxicity appears to be increased in patients over the age of 60, and in those receiving other psychotropic drugs.[872]

HYDROCARBONS. Ingestion of hydrocarbons may result in fragmentation and vacuolization of the muscle fibers with loss of cross-striations.[876] Electrocardiographic changes, arrhythmias, and cardiomegaly may occur. Involvement of the central nervous, renal, hepatic, and pulmonary systems may dominate the clinical presentation and obscure the myocardial damage, which may well contribute to the mortality of hydrocarbon ingestion.[876] The electrocardiographic changes include ST-segment and T-wave abnormalities, although patterns suggesting acute myocardial injury have been noted.[877]

The *fluorinated hydrocarbons*, commonly used as aerosol propellants, appear to be cardiac toxins, contrary to their reputation of being inert. In animal preparations, at least, the aerosol propellants cause ventricular tachyarrhythmias, depress myocardial contractility, and lower systemic vascular resistance and arterial pressure.[878] These cardiovascular effects may be involved in the sudden deaths seen in individuals who abuse aerosols for their psychotropic effect.[879]

CATECHOLAMINES. Myocarditis is frequently observed in conjunction with pheochromocytoma, and the myocardial damage has been attributed to high levels of circulating catecholamines[71a, 880] (p. 1812). Similar changes have been demonstrated in experimental animals treated with prolonged infusions of L-norepinephrine. Catecholamines may produce an acute myocarditis, with focal myocardial necrosis, inflammation, epicardial hemorrhages, tachycardia, and arrhythmias.[881, 882] Phenylpropanolamine, a sympathomimetic amine used in decongestants and appetite suppressants, may result in similar findings.[883]

A variety of mechanisms have been suggested. A direct toxic effect may be involved, or the damage may be secondary to relative tissue hypoxia because of heightened metabolic demands.[884] Alternatively, the damage may result from changes in autonomic tone, enhanced lipid mobility, calcium overload, damaging effects of catecholamine oxidation products, or increased sarcolemmal permeability.[884–888] Aspirin and dipyridamole appear to offer some protection against experimental myocardial necrosis by catecholamines, suggesting that platelet aggregation plays a major role. It has been suggested that the rare development of a myocardial infarction after prolonged stress may result from intravascular platelet thrombosis induced by catecholamines, which may lead to occlusion of a coronary artery previously narrowed by an atheroma.[888]

LEAD. The prominent features in lead poisoning generally center on the gastrointestinal and central nervous systems. However, myocardial involvement may contribute to or be the principal cause of death in some cases.[841, 889] Reported pathological changes include cloudy swelling of the myofibers, with interstitial fibrosis and edema but without much of a cellular infiltrate. Electrocardiographic changes, chest pain, atrioventricular conduction defects, and overt congestive heart failure may occur.[879, 890] The electrocardiographic and myocardial changes appear to be reversible.

CARBON MONOXIDE. Both acute and chronic carbon monoxide toxicity are common. While central nervous system findings usually dominate the clinical presentation, significant and occasionally fatal cardiac abnormalities are often present.[891] Because carbon monoxide has a higher affinity for hemoglobin than does oxygen, insufficient oxygen is transported to the tissues.[892] Thus, the cardiac toxicity is the result of myocardial hypoxia, but a direct toxic effect of the gas on myocardial mitochondria may also play a role.[893] The *histological features* include focal areas of necrosis, most marked in the subendocardium. Focal perivascular infiltrates and punctate hemorrhages are also seen.[892] The electrocardiographic changes in survivors are transient.[892] Administration of 100 per cent oxygen, bed rest, and surveillance for serious rhythm or conduction abnormalities will usually permit rapid recovery.[892]

Cardiac involvement may appear promptly after exposure or it may be delayed for up to several days. Palpitations, sinus tachycardia, and various arrhythmias, including ventricular extrasystoles and atrial fibrillation, are common.[892, 894] Bradycardia and AV block may occur in more severe cases. In patients with ischemic heart disease, angina pectoris and myocardial infarction may be precipitated. Electrocardiographic ST-segment and T-wave abnormalities are quite common. Transient left ventricular wall motion abnormalities may be present.[895]

MERCURY. Electrocardiographic abnormalities,[879] principally ST-segment depression, T-wave changes, and prolongation of the Q-T interval, are common findings in mercury poisoning. However, no specific cardiac symptoms occur.[896]

PHOSPHORUS. Ingestion of phosphorus leads to death in 30 to 50 per cent of individuals, with most deaths occurring within 36 hours.[897] The heart is dilated, with diffuse interstitial edema but without a cellular infiltrate. Electrocardiographic abnormalities occur in the majority of patients and consist of ST-segment and T-wave abnormalities, prolongation of the QRS complex and Q-T interval, and atrial arrhythmias.[897] Prominent clinical features include severe biventricular depression of contractile function, peripheral vasodilatation, and marked hypotension.

HYPOCALCEMIA. In rare patients with chronic hypocalcemia (often due to hypoparathyroidism), congestive heart failure may occur and resolve only when the serum calcium level is raised.[898–901] Rapid transfusion of citrated blood can produce hypocalcemia and profound reversible myocardial depression.[902]

HYPOPHOSPHATEMIA. A form of reversible left ventricular dysfunction may be seen with severe hypophosphatemia. Restoration of the serum phosphate level to normal results in hemodynamic recovery.[903]

HYPOMAGNESEMIA. Focal cardiac necrosis is found in experimental magnesium deficiency and may account for the supraventricular and ventricular arrhythmias and electrocardiographic changes that are seen clinically.[904, 905] The ventricular arrhythmias are particularly likely to occur when hypomagnesemia complicates digitalis toxicity.[904]

SELENIUM DEFICIENCY. Dietary deficiency of the trace element selenium appears to be one of the principal factors responsible for a form of dilated cardiomyopathy endemic to certain rural areas in China that are deficient in selenium,[906] although others have questioned the etiological role played by selenium.[907] Termed *Keshan disease*, it affects mainly children and young women and apparently is prevented by the prophylactic administration of sodium selenite tablets.[908] A similar cardiomyopathy, occasionally fatal, may be found in Occidentals subjected to prolonged parenteral hyperalimentation.[909–912]

SCORPION STING. The venom of the scorpion is mainly neurotoxic, but cardiac findings may be prominent and even fatal, particularly in children.[841, 913] Hearts are normal on gross examination with prominent microscopic changes usually but not invariably present, particularly in the subendocardial regions and papillary muscles.[914] Degeneration and necrosis of muscle fibers are noted, with interstitial edema and a mononuclear infiltrate. The histological features of scorpion sting suggest high levels of circulating catecholamines[914, 915] and are similar to those seen with experimental catecholamine infusion and in pheochromocytoma. The parasympathetic system appears to be stimulated as well.[916]

The *electrocardiogram* often initially shows tall peaked T waves that progress to inversions and ST-segment shifts. Q waves may appear, and the Q-T interval is usually prolonged. Atrial, junctional, and ventricular arrhythmias may occur. Tachycardia, hypertension, anxiety, diaphoresis, and pulmonary edema—findings resembling those of a massive catecholamine effect—are striking in many patients.[914, 915] A smaller number of patients are seen in shock with peripheral vascular collapse. Most deaths are due to pulmonary edema, presumably the result of left ventricular dysfunction. Occasionally, sudden and unexpected deaths occur in a smaller percentage of patients, presumably as a consequence of arrhythmias. Adrenergic blocking agents and the use of specific antivenom appear to be useful in the management of the cardiovascular manifestation of scorpion stings.[917, 918]

WASP AND SPIDER STINGS. Stings by the vespine wasps may lead to hypotension, circulatory collapse, and cyanosis,[919] manifestations of anaphylaxis. Occasional patients may have chest pain and clinical findings compatible with acute myocardial infarction. The mechanism of myocardial damage is unclear; perhaps it merely reflects necrosis from profound hypotension, although a direct toxic effect on the myocardium or an indirect effect on the coronary arteries may be involved.

Cardiovascular collapse may also appear after stings due to the "black widow" spider (*Latrodectus mactans*). Atrial arrhythmias, labile blood pressure, and increased urinary levels of vanillylmandelic acid suggest that the stings may result in increased catecholamine levels.[920]

SNAKE BITE. Cardiac complications are usually not prominent features of snake bites, and the clinical picture is usually dominated by the neurological, hematological, and vascular damage produced by the snakebite toxin.[921] Myocardial involvement is seen on occasion and may rarely contribute to morbidity and mortality.[841] T-wave abnormalities are the most common manifestation of myocardial involvement, although ST-segment depression, QRS prolongation, and AV conduction defects may also be seen.[922] The electrocardiographic changes are usually transient, but when persistent they are attributed to direct myocardial damage due to the toxin.[923] Death may occur from circulatory collapse in adder bites, and myocardial infarction due to hypotension and coronary artery thrombosis has been reported[924]; coronary artery vasospasm may also be involved.[925]

ARSENIC. Arsenicals are currently utilized in pesticides. Myocardial involvement may be seen in both acute and chronic poisoning; the heart may be dilated, with accumulation of pericardial fluid.[926] Multiple local and confluent areas of subepicardial and subendocardial hemorrhage are characteristic findings.[926, 927] The myocardium is usually abnormal, with evidence of a perivascular mononuclear infiltrate.

Clinically unrecognized, toxic, interstitial myocarditis[928] is reflected in T-wave inversions and ST-segment depressions, along with prolongation of the Q-T interval.[929] The electrocardiographic changes usually revert to normal within 2 to 4 weeks. The electrocardiographic abnormalities appear to resolve more rapidly when BAL (British antilewisite, dimercaprol) is utilized in therapy.[930] Death is often due to acute renal failure, although circulatory collapse may occur.[926, 927]

Industrial exposure to *arsine gas* is often rapidly fatal, with deaths due to myocardial failure and uremia.[931] The principal toxic effect of arsine is on the red blood cells, with the production of massive hemolysis. Cardiac dilatation is typically present at postmortem examination. Myocardial edema with subepicardial hemorrhage, fibrosis, cloudy swelling, and fragmentation of muscle fibers with a minimal cellular infiltrate constitute the principal histological findings. T-wave changes are common. Death from pulmonary edema usually occurs within two days of exposure.

CYCLOPHOSPHAMIDE (See also p. 1751). High doses of cyclophosphamide (120 to 240 mg/kg over 1 to 4 days) have been associated with electrocardiographic changes, congestive heart failure, and death from hemorrhagic myocarditis.[932] In the majority of patients treated a reversible decrease of QRS voltage and systolic function is seen, often asymptomatic, although more than 20 per cent may succumb owing to myopericarditis.[933, 934] The hearts are dilated, with subepicardial and subendocardial ecchymoses, and the left ventricle is thickened.[934] The myocardial damage appears to result from direct endothelial damage and resultant fibrin microthrombi in the capillaries.

PARACETAMOL. Paracetamol, a phenacetin metabolite, may result in massive liver necrosis. On occasion it also results in fatty degeneration and focal necrosis of the myocardium, typically on the second to fourth day after an overdose.[935]

THYROID HORMONE. Rare cases of sudden death have been seen with thyroid hormone abuse, and pathological examination has revealed evidence of myocarditis with focal leukocytic infiltration and fibrosis.[936]

MICONAZOLE. Anaphylaxis and cardiac arrest may be seen in patients with hematological malignancies treated with the antifungal agent miconazole.[937] The mechanism of apparent cardiotoxicity is unclear.

DISOPYRAMIDE (See also p. 631). The antiarrhythmic agent disopyramide may lead to depression of left ventricular function when given either intravenously or orally, particularly after a large loading dose, although this effect usually is seen only in patients with preexisting left ventricular dysfunction.[938, 939] In addition to an exacerbation of congestive failure, disopyramide may also precipitate profound cardiovascular collapse and death.[940]

5-FLUOROURACIL. This antineoplastic agent has rarely been associated with cardiotoxicity manifested by chest pain, electrocardiographic changes, and arrhythmia.[932, 941] Swelling of myocardial fibers has been demonstrated in an animal preparation.[942]

DAUNORUBICIN AND ADRIAMYCIN (See p. 1748).

HYPERSENSITIVITY

Hypersensitivity to a variety of agents may result in allergic reactions that involve the myocardium. In addition to anaphylaxis and serum sickness, allergies to a variety of drugs (most commonly the sulfonamides, the penicillins, and methyldopa) or other sensitizers may lead to an allergic myocarditis, characterized by eosinophilia, and a perivascular infiltration of the myocardium by eosinophils, multinucleated giant

TABLE 42–13 DRUGS REPORTED TO BE ASSOCIATED WITH HYPERSENSITIVITY MYOCARDITIS

Acetazolamide	Para-aminosalicylic acid
Amitriptyline hydrochloride	Penicillin
Amphotericin B	Phenindione
Ampicillin	Phenylbutazone
Carbamazepine	Phenytoin
Chlorthalidone	Streptomycin
Hydrochlorothiazide	Sulfadiazine
Indomethacin	Sulfisoxazole
Isoniazid	Sulfonylureas
Methyldopa	Tetracycline
Oxyphenbutazone	

From Tabercio, C. P., et al.: Myocarditis related to drug hypersensitivity. Mayo Clin. Proc. *60*:463, 1985.

cells, and leukocytes (Table 42–13). Hypersensitivity myocarditis is rarely recognized clinically and is often first discovered at postmortem examination. Since some of the clinical courses of patients are marked by sudden death (presumably arrhythmic in origin), it is likely that undiagnosed hypersensitivity myocarditis may have significant clinical effects[943] (Table 42–14). Because of the significant deleterious effects, a high index of suspicion for this condition should be maintained, particularly if there is concomitant eosinophilia.[943] Therapy includes discontinuation of the offending agent, and corticosteroids and/or immunosuppression therapy in severe cases.[943]

METHYLDOPA. This drug is widely used in the treatment of hypertension (p. 872). Although hepatitis is the most frequently encountered serious adverse reaction, sudden and unexpected death has been reported in a number of patients found at necropsy to have had an unsuspected myocarditis.[842] The *histological findings* have the characteristics of an allergic myocarditis, showing an interstitial inflammatory infiltrate with abundant eosinophils, a vasculitis, and focal myocardial necrosis.[944] Electrocardiographic changes include sinus bradycardia, sinus pauses, and first- and second-degree AV block.[945]

PENICILLIN. Allergic reactions to penicillin are fairly common, but myocardial involvement is rare.[841, 842] *Histological findings* consist of a perivascular and interstitial infiltrate composed of eosinophils, plasma cells, lymphocytes, and histiocytes.[946] Both myocardial infarction and pericarditis may occur and account for some of the electrocardiographic changes.[947] Transient electrocardiographic changes may be the only manifestation of cardiac involvement, with bradycardia, ST-segment elevation, and T-wave inversion.

SULFONAMIDES. Sulfonamides may result in myocardial damage owing to a hypersensitivity vasculitis as well as a myocarditis.[943] Fatal cases usually demonstrate an eosinophilic myocarditis, sometimes with granulomas. While usually clinically silent, severe and even fatal congestive heart failure may occur.[948] Electrocardiographic changes are usually absent, but nonspecific ST-segment and T-wave abnormalities may be seen.[860, 948]

TETRACYCLINE. Allergic reactions to antibiotics of the tetracycline class include fever, tachycardia, and first-degree AV block. Postmortem findings include cardiac dilatation, fibrinoid muscle cell degeneration, and a diffuse interstitial and perivascular infiltrate.[841, 842]

PHENINDIONE. Marked congestive heart failure with cardiomegaly and pulmonary edema has been reported following the use of phenindione. The electrocardiogram may show sinus tachycardia, low QRS voltage, and T-wave inversion.[842, 949]

TABLE 42–14 FEATURES OF DRUG-INDUCED HYPERSENSITIVITY MYOCARDITIS

Electrocardiographic changes
- Inappropriate sinus tachycardia
- Conduction delays
- ST-segment and T-wave abnormalities

Mildly elevated myocardial enzyme levels (seen in 75% of patients)
Cardiomegaly
Hemodynamic collapse
Ventricular arrhythmias
Sudden death

Adapted from Tabercio, C. P., et al.: Myocarditis related to drug hypersensitivity. Mayo Clin. Proc. *60*:463, 1985.

PHENYLBUTAZONE. Myocarditis is an uncommon complication[842] but is characterized by dyspnea, chest pain, hypotension, and extensive ST-segment elevations.[950] Pericardial effusions with a prominent perivascular infiltrate may be seen in the myocardium.[951]

ANTITUBERCULOUS DRUGS. Most reactions to antituberculous drugs consist of a fever, rash, or both, but serious and fatal cardiac reactions may occur. *Paraaminosalicylic acid* may lead to the development of interstitial edema, acute inflammatory infiltrate, refractory congestive heat failure, hypotension, and ventricular irritability.[952] It is commonly associated with transient arrhythmias or cardiac dilatation.[953]

Streptomycin has been implicated as a rare cause of myocarditis. Pathological findings may include cardiac dilatation, myocarditis with necrosis, hemorrhage, and a fibrinous pericardial effusion.[954] Clinically, it may be associated with chest pain, dyspnea, fever, and rash, followed by collapse and death.

LYME CARDITIS. Lyme disease is caused by a tickborne spirochete (*Borrelia burgdorferi*).[955] The disease is found principally in areas of tick distribution (northeastern, midwestern, and western United States),[956] with the majority of cases found in the northeastern coast. It usually begins during the summer months with a characteristic skin rash (erythema chronicum migrans), followed in weeks to months by neurological, joint, or cardiac involvement.[957, 958] The later manifestations, including carditis, have been thought to be immune-mediated, perhaps related to circulating immune complexes,[959] although the demonstration of spirochetes in the myocardium of one patient suggests that direct cardiac damage may be involved.[960]

About 10 per cent of patients with Lyme disease develop evidence of cardiac involvement, the most common manifestation being variable degrees of AV block. Syncope due to complete heart block is frequent with cardiac involvement, as are diffuse ST-segment and T-wave abnormalities.[959] Transient asymptomatic left ventricular dysfunction may be detected by radionuclide ventriculography in as many as one-third of patients, although cardiomegaly or symptoms of congestive heart failure are rare.[959] A positive gallium scan may point to suspected cardiac involvement in this disease[961, 962] (Fig. 42–32).

The value of specific therapy in Lyme carditis remains uncertain; however, it is thought that treating the early manifestations of the disease may prevent development of late complications.[963, 964] Although the skin eruption responds to tetracycline or penicillin, a beneficial effect of antibiotics on the carditis is unestablished.[959] Advanced AV block is usually treated with salicylates or prednisone, although patients with the most severe involvement (meningoencephalitis, complete AV block for longer than one week, or cardiomegaly) are treated routinely with corticosteroids. Temporary transvenous pacing may be required for up to a week in patients with complete heart block.[959]

GIANT CELL MYOCARDITIS. Giant cell myocarditis is a rare disease of unknown etiology characterized by the presence of multinucleated giant cells in the myocardium. Variously called acute isolated myocarditis and granulomatous myocarditis, this condition is typically a rapidly fatal disease, often of young to middle-aged adults.[965] *Pathological findings* are usually impressive. The ventricles are dilated, and when death is not sudden, mural thrombi may be present. A serpiginous area of myocardial necrosis may be seen involving the right as well as the left ventricle.[965, 966] Multinucleated giant cells are found, particularly at the margins of the areas of myocardial necrosis; the giant cells appear to be of macrophage, rather than myocyte origin.[966, 967] An extensive inflammatory infiltrate is present within the necrotic areas, composed of eosinophils, histiocytes, and other cells.[965, 966]

Although giant cell myocarditis appears to be associated with thymoma, systemic lupus erythematosus, and thyro-

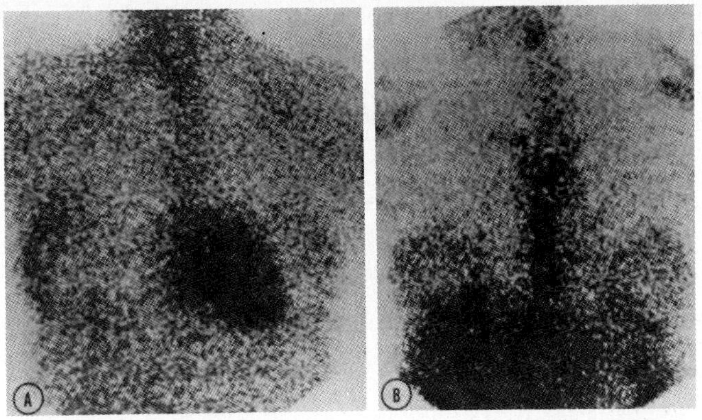

FIGURE 42–32. Gallium-67 scan in patient with Lyme disease showing striking myocardial uptake (*A*) with resolution 8 weeks later (*B*); hepatic uptake but not cardiac uptake is prominent. (From Jacobs, J. C., et al.: Lyme carditis diagnosed by gallium scan. J. Pediatr. *105*:950, 1984.)

toxicosis,[968] the cause of the disease remains obscure. In many ways the clinical features suggest a viral myocarditis except for the rapid and virulent course. However, despite careful investigation there has been no serological or bacteriological evidence of an infectious etiology.[965] Sarcoid, syphilis, and tuberculosis have all been proposed as possible causes, although these usually present distinctive histological features. It has also been suggested that the cause is an autoimmune reaction,[965, 968] although little evidence aside from the histological findings supports this view.

Both sexes are equally affected; the onset is typically rapid, with dyspnea, chest pain, orthopnea, and hypotension.[965, 969] Fever is usually present with electrocardiographic evidence of widespread myocardial involvement. Sinus tachycardia, left bundle branch block, atrial and ventricular arrhythmias, complete heart block, and findings suggesting acute myocardial necrosis may be seen.[969] Overt congestive heart failure and sudden death may occur.[965] Therapy is invariably unsuccessful, although corticosteroids and immunosuppressive agents have been used. It has been suggested that cyclosporine might be more effective.[965]

REJECTION OF THE TRANSPLANTED HEART. A major barrier to wider application of cardiac transplantation remains the problem of immunologically mediated injury as a result of rejection (p. 1664). Acute rejection is most frequent in the first 3 months after transplantation. In the immediate postoperative period, immunosuppression is accomplished with high-dose prednisone and cyclosporine.[970, 971] The findings in rejection may be clinically subtle, particularly when cyclosporine is used.[972] In the era before cyclosporine, rejection was often heralded by congestive heart failure and a decline in the QRS voltage, presumably secondary to myocardial edema secondary to the rejection process. With the use of cyclosporine, rejection is a smoldering process without prominent clinical findings, probably related to the absence of the interstitial myocardial edema that was so common in the precyclosporine era. As a consequence, the presence and severity of rejection can be evaluated only by percutaneous right ventricular endomyocardial biopsy. A biopsy specimen is usually obtained as a baseline shortly after transplantation and the procedure repeated routinely and during suspected rejection episodes. During rejection, initially there are perivascular and endocardial mononuclear cell infiltrates, which later extend into the interstitium and result in myocyte necrosis.[973, 974] A peculiar form of myocardial fibrosis of uncertain significance is found in the biopsy specimens of many heart transplant patients treated with cyclosporine.[972]

Treatment of early acute rejection by intensive immunosuppression is usually successful, although a significant number of infections and other serious complications occur as a result of the immunosuppression. Late chronic rejection is believed to be responsible for the accelerated development of atherosclerosis in the coronary arteries of the transplanted heart.[970] The use of warfarin and dipyridamole as well as of diets low in cholesterol and saturated fats has reduced the incidence of heart transplant arteriosclerosis, but it continues to be a major problem, accounting for about 50 per cent of the cardiac transplant failures after 2 years.[975]

PHYSICAL AGENTS

HEAT STROKE. This condition results from failure of the thermoregulatory center following exposure to high ambient temperature and is manifested principally by hyperpyrexia and central nervous system dysfunction. However, cardiovascular abnormalities are common. *Pathological changes* include dilatation of the right side of the heart, particularly the right atrium. Hemorrhages of the subendocardium and the subepicardium are frequently seen at necropsy and often involve the interventricular septum and posterior wall of the left ventricle. Histological findings include degeneration and necrosis of muscle fibers as well as interstitial edema.[976, 977] Possible factors responsible for myocardial damage include direct thermal injury, myocardial hypoxia secondary to circulatory collapse, decreased coronary blood flow, and metabolic abnormalities resulting from widespread injury to other organs.[976] Hypotension and circulatory collapse may occur.

Sinus tachycardia is invariably present, while atrial and ventricular arrhythmias are usually absent. Transient prolongation of the Q-T interval may be seen, along with ST-segment and T-wave abnormalities. It may take up to several months for these repolarization abnormalities to resolve.[976] P-wave abnormalities may occur, but abnormalities of the QRS complex or of atrioventricular conduction are not usually seen. Serum enzyme levels may be elevated and may reflect myocardial damage, at least in part.

HYPOTHERMIA. Low temperature may also result in myocardial damage. Cardiac dilatation may occur with epicardial petechiae and subendocardial hemorrhages.[978] Microinfarcts are present in the ventricular myocardium, and fatty changes are common.[979] The lesions are not due to the low temperature per se but appear to be the result of the circulatory collapse, hemoconcentration, capillary sludging, and depressed cellular metabolism that accompany hypothermia.

RADIATION. The employment of ionizing radiation during radiotherapy or, less commonly, after radiation accidents, may result in a variety of acute and chronic cardiac complications including pericarditis with effusion, tamponade, and constriction; coronary artery fibrosis and myocardial infarction; myocardial fibrosis; and conduction disturbances.[980–985] While the heart is thought to be one of the organs most resistant to the effects of radiation, damage to the pericardium (p. 1746), myocardium, and endocardium occurs. Although radiation probably results in some degree of tissue damage in all patients, clinically significant cardiac involvement occurs in the minority of patients.[984] Radiation-induced cardiac damage is related to the dose of radiation, the mass of heart irradiated, and the dose schedule of the radiation.

Acute cardiac damage has been studied in experimental animals, and it appears that the findings are similar in humans.[986] The initial changes are those of a pancarditis, with an exudative infiltrate of the pericardium, epicardium, myocardium, and endocardium, often with inflammation of the smaller arteries. The acute changes resolve within 48 hours, to be followed by a latent period in which there are no important pathological findings. The late cardiac damage following irradiation appears to result from a long-lasting injury of the capillary endothelial cells, which leads to cell death, capillary rupture, and microthrombi. Because of this damage to the microvasculature, ischemia results and is followed by myocardial fibrosis.[986] In addition to microvascular damage, the major epicardial coronary arteries may become narrowed.[941, 987]

Only an occasional patient manifests acute cardiac abnormality clinically with radiation therapy; typically this consists of acute pericarditis. A mild, transient, asymptomatic depression of left ventricular function may be seen early after radiation therapy.[981] The more common clinical expressions of radiation heart disease occur months or years after the exposure. The pericardium is the most common site of clinical involvement, with findings of chronic pericardial effusion or pericardial constriction.[986] Myocardial damage occurs less frequently[988, 989] and is characterized by myocardial fibrosis with or without endocardial fibrosis or fibroelastosis.[986] Left and/or right ventricular dysfunction at rest or with exercise appears to be a common, albeit usually asymptomatic, finding 5 to 20 years after radiation therapy, especially in those in whom the now-outmoded technique of a single anteroposterior port was used.[980, 982, 984, 990] It appears that radiation and cancer chemotherapeutic agents may act synergistically in producing myocardial damage and that withdrawal of corticosteroids may activate previously subclinical radiation injury. In experimental animals, corticosteroids and nonsteroidal antiinflammatory agents, if given early, retard the development of radiation-induced heart disease.[991]

REFERENCES

CLASSIFICATION AND ENDOMYOCARDIAL BIOPSY

1. Shabetai, R.: Cardiomyopathy: How far have we come in 25 years, how far yet to go? J. Am. Coll. Cardiol. *1*:252, 1983.
2. Brigden, W.: Uncommon myocardial diseases: The non-coronary cardiomyopathies. Lancet *2*:1179, 1957.
3. Report of the WHO/ISFC task force on the definition and classification of cardiomyopathies. Br. Heart J. *44*:672, 1980.
4. Pantely, G. A., and Bristow, J. D.: Ischemic cardiomyopathy. Prog. Cardiovasc. Dis. *27*:95, 1984.
4a. Goodwin, J. F.: The frontiers of cardiomyopathy. Br. Heart J. *48*:1, 1982.
5. Gillum, R. F.: Idiopathic cardiomyopathy in the United States, 1970–1982. Am. Heart J. *111*:752, 1986.
6. Abelmann, W. H.: Classification and natural history of primary myocardial disease. Prog. Cardiovasc. Dis. *27*:73, 1984.
7. Przybojewski, J. Z.: Endomyocardial biopsy: A review of the literature. Cathet. Cardiovasc. Diagn. *11*:287, 1985.
8. Fowles, R. E., and Mason, J. W.: Endomyocardial biopsy. Ann. Intern. Med. *97*:885, 1982.
9. Unverferth, D. V., and Baker, P. B.: Value of endomyocardial biopsy. Am. J. Med. *80*:22, 1986.
10. O'Connell, J. B., Costanzo-Nordin, M. R., Subramanian, R., and Robinson, J. A.: Dilated cardiomyopathy: Emerging role of endomyocardial biopsy. Curr. Probl. Cardiol. *11*:446, 1986.
11. Williams, G. A., Kaintz, R. P., Habermehl, K. K., Nelson, J. G., and Kennedy, H. L.: Clinical experience with two-dimensional echocardiography to guide endomyocardial biopsy. Clin. Cardiol. *8*:137, 1985.
12. French, J. W., Popp, R. L., and Pitlick, P. I.: Cardiac localization of transvascular bioptome using two-dimensional echocardiography. Am. J. Cardiol. *51*:219, 1983.
13. Baandrup, U., Florio, R. A., Rehahn, M., Richardson, P. J., and Olsen, E. G. J.: Critical analysis of endomyocardial biopsies from patients suspected of having cardiomyopathy. II. Comparison of histology and clinical/hemodynamic information. Br. Heart J. *45*:487, 1981.
14. Mason, J. W.: Endomyocardial biopsy: the balance of success and failure. Circulation *71*:185, 1985.
15. Fowles, R. E., and Mason, J. W.: Role of cardiac biopsy in the diagnosis and management of cardiac disease. Prog. Cardiovasc. Dis. *27*:153, 1984.
16. Aretz, H. T., Diagnosis of myocarditis by endomyocardial biopsy. Med. Clin. North Am. *70*:1220, 1986.

DILATED CARDIOMYOPATHY

17. Keren, A., Billingham, M. E., Weintraub, D., Stinson, E. B., and Popp, R. L.: Mildly dilated congestive cardiomyopathy. Circulation *72*:302, 1985.
18. Johnson, R. A., and Palacios, I.: Dilated cardiomyopathies of the adult. N. Engl. J. Med. *307*:1051 and 1119, 1982.
19. Fuster, V., Gersh, B. J., Giuliani, E. R., Tajik, A. J., Brandenburg, R. O., and Grye, R. L.: The natural history of idiopathic dilated cardiomyopathy. Am J. Cardiol. *47*:525, 1981.
20. Unverferth, D. V., Magorien, R. D., Moeschberger, M. L., Baker, P. B., Fetters, J. K., and Leier, C. V.: Factors influencing the one-year mortality of dilated cardiomyopathy. Am. J. Cardiol. *54*:147, 1984.
21. Hayakawa, M., Inoh, T., and Fukazaki, H.: Dilated cardiomyopathy. An echocardiographic follow-up of 50 patients. Jpn. Heart J. *25*:955, 1984.
22. Franciosa, J. A., Wilen, M., Ziesche, S., and Cohn, J. N.: Survival in men with severe chronic left ventricular failure due to either coronary heart disease or idiopathic dilated cardiomyopathy. Am. J. Cardiol. *51*:831, 1983.
23. Natural history of dilated cardiomyopathy (editorial). Lancet *1*:248, 1986.
24. Figulla, H. R., Rahlf, G., Nieger, M., Luig, H., and Kreuzer, H.: Spontaneous hemodynamic improvement or stabilization and associated biopsy findings in patients with congestive cardiomyopathy. Circulation *71*:1095, 1985.
25. Taliercio, C. P., Seward, J. B., Driscoll, D. J., Fisher, L. D., Gersh, B. J., and Tajik, A. J.: Idiopathic dilated cardiomyopathy in the young: Clinical profile and natural history. J. Am. Coll. Cardiol. *6*:1126, 1985.
26. Van der Hauwaert, L. G., Denef, B., and Dumoulin, M.: Long-term echocardiographic assessment of dilated cardiomyopathy in children. Am. J. Cardiol. *52*:1066, 1983.
27. Benjamin, I. J., Schuster, E. H., and Bulkley, B. H.: Cardiac hypertrophy in idiopathic dilated congestive cardiomyopathy: A clinicopathologic study. Circulation *64*:442, 1981.
28. Rose, A. G., and Beck, W.: Dilated (congestive) cardiomyopathy: A syndrome of severe cardiac dysfunction with remarkably few morphological features of myocardial damage. Histopathology *9*:367, 1985.
29. Miller, D. H., and Borer, J. S.: The cardiomyopathies. A pathophysiologic approach to therapeutic management. Arch. Intern. Med. *143*:2157, 1983.
30. Davies, M. J.: The cardiomyopathies: A review of terminology, pathology and pathogenesis. Histopathology *8*:363, 1984.
31. Fitchett, D. H., Sugrue, D. D., MacArthur, C. G., and Oakley, C. M.: Right ventricular dilated cardiomyopathy. Br. Heart J. *52*:25, 1984.
32. Ibsen, H. H. W., Baandrup, U., and Simonsen, E. E.: Familial right ventricular dilated cardiomyopathy. Br. Heart J. *54*:156, 1985.
33. Unverferth, D. V., Baker, P. B., Swift, S. E., Chaffee, R., Fetters, J. K., Uretsky, B. F., Thompson, M. E., and Leier, C. V.: Extent of myocardial fibrosis and cellular hypertrophy in dilated cardiomyopathy. Am. J. Cardiol. *57*:816, 1986.
34. Dick, M. R., Unverferth, D. V., and Baba, N.: The pattern of myocardial degeneration in nonischemic congestive cardiomyopathy. Hum. Pathol. *13*:740, 1982.
35. Tazelaar, H. D., and Billingham, M. E.: Leukocytic infiltrates in idiopathic dilated cardiomyopathy. A source of confusion with active myocarditis. Am. J. Surg. Pathol. *10*:405, 1986.
36. Rose, A. G., Fraser, R. C., and Beck, W.: Absence of evidence of myocarditis in endomyocardial biopsy specimens from patients with dilated (congestive) cardiomyopathy. S. Afr. Med. J. *66*:871, 1984.
37. Amorim, D. S., and Olsen, E. G. J.: Assessment of heart neurons in dilated (congestive) cardiomyopathy. Br. Heart J. *47*:11, 1982.
38. Schwarz, F., Mall, G., Zebe, H., Blickle, J., Derks, H., Manthey, J., and Kubler, W.: Quantitative morphologic findings of the myocardium in idiopathic dilated cardiomyopathy. Am. J. Cardiol. *51*:501, 1983.
39. Peters, T. J., Wells, G., Oakley, C. M., Brooksby, I. A. B., Jenkins, B. S., Webb-Peploe, M. M., and Coltart, D. J.: Enzymatic analysis of endocardial biopsy specimens from patients with cardiomyopathies. Br. Heart J. *39*:1333, 1977.
40. Hartz, A. J., Anderson, A. J., Brooks, H. L., Manley, J. C., Parent. G. T., and Barboriak, J. J.: The association of smoking with cardiomyopathy. N. Engl. J. Med. *311*:1201, 1984.
40a. Unverferth, D. V.: Dilated cardiomyopathy. Mt. Kisco, N.Y., Futura Publishing Co., 1985.
41. Goodwin, J. F.: Mechanisms in cardiomyopathies. J. Mol. Cell. Cardiol. *17*:5, 1985.
42. Shapiro, L. M., Rozkovec, A., Cambridge, G., Hallidie-Smith, K. A., and Goodwin, J. F.: Myocarditis in siblings leading to chronic heart failure. Eur. Heart J. *4*:742, 1983.
43. Kereiakes, D. J., and Parmley, W. W.: Myocarditis and cardiomyopathy. Am Heart J. *108*:1318, 1984.
44. Cassling, R. S., Linder, J., Sears, T. D., Waller, B. F., Rogler, W. C., Wilson, J. E., Kugler, J. D., Kay, D. H., Dillon, J. C., Slack, J. D., and McManus, B. M.: Quantitative evaluation of inflammation in biopsy specimens from idiopathically failing or irritable hearts: Experience in 80 pediatric and adult patients. Am. Heart J. *110*:713, 1985.
45. Zee-Cheng, C. S., Tsae, C. C., Palmer, D. C., Codd, J. E., Pennington, D. G., and Williams, G. A.: High incidence of myocarditis by endomyocardial biopsy in patients with idiopathic congestive cardiomyopathy. J. Am. Coll. Cardiol. *3*:63, 1984.
46. Parrillo, J. E., Aretz, H. T., Palacios, I., Fallon, J. T., and Block, P. C.: The results of transvenous endomyocardial biopsy can frequently be used to diagnose myocardial diseases in patients with idiopathic heart failure. Endomyocardial biopsies in 100 consecutive patients revealed a substantial incidence of myocarditis. Circulation *69*:93, 1984.
47. Fenoglio, J. J., Jr., Ursell, P. C., Kellogg, C. F., Drusin, R. E., and Weiss, M. B.: Diagnosis and classification of myocarditis by endomyocardial biopsy. N. Engl. J. Med. *308*:12, 1983.
48. Shanes, J. G., Krone, R. J., Tsai, C. C., Fischer, K., and Williams, G. A.: Mild myocardial inflammation presenting as congestive cardiomyopathy responsive to immunosuppression. Am. Heart J. *107*:798, 1984.
49. Dec, G. W. Jr., Palacios, I. F., Fallon, J. T., Aretz, H. T., Mills, J., Lee, D. C., and Johnson, R. A.: Active myocarditis in the spectrum of acute dilated cardiomyopathies. Clinical features, histologic correlates, and clinical outcome. N. Engl. J. Med. *312*:885, 1985.
50. Nippoldt, T. B., Edwards, W.D., Holmes, D. R. Jr., Reeder, G. S., Hartzler, G. O., and Smith, H. C.: Right ventricular endomyocardial biopsy: Clinicopathologic correlates in 100 consecutive patients. Mayo Clin. Proc. *57*:407, 1982.
51. MacArthur, C. G., Tarin, D., Goodwin, J. F., and Hallidie-Smith, K. A.: The relationship of myocarditis to dilated cardiomyopathy. Eur. Heart J. *5*:1023, 1984.
52. Bowles, N. E., Richardson, P. J., Olsen, E. G., and Archard, L. C.: Detection of Coxsackie B virus–specific RNA sequences in myocardial biopsy samples from patients with myocarditis and dilated cardiomyopathy. Lancet *1*:1120, 1986.
53. Regan, T. J.: Alcoholic cardiomyopathy. Prog. Cardiovasc. Dis. *27*:141, 1984.
54. Lowry, P. J., Edwards, C. W., and Nagle, R. E.: Herpes-like virus particles in myocardium of patient progressing to congestive cardiomyopathy. Br. Heart J. *48*:501, 1982.
55. O'Connell, J. B., Robinson, J. A., Henkin, R. E., and Gunnar, R. M.: Immunosuppressive therapy in patients with congestive cardiomyopathy and myocardial uptake of gallium-67. Circulation *64*:780, 1981.

56. O'Connell, J. B., Henkin, R. E., Robinson, J. A., Subramanian, R., Scanlon, P. J., and Gunnar, R. M.: Gallium-67 imaging in patients with dilated cardiomyopathy and biopsy-proven myocarditis. Circulation *70*:58, 1984.
57. O'Connell, J. B., Henkin, R. E., and Robinson, J. A.: Imaging techniques for myocardial inflammation. Ann. Clin. Lab. Sci. *16*:146, 1986.
58. O'Connell, J. B., and Henkin, R. E.: Myocardial gallium-67 imaging in dilated cardiomyopathy. Postgrad. Med. J. *61*:1132, 1985.
59. Eckstein, R., Mempel, W., and Bolte, H.-D.: Reduced suppressor cell activity in congestive cardiomyopathy and in myocarditis. Circulation *65*:1224, 1982.
60. Dilated Cardiomyopathy—an immunological tombstone? (editorial). Int. J. Cardiol. *6*:443, 1984.
61. Lowry, P. J., Thompson, R. A., and Littler, W. A.: Humoral immunity in cardiomyopathy. Br. Heart J. *50*:390, 1983.
62. Yamakawa, K., Fukuta, S., Kimura, Y., Hayashi, Y., and Kusukawa, R.: Circulating anti-heart antibodies in heart diseases detected using an immunofluorescent technique. Jpn. Circ. J. *47*:1173, 1983.
63. Maisch, B., Deeg, P., Liebau, G., and Kochsiek, K.: Diagnostic relevance of humoral and cytotoxic immune reactions in primary and secondary dilated cardiomyopathy. Am. J. Cardiol. *52*:1072, 1983.
64. Maisch, B.: Surface antigens of adult heart cells and their use in diagnosis. Basic Res. Cardiol. *80*:47, 1985.
65. Anderson, J. L., Carlquist, J. F., and Hammond, E. H.: Deficient natural killer cell activity in patients with idiopathic dilated cardiomyopathy. Lancet *2*:1124, 1982.
66. Sanderson, J. E., Koech, D., Iha, D., and Ojiambo, H. P.: T-lymphocyte subsets in idiopathic dilated cardiomyopathy. Am. J. Cardiol. *55*:755, 1985.
67. Franceschini, R., Messina, V., Petillo, A., Corazza, M., Bottaro, L., and Gianrossi, R.: Humoral immunity and lymphocyte subpopulations in patients with dilated cardiomyopathy. Int. J. Cardiol. *8*:113, 1985.
68. Anderson, J. L., Carlquist, J. F., and Higashikubo, R.: Quantitation of lymphocyte subsets by immunofluorescence flow cytometry in idiopathic dilated cardiomyopathy. Am. J. Cardiol. *55*:1550, 1985.
69. Lowry, P. J., Thompson, R. A., and Littler, W. A.: Cellular immunity in congestive cardiomyopathy. The normal cellular immune response. Br. Heart J. *53*:394, 1985.
70. Olsen, E. G. J.: Myocarditis—a case of mistaken identity? Br. Heart J. *50*:303, 1983.
71. Katz, A. M., Freston, J. W., Messineo, F. C., and Herbette, L. G.: Membrane damage and the pathogenesis of cardiomyopathies. J. Mol. Cell. Cardiol. *17*:11, 1985.
71a. Imperato-McGinley, J., Gautier, T., Ehlers, K., Zullo, M. A., Goldstein, D. S., and Vaughan, E. D., Jr.: Reversibility of catecholamine-induced dilated cardiomyopathy in a child with a pheochromocytoma. N. Engl. J. Med. *316*:793, 1987.
72. Factor, S. M., and Sonnenblick, E. H.: Hypothesis: Is congestive cardiomyopathy caused by hyperactive myocardial microcirculation (microvascular spasm)? (Editorial) Am. J. Cardiol. *50*:1149, 1982.
73. O'Connell, J. B., Fowles, R. E., Robinson, J. A., Subramanian, R., Henkin, R. E., and Gunnar, R. M.: Clinical and pathologic findings of myocarditis in two families with dilated cardiomyopathy. Am. Heart J. *107*:127, 1984.
74. Graber, H. L., Unverferth, D. V., Baker, P. B., Ryan, J. M., Baba, N., and Wooley, C. F.: Evolution of a hereditary cardiac conduction and muscle disorder: A study involving a family with six generations affected. Circulation *74*:21, 1986.
75. Michels, V. V., Driscoll, D. J., and Miller, F. A., Jr.: Familial aggregation of idiopathic dilated cardiomyopathy. Am. J. Cardiol. *55*:1232, 1985.
76. Greenlee, P. R., Anderson, J. L., Lutz, J. R., Lindsay, A. E., and Hagan, A. D.: Familial automaticity-conduction disorder with associated cardiomyopathy. Clin. Invest. *1*:33, 1986.
77. Przybojewski, J. Z., van der Walt, J. J., van Eeden, P. J., and Tiedt, F. A.: Familial dilated (congestive) cardiomyopathy. Occurrence in two brothers and an overview of the literature. S. Afr. Med. J. *66*:26, 1984.
77a. Berko, B. A., and Swift, M.: X-linked dilated cardiomyopathy. N. Engl. J. Med. *316*:1186, 1987.
78. Unverferth, D. V.: Etiologic factors, pathogenesis, and prognosis of dilated cardiomyopathy. J. Lab. Clin. Med. *106*:349, 1985.
79. Waber, L. J., Valle, D., Neill, C. DiMauro, S., and Shug, A.: Carnitine deficiency presenting as familial cardiomyopathy: A treatable defect in carnitine transport. J. Pediatr. *101*:700, 1982.
80. Bulkley, B. H.: The cardiomyopathies. Hosp. Pract. *19*:59, 1984.
81. Torp, A.: Incidence of congestive cardiomyopathy. Postgrad. Med. J. *54*:435, 1978.
82. Pasternac, A., and Bourassa, M. G.: Pathogenesis of chest pain in patients with cardiomyopathies and normal coronary arteries. Int. J. Cardiol. *3*:273, 1983.
83. Pasternac, A., Noble, J., Streulens, Y., Elie, R., Henschke, C., and Bourassa, M. G.: Pathophysiology of chest pain in patients with cardiomyopathies and normal coronary arteries. Circulation *65*:778, 1982.
84. Nitenberg, A., Foult, J. M., Blanchet, F., and Zouioueche, S.: Multifactorial determinants of reduced coronary flow reserve after dipyridamole in dilated cardiomyopathy. Am. J. Cardiol. *55*:748, 1985.
85. Unverferth, D. V., Magorien, R. D., Lewis, R. P., and Leier, C. V.: The role of subendocardial ischemia in perpetuating myocardial failure in patients with nonischemic congestive cardiomyopathy. Am. Heart J. *105*:176, 1983.
86. Boltwood, C. M., Tei, C., Wong, M., and Shah, P. M.: Quantitative echocardiography of the mitral complex in dilated cardiomyopathy: The mechanism of functional mitral regurgitation. Circulation *68*:498, 1983.
87. Huang, S. K., Messer, J. V., and Denes, P.: Significance of ventricular tachycardia in idiopathic dilated cardiomyopathy: Observations in 35 patients. Am. J. Cardiol. *51*:507, 1983.
88. von Olshausen, K., Schafer, A., Mehmel, H. C., Schwarz, F., Senges, J., and Kubler, W.: Ventricular arrhythmias in idiopathic dilated cardiomyopathy. Br. Heart J. *51*:195, 1984.
89. Holmes, J., Kubo, S. H., Cody, R. J., and Kligfield, P.: Arrhythmias in ischemic and nonischemic dilated cardiomyopathy: Prediction of mortality by ambulatory electrocardiography. Am. J. Cardiol. *55*:146, 1985.
90. Huang, S. K., Messer, J. V., and Denes, P.: Significance of ventricular tachycardia in idiopathic dilated cardiomyopathy: Observations in 35 patients. Am. J. Cardiol. *51*:507, 1983.
91. Meinertz, T., Hofmann, T., Kasper, W., Treese, N., Bechtold, H., Stienen, U., Pop, T., Leitner, E. R., Andresen, D., and Meyer, J.: Significance of ventricular arrhythmias in idiopathic dilated cardiomyopathy. Am. J. Cardiol. *53*:902, 1984.
92. Maskin, C. S., Siskind, S. J., and LeJemtel, T. H.: High prevalence of nonsustained ventricular tachycardia in severe congestive heart failure. Am. Heart J. *107*, 896, 1984.
93. Chakko, C. S., and Gheorghiade, M.: Ventricular arrhythmias in severe heart failure: Incidence, significance, and effectiveness of antiarrhythmic therapy. Am. Heart J. *109*:497, 1985.
94. McLaran, C. J., Gersh, B. J., Sugrue, D. D., Hammill, S. C., Seward, J. B., and Holmes, D. R., Jr.: Tachycardia induced myocardial dysfunction. A reversible phenomenon? Br. Heart J. *53*:323, 1985.
95. Gillette, P. C., Smith, R. T., Garson, A. Jr., Mullins, C. E., Gutgesell, H. P., Goh, T. H., Cooley, D. A., and McNamara, D. G.: Chronic supraventricular tachycardia. A curable cause of congestive cardiomyopathy. J.A.M.A. *253*:391, 1985.
96. Olsson, S. B., Blomstrom, P., Sabel, K. G., and William-Olsson, G.: Incessant ectopic atrial tachycardia: successful surgical treatment with regression of dilated cardiomyopathy picture. Am. J. Cardiol. *53*:1465, 1984.
97. Packer, D. L., Bardy, G. H., Worley, S. J., Smith, M. S., Cobb, F. R., Coleman, R. E., Gallagher, J. J., and German, L. D.: Tachycardia-induced cardiomyopathy: A reversible form of left ventricular dysfunction. Am. J. Cardiol. *57*:563, 1986.
98. Goldberg, S. J., Valdes-Cruz, L. M., Sahn, D. J., and Allen, H. D.,: Two-dimensional echocardiographic evaluation of dilated cardiomyopathy in children. Am. J. Cardiol. *52*:1244, 1983.
99. Gardin, J. M., Iseri, L. T., Elkayam, U., Tobis, J., Childs, W., Burn, C. S., and Henry, W. L.: Evaluation of dilated cardiomyopathy by pulsed Doppler echocardiography. Am. Heart J. *106*:1057, 1983.
100. Marsh, J. D., Green, L. H., Wynne, J., Cohn, P. F., and Grossman, W.: Left ventricular end-systolic pressure—dimension and stress-length relations in normal human subjects. Am. J. Cardiol. *44*:1311, 1979.
101. Iskandrian, A. S., Hakki, A. H., and Kane, S.: Resting thallium-201 myocardial perfusion patterns in patients with severe left ventricular dysfunction: Differences between patients with primary cardiomyopathy, chronic coronary artery disease, or acute myocardial infarction. Am. Heart J. *111*:760, 1986.
102. Saltissi, S., Hockings, B., Croft, D. N., and Webb-Peploe, M. M.: Thallium-201 myocardial imaging in patients with dilated and ischemic cardiomyopathy. Br. Heart J. *46*:290, 1981.
103. Dunn, R. F., Uren, R. F., Sadick, N., Bautovich, G., McLaughlin, A., Hiroe, M., and Kelly, D. T.: Comparison of thallium-201 scanning in idiopathic dilated cardiomyopathy and severe coronary artery disease. Circulation *66*:804, 1982.
104. Greenberg, J., Boucher, C. A., Okada, R. D., Murphy, J. H., Palacios, I., Pohost, G. M., and Strauss, H. W.: Incidence of regional wall motion abnormalities in primary congestive cardiomyopathy. J. Am. Coll. Cardiol. *1*:723, 1983.
105. Colucci, W., Wynne, J., Holman, B. L., and Braunwald, E.: Chronic therapy of heart failure with prazosin: A randomized double-blind trial. Am. J. Cardiol. *45*:337, 1980.
106. Engler, R., Ray, R., Higgins, C. B., McNally, C., Buxton, W. H., Bhargava, V., and Shabetai, R.: Clinical assessment and follow-up of functional capacity in patients with chronic congestive cardiomyopathy. Am. J. Cardiol. *49*:1832, 1982.
107. Wallis, D. E., O'Connell, J. B., Henkin, R. E., Costanzo-Nordin, M. R., and Scanlon, P. J.: Segmental wall motion abnormalities in dilated cardiomyopathy: A common finding and good prognostic sign. J. Am. Coll. Cardiol. *4*:674, 1984.
107a. Zucchi, R., Barsotti, A., Mariotti, R., Biadi, O., Balbarini, A., and Mariani, M.: Asynergy and left ventricular performance in dilative cardiomyopathy. Clin. Cardiol. *10*:153, 1987.
108. Opherk, D., Schwarz, F., Mall, G., Manthey, J., Baller, D., and Kubler, W.: Coronary dilatory capacity in idiopathic dilated cardiomyopathy: Analysis of 16 patients. Am. J. Cardiol. *51*:1657, 1983.
109. Pitt, B.: Evaluation of the patient with congestive heart failure and ventricular arrhythmias. Am. J. Cardiol. *57*:19B, 1986.
110. Cohn, J. N., Archibald, D. G., Ziesche, S., Franciosa, J. A., Harston, W. E., Tristani, F. E., Dunkman, W. B., Jacobs, W., Francis, G. S., Flohr, K. H., Goldman, S., Cobb, F. R., Shah, P. M., Saunders, R., Fletcher, R. D., Loeb, H. S., Hughes, V. C., and Baker, B.: Effect of vasodilator therapy on mortality in chronic congestive heart failure. Results of Veterans Administration cooperative study. N. Engl. J. Med. *314*:1547, 1986.
111. Swedberg, K., Hjalmarson, A., Waagstein, F., and Wallentin, I.: Beneficial effects of long-term beta-blockade in congestive cardiomyopathy. Br. Heart J. *44*:117, 1980.
112. Waagstein, F., Hjalmarson, A., Swedberg, K., and Wallentin, C.: Beta-blockers in dilated cardiomyopathies: They work. Eur. Heart J. *4* (Suppl. A):173, 1983.
113. Swedberg, K., Hjalmarson, A., Waagstein, F., and Wallentin, I.: Adverse effects of beta-blockade withdrawal in patients with congestive cardiomyopathy. Br. Heart J. *44*:134, 1980.
114. Fisher, M. L., Plotnick, G. D., Peters, R. W., and Carliner, N. H.: Beta

blockers in congestive cardiomyopathy. Conceptual advance or contraindication? Am. J. Med. *80*:59, 1986.
115. Engelmeier, R. S., O'Connell, J. B., Walsh, R., Rad, N., Scanlon, P. J., and Gunnar, R. M.: Improvement in symptoms and exercise tolerance by metoprolol in patients with dilated cardiomyopathy: A double-blind, randomized, placebo-controlled trial. Circulation *72*:536, 1985.
116. Bhatia, S. J., Swedberg, K., and Chatterjee, K.: Acute hemodynamic and metabolic effects of ICI 118,587 (Corwin), a selective partial beta 1 agonist, in patients with dilated cardiomyopathy. Am. Heart J. *111*:692, 1986.
117. Anderson, J. L., Lutz, J. R., Gilbert, E. M., Sorensen, S. G., Yanowitz, F. G., Menlove, R. L., and Bartholomew, M.: A randomized trial of low-dose beta-blockade therapy for idiopathic dilated cardiomyopathy. Am. J. Cardiol. 55:471, 1985.
118. Currie, P. J., Kelly, M. J., McKenzie, A., Harper, R. W., Lim, Y. L., Federman, J., Anderson, S. T., and Pitt, A.: Oral beta-adrenergic blockade with metoprolol in chronic severe dilated cardiomyopathy. J. Am. Coll. Cardiol. *3*:203, 1984.
119. Ikram, H., and Fitzpatrick, D.: Double-blind trial of chronic oral beta blockade in congestive cardiomyopathy. Lancet 2:490, 1981.
120. Ikram, H., and Fitzpatrick, M. A.: Beta blockade for dilated cardiomyopathy: The evidence against therapeutic benefit. Eur. Heart J. *4* (Suppl A):179, 1983.
121. Fowler, M. B., and Bristow, M. R.: Rationale for beta-adrenergic blocking drugs in cardiomyopathy. Am. J. Cardiol. 55:120D, 1985.
122. Alderman, J., and Grossman, W.: Are beta-adrenergic-blocking drugs useful in the treatment of dilated cardiomyopathy? Circulation *71*:854, 1985.
123. Parmley, W. W., and Chatterjee, K.: Congestive heart failure and arrhythmias: An overview. Am. J. Cardiol. 57:34B, 1986.
124. Poll D. S., Marchlinski, F. E., Buxton, A. E., Doherty, J. U., Waxman, H. L., and Josephson, M. E.: Sustained ventricular tachycardia in patients with idiopathic dilated cardiomyopathy: Electrophysiologic testing and lack of response to antiarrhythmic drug therapy. Circulation *70*:451, 1984.
125. Lapeyre, A. C., Steele, P. M., Kazmier, F. J., Chesebro, J. H., Vlietstra, R. E., and Fuster, V.: Low incidence of systemic embolism in left ventricular aneurysm—A comparison with idiopathic dilated cardiomyopathy. J. Am. Coll. Cardiol. *1*:704, 1983.
126. Kyrle, P. A., Korninger, C., Gossinger, H., Glogar, D., Lechner, K., Niessner, H., and Pabinger, I.: Prevention of arterial and pulmonary embolism by oral anticoagulants in patients with dilated cardiomyopathy. Thromb. Haemost. *54*:521, 1985.
127. Gottdiener, J. S., Gay, J. A., VanVoorhees, L., DiBianco, R., and Fletcher, R. D.: Frequency and embolic potential of left ventricular thrombus in dilated cardiomyopathy: Assessment by two-dimensional echocardiography. Am. J. Cardiol. 52:1281, 1983.
128. Gould, L., Gopalaswamy, C., Chandy, F., and Kim, B. S.: Congestive cardiomyopathy and left ventricular thrombus. Arch. Intern. Med. *143*:1472, 1983.
129. Hosenpud, J. D., McAnulty, J. H., and Niles, N. R.: Lack of objective improvement in ventricular systolic function in patients with myocarditis treated with azathioprine and prednisone. J. Am. Coll. Cardiol. *6*:797, 1985.
130. Vignola, P. H., Honuma, K., Swaye, P. S., Rozanski, J. J., Blankstein, R. L., Benson, J., Gosselin, H. J., and Lister, J. W.: Lymphocytic myocarditis presenting as unexplained ventricular arrhythmias: Diagnosis with endomyocardial biopsy and response to immunosuppression. J. Am. Coll. Cardiol. *4*:812, 1984.
131. Hassell, L. A., Fowles, R. E., and Stinson, E. B.: Patients with congestive cardiomyopathy as cardiac transplant recipients: Indications for and results of cardiac transplantation and comparison with patients with coronary artery disease. Am. J. Cardiol. *47*:1205, 1981.
132. Baldwin, J. C., and Shumway, N. E.: Cardiac transplantation. Z. Kardiol. *74*:39, 1985.
133. Baumgartner, W. H.: Role of cardiac transplantation in the management of congestive heart failure. Am. J. Med. *80*:51, 1986.
134. Walsh, T. K., and Vacek, J. L.: Ethanol and heart disease. An underestimated contributing factor. Postgrad. Med. *79*:60, 1986.
135. Clark, L. T.: Alcohol use and hypertension. Clinical considerations and implications. Postgrad. Med. *75*:273, 1984.
136. Regan, T. J.: Alcoholic cardiomyopathy. Prog. Cardiovasc. Dis. *27*:141, 1984.
137. Sacher, M. L., Siskind, S. J., and Boal, B. H.: Gated radionuclide angiocardiography in the noninvasive evaluation of a partially reversible alcoholic cardiomyopathy. Am. J. Med. *80*:1205, 1986.
138. Alexander, C. S.: Cobalt-beer cardiomyopathy. A clinical and pathological study of twenty-eight cases. Am. J. Med. *53*:395, 1972.
139. Lange, L. G., and Sobel, B. E.: Myocardial metabolites of ethanol. Circ. Res. *52*:479, 1983.
140. Cardiovascular beriberi (editorial). Lancet *1*:1287, 1982.
141. Carson, P.: Alcoholic cardiac berberi (editorial). Br. Med. J. (Clin. Res.) *284*:1817, 1982.
142. Hepp, A., Schier, H., and Kochsiek, K.: Comparative haemodynamic studies on the acute cardiac effects of alcohol in the rat and guinea pig. Eur. Heart J. *5*:85, 1984.
143. Kelbaek, H., Gjorup, T., Brynjolf, I., Christensen, N. J., and Godtfredsen, J.: Acute effects of alcohol on left ventricular function in healthy subjects at rest and during upright exercise. Am. J. Cardiol. *55*:164, 1985.
144. Lang, R. M., Borow, K. M., Neumann, A., and Feldman, T.: Adverse cardiac effects of acute alcohol ingestion in young adults. Ann. Intern. Med. *102*:742, 1985.
145. Noren, G. R., Staley, N. A., Einzig, S., Mikell, F. L., and Asinger, R. W.: Alcohol-induced congestive cardiomyopathy: An animal model. Cardiovasc. Res. *17*:81, 1983.
146. Regan, T. J., Ettinger, P. O., Lyons, M. M., Moschos, C. B., and Weisse, A. B.: Ethyl alcohol as a cardiac risk factor. Cur. Probl. Cardiol. *2*:1, 1977.
147. Knochel, J. P.: Cardiovascular effects of alcohol. Ann. Intern. Med. *98*:849, 1983.
148. Rubin, E.: Alcohol and the heart: theoretical considerations. Fed. Proc. *41*:2460, 1982.
149. Lange, L. G., and Sobel, B. E.: Impaired cardiac mitochondrial function induced by specific metabolites of ethanol: Fatty acid ethyl esters. J. Am. Coll. Cardiol. *1*:667, 1983.
150. Regan, T. J., Levinson, G. E., Oldewurtel, H. A., Frank, M. J., Weisse, A. B., and Moschos, C. B.: Ventricular function in noncardiacs with alcoholic fatty liver: Role of ethanol in the production of cardiomyopathy. J. Clin. Invest. *48*:397, 1969.
151. Tsiplenkova, V. G., Vikhert, A. M., and Cherpachenko, N. M.: Ultrastructural and histochemical observations in human and experimental alcoholic cardiomyopathy. J. Am. Coll. Cardiol. *8*:22A, 1986.
152. Burch, G. E., and Giles, T. D.: The small coronary arteries in alcoholic cardiomyopathy. Am. Heart J. *94*:471, 1977.
153. Factor, S. M.: Intramyocardial small-vessel disease in chronic alcoholism. Am. Heart J. *92*:561, 1976.
154. Weisharr, R., Sarma, J. S. M., Maruyama, Y., Fischer, R., Bertuglia, S., and Bing, R. J.: Reversibility of mitochondrial and contractile changes in the myocardium after cessation of prolonged ethanol intake. Am. J. Cardiol. *40*:556, 1977.
155. Schultheiss, H. P., Spiegel, M., and Bolte, H. D.: The effects of chronic ethanol treatment on oligomycin sensitive ATPase activity in the guinea pig heart. Basic Res. Cardiol. *80*:548, 1985.
156. Demakis, J. G., Proskey, A., Rahimtoola, S. H., Jamil, M., Sutton, G. C., Rosen, K. M., Gunnar, R. M., and Tobin, J. R., Jr.: The natural course of alcoholic cardiomyopathy. Ann. Intern. Med. *80*:293, 1974.
157. Wu, C. F., Sudhaker, M., Jaferi, G., Ahmed, S. S., and Regan, T. J.: Preclinical cardiomyopathy in chronic alcoholics: A sex difference. Am. Heart. J. *91*:291, 1976.
158. Dancy, M., Leech, G., Bland, J. M., Gaitonde, M. K., and Maxwell, J. D.: Preclinical left ventricular abnormalities in alcoholics are independent of nutritional status, cirrhosis, and cigarette smoking. Lancet *1*:1122, 1985.
159. Kelbaek, H., Eriksen, J., Brynjolf, I., Raboel, A., Lund, J. O., Munck, O., Bonnevie, O., and Godtfredsen, J.: Cardiac performance in patients with asymptomatic alcoholic cirrhosis of the liver. Am. J. Cardiol. *54*:852, 1984.
160. Ahmed, S. S., Howard, M., ten Hove, W., Leevy, C. M., and Regan, T. J.: Cardiac function in alcoholics with cirrhosis: absence of overt cardiomyopathy—myth or fact? J. Am. Coll. Cardiol. *3*:696, 1984.
161. Mathews, E. C., Gardin, J. M., Henry, W. L., Del Negro, A. A., Fletcher, R. D., Snow, J. A., and Epstein, S. E.: Echocardiographic abnormalities in chronic alcoholics with and without overt congestive heart failure. Am. J. Cardiol. *47*:570, 1981.
162. Askanas, A., Udoshi, M., and Sadjadi, S. A.: The heart in chronic alcoholism. A noninvasive study. Am. Heart J. *99*:9, 1980.
163. Kino, M., Imamitchi, H., Morigutchi, M., Kawamura, K., and Takatsu, T.: Cardiovascular status in asymptomatic alcoholics, with reference to the level of ethanol consumption. Br. Heart J. *46*:545, 1981.
164. Greenspan, A. J., and Schaal, S. F.: The "holiday heart": Electrophysiologic studies of alcohol effects in alcoholics. Ann. Intern. Med. *98*:135, 1983.
165. Rich, E. C., Siebold, C., and Campion, B.: Alcohol-related acute atrial fibrillation. A case-control study and review of 40 patients. Arch. Intern. Med. *145*:830, 1985.
166. Engel, T. R., and Luck, J. C.: Effect of whiskey on atrial vulnerability and "holiday heart." J. Am. Coll. Cardiol. *1*:816, 1983.
167. Vikhert, A. M., Tsiplenkova, V. G., and Cherpachenko, N. M.: Alcoholic cardiomyopathy and sudden cardiac death. J. Am. Coll. Cardiol. 8:3A, 1986.
168. Bashour, T. T., Fahdul, H., and Chen, T. O.: Electrocardiographic abnormalities in alcoholic cardiomyopathy. A study of 65 patients. Chest *68*:24, 1975.
169. Lacour, F., Sr., and Suire, E. M.: The diagnosis of alcohol cardiomyopathies. J. La. State Med. Soc. *130*:159, 1978.
170. McDonald, C. D., Burch, G. E., and Walsh, J. J.: Alcoholic cardiomyopathy managed with prolonged bed rest. Ann. Intern. Med. *74*:681, 1971.
171. Barborik, M., and Dusek, J.: Cardiomyopathy accompanying industrial cobalt exposure. Br. Heart J. *34*:113, 1972.
172. Manifold, I. H., Platts, M. M., and Kennedy, A.: Cobalt cardiomyopathy in a patient on maintenance haemodialysis. Br. Med. J. 2:1609, 1978.
173. Horowitz, S. F., Matza, D., and Machac. J.: Cardiotoxic effects of chemicals. Mt. Sinai J. Med. (NY) 52:650, 1985.

HYPERTROPHIC CARDIOMYOPATHY

174. Teare, R. D.: Asymmetrical hypertrophy of the heart in young adults. Br. Heart J. *20*:1, 1958.
174a. Iida, K., Yukisada, K., Sugishita, Y., Matsuda, M., Koseki, S., and Ito, I.: Impaired left ventricular rapid filling during exercise in patients with hypertrophic cardiomyopathy. Clin. Cardiol. *10*:147, 1987.
175. Morrow, A. G., and Braunwald, E.: Functional aortic stenosis: A malformation characterized by resistance to left ventricular outflow without anatomic obstruction. Circulation *20*:181, 1959.
175a. ten Cate, F. J.: Hypertrophic Cardiomyopathy. New York, Marcel Dekker, 1985.
176. Clark, C. E., Henry, W. L., and Epstein, S. E.: Familial prevalence and

genetic transmission of idiopathic hypertrophic subaortic stenosis. N. Engl. J. Med. *289*:709, 1973.
177. Maron, B. J., Nichols, P. F. 3d., Pickle, L. W., Wesley, Y. E., and Mulvihill, J. J.: Patterns of inheritance in hypertrophic cardiomyopathy: Assessment by M-mode and two-dimensional echocardiography. Am. J. Cardiol. *53*:1087, 1984.
178. Wigle, E. D., Sasson, Z., Henderson, M. A., Ruddy, T. D., Fulop, J., Rakowski, H., and Williams, W. G.: Hypertrophic cardiomyopathy. The importance of the site and the extent of hypertrophy. A review. Prog. Cardiovasc. Dis. *28*:1, 1985.
179. Nishimura, R. A., Giuliani, E. R., and Brandenburg, R. O.: Hypertrophic cardiomyopathy. Cardiovasc. Rev. Reports, *4*:931, 1983.
180. Epstein, S. E., Henry, W. L., Clark, C. E., Roberts, W. C., Maron, B. J., Ferrans, V. J., Redwood, D. R., and Morrow, A. G.: Asymmetric septal hypertrophy. Ann Intern. Med. *81*:650, 1974.
181. Maron, B. J., Gottdiener, J. S., Roberts, W. C., Henry, W. L., Savage, D. D., and Epstein, S. E.: Left ventricular outflow tract obstruction due to systolic anterior motion of the anterior mitral leaflet in patients with concentric left ventricular hypertrophy. Circulation *57*:527, 1978.
182. Come, P. C., Bulkly, B. H., Goodman, Z. D., Hutchins, G. M., Pitt, B., and Fortuin, N. J.: Hypercontractile cardiac states simulating hypertrophic cardiomyopathy. Circulation *55*:901, 1977.
183. Buxton, A. E., Morganroth, J., Josephson, M. E., Perloff, J. K., and Shelborne, J. C.: Isolated dextroversion of the heart with asymmetric septal hypertrophy. Am. Heart J. *92*:785, 1976.
184. Sommerville, J., and Becu, L.: Congenital heart disease associated with hypertrophic cardiomyopathy. Johns Hopkins Med. J. *140*:151, 1977.
185. Maron, B. J., Gottdiener, J. S., Roberts, W. C., Hammer, W. J., and Epstein, S. E.: Nongenetically transmitted disproportionate ventricular septal thickening associated with left ventricular outflow obstruction. Br. Heart J. *41*:345, 1979.
186. Sommerville, J., and Becu, L.: Congenital heart disease associated with hypertrophic cardiomyopathy. Br. Heart J. *40*:1034, 1978.
187. Abbasi, A., Slaughter, J. C., and Allen, M. W.: Asymmetrical septal hypertrophy in patients with long-term hemodialysis. Chest *74*:548, 1978.
188. Maron, B. J., Clark, C. E., Henry, W. L., Fukuda, T., Edwards, J. E., Mathews, E. C., Jr., Redwood, D. R., and Epstein, S. E.: Prevalence and characteristics of disproportionate ventricular septal thickening in patients with acquired or congenital heart disease. Echocardiographic and morphologic findings. Circulation *55*:489, 1977.
189. Larter, W. E., Allen, H. D., Sahn, D. J., and Goldberg, S. J.: The asymmetrically hypertrophied septum. Further differentiation of its causes. Circulation *53*:19, 1976.
190. Stern, A., Kessler, K. M., Hammer, W. J., Kreulen, T., and Spann, J. F.: Septal-free wall disproportion in inferior infarction: The echocardiographic differentiation from hypertrophic cardiomyopathy. Circulation *58*:700, 1978.
191. Raj., M. V. J., Srinivas, V., Graham, I. M., and Evans, D. W.: Coexistence of asymmetric septal hypertrophy and aortic valve disease in adults. Thorax *34*:91, 1979.
192. Maron, B. J., Gottdiener, J. S., and Epstein, S. E.: Patterns and significance of distribution of left ventricular hypertrophy in hypertrophic cardiomyopathy: A wide-angle two-dimensional echocardiographic study of 125 patients. Am. J. Cardiol. *48*:418, 1981.
193. Maron, B. J., Gottdiener, J. S., Bonow, R. O., and Epstein, S. E., Hypertrophic cardiomyopathy with unusual locations of left ventricular hypertrophy undetectable by M-mode echocardiography. Identification by wide-angle two-dimensional echocardiography. Circulation *63*:409, 1981.
194. Ciro, E., Nichols, P. F., III, and Maron, B. J.: Heterogeneous morphologic expression of genetically transmitted hypertrophic cardiomyopathy. Circulation *67*:1227, 1983.
195. Maron, B. J., Spirito, P., Chiarella, F., and Vecchio, C.: Unusual distribution of left ventricular hypertrophy in obstructive hypertrophic cardiomyopathy: Localized posterobasal free wall thickening in two patients. J. Am. Coll. Cardiol. *5*:1474, 1985.
196. Maron, B. J.: Asymmetry in hypertrophic cardiomyopathy: The septal to free wall thickness ratio revisited. Am J. Cardiol. *55*:835, 1985.
197. Keren, G., Belhassen, B., Sherez, J., Miller, H. I., Megidish, R., Berenfeld, D., and Laniado, S.: Apical hypertrophic cardiomyopathy: Evaluation by noninvasive and invasive techniques in 23 patients. Circulation *71*:45, 1985.
198. Vacek, J. L., Davis, W. R., Bellinger, R. L., and McKiernan, T. L.: Apical hypertrophic cardiomyopathy in American patients. Am. Heart J. *108*:1501, 1984.
199. Rovelli, E. G., Parenti, F., and Devizzi, S.: Apical hypertrophic cardiomyopathy of "Japanese type" in a Western European person. Am. J. Cardiol. *57*,358, 1986.
200. Abinader, E. G., Rauchfleisch, S., and Naschitz, J.: Hypertrophic apical cardiomyopathy: A subtype of hypertrophic cardiomyopathy. Isr. J. Med. Sci.*18*:1005, 1982.
201. Steingo, L., Dansky, R., Pocock, W. A., and Barlow, J. B.: Apical hypertrophic nonobstructive cardiomyopathy. Am. Heart J. *104*:635, 1982.
202. Bertrand, M. E., Tilmant, P. Y., Lablanche, J. M., and Thieuleux, F. A.: Apical hypertrophic cardiomyopathy: Clinical and metabolic studies. Eur. Heart J. *4*:127, 1983.
203. Kereiakes, D. J., Anderson, D. J., Crouse, L., and Chatterjee, K.: Apical hypertrophic cardiomyopathy. Am. Heart J. *105*:855, 1983.
204. Panidis, I. P., Nestico, P., Hakki, A. H., Mintz, G. S., Segal, B. L., and Iskandrian, A. S.: Systolic and diastolic left ventricular performance at rest and during exercise in apical hypertrophic cardiomyopathy. Am. J. Cardiol. *57*:356, 1986.
205. Yamaguchi, H., Ishimura, T., Nishiyama, S., Nagasaki, F., Nakanishi, S., Takatsu, F., Nishijo, T., Umeda, T., and Machii, K.: Hypertrophic nonobstructive cardiomyopathy with giant negative T waves (apical hypertrophy): Ventriculographic and echocardiographic features in 30 patients. Am. J. Cardiol. *44*:401, 1979.
206. Maron, B. J., Bonow, R. O., Seshagiri, T. N. R., Roberts, W. C., and Epstein, S. E.: Hypertrophic cardiomyopathy with ventricular septal hypertrophy localized to the apical region of the left ventricle (apical hypertrophic cardiomyopathy). Am. J. Cardiol. *49*:1838, 1982.
207. Topol, E. J., Traill, T. A., and Fortuin, N. J.: Hypertensive hypertrophic cardiomyopathy of the elderly. N. Engl. J. Med. *312*:277, 1985.
208. Bulkley, B. H., Weisfeldt, M. L., and Hutchins, G. M.: Asymmetric septal hypertrophy and myocardial fiber disarray. Features of normal, developing and malformed hearts. Circulation *56*:292, 1977.
209. Rassmussen, S., Corya, B. C., Feigenbaum, H., and Knoebel, S. B.: Detection of myocardial scar tissue by M-mode echocardiography. Circulation *57*:230, 1978.
210. Maron, B. J., Savage, D. D., Clark, C. E., Henry, W. L., Vlodaver, Z., Edwards, J. E., and Epstein, S. E.: Prevalence and characteristics of disproportionate ventricular septal thickening in patients with coronary artery disease. Circulation *57*:250, 1978.
211. Olsen, E. G. J.: The pathology of idiopathic hypertrophic subaortic stenosis (hypertrophic cardiomyopathy). A critical review. Am. Heart J. *100*:553, 1980.
212. Symons, C., Fortune, F., Greenbaum, R. A., and Dandona, P.: Cardiac hypertrophy, hypertrophic cardiomyopathy, and hyperparathyroidism—an association. Br. Heart J. *54*:539, 1985.
213. Altman, D. I., Murray, J., Milner, S., Dansky, R., and Levin, S. E.: Asymmetric septal hypertrophy and hypothyroidism in children. Br. Heart J. *54*:533, 1985.
214. Wilson, R., Gibson, T. C., Terrien, C. M., Jr., and Levy, A. M.: Hyperthyroidism and familial hypertrophic cardiomyopathy. Arch. Intern. Med. *143*:378, 1983.
215. Thompson, R., Ahmed, M., Pridie, R., and Yacoub, M.: Hypertrophic cardiomyopathy after aortic valve replacement. Am. J. Cardiol. *45*:33, 1980.
216. Shapiro, L. M., Howat, A. P., Crean, P. A., and Westgate, C. J.: An echocardiographic study of localized subaortic hypertrophy. Eur. Heart J. *7*:127, 1986.
217. Isner, J. M., Falcone, M. W., Virmani, R., and Roberts, W. C.: Cardiac sarcoma causing "ASH" and simulating coronary heart disease. Am. J. Med. *66*:1025, 1979.
218. Cabin, H. S., Costello, R. M., Vasudevan, G., Maron, B. J., and Roberts, W. C.: Cardiac lymphoma mimicking hypertrophic cardiomyopathy. Am. Heart J. *102*:466, 1981.
219. Bulkley, B. H., and Hutchins, G. M.: Pompe's disease presenting as hypertrophic myocardiopathy with Wolff-Parkinson-White syndrome. Am. Heart J. *96*:246, 1978.
220. Sedlis, S. P., Saffitz, J. E., Schwob, V. S., and Jaffe, A. S.: Cardiac amyloidosis simulating hypertrophic cardiomyopathy. Am. J. Cardiol. *53*:969, 1984.
221. Colucci, W. S., Lorell, B. H., Schoen, F. J., Warhol, M. J., and Grossman, W.: Hypertrophic obstructive cardiomyopathy due to Fabry's disease. N. Engl. J. Med. *307*:926, 1982.
222. Henry, W. L., Clark, C. E., Roberts, W. C., Morrow, A. G., and Epstein, S. E.: Differences in the distribution of myocardial abnormalities in patients with obstructive and nonobstructive asymmetric septal hypertrophy (ASH). Echocardiographic and gross anatomic findings. Circulation *50*:447, 1974.
223. Davies, M. J.: The current status of myocardial disarray in hypertrophic cardiomyopathy (editorial). Br. Heart J. *51*:361, 1984.
224. Tanaka, M., Fujiwara, H., Onodera, T., Wu, D. J., Hamashima, Y., and Kawai, C.: Quantitative analysis of myocardial fibrosis in normals, hypertensive hearts, and hypertrophic cardiomyopathy. Br. Heart J. *55*:575, 1986.
224a. Unverferth, D. V., Baker, P. B., Pearce, L. I., Lautman, J., and Roberts, W. C.: Regional myocyte hypertrophy and increased interstitial myocardial fibrosis in hypertrophic cardiomyopathy. Am. J. Cardiol. *59*:932, 1987.
225. Maron, B. J., and Roberts, W. C.: Hypertrophic cardiomyopathy and cardiac muscle cell disorganization revisited: Relation between the two and significance. Am. Heart J. *102*:95, 1981.
226. Wigle, E. D., and Silver, M. D.: Editorial: Myocardial fiber disarray and ventricular septal hypertrophy in asymmetrical hypertrophy of the heart. Circulation *58*:398, 1978.
227. Olsen, E. G.: Myocardial disarray revisited (editorial). Br. Med. J. *285*:991, 1982.
228. Bulkley, B. H., D'Amico, B., and Taylor, A. L.: Extensive myocardial fiber disarray in aortic and pulmonary atresia. Relevance to hypertrophic cardiomyopathy. Circulation *67*:191, 1983.
229. Becker, A. E., and Caruso, G.: Myocardial disarray. A critical review. Br. Heart J. *47*:527, 1982.
230. Maron, B. J.: Myocardial disorganisation in hypertrophic cardiomyopathy. Another point of view. Br. Heart J. *50*:1, 1983.
231. Isner, J. M., Maron, B. J., and Roberts, W. C.: Comparison of amount of myocardial cell disorganization in operatively excised septectomy specimens with amount observed at necropsy in 18 patients with hypertrophic cardiomyopathy. Am. J. Cardiol. *46*:42, 1980.
232. Maron, B. J., Anan, T. J., and Roberts, W. C.: Quantitative analysis of the distribution of cardiac muscle cell disorganization in the left ventricular free wall of patients with hypertrophic cardiomyopathy. Circulation *63*:882, 1981.
233. Olsen, E. G.: Anatomic and light microscopic characterization of hypertrophic obstructive and non-obstructive cardiomyopathy. Eur. Heart J. *4*:1, 1983.
233a. Maron, B. J., Wolfson, J. K., Epstein, S. E., and Roberts, W. C.: Intramural ("small vessel") coronary artery disease in hypertrophic cardiomyopathy. J. Am. Coll. Cardiol. *8*:545, 1986.
234. Kishimoto, C., Kaburagi, T., Takayama, S., Yokoyama, S., Hanyu, I., Takatsu,

Y., and Tomimoto, K.: Two forms of hypertrophic cardiomyopathy distinguished by inheritance of HLA haplotypes and left ventricular outflow tract obstruction. Am. Heart J. *105*:988, 1983.
235. Beckers, J., Vandeputte, R., Geboers, J., and DeGeest, H.: HLA complex and hypertrophic cardiomyopathy in a European population. Eur. Heart J. *6*:963, 1985.
236. Fiorito, S., Autore, C., Fragola, P. V., Purpura, M., Cannata, D., and Sangiorgi, M.: HLA-DR3 antigen linkage in patients with hypertrophic obstructive cardiomyopathy. Am. Heart J. *111*:91, 1986.
237. Gardin, J. M., Gottdiener, J. S., Radvany, R., Maron, B. J., and Lesch, M.: HLA linkage vs. association in hypertrophic cardiomyopathy. Evidence for the absence of an association in a heterogeneous caucasian population. Chest *81*:466, 1982.
238. Haugland, H., Ohm, O. J., Boman, H., and Thorsby, E.: Hypertrophic cardiomyopathy in three generations of a large Norwegian family. A clinical, echocardiographic, and genetic study. Br. Heart J. *55*:168, 1986.
239. Zezulka, A., MacKintosh, P., Jobson, S., Lowry, P., and Shapiro, L. M.: Human lymphocyte antigens in hypertrophic cardiomyopathy. Int. J. Cardiol. *12*:193, 1986.
240. Hirzel, H. O., Tuchschmid, C. R., Schneider, J., Krayenbeuhl, H. P., and Schaub, M. C.: Relationship between myosin isoenzyme composition, hemodynamics, and myocardial structure in various forms of human cardiac hypertrophy. Circ. Res. *57*:729, 1985.
241. Silverman, K. J., Hutchins, G. M., Weiss, J. L., and Moore, G. W.: Catenoidal shape of the interventricular septum in idiopathic hypertrophic subaortic stenosis: Two dimensional echocardiographic confirmation. Am. J. Cardiol. *49*:27, 1982.
242. Perloff, J. K.: Pathogenesis of hypertrophic cardiomyopathy: Hypothesis and speculation. Am. Heart J. *101*:219, 1981.
243. Bernardi, D., Bernini, L., Cini, G., Ghione, S., and Bonechi, I.: Asymmetric septal hypertrophy and sympathetic overactivity in normotensive hemodialyzed patients. Am. Heart J. *109*:539, 1985.
244. Raum, W. J., Laks, M. M., Garner, D., and Swerdloff, R. S.: Beta-adrenergic receptor and cyclic AMP alterations in the canine ventricular septum during long-term norepinephrine infusion: Implications of hypertrophic cardiomyopathy. Circulation *68*:693, 1983.
245. Koga, Y., Itaya, M., and Toshima, H.: Increased cardiovascular response to epinephrine in hypertrophic cardiomyopathy. Jpn. Heart J. *26*:727, 1985.
246. Golf, S., Myhre, E., Abdelnoor, M., Andersen, D., and Hansson, V.: Hypertrophic cardiomyopathy characterized by beta-adrenoceptor density, relative amount of beta-adrenoceptor subtypes, and adenylate cyclase activity. Cardiovasc. Res. *19*:693, 1985.
247. Olsen, E. G.: An endocrine experimental model for myofibrillar disarray as found in hypertrophic cardiomyopathy. J. Mol. Cell. Cardiol. *17*:35. 1985.
248. James, T. N., and Marshall, T. K.: De Subitaneis Mortibus. XII. Asymmetrical hypertrophy of the heart. Circulation *51*:1149, 1975.
249. Ogata, Y., Hiyamuta, K., Terasawa, M., Ohkita, Y., Bekki, H., Koga, Y., and Toshima, H.: Relationship of exercise or pacing induced ST segment depression and myocardial lactate metabolism in patients with hypertrophic cardiomyopathy. Jpn. Heart J. *27*:145, 1986.
250. Factor, S. M., Minase, T., Cho, S., Dominitz, R., and Sonnenblick, E. H.: Microvascular spasm in the cardiomyopathic Syrian hamster: A preventable cause of focal myocardial necrosis. Circulation *66*:342, 1982.
251. Lorell, B. H., Paulus, W. J., Grossman, W., Wynne, J., and Cohn, P. F.: Modification of abnormal left ventricular diastolic properties by nifedipine in patients with hypertrophic cardiomyopathy. Circulation *65*:499, 1982.
251a. Goodwin, J. F., McKenna, W. J., and Alvares, R.: Cardiomyopathies—the message for the 1980's. Part II. Postgrad. Med. J. *62*:513, 1986.
252. Pearce, P. C., Hawkey, C., Symons, C., and Olsen, E. G.: Role of calcium in the induction of cardiac hypertrophy and myofibrillar disarray. Experimental studies of a possible cause of hypertrophic cardiomyopathy. Br. Heart J. *54*:420, 1985.
253. Grossman, W., Paulus, W., and Lorell, B.: Haemodynamic evaluation of diastolic abnormalities in hypertrophic cardiomyopathy. Postgrad. Med. J. *61*:1113, 1985.
253a. Gwathmey, J. K., Warren, S., Briggs, G. M., Copelas, L., Feldman, M. D., Callahan, M., Schoen, F., Grossman, W., and Morgan, J. F.: Direct evidence for intracellular Ca^{++} overload in working myocardium from patients with hypertrophic cardiomyopathy. (Submitted for publication).
254. Pollick, C., Rakowski, H., and Wigle, E. D.: Muscular subaortic stenosis: The quantitative relationship between systolic anterior motion and the pressure gradient. Circulation *69*:43, 1984.
255. Levine, R. A., and Weyman, A. E.: Dynamic subaortic obstruction in hypertrophic cardiomyopathy: Criteria and controversy. J. Am. Coll. Cardiol. *6*:16, 1985.
256. Pollick, C., Morgan, C. D., Gilbert, B. W., Rakowski, H., and Wigle, E. D.: Muscular subaortic stenosis: the temporal relationship between systolic anterior motion of the anterior mitral leaflet and the pressure gradient. Circulation *66*:1087, 1982.
256a. Maron, B. J., Bonow, R. O., Cannon, R. O., III, Leon, M. B., and Epstein, S. E.: Hypertrophic cardiomyopathy: Interrelations of clinical manifestations, pathophysiology and therapy. N. Engl. J. Med. *316*:780, 844, 1987.
257. Murgo, J. P., Alter, B. R., Dorethy, J. F., Altobelli, S. A., and McGranahan. G. M., Jr.: Dynamics of left ventricular ejection in obstructive and nonobstructive hypertrophic cardiomyopathy. J. Clin. Invest. *66*:1369, 1980.
258. Murgo, J. P., Alter, B. R., Dorethy, J. F., Altobelli, S. A., Craig, W. E., and McGranahan, G. M., Jr.: The effects of intraventricular gradients on left ventricular ejection dynamics. Eur. Heart J. *4*:23, 1983.
259. Criley, J. M., and Siegel, R. J.: Has "obstruction" hindered our understanding of hypertrophic cardiomyopathy? Circulation 72:1148, 1985.
260. Murgo, J. P.: Does outflow obstruction exist in hypertrophic cardiomyopathy? N. Engl. J. Med. *307*:1008, 1982.
261. Braunwald, E., Lambrew, C. T., Rockoff, S. D., Ross, J., Jr., and Morrow, A. G.: Idiopathic hypertrophic subaortic stenosis. Circulation *29/30* (Suppl. IV):1, 1964.
262. Shenoy, M. M., Khanna, A., Nejat, M., Greif, E., and Friedman, S. A.: Hypertrophic cardiomyopathy in the elderly. A frequently misdiagnosed disease. Arch. Intern. Med. *146*:658, 1986.
263. Frank, S., and Braunwald, E.: Idiopathic hypertrophic subaortic stenosis. Clinical analysis of 126 patients with emphasis on the natural history. Circulation *37*:759, 1968.
264. Maron, B. J., Roberts, W. C., Edwards, J. E., McAllister, H. U., Jr., Foley, D. D., and Epstein, S. E.: Sudden death in patients with hypertrophic cardiomyopathy: Characterization of 26 patients without functional limitation. Am. J. Cardiol. *41*:803, 1978.
265. Maron, B. J., Tajik, A. J., Ruttenberg, H. D., Graham, T. P., Atwood, G. F., Victorica, B. E., Lie, J. T., and Roberts, W. C.: Hypertrophic cardiomyopathy in infants: Clinical features and natural history. Circulation *65*:7, 1982.
266. Sutton, M. G. St. J., Tajik, A. J., Smith, H. C., and Ritman, E. L.: Angina in idiopathic hypertrophic subaortic stenosis. A clinical correlation of regional left ventricular dysfunction: A videometric and echocardiographic study. Circulation *61*:561, 1980.
267. Maron, B. J., Epstein, S. E., and Roberts, W. C.: Hypertrophic cardiomyopathy and transmural myocardial infarction without significant atherosclerosis of the extramural coronary arteries. Am. J. Cardiol. *43*:1086, 1979.
268. McKenna, W., Harris, L., and Deanfield, J.: Syncope in hypertrophic cardiomyopathy. Br. Heart J. *47*:117, 1982.
269. McKenna, W., Harris, L., and Deanfield, J.: Syncope in hypertrophic cardiomyopathy. Br. Heart J. *47*:177, 1982.
270. Luisada, A. A., Frazin, L., Singhal, A., and Nunez, A.: Various types of systolic clicks in patients with muscular subaortic stenosis. Jpn. Heart J. *26*:133, 1985.
271. Chandraratna, P. A., and Aronow, W. S.: Genesis of the systolic murmur of idiopathic hypertrophic subaortic stenosis. Phonocardiographic, echocardiographic, and pulsed Doppler ultrasound correlations. Chest *83*:638, 1983.
272. Kramer, D. S., French, W. J., and Criley, J. M.: The postextrasystolic murmur response to gradient in hypertrophic cardiomyopathy. Ann. Intern. Med. *104*:772, 1986.
273. Wiener, M. W., Vondoenhoff, L. J., and Cohen, J.: Aortic regurgitation first appearing 12 years after successful septal myectomy for hypertrophic obstructive cardiomyopathy. Am. J. Med. *72*:157, 1982.
274. Maron, B. J., Wolfson, J. K., Ciro, E., and Spirito, P.: Relation of electrocardiographic abnormalities and patterns of left ventricular hypertrophy identified by 2-dimensional echocardiography in patients with hypertrophic cardiomyopathy. Am. J. Cardiol. *51*:189, 1983.
275. Henderson, M. A., Ruddy, T. D., Makowski, H., and Wigle, E. D.: Left ventricular hypertrophy by ECG in hypertrophic cardiomyopathy. J. Am. Coll. Cardiol. *1*:693, 1983.
276. Maron, B. J., Wolfson, J. K., Ciro, E., and Spirito, P.: Relation of electrocardiographic abnormalities and patterns of left ventricular hypertrophy identified by two-dimensional echocardiography in patients with hypertrophic cardiomyopathy. Am. J. Cardiol. *51*:189, 1983.
277. McKenna, W. J., Borggrefe, M., England, D., Deanfield, J., Oakley, C. M., and Goodwin, J. F.: The natural history of left ventricular hypertrophy in hypertrophic cardiomyopathy: An electrocardiographic study. Circulation *66*:1233, 1982.
278. Cosio, F. G., Moro, C., Alonso, M., de la Calzada, C. S., and Llovet, A.: The Q waves of hypertrophic cardiomyopathy: An electrophysiologic study. N. Engl. J. Med. *302*:96, 1980.
279. Touboul, P., Kirkorian, G., Atallah, G., Cahen, P., de Zuloaga, C., and Moleur, P.: Atrioventricular block and preexcitation in hypertrophic cardiomyopathy. Am. J. Cardiol. *15*:961, 1984.
280. Krikler, D. M., Davies, M. J., Rowland, E., Goodwin, J. F., Evans, R. C., and Shaw, D. B.: Sudden death in hypertrophic cardiomyopathy: Associated accessory atrioventricular pathways. Br. Med. J. *43*:245, 1980.
281. Khair, G. Z., and Bamrah, V. S.: Syncope in hypertrophic cardiomyopathy. I. Association with atrioventricular block. Am. Heart J. *110*:1081, 1985.
282. McKenna, W. J., Chetty, S., Oakley, C. M., and Goodwin, J. F.: Arrhythmia in hypertrophic cardiomyopathy: Exercise electrocardiographic and 48 hour ambulatory electrocardiographic assessment with and without beta adrenergic blocking therapy. Am. J. Cardiol. *45*:1, 1980.
283. Anderson, K. P., Stinson, E. B., Derby, G. C., Oyer, P. E., and Mason, J. W.: Vulnerability of patients with obstructive hypertrophic cardiomyopathy to ventricular arrhythmia induction in the operating room. Analysis of 17 patients. Am. J. Cardiol. *51*:811, 1983.
284. McKenna, W. J.: Arrhythmia and prognosis in hypertrophic cardiomyopathy. Eur. Heart J. *4*:225, 1983.
285. Bjarnason, I., Hardarson, T., and Jonsson, S.: Cardiac arrhythmias in hypertrophic cardiomyopathy. Br. Heart J. *48*:198, 1982.
286. Frank, M. J., Watkins, L. O., Prisant, L. M., Stefadouros, M. A., and Abdulla, A. M.: Potentially lethal arrhythmias and their management in hypertrophic cardiomyopathy. Am. J. Cardiol. *53*:1608, 1984.
287. McKenna, W. J., England, D., Doi, Y. L., Deanfield, J. E., Oakley, C., and Goodwin, J. F.: Arrhythmia in hypertrophic cardiomyopathy. I. Influence on prognosis. Br. Heart J. *46*:168, 1981.

288. Stafford, W. J., Trohman, R. G., Bilsker, M., Zaman, L., Castellanos, A., and Myerburg, R. J.: Cardiac arrest in an adolescent with atrial fibrillation and hypertrophic cardiomyopathy. J. Am. Coll. Cardiol. *7*:701, 1986.
289. Kowey, P. R., Eisenberg, R., and Engel, T. R.: Sustained arrhythmias in hypertrophic obstructive cardiomyopathy. N. Engl. J. Med. *310*:1566, 1984.
290. Kronzon, I., and Glassman, E.: Mitral ring calcification in idiopathic hypertrophic subaortic stenosis. Am. J. Cardiol. *42*:60, 1978.
291. Maron, B. J.: Echocardiographic assessment of left ventricular hypertrophy in patients with obstructive or nonobstructive hypertrophic cardiomyopathy. Eur. Heart J. *4*:73, 1983.
292. Shapiro, L. M., Kleinebenne, A., and McKenna, W. J.: The distribution of left ventricular hypertrophy in hypertrophic cardiomyopathy: Comparison to athletes and hypertensives. Eur. Heart J. *6*:967, 1985.
293. Domenicucci, S., ten Cate, F. J., Das, S. K., Serruys, P. W., Vletter, W. B., and Roelandt, J.: Extent of hypertrophy in hypertrophic cardiomyopathy: Two-dimensional echocardiographic and angiographic correlation. Eur. Heart J. *4*:67, 1983.
294. McDonnell, M. A., and Tsagaris, T. J.: Recognition and diagnosis of apical hypertrophic cardiomyopathy. Chest *84*:644, 1983.
295. Danchin, N., Voiriot, P., Godenir, J. P., Neimann, J. L., Cherrier, F., and Faivre, G.: La cardiomyopathie hypertrophique apicale: Un element du continuum des cardiomyopathies hypertrophiques. Presse Med. *14*:1645, 1985.
296. Emanuel R., Marcomichelakis, J., Withers, R., and O'Brien, K.: Asymmetric septal hypertrophy and hypertrophic cardiomyopathy. Br. Heart J. *49*:309, 1983.
297. Wicker, P., Roudaut, R., Haissaguere, M., Villega-Arino, P., Clementy, J., and Dallocchio, M.: Prevalence and significance of asymmetric septal hypertrophy in hypertension: An echocardiographic and clinical study. Eur. Heart J. *4*:1, 1983.
298. Hess, O. M., Schneider, J., Turina, M., Carroll, J. D., Rothlin, M., and Krayenbuehl, H. P.: Asymmetric septal hypertrophy in patients with aortic stenosis: An adaptive mechanism or a coexistence of hypertrophic cardiomyopathy? J. Am. Coll. Cardiol. *1*:783, 1983.
299. Wei, J. Y., Weiss, J. L., and Bulkley, B. H.: The heterogeneity of hypertrophic cardiomyopathy: An autopsy and one-dimensional echocardiographic study. Am. J. Cardiol. *45*:24, 1980.
300. Doi, Y. L., Deanfield, J. E., McKenna, W. J., Dargie, H. J., Oakley, C. M., and Goodwin, J. F.: Echocardiographic differentiation of hypertensive heart disease and hypertrophic cardiomyopathy. Br. Heart J. *44*:395, 1980.
301. Bernstein, R. F., Tei, C., Child, J. S., and Shah, P. M.: Angled interventricular septum on echocardiography: Anatomic anomaly or technical artifact? J. Am. Coll. Cardiol. *2*:297, 1983.
302. Bhandari, A. K., and Nanda, N. C.: Myocardial texture characterization by two-dimensional echocardiography. Am. J. Cardiol. *51*:817, 1983.
303. Silverman, K. J., Hutchins, G. M., Weiss, J. L., and Moore, G. W.: Catenoid shape of the interventricular septum in idiopathic hypertrophic subaortic stenosis: Two-dimensional echocardiographic confirmation. Am. J. Cardiol. *49*:27, 1982.
304. Spirito, P., and Maron, B. J.: Significance of left ventricular outflow tract cross-sectional area in hypertrophic cardiomyopathy: A two-dimensional echocardiographic assessment. Circulation *67*:1100, 1983.
305. Maron, B. J., Gottdiener, J. S., Arce, J., Rosing, D. R., Wesley, Y. E., and Epstein, S. E.: Dynamic subaortic obstruction in hypertrophic cardiomyopathy: Analysis by pulsed Doppler echocardiography. J. Am. Coll. Cardiol. *6*:1, 1985.
306. Maron, B. J., Harding, A. M., Spirito, P., Roberts, W. C., and Waller, B. F.: Systolic anterior motion of the posterior mitral leaflet: A previously unrecognized cause of dynamic subaortic obstruction in patients with hypertrophic cardiomyopathy. Circulation *68*:282, 1983.
307. Gilbert, B. W., Pollick, C., Adelman, A. G., and Wigle, E. D.: Hypertrophic cardiomyopathy: Subclassification by M mode echocardiography. Am. J. Cardiol. *45*:861, 1980.
308. Pollick, C., Morgan, C. D., Gilbert, B. W., Rakowski, H., and Wigle, E. D.: Muscular subaortic stenosis: The temporal relationship between systolic anterior motion of the anterior mitral leaflet and the pressure gradient. Circulation *66*:1087, 1982.
309. Doi, Y. L., McKenna, W. J., Oakley, C. M., and Goodwin, J. F.: "Pseudo" systolic anterior motion in patients with hypertensive heart disease. Eur. Heart J. *4*:838, 1983.
310. Maron, B. J., Gottdiener, J. S., and Perry, L. W.: Specificity of systolic anterior motion of anterior mitral leaflet for hypertrophic cardiomyopathy: Prevalence in large population of patients with other cardiac diseases. Br. Heart J. *45*:206, 1981.
311. Maron B. J., Epstein, S. E., Bonow, R. O., Wyngaarden, M. K., and Wesley, Y. E.: Obstructive hypertrophic cardiomyopathy associated with minimal left ventricular hypertrophy. Am. J. Cardiol. *53*:377, 1984.
312. Gardin, J. M., Talano, J. V., Stephanides, L., Fizzano, J., and Lesch, M.: Systolic anterior motion in the absence of asymmetric septal hypertrophy: A buckling phenomenon of the chordae tendinae. Circulation *63*:181, 1981.
313. Ballester, M., Rickards, A., Rees, S., and McDonald, L.: Systolic anterior motion of the mitral valve in hypertrophic cardiomyopathy. A cross-sectional echocardiographic study. Eur. Heart J. *4*:846, 1983.
314. Nagata, S., Nimura, Y., Beppu, S., Park, Y. D., and Sakakibara, H.: Mechanism of systolic anterior motion of mitral valve and site of intraventricular pressure gradient in hypertrophic obstructive cardiomyopathy. Br. Heart J. *49*:234, 1983.
315. Kaul, S., Tei, C., and Shah, P. M.: Interventricular septal and free wall dynamics in hypertrophic cardiomyopathy. J. Am. Coll. Cardiol. *1*:1024, 1983.
316. Venco, A., Recusani, F., and Sgalambro, A.: Diastolic movement of mitral valve in hypertrophic cardiomyopathy: An echocardiographic study. Br. Heart J. *43*:159, 1980.
317. Sabbah, H. N., Alam, M., Anbe, D. T., and Stein, P. D.: Mid-systolic closure of the aortic valve in hypertrophic obstructive cardiomyopathy: A pressure-related phenomenon induced by turbulent blood flow. Cathet. Cardiovasc. Diagn. *6*:397, 1980.
317a. Nishimura, R. A., Tajik, A. J., Reeder, G. S., and Seward, J. B.: Evaluation of hypertrophic cardiomyopathy by Doppler color flow imaging: Initial observations. Mayo Clin. Proc. *61*:631, 1986.
318. Hanrath, P., Mathey, D. G., Siegert, R., and Bleifeld, W.: Left ventricular relaxation and filling pattern in different forms of left ventricular hypertrophy: An echocardiographic study. Am. J. Cardiol. *45*:15, 1980.
319. Spirito, P., Maron, B. J., Chiarella, F., Bellotti, P., Tramarin, R., Pozzoli, M., and Vecchio, C.: Diastolic abnormalities in patients with hypertrophic cardiomyopathy: Relation to magnitude of left ventricular hypertrophy. Circulation *72*:310, 1985.
320. Gardin, J. M., Dabestani, A., Glasgow, G. A., Butman, S., Burn, C. S., and Henry, W. L.: Echocardiographic and Doppler flow observations in obstructed and nonobstructed hypertrophic cardiomyopathy. Am. J. Cardiol. *56*:614, 1985.
321. Kinoshita, N., Nimura, Y., Okamoto, M., Miyatake, K., Nagata, S., and Sakakibara, H.: Mitral regurgitation in hypertrophic cardiomyopathy. Noninvasive study by two dimensional Doppler echocardiography. Br. Heart J. *49*:574, 1983.
322. Suzuki, Y., Kadota, K., Nohara, R., Tamaki, S., Kambara, H., Yoshida, A., Murakami, T., Osakada, G., Kawai, C., Tamaki, N., Mukai, T., and Torizuka, K.: Recognition of regional hypertrophy in hypertrophic cardiomyopathy using thallium-201 emission-computed tomography: Comparison with two-dimensional echocardiography. Am. J. Cardiol. *53*:1095, 1984.
323. Nagata, S., Park, Y., Minamikawa, T., Yutani, C., Kamiya, T., Nishimura, T., Kozuka, T., Sakakibara, H., and Nimura, Y.: Thallium perfusion and cardiac enzyme abnormalities in patients with familial hypertrophic cardiomyopathy. Am. Heart J. *109*:1317, 1985.
324. Pitcher, D., Wainwright, R., Maisey, M., Curry, P., and Sowton, E.: Assessment of chest pain in hypertrophic cardiomyopathy using exercise thallium-201 myocardial scintigraphy. Br. Heart J. *44*:650, 1980.
325. Bonow, R. O., Rosing, D. R., Bacharach, S. L., Green, M. V., Kent, K. M., Lipson, L. C., Maron, B. J., Leon, M. B., and Epstein, S. E.: Effects of verapamil on left ventricular systolic function and diastolic filling in patients with hypertrophic cardiomyopathy. Circulation *64*:787, 1981.
326. Betocchi, S., Bonow, R. O, Bacharach, S. L., Rosing, D. R., Maron, B. J., and Green, M. V.: Isovolumic relaxation period in hypertrophic cardiomyopathy: Assessment by radionuclide angiography. J. Am. Coll. Cardiol. *7*:74, 1986.
327. Cannon, R. O., 3d., Schenke, W. H., Bonow, R. O., Leon, M. B., and Rosing, D. R.: Left ventricular pulsus alternans in patients with hypertrophic cardiomyopathy and severe obstruction to left ventricular outflow. Circulation *73*:276, 1986.
328. Hirota, Y., Furubayashi, K., Kaku, K., Shimizu, G., Kino, M., Kawamura, K., and Takatsu, T.: Hypertrophic nonobstructive cardiomyopathy: A precise assessment of hemodynamic characteristics and clinical implications. Am. J. Cardiol. *50*:990, 1982.
329. Pouleur, H., Rousseau, M. F., van Eyll, C., Brasseur, L. A., and Charlier, A. A.: Force-velocity-length relations in hypertrophic cardiomyopathy: Evidence of normal or depressed myocardial contractility. Am. J. Cardiol. *52*:813, 1983.
330. Falicov, R. E., and Resnekov, L.: Mid ventricular obstruction in hypertrophic obstructive cardiomyopathy. New diagnostic and therapeutic challenge. Br. Heart J. *39*:701, 1977.
331. Kishimoto, C., Kadota, K., Sakurai, T., Murakami, T., Fujita, M., and Kawai, C.: Improved evaluation of hypertrophic cardiomyopathy by biventriculography with axial projection. Am. Heart J. *110*:77, 1985.
332. Cokkinos, D. V., Krajcer, Z., and Leachman, R. D.: Coronary artery disease in hypertrophic cardiomyopathy. Am. J. Cardiol. *55*:1437, 1985.
333. Brugada, P., Bär, F. W. H. M., de Zwaan, C., Roy, D., Green, M., and Wellens, H. J. J.: "Sawfish" systolic narrowing of the left anterior descending coronary artery: An angiographic sign of hypertrophic cardiomyopathy. Circulation *66*:800, 1982.
334. Pichard, A. D., Meller, J., Teichholz, L. E., Lipnik, S., Gorlin, R., and Herman, M. V.: Septal perforator compression (narrowing) in idiopathic hypertrophic subaortic stenosis. Am. J. Cardiol. *40*:310, 1977.
335. Glancy, D. L., Shephard, R. L., Beiser, G. D., and Epstein, S. E.: The dynamic nature of left ventricular outflow obstruction in idiopathic hypertrophic subaortic stenosis. Ann. Intern. Med. *75*:589, 1971.
336. Delman, A. J., and Stein, E.: Dynamic Auscultation and Phonocardiography, Philadelphia, W. B. Saunders Company, 1979, p. 825.
337. LeJemtal, T. H., Ribner, H. S., Strom, J. A., Jordan, A., and Sonnenblick, E. H.: Lack of accentuation by the Valsalva maneuver of the murmur of idiopathic hypertrophic subaortic stenosis: Importance of monitoring the pulse. Can. Med. Assoc. J. *126*:48, 1982.
338. Bartall, H., Amber, S., Desser, K. B., and Benchimol, A.: Normalization of the external carotid pulse tracing of hypertrophic subaortic stenosis during Müller's maneuver. Chest *74*:77, 1978.
339. Angoff, G. H., Wistran, D., Sloss, L. J., Markis, J. E., Come, P. C., Zoll, P. M., and Cohn, P. F.: Value of a noninvasively induced ventricular extrasystole during echocardiographic and phonocardiographic assessment of patients with idiopathic hypertrophic subaortic stenosis. Am. J. Cardiol. *42*:919, 1978.
340. Brockenbrough, E. C., Braunwald, E., and Morrow, A. G.: A hemodynamic

technic for the detection of hypertrophic subaortic stenosis. Circulation 23:189, 1961.
341. Bourmayan, C., Razavi, A., Fournier, C., Dussaule, J. C., Baragan, J., Gerbaux, A., and Gay, J.: Effect of propranolol on left ventricular relaxation in hypertrophic cardiomyopathy: An echographic study. Am. Heart J. 109:1311, 1985.
342. Cohen, L. S., and Braunwald, E.: Amelioration of angina pectoris in idiopathic hypertrophic subaortic stenosis with beta-adrenergic blockade. Circulation 35:847, 1967.
343. Cardiomyopathies. Geneva, World Health Organization, 1984.
344. Thompson, D. S., Haqvi, N., Juul, S. M., Swanton, R. H., Coltart, D. J., Jenkins, D. S., and Webb-Peploe, M. M.: Effects of propranolol on myocardial oxygen consumption, substrate extraction and haemodynamics in hypertrophic cardiomyopathy. Br. Heart J. 44:488, 1980.
345. Alvares, R. F., and Goodwin, J. F.: Noninvasive assessment of diastolic function in hypertrophic cardiomyopathy on and off beta adrenergic blocking drugs. Br. Heart J. 48:204, 1982.
346. Shah, P. M., Adelman, A. G., Wigle, E. D., Gobel, F. L., Burchell, H. B., Hardarson, T., Curill, R., de la Calzada, C., Oakley, C. M., and Goodwin, J. F.: The natural (and unnatural) history of hypertrophic obstructive cardiomyopathy. Circ. Res. 34/35 (Suppl. II):11, 1974.
347. Goodwin, J. G., and Oakley, C. M.: Medical and surgical treatment of hypertrophic cardiomyopathy. Eur. Heart J. 4:209, 1983.
348. Canedo, M. I., Frank, M. J., and Abdulla, A. M.: Rhythm disturbances in hypertrophic cardiomyopathy: Prevalence, relation to symptoms and management. Am. J. Cardiol. 45:848, 1980.
349. Frank, M. J., Abdulla, A. M., Watkins, L. O., Prisant, L., and Stefadouros, M. A.: Long-term medical management of hypertrophic cardiomyopathy: Usefulness of propranolol. Eur. Heart J. 4:155, 1983.
350. Losse, B., Kuhn, H., Loogen, F., and Schulte, H. D.: Exercise performance in hypertrophic cardiomyopathies. Eur. Heart J. 4:197, 1983.
351. Rouleau, J.-L., Chuck, L. H. S., Hollosi, G., Kidd. P., Sievers, R. E., Wikman-Coffelt, J., and Parmley, W. W.: Verapamil preserves myocardial contractility in the hereditary cardiomyopathy of the Syrian hamster. Circ. Res. 50:405, 1982.
352. Spicer, R. L., Rocchini, A. P., Crowley, D. C., Vasiliades, J., and Rosenthal, A.: Hemodynamic effects of verapamil in children and adolescents with hypertrophic cardiomyopathy. Circulation 67:413, 1983.
353. Anderson, D. M., Raff, G. L., Ports, T. A., Brundage, B. H., Parmley, W. W., and Chatterjee, K.: Hypertrophic obstructive cardiomyopathy. Effects of acute and chronic verapamil treatment on left ventricular systolic and diastolic function. Br. Heart J. 51:523, 1984.
354. Spicer, R. L., Rocchini, A. P., Crowley, D. C., Vasiliades, J., and Rosenthal, A.: Hemodynamic effects of verapamil on children and adolescents with hypertrophic cardiomyopathy. Circulation 67:413, 1983.
355. TenCate, F. J., Serruys, P. W., Mey, S., and Roelandt, J.: Effects of short-term administration of verapamil on left ventricular relaxation and filling dynamics measured by a combined hemodynamic-ultrasonic technique in patients with hypertrophic cardiomyopathy. Circulation 68:1274, 1983.
356. Bonow, R. O, Dilsizian, V., Rosing, D. R., Maron, B. J., Bacharach, S. L., and Green, M. V.: Verapamil-induced improvement in left ventricular diastolic filling and increased exercise tolerance in patients with hypertrophic cardiomyopathy: short- and long-term effects. Circulation 72:853, 1985.
357. Bonow, R. O, Frederick, T. M., Bacharach, S. L., Green, M. V., Goose, P. W., Maron, B. J., and Rosing, D. R.: Atrial systole and left ventricular filling in hypertrophic cardiomyopathy: Effect of verapamil. Am. J. Cardiol. 51:1386, 1983.
358. Hanrath, P., Mathey, D. G., Kremer, P., Sonntag, F., and Bleifield, W.: Effect of verapamil on left ventricular isovolumic relaxation time and regional left ventricular filling in hypertrophic cardiomyopathy. Am. J. Cardiol. 45:1258, 1980.
359. Bonow, R. O., Frederick, T. M., Bacharach, S. L., Green, M. V., Goose, P. W., and Rosing, D. R.: Atrial systole and left ventricular filling in patients with hypertrophic cardiomyopathy: Effect of verapamil. J. Am. Coll. Cardiol. 1:738, 1983.
359a. Chatterjee, K.: Calcium antagonist agents in hypertrophic cardiomyopathy. Am. J. Cardiol. 59:146B, 1987.
360. Hess, O. M., Grimm, J., and Krayenbuehl, H. P.: Diastolic function in hypertrophic cardiomyopathy: Effects of propranolol and verapamil on diastolic stiffness. Eur. Heart J. 4:47, 1983.
361. Bonow, R. O, Ostrow, H. G., Rosing, D. R., Cannon, R. O. 3d, Lipson, L. C., Maron, B. J., Kent, K. M., Bacharach, S. L., and Green, M. V.: Effects of verapamil on left ventricular systolic and diastolic function in patients with hypertrophic cardiomyopathy: Pressure-volume analysis with a nonimaging scintillation probe. Circulation 68:1062, 1983.
362. Tendera, M., Polonski, L., and Kozielska, E.: Left ventricular end-diastolic pressure-volume relationships in hypertrophic cardiomyopathy. Changes induced by verapamil. Chest 84:54, 1983.
363. Bonow, R. O.: Effects of calcium-channel blocking agents on left ventricular diastolic function in hypertrophic cardiomyopathy and in coronary artery disease. Am. J. Cardiol. 55:172B, 1985.
364. Kober, G., Schmidt-Moritz, A., Hopf, R., and Kaltenbach, M.: Long-term treatment of hypertrophic obstructive cardiomyopathy—usefulness of verapamil. Eur. Heart J. 4:165, 1983.
365. Kaltenbach, M., and Hopf, R.: Treatment of hypertrophic cardiomyopathy: Relation to pathological mechanisms. J. Mol. Cell. Cardiol. 2:59, 1985.
366. Spicer, R. L., Rocchini, A. P., Crowley D. C., and Rosenthal, A.: Chronic verapamil therapy in pediatric and young adult patients with hypertrophic cardiomyopathy. Am. J. Cardiol. 53:1614, 1984.
367. Bonow, R. O, Rosing, D. R., and Epstein, S. E.: The acute and chronic effects of verapamil on left ventricular function in patients with hypertrophic cardiomyopathy. Eur. Heart J. 4:57, 1983.
368. Hanrath, P., Schluter, M., Sonntag, F., Diemert, J., and Bleifeld, W.: Influence of verapamil therapy on left ventricular performance at rest and during exercise in hypertrophic cardiomyopathy. Am. J. Cardiol. 52:544, 1983.
369. Rosing, D. R., Kent, K. M., Maron, B. J., and Epstein, S. E.: Verapamil therapy: A new approach to the pharmacologic treatment of hypertrophic cardiomyopathy. II. Effects on exercise capacity and symptomatic status. Circulation 60:1208, 1979.
370. Rosing, D. R., Condit, J. R., Maron, B. J., Kent, K. M., Leon, M. B., Bonow, R. O., Lipson, L. C., and Epstein, S. E.: Verapamil therapy: A new approach to the pharmacologic treatment of hypertrophic cardiomyopathy. III. Effects of long-term administration. Am. J. Cardiol. 48:545, 1981.
371. Epstein, S. E., and Rosing, D. R.: Verapamil: Its potential for causing serious complications in patients with hypertrophic cardiomyopathy. Circulation 64:437, 1981.
372. Lorell, B. H.: Use of calcium channel blockers in hypertrophic cardiomyopathy. Am. J. Med. 78:43, 1985.
373. Perrot, B., Danchin, N., and Terrier de la Chaise, A.: Verapamil: a cause of sudden death in a patient with hypertrophic cardiomyopathy. Br. Heart J. 51:352, 1984.
374. Paulus, W. J., Lorell, B. H., Craig, W. E., Wynne, J., Murgo, J. P., and Grossman, W.: Comparison of the effects of nitroprusside and nifedipine on diastolic properties in patients with hypertrophic cardiomyopathy: Altered left ventricular loading or improved muscle inactivation? J. Am. Coll. Cardiol. 2:879, 1983.
375. Koide, T., Kakihana, M., Takabatake, Y., Iizuka, M., Uchida, Y., Ozeki, K., Morooka, S., Kato, A., Tanaka, S., Oya, T., Momomura, S., and Murao, S.: Long-term clinical effects of calcium inhibitors in hypertrophic cardiomyopathy compared to the effect of beta-blocking agents. Jpn. Heart J. 22:87, 1981.
376. Landmark, K., Sire, S., Thaulow, E., Amlie, J. P., and Nitter-Hauge, S.: Haemodynamic effects of nifedipine and propranolol in patients with hypertrophic obstructive cardiomyopathy. Br. Heart J. 48:19, 1982.
377. Betocchi, S., Cannon, R. O. 3d, Watson, R. M., Bonow, R. O., Ostrow, H. G, Epstein, S. E., and Rosing, D. R.: Effects of sublingual nifedipine on hemodynamics and systolic and diastolic function in patients with hypertrophic cardiomyopathy Circulation. 72:1001, 1985.
378. Fedor, J. M., Stack, R. S., Pryor, D. B., and Phillips, H. R.: Adverse effects of nifedipine therapy on hypertrophic obstructive cardiomyopathy. Chest 83:704, 1983.
379. Nagao, M., Omote, S., Takizawa, A., and Yasue, H.: Effect of diltiazem on left ventricular isovolumic relaxation time in patients with hypertrophic cardiomyopathy. Jpn. Circ. J. 47:54, 1983.
380. Suwa, M., Hirota, Y., and Kawamura, K.: Improvement in left ventricular diastolic function during intravenous and oral diltiazem therapy in patients with hypertrophic cardiomyopathy: an echocardiographic study. Am. J. Cardiol. 54:1047, 1984.
381. Strauer, B. E., Atef Mahmoud, M., Bayer, F., Bohn, I., and Motz, U.: Reversal of left ventricular hypertrophy and improvement of cardiac function in man by nifedipine. Eur. Heart J. 5:53, 1984.
382. Rosing, D. R., Idanpaan-Heikkila, U., Maron, B. J., Bonow, R. O., and Epstein, S. E.: Use of calcium-channel blocking drugs in hypertrophic cardiomyopathy. Am. J. Cardiol. 55:185B, 1985.
383. Pollick, C.: Muscular subaortic stenosis. Hemodynamic and clinical improvement after disopyramide. N. Engl. J. Med. 307:997, 1982.
384. Sugrue, D. D., Dickie, S., Myers, M. J., Lavender, J. P., and McKenna, W. J.: Effects of amiodarone on left ventricular ejection and filling in hypertrophic cardiomyopathy as assessed by radionuclide angiography. Am. J. Cardiol. 54:1054, 1984.
385. McKenna, W. J., Harris, L., Rowland, E., Kleinebenne, A., Krikler, D. M., Oakley, C. M., and Goodwin, J. F.: Amiodarone for long-term management of patients with hypertrophic cardiomyopathy. Am. J. Cardiol. 54:802, 1984.
386. Maron, B. J., Wesley, Y. E., and Arce, J.: Hypertrophic cardiomyopathy compatible with successful completion of the marathon. Am. J. Cardiol. 53:1470, 1984.
387. Maron, B. J., Gaffney, F. A., Jeresaty, R. M., McKenna, W. J., and Miller, W. W.: Task force III: Hypertrophic cardiomyopathy, other myopericardial diseases and mitral valve prolapse. J. Am. Coll. Cardiol. 6:1215, 1985.
388. Chagnac, A., Rudniki, C., Loebel, H., and Zahavi, I.: Infectious endocarditis in idiopathic hypertrophic subaortic stenosis: Report of three cases and review of the literature. Chest 81:346, 1982.
388a. Kirklin, J. W., and Barratt-Boyes, B. G.: Cardiac Surgery. New York, John Wiley and Sons, 1986, pp. 1013–1030.
389. Maron, B. J., Koch, J.-P., Kent, K. M., Epstein, S. E., and Morrow, A. G.: Results of surgery for idiopathic subaortic stenosis. J. Cardiovasc. Med. 5:145, 1980.
390. Beahrs, M. M., Tajik, A. J., Seward, J. B., Giuliani, E. R., and McGoon, D. C.: Hypertrophic obstructive cardiomyopathy: Ten- to 21-year followup after partial septal myectomy. Am. J. Cardio. 51:1160, 1983.
391. Maron, B. J., Epstein, S. E., and Morrow, A. G.: Symptomatic status and prognosis of patients after operation for hypertrophic obstructive cardiomyopathy: Efficacy of ventricular septal myotomy and myectomy. Eur. Heart J. 4:175, 1983.
392. Bircks, W., and Schulte, H. D.: Surgical treatment of hypertrophic obstructive cardiomyopathy with special reference to complications and to atypical hypertrophic obstructive cardiomyopathy. Eur. Heart J. 4:187, 1983.

393. Binet, J. P., David, P., and Piot, J. D.: Surgical treatment of hypertrophic obstructive cardiomyopathies. Eur. Heart J. 2:191, 1983.
394. Koch, J.-P., Maron, B. J., Epstein, S. E., and Morrow, A. G.: Results of operation for obstructive hypertrophic cardiomyopathy in the elderly: Septal myotomy and myectomy in 20 patients 65 years of age or older. Am. J. Cardiol. *46*:963, 1980.
395. Fighali, S., Krajcer, Z., and Leachman, R. D.: Septal myomectomy and mitral valve replacement for idiopathic hypertrophic subaortic stenosis: Short- and long-term follow-up. J. Am. Coll. Cardiol. *3*:1127, 1984.
396. Redwood, D. R., Goldstein, R. E., Hirshfeld, J., Borer, J. S., Morganroth, J., Morrow, A. G., and Epstein, S. E.: Exercise performance after septal myotomy and myectomy in patients with obstructive cardiomyopathy. Am. J. Cardiol. *44*:215, 1979.
397. Borer, J. S., Bacharach, S. L., Green, M. V., Kent, K. M., Rosing, D. R., Seides, S. F., Morrow, A. G., and Epstein S. E.: Effect of septal myotomy and myectomy on left ventricular systolic function at rest and during exercise in patients with IHSS. Circulation *60*(Suppl. I):I–82, 1979.
398. Duda, A. M., Gill, C. C., Kitazume, H., Moodie, D. S., and Loop, F. D.: Surgical treatment of idiopathic hypertrophic subaortic stenosis with other cardiac pathology. Cleve. Clin. Q. *51*:27, 1984.
399. Gill, C. C., Duda, A. M., Kitazume, H., Kramer, J. R., and Loop, F. D.: Idiopathic hypertrophic subaortic stenosis and coronary atherosclerosis. Results of coronary artery bypass alone and myectomy combined with coronary artery bypass. J. Thorac. Cardiovasc. Surg. *84*:856, 1982.
400. Isner, J. M., Clarke, R. H., Pandian, N. G., Donaldson, R. F., Salem, D. N., Konstam, M. A., Payne, D. D., and Cleveland, R. J.: Laser myoplasty for hypertrophic cardiomyopathy. In vitro experience in human postmortem hearts and in vivo experience in a canine model (transarterial) and human patient (intraoperative). Am. J. Cardiol. *53*:1620, 1984.
401. Shah, D. M., and Sunderji, S. G.: Hypertrophic cardiomyopathy and pregnancy: report of a maternal mortality and review of literature. Obstet. Gynecol. Surv. *40*:444, 1985.
402. Evans-Jones, J. C.: Hypertrophic cardiomyopathy in pregnancy. J. R. Soc. Med. *76*:524, 1983.
403. Fujiwara, H., Onodera, T., Tanaka, M., Shirane, H., Kato, H., Yoshikawa, J., Osakada, G., Sasayama, S., and Kawai, C.: Progression from hypertrophic obstructive cardiomyopathy to typical dilated cardiomyopathy-like features in the end stage. Jpn. Circ. J. *48*:1210, 1984.
404. Funakoshi, M., Imamura, M., Sasaki, J., Fujino, M., Kawano, T., Sasaki, Y., Nakashima, Y., Motooka, T., Fukuda, K., Imagawa, M., et al.: Seventeen year follow-up of a patient with hypertrophic cardiomyopathy which progressed to dilated cardiomyopathy. Jpn. Heart J. *25*:805, 1984.
405. Brett, W., Brandt, P. W., Bierre, A. R., and Roche, A. H.: Progression of hypertrophic cardiomyopathy to congestive cardiomyopathy: Case report. NZ Med. J. *98*:994, 1985.
406. Yutani, C., Imakita, M., Ishibashi-Ueda, H., Hatanaka, K., Nagata, S., Sakakibara, H., and Nimura, Y.: Three autopsy cases of progression to left ventricular dilatation in patients with hypertrophic cardiomyopathy. Am. Heart J. *109*:545, 1985.
407. Spirito, P., Maron, B. J., Bonow, R. O., Epstein, S. E.: Occurrence and significance of progressive left ventricular wall thinning and relative cavity dilatation in patients with hypertrophic cardiomyopathy. Am. J. Cardiol. (*in press*).
408. Waller, B. F., Maron, B. J., Epstein, S. E., and Roberts, W. C.: Transmural myocardial infarction in hypertrophic cardiomyopathy: A cause of conversion from left ventricular asymmetry to symmetry and from normal-sized to dilated left ventricular cavity. Chest 79:461, 1981.
409. Domenicucci, S., Lazzeroni, E., Roelandt, J., ten Cate, F. J., Vletter, W. B., Arntzenius, A. C., and Das, S. K.: Progression of hypertrophic cardiomyopathy. A cross sectional echocardiographic study. Br. Heart J. *53*:405, 1985.
410. Ciro, E., Maron, B. J., Bonow, R. O., Cannon, R. O., and Epstein, S. E.: Relation between marked changes in left ventricular outflow tract gradient and disease progression in hypertrophic cardiomyopathy. Am. J. Cardiol. *53*:1103, 1984.
411. Maron, B. J., Lipson, L. C., Roberts, W. C., Savage, D. D., and Epstein, S. E.: "Malignant" hypertrophic cardiomyopathy: Identification of a subgroup of families with unusually frequent premature deaths. Am. J. Cardiol. *41*:1133, 1978.
412. Baron, B. J., Roberts, W. C., Epstein, S. E.: Sudden death in hypertrophic cardiomyopathy: A profile of 78 patients. Circulation *65*:1388, 1982.
413. McKenna, W., Deanfield, J., Faruqui, A., England, D., Oakley, C., and Goodwin, J.: Prognosis in hypertrophic cardiomyopathy: Role of age and clinical, electrocardiographic and hemodynamic features. Am. J. Cardiol. *47*:532, 1981.
414. Newman, H., Sugrue, D., Oakley, C. M., Goodwin, J. F., and McKenna, W. J.: Relation of left ventricular function and prognosis in hypertrophic cardiomyopathy: An angiographic study. J. Am. Coll. Cardiol. *5*:1064, 1985.
415. Brandenburg, R. O.: Cardiomyopathies and their role in sudden death. J. Am. Coll. Cardiol. *5*:185B, 1985.
416. Maron, B. J., Epstein, S. E., and Roberts, W. C.: Causes of sudden death in competitive athletes. J. Am. Coll. Cardiol. *7*:204, 1986.
417. Koga, Y., Itaya, K., and Toshima, H.: Prognosis in hypertrophic cardiomyopathy. Am. Heart J. *108*:351, 1984.
418. Louie, E. K., and Maron, B. J.: Hypertrophic cardiomyopathy with extreme increase in left ventricular wall thickness: Functional and morphologic features and clinical significance. J. Am. Coll. Cardiol. *8*:57, 1986.
419. McKenna, W. J., Oakley, C. M., Krikler, D. M., and Goodwin, J. F.: Improved survival with amiodarone in patients with hypertrophic cardiomyopathy and ventricular tachycardia. Br. Heart J. *53*:412, 1985.
420. McKenna, W. J., Harris, L., Perez, G., Krikler, D. M., Oakley, C., and Goodwin, J. F.: Arrhythmia in hypertrophic cardiomyopathy. II. Comparison of amiodarone and verapamil in treatment. Br. Heart J. *46*:173, 1981.

RESTRICTIVE AND INFILTRATIVE CARDIOMYOPATHIES

421. Benotti, J. R., and Grossman, W.: Restrictive cardiomyopathy. Annu. Rev. Med. *35*:113, 1984.
422. Hosenpud, J. D., and Niles, N. R.: Clinical, hemodynamic and endomyocardial biopsy findings in idiopathic restrictive cardiomyopathy. West. J. Med. *144*:303, 1986.
423. Isner, J. M., Carter, B. L., Bankoff, M. S., Pastore, J. O., Ramaswamy, K., McAdam, K. P., and Salem, D. N.: Differentiation of constrictive pericarditis from restrictive cardiomyopathy by computed tomographic imaging. Am. Heart J. *105*:1019, 1983.
424. Hirota, Y., Kohriyama, T., Hayashi, T., Kaku, K., Nishimura, H., Saito, T., Nakayama, Y., Suwa, M., Kino, M., and Kawamura, K.: Idiopathic restrictive cardiomyopathy: Differences of left ventricular relaxation and diastolic wave forms from constrictive pericarditis. Am. J. Cardiol. *52*:421, 1983.
424a. Schoenfeld, M. H., Supple, E. W., Dec, G. W., Fallon, J. T., and Palacios, I. F.: Restrictive cardiomyopathy versus constructive pericarditis: Role of endomyocardial biopsy in avoiding unnecessary thoracotomy. Circulation *75*:1012, 1987.
425. Siegel, R. J., Shah, P. K., and Fishbein, M. C.: Idiopathic restrictive cardiomyopathy. Circulation *70*:165, 1984.
426. Benotti, J. R., Grossman, W., and Cohn, P. F.: The clinical profile of restrictive cardiomyopathy. Circulation *61*:1206, 1980.
427. Navarro-Lopez, F., Llorian, A., Ferrer-Roca, O., Betriu, A., amd Sanz, G.: Restrictive cardiomyopathy in pseudoxanthoma elasticum. Chest *78*:113, 180.
428. Janos, G. G., Arjunan, K., Meyer, R. A., Engel, P., and Kaplan, S.: Differentiation of constrictive pericarditis and restrictive cardiomyopathy using digitized echocardiography. J. Am. Coll. Cardiol. *1*:541, 1983.
429. Shabetai, R.: Profiles in constrictive pericarditis, cardiac tamponade and restrictive cardiomyopathy. *In* Grossman, W. (ed.): Cardiac Catheterization and Angiography. Philadelphia, Lea and Febiger, 1974, p. 304.
430. Borer, J. S., Henry, W. L., and Epstein, S. E.: Echocardiographic observations in patients with systemic infiltrative disease involving the heart. Am. J. Cardiol. *39*:184, 1977.
431. Glenner, G. C.: Amyloid deposits and amyloidosis: The β-fibrilloses. N. Engl. J. Med. *302*:1283 and 1333, 1980.
432. Fogo, A., and Virmani, R.: Cardiac amyloidosis. Primary Cardiology *10*:54, 1984.
433. Sanchez-Ramos, J. A., Redondo-Sanchez, R., Garcia-Crespo, P., Superby-Jeldres, A., and Schuller-Perez, A.: Cardiac amyloidosis. Cardiovascular Reviews and Reports *5*:524, 1984.
434. Cornwell, G. G. 3d, Murdoch, W. L., Kyle, R. A., Westermark, P., and Pitkanen, P.: Frequency and distribution of senile cardiovascular amyloid. A clinicopathologic correlation. Am. J. Med. *75*:618, 1983.
435. Ruder, M. A., Alpert, M. A., Sanfelippo, J. F., Dix, J. D., and Whiting, R. B.: Symptomatic cardiac amyloidosis in an American family. South. Med. J. *77*:831, 1984.
436. Hodkinson, H. M., and Pomerance, A.: The clinical significance of senile cardiac amyloidosis: A prospective clinicopathological study. Q. J. Med. *46*:381, 1977.
437. Roberts, W. C., and Waller, B. F.: Cardiac amyloidosis causing cardiac dysfunction: Analysis of 54 necropsy patients. Am. J. Cardiol. *52*:137, 1983.
438. Maule, W. F., and Martin, R. H.: Primary cardiac amyloidosis: An angiographic clue to early diagnosis. Ann. Intern. Med. *98*:177, 1983.
439. Allen, D. C., and Doherty, C. C.: Sudden death in a patient with amyloidosis of the cardiac conduction system. Br. Heart J. *51*:233, 1984.
440. Eriksson, A., Eriksson, P., Olofsson, B. O., and Thornell, L. E.: The cardiac atrioventricular conduction system in familial amyloidosis with polyneuropathy. Acta Pathol. Microbiol. Immunol. Scand. *91*:343, 1983.
441. Ridolfi, R. L., Bulkley, B. H., and Hutchins, G. M.: The conduction system in cardiac amyloidosis. Clinical and pathologic features of 23 patients. Am. J. Med. *62*:677, 1977.
442. Ladefoged, C., and Rohr, N.: Amyloid deposits in aortic and mitral valves. Virchows Arch. *404*:301, 1984.
443. Saffitz, J. E., Sazama, K., and Roberts, W. C.: Amyloidosis limited to small arteries causing angina pectoris and sudden death. Am. J. Cardiol. *51*:1234, 1983.
444. Smith, R. R. L., and Hutchins, G. M.: Ischemic heart disease secondary to amyloidosis of intramyocardial arteries. Am. J. Cardiol. *44*:413, 1979.
445. Chew, C., Ziady, G. M., Raphael, M. J., and Oakley, C. M.: The functional defect in amyloid heart disease: The "stiff heart" syndrome. Am. J. Cardiol. *36*:438, 1975.
446. Kern, M. J., Lorell, B. H., and Grossman, W.: Cardiac amyloidosis masquerading as constrictive pericarditis. Cathet. Cardiovasc. Diagn. *8*:629, 1982.
447. Tyberg, T. I., Goodyer, A. V., Hurst, V. W., III, Alexander, J., and Langou, R. A.: Left ventricular filling in differentiating restrictive amyloid cardiomyopathy and constrictive pericarditis. Am. J. Cardiol. *47*:791, 1981.
448. Garcia, R., and Saleh, S. M.: Amyloidosis. Cardiovascular manifestations in five illustrative cases. Arch. Intern. Med. *121*:259, 1968.
449. Eriksson P., Karp, K., Bjerle, P., and Olofsson, B. O.: Disturbances of cardiac rhythm and conduction in familial amyloidosis with polyneuropathy. Br. Heart J. *51*:658, 1984.
450. Falk, R. H., Rubinow, A., and Cohen, A. S.: Cardiac arrhythmias in systemic amyloidosis: correlation with echocardiographic abnormalities. J. Am. Coll. Cardiol. *3*:107, 1984.

451. Olofsson, B. O., Andersson, R., and Furberg, B.: Atrioventricular and intraventricular conduction in familial amyloidosis with polyneuropathy. Acta Med. Scand. *208*:77, 1980.
452. Gray, L. W., Duca, P. R., and Chung, E. K.: Sick sinus syndrome due to cardiac amyloidosis. Cardiology *63*:212, 1978.
453. Olofsson, B. O., Eriksson, P., and Eriksson, A.: The sick sinus syndrome in familial amyloidosis with polyneuropathy. Int. J. Cardiol. *4*:71, 1983.
454. Siqueira-Filho, A. G., Cunha, C. L. P., Tajik, A. J., Seward, J. B., Schattenberg, T. T., and Giuliani, E. R.: M-mode and two-dimensional echocardiographic features in cardiac amyloidosis. Circulation *63*:188, 1981.
454a. Falk, R. H., Plehn, J. F., Deering, T., Schick, E. C., Jr., Boinay, P., Rubinow, A., Skinner, M., and Cohen, A. S.: Sensitivity and specificity of the echocardiographic features of cardiac amyloidosis. Am. J. Cardiol. *59*:418, 1987.
455. Cueto-Garcia, L., Tajik, A. J., Kyle, R. A., Edwards, W. D., Greipp, P. R., Callahan, J. A., Shub, C., and Seward, J. B.: Serial echocardiographic observations in patients with primary systemic amyloidosis: An introduction to the concept of early (asymptomatic) amyloid infiltration of the heart. Mayo Clin. Proc. *59*:589, 1984.
456. Backman, C., and Olofsson, B. O.: Echocardiographic features in familial amyloidosis with polyneuropathy. Acta Med. Scand. *214*:273, 1983.
457. Eriksson, P., Backman, C., Bjerle, P., Eriksson, H., Holm, S., and Olofsson, B. O.: Non-invasive assessment of the presence and severity of cardiac amyloidosis. A study in familial amyloidosis with polyneuropathy by cross sectional echocardiography and technetium-99m pyrophosphate scintigraphy. Br. Heart J. *52*:321, 1984.
458. Brodarick, S., Paine, R., Higa, E., and Carmichael, K. A.: Pericardial tamponade, a new complication of amyloid heart disease. Am. J. Med. *73*:133, 1982.
459. Nicolosi, G. L., Pavan, D., Lestuzzi, C., Burelli, C., Zardo, F., and Zanuttini, D.: Prospective identification of patients with amyloid heart disease by two-dimensional echocardiography. Circulation *70*:432, 1984.
460. Hongo, M., and Ikeda, S. I.: Echocardiographic assessment of the evolution of amyloid heart disease: A study with familial amyloid polyneuropathy. Circulation *73*:249, 1986.
461. Eriksson, P., Eriksson, A., Backman, C., Hofer, P. A., and Olofsson, B. O.: Highly refractile myocardial echoes in familial amyloidosis with polyneuropathy. Acta Med. Scand. *217*:27, 1985.
462. Sivaram, C. A., Jugdutt, B. I., Amy, R. W., Basualdo, C. A., Haraphongse, M., and Shnitka, T. K.: Cardiac amyloidosis: Combined use of two-dimensional echocardiography and electrocardiography in noninvasive screening before biopsy. Clin. Cardiol. *8*:511, 1985.
463. Leinonen, H., and Pohjola-Sintonen, S.: Cardiac amyloidosos. Therapeutic and diagnostic difficulties with reference to two different forms of the disease. Acta Med. Scand. *219*:125, 1986.
464. Cueto-Garcia, L., Reeder, G. S., Kyle, R. H., Wood, D. L., Seward, J. B., Naessens, J., Offord, K. P., Greipp, P. R., Edwards, W. D., and Tajik, A. J.: Echocardiographic findings in systemic amyloidosis: Spectrum of cardiac involvement and relation to survival. J. Am. Coll. Cardiol. *6*:737, 1985.
465. Carroll, J. D., Gaasch, W. H., and McAdam, K. P. W. J.: Amyloid cardiomyopathy: Characterization by a distinctive voltage/mass relation. Am. J. Cardiol. *49*:9, 1982.
466. St. John Sutton, M. D., Reicheck, N., Kastor, J. A., and Giuliani, E. R.: Computerized M-mode echocardiographic analysis of left ventricular dysfunction in cardiac amyloid. Circulation *66*:790, 1982.
467. Falk, R. H., Lee, V. W., Rubinow, A., Hood, W. B. Jr., and Cohen, A. S.: Sensitivity of technetium-99m-pyrophosphate scintigraphy in diagnosing cardiac amyloidosis. Am. J. Cardiol. *51*:826, 1983.
468. Sekiya, T., Foster, C. J., Isherwood, I., Lucas, S. B., Kahn, M. K., and Miller, J. P.: Computed tomographic appearances of cardiac amyloidosis. Br. Heart J. *51*:519, 1984.
469. Eriksson, P., Backman, C., Bjerle, P., Eriksson, A., Holm, S., and Olofsson, B. O.: Noninvasive assessment of the presence and severity of cardiac amyloidosis. A study in familial amyloidosis with polyneuropathy by cross sectional echocardiography and technetium-99m pyrophosphate scintigraphy. Br. Heart J. 52:321, 1984.
470. Wizenberg, T. A., Muz, J., Sohn, Y. H., Samlowski, W., and Weissler, A. M.: Value of positive myocardial technetium-99m-pyrophosphate scintigraphy in the noninvasive diagnosis of cardiac amyloidosis. Am. Heart J. *103*:468, 1982.
471. Saltissi, S., Kertes, P. J., and Julian, D. G.: Primary cardiac amyloidosis in a young man presenting with angina pectoris. Br. Heart J. 52:233, 1984.
472. Leinonen, H., Totterman, K. J., Korppi-Tommola, T., and Korhola, O.: Negative myocardial technetium-99m-pyrophosphate scintigraphy in amyloid heart disease associated with type AA systemic amyloidosis. Am. J. Cardiol. *15*:380, 1984.
473. Browning, M. J., Banks, R. H., Tribe, C. R., Hollingworth, P., Kingswood, C., Mackenzie, J. C., and Bacon, P. A.: Ten years' experience of an amyloid clinic—a clinicopathological survey. Q. J. Med. *54*:213, 1985.
474. Kyle, R. A., and Baynd, E. D.: Amyloidosis: Review of 236 cases. Medicine *54*:271, 1975.
475. Rubinow, A., Skinner, M., and Cohen, A. S.: Digoxin sensitivity in amyloid cardiomyopathy. Circulation *63*:1285, 1981.
476. Gertz, M. H., Skinner, M., Connors, L. H., Falk, R. H., Cohen, A. S., and Kyle, R. H.: Selective binding of nifedipine to amyloid fibrils. Am. J. Cardiol. 55:1646, 1985.
477. Griffiths, B. E., Hughes, P., Dowdle, R., and Stephens, M. R.: Cardiac amyloidosis with asymmetrical septal hypertrophy and deterioration after nifedipine. Thorax *37*:711, 1982.
478. Gertz, M. A.: Falk, R. H., Skinner, M., Cohen, A. S., and Kyle, R. A.: Worsening of congestive heart failure in amyloid heart disease treated by calcium channel-blocking agents. Am. J. Cardiol. *55*:1645, 1985.
479. Eriksson, P., and Olofsson, B. O.: Pacemaker treatment in familial amyloidosis with polyneuropathy. PACE *7*:702, 1984.
480. Taylor, W. J.: Genetic aspects of the cardiomyopathies. Prog. Med. Genet. *5*:163, 1983.
481. Desnick, R. J., Blieden, L. C., Sharp, H. L., Hofschire, P. J., and Moller, J. H.: Cardiac valvular anomalies in Fabry disease. Clinical, morphologic and biochemical studies. Circulation *54*:818, 1976.
482. Sakuraba, H., Yanagawa, Y., Igarashi, T., Suzuki, Y., Suzuki, T., Watanabe, K., Ieki, K., Shimoda, K., and Yamanaka, T.: Cardiovascular manifestations in Fabry's disease. Clin. Genetics *29*:276, 1986.
483. Goldman, M. E., Cantor, R., Schwartz, M. F., Baker, M., Desnick, R. J.: Echocardiographic abnormalities and disease severity in Fabry's disease. J. Am. Coll. Cardiol. *7*:1157, 1986.
484. Seino, Y., Vyden, J. K., Philippart, M., Rose, H. B., and Nagasawa, K.: Peripheral hemodynamics in patients with Fabry's disease. Am. Heart J. *105*:783, 1983.
485. Mehta, J., Tuna, N., Moller, J. H., and Desnick, R. J.: Electrocardiographic and vectorcardiographic abnormalities in Fabry's disease. Am. Heart J. *93*:699, 1977.
485a. Yokoyama, A., Yamazoe, M., and Shibata, A.: A case of heterozygous Fabry's disease with a short PR interval and giant negative T waves. Br. Heart J. *57*:296, 1987.
486. Cohen, I. S., Fluri-Lundeen, J., and Wharton, T. P.: Two dimensional echocardiographic similarity of Fabry's disease to cardiac amyloidosis: A function of ultrastructural analogy? JCU *11*:437, 1983.
487. Broadbent, J. C., Edwards, W. D., Gordon, H., Hartzler, G. O., and Krawisz, J. E.: Fabry cardiomyopathy in the female confirmed by endomyocardial biopsy. Mayo Clin. Proc. *56*:623, 1981.
488. Maben, P., Evans, R., Lin, J., and Vaughan, D.: Endomyocardial biopsy. J. Kansas Med. Soc. *84*:556, 1983.
489. Kramer, W., Thormann, J., Mueller, K., and Frenzel, H.: Progressive cardiac involvement by Fabry's disease despite successful renal allotransplantation. Int. J. Cardiol. *7*:72, 1985.
490. Casta, A., Hayden, K., and Wolf, W. J.: Calcification of the ascending aorta and aortic and mitral valves in Gaucher's disease. Am. J. Cardiol. *54*:1390, 1984.
491. Platzker, Y., Pisman, E. Z., Pines, A., and Kellermann, J. J.: Unusual echocardiographic pattern in Gaucher's disease. Cardiology *72*:144, 1985.
492. Wilson, E. R., Barton, N. W., and Barranger, J. H.: Vascular involvement in type 3 neuronopathic Gaucher's disease. Arch. Pathol. Lab. Med. *109*:82, 1985.
493. Buja, L. M., and Roberts, W. C.: Iron in the heart. Etiology and clinical significance. Am. J. Med. *51*:209, 1971.
494. Arnett, E. N., Nienhuis, A. W., Henry, W. L., Ferrans, V. J., Redwood, D. R., and Roberts, W. C.: Massive myocardial hemosiderosis: A structure-function conference at the National Heart and Lung Institute. Am. Heart J. *90*:777, 1975.
495. Dabestani, A., Child, J. S., Henze, E., Perloff, J. K., Schon, H., Figueroa, W. G., Schelbert, H. R., and Thessomboon, S.: Primary hemochromatosis: Anatomic and physiologic characteristics of the cardiac ventricles and their response to phlebotomy. Am. J. Cardiol. *54*:153, 1984.
496. Candell-Riera, J., Lu, L., Seres, L., Gonzalez, J. B., Batlle, J., Permanyer-Miralda, G., Garcia-del-Castillo, H., and Soler-Soler, J.: Cardiac hemochromatosis: Beneficial effects of iron removal therapy. An echocardiographic study. Am. J. Cardiol. *52*:824, 1983.
497. Valdes-Cruz, L. M., Reinecke, C., Rutkowski, M., Dudell, G. G., Goldberg, S. J., Allen, H. D., Sahn, D. J., and Piomelli, S.: Preclinical abnormal segmental cardiac manifestations of thalassemia major in children on transfusion-chelation therapy: Echographic alterations of left ventricular posterior wall contraction and relaxation patterns. Am. Heart J. *103*:505, 1982.
498. Furth, P. A., Futterweit, W., and Gorlin, R.: Refractory biventricular heart failure in secondary hemochromatosis. Am. J. Med. Sci. *290*:209, 1985.
499. Powell, L. W., and Isselbacher, K. J.: Hemochromatosis. *In* Braunwald, E., Isselbacher, K. J., Petersdorf, R. G., Wilson, J. P., Martin, J. B., and Fauci, A. S. (eds.): Harrison's Principles of Internal Medicine. New York, McGraw-Hill, 1987, p. 1632.
500. Cutler, D. J., Isner, J. M., Bracey, A. W., Hufnagel, C. A., Conrad, P. W., Roberts, W. C., Kerwin, D. M., and Weintraub, A. M.: Hemochromatosis heart disease: An unemphasized cause of potentially reversible restrictive cardiomyopathy. Am. J. Med. *69*:923, 1980.
501. Short, E. M., Winkle, R. A., and Billingham, M. E.: Myocardial involvement in idiopathic hemochromatosis. Morphologic and clinical improvement following venesection. Am. J. Med. *70*:1275, 1981.
502. Editorial: Sarcoid heart disease. Br. Med. J. *4*:627, 1972.
503. Baughman, R. P., Gerson, M., and Bosken, C. H.: Right and left ventricular function at rest and with exercise in patients with sarcoidosis. Chest *85*:301, 1984.
504. Lewin, R. F., Mor, R., Spitzer, S., Arditti, A., Hellman, C., and Agmon, J.: Echocardiographic evaluation of patients with systemic sarcoidosis. Am. Heart J. *110*:116, 1985.
505. Silverman, K. J., Hutchins, G. M., and Bulkley, B. H.: Cardiac sarcoid: A clinicopathologic study of 84 unselected patients with systemic sarcoidosis. Circulation *58*:1204, 1978.
506. Roberts, W. C., McAllister, H. A., and Ferrans, V. J.: Sarcoidosis of the heart. A clinicopathologic study of 35 necropsy patients (Group I) and review

of 78 previously described necropsy patients (Group II). Am. J. Cardiol. 63:86, 1977.
507. Burton, D. A., Kapur, S., Shapiro, S. R., Leatherbury, L., and Scott, L. P., 3rd: Fulminant cardiac sarcoidosis in childhood. Am. J. Cardiol. 58:177, 1986.
507a. Valantine, H., McKenna, W. J., Nihoyannopoulos, P., Mitchell, A., Foale, R. A., Davies, M. J., Oakley, C. M.: Sarcoidosis: a pattern of clinical and morphological presentation. Br. Heart J. 57:256, 1987.
508. Freiman, D. G.: The pathology of sarcoidosis. Semin. Roentgenol. 20:327, 1985.
509. Fleming, H. H.: Sarcoid heart disease editorial. Br. Med. J. 292:1095, 1986.
510. Lemery, R., McGoon, M. D., and Edwards, W. D.: Cardiac sarcoidosis: a potentially treatable form of myocarditis. Mayo Clin. Proc. 60:549, 1985.
511. James, T. N.: Subitaneis Mortibus. XXV. Sarcoid heart disease. Circulation 56:320, 1977.
512. Fleming, H. A.: Sarcoid heart disease. Br. Heart J. 36:54, 1974.
513. Abeler, V.: Sarcoidosis of the cardiac conducting system. Am. Heart J. 97:701, 1979.
514. Walsh, M. J.: Systemic sarcoidosis with refractory ventricular tachycardia and heart failure. Br. Heart J. 40:931, 1978.
515. Serwer, G. A., Edwards, S. B., Benson, W., Jr., Anderson, P. A. W., and Spack, M.: Ventricular tachycardia due to cardiac sarcoidosis in a child. Pediatrics 62:322, 1978.
516. Miller, A., Jackler, I., and Chuang, M.: Onset of sarcoidosis with left ventricular failure and multisystem involvement. Chest 70:302, 1976.
517. Thunell, M., Bjerle, P., Olofsson, B. O., Osterman, G., and Stjernberg, N.: Cardiopulmonary function in sarcoidosis. Acta Med. Scand. 215:215, 1984.
518. Koide, T., Itoyama, S., Kato, K., Kato, A., and Murao, S.: Cardiac sarcoidosis with 12-year survival. Jpn. Heart J. 23:263, 1982.
519. Ahmed, S. S., Rozefort, R., Taclob, L. T., and Brancato, R. W.: Development of ventricular aneurysm in cardiac sarcoidosis. Angiology 28:323, 1977.
520. Verkleeren, J. L., Glover, M. U., Bloor, C., and Joswig, B. C.: Cardiac tamponade secondary to sarcoidosis. Am. Heart J. 106:601, 1983.
520a. Kirklin, J. W., and Barratt-Boyes, B. G.: Cardiac Surgery. New York, John Wiley and Sons, 1986, pp. 1419–1426.
521. Thunell, M., Bjerle, P., and Stjernberg, N.: ECG abnormalities in patients with sarcoidosis. Acta Med. Scand. 213:115, 1983.
522. Cepin, D., McDonough, M., and James, F.: Cardiac sarcoidosis. A case with unusual manifestation. Arch. Intern. Med. 143:142, 1983.
523. Lorell, B., Alderman, E. L., and Mason, J. W.: Cardiac sarcoidosis. Diagnosis with endomyocardial biopsy and treatment with corticosteroids. Am. J. Cardiol. 42:143, 1978.
524. Kinney, E. L., Jackson, G. L., Reeves, W. C., and Zelis, R.: Thallium-scan myocardial defects and echocardiographic abnormalities in patients with sarcoidosis without clinical cardiac dysfunction. An analysis of 44 patients. Am. J. Med. 68:497, 1980.
525. Forman, M. B., Sandler, M. P., Sacks, G. A., Kronenberg, M. W., and Powers, T. A.: Radionuclide imaging in myocardial sarcoidosis. Demonstration of myocardial uptake of technetium pyrophosphate 99m and gallium. Chest 83:578, 1983.
526. Tornling, G., Olsson, G., and von Unge, A.: Ventricular fibrillation in myocardial sarcoidosis. Eur. J. Respir. Dis. 66:347, 1985.
527. Stein, E., Stimmel, B., and Siltzbach, L. E.: Clinical course of cardiac sarcoidosis. Ann. N.Y. Acad. Sci. 278:470, 1976.
528. Ishikawa, T., Kondoh, H., Nakagawa, S., Koiwaya, Y., and Tanaka, K.: Steroid therapy in cardiac sarcoidosis: Increased left ventricular contractility concomitant with electrocardiographic improvement after prednisolone. Chest 85:445, 1984.
529. Becker, B. J. P., Chatgidakis, C. B., and Van Lingen, B.: Cardiovascular collagenosis with parietal endocardial thrombosis. A clinicopathological study of forty cases. Circulation 7:345, 1953.
530. Davies, J. N. P., and Coles, R. M.: Some considerations regarding obscure disease affecting the mural endocardium. Am. Heart J. 59:606, 1960.
531. Goodwin, J. F.: Endomyocardial disease—clinical features. Postgrad. Med. J. 59:154, 1983.
532. Cherian, G., Vijayaraghavan, G., Krishnaswami, S., Sukumar, I. P., John, S., Jairaj, P. S., and Bhaktaviziam, A.: Endomyocardial fibrosis: Report on the hemodynamic data in 29 patients and review of the results of surgery. Am. Heart J. 105:659, 1983.
533. Acquatella, H., Schiller, N. B., Puigbo, J. J., Gomez-Mancebo, J. R., Suarez, C., and Acquatella, G.: Value of two-dimensional echocardiography in endomyocardial disease with and without eosinophilia. A clinical and pathological study. Circulation 67:1219, 1983.
534. Cherian, K. M., John, T. A., and Abraham, K. A.: Endomyocardial fibrosis: Clinical profile and role of surgery in management. Am. Heart J. 105:706, 1983.
535. Olsen, E. G.: Pathological aspects of endomyocardial fibrosis. Postgrad. Med. J. 59:135, 1983.
536. Davies, J., Spry, C. J. F., Vijayaraghaven, G., and De Souza, J. A.: A comparison of the clinical and cardiological features of endomyocardial disease in temperate and tropical regions. Postgrad. Med. J. 59:179, 1983.
537. Spry, C. J. F., Tai, P. C., and Davies, J.: The cardiotoxicity of eosinophils. Postgrad. Med. J. 59:147, 1983.
538. Olsen, E. G., and Spry, C. J.: Relation between eosinophilia and endomyocardial disease. Prog. Cardiovasc. Dis. 27:241, 1985.
539. Fauci, A. S., Harley, J. B., Roberts, W. C., Ferrans, V. J., Gralnick, H. R., and Bjornson, B. H.: NIH conference. The idiopathic hypereosinophilic syndrome. Clinical, pathophysiologic, and therapeutic considerations. Ann. Intern. Med. 97:78, 1982.
540. Spry, C. J., Weetman, A. P., Olsson, I., Tai, P. C., and Olsen, E. G.: The pathogenesis of eosinophilic endomyocardial disease in patients with carcinomas of the lung. Heart Vessels 1:162, 1985.
541. Harley, J. B., Fauci, A. S., and Gralnick, H. R.: Noncardiovascular findings associated with heart disease in the idiopathic hypereosinophilic syndrome. Am. J. Cardiol. 52:321, 1983.
542. Spry, C. J.: The hypereosinophilic syndrome: Clinical features, laboratory findings and treatment. Allergy 37:539, 1982.
543. Lanham, J. G., Cooke, S., Davies, J., and Hughes, G. R. V.: Endomyocardial complications of the Churg-Strauss syndrome. Postgrad. Med. J. 61:341, 1985.
544. Andy, J. J.: Helminthiasis, the hypereosinophilic syndrome and endomyocardial fibrosis: Some observations and an hypothesis. Afr. J. Med. Med. Sci. 12:155, 1983.
545. Date, A., Parameswaran, A., and Bhaktaviziam, A.: Renal lesions in the obliterative cardiomyopathies: Endomyocardial fibrosis and Löffler's endocarditis. J. Pathol. 140:113, 1983.
546. Gottdiener, J. S., Maron, B. J., Schooley, R. T., Harley, J. B., Roberts, W. C., and Fauci, A. S.: Two-dimensional echocardiographic assessment of the idiopathic hypereosinophilic syndrome. Anatomic basis of mitral regurgitation and peripheral embolization. Circulation 67:572, 1983.
547. Rodger, J. C., Irvine, K. C., and Lerski, R. A.: Echocardiography in Löffler's endocarditis. Br. Heart J. 46:110, 1981.
548. Acquatella, H.: Two-dimensional echocardiography in endomyocardial disease. Postgrad. Med. J. 59:157, 1983.
549. Davies, J., Gibson, D. G., Foale, R., Heer, K., Spry, C. J., Oakley, C. M., and Goodwin, J. F.: Echocardiographic features of eosinophilic endomyocardial disease. Br. Heart J. 48:434, 1982.
550. Kim, C. H., Vlietstra, R. E., Edwards, W. D., Reeder, G. S., and Gleich, G. J.: Steroid-responsive eosinophilic myocarditis: diagnosis by endomyocardial biopsy. Am. J. Cardiol. 53:1472, 1984.
551. Davies, J., Spry, C. J., Sapsford, R., Olsen, E. G., de Perez, G., Oakley, C. M., and Goodwin, J. F.: Cardiovascular features of 11 patients with eosinophilic endomyocardial disease. Q. J. Med. 52:23, 1983.
552. Blake, D. P., Palmer, I. E., and Olinger, G. N.: Mitral valve replacement in idiopathic hypereosinophilic syndrome. J. Thorac. Cardiovasc. Surg. 89:630, 1985.
553. Fournial, G., Schlanger, R., Berthoumieu, F., Pris, J., Marco, J., and Eschapasse, H.: Surgery for cardiac complications caused by endocardial mural fibrin deposits in a hypereosinophilic syndrome. Circulation 65:1010, 1982.
554. Hutt, M. S.: Epidemiology aspects of endomyocardial fibrosis. Postgrad. Med. J. 59:142, 1983.
555. Lengyel, M., Arvay, A., and Palik, I.: Massive endocardial calcification associated with endomyocardial fibrosis. Am. J. Cardiol. 56:815, 1985.
556. Krishnaswami, H., Date, A., Bhaktaviziam, A., Krishnaswami, S., and Cherian, G.: Electron microscopic changes in tropical endomyocardial fibrosis. Trans. R. Soc. Trop. Med. Hyg. 78:205, 1984.
557. Jaiyesimi, F.: Observations on the so-called non-specific electrocardiographic changes in endomyocardial fibrosis. East Afr. Med. J. 59:56, 1982.
558. Candell-Riera, J., Permanyer-Miralda, G., and Soler-Soler, J.: Echocardiographic findings in endomyocardial fibrosis. Chest 82:88, 1982.
559. Pawzy, M. E., Ziady, G., Halim, M., Guindy, R., Mercer, E. N., and Feteih, N.: Endomyocardial fibrosis: Report of eight cases. J. Am. Coll. Cardiol. 5:983, 1985.
560. Sasidharan, K., Kartha, C. C., Balakrishnan, K. G., and Valiathan, M. S.: Early angiographic features of right ventricular endomyocardial fibrosis. Cardiology 70:127, 1983.
561. Balakrishnan, K. G., Sasidharan, K., Venkitachalam, C. G., and Sapru, R. P.: Coronary angiographic features in endomyocardial fibrosis. Cardiology 70:121, 1983.
562. Galbut, D. L., Benson, J., Blankstein, R. L., Vignola, P. A., and Gentsch, T. O.: Endomyocardial fibrosis. Preoperative diagnosis and surgical therapy. Chest 84:779, 1983.
563. Gonzalez-Lavin, L., Friedman, J. P., Hecker, S. P., and McFadden, P. M.: Endomyocardial fibrosis: Diagnosis and treatment. Am. Heart J. 105:699, 1983.
564. Bertrand, E., Chauvet, J., Assamoi, M. O., Charles, D., Ekra, E., Dienot, B. B., Caileau, G., Burdin, J., Longchaud, A., Millet, P., Ravinet, L., Quattara, K., Coulibaly, A. O., and Metras, D.: Results, indications and contra-indications of surgery in restrictive endomyocardial fibrosis: Comparative study on 31 operated and 30 non-operated patients. East Afr. Med. J. 62:151, 1985.
565. Metras, D., Coulibaly, A. O., and Ouattara, K.: The surgical treatment of endomyocardial fibrosis: Results in 55 patients. Circulation 72:II274, 1985.
566. Valiathan, M. S., Sankarkumar, R., Balakrishnan, K. G., and Mohansingh, M. P.: Surgical palliation for endomyocardial fibrosis: Early results. Thorax 38:421, 1983.
567. Moraes, C. R., Buffolo, E., Lima, R., Victor, E., Lira, V., Escobar, M., Rodrigues, J., Saraiva, L., and Andrade, J. C.: Surgical treatment of endomyocardial fibrosis. J. Thorac. Cardiovasc. Surg. 85:738, 1983.
568. Balakrishnan, K. G., Venkitachalam, C. G., Pillai, V. R., Subramanian, R., and Valiathan, M. S.: Postoperative evaluation of endomyocardial fibrosis. Cardiology 73:73, 1986.
569. Metras, D., Ouezzin-Coulibaly, A., Ouattara, K., Bertrand, E., and Chauvet, J.: Endomyocardial fibrosis masquerading as rheumatic mitral incompetence. A report of six surgical cases. J. Thorac. Cardiovasc. Surg. 86:753, 1983.
570. Russo, P. H., Wright, J. E., Ho, S. Y., Maneksa, J. R., and Clitsakis, D.: Endocardectomy for the surgical treatment of endocardial fibrosis of the left ventricle. Thorax 40:621, 1985.
571. Metras, D., Ouattara, K., Coulibaly, A. O., and Touze, J. E.: Left endomyocardial fibrosis with severe mitral insufficiency; the case for mitral valve repair. A report of 4 cases. Thorac. Cardiovasc. Surg. 31:297, 1983.
572. Ferrans, V. J., and Roberts, W. C.: The carcinoid endocardial plaque. An ultrastrucural study. Hum. Pathol. 7:387, 1976.
573. Ross, E. M., and Roberts, W. C.: The carcinoid syndrome: Comparison of 21

necropsy subjects with carcinoid heart disease to 15 necropsy subjects without carcinoid heart disease. Am. J. Med. 79:339, 1985.
574. Grahame-Smith, D. G.: The carcinoid syndrome. *In* Bondy, P. K., and Rosenberg, L. E. (eds.): Metabolic Control and Disease. 9th ed. Philadelphia, W. B. Saunders Company, 1980, p. 1703.
575. Topol, F., and Fortuin, N. J.: Coronary artery spasm and cardiac arrest in carcinoid heart disease. Am. J. Med. 77:950, 1984.
576. Hendel, N., Leckie, B., and Richards, J.: Carcinoid heart disease: Eight-year survival following tricuspid valve replacement and pulmonary valvotomy. Ann. Thorac. Surg. *30*:391, 1980.
577. Artaza, A., Beiner, J. H., Gonzalez, M., Aranda, I., deTeresa, E. G., and Pulpon, L. H.: Carcinoid heart disease: Report of a case secondary to a pure carcinoid tumor of the ovary. Eur. Heart J. *6*:800, 1985.
578. Gutman, J. M., and Schiller, N. B.: Carcinoid heart disease: Diagnostic usefulness of echocardiography. Primary Cardiology 9:130:1983.
579. Tornebrandt, K., Eskilsson, J., and Nobin, H.: Heart involvement in metastatic carcinoid disease. Clin. Cardiol. *9*:13, 1986.
580. Marin-Huerta, E., Navascues, I., Palomegue, C. F., Nunez, A., Cobos, M. A., and Asin, E.: Carcinoid heart disease: A Doppler echocardiographic report. Eur. Heart J. *6*:806, 1985.
581. Reid, C. L., Chandraratna, P. A., Kawanishi, D. I., Pitha, J. V., and Rahimtoola, S. H.: Echocardiographic features of carcinoid heart disease. Am. Heart J. *107*:801, 1984.
582. Taber, M., Askenazi, J., Ribner, H., Kumar, S., and Lesch, M.: The tricuspid valve in carcinoid syndrome. An echocardiographic study. Arch. Intern. Med. *143*:1033, 1983.
583. Forman, M. B., Byrd, B. F., 3rd, Oates, J. A., and Robertson, R. M.: Two-dimensional echocardiography in the diagnosis of carcinoid heart disease. Am. Heart J. *107*:492, 1984.
584. Davies, M. K., Lowry, P. J., and Littler, W. A.: Cross sectional echocardiographic feature in carcinoid heart disease. A mechanism for tricuspid regurgitation in this syndrome. Br. Heart J. *51*:355, 1984.
585. Howard, R. J., Drobac, M., Rider, W. D., Keane, T. T., Finlayson, J., Silver, M. D., Wigle, E. D., and Rakowski, H.: Carcinoid heart disease: Diagnosis by two-dimensional echocardiography. Circulation *66*:1059, 1982.
586. Zinner, M. J., Yeo, C. J., and Jaffe, B. M.: The effect of carcinoid levels of serotonin and substance P on hemodynamics. Ann. Surg. *199*:197, 1984.
587. DiSesa, V. J., Mills, R. M., Jr., and Collins, J. J., Jr.: Surgical management of carcinoid heart disease. Chest *88*:789, 1985.

MYOCARDITIS

588. Miller, B. R., Vohr, F. H., Christian, F. V., and Singh, H. K.: Cardiac valvular replacement in carcinoid heart disease. Am. J. Med. *75*:896, 1983.
589. Reyes, M. P., and Lerner, A. M.: Coxsackievirus myocarditis—with special reference to acute and chronic effects. Prog. Cardiovasc. Dis. *27*:373, 1985.
590. James, T. N.: Myocarditis and cardiomyopathy (editorial). N. Engl. J. Med. *308*:39, 1983.
591. James, T. N., Schlant, R. C., and Marshall, T. K.: De Subitaneis Mortibus. XXIX. Randomly distributed focal myocardial lesions causing destruction in the His bundle or a narrow origin left bundle branch. Circulation *57*:816, 1978.
592. Kawai, C., and Kishimoto, C.: Viral myocarditis and dilated cardiomyopathy—an experimental study with special reference to immunological behavior of T and B-lymphocytes. Postgrad. Med. J. *61*:1125, 1985.
593. Matsumori, A., and Kawai, C.: An animal model of congestive (dilated) cardiomyopathy: Dilatation and hypertrophy of the heart in the chronic stage in DBA/2 mice with myocarditis caused by encephalomyocarditis virus. Circulation *66*:355, 1982.
594. Strain, J. E., Grose, R. M., Factor, S. M., and Fisher, J. D.: Results of endomyocardial biopsy in patients with spontaneous ventricular tachycardia but without apparent structural heart disease. Circulation *68*:1171, 1983.
595. Kishimoto, C., Kuribayashi, K., Masuda, I., Tomioka, N., and Kawai, C.: Immunologic behavior of lymphocytes in experimental viral myocarditis: Significance of T lymphocytes in the severity of myocarditis and silent myocarditis in BALB/c-nu/nu mice. Circulation *71*:1247, 1985.
596. Maisch, B., Bulowius, U., Schmier, K., Klopf, D., Koper, D., Sibelis, T., and Kochsiek, K.: Immunological cellular regulator and effector mechanisms in myocarditis. Herz *10*:8, 1985.
597. Saphir, O., Wile, S. A., and Reingold, J. M.: Myocarditis in children. Am. J. Dis. Child. *67*:294, 1944.
598. Saphir, O.: Myocarditis: A general review with an analysis of two hundred and forty cases. Arch. Pathol. *32*:1000, 1941; *33*:88, 1942.
599. Stevens, P. J., and Underwood Ground, K. E.: Occurrence and significance of myocarditis in trauma. Aerospace Med. *41*:776, 1970.
600. Karjalainen, J., and Heikkila, J.: "Acute pericarditis:" Myocardial enzyme release as evidence for myocarditis. Am. Heart J. *111*:546, 1986.
601. Gore, I., and Saphir, O.: Myocarditis: A classification of 1402 cases. Am. Heart J. *34*:827, 1947.
602. Fine, I., Brainerd, H., and Sokolow, M.: Myocarditis in acute infectious diseases: A clinical and electrocardiographic study. Circulation 2:859, 1950.
603. Lim, C. H., Toh, C. C. S., Chia, B-L., and Low, L-P.: Stokes-Adams attacks due to acute nonspecific myocarditis. Am. Heart J. *90*:172, 1975.
604. Reeves, W. C., Jackson, G. L., Flickinger, F. W., Divee, H. G., Schwiter, E. J., Werner, J., Whitesell, L., Bidde, M. A., Copenhover, G., Shaikh, B. S., and Zelis, R.: Radionuclide imaging of experimental myocarditis. Circulation *63*:640, 1981.
605. Matsumori, A., Kadota, K., and Kawai, C.: Technetium-99m pyrophosphate uptake in experimental viral perimyocarditis. Sequential study of myocardial uptake and pathologic correlates. Circulation *61*:802, 1980.
606. Daly, K., Richardson, P. J., Olsen, E. G., Morgan-Capner, P., McSorley, C., Jackson, G., and Jewitt, D. E.: Acute myocarditis. Role of histological and virological examination in the diagnosis and assessment of immunosuppressive treatment. Br. Heart J. *51*:30, 1984.
606a. Bowles, N. E., Olsen, E. G. J., Richardson, P. J., and Archard, L. C.: Detection of coxsackie B virus–specific RNA sequences in myocardial biopsy samples from patients with myocarditis and dilated cardiomyopathy. Lancet *1*:1120, 1986.
607. Pearce, J. H.: Heart disease and filtrable virus. Circulation *21*:448, 1960.
608. Fenoglio, J. J., Ursell, P. C., Kellogg, C. F., Drusin, R. E., and Weiss, M. B.: Diagnosis and classification of myocarditis by endomyocardial biopsy. N. Engl. J. Med. *308*:12, 1983.
609. Mason, J. W., Billingham, M. E., and Ricci, D. R.: Treatment of acute inflammatory myocarditis assisted by endomyocardial biopsy, Am. J. Cardiol. *45*:1037, 1980.
610. Costanzo-Nordin, M. R., Reap, E. A., O'Connell, J. B., Robinson, J. A., and Scanlon, P. J.: A nonsteroid anti-inflammatory drug exacerbates Coxsackie B3 murine myocarditis. J. Am. Coll. Cardiol. *6*:1078, 1985.
611. Rezkalla, S., Khatib, G., and Khatib, R.: Coxsackievirus B3 murine myocarditis: Deleterious effects of nonsteroidal anti-inflammatory agents. J. Lab. Clin. Med. *107*:393, 1986.
612. O'Connell, J. B., Reap, E. A., and Robinson, J. A.: The effects of cyclosporine on acute murine Coxsackie B3 myocarditis. Circulation *73*:353, 1986.
613. Monrad, E. S., Matsumori, A., Murphy, J. C., Fox, J. G., Crumpacker, C. S., and Abelmann, W. H.: Therapy with cyclosporine in experimental murine myocarditis with encephalomyocarditis virus. Circulation *73*:1058, 1986.
614. Matsumori, A., Wang, H., Abelmann, W. H., and Crumpacker, C. S.: Treatment of viral myocarditis with ribavirin in an animal preparation. Circulation *71*:834, 1985.
615. Norris, D., and Loh, P. C.: Coxsackie virus myocarditis: Prophylaxis and therapy with an interferon stimulator. Proc. Soc. Exp. Biol. Med. *142*:133, 1973.
616. Levine, H. D.: Virus myocarditis: A critique of the literature from clinical, electrocardiographic, and pathologic standpoints. Am. J. Med. Sci. *277*:132, 1979.
617. Price, R. A., Garcia, J. H., and Rightsel, W. A.: Choriomeningitis and myocarditis in an adolescent with isolation of Coxsackie B-5 virus. Am. J. Clin. Pathol. *53*:825, 1970.
618. Desa'Neto, A., Bullington, D., Bullington, R. H., Desser, K. B., and Benchimol, A.: Coxsackie B5 heart disease. Demonstration of inferolateral wall myocardial necrosis. Am. J. Med. *68*:205, 1980.
619. Saffitz, J. E., Schwartz, D. J., Southworth, W., Murphree, S., Rodriguez, E. R., Ferrans, V. J., and Roberts, W. C.: Coxsackie viral myocarditis causing transmural right and left ventricular infarction without coronary narrowing. Am. J. Cardiol. *52*:644, 1983.
620. O'Neill, D., McArthur, J. D., Kennedy, J. H., and Clements, G.: Myocardial infarction and the normal arteriogram—possible role of viral myocarditis. Postgrad. Med. J. *61*:485, 1985.
621. Costanzo-Nordin, M. R., O'Connell, J. B., Subramanian, R., Robinson, J. A., and Scanlon, P. J.: Myocarditis confirmed by biopsy presenting as acute myocardial infarction. Br. Heart J. *53*:25, 1985.
622. Kron, J., Lucas, L., Lee, T. D., and McAnulty, J.: Myocardial infarction following an acute viral illness. Arch. Intern. Med. *143*:1466, 1983.
623. Ray, C. G., Portman, J. N., Stamm, S. J., and Hickman, R. O.: Hemolytic-uremic syndrome and myocarditis. Association with coxsackievirus B infection. Am. J. Dis. Child. *122*:418, 1970.
624. Smith, W. G.: Coxsackie B myopericarditis in adults. Am. Heart J. *80*:34, 1970.
625. Hirschman, S. F., and Hammer, G. S.: Coxsackie virus myopericarditis. A microbiological and clinical review. Am. J. Cardiol. *34*:224, 1974.
626. Ikaheimo, M. J., and Takkunen, J. T.: Echocardiography in acute infectious myocarditis. Chest *89*:100, 1986.
627. Nieminen, M. A., Heikkila, J., and Karjalainen, J.: Echocardiography in acute infectious myocarditis: Relation to clinical and electrocardiographic findings. Am. J. Cardiol. 53:1331, 1984.
628. Rozkovec, A., Cambridge, G., King, M., and Hallidie-Smith, K. A.: Natural history of left ventricular function in neonatal Coxsackie myocarditis. Pediatr. Cardiol. *6*:151, 1985.
629. Sainani, G. S., Dekate, M. P., and Rao, C. P.: Heart disease caused by Coxsackie virus B infection. Br. Heart J. *37*:819, 1975.
630. Read, R. B., Ede, R. J., Morgan-Capner, P., Moscoso, G., Portmann, B., and Williams, R.: Myocarditis and fulminant hepatic failure from coxsackievirus B infection. Postgrad. Med. J. *61*:749, 1985.
631. O'Connell, J. B., Robinson J. A.: Coxsackie viral myocarditis. Postgrad. Med. J. *61*:1127, 1985.
632. Editorial: Acute myocarditis and its sequelae. Br. Med. J. *3*:783, 1972.
633. Bell, E. J., and Grist, N. R.: Echoviruses, carditis and acute pleurodynia. Am. Heart J. *82*:133, 1971.
634. Bell, E. J., and Grist, N. R.: Echovirus, carditis and acute pleurodynia. Lancet *1*:326, 1970.
635. Schleissner, L. A., Fiala, M., Imagawa, D. T., and Casaburi, R.: Application of systolic time intervals to acute cardiomyopathy with echovirus 2. Chest *69*:563, 1976.
636. Henson, D., and Nufson, M. A.: Myocarditis and pneumonitis with type 21 adenovirus infection. Association with fatal myocarditis and pneumonitis. Am. J. Dis. Child *121*:334, 1971.
637. Verel, D., Warrack, A. J. N., Potter, C. W., Ward, C., and Rickards, D. F.:

Observations on the A_2 England influenza epidemic: A clinicopathological study. Am. Heart J. *92*:290, 1976.
638. Coltman, C. A., Jr.: Influenza myocarditis: Report of a case with observations on serum glutamic oxaloacetic transaminase. J.A.M.A. *180*:204, 1962.
639. Adams, C. W.: Postviral myopericarditis associated with the influenza virus. Am. J. Cardiol. *4*:56, 1959.
640. Noren, G. R., Tobin, J. D., Jr., Staley, N. A., Asinger, R. W., and Einzig, S.: Association of varicella, myocarditis, and congestive cardiomyopathy. Pediatr. Cardiol. *3*:53, 1982.
641. Coppack, S. W., Doshi, R., and Ghose, A. R.: Fatal varicella in a healthy young adult. Postgrad. Med. J. *61*:529, 1985.
642. Hackel, D. B.: Myocarditis in association with varicella. Am. J. Pathol. *29*:369, 1953.
643. Hildes, J. A., Schaberg, A., and Alcock, A. J. W.: Cardiovascular collapse in acute poliomyelitis. Circulation *12*:986, 1955.
644. Dunne, J. W., Harper, C. G., and Hilton, J. M.: Sudden infant death syndrome caused by poliomyelitis. Arch. Neurol. *41*:775, 1984.
645. Teloth, H. A.: Myocarditis in poliomyelitis. Arch. Pathol. 55:408, 1953.
646. Weinstein, L., and Shelokov, A.: Cardiovascular manifestations of acute poliomyelitis. N. Engl. J. Med. *244*:281, 1951.
647. Mohammed, I., and Carlisle, R.: Cardiac and renal involvement in mumps. West Afr. Med. J.: *20*:367, 1971.
648. Roberts, W. C., and Fox, S. M., III: Mumps of the heart: Clinical and pathologic features. Circulation *32*:342, 1965.
649. Bengtsson, E., and Orndahl, G.: Complications of mumps with special reference to the incidence of myocarditis. Acta Med. Scand. *149*:381, 1954.
650. Arita, M., Ueno, Y., and Masuyama, Y.: Complete heart block in mumps myocarditis. Br. Heart J. *46*:342, 1981.
651. Saphir, O., Amromin, G. D., and Yokoo, H.: Myocarditis in viral (epidemic) hepatitis. Am. J. Med. Sci. *231*:168, 1956.
652. Bell, H.: Cardiac manifestations of viral hepatitis. J.A.M.A. *218*:387, 1971.
653. Ursell, P. C., Habib, A., Sharma, P., Mesa-Tejada, R., Lefkowitch, J. H., and Fenoglio, J. J., Jr.: Hepatitis B virus and myocarditis. Hum. Pathol. *15*:481, 1984.
654. Nagaratnam, N., deSilva, D.P.K.M., and Gunawardene, K. R. W.: Myocardial involvement in infectious hepatitis. Postgrad. Med. J. *47*:785, 1971.
655. Mahapatra, R. K., and Ellis, G. H.: Myocarditis and hepatitis B virus. Angiology *36*:116, 1985.
656. Fink, L., Reichek, N., and Sutton, M. G. St.J.: Cardiac abnormalities in acquired immune deficiency syndrome. Am. J. Cardiol. *54*:1161, 1984.
657. Cammarosano, C., and Lewis, W.: Cardiac lesions in acquired immune deficiency syndrome (AIDS). J. Am. Coll. Cardiol. *5*:703, 1985.
658. Lewis, W., Lipsick, J., and Cammarosano, C.: Cryptococcal myocarditis in acquired immune deficiency syndrome. Am. J. Cardiol. *55*:1240, 1985.
659. Moskowitz, L., Hensley, G. T., Chan, J. C., and Adams, K.: Immediate causes of death in acquired immunodeficiency syndrome. Arch. Pathol. Lab. Med. *109*:735, 1985.
660. Silver, M. A., Macher, M. A., Reichert, C. M., Levens, D. L., Parrillo, J. E., Longo, D. L., and Roberts, W. C.: Cardiac involvement by Kapsoi's sarcoma in acquired immune deficiency syndrome (AIDS). Am. J. Cardiol. 53:983, 1984.
661. Webster, B. H.: Cardiac complications of infectious mononucleosis: A review of the literature and report of five cases. Am. J. Med. Sci. *234*:62, 1957.
662. Frishman, W., Kraus, M. E., Zabkar, J., Brooks, V., Alonso, D., and Dixon, L. M.: Infectious mononucleosis and fatal myocarditis. Chest 72:535, 1977.
663. Miller, R., Ward, C., Amsterdam, E., Mason, D. T., and Zelis, R.: Focal mononucleosis myocarditis simulating myocardial infarction. Chest *63*:102, 1973.
664. Hudgins, J. M.: Infectious mononucleosis complicated by myocarditis and pericarditis. J.A.M.A. *235*:2626. 1976.
665. Goldfinger, D., Schreiber, W., and Wosika, P. H.: Permanent heart block following German measles. Am. J. Med. *2*:320, 1947.
666. Kriseman, T.: Rubella myocarditis in a 9-year-old patient. Clin. Pediatr. *23*:240, 1984.
667. Goldfield, M., Bayer, N. H., and Weinstein, L.: Electrocardiographic changes during the course of measles. J. Pediatr. *46*:30, 1955.
668. Degen, J. A.: Visceral pathology in measles: A clinico-pathologic study of 100 cases. Am. J. Med. Sci. *194*:104, 1937.
669. Weinstein L.: Cardiovascular manifestations in some of the common infectious diseases. Mod. Concepts Cardiovasc. Dis. *23*:229, 1954.
670. Wilson, R. S., Morris, T. H., and Rossell Rees, J.: Cytomegalovirus myocarditis. Br. Heart J. *34*:865, 1972.
671. Wink, K., and Schmitz, H.: Cytomegalovirus myocarditis. Am. Heart J. *100*:667, 1980.
672. Tuila, E., and Leinikki, P.: Fatal cytomegalovirus infection in a previously healthy boy with myocarditis and consumption coagulopathy as presenting signs. Scand. J. Infect. Dis. *4*:57, 1972.
673. Milei, J., and Bolomo, N. J.: Myocardial damage in viral hemorrhagic fevers. Am. Heart J. *104*:1385, 1982.
674. Obeyesekere, I., and Herman, Y.: Arbovirus heart disease: Myocarditis and cardiomyopathy following dengue and chikungunya fever—a follow-up study. Am. Heart J. *85*:186, 1973.
675. Nagaratham, N., Siripala, K., and deSilva, N.: Arbovirus (dengue type) as a cause of acute myocarditis and pericarditis. Br. Heart J. *35*:204, 1973.
676. Obeyesekere, I., and Herman, Y.: Myocarditis and cardiomyopathy after arbovirus infections (dengue and chikungunya fever). Br. Heart J. *34*:821, 1972.
677. Anderson T., Foulis, M. A., Grist, N. R., and Landsman, J. B.: Clinical and laboratory observations in a smallpox outbreak. Lancet *1*:1248, 1951.
678. Matthews, A. W., and Griffiths, I. D.: Post-vaccinal pericarditis and myocarditis. Br. Heart J. *36*:1043, 1974.
679. Finlay-Jones, L. R.: Fatal myocarditis after vaccinations for smallpox. N. Engl. J. Med. *270*:41, 1964.
680. Connell, D. E.: Myocardial degeneration in yellow fever. Am. J. Pathol. *4*:431, 1928.
681. Gills, T. D., and Gohd, R. S.: Respiratory syncytial virus and heart disease. A report of two cases. J.A.M.A. *236*:1128, 1976.
682. Bairan, A. C., Cherry, J. D., Fagan, L. F., and Coff, J. E., Jr.: Complete heart block and respiratory syncytial virus infection. Am. J. Dis. Child. *127*:264, 1974.
683. Menahem, S., and Uren, E. C.: Respiratory syncytial virus and heart block—cause and effect? Aust. NZ J. Med. *15*:55, 1985.
684. Lewes, D., Rainsford, D. J., and Lane, W. F.: Symptomless myocarditis and myalgia in viral and *Mycoplasma pneumoniae* infections. Br. Heart J. *36*:924, 1974.
685. Chen, S. C., Tsai, C. C., and Nouri, S.: Carditis associated with *Mycoplasma pneumoniae* infection. Am. J. Dis. Child. *140*:471, 1986.
686. Sands, M. J., Jr., Satz, J. E., Turner, W. E., and Soloff, L. A.: Pericarditis and perimyocarditis associated with active *Mycoplasma pneumoniae* infection. Ann. Intern. Med. *86*:544, 1977.
687. Pickens, S., and Catterall, J. R.: Disseminated intravascular coagulation and myocarditis associated with *Mycoplasma pneumoniae* infection. Br. Med. J. *1*:1526, 1978.
688. Dymock, I. W., Lawson, J. M., MacLennan, W. J., and Ross, C. A. C.: Myocarditis associated with psittacosis. Br. J. Clin. Pract. *25*:240, 1971.
689. Sutton, G. C., Morrissey, R. A., Tobin, J. R., Jr., and Anderson, T. V.: Pericardial and myocardial disease associated with serologic evidence of infection by agents of the psittacosislymphogranuloma venereum group (Chlamydiaceae). Circulation *36*:830, 1967.
690. Ognibane, A. J., O'Leary, D. S., Czarnocki, S. W., Flannery, E. P., and Grove, R. B.: Myocarditis and disseminated intravascular coagulation in scrub typhus. Am. J. Med. Sci. *262*:233, 1971.
691. Brown, G. W., Shirai, A., Jegathesan, M., Burke, D. S., Twartz, J. C., Saunders, J. P., and Huxsoll, D. L.: Febrile illness in Malaysia—an analysis of 1,629 hospitalized patients. Am. J. Trop. Med. Hyg. *33*:311, 1984.
692. Marin-Garcia, J., and Barrett, F. F.: Myocardial function in Rocky Mountain spotted fever: Echocardiographic assessment. Am. J. Cardiol. *51*:341, 1983.
693. Marin-Garcia, J., and Mirvis, D. M.: Myocardial disease in Rocky Mountain spotted fever: Clinical, functional, and pathologic findings. Pediatr. Cardiol. *5*:149, 1984.
694. Marin-Garcia, J.: Left ventricular dysfunction in Rocky Mountain spotted fever. Clin. Cardiol. *6*:501, 1983.
695. Sheridan, P., MacCraig, J. N., and Hart, R. J. C.: Myocarditis complicating Q fever. Br. Med. J. *2*:155, 1974.
696. Barraclough, D., and Popert, A. J.: Q fever presenting with paroxysmal ventricular tachycardia. Br. Med. J. 2:423, 1975.
697. Maisch, B.: Rickettsial perimyocarditis—a follow-up study. Heart Vessels *2*:55, 1986.
698. Koster, F. T., Williams, J. C., and Goodwin, J. S.: Cellular immunity in Q fever: specific lymphocyte unresponsiveness in Q fever endocarditis. J. Infect. Dis. *152*:1283, 1985.
699. Taheinia, A. C.: Electrocardiographic abnormalities and serum transaminase levels in diphtheritic myocarditis. J. Pediatr. *75*:1008, 1969.
700. Riley, H. D., Jr., and Weaver, T. S.: Cardiovascular and nervous system complications of diphtheria. Am. Pract. *3*:536, 1952.
701. Collier, R. J., and Pappenheimer, A. M.: Studies on the mode of action of diphtheria toxin. J. Exp. Med. *120*:1007; 1018, 1964.
702. Ledbetter, M. K., Cannon, A. B., and Costa, A. F.: The electrocardiogram in diphtheritic myocarditis. Am. Heart. J. *68*:599, 1964.
703. Matisonn, R. E.: Successful electrical pacing for complete heart block complicating diphtheritic myocarditis. Br. Heart J. *38*:423, 1976.
704. Thisyakorn, U., Wongvanich, J., and Kumpens, V.: Failure of corticosteroid therapy to prevent diphtheritic myocarditis or neuritis. Pediatr. Infect. Dis. *3*:126, 1984.
705. Ramos, H. C., Elias, P. R., Barrucand, L., and Da Silva, J. H.: The protective effect of carnitine in human diphtheric myocarditis. Pediatr. Res. *18*:815, 1984.
706. Sanders, V., and Misanik, L. F.: Salmonella myocarditis: Report of a case with ventricular rupture. Am. Heart J. *68*:682, 1964.
707. Siwach, S. B., and Nand, N.: Cardiovascular complications of enteric fever. Angiology *34*:436, 1983.
708. Shilkin, K. B.: *Salmonella typhimurium* pancarditis. Postgrad. Med. J. *45*:40, 1969.
709. Le-Van-Diem, A. K.: Typhoid fever with myocarditis. Am. J. Trop. Med. Hyg. *23*:218, 1974.
710. Mainzer, F.: Electrocardiographic study of typhoid myocarditis. Br. Heart J. 9:145, 1947.
711. Wallis, P. J., Branfoot, A. C., and Emerson, P. H.: Sudden death due to myocardial tuberculosis. Thorax *39*:155, 1984.
712. Ratanarapee, S., Bovornkitti, S., and Eungprabhant, V.: Tuberculous myocarditis: A report of two cases. J. Med. Assoc. Thai *68*:155, 1985.
713. Auerbach, O., and Guggenheim, A.: Tuberculosis of the myocardium: A review of the literature and a report of six new cases. Q. Bull. Sea View Hosp. *2*:264, 1937.
714. Horn, H., and Saphir, O.: The involvement of the myocardium in tuberculosis. A review of the literature and report of 3 cases. Am. Rev. Tuberc. *32*:492, 1935.
715. Rosenbaum, H., and Linn, H. J.: Tuberculosis of myocardium. Am. J. Clin. Pathol. *18*:162, 1948.
716. Gore, I.: Myocarditis in infectious diseases. Am. Pract. *1*:292, 1947.
717. Brody, A., and Smith, L. W.: Visceral pathology in scarlet fever and related streptococcal infections. Am. J. Pathol. *12*:373, 1936.

718. Hardman, J. M., and Earle, K. M.: Myocarditis in 200 fatal meningococcal infections. Arch. Pathol. *87*:318, 1969.
719. d'Agati, V., and Marangoni, B. A.: The Waterhouse-Friderichsen syndrome. N. Engl. J. Med. *232*:1, 1945.
720. Monsalve, F., Rucabado, L., Salvador, A., Bonastre, J., Cunat, J., and Rauno, M: Myocardial depression in septic shock caused by meningococcal infection. Crit. Care Med. *12*:1021, 1984.
721. Roberts, W. C., and Beard, G. W.: Gas gangrene of the heart in clostridial septicemia. Am. Heart J. *74*:482, 1967.
722. Guneratre, P.: Gas gangrene (abscess) of heart. N.Y. State J. Med. *75*:1766, 1975.
723. Castellani Pastoris, M., Nigro, G., and Middulla, M.: Arrhythmia or myocarditis: A novel clinical form of *Legionella pneumophila* infection in children without pneumonia. Eur. J. Pediatr. *144*:157, 1985.
724. Gross, D., Willens, H., and Zeldis, S. M.: Myocarditis in Legionnaire's disease. Chest *79*:232, 1981.
725. Friedland, L., Syndman, D. R., Weingarden, A. S., Hedges, T. R. 3d., Brown, R., and Busky, M.: Ocular and pericardial involvement in Legionnaires' disease. Am. J. Med. *77*:1105, 1984.
726. Gur, H., Gefel, D., and Tur-Kaspa, R.: Transient electrocardiographic changes during two episodes of relapsing brucellosis. Postgrad. Med. J. *60*:544, 1984.
727. Lubani, M., Sharda, D., and Helin, I.: Cardiac manifestations in brucellosis. Arch. Dis. Child. *61*:569, 1986.
728. McAllister, H. A., and Fenoglio, J. J.: Cardiac involvement in Whipple's disease. Circulation *52*:152, 1975.
729. James, T. N., and Bulkley, B. H.: Abnormalities of the coronary arteries in Whipple's disease. Am. Heart J. *105*:481, 1983.
730. Morrison, D. A., Gay, R. G., Feldshon, D., and Sampliner, R. E.: Severe pulmonary hypertension in a patient with Whipple's disease. Am. J. Med. *79*:263, 1985.
731. Keinath, R. D., Merrell, D. E., Vlietstra, R., and Dobbins, W. O., 3rd: Antibiotic treatment and relapse in Whipple's disease. Long-term follow-up of 88 patients. Gastroenterology *88*:1867, 1985.
732. Feldman, M.: Whipple's disease. Am. J. Med. Sci. *291*:56, 1986.
733. Doscia, J, L., Fisco, J. M., and Brace, W. T.: Complete heart block due to a solitary gumma. Am. J. Cardiol. *13*:553, 1964.
734. Spain, D. M., and Johannsen, M. W.: Three cases of localized gummatous myocarditis. Am. Heart J. *241*:689, 1942.
735. Boss, J. H., Leffkowitz, M., and Freud, M.: Unusual manifestations of syphilitic cardiovascular disease. Ann. Intern. Med. *55*:824, 1961.
736. Saphir, O.: Syphilitic myocarditis. Arch. Pathol. *13*:266, 1932.
737. Arean, V. M.: Leptospiral myocarditis. Lab. Invest. *6*:462, 1957.
738. Edwards, G. A., and Damm, B. M.: Human leptospirosis. Medicine *39*:117, 1960.
739. Sodeman, W. A., and Kellough, J. H.: The cardiac manifestations of Weil's disease. Am. J. Trop. Med. *31*:479, 1957.
740. Ram, P., and Chandra, M. S.: Unusual electrocardiographic abnormality in leptospirosis: Case reports. Angiology *36*:477, 1985.
741. Winearls, C. G., Chan, L., Coghlan, J. D., Ledingham, J. G., and Oliver, D. U.: Acute renal failure due to leptospirosis: Clinical features and outcome in six cases. Q. J. Med. *53*:487, 1984.
742. Wengrower, D., Knobler, H., Gillis, S., and Chajek-Shaul, T.: Myocarditis in tick-borne relapsing fever. J. Infect. Dis. *149*:1033, 1984.
743. Atkinson, J. B., Robinsowitz, M., McAllister, H. H., Jr., Forman, M. B., and Virmani, R.: Cardiac infections in the immunocompromised host. Cardiol. Clin. *2*:671, 1984.
744. Williams, A. H.: Aspergillus myocarditis. Am. J. Clin. Pathol. *61*:247, 1974.
745. Cade, J. F.: Pulmonary aspergillosis with myocarditis. Med. J. Aust. *1*:581, 1966.
746. Zoeckler, S. J.: Cardiac actinomycosis: A case report and survey of the literature. Circulation *3*:854, 1951.
747. Edwards, A. C.: Actinomycosis in children: A review of the literature and report of cases. Am. J. Dis. Child. *41*:1419, 1931.
748. Martin, D. S., and Smith, D. T.: Blastomycosis (American blastomycosis, Gilchrist's disease). I. A review of the literature. Am. Rev. Tuberc. *39*:275, 1939.
749. Baker, R. D., and Brian, E. W.: Blastomycosis of the heart: Report of two cases. Am. J. Pathol. *13*:139, 1937.
750. Hutter, R. V. P., and Collins, H. S.: The appearance of opportunistic fungus infections in a cancer hospital. Lab. Invest. *11*:1035, 1962.
751. Jones, I., Nassau, E., and Smith, P.: Cryptococcosis of the heart. Br. Heart J. *27*:462, 1965.
752. Van Kirk, J. E., Simon, A. B., and Armstrong, U. R.: Candida myocarditis causing complete atrioventricular block, J.A.M.A. *227*:931, 1974.
753. Atkinson, J. B., Connor, D. H., Robinowitz, M., McAllister, H. H., and Virmani, R.: Cardiac fungal infections: Review of autopsy findings in 60 patients. Hum. Pathol. *15*:935, 1984.
754. Reingold, I. M.: Myocardial lesions in disseminated coccidioidomycosis. Am. J. Clin. Pathol. *20*:1044, 1950.
755. Larson, R., and Schert, R. E.: Coccidioidal pericarditis. Circulation *7*:211, 1953.
756. Merchant, R. K., Louria. D. B., Geisler, P. H., Edgcomb, J. H., and Utz, S. P.: Fungal endocarditis: Review of the literature and report of three cases. Ann. Intern. Med. *48*:242, 1958.
757. Owen, G. E., Scherr, W. N., and Segre, E. J.: Histoplasmosis involving the heart and great vessels. Am. J. Med. *32*:552, 1962.
758. Mendoza, I., Camardo, J., Moleiro, F., Castellanos, A., Medina, V., Gomez, J., Acquatella, H., Casal, H., Tortoledo, F., and Puigbo, J.: Sustained ventricular tachycardia in chronic chagasic myocarditis: Electrophysiologic and pharmacologic characteristics. Am. J. Cardiol. *57*:423, 1986.
759. Rosenbaum, M. B.: Chagasic myocardiopathy. Progr. Cardiovasc. Dis. *7*:199, 1964.
760. Hudson, L., and Britten, V.: Immune response to South American trypanosomiasis and its relationship to the Chagas' disease. Br. Med. Bull. *41*:175, 1985.
761. Figueiredo, F., Marin-Neto, J. A., and Rossi, M. A.: The evolution of experimental *Trypanosoma cruzi* cardiomyopathy in rabbits: Further parasitological, morphological and functional studies. Int. J. Cardiol. *10*:277, 1986.
762. Editorial: Chagas' disease: Potential for immunoprophylaxis. Lancet *1*:466, 1980.
763. Ribeiro Dos Santos, R., and Hudson, L.: *Trypanosoma cruzi*: Binding of parasite antigens to mammalian cell membranes. Parasite Immunol. *2*:1, 1980.
764. Mott, K. E., and Hagstrom, J. W. C.: The pathologic lesions of the cardiac autonomic nervous system in chronic Chagas' myocarditis. Circulation *31*:273, 1965.
765. Pereira Barretto, A. C., Mady, C., Arteaga-Fernandez, E., Stolf, N., Lopes, E. A., Higuchi, M. L., Bellotti, G., and Pileggi, F.: Right ventricular endomyocardial biopsy in chronic Chagas' disease. Am. Heart J. *111*:307, 1986.
766. Mady, C., Pereira-Barretto, A. C., Ianni, B. M., Lopes, E. A., and Pileggi, F.: Right ventricular endomyocardial biopsy in undetermined form of Chagas' disease. Angiology *35*:755, 1984.
767. Teixeira, A. R. L.: Chagas' disease: Trends in immunological research and prospects for immunoprophylaxis. Bull. WHO *57*:697, 1979.
768. Acosta, A. M., and Santos-Buch, C. A.: Autoimmune myocarditis induced by *Trypanosoma cruzi*. Circulation *71*:1255, 1985.
769. Morato, M. J., Brener, Z., Cancado, J. R., Nunes, R. M., Chiari, E., and Gazzinelli, G.: Cellular immune responses of chagasic patients to antigens derived from different *Trypanosoma cruzi* strains and clones. Am. J. Trop. Med. Hyg. *35*:505, 1986.
770. d'Imperior Lima, M. R., Eisen, H., Minoprio, P., Joskowicz, M., and Coutinho, A.: Pesistence of polyclonal B cell activation with undetectable parasitemia in late stages of experimental Chagas' disease. J. Immunol. *137*:353, 1986.
771. Puigbó, J. J., Valecillos, R., Hirschhault, E, Giordano, H., Boccalandro, I., Suarez, C., and Aparicio, J. M.: Diagnosis of Chagas' cardiomyopathy. Non-invasive techniques. Postgrad. Med. *53*:527, 1977.
772. Miles, M. A., Cedillos, R. A., Povoa, M. M., De Souza, A. A., Prata, A., and Macedo, V.: Do radically dissimilar *Trypanosoma cruzi* strains (zymodemes) cause Venezuelan and Brazilian forms of Chagas' disease? Lancet *1*:1338, 1981.
773. Oliveira, J. S. M.: A natural human model of intrinsic heart nervous system denervation: Chagas' cardiopathy. Am. Heart J. *110*:1092, 1985.
774. Oliveira, J. S. M., Oliveira, J. A. M., Frederigue, V., Jr., and Filho, E. C. L.: Apical aneurysm of Chagas' heart disease. Br. Heart J. *46*:432, 1981.
775. Rossi, M. A., Goncalves, S., and Ribeiro-dos-Santos, R.: Experimental *Trypanosoma cruzi* cardiomyopathy in BALB/c mice. The potential role of intravascular platelet aggregation in its genesis. Am. J. Pathol. *114*:209, 1984.
776. Andrade, Z. A., Andrade, S. G., Oliveira, G. B., and Alonso, D. R.: Histopathology of the conducting tissue of the heart in Chagas' myocarditis. Am. Heart J. *95*:316, 1978.
777. Amorim, D. S., Manco, J. C., Gallo, L. Jr., and Marin-Neto, J. A.: Chagas' heart disease as an experimental model for studies of cardiac autonomic function in man. Mayo Clin. Proc. *57*:48, 1982.
778. Marin-Neto, J. A., Maciel, B. C., Gallo Junior, L., Junqueira Junior, L. F., and Amorim, D. S.: Effect of parasympathetic impairment on the haemodynamic response to handgrip in Chagas's heart disease. Br. Heart J. *55*:204, 1986.
779. Junqueira, L. F. Jr., Gallo, L. Jr., Manco, J. C., Marin-Neto, J. A., and Amorim, D. S.: Subtle cardiac autonomic impairment in Chagas' disease detected by baroreflex sensitivity testing. Braz. J. Med. Biol. Res. *18*:171, 1985.
780. Maguire, J. H., Mott, K. E., Lehman, J. S., Hoff, R., Muniz, T. M., Guimaraes, A. C., Sherlock, I., and Morrow, R. H.: Relationship of electrocardiographic abnormalities and seropositivity to *Trypanosoma cruzi* within a rural community in Northeast Brazil. Am. Heart J. *105*:287, 1983.
781. Maguire, J. H., Mott, K. E., Hoff, R., Guimaraes, A., Franca, J. T., Almeida de Souza, J. A., Ramos, N. B., and Sherlock, I. A.: A three-year follow-up study of infection with *Trypanosoma cruzi* and electrocardiographic abnormalities in a rural community in northeast Brazil. Am. J. Trop. Med. Hyg. *31*:42, 1982.
782. Chiale, P. A., Przybylski, J., Laino, R. A., Halpern, M. S., Sanchez, R. A., Gafrieli, A., Elizari, M. V., and Rosenbaum, M. B.: Electrocardiographic changes evoked by ajmaline in chronic Chagas' disease without manifest myocarditis. Am. J. Cardiol. *49*:14, 1982.
783. Pimenta, J., Miranda, M., and Pereira, C. B.: Electrophysiologic findings in long-term asymptomatic chagasic individuals. Am. Heart J. *106*:374, 1983.
784. Pereira, M. H., Brito, F. S., Ambrose, J. A., Pereira C. B., Levi, G. C., Neto, V. A., and Martinez, E. E.: Exercise testing in the latent phase of Chagas' disease. Clin. Cardiol. *7*:261, 1984.
785. Oliveira, J. S., Correa De Araujo, R. R., Navarro, M. A., and Muccillo, G.: Cardiac thrombosis and thromboembolism in chronic Chagas' heart disease. Am. J. Cardiol. *52*:147, 1983.
786. Combellas, I., Puigbo, J. J., Acquatella, H., Tortoledo, F., and Gomez, J. R.: Echocardiographic features of impaired left ventricular diastolic function in Chagas's heart disease. Br. Heart J. *53*:298, 1985.
787. Caeiro, T., Amuchastegui, L. M., Moreyra, E., and Gibson, D. G.: Abnormal left ventricular diastolic function in chronic Chagas' disease: An echocardiographic study. Int. J. Cardiol. *9*:417, 1985.

788. Arreaza, N., Puigbo, J. J., Acquatella, H., Casal, H., Giordano, H., Valecillos, R., Mendoza, I., Perez, J. F., Hirschhaut, E., and Combellas, I.: Radionuclide evaluation of left-ventricular function in chronic Chagas' cardiomyopathy. J. Nucl. Med. *24*:563, 1983.
789. Hammermeister, K. E., Caeiro, T., Crespo, E., Palmero, H., and Gibson, D. G.: Left ventricular wall motion in patients with Chagas's disease. Br. Heart J. *51*:70, 1984.
790. Carrasco, H. A., Medina, M., Inglessis, G., Fuenmayor, A., Molina, C., and Davila, D.: Right ventricular function in Chagas disease. Int. J. Cardiol. *2*:325, 1983.
791. Carrasco, H. A., Barboza, J. S., Inglessis, G., Fuenmayor, A., and Molina, C.: Left ventricular cineangiography in Chagas' disease: Detection of early myocardial damage. Am. Heart J. *104*:595, 1982.
792. Carrasco, H. A., Barboza, J. S., Inglessis, G., Fuenmayor, A., and Molina, C.: Left ventricular cineangiography in Chagas' disease: Detection of early myocardial damage. Am. Heart J. *104*:595, 1982.
793. Factor, S. M., Cho, S., Wittner, M., and Tanowitz, H.: Abnormalities of the coronary microcirculation in acute murine Chagas' disease. Am. J. Trop. Med. Hyg. *34*:246, 1985.
794. Higashi, G. I.: Immunodiagnostic tests for protozoan and helminthic infections. Diagn. Immunol. 2:2, 1984.
795. Araujo, F., Chiari, E., and Dias, J. C. P.: Demonstration of *Trypanosoma cruzi* antigen in serum from patients with Chagas' disease. Lancet *1*:246, 1981.
796. Espinosa, R., Carrasco, H. A., Belandria, F., Fuenmayor, A. M., Molina, C., Gonzalez, R., and Martinez, O.: Life expectancy analysis in patients with Chagas' disease: Prognosis after one decade (1973–1983). Int. J. Cardiol. 8:45, 1985.
797. Apt, W., Arribada, A., Cabrera, L., and Sandoval, J.: Natural history of chagasic cardiopathy in Chile. Follow-up of 71 cases after 4 years. J. Trop. Med. Hyg. *86*:217, 1983.
798. Schofield, C. J.: Control of Chagas' disease vectors. Br. Med. Bull. *41*:187, 1985.
799. Marsden, P. D.: Selective primary health care: strategies for control of disease in the developing world. XVI. Chagas' disease. Rev. Infect. Dis. *6*:855, 1984.
800. Carrasco, H. A., Vicuna, A. V., Molina, C., Landaeta, A., Reynosa, J., Vicuna, N., Fuenmayor, A., and Lopez, F.: Effect of low oral doses of disopyramide and amiodarone on ventricular and atrial arrhythmias of chagasic patients with advanced myocardial damage. Int. J. Cardiol. 9:425, 1985.
801. Haedo, A. H., Chiale, P. A., Bandieri, J. D., Lazzari, J. O., Elizari, M. V., and Rosenbaum, M. B.: Comparative antiarrhythmic efficacy of verapamil, 17-monochloracetylaimaline, mexiletine and amiodarone in patients with severe chagasic myocarditis: Relation with the underlying arrhythmogenic mechanisms. J. Am. Coll. Cardiol. 7:1114, 1986.
802. Rosenbaum, M. B., Chiale, P. A., Haedo, A., Lazzari, J. O., and Elizari, M. V.: Ten years of experience with amiodarone. Am. Heart J. *106*:957, 1983.
803. Chiale, P. A., Halpern, M. S., Nau, G. J., Tambussi, A. M., Przybylski, J., Lazzari, J. O., Elizari, M. V., and Rosenbaum, M. B: Efficacy of amiodarone during long-term treatment of malignant ventricular arrhythmias in patients with chronic chagasic myocarditis. Am. Heart J. *107*:656, 1984.
804. Bellotti, G., Silva, L. A., Esteves Filho, A., Rati, M., de Moraes, A. V., Ramires, J. A., da Luz, P., and Pileggi, F.: Hemodynamic effects of intravenous administration of amiodarone in congestive heart failure from chronic Chagas' disease. Am. J. Cardiol. *52*:1046, 1983.
805. Francis, T. I.: Visceral complications of Gambian trypanosomiasis in a Nigerian. Trans. R. Soc. Trop. Med. Hyg. *66*:140, 1972.
806. deRaadt, P., and Koten, J. W.: Myocarditis in rhodesiense trypanosomiasis. East Afr. Med. J. *45*:128, 1968.
807. Poltera, A. A., Cox, N., and Owor, R.: Pancarditis affecting the conducting system and all valves in human African trypanosomiasis. Br. Heart J. *38*:827, 1976.
808. Jehn, U., Fink, M., Gundlach, P., Schwab, W. D., Bise, K., Deckstein, W. D., and Wilske, B.: Lethal cardiac and cerebral toxoplasmosis in a patient with acute myeloid leukemia after successful allogenic bone marrow transplantation. Transplantation *38*:430, 1984.
809. Van der Horst, R., Kleverman, P., Schonland, M., and Gotsman, M.: Fatal myocardial necrosis probably due to toxoplasma myocarditis. S. Afr. Med. J. *46*:949, 1972.
810. Permanyer-Miralda, G., Sagrista-Sauleda, J., and Soler-Soler, J.: Primary acute pericardial disease: A prospective series of 231 consecutive patients. Am. J. Cardiol. *56*:623, 1985.
811. Leak, D., and Meghji, M.: Toxoplasmic infection in cardiac disease. Am. J. Cardiol. *43*:841, 1979.
812. Sagrista-Sauleda, J., Permanyer-Miralda, G., Juste-Sanchez, C., de Buen-Sanchez, M. L., Pujadas-Capmany, R., Arcalis-Arce, L., and Soler-Soler, J.: Huge chronic pericardial effusion caused by *Toxoplasma gondii*. Circulation *66*:895, 1982.
813. Mary, A. S., and Hamilton, M.: Ventricular tachycardia in a patient with toxoplasmosis. Br. Heart J. *35*:349, 1973.
814. McGregor, C. G., Fleck, D. G., Nagington, J., Stovin, P. G., Cory-Pearce, R., and English, T. A.: Disseminated toxoplasmosis in cardiac transplantation. J. Clin. Pathol. *37*:74, 1984.
815. Rojas, R. A., and Deza, D.: Cardiac changes in malarial patients. Am. Heart J. *33*:702, 1947.
816. Merkel, W. C.: *Plasmodium falciparum* malaria: The coronary and myocardial lesions observed at autopsy in two cases of acute fulminating *Plasmodium falciparum* infection. Arch. Pathol. *41*:290, 1946.
817. Herrera, J. M.: Cardiac lesions in vivax malaria: Study of a case with coronary and myocardial damage. Arch. Inst. Cardiol. Mex. *30*:26, 1960.
818. Simonson, E., and Keys, A.: Experimental malaria in man. III. The changes in the electrocardiogram. J. Clin. Invest. *29*:68, 1950.
819. Wessel, H. U., Sommers, H. M., Cugell, D. W., and Paul, M. H.: Variants of cardiopulmonary manifestations of Manson's schistosomiasis: Report of two cases. Ann. Intern Med. *62*:757, 1965.
820. Bedford, D. E., Aidaros, S. M., and Girgis, B.: Bilharzial heart disease in Egypt: Cor pulmonale due to bilharzial pulmonary endarteritis. Br. Heart J. *8*:87, 1946.
821. Zahawi, S., and Shukri, N.: Histopathology of fatal myocarditis due to ectopic schistosomiasis. Trans. R. Soc. Trop. Med. Hyg. *50*:166, 1956.
822. Kean, B. H., and Breslou, R. C.: Parasites of the Human Heart. New York, Grune and Stratton, 1964.
823. Africa, C. M., Garcia, E. Y., and DeLeon, W.: Intestinal heterophyiasis with cardiac involvement. A contribution to the etiology of heart failure. J. Philipp. Isl. Med. Assoc. *15*:358, 1935.
824. Helimsky, A. M.: Cysticercosis of the brain, heart and skeletal muscles. Med. Parazitol. (Mosk.) *31*:610, 1962.
825. Goldsmid, J. M.: Two unusual cases of cysticercosis in man in Rhodesia. J. Helminthol. *40*:331, 1966.
826. Ibarra-Perez, C., Fernandez-Diez, J., and Rodriguez-Trujillo, F.: Myocardial cysticercosis: Report of two cases with coexisting heart disease. South. Med. J. *65*:484, 1972.
827. Kostucki, W., van Kuyk, M., and Cornil, A.: Changing echocardiographic features of a hydatid cyst of the heart. Br. Heart J. *54*:224, 1985.
828. Limacher, M. C., McEntee, C. W., Attar, M., Nelson, J. G., DeBakey, M. E., and Quinones, M. A.: Cardiac echinococcal cyst: diagnosis by two-dimensional echocardiography. J. Am. Coll. Cardiol. *2*:574, 1983.
829. Erol, C., Candan, I., Akalin, H., Sonel, A., and Kervancioglu, C.: Cardiac hydatid cyst simulating tricuspid stenosis. Am. J. Cardiol. *56*:833, 1985.
830. Franquet, T., Lecumberri, F., and Joly, M.: Hydatid heart disease. Br. J. Radiol. *57*:171, 1984.
831. Przybojewski, J. Z.: Primary cardiac hydatid disease. A case report. S. Afr. Med. J. *65*:438, 1984.
832. Malouf, J., Saksouk, F. A., Alam, S., Rizk, G. K., and Dagher, I.: Hydatid cyst of the heart: Diagnosis by two-dimensional echocardiography and computed tomography. *109*:605, 1985.
833. Oliver, J M., Benito, L. P., Ferrufino, O., Sotillo, J. F., and Nunez, L.: Cardiac hydatid cysts diagnosed by two-dimensional echocardiography. Am. Heart J. *104*:164, 1982.
834. Editorial: Medical treatment of hydatid disease. Br. Med. J. 2:563, 1979.
835. Becroft, D. M. O.: Infection by the dog roundworm *Toxocara canis* and fatal myocarditis. N. Engl. J. Med. *63*:729, 1964.
836. Friedman, S., and Hervada, A. R.: Severe myocarditis with recovery in a child with visceral larva migrans. J. Pediatr. *56*:91, 1960.
837. Barr, R.: Human trichinosis: Report of four cases, with emphasis on central nervous system involvement, and a survey of 500 consecutive autopsies at the Ottawa Civic Hospital. Can. Med. Assoc. J. *95*:912, 1966.
838. Ursell, P. C., Habib, A., Babchick, O., Rottolo, R., Despommier, D., and Fenoglio, J. J.: Myocarditis caused by *Trichinella spiralis* (letter). Arch. Pathol. Lab. Med. *108*:4, 1984.
839. Grey, D. F., Morse, B. S., and Phillips, W. F.: Trichinosis with neurologic and cardiac involvement: Review of the literature and report of three cases. Ann. Intern. Med. *57*:230, 1962.
840. Solarz, S. D.: An electrocardiographic study of one hundred and fourteen consecutive cases of trichinosis. Am. Heart J. *34*:230, 1947.
841. Van Stee, E. W. (ed.): Cardiovascular Toxicology. New York, Raven Press, 1982, 388 pp.
842. Bristow, M. R. (ed.): Drug-Induced Heart Disease. Amsterdam, Elsevier Press, 1980, 476 pp.
843. Kossowsky, W. H., and Lyon, A. P.: Cocaine and acute myocardial infarction. A probable connection. Chest *86*:729, 1984.
844. Barth, C. W., 3rd, Bray, M., and Roberts, W. C.: Rupture of the ascending aorta during cocaine intoxication. Am. J. Cardiol. *57*:496, 1986.
845. Nanji, A. H., and Filipenko, J. D.: Asystole and ventricular fibrillation associated with cocaine intoxication. Chest *85*:132, 1984.
846. Boag, F., and Havard, C. W.: Cardiac arrhythmia and myocardial ischemia related to cocaine and alcohol consumption. Postgrad. Med. J. *61*:997, 1985.
847. Cregler, L. L., and Mark, H.: Relation of acute myocardial infarction to cocaine abuse. Am. J. Cardiol. *56*:794, 1985.
848. Pasternack, P. F., Colvin, S. B., and Baumann, F. G.: Cocaine-induced angina pectoris and acute myocardial infarction in patients younger than 40 years. Am. J. Cardiol. *55*:84, 1985.
849. Weiss, R. J.: Recurrent myocardial infarction caused by cocaine abuse. Am. Heart J. *111*:793, 1986.
850. Simpson, R. W., and Edwards, W. D.: Pathogenesis of cocaine-induced ischemic heart disease. Autopsy findings in a 21-year-old man. Arch. Pathol. Lab. Med. *110*:479, 1986.
851. Schachne, J. S., Roberts, B. H., and Thompson, P. D.: Coronary-artery spasm and myocardial infarction associated with cocaine use (letter). N. Engl. J. Med. *310*:1665, 1984.
852. Howard, R. E., Hueter, D. C., and Davis, G. J.: Acute myocardial infarction following cocaine abuse in a young woman with normal coronary arteries. J.A.M.A. *254*:95, 1985.
853. Cregler, L. L., and Mark, H.: Cardiovascular dangers of cocaine abuse. Am. J. Cardiol. *57*:1185, 1986.
854. Nahas, G., Trouve, R., Demus, J. R., and von Sitbon, M.: A calcium-channel blocker as antidote to the cardiac effects of cocaine intoxication (letter). N. Engl. J. Med. *313*:519, 1985.
855. Levin, R., Burtt, D. M., Levin, W. A., and Ginsberg, M. B.: Ventricular fibrillation in a tetraplegic patient who had a therapeutic level of a tricyclic antidepressant. Case Report. Paraplegia 23:354, 1985.
856. Veith, R. C., Raskind, M. A., Caldwell, J. H., Barnes, R. F., Gumbrecht,

G., and Ritchie, J. L.: Cardiovascular effects of tricyclic antidepressants in depressed patients with chronic heart disease. N. Engl. J. Med. *306*:954, 1982.
857. Horowitz, J. D.: Drug Therapy. Drugs that induce heart problems. Which agents? What effects? J. Cardiovasc. Med. *8*:308, 1983.
858. Glassman, A. H.: Cardiovascular effects of tricyclic antidepressants. Annu. Rev. Med. *35*:503, 1984.
859. Orme, M. L.: Antidepressants and heart disease (editorial). Br. Med. J. *289*:1, 1984.
860. Surawicz, B., and Lasseter, K. C.: Effect of drugs on the electrocardiogram. Prog. Cardiovasc. Dis. *13*:26, 1970.
861. Fowler, N. O., McCall, D., Chou, T. C., Holmes, J. C., and Hanenson, I. B.: Electrocardiographic changes and cardiac arrhythmias in patients receiving psychotropic drugs. Am. J. Cardiol. *37*:223, 1976.
862. Raehl, C. L., Patel, A. K., and LeRoy, M.: Drug-induced torsade de pointes. Clin. Pharm. *4*:675, 1985.
863. Liberatore, M. A. and Robinson, D. S.: Torsade de pointes: a mechanism for sudden death associated with neuroleptic drug therapy? J. Clin. Psychopharmacol. *4*:143, 1984.
864. Burda, D. C.: Electrocardiographic abnormalities induced by thioridazine (Mellaril). Am. Heart J. *76*:153, 1968.
865. Raisfeld, I. H.: Cardiovascular complications of antidepressant therapy. Interactions at the adrenergic neuron. Am. Heart J. *83*:129, 1972.
866. Murphy, M. L., Bullock, R. T., and Pearce, M. B.: The correlation of metabolic and ultrastructural changes in emetine myocardial toxicity. Am. Heart J. *87*:105, 1974.
867. Sanghri, L. M., and Mathur, B. B.: Electrocardiogram after chloroquine and emetine. Circulation *32*:281, 1965.
868. Harbin, A. D., Gerson, M. C., and O'Connell, J. B.: Simulation of acute myopericarditis by constrictive pericardial disease with endomyocardial fibrosis due to methysergide therapy. J. Am. Coll. Cardiol. *4*:196, 1984.
869. Michael, T. A. D., and Arivazzadek, S.: The effects of acute chloroquine poisoning with special reference to the heart. Am. Heart J. *79*:831, 1970.
869a. Ratliff, N. B., Estes, M. L., Myles, J. L., Shirey, E. K., and McMahon, J. T.: Diagnosis of chloroquine cardiomyopathy by endomyocardial biopsy. N. Engl. J. Med. *316*:191, 1987.
870. Chulay, J. D., Spencer, H. C., and Mugambi, M.: Electrocardiographic changes during treatment of leishmaniasis with pentavalent antimony (sodium stibogluconate). Am. J. Trop. Med. Hyg. *34*:702, 1985.
871. Honey, M.: The effects of sodium antimony tartrate on the myocardium. Br. Heart J. *22*:601, 1960.
872. Mitchell, J. E., and Mackenzie, T. B.: Cardiac effects of lithium therapy in man: A review. J. Clin. Psychiatry *43*:47, 1982.
873. Montalescot, G., Levy, Y., Farge, D., Brochard, L., Fantin, B., Arnoux, C., and Hatt, P. Y.: Lithium causing a serious sinus-node dysfunction at therapeutic doses. Clin. Cardiol. *7*:617, 1984.
874. Martin, C. A., and Piascik, M. T.: First degree A-V block in patients on lithium carbonate. Can. J. Psychiatry *30*:114, 1985.
875. Arana, G. W., Dupont, R. M., and Clawson, L. D.: Is there clinical evidence that lithium toxicity can induce myocarditis? J. Clin. Psychopharmacol. *4*:364, 1984.
876. James, F. W., Kaplan, S., and Benzing, G., III: Cardiac complications following hydrocarbon ingestion. Am. J. Dis. Child *121*:431, 1971.
877. Steiner, M. H.: Syndromes of kerosene poisoning in children. Am. J. Dis. Child. *74*:32, 1947.
878. Harris, W. S.: Toxic effects of aerosol propellants on the heart. Arch. Intern. Med. *131*:162, 1973.
879. Rosenman, K. D.: Cardiovascular disease and work place exposures. Arch. Environ. Health. *39*:218, 1984.
880. Bagnell, W. E., Salway, S. G., and Jackson, E. W.: Phaeochromocytoma with myocarditis managed with *l*-methyl-*p*-tyrosine. Postgrad. Med. J. *52*:653, 1976.
881. Szakacs, J. E., and Mehlman, B.: Pathologic changes induced by *l*-norepinephrine: Quantitative aspects. Am. J. Cardiol. *5*:619, 1960.
882. Ferry, D. R., Henry, R. L., and Kern, M. J.: Epinephrine-induced myocardial infarction in a patient with angiographically normal coronary arteries. Am. Heart. J. *111*:1193, 1986.
883. Pentel, P. R., Mikell, F. L., and Zavoral, J. H.: Myocardial injury after phenylpropanolamine ingestion. Br. Heart J. *47*:51, 1982.
884. Rona, G.: Cathecholamine cardiotoxicity. J. Mol. Cell Cardiol. *17*:291, 1985.
885. Panagia, V., Pierce, G. N., Dhalla, K. S., Ganguly, P. K., Beamish, R. E., and Dhalla, N. S.: Adaptive changes in subcellular calcium transport during catecholamine-induced cardiomyopathy. J. Mol. Cell. Cardiol. *17*:411, 1985.
886. Downing, S. E., and Lee, J. C.: Contribution of alpha-adrenoceptor activation to the pathogenesis of norepinephrine cardiomyopathy. Circ. Res. *52*:471, 1983.
887. Opie, L. H., Walpoth, B., and Barsacchi, R.: Calcium and catecholamines: Relevance to cardiomyopathies and significance in therapeutic strategies. J. Mol. Cell. Cardiol. *17*:21, 1985.
888. Haft, J. I., Gershengorn, K., Kranz, P. D., and Oestreicher, R.: Protection against epinephrine-induced myocardial necrosis by drugs that inhibit platelet aggregation. Am. J. Cardiol. *30*:838, 1972.
889. Kline, T. S.: Myocardial changes in lead poisoning. Am. J. Dis. Child. *99*:48, 1960.
890. Freeman, R.: Reversible myocarditis due to chronic lead poisoning in childhood. Arch. Dis. Child. *40*:389, 1965.
891. Kurppa, K., Hietanen, E., Klockars, M., Partinen, M., Rantanen, J., Ronnemaa, T., and Viikari, J.: Chemical exposures at work and cardiovascular morbidity. Atherosclerosis, ischemic heart disease, hypertension, cardiomyopathy and arrhythmias. Scand. J. Work Environ. Health *10*:381, 1984.
892. Anderson, R. F., Allensenarth, D. C., and DeGroot, W. J.: Myocardial toxicity from carbon monoxide poisoning. Ann. Intern. Med. *67*:1172, 1967.
893. Hayes, J. M., and Hall, G. V.: The myocardial toxicity of carbon monoxide. Med. J. Aust. *1*:865, 1964.
894. Shafer, N., Smilay, M. G., and MacMillan, F. P.: Primary myocardial disease in man resulting from acute carbon monoxide poisoning. Am. J. Med. *38*:316, 1965.
895. Corya, B. C., Black, M. J., and McHenry, P. L.: Echocardiographic findings after acute carbon monoxide poisoning. Br. Heart J. *38*:712, 1976.
896. Dahhan, S. S., and Orfaly, H.: Electrocardiographic changes in mercury poisoning. Am. J. Cardiol. *14*:178, 1964.
897. Talley, R. C., Tinhart, J. W., Trevino, A. J., Moore, C., and Beller, B. M.: Acute elemental phosphorus poisoning in man: Cardiovascular toxicity. Am. Heart J. *84*:139, 1972.
898. Connor, T. B., Rosen, B. L., Blaustein, M. P., Applefeld, M. M., and Doyle, L. A.: Hypocalcemia precipitating congestive heart failure. N. Engl. J. Med. *307*:869, 1982.
899. Giles, T. D., Iteld, B. J., and Rives, K. L.: The cardiomyopathy of hypoparathyroidism. Chest *79*:225, 1981.
900. Levine, S. N., and Rheams, C. N.: Hypocalcemic heart failure. Am. J. Med. *78*:1033, 1985.
901. Rimailho, A., Bouchard, P., Schaison, G., Richard, C., and Auzepy, P.: Improvement of hypocalcemic cardiomyopathy by correction of serum calcium level. Am. Heart J. *109*:611, 1985.
902. Bashour, T. T., Ryan, C., Kabbani, S. S., and Crew, J.: Hypocalcemic acute myocardial failure secondary to rapid transfusion of citrated blood. Am. Heart J. *108*:1040, 1984.
903. Berkelhammer, C., and Bear, R. A.: A clinical approach to common electrolyte problems: 3. Hypophosphatemia. Can. Med. Assoc. J. *130*:17, 1984.
904. Berkelhammer, C., and Bear, R. A.: A clinical approach to common electrolyte problems. 4. Hypomagnesemia. Can. Med. Assoc. J. *132*:360, 1985.
905. Iseri, L. T., and French, J. H.: Magnesium: nature's physiologic calcium blocker. Am. Heart J. *108*:188, 1984.
906. Editorial: Selenium in the heart of China. Lancet *2*:889, 1979.
907. Li, G. S., Wang, F., Kang, D., and Li, C.: Keshan disease: An endemic cardiomyopathy in China. Hum. Pathol. *16*:602, 1985.
908. Keshan Disease Research Group of the Chinese Academy of Medical Sciences: Observations on the effect of sodium selenite in prevention of Keshan disease. Chin. Med. J. (Engl.) 92:471, 1979.
909. Johnson, R. A., Baker, S. S., Fallon, J. T., Maynard, E. P., III, Ruskin, J. N., Wen, A., Ge, K., and Cohen, H. J.: An occidental case of cardiomyopathy and selenium deficiency. N. Engl. J. Med. *304*:1210, 1981.
910. Fleming, C. R., Lie, J. T., McCall, J. T., O'Brien, J. F., Baillie, E. E., and Thistle, J. L.: Selenium deficiency and fatal cardiomyopathy in a patient on home parenteral nutrition. Gastroenterology *83*:689, 1982.
911. Selenium perspective (editorial). Lancet *1*:685, 1983.
912. Quercia, R. A., Korn, S., O'Neill, D., Dougherty, J. E., Ludwig, M., Schweizer, R., and Sigman, R.: Selenium deficiency and fatal cardiomyopathy in a patient receiving long-term home parenteral nutrition. Clin. Pharm. *3*:531, 1984.
913. Santhanakrishnan, B. R., and Gajalakshmi, B. S.: Pathogenesis of cardiovascular complications in children following scorpion envenoming. Ann. Trop. Paediatr. *6*:117, 1986.
914. Murthy, K. R. K., Billimoria, F. R., Khopkar, M., and Dave, K. N.: Acute hyperglycaemia and hyperkalaemia in acute myocarditis produced by scorpion (*Buthus tamulus*) venom injection in dogs. Indian Heart. J. *38*:71, 1986.
915. Bisarya, B. N., Vasavada, J. P., Bhatt, A., Nair, P. N. R., and Sharma, V. R.: Hemiplegia and myocarditis following scorpion bite (a case report). Indian Heart J. *29*:97, 1977.
916. Gueron, M., Adolph, R. J., Grupp, I. L., Gabel, M., Grupp, G., and Fowler, N. O.: Hemodynamic and myocardial consequences of scorpion venom. Am. J. Cardiol. *45*:979, 1980.
917. Rachesky, I. J., Banner, W. Jr., Dansky, J., and Tong, T.: Treatments for *Centruroides exilicauda* envenomation. Am. J. Dis. Child. *138*:1136, 1984.
918. Amitai, Y., Mines, Y., Aker, M., and Goitein, K.: Scorpion sting in children. A review of 51 cases. Clin. Pediatr. *24*:136, 1985.
919. Levine, H. D.: Acute myocardial infarction following wasp sting: Report of two cases and critical survey of the literature. Am. Heart J. *91*:365, 1976.
920. Weitzman, S., Margulis, G., and Lehmann, E.: Uncommon cardiovascular manifestations and high catecholamine levels due to "black widow" bite. Am. Heart J. *93*:89, 1977.
921. Reid, H. A.: Snakebite in the tropics. Br. Med. J. *3*:359, 1968.
922. Weiser, E., Wollberg, Z., Kochva, E., and Lee, S. Y.: Cardiotoxic effects of the venom of the burrowing asp, *Atractaspis engaddensis (Atractaspididae, Ophidia)*. Toxicon *22*:767, 1984.
923. Reid, H. A., Thean, P. C., Chan, K. E., and Baharom, A. R.: Clinical effects of bites by Malayan viper (*Ancistrodon rhodostoma*). Lancet *1*:617, 1963.
924. Chadha, J. S., Ashby, D. W., and Brown, J. O.: Abnormal electrocardiogram after adder bite. Br. Heart J. *30*:138, 1968.
925. Lee, S. Y., Lee, C. Y., Chen, Y. M., and Kochva, E.: Coronary vasospasm as the primary cause of death due to the venom of the burrowing asp, *Atractaspis engaddensis*. Toxicon *24*:285, 1986.
926. Weinberg, S. L.: The electrocardiogram in acute arsenic poisoning. Am. Heart J. *60*:971, 1960.
927. Barry, K. G., and Herndon, E. G., Jr.: Electrocardiographic changes associated with acute arsenic poisoning. Med. Ann. D.C. *31*:25, 1962.

928. Wenzel, D. G.: Drug-induced cardiomyopathies. J. Pharm. Sci. *56*:1209, 1967.
929. Zaloga, G. P., Deal, J., Spurling, T., Richter, J., and Chernow, B.: Unusual manifestations of arsenic intoxication. Am. J. Med. Sci. *289*:210, 1985.
930. Glazener, F. S., Ellis, J. G., and Johnson, P. K.: Electrocardiographic findings with arsenic poisoning. Calif. Med. *109*:158, 1968.
931. McKinstry, W. J., and Hicks, V. M.: Emergency-arsine poisoning. Arch. Intern. Med. *100*:34, 1957.
932. Kantrowitz, N. E., and Bristow, M. R.: Cardiotoxicity of antitumor agents. Prog. Cardiovasc. Dis. *27*:195, 1984.
933. Cazin, B., Gorin, N. C., Laporte, J. P., Gallet, B., Douay, L., Lopez, M., Najman, A., and Duhamel, G.: Cardiac complications after bone marrow transplantation. A report on a series of 63 consecutive transplantations. Cancer *57*:2061, 1986.
934. Gottdiener, J. S., Appelbaum, F. R., Ferrans, V. J., Deisseroth, A., and Ziegler, J.: Cardiotoxicity associated with high-dose cyclophosphamide therapy. Arch. Intern. Med. *141*:758, 1981.
935. Sanerkin, N. G.: Acute myocardial necrosis in paracetamol poisoning. Br. Med. J. *3*:478, 1971.
936. Bhasin, S., Wallace, W., Lawrence, J. B., and Lesch, M.: Sudden death associated with thyroid hormone abuse. Am. J. Med. *71*:887, 1981.
937. Fainstein, V., and Bodey, G. P.: Cardiorespiratory toxicity due to miconazole. Ann. Intern. Med. *93*:432, 1980.
938. Kowey, P. R., Friedman, P. L., Podrid, P. J., Zielonka, J., Lown, B., Wynne, J., and Holman, B. L.: Use of radionuclide ventriculography for assessment of changes in myocardial performance by disopyramide phosphate. Am. Heart J. *104*:769, 1982.
939. Gottdiener, J. S., Dibianco, R., Bates, R., Sauerbrunn, B. J., and Fletcher, R. D.: Effects of disopyramide on left ventricular function: assessment by radionuclide cineangiography. Am. J. Cardiol. *51*:1554, 1983.
940. Morady, F., Scheinman, M. M., and Desai, J.: Disopyramide. Ann. Intern. Med. *96*:337, 1982.
941. Lancaster, L. D. and Ewy, G. A.: Cardiac consequences of malignancy and their treatment. Adv. Intern. Med. *30*:275, 1984.
942. Vorobiof, D. A.: Cardiotoxicity of 5-fluorouracil. A case report. South Africa Med. J. *61*:634, 1982.
943. Taliercio, C. P., Olney, B. A., and Lie, J. T.: Myocarditis related to drug hypersensitivity. Mayo Clin. Proc. *60*:463, 1985.
944. Mullick, F. G., and McAllister, H. A.: Myocarditis associated with methyldopa therapy. J.A.M.A. 237:1699, 1977.
945. Sadjadi, S. A., Leghari, R. U., and Berger, A. R.: Prolongation of the PR interval induced by methyldopa. Am. J. Cardiol. *54*:675, 1984.
946. Plafker, J.: Penicillin-related nephritis and myocarditis: A case report. South. Med. J. *64*:852, 1971.
947. Schoenivetter, A. H., and Silber, E. N.: Penicillin hypersensitivity, acute pericarditis, and eosinophilia. J.A.M.A. *191*:672, 1965.
948. MacSearraegh, E. T. M., and Patel, I. C. M.: Cardiomyopathy as a complication of sulphonamide therapy. Br. Med. J. 3:33, 1968.
949. Kerwin, A. J.: Fatal myocarditis due to sensitivity to phenindione. Can. Med. Assoc. J. *90*:1418, 1964.
950. Hodge, P. R., and Lawrence, J. R.: Two cases of myocarditis associated with phnylbutazone therapy. Med. J. Aust. *1*:640, 1957.
951. Edelstein, J. M.: Butazolidin angiitis and periangiitis simulating Aschoff nodule. Am. Heart J. *69*:573, 1965.
952. Barrett, D. A., II, Dalldorf, F. G., Barnwell, W. H., II, and Hudson, R. P.: Allergic giant cell myocarditis complicating tuberculosis chemotherapy. Arch. Pathol. *91*:201, 1971.
953. Hubaytar, R. T., and Simpson, D. G.: Atrial fibrillation due to hypersensitivity due to para-aminosalicylic acid. Am. Rev. Respir. Dis, *86*:720, 1962.
954. Chatterjee, S. S., and Thakre, M. W.: Fiedler's myocarditis; Report of a fatal case following intramuscular injection of streptomycin. Tubercle *39*:240, 1958.
955. Steere, A. C., Taylor, E., Wilson, M. L, Levine, J. F., and Spielman, A.: Longitudinal assessment of the clinical and epidemiological features of Lyme disease in a defined population. J. Infect. Dis. *154*:295, 1986.
956. Schmid, G. P., Horsley, R., Streere, A. C., Hanrahan, J. P., Davis, J. P., Bowen, G. S., Osterholm, M. T., Weisfeld, J. S., Hightower, A. W., and Broome, C. V.: Surveillance of Lyme disease in the United States, 1982. J. Infect. Dis. *151*:1144, 1985.
957. Steere, A. C., Malawista, S. E., Bartenhagen, N. H., Spieler, P. N., Newman, J. H., Rahn, D. W., Hutchinson, G. J., Green, J., Snydman, D. R., and Taylor, E.: The clinical spectrum and treatment of Lyme disease. Yale J. Biol. Med. *57*:453, 1984.
958. Steere, A. C., Malawista, S. E., Newman, J. H., Spiebler, P. N., and Bartenhagen, N. H.: Antibiotic therapy in Lyme disease. Ann. Intern. Med. *93*:1, 1980.
959. Steere, A. C., Batsford, W. P., Weinberg, M., Alexander, J., Berger, H. J., Wolfson, S., and Malawista, S. E.: Lyme carditis: Cardiac abnormalities of Lyme disease. Ann. Intern. Med. *93*:8, 1980.
960. Marcus, L. C., Steere, A. C., Duray, P. H., Anderson, A. E., and Mahoney, E. B.: Fatal pancarditis in a patient with coexistent Lyme disease and babesiosis. Demonstration of spirochetes in the myocardium. Ann. Intern. Med. *103*:374, 1985.
961. Alpert, L. I., Welch, P., and Fisher, N.: Gallium-positive Lyme disease myocarditis. Clin. Nucl. Med. *10*:617, 1985.
962. Jacobs, J. C., Rosen, J. M., and Szer, I. S.: Lyme myocarditis diagnosed by gallium scan. J. Pediatr. *105*:950, 1984.
963. Steere, A. C., Hutchinson, G. J., Rahn, D. W., Sigal, L. H., Craft, J. E., DeSanna, E. T., and Malawista, S. E.: Treatment of the early manifestations of Lyme disease. Ann. Intern. Med. *99*:22, 1983.
964. Hansen, K., and Madsen, J. K.: Myocarditis associated with tick-borne *Borrelia burgdorferi* infection (letter). Lancet *1*:1323, 1986.
965. Wilson, M. S., Barth, R. F., Baker, P. B., Unverferth, D. V., and Kolibash, A. J.: Giant cell myocarditis. Am. J. Med. 79:647, 1985.
966. Theaker, J. M., Gatter, K. C., Heryet, A., Evans, D. J., and McGee, J. O.: Giant cell myocarditis: Evidence for the macrophage origin of the giant cells. J. Clin. Pathol. 38:160, 1985.
967. Rabson, A. B., Schoen, F. J., Warhol, M. J., Mudge, G. H., and Collins, J. J., Jr.: Giant cell myocarditis after mitral valve replacement: case report and studies of the nature of giant cells. Hum. Pathol. *15*:585, 1984.
968. Kloin, J. E.: Pernicious anemia and giant cell myocarditis. New association. Am. J. Med. 78:355, 1985.
969. McFalls, E. O., Hosenpud, J. D., McAnulty, J. H., Kron, J., and Niles, N. R.: Granulomatous myocarditis. Diagnosis by endomyocardial biopsy and response to corticosteroids in two patients. Chest 89:509, 1986.
970. Modry, D. L., Oyer, P. E., Jamieson, S. W., Stinson, E. B., Baldwin, J. C., Reitz, B. A., Dawkins, K. D., McGregor, C. G., Hunt, S. A., Moran, M., Myers, B., and Shumway, N. E.: Cyclosporine in heart and heart-lung transplantation. Can. J. Surg. 28:274, 1985.
971. Goldman, M. H., Barnhart, G., Mohanakumar, T., Wetstein, L., Szentpetery, S., Wolfgang, T. C., and Lower, R. R.: Cyclosporine in cardiac transplantation. Surg. Clin. North Am. *65*:637, 1985.
972. Cohen, D. J., Loertscher, R., Rubin, M. F., Tilney, N. L., Carpenter, C. B., and Strom, T. B.: Cyclosporine: a new immunosuppressive agent for organ transplantation. Ann. Int. Med. *101*:667, 1984.
973. Zeevi, A., Fung, J., Zerbe, T. R., Kaufman, C., Rabin, B. S., Griffith, B. P., Hardesty, R. L., and Duquesnoy, R. J.: Allospecificity of activated T cells grown from endomyocardial biopsies from heart transplant patients. Transplantation *41*:620, 1986.
974. Sibley, R. K., Olivari, M. T., Ring, W. S., and Bolman, R. M.: Endomyocardial biopsy in the cardiac allograft recipient. A review of 570 biopsies. Ann. Surg. *203*:177, 1986.
975. Palmer, D. C., Tsai, C. C., Roodman, S. T., Codd, J. E., Miller, L. W., Sarafian, J. E., and Williams, G. A.: Heart graft arteriosclerosis. Transplantation 39:385, 1985.
976. Kew, M. C., Tucker, R. B. K., Bersohn, I., and Seftel, H. C.: The heart in heatstroke. Am. Heart J. 77:324, 1969.
977. Malamud, N., Haymaker, W., and Luster, R. F.: Heatstroke: A clinicopathological study of 125 fatal cases. Milit. Surg. *99*:397, 1946.
978. Duguid, H., Simpson, R. G., and Stowers, R. G.: Accidental hypothermia. Lancet 2:1213, 1961.
979. Read, A. E., Ainslie-Smith, D., Gough, K. R., and Holmes, R.: Pancreatitis and accidental hypothermia. Lancet 2:1219, 1961.
980. Burns, R. J., Bar-Shlomo, B. Z., Druck, M. N., Herman, J. G., Gilbert, B. W., Perrault, D. J., and McLaughlin, P. R.: Detection of radiation cardiomyopathy by gated radionuclide angiography. Am. J. Med. *74*:297, 1983.
981. Ikaheimo, M. J., Niemela, K. O., Linnaluoto, M. M., Jakobsson, M. J., Takkunen, J. T., and Tasknen, P. J.: Early cardiac changes related to radiation therapy. Am. J. Cardiol. *56*:943, 1985.
982. Gottdiener, J. S., Katin, M. J., Borer, J. S., Bacharach, S. L., and Green, M. V.: Late cardiac effects of therapeutic mediastinal irradiation. Assessment by echocardiography and radionuclide angiography. N. Engl. J. Med. *308*:569, 1983.
983. Kereiakes, D. J., Morady, F. M., and Ports, T. A.: High-degree atrioventricular block after radiation therapy. Am. J. Cardiol. *51*:1233, 1983.
984. Applefeld, M. M., and Wiernik, P. H.: Cardiac disease after radiation therapy for Hodgkin's disease: Analysis of 48 patients. Am. J. Cardiol. *51*:1679, 1983.
985. Totterman, K. J., Pesonen, E., and Siltanen, P.: Radiation-related chronic heart disease. Chest 83:875, 1983.
986. Stewart, J. R., and Fajardo, C. F.: Radiation-induced heart disease. Clinical and experimental aspects. Radiol. Clin. North Am. 9:511, 1971.
987. Brosius, F. C., III, Waller, B. F., and Roberts, W. C.: Radiation heart disease: Analysis of 16 young (aged 15 to 33 years) necropsy patients who received over 3,500 rads to the heart. Am. J. Med. *70*:519, 1981.
988. Gottdiener, J. S. Katin, M. J., Borer, J. S., Bacharach, S. L., and Green, M. V.: Late cardiac effects of therapeutic mediastinal irradiation. Assessment by echocardiography and radionuclide ventriculography. N. Engl. J. Med. *308*:569, 1983.
989. Burns, R. J., Bar-Shlomo, B-Z., Druck, M. N., Herman, J. G., Gilbert, B. W., Perrault, D. J., and McLaughlin, P. R.: Detection of radiation cardiomyopathy by gated radionuclide angiography. Am. J. Med. *74*:297, 1983.
990. Perrault, D. J., Levy, M., Herman, J. D., Burns, R. J., Bar-Shlomo, B. Z., Druck, M. N., Wu, W. Q., McLaughlin, P. R., and Gilbert, B. W.: Echocardiographic abnormalities following cardiac radiation. J. Clin. Oncol. 3:546, 1985.
991. Reeves, W. C., Cunningham, D., Schwiter, E. J., Abt, A. Skarlatos, S., Wood, M. A., and Whitesell, L.: Myocardial hydroxyproline reduced by early administration of methylprednisolone or ibuprofen to rabbits with radiation-induced heart disease. Circulation 65:924, 1982.

43 PRIMARY TUMORS OF THE HEART

by WILSON S. COLUCCI, M.D., and
EUGENE BRAUNWALD, M.D.

"A diagnosis is easy as long as you think of it."
SOMA WEISS

The incidence of primary tumors of the heart* in autopsy series ranges from 0.0017 to 0.28 per cent.[1–5] Thus, these tumors are far less common than metastatic tumors to the heart.[6] The diagnosis is further complicated by an extraordinary variety of nonspecific clinical signs and symptoms that are capable of masquerading as many other more common cardiovascular and systemic diseases (Table 43–1). Prior to the advent of modern cardiopulmonary bypass surgical techniques, the correct antemortem diagnosis of an intracardiac tumor was largely academic, since effective therapy was not possible. However, now that many cardiac tumors are curable by operation, it is critically important to establish this diagnosis whenever possible. During the last decade, major advances in noninvasive cardiovascular diagnostic techniques have greatly facilitated this task, and it is now possible safely and readily to screen patients suspected of having a cardiac tumor, in many cases arriving at a definitive diagnosis preoperatively. Nevertheless, a high index of suspicion remains the most important element in diagnosing a cardiac tumor.

HISTORICAL PERSPECTIVE

Although primary tumors of the heart have been recognized since at least as early as the sixteenth century,[7] a correct antemortem diagnosis was not recorded until 1934.[8] The modern era of diagnosis began with the development of angiography, which permitted the visualization of cardiac tumors during life, and, in 1952, Goldberg et al. reported the first angiographic diagnosis of a left atrial myxoma.[9]

Before the development of modern open-heart surgical techniques, there were only rare reports of the successful removal of cardiac tumors, most on the epicardial surface.[10] Prior to the use of cardiopulmonary bypass, most attempts to remove intracardiac tumors were unsuccessful. In 1954, Crafoord performed the first successful excision of an intracardiac tumor, a left atrial myxoma, utilizing total cardiopulmonary bypass under direct vision.[11] The successful surgical excision of a wide variety of cardiac tumors is now possible, and in many instances a complete cure has been achieved.[12–16]

Advances in the field of noninvasive cardiovascular diagnosis have had a major impact on the ability of physicians to recognize correctly cardiac tumors ante mortem. A cardiac tumor was first demonstrated by M-mode echocardiography in 1959,[17] and, subsequently, echocardiography has become the cornerstone of the noninvasive diagnosis of cardiac tumors. Two-dimensional echocardiography has proved to be extremely useful and, in most situations, superior to M-mode echocardiography.[18, 19] Newer diagnostic methods, including radionuclide gated blood pool scanning[20, 21]; digital subtraction angiography, often employing intravenous injection of contrast medium (p. 357)[22]; and computed tomography[23–27] (p. 365), have been shown to be of value in the diagnosis of cardiac tumors. Most recently, magnetic resonance imaging (p. 374) has also been shown to be particularly effective in the detection and the precise anatomical characterization of cardiac tumors.[28–31] Not surprisingly, the widespread use of cross-sectional echocardiography, as well as some of these newer noninvasive methods, has resulted in a substantial increase in the detection of patients with primary cardiac tumors, many of whom are symptomatic.[19] Thus, during the past quarter century it has become possible to diagnose and successfully treat the majority of primary cardiac tumors. An appreciation of the clinical features, therefore, is now of far greater importance than heretofore.

CLINICAL PRESENTATION (Table 43–1)

SYSTEMIC FINDINGS. Cardiac tumors, particularly cardiac myxoma, can produce a broad array of systemic (i.e., noncardiac) findings, including fever, cachexia, malaise, arthralgias, Raynaud's phenomenon, rash, clubbing, and episodic bizarre behavior,[32–34] as well as systemic and pulmonary emboli. A variety of laboratory findings has been reported, including hypergammaglobulinemia, an elevated erythrocyte sedimentation rate, thrombocytosis, thrombocytopenia, polycythemia, leukocytosis, and anemia.[32–36] The mechanism by which cardiac tumors cause these systemic manifestations is not known with certainty, but it has been attributed to secretory products of the tumor or to tumor necrosis.[31, 32, 37] An immunological basis for the systemic manifestations is suggested by the finding of an increased titer of antimyocardial antibodies in a patient with a myxoma and a fall in the titer following surgical removal of the tumor.[38] A case of multiple myeloma has been attributed to continuous immunological stimulation by a left atrial myxoma.[39] Because the cardiac findings

*Tumors arising elsewhere in the body and metastasizing to the pericardium and heart are discussed in Chap. 44 (Pericardial Disease) and Chap. 55 (Hematologic-Oncologic Disorders, Coagulation, and Heart Disease).

TABLE 43–1 SYMPTOMS AND SIGNS OF CARDIAC MYXOMA

SYMPTOM	INCIDENCE %
Dyspnea on exertion	>75
Paroxysmal dyspnea	~25
Fever	~50
Weight loss	~25
Severe dizziness/syncope	~20
Sudden death	~15
Hemoptysis	~15
SIGN	**INCIDENCE %**
Mitral diastolic murmur	~75
Mitral systolic murmur	~50
Pulmonary hypertension	~70
Right heart failure	~70
Pulmonary emboli	~25
Anemia	>33
Elevated ESR	>33
Third heart sound (tumor plop)	>33
Atrial fibrillation	~15
Elevated globulins	~10
Clubbing	~5
Raynaud's phenomenon	<5

ESR = Erythrocyte sedimentation rate.
From Fisher, J.: Cardiac myxoma. Cardiovasc. Rev. Rep. 9:1195, 1983.

are nonspecific and may be subtle or absent, it is not unusual for these systemic findings to lead to a diagnosis of collagen vascular disease, infection, or noncardiac malignant disease.[40–43] Rarely, myxomas may be superinfected by bacteria or fungi.[44, 45]

EMBOLIC PHENOMENA. The embolization of tumor fragments or of thrombi from the surface of a tumor is a frequent and often dramatic clinical occurrence.[46–54] Although myxomas are the source of most tumor emboli because of the combination of their friable consistency and intracavitary location, other types of cardiac tumors occasionally may embolize.

The distribution of tumor emboli depends upon the location of the tumor and the presence or absence of intracardiac shunts. Left-sided tumors embolize to the systemic circulation, resulting in infarction and hemorrhage of viscera, including the heart,[53] as well as peripheral limb ischemia and vascular aneurysms.[34, 42, 47, 48, 52, 54] The diagnosis of an intracardiac tumor may be made after histological examination of systemic embolic material,[46, 47, 49] and therefore it is of critical importance to make every effort to recover and examine embolic material. In some cases, particularly when petechiae are present, biopsy of skin or muscle[34] may demonstrate intravascular tumor emboli.

Multiple systemic emboli may mimic systemic vasculitis[34, 40, 42, 43] or infective endocarditis,[41] especially when associated with other manifestations of a systemic illness such as fever, weight loss, arthralgias, elevated erythrocyte sedimentation rate, and elevated serum gamma globulins. The finding at angiography of multiple vascular aneurysms secondary to tumor emboli in the cerebral, renal, femoral, and coronary arteries is not infrequent,[52] and may lead to the mistaken diagnosis of polyarteritis nodosa.[42] The neurological consequences of embolization include transient ischemic attacks, seizures, syncope, and cerebral, cerebellar, brain stem, spinal cord, or retinal infarction.[48, 52, 54] The neurological event may occasionally be the first or only clinical manifestation of a cardiac tumor. An embolic stroke in a young person without evidence of cerebrovascular disease, particularly in the presence of sinus rhythm, should raise the possibility of intracardiac myxoma, as well as infective endocarditis (p. 1107) and prolapse of the mitral valve (p. 1045).

Right-sided cardiac tumors, and left-sided cardiac tumors proximal to left-to-right intracardiac shunts, may result in pulmonary emboli.[50, 51, 55] Indeed, serious pulmonary hypertension and secondary cor pulmonale due to chronic recurrent pulmonary emboli from a right atrial myxoma have been noted.[51] Clinically, the findings may be indistinguishable from pulmonary emboli secondary to venous thromboembolism (p. 1578). Although the findings on chest roentgenogram are nonspecific,[56] perfusion lung scanning in such patients may be atypical of pulmonary embolism in two respects: (1) The tumor-produced perfusion defects may remain static for long periods, as opposed to typical pulmonary embolic disease in which the defects usually resolve over the course of a few weeks; and (2) there may be complete absence of flow to one lung in the presence of completely normal perfusion of the opposite lung, a pattern unusual with typical pulmonary emboli.[56]

CARDIAC MANIFESTATIONS

The specific signs and symptoms produced by tumors are more closely related to their precise anatomical location than to their histological types.[57] Thus, it is useful to consider the constellation of findings which is typical of each location. The presentation of *pericardial tumors* is considered on page 1515 and will not be discussed here except to point out that primary tumors of the myocardium and endocardium may extend into the pericardial space and produce many of the clinical manifestations of pericardial tumors, including hemorrhagic pericardial effusion and compression of the heart by the effusion or the tumor itself.

MYOCARDIAL TUMORS. When clinically apparent, myocardial tumors most commonly result in disturbances of conduction or rhythm,[56–60] the precise nature of which is determined by the location of the tumor. Thus, tumors in the area of the atrioventricular node, typically angiomas and mesotheliomas, may produce atrioventricular (AV) conduction disturbances, including complete heart block and asystole, and can lead to sudden death.[58, 59] A wide variety of arrhythmias may be produced, including atrial fibrillation or flutter, paroxysmal atrial tachycardia with or without block, nodal rhythm, ventricular premature beats, ventricular tachycardia,[60] and ventricular fibrillation.[57] Intramural tumors may also produce symptoms by virtue of their size and location. Impairment of ventricular performance may simulate congestive, restrictive, or hypertrophic cardiomyopathy (Chap. 42).[58, 61] Myocardial rupture rarely may result from tumor infiltration of the myocardial wall.

LEFT ATRIAL TUMORS. Mobile, pedunculated, left atrial tumors may prolapse to variable degrees into the mitral valve orifice, resulting in obstruction to atrioventricular blood flow and, frequently, mitral regurgitation. The resultant signs and symptoms often mimic those of mitral valve disease,[57, 62] especially mitral stenosis (Chap. 33), and include dyspnea, orthopnea, paroxysmal nocturnal dyspnea, acute pulmonary edema, cough, hemoptysis, chest pain, peripheral edema, and fatigue. However, weight loss, pallor, syncope, and sudden death—manifestations uncommon for mitral valve disease—also occur. It is not unusual for the symptoms to be sudden in onset, intermittent, and related to the patient's body position.[57, 62] Although the majority of symptoms produced by left atrial tumors are nonspecific, the occurrence of paroxysmal symptoms that arise characteristically in a particular body position and are out of proportion to the clinical findings should raise the possibility of a left atrial tumor. The most common primary cardiac tumor presenting in the left

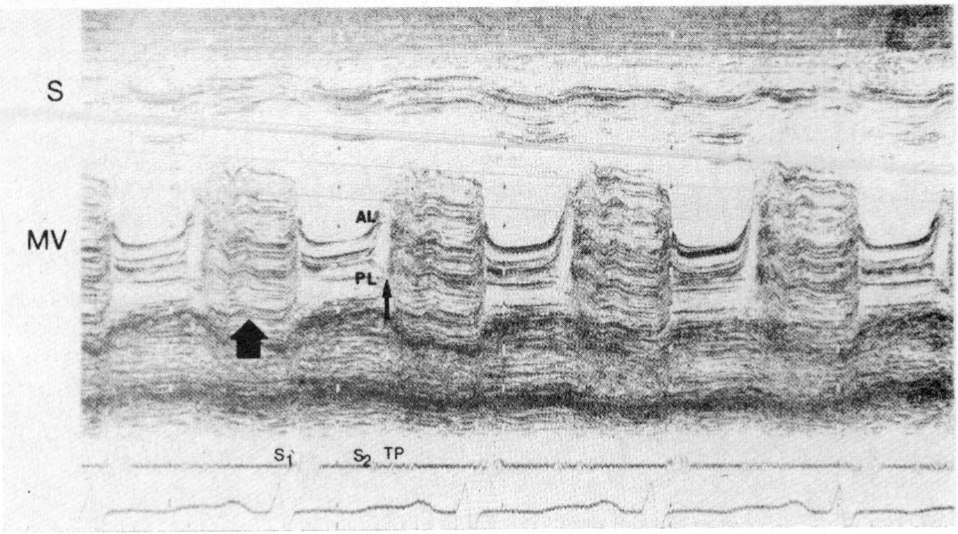

FIGURE 43–1. Simultaneous M-mode echocardiogram and phonocardiogram of a left atrial myxoma. The left atrial myxoma (thick arrow) prolapses into the mitral valve orifice during diastole, and appears as a dense collection of echoes posterior to the anterior leaflet (AL) of the mitral valve (MV). The appearance of the left atrial myxoma within the mitral valve orifice (thin arrow) correlates with a low-pitched sound, termed the tumor "plop" (TP). S = intraventricular septum; PL = posterior leaflet of the mitral valve; S_1 = first heart sound; S_2 = second heart sound. (From Salcedo, E. E., et al.: Echocardiographic findings in 25 patients with left atrial myxoma. Reprinted by permission of the American College of Cardiology. J. Am. Coll. Cardiol. *1*:1162, 1983.)

atrium is the benign myxoma, the large majority of which are solitary.

Physical examination may disclose signs of pulmonary congestion, an S_4, a loud S_1 which is often widely split, a holosystolic murmur which is loudest at the apex and resembles mitral regurgitation, and a diastolic murmur resulting from the obstruction to flow through the mitral orifice produced by the tumor. The loud S_1 that occurs in patients with left atrial myxoma may be due to the late onset of mitral valve closure (p. 44) resulting from prolapse of the tumor through the mitral valve orifice.[63] Consequently the left ventricular–left atrial pressure crossover occurs at a higher pressure, as in patients with mitral stenosis or a short P-R interval. It has been suggested that the finding of a loud S_1 in the absence of a short P-R interval or a mitral diastolic murmur should raise the consideration of a left atrial tumor.[63] In many cases an early diastolic sound, termed a tumor plop, can be identified (Fig. 43–1). It is thought to be produced as the tumor strikes the endocardial wall or as its excursion is abruptly halted[64] (Fig. 3–15, p. 51). Although in most cases the tumor plop occurs later than the opening snap of the mitral valve and earlier than the S_3, it is not surprising that this sound is frequently confused with the opening snap or the S_3.

RIGHT ATRIAL TUMORS. Right atrial tumors frequently produce symptoms of right heart failure, including fatigue, peripheral edema, ascites, hepatomegaly, and prominent *a* waves in the jugular venous pulse.[55, 57] The average time interval from the symptomatic presentation to the correct diagnosis of right atrial tumor is 3 years.[65] The development of right heart failure may be rapidly progressive and is often associated with new systolic or diastolic murmurs or both.[56, 66] The murmurs are generally the result of tumor obstruction to tricuspid valve flow or of tricuspid regurgitation caused by tumor interference with valve closure or valve destruction caused directly or indirectly by the tumor.[67] It is not surprising that right atrial tumors have been misdiagnosed as Ebstein's anomaly of the tricuspid valve, constrictive pericarditis, tricuspid stenosis, carcinoid syndrome, superior vena caval syndrome, and cardiomyopathy (Table 43–2). Pulmonary embolism and pulmonary hypertension occur and may simulate classic thromboembolic disease.[51, 55, 56] Right atrial hypertension may cause right-to-left shunting through a patent foramen ovale, with systemic hypoxia, cyanosis, clubbing, and polycythemia.[56, 68] Whereas myxomas occur much more commonly in the left atrium than the right atrium, sarcomas occur more commonly in the right atrium.[55]

Physical examination may reveal peripheral edema, evidence of superior vena caval obstruction, hepatomegaly, and ascites. An early diastolic rumbling murmur, alone or in combination with a holosystolic murmur secondary to tricuspid regurgitation, may demonstrate respiratory or positional variation. Because of the rarity of *isolated* rheumatic tricuspid valvular disease, the lack of other valvular findings should raise the question of a right atrial tumor. A protodiastolic tumor plop has been described and is thought to be similar in etiology to that produced by the left atrial tumor.[69] The jugular venous pressure may be elevated, and a prominent *a* wave and steep *y* descent have been described.[70]

RIGHT VENTRICULAR TUMORS. Right ventricular tumors often present with right heart failure as a result of obstruction to right ventricular filling or outflow. Clinical mani-

TABLE 43–2 CONDITIONS OFTEN CONFUSED WITH ATRIAL MYXOMA

Left atrium
Rheumatic mitral valve disease (MS, MR)
Pulmonary hypertension (primary, or secondary to mitral valve disease or LV failure)
Intrinsic lung disease
Cerebrovascular disease (CVA, TIA)
Endocarditis
Rheumatic fever
Myocarditis
Vasculitis (polyarteritis, lupus erythematosus)
Right atrium
Rheumatic tricuspid valve disease (TS, TR)
Ebstein's anomaly
Atrial septal defect
Pulmonary hypertension
Pulmonary emboli
Constrictive pericarditis
Pleuropericarditis (rub)
Carcinoid heart disease
Cardiomyopathy
Right ventricle
Pulmonic stenosis
Infundibular stenosis
Pulmonary emboli
Pulmonary hypertension
Left ventricle
Aortic stenosis
Subaortic stenosis
Cerebrovascular disease
Mural thrombus

MS = mitral stenosis; MR = mitral regurgitation; LV = left ventricular; CVA = cerebrovascular accident; TIA = transient ischemic attack; TS = tricuspid stenosis; TR = tricuspid regurgitation.

From Fisher, J.: Cardiac myxoma. Cardiovasc. Rev. Rep. 9:1195, 1983.

festations include peripheral edema, hepatomegaly, ascites, shortness of breath, syncope, and sudden death.[71]

A systolic ejection murmur at the left sternal border is usually found on physical examination.[72] A presystolic murmur[73] and a diastolic rumble[57] have been noted and are thought to be due to obstruction of the tricuspid valve. An S_3 may be audible, and a low-pitched diastolic sound that coincides with the maximal anterior excursion of the tumor has been ascribed either to tumor or to late closure of the pulmonary valve.[71] P_2 is often delayed, and its intensity may be normal, decreased, or increased. Tumor emboli to the pulmonary arteries may result in pulmonary hypertension, and the presence of tumor in the pulmonic valve orifice may lead to pulmonary regurgitation. The jugular veins are frequently distended with a prominent *a* wave and may demonstrate a Kussmaul's sign (p. 20).[72]

The cardiac findings often lead to a diagnosis of pulmonic stenosis, restrictive cardiomyopathy, or tricuspid regurgitation.[71–74] Whereas pulmonic stenosis is often asymptomatic and slowly progressive, the symptoms of right ventricular tumors are often rapidly progressive, and there is no poststenotic dilatation or systolic ejection click.

LEFT VENTRICULAR TUMORS. When left ventricular tumors are predominantly intramural in location, they are often asymptomatic, or they may present as conduction disturbances, arrhythmias, or interference with ventricular function. However, when the tumor also has a significant intracavitary component, there may be obstruction to left ventricular outflow, resulting in syncope and findings consistent with left ventricular failure. Atypical chest pain has also been reported and in some cases may reflect obstruction of a coronary artery either directly by tumor involvement or as a result of a tumor embolus to the coronary artery.

On physical examination a systolic murmur may be noted, and both the murmur and the blood pressure may vary with position.[75] Left ventricular tumors may simulate the findings of aortic stenosis, subaortic stenosis, hypertrophic cardiomyopathy,[61] endocardial fibroelastosis, and coronary artery disease.[76]

BENIGN VERSUS MALIGNANT TUMORS

The types of benign and malignant mesenchymal tumors that may develop in the heart are typical of those occurring in any mass of striated muscle and connective tissue. Although the exact incidence of each specific tumor type cannot be stated, about 75 per cent of all cardiac tumors are benign histologically and the remainder are malignant.[3, 4] The majority of benign cardiac tumors are myxomas, followed in frequency by a wide variety of other tumors (Table 43–3). Almost all malignant cardiac tumors are sarcomas, and of these the angiosarcoma and rhabdomyosarcoma are the most common forms.

Although it is often difficult or impossible to differentiate histologically benign from malignant tumors prior to operation, certain findings may be helpful. Characteristics suggestive of malignancy include the presence of distant metastases, local mediastinal invasion, evidence of rapid growth in tumor size, hemorrhagic pericardial effusion, precordial pain, location of the tumor on the right side of the heart or on the atrial free wall,[77] evidence of combined intramural and intracavitary location,[78] and extension into the pulmonary veins. Benign tumors are more likely to occur on the left side of the interatrial septum and to grow slowly. Although benign tumors do not metastasize, distant tumor emboli may mimic peripheral or pulmonary metastases. The preoperative differentiation between benign and malignant tumors may occasionally be made by examination of peripheral tumor emboli recovered by arteriotomy or by biopsy of skin or muscle.[46, 47, 49]

TABLE 43–3 RELATIVE INCIDENCE OF TUMORS OF THE HEART

Type	Number	Per Cent
Benign		
Myxoma	130	30.5
Lipoma	45	10.5
Papillary fibroelastoma	42	9.9
Rhabdomyoma	36	8.5
Fibroma	17	4.0
Hemangioma	15	3.5
Teratoma	14	3.3
Mesothelioma of the AV node	12	2.8
Granular cell tumor	3	—
Neurofibroma	3	—
Lymphangioma	2	—
Subtotal	319	75.1
Malignant		
Angiosarcoma	39	9.2
Rhabdomyosarcoma	26	6.1
Fibrosarcoma	14	3.3
Malignant lymphoma	7	1.6
Extraskeletal osteosarcoma	5	—
Neurogenic sarcoma	4	—
Malignant teratoma	4	—
Thymoma	4	—
Leiomyosarcoma	1	—
Liposarcoma	1	—
Synovial sarcoma	1	—
Subtotal	106	24.9
TOTAL	425	100.0

Modified from McAllister, H. A., and Fenoglio, J. J.: Tumors of the cardiovascular system. *In* Atlas of Tumor Pathology. Washington, D.C., Armed Forces Institute of Pathology, 1978. Fasc. 15, 2nd series.

BENIGN CARDIAC TUMORS

Myxomas

As already pointed out, myxomas are the most common type of primary cardiac tumor, composing 30 to 50 per cent of the total in most pathological series.[3, 4, 79] Ninety-three per cent of myxomas have been reported to occur sporadically.[80] The mean age of patients with sporadic myxoma is 51 years, and 76 per cent occur in females.[81] However, myxomas have been described in patients ranging in age from 3 to 83 years and are now not infrequently diagnosed in elderly patients in whom the symptoms and signs of cardiac tumor may have been attributed to other causes for a substantial time.[82] Approximately 86 per cent of myxomas occur in the left atrium, and over 90 per cent are solitary.[81] In the left atrium, the usual site of attachment is in the area of the fossa ovalis. Myxomas also may occur in the right atrium, and less often still, in the right or left ventricle. Multiple tumors may occur in the same chamber or in a combination of chambers.[82–85] Although myxomas may occasionally be found on the posterior left atrial wall, tumors presenting in this location should raise the suspicion of a malignant tumor. Myxomas of the mitral valve have been reported.[86]

The clinical signs and symptoms produced by cardiac myxomas include nonspecific manifestations as discussed above, embolization, and mechanical interference with cardiac function (Table 43–1). Not surprisingly, the symptoms produced by cardiac myxomas may simulate a wide variety of other cardiac and noncardiac conditions (Table 43–2). The clinical presentation of cardiac myxomas in 130 patients reviewed at the Armed Forces Institute of Pathology is summarized in Table 43–5.

FAMILIAL MYXOMAS. These tumors may be familial, and if so, they appear to be transmitted in an autosomal dominant manner.[80, 81, 87] In addition, some patients with myxoma may have a syndrome that involves a complex of abnormalities including lentigines or pigmented nevi or both, primary nodular adrenal cortical disease with or without Cushing's syndrome, myxomatous mammary fibroadenomas, testicular tumors, and pituitary adenomas with gigantism or acromegaly[88–93] (Fig. 43–2). Patients may have two or more components of this complex, and generally the first component is diagnosed at a relatively young age (mean age, 18 years). Certain aspects of this syndrome have been referred to as the NAME syndrome (*n*evi, *a*trial myxoma, *m*yxoid neurofibroma, *e*phelides)[91] or the LAMB syndrome (*l*entigines, *a*trial *m*yxoma and *b*lue nevi).[89] The majority of patients so far described have had cardiac myxomas.

Taken together, familial myxoma or the complex of findings described above constitutes approximately 7 per cent of all myxomas.[80, 80a] Compared to patients with sporadic myxoma, these patients are younger (mean age, 20's), are more likely to have multiple myxomas involving chambers other than the left atrium, and are more likely to have recurrence of myxomas postoperatively[80] (Table 43–4). Such "recurrences" most likely represent the multicentric nature of this disease. When multiple myxomas occur simultaneously they are referred to as synchronous, whereas multiple myxomas presenting at different times are referred to as metasynchronous.[80]

Because cardiac myxomas may be familial,[87] routine echocardiographic screening of first degree relatives is appropriate, particularly if the patient is young or has multiple tumors. In patients with a familial history or other components of the syndrome described above, a careful search should be made preoperatively for multiple cardiac myxomas. In addition, these patients should be observed closely postoperatively for the development of other tumors (metasynchronous), which occurs in 12 to 22 per cent of such patients.[80]

PATHOLOGY. The pathological features of myxoma are similar to those of an organized thrombus, a finding that has led to the suggestion that myxomas are not true neoplasms but may represent one form of organization of an endocardial thrombus.[94] Although most investigators favor the view that myxomas are a true neoplastic process,[3, 4, 95] the cellular origin of the myxoma is not entirely agreed upon. Histological, ultrastructural, and immunohistochemical evidence indicating considerable cellular heterogeneity within the tumor has been interpreted as support for the thesis that myxomas originate by divergent differentiation of mesenchymal cells.[96–99] Likewise, when cardiac myxomas are grown in tissue culture a distinctive polygonal cell results that has the characteristics of a multipotential mesenchymal cell.[100] Some investigators, however, have suggested an origin from endocardial cells.[101] Although histologically benign, myxomas may rarely exhibit malignant biological behavior with invasion of the interatrial septum.[102] Occasional reports suggest that myxomas may have a malignant counterpart[103] as well as the ability to implant and grow at distant foci such as the brain or bone.[104, 105]

Grossly, myxomas are generally pedunculated, with a fibrovascular stalk. Most sessile tumors probably represent the base of the pedicle, which remains after the body has embolized.[3] The tumors average 4 to 8 cm in diameter, although tumors of up to 15 cm have been reported. Most myxomas are gelatinous and polypoid, although they may also be smooth and round with a glistening surface; areas of hemorrhage are not unusual (Fig. 43–3).

By *light microscopy*, the cells are uniform, small, and polygonal with round or oval nuclei and a moderate amount of cytoplasm. The cells are surrounded by myxomatous stroma composed predominantly of an eosinophilic matrix which appears to be composed of an acid mucopolysac-

TABLE 43–4 FEATURES OF SPORADIC, "COMPLEX,"* AND FAMILIAL CARDIAC MYXOMA

	Sporadic	"Complex"	Familial
Mean age (yr)	53	26	25
Single left atrial site (%)	76	30	37
Multiple (%)	1	53	30
Recurrent (%)	1–3	22	12

*Complex of myxomas, spotty pigmentation, and endocrine overactivity.
From McCarthy, P. M., et al.: The significance of multiple, recurrent, and "complex" cardiac myxomas. J. Thorac. Cardiovasc. Surg. *91*:389, 1986.

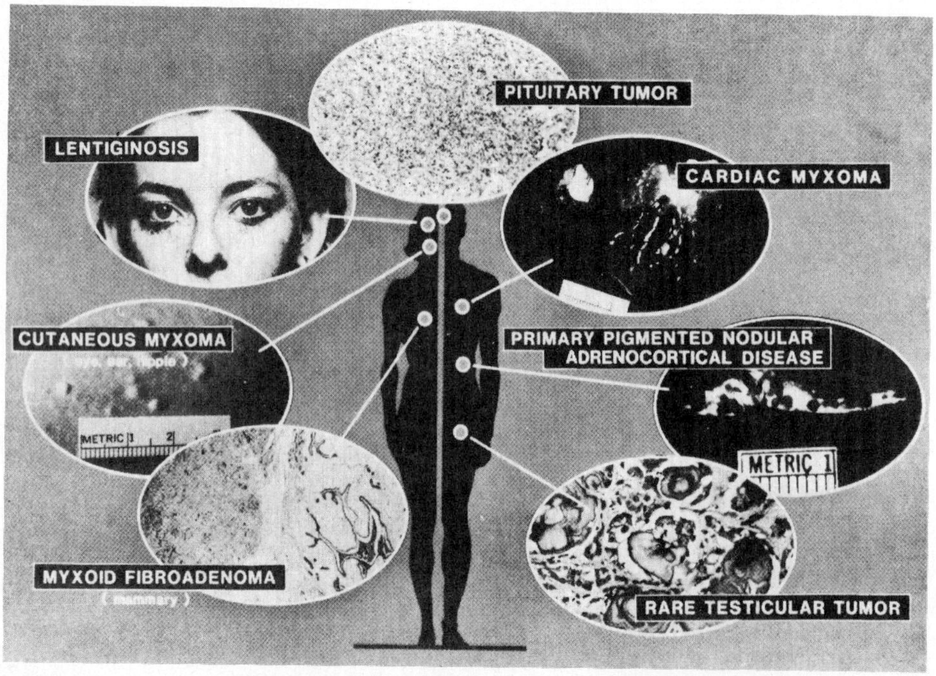

FIGURE 43–2. Clinical elements which may be found in patients with "complex" myxomas. The biological behavior of cardiac myxomas associated with this syndrome differs from that of the more common solitary myxoma. In these patients cardiac myxomas tend to occur at a younger age, are more likely to be familial, and the incidence of multiple and recurrent tumors is higher. (From McCarthy, P. M., et al.: The significance of multiple, recurrent, and "complex" cardiac myxomas. J. Thorac. Cardiovasc. Surg. *91*:389, 1986.)

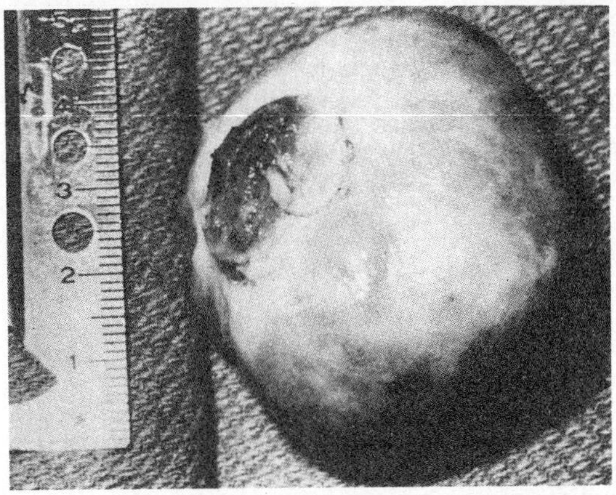

FIGURE 43–3. Gross pathological specimen of a left atrial myxoma removed at operation. The myxoma had a smooth, glistening capsule and measured approximately 5 cm in diameter. By two-dimensional echocardiography, the tumor was seen to prolapse into the left ventricle during diastole. (From Salcedo, E. E., et al.: Echocardiographic findings in 25 patients with left atrial myxoma. Reprinted by permission of the American College of Cardiology. J. Am. Coll. Cardiol. *1*:1162, 1983.)

charide similar to chondroitin C.[3] The cells and the stroma are frequently positive with periodic acid-Schiff stain, whereas only stroma is stained with alcian blue stain. Elastic fibers, reticular fibers, smooth muscle cells, collagen, calcium, and bone may be seen. Other cellular elements include lymphocytes, plasma cells, mast cells, histiocytes, and, rarely, fibrocytes. Thin-walled vessels simulating primitive capillaries are present. The surface of the tumor consists of the typical myxoma cells and, in some cases, thrombus.

On *electron microscopic examination,* the myxoma cells demonstrate areas of intracellular junctions (zonulae adherentes), single nuclei with finely dispersed chromatin and nucleoli, rough endoplasmic reticulum, free ribosomes, mitochondria, Golgi complexes, and cytoplasmic filaments.[3, 95, 106] On examination with scanning electron microscopy, myxomas are covered by endothelium and possess endothelium-lined crevices and clefts, features not seen in atrial thrombus.[107]

PAPILLARY TUMORS OF HEART VALVES. Papillary tumors of the cardiac valves and adjacent endocardium are found, not uncommonly, post mortem and may be identified during life by two-dimensional echocardiography.[3, 108] Although the clinical significance of these lesions is debated, there is evidence that they have the potential to cause valvular dysfunction and embolize to vital structures.[3, 108, 109] These lesions have a characteristic frond-like appearance, may be up to 3 or 4 cm in diameter, are single or multiple, and may occur on any valve; most often the ventricular surface of semilunar valves and the atrial surface of AV valves are affected. Rarely, they may be present on papillary muscle, chordae tendineae, or endocardium.[110] The tricuspid valve is most commonly involved in children and the mitral and aortic valves in adults.[4] Histologically the tumor is covered by endothelium that surrounds a core of loose connective tissue consisting of an acid

TABLE 43–5 CLINICAL PRESENTATION OF CARDIAC MYXOMA IN 130 PATIENTS*

Signs and symptoms of mitral valve disease	57
Embolic phenomena	36
No cardiac symptoms—incidental finding	16
Signs and symptoms of tricuspid valve disease	6
Sudden unexpected death	5
Pericarditis	4
Myocardial infarction	3
Signs and symptoms of pulmonary valve disease	2
Fever of undetermined origin	2

*One patient with multiple myxomas had signs and symptoms of mitral and tricuspid valve disease.

From McAllister, H. A., and Fenoglio, J. J.: Tumors of the cardiovascular system. *In* Atlas of Tumor Pathology. Washington, D.C., Armed Forces Institute of Pathology, 1978. Fasc. 15, 2d series.

mucopolysaccharide matrix, smooth muscle cells, and collagen and elastic fibers.[4] The pathogenesis of these lesions is unsettled, but it appears that they may originate from organized mural thrombi.[3, 91, 110] Papillary tumors are generally distinguished from *Lambl's excrescences*, which are ubiquitous acellular deposits covered by a single layer of endothelium and found on heart valves at the site of endothelial damage in over 70 per cent of adults.[3]

RHABDOMYOMAS. These are the most common cardiac tumors of infants and children, the large majority occurring in patients younger than 1 year.[111] Morphological evidence suggests that rhabdomyomas are actually myocardial hamartomas rather than true neoplasms.[112] Consistent with this view is the complete lack of any mitotic activity[111] and the observation at the ultrastructural level that the characteristic glycogen-laden cells are typical of immature myocytes[112] and are strongly associated with tuberous sclerosis, a familial syndrome characterized by hamartomas in several organs, epilepsy, mental deficiency, and adenoma sebaceum. Alternatively, it has been suggested that rhabdomyomas may represent a nodular form of a diffuse cardiac glycogen storage disease.[113]

One-third to one-half of patients with cardiac rhabdomyomas are found at autopsy to have tuberous sclerosis; adenoma sebaceum and benign kidney tumors (angiomyolipomas and hamartomas) are seen less frequently.[111] Conversely, approximately 50 per cent or more of patients having tuberous sclerosis but no signs or symptoms of cardiac disease have been shown to have findings on echocardiography that are consistent with rhabdomyoma.[114, 115] Rhabdomyomas causing significant intracavitary obstruction may result in death within the first 24 hours of life, whereas patients with less severe involvement may remain asymptomatic, or the tumor may become apparent during infancy or early childhood.[111]

Rhabdomyomas invariably involve the ventricles, affecting the left and right sides equally. Ninety per cent are multiple, and in 30 per cent there is involvement of at least one of the atria. Approximately 50 per cent of rhabdomyomas are large enough to cause significant obstruction of a cardiac chamber or valvular orifice.[111, 116] Nonspecific clinical manifestations—including cardiomegaly, right or left ventricular failure or both, an S_3, S_4, and systolic or diastolic murmurs—may mimic mitral stenosis, mitral atresia, aortic stenosis, subaortic stenosis, and infundibular pulmonic stenosis.[117]

Rhabdomyomas are yellow-gray and range from 1 mm to several centimeters in diameter. The microscopic hallmark, termed the spider cell, is a cell containing a central cytoplasmic mass that is suspended by fine fibrillar processes radiating to the periphery, thus giving the appearance of a spider hanging in a net.[3] The cytoplasm is rich in glycogen and stains positively with periodic acid-Schiff reagent.[3] Electron microscopy demonstrates myofibrils, cytoplasmic and mitochondrial glycogen, and apparent intercellular junctions similar to intercalated disks.[111]

FIBROMAS AND HAMARTOMAS. Fibromas are benign, connective tissue tumors that occur predominantly in children. The majority occur before the age of 10 years, and about 40 per cent are diagnosed in infants less than 1 year of age.[118] Males and females appear equally affected. Fibromas constitute the second most common type of primary cardiac tumor occurring in infants and children.[118, 119] Whether fibromas represent hamartomas or true neoplasms is debated.[119] The histological criteria for diagnosis are not uniformly agreed upon, and therefore several designations are employed, including fibromyxoma, fibroelastic hamartoma, embryonic mesenchymoma, fibroma, and fibrous rhabdomyoma.[82]

Almost all fibromas occur within the ventricular myocardium—most frequently within the anterior free wall of the left ventricle or the interventricular septum and much less often in the posterior left ventricular wall or right ventricle. Typically, they are gray, firm, circumscribed, not capsulated, and range in size from 3 to 7 cm. Grossly, they resemble fibroids and exhibit a whorled appearance on cut sections. Microscopically, cardiac fibromas consist of elongated fibroblasts admixed with fibrous tissue consisting of collagen and elastic fibers. Their cellularity is variable, and mitotic figures are rarely, if ever, seen. Fibrous tissue is intermingled with adjacent myocardial fibers at the margins of the lesion.[119] Calcification and islands of bone formation may be seen microscopically and occasionally radiographically. The *Gorlin syndrome,* the main features of which are multiple nevoid basal cell carcinomas, cysts of the jaw, and skeletal abnormalities, may be associated in some cases with cardiac tumors, either fibromas or fibrous histiocytomas.[120]

Although fibromas may be incidental findings at postmortem examination, approximately 70 per cent at some time show signs or symptoms due to mechanical interference with intracardiac flow, ventricular contraction, or conduction disturbances.[3] Clinical manifestations are protean and include murmurs, atypical chest pain, congestive heart failure and signs of subaortic stenosis, valvular or infundibular pulmonic stenosis with right ventricular hypertrophy, tricuspid stenosis, conduction disturbances, ventricular tachycardia,[60] and sudden death. As in the case of rhabdomyomas, the increased usage of echocardiography has resulted in the not infrequent detection of cardiac fibromas in patients without cardiac signs or symptoms.[121, 122]

LIPOMAS AND LIPOMATOUS HYPERTROPHY OF THE ATRIAL SEPTUM. Lipomas occur at all ages and with equal frequency in both sexes. Most range in diameter from 1 to 15 cm, although some have been reported to weigh more than 2 kg.[123] Most tumors are sessile or polypoid and occur in the subendocardium or subpericardium, although about one-fourth are completely intramuscular.[2] Subendocardial tumors with intracavitary extension produce symptoms that are characteristic of their location, whereas subepicardial tumors may cause compression of the heart and pericardial effusion. The most common chambers affected are the left ventricle, right atrium, and interatrial septum.[4] Intramural tumors may be asymptomatic or result in arrhythmias, AV or intraventricular conduction disturbances, or mechanical interference[124] Many tumors are clinically silent and are found only at autopsy or become apparent on a routine chest roentgenogram.

Microscopically, the lesions are usually well encapsulated, composed of typical mature fat cells, and occasionally contain fibrous connective tissue (fibrolipoma), muscular tissue (myolipoma), or vacuolated brown fat resembling a hibernoma.

Whereas lipomas are true neoplasms, a condition termed *lipomatous hypertrophy of the interatrial septum* represents the occurrence of an accumulation of mature adipose tissue within the interatrial septum.[119–121] These lesions range from 1 to 6.5 cm in dimension, most often protrude into the right atrium, and are more common in obese, elderly, or female patients.[125] A variety of atrial arrhythmias have been attributed to these lesions, but a cause-and-effect relationship has been difficult to establish.[125–127] Since this lesion may occasionally be detected by cineangiography, echocardiography, computed tomography,[121] or other diagnostic techniques, the major clinical dilemma is the differential diagnosis and treatment of an intraatrial filling defect.

ANGIOMAS. Benign vascular tumors, including hemangiomas, lymphangiomas, and angioreticulomas, are extremely rare.[128] Anatomically, they may occur in any part of the heart, but usually are intramural, often in the interventricular septum or AV node, where they may cause complete heart block and sudden death.[129] Cardiac tamponade due to hemopericardium may be the presenting clinical syndrome. More commonly found in the right heart chambers, hemangiomas are generally sessile or polypoid subendocardial nodules ranging from 2 to 3.5 cm in diameter. Histologically, the tumors consist of endothelium-lined spaces which may contain blood, lymph, or thrombi; they are classified according to the predominant type of proliferating vascular channel.

TERATOMAS. These tumors, which contain elements of all three germ cell layers, occur within the heart less frequently than in the anterior mediastinum. Teratomas are generally observed in children,[130] and when located within the heart, they occur predominantly within the right atrium, right ventricle, or the interatrial or interventricular septum.[130] Angiography, computed tomography (p. 350), radionuclide imaging, and two-dimensional echocardiography all appear useful in establishing the diagnosis.

BENIGN CYSTIC TUMORS. Benign cystic tumors are small lesions, generally less than 15 mm, that are found in the area of the AV node.[58, 59] These lesions are characterized by tubules and cysts lined by flat or cuboidal cells that are devoid of mitotic activity, but may have secretory function. The embryogenic basis and histological classification of these lesions has been controversial,[131, 132] as reflected by the variety of terms by which they are called in the literature, including lymphangioendothelioma, mesothelioma, and congenital polycystic tumor.[132]

These lesions present during the first or second decade, exhibit a marked female predominance, and are frequently noted at the time of puberty or pregnancy, thus suggesting a hormonal role in their development and expression. Because of their location in the area of the AV node, they most often present as progressive heart block, syncope, or sudden death, although many are asymptomatic and consistent with a long life. Ventricular tachycardia progressing to ventricular fibrillation has been observed, perhaps explaining the poor results obtained with cardiac pacemakers in this condition.[58]

Epithelium-lined cysts are extremely rare lesions which are usually an incidental postmortem finding.[2, 4] They are 4 to 25 mm in diameter and are lined with cuboidal or columnar ciliated epithelium.

ENDOCRINE TUMORS OF THE HEART. Approximately 2 per cent of *paragangliomas* are intrathoracic, and of these most are located in the posterior mediastinum. However, these tumors can also occur in close association with the left atrial or left ventricular epicardium, where they are thought to have arisen from sympathetic fibers to the myocardium or coronary vasculature or from ectopic chromaffin cells.[133] More rarely still, paragangliomas may arise within the interatrial septum.[134, 135] Tumors in any of these locations may secrete catecholamines and therefore can be associated with signs and symptoms characteristic of pheochromocytoma (p. 1812).[133–135]

Rarely, benign *thyroid tumors* arise within the heart, presumably from ectopic rests of thyroid tissue.[136–138] These tumors most often arise from the interventricular septum and present, not infrequently, as obstruction to right ventricular outflow.

MALIGNANT CARDIAC TUMORS

About one-fourth of all cardiac tumors exhibit typically malignant histological characteristics and invasive behavior[2–4] (Table 43–3). Virtually all of these are sarcomas, thus making these tumors second in overall frequency only to myxomas. Sarcomas may occur at any age, but are most common between the third and fifth decades and show no sex preference. In decreasing order of frequency the sites involved are the right atrium, left atrium, right ventricle, left ventricle, and interventricular septum.

Sarcomas derive from mesenchyme and therefore may display a wide variety of morphological types which may be subtyped as angiosarcoma, rhabdomyosarcoma, fibrosarcoma, and lymphosarcoma.[4]

From a clinical viewpoint, sarcomas characteristically display a rapidly downhill course. Death most often occurs from a few weeks to 2 years after the onset of symptoms. These tumors proliferate rapidly and generally cause death through widespread infiltration of the myocardium, obstruction of flow within the heart, or distant metastases. About 75 per cent of all patients with cardiac sarcomas have pathological evidence of distant metastases at the time of death.[139] The most frequent sites are the lungs, thoracic lymph nodes, mediastinum, and vertebral column; less often the liver, kidneys, adrenals, pancreas, bone, spleen, and bowel are involved.

The cardiac findings are determined primarily by the location of the tumor and by the extent of intracavitary obstruction. Typical presentations include progressive, unexplained, congestive heart failure, particularly of the right side; precordial pain; pericardial effusion; tamponade; arrhythmias; conduction disturbances; obstruction of the venae cavae; and sudden death. Tumors limited to the myocardium without intracavitary extension may produce no cardiac symptoms or may cause arrhythmias and conduction disturbances. Because of the rapid growth potential of sarcomas, they commonly extend into the cardiac chambers, the pericardial space, or both. In about 20 per cent of cases, the tumor is sessile or polypoid.[140] When there is extension into the pericardial space, hemorrhagic pericardial effusion is common, and tamponade may occur. Because the right side of the heart is most commonly affected, sarcomas frequently cause signs of right heart failure as a result of obstruction of the right atrium, right ventricle, or tricuspid or pulmonic valves. In addition, obstruction of the superior vena cava may result in swelling of the face and upper extremities, whereas obstruction of the inferior vena cava may result in visceral congestion.

ANGIOSARCOMAS. Included within this category are malignant hemangioendotheliomas, angiosarcomas, Kaposi's sarcomas, angioreticuloendotheliomas, and cavernous angiosarcomas.[4, 141, 142] All 40 patients in one series were adults.[141] In distinction to most other cardiac sarcomas, in which the sex distribution is equal, there appears to be a 2:1 male-to-female ratio among patients with angiosarcomas. These tumors have a striking predilection for the right atrium, most often arising from the interatrial septum,[143] and may be infiltrative or polypoid in nature. Microscopically, angiosarcomas are characterized by ill-defined anastomotic vascular channels lined with atypical, often heaped-up, endothelial cells.[144] By electron microscopy, immature endothelial cells, primitive pericytes, and undifferentiated mesenchymal cells may be identified.[145] Associated cavernous hemangiomas of the liver have been reported.[2]

RHABDOMYOSARCOMAS. These are tumors of striated muscle which most often diffusely infiltrate the myocardium but which may also, on occasion, form a polypoid extension into the cardiac chambers and therefore have been clinically mistaken for myxoma.[2] Rhabdomyoblasts are the histological hallmark of this tumor, and 20 to 30 per cent of the tumors have cross-striations.[4] "Strap cells," "tennis racquet cells," and "spider cells" with periodic acid-Schiff-positive cytoplasm may be seen.

FIBROSARCOMAS. Fibrosarcomas of the heart resemble the soft, whitish "fish flesh" characteristic of this tumor type elsewhere in the body. They may contain areas of hemorrhage and necrosis and extensively infiltrate the heart, often involving more than one cardiac chamber. A thrombus may form in an obstructed pulmonary vein or the vena cava or over the mural surface of the tumor.[3]

LYMPHOSARCOMAS. Although cardiac involvement of systemic lymphoma has been reported in 25 to 36 per cent of cases, primary lymphosarcoma involving only the heart or pericardium appears to be much less common.[146] Myocardial infiltration by lymphoma may be nodular or diffuse, and the clinical syndrome of hypertrophic cardiomyopathy has been mimicked.[147]

PULMONARY ARTERY SARCOMAS. Sarcomas of the pulmonary artery trunk, main branches, or pulmonic valve may present as tumor emboli to the lungs or as right ventricular outflow obstruction.[148, 149] These tumors may originate from undifferentiated tissue of the bulbis cordis, usually present after the fourth decade, and show a 2:1 female predominance.[149] Typical symptoms include dyspnea, chest pain, cough, and hemoptysis and may be associated with radiographic findings of a pulmonary hilar mass or cardiomegaly. Right ventricular injection of contrast material helps to delineate the tumor. Although most reported cases were diagnosed post mortem, it is likely that early diagnosis, surgical resection, and possibly chemotherapy may have an impact on survival of patients with this tumor.[149]

DIAGNOSTIC TECHNIQUES

Although certain clinical manifestations may be suggestive of a cardiac tumor, no clinical finding or set of findings is pathognomonic. Furthermore, the majority of cardiac tumors produce signs and symptoms typical of the common forms of heart disease. The development of modern diagnostic methods has had a major impact on the diagnosis and hence the natural history of cardiac tumors. Whereas only 20 years ago the diagnosis of a cardiac tumor was rarely made antemortem, it is now not unusual for cardiac tumors to be diagnosed and cured in patients who are totally asymptomatic or without signs of cardiovascular disease.[150] Although cardiac catheterization made possible the definitive preoperative diagnosis of cardiac tumors, it was not until the advent of echocardiography that it was feasible to evaluate all patients suspected of this diagnosis. Both M-mode and two-dimensional echocardiography are effective screening techniques. However, two-dimensional echocardiography is more sensitive and provides considerably more information regarding the site of tumor attachment, pattern of tumor movement, and size. In many centers, the information provided by two-dimensional echocardiography (p. 129), computed tomography (CT) (p. 365), or magnetic resonance imaging (MRI) (p. 374) is considered sufficient to proceed directly to surgery without cardiac catheterization and angiography. M-mode echocardiography alone does not provide adequate information in the majority of cases to proceed to surgery. Catheterization and angiography should not be omitted in the absence of a technically adequate two-dimensional echocardiographic study, CT, or MRI that have visualized all four cardiac chambers.

It is imperative that noninvasive evaluation, preferably by two-dimensional echocardiography (or CT or MRI), be performed whenever cardiac catheterization is planned and the diagnosis of cardiac tumor is considered. Thus, when left atrial myxoma is suspected, it is safest to visualize the left atrium by injecting the contrast agent into the pulmonary artery and filming during the levophase. It is particularly important to avoid the transseptal approach, since this risks dislodgement of fragments of tumor that may be attached in the region of the fossa ovalis. Furthermore, since cardiac tumors may be multiple and present in more than one chamber, all four chambers should be visualized noninvasively prior to cardiac catheterization whenever possible. Because the diagnosis of cardiac tumor may be missed at cardiac catheterization, it has been suggested that echocardiography be performed routinely before cardiac catheterization, particularly in patients with the clinical diagnosis of mitral stenosis.

RADIOLOGICAL EXAMINATION

Cardiac tumors may display several findings on plain chest roentgenograms. These include alterations in cardiac contour, changes in overall cardiac size, specific chamber enlargement, alterations in pulmonary vascularity, and intracardiac calcification.[151, 152] The cardiac contour may be normal, may display generalized or specific chamber enlargement that mimics virtually any type of valvular heart disease, or may demonstrate a bizarre appearance. Pericardial effusions are rather common and generally indicate invasion of the pericardial space by a malignant tumor. Mediastinal widening, due to hilar and paramediastinal adenopathy, may indicate spread of a malignant cardiac tumor.[151] A bumpy, irregular, or fuzzy cardiac border may be seen when the pericardium is involved. Cardiac enlargement may reflect rapid tumor growth, particularly in the case of sarcomas, whereas specific chamber enlargement is frequently due to intracavitary obstruction, particularly by pedunculated tumors such as myxomas. Thus, left atrial myxoma may produce the radiological pattern characteristic of mitral stenosis. Occasionally a large tumor mass displaces the heart and may simulate enlargement of a specific chamber.

Calcification visible by roentgenographic methods may occur with several types of cardiac tumor, including rhabdomyomas, fibromas, hamartomas, teratomas, myxomas, and angiomas.[152] Visualization of intracardiac calcium in an infant or a child is unusual and should immediately raise the question of an intracardiac tumor. Cardiac fluoroscopy and laminography may be helpful in differentiating calcification of cardiac tumor from that of other structures, such as cardiac valves, coronary arteries, pericardium, and mural thrombus. Occasionally, calcified atrial polypoid tumors may be seen to prolapse into the ventricle during diastole.[153] Fluoroscopy is also useful in differentiating cardiac tumor from ventricular aneurysm, both of which may result in a localized protrusion on plain chest roentgenograms. However, on fluoroscopic examination, cardiac tumors do not display the paradoxical motion during ventricular contraction that is characteristic of ventricular aneurysm.

NONINVASIVE METHODS

ECHOCARDIOGRAPHY

M-Mode Echocardiography. This technique has been extensively used in the diagnosis and evaluation of cardiac tumors. This technique is most useful for recognizing pedunculated tumors of the left atrium, primarily left atrial myxomas, and is generally less sensitive for the detection of intramural and sessile tumors.

Left atrial tumors are often pedunculated myxomas that traverse the mitral valve during diastole. Thus, during diastole when the tumor extends into the AV canal, a mass of echoes is visualized behind the anterior leaflet of the mitral valve (Fig. 43–1). During systole, the mitral valve is closed, the tumor is confined to the left atrium, and therefore the mass of echoes is no longer seen in the AV canal. Posterior descent of the anterior mitral leaflet may also be slow as a result of mechanical interference by the tumor. In some cases the tumor is less mobile and therefore may not traverse the mitral orifice; it may be detected only if the left atrium is carefully imaged from several different angles.[154] It has been suggested that to diagnose left atrial tumors reliably the ultrasound beam should be directed in turn (1) through both leaflets of the mitral valve, (2) through the aorta and left atrium, (3) in an intermediate direction through the anterior mitral leaflet and left atrium, and (4) caudally, with a suprasternal transducer position.[154]

Right atrial tumors (p. 1472) generally appear as echoes behind the tricuspid valve, prolapsing into the right ventricle during diastole.[55, 67] Because myxomas frequently occur biatrially, it is vital that when the diagnosis of myxoma is suspected the echocardiographic examination be thorough and include both atria.

Ventricular tumors are less frequently diagnosed by M-mode echocardiography.[84, 155] Left ventricular tumors may be visualized as a mass of echoes interposed between the interventricular septum and the anterior leaflet of the mitral valve, and are present during both systole and diastole. Large left ventricular tumors may cause apparent filling of the left ventricular cavity by an echo-dense mass. *Right ventricular tumors* may be visualized as intracavitary echoes in the right ventricle and, in addition, may result in a paradoxical square wave motion of the interventricular septum.[73, 156] Although reverberations produced by a right ventricular mass may be imaged in a position posterior to the tricuspid valve, the right atrial cavity is free of echoes in such cases.[156]

Two-Dimensional Echocardiography (See Fig. 5–108, p. 130). This technique provides substantial advantages over conventional M-mode echocardiography for the diagnosis and preoperative evaluation of intracardiac tumors.[19, 157–159] In the majority of cases of cardiac tumors, the information provided by two-dimensional echocardiography provides adequate information regarding tumor size, attachment, and mobility to allow operative resection without preoperative angiography. This technique is sensitive for detection of small tumors and is especially useful for detection of left ventricular tumors and tumors that do not prolapse through the mitral or tricuspid valve orifices.

According to a recently proposed echocardiographic classification system for left atrial myxomas, Class I tumors are small and prolapse through the mitral valve; Class II tumors are small and nonprolapsing; Class III tumors are large and prolapse; and Class IV tumors are large and nonprolapsing.[160] The increased sensitivity of two-dimensional echocardiography makes possible the diagnosis of cardiac tumors in neonates and in utero.[161] The improved diagnostic power and widespread use of two-dimensional echocardiography have resulted in an increase in the detection of primary cardiac tumors, in many cases prior to the onset of clinical signs or symptoms.

Two-dimensional echocardiography may facilitate the differentiation between left atrial thrombus and myxoma, because the former typically produces a layered appearance and is generally situated in the posterior portion of the atrium, whereas the latter is often mottled in appearance and rarely occurs in the posterior portion of the atrium. In some atrial myxomas, areas of echolucency may be seen within the tumor mass, corresponding to areas of hemorrhage within the tumor. Since these areas of echolucency are not found in thrombotic or infective lesions, this finding may be of value in the differential diagnosis of an intraatrial mass. Continuous-mode Doppler ultrasonography may be useful for evaluating the hemodynamic consequences of valvular obstruction or incompetence caused by cardiac tumors.[162]

RADIONUCLIDE IMAGING. Gated blood pool scanning has been used to identify atrial, ventricular, and intramural tumors.[20, 21] Radionuclide ventriculography generally has a lower rate of resolution than does echocardiography or contrast injection angiography and therefore may be less sensitive for the detection of small filling defects. However, radionuclide ventriculography may provide clear visualization of filling defects in some cases when other methods are nondiagnostic, particularly in the case of ventricular or intramural tumors. In some cases, gated blood pool scanning may provide more detailed information regarding myocardial geometry and tumor size and location than that obtained by echocardiography.[20] Mobile left atrial tumors may be seen to prolapse into the left ventricle during diastole.[20] Thus, gated blood pool scanning may, in some cases, provide information complementary to that obtained by echocardiography. In some cases in which the cardiac tumor was not evident by routine static or dynamic radionuclide imaging, it has been possible to delineate the tumor and its movement during a cardiac cycle by use of a computer-generated composite functional image.[21]

COMPUTED TOMOGRAPHY. Computed tomography of the heart has been used to demonstrate cardiac tumors[23–27] (Figs. 43–4, and 12–13, p. 365). Although more experience will be necessary to establish its role, certain advantages are already apparent. These include a high degree of tissue discrimination, which may allow definition of the degree of intramural tumor extension; evaluation of the extracardiac structures; and the ability to construct images in any plane. Resolution appears to be improved substantially by gating the computed tomographic acquisition to

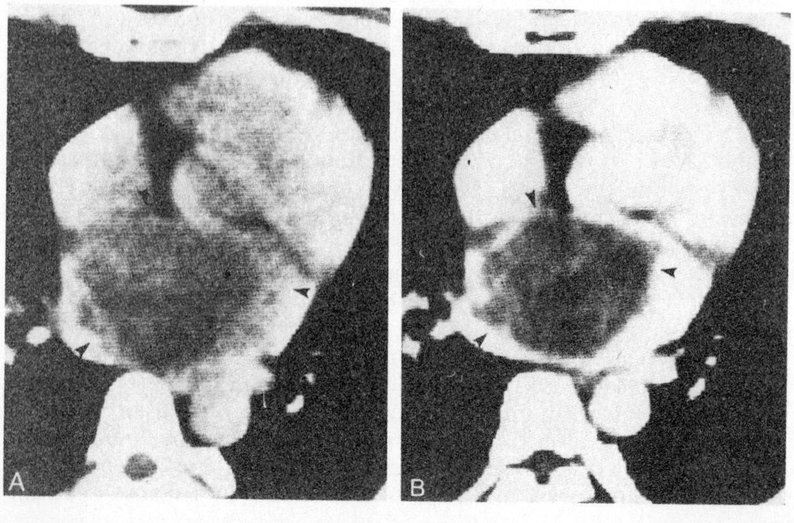

FIGURE 43–4. Demonstration of a left atrial myxoma by computed tomography. The tumor is seen as a smooth mass in the left atrium (arrows). *A*, Precontrast; *B*, Postcontrast. (From Tsuchiya, F., et al.: CT findings of atrial myxoma. Radiology *151*:139, 1984.)

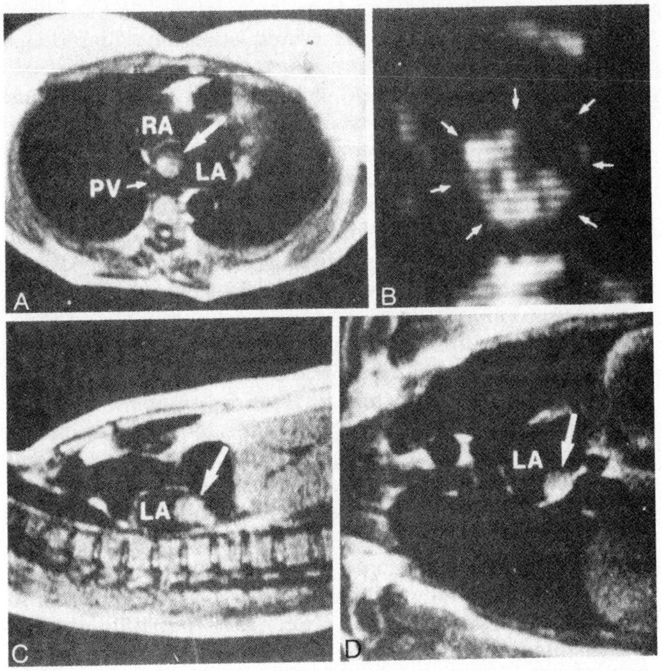

FIGURE 43–5. The appearance of a large left atrial myxoma by magnetic resonance imaging. Imaging was gated to the electrocardiogram and was performed at end systole. Images were acquired in the transverse (*A, B*), sagittal (*C*), and coronal (*D*) planes. (From Pflugfelder, P. W., et al.: Detection of atrial myxoma by magnetic resonance imaging. Am. J. Cardiol. *55*:42, 1985.)

the cardiac cycle.[27] At present CT appears to be most useful in the evaluation of suspected tumors of the heart to determine the degree of myocardial invasion and the involvement of pericardial and extracardiac structures.

MAGNETIC RESONANCE IMAGING MRI may be of considerable value in the detection and delineation of cardiac tumors[28–31] and in some cases may depict the size, shape, and surface characteristics of the tumor more clearly than two-dimensional echocardiography.[28, 30] The larger field of view with MRI (Figs. 43–5, 12–34, and 12–35, p. 374) provides better definition of tumor prolapse, secondary valve obstruction, and cardiac chamber size than does two-dimensional echocardiography.

OTHER NONINVASIVE METHODS. Cardiac tumors cannot be diagnosed by phonocardiography, apexcardiography, or jugular venous or carotid pulse analysis. However, when valvular or myocardial disease is suspected on clinical grounds, certain atypical findings may raise the question of cardiac tumor. The intensity of the systolic or diastolic murmur caused by a left atrial myxoma is often exquisitely sensitive to positional change, a finding atypical of valvular heart disease. S_1 may be delayed as a consequence of an elevated left atrial pressure, as in mitral stenosis (p. 44). It is often intense and widely split, and an early systolic sound may occur, representing tumor movement toward the atrium during systole.[163] In addition, a tumor "plop" may be present about 100 msec after S_2, which appears to result from the sudden tension of the tumor stalk as it prolapses into the left ventricle during diastole or from the tumor striking the myocardium[64] (Figs. 43–1 and 3–15, p. 51). The tumor plop *precedes* the end of the rapid filling wave of the apexcardiogram and can thereby be differentiated from an S_3; as noted, it usually occurs later than an opening snap. Systolic time intervals are usually consistent with a reduced stroke volume (p. 54). Apexcardiography often shows a deep notch on the upstroke which occurs at the time of extrusion of the tumor through the mitral valve in early systole.

Right atrial tumors may also result in a widely split S_1 and an early systolic sound. The S_2 may be paradoxically split as a result of early pulmonic valve closure.[164] A tumor plop and systolic and diastolic murmurs which are increased by inspiration may also occur with right atrial tumors.[163] The jugular venous pulse tracing may reflect obstruction of the tricuspid orifice, demonstrating an accentuated *a* wave, attenuation of the *x* descent, or an early, broad *v* wave.[163]

ANGIOGRAPHY

Cardiac catheterization and selective angiocardiography are not necessary in all cases of cardiac tumors, since, as discussed above, in many cases adequate preoperative information may be obtained by echocardiography, CT, or MRI. However, several circumstances exist in which the risk and expense of cardiac catheterization are outweighed by the supplemental information it may provide. These situations include cases in which (1) noninvasive evaluation has not been fully adequate in defining tumor location or attachment; (2) all four cardiac chambers have not been adequately visualized noninvasively; (3) a malignant cardiac tumor is considered likely; or (4) other cardiac lesions may coexist with a cardiac tumor and possibly dictate a different surgical approach. For instance, when a malignant cardiac tumor is suspected, cardiac angiography may provide valuable information regarding the degree of myocardial, vascular, and/or pericardial invasion. Likewise, in certain cases, such as the presence of pulmonary hypertension or the coexistence of significant valvular or coronary artery lesions, cardiac catheterization and angiography may provide information that significantly affects the surgical approach.

The major angiographic findings in patients with cardiac tumors include (1) compression or displacement of cardiac chambers or large vessels, (2) deformity of cardiac chambers, (3) intracavitary filling defects, (4) marked variations in myocardial thickness, (5) pericardial effusion, and (6) local alterations in wall motion.[151, 152] Displacement of the cardiac chambers or the great vessels without deformation of the internal contour may be observed in both benign and malignant tumors, whereas deformation of a cardiac chamber usually indicates an infiltrating malignant lesion.[152] The most frequent angiographic findings are intracavitary filling defects, which may be either fixed or mobile. Fixed defects may be lobulated or appear as a coarse nodularity of the myocardium often difficult to distinguish from a mural thrombus. Such defects may reflect endocardial tumors with broad attachments or intramural tumors with intracavitary extension. Mobile intracavitary defects are usually pedunculated tumors, typically myxomas, although the stalk may be difficult to visualize. Such tumors may prolapse into the AV valve orifice during diastole or, in the case of ventricular tumors, into the left ventricular outflow tract during systole. An atrial ball thrombus may mimic a pedunculated tumor, but is more likely to be associated with clot in the atrial appendage.

A localized increase in myocardial wall thickness, especially when accompanied by a pericardial effusion, suggests an infiltrating malignant tumor. It is often difficult to differentiate myocardial thickening from pericardial effusion, but this may be aided by observation of the thickness of the right atrial wall. Since the right atrial wall is seldom infiltrated by tumor, the finding of right atrial thickening to greater than 5 mm suggests a pericardial effusion.[152] In myocardial infiltration, localized areas of disordered wall motion may also be noted by cineangiography. Coronary arteriography may in some cases allow visualization of the vascular supply of the tumor, thus demarcating the extent of tumor invasion, the source of its blood supply, and its relation to the coronary arteries.[165, 166] However, the vascular pattern of cardiac tumors has not proved to be a useful sign of malignancy.[152]

False-negative angiographic studies generally occur when the diagnosis is not suspected prior to catheterization. False-positive studies are most often the result of thrombus, but may also be produced by many entities,

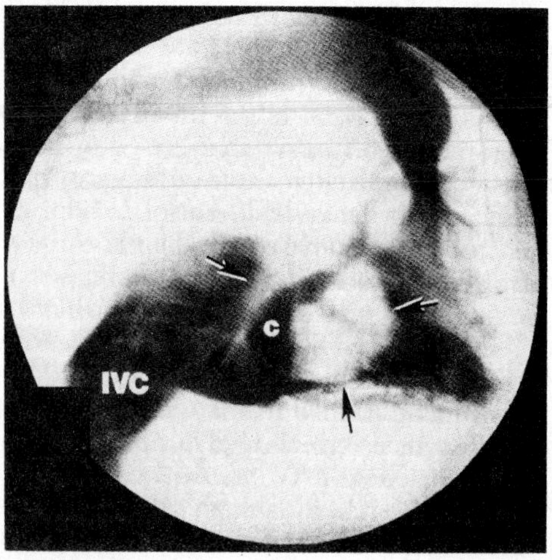

FIGURE 43–6. Demonstration of a hemangiosarcoma of the right atrium by digital subtraction angiography. Contrast medium (20 cc) was injected into the right atrium. (From Gilbreath, P., et al.: Demonstration of intracardiac neoplasm by digital subtraction angiography. Noninvasive Medical Imaging *1*:205, 1984.)

such as streaming of nonopaque venous blood, a hematoma in the atrial septum, an aneurysm of the muscular or membranous ventricular septum, Bernheim syndrome, congenital septal dysplasia, and hydatid cysts of the interventricular septum.[152, 167]

The major risk of angiography is peripheral embolization due to dislodgement of a fragment of tumor or of an associated thrombus.[152, 168] Therefore, the thorough evaluation of all cardiac chambers by *noninvasive* methods prior to catheterization is to be recommended in patients suspected of having cardiac tumors so that contrast material can be injected into the chamber proximal (upstream) to the location of the tumor. The transseptal approach to the left atrium (p. 246) is particularly hazardous because of the frequent occurrence of left atrial myxomas in the region of the fossa ovalis.

Growing experience with digital subtraction angiography (p. 356) indicates that it can provide important diagnostic information in patients with atrial or ventricular tumors having intracavitary projections (Fig. 43–6). The ability to image intracavitary structures during injection of contrast material from a remote site eliminates the risk of catheter-induced tumor embolization and may play an important role in the diagnosis and characterization of a cardiac tumor, particularly in patients in whom echocardiography is not technically satisfactory.

TREATMENT AND PROGNOSIS

BENIGN TUMORS

Operative excision is the treatment of choice for most benign cardiac tumors and in many cases results in a complete cure.[12, 15, 169] Although many tumors are histologically benign, all cardiac tumors are potentially lethal as a result of intracavitary or valvular obstruction, peripheral embolization, and disturbances of rhythm or conduction. Unfortunately, it is not unusual for patients to die or experience a major complication while awaiting operation, and therefore it is mandatory to carry out the operation promptly after the diagnosis has been established.[170]

Although some epicardial tumors may be removed without the aid of extracorporeal circulation, most intramural and intracavitary tumors must be excised under direct vision, with use of the heart-lung machine. Closed approaches, although occasionally used in the past, are not now recommended because of increased risk of dislodging tumor fragments. In addition, excision cannot be as complete, and adequate inspection of the other cardiac chambers for additional tumors is not possible.

The dislodgement of tumor fragments constitutes a major risk of operation and may result in peripheral emboli or the dispersion of micrometastases, which may seed peripherally. To reduce this risk, manipulation of the heart prior to cardiopulmonary bypass should be minimized. Some surgeons recommend that venous cannulation for cardiopulmonary bypass be performed via the femoral or azygous vein rather than through the right atrium to avoid dislodging an unsuspected right atrial tumor.[168] In addition, the tumor should be removed en bloc when possible, and the chamber then irrigated well with saline.

ATRIAL MYXOMAS. Numerous reports document complete cure of left and right atrial myxomas with follow-up periods of 10 to 15 years.[13–16, 170, 171] In about 1 to 5 per cent of cases a recurrence or second cardiac myxoma has been reported following resection of the initial myxoma.[80, 172] Possible causes of the second tumor include incomplete excision of the original tumor with regrowth, growth from a second "pretumorous" focus, i.e., metasynchronous, or intracardiac implantation from the original tumor. Because of the first two possibilities, some surgeons have advocated excision of the entire region of the fossa ovalis and repair of the resultant atrial septal defect to remove presumably high concentrations of "pretumor" cells thought to be located in that region. Other surgeons have reported equally successful long-term recurrence-free periods with simple excision of the tumor and a small rim at the base.[13–15, 80] It now appears that in approximately 7 per cent of patients with (1) a familial history of cardiac myxoma, (2) features of the complex of lentigines and other abnormalities described on p. 1474, or (3) synchronous tumor appearance (i.e., multiple tumors at the time of presentation), the incidence of a second tumor occurring at some time in the future is in the range of 12 to 22 per cent, as compared to approximately 1 per cent for patients with sporadic atrial myxoma.[80] It is believed that tumor recurrence in these cases is from a second pretumorous focus of cells. In these high-risk patients, a careful search for multiple tumors preoperatively and more extensive resection of the underlying endocardium, atrial septum, or both is recommended. Careful echocardiographic follow-up for detection of metasynchronous tumors is recommended[80] in all patients following resection of a myxoma. Regardless of the extent of tumor resection performed, such patients should receive periodic long-term follow-up by cross-sectional echocardiography.

OTHER BENIGN TUMORS. Although the majority of operations for cardiac tumors have been performed for atrial myxomas owing to their high frequency, successful excision has also been reported for ventricular myxomas, as well as most other types of benign cardiac tumor, including rhabdomyoma, hamartoma, fibroma, lipoma, hemangioma, and papillary fibroelastoma.[60, 117, 119, 129, 173–178] The major surgical considerations in excision of ventricular tumors include preservation of adequate ventricular myocardium, maintenance of proper atrioventricular valve function, and preservation of as much of the conduction system as possible. Often, however, papillary muscles, chordae tendineae, or the AV conduction system must be sacrificed during the resection of a tumor, thereby necessitating replacement of the atrioventricular valve, implantation of a pacemaker, or both.

MALIGNANT TUMORS

Operation is not an effective treatment for the great majority of primary malignant tumors of the heart because of the large mass of cardiac tissue involved or the presence of metastases. The major role for surgery in such cases is to establish a diagnosis in order to exclude the possibility of a curable benign tumor. Nevertheless, in some cases palliation of hemodynamics and/or constitutional symptoms and extension of life may be achieved by aggressive therapy. Survivals of from 1 to 3 years have been reported following partial resection, chemotherapy, radiation therapy, or various combinations of these modalities.[77, 145, 179–182] In some instances, localized recurrences have been eliminated by multiple operations. Some success in palliation of symptoms has been reported following the combination of chemotherapy and radiation therapy[182] and radiation therapy alone.[183] Lymphosarcoma of the heart frequently responds to chemotherapy, radiation therapy, or both.[184, 185] Unfortunately, many other reports indicate a failure to alter the course of cardiac sarcomas despite various combinations of surgery, chemotherapy, and radiation therapy.

REFERENCES

HISTORICAL PERSPECTIVE

1. Straus, R., and Merliss, R.: Primary tumors of the heart. Arch. Pathol. *39*:74, 1945.
2. Fine, G.: Neoplasms of the pericardium and heart. *In* Gould, S. E. (ed.): Pathology of the Heart and Blood Vessels. Springfield, Ill., Charles C Thomas, 1968, p. 851.
3. Heath, D.: Pathology of cardiac tumors. Am. J. Cardiol. *21*:315, 1968.
4. Lammers, R. J., and Bloor, C. M.: Pathology of cardiac tumors. *In* Kapoor, A. S. (ed.): Cancer of the Heart. New York, Springer-Verlag, 1986, p. 1.
5. Urba, W. J., and Longo, D. L.: Primary solid tumors of the heart. *In* Kapoor, A. S. (ed.): Cancer of the Heart. New York, Springer-Verlag, 1986, p. 62.
6. Smith, C.: Tumors of the heart. Arch. Pathol. Lab. Med. *110*:1, 1986.
7. Mahaim, I.: Les Tumeurs et les Polypes de Coeur: Étude Anatomo-Cliniqué. Paris, Masson, 1945.
8. Barnes, A. R., Beaver, D. C., and Snell, A. M.: Primary sarcoma of the heart: Report of a case with E. C. G. and pathological studies. Am. Heart J. 9:480, 1934.
9. Goldberg, H. P., Glenn, F., Dotter, C. T., and Steinberg, I.: Myxoma of the left atrium. Diagnosis made during life with operative and postmortem findings. Circulation *6*:762, 1952.
10. Beck, C. S.: An intrapericardial teratoma and a tumor of the heart: Both removed operatively. Ann. Surg. *116*:161, 1942.
11. Crafoord, C. L.: Case report. *In* Lam, C. R. (eds.): Proceedings. International Symposium on Cardiovascular Surgery. Philadelphia, W. B. Saunders Company, 1955, p. 202.
12. Eckstein, R., Gossner, W., and Rienmuller, R.: Primary malignant fibrous histiocytoma of the left atrium. Surgical and chemotherapeutic management. Br. Heart J. 52:354, 1984.
13. Reece, I. J., Cooley, D. A., Frazier, O. H., Hallman, G. L., Powers, P. L., and Montero, C. G.: Cardiac tumors. Clinical spectrum and prognosis of lesions other than classical benign myxoma in 20 patients. J. Thorac. Cardiovasc. Surg. 88:439, 1984.
14. Hanson, E. C., Gill, C. C., Razavi, M., and Loop, F. D.: The surgical treatment of atrial myxomas. Clinical experience and late results in 33 patients. J. Thorac. Cardiovasc. Surg. *89*:298, 1985.
15. Guiloff, A. K., Flege, J. B., Callard, G. M., Dunn, E. J., Wilson, J. M., and Wright, C. B.: Surgery of left atrial myxomas. Report of eleven cases and review of literature. J. Cardiovasc. Surg. 27:194, 1986.
16. Cooley, D. A.: Surgical management of cardiac tumor. *In* Kapoor, A. S. (ed.): Cancer of the Heart. New York, Springer-Verlag, 1986, p. 126.
17. Effert, S., and Domanig, E.: The diagnosis of intra-atrial tumor and thrombi by the ultrasonic echo method. Ger. Med. Mon. *4*:1, 1959.
18. Come, P. C., Kurland, G. S., and Vine, H. S.: Two dimensional echocardiography in differentiating right atrial and tricuspid valve mass lesions. Am. J. Cardiol. *44*:1207, 1979.
19. Fyke, F. E., Seqard, J. B., Edwards, W. D., Miller, F.A., Reeder, G. S., Schattenberg, T. T., Schub, C., and Tajik, A. J.: Primary cardiac tumors: Experience with 30 consecutive patients since the introduction of two-dimensional echocardiography. J. Am. Coll. Cardiol. 5:1465, 1985.
20. Pohost, G. M., Pastore, J. O., McKusick, K. A., Chiotellis, P. N., Kapeliakis, G. Z., Myers, G. S., Dinsmore, R. E., and Block, P. C.: Detection of left atrial myxoma by gated radionuclide cardiac imaging. Circulation 55:88, 1977.
21. Bough, E., Bodem, W., Gandsman, E., Benham, I., McEnany, M., and Shulman, R.: Radionuclide diagnosis of left atrial myxoma with computer-generated functional images. Am. J. Cardiol. 52:1365, 1986.
22. Tamari, I., Goldberg, H. L., Moses, J. W., Fisher, J., and Borer, J. S.: Left atrial myxoma: Diagnosis by digital substraction intravenous angiography. Cathet. Cardiovasc. Diagn. *12*:26, 1986.
23. Huggins, T. J., Huggins, M. J., Schnapf, D. J., Brott, W. H., Sinnott, R. C., and Shawl, F. A.: Left atrial myxoma: Computed tomography as a diagnostic modality. J. Comput. Assist. Tomogr. *4*:253, 1980.
24. Godwin, J. D., Axel, L., Adams, J. R., Schiller, N. B., Simpson, P. C., Jr., and Gertz, E. W.: Computed tomography: A new method for diagnosing tumor of the heart. Circulation *63*:448, 1981.
25. Kawai, N., Sotobata, I., Iwase, M., Shiki, K., Yokota, M., Kondo, K., Iwamura, N., and Tsuchida, T.: Evaluation of left atrial myxoma with transmission computed tomography. Am. Heart J. *109*:1116, 1985.
26. Cornalba, G., and Dore, R.: Cardiac tumor associated with tuberous sclerosis. CT Diagnosis. Comput. Assist. Tomogr. 9:809, 1985.
27. Jack, C. M., Cleland, J., and Geddes, J. S.: Left atrial rhabdomyosarcoma and the use of digital gated computed tomography in its diagnosis. Br. Heart J. 55:305, 1986.
28. Amparo, E. G., Higgins, C. B., Farmer, D., Gamsu, G, and McNamara, M.: Gated MRI of cardiac and paracardiac masses: Initial experience. A. J. R. *143*:1151, 1984.
29. Pizzarello, R. A., Goldberg, S. M., Goldman, M. A., Gottesman, R., Fetten, J. V., Brown, N., Kahn, E. I., and Stein, H. L.: Tumor of the heart diagnosed by magnetic resonance imaging. J. Am. Coll. Cardiol. *5*:989, 1985.
30. Go, R. T., O'Donnell, J. K., Underwood, D. A., Feiglin, D. H., Salcedo, E. E., Pantoja, M., MacIntyre, W. J., and Meaney, T. F.: Comparison of gated cardiac MRI and 2D echocardiography of intracardiac neoplasms. A. J. R. *145*:21, 1985.
31. Levine, R. A., Weyman, A. E., Dinsmore, R. E., Southern, J., Rosen, B. R., Guyer, D. E., Brady, T. J., and Okada, R. D.: Noninvasive tissue characterization: Diagnosis of lipomatous hypertrophy of the atrial septum by nuclear magnetic resonance imaging. J. Am. Col. Cardiol. 7:688, 1986.

CLINICAL PRESENTATION

32. Goodwin, J. F.: Symposium on cardiac tumors. The spectrum of cardiac tumors. Am. J. Cardiol. *21*:307, 1968.
33. MacGregor, G. A., and Cullen, R. A.: The syndrome of fever, anaemia and high sedimentation rate with an atrial myxoma. Br. Med. J. *5*:158, 1959.
34. Huston, K. A., Combs, J. J., Lie, J. T., and Guiliani, E. R.: Left atrial myxoma simulating peripheral vasculitis. Mayo Clin. Proc. *53*:752, 1978.
35. Levinson, J. P., and Kincaid, O. W.: Myxoma of the right atrium associated with polycythemia. N. Engl. J. Med. *264*:1187, 1961.
36. Vuopio, P., and Nikkila, E. A.: Hemolytic anemia and thrombocytopenia in a case of left atrial myxoma associated with mitral stenosis. Am. J. Cardiol. *17*:585, 1966.
37. Boss, J. H., and Bechar, M.: Myxoma of the heart. Report based on four cases. Am. J. Cardiol. 3:823, 1959.
38. Curry, H. L. F., Mathews, J. A., and Robinson, J.: Right atrial myxoma mimicking a rheumatic disorder. Br. Med. J. *1*:542, 1967.
39. Graham, S. L., and Sellers, A. L.: Atrial myxoma with multiple myeloma. Arch. Intern. Med. *139*:116, 1979.
40. Kaminsky, M. E., Ehlers, K. H., Engle, M. A., Klein, A. A., Levin, A. R., and Subramanian, V. A.: Atrial myxoma mimicking a collagen disorder. Chest 75:93, 1979.
41. Rajpal, R. S., Leibsohn, J. A., Liekweg, W. G., Gross, C. M., Olinger, G. N., Rose, H. D., and Bamrah, V. S.: Infected left atrial myxoma with bacteremia simulating infective endocarditis. Arch. Intern. Med. *139*:1176, 1979.
42. Leonhardt, E. T. G., and Kullenberg, K. P. G.: Bilateral atrial myxomas with multiple arterial aneurysms—A syndrome minimicking polyarteritis nodosa. Am. J. Med. *62*:792, 1977.
43. Byrd, W. E., Matthews, O. P., and Hunt, R. E.: Left atrial myxoma presenting as a systemic vasculitis. Arthritis Rheum. *23*:240, 1980.
44. Quinn, T. J., Condini, M. A., and Harris, A. A.: Infected cardiac myxoma. Am. J. Cardiol. 53:381, 1984.
45. Transden, T. M., Prichard, J. G., and Storz, S. O.: *Streptococcus viridans* bacteremia associated with atrial myxoma. Am. Heart J. *110*:180, 1985.
46. Silverman, J., Olwin, J. S., and Graettinger, J. S.: Cardiac myxomas with systemic mobilization. Circulation *26*:99, 1962.
47. Koikkalainen, K., Kostiainen, S., and Luosto, R.: Left atrial myxoma revealed by femoral embolectomy. Scand. J. Thorac. Cardiovasc. Surg. *11*:33, 1977.
48. Yufe, R., Karpati, G., and Carpenter, S.: Cardiac myxoma: A diagnostic challenge for the neurologist. Neurology *26*:1060, 1976.
49. Schweiger, M. J., Hafer, J. G., Jr., Brown, R., and Gianelly, R. E.: Spontaneous cure of infected left atrial myxoma following embolization. Am. Heart J. 99:630, 1980.
50. Gonzalez, A., Altieri, P. I., Marquez, E., Cox, R. A., and Castillo, M.: Massive pulmonary embolism associated with a right ventricular myxoma. Am. J. Med. *69*:795, 1980.
51. Heath, D., and Mackinnon, J.: Pulmonary hypertension due to myxoma of the right atrium. With special reference to the behavior of emboli of myxoma in the lung. Am. Heart J. *68*:227, 1964.
52. Semb, B. K., Wexels, J. C., Vatne, K., and Bjornstad, P. G.: Angiographic and echocardiographic observations in surgical patients with atrial myxoma. Cardiovasc. Intervent. Radiol. 8:119, 1985.
53. Rath, S., Har-Zahav, Y., Battler, A., Argeranat, O., and Neufeld, H. N.: Coronary arterial embolus from left atrial myxoma. Am. J. Cardiol. *54*:1392, 1984.
54. Branch, C. L., Jr., Laster, D. W., and Kelley, D. L., Jr.: Left atrial myxoma with cerebral emboli. Neurosurgery *16*:675, 1985.

55. Panidis, I. P., Kotler, M. N., Mintz, G. S., and Ross, J.: Clinical and echocardiographic features of right atrial masses. Am. Heart J. *107*:745, 1984.
56. Muroff, L. R., and Johnson, P. M.: Right atrial myxoma presenting as nonresolving pulmonary emboli: Case report. J. Nucl. Med. *17*:890, 1976.
57. Harvey, W. P.: Clinical aspects of cardiac tumors. Am. J. Cardiol. *21*:328, 1968.
58. James, T. N., and Galakhov, I.: De subitaneis mortibus XXVI. Fatal electrical instability of the heart associated with benign congenital polycystic tumor of the atrioventricular node. Circulation *56*:667, 1977.
59. Nishida, K., Kamijima, G., and Nagayama, T.: Mesothelioma of the atrioventricular node. Br. Heart J. *53*:468, 1985.
60. Iwa, T., Kamata, E., Misaki, T., Ishida, K., and Okada, R.: Successful surgical ablation of reentrant ventricular tachycardia caused by myocardial fibroma. J. Thorac. Cardiovasc. Surg. *87*:469, 1984.
61. Cabin, H. S., Costello, R. M., Vasudevan, G., Mauron, B. J., and Roberts, W. C.: Cardiac lymphoma mimicking hypertrophic cardiomyopathy. Am. Heart J. *102*:466, 1981.
62. Greenwood, W. F.: Profile of atrial myxoma. Am. J. Cardiol. *21*:367, 1968.
63. Gershlick, A. H., Leech, G., Mills, P. G., and Leatham, A.: The loud first heart sound in left atrial myxoma. Br. Heart J. *52*:403, 1984.
64. Bass, N. M., and Sharratt, G. J. P.: Left atrial myxoma diagnosed by echocardiography with observations on tumor movement. Br. Heart J. *35*:1332, 1973.
65. Hansen, J. F., Lyngborg, K., Andersen, M., and Wennevoid, A.: Right atrial myxoma. Acta Med. Scand. *186*:165, 1969.
66. Goldschlager, A., Popper, R., Goldschlager, N., Gerbode, F., and Prozan, G.: Right atrial myxoma with right to left shunt and polycythemia presenting as congenital heart disease. Am. J. Cardiol. *30*:82, 1972.
67. Waxler, E. B., Kawai, N., and Kasparian, H.: Right atrial myxoma: Echocardiographic, phonocardiographic and hemodynamic signs. Am. Heart J. *82*:251, 1972.
68. Talley, R. C., Baldwin, B. J., Symbas, P. N., and Nutter, D. O.: Right atrial myxoma. Unusual presentation with cyanosis and clubbing. Am. J. Med. *48*:256, 1970.
69. Massumi, R.: Bedside diagnosis of right heart myxomas through detection of palpable tumor shocks and audible plops. Am. Heart J. *105*:303, 1983.
70. Saunerstedt, R., Varnauskas, E., Paulin, S., Linder, E, Ljunggren, H., and Werko, L.: Right atrial myxoma. Report of a case and review of the literature. Am. Heart J. *64*:243, 1962.
71. Hada, Y., Wolfe, C., Murry, C. F., and Craige, E.: Right ventricular myxoma. Case report and review of phonocardiographic and auscultatory manifestations. Am. Heart J. *100*:871, 1980.
72. Goldstein, S., and Mahoney, E. B.: Right ventricular fibrosarcoma causing pulmonic stenosis. Am. J. Cardiol. *17*:570, 1966.
73. Sasse, L., Lorentzen, D., and Alvarez, H.: Paradoxical septal motion secondary to right venticular tumor. J.A.M.A. *234*:955, 1975.
74. Mahoney, L., Schieken, R. M., and Doty, D.: Cardiac rhabdomyoma simulating pulmonic stenosis. Cathet. Cardiovasc. Diagn. *5*:385, 1979.
75. de Paiva, E. C., Maciera-Coelko, E., Amram, S. S., Duarte, C., and Coelho, E.: Intracavitary left ventricular myxoma. Am. J. Cardiol. *20*:260, 1967.
76. Hoen, A. G., and Ellis, E. J.: Intramural fibroma of the heart. Am. J. Cardiol. *17*:579, 1966.
77. Mich, R. J., Gillam, L. D., and Weyman, A. E.: Osteogenic sarcomas mimicking left atrial myxomas: Clinical and two-dimensional echocardiographic features. J. Am. Coll. Cardiol. *6*:1422, 1985.
78. Reynard, J. S., Jr., Gregoratos, G., Gordon, M. J., and Bloor, C. M.: Primary osteosarcoma of the heart. Am. Heart J. *109*:598, 1985.
79. Bulkley, B. H., and Hutchins, G. M.: Atrial myxomas: A fifty year review. Am. Heart J. *97*:639, 1979.
80. McCarthy, P. M., Piehler, J. M., Schaff, H. V., Pluth, J. R., Orszulak, T. A., Vidaillet, H. J., Jr., and Carney, J. A.: The significance of multiple, recurrent, and "complex" cardiac myxomas. Thorac. Cardiovasc. Surg. *91*:389, 1986.
80a. Vidaillet, H. J., Jr., Seward, J. B., Fyke, F. E., Su, W. P. D., and Tajik, A. J.: "Syndrome myxoma": a subset of patients with cardiac myxoma associated with pigmented skin lesions and peripheral and endocrine neoplasms. Br. Heart J. *57*:247, 1987.
81. Carney, J. A.: Differences between nonfamilial and familial cardiac myxoma. Am. J. Surg. Pathol. *9*:53, 1985.
82. Davison, E. T., Mumford, D., Zaman, Q., and Horowitz, A.: Left atrial myxoma in the elderly. Report of four patients over the age of 70 and review of the literature. J. Am. Geriatr. Soc. *34*:229, 1986.
83. Imperio, J., Summers, D., Krasnow, N., and Piccone, V. A., Jr.: The distribution pattern of biatrial myxomas. Ann. Thorac. Surg. *29*:469, 1980.
84. Morgan, D. L., Palazola, J., Reed, W., Bell, H. H., Kindred, L. H., and Beauchamp, G. D.: Left heart myxomas. Am. J. Cardiol. *40*:611, 1977.
85. Dashkoff, N., Boersma, R. B., Nanda, N. C., Gramiak, R., Anderson, M. N., and Subramanian, S.: Bilateral atrial myxomas. Echocardiographic considerations. Am. J. Med. *65*:361, 1978.
86. Gosse, P., Herpin, D., Roudaut, R., Malergue, M. C., Longy, M., Baudet, E., and Dallocchio, M.: Myxoma of the mitral valve diagnosed by echocardiography. Am. Heart J. *111*:803, 1986.
87. Powers, J. C., Falkoff, M., Heinle, R. A., Nanda, N. C., Ong, L. S., Weiner, R. S., and Barold, S. S.: Familial cardiac myxoma. Emphasis on unusual clinical manifestations. J. Thorac. Cardiovasc. Surg. *77*:782, 1979.
88. Carney, J. A., Gordon, J., Carpenter, P. C., Shenoy, B. V., and Go, L. V.: The complex of myxomas, spotty pigmentation, and endocrine overactivity. Medicine *64*:270, 1985.
89. Rhodes, A. R., Silverman, R. A., Harrist, T. J., and Perez-Atayde, A. R.: Mucocutaneous lentigines, cardiomucocutaneous myxomas, and multiple blue nevi: The "LAMB" syndrome. Am. Acad. Dermatol. *10*:72, 1984.
90. Peterson, L. L., and Serrill, W. S.: Lentiginosis associated with a left atrial myxoma. Am. Acad. Dermatol. *10*:337, 1984.
91. Vidaillet, H. J., Jr., Seward, J. B., Fyke, E., and Tajik, A. J.: Name syndrome (nevi, atrial myxoma, myxoid neurofibroma, ephelides): A new and unrecognized subset of patients with cardiac myxoma. Minn. Med. *67*:695, 1984.
92. Carney, J. A., Hruska, L. S., Beauchamp, G. D., and Gordon, H.: Dominant inheritance of the complex of myxomas, spotty pigmentation and endocrine overactivity. Mayo Clin. Proc. *61*:165, 1986.
93. Michels, V. V.: A new inherited syndrome with cardiac, cutaneous, and endocrine involvement. Mayo Clin. Proc. *61*:224, 1986.
94. Sayler, W. R., Page, D. L., and Hutchins, G. M.: The development of cardiac myxomas and papillary endocardial lesions from mural thrombus. Am. Heart J. *89*:4, 1975.
95. Ferrans, V. J., and Roberts, W. C.: Structural features of cardiac myxomas. Hum. Pathol. *4*:111, 1973.
96. Tanimura, A., Tanaka, S., Kitazono, M., and Kosuga, K: The surface lining cells of cardiac myxoma. Light, electron microscopic and immunohistochemical observation. Acta Pathol. Jpn. *35*:667, 1986.
97. Boxer, M. E.: Cardiac myxoma: An immunoperoxidase study of histogenesis. Histopathology *8*:861, 1984.
98. Landon, G., Ordonez, N. G., and Guarda, L. A.: Cardiac myxomas. An immunohistochemical study using endothelial, histiocytic, and smooth-muscle cell markers. Arch. Pathol. Lab. Med. *110*:116, 1986.
99. McComb, R. D.: Heterogeneous expression of factor VIII/von Willebrand factor by cardiac myxoma cells. Am. J. Surg. Pathol. *8*:539, 1984.
100. Powers, J. C., Falkoff, M., Heinle, R. A., Nanda, N. C., Ong, L. S., Weiner, R. S., and Barold, S. S.: Familial cardiac myxoma: Emphasis on unusual clinical manifestations. J. Thorac. Cardiovasc. Surg. *77*:782, 1979.
101. Takagi, M.: Ultrastructural and immunohistochemical characteristics of cardiac myxoma. Acta Pathol. Jpn. *34*:1099, 1984.
102. Hannah, H, Eisemann, G., Hiszcyniskyj, R., Wimsky, M., and Cohen, R.: Invasive atrial myxoma. Documentation of malignant potential of cardiac myxoma. Am. Heart J. *104*:881, 1982.
103. Chen, K. T.: Carcinosarcoma of the heart. Am. Surg. Oncol. *27*:48, 1984.
104. Seo, I. S., Warner, T. F. C. S., Colyer, R. A., and Winkler, F. R.: Metastasizing atrial myxoma. Am. J. Surg. Pathol. *4*:391, 1980.
105. Budzilovich, G., Aleksic, S., Greco, A., Fernandez, J., Harris, J., and Finegold, M.: Malignant cardiac myxoma with cerebral metastases. Surg. Neurol. *11*:461, 1979.
106. Feldman, P. S., Horvath, E., and Kovacs, K.: An ultrastructural study of seven cardiac myxomas. Cancer *40*:2216, 1977.
107. Wold, L. E., and Lie, J. T.: Scanning electron microscopy of intracardiac myxoma. Mayo Clin. Proc. *56*:198, 1981.
108. Topol, E. J., Bierm, R. O., and Reitz, B. A.: Cardiac papillary fibroelastoma and stroke. Am. J. Med. *80*:129, 1986.
109. Pomerance, A.: Papillary "tumours" of the heart valves. J. Pathol. Bacteriol. *81*:135, 1961.
110. Lichtenstein, H. L., Lee, J. C. K., and Stewart, S.: Papillary tumor of the heart: Incidental finding at surgery. Hum. Pathol. *10*:473, 1979.
111. Fenoglio, J. J., McAllister, H. A., and Ferrans,, V. J.: Cardiac rhabdomyoma: A clinicopathologic and electron microscopic study. Am. J. Cardiol. *38*:241, 1976.
112. Bruni, C., Prioleau, P. G., Ivey, H. H., and Nolan, S. P.: New fine structural features of cardiac rhabdomyoma: A case report. Cancer *46*:2068, 1980.
113. Shrivastava, S., Jacks, J. J., White, R. S., and Edwards, J. E.: Diffuse rhabdomyomatosis of the heart. Arch. Pathol. Lab. Med. *101*:78, 1977.
114. Bass, J. L., Breningstall, G. N., and Swaiman, K. F.: Echocardiographic incidence of cardiac rhabdomyoma in tuberous sclerosis. Am. J. Cardiol. *55*:137, 1985.
115. Gibbs, J. L.: The heart and tuberous sclerosis. An echocardiographic and electrocardiographic study. Br. Heart J. *54*:596, 1985.
116. Howanitz, E. P., Teske, D. W., Qualman, S. J., Finck, S., and Kilman, J. W.: Pedunculated left ventricular rhabdomyoma. Ann. Thorac. Surg. *41*:443, 1986.
117. Mair, D. D., Titus J. L., Davis, G. D., and Ritter, D. G.: Cardiac rhabdomyoma simulating mitral atresia. Chest *71*:102, 1977.
118. Van der Hauwaert, L. G.: Cardiac tumours in infancy and childhood. Br. Heart J. *33*:125, 1971.
119. Feldman, P. S., and Meyer, M. W.: Fibroelastic hamartoma (fibroma) of the heart. Cancer *38*:314, 1976.
120. Jones, K. L., Wolf, P. L., Jensen, P., Dittrich, H., Benirschke, K., and Bloor, C.: The Gorlin syndrome: A genetically determined disorder associated with cardiac tumor. Am. Heart J. *111*:1013, 1986.
121. Takahashi, K., Imamura, Y., Ochi, T., Hamada, M., Ito, T., Hiwada, K., and Kokubu, T.: Echocardiographic demonstration of an asymptomatic patient with left ventricular fibroma. Am. J. Cardiol. *53*:981, 1984.
122. deRuiz, M., Potter, J. L., Stavinoha, J., Flournoy, J. G., and Sullivan, B. M.: Real-time untrasound diagnosis of cardiac fibroma in a neonate. J. Ultrasound Med. *4*:367, 1985.
123. Moulton, A. L., Jaretzki, A., 3rd, Bowman, F. O., Jr., Silverstein, E. F., and Bregman, D.: Massive lipoma of the heart. N.Y. State J. Med. *76*:1820, 1976.
124. Reyes, L. H., Rubio, P. A., Korompai, F. L., and Guinn, G. A.: Lipoma of the heart. Int. Surg. *61*:179, 1976.
125. Prior, J. T.: Lipomatous hypertrophy of cardiac interatrial septum. Arch. Pathol. *78*:11, 1964.
126. Hutter, A. M., Jr., and Page, D. L.: Atrial arrhythmias and lipomatous hypertrophy of the cardiac interatrial septum. Am. Heart J. *82*:16, 1971.
127. Simons, M., Cabin, H. S., and Jaffer, C. C.: Lipomatous hypertrophy of the

atrial septum: Diagnosis by combined echocardiography and computerized tomography. Am. J. Cardiol. 54:465, 1984.

128. Tabry, I. F., Nasser, V. H., Rizk, G., Touma, A., and Dagher, I. K.: Cavernous hemangioma of the heart: Case report and review of the literature. J. Thorac. Cardiovasc. Surg. 69:415, 1975.

MALIGNANT CARDIAC TUMORS

129. Grant, R. T., and Camp, P. D.: A case of complete heart block due to an arterial angioma. Heart 16:137, 1933.
130. Cox, J. N., Friedli, B., Mechmeche, M., Ismail, M. B., Oberhaensli, I., and Faidutti, B.: Teratoma of the heart. Virchows Arch. (A) 402:163, 1983.
131. Duray, P. H., Mark, E. J., Barwick, K. W., Madri, J. A., and Strom, R. L.: Congenital polycystic tumor of the atrioventricular node. Arch. Pathol. Lab. Med. 109:30, 1985.
132. Linder, J., Shelburne, J. D., Sorge, J. P., Whalen, R. E., and Hackel, D. B.: Congenital endodermal heterotopia of the atrioventricular node: Evidence for the endodermal origin of so-called mesotheliomas of the atrioventricular node. Hum. Pathol. 15:1093, 1984.
133. David, T. E., Lenkei, S. C., Marquez-Julio, A., Goldberg, J. A., and Meldrum, D. A.: Pheochromocytoma of the heart. Ann. Thorac. Surg. 41:98, 1986.
134. Awoke, S., and Perlstein, R. S.: Dopamine- and norepinephrine-secreting intrapericardial pheochromocytoma in a normotensive patient. South. Med. J. 78:994, 1985.
135. Hodgson, S. F., Sheps, S. G., Subramanian, R., Lie, J. T., and Carney, J. A.: Catecholamine-secreting paraganglioma of the interatrial septum. Am. J. Med. 77:157, 1984.
136. Rogers, W. M., and Keston, H. D.: A thyroid mass in the ventricular septum obstructing the right ventricular outflow tract and producing a murmur. J. Cardiovasc. Surg. 4:175, 1983.
137. Lo, H. M., Tseng, Y. Z., Tseng, C. D., Chu, S. H., Chuang, S. M., and Wu, T. L.: Intracardiac goiter: A cause of right ventricular outflow obstruction and successful operative therapy. Am. J. Cardiol. 53:976, 1984.
138. Shemin, R. J., Marsh, J. D., and Schoen, F. J.: Benign intracardiac thryoid mass causing right ventricular outflow tract obstruction. Am. J. Cardiol. 56:828, 1985.
139. Whorton, C. M.: Primary malignant tumor of the heart. Cancer 2:245, 1949.
140. Goldberg, H. P., and Steinberg, I.: Primary tumors of the heart. Circulation 11:963, 1955.
141. Glancy, L., Morales, J. B., and Roberts, W. C.: Angiosarcoma of the heart. Am. J. Cardiol. 21:413, 1968.
142. Janigan, D. T., Husain, A., and Robinson, N. A.: Cardiac angiosarcomas. A review and a case report. Cancer 57:852, 1986.
143. Rossi, N. P., Kioschos, J. M., Ascenbrener, C. A., and Ehrenhaft, J. L.: Primary angiosarcoma of the heart. Cancer 37:891, 1976.
144. Panella, J. S., Paige, M. L., Victor, T. A., Semerdjian, R. A., and Hueter, D. C.: Angiosarcoma of the heart. Diagnosis by echocardiography. Chest 76:221, 1979.
145. Yang, H.-Y., Wasielewski, J. F., Lee, E., and Paik, Y. K.: Angiosarcoma of the heart: Ultrastructural study. Cancer 47:72, 1981.
146. Roberts, W. C., Glancy, D. L., and DeVita, V. T., Jr.: Heart in malignant lymphoma. A study of 196 autopsy cases. Am. J. Cardiol. 22:85, 1968.
147. Fiester, R. F.: Reticulum cell sarcoma of the heart. Arch. Pathol. 99:80, 1975.
148. Smookler, B., Marsh, H., and Roberts, W. C.: Primary sarcoma of the pulmonary trunk and/or right left main pulmonary artery. Am. J. Med. 63:263, 1977.
149. Bleisch, N., and Kraus, F.: Polypoid sarcoma of the pulmonary trunk. Cancer 46:314, 1980.

DIAGNOSTIC TECHNIQUES

150. Oldershaw, P. J., Sutton, M. St. J., and Gibson, R. V.: Long asymptomatic period of atrial myxomas. Thorax 35:70, 1980.
151. Steiner, R. E.: Radiologic aspects of cardiac tumors. Am. J. Cardiol. 21:344, 1968.
152. Abrams, H. L., Adams, D. F., and Grant, H. A.: The radiology of tumors of the heart. Radiol. Clin. North Am. 9:299, 1971.
153. Buenger, R., Ogelsby, P., and Egbert, H.: Calcified polyp of the heart. Radiology 67:531, 1956.
154. Petsas, A. A., Gottlieb, S., Kingsley, B., Segal, B. L., and Myerburg, R. J.: Echocardiographic diagnosis of left atrial myxoma. Usefulness of suprasternal approach. Br. Heart J. 38:627, 1976.
155. Sabot, G., Fauvel, J. M., and Bounhoure, J. P.: Echocardiographic diagnosis of mobile left ventricular tumour. Br. Heart J. 42:113, 1979.
156. Nanda, N. C., Barold, S. S., Gramiak, R., Ong, L. S., and Heinle, R. A.: Echocardiographic features of right ventricular outflow tumor prolapsing into the pulmonary artery. Am. J. Cardiol. 40:272, 1977.
157. Green, S. E., Joynt, L. E., Fitzgerald, P. J., Rubenson, D. S., and Popp, R. L.: In vivo ultrasonic tissue characterization of human intracardiac masses. Am. J. Cardiol. 51:231, 1983.
158. Duncan, W. J., Rowe, R. D., Freedom, R. M., Izukawa, T., and Olley, P. M.: Space-occupying lesions of the myocardium: Role of two-dimensional echocardiography in detection of cardiac tumors in children. Am. Heart J. 104:780, 1982.
159. Abramowitz, R., Majdan, J. F., Plzak, L. F., and Berger, B. C.: Two-dimensional echocardiographic diagnosis of separate myxomas of both the left atrium and left ventricle. Am. J. Cardiol. 53:37, 1984.
160. Charuzi, Y., Bolger, A., Beeder, C., and Lew, A. S.: A new echocardiographic classification of left atrial myxoma. Am. J. Cardiol 55:614, 1985.
161. Dennis, M. A., Appareti, K., Manco-Johnson, M. L., Clewell, W., and Wiggins, J.: The echocardiographic diagnosis of multiple fetal cardiac tumors. Ultrasound Med. 4:327, 1985.
162. Panidis, I. P., Mimtz, G. S., and McAllister, M.: Hemodynamic consequences of the left atrial myxomas as assessed by Doppler ultrasound. Am. Heart J. 111:927, 1986.
163. Tavel, M. E.: Clinical Phonocardiography and External Pulse Recording. 2nd ed. Chicago, Year Book Medical Publishers, 1972, pp. 248–249.
164. Kaufmann, G., Rutishauser, W., and Hegglin, R.: Heart sounds in atrial tumors. Am. J. Cardiol. 8:350, 1961.
165. Singh, R. N., Burkholder, J. A., and Magovern, G. J.: Coronary arteriography as an aid in left atrial myxoma diagnosis. Cardiovasc. Intervent. Radiol. 7:40, 1984.
166. Weyne, A. E., Heyndrickx, G. R., Cuvelier, C. C., Afshrift, M. B., Kunnen, M. F., and Derom, F. E.: Cardiac imaging techniques in the diagnosis of angiosarcoma of the heart; report of two cases. Postgrad. Med. J. 61:271, 1985.
167. Wollenweber, G., Giuliani, E. R., Harrison, C. E., and Kincaid, O. W.: Pseudotumors of the right heart. Arch. Intern. Med. 121:169, 1968.
168. Pendyck, F., Pierce, E. C., Baron, M. G., and Lukban, S. B.: Embolization of left atrial myxoma after transseptal cardiac catheterization. Am. J. Cardiol. 30:569, 1972.

TREATMENT AND PROGNOSIS

169. Becker, R. C., Loeffler, J. S., Leopold, K. A., and Underwood, D. A.: Primary tumors of the heart: A review with emphasis on diagnosis and potential treatment modalities. Semin. Surg. Oncol. 1:161, 1985.
170. Semb, B. K.: Surgical considerations in the treatment of cardiac myxoma. J. Thorac. Cardiovasc. Surg. 87:251, 1984.
171. Marvasti, M. A., Obeid, A. I., Potts, J. L., and Parker, F. B.: Approach in the management of atrial myxoma with long-term follow-up. Ann. Thorac. Surg. 38:53, 1984.
172. Gray, I. R., and Williams, W. G.: Recurring cardiac myxoma. Br. Heart J. 53:645, 1985.
173. Parks, F. R., Adams, F., and Longmire, W. P.: Successful excision of a left ventricular hamartoma. Circulation 26:1316, 1962.
174. Etches, P. C., Gribbin, B., and Gunning, A. J.: Echocardiographic diagnosis and successful removal of cardiac fibroma in 4-year old child. Br. Heart J. 43:360, 1980.
175. Goldman, S. Lortscher, R., and Pappas, G.: Surgical treatment for rhabdomyoma of the right atrium causing arrhythmias. J. Thorac. Cardiovasc. Surg. 89:802, 1985.
176. Corno, A., deSimone, G., Catena, G., and Marcelletti, C.: Cardiac rhabdomyoma: Surgical treatment in the neonate. Thorac. Cardiovasc. Surg. 87:1984.
177. Foster, E. D., Spooner, E. W., Farina, M. A., Shaker, R. M., and Alley, R. D.: Cardiac rhabdomyoma in the neonate: Surgical treatment. Ann. Thorac. Surg. 37:249, 1984.
178. Orringer, M. B., Sisson, J. C., Glazer, G., Shapiro, B., Francis, I., Behrendt, D. M., Thompson, N. W., and Lloyd, R. V.: Surgical treatment of cardiac pheochromocytomas. J. Thorac. Cardiovasc. Surg. 89:753, 1985.
179. Marvasti, M. A., Bove, E. L., Obeid, A. I., Bowser, M. A., and Parker, F. B., Jr.: Primary osteosarcoma of left atrium: Complete surgical excision. Ann. Thorac. Surg. 40:402, 1985.
180. Sharma, S., Tendolkar, A., and Parulkar, G. B.: Angiosarcoma of the heart. Am. Heart J. 109:601, 1985.
181. Vergnon, J. M., Vincent, M., Perinetti, M., Loire, R., Cordier, J. F., and Brune, J.: Chemotherapy of metastatic primary cardiac sarcomas. Am. Heart J. 110:682, 1985.
182. Hollingworth, J. H., and Sturgill, B. C.: Treatment of primary angiosarcoma of the heart. Am. Heart J. 78:254, 1969.
183. Allaire, F. J., Grimm, C. A., Taylor, L. M., and Pfaff, J. P.: Primary hemangioendothelioma of the heart. Rocky Mt. Med. J. 61:34, 1964.
184. Terry, L. N., and Kilgerman, M. M.: Pericardial and myocardial involvement by lymphomas and leukemias. The role of radiotherapy. Cancer 25:1003, 1970.
185. Garfein, O. B.: Lymphosarcoma of the right atrium: Angiographic and hemodynamic documentation of response to chemotherapy. Arch. Intern. Med. Med. 135:325, 1975.

44 PERICARDIAL DISEASE

by BEVERLY H. LORELL, M.D., and EUGENE BRAUNWALD, M.D.

ANATOMY

The pericardium forms a strong flask-shaped sac with short tube-like extensions that enclose the origins of the aorta and its junction with the aortic arch, the pulmonary artery where it branches, the proximal pulmonary veins, and the venae cavae. Fibrous tissue of the pericardium actually blends with adventitia of the great arteries to form strong attachments. In addition, the pericardium has firm ligamentous attachments anteriorly to the sternum and xiphoid process, posteriorly to the vertebral column, and inferiorly to the diaphragm.[1,2]

The human pericardium receives its arterial blood supply from small branches of the aorta and internal mammary and musculophrenic arteries. The pericardium is innervated by the vagus, left recurrent laryngeal nerve, and esophageal plexus and also has rich sympathetic innervation from the stellate and first dorsal ganglia and the cardiac, aortic, and diaphragmatic plexuses. The phrenic nerves course over the pericardium en route to the diaphragm. The afferent nerves responsible for pain perception appear to be transmitted via the phrenic nerve entering the spinal cord at C4 to C5.[3] Recent studies suggest that peripheral sensory fibers which enter the dorsal root ganglia at C8 to T2 supply both the brachial plexus and the pericardium; this provides a possible morphological explanation for referred pericardial pain.[4]

THE TWO LAYERS OF THE PERICARDIUM. The pericardium is composed of a fibrous outer layer and an inner serous membrane that has a single layer of mesothelial cells. The inner serous layer is intimately attached to the surface of the heart and epicardial fat to form the *visceral pericardium,* and this inner serous membrane reflects back on itself to line the outer fibrous layer to form the *parietal pericardium.* The pericardium has two major serosal tunnels: the *transverse sinus,* which lies posterior to the great arteries and anterior to the atria and superior vena cava, and the *oblique sinus,* which lies posterior to the left atrium so that the posterior left atrial wall is actually separated from the pericardial space. The anatomy of these pericardial recesses is important because they may be misinterpreted as aortic dissection or mediastinal masses on computed tomographic or magnetic resonance scans.[5] The serous visceral pericardium is attached to the parietal pericardium by delicate connective tissue with elastin fibers. The parietal pericardium is composed of collagen fibers interlaced with extensive elastic fibers, which are wavy during childhood and become progressively straighter with age, suggesting that pericardia in the young are more compliant than those of the elderly.

ELECTRON MICROSCOPY. This reveals that exuberant microvilli and long, single cilia project from the serous mesothelium composing the visceral pericardium and the inner lining of the parietal pericardium (Fig. 44–1),[6] and increase markedly the surface area available for fluid

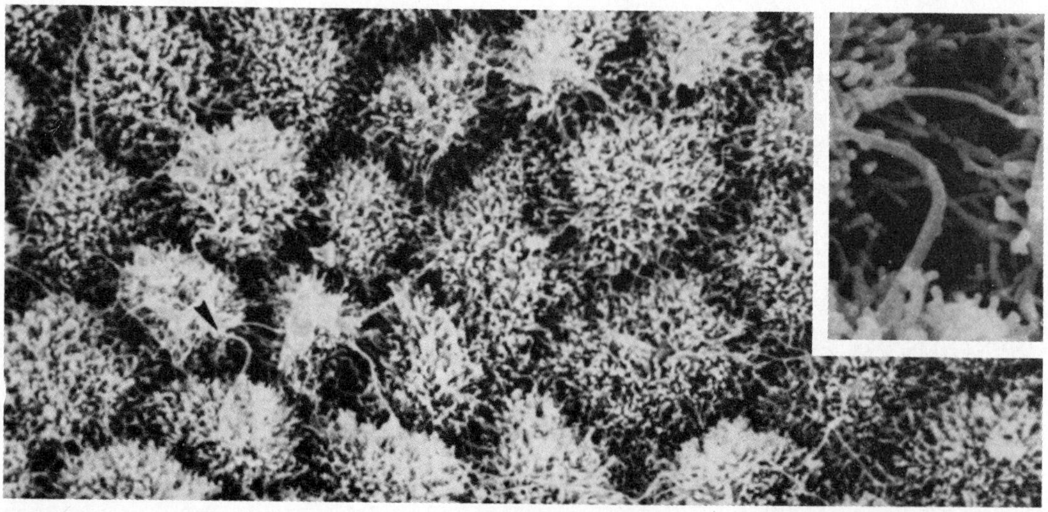

FIGURE 44–1. Scanning electron micrograph of human parietal pericardium. The mesothelial cells are covered with microvilli, and individual long cilia (arrow) are also present. Insert shows cilia at higher magnification. (From Ishihara, T., et al.: Histologic and ultrastructural features of normal human parietal pericardium. Am. J. Cardiol. *46*:744, 1980.)

transport. Both microvilli and cilia provide a specialized surface to permit movement of the pericardial membranes over each other during each cardiac cycle and to permit the pericardium to accommodate changes in cardiac shape during contraction.

PERICARDIAL FLUID. The human pericardium normally contains up to 50 ml of clear fluid.[7] The visceral pericardium is believed to be the source of normal pericardial fluid and of excessive fluid in disease states. Normal pericardial fluid appears to be an ultrafiltrate of plasma, since electrolytes are present in pericardial fluid in concentrations compatible with such an ultrafiltrate; protein concentrations are about one-third those of the plasma, and albumin is present in a higher ratio in pericardial fluid, reflecting its lower molecular weight.[8] Pericardial fluid also contains phospholipids, which serve as a lubricant to reduce friction between the surfaces of the parietal pericardium and the visceral pericardium.[9] Current data suggest that drainage of the pericardial space occurs both by the thoracic duct via the parietal pericardium and by the right lymphatic duct via the right pleural space.

FUNCTIONS OF THE PERICARDIUM

The pericardium's ligamentous attachments help to fix the heart anatomically and prevent excessive motion with changes in body position. The pericardium also reduces friction between the heart and surrounding organs and provides a barrier against the extension of infection and malignancy from contiguous organs to the heart itself. The role of the pericardium in the regulation of the circulation is controversial, since congenital absence of the pericardium is not associated with overt disturbances of cardiac function. However, observations in both dogs and man indicate that the pericardium may play a role in (1) the distribution of hydrostatic forces on the heart, (2) the prevention of acute cardiac dilatation, and (3) diastolic coupling of the two ventricles (p. 1486).

The normal pericardium is stiff, and the relationship between pressure within the pericardium and total intrapericardial volume, which is the sum of the volume of the heart itself and the reserve volume of the surrounding pericardial sac, appears as a steep curve when plotted on a graph.[3] Thus, once the pericardium is filled, intrapericardial pressure rises sharply as volume is increased (Fig. 44–2). Normally, the pericardial sac is filled with a thin film of fluid distributed throughout the pericardial space in such a way that the pericardial reserve volume is not

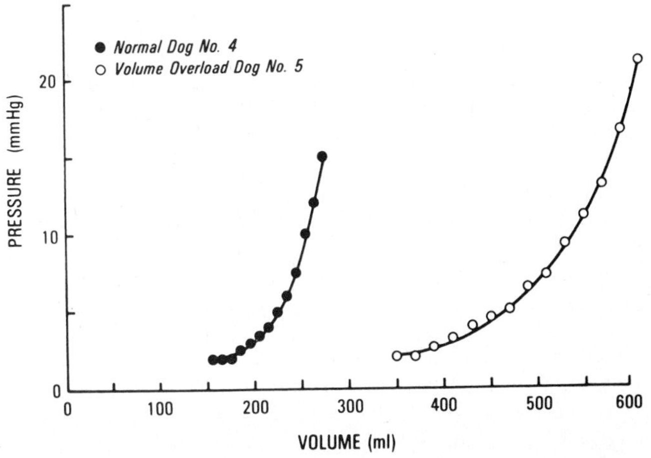

FIGURE 44–2. Pericardial pressure-volume curves from a normal dog (left) and from a dog with chronic volume overload (right). Note the normal pressure-volume curve (right) is initially flat but becomes extremely steep as total volume within the pericardium increases. In response to chronic cardiac dilatation, the pericardium enlarges in size and mass such that the pericardium can accommodate a large volume at low pressure (right curve). (From Freeman, G. L., and LeWinter, M. M.: Pericardial adaptations during chronic dilation in dogs. Circ. Res. *54*:294, 1984, by permission of the American Heart Association, Inc.)

exceeded. This permits respiratory and postural changes in cardiac volume and total intrapericardial volume to occur without significant changes in intrapericardial pressure. When measured with a fluid-filled or micromanometer-tipped catheter, pericardial pressure is nearly equal to intrapleural pressure and varies from −5 to +5 cm H_2O during the respiratory cycle.[10, 11]

INTRAPERICARDIAL PRESSURE. Pericardial pressure is a determinant of the *transmural distending pressure* of the cardial chambers and thereby contributes to the operation of the Frank-Starling mechanism in the beat-to-beat regulation of stroke volume (p. 405). The transmural distending pressure of either ventricle is the difference between intracardiac and intrapericardial pressures and is independent of gravity. For example, when left ventricular end-diastolic pressure is +5 mm Hg and intrapericardial pressure is −2 mm Hg, relative to atmosphere—the actual ventricular distending pressure—is 5 − (−2) = 7 mm Hg. Studies using micromanometer pressure measurements support the view that pericardial pressure is usually very low and thus exerts only a small influence on the average transmural distending pressure of the heart as long as pericardial reserve volume is not exceeded by volume loading.[11] Even under normal conditions, however, the pericardium does influence the pattern of venous return and ventricular filling, which occurs in every cardiac cycle. Ventricular ejection is accompanied by abrupt descent of the atrioventricular junction (the "base" of the heart) and a reduction in right atrial pressure, manifested by the x descent* in the right atrial pressure pulse as well as by a decline in intrapericardial pressure. These changes result in a surge of venous return during systole, particularly when ventricular and pericardial pressures are increased.[12] Brecher has shown that the acceleration of venous return during systolic ejection is diminished by opening of the pericardium.[13]

When the volume of the heart or other contents of the pericardial sac increase and exceed the elastic limits of the pericardium, during diastole the heart is shifted to the steep portion of the curve relating intrapericardial pressure and volume, resulting in marked increases in intrapericardial and intracardiac pressures. However, the difference between the two pressures, i.e., the transmural pressure, usually declines. In the extreme case of cardiac tamponade, in which both intrapericardial and intracardiac pressures are markedly increased, the transmural pressure distending the ventricles may fall precipitously, resulting in decreased ventricular diastolic volumes and preload. Taken together, these findings indicate that changes in intrapericardial pressure modestly modulate the regulation of stroke volume by ventricular preload, i.e., the Frank-Starling mechanism, and exert a substantial influence only at higher ventricular and pericardial pressures.

This classic view has been seriously challenged by Smiseth and coworkers,[14] who contend that the use of either fluid-filled or micromanometer catheters underestimates pericardial pressure and its influence on transmural distending pressures in normal hearts. They have shown in dogs that the measurement of the surface contact pressure of the pericardium against the heart using a flat balloon is more accurate than a fluid-filled catheter in estimating the actual pericardial pressure (the fall in left ventricular pressure observed immediately after opening of the pericardium in the absence of any change in chamber volume). Observations from dogs and from humans indicate that when the amount of fluid in the pericardial sac is small, pericardial pressure measured in this way is much higher than intrathoracic pressure or

---

*It is recognized that the descent in venous pressure after the *a* wave is usually termed the *x* descent and, after the *c* wave, the *x′* descent. In this chapter, the major systolic venous pressure descent after the *a* and *c* waves will be termed the *x* descent.

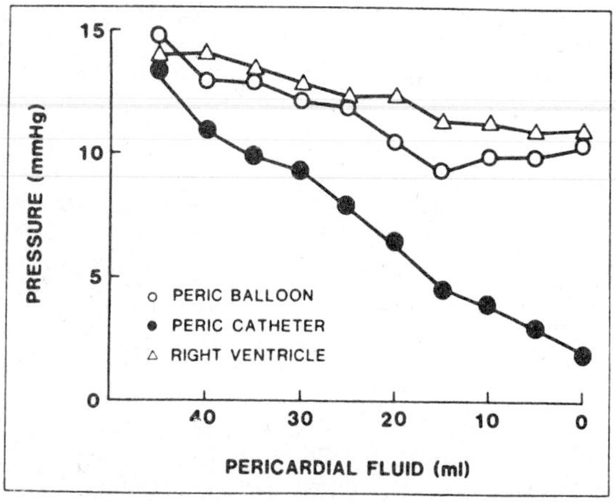

FIGURE 44–3. Pericardial pressure measured by a flat balloon (open circles) and a fluid-filled end-hole catheter (closed circles) during the infusion and withdrawal of saline from a dog's pericardial sac. When a substantial volume of fluid is present, both techniques of pressure measurement yield similar measurements of pericardial pressure. As the pericardium is emptied of fluid, measurements made with a standard end-hole catheter indicate that pericardial pressure falls to a value near zero when the pericardial sac is dry. In contrast, when the pericardial sac is dry, pericardial pressure measured with a flat balloon is considerably higher and is similar to right ventricular diastolic pressure (triangles). (From Smith, E. R., et al.: Mechanism of action of nitrates. Am. J. Med. *76*:14, 1984.)

pericardial pressure measured with a fluid-filled or micromanometer catheter, whereas pericardial pressures measured by either a balloon or fluid-filled catheter are similar when a substantial volume of pericardial fluid is present (Fig. 44–3).[15, 16] This analysis indicates that left ventricular transmural pressure in normal hearts should be estimated by subtracting right atrial pressure rather than intrathoracic pressure. It also suggests that the transmural distending pressure of the normal right ventricle is extremely small.

LIMITATION OF CARDIAC DISTENTION. The relatively nondistensible pericardium may help to limit acute distention of the heart. This was appreciated as early as 1898 by Claude Bernard, who used a pump to increase pressure in excised hearts with and without the pericardium and noted that hearts unsupported by the pericardium ruptured at lower pressures than did hearts with intact pericardia.[17] More recent studies in dogs have suggested that the pericardium may restrain left ventricular filling, so that ventricular volume is greater at any given ventricular pressure with the pericardium removed than with the pericardium intact.[18–20] In addition, acute changes in intracardiac and total intrapericardial volume result in an upward shift of the left ventricular pressure-volume relationship, which is in part mediated by the restraining effect of the pericardium.

Thus, Shirato and coworkers demonstrated that acute volume loading with dextran in dogs with intact pericardia resulted in an upward shift in the left ventricular pressure-segment length relationship, i.e., left ventricular pressure was higher at any given segment length while the reduction of venous return and cardiac volume by means of nitroprusside administration shifted the curves downward toward control levels.[21] This occurred because nitroprusside and other vasodilators that decrease right heart filling reduce the total volume occupied by the heart within the pericardial space and thus reduce the restraining of the left ventricle by the pericardium; in turn, this causes a downward shift of the left ventricular pressure-volume relationship so that a given left ventricular volume is associated with a lower left ventricular diastolic pressure. After pericardiectomy, volume loading resulted in a rightward shift in the pressure-segment length relationship[22] and, after nitroprusside, a leftward shift along a single curve. When the effect of the pericardium was eliminated by plotting left ventricular transmural pressure versus segment length, the points during all interventions also fell along a single curve.

Refsum et al. investigated the role of the pericardium in the mechanism of shifts in the left ventricular pressure-volume relationship by infusing saline both intravenously and into the pericardial sac in closed-chest dogs in which intrapericardial and cardiac volumes were assessed by computed tomography.[23] Acute upward shifts in the left ventricular diastolic pressure-volume relationship during volume loading were due to elevations in intrapericardial pressure induced by increases in total intrapericardial volume.

A restraining effect of the pericardium has also been observed early in the course of chronic volume overloading induced by formation of arteriovenous shunts in dogs prior to enlargement of the pericardium by stretch or hypertrophy, but this restraining effect was not apparent in dogs studied late during the course of chronic volume overload.[24] This occurs because chronic left ventricular enlargement and hypertrophy are accompanied by an increase in the compliance of the pericardial chamber and an increase in total pericardial volume due to the addition of new pericardial tissue.[25] Furthermore, this restraining effect of the pericardium is minor if acute volume overload, such as that caused by mitral regurgitation, results in a rise in left atrial pressure without a substantial rise in right atrial pressure.[26]

These observations suggest that shifts in the left ventricular intracavity pressure-volume relation following volume loading or vasodilator administration are largely due to changes in intrapericardial pressure.[27, 28] However, the pericardium does not affect *intrinsic myocardial compliance* nor does it account for changes in the left ventricular diastolic pressure-volume relationship observed during ischemia.[29]

VENTRICULAR INTERDEPENDENCE. The pericardium also contributes to diastolic coupling between the two ventricles, i.e., to ventricular interdependence. The distention of one ventricle alters the distensibility of the other, even in the absence of the pericardium.[30–33] This effect appears to be mediated in part by shared encircling muscle bands and by the interventricular septum, which tends to bulge into the left ventricle, causing a change in the shape of the left ventricle when the right ventricle is distended.[34] In the absence of the pericardium, large increases in right ventricular volume and pressure are required to cause an appreciable increase in left ventricular filling pressure.[35, 36] In contrast, the presence of an intact pericardium markedly accentuates the coupling between ventricular diastolic pressures.[37–40] When right ventricular volume and pressure are increased with the pericardium intact, right and left ventricular filling pressures are closely correlated and left ventricular volume is smaller than in the absence of the pericardium, when cardiac distensibility is primarily related to properties of the myocardium.[40] This effect of the pericardium on diastolic ventricular interaction is present at normal filling pressures and becomes of increasing importance at high right ventricular filling pressures.[35] During volume loading in normal conscious dogs, it has been shown that pericardial pressure exerts a disproportionately greater effect on the thin-walled right ventricle.

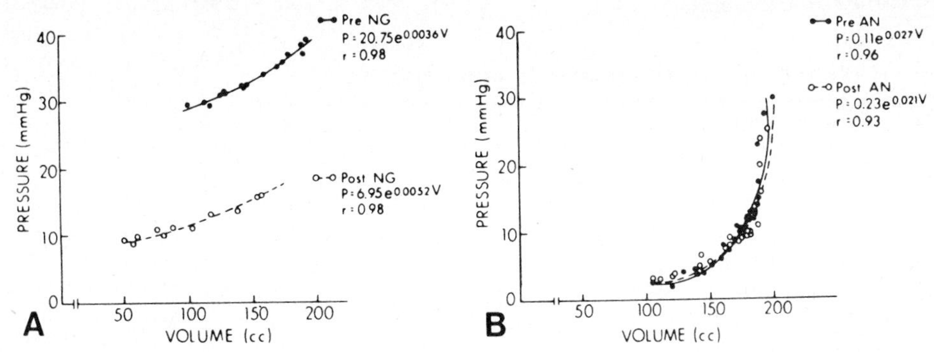

FIGURE 44–4. Left ventricular pressure-volume curves in man (*A*) before and after nitroglycerin (NG) and (*B*) before and after amyl nitrite (AN). Nitroglycerin, which causes venodilation and reduces total intrapericardial volume, shifts the curve downward and leftward. In contrast, the curves before and after amyl nitrite, which causes arterial dilation, can be superimposed. (From Ludbrook, P. A., et al.: Influence of right ventricular hemodynamics on left ventricular diastolic pressure-volume relations in man. Circulation *59*:21, 1979, by permission of the American Heart Association, Inc.)

This suggests that the pericardium couples diastolic function of the two ventricles via its influence on right ventricular filling and geometry, which affects the left ventricle through series interaction.[11]

Although normal pericardium does not appear to contribute importantly to the interaction of the ventricles during systole at normal filling pressures,[41] it does influence systolic function during conditions of volume expansion.[20, 42] Kanazawa et al.[42] showed that whereas removal of the pericardium in dogs caused insignificant changes in stroke volume, removal of the pericardium during volume loading caused a substantial increase in stroke volume associated with an increase in end-diastolic segment length and systolic excursion. Although pericardial pressure was not measured, it is likely that this increase in stroke volume was due to the Frank-Starling mechanism via an increase of the transmural distending pressure of the ventricle following removal of the pericardium. Further, during volume overload, the pericardium caused an upward shift in the left ventricular end-systolic pressure-volume relationship in the absence of a change in inotropic state. The pericardium also appears to limit maximal oxygen consumption by limiting stroke volume and cardiac output during maximal exercise in conscious dogs.[43] These observations suggest that the normal pericardium exerts a restraining effect and modifies ventricular interaction during systole at high ventricular filling pressures.

In *summary*, there is experimental evidence that the pericardium limits acute distention of the heart, mediates changes in the relationship between ventricular pressure and volume, and enhances the effect that distention of one ventricle has on the diastolic pressure-volume relationships of the contralateral ventricle.

FUNCTIONS OF THE PERICARDIUM IN MAN. There is evidence in man that the restraining effects of the pericardium are clinically relevant. First, in humans after pericardiotomy, there is a downward shift of the left ventricular pressure-volume curve that is increasingly apparent as left ventricular volume increases.[44] In addition, angiotensin, nitroprusside, and nitroglycerin infusions, which alter intracardiac volume, cause acute shifts in the left ventricular diastolic pressure-volume relation,[45–47] an effect which probably depends on the presence of the pericardium. The downward shift in the left ventricular pressure-volume curve that occurs during nitroglycerin administration in humans is not observed with amyl nitrite, which alters aortic pressure but has little acute effect on intrapericardial volumes (Fig. 44–4).[48] After pericardiotomy and loss of the restraining effect of the pericardium, the human left ventricular pressure-volume curve is not altered by nitroprusside administration.[49] These observations indicate that the beneficial effects of interventions such as nitroprusside infusion, in which an augmentation of stroke volume may be observed at a lower ventricular filling pressure, are in part due to an alteration of *apparent* cardiac distensibility mediated by reducing the restraining effect of the pericardium.[50]

The pericardium may also provide a significant restraining effect on acute cardiac dilatation during acute volume loading in humans. Extrapolating the findings of dog experiments may underestimate the restraining effect of the human pericardium during acute volume loading because normal human pericardium is about seven times thicker and shows much greater viscous responses than canine pericardium.[51] Thus, volume overload due to acute mitral regurgitation is sometimes associated with striking elevation and equilibration of diastolic pressures in all four cardiac chambers similar to that observed in constrictive pericardial disease (p. 1501), but these findings do not appear to be present in patients with chronic volume overload.[52] Similarly, acute right ventricular infarction is sometimes associated with elevation and equilibration of diastolic right and left ventricular pressures[53] that have been shown experimentally to be related to the elevation of intrapericardial pressure.[54] The effect of the pericardium on the coupling between right and left ventricular pressures in man is dramatically illustrated by the pathophysiology of pericardial tamponade (p. 1492).

ACUTE PERICARDITIS

Acute pericarditis is a syndrome caused by inflammation of the pericardium and characterized by chest pain, a pericardial friction rub, and serial electrocardiographic abnormalities. The incidence of pericardial inflammation detected in several autopsy series ranges from 2 to 6 per cent, whereas pericarditis is diagnosed clinically in only about 1 out of 1000 hospital admissions. This suggests that pericarditis is frequently inapparent clinically, although it may occur in the presence of a vast number of medical and surgical disorders (Table 44–1). The most common causes of the syndrome of acute pericarditis include idiopathic or viral pericarditis, uremia, bacterial infection, acute myocardial infarction, tuberculosis, neoplasm, and trauma.[55] All types of pericarditis are more common in

TABLE 44–1 ETIOLOGIES OF PERICARDITIS

1. **Idiopathic** (nonspecific)
2. **Viral infections**: Coxsackie A virus, Coxsackie B virus, echovirus, adenovirus, mumps virus, infectious mononucleosis, varicella, hepatitis B
3. **Tuberculosis**
4. **Acute bacterial infection**: pneumococcus, staphylococcus, streptococcus, gram-negative septicemia, *Neisseria meningitidis, Neisseria gonorrhoeae*, tularemia, *Legionella pneumophila*
5. **Fungal infections**: histoplasmosis, coccidioidomycosis, *Candida*, blastomycosis
6. **Other infections**: toxoplasmosis, amebiasis, mycoplasma, *Nocardia*, actinomycosis, echinococcosis, Lyme disease
7. **Acute myocardial infarction**
8. **Uremia**: untreated uremia; in association with hemodialysis
9. **Neoplastic disease**: lung cancer, breast cancer, leukemia, Hodgkin's disease, lymphoma
10. **Radiation**
11. **Autoimmune disorders**: acute rheumatic fever, systemic lupus erythematosis, rheumatoid arthritis, scleroderma, mixed connective tissue disease, Wegener's granulomatosis, polyarteritis nodosa
12. **Other inflammatory disorders**: sarcoidosis, amyloidosis, inflammatory bowel disease, Whipple's disease, temporal arteritis, Behçet's disease
13. **Drugs**: hydralazine, procainamide, diphenylhydantoin, isoniazid, phenylbutazone, dantrolene, doxorubicin, methysergide, penicillin (with hypereosinophilia)
14. **Trauma**: including chest trauma; hemopericardium following thoracic surgery, pacemaker insertion, cardiac diagnostic procedures; esophageal rupture; pancreatic-pericardial fistula
15. **Delayed postmyocardial-pericardial injury syndromes**:
    a. Postmyocardial infarction (Dressler) syndrome
    b. Postpericardiotomy syndrome
16. **Dissecting aortic aneurysm**
17. **Myxedema**
18. **Chylopericardium**

men than in women and in adults compared with young children. The relative frequency of causes of pericarditis depend on the clinical setting. Presumed viral or idiopathic pericarditis is common in an outpatient setting, while pericarditis related to trauma, neoplasm, and uremia is seen more frequently in tertiary hospitals.

The *pathological changes* of acute pericarditis are those of acute inflammation, including the presence of polymorphonuclear leukocytes, increased pericardial vascularity, and deposition of fibrin. Inflammation may also involve the superficial myocardium, and fibrinous adhesions may form between the pericardium and epicardium and between the pericardium and adjacent sternum and pleura. The visceral pericardium may also react to acute injury by exudation of fluid. The pathological and clinical features of specific etiologies of pericarditis are discussed later in this chapter. This section will focus on clinical features common to acute pericarditis of many causes.

HISTORY. *Chest pain* is frequently the chief complaint of patients with acute pericarditis; its quality and location are variable (Table 44–2). Pain is often localized to retrosternal and left precordial regions and frequently radiates to the trapezius ridge and neck. Occasionally, it may be localized to the epigastrium, mimicking an acute abdomen, or have a dull or oppressive quality, with radiation to the left arm similar to the ischemic pain of myocardial infarction. The pain is often aggravated by lying supine, coughing, deep inspiration, and swallowing and is eased by sitting up and leaning forward. Sometimes it is noted with each heartbeat. The pain associated with pericarditis may arise from inflammation of both the pericardium and the adjacent pleura, accounting for the pleuritic nature of the discomfort. Pericardial pain may also be provoked by stretch of the pericardial sac due to the presence of intrapericardial fluid.

Acute pericarditis may also cause *dyspnea*. This symptom is related in part to the need to breathe shallowly to avoid pericardiopleuritic chest pain. Dyspnea may be aggravated by the presence of fever or by the development of a large pericardial effusion that compresses adjacent bronchi and pulmonary parenchyma. Additional symptoms such as cough, sputum production, or weight loss may be due to an underlying systemic disease such as tuberculosis or uremia.

PHYSICAL EXAMINATION. The *pericardial friction rub* is the pathognomonic physical finding of acute pericarditis. It is a scratching, grating, high-pitched sound, described by Laennec's associate Victor Collin as "the squeak of leather of a new saddle under the rider." Although the sound is believed to arise from friction between the roughened pericardial and epicardial surfaces, a loud pericardial rub may be heard in the presence of scant or large pericardial effusions.[56] The pericardial friction rub is classically described as having three components that are related to cardiac motion during atrial systole (presystole), ventricular systole, and rapid ventricular filling in early diastole. Spodick's prospective analysis of the pericardial friction rub revealed that the presystolic component is present in about 70 per cent of cases, while a ventricular systolic component is the loudest and most easily heard component, present in almost all cases.[57] The rapid diastolic filling component is detected less frequently and may be slurred into that of atrial contraction, resulting in a biphasic "to-and-fro" rub. In this series, a true three-component rub was detected about half the time and at the lower left sternal border. The single-component rub is the least common but is likely to be the auscultatory finding in patients with atrial fibrillation.

An important feature of the pericardial friction rub is that it is often evanescent and may change in quality from one examination to the next. Detection of the rub is aided by listening with the stethoscope diaphragm applied firmly to the chest at the lower left sternal border during inspiration and full expiration with the patient sitting up and leaning forward. Occasionally, a rub may be detected with the patient lying supine with arms extended above the head during inspiration or suspended respiration. The single-component pericardial friction rub may be mistaken for a systolic murmur or tricuspid or mitral regurgitation. A pericardial rub may also be confused with the crunch of air in the mediastinum or the artifact of skin scratching

TABLE 44–2 PERICARDIAL VERSUS ISCHEMIC PAIN

	ISCHEMIA	PERICARDITIS
Location	Retrosternal; left shoulder, arm	Precordium; left trapezius ridge
Quality	Pressure, burning, buildup	Sharp, pleuritic; or dull, oppressive
Thoracic motion	No effect	Increased by breathing, rotating thorax
Duration	Angina; 1 or 2 to 15 min Unstable angina: ½ hr to hrs	Hours or days
Effort	Stable angina: usually Unstable angina or infarction: usually not	No relation
Posture	No effect; may sit, belch, use Valsalva or knee-chest position for relief	Leaning forward for relief; aggravated by recumbency

From Fowler N. O.: Acute pericarditis. *In* Fowler, N. O. (ed.): The Pericardium in Health and Disease. Mt. Kisco, NY, Futura Publishing Co., 1985, p. 158.

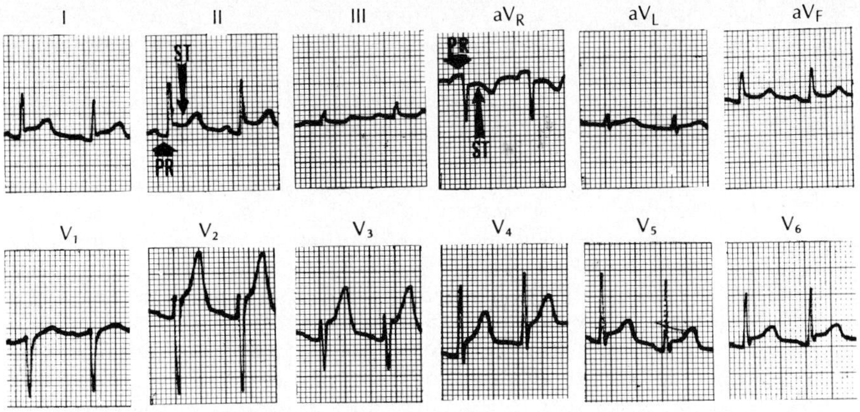

FIGURE 44–5. Stage 1 electrocardiographic changes of acute pericarditis with diffuse ST-segment elevations (*long arrow*) in all leads except aVr. Depression of the P-R segment (*short arrow*) is present in lead II and the left chest leads, with reciprocal P-R segment elevation in aVr. (From Goldberger, A. L.: Myocardial Infarction: Electrocardiographic Differential Diagnosis. 3rd ed. St. Louis, C. V. Mosby, 1984, p. 181.)

against the stethoscope. Pericardial friction rubs may be differentiated from murmurs by (1) the use of exercise to permit detection of a classic three-component rub, (2) the failure of a rub to radiate widely or to vary in timing and duration with inspiration or change in posture in a manner characteristic of regurgitant murmurs, and (3) by the confirmatory finding of typical electrocardiographic changes of pericarditis.

ELECTROCARDIOGRAM. Serial electrocardiograms are extremely helpful in confirming the diagnosis of acute pericarditis. Electrocardiographic changes can occur a few hours or days after the onset of pericardial pain, and the electrocardiographic diagnosis of acute pericarditis is made by detecting the serial appearance of *four stages of abnormalities* of the ST segments and T waves (Fig. 44–5).[58, 59] The etiology of these changes is believed to be related to an actual current of injury caused by superficial myocardial inflammation or epicardial injury.[59]

There are four stages in the electrocardiographic evolution of acute pericarditis (Table 44–3). Stage I electrocardiographic changes accompany the onset of chest pain and are virtually diagnostic of acute pericarditis (Fig. 7–13, p. 190). These comprise ST-segment elevation, which, unlike the pattern of ST-segment elevation in acute myocardial infarction, is concave upward and usually present in all leads except aVr and V_1.[59] The T waves are usually *upright* in the leads with ST-segment elevation. Stage II occurs several days later and represents the return of ST segments to baseline, accompanied by T-wave flattening. This change in the ST segments usually occurs prior to the appearance of T-wave inversion. In contrast, T waves in acute myocardial infarction often become inverted *before* the ST segments return to baseline. Stage III is characterized by inversion of the T waves so that the T-wave vector becomes directed opposite to the ST-segment vector. T-wave inversion is generally present in most leads and is not associated with the loss of R-wave voltage or the appearance of Q waves. These features help to differentiate this stage of nonspecific T-wave inversion from changes associated with the evolution of transmural or subendocardial myocardial infarction. Stage IV represents the reversion of T-wave changes to normal, which may occur up to weeks or months later. T-wave inversion may occasionally persist indefinitely in patients with chronic pericardial inflammation due to tuberculosis, uremia, or neoplastic pericardial disease.

Electrocardiographic abnormalities appear in about 90 per cent of cases of acute pericarditis, and the finding of typical Stage I changes or a classic evolution of all four stages can be diagnostic even when other clinical features of pericarditis are misleading. All four stages can be detected in about 50 per cent of patients with acute pericarditis. In addition, depression of the P-R segment occurs in about 80 per cent of patients with acute pericarditis.[58] Depression of the P-R segment occurs during the early stages of ST-segment elevation or T-wave inversion, is usually present in both limb and precordial leads, and may reflect abnormal atrial repolarization due to atrial inflammation.

Variations of the patterns described above are present in slightly less than 50 per cent of patients with pericarditis and include (1) isolated P-R segment depression, (2) the absence of one or more stages of the ST-segment and T-wave changes, (3) evolution of Stage I (ST-segment elevation) directly to Stage IV (reversion of T waves to normal), (4) persistence of T-wave inversion, (5) appearance of ST-segment changes in only a few leads, (6) appearance of marked T-wave inversion before the ST-segments have returned to baseline, and (7) the absence of any serial electrocardiographic changes whatsoever.[60] Regional ST-segment deviation may be confused with electrocardiographic changes of regional myocardial ischemia.

TABLE 44–3 FOUR-STAGE ("TYPICAL") ECG EVOLUTION OF ACUTE PERICARDITIS

Sequence	Leads of "Epicardial" Derivation (I, II, aV_L, aV_F, V_{3-6})			Leads Reflecting "Endocardial" Potential aV_R, often V_1, sometimes V_2		
Stage	**J-ST***	**T waves**	**PR segment**	**ST segment**	**T waves**	**PR segment**
I	Elevated	Upright	Depressed or isoelectric	Depressed	Inverted	Elevated or isoelectric
II early	Isoelectric	Upright	Isoelectric or depressed	Isoelectric	Inverted	Isoelectric or elevated
II late	Isoelectric	Low to flat to inverted	Isoelectric or depressed	Isoelectric	Shallow to flat to upright	Isoelectric or elevated
III	Isoelectric	Inverted	Isoelectric	Isoelectric	Upright	Isoelectric
IV	Isoelectric	Upright	Isoelectric	Isoelectric	Inverted	Isoelectric

*J-ST = junction of S (or T) wave with the end of the QRS complex.
Modified from Spodick, D. H.: Electrocardiographic changes in acute pericarditis. Am. J. Cardiol. 33:470, 1974.

In addition to the features described above that help to distinguish the ST-segment changes of pericarditis from those of acute myocardial infarction, the changes of Stage I must also be differentiated from the electrocardiographic variant of normal early repolarization (p. 204).[61] This pattern is usually seen in young males, in whom the clinical syndrome of pain and dyspnea suggesting acute pericarditis is absent; P-R segment depression is occasionally present but is uncommon, and most importantly, the electrocardiogram does not evolve through a pattern of the return of ST segments to baseline followed by T-wave inversion. An ST segment/T wave ratio greater than 0.25 in lead V_6 also appears to discriminate patients with acute pericarditis from those with the normal variant of early repolarization.[62]

Sinus tachycardia is common and may be present in the absence of other contributing factors, such as fever or hemodynamic compromise.[63] Other atrial arrhythmias are very infrequent in uncomplicated acute pericarditis and when present suggest underlying myocardial disease.[64] Atrioventricular block, bundle branch block, and ventricular tachycardia are not features of acute pericarditis, and these findings suggest the presence of extensive myocardial inflammation, fibrosis, or acute ischemia.

OTHER LABORATORY FINDINGS. The *chest roentgenogram* is of little value in the diagnosis of uncomplicated acute pericarditis. If acute pericarditis is complicated by the appearance of a large pericardial effusion, the chest roentgenogram may show both enlargement and changes in configuration of the cardiac silhouette. The chest roentgenogram may provide clues to the underlying etiology of acute pericarditis as in the case of pericarditis secondary to tuberculosis or malignancy. Pleural effusions occur in about one-fourth of patients with pericarditis and are usually left pleural effusions in contrast with findings in patients with heart failure in whom right pleural effusions predominate.[65]

The *echocardiogram* is the most sensitive and accurate tool in the detection and quantification of pericardial fluid and is discussed on pages 127 to 129. Technetium-99m pyrophosphate scans[66] and gallium radionuclide scans have also been reported to be useful in detecting acute pericarditis,[67] but their sensitivity and specificity is not known.

Acute pericarditis is often associated with nonspecific indicators of inflammation, including leukocytosis and elevation of the sedimentation rate. Although cardiac isoenzymes are usually normal, modest elevation of the MB fraction of creatine phosphokinase may occur in the presence of epicardial inflammation accompanying acute pericarditis.[68–70] For this reason, cardiac isoenzymes cannot always be used to differentiate between acute pericarditis and acute myocardial infarction.

On the basis of the history (including that of recent travel), physical examination, and the clinical setting in which pericarditis occurs, some patients may require more extensive diagnostic tests to clarify the possibility of an underlying systemic disease. Because of the serious consequences of missing the diagnosis of tuberculous pericarditis, screening for tuberculosis with a tuberculin skin test and a control skin test to exclude anergy is reasonable for all patients suspected of having acute pericarditis. Other diagnostic tests that may be indicated in individual patients are necessary according to the clinical presentation: (1) blood cultures to exclude associated possible infective endocarditis and bacteremia; (2) acute and convalescent cultures of blood, urine, throat, and feces (if available from the hospital laboratory) to evaluate a suspected viral etiology; (3) fungal serological tests to evaluate a suspected fungal etiology in patients from endemic areas or in immunocompromised patients; (4) ASO titer in children with suspected rheumatic fever; (5) cold agglutinins to exclude a mycoplasma etiology; (6) heterophil antibody test to exclude infectious mononucleosis; (7) immunofluorescent antibody titers for toxoplasmosis; (8) TSH, T_4, and T_3 to exclude hypothyroidism; (9) BUN and creatinine to exclude uremic etiology; and (10) antinuclear antibody titer (ANA) and rheumatoid factor to exclude systemic lupus erythematosus and rheumatoid arthritis.

The issue of the additional diagnostic yield of pericardiocentesis or pericardial biopsy has been addressed by a prospective study of 231 patients with acute pericarditis of inapparent cause.[71] Noninvasive clinical and laboratory studies as described above were done in all patients. A diagnostic pericardiocentesis was done if clinical illness and an effusion lasted more than 1 week, followed by diagnostic biopsy if clinical illness lasted more than 3 weeks. This strategy yielded a diagnosis in 14 per cent of patients, which in the majority warranted specific therapy (bacterial pericarditis, tuberculosis, toxoplasmosis, unsuspected malignancy). The diagnostic yield was substantial when pericardiocentesis or pericardiectomy with biopsy was done to relieve cardiac tamponade (39 per cent and 54 per cent, respectively), and 5 per cent when these procedures were done only for diagnostic reasons. This experience suggests that there is a higher likelihood of establishing an etiological diagnosis in patients who develop cardiac tamponade than in those with uncomplicated acute pericarditis, and *therapeutic pericardiocentesis or pericardiectomy should always be accompanied by a rigorous examination of fluid or tissue* for occult malignancy or infection. In the immunocompetent patient with uncomplicated acute pericarditis, diagnostic pericardiocentesis or biopsy is usually unwarranted.

MANAGEMENT. The first step in the management of acute pericarditis consists of establishing whether the pericarditis is related to an underlying problem that requires specific therapy. Nonspecific therapy of an initial episode of pericarditis should include bed rest until pain and fever have disappeared, since activity may cause worsening of symptoms. Observation in the hospital is warranted for almost all patients with acute pericarditis to exclude an associated myocardial infarction or a pyogenic process and to watch for the development of tamponade.

The pain of pericarditis usually responds to nonsteroidal antiinflammatory agents such as aspirin (650 mg orally every 3 to 4 hours) or indomethacin (25 to 50 mg orally four times daily). When pain is severe and does not respond to this therapy within 48 hours, corticosteroids may be employed. If prednisone is used, large doses, such as 60 to 80 mg daily in divided doses, should be given. After 5 to 7 days, if the patient has been free of symptoms for several days, antiinflammatory agents should be tapered. Owing to the adverse consequences of long-term steroid therapy, it is desirable to avoid their use for pain control whenever possible. When long-term steroid administration is needed to control pain and other evidence of inflammation, alternate-day therapy should be attempted. Patients in whom steroids cannot be discontinued may tolerate tapering of steroids and weaning to nonsteroidal antiinflammatory agents.

Antibiotics should be used only to treat documented purulent pericarditis. Oral anticoagulants should not be administered during the acute phase of pericarditis of any cause. If anticoagulants must be continued owing to the presence of a mechanical prosthetic heart valve, we recommend the use of intravenous heparin, which can be promptly reversed with protamine, and both physical examination and echocardiography should be performed at regular intervals to watch closely for the development of a pericardial effusion under pressure.

NATURAL HISTORY. Viral pericarditis, idiopathic pericarditis, post-myocardial infarction pericarditis, or the post-pericardiotomy syndrome are usually self-limited; clinical and laboratory signs of inflammation abate after 2 to 6 weeks. The most troublesome complication is the development of recurrent episodes of pericardial inflammation at intervals of weeks or months after the initial episode. Although cardiac tamponade is uncommon, disabling chest pain associated with fever may recur over a period of years and require steroid administration for pain relief.[72] Pericardiectomy is not always followed by relief of pain.

Pericarditis can also be complicated by the development of disabling or life-threatening hemodynamic complications due to cardiac compression. These include (1) the development of a pericardial effusion under pressure, resulting in cardiac tamponade; (2) the development of fibrosis and/or calcification of the pericardium, resulting in constrictive physiology; and (3) a combination of both effusive and constrictive pericardial disease.

PERICARDIAL EFFUSION

Pericardial effusion may develop as a response to injury of the parietal pericardium with all causes of acute pericarditis. It may be clinically silent, but if the accumulation of fluid causes intrapericardial pressure to increase, resulting in cardiac compression, the symptoms of cardiac tamponade develop. The development of increased intrapericardial pressure secondary to a pericardial effusion depends on several factors: (1) the absolute volume of the effusion, (2) the rate of fluid accumulation, and (3) the physical characteristics of the pericardium. The pericardial space in humans normally contains between 15 and 50 ml of fluid. If additional fluid accumulates slowly, the pericardium stretches; the pericardial sac can accommodate up to 1 to 2 liters without elevation of intrapericardial pressure. However, the normal unstretched pericardial sac can accommodate the rapid addition of only 80 to 200 ml of fluid and still remain on the flat portion of the curve relating intrapericardial pressure and volume (Fig. 44–2, p. 1485). If additional fluid is added rapidly to a volume exceeding about 150 to 200 ml, a marked rise of intrapericardial pressure occurs. Intrapericardial pressure may also increase markedly after the accumulation of a smaller amount of fluid if the pericardium is excessively stiff because of fibrosis or tumor infiltration.

PERICARDIAL EFFUSION WITHOUT CARDIAC COMPRESSION

HISTORY. Patients who develop a pericardial effusion without elevation of intrapericardial pressure may have no symptoms whatsoever. Occasionally these patients complain of a constant oppressive dull ache or pressure in the chest. Large pericardial effusions may cause symptoms by mechanical compression of adjacent structures including dysphagia from esophageal compression, cough due to bronchial/tracheal compression, dyspnea from lung compression with subsequent atelectasis, hiccups due to phrenic nerve compression, or hoarseness due to recurrent laryngeal nerve compression. Nausea and a sense of abdominal fullness may occur from pressure on adjacent abdominal viscera.

PHYSICAL EXAMINATION. A small pericardial effusion in the absence of an increase in intrapericardial pressure may result in no specific physical findings, whereas a large effusion may produce several characteristic physical findings. First, the heart sounds may be muffled owing to the interposition of fluid between the chest wall and the cardiac chambers. Compression of the base of the left lung by pericardial fluid produces *Ewart's sign*, a patch of dullness on auscultation beneath the angle of the left scapula. Rales may be heard over the lung fields secondary to compression of lung parenchyma. Abnormalities of the arterial pulse, systemic blood pressure, and jugular venous pulse do not occur when a large pericardial effusion is present without significant elevation of the intrapericardial pressure.

CHEST ROENTGENOGRAM. Enlargement of the cardiac silhouette usually does not occur until at least 250 ml of fluid have accumulated in the pericardial space. Therefore, a normal or unchanged chest roentgenogram does not exclude the presence of a hemodynamically important pericardial effusion. This examination may suggest the presence of a pericardial effusion if there is a rapid increase in the size of the cardiac silhouette in the presence of clear lung fields (Fig. 6–43, p. 166). In some cases the heart may assume a globular or waterbottle shape, blurring the contours along the left cardiac border and obscuring the hilar vessels. Loculated effusions may have a cystlike appearance (Fig. 44–6). The parietal pericardial and epicardial fat layers are normally separated by 1 to 2 mm. The presence of an effusion may result in more marked separation of the pericardial fat lines, apparent on high-quality frontal or lateral chest films in about 25 per cent of patients with pericardial effusions.[73] *Fluoroscopy* may reveal absent or weak pulsations and the absence of any changes in the size and shape of the cardiac silhouette

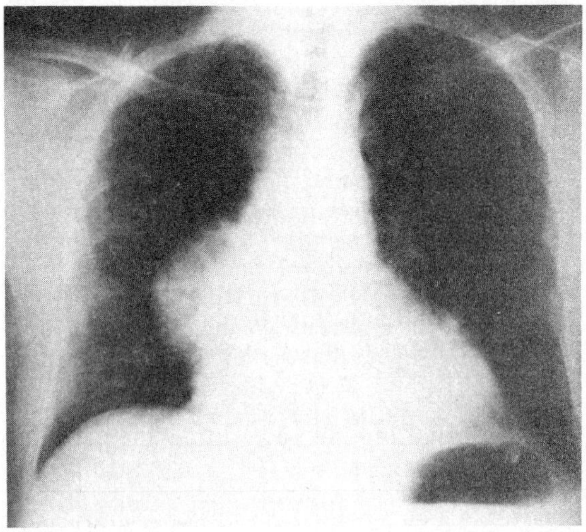

FIGURE 44–6. Posteroanterior chest roentgenogram from a patient with recurrent pericarditis and a loculated pericardial effusion which was subsequently drained surgically. In this patient, the loculated pericardial effusion simulated the roentgenographic appearance of a pericardial cyst.

during inspiration. These findings are especially useful in the cardiac catheterization laboratory when possible perforation of the heart is suspected.

Radionuclide scanning with technetium-labeled aggregates of albumin has also been used to label blood within the heart, liver, and lungs simultaneously. The presence of an abnormal unlabeled space between the heart and the adjacent liver and lungs suggests the presence of a pericardial effusion.[74] *Computed tomography* (p. 364) has also been used to image pericardial effusions,[75, 76] and *magnetic resonance imaging* can identify effusions, differentiate fluid from epicardial fat, and delineate other pathology including pericardial thickening and intrapericardial masses[77] (Fig. 12–32, p. 373).

ELECTROCARDIOGRAM. The electrocardiogram may reveal the nonspecific findings of a reduction in QRS voltage and flattening of the T waves as fluid accumulates within the pericardial space.[78] Electrical alternans (p. 214) suggests the presence of a massive pericardial effusion and cardiac tamponade.

ECHOCARDIOGRAPHY (See also p. 127). This technique is the most accurate, rapid, and widely used technique for evaluating a pericardial effusion, in following the accumulation or resolution of fluid over time, and in assessing the functional status of the cardiac valves and myocardium. Recognition of pericardial fluid depends on the acoustical differences among the pericardium, cardiac muscle, and pericardial fluid. Accumulation of pericardial fluid results in the appearance of an echo-free space between the posterior left ventricular wall and posterior parietal pericardium and between the anterior wall of the right ventricle and adjacent echoes of the parietal pericardium and chest wall.[79, 79a] Posterior and anterior epicardial fat can simulate this echocardiographic appearance of a pericardial effusion.[80] M-mode echocardiography appears to be sufficiently sensitive to detect as little as 20 ml of pericardial fluid.[81]

Although the quantification of pericardial effusions by echocardiography is not precise, several guidelines of assessment are helpful. Very small effusions are likely to be imaged only posteriorly, with separation of the pericardial and epicardial echoes only in systole. Small- to moderate-sized effusions are likely to be imaged only posteriorly, with the presence of an echo-free space throughout the cardiac cycle. Pericardial effusions of approximately 300 ml can usually be imaged both anteriorly and posteriorly. Moderate-to-large effusions may be associated with excessive swinging motion of the heart and the false-positive appearance of mitral valve prolapse and anterior septal motion. Normally, the echo-free space representing a pericardial effusion disappears behind the left atrium owing to the absence of fluid in the oblique pericardial sinus. However, in massive effusions, fluid may also collect in the oblique sinus, resulting in an echo-free space behind the left atrium as well as the left ventricle.

M-mode echocardiography is usually adequate to diagnose pericardial effusion, but occasionally the diagnosis may be confused with a left pleural effusion, giant left atrium, pulmonary infiltrate, and retrograde hiatal hernia. Two-dimensional echocardiography is particularly useful in a loculated pericardial effusion[82] (Figs. 5–102 to 105, pp. 127 to 128). Blood in the pericardial space can often be differentiated from an effusion of lower acoustical density.[83] Two-dimensional echocardiography is useful in identifying rapidly the presence of hemopericardium with or without thrombus formation secondary to cardiac invasive procedures.[84]

MANAGEMENT. The clinical significance of any pericardial effusion depends on (1) the presence or absence of hemodynamic embarrassment due to increased intrapericardial pressure and (2) the presence and nature of the underlying systemic disease. The use of echocardiography to establish the diagnosis of a pericardial effusion is warranted in suspected cases of acute pericarditis, since presence of an effusion is suggestive, although not diagnostic, of pericardial inflammation. Pericardiocentesis (p. 1498) is *not* indicated unless there is evidence of cardiac compression caused by cardiac tamponade or unless analysis of pericardial fluid is essential to establish a diagnosis such as acute bacterial pericarditis.

Chronic Pericardial Effusions

Chronic pericardial effusions persisting for more than 6 months may occur in any form of pericardial disease. Often they are surprisingly well tolerated, with no symptoms of cardiac compression, and are discovered when a routine chest roentgenogram discloses an unexpectedly large cardiac silhouette. Chronic pericardial effusions are particularly likely to be found in patients with previous idiopathic or viral pericarditis, uremic pericarditis, and pericarditis secondary to myxedema or neoplasm. The management of chronic pericardial effusion depends in part on the cause. Stable and apparently idiopathic effusions in asymptomatic patients usually require no specific treatment except for avoidance of anticoagulants.

PERICARDIAL EFFUSION WITH CARDIAC COMPRESSION: CARDIAC TAMPONADE

An increase in intrapericardial pressure secondary to fluid accumulation within the pericardial space results in cardiac tamponade, which is characterized by (1) an elevation of intracardiac pressures, (2) progressive limitation of ventricular diastolic filling, and (3) a reduction of stroke volume.

PATHOPHYSIOLOGY

As already noted, intrapericardial pressure is normally very close to intrapleural pressure and several millimeters of mercury lower than right and left ventricular diastolic pressures. When the addition of fluid into the pericardial space causes intrapericardial pressure to rise to the level of the right atrial and right ventricular diastolic pressures, the transmural pressure distending these chambers declines to close to zero and cardiac tamponade occurs.[85] The rise of right atrial and intrapericardial pressures is less marked in the presence of hypovolemia; therefore, cardiac tamponade may be masked when hypovolemia is present. Further accumulation of intrapericardial fluid causes both intrapericardial and right ventricular diastolic pressures to rise together to the level of left ventricular diastolic pressure, and subsequently all three pressures rise together associated with a fall in systemic arterial pressure. If left ventricular diastolic pressure is markedly elevated owing to preexisting left ventricular disease, cardiac tamponade occurs when right atrial and right ventricular diastolic and pericardial pressures equalize but at a lower level than the left ventricular diastolic pressure.[86]

Equalization of intrapericardial and ventricular filling pressures results in markedly diminished transmural distending pressures and diastolic volumes of both ventricles and a fall in stroke volume.[85, 87–90] The reduction in stroke volume is initially compensated for by reflex increases in adrenergic tone; both tachycardia and increases in ejection fraction initially help to maintain forward cardiac output.[85, 91] The importance of the adrenergic support of the heart is reflected in the finding that when beta-adrenoceptor blockade is carried out in cardiac tamponade, ejection fraction and stroke volume decline.[90] As cardiac tamponade develops and systemic vascular resistance increases so that, at first, systemic arterial pressure is maintained at the expense of cardiac output. Acute increases in pericardial volume and pressure also reflexly induce a marked decrease in urinary sodium excretion.[92] With severe cardiac tamponade, as cardiac output declines, compensatory mechanisms are no longer sufficient to maintain systemic arterial pressure, and perfusion of vital organs becomes impaired[91]; reduced coronary perfusion causes selective hypoperfusion of the subendocardium.[93, 94] The addition of myocardial ischemia during cardiac tamponade could further compromise left ventricular stroke volume. In extreme cardiac tamponade, transmural diastolic ventricular pressures may actually be less than zero, suggesting that ventricular filling occurs by diastolic suction.[95] Sinus bradycardia, mediated by the cardiac depressor branches of the vagus nerve and by the nonvagal mechanism of sinoatrial node ischemia, may also occur during severe cardiac tamponade.[96, 97] Profound bradycardia often occurs during severe hypotension and precedes the development of electrical and mechanical dissociation and death.[98]

Cardiac tamponade also alters the dynamics of systemic venous return and cardiac filling. Normally, one surge of systemic venous return occurs during ventricular ejection coincident with the systolic *x* descent of the venous pressure pulse, and a second surge occurs during right atrial emptying with the opening of the tricuspid valve in diastole, corresponding to the *y* descent. In cardiac tamponade, the heart is compressed throughout the cardiac cycle. During ejection, intracardiac volume decreases, resulting in a transient fall in both intrapericardial and right atrial pressures, manifested as the *x* descent, which is accompanied by a surge of systemic venous return into the right atrium. However, in diastole, the total volume within the pericardial space remains elevated despite opening of the tricuspid valve. Intrapericardial pressure remains elevated and is equal to, or exceeds, early diastolic right atrial pressure so that transmural distending pressure is close to zero. As a result, the usual surge of systemic venous return during early diastole is abolished, right atrial emptying is impeded, and the right atrium is compressed or partially collapsed during diastole. These events are graphically reflected in the right atrial or systemic venous waveform in cardiac tamponade, in that the systolic *x* descent is prominent while the diastolic *y* descent is usually absent or attenuated.

Hemodynamic deterioration during cardiac tamponade is dependent critically on atrial compression during diastole with the secondary impairment of cardiac filling. Fowler and Gabel[99] studied regional cardiac tamponade in dogs and showed that isolated tamponade of the right or left ventricle is inconsequential and that a substantial fall in cardiac output and aortic pressure only occurs when the atria (and intrapericardial veins) are also compressed. Compression of the right atrium is likely to be more important than left atrial compression because pericardial fluid is often not present behind the left atrium during cardiac tamponade. Also, echocardiographic studies of patients with cardiac tamponade indicate that right atrial diastolic collapse is uniformly present while left atrial and right ventricular diastolic collapse is variable.[100] For example, right ventricular collapse may be absent in pericardial tamponade in the presence of severe right ventricular hypertrophy.[101]

During the development of tamponade, collapse of the right atrium and right ventricle initially occurs only in early diastole in association with delayed diastolic filling of the right ventricle and a modest fall in cardiac output without hypotension or overt hemodynamic deterioration (Fig. 44–7).[101, 102] Pandiastolic right atrial and ventricular collapse indicates that pericardial pressure equals or exceeds right atrial and ventricular pressures throughout diastole so that the ventricles may fill only during atrial systole. This stage is accompanied by a severe reduction in ventricular volumes, a failure of compensatory mechanisms, and hypotension.[101, 102] In this setting, pulsus alternans may occur due to beat-to-beat variation in right ventricular output and left ventricular filling.[102] During hypovolemia with low right heart pressures, right ventricular collapse occurs at low intrapericardial pressures while volume expansion delays the development of right ventricular diastolic collapse and hemodynamic deterioration until a higher intrapericardial pressure is achieved.[102, 103] Singh et al.[104] have obtained simultaneous hemodynamic and two-dimensional echocardiographic measurements in patients undergoing pericardiocentesis, and have shown that hemodynamic improvement first occurs at the point of disappearance of right ventricular diastolic collapse which is followed by further improvement in cardiac output and the subsequent disappearance of right atrial collapse during continued pericardiocentesis.

PULSUS PARADOXUS. Inspiration and the transmission of negative intrathoracic pressure to the pericardial space alter further the dynamics of right and left ventricular filling and are responsible for pulsus paradoxus, the inspiratory fall of aortic systolic pressure greater than 10 mm Hg (Fig. 44–8). The finding of weakening of the arterial

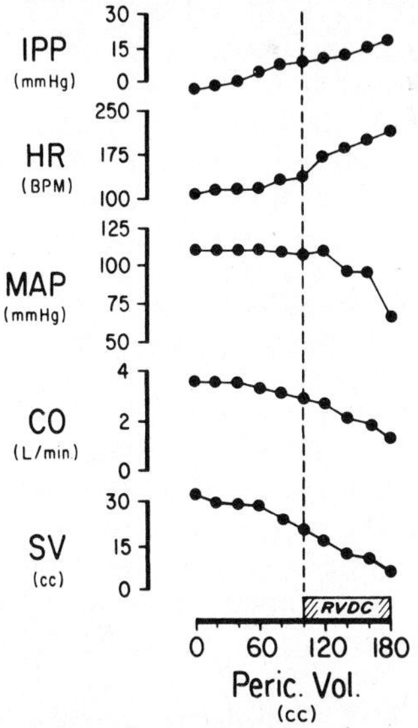

FIGURE 44–7. Hemodynamic measurements from a dog with experimental cardiac tamponade in which two-dimensional echocardiograms showed right ventricular diastolic collapse (RVDC). Mean intrapericardial pressure (IPP) continuously rose as pericardial volume increased, accompanied by a progressive decline of stroke volume (SV). At the time when RVDC was first detected, mean arterial pressure (MAP) was well-preserved, cardiac output (CO) had only modestly declined, and a compensatory increase in heart rate (HR) was present. Mean arterial pressure fell rapidly late in the course of cardiac tamponade in the decompensated phase. (From Leimgruber, P. P., et al.: The hemodynamic derangement associated with right ventricular diastolic collapse in cardiac tamponade: An experimental echocardiographic study. Circulation *68*:612, 1983, by permission of the American Heart Association, Inc.)

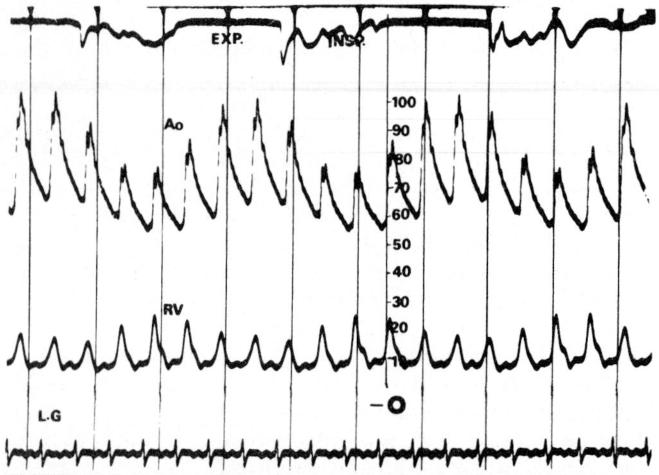

FIGURE 44–8. Recording of aortic (Ao) and right ventricular (RV) pressures in a patient with cardiac tamponade complicated by hypovolemia. *Pulsus paradoxus* is evident as a marked inspiratory decline in aortic systolic and pulse pressures during inspiration (INSP). RV pressure variation is out of phase with aortic pressure. Note that the RV waveform does *not* show a dip-and-plateau configuration. (From Shabetai, R., et al.: The hemodynamics of cardiac tamponade and constrictive pericarditis. Am. J. Cardiol. *26*:480, 1970.)

pulse during inspiration was described by Kussmaul in 1873 as the apparent paradox of the disappearance of the pulse during inspiration despite persistence of the heartbeat. It should be emphasized that pulsus paradoxus is in fact an exaggeration of the normal inspiratory decline of left ventricular stroke volume by about 7 per cent and of systemic arterial pressure by 3 per cent.[105] Inspiration is normally accompanied by an increase in diastolic dimensions of the right ventricle, a small decrease in left ventricular dimension, and increased velocity of flow from the venae cavae into the right atrium.[106, 107] Pulsus paradoxus in cardiac tamponade appears to result from an exaggeration of these normal findings.

Measurement of intracardiac pressures and flow during experimental tamponade[108] and in man during cardiac tamponade[105, 109, 110] have demonstrated that inspiration is associated with falls in intrapericardial and right atrial pressures, which results in augmentation of flow from the venae cavae into the right atrium and right ventricle and augmentation of pulmonary artery flow and pulmonary artery systolic pressure. The increase in venous return flow during inspiration results in a marked and exaggerated increase in right ventricular dimensions accompanied by a reduction in left ventricular dimensions and flattening and displacement of the septum toward the left ventricle.[111] On the left side of the heart, atrial and ventricular diastolic pressures fall, accompanied by a fall in aortic flow and systolic arterial pressure.[105, 110, 111] *Thus, pulsus paradoxus in cardiac tamponade is critically dependent on the inspiratory augmentation of systemic venous return and right ventricular filling.*

Shabetai et al. demonstrated that when experimental cardiac tamponade was induced in dogs, pulsus paradoxus did not develop when either the right heart was bypassed or right ventricular volume was strictly controlled.[108] These experiments also demonstrated that inspiratory pooling of blood within the lungs or traction on the heart by the diaphragm were not essential mechanisms of pulsus paradoxus in cardiac tamponade. Thus, these observations indicate that pulsus paradoxus in cardiac tamponade depends on the inspiratory expansion of right heart filling at the expense of left heart filling (Fig. 44–9).

However, competition for a "fixed space" within the pericardium is not the entire mechanism accounting for pulsus paradoxus, since the cyclic variations in pulmonary artery and aortic pressures are not precisely 180 degrees out of phase. The presence of pulsus paradoxus also indicates a marked reduction of left ventricular diastolic volume so that the left ventricle may be operating on the steep ascending limb of the Starling curve and a small inspiratory reduction of left ventricular filling results in marked depression of left ventricular stroke volume and systolic pressure.[112] Pulsus paradoxus is occasionally observed in constrictive pericarditis and restrictive heart disease, and the latter mechanism may account for its presence in these disorders.

Pulsus paradoxus has also been observed in severe lung disease and massive pulmonary embolism.[113, 114] Under these circumstances, pulsus paradoxus is probably related both to the transmission of excessively negative intrathoracic pressure during inspiration to the aorta, inspiratory pooling of right ventricular stroke volumes in the lungs, and exaggerated right heart filling with an associated decrease in left heart filling during inspiration. Pulsus paradoxus may be absent in cardiac tamponade when left ventricular hypertrophy or heart failure causes a marked elevation of left ventricular diastolic pressure so that the

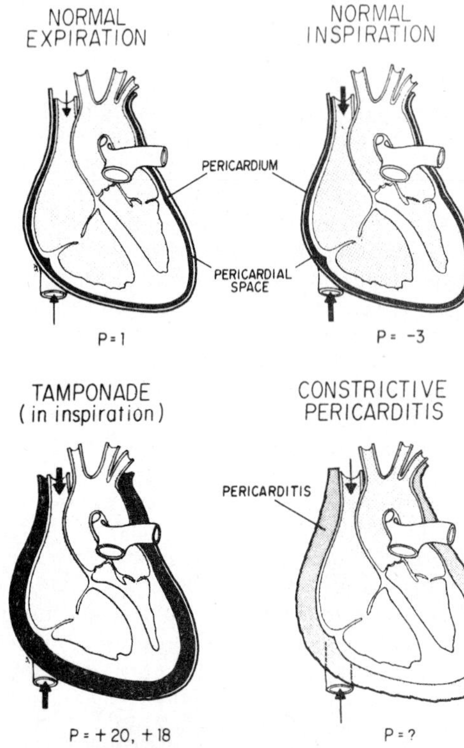

FIGURE 44–9. Schematic illustration of the hemodynamic effects of respiration. In the normal heart (*upper panel*), inspiration results in a fall in intrathoracic and intrapericardial pressure from +1 to −3 mm Hg, which causes an increase in venous return (heavy black arrows) and a slight increase in right ventricular size at the expense of a slight decrease in left ventricular size due to displacement of the interventricular septum from right to left. During cardiac tamponade (*lower left panel*), inspiration causes a fall in the elevated intrapericardial pressure from +20 to + 18 mm Hg. Although both the right and left heart volumes are diminished owing to compression by the pericardial effusion, the inspiratory fall in intrapericardial pressure results in an increase in venous return (heavy black arrow), an increase in right heart volume due to septal bulging, and a further decrease in left heart volume. In constrictive pericarditis (*lower right panel*), the inspiratory fall in intrathoracic pressure is not transmitted to the heart, since the pericardial space is obliterated. For this reason, there is minimal or no increase in venous return (light black arrows) during inspiration. (From Shabetai, R.: The Pericardium. New York, Grune and Stratton, 1981, p. 244).

two ventricles are unequally compressed,[86] in atrial septal defect when the increase in systemic venous return during inspiration is shared between the two sides of the heart,[115] in aortic regurgitation when there is a major component of left ventricular filling that is independent of respiratory variation, and in the presence of pulmonary hypertension which impedes the inspiratory increase in right ventricular filling.

ETIOLOGY

Cardiac tamponade may occur with almost any cause of pericarditis and may exist in either an acute or a chronic form. The distribution of etiologies of acute cardiac tamponade in a city hospital between 1963 and 1980 is given in Table 44–4.[116] In this series the most frequent causes of cardiac tamponade were neoplasm and idiopathic or viral pericarditis, followed by pericarditis associated with myocardial infarction, invasive cardiac diagnostic procedures, purulent bacterial infection, and tuberculosis.

CLINICAL MANIFESTATIONS

The triad of (1) a decline in systemic arterial pressure; (2) elevation of systemic venous pressure; and (3) a small, quiet heart was described by the thoracic surgeon Claude S. Beck in 1935.[117] These three features are typical of cardiac tamponade from intrapericardial hemorrhage due to penetrating heart wounds, aortic dissection, and intrapericardial rupture of an aortic or cardiac aneurysm. This syndrome develops when the pericardium is not enlarged or stretched, so that the addition of less than 200 ml of fluid or blood causes intrapericardial pressure to rise abruptly to above 20 to 30 mm Hg. In cases that are not immediately fatal, both cardiac output and arterial pressure fall, accompanied by tachycardia and tachypnea. The patient may be stuporous or agitated and restless, and the additional important finding of pulsus paradoxus may be difficult to appreciate when profound hypotension is present. Jugular venous pressure is usually markedly elevated. Precordial heart activity is usually not palpable and heart sounds are distant or inaudible. Cold, clammy extremities and anuria may be present.

Patients in whom cardiac tamponade develops slowly differ from those with cardiac tamponade due to cardiac penetration or rupture. In the setting of more slowly developing cardiac tamponade, patients usually appear acutely ill but not in extremis and the major complaint is usually dyspnea.[116] Chest pain may also be present. In patients with chronic development of tamponade, additional systemic symptoms may include weight loss, anorexia, and profound weakness.

TABLE 44–4 COMMON ETIOLOGIES OF CARDIAC TAMPONADE

Disorder	%
Malignant disease	32
Idiopathic pericarditis	14
Uremia	9
Acute cardiac infarction (receiving heparin)	9
Diagnostic procedures with cardiac perforation	7.5
Bacterial	7.5
Tuberculosis	5
Radiation	4
Myxedema	4
Dissecting aortic aneurysm	4
Postpericardiotomy syndrome	2
Systemic lupus erythematosus	2
Cardiomyopathy (receiving anticoagulants)	2

Modified from Guberman, B. A., et al.: Cardiac tamponade in medical patients. Circulation *64*:633, 1981, by permission of the American Heart Association, Inc.

The most common *physical finding* in a series of 56 medical patients with cardiac tamponade was *jugular venous distention.*[116] In addition to absolute elevation of the systemic venous pressure, a characteristic waveform consisting of a prominent systolic *x* descent and absent diastolic *y* descent can often be appreciated at the bedside. Other common physical findings include tachypnea (80 per cent), tachycardia (77 per cent), pulsus paradoxus (77 per cent), pulsus paradoxus with total inspiratory disappearance of the brachial pulse and Korotkoff sounds (23 per cent), pericardial friction rub (29 per cent), hepatomegaly (55 per cent), and diminished heart sounds (34 per cent). It is noteworthy that systolic arterial hypotension, consisting of a systolic pressure less than 100 mm Hg, was present in a minority (36 per cent), and the majority of patients were alert, with warm extremities and preserved urine output.[116]

The finding of *pulsus paradoxus* is critical in making the diagnosis of cardiac tamponade, since most patients with slowly developing cardiac tamponade do not have the classical physical findings of a small, quiet heart and severe hypotension.[116] Pulsus paradoxus can be detected on physical examination as an inspiratory decrease in the amplitude of the palpated pulse in the femoral or carotid arteries. Total paradox, i.e., complete disappearance of the palpated pulse during inspiration, occurs during very severe cardiac tamponade or tamponade combined with hypovolemia. The magnitude of the paradoxical pulse can be accurately quantified by means of an intraarterial catheter but may be estimated by cuff sphygmomanometry. The cuff should be inflated 20 mm Hg above systolic pressure and slowly deflated until the Korotkoff sounds are heard only during expiration. The cuff should then be deflated to the point at which Korotkoff sounds are heard equally well in inspiration and expiration. The difference between these pressures is the estimated magnitude of pulsus paradoxus.

Other disorders with systemic venous distention, pulsus paradoxus, and clear lungs that can be confused with cardiac tamponade include obstructive pulmonary disease,[114] constrictive pericarditis, restrictive cardiomyopathy, and massive pulmonary embolism.[113] Pulsus paradoxus is occasionally noted during severe hypovolemia due to hemorrhagic or septic shock, but jugular venous distention is usually absent.[118] Cardiac tamponade may be confused with shock due to right ventricular infarction with jugular venous distention and clear lungs.[53] However, the hemodynamics of right ventricular infarction are more like those of constrictive physiology than of tamponade (p. 1501).

The clinical findings may be further modified in patients with so-called *low-pressure cardiac tamponade*[119] who are normotensive and in whom the physical examination is normal except for moderate elevation of jugular venous pressure to about 5 to 15 mm Hg. This syndrome represents an early stage in the development of cardiac tamponade in which accumulation of a pericardial effusion causes intrapericardial pressure to rise and equilibrate with low right heart diastolic filling pressures. Pericardiocentesis reduces intrapericardial pressure and causes the separation of right atrial and intrapericardial pressures. Low-pressure cardiac tamponade has been reported in patients with tuberculosis and neoplastic pericarditis and is often associated with severe dehydration.

Tension pneumopericardium causes hemodynamic changes similar to those of acute hemorrhagic cardiac tamponade.[120] It is being increasingly recognized as a cause of cardiac tamponade with a high mortality in infants during mechanical ventilation, and in adults due to penetrating chest trauma, gastric and esophageal rupture, gas production from contiguous infection, and diagnostic procedures such as sternal bone marrow aspiration.[121] Characteristic

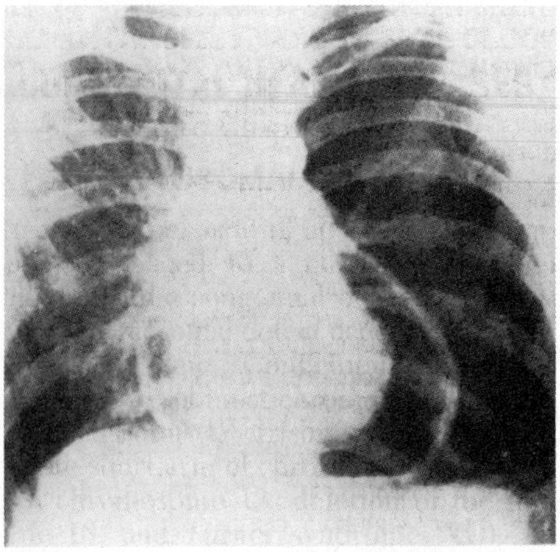

FIGURE 44–10. Posteroanterior chest roentgenogram from a patient with pneumopericardium. The heart is completely surrounded by air, and the pericardium can be seen as a thin stripe of soft tissue density. (From Cummings, R. G., et al.: Pneumopericardium resulting in cardiac tamponade. Ann. Thorac. Surg. *37*:511, 1984.)

clinical findings include muffled heart sounds, bradycardia, and shifting tympany over the precordium. Unique auscultatory findings can be detected including a metallic cracking sound, and the "bruit de moulin," which was described in the first report of pneumopericardium in 1844 by Bricheteau as "the noise made by floats of a mill wheel as they strike the water,"[122] and which indicates the presence of both air and fluid in the pericardial space.

CHEST ROENTGENOGRAM. There are no roentgenographic features diagnostic of cardiac tamponade. The heart may appear completely normal in size in cardiac tamponade that develops from acute hemopericardium due to cardiac rupture or laceration. On the other hand, if an effusion accumulates slowly to more than 250 ml, the cardiac silhouette may be enlarged (Fig. 6–43*A*, p. 166). Other roentgenographic findings may include obscuring of vessels at the hilum, a globular or waterbottle configuration of the heart, clear lungs, and separation of epicardial and pericardial fat pads. These findings suggest the presence of a large pericardial effusion but supply no information about its hemodynamic significance. In patients with cardiac tamponade due to tension pneumopericardium, the chest roentgenogram usually shows that the heart is surrounded by air delineated by a stripe of soft tissue extending up the aorta consisting of the pericardium (Fig. 44–10).

ELECTROCARDIOGRAM. The electrocardiographic abnormalities seen in acute cardiac tamponade include those of acute pericarditis and pericardial effusion per se (p. 1489). The development of electrical alternans[123] is a more specific indicator of pericardial tamponade and reflects pendular swinging of the heart within the pericardial space.[124] This may not be the only mechanism, because two-dimensional echocardiographic findings suggest that electrical alternans may be related to a beat-to-beat alteration of right and left ventricular filling.[102] Electrical alternans may also occur in constrictive pericarditis, in tension pneumothorax, after myocardial infarction, and with severe cardiac muscle dysfunction. However, the appearance of electrical alternans in a patient with a known pericardial effusion is highly suggestive of cardiac tamponade—a finding that has been confirmed in experimental cardiac tamponade.[125] Electrical alternans of the QRS complex may occur in a 2:1 or 3:1 pattern. Alternans is usually limited to the QRS complex, but alternans of the P wave, QRS complex, and T wave may rarely occur and appears to be limited to extreme cardiac tamponade,[126] often in association with neoplastic or tuberculous effusion. Both the abnormal heart motion within the pericardial sac and electrical alternans disappear when pericardial fluid is aspirated.

ECHOCARDIOGRAM (See also p. 127). In patients with jugular venous distention and the possibility of cardiac tamponade, echocardiography is extremely useful and should be performed prior to consideration of pericardiocentesis. In the rare instance of a patient who is in extremis from the extremely rapid development of cardiac tamponade, the physician may have to rely on the history and physical findings to make a judgment about the need for pericardiocentesis. If echocardiography is readily available and the patient with suspected cardiac tamponade is not moribund, obtaining an echocardiogram will increase the likelihood of diagnosing cardiac tamponade correctly and prevent inappropriate and potentially lethal attempts at pericardiocentesis or pericardiotomy. First, the echocardiogram helps to document the presence and magnitude of a pericardial effusion (Fig. 5–106, p. 129). The absence of echocardiographic evidence of a pericardial effusion virtually excludes the diagnosis of cardiac tamponade (with the important exception of the postoperative cardiac surgery patient in whom loculated fluid or thrombus may cause cardiac compression). Second, the echocardiogram rapidly can differentiate cardiac tamponade from other causes of systemic venous hypertension and hypotension, including constrictive pericarditis, cardiac muscle dysfunction, and right ventricular infarction. The appearance of dense echoes in the pericardial space extrinsic to the pericardium suggests the presence of material other than free fluid.[83, 84] Echocardiograms can often detect both massive extracardiac hematoma and extrinsic compression of the heart by tumor,[127] which can cause cardiac compression with the physiology of cardiac constriction or cardiac tamponade.

The M-mode and two-dimensional echocardiogram can provide additional clues that a pericardial effusion is associated with cardiac tamponade. These important features include a marked reduction in the E-to-F slope and excursion of the anterior mitral valve leaflet, and early systolic notching of the anterior right ventricular wall. The presence of pulsus paradoxus is associated with sudden leftward motion of the septum during inspiration[128] and an exaggerated increase in right ventricular size with a reciprocal decrease in left ventricular size.[129, 130] When the inspiratory reduction in left ventricular filling is extreme, the aortic valve may close prematurely or fail to open[131] and mitral valve opening may be delayed until atrial systole.

Diastolic right atrial and right ventricular compression or collapse occur early during the development of cardiac tamponade (Fig. 44–11).[100–104] Left atrial diastolic collapse can also occur when pericardial fluid is present behind the left atrium.[100] Right ventricular diastolic collapse appears to be more predictive of cardiac tamponade than pulsus paradoxus, particularly during hypervolemia,[132, 133] but it may be absent in the presence of right ventricular hypertrophy.[101, 102, 132] Thus, the echocardiographic findings of a pericardial effusion, an inspiratory increase in right ventricular dimensions, and right atrial and ventricular diastolic collapse strongly suggest the diagnosis of cardiac tamponade. However, these changes are not 100 per cent sensitive or specific,[100, 102, 104, 132] and experimental studies indicate that a single echocardiogram cannot always predict the presence or severity of cardiac tamponade.[134]

OTHER LABORATORY TESTS. *Radionuclide* and *contrast angiography* can also detect right ventricular and right

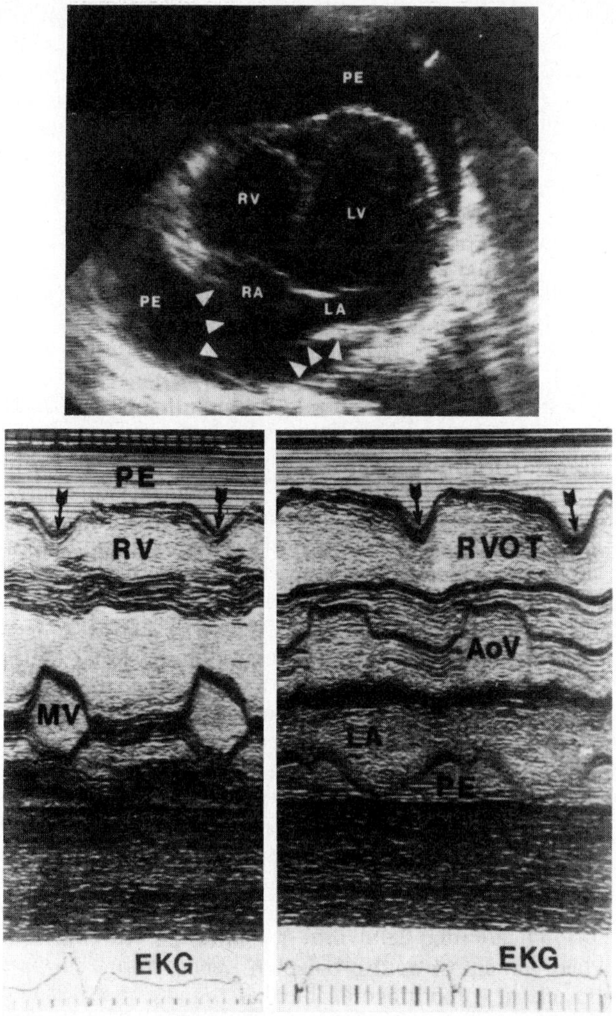

FIGURE 44–11. Two-dimensional (*upper panel*) and M-mode (*lower panels*) echocardiograms from a patient with a malignant pericardial effusion and cardiac tamponade. The two-dimensional image shows a large pericardial effusion (PE) adjacent to the borders of the right ventricle (RV), right atrium (RA), and left ventricle (LV). The effusion is sufficiently large that fluid is also present behind the left atrium (LA). Diastolic compression (white arrows) of both the right and left atria is present. The M-mode images also show striking diastolic compression (dark arrows) of the right ventricle during diastole when the mitral valve (MV) is open, and compression of the right ventricular outflow tract (RVOT) in early-to-mid diastole after aortic valve (AoV) closure.

atrial collapse and compression of the superior vena cava as it enters the pericardium,[135, 136] but these findings, while suggestive of cardiac tamponade, also lack complete sensitivity and specificity. Therefore, it must be emphasized that cardiac tamponade is a clinical—not an echocardiographic or a radionuclide—diagnosis that is established definitively by documentation of the elevation and equilibration of intrapericardial and right atrial pressures and the reversal of these findings by evacuation of pericardial fluid.

CARDIAC CATHETERIZATION

Cardiac catheterization is invaluable in establishing the hemodynamic importance of a pericardial effusion. Except in extreme emergencies—situations in which the patient is moribund—we prefer to catheterize the right heart and measure pressure in the pericardial space in conjunction with pericardiocentesis. Cardiac catheterization (1) provides absolute confirmation of the diagnosis of cardiac tamponade, (2) quantitates the magnitude of hemodynamic compromise, (3) guides pericardiocentesis by documenting that pericardial aspiration is associated with hemodynamic improvement, and (4) permits the detection of coexisting hemodynamic problems including left ventricular failure, effusive-constrictive pericarditis (p. 1508), and unsuspected pulmonary hypertension in patients with malignant effusions.

Cardiac catheterization typically demonstrates elevation of right atrial pressure with a characteristic prominent systolic x descent and a diminutive or absent diastolic y descent. When intrapericardial and right atrial pressures are recorded simultaneously, both are elevated and virtually identical (Fig. 44–12); both pressures fall during inspiration, and intrapericardial pressure may fall slightly below right atrial pressure during systolic ejection at the time of the x descent. If intrapericardial pressure is not elevated, and if right atrial and intrapericardial pressures are not virtually identical, the diagnosis of cardiac tamponade must be reconsidered.

Right ventricular diastolic pressure is elevated and equal to right atrial and intrapericardial pressures and lacks the dip-and-plateau configuration characteristic of constrictive pericarditis (p. 1506). Since right ventricular and pulmonary artery systolic pressures are equal to the pressure developed by the right ventricle plus the intrapericardial pressure, right ventricular and pulmonary artery systolic

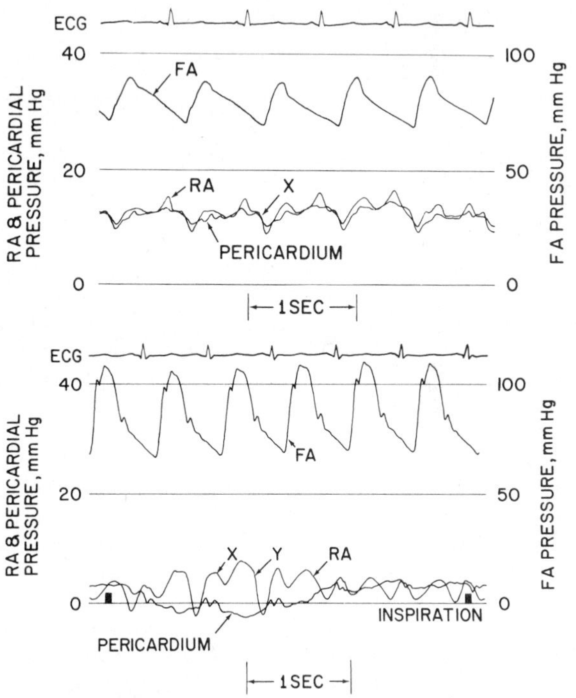

FIGURE 44–12. Simultaneous right atrial (RA) and intrapericardial pressures (scale 0 to 40 mm Hg) and femoral artery (FA) pressure (scale 0 to 100 mm Hg) from a patient with decompensated cardiac tamponade. Before pericardiocentesis (*upper panel*), systemic hypotension is present, and there is elevation and equalization of right atrial and intrapericardial pressures. Note that a systolic x descent is present, but the diastolic y descent is absent, suggesting that right atrial emptying is impeded by compression of the right ventricle in early diastole. After aspiration of about 300 ml of pericardial fluid (*lower panel*), cardiac tamponade is relieved as shown by the restoration of intrapericardial pressure to zero, the restoration of right atrial pressure to a normal level, and the improvement in systemic arterial pressure. The right atrial tracing shows the appearance of a diastolic y descent, which indicates the relief of cardiac compression and restoration of normal right atrial emptying in early diastole. Although this degree of fluid aspiration relieved tamponade physiology, a further 1500 ml of fluid was subsequently aspirated from the pericardial space. (From Lorell, B. H., and Grossman, W.: Profiles in constrictive pericarditis, restrictive cardiomyopathy, and cardiac tamponade. In Grossman, W. [ed.]: Cardiac Catheterization and Angiography. Philadelphia, Lea & Febiger, 1986, p. 440.)

pressures are usually moderately elevated in the range of 35 to 50 mm Hg. In the case of severe cardiac compression, right ventricular systolic pressure may be reduced and only slightly higher than right ventricular diastolic pressure.

Usually, the pulmonary capillary wedge pressure and left ventricular diastolic pressure are elevated and equal to intrapericardial pressure when recorded simultaneously. However, in patients with severe underlying left ventricular dysfunction and marked elevation of the left ventricular diastolic pressure, cardiac tamponade can be present when intrapericardial and right atrial pressures are equal but lower than left ventricular diastolic pressure.[86] Depending on the severity of cardiac compression, left ventricular systolic and aortic pressures may be normal or reduced.

Pulsus paradoxus can be easily documented by intraarterial catheterization and pressure measurement. Simultaneous recording of systemic arterial and right ventricular pressures shows that the inspiratory pressure variation is out of phase (Fig. 44–8). Stroke volume is usually markedly depressed. Cardiac output may be normal, owing to the compensatory effect of tachycardia, or it may be markedly reduced when cardiac tamponade is severe; systemic vascular resistance is usually elevated.

Angiographic studies are not essential if echocardiographic findings suggestive of cardiac tamponade were obtained prior to cardiac catheterization. In an otherwise normal heart, right and left ventricular end-diastolic volumes are usually reduced with normal or increased ejection fractions.

Aspiration of pericardial fluid results initially in the lowering of the identical intrapericardial, right atrial, right ventricular, and left ventricular diastolic pressures, followed by a fall of intrapericardial pressure below right atrial pressure and reappearance of the *y* descent in the right atrial waveform (Fig. 44–12). Further aspiration causes intrapericardial pressure to fall to a mean level of zero and to fluctuate with changes in intrathoracic pressure. Since the pressure-volume curve of the pericardium is steep, the initial aspiration of 50 to 100 ml of pericardial fluid usually leads to a striking reduction in intrapericardial pressure, a striking improvement in systemic arterial pressure and cardiac output, and the abolition of pulsus paradoxus.

If intrapericardial pressure falls to zero or becomes negative and right atrial pressure remains elevated, *effusive-constrictive pericarditis* (p. 1508) should be strongly considered, especially in patients with underlying neoplasms or prior radiation. Other causes of continued elevation of right atrial pressure after successful pericardiocentesis include the coexistence of cardiac tamponade and (1) preexisting left ventricular dysfunction causing, in turn, pulmonary hypertension and right atrial hypertension, (2) tricuspid valve disease, (3) right ventricular failure, and (4) restrictive cardiomyopathy.

The distinction between cardiac tamponade and the superior vena caval syndrome must always be made in patients with neoplastic disease in whom these lesions may occur individually or together. In patients with obstruction of the superior vena cava, cardiac tamponade may be suspected from the presence of elevated jugular venous pressure and pulsus paradoxus due to respiratory distress. In this condition (without accompanying cardiac tamponade) pressure in the superior vena cava is markedly elevated, with dampened pulsations, and exceeds right atrial and inferior vena caval pressures. If elevation of jugular venous pressure persists after relief of cardiac tamponade in patients with neoplastic disease, obstruction of the superior vena cava—as reflected in a pressure gradient between the superior vena cava and right atrium—should be sought. Superior vena caval obstruction may be amenable to radiation therapy.

PERICARDIOCENTESIS

Hemodynamic support during preparation of the patient for pericardiocentesis or pericardiotomy should include administration of intravenous fluid, blood, plasma, or saline. The rationale for volume expansion is that it has been shown to delay the appearance of right ventricular diastolic collapse and hemodynamic deterioration.[102, 103] In experimental cardiac tamponade, administration of norepinephrine and isoproterenol[137] has produced an increase in cardiac output. The vasodilators hydralazine and nitroprusside have also been employed in experimental cardiac tamponade to promote an increase in cardiac output secondary to the reduction of elevated systemic resistance.[138, 139] The administration of vasodilators in conjunction with volume expansion must be done with extreme caution in patients with cardiac tamponade because it may be hazardous in patients with borderline or frank hypotension. Positive-pressure ventilation should be avoided whenever possible, since it has been shown to depress cardiac output further in patients with cardiac tamponade.[140]

Pericardial fluid under pressure causing tamponade can be evacuated by (1) percutaneous pericardiocentesis using a needle or catheter, (2) pericardiotomy via a subxiphoid incision, or (3) partial or extensive surgical pericardiectomy. Considerable controversy exists regarding the exact indications for pericardiocentesis,[141] although the procedure has been performed extensively since its initial demonstration in 1840 by the Viennese physician Franz Schuh. The benefits of pericardiocentesis include the rapid relief of cardiac tamponade and the opportunity to obtain accurate hemodynamic measurements before and after pericardial aspiration. The major risk of percutaneous pericardiocentesis is laceration of the heart, coronary arteries, or lung. Prior to the 1970's, pericardiocentesis was usually performed blindly at the bedside using a sharp needle without hemodynamic or echocardiographic monitoring, and the risk of death or life-threatening complications appeared to be as high as 20 per cent.[141]

The technique has changed somewhat, and the modern approach is exemplified by the Stanford experience in 123 patients.[142] In the majority of patients, pericardiocentesis was performed by a cardiologist in the cardiac catheterization laboratory using a subxiphoid approach under fluoroscopic guidance with hemodynamic and electrocardiographic monitoring. In this experience, five deaths occurred in association with pericardiocentesis; nonfatal hemopericardium developed in an additional five patients. Pericardiocentesis in this study was successful in obtaining pericardial fluid in 106 of 123 patients. Importantly, the probability of success in safely obtaining fluid was directly related to the size of the pericardial effusion, since fluid was obtained in 93 per cent of patients with large effusions located both anteriorly and posteriorly on echocardiogram but in only 58 per cent with a small posterior pericardial effusion. In 23 patients a specific etiological diagnosis was possible from analysis of the pericardial fluid. Cardiac tamponade was successfully relieved by pericardiocentesis in 61 per cent, while the remainder required subsequent surgical drainage owing to either failure to relieve tamponade or recurrence after pericardiocentesis. Surgery was most frequently required in patients with acute traumatic hemopericardium. An unsuspected physiological cause of increased systemic venous pressure other than simple cardiac tamponade was documented in 40 per cent of the patients studied, including effusive-constrictive pericarditis in 17 per cent, congestive heart failure in 16 per cent, and coexisting neoplastic superior vena caval obstruction in 5 per cent. Similar experiences with pericardiocentesis have been reported by others.[143–145]

Two-dimensional echocardiography is useful in guiding pericardiocentesis. Callahan et al.[146] have reported their experience in 132 consecutive pericardiocenteses guided by two-dimensional echocardiography. Pericardiocentesis was successful in obtaining pericardial fluid in 95 per cent of the procedures. In this experience there were no deaths, one pneumothorax, and three minor complications. Partial or complete surgical pericardiectomy was subsequently required in 25 per cent of patients for recurrent effusion, chronic relapsing pericarditis, or effusive-constrictive disease.

Thus, pericardiocentesis is now safer than it was a decade ago, and the procedure, when performed by an experienced operator, is associated with only about a 0 to 5 per cent risk of development of a life-threatening complication. The procedure is most likely to be successful and uncomplicated when performed in patients with clear-cut echocardiographic evidence of a large effusion with an anterior clear space of 10 mm or more. Cardiac tamponade associated with malignant pericardial effusion or prior radiation therapy can often be managed with pericardiocentesis alone or with a combination of pericardiocentesis, radiation therapy, and local or systemic chemotherapy.[142] This therapeutic approach may be preferable in patients with advanced malignancy when it is desirable to avoid major surgery that is not definitive.

These experiences with pericardiocentesis[142–145] suggest that the procedure should usually be performed in conjunction with hemodynamic measurements, including right heart and intrapericardial pressures, in order to document the presence of the physiological changes of cardiac tamponade before attempted pericardiocentesis and to exclude other important coexisting causes of elevated jugular venous pressure, such as effusive-constrictive disease, superior vena caval obstruction, and left ventricular failure. There is rarely justification for performing blind-needle pericardiocentesis at the bedside in the absence of optimal hemodynamic monitoring or of a previous echocardiogram documenting the presence of a large anterior and posterior effusion.

Pericardiocentesis is likely to be either complicated or unsuccessful in improving hemodynamics in patients with (1) acute traumatic hemopericardium in which blood enters the pericardial space as rapidly as it can be aspirated, (2) a small pericardial effusion judged to be less than 200 ml in size, (3) absence of an anterior effusion on the basis of echocardiogram, (4) a loculated effusion, or (5) clot and fibrin as well as fluid filling the mediastinal or pericardial space postoperatively. Acute hemopericardium secondary to laceration, puncture of the heart, or leaking left ventricular or aortic aneurysm is likely to recur rapidly after needle drainage. Pericardiocentesis should be used only as an emergency temporizing measure before surgical pericardial exploration in which repair of the heart or aorta may be necessary.[147] Surgical drainage is also usually preferred in patients with tamponade caused by purulent pericarditis to permit extensive drainage and in patients with suspected or known tuberculous pericarditis to permit bacteriological and histological examination of pericardial biopsy specimens. A very rare complication which may occur after the relief of cardiac tamponade is the development of sudden ventricular dilation[148] and acute pulmonary edema.[149] The mechanism is probably a sudden increase in venous return following the relief of pericardial compression in the presence of underlying ventricular dysfunction.

COMBINED CATHETERIZATION AND PERICARDIOCENTESIS

We prefer the following method of combined catheterization and pericardiocentesis, which allows documentation of increased intrapericardial pressure and assessment of hemodynamic improvement after pericardiocentesis.[150] In contrast to traditional bedside sharp-needle pericardiocentesis, this method utilizes a soft catheter for pericardial aspiration and thus eliminates the prolonged presence of a sharp needle in the pericardial sac, thereby minimizing the risk of cardiac laceration. If possible, pericardiocentesis should be performed in a cardiac procedure laboratory in which radiographic and hemodynamic monitoring facilities are optimal and by cardiologists experienced with hemodynamic measurements and the procedure itself. Before the procedure, the patient's blood should be typed and crossmatched and the cardiac surgery team alerted.

CARDIAC CATHETERIZATION. Pericardiocentesis is performed after the recording of baseline hemodynamic variables and cardiac output. Since the equilibration of right and left ventricular diastolic pressures is an important feature of cardiac tamponade, it is often desirable to catheterize both sides of the heart and to record right atrial and right ventricular pressures simultaneously with left ventricular pressure. Care should be taken to use equisensitive transducers and to avoid an underdamped catheter-transducer system. Before pericardiocentesis, the transducer system that will be used to record intrapericardial pressure should be leveled with the other transducers, calibrated, and connected to a short length of fluid-filled tubing and a stopcock.

PERICARDIOCENTESIS. The procedure is best carried out with the patient's thorax and head tilted up, which enhances the pooling of the effusion anteriorly and inferiorly. Although multiple sites have been advocated for pericardiocentesis, we strongly prefer the subxiphoid route, since it is extrapleural and avoids the coronary, pericardial, and internal mammary arteries. The skin is shaved, cleansed, and prepared in aseptic fashion, and the skin and subcutaneous tissue are anesthetized with 1 per cent lidocaine. The skin is pierced with a No. 11 blade, 0.5 cm below and to the left of the xiphoid process, and the subcutaneous tissues are spread with a small curved clamp. A long, 8-inch, thin-walled 16- to 18-gauge pointed needle is attached via stopcock to a hand-held syringe containing 1 per cent lidocaine. One port of the stopcock is connected to the short length of fluid-filled tubing and the transducer that will be used to measure pericardial pressure (Fig. 44–13). The thin-walled needle commonly used for lumbar puncture is not adequate because its long sharp bevel poses some hazard. The metal hub of the needle may be attached by a sterile connector to the V lead of an electrocardiographic machine, and the electrocardiogram should be continuously recorded. It is essential that the electrocardiographic apparatus have equipotential grounding with no chance of a current wave that could induce ventricular fibrillation. If this condition cannot be assured, it is safer to omit electrocardiographic monitoring from the needle.

The needle is directed posteriorly until the tip passes posterior to the bony cage. The hub of the needle is then pressed toward the diaphragm and the needle is advanced with a 15-degree posterior tilt, either directly toward the patient's head or toward the right or left shoulder. As the needle is smoothly and slowly advanced, the operator periodically attempts to aspirate fluid and then injects a small amount of lidocaine to clear the needle and to provide anesthesia of the deep tissues. The needle is advanced until the pericardial membrane is felt to "give" and pericardial fluid is aspirated or until ST-segment elevation and ventricular premature beats appear on the electrocardiogram, indicating that the needle has reached the epicardium. In the latter case, the needle is promptly and smoothly withdrawn while the operator attempts to aspirate pericardial fluid until the needle lies within the fluid-filled pericardial space and the ECG changes disappear. If fluid cannot be freely aspirated, the needle is slowly withdrawn out of the body, avoiding lateral motion; the needle is flushed and the procedure repeated.

If hemorrhagic fluid is freely aspirated, and it is not clear whether the needle is in the ventricle, atrium, or pericardial space, a few milliliters of contrast medium may be injected under fluoroscopic observation. If the contrast medium instantly swirls and disappears, the needle is

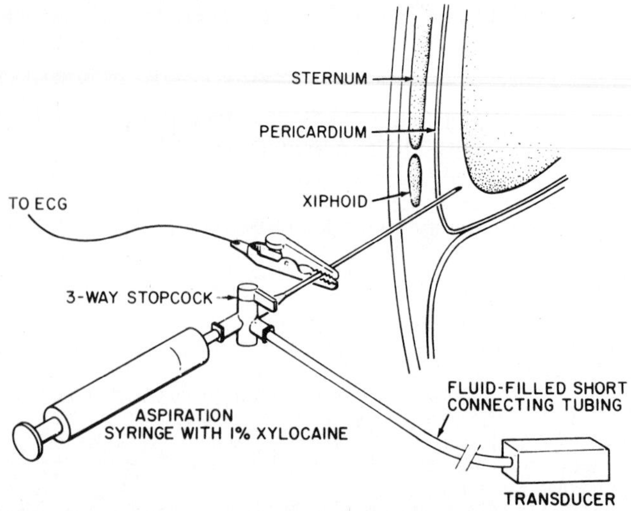

FIGURE 44–13. Pericardiocentesis using the subxiphoid approach, which avoids the major epicardial vessels. A hollow needle, which is attached via a stopcock to an aspiration syringe and to a short length of connecting tubing to a transducer, is used to enter the pericardial space. When fluid is initially aspirated, the pressure waveform at the needle tip should be briefly examined to confirm that the needle tip is in the pericardial space. A floppy-tipped guidewire is then passed through the hollow needle, the needle is exchanged for a soft flexible catheter with end- and side-holes to facilitate safe and thorough drainage of the pericardial sac. (From Lorell, B. H., and Grossman, W.: Profiles in constrictive pericarditis, restrictive cardiomyopathy, and cardiac tamponade. In Grossman, W. [ed.]: Cardiac Catheterization and Angiography. Philadelphia, Lea and Febiger, 1986, p. 436.)

within a cardiac chamber; in contrast, the appearance of sluggish layering of contrast medium inferiorly indicates that the needle is correctly positioned. When fluid can be freely aspirated, the stopcock is turned into its transducer, and needle tip and phasic right atrial pressures are simultaneously displayed. If the needle tip is in the pericardial space, pericardial and right atrial pressures should be equal with identical waveforms. A soft, floppy-tip guidewire is then passed through the hollow needle so that its tip lies within the pericardial space, as confirmed by fluoroscopy. A soft Teflon catheter with multiple sideholes and an end hole (i.e., a Teflon Gensini catheter) is advanced over the guidewire, the guidewire is removed, and a few milliliters of fluid are aspirated. The catheter is then promptly connected to the prepared transducer, and intrapericardial pressure is recorded simultaneously with right atrial and systemic arterial pressures to document the presence of cardiac tamponade.

HANDLING OF THE PERICARDIAL FLUID. Fluid samples are then aspirated from the catheter and sent for analysis of protein, amylase, glucose, and cholesterol content; hematocrit and white blood cell count; and bacteriological culture for aerobic and anaerobic bacteria, tuberculosis, and fungi. In most cases, a generous sample of fluid should also be sent in a heparinized container for cytological examination.

POST-PERICARDIOCENTESIS MEASUREMENT. Right atrial, systemic arterial, and intrapericardial pressures should be recorded periodically as aliquots of fluid are removed—not only until intrapericardial pressure falls to zero but until no further fluid can be aspirated; intrapericardial pressure may return to normal levels after removal of only 50 to 100 ml of fluid in the presence of an effusion of 1 to 2 liters. When no further fluid can be aspirated or drained, cardiac output and systemic arterial pressure as well as right atrial, right ventricular, and left ventricular pressures should be recorded, the last three simultaneously. The jugular veins should also be examined.

DOCUMENTATION OF SUCCESSFUL PERICARDIOCENTESIS. Successful relief of cardiac tamponade is documented by (1) the fall of intrapericardial pressure to levels of -3 and $+3$ mm Hg, (2) the fall of elevated right atrial pressure and separation between right and left heart filling pressure, (3) augmentation of cardiac output, and (4) disappearance of pulsus paradoxus. The presence of continued elevation and equilibration of right and left ventricular diastolic pressures with the appearance of a prominent *y* descent in the right atrial pressure tracing strongly suggests the presence of a constricting pericardium due to effusive-constrictive pericarditis (p. 1508). Jugular venous distention despite a fall in right atrial pressure should raise the question of coexisting superior vena caval obstruction, particularly in patients with known or suspected malignant disease.

Some investigators have advocated the routine injection of a small volume of CO_2 or air into the pericardial space to outline the pericardium at the end of the procedure. This procedure has not been shown to be of aid in identifying unsuspected tumor masses,[142] and we do not advocate it. When the pericardial space is nearly obliterated, there is also the risk of injecting gas into a pleural cavity or cardiac chamber or the production of air tamponade.

POSTPERICARDIOCENTESIS MANAGEMENT. It is often desirable to leave the intrapericardial catheter in place for several hours to permit repeated aspiration of fluid if cardiac tamponade recurs or to allow instillation of a nonabsorbable corticosteroid or antineoplastic agent. The catheter may be sutured securely to the skin and attached via a three-way stopcock to a closed drainage system with a water seal. If the fluid is hemorrhagic or rich in fibrin, the catheter must be cleared frequently with a few milliliters of fluid. Dilute heparin may be instilled into the catheter to prevent clotting. The catheter should usually be removed after 24 to 48 hours because of the risk of introducing infection and producing iatrogenic purulent pericarditis. However, in some patients, continuous catheter drainage for several days has been reported to be necessary and effective in relieving cardiac tamponade.[146, 151, 152] Percutaneous pericardial drainage in infants and children can be done without complications using a modification of this approach in which a catheter is inserted over a curved guidewire into the pericardial space under fluoroscopic control.[152]

Following pericardiocentesis, the majority of patients should be observed for about 24 hours in an intensive care setting for recurrence of cardiac tamponade. It is frequently helpful to obtain an echocardiogram soon after pericardiocentesis to establish the appearance of the heart and pericardium following aspiration. Percutaneous pericardial biopsy is not recommended because of the risk of lacerating the pericardium, pleura, or ventricular wall.

PERICARDIECTOMY AND PERICARDIOTOMY

Surgical evacuation of pericardial fluid under pressure can be accomplished for patients who do not require extensive pericardial excision with the *subxiphoid limited pericardiotomy,* initially performed in 1829 by Larrey, a surgeon in Napoleon's army.[153] Subxiphoid pericardiotomy can sometimes be performed under local anesthesia. After a small longitudinal incision is made below the xiphoid process through the linea alba, the diaphragm and pericardium are dissected away from the sternum, and the diaphragm is retracted inferiorly to permit direct exposure of the anterior pericardium. The pericardium is visualized, a small incision is made in the pericardium, a small segment of pericardium is resected for drainage, and a tube is inserted into the pericardial space for extrathoracic drainage into a sterile container by gravity.

The use of the term *creation of a subxiphoid pericardial window*[147, 154] to describe this operation should probably be avoided because it produces confusion with a limited pericardiectomy, which is often referred to as creation of a pleuropericardial window or pericardial window. A *limited pericardiectomy*[155] via a left hemithorax drains the pericardial cavity into the left hemithorax, and all accessible pericardial tissue is not excised. In a *complete pericardiectomy* the pericardium is resected from the right phrenic nerve to the left pulmonary veins (sparing the left phrenic nerve) and from the great vessels to the mid-diaphragm, while a partial pericardiectomy is limited by the great vessels.[156]

The relative efficacy of these approaches has been reviewed in two large series.[155, 156] The overall 30-day surgical mortality ranged from 12.5 to 15.5 per cent and was higher in patients with malignant effusions than benign ones. The subxiphoid pericardiotomy has some advantages over extensive formal pericardiectomy in that it is simpler and quicker, permits both drainage of pericardial fluid and examination of a small pericardial biopsy specimen, and can usually be performed safely in critically ill patients. However, this approach is associated with a significantly higher potential for the need of reoperation for recurrent tamponade or constrictive disease within a few months after surgery in comparison with complete pericardiectomy.[155] This suggests that the less invasive subxiphoid pericardiotomy should be chosen as a palliative procedure in patients who are critically ill with limited expected survival. The left thoracotomy partial pericardiectomy appears to offer none of the advantages of the subxiphoid pericardiotomy and is associated with higher operative mortality.[156] Complete pericardiectomy is usually recommended for the surgical treatment of patients with effusive pericardial disease who are in good general condition and who are expected to survive more than a few months.

PERICARDIOSCOPY. This procedure, using a flexible fiberoptic bronchoscope, has been reported as an adjunct to subxiphoid pericardiotomy following the drainage of the effusion in the operating room.[157, 158] Pericardioscopy permits visualization of the parietal pericardium and epicardium on the anterior, posterior, and inferior surfaces of the heart, and allows selective biopsies beyond the small region of pericardium that is usually accessible with a subxiphoid incision.

CONSTRICTIVE PERICARDITIS

Constrictive pericarditis is present when a fibrotic, thickened, and adherent pericardium restricts diastolic filling of the heart. It usually begins with an initial episode of acute pericarditis characterized by fibrin deposition, often with a pericardial effusion which may not be detectable clinically. This then progresses slowly to a subacute stage of organization and resorption of the effusion, followed by a chronic stage consisting of fibrous scarring and thickening of the pericardium with obliteration of the pericardial space. In the majority of cases, the visceral and parietal layers become completely fused; however, in a few cases, the constricting process is produced primarily by the visceral pericardium (epicardium). In the chronic stage of constrictive pericarditis, calcium deposition may contribute to thickening and stiffening of the pericardium. Constrictive pericarditis is usually a symmetrical scarring process that produces uniform restriction of the filling of all heart chambers. Exceptional cases of strictly localized pericardial thickening have been reported, including constricting bands in the atrioventricular groove surrounding the semilunar valve rings, or in the aortic groove, right ventricular outflow tract, and venae cavae.[159, 160]

PATHOPHYSIOLOGY

In classic constrictive pericarditis, a heavily fibrosed or calcified pericardium restricts diastolic filling of all chambers of the heart and determines its diastolic volume.[91] The symmetrical constricting effect of the pericardium results in elevation and equilibrium of diastolic pressures in all four cardiac chambers (as well as of pulmonary capillary wedge pressures). In early diastole when intracardiac volume is less than that defined by the stiff pericardium, diastolic filling is unimpeded, and early diastolic filling occurs abnormally rapidly because venous pressure is elevated. Rapid early diastolic filling is abruptly halted when the intracardiac volume reaches the limit set by the noncompliant pericardium.

Instantaneous plots of ventricular volume versus time in patients with constrictive pericarditis have shown that virtually all filling of the ventricle occurs very early in diastole. This abnormal pattern of diastolic filling is reflected in the characteristic dip-and-plateau waveforms in both right and left ventricles (Fig. 44–14). The rapid rise in pressure after the early diastolic dip corresponds to the period of rapid diastolic filling, while the plateau phase corresponds to the period of mid and late diastole when there is little additional expansion of the ventricular volume. Since the atria are equilibrated with the ventricles in early diastole, the jugular venous waveform and right and left atrial waveforms show a prominent and deep diastolic y descent. The systolic x descent is usually also present, and the venous waveform may therefore exhibit a characteristic "M" or "W" configuration.

A bimodal pattern of systemic venous return occurs in constrictive pericarditis with an acceleration of systemic venous blood flow from the venae cavae into the right atrium during both ventricular systolic ejection and early diastole. The greatest acceleration of venous blood flow occurs during early diastole simultaneous with the y descent. This contrasts with the normal filling pattern, in which a bimodal pattern of systemic venous return also is present, but the major surge of venous return occurs during systole. The pattern of systemic venous return in constrictive pericarditis also contrasts with that in cardiac tamponade. Cardiac compression is present throughout diastole in cardiac tamponade, so that the diastolic surge

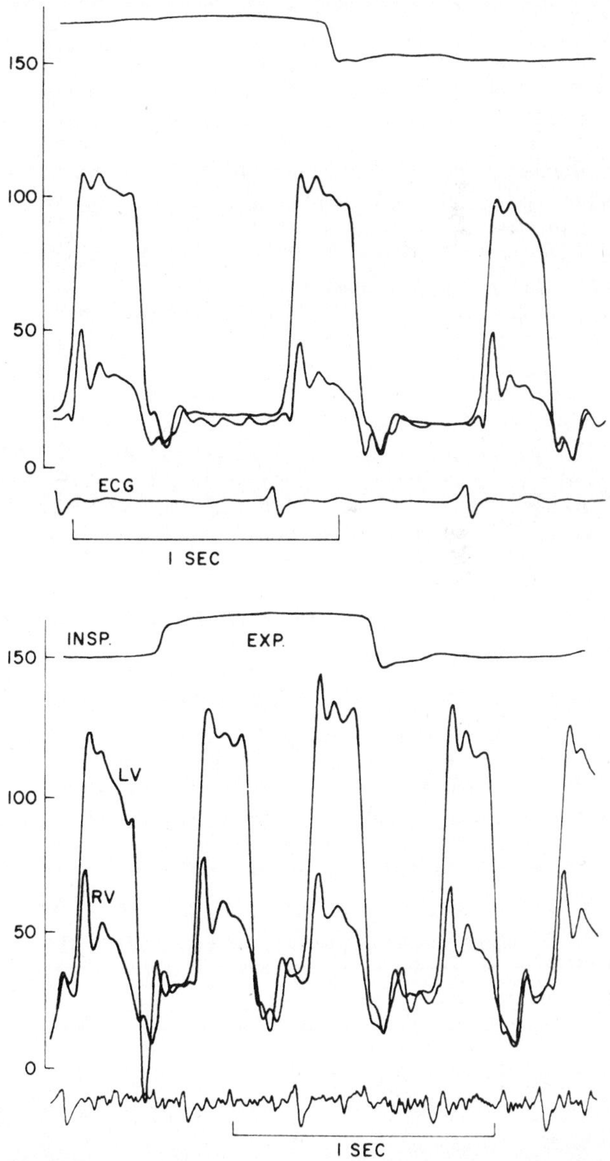

FIGURE 44–14. Simultaneous right ventricular (RV) and left ventricular (LV) pressure recordings in a patient with constrictive pericarditis. *Upper panel,* Equilibration of right and left ventricular diastolic pressures, and a characteristic dip-and-plateau contour of the diastolic waveforms. *Lower panel,* Tachycardia induced by bicycle exercise obscures the diastolic plateau, although diastolic pressures remain equilibrated. (From Shabetai, R.: The Pericardium. New York, Grune and Stratton, 1981, p. 181.)

of venous return is blunted and the venous pressure tracing shows an absent or attenuated diastolic y descent and a predominant x descent.

Another striking abnormality of constrictive pericarditis is the failure of intrathoracic pressure changes during respiration to be transmitted to the pericardial space and intracardiac chambers. As a consequence, during inspiration, systemic venous and right arterial pressures (in relation to atmosphere) do not fall and venous flow into the right atrium does not increase, in contrast to the situation in normal subjects and patients with cardiac tamponade (Fig. 44–9). In some patients, systemic venous pressure may actually increase with inspiration, i.e., *Kussmaul's sign*. This finding is not specific for constrictive pericarditis and may occur in other disorders such as chronic right ventricular failure and restrictive cardiomyopathy, in which right atrial and systemic venous pressures also are markedly elevated. However, Kussmaul's sign does *not* occur in acute cardiac tamponade, in which the inspiratory fall in intrathoracic pressure is transmitted to the fluid-filled pericardial space.[161] Pulsus paradoxus is less common in constrictive pericarditis than in cardiac tamponade, in which the mechanism is thought to be largely the exaggerated increase in right ventricular filling during inspiration at the expense of left ventricular filling. The presence of an inspiratory fall in arterial pressure greater than 10 mm Hg suggests the presence of a tense pericardial effusion or coexisting pulmonary disease.[87]

CONSEQUENCES OF PERICARDIAL CONSTRICTION. Restriction of diastolic filling ultimately results in compensatory renal retention of sodium and water that contributes further to the increase in systemic venous pressure and initially serves to maintain diastolic filling of the ventricles despite pericardial compression. In some cases, the pericardial scar is so dense that diastolic ventricular volumes are reduced. When right and left ventricular preload are substantially reduced, stroke volume and cardiac output fall despite compensatory tachycardia. The presence of reduced cardiac output, tachycardia, and elevated right and left heart filling pressures may simulate myocardial failure, and classic ventricular performance curves may show a reduced left ventricular stroke volume relative to an elevated left ventricular filling pressure. However, it must be emphasized that systolic contraction of the ventricles and the intrinsic contractile state of the myocardium are usually normal or nearly so.[162] In severe cases of constrictive pericarditis, myocardial systolic function may also be depressed because of myocardial atrophy, fibrosis, or compression of superficial coronary arteries in the fibrotic pericardium resulting in myocardial ischemia.[163–165] Although the presence of coexisting myocardial dysfunction secondary to the latter process (or of any etiology) is usually a factor predictive of a poor outcome after pericardiectomy (p. 1507), a striking improvement of left ventricular ejection fraction may occasionally occur after the stripping of a fibrotic and thick pericardium.[166]

Pathophysiological and hemodynamic findings in patients with subacute noncalcific pericarditis which causes *elastic compression of the heart* may differ from those in patients with chronic constrictive pericarditis in whom the pericardium resembles a rigid shell. Hancock has suggested that the presence of a thick fluid-fibrin layer in the process of organization leads to relatively elastic compression of the heart, which may be compared to "wrapping the heart tightly with rubber bands."[161] The pathophysiological disturbance caused by this nonrigid fibroelastic form of constrictive pericarditis is similar to that in cardiac tamponade, since fibroelastic constriction compresses the heart continuously throughout the cardiac cycle, and respiratory changes in intrathoracic pressure usually are transmitted to the cardiac chambers.[167] Thus, patterns of ventricular filling and waveforms in the subacute form of fibroelastic compression tend to resemble those of cardiac tamponade rather than of constrictive pericarditis, and include a systemic venous waveform with a predominant x descent, an inconspicuous early diastolic dip in the ventricular waveform, an inspiratory fall in systemic venous and right atrial pressures, and the presence of pulsus paradoxus (Table 44–5).

ETIOLOGY. Tuberculosis was formerly a leading cause of constrictive pericarditis.[168,169] This is still true in developing nations, whereas with the advent of antituberculosis therapy this disease now accounts for 15 per cent or fewer of cases in developed nations.[7] The largest number of cases of constrictive pericarditis today are of unknown etiology and attributed to earlier clinically inapparent viral pericarditis.[170] Other nontubercular causes include chronic renal failure treated with hemodialysis (p. 1514), connective tissue disorders including rheumatoid arthritis and systemic lupus erythematosus (pp. 1525 and 1720), and neoplastic pericardial infiltration or encasement of the heart mostly commonly caused by lung cancer, breast cancer, Hodgkin's disease, and lymphoma (p. 1515).

Constrictive pericarditis may also occur months to years after mediastinal irradiation, especially during therapy for breast cancer or Hodgkin's disease (p. 1517). Constrictive pericarditis can develop after incomplete drainage of purulent pericarditis (p. 1512), and as a complication of fungal infections (p. 1513) and parasitic infections (p. 1514). It is being increasingly recognized as a complication of cardiac surgery and cardiac procedures involving hemopericar-

TABLE 44–5 CLINICAL AND HEMODYNAMIC FEATURES OF COMPRESSIVE PERICARDIAL DISEASE

	Cardiac Tamponade	Subacute "Elastic" Constriction	Chronic "Rigid" Constriction
Duration of symptoms	Hours to days	Weeks to months	Months to years
Chest pain, friction rub	Usual	Recent past	Remote
Pulsus paradoxus	Prominent	Usually prominent	Slight or absent
Kussmaul's sign	Absent	Usually absent	Often present
Early diastolic knock	Absent	Usually absent	Often present
Heart size on chest roentgenogram	Usually enlarged	Usually enlarged	Usually normal, sometimes enlarged
Pericardial calcification	Absent	Rare	Often present
Abnormal P waves or atrial fibrillation	Absent	Absent	Often present
Venous (right atrial) waveform	X or Xy	Xy or XY	XY or xY
Pericardial effusion	Always present	Often present	Absent

X and Y = prominent x and y descents, respectively, x and y = inconspicuous x and y descents.
Modified from Hancock, E. W.: On the elastic and rigid forms of constrictive pericarditis. Am. Heart J. *100*:917, 1980.

dium (p. 1523).[171] Constrictive pericarditis may occasionally follow pericarditis associated with acute myocardial infarction and the postpericardiotomy syndrome.

CONSTRICTIVE PERICARDITIS IN CHILDREN. Constrictive pericarditis is far less common in children than in adults and may rarely occur following a viral syndrome in a child mistakenly thought to have hepatitis or a protein-losing enteropathy. When constrictive pericarditis occurs in young children, tuberculosis should be strongly considered since it has been shown to be a proved or highly likely cause in 56 per cent of 84 children with constrictive pericarditis reported in the literature.[172] Nontraumatic hemopericardium has been reported in children and young adults with congenital bleeding disorders complicated by a second process such as endocarditis or viral syndrome, and constrictive pericarditis has occurred following pericardial bleeding caused by congenital afibrinogenemia.[173] The newly described familial syndrome of pericarditis, arthritis, and camptodactyly (flexion contractures) is an uncommon cause of constrictive pericarditis in children and young adults.[174] An uncommon congenital cause of constrictive pericarditis is *mulibrey nanism,* an autosomal recessive disorder characterized by dwarfism, constrictive pericarditis, abnormal fundi, and fibrous dysplasia of the long bones.[175]

CLINICAL FEATURES

The principal clinical features of severe chronic constrictive pericarditis were vividly described by Cheevers of Guy's Hospital in 1842.[176] In patients in whom systemic venous and right atrial pressures are modestly elevated (10 to 15 mm Hg), left ventricular filling pressure is also usually only modestly elevated. In this setting, symptoms secondary to systemic venous congestion such as edema, abdominal swelling, and discomfort resulting from ascites and passive hepatic congestion may predominate. Vague abdominal symptoms such as postprandial fullness, dyspepsia, flatulence, and anorexia may also be present. When both right and left heart filling pressures are elevated to the level of 15 to 30 mm Hg, symptoms of pulmonary venous congestion, such as exertional dyspnea, cough, and orthopnea, are present. Pleural effusions and elevation of the diaphragm due to ascites may also contribute to dyspnea. Severe fatigue, weight loss, and muscle wasting suggest the presence of a fixed or reduced cardiac output.

PHYSICAL EXAMINATION. The single most important finding is elevation of jugular venous pressure. If the neck is examined casually, or if the patient is examined supine so that jugular venous pressure is measured above the angle of the jaw, this important clue to the presence of constrictive pericarditis may be missed. A prominent feature of the elevated jugular venous pressure is the rapidly collapsing negative wave of the diastolic y descent.[177] In patients in sinus rhythm, both x and y descents can be distinguished; the x descent is synchronous while the diastolic y is out of phase with the carotid pulse. These features may be difficult to detect in patients with tachycardia, tachypnea, or arrhythmia. It may also be difficult to distinguish between right heart failure due to tricuspid regurgitation and chronic constrictive pericarditis by neck vein examination at the bedside. The finding of Kussmaul's sign (an inspiratory increase in systemic venous pressure) is difficult to appreciate at the bedside and may be confused with exaggerated amplitude of the venous waves during inspiration.

The arterial pulse may be normal or show a diminished pulse pressure. Severe pulsus paradoxus is uncommon in rigid constrictive pericarditis unless pericardial fluid under pressure is also present.[171] Systolic retraction of the apical impulse occurs in the majority of patients and usually consists of an unobtrusive diffuse precordial movement.[178]

Auscultatory Findings. The most impressive abnormality during auscultation is the *diastolic pericardial knock*, an early diastolic sound that is often heard along

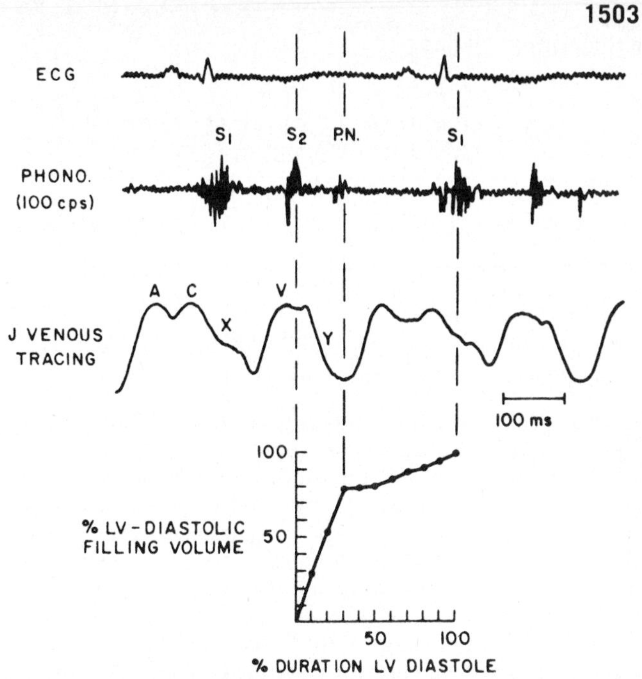

FIGURE 44–15. Electrocardiogram (ECG), phonocardiogram (PHONO), jugular venous pulse tracing, and left ventricular (LV) diastolic filling curve in a patient with constrictive pericarditis and pericardial knock (PN). The pericardial knock occurs simultaneously with the nadir of the diastolic *y* descent and sudden plateau of the LV filling curve. (From Tyberg, T. I., et al.: Genesis of pericardial knock in constrictive pericarditis. Am. J. Cardiol. 46:570, 1980.)

the left sternal border in rigid constrictive pericarditis, is infrequently heard in subacute constrictive pericarditis of the fibroelastic variety, and is not heard in pure cardiac tamponade.[161] The pericardial knock usually occurs 0.09 to 0.12 second after A_2 and corresponds in timing to the sudden cessation of ventricular filling and the premature diastolic plateau of the diastolic ventricular volume curve (Fig. 44–15).[179] The pericardial knock tends to occur earlier and to have a higher acoustic frequency than the typical S_3 gallop sound, and therefore it may be confused with the opening snap of mitral stenosis. Widening of the aortic and pulmonic components of the second heart sound may occur in constrictive pericarditis. This is attributed to a fixed right ventricular stroke volume during inspiration due to pericardial compression as well as the presence of premature aortic valve closure due to a transitory inspiratory decrease in left ventricular stroke volume.

Extracardiac Findings. Hepatomegaly is usually present and prominent hepatic pulsations which conform to the jugular venous pulse can be detected in 70 per cent of patients (Fig. 2–6, p. 19).[180] Other evidence of hepatic dysfunction secondary to passive liver congestion and diminished cardiac output includes ascites, icterus, spider angiomas, and palmar erythema. In young patients with competent venous valves, edema of the extremities may be noticeably absent in the presence of marked abdominal distention. Older patients with longstanding constrictive pericarditis may have enormous ascites and massive swelling of the scrotum, thighs, and calves. In contrast, the upper torso and arms may show evidence of marked muscle wasting and cachexia.

CHEST ROENTGENOGRAM (See also p. 166). The cardiac silhouette may be small, normal, or enlarged. Cardiac enlargement may be apparent due to coexisting pericardial effusion, the contribution of an enormously thickened pericardium, or preexisting cardiac chamber enlargement or hypertrophy. The right superior mediastinum may be prominent due to engorgement of the superior vena cava, and left atrial enlargement is common.[181] Extensive calci-

TABLE 44–6 RADIOLOGICAL FEATURES OF CONSTRICTIVE PERICARDITIS

Normal heart size	33%
Enlarged heart	67%
Calcified pericardium	43%
Pleural effusion	83%
Pulmonary venous congestion	86%
Left atrial enlargement	85%

Modified from Pulvaneswary, M., et al.: Constrictive pericarditis. Clinical, hemodynamic, and radiologic correlation. Australas. Radiol. 26:53, 1982.

fication of the pericardium is present in approximately half the patients and raises the possibility of a tubercular etiology. However, this finding is not specific for constrictive pericarditis in that a calcified pericardium is not necessarily a constricted one. Calcification of the pericardium is often detected on the lateral chest film in the atrioventricular groove or along the anterior and diaphragmatic surfaces of the right ventricle. Fluoroscopy may be helpful in distinguishing pericardial calcification from calcium within the wall of a myocardial aneurysm or thrombus or within the mitral or aortic valves, mitral annulus, or coronary arteries. Pleural effusions are present in the majority of patients. Since left atrial pressure is commonly elevated to between 15 to 30 mm Hg, there may be evidence of redistribution of blood flow, while Kerley's B lines or infiltrates suggestive of frank pulmonary edema are rare (Table 44–6).

ELECTROCARDIOGRAM. Electrocardiographic findings include low QRS voltage, generalized T-wave inversion or flattening, and left atrial abnormalities suggestive of P mitrale (Fig. 44–16).[59] Atrial fibrillation occurs in less than half the patients with constrictive pericarditis and is thought to be related to longstanding elevation of atrial pressures and atrial enlargement. In a postmortem study of constrictive pericarditis, Levine noted that atrioventricular block, intraventricular conduction defects, and pseudoinfarction patterns with deep wide Q waves seemed to be related to an extension of calcification into the myocardium and around the coronary arteries, compromising coronary blood flow.[164] An unusual pattern of right ventricular hypertrophy and right-axis deviation may be present in about 5 per cent of patients due to dense pericardial scar overlying the right ventricular outflow tract.[182]

ECHOCARDIOGRAM (See also p. 128). One distinct M-mode echocardiographic pattern of pericardial thickening in constrictive pericarditis consists of two parallel lines representing the visceral and parietal pericardia separated by a clear space of at least 1 mm; another consists of

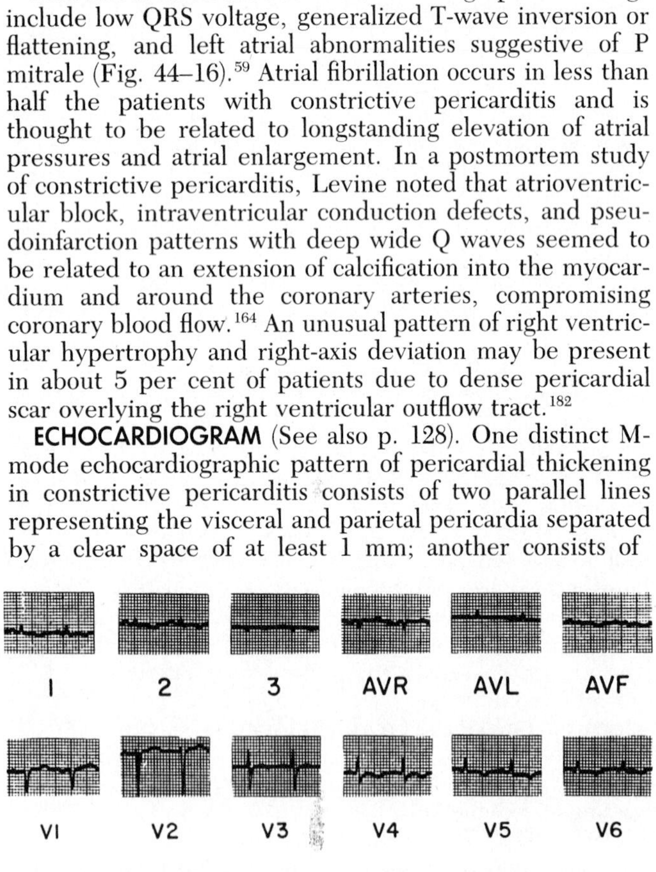

FIGURE 44–16. Electrocardiogram of a patient with constrictive pericarditis, showing low-voltage QRS complexes in the limb leads and in the left precordial leads. Diffuse nonspecific T-wave abnormalities are present. (Reproduced by permission from Fowler, N. O.: Constrictive pericarditis. *In* Fowler, N. O. [ed.]: The Pericardium in Health and Disease. Mt. Kisco, NY, Futura Publishing Co., 1985, p. 312.)

multiple dense echoes.[183] Extreme respiratory variation in the depth of the pulmonic valve *a* wave[184] and premature pulmonic valve opening secondary to a high right ventricular early diastolic pressure may be present[185]; however, these changes are also seen in other disorders with high right ventricular early diastolic pressure, such as tricuspid and pulmonic regurgitation. Other M-mode echocardiographic abnormalities include abrupt posterior motion of the interventricular septum in early diastole, coinciding with the pericardial knock, and abrupt posterior motion during atrial systole[186] (Fig. 5–106, p. 129). Engel et al.[187] recently reviewed M-mode echocardiograms from 40 patients with proven constrictive pericarditis and 40 normal subjects. They observed that normal left ventricular size, left atrial enlargement, flattened diastolic ventricular wall motion, and abnormal septal motion were present in most patients, but no single feature was diagnostic of constrictive pericarditis. Computer-assisted digitization of M-mode echocardiograms may be useful in distinguishing the abnormal rapid early diastolic filling of constrictive pericarditis from the more delayed filling pattern of restrictive cardiomyopathy.[188]

Two-dimensional echocardiography in constrictive pericarditis has been reported to show an immobile and dense appearance of the pericardium, bulging of the interventricular septum into the left ventricle during inspiration, prominent early diastolic filling, and dilatation of the hepatic veins and inferior vena cava.[189] Intense and spontaneous contrast in the inferior vena cava can also be seen.[190] Further studies in an experimental dog model and in patients have confirmed that two-dimensional echocardiography can demonstrate abnormal early diastolic filling but greatly overestimates pericardial thickness.[191]

COMPUTED TOMOGRAPHY AND MAGNETIC RESONANCE IMAGING. Computed tomography (CT) has also emerged as a valuable tool in the evaluation of suspected constrictive pericarditis (Fig. 44–17) (see also Figs. 12–11, p. 364 and 12–12, p. 365). This technique is especially useful in identifying pericardial thickening and geometry and in identifying other findings compatible with constrictive pericarditis, including dilation of the venae cavae and deformation of the right ventricle.[192–194] Nonvisualization of the left ventricular posterolateral wall by CT suggests coexisting myocardial fibrosis or atrophy and predicts a poor outcome following pericardiectomy.[195] The early experience with magnetic resonance imaging (MRI) in patients with constrictive pericarditis suggests that it can detect findings suggestive of constrictive pericarditis including pericardial thickening, dilatation of the venae cavae and hepatic veins, and narrowing of the right ventricle (Fig. 44–18)[196] (see also Fig. 12–32, p. 373).

OTHER LABORATORY FINDINGS. Chronic elevation of right atrial pressure causing passive congestion of the liver, kidneys, and gastrointestinal tract may cause other abnormal laboratory findings. These include depressed serum albumin, elevated serum globulin, elevated conjugated and unconjugated serum bilirubin, and abnormal hepatocellular function tests. In patients with hepatomegaly and ascites, liver biopsy may show histological features similar to the Budd-Chiari syndrome, including hepatic venule thrombi and ductular proliferation.[197] Protein-losing enteropathy may be evident from the presence of albumin in the stool and lymphangiectasis on small bowel biopsy.[198] Elevated systemic venous pressure may also produce variable degrees of albuminuria as well as pronounced protein loss consistent with the nephrotic syndrome.[199] Nonspecific evidence of the presence of chronic disease such as a normocytic and normochromic anemia may be found.

DIFFERENTIAL DIAGNOSIS. Constrictive pericarditis

should be suspected in patients with jugular venous distention, unexplained cardiac enlargement, hepatomegaly, systemic edema, or ascites. It must be distinguished from superior vena caval obstruction, nephrotic syndrome, hepatic and intraabdominal disease due to malignancy, and other cardiac causes of right atrial hypertension including restrictive cardiomyopathy (p. 1430), triscupid stenosis (p. 1069), tricuspid regurgitation (p. 1072), hypertrophic cardiomyopathy (p. 1418), and right atrial myxoma (p. 1472). Patients with constrictive pericarditis may be extremely difficult to distinguish from those with restrictive physiology due to amyloidosis, hemochromatosis,[200] and the hypereosinophilic syndrome which may involve pericardium as well as the myocardium.[201, 202] Both constrictive pericarditis and restrictive cardiomyopathy may show the electrocardiographic changes of atrial fibrillation, left atrial abnormalities, and diffuse low QRS voltage with T-wave flattening. The presence of atrioventricular block and conduction disturbances simulating myocardial infarction favors the diagnosis of restrictive cardiomyopathy. Echocardiography in some patients with restrictive cardiomyopathy may show abnormal thickening of the ventricular myocardium or a peculiar "sparkling" appearance when amyloidosis is present.[203] The simultaneous use of electrocardiography and echocardiography to demonstrate a reduction of the voltage:mass ratio has been described in patients with amyloid restrictive cardiomyopathy in whom diffuse low QRS voltage is associated with increased thickness of the left ventricular wall due to amyloid deposition.[204]

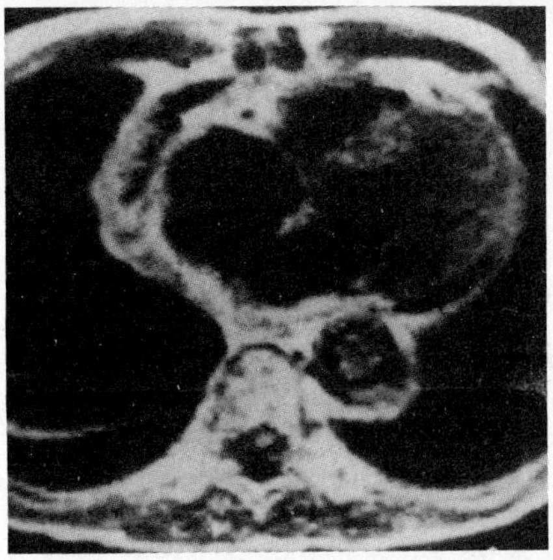

FIGURE 44–18. Magnetic resonance image from a patient with constrictive uremic pericarditis shows irregular thickening of the visceral and parietal pericardial layers, which are separated by low-intensity fluid, overlying the enlarged right atrium. Pericardial fluid is also present behind the left ventricle, which is hypertrophied. (From Soulen, R. L., et al.: Magnetic resonance imaging of constrictive pericardial disease. Am. J. Cardiol. *55*:480, 1985.)

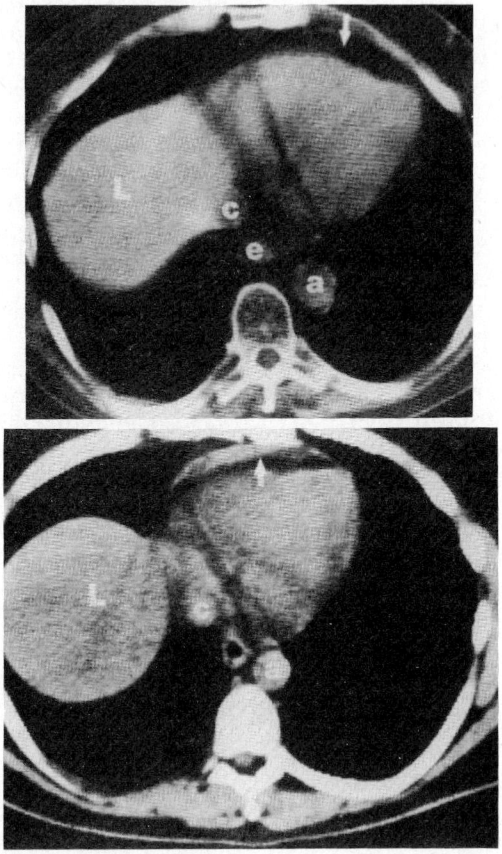

FIGURE 44–17. Computed tomographic scans from a normal adult (*top*) and from a patient with constrictive pericarditis (*bottom*). The normal pericardium (arrow, top) has the appearance of a faint, pencil-thin line outlined by low-density epicardial and mediastinal fat. The pericardium from the patient with constrictive pericarditis (arrow, bottom) appears markedly thickened. Both scans were obtained at the level of the right hemidiaphragm where the dome of the liver (L), the esophagus (e), inferior vena cava (c), and the descending thoracic aorta (a) can be seen. (From Sutton, F. J., et al.: The role of echocardiography and computed tomography in the evaluation of constrictive pericarditis. Am. Heart J. *109*:350, 1985.)

In the presence of findings suggestive of constrictive pericarditis, right and left heart catheterization should be performed to document the presence of constrictive physiology and to exclude other causes of right atrial hypertension. Diuresis should be avoided before catheterization since hypovolemia may obscure the characteristic hemodynamic findings. Cardiac catheterization and angiography, often with endomyocardial biopsy, are usually helpful in discriminating constrictive pericarditis from restrictive cardiomyopathy in many patients, but, in a minority, an exploratory thoracotomy may be required.

CARDIAC CATHETERIZATION AND ANGIOGRAPHY

Cardiac catheterization is useful in the assessment of patients suspected of having constrictive pericarditis (1) to document the presence of elevation and equilibrium of diastolic filling pressures, (2) to assess the effects of constrictive pericarditis on stroke volume and cardiac output, (3) to evaluate myocardial systolic function, (4) to assist in the difficult discrimination between constrictive pericarditis and restrictive cardiomyopathy, and (5) to exclude compression of the coronary arteries by the fibrotic pericardium.

Catheterization of both the right and left ventricles should be performed to permit the simultaneous recording of right and left heart filling pressures. Typical findings include the elevation and virtual identity (within 5 mm Hg) of right atrial, right ventricular diastolic, left atrial (pulmonary capillary wedge), and left ventricular diastolic pressures before the *a* wave. Right atrial pressure is characterized by a preserved systolic *x* descent, a prominent early diastolic *y* descent, and *a* and *v* waves that are small and equal in height and result in the typical "M" or "W" configurations (Fig. 44–19). Both the right and left ventricular diastolic pressures show an early diastolic dip followed by a pressure plateau.[91, 150] This sign may be obscured by the presence of tachycardia, although the equilibration of diastolic pressures persists during exercise (Fig. 44–20), and the damping effect of connecting tubes or bubbles within the catheters and transducers. Right ventricular and pulmonary artery systolic pressures are usually modestly elevated, in the range of 35 to 40 mm

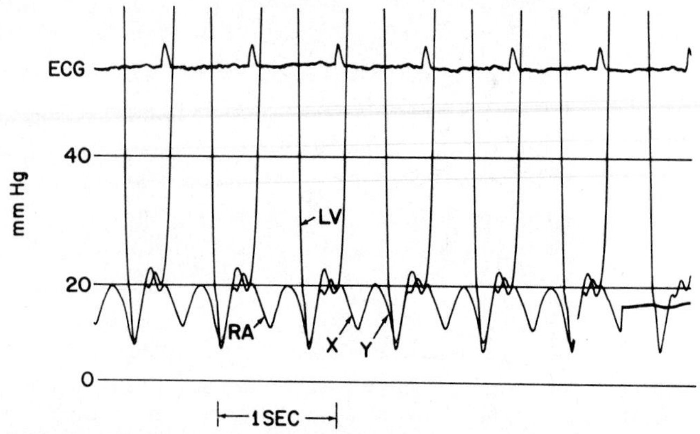

FIGURE 44–19. Simultaneous left ventricular (LV) and right atrial (RA) pressure recordings from a patient with constrictive pericarditis which show that both pressures are elevated and virtually equal throughout diastole. The prominent diastolic *y* descent in the right atrial waveform indicates that right atrial emptying is rapid and unimpeded in early diastole. In contrast, the *y* descent is absent or attenuated in cardiac tamponade because cardiac compression limits right ventricular filling throughout diastole. (From Lorell, B. H., and Grossman, W.: Profiles in constrictive pericarditis, restrictive cardiomyopathy, and cardiac tamponade. In Grossman, W. [ed.]: Cardiac Catheterization and Angiography. Philadelphia, Lea and Febiger, 1986, p. 440.)

Hg, and rarely exceed 60 mm Hg. When hemodynamics at rest are unremarkable, the rapid infusion of about 1000 ml of warmed saline over 6 to 8 minutes may unmask these findings in the occasional patient with *occult constrictive pericarditis.*[205, 206]

Careful recordings during respiration show that mean right atrial pressure fails to decrease normally or actually rises during inspiration (a hemodynamic correlate of Kussmaul's sign). Since inspiration is associated with the transient pooling of blood within the pulmonary bed and a reduction in right ventricular afterload, inspiration causes a fall in pulmonary artery and right ventricular systolic pressures, pulmonary capillary wedge pressure, and left ventricular diastolic pressure. Because constrictive pericarditis is not associated with marked inspiratory swings in right ventricular filling, pulsus paradoxus is usually absent or less prominent than that observed in cardiac tamponade. Both cardiac output and stroke volume are low-normal or depressed.[150] When they are depressed, compensatory tachycardia and elevation of systemic vascular resistance may be found.

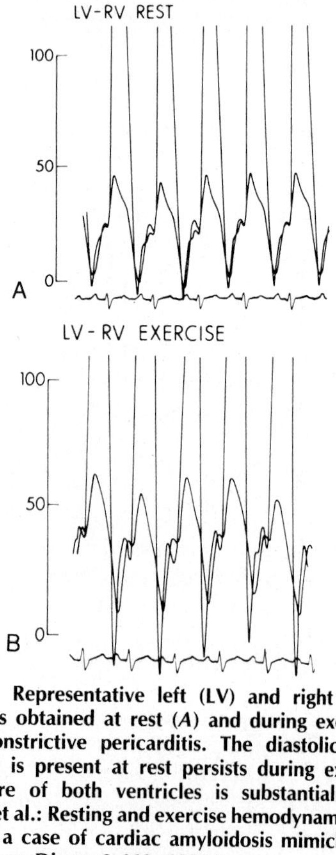

FIGURE 44–20. Representative left (LV) and right ventricular (RV) pressure tracings obtained at rest (*A*) and during exercise (*B*) from a patient with constrictive pericarditis. The diastolic equalization of pressures which is present at rest persists during exercise when the diastolic pressure of both ventricles is substantially higher. (From Robbins, M. A., et al.: Resting and exercise hemodynamics in constrictive pericarditis and a case of cardiac amyloidosis mimicking constriction. Cathet. Cardiovasc. Diagn. 9:463, 1983.)

The *left ventricular angiogram* usually demonstrates that left ventricular end-systolic and end-diastolic volumes are normal or decreased. In the absence of myocardial fibrosis or inflammation, both isovolumetric and ejection-phase indices of systolic function (Chap. 15) are normal.[207] Venous angiography may demonstrate superior vena caval dilatation and straightening of the right heart border; pericardial thickening may be detectable. These findings contrast with those of cardiac tamponade in which diastolic compression of the superior vena cava and right atrium is present. Coronary angiography may demonstrate that the coronary arteries are within the cardiac silhouette rather than on the surface of the heart, and diastolic pinching or external compression of the coronary arteries may be detected occasionally.[208, 209]

HEMODYNAMIC DIFFERENTIATION AMONG CONSTRICTIVE PERICARDITIS, CARDIAC TAMPONADE, AND RESTRICTIVE CARDIOMYOPATHY (See also p. 1492). Although both constrictive pericarditis and tamponade are characterized by elevation and equilibrium of right and left ventricular diastolic pressures, several hemodynamic features differ. In contrast to patients with constrictive pericarditis, patients with cardiac tamponade demonstrate (1) pulsus paradoxus, often marked, (2) a fall in right atrial pressure during inspiration, (3) elevation of intrapericardial pressure, (4) a right atrial pressure tracing with a predominant *x* descent and an attenuated or absent *y* descent, and (5) lack of a prominent dip-and-plateau pattern in the right and left ventricular pressure pulses.

The findings of cardiac catheterization help to differentiate some but not all patients with constrictive pericarditis from those with *restrictive cardiomyopathy* (p. 1431) due to amyloidosis, hemochromatosis, or other causes (Table 44–7). In both conditions, right and left ventricular diastolic pressures are elevated, stroke volume and cardiac output are depressed, left ventricular end-diastolic volume is normal or decreased, and diastolic filling is impaired. A diagnosis of restrictive cardiomyopathy is more likely when marked right ventricular systolic hypertension is present (pressure > 60 mg Hg), and left ventricular diastolic pressure exceeds right ventricular diastolic pressure at rest or during exercise by more than 5 mm Hg.[210] However, in some patients with restrictive cardiomyopathy, hemodynamics at rest and during exercise may be indistinguishable from constrictive pericarditis, with equilibration of right and left ventricular diastolic pressures and a predominant dip-and-plateau pattern in the ventricular waveforms.[150, 211–213]

On angiography, straightening of the right heart border may be present in both conditions, and thickening of the heart border may be detected because of either pericardial or myocardial thickening.[214] Decreased motion of the right ventricular free wall occurs in both conditions, while normal motion of the crista supraventricularis is usually present in constrictive pericarditis but not in restrictive cardiomyopathy.[215]

The finding of a depressed left ventricular ejection

TABLE 44–7 CONSTRICTIVE PERICARDITIS VERSUS RESTRICTIVE CARDIOMYOPATHY

	Constrictive Pericarditis	Restrictive Cardiomyopathy
S_3 gallop	Absent	May be present
Pericardial knock	May be present	Absent
Palpable systolic apical impulse	Absent	May be present
Pericardial calcification	Present 50%	Absent
Pulsus paradoxus	May be present	May be present
Equal RV and LV diastolic pressures	Usually present	LV > RV
Rate of LV filling	80% in first half of diastole	40% in first half of diastole
PEP/LVET	Av. 0.31	Av. 0.48 (congestive failure)
CAT scan, echo, MRI	Thickened pericardium	Normal pericardium

Modified from Fowler, N. O.: Constrictive pericarditis. *In* Fowler, N. O. (ed.): The Pericardium in Health and Disease. Mt. Kisco, NY, Futura Publishing Co., 1985, p. 319.

fraction in the presence of a small heart has been suggested as a diagnostic feature of restrictive cardiomyopathy.[214] However, the left ventricular ejection fraction may be normal in some patients with restrictive cardiomyopathy and, conversely, is occasionally reduced in patients with constrictive pericarditis.[211, 212] Frame-by-frame analysis of left ventricular filling has been suggested as a method for differentiating between constrictive pericarditis and restrictive cardiomyopathy.[216] In constrictive pericarditis, early diastolic filling tends to be excessively rapid in contrast to restrictive cardiomyopathy, in which early diastolic filling is slower than normal.

Endomyocardial biopsy has also proved useful in documenting the presence of amyloidosis and other forms of infiltrative myocardial disease in patients in whom constrictive pericarditis and restrictive cardiomyopathy could not be differentiated at cardiac catheterization.[211, 216a] However, normal findings on endomyocardial biopsy do not exclude the presence of a restrictive cardiomyopathy.[212] Furthermore, a pericardial effusion may on occasion coexist with amyloid heart disease.[217, 218] Computed tomography and magnetic resonance imaging are enormously valuable in differentiating between constrictive pericarditis and restrictive cardiomyopathy. In an ever-decreasing minority of patients, exploratory thoracotomy with careful examination of both pericardial and myocardial biopsy specimens is warranted to differentiate constrictive pericarditis, a condition that is usually treatable surgically, from restrictive cardiomyopathy, in which treatment is usually expectant.

MANAGEMENT

Constrictive pericarditis is a progressive disease without spontaneous reversal of either pericardial thickening or abnormal symptoms and hemodynamics. A minority of patients may survive for many years with moderate jugular venous distention and peripheral edema that is controlled by the judicious use of diet and diuretics. The majority of patients who are symptomatic and come to medical attention, however, become progressively more disabled by weakness, ascites, and peripheral edema and subsequently suffer the complications of severe cardiac cachexia. Treatment for constrictive pericarditis is complete resection of the pericardium, which achieves excision of the pericardium from the anterior and inferior surfaces of the right ventricle and the diaphragmatic and anterolateral surfaces of the left ventricle extending to the great vessels and to or across the atrioventricular grooves. The use of a median sternotomy rather than a left thoracotomy and of cardiopulmonary bypass permits greater mobilization of the heart.[219] Performance of pericardiectomy earlier in the course of the disease before appearance of cardiac cachexia and dense pericardial calcification has been a useful development.

In 1980, Culliford et al. reported an operative mortality of 15 per cent with a range of 6 to 25 per cent in over 300 reported cases of pericardiectomy.[220] In over 400 cases reported in 7 series since 1981, the average operative mortality was 12 per cent and ranged from 7 to 14 per cent.[154, 155, 221–225] A low-output syndrome occurred in 14 to 28 per cent of patients in the immediate postoperative period, and risk factors predictive of in-hospital mortality and low-output syndrome include the degree of preoperative disability (functional Class III or IV) and severity of constriction as indicated by a marked elevation of right ventricular end-diastolic pressure.[221, 224] Symptomatic improvement can be expected in about 90 per cent of survivors.[220–222, 224] Careful actuarial analysis of long-term survival has been available in large series from the Mayo Clinic[221] and Stanford,[224] which have reported a 5-year survival of 84 and 74 per cent, respectively. Long-term survival does not appear to be influenced by age, choice of median sternotomy or left thoracotomy, or low-output syndrome postoperatively. However, overall outcome is unfavorably influenced by the presence of functional Class IV preoperatively, diuretic use, renal insufficiency in the preoperative state, and the presence of radiation pericarditis.[211, 224] These considerations indicate that pericardiectomy should be performed early in the course of symptomatic patients with constrictive pericarditis since the development of severe clinical disability is associated with a poor surgical outcome.

Pericardiectomy probably should *not* be attempted routinely in very elderly patients with severe liver dysfunction, cachexia, densely calcified pericardium, and massive cardiac enlargement indicative of underlying myocardial damage, or in patients with a limited life expectancy. Patients with known or suspected tubercular pericarditis should be treated with combined antituberculosis drugs for 1 to 4 weeks prior to operation, depending on the urgency of the situation; if the diagnosis is confirmed, these drugs should be continued for 6 to 12 months after pericardiectomy.

Marked hemodynamic and symptomatic improvement is apparent in some patients immediately after operation. In others, symptomatic improvement and resolution of elevated jugular venous pressure and abnormal filling patterns may be delayed for weeks to months.[226] This delayed or inadequate response to pericardiectomy has been attributed to incomplete pericardial resection, myocardial damage by the inflammatory process,[221, 224, 227] and development of recurrent cardiac compression by mediastinal inflammation and fibrosis.[228, 229] Unrecognized constriction by an epicardial peel (visceral pericardium) may be responsible for a poor response to pericardiectomy.[230, 231] The importance of visceral constriction has also been underscored by the Stanford experience in which 59 per cent of patients had involvement of the visceral pericardium (epicardium) and required visceral decortication.[224] Consideration should be given to epicardial dissection when there is little change in size of the heart or fall in intracardiac pressures after removal of the parietal pericardial layer.[221]

EFFUSIVE-CONSTRICTIVE PERICARDITIS

In effusive-constrictive pericarditis a tense pericardial effusion exists in the presence of visceral pericardial constriction.[232, 233] The hallmark of this condition is continued elevation of right atrial pressure after the aspiration of pericardial fluid and restoration of intrapericardial pressure to zero. This entity may represent a stage in the development of classic constrictive pericarditis. The most common causes of effusive-constrictive pericarditis are the same as for chronic constrictive pericarditis (p. 1502) and include idiopathic or presumed viral pericarditis, tuberculosis, neoplastic infiltration of the pericardium, and mediastinal irradiation.[233, 234] *Symptoms* are nonspecific and include atypical chest pain and a heavy sensation over the precordium; in advanced cases, exertional dyspnea may be present.

The *physical findings* usually resemble those of cardiac tamponade, including pulsus paradoxus, a normal or diminished pulse pressure, and jugular venous distention with a predominant *x* descent and an attenuated or absent *y* descent. The chest roentgenogram usually shows cardiac enlargement consistent with the presence of a pericardial effusion, and the electrocardiogram may show nonspecific ST- and T-wave abnormalities or diffuse low QRS voltage. Both M-mode and two-dimensional echocardiograms may show a pericardial effusion sandwiched between thickened pericardial membranes with fibrinous pericardial bands.[235]

DIAGNOSIS. Although effusive-constrictive pericarditis can be suspected on clinical grounds, the diagnosis is made by recording right heart and intrapericardial pressures both before and after pericardiocentesis.[233, 234] Prior to pericardiocentesis, the physiology of cardiac tamponade may be present (p. 1492) with elevation and equilibration of intrapericardial, right atrial, right ventricular, and left ventricular diastolic pressures. The right atrial pressure tracing usually shows a prominent *x* descent and an inspiratory fall in right heart filling pressure. Pericardiocentesis with restoration of intrapericardial pressure to zero may reduce pulsus paradoxus and improve cardiac output, but it does not restore the hemodynamics entirely to normal. After pericardiocentesis, there is persistent elevation and equilibration of right atrial and right and left ventricular diastolic pressures. The waveforms convert to a pattern like that in constrictive pericarditis, with a prominent *y* descent in the right atrial pressure tracing, a dip-and-plateau pattern in the right ventricular pressure, and the absence of respiratory variation in right heart filling pressures.

MANAGEMENT. Pericardiocentesis may be useful in transiently improving systemic arterial pressure and cardiac output. However, persistent constriction after successful pericardiocentesis indicates the presence of a thickened, constrictive visceral pericardium and the need for further intervention. Treatment consists of total parietal and visceral pericardiectomy[231, 233] and specific therapy for underlying malignancy or tuberculosis, if present.

SPECIFIC FORMS OF PERICARDITIS

VIRAL PERICARDITIS

ETIOLOGY AND PATHOGENESIS. The viruses that most commonly cause acute pericarditis are Coxsackie virus group B and echovirus type 8.[236] Although viral pericarditis appears to be uncommon in young children, coxsackie A9 has been reported as a cause of pericarditis in neonates.[237] Other viruses responsible for acute pericarditis include those that cause myocarditis (Table 42–12, p. 1442) and includes mumps, influenza, infectious mononucleosis, poliomyelitis, varicella, and hepatitis B.[238–241] Infectious mononucleosis may cause acute myopericarditis with the complications of cardiac tamponade, constrictive pericarditis, and severe chest pain.[239] Varicella (chickenpox) may be associated with the complications of both severe viral pneumonia and acute pericarditis.[240] *Mycoplasma pneumoniae*, an important cause of adult nonbacterial pneumonia, also rarely causes myopericarditis.[242] Cytomegalovirus and other unusual pathogens may cause pericarditis in immunocompromised patients,[243] including those with the acquired immunodeficiency syndrome (AIDS).[244, 245] There are no clinical features that distinguish acute viral pericarditis from idiopathic pericarditis, and it is likely that many cases of community-acquired idiopathic pericarditis are due to unrecognized viral infections. The seasonal peak incidence of idiopathic pericarditis is in the spring and fall, which coincides with the increased incidence of enterovirus epidemics.

PATHOLOGY. Viral pericarditis causes inflammation of the visceral and parietal pericardial membranes, with infiltration first of polymorphonuclear leukocytes and then of lymphocytes around small vessels. Fibrin is deposited in the pericardial space, giving the pericardium a shaggy, reddened appearance. In some cases, the inflammation may result in a serous, serofibrinous, suppurative, or hemorrhagic effusion with a predominance of lymphocytes. Both echo- and Coxsackie viruses may produce suppurative effusions that resolve by organization, formation of thick adhesions, calcification, and thickening of the pericardium, resulting in constrictive pericarditis.[246]

CLINICAL FINDINGS. A prodromal syndrome of an upper respiratory tract infection that may be described as a "cold" or the "flu" within the preceding weeks is frequently reported by patients with viral pericarditis. The clinical features of viral pericarditis are similar to those of acute pericarditis of many causes which were described earlier (p. 1487). Viral or idiopathic pericarditis should be suspected in young or otherwise healthy adults with a characteristic prodromal illness and a syndrome of acute pericardial pain. It must be differentiated from pericarditis due to trauma, purulent pericardial infection, myocarditis, and systemic lupus erythematosus. In older patients, pericarditis due to rheumatoid disorders, myocardial infarction, tuberculosis, or neoplasm should be investigated before a viral etiology is presumed. The diagnosis of viral infection is strongly supported by the finding of a greater than fourfold rise in serial neutralizing viral antibody titers during the initial 3 weeks of illness.[87] It is rarely productive to attempt to isolate virus from blood, pericardial fluid, pleural fluid, or stool. The development of reverse immunoassays (RIA's) of antibodies to enteroviruses holds promise for studies of the role of these viruses in acute pericarditis. In one series positive Coxsackie B-specific IgM RIA titers were detected in 97 per cent of 30 patients with proved enterovirus infections and in 49 per cent of 37 patients with idiopathic myopericarditis, while positive responses were rare in control specimens from normal subjects.[247] Pericarditis due to infectious mononucleosis is suggested in the clinical setting of the young patient with high fever, adenopathy, sore throat, and positive heterophil test.

In a patient with a viral illness, the diagnosis of suspected pericarditis is confirmed clinically by the finding of a characteristic pericardial friction rub. Serial electrocardiographic changes of acute pericarditis (p. 1489) are not specific for the etiology of either viral or idiopathic pericarditis; however, the appearance of characteristic electrocardiographic changes may lead to the recognition of pericardial involvement in patients with a viral upper respiratory tract infection. Echocardiographic documentation of a pericardial effusion is also supportive evidence of pericardial inflammation in a patient with a viral upper respiratory tract infection and chest pain. Other laboratory findings suggestive of inflammation but not diagnostic of pericarditis include elevation of the sedimentation rate and leukocytosis. Cardiac isoenzymes are frequently abnormally elevated and suggest the presence of extensive associated epicarditis or myocarditis.[68–70]

Acute viral or idiopathic pericarditis is usually a short, dramatic, self-limited illness lasting 1 to 3 weeks. Important complications of acute viral or idiopathic pericarditis include (1) associated myocarditis, (2) recurrent pericarditis, (3) pericardial effusion with cardiac tamponade, and (4) the late development of constrictive pericarditis. Acute myocarditis, which may develop in association with pericarditis due to any of the viruses causing acute pericarditis (p. 1442) may result in acute congestive heart failure, arrhythmias or conduction disturbances, and cardiac enlargement that usually resolves completely or uncommonly leads to the development of a chronic congestive cardiomyopathy.

Pericarditis may recur several weeks later in about 15 to 40 per cent of patients, and a small number of patients develop disabling recurrences over months to years that are extremely difficult to manage.[72] These recurrences of pericardial pain may be due to an immunological response to the initial viral injury rather than recurrent viral infections of the pericardium. This hypothesis is supported by detailed observations in a patient with severe recurrent pericarditis whose neutralizing antibody titers against Coxsackie B rose only during the first attack and in whom interferon successfully inhibited recurrent pericarditis.[248]

MANAGEMENT. Treatment is directed against symptoms, with close observation for the development of cardiac tamponade or myocarditis early in the patient's course. For these reasons, most patients with an initial acute episode of pericarditis should be observed in the hospital. Bed or chair rest is warranted, and the avoidance of excessive motion and exercise helps to relieve pericardial pain and dyspnea. Pericardial pain and fever usually respond to nonsteroidal antiinflammatory agents and occasionally require steroids. Patients may be discharged from the hospital when fever and pericardial pain have disappeared and any pericardial effusion that was present has decreased in size. However, patients should be examined at regular intervals over the next few weeks to look for the complications of effusive-constrictive pericarditis and at longer intervals for the development of late constrictive pericarditis. Patients who develop tachyarrhythmias or acute conduction defects suggestive of myocardial involvement warrant close observation and electrocardiographic monitoring.

Recurrent pericarditis may require the reinstitution of antiinflammatory drug therapy with titration to the minimum dose needed to relieve symptoms, followed by gradual tapering of the drug over several weeks to months. Pericardiectomy is occasionally needed for relief of severe recurrent pericardial pain in patients who cannot be weaned from steroids or other antiinflammatory drugs but is not always followed by relief of pain.[72]

TUBERCULOUS PERICARDITIS

ETIOLOGY AND PATHOGENESIS. In industrialized nations, the incidence of tuberculosis pericarditis has decreased within the past 3 decades as a result of effective chemotherapy and public health surveillance. In this setting, it is now a very uncommon cause of acute pericarditis. In a series of 231 consecutive patients who were evaluated prospectively using a rigorous protocol which included pericardiocentesis and biopsy, tuberculosis was diagnosed in only 4 per cent of patients and in 7 per cent of the subset who developed cardiac tamponade.[71] Similarly, tuberculous pericarditis was reported in none of 145 patients who required pericardial drainage[156] and in only 6 per cent of 231 patients who underwent pericardiectomy for chronic constriction[221] at the Mayo Clinic. The incidence of tuberculous pericarditis among patients with pulmonary tuberculosis ranges from about 1 to 8 per cent.[249] The disease continues to be important in immunosuppressed patients and among the underprivileged, including South and West African blacks, the black poor of the United States, and Asian and African immigrants.[250–252] For example, in Transkei, South Africa, tuberculous pericarditis is the second most common cause of "heart failure" after rheumatic heart disease.[251]

Tuberculous pericarditis usually develops by retrograde spread from peribronchial, peritracheal, or mediastinal lymph nodes or by early hematogenous spread from the primary tuberculous infection. Less commonly, the pericardium is involved by the breakdown and contiguous spread of a necrotic tuberculous lesion in the lung, pleura, or spine or by hematogenous spread from distant secondary genitourinary or skeletal infections.[253, 254] Pericarditis can also be caused by atypical mycobacteria,[255] which has been reported in association with the acquired immune deficiency syndrome.[245]

PATHOLOGY. Tuberculous pericarditis usually begins with diffuse fibrin deposits, granuloma formation, and the presence of viable acid-fast bacilli.[253] A pericardial effusion then develops, which may be serous but more often contains some blood with a protein content exceeding 2.5 gm/dl. Although polymorphonuclear leukocytes are present early in the development of the effusion, they are later replaced by lymphocytes, monocytes, and plasma cells. Both complement-fixing antimyolemmal and antimyosin-type antibodies have been demonstrated in about 75 per cent of patients with acute tuberculous pericarditis in contrast to the much lower incidence in patients with viral pericarditis or constrictive pericarditis due to tuberculosis, which suggests that cytolysis mediated by antimyolemmal antibodies may contribute to the development of exudate tuberculous pericarditis.[256] A tuberculous pericardial effusion usually develops very slowly and therefore does not cause hemodynamic complications; however, when it accumulates rapidly, even a small effusion may produce cardiac tamponade. As the effusion is absorbed, the pericardium thickens, granulomas proliferate, and a thick coat of fibrin is deposited on the parietal pericardium. At this stage, viable acid-fast bacilli may no longer be present, but caseation may develop and penetrate the myocardium. Finally, fibrous pericarditis develops as the granulomatous reaction is replaced by fibrous tissue and collagen. These changes are followed by the accumulation of cholesterol crystals and the development of pericardial calcification. Constrictive pericarditis develops in almost all patients with untreated tuberculous pericarditis and in about half or less of the patients who receive antituberculosis chemotherapy.[257, 258]

CLINICAL MANIFESTATIONS. Tuberculous pericarditis is usually detected clinically either in the effusive stage or late, i.e., after the development of constrictive pericarditis. It usually develops slowly, with nonspecific systemic symptoms such as fever, night sweats, fatigue, and dyspnea.[251, 257, 258] In South Africa, right upper abdominal aching due to liver congestion is common in patients with effusive tuberculous pericarditis.[251, 257] A torpid course is not invariably present, and an acute illness of less than 2 weeks' duration was described in 4 of 9 patients in whom tuberculous pericarditis was diagnosed during a prospective evaluation of acute pericarditis.[71] Severe pericardial pain of acute onset characteristic of viral and idiopathic pericarditis is uncommon in tuberculous pericarditis.[251, 258] Heavy sputum production, cough, and hemoptysis—clues to the presence of cavitary pulmonary tuberculosis—are usually absent.

Abnormalities on *physical examination* usually include fever, sinus tachycardia, and a pericardial friction rub. In South African patients with tuberculous pericardial effusion, evidence of chronic cardiac compression that mimics heart failure is by far the most common presentation. In a series of 88 patients with effusive tuberculous pericarditis, jugular venous distention was present in 88 per cent, hepatomegaly in 95 per cent, and ascites in 73 per cent, whereas a pericardial friction rub was heard in only 18 per cent.[251] If the complications of cardiac tamponade or effusive-constrictive pericarditis are present, the physical examination may reveal edema, jugular venous distention, pulsus paradoxus, distant heart sounds, hepatomegaly, and ascites. The *chest roentgenogram* usually shows an enlarged cardiac silhouette, and pleural effusions may be detected in about half the patients. However, the apices and hila of the lung are usually normal, and pulmonary infiltrates or calcification are present in a minority of the patients.

The *clinical presentation* of patients who develop chronic constrictive pericarditis differs from that of acute or subacute effusive tuberculous pericarditis. Dramatic symptoms such as high fever, night sweats, and precordial pain are uncommon. Findings compatible with severe chronic systemic venous congestion with low cardiac output predominate; these include jugular venous distention, hypotension with a narrow pulse pressure, abdominal distention, edema, and muscle wasting. Dyspnea related to large pleural effusions is common.[251, 257, 259]

During the transition from effusion to constrictive pericarditis, dense, frondlike echoes may be appreciated in the pericardial space; however, these findings may also be seen in malignant pericarditis.[260] Gallium-67 uptake in the pericardium is a nonspecific indicator of pericardial inflammation and can occur in tuberculous, purulent, and acute nonspecific pericarditis.[261]

DIAGNOSIS. Tuberculous pericarditis should be suspected in patients with fever and unexplained cardiomegaly, particularly those who are susceptible to tuberculosis, i.e., the underprivileged or immunosuppressed. It is noteworthy that tuberculous pericarditis may develop during chemotherapy for pulmonary tuberculosis.[262] In a minority of patients with pericarditis, a definitive diagnosis of a tuberculous origin may be made by culture or histological demonstration of tuberculosis outside the pericardium (sputum, gastric washings, pleural fluid, liver or bone marrow biopsy). A definitive diagnosis can be made by isolation of the bacillus from the pericardial fluid or pericardial biopsy. It is difficult to establish a definitive bacteriological diagnosis because of (1) the low yield of the bacillus when pericardial fluid is examined by acid-fast stain or microscopy; (2) failure of the bacillus to grow on appropriate media or in guinea pigs, even in patients with known tuberculous pericardial effusion; and (3) the need to observe bacterial cultures for at least 8 weeks. The probability of obtaining a definitive diagnosis is greatest if both pericardial fluid and a pericardial biopsy specimen are examined early in the effusive stage.[263] However, it must be emphasized that a negative pericardial biopsy does not exclude tuberculous pericarditis, since in some patients examination of the entire pericardium removed at pericardiectomy or autopsy is required to demonstrate clear-cut evidence of tuberculosis.[264] Furthermore, the finding of granulomas and caseous material without viable bacilli is also not diagnostic of tuberculous pericarditis, since these findings can be present in chronic pericardial disease due to rheumatoid arthritis and sarcoidosis.[170]

It may be necessary to make a presumptive clinical diagnosis of tuberculous pericarditis in severely ill patients with a large hemorrhagic pericardial effusion, a positive tuberculin skin test, and systemic symptoms such as weight loss and anorexia, even when examinations of the pericardial fluid and biopsy do not reveal tuberculosis. In such patients, clinical improvement may occur after initiation of antituberculosis chemotherapy. It should be emphasized that the tuberculin skin test *alone* is not a reliable indicator of tuberculous pericarditis since it may be negative in as many as 30 per cent of patients with documented tuberculosis due to anergy,[71] and is positive in about 30 to 40 per cent of patients with acute idiopathic pericarditis and benign natural history.[71, 170] Making a presumptive clinical diagnosis of tuberculous pericarditis requires exquisite judgment, since on the one hand treatment should not be withheld from the seriously ill patient, while on the other it is not prudent to commit patients with nontuberculous effusions to a prolonged course of multiple-drug antituberculosis therapy. The systematic approach suggested by Permanyer-Miralda et al. appears to have a high likelihood of identifying patients with tuberculous pericarditis with a very low risk of either missing active tuberculosis or inappropriately applying blind antituberculous therapy.[71] In patients with acute pericarditis of unknown cause, baseline clinical and laboratory studies including a tuberculin skin test are obtained, and treatment with bed rest and nonsteroidal antiinflammatory agents is begun. Pericardiocentesis is performed in the presence of cardiac tamponade or for clinical illness lasting more than 1 week with echocardiographic evidence of an effusion; at this stage, sputum and gastric aspirate samples are examined for tubercle bacilli. Surgical biopsy of the pericardium is done in (1) patients undergoing surgical relief of cardiac tamponade, and (2) as a diagnostic test in patients with clinical illness of more than 3 weeks' duration after hospitalization; blind antituberculosis treatment is considered if fever and pericardial effusion persist for more than 5 weeks after initiation of this protocol. This strategy remains to be validated in other populations.

MANAGEMENT. In the era before antituberculosis chemotherapy, tuberculous pericarditis was rapidly fatal, with a mortality rate greater than 80 per cent; the remaining patients had a protracted course of months to years with a frequently fatal outcome due to miliary tuberculosis or constrictive pericarditis. Since the introduction of early chemotherapy, mortality from acute tuberculous pericarditis has fallen to less than 50 per cent, but the effectiveness of antituberculosis chemotherapy in preventing the development of constrictive pericarditis is controversial.[250, 257, 258]

Treatment of tuberculous pericarditis includes hospitalization with bed rest and particular attention to findings on physical examination, electrocardiography, and echocardiography that suggest the development of an enlarging pericardial effusion and tamponade. Initial chemotherapy should usually consist of a three-drug regimen, ordinarily isoniazid (300 mg/day), rifampin (600 mg/day), pyrazinamide (2 gm/day), and streptomycin 1 gm or ethambutol 15 mg/kg/day. The use of corticosteroids has been advocated to reduce pericardial inflammation and enhance resorption of pericardial effusion, but there is no conclusive evidence that steroids reduce the risk of developing tuberculous constrictive pericarditis.[258, 265] We believe that corticosteroids should be reserved for critically ill patients with recurrent large effusions who do not respond to antituberculosis drugs alone.

In patients with documented cardiac tamponade or with a large pericardial effusion apparent on echocardiogram, the effusion should be drained initially by percutaneous pericardiocentesis with continued catheter drainage. *Pericardiectomy* should be performed after 4 to 6 weeks of antituberculosis drug therapy if patients develop large recurrent effusions or cardiac compression due to effusive-constrictive disease or constrictive pericarditis.[249–251, 265] Pericardiectomy should be performed early in the course of patients with clinical and hemodynamic evidence of chronic cardiac compression with anticipation of a good outcome. In a South African study of 113 patients with severe constrictive tuberculous pericarditis, 97 per cent were discharged from the hospital; in the majority, hepatomegaly and edema promptly resolved, whereas resolution of venous congestion required 2 to 3 months in some patients.[259] Mortality is high among patients who undergo pericardiectomy at the late stage of calcific pericardial constriction.[250, 259]

BACTERIAL (PURULENT) PERICARDITIS

Although the clinical spectrum of bacterial purulent pericarditis has changed over the past 4 decades, mortality remains high. Since the introduction of antibiotics in the 1940's, the incidence of bacterial pericarditis detected at autopsy has decreased.[266, 267] Prior to 1943, purulent pericarditis occurred primarily as a complication of pneumococcal pneumonia or empyema, and uncontrolled pleuropulmonary disease due to staphylococci or streptococci. During the antibiotic era there has been a decline in the incidence of pneumococcal and streptococcal pericarditis, although these organisms continue to cause life-threatening pericarditis.[268, 269] The incidence of hospital-acquired penicillin-resistant staphylococcal pericarditis in post-thoracotomy patients has increased, and there is a widened spectrum of organisms responsible for bacterial pericarditis, including the gram-negative bacilli (*Proteus, E. coli, Pseudomonas, Klebsiella*),[267] *Brucella melitensis*,[270] *Salmonella* species,[271, 272] *Neisseria gonorrhoeae*,[273] *Hemophilus influenzae*,[274] *Francisella tularensis*,[275] anaerobic organisms,[276, 277] and other unusual pathogens.[278–281] It is now established that *Neisseria meningitidis*, particularly from serogroup C, can cause either primary infection of the pericardium in the absence of meningitis or secondary pericarditis complicating meningitis and sepsis.[282] *Legionella pneumophila*, the causative organism in Legionnaire's disease, has been reported as a cause of purulent pericarditis associated with pneumonia and as a primary infection.[283, 284] Important predisposing factors for the development of purulent pericarditis include a preexisting pericardial effusion as in uremic pericarditis, as well as immunodepression due to burns, immunotherapy, lymphoma, or leukemia, or acquired immunodeficiency syndrome.[244, 245]

The routes of pericardial infection have also changed. Direct pulmonary extension of bacterial pneumonia or empyema now accounts for only about 20 per cent of cases of purulent pericarditis.[277] Today, purulent pericarditis tends to occur in adults via (1) contiguous spread from an early postoperative infection after thoracic surgery or trauma, (2) infection related to infective endocarditis, (3) extension from a subdiaphragmatic suppurative source, and (4) hematogenous spread during bacteremia. In patients with endocarditis, bacterial pericarditis is a life-threatening complication which is detected antemortem in about 1 out of 25 patients with endocarditis,[285] in about 1 out of 8 patients with endocarditis studied at autopsy, and in a higher percentage of those with staphylococcal endocarditis.[267] In such patients, bacterial pericarditis may develop by (1) extension from a valve ring abscess, (2) rupture of an aneurysm, (3) extension from a myocardial abscess, or (4) septic coronary embolus (Fig. 44–21).[286] An infected myocardial infarction or aortic aneurysm may also be a source for the development of purulent bacterial pericarditis.[287]

In *children*, the most common organisms responsible for purulent pericarditis include *Staphylococcus aureus* followed by *Hemophilus influenzae* and *Neisseria meningitidis*.[288–290] *Hemophilus influenzae* pericarditis has been increasingly recognized in young children and is usually characterized by a mild prodromal illness followed by the rapid development of cardiac compression and death due to pericardial effusion.[289] Pediatric illnesses associated with the development of bacterial pericarditis include pharyngitis, pneumonia, meningitis, otitis media, impertigo, endocarditis, and bacterial arthritis.[290] The development of bacterial pericarditis in infants and children carries a mortality approaching 70 per cent, depending on the organism, and the risk of the extremely rapid development of constrictive pericarditis.[291] The high mortality rate in children appears to be markedly reduced by early diagnosis and combined treatment with parenteral antibiotics and open surgical pericardial drainage, if effusion recurs after initial pericardiocentesis.[288–291]

PATHOLOGY. Bacterial pericarditis is usually frankly suppurative by the time it is detected clinically. The inflammation may result in organization and dense adhesions with a loculated pericardial effusion followed by

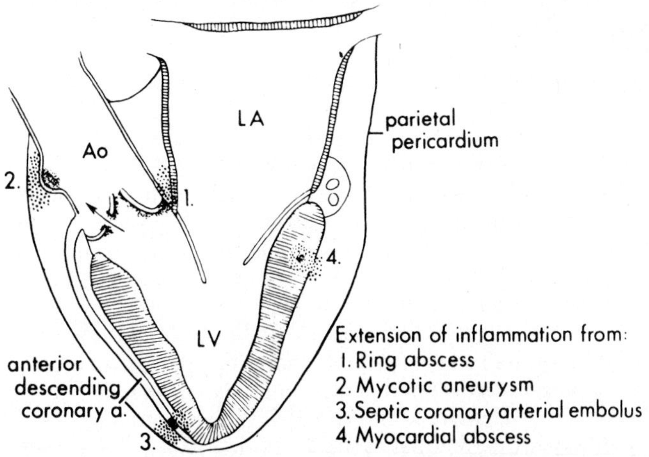

FIGURE 44–21. Schematic representation of the pathogenesis of pericarditis in infective endocarditis. Ao = aorta; LV = left ventricle; LA = left atrium. (From Roberts, W. C., and Spray, T. L.: Pericardial heart disease: A study of its causes, consequences, and morphologic features. *In* Spodick, D. H. [ed.]: Pericardial Diseases. Philadelphia, F. A. Davis Co., 1976, p. 31.)

obliteration of the pericardial space, thickening, and eventual calcification of the pericardium. In some patients, the inflammation may involve the adjacent sternum, pleura, and diaphragm with formation of dense adhesions between the parietal pericardium and contiguous structures.

CLINICAL FEATURES. Bacterial pericarditis is usually an acute fulminant illness of only a few days' duration. In one series,[277] the mean duration of symptoms before hospitalization was only 3 days. High fevers, shaking chills, night sweats, and dyspnea are common. In most patients the symptom of typical pericardial chest pain is absent. Although tachycardia is present in nearly all patients, a pericardial friction rub is present in less than half. In many cases, the pericarditis remains unsuspected because of the dominant presence of symptoms and signs related to an underlying known infection, such as pneumonia or mediastinitis following complicated thoracic surgery or trauma. The appearance of new jugular venous distention and pulsus paradoxus may be the first evidence of pericardial involvement, and these ominous signs reflect the development of cardiac tamponade due to the acute accumulation of suppurative fluid under pressure. In one series, cardiac tamponade developed acutely in 38 per cent of patients with previously unsuspected purulent pericarditis, and contributed to death in the majority.[277]

LABORATORY FINDINGS. These usually include leukocytosis with a marked leftward shift. The *chest roentgenogram* usually shows enlargement of the cardiac shadow and, less commonly, widening of the mediastinum. In most cases the roentgenogram shows evidence of underlying pneumonia, empyema, or mediastinitis without overt evidence of pericardial involvement. Electrocardiographic changes typically include ST-segment and T-wave changes characteristic of pericarditis in the majority of patients.[269, 277] The appearance of electrical alternans suggests the possibility of cardiac tamponade. In patients with suspected infective endocarditis, the appearance of a prolonged P-R interval, atrioventricular dissociation, or bundle branch block is strong evidence of extension of infection from the valve ring into the adjacent myocardium—an important predisposing factor for the development of pericarditis, especially in patients with staphylococcal endocarditis.[277]

Pericardial fluid usually shows polymorphonuclear leukocytosis and sometimes frank pus. Pericardial glucose levels are usually depressed and the protein content is elevated; lactate dehydrogenase values may also be markedly elevated.

Purulent pericarditis should be suspected in a debilitated patient with unexplained high spiking fevers, dyspnea, markedly elevated white blood cell count, and an increase in the size of the cardiac silhouette on chest roentgenogram. The key to the diagnosis, which unfortunately is frequently not made before death, is a high index of suspicion. An echocardiogram should be promptly obtained to look for evidence of a new pericardial effusion and/or loculation of fluid with adhesions.

A special comment is warranted about pericarditis associated with meningococcal infection. The pericardium may become infected early during meningococcal sepsis (in the presence or absence of meningitis) causing purulent pericarditis with cardiac tamponade, as described above.[282] In these cases, the pericardial fluid is frankly purulent and viable organisms usually can be isolated. In addition, sterile pericarditis may occur late in the convalescent period in association with arthritis, pleuritis, and ophthalmitis. This syndrome appears to have an immunological etiology, does not require further antibiotic therapy if the primary infection has been adequately treated, and responds to anti-inflammatory agents. A febrile, self-limited polyserositis with pericarditis has also been reported after effective treatment of sepsis due to *Staphylococcus aureus*.[293]

MANAGEMENT. Despite the lower incidence of purulent bacterial pericarditis in the antibiotic era, overall survival continues to be extremely poor, averaging about 30 per cent in modern series.[266, 277, 292] The poor prognosis stems in large part from failure of clinical diagnosis before death. In patients treated only with antibiotics without pericardial drainage, the rapid unsuspected development of a large pericardial effusion may result in sudden cardiovascular collapse and death due to cardiac tamponade. The high mortality from purulent pericarditis can be reduced substantially through the institution of both appropriate parenteral antibiotic therapy and early complete surgical drainage. The survival rate when the disease is recognized early and managed appropriately is about 50 per cent.[266, 277, 292] Early surgical drainage of the pericardium also helps to prevent the complication of constrictive pericarditis.

The suspicion that purulent pericardial fluid is present should mandate exploration of the pericardial space. This may be done by percutaneous pericardiocentesis *only* if there is echocardiographic evidence of a large anterior and posterior pericardial effusion that may be safely tapped or, preferably, by a generous subxiphoid pericardiotomy with thorough pericardial drainage.

Both pericardial fluid and pericardial tissue should be immediately studied by an experienced examiner using Gram-stained, acid-fast, and fungal smears. The fluid should then be cultured for aerobic and anaerobic bacteria with appropriate antibiotic sensitivity testing, and for fungi and tuberculosis. Pericardial fluid should also be examined for white blood cell count and differential, hematocrit, and glucose and protein content. Cultures of blood, sputum, and recent surgical wounds should also be obtained.

Results of Gram staining of the pericardial fluid should be used in the selection of antibiotic therapy. If the effusion is purulent but no organisms can be easily identified and tuberculosis is not considered likely, therapy should be initiated with both a semisynthetic antistaphylococcal antibiotic and an aminoglycoside. Depending on the results of the cultures of the pericardial fluid and blood, antibiotic therapy may then be modified. High concentrations of antibiotics can be achieved in pericardial fluid, so that instillation of antibiotics into the pericardial space is not warranted.[294] However, systemic antibiotics alone are inadequate treatment, and prompt and thorough surgical drainage of the pericardium is essential in almost all patients with bacterial pericarditis.[266, 270, 288, 289] Percutaneous aspiration of a large effusion may be extremely helpful in making an initial bacteriological diagnosis and initiating therapy, and is sometimes effective in preventing recurrent effusion.[295] However, purulent pericardial effusions are likely to recur and more extensive surgical drainage may be needed in some patients after antibiotic therapy has been initiated. Open drainage, through creation of a subxiphoid pericardiotomy, is usually adequate when the diagnosis is made early and when the pericardial fluid is thin and the pericardium minimally thickened. This procedure is also the preferred route of drainage in severely disabled patients, since it can be performed under local anesthesia and avoids the pleural cavities. In a patient with a thick purulent effusion and dense adhesions with loculation, extensive pericardiectomy is needed to achieve adequate drainage and to prevent development of constrictive pericarditis,[267, 269, 277, 288, 291] which can occur very early after presentation.[296]

FUNGAL AND PARASITIC PERICARDITIS

ETIOLOGY AND PATHOPHYSIOLOGY. Histoplasmosis is the most common cause of fungal pericarditis. This diagnosis should be considered in young otherwise healthy patients suspected of having acute viral or tuberculous pericarditis who live in the Ohio or Mississippi River Valley or the Western Appalachians, where the fungus is endemic.[297] In these areas, histoplasmosis is acquired by inhalation of spores during small rural outbreaks from bird or bat droppings and during major urban outbreaks related to excavation and building demolition. Coccidioidomycosis pericarditis occurs in patients who have inhaled chlamydospores from soil or dust in areas of the southwestern United States (particularly the San Joaquin Valley), and Argentina, where it is endemic.[298–300] Other fungal infections responsible for pericarditis include aspergillosis, blastomycosis, and those caused by *Candida albicans* and *Candida tropicalis*.[301, 302] Groups at increased risk for the development of fungal pericarditis consequent to disseminated infection include drug addicts and patients who are immunosuppressed or who have received potent broad-spectrum antibiotics.[277, 301]

Histoplasmosis pericarditis most commonly develops as a noninfectious inflammatory response to infection confined to adjacent mediastinal lymph nodes, and rarely by direct or hematogenous infection in patients with disseminated infection.[297, 303, 304] The isolation of organisms from pericardial fluid is unusual, and its predilection for young immunocompetent males suggests that self-limited histoplasmosis pericarditis usually represents a sterile immune reaction. Pericarditis due to fungi other than histoplasmosis may occur as a complication of open heart surgery in adults and children, owing to spread from contiguous infected lymph nodes or pulmonary lesions, or as a result of hematogenous dissemination in immunosuppressed patients with fungal sepsis.

PATHOLOGY. Pericardial fluid may accumulate extremely rapidly and in massive quantities in patients with histoplasmosis. The fluid can be serous or hemorrhagic with an elevated protein content and polymorphonuclear leukocytosis. In cases of fungal pericarditis due to agents other than *Histoplasma,* exudative pericardial effusions may accumulate more slowly, so that an effusion may be present for months. Histoplasmosis and other fungal pericardial effusions occasionally become organized, with pericardial thickening, the appearance of granulomas and multinucleated giant cells, and the development of a constricting, calcified pericardium.[297, 303, 304]

Histoplasmosis in patients with disseminated infection may rarely cause infection of the myocardium and endocardium as well as of the pericardium.[304] Similarly, aspergillosis and coccidioidomycosis may cause pericarditis in the context of pulmonary infection, endocarditis, and myocardial abscess. Therefore, cardiac decompensation in patients with fungal pericarditis may be due either to the presence of cardiac compression from a pericardial effusion or a constricting pericardium or to an underlying myocardial infection.

CLINICAL FEATURES

Histoplasmosis Pericarditis. The course of this illness is now better understood because of two large urban outbreaks in which 6.3 per cent of 712 clinically recognized cases involved acute pericarditis.[297] Almost all of the patients had a preceding respiratory illness and manifested pericardial pain and typical electrocardiographic changes. The chest roentgenogram was always abnormal, an enlarged cardiac silhouette was present in 95 per cent, and pleural effusions and intrathoracic adenopathy were present in two-thirds of the patients. Notably, the "classic" manifestations of histoplasmosis and acute self-limited disseminated infection or severe cavity pulmonary infection were absent. However, over 40 per cent of patients had hemodynamic compromise or frank cardiac tamponade consistent with other reports.[297, 304] Histoplasmosis pericarditis can rarely occur in the less common setting of severe prolonged disseminated infection evident by fever, anemia, leukopenia, and the syndrome of pneumonitis progressing to pulmonary cavitation, massive hepatomegaly, meningitis, myocarditis, or endocarditis, Severe disseminated infections are especially likely to occur in young infants, elderly males, and immunosuppressed patients.

Coccidioidomycosis Pericarditis. This condition does not occur in the brief self-limited influenzalike form of the infection but is instead a complication of the progressive disseminated form of coccidioidomycosis.[298, 299] Blacks, Filipinos, and Chicanos appear to be especially vulnerable to the development of disseminated coccidioidomycosis. These patients are usually chronically ill and debilitated, with fever, weight loss, and the complications of pulmonary cavitations with lymphadenopathy, osteomyelitis, and meningitis. In immunocompromised patients, the insidious appearance of symptoms of fungal pericarditis and underlying myocardial infection may initially be overlooked because attention is focused on symptoms related to underlying lymphoma, leukemia, or known valvular endocarditis. Physical findings suggestive of cardiac compression (jugular venous distention, hypotension, pulsus paradoxus) may be the first clues to the diagnosis of fungal pericarditis.

DIAGNOSIS. In young and otherwise healthy adults with evidence of pericarditis, a presumptive clinical diagnosis of *histoplasmosis pericarditis* can be made on the basis of (1) residence or travel in an endemic area, (2) an elevated complement-fixation titer of at least 1:32, and (3) a positive immunodiffusion test.[297] Most patients do not show a progressive rise in titer because pericarditis usually occurs after initial mild or asymptomatic pneumonitis such that titers are high when first measured. Histoplasmin skin tests are not helpful and their use may falsely elevate antibody titers.[297] Histoplasma may be isolated from invasive biopsies of mediastinal nodes, but cultures or methenamine silver stains rarely identify the organism in extrapulmonary sites such as the liver, bone marrow, and pericardium in patients with benign, self-limited form of pericarditis. Histoplasmosis pericarditis which occurs in the setting of severe disseminated infection must be differentiated from sarcoidosis, tuberculosis, Hodgkin's disease, and brucellosis. Histological tissue examination and culture are important in the diagnosis of disseminated progressive histoplasmosis. In this setting the organism may be isolated from extrapericardial sites such as the bone marrow, exudate from ulcers, or sputum by inoculation on Sabouraud's medium or by guinea pig inoculation with subsequent subculture of the spleen.

A presumptive diagnosis of *coccidioidomycosis pericarditis* is made in a patient with pericarditis who has (1) a history of dust exposure in an endemic area in the southwestern United States, California Central Valleys, or South America; (2) a characteristic clinical picture of disseminated coccidioidomycosis involving the lungs and other organs; (3) the appearance of a positive serum precipitin test early in the infection followed by a rising positive complement-fixation antibody titer; and (4) microscopic evidence of the characteristic spherule in biopsy material. A definitive diagnosis is made by culture identification of the organism on Sabouraud's medium. Coccidioidin skin tests are often negative in the presence of progressive disseminated disease. If pericarditis due to other fungal organisms is suspected, appropriate complement-fixing antibody titers should be measured. Depending on the clinical setting it may be imporant to obtain pericardial fluid and a pericardial biopsy specimen. It must be emphasized that the microscopic finding of granulomas alone is nonspecific and may occur in tuberculosis, fungal and parasitic infections, and sarcoid involvement of the pericardium. Therefore, histological documentation of the characteristic apperance of the fungus and subsequent culture identification are important.

MANAGEMENT. Histoplasmosis pericarditis is generally a benign illness which resolves within 2 weeks and does not require treatment with amphotericin B.[297] Nonsteroidal antiinflammatory drugs or steroids appear to shorten the duration of chest pain, fever, pericardial friction rub, and effusion.[297] Patients should always be hospitalized, because histoplasmosis may cause the rapid development of massive effusions with acute cardiac tamponade that require emergency pericardiocentesis or pericardiectomy.[297, 304] Although pericardial calcification and pericardial constriction have been reported in histoplasmosis pericarditis, these complications are uncommon.[303] Intravenous amphotericin B is required only for patients with histoplasmosis pericarditis and severe systemic disease.

In nonhistoplasmosis fungal pericarditis, spontaneous remissions do not occur; infection progresses until the patient dies either of the underlying disease or of fungal pericardial and myocardial involvement. Drug therapy for pericarditis associated with disseminated coccidioidomycosis, aspergillosis, and blastomycosis consists of prolonged intravenous therapy with amphotericin B. The South American form of blastomycosis may require the addition of a sulfonamide. *Candida pericarditis* associated with fungal sepsis and disseminated infection is treated with amphotericin B, 5-fluorocytosine, and miconazole.[305] In many cases of nonhistoplasmosis fungal pericarditis, chronic pericardial fungal infection progresses to severe pericardial constriction or, less commonly, cardiac tamponade. Therefore, depending on the patient's underlying medical condition, pericardiectomy is usually indicated. Intrapericardial instillation of antifungal agents has not proved helpful in these diseases. The marked toxicity associated with prolonged amphotericin B administration underscores the importance of making a definitive diagnosis after histological examination or culture.

Pericarditis may also be caused by *Actinomyces israelii* and *Nocardia asteroides,* which are intermediate forms between fungi and bacteria.[306, 307]

PARASITIC PERICARDITIS. The parasite *Toxoplasma gondii,* which is usually acquired by accidental cyst ingestion in endemic areas, is a cause of myocarditis, acute pericarditis, and chronic pericardial effusion.[308] The prevalence of toxoplasma as a cause of acute pericarditis of unknown origin may be underestimated.[71] Other parasitic causes include amebiasis,[309, 310] schistosomiasis,[311] and echinococcosis.[312] Very rare causes of parasitic pericarditis include dracunculosis,[313] cysticercosis, and filariasis.[314] These unusual pathogens rarely cause acute cardiac tamponade but may cause chronic constrictive pericarditis. The spirochetes *Borrelia burgdorferi* and *Babesia microti* are newly recognized as a cause of fatal myopericarditis in association with Lyme disease.[315]

PERICARDITIS FOLLOWING ACUTE MYOCARDIAL INFARCTION (See also p. 1286)

Pericarditis occurs during the first few days after acute myocardial infarction in about 7 per cent of patients. The incidence of early postmyocardial infarction pericarditis varies from 6 to 23 per cent, although a much higher incidence is detected at autopsy.[316–321] Almost all patients with acute transmural myocardial infarction are found to have evidence of a localized fibrinous pericarditis overlying the infarction at autopsy. Fibrinous pericarditis occurs in about 1 of 10 patients with subendocardial infarction at postmortem examination.[322] Pericarditis is more prevalent in anterior than in inferior infarction in most series[317, 318] and also occurs after lateral and predominant right ventricular infarction. Other forms of pericardial involvement after myocardial infarction include acute pericardial hemorrhage secondary to cardiac rupture (p. 1538) and the late occurrence of the Dressler syndrome (p. 1521).

CLINICAL FEATURES. Pericarditis is recognized clinically by the appearance of a pericardial friction rub and pericardial chest pain between 12 hours and 10 days after acute myocardial infarction. However, in most patients with postinfarction pericarditis, a pericardial friction rub and pericardial chest pain appear on the second or third day after infarction.[316, 318, 320] There is usually a slight temperature elevation. Appearance of a new friction rub more than 10 days after acute infarction probably represents the onset of Dressler syndrome (p. 1521) or pericarditis complicating a second infarction. Since pericardial friction rubs are notoriously evanescent, serial auscultatory evaluation of patients in various positions in a quiet room is important for detection. Pericardial rubs with a single systolic component heard near the apex may be confused with a new murmur of mitral regurgitation due to papillary muscle dysfunction or rupture. Postinfarction pericarditis does not directly cause hemodynamic deterioration unless a pericardial effusion under pressure develops, causing cardiac tamponade.

In recent series of patients with early postinfarction pericarditis,[318] and of patients with acute infarction and pericardial effusion,[323] the use of heparin did not appear to be associated with increased risk. However, hemorrhagic cardiac tamponade related to the use of anticoagulants has been reported as a rare complication in patients with postinfarction pericarditis.[324–326] *Constrictive pericarditis* has been reported as a sequel of hemopericardium after infarction.[327, 328] Acute thrombolytic therapy of acute infarction with streptokinase or tissue plasminogen activator followed by intravenous heparin has not yet been reported to promote the development of hemopericardium after infarction.

The typical diagnostic electrocardiographic changes of acute pericarditis are extremely rare in early postinfarction pericarditis,[320] and the electrocardiogram *cannot* be used to confirm the diagnosis in this setting.

ECHOCARDIOGRAPHY. The finding of a small pericardial effusion in the absence of hemodynamic compromise is also not pathognomonic of acute postinfarction pericarditis. Galve et al. recently found that a small pericardial effusion could be detected in 28 per cent of patients early after acute infarction in comparison with 8 per cent of asymptomatic patients with unstable angina and 5 per cent of normal subjects.[323] The presence of a pericardial effusion correlates well with the presence of extensive infarction and congestive failure, but not with clinical pericarditis evident as a pericardial rub or pain. Both a high Killip classification[317, 318] and atrial tachyarrhythmias appear to be more common in patients with pericarditis following infarction.[329, 330] However, the appearance of acute postinfarction pericarditis per se does not appear to affect adversely the mortality after acute infarction.[317, 318, 320]

DIFFERENTIAL DIAGNOSIS. Postinfarction pericarditis without cardiac compression must be differentiated from acute stress ulcer, acute pulmonary embolus, and, most importantly, recurrent myocardial ischemia. Myocardial ischemic pain usually can be differentiated from the pain of postinfarction pericarditis by (1) obvious amelioration of the pain by nitroglycerin and (2) the appearance of new regional ST-segment and T-wave changes with reciprocal changes.

CARDIAC TAMPONADE. The development of cardiac tamponade in patients with myocardial infarction may be related to pericardial hemorrhage secondary to pericarditis or to myocardial rupture within the first 3 days after infarction. Both situations may be associated with cardiovascular collapse, the appearance of dense echoes in the pericardial space on echocardiography, and an abrupt increase in heart size on the chest roentgenogram. Pericardiocentesis may successfully relieve postinfarction hemorrhagic cardiac tamponade in occasional patients.[331] Massive cardiac hemorrhage secondary to cardiac rupture is usually followed by the rapid development of electromechanical dissociation and death despite successful aspiration of the pericardial space, although survivors have been reported after subacute rupture.[332]

Acute cardiac tamponade secondary to postinfarction pericarditis must also be differentiated from cardiogenic shock without intrapericardial hemorrhage due to an acute ventricular septal defect or mitral regurgitation. In the setting of an inferior myocardial infarction, the appearance of hypotension, pulsus paradoxus, and jugular venous distention may be related to massive right ventricular infarction rather than to cardiac tamponade.[53, 54] Echocardiographic findings of right ventricular enlargement without a significant pericardial effusion, and catheterization findings suggestive of constrictive physiology (right atrial waveform with steep *y* descent) rather than cardiac tamponade (right atrial waveform with attenuated *y* descent), help to differentiate these entities and prevent possibly disastrous attempts at pericardiocentesis.

MANAGEMENT. Postinfarction pericarditis may produce mild symptoms that require no specific therapy or severe chest pain that persists for several days. If the pain is severe, high-dose aspirin will relieve pain within 48 hours in most patients. A short course of prednisone may be required in patients whose pain does not improve after a 48-hour trial of nonsteroidal antiinflammatory agents.[318, 333]

There is experimental evidence that indomethacin, ibuprofen, and multiple large doses of corticosteroids interfere with the conversion of the myocardial infarct into a scar, so that marked thinning of the myocardial wall occurs.[334, 335] Myocardial rupture has been observed in a patient during ibuprofen use for postinfarction pericarditis.[336] Although the clinical importance of these findings is not clear, they suggest that steroids and nonsteroidal antiinflammatory drugs should be employed with caution in patients with acute myocardial infarction. Fortunately, aspirin does not appear to cause any of these adverse effects, and postinfarction pericarditis usually responds well to aspirin. Accordingly, we favor use of this drug.

UREMIC PERICARDITIS (See also p. 1840)

ETIOLOGY. Pericarditis is a frequent and serious complication of chronic renal failure. Bright noted the presence of pericarditis in 8 per cent of autopsied patients with chronic renal failure reported in 1836 from Guy's Hospital.[337] Before the advent of dialysis uremic pericarditis was detected in about half the patients with untreated chronic renal failure and was usually a harbinger of death. Uremic pericarditis is now detected clinically in up to 20 per cent of uremic patients who require chronic dialysis.[338, 339] Uremic pericarditis tends to be a complication occurring either before initiation of dialysis or during the first few months of therapy.

The etiology of uremic pericarditis is unknown. Viral causes have been proposed,[340] but there is no consistent evidence to suggest a viral etiology in the majority of cases of uremic pericarditis. Specific etiologies, including purulent bacterial infections, are common in patients with uremic pericarditis,[339] and it is unwise to assume that pericarditis in a patient with severe renal disease is simply related to uremia. Toxic catabolic nitrogen metabolites and secondary hyperparathyroidism have been suggested mechanisms responsible for uremic pericarditis. This hypothesis is supported by the observations that uremic pericarditis is rare in patients with acute mild renal failure and that uremic pericarditis often improves with initiation of dialysis in previously untreated patients. However, there is no clear correlation between the development of pericarditis and the levels of catabolic metabolites in uremic patients.[39, 341] It has also been proposed that pericarditis in dialysis patients may reflect an immunological response. Some support for this hypothesis comes from the observations that 64 per cent of 25 patients with chronic uremia and pericarditis had complement-fixing antimyolemmal antibodies with cytolytic properties for cardiac tissue, whereas antimyocardial antibodies were rarely detected in patients with acute renal failure due to surgery or trauma.[342] It is possible that etiological factors in nondialyzed patients differ from those in patients undergoing regular dialysis. In the latter group, systemic and regional heparinization during dialysis itself may exacerbate uremic pericarditis by promoting the tendency of vascular pericardial granulation tissue to bleed into the pericardial space.

PATHOLOGY. Acute uremic pericarditis is characterized by the appearance of shaggy, hemorrhagic, fibrinous exudate on both parietal and visceral pericardial surfaces with little acute inflammatory cellular reaction. In some patients, the friable pericardial surface may bleed, giving rise to hemorrhagic pericardial effusion. Subacute or chronic constrictive pericarditis may develop, coincident with organization of the effusion and formation of thick adhesions within the pericardial space.[343]

CLINICAL FEATURES. The development of pericarditis in patients undergoing dialysis is of clinical importance, since it may (1) cause disability or life-threatening cardiac tamponade in patients who are otherwise well-compensated on dialysis, (2) compromise the status of patients who are candidates for renal transplantation, and (3) cause hemodynamic complications during routine dialysis. Patients with uremic pericarditis usually come to medical attention because of the development of chest pain. A pericardial friction rub is present on initial presentation in nearly 90 per cent of patients.[339, 344] Fever, leukocytosis, and tachycardia are frequent but nonspecific findings. Dyspnea and cardiac enlargement on the chest roentgenogram are common, but these findings can be related to underlying myocardial dysfunction and volume overload.

Uremic pericarditis with a large pericardial effusion may first come to clinical attention when an otherwise asymptomatic patient becomes hypotensive and confused upon fluid removal during ultrafiltration. This occurs because volume depletion may cause an abrupt fall in systemic blood pressure when ventricular filling is already compromised by the presence of a large, tense pericardial effusion. Uremic pericarditis can also present as acute or subacute tamponade with the findings of jugular venous distention, hypotension, and pulsus paradoxus.

ECHOCARDIOGRAPHY. The role of echocardiography in the diagnosis of uremic pericarditis merits critical attention. The presence of a small pericardial effusion is common in uremic patients, and in the absence of typical pericardial pain and friction rubs it is not diagnostic of pericarditis. Asymptomatic pericardial effusions of small to moderate size occur in between 36 to 62 per cent of uremic patients who require dialysis and appear to be related to volume overload and clinical congestive heart failure.[345, 346] On the other hand, the presence of a large anterior and posterior pericardial effusion in patients with uremic pericarditis is associated with a high likelihood of requiring intervention to relieve tamponade.[339, 345] The presence of a large pericardial effusion in association with echocardiographic findings of right atrial and right ventricular collapse suggests cardiac tamponade in a patient with uremic pericarditis.

CARDIAC CATHETERIZATION. This procedure is recommended in patients who are suspected of having cardiac tamponade because of development of intolerance of dialysis, hypotension, or dyspnea and in whom echocardiography reveals only a small to moderate effusion. Prior to consideration of pericardiocentesis or pericardiectomy, it is important to document that these clinical findings are indeed related to the hemodynamics of cardiac tamponade (elevation and equilibration of pericardial, right and left heart filling pressures) rather than to underlying congestive cardiomyopathy, ischemic heart disease, or excessively vigorous ultrafiltration. It must be remembered that pulsus paradoxus may be absent in uremic patients with cardiac tamponade and coexisting left ventricular failure and elevated left ventricular filling pressures.

MANAGEMENT. Patients with symptomatic pericarditis which develops before initiation of dialysis almost always respond to vigorous dialysis.[338, 339, 345] In contrast, less than half of patients with asymptomatic pericardial effusions show resolution of the effusion after initiation of dialysis.[345] No treatment is required for small, asymptomatic pericardial effusions that can be followed simply by serial echocardiography.[346] Treatment of symptomatic uremic pericarditis which develops in patients already undergoing dialysis is controversial, and multiple approaches have been advocated. About two-thirds of patients who develop effusive uremic pericarditis following the initiation of dialysis will respond to a program of intensification of dialysis and regional heparinization. The remainder are likely to require operative drainage of the pericardium.[338, 339, 347, 348] Factors which predict that the strategy of intensive dialysis is likely to fail include the presence of large anterior and posterior effusions, high fever, leukocytosis with a left shift, hypotension, and jugular venous distention.[349]

Nonsteroidal antiinflammatory drugs have been widely advocated as therapy for patients with uremic pericarditis. A randomized and double-blinded comparison of indomethacin and placebo in symptomatic patients with uremic pericarditis showed that indomethacin reduced the duration of fever, but it had no significant effect on the duration of chest pain, pericardial rub, pericardial effusion, or need for relief of tamponade which occurred in 20 per cent of patients.[350] The complications of long-term steroid administration limit its usefulness in the treatment of recurrent uremic pericarditis.

Pericardiocentesis. This procedure followed by the insertion of an indwelling catheter and the instillation of a nonresorbable steroid into the epicardial space has also been advocated,[351, 352] but this procedure has been complicated by the development of purulent pericarditis.[353] A single pericardiocentesis followed by a one-time instillation of triamcinolone appears to be effective and may eliminate the need for prolonged catheter drainage.[354] Although repetitive pericardiocenteses with low morbidity and mortality have been reported in uremic patients,[355, 356] other investigators have reported a substantial mortality as a consequence of pericardiocentesis.[339] The presence of a friable visceral pericardium may increase the risk of traumatic intrapericardial hemorrhage in uremic pericarditis, and many patients are also compromised by the presence of left ventricular dysfunction. These considerations warrant special caution during the performance of pericardiocentesis in uremic patients. This procedure should probably be carried out only by experienced personnel in an optimal environment, with echocardiographic documentation that a large anterior and posterior effusion is present that can be safely aspirated.

SURGICAL TREATMENT. In uremic patients with pericardial effusions, a subxiphoid pericardiostomy or limited pericardiectomy (window) performed through a left thoracotomy are effective in relieving cardiac tamponade and do not appear to be associated with an appreciable risk of developing recurrent effusions or constriction.[357, 358]

Early surgical intervention in uremic patients with a large pericardial effusion has been advocated as a prophylactic measure to prevent the development of cardiac tamponade and to allow the procedure to be carried out at a time when the patient's condition is clinically stable. We believe that this approach is excessively aggressive, since many symptomatic uremic patients with pericardial effusions respond well to intensification of dialysis.

We advocate that the patient whose condition is hemodynamically unstable with hemodynamic evidence of cardiac tamponade and echocardiographic evidence of a large anterior and posterior effusion be treated by percutaneous pericardiocentesis with continued catheter drainage of the pericardial sac for 24 to 48 hours. Subxiphoid pericardiotomy or limited pericardiectomy is reserved for patients with hemodynamic instability associated with recurrent pericardial effusions following pericardiocentesis or loculated pericardial effusions.

NEOPLASTIC PERICARDITIS (See also p. 1744)

PATHOLOGY. At autopsy, the pericardium is involved in 5 to 10 per cent of patients with malignant neoplasm.[359–361] Lung cancer, breast cancer, leukemia, Hodgkin's disease, and non-Hodgkin's lymphoma account for about 80 per cent of reported cases of malignant pericarditis. Other malignancies reported to lead to pericardial involvement include gastrointestinal cancer, ovarian cancer, sarcomas, and melanoma.[362–369] In children the most common etiologies are non-Hodgkin's lymphoma, neuroblastoma, sarcomas, and Wilms' tumor.[368] Primary malignancies of the pericardium are rare and are predominantly due to mesothelioma, including that arising after asbestos and fiber glass exposure, and, less frequently, malignant fibrosarcoma, angiosarcoma, and benign and malignant teratomas.[370–373, 373a] Cathecholamine-secreting pheochromocytoma is a rare primary neoplasm of the pericardium[374] (Fig. 12–34, p. 374).

Pericardial metastases may involve the heart in several ways: (1) extension and attachment to the pericardium of a malignant mediastinal mass, (2) nodular tumor deposits from hematogenous or lymphatic spread, (3) diffuse pericardial thickening and infiltration with tumor, and (4) local infiltration of the pericardium.[365, 375] In the majority of cases, the epicardium and myocardium are not involved.

Neoplastic pericarditis may cause several syndromes of cardiac compression. Neoplastic involvement of the pericardium may result in serosanguinous or hemorrhagic effusions which may develop extremely rapidly, causing acute or subacute cardiac tamponade. Pericardial involvement by tumors such as sarcomas, mesotheliomas, and melanomas can also erode the cardiac chamber or intrapericardial blood vessels, causing acute pericardial distention and abruptly fatal cardiac tamponade. A rare cause of hemorrhagic effusion and cardiac tamponade is intrapericardial extramedullary hematopoiesis associated with preleukemic conditions.[376, 377] Cardiac compression may also occur as a consequence of the development of both a thickened pericardium and a pericardial effusion under pressure (effusive-constrictive pericarditis), or it may be caused by thickening of the pericardium produced by tumor encasement of the heart, causing the physiology of constrictive pericarditis.[127, 233, 234, 378]

Not all pericardial effusions associated with mediastinal cancer are malignant. Asymptomatic pericardial effusions are common in patients with mediastinal lymphoma and Hodgkin's disease.[379] These evanescent effusions are frequently detected during staging procedures, and presumably develop because of impaired lymphatic drainage.

CLINICAL FEATURES. Neoplastic pericarditis is often asymptomatic and detected only as an incidental finding at autopsy. However, it is the most common specific etiology of acute pericarditis in developed countries. In a prospective series of patients with acute pericarditis of unknown cause, a diagnostic protocol revealed an unsuspected malignant etiology in 5 per cent of patients.[71] In patients with undiagnosed cancer or leukemia, cardiac tamponade can be the initial manifestation.[362, 380–382] In patients with known malignancy, symptoms resulting from pericardial involvement may be incorrectly attributed to the underlying neoplasm, so that malignant pericarditis is not suspected until symptoms and signs of severe cardiac compression appear.

In patients with malignant pericarditis, dyspnea is by far the most common symptom.[362, 366, 383] Other frequent symptoms and physical findings include chest pain, cough, orthopnea and hepatomegaly. Distant heart sounds and a pericardial friction rub are rarely detected, which may be due in part to a low index of suspicion.[362, 383] In the majority of patients, the diagnosis is made only when there is evidence of cardiac compression or frank cardiac tamponade, manifest as jugular venous distention, pulsus paradoxus, and hypotension. These findings occur more frequently with neoplastic pericarditis than in patients with an underlying neoplasm and idiopathic or radiation-induced pericarditis.[362]

The *chest roentgenogram* is abnormal in more than 90 per cent of patients with malignant pericarditis and may show a pleural effusion, cardiac enlargement, mediastinal widening, a hilar mass, or, less commonly, an irregular nodular contour of the cardiac silhouette.[362, 366] The *electrocardiogram* is usually abnormal but nonspecific, showing tachycardia, ST- and T-wave changes, low QRS voltage, and occasionally atrial fibrillation. In occasional patients, persistent tachycardia or electrocardiographic changes are the initial findings which lead to the diagnosis.[383] Electrocardiographic findings which are rarely seen in pericarditis, such as atrioventricular conduction disturbances, suggest malignant invasion of the myocardium and conduction system.

DIAGNOSIS. Patients with cancer and pericarditis deserve a careful and systematic evaluation, and these patients should not be summarily assumed to have a preterminal condition. The diagnosis of malignant pericarditis depends on both documentation of pericardial inflammation and substantiation that pericarditis is due to neoplasm. It is often not appreciated that, in approximately half the patients with neoplastic disease, symptomatic pericarditis has a nonmalignant etiology, most commonly prior radiation or idiopathic causes.[142, 362] Many patients with advanced neoplastic disease are immunosuppressed as a consequence of their malignancy and/or therapy and are therefore also at risk for tuberculous and fungal pericarditis. Acute pericarditis has also been rarely reported as a complication of the intravenous administration of the chemotherapeutic agents Adriamycin and Daunorubicin. In patients with acquired immunodeficiency syndrome, the differential diagnosis is complex and includes involvement of the pericardium with Kaposi's sarcoma as well as opportunistic infections with fungus or atypical acid-fast bacilli.[244, 245, 306]

Neoplastic pericarditis with cardiac compression must be differentiated from other causes of jugular venous distention, hepatomegaly, and peripheral edema in cancer patients. The most important of these are (1) underlying left ventricular dysfunction secondary to prior cardiac disease or Adriamycin cardiac toxicity, (2) superior vena caval obstruction, (3) malignant hepatic involvement with portal hypertension, and (4) lymphangitic tumor spread in the lungs with secondary pulmonary hypertension.

Echocardiography often provides critical information about the presence and size of a pericardial effusion and the thickness and motion of the pericardium, and may suggest the presence of abnormal diastolic filling of the heart due to cardiac compression. Two-dimensional echocardiography may be helpful in the detection of irregular undulating masses that protrude into the pericardial space and suggest the presence of pericardial metastases.[384] Computed tomography and magnetic resonance imaging can also detect the presence of pericardial effusions, and, in some instances, may give added information regarding the presence and location of space-occupying masses within the pericardium and adjacent mediastinum and lungs (Fig. 44–22).[385, 386]

We recommend that pericardiocentesis using the catheter drainage technique in conjunction with cardiac catheterization (p. 1499) should be performed in cancer patients with suspected cardiac tamponade in whom a large pericardial effusion is documented by echocardiography. Two additional diagnoses should always be systematically evaluated during cardiac catheterization in these patients. First, superior vena caval obstruction may coexist with malignant cardiac tamponade and contribute to the development of facial edema and jugular venous distention and should be systemically excluded at cardiac catheterization in cancer patients.[142, 362] Second, cyanosis, hypoxemia, and elevation of the pulmonary vascular resistance are not features of cardiac tamponade, and pulmonary microvas-

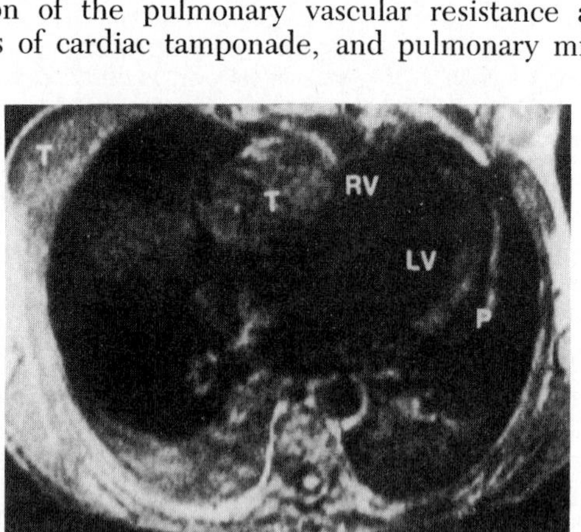

FIGURE 44–22. Magnetic resonance image of a large tumor mass (T) adjacent to the right ventricle (RV) from a patient with a metastatic sarcoma. A pericardial effusion (P) is apparent along the border of the left ventricular free wall (LV). Multiple small pleural tumors are also evident. (From Pizzarello, R. A., et al.: Tumor of the heart diagnosed by magnetic resonance imaging. J. Am. Coll. Cardiol. 5:989, 1985. Reprinted with permission from the American College of Cardiology.)

cular tumor (lymphangitic tumor) should be strongly suspected in the patient with these findings or persistent dyspnea following pericardiocentesis. Support for this diagnosis can be provided through cytological analysis by obtaining, at the same setting as pericardiocentesis and right heart catheterization, a sample of blood from the pulmonary capillary wedge position using the right heart catheter.[387]

The gross appearance of the pericardial fluid does not differentiate between neoplastic, radiation, or idiopathic etiologies. Since treatment strategies differ, it is necessary to carry out a meticulous cytological examination of pericardial fluid in an attempt to differentiate malignant pericarditis from radiation-induced or idiopathic pericarditis. Cytological examination of pericardial fluid is diagnostic of a malignancy in about 85 per cent of cases of malignant pericarditis.[142, 362, 388–390] False-negative cytological diagnoses are uncommon in carcinomatous pericarditis but occur more commonly with involvement by lymphoma or mesothelioma.[142, 362, 390] The measurement of carcinoembryonic antigen (CEA) may add to the diagnostic yield of the examination of pericardial fluid in patients with suspected malignant pericarditis.[391] In patients strongly suspected of having neoplastic pericarditis, open pericardial biopsy may be required if the cytological examination of pericardial fluid is negative. If a sufficiently large biopsy specimen is obtained, open pericardial biopsy should provide a histological diagnosis in up to 90 per cent of cases.[388] However, false-negative diagnoses may occur if only a small tissue sample is obtained, and in critically ill patients open pericardial biopsy is not without risk.[362]

In patients with echocardiographic evidence of a thickened pericardium and the physical findings of cardiac compression (jugular venous distention, edema, ascites, and hepatomegaly), cardiac catheterization is useful for documenting the presence of constrictive physiology before a decision is made to proceed with aggressive surgical intervention, i.e., extensive pericardiectomy.

NATURAL HISTORY. If cardiac tamponade can be avoided or successfully treated, the mere presence of neoplastic pericarditis does not imply that death is imminent. Since lung cancer and breast cancer are by far the most common causes of malignant pericarditis with cardiac tamponade, both the management strategy and subsequent natural history usually depend on the type of underlying malignancy. The natural history of neoplastic pericarditis in patients treated for cardiac tamponade was studied using a Kaplan-Meier analysis in two series.[156, 362] In both series, the mean survival was 4 months, with 25 per cent of patients surviving 1 year. However, the outcome of patients with malignant pericarditis due to breast cancer was strikingly better than that of patients with lung cancer. Following surgical treatment of cardiac tamponade in lung cancer patients, the mean survival was only 3.5 months in contrast with breast cancer patients in whom mean survival was 9 months with survivorship extending to more than 5 years.[156] A similar prolonged survival in patients with malignant effusion due to breast cancer has been reported by others.[362, 390, 392]

MANAGEMENT. Decisions about the management of neoplastic pericardial effusion depend on the patient's general condition, the presence or absence of clinical manifestations related to cardiac compression, and the prognosis and treatment options available for the specific histology and stage of the underlying malignancy. At one extreme are debilitated patients with end-stage malignant disease who have no promising treatment option for the underlying malignancy and a bleak prognosis. In this setting, diagnostic procedures should be as brief and painless as possible, and intervention should be directed toward alleviation of symptoms with a goal of improving the quality of the remaining days or weeks of life. In these patients, pericardiocentesis with catheter drainage is indicated for immediate relief of severe dyspnea, chest pain, or orthopnea. If cardiac tamponade recurs, palliation can be achieved by a subxiphoid pericardiotomy.[156, 393] The more invasive and debilitating partial pericardiectomy (window) done via a left thoracotomy has also been advocated,[394] but this procedure appears to have no palliative advantage over a subxiphoid pericardiotomy and should rarely be done in patients with end-stage malignancy.[156] When the general prognosis of the patient is better, several more aggressive treatment options are available, the goals of which are (1) relief of cardiac tamponade, (2) prevention of recurrence of the malignant effusion, and (3) treatment or prevention of constrictive pericardial disease.

In patients with asymptomatic pericardial effusion who have a treatment option of effective chemotherapy or hormonal therapy directed against the underlying malignancy, treatment with systemic agents alone can be attempted while progression of the effusion is observed by means of echocardiography. In patients with cardiac tamponade and large effusions secondary to neoplastic pericarditis, pericardiocentesis with catheter drainage in combination with systemic chemotherapy can be attempted.[142, 362, 383] The instillation of chemotherapeutic agents or radioisotopes into the pericardial space following pericardiocentesis and catheter drainage has been advocated with the aim of sclerosis of the pericardial membranes and obliteration of the pericardial space.[383, 395] However, there is no convincing evidence to date from either a large collective experience or prospective trial to indicate that instillation of intrapericardial drugs alters the outcome after thorough pericardial drainage. Side effects of instillation of intrapericardial agents include chest pain, nausea, and fever.

External-beam radiation therapy is an important option for patients with radiosensitive tumors who have not yet received extensive mediastinal or cardiac radiation as a treatment modality. Approximately half the patients with malignant pericarditis due to a variety of primary tumors have responded to this form of treatment.[396, 397] In one series, malignant pericardial effusion improved significantly in 11 of 16 patients with breast cancer, while six of seven patients with malignant pericarditis secondary to leukemia or lymphoma improved with cardiac radiation.[397]

In cancer patients whose general condition is good who develop recurrent symptomatic effusion after pericardiocentesis, a limited subxiphoid pericardiotomy should probably not be chosen when the goal is definitive therapy. The large experience at the Mayo Clinic indicates that this procedure has a much higher potential for being followed by recurrent tamponade, constriction, or reoperation than does extensive pericardiectomy, and that recurrent tamponade almost always occurs in less than a year after operation.[142] Since one out of four patients with malignant effusive pericarditis is likely to survive at least a year, extensive surgical pericardiectomy should be strongly considered in cancer patients with recurrent effusions or pericardial constriction due to breast cancer or other malignancies who have potential response to systemic cancer therapy or a good prognosis (one or more years of expected survival) relative to the underlying malignancy.

RADIATION PERICARDITIS

ETIOLOGY. Radiation injury to the heart and pericardium is an important complication of radiation therapy used in the treatment of breast carcinoma, Hodgkin's disease, and non-Hodgkin's lymphoma. Factors which influence the development of radiation-induced heart disease include (1) the radiation dosage; (2) the duration of therapy; (3) the volume of the heart included in the radiation field; (4) the use of a cobalt-60 source, with inhomogeneous dose distribution, in comparison with a linear accelerator source; and (5) anterior weighting of the radiation dose.[398] When at least 60 per cent of the cardiac silhouette is included within the treatment beam, as occurs in mantle field therapy of patients with Hodgkin's disease, the risk of radiation-induced pericarditis is about 5 to 7 per cent when a dosage below 4000 rads is delivered over 4 weeks, and rises sharply in incidence above this dosage.[398–401] When the whole pericardium is included in the field, the incidence of pericarditis is about 20 per cent, while the use of a subcarinal block that shields the heart decreases the risk to about 2.5 per cent.[400] In patients with Hodgkin's disease who receive radiation therapy using a cobalt-60 source or anterior weighting of the beam, which results in a higher dosage to the pericardium under the entry surface, the incidence of pericarditis rises to about 20 per cent[402, 403] and approaches 50 per cent when a fluid challenge is used to unmask occult constrictive pericarditis.[404] In breast cancer radiation therapy in which the volume of the heart included in the field usually is less than 30 per cent, the incidence of radiation-induced pericarditis is less than 5 per cent, with a tolerance for up to 6000 rads given over 6 weeks.[398]

Pericardial injury may occur during the course of treatment or, more commonly, months later. In one series, in 92 per cent of cases involving pericardial effusions, the complication occurred within 12 months after completion of the course of radiation therapy.[402] However, it is now recognized that radiation pericarditis manifested as chronic pericardial effusion or constrictive pericarditis may become apparent many years after radiation therapy.[398, 401, 403–406]

PATHOLOGY. Radiation pericarditis is associated with fibrin deposition and pericardial fibrosis (Fig. 44–23). The acute inflammatory stage may be accompanied by a pericardial effusion that may be serous, serosanguineous, or hemorrhagic with a high protein and lymphocyte content.[398] The inflammation and initial effusion may resolve spontaneously, or the effusion may organize and progress to a stage of dense fibrinous adhesions with gradual obliteration of the pericardial space, thickening of the pericardium, and proliferation of small blood vessels within the pericardium associated with a chronic pericardial effusion or a constricting pericardium. The visceral pericardium may also become fibrotic and thickened, and radiation pericarditis is a common cause of effusive-constrictive pericardial disease.[233] Radiation injury represents an important cause of constrictive pericarditis in children, in whom this condition is relatively uncommon.[407]

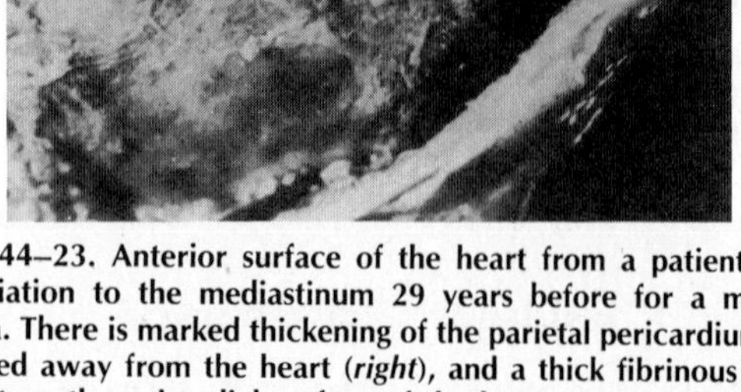

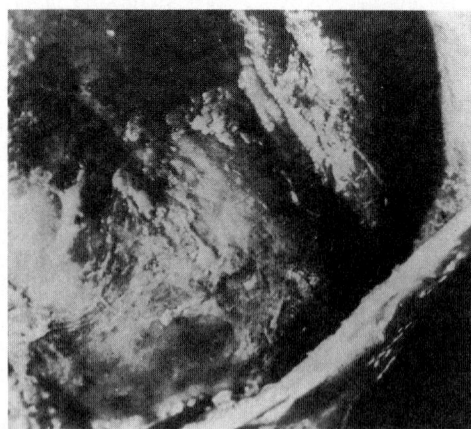

FIGURE 44–23. Anterior surface of the heart from a patient treated with radiation to the mediastinum 29 years before for a malignant thymoma. There is marked thickening of the parietal pericardium which is reflected away from the heart (*right*), and a thick fibrinous exudate is present on the epicardial surface of the heart. (From Stewart, J. R., and Fajardo, L. F.: Radiation-induced heart disease. Prog. Cardiovasc. Dis. *27*:173, 1984.)

It is important to recognize that radiation may occasionally injure the heart itself, causing interstitial myocardial fibrosis, valvular thickening, endothelial proliferation and fibrotic thickening of small intramyocardial arteries, and, possibly, premature atherosclerosis of the epicardial coronary arteris.[398, 408]

CLINICAL FEATURES. Acute pericarditis due to irradiation is not frequently evident clinically. It usually occurs in the context of irradiation of bulky mediastinal tumor adjacent to the pericardium, which suggests that acute pericarditis is largely related to inflammatory necrosis of the adjacent tumor.[398] Patients may manifest a syndrome of acute pericarditis consisting of fever, pericardial pain, anorexia, malaise, a pericardial friction rub, and electrocardiographic abnormalities. Acute pericarditis which occurs during radiation therapy usually abates rapidly, does not preclude completion of planned treatment, and does not correlate well with the risk of late pericardial damage.

In the delayed form of pericardial injury, the onset of symptoms is usually within 12 months but varies from 4 months to more than 20 years. It may be manifested as the syndrome of acute idiopathic pericarditis or as an asymptomatic pericardial effusion with a coexisting pleural effusion on the chest roentgenogram. In about half of the patients, there is some degree of cardiac compression associated with dyspnea, jugular venous distention, and pulsus paradoxus due to delayed chronic pericardial effusion. This importance of this mode of presentation is underscored by the fact that radiation-induced pericardial effusion now accounts for the diagnosis in 10 per cent of patients who undergo surgical drainage of the pericardium.[155, 156] In the Stanford experience,[398] about 20 per cent developed chronic pericarditis which required pericardiectomy. Such patients may present years after radiation therapy with the insidious onset of fatigue, dyspnea, systemic edema, and jugular venous distention due to the development of constrictive pericarditis.[406, 407, 409] The clinical recognition and consequences of this delayed form of pericardial injury have become increasingly important as patients with breast cancer and Hodgkin's disease have had prolonged survival and cures.

DIAGNOSIS. Radiation-induced pericarditis with a pericardial effusion is most often confused with pericarditis due to the underlying malignancy. However, patients with malignant pericardial effusion are more likely to have massive effusions and cardiac tamponade, and cytological examination of pericardial fluid can identify a malignant origin in about 85 per cent of cases.[362] When symptoms referable to the pericardium occur years after apparently successful treatment of Hodgkin's disease or lymphoma, the pericarditis is much more likely to be related to radiation injury than to recurrent mediastinal malignancy. Occasionally, histological examination of the pericardium may be required to differentiate between these two entities.

MANAGEMENT. Patients in whom an asymptomatic pericardial effusion develops after radiation therapy may be followed by physical examination and serial echocardiography without the institution of specific therapy. Percutaneous pericardiocentesis should be limited to the treatment of cardiac tamponade or to drainage of a large pericardial effusion when cytological examination is required for management. Systemic corticosteroids should be reserved for patients with severe intractable pain or life-threatening effusive disease due to the well-documented risk of unmasking latent radiation-induced lung or heart injury when steroids are withdrawn.[410]

Pericardiectomy is required for that small number of symptomatic patients with large recurrent pericardial effusion, severe effusive-constrictive pericarditis, or constrictive pericarditis. The surgical experience at the Mayo Clinic has shown that late constriction developed in 75 per cent of patients with radiation-induced pericarditis who underwent drainage with a limited left thoracic partial pericardiectomy (window).[156] These data are supported by the Stanford experience and others.[155, 224] They suggest that extensive pericardiectomy should be performed in patients with severe effusive or effusive-constrictive radiation-induced pericarditis whose prognosis is otherwise favorable. Actuarial analysis has shown that the 5-year survival rate after pericardiectomy for postirradiation pericarditis was 51 per cent, which is less than the 83 per cent 5-year survival rate of other patients who underwent pericardiectomy.[224] Factors which contribute to a poor outcome include the failure to resect a constricting visceral pericardium (epicardium), and underlying myocardial injury.[224, 411]

PERICARDITIS RELATED TO HYPERSENSITIVITY OR AUTOIMMUNITY

Acute Rheumatic Fever (See also p. 1706)

During the 19th century, acute rheumatic fever was believed to be the most common cause of pericarditis, and it was recognized that rheumatic pericarditis could occur independently of overt endocarditis.[412] The condition is now uncommon, but occasionally the development of a pericardial friction rub or effusion is the initial clue to the presence of rheumatic carditis.

PATHOPHYSIOLOGY. Rheumatic pericarditis is characterized by fibrin deposition that can be accompanied by a fibrinous, serofibrinous, or purulent exudate.[412] The pericardial reaction usually resolves spontaneously. The deposition of IgG, IgM, and complement on the pericardial surface during active pericarditis has been reported,[413] but it is still unclear whether pericarditis occurs as an immune-mediated mechanism or simply as nonspecific inflammation associated with the underlying myocarditis. The development of chronic calcification and constrictive pericarditis, although reported, is very unusual.[414]

CLINICAL FEATURES. Rheumatic pericarditis usually occurs at the onset of the initial episode of acute rheumatic fever and may be asymptomatic or associated with typical pericardial pain and other symptoms of acute rheumatic fever, including fever, malaise, and arthralgias (p. 1711). When present, pericarditis usually indicates an extensive pancarditis. The diagnosis of rheumatic pericarditis is based on the presence of typical pericardial chest pain (p. 1488), a pericardial friction rub, or echocardiographic evidence of a pericardial effusion in association with the usual serological and clinical criteria for acute rheumatic fever (p. 1713). The development of pericarditis in children, which is otherwise unusual in this age group, should prompt a rigorous search for evidence of acute rheumatic fever. The combination of pericarditis, fever, arthralgias, and rash in a child or young adult may be mistaken for a viral exanthem, infectious endocarditis, juvenile rheumatoid arthritis, systemic lupus erythematosus, Henoch-Schönlein purpura, Crohn's disease, or sickle cell crisis.

MANAGEMENT. The treatment of rheumatic pericarditis is that of acute rheumatic fever and includes bed rest and penicillin as well as digoxin if myocardial failure is present. Chest pain associated with rheumatic pericarditis should be treated with aspirin, as described on page 1715. Rarely, corticosteroids are required. Small or moderate-sized pericardial effusions usually resolve spontaneously, and pericardiocentesis should not be performed solely for diagnostic reasons in a patient with documented acute rheumatic fever.

Pericarditis Associated with Systemic Lupus Erythematosus (See also p. 1721)

Pericarditis usually occurs during flare-ups of disease activity in patients with systemic lupus erythematosus (SLE) and is the most common cardiovascular manifestation of the disease.[415] Pericarditis is detected clinically in about 20 to 40 per cent of these patients during the course of their disease.[415, 416] Echocardiographic abnormalities can be detected in a higher percentage of these patients, but the clinical significance of this is unclear.[416, 417] The prevalence of pericarditis in autopsied patients ranges from 43 to 100 per cent, and averages 62 per cent, whereas the prevalence of myocarditis in autopsy series is about 40 per cent.[418, 419] The inflammatory process may cause fibrinous or effusive pericarditis with the rare occurrence of pathognomonic hematoxylin bodies in the visceral pericardium. Pericardial fluid may be serous or grossly hemorrhagic with a high protein content, low glucose content, and white cell count below 10,000/mm^3 (composed primarily of polymorphonuclear leukocytes). Low pericardial fluid complement levels relative to normal serum values have been reported. However, caution must be used in interpreting this finding, since total hemolytic complement levels appear to be normally low in pericardial fluid.[415, 420] Cardiac tamponade occurs in less than 10 per cent of patients with SLE and clinically recognized pericarditis, while the development of constrictive pericarditis has been reported but is extremely rare.[421, 422] Pericarditis due to SLE may be accompanied by other cardiac lesions, including verrucous endocarditis, inflammation and necrosis involving the conduction system, and coronary artery vasculitis.[415, 418]

CLINICAL FEATURES. Pericarditis should be suspected when patients with SLE develop pleuritic chest pain, a pericardial rub, and an enlarging cardiac silhouette on the chest roentgenogram.[415] Electrocardiographic abnormalities are those characteristic of acute pericarditis. Since pericarditis usually occurs during periods of active disease, there is typically evidence of increased disease activity on blood tests for complement-fixation levels, antinuclear antibodies, LE cell preparations, and sedimentation rate. The chest roentgenogram may show enlargement of the cardiac silhouette, pleural effusions, and parenchymal infiltrates. The *echocardiogram* may show evidence of a new pericardial effusion, suggesting the presence of pericardial inflammation. Since many patients with SLE are treated with corticosteroids and immunosuppressive and cytotoxic agents, a careful physical examination, blood cultures, and tuberculin skin test should be performed to search for evidence of purulent, fungal, or tuberculous pericarditis. Except when purulent pericarditis is strongly suspected, it is not necessary to confirm the clinical diagnosis of SLE pericarditis by performing pericardiocentesis.

MANAGEMENT. In the majority of patients, pericarditis subsides when the systemic disease becomes inactive following treatment with corticosteroids or immunotherapy.

The usual complication of cardiac tamponade can ordinarily be treated with pericardiocentesis and usually does not require surgical intervention (i.e., pericardiotomy or pericardiectomy). However, since the development of acute cardiac tamponade is unpredictable, symptomatic patients with SLE pericarditis should be hospitalized and kept under close observation.

Rheumatoid Arthritis (See also p. 1719)

Rheumatoid pericarditis was first described by Charcot, who observed pericardial fibrosis in four of nine autopsied patients.[423] Although pericarditis is detected at autopsy in up to 50 per cent of patients with rheumatoid arthritis (RA), the clinical incidence of symptomatic pericarditis is less than 10 per cent.[424–426] On the basis of echocardiographic criteria for the presence of a pericardial effusion, possible pericarditis has been detected in 50 per cent of patients with chronic nodular RA, in 15 per cent of patients with nonnodular RA and in no patients of comparable age with osteoarthritis.[427] Pericarditis tends to appear in patients with other evidence of severe RA, including extensive joint deformity, subcutaneous rheumatoid nodules, pneumonitis, and positive serum rheumatoid factor. Rheumatoid pericarditis in adults can cause cardiac tamponade and has become recognized as a cause of effusive-constrictive pericarditis and constrictive pericarditis.[233, 424, 428, 429] Pericarditis, and the complication of cardiac tamponade, may occur with or without evidence of active joint involvement in children with juvenile RA[430] and in adults with juvenile RA (adult Still's disease).[431, 432]

PATHOLOGY. Typical pathological changes in the pericardium are those of nonspecific fibrous thickening of the visceral and parietal pericardium with adhesions. Rarely, small, necrotic granulomatous nodules are detected on the epicardial surface that are histologically identical to the subcutaneous rheumatoid nodule. Pericardial effusions, whose characteristics are similar to those of pleural effusions associated with RA pericarditis, are usually serous or hemorrhagic, with greater than 5 gm/dl of protein, glucose levels less than 45 mg/dl, high cholesterol levels, and white blood cell counts ranging from 20,000 to 90,000/mm^3.[424, 425] Soluble immune complexes, positive latex-fixation titers, and low complement levels in the pericardial fluid have also been described.[433] Acute pericarditis may progress to cause diffusely constricting fibrotic pericarditis and can coexist with other cardiac lesions, including granulomatous aortic and mitral valve deformity causing chronic mitral or aortic regurgitation.

CLINICAL FEATURES. RA is often associated with fever, precordial chest pain, and dyspnea in association with a pericardial friction rub.[433] Pericarditis commonly coexists with an exacerbation of joint inflammation and pleuritis, manifest on the chest roentgenogram as a unilateral or bilateral pleural effusion in about 65 per cent of cases.[433] The electrocardiogram usually shows nonspecific ST-segment and T-wave changes. The presence of atrioventricular block in patients with rheumatoid pericarditis probably reflects rheumatoid myocardial involvement (p. 1719). On echocardiography a pericardial effusion is present in approximately half the patients with nodular RA,[434, 435] but its presence does not always correlate with the existence of symptomatic pericarditis.

Although rheumatoid pericarditis is usually self-limited and benign, cardiac tamponade may develop abruptly in 3 to 25 per cent of patients[424, 429] and has been reported as a complication of sudden steroid withdrawal.[435] An uncommon but major complication is the rapid onset of subacute effusive-constrictive pericarditis.[424, 428, 429] The development of chronic constrictive pericarditis is a well-recognized complication which is more prevalent in males than females.[436, 437]

MANAGEMENT. Patients with symptomatic pericarditis may be treated with aspirin or other nonsteroidal antiinflammatory agents, as described on page 1490. Pericardiocentesis is indicated for relief of a large anterior-posterior effusion causing cardiac tamponade. There is no clear evidence that steroids alter the natural history of effusions or prevent the development of the constrictive pericarditis. There is now an extensive experience in the surgical management of rheumatoid pericarditis, and patients with connective tissue disorders (predominantly RA) now comprise about 10 to 20 per cent of patients undergoing pericardiectomy.[222, 224] In patients with documented effusive-constrictive or constrictive pericarditis, pericardiectomy can provide gratifying hemodynamic and symptomatic improvement.[224, 424, 428, 429, 436, 437]

Scleroderma Pericarditis (See also p. 1723)

Pericardial involvement is found at autopsy in about 50 per cent of patients with progressive systemic sclerosis (scleroderma), while pericarditis is detected clinically in about 10 per cent of patients.[438–440] While the pathogenesis of scleroderma pericarditis is unknown, it has been suggested that increased collagen formation by fibroblasts, in combination with tissue hypoxia, may result in aberrant collagen metabolism. Histological changes consist of nonspecific fibrotic pericardial thickening with adhesions and perivascular inflammatory cells. Although pericardial effusions can be detected by means of echocardiography in about 40 per cent of patients with scleroderma, in the majority of patients a pericardial effusion is not associated with symptoms.[441]

When present, the pericardial effusion is straw-colored and characterized by a protein content greater than 5 gm/dl, low cell count, and (in contrast to the characteristics of pericardial effusions in SLE and RA) the absence of autoantibodies, low complement levels, and immune complexes. Pericardial involvement is often associated with sclerodermatous infiltration of the heart, causing a restrictive cardiomyopathy.[440]

Scleroderma pericardial disease may be manifested as an acute syndrome resembling viral myocarditis, with fever, chest pain, and pericardial friction rub, and nonspecific electrocardiographic ST- and T-wave changes.[439] Other patients develop a chronic pericardial effusion or pericardial constriction with symptoms of right and left atrial hypertension, cardiomegaly and pleural effusions on the chest roentgenogram, and low QRS voltage on the electrocardiogram.

MANAGEMENT. There is no definitive treatment for scleroderma pericarditis. Patients with the syndrome of acute pericarditis may be treated with aspirin, as described on page 1490. Rarely, pericardial effusions with cardiac tamponade may develop, necessitating pericardiocentesis.[442] Patients with constrictive pericarditis may require pericardiectomy. Severe recurrent constrictive pericarditis has also been reported as a complication of idiopathic retroperitoneal and mediastinal fibrosis, which are regional expressions of a systemic sclerosing disease.[443] It is especially important to perform cardiac catheterization in patients with scleroderma and suspected cardiac tamponade or constrictive pericarditis, since dyspnea and systemic venous hypertension may be related to sclerodermatous involvement of the pericardium or myocardium or to pulmonary hypertension secondary to pulmonary fibrosis. The development of symptomatic pericarditis in patients with scleroderma is ominous, since the 5-year survival rate is about 25 per cent when isolated pericardial or other cardiac involvement is present and about 75 per cent in patients without heart, lung, or kidney involvement.[444]

Pericarditis in Other Connective Tissue Disorders

Acute pericarditis with pericardial effusions occurs in about 30 per cent of patients with mixed connective tissue and may coexist with other cardiac abnormalities including myocarditis and intimal hyperplasia of the coronary arteries.[445, 446]

Pericarditis may rarely develop in other connective tissue disorders, including the Sjögren syndrome, dermatomyositis, ankylosing spondylitis, the Reiter syndrome, Wegener's granulomatosis, the Felty syndrome, and severe serum sickness.[447–450] Pericarditis associated with polyarteritis nodosa may occur in patients who are hepatitis B antigen-positive. It also occurs in disorders of possible autoimmune etiology, including temporal arteritis,[451] inflammatory bowel disease,[452] Kawasaki's disease,[453] familial Mediterranean fever, Whipple's disease,[454] celiac disease,[455] Behcet's disease, and myasthenia gravis.[456] Amyloidosis is well known as a cause of infiltrative restrictive myopathy, the hemodynamics of which may mimic constrictive pericarditis (p. 1501), but it may also involve the pericardium and cause pericardial effusions.[217, 218]

Cardiac involvement is present at autopsy in about 25 per cent of patients with sarcoidosis and can involve the pericardium in the absence of significant myocardial infiltration.[457] Sarcoidosis can be a rare cause of cardiac tamponade and constrictive pericarditis[458–460]; in the latter case, the findings of pericardial thickening with noncaseating granulomas may cause confusion with tuberculous or fungal pericarditis (Fig. 44–24).[170, 458–460]

Drug- and Toxin-Related Pericarditis

Pericarditis occurs in about 25 per cent of patients with procainamide-related and 2 per cent of those with hydralazine-related development of the drug-induced SLE syndrome.[461] In these patients, pericarditis may occasionally be complicated by the development of cardiac tamponade or the rapid development of pericardial constriction.[462] Other drugs that may produce pericarditis in association with the drug-induced syndrome of SLE include reserpine, methyldopa, isoniazid, and diphenylhydantoin.[463]

Other drugs appear to produce pericarditis through separate mechanisms. Pericarditis has been reported as a complication of a hypersensitivity reaction with peripheral eosinophilia after administration of penicillin[464] and cromolyn sodium.[465] The mechanisms of drug-induced pericarditis following administration of 6-amino-D-psicofuranosylpurine,[466] minoxidil,[467] and dantrolene sodium[468] are not understood. Methysergide is well-recognized as a cause of constrictive pericarditis as part of a generalized process of mediastinal fibrosis.[469] The anthracycline neoplastic agents doxorubicin and Daunorubicin may cause acute pericarditis as well as myocardial inflammation,[470] and pericarditis has also been reported in association with the use of cytosine arabinoside.[471, 472] Pericarditis has also been reported as a foreign body reaction to the presence of silicone[473] and talc[474] within the pericardial space, in association with cardiac iron deposition in thalassaemia,[475] and as a toxic response to scorpionfish sting.[476]

Acute drug-related pericarditis usually resolves when the offending drug is discontinued, and improvement may be accelerated by the administration of corticosteroids. The rare development of chronic constrictive pericarditis may be treated by pericardiectomy.

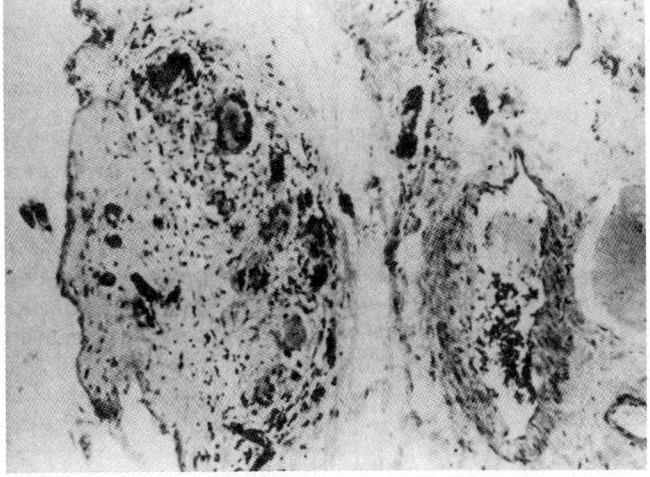

FIGURE 44–24. Photomicrograph of a pericardial biopsy from a patient with cardiac tamponade secondary to cardiac sarcoidosis which shows a noncaseating granuloma with several giant cells (× 250 magnification). (From Verkleeren, J. L., et al.: Cardiac tamponade secondary to sarcoidosis. Am. Heart J. *106*:601, 1983.)

Postmyocardial Infarction Syndrome (Dressler Syndrome)

The Dressler syndrome is an acute illness with fever, pericarditis, and pleuritis, possibly of autoimmune origin, that occurs weeks to months after an acute myocardial infarction.[477] Today, a distinction is usually made between acute postinfarction pericarditis, which occurs during the first week after infarction (p. 1514) and Dressler syndrome, which usually appears 2 to 3 weeks after infarction, with a range of 1 week to several months. Dressler estimated that this syndrome occurred in up to 4 per cent of patients after acute myocardial infarction[478]; however, a more recent series from the same hospital indicates that the incidence of Dressler syndrome has markedly decreased.[318]

ETIOLOGY. The etiology of this syndrome is unknown. The association of symptoms and the appearance of antimyocardial antibodies has led to the hypothesis that an autoimmune mechanism, with or without a latent viral infection, is the etiology.[479, 480] Some workers have concluded that the development of antimyocardial antibodies is not specific for the presence of Dressler syndrome.[318, 481] Leakage of blood into the pericardial space is another proposed mechanism, and the current lower incidence of the syndrome may reflect less use of oral anticoagulants in the postinfarction period.[318] It is likely that there are common factors in the pathogenesis of Dressler syndrome and the postpericardiotomy syndrome (p. 1522), both of which share the following features: (1) an initial insult of endothelial cell injury and entry of blood into the pericardial space; and (2) a delayed response after the initial insult, consisting of fever and inflammation of the pericardial surfaces; (3) the development of antiheart antibodies; (4) a dramatic response to antiinflammatory agents; and (5) a tendency for recurrence.

PATHOLOGY. The histology of the pericardium usually reveals a nonspecific inflammation with fibrin deposition. In contrast to the acute pericarditis following myocardial infarction in which pericardial inflammation is often patchy, overlying the regions of infarction, the pericarditis in Dressler syndrome is usually diffuse.

CLINICAL FEATURES. Patients characteristically have severe malaise, fever, chest pain, and pleurisy.[482] The chest pain may be severe enough initially to cause both patient and physician to consider that it is caused by a second myocardial infarction. Dressler syndrome is occasionally the initial presentation of a previously undiagnosed infarction.[483] Physical examination often discloses a pericardial friction rub and sometimes a pleural friction rub as well. The *chest roentgenogram* commonly reveals an enlarged cardiac silhouette secondary to pericardial effusion associated with pleural effusions[478] and, occasionally, transient pulmonary infiltrates. The echocardiographic evidence of a pericardial effusion in the absence of other symptoms is not diagnostic of Dressler syndrome, since asymptomatic pericardial effusions occur in about one of four patients following myocardial infarction.[323] Electrocardiographic abnormalities usually consist of serial ST-segment and T-wave changes strongly suggestive of acute pericarditis, but the electrocardiogram may not be helpful in patients with persistent repolarization abnormalities following infarction. Blood tests usually reveal the nonspecific findings of an increased erythrocyte sedimentation rate and peripheral leukocytosis. Tests for antimyocardial antibodies are not widely available or established as a means of confirming the diagnosis.

Dressler syndrome can usually be differentiated from recurrent myocardial infarction by (1) the characteristics of the chest pain and its failure to improve with nitroglycerin, (2) the absence of new Q waves on the electrocardiogram, and (3) the absence of a marked rise in the creatine kinase isoenzyme (CK-MB) band. Small increases in cardiac enzyme levels may occur in pericarditis when the underlying epicardium is involved. Dressler syndrome must also be distinguished from hemorrhagic pericarditis secondary to chronic systemic anticoagulation.

MANAGEMENT. A single episode of Dressler syndrome is usually self-limited, but the syndrome does tend to recur. The initial syndrome usually warrants hospital admission and observation for development of pericardial effusion or cardiac tamponade.[484] Oral anticoagulants should be discontinued because of the risk of pericardial hemorrhage. As in other patients with acute pericarditis, patients who are severely symptomatic with fever and chest pain usually benefit from bed rest and treatment with aspirin or a nonsteroidal antiinflammatory agent. Recurrent episodes of Dressler syndrome may respond only to corticosteroids and occasionally require complete pericardiectomy for relief of intractable pericardial pain or prevention of recurrence. Cardiac tamponade in the absence of anticoagulant therapy, although uncommon, has been reported,[484] and can usually be managed with pericardiocentesis. Constrictive pericarditis is an extremely rare complication of Dressler syndrome that may be relieved by pericardiectomy.[485, 486]

Postpericardiotomy Syndrome

ETIOLOGY. Postpericardiotomy syndrome is identified by the appearance of fever, pericarditis, and pleuritis more than a week after a cardiac operation in which the pericardium has been opened and manipulated. This syndrome was first recognized in patients after mitral valvulotomy for rheumatic heart disease, and it was initially believed to represent a reactivation of rheumatic fever.[487] Subsequently it was realized that the syndrome could occur following cardiac operations in patients without rheumatic heart disease and that the common denominator appeared to be wide incision and manipulation of the pericardium.[488] An identical clinical syndrome has been reported following cardiac perforation by a catheter or transvenous pacemaker, blunt chest trauma, percutaneous diagnostic left ventricular puncture, and epicardial pacemaker implantation.[489] The incidence of postpericardiotomy syndrome following cardiac surgery ranges from 10 to 40 per cent in various series, and is higher in children than in adults.[490–492] The observation of a 31 per cent incidence of postpericardiotomy syndrome in patients undergoing cardiac surgery for the Wolff-Parkinson-White syndrome clearly indicates that pericardial damage prior to surgery is not a contributing factor.[492] Furthermore, pericardial drainage techniques do not appear to affect the frequency of development of the syndrome after cardiac surgery.[493]

Analogous to the Dressler syndrome, the etiology of postpericardiotomy syndrome is hypothesized to be an autoimmune reaction directed against the epicardium, possibly in concert with a new or reactivated viral infection. Studies by Engle and colleagues have demonstrated that antiheart antibodies appear in the serum of some patients who undergo pericardiotomy and that there is a positive correlation between the level of the titers and the incidence of the syndrome.[491] Approximately 70 per cent of patients with the postpericardiotomy syndrome and high antiheart antibody titers also develop a fourfold or higher rise in titer against one or more viral antigens, while in patients without the postpericardiotomy syndrome, a rise in viral titers occurs in only 8 per cent of those with negative antiheart antibody titers and in only 19 per cent of those with low levels of antiheart antibody titers. These findings suggest that viral infection may be a triggering or permissive factor. The postpericardiotomy syndrome is rare in children under 2 years of age who undergo cardiac surgery, a finding that may be related to the short exposure time to viruses or to the persistence of protective maternal antibodies transmitted via the placenta. The development of pleuritis and pleural effusions is believed to reflect involvement of the pleura adjacent to the inflamed pericardium; involvement of serous membranes distant from the heart is uncommon.

PATHOLOGY. There are no pathognomonic histological features of postpericardiotomy syndrome. The presence of blood in the pericardial space adjacent to an injured epicardium may result in the later development of pericardial adhesions, thickening of the pericardial membranes, and occasionally fibrinous obliteration of the pericardial space, causing pericardial constriction. Pericardial effusions in patients with postpericardiotomy syndrome may be straw-colored, serosanguineous, or frankly hemorrhagic, with a protein content higher than 4.5 gm/dl and a white blood cell count between 3000 and 8000/mm^3 (composed of both lymphocytes and granulocytes).[494]

CLINICAL FEATURES. Patients typically develop an acute illness characterized by fever, malaise, and chest pain that usually begins during the second or third postoperative week (Fig. 44–25). In some cases, the fever may reflect a continuation of the more common problem of fever in the first week after operation. The chest pain is typical of acute pericarditis (p. 1488) and often has a pleuritic quality. Nonspecific signs of inflammation including an elevated sedimentation rate and polymorphonuclear leukocytosis may also be present.

Physical examination often reveals a pericardial friction rub. It should be noted that the friction rub present in almost all patients during the first few days after cardiac surgery disappears in most patients who do not develop postpericardiotomy syndrome by the end of the first post-

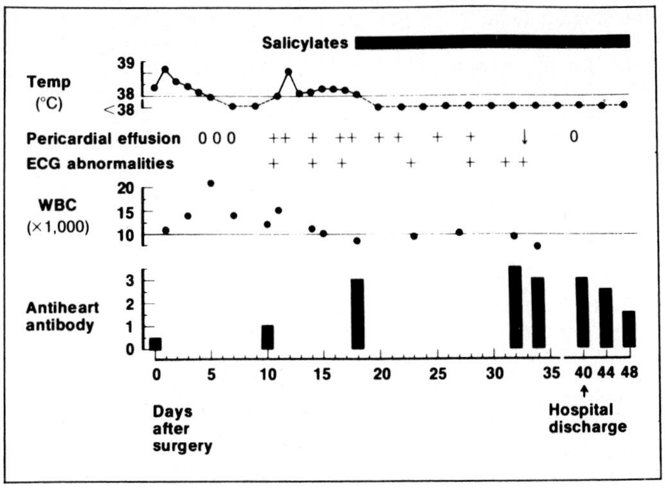

FIGURE 44–25. Representative clinical course of a child with the postpericardiotomy syndrome following cardiac surgery. Note that a febrile illness associated with effusive pericarditis, electrocardiographic changes, and leukocytosis began about 10 days after surgery. The administration of salicylates was followed by prompt relief of fever and pericarditis. The antiheart antibody titer, which was initially high, subsequently declined. (From Engle, M. A., et al.: The postpericardiotomy syndrome. 25 years' experience. J. Cardiovasc. Med. *4*:321, 1984.)

operative week. The *chest roentgenogram* demonstrates left-sided or bilateral pleural effusions in about two-thirds of patients, pulmonary infiltrates in about one-tenth, and transient enlargement of the cardiac silhouette in half.[492] *Electrocardiography* may show nonspecific ST-segment and T-wave changes and a variety of episodic tachyarrhythmias. *Echocardiography* is useful in monitoring the appearance and size of a pericardial effusion, and in detecting evidence of cardiac compression such as right atrial collapse. However, it should be noted that pericardial effusions are extremely common after cardiac surgery, and occur in 56 to 84 per cent of patients within the first 10 days after cardiac surgery.[495, 496] Thus, the diagnosis of postpericardiotomy syndrome is made on clinical grounds on the basis of recognition of the distinctive features of the syndrome in the postoperative patient. Other causes of postoperative fever, particularly infection (including the viral-induced postperfusion syndrome of atypical lymphocytosis, fever, and hepatosplenomegaly), must be excluded.[497]

MANAGEMENT. The postpericardiotomy syndrome is a self-limited but often prolonged and disabling illness. Fever and severe chest pain are usually relieved by aspirin or nonsteroidal antiinflammatory drugs. Corticosteroids should be reserved for patients in whom fever and chest pain are not relieved within 48 hours by other antiinflammatory agents. Recurrences tend to appear during the first 6 months after surgery.

Cardiac tamponade is an important and well-recognized complication of the postpericardiotomy syndrome.[494, 498–500] In one large recent series of adult patients who survived cardiac surgery, almost 1 per cent developed cardiac tamponade an average of 49 days after surgery—in association with fever, a pericardial friction rub, and pericardial chest pain typical of the postpericardiotomy syndrome.[494] In contrast to the important role of anticoagulation in *early* postoperative bleeding after cardiac surgery, the use of anticoagulants did not appear to be a prerequisite for the development of cardiac tamponade in association with the postpericardiotomy syndrome. Cardiac tamponade can be managed conservatively by pericardiocentesis followed by the administration of antiinflammatory agents.[494] Patients with recurrent tamponade require surgical drainage and pericardiectomy. Percutaneous pericardiocentesis should not be attempted in patients with echocardiographic evidence of only a small posterior effusion, a loculated effusion, or an effusion with dense echoes suggesting the presence of both thrombus and free fluid. Constrictive pericarditis is a rare complication that may occur months to years after the postpericardiotomy syndrome.

Postoperative Hemopericardium

Acute cardiac tamponade and pericardial constriction in the absence of typical features of the postpericardiotomy syndrome also occur secondary to hemopericardium following cardiac surgery and perforation of the heart during cardiac catheterization (including transseptal left heart catheterization), pacemaker insertion, pericardiocentesis, valvuloplasty, and coronary artery angioplasty.[501–504] Acute pericarditis without frank cardiac perforation has been reported in 0.5 per cent of 981 patients who underwent angioplasty, and this complication may be secondary to occult epicardial-pericardial hematoma formation.[505] In some patients, cardiac tamponade following invasive cardiac procedures and cardiac surgery has been successfully managed with pericardiocentesis.[494, 506] However, the development of early and late postoperative tamponade is usually due to the combination of free fluid and organizing thrombus, which requires open surgical drainage of the pericardial space. Localized compression of the heart has also been reported as a complication of the postoperative cardiac tamponade.[507]

Constrictive pericarditis is being increasingly recognized as a complication of cardiac surgery and may occur in patients in whom the pericardium is left open but in situ.[154, 508–513] The time interval between the cardiac operation and the definitive diagnosis usually is about a year, but severe effusive-constrictive pericarditis has been reported as early as 2 to 6 weeks after operation.[513, 514] In a review of 5207 adults who underwent cardiac surgery, 0.2 per cent (11 patients) developed constrictive pericarditis documented by cardiac catheterization an average of 82 days after operation.[512] Important clinical features in these patients include dyspnea, jugular venous distention, pedal edema, and increased roentgenographic heart size, while echocardiographic evidence of pericardial thickening with a posterior pericardial effusion was detected in the majority. These patients were found to have hemorrhage-induced fibrosis of the pericardium, usually associated with a posterior organized hematoma.[512] The majority improved after undergoing extensive pericardiectomy. Povidone iodine irrigation of the heart is postulated to be a triggering factor in some patients.[510, 512] This factor has been absent in other reports, and it is likely that intrapericardial hemorrhage and serosal injury are also contributing factors.[513] There is now strong evidence that postoperative constrictive pericarditis can involve bypass grafts and contribute to premature graft closure as well as damage to grafts during pericardiectomy.[514–517]

OTHER FORMS OF PERICARDIAL DISEASE

Myxedema Pericardial Disease

Myxedema is frequently associated with a myopathy; pericardial effusion also occurs in up to one-third of patients.[518–520] Since myxedematous patients frequently have ascites, pleural effusions, and uveal edema, it has been suggested that pericardial effusion may be related to a combination of sodium and water retention, slow lymphatic drainage, and increased capillary permeability with protein extravasation.[521] The pericardial fluid is usually clear or straw-colored, with elevated protein and cholesterol concentrations and few leukocytes or red blood cells. Pericardial fluid usually accumulates very slowly and may achieve enormous volumes of 5 to 6 liters. Occasionally, the pericardial effusion may resemble a viscous jelly rather than a clear fluid.

Myxedematous pericardial effusions usually do not cause symptoms. Often attention is called to the heart by the finding of marked cardiomegaly on a chest roentgenogram, and a large pericardial effusion is occasionally the presenting feature of hypothyroidism.[522, 523] Since infants and elderly patients with hypothyroidism may be asymptomatic, this etiology should always be excluded in these patients with a pericardial effusion of unknown cause. The *electrocardiogram* often shows nonspecific abnormalities, including low QRS voltage and flattened or inverted T waves due to either myxedematous heart disease or pericardial effusion. Myxedematous patients with cardiac compression from a pericardial effusion may show the absence of the expected compensatory tachycardia.

Myxedematous pericardial effusions tend to regress slowly and ultimately disappear over a period of months after patients have been treated with thyroid replacement and have returned to the euthyroid state.[518, 519, 522, 523] Cardiac tamponade has been reported, but it is a rare complication.[522, 524, 525]

Cholesterol Pericarditis

Cholesterol pericarditis results from pericardial injury associated with deposition of cholesterol crystals and a mononuclear cell inflammatory reaction consisting of foam cells, macrophages, and giant cells. The presence of cholesterol crystals in the pericardial space is believed to provoke a chronic inflammatory response that results in effusion and may ultimately lead to the development of constrictive pericarditis. A pericardial effusion that contains microscopic cholesterol crystals typically has a glittering "gold" appearance. The similarities in the lipid and cholesterol contents of pericardial fluid and serum in some patients with cholesterol pericarditis suggest that simple transudation may explain the high cholesterol content in the pericardial space.

MANAGEMENT. This includes the detection and treatment of any underlying predisposing condition associated with the development of cholesterol pericarditis, such as tuberculous, rheumatoid, or myxedematous pericarditis or hypercholesterolemia. However, in the majority of cases, cholesterol pericarditis occurs in the absence of a clear underlying disease.[526] Although cholesterol pericardial effusions are usually large, because they develop slowly, they rarely cause cardiac tamponade. Pericardiectomy is indicated in the unlikely event of cardiac tamponade as well as in the treatment of massive cholesterol pericardial effusion, which may cause dyspnea and chest pain.[527] The development of constrictive pericarditis requiring pericardiectomy is rare.[528]

Chylopericardium

Idiopathic chylopericardium is rare, and chylopericardium is usually associated with mechanical obstruction of the thoracic duct or its drainage into the left subclavian vein resulting from (1) surgical or traumatic rupture of the thoracic duct or (2) lymphatic blockage by neoplasm, tuberculosis, or congenital lymphangiomatosis.[529, 530] Thoracic duct obstruction with failure of adequate collateral drainage then results in reflux of chyle through lymphatics draining the pericardium. Most patients with chylopericardium are asymptomatic and come to clinical attention when a large, slowly accumulating pericardial effusion is detected on chest roentgenogram or echocardiogram. The presence of a connection between a damaged thoracic duct and the pericardial space can be established by lymphangiography and radionuclide lymphangiography with technetium-99m antimony sulfur colloid, as well as by the recovery of ingested Sudan III, a lipophilic dye, from pericardial aspirate.[529, 530] Computed tomography may demonstrate a density compatible with fat in the pericardial space.[531] The pericardial fluid is usually milky white with a high cholesterol and triglyceride content, a protein content greater than 3.5 gm/dl, and microscopic fat droplets demonstrated with a Sudan III stain.[530] Lymphopericardium, which is due to pericardial angiomas as part of a generalized lymphangiectasis, is characterized by clear pericardial fluid.

Cardiac tamponade and constrictive pericarditis are rare complications.[529, 531] The management of symptomatic chylopericardium consists of efforts to reduce the likelihood of recurrence. These include ingestion of a diet rich in medium-chain triglycerides or, if this is unsuccessful, in ligation of the thoracic duct, and parietal pericardiectomy to evacuate chylous fluid and prevent reaccumulation.[530, 532]

Traumatic Pericarditis (See also p. 1536)

In addition to penetrating or nonpenetrating cardiac trauma (Chap. 45), other important causes of traumatic pericarditis include rupture of the esophagus into the pericardial space, which may occur from esophageal erosion secondary to esophageal carcinoma or sudden rupture of the esophageal contents into the pericardial space in Boerhaave's syndrome, or as a complication of esophagogastrectomy. Traumatic pericarditis due to esophageal rupture is usually followed by intense erosive pericardial inflammation and infection. Esophageal rupture or perforation may also be followed by the development of the esophagopericardial fistula.[533] These disorders require immediate surgical intervention and are associated with a high mortality. Pericarditis may also occur secondary to pancreatitis associated with a pericardial effusion with high amylase content and, rarely, the development of cardiac tamponade or a pancreatic-pericardial fistula.[534, 535]

Pericardial trauma may also give rise to unusual traumatic syndromes, including cardiovascular collapse following herniation of the heart through a tear in the pericardium, mimicking congenital partial absence of the pericardium with cardiac subluxation,[536] and intrapericardial diaphragmatic hernia.[537] Life-threatening cardiac herniation may also occur following radical left pneumonectomy with partial pericardial resection.[538]

Pericardial Cysts

Pericardial cysts are rare developmental anomalies and are typically located at the right costophrenic angle.[539] Unusual locations include the left costophrenic angle, hilum, and superior mediastinum at the level of

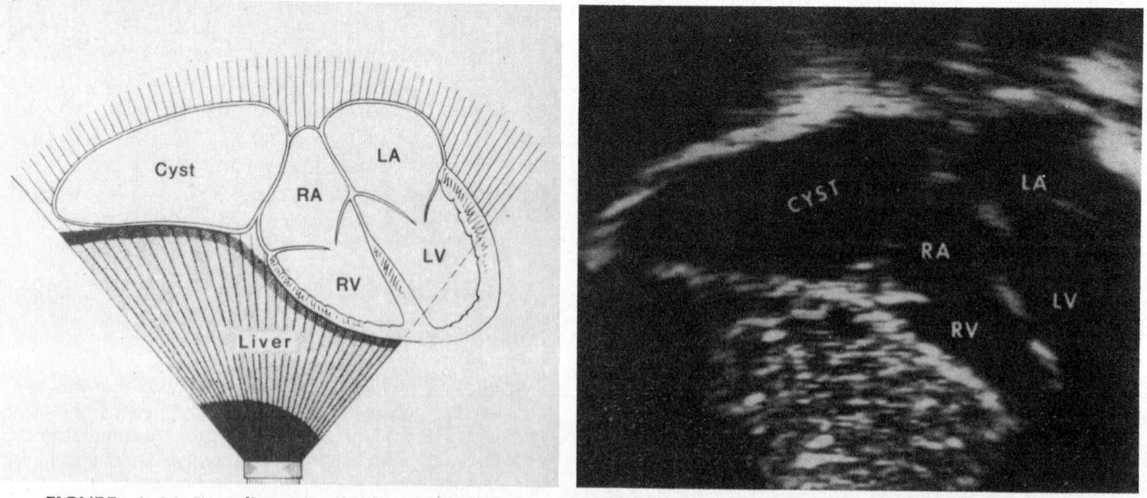

FIGURE 44–26. Two-dimensional subcostal echocardiographic appearance of a well-demarcated benign pericardial cyst adjacent to the right atrial (RA) wall. (From Hynes, J. K., et al.: Two-dimensional echocardiographic diagnosis of pericardial cyst. Mayo Clin. Proc. *58*:60, 1983.)

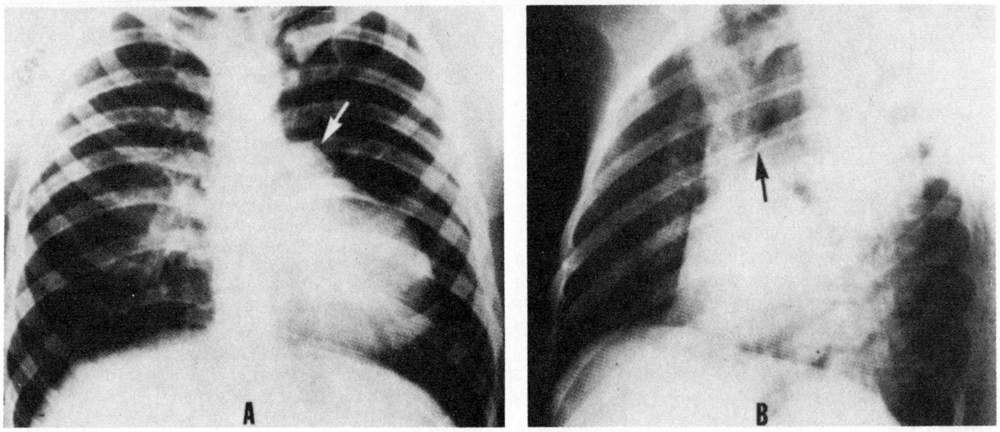

FIGURE 44–27. Chest roentgenograms in a patient with total absence of the left pericardium in posteroanterior (*A*) and left anterior oblique views (*B*). The heart is shifted leftward, and the pulmonary artery segment is prominent (white arrow). There is a tongue of lung between the aorta and main pulmonary artery (black arrow). (From Nassar, W. K., et al.: Congenital absence of left pericardium. Circulation *34*:100, 1966, by permission of the American Heart Association, Inc.)

the aortic arch. They are usually unilocular and filled with clear liquid, giving rise to the term "spring-water cysts."

Pericardial cysts usually do not cause symptoms or unusual physical findings. Rarely, chest pain may occur owing to torsion of the cyst. These lesions typically come to medical attention as an unsuspected finding on a chest roentgenogram of a round, sharply defined mass along the right cardiac border. The size of the cyst may vary over time.[540, 541] In most cases, a cyst can be differentiated from a solid tumor or aneurysm by two-dimensional echocardiography or computerized tomography (Fig. 44–26).[541] When a suspected pericardial cyst is present in an unusual location, angiography may occasionally be needed to discriminate a cyst from an aneurysm or pseudoaneurysm. Pericardial cysts located at the right costophrenic angle can be accurately diagnosed and treated by percutaneous aspiration under fluoroscopic guidance.[542] Because long-term follow-up studies have shown that most asymptomatic patients do not develop symptoms, most patients should be managed conservatively, without surgical exploration.[543]

Other benign developmental abnormalities of the pericardium include benign intrapericardial teratomas and intrapericardial bronchial cysts, which can be identified by computed tomography.[544]

Congenital Absence and Defects of the Pericardium

Congenital absence of the pericardium was first described anatomically by Realdus Columbus in 1559, but its antemortem detection did not occur until 1959.[545] This anomaly usually involves a partial defect of the left-sided pericardium which is potentially lethal; total or partial absence of the right-sided pericardium is extremely rare.[546] There is a 3:1 male-to-female predominance among patients with pericardial defects, and about 30 per cent have other congenital anomalies, including atrial septal defect, bicuspid aortic valve, bronchogenic cysts, or pulmonic sequestration.[547] A familial occurrence of congenital absence of the pericardium has been reported.[548]

TOTAL ABSENCE OF THE PERICARDIUM. This is usually associated with no symptoms. Occasionally the patient may complain of chest discomfort and palpitations. The etiology of these symptoms is unknown, but they may be related to torsion of the great vessels due to excess mobility of the heart. Most asymptomatic patients come to medical attention because of an unexplained heart murmur or abnormal chest roentgenogram.

Clinical features of patients with total absence of the left pericardium include widened splitting of the second heart sound, a hyperdynamic precordial impulse, leftward displacement of the apical impulse, and a systolic murmur at the upper left sternal border that may be related to turbulent blood flow in an unusually mobile heart. Electrocardiographic abnormalities include right-axis deviation due to levoposition of the heart, incomplete right bundle branch block, clockwise displacement of the QRS transition zone of the precordial leads, and tall and peaked P waves in the right precordial leads.[547, 549]

The standard posteroanterior view of the chest roentgenogram reveals marked leftward displacement of the cardiac silhouette (Fig. 44–27), prominence of the main pulmonary artery, and interposition of radiolucent lung tissue between the aorta and main pulmonary artery or between the left hemidiaphragm and inferior cardiac border. This anomaly must be differentiated from other conditions that cause prominence of the left hilum or pulmonary artery on the standard chest film,

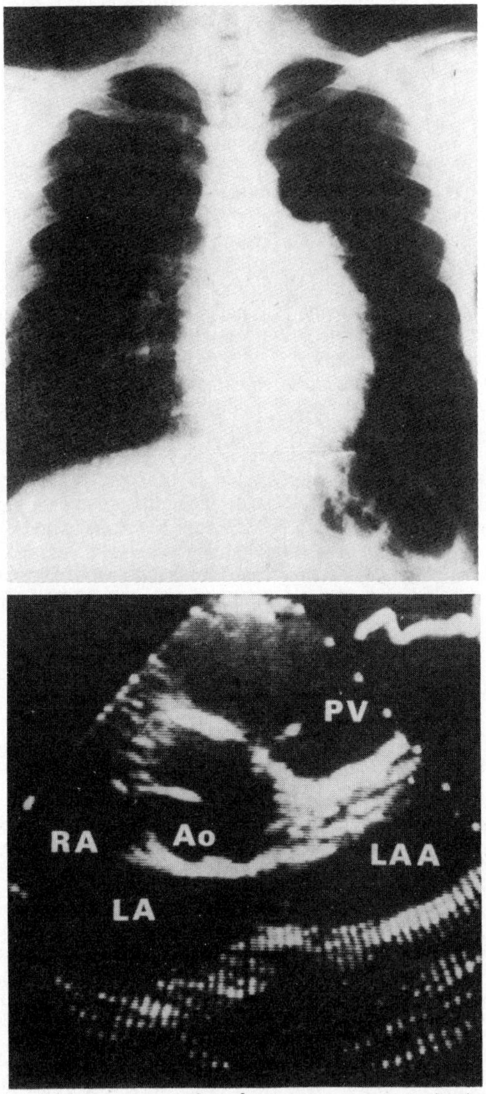

FIGURE 44–28. Anteroposterior chest roentgenogram (*top*) and two-dimensional parasternal short axis echocardiogram (*bottom*) from a patient with the potentially lethal condition of partial absence of the left pericardium. The chest roentgenogram shows prominence of the left hilum. The echocardiogram suggests that the left atrium (LA) communicates with a giant left atrial appendage (LAA) which appears to encircle the pulmonary trunk (PV = pulmonary valve; RA = right atrium; Ao = aorta). This appearance is caused by protrusion of the left atrial appendage through the partial defect in the pericardium. (From Ruys, F., et al.: Expansion of the left atrial appendage is a distinctive cross-sectional echocardiographic feature of congenital defect of the pericardium. Eur. Heart J. *4*:738, 1983.)

including pulmonic valve stenosis, atrial septal defect, idiopathic dilatation of the pulmonary artery, and hilar adenopathy.

M-mode echocardiographic findings simulate those seen in right ventricular volume overload, including dilatation of the right ventricle and paradoxical anterior motion of the septum in systole, which is an artifact related to exaggerated cardiac rotation. Two-dimensional echocardiography can demonstrate a localized bulge of the left ventricular contour and the drop-off of pericardial echoes.[550, 551] Radionuclide perfusion imaging can be used to confirm the diagnosis by the demonstration of a wedge of lung tissue between the heart and left hemidiaphragm[552]; computed tomography and magnetic resonance imaging can also be used to detect absence of the left pericardium.[553]

Findings at cardiac catheterization are usually normal. Diagnostic left pneumothorax has been used in the past to outline the pericardium, but this procedure is not without risk and is now rarely needed to make the diagnosis of complete absence of the left pericardium if radiological and echocardiographic findings are compatible with the diagnosis. Cardiac catheterization with angiography is indicated only if there is a strong suspicion of associated congenital anomalies requiring surgical correction. Usually no specific therapy is required for management of complete absence of the left-sided pericardium.

PARTIAL PERICARDIAL DEFECTS. When located on the left side, these congenital defects may be complicated by herniation of the left atrial appendage, atrium, or left ventricle through the defect, associated with chest pain, syncope, and sudden death from cardiac strangulation.[554, 555] The chest roentgenogram usually shows the nonspecific finding of prominence of the upper portion of the left heart border which must be distinguished from pulmonary artery dilation or aneurysm of the left atrial appendage. Two-dimensional echocardiography is helpful in demonstrating dilation and exaggerated motion of the left atrial appendage which extends anterior to the pulmonary artery (Fig. 44–28).[556] Pulmonary artery angiography with follow-through of contrast opacification of the left heart is the standard method of definitively demonstrating herniation of the left atrium or left atrial appendage beyond the left heart border.[556]

The even rarer anomaly of *partial right-sided pericardial defect* may be associated with inspiratory right-sided chest pain secondary to herniation of the right atrium and right ventricle through the defect or herniation of lung into the pericardial cavity. The chest roentgenogram may show an unusual protuberance of the right heart border, and technetium-99m cardiac blood pool imaging may demonstrate that the abnormal contour of the right heart border fills simultaneously with the right atrium.[557] Right atrial angiography in the left anterior oblique projection is helpful in documenting herniation of the right atrium and right ventricle through the pericardial defect. Surgical treatment of partial left- or right-sided pericardial defects is usually indicated to relieve symptoms and prevent cardiac strangulation. The defect may be approached by excision of the atrial appendage, pericardioplasty, or pericardiectomy.[558]

REFERENCES

ANATOMY AND FUNCTIONS

1. Holt, J. P.: The normal pericardium. Am. J. Cardiol. *26*:455, 1970.
2. Shabetai, R.: Function of the Pericardium. In Fowler, N. D. (ed.): The Pericardium in Health and Disease. Mt. Kisco, N.Y., Futura Publishing Co., 1985, pp. 19–20.
3. Capps, J. A.: Pain from the pleura and pericardium. Res. Publ. Assoc. Res. Nerv. Ment. Dis. *23*:263, 1943.
4. Alles, A., and Dom, R. M.: Peripheral sensory nerve fibers that dichotomize to supply the brachium and the pericardium in the rat. Brain Res. *342*:382, 1985.
5. Levy-Ravetch, M., Auh, Y. H., Rubenstein, W. A., Whalen, J. P., Kazam, E.: Computed tomography of the pericardial recesses. Am. J. Roentgenol. *144*:707, 1985.
6. Ishihara, T., Ferrans, V. J., Jones, M., Boyce, S. W., Kawanami, O., and Roberts, W. C.: Histologic and ultrastructural features of normal human parietal pericardium. Am. J. Cardiol *46*:744, 1980.
7. Roberts, W. C., and Spray, T. L.: Pericardial heart disease: A study of its causes, consequences and morphologic features. *In* Spodick, D. H. (ed.): Pericardial Diseases. Philadelphia, F. A. Davis Co., 1976, pp. 11–65.
8. Gibson, A. T., and Segal, M. B.: A study of the composition of pericardial fluid, with special reference to the probable mechanism of fluid formation. J. Physiol. (Lond.) *277*:367, 1978.
9. Hills, B. A., and Butler, B. D.: Phospholipids identified on the pericardium and their ability to impart boundary lubrication. Ann. Biomed. Eng. *13*:573, 1985.
10. Morgan, B. C., Guntheroth, W. C., and Dillard, D. H.: The relationship of pericardial to pleural pressure during quiet respiration and cardiac tamponade. Circ. Res. *16*:493, 1965.
11. Tyson, G. S., Jr., Maier, G. W., Olsen, C. O., Davis, J. W., and Rankin, J. S.: Pericardial influences on ventricular filling in the conscious dog. Circ. Res. *54*:173, 1984.
12. Holt, J. P., Rhode, E. A., and Kines, H.: Pericardial and ventricular pressure. Circ. Res. *8*:1171, 1960.
13. Brecher, G. A.: Venous Return. New York, Grune and Stratton, 1956.
14. Smiseth, O. A., Frais, M. A., Kingma, I., Smith, E. R., and Tyberg, J. V.: Assessment of pericardial constraint in dogs. Circulation 71:158, 1985.
15. Smiseth, O. A., Frais, M. A., Kingma, I., White, A. V. M., Knudtson, M. L., Cohen, J. M., Manyari, D. E., Smith, E. R., and Tyberg, J. V.: Assessment of pericardial constraint: The relation between right ventricular filling pressure and pericardial pressure measured after pericardiocentesis. J. Am. Coll. Cardiol. *7*:307, 1986.
16. Tyberg, J. V., Taichman, G. C., Smith, E. R., Douglas, N. W., Smiseth, O. A., and Keon, W. J.: The relationship between pericardial pressure and right atrial pressure: an intraoperative study. Circulation *73*:428, 1986.
17. Bernard, H. L.: The functions of the pericardium. J. Physiol. *22*:43, 1898.
18. Bartle, S. H., Hermann, H. J., Cavo, J. W., Moore, R. A., and Costenbader, J. M.: Effect of the pericardium on left ventricular volume and function in acute hypervolaemia. Cardiovasc. Res. *2*:248, 1968.
19. Spotnitz, H. M., and Kaiser, G. A.: The effect of the pericardium on pressure-volume relations in the canine left ventricle. J. Surg. Res. *11*:375, 1971.
20. Stokland, O., Miller, M. M., Lekven, J., and Ilebekk, A.: The significance of the intact pericardium for cardiac performance in the dog. Circ. Res. *47*:27, 1980.
21. Shirato, K., Shabetai, R., Bhargave, V., Franklin, D., and Ross, J., Jr.: Alteration of the left ventricular diastolic pressure-segment length relation produced by the pericardium. Circulation *57*:1191, 1978.
22. Crawford, H. H., Badke, F. R., and Amon, K. W.: Effect of the undisturbed pericardium on left ventricular size and performance during acute volume loading. Am. Heart J. *105*:267, 1983.
23. Refsum, H., Junemann, M., Lipton, M. J., Skioldebrand, C., Carlsson, E., and Tyberg, J. V.: Ventricular diastolic pressure-volume relations and the pericardium. Circulation *64*:997, 1981.
24. LeWinter, M. M., and Pavelec, R.: Influence of the pericardium on left ventricular end-diastolic pressure-segment relations during early and later stages of experimental chronic volume overload in dogs. Circ. Res. *50*:501, 1982.
25. Freeman, G. L., and LeWinter, M. M.: Pericardial adaptations during chronic cardiac dilation in dogs. Circ. Res. *54*:294, 1984.
26. Freeman, G. L., and LeWinter, M. M.: Role of parietal pericardium in acute severe mitral regurgitation in dogs. Am. J. Cardiol. *54*:217, 1984.
27. Bhargava, V., Shabetai, R., Ross, J., Jr., Shirato, K., Pavelec, R. S., and Mason, P. A.: Influence of the pericardium on left ventricular diastolic pressure-volume curves in dogs with sustained volume overload. Am. Heart J. *105*:995, 1983.
28. Smiseth, O. A., Refsum, H., Junemann, M., Sievers, R. E., Lipton, M. J., Carlsson, E., and Tyberg, J. V.: Ventricular diastolic pressure-volume shifts during acute ischemic left ventricular failure in dogs. J. Am. Coll. Cardiol. *3*:966, 1984.
29. Serizawa, T., Carabello, B. A., and Grossman, W.: Effect of pacing-induced ischemia on left ventricular diastolic pressure-volume relations in dogs with coronary stenosis. Circ. Res. *46*:430, 1980.
30. Taylor, R. R., Covell, J. W., Sonnenblick, E. H., and Ross, J., Jr.: Dependence of ventricular distensibility on filling of the opposite ventricle. Am. J. Physiol. *213*:711, 1967.
31. Laks, M. M., Garner, D., and Swan, H. J. C.: Volumes and compliances measured simultaneously in the right and left ventricles of the dog. Circ. Res. *20*:565, 1967.
32. Elzinga, G., Van Grondelle, R., Westerhof, N., and Van Den Bos, G. C.: Ventricular interference. Am. J. Physiol. *226*:941, 1974.
33. Santamore, W. P., Lynch, P. R., Meier, G., Heckman, J., and Bove, A. A.: Myocardial interaction between the ventricles. J. Appl. Physiol. *41*:362, 1976.
34. Brinker, J. A., Weiss, J. L., Lappe, D. L., Rabson, J. L., Summer, W. R., Permutt, S., and Weisfeldt, M. L.: Leftward septal displacement during right ventricular loading in man. Circulation *61*:626, 1980.
35. Spadaro, J., Bing, O. H., Gaasch, W. H., and Weintraub, R. M.: Pericardial modulation of right and left ventricular diastolic interaction. Circ. Res. *48*:233, 1981.
36. Lorell, B. H., Palacios, I., Daggett, W. M., Jacobs, M. L., Fowler, B. N., and Newell, J. B.: Right ventricular distention and left ventricular compliance. Am. J. Physiol. *240*:H87, 1981.
37. Janicki, J. S., and Weber, K. T.: The pericardium and ventricular interaction, distensibility, and function. Am. J. Physiol. 238:H494, 1980.
38. Shirato, K., Kanazawa, M., Ishikawa, K., Nakajima, T., and Takishma, T.: The effect of the percardium on the diastolic properties of the heart. Jpn. Circ. J. *46*:113, 1982.
39. Maruyama, Y., Ashikawa, K., Isoyama, S., Kanatsuke, H., Ino-Oka, E., and Takishima, T.: Mechanical interactions between four heart chambers with and without the pericardium in canine hearts. Circ. Res. *50*:86, 1982.
40. Glantz, S. A., Misbach, G. A., Moores, W. Y., Mathey, D. G., Levken, J., Stowe, D. F., Parmley, W. W., and Tyberg, J. V.: The pericardium substantially affects the left ventricular diastolic pressure-volume relationship in the dog. Circulation *42*:433, 1978.
41. Mangano, D. T.: The effect of the pericardium on ventricular systolic function in man. Circulation *61*:352, 1980.
42. Kanazawa, M., Shirato, K., Ishikawa, K., Nakajima, T., Haneda, T., and Takishima, T.: The effect of pericardium on the end-systolic pressure-segment length relationship in canine left ventricle in acute volume overload. Circulation *68*:1290, 1983.
43. Stray-Gendersen, J., Musch, T. I., Haidet, G. C., Swain, D. P., Ordway, G. A., and Mitchell, J. A.: The effect of pericardiectomy on maximal oxygen

consumption and maximal cardiac output in untrained dogs. Circ. Res. 58:523, 1986.
44. Ringertz, H. G., Misbach, G. A., and Tyberg, J. V.: Effect of the normal pericardium on the left ventricular diastolic pressure-volume relationship. Acta Radiol. 22:529, 1981.
45. Alderman, E. L., and Glanz, S. A.: Acute hemodynamic interventions shift the diastolic pressure-volume curve in man. Circulation *54*:662, 1976.
46. Brodie, B. R., Grossman, W., Mann, T., and McLaurin, L. P.: Effects of sodium nitroprusside on left ventricular diastolic pressure-volume relations. J. Clin. Invest. *59*:59, 1977.
47. Ludbrook, P. A., Byrne, J. D., Kurnik, P. B., and McKnight, R. C.: Influence of reduction of preload and afterload by nitroglycerin on left ventricular diastolic pressure-volume relations and relaxation in man. Circulation *56*:937, 1977.
48. Ludbrook, P. A., Byrne, J. D., and McKnight, R. C.: Influence of right ventricular hemodynamics on left ventricular diastolic pressure-overload relations in man. Circulation *59*:21, 1979.
49. Wong, C. Y., and Spotnitz, H. M.: Effects of nitroprusside on end-diastolic pressure-diameter relations of the human left ventricle after pericardiotomy. J. Thorac. Cardiovasc. Surg. *82*:350, 1981.
50. Ross, J., Jr.: Acute displacement of the diastolic pressure-volume curve of the left ventricle: Role of the pericardium and the right ventricle. Circulation *59*:32, 1979.
51. Lee, M. J., and Boughner, D. R.: Mechanical properties of human pericardium. Circ. Res. *57*:475, 1985.
52. Bartle, S. H., and Hermann, H. J.: Acute mitral regurgitation in man. Hemodynamic evidence and observations indicating an early role for the pericardium. Circulation *36*:839, 1967.
53. Lorell, B. H., Leinbach, R. C., Pohost, G. M., Gold, H. K., Dinsmore, R. E., Hutter, A. M., Jr., Pastore, J. O., and DeSanctis, R. W.: Right ventricular infarction. Am. J. Cardiol. *43*:465, 1979.
54. Goldstein, J. A., Vlahakes, G. H., Verrier, E. D., Schiller, N. B., Tyberg, J. V., Ports, T. A., Parmley, W. W., and Chatterjee, K.: The role of right ventricular systolic dysfunction and elevated intrapericardial pressure in the genesis of low output in experimental right ventricular infarction. Circulation *65*:513, 1982.

ACUTE PERICARDITIS

55. Sodeman, W. A., and Smith, R. H.: A re-evaluation of the diagnostic criteria for acute pericarditis. Am. J. Med. Sci. *235*:672, 1958.
56. Markiewicz, W., Brik, A., Brook, G., Edoute, Y., Monakier, I., and Markiewicz, Y.: Pericardial rub in pericardial effusion: Lack of correlation with amount of fluid. Chest *77*:643, 1980.
57. Spodick, D. H.: Pericardial rub: Prospective, multiple observer investigation of pericardial friction rub in 100 patients. Am. J. Cardiol. *35*:357, 1975.
58. Spodick, D. H.: Diagnostic electrocardiographic sequences in acute pericarditis: Significance of PR segment and PR vector changes. Circulation *48*:575, 1973.
59. Surawicz, B., and Lasseter, K. C.: Electrocardiogram in pericarditis. Am. J. Cardiol. *26*:471, 1970.
60. Bruce, M. A., and Spodick, D. H.: Atypical electrocardiogram in acute pericarditis: Characteristics and prevalence. J. Electrocardiol. *13*:61, 1980.
61. Wanner, W. R., Schaal, S. F., Bashore, T. M., Norton, V. J., Lewis, R. P., and Fulkerson, P. K.: Repolarization variant vs. acute pericarditis. A prospective electrocardiographic and echocardiographic evaluation. Chest *83*:180, 1983.
62. Ginzton, L. E., and Laks, M. M.: The differential diagnosis of acute pericarditis. Circulation *65*:1004, 1982.
63. Dressler, N.: Sinus tachycardia complicating and outlasting pericarditis. Am. Heart J. *72*:422, 1966.
64. Spodick, D. H.: Frequency of arrhythmias in acute pericarditis determined by Holter monitoring. Am. J. Cardiol. *53*:842, 1984.
65. Weiss, J. M., and Spodick, D. H.: Association of left pleural effusion with pericardial disease. N. Engl. J. Med. *308*:696, 1983.
66. Olson H. G., Lyons, K. P., Aronow, W. S., Kuperus, J., Orlando, J. R., and Waters, H. J.: Technetium-99m stannous pyrophosphate myocardial scintigrams in pericardial disease. Am. Heart J. *99*:459, 1980.
67. Martin, P., Devriendt, J., Goffin, Y., and Verhas, M.: Gallium-67 scintigraphy in fibrinous pericarditis associated with bacterial endocarditis. Eur. J. Nucl. Med. *7*:192, 1982.
68. Tiefenbrunn, A. J., and Roberts, R.: Elevation of plasma MB creatine kinase and the development of new Q waves in association with pericarditis. Chest *77*:438, 1980.
69. Karjalainen, J., and Heikkila, J.: Acute pericarditis: Myocardial enzyme release as evidence of myocarditis. Am. Heart J. *111*:546, 1986.
70. Marmor, A., Grenadir, E., Keidar, A., Edward, S., and Palant, A.: The MB fraction of creatine phosphokinase: An indicator of myocardial involvement in acute pericarditis. Arch. Intern. Med. *139*:819, 1979.
71. Permanyer-Miralda, G., Sagrista-Sauleda, J., and Soler-Soler, J.: Primary acute pericardial disease: A prospective series of 231 consecutive patients. Am. J. Cardiol. *56*:623, 1985.
72. Fowler, N. O., and Harbin, A. D.: Recurrent pericarditis: Follow-up of 31 patients. J. Am. Coll. Cardiol. *7*:300, 1986.

PERICARDIAL EFFUSION

73. Carsky, E. W., Mauceri, R. A., and Azimi, F.: The epicardial fat pad sign: Analysis of frontal and lateral chest radiographs in patients with pericardial effusion. Radiology *137*:303, 1980.
74. Mattsson, O.: Scintigraphy of pericardial effusion. Acta Radiol. Diag. *17*:737, 1976.
75. Silverman, P. M., Harell, G. S., and Korobkin, M.: Computed tomography of the abnormal pericardium. Am. J. Radiol. *140*:1125, 1983.
76. Gouliamos, A., Andreou, J., Steriotis, J., Kalovidouris, A., Vlahos, L., and Papavassilou, C.: Detection of pericardial disease by computed tomography. Clin. Radiol. *35*:397, 1984.
77. Stark, D. D., Higgins, C. B., Lanzer, P., Lipton, M. J., Schiller, N., Crooks, L. E., Botvinick, E. B., and Kaufman, L.: Magnetic resonance of the pericardium: Normal and pathologic findings. Radiology *150*:469, 1984.
78. Unverferth, D. V., Williams, T. E., and Fulkerson, P. K.: Electrocardiographic voltage in pericardial effusion. Chest *75*:157, 1979.
79. Feigenbaum, H.: Echocardiographic diagnosis of pericardial effusion. Am. J. Cardiol. *26*:475, 1970.
79a. Crandell-Riera, J., Del Castillo, G., Permanyer-Miralda, G., and Soler-Soler, J.: Pericardial effusion: Diagnostic value of the subcostal acoustic window (inferior vena cava–right atrial projection). Clin. Cardiol. *10*:262, 1987.
80. Rifkins, R. D., Isner, J. M., Carter, B. L., and Bankoff, M. S.: Combined posterioranterior subepicardial fat pad simulating the echocardiographic diagnosis of pericardial effusion. J. Am. Coll. Cardiol. *3*:1333, 1984.
81. Horowitz, M. S., Schultz, C. S., and Stinson, E. B.: Sensitivity and specificity of echocardiographic diagnosis of pericardial effusion. Circulation *50*:239, 1974.
82. Friedman, M. J., Sahn, D. J., and Haber, K.: Two-dimensional echocardiography and B-mode ultrasonography for the diagnosis of loculated pericardial effusion. Circulation *60*:1644, 1979.
83. Lopez-Sendon, J., Garcia-Fernandez, M. A., Coma-Canella, I., Silvestre, J., de Miguel, E., and Jadraque, L. M.: Identification of blood in the pericardial cavity in dogs by two-dimensional echocardiography. Am. J. Cardiol. *53*:1194, 1984.
84. Iliceto, S., Antonelli, G., Sorino, M., Calabrese, P., Biasco, G., and Risson, P.: Two-dimensional echocardiographic recognition of complications of cardiac invasive procedures. Am. J. Cardiol. *53*:846, 1984.
85. Fowler, N. O.: Physiology of cardiac tamponade and pulsus paradoxus. Physiological, circulatory, and pharmacologic responses in cardiac tamponade. Mod. Conc. Cardiovasc. Dis. *47*:115, 1978.
86. Reddy, P. S., Curtiss, E. I., O'Toole, J. D., and Shaver, J. A.: Cardiac tamponade: Hemodynamic observations in man. Circulation *58*:265, 1978.
87. Spodick, D. H.: The normal and diseased pericardium: Current concepts of pericardial physiology, diagnosis, and treatment. J. Am. Coll. Cardiol. *1*:240, 1983.
88. Craig, R. J., Walen, R. E., Behar, V. S., and McIntosh, H. D.: Pressure and volume changes of the left ventricle in acute pericardial tamponade. Am. J. Cardiol. *22*:65, 1968.
89. Manyari, D. E., Kostuk, W. J., and Purves, P.: Effect of pericardiocentesis on right and left ventricular function and volumes in pericardial effusion. Am. J. Cardiol. *52*:159, 1983.
90. Pegram, B. L., Kardon, M. B., and Bishop, V. S.: Changes in left ventricular internal diameter with increasing pericardial pressure. Cardiovasc. Res. *9*:707, 1975.
91. Shabetai, R., Fowler, N. O., and Guntheroth, W. G.: The hemodynamics of cardiac tamponade and constrictive pericarditis. Am. J. Cardiol. *26*:480, 1970.
92. Osborn, J. L., and Lawton, M. T.: Neurogenic antinatiuresis during development of acute cardiac tamponade. Am. J. Physiol. *250*:H195, 1986.
93. Wechsler, A. S., Auerbach, B. J., Graham, T. C., and Sabiston, D. C.: Distribution of intramyocardial blood flow during pericardial tamponade: Correlation with microscopic anatomy and intrinsic myocardial contractility. J. Thorac. Cardiovasc. Surg. *68*:847, 1974.
94. Frank, M. J., Nadimi, M., Lesniak, L. J., Hilmi, K. I., and Levinson, G. E.: Effects of cardiac tamponade on myocardial performance, blood flow and metabolism. Am. J. Physiol. *220*:179, 1971.
95. Brecher, G. A.: Critical review of recent work on ventricular diastolic suction. Circ. Res. *6*:554, 1958.
96. Kostreva, D. R., Castaner, A., Pedersen, D. H., and Kampine, J. P.: Nonvagally mediated bradycardia during cardiac tamponade or severe hemorrhage. Cardiology *68*:65, 1981.
97. Castaner, A., Kostreva, D. R., and Kampine, J. P.: Changes in autonomic nerve activity during acute cardiac tamponade. Cardiology *66*:163, 1980.
98. Friedman, H. S., Gomes, J. A., Tardio, A. R., and Haft, J. I.: The electrocardiographic features of acute cardiac tamponade. Circulation *50*:260, 1974.
99. Fowler, N. O., and Gabel, M.: The hemodynamic effects of cardiac tamponade: Mainly the result of atrial, not ventricular, compression. Circulation *71*:154, 1985.
100. Kronton, I., Cohen, M. L., and Winer, H. E.: Diastolic atrial compression: a sensitive echocardiographic sign of cardiac tamponade. J. Am. Coll. Cardiol. *2*:770, 1983.
101. Leimgruber, P. P., Klopfenstein, H. S., Wann, L. S., and Brooks, H. L.: The hemodynamic derangement associated with right ventricular diastolic collapse in cardiac tamponade: An experimental echocardiographic study. Circulation *68*:612, 1983.
102. Gaffney, F. A., Keller, A. M., Peshock, R. M., Lin, J., and Firth, B. G.: Pathophysiologic mechanisms of cardiac tamponade and pulsus alternans shown by echocardiography. Am. J. Cardiol. *53*:1162, 1984.
103. Klopfenstein, H. S., Cogswell, T. L., Bernath, G. A., Wann, L. S., Tipton, R. K., Hoffman, R. G., and Brooks, H. L.: Alternations in intravascular volume affect the relation between right ventricular diastolic collapse and the hemodynamic severity of cardiac tamponade. J. Am. Coll. Cardiol. *6*:1057, 1985.
104. Singh, S., Wann, L. S., Schuchard, G. H., Klopfenstein, H. S., Leimgruber, P. P., Keelan, M. H., Jr., and Brooks, H. L.: Right ventricular and right atrial collapse in patients with cardiac tamponade—a combined echocardiographic and hemodynamic study. Circulation *70*:966, 1984.
105. Ruskin, J., Bache, R. J., Rembert, J. C., and Greenfield, J. C., Jr.: Pressure-

flow studies in man: Effect of respiration on left ventricular stroke volume. Circulation *48*:79, 1973.
106. Goldblatt, A., Harrison, D. C., Glick, G., and Braunwald, E.: Studies on cardiac dimensions in intact, unanesthetized man. II. Effects of respiration. Circ. Res. *13*:448, 1963.
107. Wexler, L., Bergel, D. H., Gabe, I. T., Makin, G. S., and Mills, C. J.: Velocity of blood flow in normal human venae cavae. Circ. Res. *23*:349, 1968.
108. Shabetai, R., Fowler, N. O., Fenton, J. C., and Masangkay, M.: Pulsus paradoxus. J. Clin. Invest. *44*:1882, 1965.
109. Shabetai, R., Fowler, N. O., and Gueron, M.: The effects of respiration on aortic pressure and flow. Am. Heart J. *65*:525, 1963.
110. Gabe, I. T., Mason, D. T., Gault, J. H., Ross, J., Jr., Zelis, R., Mills, C. J., Braunwald, E., and Schillingford, J. P.: Effect of respiration on venous return and stroke volume in cardiac tamponade. Br. Heart J. *32*:592, 1970.
111. Settle, H. P., Adolph, R. J., Fowler, N. O., Engel, P., Agruss, N. S., and Levenson, N. I.: Echocardiographic study of cardiac tamponade. Circulation *56*:951, 1977.
112. Friedman, H. S., Sakurai, H., and Lajam, F.: Pulsus paradoxus: A manifestation of marked reduction of left ventricular end-diastolic volume in cardiac tamponade. J. Thorac. Cardiovasc. Surg. *79*:74, 1980.
113. Cohen, S. I., Kupersmith, J., Aroesty, J., and Rowe, J. W.: Pulsus paradoxus and Kussmaul's sign in acute pulmonary embolism. Am. J. Cardiol. *32*:271, 1973.
114. Settle, H. P., Jr., Engel, P. J., Fowler, N. O., Allen, J. M., Vassolo, C. L., Hackworth, J. N., Adolph, R. J., and Eppert, D. C.: Echocardiographic study of the paradoxical arterial pulse in chronic obstructive lung disease. Circulation *62*:1297, 1980.
115. Winer, H. E., and Kronzon, I.: Absence of paradoxical pulse in patients with cardiac tamponade and atrial septal defects. Am. J. Cardiol. *44*:378, 1979.
116. Guberman, B. A., Fowler, N. O., Engel, P. J., Gueron, M., and Allen, J. M.: Cardiac tamponade in medical patients. Circulation *64*:633, 1981.
117. Beck, C. S.: Two cardiac compression triads. J.A.M.A. *104*:714, 1935.
118. Cohn, J. N., Pinkerson, A. L., and Tristani, F. E.: Mechanism of pulsus paradoxus in clinical shock. J. Clin. Invest. *46*:1744, 1967.
119. Antman, E. M., Cargill, V., and Grossman, W.: Low-pressure cardiac tamponade. Ann. Intern. Med. *91*:403, 1979.
120. Reed, J. R., and Thomas, W. P.: Hemodynamics of progressive pneumopericardium in the dog. Am. J. Vet. Res. *45*:301, 1984.
121. Cummings, R. G., Wesly, R. L. R., Adams, D. H., and Lowe, J. E.: Pneumopericardium resulting in cardiac tamponade. Ann. Thorac. Surg. *37*:511, 1984.
122. Bricheteau: Observat d'hydropneumopercarde accompane d'un fluctuation perceptible a l'orielle. Arch. Gen. Med. *4*:334, 1844.
123. Littmann, D., and Spodick, D. H.: Total electrical alternation in pericardial disease. Circulation *17*:912, 1958.
124. Usher, B. W., and Popp, R. L.: Electrical alternans: Mechanism in pericardial effusion. Am. Heart J. *83*:459, 1972.
125. Friedman, H. S., Lajam, F., Calderon, J., Zaman, Q., Marino, N. D., and Gomes, J. A.: Electrocardiographic features of experimental cardiac tamponade in closed-chest dogs. Eur. J. Cardiol. *6*:311, 1977.
126. Spodick, D. H.: Acute cardiac tamponade: Pathologic physiology, diagnosis and management. Progr. Cardiovasc. Dis. *10*:64, 1967.
127. Wynne, J., Markis, J. E., and Grossman, W.: Extrinsic compression of the heart by tumor masquerading as cardiac tamponade. Cathet. Cardiovasc. Diag. *4*:81, 1978.
128. Cosio, F. G., Martinez, J. P., Serrano, C. M., Calzada, C. S., and Alcaire, C. C.: Abnormal septal motion in cardiac tamponade with pulsus paradoxus. Echocardiographic and hemodynamic observations. Chest *71*:787, 1977.
129. Kronzon, I., Cohen, M. J., and Winer, H. E.: Contribution of echocardiography to the understanding of the pathophysiology of cardiac tamponade. J. Am. Coll. Cardiol. *1*:1180, 1983.
130. D'Cruz, I. A., Cohen, H. C., Prabhus, R., and Glick, G.: Diagnosis of cardiac tamponade by echocardiography (changes in mitral valve motion and ventricular dimensions with special reference to paradoxical pulse). Circulation *52*:460, 1975.
131. Shindler, D. M., Reddy, K., Shindler, O. I., and Kostis, J. B.: Failure of the aortic valve to open during inspiration in cardiac tamponade. Chest *82*:797, 1982.
132. Singh, S., Wann, L. S., Klopfenstein, H. S., Hartz, A., and Brooks, H. L.: Usefulness of right ventricular diastolic collapse in diagnosing cardiac tamponade and comparison to pulsus paradoxus. Am. J. Cardiol. *57*:652, 1986.
133. Cogswell, T. L., Bernath, G. A., Wann, L. S., Hoffman, R. G., Brooks, H. L., and Klopfenstein, H. S.: Effects of intravascular volume on the value of pulsus paradoxus and right ventricular diastolic collapse in predicting cardiac tamponade. Circulation *72*:1076, 1985.
134. Martins, J. B., and Kerber, R. E.: Can cardiac tamponade be diagnosed by echocardiography? Circulation *60*:737, 1979.
135. Uren, R. F., McLaughlin, A. F., and Cormack, J.: Cardiac tamponade: Accurate diagnosis by radionuclide angiography. Aust. N.Z.J. Med. *10*:414, 1980.
136. Miller, S. W., Feldman, L., Palacios, I., Dinsmore, R. E., Newell, J. B., Gillam, L., and Weyman, A. E.: Compression of the superior vena cava and right atrium in cardiac tamponade. Am. J. Cardiol. *50*:1287, 1982.
137. Fowler, N. O., and Holmes, J. C.: Hemodynamic effect of isoproterenol and norepinephrine in acute cardiac tamponade. J. Clin. Invest. *48*:502, 1969.
138. Gascho, J. A., Martins, J. B., Marcus, M. L., and Kerber, R. E.: Effects of volume expansion and vasodilators in acute pericardial tamponade. Am. J. Physiol. *240*:H49, 1981.
139. Kerber, R. E., Jascho, J. A., Litchfield, R., Wolfson, P., Ott, D., and Pandian, N. J.: Hemodynamic effects of volume expansion and nitroprusside compared with the pericardiocentesis in patients with cardiac tamponade. N. Engl. J. Med. *307*:929, 1982.
140. Moller, C. T., Schoonbee, C. G., and Rosendorff, C.: Hemodynamics of cardiac tamponade during various modes of ventilation. Br. J. Anaesth. *51*:409, 1979.
141. Kilpatrick, Z. M., and Chapman, C. B.: On pericardiocentesis. Am. J. Cardiol. *16*:722, 1965.
142. Krikorian, J. G., and Hancock, E. W.: Pericardiocentesis. Am. J. Med. *65*:808, 1978.
143. Wong, B., Murphy, J., Chang, E. J., Hassenein, K., and Dunn, M.: The risk of pericardiocentesis. Am. J. Cardiol. *44*:1110, 1979.
144. Kaiser, E., and Loewenneck, H.: Pericardial puncture. The most favorable anatomical approach. Munch. Med. Wochenschr. *123*:1697, 1981.
145. Heilerh, B., Anderes, U., and Follath, F.: Diagnosis and therapy of cardiac tamponade. An analysis of 50 patients. Schweiz. Med. Wochenschr. *111*:735, 1981.
146. Callahan, J A., Seward, J. B., Nishimura, R. A., Miller, F. A., Reeder, G. S., Shub, C., Callahan, M. J., Schattenberg, T. T., and Tajik, A. J.: Two-dimensional echocardiographically guided pericardiocentesis: experience in 117 consecutive patients. Am. J. Cardiol. *55*:476, 1985.
147. Aron, D. V., Richardson, J. D., Webb, G., Grover, F. L., and Trinkle, J. K.: Subxiphoid pericardial window in patients with suspected traumatic pericardial tamponade. Ann. Thorac. Surg. *23*:545, 1977.
148. Armstrong, N. F., Feigenbaum, H., and Dillon, J. C.: Acute right ventricular dilation and echocardiographic volume overload following pericardiocentesis for relief of cardiac tamponade. Am. Heart J. *107*:1266, 1984.
149. Shenoy, M. M., Dhar, S., Gittin, R., Sinha, A. K., and Sabado, M.: Pulmonary edema following pericardiectomy for cardiac tamponade. Chest *86*:647, 1984.
150. Lorell, B. H., and Grossman, W.: Profiles in constrictive pericarditis, restrictive cardiomyopathy, and cardiac tamponade. *In* Grossman, W. (ed.): Cardiac Catheterization and Angiography. 3rd ed. Philadelphia, Lea and Febiger, 1986, pp. 427–445.
151. Erdman, S., Levinsky, L., Derivi, E., and Levy, M. J.: Closed pericardial drainage for relief of cardiac tamponade. Thorac. Cardiovasc. Surg. *34*:66, 1986.
152. Lock, J. E., Bass, J. L., Kulif, T. J., and Fuhrman, B. P.: Chronic percutaneous pericardial drainage with modified pigtail catheters in children. Am. J. Cardiol. *53*:1179, 1984.
153. Larrey, D. J.: New surgical procedure to open the pericardium and determine the cause of fluid in its cavity. Clin. Chirurg. *36*:393, 1829.
154. Miller, J. I., Mansour, K. A., and Hatcher, C. R., Jr.: Pericardiectomy: current indications, concepts, and results in a university center. Ann. Thorac. Surg. *34*:40, 1982.
155. Palatianos, G. M., Thurer, R. J., and Kaiser, G. A.: Comparison of effectiveness and safety of operations on the pericardium. Chest *88*:30, 1985.
156. Piehler, J. M., Pluth, J. R., Schaff, H. V., Danielson, G. K., Orszulak, T. A., and Puga, F. J.: Surgical management of effusive pericardial disease. J. Thorac. Cardiovasc. Surg. *90*:506, 1986.
157. Little, A. G., and Ferguson, M. K.: Pericardioscopy as adjunct to pericardial window. Chest *89*:53, 1986.
158. Kondos, G. T., Rich, S., and Levitsky, S.: Flexible fiberoptic bronchoscopy for the diagnosis of pericardial disease. J. Am. Coll. Cardiol. *7*:432, 1986.

CONSTRICTIVE PERICARDITIS

159. Chesler, E., Matha, A. S., Matisonn, R. E., and Rogers, M. N. A.: Subpulmonic stenosis as a result of noncalcific pericarditis. Chest *69*:425, 1976.
160. Nishimura, R. A., Kazmier, F. J., Smith, H. C., and Danielson, G. K.: Right ventricular outflow obstruction caused by constrictive pericardial disease. Am. J. Cardiol. *55*:1447, 1985.
161. Hancock, E. W.: Constrictive pericarditis: Modern view of diagnosis and managment. J. Cardiovasc. Med. *41*:367, 1980.
162. Gaasch, W. H., Peterson, K. L., and Shabetai, R.: Left ventricular function in chronic constrictive pericarditis. Am. J. Cardiol. *34*:107, 1974.
163. Dines, D. E., Edwards, J. E., and Burchell, H. B.: Myocardial atrophy in constrictive pericarditis. Proc. Staff Meet. Mayo Clin. *33*:93, 1958.
164. Levine, H. D.: Myocardial fibrosis in constrictive pericarditis. Electrocardiographic and pathologic observations. Circulation *48*:1268, 1973.
165. Gregory, M. A., Whitton, I. D., and Cameron, E. W.: Myocardial ischemia in constrictive pericarditis: A morphometric and electron microscopic study. Br. J. Exp. Pathol. *65*:365, 1984.
166. Nichols, D. A., and Peter, R. H.: Constrictive pericarditis as a late complication of meningococcal pericarditis. Am. J. Cardiol. *55*:1442, 1985.
167. Hancock, E. W.: On the elastic and rigid forms of constrictive pericarditis. Am. Heart J. *100*:917, 1980.
168. Paul, O., Castleman, B., and White, P. D.: Chronic constrictive pericarditis: A study of 53 cases. Am. J. Med. Sci. *216*:361, 1948.
169. Andrews, G. W. S., Pickering, G. W., and Sellors, T. H.: The aetiology of constrictive pericarditis with special reference to tuberculous pericarditis, together with a note on polyserositis. Q. J. Med. *17*:291, 1948.
170. Blake, S., Bonar, S., O'Neill, H., Hanly, P., Drury, I., Flanagan, M., and Garrett, J.: Aetiology of chronic constrictive pericarditis. Br. Heart J. *50*:273, 1983.
171. Fowler, N. O.: Constrictive pericarditis: New aspects. Am. J. Cardiol. *50*:1014, 1982.

172. Van der Horst, R. L.: Pericardial calcification in childhood. Cardiovasc. Radiol. *1*:265, 1978.
173. Bonische, C. H., and Jaffe, J. P.: Spontaneous severe constrictive pericarditis in congenital afibrinogenemia: Mechanism, evaluation and successful surgical management. Am. Heart J. *101*:503, 1981.
174. Laxer, R. M., Cameron, B. J., Chaisson, D., Smith, C. R., and Stein, L. D.: The camptodactyly-arthropathy-pericarditis syndrome: Case report and literature review. Arthritis Rheum. *29*:439, 1986.
175. Voorhees, M. L., Husson, G. S., and Blackman, M. S.: Growth failure with pericardial constriction. The syndrome of mulibrey nanism. Am. J. Dis. Child. *130*:1146, 1976.
176. Cheevers, N.: Observations on the disease of the orifice and valves of the aorta. Guy's Hosp. Rep. *7*:387, 1842.
177. Hancock, E. W.: Constrictive pericarditis. Clinical clues to diagnosis. J.A.M.A. *232*:176, 1975.
178. Blake, S.: The clinical diagnosis of constrictive pericarditis. Am. Heart J. *106*:432, 1983.
179. Tyberg, T. I., Goodyer, A. V. N., and Langou, R. A.: Genesis of pericardial knock in constrictive pericarditis. Am. J. Cardiol. *46*:570, 1980.
180. Manga, P., Vythilingum, S., and Mitha, A. S.: Pulsatile hepatomegaly in constrictive pericarditis. Br. Heart J. *52*:465, 1984.
181. Plus, G. E., Brower, A. J., and Clagett, O. T.: Chronic constrictive pericarditis: Roentgenologic findings in 35 surgically proved cases. Proc. Staff Meet. Mayo Clin. *32*:555, 1957.
182. Chesler, E., Mitha, A. S., and Matisonn, R. E.: The ECG of constrictive pericarditis—Pattern resembling right ventricular hypertrophy. Am. Heart J. *91*:420, 1979.
183. Schnittger, I., Bowden, R. E., Abrams, J., and Popp, R. L.: Echocardiography: Pericardial thickening and constrictive pericarditis. Am. J. Cardiol. *42*:388, 1978.
184. Doi, Y. L., Sugiura, T., and Spodick, D. H.: Motion of pulmonic valve and constrictive pericarditis. Chest *80*:513, 1981.
185. Tanaka, C. N., Nishimoto, M., Takeuchi, K., Fukukawa, K., Kawai, S., and Oku, H.: Presystolic pulmonic valve opening in constrictive pericarditis. Jpn. Heart J. *20*:419, 1979.
186. Tei, C., Child, J. S., Tanaka, H., and Shah, P. M.: Atrial systolic notch on the interventricular septal echogram: An echocardiographic sign of constrictive pericarditis. J. Am. Coll. Cardiol. *1*:907, 1983.
187. Engel, P. J., Fowler, N. O., Tei, C. W., Shah, P. M., Driedger, H. J., Shabetai, R., Harbin, A. D., and Franch, R. H.: M-mode echocardiography in constrictive pericarditis. J. Am. Coll. Cardiol. *6*:471, 1985.
188. Janos, G. G., Arjunan, K., Meyer, R. A., Engel, P., and Kaplan, S.: Differentiation of constrictive pericarditis and restrictive cardiomyopathy using digitized echocardiography. J. Am. Coll. Cardiol. *1*:541, 1983.
189. Lewis, B. S.: Real time two-dimensional echocardiography in constrictive pericarditis. Am. J. Cardiol. *49*:1789, 1982.
190. Hjemdahl-Monson, C. E., Daniels, J., Kaufman, D., Stern, E. H., Teichholz, L. E., and Meltzer, R. S.: Spontaneous contrast in the inferior vena cava in a patient with constrictive pericarditis. J. Am. Coll. Cardiol. *4*:165, 1984.
191. Pandian, N. G., Skorton, D. J., Kieso, R. A., and Kerber, R. E.: Diagnosis of constrictive pericarditis by two-dimensional echocardiography: studies in an new experimental model and in patients. J. Am. Coll. Cardiol. *4*:1164,1984.
192. Doppman, J. L., Reinmuller, R., Lissner, J., Cyran, J., Bolte, H. D., Strauer, B. E., and Hellwig, H.: Computed tomography in constrictive pericardial disease. J. Comput. Assist. Tomogr. *5*:1, 1981.
193. Sutton, F. J., Whitney, N. O., and Applefeld, M. M.: The role of echocardiography and computed tomography in the evaluation of constrictive pericarditis. Am. Heart J. *109*:350, 1985.
194. Nishimura, R. A., Connolly, D. C., Parkin, T. W., and Stanson, A. W.: Constrictive pericarditis: Assessment of current diagnostic procedures. Mayo Clin. Proc. *60*:397, 1985.
195. Reinmuller, R., Doppman, J. L., Lossner, J., Kemkes, B. M., and Strauer, B. E.: Constrictive pericardial disease: prognostic significance of a nonvisualized left ventricular wall. Radiology *156*:753, 1985.
196. Soulen, R. L., Stark, D. D., and Higgins, C. B.: Magnetic resonance imaging of constrictive pericardial disease. Am. J. Cardiol. *55*:480, 1985.
197. Solano, F. X., Young, E., Talamo, T. S., and Dekker, A.: Constrictive pericarditis mimicking Budd-Chiari syndrome. Am. J. Med. *80*:113, 1986.
198. Wilkinson, P., Pinto, B., and Senior, J. R.: Reversible protein-losing enteropathy with intestinal lymphangiectasia, secondary to chronic constrictive pericarditis. N. Engl. J. Med. *273*:1178, 1965.
199. Pastor, B. H., and Cahn, M.: Reversible nephrotic syndrome resulting from constrictive pericarditis. N. Engl. J. Med. *262*:872, 1960.
200. Wasserman, A. J., Richardson, D. W., Baird, C. L., and Wyso, E. M.: Cardiac hemochromatosis simulating constrictive pericarditis. Am. J. Med. *32*:316, 1962.
201. Arrillo, J. E., Borer, J. S., Henry, W. L., Wolff, S. M., and Fauci, A. S.: The cardiovascular manifestations of the hypereosinophilic syndrome. Am. J. Med. *67*:572, 1979.
202. Virmani, R., Chun, P. K. C., Dunn, B. E., Hartmen, D., and McAllister, H. A.: Eosinophilic constrictive pericarditis. Am. Heart J. *107*:803, 1984.
203. Siguera-Filho, A. G., Cunha, C. L. P., Tajik, A. J., Seward, J. B., Schattenberg, T. T., and Giuliani, E. R.: M-mode and two-dimensional echocardiographic features in cardiac amyloidosis. Circulation *63*:188, 1981.
204. Carroll, J. D., Gaasch, W. H., and McAdam, K. P. W. J.: Amyloid cardiomyopathy: Characterization by a distinctive voltage/mass ratio. Am. J. Cardiol. *49*:9, 1982.
205. Bush, C. A., Stang, J. M., Wooley, C. G., and Kilman, J.: Occult constrictive pericardial disease. Diagnosis by rapid volume expansion and correction by pericardiectomy. Circulation *56*:924, 1977.
206. Kilman, J. W., Bush, C. A., Wooley, C. G., Stang, J. M., Teply, J., and Baba, N.: The changing spectrum of pericardiectomy for chronic pericarditis: Occult constrictive pericarditis. J. Thorac. Cardiovasc. Surg. *74*:668, 1977.
207. Lewis, B. S., and Gotsman, M. S.: Left ventricular function in systole and diastole in constrictive pericarditis. Am. Heart J. *86*:23, 1973.
208. Alexander, J., Kelley, M. J., Cohen, L. S., and Langou, R. A.: The angiographic appearance of the coronary arteries in constrictive pericarditis. Radiology *131*:609, 1979.
209. Goldberg, E., Stein, J., Berger, M., and Berdoff, R. L.: Diastolic segmental coronary artery obliteration in constrictive pericarditis. Cathet. Cardiovasc. Diagn. *7*:197, 1981.
210. Meaney, E., Shabetai, R., and Bhargava, V.: Cardiac amyloidosis, constrictive pericarditis and restrictive cardiomyopathy. Am. J. Cardiol. *38*:547, 1976.
211. Swanton, R. H., Brooksby, I. A. B., Davies, M. J., Coltart, D. J., Jenkins, B. S., and Webb-Peploe, M. M.: Systolic and diastolic ventricular function in cardiac amyloidosis. Studies in six cases diagnosed with endomyocardial biopsy. Am. J. Cardiol. *39*:658, 1977.
212. Benotti, J. R., Grossman, W., and Cohn, P. F.: Clinical profile of restrictive cardiomyopathy. Circulation *61*:1206, 1980.
213. Robbins, M. A., Pizzarello, R. A., Stechel, R. P., Chiaramida, S. A., and Gulotta, S. J.: Resting and exercise hemodynamics in constrictive pericarditis and a case of cardiac amyloidosis mimicking constriction. Cathet. Cardiovasc. Diagn. *9*:463, 1983.
214. Chew, C., Ziady, G., Raphael, M. J., and Oakley, C. M.: The functional defect in amyloid heart disease. Am. J. Cardiol. *36*:438, 1975.
215. Chang, L. W., and Grollman, J. H., Jr.: Angiographic differentiation of constrictive pericarditis and restrictive cardiomyopathy due to amyloidosis. Am. J. Radiol. *130*:451, 1978.
216. Tyberg, T. I., Goodyer, A. V. N., Hurst, V. W., Alexander, J., and Langou, R. A.: Left ventricular filling in differentiating restrictive amyloid cardiomyopathy and constrictive pericarditis. Am. J. Cardiol. *47*:791,1981.
216a. Schoenfeld, M. H., Supple, E. W., Dec, G. W., Fallon, J. T., and Palacios, I. F.: Restrictive cardiomyopathy versus constrictive pericarditis: Role of endomyocardial biopsy in avoiding unnecessary thoracotomy. Circulation *75*:1012, 1987.
217. Broadarick, S., Paine, R., Higa, E., and Carmichael, K. A.: Pericardial tamponade—A new complication of amyloid heart disease. Am. J. Med. *73*:133,1982.
218. Kern, M. J., Lorell, B. H., and Grossman, W.: Cardiac amyloidosis masquerading as constrictive pericarditis. Cathet. Cardiovasc. Diagn. *8*:629,1982.
219. Copeland, J. G., Stinson, E. B., Griepp, R. B., and Shumway, N. E.: Surgical treatment of chronic constrictive pericarditis using cardiopulmonary bypass. J. Thorac. Cardiovasc. Surg. *69*:236, 1975.
220. Culliford, A. T., Lipton, M., and Spencer, F. C.: Operation for chronic constrictive pericarditis: Do the surgical approach and degree of pericardial resection influence the outcome significantly? Ann. Thorac. Surg. *29*:146, 1980.
221. McCaughlin, B. C., Schaff, H. V., Piehler, J. M., Danielson, G. K., Orszulak, T. A., Puga, F. J., Pluth, J. R., Connolly, D. C., and McGoon, D. C.: Early and late results of pericardiectomy for constrictive pericarditis. J. Thorac. Cardiovasc. Surg. *89*:340, 1985.
222. Robertson, J. M., and Mulder, D. G.: Pericardiectomy: A changing scene. Am. J. Surg. *148*:86, 1984.
223. Aagaard, M. T., and Haraldsted, V. Y.: Chronic constrictive pericarditis treated with total pericardiectomy. Thorac. Cardiovasc. Surg. *32*:311, 1984.
224. Siefert, F. C., Miller, C. D., Oesterle, S. N., Oyer, P. E., Stinson, E. B., and Shumway, N. E.: Surgical treatment of constrictive pericarditis: analysis of outcome and diagnostic error. Circulation *72*(Suppl. II):264, 1985.
225. Ferson, P. F., and Bahnson, H. T.: Surgical treatment of constrictive pericarditis. Cardiov. Reviews and Reports *4*:1103, 1983.
226. Viola, A. R.: The influence of pericardiectomy on the hemodynamics of chronic constrictive pericarditis. Circulation *48*:1038, 1973.
227. Dalton, J. C., Pearson, R. J., and White, P. D.: Constrictive pericarditis: A review and long-term followup of 78 cases. Ann. Intern. Med. *45*:445, 1956.
228. Pick, R. A., Joswig, B. C., and Bloor, C. M.: Recurrent cardiac constriction after pericardiectomy. Arch. Intern. Med. *144*:2061, 1984.
229. Kashani, I. A., Higgins, C. B., and Utley, J. R.: Inflammatory constriction following complete pericardiectomy in tuberculous constrictive pericarditis. Clin. Pediatr. *22*:219, 1983.
230. Harrington, S. W.: Chronic constrictive pericarditis. Partial pericardiectomy and epicardiolysis in 24 cases. Ann. Surg. *120*:468, 1944.
231. Walsh, T. J., Baughman, K. L., Gardner, T. J., and Bulkley, B. H.: Constrictive epicarditis as a cause of delayed or absent response to pericardiectomy. J. Thorac. Cardiovasc. Surg. *83*:126, 1982.
232. Spodick, D. H., and Kumar, S.: Subacute constrictive pericarditis with cardiac tamponade. Dis. Chest *54*:62, 1968.
233. Hancock, E. W.: Subacute effusive constrictive pericarditis. Circulation *43*:183, 1971.
234. Mann, T., Brodie, B. R., Grossman, W., and McLaurin, L.: Effusive-constrictive hemodynamic pattern due to neoplastic involvement of the pericardium. Am. J. Cardiol. *41*:781, 1978.
235. Martin, R. P., Bowden, R., Filly, K., and Popp, R. L.: Intrapericardial abnormalities in patients with pericardial effusion. Circulation *61*:568, 1980.

SPECIFIC FORMS OF PERICARDITIS

236. Brodie, H. R., and Marchessault, V.: Acute benign pericarditis caused by Coxsackie virus group B. N. Engl. J. Med. *262*:1278, 1960.
237. Talsma, M., Vegtinh, M., and Hess, J.: Generalized Coxsackie A9 infection in a neonate presenting with pericarditis. Br. Heart J. *52*:683, 1984.

238. Kleinfeld, M., Milles, S., and Lidsky, M.: Mumps pericarditis: Review of the literature and report of a case. Am. Heart J. *55*:153, 1958.
239. Cheng, T. C.: Severe chest pain due to infectious mononucleosis. Postgrad. Med. *73*:149, 1983.
240. Williams, A. J., Freemont, A. J., and Barnett, D. B.: Pericarditis and arthritis complicating chicken pox. Br. J. Clin. Pract. *37*:226, 1983.
241. Adler, R., Takahashi, M., and Wright, H. T. Jr.: Acute pericarditis associated with hepatitis B infection. Pediatrics *61*:716, 1978.
242. Linz, D. H., Tolle, S. W., and Elliot, D. L.: *Mycoplasma pneumoniae*. Experience at a referral center. West. J. Med. *140*:895, 1984.
243. Etienne, J., Matillon, Y., Lehot, L. L., Brune, J., and Chomel, J. J.: Discovery of cytomegalovirus in pericarditis fluid from a patient with neoplasm. Infection *10*:102, 1982.
244. Cammarosano, C., and Lewis, W.: Cardiac lesions in acquired immune deficiency syndrome (AIDS). J. Am. Coll. Cardiol. *5*:703, 1985.
245. Cohen, I. S., Anderson, D. W., Virmani, R., Reen, B. M., Macher, A. M., Sennesh, J., DiLorenzo, P., and Redfield, R. R.: Congestive cardiomyopathy in association with the acquired immunodeficiency syndrome. N. Engl. J. Med. *315*:628, 1986.
246. Cooper, D. K. C., and Sturridge, M. F.: Constrictive pericarditis following Coxsackie virus infection. Thorax *31*:472, 1976.
247. Frisk, G., Torfason, E. G., and Diderholm, H.: Reverse immunoassays of IgM and IgG antibodies to Coxsackie B viruses in patients with acute myopericarditis. J. Med. Virol. *14*:191, 1984.
248. Yoneda, S., Ohte, N., Samoto, T., Kobayashi, T., Fudemoto, Y., and Wada, A.: Two cases of viral myocarditis and one case of viral pericarditis. Jpn. Circ. J. *46*:1222, 1982.
249. Larneu, A. J., Tyers, G. F., Williams, E. H., and Derrick, J. R.: Recent experience with tuberculous pericarditis. Ann. Thorac. Surg. *29*:464, 1980.
250. Desai, H. N.: Tuberculous pericarditis: A review of 100 cases. S. Afr. Med. J. *55*:877, 1979.
251. Strang, J. I. G.: Tuberculous pericarditis in Transkei. Clin. Cardiol. *5*:667, 1984.
252. Gooi, H. C., and Smith, J. M.: Tuberculous pericarditis in Birmingham. Thorax *33*:94, 1978.
253. Peel, A. A. F.: Tuberculous pericarditis. Br. Heart J. *10*:195, 1948.
254. Auerbach, O.: Pleural, peritoneal, and pericardial tuberculosis. Am. Rev. Tuberc. *61*:845, 1950.
255. Palmer, J. A., and Watanakunakorn, C.: *Mycobacterium kansasii* pericarditis. Thorax *39*:876, 1984.
256. Maisch, B., Maisch, S., and Kocksiek, K.: Immune reactions in tuberculous and chronic constrictive pericarditis. Am. J. Cardiol. *50*:1007, 1982.
257. Schrire, V.: Experience with pericarditis of Groote Schuur Hospital, Cape Town: An analysis of one hundred and sixty cases over a six-year period. S. Afr. Med. J. *33*:810, 1959.
258. Hageman, J. H., D'Esopo, N. D., and Glenn, W. W. L.: Tuberculosis of the pericardium: A long-term analysis of forty-four cases. N. Engl. J. Med. *270*:327, 1964.
259. Fennell, W. M. P.: Surgical treatment of constrictive tuberculous pericarditis. S. Afr. Med. J. *62*:353, 1982.
260. Chia, B. L., Choo, M., Tan, A., and Ee, B.: Echocardiographic abnormalities in tuberculous pericardial effusion. Am. Heart J. *107*:1034, 1984.
261. Lin, D. S., and Tipton, R. E.: Ga-67 cardiac uptake. Clin. Nucl. Med. *8*:603, 1983.
262. Hirasing, R. A., and Van Bel, F.: Tuberculous pericarditis developing during chemotherapy. Eur. J. Resp. Dis. *63*:73, 1982.
263. Barr, J. F.: The use of pericardial biopsy in establishing etiologic diagnosis in acute pericarditis. Arch. Intern. Med. *96*:693, 1955.
264. Cheitlin, M. D., Serfos, L. J., Sbar, S. S., and Glosser, S. P.: Tuberculous pericarditis: Is limited pericardial biopsy sufficient for diagnosis? Am. Rev. Resp. Dis. *98*:287, 1968.
265. Rooney, J. J., Crocco, J. A., and Lyons, H. A.: Tuberculous pericarditis. Ann. Intern. Med.*72*:73, 1970.
266. Boyle, J. D., Pearce, M. L., and Guz, L. B.: Purulent pericarditis. Review of literature and report of eleven cases. Medicine *40*:119, 1961.
267. Klacsmann, P. B., Bulkley, B. H., and Hutchins, G. M.: The changed spectrum of purulent pericarditis. An 86 year autopsy experience in 200 patients. Am. J. Med. *63*:666, 1977.
268. Berk, S. L., Rice, P. A., Reynolds, C. A., and Finland, M.: Pneumococcal pericarditis: A persisting problem in contemporary diagnosis. Am. J. Med. *70*:247, 1981.
269. Kauffman, C. A., Watanakunakorn, C., and Phair, J. P.: Purulent pneumococcal pericarditis: A continuing problem in the antibiotic era. Am. J. Med. *54*:743, 1973.
270. Ugartemendia, M. C., Curos-Abadal, A., Pujol-Rakosnik, M., Pujadas-Capmany, R., Escriva-Montserrat, E., and Jane-Pesquer, J.: *Brucella melitensis* pericarditis. Am. Heart J. *109*:1108, 1985.
271. Levin, H. S., and Hosier, D. M.: *Salmonella* pericarditis. Report of a case and review of the literature. Ann. Intern. Med. *55*:817, 1961.
272. Haggman, D. L., Rehm, S. J., Moodie, D. S., and MacKenzie, A. H.: Nontyphoidal *Salmonella* pericarditis: A case report and review of the literature. Pediatr. Infect. Dis. *5*:259, 1986.
273. Vietzke, W. M.: Gonococcal arthritis with pericarditis. Arch. Intern. Med. *117*:270, 1966.
274. Buckingham, T. A., Wilner, G., and Sugar, S. J.: *Hemophilus influenzae* pericarditis in adults. Arch. Intern. Med. *143*:1809, 1983.
275. Evans, M. E., Gregory, D. W., Schaffner, W., and McGee, Z. A.: Tularemia: A 30-year experience with 88 cases. Medicine *64*:251, 1985.
276. Finley, R. W., and Marr, J. J.: Anaerobic bacterial abscess following myocardial infarction. Am. J. Med. *78*:513, 1985.
277. Rubin, R. H., and Moellering, R. C., Jr.: Clinical, microbiologic, and therapeutic aspects of purulent pericarditis. Am. J. Med. *59*:68, 1975.
278. Holoshitz, J., Schneider, M., Yaretsky, A., Bernheim, J., and Klajman, A.: *Listeria monocytogenes* pericarditis in a chronically hemodialyzed patient. Am. J. Med. Sci. *288*:34, 1984.
279. Kahn, M. Y.: Subacute constrictive pericarditis from *Serratia marcescens*. Hum. Pathol. *14*:1089, 1983.
280. Hanson, G., and Engel, P. J.: Purulent pericarditis caused by beta-hemolytic group C streptococcus. Arch. Intern. Med. *414*:1351, 1981.
281. Lieber, I. H., Rensimer, E. R., and Ericsson, C. D.: *Campylobacter* pericarditis in hypothyroidism. Am. Heart J. *102*:462, 1981.
282. Blaser, M. J., Reingold, A. L., Alsever, R. N., and Hightower, A.: Primary meningococcal pericarditis: A disease of adults associated with serogroup C *Neisseria meningitidis*. Rev. Infect. Dis. *6*:625, 1984.
283. Mayock, R., Skate, B., and Kohler, R. B.: *Legionella pneumophila* pericarditis proven by culture of pericardial fluid. Am. J. Med. *75*:534, 1983.
284. Nelson, D. P., Rensimer, E. B., and Raffin, T. A.: *Legionella pneumophila* pericarditis without pneumonia. Arch. Int. Med. *145*:926, 1985.
285. Pititalot, J. P., Allal, J., Thomas, P., Poupet, J. Y., Rossi, F., Barraine, B., Giraudon, B., and Sudre, Y.: Cardiac complications of infectious endocarditis. Ann. Med. Interne (Paris) *136*:539, 1985.
286. Weinstein, L.: Life-threatening complications of infective endocarditis and their management. Arch. Intern. Med. *146*:953, 1986.
287. Olson, L. J., Edwards, W. D., Olney, B. A., Orszulak, T. A., and Josa, M.: Hemorrhagic cardiac tamponade: a clinicopathologic correlation. Mayo Clin. Proc. *59*:785, 1984.
288. Morgan, R. J., Stephenson, L. W., Woolf, P. K., Edie, R. N., and Edmunds, L. H., Jr.: Surgical treatment of purulent pericarditis in children. J. Thorac. Cardiovasc. Surg. *85*:527, 1983.
289. Fyfe, D. A., Hagler, D. J., Puga, F. J., and Driscoll, D. J.: Clinical and therapeutic aspects of *Hemophilus influenzae* pericarditis in pediatric patients. Mayo Clin. Proc. *59*:415, 1984.
290. Hier-Madsen, K., Suanamaki, K. I., Wulff, J., Kjller, S., and Jensen, C.: Purulent pericarditis in children. Review and case report. Scand. J. Thorac. Cardiovasc. Surg. *19*:185, 1985.
291. Chun, P. K., and Rocchini, A. P.: Occult constrictive pericarditis in infancy. Chest *778*:648, 1980.
292. Gould, K., Barnett, J. A., and Sanford, J. P.: Purulent pericarditis in the antibiotic era. Arch. Intern. Med. *134*:923, 1974.
293. Miller, G. C., and Witham, A. C.: Delayed febrile pleuropericarditis after sepsis. Ann. Intern. Med. *79*:194, 1973.
294. Tan, J. S., Holmes, J. C., Fowler, N. O., Manitsas, G. T., and Phair, J. P.: Antibiotic levels in pericardial fluid. J. Clin. Invest. *53*:7, 1974.
295. Biancaniello, T. M., Anagnostipoulos, C. E., Bernstein, H. E., and Proctor, C.: Purulent meningococcal pericarditis: Chronic percutaneous drainage with a modified catheter aided by echocardiography. Clin. Cardiol. *8*:542, 1985.
296. Laaban, J. P., d'Orbcastel, O. R., Prudent, J., deFenoyl, O., and Rochemaure, J.: Primary pneumococcal pericarditis complicated by acute constriction. Intensive Care Med. *10*:155, 1984.
297. Wheat, L. J., Stein, L., Corya, B. C., Wass, J. L., Norton, J. A., Grider, K., Slama, T. G., French, M. L., and Kohler, R. B.: Pericarditis as a manifestation of histoplasmosis during two large urban outbreaks. Medicine *62*:110, 1983.
298. Larsen, R., and Scherb, R. E.: Coccidioidal pericarditis. Circulation *7*:211, 1953.
299. Chapman, M. G., and Kaplan, L.: Cardiac involvement in coccidioidomycosis. Am. J. Med. *23*:87, 1957.
300. Gronemeyer, M. G., Weissfeld, A., S., and Sonnenwirth, A. C.: Cardiac involvement in coccidioidomycosis. Am J. Med. *23*:87, 1957.
301. Walsh, T. J., and Bulkley, B. J.: Aspergillus pericarditis: Clinical and pathologic features in the immunocompromised patient. Cancer *49*:48, 1982.
302. Ross, E. M., Macher, A. M., and Roberts, W. C.: *Aspergillus fumigatus* thrombi causing total occlusion of both coronary arterial ostia, all four major coronary arteries and coronary sinus and associated with purulent pericarditis. Am. J. Cardiol. *56*:499, 1985.
303. Kleger, H. L., and Fisher, E. R.: Fibrocalcific constrictive pericarditis due to *Histoplasma capsulatum*. N. Engl. J. Med. *267*:593, 1962.
304. Prager, R. L., Burney, D. P., Waterhouse, G., and Bender, H. W., Jr.: Pulmonary, mediastinal, and cardiac presentations of histoplasmosis. Ann. Thorac. Surg. *30*:385, 1980.
305. Eng, R. J., Sen, P., Browne, K., and Louria, D. B.: *Candida* pericarditis. Am. J. Med. *70*:867, 1981.
306. Holtz, H. A., Lavery, D. P., and Kapila, R.: *Actinomycetales* infection in the acquired immunodeficiency syndrome. Ann. Intern. Med. *102*:203, 1985.
307. Ramsdale, D. R., Gautam, P. C., Perera, B., and Charles, R. G.: Cardiac tamponade due to actinomycosis. Thorax *39*:473, 1984.
308. Sagrista-Sauleda, J., Permanyer-Miralda, G., Juste-Sanchez, C., De Buen-Sanchez, M. L., Pujadas-Capmany, R., Arcalis-Arce, L., and Soler-Soler, J.: Huge chronic pericardial effusion caused by *Toxoplasma gondii*. Circulation *66*:895, 1982.
309. Bansal, B. C., and Gupta, D. S.: Amoebic pericarditis. Postgrad. Med. J. *47*:678, 1971.
310. Adeyamo, A. O., and Aderounmu, A.: Intrathoracic complications of amoebic liver abscess. J. Roy. Soc. Med. *73*:17, 1984.
311. van der Horst, R.: Schistosomiasis of the pericardium. J. R. Soc. Trop. Med. Hygiene *73*:243, 1979.

312. Chens, W.: Hydatid cysts in the pericardium—A new case and review of the literature. J. Thorac. Cardiovasc. Surg. *30*:56, 1982.
313. Kinare, S. G., Parulkar, G. B., and Sen, P. K.: Constrictive pericarditis resulting from dracunculosis. Br. Med. J. *1*:845, 1962.
314. Charon, A., and Sinha, K.: Constrictive pericarditis following filiariasis. Indian Heart J. *25*:213, 1973.
315. Marcus, L. C., Steere, A. C., Duray, P. H., Anderson, A. E., and Mahoney, E. B.: Fatal pancarditis in a patient with coexistent Lyme disease and babesiosis. Intern. Med. *103*:374, 1985.
316. Thadani, U., Chopra, M. P., Aber, C. P., and Portal, R. W.: Pericarditis after acute myocardial infarction. Br. Med. J. *2*:135, 1971.
317. Dubois, C., Smeets, J. P., Demoulin, J. C., Pierard, L., Henrad, L., Preston, L., and Kulbertus, H. E.: Frequency and clinical significance of pericardial friction rubs in the acute phase of myocardial infarction. Eur. Heart J. *6*:766, 1985.
318. Lichstein, E., Arsura, E., Hollander, G., Greengart, A., and Sanders, M.: Current incidence of postmyocardial infarction (Dressler's) syndrome. Am. J. Cardiol. *50*:1269, 1982.
319. Toole, J. C., and Silverman, M. E.: Pericarditis of acute myocardial infarction. Chest *67*:647, 1975.
320. Krainin, F. M., Flessas, A. P., and Spodick, D. H: Infarction-associated pericarditis. N. Engl. J. Med. *311*:1211, 1984.
321. Khan, A. J.: Pericarditis of myocardial infarction: Review of the literature with case presentation. Am. Heart J. *90*:788, 1975.
322. Levine, H. D.: Subendocardial infarction in retrospect: Pathologic, cardiographic, and ancillary features. Circulation *72*:790, 1985.
323. Galve, E., Garcia-del-Castillo, H., Evangelista, A., Batlle, J., Permanyer-Miralda, G., and Soler-Soler, J.: Pericardial effusion in the course of myocardial infarction: Incidence, natural history, and clinical relevance. Circulation *73*:294, 1986.
324. Anderson, M. W., Christensen, N. A., and Edwards, J. E.: Hemopericardium complicating myocardial infarction in the absence of cardiac rupture. Arch. Intern. Med. *90*:634, 1952.
325. Aarseth, S., and Lange, H. F.: The influence of anticoagulant therapy on the occurrence of cardiac rupture and hemopericardium following heart infarction. I. A study of 89 cases of hemopericardium. Am. Heart J. *56*:250, 1958.
326. Lange, H. F., and Aarseth, S.: The influence of anticoagulant therapy on the occurrence of cardiac rupture and hemopericardium following heart infarction. II. A controlled study of a selected treated group based on 1044 autopsies. Am. Heart J. *56*:257, 1958.
327. Karim, A. M., and Solomon, J.: Constrictive pericarditis after myocardial infarction. Am. J. Med. *79*:389, 1985.
328. Low, R. I., Arthur, A., Kelly, P. B., and Takeda, P. A.: Clotted hemopericardium post myocardial infarction presenting as effusive constrictive pericarditis. Am. Heart J. *109*:905, 1985.
329. Liberthson, R. R., Salisbury, K. W., and Hutter, A. M., Jr.: Atrial tachyarrhythmias in acute myocardial infarction. Am. J. Med. *60*:956, 1976.
330. Liem, K. L., Durrer, D., and Lie, K. L.: Pericarditis in acute myocardial infarction. Lancet *2*:1004, 1975.
331. Limaye, S. B., and Stubberfield, J.: Cardiac tamponade following infarction: management with pericardiocentesis and surgery. Aust. N. Z. J. Med. *15*:446, 1985.
332. Dvorak, K., and Cerny, J.: Long-term survival of subacute cardiac rupture with tamponade in acute myocardial infarction, without surgical intervention (the role of pericardiocentesis). Cor. Vasa. *21*:233, 1979.
333. Berman, J., Haffajee, C. I., and Alpert, J. S.: Therapy of symptomatic pericarditis after myocardial infarction: Retrospective and prospective studies of aspirin, indomethacin, prednisone, and spontaneous resolution. Am. Heart J. *101*:750, 1981.
334. Hammerman, H., Kloner, R. A., Schoen, F. J., Brown, E. J., Hale, S., and Braunwald, E.: Indomethacin induced scar thinning following experimental myocardial infarction. Circulation *67*:1290, 1983.
335. Brown, E. J., Kloner, R. A., Schoen, F. J., Hammerman, H., Hale, S., and Braunwald, E.: Scar thinning due to ibuprofen administration following experimental myocardial infarction. Am. J. Cardiol. *51*:877, 1983.
336. Boden, W. E., and Sadaniantz, A.: Ventricular septal rupture during ibuprofen therapy for pericarditis after acute myocardial infarction. Am. J. Cardiol. *55*:1631, 1985.
337. Bright, R.: Tabular view of the morbid appearance in 100 cases connected with albuminous urine: With observations. Guy's Hosp. Rep. *1*:380, 1836.
338. Renfrew, R., Buselmeier, T. J., and Kjeilstrand, C. M.: Pericarditis and renal failure. Ann. Rev. Med. *31*:345, 1980.
339. Luft, L. C., Gilman, J. K., and Weyman, A. E.: Pericarditis in the patient with uremia: Clinical and echocardiographic evaluation. Nephron *25*:160, 1980.
340. Osanloo, E., Shalhoub, R. J., Cioffi, R. F., and Parker, R. H.: Viral pericarditis in patients receiving hemodialysis. Arch. Intern. Med. *139*:310, 1979.
341. Shabetai, R.: Uremia, dialysis, and metabolic causes of pericardial disease. *In* The Pericardium. New York, Grune and Stratton, 1981, pp. 385–389.
342. Maisch, B., and Kochsiek, K.: Humoral immune reactions in uremic pericarditis. Am. J. Nephrol. *3*:264, 1983.
343. Lindsay, J., Jr., Crawley, I. S., and Callaway, G. M.: Chronic constrictive pericarditis following uremic hemopericardium. Am. Heart J. *79*:390, 1970.
344. Comty, C. M., Cohen, S. L., and Shapiro, F. L.: Pericarditis in the patient with uremia: Clinical and echocardiographic evaluation. Nephron *25*:160, 1980.
345. Frommer, J. P., Young, J. B., and Ayus, J. C.: Asymptomatic pericardial effusion in uremic patients: Effect of long-term dialysis. Nephron *39*:296, 1985.
346. Yoshida, K., Shiina, A., Asano, Y., and Hosoda, S.: Uremic pericardial effusion: Detection and evaluation of uremic pericardial effusion by echocardiography. Clin. Nephrol. *13*:260, 1980.
347. Masson, J. F., Maes, M. L., and Zilberman, C.: Pericarditis in chronic renal insufficiency treated by periodic hemodialysis. Rev. Med. Intern. *2*:447, 1981.
348. Kwasnik, E. M., Koster, J. K., Lazarus, J. M., Sloss, L. J., Mee, R. B. B., Cohn, L. H., and Collins, J. J.: Conservative management of uremic pericardial effusions. J. Thorac. Cardiovasc. Surg. *76*:629, 1978.
349. Rotler, M. N., and Swartz, C.: Predicting success of intensive dialysis in the treatment of uremic pericarditis. Am. J. Med. *76*:38, 1984.
350. Spector, D., Alfred, H., Seidlecki, M., and Briefel, G.: A controlled study of the effect of indomethacin in uremic pericarditis. Kidney Int. *24*:663, 1983.
351. Buselmeir, T. J., Davin, T. D., and Simmons, R. L.: Treatment of intractable uremic pericardial effusion: Avoidance of pericardiectomy with local steroid instillation. J.A.M.A. *240*:1358, 1978.
352. Fuller, T. J., Knochel, J. P., Brennan, J. P., Fetner, C. D., and White, M. G.: Reversal of intractable uremic pericarditis by triamcinolone hexacetonide. Arch. Intern. Med. *136*:979, 1976.
353. Feinroth, M. V., Goldstein, E. J., Josephson, A., and Freidman, E. A.: Infection complicating intrapericardial steroid instillation in uremic pericarditis. Clin. Nephrol. *15*:331, 1981.
354. Quigg, R. J., Idelson, B. A., Yoburn, D. C., Hymes, J. L., Schick, E. G., and Bernard, D. B.: Local steroids in dialysis-associated pericardial effusion. Arch. Intern. Med. *145*:2249, 1985.
355. Silverberg, S., Oreopoulos, D. G., Wise, D. J., Uden, D. E., Meindok, H., Jones, M., Rapaport, A., and deVeber, G. A.: Pericarditis in patients undergoing long-term hemodialysis and peritoneal dialysis. Am. J. Med. *63*:874, 1977.
356. Beaudry, C., Nakamoto, S., and Koloff, W. J.: Uremic pericarditis and cardiac tamponade in chronic renal failure. Ann. Intern. Med. *64*:990, 1966.
357. Frame, J. R., Lucas, S. K., Pederson, J. A., and Elkins, R. C.: Surgical treatment of pericarditis in the dialysis patient. Am. J. Surg. *146*:300, 1983.
358. Prager, R. L., Wilson, C. H., and Bender, H. W., Jr.: The subxiphoid approach to pericardial disease. Ann. Thorac. Surg. *34*:6, 1982.
359. DeLoach, J. F., and Haynes, J. W.: Secondary tumors of the heart and pericardium. Arch. Intern. Med. *91*:224, 1953.
360. Goudie, R. B.: Secondary tumors of the heart and pericardium. Br. Heart J. *17*:183, 1955.
361. Scott, R. W., and Garvin, C. F.: Tumors of the heart and pericardium. Am. Heart J. *17*:431, 1939.
362. Posner, M. R., Cohen, G. I., and Skarin, A. T.: Pericardial disease in patients with cancer. Am. J. Med. *71*:407, 1981.
363. Roberts, W. C., Bodey, G. P., and Wertlake, P. T.: The heart in acute leukemia: A study of 420 autopsy cases. Am. J. Cardiol. *21*:388, 1968.
364. Roberts, W. C., Glancy, D. L., and DeVita, V. T.: Heart in malignant lymphoma (Hodgkin's disease, lymphosarcoma, reticulum cell sarcoma and mycosis fungoides): A study of 196 autopsy cases. Am. J. Cardiol. *22*:85, 1968.
365. Gassman, H. S., Meadows, R., and Baker, L. A.: Metastatic tumors of the heart. Am. J. Med. *19*:357, 1955.
366. Thurber, D. L., Edwards, J. E., and Achor, R. W.: Secondary malignant tumors of the pericardium. Circulation *26*:228, 1962.
367. Cohen, G. U., Perry, T. M., and Evans, J. M.: Neoplastic invasion of the heart and pericardium. Ann. Intern. Med. *42*:1238, 1955.
368. Chan, H. S., Sonley, M. J., Moes, C. A., Daneman, A., Smith, C. R., and Martin, D. J.: Primary and secondary tumors of childhood involving the heart, pericardium, and great vessels. Cancer *56*:825, 1985.
369. Glancy, D. L., and Roberts, W. C.: The heart in malignant melanoma: A study of 70 autopsy cases. Am. J. Cardiol. *21*:555, 1968.
370. Sytman, A. L., and MacAlpin, R. N.: Primary pericardial mesothelioma: Report of two cases and review of the literature. Am. Heart J. *81*:760, 1971.
371. Harveit, F., Brubakk, O., and Roksted, K.: Pericardial angiomatosis. Acta Med. Scand. *199*:519, 1976.
372. Poole-Wilson, P. A., Farnsworth, A., Braimbridge, M. V., and Pambakian, H.: Angiosarcoma of pericardium. Problem in diagnosis and management. Br. Heart J. *38*:240, 1976.
373. Churg, A., Warnock, M. L., and Bensch, K. G.: Malignant mesothelioma arising after direct application of asbestos and fiber glass to the pericardium. Am. Rev. Resp. Dis. *118*:419, 1978.
373a. Llewellyn, M. J., Atkinson, M. W., and Fabri, B.: Case report—Pericardial constriction caused by primary mesothelioma. Br. Heart J. *57*:54, 1987.
374. Awoke, S., and Perlstein, R. S.: Dopamine- and norepinephrine-secreting intrapericardial pheochromocytoma in a normotensive patient. South. Med. J. *78*:994, 1985.
375. Kline, J. K.: Cardiac lymphatic involvement by metastatic tumor. Cancer *29*:799, 1972.
376. Vilaseca, J., Arnau, J. M., Tallada, N., Bernado, L., Lopez-Vivancos, J., and Guardia, J.: Agnogenic myeloid metaplasia presenting as massive pericardial effusion due to extramedullary hematopoesis. Acta Haematol. *73*:239, 1985.
377. Haedersdal, C., Hasselbalch, H., Devantier, A., and Saunamaki, K: Pericardial haematopoesis with tamponade in myelofibrosis. Scand. J. Haematol. *34*:270, 1985.
378. Donnelly, M. S., Weinberg, D. S., Skarin, A. T., and Levine, H. D.: Sick sinus syndrome with seroconstrictive pericarditis in malignant lymphoma involving the heart: A case report. Med. Pediatr. Oncol. *9*:273, 1981.
379. Markiewicz, W., Gladstein, E., London, E. J., and Popp, R. L.: Echocardiographic detection of pericardial effusion and pericardial thickening in malignant lymphoma. Radiology *123*:161, 1977.
380. Fraser, R. S., Viloria, J. B., and Wang, N. S.: Cardiac tamponade as a presentation of extracardiac malignancy. Cancer *45*:1697, 1980.
381. Chu, J. Y., Demello, D., O'Connor, D. M., and Chen, S. C.: Pericarditis as the presenting manifestation of acute nonlymphocytic leukemia in a young child. Cancer *52*:322, 1983.
382. Lopez, J. M, Delgado, J. L, Tovar, E., and Gonzalez, A. G.: Massive

pericardial effusion produced by extracardiac malignant neoplasms. Arch. Intern. Med. *143*:1815, 1983.
383. Theologides, A.: Neoplastic cardiac tamponade. Semin. Oncol. *5*:181, 1978.
384. Chandraratna, P. A. N., and Aronow, W. S.: Detection of pericardial metastases by cross-sectional echocardiography. Circulation *63*:197, 1981.
385. Gouliamos, A., Andreou, J., Steriotis, J., Kalovidouris, A., Vlahos, L., and Papavassiliou, C.: Detection of pericardial heart disease by computed tomography. Clin. Radiol. *35*:397, 1984.
386. Pizzarello, R. A., Goldberg, S. M., Goldman, M. A., Gottesman, R., Felten, J. V., Brown, N., Kahn, E. I., and Stein, H. L.: Tumor of the heart diagnosed by magnetic resonance imaging. J. Am. Coll. Cardiol. *5*:989, 1985.
387. Masson, R. G., and Ruggieri, J.: Pulmonary microvascular cytology. Chest *88*:908, 1985.
388. Zipf, R. E., Jr., and Johnston, W. W.: The role of cytology in the evaluation of pericardial effusion. Chest *62*:593, 1972.
389. King, D. T., and Nieberg, R. K.: The use of cytology to evaluate pericardial effusions. Ann. Clin. Lab. Sci. *9*:18, 1979.
390. Yazdi, H. M., Hajdu, S. I., and Melamed, M. R.: Cytopathology of pericardial effusions. Acta Cytol. J. *24*:401, 1980.
391. Tatsuda, M., Yamamura, H., Yamamoto, R., Ichii, M., Iishi, H., and Noguchi, S.: Carcinoembryonic antigens in the pericardial fluid of patients with malignant pericarditis. Oncology *41*:328, 1984.
392. Bitran, J. D., Evans, R., and Brown, C.: The management of cardiac tamponade in patients with breast cancer. J. Surg. Oncol. *27*:42, 1984.
393. Hankins, J. R., Satterfield, J. R., Aisner, J., Wiernik, P. H., and McLaughlin, J. S.: Pericardial window for malignant pericardial effusion. Ann. Thorac. Surg. *30*:465, 1980.
394. Hill, G. J., and Cohen, B. I.: Pleural pericardial window for palliation of cardiac tamponade due to cancer. Cancer *26*:81, 1970.
395. Mauch, P. E.: Treatment of malignant pericardial effusions. *In* DeVita, V. T., Hellman, S., and Rosenberg, S. A. (eds.): Cancer: Principles and Practice of Oncology. 2nd ed. Philadelphia, J. B. Lippincott Co., 1982, pp. 1571–1573.
396. Terry, L. H., and Kligerman, M. M.: Pericardial and myocardial involvement in lymphomas and leukemias—the role of radiotherapy. Cancer *25*:1003, 1970.
397. Cham, W. C., Freiman, A. H., and Carstens, P. H. B.: Radiation therapy of cardiac and pericardial metastases. Ther. Radiol. *114*:701, 1975.
398. Stewart, J. R., and Fajardo, L. F.: Radiation-induced heart disease: An update. Prog. Cardiovasc. Dis. *27*:173, 1984.
399. Stewart, J. R., Cohn, K. E., and Fajardo, L. F.: Radiation-induced heart disease: A study of twenty-five patients. Radiology *89*:302, 1967.
400. Carmel, R. J., and Kaplan, H. S.: Mantle irradiation in Hodgkin's disease. Cancer *37*:2813, 1976.
401. Mills, S. B., Baglan, R. J., Kurichety, P., Prasad, G., Lee, J. Y., and Moller, R.: Symptomatic radiation-induced pericarditis in Hodgkin's disease. Int. J. Radiat. Oncol. Biol. Phys. *10*:2061, 1984.
402. Martin, R. G., Ruckdeschel, J. C., Chang, P., Byhardt, R., Bouchard, R. J. and Wiernik, P. H.: Radiation-related pericarditis. Am. J. Cardiol. *35*:216, 1975.
403. Coltart, R. S., Roberts, J. T., Thom, C. H., and Petch, M. C.: Severe constrictive pericarditis after single 16 MeV anterior mantle irradiation for Hodgkin's disease. Lancet *1*:488, 1985.
404. Applefeld, M. M., Slawson, R. G., Spicer, K. M., and Singleton, R. T.: Long-term cardiovascular evaluation of patients with Hodgkin's disease treated by thoracic mantle radiation therapy. Cancer Treat. Rep. *66*:1003, 1982.
405. Applefeld, M. M., Slawson, R. G., Hall-Craigs, M., Green, D. C., Singleton, R. T., and Wiernik, P. H.: Delayed pericardial disease after radiotherapy. Am. J. Cardiol. *47*:210, 1981.
406. Haas, J.: Symptomatic constrictive pericarditis developing 45 years after radiation therapy to the mediastinum. Am. Heart J. *77*:89, 1969.
407. Greenwood, R. D., Rosenthal, A., Cassedy, R., Jaffe, N., and Nadas, A. S.: Constrictive pericarditis in childhood due to mediastinal irradiation. Circulation *50*:1033, 1974.
408. Brosius, F. C., Waller, B. F., and Roberts, W. C.: Radiation heart disease. Am. J. Med. *70*:519, 1981.
409. Steinberg, I.: Effusive-constrictive pericarditis: Two cases illustrating value of angiocardiography in diagnosis. Am. J. Cardiol. *19*:343, 1976.
410. Castellino, R. A., Gladstein, E., and Turbow, M. M.: Latent radiation injury of lungs or heart activated by steroid withdrawal. Ann. Intern. Med. *80*:593, 1974.
411. Morton, D. L., Kagan, A. R., Roberts, W. C., O'Brien, K. P., Holmes, E. C., and Adkins, P. C.: Pericardiectomy for radiation-induced pericarditis with effusion. Ann. Thorac. Surg. *8*:195, 1969.
412. Osler, W.: The Principles and Practice of Medicine. New York, D. Appleton and Company, 1892, p. 273.
413. Persellin, S. T., Ramirez, G., and Moatamed, F.: Immunopathology of rheumatic pericarditis. Arthritis Rheum. *25*:1054, 1982.
414. Przybojewski, J. Z.: Rheumatic constrictive pericarditis. A case report and review of the literature. S. Afr. Med. J. *59*:682, 1981.
415. Ansari, A., Larson, P. H., and Bates, H. D.: Cardiovascular manifestations of systemic lupus erythematosus: Current perspective. Prog. Cardiovasc. Dis. *27*:421, 1985.
416. Badvi, E., Garcia-Rubi, D., Robles, E., Jiminez, J., Juan, L., Deleze, M., Dias, A., and Nimta, G.: Cardiovascular manifestations in systemic lupus erythematosus. Prospective study of 100 patients. Angiology *36*:431, 1985.
417. Chang, R. W.: Cardiac manifestation of systemic lupus erythematosus. Clin. Rheum. Dis. *8*:197, 1982.
418. Doherty, N. E., and Siegel, R. J.: Cardiovascular manifestations of systemic lupus erythematosus. Am. Heart J. *110*:1257, 1985.
419. Bulkley, B. H., and Roberts, W. C.: The heart in systemic lupus erythematosus and the changes induced in it by corticosteroid therapy. Am. J. Med. *58*:243, 1975.
420. Kinney, E., Wynn, J., Hinton, D. M., Demers, S. L., O'Neill, M., Parr, G., Ward, S., and Zelis, R.: Pericardial-fluid complement. Normal values. Am. J. Clin. Pathol. *72*:972, 1979.
421. Jacobsen, E. J., and Reza, M. J.: Constrictive pericarditis in systemic lupus erythematosus. Demonstration of immunoglobulins in the pericardium. Arthritis Rheum. *21*:972, 1978.
422. Starkey, R. H., and Hahn, B. H.: Rapid development of constrictive pericarditis in a patient with systemic lupus erythematosus. Chest *63*:448, 1973.
423. Charcot, J. M.: Clinical lecture on senile and chronic diseases. London, Sydenham Society, 1891, pp. 172–175.
424. Thadani, U., Iveson, J. M., and Wright, V.: Cardiac tamponade, constrictive pericarditis and pericardial resection in rheumatoid arthritis. Medicine *54*:261, 1975.
425. Casademont, M., and Casademont, J.: Pleuropericarditis in rheumatic disease. Cardiovasc. Rev. Reports *5*:161, 1984.
426. Gordon, D. A., Stein, J. N., and Broder, I.: Extra-articular features of rheumatoid arthritis: A systemic analysis of 127 cases. Ann. Intern. Med. *58*:102, 1963.
427. Bacon, P. A., and Gibson, D. G.: Cardiac involvement in rheumatoid arthritis; an echocardiographic study. Ann. Rheum. Dis. *31*:426, 1972.
428. John, J. T., Jr., Hough, A., and Sergent, J. S.: Pericardial disease in rheumatoid arthritis. Am. J. Med. *66*:385, 1979.
429. Burney, D. P., Martin, C. E., Thomas, C. S., Fisher, R. D., and Bender, H. W., Jr.: Rheumatoid pericarditis. Clinical significance and operative management. J. Thorac. Cardiovasc. Surg. *77*:511, 1979.
430. Alukal, M. K., Costello, P. B., and Green, F. A.: Cardiac tamponade in systemic juvenile rheumatoid arthritis requiring emergency pericardiectomy. J. Rheumatol. *11*:222, 1984.
431. Esdaile, J. M., Tannenbaum, H., and Hawkins, D.: Adult Still's disease. Am. J. Med. *68*:825, 1980.
432. Jamieson, T. W.: Adult Still's disease complicated by cardiac tamponade. J.A.M.A. *249*:2065, 1983.
433. Franco, A. E., Levine, H. D., and Hall, A. P.: Rheumatoid pericarditis. Ann. Intern. Med. *7*:837, 1972.
434. Parkash, R., Atassi, A., Poske, R., and Rosen, K. M.: Prevalence of pericardial effusion and mitral valve involvement in patients with rheumatoid arthritis without cardiac symptoms. N. Engl. J. Med. *289*:597, 1973.
435. Mathew, P. K.: Pericardial tamponade secondary to sudden steroid withdrawal in chronic rheumatoid arthritis. Chest *75*:532, 1977.
436. Thould, A. K.: Constrictive pericarditis in rheumatoid arthritis. Ann. Rheum. Dis. *45*:89, 1986.
437. Keith, T. A.: Chronic constrictive pericarditis in association with rheumatoid disease. Circulation *25*:477, 1962.
438. Nassar, W. K., Miskin, M. E., and Rosenbaum, D.: Pericardial and myocardial disease in progressive systemic sclerosis. Am. J. Cardiol. *22*:538, 1968.
439. McWhorter, J. E., and LeRoy, E. C.: Pericardial disease in scleroderma (systemic sclerosis). Am. J. Med. *57*:566, 1974.
440. Bulkley, B. H., Rjdolfi, R. T., Salyer, W. R., and Hutchins, G. M.: Myocardial lesions of progressive systemic sclerosis. Circulation *53*:483, 1976.
441. Smith, J. W., Clements, P. J., Levisman, J., Furst, D., and Foss, M.: Echocardiographic features of progressive systemic sclerosis. Am. J. Med. *66*:28, 1979.
442. Uhl, G. S., and Kippes, G. M.: Pericardial tamponade in systemic sclerosis (scleroderma). Br. Heart J. *42*:345, 1979.
443. Hanley, P. C.: Constrictive pericarditis associated with combined retroperitoneal and mediastinal fibrosis. Mayo Clin. Proc. *59*:300, 1984.
444. Medsger, T. A., Jr., Masi, A. T., and Rodnan, G. P.: Survival with systemic sclerosis (scleroderma). A life-table analysis of clinical and demographic factors in 309 patients. Ann. Intern. Med. *75*:369, 1971.
445. Alpert, M. A., Goldberg, S. H., Singsen, B. H., Durham, J. B., Sharp, G. C., Ahmad, M., Madigan, N. P., Hurst, D. P., and Sullivan, W. D.: Cardiovascular complications of mixed connective tissue disease in adults. Circulation *69*:1182, 1983.
446. Badvi, E., Robles, S. E., Garcia, R. D., and Mintz, S. G.: Cardiovascular manifestations in mixed connective tissue disease in adults. Arch. Inst. Cardiol. Mex. *54*:493, 1984.
447. Schiavone, W. A., Ahmad, M., and Ockner, S. A.: Unusual cardiac complications of Wegner's granulomatosis. Chest *88*:745, 1985.
448. Csonka, G. W., and Oates, J. K.: Pericarditis and electrocardiographic changes in Reiter's syndrome. Br. Med. J. *1*:866, 1957.
449. Goldman, M. J., and Lau, F. Y. K.: Acute pericarditis associated with serum sickness. N. Engl. J. Med. *250*:278, 1954.
450. Shapiro, L., and Buckingham, R. B.: Septic rheumatoid pericarditis complicating Felty's syndrome. Arthritis Rheum. *24*:1435, 1981.
451. Dupond, J. L., and Leconte-des-Floris, R.: Temporal arteritis manifested as an acute febrile pericarditis. J.A.M.A. *247*:2731, 1982.
452. Patwardian, R. V., Heilpern, R. J., Brewster, A. C., and Darrah, J. J.: Pleuropericarditis: An extraintestinal complication of inflammatory bowel disease. Arch. Intern. Med. *143*:94, 1983.
453. Laane, B. F.: Infantile polyarteritis nodosa or mucocutaneous lymph node syndrome (Kawasaki disease). Arteritis associated with aneurysm, thromboses and rupture of the coronary artery with cardiac tamponade. Tijdschr. Nor. Laegeforen *101*:1583, 1981.
454. Crake, T., Sandie, G. I., Crisp, A. J., and Record, C. O.: Constrictive pericarditis and intestinal hemorrhage due to Whipple's disease. Postgrad. Med. J. *59*:194, 1983.

455. Dawes, P. T., and Atherton, S. T.: Coeliac disease presenting as recurrent pericarditis. Lancet *1*:1021, 1981.
456. Wanner, W. R., Williams, T. E., Fulkerson, P. K., Mendell, J. R., and Leier, C. V.: Postoperative pericarditis following thymectomy for myasthenia gravis. A prospective study. Chest *83*:647, 1983.
457. Silverman, K. J., Hutchins, G. M., and Bulkley, B. H.: Cardiac sarcoid: A clinicopathologic study of 84 unselected patients with systemic sarcoidosis. Circulation *58*:1204, 1978.
458. Verkleeren, J. L., Glover, M. V., Bloor, C., and Joswig, B. C.: Cardiac tamponade secondary to sarcoidosis. Am. Heart J. *106*:601, 1983.
459. Hiss, H. P.: Pleuropericarditis in sarcoidosis. South. Med. J. *79*:258, 1986.
460. Garrett, J., O'Neill, H., and Blake, S.: Constrictive pericarditis associated with sarcoidosis. Am. Heart J. *107*:394, 1984.
461. Alarcon-Segovia, D.: Drug-induced lupus syndromes. Mayo Clin. Proc. *44*:664, 1969.
462. Browning, C. A., Bishop, R. L., Heilpern, R. J., Singh, J. B., and Spodick, D. H.: Accelerated constrictive pericarditis in procainamide-induced systemic lupus erythematosus. Am. J. Cardiol. *53*:376, 1984.
463. Harrington, T. M., and Davis, D. E.: Systemic lupus-like syndrome induced by methyldopa therapy. Chest *79*:696, 1981.
464. Schoenwetter, A. H., and Silber, E. N.: Penicillin hypersensitivity, acute pericarditis and eosinophilia. J.A.M.A. *191*:136, 1965.
465. Slater, E. E.: Cardiac tamponade and peripheral eosinophilia in a patient receiving cromolyn sodium. Chest *73*:878, 1978.
466. Yates, R. C., and Olson, K. B.: Drug-induced pericarditis. Report of three cases due to 6-amino-9-D-psicofuranosylpurine. N. Engl. J. Med. *265*:274, 1961.
467. Krehlik, J. M., Hindson, D. A., Crowley, J. J., Jr., and Knight, L. L.: Minoxidil-associated pericarditis and fatal cardiac tamponade. West. J. Med. *143*:527, 1985.
468. Miller, D. H., and Haas, L. F.: Pneumonitis, pleural effusion and pericarditis following treatment with dantrolene. J. Neurol. Neurosurg. Psychol. *47*:553, 1984.
469. Harbin, A. D., Gerson, M. C., and O'Connell, J. B.: Simulation of acute myopericarditis by constrictive pericardial disease with endomyocardial fibrosis due to methysergide therapy. J. Am. Coll. Cardiol. *4*:196, 1984.
470. Bristow, M. R., Thomspon, P. D., Martin, R. P., Mason, J. W., Billingham, M. E., and Harrison, D. C.: Early anthracycline toxicity. Am. J. Med. *65*:823, 1978.
471. Vaickus, L., and Letendre, L.: Pericarditis induced by high-dose cytarabine therapy. Arch. Intern. Med. *144*:1868, 1984.
472. Cazin, B., Gorin, N. C., Laporte, J. P., Gallet, B., Dovay, L., Lopez, M., Najman, A., and Duhamel, G.: Cardiac complications after bone marrow transplantation. Cancer *57*:2061, 1986.
473. Ratliff, N. B., McMahon, J. T., Shirey, E. K., and Groves, L. K.: Silicone pericarditis. Cleveland Clin. Q. *51*:185, 1984.
474. Fraker, T. D., Jr., Walsh, T. E., Morgan, R. J., and Kim, K.: Constrictive pericarditis after the Beck operation. Am. J. Cardiol. *54*:931, 1984.
475. Sonokul, D., Parcharee, P., Wasi, P., and Fucharoen, S.: Cardiac pathology in 47 patients with beta-thalassaemia/haemoglobin E. Southeast Asian J. Trop. Med. Public Health *15*:554, 1984.
476. Abdun Nur, D., Marcus, C. S., and Russell, F. E.: Pericarditis associated with scorpionfish (*Scorpaena buttata*) sting. Toxicon *19*:579, 1981.
477. Dressler, W.: A postmyocardial infarction syndrome. Preliminary report of a complication resembling idiopathic recurrent benign pericarditis. J.A.M.A. *160*:1379, 1956.
478. Dressler, W.: The post-myocardial infarction syndrome. A report of 44 cases. Arch. Intern. Med. *103*:28, 1959.
479. Davies, A. M., and Gery, I.: The role of autoantibodies in heart disease. Am. Heart J. *60*:669, 1960.
480. Van der Geld, H.: Anti-heart antibodies in the post-pericardiotomy and the post-myocardial infarction syndrome. Lancet 2:617, 1964.
481. Liem, K. L., ten Veen, J. H., Lie, K. I., Feltkamp, T. E. W., and Durrer, D.: Incidence and significance of heart muscle antibodies in patients with acute myocardial infarction and unstable angina. Acta Med. Scand. *206*:473, 1971.
482. Weiser, N. J., Kantor, M., and Russell, H. K.: Post-myocardial infarction syndrome. Circulation *20*:371, 1959.
483. Streifer, J., Pitlik, S., Dux, S., Perry, G., Heilman, C., Greenwald, M., and Rosenfeld, J. B.: Dressler's syndrome after right ventricular infarction. Postgrad. Med. J. *60*:298, 1984.
484. Hertzeanu, H., Almog, C., and Algom, M.: Cardiac tamponade in Dressler's syndrome. Cardiology *70*:31, 1983.
485. Goldhaber, S. Z., Lorell, B. H., and Green, L. H.: Constrictive pericarditis. A case requiring pericardiectomy following Dressler's postmyocardial infarction syndrome. J. Thorac. Cardiovasc. Surg. *81*:793, 1981.
486. Haiat, R., Desoutter, P., Stolitz, J. P., Chousterman, M., Cattan, P., and Gandjbaklich, I.: Constrictive pericarditis secondary to myocardial infarction. Arch. Mal. Coeur *74*:1349, 1981.
487. Soloff, L. A., Zatuchni, J., Janton, D. H., O'Neill, T. J. E., and Glover, R. P.: Reactivation of rheumatic fever following mitral commissurotomy. Circulation *8*:481, 1953.
488. Engle, M. A., and Ito, T.: The postpericardiotomy syndrome. Am. J. Cardiol. *7*:73, 1961.
489. Peters, R. W., Scheinman, M. M., Raskin, S., and Thomas, A. N.: Unusual complications of epicardial pacemakers. Am. J. Cardiol. *45*:1088, 1980.
490. Livelli, F. D., Jr., Johnson, R. A., McEnany, M. T., Sherman, E., Newell, J., Block, P. C., and DeSanctis, R. W.: Unexplained in-hospital fever following cardiac surgery: Natural history, relationship to postpericardiotomy syndrome and a prospective study of therapy with indomethacin versus placebo. Circulation *57*:968, 1978.
491. Engle, M. A., Gay, W. A., Jr., Zabriskie, J. B., and Senterfit, L. B.: The postpericardiotomy syndrome: 25 years' experience. J. Cardiovasc. Med. *4*:321, 1984.
492. Kaminsky, M. E., Rodan, B. A., Osborne, D. R., Chen, J. T. T., Sealy, W. C. and Putman, C. E.: Postpericardiotomy syndrome. Am. J. Radiol. *138*:503, 1982.
493. DeSaulniers, D., Gervais, N., and Rouleau, J.: Does pericardial drainage decrease the frequency of the postpericardiotomy syndrome? Can. J. Surg. *24*:265, 1981.
494. Ofori-Krakye, S. K., Tyberg, T. I., Geha, A. S., Hammond, G. L., Cohen, L. S., and Langou, R. A.: Late cardiac tamponade after open heart surgery: Incidence, role of anticoagulants in its pathogenesis and its relationship to the postpericardiotomy syndrome. Circulation *63*:1323, 1981.
495. Weitzman, L. B., Tinkler, W. P., Kronzon, I., Cohen, M. L., Glassman, I., and Spencer, F. C.: The incidence and natural history of pericardial effusion after cardiac surgery—an echocardiographic study. Circulation *69*:506, 1984.
496. Stevenson, L. W., Child, J. S., Laks, H., and Kern, L.: Incidence and significance of early pericardial effusions after cardiac surgery. Am. J. Cardiol. *54*:848, 1984.
497. Wheller, E. O., Turner, J. D., and Scannell, J. G.: Fever, splenomegaly, and atypical lymphocytes. A syndrome observed after cardiac surgery utilizing a pump oxygenator. N. Engl. J. Med. *266*:454, 1962.
498. Berger, R. L., Loveless, G., and Warner, O.: Delayed and latent postcardiotomy tamponade: Recognition and nonoperative treatment. Ann. Thorac. Surg. *12*:22, 1971.
499. McCabe, J. C., Engle, M. A., and Ebert, P. A.: Chronic pericardial effusion requiring pericardiectomy in the postpericardiotomy syndrome. J. Thorac. Cardiovasc. Surg. *67*:814, 1974.
500. King, T. E., Jr., Stelzner, T. J., and Sahn, S. A.: Cardiac tamponade complicating the postpericardiotomy syndrome. Chest *83*:500, 1983.
501. Gehl, L., Iskandrian, A. S., Goel, I., Mintz, G. S., Kimbiris, D., Bemis, C. E., Mundth, E. D., and Segal, B. L.: Cardiac perforation with tamponade during cardiac catheterization. Cathet. Cardiovasc. Diagn. *8*:293, 1982.
502. B-Lundqvist, C., Olsson, S. B., and Varnauskas, E.: Transseptal left heart catheterization: A review of 278 studies. Clin. Cardiol. *9*:21, 1986.
503. Foster, C. J., Constrictive pericarditis complicating an endocardial pacemaker. Br. Heart J. *47*:497, 1982.
504. Goldbaum, T. S., Jacob, A. S., Smith, D. F., Pichard, A., and Lindsay, J., Jr.: Cardiac tamponade following percutaneous transluminal coronary angioplasty. Cathet. Cardiovasc. Diagn. *11*:413, 1985.
505. Slack, J. D., Pickerton, C. A., and Nassar, W. K.: Acute pericarditis after percutaneous transluminal coronary angioplasty. Am. J. Cardiol. *55*:843, 1985.
506. Lindenau, K. F., Warnke, H., and Bergmann, U.: Cardiac tamponade following open heart surgery. Zentralbl. Chir. *104*:1345, 1979.
507. Marx, P., Jaffe, C., Laks, H., and Wolfson, S.: Delayed post-cardiac-surgery tamponade producing localized right atrial compression. Cathet. Cardiovasc. Diagn. *7*:275, 1981.
508. Kanakis, C., Sheikh, A. I., and Rosen, K. M.: Constrictive pericardial disease following mitral valve replacement. Chest *79*:593, 1981.
509. Little, W. C., Primm, R. K., Karp, R. B., and Hood, W. P., Jr.: Clotted hemopericardium with the hemodynamic characteristics of constrictive pericarditis. Am. J. Cardiol. *45*:386, 1980.
510. Marsa, R., Mehta, S., Willis, N., and Bailey, L.: Constrictive pericarditis after myocardial revascularization: Report of three cases. Am. J. Cardiol. *44*:177, 1979.
511. Cohen, M. V., and Greenberg, M. A.: Constrictive pericarditis: Early and late complication of cardiac surgery. Am. J. Cardiol. *43*:657, 1979.
512. Kutcher, M. A., King, S. B., Alimurung, B. N., Craver, J. M., and Logue, R. B.: Constrictive pericarditis as a complication of cardiac surgery: Recognition of an entity. Am. J. Cardiol. *50*:742, 1982.
513. Ng, A. S. H., Dorosti, K., and Sheldon, W. C.: Constrictive pericarditis following cardiac surgery—Cleveland Clinic experience: Report of 12 cases and review. Cleveland Clin. Q. *50*:39, 1984.
514. Ribiero, P., Sapsford, R., Evans, T., Parcharidis, G., and Oakley, C.: Constrictive pericarditis as a complication of coronary artery bypass surgery. Br. Heart J. *51*:205, 1984.
515. Kabbani, S. S., Bashour, T., Ellertson, D. G., Geiger, J., Hanna, E. S., and Cheng, T. O.: Constrictive pericarditis following myocardial revascularization: A possible cause of graft occlusion. Am. Heart J. *110*:493, 1985.
516. Bewtra, C., and Schultz, R. D.: Constrictive calcific pericarditis following coronary arterial bypass surgery. Hum. Pathol. *16*:522, 1985.
517. Halon, D. A., Koren, G., Kriwisky, M., Applebaum, A., and Gotsman, M. S.: Constrictive pericarditis following coronary artery bypass grafting in a patient with chronic asymptomatic pericardial disease. Cardiology *70*:280, 1983.
518. Kerber, R. E., and Sherman, B.: Echocardiographic evaluation of pericardial effusion in myxedema. Incidence and biochemical and clinical correlations. Circulation *52*:823, 1975.
519. Kern, R. A., Soloff, L. A., Snope, W. J., and Bello, C. T.: Pericardial effusion: A constant, early, and major factor in the cardiac syndrome of hypothyroidism (myxedema heart). Am. J. Med. Sci. *217*:609, 1949.
520. Hardisty, C. A., Naik, D. R., and Munro, D. S.: Pericardial effusion in hypothyroidism. Clin. Endocrinol. *13*:349, 1980.
521. Parving, H., Hansen, J. M., Nielsen, S. V., Rossing, N., Munck, O., and Lassen, N. A.: Mechanisms of edema formation in myxedema-increased protein extravasation and relatively slow lymphatic drainage. N. Engl. J. Med. *301*:460, 1981.
522. Zimmerman, J., Yahalom, J., and Bar-On, H.: Clinical spectrum of pericardial effusion as the presenting feature of hypothyroidism. Am. Heart J. *106*:770, 1983.

523. Williams, L. H. P., Jayatunga, R., and Scott, O.: Massive pericardial effusion in a hypothyroid child. Br. Heart J. *51*:231, 1984.
524. Das, S., Lieberman, A. N., and Schussler, G. C.: Prolonged persistence of a large pericardial effusion and hemodynamic evidence of cardiac tamponade during treatment of myxedema. Clin. Cardiol. *5*:459, 1982.
525. Smolar, E. N., Rubin, J. E., Avramides, A., and Carter, A. C.: Cardiac tamponade in primary myxedema and review of the literature. Am. J. Med. Sci. *272*:345, 1976.
526. Rosenbau, D. L., and Yu, P. N.: Idiopathic cholesterol pericarditis with effusion. Am. Heart J. *70*:515, 1965.
527. Ridenhouse, C. E., and Kiphart, R. J.: Idiopathic cholesterol pericarditis treatment with pericardiectomy. Ann. Thorac. Surg. *4*:360, 1967.
528. Stanley, R. J., Subramanian, R., and Lie, J. T.: Cholesterol pericarditis teminating as constrictive calcific pericarditis. Follow-up study of patient with 40-year history of disease. Am. J. Cardiol. *46*:511, 1980.
529. Bhatt, M. A., Ferrante, J. W., Gielchinsky, I., and Norman, J. C.: Pleuropulmonary and skeletal lymphangiomatosis with chylothorax and chylopericardium. Ann. Thorac. Surg. *40*:398, 1985.
530. Rose, D. M., Colvin, S. B., Danilowicz, D., and Isom, O. W.: Cardiac tamponade secondary to chylopericardium following cardiac surgery: Case report and review of the literature. Ann. Thorac. Surg. *34*:333, 1982.
531. Morishita, Y., Taira, A., Furoi, A., Arima, S., and Tanaka, H.: Constrictive pericarditis secondary to primary chylopericardium. Am. Heart J. *109*:373, 1985.
532. Pollard, W. M., Schuchmann, G. F., and Bowen, T. E.: Isolated chylopericardium after cardiac operations. J. Thorac. Cardiovasc. Surg. *81*:943, 1981.
533. Kottinen, M. P., Pitkaranta, P. P., Heikkinen, L. O., Talja, M. T., and Ala-Kulju, K. V.: Esophago-pericardial fistula. A case report and review of the literature. Thorac. Cardiovasc. Surg. *33*:341, 1985.
534. Davidson, E. D., Horney, J. T., and Salter, P. P.: Internal pancreatic fistula to the pericardium and pleura. Surgery *85*:478, 1979.
535. Withrington, R., and Collins, P.: Cardiac tamponade in acute pancreatitis. Thorax *35*:959, 1980.
536. Clifford, R. P., and Gill, K. S.: Traumatic rupture of the pericardium with dislocation of the heart. Injury *16*:123, 1984.
537. Callejas, M. A., Mestres, C. A., Catalan, M., and Sanchez-Lloret, J.: Traumatic intrapericardial diaphragmatic rupture. Thorac. Cardiovasc. Surg. *32*:376, 1984.
538. Cassorla, L., and Katz, J. A.: Management of cardiac herniation after intrapericardial pneumonectomy. Anesthesiology *60*:362, 1984.
539 Feigin, D. S., Fenoglio, J. J., McAllister, H. A., and Madewell, J. E.: Pericardial cysts: A radiologic-pathologic correlation and review. Radiology *125*:15, 1977.
540. Kruger, S. R., Michaud, J., and Cannom, D. S.: Spontaneous resolution of a pericardial cyst. Am. Heart J. *109*:1390, 1985.
541. Hynes, J. K., Tajik, A. J., Osborn, M. J., Orszulak, T. A., and Seward, J. B.: Two-dimensional echocardiographic diagnosis of pericardial cyst. Mayo Clin. Proc. *58*:60, 1983.
542. Klatte, E. C., and Yune, H. Y.: Diagnosis and treatment of pericardial cysts. Radiology *104*:541, 1972.
543. Unverferth, D. V., and Wooley, C. F.: The differential diagnosis of paracardiac lesions: Pericardial cysts. Cathet. Cardiovasc. Diagn. 5:31, 1979.
544. Moncada, R., Baglia, K., Moguillansky, S. J., Subramanian, R., Demos, T. C., Lozada, C., Bianchi, G., and Ow, E. P.: CT diagnosis of congenital intrapericardial masses. J. Comput. Assist. Tomogr. 9:56, 1985.
545. Ellis, K., Leeds, N. E., and Himmelstein, A.: Congenital deficiencies in partial percardium: Review of two new cases including successful diagnosis by plain roentgenography. Am. J. Roentgenol. *82*:125, 1959.
546. Nassar, W. K., Helman, C., Tavel, M. E., Feigenbaum, H., and Fisch, C.: Congenital absence of the left pericardium. Circulation *41*:469, 1970.
547. Morgan, J. R., Rogers, A. K., and Forker, A. D.: Congenital absence of the left pericardium. Ann. Intern. Med. *74*::370, 1971.
548. Taysi, K., Hartmann, A. F., Shackelford, G. D., and Sundarum, V.: Congenital absence of the pericardium in a family. Am. J. Med. Genet. *21*:77, 1985.
549. Inoue, H., Fujii, J., Mashima, S., and Marao, S.: Pseudo right atrial overloading pattern in complete defect of the left pericardium. J. Electrocardiol. *14*:413, 1981.
550. Kansal, S., Roitman, D., and Sheffield, L. T.: Two-dimensional echocardiography of congenital absence of pericardium. Am. Heart J. *109*:912, 1985.
551. Candan, I., Erol, C., and Sonel, A.: Cross sectional echocardiographic appearance in presumed congenital absence of the left pericardium. Br. Heart J. *55*:405, 1986.
552. D'Altoria, R. A., and Caro, J. Y.: Congenital absence of the left pericardium detected by imaging of the lung: Case report. J. Nucl. Med. *18*:267, 1977.
553. Gutierrez, F. R., Shackelford, G. D., McKnight, R. C., Levitt, R. G., and Hartmann, A.: Diagnosis of congenital absence of left pericardium by MR imaging. J. Comput. Assist. Tomogr. 9:551, 1985.
554. Saito, R., and Hotta, F.: Congenital pericardial defect associated with cardiac incarceration: Case report. Am. Heart J. *100*:866, 1980.
555. Jones, J. W., and McManus, B. M.: Fatal cardiac strangulation by congenital partial percardial defect. Am. Heart J. *107*:183, 1984.
556. Ruys, F., Paulus, W., Stevens, C., and Brutsaert, D.: Expansion of the left atrial appendage is a distinctive cross-sectional echocardiographic feature of congenital defect of the pericardium. Eur. Heart J. *4*:738, 1983.
557. Minocha, G. K., Falicov, R. E., and Nijensohn, E.: Partial right-sided congenital pericardial defect with herniation of the right atrium and right ventricle. Chest *76*:484, 1979.
558. Bernal, J. M., Lepiedra, J. O., Gonzalez, I., Saez, A., Pastor, E., and Miralles, P. J.: Angiographic demonstration of a partial defect of the pericardium with herniation of the left atrium and ventricle. J. Cardiovasc. Surg. *27*:344, 1986.

45 TRAUMATIC HEART DISEASE

by PETER F. COHN, M.D., and
EUGENE BRAUNWALD, M.D.

THE PROBLEM IN PERSPECTIVE

Unfortunately, traumatic heart disease is still regarded as an uncommon and even esoteric form of heart disease of interest primarily to emergency physicians or those in the military service. That this is not the case is attested to by the statistics—violent injury accounts for the majority of deaths in persons under 40 years of age,[1] and among these victims cardiac trauma is one of the leading causes of death.[2, 3] Reports of increasing traumatic heart disease in civilians may be attributed to the accelerating mechanization of contemporary life—especially in the work place and on the roads. For example, chest injuries are directly responsible for more than 25 per cent of the 50,000 to 60,000 deaths that result annually from automobile accidents and contribute significantly to another 25 per cent of these deaths.[4] The increasing frequency of physical violence has also resulted in a corresponding increase in the incidence of traumatic heart disease, especially in *young adult males*. These are the most frequent victims, since they are more likely to have automobile and motorcycle accidents, to incur injuries while performing heavy labor, and to be involved in or victims of acts of physical violence.

There is, regrettably, no evidence that the frequency of these mishaps is declining or even approaching a plateau. At Boston City Hospital, for example, the annual incidence of penetrating wounds of the heart rose from 2.8 cases during the period from 1956 through 1964 to 8.0 cases from 1965 through 1976.[5] In addition, the incidence of medically related cardiac trauma is also rising, such as increased use of intravascular and intracardiac catheters leading to penetrating injuries of the heart and great vessels, and resuscitative cardiac massage causing a variety of nonpenetrating injuries of these organs.

The two principal, immediate consequences of cardiac injury are *exsanguinating hemorrhage* and *cardiac tamponade*. Effective treatment has resulted in an increasing number of immediate survivors, and later sequelae—including myocardial infarction, aneurysm, pseudoaneurysm, ventricular septal defect, valvular damage, recurrent pericarditis, and constrictive pericarditis—are becoming far more common. Serious cardiac trauma is frequently overlooked in patients with nonpenetrating injury, particularly when other structures such as the thoracic cage and lungs are obviously damaged. Such oversight can be tragic, because the lethal consequences of cardiac injury may suddenly emerge after the more superficial injuries have been attended to. Clearly, a much higher index of suspicion of this possibility is necessary if the increasing magnitude of this problem is to be halted and reversed.

NONPENETRATING CARDIAC INJURY

Nonpenetrating injuries result from the effects of external physical forces, but it is important to recognize that these forces need not necessarily be applied directly to the chest, since injuries to the heart and great vessels may also occur with trauma to other parts of the body. Parmley et al. have summarized the mechanisms of nonpenetrating injuries to the heart as follows: (1) direct force against the chest; (2) bidirectional force against the thorax; (3) indirect forces resulting in a marked increase in intravascular pressure, as from sudden compression in the abdomen and lower extremities; (4) decelerative forces; (5) blast forces; (6) concussive forces; and (7) combinations of these.[6]

The most common cause of nonpenetrating injury in civilian life is probably that directly related to *vehicular impact*, either by direct compression, usually with the steering wheel squeezing the heart between the sternum and the spine, or by indirect compression. Causes of nonpenetrating injuries other than automobile and motorcycle accidents include direct blows to the chest by any kind of blunt object or missile, such as a clenched fist or even various kinds of sporting equipment, as well as by the kicks of animals, falls, and cardiac resuscitative procedures. Fractures of the bony structures of the chest wall are *not* necessary accompaniments of cardiac injury in any of these situations. This point is of critical importance, since *the absence of such obvious injuries following trauma should by no means exclude the possibility of nonpenetrating injury to the heart*. The clinical manifestations may not be apparent for days or even weeks after the accident.[7]

Pathological findings following nonpenetrating cardiac injury usually include some degree of *pericarditis*, which may be associated with the late development of *pericardial constriction*. Changes in the heart itself range from minute ecchymotic areas in the subepicardium or subendocardium to transmural contusions with edematous, fragmented, or

TABLE 45–1 TYPES OF CARDIAC INJURY FROM BLUNT TRAUMA

A. Myocardium
  1. Contusion
  2. Laceration
  3. Rupture
  4. Septal perforation
  5. Aneurysm, pseudoaneurysm
  6. Hemopericardium, tamponade
  7. Thrombosis, systemic embolism
B. Pericardium
  1. Pericarditis
  2. Postpericardiotomy syndrome
  3. Constrictive pericarditis
  4. Pericardial laceration
  5. Hemorrhage
  6. Cardiac herniation
C. Endocardial structures
  1. Rupture of papillary muscle
  2. Rupture of chordae tendineae
  3. Rupture of atrioventricular and semilunar valves
D. Coronary artery
  1. Thrombosis
  2. Laceration
  3. Fistula

From Jackson, D. H., and Murphy, G. W.: Nonpenetrating cardiac trauma. Mod. Conc. Cardiovasc. Dis. *45*:123, 1976, by permission of the American Heart Association, Inc.

necrotic muscle fibers, surrounded at first by red blood cells and invaded soon thereafter by polymorphonuclear leukocytes. The external appearance of the heart may be misleading in the case of nonpenetrating injury, since large areas of intramural contusion, including involvement of the interventricular septum, may not be apparent.[4, 8] In patients who survive the injury, healing is by scar formation resembling that following acute myocardial infarction, and

TABLE 45–2 NONPENETRATING CARDIAC TRAUMA

Type and/or Site of Injury	Number of Cases	Cases Combined with Aortic Rupture	Total
Rupture	273	80	353
Right ventricle	56	10	66
Left ventricle	46	13	59
Right atrium	35	6	51
Left atrium	24	2	26
IV septum	25(20*)	7(4*)	30(24*)
IA septum	18(10*)	5(3*)	25(13*)
Multiple chamber	69	37	106
ruptures			128
Contusion/laceration	105	24	
Pericardial laceration	18	18	36
Hemopericardium	13	12	25
Valvular laceration/rupture	1(2†)	0(4†)	1(6†)
Aortic valve	1(1†)	0(2†)	1(3†)
Pulmonic valve	0(4†)	0	0(4†)
Tricuspid valve	0(8†)	0	0(8†)
Mitral valve	0(8†)	0(1†)	0(9†)
Mitral and tricuspid valves	0(1†)	0(1†)	0(2†)
Coronary artery laceration/rupture	0(7†)	1(2†)	1(9†)
Papillary muscle laceration/rupture	1(23†)	0	1(23†)
TOTAL	411	135	546

Numbers in parentheses indicate more significant associated cardiac injuries (tabulated in another column).
*Associated with other sites of cardiac rupture.
†Combined with cardiac rupture or other cardiac injury.
From Parmley, L. F., et al.: Nonpenetrating traumatic injury of the heart. Circulation *18*:371, 1958, by permission of the American Heart Association, Inc.

post-traumatic aneurysms resembling postinfarction aneurysms may develop. The types of cardiac injury resulting from blunt (nonpenetrating) trauma are listed in Table 45–1, the most severe forms being rupture of the aortic or mitral valve and rupture of the interventricular septum or even of the free wall of a cardiac chamber. These injuries are frequently fatal, but fortunately they constitute only a small fraction of all nonpenetrating injuries (Table 45–2).

Pericardium

(See p. 1491)

Injury to the pericardium in blunt trauma may range from contusion to laceration or rupture. Whether the pericardium tears or not, some degree of traumatic pericarditis is found at autopsy or operation in most patients sustaining severe blunt trauma of the chest, especially of the precordial area. Parmley et al. reported pericardial laceration or rupture in 249 of 546 autopsy cases of nonpenetrating trauma to the heart,[6] but it should be noted that this rarely occurs as an isolated lesion (Table 45–2) and is usually associated with cardiac contusion and even more serious cardiac injury. On the basis of a series of experiments in a canine model, in which 14 of 18 dogs receiving sublethal blunt chest trauma developed pericardial rents, DeMuth et al. suggested that a higher frequency of pericardial tears than is generally appreciated occurs in survivors of chest trauma.[9] Herniation of the heart or a portion of it through the defect may result from such injuries.[10] Clinically, a rent in the pericardium can occur as a consequence of blunt trauma, and delayed herniation of the heart through the rent may then acutely compromise circulatory function.[11]

CLINICAL FEATURES AND DIAGNOSIS. Clinically, traumatic pericarditis is manifested by the development of a typical pericardial friction rub and ST-T–wave changes on the electrocardiogram characteristic of pericarditis (p. 1489). During and immediately following the acute episode, the major problem is not the pericarditis itself but its most common complications, i.e., hemopericardium and resultant tamponade, discussed on p. 1492. Commonly, the patient is restless, with hypotension, oliguria or anuria, distant heart sounds, and pulsus paradoxus. There is usually diffuse low voltage on the electrocardiogram. Pericardial fluid on the echocardiogram (p. 127) is a key finding.[12]

TREATMENT AND PROGNOSIS. As a rule, uncomplicated pericarditis simply resolves. Tamponade, however, requires emergency operative treatment, as discussed below. Recurrent pericardial effusions sometimes associated with chest pain and fever, i.e., the so-called postcardiotomy syndrome, occur in a small number of patients. The etiology of this syndrome is not clear (p. 1522). Although patients with recurrent effusion usually respond to aspirin or nonsteroidal antiinflammatory agents, occasionally glucocorticosteroids are necessary. *Constrictive pericarditis* (p. 1501) occurs as a rare complication of traumatic pericarditis, with or without recurrent effusions.

Myocardium

As early as 1935 experimental studies stressed the vulnerability of the heart to blunt trauma.[13] More recently, a method of producing a standard, graded, isolated injury to the myocardium through the intact chest wall of anesthetized dogs using a captive-bolt handgun or an air-pressurized impactor with energy transferred through a metal disc has been described.[14–16] As the power was increased, the degree of injury became correspondingly more severe. The first level of energy produced only arrhythmias, intermediate levels produced varying degrees of hematoma associated with impairment of ventricular function, and the highest level of energy was nearly always fatal. The earliest changes could be assessed with two-dimensional echocardiography and then confirmed pathologically.[16] With trauma to the left side of the chest, abnormalities were mostly in the anterolateral wall of the left ventricle; trauma to the right chest produced septal and right ventricular wall contusion.

Since the consequences of nonpenetrating injury to the myocardium vary in intensity from mild contusion to cardiac rupture, it is not surprising that clinical manifestations also vary proportionately and that a high index of suspicion is often necessary for their recognition in all but the most obvious cases.[17, 18] In patients with preexisting ischemic, valvular, or myopathic heart disease, the added insult of the myocardial trauma can be more serious than a comparable injury in a normal person.

CONTUSION. Myocardial contusion usually produces no significant symptoms and often goes unrecognized.[18a] At times, manifestations of the injury are masked by injury to the chest wall or other organs.[18b] This is important because as many as 75 per cent of patients with myocardial contusion can have signs of external chest injury.[19] Thus, as is the case with any condition, there is a higher frequency of diagnosis of cardiac contusion associated with increasing awareness of the lesion.

Clinical Features and Diagnosis. The most common symptom of myocardial contusion is precordial pain resembling that of myocardial infarction, but the pain from other sites of chest trauma can confuse the clinical picture.[18, 19] As with myocardial infarction, nitroglycerin and related drugs have little effect in relieving the pain. The *electrocardiogram* probably represents one of the most helpful tools for recognizing contusion of the left ventricle. Either nonspecific ST-T abnormalities or the classic findings of pericarditis are the most common changes noted. Initially, electrocardiographic signs of deeper injury to the myocardium, i.e., pathological Q waves, may be dwarfed by pericardial inflammation; only as the latter subsides does injury to the myocardium become more evident. However, because the possibility of cardiac trauma is not considered, an electrocardiogram is often not recorded immediately on patients with chest injuries and the diagnosis may be missed. Just as in acute myocardial infarction, serial findings, i.e., the evolution of Q waves and the subsidence of the ST-segment and T-wave abnormalities, are of critical importance. The sensitivity and specificity of electrocardiographic findings are less than 100 per cent, however; hence the need for additional tests.

Since *serum enzyme levels* may be elevated by trauma to noncardiac as well as to cardiac tissue, they too are of limited diagnostic value. With the widespread availability of reliable measurements of the MB band of creatine kinase (CK), the cardiospecific isoenzyme of creatine kinase, the presence or absence of cardiac necrosis can be better documented in patients with blunt trauma.[21, 22] Indeed, with the electrocardiogram and CK-MB as screening tests, the detection of myocardial contusion has increased from 7 to 17 per cent in patients with blunt chest trauma presenting to the Henry Ford Hospital.[23] However, false-positive elevations of the CK-MB isoenzyme can also be seen if the total CK is greater than 20,000 units; this can occur after massive body injury.

Another potentially important diagnostic tool is *radionuclide imaging* (Chap. 11).[24] Myocardial perfusion is reduced in areas of myocardial contusion.[21, 22] Chiu et al. have used technetium-labeled pyrophosphate to demonstrate images of positive uptake that were then correlated with postmortem angiograms showing extravasation of contrast material.[25] Images usually became negative 1 week after the trauma. Contused myocardium concentrates ^{99m}Tc-pyrophosphate in amounts comparable to those observed in ischemic injury. Scanning following injection of

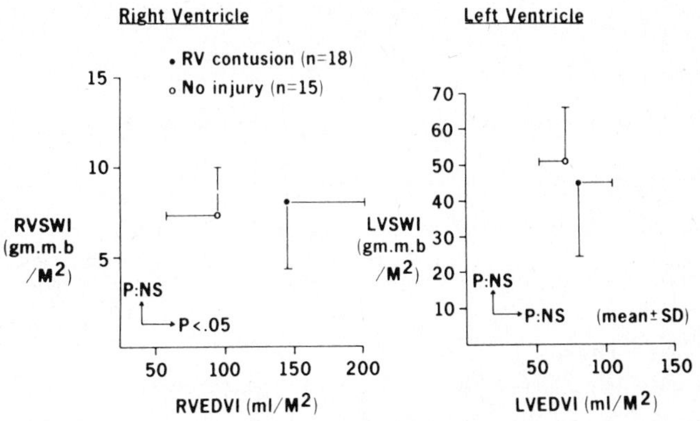

FIGURE 45–1. Left and right ventricular (LV and RV) myocardial function curves in 43 patients who sustained acute myocardial contusion complicating blunt chest injury. Patients with RV contusion (●) maintained an RV stroke work index (RVSWI) similar to that of patients without RV contusion (○) by virtue of a larger RV end-diastolic volume index (RVEDVI) (preload). Hence, RV performance was well-maintained albeit at a greater preload and the two groups of patients appeared to have identical LV function. NS = not significant; SD = standard deviation. (From Sutherland, G. R., et al.: Hemodynamic adaptation to acute myocardial contusion complicating blunt chest injury. Am. J. Cardiol. *57*:291, 1986.)

radioactive thallium to detect areas of reduced perfusion and of labeled pyrophosphate to locate areas of recent necrosis may be expected to identify patients with myocardial damage following blunt trauma, to localize this damage, and to indicate the extent of the damage. Radionuclide ventriculography often shows a reduced ventricular ejection fraction in such patients.[26] These tests show changes similar to those observed in patients with acute myocardial infarction (Chap. 11). Sutherland et al.[26] used gated radionuclide ventriculography to define focal defects in ventricular wall motion. They subgrouped the 43 patients whom they studied into those with right ventricular abnormalities (18), left ventricular abnormalities (4), biventricular abnormalities (6), and neither kind (15). They described the state of right ventricular pump function using modified ventricular function curves and found it to be surprisingly well preserved (Fig. 45–1).

In addition to identifying pericardial effusion, *two-dimensional echocardiography* is also useful in evaluating cardiac injuries, including myocardial contusion. Such findings as abnormal wall motion and chamber enlargement can be detected with this technique.[12, 27] Echocardiography is useful when the patient with suspected cardiac injury first undergoes testing, as well as after emergency thoracotomy and cardiac repair in an effort to detect residual cardiac damage. A recommended decision schema for evaluating cardiac injury immediately after early cardiorrhaphy is depicted in Figure 45–2. (When confirmed with pulsed-Doppler echocardiography, intracardiac shunts and regurgitant lesions can be demonstrated.)

A wide variety of *arrhythmias* is common with areas of extensive contusion,[28] and ventricular tachycardia that degenerates into ventricular fibrillation represents a frequent cause of death in these patients. The precise mechanism responsible for these arrhythmias has not been defined, but in the dog, increasing frequencies of ventricular premature beats were observed with increasing grades of trauma.[14] In addition, both atrioventricular and intraventricular conduction defects, as well as sinus node dysfunction, are seen.[29, 30] In contrast to acute myocardial infarc-

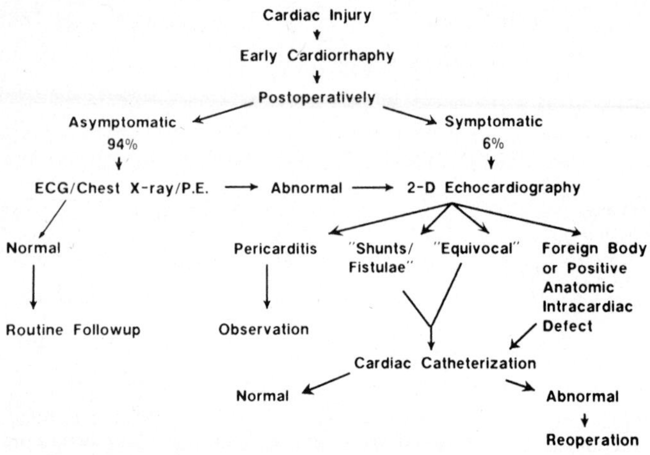

FIGURE 45–2. A recommended decision schema for post-traumatic cardiac evaluation. Following cardiac injury repair is generally carried out by simple cardiorrhaphy. This algorithm shows a suggested approach to detect residual damage following emergency cardiorrhaphy. (From Mattox, K. L., et al.: Cardiac evaluation following heart injury. J. Trauma *25*:758, © by Williams and Wilkins, 1985.)

tion, cardiac contusion rarely leads to severe *heart failure* unless massive damage to a valve or rupture of the interventricular septum has occurred. However, some impairment of right and/or left ventricular function, as reflected in depressed ejection fractions and ventricular function (myocardial performance) curves, may be found.[26, 32] In the animal model, alcohol ingestion potentiates the effect of blunt trauma on the myocardium.[33] This gives added strength to the warning not to mix drinking and driving.

Treatment and Prognosis. Treatment of myocardial contusion has traditionally involved a 4- to 6-week period of bed rest with progressive ambulation thereafter. However, in this era of progressively earlier ambulation for patients with myocardial infarction, a more aggressive approach appears to be reasonable after several days of close observation, as with an infarction. From the point of view of physical activity, we recommend treating these patients in a manner similar to those with acute myocardial infarction with comparable extent of myocardial damage (Chap. 41). *Treatment with anticoagulants is contraindicated*, however, since it may precipitate or exacerbate intramyocardial or intrapericardial hemorrhage. Atrial fibrillation, when present, usually reverts to sinus rhythm spontaneously. If it does not, digitalis glycosides may be used to slow the ventricular rate and may also cause reversion to sinus rhythm. Chest pain is best treated with analgesics.

The prognosis for complete or partial recovery is generally excellent, but these patients require careful followup, since late complications, ranging from ventricular arrhythmias to cardiac rupture, may occur.[33a] Coronary occlusion,[34, 35] sinus of Valsalva–right atrial fistula,[36] and cardiac aneurysms[37] are occasional sequelae, and there is no agreement about whether or not surgical resection of the last-named is required.[38] It is our policy to use the presence of heart failure as an indication for operation of aneurysms analogous to that in patients with postinfarct aneurysms (p. 1374).

Although many analogies can be drawn between the cardiac necrosis caused by trauma and that caused by coronary artery disease, a number of critically important differences must be emphasized. Patients with acute myocardial infarction generally have diffuse, obstructive, gradually progressive coronary artery disease, are frequently middle-aged or elderly, and may have underlying heart disease such as that secondary to prolonged hypertension or diabetes mellitus; patients with traumatic myocardial contusion generally have normal coronary vessels and only a discrete area of myocardial damage; most often, they are young and without underlying cardiovascular illness. Hence, the long-term prognosis in patients with myocardial necrosis secondary to trauma tends to be far better, *if they survive the acute episode.*

CARDIAC RUPTURE. There appear to be two mechanisms of cardiac rupture: (1) acute laceration due to compression of the heart by direct force,[38a] and (2) contusion and hemorrhage that proceed to necrosis, softening, and rupture several days following the trauma. Rupture of a cardiac chamber usually, but not always, results in immediate death. However, Bright and Beck reported that 30 of 152 patients with ventricular rupture survived 30 minutes or longer after the initial trauma.[13] It is this minority of patients that must be assessed and treated immediately in the emergency room setting.

Clinical Features and Diagnosis. In the patient who survives the first few minutes of cardiac rupture, the clinical picture of cardiac tamponade described above is common. Although ventricular rupture is far more common than is atrial rupture,[4] the latter occurs particularly following automobile accidents.[39] Rupture of the interventricular septum should be suspected in patients who develop severe congestive heart failure immediately or within several days of the trauma, together with a new holosystolic murmur along the left sternal border; however, trauma to the mitral valve apparatus, which may be manifested with a similar picture clinically, must be excluded. On the basis of a series of 546 autopsy cases of nonpenetrating injury to the heart, the incidence of rupture of the ventricular septum has been estimated by Parmley et al. to be a little more than 5 per cent, with a similar number of patients experiencing rupture of the atrial septum (Table 45–2).[6] These lesions may occur without other serious cardiac injuries, but occasionally other abnormalities are present, including valve cusp perforations and a variety of intracardiac shunts.[40] Although the predilection for perforation of the ventricular septum is highest at the apex, any portion of the muscular septum may be involved, and multiple perforations are not uncommon. The diagnosis of ventricular septal defect and of damage to the mitral valve apparatus can be confirmed by means of catheterization, demonstration of an oxygen step-up in the right ventricle, left ventricular angiography,[41] as well as by pulsed-Doppler echocardiography.[27]

Treatment and Prognosis. Patients with external rupture of the heart obviously require emergency operation if they are to have any chance of survival. Although surgery should not be postponed, pericardiocentesis and expansion of the intravascular volume can be carried out while the most rapid preparations possible for operation are undertaken. Successful surgical treatment of external cardiac rupture has been reported in a small number of cases.[42] In contrast, patients with rupture of the interventricular septum do not always require emergency operation. Indeed, many defects are small, with minimal left-to-right shunts, and may even heal spontaneously. If heart failure subsequently develops, as occurs in many patients, surgical correction should be carried out promptly and is often successful.

COMPLICATIONS OF CARDIAC RESUSCITATION

In 1960, Kouwenhoven et al. described the technique of closed-chest (external) cardiac massage, and this tech-

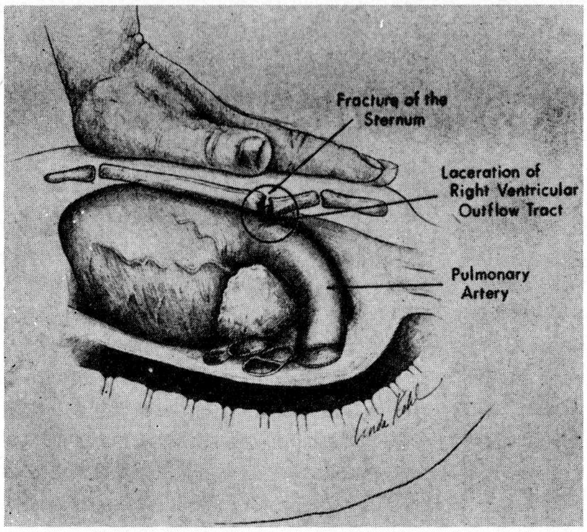

FIGURE 45–3. Schematic diagram showing the mechanism and site of laceration of the right ventricular outflow tract during external cardiac massage. (From Sethi, G. K., et al.: Complications of external cardiac massage. Report of a case of laceration of right ventricular outflow tract. J. Cardiovasc. Surg. *18*:187, 1977.)

nique quickly replaced open-chest massage in the management of cardiac arrest.[43] This procedure is generally thought to be safe and simple—so much so that it is included as part of the cardiopulmonary resuscitation technique taught to laymen. What is not sufficiently appreciated is that the procedure itself can often result in serious complications, which may go unrecognized because many of the patients succumb to the cardiac arrest itself. Even at postmortem examination, the complications may be improperly attributed to the underlying cardiac disease.

Rupture of the left ventricle is a more common complication of cardiac massage than rupture of the right ventricle (Fig. 45–3). However, rupture of either chamber may occur and may be life-threatening if the patient survives the cardiac dysrhythmia that necessitated massage in the first place. In a series of autopsies on 60 patients in whom external cardiac massage had been carried out, Adelson observed four instances of laceration of the left ventricle and one each of the left atrium and cardiac vein.[44] Since in most instances external resuscitation is performed for patients with myocardial infarction, it may not always be clear whether the left ventricular rupture preceded or occurred as a consequence of the massage.

Rupture of right ventricular papillary muscles with acute tricuspid regurgitation has also been reported as a complication of closed-chest cardiac massage,[45] as has rupture of the atria and aorta and dissecting hematoma of a coronary artery,[46] plus a variety of noncardiovascular traumatic lesions, such as fracture of the sternum, hemothorax, pneumothorax, and laceration of abdominal organs. Because of the efficacy of cardiopulmonary resuscitation and its increasing use by paramedical personnel and laymen,[47] an increasing number of such complications may be anticipated in the future. This increased incidence will be stemmed only by extensive and repeated educational programs for all individuals likely to employ this technique.

PENETRATING CARDIAC INJURY

In their review, Karrel et al.[48] noted the long medical history of penetrating cardiac wounds, which have been recorded since 3000 B.C. Up to the end of the nineteenth century, this type of wound was thought to be invariably fatal.

Penetrating cardiac injuries occurring in civilian life are due to a variety of objects, such as bullets, knives, ice picks, and the like,[49, 50] but they may also be due to the inward displacement of ribs or sternal fragments accompanying chest injuries. The chamber most commonly involved in this type of injury is the right ventricle because of its anterior position, followed, in descending order of frequency, by the left ventricle, the right atrium, and the left atrium.[50] However, penetrating wounds of the precordium are not the only types of wounds that may result in cardiac injury. Occasionally, wounds of other areas of the chest, as well as of the neck and upper abdomen, are associated with penetration of the heart. In addition, intravenous or intracardiac catheters may fracture and become impaled within the walls of a great vessel or cardiac chamber (Chap. 9). Migration of an indwelling venous catheter into the pulmonary artery, which may ultimately lead to perforation of this vessel, is another complication that has increased in frequency with its widespread use in intensive care units. Formerly, thoracotomy was necessary to remove these catheter fragments, but noninvasive snare and other devices are now available for this purpose.[51, 52]

Perforation of the right ventricle with a transvenous pacing electrode is not uncommon, but tamponade is rare. During cardiac catheterization, perforation of the thin-walled right atrium or outflow tract of the right ventricle has been reported. Such patients usually require only careful observation, but when tamponade occurs, immediate drainage is mandatory.[53] Coronary angioplasty[54] and endomyocardial biopsy[55] can also result in tamponade. Dissection of the aorta or arch vessels has been reported as a complication of retrograde arterial catheterization and occasionally is also severe enough to require operative intervention.

Penetrating wounds of the heart often result in laceration of the pericardium, sometimes occurring alone but usually associated with laceration of the myocardium itself. One or more chambers but also the cardiac valves and their accessory structures, as well as the interventricular and interatrial septa, may be perforated. Cardiac tamponade resulting from pneumopericardium has been reported.[56] When laceration of the pericardium occurs as an isolated lesion, acute compromise of cardiac function resulting from herniation of the heart may be the presenting manifestation. Occasionally, low-velocity missiles may penetrate the cardiac chambers but may be retained within the myocardium.

The most common penetrating injuries resulting from physical violence are stab and gunshot wounds.[57, 58] The former do not necessarily cause extensive cellular destruction adjacent to the wound; they resemble surgical incisions, and transmural wounds in the thick-walled left ventricle may actually seal quickly without disastrous consequences. In contrast, bullet wounds are associated with bleeding that is not usually self-limited and extensive cellular destruction in and adjacent to the path of the bullet. When a coronary artery is lacerated or perforated, myocardial infarction may ensue.

CLINICAL FEATURES AND DIAGNOSIS. The clinical picture of a penetrating wound of the heart depends on several factors, including the object responsible for the injury (i.e., bullet, knife, ice pick), the size of the wound, and the precise location of the structures injured. Pericardial laceration occurring by itself is uncommon and of relatively little significance, unless infection supervenes. Rather, the injuries to underlying cardiac structures usually determine the clinical presentation, course, and choice of treatment. However, the nature of the pericardial wound is important, i.e., whether or not the wound is open and allows free drainage of intrapericardial blood. If the pericardium remains open and extravasated blood can pass freely into the pleural cavities or mediastinum, cardiac tamponade will not develop, at least initially, and the presenting signs and symptoms will be those of hemorrhage and hemothorax. On the other hand, if the pericardium does *not* permit free drainage, because its opening has been obliterated by a blood clot, adjacent lung tissue, or other structures, or because a flap develops in the pericardial rent, immediate exsanguination may be averted, but tamponade may occur minutes or hours later. In some instances, blood accumulates both intra- and extrapericardially.

Whether the hemorrhage is intra- or extrapericardial, its severity can often be surmised from the clinical picture. Traumatic penetrating lesions of the heart are usually associated with injuries to the lungs and other organs, which may predominate at first; a high index of suspicion of cardiac penetration is necessary when patients are evaluated following thoracic or upper abdominal trauma. Though extensive injuries to the pericardium and underlying heart are usually immediately fatal or result in shock, delayed clinical manifestations of cardiac injury as a result of hemorrhage, infection, retained foreign bodies, or arrhythmias may become apparent after the other bodily injuries have been attended to. Failure to give serious consideration to the possibility that *cardiac* damage has occurred in a patient with obvious noncardiac trauma may lead to an unanticipated catastrophe.

Although echocardiography is extremely valuable in the recognition of pericardial effusion[12, 27] (p. 127), foreign

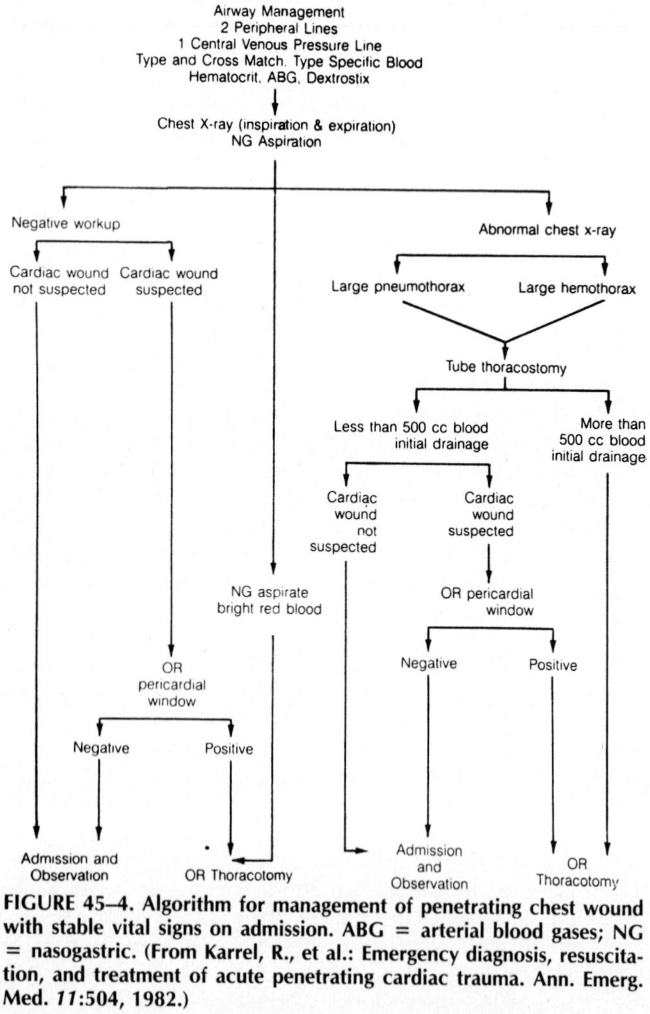

FIGURE 45–4. Algorithm for management of penetrating chest wound with stable vital signs on admission. ABG = arterial blood gases; NG = nasogastric. (From Karrel, R., et al.: Emergency diagnosis, resuscitation, and treatment of acute penetrating cardiac trauma. Ann. Emerg. Med. *11*:504, 1982.)

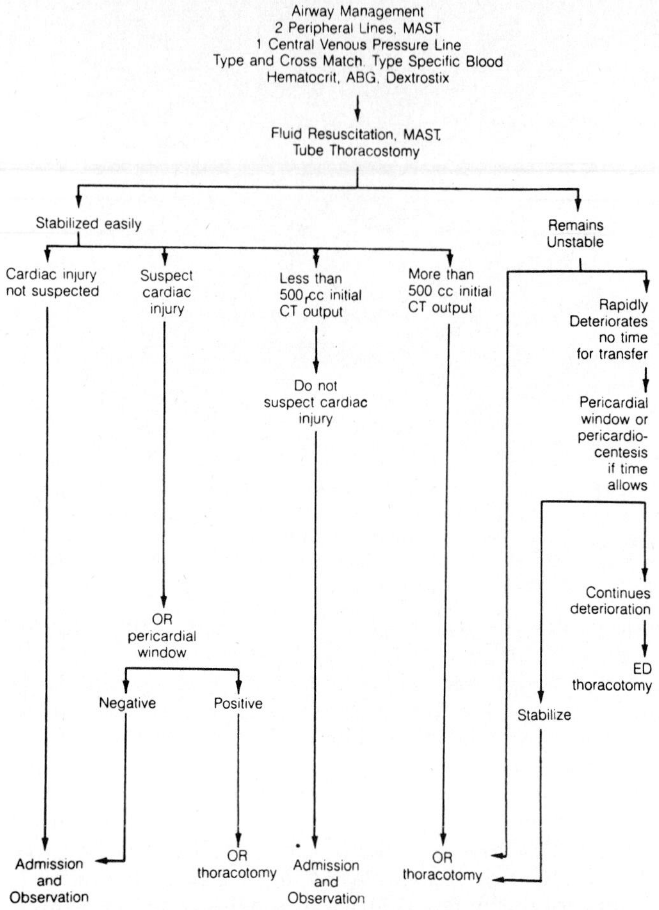

FIGURE 45–5. Algorithm for penetrating chest wound with unstable vital signs on admission. MAST = military anti-shock trousers. (From Karrel, R., et al.: Emergency diagnosis, resuscitation, and treatment of acute penetrating cardiac trauma. Ann. Emerg. Med. *11*:504, 1982.)

bodies in the heart,[59] and intracardiac shunts (with Doppler echocardiography),[12, 27, 60, 61] it is not always readily available in an emergency setting. When agitation, cool and clammy skin, neck vein distention, pulsus paradoxus, and other classic findings of tamponade (considered earlier) are present, the diagnosis can be relatively simple; in patients without such typical findings, the clinical picture may be attributed to blood loss, especially since volume expansion can improve the hemodynamic state at least temporarily. Whether or not pericardiocentesis should be performed as a diagnostic test is controversial.[48] If nonclotting blood is obtained, the diagnosis of hemopericardium is confirmed, and the accompanying decompression may constitute effective, albeit temporary, initial treatment. If the pericardiocentesis is negative, however, cardiac tamponade cannot be ruled out. Since, as discussed below, the primary management in any event is thoracotomy, it seems pointless to waste valuable time with pericardial aspiration unless there is doubt regarding the diagnosis.

TREATMENT. The definitive treatment of cardiac wounds *accompanied by severe hemorrhage* is immediate thoracotomy and cardiorrhaphy.[61a] Although multiple pericardiocenteses are no longer considered a substitute for thoracotomy in the treatment of cardiac wounds associated with cardiac tamponade, there may still be a role for pericardial aspiration *while the patient is being prepared for operation.* Algorithms for management of patients with penetrating chest wounds—with either stable or unstable vital signs—have been proposed by Karrel et al.[48] (Figs. 45–4 and 45–5). The availability in many hospitals of surgical teams and equipment for cardiopulmonary bypass has permitted the safe and effective repair of many penetrating injuries of the heart. Marshall and associates[58] described a 10½-year experience with 47 patients admitted after penetrating cardiac trauma (stab wounds and gunshot wounds); 46 underwent immediate surgery and 10 died. The one patient who refused surgery also died, resulting in a total mortality of 11/47, or 23 per cent. Mortality was 26 per cent in patients with shunts and 15 per cent for those with tamponade. These figures are in agreement for those reported in other recent series.[48]

The decision for or against thoracotomy must, of course, depend on the setting in which the patient is encountered, the availability and skill of the surgical team, and facilities for cardiopulmonary bypass, all measured against the gravity of the clinical picture. Even in hospitals without the facilities of cardiopulmonary bypass, treatment of penetrating injuries of the heart may be very successful.[57]

Occasionally, thoracotomy may be performed in moribund patients for whom general anesthesia is unnecessary. However, every effort must be made to maintain adequate ventilation. Administration of antibiotics and tetanus prophylaxis should also be instituted as routine measures. Operative treatment includes repair of the pericardium, myocardium, aorta, and valves as well as of any lacerations of the coronary arteries. At operation, the heart and great vessels should be thoroughly examined for the presence of multiple wounds. When the bullet has penetrated the anterior wall of the heart, the posterior wall should always be inspected for an exit wound before the chest is closed. Many victims of penetrating cardiac injury, young and otherwise in good health, can withstand relatively long periods of hypoperfusion without irreversible brain, renal, or cardiac damage. Therefore, one should err on the side of aggressive attempts at resuscitation in patients who arrive moribund in the operating room. Retained foreign bodies in the heart are less of a problem in civilian than in military injuries, because shootings in civilian life usually occur at short range and thus result in through-and-through wounds.

There is disagreement concerning whether or not retained foreign bodies should be removed. Certainly, if the projectile is accessible, it should be removed; echocardiography (Fig. 45–6) can be helpful in locating foreign bodies.[59] If deemed not dangerous, they can probably be left in place, although there is some risk of later infection, pain, aneurysm formation, or migration of the foreign body.[62, 63] In addition, dealing with a patient who is preoccupied with the knowledge that he has a foreign body retained in or close to the heart may present some difficulty; indeed, anxiety can become excessive, impairing the patient's function more than the physical damage and, occasionally, becoming an indication for reoperation and extraction of the object. The serious consequences of a foreign body embolus from the left ventricle also encourages a more aggressive surgical policy toward foreign bodies lodged in that chamber than in the right ventricle. Foreign bodies embedded at strategic points in great vessels may erode the vessel and cause potentially severe hemorrhage or may embolize and should, if possible, be removed.

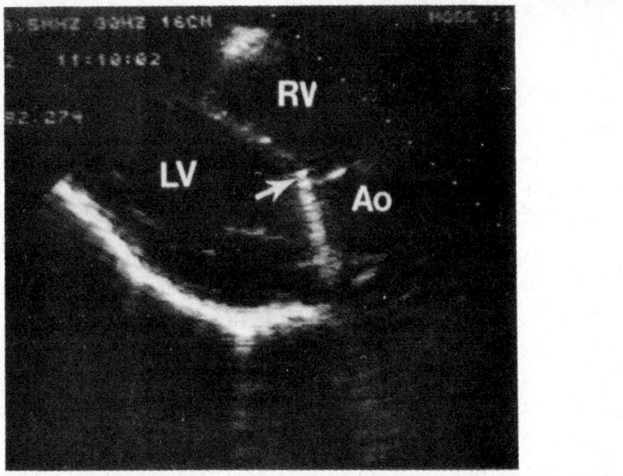

FIGURE 45–6. Two-dimensional echocardiographic image in the left parasternal long-axis view. A bullet fragment (arrow) is located high in the interventricular septum and has the typical appearance of such missiles with dense trailing reverberations. Ao = aortic root; LV = left ventricle; RV = right ventricle. (From Hassett, A., et al.: Utility of echocardiography in the management of patients with penetrating missile wounds of the heart. Reprinted with permission of the American College of Cardiology. J. Am. Coll. Cardiol. *7*:1151, 1986.)

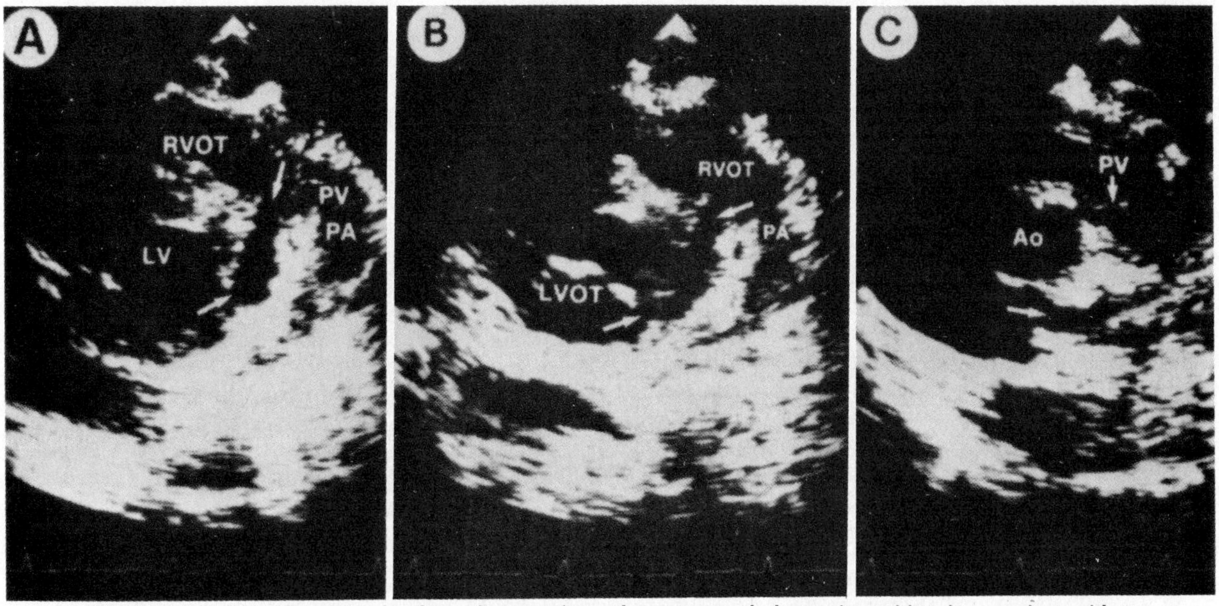

FIGURE 45–7. Two-dimensional echocardiogram from the parasternal short-axis position in a patient with a ventricular septal defect caused by knife stabbing. *A*, A defect is seen in the interventricular septum (arrows) between the left ventricle (LV) and the right ventricular outflow tract (RVOT) just proximal to the pulmonary valve (PV). *B*, At a slightly higher level the defect originates in the left ventricular outflow tract (LVOT) and exits in the distal right ventricular outflow tract. *C*, At an even higher level, but just below the aorta (Ao) and left atrium, a portion of the defect is seen (arrow). PA = pulmonary artery. (From Goldfarb, M. S., et al.: Two-dimensional Doppler echocardiographic diagnosis of a traumatic intracardiac shunt. Am. J. Cardiol. *57*:494, 1986.)

Late complications of penetrating wounds of the heart are quite common and include post-traumatic pericarditis and infection as well as arrhythmias, ventricular septal defect, and ventricular aneurysm.

PROGNOSIS. The outlook following a penetrating wound depends, first and foremost, on the extent of the injury. Gunshot wounds of the heart are more usually fatal than are stab wounds, while among the latter, knife wounds are more serious than are ice pick wounds. Salvage rates are lower in patients with extrapericardial hemorrhage compared with tamponade and also with penetrating wounds involving thin-walled structures such as the atria or the pulmonary artery, since they rarely seal off spontaneously, whereas injury to the ventricles is associated with distinctly higher survival. The state of consciousness and the extent of damage to the central nervous system, if any, at the time the patient presents to the hospital also affect prognosis. It is clear that delay in performing the initial thoracotomy also adversely influences the chances for survival.

Rupture of the interventricular septum is often a late complication of penetrating injury as it is with blunt injury (Fig. 45–7). Asfaw et al. described 12 patients with stab wounds who presented with cardiac tamponade and who had epicardial and pericardial wounds which were repaired at thoracotomy.[64] Days to years later, septal defects were diagnosed, but only four patients were symptomatic enough to warrant subsequent reoperation for closure of the defect.

INJURIES TO CARDIAC VALVES, PAPILLARY MUSCLES, AND CHORDAE TENDINEAE

Reports of injuries to the cardiac valves and their accessory structures date back to the late nineteenth century. Patients with preexisting valvular heart disease may be at higher risk than those with normal valves for the development of valvular injury following blunt trauma. Parmley et al. reported a 9 per cent incidence of valvular injury in their report of 546 cases of nonpenetrating chest trauma (Table 45–2).[6] Damage to the aortic valve is by far the most common of these lesions (Fig. 45–8). (Parmley's series appears to be an exception in this regard.) This is followed, in order, by damage to the mitral and tricuspid valves, presumably owing to the higher pressures generated by blunt trauma to the aorta. The aortic valve is probably most vulnerable to damage early in diastole, when the ventricle and aorta are nearly full.[65] Indeed, sustained damage of the aortic valve should be suspected in any patient without a history of heart disease who presents with a heart murmur after severe blunt trauma to the chest. Damage to cardiac valves may also occur as a consequence of penetrating wounds of the heart, but, in contrast to the damage caused by nonpenetrating injury, these are rarely solitary lesions.[66] Blunt chest trauma has also been reported to cause bioprosthetic valve dysfunction.[67–69]

CLINICAL FEATURES AND DIAGNOSIS. New, loud, musical murmurs are characteristic of injury to the valves and their supporting structures. The combination of a high-pitched diastolic blowing murmur with a widened pulse pressure following blunt trauma to the chest suggests rupture of the *aortic valve*. The murmur and the hemodynamic consequences of the rupture may not appear for several days following the trauma. Aortic regurgitation may also occur transiently owing to perivalvular edema or hemorrhage.

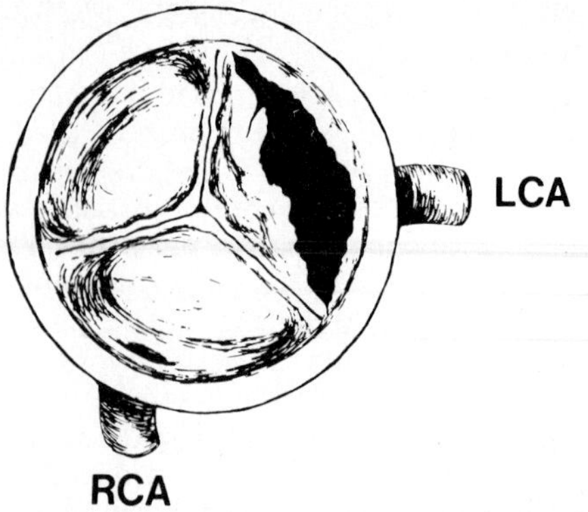

FIGURE 45–8. Diagram showing avulsion of the left coronary cusp of the aortic valve due to blunt chest trauma. (From Devineni, R., and McKenzie, F. N.: Avulsion of a normal aortic valve cusp due to blunt chest injury. J. Trauma *24*:910, © by Williams and Wilkins, 1984.)

Rupture of the *mitral valve* or of a papillary muscle appears to occur as a consequence of sudden obstruction to left ventricular outflow due to blunt injury in early diastole. It is usually associated with the development of precordial pain and a loud, harsh holosystolic murmur that radiates to the apex. Fulminant pulmonary edema quickly develops; those patients with lesser degrees of regurgitation due to torn leaflets or chordae tendineae may remain compensated for longer periods of time, although they may eventually show signs of decompensation.

Rupture of the *tricuspid valve* is rare[70] and more benign than mitral valve rupture, with symptoms ranging from fatigue to ascites and edema. Physical findings can be striking, with prominent systolic venous pulsations, hepatic pulsations, and a typical holosystolic murmur with inspiratory accentuation.

TREATMENT AND PROGNOSIS. The prognosis depends largely on the severity of the regurgitation. Since the lesion usually develops suddenly, the ventricle does not have the opportunity to adapt to this burden, as it does in most forms of chronic valvular regurgitation. Obviously, the baseline condition of the ventricle prior to the trauma and the presence of other injuries occurring simultaneously affect the heart's ability to tolerate the insult. When effective surgical treatment is possible, survival without the need for operation is not uncommon in patients with mild or moderate regurgitation. With severe left ventricular failure due to a ruptured mitral valve or papillary muscle, however, early surgery is mandatory, and replacement of the valve is usually preferred over valvuloplasty. This is also usually true with aortic valve damage,[71] but some have advocated valvuloplasty[69] when this will abolish or greatly reduce the regurgitation.

It must be appreciated that the diagnosis of acute left ventricular failure may be difficult immediately after serious trauma, because fractured ribs and pulmonary contusions may be blamed for the shortness of breath and dyspnea. When left ventricular failure develops slowly or the lesion is not hemodynamically significant, as with lesser degrees of injury, medical therapy may suffice. Hemorrhage into a papillary muscle may cause late necrosis and delayed rupture, and these patients must be observed carefully.

Post-traumatic *tricuspid* regurgitation appears to have a more benign course, and many patients survive for long periods with supportive treatment. However, when failure does occur, valve replacement is the procedure of choice.

INJURIES TO THE CORONARY ARTERIES

Transmural myocardial infarctions have been reported following blunt trauma, but angiographic confirmation of coronary obstruction is rare, and, when found, its relationship to preexisting coronary atherosclerosis may be difficult to determine. When infarction occurs, it may not be clear whether it results directly from myocardial contusion, from trauma to a coronary artery, or from some combination of these two processes. In many cases of myocardial infarction, preexisting coronary artery disease has been present, and it is reasonable to postulate that the injury dislodges a plaque, which then obstructs the vessel completely.[72] However, it is also possible that a normal coronary artery becomes occluded, by either a traumatically induced intimal tear or hemorrhage. Indeed, coronary arteriography has provided strong evidence that myocardial infarction follows blunt chest trauma in previously asymptomatic persons with normal vessels except for complete obstruction of the vessel supplying the infarcted area.[73, 74] The complications of myocardial infarction—arrhythmias, pump failure, and late development of aneurysms—are similar when the lesion has an atherosclerotic basis, and treatment is similar as well. However, it may be anticipated that *following survival from the initial episode, the long-term prognosis will be more favorable in patients with traumatic damage of a coronary artery,* because the remaining vessels are usually normal. There are exceptions, however.[75]

Left ventricular *aneurysms and pseudoaneurysms* following injury to the coronary arteries can lead to ventricular rupture, cardiac failure, embolism, or arrhythmia. Operative intervention is indicated, particularly in the presence of a pseudoaneurysm, in which the myocardium has actually ruptured but in which a thrombus, fibrous tissue, and/or pericardium prevent exsanguination, since external rupture—an event which is usually fatal—is likely to occur ultimately if the condition is left untreated. Pseudoaneurysm can often be differentiated from true aneurysm by contrast or radionuclide angiography.

Formation of an *arteriovenous fistula* is an unusual complication of traumatic damage of a coronary artery.[76] Injury to the right coronary artery is more commonly followed by an arteriovenous fistula than is injury to the left. The venous side of the fistula may be the coronary sinus, the great cardiac vein (Fig. 45–9), the right atrium, or the right ventricle; in the last instance, the fistula should be termed an "arteriocameral fistula." The murmur in traumatic coronary arteriovenous or arteriocameral fistula is usually loud, widely radiating, and continuous; the electrocardiogram frequently shows transmural myocardial infarction, and the roentgenogram exhibits cardiomegaly with increased pulmonary vascularity. In patients who do not undergo surgical repair, symptoms of congestive heart failure and chest pain are frequent unless the shunt is minimal.

Espada et al. reported nine patients with *coronary artery lacerations* among a series of 76 penetrating wounds of the heart, including seven patients with stab wounds and two with gunshot wounds.[77] As might be anticipated, the left anterior descending coronary artery is the vessel most commonly involved, and at operation, the treatment of choice is suture-ligation of the cut vessel with coronary artery bypass grafting if the lacerated vessel is large and the lesion is a proximal one. Angiography is not advised in the emergency setting, as it is with nonpenetrating trauma. However, postoperative angiography is useful in localizing the presence of possible residual injuries such as a coronary arteriocameral fistula.

INJURIES TO THE GREAT VESSELS

(See also p. 1569)

Rupture of the aorta is one of the most common traumatic lesions involving the heart or great vessels. The first case of rupture of the aorta due to *blunt* trauma was reported by Vesalius in 1557 and its relative frequency is reflected in the finding that in one of every six automobile accident victims dying from blunt chest trauma the aorta is ruptured.[78] To a lesser extent, aortic rupture also occurs with falls from heights and other types of crushing injuries.[78a] Rupture occurs in the isthmus in 90 per cent of cases. Multiple tears may be present in some patients, and in others the edges of the torn aorta may be separated by several centimeters, producing a mediastinal hematoma or pseudoaneurysm.

It has been estimated that 10 to 20 per cent of patients with ruptured aorta live long enough to be treated successfully under ideal circumstances, which include a high level of awareness of the possibility of aortic rupture in victims of automobile accidents as well as a well-coordinated team approach.[79] As with cardiac injury, rupture of the aorta may be overshadowed by injuries to other organs, and the diagnosis may be overlooked.[80] Common clinical and radiological findings are listed in Table 45–3. Patients with aortic rupture often complain of pain in the back in addition to the chest, similar to that in patients with aortic dissection (p. 1555). If the expanding mediastinal hematoma or false aneurysm narrows the aortic lumen, or if the torn intima and media cause partial aortic obstruction, ischemia of the spinal cord and kidneys may ensue. A systolic murmur may be heard in the midscapular region, and widening of the superior mediastinum is visible on the chest roentgenogram (Fig. 46–23, p. 1569).[81, 82]

A diagnostic triad that occurs in well over half the cases of ruptured aorta consists of (1) increased arterial pressure and pulse amplitude in the upper extremities, (2) decreased pressure and pulse amplitude in the lower extremities, and (3) radiological evidence of widening of the superior mediastinum.[81, 83] Chronic rupture of the aorta may be manifested by hoarseness, dysphagia, and cough. The diagnosis can be confirmed by aortography, which should be performed as soon as the nature of the injury is suspected. Aortography is essential for diagnosing and localizing the injury; the entire thoracic aorta and its branches should be visualized so as not to overlook a rupture occurring at an unusual site or multiple sites of rupture (Fig. 45–10).[84]

Penetrating trauma to the great vessels, which is usually the result of bullet or stab wounds, occurs most commonly in conjunction with cardiac wounds. Cardiac tamponade is a frequent complication of injury to the intrapericardial segment of one of the great vessels, but when it is extrapericardial, massive hemothorax is usually the presenting finding. The superior vena cava, trachea, or esophagus or some combination of these structures may be compressed if a large mediastinal hematoma forms as a result of bleeding. Injury to the innominate or carotid arteries may compress these vessels, with resultant neurological signs. An arteriovenous fistula may develop with symptoms of conges-

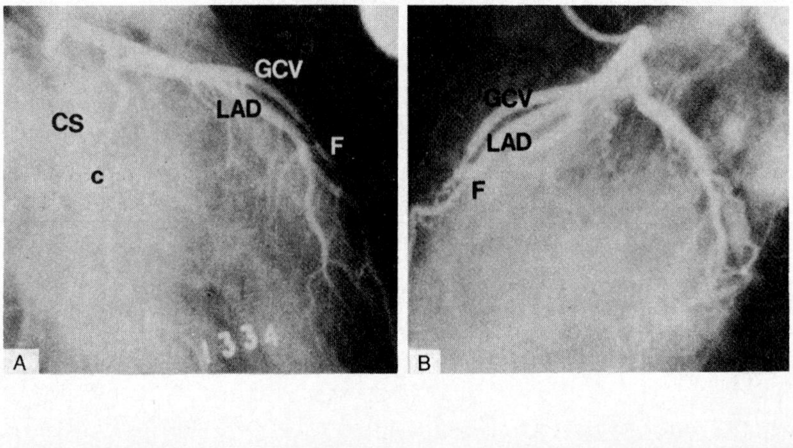

FIGURE 45–9. Left coronary arteriograms (*A*) in the right anterior oblique projection and (*B*) in the left anterior oblique projection in a patient six weeks after a penetrating chest injury. The fistula (F) can be seen arising from the second diagonal branch of the left anterior descending coronary artery (LAD) with early opacification of the great cardiac vein (GCV) and coronary sinus (CS). C = circumflex branch. (From Martin, R., et al.: Late pericardial tamponade and coronary arteriovenous fistula after trauma. Br. Heart J. *55*:216, 1986.)

TABLE 45–3 CLINICAL AND RADIOLOGICAL FINDINGS IN PATIENTS WITH AORTIC INJURY

A. CLINICAL FINDINGS	PERCENTAGE OF PATIENTS
Bone fractures (other than ribs)	75
External evidence of thoracic injury	66
Upper extremity hypertension	30–45
Systolic murmur	20–45
Dyspnea	10
Paralysis	10
Back pain	7
Dysphagia	4

B. RADIOLOGIC FINDINGS	PERCENTAGE OF PATIENTS
Abnormal aortic outline	100
Mediastinal widening	50–100
NG tube displaced to right	100
Displaced SVC	85
Left apical cap	65–93
Opacification of AP clear space	60
First or second rib fractures	50
Depressed left bronchus	35–80
Pneumothorax/pneumomediastinum	35–50
Hemothorax	20–65
Displaced right paraspinous line	15–55
Pulmonary contusion	15–50
Displaced left paraspinous line	15–25
Deviation of trachea to right	10–55

SVC = superior vena cava; NG = nasogastric; AP = anteroposterior.
Adapted from Barcia, T. C., and Livoni, J. P.: Indications for angiography in blunt thoracic trauma. Radiology *147*:15, 1983.

tive heart failure accompanied by a systolic or, more commonly, a continuous murmur.[85] These fistulous connections may also involve the systemic and pulmonary vessel.[86]

Penetrating injury to the great vessels should be suspected in any patient in whom a projectile traverses the mediastinum and is suggested by radiological evidence of a widened mediastinum. Aortography should be performed immediately, provided that emergency thoracotomy for shock or tamponade can be deferred briefly. Immediate operation, sometimes using a heparinized shunt between the ascending and descending aorta, should be carried out as soon as the diagnosis of thoracic aortic disruption has been established.[87] At the time of operation, the widest possible exposure is recommended. Pickard et al.

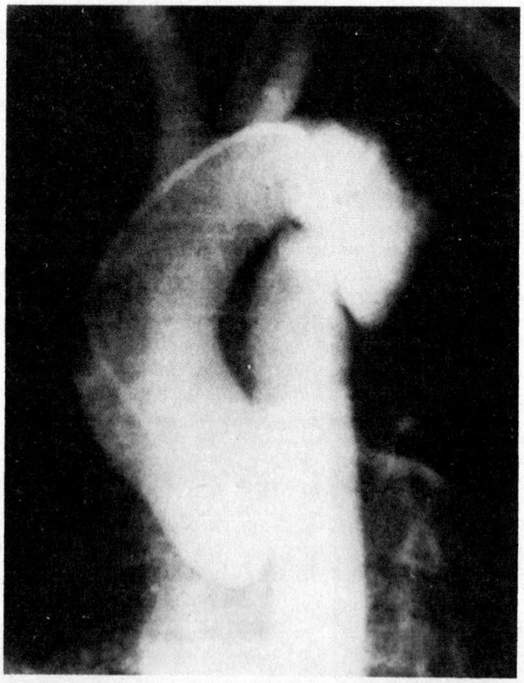

FIGURE 45–10. In a 27-year-old male, acute false and irregular aneurysm of the thoracic aorta just distal to the left subclavian artery. (Reproduced with permission from Andresen, J., and Axelsen, F.: Traumatic rupture of the thoracic aorta. Scand. J. Thorac. Cardiovasc. Surg. *14*:281, 1980.)

described their experience with 22 patients with transection of the descending thoracic aorta secondary to blunt trauma who reached the hospital alive; five patients died shortly after admission, three died in the operating room, three died within 30 days of operation, and one died more than 1 year after the injury.[88] Ten patients were long-term survivors. A Dacron tube graft was utilized to bridge the defect in the majority of patients.

In order to avoid the problem inherent in heparinization, i.e., bleeding from what are often multiple sites of trauma, tears of the descending thoracic aorta may often be repaired without cardiopulmonary bypass by simple aortic cross-clamping, as long as the cross-clamp time is restricted to less than 30 minutes.[89, 90] An experienced surgeon can interpose a graft into the aorta with a total occlusion time ranging from 13 to 21 minutes, and ischemic injury to the spinal cord or kidneys should not occur. This technique may be aided by the intravenous administration of nitroprusside, which can maintain proximal aortic systolic pressure below 140 mm Hg.

Antiadrenergic agents such as guanethidine, reserpine, and propranolol, which have been utilized in the treatment of spontaneous dissection of the aorta (p. 1519), may also have a role in treatment of patients with aortic rupture if, for logistical reasons, operation must be deferred.

REFERENCES

THE PROBLEM IN PERSPECTIVE

1. Committee on Trauma and Committee on Shock: Accidental death and disability: The neglected diseases of modern society. Washington, D.C., National Academy of Sciences, 1965, p. 5.
2. Cheitlin, M. D.: Cardiovascular trauma, part I (key references). Circulation *65*:1529, 1982.
3. Cheitlin, M. D.: Cardiovascular trauma, part II (key references). Circulation *66*:244, 1982.
4. Mayfield, W., and Hurley, E. J.: Blunt cardiac trauma. Am. J. Surg. *148*:162, 1984.
5. Sherman, M. M., Saini, V. K., Yarnoz, M. D., Ramp, J., Williams, L. F., and Berger, R. L.: Management of penetrating heart wounds. Am. J. Surg. *135*:553, 1978.

NONPENETRATING CARDIAC INJURY

6. Parmley, L. F., Manion, W. C., and Mattingly, T. W.: Nonpenetrating traumatic injury of the heart. Circulation *18*:371, 1958.
7. MacKintosh, A. F., and Fleming, H. A.: Cardiac damage presenting late after road accidents. Thorax *36*:811, 1981.
8. Rothstein, R. J.: Myocardial contusion. J.A.M.A. *250*:2189, 1983.
9. DeMuth, W. E., Lerner, E. H., and Liedtke, A. J.: Nonpenetrating injury of the heart: An experimental model. J. Trauma *13*:639, 1973.
10. Clifford, R. P., and Gill, K. S.: Traumatic rupture of the pericardium with dislocation of the heart. Injury *16*:123, 1984.
11. King, J. B., and Sapsford, R. N.: Acute rupture of the pericardium with delayed dislocation of the heart: A case report. Injury 9:303, 1978.
12. Miller, F. A., Jr., Seward, J. B., Gersh, B. J., Tajik, A. J., and Mucha, P., Jr.: Two-dimensional echocardiographic findings in cardiac trauma. Am. J. Cardiol. *50*:1022, 1982.
13. Bright, E. F., and Beck, C. S.: Nonpenetrating wounds of the heart: Clinical and experimental studies. Am. Heart J. *10*:293, 1935.
14. Lau, V.-K., Viano, D. C., and Doty, D. B.: Experimental cardiac trauma—Ballistics of a captive bolt pistol. J. Trauma *21*:39, 1982.
15. Stein, P. D., Sabbah, H. N., Viano, D. C., and Vostal, J. J.: Response of the heart to nonpenetrating cardiac trauma. J. Trauma *22*:364, 1982.
16. Pandian, N. G., Skorton, D. J., Doty, D. B., and Kerber, R. E.: Immediate diagnosis of acute myocardial contusion by two-dimensional echocardiography: Studies in a canine model of blunt chest trauma. J. Am. Coll. Cardiol. *2*:488, 1983.
17. Gay W.: Blunt trauma to the heart and great vessels. Surgery *91*:507, 1982.
18. Tenzer, M. L.: The spectrum of myocardial contusion: A review. J. Trauma *25*:620, 1985.
18a. Cometta, A., Chiolero, R., and Freeman, J.: Cardiac contusions in nonpenetrating chest injuries. Schweiz. Med. Wochenschr. *116*:559, 1986.
18b. Frazee, R. C., Mucha, P., Jr., Farnell, M. B., and Miller, F. A., Jr.: Objective evaluation of blunt cardiac trauma. J. Trauma *26*:510, 1986.
19. Snow, N., Richardson, J. D., and Flint, L. M., Jr.: Myocardial contusion: Implications for patients with multiple traumatic injuries. Surgery *92*:744, 1982.
20. Potkin, R. T., Werner, J. A., Trobaugh, G. B., Chestnut, C. H., III, Carrico, C. J., Hallstrom, A., and Cobb, L. A.: Evaluation of noninvasive tests of cardiac damage in suspected cardiac contusion . Circulation *66*:627, 1982.
21. Potkin, R. T., Werner, J. A., Trobaugh, G. B., Chestnut, C. H., III., Carrico, C. J., Hallstrom, A., and Cobb, L. A.: Evaluation of noninvasive tests of cardiac damage in suspected cardiac contusion. Circulation *66*:627, 1982.
22. Kumar, S. A., Puri, V. K., Mittal, V. K., and Cortez, J.: Myocardial contusion following nonfatal blunt chest trauma. J. Trauma *23*:327, 1983.
23. Torres-Mirabal, P., Gruenberg, J. C., Brown, R. S., and Obeid, F. N.: Spectrum of myocardial contusion. Am. Surg. *48*:383, 1982.
24. McConnell, B. J., McConnell, R. W., and Guiberteau, M. J.: Radionuclide imaging in blunt trauma. Radiol. Clin. North Am. *19*:37, 1981.
25. Chiu, C. L., Roelofs, J. D., Go, R. T., Doty, D. B., Rose, E. F., and Christie, J. H.: Coronary angiographic and scintigraphic findings in experimental cardiac contusion. Radiology *116*:679, 1975.
26. Sutherland, G. R., Cheung, H. W., Holliday, R. L., Driedger, A. A., and

Sibbald, W. J.: Hemodynamic adaptation to acute myocardial contusion complicating blunt chest injury. Am. J. Cardiol. 57:291, 1986.
27. Mattox, K. L., Limacher, M. C., Feliciano, D. V., Colosimo, L., O'Meara, M. E., Beall, A. C., Jr., and DeBakey, M. E.: Cardiac evaluation following heart injury. J. Trauma 25:758, 1985.
28. Fox, K. M., Rowland, E., Krikler, D. M., Bentall, H. H., and Goodwin, J. F.: Electrophysiological manifestations on nonpenetrating cardiac trauma. Br. Heart J. 43:458, 1980.
29. Brennan, J. A., Field, J. M., and Liedtke, A. J.: Reversible heart block following nonpenetrating chest trauma. J. Trauma 19:784, 1979.
30. Bognolo, D. A., Rabow, F. I., Vijayanagar, R. R., and Eckstein, P. F.: Traumatic sinus node dysfunction. Ann. Emerg. Med. 11:319, 1982.
31. Évora, P. R. B., Ribeiro, P. J. F., Brasil, J. C. F., Otaviano, A. G., Amaral, F. T. V., Reis, C. L., Secches, A. L., and Marin-Neto, J. A.: Late surgical repair of ventricular septal defect due to nonpenetrating chest trauma: Review and report of two contrasting cases. J. Trauma 25:1007, 1985.
32. Torres-Mirabal, P., Gruenberg, J. C., Talbert, J. G., and Brown, R. S.: Ventricular function in myocardial contusion: A preliminary study. Crit. Care Med. 10:19, 1982.
33. Desiderio, M. A.: The potentiation of the response to blunt cardiac trauma by ethanol in dogs. J. Trauma 26:467, 1986.
33a. Watt, A. H., and Stephens, M. R.: Myocardial infarction after blunt chest trauma incurred during rugby football that later required cardiac transplantation. Br. Heart J. 55:408, 1986.
34. Wainwright, R. J., Edwards, A. C., Maisey, M. N., and Sowton, E.: Early occlusion and late stricture of normal coronary arteries following blunt chest trauma. Chest 78:796, 1980.
35. Espinosa, R., Badui, E., Castaño,, R., and Madrid, R.: Acute posterior wall myocardial infarction secondary to football chest trauma. Chest 88:928, 1985.
36. DeSa'Neto, A., Padnick, M. B., Desser, K. B., and Steinhoff, N. G.: Right sinus of valsalva-right atrial fistula secondary to nonpenetrating chest trauma. Circulation 60:205, 1979.
37. Rheuban, K. S., Tompkins, D. G., Nolan, S. P., Berger, B., Martin, R., and Schneider, J. A.: Myocardial necrosis and ventricular aneurysm following closed chest injury in a child. J. Trauma 21:170, 1981.
38. Candell, J., Valle, V., Payá, J., Cortadellas, J., Esplugas, E., and Rius, J.: Post-traumatic coronary occlusion and early left ventricular aneurysm. Am. Heart J. 97:509, 1979.
38a. Getz, B. S., Davies, E., Steinberg, S. M., Beaver, B. L., and Koenig, F. A.: Blunt cardiac trauma resulting in right atrial rupture. J.A.M.A. 255:761, 1986.
39. Smith, J. M., III, Grober, F. L., Marcos, J. J., Arom, K. V., and Trinkle, J. K.: Blunt traumatic rupture of the atria. J. Thorac. Cardiovasc. Surg. 71:617, 1976.
40. Hines, G. L., Doyle, E., and Acinapura, A. J.: Post-traumatic ventricular septal defect, mitral insufficiency, and multiple coronary cameral fistulas. J. Trauma 17:234, 1977.
41. Pickard, L. R., Mattox, K. L., and Beall, A. C., Jr.: Ventricular septal defect from blunt chest injury. J. Trauma 20:329, 1980.
42. Williams, J. B., Silver, D. G., and Laws, H. L.: Successful management of heart rupture from blunt trauma. J. Trauma 21:534, 1981.
43. Kouwenhoven, W. B., Jude, J. R., and Knickerbocker, G. G.: Closed chest cardiac massage. J.A.M.A. 173:1064, 1966.
44. Adelson, L.: A clinicopathologic study of the anatomic changes in the heart resulting from cardiac massage. Surg. Gynecol. Obstet. 104:513, 1957.
45. Gerry, J. L., Bulkley, B. H., and Hutchins, G. M.: Rupture of the papillary muscle of the tricuspid valve. A complication of cardiopulmonary resuscitation and a rare cause of tricuspid insufficiency. Am. J. Cardiol. 40:825, 1977.
46. Baker, P. B., Keyhani-Rofagha, S., Graham, R. L., and Sharma, H. M.: Dissecting hematoma (aneurysm) of coronary arteries. Am. J. Med. 80:317, 1986.
47. Ewy, G. A.: Current status of cardiopulmonary resuscitation. Mod. Conc. Cardiovasc. Dis. 53:43, 1984.

PENETRATING CARDIAC INJURY

48. Karrel, R., Shaffer, M. A., and Franaszek, J. B.: Emergency diagnosis, resuscitation, and treatment of acute penetrating cardiac trauma. Ann. Emerg. Med. 11:504, 1982.
49. Symbas, P. N.: Chest trauma: What injury, what treatment approach? J. Cardiovasc. Med. 6:989, 1981.
50. Fallahnejad, M., Kutty, A. C. K., and Wallace, H. W.: Secondary lesions of penetrating cardiac injuries. Ann. Surg. 191:228, 1980.
51. Bloomfield, D. A.: The nonsurgical retrieval of intracardiac foreign bodies—An international survey. Cathet. Cardiovasc. Diagn. 4:1, 1978.
52. Auge, J. M., Oriol, A., Serra, C., and Crexells, C.: The use of pigtail catheters for retrieval of foreign bodies from the cardiovascular system. Cathet. Cardiovasc. Diagn. 10:625, 1984.
53. Gehl, L., Iskandriann, A. N., Goel, I., Mintz, G. S., Kimbiris, D., Bemis, C. E., Mundth, E. D., and Segal, B. L.: Cardiac perforation with tamponade during cardiac catheterization. Cathet. Cardiovasc. Diagn. 8:293, 1982.
54. Goldbaum, T. S., Jacob, A. S., Smith, D. F., Pichard, A., and Lindsay, J., Jr.: Cardiac tamponade following percutaneous transluminal coronary angioplasty: Four case reports. Cathet. Cardiovasc. Diagn. 11:413, 1985.
55. Przybojewski, J. Z.: Endomyocardial biopsy: a review of the literature. Cathet. Cardiovasc. Diagn. 11:287, 1985.
56. Cummings, R. G., Wesly, R. L. R., Adams, D. H., and Lowe, J. E.: Pneumopericardium resulting in cardiac tamponade. Ann. Thoracic Surg. 37:511, 1984.
57. Wilder, J. R., Dhar, N., Kudchadkar, A., and Kryger, S.: Penetration injury to the heart. J.A.M.A. 244:2080, 1980.
58. Marshall, W. G., Jr., Bell, J. L., and Kouchoukos, N. T.: Penetrating cardiac trauma. J. Trauma 24:147, 1984.
59. Hassett, A., Moran, J., Sabiston, D. C., and Kisslo, J.: Utility of echocardiography in the management of patients with penetrating missile wounds of the heart. J. Am. Coll. Cardiol. 7:1151, 1986.
60. Miller, J. T., Richards, K. L., Miller, J. F., and Crawford, M. H.: Doppler echocardiographic determination of the cause of a systolic murmur following penetrating chest trauma. Am. Heart J. 111:988, 1986.
61. Goldfarb, M. S., Walpole, H. T., Jr., Landolt, C. C., McIntyre, A. B., and Felner, J. M.: Two-dimensional Doppler echocardiographic diagnosis of a traumatic intracardiac shunt. Am. J. Cardiol. 57:494, 1986.
61a. Martin, L. F., Mavroudis, C., Dyess, D. L., Gray, L. A., Jr., and Richardson, J. D.: The first 70 years' experience managing cardiac disruption due to penetrating and blunt injuries at the University of Louisville. Am. Surg. 52:14, 1986.
62. Moncada, R., Matuga, T., Unger, E., Freeark, R., and Pizarro, A.: Migratory trauma—cardiovascular foreign bodies. Circulation 57:186, 1978.
63. Alsofrom, D. J., Marcus, N. H., Seigel, R. S., Talbot, W. A., Akl, B. F., Schiller, W. R., and Sklar, D. P.: Shotgun pellet embolization from the chest to the middle cerebral arteries. J. Trauma 22:155, 1982.
64. Asfaw, I., Thoms, N. W., and Arfulu, A.: Interventricular septal defects from penetrating injuries of the heart. A report of 12 cases and review of the literature. J. Thorac. Cardiovasc. Surg. 69:450, 1975.
65. Morritt, G. N., Taylor, N. C., Miller, H. C., and Walbaum. P. R.: Traumatic aortic regurgitation. J. R. Coll. Surg. (Edinb.) 24:87, 1979.
66. Rustad, D. G., Hopeman, A. R., Murr, P. C., and VanWay, C. W., III: Aorta-cardiac fistula with aortic valve injury from penetrating trauma. J. Trauma 26:266, 1986.
67. Reinfeld, H. B., Agatston, A. S., Robinson, M. J., and Hildner, F. J.: Bioprosthetic mitral valve dysfunction following blunt chest trauma. Am. Heart J. 111:800, 1986.
68. Mazzucco, A., Rizzoli, G., Faggian, G., Aru, G., Bortolotti, U., Sorbara, C., and Chioin, R.: Acute mitral regurgitation after blunt chest trauma. Arch. Intern. Med. 143:2326, 1983.
69. Rumisek, J. D., Robonowitz, M., Virmani, R., Barry, M. J., and Steudel, W. T.: Bioprosthetic heart valve rupture associated with trauma. J. Trauma 26:276, 1986.
70. Eskilsson, J.: Tricuspid insufficiency caused by nonpenetrating chest trauma: Report of two cases diagnosed by Doppler cardiography. Acta Med. Scand. 218:347, 1985.
71. Kimbler, R. W., Stokes, J. P., and Barnhorst, D. A.: The surgical treatment of traumatic rupture of the aortic valve. Report of a case after blunt trauma. J. Trauma 17:168, 1977.
72. Roberts, W. C., and Maron, B. J.: Sudden death while playing professional football. Am. Heart J. 102:1061, 1981.
73. Pifarre, R., Grieco, J., Garibaldi, A., Sullivan, H. J., Montoya, A., and Bakhos, A.: Acute coronary artery occlusion secondary to blunt chest trauma. J. Thorac. Cardiovasc. Surg. 83:122, 1982.
74. Vlay, S. C., Blumenthal, D. S., Shoback, D., Fehir, K., and Bulkley, B. H.: Delayed acute myocardial infarction after blunt chest trauma in a young woman. Am. Heart J. 100:907, 1980.
75. Watt, A. H., and Stephens, M. R.: Myocardial infarction after blunt chest trauma incurred during rugby football that later required cardiac transplantation. Br. Heart J. 55:408, 1986.
76. Martin, R., Mitchell, A., and Dhalla, N.: Late pericardial tamponade and coronary arteriovenous fistula after trauma. Br. Heart J. 55:216, 1986.
77. Espada, R., Whisennard, H. H., Mattox, K. L., and Beall, A. C., Jr.: Surgical management of penetrating injuries to the coronary arteries. Surgery 78:755, 1975.
78. Greendyke, R. M.: Traumatic rupture of the aorta. Special reference to automobile accidents. J.A.M.A. 195:527, 1966.
78a. Shaikh, K. A., Schwab, C. W., and Camishion, R. C.: Aortic rupture in blunt trauma. Am. Surg. 52:47, 1986.
79. Ayella, R. J., Hankins, J. R., Turney, S. Z., and Cowley, R. A.: Ruptured thoracic aorta due to blunt trauma. J. Trauma 17:199, 1977.
80. Barcia, T. C., and Livoni, J. P.: Indications for angiography in blunt thoracic trauma. Radiology 147:15, 1983.
81. Puijlaert, C. B. A. J.: Roentgen diagnosis of traumatic rupture of the aorta, Radiologia Clin. 45:217, 1976.
82. Gundry, S. R., Burney, R. E., Mackenzie, J. R., Wilton, G. P., Whitehouse, W. M., Wu, S.-C., and Kirsh, M.: Assessment of mediastinal widening associated with traumatic rupture of the aorta. J. Trauma 23:293, 1983.
83. Symbas, P. N., Tyras, D. H., Ware, R. E., and Hatcher, C. R., Jr.: Rupture of the aorta. A diagnostic triad. Ann. Thorac. Surg. 15:405, 1973.
84. Kirsh, M. M., Orringer, M. B., Behrendt, D. M., Mills, L. J., Tashjian, J., and Sloan, H.: Management of unusual traumatic ruptures of the aorta. Surg. Gynecol. Obstet. 146:365, 1978.
85. Machiedo, G. W., Jain, K. M., Swan, K. G., Petrocelli, J. C., and Blackwood, J. M.: Traumatic aorto-caval fistula. J. Trauma 23:243, 1983.
86. Arom, K. V., and Lyons, G. W.: Traumatic pulmonary arteriovenous fistula. J. Thorac. Cardiovasc. Surg. 70:918, 1975.
87. Akins, C. W., Buckley, M. J., Daggett, W., McIlduff, J. B., and Austen, W. G.: Acute traumatic disruption of the thoracic aorta: A ten-year experience. Ann. Thorac. Surg. 31:305, 1981.
88. Pickard, L. R., Mattox, K. L., Espada, R., Beall, A. C., and DeBakey, M. E.: Transection of the descending thoracic aorta secondary to blunt trauma. J. Trauma 17:749, 1977.
89. Vasko, J. S., Raess, D. H., Williams, T. E., Jr., Kakos, G. S., Kilman, J. W., Meckstroth, C. V., Cattaneo, S. M., and Klassen, K. P.: Nonpenetrating trauma to the thoracic aorta. Surgery 82:400, 1977.
90. Turney, S. Z., Attar, S., Ayella, R., Cowley, R. A., and McLaughlin, J.: Traumatic rupture of the aorta. A five-year experience. J. Thorac. Cardiovasc. Surg. 72:727, 1976.

46 DISEASES OF THE AORTA

by KIM A. EAGLE, M.D., and
ROMAN W. DE SANCTIS, M.D.

THE NORMAL AORTA

FUNCTION. Appropriately called by the ancients "the greatest artery," the aorta is admirably crafted for its task. This thin but large and remarkably tough vessel must absorb the impact of 2.5 to 3 billion heartbeats in an average lifetime while carrying roughly 200,000,000 liters of blood to the body.

Arteries can be categorized as either "conductance" or "resistance" vessels. Conductance vessels are the conduits for blood, and the aorta is the ultimate conductance vessel. It is composed of three layers: a thin, inner tunica intima; a thick middle layer, the tunica media; and a rather thin outer layer, the tunica adventitia. The strength of the aorta lies in the tunica media, which is composed of laminated but intertwining sheets of elastic tissue arranged in a spiral fashion so as to afford maximum tensile strength. As thin as it is, the wall of the aorta can withstand the experimental pressure of thousands of millimeters of mercury without bursting. In contrast to peripheral arteries, the aortic media contains very little smooth muscle, although there is a network of some smooth muscle and collagen between the elastic layers. This tremendous accretion of elastic tissue in the aorta gives it not only great tensile strength but also elasticity, which serves a vital circulatory role. The aortic intima is a thin, delicate layer lined by endothelium and easily traumatized. The adventitia contains mainly collagen but also houses the important vasa vasorum and lymphatics, which nourish the aortic wall.

As systole develops, part of the force generated by the contracting ventricle is converted into potential energy stored in the wall of the aorta as it is distended by the blood ejected into it. In diastole, this potential energy in the stretched aortic wall is transformed into kinetic energy as the resilient aorta decompresses, and the force that is created acts against the column of blood contained within the lumen. With a competent aortic valve proximally, the blood is propelled distally into the arterial bed. Thus, the aorta plays a major role in keeping the blood circulating after it is delivered into the aorta by the heart. The pulse wave itself with its milking effect is transmitted along the aorta to the periphery at a speed of about 5 meters per second. This is much faster than the velocity of the intraluminal blood, which travels only 40 to 50 cm per second.

The systolic pressure developed within the aorta is a function of the volume of blood ejected into the aorta, the compliance or distensibility of the aorta, and the resistance to blood flow. Resistance is determined primarily by the tone in the peripheral muscular arteries and arterioles and to a slight extent by the inertia of the column of blood in the aorta when systole commences. The aorta and its branches tend to stiffen with age, accounting for the increase in systolic blood pressure with advancing age.

In addition to its conductance and pumping functions, the aorta plays a role in the control of systemic vascular resistance and heart rate. Pressure-responsive receptors analogous to those in the carotid sinus lie in the ascending aorta and the aortic arch and send afferent signals to the vasomotor center in the brain stem by way of the vagus nerves. Raising the aortic pressure causes reflex bradycardia and reduction of systemic vascular resistance, whereas lowering the pressure increases the heart rate and systemic resistance.

ANATOMICAL CONSIDERATIONS. The *ascending aorta* in a normal adult is about 3 cm wide at its origin from the base of the heart and extends 5 to 6 cm cephalad to join the aortic arch. Normally, the ascending aorta lies just to the right of the midline. Its proximal portion is within the pericardial cavity. Nearby structures include the pulmonary trunk in front and the left atrium, right pulmonary artery, and right main stem bronchus behind.

The *arch of the aorta* gives rise to all the brachiocephalic vessels. It courses slightly leftward in front of the trachea and then proceeds dorsally and inferiorly above the left main stem bronchus to the left of the trachea and esophagus. The arch assumes almost a directly anteroposterior orientation in the superior mediastinum. Other closely related structures are the left phrenic and vagus nerves to the left of the arch; inferiorly lie the bifurcation of the pulmonary trunk and most of the left lung. The left recurrent laryngeal nerve also loops underneath it distally.

The *descending thoracic aorta* is the continuation of the aorta beyond the arch. It lies in the posterior mediastinum to the left of the vertebral column, gradually courses in front of the vertebral column as it descends, occupying a position behind the esophagus, and passes through the diaphragm, usually at the level of the 12th thoracic vertebra.

A small but important segment called the *aortic isthmus* is the point at which the arch and descending thoracic aorta join. This is where coarctations of the aorta are usually located, and it is also the point at which the mobile portion of the aorta—the ascending aorta and arch—becomes relatively fixed to the thorax by the pleural reflections, intercostal arteries, and left subclavian artery. The aorta is especially vulnerable to trauma at this point.

The *abdominal aorta* forms the continuation of the thoracic aorta, giving off the important splanchnic vessels and ending in the aortic bifurcation at the level of the 4th lumbar vertebra.

EXAMINATION OF THE AORTA

Unless the aorta is abnormally enlarged, the only location at which it can be palpated is in the abdomen. The ease with which it can be felt depends largely on the body habitus and on the pulse pressure; it is readily felt in thin individuals. It is quite sensitive to pressure. Auscultation usually is unrevealing in aortic diseases, except for occasional bruits at sites of narrowing of the aorta or its tributary branches. Diseases of the proximal ascending aorta sometimes involve the aortic valve, with resultant aortic insufficiency.

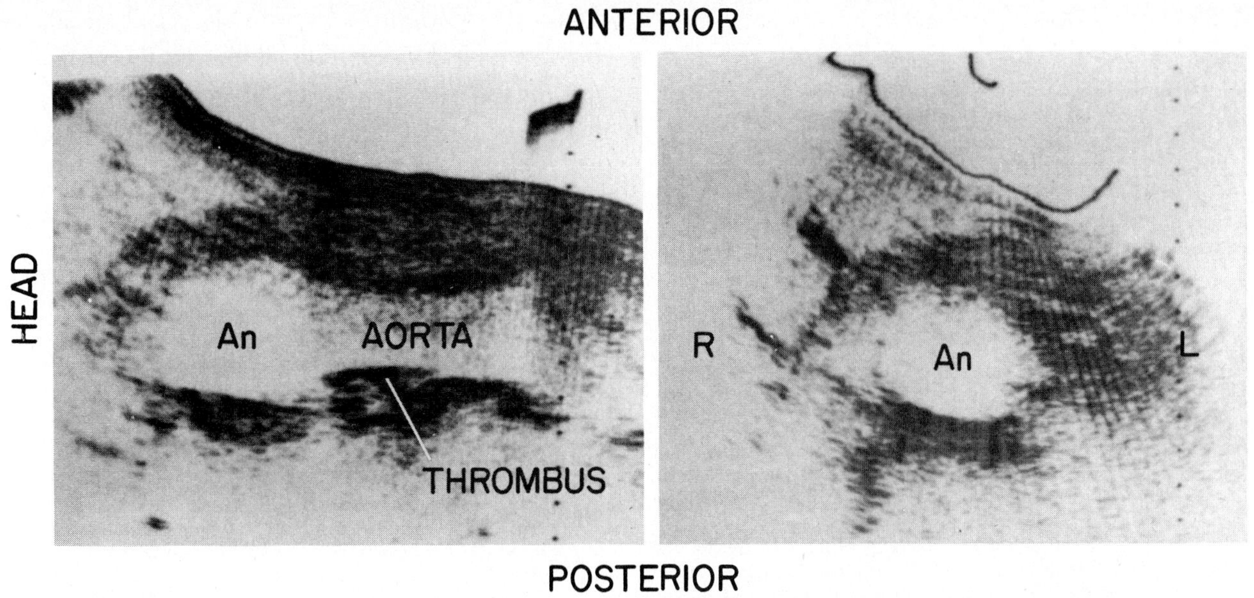

FIGURE 46–1. Cross-sectional echocardiograms of an abdominal aortic aneurysm in a 62-year-old man. *Left*, Lateral view showing a 5-cm aneurysm (An), with dilatation of the aorta distal to the aneurysm. The widened aorta is visualized down to the aortic bifurcation. Note the thrombus in the wall of the aneurysm. The dense echoes between the aneurysm and skin are made up of subcutaneous fat, muscle, and mesenteric contents. *Right*, Echogram with the ultrasound beam oriented in the anteroposterior direction showing the aneurysm clearly. R and L indicate the patient's right and left sides. The distance between each of the dots aligned vertically on the right in both scans represents 1 cm. (Courtesy of Rob Kirkpatrick, M.D., Department of Radiology, Massachusetts General Hospital, Boston.)

Chest roentgenography and fluoroscopy are valuable and simple procedures for assessing the aorta. Normally, the ascending aorta is not visible on the direct anteroposterior chest roentgenogram. The aortic arch is seen as the aortic "knob" or "knuckle" in the superior mediastinum just to the left of the vertebral column (Fig. 6–1, p. 141). The edge of the descending thoracic aorta can often be recognized to the left of the spine.

On the lateral chest roentgenogram, the proximal ascending aorta can be seen as an indistinct shadow in the middle mediastinum arising from the base of the heart. The ascending aorta and arch are best demonstrated in a left anterior oblique projection—a view that should always be included when disease of the thoracic aorta is suspected (Fig. 6–12, p. 149).

Calcification in the aortic knob is often present, particularly in older people and patients with hypertension. It has little significance. Arteriosclerosis often results in extensive aortic calcification. The location of aortic calcification is useful in the differential diagnosis of aortic disease. For example, syphilis usually causes calcification of the ascending aorta predominantly, whereas arteriosclerotic calcification is ordinarily densest in the arch and the descending thoracic and abdominal aorta. Aneurysms of the abdominal aorta can often be seen radiographically if they are calcified. A lateral film of the abdomen is the most useful view for demonstrating them.

Normally, the aorta tends to elongate and widen slightly with age, a process which is accelerated by hypertension. Aneurysms, of course, appear as localized dilatations of the aorta. It is sometimes difficult to distinguish aneurysms from other mediastinal masses. In such cases fluoroscopy or real-time ultrasound may be very helpful by showing the presence or absence of pulsations in the mass.

Angiographic study of the aorta is of critical importance in the evaluation of aortic diseases. Aneurysms, aortic dissections, and occlusive disease of the aorta and its arterial branches can usually be readily demonstrated by a contrast study. With technical improvements in digital subtraction angiography (p. 356), performed by venous injection of contrast material, adequate aortic definition should be possible while obviating catheterization of the aorta. However, this technique is currently limited by poor spatial resolution, artifacts caused by patient movement, and difficulty in defining anatomical detail because of overlapping blood vessels.[1, 2]

Ultrasonography is a very important tool in the diagnosis of aortic diseases (p. 131). The presence or absence of an

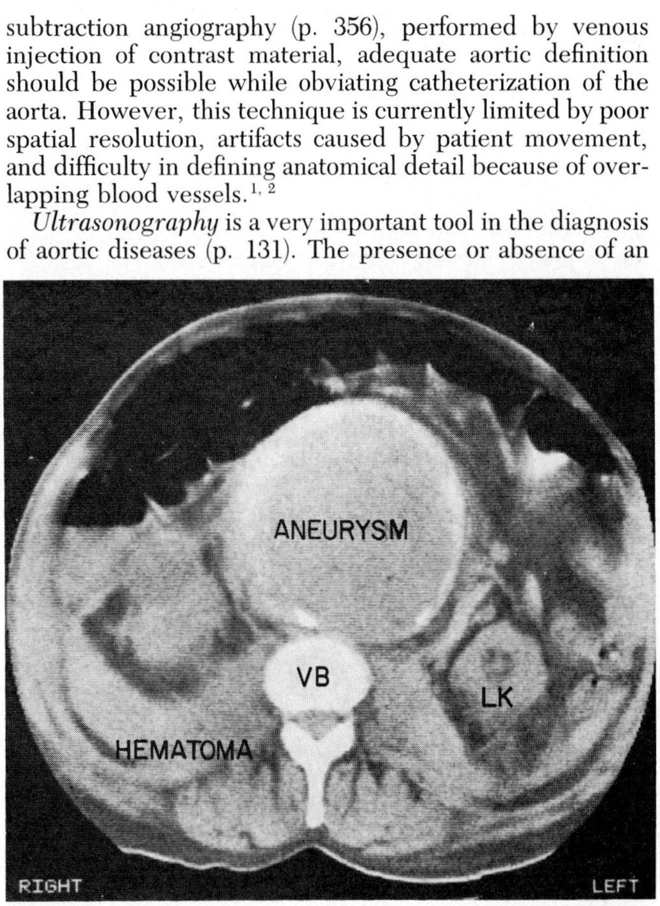

FIGURE 46–2. Abdominal CT scan showing a large, leaking abdominal aortic aneurysm. The aneurysm measures approximately 11 cm in diameter and abuts the vertebral body (VB) posteriorly. The light areas in the periphery of the aneurysm are calcific deposits in the aortic wall. The lower pole of the left kidney is identified (LK), and behind the right kidney is a retroperitoneal hematoma. (Courtesy of Jack Wittenberg, M.D., Department of Radiology, Massachusetts General Hospital, Boston.)

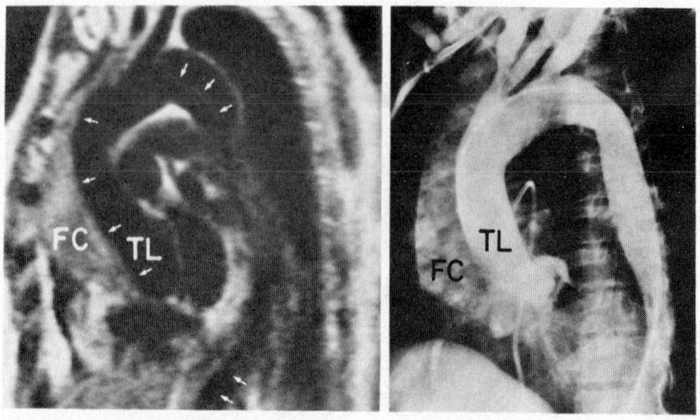

FIGURE 46–3. Nuclear magnetic resonance image in long axis (left), with corresponding aortogram (right) in a 55-year-old woman with a Type A dissection. The arrows indicate the partition between the false channel (FC) of the dissection and the true lumen (TL) of the aorta. The dissection extends into the descending thoracic aorta. The false channel shows up densely in the NMR scan because of stagnant blood flow within it. (Courtesy of Robert E. Dinsmore, M.D., Chief of Cardiac Radiology, Massachusetts General Hospital, Boston. NMR scan from Dinsmore, R. E., et al., A. J. R. 146:1286, 1986.)

abdominal aortic aneurysm can be definitively established by this simple noninvasive technique. In particular, cross-sectional (two-dimensional) echocardiography is extremely accurate in both diagnosing and sizing abdominal aortic aneurysms (Fig. 46–1) and can also provide valuable information about the location and size of aortic root aneurysms.[3–5]

Computed tomographic scanning of the body (CT scan), enhanced by intravenous injection of contrast material, is being used increasingly for noninvasive visualization of the aorta (Fig. 46–2, and Fig. 12–20, p. 367). CT scans are particularly useful for the diagnosis and sizing of thoracic and abdominal aortic aneurysms and for the diagnosis of aortic dissection and traumatic aneurysms of the aorta.[5–8, 8a, 8b] In determining the size of abdominal aortic aneurysms, the CT scan is as accurate as ultrasonography, if not more so. Magnetic resonance imaging (MRI) is another promising noninvasive technique for evaluating aortic disease (Fig. 12–39, p. 376). It has advantages over CT scanning in that imaging can be performed in multiple planes (i.e., coronal and sagittal planes) and contrast agents are unnecessary. Early studies confirm its accuracy in locating and sizing aortic aneurysms and dissections (Fig. 46–3).[9–12, 12a, 12b]

PATHOGENESIS OF DISEASES OF THE AORTA

Diseases of the aorta are either congenital or acquired. Congenital defects in turn are either gross anatomical abnormalities, such as coarctation, right aortic arch, anomalous arterial branches, double aortic arches, and so on, or histological disorders, such as degenerative abnormalities in the aortic wall that predispose to later problems (e.g., cystic medial degeneration in the Marfan syndrome and other inherited connective tissue disorders).

The only congenital gross anatomical disease considered in this chapter is pseudocoarctation (p. 1568). *Coarctation* is discussed on pages 848, 929, and 994. All other conditions discussed either are acquired or result from congenital histological changes in the aortic wall.

Acquired diseases of the aorta are primarily the result of degenerative changes in the aortic wall. Prominent among the factors which lead to this degeneration are aging, arteriosclerosis, hypertension, and specific infectious, inflammatory, or autoimmune diseases that involve the aorta focally or diffusely. Some of these processes may affect the aortic root, with resultant aortic insufficiency, or the major arterial branches arising from the aorta. The importance of the velocity at which blood is ejected from the left ventricle (dV/dt) as a major shearing stress on the aortic wall has also been emphasized as promoting aortic dissection.

Arteriosclerosis is especially important in the pathogenesis of aortic aneurysms. Hypertension may be particularly important in causing diseases of the aorta. Experimental work suggests that hypertension leads to structural aortic changes that may accelerate medial degeneration in certain patients; may decrease the blood flow in the vasa vasorum, with resultant ischemia of the aortic wall; and may initiate a response that stiffens the aorta and serves to perpetuate the hypertensive state. Although some degree of aortic medial degeneration is common with aging, the extent and severity of these changes are much greater in hypertensive individuals.[13–15]

ARTERIOSCLEROTIC AORTIC ANEURYSMS

ABDOMINAL AORTIC ANEURYSMS

Approximately three-fourths of all arteriosclerotic aortic aneurysms are confined to the abdominal aorta. Normally, in the adult, the aorta measures 2 cm in diameter at the level of the celiac axis and 1.8 cm just below the renal arteries; it then tapers slightly to the iliac vessels. Most abdominal aneurysms arise in the area between the renal arteries and the aortic bifurcation. Clinically significant aneurysms measure 4 cm or more in diameter.

ETIOLOGY AND PATHOGENESIS. Abdominal aortic aneurysms arise in areas of dense atherosclerosis. The atherosclerotic process erodes the aortic wall, destroying the medial elastic elements.[15a] This causes weakening of the aortic wall and eventually leads to fusiform or, rarely, saccular dilatation of the abdominal aorta. As the aorta widens, tension in the wall of the aorta rises in accordance with Laplace's law, which states that tension is proportional to the product of pressure and radius. Further widening results in greater tension, which in turn leads to acceleration in the rate of enlargement of the aneurysm. A vicious circle is thus established and produces dilatation that is often rapidly progressive. Hypertension may also contribute to the pathogenesis of these aneurysms.

Most abdominal aortic aneurysms arise just below the renal arteries and extend to, and often involve, the aortic bifurcation. Only 2 to 5 per cent of abdominal aortic aneurysms are suprarenal, and these usually result from the distal extension of a thoracic aneurysm into the abdomen. As aneurysms expand they may compress contiguous structures. Laminated thrombi frequently form in areas of stagnant flow within the aneurysm. Thrombotic and arteriosclerotic debris may embolize distally (p. 1570) and compromise the circulation of tributary arteries. Finally, the aneurysm may rupture. Of those aneurysms which do rupture, 80 per cent rupture retroperitoneally, and most of the remainder rupture into the periotoneal cavity, causing rapid circulatory collapse.[16] Rarely, an aneurysm may rupture into the inferior vena cava, iliac vein, or renal vein.[17, 18]

CLINICAL MANIFESTATIONS. The majority of abdominal aneurysms are asymptomatic and are discovered on routine physical examination or on a routine abdominal roentgenogram.[19] Aneurysms may cause a sense of fullness in the epigastrium. If pain is present, it is usually located in the hypogastrium and lower back. The pain is usually steady, with a gnawing quality, and may last for hours or days at a time. In contrast to musculoskeletal back pain, it is not affected by movement, although patients may be more comfortable in certain positions, such as with the legs drawn up. Some astute patients may suspect an aneurysm by recognizing an abnormal pulsation of the aorta, as when lying down reading a book perched on the abdomen. Expansion and impending rupture are heralded by the development of pain, often of sudden onset, which is characteristically constant, severe, and located in the back or lower abdomen, sometimes with radiation into groin, buttocks, or legs. Actual rupture is associated with the abrupt onset of back pain with abdominal pain and tenderness. Most patients have a palpable, pulsatile abdominal mass and many are hypotensive.[20]

Many aneurysms can be detected on physical examination, although even large aneurysms may be difficult or impossible to detect in obese individuals. When palpable, a pulsatile mass extending variably from between the xiphoid process to the umbilicus may be appreciated. Owing to difficulty in distinguishing the abdominal aorta from surrounding structures by palpation, the size of an aneurysm tends to be overestimated on physical examination. Moreover, it may sometimes be difficult to differentiate a tortuous, ectatic aorta from true aneurysmal dilatation. Aneurysms are often sensitive to palpation and may be quite tender if they are rapidly expanding or about to rupture. Aneurysms should always be palpated cautiously, particularly if they are tender.[21]

Associated occlusive arterial disease is sometimes present in the femoral pulses and distal pulses in the legs or feet. Bruits arising from associated narrowed arteries may be heard over the aneurysm. Rarely, an aneurysm may expand in such a way to occlude the inferior vena cava or one of the iliac veins, resulting in venous congestion and edema in one or both legs. Occasionally an arteriovenous fistula may be formed by spontaneous rupture into the inferior vena cava, iliac vein, or renal vein and a syndrome of hemodynamic collapse and acute high-output cardiac failure results.[18, 21a]

Patients who suffer rupture of an abdominal aortic aneurysm are critically ill.[21b] Hemorrhagic shock may ensue rapidly and is manifested by hypotension, vasoconstriction, mottled skin, diaphoresis, mental obtundation, oliguria, and terminally by arrhythmias and cardiac arrest.[20] Retroperitoneal hemorrhage may be signaled by hematomas in the flanks and groin. Rupture into the abdominal cavity may result in abdominal distention, whereas rupture into the duodenum presents as massive gastrointestinal hemorrhage.

DIAGNOSIS AND SIZING OF ANEURYSMS. Currently, aneurysms may be detected and their size estimated by seven methods: (1) physical examination, (2) routine roentgenography, (3) abdominal cross-sectional echocardiography, (4) abdominal aortic angiography, (5) digital subtraction angiography, (6) CT scan, and (7) MRI.

Brewster and colleagues have carefully compared results on physical examination, routine roentgenography, two-dimensional echocardiography, and aortic angiography for sizing abdominal aortic aneurysms.[22] *Physical examination* is clearly the least accurate. *Lateral x-ray examination* of the lumbar spine is inexpensive and reliably detects the outline of the aneurysm if its wall is calcified (Fig. 46–4). However, this is not the case in at least one-fourth of all patients with aneurysms, so that these cannot be visualized radiographically.[23] *Cross-sectional ultrasound* is very accurate and is easily and atraumatically performed (Fig. 46–1). Refinements in ultrasonic techniques have permitted precise definition of the aortic adventitial border. Thus, abdominal ultrasound is currently the simplest and best way to detect and size an abdominal aortic aneurysm.

Abdominal aortic angiography is less accurate in predicting size because the full width of an aneurysm may be masked by the presence of nonopacified mural thrombus (Fig. 46–5). Moreover, angiography carries with it a small but definite risk of complications, including hematoma, localized dissection, infection, embolization, and renal failure. Nevertheless, when angiography is performed in experienced hands, morbidity from the procedure is minimal, and valuable information is often gleaned from it. Thus, in a survey of 190 patients, angiography of the aorta and distal circulation resulted in only minor complications in 2 per cent; averted an incorrect diagnosis in 11 per cent; revealed extension of the aneurysm above the renal arteries in 5 per cent; showed renal artery stenosis in 22 per cent and atypical renal arterial anatomy in 17 per cent; delineated significant occlusive vascular disease in 48 per cent; and demonstrated associated aneurysms of the iliac, hypogastric, femoral, and popliteal vessels in 50 per cent.[24] Thus, aortography—if performed by experienced angiographers—is currently recommended for patients in whom

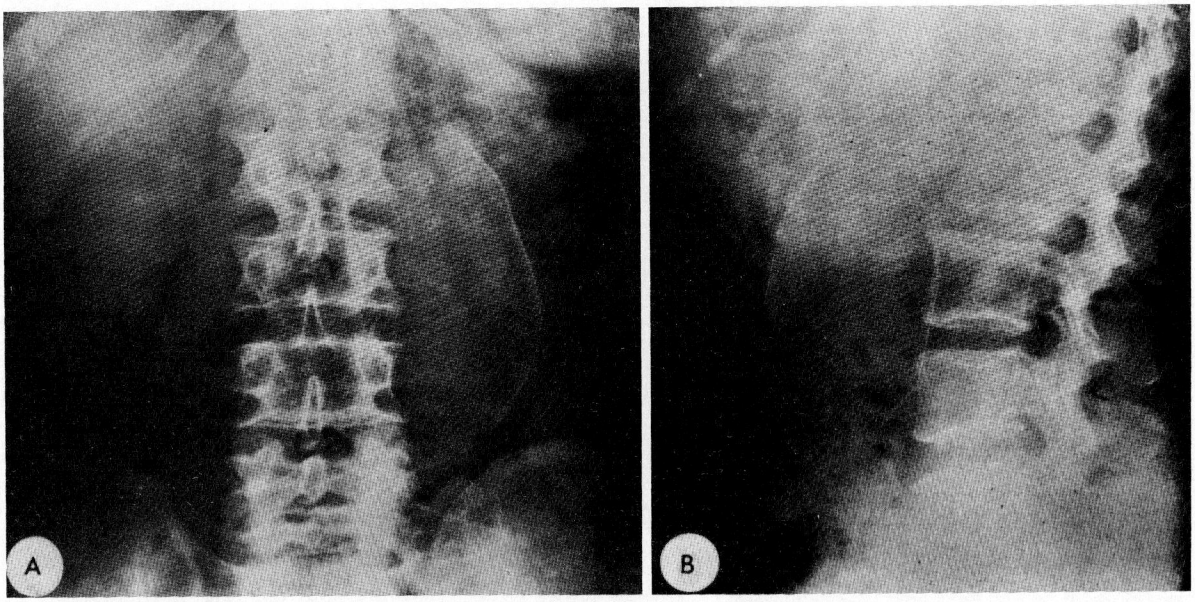

FIGURE 46–4. Anteroposterior (*A*) and lateral (*B*) views of the lumbar spinal column and the abdomen, disclosing a soft tissue mass with curvilinear calcification. (From Estes, J. E., Jr.: Abdominal aortic aneurysm: A study of one hundred and two cases. Circulation *2*:261, 1950, by permission of the American Heart Association, Inc.)

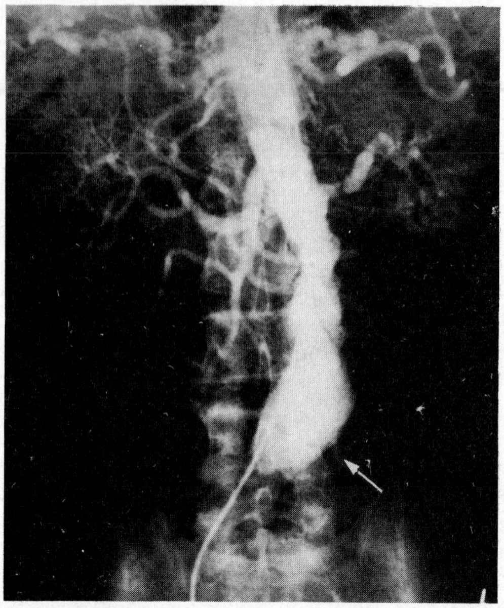

FIGURE 46–5. Abdominal aortogram showing an abdominal aortic aneurysm in a 64-year-old man. The aneurysm measures almost 6 cm in diameter and is wider than it appears because of a laminated thrombus in its wall. A faint rim of calcification outlining the left side of the aneurysm can be seen (arrow). The left renal artery is significantly narrowed. (Courtesy of Christos Athanasoulis, M.D., and Arthur Waltman, M.D., Section of Vascular Radiology, Massachusetts General Hospital, Boston.)

there is any question of a correct diagnosis, for hypertensive patients with possible renal arterial disease, when the extent of the aneurysm is unclear, and for patients with suspected associated occlusive or aneurysmal diseases. In fact, at our institution, it is done routinely in most patients under consideration for surgery in order to facilitate perioperative management.

Experience with *digital subtraction angiography* (p. 356) is still being accumulated, and it is hoped that this technique will eventually yield information as detailed as that provided by aortography, while eliminating the need for intraarterial injection. *CT scanning* may prove to be as useful as or even more accurate than ultrasound in the diagnosis and measurement of abdominal aortic aneurysms (Fig. 46–2). Additional advantages over ultrasound are that it provides better definition of the intraluminal characteristics of the aneurysm and relationships to surrounding structures such as renal arteries, retroperitoneum, and spine.[6] It also provides potentially useful information about other abdominal organs.[5, 6] On the other hand, it does involve the use of radiation and is more costly and time-consuming than ultrasound. Studies of MRI (p. 376) (Fig. 46–3) demonstrate close correlation between this technique and both CT scanning and ultrasound with regard to estimating the size of aneurysms and their relationship to the renal and iliac arteries. Its major limitations include prolonged imaging time and a greater cost. For these reasons, ultrasound remains the procedure of choice for the screening of patients with suspected aneurysms.

NATURAL HISTORY. There is a crucial relationship between the size of aneurysms and their natural history, which is why it is so important to determine their width. Half of all aneurysms greater than 6 cm in diameter rupture within 1 year, compared with 15 to 20 per cent of aneurysms less than 6 cm.[25] In a review of 24,000 consecutive autopsies, Darling et al. found that in aneurysms 10 cm or larger the incidence of rupture was 60 per cent; for those 7 to 10 cm the incidence was 45 per cent; and for those measuring 4 to 7 cm the rate was 25 per cent.[26] The time course of aneurysm growth and rupture is hard to judge in such studies because so many patients succumb to complications of associated arteriosclerosis elsewhere, especially of the cerebrovascular and coronary arteries. Recent studies suggest an "average" aneurysm expansion rate of 0.4 to 0.5 cm in diameter per year. Larger aneurysms appear to enlarge slightly more rapidly.[27, 28]

SURGICAL MANAGEMENT. At present, elective surgery is advised for all abdominal aortic aneurysms 6 cm in diameter or wider, assuming that surgical risks are not prohibitive because of other medical problems. The management of asymptomatic aneurysms less than 6 cm in diameter remains controversial. Pasch and coworkers have argued that elective resection of such lesions would result in the saving of lives and is economically attractive because it obviates the tremendously costly care associated with aneurysm rupture.[29] Cooley has argued that improvements in surgical management of acute rupture now allow salvage of nearly 80 per cent of patients,[30] but the experience of other would appear to favor elective resection of aneurysms larger than 4 cm in otherwise good surgical candidates.[25, 26] In poor-risk patients with aneurysms of 4 to 6 cm, close follow-up is advised, with immediate surgery if the aneurysm is expanding or shows signs of impending rupture, such as the sudden onset of pain.

Surgery consists of resection of the aneurysm and insertion of a synthetic prosthesis, usually of Dacron. Sometimes a simple tube graft is all that is necessary, although frequently the operation must be carried distally into one or both iliac vessels in order to excise the aneurysm completely. With large aneurysms, much of the wall of the aneurysm may be left in situ ("intrasaccular" approach of Creech). This reduces the need for extensive dissection, thereby decreasing aortic cross-clamping time, and has significantly ameliorated the problem of postoperative sexual dysfunction.

Expanding or ruptured abdominal aortic aneurysms are true surgical emergencies. In the case of rupture, patients can sometimes be stabilized by using a compression G-suit, a garment which may diminish the rate of bleeding by exerting counterforce externally against the abdomen. However, operation must be undertaken as soon as possible.

Perioperative Management. Advances in perioperative management have improved survival rates in patients undergoing surgical resection of abdominal aortic aneurysms. Many of these patients have significant heart disease, and monitoring of arterial blood pressure, cardiac output, cardiac filling pressures, and urine output may help enormously in their operative management.[31] These measurements provide a valuable guide to volume replacement. So-called "declamping shock" has been virtually eliminated by volume replacement guided by monitored pressures.[32] This term is applied to a syndrome characterized by marked hypotension upon release of the aortic cross clamp at the completion of surgery; the cause is believed to be pooling of blood in the dilated distal vascular bed and release of vasodepressor substances that have accumulated during surgery distal to the aortic clamp. The use of vasodilators such as nitroprusside or intravenous nitroglycerin may also improve and protect cardiac function by attenuating the changes in left ventricular afterload caused by clamping and unclamping the aorta.[33] Administration of mannitol and potent loop diuretics such as intravenous furosemide has reduced the frequency of postoperative renal failure.[34] The occurrence of renal failure postoperatively in patients with ruptured abdominal aortic aneurysms has correlated with very poor survival rates.[35] Autotransfusion has led to less frequent occurrence of hepatitis and fewer transfusion reactions,[36] and antibiotic coverage has reduced the frequency of infections. Hypothermia has been better controlled, and better understanding of the clotting system has improved management of hemostasis.[37]

Many patients with abdominal aortic aneurysms are heavy smokers and have serious chronic obstructive lung disease. Such patients have benefited greatly from improvements in postoperative respiratory care. Preoperative preparation of pulmonary patients is also important, and smokers should abstain from tobacco use for at least 1 month prior to surgery.

If there is evidence of carotid artery disease in patients facing elective aneurysm resection, preoperative evaluation and surgery for critical carotid stenoses, if indicated, have resulted in fewer strokes. In patients with severe coronary artery disease, it may be important to evaluate the extent of coronary narrowing prior to aneurysm resection. Since half the perioperative deaths in this setting are due to myocardial infarction,[38] Hertzer and others have recommended routine coronary angiography and selective coronary bypass surgery before aneurysm resection in patients with severe correctable coronary disease.[39] Studies by Boucher et al.[40] and Eagle et al.[41] have suggested that dipyridamole-thallium cardiac scanning (p. 329) may be an effective noninvasive means of identifying patients at highest risk for perioperative ischemic events. It is in this subgroup that coronary angiography and selective bypass surgery is likely to be most helpful. Others have evaluated exercise stress testing[42] (Chap. 8) and gated blood pool scanning[43] to identify patients at high risk.

In cases of associated renal artery stenosis with renin-dependent hypertension or severe stenosis jeopardizing renal function, simultaneous renal artery reconstruction is often performed.[44]

OPERATIVE RISK. The risk of operation obviously depends on the general status of the patient and on whether or not the aneurysm has ruptured. Prompt recognition and immediate operation for patients with rupture have markedly improved survival rates. In low-risk patients, the mortality from the elective resection of abdominal aortic aneurysms should be 2 to 5 per cent. With expanding aneurysms, mortality is 5 to 15 per cent, and with rupture, mortality has reached a plateau at approximately 50 per cent, the major determinant of survival being the speed with which surgery is accomplished.[34, 37, 44–48]

Age and preexisting cardiac, pulmonary, cerebrovascular, and/or renal diseases all add to the risk of operation. Congestive heart failure, diabetes, and evidence of coronary artery disease are particularly important, whereas advanced age per se should not be a definite contraindication to surgery in an otherwise healthy patient.[41, 49]

An alternative to aneurysmectomy for patients at very high risk has been reported by Karmody et al.[50] This group has combined thrombosis of the aortic aneurysm with right axillary to bilateral femoral artery bypass conduits. Thrombosis of the aneurysm usually followed the interruption of flow below the aortic bifurcation achieved by ligation of the iliac outflow vessels. If the aneurysm did not thrombose within 72 hours, the iliac outflow vessels responsible for continued patency were identified by angiography and were occluded by intraarterial injection of bucrylate. Although the perioperative and late mortality in these patients was high (17 deaths among 42 patients), the deaths were related mostly to associated diseases and not to the operative procedure itself.

The statistics showing better survival with elective resection of aneurysms are impressive. From several reports, the 5-year survival rate is only 5 to 10 per cent in patients with unexcised aneurysms larger than 6 cm compared with over 50 per cent for those who undergo resection and 80 per cent for the age-matched "normal" population. *Late* survival is unaffected by whether the aneurysm was electively resected, acute, or ruptured.[48] With aneurysms smaller than 6 cm, the 5-year unoperated survival rate is about 50 per cent, as opposed to 60 to 70 per cent for those who undergo resection.[21, 51, 52]

COMPLICATIONS. The rate of late complications of aneurysmectomy has been reported to be around 10 per cent.[53, 54] These complications include stenosis or occlusion of the prosthetic graft, false aneurysm formation, enteric fistula formation, infection, and rupture. Patients with graft occlusion usually have evidence of prior distal vascular disease that impedes aortic runoff. *Occlusions* occur mainly at the sites of anastomosis, and patients usually develop ischemic symptoms distal to the graft site. These stenoses may be amenable to correction by balloon catheter angioplasty.[55] *False aneurysms* may be caused by infection, but others arise spontaneously and present as expanding masses in the groin, abdomen, or lower back. *Enteric fistulas* are caused by rupture of the graft into the duodenum, resulting in gastrointestinal hemorrhage, and are associated with a high mortality. This complication can occur anywhere from 1 day to several years after operation, and the diagnosis must be suspected in any patient who has undergone abdominal aneurysmectomy and who presents with melena, hematemesis, hematochezia, or abdominal pain.[18, 56, 57] Recognition is obtained by gastrointestinal series, endoscopy, colonoscopy, or angiography. *Infections* most commonly are seen as a painful or tender groin mass, with or without a draining sinus. Recommended therapy involves administration of antibiotics, removal of the infected prosthetic material, and reestablishment of the circulation by an alternate route, usually axillofemoral bypass.

Attention has been called to the occasional occurrence of *colonic ischemia* following aneurysm surgery, caused by the intraoperative sacrifice of the inferior mesenteric artery in patients with concomitantly diseased superior or mesenteric and hypogastric arteries, resulting in inadequate perfusion of the colon.[58] This complication is best avoided by paying careful attention to collateral blood flow to the colon, maintaining adequate blood pressure during surgery, and handling the distal colon carefully at the time of operation. If necessary, reimplantation of the inferior mesenteric artery can be performed if collateral circulation is inadequate. Doppler ultrasound measurement of inferior mesenteric arterial flow or direct measurement of the inferior mesenteric arterial stump pressure may be useful in identifying patients likely to benefit from such reimplantation.[58]

THORACIC AORTIC ANEURYSMS

About one-fourth of all arteriosclerotic aneurysms involve the thoracic aorta.[59] Dilatation may occur anywhere along the thoracic aorta—that is, the ascending segment, the arch, or the descending portion; the latter two sites are the more common ones. This contrasts with leutic aneurysms, which are located predominantly in the ascending aorta. Sometimes the entire aorta is ectatic, with localized aneurysms at many sites in both the thoracic and the abdominal aorta. Aneurysms of the descending thoracic aorta not infrequently extend into the abdominal aorta, creating a thoracoabdominal aneurysm.

PATHOGENESIS. The pathogenesis of arteriosclerotic aneurysms is identical to that of aneurysms in the abdominal aorta. The arteriosclerotic process leads to weakening of the aortic wall, medial degeneration, and localized dilatation. Hypertension often coexists and contributes to both undermining the strength of the aortic wall and expansion of the aneurysm. In the thorax, localized saccular aneurysms are somewhat more common than circumferential or fusiform aneurysms. The natural history of thoracic aneurysms differs somewhat from that of abdominal aortic aneurysms in that spontaneous rupture without warning is less common, because evidence of a growing thoracic aneurysm is usually afforded by symptoms caused by compression of the surrounding structures.[60]

CLINICAL MANIFESTATIONS. Thoracic aneurysms are frequently associated with widespread atherosclerosis, particularly of the renal, cerebral, and coronary arteries. In fact, the consequences of arterial obliterative disease in these other areas may dominate the clinical picture.

Symptoms and signs of thoracic aneurysms are related to their size and location and are caused primarily by their impingement upon adjacent structures. Thus, tracheal deviation, wheezing, cough, dyspnea, stridor, hemoptysis, recurrent pneumonitis, and intrapulmonary hemorrhage are the direct result of compression of the tracheobronchial tree and contiguous lung, especially the left main stem bronchus, by aneurysms of the descending thoracic aorta. Occasionally, an asymptomatic arch aneurysm will be visible or palpable rising above the suprasternal notch. Hoarseness may follow compression of the recurrent laryngeal nerve. Arch aneurysms sometimes produce a tracheal tug. Dysphagia arises from pressure against the nearby esophagus. The superior vena caval syndrome can develop as a consequence of obstruction of venous return from the superior vena cava or innominate veins.

Pain is due to compression and erosion of adjacent musculoskeletal structures. It is usually steady and boring—occasionally pulsating—and may be extremely severe. Erosion of the sternum and right thoracic cage may result from large aneurysms of the ascending aorta, while erosion of the vertebral column and posterior left ribs may result from descending thoracic aortic aneurysms. Visible and pulsatile masses are evident when aneurysms reach and begin to erode through the chest wall. Rupture of an aneurysm is heralded by the dramatic onset of excruciating pain, usually in the area where some pain had existed previously.

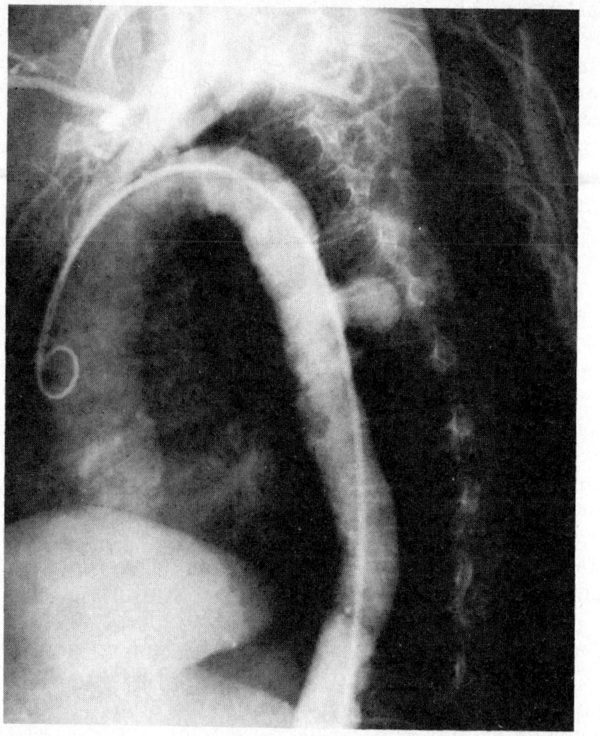

FIGURE 46–6. A localized saccular aneurysm in the descending thoracic aorta is clearly shown in the aortic angiogram of this 62-year-old man. The aneurysm had leaked, and a faint halo caused by the hematoma can be seen surrounding the aneurysm. The routine chest film appeared normal in this patient. (Courtesy of Christos Athanasoulis, M.D., and Arthur Waltman, M.D., Section of Vascular Radiology, Massachusetts General Hospital, Boston.)

DIAGNOSIS. Most thoracic aortic aneurysms are readily visible on chest roentgenograms, with fluoroscopy helping to differentiate an aneurysm from other types of mediastinal masses, such as neoplasms. However, some aneurysms are small, especially saccular aneurysms, which may rupture without having been visible on chest roentgenogram (Fig. 46–6).

Aortic angiography is clearly the definitive procedure for outlining an aneurysm, to make a diagnosis, and to reveal the anatomical features of the aneurysm (Fig. 46–7). It should be performed in all patients under consider-

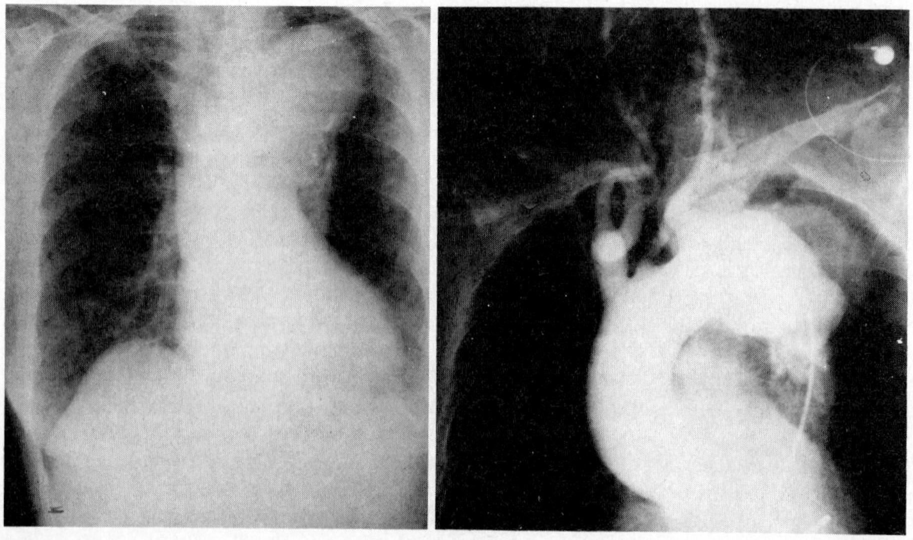

FIGURE 46–7. *Left,* Posteroanterior chest roentgenogram in a 66-year-old woman with an arteriosclerotic aneurysm of the descending thoracic aorta. *Right,* Aortographic appearance in the left oblique anterior projection. The aneurysm arises just at the site of origin of the left subclavian artery. Thrombus is evident in the outer wall of the aneurysm on the angiogram. (Courtesy of Christos Athanasoulis, M.D., and Arthur Waltman, M.D., Section of Vascular Radiology, Massachusetts General Hospital, Boston.)

ation for surgical repair. Although digital subtraction angiography continues to undergo evaluation as an alternative to conventional angiography, its inability to define the anatomy of small arteries (such as coronary arteries) and susceptibility to motion artifact limit its general application at this time.[2] CT scanning (Fig. 12–21, p. 368) enhanced by the use of a contrast medium can be used to identify and size aneurysms of both the ascending and the descending thoracic aorta.[6–8] Alternatively, significant aneurysms of either the ascending or the descending thoracic aorta can be defined by cross-sectional echocardiography, but in the thoracic aorta, unlike the abdominal aorta, this technique is not as accurate as the CT scan, especially in the descending thoracic aorta.[61] MRI is a promising technique that does not require administration of contrast agents. It appears to be as reliable as CT scanning in identifying thoracic aneurysms.[9, 11]

NATURAL HISTORY. Data for the true natural history of arteriosclerotic thoracic aortic aneurysms are somewhat scanty, but, as with abdominal aneurysms, ultimate survival is related to the size of the aneurysms. Thoracic aneurysms greater than 7 cm in diameter are more prone to rupture than are smaller ones.[60] Aneurysms that indicate expansion by producing symptoms of compression of surrounding structures are obviously diagnosed and treated earlier than aneurysms at "silent" sites. As noted, thoracic aneurysms are frequently associated with severe generalized arteriosclerosis, and many patients die of complications of arteriosclerosis before an aneurysm can rupture. When aneurysms do pursue a natural course, it has been found that symptomatic aneurysms are more prone to rupture than are asymptomatic ones. In the classic natural history study by Joyce et al., patients with symptomatic thoracic aneurysms had a 27 per cent 5-year survival compared with 58 per cent in asymptomatic patients. A third of the deaths were attributed to rupture, while more than half were caused by complications of arteriosclerosis unrelated to the aneurysm.[62]

MANAGEMENT. Historically, surgical therapy once consisted of the introduction of long lengths of thrombogenic wire into an aneurysm, with the resultant thrombus buttressing the wall of the aneurysm. Direct wrapping of the aneurysm has also been tried. Currently, surgical excision is the procedure of choice whenever possible and is advised for aneurysms measuring 7 cm or more in diameter in the ascending and descending thoracic aorta. Clearly, even smaller aneurysms should be resected if they are producing symptoms. The aggressiveness with which surgical repair is undertaken depends greatly upon the general condition of the patient. The surgical procedure must be tailored to the specific aneurysm. Saccular aneurysms can sometimes be excised directly without resection of the aorta. Fusiform aneurysms in the ascending and descending thoracic aorta are best resected and replaced with a prosthetic tubular sleeve of appropriate size. Total cardiopulmonary bypass is necessary for the removal of ascending aortic aneurysms, and partial bypass to support the circulation distal to the aneurysm is often advisable in resection of descending thoracic aortic aneurysms. A temporary shunt (Gott shunt) may be used from the proximal aorta to the aorta beyond the aneurysm to divert blood around the site of the aneurysm while it is being repaired,[63] although the use of such adjuncts is less important than are the nature and extent of the aneurysm in determining the incidence of postoperative complications.[64]

The use of a composite graft consisting of a Dacron tube with a prosthetic aortic valve sewn into one end represents a major advance in the therapy of proximal aortic aneurysms extending to the aortic annulus and associated with aortic regurgitation. The valve and graft are sewn into the annulus, and the coronary arteries reimplanted into the Dacron graft.[65] (Fig. 46–16).

Fusiform aneurysms of the arch have been successfully excised surgically; however, the risks of operation in this area are high. Arch aneurysmectomy requires excision of the aneurysm and in some instances reimplantation of all the brachiocephalic vessels. Perfusion by local cannulation of each of these important arteries is necessary while they are being reimplanted. Alternatively, resection of the aneurysm using profound hypothermia and circulatory arrest, a technique that is becoming increasingly favored by many surgical groups, has been used successfully.[66, 67]

Surgical results have improved considerably in recent years, with most major centers reporting a nearly 90 per cent survival rate for the elective resection of ascending and descending thoracic aortic aneurysms.[65, 68] Moreno-Cabral reported the results of operation in 214 patients with arteriosclerotic aneurysms of the ascending aorta. There was a 94 per cent early and an 80 per cent late survival rate.[69] In a report on 82 patients with thoracoabdominal aneurysms, the survival rate was 94 per cent.[70]

Major complications of the operation are technical, especially hemorrhage from tearing of the diseased aorta. A catastrophic complication of resection of descending thoracic aortic aneurysms is paraplegia from inadvertent interruption of the arterial blood supply to the spinal cord. This problem has been reduced considerably by maintaining distal aortic perfusion during surgery; by reducing the period of aortic cross clamping; by removal of minimal segments of aorta with the attendant intercostal arteries, especially in the areas of T7 through T9; by prompt treatment of hypertension in the proximal aorta, which elevates cerebrospinal fluid pressure, thus reducing collateral blood flow to the spinal cord; and possibly by perfusion cooling of the spinal cord during surgery.[71–73] Recent studies report that the spinal cord is injured in at least 5 per cent of patients despite these and other precautions.[65, 68, 74] Complications of associated arteriosclerosis, such as myocardial infarction, cerebrovascular infarcts, and renal failure, often manifest themselves under the massive physiological stress of surgery. The most frequent causes of early postoperative deaths are myocardial infarction, hemorrhage, respiratory failure, and sepsis. Advanced age, emergency operation, prolonged aortic cross-clamp time, extent of aneurysm, and intraoperative hypotension are the most important factors determining early perioperative morbidity and mortality.[69] Late postoperative deaths are usually associated with cardiac complications or aneurysm rupture.[69] The latter may represent aneurysm formation at the graft margins or formation of aneurysms at other aortic sites.[68]

Many patients with arteriosclerotic aneurysms are heavy smokers, and pulmonary complications are frequent. The left lung may be severely traumatized by compression during resection of large aneurysms of the descending thoracic aorta, a complication which may seriously jeopardize the patient, particularly if there is underlying pulmonary disease.

Widespread aneurysmal dilatation of the aorta often precludes operation, although there are reports of successful surgical replacement of essentially the entire diseased thoracic and abdominal aorta. Associated diseases—especially pulmonary—preclude any operation in still others. Although it seems logical to reduce blood pressure vigorously in patients with aneurysms and to reduce the velocity of ventricular ejection, the long-term impact of such therapy on retarding the expansion of aneurysms and improving survival is unknown.

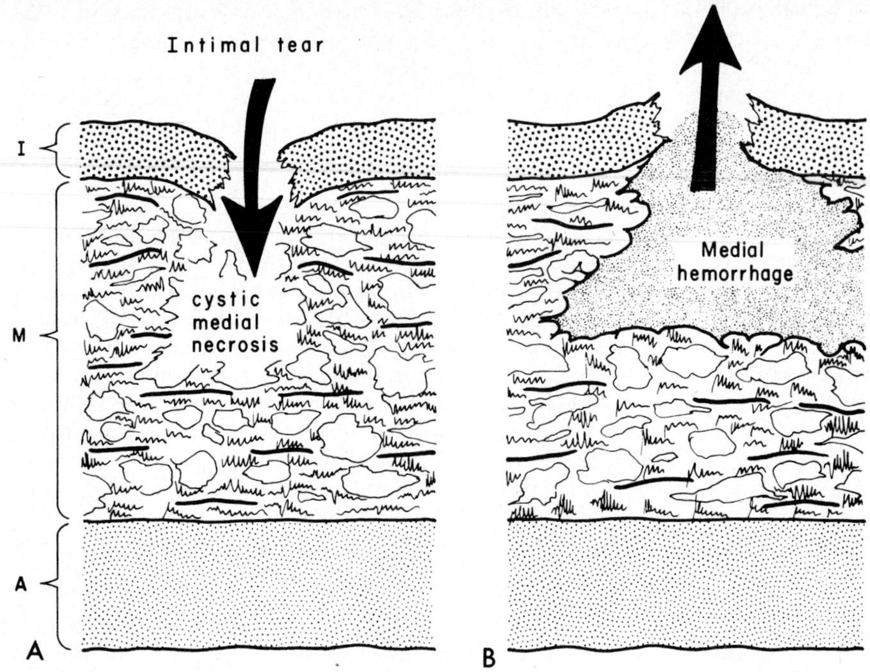

FIGURE 46–8. Proposed mechanisms of initiation of aortic dissection. In both cases, cystic medial necrosis is present. In *A*, an intimal tear is the initial event, allowing aortic blood to enter the media. In *B*, the primary event is hemorrhage into the media, with secondary rupture of the overlying intima. I = intima; M = media; A = adventitia.

AORTIC DISSECTION

Acute aortic dissection is a relatively common catastrophic illness and occurs at the rate of at least 2000 new cases per year in the United States.[75–77] Over the past two decades, great strides have been made in the diagnosis and the medical and surgical treatment of this highly lethal disease.[77a] It has been cogently pointed out that the term *dissecting hematoma* describes this entity more accurately than does the commonly used term dissecting aneurysm. More recently, the simpler term *aortic dissection* has gained favor.

Aortic dissection is caused by the sudden development of a tear in the aortic intima, opening the way for a column of blood driven by the force of the arterial pressure to enter the aortic wall, destroying the media and stripping the intima from the adventitia for variable distances along the length of the aorta.[78] It is uncertain whether the primary event in aortic dissection is rupture of the intima, with secondary dissection into the media, or hemorrhage within a diseased media followed by disruption of the subjacent intima and subsequent propagation of the dissection through the intimal tear (Fig. 46–8). However, occasional cases of extensive aortic dissection can occur without any identifiable intimal tear.

The manifestations of aortic dissection in any given patient are determined by its path as it progresses through the aorta. Thus, the circulation of any major artery arising from the aorta may be compromised; disruption of the support of the aortic valve by extension into the aortic root may cause aortic incompetence; and finally the dissecting column may rupture through the adventitia anywhere along the aorta, although the two most common sites of rupture are the pericardial space and the left pleural cavity.

CLASSIFICATION. Most classification schemes for aortic dissection are based upon the fact that over 95 per cent of all dissections arise in one of two locations: (1) the ascending aorta within several centimeters of the aortic valve; and (2) the descending thoracic aorta, usually just beyond the origin of the left subclavian artery at the site of the ligamentum arteriosum.[76] The widely used classification of DeBakey et al. recognizes three groups (Fig. 46–9).[79] Types I and II both begin in the ascending aorta; Type I extends beyond the ascending aorta and arch, whereas Type II is confined to the ascending aorta. Type III originates in the descending thoracic aorta and usually propagates distally for a variable distance; more rarely, it extends retrograde into the arch and ascending aorta. In Type IIIa dissection, the process is limited to the thoracic aorta, while a IIIb designation connotes extension of the dissection below the diaphragm.[79]

Still another classification, based upon approach to therapy and proposed by Daily et al., delineates two types, A and B.[80] Type A includes all proximal dissections and those distal dissections that extend retrograde to involve the arch and ascending aorta; Type B refers to all other distal dissections without proximal extension.

Since the behavior and management of Types I and II dissections are similar, many investigators, including ourselves, have adopted a simple two-category classification into "proximal" (DeBakey Types I and II) and "distal" (DeBakey Type III) dissections.[81] "Ascending" and "descending" have also been used synonymously with "proximal" and "distal." Proximal dissections occur more frequently than distal dissections in a ratio of almost two to one in autopsy series.[82] However, because proximal dissections are more rapidly lethal, many clinical series report larger numbers of patients with distal than proximal dissection.[81, 83]

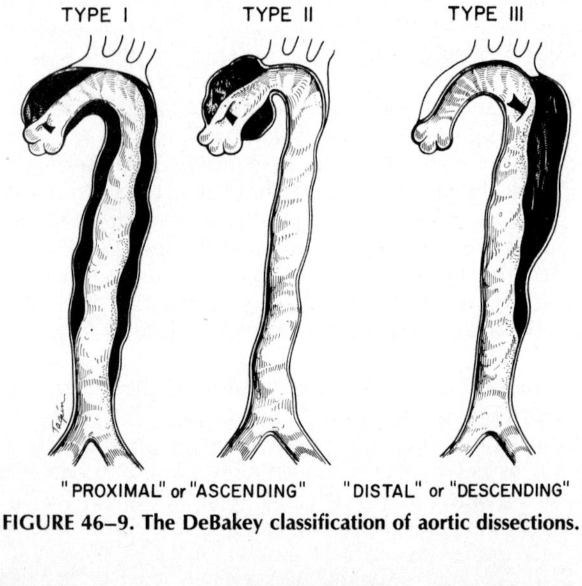

FIGURE 46–9. The DeBakey classification of aortic dissections.

Occasional other sites of origin are the aortic arch and the abdominal aorta. Furthermore, individual arteries may be the locus of isolated dissection, especially the coronary and carotid arteries.[84, 85]

ETIOLOGY AND PATHOGENESIS. Degeneration of the aortic media is believed to be the prerequisite for the development of aortic dissection.[76–78, 86] Usually, this consists of deterioration of the collagen and elastic tissue, often with cystic changes. This process, termed cystic medial necrosis or degeneration, most often is the result of chronic stress against the aortic wall, such as might occur with longstanding hypertension. Indeed, hypertension is an important contributing factor to aortic dissection and is found in well over half of all cases, especially those of distal dissection.

Although some degree of medial degeneration is part of the normal aging process in the aorta, these changes are qualitatively and quantitatively much greater in patients with aortic dissection. Cystic medial degeneration is an intrinsic feature of the hereditary defects of connective tissue, especially the Marfan (p. 1725) and Ehlers-Danlos (p. 1727) syndromes. Indeed, aortic dissection—especially proximal dissection—is a frequent and serious complication of the Marfan syndrome. However, cystic medial degeneration and aortic dissection may occur in the absence of an associated phenotypic syndrome.[87] Certain congenital cardiovascular abnormalities, especially coarctation of the aorta and bicuspid aortic valves, predispose to aortic dissection. A combination of bicuspid aortic valve, cystic medial degeneration, and aortic root dissection in the absence of the Marfan syndrome has been described.[88] Recent reports of aortic dissection in patients with Noonan syndrome and Turner syndrome have also appeared.[89, 90] Cystic medial degeneration appears to be a common theme in all these patients.

An unexplained relationship exists between pregnancy and aortic dissection (p. 1858). About half of all aortic dissections in women under the age of 40 occur during pregnancy, usually in the last trimester.[91] Isolated coronary artery dissection also usually occurs during pregnancy.

In older patients, dissections occasionally originate by way of perforation through an intimal atheromatous plaque. Trauma almost never causes a classic aortic dissection, although a localized tear in the region of the aortic isthmus is not uncommon following massive chest trauma. Rarely, dissection of the aorta is a complication of other forms of vasculitis, including granulomatous arteritis (p. 1565).

Although strenuous physical exertion and emotional stress have been linked to aortic dissection, such a relationship is not usual. In a series of 124 cases of aortic dissection that we reviewed, we found such a history in only 14 per cent.[81]

The role played by chemicals toxic to connective tissue in the etiology of dissecting aneurysm in human beings is unknown. It is well known that the seeds of *Lathyrus odoratus* (sweet pea), which contain aminopropionitrile, cause cystic medial degeneration and aortic dissection in rats.[92] We have encountered a proximal dissection in a young man with no obvious predisposing factors other than prolonged industrial exposure to dimethyl hydrazine, a connective tissue toxin.[81]

CLINICAL MANIFESTATIONS

Aortic dissection afflicts men more frequently than women in a ratio of approximately two to one and has a peak incidence in the sixth and seventh decades, with a range from childhood well into the 90's.[93] Patients with proximal dissection are on the average somewhat younger. By far the most common presenting symptom of aortic dissection is *severe pain*, which is found in over 90 per cent of cases.[94] In fact, those patients without pain usually have suffered some disturbance of consciousness as a result of the dissection that renders them unable to perceive pain. Nonetheless, painless dissection can and does occur rarely.[95]

Cataclysmic in onset, the pain of aortic dissection is often as severe at its inception as it ever becomes. This feature contrasts with that of myocardial infarction, where the pain usually has a crescendo-like onset. The pain of dissection may be all but unbearable, forcing the patient to writhe in agony or to pace restlessly in an attempt to gain some measure of relief. Several features of the pain may arouse suspicion of aortic dissection. The quality of the pain as described by the patient is often morbidly appropriate to the actual event. Adjectives such as "tearing," "ripping," and "stabbing" are frequently used. Another important characteristic of the pain of aortic dissection is its tendency to migrate from the point of its origin to other sites, following the path of the dissecting hematoma as it extends through the aorta. This feature was noted in 70 per cent of our cases.[81] Vasovagal manifestations, such as a drenching sweat, apprehension, nausea, vomiting, and faintness, are common at the outset.

The location of pain may be of some help in suggesting the site of origin.[81] Pain felt maximally in the anterior thorax is more frequent with proximal dissection, whereas pain that is most severe in the interscapular area is much more common with a distal site of origin. Although pain may be felt simultaneously in the anterior and posterior chest with both proximal and distal dissection, the *absence* of posterior interscapular pain strongly militates against a distal dissection, since over 90 per cent of patients with distal dissection report some back pain. Pain in the neck, throat, jaw, or teeth often occurs in dissections that involve the ascending aorta or arch.

Less common modes of presentation include congestive heart failure with or without associated chest pain, cerebrovascular accidents, syncope, paraplegia, and pulse loss with or without ischemic pain. Heart failure usually results from severe aortic regurgitation secondary to the dissection. The occurrence of syncope in aortic dissection may bear special significance. Syncope without focal neurological signs occurred in 6 of 124 patients in our series. In each case, there was evidence for rupture of the dissection into the pericardial cavity with cardiac tamponade.[81]

Diagnosis

PHYSICAL FINDINGS. The diagnosis of aortic dissection can often be made with reasonable assurance from the *physical examination* alone. Patients with aortic dissection may appear to be in shock; however, the blood pressure when measured is frequently elevated. More than half the patients with distal dissection are hypertensive on initial presentation. Hypotension usually results from cardiac tamponade; intrapleural or intraperitoneal rupture; or dissection of the brachiocephalic vessels resulting in "pseudohypotension," i.e., the inability to measure the blood pressure accurately because of occlusion of the brachial arteries.

Those physical findings most typically associated with aortic dissection, namely, pulse deficits, aortic insufficiency, and neurological manifestations, are more characteristic of proximal than distal dissection. Pulse abnormalities, which include the absence, diminution, or reduplication of pulses, occur in approximately one-half of patients with proximal dissection and most commonly involve the brachiocephalic vessels. Pulse deficits are much less common in patients with distal dissection and tend to involve the left subclavian and femoral arteries, although the femoral vessels are equally affected by the distal propagation of a proximal dissection. Pulses may be lost either by direct compression of the lumen of an artery through extension of the dissection into it or by blockade due to a flap of intima overlying the vessel orifice. Rarely, intimointimal intussusception may occur.[96] Whatever the cause, pulse deficits in aortic dissection may be transitory, owing to decompression of the hematoma by distal reentry into the true lumen or by movement of the intimal flap away from the occluded orifice.

Aortic regurgitation is an important feature of proximal dissection and occurs in over 50 per cent in most series.[97] It was present in two-thirds of our patients with proximal dissection.[81] When aortic regurgitation is present in patients with distal dissection, it most commonly antedates the dissection and results from preexisting dilatation of the aortic root due to severe hypertension or annuloaortic ectasia. The murmur of aortic regurgitation in aortic dissection often has a musical quality and may be heard better along the right than the left sternal border. It may wax and wane, the intensity varying directly with the height of the arterial blood pressure. Depending upon the severity of the regurgitation, other peripheral signs of aortic incompetence may be present, such as collapsing pulses and a wide pulse pressure. There are three mechanisms of aortic regurgitation in proximal dissection (Fig. 46–10): First, the dissection may dilate the aortic root, widening the annulus so that aortic leaflets are unable to coapt in diastole; second, in an asymmetrical dissection, pressure from the dissecting hematoma may depress one leaflet below the line of closure of the others; and third, the annular support of the leaflets or the leaflets themselves may be torn so as to render the valve incompetent.

As noted, patients with proximal dissection sometimes have heart failure, which is almost always due to the sudden onset of severe aortic insufficiency. In rare cases, the congestive failure may be so severe as to mask the murmur and other usual signs of aortic regurgitation. In a few such patients whom we have encountered, the presence of disproportionately bounding pulses in the face of severe heart failure, coupled with a history highly suggestive of aortic dissection, served as a clue to the correct diagnosis.

Neurological deficits associated with aortic dissection include cerebrovascular accidents, ischemic peripheral neuropathy, ischemic paraparesis, and disturbances of consciousness. Each of these is more common with proximal dissection, but deficits in the lower extremities are equally frequent in proximal and distal dissection.

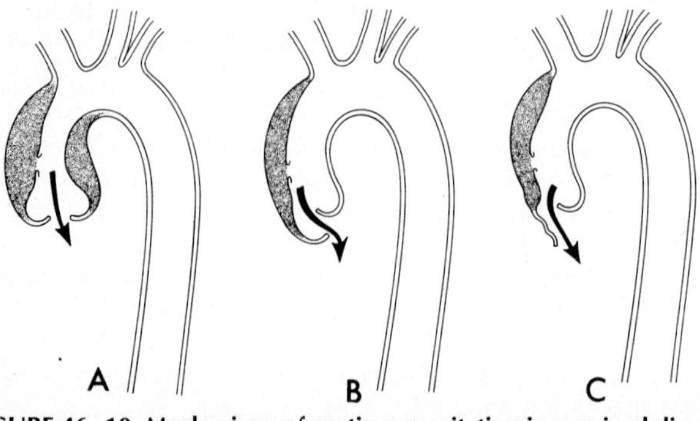

FIGURE 46–10. Mechanisms of aortic regurgitation in proximal dissecting aortic aneurysm. *A*, A circumferential tear pulls the annulus apart, preventing the leaflets from coapting. *B*, With asymmetrical dissection, pressure from the hematoma depresses one leaflet below the line of closure of the other. *C*, The annular support is disrupted, resulting in a flail aortic leaflet and aortic regurgitation.

Other occasionally encountered clinical manifestations of aortic dissection include pulsation of one of the sternoclavicular joints, Horner syndrome due to compression of the superior cervical sympathetic ganglion, vocal cord paralysis and hoarseness from pressure against the left recurrent laryngeal nerve, superior mediastinal syndrome from superior vena caval compression,[98] pulsating neck masses, tracheal or bronchial compression with bronchospasm,[76] hemorrhage into the tracheobronchial tree with hemoptysis,[99] hematemesis due to perforation into the esophagus,[100] heart block from retrograde burrowing of a dissection into the interatrial septum and thence down to the AV node,[101] and a continuous murmur due to rupture into the right atrium or ventricle.[102] Pleural effusions result from rupture of the dissection into one of the pleural spaces—usually the left—or simply from an exudative inflammatory reaction around the involved aorta. Additional complications may result from occlusion of important arteries by the dissection. Mesenteric infarction, renal infarction with severe renovascular hypertension, and myocardial infarction (seen in 1 to 2 per cent of patients with proximal dissection) are among the more serious occlusive events. Occasionally, high fever results, presumably from the release of pyrogenic substances from the hematoma or from associated effusions.

A variety of conditions may mimic aortic dissection. These include myocardial infarction, acute aortic regurgitation without dissection, thoracic nondissecting aneurysm, musculoskeletal pain, mediastinal tumors, pericarditis, and coronary insufficiency.[103] Confusion usually arises in these conditions when chest pain suggesting aortic dissection is coincidentally associated with other clinical manifestations of that entity, such as aortic regurgitation, deficient pulses, neurological abnormalities, or an abnormally widened aortic contour.[103]

Routine laboratory studies are not very helpful in making the diagnosis of aortic dissection. Anemia may develop from significant hemorrhage or sequestration of blood in the false channel. A mild to moderate polymorphonuclear leukocytosis (10,000 to 14,000/mm^3) is common. Lactic acid dehydrogenase (LDH) and bilirubin levels are sometimes elevated because of hemolysis of blood trapped within the false lumen. Serum glutamic oxaloacetic transaminase (SGOT) and creatine phosphokinase (CK or CK-MB) values are usually normal. Disseminated intravascular coagulation has been reported rarely.[104] The electrocardiogram frequently shows left ventricular hypertrophy from preexistent hypertension and usually the absence of acute ischemic changes. The absence of electrocardiographic changes of myocardial ischemia or infarction in a patient with severe chest pain is a helpful point in the differential diagnosis from myocardial infarction.

IMAGING TECHNIQUES: ULTRASOUND, CT, AND MRI. Diagnostic ultrasound (M-mode), in combination with cross-sectional (2-D) echocardiography, is helpful in the detection of a proximal dissection by revealing a widened aortic root, with delineation of the dissecting hematoma[105–107, 107a] (Fig. 46–11). CT scanning with contrast injection (Fig. 12–20, p. 367) is quite accurate in defining both ascending and descending dissections, provided there is identification of a false lumen to distinguish the dissection from a fusiform aneurysm.[107, 108] Although two-dimensional echocardiography and CT clearly offer the advantage of noninvasive diagnosis,[109, 109a] angiography is generally required to define the full extent of the dissection, to

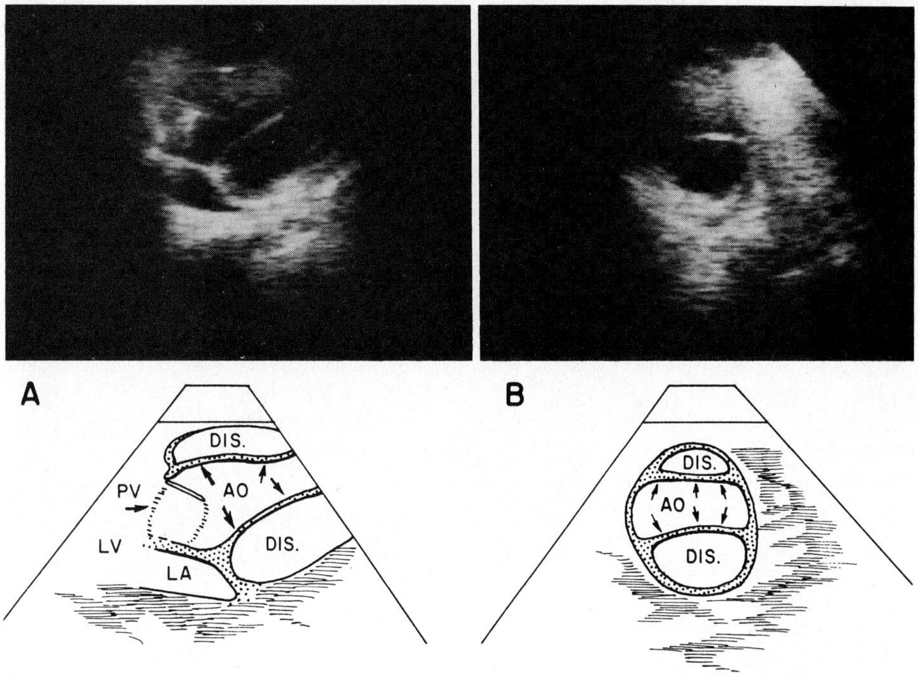

FIGURE 46–11. Cross-sectional echogram of the proximal aorta in a 63-year-old woman with dissection of the proximal aorta occurring 12 years after implantation of a Starr-Edwards aortic valve prosthesis. *A*, Parasternal long-axis recording. *B*, Short-axis recording. The actual recordings are shown above, and diagrammatic representations of the findings are pictured below. The echodense prosthetic valve (PV) is easily seen on the long-axis recording. Surrounding the aorta (AO) is the false channel of the dissection (DIS). (From Weyman, A. E.: Cross-sectional Echocardiography. Philadelphia, Lea and Febiger, 1982.)

outline the relationship of the dissection to the major aortic branches, to evaluate aortic valve competency, and to identify the site of the intimal tear. Thus, these noninvasive techniques—especially the CT scan—may be most useful in the long-term follow-up of treated patients with aortic dissection to detect evidence of localized aneurysm formation.[110, 111] Chest roentgenography and aortic angiography provide the most substantive laboratory tests for initial suspicion and definitive diagnosis, respectively. Chest roentgenography almost always reveals an abnormally widened aortic contour.[112] A localized bulge may overlay the site of origin, and the aortic silhouette may be widened wherever the dissection extends. If the aortic knob is calcified, separation of the intimal calcification from the adventitial border exceeding 1 cm (the "calcium sign") is virtually pathognomonic of aortic dissection (Fig. 46–12). Tracheal deviation or a left pleural effusion may be seen. Comparison with previous films is most helpful. On the other hand, it is possible for extensive aortic dissection to occur without radiographic abnormalities.

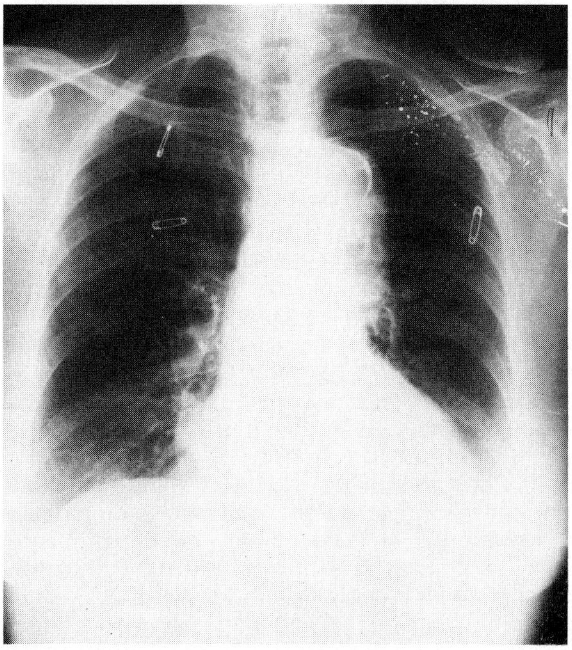

FIGURE 46–12. "Calcium sign" in distal dissection in an 80-year-old woman with longstanding hypertension. Note the marked separation of the calcification in the aortic knob and descending thoracic aorta from the outer wall of the aorta. This distance is normally no greater than 0.5 cm.

Fluoroscopy of the aorta may suggest aortic dissection in that pulsations in the abnormally widened aorta are diminished or absent over an area of dissection. This contrasts with the exaggerated pulsations usually seen in a true aneurysm. The role which MRI will play in the evaluation and follow-up of patients with suspected or proven aortic dissection is uncertain. Preliminary studies are encouraging (Fig. 12–39, p. 376), showing the technique's ability to identify the intimal tear in most patients and to classify the dissection as proximal or distal. Its inability to assess aortic valve competence and coronary artery anatomy prevent its being a substitute for angiography. Unlike CT scanning, it does not require administration of potentially toxic contrast material. However, both prolonged imaging time and cost are limiting features (Fig. 46–3).[9–12, 113]

AORTIC ANGIOGRAPHY. The single most important study in the diagnosis of aortic dissection is *aortic angiography*. Although originally performed by injection of contrast material into the pulmonary artery, with aortic opacification following the pulmonary venous phase, retrograde angiography is now the method of choice. The hazards of this approach have proved minimal, provided the catheter is carefully inserted and contrast material is not injected into the false channel. Aortic angiography has three objectives: (1) to establish a definite diagnosis, (2) to identify the site of origin of the dissection, and (3) to delineate the extent of the dissection and the distal circulation to vital organs (Figs. 46–13 and 46–14).

One additional feature to be assessed by angiography is the degree to which the false channel is opacified. There is evidence that the prognosis in medically treated patients is better in those with a nonopacified false channel, presumably an indication of thrombus formation in the channel that may serve to buttress the wall of the dissected aorta.[114] Although highly accurate, angiography is not without occasional pitfalls in the detection of aortic dissection.[103] Angiography may fail to show a dissection if there is faint opacification of the false lumen, unusual tearing of the

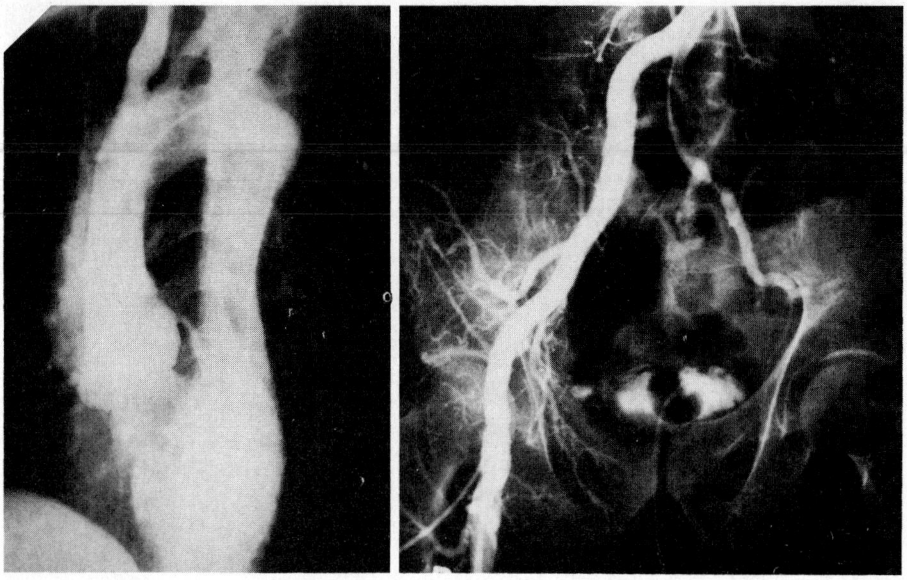

FIGURE 46–13. *Left,* Thoracic aortogram in the left anterior oblique projection showing a dissection beginning in the ascending aorta and spiraling through the aortic arch into the descending aorta. The false lumen can be faintly visualized. *Right,* Angiogram of the distal aorta showing virtual obstruction of the left iliac artery by the dissection. (Courtesy of Christos Athanasoulis, M.D., and Arthur Waltman, M.D., Section of Vascular Radiology. Massachusetts General Hospital, Boston.)

intima, a small and localized dissection, or equal simultaneous opacification of both channels.[115] Nevertheless, when properly obtained and interpreted, angiograms provide a definite diagnosis in almost every case, and the procedure is well tolerated by even critically ill patients.

MANAGEMENT

Therapy for aortic dissection is directed at halting the progression of the dissecting hematoma, since fatal complications arise not from the intimal tear itself but rather from the subsequent course taken by the dissection.[116]

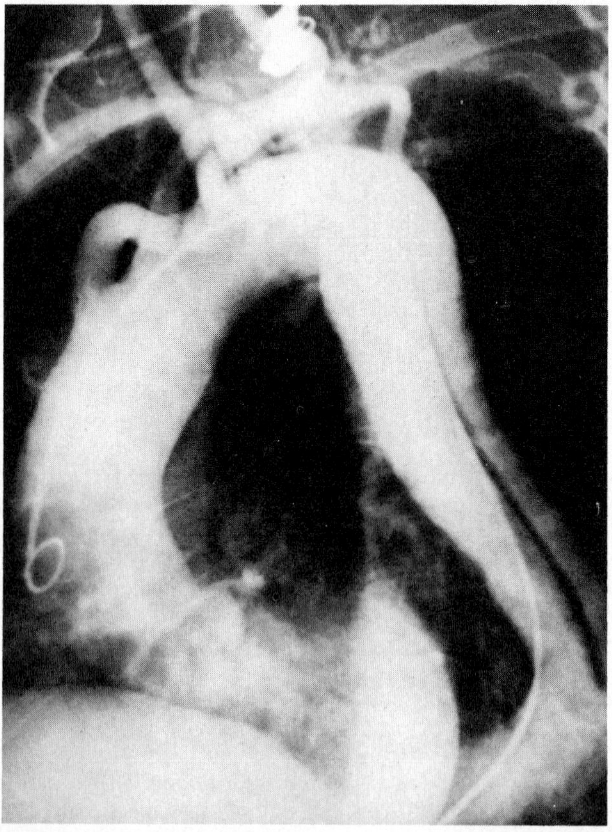

FIGURE 46–14. Left oblique anterior view of the aorta outlined angiographically showing a distal aortic dissection in a 63-year-old man. The true and false channels are clearly seen. The false channel is heavily opacified.

Without treatment, aortic dissection is highly fatal. In a collective review of long-term survival in untreated aortic dissection, more than one-fourth of all patients were dead within 24 hours, more than one-half died within the first week, more than three-fourths died within 1 month, and more than 90 per cent died within 1 year.[117]

The first surgical approach to aortic dissection was the so-called fenestration procedure in which the dissected aorta was incised and a distal communication was created between the true and false channels, thereby decompressing the false lumen.[118, 119] Definitive surgical therapy was pioneered by DeBakey and colleagues in the early 1950's.[120] Its principles are to excise the intimal tear, obliterate the false channel by oversewing aortic edges, reconstitute the aorta with or without interposition of a synthetic graft, and restore aortic valve competence by resuspension of the displaced aortic leaflets or by prosthetic aortic valve replacement in the case of proximal dissection.

In the midst of growing enthusiasm for surgical therapy, aggressive medical treatment of aortic dissection was first advocated by Wheat, Palmer, and collaborators.[121] They established two goals for pharmacological therapy: (1) reduction of the systolic blood pressure, and (2) diminution of the velocity of left ventricular ejection (dV/dt), which is thought to be a major stress acting upon the aortic wall that contributes to the genesis and propagation of aortic dissection. Originally introduced for patients too ill to withstand surgery, medical therapy now forms the basis for the initial treatment of virtually all patients with aortic dissection prior to definitive diagnosis by angiography and serves as primary long-term therapy in an additional subset of patients.

EARLY EMERGENCY TREATMENT. All patients in whom there is a strong suspicion of aortic dissection should be admitted immediately to an intensive care unit, where blood pressure, cardiac rhythm, central venous pressure, urine output, and, when necessary, pulmonary wedge pressure and cardiac output can be monitored. Initial therapeutic goals are the elimination of pain and the reduction of systolic blood pressure to 100 to 120 mm Hg (mean of 60 to 75 mm Hg) or to the lowest level commensurate with adequate vital organ (cardiac, renal, and cerebral) perfusion. Simultaneously, arterial dV/dt, which reflects the velocity of left ventricular ejection, should be reduced by beta-adrenoceptor blockade regardless of whether systolic hypertension or pain is present.

For acute reduction of arterial pressure, the potent

vasodilator sodium nitroprusside is very effective, mixed as 50 to 100 mg in 500 ml of 5 per cent dextrose in water and infused initially at 25 to 50 μg/min, with dosages varying according to blood pressure response. Side effects include nausea, restlessness, somnolence, hypotension, and cyanide or thiocyanate toxicity, which can develop after more than 48 hours of continuous use. Sodium nitroprusside alone can cause an increase in dV/dt, which can potentially contribute to propagation of the dissection.[122] Thus, adequate simultaneous beta-adrenoceptor blockade is essential when this drug is used.[123]

If sodium nitroprusside is ineffective or poorly tolerated, the ganglionic blocking agent trimethaphan (Arfonad), mixed as 500 mg to 2.0 gm in 500 ml of 5 per cent glucose and water, is used. The initial infusion rate is 1 mg/min, with the dose titrated against the blood pressure response, which is enhanced by the orthostatic maneuver of elevating the head of the bed. Limitations in the use of this powerful agent include severe hypotension, tachyphylaxis, somnolence, and sympathoplegia with urinary retention, constipation, ileus, and pupillary dilation. In contrast to sodium nitroprusside, trimethaphan depresses dV/dt, which should provide a relative advantage in the treatment of aortic dissection. However, its unpleasant side effects and rapid tachyphylaxis have relegated this drug to a position of second choice in acute therapy in most centers.

To reduce dV/dt acutely, propranolol or a comparable intravenous beta blocker should be used in incremental doses of 1 mg intravenously every 5 minutes until there is evidence of satisfactory beta blockade, usually indicated by a pulse rate of 60 to 80 beats/min in the acute setting. A test dose of 0.5 mg intravenously is advised. The maximum initial total dose should not exceed 0.15 mg/kg. Additional propranolol should be given intravenously every 4 to 6 hours in order to maintain adequate beta blockade, as reflected in heart rate, usually in dosages somewhat lower than the initial amount, i.e., 2 to 6 mg. In chronic stable dissection, propranolol (or an alternative beta blocker) can be started orally, using 20 to 40 mg every 6 hours. Propranolol is contraindicated in the presence of bradycardia, asthma, or heart failure. Since propranolol was the first generally available beta-adrenoceptor blocking drug, it is the one that has been used most widely in aortic dissection. However, there is good reason to believe that other beta blockers are equally effective if used in equivalent doses. In particular, those which are cardioselective, such as atenolol and metoprolol, may be preferable in patients with chronic obstructive lung disease or a history of bronchial asthma.

An alternative drug to reduce both blood pressure and dV/dt acutely is reserpine, 1 to 2 mg intramuscularly every 4 to 6 hours. Side effects of reserpine are drowsiness, depression, and peptic ulceration from the stimulation of hydrochloric acid secretion by the stomach. The latter risk can be minimized by concomitant administration of cimetidine or rantidine.

The role of calcium-channel antagonists in the treatment of aortic dissection is not yet fully defined, but initial experience with them is encouraging. Use of these agents in managing hypertensive crisis has been favorable (p. 880).[124] A recent report noted successful use of sublingual nifedipine to treat refractory hypertension in a patient with aortic dissection.[125] The combined vasodilator and negative inotropic effects of such drugs appear ideally suited for this disease, although further studies are needed. Once stabilized, the patient should undergo angiography for a definitive diagnosis. Angiography should be performed as soon as possible after admission, unless a life-threatening complication such as aortic rupture, free aortic regurgitation, cardiac tamponade, or compromise of a vital organ has supervened. If any of these potentially lethal problems arises, surgery must be undertaken immediately, with angiography performed if possible while the operating room is being readied.

DEFINITIVE SUBSEQUENT THERAPY. Despite minor variations from center to center, a reasonable consensus as to the definitive therapy of aortic dissection has evolved over the past two decades. Although either medical or surgical therapy can be associated with an extremely successful outcome, it can be generally stated that *surgical results are superior to medical results in acute proximal dissection*, and, conversely, *medical therapy offers a relative advantage over surgery in most cases of uncomplicated acute distal dissection.*[126–132] These differences are based largely upon the disparate natural history of proximal and distal disease. Even minute progression of a proximal dissection poses potentially devastating consequences such as pulse loss, aortic regurgitation, neurological compromise, or cardiac tamponade. Thus, immediate surgical repair promises a better outcome. In contrast, patients with distal dissection are for the most part older and have a relatively increased incidence of advanced atherosclerotic or cardiopulmonary disease, thus rendering their surgical risks considerably higher. Medical therapy has proved to be quite effective in this group. Agreement on these principles is not unanimous, however, and Miller et al. advocate the surgical treatment of all acute dissections, both proximal and distal.[132]

Recent studies report a hospital survival of approximately 75 per cent for patients with acute proximal dissection treated surgically and 80 per cent for those with acute distal dissection treated medically. Hospital survival for patients with chronic dissection (defined as presentation 2 weeks or more after the onset of dissection) treated either surgically—usually because of aortic insufficiency or an enlarging aneurysm—or medically is approximately 90 per cent.[130–134] The somewhat poorer results for surgically treated patients with acute dissection are mostly attributable to complications that have already occurred as a result of the dissection prior to definitive therapy.[131] The better survival in patients with chronic dissection derives from this same principle, i.e., they have already selected themselves out as a group destined to do well because they have survived the initial high mortality that occurs within the first 2 weeks of onset of the dissection.[129–131] The results of long-term follow-up will be discussed below.

The generally advocated *indications for definitive surgical therapy* are summarized in Table 46–1. Note that occasional patients with proximal dissection who refuse surgery or for whom surgery is contraindicated by age or

TABLE 46–1 INDICATIONS FOR DEFINITIVE SURGICAL AND MEDICAL THERAPY IN AORTIC DISSECTION

Surgical
1. Treatment of choice for acute proximal dissection
2. Treatment for acute distal dissection complicated by the following:
   a. Progression with vital organ compromise
   b. Rupture or impending rupture (e.g., saccular aneurysm formation)
   c. Aortic regurgitation (rare)
   d. Retrograde extension into the ascending aorta
   e. Dissection in Marfan's syndrome

Medical
1. Treatment of choice for uncomplicated distal dissection
2. Treatment for stable, isolated arch dissection
3. Treatment of choice for stable chronic dissection (uncomplicated dissection presenting 2 weeks or later after onset)

*Some authors advise surgical therapy for all distal dissections.[132]

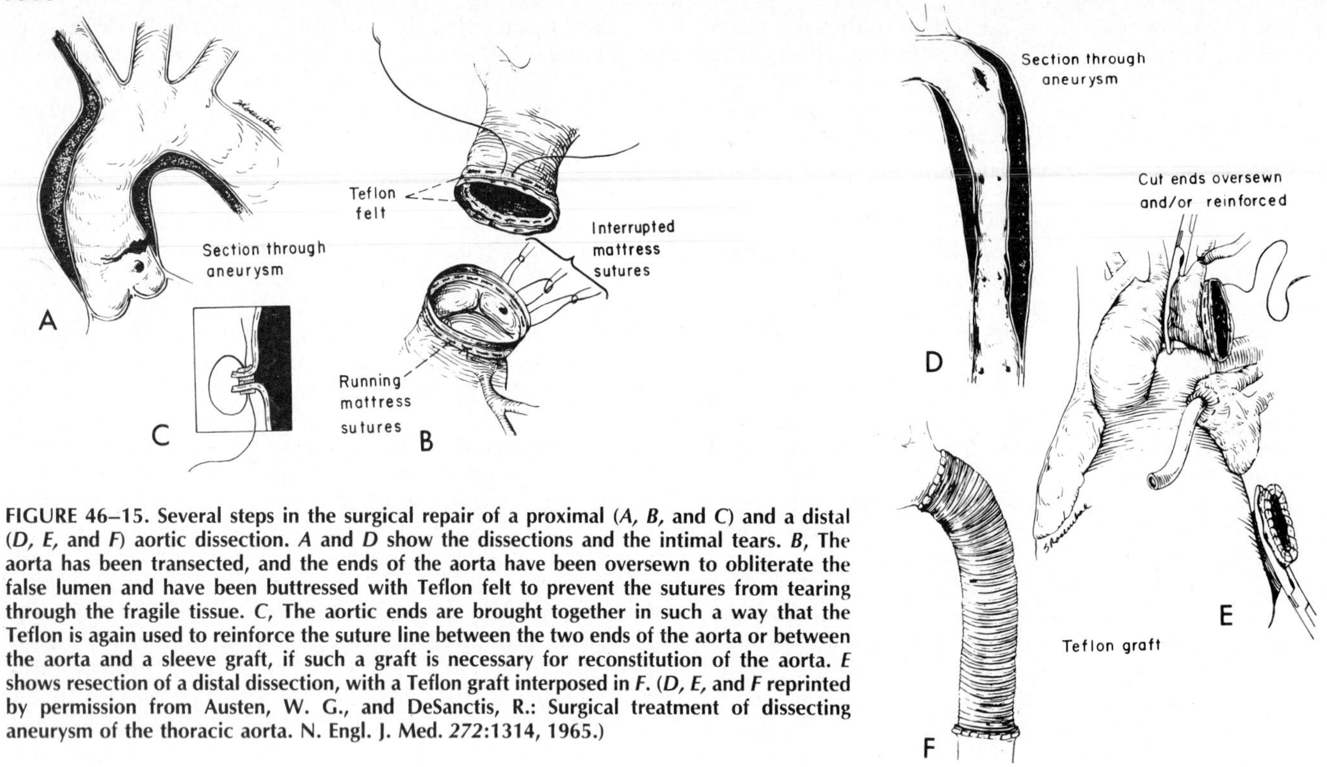

FIGURE 46–15. Several steps in the surgical repair of a proximal (*A, B,* and *C*) and a distal (*D, E,* and *F*) aortic dissection. *A* and *D* show the dissections and the intimal tears. *B,* The aorta has been transected, and the ends of the aorta have been oversewn to obliterate the false lumen and have been buttressed with Teflon felt to prevent the sutures from tearing through the fragile tissue. *C,* The aortic ends are brought together in such a way that the Teflon is again used to reinforce the suture line between the two ends of the aorta or between the aorta and a sleeve graft, if such a graft is necessary for reconstitution of the aorta. *E* shows resection of a distal dissection, with a Teflon graft interposed in *F.* (*D, E,* and *F* reprinted by permission from Austen, W. G., and DeSanctis, R.: Surgical treatment of dissecting aneurysm of the thoracic aorta. N. Engl. J. Med. *272*:1314, 1965.)

prior debilitating illness can be treated successfully by medical therapy. Moreover, both early and late medical therapy are usually required in *all* patients, including those treated surgically, to provide stabilization initially and to protect against redissection subsequently.

SURGICAL THERAPY. Although the precise timing of surgery in patients without life-threatening complications is somewhat controversial, prompt repair is generally recommended to prevent even minimal progression of the hematoma that might lead to further complications. Surgical risk for all patients is obviously increased by age; associated diseases, especially pulmonary emphysema; aneurysm leakage; cardiac tamponade; shock; or vital organ compromise, such as myocardial infarction, cerebrovascular accident, and particularly renal failure.[132]

As noted, the usual objectives of definitive surgical therapy are excision of the intimal tear and obliteration of entry into the false lumen by suturing together the edges of the dissected aorta proximally and distally. Aortic continuity is then reestablished either by joining the edges of the aorta directly or, more commonly, by interposing a prosthetic sleeve graft between the two ends of the aorta (Fig. 46–15). Determining the routes of perfusion of vital organs distal to the surgical site by angiography may be of importance. For example, one or both renal arteries occasionally are found to be fed from the false lumen, in which case the false channel in the distal end of the surgically transected aorta might be left unclosed

Miller et al. advocate a different philosophy with regard to dissections involving the proximal aorta (their Type A). In such patients, regardless of the site of the intimal tear, they recommend surgical repair of the proximal aorta to prevent proximal extension and rupture into the pericardial cavity.[132] This is their surgical policy even if the dissection originates in the distal aorta and extends proximally. Whether this is in fact the best approach is as yet unresolved.

When aortic regurgitation complicates aortic dissection, simple decompression of the false channel may be all that is necessary to resuspend the leaflets and restore valvular competence. However, most surgeons have become increasingly aggressive about replacing the aortic valve with a prosthesis if it appears that even moderate aortic regurgitation will be present after the leaflets are decompressed, thus avoiding the high risk of having to replace the aortic valve with a second operation through a diseased aorta at some later date.

For repair of a proximal dissection, total cardiopulmonary bypass is necessary. On occasion, because of extensive dissection of the aorta, it may be difficult to find a safe site for placement of a perfusion cannula. In rare cases, we have had to abandon plans for surgical repair of a proximal dissection for this reason. In the repair of dissections of the descending thoracic aorta, support of the distal circulation may be necessary and can be achieved either by partial left heart bypass or by using a conduit that carries blood from the proximal to the distal aorta, circumventing the site of the dissection.

The actual operative procedure itself, in aortic dissection, is technically demanding. The wall of the diseased aorta is often friable, and the repair must be performed with meticulous care. The use of Teflon felt to buttress the wall and prevent sutures from tearing through the fragile aorta has represented a significant technical advance (Fig. 46–15*B*). An alternate surgical approach consists of the wrapping of an unstable arch dissection with Dacron.[135] Bleeding, infection, and pulmonary or renal insufficiency constitute the most common early complications of surgical therapy. Spinal cord ischemia with resultant paraplegia due to inadvertent interruption of blood supply from the anterior spinal or intercostal arteries is a rare but dreaded consequence. Late complications include progressive aortic regurgitation if the aortic valve has not been replaced, localized aneurysm formation, and redissection at the original site of repair or at an independent secondary site.[136]

Several innovative techniques for high-risk patients have been reported. One utilizes an intraluminal sutureless prosthesis for patients with friable thoracic aortic tissue.[137]

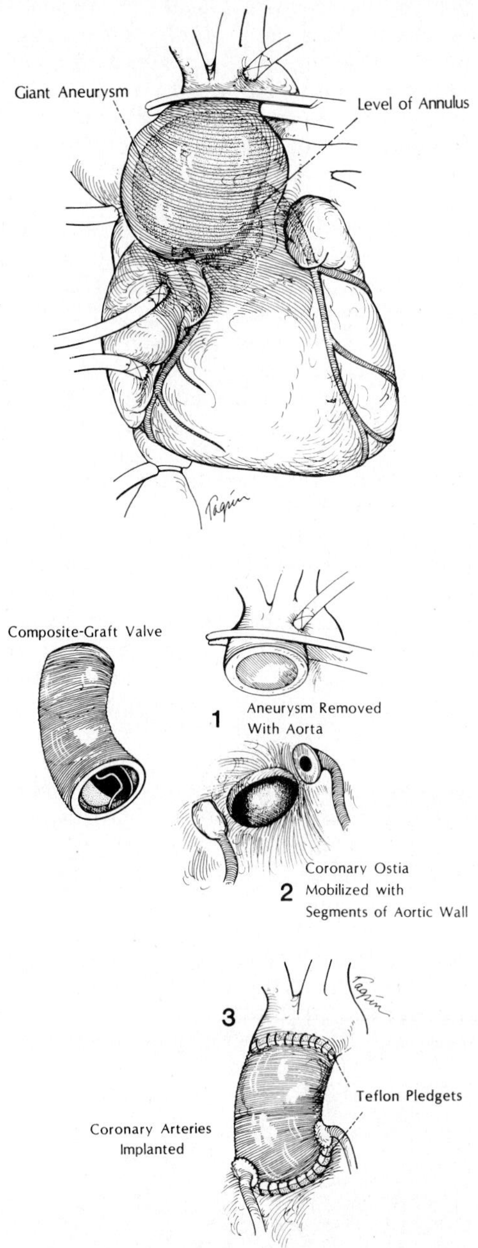

FIGURE 46–16. Technique for the composite graft replacement of an aneurysm of the ascending aorta. *Top*, The aneurysm is shown, involving the sinuses of Valsalva. The patient is on total cardiopulmonary bypass. *Bottom*, The composite graft is shown, with a low profile, tilting-disc prosthesis attached to its inferior end. (1) The aneurysm is resected with the aortic valve; (2) The coronary ostra have been excised, and mobilized with a button of aortic wall; (3) The composite graft has been secured into place using Teflon felt reinforcement for the suture line, and the coronary arteries have been reimplanted as the graft. In the method of Bentall, the composite graft is sewn inside the incised aneurysm, which is left in situ. The coronary ostra are then anastomosed directly to the graft.

The other, applied especially to distal but also to proximal dissection, consists of bypassing the dissected aorta with a Dacron sleeve, ligating the aorta at the site of proximal extension of the dissection, and creating reversal of flow in the distal aorta to perfuse the major arterial branches arising from the dissected segment.[138] Both techniques have been used in only small numbers of patients, and long-term follow-up is lacking.

In proximal dissection, when the aorta is fragile and badly torn, replacement of the aorta and the aortic valve using a composite graft into which the coronary arteries are reimplanted has been a valuable technique (Fig. 46–16).[63]

MEDICAL THERAPY. Indications for *definitive* medical therapy are summarized in Table 46–1. Clearly, operation must be performed if there is medical failure, such as rupture or impending rupture, progression of the dissection with vital organ compromise, aortic regurgitation, or inability to control pain or blood pressure with drugs. Although we prefer medical therapy for low-risk patients with stable distal dissection, some centers advise surgery in this group as well.[130, 136] Unfortunately, controlled studies of medically versus surgically treated patients with distal dissection and comparable surgical risks are lacking. Because of the extreme difficulty of the operation involved with aortic arch dissections, medical therapy is usually advocated in those rare dissections which originate in the arch, with operative intervention reserved for serious complications that might occur on medical treatment.

Medical therapy is recommended for patients with chronic dissection, defined as a stable aortic dissection that has occurred 2 or more weeks prior to presentation, unless, of course, aortic regurgitation related to the dissection becomes hemodynamically significant.

Complications of medical therapy include severe hypotension related to the drugs, with possible precipitation of acute tubular necrosis, cerebrovascular accident, or myocardial infarction.[131] Some of the drugs may cause somnolence and depression, and the specific side reactions and problems of each particular drug regimen must be anticipated.

Late follow-up of patients leaving the hospital with treated aortic dissection shows an actuarial survival rate not much worse than that of individuals of comparable age without dissection; there are no significant differences between patients with proximal vs. distal dissection, acute vs. chronic dissection, or medical vs. surgical treatment.[131] Thus, initially successful surgical or medical therapy for aortic dissection is usually sustained on long-term follow-up. Late complications include redissection, regurgitation, and localized saccular aneurysm formation.

Long-term medical therapy to control hypertension and reduce dV/dt is indicated for all patients who have sustained an aortic dissection, regardless of whether they have received definitive surgical or medical therapy. Systolic blood pressure should be controlled at or below a level of 130 to 140 mm Hg, or even lower if tolerated. Preferred agents are those with a negative inotropic as well as hypotensive effect, such as beta blockers, methyldopa, clonidine, or reserpine, together with a diuretic. Hydralazine and minoxidil increase cardiac output and arterial dV/dt and should be used only in the presence of adequate beta blockade. The value of calcium-channel blocking drugs in treating aortic dissection appears promising.[124, 125] Similarly, angiotensin-converting enzyme inhibitors (captopril and enalopril) are powerful hypotensive agents. Although there is as yet little or no experience with them in aortic dissection, they should also prove to be useful.

Follow-up of patients who have sustained an aortic dissection should include careful and repeated physical examinations; periodic chest roentgenograms, CT scans, or, when available, high-resolution digital subtraction angiography may also be useful in long-term follow-up for evidence of localized aortic aneurysm formation. MRI also promises to be a valuable tool for the follow-up of patients with aortic dissection, although long-term follow-up studies of this technique are not yet available.[9–12, 113]

ANNULOAORTIC ECTASIA

In a number of patients with pure aortic regurgitation the cause is idiopathic dilatation of the proximal aorta and the aortic annulus. The term annuloaortic ectasia was first used by Ellis et al. in 1961 to describe this clinicopathological condition.[139] The entity has been subsequently recognized with increasing frequency and makes up about 5 to 10 per cent of the population of patients who currently undergo aortic valve replacement for pure aortic regurgitation.

ETIOLOGY AND PATHOGENESIS. The common pathological feature shared by patients with annuloaortic ectasia is that of severe degenerative changes (usually cystic medial necrosis) in the wall of the afflicted aorta. Some degree of cystic medial necrosis with annuloaortic ectasia is found in virtually all cases of Marfan syndrome.[140, 141] In fact, it can be severe and is a frequent cause of death from fatal aortic rupture or dissection in this syndrome (p. 1725). There is some evidence to suggest that abnormalities in collagen cross linkage may play a role in this phenomenon,[142] while others have identified abnormalities in elastin in these patients.[143] In most reported series of patients with annuloaortic ectasia, however, patients with classic Marfan syndrome have been excluded. Careful examination of patients with this condition usually reveals that about one-fourth to one-half have other stigmata of Marfan syndrome, indicating that many patients represent a forme fruste of that connective tissue disorder. In a clinicogenetic study of 18 patients with severe aortic regurgitation and dilatation of the ascending aorta but without other evidence of the Marfan syndrome except on pathological examination of the aorta, Emanuel et al. reported that 37.3 per cent of 126 first-degree relatives whom they examined had one or more stigmata of Marfan syndrome.[144] Thus, it appears that many of these patients have primarily the aortic abnormalities of Marfan syndrome without the other manifestations of the disease. In summary, then, patients with annuloaortic ectasia appear to fall into three groups: (1) those with classic Marfan syndrome, (2) those with a forme fruste of Marfan syndrome, and (3) those with cystic medial necrosis and no obvious underlying cause.

As the media degenerates, the aorta widens. The aortic root is involved, and the annulus dilates, drawing the aortic leaflets apart and eventually making it impossible for the leaflet edges to meet in diastole; aortic regurgitation ensues. The weakened aorta may dissect and this may aggravate the aortic regurgitation.

CLINICAL MANIFESTATIONS. Men predominate over women in virtually all series by a ratio of anywhere between 2 and 8 to 1. Patients without obvious Marfan syndrome usually are encountered in the fourth, fifth, and sixth decades with progressively more severe aortic regurgitation. Patients with the classic Marfan syndrome or a forme fruste are generally younger. Some patients with annuloaortic ectasia experience sudden onset and rapid progression of symptoms, which sometimes but not always are due to severe aortic regurgitation secondary to aortic dissection. In the study of Lemon and White, recent aortic root dissection was found in 11 of 25 patients with annuloaortic ectasia who came to surgery.[145] All 11 of these patients had experienced chest pain before operation, although chest pain was also present in several patients without aortic dissection.

The physical examination may reveal abnormal pulsation of the dilated aorta over the 2nd and 3rd right intercostal spaces, especially if the examination is done with the patient sitting and in full expiration. We have seen three patients with annuloaortic ectasia who had pulsation of the right sternoclavicular joint.

There is nothing unique about the signs of aortic regurgitation in patients with annuloaortic ectasia as opposed to those with regurgitation from other causes, except for the greater intensity of the diastolic murmur to the right of the sternum in the former group and to the left in patients with a primary valvular abnormality. Lemon and White did find that the two features—acute or subacute development of symptoms and the presence of chest pain—were more frequent in the group of patients with annuloaortic ectasia than in those with pure valvular aortic regurgitation, presumably on a rheumatic basis.[145] Features of Marfan syndrome should be sought and may be obvious, subtle, or absent.

The chest film usually shows a grossly dilated aortic root and ascending aorta with left ventricular enlargement proportionate to the severity of aortic regurgitation. Calcification in the aortic valve and dilated aorta is usually absent. Echocardiography, CT scan, or MRI demonstrate an abnormally widened aortic root. The huge aorta and aortic regurgitation are easily demonstrated angiographically. Lemon and White identified three types of angiographic aortic enlargement: (1) "pear-shaped" enlargement (56 per cent) (Fig. 46–17), (2) diffuse symmetrical dilatation (27 per cent), and (3) dilatation limited to the sinuses of Valsalva (6 per cent).[146] In our own unpublished experience, aneurysmal dilatation of the sinuses of Valsalva is typically seen in those with Marfan syndrome. The mean maximal aortic diameter in Lemon and White's patients was 7.6 ± 2.7 cm and ranged from 4.8 to 15 cm. This is two to five times the normal aortic diameter. Because dissections are characteristically small, circumscribed, and confined to the ascending aorta, they may not be easy to identify angiographically.

MANAGEMENT. Surgical correction using total cardiopulmonary bypass is usually undertaken for relief of the aortic regurgitation when it is severe and responsible for symptoms of left ventricular failure or when the left ventricle or ascending aorta is increasing in size. However, in addition to replacing the aortic valve, resection of the aneurysmal aorta with insertion of a prosthetic (Dacron or Teflon) graft is generally required. Some surgeons advise sewing an artificial aortic valve to one end of a long prosthetic sleeve and suturing this in place from the aortic annulus at one end to the ascending aorta where it narrows

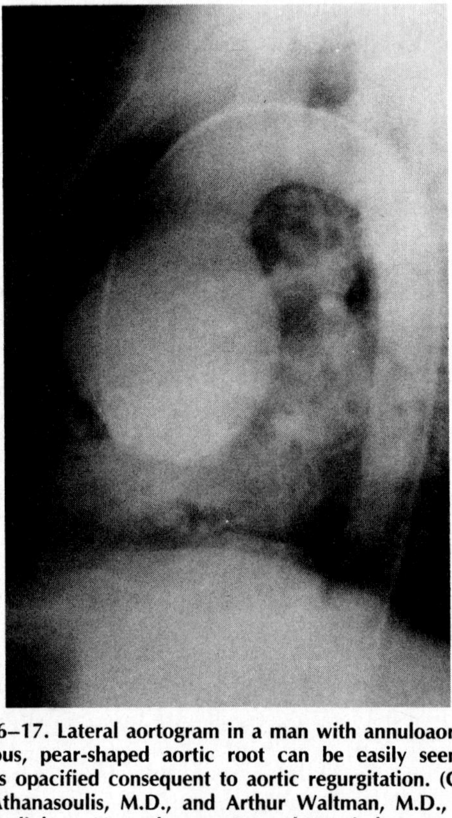

FIGURE 46–17. Lateral aortogram in a man with annuloaortic ectasia. The bulbous, pear-shaped aortic root can be easily seen. The left ventricle is opacified consequent to aortic regurgitation. (Courtesy of Christos Athanasoulis, M.D., and Arthur Waltman, M.D., Section of Vascular Radiology, Massachusetts General Hospital, Boston.)

beyond the aneurysm at the other. This reconstruction necessitates reimplantation of the coronary arteries (Fig. 46–16). In fact, with aneurysmal sinuses of Valsalva, the coronary ostia may be carried cephalad by the enlarging sinuses, again necessitating ligation and reimplantation of the coronary arteries or the construction of saphenous vein bypass conduits from the aorta to the ligated coronary arteries. Because of the magnitude of the operation and the frequently friable tissues that make operation difficult, the risks of failure of aortic valve replacement and aneurysm resection are between 10 and 15 per cent in most centers; 5- and 10-year survival rates have been reported at 77 per cent and 57 per cent, respectively.[147] Gott et al. reported a 90 per cent 8-year survival in 49 patients operated on for ascending aortic aneurysms associated with Marfan syndrome.[148] A recommendation for elective repair of the aorta in patients with Marfan syndrome and aortic root diameter greater than 6.0 cm was made.[148] However, this policy remains controversial.[149] The relative risk of dissection, based on aortic site, appears to be variable. In an echocardiographic study, 3 of 11 patients with annuloaortic ectasia developed dissection during a mean follow-up of 18 months. All three had aortic root diameters exceeding 5.0 cm; however, four other patients also had aortic diameters greater than 5.0 cm but dissection did not develop.[146]

Although postoperative results in survivors may be excellent, there is a disturbing occurrence of late sudden deaths, mostly from aortic dissection.[150] However, death from progressive heart failure and sudden cardiac deaths also occur.

AORTIC ARTERITIS SYNDROMES

Takayasu's Arteritis

This peculiar arteritis was first noted in 1908 by the Japanese ophthalmologist Takayasu, who described a young woman with cataracts and unusual wreathlike arteriovenous anastomoses surrounding the optic papillae. In discussing this case, Takayasu's colleagues called attention to two patients with similar ocular findings who also had absent radial pulses. Subsequently, this disease entity has been described by a variety of terms which reflect some of its many features, such as "aortic arch syndrome," "pulseless disease," "reversed coarctation," "occlusive thromboaortopathy," "young female arteritis," as well as Takayasu's arteritis.

DESCRIPTION, PATHOPHYSIOLOGY, AND ETIOLOGY. This disease occurs worldwide, although the majority of cases have been reported from Asia and Africa and most large series consist of Orientals, with a heavy predilection for women.[152]

The basic pathological process is that of marked intimal proliferation and fibrosis and fibrous scarring and degeneration of the elastic fibers of the media, with round cell infiltration of variable intensity. However, fibrosis predominates over cellular reaction. The adventitia and intima become markedly thickened and vasa vasorum are destroyed. In its advanced cicatricial stage, the gross appearance of the aorta strikingly resembles the tree-bark–like appearance of luetic aortitis. The proliferative process leads to obliterative luminal changes in the aorta and involved arteries. Localized aneurysm formation, poststenotic dilatation, and calcification in the aortic and arterial walls are late complications.[153] The process most often involves the arch of the aorta and its major branches, usually with changes that are most marked at the points of origin of the arteries from the aorta. It may present as multisegmental aortic disease with areas of normal wall between affected sites, diffuse involvement of the aorta, or predominantly disease of individual arteries arising from the aorta. The pulmonary arterial tree may also be affected. In a report from the United States, the most frequently affected arteries were the subclavian (90 per cent of cases), carotid (45 per cent), vertebral (25 per cent), and renal (20 per cent).[154] In another series from the United States, the subclavian arteries, mesenteric arteries, and abdominal aorta were most commonly involved, each in nearly 80 per cent of cases.[155]

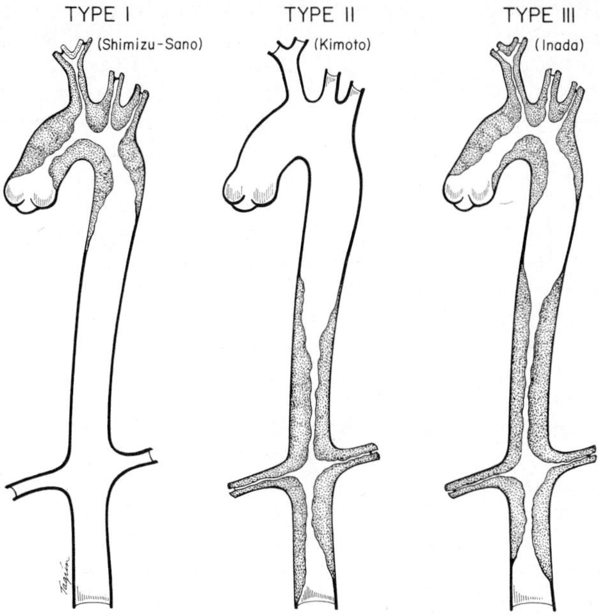

FIGURE 46–18. Types of Takayasu's arteritis. Type I involves primarily the aortic arch and brachiocephalic vessels. Type II affects the thoracoabdominal aorta and particularly the renal arteries. Type III combines features of both Types I and II. Types I and III may be complicated by aortic regurgitation. The eponyms for each type are noted.

Ueno et al. have subdivided the disease into three types, depending upon the sites of involvement[156] (Fig. 46–18). Type I involves primarily the aortic arch and its branches; Type II spares the aortic arch, involving the thoracoabdominal aorta and its branches; Type III combines features of both. Lupi-Herrera and colleagues have suggested a fourth category, Type IV, in which there is pulmonary arterial involvement.[152] In their series of 107 cases, the incidences of the various types were 8, 11, 65, and 45 per cent for Types I, II, III, and IV, respectively (including several patients in the other groups).

A specific etiology for Takayasu's arteritis has not been forthcoming.[154] It has been linked to rheumatic fever, streptococcal infections, rheumatoid arthritis, and other collagen vascular diseases. Although giant cells are occasionally found in pathological specimens of vessels involved by the disease, the entity seems clearly distinct from giant cell arteritis, which affects predominantly patients over the age of 50 and involves mainly medium-sized muscular arteries. Although the aortic scarring of advanced Takayasu's arteritis resembles that of syphilis, nothing else suggests a causal relationship. Some investigators have reported a strikingly higher incidence of tuberculin skin reactivity to both *Mycobacterium tuberculosis* and atypical mycobacteria in patients with Takayasu's arteritis compared with the general population, raising the possibility of a relationship to tuberculosis,[157] but this observation has not been confirmed.[155] Although antiaortic antibodies have been detected in patients with this disease, their etiological role is uncertain. Overall, the bulk of evidence favors an autoimmune etiology. It is likely that the arteritis represents the final common pathological expression of a number of different antigenic stimuli in susceptible patients. An association between Takayasu's arteritis and certain HLA subtypes has been reported,[158] although the importance of the association remains unclear.[154, 155]

CLINICAL MANIFESTATIONS. The disease affects women more frequently than men, in a ratio of 8 to 1. In as many as three-fourths of cases, onset is in the teenage years, although cases beginning in infancy or late middle age have been reported.[152, 160, 161] More than half the patients with this disease develop an initial systemic illness characterized by symptoms such as fever, anorexia, malaise, weight loss, night sweats, arthralgias, pleuritic pain, and fatigue. Localized pain and tenderness may be noted over affected arteries. This phase subsides, and these patients—as well as those who do not go through this so-called initial "systemic phase"—after a latent period of variable duration show symptoms and signs referable to the obliterative and inflammatory changes in the vessels. These late manifestations include diminished or absent pulses in 96 per cent, bruits in 94 per cent, hypertension in 74 per cent, and heart failure in 28 per cent.[152] The retinopathy originally described by Takayasu is seen in only about 25 per cent and is usually associated with carotid arterial involvement. The ocular process may lead to retinal detachment and loss of vision.

Patients with Types I and III manifest those findings which are considered to be most typical of this disease, namely "reversed" coarctation of the aorta with absent or diminished upper body pulses and barely detectable blood pressure in the arms, higher pressures in the lower extremities, bruits overlying diseased arteries, manifestations of ischemia at various affected sites, and syncope. Patients with Type II arteritis may have abdominal angina and claudication of the limbs but also tend to develop hypertension because of renal arterial involvement. In fact, hypertension is an extremely important complication of this disease, and it may be difficult to recognize because of the diminished pulsations in the arms. Hypertension appears to arise through several mechanisms, the two most important of which are hemodynamically significant acquired coarctation of the aorta and renal artery stenosis. Decreased aortic capacitance and reduced baroreceptor reactivity may be contributory.[162, 163]

Heart failure, when present, is usually seen in very young patients and appears to be a consequence of systemic hypertension. Rarely, aortic regurgitation can also contribute to congestive failure and is due to severe hypertension or to inflammation with scarring of the aortic valve by the inflammatory process.[164] The ostia and proximal segments of the coronary arteries can be affected, resulting in angina or myocardial infarction.[165] Rarely, aneurysms are palpable or arteriovenous fistulas occur.[160] Takayasu's arteritis may be a common cause of atypical coarctation syndromes in adults.[166] The frequent absence of antecedent systemic symptoms and the more equal sex distribution of this form of the disease have been stressed. It is also believed that Takayasu's arteritis may be responsible for some cases of what appear to be primary pulmonary hypertension.[167]

Laboratory abnormalities during the systemic phase are frequent.[155, 157] The sedimentation rate is elevated, and a low-grade leukocytosis and mild anemia of chronic disease are common. These return toward normal when the systemic phase resolves. IgG or IgM values are elevated in more than half the patients. Immune complexes are infrequently present.[154] Other serological abnormalities are common but not specific. These include elevated levels of C-reactive protein, increased antistreptolysin-O titers, the occasional presence of rheumatoid factor and antinuclear antibodies, and elevated fibrinogen levels.[168]

Chest roentgenograms are usually unrevealing, although a rim of calcification is sometimes seen in the walls of the affected arteries. Arteriography reveals typical findings of an irregular intimal surface, with stenosis of the aorta or its tributary arteries, poststenotic dilatations, saccular aneurysms, and even complete occlusion of vessels (Fig. 46–19). Lande and Rossi have described the affected thoracic aorta as having a typical, narrowed, "rat-tail" angiographic appearance (Fig. 46–20).[169]

TREATMENT AND PROGNOSIS. Adrenal corticosteroids are often effective in relieving constitutional symptoms and

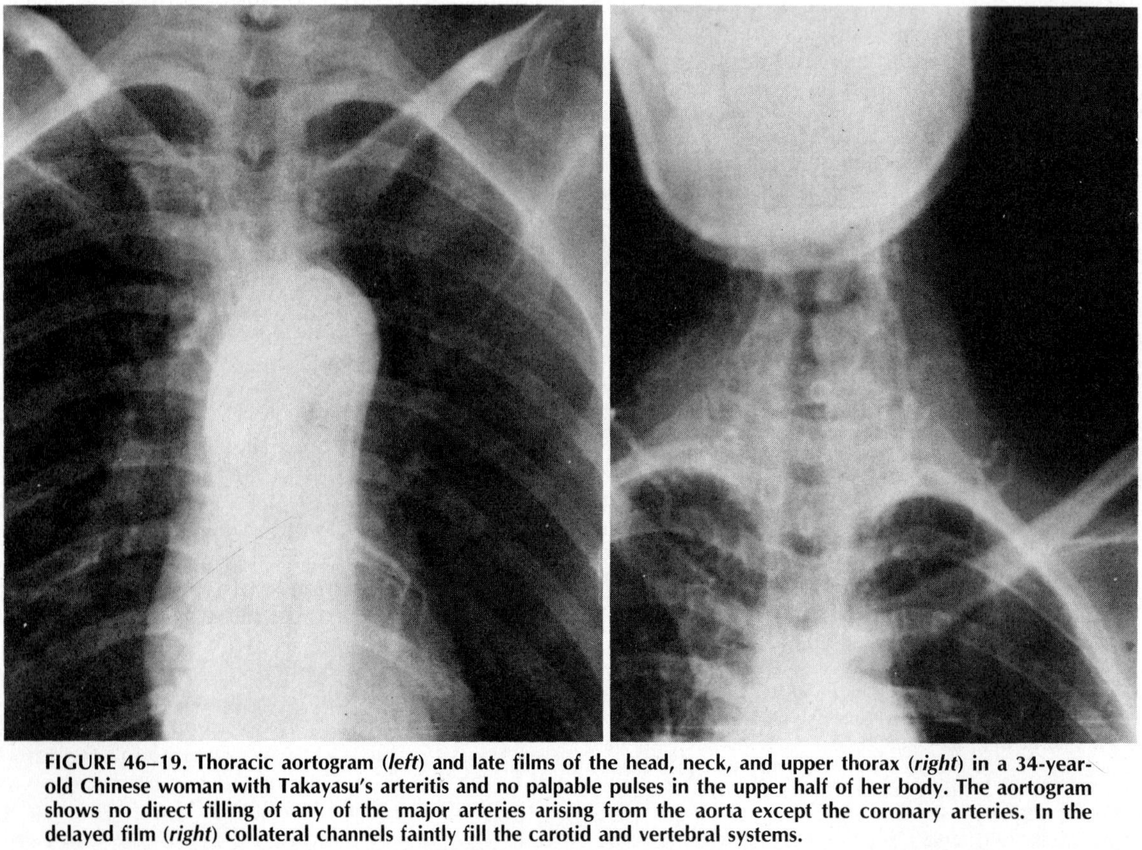

FIGURE 46–19. Thoracic aortogram (*left*) and late films of the head, neck, and upper thorax (*right*) in a 34-year-old Chinese woman with Takayasu's arteritis and no palpable pulses in the upper half of her body. The aortogram shows no direct filling of any of the major arteries arising from the aorta except the coronary arteries. In the delayed film (*right*) collateral channels faintly fill the carotid and vertebral systems.

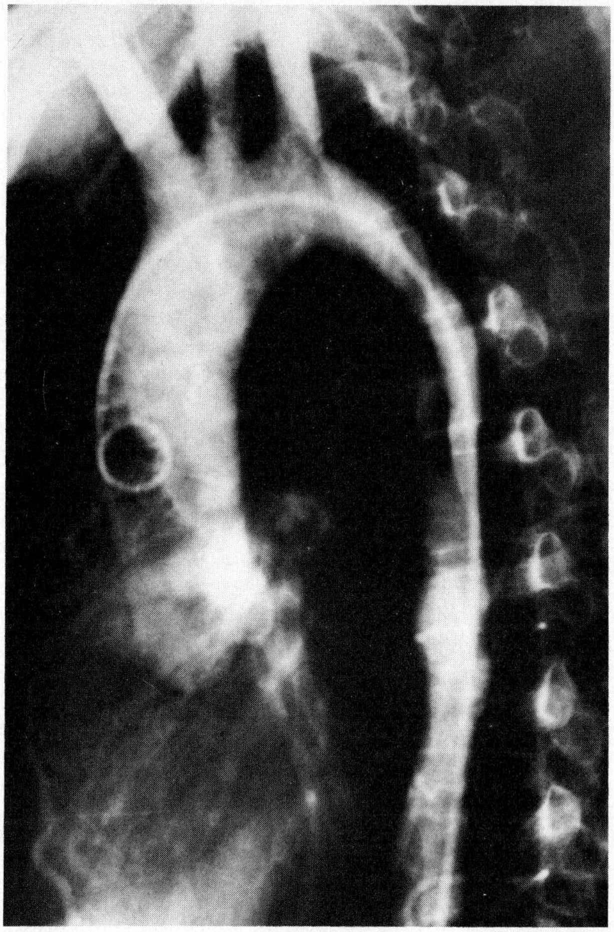

FIGURE 46–20. Aortogram in a 28-year-old Korean man with the clinical features of coarctation of the aorta that proved to be the result of Takayasu's arteritis. Note the typical "rat-tail" angiographic appearance of the descending thoracic aorta.

halting disease progression in patients with the systemic phase of the disease.[154, 155] Fever, malaise, and fatigue are often dramatically relieved by steroids, and the sedimentation rate, which is a sensitive indicator of the activity of the disease, falls toward normal. In patients with continued systemic symptoms and/or documented disease progression, cyclophosphamide can be added. This usually results in clinical improvement and the ability to reduce corticosteroids to every other day dosing.[156] The recommended dose of cyclophosphamide is 2 mg/kg/day, adjusted to maintain the peripheral leukocyte count above 3000/mm^3. Anticoagulant drugs, including those of the warfarin family, and drugs that inhibit platelet function, such as aspirin and dipyridamole, are recommended both to treat transient ischemic symptoms and to prevent progression of the disease. Their efficacy is not established. Aggressive treatment of hypertension, when present, is important. In cases related to renovascular disease, the angiotensin-converting enzyme inhibitors may be particularly effective.[170, 170a] A variety of *surgical treatments* may be needed to deal with late complications of Takayasu's arteritis,[154, 155, 171, 172, 172a] including endarterectomy, bypass of obstructed arteries (especially the renal arteries), resection of localized coarctations, excision of saccular aneurysms, and, rarely, aortic valve replacement. Successful use of percutaneous transluminal angioplasty for dilation of stenotic lesions in carotid, subclavian, renal, and mesenteric arteries has also been reported.[155, 173]

The course of the disease is unpredictable, but slow progression over a period of months to years is usual. Morbidity and mortality depend upon the presence or absence of severe complications, which include retinopathy, secondary hypertension, aortic regurgitation, and aortic or arterial aneurysms. In one series, uneventful survival over 7 years was 97 per cent in patients without major complications compared with 59 per cent in patients with complications.[174] Heart failure and cerebrovascular accidents are common causes of death. However, the combination of corticosteroid therapy, cytotoxic agents, and surgery when needed have led to 5-year survival rates that now may approximate 100 per cent.[154, 155]

GIANT CELL ARTERITIS

This disease of unknown cause is predominantly found in elderly people and characteristically involves medium-sized arteries. However, the aorta and its major branches are affected in about 15 per cent of cases.[175] The disease is also referred to as "granulomatous arteritis," "cranial" or "temporal" arteritis, and "arteritis of the aged." It is closely allied to a syndrome characterized by diffuse muscular aching and stiffness called polymyalgia rheumatica.

PATHOPHYSIOLOGY AND ETIOLOGY. The many names given this disease describe its important features. The characteristic pathological lesion that distinguishes it from other arteritis syndromes is granulomatous inflammation of the media of small- to medium-caliber arteries, about the size of the temporal artery, with special predilection for vessels of the head and neck.[175a] In addition to granulomas, an inflammatory infiltrate is usually found, composed largely of eosinophils, plasma cells, and other mononuclear cells. Endarteritis is not an important feature, but the mural involvement can lead to obstruction of involved arteries. Rarely, the aortic wall may be weakened by the inflammatory process, leading to localized aneurysm formation, aortic annular dilatation, and aortic regurgitation.[176]

Involvement of the aorta[176b] and its major tributaries, when it occurs, usually coexists with the more classic and prevalent syndromes of temporal arteritis and polymyalgia rheumatica although the aorta may rarely serve as the primary target of this disease.

The etiology of giant cell arteritis is unknown, although the generalized systemic manifestations of the disease and its occasional apparent temporal relationship to prior immunization or a viral illness suggest a possible infectious or autoimmune origin.[177] Klein et al. point out that involvement of aorta and larger arteries may often arise as corticosteroid therapy for the more classic forms of this disease is being tapered.[175]

CLINICAL MANIFESTATIONS. Giant cell arteritis typically affects patients over the age of 50 and occurs predominantly in women. The classic presentation is a triad of severe headache, marked malaise, and fever. Other constitutional symptoms are common and include anorexia, weight loss, lassitude, myalgias, and night sweats. Headaches are often intense and almost unbearable. Headache typically occurs over involved arteries, usually the temporal arteries but occasionally the occipital region. The area around the arteries is exquisitely sensitive to pressure, and complaints such as being unable to rest the head comfortably against a pillow, wear a hat, or comb one's hair are common. Claudication in the jaw muscles while chewing occurs in up to two-thirds of patients and is considered most suggestive of the diagnosis.[178] A serious complication that may occur anywhere in the course of the disease is the onset of blindness from involvement of the ophthalmic artery—blindness that is often irreversible. Visual symptoms ranging from blurring to diplopia and visual loss occur in 25 to 50 per cent of patients.[178] In its milder forms, patients may complain only of generalized muscular aches and pains and unusual fatigue, the syndrome of polymyalgia rheumatica. Blindness in these cases is uncommon. Polymyalgia rheumatica is seen in nearly 40 per cent of patients with giant cell arteritis.[179, 180]

On rare occasions, consequences of involvement of the aorta or its major tributaries may be the first manifestations of the disease, although more typically, when such involvement occurs, it is part of the more generalized syndrome. However, when aortic or major branch disease is present, the symptoms are similar to those of Takayasu's arteritis and are the result of ischemia in the structures supplied by the involved arteries. Specifically, symptoms may include claudication of either upper or lower extremities, paresthesias, Raynaud's phenomenon, abdominal angina, coronary ischemia, transient cerebral ischemic attacks, and aortic arch and great vessel "steal" syndromes. More rarely, aortic aneurysms, aortic regurgitation, and aortic dissection may occur.[181] Interestingly, renal artery involvement is almost never seen, in contrast with Takayasu's arteritis.[175] Rarely, death can occur from aortic rupture or dissection.

On *physical examination*, fever is almost universal and patients appear ill. Involved vessels are thickened and very tender. Indeed, an experienced examiner can make the diagnosis of temporal arteritis with virtual certainty at the bedside simply by palpating an indurated, beaded, tender, temporal artery. Pulses may be lost, and bruits may occur over sites of arterial occlusion. Signs of aortic regurgitation are rarely present.

Laboratory tests may be helpful in making the diagnosis. A very high sedimentation rate is virtually a sine qua non for this disease and is a valuable guide to the activity of the process. A moderate normochromic, normocytic anemia is the rule. Acute phase reactants such as alpha$_2$ globulin are increased, and IgG and C3, and C4 (complement) levels are often elevated.[182]

The *diagnosis* is confirmed by biopsy of an involved artery, usually the temporal artery. In cases of larger vessel and aortic involvement, angiography may serve to differentiate arteritis from arteriosclerosis by the following features, as described by Klein et al.: (1) long, smooth, tapering stenosis alternating with segments of normal or even slightly increased diameter; (2) the absence of irregular ulcerated atheromatous plaques seen in profile; and (3) the more typical anatomical distribution of arteritis to include the subclavian, axillary, and brachial arteries.[175]

MANAGEMENT. High-dose steroid therapy, e.g., 60 to 80 mg of prednisone per day, is recommended in all patients with granulomatous arteritis. The intent of therapy is not only to reverse the disease but also to prevent progression, especially in the ophthalmic arteries in order to prevent blindness. With constitutional symptoms and the sedimentation rate used as a guide, steroids can usually be reduced gradually to a maintenance dose of 5 to 15 mg/day (or every other day) for 1 to 2 years. The overall course is one of progressive improvement and eventual complete resolution. However, in many patients, the course of the disease may be protracted for months or years. Very rarely, surgical resection of an expanding aneurysm or replacement of a regurgitant aortic valve is necessary.[176, 181]

OTHER ARTERITIS SYNDROMES

In addition to the aortic inflammation of Takayasu's and giant cell arteritis, isolated aortic regurgitation due to dilatation of the aortic valve ring with associated aortic root involvement may occur during the course of ankylosing spondylitis, psoriatic arthritis, arthritis associated with ulcerative colitis, relapsing polychondritis, and Reiter's syndrome (Chap. 54).[183–185] In addition, aneurysms of the aorta, pulmonary artery, and other major vessels can complicate Behçet's syndrome.[186]

Reported instances of aortitis complicating each of these diseases are rare. For example, it is seen in 1 to 4 per cent of patients with ankylosing spondylitis (p. 1713), and only a small number of well-described cases of Reiter's syndrome with aortic regurgitation have been documented (p. 1714). Nevertheless, the symptoms of aortic regurgitation and resultant heart failure may eventually dominate the clinical picture. In each case of arthritis-associated aortitis, the underlying arthritic disease is particularly fulminant and prolonged, and multiple extraarticular features are usually manifest.

PATHOLOGICAL FEATURES. These appear to be similar in each of the above diseases. In the early stages of inflammation there is marked dilatation of the aortic valve ring with patchy elastic tissue disruption, an active inflammatory cell infiltrate, and subendothelial fibrosis.[183] These changes are most marked in the aortic root. Later, the proximal ascending aorta appears similar to that in luetic aortitis, with intimal thickening, coarse granular plaque formation, and characteristic obliterative endarteritis of the vasa vasorum. The aortic root dilates but usually without frank aneurysm formation. Early, the aortic valve cusps remain essentially normal and later become thickened and retracted, presumably as a result of the incompetence that arises from root dilatation. Echocardiographic data suggest that patients with subclinical aortitis may be identified by the presence of subaortic fibrous ridging or marked leaflet thickening, even when aortic root dimensions are normal.[187]

The clinical features are those of aortic regurgitation and resemble those of annuloaortic ectasia. However, it is worth noting that the course of this disease is variable. Some patients exhibit a rapid progressive course of cardiac decompensation, whereas others have a more indolent and stable natural history. Thus, the development of aortic regurgitation does not necessarily signify an irreversible downhill course. There is some evidence that the inflammation of the aortic root may be episodic; worsening of aortic regurgitation may also pursue an intermittent course.

Treatment consists of that required for the underlying arthritis or other disease. Aortic valve replacement should be performed when indicated, although special problems may be encountered in these patients. For example, pulmonary function is often impaired in ankylosing spondylitis as a result of rigidity of the thoracic spine and chest wall. In the rare patient with ulcerative colitis who requires aortic valve replacement, a porcine valve is recommended so that anticoagulation will be unnecessary. In contrast to annuloaortic ectasia, replacement of the ascending aorta itself is almost never necessary.

CARDIOVASCULAR SYPHILIS

Once accounting for 5 to 10 per cent of all cardiovascular deaths, syphilitic disease of the heart and aorta has become a relative rarity in most major medical centers today as a result of aggressive antibiotic treatment of lues in its early stages. Cardiovascular complications occur in approximately 10 per cent of cases of untreated lues. The latent period may extend from 5 to 40 years after the initial spirochetal infection, with a usual time of 10 to 25 years.

PATHOLOGY. The consequences of lues are the direct results of spirochetal infection of the aortic media, thought to occur usually during the secondary phase of the disease, with subsequent inflammation and scarring of the aortic wall. Although the aorta may be invaded anywhere along its course, the most common location is the ascending aorta. It is postulated that this area has a proclivity for syphilitic involvement because it is richer in lymphatics than any other portion of the aorta. The muscular and elastic tissues of the media are destroyed by the spirochetes and the resultant inflammatory process and are replaced by vascular fibrous tissue.

The aortic wall becomes progressively weakened by the inflammatory process, and it may become calcified. Such weakening leads to aneurysmal dilatation. The overlying intima becomes furrowed and wrinkled and is covered with large plaques of a glistening, pearly material. This accounts for the "tree-bark" appearance of the involved aorta characteristic of luetic aortitis.

The infection may extend into the aortic root, resulting in aortic regurgitation due to dilatation of the aortic annulus and separation of the aortic valve commissures. Luetic aortic regurgitation is usually associated with an aortic aneurysm. An obliterative endarteritis may also obstruct the ostia of the coronary arteries. The scarring and injury from lues may progress long after the spirochetal organisms have been eradicated.

There are four categories of syphilitic heart disease[188]: (1) uncomplicated syphilitic aortitis, (2) syphilitic aortic aneurysm, (3) syphilitic aortic valvulitis with aortic regurgitation, and (4) syphilitic coronary ostial stenosis. Based on autopsy studies, about one-third of patients with cardiovascular lues are "asymptomatic," i.e., they have postmortem pathological evidence of luetic involvement of the aortic wall without clinical manifestations. About half have a significant aortic aneurysm, and, of these, one-half to one-third have associated aortic regurgitation. Five to 10 per cent will have essentially pure aortic regurgitation, and 26 per cent will have significant luetic coronary ostial stenosis, often in association with aortic regurgitation or an aortic aneurysm.

CLINICAL MANIFESTATIONS. Luetic aneurysms can arise anywhere along the aorta (including the abdomen[189]), but the most typical location is in the ascending aorta. They are usually saccular but may be fusiform. In the absence of aortic regurgitation, aneurysms may undergo significant enlargement without producing symptoms. Eventually, an aneurysm may expand enough to reach, compress, and even erode contiguous structures, particularly the sternum and anterior right thoracic cage in the case of aneurysms of the ascending aorta. A thrusting, pulsating mass may be seen and palpated. Erosion of the bony structures of the chest wall causes pain at the point of involvement. Ascending aortic aneurysms and those involving the arch may produce a tracheal tug, stridor, and dysphagia. Aneurysms elsewhere may cause symptoms from compression of adjacent structures similar to those of any type of aneurysm located in the same area, such as hoarseness from compression of the left recurrent laryngeal nerve and cough from pressure against the left main stem bronchus in the case of aneurysms of the descending thoracic aorta.

Luetic aortic regurgitation tends to occur in older patients with luetic cardiovascular disease, presumably because the disease has been present longer in these individuals.[190] The earliest auscultatory sign of luetic aortic valve involvement is a tambour-like aortic closure sound. Because of the dilated aortic root, the murmur of luetic aortic regurgitation may be more prominent along the right sternal edge rather than the left, which is usually the case with rheumatic aortic regurgitation. It is often musical in quality and in rare instances of aortic cusp eversion may be particularly loud, with an associated thrill.

Because there is often considerable calcification in the aortic annulus, stiffness of the base of the aortic leaflets, and usually a dilated proximal aorta, a loud systolic ejection murmur, sometimes with a thrill, is often present in luetic aortic valve disease in the absence of any significant aortic stenosis. Also, a loud, slapping systolic ejection sound is sometimes caused by sudden distention of the dilated aorta in early systole.

Luetic aortic regurgitation is often associated with an aneurysm of the ascending aorta. Because of concomitant coronary ostial stenosis, angina pectoris may be particularly troublesome. Atrial fibrillation is seen more commonly than in other types of pure aortic regurgitation. Otherwise, the signs and symptoms are typical for those of aortic regurgitation.

DIAGNOSIS. Usually, there is a history of syphilis, and other manifestations of tertiary lues are found in 10 to 30 per cent of patients with cardiovascular syphilis. Fifteen to 30 per cent of patients have negative routine serological tests for syphilis (Wasserman, Hinton, Kahn, Venereal Disease Research Laboratories [VDRL], and Kolmer). On the other hand, serological tests directed against a specific treponema antigen, such as the *Treponema pallidum* immobilization (TPI) test or the fluorescent treponemal antibody absorption (FTA-ABS) test, are almost invariably positive. The chest roentgenogram may afford extremely valuable clues to the diagnosis of luetic aortitis. In sharp contrast to arteriosclerosis, calcification in the ascending aorta proximal to the brachiocephalic vessels is almost always much more extensive than that elsewhere.

Angiography may delineate the aneurysm (Fig. 46–21) and help to quantify the severity of aortic regurgitation. In patients suspected of having coronary ostial stenosis and in any patient with cardiovascular syphilis in whom surgical correction is contemplated, the coronary artery anatomy—and particularly the ostia—should be visualized by angiography if possible.

TREATMENT. All patients with syphilis, including cardiovascular syphilis, who are seen 1 year or more after the

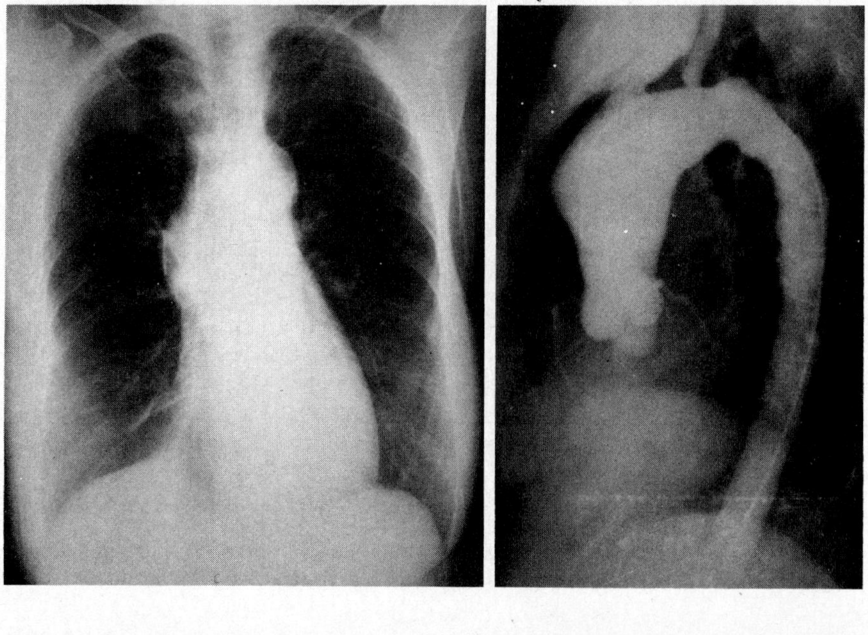

FIGURE 46–21. Films obtained from a 58-year-old woman with luetic aortitis. *Left,* Posteroanterior chest film showing an aneurysm of the ascending aorta with a faint rim of calcification. *Right,* Angiographic appearance of the aneurysm in the lateral view. (Courtesy of Christos Athanasoulis, M.D., and Arthur Waltman, M.D., Section of Vascular Radiology, Massachusetts General Hospital, Boston.)

initial contact should be given a course of antibiotic therapy aimed at curing the spirochetal infection. Penicillin is still the most effective antibiotic and is given as benzathine penicillin G (Bicillin), 2.4 million units intramuscularly weekly for 3 weeks (total of 7.2 million units). For patients allergic to penicillin, the recommended therapy is tetracycline, 500 mg orally four times daily for 30 days. In penicillin-allergic patients who cannot tolerate tetracycline, the penicillin allergy should be confirmed. In such patients, the alternative regimen is erythromycin, 500 mg orally four times daily for 30 days. Compliance and serological follow-up must be confirmed, especially with the latter regimen.[191] The effectiveness of treatment can be monitored by a decrease in VDRL titer, with the desired result being a fourfold reduction in titer in 12 to 24 months.

Although a course of antibiotics is recommended in any previously untreated patient with cardiovascular syphilis, even those with a negative serology, there is no good evidence that such treatment reverses, or even halts, the progression of aortitis or aortic regurgitation. In cases of cardiovascular syphilis, cerebrospinal fluid examination should also be performed, and, if positive, this too should be followed to assure the adequacy of therapy. Since the efficacy of antibiotics other than penicillin against syphilis is not well studied beyond 1 year, close follow-up of patients treated with these alternative modes is necessary.

Indications for excision of the luetic aneurysms are similar to those for other thoracic aortic aneurysms (p. 1553): a diameter of 7 cm or larger or an aneurysm of any size that produces symptoms or is expanding rapidly. Since many luetic aneurysms are saccular, aneurysmorrhaphy is occasionally adequate. However, since ongoing aortitis and scarring are possible, it is probably wiser to replace as much as possible of the diseased aorta with a prosthetic graft. Prosthetic replacement of the aortic valve is indicated for significant aortic regurgitation, and the results are as good as in aortic regurgitation of other causes. Since the coronary artery disease of syphilis is usually ostial, a localized endarterectomy at the orifices of the coronary arteries may be possible. If an adequate lumen cannot be obtained by endarterectomy, bypass may be necessary.[192]

PSEUDOCOARCTATION

Pseudocoarctation of the aorta is a rare condition resulting from elongation of the aortic arch, with redundancy and kinking of the aorta just distal to the origin of the left subclavian artery at the level of the ligamentum arteriosum.[193, 194] Other terms used to describe this entity have included "mild coarctation," "atypical coarctation," or "subclinical coarctation." The etiology is believed to be congenital, with a lack of compression and fusion of certain of the segments of the dorsal aortic root and fourth arch.[195] It is of interest that the incidence and distribution of associated cardiac anomalies parallel those seen in true coarctation. These anomalies include bicuspid aortic valve, sinus of Valsalva aneurysms, ventricular septal defect, corrected transposition, and Turner syndrome.[196, 196a]

CLINICAL MANIFESTATIONS. The pressure gradient across the deformed area is usually trivial or absent. Thus, the clinical features of true coarctation—upper extremity hypertension, lower extremity hypotension, and the development of collateral arterial circulation—are absent. Physical findings are often those of the associated lesions, although a murmur is sometimes heard over the aortic kink in the interscapular area. With mild degrees of obstruction, blood pressure in the lower extremities may be slightly reduced, and there may be a subtle pulse lag between the radial and femoral arteries.

The entity can usually be recognized on chest roentgenography. The typical appearance is that of a double, rounded density in the left superior mediastinum. Pitfalls in interpreting the x-ray films are common. The upper density, though relatively translucent, represents the uppermost extension of redundant aorta and is often mistaken for tumor or aneurysm. The lower density is the area of the aorta involved by poststenotic dilatation, and it is often misinterpreted as the aortic knob. Calcification may occur in the area of narrowing. Angiography confirms the diagnosis.

SIGNIFICANCE. Problems may arise in pseudocoarctation from the formation of aneurysms either proximal or distal to the kink (Fig. 46–22). Associated aneurysms of the left subclavian artery have been

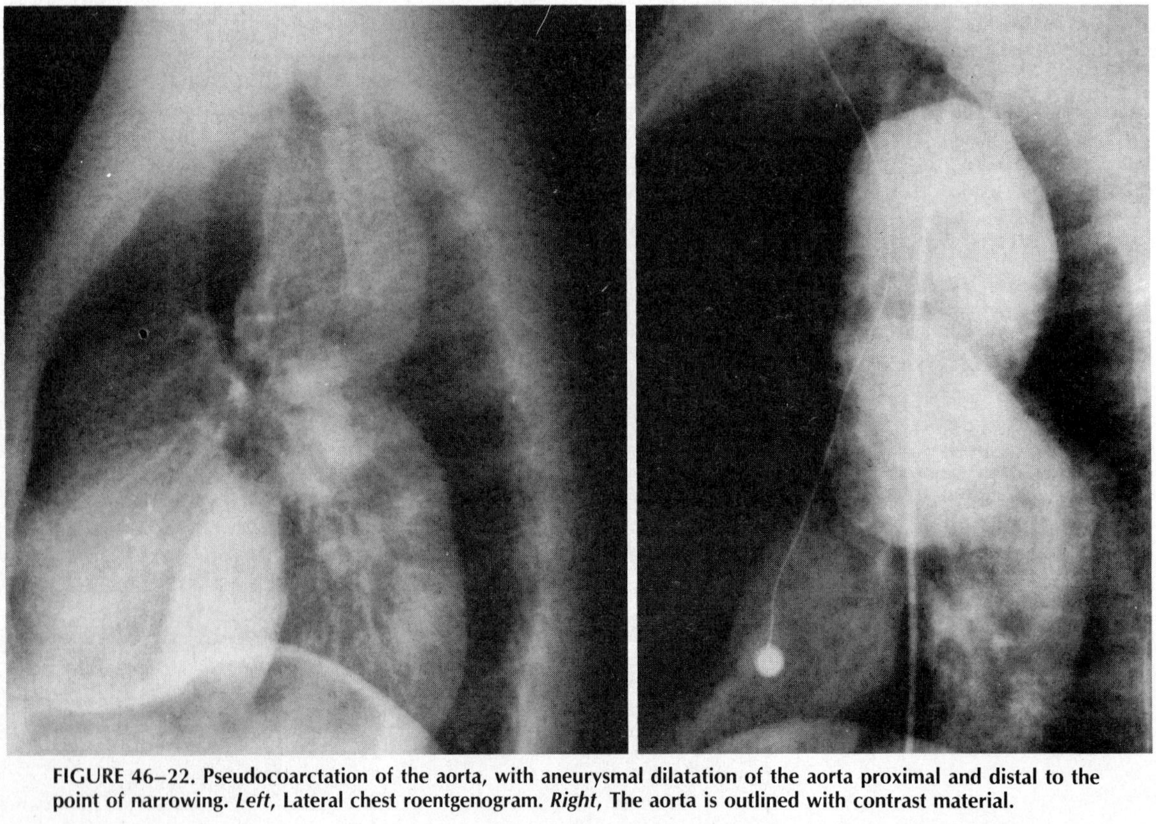

FIGURE 46–22. Pseudocoarctation of the aorta, with aneurysmal dilatation of the aorta proximal and distal to the point of narrowing. ***Left,*** Lateral chest roentgenogram. ***Right,*** The aorta is outlined with contrast material.

reported.[197] Rarely, thrombus forms at the site of atheromatous degeneration and calcification in the kinked segment.[198] Complete thrombosis can produce a picture mimicking true coarctation, although collateral arterial circulation is notably absent. Thrombus can also propagate directly into tributary vessels or embolize distally. The left subclavian artery is particularly vulnerable because of its proximity to the pseudocoarctation. Infection at the site of aortic narrowing is a rare problem.

TREATMENT. Therapy is necessary only for complications of pseudocoarctation. In the absence of complications, surgical resection is not indicated.[199] If a bruit or pressure gradient is present over an area of pseudocoarctation, antibiotic prophylaxis for endocarditis should be given before dental or surgical procedures.

AORTIC TRAUMA

(See also p. 1543)

BLUNT TRAUMA

Aortic injuries are associated with severe blunt trauma,[199a] and they are far from rare. In one autopsy series of fatal automobile accidents, rupture of the aorta was found in one-sixth of all victims.[200]

ETIOLOGY AND PATHOGENESIS. Aortic trauma most commonly results from injuries associated with sudden high-speed deceleration upon impact, such as that resulting from motor vehicle accidents, blast injuries, cave-ins, crush injuries, or severe falls.[200–202] The abrupt deceleration of the body as it crashes to a sudden stop creates enormous shearing forces which act maximally at those points where a highly mobile portion of the aorta joins a fixed segment. Less frequently, pressure or blast injuries may produce rupture of the aorta, believed to be caused by an acute increase in intraaortic pressure generated by the compression of blood contained within the aorta and further increased by the force imparted by cardiac systole.

Although the aorta may be torn anywhere along its length, the most frequent point of rupture (the site in 90 per cent of cases) is in the aortic isthmus at the site of insertion of the ligamentum arteriosum, just distal to the origin of the left subclavian artery. Here, the relatively mobile descending thoracic aorta sweeps dorsally to become fixed to the thoracic cage by the ligamentum arteriosum, the intercostal arteries, and the left subclavian artery. The injury may vary from a minuscule rent in the aortic wall to a complete circumferential transection of all three layers of the aorta. In a series of 296 cases of aortic trauma studied by Parmley et al., a circumferential tear was evident in 80 per cent.[201] If the aorta is partially transected and the patient survives, a localized saccular aneurysm or pseudoaneurysm may subsequently develop at the site of the tear. Pseudoaneurysms may also form between the two ends of a totally transected aorta.

In addition to the aortic isthmus, other areas of injury include the supravalvular portion of the ascending aorta; the innominate artery, which may be avulsed from the aorta; the aortic arch; other portions of the descending thoracic aorta; the abdominal aorta; and combinations of these.[203]

CLINICAL MANIFESTATIONS. The diagnosis of aortic trauma is often obscured by the presence of other serious injuries, such as central nervous system damage, visceral injury, and multiple skeletal fractures.[204] About two-thirds of patients with aortic rupture have clear-cut evidence of other thoracic trauma, such as chest or cardiac contusions, rib or vertebral fractures, pulmonary contusions, and hemorrhagic pleural effusions. The remaining one-third are surprisingly free of overt evidence of chest-wall injury.[205]

Few symptoms are directly attributable to the aortic trauma per se. Pressure from a localized hematoma can cause dyspnea and stridor from tracheal or bronchial compression, dysphagia from esophageal compression, or superior vena caval syndrome from caval compression. Although it is uncommon, the syndrome of so-called "acute coarctation" with upper extremity hypertension, reduced blood pressure in the lower extremities, a systolic murmur over the precordium or in the interscapular area, and a palpable radial-femoral pulse lag is virtually classic for the diagnosis. An interscapular systolic bruit may be heard.

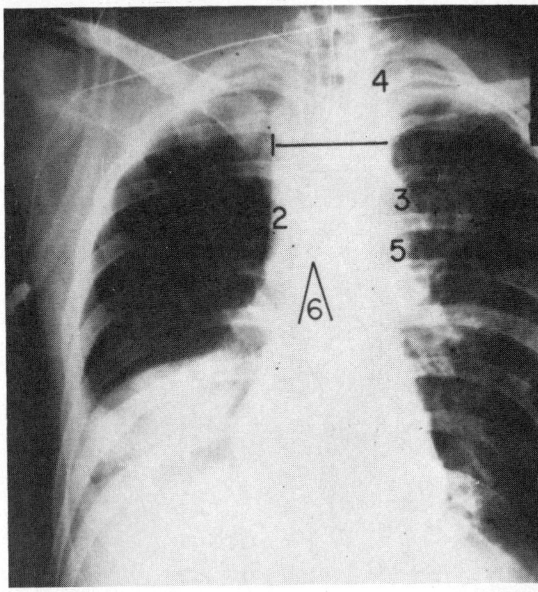

FIGURE 46–23. Aortic trauma. Roentgenographic characteristics of rupture of the proximal descending thoracic aorta in the supine anteroposterior projection (film-to-tube distance = 40 inches). The M/C ratio is 0.32. See text for key to numbers. (From Marsh, D. G., and Sturm, J. T.: Traumatic aortic rupture: Roentgenographic indications for angiography. Ann. Thorac. Surg. *21*:337, 1976.)

Otherwise, the physical examination is relatively unrevealing. Localized aneurysms developing in the aortic isthmus late after trauma may cause hoarseness, cough, and dysphagia from compression of the adjacent recurrent laryngeal nerve, bronchus, and esophagus.

DIAGNOSIS. Because the diagnosis is so frequently overshadowed by the presence of other severe injuries, rupture of the aorta is often overlooked. A *high index of suspicion is crucial, and evidence of aortic trauma should be sought in any patient with severe bodily injuries.* In the absence of classic physical findings—a common situation—the diagnosis is best suspected from the chest roentgenogram, which, if properly obtained and interpreted, is abnormal in over 90 per cent of patients with traumatic aortic rupture. Marsh and Sturm have delineated criteria for rupure of the aorta based upon a 40-degree anteroposterior supine chest film. The numbers on Figure 46–23 correspond to these criteria: (1) mediastinum measuring greater than 8 cm at the level of the aortic knob, (2) shift of the trachea toward the right, (3) blurring of the normally sharp outline of the aorta, (4) obliteration of the medial aspect of the apex of the upper lobe of the left lung, (5) opacification of the clear space between the aorta and pulmonary artery, and (6) depression of the left main stem bronchus below 40 degrees.[206] In a follow-up report, these authors identified indistinct aortic contour, opacification of the clear space between aorta and pulmonary artery, and mediastinal widening (mean diameter = 9.4 cm) as the most sensitive markers for aortic injury.[207] Others have contended that deviation of the trachea (or a nasogastric tube) to the right and depression of the main left bronchus are most sensitive.[208] The concept of increased mediastinal width compared to chest width (m/c ratio) has also been advocated as a helpful sign for quantifying the magnitude of mediastinal widening and likelihood of aortic injury.[209] While any m/c ratio greater than 0.20 is considered abnormal, the specificity of the test for identifying patients with aortic injury increases from less than 25 per cent to nearly 90 per cent when the ratio is greater than 0.28. In cases of thoracic trauma, as the ratio increases from 0.25 to 0.28, the threshold for performing angiography should be lower;

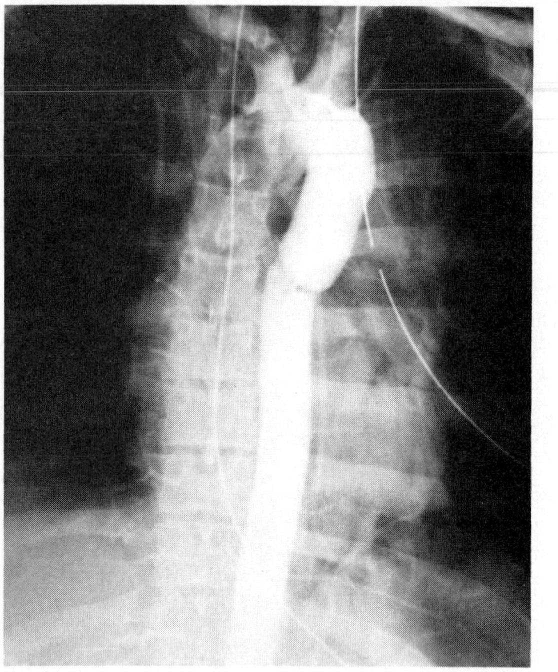

FIGURE 46–24. Thoracic aortogram in a 26-year-old man injured in a motor vehicle accident, showing traumatic transection of the aorta. The site of the tear can be clearly seen. (Courtesy of Robert Dinsmore, M.D., Massachusetts General Hospital, Boston.)

whenever the m/c ratio exceeds 0.28, additional studies should be carefully considered. CT scanning with contrast injection may confirm the diagnosis and should be performed as expeditiously as possible in a stable patient who has sustained severe chest trauma. Should the diagnosis remain in question or if the patient is unstable, the threshold for performing angiography in suspected cases should be low (Fig. 46–24 and Fig. 45–10, p. 1544).

COURSE AND PROGNOSIS. Approximately 80 per cent of patients with aortic rupture die instantly, although usually from other injuries, such as massive hemorrhage from other sites, trauma to other vital organs, or brain damage. Of those who survive the initial event, death often occurs within the first week from progressive hemorrhage at the site of the aortic tear. However, even with complete transection of the aorta, patients may be remarkably stable. About 2 to 5 per cent of patients with partial tears of the aorta go on to develop a localized aneurysm or pseudoaneurysm over a period of months or years, usually anterior to the aortic isthmus. This may either remain stable or ultimately expand. Such traumatic aneurysms frequently calcify or may become infected.[210]

TREATMENT. The treatment of aortic trauma is operative repair, which should be undertaken as soon as possible once the condition is recognized. Occasionally, other serious injuries make it necessary to delay operation in order to stabilize the patient, but even in the face of other severe trauma, surgery should be performed if there is evidence of progressive hemorrhage from the aorta. Rupture of the aorta is usually treated by resecting the torn segment of the aorta and interposing a prosthetic graft between the two ends of the aorta. It may be necessary to support the distal circulation with a pump oxygenator or conduit bypass from the proximal to the distal aorta around the rupture in order to avoid ischemic damage to the spinal cord, abdominal viscera, and kidneys.[211] Prompt recognition and operation for a ruptured aorta has resulted in survival of nearly 70 per cent of patients with this injury who reach the hospital alive.[204, 211, 212]

In cases of localized saccular aneurysms developing late after trauma, surgical excision is advised if the patient is an otherwise reasonable operative candidate. Long-term follow-up of patients with such lesions indicates that about half the aneurysms slowly expand and may even rupture. Surgery is curative and can be undertaken at a small risk (1 to 3 per cent).

PENETRATING TRAUMA

Penetrating trauma of the aorta or any of its major arterial trunks is caused by puncture or laceration by missiles or knives, particularly bullet and stab wounds. Massive hemorrhage, often leading to rapidly fatal exsanguination, ensues. The consequences of the trauma depend upon the site and severity of perforation. Thus, perforation of the aorta within the pericardial sac may lead to cardiac tamponade. Perforation of the aorta elsewhere may cause massive hemorrhage, with compression of surrounding structures by the hematoma, such as the vena cava, tracheobronchial tree, and esophagus. Occlusion of a lacerated artery itself or of adjacent vessels may occur, producing focal signs and symptoms such as loss of the right carotid and brachial pulses, with right hemispheric neurological signs in the case of occlusion of the innominate artery. Occasionally, simultaneous penetration of an adjacent artery and vein may cause an arteriovenous fistula, with a resultant continuous murmur, wide pulse pressure, and increased cardiac output.[213, 214]

MANAGEMENT. Immediate surgical repair should be undertaken in any patient suspected of having a penetrating wound of the aorta, i.e., one with a missile or stab wound of the chest associated with a wide mediastinum on roentgenogram. If the patient's condition allows it, emergency angiography can usually pinpoint the site of perforation. However, in most patients who survive to reach the hospital, immediate operation for closure of the wound and evacuation of the hematoma is necessary. Similarly, laceration or penetrating wounds of arteries require urgent surgical correction.

AORTIC THROMBOEMBOLIC DISEASE

AORTIC EMBOLISM

Between 10 and 25 per cent of peripheral arterial emboli affect the aortic bifurcation, resulting in what are termed "saddle emboli." At least 90 per cent of these emboli originate within the chambers of the left side of the heart; 5 per cent come from the aorta itself, usually from thrombus overlying an arteriosclerotic plaque; and the remainder come from undetermined sites.[215] Rarely, paradoxical systemic embolism from the venous circulation occurs through a patent foramen ovale or atrial septal defect. Conditions that predispose to peripheral embolism are myocardial infarction with mural thrombus, ventricular aneurysm, prosthetic valves, congestive cardiomyopathy, and atrial fibrillation, especially in patients with rheumatic mitral stenosis. So-called "marantic endocarditis" is occasionally encountered in chronically ill patients, especially those with malignant disease, and consists of sterile intracardiac thrombi that may dislodge and travel to distal sites. Other less frequent conditions that serve to cause arterial emboli are left atrial myxomas and acute and subacute bacterial endocarditis. Emboli in endocarditis are usually small, although large emboli are seen in acute bacterial endocarditis and fungal (*Candida*) endocarditis. An increased tendency to thromboembolism is encountered in women taking contraceptive pills and estrogens; in patients with malignant diseases, particularly carcinoma of the pancreas; and, rarely, in patients with antithrombin III deficiency.[216]

CLINICAL MANIFESTATIONS. Aortic bifurcation embolism is heralded by the sudden onset of excruciating pain in both legs. The pain usually extends distally from the midthigh area, but can also involve the buttocks, lumbosacral area, and perineum. Associated with the intense pain are numbness, symmetrical weakness, and paresthesias. Schatz and Stanley have summarized in alliteration this classic presentation as "*p*ain, *p*aralysis, *p*aresthesias, *p*ulselessness, and *p*allor."[217]

Examination reveals cold, pale extremities that are cyanotic and often exhibit a mottled, reticulated, reddish-blue appearance. These changes may progress to the blue-black color of gangrene, beginning first in the toes and extending proximally. Pulses are absent below the abdominal aorta. Initially sluggish, capillary filling is ultimately absent. Signs of ischemic neuropathy are present and include diminished or absent deep tendon reflexes, symmetrical weakness, and loss of all modalities of sensation, usually with demarcation at the level of the midthigh. If ischemia persists long enough, there may be myonecrosis with the release of products of muscle breakdown into the bloodstream, causing shock, hypotension, hyperkalemia, myoglobinuria, and acute tubular necrosis. Sepsis may add a serious further dimension to an already desperate problem. If perfusion is not reestablished within hours, death is almost inevitable.

The *differential diagnosis* includes acute aortic thrombosis from arteriosclerotic disease and dissecting aortic aneurysm. With thrombosis, there is usually a history of prior claudication, and an embolic source is lacking. With aortic dissection, a history of severe chest or back pain and an abnormal aortic contour on chest x-ray film usually provide distinguishing features.

The diagnosis is confirmed by angiography. However, most investigators advise prompt surgical intervention without angiography if the diagnosis is strongly suspected, since a delay could lead to irreversible ischemic damage to the limbs.

THERAPY. Most emboli can be removed by using Fogarty balloon-tipped catheters inserted through a transfemoral arterial approach under local anesthesia. In addition to retrieving the embolic material, passage of the Fogarty catheters into the distal arterial bed may result in the removal of any thrombus that may have formed as a result of the stagnant flow beyond the embolus. If the embolus cannot be retrieved with Fogarty catheters, removal by direct transabdominal aortotomy is necessary. Operative mortality ranges from 15 to 30 per cent, with death due to the underlying cardiac disease; limb salvage is estimated at 80 to 90 per cent in most series.[218] Anticoagulation with constant intravenous heparin is instituted upon completion of the operation and is continued until therapeutic levels are achieved with one of the warfarin sodium family of drugs. Depending upon the clinical situation, long-term anticoagulant therapy using warfarin or antiplatelet agents may be required. Reembolization may occur in up to 25 per cent of patients, and some series suggest a reduced incidence if long-term anticoagulants are used.[219] Using the transfemoral approach, surgery can be carried out with a low mortality even in patients whose other disease makes them poor operative risks. Limbs are almost uniformly salvaged if operation is undertaken promptly. All embolic debris should be cultured and examined microscopically. Left atrial myxomas are sometimes first recognized by the pathological examination of embolic specimens.

AORTIC THROMBOSIS

Rarely, primary thrombosis of the distal abdominal aorta may be seen as a result of atheromatous disease or in rare patients with antithrombin III deficiency. In such patients, treatment is generally surgical, although an occasional case of successful balloon catheter dilatation has been reported.[216, 220, 221] Studies in experimental animals using tissue plasminogen activator (t-PA) for the treatment of aortic thrombotic occlusion suggest that this modality may have a potential role in treating patients with both peripheral emboli and aortic thrombosis.[222] This agent awaits FDA approval, however.

ATHEROMATOUS EMBOLI

Embolism of atheromatous debris from the disruption of arteriosclerotic plaques in the aorta or its major arterial trunks has been noted with increasing frequency. Usually, such embolism takes the form of showers of microemboli, each between 150 and 600 μm in size, into small arterial branches—an entity that is also termed "cholesterol embolism." However, obstruction of large arteries by embolic arteriosclerotic material may also occur. By far the most common cause of cholesterol embolism is surgery that involves manipulation of an atherosclerotic aorta. Thus, atheromatous embolism into the renal and splanchnic vascular beds is common after major abdominal vascular procedures, particularly resection of abdominal aortic aneurysms. Embolism of atheromatous material also occurs as an occasional complication of intraarterial cannulation, cardiac catheterization, and cardiopulmonary bypass. In addition to these iatrogenic causes, however, spontaneously occurring cholesterol embolism is encountered, particularly from the aorta into the femoral-popliteal system. Studies have suggested a causal relationship between cholesterol embolism and anticoagulant therapy, especially long-term anticoagulation with warfarin sodium–type drugs. Presumably, anticoagulation promotes hemorrhage into plaques, leading to their disruption, or prevents the formation of protective thrombus over ulcerated plaques. Finally, atheromatous embolism has followed blunt trauma to the aorta.[223]

CLINICAL MANIFESTATIONS. The consequences of cholesterol embolism depend upon the vascular bed involved as well as the extent to which the small arterial vessels are occluded. Two important complications of cholesterol embolism following abdominal aortic surgery are pancreatitis and renal failure from diffuse microinfarction of the pancreas and kidneys, respectively. Renal failure may be severe and irreversible (p. 1835). Occasionally, cholesterol embolism has been implicated as a cause of severe renovascular hypertension. Gastrointestinal hemorrhage from microinfarction of abdominal viscera is also encountered. Showers of atheromatous emboli may affect the cerebral circulation, producing either focal neurological defects or a diffuse encephalopathic picture. In such cases, shiny cholesterol particles are sometimes visible in the retinal arteries.[224]

Spontaneously occurring cholesterol embolism in the lower extremities is manifested by bilateral pain, livedo reticularis, and purpuric and ecchymotic lesions in the lower legs, feet, and toes. These manifestations may be paroxysmal as emboli intermittently dislodge from their sites of origin. Skin necrosis and ischemic gangrene are common, especially in the toes ("blue toe syndrome").[225] In the face of this clinical evidence of severe ischemia, arterial pulses are characteristically well preserved unless there is coincidental peripheral vascular disease.

The clinical picture may mimic that of a vasculitis or septic embolism from neisserial organisms—especially meningococcemia—or bacterial endocarditis. The absence of fever and other signs of systemic illness and the localized distribution of the lesions serve to distinguish cholesterol embolism from these other entities. The diagnosis has been made by muscle biopsy, which may show cholesterol particles in the arterioles.

THERAPY. For the most part, there is no specific treatment for cholesterol microembolism. Careful attention to the prevention of necrosis and infection in the involved extremities is important. Although the amputation of gangrenous digits is occasionally necessary, the ultimate prognosis for recovery is quite good, unless embolism is frequent and recurrent. Pancreatitis often subsides, even though it may be severe. Renal failure may be irreversible.

The use of anticoagulants in the prevention of further embolism is controversial, with some investigators advocating that they be given and others contending that they promote further atheromatous emboli. Overall, it appears that they are not of much value. In instances of recurrent atheromatous embolism, it may be possible to pinpoint the source of the cholesterol particles by angiography and to perform an endarterectomy or to excise the involved segment and replace it with a prosthetic graft.

AORTIC BACTERIAL INFECTIONS

The term "infected aneurysm" has gradually replaced the original designation of "mycotic aneurysm" used by Osler to define any localized dilation caused by sepsis in the wall of the aorta or any artery and thus to avoid confusion with infections of truly fungal origin. Infection can cause virtually any kind of aneurysmal dilatation, including fusiform, saccular, and false aneurysms. Rupture into the venous system may cause arteriovenous fistulas. Alternatively, infection may arise within preexisting arteriosclerotic aneurysms. Infected aortic aneurysms are rare, with only 1.2 cases per year recently being reported from a large general hospital.[226]

PATHOGENESIS. Vascular infection may arise by any of three different mechanisms. First, septic emboli from bacterial endocarditis or diffuse bacteremia may infect normal or diseased tissue. This mechanism of infection has become less frequent owing to the widespread use of effective antibiotics for the control of septicemia. Second, there may be contiguous spread from adjacent abscesses, infected lymph nodes, empyema, and so on. This is the usual cause for rare cases of tuberculous vascular involvement. Third, sepsis may be introduced directly from an external source, such as trauma, intravenous injections, or surgery. The incidence of this type of infection is increasing because of more frequent motor vehicle accidents, the widespread use of intravenous narcotics by drug addicts, and the performance of more intravascular procedures that may produce a portal for infection, such as intraarterial catheterization and intraaortic balloon counterpulsation. With this type of sepsis, the peripheral arteries are obviously more frequently involved than the aorta per se.

Although virtually any organism may infect the arterial tree, certain bacteria seem to have a proclivity for this type of infection. In particular, this is true of the *Salmonella* group, which tends to infect arteriosclerotic aneurysms. *Staphylococcus aureus* was the most common organism identified in a recent series, followed by *Salmonella*.[227]

CLINICAL MANIFESTATIONS. Most patients with infected aortic aneurysms are febrile; the height of the fever depends upon the severity of infection, the organism, and the site of the infection. Extremely high fever and rigors are common. Symptoms may arise from localized expansion of an infected aneurysm, such as dysphagia from esophageal compression and pain in areas contiguous to the infected sac. If palpable, infected aneurysms are almost always tender. A tender and pulsatile mass in a febrile patient should be considered an infected aneurysm until proved otherwise. Jarrett et al. have suggested that infected aortic aneurysms can be differentiated from sterile ones by the presence of fever, relative preponderance in women, tenderness, lack of calcification, and a tendency for early vertebral erosion.[226] With tuberculous involvement, evidence is almost always seen on the chest x-ray.[228] This, coupled with a pulsating mass lesion, should elicit the correct diagnosis.

Sepsis in more peripheral arteries presents most commonly as fever with a palpable, painful, pulsating mass. Symptoms of compression of contiguous structures may also be present, such as arterial regurgitation or a neuropathy. Small abscesses in the distribution of the artery are often seen in staphylococcal infections. The most common sites for infected aneurysms are the following arteries: femoral, abdominal aorta, superior mesenteric, brachial, iliac, and carotid arteries. Together, the femoral arteries and abdominal aorta account for nearly 70 per cent of all mycotic aneurysms.[227]

Leukocytosis, an elevated sedimentation rate, and positive blood cultures are present in most cases. Commonly reported organisms other than *Staphylococcus aureus* and *Salmonella* species are other gram-positive and gram-negative organisms, such as pneumococcus, *Pseudomonas*, and anaerobes, but these are found less frequently. Rarely, fungal infections with *Candida* or *Aspergillus* may occur. Localization of suspected infected aneurysms in a patient with sepsis can be aided by angiography. Valuable information can sometimes be obtained from ultrasound, gallium, and CT scans.

The natural history of infected aneurysms is that of progressive expansion, thinning of the aneurysm wall, and eventual rupture. Jarrett et al. found a more rapid progression in patients with gram-negative infections.[226]

THERAPY. Treatment is always surgical excision combined with appropriate antibiotic or antituberculous chemotherapy. Wide excision of infected tissue is advised.[226, 227] Usually a prosthetic tube graft must be inserted if the aorta or a major artery is involved. Early recognition and therapy clearly alter the outcome favorably.

AORTIC TUMORS

One review cites 21 cases of primary aortic tumors recorded in the world's literature.[229] Clearly, secondary tumors can arise from direct extension and invasion from adjacent lung or abdominal neoplasms or from embolic spread. Histologic types include fibrosarcoma (most commonly), fibromyxosarcoma, myxosarcoma, fibromyxoma, angiosarcoma, malignant fibrous histiocytoma, leiomyosarcoma, and endothelioma.[230] In the 21 cases of primary aortic tumors, the age of the patients ranged from infancy to 70 years, with a mean of 53 years; sex distribution was equal. Presentation in over half the cases consisted of pain with proximal hypertension due to the acquired coarctation, decreased femoral pulses, fever, claudication, and occasionally bruits. Diagnosis is made by the usual noninvasive or angiographic techniques, with key features being the irregular appearance of the lumen and lack of enlargement of the outer diameter of the aorta.

REFERENCES

EXAMINATION OF THE AORTA

1. Feldman, L.: Digital subtraction angiography of the chest. Clin. Chest Med. 5:313, 1984.
2. Grossman, L. B., Buonocore, E., Modic, M. T., and Meaney, T. F.: Digital subtraction angiography of the thoracic aorta. Radiology *150*:323, 1984.
3. Ferrucci, J. T., Jr.: Body ultrasonography. N. Engl. J. Med. *300*:538, 590, 1979.
4. DeMaria, A. N., Bommer, W., Neumann, A., Weinert, L., Bogren, H., and Mason, D. T.: Identification and localization of aneurysms of the ascending aorta by cross-sectional echocardiography. Circulation *59*:755, 1979.
5. Meyer, J. F., and Wall, H. N., Jr.: Ultrasonic evaluation of the aorta. *In* Lindsay, J., Jr., and Hurst, J. W. (eds.): The Aorta. New York, Grune and Stratton, 1979, p. 345.
6. Brundage, B. H., Rich, S., and Spigos, D.: Computed tomography of the heart and great vessels: Present and future. Ann. Intern. Med. *101*:801, 1984.
7. Goodman, L. R., and Teplick, S. K.: Computed tomography in acute cardiopulmonary disease. Radiol. Clin. N. Am. *21*:741, 1983.
8. Moncada, R., Demos, T. C., and Churchill, R.: Detecting disease of the aorta by computed tomography. J. Cardiovasc. Med. *8*:186, 1983.
8a. Singh, H., Fitzgerald, E., and Ruttley, M. S.: Computed tomography: The investigation of choice for aortic dissection? Br. Heart J. *56*:171, 1986.
8b. White, R. D., Lipton, M. J., Higgins, C. B., Federle, M. P., Pogany, A. C., Kerland, R. K., Jr., Thaxton, T. S., Turley, K.: Noninvasive evaluation of suspected thoracic aortic disease by contrast-enhanced computed tomography. Am. J. Cardiol. *57*:282, 1986.
9. Dinsmore, R. E., Liberthson, R. R., Wismer, G. L., Miller, S. W., Liu, P., Thompson, R., McLoud, T. C., Marshall, J., Saini, S., Stratemeier, E. J., Okada, R. D., and Brady, T. J.: Magnetic resonance imaging of thoracic aortic aneurysms: Comparison with other diagnostic techniques. A. J. R. *146*:309, 1986.
10. Valk, P. E., Hale, J. D., Kaufman, L., Crooks, L. E., and Higgins, C. B.: MR imaging of the aorta with three dimensional vessel reconstruction: Validation by angiography. Radiology *157*:721, 1985.
11. Glazer, H. S., Gutierrez, F. R., Levitt, R. E., Lee, J. K., and Murphy, W. A.: The thoracic aorta studied by MR imaging. Radiology *157*:149, 1985.
12. Goldman, A. P., Kotler, M. N., Scanlon, M. H., Ostrum, B., Parameswaran, R., and Parry, W. R.: The complementary role of magnetic resonance imaging, Doppler echocardiography, and computed tomography in the diagnosis of dissecting thoracic aneurysms. Am. Heart J. *111*:970, 1986.
12a. Mossard, J. M., Baruthio, J., Germain, P., Favier, J. P., Wahl, P., Chambron, J., and Sacrez, A.: Nuclear magnetic resonance in the diagnosis of aortic diseases. Arch. Mal. Coeur. *79*:456, 1986.
12b. Goldman, A. P., Kotler, M. N., Scanlon, M. H., Ostrum, B. J., Parameswaran, R., and Parry, W. R.: Magnetic resonance imaging and two-dimensional echocardiography. Alternative approach to aortography in diagnosis of aortic dissecting aneurysm. Am. J. Med. *80*:1225, 1986.

PATHOGENESIS OF DISEASES OF THE AORTA

13. Iwatsuki, K., Cardinale, G. J., Spector, S., and Udenfriend, S.: Reduction of blood pressure and vascular collagen in hypertensive rats by β-aminopropionitrile. Proc. Natl. Acad. Sci. USA *74*:360, 1977.
14. Schlatmann, T. J. M., and Becker, A. E.: Pathogenesis of dissecting aneurysm of the aorta. Am. J. Cardiol. *39*:21, 1977.
15. Heistad, D. D., Marcus, M. L., Law, E. G., Armstrong, M. L., Ehrhardt, J. C., and Abboud, F. M.: Regulation of blood flow to the aortic media in dogs. J. Clin. Invest. *62*:133, 1978.
15a. Thurmond, A. S., and Semler, H. J.: Abdominal aortic aneurysm: Incidence in a population at risk. J. Cardiovasc. Surg. (Torino) *27*:457, 1986.

ARTERIOSCLEROTIC AORTIC ANEURYSMS

16. Darling, R. C.: Ruptured arteriosclerotic abdominal aortic aneurysms. Am. J. Surg. *119*:397, 1970.
17. Rantakokko, V., Havia, T., Inberg, M. V., and Vänttinen, E.: Abdominal aortic aneurysms: A clinical and autopsy study of 408 patients. Acta Chir. Scand. *149*:151, 1983.
18. Astarita, D., Filippone, D. R., and Cohn J. D.: Spontaneous major intra-abdominal arteriovenous fistulas: A report of several cases. Angiology *36*:656, 1985.
19. Bickerstaff, L. K., Hollier, L. H., Van Peenen, H. J., Melton, L. J., Pairolero, P. C., and Cherry, K. J.: Abdominal aortic aneurysms: The changing natural history. J. Vasc. Surg. *1*:6, 1984.
20. Crew, J. R., Bashour, T. T., Ellertson, D., Hanna, E. S., and Bilal, M.: Ruptured abdominal aortic aneurysms: Experience with 70 cases. Clin. Cardiol. *8*:433, 1985.
21. Hertzer, N. R., and Beven, E. G.: Abdominal aortic aneurysm. Postgrad. Med. *61*:72, 1977.
21a. Jenkins, A. M., Ruckley, C. V., and Nolan, B.: Ruptured abdominal aortic aneurysm. Br. J. Surg. *73*:395, 1986.
21b. Martinussen, H. J., Lolk, A., Rohr, N., Jensen, U. H., and Svendsen, V.: Ruptured abdominal aortic aneurysm with fistula into the inferior vena cava. J. Cardiovasc. Surg. (Torino) *27*:298, 1986.
22. Brewster, D. C., Darling, R. C., Raines, J. K., Sarno, R., O'Donnell, T. F., Ezpeleta, M., and Athanasoulis, C.: Assessment of abdominal aortic aneurysm size. Circulation *56*:164, 1977.
23. Retief, P. J., and Loubser, J. S.: Diagnosis and treatment of abdominal aortic aneurysm. A report of 82 cases. S. Afr. Med. J. *56*:67, 1979.
24. Brewster, D. C., Retana, A., Waltman, A. C., and Darling, R. C.: Angiography in the management of aneurysms of the abdominal aorta. Its value and safety. N. Engl. J. Med. *292*:822, 1975.
25. Gliedman, M. L., Ayers, W. B., and Vestal, B. L.: Aneurysms of the abdominal aorta and its branches: A study of untreated patients. Ann. Surg. *217*:1537, 1982.
26. Darling, R. C., Messina, C. R., Brewster, D. C., and Ottinger, L. W.: Autopsy study of unoperated abdominal aortic aneurysms. The case for early resection. Circulation *56*(Suppl. II):161, 1977.
27. Delin, A., Ohlsén, H., and Swedenborg, J.: Growth rate of abdominal aortic aneurysms as measured by computed tomography. Br. J. Surg. *72*:530, 1985.
28. Bernstein, E. F., and Chan, E. L.: Abdominal aortic aneurysm in high risk patients. Ann. Surg. *200*:255, 1985.
29. Pasch, A. R., Ricotta, J. J., May, A. G., Green, R. M., and DeWeese, J. E.: Abdominal aortic aneurysm: The case for elective resection. Circulation *70*(Suppl. I):1, 1984.
30. Cooley, D. A., and Carmichael, M. J.: Abdominal aortic aneurysm. Circulation *70*(Suppl. I):5, 1984.
31. Attia, R. R., Murphy, J. D., Snider, M., Lappas, D. G., Darling, R. C, and Lowenstein, E.: Myocardial ischemia due to infrarenal aortic cross-clamping during aortic surgery in patients with severe coronary artery disease. Circulation *53*:961, 1976.
32. Bush, H. L., Jr., LoGerfo, F. W., Weisel, R. D., Mannick, J. A., and Hechtman, H. B.: Assessment of myocardial performance and optimal volume loading during elective abdominal aortic resection. Arch. Surg. *112*:1301, 1977.
33. Shenaq, S. A., Chelly, J. E., Karlberg, H., Cohen, E., and Crawford, E. S.: Use of nitroprusside during surgery for thoracoabdominal aortic aneurysm. Circulation *70*(Suppl. I):7, 1984.
34. Thompson, J. E., Hollier, L. H., Patman, R. D., and Persson, A. V.: Surgical management of abdominal aortic aneurysms: Factors influencing mortality and morbidity—A 20-year experience. Ann. Surg. *181*:654, 1975.
35. Cullen, D. J., Ferrara, L. C., Briggs, B. A., Walker, P. F., and Grehert, J.: Survival, hospitalization charges and follow-up results in critically ill patients. N. Engl. J. Med. *294*:982, 1976.
36. Brener, B. J., Raines, J. K., and Darling, R. C.: Intraoperative autotransfusion in abdominal aortic resections. Arch. Surg. *107*:78, 1973.
37. Levin, P. M., Shore, E. H., Treiman, R. L., and Foran, R. F.: Ruptured abdominal aortic aneurysms. Surgical treatment. West J. Med. *123*:431, 1975.
38. Hertzer, N. R.: Fatal myocardial infarction following abdominal aortic aneurysm resection. Three hundred forty-three patients followed 6–11 years postoperatively. Ann. Surg. *192*:671, 1980.
39. Hertzer, N. R., Bevin, E. G., Young, J. R., O'Hara, P. J., Ruschhaupt, W. F., Graor, R. A., DeWolfe, V. G., and Maljovec, L. C.: Coronary artery disease in peripheral vascular patients. Ann. Surg. *199*:223, 1984.
40. Boucher, C. A., Brewster, D. C., Darling, R. C., Okada, R. D., Strauss, H. W., and Pohost, G. M.: Determination of cardiac risk by dipyridamole-thallium imaging before peripheral vascular surgery. N. Engl. J. Med. *312*:389, 1985.
41. Eagle, K. A., Singer, D. E., Brewster, D. C., Darling, R. C., Mulley, A. G., and Boucher, C. A.: Dipyridamole thallium scans in the preoperative evaluation of patients undergoing vascular surgery. Clin. Res. *34*:815A, 1986.
42. Leppo, J., Plaja, J., Gionet, M., Tumolo, J., Paraskos, J., and Cutler, B.: The noninvasive evaluation of cardiac risk prior to vascular surgery. Circulation 72(Suppl. III):147A, 1985.
43. Pasternack, P. F., Imparato, A. M., Riles, T. S., Baumann, E. G., Bear G., Lamparello, P. J., Benjamin, D., Sanger, J., and Kramer, E.: The value of radionuclide angiogram in the prediction of perioperative myocardial infarction in patients undergoing lower extremity revascularization procedures. Circulation 72(Suppl. II):13, 1985.
44. Brewster, D. C., Bluth, J., Darling, R. C., and Austen, W. G.: Combined aortic and renal artery reconstruction. Am. J. Surg. *131*:457, 1976.
45. Crawford, E. S., Saleh, S. A., Babb, J. W., III, Glaeser, D. H., Vaccaro, P. S., and Silvers, A.: Infrarenal abdominal aortic aneurysm: Factors influencing survival after operation performed over a 25-year period. Ann. Surg. *193*:699, 1981.
46. Ottinger, L. W.: Ruptured arteriosclerotic aneurysms of the abdominal aorta: Reducing mortality. J.A.M.A. *233*:147, 1975.
47. Darling, R. C., and Brewster, D. C.: Elective treatment of abdominal aortic aneurysms. World J. Surg. *4*:661, 1980.
48. Fielding, J. W. L., Black, J., Ashton, F., Slaney, G., and Campbell, D. J.: Diagnosis and management of 528 abdominal aortic aneurysms Br. Med. J. *283*:355, 1981.
49. O'Donnell, T. F., Darling, R. C., and Linton, R. R.: Is 80 years too old for aneurysmectomy? Arch. Surg. *111*:1250, 1976.
50. Karmody, A. M., Leather, R. P., Goldman, M., Corson, J. D., and Shah, D. M.: The current position of nonresective treatment for abdominal aortic aneurysm. Surgery *94*:591, 1983.
51. Baker, A. G., and Roberts, B.: Long-term survival following abdominal aortic aneurysmectomy. J.A.M.A. *212*:445, 1970.
52. Soreide, O., Lillestol, J., Christensen, O., Gromsgaard, L., Myhre, H. O., Solheim, K., and Trippestad, A.: Abdominal aortic aneurysms: Survival analysis of four hundred thirty-four patients. Surgery *91*:188, 1982.
53. Plate, G., Hollier, L. A., O'Brien, P., Pairolero, P. C., Cherry, K. J., and Kazmier, F. J.: Recurrent aneurysms and late vascular complications following repair of abdominal aortic aneurysms. Arch. Surg. *120*:590, 1985.
54. Hollier, L. A., Plate, G., O'Brien, P., Kazmier, F. J., Gloviczki, P., Pairolero, P. C., and Cherry, K. J.: Late survival after abdominal aortic aneurysm repair: Influence of coronary artery disease. J. Vasc. Surg. *1*:290, 1984.

55. Mitchell, E., Kadir, S., Kaufman, S. L., Chang, R., Williams, G. M., Kan, S., and White, R. I.: Percutaneous transluminal angioplasty of aortic graft stenoses. Radiology *149*:439, 1983.
56. O'Donnell, T. F., Scott, G., Shepard, A., Mackey, W., Deterling, R. A., and Callow, A. D.: Improvements in the diagnosis and management of aortoenteric fistula. Am. J. Surg. *149*:481, 1985.
57. Kierman, P. D., Pairolero, P. C., Hubert, J. P., Jr., Mucha, P., Jr., and Wallace, R. B.: Aortic graft-enteric fistula. Mayo Clin. Proc. *55*:731, 1980.
58. Ernst, C. B.: Prevention of intestinal ischemia following abdominal aortic reconstruction. Surgery *93*:102, 1983.
59. Lindsay, J., Jr.: Thoracic aneurysms. *In* Lindsay, J., Jr., and Hurst, J. W. (eds.): The Aorta. New York, Grune and Stratton, 1979, p. 121.
60. Collins, J. J., Koster, J. K., Cohn, L. H., and Van Devanter, S. H.: Common aortic aneurysms: when to intervene. J. Cardiovasc. Med. *8*:245, 1983.
61. Iliceto, S., Antonelli, G., Biasco, G., and Rizzon, P.: Two-dimensional echocardiographic evaluation of aneurysms of the descending thoracic aorta. Circulation *66*:1045, 1982.
62. Joyce, J. W., Fairbairn, J. F., Kincaid, O. W., and Juergens, J. L.: Aneurysms of the thoracic aorta—A clinical study with special reference to prognosis. Circulation *29*:176, 1964.
63. Culliford, A. T., Ayvaliotis, B., Shemin, R., Colvin, S. B., Isom, W., and Spencer, F. C.: Aneurysms of the descending aorta. J. Thorac. Cardiovasc. Surg. *85*:98, 1983.
64. Livesay, J. J., Cooley, D. A., Ventimiglia, R. A., Montero, C. G., Warrian, R. K., Brown, D. M., and Duncan, J. M.: Surgical experience in descending thoracic aneurysmectomy with and without adjuncts to avoid ischemia. Ann. Thorac. Surg. *39*:37, 1985.
65. Cabrol, C., Pavie, A., Mesnildrey, P., Gandjibakhch, I., Laughlin, L., Bors, V., and Corcos, T.: Long-term results with total replacement of the ascending aorta and reimplantation of the coronary arteries. J. Thorac. Cardiovasc. Surg. *91*:17, 1986.
66. Antunes, M. J., Colson, P. R., and Kinsley, R. H.: Hypothermia and circulatory arrest for surgical resection of aortic arch aneurysms. J. Thorac. Cardiovasc. Surg. *86*:576, 1983.
67. Crawford, E. S., and Snyder, D. M.: Treatment of aneurysms of the aortic arch. J. Thorac. Cardiovasc. Surg. *85*:237, 1983.
68. Pressler, V., and McNamara, J. J.: Aneurysms of the thoracic aorta. J. Thorac. Cardioivasc. Surg. *89*:50, 1985.
69. Moreno-Cabral, C. E., Miller, C., Mitchell, S., Stinson, E. B., Oyer, P. E., Jamieson, S. W., and Shumway, N. E.: Degenerative and atherosclerotic aneurysms of the thoracic aorta. J. Thorac. Cardiovasc. Surg. *88*:1020, 1984.
70. Crawford, E. S., Snyder, D. M., Cho, G. C., and Roehm, J. O. F., Jr.: Progress in treatment of thoracoabdominal and abdominal aortic aneurysms involving celiac, superior mesenteric, and renal arteries. Ann. Surg. *188*:404, 1978.
71. Crawford, E. S., and Rubio, P. A.: Reappraisal of adjuncts to avoid ischemia in the treatment of aneurysms of descending thoracic aorta. J. Thorac. Cardiovasc. Surg. *66*:693, 1973.
72. Wakabayashi, A., and Connolly, J. E.: Prevention of paraplegia associated with resection of extensive thoracic aneurysms. Arch. Surg. *111*:1186, 1976.
73. Coles, J. G., Wilson, G. J., Sima, A. F., Klement P., Tait, G. A., Williams, W. G., and Baird, R. J.: Intraoperative management of thoracic aortic aneurysms. J. Thorac. Cardiovasc. Surg. *85*:292, 1983.
74. Laschinger, J. C., Cunningham, J. N., Nathan, I. N., Knopp, E. A., Cooper, M. M., and Spencer, F. C.: Experimental and clinical assessment of the adequacy of partial bypass in maintenance of spinal cord blood flow during operations on the thoracic aorta. Ann. Thorac. Surg. *36*:416, 1983.

AORTIC DISSECTION

75. Wheat, M. W., Jr.: Acute dissecting aneurysms of the aorta: Diagnosis and treatment—1979. Am. Heart J. *99*:373, 1980.
76. Roberts, W. C.: Aortic dissection: Anatomy, consequences, and causes. Am. Heart J. *101*:195, 1981.
77. Doroghazi, R. M., and Slater, E. E. (eds.): Aortic Dissection. New York, McGraw-Hill Book Co., 1983.
77a. Cooke, J. P., and Safford, R. E.: Progress in the diagnosis and management of aortic dissection. Mayo Clin. Proc. *61*:147, 1986.
78. Wheat, M. W., Jr.: Pathogenesis of aortic dissection. *In* Doroghazi, R. M., and Slater, E. E. (eds.): Aortic Dissection. New York, McGraw-Hill Book Company, 1983, p. 55.
79. DeBakey, M. E., McCollum, C. H., Crawford, E. S., Morris, G. C., Howell, J., Noon, G. P., and Lawrie, G.: Dissection and dissecting aneurysms of the aorta: Twenty year follow-up of five hundred twenty-seven patients treated surgically. Surgery *92*:1118, 1982.
80. Daily, P. O., Trueblood, H. W., Stinson E. B., Wuerflein, R. D., and Shumway, N. E.: Management of acute aortic dissection. Ann. Thorac. Surg. *10*:237, 1970.
81. Slater, E. E., and DeSanctis, R. W.: The clinical recognition of dissecting aortic aneurysm. Am. J. Med. *60*:625, 1976.
82. Larson, E. W., and Edwards, W. D.: Risk factors for aortic dissection: A necropsy study of 161 cases. Am. J. Cardiol. *53*:849, 1984.
83. Leonards, J. C., and Hasleton, P. S.: Dissecting aortic aneurysms: A clinicopathological study. Q. J. Med. *48*:55, 1979.
84. Bulkley, B. H., and Roberts, W. C.: Dissecting aneurysm (hematoma) limited to coronary artery. Am. J. Med. *55*:747, 1973.
85. Hochberg, F. H., Bean, C., Fisher, C. M., and Roberson, G. H.: Stroke in a 15-year-old girl secondary to terminal carotid dissection. Neurology *25*:725, 1975.
86. Dalen, J. E., Pape, L. A., Cohn, L. H., Koster, J. K., and Collins, J. J.: Dissection of the aorta: Pathogenesis, diagnosis, and treatment. Prog. Cardiovasc. Dis. *23*:237, 1980.
87. Loeppky, C. B., Alpert, M. A., Hamel, P. C., Martin, R. H., and Saab, S. B.: Extensive aortic dissection from combined-type cystic medial necrosis in a young man without predisposing factors. Chest *79*:116, 1981.
88. McKusick, V. A., Logue, R. B., and Bahnson, H. T.: Association of aortic valvular disease and cystic medial necrosis of the ascending aorta; report of four instances. Circulation *16*:188, 1957.
89. Shachter, N., Perloff, J. K., and Mulder, D. G.: Aortic dissection in Noonan's syndrome. Am. J. Cardiol. *54*:464, 1984.
90. Price, W. H., and Wilson J.: Dissection of the aorta in Turner's syndrome. J. Med. Genetics *20*:61, 1983.
91. Pumphrey, C. W., Fay, T., and Weir, I.: Aortic dissection during pregnancy. Br. Heart J. *55*:106, 1986.
92. Ponseti, I. V., and Baird, W. A.: Scoliosis and dissecting aneurysm of the aorta in rats fed with *Lathyrus odoratus* seeds. Am. J. Pathol. *28*:1059, 1952.
93. Fikar, C. R., Amrhein, J. A., Harris, J. P., and Lewis, E. R.: Dissecting aortic aneurysm in childhood and adolescence. Clin. Pediatr. *20*:578, 1981.
94. Slater, E. E.: Aortic dissection: Presentation and diagnosis. *In* Doroghazi, R. M., and Slater, E. E. (eds.): Aortic Dissection. New York, McGraw-Hill Book Company, 1983, p. 61.
95. Cohen, S., and Littman, D.: Painless dissecting aneurysm of the aorta. N. Engl. J. Med. *271*:143, 1964.
96. Symbas, P. N., Kelly, T. F., Vlasis, S. E., Drucker, M. H., and Arensberg, D.: Intimo-intimal intussusception and other unusual manifestations of aortic dissection. J. Thorac. Cardiovasc. Surg. *79*:926, 1980.
97. Hirst, A. E., and Gore, I.: The etiology and pathology of aortic regurgitation. *In* Doroghazi, R. M., and Slater, E. E. (eds.): Aortic Dissection. New York, McGraw Hill Book Company, 1983, p. 13.
98. Riley, D. J., Liv, R. T., and Saxanoff, S.: Aortic dissection: A rare cause of the superior vena cava syndrome. J. Med. Soc. N. J. *78*:187, 1981.
99. McCarthy, C., Dickson, G. H., Besterman, E. M. M., Bromley, L. L., and Thompson, A. E.: Aortic dissection with rupture through ductus arteriosus into pulmonary artery. Br. Heart J. *34*:284, 1972.
100. Roth, J. A., and Parekh, M. A.: Dissecting aneurysms perforating the esophagus. N. Engl. J. Med. *299*:776, 1978.
101. Thiene, G., Rossi, L., and Becker, A. E.: The atrioventricular conduction system in dissecting aneurysm of the aorta. Am. Heart J. *98*:447, 1979.
102. Morris, A. L., and Barwinsky, J.: Unusual vascular complications of dissecting thoracic aortic aneurysm. Cardiovasc. Radiol. *1*:95, 1978.
103. Eagle, K. A., Quertermous, T., Kritzer, G. A., Newell, J. B., Dinsmore, R., Feldman, L., and DeSanctis, R. W.: Spectrum of conditions initially suggesting acute aortic dissection but with negative aortograms. Am. J. Cardiol. *57*:322, 1986.
104. ten Cate, J. W., Timmers, H., and Becker, A. E.: Coagulopathy in ruptured or dissecting aortic aneurysms. Am. J. Med. *59*:171, 1975.
105. Granato, J. E., Dee, P., and Gibson, R. S.: Utility of two-dimensional echocardiography in suspected ascending aortic dissection. Am J. Cardiol. *56*:123, 1985.
106. Victor, M. F., Mintz, G. S., Kotler, M. N., Wilson, A. R., and Segal, B. L.: Two dimensional echocardiographic diagnosis of aortic dissection. Am. J. Cardiol. *48*:1155, 1981.
107. Perez, J. E.: Noninvasive diagnosis: Computed tomography and ultrasound. *In* Doroghazi, R. M., and Slater, E. E. (eds.): Aortic Dissection. New York, McGraw-Hill Book Company, 1983, p. 133.
107a. Iliceto, S., Nanda, N. C., Rizzon, P., Hsuing, K. C., Goyal, R. G., Amico, A., and Strino, M.: Color Doppler evaluation of aortic dissection. Circulation *75*:748, 1987.
108. Thorsen, M. K., San Dretto, M. A., Lawson, T. L., Foley, W. D., Smith, D., and Berland L. L.: Dissecting aortic aneurysms: Accuracy of computed tomographic diagnosis. Radiology *148*:773, 1983.
109. Smith, D. C., and Jang, G. C.: Radiological diagnosis and aortic dissection. *In* Doroghazi, R. M., and Slater, E. E. (eds.): Aortic Dissection. New York, McGraw-Hill, 1983, p. 71.
109a. Vasile, N., Mathieu, D., Keita, K., Lellouche, D., Bloch, G., and Cachera, J. P.: Computed tomography of thoracic aortic dissection: Accuracy and pitfalls. J. Comput. Assis. Tomogr. *10*:211, 1986.
110. Turley, K., Ullyot, D. J., Godwin J. D., Wilson, J. M., Lipton, M., Carlsson, E., and Ebert, P. A.: Repair of dissection of the thoracic aorta. Evauation of false lumen utilizing computed tomography. J. Thorac. Cardiovasc. Surg. *81*:61, 1981.
111. Godwin, J. D., Turley, K., Herfkens, R. J., and Lipton, M. J.: Computed tomography for follow-up of chronic aortic dissections. Radiology *139*:655, 1981.
112. Earnest, F., IV, Muhm, J. R., and Sheedy, P. F., II: Roentgenographic findings in thoracic aortic dissection. Mayo Clin. Proc. *54*:43, 1979.
113. Amparo, E. G., Higgins, C. B., Hricak, L., and Sollitto, R.: Aortic dissection: Magnetic resonance imaging. Radiology *155*:399, 1985.
114. Dinsmore, R. E., Willerson, J. T., and Buckley, M. J.: Dissecting aneurysm of the aorta. Aortographic features affecting prognosis. Diagn. Radiol. *105*:567, 1972.
115. Shuford, W. H., Sybers, R. G., and Weens, H. S.: Problems of the aortographic diagnosis of dissecting aneurysms of the aorta. N. Engl. J. Med. *280*:225, 1969.
116. Collins, J. J., Jr., Koster, J. K., Jr., Cohn, L. H., and VanDevanter S. H.: Common aortic aneurysms: When to intervene. J. Cardiovasc. Med. *8*:245 1983.

117. Anagnostopoulos, C. E., Prabhakar, M. J. S., and Kittle, C. F.: Aortic dissections and dissecting aneurysms. Am. J. Cardiol. *30*:263, 1972.
118. Gurin, D., Bulmer, J. W., and Derby, R.: Dissecting aneurysms of the aorta. Diagnosis and operative relief of acute arterial obstructions due to this course. N.Y. State J. Med. *35*:1200, 1935.
119. Shaw, R. W.: Acute dissecting aortic aneurysms: Treatment by fenestration of the internal wall of the aneurysm. N. Engl. J. Med. *253*:331, 1955.
120. DeBakey, M. E., Cooley, D. A., and Creech, O., Jr.: Surgical considerations of dissecting aneurysms of the aorta. Ann. Surg. *142*:586, 1955.
121. Wheat, M. W., Jr., Palmer, R. F., Bartley, T. D., and Seelman, R. C.: Treatment of dissecting aneurysms of the aorta without surgery. J. Thorac. Cardiovasc. Surg. *50*:364, 1965.
122. Palmer, R. F., and Lasseter, K. C.: Nitroprusside and aortic dissecting aneurysm (letter). N. Engl. J. Med. *294*:1403, 1976.
123. Wheat, M. W.: Intensive drug therapy. *In* Doroghazi, R. M., and Slater, E. E. (eds.): Aortic Dissection. New York, McGraw-Hill Book Company, 1983, p. 165.
124. Frishman, W. B., Weinberg, P., Peled, H. B., Kimmel, B., Charlap, S., and Beer, N.: Calcium entry blockers for the treatment of severe hypertension and hypertensive crisis. Am. J. Med. *77*(Suppl. 2B):35, 1984.
125. White, S. R., and Hall, J.B.: Control of hypertension with nifedipine in the setting of aortic dissection. Chest *88*:781, 1985.
126. Anagnostopoulos, C. E., Athanasuleas, C. L., Garrick, T. R., and Paulissian, R.: Acute Aortic Dissections. Baltimore, University Park Press, 1975.
127. Appelbaum, A., Karp, R. B., and Kirklin, J. W.: Ascending versus descending aortic dissections. Ann. Surg. *183*:296, 1976.
128. Reul, G. J., Jr., Cooley, D. A., Hallman, G. L., Reddy, S. B., Kyger, E. R., III, and Wukasch, D. C.: Dissecting aneurysm of the descending aorta—Improved surgical results in 91 patients. Arch. Surg. *110*:632, 1975.
129. Kidd, J. N., Reul, G. J., Jr., Cooley, D. A., Sandiford, F. M., Kyger, E. R., III, and Wukasch, D. C.: Surgical treatment of aneurysms of the ascending aorta. Cardiovasc. Surg. *54*(Suppl.):118, 1976.
130. Miller, D. C., Stinson, E. B., Oyer, P. E., Rossiter, S. J., Reitz, B. A., Griepp, R. B., and Shumway, N. E.: The operative treatment of aortic dissections: Experience with 125 patients over a sixteen year period. J. Thorac. Cardiovasc. Surg. *78*:365, 1979.
131. Doroghazi, R. M., Slater, E. E., DeSanctis, R. W., Buckley, M. J., Austen, W. G., and Rosenthal, S.: Long-term survival of patients treated with aortic dissection. J. Am. Coll. Cardiol. *3*:1026, 1984.
132. Miller, D. C., Mitchell, R. C., Oyer, P. E., Stinson, E. B., Jamieson, S. W., and Shumway, N. E.: Independent determinants of operative mortality for patients with aortic dissections. Circulation *70*(Suppl. I):153, 1984.
133. Vecht, R. J., Besterman, E. M. M., Bromley, L. L., Eastcott, H. H. G., and Kenyon, J. R.: Acute dissection of the aorta: Long-term review and management. Lancet *1*:110, 1980.
134. Cachera, J. P., Vouhe, P. R., Loisance, D. Y., Menu, P., Poulain, H., Bloch, G., Vasile, N., Aubry, P., and Galey, J. J.: Surgical management of acute dissections involving the ascending aorta. J. Thorac. Cardiovasc. Surg. *82*:576, 1981.
135. Kolff, J., Bates, R. J., Balderman, S. C., Shenkoya, K., and Anagnostopoulos, C. E.: Acute aortic arch dissection: Reevaluation of the indication for medical and surgical therapy. Am. J. Cardiol. *39*:727, 1977.
136. Haverich, A., Miller, D. C., Scott, W. C., Mitchell, R. S., Oyer, P. E., Stinson, E. B., and Shumway, N. E.: Acute and chronic aortic dissections—determinants of long-term outcome for operative survivors. Circulation *72*(Suppl. II):22, 1985.
137. Lemole, G. M., Strong, M. D., Spagna, P. M., and Karmilowicz, N. P.: Improved results for dissecting aneurysms: Intraluminal sutureless prosthesis. J. Thorac. Cardiovasc. Surg. *83*:249, 1982.
138. Carpentier, A., Deloche, A., Fabiani, J. N., Chauvaud, S., Relland, J., Nottin, R., Vouhe, P., Massoud, H., and Dubost, C.: New surgical approach to aortic dissection: Flow reversal and thromboexclusion. J. Thorac. Cardiovasc. Surg. *81*:659, 1981.

ANNULOAORTIC ECTASIA

139. Ellis, P. R., Cooley, D. A., and DeBakey, M. E.: Clinical consideration and surgical treatment of annulo-aortic ectasia. J. Thorac. Cardiovasc. Surg. *42*:363, 1961.
140. Lindsay, J., Jr.: The Marfan syndrome and idiopathic cystic medial degeneration. *In* Lindsay, J., Jr., and Hurst, J. W. (eds.): The Aorta. New York, Grune and Stratton, 1979, p. 263.
141. Pyeritz, R. E., and McKusick, V. A.: The Marfan syndrome: Diagnosis and management. N. Engl. J. Med. *300*:772, 1979.
142. Boucek, R. J., Noble, N. L., Gunja-Smith, Z., and Butler, W. T.: The Marfan syndrome: A deficiency of chemically stable collagen cross links. N. Engl. J. Med. *305*:998, 1981.
143. Abraham, P. A., Perejda, A. J., Carnes, W. H., and Uitto, J.: Marfan syndrome: Demonstration of abnormal elastin in the aorta. J. Clin. Invest. *70*:1245, 1982.
144. Emanuel, R., Ng, R. A. L., Marcomichelakis, J., Moores, E. C., Jefferson, K. E., Macfaul, P. A., and Withers, R.: Formes frustes of Marfan's syndrome presenting with severe aortic regurgitation. Clinicogenetic study of 18 families. Br. Heart J. *39*:190, 1977.
145. Lemon, D. K., and White, C. W.: Annuloaortic ectasia: Angiographic, hemodynamic and clinical comparison with aortic valve insufficiency. Am. J. Cardiol. *41*:482, 1978.
146. Fox, R., Ren, J., Pandis, J. P., Kotler, M. N., Mintz, G. S., and Ross, R.: Annuloaortic ectasia: A clinical and echocardiographic study. Am. J. Cardiol. *54*:177, 1984.
147. Miller, D. C., Stinson, E. B., Oyer, P. E., Moreno-Cabral, R. J., Reitz, B. A., Rossiter, S. J., and Shumway, N. E.: Concomitant resection of ascending aortic aneurysm and replacement of the aortic valve. J. Thorac. Cardiovasc. Surg. *79*:388, 1980.
148. Gott, V. L., Pyeritz, R. E., Magovern, G. J., Jr., Cameron, D. E., and McKusick, V. A.: Surgical treatment of aneurysms of the ascending aorta in the Marfan syndrome. Results of composite-graft repair in 50 patients. N. Engl. J. Med. *314*:1070, 1986.
149. Pyeritz, R. E., Gott, V. L., McDonald, G. R., Achuff, S. C., Brinker, J. A., Haller, J. A., and Hutchins, G. M.: Surgical repair of the Marfan aorta: Technique, indications, and complications. Johns Hopkins Med. J. *151*:71, 1982.
150. Crawford, E. S.: Marfan's syndrome; broad spectral surgical treatment cardiovascular manifestations. Ann. Surg. *198*:487, 1983.

AORTIC ARTERITIS SYNDROMES

151. Takayasu, M.: Case with unusual changes of the central vessels in the retina. Acta Soc. Ophthalmol. Jpn. *12*:554, 1908.
152. Lupi-Herrera, E., Sanchez-Torres, G., Marcushamer, J., Mispireta, J., Horowitz, S., and Espino Vela, J.: Takayasu's arteritis. Clinical study of 107 cases. Am. Heart J. *93*:94, 1977.
153. Lande, A., and LaPorta, A.: Takayasu arteritis—An arteriographic-pathological correlation. Arch. Pathol. Lab. Med. *100*:437, 1976.
154. Shelhamer, J. H., Volkman, D. J., Parillo, J. E., Lawley, T. J., Johnston, M. R., and Fauci, A. S.: Takayasu's arteritis and its therapy. Ann. Intern. Med. *103*:121, 1985.
155. Hall, S., Barr, W., Lie, J. T., Stanson, A. W., Kazmier, F. J., and Hunder, G. G.: Takayasu arteritis. Medicine *64*:89, 1985.
156. Ueno, A., Awane, G., and Wakahayachi, A.: Successfully operated obliterative brachiocephalic arteritis (Takayasu) associated with the elongated coarctation. Jpn. Heart J. *8*:538, 1967.
157. Nakao, K., Ikeda, M., Kimata, S., Nhtani, H., Miyahara, M., Ishimi, Z., Hashiba, K., Takeda, Y., Ozawa, T., Matsushita, S., and Kuramochi, M.: Takayasu's arteritis—Clinical report of eighty-four cases and immunological studies of seven cases. Circulation *35*:1141, 1967.
158. Volkman, D. J., Mann, D. L., and Fauci, A. S.: Association between Takayasu's arteritis and a B-cell alloantigen in North Americans. N. Engl. J. Med. *306*:464, 1982.
159. Numano, F., Isohisa, I., Egami, M., Ohta, M., and Sasazuki, T.: HLA-DR MT and MB antigens in Takayasu disease. Tissue Antigens *21*:208, 1983.
160. Gronemeyer, P. S., and deMello, D. E.: Takayasu's disease with aneurysm of right common iliac artery and iliocaval fistula in a young infant: Case report and review of the literature. Pediatrics *69*:626, 1982.
161. Morooka, S., Saito, Y., Nonaka, Y., Gyotoku, Y., and Sugimoto, T.: Clinical features of aortitis syndrome in Japanese women older than 40 years. Am. J. Cardiol. *53*:859, 1984.
162. Swinton, N. W., and Cook, G. A.: Systolic hypertension and cardiac mortality of Takayasu's aortoarteritis. Angiology *27*:568, 1976.
163. Takishita, A., Tanaka, S., Orita, G., Kanaide, H., and Nakamura, M.: Baroflex sensitivity in patients with Takayasu's aortitis. Circulation *55*:803, 1977.
164. Akikusa, B., Kondo, Y., and Muraki, N.: Aortic insufficiency caused by Takayasu's arteritis without usual clinical features. Arch. Pathol. Lab. Med. *105*:650, 1981.
165. Cipriano, P. R., Silverman, J. F., Perlroth, M. G., Griepp, R. B., and Wexler, L.: Coronary arterial narrowing in Takayasu's aortitis. Am. J. Cardiol. *39*:744, 1977.
166. Slater, E. E., and Fallon, J. T.: Upper extremity hypertension in a 28-year-old Korean man. Case Records of the Massachusetts General Hospital. N. Engl. J. Med. *299*:1002, 1978.
167. Lupi, H. E., Sanchez, T. G., Horwitz, S., and Gutierrez, F. E.: Pulmonary artery involvement in Takayasu's arteritis. Chest *67*:69, 1975.
168. Kanaide, H., Takeshita, A., and Nakamura, M.: Etiologic aspects of coagulopathy in Takayasu's aortitis. Am. Heart J. *104*:1039, 1982.
169. Lande, A., and Rossi, P.: The value of total aortography in the diagnosis of Takayasu's arteritis. Radiology *114*:287, 1975.
170. Grossman, E., Morag, B., Nussinovitch, N., Boichis, H., Knecht, A., and Rosenthal, T.: Clinical use of captopril in Takayasu's disease. Arch. Intern. Med. *144*:95, 1984.
170a. Huddle, K. R., Doodha, M. I., and Mackenzie, M.: Captopril in the treatment of renovascular hypertension secondary to Takayasu's arteritis. S. Afr. Med. J. *69*:58, 1986.
171. Bloss, R. S., Duncan, J. M., Cooley, D. A., Leatherman, L. L., and Schnee, M. J.: Takayasu's arteritis: Surgical considerations. Ann. Thorac. Surg. *27*:574, 1979.
172. Duncan, J. M., and Cooley, D. A.: Surgical consideration in aortitis with special amphasis on Takayasu's arteritis. Texas Heart Inst. J. *10*:233, 1983.
172a. Pajari, R., Hekeli, P., and Harjola, P. T.: Treatment of Takayasu's arteritis: An analysis of 29 operated patients. Thorac. Cardiovasc. Surg. *34*:176, 1986.
173. Hodgins, G. W., and Dutton, J. W.: Transluminal dilatation of Takayasu's arteritis. Can. J. Surg. *27*:355, 1984.
174. Ishikawa, K.: Survival and morbidity after diagnosis of occlusive thromboaortopathy (Takayasu's disease). Am. J. Cardiol. *47*:1026, 1981.
175. Klein, R. G., Hunder, G. G., Stanson, A. W., and Sheps, S. G.: Large artery involvement in giant cell (temporal) arteritis. Ann. Intern. Med. *83*:806, 1975.
175a. Vincent, F. M., and Vincent, T.: Bilateral carotid siphon involvement in giant cell arteritis. Neurosurgery *18*:773, 1986.
176. Austen, W. G., and Blennerhassett, M. B.: Giant cell aortitis causing an aneurysm of the ascending aorta and aortic regurgitation. N. Engl. J. Med. *272*:80, 1965.

176a. Perruquet, J. L., Davis, D. E., and Harrington, T. M.: Aortic arch arteritis in the elderly. An important manifestation of giant cell arteritis. Arch. Intern. Med. *146*:289, 1986.
177. Ghose, M. K., Shensa, S., and Lerner, P. I.: Arteritis of the aged (giant cell arteritis) and fever of unexplained origin. Am. J. Med. *60*:429, 1976.
178. Huston, K. A., and Hunder, G. G.: Giant cell (cranial) arteritis: A clinical review. Am. Heart J. *100*:99, 1980.
179. Calamia, K. T., and Hunder, G. G.: Clinical manifestations of giant cell (temporal) arteritis. Clin. Rheum. Dis. *6*:389, 1980.
180. Chuang, T., Hunder, G. G., Ilstrup, D. M., and Kurland, L. T.: Polymyalgia rheumatica. Ann. Intern. Med. 97:672, 1982.
181. Salisbury, R. S., and Hazleman, B. L.: Successful treatment of dissecting aortic aneurysm due to giant cell arteritis. Ann. Rheum. Dis. *40*:507, 1981.
182. Malmvall, B. E., and Bengtsson, B. A.: Serum levels of immunoglobin and complement in giant cell arteritis. J.A.M.A. *236*:1876, 1976.
183. Paulus, H. E., Pearson, C. M., and Pitts, W.: Aortic insufficiency in five patients with Reiter's syndrome. A detailed clinical and pathologic study. Am. J. Med. *53*:464, 1972.
184. Muna, W. F., Roller, D. H., Craft, J., Shaw, R. K., and Ross, A. M.: Psoriatic arthritis and aortic regurgitation. J.A.M.A. *244*:363, 1980.
185. Morgan, S. H., Asherson, R. A., and Hughes, G. V.: Distal aortitis complicating Reiter's syndrome. Br. Heart J. *52*:115, 1984.
186. Park, J. H., Han, M. C., and Bettman, M. A.: Arterial manifestations of Behçet disease. A. J. R. *143*:821, 1984.
187. LaBresh, K. A., Lally, E. V., Sharma, S. C., and Ho, G.: Two-dimensional echocardiographic detection of preclinical aortic root abnormalities in rheumatoid variant diseases. Am. J. Med. *78*:908, 1985.

CARDIOVASCULAR SYPHILIS

188. Heggtveit, H. A.: Syphilitic aortitis. A clinicopathologic autopsy study of 100 cases, 1950 to 1960. Circulation *29*:346, 1964.
189. Kampmeier, R. H.: Aneurysm of the abdominal aorta. A study of 73 cases. Am. J. Med. Sci. *192*:97, 1936.
190. Prewitt, T. A.: Syphilitic aortic insufficiency. Its increased incidence in the elderly. J.A.M.A. *211*:637, 1970.
191. Center for Disease Control Recommended Treatment Schedules, 1985. The Sexually Transmitted Diseases Advisory Committee. Morbid. Mortal. Weekly Rep. *34*:94s, 1985(Suppl. 4S).
192. Duncan, J. M., and Cooley, D. A.: Surgical considerations in aortitis—syphilitic and other forms of aortitis. Texan Heart Inst. J. *10*:337, 1983.
193. Steinberg, I.: Anomalies (pseudocoarctation) of the arch of the aorta—Report of 8 new and review of 8 previously published cases. A. J. R. *88*:73, 1962.
194. Brinsfield, D. E., Shuford, W. M., Plauth, W. H., Jr., and Sybers, R. G.: Congenital anomalies of the aorta. *In* Lindsay, J., Jr., and Hurst, J. W. (eds.): The Aorta. New York, Grune and Stratton, 1979, p. 271.
195. Lavin, N., Mehta, S., Liberson, M., and Pouget, J. M.: Pseudocoarctation of the aorta. An unusual variant with coarctation. Am. J. Cardiol. *24*:584, 1969.
196. Lajos, T. Z., Meckstroth, C. V., Klassen, K. P., and Sherman, N. J.: Pseudocoarctation of the aorta. A variant or an entity? Chest *58*:571, 1970.
196a. Wolf, W. J.: Pseudocoarctation of the aortic arch in a patient with Turner's syndrome. Clin. Cardiol. *9*:A5, 1986.
197. Bahabozorgui, S., Bernstein, R. G., and Frater, R. W. M.: Pseudocoarctation of the aorta associated with aneurysm formation. Chest *60*:616, 1971.
198. Bland, E. F., and Castleman, B.: Vascular collapse in a woman with an unusual calcified ring in the aortic arch. N. Engl. J. Med. *280*:1466, 1969.
199. Prian, G. W., Kinard, S. A., Read, C. T., and Diethrich, E. B.: Pseudocoarctation: Diagnosis, etiology, natural history with emphasis on timing and technique of surgical correction. Vasc. Surg. *6*:198, 1972.
199a. Shaikh, K. A., Schwab, C. W., Camishion, R. C.: Aortic rupture in blunt trauma. Am. Surg. *52*:47, 1986.

AORTIC TRAUMA

200. Greendyke, R. M.: Traumatic rupture of aorta: Special reference to automobile accidents. J.A.M.A. *195*:527, 1966.
201. Parmley, L. F., Mattingly, T. W., Manion, W. C., and Jahnke, E. J.: Nonpenetrating traumatic injury of the aorta. Circulation *17*:1086, 1958.
202. Fleming, A. W., and Green, D. C.: Traumatic aneurysms of the thoracic aorta: Report of 43 patients. Ann. Thorac. Surg. *18*:91, 1974.
203. Faro, R. S., Monson, D. O., Weinberg, M., and Javid, H.: Disruption of aortic arch branches due to non-penetrating chest trauma. Arch. Surg. *118*:1333, 1983.
204. Sturm, J. T., Billiar, T. R., Dorsey, J. S., Luxenberg, M. G., and Perry, J. F.: Risk factors for survival following surgical treatment of traumatic aortic rupture. Ann. Thorac. Surg. *39*:418, 1985.
205. Jang, G. C., Brody, W. R., and Dinsmore, R. E.: Radiologic diagnosis of aortic disease. *In* Lindsay, J., Jr., and Hurst, J. W. (eds.): The Aorta. New York, Grune and Stratton, 1979, p. 295.
206. Marsh, D. G., and Sturm, J. T.: Traumatic aortic rupture: Roentgenographic indications for angiography. Ann. Thorac. Surg. *21*:337, 1976.
207. Sturm, J. T., Olson, F. R., and Cicero, J. J.: Chest roentgenographic findings in 26 patients with traumatic rupture of the thoracic aorta. Ann. Emerg. Med. *12*:598, 1983.
208. Woodring, J. H., and Dillon, M. L.: Radiographic manifestations of mediastinal hemorrhage from blunt chest trauma. Ann. Thorac. Surg. *37*:171, 1984.
209. Stark, P.: Traumatic rupture of the thoracic aorta: A review. Crit. Rev. Diag. Imaging *21*:229, 1983.
210. Schwartz, M. L., Fisher, R., Sako, Y., Castaneda, A. R., Grage, T. B., and Nicoloff, D. M.: Post-traumatic aneurysms of the thoracic aorta. Surgery *78*:589, 1975.
211. Akins, C. W., Buckley, M. J., Daggett, W., McIlduff, J. B., and Austen, W. G.: Acute traumatic disruption of the thoracic aorta: A ten-year experience. Ann. Thorac. Surg. *31*:305, 1981.
212. Stiles, Q. R., Cohlmia, G. S., Smith, J. H., Dunn, J. T., and Yellin, A. E.: Management of injuries of the thoracic and abdominal aorta. Am. J. Surg. *150*:132, 1985.
213. Haskell, R. J., French, W. J., and Harley, D. P.: Traumatic aorto-right ventricular fistula presenting with a diastolic murmur. Am. Heart J. *109*:1110, 1985.
214. Snow, N., and Johnson, P.: Traumatic fistula between the descending thoracic aorta and left main pulmonary artery. J. Trauma *25*:263, 1985.

AORTIC THROMBOEMBOLIC DISEASE

215. Heiskell, C. A., and Conn, J., Jr.: Aortoarterial emboli. Am. J. Surg. *132*:4, 1976.
216. Shapiro, M. E., Rodvien, R., Bauer, K. A., and Salzman, E. W.: Acute aortic thrombosis in antithrombin III deficiency. J.A.M.A. *245*:1759, 1981.
217. Schatz, I. J., and Stanley, J. C.: Saddle embolus of the aorta. J.A.M.A. *235*:1262, 1976.
218. Thompson, J. E., and Garrett, W. V.: Peripheral-arterial surgery. N. Engl. J. Med. *302*:491, 1980.
219. Busuttil, R. W., Keehan, G., Milliken, J., Paredero, V. M., Baker, J. J., Machleder, H. I., Moore, W.S., and Barker, W. S.: Aortic saddle embolus. Ann. Surg. *197*:698, 1983.
220. Tegtmeyer, C. J., Wellons, H. A., and Thompson, R. N.: Balloon dilation of the abdominal aorta. J.A.M.A. *244*:2636, 1980.
221. Deriu, G. P., and Ballotta, E.: Natural history of ascending thrombosis of the aorta. Am. J. Surg. *145*:652, 1983.
222. Topol, E. J., Ciuffo, A. A., Pearson, T. A., Dillman, J., Builder, S., Grossbard, E., Weisfeldt, M., and Bulkley, B. H.: Thombolysis with recombinant tissue plasminogen activator in atherosclerotic thrombotic occlusion. J. Am. Coll. Cardiol. *5*:85, 1985.

ATHEROMATOUS EMBOLI

223. Hertzer, N. R.: Peripheral atheromatous embolization following blunt abdominal trauma. Surgery *82*:244, 1977.
224. Coppetto, J. R., Lessell, S., Greco, T. P., and Eisenberg, M. S.: Diffuse disseminated atheroembolism. Arch. Ophthalmol. *102*:255, 1984.
225. Fisher, D. F., Clagett, G. P., Brigham, R. A., Orecchia, P. M., Youkey, J. R., Aronoff, R. J., Fry, R. E., and Fry, W. J.: Dilemmas in dealing with the blue toe syndrome: Aortic vs. peripheral source. Am. J. Surg. *148*:836, 1984.

AORTIC BACTERIAL INFECTIONS

226. Jarrett, F., Darling, R. C., Mundth, E. D., and Austen, W. G.: Experience with infected aneurysms of the abdominal aorta. Arch. Surg. *110*:1281, 1975.
227. Brown, S. L., Busuttil, R. W., Baker, J. D., Machleder, H. I., Moore, W. S., and Barker, W. F.: Bacteriologic and surgical determinants of survival in patients with mycotic aneurysms. J. Vasc. Surg. *1*:541, 1984.
228. Felson, B., Akers, P. V., Hall, G. S., Schreiber, J. T., Greene, R. E., and Pedrosa, C. S.: Mycotic tuberculous aneurysm of the thoracic aorta. J.A.M.A. *237*:1104, 1977.

AORTIC TUMORS

229. Chen, K. T. K.: Primary malignant fibrous histiocytoma of the aorta. Cancer *48*:840, 1981.
230. Schmid, E., Port, J. S., Carroll, R. M., and Friedman, N. B.: Primary metastasizing aortic endothelioma. Cancer *54*:1407, 1984.

47 PULMONARY EMBOLISM

by SAMUEL Z. GOLDHABER, M.D., and
EUGENE BRAUNWALD, M.D.

Pulmonary embolism (PE) accounts for an estimated 300,000 hospitalizations and as many as 50,000 deaths annually. During the past decade, this mortality rate has not declined.[1] PE may be elusive and, despite advances in diagnostic imaging, commonly goes undetected until postmortem examination.[2, 3] Therefore, prompt and accurate *diagnosis* remains the most important step toward managing this illness. In addition, new therapeutic measures are needed to decrease the mortality rate, and efforts to utilize pharmacological and mechanical prophylaxis must be renewed.

FACTORS THAT PREDISPOSE TO PULMONARY EMBOLISM

In 1856, Rudolf Virchow postulated that a triad of factors led to intravascular coagulation: (1) local trauma to the vessel wall, (2) hypercoagulability, and (3) stasis.[4] One useful approach to classifying hypercoagulable states is to consider them as either primary or secondary.[5] Primary hypercoagulable states require laboratory demonstration of specific abnormalities, whereas secondary states are clinical conditions associated with an increased risk for PE.

HYPERCOAGULABLE STATES

PRIMARY HYPERCOAGULABLE STATES. Antithrombin III (AT-III) is the major inhibitor of thrombin (which converts circulating fibrinogen to fibrin clot) and other activated clotting factors (Fig. 47–1). The most frequent manifestations of *AT-III deficiency* are recurrent PE and DVT.[5] *Deficiencies of protein C* (which consumes factors Va and VIIIa and also stimulates fibrinolysis)[6] *and protein* S (a cofactor for activated protein C) also predispose to recurrent venous thromboembolism at a young age. *Defective fibrinolysis*, whether due to defective release of tissue plasminogen activator (t-PA)[7] or an excess of t-PA inhibitor,[8] is also associated with venous thrombosis. "*Lupus anticoagulant*," usually encountered in patients without lupus, is often associated with a prolonged partial thromboplastin time (PTT) but paradoxically increases the risk of venous thromboembolism.[9, 10, 10a] Investigation of potential primary hypercoagulable states (Table 47–1) has the highest yield in patients younger than 45 years old who have "idiopathic" PE or deep venous thrombosis (DVT). Among such patients, as many as one-third may have an identifiable disorder related to defective fibrinolysis or deficiencies in protein C, protein S, or AT-III.[11]

SECONDARY HYPERCOAGULABLE STATES. Some of the most readily recognized risk factors for PE occur in *secondary* hypercoagulable states (Table 47–1), in which the molecular mechanisms causing thrombosis are not known as they are in the primary conditions. When investigating the possibility of PE, clinicians may find the presence of these clinical conditions to be more useful than symptoms and signs of PE, which are often nonspecific. Among hospitalized patients, the most common setting for PE is the *recent surgical procedure*, in which vessel trauma is combined with immobilization. *Obesity*, with its associated venous stasis, may be a long-term risk factor for PE[12] and may also increase the risk of PE among hospitalized patients undergoing surgery. *Cancer* is another well-established risk factor for PE. Patients with known malignancy in whom PE is suspected may have either thrombotic or tumor emboli. Furthermore, PE[13] or DVT[14] in patients without overt cancer may herald the presence of occult malignancy that will become manifest clinically within the next several years. This suggests that patients with venous thromboembolism should be screened and followed carefully for cancer when no etiology for the PE or DVT is clinically apparent.[15] PE is also associated with *oral contraceptive use*[16] and *pregnancy*, particularly among women confined to bed because of preeclampsia or eclampsia or those who have had a cesarean section.[17]

Indwelling central venous lines can be a nidus for right atrial thrombus that serves as a source of PE. These catheters are being used with increasing frequency to

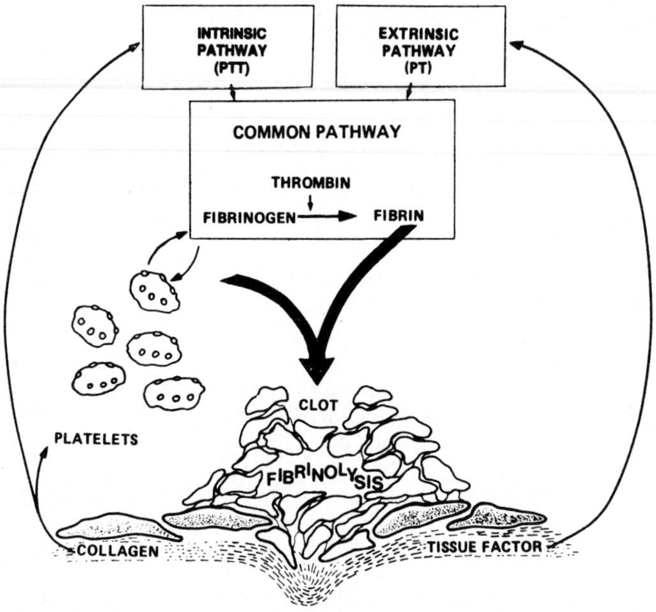

FIGURE 47–1. Simplified scheme of the hemostatic system, showing interaction of vessel wall, platelets, coagulation pathways, and fibrinolytic system. Not shown are regulatory and inhibitory mechanisms. (From Stead, R. B.: Regulation of hemostasis. *In* Goldhaber, S. Z. [ed.]: Pulmonary Embolism and Deep Venous Thrombosis. Philadelphia, W. B. Saunders Company, 1985, p. 28.)

provide alimentation for chronically ill patients and as venous access for long-term cancer chemotherapy protocols (Fig. 47–2). An increasing number of reports have also noted large right atrial thrombi due to acute myocardial infarction, congestive heart failure, atrial fibrillation, or a combination of predisposing factors.[18] In fact, the detection of right atrial thrombus (usually with two-dimensional echocardiography) in most cases should prompt a search for concomitant PE.

TABLE 47–1 HYPERCOAGULABLE STATES

Clinical Indicators of a Primary Hypercoagulable State
Family history of thrombosis
Recurrent thrombosis without apparent precipitating factors
Thrombosis at unusual anatomical sites
Thrombosis at early age
Secondary Hypercoagulable States
Abnormalities of coagulation and fibrinolysis
Malignancy
Pregnancy
Use of oral contraceptives
Infusion of prothrombin complex concentrates
Nephrotic syndrome
Abnormalities of platelets
Myeloproliferative disorders
Paroxysmal nocturnal hemoglobinuria
Hyperlipidemia
Diabetes mellitus
Heparin-induced thrombocytopenia
Abnormalities of blood vessels and rheology
Conditions promoting venous stasis (immobilization, obesity, advanced age, postoperative state)
Artificial surfaces
Vasculitis and chronic occlusive arterial disease
Homocystinuria
Hyperviscosity (polycythemia, leukemia, sickle cell disease, leukoagglutination, increased serum viscosity)
Thrombotic thrombocytopenic purpura

From Schafer, A. I.: The hypercoagulable states. Ann. Intern. Med. *102*:818 and 824, 1985.

DEEP VENOUS THROMBOSIS

RELATIONSHIP OF DVT TO PE. Although the risk of PE among patients with DVT proximal to the calf is high (approximately 35 to 50 per cent), this risk is lower when DVT remains confined to calf veins.[18a, 19] In contrast to proximal leg DVT, superficial thrombophlebitis[20] and upper extremity thrombosis are rarely associated with PE.

DIAGNOSIS OF DVT. DVT often occurs without any symptoms or signs. When present, however, the major symptoms are leg pain, tenderness, and swelling, while the major signs are leg edema, discomfort in the calf upon forced dorsiflexion of the foot (Homans' sign), venous distention of subcutaneous vessels, discoloration, and a palp-

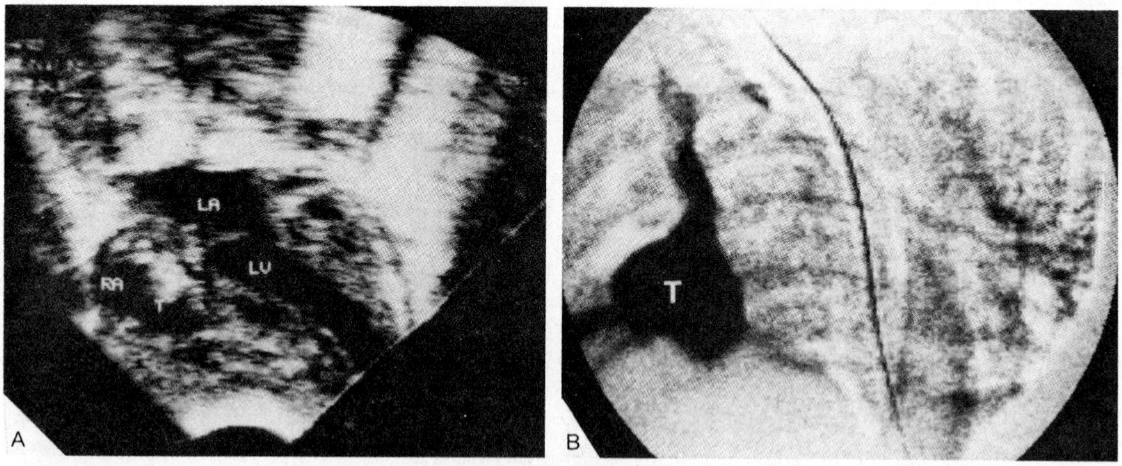

FIGURE 47–2. *A*, Two-dimensional echocardiogram from the subxiphoid position in a 9-month-old boy with *Staphylococcus epidermidis* septicemia and a central hyperalimentation line. A large thrombus (T) can be seen low in the right atrium (RA), just above the tricuspid valve. The mass, acting as a partial ball-valve thrombus, obstructed right ventricular outflow. LA = left atrium; LV = left ventricle. *B*, Digital subtraction angiogram, with contrast material injected through the hyperalimentation catheter. With the catheter tip in the superior aspect of the RA, contrast enters a large cavitary RA thrombus (T), which acts as a cul-de-sac. Thus, contrast cannot be seen in the RA or right ventricle. This thrombus is an ominous nidus for potential pulmonary embolization. (From Fulton, D. R.: Venous thromboembolism in children. *In* Goldhaber, S. Z. [ed.]: Pulmonary Embolism and Deep Venous Thrombosis. Philadelphia, W. B. Saunders Company, 1985, p. 249.)

able cord (i.e., thrombus). Unfortunately, these symptoms and signs are not specific for DVT, so that diagnoses based on clinical findings are often incorrect.[21] Therefore, clinical suspicion of DVT should prompt definitive radiological evaluation.

Leg Phlebography. This technique remains the most accurate modality to establish or exclude DVT. Despite its high cost, invasive nature, and occasional complications, leg phlebography is generally safe, rapid, and reliable, and we use it routinely to diagnose DVT at our institution.[22, 78]

Impedance Plethysmography (IPG). IPG is the most widely used noninvasive test to detect DVT. IPG measures changes in electrical resistance caused by obstruction to venous outflow.[23] Two recent large-scale studies have suggested that serial IPG testing repeated three to six times over 10 to 14 days will accurately detect calf-vein DVT that extends proximally.[24, 25] Serial IPG studies appear as useful as the combination of IPG plus leg scanning using iodine-125–labeled fibrinogen.[26] Other noninvasive approaches include venous Doppler ultrasound examination and phleborheography, used alone[27] or in combination.[28]

TREATMENT OF DVT. For all cases of DVT proximal to the calf and for symptomatic calf DVT,[29] the preferred treatment is initial heparin anticoagulation followed by warfarin therapy. In our institution, we treat almost all patients who have venographically documented DVT. This is true even though asymptomatic DVT limited to the calf need not be treated with anticoagulation as long as serial noninvasive monitoring for 2 weeks after diagnosis confirms that the clot has not extended proximally. Anticoagulation will reduce the risk of proximal propagation of clot and subsequent PE. Usually, therapy is initiated with a continuous intravenous infusion of heparin, because this appears to be more efficacious than intermittent subcutaneous administration.[30]

During chronic anticoagulation with conventional dosages of warfarin, bleeding complications are frequent despite scrupulous laboratory monitoring and clinical surveillance. However, it appears that less intensive warfarin therapy effectively treats proximal DVT and is associated with a reduced risk of hemorrhage compared with standard-dose warfarin.[31] A cost-effectiveness analysis has also indicated that low-dose warfarin is advantageous compared with other strategies for the long-term treatment of proximal DVT.[32]

PROGNOSIS OF DVT. Although chronic anticoagulation (usually for 3 months) is prescribed to avert recurrent venous thromboembolism, the optimal length of such treatment is unknown. One-fifth of patients with DVT may experience a recurrence despite 3 months of anticoagulation.[33] Therefore, in our own practice, we anticoagulate patients with no long-term risk factors for 6 months, with PT maintained at 14 to 16 seconds. For those patients with risk factors such as massive obesity, cancer, or previous DVT, anticoagulants are given for an indefinite period of time.

PATHOPHYSIOLOGY OF PULMONARY EMBOLISM

When venous thrombi become dislodged from their site of formation, they flow through the venous system to the pulmonary arterial circulation. If an embolus is extremely large, it may lodge at the bifurcation of the pulmonary artery, forming a "saddle embolus" (Fig. 47–3*A*). More commonly, a major pulmonary vessel will be occluded (Fig. 47–3*B*).[34]

The pathophysiological response to acute PE depends upon the extent to which pulmonary artery blood flow is obstructed, preexisting cardiopulmonary disease, and the release of vasoactive humoral factors from activated platelets that accumulate at the site of new clot (p. 1759). In patients without prior cardiopulmonary disease, right ventricular afterload increases when pulmonary artery obstruction reduces the pulmonary vascular bed by 25 per cent or more. To compensate for this impairment, right ventricular and pulmonary artery pressures rise. The previously normal right ventricle can generate a maximum pulmonary artery systolic pressure of approximately 40 mm Hg. As right ventricular afterload increases acutely, this chamber dilates (leading in turn to tricuspid regurgitation) and becomes hypokinetic. These findings can be observed on two-dimensional (Fig. 47–4) and Doppler echocardiography, which can be used to estimate pulmonary artery

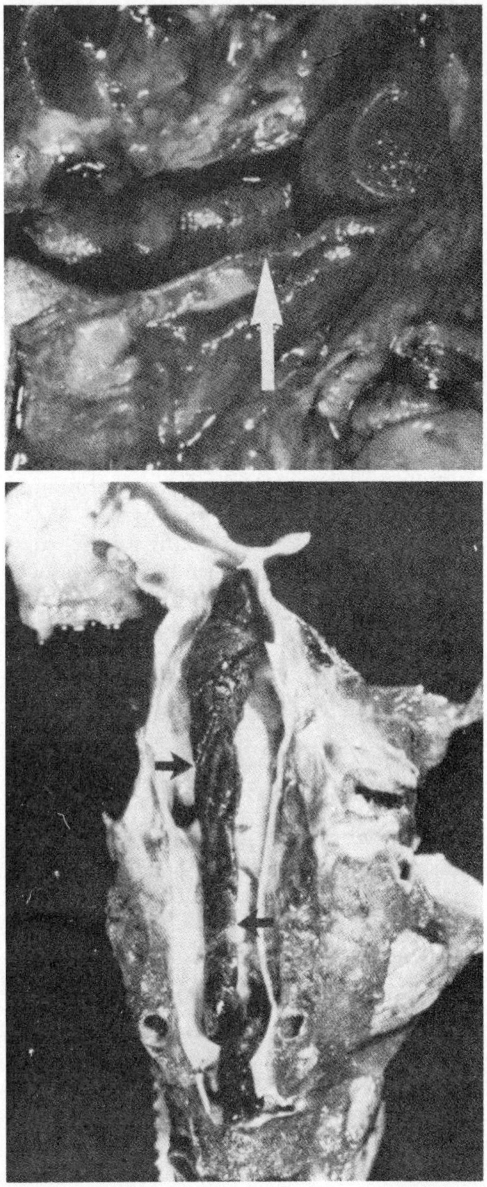

FIGURE 47–3. *Top,* **Saddle embolus at the bifurcation of the pulmonary artery.** *Bottom,* **Pulmonary embolus in left lower lobe pulmonary artery, with minimal attachment to the wall of the vessel. The embolus was dark red, typical of venous thrombi, and had indentations believed to represent impressions of the venous valves (arrows). (From Godleski, J. J.: Pathology of deep venous thrombosis and pulmonary embolism.** *In* **Goldhaber, S. Z. [ed.]: Pulmonary Embolism and Deep Venous Thrombosis. Philadelphia, W. B. Saunders Company, 1985, p. 17.)**

pressure. As the right ventricle fails, right atrial pressure rises and cardiogenic shock ensues. When cardiac function has been compromised by previous cardiopulmonary illness, relatively smaller emboli obstructing only one or two pulmonary segments can exert a similar hemodynamic effect.

Although preload, afterload, heart rate, and contractility have traditionally been considered the determinants of left ventricular systolic performance (Chap. 13), acute increases in right ventricular pressure can also affect left ventricular function. In a canine model, acutely induced moderate right ventricular hypertension displaces the interventricular septum toward the left ventricle (Fig. 61–10, p. 1880). Therefore, during pressure overload of the right ventricle, the anatomical juxtaposition of the two ventricles (i.e., ventricular interdependency) results in decreased left ventricular diastolic filling and end-diastolic volume[35] and an *apparent* change in left ventricular distensibility.

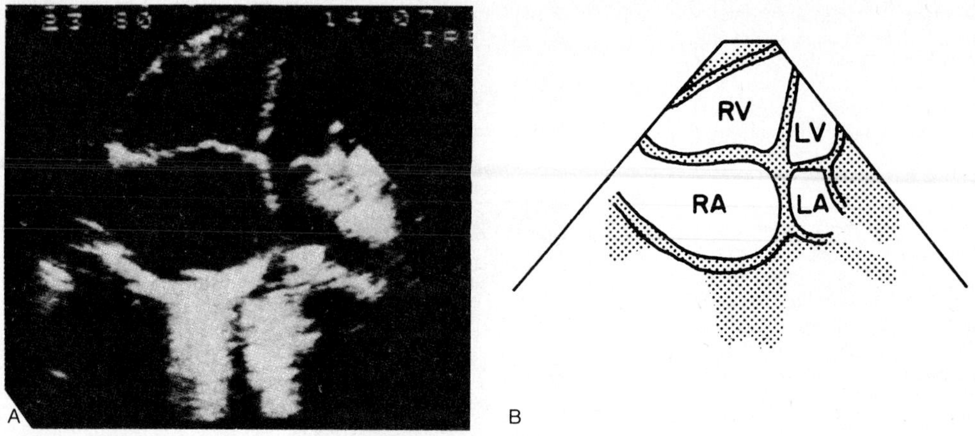

FIGURE 47–4. Apical four-chamber two-dimensional echocardiogram (*A*) and schematic drawing (*B*) from a patient with massive pulmonary embolism. There is marked dilatation of the right atrium (RA) and right ventricle (RV). (The apparent mass in the region of the left atrium [LA] is an imaging defect.) (From Hoagland, P. M.: Massive pulmonary embolism. *In* Goldhaber, S. Z. [ed.]: Pulmonary Embolism and Deep Venous Thrombosis. Philadelphia, W. B. Saunders Company, 1985, p. 187.)

After embolization, the release of neurohumoral factors causes vasoconstriction and bronchospasm that can adversely affect outcome. Experimental studies suggest that during acute PE the two most important vasoactive humoral factors are serotonin[36] and thromboxane A_2 (TxA_2).[37] Serotonin, a potent neural and smooth muscle agonist, is stored primarily in the dense bodies of platelets and mediates bronchospasm in the small airways, either by direct bronchial smooth muscle constriction or by stimulating a neural reflex that induces bronchospasm. Activated platelets also secrete TxA_2, a potent vasoconstrictor and bronchoconstrictor.

DIAGNOSIS OF PULMONARY EMBOLISM

CLINICAL PRESENTATION

Clinical suspicion of PE is of paramount importance to guide diagnostic testing. *Overdiagnosis* as well as *underdiagnosis* can occur without the judicious use of radiological imaging to detect PE. In various autopsy series, rates of overdiagnosis ranged from 32 to 62 per cent, and the rate of underdiagnosis has been reported to be as high as 84 per cent.[38] In the Urokinase-Streptokinase Pulmonary Embolism Trial (UPET), clinical symptoms and signs were tabulated in 327 patients with angiographically documented PE (Table 47–2).[39] Because symptoms and signs often do not help to discriminate between patients with true PE and those with no evidence of PE on the arteriogram,[40] the physician should pursue the diagnosis by radionuclide scanning or angiography in virtually all cases in which PE is suspected.

DIFFERENTIAL DIAGNOSIS. The differential diagnosis depends upon whether patients have other major medical problems that require hospitalization (Table 47–3). When *established pneumonia* (with an infiltrate on chest x-ray), *congestive heart failure*, or *myocardial infarction* does not respond to appropriate therapy, it may be prudent to rule out coexisting PE. *Recurrent PE* can increase pulmonary artery pressure and may be mistaken for *primary pulmonary hypertension* (p. 805).[41] Although these two conditions share many common features, certain other features can be used to differentiate them (Table 47–4).

TABLE 47–2 SYMPTOMS AND SIGNS IN 327 PATIENTS WITH PULMONARY EMBOLISM

Symptoms	
Dyspnea	84%
Pleuritic chest pain	74%
Apprehension	59%
Cough	53%
Hemoptysis	30%
Diaphoresis	36%
Syncope	13%
Signs	
Tachypnea (RR > 16/min)	92%
Rales	58%
Accentuated second heart sound	53%
Tachycardia (HR > 100/min)	44%
Fever (Temp > 37.8°C)	43%
Phlebitis	32%
Cyanosis	19%

From Bell, W. R., Simon, T. L., and DeMets, D. L.: The clinical features of submassive and massive pulmonary emboli. Am. J. Med. 62:355, 1977. (Data based on the Urokinase-Streptokinase Pulmonary Embolism Trial.)

Clinical Syndromes of PE

MASSIVE PE. This can be defined as sufficient obstruction of pulmonary arterial blood flow to cause an increase in right ventricular afterload and consequent elevation of pulmonary arterial systolic pressure. Such patients are at highest risk for sudden death from PE or, over the long term, for chronic pulmonary hypertension due to pulmonary arterial clot that has failed to lyse. The most common features that suggest this diagnosis are syncope, cor pulmonale, cardiogenic shock, or cardiac arrest (particularly with electromechanical dissociation), often preceded by dyspnea or pleuritic chest pain. When syncope occurs,[42] it may at times be due to associated vagal bradyarrhythmias.[43] Patients also frequently display tachycardia, tachypnea, and cyanosis with distended neck veins; cardiogenic shock (Chap. 19) may be present or incipient. The differential diagnosis may include septic shock, superior vena caval syndrome, pericardial tamponade (p. 1492), constrictive pericarditis (p. 1501), and right ventricular infarction. When massive PE is suspected, right heart catheterization and pulmonary angiography provide valuable baseline information. If angiographic results are normal, catheterization may indicate alternative diagnoses.

SUBMASSIVE PE. This can be defined as embolism to one or more pulmonary segments *not* accompanied by elevations in right ventricular and pulmonary artery systolic pressures. The most frequent symptoms are dyspnea and pleuritic chest pain. Although these patients are not likely to succumb to an acute episode, unlysed thrombus in the pulmonary arteries could eventually lead to chronic pulmonary hypertension.

TABLE 47–3 DIFFERENTIAL DIAGNOSIS OF PULMONARY EMBOLISM

Outpatients
- Pleurodynia
- Costochondritis
- "Early pneumonia" not evident on chest x-ray
- Rib fracture

Outpatients or Inpatients
- Myocardial infarction
- Asthma
- Chronic obstructive pulmonary disease
- Established pneumonia with infiltrate on chest x-ray
- Congestive heart failure
- Pneumothorax

PULMONARY INFARCTION. With occlusion of small peripheral pulmonary arteries, bronchoconstriction frequently occurs, and collateral blood flow via the bronchial arteries may not be preserved, leading to pulmonary infarction. The clinical diagnosis of pulmonary infarction due to PE cannot be established unless an infiltrate is present on chest x-ray and the usual criteria for PE on lung scan or pulmonary angiography are met. The primary alternative diagnosis based on clinical presentation is pneumonia. Some PE patients with pulmonary infarction present with hemoptysis; virtually all experience intense pleuritic pain but tend to have a unilateral, distal embolism that is less extensive on angiography than in PE patients without pulmonary infarction.[44, 45] Typically, symptoms and signs develop 3 to 7 days after the onset of embolism. Aside from anticoagulation, treatment is supportive and usually requires substantial and prolonged narcotic analgesia.

CHRONIC PULMONARY HYPERTENSION. Recurrent PE may cause chronic pulmonary hypertension associated with a clinical syndrome of progressive right heart failure and cor pulmonale. This condition tends to develop insidiously when PE is either not diagnosed or treated inadequately. On examination, new or changing heart murmurs may be heard and the lung fields may be clear despite the presence of dyspnea, cyanosis, peripheral edema, and ascites.[46] The degree of dyspnea appears to correlate with the elevation in pulmonary artery pressure.[47] Chronic pulmonary hypertension due to recurrent PE is a feared complication of venous thromboembolism and has a poor prognosis. (It is hypothesized that the use of thrombolytic agents to treat PE may reduce the incidence of this complication.) Nevertheless, it is important to recognize this clinical syndrome[48] so that these patients can be evaluated for potential pulmonary thromboendarterectomy (see below, p. 1591).

LESS COMMON PRESENTATIONS OF PE (Table 47–5). Unusual manifestations of PE can make clinical recognition particularly difficult. It is also important to consider the possibility of *nonthrombotic* PE.[49]

TABLE 47–4 PRIMARY PULMONARY HYPERTENSION (PPH) VS. RECURRENT PE

SIMILARITIES		
Symptoms	Fatigue, dyspnea on exertion—most common Chest pain, syncope, hemoptysis, cyanosis—also common	
Clinical course	Progressive dyspnea, right heart failure	
Hemodynamics	Elevated right heart pressures, normal pulmonary capillary wedge pressure	
DIFFERENCES		
	PPH	*Recurrent PE*
Age	20 to 40 years	> 50 years
Female:male ratio	4:1	1:1
Clinical course	Continued downhill	Downhill, with stabilization between episodes
Lung scan	No segmental perfusion defects	Segmental or larger perfusion defects
Pulmonary artery systolic pressure	>60 mm Hg	< 60 mm Hg
Pulmonary arteriogram	"Pruning"	Intraluminal filling defects
Confounding problems with arteriogram	Thrombi may occur on or distal to PPH lesions	"Pruning," a common angiographic finding in PPH, can also indicate PE. Arteriogram may not show emboli late in the clinical course.
Diagnostic alternatives	Open lung biopsy	Pulmonary angioscopy
Therapy	Isoproterenol Hydralazine Nifedipine Anticoagulation	Pulmonary angioscopy Anticoagulation IVC interruption Thromboendarterectomy

From Goldhaber, S. Z.: Strategies for diagnosis. *In* Goldhaber, S. Z. (ed.): Pulmonary Embolism and Deep Venous Thrombosis. Philadelphia, W. B. Saunders Company, 1985, p. 89.

NONIMAGING MODALITIES

ARTERIAL BLOOD GASES. Hypoxemia, determined by means of arterial blood gas measurement, has traditionally been considered an important screening test for PE. Yet patients suspected of PE who are then found to have normal lung scans or pulmonary angiograms may be as hypoxemic as or more hypoxemic than those with documented PE.[50] Conversely, a high PO_2 can mistakenly dissuade the physician from pursuing the diagnosis of PE.[51] Therefore, we believe that arterial blood gases, while of value for many aspects of patient care, are not really useful in the *diagnosis* of PE.

ANALYSIS OF PLEURAL FLUID. In one prospective series, pleural effusions occurred in about half of 155 patients with PE.[52] However, this finding is nonspecific, because effusions are also common in patients with congestive heart failure, pneumonia, and cancer. Furthermore, results of pleural fluid analysis are so variable[53] that thoracentesis should not be undertaken in patients with suspected PE unless a concomitant infectious process is considered likely. If thoracentesis has been performed, thrombolytic agents should usually not be administered for 10 days.

ELECTROCARDIOGRAM. The electrocardiogram tends to show characteristic abnormalities only in patients with massive PE. Traditional manifestations of acute cor pulmonale such as $S_1Q_3T_3$ (Fig. 7–17, p. 193), right bundle

TABLE 47–5 PRESENTATIONS OF THROMBOTIC AND NONTHROMBOTIC PE

Thrombotic PE as Sole Presenting Feature (unusual manifestations)
- Fever
- Paradoxical arterial embolism
- Wheezing
- Disseminated intravascular coagulation

Sources of Nonthrombotic PE
- Tumor
- Infection
- Fat
- Amniotic fluid
- Air
- Foreign particles (e.g., bullets)
- Endogenous fluids or organs
- Parasites
- Catheters
- Silicone

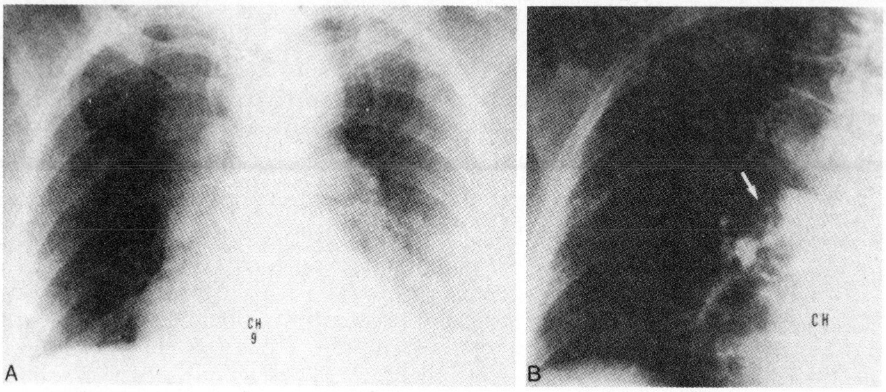

FIGURE 47–5. *A*, Chest x-ray of patient with clinical signs of pulmonary embolism showing marked oligemia (Westermark's sign) in the entire right lobe. *B*, Arteriogram from same patient showing massive saddle embolus in the right main pulmonary artery (arrow). (Courtesy of Jack L. Westcott, M.D., The New York Hospital and Cornell University Medical College.)

branch block, P pulmonale, or right-axis deviation occurred in only 26 per cent of the patients evaluated in the Urokinase Pulmonary Embolism Trial (UPET).[54] Usually, when the electrocardiogram suggests PE, the diagnosis tends to be apparent for other reasons, such as the clinical presentation.

BLOOD TESTS. To date, no rapid, inexpensive, and accurate blood test to screen for PE or DVT (analogous to the CK-MB enzyme assay used to diagnose acute myocardial infarction) has been found. The most frequently studied test is the determination of fibrin split products (FSP), also known as fibrinogen/fibrin degradation products (FDP/fdp, or FDPs).[55] FDPs have been found to be markedly increased in some patients with PE.

CONVENTIONAL IMAGING MODALITIES

CHEST ROENTGENOGRAPHY. Occlusion of a lobar or segmental artery will cause a relative local hyperlucency on plain film, with markedly diminished vascular markings (Fig. 45–5). An engorged major hilar artery on a plain film is another important clue to massive PE, especially when serial studies are available.[56] The sudden appearance of a "plump" vessel, particularly the right descending pulmonary artery,[57] strongly suggests embolic disease. In most cases, hilar signs are right-sided because cardiac and main pulmonary artery shadows make it difficult to visualize left-sided hilar signs. Abrupt tapering or termination of a vessel, termed the "knuckle sign," although rarely noted, can be diagnostic of PE.[58] Nonspecific signs include diminished volume of a lower lobe with displacement of a major fissure or elevation of a hemidiaphragm.[56] Obviously, these findings on chest roentgenography are not diagnostic, but in the proper clinical setting they may increase or even arouse suspicion.[59]

In *pulmonary infarction*, parenchymal consolidation is observed as an increased radiographic density. This finding may be due to actual tissue necrosis or to so-called reversible infarction (i.e., hemorrhage and edema) that clears within 3 to 7 days. However, if infarction leads to necrosis, the average time of resolution is about 3 weeks, usually with permanent residual fibrotic changes.[60] The classic configuration is a homogeneous wedge-shaped density in the peripheral region of the lung with a rounded, convex apex pointing toward the hilum—commonly referred to as "Hampton's hump" (Fig. 47–6).[61] *Absence* of an air bronchogram in a parenchymal consolidation is suggestive of infarction[62] as opposed to a pneumonic process; on the other hand, the *presence* of an air bronchogram is inconclusive because it is sometimes observed in patients with PE.

The chest roentgenogram may also provide an important clue that pulmonary artery hypertension is due to chronic PE when there is right-sided cardiomegaly, mosaic oligemia, or right descending pulmonary artery enlargement.[63] Overall, however, chest roentgenography is an insensitive screening test for PE. Its major diagnostic utility lies in its capacity to suggest diagnoses *other* than PE.

LUNG SCANNING. Perfusion lung scanning is the key diagnostic test in screening for PE. A normal scan essentially rules out all but trivial-sized PE and directs clinical attention to other diagnostic possibilities. Abnormal scans are usually categorized as having a low, moderate, high, or indeterminate probability for PE, but the optimal definitions of these categories have not yet been agreed upon. For patients with perfusion defects that are segmental or greater in size, normal ventilation on scintigraphy in the same areas as the perfusion defects increases the likelihood of PE. Traditionally, at the Brigham and Women's Hospital, *low probability* scans are defined as showing subsegmental perfusion defects without a ventilation study or subsegmental or larger perfusion defects with abnormal ventilation correlating with the perfusion defects (a ventilation-perfusion [$\dot{V}/\dot{Q}$] "match"). *Moderate probability* scans show multiple subsegmental perfusion defects with normal ventilation or segmental or larger perfusion defects without a ventilation study. *High probability* scans show segmental or larger perfusion defects with normal ventilation ($\dot{V}/\dot{Q}$ "mismatch"). Scans are of *indeterminate probability* when the chest x-ray either demonstrates COPD or is abnormal in the region(s) of the perfusion defect. In patients with only a single perfusion defect, reliable probability estimates are difficult to derive from currently available data.[64]

To date, Hull and colleagues have published the largest prospective study comparing abnormal ventilation-perfusion lung scans with results on pulmonary angiography

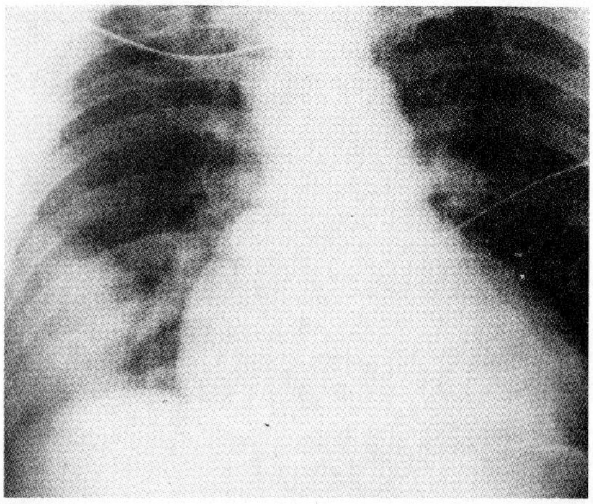

FIGURE 47–6. Posteroanterior chest x-ray of patient with pulmonary embolism showing "Hampton's hump" in right lower lung field, a homogeneous, wedge-shaped density in the peripheral lung field, convex to the hilum. (Courtesy of Jack L. Westcott, M.D., The New York Hospital and Cornell University Medical College.)

among patients suspected of having PE.[65] Their findings support the traditional definition of a *high probability* lung scan (e.g., 86 per cent accuracy) but call into question that of *low probability* scans. However, these results have been challenged owing to potential selection bias in the patient population that they studied. At Duke University Medical Center, angiographic evidence of PE was found in 15 per cent of patients with low probability scans, 32 per cent with moderate scans, 66 per cent with high probability scans, and 39 per cent with indeterminate scans[66]; however, this was also a highly selected and unrepresentative population. Data comparing lung scans and pulmonary angiograms in approximately 1000 patients are currently being analyzed from the recently completed Prospective Investigation of Pulmonary Embolism Diagnosis.

Given the limitations of lung scanning, it is worrisome if clinicians defer pulmonary angiography in favor of lung scanning, particularly when the results of the latter differ sharply from the clinical impression.[67] Therefore, in estimating the probability of PE, the physician should interpret the lung scan based on the clinical assessment of the likelihood of disease. This clinical estimate is obtained by integrating history, symptoms, signs, and results on chest roentgenogram.[68]

PULMONARY ANGIOGRAPHY

Indications. Because of the controversy surrounding the interpretation of abnormal lung scans, a diagnostic problem arises every time a patient's scan is abnormal. Should all patients (outside of a research protocol) be referred for pulmonary angiography? We think not (Fig. 47–7). When a lung scan is normal, there is generally no reason to pursue the diagnosis of PE. Instead, alternative diagnostic possibilities should be considered, such as pleuritis, pleurodynia, or costochondritis. Conversely, when ventilation-perfusion lung scanning indicates a high probability of PE and clinical suspicion is high prior to scanning, it is generally not necessary to proceed with pulmonary angiography. In most situations, multiple segmental or lobar perfusion defects in areas of normal ventilation will correspond with angiographically documented PE. However, if thrombolytic therapy or inferior vena caval interruption is being considered, one may wish to eliminate even the slightest diagnostic uncertainty by obtaining a pulmonary angiogram.

For patients with low probability scans, we do not obtain pulmonary angiograms unless clinical suspicion of PE is high, since many subsegmental and nonsegmental perfusion defects that match ventilation defects have been found to correspond with normal angiographic findings.[69, 70] In one small study of patients with low probability ventilation-perfusion scans, major short-term morbidity or death attributable to PE was not identified.[71]

In general, pulmonary angiography is reserved for patients with moderate probability or indeterminate lung scans except when clinical suspicion for PE is high despite scan results or when thrombolytic therapy or caval interruption is being considered. The use of pulmonary angiography is increasing because the limitations of lung scanning and clinical diagnosis are becoming more widely appreciated. However, unless the patient is hemodynamically unstable or empirical heparinization is absolutely contraindicated (e.g., active gastrointestinal bleeding), these studies need not be done on an emergency basis.

We do not substitute impedance plethysmography (IPG) or venography for pulmonary angiography, nor do we rely on empirical treatment with heparin followed by serial lung scanning to detect improved perfusion as a means of

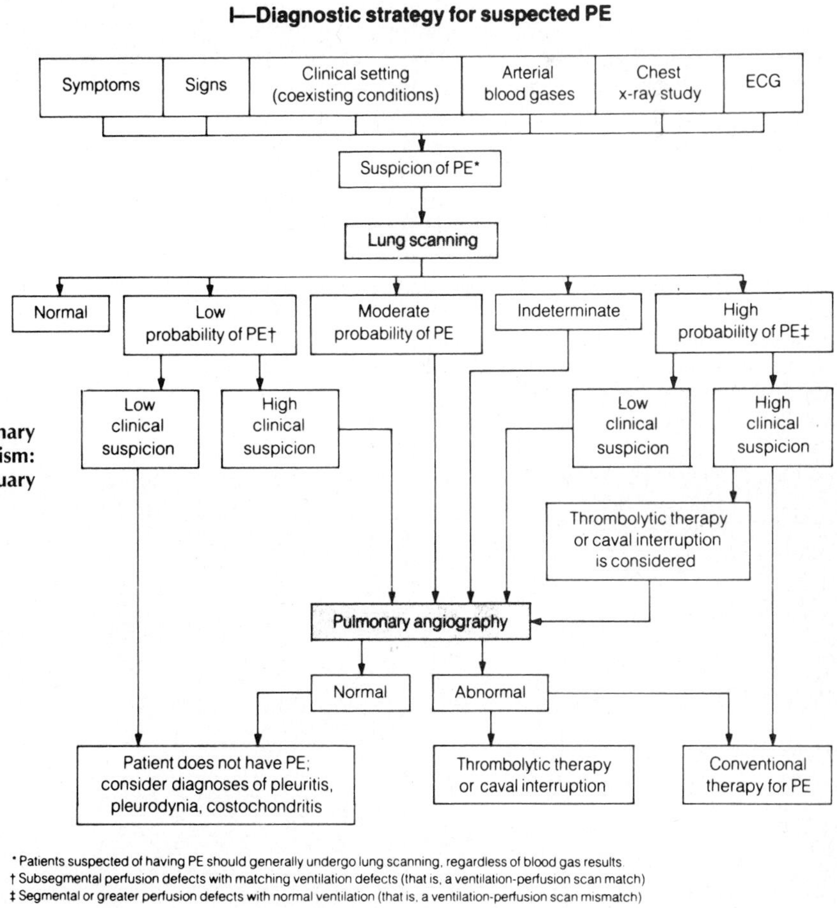

FIGURE 47–7. Diagnostic strategy in suspected pulmonary embolism. (From Goldhaber, S. Z.: Pulmonary embolism: Diagnostic and therapeutic options. Consultant, February 1986, p. 126.)

avoiding angiography, since both these strategies can be seriously misleading. In the prospective study by Hull et al., only 43 per cent of patients with positive pulmonary angiograms also had positive results on IPG. Conversely, 18 per cent of patients with normal pulmonary angiograms had positive IPG results.[65] If one argues that venography, rather than IPG, should be used to direct the workup of PE, the results would still be discordant. Of patients with positive pulmonary angiograms, only 71 per cent had positive venograms; conversely, 33 per cent of patients with normal pulmonary angiograms had positive venograms. Based on these findings, neither IPG nor venography should, in our opinion, be used to diagnose PE.

The diagnostic strategy of obtaining serial lung scans in patients suspected of PE can be misleading. For example, someone with an early viral pneumonia (and no chest x-ray infiltrate) might have a moderate probability lung scan. Advocates of serial diagnostic lung scanning would opt for deferring angiography, empirically treating with heparin, and repeating the lung scan several days later. Under most circumstances, however, the viral pneumonia would resolve spontaneously and the lung scan would revert to normal. With serial scans, such a patient would then be considered as having PE that responded to heparin therapy and long-term warfarin therapy would be undertaken. In contrast, with a negative pulmonary angiogram, this patient could be discharged from the hospital immediately, without misdiagnosis and inappropriate long-term anticoagulation.

To *summarize*, except for extenuating circumstances such as terminal illness or a history of life-threatening anaphylaxis to contrast medium, we recommend pulmonary angiography when lung scans are inconclusive (i.e., moderate or indeterminate probability for PE).[69] We also pursue angiography when our clinical suspicion for the condition is not consistent with the lung scan result. Finally, when we plan thrombolytic therapy or vena caval interruption, we prefer to obtain angiographic confirmation of the suspected diagnosis.

Performance of Pulmonary Angiography. The pulmonary angiogram is the most specific examination available for establishing the clinical diagnosis of PE and serves as the template against which other techniques and approaches are measured.[72, 78] The procedure is generally safe, except in patients who are allergic to the contrast agent or in whom right ventricular end-diastolic pressure exceeds 20 mm Hg. New contrast agents of lower osmolality are less toxic than conventional angiographic dye in patients with pulmonary hypertension.[73] In patients with markedly elevated right ventricular end-diastolic pressure, we perform superselective pulmonary angiography using a nonionic contrast agent, even though these newly developed agents are far more costly. In addition, pulmonary angiography may present a specific hazard in patients with amiodarone-induced pulmonary toxicity (p. 639), since it has been reported to cause rapidly progressive fatal adult respiratory distress syndrome.[74]

PREPARATION OF THE PATIENT. The rationale for performing this test should be carefully explained to the patient. Those with high probability lung scans should understand that there is a 10 to 15 per cent chance that they do not have PE but that this determination can be made only with pulmonary angiography.

The patient should be told that the procedure may cause discomfort. The injection of local anesthesia may cause a burning sensation prior to the initial venipuncture, and the prolonged supine position on the angiographic examination table may cause back ache. The injection of contrast medium causes a transient hot, flushed feeling coupled almost inevitably with an urge to cough. (Nonionic contrast agents have the advantage of causing a much milder heat sensation.) Patients should also be informed that pulmonary angiography usually requires between one and five sets of injections in different views (Fig. 47–8).

A history of allergy to contrast medium should be elicited. Patients should avoid heavy meals for at least 4 hours prior to angiography. Heparin can be discontinued 2 to 4 hours before the procedure. Premedication may include 25 to 50 mg of oral diphenhydramine or 5 to 10 mg of diazepam 30 to 60 minutes before the procedure; when there is a history of adverse reactions to contrast medium, high-dose steroids may be added. If true anaphylaxis to dye has occurred in the past, the decision to proceed with the study must be questioned.

THE ANGIOGRAPHIC PROCEDURE. Our preferred approach is via the right femoral vein. Percutaneous cannulation of the femoral vein (located 1 to 2 cm medial to the palpable femoral artery) permits rapid access to a large vessel and avoids the problems of using small brachial veins, which may be difficult to cannulate with a No. 7 French catheter and which are prone to venospasm. Ordinarily, right atrial, right ventricular, and pulmonary artery pressures are recorded through a pigtail catheter prior to pulmonary arteriography. Perfusion defects on the lung scan are used to determine which lung to study initially. *Selective* angiography should be used rather than main pulmonary artery injection. Once the catheter has been positioned and the patient has been placed in the desired projection, a test dose of 5 to 10 ml is administered. A plain "scout" film is then obtained to ensure satisfactory exposure and field of view. Prior to the injection, the patient should be carefully instructed about proper breathing technique and should be reminded to try to suppress the urge to cough. Filming is carried out during maximal inspiration. Twenty to 25 ml of contrast medium per second is injected for 2 seconds. The exposure rates for this phase are three per second for 3 seconds and then one per second for the pulmonary venous phase, which occurs 5 to 7 seconds after injection.[75] After the selective pulmonary artery injection, pulmonary artery pressures are rechecked to monitor a possible pulmonary hypertensive response, and systemic arterial pressure should be rechecked (with a sphygmomanometer rather than an indwelling arterial cannula) to detect potential hypotension.

The "large-film" method that we employ offers high resolution, clarity of vascular detail, and versatility in field size. An alternative approach utilizes cineangiography.[76]

Interpreting the Angiogram. PE cannot be excluded unless the vasculature appears normal on two different oblique views (Fig. 47–8). A definitive diagnosis of PE depends on visualization of a clot. Primary arteriographic

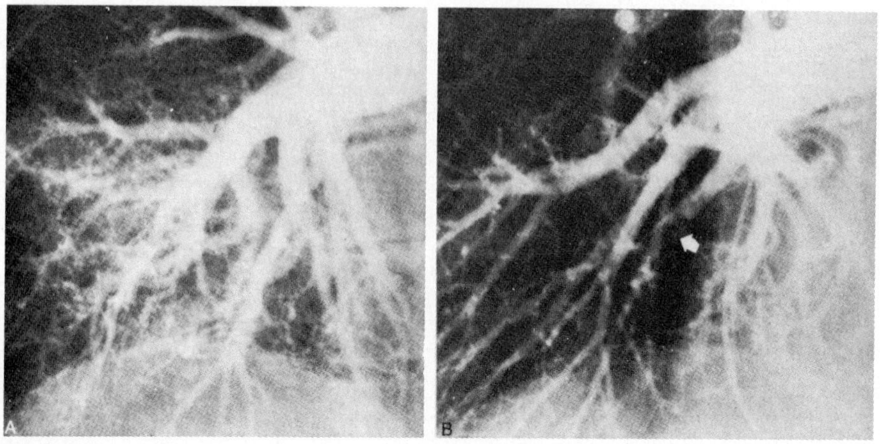

FIGURE 47–8. Selective right pulmonary arteriogram. *A*, Left posterior oblique projection of right lower lobe with normal-appearing pulmonary arteriogram due to overlap of vasculature. *B*, Right posterior oblique projection of the same area exhibiting an intravascular filling defect (arrow) in the artery to the lateral basal segment of the right lower lobe. (Courtesy of Thomas A. Sos, M.D., The New York Hospital and Cornell University Medical Center.)

signs of emboli are persistent lucent defects without obstruction to flow or a trailing edge of an intraluminal lucency if there is complete obstruction to flow distally. Secondary signs—not diagnostic in themselves but simply indicators of decreased pulmonary perfusion—include areas of avascularity or oligemia, a prolonged arterial phase, tortuosity of peripheral vessels, and delayed visualization of the pulmonary venous circulation. These signs are often associated with PE but can occur in other conditions (e.g., bronchial asthma, severe mitral stenosis with associated pulmonary hypertension, or left ventricular failure) and thus are not specific. A primary sign of embolus is mandatory to prevent false-positive diagnoses. Not all pulmonary artery filling defects or occlusions are due to PE. Other causes include pulmonary Takayasu's arteritis (p. 1563), angiosarcoma, and sarcoidosis.[77]

In *summary*, pulmonary angiography is an underutilized procedure that provides maximal diagnostic accuracy. Because the use of stiff catheters which occasionally cause perforation of the right heart and cardiac tamponade has been abandoned, morbidity at present is predominantly related to toxicity of the contrast agent rather than the catheterization. With proper technique, and judicious use of nonionic contrast agents, the mortality rate should not exceed 0.2 per cent.[78]

Other Imaging Modalities

DOPPLER ECHOCARDIOGRAPHY. The diagnosis of massive PE can sometimes be established by means of two-dimensional echocardiography (Fig. 47–9).[79] In addition to imaging the echo-dense clot, this technique also allows visualization of right atrial and right ventricular dilatation and hypokinesis (Fig. 47–4). Sagar and colleagues have suggested that the combination of the echocardiographic pulmonary reflection coefficient, the coefficient of tissue attenuation, and the range-gated Doppler estimate of intrapulmonary blood flow is accurate in detecting the presence of PE.[80]

DIGITAL SUBTRACTION PULMONARY ANGIOGRAPHY (DSA) (p. 356). Although DSA is a useful technique for diagnosing PE in patients suspected of having massive central embolism, it cannot exclude clinically important peripheral PE. Whether DSA remains a research procedure for detecting PE will depend mostly on whether further technological modifications can reduce motion artifacts and improve the images of segmental and subsegmental pulmonary arteries.[81]

COMPUTED TOMOGRAPHY (CT) (p. 360). This technique has been used to demonstrate chronic PE in patients with pulmonary hypertension (Fig. 47–10).[82] Because of the risks associated with conventional pulmonary angiography in these patients, CT should be considered as an experimental alternative diagnostic modality. It can also be used for serial noninvasive evaluation after medical thrombolysis or surgical embolectomy.

MAGNETIC RESONANCE IMAGING (MRI) (p. 368). This technique

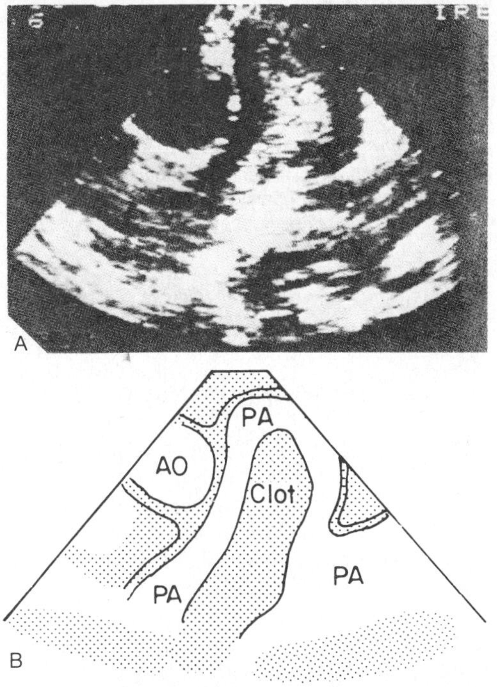

FIGURE 47–9. Two-dimensional echocardiogram in the short-axis parasternal view (*A*) and schematic drawing (*B*) showing a thrombus in the pulmonary artery in a patient with massive pulmonary embolism (seen in Figure 47–4). (From Hoagland, P. M.: Massive pulmonary embolism. *In* Goldhaber, S. Z. [ed.]: Pulmonary Embolism and Deep Venous Thrombosis. Philadelphia, W. B. Saunders Company, 1985, p. 187.)

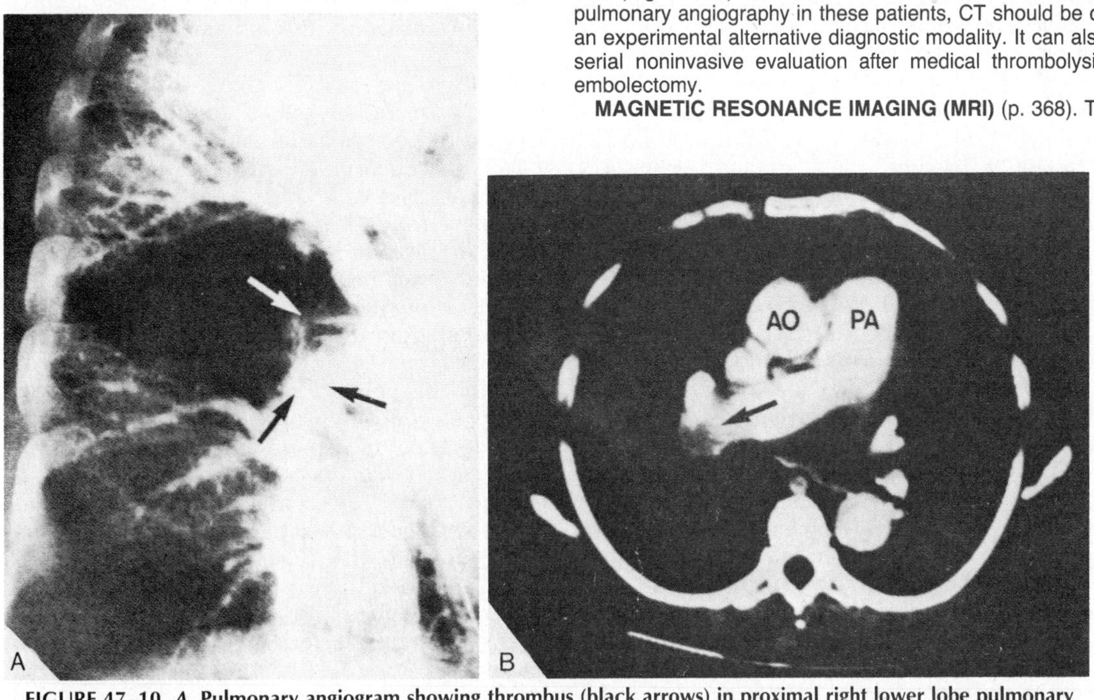

FIGURE 47–10. *A*, Pulmonary angiogram showing thrombus (black arrows) in proximal right lower lobe pulmonary artery. The most proximal portion of the thrombus is indistinct, while the upper margin can be identified as a soft tissue density (white arrow), which does not become enhanced with the injection of contrast material. *B*, The CT scan clearly visualizes a nonenhanced filling defect (arrow) in the distal right main pulmonary artery. The cross-sectional format allows excellent orientation as to the extent and localization of this proximal thrombus. (From Kereiakes, D. J., et al.: Computerized tomography in chronic thromboembolic pulmonary hypertension. Am. Heart J. *106*:1435, 1983.)

does not image rapidly flowing blood and may therefore be uniquely suited for detecting PE. Initial reports using this technique in a canine model[83] and in patients[84] have been encouraging.

INDIUM-111–LABELED PLATELET IMAGING. The physical half-life of indium-111 (2.8 days) and the biological life of the injected platelet (8 to 10 days) permit imaging of PE[85] and DVT[86] for at least 5 days after injection of the platelet suspension. Therefore, the technique is especially useful for surveillance of high-risk patients[87] and for monitoring the therapeutic response once PE and DVT have been detected and treated.[88]

FIBEROPTIC ANGIOSCOPY. After jugular venotomy and insertion of the fiberoptic angioscope into the superior vena cava, the balloon is inflated to displace blood and obtain a clear view. The angioscope is then guided with fluoroscopic assistance into the right heart and main pulmonary artery. Pulmonary artery branches as distal as segmental arteries can be examined. The technique appears to be particularly useful in patients with chronic pulmonary hypertension.[89]

TREATMENT OF PULMONARY EMBOLISM

ANTICOAGULATION

HEPARIN (See also p. 1771). Anticoagulation acts primarily to prevent further clot deposition and to allow for the body's natural fibrinolytic mechanisms to lyse clot that has already been formed. One placebo-controlled randomized trial has been carried out in PE patients.[90] The mortality rate was significantly lower among the treated patients, and the randomized trial was discontinued for ethical reasons. No randomized placebo-controlled trial with heparin has ever been undertaken in DVT.[91]

To achieve an effective antithrombotic state, a certain minimal level of heparin anticoagulation appears necessary. In practice, an effective level of heparin anticoagulation can be inferred from an activated partial thromboplastin time (PTT) that is at least 1½ times greater than the control value. Although a PTT greater than 1½ times control is probably associated with prevention of recurrent venous thromboembolism during heparin therapy, the relation between hemorrhagic risk and excessively prolonged PTT (e.g., more than 3 times control) is less well documented.[91] Nevertheless, some studies suggest a gradient between risk of bleeding and both the dose of heparin over a 24-hour period and the PTT.[92]

In the majority of studies in which continuous and intermittent infusion of heparin have been compared, the frequency of major hemorrhage was lower with continuous intravenous infusion.[92] Intermittent intravenous or subcutaneous heparin administration is disadvantageous because it temporarily paralyzes the clotting system, as reflected by wide fluctuations in the PTT. Therefore, whenever feasible, heparin therapy should be administered by continuous intravenous infusion after an initial bolus of heparin for patients with suspected acute PE.

Initiation of Heparin Therapy. Heparin is the cornerstone of treatment for acute PE. Before one initiates heparin therapy, the most important first step is to obtain a careful history. In particular, one should consider risk factors such as history of coagulopathy, thrombocytopenia, vitamin K deficiency, older age, underlying diseases, and concomitant drug therapy. If results of the history and physical examination are benign, heparin can be started prior to lung scanning or pulmonary angiography in situations when clinical suspicion of PE is high. However, if a severe bleeding problem is detected, such as active gastrointestinal bleeding, heparin therapy should be withheld and if the diagnosis of PE is confirmed, nonpharmacological treatment with interruption of the inferior vena cava (IVC) can be considered. When a potential risk of bleeding is detected in patients with documented PE, one can usually proceed cautiously with heparin. For such patients, the surgeon and angiographer should be alerted to the possible need to switch from medical to nonmedical treatment.

The dosage regimen for achieving optimal heparinization is empirical. For an average-sized adult without signs of massive PE, the usual initial dose would be a 5000-unit intravenous bolus followed by a continuous intravenous infusion at 1000 units per hour. In a patient suspected of having massive PE, the initial dose might be a 10,000-unit bolus followed by an infusion of 1500 units per hour. For maintenance heparin anticoagulation, the PTT should remain 2 to 3 times the control level and should be checked every 4 hours until the desired infusion rate is obtained. Underheparinization for established PE is of much greater concern than is a PTT that is 3½ times the control value in a patient whose risk for bleeding with heparin therapy is not particularly increased. When the PTT is less than twice the control, the continuous infusion dose should be increased rapidly. In general, the first few days of PE or DVT therapy require the highest heparin doses,[93] and regimens of 1500 to 2000 units per hour may be necessary for adequate anticoagulation.

Complications. The most important adverse effect of heparin is *hemorrhage*. Major bleeding during anticoagulation may unmask a previously silent lesion, such as bladder or colon cancer. For most cases of moderate bleeding, cessation of heparin therapy will suffice, and the PTT will usually return to normal within 2 to 3 hours. Resumption of heparin at a lower dose or alternative means of therapy will depend on the severity of the bleeding, the risk of recurrent thromboembolism, and the extent to which bleeding may have resulted from excessive anticoagulation (i.e., a PTT greater than 3 times the baseline value). In the event of life-threatening or intracranial hemorrhage, protamine sulfate should be administered at the time heparin is discontinued. Protamine, a strongly basic protein, will immediately reverse anticoagulant activity by forming a stable complex with the acidic heparin. For life-threatening hemorrhage, the usual dose is approximately 1 mg per 100 units of heparin, administered slowly (e.g., 50 mg over 10 to 30 minutes). Protamine sulfate can cause allergic reactions that vary from mild to life-threatening.[94]

Mild thrombocytopenia that may develop with heparin therapy probably represents a direct, nonimmune-mediated effect of heparin and is not associated with serious clinical consequences. *Heparin-associated thrombocytopenia*[96] (p. 1773) occurs more frequently with beef lung than with pork gut heparin.[97] When the thrombocytopenia is associated with *thrombosis*, the condition is immune-mediated and may be life-threatening. The thrombotic events are often distinctly unusual and may involve the skin[98] or major arteries,[99] such as the femoral or radial arteries.

Patients undergoing prolonged heparin therapy at relatively high doses may develop osteopenia, osteoporosis, and pathological bone fractures.[100, 101] In addition, continuous heparin infusion causes *aldosterone depression* by an unknown mechanism within 4 to 8 days after initiation of therapy.[102] In patients with a normally functioning renin-angiotensin-aldosterone axis, this is probably of no clinical significance, although serum sodium levels may drop slightly. However, it may cause clinically important hyperkalemia in certain patients, such as those with diabetes[103] or renal failure.[104]

WARFARIN SODIUM

Duration and Intensity of Therapy. Chronic anticoagulation is prescribed in PE to avert recurrent venous thromboembolism.[105] In Phase I of UPET, one-fifth of the patients enrolled in the trial suffered recurrent PE during the first 2 weeks of therapy.[106] Recurrence appeared to correlate with lack of adequate intensity of anticoagulation. Although PE patients often receive chronic oral warfarin therapy for 6 months, its optimal duration and intensity are unknown. In patients with a transiently incurred risk for the development of PE, such as an operation, the utility of continuing anticoagulation indefinitely is probably low. However, for patients with a risk factor that is irreversible (e.g., metastatic cancer) or not easily modified (e.g., massive obesity), a stronger case can be made for continuing anticoagulants indefinitely.

The American College of Chest Physicians (ACCP) in conjunction with the National Heart, Lung, and Blood Institute (NHLBI) appointed a special panel to evaluate the indications for anticoagulation in a variety of cardiovascular illnesses.[107] For venous thromboembolism (including DVT and PE) a therapeutic range for oral anticoagulation was determined in which the PT was prolonged 1.2 to 1.5 times the baseline value (using the Simplastin assay).[91] However, this recommendation, which we follow for DVT patients, is based on trials of DVT therapy, not PE (for which adequate trials are lacking). With regard to duration of therapy, the ACCP-NHLBI group recommended that patients with slowly resolving risk factors (e.g., prolonged immobilization) be treated for at least 3 months, whereas patients with tumors, AT-III or protein C deficiency, or recurrent venous thromboembolism be treated indefinitely. The panel implied that no more than 3 months of treatment was necessary for patients with risk factors that are readily reversible, such as estrogen use or transient immobilization.

We usually initiate warfarin therapy with 10 mg daily for 3 days and tend to treat patients with PE more aggressively than those with DVT, in terms of both intensity and duration of anticoagulation, maintaining the PT within the range of 16 to 20 seconds. If risk factors are transient, we treat with one year of warfarin. Otherwise, we advise indefinite anticoagulation.

Complications. The major toxic effect of warfarin is *bleeding* that tends to be proportional to the intensity of anticoagulation and may be increased by the presence of risk factors such as severe hepatic or renal disease, alcoholism, drug interactions, trauma, malignancy, and known previous bleeding sites in the gastrointestinal tract. Major life-threatening bleeding requires immediate treatment with enough fresh frozen plasma (FFP) (usually 2 units) to normalize the PT and achieve immediate hemostasis. To treat less serious bleeding, vitamin K may be administered parenterally; a dose of 10 mg subcutaneously or intramuscularly will usually reverse the effects of warfarin in 6 to 12 hours. However, this approach will make the patient relatively refractory to warfarin for up to 2 weeks, so that reinstitution of warfarin becomes more difficult. Minor bleeding with a prolonged PT may merely require interruption of warfarin therapy, with or without administration of FFP, until the PT has returned to the therapeutic range.[108] If bleeding occurs when the PT is within the therapeutic range, occult malignancy should be suspected and ruled out. Evaluation of patients with minor bleeding and a PT above the therapeutic range is less productive.

Warfarin-induced *skin necrosis*[109] is a rare but important complication that may be related to a warfarin-induced reduction of protein C.[107] In patients suspected of protein C deficiency, warfarin should be initiated with a lower dose than usual (e.g., 5 mg daily), with full heparin anticoagulation maintained until warfarin's therapeutic effect is achieved.

During pregnancy, heparin should be used instead of warfarin because warfarin is associated with a 10-fold higher rate of congenital anomalies.[95]

THROMBOLYTIC THERAPY

Streptokinase and Urokinase (First-Generation Agents)

(See also p. 1778)

Streptokinase (SK) and urokinase (UK) are proteins that indirectly (SK) or directly (UK) activate endogenous plasminogen to form plasmin, which actually lyses clot that has recently formed (Fig. 47–1). In almost all patients a lytic state will rapidly develop with SK or UK. For SK, the standard regimen to treat PE is 250,000 IU over 30 minutes followed by 100,000 IU per hour for 24 hours. For UK, the standard dose is 4400 IU/kg (i.e., 2000 IU/lb) over 10 minutes followed by 4400 IU/kg/hr (i.e., 2000 IU/lb/hr) for 12 to 24 hours. Although single-bolus therapy with UK has been proposed and appears promising,[110] experience with regimens such as 15,000 IU/kg over 10 minutes has been limited.[111]

Laboratory monitoring is directed toward verifying that the lytic state has been achieved, which is required for drug efficacy. In the presence of a lytic state, there is no need to titrate the dose. The lytic state can be verified by measuring increases in fibrin degradation products, thrombin time, whole blood euglobulin lysis time, PT, or PTT. The most sensitive, widely available test is the *thrombin time* (Table 47–6). Any *one* of these tests will suffice if the

TABLE 47–6 LABORATORY TESTS FOR MONITORING FIBRINOLYTIC THERAPY

Test	Rationale	Disadvantage
Thrombin time	Sensitive screening for hypofibrinogenemia and circulating fibrin degradation products; simple and rapid	Extremely sensitive to heparin
Plasma fibrinogen	Major plasma substrate of plasmin	Controversy exists regarding which assay for fibrinogen is most appropriate
Fibrin(ogen) degradation products; also termed fibrin split products	Specific for plasmin lysis of fibrinogen and/or fibrin	Pretreatment value may be elevated
Lysis time (plasma or whole blood)	Direct measure of the lytic state	Specialized time-consuming study that is usually not readily available
Prothrombin time; partial thromboplastin time	Will detect increased fibrin split products, hypofibrinogenemia; widely available	Less sensitive and specific than thrombin time

Modified from Stead, R. B.: Clinical pharmacology. *In* Goldhaber, S. Z. (eds.): Pulmonary Embolism and Deep Venous Thrombosis. Philadelphia, W. B. Saunders Company, 1985, p. 112.

pretreatment value is normal and if a value obtained 4 or more hours after the initiation of fibrinolytic therapy is abnormal. In general, the dose of the lytic agent can be doubled if a lytic state cannot be documented using conventional doses. Interestingly, the risk of bleeding from SK and UK has not been shown to correlate with any specific laboratory abnormality nor with the dose of the lytic agent.[94]

INDICATIONS AND CONTRAINDICATIONS. Whereas heparin acts primarily to prevent thrombus extension, thrombolytic agents promote dissolution of recently formed clots. Only three randomized trials comprising a total of 210 patients have compared SK or UK with heparin for PE treatment.[106, 112, 113]

In these trials, no reduction in mortality from PE was apparent with SK or UK, even though clots lysed more quickly when these agents were used. In two of the three studies, bleeding complications occurred more often after thrombolysis.[106, 113] Increases in pulmonary capillary diffusing capacity were demonstrated on follow-up in patients treated with SK or UK for PE compared with heparin-treated patients.[114] However, the clinical significance of these improvements in pulmonary parameters is unclear. In a nonrandomized study, seven patients treated for massive PE with UK therapy followed by heparin were later assessed and found to have sustained improvement of rest and exercise pulmonary hemodynamics.[115]

Many patients suspected of having PE will be receiving heparin by continuous infusion while undergoing diagnostic evaluation. After a definitive diagnosis is established, the physician must decide whether to continue heparin anticoagulation or to interrupt heparin treatment for a course of thrombolytic therapy. For patients with venous thromboembolism, the risk-to-benefit ratio of thrombolytic agents is highest in those with massive PE; however, patients with moderate-sized or large emboli may also benefit from this treatment. Heparin should be discontinued several hours before thrombolytic therapy is initiated. Physical handling of the patient and arterial and venous punctures should be minimized because no thrombolytic agent can discriminate between "bad" clot due to PE and "good" clot required for normal hemostasis. Whenever possible, simultaneous administration of platelet-active drugs should be avoided. Upon discontinuing SK or UK, heparin can be given by continuous infusion without a loading dose when the thrombin time decreases to approximately twice the control value. Contraindications to the use of SK or UK include intracranial disease, recent surgery, or trauma (Table 47–7).

TABLE 47–7 CONTRAINDICATIONS TO THROMBOLYTIC THERAPY

Absolute Contraindications	
History of hemorrhagic stroke	
Intracranial neoplasm	
Cranial surgery or head trauma within 14 days	
Relative Contraindications	
Major thoracic or abdominal surgery	Within 7 to 10 days
Cardiopulmonary resuscitation	Within 7 to 10 days
Biopsy or invasive procedure in a location inaccessible to external compression	Within 7 to 10 days
Parturition	
Coagulation defects (thrombocytopenia, coagulation factors deficiency)	
Uncontrolled severe hypertension	
Cerebrovascular accident (nonhemorrhagic)	

COMPLICATIONS. Trivial superficial oozing at venipuncture or arterial catheter insertion sites may be considered an index of drug efficacy rather than a complication of thrombolytic therapy. Such bleeding can be controlled with manual compression followed by a pressure dressing. In the UPET, severe bleeding, defined as the need for transfusion of more than 2 units of blood or a decrease in hematocrit of more than 10 points, occurred in 22 of the 82 (27 per cent) UK-treated patients in Phase I. The large amount of blood drawn during the first 24 hours of Phase I (about 200 ml) contributed to the fall in hematocrit; during Phase II, fewer patients (12 per cent) had severe bleeding. In many instances, bleeding occurred at the vascular puncture sites for pulmonary angiography.

Of greatest concern is the risk of intracranial bleeding, which occurs in one or two of every 1000 patients treated with thrombolytic therapy. Retroperitoneal hemorrhage can also be life-threatening because the bleeding is often sustained, brisk, and difficult to diagnose. This complication can occur during femoral catheterization if an artery is inadvertently punctured above the inguinal ligament. Genitourinary and other internal bleeding can generally be well managed; however, if internal bleeding is excessive, therapy should be discontinued. If bleeding is brisk or potentially life-threatening, fresh frozen plasma (FFP) should be administered to restore depleted plasma fibrinogen, factor V, and factor VIII—all of which will have been digested by the circulating plasmin. An alternative to FFP is cryoprecipitate, which contains factor VIII and fibrinogen.[116] Minor allergic reactions due to SK occur occasionally and are manifested by fever and chills. To suppress this reaction, steroids and diphenhydramine (Benadryl) can be administered prophylactically.

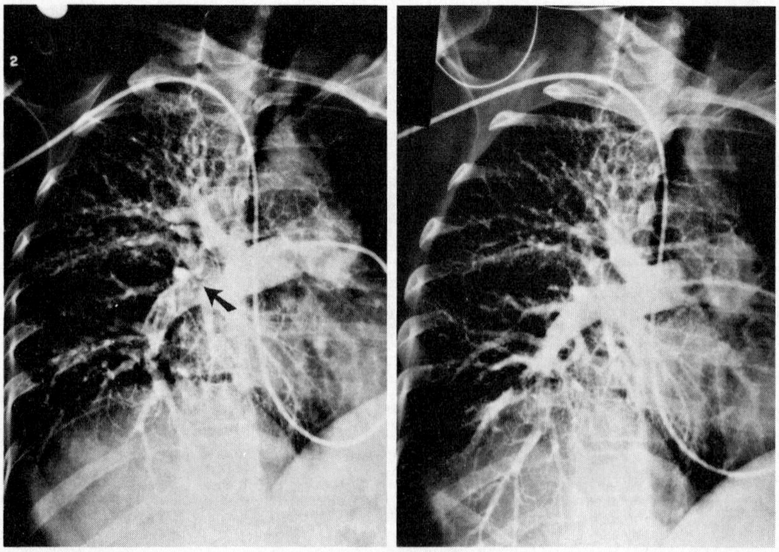

FIGURE 47–11. ***Left,*** **Right anterior oblique pulmonary angiogram of a 43-year-old woman. A large embolus can be seen in the right pulmonary artery (arrow).** ***Right,*** **After a 2-hour infusion of rt-PA, resolution is marked, with minimal residual thrombus in segmental branches. (From Goldhaber, S. Z., et al.: Acute pulmonary embolism treated with tissue plasminogen activator. Lancet** ***2:*****886, 1986.)**

Tissue Plasminogen Activator (t-PA)

(See also p. 1778)

In experimental canine and rabbit models of venous thrombosis, t-PA caused more fibrin-specific thrombolysis and less hemorrhage than did either UK or SK.[117, 118] These experiments have served as the basis for clinical use of t-PA in patients with venous thromboembolism. Its use in acute PE was first reported in a 63-year-old man with massive PE (documented angiographically) who had undergone renal transplantation 5 weeks before rt-PA treatment[119]; 30 mg (0.5 mg/kg) of rt-PA was infused over 90 minutes through a catheter inserted into the right ventricle.

In the authors' investigation, the short-term efficacy and safety of acutely administered rt-PA in acute PE[120, 121, 121a] were studied. Of 47 patients with angiographically documented PE, 44 had significant clot lysis after 2 to 6 hours of rt-PA administered through a peripheral vein (Fig. 47–11). Average pulmonary artery pressures decreased significantly after rt-PA therapy, and lung scanning indicated marked improvement in pulmonary perfusion after treatment.[122] In some patients, right ventricular dysfunction and tricuspid regurgitation were documented by Doppler echocardiography prior to treatment but resolved rapidly after rt-PA therapy.[123] Plasma fibrinogen levels decreased 42 per cent from baseline, and superficial oozing from venipuncture or arterial puncture sites, readily controlled with manual compression and pressure dressings, was common. Two patients had major hemorrhagic complications that required surgical intervention (pericardial tamponade and hemorrhage from a pelvic tumor) followed by an uneventful recovery.

In Phase I of the UPET, approximately 24 hours after initiation of therapy, only 4 per cent of the heparin-treated patients showed moderate or marked *qualitative improvement* in angiographically demonstrated clot lysis compared with 42 per cent of the UK-treated patients. With rt-PA, 83 per cent demonstrated moderate or marked improvement by 6 hours. The rate of major bleeding with rt-PA was 5 per cent compared with 27 per cent for UK-treated patients in Phase I of the UPET and 12 per cent in Phase II.[106, 124] Such historical comparisons can only be undertaken with extreme caution and do not obviate the need for randomized trials of rt-PA vs. UK to assess efficacy and safety. Furthermore, it is evident that rt-PA is only relatively fibrin-selective (p. 1779).[125] It is not surprising that rt-PA can cause minor bleeding, since no thrombolytic agent, whether fibrin-specific or not, can distinguish between the clot of acute PE and fibrin plugs at fresh arterial or venipuncture sites.

ANTICOAGULATION VS. THROMBOLYTIC THERAPY

Standard therapy for PE has employed heparin anticoagulation followed by warfarin, without thrombolytic therapy. The rationale for anticoagulation therapy is to provide prophylaxis against additional thromboembolic events while natural fibrinolytic mechanisms gradually lyse the previously formed pulmonary artery clot(s). In contrast, the rationale for thrombolytic therapy (followed by anticoagulation) is that thrombolysis actively dissolves clot that has already formed, thereby restoring cardiopulmonary function to normal as quickly as possible. Thrombolysis relieves the obstruction to pulmonary artery blood flow and thus improves right ventricular function, reduces pulmonary artery pressures, and improves pulmonary perfusion. Lytic therapy may also improve pulmonary function over the long term,[114] help prevent the development of chronic pulmonary hypertension, and reduce the source of the embolus in the peripheral venous system as well as in the pulmonary artery, thereby preventing recurrent PE.

For patients with major PE who are treated with anticoagulants alone, pulmonary artery clot may fail to resolve in 75 per cent of patients after 1 to 4 weeks[126] and in 50 per cent after 4 months[127] of follow-up. In the UPET, the UK-treated patients initially exhibited significantly greater hemodynamic and anatomical improvement than the heparin-treated patients. However, within 7 days, no difference between the two groups could be demonstrated on lung scans.[106] Unfortunately, no large-scale trial has yet been undertaken to determine whether thrombolytic therapy can reduce the mortality and recurrent PE rate compared with standard heparin treatment.

Although the Food and Drug Administration approved SK and UK in 1977 to treat PE, these agents are used only rarely for this condition, probably because of fear of bleeding complications. In 1980, an NIH Consensus Development Conference[128] concluded that thrombolytic therapy was not being utilized often enough for patients with PE who (1) had obstruction of blood flow to a lobe or multiple pulmonary segments or (2) were hemodynamically compromised, regardless of the anatomical size of the PE. Nevertheless, use of thrombolytic therapy for PE has continued to languish. As of this writing, outside of a research setting, we advocate thrombolytic therapy primarily to treat massive PE, defined as PE involving at least two lobar arteries or anatomically smaller PE associated with acute pulmonary hypertension. We also use thrombolytic therapy when a patient with submassive PE is not showing improvement with heparin therapy (Fig. 47–12).

ADJUNCTIVE MEDICAL THERAPY

Although the cornerstone of PE treatment involves anticoagulation or thrombolysis, adjunctive measures are also useful. Hypoxia should be treated with supplemental oxygen. In most cases, 2 to 4 liters of oxygen via nasal prongs will suffice. Discomfort due to PE can be intense and can cause chest wall splinting, making the patient susceptible to pneumonia and increased hypoxia owing to poor ventilation. Therefore, pain should be controlled. Although the pleuritic pain of PE often has an inflammatory

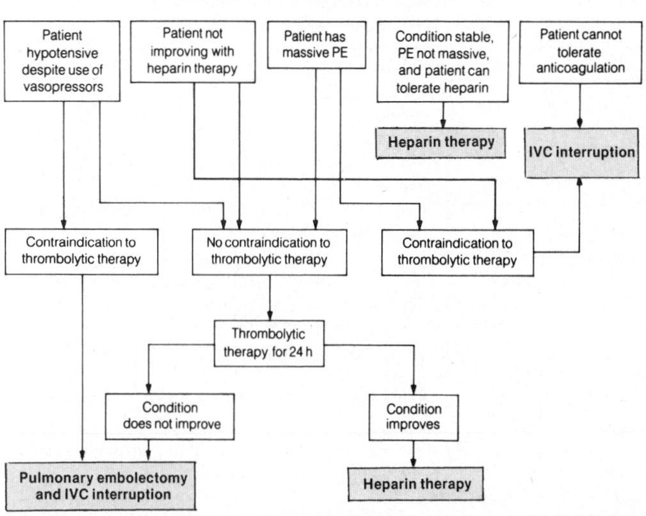

FIGURE 47–12. Therapeutic strategy once pulmonary embolism is diagnosed. (From Goldhaber, S. Z.: Pulmonary embolism: Diagnostic and therapeutic options. Consultant, February 1986, p. 127.)

component, most patients can be managed satisfactorily with narcotics rather than with antiinflammatory agents, since all the latter adversely affect platelet function and may predispose to bleeding during anticoagulant or thrombolytic therapy. If excessive use of narcotics precipitates carbon dioxide retention, the deleterious effect on respiratory depression can be readily reversed with naloxone. Fever often accompanies PE and not only should be suppressed with acetaminophen but should also lead to a search for accompanying infection, particularly pneumonia.

INFERIOR VENA CAVAL (IVC) INTERRUPTION

LIGATION. The primary purpose of IVC interruption is to prevent recurrent PE in patients with an absolute contraindication to anticoagulation (e.g., active gastrointestinal bleeding or hemorrhagic stroke) (Table 47–8). However, no randomized clinical trial has examined medical therapy compared with IVC interruption nor has any study been done to compare the different modes of IVC interruption (i.e., ligation, external clips, filters).[129] Certain disadvantages of these devices should be recognized. First, the manufacturers of umbrellas and filters recommend that anticoagulation be continued as adjunctive therapy during and after IVC interruption to help prevent thrombosis at the site of the device. Second, if the device becomes occluded with thrombus, large paravertebral venous collateral channels will quickly develop and permit recurrent embolization. Third, it is unknown whether the currently employed interruption devices will cause long-term complications (e.g., perforation or migration). All other implanted devices, whether they be heart valves, pacemakers, or artificial hips, have a lifespan beyond which they require replacement or revision. Therefore, indications for IVC interruption in relatively young patients should be particularly stringent.

There are three possible indications for complete ligation of the inferior vena cava. One is *septic embolization*, since these emboli are usually small and would pass through all contemporary devices that maintain partial caval patency. In the presence of intravascular sepsis, no foreign material should be placed in the inferior vena cava. However, small emboli should theoretically have little difficulty traversing the collateral circulation around the ligated vessel, and patients with septic pelvic thrombophlebitis can almost always be treated successfully with heparin anticoagulation and antibiotics alone.[130] The second possible use of ligation is in the rare case of documented or potential *paradoxical embolization* because of the devastating neurological effects of even a small paradoxical embolus.[131] A third indication for ligation is the need for reoperation because *an intracaval device has migrated* to an incorrect position.[132]

TABLE 47–8 INDICATIONS FOR INTERRUPTION OF INFERIOR VENA CAVA

Generally accepted indication ↓

(1) Pulmonary embolism or extensive deep venous thrombosis and acute contraindication for anticoagulation
(2) Major bleeding upon anticoagulation for embolism or venous thrombosis
(3) Recurrent embolism leading to hemodynamic compromise
(4) Failure of adequate anticoagulation to prevent recurrent thromboembolic disease
(5) Chronic cor pulmonale for multiple pulmonary emboli
(6) Septic embolization
(7) Embolectomy
(8) Embolism of any cause leading to a period of hemodynamic compromise
(9) Massive pulmonary embolism in the absence of reversible predisposing condition

Controversial indication

From Hoagland, P. M.: Massive pulmonary embolism. *In* Goldhaber, S. Z. (ed.): Pulmonary Embolism and Deep Venous Thrombosis. Philadelphia, W. B. Saunders Company, 1985, p. 201.

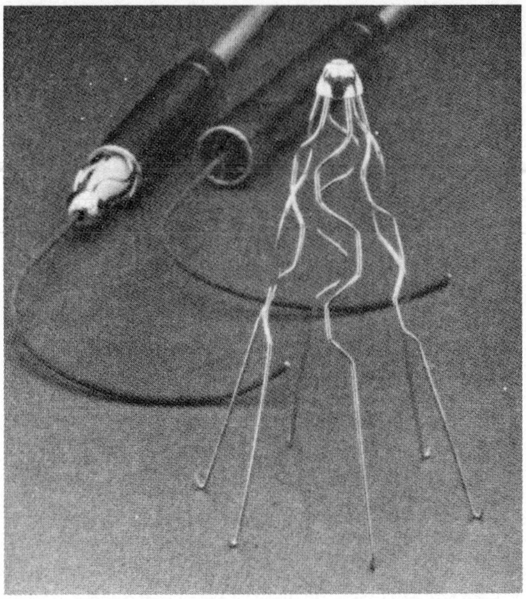

FIGURE 47–13. Kimray-Greenfield vena caval filter device. (From Hoagland, P. M.: Massive pulmonary embolism. *In* Goldhaber, S. Z.: Pulmonary Embolism and Deep Venous Thrombosis. Philadelphia, W. B. Saunders Company, 1985, p. 203.)

EXTERNAL CLIPS. If a laparotomy is performed, the external clip, such as the Adams-DeWeese device, is preferred to ligation because of its fewer hemodynamic and venous complications and the low frequency of recurrent pulmonary embolization.[133]

TRANSVENOUS DEVICES. Transvenous umbrellas or filters can be placed through a venotomy under angiographic control, using local rather than general anesthesia. Three major transvenous devices exist. The *Hunter detachable balloon occluder* may be used in the rare situation in which a patient requires total interruption of the IVC via the transvenous route.[134] Although the first clinically popular transvenous filter was the *Mobin-Uddin filter system* introduced in 1967,[135] most surgeons and angiographers prefer the more recent *Kimray-Greenfield filter* (Fig. 47–13). The latter device is cone-shaped so that it may be 80 per cent filled with clot and lead to only a 64 per cent reduction in effective cross-sectional area. It has a higher patency rate and, probably as a consequence, a lower rate of venous sequelae than the Mobin-Uddin umbrella.[136, 137] When necessary, the Kimray-Greenfield filter can be placed above the renal veins. (However, it is usually placed at the level of L3.) Whereas the Mobin-Uddin filter must be inserted through the internal jugular vein, the Kimray-Greenfield device can be placed via either the femoral or the internal jugular vein. Femoral vein insertion can be performed percutaneously and therefore the procedure is being carried out with increasing frequency by angiographers.[138] Like any procedure, the Greenfield filter has potential complications, including recurrent PE due to extension of thrombus from the filter's surface[139] and distal migration of the filter.[140]

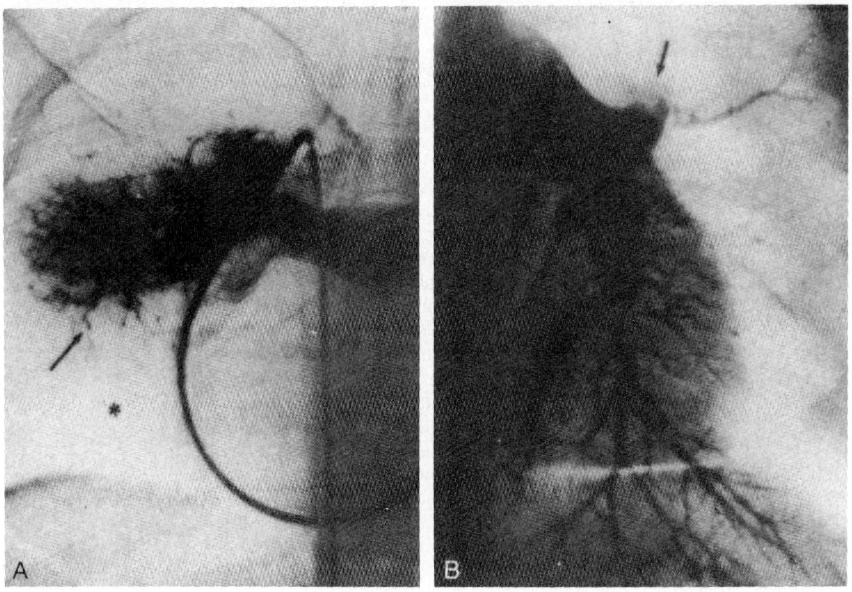

FIGURE 47–14. Preoperative angiogram (*A* and *B*) representing the classic arteriographic findings in chronic pulmonary embolism. *A*, Tapered arterial defects can be seen in distal pulmonary arteries (arrow), indicating chronic emboli. Total obstruction of the right lower lobe pulmonary artery has led to oligemia (asterisk). Segmental occlusion of right upper lobe pulmonary artery is also present. *B*, Proximal dilation of main pulmonary artery. Note the plaque in the left upper lobe pulmonary artery (small arrow) and the residual web in the left lower lobe artery (large arrow). This represents a partially resolved chronic pulmonary embolism. (From Chitwood, W. R., et al.: Surgical management of chronic pulmonary embolism. Ann. Surg. *201*:11, 1985.)

Indications for Placement of IVC Interruption Devices

Patients to whom we recommend IVC interruption are selected carefully (Fig. 47–12). We advise interruption (almost always with a percutaneously inserted Kimray-Greenfield filter) when a patient with PE cannot tolerate anticoagulation or when adequate anticoagulation does not prevent recurrent PE. However, we do not employ these devices prophylactically in patients who have sustained a single large pulmonary embolus but who can tolerate thrombolysis or anticoagulation.

PULMONARY EMBOLECTOMY

Pulmonary embolectomy can be utilized to treat PE in two different clinical settings: (1) during acute PE in the critically ill patient (e.g., when PE is associated with shock), and (2) to treat disabling dyspnea in patients with chronic pulmonary hypertension due to occult or recurrent PE. The fiberoptic angioscope can be used as an adjunct to visualize the pulmonary arteries during the procedure.[141] In patients with persistent right ventricular failure despite embolectomy, pulmonary artery counterpulsation with a balloon pump may be useful.[142]

ACUTE PE. Both transvenous pulmonary catheter suction embolectomy[143, 143a] and open pulmonary embolectomy[144] are associated with a high mortality rate and should be reserved for patients in extremis in whom thrombolytic therapy is contraindicated or is failing (Fig. 47–12).

CHRONIC PULMONARY HYPERTENSION. Recurrent PE can lead to chronic, persistent pulmonary artery clot (Fig. 47–14), with attendant pulmonary hypertension, dyspnea, and cor pulmonale. This major complication occurs most often when the diagnosis of PE is initially overlooked and anticoagulation is withheld for months or even years.[145] However, chronic obstruction of the pulmonary arteries can occur despite prompt anticoagulation.[146] Chronic pulmonary hypertension due to PE is usually refractory to anticoagulants and thrombolytic agents but can sometimes be managed with pulmonary embolectomy. Utley[147, 148] and Sabiston[149] and their coworkers have reported the largest series of such patients. Surgical success leads to a dramatic reduction in symptoms, with associated improvements noted on lung scanning and pulmonary angiography. The results of embolectomy tend to be most successful when an embolized thrombus can be removed in large segments that form a cast of the pulmonary vascular tree (Fig. 47–15).

INDICATIONS FOR PULMONARY EMBOLECTOMY. Despite progress in the technique of pulmonary embolectomy for PE, we regard this operation as a treatment of last resort (Fig. 47–12). For acute massive PE, thrombolytic therapy should be attempted first unless there is an absolute contraindication to its use. For chronic PE, we would not recommend embolectomy unless progressive incapacity due to chronic pulmonary hypertension is well documented. The potential for postoperative rehabilitation must be good, and candidates must be willing to accept the risk of death or of failure to improve that accompanies this "high-stakes" operation.

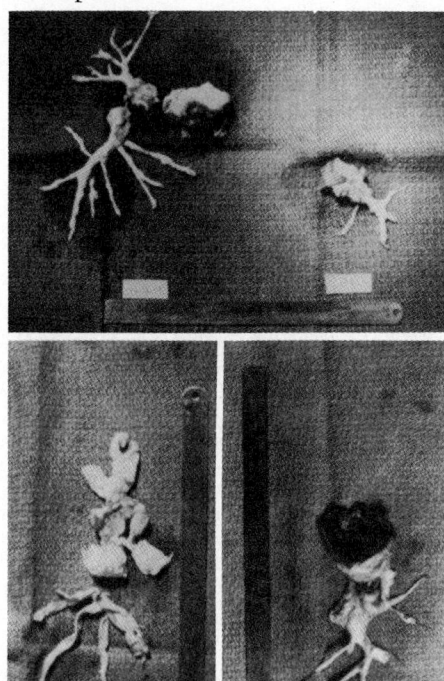

FIGURE 47–15. Large segments of chronic organized clot that were removed from the pulmonary arteries of two patients with excellent results (i.e., they advanced from New York Heart Association functional class IV to I). Both patients had had complete obstruction of one pulmonary artery and partial obstruction of the other. (From Utley, J. R.: Pulmonary thromboendarterectomy. *In* Goldhaber, S. Z. [ed.]: Pulmonary Embolism and Deep Venous Thrombosis. Philadelphia, W. B. Saunders Company, 1985, p. 278.)

PREVENTION OF PULMONARY EMBOLISM

PHARMACOLOGICAL AGENTS

CONVENTIONAL APPROACHES

Low-Dose Heparin. The most comprehensive randomized controlled trial of low-dose heparin (5000 units of subcutaneous heparin 2 hours preoperatively and every 8 hours thereafter for 7 days) as postoperative prophylaxis against fatal PE was organized by Kakkar in the International Multicentre Trial (IMT) involving 4121 patients.[150] Eligible patients were over age 40 years and were scheduled to undergo *elective* major surgery. Of the autopsied subjects, 16 controls died of PE versus only two patients in the heparin group. Although more wound hematomas occurred among heparin-treated patients, the number of deaths due to hemorrhage was not increased among those who received heparin. Collins and Peto have reviewed data from about 50 smaller randomized controlled trials with approximately 8,000 patients that have confirmed the IMT result.[151] Fatal PE occurred in 33 controls as opposed to 10 of the heparin-treated patients. The latter group also had about one-third as many instances of DVT as control patients, regardless of whether they underwent general, urological, elective, orthopedic, or traumatic orthopedic surgery.

Dextran. This substance has been used for thromboembolism prophylaxis because it reportedly impairs platelet function by causing decreased platelet aggregability. Dextran 40, with a mean molecular weight of 40,000 (known also as low molecular weight dextran), is approved for prophylaxis against venous thromboembolism. Potential adverse effects include anaphylaxis, volume overload, nephrotoxicity, and (ironically) bleeding.

Warfarin. In patients at high risk for DVT or PE (e.g., a patient with prior DVT or PE), warfarin may be an appropriate agent to consider in the setting of hip surgery.[152]

Aspirin. The 1986 NIH Consensus Development Conference report concluded specifically that aspirin is not efficacious in the prophylaxis of venous thromboembolism.[153]

NEWER APPROACHES

Adjusted Low-Dose Heparin. Two research groups have suggested that among hip surgery patients, adjusted doses of subcutaneous heparin might prevent DVT more effectively than a fixed-dosage schedule.[154,155] These initial results require confirmation by other investigators.[156]

Heparin-Dihydroergotamine (H-DHE). Dihydroergotamine is a parenterally administered hydrogenated ergot preparation that exerts a selective vasoconstrictive effect on veins and venules with little or no effect on arteries and arterioles, thereby counteracting venous stasis and accelerating venous return from the legs. In an overview of 17 trials, it appears that H-DHE is more effective than either drug alone in the prophylaxis of venous thromboembolism.[157] In 1985, the FDA approved one fixed dose of heparin (5000 U) combined with 0.5 mg of DHE (Embolex). The drug is administered subcutaneously beginning 2 hours before surgery and then every 12 hours for 5 to 7 days. This regimen has been shown to be more efficacious than heparin alone in general surgery[158] and in orthopedic surgery.[159] In a multicenter study of 8001 orthopedic surgery patients, H-DHE was found to be as effective as but considerably safer than dextran 70 for preventing fatal postoperative PE.[160] The DHE component may decrease the possibility of excessive bleeding in patients receiving H-DHE. However, because of its vasoconstricting effect, H-DHE should not be administered to patients undergoing vascular surgery or to those with suspected bowel ischemia or coronary artery disease. The unique niche for H-DHE may be among patients with a higher than average risk for venous thromboembolism, such as those undergoing cancer or orthopedic surgery.

Low Molecular Weight Heparin (LMWH). LMWH, not yet commercially available, has two major potential advantages over unfractionated heparin: (1) a lower frequency of heparin-associated thrombocytopenia and (2) effective prophylaxis with administration only once daily. In a double-blind British study comparing LMWH with unfractionated heparin among 295 patients undergoing elective major abdominal surgery, the rate of DVT as detected on leg scanning with ^{125}I-labeled fibrinogen was 2.5 per cent among those who received LMWH compared with 7.5 per cent among those who received unfractionated heparin ($p < 0.05$).[161] LMWH is also very effective in preventing DVT among patients undergoing elective hip surgery.[162]

MECHANICAL MEASURES

GRADED ELASTIC COMPRESSION STOCKINGS. The most popular type of graded elastic compression is called a TED (*t*hromboem*b*olism-*d*eterrent) stocking. Pressure exerted by the TED stocking is graded: 18 mm Hg at the ankle, 14 mm Hg at midcalf, 8 mm Hg in the popliteal region, 10 mm Hg at the lower thigh, and 8 mm Hg at the upper thigh. Most studies evaluating TED stockings have shown that they reduce but do not eliminate DVT in the postoperative period.[152]

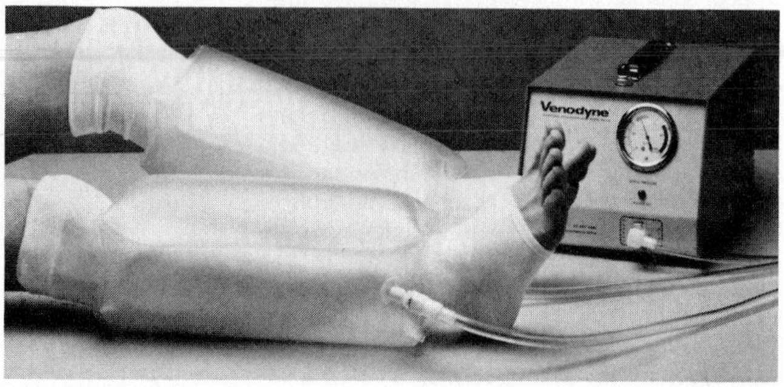

FIGURE 47–16. Calf muscle compression designed to prevent deep venous thrombosis is achieved with inflatable stockings fitted to both legs just after operation. (Courtesy of Lyne-Nicholson, Inc., Venodyne Systems, Needham Heights, Massachusetts.)

INTERMITTENT PNEUMATIC COMPRESSION (IPC). Intermittent external calf-muscle compression (Fig. 47–16) has become an increasingly popular nonpharmacological method for preventing postoperative DVT. Most studies of this technique have shown a favorable effect in preventing postoperative DVT. Some of these devices can be worn under plaster casts. In nonorthopedic operations in which bleeding must be minimized (e.g., neurosurgery), intermittent calf-muscle compression may be the perioperative prophylactic method of choice.[152]

INFERIOR VENA CAVAL (IVC) INTERRUPTION. Only under exceptional circumstances should IVC interruption be used prophylactically as a preoperative measure. Patients must be at extraordinarily high risk for PE (e.g., recent prior PE) *and* must have an absolute contraindication to pharmacological prophylaxis (e.g., active gastrointestinal bleeding, chemotherapy-induced thrombocytopenia, or neurosurgery).

COMBINED MODALITIES. Graded compression stockings help prevent venous thromboembolism and are virtually risk-free. Unfortunately, many physicians and surgeons rely *solely* on early ambulation and graded compression stockings to prevent PE and DVT. This strategy toward prophylaxis is injudicious.[163] Recently, an overview of 45 trials of venous thromboembolism prophylaxis in patients undergoing general thoracoabdominal, gynecological, or prostate surgery (excluding those studies in which all patients were being operated on for malignant disorders) indicated that the rate of DVT, as detected by fibrinogen scanning, was lowest (6 per cent) when low-dose heparin was used *in combination with* graded compression stockings. In contrast, in controls who received no therapy, the rate of DVT was 27 per cent; in those treated only with low-dose heparin, it was 10 per cent.[164]

RECOMMENDED APPROACH TO PROPHYLAXIS OF PULMONARY EMBOLISM

The 1986 NIH Consensus Development Conference on Prevention of Venous Thrombosis and PE has issued recommendations for many specific conditions.[153]

Surgical Patients

GENERAL SURGERY. Among patients over the age of 40, the average frequency of DVT is 25 per cent based on fibrinogen scanning and 19 per cent based on venography in control patients who do not receive prophylaxis. Clinically significant PE occurs in approximately 1.6 per cent of the general surgical population.[153] The NIH Consensus statement recommends prophylaxis in *all* general surgical patients when any *one* of the following criteria apply:

TABLE 47–9 AN APPROACH TO PROPHYLAXIS OF VENOUS THROMBOEMBOLISM

TYPE OF OPERATION OR CONDITION	AVERAGE-RISK PATIENT	HIGH-RISK PATIENT (E.G., HISTORY OF PRIOR PE OR DVT)
General surgery (or urological or gynecological surgery)	Graded compression stockings *PLUS* low-dose SC heparin	Graded compression stockings *PLUS* heparin-dihydroergotamine
Orthopedic surgery	Graded compression stockings or IPC *PLUS* adjusted-dose SC heparin	Graded compression stockings or IPC *PLUS* warfarin
Pregnancy	Exercise	Exercise *PLUS* graded compression stockings *PLUS* periodic noninvasive testing of the legs
Neurosurgery	IPC	IPC

IPC = intermittent pneumatic compression; SC = subcutaneous.

- 40 years of age or older, *or*
- undergoing a surgical procedure of more than 1 hour's duration, *or*
- obesity, *or*
- cancer, *or*
- prior PE or DVT

The recommended modality is heparin, 5,000 units subcutaneously every 8 to 12 hours, beginning prior to surgery and continuing at least until the patient is ambulatory. Alternative prophylactic modalities include dextran, IPC or graded compression stockings, and H-DHE. Our approach to prophylaxis consists of graded compression stockings for all patients in conjunction with low-dose heparin for patients at average risk and H-DHE (if no contraindications exist) for those at higher risk (Table 47–9).

ORTHOPEDIC SURGERY. In hip surgery and knee reconstruction, DVT rates range from 45 to 70 per cent. Among hip surgery patients, the frequency of fatal PE is 1 to 3 per cent.[153] Efforts at prophylaxis have been least successful among patients undergoing elective or emergency hip surgery. The NIH panel recommends any of the following modalities: low-dose warfarin, dextran, adjusted-dose heparin, or mechanical measures. With this in mind, our approach includes mechanical methods along with adjusted-dose heparin in patients at average risk; for high-risk patients, we favor mechanical measures plus warfarin prophylaxis. If the FDA approves H-DHE for prophylaxis in hip surgery patients, we will utilize this modality (except when contraindicated) in addition to mechanical measures.

UROLOGICAL SURGERY. The overall risk of venous thromboembolism in urological surgery is 25 per cent, similar to that in general surgery. Open prostatectomy is associated with a rate of DVT of 40 per cent, whereas for transurethral prostatectomy this rate is 10 per cent.[153] The NIH panel recommends low-dose heparin. Our practice for urological patients is the same as for general surgical patients, i.e., graded compression stockings combined with low-dose heparin for patients at average risk.

PREGNANCY AND GYNECOLOGICAL SURGERY. Although the NIH panel endorses low-dose heparin for pregnant women at risk, the high rate of stillbirths and reports of bone demineralization among heparin-treated pregnant women has led us to withhold pharmacological prophylaxis. Instead, in addition to graded compression stockings, we recommend that pregnant women with previous venous thromboembolism (or other major risk factors) engage in at least 30 minutes of daily exercise and undergo periodic noninvasive testing of the legs (with impedance plethysmography or phleborheography) for early detection of venous thrombosis. The guidelines for prophylaxis in gynecological surgery are the same as for general surgery. Patients with gynecological cancer should be considered at high risk for venous thromboembolism and may benefit more from H-DHE or IPC[165] than from low-dose heparin.[166]

NEUROSURGERY. The risk of PE and DVT in neurosurgical patients is similar to that in other surgical high-risk groups. For patients with intracranial or spinal cord lesions, even minor bleeding could have disastrous consequences. Therefore, IPC is recommended.

Medical Patients

The general medical population has been the least studied group with regard to DVT. These patients are frequently immobilized for prolonged periods; those who have cancer are likely to be in a hypercoagulable state. With the renewed interest in thrombolytic therapy followed by heparin anticoagulation for patients with *acute myocardial infarction*, the issue of DVT and PE prophylaxis has become a secondary concern. Patients with *unstable angina* treated with IPC or fixed low-dose heparin (5,000 units subcutaneously every 12 hours) may have fewer episodes of venous thromboembolism than those who receive only graded compression stockings.[167] For *nonhemorrhagic stroke*, the frequency of DVT can be reduced with low-dose subcutaneous heparin. For those patients found to have *hemorrhagic stroke*, IPC appears to be useful.[152]

Cost-Effectiveness

Routine prophylaxis of venous thromboembolism is much more cost-effective than is routine surveillance.[168, 169] Among general surgical patients, use of graded compression stockings appears particularly cost-effective,[170] whereas among orthopedic surgical patients, IPC appears most cost-effective.[171]

REFERENCES

FACTORS THAT PREDISPOSE TO PULMONARY EMBOLISM

1. Wessler, S.: Prevention of venous thromboembolism: Rationale, practice, and problems. NIH Consensus Development Conference on Prevention of Venous Thrombosis and Pulmonary Embolism, 1986.
2. Goldman, L., Sayson, R., Robbins, S., Cohn, L. H., Bettmann, M., and Weisberg, M.: The value of the autopsy in three medical eras. N. Engl. J. Med. *308*:1000, 1983.
3. Puxty, J. A. H., Hornan, M. A., and Fox, R. A.: Necropsies in the elderly. Lancet *1*:1262, 1983.
4. Virchow, R.: Gesammelte Abhandlungen zur Wissenschaftlichen Medizin. Frankfurt, Meidinger Sohn, 1856, p. 219.
5. Schafer, A. I.: The hypercoagulable states. Ann. Intern. Med. *102*:814, 1985.
6. Clouse, L. H., and Comp, P. C.: The regulation of hemostasis: The protein C system. N. Engl. J. Med. *314*:1298, 1986.
7. Stead, N. W., Bauer, K. A., Kinney, T. R., Lewis, J. G., Campbell, E. E., Shifman, M. A., Rosenberg, R. D., and Pizzo, S. V.: Venous thrombosis in a family with defective release of vascular plasminogen activator and elevated plasma factor VIII/von Willebrand's factor. Am. J. Med. *74*:33, 1983.
8. Pizzo, S. V., Fuchs, H. E., Doman, K. A., Petruska, D. B., and Berger, H., Jr.: Release of tissue plasminogen activator and its fast-acting inhibitor in defective fibrinolysis. Arch. Intern. Med. *146*:188, 1986.
9. Feinstein, D. I.: Lupus anticoagulant, thrombosis, and fetal loss. N. Engl. J. Med. *313*:1348, 1985.
10. Branch, D. W., Scott. J. R., Kochenour, N. K., and Hershgold, E.: Obstetric complications associated with the lupus anticoagulant. N. Engl. J. Med. *313*:1322, 1985.

10a. Petri, M., Rheinschmidt, M., Whiting-O'Keefe, Q., Hellmann, D., and Corash, L.: The frequency of lupus anticoagulant in systemic lupus erythematosus. A study of sixty consecutive patients by activated partial thromboplastin time, Russell viper venom time, and anticardiolipin antibody level. Ann. Intern. Med. *106*:524, 1987.

11. Scharrer, I., and Hach, V.: The Frankfurt Idiopathic Thrombosis Project—Investigation of 870 juvenile patients with venous thrombosis or hereditary fibrinolysis and coagulation disorders. Fibrinolysis Suppl I (Abstract #160), 1986.
12. Goldhaber, S. Z., Savage, D. D., Garrison, R. J., Castelli, W. P., Kannel, W. B., McNamara, P. M., Gherardi, G., and Feinleib, M.: Risk factors for pulmonary embolism: The Framingham Study. Am. J. Med. *74*:1023, 1983.
13. Gore, J. M., Appelbaum, J. S., Greene, H. L., Dexter, L., and Dalen, J. E.: Occult cancer in patients with acute pulmonary embolism. Ann. Intern. Med. *96*:556, 1982.
14. Goldberg, R. J., Seneff, M., Gore, J. M., Anderson, F. A., Jr., Greene, H. L., Wheeler, H. B., and Dalen, J. E.: Occult malignancy in patients with deep venous thrombosis. Arch. Intern. Med. *147*:251, 1987.
15. Goldhaber, S. Z., Buring, J. E., and Hennekens, C. H.: Cancer and venous thromboembolism. Arch. Intern. Med. *147*:216, 1987.
16. Stolley, P. D., Tonascia, J. A., Tockman, M. S., Sartwell, P. E., Rutledge, A. H., and Jacobs, M. P.: Thrombosis with low-estrogen oral contraceptives. Am. J. Epidemiol. *102*:197, 1975.
17. Treffers, P. E., Huidekoper, B. L., Weenink, G. H., and Kloosterman, G. J.: Epidemiologic observations of thrombo-embolic disease during pregnancy and in the puerperium, in 56,022 women. Int. J. Gynaecol. Obstet. *21*:327, 1983.
18. Farfel, Z., Shecter, M., Vered, Z., Rath, S., Goor, D., and Gafni, J.: Review of echocardiographically diagnosed right heart entrapment of pulmonary emboli-in-transit with emphasis on management. Am. Heart J. *113*:171, 1987.
18a. Dorfman, G. S., Cronan, J. J., Tupper, T. B., Messersmith, R. N., Denny, D. F., and Lee, C. H.: Occult pulmonary embolism: A common occurrence in deep venous thrombosis. A.J.R. *148*:263, 1987.
19. Moser, K. M., and LeMoine, J. R.: Is embolic risk conditioned by location of deep venous thrombosis? Ann. Intern. Med. *94*:439, 1981.
20. Husni, E. A., and Williams, W. A.: Superficial thrombophlebitis of lower limbs. Surgery *91*:70, 1982.
21. Hull, R., Hirsh, J., Sackett, D. L., and Stoddart, G.: Cost effectiveness of clinical diagnosis, venography, and noninvasive testing in patients with symptomatic deep-vein thrombosis. N. Engl. J. Med. *304*:1561, 1981.
22. Bettmann, M. A.: Leg phlebography. Postgrad. Radiol. *1*:127, 1981.
23. Wheeler, H. B.: A modern approach to diagnosing deep venous thrombosis. J. Cardiovasc. Med. *5*:217, 1980.
24. Hull, R. D., Hirsh, J., Carter, C. J., Jay, R. M., Ockelford, P. A., Buller, H. R., Turpie, A. G., Powers, P., Kinch, D., Dodd, P. E., Gill, G. J., Leclerc, J. R., and Gent, M.: Diagnostic efficacy of impedance plethysmography for clinically suspected deep-vein thrombosis: A randomized trial. Ann. Intern. Med. *102*:21, 1985.
25. Huisman, M. V., Buller, H. R., ten Cate, J. W., and Vreeken, J.: Serial impedance plethysmography for suspected deep venous thrombosis in outpatients. The Amsterdam General Practitioner Study. N. Engl. J. Med. *314*:823, 1986.
26. Hull, R. D., Carter, C. J., Jay, R. M., Ockelford, P. A., Hirsh, J., Turpie, A. G., Zielinsky, A., Gent, M., and Powers, P. J.: The diagnosis of acute, recurrent, deep-vein thrombosis: A diagnostic challenge. Circulation *67*:901, 1983.
27. Comerota, A. J., White, J. V., and Katz, M. L.: Diagnostic methods for deep vein thrombosis: Venous Doppler examination, phleborheography, iodine-125 fibrinogen uptake, and phlebography. Am. J. Surg. *150*(4A):14, 1985.
28. Ouriel, K., Whitehouse, W. M., Jr., and Zarins, C. K.: Combined use of Doppler ultrasound and phleborheography in suspected deep venous thrombosis. Surg. Gynecol. Obstet. *159*:242, 1984.
29. Lagerstedt, C. I., Olsson, C.-G., Fagher, B. O., Oqvist, B. W., and Albrechtsson, U.: Need for long-term anticoagulant treatment in symptomatic calf-vein thrombosis. Lancet 2:515, 1985.
30. Hull, R. D., Raskob, G. E., Hirsh, J., Jay, R. M., Leclerc, J. R., Geerts, W. H., Rosenbloom, D., Sackett, D. L., Anderson, C., Harrison, L., and Gent, M.: Continuous intravenous heparin compared with intermittent subcutaneous heparin in the initial treatment of proximal-vein thrombosis. N. Engl. J. Med. *315*:1109, 1986.
31. Hull, R., Hirsh, J., Jay, R., Carter, C., England, C., Gent, M., Turpie, A. G. G., McLoughlin, D., Dodd, P., Thomas, M., Raskob, G., and Ockelford, P.: Different intensities of oral anticoagulant therapy in the treatment of proximal-vein thrombosis. N. Engl. J. Med. *307*:1676, 1982.
32. Hull, R. D., Raskob, G. E., Hirsh, J., and Sackett, D. L.: A cost-effectiveness analysis of alternative approaches for long-term treatment of proximal venous thrombosis. J.A.M.A. *252*:235, 1984.
33. Hull, R. D., Carter, C. J., Jay, R. M., Ockelford, P. A., Hirsh, J., Turpie, A. G., Zielinsky, A., Gent, M., and Powers, P. J.: The diagnosis of acute, recurrent deep-vein thrombosis: A diagnostic challenge. Circulation *67*:901, 1983.
34. Godleski, J. J.: Pathology of deep venous thrombosis and pulmonary embolism. *In* Goldhaber, S. Z. (ed.): Pulmonary Embolism and Deep Venous Thrombosis. Philadelphia, W. B. Saunders Company, 1985, p. 11.
35. Visner, M. S., Arentzen, C. E., O'Connor, M. D., Larson, E. V., and Anderson, R. W.: Alterations in left ventricular three-dimensional dynamic geometry during acute right ventricular hypertension in the conscious dog. Circulation *67*:353, 1983.
36. Manny, J., and Hechtman, H. B.: Vasoactive humoral factors. *In* Goldhaber, S. Z. (ed.): Pulmonary Embolism and Deep Venous Thrombosis. Philadelphia, W. B. Saunders Company, 1985, p. 283.
37. Utsunomiya, T., Krausz, M., Levine, L., Shepro, D., and Hechtman, H. B.: Thromboxane mediation of cardiopulmonary effects of embolism. J. Clin. Invest. *70*:361, 1982.
38. Goldhaber, S. Z.: Strategies for diagnosis. *In* Goldhaber, S. Z. (ed.): Pulmonary Embolism and Deep Venous Thrombosis. Philadelphia, W. B. Saunders Company, 1985, p. 79.
39. Bell, W. R., Simon, T. L., and DeMets, D. L.: The clinical features of submassive and massive pulmonary emboli. Am. J. Med. *62*:355, 1977.
40. Stein, P. D., Willis, P. W. III, and DeMets, D. L.: History and physical examination in acute pulmonary embolism in patients without preexisting cardiac or pulmonary disease. Am. J. Cardiol. *47*:218, 1981.
41. Rich, S., Pietra, G. G., Kieras, K., Hart, K., and Brundage, B. H.: Primary pulmonary hypertension: Radiographic and scintigraphic patterns of histologic subtypes. Ann. Intern. Med. *105*:499, 1986.
42. Thames, M. D., Alpert, J. S., and Dalen, J. E.: Syncope in patients with pulmonary embolism. J.A.M.A. *238*:2509, 1977.
43. Simpson, R. J., Jr., Podolak, R. P., Mangano, C. A., Jr., Foster, J. R., and Dalldorf, F. G.: Vagal syncope during recurrent pulmonary embolism. J.A.M.A. *249*:390, 1983.
44. Dalen, J. E., Haffajee, C. I., Alpert, J. S., Howe, J. P. III, Ockene, I. S., and Paraskos, J. A.: Pulmonary embolism, pulmonary hemorrhage and pulmonary infarction. N. Engl. J. Med. *296*:1431, 1977.
45. Tsao, M.-S., Schraufnagel, D., and Wang, N.-S.: Pathogenesis of pulmonary infarction. Am. J. Med. *72*:599, 1982.
46. Hollister, L. E., and Cull, V. L.: The syndrome of chronic thrombosis of the major pulmonary arteries. Am. J. Med. *21*:312, 1956.
47. Wilhelmsen, L., Hagman, M., and Werko, L.: Recurrent pulmonary embolism—Incidence, predisposing factors and prognosis. Acta Med. Scand. *192*:565, 1972.
48. Sutton, G. C., Hall, R. J. C., and Kerr, I. H.: Clinical course and late prognosis of treated subacute massive, acute minor, and chronic pulmonary thromboembolism. Br. Heart J. *39*:1135, 1977.
49. Adler, D. S.: Nonthrombotic pulmonary embolism. *In* Goldhaber, S. Z. (ed.): Pulmonary Embolism and Deep Venous Thrombosis. Philadelphia, W. B. Saunders Company, 1985, p. 209.
50. Branch, W. T., Jr., and McNeil, B. J.: Analysis of the differential diagnosis and assessment of pleuritic chest pain in young adults. Am. J. Med. *75*:671, 1983.
51. Robin, E. D.: Overdiagnosis and overtreatment of pulmonary embolism: The emperor may have no clothes. Ann. Intern. Med. *87*:775, 1977.
52. Bynum, L. J., and Wilson, J. E. III: Radiographic features of pleural effusions in pulmonary embolism. Am. Rev. Respir. Dis. *117*:829, 1978.
53. Bynum, L. J., and Wilson, J. E. III: Characteristics of pleural effusions associated with pulmonary embolism. Arch. Intern. Med. *136*:159, 1976.
54. Stein, P. D., Dalen, J. E., McIntyre, K. M., Sasahara, A. A., Wenger, N. K., and Willis, P. W. III: The electrocardiogram in acute pulmonary embolism. Prog. Cardiovasc. Dis. *17*:247, 1975.
55. Rickman, F. D., Handin, R., Howe, J. P., Alpert, J. S., Dexter, L., and Dalen, J. E.: Fibrin split products in acute pulmonary embolism. Ann. Intern. Med. *79*:664, 1973.
56. Kerr, I. H., Simon, G., and Sutton, G. C.: The value of the plain radiograph in acute massive pulmonary embolism. Br. J. Radiol. *44*:751, 1971.
57. Palla, A., Donnamaria, V., Petruzzelli, S., Rossi, G., Riccetti, G., and Giuntini, C.: Enlargement of the right descending pulmonary artery in pulmonary embolism. A.J.R. *141*:513, 1983.
58. Williams, J. R., and Wilcox, W. C.: Pulmonary embolism: Roentgenographic and angiographic considerations. A.J.R. *89*:333, 1963.
59. Markisz, J. A.: Radiologic and nuclear medicine diagnosis. *In* Goldhaber, S. Z. (ed.): Pulmonary Embolism and Deep Venous Thrombosis. Philadelphia, W. B. Saunders Company, 1985, p. 41.
60. Fleischner, F. G.: Roentgenology of the pulmonary infarct. Semin. Roentgenol. *2*:61, 1967.
61. Hampton, A. O., and Castleman, B.: Correlation of postmortem chest teleroentgenograms with autopsy findings with special reference to pulmonary embolism and infarction. A.J.R. *43*:305, 1940.
62. Bachynski, J. E.: Absence of the air bronchogram sign: A reliable finding in pulmonary embolism with infarction or hemorrhage. Radiology *100*:547, 1971.
63. Woodruff, W. W. III, Hoeck, B. E., Chitwood, W. R., Jr., Lyerly, H. K., Sabiston, D. C., Jr., and Chen, J. T. T.: Radiographic findings in pulmonary hypertension from unresolved embolism. A.J.R. *144*:681, 1985.
64. McNeil, B. J.: Ventilation-perfusion studies and the diagnosis of pulmonary embolism: Concise communication. J. Nucl. Med. *21*:319, 1980.
65. Hull, R. D., Hirsh, J., Carter, C. J., Raskob, G. E., Gill, G. J., Jay, R. M., Leclerc, J. R., David, M., and Coates, G.: Diagnostic value of ventilation-perfusion lung scanning in patients with suspected pulmonary embolism. Chest *88*:819, 1985.
66. Braun, S. D., Newman, G. E., Ford, K., Miller, G. A., Coleman, R. E., and Dunnick, N. R.: Ventilation-perfusion scanning and pulmonary angiography: Correlation in clinical high-probability pulmonary embolism. A.J.R. *143*:977, 1984.
67. Marsh, J. D., Glynn, M. A., and Torman, H. A.: Pulmonary angiography: Application in a new spectrum of patients. Am. J. Med. *75*:763, 1983.
68. Frankel, N., Coleman, R. E., Pryor, D. B., Sostman, D., and Ravin, C. E.: Utilization of lung scans by clinicians. J. Nucl. Med. *27*:366, 1986.
69. Dawley, D. L., and Goldhaber, S. Z.: Impact of lung scanning on the management of suspected pulmonary embolism. Am. Heart J. *In press.*
70. Cheely, R., McCartney, W. H., Perry, J. R., Delany, D. J., Bustad, L., Wynia, V. H., and Griggs, T. R.: The role of noninvasive tests versus pulmonary angiography in the diagnosis of pulmonary embolism. Am. J. Med. *70*:17, 1981.

71. Lee, M. E., Biello, D. R., Kumar, B., and Siegel, B. A.: "Low-probability" ventilation-perfusion scintigrams: Clinical outcomes in 99 patients. Radiology *156*:497, 1985.
72. Mills, S. R., Jackson, D. C., Older, R. A., Heaston, D. K., and Moore, A. U.: The incidence, etiologies, and avoidance of complications of pulmonary angiography in a large series. Radiology *136*:295, 1980.
73. McCracken, S., and Bettmann, M.: Current status of ionic and non-ionic intravascular contrast media. Postgrad. Radiol. *3*:345, 1983.
74. Wood, D. L., Osborn, M. J., Rooke, J., and Holmes, D. R.: Amiodarone pulmonary toxicity: Report of two cases associated with rapidly progressive fatal adult respiratory distress syndrome after pulmonary angiography. Mayo Clin. Proc. *60*:601, 1985.
75. Dotter, C. T., and Rosch, J.: Pulmonary angiography: Technique. *In* Abrams, H. L. (ed.): Abrams Angiography: Vascular and Interventional Radiology. Boston, Little, Brown and Co., 1983, p. 707.
76. Benotti, J. R., and Grossman, W.: Pulmonary angiography. *In* Grossman, W. (ed.): Cardiac Catheterization and Angiography. Philadelphia, Lea and Febiger, 1986, p. 213.
77. Cassling, R. J., Lois, J. F., and Gomes, A. S.: Unusual pulmonary angiographic findings in suspected pulmonary embolism. A.J.R. *145*:995, 1985.
78. Kramer, F. L., Teitelbaum, G., and Merli, G. J.: Panvenography and pulmonary angiography in the diagnosis of deep venous thrombosis and pulmonary thromboembolism. Radiol. Clin. North Am. *24*:397, 1986.
79. Kasper, W., Meinertz, T., Henkel, B., Eissner, D., Hahn, K., Hofmann, T., Zeiher, A., and Just, H.: Echocardiographic findings in patients with proved pulmonary embolism. Am. Heart J. *112*:1284, 1986.
80. Sagar, K. B., Rhyne, T. L., and Greenfield, L. J.: Echocardiographic tissue characterization and range-gated Doppler ultrasound for the diagnosis of pulmonary embolism. Circulation *67*:365, 1983.
81. Pond, G. D.: Pulmonary digital subtraction angiography. Radiol. Clin. North Am. *23*:243, 1985.
82. Kereiakes, D. J., Herfkens, R. J., Brundage, B. H., Gamsu, G., and Lipton, M. J.: Computerized tomography in chronic thromboembolic pulmonary hypertension. Am. Heart J. *106*:1432, 1983.
83. Gamsu, G., Hirji, M., Moore, E. H., Webb, W. R., and Brito, A.: Experimental pulmonary emboli detected using magnetic resonance. Radiology *153*:467, 1984.
84. Moore, E. H., Gamsu, G., Webb, H. R., and Stulbarg, M. S.: Pulmonary embolus: Detection and follow-up using magnetic resonance. Radiology *153*:471, 1984.
85. Ezekowitz, M. D., Eichner, E. R., Scatterday, R., and Elkins, R. C.: Diagnosis of a persistent pulmonary embolus by indium-111 platelet scintigraphy with angiographic and tissue confirmation. Am. J. Med. *72*:839, 1982.
86. Ezekowitz, M. D., Pope, C. F., Sostman, H. D., Smith, E. O., Glickman, M., Rapoport, S., Sniderman, K. W., Friedlaender, G., Pelker, R. B., Taylor, F. B., and Zaret, B. L.: Indium-111 platelet scintigraphy for the diagnosis of acute venous thrombosis. Circulation *73*:668, 1986.
87. Clarke-Pearson, D. L., Coleman, R. E., Siegel, R., Synan, I. S., and Petry, N.: Indium-111 platelet imaging for the detection of deep venous thrombosis and pulmonary embolism in patients without symptoms after surgery. Surgery *98*:98, 1985.
88. Ezekowitz, M. D., Pope, C. F., and Smith, E. O.: Indium-111 platelet imaging. *In* Goldhaber, S. Z. (ed.): Pulmonary Embolism and Deep Venous Thrombosis. Philadelphia, W. B. Saunders Company, 1985, p. 261.
89. Shure, D., Gregoratos, G., and Moser, K. M.: Fiberoptic angioscopy: Role in the diagnosis of chronic pulmonary arterial obstruction. Ann. Intern. Med. *103*:844, 1985.

TREATMENT OF PULMONARY EMBOLISM

90. Barritt, D. W., and Jordan, S. C.: Anticoagulant drugs in the treatment of pulmonary embolism. A controlled trial. Lancet *1*:1309, 1960.
91. Hyers, T. M., Hull, R. D., and Weg, J. G.: Antithrombotic therapy for venous thromboembolic disease. Chest *89*:26s, 1986.
92. Kelton, J. G., and Hirsh, J.: Bleeding associated with antithrombotic therapy. Semin. Hematol. *17*:259, 1980.
93. Beaver, B. L., Young, D., and Satiani, B.: Prediction of heparin requirements in acute thromboplastic venous disease. Arch. Surg. *120*:436, 1985.
94. Stead, R. B.: Clinical pharmacology. *In* Goldhaber, S. Z. (ed.): Pulmonary Embolism and Deep Venous Thrombosis. Philadelphia, W. B. Saunders Company, 1985, p. 99.
95. Hall, J. G., Pauli, R. M., and Wilson, K. M.: Maternal and fetal sequelae of anticoagulation during pregnancy. Am. J. Med. *68*:122, 1980.
96. Bell, W. R., Tomasulo, P. A., Alving, B. M., and Duffy, T. P.: Thrombocytopenia occurring during the administration of heparin: A prospective study in 51 patients. Ann. Intern. Med. *85*:155, 1976.
97. Powers, P. J., Kelton, J. G., and Carter, C. J.: Studies on the frequency of heparin-associated thrombocytopenia. Thrombosis Res. *33*:439, 1984.
98. Kelly, R. A., Gelfand, J. A., and Pincus, S. H.: Cutaneous necrosis caused by systemically administered heparin. J.A.M.A. *246*:1582, 1981.
99. Cimo, P. L., Moake, J. L., Weinger, R. S., Ben-Menachem, Y., and Khalil, K. G.: Heparin-induced thrombocytopenia: Association with a platelet aggregating factor and arterial thromboses. Am. J. Hematol. *6*:125, 1976.
100. Squires, J. W., and Pinch, L. W.: Heparin-induced spinal fractures. J.A.M.A. *241*:2417, 1979.
101. de Swiet, M., Ward, P. D., Fidler, J., Horsman, A., Katz, D., Letsky, E., Peacock, M., and Wise, P. H.: Prolonged heparin therapy in pregnancy causes bone demineralization. Br. J. Obstet. Gynaecol. *90*:1129, 1983.
102. O'Kelly, R., Magee, F., and McKenna, T. J.: Routine heparin therapy inhibits adrenal aldosterone production. J. Clin. Endocrinol. Metab. *56*:108, 1983.
103. Phelps, K. R., Oh, M. S., and Carroll, H. J.: Heparin-induced hyperkalemia: Report of a case. Nephron *25*:254, 1980.
104. Leekey, D., Gantt, C., and Lim, V.: Heparin-induced hypoaldosteronism—Report of a case. J.A.M.A. *246*:2189, 1981.
105. Coon, W. W., and Willis, P. W. III: Thromboembolic complications during anticoagulant therapy. Arch. Surg. *105*:209, 1972.
106. Urokinase Pulmonary Embolism Trial: A National Cooperative Study. Circulation *47* and *48*(II):1, 1973.
107. American College of Chest Physicians and the National Heart, Lung, and Blood Institute National Conference on Antithrombotic Therapy. Arch. Intern. Med. *146*:462, 1986.
108. Michaels, L.: Incidence of thromboembolism after stopping anticoagulant therapy. Relationship to hemorrhage at the time of termination. J.A.M.A. *215*:595, 1971.
109. Broekmans, A. W., Bertina, R. M., Leoliger, E. A., Hoffmann, V., and Klingemann, H. G.: Protein C and the development of skin necrosis during anticoagulant therapy. Thromb. Haemost. *49*:251, 1983.
110. Dickie, K. J., de Groot, W. J., Cooley, R. N., Bond, T. P., and Guest, M. M.: Hemodynamic effects of bolus infusion of urokinase in pulmonary thromboembolism. Am. Rev. Respir. Dis. *109*:48, 1974.
111. Petitpretz, P., Simmoneau, G., Cerrina, J., Musset, D., Dreyfus, M., Vandenbroek, M.-D., and Duroux, P.: Effects of a single bolus of urokinase in patients with life-threatening pulmonary emboli: A descriptive trial. Circulation *70*:861, 1984.
112. Tibbutt, D. A., Davies, J. A., Anderson, J. A., Fletcher, E. W. L., Hamill, J., Holt, J. M., Thomas, M. L., Lee, G. de J., Miller, G. A. H., Sharp, A. A., and Sutton, G. C.: Comparison by controlled clinical trial of streptokinase and heparin in treatment of life-threatening pulmonary embolism. Br. Med. J. *1*:343, 1974.
113. Ly, B., Arnesen, H., Eie, H., and Hol, R.: A controlled clinical trial of streptokinase and heparin in the treatment of major pulmonary embolism. Acta Med. Scand. *203*:465, 1978.
114. Sharma, G. V. R. K., Burleson, V. A., and Sasahara, A. A.: Effect of thrombolytic therapy on pulmonary-capillary blood volume in patients with pulmonary embolism. N. Engl. J. Med. *303*:842, 1980.
115. Schwartz, F., Stehr, H., Zimmermann, R., Manthey, J., and Kubler, W.: Sustained improvement of pulmonary hemodynamics in patients at rest and during exercise after thrombolytic treatment of massive pulmonary embolism. Circulation *71*:117, 1985.
116. Schrier, S. L.: Transfusion therapy. *In* Rubinstein, E., and Federman, D. D. (eds.): Scientific American Medicine. New York, Scientific American Inc., *5* (x):1–10, July, 1985.
117. Matsuo, O., Rijken, D. C., and Collen, D.: Thrombolysis by human tissue plasminogen activator and urokinase in rabbits with experimental pulmonary embolus. Nature *291*:590, 1981.
118. Agnelli, G., Buchanan, M. R., Fernandez, F., Boneau, R., Van Ryn, J., Hirsh, J., and Collen, D.: A comparison of the thrombolytic and hemorrhagic effects of tissue-type plasminogen activator and streptokinase in rabbits. Circulation *72*:178, 1985.
119. Bounameaux, H., Vermylen, J., and Collen, D.: Thrombolytic treatment with recombinant tissue-type plasminogen activator in a patient with massive pulmonary embolism. Ann. Intern. Med. *103*:64, 1985.
120. Goldhaber, S. Z., Vaughan, D. E., Markis, J. E., Selwyn, A. P., Meyerovitz, M. F., Loscalzo, J., Kim, D. S., Kessler, C. M., Dawley, D. L., Sharma, G. V. R. K., Sasahara, A., Grossbard, E. B., and Braunwald, E.: Acute pulmonary embolism treated with tissue plasminogen activator. Lancet *2*:886, 1986.
121. Goldhaber, S. Z., Markis, J. E., Kessler, C. M., Meyerovitz, M. F., Kim, D., Vaughan, D. E., Selwyn, A. P., Loscalzo, J., Dawley, D. L., Sharma, G. V. R. K., Sasahara, A., Grossbard, E. B., and Braunwald, E.: Perspectives on treatment of acute pulmonary embolism with tissue plasminogen activator. Semin. Thromb. Hemostas. *13*:221, 1987.
121a. Goldhaber, S. Z., Meyerovitz, M. F., Markis, J. E., Kin, D., Kessler, C. M., Sharma, G. V. R. K., Vaughan, D. E., Selwyn, A. P., Dawley, D. L., Loscalzo, J., Sasahara, A., Grossbard, E. B., and Braunwald, E.: Thrombolytic therapy of acute pulmonary embolism: Current status and future potential. J. Am. Coll. Cardiol. (in press.)
122. Markis, J. E., Goldhaber, S. Z., Kim, D. S., Palla, A., Parker, J. A., and Braunwald, E.: Early improved pulmonary perfusion after intravenous recombinant tissue plasminogen activator for acute pulmonary embolism. Circulation *74*:II-127, 1986 (abstract).
123. Come, P. C., and Markis, J. E.: Reversal of right ventricular dysfunction in patients with acute pulmonary embolism after treatment with intravenous tissue plasminogen activator (abstract). J. Am. Coll. Cardiol. *9*:40A, 1987.
124. Urokinase-Streptokinase Embolism Trial: Phase 2 results. A cooperative study. J.A.M.A. *229*:1606, 1974.
125. Sobel, B. E., Gross, R. W., and Robison, A. K.: Thrombolysis, clot selectivity, and kinetics. Circulation *70*:160, 1984.
126. Dalen, J. E., Banas, J. S., Brooks, H. L., Evans, G. L., Paraskos, J. A., and Dexter, L.: Resolution rate of acute pulmonary embolism in man. N. Engl. J. Med. *280*:1194, 1969.
127. Tow, D. E., and Wagner, N. H., Jr.: Recovery of pulmonary artery flow in patients with pulmonary embolism. N. Engl. J. Med. *276*:1053, 1967.
128. Thrombolytic Therapy in Thrombosis: A National Institutes of Health Consensus Development Conference. Ann. Intern. Med. *93*:141, 1980.
129. Goldhaber, S. Z., Buring, J. E., Lipnick, R. J., and Hennekens, C. H.: Interruption of the inferior vena cava by clip or filter. Am. J. Med. *76*:512, 1984.

130. Josey, W. E., and Staggers, S. R.: Heparin therapy in septic pelvic thrombophlebitis. A study of 46 cases. Am. J. Obstet. Gynecol. *120*:228, 1974.
131. Toole, A. L., Lowman, R., and Stern, H.: Pulmonary embolism and intracardiac shunt. A unique indication for operation. Ann. Thorac. Surg. *22*:296, 1976.
132. Hoagland, P. M.: Massive pulmonary embolism. *In* Goldhaber, S. Z. (ed.): Pulmonary Embolism and Deep Venous Thrombosis. Philadelphia, W. B. Saunders Company, 1985, p. 179.
133. Askew, A. R., and Gardner, A. M. N.: Long term follow-up of partial caval occlusion by clip. Am. J. Surg. *140*:441, 1980.
134. Hunter, J. A., DeLaria, G. A., Goldin, M. D., Javid, H., Najafi, H., and Serry, C.: Requirements for a method of transvenous inferior vena cava interruption. Arch. Surg. *115*:1324, 1980.
135. Mobin-Uddin, K., Utley, J. R., and Bryant, L. R.: The inferior vena cava umbrella filter. Prog. Cardiovasc. Dis. *17*:391, 1975.
136. McIntyre, A. B., McCready, R. A., Hyde, G. L., and Mattingly, W.: A ten year follow-up study of the Mobin-Uddin filter for vena cava interruption. Surg. Gynecol. Obstet. *158*:513, 1984.
137. Greenfield, L. J.: Current indications for and results of Greenfield filter placement. J. Vasc. Surg. *1*:502, 1984.
138. Denny, D. F., Cronan, J. J., Dorfman, G. S., and Esplin, C.: Percutaneous Kimray-Greenfield filter placement by femoral vein puncture. A.J.R. *145*:827, 1985.
139. Braun, T. I., and Goldberg, S. K.: An unusual thromboembolic complication of a Greenfield vena caval filter. Chest 87:127, 1985.
140. Sidawy, A. N., and Menzoian, J. D.: Distal migration and deformation of the Greenfield vena cava filter. Surgery 99:369, 1986.
141. Beckman, D., Solmos, B., Herad, G., and Siderys, H.: Intraoperative pulmonary angioscopy using the flexible fiberoptic choledochoscope. Ann. Thorac. Surg. *41*:563, 1986.
142. Gold, J. P., Shemin, R. J., DiSesa, V. J., Cohn, L., and Collins, J. J., Jr.: Balloon pump support of the failing right heart. Clin. Cardiol. *8*:599, 1985.
143. Moore, J. H., Jr., Koolpe, H. A., Carabasi, R. A., Yang, S. L., and Jarrell, B. E.: Transvenous catheter pulmonary embolectomy. Arch. Surg. *120*:1372, 1985.
143a. Feitelberg, S. P., Kahn, S. E., Kotler, M. N., Cope, C., Nakhjavan, F. K., and Lippmann, M.: Transfemoral embolectomy for massive pulmonary embolus and associated myocardial infarction. Am. Heart J. *113*:819, 1987.
144. Greenfield, L. J.: Vena caval interruption and pulmonary embolectomy. Clin. Chest Med. 5:495, 1984.
145. Riedel, M., Stanek, V., Widimsky, J., and Prerovsky, I.: Long-term follow-up of patients with pulmonary thromboembolism. Late prognosis and evolution of hemodynamic and respiratory data. Chest *81*:151, 1982.
146. Benotti, J. R., Ockene, I. S., Alpert, J. S., and Dalen, J. E.: The clinical profile of unresolved pulmonary embolism. Chest *84*:669, 1983.
147. Moser, K. M., Spragg, R. G., Utley, J., and Daily, P. O.: Chronic thrombotic obstruction of major pulmonary arteries: Results of thromboendarterectomy in 15 patients. Ann. Intern. Med. 99:299, 1983.
148. Utley, J. R.: Pulmonary thromboendarterectomy. *In* Goldhaber, S. Z. (ed.): Pulmonary Embolism and Deep Venous Thrombosis. Philadelphia, W. B. Saunders Company, 1985, p. 275.
149. Chitwood, W. R., Jr., Lyerly, H. K., and Sabiston, D. C., Jr.: Surgical management of chronic pulmonary embolism. Ann. Surg. *201*:11, 1985.

PREVENTION OF PULMONARY EMBOLISM

150. An International Multicentre Trial: Prevention of fatal postoperative pulmonary embolism by low doses of heparin. Lancet 2:45, 1975.
151. Collins, R., and Peto, R.: Statistical overviews of trials in perioperative heparin. Presented at the 1986 NIH Consensus Development Conference on Prevention of Venous Thrombosis and Pulmonary Embolism.
152. Goldhaber, S. Z.: Prevention of venous thromboembolism. *In* Goldhaber, S. Z. (ed.): Pulmonary Embolism and Deep Venous Thrombosis. Philadelphia, W. B. Saunders Company, 1985, p. 135.
153. NIH Consensus Development Statement. Prevention of venous thrombosis and pulmonary embolism. J.A.M.A. *256*:744, 1986.
154. Poller, L., Taberner, D. A., Sandilands, D. G., and Galasko, C. S. B.: An evaluation of APTT monitoring of low-dose heparin dosage in hip surgery. Thromb. Haemost. *47*:50, 1982.
155. Leyvraz, P. F., Richard, J., Bachmann, F., Van Melle, G., Treyvand, J.-M., Livio, J.-J., and Candardjis, G.: Adjusted versus fixed-dose subcutaneous heparin in the prevention of deep-vein thrombosis after total hip replacement. N. Engl. J. Med. *309*:954, 1983.
156. Salzman, E. W.: Progress in preventing venous thromboembolism. N. Engl. J. Med. *309*:980, 1983.
157. Gent, M., and Roberts, R. S.: A meta-analysis of the studies of dihydroergotamine plus heparin in the prophylaxis of deep vein thrombosis. Chest 89:396S, 1986.
158. The Multicenter Trial Committee: Dihydroergotamine-heparin prophylaxis of postoperative deep vein thrombosis. A multicenter trial. J.A.M.A. *251*:2960, 1984.
159. Beisaw, N. E., Comerota, A. J., Groth, H. E., Merli, G. J., Weitz, H. H., Zimmerman, R. C., DiSerio, F. J., and Sasahara, A. A.: A controlled, prospective, randomized, multicenter trial of DHE/heparin in the prevention of DVT following total hip replacement. J. Bone Joint Surg. 1987; *in press.*
160. Gruber, U. F.: Prevention of fatal postoperative pulmonary embolism by heparin dihydroergotamine or Dextran 70. Br. J. Surg. *69*:S54, 1982.
161. Kakkar, V. V.: Prevention of post-operative venous thromboembolism by a new low molecular weight heparin fraction. Nouv. Rev. Fr. Hematol. *26*:277, 1984.
162. Turpie, A. G. G., Levine, M. N., Hirsh, J., Carter, C. J., Jay, R. M., Powers, P. J., Andrew, M., Hull, R. D., and Gent, M.: A randomized controlled trial of low-molecular-weight heparin (enoxaparin) to prevent deep-vein thrombosis in patients undergoing elective hip surgery. N. Engl. J. Med. *315*:925, 1986.
163. Kakkar, V. V., and Adams, P. C.: Preventive and therapeutic approach to venous thromboembolic disease and pulmonary embolism—Can death from pulmonary embolism be prevented? J. Am. Coll. Cardiol. *8*:146B, 1986.
164. Colditz, G. A., Tuden, R. L., and Oster, G.: Rates of venous thrombosis after general surgery: Combined results of randomized clinical trials. Lancet 2:143, 1986.
165. Clarke-Pearson, D. L., Synan, I. S., Hinshaw, W. M., Coleman, E., and Creasman, W. T.: Prevention of postoperative venous thromboembolism by external pneumatic calf compression in patients with gynecologic malignancy. Obstet. Gynecol. *63*:92, 1984.
166. Clarke-Pearson, D. L., DeLong, E. R., Synan, I. S., and Creasman, W. T.: Complications of low-dose heparin prophylaxis in gynecologic oncology surgery. Obstet. Gynecol. *64*:689, 1984.
167. Salzman, E. W., Sobel, M., Lewis, J., Sweeney, J., Hussey, S., and Kurland, G.: Prevention of venous thromboembolism in unstable angina pectoris. N. Engl. J. Med. *306*:991, 1982.
168. Salzman, E. W., and Davies, G. C.: Prophylaxis of venous thromboembolism. Analysis of cost effectiveness. Ann. Surg. *191*:207, 1979.
169. Hull, R. D., Hirsh, J., Sackett, D. L., and Stoddart, G. L.: Cost-effectiveness of primary and secondary prevention of fatal pulmonary embolism in high-risk surgical patients. Can. Med. Assoc. J. *127*:990, 1982.
170. Oster, G., Tuden, R. L., and Colditz, G. A.: Prevention of venous thromboembolism after general surgery: A cost-effectiveness analysis of alternative approaches to prophylaxis. Am. J. Med. *82*: *In press*, 1987.
171. Oster, G., Tuden, R. L., and Colditz, G. A.: A cost-effectiveness analysis of prophylaxis against deep-vein thrombosis in major orthopedic surgery. J.A.M.A. 257:203, 1987.

48 COR PULMONALE

by E. REGIS McFADDEN, Jr., M.D., and
EUGENE BRAUNWALD, M.D.

According to the World Health Organization, the chronic form of cor pulmonale is composed of some combination of hypertrophy and dilatation of the right ventricle secondary to pulmonary hypertension; the latter is caused by disease of the pulmonary parenchyma and/or pulmonary vascular system between the origins of the main pulmonary artery and the entry of the pulmonary veins into the left atrium.[1] Acute cor pulmonale is defined as acute right heart strain or overload resulting from the pulmonary hypertension usually due to massive pulmonary embolism.[2] Cor pulmonale includes many disease states with diverse etiologies, pathophysiological mechanisms, and clinical characteristics that have in common only a disturbance of the pulmonary circulation. This chapter focuses on those conditions (with the exclusion of primary pulmonary hypertension, Chap. 26, and pulmonary thromboembolism, Chap. 47), that act directly on the pulmonary vessels, both acutely and chronically, and those that produce pulmonary hypertension by acting primarily on the gas-exchanging, neuromuscular, and ventilatory control functions of the respiratory system.

ANATOMICAL AND PATHOPHYSIOLOGICAL CORRELATES

RIGHT VENTRICULAR ANATOMY

In the first 3 months of life in infants born at, or near, sea level, the right ventricle is larger and heavier and has a greater end-diastolic volume than the left.[3,7] With advancing age, the left ventricle becomes dominant, and in the adult, the right ventricular wall is relatively thin and has a crescentic configuration on cross section. However, in high-altitude dwellers, the situation is different. The degree of right ventricular preponderance, both at birth and for the first 3 months of life, is greater than that seen in low-altitude residents, and the normal regression in size is so delayed that right ventricular enlargement can persist through the first decade.[6] In native adults living above 12,000 feet, 93 per cent of the hearts in a necropsy series showed some degree of right ventricular enlargement.[8] These morphological findings have a close relationship with the hemodynamic characteristics of individuals at high altitudes and can be related to the degree of pulmonary arterial hypertension.[9]

Several methods are used to ascertain the characteristics, presence, and severity of right ventricular hypertrophy; the two traditional methods involve the measurement of ventricular weight and wall thickness. Many investigators believe that wall thickness determinations are not sufficiently precise. Fulton et al. have provided weight criteria that are used widely.[10] In their technique, the right ventricle is dissected free, and the septum is weighed together with the left ventricle. Right ventricular weight can then be described in absolute terms or as a ratio of the left ventricle (LV) plus the septum (S), i.e., (LV + S)/RV. Using these criteria, a heart is considered normal only if the total ventricular weight is less that 250 gm, the free wall of the right ventricle weighs less than 65 gm, and the ratio of (LV + S)/RV is between 2.3:1 and 3.3:1. If left ventricular hypertrophy is also present, the ratio may be within normal limits or even raised. Using this method, Mitchell and colleagues found that the upper limits of normal (as defined by the mean plus 2 standard deviations) in men 40 or more years of age at death were 69 gm for the right ventricle and 203 gm for the left ventricle plus septum. These observers also noted that in their study right ventricular thickness was a relatively poor index of hypertrophy.[11]

Others have determined muscle fiber size morphometrically and found the distribution of myocardial fiber diameters to be uniform, with a distinct bell-shaped distribution noted for the right ventricle, left ventricle, and septum.[12] In cases of pure right ventricular hypertrophy, the distribution always shifted so that the mean diameter of the muscle fibers from the right ventricle exceeded that of the septum or normal left ventricle. An example of an enlarged right ventricle in cor pulmonale is shown in Figure 48–1.

RIGHT VENTRICULAR FUNCTION

Because right ventricular hypertrophy occurs most commonly in association with longstanding elevations in pulmonary arterial pressures, an analogy has often been made between the left ventricle in systemic hypertension and the right ventricle in pulmonary hypertension. Since there is no fundamental difference in either the configuration or the pumping action of the two ventricles before birth, the differences that exist in the adult have been attributed to the flow resistance in the respective circulations.[13] As al-

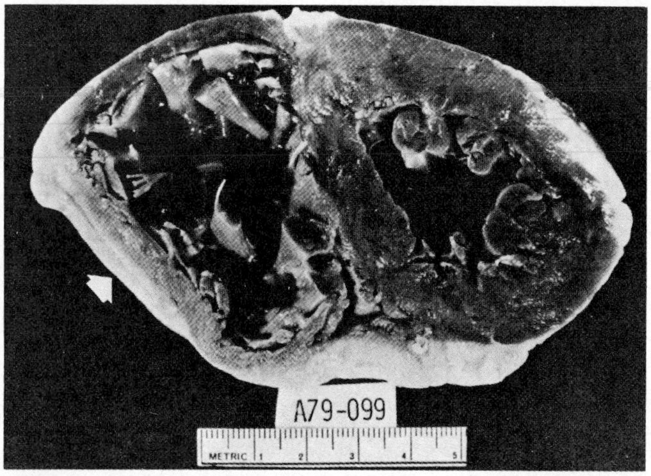

FIGURE 48–1. Cor pulmonale, heart cut in cross section. Notice the rounded contour of the right ventricular cavity (indicated by arrow), which is typical of dilation. The normal right ventricle is a crescent-shaped thin-walled structure. Both hypertrophy and dilatation of the right ventricle are present in this case. (From Taylor, W. E.: Pathology of pulmonary heart disease. *In* Rubin, L. J. [ed.]: Pulmonary Heart Disease. Boston, Martinus Nijhoff, 1984, p. 65.)

ready noted, the normal adult right ventricle has thin walls and a crescent shape; its pumping action is akin to that of a bellows working in series with a low-pressure circuit, in contrast to the concentric contraction of the left ventricle.[13, 13a] The right ventricle is more compliant,[14] and in comparison with the left it is better able to handle an increase in a volume than a pressure load. The evidence in support of this statement is derived in the main from animal data[15-18] (Fig. 48–2), which contrasts the effects of increasing preload and afterload on right and left ventricular function. In the left-hand panel, stroke volume is plotted as a function of various afterloads that were produced by actively constricting the main pulmonary artery and aorta in the dog.[15, 16] Small increments in pulmonary artery pressure are associated with sharp decreases in right ventricular stroke volume. In contrast, the left ventricle, which normally works against high initial pressures, continues to maintain stroke volume despite substantial increases in systemic arterial pressure.

The right-hand portion of this figure demonstrates the effects of increasing preload. These ventricular function curves (Chap. 13) were obtained by volume infusions into the atria of dogs.[18] Note the marked differences in the respective ventricular stroke work that occur as right and left atrial pressures are increased. For a fourfold elevation in filling pressure (i.e., from 5 to 20 cm H_2O), the increase in left ventricular work was approximately five times that of the right.

In response to chronic pressure loads, significant changes develop in the configuration, mass, and functional characteristics of the right ventricle. The rate at which these occur in humans and the magnitude of the pressures needed to produce them are unknown. However, animal studies indicate that alterations in structure and function can be quite rapid following experimental outflow tract obstruction. Spann et al. observed a 71 per cent increase in right ventricular weight in cats 2 days after the pulmonary artery was banded, and within a month weight had risen to 2.5 times the normal value.[19] This increase was not from an elevation in cardiac tissue water, since the wet to dry weight ratios were not significantly different from normal. It is doubtful that the response is as rapid in humans.

The lumen of the main pulmonary artery can be reduced acutely by 60 to 80 per cent before aortic pressure declines.[20-22] Because these experiments ignored the effects of neurohumoral compensations that support the systemic circulation, the impression has arisen that the acute right ventricular response is an abrupt, all-or-none event. However, as suggested in Figure 48–2, right ventricular decompensation is really a continuum.[15, 18] At right ventricular systolic pressures of 60 to 80 mm Hg, right ventricular dilatation and failure occur with systemic hypotension and hypoperfusion.[23] The rate and/or absolute level of outflow tract obstruction at which these alterations develop can be greatly amplified or attenuated by respectively decreasing or increasing right coronary artery blood flow.[23] The relative roles played by changes in coronary blood flow in acute right heart failure in humans have yet to be determined.

PULMONARY VASCULAR ANATOMY

DEVELOPMENT. Embryologically, the primitive main pulmonary artery and its main right and left branches are derived from the aortic sac, whereas the peripheral pulmonary arteries arise from a network of vessels around the bronchial bud.[24] Each pulmonary artery forms a close relationship with a stem bronchus and provides an arterial partner for each new airway ramification. This branching pattern of airways and arteries is complete all the way out to the preacinar region by week 16 of intrauterine life, and further growth occurs only in dimensions.[25]

At birth the alveolar region is represented by primitive air sacs, and during early childhood the acini grow rapidly by budding new alveoli from respiratory bronchioli, alveolar ducts, and more distal air spaces.[26, 27] New arteries and veins continue to develop up to the 18th month of life and then increase in size with further age.[26] These vessels follow the course of the alveoli and not the airway. By the age of 8 years the number of alveoli and blood vessels reaches that of the adult.[26]

It has been traditionally held that the branching pattern and course

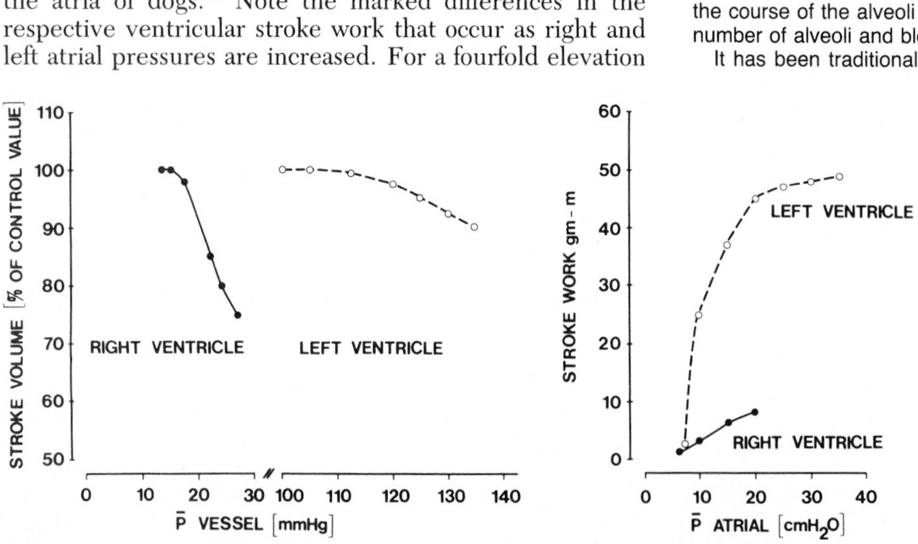

FIGURE 48–2. Effects of increasing preload and afterload on right and left ventricular function. The data in the left panel were obtained by constricting the main pulmonary artery and aorta in dogs. The right panel demonstrates the effect of increasing preloads.

of the airways and pulmonary arteries always parallel each other, at least within the alveolar region. However, it is now recognized that an irregular branching pattern from the hilum to the level of the capillaries exists with so-called "axial" or "conventional" arteries following the airways and supernumerary arteries, which are side branches arising from the main arteries but without a corresponding airway.[28] Two types of supernumerary vessels have been recognized: aberrant and accessory. An *aberrant* artery arises independently of any airway but then joins one downstream and branches with it. An *accessory* artery branches independently of any airway and usually enters the periphery of a respiratory unit. The supernumerary vessels contribute significantly to the total cross-sectional area of the vascular bed, particularly during recruitment, as discussed below.

WALL STRUCTURE. Starting from the main pulmonary artery and proceeding distally toward the capillaries, four structural regions can be identified: elastic, muscular, partially muscular, and nonmuscular.[28] In keeping with its embryological derivation, the main pulmonary artery and the first five generations are elastic in nature but less so than the aorta and major systemic arteries. These vessels by definition have more than five elastic laminae in their media and are over 2000 μm in diameter in the adult. In the axial pathway, the next three generations are said to be transitional.

Muscular arteries have between 2 and 5 elastic laminae and a continuous muscle coat. These arteries form the majority of vessels in the lung and are found in a diameter range of 150 to 2000 μm in the adult. The medial muscle coat is very thin compared with the arterioles in the systemic circulation. These vessels give way to partially muscular arteries in which the muscle is arranged in a spiral so that in cross section it appears as a crescent, with the rest of the wall being like a capillary. Nonmuscular arteries are larger than capillaries and range from 30 to 75 μm in diameter in adults. Partially muscular and nonmuscular arteries all lie within the alveolar units in adults. The smallest muscular and partially muscular ones are thought to represent the resistance arteries.[28]

Although there is great variation in the sizes of arteries that accompany conducting airways such as lobar bronchi, those that follow the respiratory bronchi and alveolar ducts are muscular or partially so.[28] The implications for function of these observations are severalfold. It is known that gas exchange occurs in respiratory bronchi and alveolar ducts through the arteries that accompany these structures.[29] When this information is coupled with the fact that hypoxia acts directly to constrict muscular arteries, it is apparent that this area of the lung has the propensity for active control of pulmonary blood flow. Further, since the spiral of muscle in the partially muscular arteries is directly contiguous with the muscle encircling the larger vessels, retrograde propagation of the hypoxic stimulus can occur in the intracellular pathways of the muscle syncytium,[28] and a wider and more severe response can develop.

INNERVATION. In further contrast to the peripheral circulation, it has proved difficult to demonstrate a nerve supply in the pulmonary circulation. Evidence suggests that although both adrenergic and cholinergic fibers are present, they are sparse in comparison with those innervating systemic vessels of similar size, and their distribution tends to be concentrated in the larger vessels at the hilum.[29, 30]

In *summary,* the structure of the pulmonary circulation is in keeping with its hemodynamics. The thin-walled, sparsely innervated vessels which contain relatively small amounts of smooth muscle (Fig. 26–4*A*, p. 798) do not favor the development of marked vasomotor responses, and, indeed, vasoconstriction *alone* is not sufficient to overload the right ventricle to the point of producing acute cor pulmonale.[31] Consequently, mechanical obstruction of the pulmonary circulation can be inferred when there is acute cor pulmonale, and structural alterations in the pulmonary vascular bed must be present in the chronic form.

PHYSIOLOGY OF THE PULMONARY CIRCULATION

(See also Chapter 26)

The physiology of the pulmonary circulation is unique from several standpoints. Most of this vascular bed is contained within the parenchyma of the lung, and thus the vessels are subjected to external distending and compressive forces which can act independently of any intrinsic properties of the vessels themselves. In addition, the pulmonary circulation is in series with a pump capable of developing only low pressures, yet it must accommodate the entire cardiac output under all states of physical activity. Consequently, it must adjust to wide variations in blood flow without much change in pressure so as not to overload the right ventricle.

PRESSURE-VOLUME RELATIONSHIPS. Historically, it has been thought that the pulmonary circulation is highly distensible and that the vessels dilate to accommodate increases in cardiac output and, in this manner, prevent an increase in pulmonary artery pressure in high-flow states.[32, 33] However, actual measurements of the compliance of the pulmonary vessels have shown that this vascular bed is significantly stiffer than its systemic counterpart,[34, 35] and only small increments in blood volume can be accepted by the large pulmonary vessels.[36-39] It has subsequently been demonstrated that a major mechanism to accommodate increased blood volume is the recruitment of previously unperfused vessels.[34, 40] Morphological evidence suggests that both recruitment and distention occur with an increase in pulmonary blood flow and that the transmural pressures to which the vessel is subjected are what determines which one predominates.[41] In superior portions of the lung where the vessels are collapsed or where alveolar pressure is greater than pulmonary venous pressure, recruitment appears to be the major mechanism. Distention is more important in dependent portions of the lung in which pulmonary venous pressure is greater than alveolar pressure (see below)[29] (Fig. 18–5, p. 548).

PRESSURE-FLOW RELATIONSHIPS. Evaluation of the pressure-flow relationships of the pulmonary circulation in normal humans at any given lung volume demonstrates a hyperbolic configuration in which large changes in pulmonary blood flow are associated with small elevations in pulmonary artery pressure (Fig. 48–3*A*). The net result is

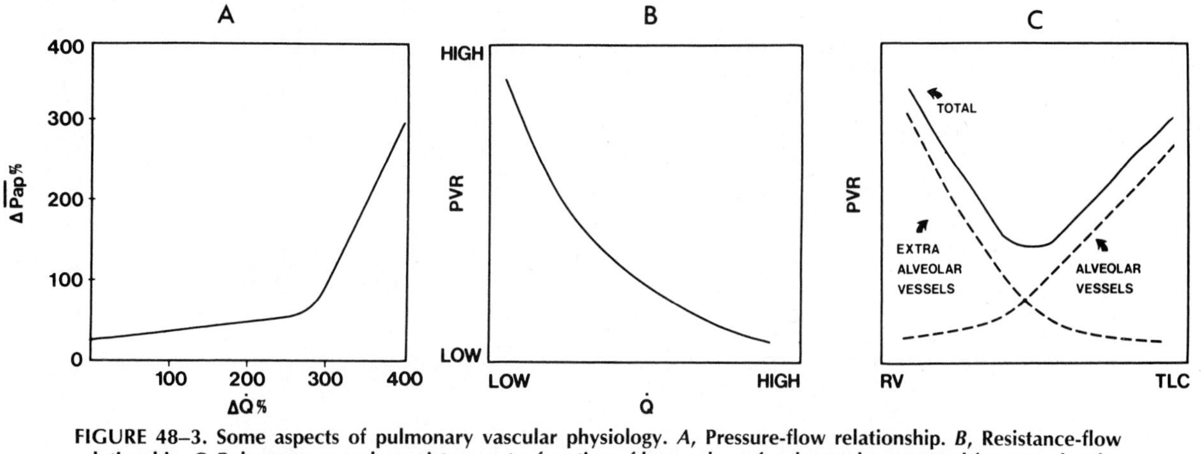

FIGURE 48–3. Some aspects of pulmonary vascular physiology. *A*, Pressure-flow relationship. *B*, Resistance-flow relationship. *C*, Pulmonary vascular resistance as a function of lung volume for the total system and for extraalveolar and alveolar vessels. △PAP = per cent change of mean pulmonary artery pressure from control; △Q = per cent change in cardiac output; 100 = normal cardiac output; RV = residual volume; TLC = total lung capacity.

that as flow increases, pulmonary vascular resistance decreases (Fig. 48–3*B*).[31] Consequently, irrespective of whether distention or recruitment occurs, both mechanisms subserve the necessity of maintaining a low pressure circuit during situations of increased blood flow.

A U-shaped curve describes pulmonary vascular resistance as a function of lung volume (Fig. 48–3*C*).[38] At the extremes of lung volume of full inflation and deflation, vascular resistance is high, and it reaches its nadir at about the resting end-expiratory position (i.e., at functional residual capacity). These findings can be explained by considering the geometry assumed by the alveolar and intrapulmonic but extraalveolar vessels in response to the transmural pressures to which they are exposed.

Because the pulmonary vessels are within the substance of the lung, their dimensions reflect the forces exerted upon them by the pulmonary parenchyma. At low lung volumes, the extraalveolar vessels tend to collapse because radial traction no longer supports them. Simultaneously, the alveolar vessels are pulled open by the increased recoil forces generated by the tendency of the alveoli to become smaller. As the lung is inflated to volumes above functional residual capacity, the larger vessels tend to be pulled open, but there is now a progressive increase in the resistance of the small vessels as they are squeezed and lengthened by enlarging alveoli. In addition to this deformation, alterations in alveolar pressure can also dynamically influence the lumina of small vessels. When alveolar pressure is positive, as it is during expiration or with the Valsalva maneuver, vessels are compressed. Alternatively, with negative pressure, as with inspiration or the Mueller maneuver, small vessels are subjected to a proportional distending pressure. It is therefore apparent that alveolar pressure can play a critical role in determining the distribution of pulmonary blood flow and, accordingly, gas exchange.

DETERMINANTS OF PULMONARY GAS EXCHANGE

DISTRIBUTION OF PULMONARY BLOOD FLOW. In the normal human in the upright position, blood flow per unit volume of lung steadily increases from the apex to the base, with flow at the apex being virtually nil.[42, 43] This distribution is affected by changes of posture and by exercise. When a subject is in the supine position, apical blood flow increases but the basal flow remains virtually unchanged, with the result that the distribution from apex to base becomes almost uniform. In this posture, however, flow in the posterior or dependent regions exceeds that in the anterior parts. During mild exercise in the upright position, flow to both the upper and the lower zones increases but more to the upper, so that flow becomes more evenly distributed.

West,[42, 43] and Permutt and Riley[44] have independently demonstrated that the pressure-flow relationships through the lung can be analogous to those of a "waterfall" or Starling resistor. The basic point of these studies is that the effective pressure drop in the pulmonary vasculature is not always the difference between inflow (pulmonary artery) and outflow (left atrial) pressures but often is between the inflow pressure and the closing pressure of small vessels downstream.

In normal human lungs pulmonary arterial and venous pressures both increase from superior to dependent regions because of hydrostatic effects resulting from gravity acting on the blood.[42, 43] However, alveolar pressures remain essentially constant throughout the lung. Alveolar pressure exceeds venous pressure at a more dependent portion of the lung than does arterial pressure. This results in distribution of blood flow to three major areas (Fig. 18–5, p. 548). In the most superior area (zone I) no flow occurs because alveolar pressure exceeds pulmonary arterial pressure. Presumably, this is because thin-walled collapsible vessels are directly exposed to alveolar pressure. In humans, the pulmonary artery pressure is sufficiently high to bring blood to the apex of the lung so that no zone I is present under normal conditions. It can develop, however, if pulmonary artery pressure falls or if alveolar pressure is elevated, as it is in obstructive airway disease. In the middle zone (zone II), arterial pressure exceeds alveolar pressure, but the latter is greater than venous pressure. Here, flow through the capillaries is proportional to the difference between arterial and alveolar pressure. In the lowest zone, zone III, venous pressure exceeds alveolar pressure, the vessels are held open, and flow is determined in the usual way by the arterial-venous pressure difference. A small zone of reduced flow at the very base of the lung has also been observed and attributed to a possible increase in the interstitial pressure as a consequence of the reduced expansion of the lung parenchyma in the lower zone. This has, therefore, been called zone IV. There is still some uncertainty about the cause of the reduced flow in this area, but the concept of reduction in flow caused by an increased interstitial pressure is almost certainly important in mitral stenosis and may be responsible for the reduction in basilar blood flow observed in that condition.

Distribution of Ventilation

The distribution of ventilation, like that of perfusion, decreases from base to apex in the normal lung, but the rate of change is only about one-third that seen with blood flow.[42] Here, too, gravity plays a role, and changes in posture have an influence. Thus, when normal subjects lie supine, the difference in ventilation between the anatomical upper and lower zones is abolished,[42] and in the inverted lung, the apex ventilates better than the base, so the normal pattern is reversed.

Evaluation of the relative rates of expansion of the upper and lower zones in the upright position reveals different patterns of distribution, depending upon the lung volume from which inspiration is initiated.[45] As a consequence of the effect of gravity and the shape of the pressure-volume curve of the lung, when a normal subject takes a breath from functional residual capacity (FRC), ventilation is preferentially distributed to the dependent lung zones. Since blood flow in the resting state is also preferentially distributed to this area, this matching of ventilation to perfusion in different body positions insures efficient gas exchange under a variety of physiological conditions.

If breathing takes place at lung volumes lower than FRC, the distribution of ventilation is quite different. Because of closure of dependent airways, the most inferior portions of the lung do not ventilate, and all of the inspired gas goes preferentially to the upper zones. The phenomenon of airway closure at low lung volumes has major physiological significance and can produce substantial alterations in ventilation-perfusion relationships and arterial hypoxia.[46, 47]

Ventilation-Perfusion Ratios

Ventilation-perfusion (V_A/Q) ratios are important because they are the determinants of the gas exchange that occurs in any part of the lung, and thereby they affect the overall efficiency of the lungs in taking up oxygen and eliminating carbon dioxide.[42] The partial pressure of oxygen in the alveolar gas (and therefore in the end-capillary blood) is set by a balance between the rate of removal by the blood and its rate of replenishment by ventilation. If ventilation is gradually reduced and perfusion maintained to an alveolus, oxygen tension falls and carbon dioxide tension rises. The limit is reached when the unit is not ventilated at all, and the pulmonary venous oxygen and carbon dioxide will be those of mixed venous blood. This is a $\dot{V}_A/\dot{Q}$ relationship of zero and corresponds to the situation in which there is a true anatomical pulmonary arteriovenous shunt, e.g., a pulmonary arteriovenous fistula or a functional one such as produced by atelectasis. By contrast, if perfusion to a normally ventilating alveolus is gradually reduced, the oxygen tension in the venous blood draining this alveolus rises and the partial pressure of carbon dioxide falls. The limit now occurs when the unit is unperfused. This is a $\dot{V}_A/\dot{Q}$ of infinity and is seen in situations in which blood supply is disrupted, such as by pulmonary emboli or other disease in which occlusion of the pulmonary arterial circulation occurs. Between these two extreme examples, a wide range of $\dot{V}_A/\dot{Q}$ abnormalities is possible.

The alveoli hypoventilated in relation to their perfusion (i.e., low $\dot{V}_A/\dot{Q}$ ratio) cause hypoxemia, and their presence has the same effect as mixing venous and arterial blood. This is termed venous admixture or "wasted blood" and is evaluated clinically by determining the oxygen tension difference between ideal alveolar gas and arterial blood. Normally, venous admixture or "shunt effect" is only about 2 to 3 per cent of the cardiac output, but in severe disease it may rise to 30 per cent or more. The normal alveolar arterial difference of oxygen (A-aDO_2) is 20 mm Hg or less.[48, 49]

The alveoli which are hyperventilated in relation to their perfusion (i.e., high $\dot{V}_A/\dot{Q}$ ratio) mainly affect CO_2 elimination. They behave as if part of the inspired gas bypassed the alveoli, so this effect has been called "wasted ventilation" or an increase in "physiological dead space." It is evaluated by comparing mixed expired and arterial CO_2, using the Bohr equation. Normally the physiological dead space is less than 30 per cent of the tidal volume.[49, 50] In severe lung disease it can rise to 50 per cent or more. Every pathological condition that directly affects the pulmonary parenchyma or its vascular bed results in mismatched ventilation and blood flow. Consequently, this abnormality is by far the most common cause of arterial hypoxemia in disease states. Both venous admixture and physiological dead space are typically increased in chronic obstructive and infiltrative lung diseases. In pulmonary thromboembolism an increase in dead space predominates.

In many pulmonary parenchymal diseases, blood supply to poorly ventilating areas tends to be reduced, so that the $\dot{V}_A/\dot{Q}$ ratios are not as low as they would otherwise be. One reason for this is that the local pathological process tends to disturb both ventilation and perfusion by its mechanical effects. Another is local hypoxic vasoconstriction, which shunts blood away from the involved alveoli.[51-53] In the case of thromboembolic phenomena, the regional decreases in CO_2 concentration that occur cause local increases in the resistance of small airways and thus reduce ventilation to the affected region.

Other Causes of Abnormal Arterial Blood Gases

In addition to $\dot{V}_A/\dot{Q}$ inequalities, there are four other causes of arterial hypoxemia: (1) anatomical right-to-left intracardiac or intrapulmonary shunts usually caused by congenital heart disease (Chaps. 30 and 31); (2) reductions in the inspired concentration of oxygen; (3) defects in the diffusion of oxygen from the alveolus to the blood; and (4) alveolar hypoventilation.

Although it was originally thought that measurements of the *diffusing capacity* of the lung for oxygen demonstrated a specific impairment in molecular oxygen transfer across a thickened membrane (i.e., alveolar capillary block), it is now appreciated that single breath tests of diffusing capacity that employ carbon monoxide are profoundly influenced by three variables: (1) the surface area available for diffusion, (2) the volume of blood within the capillaries, and (3) the rate of combination of CO and hemoglobin.[54] Other factors, such as the molecular path for diffusion and the stratified heterogeneity of gas mixtures, also play a role.[55] In addition to the above, steady-state methods are also influenced by regional $\dot{V}_A/\dot{Q}$ relationships.[54] Thus, these techniques do not measure the thickness of the alveolar-capillary membrane, and in any disease associated with a loss of elastic recoil (loss of surface area through disruption of alveolar walls), marked $\dot{V}_A/\dot{Q}$ heterogeneities or loss of capillary bed will be associated with a reduced "diffusing capacity." Even so, the effect that this has on gas exchange is, at most, small.

ALVEOLAR HYPOVENTILATION. This is a condition in which insufficient gas exchange occurs to meet metabolic demands. It can result from many causes: severe $\dot{V}_A/\dot{Q}$ inequalities; reduced drive from the respiratory center so that the patient "will not breathe"; failure of the patient's respiratory system to act on the information sent from the central nervous system because of severe intrinsic pulmonary disease; or abnormalities of the neuromuscular apparatus of the chest wall or diaphragm.[56] In the latter cases the patient "cannot breathe." Regardless of cause, the cardinal features of the arterial blood are hypoxemia and hypercapnia, and both must be present to establish the diagnosis. The various diseases associated with alveolar hypoventilation and the mechanisms by which it comes about in each are discussed as examples of chronic cor pulmonale later in this chapter.

EFFECTS OF ALVEOLAR GAS TENSIONS ON THE PULMONARY CIRCULATION

HYPOXIA. The most potent stimulus for the development of pulmonary vasoconstriction is alveolar hypoxia.[29, 51, 52, 57] Although acute vasoconstriction appears when the alveolar pO_2 is 60 mm Hg or lower, this response is found only in approximately two-thirds of normal subjects.[58] It is speculated that the subjects who respond to hypoxemia with pulmonary vasoconstriction are those who would be prone to develop chronic cor pulmonale if they developed a disease that interfered with effective alveolar ventilation.[59] The pulmonary constrictor response to hypoxia appears to be locally mediated since it can be elicited both in denervated lungs and isolated perfused lungs (Fig. 26–2, p. 795).

ACIDOSIS. This has also been shown to produce significant increases in pulmonary vascular resistance as well as to act synergistically with hypoxia.[60] In contrast, an increase in arterial pCO_2 seems to exert no direct effect. Instead it seems to operate by way of the increase in hydrogen ion concentration that it induces. The interaction of hypoxia and acidemia is clinically important; these two conditions frequently coexist, and their interplay follows a predictable pattern (Fig. 48–4). At minor degrees of oxygen unsaturation, pulmonary artery pressure is relatively insensitive to hydrogen ion concentration, whereas it is extremely sensitive at high levels of unsaturation. On the other hand, when the pH is high, the pressor effect of hypoxia is blunted.

Although the localization of the pulmonary vascular pressor response within the lung is still controversial, most studies indicate that it occurs in partially muscular arteries less than 200 μm in diameter.[28, 51, 53, 61] The mechanism by which hypoxia causes pulmonary arterial smooth muscle to constrict is unclear.

However, the available information points toward two major alternatives: an indirect effect by which hypoxia might cause endothelial cells to generate various eicosanoids, or other cells in the pulmonary parenchyma to release vasoactive substances (e.g., histamine from mast cells) or a direct effect of hypoxia on pulmonary arterial smooth muscle. Other influences may enhance hypoxic pulmonary vasoconstriction. For example, it is possible that extrapulmonic reflexes or the adrenergic neurotransmitter norepinephrine may augment the pressor response.

PULMONARY HYPERTENSION. The precise mechanism by which the resting tone of the pulmonary circulation is controlled is unknown. The smooth muscle and connective tissue elements in the walls of the vessels certainly contribute. However, the relative roles of other potential controlling factors such as the neuropeptides of the non-

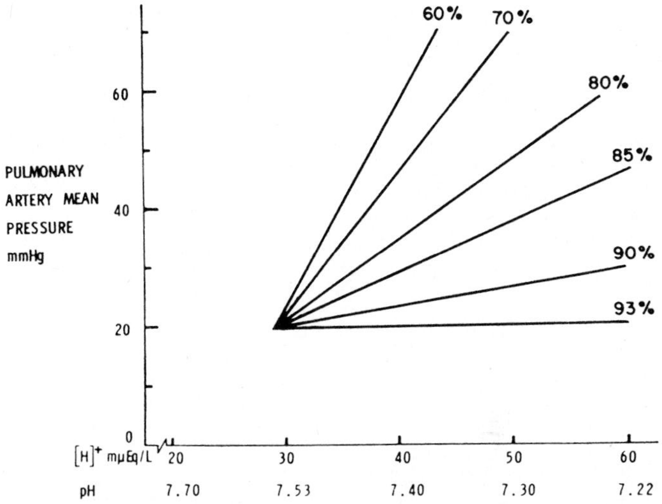

FIGURE 48–4. Relationship of arterial oxygen saturation and hydrogen ion concentration to pulmonary artery pressure. (From Enson, Y., et al.: The influence of hydrogen ion concentration and hypoxia on the pulmonary circulation. J. Clin. Invest. *43*:1146, 1964.)

adrenergic-noncholinergic nervous system, or locally formed or circulating mediators such as the eicosanoids (prostacyclin, thromboxane, leukotrienes), catecholamines (epinephrine, norepinephrine), and autacoids (histamine, bradykinin), have yet to be explored.[62]

Vasoconstriction produces an acute rise in pressure, and it is now known that continuing constriction with pulmonary hypertension of even a few days' duration is associated with structural changes in the vessels.[28] Luminal narrowing is brought about by an increase in the thickness of the medial coat, endothelial swelling, and hypertrophy, and the appearance of muscle at more peripheral levels than normal. With continued insult a reduction in cross-sectional area of the vascular bed develops in association with an increase in right ventricular weight. Although these structural and functional changes occur with all forms of pulmonary hypertension, different time sequences of development or ultrastructural patterns may be seen with different disease processes.

CHRONIC COR PULMONALE

INCIDENCE

Because of its association with chronic lung disease, chronic cor pulmonale is believed to be a common type of heart disease.[1, 5, 7, 63] The U.S. public health service estimates that chronic lung disease affects 47 million people in the United States alone and accounts for over 80,000 deaths every year.[64] Although precise figures on the prevalence of cor pulmonale are lacking, it is possible to appreciate the potential magnitude of the problem by recognizing that chronic bronchitis and emphysema are its most common causes and that these two diseases result in approximately 30,000 deaths per year.[64a] In one study in England, cor pulmonale was responsible for 30 to 40 per cent of all clinical cases of heart failure, of a total of 487 cases of cardiac disease,[65] and in the United States 10 to 30 per cent of hospital admissions for congestive heart failure are due to cor pulmonale.[66] Most patients are 45 years of age or older, and men are affected more frequently than women.

The presence of pulmonary hypertension and chronic respiratory disease contributes significantly to mortality. The available data suggest that the severity of pulmonary hypertension correlates more closely with survival than any other variable studied[67-69] (Fig. 48–5). Patients with severe airway obstruction ($FEV_1 < 1.0$ liters) without pulmonary hypertension have much greater longevity than those without this finding. In the study of Burrows and colleagues,[67] no patient with a pulmonary vascular resistance greater than 550 dynes-sec-cm^{-5} survived 3 years. Similarly, in Bishop's study[68] mortality rates increased progressively as pulmonary pressures rose. In the latter investigation, less than 10 per cent of patients with a mean pulmonary artery pressure of 45 mm Hg or more survived 5 years. Finally, Traver et al.[69] in a study on patients with obstructive lung disease found a 50 per cent mortality rate of 7 years in patients with cor pulmonale and 13.5 years in those without cor pulmonale.

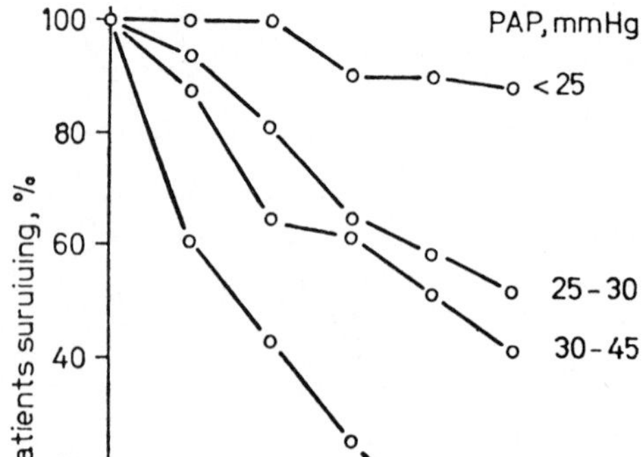

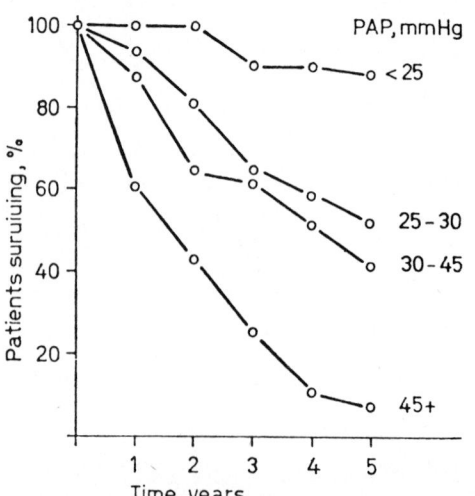

FIGURE 48–5. Correlation between survival and mean pulmonary arterial pressure in patients with chronic bronchitis. (From Bishop, J. M.: Hypoxia and pulmonary hypertension in chronic bronchitis. Prog. Resp. Res. 9:10, 1975.)

ETIOLOGY

There are many causes of cor pulmonale. Any disease that affects ventilatory mechanics, gas exchange, or the vascular bed either directly, through intrapulmonic events, or indirectly, via its effect on ventilatory control or the neuromuscular apparatus of respiration, may cause cor pulmonale. Since this is true of essentially all primary pulmonary disorders, the development of cor pulmonale simply indicates that the primary disease was sufficiently advanced to raise pulmonary artery pressure, cause right ventricular hypertrophy, and impair right ventricular function. Fortunately, most disorders affect too small a segment of the lungs or are too circumscribed in their effects on gas exchange to initiate the chain of events that leads to right ventricular hypertrophy and failure. A list of the various disease categories commonly associated with cor pulmonale, along with some specific examples of each process, is presented in Table 48–1.

PATHOPHYSIOLOGY

FACTORS CONTRIBUTING TO THE DEVELOPMENT OF PULMONARY HYPERTENSION (Fig. 48–6). The most important pathogenetic mechanisms that produce abnormalities in right ventricular structure and function are pulmonary hypertension and abnormal concentrations of blood gases that directly modify myocardial performance.[70] As already noted, the normal pulmonary circulation is a low-resistance system with considerable reserve; therefore, substantial reductions in the size of the effective vascular bed must occur before pulmonary hypertension develops and becomes sustained. The pathogenetic sequence is unknown, and probably a number of mechanisms interact to produce pulmonary hypertension. Any theory regarding the development of cor pulmonale must take into account the effects of the anatomical loss of vessels, i.e., anatomical restriction of the pulmonary vascular bed, pulmonary arteriolar constriction, increased blood viscosity, and increased blood flow, although their relative roles have not been clearly defined.[63]

It has long been thought that the essential pathology in

TABLE 48–1 ETIOLOGIES OF PULMONARY HEART DISEASE

1. Diseases affecting air passages of the lung and alveoli
   a. Chronic obstructive pulmonary diseases
   b. Cystic fibrosis
   c. Congenital developmental defects
   d. Infiltrative or granulomatous diseases
      (1) Idiopathic pulmonary fibrosis
      (2) Sarcoidosis
      (3) Pneumoconiosis
      (4) Scleroderma
      (5) Mixed connective tissue disease
      (6) Systemic lupus erythematosus
      (7) Rheumatoid arthritis
      (8) Polymyositis
      (9) Eosinophilic granuloma
      (10) Malignant infiltration
      (11) Radiation
   e. Upper airways obstruction
   f. Pulmonary resection
   g. High-altitude disease
2. Diseases affecting thoracic cage movement
   a. Kyphoscoliosis
   b. Thoracoplasty
   c. Pleural fibrosis
   d. Neuromuscular weakness
   e. Sleep apnea syndromes
   f. Idiopathic hypoventilation
3. Diseases affecting the pulmonary vasculature
   a. Primary diseases of the arterial wall
      (1) Primary pulmonary hypertension
      (2) Granulomatous pulmonary arteritis
      (3) Toxin-induced pulmonary hypertension
         a) Aminorex fumarate
         b) Intravenous drug abuse
      (4) Chronic liver disease
      (5) Peripheral pulmonic stenosis
   b. Thrombotic disorders
      (1) Sickle cell diseases
      (2) Pulmonary microthrombi
   c. Embolic disorders
      (1) Thromboembolism
      (2) Tumor embolism
      (3) Other embolism (amniotic fluid, air)
      (4) Schistosomiasis and other parasites
4. Pressures on pulmonary arteries by mediastinal tumors, aneurysms, granulomata, or fibrosis

From Rubin, L. J.: Introduction. Pulmonary Heart Disease. Boston, Martinus Nijhoff, 1984, p. 1.

chronic cor pulmonale is a *physical loss of vessels*, leading to a restricted vascular bed. Although it is certainly true that this mechanism contributes to the pulmonary hypertension observed in vascular occlusion resulting from multiple pulmonary emboli, aplasia, or extensive excision of lung tissue,[21, 57] other factors also must be considered since emphysema, a disease in which alveolar vessels are widely destroyed, is typically associated with resting pulmonary hypertension and cor pulmonale only late in its course.[72] Thus, a decrease in the anatomical extent of the pulmonary vascular bed does not play a major role in the development of pulmonary hypertension unless the reduction is extreme. However, other processes (i.e., a constricted vascular bed) can *decrease the effective cross-sectional area without a loss of vessels*. The effective area can be reduced by arteriolar constriction secondary to alveolar hypoxemia and acidosis[57, 59, 60, 62] and by the various pathological changes responsible for pulmonary hypertension[28, 73-75] (Chap. 26).

The potent vasoconstricting influence resulting from alveolar hypoxia is shared by the disease entities responsible for chronic cor pulmonale and listed in Table 48–1. The resulting pulmonary hypertension, when persistent, can make the vessels rigid and reduce their lumina by producing intimal thickening, inflammatory changes, and medial hypertrophy.[28]

Intimal thickening of the pulmonary arterioles, regardless of its mechanism, often has a patchy distribution and is a frequent postmortem finding in patients beyond the age of 40 years who were free of pulmonary hypertension during life.[76] Therefore, the extent must be great to account for the perpetuation or worsening of pulmonary hypertension. Intimal thickening can be both a cause and a result of pulmonary hypertension. The reversibility of this process is unknown, but the fibrotic component is presumably permanent. Inflammatory changes vary from cellular infiltrates to fibrinoid necrosis and fibrosis. Most often these types of alterations are found in diffuse inflammatory lung lesions or with systemic illness with vasculitis. However, they have been noted secondary to pulmonary hypertension of any cause.[74, 76] Hypertrophy and hyperplasia of the smooth muscle in the media of the arterioles are regular findings in longstanding pulmonary hypertension and have been found to be reversible to some extent.[28, 73-75]

Some insight into the time course of the pathological changes in the pulmonary circulation and their effects can be gained from studies in experimental animals. The available data indicate that chronic pulmonary hypertension can be produced in many species with either normobaric or hypobaric hypoxia. In the rat, for example, resting pulmonary vascular pressures begin to rise within 3 days of exposure to hypoxia, and they double by 10 days. Striking changes take place in the vessels over this interval. According to Meyrick and Reid,[28] the timing and severity of the increase in pressure correlates most closely with a reduction in cross sectional area of the precapillary vessels in the microcirculation. New muscle appears in smaller and more peripheral arteries than normal, and fewer of them fill with barium sulfate, indicating a reduction in effective luminal size. In the large muscular arteries, all

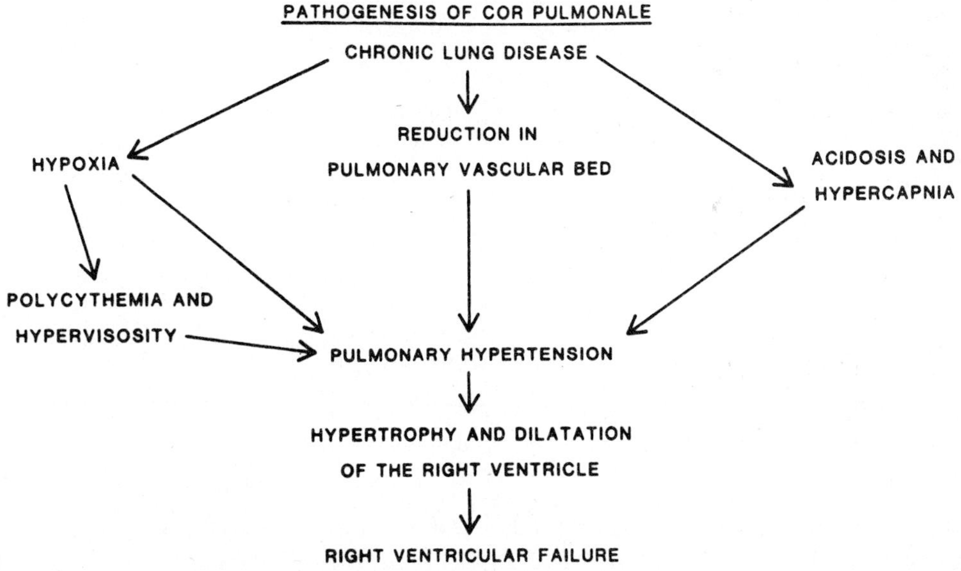

FIGURE 48–6. Pathogenesis of cor pulmonale. (From Summer, W. R.: Acute cor pulmonale. In Rubin, L. J. [ed.]: Pulmonary Heart Disease. Boston, Martinus Nijhoff, 1984, p. 285.)

three coats of the wall hypertrophy, resulting in an increase in medial thickness. The changes in the larger vessels plateau before those in the periphery are complete.

Once the vascular remodeling has occurred, removal of the stimulus results in incomplete recovery, and although right ventricular weight and pulmonary artery pressures fall, they do not reach baseline values. The reasons for this are that the structural changes in the vessels do not resolve completely. Even 2 months after returning to a normoxic environment, vascular remodeling is incomplete and remnants of the acute changes in both large and small vessels remain.

The *structural* changes induced by hypoxia are believed to account for half of the rise in pulmonary artery pressure that persists when the patient breathes room air. These changes also set the stage for further reactivity. Acute hypoxia superimposed on a vascular bed in which structural remodeling has occurred is known to produce a greater hemodynamic effect than that seen in a normal circulation.[28]

An *increase in the viscosity of blood* has been shown experimentally to raise pulmonary vascular resistance.[77] Viscosity is generally elevated as a result of chronic hypoxemia stimulating red cell production through erythropoietin release. It represents an adaptation that tends to restore arterial oxygen delivery. However, the compensatory mechanism is useful only up to a point, because at very high levels of hematocrit, the high viscosity of the blood can impair capillary flow.[78] With high hematocrits the shear rates are low, and as the blood flow slows in the capillaries, viscosity increases even further, requiring a greater driving pressure. In experimental animals polycythemia contributes significantly to the rise in pulmonary resistance during both acute hypoxia and recovery.[28] These considerations have served as the rationale for phlebotomy in selected patients with cor pulmonale.

The final traditional factor that has been proposed as contributing to pulmonary hypertension is an increase *in pulmonary blood flow.* Extensive intimal hypertrophy and pathological medial necrosis have been created in the pulmonary circulation of animals by anastomosing a pulmonary artery either to the aorta or to one of its main branches.[79] Although studies demonstrate that collateral channels develop between the bronchial and pulmonary vascular beds in chronic obstructive pulmonary disease,[80, 81] except in the case of bronchiectasis these channels are seldom large enough to contribute importantly to pulmonary hypertension.[81] As discussed below, increased cardiac output can raise pulmonary pressures in patients with both constricted and restricted vascular beds.

One area in which high pulmonary blood flow appears to play an important role in the development of elevated pulmonary artery pressure and resistance is in congenital heart diseases associated with left-to-right shunts[82] (p. 802). Once established, the anatomical changes in the pulmonary vascular bed may not be completely reversible, even when pulmonary blood flow is restored to normal surgically. Morphological examination of the lungs of patients with congenital cardiac diseases and high pulmonary flow shows a gradation of pathological changes that reflects the duration and severity of the condition[82, 83] (p. 803).

It is not clear how the above-described pathogenetic mechanisms interrelate in the development of pulmonary hypertension. It is easy to appreciate that the loss of vessels and diffuse constriction of the arterioles with its attendant pathological changes in their walls and lumina can combine to cause a reduction of the pulmonary vascular bed, which in turn causes an increase in pulmonary vascular resistance. However, these changes need not be manifested at rest as an elevated pulmonary artery pressure. As shown in Figure 48–3, the normal pulmonary vascular bed has the ability to accept large increases in flow without marked increases in pressure, probably through the recruitment of parallel vascular channels. In the case of a restricted vascular bed, this reserve is lost and the patients' physiological response is as though they were starting at the bend of the normal pressure-flow relationship (Fig. 48–7). The importance of hypoxia as a determinant of pulmonary artery pressure is demonstrated in Figure 48–8.

Under these circumstances pressure can rise dramatically with exercise or any other condition that causes pulmonary blood flow to increase (Fig. 48–9). With time

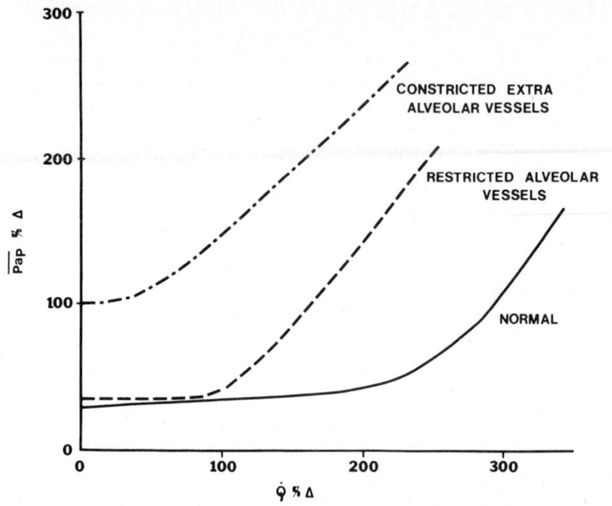

FIGURE 48–7. Pressure-flow relationship of normal, restricted, and constricted pulmonary vascular beds. The vertical axis indicates the percentage of change in mean pulmonary artery pressure (PAP % △), whereas the horizontal scale shows the percentage of change in cardiac output (Q̇ % △). In both instances 100% = normal, basal level.

and progression of the underlying disease as the secondary changes in the vessels develop, further raising pulmonary vascular resistance, pulmonary artery pressure becomes elevated, even at rest. The pressure-flow relationship (Fig. 48–3A) is shifted upward and to the left, as in a constricted bed, so that small increments in flow produce large in-

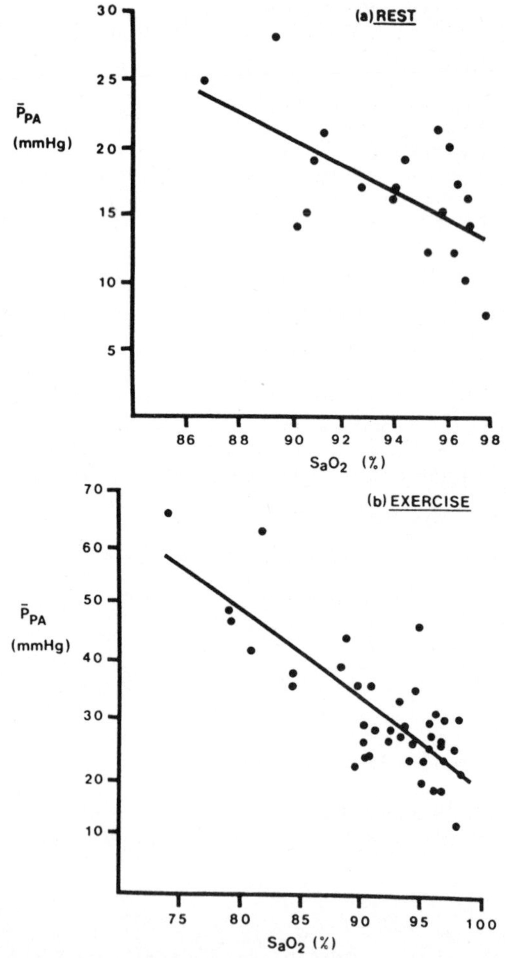

FIGURE 48–8. The correlation between arterial oxygen saturation (SaO_2) and pulmonary artery pressures ($\bar{P}_{pa}$) at rest and on exercise in patients with chronic obstructive lung disease. (From Stewart, R. I., et al.: Cardiac output during exercise in patients with COPD. Chest *89*:199, 1986.)

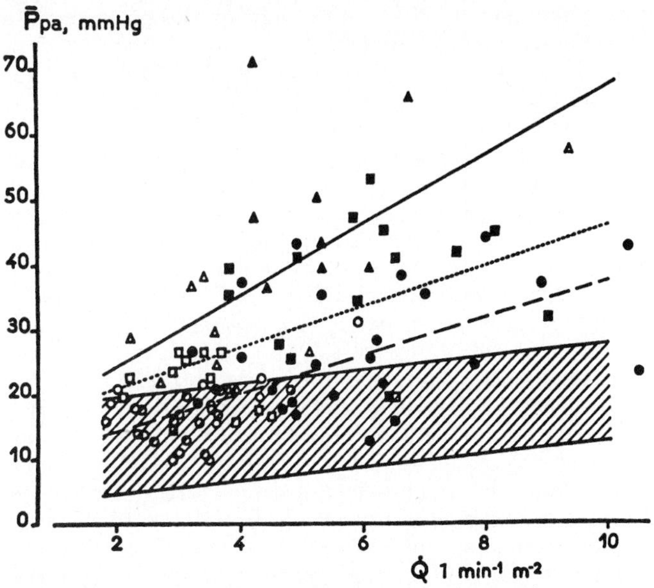

FIGURE 48–9. The relationship between cardiac index (Q̇) and mean pulmonary artery pressure ($\bar{P}_{pa}$) at rest (open symbols) and during exercise (closed symbols). Patients with chronic bronchitis are shown in circles. Patients with chronic bronchitis and a history of right heart failure are shown as squares. Patients with chronic bronchitis and clinical right heart failure are shown as triangles. Hatched area represents 95 per cent confidence interval of normal values. The increase in $\bar{P}_{pa}$ is larger at any given Q̇ as patients deteriorate and develop cor pulmonale. (From Fowler, N. O., Wescott, R. N., Scott, R. C., and Hess, E.: The cardiac output in chronic cor pulmonale. Circulation 6:888, 1952, by permission of the American Heart Association, Inc.)

creases in pressure over the entire range of cardiac outputs. It may be inferred that small increases in output are accompanied by large increases in right ventricular work. Increases in viscosity, collateral blood flow, hypoxemia, and acidemia worsen the situation by further increasing pulmonary artery pressure.

The data to support this general picture are derived from observations on the response to exercise of patients with chronic bronchitis (constricted vascular bed) and emphysema (restricted vascular bed).[67, 84, 85] In the former, pulmonary diffusing capacity *increases normally* with increases in cardiac output with exercise, and the work capacity of these patients is limited by the state of their pulmonary mechanics and resulting gas exchange. It appears that the ability to dilate extraalveolar vessels normally and recruit alveolar vessels is reasonably intact, although pulmonary artery pressure rises. In contrast, in patients with emphysema without resting pulmonary hypertension, diffusing capacity *does not increase normally* with exercise. The total oxygen uptake of these patients is limited by insufficient effective alveolar-capillary surface rather than by cardiac output of ventilation, and recruitment of alveolar vessels is severely curtailed.[84]

RIGHT VENTRICULAR DYNAMICS. The hemodynamic findings in cor pulmonale depend to some extent on the cause and duration of the underlying pathological process. Patients with relatively mild obstructive lung disease without severe hypoxemia generally have normal mean right atrial and right ventricular end-diastolic pressures, normal or low cardiac outputs, normal or slightly elevated pulmonary artery pressures, and slightly elevated pulmonary vascular resistances at rest.[18, 67, 86-88] Right ventricular ejection fractions, as determined by radionuclide angiography, tend to be normal.[89, 90] With exercise, pulmonary artery pressure rises further, right ventricular stroke work increases (Fig. 48–9), and right ventricular ejection fractions fall.[89, 90] Relating end-diastolic pressure to stroke work suggests that these patients function on an extension of the normal right ventricular function curve.[91] These findings need not be accompanied by clinical or electrocardiographic evidence of right ventricular hypertrophy,[87] although evidence of right ventricular enlargement may be seen on two-dimensional echocardiography. However, acute right ventricular failure can develop in these patients if respiratory failure, hypoxia, and further elevation of pulmonary artery pressure are precipitated by a pulmonary infection.

Progression of the airway obstruction tends to accentuate these findings. As the ventilatory impairment worsens, the hemodynamic alterations follow suit. At the stage when severe chronic hypoxemia develops, usually in association with chronic hypercapnia, there is moderate pulmonary hypertension at rest, which becomes more severe during exercise in association with abnormal right ventricular filling pressures and function[67-69, 89-92] (Figs. 48–9 and 48–10). Cardiac output tends to be normal or even slightly elevated at rest but increases little with exercise when the patient breathes room air; oxygen administration, however, may lower pulmonary artery pressure and raise the right ventricular ejection fraction.[92] Systolic pulmonary artery pressures can reach levels of 80 mm Hg, and these patients are likely to show the clinical and electrocardiographic changes usually ascribed to cor pulmonale. Failure of the right ventricle is associated with an expanded circulating blood volume. However, in contrast to left ventricular failure, the pulmonary blood volume/total volume ratio remains essentially normal (approximately 1 to 10) even though red cell mass may be considerably increased.[87] Both circulating plasma volume and lung water increase,[93, 94] and both have been shown to decrease as pulmonary artery pressure is lowered with therapy.

LEFT VENTRICULAR DYNAMICS. Abnormally elevated pulmonary venous pressures, with or without overt left

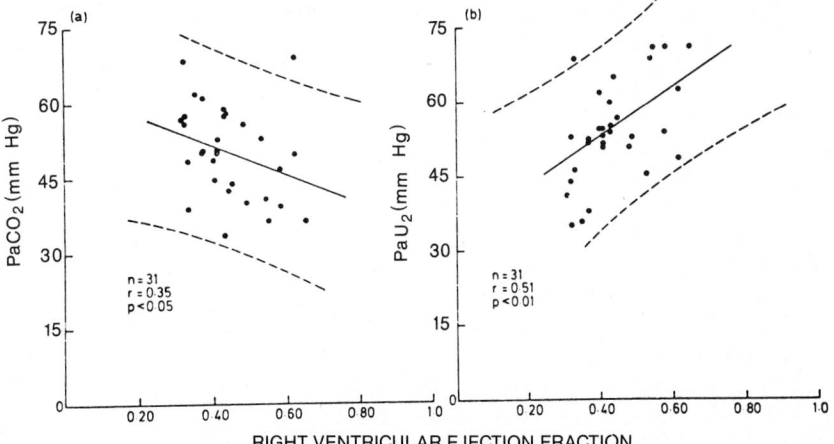

FIGURE 48–10. Relationship between arterial carbon dioxide (P_{CO_2}) (left panel) and arterial oxygen tension (P_{O_2}) (right panel) and right ventricular ejection fraction in patients with chronic bronchitis and emphysema. These data represent air breathing at rest. (From Flenley, D. C., and Muir, A. L.: Cardiovascular effects of oxygen therapy for pulmonary arterial hypertension. Clin. Chest Med. *4*:297, 1983.)

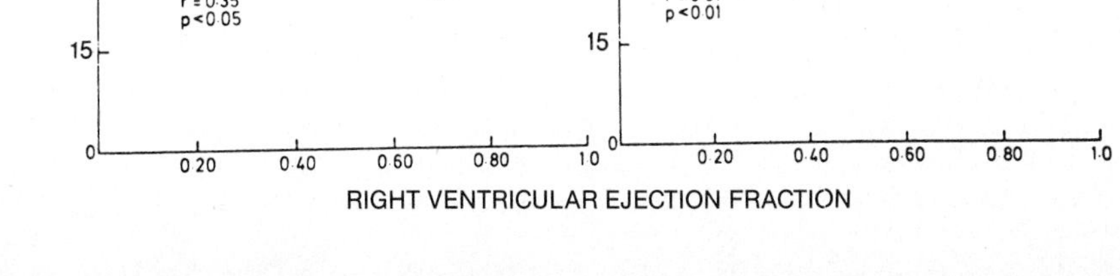

ventricular failure, invariably produce alterations in pulmonary mechanics and gas exchange, even in patients with normal lungs (Chapter 61). Consequently, left ventricular dysfunction could have deleterious effects in cor pulmonale. Controversy persists about whether the disease affecting the lungs and right ventricle in these patients produces left ventricular disease, or whether the latter results from independent causes. Evidence exists that many patients with cor pulmonale who are over the age of 65 are hypertensive and have reduced left ventricular compliance and/or have regional left ventricular wall motion disorders secondary to ischemic heart disease.

The view that disorders of the right ventricle may result in left ventricular disease has gained support from several sources. Animal experiments have shown that (1) right ventricular failure following banding of the pulmonary artery leads to similar morphological and biochemical changes in both cardiac chambers and to reduced contractility of the left ventricle,[95-97] (2) in both isolated hearts and intact animals alterations in right ventricular compliance or dimensions also change the mechanical properties of the left ventricle, perhaps acting in part through changes in the thickness or position of the interventricular septum (Fig. 61–10, p. 1880)[14, 98, 99] and (3) cattle at high altitude with severe pulmonary hypertension have increased left ventricular end-diastolic pressures.[100] Although these observations are provocative, their relevance to human disease is uncertain.

Autopsy studies have shown that left ventricular hypertrophy occurs in some patients with cor pulmonale,[101-103] and left ventricular dysfunction of varying degrees has been observed in vivo.[95, 103-105] In all of these investigations, none of the usual etiologies of left ventricular disease were apparent. Thus, it appears that the structure and function of the left ventricle can become abnormal in association with the pathogenetic mechanisms underlying cor pulmonale. However, this is probably a very uncommon occurrence and the weight of current evidence indicates that cor pulmonale usually does not seriously impair left ventricular performance.[67, 91, 102, 106-112] When abnormalities have been found, they could be explained either by a reduction in right ventricular stroke volume causing diminished left-sided filling or by independent disease processes such as coronary artery disease[95, 112] with experimental hypoxemia. However, given the heterogeneity of the population with cor pulmonale and the variance of its natural history, the controversy will undoubtedly continue.

CLINICAL MANIFESTATIONS

As with other aspects of cor pulmonale, the clinical, radiological, therapeutic, and prognostic features are strongly influenced by the underlying disease process responsible for the pulmonary hypertension.[111] Without doubt, the diseases that affect the pulmonary parenchyma, the intrathoracic airways, or both account for the vast majority of cases of cor pulmonale.

Chronic Obstructive Pulmonary Disease (COPD)[111a]

COPD, by far the most common form of pulmonary parenchymal disease responsible for chronic pulmonary hypertension, consists of chronic bronchitis, emphysema, and bronchial asthma. However, atopic asthma does *not* produce chronic cor pulmonale[72] and intrinsic, or nonatopic, asthma is often a variant of chronic bronchitis; in this discussion, COPD refers only to chronic bronchitis and emphysema exclusively.

In most patients with COPD, chronic bronchitis and emphysema coexist, but cor pulmonale is restricted to those with functionally significant airway disease with or without emphysema.[72] This admixture has given rise to a great deal of confusion in terminology in the literature, and until the matter was sorted out by Burrows and colleagues[113] and Mitchell and Filley,[114] the terms bronchitis and emphysema were frequently considered to be synonymous. Additional observations uncovered fundamental differences in the clinical, physiological, and pathological features of the two conditions and laid the groundwork for a better understanding of these diseases.

CHRONIC BRONCHITIS. It is possible to think of COPD as a continuum, with chronic bronchitis at one extreme and emphysema at the other and the majority of patients having features of both conditions. The distinctions between the two groups are presented in Table 48–2. In the chronic bronchitis variety ("blue bloater," "nonfighter"), chronic cough with sputum production, frequently recurring chest infection, secondary erythrocytosis, and repeated bouts of right heart failure are common. Physiologically, the patients have hypoxemia and hypercapnia at rest, normal diffusion capacity, and elevated residual volume, functional residual capacity, and airway resistance, with relatively normal values for total lung capacity and pulmonary compliance. Maximum flow rates and forced

TABLE 48–2 COMPARISON OF THE CLINICAL AND PHYSIOLOGICAL FEATURES OF EMPHYSEMA AND CHRONIC BRONCHITIS

	EMPHYSEMA	CHRONIC BRONCHITIS
SYNONYMS	Pink puffer Fighter	Blue bloater Nonfighter
SIGNS AND SYMPTOMS		
Cough and sputum	Scant	Marked
Dyspnea at rest	Marked	Usually absent
Recurrent chest infections	Unusual	Frequent
Habitus	Often thin, wasted	Often obese
Cyanosis	No	Yes
Edema	No	Yes
Increased AP diameter of thorax	Marked	Mild
Hyperresonance to percussion	Marked	Mild
Breath sounds	Absent to depressed	Rales and rhonchi
Chest x-ray	Hyperinflation; no cardiomegaly	No hyperinflation; cardiomegaly
Electrocardiogram	RVM uncommon	RVM common
PULMONARY GAS EXCHANGE		
Hematocrit	Normal	Elevated
P_aO_2	Slight reduction	Marked reduction
P_aCO_2	Low or normal	Elevated
Diffusing capacity	Markedly decreased	Normal or slightly reduced
PULMONARY MECHANICS		
Expiratory flow rates	Reduced	Reduced
Elastic recoil	Markedly reduced	Normal or slightly reduced
Lung volume	Marked hyperinflation	Mild hyperinflation
PULMONARY CIRCULATION		
Pulmonary hypertension at rest	None or mild	Marked
with exercise	Moderate	Marked
Right heart failure	Terminal	Repeated

expiratory volumes are abnormally depressed. The chest roentgenogram shows moderately hyperinflated lungs, increased bronchovascular markings, and sometimes cardiomegaly.

The basic abnormality is widespread but regionally unequal airway obstruction that results in mismatched $\dot{V}_A/\dot{Q}$ relationships. In regions of low $\dot{V}_A/\dot{Q}$ ratios, pulmonary arterial constriction on the basis of hypoxia, and/or acidosis occurs. With progression, alveolar hypoventilation develops, the vascular bed becomes constricted, and the pulmonary artery pressure at rest rises.

In the emphysematous type ("pink puffer," "fighter"), dyspnea is the dominant symptom, while cough and sputum production are considerably less prominent. Erythrocytosis is uncommon, and right heart failure tends to occur as a terminal event. In keeping with the hyperventilation, the alveolar-arterial gradient for oxygen is abnormally elevated, but arterial oxygen tension is usually normal or only slightly depressed; hypocapnia is common. Standard spirometric indices cannot differentiate this group from those with chronic bronchitis, since the degree of obstruction as measured by this technique may be similar. However, the pink puffer has abnormally low diffusing capacity, and greatly increased lung volumes and pulmonary compliance. Roentgenograms of the chest reveal marked pulmonary hyperinflation with flattened diaphragms, oligemia of the peripheral lung fields, and a small heart. With the onset of cor pulmonale, the prominence of the vascular markings increases, but right ventricular enlargement may be difficult to observe.

Although there is some airway disease in this condition, the primary pathological defect is widespread destruction of alveolar septa. As a result, the surface area for gas exchange is lost more or less in proportion to alveolar vessels, and arterial gas tensions can be reasonably well maintained for a period of time by increasing ventilation. However, the destruction of the parenchyma results in loss of lateral traction of small airways so that they narrow and collapse. Then the regional distribution of inspired air becomes more impaired, with resultant worsening of the abnormalities in $\dot{V}_A/\dot{Q}$ ratios. These patients initially have a restricted vascular bed, with normal or near-normal pulmonary artery pressures at rest. As their disease process worsens with the development of airway disease and further deterioration of gas exchange, secondary changes in the vasculature occur and resting pulmonary artery hypertension and cor pulmonale develop.

CLINICAL MANIFESTATIONS OF COR PULMONALE WITH HEART FAILURE. These include increasing dyspnea; paroxysmal cough, occasionally with syncope; and fluid retention with edema and sometimes ascites. The distended neck veins exhibit prominent *a* and *v* waves and do not collapse with inspiration. Central cyanosis is frequently present, and hypoxemia, as measured by arterial oxygen saturation, correlates with the pulmonary artery pressure[115] (Fig. 48–8). Right ventricular hypertrophy is indicated by a palpable parasternal or subxiphoid heave. On auscultation, an S3 gallop, accentuated by inspiration, and a loud pulmonic second sound are frequently present. A holosystolic murmur along the lower left parasternal edge, accentuated by inspiration, usually indicates tricuspid regurgitation; its presence can be confirmed by Doppler echocardiography.[116] These cardiac findings can be evanescent and can develop quickly when acute respiratory failure is superimposed on COPD. Radionuclide techniques have shown that right ventricular ejection fractions are correlated positively with arterial oxygen tension and inversely with arterial pCO_2[117] (Fig. 48–10). Examination of the lungs reveals diffuse inspiratory and expiratory rhonchi and wheezes, and the liver is enlarged and frequently pulsatile. If acute respiratory failure is present in addition, papilledema, confusion, a hyperkinetic circulation, and asterixis may also be present.

It is important to recognize that the hypoxemia of patients with COPD may be profoundly worsened during sleep.[118] This phenomenon may cause a further rise in pulmonary artery pressure and nocturnal cardiac arrhythmias.[119, 120] The possible pathogenetic role of these phenomena in the development of cor pulmonale is discussed below.

Treatment

The management of cor pulmonale in COPD is to relieve pulmonary hypertension by improving gas exchange.[120, 121] This is accomplished by reducing bronchial smooth muscle constriction, promoting drainage of retained secretions, treating respiratory tract infections, and providing supplemental oxygen. The first two goals can be achieved simultaneously with the use of bronchodilators. In addition to relieving smooth muscle spasm, the sympathomimetics also increase mucociliary transport.[122] The net effect of these measures is to reduce airway obstruction and improve the regional distribution of inspired air and, in that manner, $\dot{V}_A/\dot{Q}$ relationships. Methylxanthines may provide benefits above and beyond the usual bronchodilatation, for this class of compounds has been reported to produce favorable hemodynamic effects as well. In one study the intravenous administration of aminophylline in patients with cor pulmonale was shown to reduce mean pulmonary artery and right and left ventricular end-diastolic pressures significantly without inducing a change in the cardiac index,[123] and in another, right and left ventricular ejection fractions were increased.[124]

The administration of supplemental oxygen in a controlled fashion represents a major advance in the treatment of cor pulmonale. In acute respiratory failure, supplemental oxygen results in prompt and often dramatic improvement in pulmonary hemodynamics.[67] In patients with progressive right ventricular hypertrophy or recurrent heart failure from cor pulmonale associated with severe hypoxemia ($PaO_2 < 50$ mm Hg) and severe pulmonary hypertension, marked improvement has been found when oxygen was administered for 12 to 15 hours per day.[125, 126] Two major controlled studies of different aspects of long-term oxygen therapy in patients with COPD have been carried out. The U.S. (NIH-sponsored) Nocturnal Oxygen Therapy Trial[127] sought to determine if oxygen given for 19 hours a day improved survival over that observed with predominant nocturnal therapy (12 hr/day). The English (MRC) trial, on the other hand, sought to discover whether oxygen administration for 15 to 24 hours of the day had a positive effect on survival as compared with no oxygen.[128] The composite data are contained in Figure 48–11. Survival was the poorest in those who did not receive supplemental oxygen and the best in those who received it for the longest portion of the day. The criteria most commonly used to initiate chronic oxygen therapy are an arterial oxygen tension of 55 mm Hg or less, hematocrit 55 per cent or more, P pulmonale on ECG, and systemic edema. The inspired oxygen concentration is adjusted to produce a pO_2 of 60 mm Hg or greater. If chronic oxygen therapy is contemplated, it is *mandatory* to demonstrate that the supplemental oxygen does not result in worsening of alveolar hypoventilation with progressive hypercapnia.

Another means of reducing pulmonary artery pressure that is gaining widespread use is afterload reduction with vasodilators. This approach assumes that the right ventricular failure results from increased afterload and that a

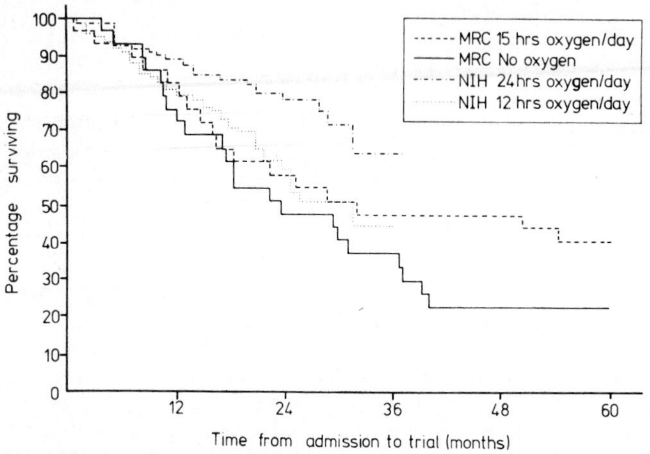

FIGURE 48–11. Survival curves in the MRC (British) and NIH (U.S.) long-term oxygen therapy trials in patients with severe hypoxemia and cor pulmonale. (From Flenley, D. C., and Muir, A. L.: Cardiovascular effects of oxygen therapy for pulmonary arterial hypertension. Clin. Chest Med. *4*:297, 1983.)

significant feature of the latter is related to active vasoconstriction.[129] A beneficial effect is defined as a reduction of 20 per cent or more in pulmonary vascular resistance in association with an unchanging or increased cardiac output and a decreased or unchanged pulmonary artery pressure.[129]

A number of drugs have been tried with varying degrees of effectiveness: isoproterenol,[130] phentolamine, [131] diazoxide,[132] prazosin,[133] hydralazine,[134, 135] and the calcium antagonists diltiazem and nifedipine.[136-138] These have all been reported to improve pulmonary vascular hemodynamics. Hydralazine (Fig. 48–12) and nifedipine appear to be particularly beneficial and have been found to reduce pulmonary vascular resistance and increase cardiac output in patients with pulmonary hypertension from various causes[134-139] (p. 813). Nifedipine has also been shown to inhibit hypoxic vasoconstriction in patients with acute respiratory failure.[138]

In patients with chronic obstructive lung disease, vasodilators should be reserved until conventional therapy with oxygen and bronchodilators has been shown to be ineffective. When they are given, it is mandatory that objective monitoring be undertaken to watch for adverse responses, i.e., worsening hypoxemia and systemic hypotension.[140]

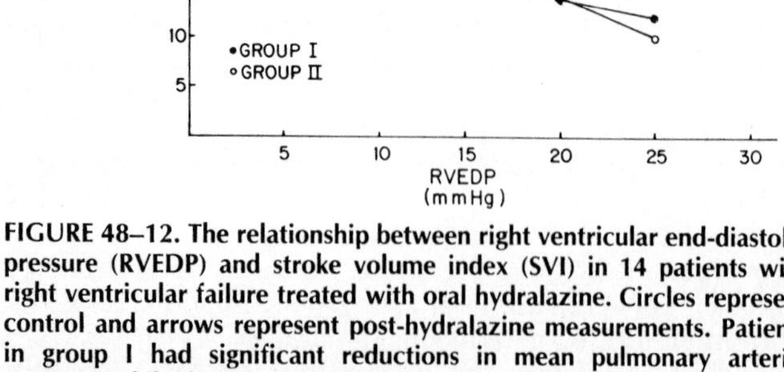

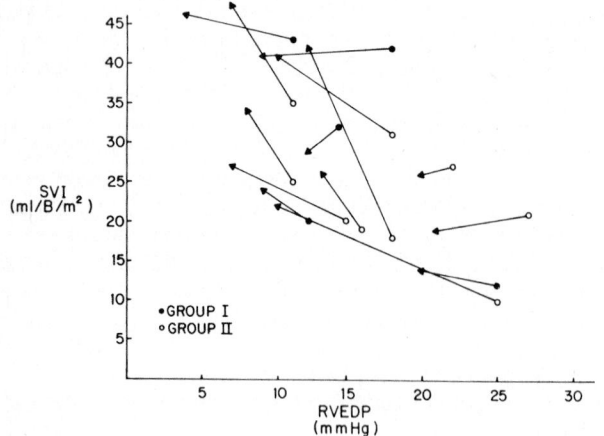

FIGURE 48–12. The relationship between right ventricular end-diastolic pressure (RVEDP) and stroke volume index (SVI) in 14 patients with right ventricular failure treated with oral hydralazine. Circles represent control and arrows represent post-hydralazine measurements. Patients in group I had significant reductions in mean pulmonary arterial pressure, while those in group II did not. (From Rubin LJ: Cardiovascular effects of vasodilator therapy for pulmonary arterial hypertension. Clin. Chest Med., *4*:309, 1983.)

The indications for the use of other ancillary therapeutic measures such as phlebotomy, diuretics, and cardiac glycosides are considerably less clear. In the case of phlebotomy, most older studies have demonstrated an improvement in the subjective complaints related to vascular engorgement but no evidence of improvement in pulmonary gas exchange, mechanics, or hemodynamics has been found.[141, 142] Newer evidence, however, suggests that erythropheresis in patients with secondary polycythemia and cor pulmonale reduces blood viscosity and improves right ventricular function.[143, 144] Diuretics are commonly used for cor pulmonale with failure, and, although there is little question of their effectiveness in relieving fluid retention, there are scant data to demonstrate that they improve pulmonary hemodynamics or gas exchange in the absence of left ventricular decompensation. Excessive use, particularly of potent agents, can aggravate the loss of H^+ and Cl^- induced by chronic hypercapnia and cause a severe metabolic alkalosis. Hence, they should be used sparingly.

The use of cardiac glycosides in patients with cor pulmonale is quite controversial. Digitalis apparently is effective in raising cardiac output in patients with cor pulmonale at rest but only at the expense of concomitant increases in pulmonary artery pressures. The consensus is that there is no clear-cut evidence that cardiac glycosides are of substantial benefit unless left ventricular failure coexists.[145] Sympathomimetics, such as terbutaline, may, in addition to their beneficial effects on the tracheobronchial tree, exert a positive inotropic effect.[146]

The *prognosis* of cor pulmonale in patients with COPD is difficult to state with certainty, for it is inextricably linked to the underlying disorder. When cor pulmonale develops in patients with emphysema, life expectancy is quite short, yet patients with bronchitis usually tolerate three to five episodes of failure before ultimately succumbing to their disease. Although long-term survival has been reported following the onset of cor pulmonale with heart failure, the 2- to 3-year survival rate ranges from 33 to 50 per cent,[147-150] but it may be improved with continuous oxygen therapy.

In both the NIH and MRC trials cited above, pulmonary vascular resistance and pulmonary artery pressure either declined or remained constant in those patients treated with oxygen, suggesting a stabilization of the disease process. In those not so treated, mean pulmonary pressure and total pulmonary vascular resistance rose 3 mm Hg and 100 dynes-sec-cm^{-5} per year, respectively.

Chronic Suppurative Pulmonary Disease

The two prime examples of chronic suppurative disease associated with chronic cor pulmonale are bronchiectasis and cystic fibrosis.

BRONCHIECTASIS. This chronic inflammatory disease is characterized clinically by cough and the production of copious amounts of purulent sputum and pathologically by cylindrical and saccular dilatation of airways.[151, 152] In the majority of patients one can elicit a history of pneumonia developing as a complication of measles, pertussis, or some other contagious disease of childhood. It is thought that bacterial pneumonia and associated atelectasis are responsible for the destruction and dilatation of the bronchial walls. A small percentage of cases are associated with congenital defects such as Kartagener triad (p. 1628) and either congenital or acquired defects in immune mechanisms. Cor pulmonale develops in far-advanced cases in which destruction of lung tissue and fibrosis are extensive. The mechanism for pulmonary hypertension is believed to be capillary loss, hypoxia, and increased bronchial-pulmonary collateral blood flow. Formerly this was a relatively common affliction, but bronchiectasis has decreased considerably in incidence during the past two decades.

CYSTIC FIBROSIS. This genetic (autosomal recessive) defect is characterized by the secretion from exocrine glands of thick, tenacious mucus in which the mucopolysaccharide content is relatively insoluble and easily denatured. The lungs are involved to some extent in virtually all patients with the disease, and the thick mucus throughout the tracheobronchial tree partially or completely obstructs air passages, giving rise to focal atelectasis, pneumonia, bronchiectasis, and abscess formation.[153] Cor pulmonale is an important feature in the natural history, and it contributes to 70 per cent of the deaths.[154] Clinical recognition of the cardiac involvement in cystic fibrosis can be difficult in the early stage of the disease. Many investigators employ noninvasive radionuclide and/or echocardiography to improve detection.[155] One group has developed an echocardiographic scoring system that provides a method for assessing the progression of the cardiac involvement and for evaluating prognosis.[156] Physiological studies have suggested that hypoxia is the principal stimulus to the production of pulmonary hypertension, and pathological data have supported this.[157, 157a, 158] In the past, the development of cardiac failure usually presaged death within a few months. In recent years, however, the prognosis has been improving, and a number of patients have survived for considerable periods. These patients have been maintained on a vigorous, comprehensive, pulmonary care program with postural drainage, antibiotics, and bronchodilators.

Restrictive Lung Diseases

This category encompasses a multitude of diseases which have in common a destruction of functioning pulmonary parenchyma with restriction of the pulmonary vascular bed. The latter results from a physical loss of vessels as well as from intrinsic abnormalities in the lumina and walls of those remaining. Essentially, five processes alone or in combination can produce this effect: (1) diffuse interstitial, (2) diffuse alveolar, (3) mixed alveolar-interstitial, (4) chest wall and pleural, and (5) extensive resection of lung tissue with disease in the residual parenchyma. Specific examples of the first three categories are sarcoidosis, radiation fibrosis, connective tissue disorders with primary or secondary lung involvement, fibrosing alveolitis, alveolar proteinosis, pneumoconiosis, and progressive massive fibrosis. The prototypes for the fourth and fifth categories are thoracoplasty for chronic tuberculosis and surgical resections for granulomatous disease or bronchiectasis.

Pulmonary parenchymal disease, especially when complicated by fibrosis of tissue and secondary vascular changes, can lead to severe pulmonary hypertension. As with the other conditions with a restricted vascular bed, the pulmonary hypertension is initially confined to circumstances in which the cardiac output is elevated. As the vascular bed becomes further restricted and the vessels stiffen, pulmonary hypertension persists at rest and intensifies with increased blood flow. As long as hypoxemia remains mild, pulmonary hypertension is modest, but cor pulmonale develops with respiratory failure. Fortunately, the sequence is not inevitable in most patients with these problems. If the pathological process stabilizes, as is often the case, the patient is left with modest pulmonary hypertension at rest, which is usually well tolerated.[57]

In these diseases, the lungs are stiff, with reduced volumes, and minute ventilation is high, with or without an elevated alveolar ventilation. Arterial oxygen tension is usually moderately reduced at rest, but severe hypoxemia may develop with exercise. The diffusing capacity is low and fails to increase normally as cardiac output is increased. In contrast to the chronic obstructive syndromes, the correlation between arterial blood gases and pulmonary artery pressure is poor[159] and there seems to be a parallel deterioration in pulmonary mechanics and hemodynamics.[160] As a general rule, when the vital capacity is greater than 80 per cent of normal, hemodynamics are normal. When vital capacity is between 50 and 80 per cent, vascular resistance is increased and pulmonary artery pressure in the resting state is at the upper limits of normal. When vital capacity is below 50 per cent, pulmonary hypertension is usually present at rest. The role of hypoxic vasoconstriction in these patients has been difficult to clarify. Experimental evidence indicates that the ability of the pulmonary vasculature to respond to alveolar hypoxia is abnormal in diseased regions, so that when hypoxia does occur, blood is shifted toward the affected areas, thus worsening net gas exchange.[16] In any event, the development of severe hypoxemia and carbon dioxide retention heralds the onset of right ventricular failure, which is usually seen late in the course.

In keeping with the pathophysiology, the prominent symptoms of restrictive lung disease are tachypnea at rest and severe dyspnea on exertion. Fine inspiratory rales are found, along with the previously mentioned signs of pulmonary hypertension and right ventricular hypertrophy and/or failure. Early in the course of patients with pulmonary fibrosis, glucocorticoids or immunosuppressive drugs may be helpful if noninfectious inflammatory processes are believed to be present. In the late stages with extensive pulmonary fibrosis, these modalities are unsuccessful; all that can be offered is continuous oxygen therapy, diuretics, and cardiac glycosides. Vasodilator therapy is still experimental but may offer some hope in selected patients.[129] Although many of the diseases in this category progress slowly, once cor pulmonale develops the prognosis is grim.

Disorders of the Neuromuscular Apparatus and Chest Wall

These disorders have in common the mechanical failure of the bellows apparatus, through weakness or paralysis of the respiratory muscles or through distortion of the geometry of the thorax. Several factors contribute to the development of cor pulmonale.

FAILURE OF THE NEUROMUSCULAR APPARATUS. Respiratory muscle weakness can result from generalized diseases of muscles such as myopathic infiltrating diseases or muscular dystrophy, but it more commonly follows a neurological disorder, such as a cord lesion at or below the third cervical vertebra, amyotrophic lateral sclerosis, myasthenia gravis, poliomyelitis, or Guillain-Barré syndrome.[162] In all of these diseases, the primary derangement is *generalized alveolar hypoventilation* from mechanical impedance to the movement of the rib cage, diaphragm, or both. The lungs and airways are usually not diseased, although they can become so with retained secretions and multiple aspirations. Although acute respiratory failure is common in these diseases, for cor pulmonale to develop in response to the hypoxic and hypercapneic stimuli the disorder must be chronic; consequently, this complication tends to be seen more often with cord lesions than with the other conditions just noted. Mechanical ventilatory support is the only treatment for the hypoventilation; a cuirass type of respirator is effective in these patients. Along with this, vigorous bronchial toilet facilitates the impaired handling of secretions that frequently coexists.

Bilateral diaphragmatic paralysis is an uncommon but insidious and frequently missed cause of cor pulmonale.[163] In the upright position ventilation may be normal or almost so, but with assumption of the supine position gas exchange deteriorates. The diagnosis may be suspected in the patient with supine breathlessness, a disturbed sleep pattern, paradoxical (i.e., inward) motion of the abdomen on inspiration, and a low vital capacity in the erect position. Treatment consists of assisting ventilation when the patient is supine or during sleep. This can easily be accomplished under most circumstances with a rocking bed. When this is inadequate, electrical pacing of the diaphragm may be used.[164] Occasionally, diaphragmatic fatigue can contribute to the respiratory failure of COPD.[165] Bilateral diaphragmatic paralysis can occur following cardiac surgery.[166] The use of ice cardioplegia can damage the phrenic nerves and result in respiratory failure that becomes manifest as soon as the patient is removed from the ventilator postoperatively. Usually this complication is transitory and diaphragmatic function returns.

CHEST-WALL DISORDERS. The common congenital or acquired abnormalities that distort the geometry of the thoracic cage include kyphoscoliosis, pectus excavatum, pectus carinatum, and ankylosing spondylitis; of these only kyphoscoliosis is associated with cor pulmonale.[167] Kyphosis refers to any posterior angulation of the spine, and scoliosis consists of a lateral displacement with at least one compensatory curve in the opposite direction. Of these two processes, a kyphotic angle exceeding 100 degrees or an angle of scoliosis in excess of 120 degrees may be associated with cor pulmonale.[168] Such marked structural abnormalities of the thorax lead to abnormal positioning and functioning of the respiratory muscles, compression of the lung and pulmonary vasculature, and abnormal gas exchange.[168, 169] In addition, it has been suggested that scoliosis interferes with the growth and development of alveoli and pulmonary arteries[170]; dyspnea is the major symptom of these disorders.

Therapy is directed toward avoiding complicating infections; episodes of acute respiratory failure are treated with mechanical ventilation. Surgical improvement of the thoracic deformity is not often associated with a commensurate change in cardiorespiratory function.[171]

Inadequate Ventilatory Drive

The common denominator in this category is a depressed output from the respiratory center, with resultant generalized alveolar hypoventilation. Cor pulmonale is then the result of pulmonary hypertension caused by chronic hypoxemia and acidemia.

OBESITY-HYPOVENTILATION SYNDROME. The association of extreme obesity with alveolar hypoventilation was originally made by Sir William Osler; Burwell et al. subsequently coined the term "pickwickian syndrome" to describe the combination of obesity, somnolence, plethora, and edema.[172] Despite many investigations, the pathogenesis of the hypoventilation in this syndrome remains obscure.[173] Excessive reduction of chest-wall compliance and muscle weakness secondary to obesity may account for part, but many extremely obese individuals with these defects do not hypoventilate. These patients may have abnormally low ventilatory responses to hypercapneic and

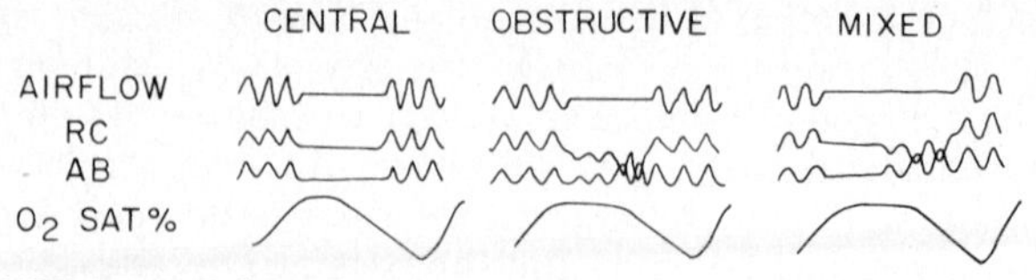

FIGURE 48–13. Schematic representation of the three patterns of apnea that develop during sleep in humans. RC and AB represent ribcage and abdominal displacement, respectively. O_2 sat = oxygen saturation. In each type, airflow at the nose and mouth are absent, indicating apnea. In central apneas, respiratory efforts as measured by the movement of the ribcage and abdomen are absent. During obstructive apneas the efforts by the chest wall muscles are present throughout the entire episode. In mixed apneas, both central and obstructive patterns are present. (From Strohl, K. P., et al.: Physiologic basis of therapy for sleep apnea. Am. Rev. Resp. Dis. *134*:791, 1986.)

anoxic stimulation, which improve with treatment.[174] Consequently, hyposensitivity of the respiratory center with dispersed ventilatory drive, whether acquired or preexistent, is probably a background factor.

The primary *treatment* of this disorder consists of weight reduction. The respiratory stimulant progesterone and its congeners have been shown to increase alveolar ventilation so that hypoxemia, hypercapnia, and cor pulmonale all improve substantially.[175, 176] This may prove to be a useful adjunct until weight is reduced. If the respiratory and cardiac failure are life-threatening, ventilatory assistance may be required.

SLEEP APNEA SYNDROME. After the description of the pickwickian syndrome, variant manifestations such as periodic respirations and hypersomnia were recognized, and it soon became apparent that patients with disturbed respirations during sleep could develop pulmonary hypertension and cor pulmonale.[177] This has been designated the sleep apnea syndrome. Three types of patterns have been recorded (Fig. 48–13): *central apnea*, in which airflow stops in conjunction with cessation of all respiratory muscle effort; (2) *obstructive apnea*, in which upper airway obstruction causes airflow to cease despite continuing or increasing efforts of the inspiratory muscles. The obstruction is believed to result from relaxation or discoordination of the buccal and pharyngeal muscles, from collapse of the walls of the pharynx due to failure of the genioglossus muscle, from greatly enlarged tonsils or adenoids, from backward movement of the tongue during sleep, and from narrowing of the upper airway secondary to marked obesity,[178a] and (3) *mixed apnea*, in which airflow and respiratory effort stop early in the episode, followed by a resumption of unsuccessful respiratory effort.[177, 178]

The apneic periods, which can occur 40 to 60 times per hour,[178] are associated with phasic hypoxemia and hypercapnia. Alterations in gas exchange are quite severe and the pO_2 can reach values of 20 to 25 mm Hg with saturations below 50 per cent. Pulmonary artery pressures rise with each apneic period, and with repetitive episodes the pressures progressively increase throughout the night[174] (Fig. 48–14). Hence, pulmonary hypertension is most severe in the morning. During the day the pressures fall only to rise again with sleep the next night. Eventually hypoxemia, hypercapnia, and pulmonary hypertension become permanent and gradually worsen while the patient is awake.

In association with the fluctuation in gas exchange patients have severe brady- and tachyarrhythmias.[179] The former occurs during periods of apnea while the latter begins with the onset of breathing. The type of arrhythmias found consist of sinus bradycardia, sinus arrest, long asystolic periods (ranging from 2 to 13 seconds), sinoatrial block, premature atrial contractions, atrial fibrillation, ventricular premature beats with bigeminy and trigeminy,

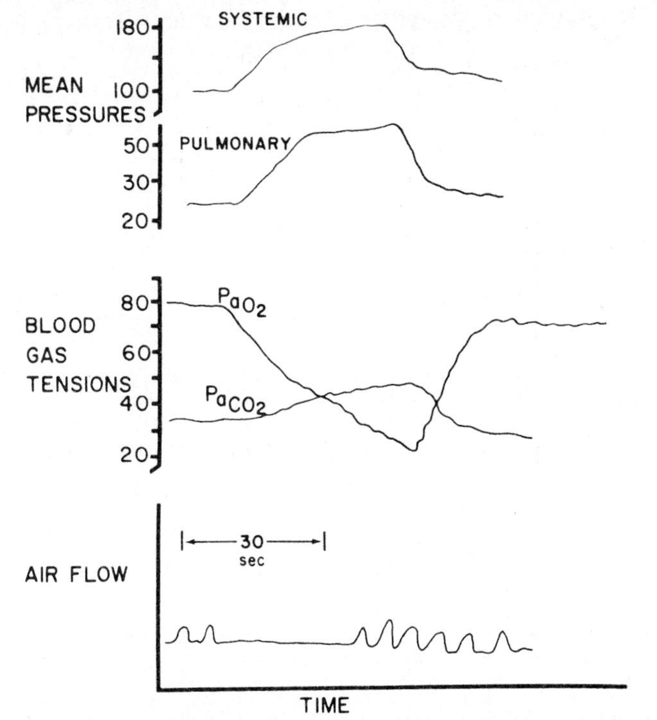

FIGURE 48–14. Schematic representation of hemodynamic and blood gas events during an apnea. Respiratory pauses are associated with a fall in PaO_2 that generally exceeds the rise in $PaCO_2$. The combined hypoxia and hypercapnia are probably responsible for the rise in pulmonary arterial pressure which occurs with each apnea. Note that baseline pulmonary arterial pressure is slightly higher following the apneic episode. (From Weil, J. V.: Pulmonary hypertension and cor pulmonale in hypoventilating patients. *In* Weir, E. K., and Reeves, J. T. [eds.]: Pulmonary Hypertension. Mount Kisco, N.Y., Futura Publishing Co., 1984, p. 321.)

multifocal premature beats, and ventricular tachycardia.[179, 180, 180a] Pulmonary capillary wedge pressures may also increase during periods of apnea.[181] The clinical symptomatology differs depending on the type, frequency, and intensity of the abnormal, sleep-related respiratory pattern.

The patient rarely reaches the deep stages of sleep because of hypoxic arousal and so is chronically sleep-deprived. The other common clinical manifestations are loud snoring, abnormal behavior during sleep (somnambulism, tremors, or myoclonus), altered states of consciousness, nocturnal enuresis, morning headache, daytime hypersomnolence, hypnagogic hallucinations, and systemic hypertension (Fig. 48–15). The majority of patients with sleep apnea are *not obese* and ventilate normally when awake. Patients with obstructive apnea tend to have less severe hypoventilation and fewer hemodynamic abnormalities than patients with the other varieties. The diagnosis is readily established by performing polysomnography during sleep.

The etiology of sleep apnea is unknown. The weight of current evidence indicates that obstructive apneas occur because of occlusion of the upper airway in the region of the pharynx.[178] Central apneas, on the other hand, may have multiple mechanisms including sleep-induced alteration in respiratory muscle drive, depressed central ventilatory output, and/or a change in the thresholds for sleep and/or arousal.[178]

Management. Although treatment depends upon the type of apnea present, certain precautions transcend type. Sedatives and antihistamines should be assiduously avoided or withdrawn and oxygen should be used with caution. Death has followed the use of both narcoleptics and uncontrolled oxygen administration.[178] Treatment of central apnea consists of respiratory stimulants or nocturnal ventilatory support with respirators.[178] Phrenic nerve or diaphragmatic pacing has also been recommended.[164] In obstructive apnea, tracheostomy and nasal CPAP (continuous positive airway pressure applied to the nose during sleep) are the most commonly employed therapeutic modalities.[178] The former bypasses the area of obstruction while the latter is believed to act as a pneumatic splint that prevents upper airway collapse. In an obese patient with obstructive apnea, weight reduction may obviate the need for a permanent tracheal cannula. Removal of enlarged tonsils and/or adenoids or surgical enlargement of the entrance to the airway may be enormously helpful. Nocturnal oxygen therapy may be helpful in some patients by reducing the duration of the apneic periods and decreasing the related arrhythmias but, as already indicated, should be used with care.[183]

PRIMARY ALVEOLAR HYPOVENTILATION. Generalized alveolar hypoventilation in the absence of obesity or intrinsic disease of the lungs, chest wall, or neuromuscular apparatus has been ascribed to a failure of the autonomic control of ventilation. Most cases are acquired and are seen following encephalitis, brain stem surgery, meningitis, and the like, but congenital occurrence has been reported.[184] In this rare condition, the respiratory center does not respond normally to its chemical stimuli, and the patient has a flat or markedly depressed ventilatory—carbon dioxide response curve. However, an affected patient can improve alveolar ventilation and restore the arterial oxygen and carbon dioxide to normal by voluntary hyperventilation. This syndrome has been called *Ondine's curse*. The pathogenesis and treatment are similar to that outlined for other forms of generalized alveolar hypoventilation. An interesting therapeutic development is long-term pacing of the diaphragm by means of electrical stimulation of the phrenic nerves.[164]

CHRONIC MOUNTAIN SICKNESS. Some acclimatized residents of high altitudes suffer a transient loss of their adaptation after short stays at sea level and, upon return to altitude, develop acute pulmonary edema with circula-

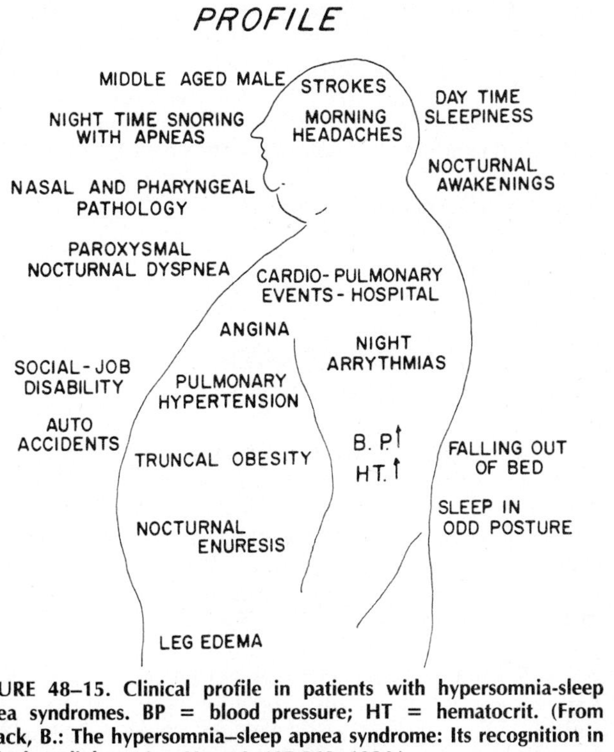

FIGURE 48–15. Clinical profile in patients with hypersomnia-sleep apnea syndromes. BP = blood pressure; HT = hematocrit. (From Burack, B.: The hypersomnia–sleep apnea syndrome: Its recognition in clinical cardiology. Am. Heart J. *107*:543, 1984.)

tory and electrocardiographic changes similar to those seen in acute cor pulmonale[185] (p. 193). Some persons remaining at high altitude lose their acclimatization and develop signs and symptoms of generalized alveolar hypoventilation with chronic cor pulmonale. This syndrome is variously called *chronic mountain sickness, soroche*, or *Monge disease.*[186] The mechanism for the hypoventilation is unknown, but Severinghaus et al. have postulated that it is due to an adaptation or desensitization of the hypoxic chemoreceptors in the carotid body to chronic hypoxia.[187] The only treatment is removal of the patient to sea level, where pulmonary artery pressure usually falls acutely. With prolonged residence at sea level polycythemia disappears, and there is believed to be some involution of the structural changes of the pulmonary vessels.

UPPER AIRWAY OBSTRUCTION. Obstruction of the upper airways may be responsible for an inadequate ventilatory drive, global alveolar hypoventilation, and cor pulmonale. For the most part this occurs in children, especially black children, who have enlarged tonsils and adenoids.[188] Other causes include vascular ring (p. 966), macroglossia, micrognathia, laryngotracheomalacia, laryngeal web, Crouzon disease, Hurler syndrome, and severe Pierre Robin syndrome,[189, 190] but it can also develop with obstruction during sleep in both children and adults.[182] The mechanism for the hypoventilation is not clear. It has been suggested that an abnormally reactive pulmonary vascular bed, a defect in the central control of respiration, and an interference with normal sleep physiology, as in the sleep apnea syndrome, may play a part, singly or in combination. There is little direct evidence for the first mechanism. However, it is known that ventilatory responsiveness to carbon dioxide is blunted in these patients and that it does not return to normal following therapy.[191]

The clinical features may mimic asthma, but more often the patients display somnolence, respiratory stridor, and recurrent respiratory tract infections. Treatment consists of surgical removal of the obstruction.

PULMONARY VASCULAR DISORDERS (see also Chap. 26). This category consists of diseases that primarily affect the pulmonary vasculature, with minimal or no parenchymal involvement. These diseases represent the most straightforward pathogenetic sequence in which pulmonary hypertension and right ventricular overloading are consequences of a progressive increase in pulmonary vascular resistance resulting from gradual obliteration of the blood vessels. In addition to their pathophysiology, these diseases also share in common the symptom of dyspnea and strikingly high pulmonary artery pressures, despite the fact that both vital capacity and pulmonary gas exchange may be only minimally impaired.[192] The latter finding is frequently of considerable diagnostic importance.

NONINVASIVE ASSESSMENT OF COR PULMONALE

ELECTROCARDIOGRAPHIC FINDINGS (Table 48–3). In the past, the use of the electrocardiogram to make the diagnosis of cor pulmonale has centered largely, if not exclusively, on the electrocardiographic demonstration of right ventricular hypertrophy (p. 192). The classic criteria of a shift of the mean QRS axis to the right (right axis deviation greater than + 110 degrees), an R:S ratio in V_1 greater than 1, and an R:S ratio in V_6 of less than 1 were derived from patients with congenital heart disease[193, 194] and have proved to be relatively poor criteria of cor pulmonale in patients with chronic obstructive lung disease.[195, 196] The reason is that right ventricular hypertrophy per se is a late manifestation in these syndromes and occurs only after repeated dilatation of the ventricle.[197]

Kilcoyne and associates studied 200 patients with chronic obstructive lung disease and were able to demonstrate that when the arterial oxygen saturation fell below 85 per cent and mean pulmonary pressure was 25 mm Hg or greater, one or more of the following changes would develop in the electrocardiogram: (1) a rightward shift of the mean QRS axis of 30 degrees or more from its previous position; (2) inverted, biphasic, or flattened T waves in the right

TABLE 48–3 ELECTROCARDIOGRAPHIC CHANGES IN COR PULMONALE

ECG Criteria for Cor Pulmonale** without **Obstructive Disease** of the **Airways*	
1.	Right-axis deviation with a mean QRS axis to the right of + 110°
2.	R/S amplitude ratio in $V_1 > 1$
3.	R/S amplitude ratio in $V_6 < 1$
4.	Clockwise rotation of the electrical axis
5.	P-pulmonale pattern
6.	S_1Q_3 or $S_1S_2S_3$ pattern
7.	Normal-voltage QRS
***ECG Changes in Chronic Cor Pulmonale with Obstructive Disease of the Airways*†**	
1.	Isoelectric P waves in lead I or right-axis deviation of the P vector
2.	P-pulmonale pattern (an increase in P-wave amplitude in II, III, aV_f)
3.	Tendency for right-axis deviation of the QRS
4.	R/S amplitude ratio in $V_6 < 1$
5.	Low-voltage QRS
6.	S_1Q_3 or $S_1S_2S_3$ pattern
7.	Incomplete (and rarely complete) right bundle branch block
8.	R/S amplitude ratio in $V_1 > 1$
9.	Marked clockwise rotation of the electrical axis
10.	Occasional large Q wave or QS in the inferior or midprecordial leads, suggesting healed myocardial infarction

*Any one of the first three criteria suffices to raise suspicion of right ventricular hypertrophy. The diagnosis becomes more certain if two or more of these findings are present (2 and 7). The last four criteria commonly occur in cor pulmonale secondary to primary alveolar hypoventilation interstitial disease of the lung, or pulmonary vascular disease.

†The first seven criteria are suggestive but nonspecific; the last three are more characteristic of cor pulmonale in obstructive disease of the airways.

Reproduced with permission from Holford, F. D.: The electrocardiogram in lung disease. *In* Fishman, A. P. (ed.): Pulmonary Diseases and Disorders. New York, McGraw-Hill Book Co., 1980, p. 140.

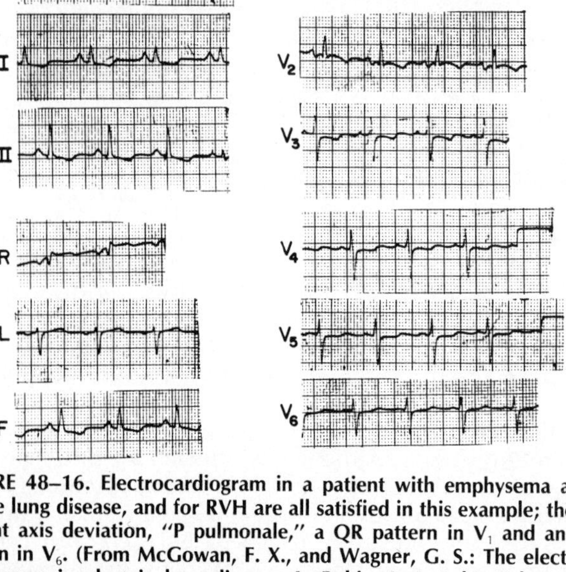

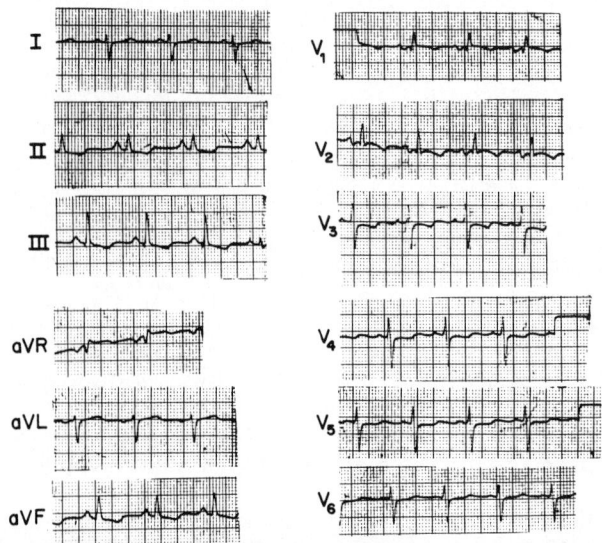

FIGURE 48–16. Electrocardiogram in a patient with emphysema and diffuse lung disease, and for RVH are all satisfied in this example; there is right axis deviation, "P pulmonale," a QR pattern in V_1 and an rS pattern in V_6. (From McGowan, F. X., and Wagner, G. S.: The electrocardiogram in chronic lung disease. *In* Rubin, L. J. [ed.]: Pulmonary Heart Disease. Boston, Martinus Nijhoff, 1984, p. 117.)

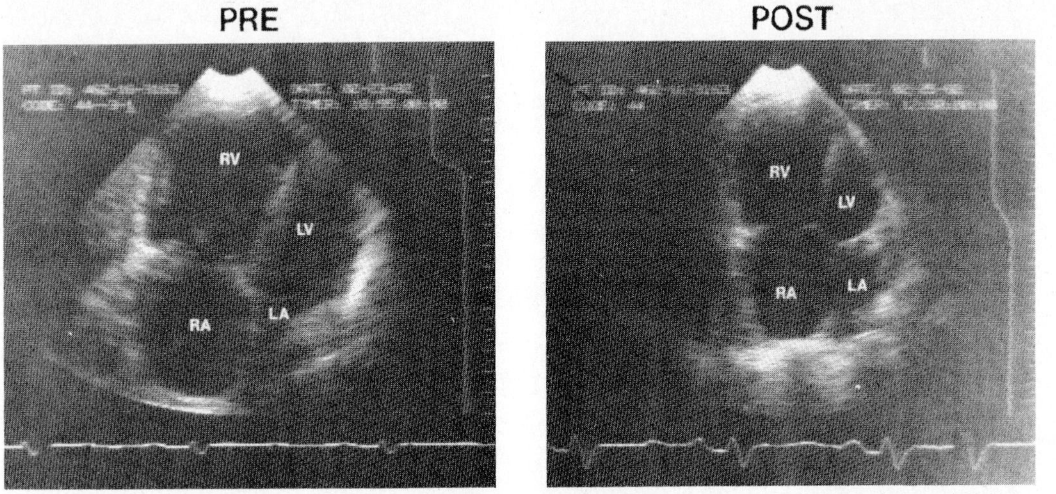

FIGURE 48–17. Echocardiogram from a 47-year-old man with pulmonary hypertension before (*left*) and 48 hours after (*right*) beginning therapy with nifedipine. The right atrium and right ventricle are greatly increased in size before treatment and are reduced in size by therapy. (From Rubin, L. J.: Cardiovascular effects of vasodilator therapy for pulmonary arterial hypertension. Clin. Chest Med. *4*:309, 1983.)

precordial leads; (3) depressed ST segments in leads II, III, and aV_f; and (4) incomplete or complete right bundle branch block.[196] With an increase in arterial saturation, these alterations disappeared. The T-wave changes in the right precordial leads and the axis shifts to the right occurred with only modest elevations of pulmonary artery pressure, but if these elevations became more severe, and if recurrences were frequent, then the rightward rotation of the QRS axis and the T-wave changes in the right precordial leads tended to become persistent. If pulmonary function were not improved, true right-axis deviation (a frontal plane axis greater than + 90 degrees) and increased R-wave voltage in the right precordial leads developed (Fig. 48–16). Once the latter occurred, the electrocardiogram was less likely to mirror any physiological variability, as reversion of the increased voltage to normal rarely occurred after improvements in arterial blood gases.

Other studies have suggested that clockwise rotation, right-axis deviation, a qR pattern in aV_r, and electrocardiographic evidence of right atrial enlargement, in that order, would also point to right ventricular hypertrophy in patients with chronic cor pulmonale (Chap. 7). Occasionally in chronic obstructive lung disease the mean QRS axis may be directed posteriorly, superiorly, and to the right so that there is apparent left-axis deviation in the standard limb leads. This pattern, along with low voltage, is most often associated with emphysema.

Electrocardiographic features of prognostic importance in severe chronic bronchial obstruction have been outlined by Kok-Jensen.[198] In a study of 288 patients, survival was found to be very poor in patients with a QRS axis of +90 to +180 degrees and an amplitude of the P wave in lead II of 0.20 mV or more; only 37 and 42 per cent, respectively, of the patients with these changes were alive after 4 years.

The vectorcardiogram has been correlated with hemodynamics in patients with chronic obstructive pulmonary disease and a linear correlation has been found between terminal rightward QRS forces and mean pulmonary pressures during exercise. Since in one such correlation[199] no patient met the electrocardiographic criteria for right ventricular hypertrophy, it was suggested that the vectorcardiogram may be more selective in identifying early hemodynamic abnormalities in the pulmonary circulation.

OTHER NONINVASIVE ASSESSMENT OF RIGHT VENTRICULAR FUNCTION. Other potentially useful techniques are echocardiography and radionuclide imaging. The use of M-mode echocardiography in adults with obstructive airway disease has tended to be disappointing because the pulmonary hyperinflation associated with these conditions frequently precludes adequate visualization of the cardiac valves and chambers. Two-dimensional techniques, however, can overcome this deficiency and permit visualization of right ventricular dimensions and wall thickness (Fig. 48–17). These parameters are markedly influenced by the state of ventricular function and correlate well with radionuclide parameters of size and function.[200] Various echocardiographic techniques are now available for the noninvasive assessment of pulmonary artery pressure, which are discussed on page 100. The most useful of these appears to be Doppler echocardiographic assessment of the velocity of tricuspid regurgitant blood flow, which when utilized in the Bernoulli equation can be used to determine the right ventricular–right atrial pressure gradient. When this is added to the right atrial pressure, which is assessed clinically, the pulmonary artery systolic pressure can be estimated.

A frequently used radionuclide for right ventricular imaging is thallium-201. The distribution of this isotope is a function of regional myocardial blood flow and myocardial mass, and so only the left ventricle tends to be visualized at rest. When the right ventricle is imaged at rest, hypertrophy and dysfunction of the right ventricle are usually present.[201]

REFERENCES

ANATOMICAL AND PATHOPHYSIOLOGICAL CORRELATES

1. Chronic cor pulmonale: Report of an expert committee. Wld. Hlth. Org. Tech. Rep. Ser. *213*:1, 1961.
2. McGinn, S., and White, P. D.: Acute cor pulmonale resulting from pulmonary embolism. J.A.M.A. *104*:1473, 1935.
3. Lewis, T.: Observations upon ventricular hypertrophy with especial reference to preponderance of one or other chamber. Heart *5*:367, 1914.
4. Emery, J. L., and Mithal, A.: Weight of cardiac ventricles at and after birth. Br. Heart J. *23*:313, 1961.
5. Keen, E. N.: The post-natal development of the human cardiac ventricles. J. Anat. *89*:484, 1955.
6. Arias-Stella, J., and Recavarren, S.: Right ventricular hypertrophy in native children living at high altitude. Am. J. Pathol. *41*:55, 1962.
7. Mathew, R., Thilenius, O. G., and Arcilla, R. A.: Comparative response of right and left ventricles to volume overload. Am. J. Cardiol. *38*:239, 1976.
8. Recavarren, S., and Arias-Stella, J.: Right ventricular hypertrophy in people born and living at high altitudes. Br. Heart J. *26*:806, 1964.
9. Penaloza, D., Sime, F., Banchero, N., Gamboa, R., Cruz, J., and Martico-Rena, E.: Pulmonary hypertension in healthy men born and living at high altitudes. Am. J. Cardiol. *11*:150, 1963.
10. Fulton, R. M., Hutchinson, E. C., and Jones, A. M.: Ventricular weight in cardiac hypertrophy. Br. Heart J. *14*:413, 1952.

11. Mitchell, R. S., Stanford, R. E., Silvers, G. W., and Dart, G.: The right ventricle in chronic airway obstruction: A clinicopathologic study. Am. Rev. Respir. Dis. *114*:147, 1976.
12. Ishikawa, S., Fattal, G. A., Popiewicz, J., and Wyatt, J. P.: Functional morphometry of myocardial fibers in cor pulmonale. Am. Rev. Respir. Dis. *105*:358, 1972.
13. Brecher, G. A., and Galletti, P. M.: Functional anatomy of cardiac pumping. *In* Hamilton, A. F., and Dow, P. (eds.): Handbook of Physiology; Circulation. Vol. II. Washington, D.C., American Physiological Society, 1963, p. 759.
13a. Visner, M. S., Arentzen, C. E., O'Connor, M. J., Larson, E. V., and Anderson, R. W.: Alterations in left ventricular three-dimensional dynamic geometry and systolic function during acute right ventricular hypertension in the conscious dog. Circulation *67*:353, 1983.
14. Laks, M. M., Garner, D., and Swan, H. J. C.: Volumes and compliances measured simultaneously in the right and left ventricles of the dog. Circ. Res. *20*:565, 1967.
15. Abel, F. L., and Waldhausen, J. A.: Effects of alterations in pulmonary vascular resistance on right ventricular function. J. Thorac. Cardiovasc. Surg. *54*:886, 1967.
16. Abel, F. L.: Effects of alterations in peripheral resistance on left ventricular function. Proc. Soc. Exp. Biol. Med. *120*:52, 1965.
17. Morrison, D., Goldman, S., Wright, A. L., Henry, R., Sorenson, S., Caldwell, J., and Ritchie, J.: The effect of pulmonary hypertension on systolic function of the right ventricle. Chest *84*:250, 1983.
18. Sarnoff, S. J., and Berglund, E.: Ventricular function. I. Starling's law of the heart studied by means of simultaneous right and left ventricular function curves in the dog. Circulation *9*:706, 1954.
19. Spann, J. R., Buccino, R. A., Sonnenblick, E. H., and Braunwald, E. B.: Contractile state of cardiac muscle obtained from cats with experimentally produced ventricular hypertrophy and heart failure. Circ. Res. *21*:341, 1967.
20. Haggart, G. E., and Walker, A. M.: The physiology of pulmonary embolism as disclosed by quantitative occlusion of the pulmonary artery. Arch. Surg. *6*:764, 1923.
21. Gibbond, J. H., Hopkinson, M., and Churchill, E. D.: Changes in the circulation produced by gradual occlusion of the pulmonary artery. J. Clin. Invest. *11*:543, 1932.
22. Fineberg, M. H., and Wiggens, C. J.: Compensation and failure of the right ventricle. Am. Heart J. *11*:255, 1936.
23. Brooks, H., Kirk, E. S., Vokonas, P. S., Urschel, C. W., and Sonnenblick, E. H.: Performance of the right ventricle under stress: Relation to right coronary flow. J. Clin. Invest. *50*:2176, 1971.
24. Krahl, V. E.: Anatomy of the mammalian lung. *In* Fenn, O. W., and Rahn, H. (eds.): Handbook of Physiology; Respiration. Vol. I. Washington, D.C., American Physiological Society, 1964, p. 224.
25. Hislop, A., and Reid, L.: Intrapulmonary arterial development during fetal life—branching pattern and structure. J. Anat. *113*:35, 1972.
26. Davies, G. M., and Reid, L.: Growth of the alveoli and pulmonary arteries in childhood. Thorax *25*:669, 1975.
27. Boyden, E. A., and Tompsett, D. H.: The changing patterns in the developing lungs of infants. Acta Anat. *61*:164, 1965.
28. Meyrick, B., and Reid, L.: Pulmonary hypertension: Anatomic and physiologic correlations. Clin. Chem. Med. *4*:199, 1983.
29. Fishman, A. P.: Regulation of the pulmonary circulation. *In* Fishman, A. P. (ed.): Pulmonary Diseases and Disorders. New York, McGraw-Hill Book Co., 1980, p. 397.
30. Hebb, C.: Motor innervation of the pulmonary blood vessels of mammals. *In* Fishman, A. P., and Hecht, H. H. (eds.): The Pulmonary Circulation and the Interstitial Space. Chicago, University of Chicago Press, 1969, p. 195.
31. Fishman, A. P.: Dynamics of the pulmonary circulation. *In* Hamilton, W. F., and Dow, P. (eds.): Handbook of Physiology; Circulation. Vol. II, Washington, D.C., American Physiological Society, 1963, p. 1667.
32. Bard, P.: The pulmonary circulation and respiratory variations in the systemic circulation. *In* Bard, P. (ed.): Medical Physiology. St. Louis, C. V. Mosby, 1961, p. 231.
33. Brofman, B. L., Charms, B. L., Kohn, P. M., Elder, J., Newman, R., and Rizika, M.: Unilateral pulmonary artery occlusion in man. Control Studies. J. Thorac. Surg. *34*:206, 1957.
34. Guyton, A. C.: Circulatory Physiology: Cardiac Output and Its Regulation. Philadelphia, W. B. Saunders Company, 1963.
35. Maseri, A., Caldini, P., Howard, P., Joshi, R. C., Permutt, S., and Zierler, K. L.: Determinants of pulmonary vascular volume—recruitment versus distensibility. Circ. Res. *31*:218, 1972.
36. Lanari, A., and Agrest, A.: Pressure-volume relationship in the pulmonary vascular bed. Acta Physiol. Lat. Am. *4*:116, 1954.
37. Caro, C. G.: Extensibility of blood vessels in isolated rabbit lung. J. Physiol. (Lond.) *178*:193, 1865.
38. Howell, J. B. L., Permutt, S., Proctor, D. F., and Riley, R. L.: Effect of inflation of the lung on different parts of the pulmonary vascular bed. J. Appl. Physiol. *16*:71, 1961.
39. Engelberg, J., and DuBois, A. B.: Mechanics of pulmonary circulation in isolated rabbit lungs. Am. J. Physiol. *186*:401, 1959.
40. Maseri, A., Caldini, P., Permutt, S., and Zierler, K. L.: Pressure volume relationship in the pulmonary circulation. *In* Widimsky, J., Daum, S., and Herzog, H. (eds.): Progress in Respiration Research. Vol. 5, Basel, S. Karger, 1970, p. 53.
41. Glazier, J. B., Hughes, J. M. B., Maloney, J. E., and West, J. B.: Measurements of capillary dimensions and blood volume in rapidly frozen lungs. J. Appl. Physiol. *26*:65, 1969.
42. West, J. B.: Ventilation/Blood Flow and Gas Exchange. 2nd ed. Philadelphia, F. A. Davis Co., 1970.
43. West, J. B.: The use of radioactive materials in the study of lung function. *In* Fishman, A. P. (ed.): Pulmonary Diseases and Disorders. New York, McGraw-Hill Book Co., 1980, p. 378.
44. Permutt, S., and Riley, R. L.: Hemodynamics of collapsible vessels with tone: The vascular waterfall. J. Appl. Physiol. *18*:924, 1963.
45. Klocke, R. A.: Intrapulmonary distribution of air and blood. *In* Fishman, A. P. (ed.): Pulmonary Diseases and Disorders. New York, McGraw-Hill Book Co., 1980, p. 373.
46. LeBlanc, P., Ruff, F., and Milic-Emili, J.: Effect of age and body position on airway closure in man. J. Appl. Physiol. *28*:448, 1970.
47. Craig, D. B., Wahba, W. M., Don, H. F., Coutre, J. G., and Becklake, M. R.: Closing volume and its relationship to gas exchange in seated and supine position. J. Appl. Physiol. *31*:717, 1971.
48. Lenfant, C.: Measurements of ventilation-perfusion distribution with alveolar-arterial differences. J. Appl. Physiol. *18*:1090, 1963.
49. Raine, J. M., and Bishop, J. M.: A-a difference in O_2 tension and physiologic dead space in normal man. J. Appl. Physiol. *18*:284, 1963.
50. Severinghaus, J. W., and Stupfel, M.: Alveolar dead space as an index of distribution of blood flow in pulmonary capillaries. J. Appl. Physiol. *10*:335, 1957.
51. Fishman, A. P.: Respiratory gases in the regulation of the pulmonary circulation. Physiol. Rev. *41*:214, 1961.
52. Fishman, A. P.: Hypoxia and its effects on the pulmonary circulation. Circ. Res. *38*:221, 1976.
53. Bergofsky, E. H.: Mechanisms underlying vasomotor regulation of regional pulmonary blood flow in normal and disease states. Am. J. Med. *57*:378, 1974.
54. Bates, D. V., Macklem, P. T., and Christie, R. V.: Respiratory Function in Disease, 2nd ed. Philadelphia, W. B. Saunders Company, 1971, p. 75.
55. Engel, L. A., and Macklem, P. T.: Gas mixing and distribution in the lung. *In* Widdicombe, J. G. (ed.): Respiratory Physiology II. International Review of Physiology. Vol. 14. Baltimore, University Park Press, 1977, p. 37.
56. Sykes, M. K., McNicol, M. W., and Campbell, E. J. M.: Respiratory Failure. Oxford, Blackwell Scientific Publications, 1971, p. 56ff.
57. Fishman, A. P.: Cor pulmonale. Am. Rev. Respir. Dis. *114*:775, 1976.
58. Fowler, K. T., and Read, J.: Effect of alveolar hypoxia on zonal distribution of pulmonary blood flow. J. Appl. Physiol. *18*:244, 1963.
59. Lindsay, D. A., and Reed, J.: Pulmonary vascular responsiveness in the prognosis of chronic obstructive lung disease. Am. Rev. Respir. Dis. *105*:242, 1972.
60. Enson, Y., Guintini, C., Lewis, M. L., Morris, T. Q., Ferrer, I. M., and Harvey, R. M.: The influence of hydrogen ion concentration and hypoxia on the pulmonary circulation. J. Clin. Invest. *43*:1146, 1964.
61. Bergofsky, E. H., Haas, F., and Procelli, R. J.: Determination of the sensitive vascular sites from which hypoxia and hypercapnia elicit rises in pulmonary arterial pressure. Fed. Proc. *27*:1420, 1968.
62. Bergofsky, E. H.: Humoral control of the pulmonary circulation. Ann. Rev. Physiol. *42*:221, 1980.

CHRONIC COR PULMONALE

63. Fishman, A. P.: Cor pulmonale. *In* Fishman, A. P. (ed.): Pulmonary Diseases and Disorders. New York, McGraw-Hill Book Co., 1980, p. 853.
64. U. S. Department of Health and Human Services, National Heart, Lung and Blood Institute, Division of Lung Diseases: Progress report, 1980, p. 121.
64a. Respiratory Disease. Task force report on prevention, control and education. Washington, D.C., U.S. Department of Health, Education and Welfare, Public Health Service, National Institute of Health, 1977, p. 83.
65. Stuart-Harris, C. H., Twidle, R. H. S., and Clifton, M. A.: Hospital study of congestive heart failure with special reference to cor pulmonale. Br. Med. J. *2*:201, 1959.
66. Inter-Society Commission for Heart Disease Resources: Primary prevention of pulmonary heart disease. Circulation *41*:A-17, 1970.
67. Burrows, B., Kettel, L. J., Niden, A. H., Rabinowitz, M., and Diener, C. F.: Patterns of cardiovascular dysfunction in chronic obstructive lung disease. N. Engl. J. Med. *286*:912, 1972.
68. Bishop, J. M.: Hypoxia and pulmonary hypertension in chronic bronchitis. Prog. Resp. Dis. *9*:10, 1975.
69. Traver, G. A., Cline, M. G., Burrows, B.: Predictors of mortality in chronic obstructive pulmonary disease. Am. Rev. Respir. Dis. *119*:895, 1979.
70. Berbel, L. N., and Miro, R. E.: Pulmonary hypertension in the pathogenesis of cor pulmonale. Cardiovasc. Rev. *4*:359, 1983.
71. Rubin, L. J.: Pulmonary Hypertension Secondary to Lung Disease. *In* Weir, E. K., and Reeves, J. T. (eds.): Pulmonary Hypertension. Mount Kisco, N.Y., Futura Publishing Company, Inc., 1984, p. 291.
72. Thurlbeck, W. M., Henderson, J. A., Fraser, R. G., and Bates, D. V.: Chronic obstructive lung disease. A comparison between clinical, roentgenologic, functional and morphologic criteria in chronic bronchitis, emphysema, asthma and bronchiectasis. Medicine *48*:81, 1970.
73. Edwards, J. E.: Pathology of chronic pulmonary hypertension. Pathol. Annu. *9*:1, 1974.
74. Wagenvoort, C. A., and Wagenvoort, N.: Hypoxic pulmonary vascular lesions in man at high altitude and in patients with chronic respiratory disease. Pathol. Microbiol. *39*:276, 1973.
75. Semmens, M., and Reid, L.: Pulmonary arterial muscularity and right ventricular hypertrophy in chronic bronchitis and emphysema. Br. J. Dis. Chest. *68*:253, 1974.
76. Wagenvoort, C. A., Heath, D., and Edwards, J. E.: The Pathology of the Pulmonary Vasculature. Springfield, Ill., Charles C Thomas, 1964.
77. Roos, A.: Poiseuille's law and its limitation in vascular systems. *In* Grover, R. F. (ed.): Progress in Research in Emphysema and Chronic Bronchitis. Basel, Karger, 1963, p. 32.
78. Wells, R. E., and Merrill, E. W.: Influence of flow properties of blood upon viscosity hematocrit relationships. J. Clin. Invest. *41*:1591, 1962.

79. Rendas, A., Lennar, S., and Reid, L.: Aorto-pulmonary shunts in growing pigs: Functional and structural assessment of the changes in the pulmonary circulation. J. Thorac. Cardiovasc. Surg. *77*:109, 1979.
80. Balchum, O. J., Jung, R. C., Turner, A. F., and Jacobson, G.: Pulmonary artery to vein shunts in obstructive pulmonary disease. Am. J. Med. *43*:178, 1967.
81. Boushy, S. F., North, L. B., and Trice, J. A.: The bronchial arteries in chronic obstructive pulmonary disease. Am. J. Med. *46*:506, 1969.
82. Meyrick, B., and Reid, L.: Ultrastructural findings in lung biopsy material from children with congenital heart defects. Am. J. Pathol. *101*:527, 1980.
83. Rabinovitz, M., Haworth, S., Vanck, Z., Zawter, G., Castaneda, A. R., Nadas, A. S., and Reid, L. M.: Early pulmonary vascular changes in congenital heart disease studied in biopsy tissue. Hum. Pathol. *11*:499, 1980.
84. Marcus, J. H., McLean, R. L., Duffell, G. M., and Ingram, R. H.: Exercise performance in relation to the pathophysiologic type of chronic obstructive pulmonary disease. Am. J. Med. *49*:14, 1970.
85. Harris, P., Segal, N., and Bishop, J. M.: The relation between pressure and flow in the pulmonary circulation in normal subjects and in patients with chronic bronchitis and mitral stenosis. Cardiovasc. Res. *2*:73, 1968.
86. Seibold, H., Henze, E., Kohler, J., Roth, J., Schmidt, A., and Adam, W.: Right ventricular function in patients with chronic obstructive pulmonary disease. Klin. Wochenschr. *63*:1041, 1985.
87. Kawakami, Y., Kishi, F., Yamamoto, H., and Miyamoto, K.: Relation of oxygen delivery, mixed venous oxygenation and pulmonary hemodynamics to prognosis in chronic obstructive pulmonary disease. N. Engl. J. Med. *308*:1045, 1983.
88. Bergofsky, E. H.: Tissue oxygen delivery and cor pulmonale in chronic obstructive pulmonary disease. N. Engl. J. Med. *308*:1092, 1983.
89. Berger, H. S., Matthay, R. A., Loke, J., Marshall, R. C., Gottschalk, A., and Zaret, B. L.: Assessment of cardiac performance with quantitative radionuclide angiocardiography: Right ventricular ejection fraction with reference to findings in chronic obstructive pulmonary disease. Am. J. Cardiol. *41*:897, 1978.
90. Olvey, S. K., Redufo, L. A., Stevens, P. M., Deaton, W. J., and Miller, R. R.: First pass radionuclide assessment of right and left ventricular ejection fraction in chronic pulmonary disease. Effect of oxygen upon exercise response. Chest *78*:4, 1980.
91. Khaja, F., and Parker, J. D.: Right and left ventricular performance in chronic obstructive lung disease. Am. Heart J. *82*:319, 1971.
92. Stewart, R. I., and Lewis, C. M.: Cardiac output during exercise in patients with COPD. Chest *89*:199, 1986.
93. Samet, P., Fritts, H. W., Jr., Fishman, A. P., and Cournand, A.: The blood volume in heart disease. Medicine *36*:211, 1957.
94. Turino, G. M., Edelman, N. H., Richards, E. C., and Fishman, A. P.: Extravascular lung water in cor pulmonale. Bull. Physiol. Pathol. Respir. *4*:47, 1968.
95. Meerson, F. Z.: The myocardium in hyperfunction, hypertrophy, and heart failure. Circ. Res. *25*(Suppl. *2*):1, 1969.
96. Chidsey, C. A., Kaiser, G. A., Sonnenblick, E. H., Spann, J. F., and Braunwald, E.: Cardiac norepinephrine stores in experimental heart failure in the dog. J. Clin. Invest. *43*:2386, 1964.
97. Chandler, B. M., Sonnenblick, E. H., Spann, J. F., Jr., and Pool, P. E.: Association of depressed myofibrillar adenosine triphosphatase and reduced contractility in experimental heart failure. Circ. Res. *21*:717, 1967.
98. Kelly, D. T., Spotnitz, H. M., Beiser, G. D., Pierce, J. E., and Epstein, S. E.: Effects of chronic right ventricular volume and pressure loading on left ventricular performance. Circulation *44*:403, 1971.
99. Stool, E. W., Mullins, C. B., Leshin, S. J., and Mitchell, J. H.: Dimensional changes of the left ventricle during acute pulmonary arterial hypertension in dogs. Am. J. Cardiol. *33*:868, 1974.
100. Hecht, H. H., Kuida, H., and Tsagaris, T. J.: Brisket disease. IV. Impairment of left ventricular function in a form of cor pulmonale. Trans. Assoc. Am. Physicians *75*:263, 1962.
101. Fluck, D. C., Chandrasekar, R. G., and Gardner, F. U.: Left ventricular hypertrophy in chronic bronchitis. Br. Heart J. *28*:92, 1966.
102. Murphy, M. L., Adamson, J., and Hutcheson, F.: Left ventricular hypertrophy in patients with chronic bronchitis and emphysema. Ann. Intern. Med. *81*:307, 1974.
103. Rao, S. B., Cohn, K. E., Eldridge, F. L., and Hancock, E. W.: Left ventricular failure secondary to chronic pulmonary disease. Am. J. Med. *45*:229, 1968.
104. Jezek, V., and Schrijen, F.: Left ventricular function in chronic obstructive pulmonary disease with and without cardiac failure. Clin. Sci. Mol. Med. *45*:267, 1973.
105. Seibold, H., Roth, U., Lippert, R., Kohler, J., Wieshammer, S., Henze, E., and Stanch, M.: Left heart function in chronic obstructive lung disease. Klin. Wochenschr. *64*:433, 1986.
106. Frank, M. J., Weisser, A. B., Moschos, C. B., and Levinson, G. E.: Left ventricular function, metabolism, and blood flow in chronic cor pulmonale. Circulation *48*:798, 1973.
107. Williams, J. F., Childress, R. H., Boyd, D. L., Higgs, L. M., and Behnke, R. H.: Left ventricular function in patients with chronic obstructive pulmonary disease. J. Clin. Invest. *47*:1143, 1968.
108. Unger, K., Shaw, D., Karliner, J. S., Crawford, M., O'Rourke, R. A., and Moser, K. M.: Evaluation of left ventricular performance in acutely ill patients with chronic obstructive lung disease. Chest *68*:135, 1975.
109. Steele, P., Ellis, J. H., Jr., Van Dyke, D., Sutton, F., Creagh, E., and Davies, H.: Left ventricular ejection fraction in severe chronic obstructive airways disease. Am. J. Med. *59*:21, 1975.
110. Christianson, L. C., Shah, A., and Fisher, V. J.: Quantitative left ventricular cineangiography in patients with chronic obstructive pulmonary disease. Am. J. Med. *66*:399, 1979.
111. Gabinski, C., Courty, G., Besse, P., and Castaing, R.: Left ventricular function in chronic obstructive lung disease. Bull. Eur. Physiopathol. Resp. *15*:755, 1979.
111a. Rubin, L. J.: Clinical Evaluation. *In* Rubin, L. J. (ed.): Pulmonary Heart Disease. Boston, Martinus Nijhoff, 1984, p. 107.
111b. Murphy, M. L., and Bone, R. C.: Cor Pulmonale in Chronic Bronchitis and Emphysema. Mount Kisco, N.Y., Futura Publishing Co., 1984, 276 pp.
112. Slutsky, A., Hooper, W., Ackerman, W., Ashburn, W., Gerber, R., Moser, K., and Karliner, J.: Evaluation of left ventricular function in chronic pulmonary disease by exercise gated equilibrium radionuclide angiography. Am. Heart J. *101*:414, 1981.
113. Burrows, B., Fletcher, C. M., Heard, B. E., Jones, N. L., and Wootliff, S. S.: Emphysematous and bronchial types of chronic airways obstruction: Clinico-pathological study of patients in London and Chicago. Lancet *1*:830, 1966.
114. Mitchell, R. S., and Filley, G. F.: Chronic obstructive bronchopulmonary disease. I. Clinical features. Am. Rev. Respir. Dis. *89*:360, 1964.
115. Bishop, J. M., and Grass, K. W.: Use of other physiologic variables to predict pulmonary artery pressure in patients with chronic respiratory distress. Multicenter study. Eur. Heart J. *2*:509, 1981.
116. Venditho, M. A., Pisano, D., Simelans, J. P., and Dickerson, C. N.: The incidence of tricuspid valvular regurgitation in patients with severe chronic obstructive pulmonary disease as determined by two-dimensional echocardiography. JAMA *84*:264, 1984.
117. Flenley, D. C., and Muir, A. L.: Cardiovascular effects of oxygen therapy for pulmonary arterial hypertension. Clin. Chem. Med. *4*:297, 1983.
118. Douglas, N. J., Calvertey, P. M. A., Leggett, R. J. E., Brash, H. M., Flenley, D. C., and Brezinsua, V.: Transient hypoxemia during sleep in chronic bronchitis and emphysema. Lancet *1*:1, 1979.
119. Tinlapun, V. G., and Mir, M. A.: Nocturnal hypoxemia and associated electrocardiographic changes in patients with chronic obstructive airway disease. N. Engl. J. Med. *306*:125, 1982.
120. Ingram, R.: Chronic bronchitis, emphysema, and chronic airways obstruction. *In* Braunwald, E., et al. (eds.): Harrison's Principles of Internal Medicine. 11th ed. New York, McGraw-Hill Book Co., 1987, p. 1087.
121. Rubin, L. J., and Peter, R. H.: Therapy of Pulmonary Heart Disease. *In* Rubin, L. J. (ed.) Pulmonary Heart Disease. Boston, Martinus Nijhoff, 1984, p. 325.
122. McFadden, R. E., Jr.: Inhaled Aerosol Bronchodilators. Baltimore, Williams and Wilkins, 1986, p. 99.
123. Parker, J. O., Kelkar, K., and West, R. S.: Hemodynamic effects of aminophylline in cor pulmonale. Circulation *33*:17, 1966.
124. Matthay, R. A., Berger, H. J., Locke, J., Gottschalk, A., and Zaret, B. L.: Effect of aminophylline upon right and left ventricular performance in chronic obstructive pulmonary disease. Noninvasive assessment by radionuclide angiocardiography. Am. J. Med. *65*:903, 1978.
125. Burrows, B.: Arterial oxygenation and pulmonary hemodynamics in patients with chronic airways obstruction. (Proceedings of Conference on the Scientific Basis of Respiratory Therapy.) Am. Rev. Respir. Dis. *110*:64, 1974.
125a. Shepard, J. W., Garrison, M. W., Grithin, D. H., Evans, R., and Schweitzer, P. K.: Relationship of ventricular ectopy to nocturnal oxygen desaturation in patients with chronic obstructive pulmonary disease. Am. J. Med. *78*:28, 1985.
126. Morrison, D., Caldwell, J., Lakshminaryan, S., Ritchie, J. L., and Kennedy, J. W.: The acute effects of low flow oxygen and isosorbide dinitrate on left and right ventricular ejection fractions in chronic obstructive pulmonary disease. J. Am. Coll. Cardiol. *2*:652, 1983.
127. Nocturnal Oxygen Therapy Trial Group. Continuous or nocturnal oxygen therapy in hypoxemic chronic obstructive lung disease. A clinical trial. Ann. Intern. Med. *93*:391, 1980.
128. MRC Working Party: Long-term ancillary oxygen therapy in chronic hypoxic cor pulmonale complicating chronic bronchitis and emphysema. A clinical trial. Lancet *1*:681, 1981.
129. Rubin, L. J.: Cardiovascular effects of vasodilator therapy for pulmonary arterial hypertension. Clin. Chest. Med. *4*:309, 1983.
130. Lupi-Herrera, E., Bialostozky, D., and Sobrino, A.: The role of isoproterenol in pulmonary artery hypertension of unknown etiology. Chest *79*:292, 1981.
131. Ruskin, J., and Hutter, A. M.: Primary pulmonary hypertension treated with oral phentolamine. Ann. Intern. Med. *90*:772, 1979.
132. Klinke, W. P., and Gilbert, J. A. L.: Diazoxide in primary pulmonary hypertension. N. Engl. J. Med. *302*:91, 1980.
133. Vik-Mo, H., Walde, N., Jentoft, H., and Halvorsen, F. J.: Improved haemodynamics but reduced arterial blood oxygenation at rest and during exercise after long-term oral prazosin therapy in chronic cor pulmonale. Eur. Heart J. *6*:1047, 1985.
134. Rubin, L. J., Handel, F., and Peter, R. H.: The effects of oral hydralazine on right ventricular and diastolic pressure in patients with right ventricular failure. Circulation *65*:1369, 1982.
135. Brent, B. N., Berger, J., Matthay, R. A., Mahler, D., Pytlik, L., and Zaret, L.: Contrasting acute effects of vasodilators (nitroglycerin, nitroprusside and hydralazine) on right ventricular performance in patients with chronic obstructive pulmonary disease and pulmonary hypertension: A combined radionuclide-hemodynamic study. Am. J. Cardiol. *51*:1682, 1983.
136. Singh, H., Ebejer, M. J., Higgins, D. A., Henderson, A. H., and Campbell, I. A.: Acute haemodynamic effects of nifedipine at rest and during maximum exercise in patients with chronic cor pulmonale. Thorax *40*:910, 1985.
137. Crevey, B. J., Dantzker, D. R., Bower, J. S., Popat, K. D., and Walker, S. D.: Hemodynamic and gas exchange effects of intravenous diltiazem in patients with pulmonary hypertension. Am. J. Cardiol. *49*:578, 1982.
138. Simonneau, G., Escourrou, P., Duroux, P., and Lockhart, A.: Inhibition of hypoxic pulmonary vasoconstriction by nifedipine. N. Engl. J. Med. *304*:1582, 1981.

139. Rubin, L. J.: Cardiovascular Effects of Vasodilator Therapy for Pulmonary Arterial Hypertension. Clin. Chest Med. *4*:309, 1983.
140. Packer, M., Greenberg, B., Massiz, B., and Dash, H.: Deleterious effects of hydralazine in patients with pulmonary hypertension. N. Engl. J. Med. *306*:1326, 1982.
141. Dayton, L. M., McCullough, R. E., Scheinhorn, D. J., and Weil, J. V.: Symptomatic and pulmonary response to acute phlebotomy in secondary polycythemia. Chest *68*:785, 1975.
142. Rakita, L., Gillespie, D. G., and Sancetta, S. M.: The acute and chronic effects of phlebotomy on general hemodynamics and pulmonary function of patients with secondary polycythemia associated with pulmonary emphysema. Am. Heart J. *70*:466, 1965.
143. Wallis, P. J. W., Skehan, J. D., Newland, A. C., Wedzicha, J. A., Mills, P. G., and Empey, D. W.: Effect of erythropheresis on pulmonary hemodynamics and O_2 transport in patients with secondary polycythemia and cor pulmonale. Clin. Sci. *70*:91, 1986.
144. Erickson, A. D., Golden, W. R., Claunch, B. C., Donat, W. E., and Kaemmerlen, J. T.: Acute effects of phlebotomy on right ventricular size and performance in polycythemic patients with chronic obstructive pulmonary disease. Am. J. Cardiol. *52*:163, 1983.
145. Mathur, P. N., Powles, A. C. P., Pugsley, S. O., McEwan, M. P., and Campbell, E. J. M.: Effect of digoxin on right ventricular function in severe chronic airway obstruction. Ann. Intern. Med. *95*:283, 1981.
146. Sunderrajan, E. V., Byron, W. A., McKenzie, W. N., Hurst, D. J., Allegro, M. M., Thakur, V. M., and Holmes, R. A.: The effect of terbutaline on cardiac function in patients with stable chronic obstructive lung disease. JAMA *250*:2151, 1983.
147. Gottlieb, L. S., and Balchum, O. J.: Course of chronic obstructive pulmonary disease following first onset of respiratory failure. Chest *63*:5, 1973.
148. Stevens, P. M., Terplan, M., and Knowles, J. H.: Prognosis of cor pulmonale. N. Engl. J. Med. *269*:1289, 1963.
149. Burrows, B., and Earle, R. H.: Course and prognosis of chronic obstructive lung disease. A prospective study of 200 patients. N. Engl. J. Med. *280*:397, 1969.
150. Mitchell, R. S., Webb, N. C., and Filley, G. F.: Chronic obstructive lung disease. III. Factors influencing prognosis. Am. Rev. Respir. Dis. *89*:878, 1964.
151. Glauser, E. M., Cook, C. D., and Harris, C. B. C.: Bronchiectasis. A review of 187 cases in children with follow-up pulmonary function studies in 58. Acta Paediatr. Scand. (Suppl.) *165*:1, 1966.
152. Reid, L.: Reduction in bronchial subdivisions in bronchiectasis. Thorax *5*:233, 1950.
153. Colten, H. R.: Cystic fibrosis. *In* Braunwald, E., et al. (eds.): Harrison's Principles of Internal Medicine. 11th ed. New York, McGraw-Hill Book Co., 1987, p. 1085.
154. Moss, A. J.: The cardiovascular system in cystic fibrosis. Pediatrics *70*:728, 1982.
155. Moskowitz, W. B., Gewitz, M. H., Heyman, S., Ruddy, R. M., and Scanlin, T. F.: Cardiac involvement in cystic fibrosis: Early noninvasive detection and vasodilator therapy. Ped. Pharmacol. *5*:139, 1985.
156. Lester, L. A., Egge, A. C., Hubbard, V. S., Camerini-Otero, C. S., and Fink, R. J.: Echocardiography in cystic fibrosis: A proposed scoring system. J. Pediatr. *97*:742, 1980.
157. Ryland, D., and Reed, L.: The pulmonary circulation in cystic fibrosis. Thorax *30*:285, 1975.
157a. Benesova, D., Voriskova, M., Hrobonova, V., and Vavrova, V.: Cardiovascular complications of cystic fibrosis. Cesk. Pediatr. *38*:458, 1983.
158. Sahilahti, E., and Rapola, J.: Frequent myocardial lesions in Schwachman's syndrome. Eight fatal cases among 16 Finnish patients. Acta Paediatr. Scand. *73*:642, 1984.
159. Emirgil, C., Sobol, B. J., Herbert, W. H., and Trout, K.: The lesser circulation in pulmonary fibrosis secondary to sarcoidosis and its relationship to respiratory function. Chest *60*:371, 1971.
160. Enson, Y., Thomas, H. M., III, Bosken, C. H., Wood, J. A., LeRoy, E. C., Blanc, W. A., Wigger, H. J., and Harvey, R. M.: Pulmonary hypertension in interstitial lung disease: Relationship of vascular resistance to abnormal lung structure. Trans. Assoc. Am. Physicians *88*:248, 1975.
161. Irwin, R. S., Martinez-Gonzalez-Rio, J., Thomas, H. M., III, and Fritts, H. W., Jr.: The effect of granulomatous pulmonary disease in dogs on the response of the pulmonary circulation to hypoxia. J. Clin. Invest. *60*:1258, 1977.
162. Keltz, H.: The effect of respiratory muscle dysfunction on pulmonary function in patients with neuromuscular disease. Am. Rev. Respir. Dis. *91*:934, 1965.
163. Newsom Davis, J., Goldman, M., Loh, L., and Casson, M.: Diaphragm function and alveolar hypoventilation. Q. J. Med. *45*:87, 1976.
164. Glenn, W. W. L., Holcomb, W. C., Hogan, J., Matano, I., Gee, J. B. L., Motoyama, E. K., Kim, C. S., Poirier, R. S., and Forbes G.: Diaphragm pacing by radiofrequency transmission in the treatment of chronic ventilatory insufficiency: Present status. J. Thorac. Cardiovasc. Surg. *66*:505, 1973.
165. Aubier, M., DeTroyer, A., Sampson, M., Macklem, P. T., and Roussos, C.: Aminophylline improves diaphragmatic contractility. N. Engl. J. Med. *305*:249, 1981.
166. Chandler, K. W., Rozas, C. J., Kory, R. C., and Goldman, A. L.: Bilateral diaphragmatic paralysis complicating local cardiac hypothermia during open heart surgery. Am. J. Med. *77*:243, 1984.
167. Bergofsky, E. H.: Respiratory failure in disorders of the thoracic cage. Am. Rev. Respir. Dis. *119*:643, 1979.
168. Bergofsky, E. H., Turino, G. M., and Fishman, A. P.: Cardiorespiratory failure in kyphoscoliosis. Medicine *38*:263, 1959.
169. Bjure, J., Grimby, G., Kasalicky, J., Lindh, M., and Nachemson, A.: Respiratory impairment and airway closure in patients with untreated idiopathic scoliosis. Thorax *25*:451, 1970.
170. Davies, G., and Reid, L.: Effect of scoliosis on growth of alveoli and pulmonary arteries and on the right ventricle. Arch. Dis. Child. *46*:623, 1971.
171. Westgate, H. D., and Moe, J. H.: Pulmonary function in kyphoscoliosis before and after correction by the Harrington instrumentation method. J. Bone Joint Surg. *51*:935, 1969.
172. Burwell, C. S., Robin, E. D., Whaley, R. D., and Bickelman, A. G.: Extreme obesity associated with alveolar hypoventilation—A Pickwickian syndrome. Am. J. Med. *21*:811, 1956.
173. Rochester, D. F., and Enson, Y.: Current concepts in the pathogenesis of the obesity-hypoventilation syndrome. Am. J. Med. *57*:402, 1974.
174. Weil, J. V.: Pulmonary hypertension and cor pulmonale in hypoventilating patients. *In* Weir, E. K., and Reeves, J. T. (eds.): Pulmonary Hypertension. Mount Kisco, N.Y., Futura Publishing Co., 1984, p. 321.
175. Lyons, H. A., and Huang, C. T.: Therapeutic use of progesterone in alveolar hypoventilation associated with obesity. Am. J. Med. *44*:881, 1968.
176. Sutton, F. D., Zwillich, C. W., Creagh, C. E., Pierson, D. J., and Weil, J. V.: Progesterone for outpatient treatment of pickwickian syndrome. Ann. Intern. Med. *83*:476, 1975.
177. Cherniack, N. S.: Respiratory dysrhythmias during sleep. N. Engl. J. Med. *305*:325, 1981.
178. Strohl, K. P., Cherniack, N. S., and Gather, B.: Physiologic basis of therapy in sleep apnea. Ann. Rev. Respir. Dis. *134*:791, 1986.
179. Burrek, B.: The hypersomnia-sleep apnea syndrome: Its recognition in clinical cardiology. Am. Heart J. *107*:543, 1984.
180. Guilleminault, C., Cannally, S. J., and Winkler, R. A.: Cardiac arrhythmia and conduction disturbances during sleep in 400 patients with sleep apnea syndrome. Am. J. Cardiol. *52*:490, 1983.
180a. Peiser, J., Ovnat, A., Uwyyed, K., Lavie, P., and Charuzi, I.: Cardiac arrhythmias during sleep in morbidly obese sleep-apneic patients before and after gastric bypass surgery. Clin. Cardiol. *8*:519, 1985.
181. Buda, A. J., Schroeder, J. S., and Guilleminault, C.: Abnormalities of pulmonary wedge pressures in sleep-induced apnea. Int. J. Cardiol. *1*:67, 1981.
182. Glenn, W. W. L., Gee, J. B. L., Cole, D. R., Farmer, W. C., Shaw, R. K., and Beckman, C. B.: Combined central alveolar hypoventilation and upper airway obstruction. Treatment by tracheostomy and diaphragm pacing. Am. J. Med. *64*:50, 1978.
183. Martin, R. J., Sanders, M. H., Gray, B. A., and Pennock, B. E.: Acute and long-term ventilatory effects of hyperoxia in the adult sleep apnea syndrome. Am. Rev. Respir. Dis. *125*:175, 1982.
184. Mellins, R. B., Balfour, H. H., Jr., Turino, G. M., and Winters, R. W.: Failure of automatic control of ventilation (Ondine's curse). Medicine *49*:487, 1970.
185. Penaloza, D., and Sime, F.: Circulatory dynamics during high altitude pulmonary edema. Am. J. Cardiol. *23*:369, 1969.
186. Penaloza, D., and Sime, F.: Chronic cor pulmonale due to loss of altitude acclimatization (chronic mountain sickness). Am. J. Med. *50*:728, 1971.
187. Severinghaus, J. W., Bainton, C. R., and Carcelen, A.: Respiratory insensitivity to hypoxia in chronically hypoxic man. Respir. Physiol. *1*:308, 1966.
188. Bland, J. W., Edwards, F. K., and Brainsfield, D.: Pulmonary hypertension and congestive heart failure in children with chronic upper airway obstruction. New concepts and etiologic factors. Am. J. Cardiol. *23*:830, 1969.
189. Noonan, J. A.: Pulmonary heart disease. Pediatr. Clin. North Am. *18*:1255, 1971.
190. Johnson, G. M., and Todd, D. W.: Cor pulmonale in severe Pierre Robin syndrome. Pediatrics *65*:152, 1980.
191. Ingram, R. H., Jr., and Bishop, J. B.: Ventilatory response to carbon dioxide after removal of chronic upper airway obstruction. Am. Rev. Respir. Dis. *102*:645, 1970.
192. Williams, M. H., Jr., Adler, J. J., and Colp, C.: Pulmonary function studies as an aid in the differential diagnosis of pulmonary hypertension. Am. J. Med. *47*:378, 1969.
193. McGowan, F. X., and Wagner, G. S.: The Electrocardiogram in Chronic Lung Disease. *In* Rubin, L. J. (ed.): Pulmonary Heart Disease. Boston, Martinus Nijhoff, 1984, p. 117.
194. Goodwin, J. F., and Abdin, Z. N.: The cardiogram of congenital and acquired right ventricular hypertrophy. Br. Heart J. *21*:523, 1959.
195. Phillips, R. W.: The electrocardiogram in cor pulmonale secondary to pulmonary emphysema: A study of 18 cases proved by autopsy. Am. Heart J. *56*:352, 1958.
196. Kilcoyne, M. M., Davis, A. L., and Ferrer, M. I.: A dynamic electrocardiographic concept useful in the diagnosis of cor pulmonale. Circulation *42*:903, 1970.
197. Holford, F. D.: The electrocardiogram in lung diseases. *In* Fishman, A. P. (ed.): Pulmonary Diseases and Disorders. New York, McGraw-Hill Book Co., 1980, p. 139.
198. Kok-Jensen, A.: Simple electrocardiographic features of importance for prognosis in severe chronic bronchial obstruction. Scand. J. Respir. Dis. *56*:273, 1975.
199. Wilson, J. R., Mason, U. G., Bahler, R. C., Chester, E. H., Picken, J. J., and Baum, G. L.: Vectorcardiographic detection of early hemodynamic abnormalities in chronic obstructive pulmonary disease. Chest *76*:160, 1979.
200. Starling, M. R., Crawford, M. H., Sorensen, S. G., and O'Rourke, R. A.: A new two-dimensional echocardiographic technique for evaluating right ventricular size and performance in patients with obstructive lung disease. Circulation *66*:612, 1982.
201. Shuk, J. W., Walder, J., Oetgen, W., and Thomas, H. M.: Right ventricular visualization by thallium 201 myocardial scintigraphy in chronic obstructive pulmonary disease. South. Med. J. *78*:1435, 1985.

PART IV BROADER PERSPECTIVES ON HEART DISEASE AND CARDIOLOGIC PRACTICE

49 GENETICS AND CARDIOVASCULAR DISEASE

by JOSEPH L. GOLDSTEIN, M.D., and MICHAEL S. BROWN, M.D.

GENERAL PRINCIPLES OF CARDIOVASCULAR GENETICS

As with diseases affecting other body systems, genetic factors play a significant role in the pathogenesis of most diseases of the heart. In some disorders, such as the Marfan syndrome and familial hypercholesterolemia, the genetic effects are relatively clearly discernible and easy to analyze. In other diseases, such as most forms of congenital heart disease, the role of hereditary factors, although demonstrable, is less clear-cut, and the fundamental genetic mechanisms remain obscure.

In this chapter, the general principles of hereditary disease as they apply to the major forms of heart disease are first reviewed. This is followed by a discussion of those disorders of the cardiovascular system for which a clear-cut genetic etiology has been demonstrated. In discussing a disorder, the major emphasis has been placed on the genetic aspects rather than on the clinical features, which are discussed elsewhere in this book.

MOLECULAR BASIS OF GENE EXPRESSION. All hereditary information is transmitted from parent to offspring through the inheritance of deoxyribonucleic acid (DNA). *DNA* is a linear polymer composed of purine and pyrimidine bases, the sequence of which ultimately determines the sequence of amino acids in every protein molecule made by the body. The four types of bases in DNA are arranged in groups of three, each group forming a code word or codon that signifies a particular amino acid. A *gene* represents the sequence of bases in DNA that codes for the amino acid sequence of a single polypeptide chain of a protein molecule.[1] The gene is the basic unit of heredity that is transmitted to each offspring during the formation of sperm and ova. Each gene contains the coding information that specifies the sequence of amino acids in one protein chain (for review, see reference 1). It is estimated that the amount of DNA in the nucleus of each human cell is sufficient to code for 100,000 proteins. The genes are arranged in linear sequence organized into rod-shaped bodies called *chromosomes.* Each human cell contains 46 chromosomes, arranged in 23 pairs, one member of each pair having been derived from each of the individual's parents. Thus, each individual inherits two copies of each chromosome and hence two copies of each gene. The site at which a gene is located on a particular chromosome is termed the *genetic locus.* When a gene occupying a genetic locus exists in two or more different forms, these alternate forms of the gene are referred to as *alleles.*

A given gene always resides at a specified genetic locus on one particular chromosome. For example, the genetic locus for the human Rh blood group is on chromosome No. 1; at this chromosomal site in each individual there are two Rh genes, one on chromosome No. 1 derived from the mother and the other on chromosome No. 1 derived from the father. When both genes at the same genetic locus are identical, the individual is a *homozygote.* When the two genes differ (i.e., two alleles are present at the locus), the individual is a *heterozygote.* Each individual is homozygous at some loci and heterozygous at others.

Considerable progress has been made in recent years in delineating the human gene map. The chromosomal location of more than 750 genes is now known.[2]

MUTATION AS THE ORIGIN OF GENETIC DISEASE. A *mutation* is a stable, heritable alteration in DNA. Although the causes of mutation in human beings are largely unknown, a variety of environmental agents, such as radiation, viruses, and chemicals, are among the factors that are implicated.

Mutations can involve a visible alteration in the structure of a chromosome, such as a deletion or translocation of a portion of a chromosome, or they can involve a minute change in one of the purine or pyrimidine bases of a single gene. Most commonly, such "point" mutations consist of the substitution of one base for another, thus changing the meaning of the codon containing that base; hence, their designation as *missense mutations.* Of all of the human mutations so far elucidated, the vast majority involve such single-base changes. These missense mutations cause the substitution of one amino acid for another in the protein specified by the mutant gene. Such substitution can have little effect on the function of the protein, or it can totally eliminate all function. If the protein that is involved happens to be an enzyme, the loss of function may produce a metabolic disease.

CELLULAR MECHANISM BY WHICH MUTANT GENES PRODUCE DISEASES. Critical to the modern understanding of heredity is the concept that the only information transmitted from generation to generation is the sequence of bases in DNA and that these sequences, in turn, specify only the primary structure of RNA and protein molecules. All other chemical reactions within a cell—such as the synthesis of complex lipids and carbohydrates, the formation of membranes and other cellular organelles, the accumulation and partitioning of inorganic ions, and so on—occur as a secondary consequence of the action of specific proteins. Many of these proteins are enzymes that catalyze the biochemical conversion of one molecule into another. Others are structural proteins, such as collagen and elastin, and still others are regulatory proteins that dictate how much of each enzyme and each structural protein is to be made.

Since proteins are the cellular molecules the structures of which are encoded by genes, mutations in genes exert their deleterious effects by altering the structure of enzymes, structural proteins, or regulatory proteins. Thus, in a disease like Pompe disease (Type II glycogen storage disease) (see p. 1013), massive accumulation of glycogen in the heart is due not to a primary structural abnormality in the polysaccharide glycogen but to a structural abnormality in a protein, acid maltase, a lysosomal enzyme that is required to degrade glycogen.

GENETIC HETEROGENEITY. This exists when two or more mutations can produce a similar clinical syndrome. It is now believed that most, if not all, hereditary diseases, when carefully analyzed, will be shown to be genetically heterogeneous.[3]

Genetic heterogeneity may result from the existence of mutations at a single genetic locus (allelic mutations) or from mutations at different genetic loci (nonallelic mutations). In some cases of heterogeneity, not merely does the genetic locus differ but the mode of inheritance will also differ. For example, atrial septal defect can be inherited by an autosomal dominant mechanism in some families and by a multifactorial mechanism in other families.

CATEGORIES OF GENETIC DISORDERS AFFECTING THE CARDIOVASCULAR SYSTEM

Genetic diseases of the cardiovascular system, like all genetic disorders, generally fall into one of three categories:

1. *Chromosomal disorders* involve the lack, excess, or abnormal arrangement of one or more chromosomes, producing excessive or deficient genetic material and affecting many genes.
2. *Mendelian* or *single-gene disorders* are determined primarily by a single mutant gene that is transmitted to offspring in a predictable way. As a result, these disorders display simple (mendelian) inheritance patterns which can be classified into autosomal dominant, autosomal recessive, or X-linked types.
3. *Multifactorial disorders* are caused by an interaction of multiple genes and multiple exogenous or environmental factors. Although many of these multifactorial disorders, such as coronary artery disease (CAD) and most types of congenital heart disease, "run in families," the inheritance pattern is complex and unpredictable. In general, the risk to relatives is much less than that seen in the single-gene disorders. As discussed below, each of these three categories of genetic disease presents different problems with respect to causation, prevention, diagnosis, genetic counseling, and treatment.

CHROMOSOMAL DISORDERS

As noted, the number of chromosomes in normal individuals is 46, of which 44 represent the 22 pairs of *autosomes* and the other 2 are the *sex chromosomes.* Females have 2 X chromosomes (XX) and males have 1 X chromosome and 1 Y chromosome (XY). Each of the 22 pairs of autosomes and the 2 sex chromosomes can be identified microscopically on the basis of size, location of the centromere (which divides the chromosome into arms of equal or unequal length), and the unique banding pattern (which is determined after treatment with special dyes and proteolytic enzymes).

Of the two most common chromosomal disorders causing heart disease, one results from an extra chromosome and the other results from a deficiency of one chromosome. Trisomy 21 (Down syndrome or mongolism) is characterized by the presence of three rather than two copies of chromosome 21, and the common form of Turner syndrome is characterized by the presence of one X chromosome rather than two X's or an X and a Y. The abnormality in both of these disorders appears to arise through *nondisjunction*, either during meiosis in one parent (i.e., in spermatogenesis or oogenesis) or in the first mitotic cleavage of the zygote. In meiotic nondisjunction, a pair of chromosomes does not separate normally so that both members of the pair (or none) pass into one gamete. When an additional copy of the chromosome is added during fertilization, three copies of the same chromosome (or only one) are in the new zygote instead of the pair found in normal persons.

The detected frequency of chromosomal aberrations among unselected newborn infants is 1 in 200 (0.5 per cent), whereas among first trimester spontaneous abortions the frequency of chromosomal defects is as high as 50 per cent. Thus, the vast majority of chromosomal abnormalities are lost in early fetal life. In most instances chromosomal disorders occur as new mutations; both parents are usually normal, and the risk of recurrence to relatives is usually low.

SINGLE-GENE DISORDERS

Disorders caused by the transmission of a single mutant gene show one of three simple (or mendelian) patterns of inheritance: (1) autosomal dominant, (2) autosomal recessive, or (3) X-linked. The distinction between "dominant" and "recessive" must be understood as one of convenience in pedigree analysis rather than as necessarily implying a fundamental difference in genetic mechanism. The term *dominant* implies that a mutation will be clinically manifest when an individual has a single dose of this mutation (or is *heterozygous* for it), whereas the term *recessive* implies that a double dose (or *homozygosity*) is required for clinical detection. Genes themselves are never dominant or recessive; their effects, however, produce clinical patterns that are classified as dominant or recessive.

The demonstration that a particular syndrome shows one of the three mendelian patterns of inheritance implies that its pathogenesis, no matter how complex, is due to an abnormality in a single protein molecule. For example, in the Marfan syndrome (pp. 1630 and 1727), all the clinical manifestations, which include such seemingly unrelated disturbances as ectopia lentis, scoliosis, arachnodactyly, and dissecting aneurysm, are the physiological consequences of a single abnormal protein that is encoded by a single abnormal gene. In many mendelian disorders, especially in those with dominant inheritance, it is not yet possible to demonstrate directly the protein that is primarily altered by the mutation. In such cases, only the distal physiological effects of the mutation are recognizable. Nevertheless, it is safe to assume that a single primary defect exists whenever a disease is transmitted by a single gene mechanism and that the various manifestations of the disease can all be related to the mutational event by a more or less complicated "pedigree of causes."

AUTOSOMAL DOMINANT DISORDERS. Dominant diseases are those manifest in the heterozygous state, i.e., when only one abnormal gene (*mutant allele*) is present and the corresponding partner allele on the homologous chromosome is normal. The gene responsible for an autosomal dominant disorder is located on 1 of the 22 autosomes; thus, both males and females can be affected. Since alleles segregate independently at meiosis, there is a one in two chance that the offspring of an affected heterozygote will inherit the mutant allele and, similarly, a one in two chance of his or her inheriting the normal allele.

The following features are characteristic of autosomal dominant inheritance: (1) Each affected individual has an affected parent (unless the condition arose by a new mutation in the individual or is mildly expressed in the affected parent); (2) an affected individual will bear, on the average, both normal and affected offspring in equal proportions; (3) normal children of an affected individual will have only normal offspring; (4) men and women are affected in equal proportion; (5) each sex is equally likely to transmit the condition to male and female offspring, with male-to-male transmission occurring; and (6) vertical transmission of the condition through successive generations occurs, especially when the trait does not impair reproductive capacity.

Although half the offspring of an individual with an autosomal dominant condition will inherit the disease, it is not necessarily true that each affected person must have an affected parent. In every autosomal dominant disease a certain proportion of affected persons owe the disorder to a new mutation rather than to an inherited mutation. The parent in whose germ cells the new mutation arose will be clinically normal. Likewise, the siblings of the affected individual will be normal, since the mutation will affect only a single germ cell. However, the affected individual will transmit the disease and half of his or her children will be affected.

The proportion of patients with dominant disorders who represent new mutations is inversely proportional to the effect of the disease on *biological fitness*. Biological fitness refers to the ability of an affected individual to produce children who survive to adult life and reproduce. In the extreme case, if a dominant mutation produces absolute infertility, then all observed cases would of necessity represent new mutations, and it would be impossible to prove the genetic transmission of the trait. In less severe disorders, as in the Marfan syndrome, the cardiac disease reduces biological fitness to about 85 per cent of normal, and the proportion of cases due to new mutations is about 15 per cent.

Before it is concluded that a dominant disorder in a given patient with unaffected parents is the result of a new mutation, two other considerations are important: (1) the possibility that the gene may be carried by one parent in whom the disease is of low expressivity (discussed below), and (2) the possibility that extramarital paternity may have occurred, which is found in about 3 to 5 per cent of randomly studied children in the United States.

Most autosomal dominant disorders show two characteristic features that are not usually seen in recessive syndromes: (1) *delayed age of onset*, and (2) *variability in clinical expression*. Delayed age of onset is seen in such disorders as myotonic dystrophy (p. 1787) and hypertrophic obstructive cardiomyopathy (p. 1418). These disorders typically do not become manifest clinically until adult life, even though the mutant gene is present from the time of conception. Variability in clinical expression is illustrated dramatically by the Holt-Oram syndrome (discussed below). Patients in the same family inheriting the same abnormal gene may have any one of the following:

(1) atrial septal defect and a skeletal abnormality of the upper extremity, (2) only atrial septal defect, or (3) only a skeletal abnormality of the upper extremity. This diversity in clinical manifestations makes it difficult to recognize that each family member suffers from the same genetic abnormality.

Since dominant mutations involve a type of gene product that in a 50 per cent deficiency is capable of producing clinical symptoms in heterozygotes, the responsible mutations are likely to involve abnormalities in two classes of proteins: (1) those that regulate complex metabolic pathways, such as membrane receptors and rate-limiting enzymes in pathways under feedback control, and (2) key structural proteins, such as those involved in connective tissue formation. At present, however, the basic biochemical defects have been identified in only a handful of the known autosomal dominant disorders.

Examples of autosomal dominant disorders that involve the cardiovascular system include the Holt-Oram syndrome, the Noonan syndrome, the Marfan syndrome, hypertrophic obstructive cardiomyopathy, and familial hypercholesterolemia.

AUTOSOMAL RECESSIVE DISORDERS. Autosomal recessive conditions are clinically apparent only in the homozygous state, i.e., when both alleles at a particular genetic locus are mutant alleles. The gene responsible for an autosomal recessive disorder is located on 1 of the 22 autosomes; thus, both men and women can be affected.

The following features are characteristic of autosomal recessive inheritance: (1) the parents are clinically normal; (2) only siblings are affected and vertical transmission does not occur; and (3) men and women are affected in equal proportions.

The relative infrequency of recessive genes in the population and the requirement that two abnormal genes be present for clinical expression combine to create special conditions for autosomal recessive inheritance: (1) If a husband and a wife are both carriers for the same autosomal recessive gene, 25 per cent of the children will be normal, 50 per cent will be heterozygous carriers, and 25 per cent will be homozygous and affected with the disease; (2) if an affected individual marries a heterozygote (as may occur with consanguineous marriage), half the children will be affected, and a pedigree simulating dominant inheritance would result; (3) if two individuals with the same recessive disease marry, all of their children will be affected; and (4) the more infrequent the mutant gene in the population, the stronger the likelihood that affected individuals will be the product of consanguineous matings.

In general, consanguinity is an infrequent finding clinically in most families with recessive diseases in the United States. This is because the background rate for consanguinity in the general population is very low. Thus, in most of the United States (as opposed to areas with relative geographical isolation, such as northern Norway, Switzerland, and so on), a disorder must be extremely rare before it is associated with an important frequency of consanguinity. For example, consanguinity is expected in a large proportion of families having children with very rare disorders such as the Kartagener syndrome and mulibrey nanism.

The clinical picture in autosomal recessive disorders tends to be more uniform than that of dominant diseases, and onset often occurs early in life. As a general rule, recessive disorders are more commonly diagnosed in children, whereas dominant diseases are more frequently encountered in adults.

Inasmuch as only one of four children in a sibship is expected to be affected with a recessive disease, multiple cases in a family may not occur. This is especially true in a society in which small families are common. Consider, for example, 16 families in which both parents are heterozygous for the same recessive disorder. If each family has 2 children, 9 of the families will have no affected children, 6 will have 1 affected and 1 normal child, and only 1 of the 16 families will have 2 affected children. Thus, in the United States, physicians will usually see sporadic or isolated cases of a recessive disorder without an affected sibling to alert them to the possibility of a genetic etiology. Fortunately, because of the relatively uniform clinical picture of recessive disorders and because most can be diagnosed by biochemical tests, the correct diagnosis can usually be made even when no other members of a family are clinically affected.

The basic biochemical lesions underlying many autosomal recessive disorders have been identified. Of the three types of proteins in which mutations could occur (i.e., enzymes, structural proteins, and regulatory proteins), the most easy to study have been the enzymes. A mutation that destroys the catalytic activity of an enzyme generally does not impair the health of a heterozygote (i.e., an individual who has one mutant allele specifying a functionless enzyme and one normal allele on the partner chromosome specifying a normal enzyme). In this situation each cell in the body usually produces about 50 per cent of the normal number of active enzyme molecules. However, metabolic regulatory mechanisms avert any clinical consequences of this 50 per cent deficiency, and so heterozygotes are usually clinically normal. On the other hand, when an individual inherits functionless alleles at both loci specifying an enzyme, the reduction in enzyme activity is too great for any compensatory mechanism to overcome, and a disease results. Thus, heterozygotes for homocystinuria, in which patients have half the normal activity of cystathionine synthase, are clinically asymptomatic because the body compensates for the half-normal level of the enzyme by raising the homocystine concentration approximately twofold. Under these conditions a normal amount of homocystine can be metabolized and no symptoms occur. On the other hand, the homozygote for homocystinuria has such a severe reduction in cystathionine synthase activity that enormous levels accumulate within the blood and tissues, causing thrombotic events at a young age.

Examples of autosomal recessive disorders involving the heart include Pompe disease (pp. 1013 and 1632), the Kartagener syndrome (p. 1628), homocystinuria, and the Jervell and Lange-Nielsen syndrome (p. 1635).

X-LINKED DISORDERS. The genes responsible for one class of disorders are located on the X chromosome, and thus the clinical risk and severity of the disease are different for the two sexes. Since a woman has two X chromosomes, she may be either heterozygous or homozygous for the mutant gene, and the trait may therefore demonstrate either recessive or dominant expression. Men, on the other hand, have only one X chromosome, so they can be expected to display the full syndrome whenever they inherit the gene, regardless of whether the gene behaves as a recessive or as a dominant trait in a woman. Thus, the terms *X-linked dominant* or *X-linked recessive* refer only to the expression of the gene in women.

An important feature of all X-linked inheritance is the absence of male-to-male (i.e., father-to-son) transmission of the trait. This follows from the fact that a man must always contribute his Y chromosome to his sons; hence, he can never contribute his X chromosome. On the other hand, a man contributes his X chromosome to all of his daughters.

The characteristic features of X-linked recessive inheritance are as follows: (1) In contrast to the vertical transmission in dominant traits (parents and children affected) and the horizontal transmission in autosomal recessive traits (siblings affected), the pedigree pattern in X-linked recessive traits tends to be oblique because of the occurrence of the trait in the sons of normal carrier sisters of affected males (uncles and nephews affected); (2) male offspring of carrier women have a 50 per cent chance of being affected; (3) all female offspring of affected males are carriers; (4) affected males do not transmit the trait to any offspring; and (5) affected homozygous females occur only when an affected male marries a carrier female.

Examples of X-linked recessive disorders involving the heart include Duchenne muscular dystrophy (p. 1782), Fabry disease (p. 1434), and the Hunter syndrome (p. 1729).

MULTIFACTORIAL GENETIC DISEASES

Most of the common diseases of the heart, such as coronary artery disease and congenital heart disease, have long been known to "run in families." They fit best into the category of *multifactorial genetic diseases*. The genetic element in these disorders rarely manifests itself in an all-or-none fashion as it does in the single-gene disorders and in chromosomal aberrations. Instead, the interaction of multiple genes with multiple environmental factors produces the familial aggregation.[4]

In the multifactorial genetic diseases, there is a *polygenic component* consisting of multiple genes that interact in a cumulative fashion. An individual inheriting the right combination of these genes passes beyond a "threshold of risk," at which point an *environmental component* determines whether or not and to what extent he or she is clinically affected. For another individual in the same family to express the same syndrome, he must inherit the same or a very similar combination of genes. Since the first-degree relatives of an affected individual (i.e., parents, siblings, and offspring) each share half his genes, they are all at increased risk of exhibiting the same polygenic syndrome. Second-degree relatives (uncles, aunts, and grandparents) share on the average one-fourth of an individual's genes $(1/2)^2$, and third-degree relatives (cousins) share one-eighth $(1/2)^3$. Thus, as the degree of relation becomes more distant, the likelihood of a relative inheriting the same combination of genes becomes less. Moreover, the chance of any relative inheriting the right combination of risk genes decreases as the number of genes required for the expression of a given trait increases.

Since the precise number of genes responsible for polygenic traits is unknown, one cannot calculate the precise risk of inheritance for a relative of an affected individual. Rather, one must rely on empirical risk figures (i.e., a direct tally of the proportion of affected relatives in previously reported families). In contrast to the single-gene disorders, in which 25 or 50 per cent of the first-degree relatives of an affected proband are at genetic risk, multifactorial genetic disorders generally affect no more than 5 to 10 per cent of first-degree relatives. Moreover, in contrast to mendelian traits, the recurrence risk of multifactorial conditions varies from family to family, and its estimation is significantly influenced by two factors: (1) the number of affected persons already present in the family, and (2) the severity of the disorder in the index case. The larger the number of affected relatives and the more severe their disease, the higher the risk to other relatives.

The hypothesis of a polygenic component in the inheritance of multifactorial diseases has been given a sound basis in recent years by the demonstration that at least one-third of all gene loci harbor different alleles that vary among individuals. Such a large degree of variation in normal genes, such as those that specify blood groups and the HLA system, undoubtedly provides the substratum for variations in genetic predisposition with which environmental factors can interact. Such variation among a normal gene is termed a *polymorphism*. An important observation of recent years has been the finding that certain alleles at the HLA loci predispose individuals to certain specific diseases. For example, if one inherits the B-27 allele at the HLA-B locus, one has a 120-fold greater chance for developing ankylosing spondylitis than an individual who lacks this allele. Ankylosing spondylitis remains a multifactorial disease, however, because its development clearly requires one or more other factors in addition to the B-27 allele. Thus, fewer than 15 per cent of people who inherit this allele develop this disease.

Multifactorial disorders are heterogeneous in the sense that the relative contribution of the polygenic factors ("risk genes") and environmental factors to the etiology will vary greatly from patient to patient. However, it is important to remember that among common phenotypes that are largely multifactorial, there will often be a small proportion in whom the phenotype is created by major mutant genes. For example, although coronary artery disease is usually of multifactorial etiology, about 5 per cent of subjects with premature myocardial infarctions are heterozygotes for familial hypercholesterolemia, a single-gene disorder that produces atherosclerosis in the absence of any other predisposing factor.[5] Similarly, in a small proportion of patients with other common cardiovascular diseases such as atrial septal defect, the condition is not multifactorial but determined by a single gene, as in the Holt-Oram syndrome.

GENE ACTION AND THE CARDIOVASCULAR SYSTEM

The existence of a gene affecting a specific cardiac function is frequently inferred from genetic analysis of pedigrees showing mendelian inheritance of a heart disorder. The function of the gene is deduced by analysis of the defect produced in family members who carry a mutant allele. Since at least 50 simply inherited disorders of the heart and vasculature are currently recognized (composing about 5 per cent of all mendelian disorders currently known to exist in humans),[6] there must be at least 50 genes and hence 50 protein molecules that affect cardiac function in a major way. Mutation of these genes produces cardiac dysfunction, which can be manifest clinically at several levels, including congenital cardiac malformations, derangement of the connective tissue elements of the heart and vascular system, cardiomyopathies, cardiac arrhythmias and conduction defects, pericarditis, cardiac tumors, and coronary artery disease. The nature of the proteins specified by these 50 critical genes is generally unknown.

The single-gene–determined disorders of the heart may potentially provide investigative models for unraveling the complexities of cardiovascular physiology and biochemistry. Most significant has been the use of the familial hypercholesterolemia syndrome to delineate a mechanism by which human cholesterol metabolism is regulated.[7] Inasmuch as several mendelian disorders that affect cardiac muscle structure (such as hypertrophic obstructive cardiomyopathy) are now recognized, it is predictable that the elucidation of the basic defect in each of them will provide biochemical information necessary to define the basis of human structural abnormalities, such as cardiac hypertrophy.

GENETIC COUNSELING IN CARDIOLOGY

THE FAMILY HISTORY

When caring for a patient with a possible genetic disorder involving the heart, the physician begins by taking a careful *family history* and by carrying out a *family evaluation.* The first step involves obtaining certain information on the *proband* or *index case* (i.e., the clinically affected person who has brought the family to attention) and on each of the patient's *first-degree relatives* (i.e., the parents, sibs, and offspring of the proband). This information includes the given name, surname, and maiden name; birth date or current age; age at death, whether an autopsy was performed, and cause of death; and presence of any disease or defect. Ideally, the family history should also include the name and address of the individuals' physicians and the hospitals to which they were admitted.

The second step includes asking six questions designed to survey the family for the presence of disease:

1. Is there any relative with an identical or similar trait?
2. Is there any relative with a trait that is absent in the proband but that is known to occur in some patients with the same disease? This question requires that the physician have some knowledge about the manifestations of the disease in question. For example, when obtaining the family history from a proband with dissecting aneurysm possibly caused by the Marfan syndrome, one should ask about the occurrence of eye abnormalities, cardiac abnormalities, and skeletal abnormalities in the proband's relatives.
3. Is there any relative with a trait that is recognized to be genetically determined? The purpose of this question is to ascertain the occurrence of hereditary disease in the family even though the patients may not consider themselves to be involved.
4. Is there any relative with an unusual disease, or has any relative died of a rare condition? The purpose of this question is to identify a condition that might be genetically determined though not recognized as such by the patient. In addition, this question may help to identify conditions in relatives that might be etiologically related to the patient's problem. For example, a patient with a cardiac tumor should be suspected of having underlying tuberous sclerosis if he or she has a brother with adenoma sebaceum and mental retardation, both of which can be manifestations of the tuberous sclerosis gene.
5. Is there any consanguinity in the family? Not only should this inquiry be made directly, but, in addition, one should ask whether common last names appear in the families of husband and wife. Consanguineous marriage may be the source of a rare autosomal recessive syndrome, such as Pompe disease, and sometimes its presence in the family may not be known by the proband.
6. What is the ethnic origin of the family? Persons of certain ethnic origins have an increased chance of certain genetic diseases. Mulibrey nanism (p. 1620) is one example of a familial heart disease that occurs with increased frequency in a specific ethnic group, the Finns.

The third step involves an examination of available family members, both those affected and those believed to be unaffected.

RETROSPECTIVE GENETIC COUNSELING

The prevention of hereditary cardiac diseases requires the identification of matings that are capable of producing defective offspring. These may be matings in which one of the two individuals is carrying a dominant or X-linked gene mutation or matings in which both individuals are carriers of a deleterious recessive gene. Such individuals are usually identified through an affected child or near relative, in which case retrospective genetic counseling can be provided.

When advising family members about the risk of transmitting a disorder that has already affected someone in the family, the first step is to be certain of the *correct diagnosis*—in particular, to make certain that the problem in question is really of genetic origin. This is especially important in cardiac disorders that may have both genetic and nongenetic causes. For example, some cases of patent ductus arteriosus are caused by a multifactorial genetic mechanism, whereas others are caused by rubella (p. 897). Second, if the disease has a hereditary element, one must consider the possibility of *genetic heterogeneity*, a situation in which clinically similar genetic disorders show varying patterns of inheritance. For example, there are two types of atrial septal defect that resemble each other closely: a rare form showing autosomal dominant inheritance, as in the Holt-Oram syndrome (pp. 892 and 1627), and a common form having a multifactorial etiology.

To estimate the *recurrence risk*, one must consider what is known of the genetic mechanisms determining the relevant disorder. When more than one genetic mechanism exists, or when environmental factors can cause clinically indistinguishable traits, then the *relative probabilities* of the different mechanisms operating in the particular family are computed. For conditions determined by simple mendelian inheritance, there is no difficulty in predicting the probability of an offspring being affected, provided the genotypes of the parents can be recognized. Identification of the parental genotype is easiest for autosomal recessive and X-linked disorders, since the basic lesions in these two forms of mendelian inheritance usually involve simple enzyme deficiencies for which biochemical tests are now available.

Identification of the parental genotype is considerably more difficult for autosomal dominant disorders, since the basic defect is known for only a few. Thus, diagnosis of the heterozygote for a dominant disorder depends almost exclusively on the clinical evaluation and a careful pedigree analysis. In counseling a family in which one relative is affected with a dominant disorder, it is important that appropriate clinical examination of all first-degree relatives and appropriately selected distant relatives be carried out. If relatives appear unaffected, one must constantly consider the possibility that the clinical symptoms may be masked by *delayed age of onset* and *variability in expression.* When no relatives are affected, the possibility of a new dominant mutation must be entertained. The probability of a case of an autosomal dominant disorder being the result of a new mutation is inversely proportional to the reproductive fitness of the disorder.

In advising families about multifactorial genetic diseases in which the inheritance pattern is not clear-cut, such as premature coronary artery disease, the physician must resort to empirical risk estimates that have been derived from retrospectively assembled data (see Chap. 36).

Once the parental genotypes are determined, the genetic prognosis is usually presented in terms of probability that a given couple will produce an affected offspring. The physician providing genetic counseling must make certain that the couple understands not only the meaning of such absolute risk figures but also the severity of the disease and the variability in clinical expression. In other words, in dealing with a disorder such as the Noonan syndrome, it is important not only that the parents realize that they have a 50 per cent risk of producing a child with this disorder but also that they know that a certain proportion of patients with the disorder have severe disease, a certain proportion have mild disease, and so on. They should also have an understanding of the potential impact of the disease on their family. Thus, a disease that is lethal at birth might be classified by some as more "severe" than one that is lethal at age 16, but the latter is likely to have a much more profound impact on the family.

Although different families initially react in different ways to the same risk, most couples who seek genetic advice can be expected to take a responsible course of action that is based on the information quoted. Thus, the physician avoids giving direct advice to the couple concerning whether they "should" or "should not" have children. For serious genetic disease, it has been observed that when the recurrence risk is high, i.e., equal to or greater than 1 in 10, most parents are deterred from planning further children. When the risks are low, i.e., less than 1 in 10, most parents continue with additional pregnancies.[8]

PRENATAL DIAGNOSIS

The use of transabdominal amniocentesis permits diagnosis of certain genetic diseases at an early enough stage to terminate the pregnancy to prevent the birth of a defective child. This procedure allows high-risk couples the opportunity to have unaffected children, provided they are willing to have the pregnancy terminated in the event that an abnormal fetus is detected.[3, 9]

Prenatal diagnosis usually requires obtaining amniotic fluid at week 16 of gestation, centrifuging the fluid to obtain fetal amniotic cells, and culturing the fetal cells in vitro. The culture process requires about 3 weeks. By this means the karyotype of the fetus can be determined to ascertain fetal sex and to detect various chromosomal aberrations, such as Down syndrome. Moreover, many inborn errors of metabolism can be detected by suitable assays of specific enzyme activities or restriction length DNA polymorphisms linked to the locus of interest. If the precise molecular defect is known at the DNA level, prenatal diagnosis can be made with radioactive DNA or RNA probes that hybridize specifically to the abnormal gene in the cultured fetal cells.

A promising new approach to prenatal diagnosis has recently been introduced. This approach, called *chorionic villus sampling*, permits the detection of genetic abnormalities between the 9th and 12th week of gestation. A catheter is passed through the cervix into the placenta in order to obtain a sample of developing chorionic villi, which consists of a mixture of trophoblastic and mesenchymal cells. A single aspiration yields enough tissue to perform studies of chromosomes, enzyme assays, or DNA polymorphisms. Ongoing clinical trials suggest that this technique is relatively safe with a miscarriage rate of no more than 4 per cent.

In addition to the use of amniotic cells and chorionic villus sampling for prenatal diagnosis, other methods such as fetoscopy and radiology can be employed. For example, the Ellis–van Creveld syndrome and the Holt-Oram syndrome can be diagnosed in utero by ultrasonographic visualization of the accompanying upper limb abnormality. Table 49–1 lists those genetic disorders affecting the cardiovascular system for which prenatal diagnosis is currently feasible.

TABLE 49–1 GENETIC DISORDERS AFFECTING THE HEART FOR WHICH PRENATAL DIAGNOSIS IS FEASIBLE

Disorder	Expression in Cultured Amniotic Fluid Cells	Detectable Abnormality
Down syndrome	Yes	Trisomy 21 or unbalanced 14/21 translocation by karyotype
Ellis-van Creveld syndrome	No	Visualization of bilateral polydactyly by fetoscopy
Duchenne muscular dystrophy	Yes	Restriction length DNA polymorphism linked to *Duchenne muscular dystrophy* locus
Myotonic dystrophy	No	Gene for *myotonic dystrophy* closely linked with *secretor* gene, the product of which is present in amniotic fluid
Ehlers-Danlos, Type IV	Yes	Deficient synthesis of Type III collagen
Homocystinuria	Yes	Deficiency of cystathionine synthase
Pompe disease	Yes	Deficiency of lysosomal acid maltase
Homozygous familial hypercholesterolemia	Yes	Deficiency of receptors for low-density lipoprotein
Cholesterylester storage disease	Yes	Deficiency of lysosomal acid lipase
Fabry disease	Yes	Deficiency of α-galactosidase A
Mucopolysaccharidoses		
Type I-H, Hurler syndrome	Yes	Deficiency of α-L-iduronidase
Type I-S, Scheie syndrome	Yes	Deficiency of α-L-iduronidase
Type I-H/S, Hurler-Scheie compound	Yes	Deficiency of α-L-iduronidase
Type II, Hunter syndrome	Yes	Deficiency of sulfoiduronide sulfatase
Type IV, Morquio syndrome	Yes	Deficiency of *N*-acetylhexosamine sulfate sulfatase
Type VI, Maroteaux-Lamy syndrome	Yes	Deficiency of arylsulfatase B
Mucolipidosis, Type III	Yes	Deficiency of *N*-acetylglucosamine-1-phosphotransferase

GENETICS OF SPECIFIC FORMS OF CARDIOVASCULAR DISEASE

CONGENITAL HEART DISEASES

(See also Chaps. 30 and 31)

CHROMOSOMAL DISORDERS

Approximately 5 per cent of all congenital heart malformations can be traced to a chromosomal aberration.[10] Virtually all cases of a congenital heart malformation associated with a chromosomal defect occur as part of a multiple malformation syndrome. Congenital heart disease is a characteristic feature of most chromosomal disorders, such as trisomy 13, trisomy 18, trisomy 21 (Down syndrome), deletion of the short arm of chromosome 4, deletion of the long arm of chromosome 13, deletion of the long arm of chromosome 18, and Turner syndrome (XO). A chromosomal syndrome that does *not* show an increased frequency of congenital heart disease is the Klinefelter syndrome (XXY). A discussion follows of the two chromosomal syndromes that most commonly cause congenital heart disease, Down syndrome and Turner syndrome.

DOWN SYNDROME. The trisomy 21 form of Down syndrome (mongolism) is the most common human chromosomal aberration, occurring in approximately 1 in every 600 neonates. Congenital heart disease, which is found in as many as 50 per cent of patients with this disorder, constitutes a major source of morbidity and mortality.[11–14]

The two most common cardiac lesions in Down syndrome are ventricular septal defect and endocardial cushion defect. Among patients with the complete form of endocardial cushion defect, those with Down syndrome account for about 50 per cent.[14] Secundum atrial septal defect, tetralogy of Fallot, and isolated patent ductus arteriosus are also observed in patients with Down syndrome. Transposition of the great arteries and coarctation of the aorta are rarely seen. Most patients having Down syndrome with congenital heart disease have a single lesion. However, as many as 30 per cent of those with heart disease may have multiple cardiac defects.[13]

The decision to repair surgically a congenital heart lesion in a patient with Down syndrome is often a complicated one. Factors to be considered include the seriousness of the defect; whether the patient is living at home or with relatives or is institutionalized; and the patient's degree of cooperation. Although it is generally believed that patients with Down syndrome are poor operative candidates because of their increased susceptibility to infections, recent surgical follow-up studies suggest that their postoperative mortality is no higher than that of a non–Down syndrome population with similar cardiac lesions.[11, 15]

The most important factor in preventing the birth of a child with the trisomy 21 form of Down syndrome is maternal age. A marked increase in incidence occurs in children born to older mothers,[16, 17] as shown in Table 49–2.

TABLE 49–2 RISK OF HAVING A CHILD WITH DOWN SYNDROME AS A FUNCTION OF MATERNAL AGE

Maternal Age	Estimated Risk
< 20 years	1 in 1800
20–29 years	1 in 1200
30–34 years	1 in 750
35–39 years	1 in 250
40–44 years	1 in 80
≥ 45 years	1 in 25

The recurrence risk to a couple who has had one child with the trisomy 21 form of Down syndrome is 2 per cent, i.e., there is a 1 in 50 chance that the next child will also have the trisomy 21 form of Down syndrome.[16] The recurrence risk is 2 per cent regardless of whether the mother is young (age 20) or old (age 45).[16] All women who are 36 years of age and older and all women who have had one child with trisomy 21 Down syndrome should have each of their subsequent pregnancies monitored by amniocentesis for a prenatal diagnosis.

The trisomy 21 aberration accounts for virtually all cases of Down syndrome in infants born to women above age 30 and for 90 per cent of all cases in those born to women below age 30. The remaining 10 per cent of patients with Down syndrome born to women below age 30 have a translocation form. On karyotype analysis, such patients have the normal number of 46 chromosomes, including 2 normal chromosomes No. 21, 1 normal chromosome No. 14, and an unpaired large chromosome that represents an extra chromosome No. 21 that is joined to 1 chromosome No. 14. There are no clinical differences between children with the trisomy 21 form of Down syndrome and those with the translocation form.

Karyotypes of the parents of children with the translocation form of Down syndrome exhibit one of the following:

1. In about 90 per cent of cases, both parents have normal karyotypes, so the translocation is assumed to have originated during gametogenesis, and the risk of recurrence is no more than 2 per cent to subsequent children.
2. In 10 per cent of cases one of the parents will have an abnormal karyotype consisting of 45 chromosomes with 1 normal chromosome No. 14, 1 normal chromosome No. 21, and a large chromosome that contains fused copies of both the 14 and 21 chromosomes.

About 5 to 20 per cent of the live-born offspring of an individual who is a "balanced" translocation carrier for the 14/21 chromosome will have Down syndrome, depending on whether the father (5 per cent) or the mother (20 per cent) carries the "balanced" translocation.[16] Other types of translocation occur, but these are much less frequent. Overall, the inherited translocation form of Down syndrome is extremely rare, especially compared with the trisomy 21 form of the disorder. Nevertheless, it is important to identify all such cases so that the pregnancies of all family members who are translocation carriers can be appropriately monitored by amniocentesis.

TURNER SYNDROME (See pp. 994 and 995). Turner syndrome is characterized by the occurrence in a phenotypic female of the following clinical features: shortness of stature, amenorrhea due to gonadal dysgenesis, shield-shaped chest, pigmented nevi, webbing of the neck, cubitus valgus, shortening of metacarpals and metatarsals, renal abnormalities, and cardiovascular abnormalities. In about 60 per cent of patients with these clinical features, all the cells in the body will be deficient in one of the two X chromosomes (45,X form). The remaining 40 per cent of patients include individuals who have a mixture of cells, some of which show the 45,X karyotype and some of which show the normal karyotype (45,X/46,XX mosaicism), and individuals whose cells show structural abnormalities in one of the two X chromosomes (such as a single isochromosome X or a single ring X chromosome). Patients with the 45,X/46,XX form of Turner syndrome are often less severely clinically involved and may be nearly normal.

Most fetuses with the 45,X form of Turner syndrome die in utero and are aborted spontaneously. Recent studies indicate that the 45,X chromosomal abnormality occurs in as many as 5 per cent of all spontaneous abortions and in about 1 in 2500 female live births.[18]

Cardiovascular abnormalities occur in 35 to 50 per cent of all patients with the 45,X form of Turner syndrome.[19–22] Coarctation of the aorta is by far the most common abnormality that is encountered, accounting for 70 per cent of all cardiac anomalies. Other congenital malformations are occasionally seen, including bicuspid aortic valve, hypertrophic obstructive cardiomyopathy, ventricular septal defect, prolapse of the mitral valve, and dextrocardia.[19–23] Stenosis of the pulmonic valve is rarely, if ever, seen in Turner syndrome. This is in striking contrast to findings in the superficially similar Noonan syndrome, in which coarctation of the aorta is rarely encountered and stenosis of the pulmonic valve is the cardinal cardiac manifestation[22] (discussed below).

Patients with Turner syndrome caused by an isochromosome X or a ring X differ clinically from patients with the 45,X karyotype in that webbing of the neck and coarctation of the aorta are absent.[19, 21] In patients with mosaic Turner syndrome, coarctation of the aorta occurs, but its frequency is considerably less than in the 45,X patients.

Adults with Turner syndrome are prone to systemic hypertension. This association between Turner syndrome and hypertension occurs in the absence of coarctation of the aorta and appears to be unrelated to the karyotypic abnormality.[19] The mechanism underlying the hypertension has not been defined.

Family studies have revealed a high frequency of both diabetes mellitus and thyroid autoantibodies in the chromosomally normal relatives of patients with Turner syndrome.[19] These findings have suggested that a genetic tendency to autoantibody formation in parents may predispose to the occurrence of chromosomal abnormalities in their offspring.

Advanced maternal age does not appear to predispose to offspring with Turner syndrome, unlike Down syndrome. Once a couple has had one child with Turner syndrome, the recurrence risk to subsequent offspring is virtually zero.

SINGLE-GENE DISORDERS

At least eight forms of congenital heart disease are now recognized to be caused by single-gene mutations. Together, these eight disorders account for about 5 per cent of all forms of congenital heart disease. In six of these disorders, the responsible mutation causes a multisystem syndrome of which congenital heart disease is only one component. Each of these mutations presumably disrupts the function of a single protein the action of which is necessary for several developmental events, including normal embryogenesis of the heart. Virtually nothing is known of how these mutant genes act at the molecular and cellular level.

The identification of any one of these eight single-gene disorders in a given individual enables the cardiologist to apply knowledge of the genetics of the syndrome to the identification of further cases in the same family and to provide genetic counseling to appropriate family members.

NOONAN SYNDROME (See also p. 942). The eponym Noonan syndrome describes a common clinical entity characterized by shortness of stature, mild mental retardation, a unique facial appearance (Fig. 49–1), webbing of the neck, cryptorchidism, renal anomalies, and congenital heart disease.[24–29] Skeletal deformities are also frequent, including scoliosis and pectus carinatum. Affected individuals superficially resemble patients with Turner syndrome in that shortness of stature, webbing of the neck, cubitus valgus, skeletal anomalies, renal abnormalities, and congenital heart disease are present in both disorders. Because of these clinical similarities, Noonan syndrome has frequently been referred to in the literature as male "Turner syndrome," "Turner phenotype with normal chromosomes," and XX and XY "Turner phenotype."[24–28]

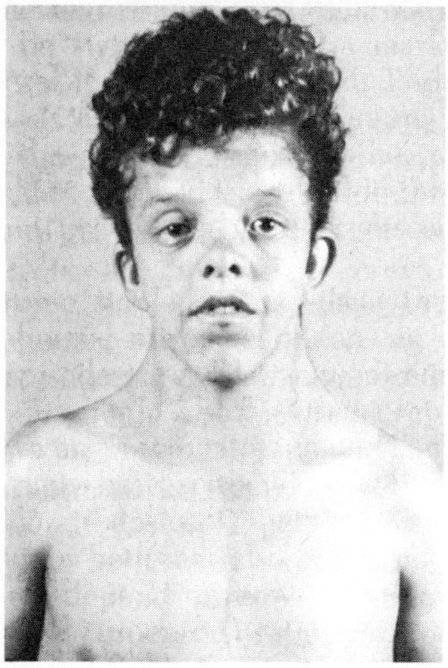

FIGURE 49–1. Eighteen-year-old boy with the Noonan syndrome. The facial abnormalities consist of curly hair, epicanthal folds, ptosis of eyelids, hypertelorism, strabismus, small chin, and low-set ears with abnormal auricles. Webbing of the neck is also evident.

However, several striking genetic and clinical differences between Noonan syndrome and Turner syndrome clearly separate these two disorders as distinct entities. (1) In contrast to Turner syndrome, in Noonan syndrome both males and females are affected and the karyotype in both sexes is normal;[24–28] (2) coarctation of the aorta, which rarely occurs in Noonan syndrome, is the most frequent cardiac lesion in Turner syndrome; conversely, *pulmonic stenosis*, which does not occur in Turner syndrome, is the most common cardiac lesion in Noonan syndrome;[23–31] and (3) Noonan syndrome is determined by a single mutant gene inherited as an autosomal dominant trait.[25, 27, 28, 32–34]

Approximately 50 per cent of patients with Noonan syndrome have congenital heart disease.[25, 29] The most common lesion is valvular pulmonary stenosis, occurring in about 60 per cent of those patients who have a congenital cardiac malformation. The stenotic pulmonic valve is frequently dysplastic. Characteristically, the annulus is of normal size, but the cusps are thickened and immobile.[23–31] The electrocardiogram is often different from the pattern usually seen in pulmonary valve stenosis: Left anterior hemiblock is common, and a deep S wave is frequently present in the precordial leads.[11, 23]

Atrial septal defect and hypertrophic cardiomyopathy occur in about 20 per cent of patients with Noonan syndrome who have congenital heart disease. The cardiomyopathy frequently produces an eccentric hypertrophy of the left ventricle that can easily be missed during cardiac catherization limited to the right side of the heart.[35–38] Although the majority of patients show a single heart defect, some show a combination of pulmonary stenosis and either atrial septal defect or hypertrophic cardiomyopathy.

In addition to anomalies of the heart itself, abnormalities

of the systemic arteries have been reported in patients with Noonan syndrome. These include fistulas of the coronary arteries, peripheral pulmonic stenosis, anomalous pulmonary venous septum, hemangiomas, peripheral lymphedema, and intestinal lymphangiectasis.[31]

Patients with Noonan syndrome undergoing cardiac surgery are particularly vulnerable to several complications: (1) technical difficulties because of the dysplastic nature of the pulmonic valve, sometimes necessitating total valve replacement—a formidable problem in infants and young children; (2) difficulty in establishing outflow drainage during total cardiopulmonary bypass because of the systemic venous anomalies; (3) increased risk of malignant hyperpyrexia during general anesthesia; and (4) development of persistent chylothorax because of pulmonary lymphangiectasis.[31]

The evidence for a genetic etiology of Noonan syndrome is provided by its occurrence in multiple siblings and in multiple generations of the same family. Family studies are consistent with autosomal dominant inheritance of a single mutant gene.[25, 27, 28, 32–34] Figure 49–2 shows a pedigree of a family with Noonan syndrome: The mutant gene segregated through three generations, and one affected woman had affected children with two different husbands. As with most autosomal dominant traits, the Noonan syndrome gene shows a marked variation in its clinical expression; some affected individuals show only minor abnormalities (such as epicanthal folds and low-set ears), whereas others in the same family show the full syndrome with severe congenital heart disease.

Although male-to-male transmission of the mutant gene has been documented in several pedigrees,[25, 32–34] most affected men, unlike affected women, show a deficiency in the number of offspring. This deficiency can be attributed to two factors: (1) Males appear to have a higher frequency of severe cardiac lesions than do females and therefore have less chance of surviving to reproductive age, and (2) about 75 per cent of affected males have bilateral cryptorchidism, whereas the affected females appear to have normal gonadal function.[24–34] This striking diminution in reproductive fitness in males with Noonan syndrome is consistent with the clinical observation that as many as 50 per cent of all cases of Noonan syndrome are sporadic cases. Such sporadic cases presumably represent new mutations.

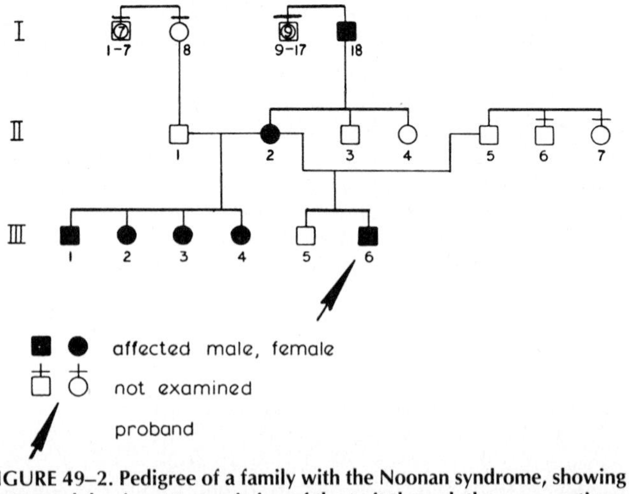

FIGURE 49–2. Pedigree of a family with the Noonan syndrome, showing autosomal dominant transmission of the trait through three generations. Note that II-2 had affected children by two different husbands. (From Baird, P. A., and De Jong, B. P.: Noonan's syndrome [XX and XY Turner phenotype] in three generations of a family. J. Pediatr. *80*:110, 1972.)

It has been only twenty years since Noonan syndrome was recognized as a distinct clinical and genetic entity separate from Turner syndrome. Nevertheless, in this short time more than 500 cases of Noonan syndrome have been reported. It has been estimated that the disorder may occur more frequently than 1 in 1000 persons in the population.[25, 39] The basic defect underlying Noonan syndrome is unknown. If it follows the pattern of other extremely common genetic diseases, it will ultimately be found to be genetically heterogeneous in that several different mutations will be able to cause a similar clinical syndrome.

In view of the high frequency of Noonan syndrome, the cardiologist should have a high index of suspicion of this disorder whenever a patient with congenital pulmonic stenosis is encountered. Attribution of this lesion to Noonan syndrome may be difficult, especially since 50 per cent of the cases may represent new mutations and thus the patients may exhibit a negative family history. The diagnosis is made even more difficult because many of the patients with documented Noonan syndrome have only mild facial abnormalities. Webbing of the neck, shortness of stature, and associated skeletal abnormalities may be absent. The almost-invariant associated lesions are eye abnormalities (mostly ptosis, hypertelorism, and epicanthus), so the physician should consider the presumptive diagnosis of Noonan syndrome whenever a patient with pulmonic stenosis and one of these eye abnormalities is seen. In these cases, all first-degree relatives should be examined for the presence of mild facial abnormalities of the Noonan type as well as for occult cardiac lesions, especially pulmonic stenosis. The importance of making the diagnosis of Noonan syndrome lies in the ability of the physician to advise the patient that half of his or her children will be similarly affected.

LEOPARD SYNDROME. The LEOPARD syndrome is a rare, single gene–determined complex of congenital malformations affecting the cardiovascular system, the skin, the inner ear, and somatic and sexual development.[40–42] The cardinal features of the disorder are embodied in the mnemonic device LEOPARD: *L*, lentigenes; *E*, electrocardiographic conduction defects; *O*, ocular hypertelorism; *P*, pulmonic valve stenosis; *A*, abnormalities of genitals; *R*, retardation of growth, and *D*, deafness, sensorineural.[40]

Cardiac abnormalities, a common feature of the disorder, consist of anatomical malformations as well as electrocardiographic conduction defects. Stenosis of the pulmonic valve appears to be the most frequently encountered cardiac lesion. It may exist as an isolated anomaly or it may be combined with aortic stenosis. Other cardiac defects that have been reported include endocardial fibroelastosis and hypertrophic cardiomyopathy.[40–44] The cardiac disease characteristically appears early in childhood and usually runs a progressive course. The most common electrocardiographic defects include prolonged P-R interval, left anterior hemiblock, widening of the QRS, and complete heart block. The functional significance of these electrocardiographic abnormalities is highly variable from patient to patient, being well tolerated in some or sufficiently serious to produce sudden death in others.

The most distinctive and striking feature of the syndrome, and the one that is diagnostic when present, is the occurrence of numerous lentigenes. These small (up to 5 mm in diameter), dark-brown spots, which spare only the mucosal surfaces, are most concentrated over the neck and upper extremities (Fig. 49–3). In some patients, the lentigenes are present at the time of birth, whereas in others they appear shortly after birth. In all patients, the number increases with age. Lentigenes differ from freckles in

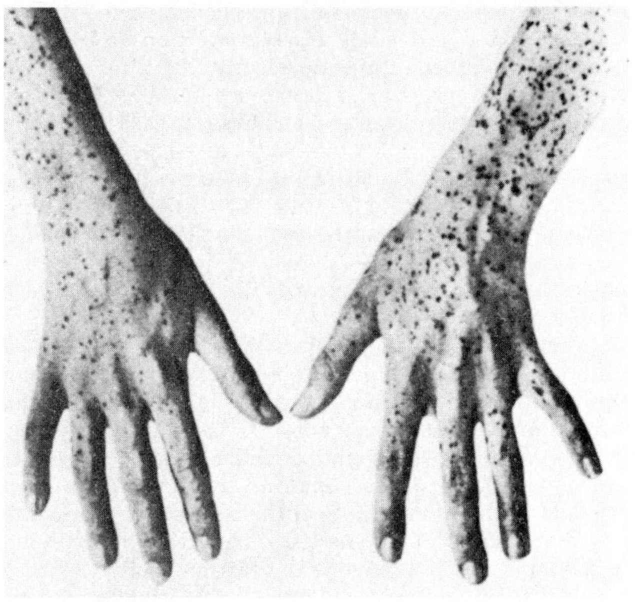

FIGURE 49–3. Skin of a 16-year-old boy with the LEOPARD syndrome covered with numerous deeply pigmented lentigines. (From Polani, P. E., and Moynahan, E. J.: Progressive carciomyopathic lentiginosis. Q. J. Med. *41*:205, 1972.)

several respects: (1) They appear before age 5, whereas freckles usually appear at 6 to 8 years of age; (2) they do not increase in numbers with exposure to sunlight, whereas freckles do; and (3) microscopically, the quantity of melanocytes and the distribution of melanin in the pigmented and adjacent nonpigmented skin differ.[40]

The LEOPARD syndrome is inherited as an autosomal dominant trait. The clinical findings are highly variable from patient to patient, both within the same family as well as between affected individuals from different families. The most frequently encountered manifestations of the mutant gene are those relating to the cardiovascular system, occurring in at least 95 per cent of affected subjects. About 80 per cent have lentigenes. Deafness and abnormalities of genitals (hypospadias and undescended testes in the male) occur in about 20 per cent of patients.

The population frequency of the gene causing the LEOPARD syndrome is very low. Nothing is currently known about the relative proportion of cases arising from familial transmission of the mutant gene versus those arising from new mutations. Moreover, nothing is known regarding the biochemical action of the mutant gene.

HOLT-ORAM SYNDROME (See also p. 1627). Although atrial septal defect almost always occurs as a sporadic disorder, there are occasional families in which the pedigree pattern suggests the operation of a single mutant gene. The Holt-Oram syndrome and familial atrial septal defect with prolonged atrioventricular (AV) conduction are two examples of rare autosomal dominant disorders that are hidden among the more common sporadic cases of atrial septal defect.

The cardinal clinical manifestation of the Holt-Oram syndrome is the occurrence of an upper limb deformity in a patient with congenital heart disease.[45–50] Atrial septal defect of the secundum type is the most frequently encountered congenital heart malformation in affected individuals. This is usually accompanied by one or more electrocardiographic abnormalities, such as first-degree atrioventricular block, right bundle branch block, or bradycardia. Ventricular septal defect is the second most commonly encountered congenital heart lesion. Although virtually any form of congenital heart disease has been reported to occur in the syndrome, 70 per cent of affected individuals have either an atrial septal defect or a ventricular septal defect.

Many different upper limb deformities have been observed in association with the congenital heart disease in the Holt-Oram syndrome.[51] These limb deformities are typically bilateral but not necessarily symmetrical. If asymmetry is present, the skeletal lesions are usually more severe on the left side.[47] The most characteristic anomaly involves the thumbs. They may be absent, hypoplastic, triphalangeal, or finger-like. The last-named anomaly is referred to as "digitalization of the thumbs." The radius and the forearm are variably involved, the defects ranging in different patients from absent or hypoplastic radii to phocomelia.

Although deformities of the thumb are the best known features of the Holt-Oram syndrome, they do not occur in every case, nor are they pathognomonic.[51, 52] Bilateral thumb abnormalities may also occur in the Diamond-Blackfan syndrome, in Fanconi anemia, or in thalidomide embryopathy. The most frequently encountered and specific upper limb abnormalities—namely, the presence of an abnormal scaphoid bone and/or accessory carpal bones—are detected on radiographs of the wrists. Various abnormalities also occur in the shoulder. The most common finding is a rotation of the scapula. Deformities of the humeral head and accessory ossicles around the shoulder have also been frequently noted.[51, 52]

As in many dominantly inherited syndromes, individuals inheriting the Holt-Oram gene show varying degrees of clinical involvement. Intrafamilial variability appears to be as great as interfamilial variability.[45–50] The penetrance of the Holt-Oram gene is nearly 100 per cent, i.e., all individuals who inherit the gene manifest one or more clinical abnormalities, and this can be shown provided that appropriate studies, including wrist radiographs and electrocardiograms, are performed.[49] In about 60 per cent of cases, one of the parents is affected. The other 40 per cent of cases occur sporadically and apparently represent new mutations occurring in the germ cells of one of the parents.[47] Although the biochemical action of the mutant gene has not been defined, it presumably acts by disrupting a critical embryonic event common to the formation of the upper limbs and the heart. Recent studies suggest that it may be possible to diagnose the disorder in utero by ultrasonographic detection of the upper limb abnormality. One at-risk fetus was examined by ultrasound at 14 weeks of gestation and shown to have bilateral absence of the radii and several finger digits.[53]

The population frequency of the Holt-Oram syndrome has not been determined. However, the disorder is probably greatly underdiagnosed, with most cases being mistakenly considered as "garden-variety" atrial septal defects. The importance of separating the patient with the Holt-Oram syndrome from those cases of atrial septal defect that are not determined by a single-gene mechanism cannot be overemphasized. If the patient has Holt-Oram syndrome, then 50 per cent of the first-degree relatives (i.e., offspring, siblings, and parents) will be affected. In contrast, if a patient has a sporadic type of atrial septal defect, only about 3 per cent of the first-degree relatives would be affected. Thus, genetic counseling is quite different in these two situations.

FAMILIAL ATRIAL SEPTAL DEFECT WITH PROLONGED AV CONDUCTION. The syndrome of atrial septal defect with prolonged AV conduction represents a second example (the first being the Holt-Oram syndrome) of a single-gene–determined form of atrial septal defect. Pedigree studies of at least 20 large families leave little doubt about the autosomal dominant inheritance of this disorder.[54–56]

The mutant gene shows a high degree of penetrance, and there is surprisingly little pleiotropy. That is, the mutant gene appears to cause only atrial septal defect and an abnormality of the AV conduction system. The latter is manifest clinically as either first- or second-degree heart block. Rarely, complete heart block occurs.

In the absence of a biochemical marker for the mutant gene, the diagnosis can be made only through careful clinical examination of family members of suspected cases. "Garden-variety" atrial septal defect can be excluded both by a family pedigree showing dominant inheritance and by electrocardiographic evidence of AV conduction block. The Holt-Oram syndrome can be ruled out by a normal clinical and radiological examination of the upper extremities.

ELLIS–VAN CREVELD SYNDROME. The Ellis–van Creveld syndrome constitutes a rare form of congenital heart disease that is inherited as an autosomal recessive trait. Affected individuals manifest abnormalities not only of the heart but also of the skeletal system, the nails, and the mouth.[57–59]

Congenital heart disease occurs in 50 to 60 per cent of patients and frequently causes deaths in infancy. The most common cardiac lesion involves the atrium, producing either a single atrium or a large atrial septal defect. The atrial lesion may occur alone, or it may be associated with another cardiac defect, such as aortic atresia, hypoplastic ascending aorta, or hypoplastic left ventricle.

The skeletal findings in the Ellis–van Creveld syndrome are characteristic. The patients have an abnormally small stature that is present from the time of birth. They exhibit a particularly striking shortening in the distal parts of the extremities. Bilateral polydactyly and fusion of the carpal bones are also present. Additional findings include the presence of hypoplastic nails and several oral abnormalities, including labiogingival adherences, accessory frenula, and hypodontia.

About half of affected individuals die in early infancy as a result of cardiorespiratory problems. The majority of survivors have normal intelligence. Eventual adult stature is in the range of 45 to 60 inches (115 to 150 cm).

Although the Ellis–van Creveld syndrome is an extremely rare disorder in the general population, it occurs with high frequency in certain isolated groups. As a result, the genetics of the disease have been well delineated.[58] The following observations support an autosomal recessive inheritance pattern: (1) The disorder occurs with equal frequency in males and females; (2) only siblings are affected in a given family; and (3) about one-third of all cases result from parental consanguinity. Most cases of the disorder in the United States occur in the Old Order Amish, an inbred religious isolate in Lancaster County, Pennsylvania, in which 13 per cent of the population carries the mutant gene.[58]

The underlying biochemical defect responsible for the Ellis–van Creveld syndrome has not yet been identified. Nonetheless, since affected individuals always manifest bilateral polydactyly of the hands, it is possible to make a prenatal diagnosis in pregnancies at risk by inspecting the fetus in utero, using fetoscopy to determine whether or not polydactyly is present.[60]

SUPRAVALVULAR AORTIC STENOSIS (See also p. 937). Supravalvular aortic stenosis can occur as an isolated congenital anomaly and as a component of two different clinical entities: (1) as a nonfamilial syndrome resulting from fetal hypercalcemia and characterized by elfin facies (antiverted nostrils, patulous lips, and small chin), mental retardation, dental anomalies, and congenital supravalvular aortic stenosis[61]; and (2) a familial syndrome transmitted as an autosomal dominant trait and characterized by the presence of pulmonary and systemic arterial stenoses in the *absence* of mental retardation and elfin facies.[62–65] Although these two syndromes are often discussed in textbooks as representing a "spectrum of the same disease," they are clinically and genetically distinct disorders. Since the first syndrome is not transmitted by a single-gene mechanism but rather results from excessive exposure or excessive hypersensitivity of fetal tissues to vitamin D, it will not be discussed further.

Patients with familial supravalvular aortic stenosis can exhibit a wide range of arterial abnormalities. Although supravalvular aortic stenosis is the "typical" lesion, many affected individuals have stenosis of the pulmonary artery (peripheral or supravalvular), brachiocephalic arterial stenosis, hypoplasia or coarctation of the descending aorta, and dilatation and tortuosity of the coronary arteries. Like most dominant traits, the mutant gene is variably expressed even among affected persons in the same family.

Most patients initially come to medical attention because of an asymptomatic heart murmur. Clinical signs of dyspnea, angina pectoris, syncope, or claudication do not usually begin until after age 20 years. Those patients who manifest coarctation of the descending aorta may show signs of hypertension. Since affected individuals are at risk for bacterial endocarditis and should receive antibiotics at appropriate times, it is important to identify all affected relatives as early in life as possible.

KARTAGENER SYNDROME. Kartagener syndrome consists of the triad of sinusitis, bronchiectasis, and situs inversus with dextrocardia.[66–69] The disorder is inherited as an autosomal recessive trait; males and females are affected with equal frequency. In addition to the classic triad mentioned above, affected males are infertile as a result of immobile spermatozoa.

Since individuals with Kartagener syndrome are homozygous for a mutant gene, the clinical course is remarkably uniform among affected persons. Cases in these individuals initially come to attention in infancy because of mucopurulent nasal discharge and repeated bouts of upper respiratory infections, otitis media, and pneumonia. By the preschool years, most patients exhibit persistent sinusitis, chronic bronchitis, and bronchiectasis. As many as 90 per cent of affected individuals have complete situs inversus, a mirror image reversal of internal organs due to a sinistral instead of a dextral rotation of the viscera occurring between days 10 and 15 of gestation.

In most affected individuals, dextrocardia is the only cardiac manifestation. Occasionally, one or more associated cardiac anomalies are present, such as transposition of the great arteries and trilocular or bilocular heart.

Kartagener syndrome occurs in about 1 person in 68,000. Of all persons with bronchiectasis, about 1.4 per cent have Kartagener syndrome, and of all persons with situs inversus, about 15 per cent have Kartagener syndrome.[70] The occurrence of this disorder in multiple siblings, male as well as female; the absence of any manifestations in the parents or in the children of affected individuals; and the presence of a higher than average frequency of consanguinity among the parents of affected individuals all support an autosomal recessive mode of inheritance.

The nature of the primary genetic defect in the Kartagener syndrome has been elucidated by electron microscopic investigation of a ciliated mucosal biopsy or of an ejaculate. These studies show that the nonmotile cilia and sperm obtained from affected individuals are structurally

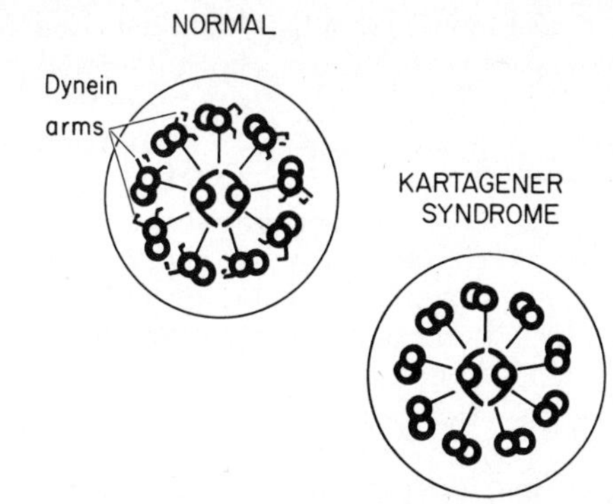

FIGURE 49–4. Schematic drawing of electron micrographs of cross sections through spermatozoa (or respiratory cilia), showing the location of dynein arms in normal cells and their absence in cells from a patient with the Kartagener syndrome. Normal motile spermatozoa and respiratory cilia possess nine micro-tubular doublets, each of which contains two dynein arms.

normal in most respects. However, the so-called dynein arms are abnormal.[66, 70] Dynein arms are protein structures that normally form temporary cross bridges between adjacent microtubules in cilia and sperm tails (Fig. 49–4). The dynein arms play a role analogous to that of myosin in muscle in that they allow the sliding of the microtubules upon each other to generate movements of cilia and sperm.

Several different mutations can produce the Kartagener syndrome. In all cases the mutant gene disrupts the synthesis either of the dynein protein itself or of a protein that binds dynein to the microtubules,[66, 70] causing any one of several types of morphological abnormalities in the ciliary axoneme: missing dynein arms (Fig. 49–4), abnormally short dynein arms, short spokes with no central sheath, missing central microtubules, or displacement of one of the nine peripheral microtubular doublets. The presence of any one of these abnormalities in the ciliary axoneme can presumably produce immobility of sperm and respiratory cilia, accounting for the clinical findings of infertility, sinusitis, and bronchiectasis. The molecular basis of the situs inversus is less certain, but it is reasonable to suppose that a malrotation of the visceral tissues occurs in the embryo when the ciliary movements of visceral epithelia do not occur.

PRIMARY PULMONARY HYPERTENSION (See also p. 805). Primary pulmonary hypertension is a disorder characterized by increased arterial pressure in the pulmonary circulation caused by changes that appear to be intrinsic to the pulmonary vasculature. Although most cases are sporadic, a familial form also occurs.[71–76] The mode of inheritance appears to be autosomal dominant. Many large pedigrees showing vertical transmission through three generations have been reported.[71–76] Onset of symptoms occurs from early childhood to middle age. Except for a history of family involvement, affected individuals show no unique clinical features that allow them to be distinguished from patients with nongenetic forms of primary pulmonary hypertension. However, the presence of the disorder in a man should be a clue to the familial form, since the nongenetic forms occur much more frequently in women than in men.

MULTIFACTORIAL DISORDERS

The chromosomal abnormalities and single-gene disorders that produce congenital heart disease account for no more than 5 to 10 per cent of all cases of congenital heart disease.[10] The remaining "garden-variety" cases are believed to result from developmental defects involving multiple genes and possibly environmental factors. Hence, the genetic predisposition in most cases of congenital heart disease is multifactorial.[77–79]

In general, congenital heart defects produced by chromosomal errors (as in Down syndrome) and by single-gene mutations (as in Noonan syndrome and Kartagener syndrome) are a part of a multisystem disorder. On the other hand, congenital heart defects with multifactorial inheritance typically occur as discrete lesions that are not part of a multisystem disorder.

As in other disorders showing multifactorial inheritance, the recurrence risk to first-degree relatives of a patient with a "garden-variety" type of congenital heart disease is considerably less than the 25 to 50 per cent risk that occurs in single-gene disorders. Although the relative risk to the siblings and offspring of such a patient is 3 to 40 times the estimated population frequency, the overall absolute risk for these first-degree relatives is low, in the range of 1 to 4 per cent.[77, 80] Table 49–3 lists the expected recurrence risk for siblings and offspring of patients with the 14 most common forms of congenital heart disease. Although these empirical data are useful in the genetic counseling of families that have had only one child with a congenital heart lesion, they do not apply in families with more than one affected person. When two first-degree relatives are affected, the recurrence risk in subsequent offspring doubles or triples; with three affected, the risks reach 10 to 20 per cent. When the first case is diagnosed in a given

TABLE 49–3 EMPIRICAL RECURRENCE RISKS FOR SIBLINGS AND OFFSPRING OF PROBANDS WITH CONGENITAL HEART LESIONS

	Risk to Siblings		Risk to Offspring	
Abnormality in Proband	Number Affected/ Total Number	Per Cent	Number Affected/ Total Number	Per Cent
Ventricular septal defect	28/672	4.2	7/174	4.0
Patent ductus arteriosus	18/516	3.5	6/139	4.3
Tetralogy of Fallot	11/366	3.0	6/141	4.2
Atrial septal defect	11/380	2.9	5/199	2.7
Pulmonic stenosis	10/375	2.7	4/111	3.6
Aortic stenosis	8/361	2.2	4/103	3.9
Coarctation of aorta	5/281	1.8	7/253	2.7
Transposition of great vessels	4/229	1.7		
Atrioventricular canal	4/151	2.6		
Tricuspid atresia	1/98	1.0		
Ebstein anomaly	1/105	1.0		
Truncus arteriosus	1/86	1.2		
Pulmonic atresia	1/80	1.3		
Hypoplastic left heart	8/370	2.2		

Modified from Nora, J. J., and Nora, A. H.: Circulation 57:205–213, 1978; Nora, J. J., McGill, C. W., and McNamara, D. G.: Teratology 3:325–330, 1970; and Nora, J. J., Dodd, P. F., Hattwick, M. A. W., et al.: J.A.M.A. 209:2052–2053, 1969. Copyright 1969, American Medical Association.

family, it is not possible to predict whether that family is at risk for multiple occurrences of congenital heart disease.

HEREDITARY DISORDERS OF CONNECTIVE TISSUE

(See also Chapter 54)

The hereditary disorders of connective tissue are a group of diseases in which the predominant pathological condition involves either the fibrous elements (such as collagen and elastin) or the nonfibrous elements (such as the mucopolysaccharide ground substance) of connective tissue throughout the body.[81] Since collagen, elastin, and mucopolysaccharides are all essential components of arteries and heart valves, it is not surprising that mutations affecting either the structure or the metabolism of these macromolecules would produce abnormalities in cardiac function. We now recognize 17 different hereditary connective tissue disorders in which cardiac involvement is a prominent feature. Each of these disorders is determined by a single-gene mechanism. The major clinical and genetic aspects of these disorders are summarized in Table 49–4.

As evident from this table, four types of cardiovascular disease—premature coronary artery disease, aortic regurgitation, mitral regurgitation, and abnormalities in the peripheral arteries—occur with high frequency in patients with the hereditary disorders of connective tissue. Of the 17 disorders listed in Table 49–4, 7 cause premature coronary artery disease (alkaptonuria, homocystinuria, pseudoxanthoma elasticum, idiopathic arterial calcification of infancy, Hurler syndrome, Hurler-Scheie compound, and Hunter syndrome), and 9 cause aortic or mitral regurgitation or both (Marfan syndrome, familial mitral valve prolapse syndrome, osteogenesis imperfecta, Hurler syndrome, Hurler-Scheie compound, Hunter syndrome, Morquio syndrome, Maroteaux-Lamy syndrome, and Type III mucolipidosis).

The Marfan syndrome and familial mitral valve prolapse syndrome are relatively common and are frequently encountered by cardiologists. Their genetic aspects are discussed here in detail. The 15 other inborn disorders listed in Table 49–4 are rare, each having a population frequency of 1 in 40,000 to 100,000 persons, and are not considered further in this chapter. Pertinent references in the literature are provided in the table.

MARFAN SYNDROME (See also p. 1725). Marfan syndrome is a generalized disorder of connective tissue that is inherited as an autosomal dominant trait. The cardinal manifestations consist of abnormalities of the eye (high-grade myopia and ectopia lentis), of the skeletal system (gangling habitus, arachnodactyly, pectus excavatum, and pectus carinatum), and of the cardiovascular system. In individual patients, all manifestations may not be present.[81]

Cardiac abnormalities occur in at least 60 per cent of affected adults.[81–83] The major cardiovascular lesion in adults is a dilatation of the aortic ring, the sinuses of Valsalva, and the ascending thoracic aorta. Stretching of the aortic valve leads ultimately to aortic regurgitation, aortic dissection (p. 1727), or both.

Among 505 unselected cases of aortic dissection, 74 occurred in patients under age 40. Twelve of these younger patients (16 per cent) had Marfan syndrome.[108] Aortic dissection is the most serious complication. Together with the other aortic valve abnormalities, it represents the leading cause of death. Most of the patients are young (in the early 30's) and in good health when dissection occurs.[109] Two approaches to prevention of aortic dissection in Marfan patients have been suggested. First, propranolol may be useful in preventing aortic dissection by reducing dP/dt to low-normal levels.[110] Second, prophylactic composite aortic graft-valve repair has been performed with low operative and long-term mortality in asymptomatic patients when their aortic aneurysms reach a diameter of 6 cm.[111]

Pregnancy greatly increases the risk of aortic dissection and rupture and hence poses a serious risk to life.[112] Although the basic defect leading to the weakening of the aortic wall is unknown, histological studies show a striking loss of elastic fibers in the media of the damaged aortic segment.[81]

Mitral regurgitation is a frequently encountered cardiac abnormality in affected adults.[81–83] The mitral regurgitation is usually due to redundant cusps and chordae tendineae, producing a "floppy" prolapsed mitral valve (p. 1045). Cineangiography usually shows retroversion of a redundant posterior mitral valve leaflet with regurgitation occurring in late systole. These patients typically manifest a late systolic murmur with or without mid- to late systolic clicks. In some patients the mitral regurgitation is severe and functionally significant. On the basis of echocardiographic findings, mitral prolapse may be more common than aortic regurgitation. Massive calcification of the mitral annulus is occasionally seen.[113] Less common complications include cystic disease of the lung, recurrent spontaneous pneumothorax, and bacterial endocarditis, which may be superimposed on minor changes of the heart valves.[81]

The cardiac manifestations of Marfan syndrome are more subtle and less severe in children than in adults.[83] The most common cardiac lesion in the pediatric age group is an isolated mitral regurgitation that is usually asymptomatic but can be very severe. In contrast to Marfan adults, affected children rarely manifest signs of aortic root disease. However, when aortic regurgitation is present, the patients show a rapidly deteriorating course. The overall mortality in one large study of children with Marfan syndrome was as high as 14 per cent.[83]

Although the basic defect has not been identified, the genetics of Marfan syndrome are well understood.[81] The disorder is inherited as an autosomal dominant trait with marked variability in clinical expression. In about 85 per cent of cases, one of the parents is affected. The other 15 per cent of cases occur sporadically and apparently represent new mutations occurring in the germ cells of one of the parents.[114] The average age of the fathers of those with sporadic cases is 7 years higher than that of the fathers of those having inherited cases. These data suggest that the new mutations occur in the father's germ cells and that their frequency increases with paternal age.[114]

Relatives at 50 per cent risk for having Marfan syndrome frequently request that studies be performed on them to determine whether they have it and are thus at risk of passing the mutant gene to their children. This may pose a problem for the physician, since some affected patients are asymptomatic and show no obvious features of the syndrome. Nevertheless, subtle manifestations can be detected in a high proportion of asymptomatic Marfan syndrome patients by three studies: echocardiography (looking for prolapse of the mitral valve and aortic root dilation), anthropometrical evaluation (measuring the upper and lower body segments), and ophthalmological examination (searching for ectopia lentis).[115, 116]

MITRAL VALVE PROLAPSE SYNDROME (See also p. 1045). Familial mitral valve prolapse syndrome is an autosomal dominant disorder characterized by ballooning or prolapse of the posterior mitral valve leaflet, which

TABLE 49–4 HEREDITARY DISORDERS OF CONNECTIVE TISSUE WITH CARDIOVASCULAR INVOLVEMENT

Disorder	Major Clinical Manifestations		Cardiovascular Involvement in Affected Subjects (Per Cent)	Typical Age of Onset of Cardiovascular Abnormality	Primary Biochemical Defect	Mechanism of Inheritance	References
	Cardiovascular	Noncardiovascular					
Marfan syndrome	Aortic aneurysm and rupture, mitral regurgitation	Ectopia lentis, gracile habitus, arachnodactyly	50–70	Young adult	Not known	Dominant	81–83
Familial midsystolic click syndrome	Late systolic murmur, midsystolic clicks, abnormal EKG, mitral valve prolapse	None	100	Young adult	Not known	Dominant	84–87
Osteogenesis imperfecta	Aortic regurgitation	Multiple fractures, blue sclerae, otosclerosis, and deafness	Rare	Adult	Deficient synthesis of Type I collagen	Dominant	81
Ehlers-Danlos Type IV*	Rupture of aorta and other large arteries	Severe bruisability, rupture of bowel, minimal joint laxity	>95	Young adult	Deficient synthesis of Type III collagen	Dominant	81, 88–91
Cutis laxa, recessive form	Peripheral pulmonic stenosis, arterial aneurysms	Pendulous skin, hernias, severe emphysema	50	Infancy	Not known	Recessive	92
Alkaptonuria	Calcific aortic stenosis, generalized atherosclerosis	Black urine, pigmentation of cartilage, degenerative joint changes	50–75	Adult	Deficiency of homogentisic acid oxidase	Recessive	81
Homocystinuria*	Arterial and venous thrombosis, myocardial infarction, pulmonary embolism	Ectopia lentis, osteoporosis, mental retardation	>95	Young adult	Deficiency of cystathionine synthase	Recessive	81, 93–96
Pseudoxanthoma elasticum	Coronary artery disease, claudication, hypertension	Peau d'orange skin, retinal angioid streaks, gastrointestinal bleeding	50	Young adult	Not known	Dominant and recessive forms	81, 97–101
Idiopathic arterial calcification of infancy	Death from myocardial infarction in first 5 months of life, generalized calcification of peripheral arteries	None	100	Neonates	Not known	Recessive	102, 103
Mucopolysaccharidoses*					Abnormal degradation of mucopolysaccharidoses due to:		81, 104, 105
Type I-H, Hurler syndrome*	Aortic and mitral regurgitation, coronary artery disease, cardiomyopathy	Corneal clouding, coarse features, mental retardation, early death	50–75	Before age 2	Deficiency of α-L-iduronidase (I-H allele)	Recessive	81, 104, 105
Type I-S, Scheie syndrome	Aortic regurgitation	Stiff joints, normal intelligence, corneal clouding	>95	Adult	Deficiency of α-L-iduronidase (I-S allele)	Recessive	81, 104, 105
Type I-H/S, Hurler-Scheie compound*	Aortic and mitral regurgitation	Phenotype intermediate between Hurler and Scheie syndromes	>95	Young adult	Deficiency of α-L-iduronidase (I-H and I-S alleles)	Recessive; genetic compound of Type I-H and I-S alleles	81, 104, 105
Type II, Hunter syndrome (severe)*	Aortic and mitral regurgitation, coronary artery disease, cardiomyopathy	No corneal clouding; milder course than in Type I-H, but death before age 15	>95	Childhood	Deficiency of sulfoiduronide sulfatase (severe allele)	X-linked	81, 104, 105
Type II, Hunter syndrome (mild)*	Aortic and mitral regurgitation, coronary artery disease	Survival to 30's and 50's, fair intelligence	>95	Young adult	Deficiency of sulfoiduronide sulfatase (mild allele)	X-linked	81, 104, 105
Type IV, Morquio syndrome*	Aortic regurgitation	Severe bone changes with gibbus and dwarfism, corneal clouding, normal intelligence	>75	Young adult	Deficiency of *N*-acetylhexosamine sulfate sulfatase	Recessive	81, 104, 105
Type VI, Maroteaux Lamy syndrome*	Aortic and mitral regurgitation	Corneal clouding, severe osseous changes, normal intelligence	>95	Childhood	Deficiency of arylsulfatase B	Recessive	81, 104, 105
Mucolipidosis, Type III (pseudo-Hurler polydystrophy)*	Aortic and mitral regurgitation	Claw hand and stiff joints, coarse facies, kyphoscoliosis, corneal clouding, carpal tunnel syndrome, low normal intelligence	>95	Young adult	Deficiency of *N*-acetylglucosamine-1-phosphotransferase	Recessive	81, 106, 107

*Prenatal diagnosis is possible.

produces a midsystolic click and a late systolic murmur.[84–87] Since the initial delineation of the syndrome in 1963, myriad reports have appeared in the literature describing patients with this disorder. However, most of these reports have failed to take into account that prolapse of the mitral valve per se is etiologically a heterogeneous entity and that the dominantly inherited syndrome constitutes only one of its many causes.

A syndrome virtually identical to familial mitral valve prolapse syndrome has also been described in patients with Marfan syndrome, Turner syndrome, Ehlers-Danlos syndrome, hypertrophic obstructive cardiomyopathy, acute rheumatic fever, and coronary artery disease; following mitral commissurotomy; and in association with ruptured chordae tendineae and secundum atrial septal defect.[84, 85] In these last-named disorders, prolapse of the mitral valve is considered a secondary phenomenon that results from a variety of abnormalities involving the mitral leaflets, chordae tendineae, papillary muscles, or mitral annulus. The clinical significance of the valvular dysfunction is usually subordinate to that of the primary disease process.

In contrast to the secondary causes of prolapse of the mitral valve, in familial mitral valve prolapse syndrome, the pathological condition of the mitral valve almost always consists of a myxomatous degeneration.[84, 85] Microscopy of involved leaflets shows replacement of the central fibrous tissue by metachromatically staining, loose, myxomatous material accompanied by fibroelastic thickening of the adjacent endocardium.[84]

A large degree of clinical variability appears in families affected with familial mitral valve prolapse syndrome. Affected females more often show clinical signs than do affected males. Symptoms of prolapse of the mitral valve can develop at any age and can range from mild to severe. Common presentations include palpitations, presyncope, syncope, chest pain, dyspnea, and/or fatigue.[84, 85] The palpitations are usually due to atrial or ventricular arrhythmias. Sudden death is presumably due to ventricular arrhythmias. The major auscultatory findings typically consist of a nonejection click in midsystole or a late systolic murmur heard best at the cardiac apex or both.[84, 85] Diagnosis can be confirmed by echocardiography or ventricular cineangiography. The major complications of the syndrome include bacterial endocarditis, severe mitral insufficiency, and life-threatening arrhythmias.[84, 85]

The population frequency of the primary form of prolapse of the mitral valve has been reported to be as high as 6 to 17 per cent among apparently healthy young women.[117, 118] These estimates, if correct, place prolapse of the mitral valve among the commonest of all cardiac abnormalities. Although an autosomal dominant mechanism appears to account for mitral valve prolapse in certain families,[84–87] the exact proportion of patients with the primary syndrome who owe their disease to a single mutant gene is unknown. Genetic studies designed to answer this question are made difficult by the presence of silent or asymptomatic prolapse in some subjects who are known to possess the abnormal gene.

CARDIOMYOPATHIES

At least 10 single-gene–determined forms of cardiomyopathy are currently recognized. In some of these disorders, the myocardial disease dominates the clinical picture, as in Pompe disease, familial hypertrophic obstructive cardiomyopathy, and familial dilated cardiomyopathy. In some, the cardiomyopathy occurs as part of a generalized metabolic disease, as in hemochromatosis and familial amyloidosis. In others, the cardiomyopathy occurs as part of a neuromyopathic syndrome, as in myotonic dystrophy, Duchenne muscular dystrophy, and Friedreich's ataxia.

POMPE DISEASE (TYPE II GLYCOGEN STORAGE DISEASE) (See also p. 1013). Pompe disease is a rare inborn error of glycogen metabolism that results from an absence of the lysosomal enzyme acid α-1,4-glucosidase.[119] Once synthesized in cells, glycogen is degraded by several mechanisms, one of which involves a nonlysosomal phosphorylytic pathway that converts glycogen to glucose-6-phosphate. The other pathway involves hydrolysis of the glycogen to glucose within lysosomes. In the absence of the lysosomal acid maltase, large amounts of glycogen accumulate within lysosomes of tissues throughout the body, including the heart. Since the nonlysosomal phosphorylytic pathway of glycogen breakdown is normal in Pompe disease, carbohydrate metabolism is normal and hypoglycemia does not occur.

The massive accumulation of glycogen in body tissues in Pompe disease leads to a characteristic clinical picture that becomes apparent within the first few months of life. Affected infants typically have feeding difficulty, inadequate weight gain, respiratory difficulty, hypotonia, atrophy of subcutaneous fat, enlarged tongue, and congestive heart failure.[119] Death from cardiac failure invariably occurs within the first year of life. The cardiomyopathy of Pompe disease is characterized by the absence of significant heart murmurs, the presence of massive cardiomegaly on chest roentgenograms, and the presence of several distinctive electrocardiographic findings. The latter include a short P-R interval (0.05 to 0.09 sec) and huge QRS complexes.[120]

Pompe disease is inherited as an autosomal recessive trait. The gene coding for lysosomal acid α-1,4-glucosidase is located on chromosome 17.[121] Because the disorder is quite rare (occurring with a population frequency of less than 1 in 100,000 persons[122]), about 20 per cent of affected cases are associated with parental consanguinity. As in most recessive disorders, the heterozygous parents manifest no detectable clinical abnormalities. Inasmuch as the lysosomal acid α-1,4-glucosidase enzyme is normally present in cultured amniotic fluid cells, prenatal diagnosis of homozygous affected fetuses is feasible and has successfully been carried out in couples who have a 25 per cent recurrence risk for having a second child with Pompe disease.

FAMILIAL HYPERTROPHIC OBSTRUCTIVE CARDIOMYOPATHY (See also p. 1418). Familial hypertrophic obstructive cardiomyopathy is determined by an autosomal dominant mechanism. Recent studies of both the asymptomatic and the symptomatic relatives of patients with clinically apparent cases have demonstrated that asymmetrical septal hypertrophy, often without outflow obstruction, represents the most constant and characteristic feature of this disorder.[123–125] Asymmetrical septal hypertrophy is detected by echocardiography and is defined as the presence of a ventricular septum that is at least 30 per cent thicker than the posterobasal wall of the left ventricle.[124]

In one recent genetic analysis of 70 affected individuals, the disease appeared to be inherited as an autosomal dominant trait in 56 per cent of the families.[123] It is not clear at this point whether the remaining 44 per cent of affected individuals owe their disease to new mutations or whether they have a different mechanism for the obstructive cardiomyopathy. In families with the dominantly inherited disease, the mutant gene appears to be fully penetrant; that is, virtually all individuals who inherit the gene show asymmetrical septal hypertrophy. Nevertheless, the resulting clinical manifestations are variable from patient to patient.[123–125] In full-blown cases of hypertrophic obstructive cardiomyopathy, the asymmetrical septal hypertrophy progresses to ventricular outflow tract obstruction, and this, in turn, leads to the clinical findings of dyspnea, fatigability, angina, syncope, palpitations due to arrhythmias, and sudden death.[126] Patients with the complete syndrome, who typically come to medical attention between the ages of 20 and 30 years, probably represent no more than 20 per cent of all individuals affected with familial hypertrophic obstructive cardiomyopathy.[124] The other 80 per cent of subjects who have inherited the mutant gene show echocardiographic evidence of asymmetrical septal hypertrophy but manifest no clinical abnormalities (about 20 per cent of gene carriers) or show nonspecific electrocardiographic and auscultatory findings that are nondiagnostic (60 per cent of gene carriers).[124]

Many large pedigrees with familial hypertrophic obstructive cardiomyopathy have been reported in the literature, providing abundant evidence for autosomal dominant transmission.[126–129] The most impressive pedigree to date is that of a French-Canadian kindred in which the genealogical survey was extended to the original immigrant from France in the 1600's.[128] In family studies, echocardiography has demonstrated that 93 per cent of probands have an affected parent,[124] thus implying that no more than 7 per cent of cases of hypertrophic obstructive cardiomyopathy represent new mutations. This estimate agrees well with estimates of the limited extent to which this disorder reduces reproductive fitness.

A subgroup of families with unusually frequent premature deaths (termed "malignant" hypertrophic cardiomyopathy) has recently been identified.[129] Of the 69 first-degree relatives in these 8 families, 41 had clinical evidence of hypertrophic cardiomyopathy and 32 (78 per cent of those affected) died of heart disease before 50 years of age. Sudden and unexpected death occurred in 23 of the 32 patients.

The basic biochemical defect is unknown. Discovery of the mechanism of action of the mutant gene will undoubtedly provide insight into the biochemical and cellular basis of ventricular hypertrophy.

FAMILIAL CARDIOMYOPATHY (See also p. 1414). The designation familial cardiomyopathy is used to refer to an ill-defined and undoubtedly heterogeneous group of entities having the common denominators of cardiomegaly, congestive cardiomyopathy, and familial occurrence, suggestive of autosomal dominant inheritance. The major clinical manifestations of familial cardiomyopathy include cardiomegaly, congestive heart failure, arrhythmias, syncope, and sudden death. Angina pectoris and embolic episodes are also frequently noted. Electrocardiographic abnormalities, which include rhythm disturbances, left ventricular hypertrophy, intraventricular conduction defects, abnormal Q waves, and the Wolff-Parkinson-White pattern, are often present in affected individuals many years prior to signs of clinical deterioration.[130–135]

The prognosis is highly variable from person to person. Some affected individuals remain asymptomatic except for electrocardiographic abnormalities. Others die of intractable heart failure or of arrhythmias as young adults.[131] Histological examination of affected hearts typically reveals diffuse fibrosis with severe hypertrophy of the remaining muscle fibers.[130–135]

Although the autosomal dominant inheritance of familial cardiomyopathy is beyond doubt in certain pedigrees, there are no unique clinical manifestations of the mutant gene. Thus, in the patient who has a congestive cardiomyopathy and whose family history is not informative, it is difficult to know whether there is a 50 per cent risk of transmitting the disorder to children or whether the cardiomyopathy has a nongenetic etiology. X-linked transmission of dilated cardiomyopathy has also been reported.[135a]

IDIOPATHIC HEMOCHROMATOSIS (See also p. 1739). Idiopathic hemochromatosis is a hereditary multisystem disorder characterized by the deposition of iron in the liver, pancreas, skin, and heart.[136, 137] Clinical manifestations consist of cirrhosis, diabetes mellitus, hyperpigmentation, hypogonadism, cardiomyopathy, and a high incidence of hepatoma. The clinical manifestations are delayed for many years until iron overload has caused significant tissue damage and organ failure. The average diet in America allows a maximal routine iron balance of about 4 mg/per day in males.[137] The average age of overt clinical presentation is usually 40 years or older. Diagnosis is confirmed by the finding of an elevated serum iron concentration (> 180 μg per cent), an elevated transferrin saturation (> 80 per cent), an elevated serum ferritin level (> 900 ng/ml), and an increase in the hepatic iron content (> 600 μg/100 mg dry weight) in the absence of known causes of exogenous iron overload.

The major cardiac findings are rhythm and conduction disturbances and biventricular congestive heart failure, which occur separately or together.[136] The commonest arrhythmias are ventricular extrasystoles, paroxysmal atrial tachycardia and fibrillation, and atrioventricular block. The clinical manifestations of congestive failure include dyspnea, edema, ascites, and a large, globular cardiac silhouette on chest roentgenograms. Rarely, hemochromatosis simulates constrictive pericarditis (presumably because of the decrease in myocardial compliance caused by the iron infiltration of the myocardium), and in such patients a small or normal-sized heart is seen.

Cardiac manifestations are the presenting feature in only 15 per cent of cases, but approximately one-third of patients with hemochromatosis die from congestive heart failure.[137] Cardiac abnormalities are particularly prominent in young patients. Death usually follows within 1 year of onset. A program of repeated phlebotomy may alleviate congestive failure and increase survival in some patients.

Idiopathic hemochromatosis has long been recognized to be an inherited disorder, yet its genetics remained, until the late 1970's, a controversial subject.[138, 139] The difficulty in delineating the precise mode of inheritance arose for several reasons. First, the basic biochemical defect that causes excessive iron absorption from the intestine has not been defined, and thus no unequivocal method for identifying the genotype of affected individuals is available. Second, the phenotypic expression of the disease is highly variable and is greatly influenced by age, sex (the full-blown syndrome is 10 times more common in men than in women), and environmental factors that cause liver damage and promote iron absorption (such as alcoholism, hepatitis, and chronic malnutrition).

In some families parents are free of any evidence of disease, whereas one or more of their offspring become ill as middle-aged adults; this suggests classic autosomal recessive inheritance.[140, 141] In other families, three successive generations have been involved, suggesting autosomal dominant inheritance.[142] Recent studies, however, have pointed out that the vertical transmission of full-blown cases of hemochromatosis is rare, even though it is not unusual to find minor derangements of iron metabolism in the children, siblings, and parents of affected individuals.[137] The most reasonable genetic hypothesis is that the overt cases represent individuals who are homozygous for an abnormal gene, and the individuals with minor abnormalities in iron metabolism are heterozygous carriers.[137]

The genetic hypothesis of autosomal recessive inheritance has recently been clarified by studies of HLA genotype in affected individuals and their relatives.[141–147] The gene causing hemochromatosis is situated close to the HLA-A locus on the short arm of chromosome 6. The gene is present in the heterozygous state in 8 to 10 per cent of Caucasian populations, with 1 in 333 individuals in the population being homozygotes.

Because of the close linkage between the hemochromatosis gene and the HLA loci, siblings with overt hemochromatosis usually have identical HLA alleles on both maternal and paternal chromosomes, i.e., they have the same HLA haplotypes. The most common haplotype in kindreds with hemochromatosis involves the A-3 allele and the B-14 allele (haplotype: HLA-A-3, B-14). However, other haplotypes also occur, thus indicating that the genetic locus for hemochromatosis is clearly distinct from any of the HLA loci. Among the affected homozygotes who have the HLA-A-3 alleles, 30 per cent are homozygous for the A-3 allele, and the remaining 70 per cent are heterozygous for the A-3 allele.[137]

The reason for the association between the HLA-A-3 allele and the hemochromatosis gene is unknown. This linkage possibly suggests a common ancestral origin of the hemochromatosis gene for all affected individuals who carry the HLA-A-3 allele. For example, a mutation leading to enhanced iron absorption may have arisen adjacent to the HLA-A locus on chromosome 6 of an individual who by chance carried the A-3 allele. Because of tight linkage, the two genes have not been separated by recombination over the years, thus explaining the high frequency of HLA-A-3 alleles among affected patients.

Removal of iron by repeated venesections (weekly for 3 years and every 3 to 4 months thereafter) or treatment with an iron chelating agent, desferrioxamine, or both prolongs survival, cures the cardiomyopathy, and may arrest the cirrhosis. Thus, it is incumbent upon the physician who diagnoses a patient with idiopathic hemochromatosis to identify all affected homozygotes among the siblings. This can be done by HLA typing in conjunction with investigation of plasma iron levels, ferritin levels, and total iron-binding capacity.[137] Prophylactic venesections in asymptomatic homozygotes should prevent clinical expression of the disorder.

FAMILIAL AMYLOIDOSIS (See also p. 1431). Amyloid can affect the heart in several ways, including infiltration of the myocardium, infiltration of the walls of the coronary arteries, and deposition in the valves.[148] In most patients with cardiac amyloidosis, the condition does not appear to be inherited. Rather, it is associated with a systemic disorder, such as multiple myeloma, tuberculosis, or chronic osteomyelitis, or it occurs in a relatively high proportion of elderly people in the form of senile cardiac amyloidosis that is localized exclusively to the heart.[148, 149] On the other hand, a dominantly inherited form of primary systemic amyloidosis has been reported in several families.[150, 151] The predominant clinical feature in these families is cardiac involvement, which appears in the fifth decade of life as a restrictive cardiomyopathy, producing congestive heart failure and progressing to death in 3 to 6 years.

MYOTONIC DYSTROPHY (See also p. 1787). Myotonic dystrophy (Steinert disease) is a multisystem disorder inherited as an autosomal dominant trait.[152] The characteristic clinical features include the presence of myotonia (especially in the hands), atrophy of the muscles of the face and the sternocleidomastoids (causing the expressionless "myopathic facies"), bilateral cataracts, frontal baldness, testicular atrophy, infertility or menstrual irregularities, hyperinsulinemia, hypercatabolism of immunoglobulins, and cardiac abnormalities (Figs. 57–9, 10, and 11, pp. 1787 and 1788).

The manifestations of the cardiac disease vary from asymptomatic electrocardiographic abnormalities to overt rhythm and conduction disturbances with heart failure. Abnormal electrocardiographic patterns have been reported in over 50 per cent of affected patients.[153–156] These abnormalities include sinus bradycardia, left-axis deviation, low-voltage T waves, atrial flutter and fibrillation, and AV conduction disturbances that vary from an innocuous prolonged P-R interval to complete AV block with Stokes-Adams attacks. In general, the systemic disease, which begins in the early 20's, is present for several years before cardiac manifestations become overt. Occasionally, however, the rhythm disturbances, conduction defects, or heart failure may become the chief presenting problem and dominate the clinical picture.

The best methods for identifying asymptomatic subjects at 50 per cent risk for ultimately developing the full-blown syndrome are slit-lamp examination (for lens changes), electromyography (for myotonic discharge), and measurement of serum immunoglobulins (for low IgG levels).[157] About 25 per cent of index subjects with myotonic dystrophy owe their disease to a new mutation.[157]

The gene causing myotonic dystrophy is located on chromosome 19 and is linked to the gene *secretor*, which determines the secretion of the ABO blood group substances into blood fluids, including saliva and amniotic fluid.[158] This linkage relation makes it possible, in selected families, to perform amniocentesis for determination of secretor status of the fetus and thereby predict inheritance of the gene for myotonic dystrophy.[159]

DUCHENNE MUSCULAR DYSTROPHY (See also p. 1782). As this disorder is inherited as an X-linked recessive trait, it occurs almost exclusively in males. It characteristically begins during the first 5 years of life. Initial involvement of the pelvic girdle muscles causes lumbar lordosis, a clumsy waddling gait, and pseudohypertrophy of the calves. Progression to other muscles is rapid, and most affected boys are confined to a wheelchair or bed by age 10 years[160] (Fig. 57–1, p. 1782).

The severe and widespread nature of the skeletal muscle impairment generally overshadows the myocardial involvement, which is present in almost all cases. The electrocardiogram is characteristic in that a tall R wave in lead V_1 and deep Q waves in leads I, aV_1, and V_{5-6} are said to occur in no other form of muscular dystrophy[161] (Fig. 57–2, p. 1783). In the majority of patients with Duchenne muscular dystrophy, the distinctive electrocardiogram is the only evidence of cardiac involvement. However, progressive heart failure may develop after years of cardiac stability, and a variety of arrhythmias occur, including labile sinus tachycardia, paroxysmal ventricular tachycardia, and atrial flutter.[161] At autopsy, the heart is not enlarged or hypertrophic. The cardinal pathological findings consist of left ventricular fibrosis and an arteriopathy involving small intramural coronary arteries[161] (Fig. 57–3, p. 1784).

Although the underlying biochemical defect remains obscure, early skeletal muscle damage can be detected by release of the muscle enzyme creatine phosphokinase (CPK) into the serum, thus providing a useful diagnostic test for affected boys. Two-thirds of heterozygous carrier women also have elevated serum CPK levels, making this test useful in genetic counseling.[162] About one-sixth of asymptomatic carrier women show the distinctive electrocardiogram that is seen in affected boys.[163, 164]

The sisters of affected boys often seek genetic counseling and carrier testing before planning their families. Recent studies have demonstrated the usefulness of DNA probes for making a prenatal diagnosis of affected male fetuses. The locus that is disrupted in this disorder has been localized by recombinant DNA techniques to a region spanning 230 kilobases of DNA on the X chromosome. Approximately 10 per cent of affected patients have large deletions that map to this region, whereas the remaining 90 per cent have more subtle genetic abnormalities in this region.[165]

FRIEDREICH'S ATAXIA (See also p. 1789). Friedreich's

ataxia is a familial neuromuscular disorder, inherited as an autosomal recessive trait and characterized clinically by spinocerebellar ataxia, loss of deep tendon reflexes, skeletal deformities, and cardiomyopathy.[166] The one distinctive clinical sign is "Friedreich foot" (Fig. 57–13, p. 1789), a bilateral deformity characterized by *pes cavus* with hammertoes.

Electrocardiographic abnormalities have been found in over 90 per cent of cases and are present in young children close to the time of onset of the neurological disorder.[166–169] The most frequent electrocardiographic change is inversion of the T waves, especially in the left precordial leads but also in leads I, II, and aV_f (Figs. 57–15, p. 1790, and 57–18, p. 1791). Labile sinus tachycardia is common, and rhythm disturbances, especially atrial fibrillation and paroxysmal supraventricular tachycardia, develop in late stages of the disease. Findings suggestive of biventricular hypertrophic obstructive cardiomyopathy have also been reported.[170, 171] At autopsy, the heart shows muscle fiber hypertrophy, interstitial fibrosis, and obliterative disease of small intramural coronary arteries[169] (Fig. 57–17, p. 1791).

The parents of affected patients, who are obligate heterozygotes, do not typically have clinically significant cardiac disease but occasionally may show electrocardiographic abnormalities and asymmetrical septal hypertrophy by echocardiography.[172]

ENDOCARDIAL FIBROELASTOSIS (See also p. 1011). Endocardial fibroelastosis is a disease of infancy and early childhood characterized by thickening of the endocardium, especially of the left ventricle, with resulting cardiac hypertrophy and congestive heart failure. The primary form of the condition occurs in the absence of any other congenital cardiac abnormalities.[173, 174] Like Pompe disease, primary endocardial fibroelastosis causes congestive heart failure and early death in infancy in the absence of cyanosis or significant murmurs.

The incidence of primary endocardial fibroelastosis in the United States is relatively high: 1 case in 5000 to 6000 live births.[175] The occurrence of the disorder among male and female siblings in certain families suggests that one form of endocardial fibroelastosis is due to autosomal recessive inheritance of a mutant gene.[175–177] In addition, an X-linked form of endocardial fibroelastosis has also been described. However, the majority of cases occur sporadically, and, when all family data are subjected to genetic analysis, the proportion of affected siblings is about 7 per cent, a number that is significantly below the expected 25 per cent for simple autosomal recessive inheritance.[176–178] The simplest hypothesis and the one most consistent with available data is that primary endocardial fibroelastosis is heterogeneous in etiology, some cases having a nongenetic cause, some cases being due to autosomal recessive or X-linked recessive inheritance, and most cases having a multifactorial etiology.[176–178]

The biochemical basis of one form of autosomal recessively inherited endocardial fibroelastosis has recently been traced to a severe deficiency of plasma and tissue carnitine.[179] This discovery was made in a family in which cardiomyopathy developed in four of five children, three of whom died suddenly and were found at autopsy to have endocardial fibroelastosis. Study of the surviving affected member of the kindred and autopsy of one of the deceased siblings revealed a 90 to 95 per cent reduction in the carnitine level in plasma, heart and skeletal muscle, and liver. Treatment of the affected child with oral L-carnitine improved myocardial function and reduced the cardiomegaly. The enzymatic basis for the carnitine deficiency in this family is not known. Although other patients with generalized carnitine deficiency have been described, their major clinical manifestation typically consists of progressive skeletal myopathy rather than cardiomegaly.[180] Further studies will be necessary to determine what proportion of patients with nonfamilial and familial forms of endocardial fibroelastosis owe their disease to carnitine deficiency.

CARDIAC ARRHYTHMIAS AND CONDUCTION DEFECTS

In addition to the familial cardiomyopathies that may occur with arrhythmias or conduction defects, a number of familial syndromes that primarily affect the pacemaking and conducting tissues of the heart have been described. Although familial aggregation has been reported for virtually every type of cardiac arrhythmia and conduction defect, in most cases the available genetic data are insufficient to determine whether the defect in a given family results from a single-gene mutation or a multifactorial genetic mechanism. Evidence for a *single-gene mechanism* is compelling, however, in several distinct syndromes.

JERVELL AND LANGE-NIELSEN SYNDROME (See also p. 749). This disorder is characterized by congenital deafness, syncope, prolonged Q-T interval, and sudden death.[181–184] Affected individuals are seen typically in childhood with congenital high-tone perceptive deafness, which is bilateral and severe, and fainting spells precipitated by exertion or nervousness. The electrocardiogram shows a prolonged Q-T interval and large T waves. The syncopal attacks are believed due to episodic ventricular arrhythmias or Stokes-Adams attacks. Administration of digitalis can reduce the Q-T interval and diminish the frequency of syncopal attacks. Since syncopal attacks are usually provoked by exercise, fear, or anger, affected children should be protected from physical and mental stress. At autopsy, histological abnormalities in the artery to the sinus node and to the AV node have been demonstrated.

The cardiac and auditory abnormalities appear to represent a pleiotropic expression of a single gene abnormality, which is inherited by an autosomal recessive mechanism.[185] The incidence of consanguinity among the parents of affected subjects is increased.[182] Although the heterozygotes are clinically normal, their electrocardiograms may show a mildly prolonged Q-T interval.[182] The overall incidence of homozygous affected individuals among all deaf children is about 1 case in 100, whereas among the general population it is about 1 case in 300,000 persons.[182, 185]

ROMANO-WARD SYNDROME (See also p. 749). Romano-Ward syndrome is similar to Jervell and Lange-Nielsen syndrome in that affected individuals show a prolonged Q-T interval and an abnormal configuration of T waves on their electrocardiograms and are prone to ventricular fibrillation and sudden death.[186–190] The two syndromes are clinically and genetically distinct: Deafness is not a feature of Romano-Ward syndrome, and Romano-Ward syndrome is inherited as an autosomal dominant trait.

Patients are usually healthy except for episodes which may take one of three forms: (1) transient attacks of palpitation, numbness, or anginal chest pain without loss of consciousness; (2) sudden loss of consciousness, usually precipitated by exertion or emotional stress; or (3) sudden death. The disorder is predominantly a childhood illness, with onset usually before age 3 years. However, as in most autosomal dominant disorders, a marked variation in the degree of clinical expression occurs, and some affected subjects do not show clinical signs until age 30 years. In general, the later the age of onset, the milder the disease and the less the threat of sudden death. The molecular basis for the underlying abnormality is not known.

FAMILIAL HEART BLOCK (See also p. 967). At least two genetically distinct causes of heart block are currently recognized—one with a congenital onset and one with an adult onset. The congenital disorder is seen either at the time of birth or in early childhood as severe bradycardia due to complete AV block. The prognosis for the congenital form of familial heart block is extremely poor. Most affected individuals die in the neonatal period. Autopsy in several cases has revealed an absence of the AV node as well as an absence of myocardial fibers in the lower part of the interatrial septum.[191, 192]

Early studies suggested that congenital heart block was inherited as an autosomal recessive trait.[191, 192] However, recent reports have shown that a large proportion of infants previously diagnosed as having the autosomal recessive form of congenital heart block are offspring of mothers who have active systemic lupus erythematosus, rheumatoid arthritis, or some other connective tissue disease. The placental transfer of maternal IgG antibody directed against a tissue ribonucleoprotein antigen called Ro(SS-A) is presumed to cause damage to the fetal cardiac conduction system in utero.[193–195] In one study of congenital heart block, 14 of 22 affected children had been born to 11 mothers who had clinical or laboratory evidence of lupus.[194] Congenital heart block may thus represent a familial disease that is not genetic. The clinician should suspect the presence of lupus or a related collagen vascular disease in any mother who gives birth to an infant with congenital heart block.

Familial heart block of adult onset appears to be inherited as an autosomal dominant disorder with varying expressivity.[196–199] Affected individuals typically are seen between the ages of 30 and 50 years with one of the following conduction abnormalities: right bundle branch block alone, left-axis deviation alone, right bundle branch block and left-axis deviation, or complete heart block. Patients may also show atrial fibrillation, atrial flutter, or bidirectional tachycardia. It must be emphasized that affected individuals in the same family characteristically manifest different electrocardiographic patterns. The electrocardiogram in the adult form of familial heart block tends to show a wider QRS complex than is found in the congenital form of familial heart block. Left untreated without a pacemaker, most patients with the adult form of familial heart block ultimately develop syncopal episodes or die suddenly—hence the need for the physician to examine and treat asymptomatic relatives who are at 50 per cent genetic risk.

WOLFF-PARKINSON-WHITE SYNDROME (See also p. 685). The electrocardiographic features of this syndrome are the presence of a short P-R interval and a prolonged QRS, the latter being specifically characterized by a slurred upstroke of the R wave called a delta wave. Patients with Wolff-Parkinson-White (WPW) syndrome are especially prone to paroxysmal supraventricular tachycardia. Although the majority of patients with WPW syndrome do not have a familial disorder, a familial occurrence has been reported on numerous occasions.[200, 201] In certain families, WPW syndrome occurs as a dominantly inherited disorder with no associated cardiac defects, whereas in other families it can occur in association with a dominantly inherited form of familial cardiomyopathy.[202]

CONSTRICTIVE PERICARDITIS

(See also Chapter 44)

MULIBREY NANISM. Mulibrey nanism is a rare autosomal recessive disorder in which constrictive pericarditis is one of the cardinal manifestations. Described for the first time in 1973, the syndrome was given the name mulibrey nanism to symbolize some of these protean features. Mulibrey stands for *mu*scle, *li*ver, *br*ain, and *ey*es; nanism is derived from the Greek word for dwarf, *nanos*.[203, 204] A more appropriate name would be "constrictive pericarditis with dwarfism" to emphasize the two most prominent and consistent features of the syndrome.

Growth failure is evident at the time of birth and is progressive. Affected infants show a triangular face often with hypocephaloid skull, muscular hypotonia, a peculiar squeaky voice, and yellowish dots and pigment dispersion in the ocular fundus. Of 28 patients described in the literature, 25 have shown clinical signs of pericardial constriction, as manifested by prominent neck veins, elevated right-heart pressures on cardiac catherization, and hepatomegaly.[203–208] About 30 per cent of the affected patients so far reported have had ascites, peripheral edema, and proven pericardial constriction necessitating treatment by pericardiotomy.[203–208] Microscopic examination shows a thickened pericardium with calcium deposits but without evidence of active inflammation.[208]

Twenty-four of the 28 reported cases have come from a sparsely settled area of Finland.[203, 204] Two cases have been reported in Canadians,[206] one case in an American,[208] and one case in an Egyptian.[207] All the familial cases have been limited to siblings, and most of the single cases (three of the Finnish patients, the American patient, and the Egyptian patient) have been born to consanguineous parents. These observations strongly support autosomal recessive inheritance. The pathogenesis of this unique disorder is completely unknown.

CARDIAC TUMORS

(See also Chapter 43)

The two most common primary tumors of the heart, myxomas and rhabdomyomas, can occur with or without familial involvement. The nonfamilial cases could represent (1) the occurrence of nongenetic cases, (2) the sporadic occurrence of tumors owing to new single-gene mutations, or (3) the occurrence of only one homozygote in a sibship as in autosomal recessive inheritance. In general, patients with nonfamilial tumors tend to have a single tumor, whereas those with tumors of a genetic origin tend to have multiple tumors.

INTRACARDIAC MYXOMA (See also p. 1474). Most cases of intracardiac myxoma occur as sporadic cases without familial involvement. However, since 1971 at least five families with multiple affected members have been reported.[209–214] In three of the families, only siblings have been affected, suggesting autosomal recessive inheritance.[209–212] However, in two families autosomal dominant inheritance was suggested by the occurrence of myxomas in both a parent and one or more siblings.[213, 214] Affected individuals typically come to attention between the ages of 20 and 40 years because of syncope or signs of systemic embolization. The unique feature of the familial myxoma syndrome, as distinct from the more common nonfamilial tumor, is the presence of multiple tumors that are frequently in atypical locations, such as the pulmonic valve and the right ventricle.

RHABDOMYOMA (See also p. 1475). At least 50 per cent of patients with a single rhabdomyoma of the heart and probably all patients with multiple cardiac rhabdomyomas have tuberous sclerosis.[215] This autosomal dominant disorder is characterized clinically by the following features: adenoma sebaceum of the skin, mental retardation, epilepsy, intracranial calcifications, cutaneous findings (shagreen patches, periungual fibromas, depigmented cutaneous areas), honeycomb lung, gliomas of the brain, retinal phakomas, mixed mesodermal tumors of the kidney, and multiple cardiac rhabdomyomas.[216, 217] As in most autosomal dominant disorders, a wide range of variability in clinical expression from patient to patient occurs.

The most common clinical manifestations, present in at least 60 per cent of affected individuals, are adenoma sebaceum, epilepsy, mental retardation, shagreen patches, and depigmented cutaneous areas.[216, 217] Multiple rhabdomyomas, although highly specific for tuberous sclerosis, are a relatively infrequent manifestation, with no more than 5 per cent of affected individuals developing clinically significant cardiac tumors. Although the rhabdomyomas can occur at any age, they typically come to clinical attention in the neonatal period.[215] The typical patient with rhabdomyomas either shows signs of cardiac failure in the first few days of life or has severe arrhythmias.[215] Some rhabdomyomas may undergo neoplastic change to rhabdomyosarcoma.

CORONARY ARTERY DISEASE

(See also Chapter 36)

Evidence that genetic factors contribute to the pathogenesis of coronary atherosclerosis is based on observations of four types: (1) differences in prevalence among genetically different groups living under similar environmental circumstances[218]; (2) familial aggregation in which first-degree relatives of index coronary patients less than 60 years of age show a five- to sevenfold increased risk of death from myocardial infarction, compared with controls[219, 220]; (3) higher concordance for myocardial infarction in identical twins as opposed to fraternal twins (for female twin pairs: 44 per cent concordance for monozygotic twins and 14 per cent for dizygotic twins)[221]; and (4) association with one or more genetically determined risk factors, such as hypercholesterolemia, hypertriglyceridemia, diabetes mellitus, hypertension, obesity, personality type, and distribution of coronary vasculature.[222, 223]

In most families that seem genetically predisposed to coronary artery disease by history, the nature of the genetic factors underlying this predisposition is obscure.[224] Most patients with coronary artery disease have inherited multiple predisposing genes that interact with multiple environmental factors to produce the disease. In these patients atherosclerosis does not have a single cause. Yet treatment of one of the predisposing factors, such as mild hypertension or hypercholesterolemia, or stopping smoking, will likely slow the progression of the disease.

In some patients coronary artery disease is produced by a single abnormal gene that has a major effect. At least 13 different single-gene disorders, and hence at least 13 different mutant genes, are known to predispose to premature coronary artery disease (Table 49–5). The most common of these single-gene disorders are those that produce hyperlipidemia. At least 20 per cent of consecutively studied survivors of acute myocardial infarction manifest one of these common autosomal dominant forms of familial hyperlipidemia: familial hypercholesterolemia, familial hypertriglyceridemia, or multiple lipoprotein–type hyperlipidemia.[225] The other monogenic hyperlipidemia that predisposes to coronary artery disease, familial dysbetalipoproteinemia (Type 3 hyperlipidemia), is much less common, occurring in only about 1 in 500 unselected survivors of myocardial infarction.[225] These four monogenic forms of hyperlipidemia are discussed in the next section.

In addition to the familial hyperlipidemias, at least nine inborn errors of metabolism are seen, in which coronary narrowing and occlusion are often part of the clinical syndrome, e.g., Hunter syndrome, Hurler syndrome, homocystinuria, alkaptonuria, pseudoxanthoma elasticum,

TABLE 49–5 SINGLE-GENE DISORDERS THAT PREDISPOSE TO PREMATURE CORONARY ARTERY DISEASE

Disorder	Typical Age for Myocardial Infarction	Primary Biochemical Defect	Mechanism of Inheritance	Estimated Population Frequency	References
Familial hypercholesterolemia		Defective cell surface receptor for plasma LDL	Dominant		
Heterozygous form	Adult			1 in 500	7, 227
Homozygous form*	Childhood			1 in 1,000,000	
Multiple lipoprotein-type hyperlipidemia (Familial combined hyperlipidemia)	Adult	Not known	Dominant	1 in 200	225, 227
Familial hypertriglyceridemia	Adult	Not known	Dominant	1 in 300	225, 227
Familial dysbetalipoproteinemia	Adult	Abnormal apo E-2	Recessive	1 in 40,000	225, 227
Hurler syndrome, Type I-H mucopolysaccharidosis*	Childhood	Deficiency of α-L-iduronidase	Recessive	1 in 40,000	81, 104
Hunter syndrome, Type II mucopolysaccharidosis*	Childhood	Deficiency of sulfoiduronide sulfatase	X-linked	1 in 30,000	81, 104
Homocystinuria*	Young adult	Deficiency of cystathionine synthase	Recessive	1 in 75,000	81, 93–95
Pseudoxanthoma elasticum	Young adult	Not known	Dominant and recessive	1 in 100,000	81, 101
Alkaptonuria	Adult	Deficiency of homogentisic acid oxidase	Recessive	1 in 100,000	81
Werner syndrome	Adult	Not known	Recessive	1 in 500,000	228, 229
Fabry disease*	Young adult	Deficiency of α-galactosidase A	X-linked	1 in 40,000	230, 231
Cholesteryl ester storage disease*	Young adult	Deficiency of lysosomal acid lipase	Recessive	1 in 1,000,000	232
Arterial calcification of infancy	Neonates	Not known	Recessive	1 in 1,000,000	102, 103

*Prenatal diagnosis is possible.

Werner syndrome, idiopathic arterial calcification of infancy, cholesteryl ester storage disease, and Fabry disease (Table 49–5). The mechanism for the coronary occlusion differs for each disorder and is directly related to the action of the particular gene. For example, in the Hunter and Hurler syndromes (p. 1728), mucopolysaccharides accumulate in the coronary vessels, whereas in Fabry disease, glycolipids accumulate (p. 1428). Seven of these inborn errors are inherited as autosomal recessive traits (Table 49–5). Although the homozygous form of each condition occurs rarely, with incidences ranging from 1 to 40,000 (homocystinuria) to 1 in 500,000 (Werner syndrome), the estimated combined frequency for the heterozygous carriers of these seven genes is quite significant, involving somewhere between 1 in 30 and 1 in 100 persons in the population. It will therefore be important to determine whether any of the genes for these seven inborn errors can significantly predispose its heterozygous carriers to develop premature coronary atherosclerosis. No such data are currently available.

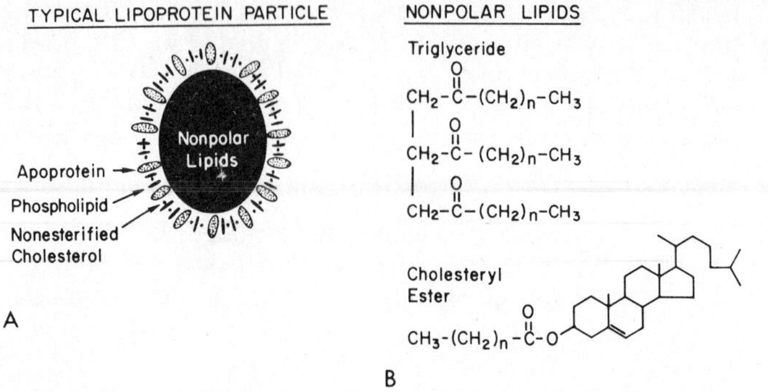

FIGURE 49–5. *A*, Diagrammatic representation of the structure of a typical plasma lipoprotein particle. The *core* of the spherical lipoprotein particle is composed of two nonpolar lipids, triglyceride and cholesteryl ester, which are present in different lipoproteins in varying amounts. The nonpolar core is surrounded by a *surface coat* composed primarily of phospholipids. Apoproteins are exposed at the surface and extend into the core. Variable amounts of unesterified cholesterol are interdigitated with the phospholipids of the surface coat. The quantitative composition of each of the different classes of lipoprotein particles in human plasma is discussed in Chapter 35. *B*, Structures of the two nonpolar lipids, triglyceride and cholesteryl ester. In order for these nonpolar lipids to be assimilated into tissues, the ester bonds between the fatty acids and either glycerol (triglycerides) or cholesterol (cholesteryl esters) must be broken by lipoprotein lipase and the lysosomal cholesteryl esterase, respectively.

SINGLE-GENE DISORDERS CAUSING HYPERLIPIDEMIA AND PREMATURE ATHEROSCLEROSIS

Four monogenic diseases exist in which hyperlipidemia results from a discrete inborn error of metabolism affecting the synthesis, degradation, or structure of a plasma lipoprotein. Each of these single-gene diseases predisposes to coronary atherosclerosis. Together, these diseases are responsible for about 20 per cent of myocardial infarctions that occur before the age of 60.[225] To provide a conceptual background for discussion of these disorders, a brief explanation of normal lipoprotein transport is necessary (for review, see references 7, 226, 233, and 234).

The plasma lipoproteins are globular particles of high molecular weight that transport triglycerides and cholesteryl esters. Each lipoprotein contains a nonpolar core in which cholesteryl ester and triglyceride molecules are packed to form an oil droplet (Fig. 49–5). Surrounding the core is a polar surface coat composed predominantly of phospholipids and unesterified cholesterol. Each lipoprotein also contains specific proteins (termed *apoproteins*) that bind to enzymes or transport proteins, directing the lipoprotein to its sites of metabolism.

The lipoproteins of human plasma can be divided into five major classes, which are discussed in detail in Chapter 36. Each of these five lipoprotein classes differs from the others in the relative proportion of cholesteryl ester and triglyceride in the core, in the nature of its apoproteins, and in density, size, and electrophoretic mobility.[235]

A model showing the salient features of plasma lipoprotein transport is illustrated in Figure 49–6. Lipoproteins transport lipids that are absorbed from the intestine (exogenous pathway) as well as those that emerge from other tissues (endogenous pathway).[7, 233, 234] Within the intestine, cholesterol and triglycerides are incorporated into large lipoprotein particles called *chylomicrons*. After they enter the bloodstream, the chylomicrons bind to an enzyme, *lipoprotein lipase*, which is adherent to capillary walls in

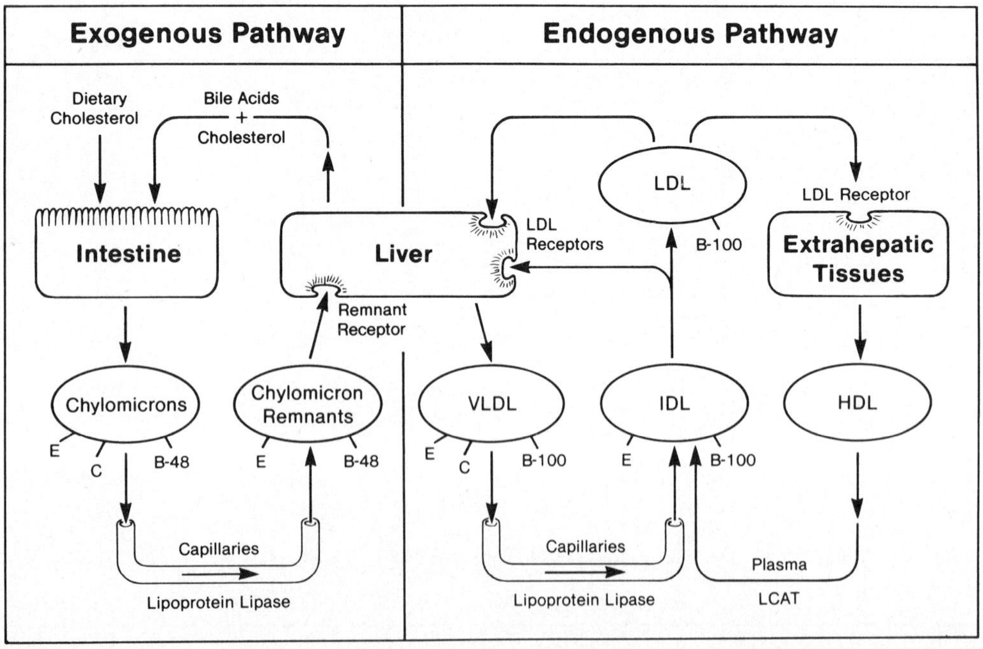

FIGURE 49–6. Model for the metabolism of plasma lipoproteins, showing the separate pathways for transport of exogenous and endogenous lipids. The details of this model are discussed in the text. CE denotes cholesteryl esters; FFA, free fatty acids; TG, triglycerides; HDL, high-density lipoprotein; IDL, intermediate-density lipoprotein; LCAT, lecithin:cholesterol acyltransferase; LDL, low-density lipoprotein; and VLDL, very low-density lipoprotein. A-1, A-2, B-48, B-100, C's and E represent apoproteins associated with the indicated lipoprotein particle. (From Brown, M. S., and Goldstein, J. L.: *In* Gilman's The Pharmacological Basis of Therapeutics. 7th ed. New York, Macmillan Publishing Co., 1985, p. 827.)

adipose tissue and muscle. This enzyme hydrolyzes the triglycerides of the chylomicrons. The liberated fatty acids enter the underlying adipocytes or muscle cells, where they are either reesterified to triglycerides for storage or oxidized for energy.

After the triglycerides are removed, the remainder of the chylomicron dissociates from the capillary wall and reenters the circulation, where it is now designated as a *chylomicron remnant*. The chylomicron remnant is relatively poor in triglyceride and enriched in cholesteryl esters. It is also enriched in an important protein called *apoprotein E*. Chylomicron remnants travel to the liver, where they are taken up with great efficiency as a result of the binding of the apoprotein E to receptors on the surface of hepatocytes. Overall, the two-step pathway of chylomicron metabolism delivers dietary triglyceride to adipose tissue and muscle and dietary cholesterol to the liver.[233, 234]

In the liver the metabolism of dietary fat and endogenously synthesized fat is coordinated to supply needed amounts of fuel and cholesterol to body tissues despite fluctuations in dietary intake. To supply cholesterol and trigylcerides to body tissues, the liver incorporates them into *very low-density lipoproteins (VLDL)*.

VLDL particles are triglyceride-rich and thus resemble chylomicrons, although they are smaller in size. The triglycerides of VLDL are removed through interaction with lipoprotein lipase. The cholesteryl ester–rich remnant of VLDL metabolism is released from the endothelial wall and reenters the circulation, where it is designated *intermediate-density lipoprotein (IDL)*. Although it is similar in structure to the chylomicron remnant, the IDL particle has a different fate. Some IDL particles are taken up by the liver as a result of binding to LDL receptors (see below). Other IDL particles remain in the circulation, where the last traces of triglyceride are removed, and the particle is converted into *low-density lipoprotein (LDL)*. During this conversion, all of the apoproteins leave the particle, with the exception of apoprotein B.[7, 234]

About two-thirds to three-fourths of the cholesterol in normal human plasma is contained within LDL particles. LDL is the particle whose elevation is most frequently related to atherosclerosis. When patients are found to have hypercholesterolemia, this is almost always due to an elevation in the number of LDL particles per milliliter of plasma.

In normal humans LDL circulates with a half-time of about 1.5 days. It is metabolized in liver and extrahepatic tissues. LDL is metabolized by at least two pathways. One pathway involves specific *LDL receptors*, which are located on the surface of liver and extrahepatic cells. The receptor recognizes the *apoprotein B* component of LDL. Binding leads to the uptake and degradation of LDL through a process called *receptor-mediated endocytosis*. This process liberates cholesterol, which all cells need for synthesis of new plasma membranes and which specialized cells need for synthesis of steroid hormones and bile acids.[236]

In normal humans the LDL receptor mediates the degradation of about two-thirds of the LDL particles that are metabolized each day. The remainder of LDL is degraded by receptor-independent pathways. Some of this degradation is believed to occur in macrophages and cells of the reticuloendothelial system, which degrade all plasma proteins. In contrast to the receptor-mediated pathway, which supplies cholesterol to cells for specific metabolic purposes, the *scavenger cell pathway* functions primarily to clear plasma of excess proteins.[7, 234, 237]

As the membranes of parenchymal cells and scavenger cells undergo turnover and as cells die and are renewed, cholesterol is released into the plasma, where it binds to *high-density lipoprotein (HDL)*. When it leaves the tissues, cholesterol is in an unesterified form. For transport in plasma, the cholesterol must be esterified; that is, a fatty acid must be attached in ester linkage to the cholesterol. This esterification reaction occurs in the plasma. The cholesterol that binds to HDL is acted upon by a circulating enzyme called *lecithin:cholesterol acyltransferase (LCAT)*. The cholesteryl esters that are formed by this enzyme are quickly transferred to VLDL and LDL particles in plasma.[237a] This completes a cycle by which extrahepatic cells take up cholesterol from LDL and then return cholesterol to new particles of LDL as they are being formed in the plasma. This continuous cycling of cholesterol into and out of tissues accounts for a large fraction of the plasma cholesterol in humans.[233, 237a] This explains why acute changes in dietary cholesterol have relatively small effects on the plasma cholesterol level, since most of the plasma cholesterol represents molecules that are cycling into and out of various tissues and not molecules that have recently been synthesized or absorbed from the diet.[233, 237a]

FAMILIAL HYPERCHOLESTEROLEMIA (See also p. 1154). Familial hypercholesterolemia is the outstanding example of a single-gene mutation that produces both hypercholesterolemia and atherosclerosis. It is one of the few examples of an autosomal dominant trait for which homozygotes exist. Heterozygotes for familial hypercholesterolemia number about 1 in 500 persons in the population, making this disease one of the most common disorders that is caused by a single mutant gene. Homozygotes for familial hypercholesterolemia are rare; they occur at a frequency of 1 in one million.[7, 227]

The inherited defect in familial hypercholesterolemia lies in the gene for the cell-surface LDL receptor. Heterozygotes inherit one mutant gene for the receptor and one normal gene. Their cells can produce only half the normal number of receptors. Homozygotes inherit two copies of the mutant gene. Their cells can produce few, if any, LDL receptors. The heterozygous and homozygous forms of the disease differ in severity. Heterozygotes have 2- to 3-fold elevations of plasma LDL, whereas homozygotes have 6- to 10-fold elevations. Heterozygotes develop myocardial infarctions typically in their 30's and 40's, whereas homozygotes usually develop mycardial infarctions before the age of 20.

Heterozygous Familial Hypercholesterolemia. At the time of birth, these individuals have two- to threefold elevation in the LDL-cholesterol level, which persists throughout life.[238] This hypercholesterolemia leads to cholesterol deposition in arteries (producing atheromas) and in tendons (producing xanthomas).

A number of studies have carefully documented the incidence of premature coronary artery disease in heterozygotes. In England, Slack found that the mean onset of coronary artery disease was 43 years for heterozygous men and 53 years for heterozygous women.[239] Eighty-five per cent of the affected males and 58 per cent of the affected females had sustained a myocardial infarction by age 60. In Denmark, Jensen et al. found that the incidence of coronary artery disease among heterozygotes over a 20-year period (32 per cent) was 25 times greater than among unaffected relatives (1.3 per cent).[240]

In the United States, familial hypercholesterolemia heterozygotes constitute about 5 per cent of all patients who have a myocardial infarction.[225] Stone et al. found that the cumulative probability of coronary artery disease by age 40 in male heterozygotes was 16 per cent.[241] By age 60 it had risen to 52 per cent, as opposed to 12.7 per cent in unaffected men. Female heterozygotes showed an incidence of coronary artery disease of 33 per cent by age 60, compared with only 9 per cent in unaffected females. Thus, despite the presence of the same genetic abnormality and similarly elevated plasma LDL levels, heterozygous women manifest coronary artery disease less often and at a later age than do heterozygous men.

Despite this marked increase in the frequency of coronary artery disease, familial hypercholesterolemia heterozygotes do *not* appear to have an increased frequency of cerebral vascular disease or of hypertension. The incidence of peripheral vascular disease is possibly elevated in familial hypercholesterolemia heterozygotes, but not in so striking a fashion as the incidence of coronary artery disease. In contrast, patients with familial dysbetalipoproteinemia (Type III hyperlipoproteinemia) have an increased incidence of both coronary artery disease and peripheral vascular disease (see below). Patients with dysbetalipoproteinemia accumulate IDL particles in plasma, whereas familial hypercholesterolemia patients accumulate LDL particles. It is possible that the LDL particles have a greater toxicity for coronary arteries than for peripheral arteries, whereas IDL particles are equally toxic for both types of vessels.

Familial hypercholesterolemia heterozygotes also have tendon xanthomas, which are nodular swellings that may involve the Achilles tendon and various tendons about the knee, elbow, and dorsum of the hand (Fig. 49–7*A*). Like the atheromas, the xanthomas consist of massive deposits of cholesterol, apparently derived from the deposition of LDL particles. The cholesterol is located as amorphous extracellular deposits as well as vacuoles within scavenger cells (macrophages) that have invaded the lesion. The latter become so swollen with lipid droplets that they are termed *foam cells*.

In familial hypercholesterolemia heterozygotes, cholesterol deposits are also formed in the soft tissue of the eyelid, producing xanthelasma, and within the cornea, producing arcus cornae (Fig. 49–7*B*). Whereas tendon xanthomas are diagnostic of familial hypercholesterolemia, xanthelasma and arcus corneae are not specific. The latter also occur in many adults with normal plasma lipid levels. The incidence of tendon xanthomas in familial hypercholesterolemia increases with age, but no more than 75 per cent of affected heterozygotes display this sign.[227]

Homozygous Familial Hypercholesterolemia. Homozygotes have marked elevations in the plasma level of LDL from birth, the plasma cholesterol level usually being six- to eightfold above normal. A unique type of planar cutaneous xanthoma is often present at birth and always develops within the first 6 years of life.[227, 242] These yellow xanthomas occur at points of trauma, such as over the knees, elbows, and buttocks. They almost always occur in the interdigital webs of the hands, particularly between the thumb and index finger (Fig. 49–7*C*). Tendon xanthomas, arcus corneae, and xanthelasma also occur in homozygotes.

Coronary artery atherosclerosis in homozygotes is rapidly progressive. Angina pectoris, myocardial infarction, or sudden death occur commonly in homozygotes between the ages of 5 and 30. One homozygote is even recorded as having had an acute myocardial infarction as early as 18 months of age. Very few homozygotes survive past age 30.[227, 243, 244]

In homozygotes, severe atherosclerosis occurs not only in the coronary arteries but also in the thoracic and

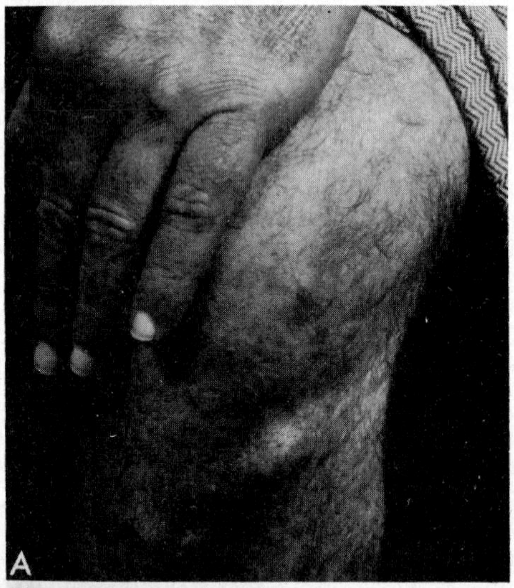

FIGURE 49–7. Forms of xanthomas and other lipid deposition frequently seen in patients with familial hypercholesterolemia. Tendon xanthomas (*A*) and arcus corneae (*B*) occur in both heterozygotes and homozygotes. Cutaneous planar xanthomas (*C*), which usually have a bright orange hue, occur in homozygotes and not in heterozygotes.

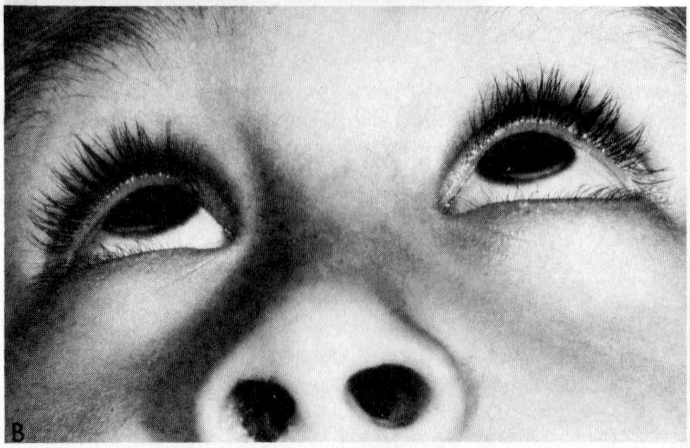

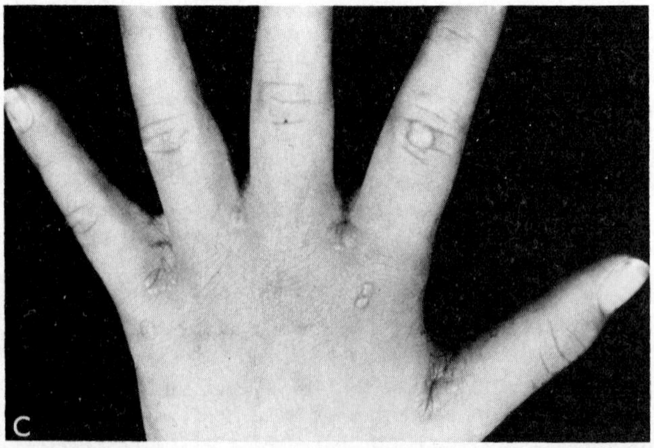

abdominal aorta as well as in the major pulmonary arteries.[227, 243, 244] Microscopic examination of the coronary and pulmonary arterial lesions in these children and young adults shows typical atherosclerotic plaques as well as a striking intimal infiltration of xanthomatous foam cells and cholesterol clefts that are reminiscent of the histological appearance of a tendon xanthoma.[243, 245] Atheromatous and xanthomatous involvement of the aortic valve is another characteristic cardiac manifestation observed in the homozygote. The deposition of cholesterol frequently produces significant aortic stenosis, which in turn causes congestive heart failure.[243–248] Necropsy has confirmed the presence of an aortic valve lesion, and in several of these cases histological studies have demonstrated cholesterol clefts and foam cells in the aortic valve cusps, at the same time excluding an associated rheumatic valvulitis or congenital bicuspid valve.[227, 243, 244]

Xanthomatous plaquing and thickening of the endocardial surfaces of the mitral valve and endocardium have also been observed in the homozygote and may explain the clinical findings of mitral regurgitation and mitral stenosis that are occasionally reported.[243, 244] Since the homozygote often has painful joints, a persistently elevated sedimentation rate (due to the high plasma LDL level), and cardiac murmurs, a misdiagnosis of acute rheumatic fever may easily be made.[249] Diffuse xanthomatous infiltration of the myocardium is occasionally mentioned as another pathological lesion in the homozygote,[243] but this has not been well documented.

In contrast to the disorders causing hypertriglyceridemia, in familial hypercholesterolemia, obesity and diabetes mellitus do not occur with increased frequency in either the homozygote or the heterozygote. A slender body habitus is the general rule.

Pathogenesis. The primary defect in familial hypercholesterolemia resides in the gene for the LDL receptor. The gene has been isolated by molecular cloning, and several of the mutations in familial hypercholesterolemia patients have been elucidated in molecular detail.[7, 250] These mutations can lead to abnormalities in any region of the LDL receptor protein. Some of the mutations totally abolish synthesis of receptors. Other mutations cause relatively subtle defects that affect only the site that binds LDL. Still other mutations can leave the binding site intact but destroy the site that allows the receptor to carry LDL into the cell. Thus, patients with familial hypercholesterolemia can have manifestations of varying severity. In general, those individuals with mutations that totally abolish the function of the gene have higher plasma cholesterol levels and a more severe clinical course than do individuals whose mutations only partially inactivate the gene.

Familial hypercholesterolemia homozygotes inherit two mutant genes at the LDL receptor locus, one from each parent. However, both mutations need not be the same. Thus, homozygotes show a spectrum of severity. In the most severe cases no functional LDL receptors are produced. These individuals with the receptor-negative phenotype remove LDL from plasma at a very sluggish rate. The lipoprotein builds up to high levels and produces atherosclerosis. Other homozygotes have at least one copy of an allele that produces some functional receptors. These individuals are said to have the receptor-defective phenotype. As a rule, these individuals also have very high plasma LDL cholesterol levels (greater than 500 mg/dl). However, they seem to have a slightly better prognosis than the receptor-negative individuals.[227] Moreover, they have the potential to respond to some forms of therapy (see below).

Heterozygotes with familial hypercholesterolemia always have one normal allele at the LDL receptor locus. Therefore, even if their mutant allele is totally nonfunctional, they are able to produce about 50 per cent of the normal number of LDL receptors. Because of this 50 per cent deficiency of LDL receptors, plasma LDL levels rise two to threefold until a new steady-state is attained in which the rate of degradation of plasma LDL equals the rate of production. However, this compensation is achieved at a severe price. The two to threefold elevation in LDL levels leads to accelerated atherosclerosis.

In heterozygotes and homozygotes the elevated LDL level causes an increase in the uptake of LDL by scavenger cells, which do not utilize the LDL receptor, and, as a consequence, LDL-cholesterol accumulates in these macrophage-like cells at various sites in the body, such as in tendon, producing xanthomas. The accelerated coronary atherosclerosis characteristic of familial hypercholesterolemia also results from the large amounts of LDL that penetrate the artery wall following endothelial damage. The large quantities of LDL that infiltrate the artery wall present a load of lipoproteins that is greater than can be cleared from the interstitial space by the scavenger cells, ultimately resulting in atherosclerosis (Chap. 35). There is also evidence that the high LDL levels may enhance the growth of the atherosclerotic plaques by accelerating the aggregation of platelets at sites of endothelial injury.[251]

Diagnosis. The finding of an isolated elevation of plasma cholesterol with a normal concentration of plasma triglycerides suggests the diagnosis of heterozygous familial hypercholesterolemia. Such an elevation in plasma cholesterol is due to an isolated elevation in the plasma concentration of LDL (Type IIA hyperlipoproteinemia) in nearly all cases. However, it must be appreciated that most individuals with Type IIA hyperlipoproteinemia have, rather than familial hypercholesterolemia, a form of polygenic hypercholesterolemia that puts them on the upper end of the bell-shaped curve for the general population.[227] As noted below, Type IIA hyperlipoproteinemia may also be caused by the disease multiple lipoprotein–type hyperlipidemia. Hypothyroidism and nephrotic syndrome can also cause Type IIA hyperlipoproteinemia.

Among individuals with a Type IIA lipoprotein pattern, those with heterozygous familial hypercholesterolemia can usually be distinguished from those with polygenic hypercholesterolemia and multiple lipoprotein–type hyperlipidemia. In familial hypercholesterolemia, the plasma cholesterol level tends to be higher than in the other two disorders. Thus, a plasma cholesterol level in the range of 350 to 400 mg/dl is much more suggestive of heterozygous familial hypercholesterolemia than of the other disorders. However, cholesterol levels of 285 to 350 mg/dl are not diagnostic and may be observed in many patients with heterozygous familial hypercholesterolemia as well as with other disorders. Tendon xanthomas do not occur typically in patients with forms of hyperlipidemia other than familial hypercholesterolemia. Other family members should be surveyed when the diagnosis is in doubt. The penetrance of the gene is extremely high in familial hypercholesterolemia, with 50 per cent of first-degree relatives showing an elevated plasma cholesterol level. Hypercholesterolemia in childhood is characteristic of familial hypercholesterolemia but not of the other aforementioned disorders.[227, 233]

A small fraction, approximately 10 per cent, of heterozygotes with familial hypercholesterolemia have, in addition to the raised cholesterol level, an elevated plasma triglyceride level (Type IIB pattern). This condition is difficult to differentiate from multiple lipoprotein–type hyperlipidemia. However, the presence of a tendon xanthoma or a hypercholesterolemic child in the family favors the diagnosis of heterozygous familial hypercholesterolemia.

The diagnosis of *homozygous familial hypercholesterolemia* can readily be established. Often a dermatologist is the first to see these patients in childhood because of obvious cutaneous xanthomas. Occasionally, the development of angina pectoris due to premature coronary atherosclerosis or a syncopal episode caused by xanthomatous aortic stenosis are the presenting features. A cholesterol level greater than 600 mg/dl with a normal triglyceride level in a nonjaundiced child suggests this diagnosis. Both parents should have heterozygous familial hypercholesterolemia with moderately elevated cholesterol levels.

The diagnosis of both heterozygotes and homozygotes with familial hypercholesterolemia can be established in specialized laboratories by direct measurement of the number of LDL receptors on freshly isolated blood lymphocytes[252, 253] or cultured skin fibroblasts.[227] The finding of an absence of LDL receptors on cultured amniotic fluid cells has permitted the diagnosis of homozygous familial hypercholesterolemia in utero.[254] With the cloning of the LDL receptor gene, it now becomes possible to diagnose familial hypercholesterolemia by hybridization studies of DNA isolated from circulating leukocytes of affected subjects.[250] However, widespread use of this technique will be limited because of the large number of different mutations in this gene that cause familial hypercholesterolemia. It is not presently feasible to screen for all potential mutations in an individual at risk.

A functional assay of LDL receptors also offers promise as a diagnostic test. Lymphocytes isolated from blood are stimulated to divide in the presence of LDL plus an inhibitor of cholesterol synthesis. Under these conditions, the rate of cell division is proportional to the number of functional LDL receptors. In one study this technique was capable of differentiating normal subjects from FH heterozygotes.[253]

Treatment. Every effort should be made to lower the plasma LDL level into the normal range, since atherosclerosis in this disorder is a consequence of the longstanding elevation of plasma LDL levels. Patients should be placed on a diet that is low in cholesterol and saturated fats and high in polyunsaturated fats (p. 1167); this usually results in a 10 to 15 per cent drop in the plasma cholesterol level.[227, 255, 256]

When dietary therapy fails to lower the cholesterol levels to the normal range, bile acid–binding resins, such as cholestyramine or colestipol (p. 1169), should be added to the regimen. These resins trap the bile acids that are secreted by the liver into the intestine and transport them into the feces. The initial result of this treatment is a dramatic loss of cholesterol from the body, since the body responds to bile acid depletion by converting additional cholesterol into bile acids. The liver also takes up more cholesterol by producing more LDL receptors. Unfortunately, subjects with familial hyperlipoproteinemia also respond to this loss of cholesterol stores with a compensatory enhancement of cholesterol synthesis by the liver, which ultimately limits the long-term success of this therapy. However, the addition of nicotinic acid may help to block this compensatory increase in hepatic cholesterol synthesis.[227, 256] The extent of reduction in plasma cholesterol level that is usually achieved in heterozygotes is in the range of 25 per cent with the combination of diet and bile acid–binding resins, and nicotinic acid allows the addition of a further lowering of the cholesterol levels. Gastrointestinal bloating, cramps, and constipation are the major side effects of bile acid–binding resins, whereas hepatotoxicity, flushing, and headaches are the major side effects of nicotinic acid. Partial ileal bypass has the same functional effect as bile acid–binding resins, i.e., it causes a loss of bile acids in the stool and results in a moderate to marked lowering of plasma cholesterol level in heterozygotes. This operation may be indicated in patients in whom drug therapy is not tolerated.

A promising new treatment consists of a class of drugs that inhibit synthesis of cholesterol in the liver by inhibiting the activity of a rate-limiting enzyme, 3-hydroxy-3-methylglutaryl coenzyme A reductase (HMG CoA reductase).[76, 255–257] The first of this class of drugs to reach advanced clinical trials is called mevinolin. It reduces plasma LDL-cholesterol levels by up to 30 per cent in heterozygotes.[258] When mevinolin is given together with a bile acid binding resin such as cholestyramine, the compensatory increase in cholesterol synthesis is blocked and plasma LDL levels fall by about 50 per cent on average.[255, 259, 260] As of this writing, the long-term safety of mevinolin has not yet been established and the drug is not yet available for general use.

A reduction of serum cholesterol is much more difficult to achieve in receptor-negative homozygotes than heterozygotes, since combination therapy consisting of diet, a bile acid–binding resin, and nicotinic acid (or mevinolin) has little effect[227, 255, 256] and ileal bypass is uniformly ineffective.[261] Portacaval anastomosis has been effective in several children[262] but must still be regarded as an experimental procedure. Plasma exchanges at monthly intervals using a continuous-flow blood cell separator will lower the cholesterol in all homozygotes[263] to about 300 mg/dl; it then gradually rises over the ensuing 4 weeks to the pretreatment level of 600 to 900 mg/dl. Plasma exchange is the treatment of choice for familial hypercholesterolemia homozygotes when facilities for carrying out this procedure on a monthly basis are available.

One 6-year-old girl with homozygous familial hypercholesterolemia has been successfully treated by combined liver and heart transplantation.[264] The new liver, with its normal complement of LDL receptors, was able to lower the plasma LDL level nearly into the normal range. The heart transplantation was necessitated because the patient had sustained several previous myocardial infarctions and suffered from congestive heart failure. Two and one-half years after this operation the patient was doing well clinically.

FAMILIAL HYPERTRIGLYCERIDEMIA. Patients with this common autosomal dominant disorder, in which the concentration of VLDL is elevated in the plasma, do not usually exhibit hypertriglyceridemia until puberty or early adulthood. The fasting plasma triglyceride level then tends to be moderately elevated and in the range of 200 to 500 mg/dl (Type IV lipoprotein pattern). Obesity, hyperglycemia, hyperinsulinemia, hypertension, and hyperuricemia occur frequently in these patients.[233, 265, 266] Xanthomas are *not* a characteristic feature.

Patients with familial hypertriglyceridemia exhibit a slightly increased incidence of atherosclerosis; affected patients constituted 5 per cent of all patients with myocardial infarction in one study.[225] It is not certain that the hypertriglyceridemia per se accounts for the increased atherosclerosis, since many patients with this condition have diabetes, obesity, and hypertension[267] and each of these features by itself may predispose to atherosclerosis.

Patients with familial hypertriglyceridemia with mild to moderate elevations of VLDL can develop a severe exacerbation when exposed to a variety of precipitating factors, such as excessive consumption of alcohol, poorly controlled diabetes, ingestion of birth control pills containing estrogen, and the development of hypothyroidism.[266, 267] The plasma triglyceride level in affected patients can rise to values in excess of 1000 mg/dl in response to any of these stimuli, and large triglyceride-laden particles with the characteristics of chylomicrons appear in the plasma. Such patients develop *mixed hyperlipidemia*, with an elevation in the concentration of both VLDL and chylomicrons (Type V lipoprotein pattern) during these exacerbations. Patients may develop eruptive xanthomas and pancreatitis whenever the concentration of chylomicrons rises to high levels. The chylomicron-like particles disappear from the plasma, and the patient returns to the basal condition, in which the concentration of triglycerides is moderately elevated when the exacerbating condition is treated.

Some of the members in certain families with the so-called "familial Type V hyperlipidemia" exhibit a severe mixed hyperlipemia even in the absence of known exacerbating factors. Only the mild form of the disease, with moderate hypertriglyceridemia and no hyperchylomicronemia (Type IV pattern), may be present in other affected individuals in the same family.[233, 266]

Pathogenesis. Familial hypertriglyceridemia is transmitted as an autosomal dominant trait, implying a mutation of a single gene. This disorder appears to be genetically heterogeneous in that patients from different families may have different mutations accounting for the hypertriglyceridemia phenotype.[233, 265, 266] No consistent abnormalities of lipoprotein structure have thus far been identified, although affected patients tend to have larger, more triglyceride-rich VLDL particles than do normal subjects and patients with other hypertriglyceridemic syndromes (see below). Some patients have an elevated production rate for VLDL-triglyceride, especially when their diets are high in carbohydrate.[268] Although many of these patients suffer from obesity and diabetes mellitus, other individuals with obesity and diabetes mellitus also overproduce VLDL but have normal plasma VLDL levels. This observation suggests that inability to catabolize the triglycerides of VLDL represents the underlying defect in patients with familial hypertriglyceridemia. Hypertriglyceridemia results when VLDL production rates become elevated owing to obesity or diabetes.[233, 266] However, lipoprotein lipase activity in plasma following the administration of heparin is generally normal.

Diabetes and obesity tend to increase VLDL-triglyceride production and hence to exacerbate hypertriglyceridemia in this syndrome, but the increased prevalence of these conditions is believed to be fortuitous. There is evidence that hypertriglyceridemia and diabetes are inherited by independent mechanisms.[269] However, the hypertriglyceridemia is much more severe when an individual inherits both the gene or genes for diabetes and the gene for hypertriglyceridemia, and such a person is more likely to come to medical attention. Similarly, an individual of normal weight with familial hypertriglyceridemia will usually have mild hypertriglyceridemia and will be less likely to come to medical attention. However, if such an individual becomes obese, the hypertriglyceridemia will worsen, and a diagnosis is more likely to be made.[233]

Diagnosis. A moderate elevation in plasma triglyceride level, together with a normal cholesterol level, suggests the possibility of familial hypertriglyceridemia. Plasma electrophoresis shows an increase in the pre-beta fraction (Type IV lipoprotein pattern). In the occasional patient who exhibits severe hypertriglyceridemia with an elevation of chylomicrons and VLDL (Type V lipoprotein pattern), the plasma shows a creamy supernatant layer (chylomicrons) and a cloudy infranatant layer (VLDL) after overnight storage in the refrigerator.[233, 266]

No simple test currently exists to determine whether an individual who has an elevation in VLDL levels with or without an elevation in chylomicrons has familial hypertriglyceridemia or hypertriglyceridemia due to some other genetic or acquired cause, such as multiple lipoprotein–type hyperlipidemia or sporadic hypertriglyceridemia. However, half of the first-degree relatives of patients with typical cases of familial hypertriglyceridemia exhibit hypertriglyceridemia, and no relatives with isolated hypercholesterolemia should be found. When the latter is present, the diagnosis of multiple lipoprotein–type hyperlipase is suggested.

Treatment. It is essential, first of all, to control all of the exacerbating conditions, including obesity. The diet should be restricted in calories, saturated fat, and alcohol. Diabetes mellitus and hypothyroidism, if present, should be treated vigorously; oral contraceptives should be avoided. However, if the above measures fail, clofibrate is usually effective.[233, 265, 266]

MULTIPLE LIPOPROTEIN–TYPE HYPERLIPIDEMIA (FAMILIAL COMBINED HYPERLIPIDEMIA). In this common disorder, inherited as an autosomal dominant trait, affected individuals in a single family characteristically show one of three different lipoprotein patterns: hypercholesterolemia (Type IIA), hypertriglyceridemia (Type IV), or both hypercholesterolemia and hypertriglyceridemia.[225, 233, 268] In this condition, hyperlipidemia is not usually present in affected patients in childhood but begins to appear at puberty and continues thereafter. The lipid elevations are often mild, and they change over time in affected individuals, often exhibiting a mildly elevated cholesterol level at one examination and/or a mildly elevated triglyceride level at another. An elevation in the incidence of myocardial infarction in affected women as well as men is characteristic, and there is usually a strong family history of premature coronary artery disease. Indeed, patients with multiple lipoprotein–type hyperlipidemia constitute about 10 per cent of all patients who have a myocardial infarction.[225] Xanthomas are not a feature of this condition. Although the incidence of obesity, hyperuricemia, and glucose intolerance is increased in affected individuals, especially those with hypertriglyceridemia, this association is not so striking as the one found with familial hypertriglyceridemia.

Pathogenesis. Since the disease is transmitted within families as an autosomal dominant trait, a mutation in a single gene is probably responsible. As would be expected with this mode of inheritance, about half of the first-degree relatives of an affected individual also have hyperlipidemia.[225, 270–275] A key feature of this condition is the great variability of blood lipids among affected individuals in the same family and, as already pointed out, in the same individual at different times. About one-third of relatives of those individuals with hyperlipidemia will have hypercholesterolemia (Type IIA lipoprotein pattern), one-third will have hypertriglyceridemia (Type IV), and the remainder both hypercholesterolemia and hypertriglyceridemia (Type IIB). The plasma lipid levels tend to hover at the 95th percentile for the population. The variability of lipoprotein phenotypes that constitutes the characteristic feature of this condition is illustrated in Figure 49–8, which shows the pedigrees of four large families affected by this disorder.

It has been postulated[225] and demonstrated[268, 276] that affected individuals have an elevated secretion rate for VLDL from the liver and that this overproduction of the apoprotein B component of VLDL may manifest itself alternatively as an elevation in plasma VLDL levels (hypertriglyceridemia), an elevation in LDL levels (hypercholesterolemia), or both, depending on the interplay of factors governing the efficiency of conversion of VLDL to LDL and the efficiency of catabolism of LDL. As in familial hypertriglyceridemia, the hyperlipidemia is worsened by diabetes, alcoholism, and hypothyroidism.

Diagnosis. There are no clinical or laboratory methods that indicate whether an individual with hyperlipidemia has the multiple lipoprotein–type disorder, since type IIA, IIB, and IV lipoprotein patterns can each occur in patients with several diseases. However, this disorder should be suspected in any individual whose hyperlipoproteinemia is mild, whose lipoprotein type changes with time, and among whose relatives multiple abnormal lipoprotein types occur (Fig. 49–8). Tendon xanthomas in the patient or relatives or the finding of hypercholesterolemia in a relative under the age of 10 years, both of which suggest the diagnosis of heterozygous familial hypercholesterolemia, exclude the diagnosis of multiple lipoprotein–type hyperlipidemia.

Treatment. Weight reduction, restriction of dietary saturated fat and cholesterol, and avoidance of alcohol and oral contraceptives are useful general measures. In addition, clofibrate is effective when the triglyceride level is elevated with or without hypercholesterolemia, while a bile acid–binding resin usually lowers an elevated cholesterol level. However, the lowering of cholesterol levels with such a drug may be accompanied by an increase in triglyceride levels that tends to negate its beneficial effects.

FAMILIAL DYSBETALIPOPROTEINEMIA (TYPE III HYPERLIPOPROTEINEMIA). The expression of this disorder, which is transmitted by a single-gene mechanism, requires the presence of a mutation in a gene encoding a plasma apolipoprotein (apo E) plus contributory environmental or genetic factors.[233, 277, 278] The plasma concentrations of cholesterol and triglycerides are both elevated because of the accumulation in plasma of remnant-like particles derived from the partial catabolism of VLDL and chylomicrons.

Clinical Features. Hyperlipidemia or any of the other clinical features of the disease are usually not manifest until after the age of 20 years. Two types of cutaneous xanthomas are characteristic of familial dysbetalipoproteinemia: xanthomata striata palmaris, which appear as orange or yellow discolorations of the palmar and digital creases, and tuberous or tuberoeruptive xanthomas, which are bulbous cutaneous xanthomas that may vary from pea- to lemon-sized and are characteristically located over the elbows and knees. Xanthelasmas of the eyelids also occur, but these are not unique to this disorder (p. 15). Patients with clinical manifestations of dysbetalipoproteinemia are often found to have hypothyroidism, obesity, or diabetes mellitus.[233, 277, 278]

Clinically, this condition is characterized by severe atherosclerosis involving the coronary arteries, the internal carotids, and the abdominal aorta and its branches. Forty-three per cent of the nearly 50 patients described by Morganroth et al.[279] had detectable vascular disease, and in the one-third who had coronary artery disease the mean age of onset was 38 years in men and about a decade later in women. Peripheral vascular disease, manifest mainly as claudication, was also found in about one-third, again appearing earlier in men than in women; cerebrovascular disease occurred in 5 of their 47 patients. Except for homozygous familial hypercholesterolemia, familial dysbetalipoproteinemia probably results in as high a risk of premature vascular disease as any form of hyperlipidemia. This diagnosis should be considered in any patient who has hyperlipidemia and peripheral vascular disease.

Pathogenesis. This form of hyperlipidemia is caused by the accumulation of relatively large lipoprotein particles that contain both triglycerides and cholesteryl esters and that resemble the remnants and IDL particles that are normally produced from the catabolism of chylomicrons and VLDL through the action of lipoprotein lipase (Fig. 49–5). These remnant particles are rapidly taken up by the liver of normal subjects, and hence they are barely detectable in plasma. However, the uptake of remnants by the

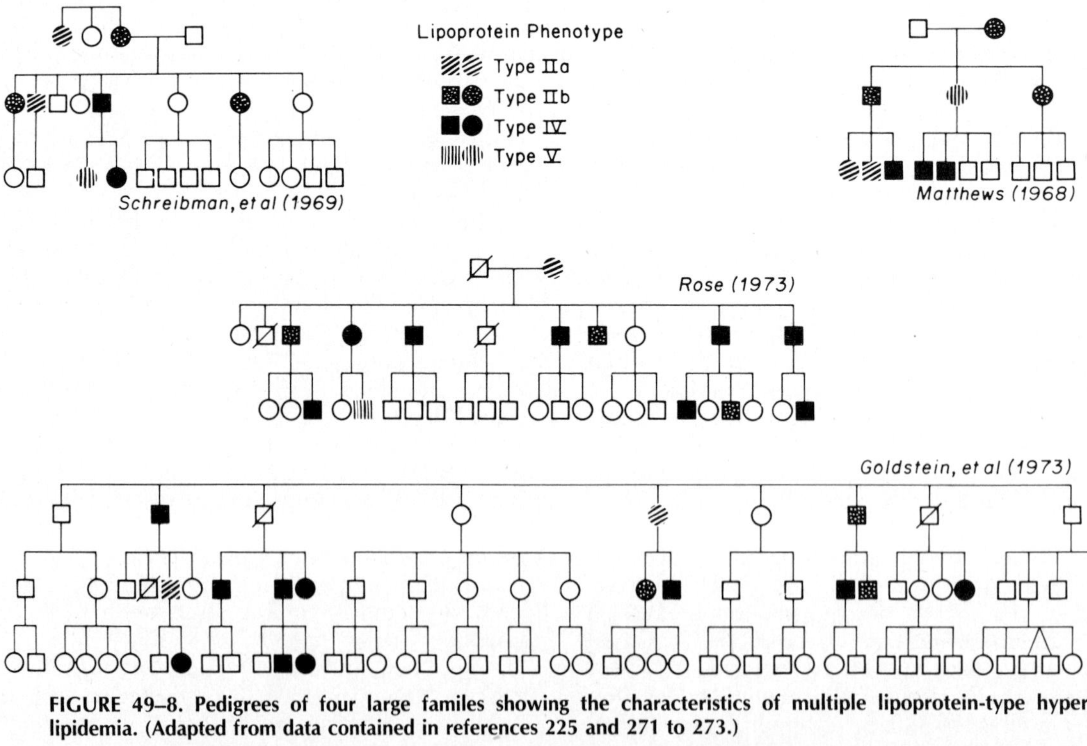

FIGURE 49–8. Pedigrees of four large familes showing the characteristics of multiple lipoprotein-type hyperlipidemia. (Adapted from data contained in references 225 and 271 to 273.)

liver is blocked in patients with familial dysbetalipoproteinemia, leading to the accumulation of high levels of these lipoproteins in plasma and deposition in tissues, producing xanthomas and atherosclerosis.[238, 277, 278]

Patients with familial dysbetalipoproteinemia are homozygous for a mutant gene specifying apoprotein E, a normal constituent of VLDL and chylomicron remnants.[278, 280] The normal function of apo E is to bind to hepatic lipoprotein receptors, an event which is necessary for the rapid hepatic uptake of IDL and chylomicron remnants.[281, 282] The apo E gene is polymorphic in the population. The three common alleles are designated apo E-2, apo E-3, and apo E-4. The apo E-3 and apo E-4 alleles code for proteins that function normally. The protein specified by the apo E-2 allele is nonfunctional. It does not bind to hepatic receptors.[278, 281]

About 1 per cent of Caucasian individuals are homozygous for the apo E-2 allele. However, only 1 in 100 of these homozygous individuals (or 1 in 10, 000 of the general population) has clear-cut familial dysbetalipoproteinemia.[272, 278, 280] The vast majority of apo E-2 homozygotes are able to compensate somehow for their defective protein. They have very slight elevations in the concentration of IDL and chylomicron remnants in plasma and are asymptomatic. The reason why 1 per cent of the apo E-2 homozygotes cannot compensate for their defect and develop severe dysbetalipoproteinemia is not known. In some families the expression of dysbetalipoproteinemia appears to require two factors: (1) homozygosity for the apo E-2 allele and (2) the independent inheritance of another form of genetic hyperlipidemia, such as familial combined hyperlipidemia or familial hypercholesterolemia.[278, 283] When either of these dominant traits is present together with apo E-2 homozygosity, the disease is expressed as familial dysbetalipoproteinemia. Other subjects with symptomatic dysbetalipoproteinemia who are apo E-2 homozygotes apparently have the clinical expression brought on by hypothyroidism or by diabetes mellitus.[277, 278, 284]

Diagnosis. Approximately 80 per cent of symptomatic patients with familial dysbetalipoproteinemia exhibit palmar or tuberous xanthomas. The diagnosis is also suggested when a moderate elevation in the plasma concentration of both cholesterol and triglyceride occurs in such a way that the absolute concentrations of cholesterol and triglyceride are nearly equal (e.g., the plasma cholesterol and triglyceride levels are both about 300 mg/dl). However, this finding is not a uniform one, since when the disease is in exacerbation, the plasma triglyceride level tends to rise much higher than the cholesterol level.

The diagnosis is strongly supported by the finding of a so-called "broad beta" band on lipoprotein electrophoresis (Type III pattern), which results from the presence of the remnant particles that migrate between beta- and pre–beta-lipoproteins and cause a distinctive smear of this region of the electrophoretogram. Two procedures that require specialized laboratories can be used to establish the diagnosis firmly. When the chemical composition of the VLDL is measured in plasma subjected to ultracentrifugation, the VLDL fraction contains abnormal remnant particles and has a relatively high ratio of cholesterol to triglyceride.[233, 265, 277] The diagnosis can be confirmed by the finding of homozygosity for expression of the apo E-2 allele after isoelectric focusing of the proteins extracted from the remnant particles.[277, 278, 280]

Treatment. A trial of l-thyroxine should be instituted if a careful search reveals any evidence of hypothyroidism. A dramatic lowering of lipid levels occurs when hypothyroidism is treated. In addition, vigorous treatment of obesity and diabetes mellitus is indicated. However, if these measures are not successful, treatment with clofibrate is indicated and usually results in a dramatic and sustained reduction in plasma lipid levels.[255, 256]

TABLE 49–6 SINGLE-GENE DISORDERS THAT PREDISPOSE TO HYPERTENSION

Disorder	Mechanism of Inheritance
Polycystic kidney disease	Dominant
Alport syndrome	Dominant
Medullary thyroid carcinoma with pheochromocytoma	Dominant
Acute intermittent porphyria	Dominant
Neurofibromatosis	Dominant
Pseudoxanthoma elasticum	Dominant and recessive
Riley-Day syndrome (dysautonomia)	Recessive
Adrenogenital syndrome, 17-hydroxylase deficiency	Recessive
Fabry disease	X-linked

HYPERTENSION

The genetics of essential hypertension are discussed on page 829. In brief, the current view is that blood pressure shows a continuous distribution, that multiple genes and multiple environmental factors act in concert to determine the level of one's blood pressure, just as the determination of intelligence and skin color is multifactorial, and that essential hypertension represents the upper end of the blood pressure distribution. Thus, the etiology of hypertension in the vast majority of patients will not be traceable to the operation of a single mutant gene. However, the physician should be aware that there are a number of rare monogenic disorders in which hypertension is a part of the clinical syndrome. These rare disorders, which often masquerade under the umbrella of essential hypertension, are listed in Table 49–6.

REFERENCES

GENERAL PRINCIPLES OF CARDIOVASCULAR GENETICS

1. Darnell, J., Lodish, H., and Baltimore, D.: Molecular Cell Biology. New York, Scientific American Books, Inc., 1986.
2. McKusick, V. A.: The morbid anatomy of the human genome: A review of gene mapping in clinical medicine. Medicine *65*:1, 1986.
3. Stanbury, J. B., Wyngaarden, J. B., Fredrickson, D. S., Goldstein, J. L., and Brown, M. S.: The Metabolic Basis of Inherited Disease. 5th ed. New York, McGraw-Hill Book Co., 1983, pp. 3, 61.
4. Vogel, F., and Motulsky, A. G.: Human Genetics: Problems and Approaches. Berlin, Springer-Verlag, 1979.
5. Goldstein, J. L., and Brown, M. S.: Familial hypercholesterolemia: A genetic receptor disease. Hospital Practice *20*:35, 1985.
6. McKusick, V. A.: Mendelian Inheritance in Man. 6th ed. Baltimore, Johns Hopkins University Press, 1983.
7. Brown, M. S., and Goldstein, J. L.: A receptor-mediated pathway for cholesterol homeostasis. Science *232*:34, 1986.
8. Carter, C. O., Roberts, J. A. F., Evans, K. A., and Buck, A. R.: Genetic clinic. Lancet *1*:281, 1971.
9. Jackson, L. G.: First-trimester diagnosis of fetal genetic disorders. Hospital Practice *20*:39, 1985.

GENETICS OF SPECIFIC FORMS OF CARDIOVASCULAR DISEASE

10. Nora, J. J., and Nora, A. H.: Recurrence risks in children having one parent with a congenital heart disease. Circulation *53*:701, 1976.
11. Noonan, J. A.: Syndromes associated with cardiac defects. *In* Engle, M. A. (ed.): Pediatric Cardiovascular Disease II. Philadelphia, F. A. Davis Co., 1981, p. 97.
12. Tandon, R., and Edwards, J. E.: Cardiac malformations associated with Down's syndrome. Circulation *47*:1349, 1973.
13. Park, S. C., Mathews, R. A., Zuberbuhler, J. R., Rowe, R. D., Neches, W. H., and Lenox, C. C.: Down syndrome with congenital heart malformation. Am. J. Dis. Child. *131*:29, 1977.
14. Greenwood, R. D., and Nadas, A. S.: The clinical course of cardiac disease in Down's syndrome. Pediatrics *58*:893, 1976.
15. Katlic, M. R., Clark, E. B., Neill, C., and Haller, J. A., Jr.: Surgical management of congenital heart disease in Down's syndrome. J. Thorac. Cardiovasc. Surg. *74*:204, 1977.

16. Mikkelsen, M., and Stene, J.: Genetic counseling in Down's syndrome. Hum. Hered. *20*:457, 1970.
17. Hook, E. B.: Estimates of maternal age-specific risks of a Down-syndrome birth in women aged 34–41. Lancet *2*:33, 1976.
18. Gerald, P. S.: Sex chromosome disorders. N. Engl. J. Med. *294*:706, 1976.
19. Engel, E., and Forbes, A. P.: Cytogenetic and clinical findings in 48 patients with congenitally defective or absent ovaries. Medicine *44*:135, 1965.
20. Schmid, W., Naef, E., Murset, G., and Prader, A.: Cytogenetic findings in 89 cases of Turner's syndrome with abnormal karyotypes. Humangenetik *24*:93, 1974.
21. Palmer, C. G., and Reichmann, A.: Chromosomal and clinical findings in 110 females with Turner syndrome. Hum. Genet. *35*:35, 1976.
22. Nora, J. J., Torres, F. G., Sinha, A. K., and McNamara, D. G.: Characteristic cardiovascular anomalies of XO Turner syndrome, XX and XY phenotype and XO/XX Turner mosaic. Am. J. Cardiol. *25*:639, 1970.
23. Van Der Hauwaert, L. G., Fryns, J. P., Dumoulin, M., and Logghe, N.: Cardiovascular malformations in Turner's and Noonan's syndrome. Br. Heart J. *40*:500, 1978.
24. Noonan, J. A.: Hypertelorism with Turner phenotype. Am. J. Dis. Child. *116*:373, 1968.
25. Mendez, H. M. M., and Opitz, J. M.: Noonan syndrome: A review. Am. J. Med. Genet. *21*:493, 1985.
26. Nora, J. J., Nora, A. H., Sinha, A. K., Spangler, R. D., and Lubs, H. A.: The Ullrich-Noonan syndrome (Turner phenotype). Am. J. Dis. Child. *127*:48, 1974.
27. Levy, E. P., Pashayan, H., Fraser, F. C., and Pinsky, L.: XX and XY Turner phenotypes in a family. Am. J. Dis. Child. *120*:36, 1970.
28. Nora, J. J., and Sinha, A. K.: Direct familial transmission of the Turner phenotype. Am. J. Dis. Child. *116*:343, 1968.
29. Nora, J. J., Lortscher, R. H., and Spangler, R. D.: Echocardiographic studies of left ventricular disease in Ullrich-Noonan syndrome. Am. J. Dis. Child. *129*:1417, 1975.
30. Caralis, D. G., Char, F., Graber, J. D., and Voigt, G. C.: Delineation of multiple cardiac anomalies associated with the Noonan syndrome in an adult and review of the literature. Johns Hopkins Med. J. *134*:346, 1974.
31. Pearl, W.: Cardiovascular anomalies in Noonan's syndrome. Chest *71*:677, 1977.
32. Qazi, Q. H., Arnon, R. G., Paydar, M. H., and Mapa, H. C.: Familial occurrence of Noonan syndrome. Am. J. Dis. Child. *127*:696, 1974.
33. Bolton, M. R., Pugh, D. M., Mattioli, L. F., Dunn, M. I., and Schimke, R. N.: The Noonan syndrome: A family study. Ann. Intern. Med. *80*:626, 1974.
34. Baird, P. A., and De Jong, B. P.: Noonan's syndrome (XX and XY Turner phenotype) in three generations of a family. J. Pediatr. *80*:110, 1972.
35. Nghiem, Q. X., Toledo, J. R., Schreiber, M. H., Harris, L. C., Lockhart, L. L., and Tyson, K. R. T.: Congenital idiopathic hypertrophic subaortic stenosis associated with a phenotypic Turner's syndrome. Am. J. Cardiol. *30*:683, 1972.
36. Phornphutkul, C., Rosenthal, A., and Nadas, A. S.: Cardiomyopathy in Noonan's syndrome. Br. Heart J. *35*:99, 1973.
37. Tanimura, A., Hayashi, I., Adachi, K., Nakashima, T., Ota, K., and Toshima, H.: Noonan syndrome with hypertrophic obstructive cardiomyopathy. Acta Pathol. Jpn. *27*:225, 1977.
38. Ehlers, K. H., Engle, M. A., Levin, A. R., and Deely, W. J.: Eccentric ventricular hypertrophy in familial and sporadic instances of 46 XX, XY Turner phenotype. Circulation *45*:639, 1972.
39. Summitt, R. L.: Turner syndrome and Noonan's syndrome. J. Pediatr. *75*:729, 1969.
40. Gorlin, R. J., Anderson, R. C., and Blaw, M.: Multiple lentigenes syndrome. Am. J. Dis. Child. *117*:652, 1969.
41. Seuanez, H., Mane-Garzon, F., and Kolski, R.: Cardio-cutaneous syndrome (the "LEOPARD" syndrome). Review of the literature and a new family. Clin. Genet. *9*:266, 1976.
42. Polani, P. E., and Moynahan, E. J.: Progressive cardiomyopathic lentiginosis. Quart. J. Med. *41*:205, 1972.
43. Hopkins, B. E., Taylor, R. R., and Robinson, J. S.: Familial hypertrophic cardiomyopathy and lentiginosis. Aust. NZ J. Med. *5*:359, 1975.
44. Somerville, J., and Bonham-Carter, R. E.: The heart in lentiginosis. Br. Heart J. *34*:58, 1972.
45. Holt, M., and Oram, S.: Familial heart disease with skeletal malformations. Br. Heart J. *22*:236, 1960.
46. Massumi, R. A., and Nutter, D. O.: The syndrome of familial defects of heart and upper extremities (Holt-Oram syndrome). Circulation *34*:65, 1966.
47. Smith, A. T., Sack, G. H., and Taylor, G. J.: Holt-Oram syndrome. J. Pediatr. *95*:538, 1979.
48. Cascos, A. S.: Genetics of atrial septal defect. Arch. Dis. Child. *47*:581, 1972.
49. Gladstone, I., and Sybert, V. P.: Holt-Oram syndrome: Penetrance of the gene and lack of maternal effect. Clin. Genet. *21*:98, 1982.
50. Zhang, K-Z., Sun, Q-B., and Cheng, T. O.: Holt-Oram syndrome in China: A collective review of 18 cases. Am. Heart J. *111*:572, 1986.
51. Poznanski, A. K., Stern, A. M., and Gall, J. C., Jr.: Skeletal anomalies in genetically determined congenital heart disease. Radiol. Clin. North Am. *9*:435, 1971.
52. Lin, A. E., and Perloff, J. K.: Upper limb malformations associated with congenital heart disease. Am. J. Cardiol. *55*:1576, 1985.
53. Muller, L. M., De Jong, G., and Van Heerden, K. M. M.: The antenatal ultrasonographic detection of the Holt-Oram syndrome. S. Afr. Med. J. *68*:313, 1985.
54. Emanuel, R., O'Brien, K., Somerville, J., Jefferson, K., and Hegde, M.: Association of secundum atrial septal defect with abnormalities of atrioventricular conduction or left axis deviation. Br. Heart J. *37*:1085, 1975.
55. Bjornstad, P. G.: Secundum-type atrial septal defect with prolonged PR interval and autosomal dominant mode of inheritance. Br. Heart J. *36*:1149, 1974.
56. Pease, W. E., Nordenberg, A., and Ladda, R. L.: Familial atrial septal defect with prolonged atrioventricular conduction. Circulation *53*:759, 1976.
57. da Silva, E. O., Janovitz, D., and de Albuquerque, S. C.: Ellis–van Creveld syndrome: Report of 15 cases in an inbred kindred. J. Med. Genet. *17*:349, 1980.
58. McKusick, V. A., Egeland, J. A., Eldridge, R., and Krusen, D. E.: Dwarfism in the Amish. I. The Ellis–van Creveld syndrome. Bull. Johns Hopkins Hosp. *115*:306, 1964.
59. Blackburn, M. G., and Belliveau, R. E.: Ellis–van Creveld syndrome. Am. J. Dis. Child. *122*:267, 1971.
60. Mahoney, M. J., and Hobbins, J. C.: Prenatal diagnosis of chondroectodermal dysplasia (Ellis–van Creveld syndrome) with fetoscopy and ultrasound. N. Engl. J. Med. *297*:258, 1977.
61. Becroft, D. M. O., and Chambers, D.: Supravalvular aortic stenosis–infantile hypercalcaemia syndrome: *In vitro* hypersensitivity to vitamin D_{52} and calcium. J. Med. Genet. *13*:223, 1976.
62. Kahler, R. L., Braunwald, E., Plauth, W. H., Jr., and Morrow, A. G.: Familial congenital heart disease. Am. J. Med. *40*:384, 1966.
63. McDonald, A. H., Gerlis, L. M., and Somerville, J.: Familial arteriopathy with associated pulmonary and systemic arterial stenoses. Br. Heart J. *31*:375, 1969.
64. Johnson, L. W., Fishman, R. A., Schneider, B., Parker, F. B., Jr., Husson, G., and Webb, W. R.: Familial supravalvular aortic stenosis. Chest *70*:494, 1976.
65. Eisenberg, R., Young, D., Jacobson, B., and Boito, A.: Familial supravalvular aortic stenosis. Am. J. Dis. Child. *108*:341, 1964.
66. Afzelius, B. A., and Mossberg, A.: The immotile-cilia syndrome including Kartagener's syndrome. *In* Stanbury, J. B., Wyngaarden, J. B., Fredrickson, D. S., Goldstein, J. L., and Brown, M. S. (eds.): The Metabolic Basis of Inherited Disease. 5th ed. New York, McGraw-Hill Book Co., 1983, p. 1986.
67. Holmes, L. B., Blennerhassett, J. B., and Austen, K. F.: A reappraisal of Kartagener's syndrome. Am. J. Med. Sci. *255*:13, 1968.
68. Hartline, J. V., and Zelkowitz, P. S.: Kartagener's syndrome in childhood. Am. J. Dis. Child. *121*:349, 1971.
69. Miller, R. D., and Divertie, M. B.: Kartagener's syndrome. Chest *62*:130, 1972.
70. Afzelius, B. A.: A human syndrome caused by immotile cilia. Science *193*:317, 1976.
71. Melmon, K. L., and Braunwald, E.: Familial pulmonary hypertension. N. Engl. J. Med. *269*:770, 1963.
72. Kingdon, H. S., Cohen, L. S., Roberts, W. C., and Braunwald, E.: Familial occurrence of primary pulmonary hypertension. Arch. Intern. Med. *118*:422, 1966.
73. Kuhn, E., Schaaf, J., and Wagner, A.: Primary pulmonary hypertension, congenital heart disease and skeletal anomalies in three generations. Jpn. Heart J. *4*:205, 1963.
74. Parry, W. R., and Verel, D.: Familial primary pulmonary hypertension. Br. Heart J. *28*:193, 1966.
75. Rogge, J. D., Mishkin, M. E., and Genovese, P. D.: The familial occurrence of primary pulmonary hypertension. Ann. Intern. Med. *65*:672, 1966.
76. Thompson, P., and McRae, C.: Familial pulmonary hypertension. Evidence of autosomal dominant inheritance. Br. Heart J. *32*:758, 1970.
77. Nora, J. J., McGill, C. W., and McNamara, D. G.: Empiric recurrence risks in common and uncommon congenital heart lesions. Teratology *3*:325, 1970.
78. Neill, C. A.: Genetics of congenital heart disease. Annu. Rev. Med. *24*:61, 1973.
79. Corone, P., Bonaiti, C., Feingold, J., Fromont, S., and Berthet-Bondet, D.: Familial congenital heart disease: How are the various types related? Am. J. Cardiol. *51*:942, 1983.
80. Nora, J. J., Dodd, P. F., McNamara, D. G., Hattwick, M. A. W., Leachman, R. D., and Cooley, D. A.: Risk to offspring of parents with congenital heart defects. J.A.M.A. *209*:2052, 1969.
81. McKusick, V. A.: Heritable Disorders of Connective Tissue. 4th ed. St. Louis, C. V. Mosby Co., 1972.
82. Hirst, A.E., Jr., and Gore, I.: Marfan's syndrome: A review. Prog. Cardiovasc. Dis. *16*:187, 1973.
83. Pan, C. W., Chen, C. C., Wang, S. P., Hsu, T. L., and Chaing, B. N.: Echocardiographic study of cardiac abnormalities in families of patients with Marfan's syndrome. J. Am. Coll. Cardiol. *6*:1016, 1985.
84. Wigle, E. D., Rakowski, H., Ranganathan, N., and Silver, M. D.: Mitral valve prolapse. Annu. Rev. Med. *27*:165, 1976.
85. Strahan, N. V., Murphy, E. A., Fortuin, N. J., Come, P. C., and Humphries, J. O.: Inheritance of the mitral valve prolapse syndrome. Discussion of a three-dimensional penetrance model. Am. J. Med. *74*:967, 1983.
86. Cooper, M. J., and Abinader, E. G.: Family history in assessing the risk for progression of mitral valve prolapse. Am. J. Dis. Child. *135*:647, 1981.
87. Hunt, D., and Sloman, G.: Prolapse of the posterior leaflet of the mitral valve occurring in eleven members of a family. Am. Heart J. *78*:149, 1969.
88. Barabas, A. P.: Heterogeneity of the Ehlers-Danlos syndrome: Description of the three clinical types and a hypothesis to explain the basic defect(s). Br. Med. J. *2*:612, 1967.
89. McKusick, V. A.: Multiple forms of the Ehlers-Danlos syndrome. Arch. Surg. *109*:475, 1974.
90. Pope, F. M., Martin, G. R., and McKusick, V. A.: Inheritance of Ehlers-Danlos type IV syndrome. J. Med. Genet. *14*:200, 1977.

91. Imahori, S., Bannerman, R. M., Graf, C. J., and Brennan, J. C.: Ehlers-Danlos syndrome with multiple arterial lesions. Am. J. Med. *47*:967, 1969.
92. Beighton, P.: The dominant and recessive forms of cutis laxa. J. Med. Genet. 9:216, 1972.
93. Schimke, R. N., McKusick, V. A., Huang, T., and Pollack, A. D.: Homocystinuria. J.A.M.A., *193*:87, 1965.
94. James, T. N., Carson, N. A. J., and Froggatt, P.: De Subitaneis Mortibus IV. Coronary vessels and conduction system in homocystinuria. Circulation *49*:367, 1974.
95. McCully, K. S.: Vascular pathology of homocysteinemia: Implications for the pathogenesis of arteriosclerosis. Am. J. Pathol. *56*:111, 1969.
96. Fleisher, L. D., Longhi, R. C., Tallan, H. H., Beratis, N. G., Hirschhorn, K., and Gaull, G. E.: Homocystinuria: Investigations of cystathionine synthase in cultured fetal cells and the prenatal determination of genetic status. J. Pediatr. *85*:677, 1974.
97. Altman, L. K., Fialkow, P. J., Parker, F., and Sagebiel, R. W.: Pseudo xanthoma elasticum: An underdiagnosed genetically heterogeneous disorder with protean manifestations. Arch. Intern. Med. *134*:1048, 1974.
98. Pope, F. M.: Autosomal dominant pseudoxanthoma elasticum. J. Med. Genet. *11*:152, 1974.
99. Wilhelm, K., and Paver, K.: Sudden death in pseudoxanthoma elasticum. Med. J. Aust. *2*:1363, 1972.
100. Schachner, L., and Young. D.: Pseudoxanthoma elasticum with severe cardiovascular disease in a child. Am. J. Dis. Child. *127*:571, 1974.
101. Bete, J. M., Banas, J. S., Jr., Moran, J., Pinn, V., and Levine, H. J.: Coronary artery disease in an 18 year old girl with pseudoxanthoma elasticum: Successful surgical therapy. Am. J. Cardiol. *36*:515, 1975.
102. Moran, J. J.: Idiopathic arterial calcification of infancy: A clinicopathologic study. Pathol. Annu. *10*:393, 1975.
103. Barson, A. J., Campbell, R. H. A., Langley, F. A., and Milner, R. D. G.: Idiopathic arterial calcification of infancy without intimal proliferation. Virchows Arch. Pathol. Anat. *372*:167, 1976.
104. Schieken, R. M., Kerber, R. E., Ionasescu, V. V., and Zellweger, H.: Cardiac manifestations of the mucopolysaccharidoses. Circulation *52*:700, 1975.
105. McKusick, V. A., and Neufeld, E. F.: The mucopolysaccharide storage diseases. *In* Stanbury, J. B., Wyngaarden, J. B., Fredrickson, D. S., Goldstein, J. L., and Brown, M. S. (eds.): The Metabolic Basis of Inherited Disease. 5th ed. New York, McGraw-Hill Book Co., 1983, p. 751.
106. Kelly, T. E., Thomas, G. H., Taylor, H. A., Jr., McKusick, V. A., Sly, W. S., Glaser, J. H., Robinow, M., Luzzatti, L., Espiritu, C., Feingold, M., Bull, M. J., Ashenhurst, E. M., and Ives, E. J.: Mucolipidosis III (pseudo-Hurler polydystrophy): Clinical and laboratory studies in a series of 12 patients. Johns Hopkins Med. J. *137*:156, 1975.
107. Neufeld, E. F., and McKusick, V. A.: Disorders of lysosomal enzyme synthesis and localization: I-cell disease and Pseudo-Hurler polydystrophy. *In* Stanbury, J. B., Wyngaarden, J. B., Fredrickson, D. S., Goldstein, J. L., and Brown, M. S. (eds.): The Metabolic Basis of Inherited Disease. 5th ed. New York, McGraw-Hill Book Co., 1983, p. 778.
108. Hirst, A. E., Jr., Johns, V. J., Jr., and Kime, S. W., Jr.: Dissecting aneurysm of the aorta: A review of 505 cases. Medicine *37*:217, 1958.
109. Murdoch, J. L., Walker, B. A., Halpern, B. L., Kuzma, J. W., and McKusick, V. A.: Life expectancy and causes of death in the Marfan syndrome. N. Engl. J. Med. *286*:804, 1972.
110. Halpern, B. L., Char, F., Murdoch, J. L., Horton, W. B., and McKusick, V. A.: A prospectus on the prevention of aortic rupture in the Marfan syndrome with data on survivorship without treatment. Johns Hopkins Med. J. *129*:123, 1971.
111. Gott, V. L., Pyeritz, R. E., Magovern, G. J., Jr., Cameron, D. E., and McKusick, V. A.: Surgical treatment of aneurysms of the ascending aorta in the Marfan syndrome. Results of composite-graft repair in 50 patients. N. Engl. J. Med. *314*:1070, 1986.
112. Elias, S., and Berkowitz, R. L.: The Marfan syndrome and pregnancy. Obstet. Gynecol. *47*:358, 1976.
113. Grossman, M., Knott, A. P., Jr., and Jacoby, W. J., Jr.: Calcified annulus fibrosis with mitral insufficiency in the Marfan syndrome. Arch. Intern. Med. *121*:561, 1968.
114. Murdoch, J. L., Walker, B. A., and McKusick, V. A.: Parental age effects on the occurrence of new mutations for the Marfan syndrome. Ann. Hum. Genet. *35*:331, 1972.
115. Emanuel, R., Ng, R. A. L., Marcomichelakis, J., Moores, E. C., Jefferson, K. E., Macfaul, P. A., and Withers, R.: Formes frustes of Marfan's syndrome presenting with severe aortic regurgitation. Clinicogenetic study of 18 families. Br. Heart J. *39*:190, 1977.
116. Payvandi, M. N., Kerber, R. E., Phelps, C. D., Judisch, G. F., El-Khoury, G., and Schrott, H. G.: Cardiac, skeletal and ophthalmologic abnormalities in relatives of patients with the Marfan syndrome. Circulation *55*:797, 1977.
117. Procacci, P. M., Savran, S. V., Schreiter, S. L., and Bryson, A. L.: Prevalance of clinical mitral-valve prolapse in 1169 young women. N. Engl. J. Med. *294*:1086, 1976.
118. Markiewicz, W., Stoner, J., London, E., Hunt, S. A., and Popp, R. L.: Mitral valve prolapse in one hundred presumably healthy young females. Circulation *53*:464, 1976.
119. Howell, R. R., and Williams, J. C.: The glycogen storage diseases. *In* Stanbury, J. B., Wyngaarden, J. B., Fredrickson, D. S., Goldstein, J. L., and Brown, M. S. (eds.): The Metabolic Basis of Inherited Disease. 5th ed. New York, McGraw-Hill Book Co., 1983, p. 119.
120. Ehlers, K. H., Hagstrom, J. W. C., Lukas, D. S., Redo, S. F., and Engle, M. A.: Glycogen-storage disease of the myocardium with obstruction to left ventricular outflow. Circulation *25*:96, 1962.
121. Ockerman, P. A.: Incidence of glycogen storage disease in Sweden. Paediatr. Scand, *61*:533, 1972.
122. D'Ancona, G. G., Wurm, J., and Croce, C. M.: Genetics of type II glycogenesis: Assignment of the human gene for acid α -glucosidase to chromosome 17. Proc. Natl. Acad. Sci. USA. *76*:4526, 1979.
123. Maron, B. J., Nichols, P. F., III, Pickle, L. W., Wesley, Y. E., and Mulvihill, J. J.: Patterns of inheritance of hypertrophic cardiomyopathy: Assessment by M-mode and two-dimensional echocardiography. Am. J. Cardiol. *53*:1087, 1984.
124. Clark, C. E., Henry, W L., and Epstein, S. E.: Familial prevalance and genetic transmission of idiopathic hypertrophic subaortic stenosis. N. Engl. J. Med. *289*:709, 1973.
125. Bjarnason, I., Jonsson, S., and Hardarson, T.: Mode of inheritance of hypertrophic cardiomyopathy in Iceland. Br. Heart J. *47*:122, 1982.
126. Braunwald, E., Lambrew, C. T., Rockoff, S. D., Ross, J., Jr., and Morrow, A. G.: Idiopathic hypertrophic subaortic stenosis. I. A description of the disease based on an analysis of 64 patients. Circulation *30*(Suppl. 4):3, 1964.
127. Horlick, L., Petkovich, N. J., and Bolton, C. F.: Idiopathic hypertrophic subvalvular stenosis. A study of a family involving four generations. Clinical, hemodynamic and pathologic observations. Am. J. Cardiol. *17*:411, 1966.
128. Pare, J. A. P., Fraser, R. G., Pirozynski, W. J., Shanks, J. A., and Stubington, D.: Hereditary cardiovascular dysplasia. A form of familial cardiomyopathy. Am. J. Med. *31*:37, 1961.
129. Maron, B. J., Lipson, L. C., Roberts, W. C., Savage, D. S., and Epstein, S. E.: "Malignant" hypertrophic cardiomyopathy: Identification of a subgroup of families with unusually frequent premature death. Am. J. Cardiol. *41*:1133, 1978.
130. Perloff, J. K.: The cardiomyopathies—current perspectives. Circulation *44*:942, 1971.
131. Kariv, I., Kreisler, B., Sherf, L., Feldman, S., and Rosenthal, T.: Familial cardiomyopathy. Am. J. Cardiol. *28*:693, 1971.
132. Whitfield, A. G. W.: Familial cardiomyopathy. Q. J. Med. *30*:119, 1961.
133. Ross, R. S., Bulkley, B. H., Hutchins, G. M., Harshey, J. S., Jones, R. A., Kraus, H., Liebman, J., Thorne, C. M., Weinberg, S. B., Weech, A. A., and Weech, A. A., Jr.: Idiopathic familial myocardiopathy in three generations: A clinical and pathologic study. Am. Heart J. *97*:170, 1978.
134. Csanady, M., and Szasz, K.: Familial cardiomyopathy. Cardiology *61*:122, 1976.
135. Boyd, D. L., Mishkin, M. E., Feigenbaum, H., and Genovese, P. D.: Three families with familial cardiomyopathy. Ann. Intern. Med. *63*:386, 1965.
135a. Berko, B. A., and Swift, M.: X-linked dilated cardiomyopathy. N. Engl. J. Med. *316*:1186, 1987.
136. Finch, S. C., and Finch, C. A.: Idiopathic hemochromatosis, an iron shortage disease. Medicine *34*:381, 1955.
137. Bothwell, T. H., Charlton, R. W., and Motulsky, A. G.: Idiopathic hemochromatosis. *In* Stanbury, J. B., Wyngaarden, J. B., Fredrickson, D. S., Goldstein, J. L., and Brown, M. S. (eds.): The Metabolic Basis of Inherited Disease. 5th ed. New York, McGraw-Hill Book Co., 1983, p. 1269.
138. Edwards, C. Q., Carroll, M., Bray, P., and Cartwright, G. E.: Hereditary hemochromatosis. N. Engl. J. Med. *297*:7, 1977.
139. Crosby, W. H.: Hemochromatosis: The unsolved problems. Semin. Hematol. *14*:135, 1977.
140. Saddi, R., and Feingold, J.: Idiopathic haemochromatosis: An autosomal recessive disease. Clin. Genet. *5*:234, 1974.
141. Simon, M., Alexandre, J-L., Bourel, M., le Marec, B., and Scordia, C.: Heredity of idiopathic haemochromatosis: A study of 106 families. Clin. Genet. *11*:327, 1977.
142. Rowe, J. W., Wands, J. R., Mexey, E., Waterbury, L. A., Wright, J. R., Tobin, J., and Andres, R.: Familial hemochromatosis: Characteristics of the precirrhotic stage in a large kindred. Medicine *56*:197, 1977.
143. Scheinberg, I. H.: The genetics of hemochromatosis. Arch. Intern. Med. *132*:126, 1973.
144. Simon, M., Bourel, M., Fauchet, R., and Genetet, B.: Association of HLA-A3 and HLA-B14 antigens with idiopathic haemochromatosis. Gut *17*:332, 1976.
145. Bomford, A., Eddleston, A. L. W. F., Kennedy, L. A., Batchelor, J. R., and Williams, R.: Histocompatibility antigens as markers of abnormal iron metabolism in patients with idiopathic haemochromatosis and their relatives. Lancet *1*:327, 1977.
146. Feller, E. R., Pont, A., Wands, J. R., Carter, E. A., Foster, G., Kourides, I. A., and Isselbacher, K. J.: Familial hemochromatosis. N. Engl. J. Med. *29*:1422, 1977.
147. Simon, M., Alexandre, J. L., Rauchet, R., Genetet, B., and Bourel, M.: The genetics of hemochromatosis, Prog. Med. Genet. *4*(new series):135, 1980.
148. Kyle, R. A., and Bayrd, E.D.: Amyloidosis: Review of 236 cases. Medicine *54*:271, 1975.
149. Andrade, C., Araki, S., Block, W. D., Cohen, A. S., Jackson, C. E., Kuroiwa, Y., McKusick, V. A., Nissism, J., Sohar, E., and Van Allen, M. W.: Hereditary amyloidosis. Arthritis Rheum. *13*:902, 1970.
150. Frederiksen, T., Gotzsche, H., Harboe, N., Kraer, W., and Mellemgaard, K.: Familial primary amyloidosis with severe amyloid heart disease. Am. J. Med. *33*:328, 1962.
151. Harrison, W. H., Jr., and Derrick, J. R.: Atrial standstill. A review and presentation of two new cases of familial and unusual nature with reference to epicardial pacing in one. Angiology *20*:610, 1969.
152. Hawley, R. J., Gottdiener, J. S., Gay, J. A., and Engel, W. K.: Families with myotonic dystrophy with and without cardiac involvement. Arch. Intern. Med. *143*:2134, 1983.
153. Church, S. C.: The heart in myotonia atrophica. Arch. Intern. Med. *119*:176, 1967.

154. Griggs, R. C., David, R. J., Anderson, D. C., and Dove, J. T.: Cardiac conduction in myotonic dystrophy. Am. J. Med. *59*:37, 1975.
155. Salomon, J., and Easley, R. M.: Cardiovascular abnormalities in myotonic dystrophy. Chest *64*:135, 1973.
156. Tanaka, N., Tanaka, H., Takeda, M., Niimura, T., Kanehisa, T., and Terashi, S.: Cardiomyopathy in myotonic dystrophy. A light and electron microscopic study of the myocardium. Jpn. Heart J. *14*:202, 1973.
157. Bundey, S., Carter, C. O., and Soothill, J. F.: Early recognition of heterozygote for the gene for dystrophia myotonica. J. Neurol. Neurosurg. Psychiatry *33*:279, 1970.
158. Shaw, D. J., Brook, J. D., Meredith, A. L., Harley, H. G., Sarfarazi, M., and Harper, P. S.: Gene mapping and chromosome 19. J. Med. Genet. *23*:2, 1986.
159. Schrott, H. G., Karp, L., and Omenn, G. S.: Prenatal prediction in myotonic dystrophy: Guidelines for genetic counseling. Clin. Genet. *4*:38, 1973.
160. Zundel, W. S., and Tyler, F. H.: The muscular dystrophies. N. Engl. J. Med. *10*:537, 596, 1965.
161. Perloff, J. K., Roberts, W. C., De Leon, A. C., Jr., and O'Doherty, D.: The distinctive electrocardiogram of Duchenne's progressive muscular dystrophy. Am. J. Med. *42*:179, 1967.
162. Moser, H., and Emery, A. E. H.: The manifesting carrier in Duchenne muscular dystrophy. Clin. Genet. *5*:271, 1974.
163. Mann, O., DeLeon, A. C., Jr., Perloff, J. K., Simanis, J., and Horrigan, F. D.: Duchenne's muscular dystrophy: The electrocardiogram in female relatives. Am. J. Med. Sci. *255*:376, 1968.
164. Emery, A. E. H.: Abnormalities of the electrocardiogram in female carriers of Duchenne muscular dystrophy. Br. Med. J. *2*:418, 1969.
165. Monaco, A. P., Bertelson, C. J., Middlesworth, W., Colletti, C-A., Aldridge, J., Fischbeck, K. H., Bartlett, R., Pericak-Vance, M. A., Roses, A. D., and Kunkel, L. M.: Detection of deletions spanning the Duchenne muscular dystrophy locus using a tightly linked DNA segment. Nature *316*:842, 1985.
166. Boyer, S. H., IV, Chisholm, A. W., and McKusick, V. A.: Cardiac aspects of Friedreich's ataxia. Circulation *25*:493, 1962.
167. Harding, A. E., and Hewer, R. L.: The heart disease of Friedreich's ataxia: A clinical and electrocardiographic study of 115 patients, with an analysis of serial electrocardiographic changes in 30 cases. Q. J. Med. *52*(new series):489, 1983.
168. Hewer, R. L.: Study of fatal cases of Friedreich's ataxia. Br. Med. J. *3*:649, 1968.
169. Perloff, J. K.: Cardiomyopathy associated with heredofamilial neuromyopathic diseases. Mod. Concepts Cardiovasc. Dis. *40*:23, 1971.
170. Smith, E. R., Sangalang, V. E., Heffernan, L. P., Welch, J. P., and Flemington, C. S.: Hypertrophic cardiomyopathy: The heart disease of Friedreich's ataxia. Am. Heart J. *94*:428, 1977.
171. Ruschhaupt, D. G., Thilenius, O. G., and Cassels, D. E.: Friedreich's ataxia associated with idiopathic hypertrophic subaortic stenosis. Am. Heart J. *84*:95, 1972.
172. Maione, S., Giunta, A., Mansi, D., Filla, A., Serino, A., Teti, G., de Falco, F. A., and Campanella, G.: Cardiac abnormalities in Friedreich's ataxia patients and first-degree relatives: Evidence of hypertrophic cardiomyopathy in obligate heterozygotes. Acta Neurol. (Naples) *35*:354, 1980.
173. Folger, G. M., Jr.: Endocardial fibroelastosis. Clin. Pediatr. *10*:246, 1971.
174. Mitchell, S. C., Froehlich, L. A., Banas, J. S., Jr., and Gilkeson, M. R.: An epidemiologic assessment of primary endocardial fibroelastosis. Am. J. Cardiol. *18*:859, 1966.
175. Vestermark, S.: Primary endocardial fibroelastosis in siblings. Acta Paediatr. *51*:94, 1962.
176. Hunter, A. S., and Keay, A. J.: Primary endocardial fibroelastosis. Arch. Dis. Child. *48*:66, 1973.
177. Westwood, M., Harris, R., Burn, J. L., and Barson, A. J.: Heredity in primary endocardial fibroelastosis. Br. Heart J. *37*:1077, 1975.
178. Chen, S., Thompson, M. W., and Rose, V.: Endocardial fibroelastosis: Family studies with special reference to counseling. J. Pediatr. *79*:385, 1971.
179. Tripp, M. E., Katcher, M. L., Peters, H. A., Gilbert, E. F., Arya, S., Hodach, R. J., and Shug, A. L.: Systemic carnitine deficiency presenting as familial endocardial fibroelastosis. N. Engl. J. Med. *305*:385, 1981.
180. Engel, A. G., and Angelini, C.: Carnitine deficiency of human skeletal muscle with associated lipid storage myopathy: A new syndrome. Science *179*:899, 1973.
181. Jervell, A., and Lange-Nielsen, F.: Congenital deaf-mutism, functional heart disease with prolongation of Q-T interval and sudden death. Am. Heart J. *54*:59, 1957.
182. Jervell, A.: Surdocardiac and related syndromes in children. Adv. Intern. Med. *17*:425, 1971.
183. Schwartz, P. J., Periti, M., and Malliani, A.: The long Q-T syndrome. Am. Heart J. *89*:378, 1975.
184. Denes, P.: Congenital and acquired syndrome of a long Q-T interval. Chest *71*:126, 1977.
185. Fraser, G. R., Froggatt, P., and Murphy, T.: Genetical aspects of the cardioauditory syndrome of Jervell and Lange-Nielsen (congenital deafness and electrocardiographic abnormalities). Ann. Hum. Genet. *28*:133, 1964.
186. Romano, C.: Congenital cardiac arrhythmia. Lancet *1*:658, 1965.
187. Ward, O. C.: A new familial cardiac syndrome in children. J. Irish Med. Assoc. *54*:103, 1964.
188. Itoh, S., Munemura, S., and Satoh, H.: A study of the inheritance pattern of Romano-Ward syndrome. Clin. Pediatr. *21*:20, 1982.
189. Van Der Straaten, P. J. C., and Bruins, C. L. D.: A family with heritable electrocardiographic QT-prolongation. J. Med. Genet. *10*:158, 1973.
190. Moothart, R. W., Pryor, R., Hawley, R. L., Clifford, N. J., and Blount, S. G., Jr.: The heritable syndrome of prolonged Q-T interval, syncope, and sudden death. Chest *70*:263, 1976.
191. Sarachek, N. S., and Leonard, J. J.: Familial heart block and sinus bradycardia. Am. J. Cardiol. *29*:451, 1972.
192. Crittenden, I. H., Latta, H., and Ticinovich, D. A.: Familial congenital heart block. Am. J. Dis. Child. *108*:104, 1964.
193. Chameides, L., Truex, R. C., Vetter, V., Rashkind, W. J., Galioto, Jr., F. M., and Noonan, J. A.: Association of maternal systemic lupus erythematosus with congenital complete heart block. N. Engl. J. Med. *297*:1204, 1977.
194. McCue, C. M., Mantakas, M. E., Tingelstad, J. B., and Ruddy, S.: Congenital heart block in newborns of mothers with connective tissue disease. Circulation *56*:82, 1977.
195. Scott, J. S., Maddison, P. J., Taylor, P. V., Esscher, E., Scott, O., and Skinner, R. P.: Connective-tissue disease, antibodies to ribonucleoprotein, and congenital heart block. N. Engl. J. Med. *309*:209, 1983.
196. Kennel, A. J., Callahan, J. A., Maloney, J. D., and Zajarilas, A.: Adult-onset familial infra-Hisian block. Am. Heart J. *102*:1447, 1981.
197. Vallianos, G., and Sideris, D. A.: Familial conduction defects. Cardiology *59*:190, 1974.
198. Amat-Y-Leon, F., Racki, A. J., Denes, P., Ten Eick, R. E., Singer, D. H., Bharati, S., Lev, M., and Rosen, K. M.: Familial atrial dysrhythmia with A-V block. Circulation *50*:1097, 1974.
199. Esscher, E., Hardell, L.-I., and Michaelsson, M.: Familial, isolated, complete right bundle-branch block. Br. Heart J. *37*:745, 1975.
200. Harnischfeger, W. W.: Hereditary occurrence of the pre-excitation (Wolff-Parkinson-White) syndrome with re-entry mechanism and concealed conduction. Circulation *19*:28, 1959.
201. Schneider, R. G.: Familial occurrence of Wolff-Parkinson-White syndrome. Am. Heart J. *78*:34, 1969.
202. Massumi, R. A.: Familial Wolff-Parkinson-White syndrome with cardiomyopathy. Am. J. Med. *43*:951, 1967.
203. Perheentupa, J., Autio, S., Leisti, S., Raitta, C., and Tuuteri, L.: Mulibrey nanism, an autosomal recessive syndrome with pericardial constriction. Lancet *2*:351, 1973.
204. Perheentupa, J., Autio, S., Leisti, S., Raitta, C., and Tuuteri, L.: Mulibrey nanism: Review of 23 cases of a new autosomal recessive syndrome. Birth Defects: Original Article Series *11*:3, 1975.
205. Tuuteri, L., Perheentupa, J., and Rapola, J.: The cardiopathy of mulibrey nanism, a new inherited syndrome. Chest *65*:628, 1974.
206. Cumming, G. R., Kerr, D., and Ferguson, C. C.: Constrictive pericarditis with dwarfism in two siblings (mulibrey nanism). J. Pediatr. *88*:569, 1976.
207. Thoren, C.: So-called mulibrey nanism with pericardial constriction. Lancet *2*:731, 1973.
208. Voorhess, M. L., Husson, G. S., and Blackman, M. S.: Growth failure with pericardial constriction. Am. J. Dis. Child. *130*:1146, 1976.
209. Krause, S., Adler, L. N., Reddy, P. S., and Magovern, G. J.: Intracardiac myxoma in siblings. Chest *60*:404, 1971.
210. Liebler, G. A., Magovern, G. J., Park, S. B., Cushing, W. J., Begg, F. R., and Joyner, C. R.: Familial myxomas in four siblings. J. Thorac. Cardiovasc. Surg. *71*:605, 1976.
211. Heydorn, W. H., Gomez, A. C., Kleid, J. J., and Haas, J. M.: Atrial myxoma in siblings. J. Thorac. Cardiovasc. Surg. *65*:484, 1973.
212. Farah, M. G.: Familial atrial myxoma. Ann. Intern. Med. *83*:358, 1975.
213. Siltanen, P., Tuuteri, L., Norio, R., Tala, P., Ahrenberg, P., and Halonen, P. I.: Atrial myxoma in a family. Am. J. Cardiol. *38*:252, 1976.
214. Powers, J. C., Falkoff, M., Heinle, R. A., Nanda, N. C., Ong, L. S., Weiner, R. S., and Barold, S. S.: Familial cardiac myxoma: Emphasis on unusual clinical manifestations. J. Thorac. Cardiovasc. Surg. *77*:782, 1979.
215. Tsakraklides, V., Burke, B., Mastri, A., Runge, W., Roe, E., and Anderson, R.: Rhabdomyomas of heart. Am. J. Dis. Child. *128*:639, 1974.
216. Lagos, J. C., and Gomez, M. R.: Tuberous sclerosis: Reappraisal of a clinical entity. Mayo Clin. Proc. *42*:26, 1967.
217. Nevin, N. C., and Pearce, W. G.: Diagnostic and genetical aspects of tuberous sclerosis. J. Med. Genet. *5*:273, 1968.

CORONARY ARTERY DISEASE

218. Epstein, F. H.: Risk factors in coronary heart disease—environmental and hereditary influences. Isr. J. Med. Sci. *3*:594, 1967.
219. Slack, J., and Evans, K. A.: The increased risk of death from ischaemic heart disease in first degree relatives of 121 men and 96 women with ischaemic heart disease. J. Med. Genet. *3*:239, 1966.
220. Rissanen, A. M., and Nikkila, E. A.: Coronary artery disease and its risk factors in families of young men with angina pectoris and in controls. Br. Heart J. *39*:875, 1977.
221. Harvald, B., and Hauge, M.: Coronary occlusion in twins. Acta. Genet. Med. Gemellol. (Roma) *19*:248, 1970.
222. Kannel, W. B., Castelli, W. P., Gordon, T., and McNamara, P. M.: Serum cholesterol, lipoproteins, and the risk of coronary heart disease. Ann. Intern. Med. *74*:1, 1971.
223. Neufeld, H. N., and Goldbourt, U.: Coronary heart disease: Genetic aspects. Circulation *67*:943, 1983.
224. ten Kate, L. P., Bowman, H., Daiger, S. P., and Motulsky, A. G.: Familial aggregation of coronary heart disease and its relation to known genetic risk factors. Am. J. Cardiol. *50*:945, 1982.
225. Goldstein, J. L., Schrott, H. G., Hazzard, W. R., Bierman, E. L., and Motulsky, A. G.: Hyperlipidemia in coronary heart disease. II. Genetic analysis

of lipid levels in 176 families and delineation of a new inherited disorder, combined hyperlipidemia. J. Clin. Invest. *52*:1544, 1973.

226. Goldstein, J. L., and Brown, M. S.: The LDL receptor defect in familial hypercholesterolemia: Implications for pathogenesis and therapy. Med. Clin. N. Am. *66*:335, 1982.
227. Goldstein, J. L., and Brown, M. S.: Familial hypercholesterolemia. *In* Stanbury, J. B., Wyngaarden, J. B., Fredrickson, D. S., Goldstein, J. L., and Brown, M. S. (eds.): The Metabolic Basis of Inherited Disease. 5th ed. New York, McGraw-Hill Book Co., 1983, p. 672.
228. Epstein, C. J., Martin, G. M., Schultz, A. L., and Motulsky, A. G.: Werner's syndrome: A review of its symptomatology, natural history, pathologic feasyndrome: A review of its symptomatology, natural history, pathologic features, genetics and relationship of the natural aging process. Medicine *45*:177, 1966.
229. Zackai, A. H., Weber, D., and Noth, R.: Cardiac findings in Werner's syndrome. Geriatrics 29:141, 1974.
230. Duncan, C., and McLeod, G. M.: Angiokeratoma corporis diffusum universale (Fabry's disease). Aust. Ann. Med. *1*:58, 1970.
231. Becker, A. E., Schoorl, R., Balk, A. G., and van der Heide, R. M.: Cardiac manifestations of Fabry's disease. Am. J. Cardiol. *36*:829, 1975.
232. Beaudet, A. L., Ferry, G. D., Nichols, B. L., Jr., and Rosenberg, H. S.: Cholesterol ester storage disease: Clinical, biochemical, and pathological studies. J. Pediatr. *90*:910, 1977.
233. Havel, R. J., Goldstein, J. L., and Brown, M. S.: Lipoproteins and lipid transport. *In* Bondy, P. K., and Rosenberg, L. E. (eds.): Diseases of Metabolism. 8th ed. Philadelphia, W. B. Saunders Company, 1980, p. 393.
234. Goldstein, J. L., Kita, T., and Brown, M. S.: Defective lipoprotein receptors and atherosclerosis: Lessons from an animal counterpart of familial hypercholesterolemia. N. Engl. J. Med. *309*:288, 1983.
235. Mahley, R. W., Innerarity, T. L., Rall, S. C., Jr., and Weisgraber, K. H.: Plasma lipoproteins: apolipoprotein structure and function. J. Lipid Res. *25*:1277, 1984.
236. Goldstein, J. L., Brown, M. S., Anderson, R. G. W., Russell, D. W., and Schneider, W. J.: Receptor-mediated endocytosis: Concepts emerging from the LDL receptor system. Ann. Rev. Cell Biol. *1*:1, 1985.
237. Deitschy, J. M., Spady, D. K., and Stange, E. F.: Quantitative importance of different organs for cholesterol synthesis and low-density lipoprotein degradation. Biochem. Soc. Trans. *11*:639, 1983.
237a. Norum, K. R., Berg, T., Helgerud, P., and Drevon, C. A.: Transport of cholesterol. Physiol. Rev. *63*:1343, 1983.
238. Kwiterovich, P. O., Jr., Levy, R. I., and Fredrickson, D. S.: Neontal diagnosis of familial type-II hyperlipoproteinemia. Lancet *1*:118, 1973.
239. Slack, J.: Risks of ischaemic heart disease in familial hyperlipoproteinaemic states. Lancet 2:1380, 1969.
240. Jensen, J., Blankenhorn, D. H., and Kornerup, V.: Coronary disease in familial hypercholesterolemia. Circulation *36*:77, 1967.
241. Stone, N. J., Levy, R. I., Fredrickson, D. S., and Verter, J.: Coronary artery disease in 116 kindred with familial type-II hyperlipoproteinemia. Circulation *49*:476, 1974.
242. Khachadurian, A. K., and Uthman, S. M.: Experiences with the homozygous cases of familial hypercholesterolemia. Nutr. Metab. *15*:132, 1973.
243. Goldstein, J. L.: The cardiac manifestations of the homozygous and heterozygous forms of familial type II hyperbetalipoproteinemia. Birth Defects: Original Article Series *8*:202, 1972.
244. Sprecher, D. L., Schaefer, E. J., Kent, K. M., Gregg, R. E., Zech, L. A., Hoeg, J. M., McManus, B., Roberts, W. C., and Brewer, H. B., Jr.: Cardiovascular features of homozygous familial hypercholesterolemia: Analysis of 16 patients. Am. J. Cardiol. *54*:20, 1984.
245. Buja, L. M., Kovanen, P. T., and Bilheimer, D. W.: Cellular pathology of homozygous familial hypercholesterolemia. Am. J. Pathol. 97:327, 1979.
246. Forman, M. B., Kinsley, R. H., DuPlessis, J. P., Dansky, R., Milner, S., and Levin, S. E.: Surgical correction of combined supravalvular and valvular aortic stenosis in homozygous familial hypercholesterolaemia. S. Afr. Med. J. *61*:579, 1982.
247. Allen, J. M., Thompson, G. R., Myant, N. B., Steiner, R., and Oakley, C. M.: Cardiovascular complications of homozygous familial hypercholesterolaemia. Br. Heart J. *44*:361, 1980.
248. Beppu, S., Minura, Y., Sakakibara, H., Nagata, S., Park, Y-D., Nambu, S., and Yamamoto, A.: Supravalvular aortic stenosis and coronary ostial stenosis in familial hypercholesterolemia: Two-dimensional echocardiographic assessment. Circulation *67*:878, 1983.
249. Glueck, C. J., Levy, R. I., and Fredrickson, D. S.: Acute tendinitis and arthritis: A presenting symptom of familial type II hyperlipoproteinemia. J.A.M.A. *206*:2895, 1969.
250. Russell, D. W., Lehrman, M. A., Südhof, T. C., Yamamoto, T., Davis, C. G., Hobbs, H. H., Brown, M. S., and Goldstein, J. L.: The LDL receptor in familial hypercholesterolemia: Use of human mutations to dissect a membrane protein. Cold Spring Harbor Symp. Quant. Biol. (*in press*).
251. Ross, R.: The pathogenesis of atherosclerosis—An update. N. Engl. J. Med. *314*:488, 1986.
252. Bilheimer, D. W., Ho, Y. K., Brown, M. S., Anderson, R. G. W., and Goldstein, J. L.: Genetics of the low density lipoprotein receptor: Diminished receptor activity in lymphocytes from heterozygotes with familial hypercholesterolemia. J. Clin. Invest. *61*:678, 1978.
253. Cuthbert, J. A., East, C. A., Bilheimer, D. W., and Lipsky, P. E.: Detection of familial hypercholesterolemia by assaying functional low-density-lipoprotein receptors on lymphocytes. N. Engl. J. Med. *314*:879, 1986.
254. Brown, M. S., Kovanen, P. T., Goldstein, J. L., Vandenberghe, K., Pryns, J. P., Eeckels, R., Van Den Berghe, H., and Cassiman, J. J.: Prenatal diagnosis of homozygous familial hypercholesterolaemia. Lancet *1*:526, 1978.
255. Brown, M. S., and Goldstein, J. L.: Drugs used in the treatment of hyperlipoproteinemias. *In* Gilman, A. G., Goodman, L. S., Rall, T. W., and Murad, F. (eds.): Goodman and Gilman's The Pharmacological Basis of Therapeutics. 7th ed. New York, Macmillan Publishing Co., 1985., p. 827.
256. Kane, J. P., and Havel, R. J.: Treatment of hypercholesterolemia. Ann. Rev. Med. *37*:427, 1986.
257. Brown, M. S., and Goldstein, J. L.: Lowering plasma cholesterol by raising LDL receptors (editorial). N. Engl. J. Med. Med. *305*:515, 1981.
258. Hoeg, J. M., Maher, M. B., Zech, L. A., Bailey, K. R., Gregg, R. E., Lackner, K. J., Fojo, S. S., Anchors, M. A., Bojanovski, M., Sprecher, D. L., and Brewer, H. B., Jr.: Effectiveness of mevinolin on plasma lipoprotein concentrations in type II hyperlipoproteinemia. Am. J. Cardiol. *57*:933, 1986.
259. Mabuchi, H., Sakai, T., Sakai, Y., Yoshimura, A., Watanabe, A., Wakasugi, T., Koizumi, J., and Takeda, R.: Reduction of serum cholesterol in heterozygous patients with familial hypercholesterolemia: Additive effects of compactin and cholestyramine. N. Engl. J. Med. *308*:609, 1983.
260. Bilheimer, D. W., Grundy, S. M., Brown, M. S., and Goldstein, J. L.: Mevinolin stimulates receptor-mediated clearance of low density lipoprotein from plasma in familial hypercholesterolemia heterozygotes. Proc. Natl. Acad. Sci. USA *80*:4124, 1983.
261. Thompson, G. R., and Gotto, A. M.: Ileal bypass in the treatment of hyperlipoproteinaemia. Lancet 2:35, 1973.
262. Starzl, T. E., Chase, H. P., Ahrens, E. H., Jr., McNamara, D. J., Bilheimer, D. W., Schaefer, E. J., Rey, J., Porter, K. A., Stein, E., Francavilla, A., and Benson, L. N.: Portacaval shunt in patients with familial hypercholesterolemia. Ann. Surg. *198*:273, 1983.
263. Thompson, G. R., Miller, J. P., and Breslow, J. L.: Improved survival of patients with homozygous familial hypercholesterolaemia treated with plasma exchange. Br. Med. J. *291*:1671, 1985.
264. Bilheimer, D. W., Goldstein, J. L., Grundy, S. C., Starzl, T. E., and Brown, M. S.: Liver transplantation provides low density lipoprotein receptors and lowers plasma cholesterol in a child with homozygous familial hypercholesterolemia. N. Engl. J. Med. *311*:1658, 1984.
265. Havel, R. J. (ed.): Symposium on lipid disorders. Med. Clin. North Am. Vol. 66, 1982, pp. 317–550.
266. Chait, A., and Brunzell, J. D.: Severe hypertriglyceridemia: Role of familial and acquired disorders. Metabolism *32*:209, 1983.
267. Schonfeld, G., and Kudzma, D. J.: Type IV hyperlipoproteinemia. Arch. Intern. Med. *132*:55, 1973.
268. Brunzell, J. D., Albers, J. J., Chait, A., Grundy, S. M., Groszek, E., and McDonald, G. B.: Plasma lipoproteins in familial combined hyperlipidemia and monogenic familial hypertriglyceridemia. J. Lipid Res. *24*:147, 1983.
269. Brunzell, J. D., Schrott, H. H., Motulsky, A. G., and Bierman, E. L.: Myocardial infarction in the familial forms of hypertriglyceridemia. Metabolism 25:313, 1976.
270. Nikkila, E. A., and Aro, A.: Family study of serum lipids and lipoproteins in coronary heart-disease. Lancet *1*:954, 1973.
271. Rose, H. G., Kranz, P., Weinstock, M., Juliano, J., and Haft, J. I.: Inheritance of combined hyperlipoproteinemia: Evidence for a new lipoprotein phenotype. Am. J. Med. *54*:148, 1973.
272. Matthews, R. J.: Type III and IV familial hyperlipoproteinemia: Evidence that these two syndromes are different phenotypic expressions of the same mutant gene(s). Am. J. Med. *44*:188, 1968.
273. Schriebman, P. H., Wilson, D. E., and Arky, R. A.: Familial type IV hyperlipoproteinemia. N. Engl. J. Med. *281*:981, 1969.
274. Glueck, C. J., Fallat, R., Buncher, C. R., Tsang, R., and Steiner, P.: Familial combined hyperlipoproteinemia: Studies in 91 adults and 95 children from 33 kindreds. Metabolism 22:1403, 1973.
275. Das, S. K., Chandra, M., Shukla, R. N., Nityanand, S., and Agarwal, S. S.: A study of familial combined hyperlipidemia in 11 families. Indian J. Med. Res. *78*:665, 1983.
276. Kissebah, A. H., Alfarsi, S., and Evans, D. J.: Low density lipoprotein metabolism in familial combined hyperlipidemia. Mechanism of the multiple lipoprotein phenotypic expression. Arteriosclerosis *4*:614, 1984.
277. Brown, M. S., Goldstein, J. L., and Fredrickson, D. S.: Familial type 3 hypercholesterolemia (dysbetalipoproteinemia). *In* Stanbury, J. B., Wyngaarden, J. B., Fredrickson, D. S., Goldstein, J. L., and Brown, M. S. (eds.): The Metabolic Basis of Inherited Disease, 5th ed. New York, McGraw-Hill Book Co., 1983, p. 655.
278. Mahley, R. W. and Angelin, B.: Type III hyperlipoproteinemia: Recent insights into the genetic defect of familial dysbetalipoproteinemia. Adv. Intern. Med. *29*:385, 1984.
279. Morganroth, J., Levy, R. I., and Fredrickson, D. S.: The biochemical, clinical, and genetic features of type III hyperlipoproteinemia. Ann. Intern. Med. *82*:158, 1975.
280. Utermann, G., Langenbeck, U., Beisiegel, U., and Weber, W.: Genetics of the apolipoprotein E system in man. Am. J. Hum. Genet. *32*:339, 1980.
281. Mahley, R. W., and Innerarity, T. L.: Lipoprotein receptors and cholesterol homeostasis. Biochim. Biophys. Acta *737*:197, 1983.
282. Brown, M. S. and Goldstein, J. L.: Lipoprotein receptors in the liver: Control signals for plasma cholesterol traffic. J. Clin. Invest. 72:743, 1983.
283. Utermann, G., Vogelberg, K. H., Steinmetz, A., Schoenborn, W., Pruin, N., Jaeschke, M., Hees, M., and Canzler, H.: Polymorphism of apolipoprotein E. II. Genetics of hyperlipoproteinemia type III. Clin. Genet. *15*:37, 1979.
284. Hazzard, W. R., and Bierman, E. L.: Aggravation of broad-beta disease (Type 3 hyperlipoproteinemia) by hypothyroidism. Arch. Intern. Med. *130*:822, 1972.

50 AGING AND CARDIAC DISEASE

by MYRON L. WEISFELDT, M.D.,
EDWARD G. LAKATTA, M.D.,
and GARY GERSTENBLITH, M.D.

CONCEPTS AND THEORIES OF AGING CHANGE

Students of cardiovascular medicine are often presented with two distinct issues concerning the burden imposed on the cardiovascular system by advanced age. The first is that represented by the aged, infirm patient with severe heart failure. At times no clear etiology can be defined and even when there is, the diagnostic and therapeutic management is often more challenging than is the case with the younger patient with the same disease. The issue presented by these patients, therefore, is that the cardiovascular limitations associated with aging itself are significant and often severe. There is also the observation represented by the elderly marathon runner, swimmer, or master athlete whose physical abilities are equal to or surpass those of persons who are 30 years younger. Such individuals suggest that if there is any limitation of cardiovascular reserve imposed by the aging process per se, it is minor. There is some evidence that age-associated musculoskeletal, pulmonary, and psychological factors are more important than cardiovascular considerations in these patients.

AGING, DISEASE, AND LIFE STYLE. Attempts to solve the dilemma posed by the seemingly varied effects of age in the two subject subsets noted above are handicapped by the additional effects of both an increasing prevalence of disease and an altered life style associated with aging. The most prevalent disease, coronary atherosclerosis, is present in up to 60 per cent of elderly individuals in Western society,[1, 2] has a profound effect on measurements of cardiovascular function during stress, but is difficult to diagnose in the absence of overt symptoms or electrocardiographic abnormalities. The most important life style variable is the status of physical activity. Studies on exercise conditioning and deconditioning have indicated that even short periods of changes in physical activity can have a profound influence on cardiovascular function.[3] Toxins from food and chemical exposure, including cumulative effects of cigarette smoking and radiation, as well as mulnutrition are other life style variables whose effects may merge into those of disease. There is considerable evidence, therefore, that changes in the prevalence of disease and altered life style variables accompanying aging may have accounted for some of the previously described alterations which have been attributed to aging alone.

In summary, changes in cardiovascular function accompanying aging in an unselected population may be due to changes in disease patterns and life style variables as well as those resulting simply from aging. Of the three, aging itself appears to be the least potent and therefore the most difficult to define. Although age-induced changes in cardiac structure, function, and neurohumoral responses do modify cardiovascular function, they are most important clinically when they are superimposed on significant disease or other cardiovascular stresses. The effects of aging *alone* on cardiovascular function should be examined in subjects who are free of cardiovascular disease and who have a relatively homogeneous level of physical conditioning. It is relatively easy to exclude individuals who have symptomatic disease, but identification of many individuals with atherosclerosis is more difficult because of its high prevalence and because it is often asymptomatic.

INTERPRETATION OF STUDIES OF AGING. The best information concerning aging comes from longitudinal, or repeated, studies of healthy individuals who have active life styles. Because longitudinal studies require a prolonged period to perform, most aging studies in humans have used cross-sectional methodology. In any aging study it is important to note that any data expressed as a ratio (e.g., cardiac index or myosin adenosine triphosphatase activity per milligram of protein) may change with age because of changes in the denominator (i.e., body mass or total protein content) rather than because of a change in the parameter itself. The interpretation of cross-sectional studies are also limited by the possibility that the older volunteers represent a subset of the general population selected for longevity and/or high motivational factors.

SPECIFIC CARDIOVASCULAR CHANGES IN AGING

Detailed studies of biochemical and anatomical changes accompanying aging have been performed. It is important, though, to assess the physiological importance of these findings. Although one step in a complex biochemical pathway may be altered with age, the alteration may have no physiological significance if that step does not limit the rate of the overall reaction. Clearly, important general conclusions about cardiovascular aging are as follows:

1. After neonatal development, the number of myocardial cells in the heart does not increase.[4]
2. There is moderate hypertrophy of left ventricular myocardium, probably in response to increased arterial vascular stiffness and dropout of myocytes.[5, 6]
3. When myocardial hypertrophy occurs, it is out of proportion to capillary and vascular growth.[7]
4. The ability of the myocardium to generate tension is well maintained as a result of prolonged duration of contraction and greater stiffness despite a modest decrease in the velocity of shortening of cardiac muscle.
5. There is a selective decrease in beta-adrenoceptor–mediated inotropic, chronotropic, and vasodilating cardiovascular responses with aging.[8]
6. Increased pericardial and myocardial stiffness and delayed relaxation during aging may limit left ventricular filling during stress.

GENERAL THEORIES OF AGING: CARDIOVASCULAR APPLICATION

As organized and discussed by Hayflick,[9] current broadly accepted theories of aging can be grouped by level of integration into genome, physiological, and organ theories. Because most work to date on the cardiovascular system is at the organ or cellular level, the latter two groups appear to be the most appropriate to review.

GENOME THEORIES. The most popular current genome theory proposes that genes are programmed for aging and/or death of the organism.[10–12] Each species as well as cells in culture have what appears to be unmodifiable general boundaries for the duration of survival. Because cardiac function with age never limits survival in the absence of disease or toxin exposure, little testing of this hypothesis is feasible in the cardiovascular system. Programmed dysfunction or cell destruction may account for neurohormonal regulatory dysfunction, but these notions are remote from the fundamental tenets of the hypothesis. Two other related genomic theories of aging are somatic mutation (related or not to environmental irradiation) and the error theories. Owing either to programmed DNA variability or to toxic agents there is an accumulation of cell components with errors in protein structure and/or sequence. The error theories may not be relevant, however, since searches for such errors have not been successful. In the heart certain aspects of function are so well maintained that it is difficult to use such a general theory to explain the relatively selective cardiovascular age changes.

PHYSIOLOGICAL THEORIES. Physiological theories of aging clearly appear more attractive as explanations for cardiovascular changes.[13–15] One, the cross-linkage theory of aging, points to the importance of time-related changes in the extracellular protein matrix, particularly of collagen and ground substance. Such changes are certainly at the basis of age-associated increases in stiffness of pericardial, valvular, and, perhaps, myocardial and vascular tissues. Secondary responses probably include myocardial hypertrophy and vascular smooth muscle changes. Neurohormonal changes would be more difficult to explain. Alternatively, physiological theories related to injury by free radicals and/or accumulation of waste products could easily explain the selectivity of aging changes in terms of selective sensitivity of specific enzymes to free radical injury or specific detrimental effects of waste product build-up, tissue by tissue.

ORGAN THEORIES. Organ theories are attractive in their simplicity and ease of understanding and demonstration. There are two major such theories: immunological and neuroendocrine.[16, 17] The *immunological theory* offers an explanation for survival duration characteristics of species in terms of programmed immunological dysfunction leading to autoimmune cellular injury but offers little to explain specific selection changes in the cardiovascular system. The *neuroendocrine theory*, perhaps in combination with the cross-linkage theory, would provide explanations for many of the observed changes in the characteristics of cardiac function with aging. In the neuroendocrine theory, changes in hypothalamic function, possibly genetically induced, lead to changes in nerves and mediators. Major alterations in physiological function and the response to stress reflect the long-term and progressive summation effects of changes in individual neurohormonal mediators.

CARDIAC MUSCLE FUNCTION IN AGING

EXCITATION-ACTIVATION-CONTRACTION COUPLING

In cardiac muscles of senescent animals, contraction and relaxation times are prolonged. (Figure 50–1*B* shows twitch recordings from adult rats [7 months] and aged rats [24 months].)[18–30] Prolonged duration of contraction and prolonged relaxation can be attributed to alterations in mechanisms that govern excitation–contraction coupling in the heart (see p. 389). Excitation of cardiac muscles results in

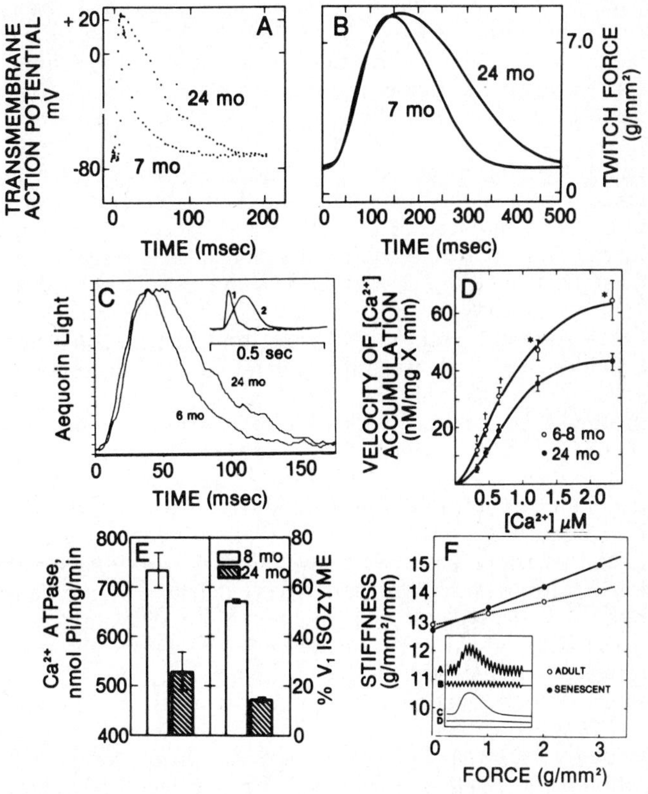

FIGURE 50–1. Representative data depicting differences in various aspects of excitation–contraction coupling mechanisms measured between young adult (6 to 9 months) and senescent (24 to 26 months) rat hearts. *A*, Transmembrane action potential[24]; *B*, isometric contraction[8]; *C*, myoplasmic [Ca^{++}] transient[13]; *D*, sarcoplasmic reticulum Ca^{++} uptake rate[25]; *E*, Ca^{++}-stimulated ATPase activity, and myosin isozyme composition (50 per cent) of the heterodimer (V_2) is included in the total percentage of V_1[26]; and *F*, dynamic stiffness, derived from the relationship of stiffness to force measurements made during the twitch. Inset shows how dynamic stiffness measurements are made. Resting force or twitch force in two sequential contractions in the presence (*upper*) and absence (*lower*) of 17 Hz sinusoidal length perturbations (<1 per cent of muscle length) is measured (see references 12 and 20 for further details). When the unperturbed signal is subtracted from the perturbed one, an approximation of force development owing only to the length perturbation at rest or throughout the time course of the muscle contraction is derived. Stiffness is the Δ force per Δ length. Dynamic stiffness in resting muscle measured across a range of resting muscle lengths (not shown) is not age related. Active dynamic stiffness (i.e., that measured during the contraction) is a linear function of force (stiffness − F + b) and is given for both age groups. An age difference is noted in the slope coefficient (0.41 ± 0.14 in the adult muscle, n = 8, versus 0.76 ± 0.05 in the senescent muscles, n = 17, p < .03), while b, the intercept, is not age related (12.9 ± 0.14 in the adult versus 12.7 ± 1.3 in the senescent muscles). (Redrawn from Spurgeon, H. A., et al.: Increased dynamic stiffness of trabeculae carneae from senescent rats. Am. J. Physiol. *232*:H373, 1977.)

a transient rise in cytosolic [Ca^{++}]. This activates myofilaments which stiffen, shorten, and produce force. The rate of decline in force or muscle lengthening reflects, in part, the rate and time course of decline in [Ca^{++}].

CALCIUM TRANSIENT (See also p. 389). The time course of the Ca^{++}–myofilament interaction is a major determinant of duration of contraction and the time course of relaxation. This is determined in part by the extent and rate of myofilament shortening during the contraction, which is itself, in part, determined by the amount of Ca^{++} bound to troponin before the onset of contraction. The extent and rate of myofilament shortening is determined, in part, by the rate of myofilament hydrolysis of adenosine triphosphate (ATP) and cross-bridge cycling rate and, in part, by the time course of the myoplasmic [Ca^{++}] transient, the duration of which is determined by sarcolemmal depolarization and by the rates of sarcoplasmic reticulum Ca^{++} release and pumping. The myoplasmic [Ca^{++}] transient that follows sarcolemmal depolarization in cardiac muscle has been monitored by injecting the chemiluminescent protein aequorin into multiple cells of that tissue and measuring the light transient that precedes contraction.[31] The duration of the myoplasmic [Ca^{++}] transient, measured as the time course of aequorin luminescence, is prolonged in isometric muscle isolated from aged versus younger adult rats (Fig. 50–1*C*). The myoplasmic free Ca^{++} transient results primarily from the sarcoplasmic reticulum Ca^{++} release and is the net result of the amount of Ca^{++} released and the extent of Ca^{++} binding to cell proteins. The rate at which the sarcoplasmic reticulum pumps Ca^{++} is diminished in hearts of senescent versus younger animals (Fig. 50–1*D*), and this appears to be a major contributor to the prolonged transient[25, 32–34] and the prolonged time course of cardiac muscle relaxation.

The transmembrane action potential of working cardiac muscle from both right and left ventricles of senescent rats[20,25] is markedly prolonged compared with young controls (Fig. 50–1*A*). The magnitude of action potential prolongation in right ventricular isometric muscle from senescent rats is as great as that in left ventricular muscle and as great as that in muscle from experimentally hypertrophied rat hearts.[35] The overshoot and level of depolarization at all relative repolarization times are also greater in older than in younger Wistar rat cardiac muscles.[20] The mechanism for the prolonged action potential (enhanced inward versus reduced outwardly directed current[s]) remains to be established. Because the diminution in sarcoplasmic reticulum Ca^{++} pumping rate in the senescent myocardium might result in less sarcoplasmic reticulum Ca^{++} loading, under some conditions at least, the amplification of the trigger for sarcoplasmic reticulum Ca^{++} release may be a requirement to maintain sufficient Ca^{++} release in the senescent myocardial cell. Some evidence for this is that in mechanically skinned cardiac cells from senescent rats, sarcoplasmic reticulum Ca^{++} release requires a greater Ca^{++} trigger than that from cells of maturing animals.[36] The larger action potential in intact senescent muscle may serve as a more effective trigger for Ca release (e.g., by way of a greater slow inward current). Alternatively, the changes in the action potential could be the result of age-related differences in sarcoplasmic reticulum Ca^{++} release (i.e., prolonged Ca^{++} transient may cause a prolonged action potential).[37]

DURATION OF CONTRACTION, RELAXATION, AND MUSCLE STIFFNESS. The prolonged time course of the myoplasmic free Ca^{++} transient may also affect other aspects of the cardiac contraction that depend on Ca^{++}–myofilament interactions (i.e., the time to peak force [Fig. 50–1*B*] and the ability of the myofilaments to shorten and stiffen at differing times after excitation). The time to peak stiffness and half relaxation time of peak stiffness are prolonged in senescent versus younger adult cardiac muscle,[24, 26, 27] probably reflecting the prolonged Ca^{++} transient and slowed Ca^{++} uptake by the sarcoplasmic reticulum. Muscle stiffness is measured as the ratio of the change in force in response to a length change. Stiffness measured in response to small sinusoidal changes in muscle length made during the contraction has been referred to as "active dynamic" stiffness (Fig. 50–1*F* inset). The active dynamic stiffness is a linear function of the force and increases as force increases with time during a contraction (Fig. 50–1*F*). The slope coefficient (α) of the active stiffness force relationship, but not its intercept, increases in senescence (Fig. 50–1*F*). Enhanced dynamic stiffness in senescent muscle is present only during contractile activation by Ca^{++}.[24, 26, 27] Aging[18, 38, 39] cannot account for the increased stiffness measured during the contraction in senescent muscles. A possible explanation for the increase in the slope stiffness during contraction is as follows: at times during contraction when force is still increasing and myoplasmic [Ca^{++}] is decreasing (see Fig. 50–1*C* inset), myoplasmic [Ca^{++}] remains higher in senescent than in younger muscles (Fig. 50–1*C*). This may result in a relative increase in Ca^{++}–myofilament interaction in senescent versus younger muscles during this phase of contraction but not at earlier times. The myofilament response to Ca^{++} is not altered with age, and neither the maximum force nor the shape of the force pCa relation differs with age.[19]

FORCE GENERATION. The amplitude of the twitch (Fig. 50–1*B*) and aequorin luminescence (Fig. 50–1*C*) do not decline in senescent muscles as long as the [Ca^{++}] in the superfusate is in the physiological range and the rate of stimulation is low. In addition, peak twitch force at relatively low rates of stimulation (6 to 48 min/liter does not differ with age across a broad range of resting lengths.[18, 20, 21, 25, 28–30, 38, 40] Postextrasystolic twitch potentiation during

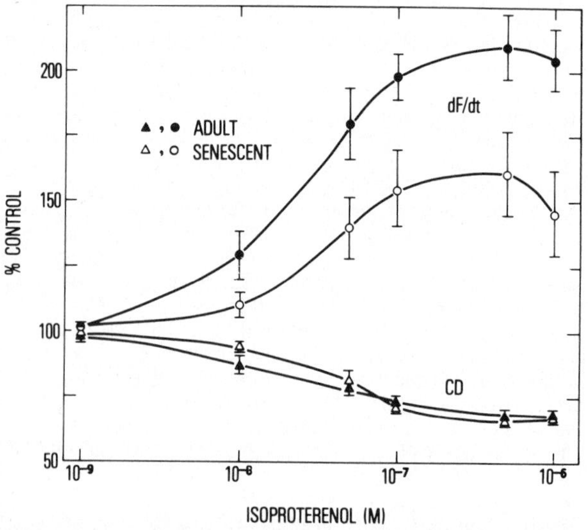

FIGURE 50–2. Effect of age on the response of the maximum rate of force development (dF/dt) and contraction duration (CD) to isoproterenol in arterially perfused interventricular septa from adult (7 to 9 months) and senescent (25 months) rats. The age difference in dose-response curves of dF/dt is significant at $p < .005$ level (regression analysis of variance, n = 6 in each age group at each isoproterenol concentration). Before isoproterenol, dF/dt was not age related, but CD was significantly prolonged in the 25-month septa. (From Guarnieri, T., et al.: Contractile and biochemical correlates of beta-adrenergic stimulation of the aged heart. Am. J. Physiol. *239*:H501, 1980.

continual paired stimulation is also preserved in senescent muscles (see Fig. 50–3*B*). The relatively low rates of stimulation required for studies in papillary muscles do not permit assessment of the extent of Ca^{++} release at rates approaching those in the rat in vivo (e.g., 300/min). In addition, the stability of isolated bulk muscle preparations require that the temperature be maintained typically at 30°C or less. The maintenance of peak twitch force at low stimulation frequencies and temperature in senescent muscle may, in part, result from the prolonged myoplasmic $[Ca^{++}]$ transient (Fig. 50–1*C*). In rat muscles bathed in physiologic $[Ca^{++}]$ in the absence of drugs, the amplitude of Ca^{++} release and twitch force decline as the stimulation frequency is increased. The magnitude of this decline is not different in senescent and young adult muscles.[31] However, in bathing medium containing higher $[Ca^{++}]$, while muscles from younger adult rats are able to produce the same Ca^{++} release and twitch force at low and higher rates of stimulation, at the higher stimulation rate, senescent muscles cannot.[31] In addition, in physiologic bathing $[Ca^{++}]$, when the coupling interval of paired stimulation is decreased below 200 msec, senescent (but not adult) muscles fail to generate a twitch response to the second stimulus.[29] These defects of the senescent muscle may be related, in part, to the diminished Ca^{++} pumping rate by sarcoplasmic reticulum in senescent muscle (Fig. 50–1*D*).

CONTRACTILE PROTEINS

A decrease in the rate of ATP hydrolysis has been observed in various contractile protein preparations isolated from the myocardium of aged as compared with younger animals.[19, 22, 23, 25, 28, 41–44] The rate and extent of this decline vary with the particular preparation studied. The Ca^{++}-activated myosin ATPase activity has been found to decline progressively with age from maturation through senescence.[22, 23, 45] Myosin ATPase activity is modulated by the myosin isozyme profile.[46] The percentage of the myosin isozyme that has the most rapid ATP hydrolytic rate (i.e., V_1 isomyosin) declines progressively with age in rats from maturation through senescence, while the proportion of the isozyme with the slowest ATP hydrolytic rate V_3 progressively increases with age.[22, 23, 45] By 24 months of age V_1 comprises less than 20 per cent of the total myosin isozyme content (Fig. 50–1*E*).

The myosin isozyme shift to a greater percentage of V_3 with aging is accompanied by a reduction in the velocity of isotonic shortening.[19, 25, 28, 44, 45] In the isometric contraction the time to peak tension and duration of the contraction are directly related to the percentage of V_3 or inversely related to the percentage of V_1.[22, 23, 45] The increase in the stiffness during the twitch in senescent versus younger adult rat cardiac muscle[18, 24] might relate to differences in isozymes. However, the impact of the isozyme composition and myosin ATPase activity on functional parameters of muscle can be overridden by other factors that modulate muscle function. For example, variations in the time course of the increase of myoplasmic free Ca^{++} with age (Fig. 50–1*C*) make it difficult to ascertain the precise role of isozyme composition or of ATPase activity on function in aged hearts because the interaction of myofilaments, and thus ATP hydrolysis, is Ca^{++}-dependent. Thus the aging rodent model in which several determinants of myocardial cell function are altered in addition to isozymes is not an optimal model to probe the specific role of altered isozyme composition on muscle function. The same consideration regarding the relationship of isozymes and function applies to rodent models of experimental hypertrophy and altered thyroid states in which, like aging, multiple factors of the excitation–contraction coupling process are altered in addition to the myosin isozymes.[35]

In *summary*, with advancing age, although the velocity of shortening of cardiac muscle is reduced and contraction and relaxation times are prolonged, peak contractile force production in many instances, as noted above, is maintained (Fig. 50–1*B*). The multiple changes that occur in cardiac excitation–activation–contraction with aging into senescence are interrelated. Many of these changes can be interpreted as adaptive. It would be incorrect, therefore, to generalize that aged myocardium exhibits compromised "contractile function."

SIMILARITIES BETWEEN AGING AND EXPERIMENTAL CARDIAC OVERLOAD IN YOUNGER ANIMALS

Many of the changes that occur in cardiac excitation–activation–contraction mechanisms with senescence in the normotensive rat also occur in the myocardium of younger animals in which experimental hypertension has caused cardiac hypertrophy.[27, 35, 41, 45–49] Thus the cardiac overload in younger hearts affects cardiac muscle in a manner that might be referred to as "accelerated aging." This raises the issue of whether the changes in cardiac muscle as reviewed above are due to the concomitant myocardial hypertrophy that accompanies senescence.[19, 27] The extent of left heart hypertrophy from adulthood to senescence is moderate.[19, 27] Hypertrophy probably contributes to but is not entirely responsible for the observed changes associated with age.

PASSIVE MUSCLE PROPERTIES

(See also p. 402)

Classic studies of muscle mechanics denote those tissue properties that do not directly depend on excitation as "passive."[50] These properties are important because they influence the rate, time course, and extent of shortening and force development. The manner in which the myofilaments are coupled to passive components of the tissue are also a determinant of the viscoelastic properties of muscle.[51, 52] Even with detailed information on the amount of collagen, its physical characteristics, and the characteristics of the network weave, direct cause–effect relationships between structural and functional alterations are difficult to substantiate.[18]

Estimation of the elastic or viscoelastic modulus is a more meaningful method of assessing passive muscle properties than measurement of resting force at L_{max} or examination of the passive length–tension curve.[53, 54] No alteration in passive viscoelastic stiffness parameters can be demonstrated.[24, 26, 27] In intact ventricles of various species, the effect of advanced age on the modulus of viscoelastic stiffness is inconclusive, with no change,[55] an increase,[56, 56a] and a decrease[57] having been observed.

PHYSICAL CONDITIONING AFFECTS SENESCENT CARDIAC MUSCLE

Chronic exercise in senescent rats abolishes prolonged contraction and reduces the active dynamic stiffness without altering myocardial mass. This chronic (5 months' duration), mild wheel-exercise protocol, which was insufficient to alter the body or heart weight in adult (6 to 9 months) and senescent (24 to 26 months) rats at sacrifice, did not alter twitch amplitude in isolated left ventricular trabecular muscle measured across a range of $[Ca^{++}]$ at either age. In the younger animals this exercise protocol was ineffective in altering the duration of contraction or dynamic stiffness measured during contraction in muscles. In senescent muscles, however, it eliminated the age-associated increase in these parameters to the levels observed in the younger adult muscle.

The reduction in both the slope stiffness coefficient and duration of contraction is consistent with an effect of exercise to reduce the duration of the myoplasmic [Ca^{++}] transient (Fig. 50–1).

A greater relative effect of chronic exercise on some other aspects of cardiac biochemistry in senescent as compared with young adult rat myocardium has also been observed. Although chronic exercise does not usually augment cytochrome *c* oxidase activity in cardiac muscle of younger animals as it does in skeletal muscle,[58] a modest augmentation of cytochrome *c* oxidase has been observed in hearts of senescent animals.[58] This was accompanied by exercise-induced increased rates of glutamate malate, palmitoylcarnitine, and succinate oxidation.[58] Thus exercise can partially reverse the decline in the oxidation rates of these substrates and in cytochrome *c* activity that occur with aging in rats.[59] Marked age-related declines in cardiac aldolase and superoxide dismutase activities in mice between 9 and 27 months are prevented by chronic exercise begun at 6 months of age and continued into old age.[60] The progressive decline in myocardial Ca^{++}-activated actomysin ATPase activity that begins during maturation (after 1 month in the rat) and progresses with advancing adult age can be retarded by a chronic (3 months) period of exercise. This relatively small beneficial effect of exercise, however, was observed only through 12 to 15 months.[60] In older animals (that begin exercise at 17 to 22 months and were sacrificed at 20 to 25 months) a decline in this ATPase occurred.[61]

DIMINISHED MYOCARDIAL RESPONSE TO BETA-ADRENOCEPTOR STIMULATION

Although the effect of beta-adrenoceptor agonists to abbreviate the duration of contraction is not age related in isolated cardiac muscle or perfused rat myocardium, their effect to enhance contractile force is diminished.[30,40] Age-related changes that are distal to the receptor–cyclase system are required to explain the diminished myocardial contractile response to isoproterenol as depicted in Figure 50–2. In the latter study neither the number of myocardial beta receptors nor their affinity for antagonists or for isoproterenol were altered with age, and neither basal levels of cyclic adenosine monophosphate (cAMP) nor the increased level achieved during the peak contractile response was age related. Furthermore, the age-related deficit in enhancement of contractility observed with isoproterenol persisted when dibutyryl cAMP was used as the agonist. Dibutyryl cAMP bypasses the receptor-cyclase system. Neither basal nor stimulated levels of protein kinase activity in the same myocardial preparations in which the contractile responses were studied were altered with age. Thus an explanation for the depressed inotropic response is that one or more steps distal to protein kinase activation differ with age. The possibilities include differences in the extent of phosphorylation of various proteins or differences in ion flux or binding that results from a given level of phosphorylation, or age differences in phosphoprotein phosphatase activity, an enzyme that dephosphorylates proteins and organelles. A 20 per cent increase in phosphoprotein phosphatase activity in the senescent heart has been measured.[40] An alternative explanation of the results of Figure 50–2 (i.e., that the [Ca^{++}]–myofilament interaction that leads to force production is altered with age) can be excluded, since in both intact and skinned preparations[19] the effect of Ca^{++} on force production, from threshold to maximum, is not altered with age.

DIMINISHED RESPONSE TO CARDIAC GLYCOSIDES IN SENESCENT MYOCARDIUM

The contractile response to ouabain is diminished in the senescent as compared with the adult myocardium (Fig. 50–3). However, the response to paired stimulation (which caused a much greater increase in contractility than ouabain) in the same muscles was *not* age-related (Fig. 50–3*B*). Thus the depressed response to ouabain of senescent muscle cannot readily be attributed to a nonspecific failure of the excitation-contraction process, to an inability of the myofilaments to generate additional force, or to a failure in energy necessary for a sustained inotropic response. The mechanism for the effect of age may be at the Na^+, K^+-ATPase receptor (i.e., an age-related difference in receptor density, ouabain binding, resultant enzyme inhibition) or in the extent of enhanced Ca^{++} loading caused by this inhibition. The relative ouabain inhibition of Na^+, K^+-ATPase in crude membrane preparations is not dependent on age over the adult range,[62] so that this particular factor cannot account for the difference seen in Figure 50–3*A*. In the intact senescent (11 to 13 years) beagle, as compared with the adult (1 to 3 years) dog, a decrement in the contractile response to acetylstrophanthidin with no difference in glycoside Na^+, K^+-ATPase inhibition has also been demonstrated.[63]

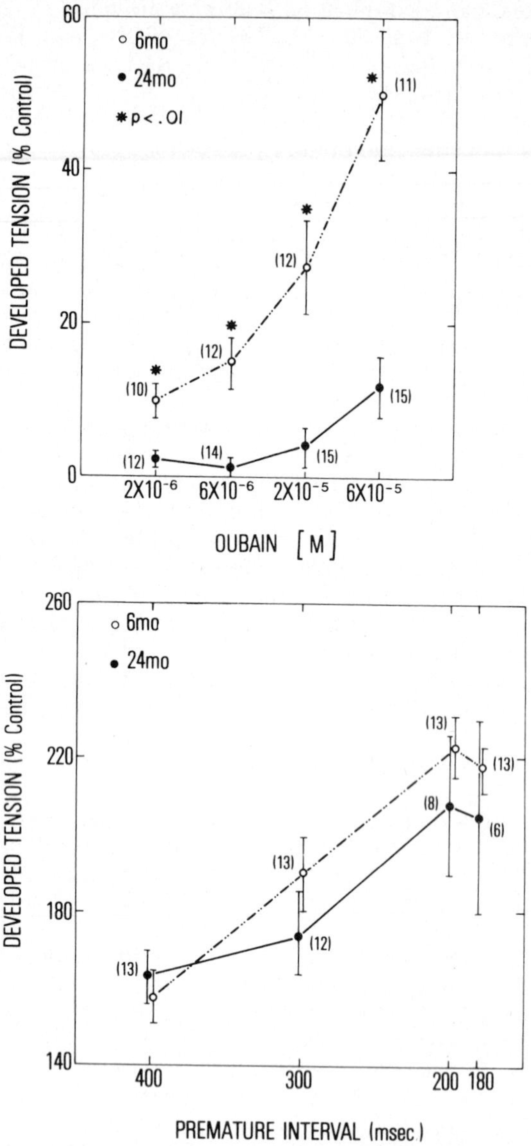

FIGURE 50–3. ***Top,*** **The effect of age of the relative increase on twitch tension in response to incremental concentrations of ouabain in isolated left ventricular trabeculae from 6- to 24-month-old rats. Before drug, twitch tension did not vary with age.** ***Bottom,*** **Same muscles show no decrease in inotropic response to post extrasystolic potentiation. (From Gerstenblith, G., et al.: Diminished inotropic responsiveness to ouabain in aged rat myocardium. Circ. Res.** ***44*****:517, 1979, by permission of the American Heart Association, Inc.)**

In *summary*, most information regarding age of the myocardium comes from studies in the rat model. Isometric force production, at least at low frequencies of stimulation, is preserved. There is no clear-cut indication that passive stiffness is increased. While the affinity of the myofibrils for Ca^{++} is preserved in senescent muscle, the inotropic responses to cardiac glycosides and beta-adrenergic stimulation are reduced. The latter may underlie, in part, the alterations in cardiodynamics (i.e., greater utilization of the Frank-Starling mechanism) during vigorous exercise in older men. In senescence, contraction is prolonged because the Ca^{++} released into the myoplasm during systole is removed more slowly than in the younger heart. A major cause of this appears to be a reduced rate of Ca^{++} sequestration by the sarcoplasmic reticulum. While the duration of the action potential is also longer in senescent than in younger cardiac muscle, its role in the prolonged contraction is less clear. The changes in the action potential could reflect age-related changes in the sarcolemmal ionic conductances or be the result of the prolonged myoplasmic Ca^{++} transient. In the older heart, myosin isozymes shift to slower forms and ATPase activity declines. These changes appear to underlie the observed decline in the velocity of shortening in senescent muscle contracting in the isotonic mode. The interrelated alterations in excitation-contraction mechanisms and myofibrillar biochemistry that occur in senescence are adaptive. The same constellation of changes is observed in the myocardium of young rats in which myocardial hypertrophy is induced by chronic hypertension or aortic banding. Some of these changes (e.g., the prolonged contraction) can be reversed by chronic exercise in senescent animals.

CARDIAC FUNCTION IN NORMAL AGING HUMANS

The effect of age on cardiac function in humans can be addressed only in the context of the population studied and the variable used to define and measure cardiac function. One of the most consistent findings in studies of the influence of aging is the large variation in the older population for nearly every cardiovascular variable. There are many older individuals whose measured performance is equal, or in some instances superior, to their middle-aged counterparts, as well as some who are considerably below the mean for their age group. This variation must be related to differences in factors other than age alone which influence cardiovascular performance. The most important of these are the presence of cardiovascular disease, primarily hypertension and coronary atherosclerosis, and physical conditioning. Therefore, the results of studies in humans must be related to the certainty of freedom from the effects of superimposed disease and the physical conditioning status of the subjects. This is particularly true when quantitating the "effect of age" on measured left ventricular performance.

ASSESSMENT OF PERFORMANCE

Another equally important consideration is the measured variable. Although maximum oxygen consumption is considered to be the best index of cardiovascular performance, there are several potential difficulties in determining the age effect on this important parameter. The first is that in order to be certain that any individual's oxygen consumption during exercise is the maximum, it is necessary to demonstrate no significant increase in oxygen consumption despite an increase in workload. This often is not found in studies of older age groups and suggests that musculoskeletal or some other noncardiovascular parameters are limiting exercise before the true maximum oxygen consumption can be achieved. Even if a plateau is reached, it is possible that age differences in muscle mass or in the ability of the muscles to extract and use oxygen may be the limiting factor rather than cardiovascular function per se. This is suggested by recent evidence that age differences in maximum oxygen consumption are minimized or abolished when the values are adjusted for lean body mass.[64]

Studies of "normal" aging have been handicapped until recently by a natural reluctance to use invasive methodology in individuals who are thought to be free of cardiovascular disease. This resulted in two major limitations in some earlier work. The first is that it was difficult to exclude individuals with occult coronary disease. This is an important consideration because the prevalence of autopsy-documented disease is much higher than the prevalence of clinically obvious disease.[65, 66] Many individuals thought to be free of coronary disease on screening using routine history, physical examination, and resting electrocardiogram undoubtedly were not. Because there is an age-related increase in the incidence of inapparent disease, many older study participants with latent coronary disease were included in study protocols. A second limitation resulting from the hesitancy to use invasive methodology was an inability to measure central circulatory function (i.e., stroke volume or its determinants, end diastolic and end systolic volumes) in relatively large numbers of volunteers. The recent introduction of nuclear cardiology techniques, specifically the use of thallium scintigraphy (p. 328) to diagnose the presence of coronary disease and gated blood pool scans (p. 317) to measure cardiac volumes during exercise, provided significant additional information concerning the effect of normal aging on cardiac function during rest and exercise stress.

HEMODYNAMICS AT REST: NO CHANGE IN STROKE VOLUME OR EJECTION FRACTION. Although invasive studies have indicated that aging is associated with a decline in cardiac output at rest,[67–69] these results may have been due to the selection of subjects not free of disease or to the methodology used. Cardiac output may increase more in younger individuals because of an age difference in the stress response to the invasive procedure itself. Several studies using noninvasive techniques have shown no age-related decrement in cardiac output, heart rate, stroke volume, or ejection fraction at rest.[70–73]

One of the more significant age-associated changes in resting cardiovascular parameters is an increase in systolic arterial pressure (Fig. 27–3, p. 822). This is probably secondary to age-associated changes in arterial stiffening, since the rise in blood pressure varies directly with vascular stiffness in different populations.[74] The increased systolic pressure is probably responsible in part for the mild left ventricular hypertrophy associated with aging (Fig. 50–4)[73, 75]; it is also seen in experimental animals as discussed earlier. This hypertrophy tends to normalize wall stress (p. 433) and may preserve indices of left ventricular function, including resting ejection fraction and the velocity of circumferential fiber shortening.[73] Apart from the increase in systolic pressure, the most striking and consistent change in resting indices is slowed and delayed early diastolic filling.[76, 77] This is probably due to prolonged cardiac muscle relaxation and is a consistent characteristic of aging which has been found in many species and experimental preparations as discussed above. Increased mitral valve stiffness may also play a role. The functional importance of this alteration under normal conditions is

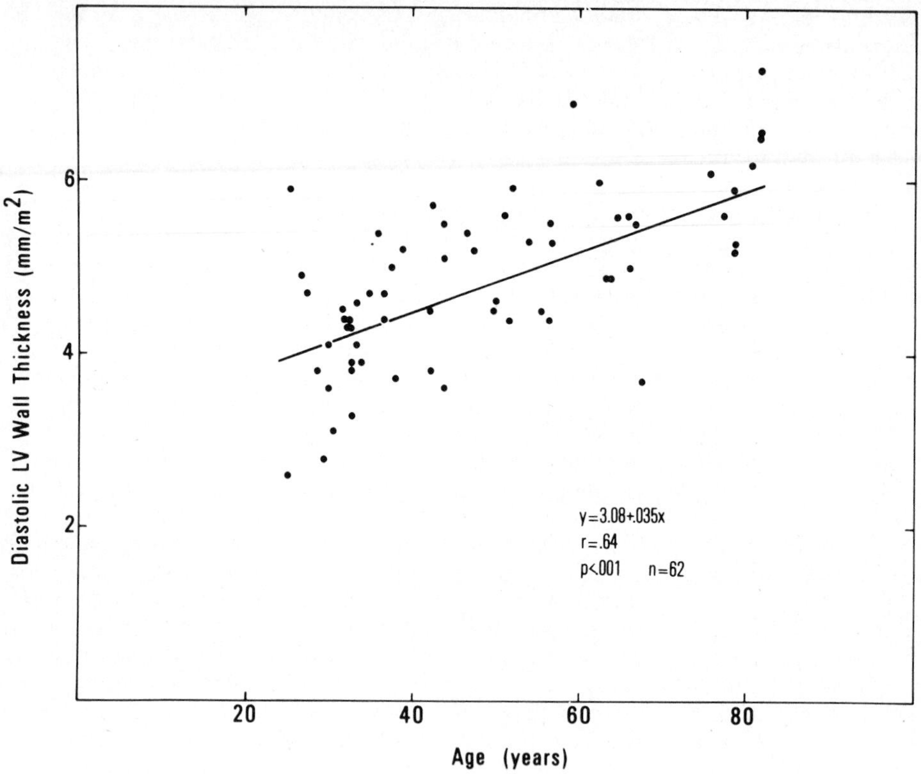

FIGURE 50–4. Linear regression plot of the relationship between age and diastolic left ventricular wall thickness (mm/M^2) in male participants of the Baltimore Longitudinal Aging Population. Increased age is associated with mild left ventricular hypertrophy. (From Gerstenblith, G., et al.: Echocardiographic assessment of a normal adult aging population. Circulation *56*:273, 1977, by permission of the American Heart Association, Inc.)

not great, since end-diastolic volume is either not age-related or slightly increased with age at rest[70, 73, 78] and during exercise.[70] However, it probably renders the older individuals more susceptible to hemodynamic compromise in the presence of a tachycardiac arrhythmic stress[79] or in the presence of superimposed ischemic or hypertensive disease, both of which independently impair diastolic filling.

HEMODYNAMICS DURING EXERCISE: NO CHANGE IN OUTPUT, LOWER HEART RATE, AND GREATER END-SYSTOLIC AND END-DIASTOLIC VOLUMES. In contrast to the subtle age effect on resting hemodynamic indices, there are more dramatic changes during exercise stress. Most investigators have reported a decline in maximum oxygen uptake and heart rate with aging,[80] even in athletes.[81] Several have reported a decline in exercise cardiac output with increasing age because of a decrease in both heart rate and stroke volume.[68, 69] In one study in individuals carefully screened to eliminate ischemic heart disease no age effect was found on cardiac output at comparable and peak workloads because an increase in stroke volume compensated for the decline in heart rate in the older individuals.[70] In this study, end-systolic and end-diastolic volumes were also measured and the increase in stroke volume was achieved by greater use of the Frank-Starling mechanism (i.e., an increase in end-diastolic volume). In younger individuals there was greater systolic emptying with a decrease in end-systolic volume, as compared with the resting values (Fig. 50–5). Ejection fraction increased more from rest to exercise in younger than in older individuals. In most older individuals free of disease, ejection fraction did increase with exercise but by only a small amount.

These age-related changes in the mechanisms used to augment cardiac output with exercise can be interpreted in the light of data showing an age-associated decrease in the inotropic,[30, 40] chronotropic,[82] and arterial vasodilating effects of catecholamine stimulation.[83, 84] During exercise, heart rate increases less in older individuals, probably because of a decreased catecholamine response (Fig. 50–5*A*). End-systolic volume (Fig. 50–5*C*) also decreases less owing to a diminished inotropic and vasodilating response to catecholamines.[84] Finally, the benefit of the Frank-Starling mechanism is unaltered with age and used effectively during exercise to maintain output through a higher stroke volume at a greater end diastolic volume (Fig. 50–5*B* and *D*).[70] The decrease in catecholamine-mediated effects during exercise is probably not caused by decreased elaboration of catecholamines, since plasma levels are higher, not lower, in humans during exercise.[85]

AGING, DISEASE, AND CARDIAC FUNCTION

ISCHEMIC HEART DISEASE

(See also Chaps. 38 and 39)

DIAGNOSIS (see p. 1320). The prevalence and severity of coronary atherosclerosis increase so dramatically with age that more than one-half of all deaths in persons aged 65 years or older are due to coronary disease and about three-fourths of all deaths from ischemic heart disease occur in the elderly.[86] The diagnosis of ischemic heart disease may be more difficult in the older individual, since the prevalence of diagnosed disease[66] is only one-third to one-half the prevalence of autopsy-documented significant atherosclerosis.[1, 65] The lack of classic symptomatology may be related to an age-associated decline in physical activity to the point at which ischemic symptoms are not present. In addition, dyspnea, rather than pain, may be the most prominent feature of the clinical picture in angina as well as infarction,[87] possibly because of the age-related changes in myocardial and pericardial compliance and diastolic relaxation discussed above. The physical examination is of limited usefulness in the diagnosis of ischemic heart disease (p. 1316). It should be remembered, however, that the transient features associated with acute ischemia (i.e., an S_4 gallop, reversed splitting of the second sound, and a systolic murmur owing to mitral regurgitation [p. 1321]) are often present in older individuals, even in the absence of ischemia.[88–90]

Stress testing (Chap. 8) is also useful in the diagnosis of an older patient with suspected coronary disease but with

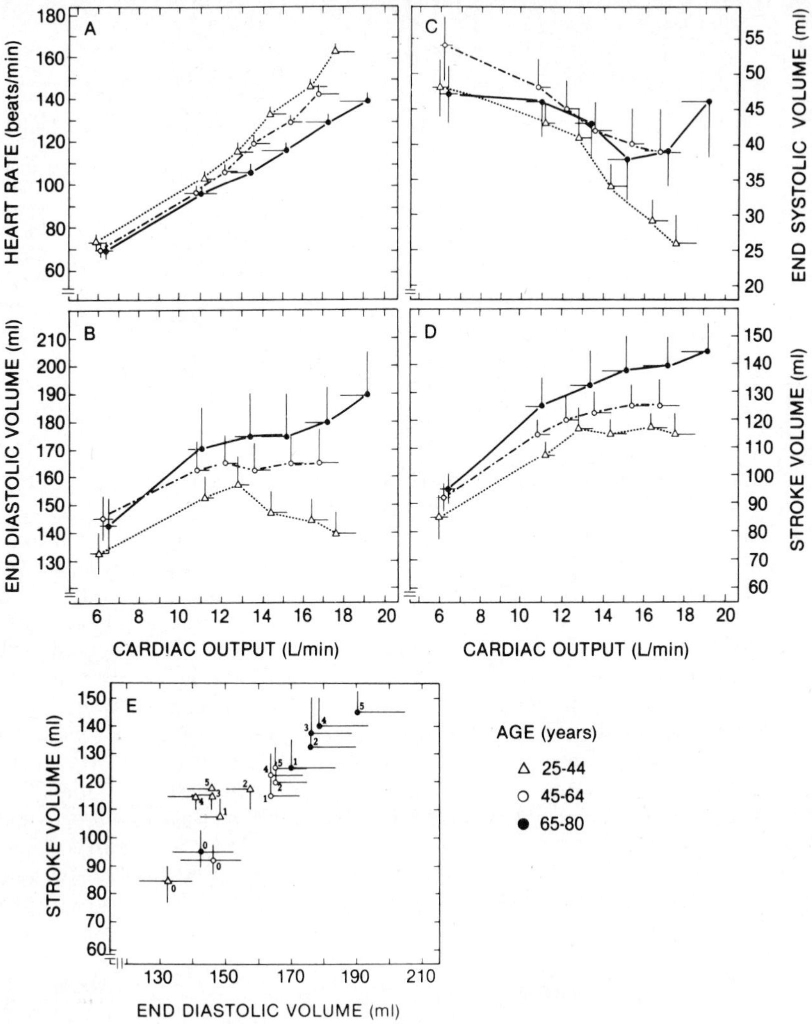

FIGURE 50–5. The relationship between cardiac output and heart rate (*panel A*), end-diastolic volume (*panel B*), end-systolic volume (*panel C*), and stroke volume (*panel D*) and the stroke volume-end diastolic volume relationship (*panel E*) at rest and during graded upright bicycle exercise measured by means of gated blood pool scans. The subjects are divided into three age groups: 25 to 44 years old (n = 22), 45 to 64 years old (n = 23), and 65 to 79 years old (n = 16). The number of subjects able to complete the exercise periods decreased with increasing workload; at a workload of 125 watts, n = 16 in group 1, n = 15 in group 2, and n = 11 in group 3. When the data were analyzed, including only those who were able to achieve the 125-watt workload a similar pattern was observed in all parameters and the significance of the age effect was unchanged. (From Rodehefer, R. J., et al.: Exercise cardiac output is maintained with advancing age in healthy human subjects: Cardiac dilatation and increased stroke volume compensate for a diminished heart rate. Circulation 69:203, 1984, by permission of the American Heart Association, Inc.)

certain caveats. The presence of resting ST-segment abnormalities or the use of digitalis, both of which are more common in the elderly, may invalidate the interpretation of the stress electrocardiogram, and in this setting stress testing using thallium scintigraphy (p. 328) is helpful. Thallium imaging is also helpful when the stress test is unexpectedly negative in an older individual whose history suggests the presence of ischemia, since the predictive accuracy of a negative test is low in a population with a high prevalence of disease. Finally, many elderly patients may not be capable of exercising to 85 to 90 per cent of their predicted maximal heart rate. In this setting a thallium scan after dipyridamole (p. 331) may provide similar diagnostic information.[91]

MANAGEMENT OF CHRONIC ISCHEMIC HEART DISEASE (See also Chap. 39). The treatment of angina in older and younger patients is similar. After diagnosis, reversible factors should be identified and treated. Of these, anemia, hyperthyroidism, hypertension, congestive heart failure, and noncompliance with medication may all be more common in the elderly. It should also be remembered that atherosclerosis is a progressive disease, and that although sometimes it has been stated that risk factor reduction is less important in the older patient, more recent evidence suggests that both successful treatment of hypertension[92, 93] and smoking cessation[94] decrease cardiovascular mortality in the elderly. The use of specific antiischemic agents is discussed below. If medical therapy fails to control symptoms adequately, percutaneous transluminal coronary angioplasty (PTCA; Chap. 40) should be considered. Although some reports indicate that in-hospital mortality associated with PTCA is higher in older than in younger patients,[95] low mortality (0.8 per cent) has also been reported, which does not differ from that in younger patients.[96] If, in patients in whom medical therapy has failed, the coronary anatomy is not suitable for PTCA, surgery should be performed. Although coronary bypass is associated with increased mortality,[97] morbidity, and duration of hospitalization, as well as increased costs in the older patient,[98] the risks of complications are decreasing[99] and long-term pain relief and survival are good[97, 100] and in most patients compare favorably with medical therapy (Fig. 50–6).[101]

MANAGEMENT OF ACUTE MYOCARDIAL INFARCTION (See also Chap. 38). The treatment of acute infarction should be undertaken with the realization that mortality, congestive heart failure, pulmonary edema, and ventricular rupture are all higher in the elderly.[102–104] It is unclear whether the increased incidence of these complications is due to intrinsic age-related changes in the response to the ischemic insult itself, poorer reserve in the remaining noninfarcted regions, perhaps owing to diminished catecholamine responsiveness, the higher prevalence of hypertension, prior myocardial damage, and/or larger infarctions. In addition to the above, important topographical changes develop hours to days after an infarction which importantly affect overall mortality and morbidity. Animal and clinical studies have defined regional dilatation and wall thinning at the site of the infarction,[105] and compensatory hypertrophy may occur in the region remote from the infarction. Age-related differences in these architectural changes accompanying an infarction could result from preexisting changes in left ventricular wall thickness,[73] peripheral impedance,[83] collagen content,[38] the capability

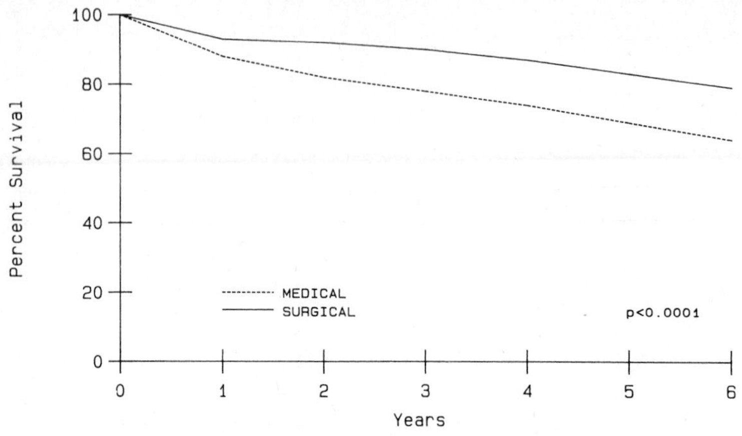

FIGURE 50–6. Cumulative 6-year survival in surgical and medical groups in 1491 patients 65 years or older from the CASS registry. Survival is adjusted for left ventricular wall motion, congestive heart failure, number of diseased vessels, number of associated medical diseases, and age at angiography. (From Gersh, B. J.: Comparison of coronary artery bypass surgery and medical therapy in patients 65 years of age or older. N. Engl. J. Med. *313*:217, 1985.)

of undergoing compensatory hypertrophy, or the inflammatory and healing response to the infarct itself.

The routine management of the older patient with an acute infarction does not differ significantly from that of the younger patient. The exception would be greater care in the administration of *lidocaine* because of central nervous system side effects (p. 625)[106] and of *heparin anticoagulation* (p. 1771) because of an increased risk of bleeding, especially in older women.[107] The elderly benefit as much as younger patients do from the secondary prevention effects of beta blockade.[108] In a Netherlands multicenter double-blind randomized trial involving more than 800 patients over the age of 60 years, oral anticoagulation was associated with a significantly lower incidence of recurrent myocardial infarction and death.[109] Successful aggressive management of complications, including septal rupture,[110] has also been reported.

ARRHYTHMIAS (See also Chap. 22)

Because of the increasing prevalence of hypertension and coronary disease, arrhythmias occur more frequently and are more often associated with hemodynamic compromise in the older age groups. In one study the incidences of supraventricular and ventricular ectopic activity (>100 beats/24 hours of ambulatory monitoring) were 26 per cent and 17 per cent, respectively, in 98 healthy subjects 60 to 85 years of age.[111] Ventricular couplets occurred in 11 per cent but ventricular tachycardia in only 4 per cent of the population. The incidence of asymptomatic ventricular tachycardia on routine treadmill testing in elderly individuals without other evidence of organic heart disease has been reported to be 4 per cent.[112] These arrhythmias were not associated with symptoms or subsequent sudden death. It should be recognized, however, that arrhythmias may be more ominous in the presence of disease. Even in the absence of disease, slowed and delayed early diastolic relaxation and filling owing to age alone[76, 77, 90] will result in greater compromised cardiac output in the older individual with a tachyarrhythmia.[79] Any compromise of cardiac output and blood pressure may in turn be associated with more critical decreases in cerebral flow in the older patient because of impaired cardiovascular reflex responses to hypotension,[78] an increased likelihood of preexisting cerebrovascular disease, and increased vascular stiffness.

The diagnosis of an arrhythmia in an older patient differs only in that the index of suspicion should perhaps be higher for any complaints relating to transient cerebral ischemia, angina, heart failure, or mental status changes. Long-term ambulatory monitoring is often useful. The urgency of therapy depends on the associated hemodynamic changes, and emergency treatment is the same in all age groups. The routine work-up should include a search for reversible precipitating factors. Some of these, including electrolyte imbalance, digitalis excess, hyperthyroidism, anemia, pulmonary embolism, and congestive heart failure, are more common in the older population. Specific therapy for the arrhythmia is guided by the severity of associated symptoms, the presence and type of underlying heart disease, and the recognition of the age-associated changes in the pharmacokinetics of the antiarrhythmic drugs as discussed below.

BRADYARRHYTHMIAS. Sinus bradycardia is often present in older individuals in the presence and absence of cardiac disease. It may be related to age-associated histological changes in the sinus node, a hypersensitive carotid sinus reflex, or medications, including digitalis, calcium- and beta-blocking drugs, and some other antihypertensives. Evaluation should be undertaken if the patient is symptomatic, and in this instance it is important to determine whether the transient symptoms are in fact caused by the bradyarrhythmia, since other causes for neurological symptoms are often present in this age group. Long-term ambulatory monitoring is most useful in this regard. If the patient is symptomatic, immediate therapy is dependent on the degree of hemodynamic compromise. Emergency temporary measures, including atropine, isoproterenol, and the insertion of a temporary pacemaker, can be used. If no reversible factors are present, the only effective long-term therapy is permanent pacing (see Chap. 23).

VALVULAR DISEASE
(See also Chap. 33)

The diagnosis of valvular disease in the elderly is often obscured by age-related but benign systolic murmurs,[90] changes in splitting of S_2, and increased stiffness of the central arteries. The latter may prevent the appearance of the slow anacrotic shoulder and small pulse pressure which would otherwise be seen in significant aortic stenosis (p. 67). The other findings, however, particularly the presence of a late-peaking systolic murmur, electrocardiographic evidence of left ventricular hypertrophy, and echocardiographic demonstration of valve narrowing and calcification all retain their significance. Doppler examination may be particularly useful in assessing the severity of obstruction (p. 100).[113] The usual etiologies are calcification of a congenitally bicuspid valve and, in those over 75 years of age, degenerative calcification.[114] Aortic valve replacement should be recommended for the usual indications (i.e., syncope, angina, and failure) and is associated with low mortality and excellent quality of life.[115, 116] The diagnosis of aortic regurgitation is not more difficult in the older age groups, but the *timing* of aortic valve replacement may be because of the often benign course of the disease. Surgery is usually recommended only for those patients who continue to be symptomatic on medical therapy. Mitral stenosis is usually due to rheumatic disease, while regurgitation can be due to rheumatic disease as well as calcification of the mitral annulus, mitral valve prolapse (at times with superimposed endocarditis), and ischemic papillary muscle dysfunction. Survival is considerably shortened in the presence of atrial fibrillation and failure,[117] and the results of mitral valve surgery are satisfactory.[118, 119]

HYPERTENSION

(See also Chap. 27)

The importance of the diagnosis and effective treatment of hypertension in the elderly cannot be overemphasized. It is the major remediable risk factor for cardiovascular morbidity and mortality, and successful therapy decreases the incidence of death and cerebrovascular events.[92, 120–122] The prevalence of hypertension, defined by a blood pressure of 160/95 or greater, is 30 per cent in elderly men,[123] and 20 per cent of the total elderly population have isolated systolic hypertension, defined by a systolic pressure exceeding 160 mm Hg and a diastolic of less than 90 mm Hg.[124] Convincing evidence of the effectiveness of therapy for even mild diastolic hypertension in the elderly is provided by the results of the Hypertension Detection and Follow-up Program Trial[92] (a 17.2 per cent reduction in mortality and 45 per cent reduction in cerebrovascular events), the Australian National Blood Pressure Study[121] (a 30 per cent reduction in trial endpoints), and, most recently, the European Working Party on High Blood Pressure in the Elderly Trial.[93] In the latter study there was a 38 per cent reduction in cardiac mortality and a 27 per cent reduction in total cardiovascular mortality using an intention-to-treat analysis.

There are no data concerning the effectiveness of therapy for isolated systolic hypertension. However, in view of the fact that systolic blood pressure is the best discriminator of risk in individuals over age 45[125] and that systolic blood pressure can be effectively controlled with minimal side effects,[126] the Joint National Committee on Detection, Evaluation, and Treatment of High Blood Pressure has recommended that therapy be instituted in the elderly with isolated systolic hypertension.[127]

Regarding specific therapy, it should be noted that thiazides have been used as the step one antihypertensive agent in all the major trials which have documented a decline in cardiovascular morbidity and mortality. There are several recent concerns, however, regarding an increase in other cardiovascular risk factors and possibly mortality in patients with baseline electrocardiographic abnormalities.[128] Although beta blockers are effective antihypertensive agents in some populations, elderly patients respond less often than do young hypertensives.[129] Calcium channel antagonists[130] and angiotensin-converting enzyme inhibitors[131] are relatively new antihypertensive agents which may be especially well suited for use in the older population. They have the potential for effectively controlling blood pressure as either single agents or in combination and may also reduce left ventricular hypertrophy. Controlled studies, however, have not been performed.

An interesting group of elderly patients with hypertensive hypertrophic cardiomyopathy has recently been described.[132] Females made up more than three-fourths of the reported group, and symptoms consisted primarily of dyspnea and chest pain. The diagnosis is made by echocardiography which shows exaggerated contractile function, small systolic and diastolic cavity dimensions, and prolonged and reduced early diastolic filling. The importance of the recognition of this patient subset is that therapy with vasodilators was associated with clinical deterioration, whereas patients treated with beta blockers or calcium antagonists were markedly improved.

DRUG USE IN THE ELDERLY

As a consequence of the increased prevalance of cardiovascular and other diseases in the elderly, the percentage of total expenditures for drugs in this age group is severalfold higher than the percentage of the total population.[133] In considering the effects of age on the pharmacokinetics and pharmacodynamics of cardiovascular agents,[134–136] it is important to note the heterogeneity of response in the older population. There are no strict age-related rules, therefore, which apply to the entire geriatric population, and it is clear that the commitment of the physician to carefully assess the therapeutic results and side effects of medical therapy must be greater in older than in younger age groups.[136a]

Although age-related changes in gastric pH and absorptive surface have been described, these have relatively unimportant effects for most cardiovascular drugs. The distribution of cardiovascular agents, however, is affected by age-associated decreases in serum albumin[136] and lean body mass[137] and increases in α_1-acid glycoproteins[138] and body fat.[137] A decrease in albumin results in increased free drug for those agents which are highly protein bound, which will, in turn, increase plasma concentrations for those agents whose metabolism is independent of the available free drug (e.g., lidocaine and propranolol). An increase in α_1-acid glycoprotein results in a decrease in the free fractions of acidic drugs such as phenytoin.[138] A change in body mass results in an increased distribution volume for fat-soluble drugs and a decreased distribution volume for water-soluble agents.

The effect of age on metabolism and excretion relates to its effect on renal and hepatic function. The influence of age on renal function has been extensively studied and results in a diminished glomerular filtration rate of 30 to 40 per cent over a broad age range,[139] as well as decreased renal tubular secretion and concentration ability. Because lean body mass decreases with age, renal function cannot be indexed using serum creatinine alone in older individuals. These changes result in decreased clearance of quinidine, procainamide, digoxin, and the water-soluble beta blocker atenolol. Diminished renal excretion of furosemide[140] results in a diminished diuretic response to this drug and presumably other agents which act on the luminal side of the kidney tubule. The effect of age on hepatic metabolism has been evaluated less extensively but is undoubtedly affected by the decrease in hepatic mass, blood flow, and activity of the microsomal fixed-function oxidizing system.[133] These changes result in increased half-lives of lidocaine and the lipid-soluble beta blockers, including propranolol.[133]

In addition to its effects on pharmacokinetics, aging may also influence the cardiac response to any given level of drug. Thus a diminished response to beta agonists,[30, 40, 84] beta blockers,[141] and digitalis preparations[62, 63] has been observed in human and/or animal models. The increased prevalence of other diseases associated with aging may render the older individual more sensitive to the side effect profile of cardiovascular agents as well. Preexisting decreased plasma volume and decreased baroreflex activity may render older patients more susceptible to the hypotensive effects of nitrates and diuretics. Preexisting conduction system disease or left ventricular dysfunction may also increase the likelihood of side effects with some beta blocker and calcium antagonist compounds.

In summary, the characterization of those cardiovascular changes in humans which are due to aging alone is difficult because of the age-related increasing prevalence of overt and latent cardiovascular disease and sedentary life style. It appears, however, that age does not significantly alter left ventricular performance except in the presence of a superimposed stress which can take the form of severe exercise or disease, particularly ischemia, a tachycardic arrhythmia, or hypertension. In these instances impaired diastolic relaxation and systolic emptying, probably related to a diminished responsiveness to beta-adrenoceptor stimulation, may occur.

The diagnostic and therapeutic principles used in the management of cardiac disease do not differ in older and younger patients. The presence of other associated diseases, changed life style habits, and altered pharmacokinetics and pharmacodynamics, however, require a more careful, skilled, conscientious, and often time-consuming application of these principles in the treatment of older patients. This is especially true in the management of hypertension, the successful treatment of which has the potential to cause an enormous reduction of cardiovascular disease and its complications. The treatment of ischemic heart disease should be adjusted to the life style of the individual patient. Nevertheless, those older patients whose life style is significantly impaired by ischemic symptoms or the side effects of medical therapy should not be denied the benefits of PTCA and bypass surgery simply because of their age.

REFERENCES

CONCEPTS AND THEORIES OF AGING CHANGE

1. Elveback, L., and Lie, J. T.: Continued high incidence of coronary artery disease at autopsy in Olmstead County, Minnesota, 1950–1979. Circulation *70*:345, 1984.
2. White, N. K., Edwards, J. E., and Dry, T. J.: The relationship of the degree of coronary atherosclerosis with age in men. Circulation *1*:645, 1950.
3. Saltin, B., Blomqvist, G., Mitchell, J. H., Johnson, R. L., Jr., Wildenthal, K., and Chapman, C. B.: Response to exercise after bed rest and after training. A longitudinal study of adaptive changes in oxygen transport and body composition. Circulation *38*(Suppl. 7): VII-1-78, 1968.
4. Moore, G. W., Hutchins, G. M., and Prito, J. C.: Cardiac hypertrophy occurs by myocyte enlargement, not repletion. Fed. Proc. *39*(Abs.):1111, 1980.
5. Weisfeldt, M. L., Wright, J. R., Shreiner, D. P., Lakatta, E. G., and Shock, N. W.: Coronary flow and oxygen extraction in perfused hearts of senescent male rats. J. Appl. Physiol. *30*:44, 1971.
6. Yin, F.C.P., Spurgeon, H. A., Rakusan, K., Weisfeldt, M. L., and Lakatta, E. G.: Use of tibial length to quantify cardiac hypertrophy: Application in the aging rat. Am. J. Physiol. *243*:H941, 1982.
7. Tomanek, R. J.: Effect of age and exercise on the extent of the myocardial capillary bed. Anat. Rec. *167*:55, 1970.
8. Gerstenblith, G., Lakatta, E. G., and Weisfeldt, M. L.: Age changes in myocardial function and exercise response. Prog. Cardiovasc. Dis *19*:1, 1976.
9. Hayflick, L.: Theories of biological aging. *In* Andres, R., Bierman, E. L., and Hazzard, W. R. (eds.): Principles of Geriatric Medicine. New York, McGraw-Hill Book Co., 1985, p. 9.
10. Roth, G. S.: Age-associated changes in hormone action: The role of receptors. *In* Schimke, R. T. (ed.): Biological Mechanisms in Aging. Washington, D.C., Department of Health and Human Services, 1980, p. 678.
11. Medvedev, Z. A.: Repetition of molecular-genetic information as a possible factor in evolutionary changes of life-span. Exp. Gerontol. 7:227, 1972.
12. Hayflick, L.: The limited in vitro life-time of human diploid cell strains. Exp. Cell. Res. *25*:585, 1961.
13. Harman, D.: The aging process. Proc. Natl. Acad. Sci. USA *78*:7124, 1981.
14. Bjorksten, J.: The crosslinkage theory of aging. Finska Kemists Medd. *80*:23, 1971.
15. Strehler, B. L.: Time, Cells and Aging. New York, Academic Press, 1977.
16. Makinodan, T., and Kay, M. B.: Age influence on the immune system. *In* Kunkel, H. G., and Dixon, Fm. J. (eds.): Advances in Immunology. Vol. 29. New York, Academic Press, 1980, p. 287.
17. Schimke, R. T. (ed): Biological Mechanisms in Aging. Conference Proceedings. Washington, D.C., Department of Health and Human Services, 1980.

CARDIAC MUSCLE FUNCTION IN AGING

18. Lakatta, E. G., and Yin, F.C.P.: Myocardial aging: Functional alterations and related cellular mechanisms. Am. J. Physiol. *242*:H927, 1982.
19. Bhatnagar, G. M., Walford, G. D., Beard, E. S., Humphreys, S. H., and Lakatta, E. G.: ATPase activity and force production in myofibrils and twitch characteristics in intact muscle from neonatal, adult, and senescent rat myocardium. J. Mol. Cell. Cardiol. *16*:203, 1984.
20. Wei, J. Y., Spurgeon, H. A., and Lakatta, E. G.: Excitation–contraction in rat myocardium: Alterations with adult aging. Am. J Physiol. *246*:H784, 1984.
21. Froehlich, J. P., Lakatta, E. G., Beard, E., Spurgeon, H. A., Weisfeldt, M. L., and Gerstenblith, G.: Studies of sarcoplasmic reticulum function and contraction duration in young adult and aged rat myocardium. J. Mol. Cell. Cardiol. *10*:427, 1978.
22. Bhatnagar, G. M., Effron, M. B., Ruano-Arroyo, G., Sprugeon, H. A., and Lakatta, E. G.: Dissociation of myosin Ca^{++}-ATPase activity from myosin isoenzymes and contractile function in rat myocardium. Fed. Proc. *44*:826, 1985.
23. Effron, M. B., Ruano-Arroyo, G., Spurgeon, H. A., Bhatnagar, G. M., and Lakatta, E. G.: Hyperthyroid state reverses prolonged contraction in rat cardiac muscle without altering myofibrillar activity. Fed. Proc. *42*:465, 1983.
24. Spurgeon, H. A., Steinbach, M. F., and Lakatta, E. G.: Chronic exercise prevents characteristic age-related changes in rat cardiac contraction. Am. J. Physiol. *244*:H513, 1983.
25. Capasso, J. M., Malhotra, A., Remily, R. M., Scheuer, J., and Sonnenblick, E. H.: Effects of age on mechanical and electrical performance of rat myocardium. Am. J. Physiol. *245*:H72, 1983.
26. Spurgeon, H. A., Thorne, P. R., Yin, F.C.P., Shock, N. W. and Weisfeldt, M. L.: Increased dynamic stiffness of trabeculae carneae from senescent rats. Am. J. Physiol. 232:H373, 1977.
27. Yin, F.C.P., Spurgeon, H. A., Weisfeldt, M. L., and Lakatta, E. G.: Mechanical properties of myocardium from hypertrophied rat hearts. A comparison between hypertrophy induced by senescence and by aortic banding. Circ. Res. *46*:292, 1980.
28. Alpert, N. R., Gale, H. H., and Taylor, N.: The effect of age on contractile protein ATPase activity and the velocity of shortening. *In* Tanz, R. D., Kavaler, F., and Roberts, J. (eds.): Factors Influencing Myocardial Contractility. New York, Academic Press, 1967, pp. 127–133.
29. Lakatta, E. G., Gerstenblith, G., Angell, C. S., Shock, N. W., and Weisfeldt, M. L.: Prolonged contraction duration in aged myocardium. J. Clin. Invest. *55*:61, 1975.
30. Lakatta, E. G., Gerstenblith G., Angell, C. S., Shock, N. W., and Weisfeldt, M. L.: Diminished inotropic response of aged myocardium to catecholamines. Circ. Res. *36*:262, 1975.
31. Orchard, C. H., and Lakatta, E. G.: Intracellular calcium transients and developed tensions in rat heart muscle. A mechanism for the negative interval-strength relationship. J. Gen. Physiol. *86*:637, 1985.
32. Narayana, N.: Differential alterations in ATP-supported calcium transport activities of sarcoplasmic reticulum and sarcolemma of aging myocardium. Biochem. Biophys. Acta *678*:442, 1981.
33. Lakatta, E. G., Capogrossi M. C., Kort, A. A., and Stern, M. D.: Spontaneous myocardial Ca oscillations: An overview with emphasis on ryanodine and caffeine. Fed. Proc. *44*:2977, 1985.
34. Heller, L. J.: Cardiac muscle mechanics from Doca- and aging spontaneous hypertensive rats. Am. J. Physiol. *235*:H82, 1978.
35. Lakatta, E. G.: Do hypertension and aging similarly affect the myocardium? Circulation *75*(Suppl. I):69, 1987.
36. Fabiato, A.: Calcium release in skinned cardiac cells: Variations with species, tissues, and development. Fed. Proc. *41*:2238, 1982.
37. Noble, D.: The surprising heart: A review of recent progress in electrophysiology. J. Physiol. *353*:1, 1984.
38. Weisfeldt, M. L., Loeven, W. A., and Shock, N. W.: Resting and active mechanical properties of trabeculae carneae from aged male rats. Am. J. Physiol. *220*:H1921, 1971.
39. Reggiani, C., Poggesi, C., Dionigi, R., Bonezzi, C., and Minelli, R.: Influenza dell'etta' sul comportasmento contrattile del miocardio ventricolare di ratto. Acta Gerontol. *25*:239, 1975.
40. Guarnieri, T., Filburn, C. R., Zitnik, G., Roth, G., and Lakatta, E. G.: Contractile and biochemical correlates of beta-adrenergic stimulation of the aged heart. Am. J. Physiol. *239*:H501, 1980.
41. Jacob, R., Kissling, G., Ebrecht, G., Holubarsch, C., Medugorac, I., and Rupp, H.: Adaptive and pathological alterations in experimental cardiac hypertrophy. *In* Chazov, E., Saks, V., and Rona, G. (eds.): Advances in Myocardiology. Vol. 4. New York, Plenum Medical, 1983, p. 55.
42. Mercadier, J-J., Lompre, A-M., Wisnewsky, C., Samuel, J-L, Bercovici, J., Swynghedauw, B., and Schwartz, K.: Myosin isoenzymic changes in several models of rat cardiac hypertrophy. Circ. Res. *49*:525, 1981.
43. Rockstein, M., Chesky, J. A., and Lopez, T.: Effects of exercise on the biochemical aging of mammalian myocardium. I. Actomyosin ATPase. J. Gerontol. *36*:294, 1981.
44. Ebrecht, G., Rupp, H., and Jacob, R.: Alterations of mechanical parameters in chemically skinned preparations of rat myocardium as a function of isoenzyme pattern of myosin. Basic Res. Cardiol. *77*:220, 1982.

45. Capasso, J. M., Malhotra, A., Scheuer, J., and Sonnenblick, E. H.: Myocardial biochemical, contractile and electrical performance after imposition of hypertension in young and old rats. Circ. Res. *58*:445, 1986.
46. Hoh, J.F.Y., and Rossmanith, G. H.: Ventricular isomyosins and the tonic regulation of cardiac contractility. *In* Stone, H. L., and Weglicki, W. B. (eds.): Pathobiology of Cardiovascular Injury. Boston, Martinus Nijhoff, 1985, p. 476.
47. Gulch R. W., Baumann, R., and Jacob, R.: Analysis of myocardial action potential in left ventricular hypertrophy of Goldblatt rats. Basic Res. Cardiol. *74*:69, 1979.
48. Capasso, J. M., Strobeck, J. E., and Sonnenblick, E. H.: Myocardial mechanical alterations during gradual onset long-term hypertension in rats. Am. J. Physiol. *241*:H435, 1981.
49. Gwanthmay, J. K., Defeo, T. T., and Morgan, J. P.: Hypertrophy-induced prolongation of intracellular Ca^{++} transients in mammalian working myocardium as detected with aequorin. Circulation *70*(Suppl. II):73, 1984.
50. Simmons, R. M., and Jewell, B. R., Mechanics and models of muscular contraction. *In* Linden, R. J. (ed.): Recent Advances in Physiology. New York, Longman, 1973, p. 87.
51. Borg, T. K., and Caulfield, J. B.: The collagen matrix of the heart. Fed. Proc. *40*:2037, 1981.
52. Borg, T. K., Ranson, W. F., Moslehy, F. A., and Caulfield, J. B.: Structural basis of ventricular stiffness. Lab. Invest. *44*:49, 1981.
53. Pinto, J. G., and Fung, Y. C.: Mechanical properties of the heart muscle in the passive state. J. Biomech. *6*:597, 1973.
54. Mirsky, I., and Laks, M. M.: Time course of changes in the mechanical properties of the canine right and left ventricles during hypertrophy caused by pressure overload. Circ. Res. *46*:530, 1980.
55. Kane, R. L., McMahon, T. A., Wagner, R. L., and Abelmann, W. H.: Ventricular elastic modulus as a function of age in the Syrian golden hamster. Circ. Res. *38*:74, 1976.
56. Templeton, G. H., Platt, M. R., Willerson, J. T., and Weisfeldt, M. L.: Influence of aging on left ventricular hemodynamics and stiffness in beagles. Circ. Res. *44*:189, 1979.
56a. Bryg, R. J., Williams, G. A., and Labovitz, A. J.: Effect of aging on left ventricular diastolic filling in normal subjects. Am. J. Cardiol. *59*:971, 1987.
57. Janz, R. F., Kubert, R. B., Mirsky, I., Korecky, B., and Taichman, G. C.: Effect of age on passive elastic stiffness of rat heart muscle. Biophys. J. *16*:281, 1976.
58. Oscai, L. B., Mole, P. A., and Holloszy, J. O.: Effects of exercise on cardiac weight and mitochondria in male and female rats. Am. J. Physiol. *220*:1944, 1971.
59. Starnes, J. W., Beyer, R. E., and Edington, D. W.: Myocardial adaptations to endurance exercise in aged rats. Am. J. Physiol. *245*:H560, 1983.
60. Steinhagen-Thiessen, E., Reznick, A. S., and Ringe, J. D.: Age dependent variations in cardiac and skeletal muscle during short and long term treadmill-running of mice. Eur. Heart J. *5*(Suppl. E):27, 1984.
61. Chesky, J. A., LaFollette, S., Travis, M., and Fortado, C.: Effects of physical training on myocardial enzyme activities in aging rats. J. Appl. Physiol. *55*:1349, 1983.
62. Gerstenblith, G., Spurgeon, H. A., Froehlich, J. P., Weisfeldt, M. L., and Lakatta, E. G.: Diminished inotropic responsiveness to ouabain in aged rat myocardium. Circ. Res. *44*:517, 1979.
63. Guarnieri, T., Spurgeon, H. A., Froehlich, J. P., Weisfeldt, M. L., and Lakatta, E. G.: Diminished inotropic response but unaltered toxicity to acetylstrophanthidin in senescent beagle. Circulation *60*:1548, 1979.

CARDIAC FUNCTION IN NORMAL AGING HUMANS

64. Fleg, J. L., and Lakatta, E. G.: Loss of muscle mass is a major determinant of the age-related decline in maximal aerobic capacity. Circulation *72*(Abs.):III-464, 1985.
65. Tejada, C., Strong, J. P., Montenegro, M. R., Restrepo, C., and Solberg, L. A.: Distribution of coronary and aortic atherosclerosis by geographic location, race and sex. Lab. Invest. *18*:509, 1968.
66. Kennedy, R. D., Andrews, G. R., and Caird, F. I.: Ischemic heart disease in the elderly. Br. Heart J. *39*:1121, 1977.
67. Brandfonbrener, M., Landowne, M., and Shock, N. W.: Changes in cardiac output with age. Circulation *12*:557, 1955.
68. Strandell, T.: Circulatory studies on healthy old men. Acta Med. Scand. *175*:1, 1964.
69. Conway, J., Wheeler, R., and Sannerstedt, R.: Sympathetic nervous activity during exercise in relation to age. Cardiovasc. Res. *5*:577, 1971.
70. Rodeheffer, R. J., Gerstenblith, G., Becker, L. C., Fleg, J. L., Weisfeldt, M. L., and Lakatta, E. G.: Exercise cardiac output is maintained with advancing age in healthy human subjects: Cardiac dilatation and increased stroke volume compensate for a diminished heart rate. Circulation *69*:203, 1984.
71. Port, S., Cobb, F. R., Coleman, E., and Jones, R. H.: Effect of age on the response of the left ventricular ejection fraction to exercise. N. Engl. J. Med. *303*:1133, 1980.
72. Proper, R., and Wall, F.: Left ventricular stroke volume measurements not affected by chronologic aging. Am. Heart J. *83*:843, 1972.
73. Gerstenblith G., Frederiksen, J., Yin, F.C.P., Fortuin, N. J., Lakatta, E. G., and Weisfeldt, M. L.: Echocardiographic assessment of a normal adult aging population. Circulation *56*:273, 1977.
74. Avolio, A. P., Fa-Quan, D., Wei-Qiang, L., Yao-Fei, L., Zhen-Dong, H., Lian-Fen, X., and O'Rourke, M. F.: Effects of aging on arterial distensibility in populations with high and low prevalence of hypertension: Comparison between urban and rural communities in China. Circulation *71*:202, 1985.
75. Sjorgen, A. L.: Left ventricular wall thickness determined by ultrasound in 100 subjects without heart disease. Chest *60*:341, 1971.
76. Gerstenblith, G., Fleg, J. L., Becker, L. C., Rodeheffer, R. J., Rogers, W. J., Weisfeldt, M. L., and Lakatta, E. G.: Maximum left ventricular filling rate in healthy individuals measured by gated blood pool scans: Effect of age. Circulation *68*:III-101, 1983.
77. Miyatake, K., Okamoto, M., Kinoshita, N., Owa, M., Nakasone, I., Sakakibara, H., and Nimura, Y.: Augmentation of atrial contribution to left ventricular inflow with aging as assessed by intracardiac Doppler flowmetry. Am. J Cardiol. *53*:586, 1984.
78. Nixon, J. V., Hallmark, H., Page, K., Raven, P. R., and Mitchell, J. H.: Ventricular performance in human hearts aged 61 to 73 years. Am. J. Cardiol. *56*:932, 1985.
79. Lima, J.A.C., Weiss, J. L., Guzman, P. A., Weisfeldt, M. L., Reid P. R., and Traill, T. A.: Incomplete filling and incoordinate contraction as mechanisms of hypotension during ventricular tachycardia in man. Circulation *68*:928, 1983.
80. Dehn, M. M., and Bruce, R. A.: Longitudinal variations in maximal oxygen intake with age and activity. J. Appl. Physiol. *33*:805, 1971.
81. Hagberg, J. M., Allen, W. K., Seals, D. R., Hurley, B. F., Easani, A. A., and Holloszy, J. O.: A hemodynamic comparison of young and older endurance athletes during exercise. J. Appl. Physiol. *58*:2041, 1985.
82. Yin, F.C.P., Raizes, G. S., Guarnieri, T., Spurgeon, H. A., Lakatta, E. G., Fortuin, N. J., and Weisfeldt, M. L.: Age associated decrease in ventricular response to hemodynamic stress during beta-adrenergic blockage. Br. Heart J. *40*:1349, 1978.
83. Yin, F.C.P., Weisfeldt, M. L., and Milnor, W. R.: The role of aortic input impedance in the decreased cardiovascular response to exercise with aging in the dog. J. Clin. Invest. *68*:28, 1981.
84. Fleisch, J. H., and Hooker, C. S.: The relationship between age and relaxation of vascular smooth muscle in the rabbit and rat. Circ. Res. *38*:243, 1976.
85. Fleg, J. L., Tzankoff, S. P., and Lakatta, E. G.: Age-related augmentation of plasma catecholamines during dynamic exercise in healthy males. J. Appl. Physiol. *59*:1033, 1985.

AGING, DISEASE, AND CARDIAC FUNCTION

86. World Health Organization. World Health Statistics Annual. Geneva, 1979.
86a. Walsh, R. A.: Cardiovascular effects of the aging process. Am. J. Med. *82*(Suppl. 1B):34, 1987.
87. MacDonald, J. B.: Presentation of acute myocardial infarction in the elderly—A review. Age Ageing *13*:196, 1984.
88. Spodick, D. H., and Quarry, V. M.: Prevalence of the fourth heart sound by phonocardiography in the absence of heart disease. Am. Heart J. *87*:11, 1974.
89. Slodki, S. J., Hussain, A. T., and Luisada, A. A.: The Q-H interval. III. A study of the second heart sound in old age. J. Am. Geriatr. Soc. *17*:673, 1969.
90. Burch, G. E., and DePasquale, N. P.: Geriatric cardiology. Am. Heart J. *78*:700, 1969.
91. Albro, P. C., Gould, K. L., Westcott, R. J., Hamilton, G. W., Ritchie, J. L., and Williams, D. L.: Noninvasive assessment of coronary stenoses by myocardial imaging during pharmacologic coronary vasodilatation. III. Clinical trial. Am. J. Cardiol. *42*:751, 1978.
92. Hypertension Detection and Follow-up Program Cooperative Group: Five-year findings of the Hypertension Detection and Follow-up Program. Mortality by race, sex, and age. J.A.M.A. *242*:2572, 1979.
93. European Working Party on High Blood Pressure in the Elderly: Mortality and morbidity results from the European Working Party on High Blood Pressure in the Elderly Trial. Lancet *1*:1349, 1985.
94. Jajich, C. L., Ostfeld, A. M., and Freeman, D. H.: Smoking and coronary heart disease mortality in the elderly. J.A.M.A. 252:2831, 1984.
95. Mock, M. B., Holmes, D. R., Vlietstra, R. E., Gersh, B. J., Detre, K. M., Kelsey, S. F., Orszulak, T. A., Schaff, H. V., Piehler, J. M., Van Raden, M. J., Passamani, E. R., Kent, K. M., and Gruentzig, A. R.: Percutaneous transluminal coronary angioplasty (PTCA) in the elderly patient: Experience in the National, Health, Lung and Blood Institute PTCA Registry. Am. J. Cardiol. *53*:89C, 1984.
96. Raizner, A. E., Hust, R. G., Lewis, J. M., Winters, W. L., Batty, J. W., and Roberts, R.: Transluminal coronary angioplasty in the elderly. Am. J. Cardiol. *57*:29, 1986.
97. Gersh, B. J., Kronmal, R. A., Schaff, H. V., Frye, R. L., Ryan, T. J., Myers, W. O., Athearn, M. W., Gosselin, A. J., Kaiser, G. C., and Killip, T.: Long-term (5 year) results of coronary bypass surgery in patients 65 years old and older: A report from the Coronary Artery Surgery Study. Circulation *68* (Suppl. 2):II-190, 1983.
98. Roberts, A. J., Woodhall, D. D., Conti, C. R., Ellison, D. W., Fisher, R., Richards, C., Marks, R. G., Knauf, D. G., and Alexander, J. A.: Mortality, morbidity, and cost-accounting related to coronary artery bypass graft surgery in the elderly. Ann. Thorac. Surg. *39*:426, 1985.
99. Elayda, M. A., Hall, R. J., Gray, A. G., Mathur, V. S., and Cooley, D. A.: Coronary revascularization in the elderly patient. J. Am. Coll. Cardiol. *3*:1398, 1984.
100. Kunis, R., Greenberg, H., Yeoh, C. B., Garfein, O. B., Pepe, A. J., Pinkernell, B. H., Sherrid, M. V., and Dwyer, E. M.: Coronary revascularization for recurrent pulmonary edema in elderly patients with ischemic heart disease and preserved ventricular function. N. Engl. J. Med. *313*:1207, 1985.
101. Gersh, B. J., Kronmal, R. A., Schaff, H. V., Frye, R. L., Ryan, T. J., Mock, M. B., Myers, W. O., Athearn, M. W., Gosselin, A. J., Kaiser, G. C., Bourassa, M. B., and Killip, T.: Comparison of coronary artery bypass surgery

and medical therapy in patients 65 years of age or older. N. Engl. J. Med. *313*:217, 1985.
102. Letting, C. A., and Silverman, M. E.: Acute myocardial infarction in hospitalized patients over age 70. Am. Heart J. *100*:331, 1980.
103. Williams, B. O., Begg, T. B., Semple, T., and McGuinness, J. B.: The elderly in a coronary care unit. Br. Med. J. 2:451, 1976.
104. Zerman, F. D., and Rodstein, M.: Cardiac rupture complicating myocardial infarction in the aged. Arch. Intern. Med. *105*:431, 1960.
105. Schuster, E. H., and Bulkley, B. H.: Expansion of transmural myocardial infarction: A pathophysiologic factor in cardiac rupture. Circulation *60*:1532, 1979.
106. Lie, K. I., Wellens, H. J., van Capelle, F. J., and Durrer, D.: Lidocaine in the prevention of primary ventricular fibrillation. N. Engl. J. Med. *291*:1324, 1974.
107. Jick, H., Sloan, D., and Borda, I. T.: Efficacy and toxicity of heparin in relation to age and sex. N. Engl. J. Med. *279*:284, 1968.
108. The Norwegian Multicenter Study Group: Timolol-induced reduction in mortality and reinfarction in patients surviving acute myocardial infarction. N. Engl. J. Med. 304:801, 1981.
109. Sixty Plus Reinfarction Study Research Group: A double-blind trial to assess long-term oral anticoagulant therapy in elderly patients after myocardial infarction. Lancet 2:990, 1980.
110. Weintraub, R. M., Thurer, R. L., Wei, J., and Aroesty, J. M.: Repair of postinfarction ventricular septal defect in the elderly. J. Thorac. Cardiovasc. Surg. *85*:191, 1983.
111. Fleg, J. L., and Kennedy, H. L.: Cardiac arrhythmias in a healthy elderly population: Detection by 24 hour ambulatory electrocardiography. Chest *81*:302, 1982.
112. Fleg, J. L., and Lakatta, E. G.: Prevalence and prognosis of exercise-induced nonsustained ventricular tachycardia in apparently healthy volunteers. Am. J. Cardiol. *54*(Abs.):762, 1984.
113. Berger, M., Berdoff, R. L., Gallerstein, P. E., and Goldberg, E: Evaluation of aortic stenosis by continuous wave Doppler ultrasound. J. Am. Coll. Cardiol. 3:150, 1984.
114. Pomerance, A.: Cardiac pathology in the elderly. *In* Noble, R. J., Rothbaum, D. A. (eds.): Geriatric Cardiology, Cardiovascular Clinics. Philadelphia, F. A. Davis Company, 1981, p. 9.
115. Hochberg, M. S., Morrow, A. G., Michaelis, L. L., McIntosh, C. I., Redwood, D. R., and Epstein, S. E.: Aortic valve replacement in the elderly. Encouraging postoperative clinical and hemodynamic results. Arch. Surg. *112*:1475, 1977.
116. Kaplan, O., Yakirevich, V., and Vidne, B. A.: Aortic valve replacement in septuagenarians. Tex. Heart Inst. J. *12*:295, 1985.
117. Caird, F. I.: Valvular heart disease. *In* Caird, F. I., Dall, J.L.C., and Kennedy, R. D. (eds.): Cardiology in Old Age. New York, Plenum Press, 1976, p. 231.
118. Hochberg, M. S., Derkae, W. M., Conkle, D. M., McIntosh, C. I., Epstein, S. E., and Morrow, A. G.: Mitral valve replacement in elderly patients. Encouraging postoperative clinical and hemodynamic results. J. Thorac. Cardiovasc. Surg. *77*:422, 1979.
119. Jamieson, W.R E., Dooner, J., Munro, A. I., Janusz, M. T., Burgess, J. J., Miyagishima, R. R., Gerein, A. N., and Allen, P.: Cardiac valve replacement in the elderly. A review of 320 consecutive cases. Circulation *64*:II-177, 1981.
120. Curb, J. D., Borhani, N. O., Schnaper, H., Kass, E., and Entwisle, G.: Detection and treatment of hypertension in older individuals. Am. J. Epidemiol. *121*:371, 1985.
121. Management Committee of the Australian Therapeutic Trial in Mild Hypertension: Treatment of mild hypertension in the elderly. Med. J. Aust. 2:398, 1981.
122. Kannel, W. B.: Blood pressure and risk of coronary heart disease: The Framingham Study. Dis. Chest 56:43, 1969.
123. Kannel, W. B., Dawber, T. R., and McGee, N. L.: Perspectives on systolic hypertension. The Framingham Study. Circulation *61*:1179, 1980.
124. Pooling Project Research Group: Relationship of blood pressure, serum cholesterol, smoking, relative weight, and ECG abnormalities to incidence of major coronary events. Final report of the Pooling Project. J. Chron. Dis. *31*:201, 1978.
125. Kannel, W. B.: Blood pressure and development of cardiovascular disease in the aged. *In* Caird, F. I., Randall, J.L.C., and Kennedy, R. D. (eds.): Cardiology in Old Age. New York, Plenum Press, 1976, p. 143.
126. Hulley, S. B., Furberg, C. D., Gurland, B., McDonald, R., Perry, H. M., Schnaper, H. W., Schoenberger, J. A., Smith, W. M., and Vogt, T. M.: Systolic Hypertension in the Elderly Program (SHEP): Antihypertensive efficacy of chlorthalidone. Am. J. Cardiol. *56*:913, 1985.
127. Joint National Committee on Detection, Evaluation, and Treatment of High Blood Pressure: The 1984 Report of the Joint National Committee on Detection, Evaluation, and Treatment of High Blood Pressure. Arch. Intern. Med. *144*:1045, 1984.
128. Multiple Risk Factor Intervention Trial Research Group: Baseline rest electrocardiographic abnormalities, antihypertensive treatment and mortality in the Multiple Risk Factor Intervention Trial. Am. J. Cardiol. *55*:1, 1985.
129. Buhler, F. R.: Age and cardiovascular response adaptation. Determinants of an antihypertensive treatment concept primarily based on beta-blockers and calcium entry blockers. Hypertension *5*:94, 1983.
130. Massie, B. M., Hirsch, A. T., Inouye, E. K., and Tubau, J. F.: Calcium channel blockers as antihypertensive agents. Am. J. Med. *77*(Suppl. 4A):135, 1984.
131. Dunn, F. G., Oigman, W., Ventura, H. O., Messerli, F. H., Kobrin, I., and Froehlich, E. D.: Enalapril improves systemic and renal hemodynamics and allows regression of left ventricular mass in essential hypertension. Am. J. Cardiol. *53*:105, 1985.
132. Topol, E. J., Traill, T. A., and Fortuin, N. J.: Hypertensive hypertrophic cardiomyopathy of the elderly. N. Engl. J. Med. *312*:277, 1984.

DRUG USE IN THE ELDERLY

133. Vestal, R. E., and Dawson, G. W.: Pharmacology and aging. *In* Finch, C. E., and Schneider, E. L. (eds.): Handbook of the Biology of Aging. 2nd ed. New York, Van Nostrand, 1985, p. 744.
134. Greenblatt, D. J., Sellers, E. M., and Shader, R. I.: Drug disposition in old age. N. Engl. J. Med. *306*:1081, 1982.
135. Sjoqvist, F., and Alvan, G.: Aging and drug disposition-metabolism. J. Chronic Dis. *36*:31, 1983.
136. Dybkaer, R., Lauritzen, M., and Krakauer, R.: Relative reference values for clinical chemical and haematological quantities in "healthy" elderly people. Acta Med. Scand. *209*:1, 1981.
136a. Covinsky, J. O.: New therapeutic modalities for the treatment of elderly patients with ischemic heart disease. Am. J. Med. 82(Suppl. 1B):41, 1987.
137. Bruce, A., Andersson, M., Arvidsson, B., and Isaksson, B.: Body composition. Prediction of normal body potassium, body water and body fat in adults on the basis of body height, body weight and age. Scand. J. Clin. Lab. Invest. *40*:461, 1980.
138. Verbeeck, R. K., Cardinal, J. A., and Wallace, S. M.: Effect of age and sex on the plasma binding of acidic and basic drugs. Eur. J. Clin. Pharmacol. *27*:91, 1984.
139. Rowe, J. W., Andres, R., Tobin, J. D., Norris, A. H., and Shock, N. W.: Age-adjusted standards for creatinine clearance. Ann. Intern. Med. *84*:567, 1976.
140. Kerremans, A. L. M., and Gribnau, F. W. J.: Changes in pharmacokinetics and in effect of furosemide in the elderly. Clin. Exp. Hypertens. [A] *5*:271, 1983.
141. Vestal, R. E., Wood, A.J.J., and Shand, D. G.: Reduced beta-adrenoceptor sensitivity in the elderly. Clin. Pharmacol. Ther. *26*:181, 1979.

51 CARDIAC SURGERY

by JOHN W. KIRKLIN, M.D.,
EUGENE H. BLACKSTONE, M.D., and
JAMES K. KIRKLIN, M.D.

Cardiac surgery is advised when the probability of survival with a useful life is greater with surgical treatment than with nonsurgical. The capability of predicting and comparing, therefore, is basic to the selection of optimal methods of management of patients as well as for scientific advances. Generally, the events being evaluated (death, return of angina, heart failure, and so on) are time-related rather than merely yes-or-no in nature, and this imposes the need for special analytic methods.[1, 2]

Ideally, cardiac surgery should have a hospital mortality approaching zero,* be curative,† and result in full functional capacity. In some patients, cure may be unattainable, and for them the operation should be palliative (provide a life expectancy and a functional capacity better than that imposed by the disease itself or by alternative methods of management). Most cardiac operations now have a low hospital mortality, and a description of the results of cardiac surgery by hospital mortality alone, or by simple description of late results, is no longer sufficient. Variables affecting the results (incremental risk factors) need identification in order to apply knowledge of results to individual patients and to improve results by neutralizing identified risk factors through discovery, new knowledge, and improved performance.

TYPES OF CARDIAC OPERATIONS

REPARATIVE. In general, reparative operations are the ones most likely to yield cure or excellent and prolonged palliation, and are least likely to require reoperation. Such operations include closure of patent ductus arteriosus, aortopulmonary window, atrial septal defect, and ventricular septal defect; the repair (opening) of mitral stenosis; and simple repair of tetralogy of Fallot. The probability of cure by these relatively simple cardiac operations can, however, be adversely affected by pre- and intraoperative conditions described below.

In some institutions, the simplest of cardiac repairs, such as pulmonary, aortic, and mitral valvotomy, and perhaps also the closure of patent ductus arteriosus, are currently being successfully accomplished with percutaneously introduced devices rather than by open operation (see pp. 1034, 1059, and 1389).

RECONSTRUCTIVE. Coronary artery bypass graft operations, transannular patches for the repair of tetralogy of Fallot, and the reconstruction of an incompetent mitral, tricuspid, or aortic valve are examples of reconstructive procedures that are inherently more complex and time consuming than simple repairs. They are not always curative procedures and reoperation may be needed, because some of them require the use of autologous, homologous, or heterologous biological or synthetic material. Others, such as the Senning type of atrial switch operation for complete transposition of the great arteries (TGA), the arterial switch operation for TGA (p. 958), and the repair of aortic coarctation, require nothing other than rearrangement of tissue in the local area. In this respect these are more likely to result in cure and infrequent necessity for reoperation.

In some reconstructive operations, an entirely new or rerouted pathway is created for pulmonary or systemic blood flow. For example, the intraventricular tunnel repair operation for double-outlet right ventricle creates a pathway from the left ventricle across the outlet portion of the right ventricle to the aorta for systemic blood flow. The

*Hospital mortality is said to approach zero when the lower 70 per cent confidence limit (CL), or interval, is less than 1 per cent and the upper CL is less than 5 per cent.

†An operation is said to be curative when the upper 70 per cent CL of postoperative survivorship, including hospital deaths, overlaps the survival of an age-sex-race matched general population.

Fontan operation for tricuspid atresia (p. 949) (and at times other conditions), in addition to closing the shunts, reroutes blood flow around the atretic tricuspid valve, to carry right atrial blood to the pulmonary artery. A valved extracardiac conduit placed between the right ventricle and the pulmonary artery for patients with tetralogy of Fallot and congenital pulmonary atresia provides a new pathway for pulmonary blood flow.

EXCISIONAL. The removal of atrial myxomas and the excision of left ventricular aneurysms are examples of excisional procedures, and in cardiac surgery they often must be accompanied by reconstructive procedures. Excisional procedures are considerably less common in cardiac surgery than in most other fields of surgery.

ABLATIVE. Treatment of the Wolff-Parkinson-White (WPW) syndrome and of intractable ventricular tachycardia by ablation of the reentry pathways (p. 645) represents an established but relatively new type of cardiac operation. In the case of WPW, the operations are usually curative since they rarely cause damage and usually provide freedom from symptoms and the need for subsequent medical therapy. The results of ablative left ventricular endocardial operations for intractable ventricular tachycardia (p. 645) can be compromised if additional damage is done to the left ventricle, whose structure and function are usually already impaired.

COMPENSATORY. Occasionally an operative procedure compensates for a cardiac condition rather than correcting it. Such operations are usually preliminary to complete repair of congenital heart disease. They may be used to provide permanent palliation in those rare instances of uncorrectable cardiac anomalies. The Blalock-Taussig subclavian to pulmonary artery shunt (p. 948), or one of its modifications, may be used to increase pulmonary blood flow in patients whose cardiac anomaly includes pulmonary stenosis and a ventricular septal defect. Pulmonary artery banding may be used to reduce pulmonary blood flow in patients with ventricular septal defect and similar conditions which result in increased pulmonary blood flow. The creation of an atrial septal defect can be life-saving in neonates with simple transposition of the great arteries and an essentially intact atrial septum. This (the Blalock-Hanlon atrial septectomy operation) was the first cardiac operation to be preempted by a percutaneous technique.[3]

Compensatory operations were useful in an earlier era, when the early (in-hospital) mortality of complete repair in certain situations, including infancy, was relatively high. They are used much less frequently today because in many institutions the incremental risks of these situations, including young age, have been neutralized. In a few situations, however, a two-stage approach, in which a compensatory operation is the first stage, is still useful.

SUBSTITUTIONAL (REPLACEMENT OR ASSISTANCE)

Valve Replacement. Replacements of cardiac valves are the most frequently performed substitutional operations. They rarely result in cure, but usually not because of failure of the biological or synthetic replacement device. More often, the operation fails to be curative because of the pre- and intraoperative conditions affecting results, as described below.[1, 4]

Biological replacement devices have the general advantage of not requiring permanent anticoagulation and the general disadvantage of limited durability (p. 1079). This disadvantage may be lessened in the future by more refined patient matching and processing of homograft valves, and more refined processing of heterograft valves. Synthetic replacement devices have the advantage of durability. They have the disadvantage of requiring permanent anticoagulation or antiplatelet therapy, and this disadvantage may continue to be difficult to overcome.

Ventricular Replacement or Assistance. Anatomical or functional total or partial replacement of the right or left ventricle separately is now possible, theoretically, under some circumstances. In skeletal muscle (such as the latissimus dorsi), the induction by repetitive electrical stimulation of the capability to perform as does cardiac muscle has been demonstrated to be feasible.[5, 6] In experimental animals, the right ventricular muscular mechanism has been replaced by a tube of prepared latissimus dorsi stimulated by a permanently implanted pacemaker[5]; no doubt this will be accomplished also in human beings. Prepared and stimulated latissimus dorsi muscle has been wrapped around the thoracic aorta as a permanent counterpulsation device and around the left ventricle as a left ventricular assist device.[6]

Artificial left ventricular assist devices have been implanted in a few patients (p. 533). However, these devices have been subject to the same problems as the total artificial heart plus the imponderableness of the function of the nonassisted right ventricle.[7]

Permanent biventricular assistance without cardiac replacement has been most successfully accomplished to date by heterotopic cardiac transplantation[8] (p. 530). Its primary indication in the United States has been elevation of pulmonary vascular resistance to such a degree that, against it, a new normal and unassisted right ventricle might not be able to generate an adequate pulmonary blood flow. It has no other advantages over cardiac replacement by orthotopic transplantation, and it has the added disadvantage that the new heart is a space-occupying lesion in the right hemothorax that sometimes compresses the right lung.

Cardiac Replacement by Transplantation. Currently, a transplanted human heart (homologous or allograft transplantation) is the most commonly used cardiac replacement device (p. 530). This procedure has been demonstrated to be technically reproducible, and the intermediate-term probability of survival has perhaps been greater for patients with it than would have been possible without it[9] (Fig. 51–1). The functional status of most patients is better after transplantation than before.

Human cardiac transplantation has two major disadvantages. One is the constant and probably life-long requirement for immunosuppressive therapy. Even with cyclosporine, episodes of rejection are not totally avoided, and side effects of the therapy cause morbidity and mortality. A second disadvantage is the relative and probably increasing scarcity of donors for cardiac transplantation in most countries of the world.[10]

Heterologous (or xenograft) cardiac transplantation has been used in at least one patient, a neonate with hypoplastic left heart syndrome, with a very short-term satisfactory result followed by death after 10 days.[11] The relative unavailability of xenograft hearts for implantation may soon be overcome by primate farms dedicated to breeding animals for heterologous cardiac transplantation, the moral justification being the same as that used in raising cattle for human consumption as food. The serious immunological problems involved in heterologous transplantation may ultimately be overcome by new knowledge, particularly in the area of acquired immunological tolerance.[12]

The question of growth of both cardiac allografts and

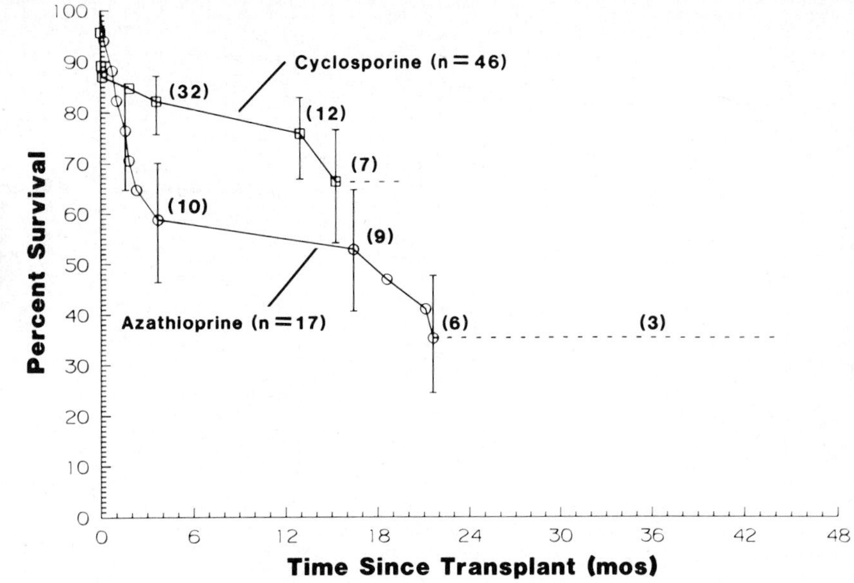

FIGURE 51–1. Stratified actuarial survival (stratification according to whether cyclosporine or azathioprine was the primary immunosuppressive agent), including hospital deaths, in a typical series of patients undergoing cardiac transplantation for a variety of pathological processes (University of Alabama at Birmingham [UAB], November 1981 to July 1985; n = 63). The vertical bars enclose the 70 per cent confidence intervals. The dashed lines indicate surviving patients observed until the end of the follow-up period.

xenografts requires further study before the results of cardiac transplantation in neonates and infants can confidently be predicted. However, the experimental studies of Bailey and colleagues do support the idea that growth of both homograft and xenograft hearts occurs.[13, 14]

Cardiac Replacement by Mechanical Devices. The totally implantable artificial heart, with an external power source (p. 533), has reached the stage of human use for cardiac replacement.[15] Whether this will continue, or whether the artificial heart will be relegated for a considerable period of time to use as a life-saving temporary cardiac replacement device, remains to be determined.[16] The disadvantages of current models of artificial hearts include (1) a continuing and important tendency to provoke thromboembolism, (2) propensity to promote bleeding tendencies because of the need for strong anticoagulant measures and possibly because of the development of consumption coagulopathies, (3) expense, and (4) the tethering of the patient to an external power source.

PREOPERATIVE CONDITIONS AFFECTING RESULTS OF CARDIAC SURGERY

CARDIAC CONDITIONS

THE LESION. In the past, the results of cardiac surgery depended considerably upon the specific cardiac lesion under treatment.[17] The hospital mortality for the repair of a foramen ovale type of atrial septal defect, for example, has approached zero in some institutions for many years, as has that for coronary artery bypass grafting, aortic valve replacement, and some other procedures. In contrast, until recently, the repair of AV canal defects, simultaneous aortic and mitral valve replacement, the Fontan operation for tricuspid atresia, the arterial switch operation for transposition of the great arteries, and other procedures have been accompanied by an appreciable hospital mortality.

Currently, the results of cardiac surgery depend very much more upon the preoperative and intraoperative conditions than upon the lesion. The repair of AV canal defects,[18] the arterial switch operation,[19] the Fontan operation,[20] and simultaneous aortic and mitral valve replacement[21] can now be performed with results quite similar to those obtained by simpler operations, when the pre- and intraoperative conditions are similar. This change has resulted from advances in the understanding of the morbid anatomy of most types of acquired and congenital heart disease, improved understanding and precision in preoperative diagnosis and evaluation, and improvement in the technical aspects of the surgery and in myocardial protection during operation.

Surgical treatment of a few lesions, however, continues to involve an increased risk of suboptimal results. In the case of a few of these (life-threatening ventricular tachycardia in patients with ischemic heart disease and anomalous origin of the left coronary artery from the pulmonary artery, for two examples), the results of operation are less than ideal (Fig. 51–2) because the lesions are invariably associated with impaired ventricular function. Advanced primary cardiomyopathy, another example, is a lesion associated with an inherently increased risk of surgery because a particular operation, cardiac replacement, is required.

VENTRICULAR STRUCTURE AND FUNCTION (SECONDARY CARDIOMYOPATHY). One of the most important limitations to the surgical treatment of heart disease is damage already sustained by the ventricles as a result of the cardiac lesion (secondary cardiomyopathy). The damage is produced by a chronic pressure or volume overload (p. 432), by acute or chronic myocardial ischemia, and uncommonly by frequent severe episodes of tachycardia. It is sometimes forgotten that the right ventricle as well as the left is subject to these damaging effects. The time required for the development of secondary right ventricular cardiomyopathy, however, is usually much longer than for secondary left ventricular cardiomyopathy, and this fact tends to obscure the existence of the former.

An early response of the heart to volume or pressure overload (or to a lesser extent chronic ischemia) is increased ventricular mass (weight). In volume overload, the increased mass represents an increased ventricular circumference without wall thinning and results in an increased ventricular volume at any given diastolic pressure. In pressure overload, the increased mass is primarily the result of increased ventricular wall thickness. The increase in mass results initially from myocardial cell hypertrophy. When the stimulus (volume or pressure overload, chronic ischemia, or prolonged tachycardia) is inordinate or prolonged, degenerative changes develop, including mitochondrial damage, sarcomere disruption, and fiber disarray.

Modest increase in ventricular mass may act as a compensatory phenomenon and preserve function. Thus in

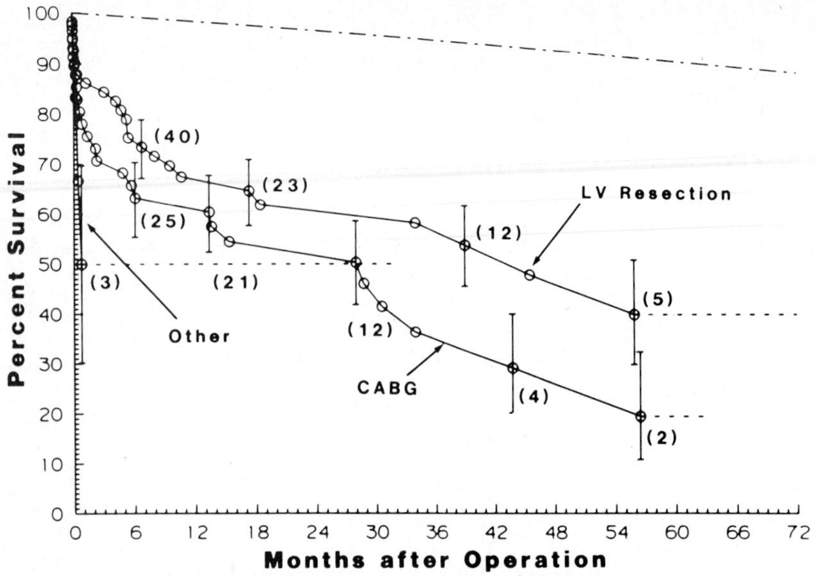

FIGURE 51–2. Stratified actuarial survival, including hospital death, after direct ablative operations for life-threatening ventricular tachycardia, with or without other procedures, in patients with ischemic heart disease (UAB; 1975 to July 1985; n = 105; deaths = 52). In addition to the direct operation for ventricular tachycardia, one group underwent left ventricular resection usually with concomitant coronary artery bypass grafting (LV resection); another group underwent coronary artery bypass grafting (CABG) because no aneurysm was present; and the third group underwent other miscellaneous procedures. (– — – = age-matched general population.)

aortic stenosis, the increased left ventricular wall thickness maintains nearly normal systolic wall stress (and thus afterload) in the face of elevated left ventricular systolic pressure.[22] When the hypertrophy no longer keeps pace with the increasing aortic stenosis and increasing ventricular systolic pressure, afterload mismatch develops and ventricular systolic and diastolic functions are adversely affected even though degenerative myocardial changes are not present. When myocardial degenerative changes then become evident, contractility becomes impaired in proportion to the extent and severity of the degenerative changes.

If only hypertrophy is present, after surgical treatment the ventricular mass usually regresses toward, but not to, normal after surgical treatment, and systolic and diastolic functions are improved and may become normal. Degenerative changes are, as far as is known, irreversible, and when they are extensive, little regression of mass occurs after surgical treatment, contractility remains impaired, and symptomatic improvement is limited. Several months or years after operation, nonregressed secondary cardiomyopathy often worsens by an unknown mechanism in spite of continuing relief of the inciting lesion, resulting in further impairment of systolic and diastolic functions, increasing symptoms, increasing ventricular electrical instability, and premature late death.

These phenomena must be considered in selecting the time of operation in most forms of congenital and acquired heart disease. When operation is deliberately delayed, the disadvantages of the progression of the secondary cardiomyopathy must be weighed against the advantages of continued medical therapy or of awaiting development of improved surgical methods.

Volume Overload (See also p. 450). Ventricular volume overload exists when the ventricular stroke volume is greater than net forward blood flow. Experimentally, the return toward but not to normal ventricular mass when volume overload has been of brief duration (less than 30 days) was demonstrated by Papadimitriou and colleagues.[23] Substantive information about the behavior of the cardiomyopathy secondary to volume overload in humans is scant, since myocardial biopsies are rarely performed in surgical patients, and late death is infrequently followed by autopsy. Inferences concerning its behavior, however, can be drawn from the observation of ventricular systolic function and functional status in patients with volume-overloaded ventricles. Patients with depressed left ventricular systolic function in whom aortic valve replacement has been carried out for aortic regurgitation, for example, have a lower 5-year survival after hospital discharge than do patients whose systolic function is normal preoperatively (Fig. 51–3*A*). In such patients, depressed preoperative exercise capacity (or increased NYHA Functional Class) still further depresses late survival (Fig. 51–3*B*).[24, 25] Poor functional capacity or depressed systolic function in the preoperative period also predisposes to lack of improvement of ventricular diastolic function late in the postoperative period.[25, 26]

Patients with atrial septal defect (ASD) slowly develop the same type of secondary cardiomyopathy in the right ventricle, because of its volume overload from the left to right shunt at atrial level. Related to this, older patients with ASD have less good right ventricular systolic function and more symptoms (Table 51–1) than younger ones, and symptomatic patients undergoing repair of ASD are older

TABLE 51–1 OLDER AGE AND DECREASED RIGHT VENTRICULAR SYSTOLIC FUNCTION IN SYMPTOMATIC PATIENTS WITH ATRIAL SEPTAL DEFECTS

Group	Age, Years (mean value)	Right Ventricular Ejection Fraction (mean value)
Asymptomatic	25	64%
Symptomatic	52	36%

From Liberthson, R. R., Boucher, C. A., Strauss, H. W., Dinsmore, R. E., McKusick, K. A., and Pohost, G. M.: Right ventricular function in adult atrial septal defect. Am. J. Cardiol. *47*:56, 1981.

TABLE 51–2 LATE POSTOPERATIVE RIGHT VENTRICULAR FUNCTION AFTER REPAIR OF ATRIAL SEPTAL DEFECT

Age at Operation (years)	n	Proportion with Near Normal RV End-Diastolic Volume
<10	11	64% (CL, 44%–81%)
>25	14	21% (CL, 10%–38%)

p = 0.04; CL = 70% confidence limits; RV = right ventricular.

From Pearlman, A. S., Borer, J. S., Clark, C. E., Henry, W. L., Redwood, D. R., Morrow, A. G., Epstein, S. E., Burn, C., Cohen, E., and McKay, F. J.: Abnormal right ventricular size and ventricular septal motion after atrial septal defect closure. Am. J. Cardiol. *41*:295, 1978.

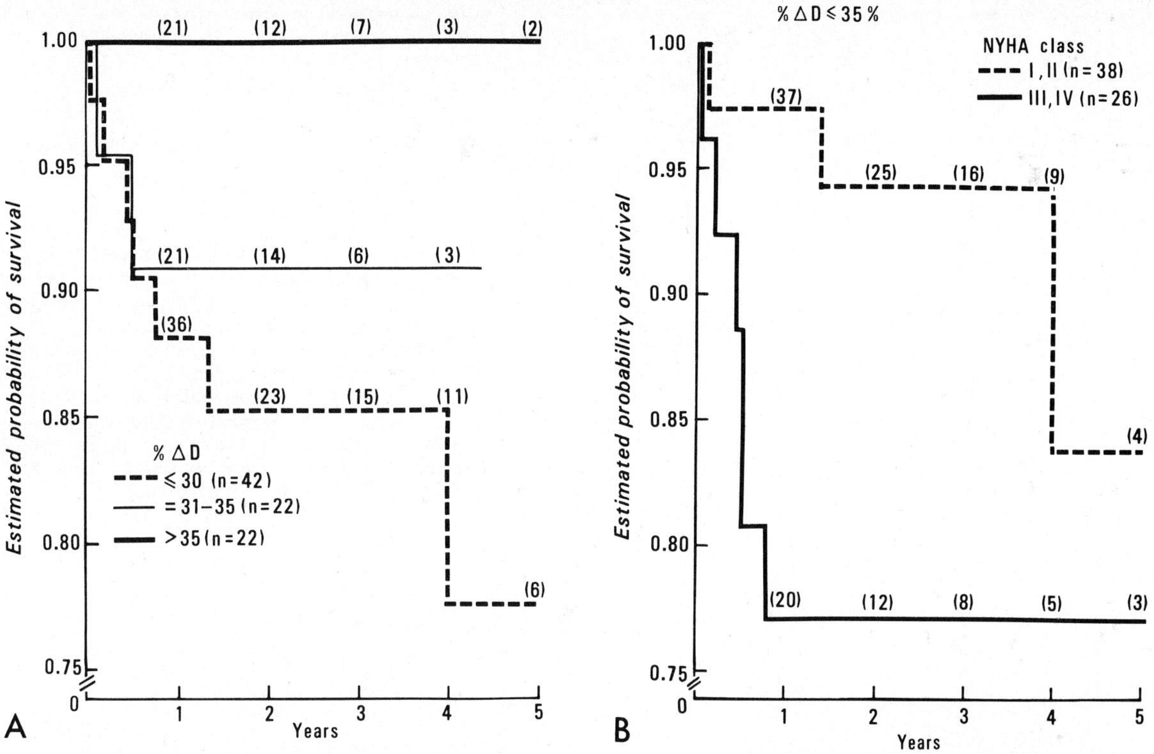

FIGURE 51–3. *A*, Relation between probability of survival after valve replacement for aortic insufficiency and preoperative per cent change of left ventricular dimension (% Δ D), an index of systolic function. Patients with low values, and thus diminished systolic function, have significantly decreased probability of survival ($p < 0.05$). (Numbers in parentheses are numbers of patients at risk at each interval.) *B*, Relation between preoperative NYHA functional classification and probability of survival after valve replacement for aortic insufficiency in patients with preoperatively depressed left ventricular systolic function. Patients in Functional Class I or II had longer survival than those in Class III or IV ($p = 0.05$). (From Cunha, C. L. P., Giuliani, E. R., Fuster, V., Seward, J. B., Brandenburg, R. O., and McGoon, D. C.: Preoperative M-mode echocardiography as a predictor of surgical results in chronic aortic insufficiency. J. Thorac. Cardiovasc. Surg. *79*:256, 1980.)

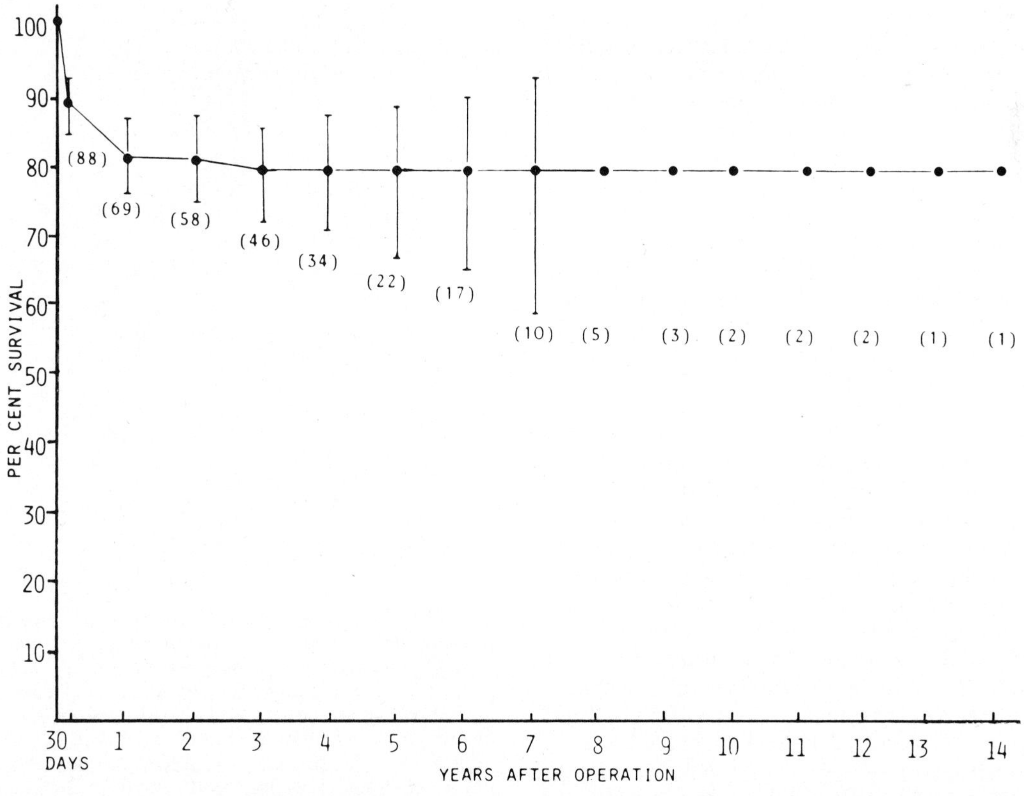

FIGURE 51–4. Actuarial survival after the Fontan repair for tricuspid atresia. Note that 93 per cent of the hospital survivors are alive up to 14 years after the repair, with death occurring rarely after the first postoperative year. (From Fontan, F., Deville, C., Quaegebeur, J., Ottenkamp, J., Sourdille, N., Choussat, A., and Brom, G. A.: Repair of tricuspid atresia in 100 patients. J. Thorac. Cardiovasc. Surg. *85*:647, 1983.)

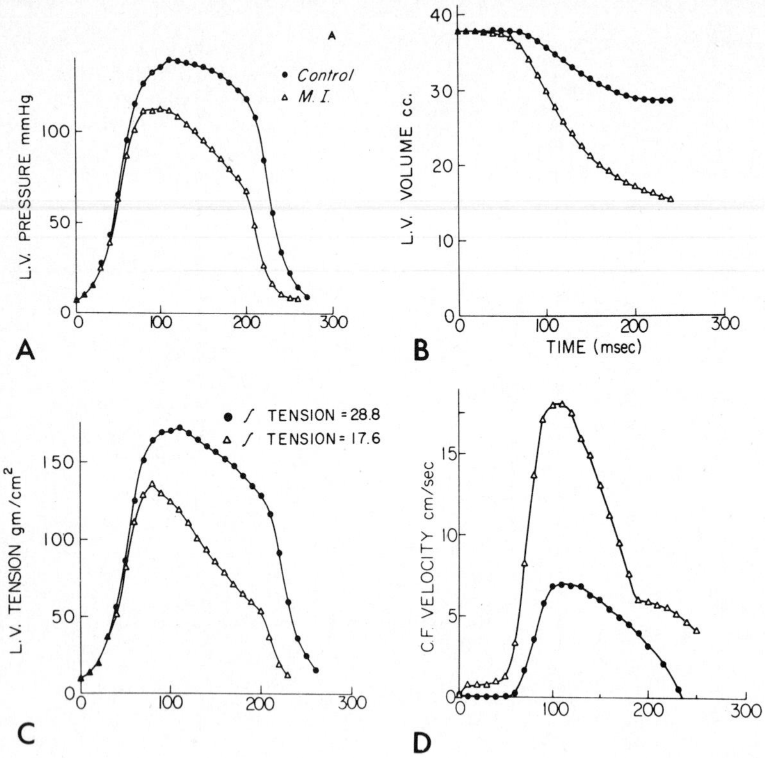

FIGURE 51–5. *A*, Experimental demonstration of the effect of mitral regurgitation on left ventricular (LV) afterload by the rapid reduction of volume during systole, *B*, and by decrease in wall tension, *C*. The result is an increase in systolic function as expressed by the mean velocity of circumferential fiber shortening (CF), *D*. (From Urschel, C. W., Covell, J. W., Sonnenblick, E. H., Ross, J., Jr., and Braunwald, E.: Myocardial mechanics in aortic and mitral valvular regurgitation: The concept of instantaneous impedance as a determinant of the performance of the intact heart. J. Clin. Invest. *47*:867, 1968.)

than are asymptomatic ones.[27] When the secondary right ventricular cardiomyopathy in patients with ASD is longstanding, it may become irreversible just as is the case in other types of secondary cardiomyopathy (Table 51–2).

Patients with tricuspid atresia (p. 949) have a volume overload of the left ventricle, since it generates pulmonary blood flow (through the ventricular septal defect and the hypoplastic and often rudimentary right ventricle into the pulmonary arteries) as well as systemic blood flow. The overload is frequently increased by the surgical creation in early life of a systemic-pulmonary artery shunt. A progressing secondary cardiomyopathy is responsible for gradual deterioration in condition of many of these patients after the second decade of life, their frequent development of increasing mitral regurgitation, and the poor response of some of them in the third and fourth decades of life to the Fontan operation. The surprisingly good long-term survival (Fig. 51–4) of individuals after the Fontan repair when it is done in the first decade of life is probably due to relief of the left ventricular volume overload as well as to ablation of cyanosis.

Other lesions resulting in chronic left or right ventricular volume overload include ventricular septal defect, aortopulmonary window, large patent ductus arteriosus, and atrioventricular septal (canal) defect.

A special situation exists when the ventricular volume overload is from mitral or tricuspid valve regurgitation, because in this setting ventricular afterload is reduced by the abnormally rapid decrease in ventricular volume and increase in wall thickness that occur during systole because of the regurgitation (Fig. 51–5).[28] The reduced ventricular afterload compensates for the developing ventricular secondary cardiomyopathy until late in the natural history of the disease. Surgical elimination of the AV valve regurgitation may unmask the secondary cardiomyopathy and show it to be more advanced than was suspected preoperatively (Fig. 51–6).

Pressure Overload (p. 431). Chronic left ventricular pressure overload is present in all forms of left ventricular outflow tract obstruction (subaortic, valvular, and supravalvular aortic stenosis), in aortic coarctation, and in systemic arterial hypertension. Chronic right ventricular pressure overload occurs in all forms of right ventricular outflow obstruction, including tetralogy of Fallot and pulmonary stenosis with intact septum. It is also present in pulmonary hypertension from any cause. The increased wall thickness

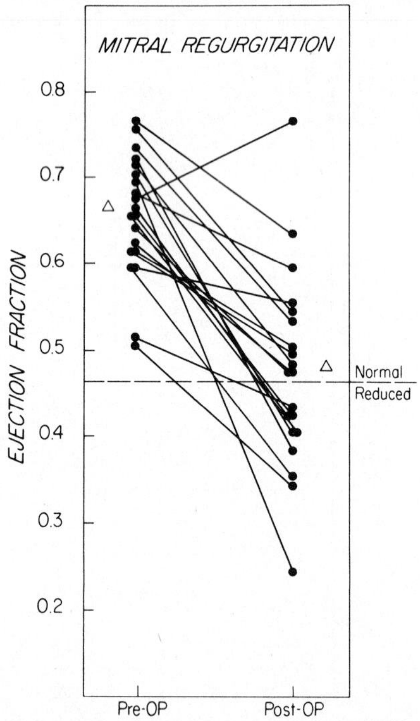

FIGURE 51–6. Ventricular systolic function (expressed as ejection fraction) before and early after mitral valve replacement for mitral regurgitation. Individual values are shown, and mean values are expressed by (△). Although all patients had an ejection fraction that was at least normal preoperatively, half had a postoperative ejection fraction below normal. (The lower limit of normal [0.50] is represented by a broken line.) All but one had a decrease in ejection fraction after operation. (From Boucher, C. A., Bingham, J. B., Osbakken, M. D., Okada, R. D., Strauss, H. W., Black, P. C., Levine, F. H., Phillips, H. R., and Pohost, G. M.: Early changes in left ventricular size and function after correction of left ventricular volume overload. Am. J. Cardiol. *47*:991, 1981.)

that develops because of a chronic pressure overload compensates for the increased intraventricular pressure by maintaining a normal afterload, the process of afterload matching.[22] Late in the course of a chronic pressure overload (Fig. 14–11, p. 434), or at birth in the case of the pressure overload produced by some kinds of congenital heart disease, the wall thickness may be insufficient to normalize ventricular afterload (a condition of afterload mismatch) and ventricular systolic function is reduced.[22, 29, 30] When such situations become chronic, the advanced secondary cardiomyopathy is associated with degenerative myocardial structural changes and reduced myocardial contractility.[31] These may not regress after surgical relief of the pressure overload.

Ischemic Damage (see Chap. 37). Ischemic damage may be existent only during a period of relative ischemia and may disappear when the metabolic demands are lessened or the regional or total myocardial blood flow increases. This type of ischemic damage may produce temporary depression of regional or ventricular contractility and/or distensibility, which results in a fall in ejection fraction and rise in left ventricular end-diastolic pressure during exercise, as well as angina pectoris in some but not all patients. When the relative ischemia is unusually prolonged or severe, myocyte cell death may occur, either massively and at one moment in one region of the myocardium (myocardial infarction) or in widely scattered small areas over a number of different moments.

A tension overload often develops in the remainder of the ventricle as a result of the effects of these regional abnormalities on the geometry of the remainder of the ventricle (an increase in ventricular volume and a resulting augmentation of wall tension, according to the law of Laplace, p. 454), with the same opportunities for development and progression of that secondary cardiomyopathy as exist in general for pressure-overloaded ventricles.

Other Secondary Cardiomyopathies. Persistent tachycardia can rapidly result in impaired ventricular function that must result from impaired myocardial structure, although the structural derangement may exist only in the form of an altered biochemical configuration within myocytes. Stopping the tachycardia, at least in the early stages, may result in reversal of the cardiomyopathy.[32]

SECONDARY SUBSYSTEM ABNORMALITIES

THE LUNGS. Preexisting abnormalities of pulmonary structure and function may prevent surgical treatment of an otherwise correctable condition, or may complicate the postoperative course. *Hypertensive pulmonary vascular disease* complicates many kinds of congenital heart disease (pp. 802 and 905). It is reversible in infants after correction of the underlying congenital cardiac malformations under most circumstances.[33, 34] However, in older patients, when it is advanced, it often persists after operation and may progress to cause premature late death. The classic description of the various stages of pulmonary vascular disease by Heath and Edwards,[35] supplemented by the more recent morphometric studies by Reid and colleagues,[36] has provided an excellent morphological understanding of the condition. Although there is a correlation between the morphology of the pulmonary vasculature and the calculated pulmonary vascular resistance, it is not sufficiently strong to allow exact prediction of the diagnosis of one from the other.[37]

When hypertensive pulmonary vascular disease becomes severe, the reactivity of the pulmonary vascular bed to physiological stimuli such as exercise disappears and an increase in pulmonary blood flow in response to exercise cannot occur. As long as there is a defect or communication between the pulmonary and systemic circulations, systemic blood flow can be augmented during exercise by right-to-left shunting, although arterial desaturation results. If the defect is closed, the opportunity for augmentation of systemic blood flow by right-to-left shunting is lost, and there is a risk of sudden death during exercise or stress resulting from an inability to increase systemic and thus coronary blood flow because of the high, nonyielding ("fixed") pulmonary vascular resistance. Therefore, pulmonary vascular disease of such severity is a contraindication to repair of the defect.

A similar but usually less severe type of pulmonary vascular disease develops gradually in patients with mitral stenosis and chronically elevated left atrial pressure. Although in unusual cases advanced morphological changes are present, more commonly there is a large element of arteriolar spasm, and pulmonary arteriolar resistance usually falls immediately after left atrial pressure is reduced by mitral valvotomy or replacement.[38]

Thrombotic occlusive lesions are a major component of pulmonary vascular disease in patients with cyanotic congenital heart disease. These occlusive lesions tend to be more extensive the more advanced the cyanotic congenital heart disease and its accompanying polycythemia.[39] In some patients, particularly those in whom congenital pulmonary atresia is a part of the malformation, congenital stenoses in the small and large branches of the pulmonary arterial tree, as well as hypertrophy of the distal pulmonary arteriolar walls, add to the hypertensive effect of the pulmonary vasculature.[40] These changes must be evaluated in toto and considered preoperatively in deciding upon the method of treatment and the probable results of cardiac surgery.

Pulmonary disease unrelated to the cardiac disease may also be present and may complicate the early and late postoperative period. The most common of these is chronic obstructive pulmonary disease. Its presence affects not only the risk of cardiac surgery, and thus the indications for it, but also postoperative management of the patient.

THE KIDNEYS (see Chap. 59). Preexisting chronic renal disease increases the risk of developing acute renal dysfunction and renal failure early in the postoperative period and thus affects patient management in this period and increases the risk of the operation.[41] Cyanotic congenital heart disease predisposes the patient to acute renal failure early postoperatively, probably because of gradually developing morphological renal abnormalities.[42] Preoperative chronic congestive heart failure likewise predisposes to acute renal failure soon after operation, most likely because of the abnormalities of renal structure and function that result from this state.

THE BLOOD. The polycythemia secondary to cyanotic congenital heart disease (pp. 903 and 1743) is overcome immediately at the start of cardiopulmonary bypass by the hemodilution that is used. However, most patients who were polycythemic preoperatively have a greater than usual tendency to bleed in the perioperative period. Special preventive measures may be required.

Longstanding congestive heart failure with hepatic congestion may reduce hepatic synthesis of normal clotting factors and thereby increase the tendency for bleeding after cardiopulmonary bypass. Because of the current prevalence of aspirin ingestion and the use of other drugs that affect platelet function, preoperative determination of bleeding time is advisable in most patients.

THE LIVER. Even mild preexisting liver disease increases the risk of acute hepatic failure early after cardiac surgery. Its presence must be taken into account in planning the

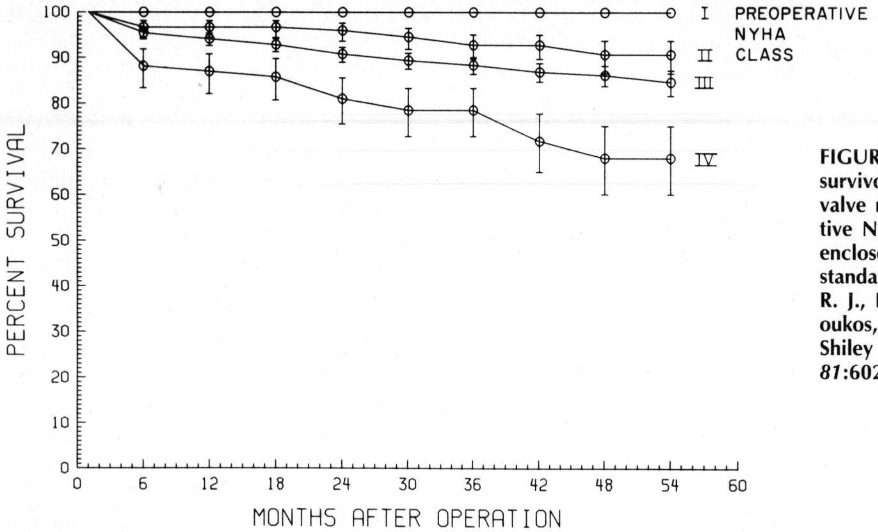

FIGURE 51–7. Actuarial survival of hospital survivors after aortic, mitral, or aortic and mitral valve replacement, according to the preoperative NYHA Functional Class. The vertical bars enclose the 70 per cent confidence limits (1 standard deviation). (From Karp, R. B., Cyrus, R. J., Blackstone, E. H., Kirklin, J. W., Kouchoukos, N. T., and Pacifico, A. D.: The Björk-Shiley valve. J. Thorac. Cardiovasc. Surg. *81*:602, 1981.)

operation and managing the patient in the early postoperative period.

THE BRAIN. Patients who have recovered from a hemiplegic episode prior to their cardiac surgery may have a temporary reappearance of the hemiplegic signs and symptoms immediately after cardiac surgery using cardiopulmonary bypass. This does not necessarily indicate that a new neurological injury has occurred, and recovery from this temporary relapse is usually rapid.

Because of the largely nonpulsatile nature of perfusion during cardiopulmonary bypass, patients with significant carotid artery stenosis may be at increased risk for ischemic neurological injury during and after operation. Thus, signs and symptoms of cerebrovascular insufficiency should be sought in adult patients with generalized atherosclerosis so that proper preoperative evaluation and intraoperative management may be employed to minimize the risk of neurological injury.

FUNCTIONAL STATE AND AGE

Advanced preoperative symptoms usually imply the presence of a secondary cardiomyopathy and impaired ventricular systolic and diastolic functions. Thus their presence affects both early and late results. As examples of the effect on early results, in infants the hospital mortality is directly related to the preoperative symptomatic state,[43] and the preoperative symptomatic state of the patient undergoing valve replacement operations (isolated or combined with other cardiac procedures) affects the probability of both early and late postoperative survival[1] (Fig. 51–7).

Both very young and very old age have been incremental risk factors for death in the earlier eras of cardiac surgery. In recent years, however, a number of studies have shown that the incremental risk of even very young age can be neutralized by proper techniques.[18, 44–46] The incremental risks of very old age have not been neutralized, but they are not sufficiently great that needed cardiac operations should be avoided in elderly patients.

INTRAOPERATIVE CONDITIONS AFFECTING RESULTS

CARDIOPULMONARY BYPASS (CPB)

CPB can be considered a safe support system for clinical cardiac surgery, judging from the fact that the hospital mortality for coronary artery bypass grafting (CABG) in recent years approaches zero. However, there are important damaging effects of CPB that contribute to in-hospital morbidity and mortality, and these must be considered in early postoperative management.

The manifestations of the damaging effects of CPB include an abnormal tendency to bleed externally and into tissues; a diffuse or whole-body "inflammatory reaction" characterized by increased capillary permeability with consequent transcapillary plasma loss, increased interstitial fluid, leukocytosis, and fever; renal dysfunction; peripheral and perhaps central vasoconstriction, which persists a variable time after CPB and results in both hemodynamic and metabolic problems; breakdown of red blood cells, resulting in hemoglobinemia, hemoglobinuria, and anemia; and perhaps increased susceptibility to infection. These all contribute to organ and subsystem dysfunction early postoperatively, a state that some investigators call "postperfusion syndrome" or "postpump syndrome." The fact that most patients convalesce normally after CPB attests only to patients' ability to compensate for these damaging effects and not to their absence. The uncommon occurrence of severe pulmonary edema without elevated left atrial pressure (p. 549), severe bleeding diatheses, and transient subtle neurological changes occasionally brings these abnormalities of CPB forcefully to attention. Much of the current residual morbidity and mortality from open heart operations are secondary to the changes produced by CPB.

The possible mechanisms for the damaging effects are the exposure of blood to an abnormal environment and altered arterial blood flow patterns. The first of these, the exposure of blood to nonendothelial surfaces, has a particularly powerful and generalized influence on the organism. This exposure has direct and indirect effects on platelets, which result in platelet clumping and embolization, a reduction in the number of platelets, a reduction in their important adhesive and aggregating properties, and a number of secondary effects.[47] Proteins are damaged by blood exposure to nonphysiological surfaces. Some degree of protein denaturation occurs, and the lipoproteins liberate free fat in the process. Fat microemboli result. Damage to proteins that are part of the humoral amplification systems has particularly complex and widespread effects. Probably an initiating event in this process is the activating of Hageman factor (Factor XII) and consequently of the cascade of the coagulation humoral amplification system, which consumes the coagulation factors to a varying degree.[47, 48] Also activated to a varying degree are the fibrinolytic system,[49] the complement system, and the kallikrein-bradykinin system.[50]

The adverse effects of activation of the complement

system may be particularly important.[51–54] This activation results in the formation of a complex of glycoproteins (C5 to C9) that aid in membrane lysis and phagocytosis. It results also in the production of powerful anaphylatoxins (among them C3a and C5a), which increase vascular permeability, cause smooth muscle contraction, mediate leukocyte chemotaxis, and facilitate leukocyte aggregation and enzyme release.[55, 56] The usefulness of these reactions as a response to localized injury is obvious, but their production in a whole-body inflammatory reaction (referred to above) may be severely detrimental. As a part of this, the anaphylatoxins stimulate polymorphonuclear aggregation, which with shear stress damage (also occurring during CPB) results in the pulmonary sequestration of leukocytes.[57, 58] This sequestration and the pulmonary endothelial injury from activated platelets probably in large measure account for the variable degree of pulmonary dysfunction seen in most patients after CPB.

Shear stresses are generated during CPB by blood pumps, suction systems, abrupt acceleration and deceleration of blood, and cavitation around the end of the arterial cannula. Shear stresses damage leukocytes[57] already subjected to other injurious effects, and also damage erythrocytes.[59] Damage to erythrocytes results in hemolysis and elevation of serum hemoglobin levels.

Part of the abnormal environment of blood is its encounter with other substances (air bubbles, bits of fibrin and tissue debris, platelet aggregates, and defoaming agents), which are incorporated into blood and may form microemboli. Thus, some degree of microembolization occurs during each operation with CPB, and this is generally greatest during the first 10 or 15 minutes of the perfusion.

Arterial blood flow patterns during CPB are variable. Most CPB for cardiac surgery is conducted with roller pumps; the arterial blood flow is nearly linear (nonpulsatile), and the arterial pressure pulse is very small. This is an alteration from the normal state, in which the arterial pulse pressure is about one-third the systolic blood pressure. However, it remains controversial whether pulsatile flow, which can be used during CPB, results in fewer functional derangements than does nonpulsatile flow.

There are some incremental risk factors that increase the probability of important clinical manifestations resulting from CPB.[54] One is the duration of CPB. In adults the probability of demonstrable structural or functional damage increases as the perfusion extends beyond about 150 minutes. Another is the age of the patient. The probability of damage appears to increase in patients under 6 months of age and even more so in those under 3 months. The probability of damage may also be greater in the very elderly. These two risk factors, duration of CPB and age, probably interact, so that in young infants the probability of demonstrable damage from more than 90 to 120 minutes of CPB seems to be as great as from over 150 minutes of CPB in adults. The cardiac defect being treated may also be influential, and preoperatively cyanotic patients seem more susceptible to the damaging effects of CPB. Other factors that may affect the probability of a demonstrable damaging effect include the perfusion flow rate, the composition of the perfusate, the oxygenating surface, and the temperature of the patient during the perfusion.

PROFOUND HYPOTHERMIA AND TOTAL CIRCULATORY ARREST

An alternative method to continuous CPB for cardiac surgery is the use of profound hypothermia and a continuous period of total circulatory arrest during the repair. The method is used routinely for infant cardiac surgery by some surgeons and by most surgeons for a few special situations at any age. This technique provides optimal surgical exposure in a field uncluttered by cannulae, which accounts for its use by many in infant cardiac surgery. In this method, the patient's body temperature is reduced to about 20°C by a sequential combination of surface cooling and then further "core cooling" by a cold perfusate during CPB[60] or by "core cooling" only. Total circulatory arrest times of 30 to 75 minutes have been used.

The hypothesis underlying the use of this method is that there is a "safe" duration of total circulatory arrest (i.e., one characterized by absence of functional or structural derangements in the early or late postoperative period) and that the "safe" duration is inversely related to body temperature during the arrest period. It is further hypothesized that hypothermia, without itself producing damage, reduces metabolic activity to the extent that the available small energy stores in the various organs maintain cell viability throughout the ischemic period of total circulatory arrest and thus allow normal structure and function to return during reperfusion. The brain is the organ most rapidly damaged by total circulatory arrest, and its "safe total circulatory arrest time" is considered the factor limiting the time of the arrest period.

Experimental data indicate that 30 minutes of total circulatory arrest at 20°C are in fact "safe."[61] Clinical experiences support this idea. However, there is uncertainty regarding the safety of longer periods of circulatory arrest. Seizures or choreoathetoid movements or both, usually but not always transient, develop in up to 10 per cent of patients subjected to longer periods of arrest. Other important evidences of brain damage, including impaired intellectual development, develop in an increasingly larger proportion of the patients as the length of total circulatory arrest is extended beyond 30 minutes and particularly when it is extended beyond 45 minutes.[62]

For these reasons, we use total circulatory arrest very infrequently in cardiac surgery, even in infants. In part this is because of concerns about the damaging effects of total circulatory arrest and in part because of the greatly improved exposure during CPB obtained by current methods of cannulation.

MYOCARDIAL PROTECTION

In the early years of cardiac surgery, little was made of the possibility that low cardiac output in the early postoperative period was related to the perioperative development of myocardial necrosis (or infarction). Then Taber and colleagues described scattered areas of myocardial necrosis estimated to involve about 30 per cent of the left ventricular myocardium in patients dying early after cardiac operations, and implicated this as the etiology of the patients' low cardiac output and death.[63] Najafi and colleagues showed that acute diffuse subendocardial myocardial infarction was a frequent finding in patients dying early after valve replacement operations and suggested that this was related to methods of intraoperative management of the myocardium.[64] When coronary artery bypass grafting began in the early 1970's, cardiologists and cardiac surgeons noted that a disturbingly high proportion of patients developed perioperatively a transmural myocardial infarct. Soon it was shown that the development of transmural myocardial infarction was not limited to patients undergoing coronary artery bypass grafting but was a complication of cardiac surgery in general.[65, 66] The rarely occurring extreme form of ischemic and/or reperfusion damage, "stone heart," was recognized at about that time.

Currently, during most cardiac operations the aorta is

clamped during at least part of the repair. This stops coronary blood flow, since the arterial input from the pump-oxygenator flows into the aorta distal to the cross-clamping. Aortic cross-clamping improves surgical exposure by stopping the coronary flow, by preventing any leakage back into the heart through the aortic valve, and by lessening and eventually stopping cardiac action. Aortic cross-clamping has the disadvantage, however, of producing immediate and global myocardial ischemia, which may lead to myocardial edema and myocardial cell damage.

Myocardial edema results in part from the same factors that increase interstitial fluid throughout the body during CPB (see earlier section). Ischemia also results in both intra- and extracellular myocardial edema. The intracellular edema is from depletion of energy stores and impairment of active membrane transport of ions and from intracellular production of new osmotically active molecules by ischemic metabolic conversion of osmotically less active larger molecules.[67] Myocardial edema, when sufficiently severe, reduces ventricular diastolic function by lessening compliance (distensibility). Ventricular diastolic function is further reduced by alterations in the intrinsic mechanical properties of the myocardium after global ischemia.[68] These changes preclude the development of a preload appropriate to the ventricular end-diastolic pressure and thereby reduce cardiac output.

Myocardial cell damage is the most important result of global myocardial ischemia, no matter what the method of myocardial protection. The amount of myocardial necrosis is a determinant of the patient's early postoperative condition and probability of survival, no doubt because of its effect on cardiac output in the early postoperative period (Fig. 51–8).

During global myocardial ischemia, the extent and severity of the alteration of myocytes depends at least upon the length of the period of cross-clamping, the temperature of the myocardium, the rapidity with which asystole develops, and the preischemic condition of the myocardium. Under particularly unfavorable circumstances, some myocytes may die during the ischemic period. Most are only damaged, however, and their ultimate survival or death depends on the specific conditions of the reperfusion as well as the extent of ischemic damage. When the ischemic damage has been marked, and the reperfusion is performed without special precautions, extensive myocardial cell death results from the reperfusion. If the conditions during reperfusion can be optimized, minimal cell death may result unless the ischemic damage has been particularly severe and prolonged. Only recently has the importance of this aspect of myocardial protection during cardiac surgery been realized, although an experimental study by Danforth and colleagues in 1960 described the favorable effect of one method of optimizing reperfusion.[69] Buckberg and colleagues have subsequently studied further the optimization of reperfusion,[70–72] and their clinical experience has been supportive of the idea that an optimized reperfusion helps to minimize myocardial damage.[73] Clearly, the events during global myocardial ischemia and reperfusion are analogous to those occurring regionally as acute myocardial infarction develops.

A number of methods for myocardial protection during cardiac surgery have been used. However, in recent years most surgeons have turned to the technique of myocardial protection with cold and cardioplegia, which greatly extends the "safe" time of global myocardial ischemia. This method takes advantage of the protective effect of cold and of sudden cessation of electromechanical activity. The data from human beings suggest that with this method no significant myocardial necrosis or permanent functional damage results from total myocardial ischemia for up to 120 minutes, if the preoperative myocardial reserves are good (i.e., NYHA Functional Class I or II). However, ventricular hypertrophy and decreased myocardial reserves (presumably present in patients preoperatively in NYHA Functional Classes III and IV) appear to shorten the safe time limits of cold cardioplegia.[1]

The cardioplegic agent most commonly used at present is potassium, in concentrations of 15 to 35 $mEq \cdot l^{-1}$. Potassium in this concentration blocks the initial "fast" (inward sodium current) phase of myocardial cellular depolarization. Even with this concentration of potassium, electromechanical activity can persist or return in the presence of agents such as catecholamines, which activate the "slow" (inward calcium and sodium current) phase of myocardial cellular depolarization on which potassium has no effect, and activate it when noncoronary collateral flow is large. Proper methodology overcomes these potential

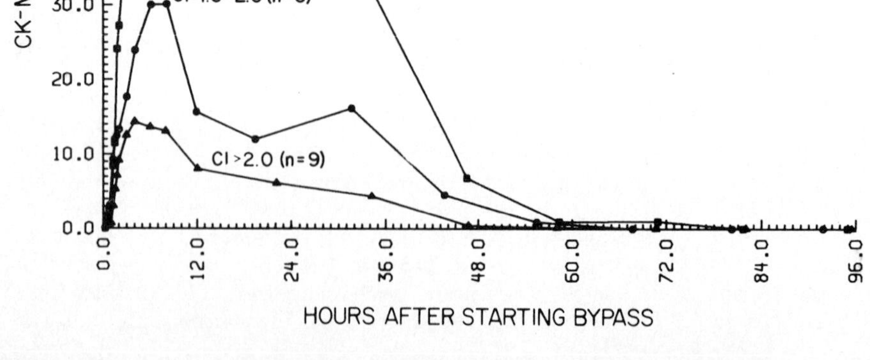

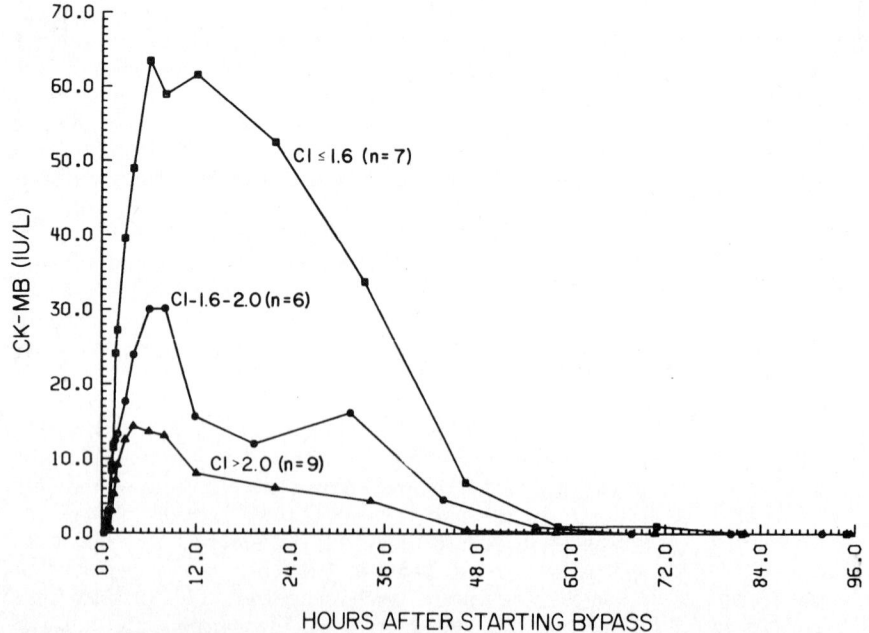

FIGURE 51–8. The relation of extent of perioperative myocardial necrosis (reflected in the blood CK-MB isoenzyme values along the vertical axis) and the early postoperative cardiac index (C1 in liters · min^{-1} · $meter^{-2}$) in 22 consecutive patients undergoing mitral valve replacement at UAB in 1975, using simple cold ischemic arrest. Geometric mean values are portrayed. Note the very high levels of CK-MB in patients with low cardiac output (1.6 or less) and the low levels in patients with large cardiac output (more than 2.0). The overall correlation of CK-MB (duration, peak, and integrated area) and cardiac index is r = −0.4 and p = 0.04. (From Kirklin, J. W., and Barratt-Boyes, B. G.: Textbook of Cardiac Surgery. New York, John Wiley and Sons, 1986, p. 87.)

problems. The cardioplegic vehicle is either asanguineous (some type of buffered electrolyte solution usually containing mannitol) or sanguineous (usually of blood from the pump-oxygenator). The cardioplegic solution is delivered into the aortic root, or directly into the coronary ostia, at a temperature of about 4°C. Infusions are repeated every 20 to 30 minutes during the ischemic period.

In spite of the experimental evidence of the advantages of an optimized reperfusion, most surgical groups currently simply release the aortic cross-clamp and allow the general body perfusion from the pump-oxygenator to reperfuse the heart. Currently it is the authors' recommendation that, when cold cardioplegia is used and the global ischemic time exceeds 30 minutes (15 minutes if ventricular hypertrophy is severe or preoperative myocardial reserves are believed to be depleted), a warm (35° to 37°C), hyperkalemic (25 to 30 mEq K^+ per liter), sanguineous solution (made simply with pump-oxygenator blood to which has been added 25 mEq K^+ as KC1 per liter) be infused into the aortic root at a pressure of 50 to 60 mm Hg for 5 minutes before the aortic cross-clamp is released. During this infusion and for about 8 to 10 minutes after the aortic cross-clamp is released, ventricular diastole persists, and then cardiac action usually begins, although atrioventricular pacing may be required for a time.

OTHER CONDITIONS AFFECTING SURGICAL RESULTS

COMPLETENESS OF REPAIR. It is sometimes forgotten that a poor hemodynamic state early in the postoperative period may be related, in part at least, to an incomplete surgical procedure (such as replacement of only one valve when two are significantly abnormal in function, very incomplete myocardial revascularization, incomplete repair of a large ventricular septal defect, the leaving of important right ventricular outflow tract obstruction in the repair of tetralogy of Fallot, and so forth). This emphasizes the need for complete knowledge of the preoperative cardiac conditions, a wise assessment of the surgical procedures needed to correct them, and a skillful and determined surgical effort to carry out a completely corrective procedure.

When in the early postoperative period the hemodynamic state is unsatisfactory, the adequacy and completeness of the surgical procedure should be assessed by whatever means are necessary. The risk of immediate reoperation and correction of any residual anatomical problem is usually less than that of treating the secondary effect of a poor hemodynamic state.

DATE OF OPERATION. Both the early and late results of cardiac operations have improved since the early days of cardiac surgery in most institutions (Fig. 51–9). Once results have become excellent in a properly organized institution, they generally stay excellent even though new personnel are gradually introduced into the system. This fact emphasizes the importance of a proper *system* for cardiac surgery and proper protocols.

This effect of date of operation upon results makes comparisons between nonconcurrent clinical experiences potentially imprecise. This is one reason that randomized trials are the ideal method for making comparisons. Appropriate statistical methods which take into account the date of operation do, however, allow useful comparisons between nonrandomized clinical experiences.

THE INSTITUTION. There are true institutional (and surgeon-to-surgeon) differences in the early and late results of cardiac surgery. These are related to variations in knowledge, technique, and experience. Since these differences are generally identified by comparisons between two or more prospective but not necessarily concurrent clinical studies involving a more or less heterogeneous population, the comparisons must be made with great care and full knowledge of the multivariate nature of the determinants of these results. For example, a preliminary comparison of the results of coronary artery bypass grafting in hospital A and in hospital B may indicate that the hospital mortality is the same in the two institutions. The conclusion might be drawn that the quality of work in the two hospitals is similar. However, analysis of the two patient populations may show a much higher proportion of patients with moderately or severely depressed left ventricular function in hospital B. Since depressed ventricular function is an incremental risk factor for hospital death, the conclusion would be that the quality of the work in hospital B was in fact superior to that in hospital A.

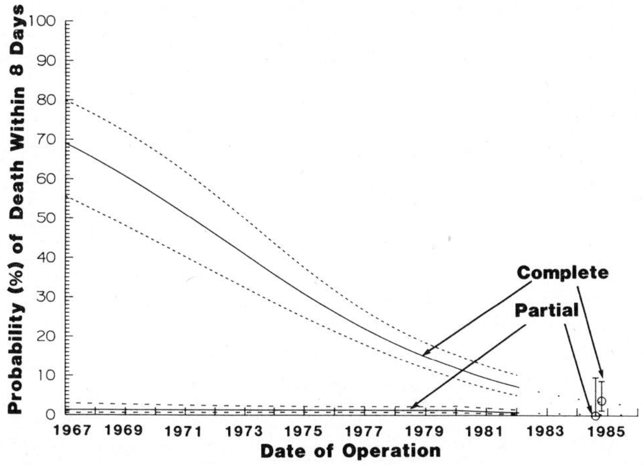

FIGURE 51–9. Nomogram of the solution of a multivariate equation describing the incremental risk factors for the repair of atrioventricular canal defects (UAB; 1967 to 1982; n = 310). The probability of death perioperatively (within the first 8 days) is on the horizontal axis and the date of operation is on the vertical axis. The dashed lines enclose the 70 per cent confidence intervals. The actual percentages of perioperative mortality (hospital deaths; UAB; January 1984 to September 1985; n = 59; 1 death) are shown to the right, on the probability line predicted by the multivariate equation based on the earlier experience; the vertical bars denote the 70 per cent confidence intervals. (From Kirklin, J. K., Blackstone, E. H., and Kirklin, J. W.: The repair of AV canal defects in infancy. Int. J. Cardiol. [*In press*].)

POSTOPERATIVE SUBSYSTEM CARE

The primary determinants of the success of a cardiac operation are events in the operating room. However, every cardiac surgical patient requires postoperative care. Unfortunately, all invasive monitoring and some that is noninvasive (for example, the recording of an electrocardiogram without proper grounding), as well as all interventions, involve risks of varying magnitude to the patient. They should, therefore, be used only when the probability of postoperative problems is greater than their inherent risks.

After cardiac operations, the combination of the basic cardiac disease, the whole-body response to cardiopulmonary bypass (CPB), the effects of the myocardial ischemic period, and the cardiac trauma of the operation create special problems. Many conceptual, scientific, and management errors are made by failing to realize that for a time after CPB and a period of global myocardial ischemia, patients are in a special biological situation to which the knowledge and rules derived for other patients may or may not apply. Fortunately, in spite of this, in many cardiac operations the risk approaches zero. Postoperative care can usually be quite simple after CPB. Yet certain situations still have an appreciable probability of hospital death or morbidity, and in them more extensive monitoring and interventions are needed.

The patient may be considered as a complex integrated system composed of a number of separate but interrelated subsystems (i.e., cardiovascular, pulmonary, renal, nervous, and alimentary). The care of such a patient can be accomplished effectively by utilizing a "subsystems analysis" approach. This commences in the operating room as CPB is being discontinued and continues into the early and late postoperative period.

An uncomplicated or normal convalescence is one devoid of any findings or events that increase the probability of hospital death or of important complications or of a suboptimal late result. As long as this pattern of normal convalescence continues, monitoring, testing, and interventions can safely be minimized. Alertness to deviations from the pattern of an uncomplicated convalescence is required, as these are an indication for greater intensity of observation and treatment.

CARDIOVASCULAR SUBSYSTEM

Convalescence can be considered normal with regard to the cardiovascular subsystem when the cardiac output is adequate for the metabolic needs of the organism. The output can be evaluated either by measuring it or by assessing its adequacy, or by both. Cardiac output may be measured by indocyanine green indicator dilution techniques, by thermodilution, or by other methods. The indocyanine green technique has the advantage that residual intracardiac shunts can be detected by the contour of the indicator dilution curve or by double-sampling techniques. The adequacy of cardiac output is assessed by evaluation of the pedal pulses and skin temperature, urine flow, and mixed venous oxygen levels, and these methods are generally highly reliable. Arterial blood pressure is ordinarily an insensitive guide to cardiac performance early in the postoperative period, chiefly because the systemic vascular resistance is often unusually high. However, arterial hypotension is always an indication for intense evaluation, and the patient cannot be considered to be convalescing normally when mean arterial blood pressure is less than 10 per cent below normal for age.

The treatment of inadequate cardiac output, once the possibility of cardiac tamponade is eliminated, is directed at increasing the output by manipulation of preload, afterload, the contractile state, and heart rate and at improving tissue oxygen levels by other means.[74] When cardiac output is low, preload is made as large as is possible by increasing blood volume until the higher of the two atrial pressures is approximately 15 mm Hg.[75] If the wall thickness of the left ventricle is unusually great, or its contractility or compliance or both are decreased, it may be helpful to take mean left atrial pressure to 20 mm Hg. When the right ventricle is the limiting one, right atrial pressure usually can advantageously be taken only to approximately 18 mm Hg. Above these levels, a fall in cardiac output often occurs.

Afterload reduction (p. 516) can often be used to improve cardiac performance early after cardiac surgery. When the left ventricular performance is the limiting one, and systemic arterial blood pressure is more than approximately 10 per cent above normal, afterload should be reduced by lowering arterial blood pressure to between normal and 10 per cent above normal, generally with intravenous nitroprusside. However, too-intensive vasodilator therapy results in coronary hypoperfusion and reduced cardiac output.[76] Rarely, in patients with severe longstanding mitral valve disease or congenital heart disease with pulmonary vascular obstructive changes, right ventricular dysfunction associated with elevated pulmonary artery pressure may limit cardiac performance, and reduction of right ventricular afterload with vasodilator agents can be attempted.

Heart rate is optimized as necessary. For patients in sinus or junctional rhythm, atrial pacing is used; if atrial fibrillation is present, ventricular pacing is used; and if AV dissociation is the rhythm, AV sequential pacing is used. If tachyarrhythmias are present, control is usually obtained by pharmacological means or by special pacing methods.[77]

If these relatively simple measures do not bring cardiac output to an adequate level, administration of catecholamines or intraaortic balloon pumping (IABP) is used. The former is chosen in infants and children, in adults without major myocardial necrosis and with only mild or moderate impairments, and in those with a contraindication to IABP. If catecholamines are indicated, dopamine (p. 524) is begun at low doses, which can be increased up to 15 $\mu g \cdot kg^{-1} \cdot min^{-1}$ if needed. When dopamine is not effective, dobutamine (p. 525) is added, using similar dosages. Epinephrine, isoproterenol, and norepinephrine are now rarely used. However, in the presence of predominantly right ventricular dysfunction and decreased or normal heart rate, isoproterenol may be the preferred drug because of its favorable effect on pulmonary vascular resistance. When catecholamines are administered and a satisfactory response obtained, 8 to 12 hours later an aggressive and persistent effort is begun gradually to reduce and finally discontinue them.

In adults, intraaortic balloon pumping (IAPB) (p. 573) is considered if adjustment of preload, afterload, and heart rate and modest doses (2.5 to 5 $\mu g \cdot kg^{-1} \cdot min^{-1}$) of dopamine do not result in adequate cardiac performance. If a strong suspicion of myocardial necrosis exists or if ventricular electrical instability is present, IABP is preferable to catecholamines as initial treatment. Intraaortic balloon pumping is a powerful treatment modality when indicated, because of its pulsatile augmentation of myocardial perfusion and reduction in left ventricular afterload.[78] When needed, the balloon pump is usually inserted in the operating room before or shortly after discontinuing cardiopulmonary bypass, using the percutaneous technique.[79] In a few institutions, temporary left ventricular assist devices have been used for extreme examples of acute left ventricular failure after cardiac surgery.[80, 81] While their use is controversial, at least some patients have survived to have a good long-term result with the use of these assist devices. Acute perioperative right ventricular failure has been managed in a few institutions by pulmonary artery balloon counterpulsation.[82] Also, temporary right ventricular assist devices have been used successfully in a very few patients.[83] Only the intraaortic balloon, however, can currently be considered a clearly useful device.

While efforts are being made to increase cardiac output, the tissue and mixed venous oxygen levels should also be raised by attention to the other variables represented in the Fick equation. The blood hemoglobin should be kept above 10 to 12 $gm \cdot dl^{-1}$ by administration of packed red blood cells or whole blood, and the PaO_2 maintained at 100 to 200 mm Hg by increasing the fractional concentration of oxygen in the inspired air. Unduly high oxygen consumption ($\dot{V}O_2$) is prevented while the patient is on a ventilator by use of sedation or paralyzing drugs, which prevent restlessness or agitation. Hyperthermia (rectal or central temperature $\geq$ 39.7°C, or 103.5°F) should be treated vigorously.

Postoperative morbidity and mortality can result from cardiac arrhythmias. These may occur when the cardiac subsystem has been otherwise functioning normally or as a complication of low cardiac output. They may be the manifestation of a severe secondary cardiomyopathy. Atrial and ventricular pacing wires, routinely placed at operation and left for 5 to 10 postoperative days, are of utmost importance in diagnosis and treatment of postoperative arrhythmias.[77]

Ventricular electrical instability, which includes premature ventricular contractions (PVC's) and ventricular tachycardia, is a potentially dangerous arrhythmia. Although controversy exists concerning the proportion of patients with PVC's who develop ventricular fibrillation, it may be that this potential exists in any patient who has significant intermittent or continuous ventricular electrical instability. Therefore, the electrocardiogram is monitored continuously for at least 48 hours in all patients, and ventricular electrical instability is treated vigorously by the methods generally used in other settings (Chap. 21).

Various atrial arrhythmias may complicate the postoperative period. Atrial fibrillation (p. 672) is treated initially with digitalis. If it persists until the seventh postoperative day in patients who have not been in atrial fibrillation preoperatively, cardioversion should usually be carried out. Atrial flutter (p. 671), formerly a difficult arrhythmia to manage postoperatively, is now usually converted to sinus rhythm by rapid atrial pacing (via the two implanted atrial wires) at the so-called critical pacing rate with sudden cessation of pacing after about 20 seconds. Digoxin is begun and continued for 6 weeks. Procainamide is begun and continued for 8 weeks, with a switch to quinidine if long-term drug therapy is indicated. Premature atrial contractions (PAC's) (p. 669) may trigger or lead to atrial fibrillation; therefore, an attempt is made to suppress them with atrial pacing, digoxin, procainamide, or quinidine. Paroxysmal supraventricular tachycardia (PSVT) is usually first treated by rapid atrial pacing and then sudden cessation. If this is unsuccessful, intravenous propranolol, verapamil, or digoxin is usually successful. If PSVT is recurrent or refractory to treatment, continuous rapid atrial pacing at approximately 100 beats faster than the intrinsic atrial rate is employed to produce and sustain a 2:1 block.[84] Patients who have had PSVT generally should receive digoxin for about 6 weeks.

When the onset of a supraventricular tachyarrhythmia is accompanied by significant hemodynamic deterioration, prompt cardioversion (p. 642) is indicated if atrial wires are not in place.

RENAL SUBSYSTEM

Convalescence after cardiac surgery can be considered uncomplicated when urine volume is "adequate." Useful but somewhat arbitrary criteria are that it be greater than 500 ml · 24 hours^{-1} · meter^{-2} or 167 ml · 8 hours^{-1} · meter^{-2} or 20 ml · hr^{-1} · meter^{-2}. Solute excretion must also be "adequate," and the convalescence is abnormal when solute excretion is insufficient to keep serum potassium levels below 5 mEq · liter^{-1}, blood urea nitrogen (BUN) levels below 40 mg · dl^{-1}, and creatinine levels below 1.5 mg · dl^{-1}. Convalescence cannot be considered normal when the urine is pink but without red blood cells early in the postoperative period, for this indicates an inordinate and potentially dangerous amount of hemolysis (free plasma hemoglobin levels > 40 mg · dl^{-1}).

As a guide to the continuing evaluation of the renal subsystem, a urinary catheter is inserted in the operating room preoperatively and left for 24 to 48 hours to monitor urine flow. Serum potassium is measured every 4 hours during the first 24 postoperative hours, and if convalescence is not normal, every 8 hours for at least the next 48 hours. Serum creatinine and BUN are measured each morning for at least the first 48 hours.

Acute renal failure after cardiac surgery is rare in adults, occurring in fewer than 0.1 per cent of patients undergoing operations such as coronary artery bypass grafting but may occur in 1 to 5 per cent of infants undergoing open intracardiac operations.[85] Although it is usually associated with low cardiac output initially, it may occur uncommonly when the other criteria of cardiac subsystem performance are satisfactory.

The probability of acute renal failure after surgery with CPB is also influenced by certain risk factors other than low cardiac output:

Young age: One reason for the apparently increased incidence in infants, noted above, is the higher proportion in this age group of seriously ill patients with low cardiac output early in the postoperative period. The immaturity of the kidney in infants and young children, resulting in less ability to concentrate the urine, may also predispose them to acute renal failure. Infants may develop more tissue hypoxia during and early after CPB than do older patients, with a resultant increased production of potassium, urea nitrogen, and other substances, some of which may be nephrotoxic.

Cyanotic heart disease: Acute renal failure is more likely to occur after operations for cyanotic heart disease.[42] A renal lesion is known to exist in many such patients preoperatively.

Preoperative impairment of renal function: This increases considerably the risk of acute renal failure in the postoperative period.[86] Therefore, a part of the preoperative evaluation should be the determination of renal function.

A long period of CPB (> 180 minutes in adults, less than this in infants and small children) probably increases the risk of acute renal failure.

Profound hypothermia and total circulatory arrest: The additional risk imposed by this is not known, nor is that of long periods of reduced flow during hypothermic CPB. However, flows 1.6 liter · min^{-1} · m^{-2} or more at 25°C and mean arterial blood pressure 30 mm Hg or more during CPB at moderate hypothermia seem adequate to minimize acute renal failure.[41]

High plasma hemoglobin level (> 40 mg · dl^{-1}) during and early after CPB probably increases the risk of acute renal failure.

Whole blood prime may be an incremental risk.

Aminoglycosides and some other antibiotics may increase the risk of acute renal failure after CPB.

Acute renal failure may develop within 12 to 48 hours after operation. Its first effect is resistant oliguria of increasing severity, resulting in very rapidly rising serum potassium levels (probably because of the acute loss of potassium from hemolyzing red blood cells and from the whole-body loss of intracellular potassium that characterizes the perioperative period in patients who have been on CPB) and more slowly rising BUN and creatinine levels. Although this form of acute renal failure is rarely the primary cause of death, it greatly complicates recovery unless effective interventions are promptly made, and is the type usually seen in infants. A less lethal form becomes apparent on the third or fourth postoperative day, and is the type usually seen in adults. This manifests itself by a progressive rise in BUN and creatinine levels, which peak at 80 to 120 and 5 to 8 mg · dl^{-1}, respectively, about 7 to 10 days postoperatively. There is often little or no oliguria, and hyperkalemia greater than 5 mEq · liter^{-1} does not usually develop. Spontaneous resolution usually follows, and as long as the patient's clinical condition is satisfactory, urine flow is adequate, and BUN and creatinine levels eventually begin to fall, dialysis is not indicated.

When oliguria occurs early postoperatively, cardiac preload performance should be optimized (see above). Intravenous furosemide ($1\ mg \cdot kg^{-1}$) is sometimes administered. If a good response is obtained, this is repeated every 6 hours for 3 days. If a response to furosemide is not obtained, the dose is doubled and then quadrupled, and then $8\ mg \cdot kg^{-1}$ is given. When the serum potassium level rises above $5.5\ mEq \cdot l^{-1}$, glucose-insulin solution is given intravenously and sodium polystyrene sulfonate (Kayexalate) enemas are used.

Unless oliguria and hyperkalemia respond to treatment within a few hours, dialysis should be carried out, especially in infants. Usually, peritoneal dialysis is used early postoperatively, particularly in infants.[86, 87] In older patients hemodialysis may be substituted for peritoneal dialysis after a few days if acute renal failure persists. With these measures many patients can be maintained in good condition until cardiac and renal functions improve and ultimately are recovered fully.

PULMONARY SUBSYSTEM

Patients are extubated after cardiac surgery as soon as the effects of the anesthetic agents have disappeared when normal convalescence is likely. In patients undergoing closed operations, including infants, this usually means extubation in the operating room. After open operations of an uncomplicated nature, such as repair of simple congenital lesions, coronary artery bypass grafting, or isolated valve replacement or valvotomy, patients (including infants) are usually extubated within 4 to 8 hours postoperatively. Following complex open operations, ventilation is usually continued at least overnight, and the patient is not extubated until the appropriate criteria are met.

While intubated, the patient is ventilated with a volume-controlled respirator that provides intermittent positive pressure breathing (IPPB). It should be equipped with valves that allow patients to breathe themselves, when they will, in between the intermittent mandatory ventilation (IMV) from the ventilator. The IMV is reduced gradually as soon as spontaneous breathing is sufficient, to accustom the patient to breathing again and to gain the hemodynamic advantages of the negative intrapleural pressures that develop during spontaneous inspiration. Positive end-expiratory pressure (PEEP) should be used in most patients, because of the studies that suggest larger lung volumes and fewer perfused but nonventilated alveoli during ventilation and smaller alveolar-arterial oxygen differences $P(A\text{-}a)O_2$ after extubation when it is used.[88] PEEP is not used in patients with chronic obstructive lung disease (for fear of air-trapping and rupturing a bulla with consequent pneumothorax), in infants who have undergone interatrial transposition of venous return, and in those undergoing Fontan's operation or a superior vena caval–right atrial anastomosis (to avoid still further elevation of jugular venous pressure). While the patient is intubated and ventilated, the inspired gases are warmed and humidified. Appropriate aspiration of the trachea, turning of the patient, and chest physiotherapy are carried out. After extubation, which should be done as soon as possible, reintubation is usually not necessary when the patient truly meets the criteria for extubation. However, when the work of breathing is excessive, when CO_2 retention is enough to produce significant respiratory acidosis, or when the patient is becoming exhausted by ventilatory efforts, reintubation is indicated. When the situation is borderline, careful observation by senior members of the team is required for proper decision-making.

OTHER SUBSYSTEMS

Abnormalities of the other subsystems are infrequent during convalescence from cardiac surgery using a pump-oxygenator. Therefore, their management is relatively straightforward.

ELECTROLYTE AND ACID-BASE DISTURBANCE. Because of the increase in extracellular fluid and total exchangeable sodium and the decrease in exchangeable potassium that develop during CPB, early postoperative fluid administration must be precise. For approximately 48 hours after operation, no sodium is administered, and $500\ ml \cdot 24\ hours^{-1} \cdot meter^{-2}$ of water (as 5 per cent glucose in water) are given intravenously.[89]

Some *metabolic acidosis* (base deficit $> 2\ mEq \cdot l^{-1}$) may be present during the early hours after intracardiac surgery, even when the patient is convalescing normally. It is left untreated if the arterial pH is 7.4 or greater and $PaCO_2$ is 30 mm Hg or more. If in this circumstance $PaCO_2$ is less than 30 mm Hg, the base deficit is treated before adjusting the $PaCO_2$ appropriately upward. When pH is less than about 7.35, the base deficit is treated. However, if convalescence is otherwise normal, treatment is delayed for 4 to 8 hours in adults and 2 to 4 hours in infants, by which time the acidosis may have cleared spontaneously. In infants particularly, it is best to avoid this additional sodium load whenever possible.

A mild *metabolic alkalosis* may be present 24 hours after operation in normally convalescing patients, probably related, in part at least, to the sodium load contained in the anticoagulant solution of the banked blood. It is self-correcting under these circumstances and is not treated.

TEMPERATURE ELEVATION. Body temperature may become severely elevated in the first 48 postoperative hours, particularly in infants, as discussed earlier. It is usually a manifestation of a profound reaction to cardiopulmonary bypass, although infection, reaction to homologous blood, or brain stem damage are other possible etiological factors. Its identification and vigorous treatment are important, because the prognosis for patients with it is otherwise poor. Whenever the usually monitored rectal temperature becomes abnormally high during the first 48 postoperative hours ($\geq$ 39.5°C, or 103°F), an esophageal thermistor should be introduced because the central ("core") temperature may be even higher than the rectal temperature under these circumstances. When the central temperature exceeds 39.7°C or 103.5°F, vigorous antipyretic measures are initiated.

Patients who are convalescing normally after cardiopulmonary bypass frequently have persistent temperature elevations ($\geq$ 38.8°C or 102°F) for 7 to 10 days after operation in the absence of infection. This finding appears to be a direct response to the effects of bypass and is a self-limiting process that does not require special therapy. Affected patients should be examined for signs of infection, but in the absence of its clinical evidence, extensive laboratory investigation is usually not warranted.

HEMORRHAGE. A bleeding tendency of some degree develops in all patients who have been on CPB, as most of the clotting factors are abnormal for a time. In spite of this, good hemostasis can be obtained in the operating room in almost all patients, although great patience and care may be required. Special hematological investigation and treatment are seldom needed, and minimal blood administration should be possible in the operating room and intensive care unit in most uncomplicated cases.

Drainage from the chest tubes is monitored postoperatively. Uncommonly, the drainage is excessive, and then prompt reoperation is indicated. Under proper circumstances, this should be necessary in only 1 or 2 per cent of patients. When rather rigorous criteria for reoperation are used, reentries are usually done within 3 to 4 hours of the patients' leaving the operating room, while the patients are in good condition, and without the disadvantages of the infusion of large volumes of homologous blood.

RESULTS OF CARDIAC SURGERY

The results of cardiac surgery are now best presented, not only in terms of the prevalence of postoperative events (death, return of angina, prosthetic valve endocarditis, and so on) but also in terms of the time of their occurrence relative to the date of operation. No longer is the simple description of "operative deaths" or "hospital deaths" sufficiently informative, since these are now generally low but also because they usually lead to underestimation of the overall early risks of operation. Incremental risk factors for the various events need identification, in part to define areas of needed research and in part for purposes of comparing and predicting so that individual patient care and programmatic planning can be on a firm scientific basis.

Methods have now been developed specifically for the purpose of studying the time-related events after cardiac surgery in this manner.[1, 2] In the case of death, an early phase of initially high but rapidly declining risk is usually present, but the early phase of risk often does not either disappear or give way to a second constant phase of risk until 3 to 12 months after operation. This invalidates the use of "hospital mortality" or "30-day mortality" as a reasonable indicator of early risks. A third phase of rising risk is present for some events after some kinds of operations. These periods of changing risk make the expression "risk per patient year" an inaccurate one.

Knowledge of the results of cardiac surgery is essential for proper patient care, since the indications for cardiac surgery are based primarily on comparison of early and late results of nonsurgical treatment (or natural history) and of surgical treatment.

CONGENITAL HEART DISEASE. The surgical closure of patent ductus arteriosus, particularly when performed in infancy, is a curative operation (see definition of curative operation, p. 1663). Likewise, when performed in infancy, repairs of ventricular septal defects, atrial septal defects, partial AV septal (canal) defects, and, if the left AV valve can be made competent, complete AV septal defects are curative operations. When the morphology of the tetralogy of Fallot allows a repair to be made in the first few years of life without the use of a transannular patch or valved extracardiac conduit, the operation is curative. When either of these must be used, the operation must be considered palliative and a second operation must be anticipated, although it may be 20 or more years away.

Tricuspid atresia, several types of conditions involving univentricular atrioventricular connections, and a few other anomalies are today best treated by the Fontan operation. Although early and intermediate-term (10 to 20 year) survival and good functional status are the usual results of this operation (Fig. 51–4), exercise capacity is limited by the absence of a ventricle between the right atrium and pulmonary artery. Thus, while the Fontan operation is palliative, it is a very good operation.

The multistage operations required for a few conditions such as aortic atresia with hypoplastic left heart syndrome and interrupted aortic arch have been shown to be initially beneficial, at least in some patients. However, there is as yet insufficient evidence of intermediate- or long-term benefits to allow their being considered either palliative or curative.

VALVULAR HEART DISEASE. Neither repair nor replacement of cardiac valves with acquired stenosis or incompetence can be considered curative operations, although they generally provide good and often long-lasting palliation (Fig. 51–10). The failure to achieve cure is usually the result of a continuing and sometimes increasing secondary cardiomyopathy, although complications from the valve replacement device or valve repair procedure and spread of the basic disease process to other valves are sometimes at fault.

ISCHEMIC HEART DISEASE. In highly favorable subsets of patients with ischemic heart disease, surgical treatment (coronary artery bypass grafting) can provide 5- or even 10-year survivals similar to those of an age-sex-race matched general population (Fig. 51–11). However, the surgical treatment of ischemic heart disease must be considered palliative rather than curative. Ultimate failure of the bypassing conduit (considerably less common when internal mammary arteries are used as conduits rather than reversed saphenous veins), progression of the arteriosclerotic coronary artery disease, and/or the presence or progression of an ischemic secondary cardiomyopathy, are generally responsible for the failure to achieve cure.

OTHER FORMS OF HEART DISEASE. The surgical ablation of the accessory AV conduction pathways usually results in the cure of the Wolff-Parkinson-White syndrome. The direct ablative operation for intractable and life-threatening ventricular tachycardia, on the other hand, results only in palliation, with the tachycardia recurring in some patients after a few years. The recurrence probably results from new arrhythmogenic foci or reentry circuits developing in the milieu of a severe secondary cardiomyopathy.

Cardiac replacement can be considered therapeutic only when cardiac transplantation from another human being is used for the replacement. To date, cardiac xenografts have functioned in humans for only a short time, and artificial hearts have been proved successful only in the early phase after insertion. Cardiac allografts transplanted from one human being to another are, however, palliative and not curative, life expectancy after cardiac transplantation being considerably less than that of an age-sex-race matched general population (Fig. 51–1).

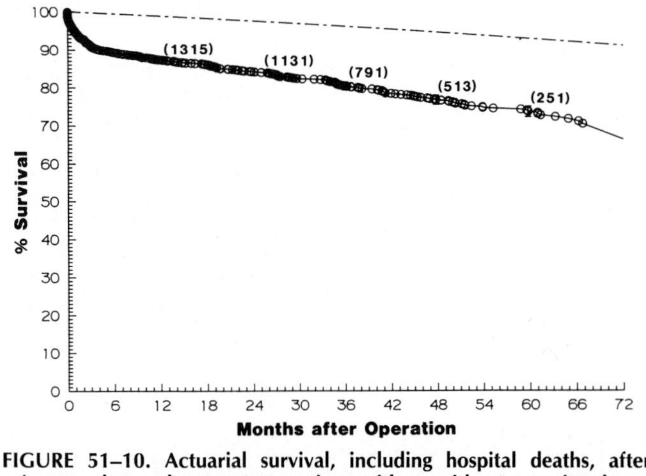

FIGURE 51–10. Actuarial survival, including hospital deaths, after primary valve replacement operations with or without associated cardiac procedures (UAB; 1975 to July 1979; n = 1533; 338 deaths). The depiction is as in the previous actuarials; the dashed-dot-dashed line is the survival of an age-sex-race matched general population.

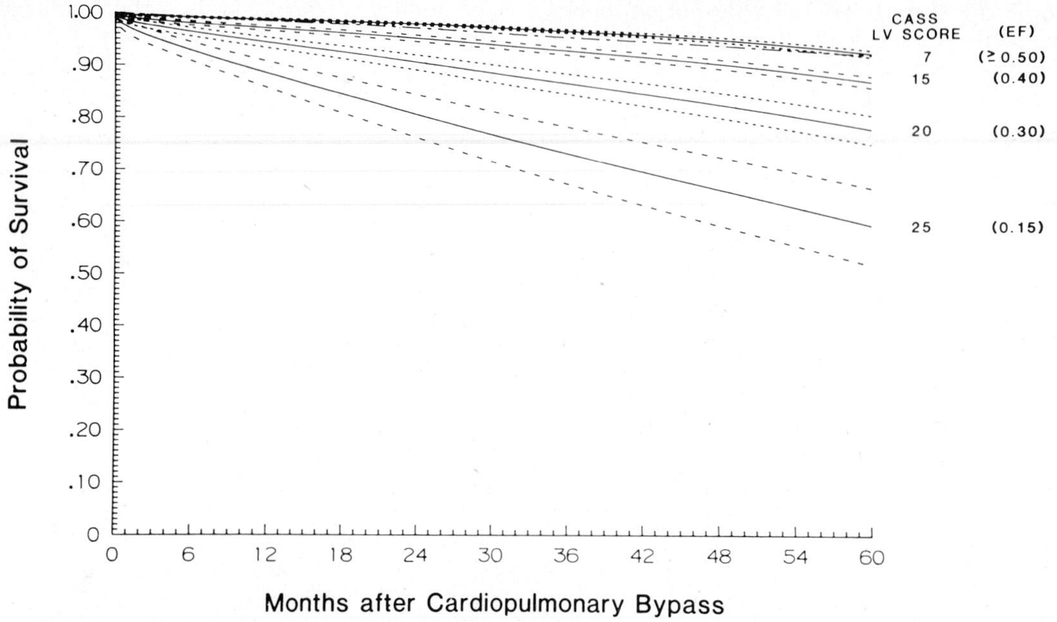

FIGURE 51–11. Nomogram of the solution of a multivariate equation (UAB; 1977 to 1981; n = 3872; 460 deaths) showing the relation between survival (including hospital deaths) after coronary artery bypass grafting, along the horizontal axis, and preoperative left ventricular function expressed as the CASS LV Score. As a reference, the corresponding ejection fraction is shown in parentheses. The dashed lines enclose the 70 per cent confidence intervals. The dash-dot-dashed line near the top is the survival of an age-sex-race matched general population. Key: CASS, Coronary Artery Surgery Study; EF, ejection fraction; LV, left ventricular. (From Kirklin, J. W., Blackstone, E. H., and Rogers, W. J.: The plights of the invasive treatment of ischemic heart disease. Reprinted with permission of the American College of Cardiology. J. Am. Coll. Cardiol. *5*:158, 1985.)

REFERENCES

1. Blackstone, E. H., and Kirklin, J. W.: Death and other time-related events after valve replacement. Circulation 72:753, 1985.
2. Blackstone, E. H., Naftel, D. C., and Turner, M. E., Jr.: The decomposition of time-varying hazard into phases, each incorporating a separate stream of concomitant information. J. Am. Stat. Assoc. *81*:615, 1986.
3. Rashkind, W. J., and Miller, W. W.: Creation of an atrial septal defect without thoracotomy: A palliative approach to complete transposition of the great arteries. J.A.M.A. *196*:991, 1966.
4. Cobanoglu, A., Grunkemeier, G. L., Aru, G. M., McKinley, C. L., and Starr, A.: Mitral replacement: Clinical experience with a ball-valve prosthesis. Ann. Surg. *202*:376, 1985.
5. Acker, M., Hammond, R., Mannion, J., Salmons, S., and Stephenson, L.: An autologous biologic pump motor: One week experience. J. Thorac. Cardiovasc. Surg. (in press).
6. Carpentier, A.: Discussion of paper by Acker et al. J. Thorac. Cardiovasc. Surg. (in press).
7. Bernhard, W. F., Gernes, D. G., Clay, W. C., Schoen, F. J., Burgeson, R., Valeri, R. C., Malaragno, A. J., and Poirier, V. L.: Investigations with an implantable, electrically actuated ventricular assist device. J. Thorac. Cardiovasc. Surg. *88*:11, 1984.
8. Barnard, C. N., Barnard, M. S., Cooper, D. K. C., Curchio, C. A., Hassoulas, J., Novitsky, D., and Wolpowitz, A.: The present status of heterotopic cardiac transplantation. J. Thorac. Cardiovasc. Surg. *81*:433, 1981.
9. Hardesty, R. L., Griffith, B. P., Trento, A., Thompson, M. E., Ferson, P. F., and Bahnson, H. T.: Mortally ill patients and excellent survival following cardiac transplantation. Ann. Thorac. Surg. *41*:126, 1986.
10. Evans, R. W., Manninen, D. L., Garrison, L. P., and Maier, A. M.: Donor availability as the primary determinant of the future of heart transplantation. J.A.M.A. *255*:1892, 1986.
11. Bailey, L. L., Nehlson-Cannarella, S. L., Concepcion, W., and Jolley, W. B.: Baboon-to-human cardiac xenotransplantation in a neonate. J.A.M.A. *254*:3321, 1985.
12. Medawar, P. B.: Immunologic tolerance. Nature *189*:14, 1961.
13. Bailey, L. L., Jang, J., Johnson, W., and Jolley, W. B.: Orthotopic cardiac xenografting in the newborn goat. J. Thorac. Cardiovasc. Surg. *89*:242, 1985.
14. Bailey, L., Roost, H., Li, Z., and Jolley, W.: Host maturation after orthotopic cardiac transplantation during neonatal life. Heart Transplantation *111*:265, 1984.
15. Kolff, J., Deeb, G. M., Cavarocchi, N. C., Riebman, J. B., Olsen, D. B., and Robbins, P. S.: The artificial heart in human subjects. J. Thorac. Cardiovasc. Surg. *87*:825, 1984.
16. Relman, A. S.: Artificial hearts—permanent and temporary. N. Engl. J. Med. *314*:644, 1986.
17. Kirklin, J. W.: A letter to Helen. J. Thorac. Cardiovasc. Surg. *78*:643, 1979.
18. Kirklin, J. W., Blackstone, E. H., Bargeron, L. M., Jr., Pacifico, A. D., and Kirklin, J. K.: The repair of AV canal defects in infancy. Int. J. Cardiol. (in press).
19. Quaegebeur, J. M., Rohmer, J., Ottenkamp, J., Buis, T., Kirklin, J. W., Blackstone, E. H., and Brom, A. G.: The arterial switch operation; an eight-year experience. J. Thorac. Cardiovasc. Surg. *92*:361, 1986.
20. Lee, C. N., Schoff, H. V., Danielson, G. K., Puga, F. J., and Driscoll, D. J.: Comparison of atriopulmonary versus atrioventricular connections for repair of tricuspid atresia. J. Thorac. Cardiovasc. Surg. (in press).
21. Kirklin, J. W., and Barratt-Boyes, B. G.: Cardiac Surgery. New York, John Wiley and Sons, 1986, pp. 431–445.
22. Ross, J.: Afterload mismatch in aortic and mitral valve disease: Implications for surgical therapy. J. Am. Coll. Cardiol. *5*:811, 1985.
23. Papadimitriou, J. M., Hopkins, B. E., and Taylor, R. R.: Regression of left ventricular dilation and hypertrophy after removal of volume overload. Circ. Res. *35*:127, 1974.
24. Karp, R. B., Cyrus, R. J., Blackstone, E. H., Kirklin, J. W., Kouchoukos, N. T., and Pacifico, A. D.: The Björk-Shiley valve. J. Thorac. Cardiovasc. Surg. *81*:602, 1981.
25. Bonow, R. O., Borer, J. S., Rosing, D. R., Henry, W. L., Pearlman, A. S., McIntosh, C. L., Morrow, A. G., and Epstein, S. E.: Preoperative exercise capacity in symptomatic patients with aortic regurgitation as a predictor of postoperative left ventricular function and long-term prognosis. Circulation *62*:1280, 1980.
26. Gault, J. H., Covell, J. W., Braunwald, E., and Ross, J., Jr.: Left ventricular performance following correction of free aortic regurgitation. Circulation *47*:773, 1970.
27. Kirklin, J. W., and Barratt-Boyes, B. G.: Cardiac Surgery. New York, John Wiley and Sons, 1986, p. 477.
28. Urschel, C. W., Covell, J. W., Sonnenblick, E. H., Ross, J., Jr., and Braunwald, E.: Myocardial mechanics in aortic and mitral valvular regurgitation: The concept of instantaneous impedance as a determinant of the performance of the intact heart. J. Clin. Invest. *47*:867, 1968.
29. Carabello, B. A., Green, L. H., Grossman, W., Cohn, L. H., Koster, J. K., and Collins, J. J., Jr.: Hemodynamic determinants of prognosis of aortic valve replacement in critical aortic stenosis and advanced congestive heart failure. Circulation *62*:42, 1980.
30. Graham, T. P., Jr., Atwood, G. F., Boerth, R. C., Boucek, R. J., Jr., and Smith, C. W.: Right and left heart size and function in infants with symptomatic coarctation. Circulation *56*:641, 1977.
31. Schwarz, F., Schaper, J., Flameng, W., and Herhlein, F. W.: Correlation between left ventricular function and myocardial ultrastructure in patients with aortic valve disease. Circulation *53* and *54* (Suppl. 11):11–67, 1976 (abstract).
32. Olsson, S. B., Blomstrom, P., Sabel, K., and William-Olsson, G.: Incessant ectopic atrial tachycardia: Successful surgical treatment with regression of dilated cardiomyopathy picture. Am. J. Cardiol. *53*:1465, 1984.
33. DuShane, J. W., and Kirklin, J. W.: Late results of the repair of ventricular septal defect on pulmonary vascular disease. *In* Kirklin, J. W. (ed.): Advances in Cardiovascular Surgery. New York, Grune and Stratton, 1973, p. 9.
34. Blackstone, E. H., Kirklin, J. W., Bradley, E. L., DuShane, J. W., and Appelbaum, A.: Optimal age and results in repair of large ventricular septal defects. J. Thorac. Cardiovasc. Surg. *72*:661, 1976.
35. Heath, D., and Edwards, J. E.: The pathology of hypertensive pulmonary vascular disease. A description of six grades of structural changes in the

pulmonary arteries with special reference to congenital cardiac septal defects. Circulation *18*:533, 1958.
36. Hislop, A., Haworth, S. G., Shinebourne, E. A., and Reid, L.: Quantitative structural analysis of pulmonary vessels in isolated ventricular septal defects in infancy. Br. Heart J. *37*:1014, 1975.
37. Kirklin, J. W., and Barratt-Boyes, B. G.: Cardiac Surgery. New York, John Wiley and Sons, 1986, p. 618.
38. Ellis, F. H., Jr., Kirklin, J. W., Parker, R. L., Burchell, H. B., and Wood, E. H.: Mitral commissurotomy. Arch. Intern. Med. *94*:774, 1954.
39. Best, P. V., and Heath, D.: Pulmonary thrombosis in cyanotic congenital heart disease without pulmonary hypertension. J. Pathol. Bacteriol. *75*:281, 1958.
40. Haworth, S. G., Rees, P. G., Taylor, J. F. N., Macartney, F. J., de Leval, M., and Stark, J.: Pulmonary atresia with ventricular septal defect and major aortopulmonary collateral arteries. Br. Heart J. *45*:133, 1981.
41. Hilberman, M., Myers, B. D., Carrier, B. J., Derby, G., Jamison, R. L., and Stinson, E. B.: Acute renal failure following cardiac surgery. J. Thorac. Cardiovasc. Surg. *77*:880, 1979.
42. Tanaka, J., Yasui, H., Nakano, E., Sese, A., Matsui, K., Takeda, Y., and Tokunaga, K.: Predisposing factors of renal dysfunction following total correction of tetralogy of Fallot in the adult. J. Thorac. Cardiovasc. Surg. *80*:135, 1980.
43. Kirklin, J. K., Blackstone, E. H., Kirklin, J. W., McKay, R., Pacifico, A. D., and Bargeron, L. M., Jr.: Intracardiac surgery in infants under age 3 months: Incremental risk factors for hospital mortality. Am. J. Cardiol. *48*:500, 1981.
44. Rizzoli, G., Blackstone, E. H., Kirklin, J. W., Pacifico, A. D., and Bargeron, L. M., Jr.: Incremental risk factors in hospital mortality rate after repair of ventricular septal defect. J. Thorac. Cardiovasc. Surg. *80*:494, 1980.
45. Studer, M., Blackstone, E. H., Kirklin, J. W., Pacifico, A. D., Soto, B., Chung, G. K. T., Kirklin, J. K., and Bargeron, L. M., Jr.: Determinants of early and late results of repair of atrioventricular septal (canal) defects. J. Thorac. Cardiovasc. Surg. *84*:523, 1982.
46. Kirklin, J. K., Blackstone, E. H., Kirklin, J. W., Pacifico, A. D., and Bargeron, L. M., Jr.: The Fontan operation: Ventricular hypertrophy, age, and date of operation as risk factors. J. Thorac. Cardiovasc. Surg. *(in press)*.
47. Kalter, R. D., Saul, C. M., Wetstein, L., Soriano, C., and Riess, R. F.: Cardiopulmonary bypass. Associated hemostatic abnormalities. J. Thorac. Cardiovasc. Surg. *77*:428, 1979.
48. Davies, G. C., Sobel, M., and Salzman, E. W.: Elevated plasma fibrinopeptide A and thromboxane B_2 levels during cardiopulmonary bypass. Circulation *61*:808, 1980.
49. Lambert, C. J., Marengo-Rowe, A. J., Leveson, J. E., Green, R. H., Theile, J. P., Geisler, G. F., Adam, J., and Mitchel, B. F.: The treatment of postperfusion bleeding using epsilon-aminocaproic acid, cryoprecipitate, fresh-frozen plasma, and protamine sulfate. Ann. Thorac. Surg. *28*:440, 1979.
50. Pang, L. M., Stalcup, S. A., Lipset, J. S., Hayes, C. J., Bowman, F. O., Jr., and Mellins, R. B.: Increased circulating bradykinin during hypothermia and cardiopulmonary bypass in children. Circulation *60*:1503, 1979.
51. Chenoweth, D. E., Cooper, S. W., Hugli, T. E., Stewart, R. W., Blackstone, E. H., and Kirklin, J. W.: Complement activation during cardiopulmonary bypass: Evidence for generation of C3a and C5a anaphylatoxins. N. Engl. J. Med. *304*:497, 1981.
52. Parker, D. J., Cantrell, J. W., Karp, R. B., Stroud, R. M., and Digerness, S. B.: Changes in serum complement and immunoglobulins following cardiopulmonary bypass. Surgery *71*:824, 1972.
53. Hammerschmidt, D. E., Stroncek, D. F., Bowers, T. K., Lammi-Keefe, C. J., Kurth, D. M., Ozalins, A., Nicoloff, D. M., Lillehei, R. C., Craddock, P. R., and Jacob, H. S.: Complement activation and neutropenia occurring during cardiopulmonary bypass. J. Thorac. Cardiovasc. Surg. *81*:370, 1981.
54. Kirklin, J. K., Westaby, S., Blackstone, E. H., Kirklin, J. W., Chenoweth, D. E., and Pacifico, A. D.: Complement and the damaging effects of cardiopulmonary bypass. J. Thorac. Cardiovasc. Surg. *86*:845, 1983.
55. Hugli, T.: Chemical aspects of the serum anaphylatoxins. Contemp. Top. Mol. Immunol. *7*:181, 1978.
56. Bjork, J., Hugli, T. E., and Smedegard, G.: Microvascular effects of anaphylatoxins C3a and C5a. J. Immunol. *134*:1115, 1985.
57. Martin, R. R.: Alterations in leukocyte structure and function due to mechanical trauma. *In* Hwang, N. H. C., Gross, D. R., and Patel, D. J. (eds.): Quantitative Cardiovascular Studies: Clinical and Research Applications of Engineering Principles. Baltimore, University Park Press, 1979, pp. 419–454.
58. Wilson, J. W.: Pulmonary morphologic changes due to extracorporeal circulation: A model for "the shock lung" at cellular level in humans. *In* Forscher, B. K., Lillehei, R. C., and Stubbs, S. S. (eds.): Shock in Low- and High-Flow States. Proceedings of a Symposium, Brook Augusta, Michigan. Amsterdam, Excerpta Medica, 1972, pp. 160–171.
59. Solen, K. A., Whiffen, J. D., and Lightfoot, E. N.: The effect of shear, specific surface, and air interface on the development of blood emboli and hemolysis. J. Biomed. Mater. Res. *12*:381, 1978.
60. Barratt-Boyes, B. G., Simpson, M. M., and Neutze, J. M.: Intracardiac surgery in neonates and infants using deep hypothermia. Circulation *61* and *62* (Suppl. III):73, 1970.
61. Treasure, T., Naftel, D. C., Conger, K. A., Garcia, J. H., Kirklin, J. W., and Blackstone, E. H.: The effect of hypothermic circulatory arrest time on cerebral function, morphology, and biochemistry. An experimental study. J. Thorac. Cardiovasc. Surg. *86*:761, 1983.
62. Wells, F. C., Coghill, S., Caplan, H. L., and Lincoln, C.: Duration of circulatory arrest does influence the psychological development of children after cardiac operation in early life. J. Thorac. Cardiovasc. Surg. *86*:823, 1983.
63. Taber, R. E., Morales, A. R., and Fine, G.: Myocardial necrosis and the postoperative low-cardiac-output syndrome. Ann. Thorac. Surg. *4*:12, 1967.
64. Najafi, H., Henson, D., Dye, W. S., Javid, H., Hunter, J. A., Callaghan, R., Eisenstein, R., and Julian, O. C.: Left ventricular hemorrhagic necrosis. Ann. Thorac. Surg. *7*:550, 1969.
65. Hultgren, H. N., Miyagawa, M., Buch, W., and Angell, W. W.: Ischemic myocardial injury during cardiopulmonary bypass surgery. Am. Heart J. *85*:167, 1973.
66. Roberts, W. C., Bulkley, B. H., and Morrow, A. G.: Pathologic anatomy of cardiac valve replacement: A study of 224 necropsy patients. Prog. Cardiovasc. Dis. *15*:539, 1973.
67. Tranum-Jensen, J., Janse, M. J., Fiolet, J. W. T., Krieger, W. J. G., D'Alnoncourt, C. H., and Durrer, D.: Tissue osmolality, cell swelling, and reperfusion in acute regional myocardial ischemia in the isolated porcine heart. Circ. Res. *49*:364, 1981.
68. Visner, M. S., Arentzen, C. E., Parrish, D. G., Larson, E. V., O'Connor, M. J., Crumbley, A. J., Bache, R. J., and Anderson, R. W.: Effects of global ischemia on the diastolic properties of the left ventricle in the conscious dog. Circulation *71*:610, 1985.
69. Danforth, W. H., Naegle, S., and Bing, R. J.: Effect of ischemia and reoxygenation on glycolytic reactions and adenosinetriphosphate in heart muscle. Circ. Res. *8*:965–971, 1960.
70. Follette, D. M., Fey, K., Buckberg, G. D., Helly, J. J., Jr., Steed, D. L., Foglia, R. P., and Maloney, J. V., Jr.: Reducing postischemic damage by temporary modification of reperfusate calcium, potassium, pH, and osmolarity. J. Thorac. Cardiovasc. Surg. *82*:221, 1981.
71. Follette, D. M., Steed, D. L., Foglia, R. P., Fey, K. H., and Buckberg, G. D.: Reduction of postischemic myocardial damage by maintaining arrest during initial reperfusion. Surg. Forum *28*:281, 1977.
72. Buckberg, G. D., Brazier, J. R., Nelson, R. L., Goldstein, S. M., McConnell, D. H., and Cooper, N.: Studies of the effects of hypothermia on regional myocardial blood flow and metabolism during cardiopulmonary bypass. I. The adequately perfused beating, fibrillating, and arrested heart. J. Thorac. Cardiovasc. Surg. *73*:87, 1977.
73. Allen, B. S., Buckberg, G. D., Schwaiger, M., Yeatman, L., Tillisch, J., Kawata, N., Messenger, J., and Lee, C.: Superiority of surgical over medical revascularization in the treatment of acute coronary occlusion. J. Thorac. Cardiovasc. Surg. *(in press)*.
74. Appelbaum, A., Blackstone, E. H., Kouchoukos, N. T., and Kirklin, J. W.: Afterload reduction and cardiac output in infants early after intracardiac surgery. Am. J. Cardiol. *39*:445, 1977.
75. Miller, D. C., Daughters, G. T., Derby, G. C., Mitchell, R. S., Ingels, N. B., Stinson, E. B., and Alderman, E. L.: Effect of early postoperative volume loading on left ventricular systolic function (including left ventricular ejection fraction determined by myocardial marker) after myocardial revascularization. Circulation 72 (Suppl. II):II-207, 1985.
76. Stinson, E. B., Holloway, E. L., and Derby, G. C.: Control of myocardial performance early after open-heart operations by vasodilator treatment. J. Thorac. Cardiovasc. Surg. *73*:523, 1977.
77. Waldo, A. L., and MacLean, W. A. H.: Diagnosis and treatment of cardiac arrhythmias following open heart surgery. Emphasis on the use of atrial and ventricular epicardial wire electrodes. Mt. Kisco, New York, Futura Publishing Co., 1980.
78. Buckley, M. J., Craver, J. M., Gold, H. K., Mundth, E. D., Daggett, W. M., and Austen, W. G.: Intra-aortic balloon pump assist for cardiogenic shock after cardiopulmonary bypass. Circulation *47* and *48* (Suppl. III):90, 1973.
79. Martin, R. S., Moncure, A. C., Buckley, M. J., Austen, G., Akins, C., and Leinback, R. C.: Complications of percutaneous intra-aortic balloon insertion. J. Thorac. Cardiovasc. Surg. *85*:186, 1983.
80. Pierce, W. S., Parr, G. V. S., Myers, J. L., Poe, W. E., Bull, A. P., and Waldhausen, J. A.: Ventricular-assist pumping in patients with cardiogenic shock after cardiac operations. N. Engl. J. Med. *305*:1606, 1981.
81. Rose, D. M., Colvin, S. B., Culliford, A. T., Isom, O. W., Cunningham, J. N., Glassman, E., and Spencer, F. C.: Late functional and hemodynamic status of surviving patients following insertion of the left heart assist device. J. Thorac. Cardiovasc. Surg. *86*:639, 1983.
82. Jett, G. K., Siwek, L. G., Picone, A. L., Applebaum, R. E., and Jones, M.: Pulmonary artery balloon counterpulsation for right ventricular failure. J. Thorac. Cardiovasc. Surg. *86*:364, 1983.
83. Dembitsky, W. P., Daily, P. O., Raney, A. A., Moores, W. Y., and Joyo, C. I.: Temporary extracorporeal support of the right ventricle. J. Thorac. Cardiovasc. Surg. *91*:518, 1986.
84. Waldo, A. L., MacLean, W. A. H., Karp, R. B., Kouchoukos, N. T., and James, T. N.: Sustained rapid atrial pacing to control supraventricular tachycardias following open heart surgery. Circulation *51* and *52* (Suppl. II):13, 1975.
85. Chesney, R. W., Kaplan, B. S., Freedom, R. M., Haller, J. A., and Drummond, K. N.: Acute renal failure: An important complication for cardiac surgery in infants. J. Pediatr. *87*:381, 1975.
86. Norman, J. C., McDonald, H. P., and Sloan, H.: The early and aggressive treatment of acute renal failure following cardiopulmonary bypass with continuous peritoneal dialysis. Surgery *56*:240, 1964.
87. Kirklin, J. W., and Barratt-Boyes, B. G.: Cardiac Surgery. New York, John Wiley and Sons, 1986, pp. 140–176.
88. Ashbaugh, D. G., and Petty, T. L.: Positive end-expiratory pressure. J. Thorac. Cardiovasc. Surg. *65*:165, 1979.
89. Sturtz, G. S., Kirklin, J. W., Burke, E. C., and Power, M. H.: Water metabolism after cardiac operations involving a Gibbon-type pump-oxygenator. I. Daily water metabolism, obligatory water losses, and requirements. Circulation *16*:988, 1957.

52 COST-EFFECTIVE STRATEGIES IN CARDIOLOGY

by LEE GOLDMAN, M.D.

The availability of an increasing number of diagnostic and therapeutic technologies, coupled with concerns over the rising costs of health care, has generated increasing interest in determining the costs and effectiveness of cardiologic care. Cost-effectiveness analysis, which initially had been used principally by economists and policy makers, is a potentially useful technique for evaluating how best to diagnose, prevent, and treat medical illnesses. Such analyses highlight the important issues that should guide the physician–decision maker. They can help in identification of gaps in knowledge and establishment of priorities for research to be carried out by clinical investigators. To appreciate the implications of the emerging literature on cost-effectiveness in cardiology, it is important to understand the basic concepts that underlie formal cost-effectiveness analysis.

QUANTITATIVE ANALYSES OF COSTS AND EFFECTIVENESS

Analysts commonly distinguish between *cost-benefit analysis*, in which both costs and benefits are expressed in the same units (such as dollars), and *cost-effectiveness analysis*, in which the costs are commonly expressed in monetary terms while the effectiveness is expressed in terms of the health benefit.[1] The health benefit commonly is measured in units such as the number of lives that are saved, the years of life gained, the quality-adjusted years of life saved,[1, 2] the days of disability avoided, or other suitable measurements.

SENSITIVITY ANALYSIS. Cost-effectiveness analyses are critically dependent on the accuracy of the assumptions on which they are based. Therefore, the analysis should include a "sensitivity analysis," in which the calculations are repeated with varying assumptions to determine whether the conclusions are altered.[1, 2] It is vital to determine whether the final conclusions are critically dependent on a tenuous estimate by determining whether reasonable variations in important assumptions make major differences in the results of the analysis.

For example, in an analysis of the cost-effectiveness of admitting patients with suspected uncomplicated acute myocardial infarction to a full-fledged coronary care unit as opposed to a nonintensive care unit bed with telemetry monitoring, it would be critical to estimate the relative difference, if any, in the rate of successful resuscitation from primary ventricular fibrillation in the two settings. The larger the estimated difference, the more cost-effective the coronary care unit would appear. If the two settings were assumed to be equally effective, the additional cost of the coronary care unit would not yield any additional effectiveness for this purpose. Since there are no randomized controlled data to address this issue, any analysis of the relative cost-effectiveness of care of patients with suspected myocardial infarction in these two settings will depend on the estimates that are made. When a sensitivity analysis was performed, the nonintensive care bed with telemetry monitoring remained the more cost-effective option for patients whose probability of acute myocardial infarction was 10 per cent or less even if it was assumed that the rate of successful resuscitation from primary ventricular fibrillation in this setting was no better than the success rate among patients seen by trained ambulance personnel within 5 minutes after onset of ventricular fibrillation in the out-of-hospital setting.[3]

THE CLINICAL DECISION TREE. Some cost-effectiveness analyses address difficult clinical problems for which no clear agreement exists, often because available data are not adequate even for the experienced clinician. In such situations, cost-effectiveness analysis may not yield clear answers, usually because the relative differences between competing strategies are small. For example, it may be difficult to decide whether or not to implant a permanent pacemaker in an elderly patient who has symptoms that are suggestive of a pacemaker-responsive arrhythmia but in whom the relationship between arrhythmia and symptoms has not been proved. The therapeutic options can be displayed using a decision tree (Fig. 52–1) that explicitly outlines the various possibilities.[4] In this decision analysis, estimates about the relative cost-effectiveness of various therapeutic strategies would depend on the patient's subjective assessment of the quality of life under different scenarios, including persistent symptoms and no pacemaker, persistent symptoms despite a pacemaker, and the pacemaker without symptoms. Since small changes in the

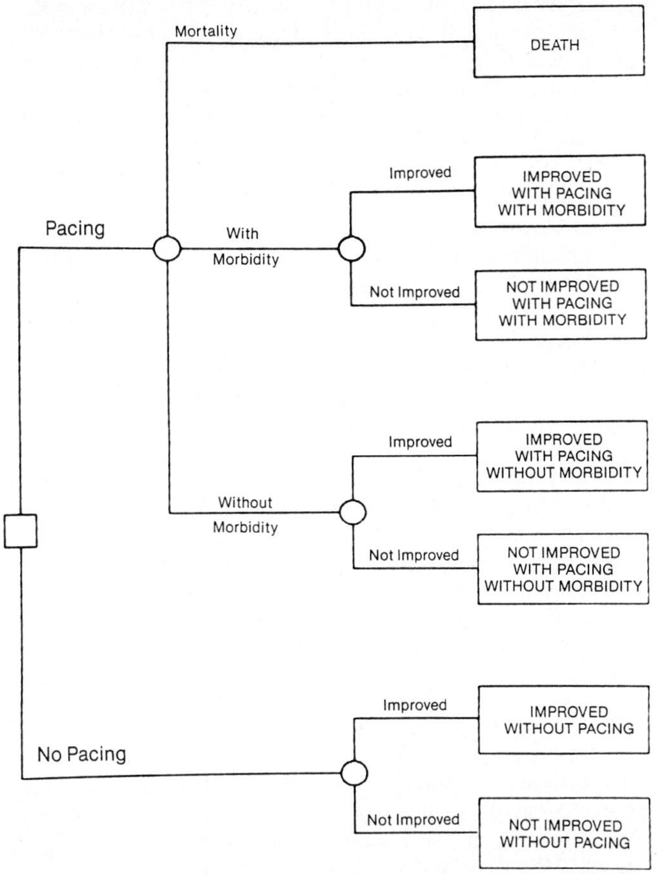

FIGURE 52–1. Decision tree for whether or not to perform empiric pacing in the elderly patient with syncope that may or may not be caused by a pacemaker-responsive arrhythmia. Branches of this decision tree explicitly detail the potential outcomes from the various options. The squares denote the outcomes of decisions that the physician must make, while the circles denote events over which the physician has no control, i.e., occur "by chance." In constructing the decision tree, physicians would use either their own judgment or use probabilities derived from the literature to estimate the likelihood of each of the events that can occur at a "chance" node. The sum of the probabilities of these chance events is always 100 per cent. In a cost-effectiveness analysis, each of the potential outcomes, as displayed in the rectangles in the right column, would be assigned a cost and a "utility." The utility would denote how highly the outcome is valued compared to perfect health, which traditionally has a value of 1.0, versus death, which traditionally has a value of 0. Cost-effectiveness calculations would compute the average expected costs and utilities for each of the various options that might be chosen by the physician, in this case the "pacing" and "no pacing" options that emanate from the initial square node. (From Kwoh, C. K., Beck, J R., and Pauker, S. G.: Repeated syncope with negative diagnostic evaluation. Med. Decis. Making *4*:351, 1984.)

assessment of quality of life under these different circumstances would alter the preferred strategy, this particular analysis could not provide a definitive solution for all cases involving this therapeutic dilemma. Nevertheless, this analysis demonstrated that empiric pacing was an attractive option in an elderly patient with unexplained syncope even when there was only about a 25 per cent chance that the syncope was caused by a pacemaker-responsive arrhythmia.

The goal of cost-effectiveness analysis is not to find the greatest possible benefit for the lowest possible cost, because it is not possible to achieve both simultaneously.[2, 5] Instead, it is necessary either to determine the resources that are available and then find the greatest possible effectiveness that can be purchased for those resources or to determine the desired effectiveness and then find the lowest cost to achieve it. In either case, it is important to have a preconceived idea of the desirable or acceptable relative ratio of cost to effectiveness. Although cost-effectiveness analyses determine the ratio of cost to effectiveness, two strategies with the same ratio may have quite different absolute costs and absolute effectiveness. For example, a program that saves 100 lives for $10,000 has the same cost-effectiveness ratio as one that saves 10,000 lives for $1,000,000, but the two programs' absolute costs and absolute effectivenesses vary 100-fold. In cost-effectiveness analyses, any potentially new strategy is usually compared with the current, or baseline, strategy by calculating the *incremental cost:incremental effectiveness* ratio.

CALCULATION OF COSTS

In determining costs, several types must be considered. *Operating costs* may include both direct costs such as salaries and indirect costs such as overhead, including utilities and maintenance. Costs can also be categorized as fixed versus variable costs. For example, the first 100 cardiac scans carried out in an imaging center may cost $100,000 for an average cost of $1000 per scan, because of the high capital costs of the equipment. However, if the laboratory were to "increase its output," the incremental cost for the next 100 scans would be much less than the average cost for the first 100 scans, because the capital costs of the equipment would be nearly the same regardless of whether 100 scans or 200 scans were performed. Thus, one could distinguish between the incremental cost of performing the second 100 scans versus the average cost of all 200 scans. In many medical analyses, true costs are not available, and charges are used in the calculation of "cost" effectiveness.[6] Since charges are often the same regardless of volume, they usually do not consider fully the important difference between average and incremental costs.

In calculating net health care costs, a useful approach is shown in Table 52–1. Unfortunately, those persons making many analyses have concentrated only on direct medical costs, without fully taking into account the other terms in the equation.

DISCOUNTING. In virtually all cost analyses, it is important to consider the time frame when costs and effects will be achieved. Since present dollars or benefits are more highly valued than a promise of future dollars or health benefits, a cost or benefit achieved immediately is more highly valued than one that is achieved later.[1] For example, one would be more willing to spend $10,000 today to prevent a death that otherwise would occur tomorrow than to spend $10,000 today to prevent a death that otherwise would occur in 10 years, even if there were no inflation and if there were no interest to be earned on the dollars. There is a preference to achieve an immediate benefit for several reasons. First, other events may intercede so that the projected future death may not occur or might be avoided as a consequence of newly available options that cost less than $10,000. Second, another illness could ter-

TABLE 52–1 CALCULATION OF NET HEALTH CARE COSTS FOR A PROGRAM

Net costs = direct medical costs*
+ health care costs associated with the adverse side effects of treatment
− savings of health care, rehabilitation, and custodial costs due to prevention or alleviation of disease
+ costs of treating disease that would not have occurred if the patient had not lived longer as a result of the original treatment

*Costs of hospitalization, physician time, medications, laboratory services, and other ancillary services.

See reference 2 for more details.

minate life during the intervening period. Also, the $10,000 might be spent during the intervening 10 years in ways that are deemed more valuable. Furthermore, there is always a lingering doubt that the money spent now will not actually achieve the desired actual effect 10 years hence. This principle, by which the promise of future events is less valued than known immediate events, is termed "discounting," and is independent of monetary inflation. It is common practice to "discount" both future costs and future benefits by about 5 per cent per year.

In discussions of cost and effectiveness, several common misconceptions often occur.[5] Cost-effective should not be equated with cost-saving, because one must often spend in order to achieve a real benefit. Although a strategy that saves money *and* achieves an equal or better outcome is obviously cost-effective, a program is also cost-effective if it yields an additional benefit that is worth the additional cost. The definition of "worth the cost" may be a somewhat arbitrary value judgment, because it is difficult to place a monetary value on years of life and productivity. In many analyses, the approximately $35,000 per year cost in 1987 dollars of renal dialysis,[7] a program that the United States has decided to support with tax dollars, has been used as the benchmark for the amount of cost that the public appears willing to bear to prolong useful life by one year.

Although physicians must be aware of the relative cost-effectiveness of various diagnostic and therapeutic options if they are to make optimal choices for their patients, decisions about the number of dollars that *should* be spent to achieve specific health care benefits will be determined ultimately by society. Physicians have a critical role to play in developing appropriate data on cost-effectiveness issues, but the individual physician's primary responsibility is to the patient, within the confines of the economic limitations that may be imposed upon both the physician and the patient by society.

One example of societal constraints on medical care expenditures is the diagnosis-related groups (DGR) system of prospective reimbursement. By defining in advance the number of dollars that a hospital will be reimbursed for the care of certain types of patients, the physician, the hospital, and the patient may all become more concerned with issues of cost-effectiveness. In an analogous manner, capitation systems, in which physicians are prepaid a fixed sum to assume the care of a patient, place an increased emphasis on the determination of cost-effective strategies.

DIAGNOSTIC TESTING

Modern cardiology includes an impressive armamentarium of diagnostic tests. Good clinical judgment, however, requires that the physician choose tests in a cost-effective manner, in which the tests individually or sequentially may lead to improved diagnosis and management. The cost-effective use of diagnostic tests requires the physician to proceed logically through evaluation of the patient, selection of diagnostic tests, integration of the test with clinical data, and formulation of management strategies.[8, 9] Each of these steps must be considered carefully for the proper utilization of diagnostic testing.

THE ESTIMATION OF CLINICAL PROBABILITIES. Regardless of the condition in question, the physician must utilize data from the medical history and physical examination to estimate the likelihood of its presence. For example, in evaluating the patient with chest pain, the physician may consider the patient's age and sex, as well as the typicality of the discomfort for angina pectoris.[10–14] The symptom may be categorized as typical angina pectoris, atypical angina pectoris, or nonanginal chest discomfort on the basis of its character, location, provocation, and response to rest or nitroglycerin (p. 1316). Similarly, in estimating the probability of the presence of hemodynamically significant aortic stenosis in an adult with a systolic murmur, one would consider factors such as the intensity, location, and radiation of the murmur, the volume and rate of upstroke of the carotid arterial pulse, and the second heart sound[15] (p. 1055). Although these estimates of clinical probabilities can be based on the judgment of an experienced physician, in some circumstances, the physician also can be aided by accumulated data from large series of patients in whom the clinical probability of conditions such as significant coronary artery disease,[13, 14] acute myocardial infarction or unstable angina pectoris,[16, 17] or hemodynamically significant aortic stenosis[15] have been determined.

ORDERING A DIAGNOSTIC TEST. When considering a test that may be ordered, the physician must determine whether the test is efficacious and sufficiently accurate for indications for which it is being considered, that no other test with acceptable efficacy is less hazardous or less expensive, and that this is the most appropriate time for ordering the test.[9, 18, 19] In one such study carried out in 1977 soon after cardiac nuclear medicine scans became clinically available, 35 per cent were found *not* to have been ordered appropriately.[18] By comparison, the rate of inappropriate ordering for M-mode echocardiograms, which had been routinely available for some time and were presumably well understood by physicians, was only 14 per cent.[19]

Tests may be ordered for such indications as to plan or monitor therapy, to establish a diagnosis, to define the extent of a known disease, to estimate prognosis, or to reassure the physician or the patient.[18–20] Although each of these indications can be a legitimate reason for ordering a diagnostic test, test results that potentially may influence therapeutic action are usually the most valued and are certainly the most cost-effective.

When assessing the accuracy of a test, one must understand terms such as sensitivity, specificity, and positive predictive value (Table 8–5, p. 235). For some tests, such as the technetium pyrophosphate scintiscan, the result is often dichotomized into "normal" versus "abnormal," even though it is understood that the precise distinction between normal and abnormal may be difficult and sometimes somewhat arbitrary. Other tests, such as the ejection fraction, are commonly reported on a continuous scale. In some circumstances, such as with the exercise electrocardiogram, a continuous result (e.g., the extent of ST-segment depression) is often dichotomized into normal or abnormal to facilitate the test's interpretation. When a continuous result is dichotomized, an increase in its sensitivity, or the likelihood of a positive test result among patients with the condition, can be obtained only at the expense of decreasing specificity, or the likelihood of a normal test result in patients without the condition.[21] For example, the sensitivity of the exercise electrocardiogram for detecting patients with coronary artery disease can be increased by reducing the depth of ST-segment depression required for a "positive" test result. However, as the definition of a "positive" test result is changed from 2 mm of ST-segment depression to 1 mm of ST-segment depression, the resulting increase in apparent sensitivity will be at the expense of a decreased specificity, because patients who have between 1 and 2 mm of ST-segment depression and who do not have coronary artery disease now will be misclassified.

In an era of cost consciousness, the physician must often be asked to decide between two tests that may offer similar types of information. For example, a radionuclide ventriculogram may provide a more accurate assessment of the left ventricular ejection fraction than can a two-dimensional echocardiogram, but the latter frequently will provide a sufficiently accurate estimate of left ventricular function to obviate the need for the more expensive radionuclide study.

The choice of tests may also depend on the timing of clinical events. For example, a technetium pyrophosphate scan can diagnose a transmural myocardial infarction (p. 341) accurately, but it is unnecessary to order such a test in patients who arrive early enough after the onset of symptoms for enzymes such as creatine kinase isoenzymes to be diagnostic. Technetium pyrophosphate scans can potentially be helpful in patients who arrive long enough after the onset of symptoms so that creatine kinase levels would have returned to normal, but even in such patients, LDH isoenzyme readings appear to be at least as accurate and far less expensive.[22, 23] Thus, technetium pyrophosphate scans usually will be helpful diagnostically in patients who arrive long enough after the acute event for creatine kinase enzymes to be unhelpful and who have other conditions, such as hemolysis or renal infarction, that make LDH isoenzyme tests unreliable.

INTEGRATING THE TEST RESULT WITH CLINICAL DATA. To use diagnostic tests efficiently, the physician should decide the threshold probability above or below which the future diagnostic or management strategy would be altered.[24, 25] For example, consider that a patient has recurrent chest pain, and on the basis of history and physical examination the physician estimates that there is a 50 per cent probability that it is caused by coronary artery disease. The physician also knows that coronary arteriography would be required to decide whether coronary artery bypass grafting or percutaneous transluminal coronary angioplasty should be carried out if coronary artery disease were present. For cost-effective test ordering, the physician then must estimate how unlikely coronary artery disease would have to be for this strategy to be altered. If the physician would proceed with catheterization provided that the probability of coronary artery disease were as low as 10 per cent (or higher) then a test such as an exercise radionuclide ventriculogram, whose negative result might reduce the probability of coronary artery disease to 30 per cent, would not be helpful in decision-making.

Threshold Approach. This concept has been called the "threshold approach"[25] to test utilization and decision-making. In essence, it indicates that a test is potentially helpful only if its result would change the pretest probability of disease to a degree that could be sufficient to alter the approach to the patient. If it is highly unlikely that the available diagnostic test could move the probability of disease across such a threshold, the test would not be very cost-effective and ordinarily would not be ordered. In some situations, however, the diagnostic threshold may be redefined because of the special characteristics of the patient at hand. For example, it would be considered important to rule out significant coronary artery disease in an otherwise healthy airline pilot who has atypical chest pain. In this situation, the combination of a normal exercise electrocardiogram and a normal exercise thallium scintiscan would make the presence of coronary disease very unlikely. However, if it were argued that the airline pilot's occupational responsibilities would require even a greater degree of certainty, it would be necessary to proceed to the test that is usually considered the benchmark, in this case, coronary arteriography, if it were necessary to be as certain as possible that coronary disease was not present.

BAYES' THEOREM. One way to understand the concepts of prior probability, thresholds, and the impact of diagnostic tests is through Bayes' theorem.[1, 8] When the prior probability (prevalence) of the disease is known in patients who are similar to the patient under consideration, and when the sensitivity and specificity of the test to be ordered

TABLE 52–2 HOW THE POSITIVE AND NEGATIVE PREDICTIVE VALUES OF THE SAME TEST VARY DEPENDING ON THE PRIOR PROBABILITY OF DISEASE

INTERPRETATION OF THE TEST RESULT WHEN 10% OF THE PATIENTS BEING TESTED HAVE THE DISEASE (PRIOR PROBABILITY = 10%)

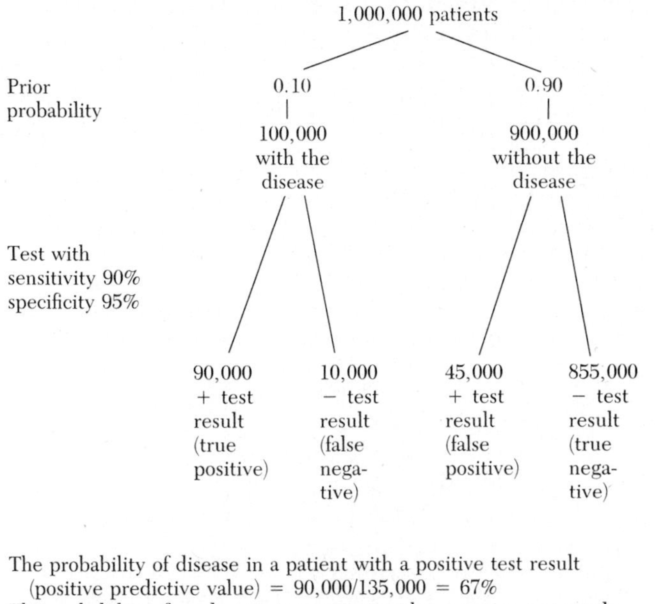

The probability of disease in a patient with a positive test result (positive predictive value) = 90,000/135,000 = 67%

The probability of no disease in a patient with a negative test result (negative predictive value) = 855,000/865,000 = 99%

INTERPRETATION OF THE TEST RESULT WHEN 50% OF THE PATIENTS BEING TESTED HAVE THE DISEASE (PRIOR PROBABILITY = 50%)

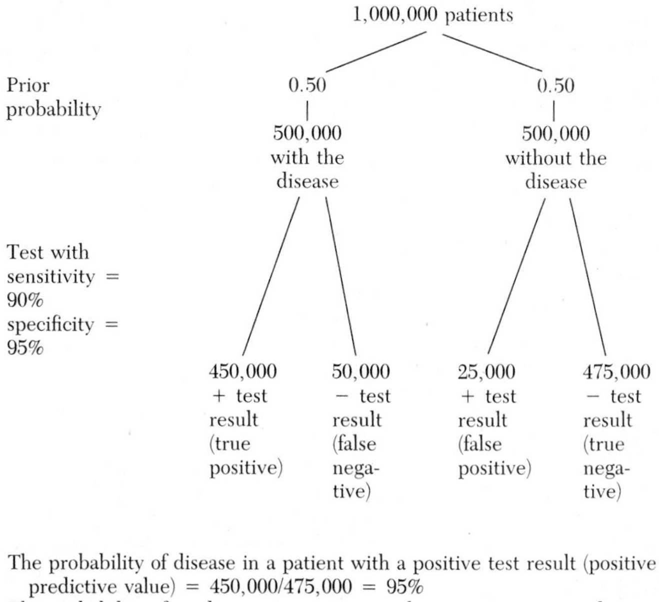

The probability of disease in a patient with a positive test result (positive predictive value) = 450,000/475,000 = 95%

The probability of no disease in a patient with a negative test result (negative predictive value) = 475,000/525,000 = 90%

From Goldman, L.: Quantitative aspects of clinical reasoning. *In* Braunwald, E., Isselbacher, K. J., Petersdorf, R. G., Wilson, J. D., Martin, J. B., and Fauci, A. S. (eds.): Harrison's Principles of Internal Medicine. New York, McGraw-Hill Book Company, 1987, p. 8.

are known, the post-test probability that the disease is present can be calculated (Table 52–2). This table emphasizes how the physician must consider both the prior (pretest) probability that the patient has a disease and the test result in estimating the post-test probability. For example, if a test has a sensitivity of 90 per cent and a specificity of 95 per cent, a patient whose prior probability of disease was 10 per cent and who has a positive test result would have a 67 per cent probability of disease after the test. By comparison, the same test result in a patient whose prior probability was 50 per cent would yield a post-test probability of 95 per cent.

A test is potentially useful if it changes the probability of disease sufficiently to cross the threshold for decision-making. Unfortunately, available data do not always provide precise guidelines for establishing such appropriate thresholds for diagnostic decision-making. Nevertheless, common clinical judgment is often a sufficient guide. For example, using pooled data from the literature,[26–35] the effects of exercise electrocardiography and exercise thallium testing can be estimated for a patient with typical angina pectoris (Fig. 52–2), a patient with atypical angina (Fig. 52–3), and a patient with presumably nonanginal chest pain (Fig. 52–4). These estimated probabilities correspond well to the actual probability of disease in patients who have been evaluated.[35]

NONINVASIVE TESTING IN PATIENTS WITH POSSIBLE ANGINA PECTORIS. The patient with symptoms typical for angina pectoris already has a high probability of coronary artery disease on the basis of the history alone (80 to 85 per cent), and the probability becomes even higher (95 per cent) if the exercise electrocardiogram is positive and becomes overwhelming (99 per cent) after a confirmatory exercise thallium scan. However, for diagnosing the presence or absence of coronary disease, the exercise thallium scan adds little to the results of the exercise test. Although the exercise thallium test may have some additional prognostic value,[36] in most situations, the results of the exercise thallium test would be unlikely to add substantial independent information regarding the diagnosis of the presence of coronary artery disease. If the exercise electrocardiogram and exercise thallium test give conflicting information, the probability of coronary artery disease in the patient with typical angina pectoris remains similar to what it was before either test was obtained (80 to 90 per cent). If both tests are negative, the patient with typical angina pectoris still has a reasonable probability of having significant coronary artery disease (30 per cent). Thus,

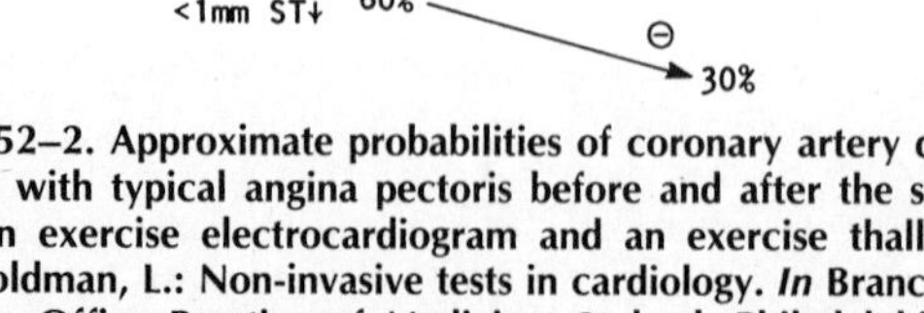

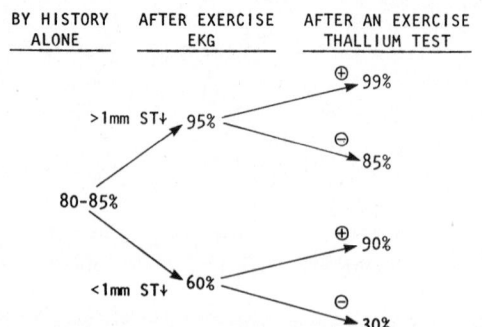

FIGURE 52–2. Approximate probabilities of coronary artery disease in a patient with typical angina pectoris before and after the sequential use of an exercise electrocardiogram and an exercise thallium test. (From Goldman, L.: Non-invasive tests in cardiology. *In* Branch, W., Jr. [ed.]: The Office Practice of Medicine. 2nd ed. Philadelphia, W. B. Saunders Company, 1987.)

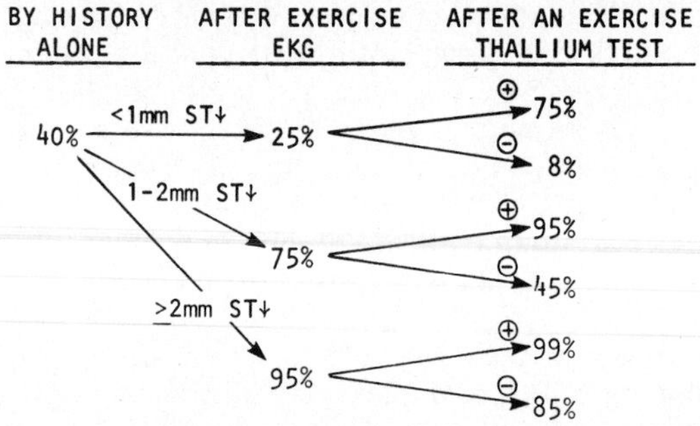

FIGURE 52–3. Approximate probabilities of coronary artery disease in a patient with atypical anginal symptoms before and after the sequential use of an exercise electrocardiogram and an exercise thallium test. (From Goldman, L.: Non-invasive tests in cardiology. *In* Branch, W., Jr. [ed.]: The Office Practice of Medicine. 2nd ed. Philadelphia, W. B. Saunders Company, 1987.)

even two negative tests have not "ruled out" coronary artery disease in a patient with typical angina to an extent to which one could simply reassure the patient, even though they imply a favorable prognosis should coronary artery disease be present (p. 1342).[36, 37] Thus, if one were trying to rule out coronary artery disease in a patient with typical angina pectoris, coronary arteriography still would be required.

In the patient with atypical angina (Fig. 52–3), positive results on both exercise electrocardiography and exercise thallium testing would raise the probability of coronary artery disease from 40 to 95 to 99 per cent. Conversely, negative results on both tests would lower the probability of coronary artery disease substantially (to 8 per cent), perhaps to a low enough level that one would not feel compelled to obtain coronary arteriography except in unusual circumstances. However, if the two tests give conflicting results, the probability of the disease has not been altered appreciably by the two tests.

In an asymptomatic subject who is in the age range in which coronary artery disease usually occurs, a strongly positive exercise electrocardiogram substantially raises the probability of coronary disease (from about 5 to 50 per cent), and a subsequent negative exercise thallium test is not sufficiently reassuring to eliminate the possibility. Thus, one cannot simply use the negative exercise thallium scan in such a patient to "prove" that the exercise electrocardiogram was a false-positive result.

It is beyond the scope of this chapter to discuss the precise guidelines for the most cost-effective use of each of the various types of cardiac diagnostic tests for each possible indication. Nevertheless, test ordering will become more cost-effective if the physician estimates the pretest probability of disease, orders the appropriate test, and properly integrates the test results with the available clinical information. A test will be helpful only to the extent that it provides nonredundant information, i.e., information above and beyond what was previously available.[12, 38, 39] It must be emphasized, however, that a test

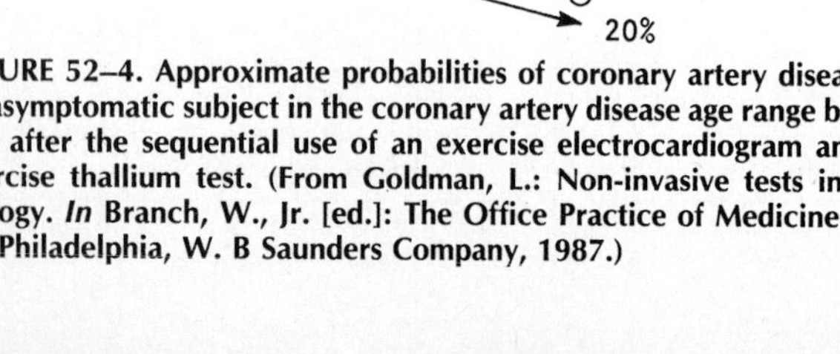

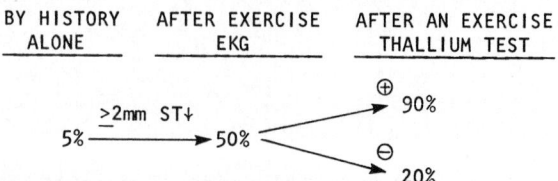

FIGURE 52–4. Approximate probabilities of coronary artery disease in an asymptomatic subject in the coronary artery disease age range before and after the sequential use of an exercise electrocardiogram and an exercise thallium test. (From Goldman, L.: Non-invasive tests in cardiology. *In* Branch, W., Jr. [ed.]: The Office Practice of Medicine. 2nd ed. Philadelphia, W. B Saunders Company, 1987.)

can add incremental information regardless of whether its result is "positive" or "negative."[40]

Cost-effective medicine requires that tests be ordered only if their incremental information will have a positive impact on patient care. The finding that major variations in test use often do not correlate with discernible differences in health outcome[41] suggests that many tests do not meet such criteria. Substantial financial savings can be realized by reducing the utilization of low or moderate cost tests as well as by reducing the utilization of expensive procedures.[42–44]

PREVENTION AND TREATMENT

Among the various preventive and therapeutic modalities in cardiology, some have been studied via formal cost-effectiveness analysis while others have been studied in a more qualitative fashion. In evaluating the cost effectiveness of any program, it must be compared to a baseline or standard current approach. In the following sections, selected data on the costs and effectiveness of several modalities for the diagnosis, prevention, and treatment of heart disease are considered.

DETECTION AND TREATMENT OF HYPERLIPIDEMIA

Substantial data indicate that the serum cholesterol level is significantly correlated with the risk of coronary artery disease (p. 1154), and after controlling for the cholesterol level, the triglyceride level is not an important independent predictor.[45, 46] The high-density lipoprotein cholesterol fraction (p. 1161) appears to be even more important than the low-density lipoprotein fraction for prediction.[46] For primary care settings, the most prudent screening technique is to obtain a total serum cholesterol level. If it is elevated, fasting levels of total cholesterol, high-density lipoprotein cholesterol, and triglycerides can be obtained to define risk more precisely and to determine the hyperlipidemia pattern to guide future dietary and perhaps drug therapy (Chap. 36).

The relationship between the intake of dietary fats and the serum cholesterol level is well established,[47, 48] and there is evidence that dietary fat intake is also correlated with the progression of coronary atherosclerosis and with long-term coronary mortality.[49, 50] The Lipid Research Clinics Coronary Primary Prevention Trial[51, 52] demonstrated that treatment with cholestyramine resulted in a 13.4 per cent reduction in the serum cholesterol level in the group randomized to treatment, whereas cholesterol levels declined by only 4.9 per cent in the randomized control group. The risk of coronary heart disease death was 24 per cent lower and the risk of myocardial infarction was 19 per cent lower in the treated group than in the control group, and the reductions in events were almost exactly what would be predicted on the basis of the reductions in serum cholesterol levels and the known association between cholesterol and event rates.[53]

Berwick and colleagues[54] estimated that screening and dietary intervention programs for hypercholesterolemia in the pediatric population would cost about $25,000 (in 1985 dollars) for 10-year-old males and $22,000 for 10-year-old females per year of life gained. If the screening was limited to children with a known family history, the cost would be about $16,000 for males and $18,000 for females per year of life saved, while for children without a family history, the figures would be about $29,000 for males and $23,000 for females. Thus, in this example, a "targeted" program, which is limited to children who are at higher risk because of a known family history, would be more cost-effective than a nontargeted program. Dietary interventions are also recommended for adults with hypercholesterolemia,[55–57] although the cost-effectiveness has not been calculated precisely.

By comparison, the cost to gain a year of life by using cholestyramine in adults who have hypercholesterolemia despite dietary measures is far higher. As calculated by Weinstein and Stason,[58] and assuming an annual treatment cost of about $2000 for cholestyramine and full compliance with treatment, the cost per year of life gained among men aged 45 to 50 years with cholesterol levels above 265 mg/dl would be about $135,000 in 1985 dollars, given a 5 per cent per year discount rate. Although treatment would be more favorable if it were restricted to men with even higher serum cholesterol levels, at the current time drug therapy cannot be considered cost-effective for patients with moderate hypercholesterolemia.

DETECTION AND TREATMENT OF HYPERTENSION

Most epidemiological data emphasize that the systolic blood pressure is an independent significant predictor of coronary heart disease but that the diastolic blood pressure is not (after controlling for the systolic blood pressure).[53] Nevertheless, it has been common practice to define the threshold for treating hypertension on the basis of the diastolic blood pressure, and virtually all treatment trials use definitions that are based on the diastolic blood pressure level.

About 20 per cent of adults in the United States have diastolic blood pressures above 95 mm Hg, and about another 10 per cent have blood pressures of 90 to 94 mm Hg.[59] There is virtually unanimous agreement that treatment of persons whose diastolic blood pressure exceeds about 105 mm Hg will reduce mortality, although the main benefit in the Veterans Administration Trials was to prevent death from conditions other than coronary heart disease.[60–62] Of course, by preventing death from strokes, congestive heart failure, and renal failure, the treatment of hypertension permits more people to survive and potentially to develop coronary heart disease.

In recent years, numerous trials have evaluated the benefit of drug treatment for mild hypertension.[63–72] Many medications that are used to treat hypertension may raise the serum cholesterol and glucose concentrations, thereby theoretically offsetting some of their blood pressure–lowering benefits. However, data suggest that the modest elevations in serum cholesterol levels and the occasional precipitation of hyperglycemia are outweighed by the predicted benefit obtained by blood pressure reduction, thus supporting the value of antihypertensive therapy.[73, 74] (Of course, it would be even more desirable to treat hypertension without raising serum cholesterol or blood sugar.)

The Australian National Blood Pressure Study[68] demonstrated that treatment of persons with diastolic blood pressure of 95 to 109 mm Hg reduced cardiovascular mortality significantly, and the reduction in incidence of coronary heart disease events was similar to what would be predicted given the reductions in blood pressure levels using projections from the Framingham equations.[73] The Hypertension Detection Follow-up Program[63–66] showed a significant 20 per cent reduction in mortality in the stepped-care group. When data from all the randomized trials of the treatment of mild to moderate hypertension are pooled, there appears to be about a 10 per cent reduction in myocardial infarction in the treated patients.[74] Treatment is predicted to have the greatest absolute ben-

TABLE 52–3 APPROXIMATE COST PER QUALITY-ADJUSTED YEAR OF LIFE GAINED BY SCREENING AND/OR TREATMENT OF HYPERTENSION (1985 DOLLARS) GIVEN EXPECTED COMPLIANCE

Treat if diastolic blood pressure 105 mm Hg or greater	$15,000
Treat if diastolic blood pressure 95–104 mm Hg	$30,000
Screen for hypertension, treat if blood pressure 95 mm Hg or greater	$31,000

See references 79, 81, and 159.

efit in patients with higher blood pressures[73] and in patients with other risk factors for coronary disease.[75] There is uncertainty, however, as to whether diuretic therapy for hypertensive men with resting electrocardiographic abnormalities would actually increase mortality[72, 76–78] (p. 862).

Weinstein and Stason[79] used data from the Framingham Heart Study to calculate the cost-effectiveness of the treatment of mild hypertension. They concluded that the reduction in direct medical care costs for stroke and coronary heart disease would offset about 22 per cent of the cost of treating moderate to severe diastolic hypertension (105 mm Hg and above) and about 15 per cent of the cost for treating mild hypertension (95 to 104 mm Hg),[79–81] an estimate similar to those made by Stokes and Carmichael.[80] The costs for a quality-adjusted year of life gained by treating or screening for hypertension were calculated using 1975 dollars but are updated using 1985 dollars in Table 52–3. It should be noted that the costs of each of these programs are less than the inflation-adjusted annual cost of hemodialysis for chronic renal failure.[7] Although hypertension detection and treatment is most cost-effective when it is performed by the patients' own physicians as part of routine medical care,[79, 81, 82] worksite programs for the detection and treatment of hypertension can more than pay for themselves by reducing direct medical costs and absenteeism.[83]

CIGARETTE SMOKING

Cigarette smoking is an independently significant correlate of the risk of developing coronary heart disease (p. 1172) and is also a major risk factor for several types of cancer. Many of these risks appear to be reversed after smokers stop smoking. Recently, Oster and colleagues[84] used data from the American Cancer Society and from other sources[85] to estimate the increase in life expectancy that could be realized by smoking cessation (Table 52–4).

Although it is not possible to design a trial in which patients are randomized to continue smoking or to guarantee smoking cessation, substantial data confirm that discontinuing smoking improves prognosis. For example, in the Multiple-Risk Factor Intervention Trial (MRFIT),[72] the enrollees who discontinued smoking had a 48 per cent reduction in coronary deaths compared with those who continued smoking, and other data confirm that quitters have lower risks than persistent smokers.[86–88]

TABLE 52–4 INCREASE IN LIFE EXPECTANCY DUE TO SMOKING CESSATION, BY SEX AND AGE AT QUITTING

	Undiscounted Increase in Years of Life Expectancy due to Smoking Cessation	
Age at Quitting*	Men	Women
35–39	5.08	3.18
40–44	4.60	2.94
45–49	4.00	2.64
50–54	3.32	2.28
55–59	2.60	1.85
60–64	1.90	1.40
65–69	1.32	0.97

*Median age used for purposes of calculation.

Adapted from Oster, G., Huse, D. M., Delea, T. E., and Colditz, G. A.: Cost effectiveness of nicotine gum as an adjunct to the physician's advice against cigarette smoking. J.A.M.A. 256:131, 1986. Copyright 1986, American Medical Association.

There are a variety of interventions to reduce smoking. On average, about 4.5 per cent of smokers will discontinue the habit for one year after receiving a physician's advice,[89–94] although the rate of quitting will be higher in more highly motivated cohorts. Nicotine gum may increase the one-year likelihood of smoking cessation by about 35 per cent, suggesting that the cost of a physician's advice plus the availability of nicotine gum per year of life saved will range from about $4250 to $6900 in men aged 35 to 69 and from about $7300 to $10,000 in women aged 35 to 69 in 1985 dollars.[84, 95–102]

Public programs are also effective, with television advertisements against smoking among the most cost effective.[103] Physicians should not be discouraged by the relatively low rate of quitting that occurs immediately after their advice, since this advice is among the most cost-effective of all the interventions and may be a necessary psychological prelude to the patient's response to subsequent interventions.[104]

OBESITY

In long-term follow-up of the Framingham cohort, obesity emerged as an independently significant risk factor for the development of coronary artery disease[105] (p. 1176). Unfortunately, it is extremely difficult for most adults to lose weight and to maintain the weight loss over the long term. Programs in schools or at the worksite commonly can help achieve weight losses of 2 to 5 kilograms at costs that are about $10 to $30 per kilogram lost, which would be highly cost-effective.[106, 107] Lay organizations such as Weight Watchers also can aid in producing similar losses at similar costs and are clearly cost-effective despite the high attrition rate.[108] More intensive weight loss programs for motivated individuals may still be very cost-effective for those persons for whom simpler measures are ineffective.[108] Although physicians may become discouraged over the ability of their patients to lose weight, the usual effects of these other programs are not substantially greater than what may sometimes be achieved simply by a physician's advice. Furthermore, it is often a physician's advice that influences patients to try other interventions that might not be considered if the physician had not identified overweight as a medical problem.

PHYSICAL ACTIVITY

Substantial data indicate that physical activity reduces coronary heart disease, partly because of its beneficial effects on other risk factors but apparently partly independently.[109–113] Unfortunately, it has been reported that less than 10 per cent of physicians recommend exercise for their patients.[114] However, many patients both want and expect their physicians to make recommendations regarding physical activity,[114] and in one survey about 25 per cent of active persons ascribed their activity in large part to the advice of a physician.[115]

Worksite exercise programs are also potentially cost-effective independent of their possible effect on the development of clinical coronary artery disease. In one study, employees in the experimental exercise program group missed fewer days of work, were more likely to remain employed, and had fewer hospital days and fewer medical claims, thus resulting in substantial health care savings.[116, 117] In fact, some employers have decided to pay their employees directly for participating in exercise programs, such as jogging. Unlike antismoking campaigns, media campaigns advocating exercise seem to encourage persons to seek out other programs in the community but not to lead to direct changes in behavior by themselves.[114, 118] Thus, it appears that a physician's encouragement of increased physical activity, especially if combined with direct guidance on how to implement the suggestion, can lead to major changes in health behavior. Although it is difficult to determine the exact degree of effectiveness to be gained for the cost, there are substantial data linking physical activity to other cardiovascular risk factors and probably independently to cardiovascular risk.[113] These data suggest that efforts to increase physical activity have the potential for being highly cost-effective.

PREVENTION OF INFECTIVE ENDOCARDITIS IN VALVULAR HEART DISEASE

(See also p. 1127)

By extrapolation from cost-effectiveness analyses,[119, 120] penicillin prophylaxis to prevent bacterial endocarditis in patients with rheumatic valvular heart disease appears to have a cost-effectiveness of about $10,000 per year of life gained. In patients with prosthetic heart valves, in whom the risk of endocarditis is higher, the cost-effectiveness is likely to be even more favorable. By comparison, two detailed cost-effectiveness analyses[119, 120] indicate that penicillin prophylaxis prior to dental work to prevent bacterial endocarditis is *not* cost-effective for patients with mitral valve prolapse (p. 1051). Using the most likely assumptions, persons are as likely to die from penicillin reactions as from endocarditis, and even given the most optimistic assumptions, it is estimated that routine pencillin prophylaxis for dental procedures in patients with mitral valve prolapse would cost over a million dollars to save a year of life. In most studies of mitral valve prolapse, the risk of endocarditis is substantially higher in patients with murmurs of mitral regurgitation,[121, 122] but it is not clear whether the cost-effectiveness in this subpopulation of patients with mitral valve prolapse is analogous to that of patients with rheumatic valvular disease.

PREHOSPITAL EMERGENCY SERVICES

(See also Chap. 24)

Prehospital emergency services range from basic life support to advanced life support services. As of 1980, more than 300 advanced life support programs, which include interventions such as defibrillation, endotracheal intubation, and intravenous or intramuscular medications, have been instituted in the United States.[123] Since about 60 per cent of patients whose death certificates list the cause of death as myocardial infarction die outside of the hospital, advances in prehospital emergency services could have a substantial impact on survival.

Prehospital emergency care appears to be extremely successful in patients who have ventricular fibrillation and who are seen very soon after cardiac arrest (p. 759). For example, in pooled data, about two-thirds of patients who are seen within 5 minutes of a ventricular fibrillation arrest survive to leave the hospital.[124] Unfortunately, many arrests are not caused by ventricular fibrillation, and even the most successful prehospital emergency services often cannot deliver care within 5 minutes. Thus, only about 15 to 20 per cent of prehospital cardiac arrest patients commonly survive to leave the hospital in even the best programs.[123, 125] These higher rates are achieved principally through advanced life support programs utilizing paramedics, which appear to increase the likelihood of reaching the hospital alive from about 19 to 34 per cent and the likelihood of being discharged alive from the hospital from 7 to 17 per cent.[123] However, the prognosis after hospital discharge of patients who were resuscitated from prehospital arrest is only about 75 per cent as high as age- and sex-matched comparison groups who have survived myocardial infarction without prehospital arrest, and it is only about 60 per cent as high as for age- and sex-adjusted members of the general population.[125]

The cost-effectiveness of prehospital emergency programs is difficult to estimate. One analysis estimated that a mobile coronary care unit has an incremental cost of about $19,000 (in 1985 dollars) per life saved above and beyond the cost of the ambulance system itself.[126] Another analysis[127] estimated that the incremental cost-effectiveness of a mobile coronary care unit was $77,000 (in 1985 dollars) per life saved and $38,000 (in 1985 dollars) per year of life saved, but this analysis included only the incremental costs of the mobile coronary care unit program and not the costs of the existing emergency medical technician and community training program to which it was added.

Analyses of the cost-effectiveness of prehospital emergency services depend on assumptions about the mean response time and the patients' prognoses, both in terms of life expectancy and in terms of quality of life and neurological impairment. For example, the longer the response time, the more likely it is that survivors of prehospital cardiac arrest will have neurological impairment. If the years of life expectancy that are gained are compromised by such neurological impairment, then the *quality* of those years of life will not be the same as the quality of the years of life that might be gained from preventive measures that delay the onset of disease. Thus, when the calculation of cost-effectiveness is adjusted for the years of life that are gained without major neurological impairment, the apparent benefit of prehospital resuscitation may be reduced. Furthermore, patients whose lives are saved by prehospital emergency services are likely to require careful medical follow-up, sometimes including expensive interventions such as coronary bypass grafting. Most studies have not clearly considered the fact that the survivors of out-of-hospital cardiac arrest will have costs other than those included in the first term of the equation in Table 52–1, such as the costs for rehabilitative and custodial care and the costs for additional diagnosis and therapy of the substantial coronary disease that may have precipitated the arrest. If these costs are taken into account, the relative cost-effectiveness of prehospital emergency services programs would be less appealing than the preceding estimates.

CORONARY CARE UNITS

Coronary care units were originally designed to provide the ready availability of resuscitative services to patients with obvious acute myocardial infarction (p. 1249). The mission of these units subsequently has been broadened substantially: patients are now admitted to rule out a myocardial infarction if there is a reasonable suspicion that one may have occurred. The interventions in these units now include prevention of arrhythmias, medical and surgical treatment of acute ischemia, treatment of severe pump failure, and procedures designed to prevent or to limit the size of the acute myocardial infarction. It is difficult, if not impossible, to disentangle each of these potential aspects of coronary care units.

HOME CARE VS CORONARY CARE. Two trials in Great Britain showed no significant difference in the survival of patients who were admitted to coronary care units compared with randomized controls who were treated at home.[128, 129] However, these studies were too small to detect the expected difference in mortality.[130] Furthermore, patients were eligible for randomization only after prolonged home observation, during which time high-risk patients were excluded and a substantial proportion of patients were actually resuscitated. Thus, these studies do not appear to apply to unselected patients coming to American hospitals. In fact, available data suggest that patients who are mistakenly discharged from the emergency room appear to have a significantly higher mortality with their acute myocardial infarctions than patients who are correctly admitted.[131]

REDUCTION OF MORTALITY IN THE CCU. If one assumes that the risk of primary ventricular fibrillation in an acute myocardial infarction is about 4.5 per cent and that the likelihood of successful resuscitation and hospital survival is about 88 per cent in coronary care units,[132] coronary care units would result in about a 4 percentage point decline in the in-hospital mortality from acute myocardial infarction compared to the pre-coronary care unit era when defibrillation could not be carried out promptly on a regular nursing unit. Data from the Minnesota area[133] document a positive effect of about this magnitude. The extent to which other intensive interventions carried out in the coronary care unit or originating from decisions made in the unit (such as intraaortic balloon counterpulsation, intravenous afterload reduction and use of beta-adrenoceptor agonists, and emergency percutaneous transluminal coronary angioplasty and coronary artery bypass grafting) contribute to a further decline in the mortality from acute myocardial infarction is less certain, even though it is clear that these interventions occasionally save individual patients. These newer, intensive interventions commonly are very costly, and they are designed to save sicker patients, which may result in fewer net years of life saved because the long-term prognosis of these sicker patients is poorer. Compared with more basic coronary care unit services, these newer, intensive interventions have higher marginal costs and lower marginal benefits. As interventions become more and more costly and save fewer and fewer lives, marginal cost-effectiveness falls, consistent with the law of diminishing returns. One can eventually approach what has been termed "flat of the curve medicine," in which the increased costs of expensive interventions yield essentially no incremental effectiveness.

It is extremely difficult to estimate the actual cost-effectiveness of coronary care units because there has never been an adequate randomized control trial in unselected patients. If the finding that the mortality is about twice as high among patients who are mistakenly discharged from the emergency room as among patients who are correctly admitted[131] is confirmed, coronary care units would be very cost-effective.

COST-EFFECTIVE ANALYSES. Because it has been difficult to estimate the cost-effectiveness of the coronary care unit overall, most analyses have concentrated on the cost-effectiveness of modifications in the original recommendation that patients with definite or suspected myocardial infarction be kept in intensive care for 3 days. For example, coronary care unit admission can be applied selectively only to patients whose probability of myocardial infarction is sufficiently high for it to be cost-effective.[3] Thus, if the probability of myocardial infarction is only 5 per cent, the incremental cost per year of life saved by admission to the coronary care unit compared with an intermediate care unit is about $194,000 (in 1985 dollars); and the cost will fall to about $46,000 (in 1985 dollars) per year of life saved if the potential for acute myocardial infarction is 20 per cent. These estimates suggest that it may be worthwhile for physicians to estimate the probability of acute myocardial infarction from clinical data or from more sophisticated calculations.[16, 17] Although data are limited, preliminary analyses suggest that the intermediate care option, which would be analogous to many "stepdown" units in which electrocardiographic monitoring and resuscitative facilities are available but in which patients do not receive intensive care nursing, is safe in patients in whom there is no indication on admission that they already need intensive care interventions.[134]

LENGTH OF STAY. The coronary care unit can also be made more cost-effective by limiting the length of stay. Data indicate that, except in patients who have recurrent ischemic pain, 24 hours is nearly always sufficient to determine whether or not a myocardial infarction has occurred.[135] Similar protocols using the electrocardiogram, the history, and serum enzyme levels substantiate that 24 hours is often a sufficient length of stay.[136] If coronary care units were used in this more cost-effective manner, the relative cost-effectiveness for patients with symptoms indicative of but not diagnostic of an acute myocardial infarction would be improved, since the original calculations noted above assumed a longer average length of stay.

When faced with a shortage of coronary care unit beds, physicians can identify correctly which patients are most in need.[137] It is estimated that coronary care units may save 20,000 lives per year and are probably responsible for about 10 to 15 per cent of the decline in coronary heart disease mortality between 1968 and 1976.[138] It is likely that coronary care units can become substantially more cost-effective by limiting admission to patients whose probability of acute myocardial infarction is at least 10 or 20 per cent and by shortening the average length of stay for patients who do not have documented myocardial infarctions or complications. Intermediate care (or "stepdown") unit admission appears to be quite cost-effective for patients whose probability of acute myocardial infarction is too high for discharge to be appropriate but not high enough for coronary care unit admission to be worthwhile.

MEDICAL THERAPY OF CORONARY ARTERY DISEASE

Although the natural history of patients with medically treated coronary artery disease appears to be improving, it is difficult to measure the impact of specific aspects of the medical treatment. The best-studied intervention is the use of "prophylactic" beta-adrenoceptor antagonists in survivors of a recent myocardial infarction. Numerous studies[139–144] have shown a substantial benefit from routine use of beta-adrenoceptor antagonists in patients who are ready for discharge after an acute myocardial infarction (p. 1288). Several studies[139, 140, 143, 145–148] indicate that the relative reduction in mortality in years 2 and 3 is similar to the 25 to 30 per cent reduction found in year 1. In the fourth, fifth, and sixth years, the benefit appears to be smaller, closer to 8 to 9 per cent.[149] Based on the costs of the medications, and the likely benefits in patients with various risks of short- and long-term complications, cost-effectiveness analysis indicates that the cost of beta-adrenoceptor antagonist therapy to save one year of life is about $3500 (in 1985 dollars) in patients at high risk for complications, about $5500 for medium-risk patients, and about $20,000 for low-risk patients. Altering the patients' age from 45 to 65 years had little effect on the analysis. These calculations suggest that beta adrenoceptor antagonist therapy in the post-myocardial infarction patient is extremely cost-effective in high- and medium-risk patients and is still rather cost-effective even in low-risk patients.[150] It is not possible as of this writing to make analogous calculations in patients with angina who have not recently survived a myocardial infarction.

CORONARY ARTERY BYPASS GRAFTING

Coronary artery bypass grafting prolongs the life of patients with left main coronary artery disease and of patients with three-vessel disease and left ventricular dysfunction.[151–153] Data on patients with less severe degrees of disease are conflicting, with the European trial[154] being the only major randomized study that showed a significant advantage for surgery among patients with two-vessel disease that included the left anterior descending artery.

In patients with marked symptoms, coronary artery bypass grafting is very efficacious in improving symptomatic status. However, several studies indicate that coronary artery bypass grafting does not, in general, improve work status[155–157] even though it improves quality of life.[155, 158] Weinstein and Stason estimated that the net cost of coronary bypass grafting is about $19,000 to $21,500 (in 1985 dollars).[159] Data also indicate that the initial investment in coronary artery bypass surgery is not offset by lower subsequent treatment costs.[160] Weinstein and Stason have also performed the most extensive cost-effectiveness analysis of coronary artery bypass grafting in patients with various symptomatic states and extents of disease[159] (Table 52–5). These calculations suggest that in patients with three-vessel disease or left main coronary artery disease, or in patients with two-vessel disease and severe angina, the cost per year of life gained from coronary bypass grafting compares favorably to the cost per year of life gained from renal dialysis in patients with chronic renal failure.

PERCUTANEOUS TRANSLUMINAL CORONARY ANGIOPLASTY

(See also Chap. 40)

The initial charges for percutaneous transluminal coronary angioplasty (PTCA) have been reported to be about 60 per cent as high as for coronary artery bypass grafting,[161–163] but this estimate included the substantial cost of the availability of standby surgery.[164] The true costs of a treatment strategy, including PTCA, must consider the immediate failure rate, the possible need for urgent coronary artery bypass grafting, and the likelihood of restenosis and its subsequent treatment. If the PTCA can be performed at a time of day when an operating suite and team normally would be "between cases," without causing them to be idle during a period when they would otherwise be in full use, the actual cost of the availability of standby surgery would be minimal and angioplasty becomes more cost-effective.

Even given the full costs of surgical standby, the expenditures for patients undergoing PTCA were significantly lower at one year than those of patients treated with coronary artery bypass grafting.[161] Since this study reported a 30 per cent immediate failure rate and a 22 per cent restenosis rate at one year, it is expected that the cost-effectiveness of PTCA will be substantially better as the initial and medium-term success rates improve.

TABLE 52–5 ESTIMATED APPROXIMATE COST PER GAIN IN ONE QUALITY-ADJUSTED YEAR OF LIFE FOR CORONARY ARTERY BYPASS GRAFTING (SEE REFERENCE 159; CALCULATIONS ARE UPDATED TO 1985 DOLLARS)

	One-Vessel Disease	Two-Vessel Disease	Three-Vessel Disease	Left Main Disease
Very mild angina	*	64,000	10,500	4,700
Mild angina	640,000	41,000	10,000	4,900
Severe angina	41,000	24,000	9,800	5,200

*Quality-adjusted life expectancy is reduced.

SUMMARY

Physicians should not view the current emphasis on cost-effective care as contradictory to excellent care. Patients should not be treated as numbers, and optimal medical care cannot be derived routinely from equations. The physician's principal responsibility is to render the best possible medical care to the patient as an individual. An understanding of the principles of cost-effectiveness should allow the physician to improve the choice of diagnostic and therapeutic strategies, and it should assist the physician's ability to determine strategies that are optimal in the aggregate and to adopt or adapt them for the individual at hand. In such a context, more cost-effective care implies better care for the individual patient as well as the conservation of resources to improve care for the population as a whole.

REFERENCES

QUANTITATIVE ANALYSES OF COSTS AND EFFECTIVENESS

1. Weinstein, M. C., and Fineberg, H. V.: Clinical Decision Analysis. Philadelphia, W. B. Saunders Company, 1980.
2. Weinstein, M. C., and Stason, W. B.: Foundations of cost-effectiveness analysis for health and medical practices. N. Engl. J. Med. *296*:716, 1977.
3. Fineberg, H., Scadden, D., and Goldman, L.: Management of patients with a low probability of acute myocardial infarction: Cost-effectiveness of alternatives to coronary care unit admission. N. Engl. J. Med. *310*:1301, 1984.
4. Kwoh, C. K., Beck, J. R., and Pauker, S. G.: Repeated syncope with negative diagnostic evaluation. To pace or not to pace? Med. Decis. Making *4*:351, 1984.
5. Doubilet, P., Weinstein, M. D., and McNeil, B. J.: Use and misuse of the term "cost effective" in medicine (Editorial). N. Engl. J. Med. *314*:253, 1986.
6. Finkler, S. A.: The distinction between cost and charges. Ann. Intern. Med. *96*:102, 1982.
7. Roberts, S. D., Maxwell, D. R., and Gross, T. L.: Cost-effective care of end-stage renal disease: A billion-dollar question. Ann. Intern. Med. *92*:243, 1980.

DIAGNOSTIC TESTING

8. Goldman, L.: Quantitative aspects of clinical reasoning. *In* Braunwald, E., Isselbacher, K. J., Petersdorf, R. G., Wilson, J. D., Martin, J. B., and Fauci, A. S. (eds.): Harrison's Principles of Internal Medicine. New York, McGraw Hill, 1986, pp. 5–12.
9. Goldman, L., and Adams, J. B.: Cost-effectiveness in medical decision making: Cardiac nuclear medicine and exercise electrocardiograms. Cardiovasc. Rev. Rep. 2:45, 1981.
10. Rifkin, R. D., and Hood, W. B.: Bayesian analysis of electrocardiographic exercise stress testing. N. Engl. J. Med. *297*:681, 1977.
11. Diamond, G. A., Staniloff, H. M., Forrester, J. S., Pollock, B. H., and Swan, H. J. C.: Computer-assisted diagnosis in the noninvasive evaluation of patients with suspected coronary artery disease. J. Am. Coll. Cardiol. *1*:444, 1983.
12. Goldman, L., Cook, E. F., Mitchell, N., Flatley, M., Sherman, H., Rosati, R., Harrell, F., Lee, K., and Cohn, P. F.: Incremental value of the exercise test for diagnosing the presence or absence of coronary artery disease. Circulation *66*:945, 1982.
13. Weiner, D. A., Ryan, T. J., McCabe, C. H., Kennedy, J. W., Schloss, M., Tristani, F., Chaitman, B. R., and Fisher, L. D.: Exercise stress testing:

Correlations among history of angina, ST-segment response and prevalence of coronary-artery disease in the coronary artery surgery study (CASS). N. Engl. J. Med. *300*:230, 1979.
14. Diamond, G. A., and Forrester, J. S.: Analysis of probability as an aid in the clinical diagnosis of coronary artery disease. N. Engl. J. Med. *300*:1350, 1979.
15. Hoagland, P. M., Cook, E. F., Wynne, J., and Goldman, L.: Value of noninvasive testing in adults with suspected aortic stenosis. Am. J. Med. *80*:1041, 1986.
16. Goldman, L., Weinberg, M., Weisberg, M., Olshen, R., Cook, E. F., Sargent, R. K., Lamas, G. A., Dennis, C., Wilson, C., Deckelbaum, L., Fineberg, H., Stiratelli, R., and the Medical House Staffs at Yale-New Haven Hospital and Brigham and Women's Hospital: A computer-derived protocol to aid in the diagnosis of emergency room patients with acute chest pain. N. Engl. J. Med. *307*:588, 1982.
17. Pozen, M. W., D'Agostino, R. B., Selker, H. P., Sytkowski, P. A., and Hood, W. B.: A predictive instrument to improve coronary care unit admission practices in acute ischemic heart disease. A prospective multicenter clinical trial. N. Engl. J. Med. *310*:1273, 1984.
18. Goldman, L., Feinstein, A. R., Batsford, W. P., Cohen, L. S., Gottschalk, A., and Zaret, B. L.: Ordering patterns and clinical impact of cardiovascular nuclear medicine procedures. Circulation *62*:680, 1980.
19. Goldman, L., Cohn, P. F., Mudge, G. H. Jr., Hashimoto, B., Sherman, H., Wynne, J., and Flatley, M.: Clinical utility and management impact of M-mode echocardiography. Am. J. Med. *75*:49, 1983.
20. Sox, H. C., Margulies, I., and Sox, C. H.: Psychologically mediated effects of diagnostic tests. Ann. Intern. Med. *95*:680, 1981.
21. McNeil, B. J., Keeler, E., and Adelstein, S. J.: Primer on certain elements of medical decision-making. N. Engl. J. Med. *293*:211, 1975.
22. Lee, T. H., and Goldman, L.: Serum enzyme assays in the diagnosis of acute myocardial infarction. Recommendations based on a quantitative analysis. Ann. Intern. Med. *105*:221, 1986.
23. Vasudevan, G., Mercer, D. W., and Varat, M. A.: Lactic dehydrogenase isoenzyme determination in the diagnosis of acute myocardial infarction. Circulation *57*:1055, 1978.
24. Pauker, S. G., and Kassirer, J. P.: Therapeutic decision-making: A cost-benefit analysis. N. Engl. J. Med. *293*:229, 1975.
25. Pauker, S. G., and Kassirer, J. P.: The threshold approach to clinical decision-making. N. Engl. J. Med. *302*:1109, 1980.
26. Goldschlager, N.: Use of the treadmill test in the diagnosis of coronary artery disease in patients with chest pain. Ann. Intern. Med. *97*:383, 1982.
27. Philbrick, J. T., Horwitz, R. I., and Feinstein, A. R.: Methodologic problems of exercise testing for coronary artery disease: Groups, analysis and bias. Am. J. Cardiol. *46*:807, 1980.
28. Gitler, B., Fishbach, M., and Steingart, R. M.: Use of electrocardiographic-thallium exercise testing in clinical practice. J. Am. Coll. Cardiol. *3*:262, 1984.
29. Hung, J., Chaitman, B. R., Lam, J., Lesperance, J., Dupras, G., Fines, P., and Bourassa, M. G.: Noninvasive diagnostic test choices for the evaluation of coronary artery disease in women: A multivariate comparison of cardiac fluoroscopy, exercise electrocardiography and exercise thallium myocardial perfusion scintigraphy. J. Am. Coll. Cardiol. *4*:8, 1984.
30. Melin, J. A., Piret, L. J., Vanbutsele, R. J. M., Rousseau, M. F., Cosyns, J., Brasseur, L. A., Beckers, C., and Detry, J. M. R.: Diagnostic value of exercise electrocardiography and thallium myocardial scintigraphy in patients without previous myocardial infarction: A Bayesian approach. Circulation *63*:1019, 1981.
31. Patterson, R. E., Horowitz, S. F., Eng, C., Rubin, A., Meller, J, Halgash, D. A., Pichard, A. D., Goldsmith, S. J., Herman, M. V., and Gorlin, R.: Can exercise electrocardiography and thallium-201 myocardial imaging exclude the diagnosis of coronary artery disease? Bayesian analysis of the clinical limits of exclusion and indications for coronary angiography. Am. J. Cardiol. *49*:1127, 1982.
32. Patterson, R. E., Eng, C., Horowitz, S. F., Gorlin, R., and Goldstein, S. R.: Bayesian comparison of cost-effectiveness of different clinical approaches to diagnose coronary artery disease. J. Am. Coll. Cardiol. *4*:278, 1984.
33. Ritchie, J. L., Zaret, B. L., Strauss, H. W., Pitt, B., Berman, D. S., Schelbert, H. R., Ashburn, W. L., Berger, H. J., and Hamilton, G. W.: Myocardial imaging with thallium-201: A multicenter study in patients with angina pectoris or acute myocardial infarction. Am. J. Cardiol. *43*:345, 1978.
34. Okada, R. D., Boucher, C. A., Strauss, H. W., and Pohost, G. M.: Exercise radionuclide imaging approaches to coronary artery disease. Am. J. Cardiol. *46*:1188, 1980.
35. Weintraub, W. S., Madeira, S. W., Bodenheimer, M. M., Seelaus, P. A., Katz, R. I., Feldman, M. S., Agarwal, J. B., Banka, V. S., and Helfant, R. H.: Critical analysis of the application of Bayes' theorem to sequential testing in the noninvasive diagnosis of coronary artery disease. Am. J. Cardiol. *54*:43, 1984.
36. Pamelia, F. X., Gibson, R. S., Watson, D. D., Craddock, G. B., Sirowatka, J., and Beller, G. A.: Prognosis with chest pain and normal thallium-201 exercise scintigrams. Am. J. Cardiol. *55*:920, 1985.
37. Gordon, D. J., Ekelund, L., Karon, J. M., Probstfield, J. L., Rubenstein, C., Sheffield, L. T., and Weissfield, L.: Predictive value of the exercise tolerance test for mortality in North American men: The Lipid Research Clinics Mortality Follow-up Study. Circulation *74*:252, 1986.
38. Goldman, L.: Noninvasive tests in cardiology. *In* Branch, W., Jr. (ed.): The Office Practice of Medicine. 2nd ed. Philadelphia, W. B. Saunders Company, 1987.
39. Harrell, F. E., Califf, R. M., Pryor, D. B., Lee, K. L., and Rosati, R. A.: Evaluating the yield of medical tests. J.A.M.A. *247*:2543, 1982.
40. Gorry, G. A., Pauker, S. G., and Schwartz, W. B.: The diagnostic importance of the normal finding. N. Engl. J. Med. *298*:486, 1978.
41. Epstein, A. M., Hartley, R. M., Charlton, J. R., Harris, C. M., Jarman, B., and McNeil, B. J.: A comparison of ambulatory test ordering for hypertensive patients in the United States and England. J.A.M.A. *252*:1723, 1984.
42. Fineberg, H. V., and Hiatt, H. H.: Evaluation of medical practices. The case for technology assessment. N. Engl. J. Med. *301*:1086, 1979.
43. Moloney, T. W., and Rogers, D. E.: Medical technology—a different view of the contentious debate over costs. N. Engl. J. Med. *301*:1413, 1979.
44. Griner, P. F., and the Medical House Staff, Strong Memorial Hospital, Rochester, New York: Use of laboratory tests in a teaching hospital: Long-term trends. Reductions in use and relative cost. Ann. Intern. Med. *90*:243, 1979.

PREVENTION AND TREATMENT

45. Hulley, S. B., Rosenman, R. H., Bawol, R. D., and Brand, R. J.: Epidemiology as a guide to clinical decisions. The association between triglyceride and coronary heart disease. N. Engl. J. Med. *302*:1383, 1980.
46. Kannel, W. B., Castelli, W. P., and Gordon, T.: Cholesterol in the prediction of atherosclerotic disease. New perspectives based on the Framingham Study. Ann. Intern. Med. *90*:85, 1979.
47. Keys, A., Anderson, J. T., and Grande, F.: Serum cholesterol response to changes in diet. IV. Particular saturated fatty acids in the diet. Metabolism *14*:776, 1965.
48. Hegsted, D. M., McGandy, R. B., Myers, M. L., and Stare, F. J.: Quantitative effects of dietary fat on serum cholesterol in man. Am. J. Clin. Nutr. *17*:281, 1965.
49. Arntzenius, A. C., Kromhout, D., Barth, J. D., Reiber, J. H. C., Bruschke, A. V. G., Buis, B., van Gent, C. M., Kempen-Voogd, N., Strikwerda, S., and van der Velde, E. A.: Diet, lipoproteins, and the progression of coronary atherosclerosis. The Leiden Intervention Trial. N. Engl. J. Med. *312*:805, 1985.
50. Kushi, L. H., Lew, R. A., Stare, F. J., Ellison, C. R., el Lozy, M., Bourke, G., Daly, L., Graham, I., Hickey, N., Mulcahy, R., and Kevaney, J.: Diet and 20-year mortality from coronary heart disease. The Ireland-Boston Diet-Heart Study. N. Engl. J. Med. *312*:811, 1985.
51. The Lipid Research Clinics Program: The Lipid Research Clinics Coronary Primary Prevention Trial results. I. Reduction in incidence of coronary heart disease. J.A.M.A. *251*:351, 1984.
52. The Lipid Research Clinics Program: The Lipid Research Clinics Coronary Primary Prevention Trial results. II. The relationship of reduction in incidence of coronary heart disease to cholesterol lowering. J.A.M.A. *251*:365, 1984.
53. Kannel, W. B., and Gordon, T. (eds.): The Framingham Study: An Epidemiologic Investigation of Cardiovascular Disease. Sections 1–32. Washington, D.C., U. S. Government Printing Office, 1970–1977.
54. Berwick, D. M., Cretin, S., and Keeler, E.: Cholesterol, Children, and Heart Disease: An Analysis of Alternatives. New York, Oxford University Press, 1980.
55. Lenfant, C.: A new challenge for America: The National Cholesterol Education Program. Circulation *73*:855, 1986.
56. Stamler, J., Wentworth, D., and Neaton, J. D.: Is relationship between serum cholesterol and risk of premature death from coronary heart disease continuous and graded? Findings in 356,222 primary screenees of the Multiple-Risk Factor Intervention Trial (MRFIT). J.A.M.A. *256*:2823, 1986.
57. The Consensus Conference, National Institutes of Health: Lowering blood cholesterol to prevent heart disease. J.A.M.A. *253*:2080, 1985.
58. Weinstein, M. C., and Stason, W. B.: Cost-effectiveness of interventions to prevent or treat coronary heart disease. Ann. Rev. Public Health *6*:41, 1985.
59. National Center for Health Statistics, U.S. Public Health Service: National Health and Nutrition Examination Survey 1976-1980. Public Use Data Tape. Hyattsville, MD, U.S. Department of Health and Human Services, 1982.
60. Veterans Administration Cooperative Study Group on Antihypertensive Agents: Effects of treatment on morbidity in hypertension. Part 1. J.A.M.A. *202*:1028, 1967.
61. Veterans Administration Cooperative Study Group on Antihypertensive Agents: Effects of treatment on morbidity in hypertension. Part 2. J.A.M.A. *213*:1143, 1970.
62. Veterans Administration Cooperative Study Group on Antihypertensive Agents: Effects of treatment on morbidity in hypertension. Part 3. Circulation *45*:991, 1972.
63. Hypertension Detection and Follow-up Program Cooperative Group: Five-year findings of the Hypertension Detection and Follow-up Program: I. Reduction in mortality of persons with high blood pressure, including mild hypertension. J.A.M.A. *242*:2562, 1979.
64. Hypertension Detection and Follow-up Program Cooperative Group: Five-year findings of the Hypertension Detection and Follow-up Program: III. Reduction in stroke incidence among persons with high blood pressure. J.A.M.A. *247*:633, 1982.
65. Hypertension Detection and Follow-up Program Cooperative Group: The effect of treatment on mortality in "mild" hypertension: Results of the Hypertension Detection and Follow-up Program. N. Engl. J. Med. *307*:976, 1982.
66. Hypertension Detection and Follow-up Program Cooperative Group: Effect of stepped care treatment on the incidence of myocardial infarction and angina pectoris: Five-year findings of the Hypertension Detection and Follow-up Program. Hypertension *6* (Suppl I):198, 1984.
67. Helgeland, A.: Treatment of mild hypertension: A five-year controlled drug trial: The Oslo study. Am. J. Med. *69*:725, 1980.
68. Australian National Blood Pressure Management Committee: The Australian therapeutic trial in mild hypertension. Lancet *1*:1261, 1980.

69. Medical Research Council Working Party: MRC trial of treatment of mild hypertension: Principal results. Br. Med. J. *291*:97, 1985.
70. Amery, A., Birkenhager, W., Brixko, P., et al.: Mortality and morbidity results from the European Working Party on High Blood Pressure in the Elderly trial. Lancet *1*:1349, 1985.
71. Coope, J., and Warrender, T. S.: Randomized trial of treatment of hypertension in the elderly in primary care. Br. Med. J. *293*:1145, 1986.
72. Multiple-Risk Factor Intervention Trial Research Group: Multiple-Risk Factor Intervention Trial: Risk factor changes and mortality results. J.A.M.A. *248*:1465, 1982.
73. Shea, S., Cook, E. F., Kannel, W. B., and Goldman, L.: Treatment of hypertension and its effect on cardiovascular risk factors: Data from the Framingham Heart Study. Circulation *71*:22, 1985.
74. Hebert, P. R., Fiebach, N. H., Eberlein, K. A., Taylor, J. O., and Hennekens, C. H.: The community-based randomized trials of pharmacologic treatment of mild-to-moderate hypertension. Am. J. Epidemiol. *in press.*
75. Freis, E. D.: Should mild hypertension be treated? (Editorial) N. Engl. J. Med. *307*:306, 1982.
76. Hollifield, J. W.: Thiazide treatment of hypertension. Effects of thiazide diuretics on serum potassium, magnesium, and ventricular ectopy. Am. J. Med. *80*(Suppl. 4A):8, 1986.
77. Helfant, R. H.: Hypokalemia and arrhythmias. Am. J. Med. *80*(Suppl. 4):13, 1986.
78. The Hypertension Detection and Follow-up Program Cooperative Research Group: The effect of antihypertensive drug treatment on mortality in the presence of resting electrocardiographic abnormalities at baseline: The HDFP experience. Circulation *70*:996, 1984.
79. Weinstein, M. C., and Stason, W. B.: Hypertension: A Policy Perspective. Cambridge, Harvard University Press, 1976.
80. Stokes, J., III, and Carmichael, D. C.: A Cost-Benefit Analysis of Model Hypertension Control. Bethesda, National Heart, Lung and Blood Institute, 1975.
81. Weinstein, M. C., and Stason, W. B.: Economic considerations in the management of mild hypertension. Ann. N. Y. Acad. Sci. *304*:424, 1978.
82. Christianson, J. B., Krishan, I., Nobrega, F. T., Davis, C. S., Smoldt, R. K., and Harris, A. M.: The Mayo Three-Community Hypertension Control Program. V. Cost-effectiveness of intervention. Mayo Clin. Proc. *56*:11, 1981.
83. Hannan, E. L., and Graham, J. K.: A cost-benefit study of hypertension screening and treatment program at the work setting. Inquiry *15*:345, 1978.
84. Oster, G., Huse, D. M., Delea, T. E., and Colditz, G. A.: Cost effectiveness of nicotine gum as an adjunct to physician's advice against cigarette smoking. J.A.M.A. *256*:1315, 1986.
85. Doll, R., and Peto, R.: Mortality in relation to smoking: Twenty years observation on male British doctors. Br. Med. J. *2*:1525, 1976.
86. Friedman, G. D., Petitti, D. B., Bawol, R. D., and Siegelaub, A. B.: Mortality in cigarette smokers and quitters. Effect of base-line differences. N. Engl. J. Med. *304*:1407, 1981.
87. Rosenberg, L., Kaufman, D. W., Helmrich, S. P., and Shapiro, S.: The risk of myocardial infarction after quitting smoking in men under 55 years of age. N. Engl. J. Med. *313*:1511, 1985.
88. Vlietstra, R. E., Kronmal, R. A., Oberman, A., Frye, R. L., and Killip, T., III.: Effect of cigarette smoking on survival of patients with angiographically documented coronary artery disease. J.A.M.A. *255*:1023, 1986.
89. Russell, M. A., Merriman, R., Stapelton, J., and Taylor, W.: Effect of nicotine chewing gum as an adjunct to general practitioners' advice against smoking. Br. Med. J. *287*:1782, 1983.
90. Russell, M. A., Wilson, C., Taylor, C., and Baker, C. D.: Effect of practitioners' advice against smoking. Br. Med. J. *2*:231, 1979.
91. Jamrozik, K., Vessey, M., Fowler, G., Wald, N., Parker, G., and Van Vunakis, H.: Controlled trial of three different antismoking interventions in general practice. Br. Med. J. *288*:1499, 1984.
92. Handel, S.: Change in smoking habits in a general practice. Postgrad. Med. J. *49*:679, 1973.
93. Pincherle, G., and Wright, H. B.: Smoking habits of business executives. Practitioner *205*:209, 1970.
94. Stewart, P. J., and Rosser, W. W.: The impact of routine advice on smoking cessation from family physicians. Can. Med. Assoc. J. *126*:1051, 1982.
95. Fagerstrom, K. O.: A comparison of psychological and pharmacological treatment in smoking cessation. J. Behav. Med. *5*:343, 1982.
96. Fee, W. M., and Stewart, M. J.: A controlled trial of nicotine chewing gum in a smoking withdrawal clinic. Practitioner *226*:148, 1982.
97. Hjalmarson, A. L.: Effect of nicotine chewing gum in smoking cessation: A randomized, placebo-controlled, double-blind study. J.A.M.A. *252*:2835, 1984.
98. Jarvik, M. E., and Schneider, N. G.: Degree of addiction and effectiveness of nicotine gum therapy for smoking. Am. J. Psychiatry *141*:790, 1984.
99. Jarvis, M. J., Raw, M., Russell, M. A., and Feyerabend, C.: Randomized controlled trial of nicotine chewing gum. Br. Med. J. *285*:537, 1982.
100. Schneider, N. G., Jarvik, M. E., Forsythe, A. B., Read, L. L., Elliott, M. L., and Schweiger, A.: Nicotine gum in smoking cessation: A placebo-controlled, double-blind trial. Addict. Behav. *8*:253, 1983.
101. British Thoracic Society: Comparison of four methods of smoking withdrawal in patients with smoking-related diseases. Br. Med. J. *286*:595, 1983.
102. Keeler, E. B., Operskalski, B. H., and Sloss, E. M.: Cost-effectiveness of health promotion programs. A report to the Henry J. Kaiser Family Foundation (Contract 85-3238).
103. Danaher, B. G., Berkanovic, E., and Gerger, B.: Mass media–based health behavior change: Televised smoking cessation program. Addict. Behav. *9*:245, 1984.
104. Health and Public Policy Committee, American College of Physicians: Methods for stopping cigarette smoking. Ann. Intern. Med. *105*:281, 1986.
105. Hubert, H. B., Feinleib, M., McNamara, P. M., and Castelli, W. P.: Obesity as an independent risk factor for cardiovascular disease: A 26-year follow-up of participants in the Framingham Heart Study. Circulation *67*:968, 1983.
106. Brownell, K. D., and Kaye, F. S.: A school-based behavior modification, nutrition, education, and physical activity program for obese children. Am. J. Clin. Nutr. *35*:277, 1982.
107. Brownell, K. D., Stunkard, A. J., and McKeon, P. E.: Weight reduction at the worksite: A promise partially fulfilled. Am. J. Psychiatry *142*:47, 1985.
108. Stunkard, A. J.: The current status of treatment for obesity in adults. *In* Stunkard, A. J., and Stellar, E. (eds.): Eating and Its Disorders. New York, Raven Press, 1984.
109. Kramsch, D. M., Aspen, A. J., Abramowitz, B. M., Kreimendahl, T., and Hood, W. B.: Reduction of coronary atherosclerosis by moderate conditioning exercise in monkeys on an atherogenic diet. N. Engl. J. Med. *305*:1483, 1981.
110. Huttunen, J. K., Lansimies, M. D., Voutilainen, E., Ehnholm, C., Hietanen, E., Penttila, I., Siitonen, O., and Rauramaa, R.: Effect of moderate physical exercise on serum lipoproteins. A controlled clinical trial with special reference to serum high-density lipoproteins. Circulation *60*:1220, 1979.
111. Gibbons, L. W., Blair, S. N., Cooper, K. H., and Smith, M.: Association between coronary heart disease risk factors and physical fitness in healthy adult women. Circulation *67*:977, 1983.
112. Kannel, W. B., Gordon, T., Sorlie, P., and McNamara, P. M.: Physical activity and coronary vulnerability: The Framingham Study. Cardiol. Dig. *6*:28, 1971.
113. Brand, R. J., Paffenbarger, R. S. Jr., Sholtz, R. I., and Kampert, J. B.: Work activity and fatal heart attacks studied by multiple logistic risk analysis. Am. J. Epidemiol. *110*:52, 1979.
114. Iverson, D. C., Fielding, J. E., Crow, R. S., and Christenson, G. M.: The promotion of physical activity in the United States population: The status of programs in medical, worksite, community, and school settings. Public Health Reports *100*:212, 1985.
115. Gilmore, A.: Canada fitness survey finds fitness means health. Can. Med. Assoc. J. *129*:181, 1983.
116. Cox, M., Shepard, R. J., and Corey, P.: Influence of an employee fitness programme upon fitness, productivity, and absenteeism. Ergonomics *24*:795, 1981.
117. Shepard, R. J., Corey, P., Renzland, P., and Cox, M.: The influence of an employee fitness and lifestyle modification upon medical care costs. Can. J. Public Health *73*:259, 1982.
118. Oldridge, N. B.: Adherence to adult exercise fitness programs. *In* Matarazzo, J. D., Miller, N. E., Herd, J. A., and Weiss, S. M. (eds.): Behaviorial Health: A Handbook of Health Enhancement and Disease Prevention. New York, John Wiley and Sons, 1984, pp. 467-487.
119. Bor, D. H., and Himmelstein, D. U.: Endocarditis prophylaxis for patients with mitral valve prolapse. A quantitative analysis. Am. J. Med. *76*:711, 1984.
120. Clemens, J. D., and Ransohoff, D. F.: A quantitative assessment of pre-dental antibiotic prophylaxis for patients with mitral valve prolapse. J. Chron. Dis. *37*:531, 1984.
121. Clemens, J. D., Horwitz, R. I., Jaffe, C. C., Feinstein, A. R., and Stanton, B. F.: A controlled evaluation of the risk of bacterial endocarditis in persons with mitral valve prolapse. N. Engl. J. Med. *307*:776, 1982.
122. Mills, P., Rose, J., Hollingsworth, J., Amara, I., and Craige, E.: Long-term prognosis of mitral valve prolapse. N. Engl. J. Med. *297*:13, 1977.
123. Eisenberg, M. S., Bergner, L., and Hallstrom, A.: Out-of-hospital cardiac arrest: Improved survival with paramedic services. Lancet 1:812, 1980.
124. Crampton, R. S., Aldrich, R. F., Gascho, J. A., Miles, J. R., and Stillerman, R.: Reduction of prehospital, ambulance, and community coronary death rates by the community-wide emergency cardiac care system. Am. J. Med. *58*:151, 1975.
125. Eisenberg, M. S., Hallstrom, A., and Bergner, L.: Long-term survival after out-of-hospital arrest. N. Engl. J. Med. *306*:1340, 1982.
126. Acton, J. P.: Evaluating public programs to save lives: The case of heart attacks. Report R-950-RC. Santa Monica, The Rand Corp., 1973.
127. Urban, N., Bergner, L., and Eisenberg, M. S.: The costs of a suburban paramedic program in reducing deaths due to cardiac arrest. Med. Care *19*:379, 1981.
128. Hill, J. D., Hampton, J. R., and Mitchell, J. R. A.: A randomized trial of home-versus-hospital management for patients with suspected myocardial infarction. Lancet *1*:837, 1978.
129. Mather, H. G., Morgan, D. C., Pearson, N. G., Read, K. L. Q., Shaw, D. B., Steed, G. R., Thorne, M. G., Lawrence, C. J., and Riley, I. S.: Myocardial infarction: A comparison between home and hospital care for patients. Br. Med. J. *1*:925, 1976.
130. Goldman, L.: Coronary care units: A perspective on their epidemiologic impact. Int. J. Cardiol. *2*:284, 1982.
131. Lee, T. H., Rouan, G., Weisberg, M. C., et al.: Patients with acute myocardial infarction sent home from the emergency room: Clinical characteristics and natural history. Am. J. Cardiol. *in press.*
132. Goldman, L., and Batsford, W. P.: Risk-benefit stratification as a guide to lidocaine prophylaxis of primary ventricular fibrillation in acute myocardial infarction: An analytic review. Yale J. Biol. Med. *52*:455, 1979.
133. Gillum, R. F., Folsom, A., Leupker, R. V., Jacobs, D. R. Jr., Kottke, T. E., Gomez-Marin, O., Prineas, R. J., Taylor, H. L., and Blackburn, H.: Sudden death and acute myocardial infarction in a metropolitan area, 1970-1980: The Minnesota Heart Survey. N. Engl. J. Med. *309*:1353, 1983.
134. Fiebach, N. H., Cook, E. F., Lee, T. H., Rouan, G., Weisberg, M., Goldman, L., and the Chest Pain Study Group: Stratified analysis of the risk of adverse outcomes in patients with myocardial infarction admitted to non-intensive care settings. Clin. Res. *34*:364A, 1986.
135. Lee, T. H., Rouan, G. W., Weisberg, M. C., Brand, D. A., Cook, E. F.,

Acampora, D., and Goldman, L.: Sensitivity of routine clinical criteria for diagnosing myocardial infarction within 24 hours of hospitalization. Ann. Intern. Med. *106*:181, 1987.
136. Mulley, A. G., Thibault, G. E., Hughes, R. A., Barnett, G. O., Reder, V. A., and Sherman, E. L.: The course of patients with suspected myocardial infarction: The identification of low-risk patients for early transfer from intensive care. N. Engl. J. Med. *302*:943, 1980.
137. Singer, D. E., Carr, P. L., Mulley, A. G., and Thibault, G. E.: Rationing intensive care—physician responses to a resource shortage. N. Engl. J. Med. *309*:1155, 1983.
138. Goldman, L., and Cook, E. F.: The decline in ischemic heart disease mortality rates. An analysis of the comparative effects of medical interventions and changes in lifestyle. Ann. Intern. Med. *101*:825, 1984.
139. Beta-Blocker Heart Attack Trial Research Group: A randomized trial of propranolol in patients with acute myocardial infarction. I. Mortality results. J.A.M.A. *247*:1707, 1982.
140. Norwegian Multicenter Study Group: Timolol-induced reduction in mortality and reinfarction in patients surviving acute myocardial infarction. N. Engl. J. Med. *304*:801, 1981.
141. Hansteen, V., Moinichen, E., Lorensten, E., et al.: One year's treatment with propranolol after myocardial infarction: Preliminary report of Norwegian Multicentre Trial. Br. Med. J. *284*:155, 1982.
142. Multicentre International Study: Improvement in prognosis of myocardial infarction by long-term beta-adrenoreceptor blockade using practolol. Br. Med. J. *3*:735, 1975.
143. Multicentre International Study: Reduction in mortality after myocardial infarction with long-term beta-adrenoceptor blockade. Br. Med. J. 2:419, 1977.
144. Yusuf, S., Peto, R., Lewis, J., Collins, R., and Sleight, P.: Beta blockade during and after myocardial infarction: An overview of the randomized trials. Prog. Cardiovasc. Dis. *27*:335, 1985.
145. Alhmark, G., and Saetre, H.: Long-term treatment with beta blockers after myocardial infarction. Eur. J. Clin. Pharmacol. *10*:77, 1976.
146. Australian and Swedish Pindolol Study Group: The effect of pindolol on the two years mortality after complicated myocardial infarction. Eur. Heart. J. *4*:367, 1983.
147. Rehnqvist, N., and Olsson, G.: Influence on ventricular arrhythmias by chronic postinfarction treatment with metoprolol. Circulation *68*:III-369, 1983.
148. Wilhelmsson, C., Vedin, J. A., Wilhelmsen, L., Tibblin, G., and Werko, L.: Reduction of sudden deaths after myocardial infarction by treatment with alprenolol. Preliminary results. Lancet 2:1157, 1974.
149. Pedersen, T. R., and the Norwegian Multicenter Study Group: Six-year follow-up of the Norwegian Multicenter Study on timolol after acute myocardial infarction. N. Engl. J. Med. *313*:1055, 1985.
150. Sia, S. T. B., Rutherford, J. D., Cook, E. F., Weinstein, M. C., and Goldman, L.: Cost-effectiveness of routine beta-blocker therapy following myocardial infarction. Circulation *74*(Suppl. II):44, 1986.
151. Takaro, T., Hultgren, H. N., Lipton, M. J., Detre, K., and Participants in the Study Group: The VA cooperative randomized study of surgery for coronary arterial occlusive disease. II. Subgroup with significant left main lesions. Circulation *54*(Suppl. III):107, 1976.
152. The Veterans Administration Coronary Artery Bypass Surgery Cooperative Study Group.: Eleven-year survival in the Veterans Administration randomized trial of coronary artery bypass surgery for stable angina. N. Engl. J. Med. *311*:1333, 1984.
153. Passamani, E., Davis, K. B., Gillispie, M. J., Killip, T., and the CASS Principal Investigators and their Associates: A randomized trial of coronary artery bypass surgery. Survival of patients with a low ejection fraction. N. Engl. J. Med. *312*:1665, 1985.
154. European Coronary Surgery Study Group: Prospective randomized study of coronary artery bypass surgery in stable angina pectoris: A progress report on survival. Circulation *65*(Suppl. II):67, 1982.
155. CASS Principal Investigators and their Associates: A randomized trial of coronary artery bypass surgery: Quality of life in patients randomly assigned to treatment groups. Circulation *68*:951, 1983.
156. Charles, E. C., Wayne, J. B., Oberman, A., Read, B. A., Haynie, C., Kouchoukos, N. T., Rogers, W. J., and Russell, R. O., Jr.: Costs and benefits associated with treatment for coronary artery disease. Circulation *66*(Suppl. III):87, 1982.
157. Gutmann, M. C., Knapp, D. N., Pollock, M. L., Schmidt, D. H., Simon, K., and Walcott, G.: Coronary artery bypass patients and work status. Circulation *66*(Suppl. III):33, 1982.
158. Kornfeld, D. S., Heller, S. S., Frank, K. A., Wilson, S. N., and Malm, J. R.: Psychological and behavioral responses after coronary artery bypass surgery. Circulation *66*(Suppl. III):24, 1982.
159. Weinstein, M. C., and Stason, W. B.: Cost-effectiveness of coronary artery bypass surgery. Circulation *66*(Suppl. III):56, 1982.
160. Hemenway, D., Sherman, H., Mudge, G. H. Jr., Flatley, M., Lindsey, N. M., and Goldman, L.: Comparative costs versus symptomatic and employment benefits of medical versus surgical treatment of stable angina pectoris. Med. Care *23*:133, 1985.
161. Reeder, G. S., Krishan, I., Nobrega, F. T., Naessens, J., Kelly, M., Christianson, J. B., and McAfee, M. K.: Is percutaneous coronary angioplasty less expensive than bypass surgery? N. Engl. J. Med. *311*:1157, 1984.
162. Jang, G. C., Block, P. C., Cowley, M. J., et al.: Relative cost of coronary angioplasty and bypass surgery in a one-vessel disease model. Am. J. Cardiol. *53*:52C, 1984.
163. Kelly, M. E., Taylor, G. J., Moses, H. W., Mikell, F. L., Dove, J. T., Batchelder, J. E., Wellons, H. A. Jr., and Schneider, J. A.: Comparative cost of myocardial revascularization: Percutaneous transluminal angioplasty and coronary artery bypass surgery. J. Am. Coll. Cardiol. 5:16, 1985.
164. Wilson, J. M., Dunn, E. J., Wright, C. B., Bailey, W. W., Callard, G. M., Melvin, D. B., Mitts, D. L., Will, R. J., and Flege, J. B., Jr.: The cost of simultaneous surgical standby for percutaneous transluminal coronary angioplasty. J. Thorac. Cardiovasc. Surg. 91:362, 1986.

PART V HEART DISEASE AND DISORDERS OF OTHER ORGAN SYSTEMS

53 GENERAL ANESTHESIA AND NONCARDIAC SURGERY IN PATIENTS WITH HEART DISEASE

by LEE GOLDMAN, M.D., MARSHALL A. WOLF, M.D., and EUGENE BRAUNWALD, M.D.

The cardiovascular system of patients undergoing general anesthesia and noncardiac surgical procedures is subject to multiple stresses owing to depression of myocardial contractility and respiration as well as fluctuations in temperature, arterial pressure (afterload), ventricular filling pressures (preload), blood volume, and activity of the autonomic nervous system. Complications of anesthesia and operation, such as hemorrhage, infection, fever, pulmonary embolism, and myocardial infarction, impose additional burdens on the cardiovascular system. The patient with cardiac disease who is compensated preoperatively may be unable to meet these increased demands during the perioperative period, in which case arrhythmias, myocardial ischemia, and/or heart failure may develop.[1, 2] As a consequence, a substantial proportion of all deaths in most series of noncardiac operations result from cardiovascular complications.

Because both the frequency and the seriousness of cardiovascular complications of general anesthesia and operation are considerably increased in the patient with known cardiovascular disease, the magnitude of these risks must be appreciated in order to decide on the advisability of noncardiac surgery in the cardiac patient. In addition, both the life expectancy and the quality of life of the patient must be taken into account. For instance, a noncardiac surgical procedure with a high risk, directed to correct a disorder which is not life-threatening, may be difficult to justify if the patient's cardiac condition precludes a survival period sufficient to allow the patient to reap the benefits of the operations. Obviously the dangers and disability of the disease for which an operation is being proposed must also be balanced against the risk of the operation itself.

ANESTHESIA

Changes in cardiovascular function during general anesthesia are due to many factors, including direct effects of the anesthetic agent(s) on the heart and indirect effects mediated primarily through the autonomic nervous system. In addition, if respiration is inadequately maintained, the resulting hypoxemia, hypercarbia, and acidosis may further depress myocardial contractility and increase cardiac irritability. The interplay of these several variables may produce changes in arterial and central venous pressures, cardiac output, and rate and rhythm. To minimize the risk of operation in the patient with a compromised cardiovascular system, it is essential to minimize these fluctuations.[3]

The choice of the anesthetic approach and the specific anesthetic agents to be used should be made by a qualified anesthesiologist, commonly after careful evaluation of the patient's medical and cardiac condition and often after consultation with the surgeon and the internist or cardiologist. Although the cardiological consultant should not expect to dictate the anesthetic approach, the quality of the consultation will be improved if the consultant appreciates the clinical pharmacology of the anesthetic agents and the effects of intubation and extubation.

GENERAL ANESTHESIA

The induction of anesthesia is usually accomplished with intravenous anesthetics. With the exception of ketamine, the agents used for the induction of anesthesia commonly lower systemic arterial pressure by about 20 to 30 per cent in healthy patients, but sometimes by a greater amount in hypertensive patients.[4] During laryngoscopy and tracheal intubation, blood pressure commonly increases by 20 to 30 mm Hg, but it may increase even more in the hypertensive patient,[4] in whom these changes in blood pressure may be associated with electrocardiographic evidence of myocardial ischemia.[5, 6] Much of this hypertensive response can be avoided by adequate topical anesthesia of the upper airways, larynx, and trachea, or by blind nasal intubation because the hypertension appears to be caused by the laryngoscopy rather than by the passage of a tube into the trachea.

INHALATION AGENTS. These agents enter the bloodstream by way of the alveoli and are excreted across the alveoli essentially unchanged. In most major operations a combination of inhalation agents and/or intravenous anesthetics are used.[3, 7]

Nitrous oxide usually causes a modest decrease of about 15 per cent in cardiac output but usually does not cause substantial hypotension because of reflex vasoconstriction (Table 53–1). Unfortunately, in many patients it is impossible to achieve full anesthesia with concentrations of nitrous oxide that also permit adequate oxygenation.

Halothane also causes a reduction in myocardial contractility, but unlike nitrous oxide, it is not associated with substantial reflex vasoconstriction. Thus, when halothane is added to nitrous oxide, there are often further reductions in arterial pressure because of reductions in cardiac output without concomitant vasoconstriction.[5] Halothane also appears to sensitize the myocardium to catecholamines, sometimes resulting in arrhythmias.

TABLE 53–1 CARDIOVASCULAR CHANGES WITH NITROUS OXIDE AND AFTER ITS ADDITION TO PREEXISTING GENERAL ANESTHETICS

	Effect			
Measurement	Nitrous Oxide	Nitrous Oxide–Halothane	Nitrous Oxide–Enflurane	Nitrous Oxide–Morphine
Blood pressure	None	Increased	None	None
Heart rate	Decreased	None	Decreased	Decreased
Cardiac output	Decreased	None	Increased	Decreased
Systemic vascular resistance	Increased	Increased	None	Increased
Central venous pressure	Increased	Increased	None	Increased

From Tarhan, S. (ed.): Cardiovascular Anesthesia and Postoperative Care. Chicago, Year Book Medical Publishers, 1982. Copyright © 1982 by Year Book Medical Publishers, Inc., Chicago.

Enflurane has properties similar to halothane but appears to result in less sensitization to catecholamines. *Isoflurane* appears to have less of a negative inotropic effect than halothane or enflurane, but it can be associated with marked decreases in systemic vascular resistance, and hence a fall in systemic blood pressure.

INTRAVENOUS ANESTHETICS. Among the narcotic analgesics, *morphine* is generally well tolerated, although it does cause venodilation, thereby decreasing preload and cardiac output. *Fentanyl* is more potent than morphine and has a shorter duration of action. Like morphine, it tends not to have major effects on myocardial contractility, but it is more likely than morphine to cause bradycardia.

Short-acting barbiturates, especially *thiopental*, often cause a fall in blood pressure because of depressive actions on myocardial contractility and sympathetic tone. In patients who have severe hypovolemia or severe cardiac dysfunction, serious reductions in cardiac output can occasionally occur after a small dose of thiopental.

Benzodiazepines can achieve adequate sedation with only mild cardiovascular depression. However, occasionally patients may become apneic or hypotensive after small doses. *Droperidol* causes vasodilation because of its alpha-adrenergic blocking action and its effect on the central nervous system.

Ketamine is unlike other commonly used intravenous anesthetics in that it does not cause cardiovascular depression. Although it may cause minimal direct myocardial depressant activity, this is commonly counterbalanced by an increase in circulating catecholamines.

MUSCLE RELAXANTS. Drugs used for muscle relaxation also may have cardiovascular effects. *Succinylcholine* can cause bradycardia, which can be reversed or prevented by the administration of atropine. In patients anesthetized with halothane, *pancuronium* and *gallamine* cause an increase in heart rate, arterial pressure, and cardiac output, while *tubocurarine* and *metocurine* result in a fall in mean arterial pressure with mild elevations in heart rate and little, if any, change in cardiac output.

SPINAL AND EPIDURAL ANESTHESIA

Spinal and epidural anesthesia cause sympathetic denervation, which produces peripheral arteriodilation and venodilation. Systemic vascular resistance may be reduced by 10 to 15 per cent. Venodilation may cause a marked reduction in right ventricular preload as a consequence of sympathetic denervation. Under these circumstances, right ventricular preload depends critically on the effects of gravity on the patient's position, and on the total blood volume (Fig. 13–31, p. 409).

REGIONAL AND LOCAL ANESTHESIA. Regional and local anesthesia cause cardiovascular effects only to the extent that the agents are absorbed into the bloodstream or where there is sympathetic blockade accompanying the local sensory block. A major concern with local or regional anesthesia is whether the technique is adequate for the planned procedure; the cardiological consultant should not underestimate the cardiovascular consequences of inadequate anesthesia.

Although it is important for the cardiological consultant to have an appreciation for the clinical pharmacology of anesthetic agents and the issues of intraoperative management, decisions about anesthetic approaches and agents should be made by the anesthesiologist. Different anesthesiologists may have preferences for different anesthetic techniques, and the anesthesiological literature clearly indicates that there is little, if any, correlation between the anesthetic route or agents and the likelihood of major clinical complications. Thus, it is the skill and experience of the anesthesiologist, including the ability to monitor hemodynamics and respond quickly, that are far more important than the specific agent that is used.

INTRAOPERATIVE HEMODYNAMICS AND ARRHYTHMIAS

During the operative procedure, it is not uncommon for systolic blood pressure to fall into the range of 95 to 105 mm Hg. Such blood pressure reductions are often brief and may respond to a lightening of the anesthesia or, in 20 to 30 per cent of patients, either to a brisk fluid challenge or the use of intravenous sympathomimetic agents. Any severe reduction in arterial pressure in patients with ischemic heart disease can reduce coronary flow and precipitate myocardial ischemia. In general, such reductions in blood pressure are not associated with major cardiac complications, such as myocardial infarction, unless they result in reductions in blood pressures which exceed approximately 33 per cent of the preoperative blood pressure and that persist for 10 or more minutes, or are more than 50 per cent below the preoperative blood pressure.[8–10] Fluids that are administered to maintain intraoperative blood pressure can potentially cause postoperative fluid overload.[11]

The risk of unplanned intraoperative hypotension is at least as great with spinal or epidural anesthesia as with general anesthesia.[12] Because spinal and epidural anesthesia are not direct myocardial depressants, they may be advantageous in patients with severe myocardial dysfunction; but even in those circumstances, well-balanced general anesthesia, sometimes including ketamine, has been used successfully.

Transient bradycardias, such as sinus bradycardia and junctional rhythm, may occur during periods of vagal stimulation. These bradyarrhythmias commonly respond to a lightening of the anesthesia or to the administration of atropine or beta-adrenoceptor agents. Tachyarrhythmias may result from hypovolemia or vasodilatation as well as from sensitization of the myocardium to catecholamines that are circulating and/or released by sympathetic nerve endings in the heart. Tachycardia is poorly tolerated by patients with mitral stenosis (p. 1024) and may cause myocardial ischemia in patients with coronary artery disease. Therapy with specific antiarrhythmic medications is usually indicated only when the arrhythmia does not respond to changes in the depth of anesthesia or to attention to problems such as hypoxemia, hypovolemia, hypotension, or the potentially precipitating surgical manipulation.

Positive-pressure ventilation during general anesthesia reduces the return of blood to the right side of the heart and tends to reduce ventricular preload. Fluid that is administered during positive-pressure ventilation will not increase preload to the extent that it would in the patient who is ventilating spontaneously. When the positive-pressure ventilation of general anesthesia ceases, ventricular preload increases, often abruptly, and hypertension or pulmonary congestion may result. Analogous physiological changes can occur with the cessation of spinal or epidural anesthesia because the venodilation caused by these agents also reduces right ventricular preload.

MONITORING. In patients with severe underlying heart disease, it is mandatory to monitor cardiac function during anesthesia,[13] including cardiac rate and rhythm and directly recorded arterial blood pressure. A radial artery line permits not only monitoring of intraarterial pressure but also frequent sampling for determination of blood gases. In the presence of peripheral vasoconstriction, indirect (cuff) blood pressure measurements may greatly underestimate true arterial pressure. Monitoring of the pulmonary artery (or, preferably, pulmonary artery wedge) pressure and cardiac output is often desirable in patients who are critically ill, who have marginal cardiovascular reserve, who are to undergo prolonged operative procedures in which major blood losses might occur, and in whom hypotensive anesthesia is to be used. Both pulmonary artery wedge pressure and cardiac output can be measured with the aid of a multiple-lumen balloon flotation catheter (Swan-Ganz) and the thermodilution method (Chap. 9). In seriously ill patients, urine output should be monitored with a Foley catheter.

THE OPERATION

Just as consultant cardiologists must understand the pharmacological effects of anesthesia, they must also recognize the physiological effects of surgery, including the direct consequences of the operation and the expected responses to postoperative recuperation.

NATURE OF THE OPERATION. Although ophthalmological surgery[14] and transurethral prostatic resection[15] are almost always safe, even in patients with a history of serious cardiac disease, general surgical mortality is often 25 to 50 per cent higher in patients with underlying cardiovascular conditions than in patients with normal cardiac function.[9, 12, 16–19] Among noncardiac surgical procedures, the highest cardiovascular complication rates are commonly associated with abdominal aortic aneurysm surgery,[20] which causes substantial myocardial stress because of aortic cross-clamping and major shifts in fluid and electrolytes. The risk of cardiac complications is also higher in other major abdominal and thoracic procedures than in procedures on the extremities, in large part because of the more difficult postoperative course. Patients who undergo surgery for aortic aneurysm, carotid arterial disease, or peripheral vascular disease often have substantial coronary artery disease as well, and the extent of the latter may be underestimated because of the limitations caused by the peripheral arterial disease.

DURATION. The duration of anesthesia is generally correlated with the risk of cardiovascular mortality and morbidity, but this is principally because the longest operations are more often on the aorta or in the abdomen or chest than on the extremities. In most series[12, 16, 19] the risk of major cardiovascular complications did not correlate with the duration of surgery after controlling for the type of surgery. However, if the operation is prolonged because of intraoperative complications, it would be expected that the risk of postoperative cardiovascular complications might increase, especially among patients with a prior myocardial infarction[9] or in situations in which the operation takes longer than 5 hours.[12]

EMERGENCY OPERATION. When surgery is carried out under emergency conditions, it is associated with a greatly increased mortality in patients with cardiovascular disease. The risk of postoperative cardiac complications, including postoperative myocardial infarction or cardiac death, is increased anywhere from 2.5- to 4-fold in emergency compared with elective surgery.[12, 18, 19] Part of this increased risk is because patients undergoing emergency surgery may often have poorly controlled or unappreciated general medical problems, such as fluid and electrolyte imbalance or hepatic dysfunction,[18] but emergency surgery appears to be an important correlate of postoperative complications, even after controlling for the underlying medical disease.[18, 21]

The application of invasive hemodynamic monitoring to noncardiac surgical procedures in patients with underlying heart disease may reduce the risk of intraoperative and postoperative cardiovascular complications. Thus the risk of a new infarction was reduced from 7.7 to 1.9 per cent when patients with a history of infarction were aggressively monitored during the period from 1977 to 1982 compared with when minimal invasive monitoring was used in the period from 1973 to 1976.[22] Although this nonrandomized study did not control for other secular changes in medical care, it should not be surprising that the application of cardiovascular anesthesiological techniques to noncardiac surgery would have a beneficial effect. Thus, in patients who have suffered a myocardial infarction within the past 3 months, who have angina that is more severe than Canadian Class II (p. 11), who have severe heart failure, or who are at high risk based on indices such as the multifactorial index of cardiac risk in noncardiac surgery,[18, 20, 23, 24] available data support the use of intraarterial and pulmonary artery catheters for careful hemodynamic monitoring. Although it has been suggested that invasive hemodynamic monitoring also be used in *all* patients over age 65 who undergo major surgery,[25] most of the benefit will be realized in the high-risk subgroups. In general, arterial and pulmonary artery pressure should not be allowed to fluctuate by more than 20 per cent of the preinduction values for longer than 5 minutes. For patients with a recent myocardial infarction or severe angina, careful monitoring should usually extend for several days into the postoperative period, especially because the risk of a postoperative myocardial infarction may not peak until about the third postoperative day.[12, 16, 22]

INFLUENCE OF UNDERLYING CARDIOVASCULAR DISEASE

ISCHEMIC HEART DISEASE

ASSESSMENT OF RISK

Clinical. Ischemic heart disease is a major determinant of perioperative morbidity and mortality. The incidence of perioperative myocardial infarction is increased 10- to 50-fold in patients who have previously suffered infarcts compared with patients who do not have a clinical history of coronary disease.

During the 1970's, several studies reported about a 30 per cent risk of reinfarction or cardiac death when patients were operated on within 3 months of the previous myocardial infarction, about a 15 per cent risk when the operation was performed 3 to 6 months after a prior infarction, and about a 5 per cent risk when the surgery was performed more than 6 months after the infarction.[9, 16, 18] However, recent data suggest that the application of invasive hemodynamic monitoring and careful regulation of oxygenation, electrolytes, volume status, and the hematocrit have markedly reduced the complication rate. For example, Wells and Kaplan[26] reported no reinfarctions in 48 patients who were operated on within 3 months after a myocardial infarction, while Rao et al.[22] reported only a 6 per cent reinfarction rate within 3 months after preoperative myocardial infarction and only a 2 per cent reinfarction rate between 3 and 6 months after a myocardial infarction.

Truly life-saving procedures must be performed regardless of the cardiac risk, and purely elective surgery should commonly be delayed for 6 months after infarction, when the cardiovascular risks will have returned to a stable, long-term baseline risk. The more difficult issue is in patients in whom the operation is not truly emergent but is also not purely elective, for example, a patient with severe symptomatic peripheral vascular disease or a patient with a potentially resectable malignancy. In such situations one would like to delay operation sufficiently long for cardiac risk to be reduced but not wait a full 6 months. Because full healing of a myocardial infarction usually takes about 4 to 6 weeks, one rational approach is to evaluate the patient with post-myocardial infarction prognostic studies, such as a submaximal exercise tolerance test,[27] and to use the patient's clinical and cardiological conditions as the guide for surgery sometime between 6 weeks and 3 months after the infarction. It should be remembered that a recent preoperative myocardial infarction will increase a patient's relative risk of reinfarction with surgery, but that the absolute risk depends on a variety of factors in addition to the timing of the infarction. Thus, patients who have good exercise tolerance and left ventricular function and who can resume normal activity levels within 6 weeks after infarction should be able to undergo surgery with relatively small absolute risks, even if their relative risk might be slightly lower if one could wait the full 6 months. By comparison, risks are likely to be substantially higher in patients who have post-infarction angina, large reversible defects on thallium scintigraphy, reduced left ventricular function, marked ST-segment depression with exercise, or other evidence of easily provokable ischemia (p. 1291). In general, one should be influenced less by whether or not a preoperative myocardial infarction was associated with the development of new Q waves than by the current state of left ventricular function and the severity of preoperative angina.

When approaching the patient with angina pectoris, the patient's current exercise tolerance should be ascertained and an assessment made as to whether the anginal pattern is stable or unstable (p. 236). Patients who are Class II by the criteria of the Canadian Cardiovascular Society[28] or the Specific Activity Scale[29, 30] can carry objects such as two grocery bags or a young child up a flight of stairs without stopping and without appreciable symptoms. In such patients most surgical procedures are generally well tolerated. Physicians should avoid relying on the *frequency* of angina because patients who voluntarily reduce their activity level may also greatly reduce their symptoms.[30] This phenomenon is especially true in patients whose surgical conditions, such as orthopedic disorders or peripheral vascular disease, limit ambulation.

Laboratory. *Exercise treadmill testing* is an objective means for assessing exercise tolerance and is especially beneficial if the history is unreliable. Unfortunately, the limited sensitivity and specificity of standard electrocardiographic exercise tolerance testing limit the use of this test for diagnosing coronary artery disease (see Chap. 8). In one study,[31] postoperative death or myocardial infarction was more common in patients with an abnormal resting electrocardiogram than in those with a normal electrocardiogram, but the results of exercise electrocardiography did not add substantially to the degree of risk separation provided by the resting electrocardiogram. It was notable, however, that five of the six patients with postoperative death or myocardial infarction could not exercise to a level of five metabolic equivalents. The prognostic value of a limited exercise tolerance in patients over age 40[31] was substantiated in persons over age 65,[32] in whom the inability to perform 2 minutes of bicycle exercise in a supine position and to raise the heart rate above 99 beats/min was an independent important predictor of cardiac complications in noncardiac surgery. Of note was that a poor exercise capacity was an independent predictor of cardiac complications, but electrocardiographic changes with exercise were not. In the latter study,[32] data from resting and exercise radionuclide ventriculography did not add important independent information for predicting perioperative cardiac risk, but the study size was too small for it to be the final word on the value of ventriculography.

In patients who are unable to exercise because of noncardiac disability (e.g., intermittent claudication or orthopedic abnormalities), dipyridamole thallium imaging (p. 331) has been extremely successful in identifying high-risk patients among selected subgroups undergoing vascular surgery.[33, 34] In one study[33] all eight postoperative ischemic events, including three myocardial infarctions, occurred in patients who had transient thallium defects precipitated by dipyridamole; there were no such events in 32 patients who had no fixed defects. Among the 16 patients with dipyridamole thallium defects, there were three myocardial infarctions and five additional patients who developed episodes of angina with ST-segment depression postoperatively.

Thus, using a combination of a careful clinical history, appropriately supplemented by exercise testing or dipyridamole thallium imaging, it is possible to identify patients whose ischemic heart disease represents a markedly increased risk for noncardiac surgery. In patients whose angina pectoris is Class III or IV, coronary arteriography, often followed by angioplasty or coronary artery bypass grafting, should be performed before nonemergent surgery. If the physiological importance of anatomical coronary artery stenoses is unclear, right atrial pacing with or without thallium injection[35] may be helpful by precipitating angina, ST-segment depression, acute elevation in the left ventricular end-diastolic pressure, or a myocardial perfusion defect on the thallium scintigram. These responses support the physiological importance of the underlying coronary disease, especially if found at heart rates of less than 100 to 120 beats/min, and would usually argue for revascularization (coronary angioplasty or bypass grafting) before major surgery.

Patients who have undergone successful coronary revascularization can undergo major noncardiac surgical procedures with a low mortality rate,[13, 36, 37] except perhaps in the first 30 days postoperatively.[38] In some circumstances both the coronary artery bypass operation and the noncardiac surgery can be performed during the course of the same procedure.[39] It must be remembered, however, that the operative mortality rate for major noncardiac surgery in patients with stable angina and a good exercise tolerance is relatively low, usually in the range of 2 per cent. At the current time there are no randomized controlled trials to assess the value of coronary artery bypass grafting preoperatively in a patient with stable angina pectoris who is about to undergo noncardiac surgery. An analysis of patients in the Coronary Artery Surgery Study registry,[40] including nonrandomized patients, showed that total operative mortality was 2.4 per cent in 458 patients who had significant coronary artery disease and underwent noncardiac surgery without prior coronary artery bypass grafting. By comparison, operative mortality was 0.9 per cent among 399 patients who had had a coronary artery bypass grafting procedure performed before noncardiac surgery. The mortality was higher in patients who had more left ventricular dysfunction or dyspnea on exertion and in patients who used nitrates, were older, and had diabetes. The risk of myocardial infarction, however, was not significantly different between the patients with and without preoperative coronary artery bypass grafting. Furthermore, if one considers the mortality associated with coronary artery bypass grafting, which was 1.4 per cent in the Coronary Artery Surgery Study, the overall mortality from combined coronary artery bypass grafting and noncardiac surgery (2.3 per cent) would be as high as for the noncardiac surgery done in the nonbypassed group (2.4 per cent). Thus the data do not argue in favor of prophylactic coronary artery bypass grafting for patients whose symptoms would not otherwise warrant revascularization, who have stable angina with a good exercise tolerance, and who do not have other factors that define a high-risk status (see below).

COMBINED CAROTID AND CORONARY ARTERY SURGERY. There is currently some controversy as to the indications for combined coronary revascularization and carotid endarterectomy in patients with coexisting coronary and carotid stenoses. It has been shown experimentally that carotid perfusion is maintained or increased during cardiopulmonary bypass,[41] thus suggesting that nonpulsatile cardiopulmonary bypass per se is unlikely to cause a stroke due to hypoperfusion. Most strokes that occur during coronary revascularization appear to be embolic in origin.[42] Combined coronary and carotid surgery can be performed at low risk,[43] but we recommend combined surgery only when there is severe bilateral or currently symptomatic carotid disease associated with unstable angina, left main coronary disease, or very symptomatic three-vessel coronary disease. If the coronary disease is stable and relatively mild, the carotid surgery should be performed first and the coronary revascularization at a later date. If the carotid disease is asymptomatic or not bilateral and severe, coronary revascularization can be performed without a proven need for prophylactic carotid surgery.[42]

USE OF BETA BLOCKERS AND CALCIUM ANTAGONISTS. Although some concern has been expressed about the use of general anesthesia in patients receiving beta-adrenoceptor agents and calcium antagonists, there are no clinical data to indicate that such medications should routinely be discontinued preoperatively. For beta-adrenoceptor agents, early concerns[44] about the safety of propranolol have been contradicted by substantial subsequent data demonstrating the safety of their use[45–47] and the dangers of discontinuing beta-adrenoceptor agents preoperatively.[48] Propranolol appears to reduce the risk of severe hypertensive episodes and ischemic electrocardiographic responses to the stresses of intubation, anesthesia, and surgery.[49, 50] In patients who rely on beta-adrenoceptor agents for the control of severe angina, the medication should be continued up to and including the morning of surgery with a small sip of water.[48] Postoperatively, the medication can be resumed orally or sometimes given through a nasogastric tube. However, intravenous propranolol should be used in patients with a prior history of severe angina that required beta-adrenoceptor agents for its control or in patients who have evidence of postoperative myocardial ischemia or otherwise unexplained hypertension or tachycardia.

Propranolol can be given as a 1-mg intravenous bolus, which is repeated up to a total loading dose of 10 mg and followed by 1 mg intravenously every 20 to 60 minutes. The second option is a 5- to 10-mg loading dose given slowly over 60 minutes, followed by a continuous intravenous infusion of 0.01 to 0.05 mg/min.[51, 52] In the future, esmolol, an ultra-short-acting beta-adrenoceptor, may be the preferred medication in doses ranging from 100 to 300 μg/kg/min after a 500 μg/kg/min loading dose.[53] If the patient suffers side effects attributable to administration of a beta blocker, treatment should be instituted with isoproterenol or dobutamine, or with glucagon, if the others are not effective.

Nifedipine can be given sublingually and nitrates can be given sublingually, topically, or intravenously, to aid in the management of the early postoperative patient with angina, but neither of these agents substitutes for beta-adrenoceptors in patients who have relied on the latter for the control of their ischemic heart disease.

HYPERTENSION

Several studies have documented that patients with hypertension have higher risks of suffering major cardiac complications during or shortly after operation than do patients who have always been normotensive. However, most, if not all, of this increased risk is because of the ischemic heart disease, left ventricular dysfunction, renal failure, or other abnormalities that often occur in patients with hypertension. Thus, in patients with mild to moderate hypertension, diastolic pressures below 110 mm Hg, and no evidence of serious end-organ damage, general anesthesia and major noncardiac surgery are generally well tolerated.[10] Halothane anesthesia may be more likely than other anesthetic agents to induce intraoperative hypotension in patients with a history of hypertension,[10] and hypertensive patients are at higher risk for labile blood pressures and for hypertensive episodes during surgery and especially just after extubation.

Although uncontrolled early studies suggested that the continuation of any hypertensive agents, especially reserpine, might increase the risk of perioperative hypotension, substantial subsequent data from more careful studies indicate that patients whose hypertension is well controlled will do at least as well, if not better, if their medications are, in fact, continued up to the time of operation.[5, 10, 54–56] Thus, although it is not mandatory to delay surgery for the weeks or months that may be required to achieve ideal blood pressure control in the stable patient with mild to moderate hypertension who has no complications of the hypertension, there is also no apparent benefit, and some potential harm, from discontinuing successful antihypertensive therapy before surgery.

Thiazide and other diuretics cause some degree of chronic volume depletion,[57, 58] and patients receiving these drugs may require more fluid administration early during the operative procedure. Guanethidine and reserpine cause depletion of norepinephrine at adrenergic nerve endings, and when hypotension develops in patients receiving these drugs and they require adrenergic agents, direct-acting agents such as norepinephrine, methoxamine, or phenylephrine should be used rather than indirect-acting agents such as ephedrine. If severe perioperative hypertension develops in a patient who has previously been receiving clonidine, and if the clonidine cannot be given orally, it can be administered intramuscularly in doses about one-half as large as the patient's usual daily dose or it can be administered topically,[59] or the patient can be treated with sublingual captopril, with methyldopa, or with a beta blocker. Although it may be desirable to continue propranolol intravenously in patients who rely on beta-adrenoceptors for the control of ischemic heart disease, it is less often necessary to use intravenous propranolol in patients who take the medicine for its antihypertensive effects. Commonly, intravenous methyldopa or, when episodes are severe, nitroprusside can be used instead.

VALVULAR HEART DISEASE

Patients with valvular heart disease undergoing anesthesia and operation are subject to many potential hazards: heart failure, infection, tachycardia, and embolization. As might be expected, patients with no or only mild limitation of activity (i.e., those in Class I or II[28–30]) tolerate operation well and probably require little more than prophylaxis for infective endocarditis (p. 1127). Those with more serious impairment of cardiac reserve (i.e., those in Class III or IV) tolerate major noncardiac surgery poorly, and their prognosis for surviving the operation is distinctly worse.[18, 19] As is the case for patients with rheumatic heart disease who face the stress of pregnancy (p. 1853), the risk of operation depends on the functional state of the heart. Patients with symptomatic critical aortic or mitral stenosis are especially prone to sudden death or acute pulmonary edema during the perioperative period; this may occur if demands on cardiac output are suddenly increased or if atrial fibrillation and a rapid ventricular rate are precipitated by anesthesia or operation. Every effort should be made to treat heart failure preoperatively. Patients with severe stenotic or regurgitant valve disease should undergo corrective valvular surgery before an elective operation, while those with severe failure who require emergency operation may benefit from intraoperative hemodynamic monitoring, afterload reduction, and preload augmentation.[60] In some patients with mitral or aortic stenosis, balloon valvuloplasty (p. 1059) may offer relief of severe obstruction at a low risk when it might not be desirable to carry out valve replacement.

HYPERTROPHIC CARDIOMYOPATHY. Patients with *hypertrophic cardiomyopathy* are intolerant of hypovolemia, which may lead to both a reduction in the elevated preload necessary to maintain cardiac output and an increase in the obstruction to left ventricular outflow (p. 1421). With careful perioperative, intraoperative, and postoperative care, however, the risk of major cardiac complications in such patients is small. In one series of 56 operations in patients with hypertrophic cardiomyopathy, there were no deaths and the only major complication was a myocardial infarction with congestive heart failure in a patient who also had underlying coronary artery disease. Intraoperative or postoperative hypotension requiring vasoconstrictors occurred in less than 10 per cent of patients.[61] It has been suggested that spinal anesthesia may be relatively contraindicated in patients with hypertrophic obstructive cardiomyopathy because of its tendency to reduce systemic vascular resistance and increase venous pooling and thereby increase the severity of obstruction to outflow.[61] Hemodynamic monitoring is not routinely required but may be helpful when these patients undergo major aortic, abdominal, or thoracic procedures.

PROSTHETIC HEART VALVES. Most patients with mechanical prosthetic heart valves receive anticoagulants on a chronic basis to prevent thromboembolic complications (p. 1079). If these medications are continued through the operative period, hemostasis, hematoma formation, and persistent postoperative bleeding may ensue. Anticoagulants can be temporarily discontinued during the perioperative period with minimal risk of thrombosis. In one study[62] no thromboembolic complications occurred in 159 patients with prosthetic valves undergoing 180 noncardiac operations when warfarin was discontinued an average of 2.9 days preoperatively and resumed 2.7 days postoperatively.[62] Using a similar approach, Katholi et al. did not observe thromboembolic complications in 25 operations on patients with prosthetic aortic valves[63]; however, two such complications occurred in the 10 patients with mitral valve prostheses when anticoagulants were discontinued for noncardiac surgery, although these patients had Kay-Shiley caged-disc valves, which are associated with a somewhat higher risk of thromboembolic complications. Because there is a distinct risk of hemorrhagic complications in patients whose anticoagulants have been discontinued for only 2 or 3 days,[62] prothrombin time should be restored to within 20 per cent of normal before one proceeds with noncardiac surgery.[64] Low molecular weight dextran can be used in the postoperative period to minimize thrombotic complications during the 2 to 3 days when the risk of hemorrhagic complications from resuming anticoagulation is relatively higher. In patients with prostheses that are at high risk for thrombosis, such as caged-disc valves, we recommend discontinuing warfarin, allowing the prothrombin time to come to within about 2 to 3 seconds of normal, using intravenous heparin until about 6 hours before the operation, restarting the heparin about 36 to 48 hours after surgery, and switching to warfarin about 2 to 5 days later.

ENDOCARDITIS PROPHYLAXIS. Patients with valvular disease and prosthetic heart valves should receive prophylactic antibiotics for surgical procedures likely to be complicated by bacteremias.[65, 66] These include incision and drainage of an infected site; oral, lower gastrointestinal, and gallbladder surgery; and genitourinary procedures. Penicillin can be used before surgery involving the upper respiratory tract, with erythromycin or vancomycin an acceptable alternative for patients with a penicillin allergy. For gastrointestinal and genitourinary surgery, which can be complicated by either enterococci or gram-negative bacteremia, gentamicin or streptomycin is required in addition to penicillin. (Suggested doses are given on p. 1127.)

The value of antibiotic prophylaxis before surgery in patients with *mitral valve prolapse* is controversial (p. 1051). Most studies indicate that patients with this condition who have murmurs of mitral regurgitation are at substantially higher risk than patients who do not have murmurs,[67, 68] and cost-effectiveness analyses argue *against* routine antibiotic prophylaxis in patients without a murmur.[69, 70] At the present time a reasonable compromise is to use antibiotic prophylaxis before surgery in patients with mitral valve prolapse who have evidence of mitral regurgitation.

CONGENITAL HEART DISEASE

Depending on the nature of the malformation, the patient with congenital heart disease may be subject to one or more potentially serious complications, such as infection, bleeding, hypoxemia, and paradoxical embolization during general anesthesia and operation. As is the case for patients with valvular heart disease, patients with congenital heart disease who are to undergo a surgical procedure require prophylaxis to prevent infective endocarditis (p. 1127). Patients with cyanotic congenital heart disease and secondary polycythemia are at increased risk of intraoperative and postoperative hemorrhage as a consequence of coagulation defects and thrombocytopenia (p. 903); this risk can be reduced with careful preoperative phlebotomy, usually to a hematocrit of 50 to 55 per cent.[71]

Patients with cyanotic congenital heart disease tolerate systemic hypotension poorly, since this increases the right-to-left shunt and the severity of hypoxemia. In one large series, induction was commonly accomplished using ketamine or fentanyl in order to avoid hypotension, and anesthesia was maintained with morphine and nitrous oxide or with large doses of fentanyl with or without nitrous oxide. Halothane in very low concentrations can be used in patients with less severe degrees of cyanosis.[72] Using careful anesthetic techniques, the risk of major anesthetic complications is extremely low even in very ill and cyanotic patients. Spinal anesthesia, which causes peripheral arterial vasodilatation and reduces venous return, can have deleterious hemodynamic effects in patients with cyanotic congenital heart disease. Occasionally, infusion of a vasoconstrictor such as phenylephrine may be required to raise systemic vascular resistance and thereby decrease the magnitude of the right-to-left shunt. Because patients with right-to-left shunts are subject to the risk of paradoxical emboli, including air emboli, meticulous techniques with regard to intravenous solutions and injections are mandatory to prevent such complications.

CONGESTIVE HEART FAILURE

Congestive heart failure is a major determinant of perioperative risk, irrespective of the nature of the underlying cardiac disorder. Mortality with surgery increases with worsening cardiac class[12, 19] and is worse in the presence of pulmonary congestion,[12] especially when a third heart sound is noted.[18, 40] Because the perioperative mortality rate appears to depend more on the patient's condition at the time of operation than on the most severe depression of cardiovascular status the patient has ever experienced, it is clearly advisable to treat the congestive heart failure before the contemplated major elective noncardiac surgery. However, because such a therapeutic regimen almost always includes a diuretic, both hypovolemia and hypokalemia are potential problems for patients treated just before operation. It is therefore desirable, if possible, to stabilize the patient's condition by treating heart failure for approximately 1 week rather than for only 1 or 2 days before the contemplated operation. Also, great care should be taken to avoid dehydration because hypovolemic patients may be especially likely to experience marked hypotension during the early phases of anesthesia. In patients over age 40 undergoing major noncardiac surgery, perioperative cardiogenic pulmonary edema will develop in about 2 per cent of patients with heart disease without prior congestive heart failure, in about 6 per cent of patients whose heart failure is well controlled, and in about 16 per cent of patients whose heart failure persists by physical examination or chest radiograph criteria before surgery.[12]

Although digitalis can counteract the myocardial depressant actions of many general anesthetic agents,[73–75] the value of digitalis in patients with congestive heart failure appears to be limited to certain subsets of patients, especially those who have a third heart sound.[76, 77] Digitalis is one of the most common causes of iatrogenic complications in hospitalized patients, and it may be associated with a higher risk of intraoperative bradyarrhythmias.[12] Therefore, preoperative digitalization is *not* recommended except in patients whose congestive heart failure is sufficiently severe that they would normally meet the criteria for chronic, long-term digitalization, based on emerging criteria[76, 77] (p. 497).

ARRHYTHMIAS

Arrhythmias are often a manifestation of underlying heart disease, and hence are frequently markers for the likelihood of perioperative cardiac complications. For example, the frequency of ventricular premature contractions correlates with left ventricular dysfunction and the severity of coronary artery disease,[78, 79] and thus frequent ventricular premature contractions in patients with coronary artery disease represent a risk factor for the development of cardiac complications.[18] Because patients who have ventricular premature contractions but no evidence of underlying heart disease on detailed examination have an apparently normal cardiac prognosis,[80] ventricular premature contractions in the *absence* of underlying heart disease should not be considered a risk factor for cardiac complications with noncardiac surgery. Atrial arrhythmias are often a manifestation of atrial enlargement, and a supraventricular rhythm other than sinus appears to be a risk factor for the development of perioperative complications.[18]

Although it would be ideal for arrhythmias to be well controlled preoperatively, the risks associated with these arrhythmias appear to be related more to the underlying cardiac disease than to the arrhythmias per se. Therefore, there currently is no evidence that asymptomatic ventricular premature contractions require aggressive preoperative control or prophylactic intraoperative suppression. Similarly, the patient with well-controlled atrial fibrillation need not be cardioverted specifically because of planned noncardiac surgery if such a management option would not otherwise be appropriate.

Patients who are most at risk for the development of postoperative supraventricular tachyarrhythmias include elderly patients undergoing pulmonary surgery, patients with subcritical valvular stenoses, and patients with prior histories of supraventricular tachyarrhythmias. Although data are less than decisive, there is a suggestion that digitalis may reduce the risk of the development of a postoperative supraventricular tachycardia in such patients,[81] and that the rate of the supraventricular tachycardia will be slower in the digitalized patient.[12, 82] Thus, we recommend prophylactic preoperative digitalization in elderly patients undergoing major pulmonary surgery, patients with subcritical valvular stenoses, and patients with a prior history of symptomatic supraventricular tachycardias, except if the latter are already taking other medications for the control of such arrhythmias.

CONDUCTION DEFECTS. The patient with *complete heart block* (p. 702) must respond to the demands for an increased cardiac output by augmenting stroke volume, but this compensatory response is prevented in many patients by a concurrent impairment of cardiac contractility. In addition, most anesthetic agents depress myocardial contractility and/or produce peripheral vasodilatation. Furthermore, anesthesia may further depress the automaticity, and therefore the ventricular rate, of the patient with heart block. Thus patients with untreated complete heart block may be unable to meet the increased demands placed on the cardiovascular system by anesthesia and operation, and a permanent or temporary pacemaker should be inserted before general anesthesia, even in asymptomatic patients (Chap. 24).

A more difficult problem is presented by the patient with *chronic bifascicular block* (p. 198).[12, 83–85] A significant fraction of patients developing this abnormality in the course of an acute myocardial infarction progress to complete heart block, often accompanied by sudden severe hemodynamic compromise (p. 1266). In several series, progression from bifascicular to complete heart block has not been documented during the perioperative period in patients without a previous history of third-degree heart block. Therefore, we do not recommend prophylactic pacemaker placement for such patients or for patients with first-degree atrioventricular (AV) block or Type I second-degree AV block (Wenckebach), although a pacemaker should always be available in the operating room for emergency placement. However, in patients who have bifascicular block, and who also have Type II second-degree AV block or a history of unexplained syncope or transient third-degree AV block, the risk of development of complete heart block is much higher, and a temporary pacemaker should be inserted preoperatively. Also, the appearance of new bifascicular block in the immediate postoperative period commonly justifies insertion of a temporary demand pacemaker, since the incidence of subsequent complete AV block is high in this group.

THE PATIENT WITH A PERMANENT PACEMAKER. When a patient with a permanent pacemaker in situ is about to undergo operation, the device should be carefully evaluated to insure that it is functioning properly preoperatively (Chap. 24). Demand pacemakers are sensitive to electromagnetic interference, such as that produced by the electrocautery, which may result in failure to pace. The danger of this potentially hazardous interaction can be reduced by placing the indifferent plate of the cautery unit as far as possible from the lead and pulse generator, and the electrocautery should be used in brief bursts rather than continuously.[86] Also, a magnet should be available in the operating room to convert the pacemaker from the demand to the fixed-rate mode. Because the cautery may also interfere with the electrocardiographic monitor and render it temporarily uninterpretable, arterial pressure should be monitored directly during the interval when the cautery is being used.

In general, a prophylactic *temporary pacemaker* should be inserted before noncardiac surgery only if the patient meets the indications for permanent pacemaker insertion[87] (see also p. 717) and the operation should not be delayed for the time required for a permanent pacemaker insertion, or if the operative course is likely to be complicated by transient bacteremia. In such situations a temporary pacemaker should be placed initially, and the permanent pacemaker can be inserted after the operation. The occasional exception is the patient who has a severe bradycardiac response to vagal stimuli and who might be difficult to manage during a major surgical procedure without a pacemaker.

GENERAL MEDICAL PROBLEMS

Patients with heart disease whose general medical status is complicated by renal insufficiency, hepatic abnormalities, hypoxemia, or electrolyte abnormalities have a higher risk of cardiac complications, presumably because these nonmedical conditions exacerbate the myocardial stress of surgery.[12] Morbidity is also higher in markedly obese patients[88] because obesity is often associated with abnormal cardiorespiratory function, metabolic function, and hemostasis. Every effort should be made to correct any general problems before surgery, and the potential long-term benefits of surgery must also be interpreted in light of the patient's general prognosis.

POSTOPERATIVE COMPLICATIONS

MYOCARDIAL INFARCTION. Seventy per cent of perioperative infarcts occur within the first 6 days, with the peak incidence by the third day.[89] The mortality rate after postoperative myocardial infarctions ranges from about 30 to 60 per cent, depending on the criteria for infarction. This time course suggests that a majority of infarctions may be more related to the postoperative recuperation than to intraoperative events. Postoperative stresses include general surgical complications, hypoxia and other pulmonary complications, fluid and electrolyte abnormalities, and the stresses of modern postoperative ambulation protocols. Substantial data indicate that prophylactic anticoagulation with low-dose heparin will reduce the risk of postoperative thromboembolic complications,[90] and such therapy is routinely indicated in most cardiac patients who undergo noncardiac surgery. In fact, such anticoagulation regimens may permit a more gradual postoperative ambulation protocol in cardiac patients, and hence possibly lower the incidence of postoperative myocardial infarction.

Myocardial infarction occurring in the perioperative period is often painless.[12, 16] Obviously, then, the incidence of perioperative infarction will be underestimated if electrocardiograms are not obtained routinely during the postoperative period. Furthermore, the electrocardiogram detects only a fraction of infarcts, and it is likely that if the incidence of infarction were determined by more sensitive methods, such as serial estimations of serum creatine kinase isoenzyme (MB fraction), it would be even higher.

HYPERTENSION. Postoperative hypertension is most likely to occur soon after the cessation of positive-pressure ventilation or in the recovery room, and it is more common after carotid endarterectomy and major abdominal vascular procedures.[10, 91, 92] Common precipitants include fluid overload after cessation of positive-pressure ventilation, hypoxemia, anxiety, and pain.[93] The principal therapeutic approaches should therefore concentrate on assuring adequate oxygenation, pain control, and fluid control. In general, supplemental oxygen, morphine, and diuretics are the mainstays of the treatment of postoperative hypertension. Nitroprusside (p. 880) is the preferred medication for severer hypertension. Intravenous hydralazine in small doses is effective for treating postoperative hypertension, but it has the potential for precipitating supraventricular tachyarrhythmias. Methyldopa will not be helpful in the emergency situation, but it may be an important part of the overall regimen because it will have its onset of effect about 4 hours after administration, at a time when one would like to be able to discontinue more vigorous intravenous antihypertensive regimens.

CONGESTIVE HEART FAILURE. Although postoperative heart failure may be precipitated by myocardial infarction or ischemia, more than half of the cases are directly caused by excess fluid administration.[11] Heart failure tends to occur soon after cessation of positive-pressure ventilation and again at about 24 to 48 hours after operation, when the fluid that was given in the perioperative period is mobilized from the extravascular sites. Diuretics, often given intravenously, sometimes supplemented by digitalis glycosides, are usually sufficient therapy for postoperative congestive heart failure.

POSTOPERATIVE ARRHYTHMIAS. Arrhythmias are common after operation and are often a manifestation of a noncardiac complication, such as bleeding, infection or an acid-base or electrolyte imbalance occurring in a patient with heart disease. Management of such arrhythmias often requires recognition and correction of extracardiac factors.

In one study of 916 patients who were in sinus rhythm throughout the course of major noncardiac surgery, 35 patients (4 per cent) developed new supraventricular tachyarrhythmias postoperatively.[94] Of these 35 patients, 46 per cent had acute cardiac conditions, 31 per cent had major infections, 29 per cent had preexisting hypotension, 26 per cent had anemia, 23 per cent had metabolic derangements, 23 per cent had received new parenteral drugs that could be implicated, and 20 per cent were hypoxic. Forty per cent of the patients required no new therapy with cardiac medications, and only two patients required electrical cardioversion; the arrhythmias of all treated patients reverted to sinus rhythm. No deaths were related to the supraventricular tachyarrhythmias per se, but half the patients in whom these arrhythmias occurred died as a result of the concurrent medical problems. Thus, a new postoperative supraventricular tachyarrhythmia should prompt a search for remediable medical problems. Direct antiarrhythmic therapy is often unnecessary and is usually secondary in importance to correction of the underlying cause of the arrhythmia.

Sinus tachycardia is the most common rhythm disturbance in the postoperative patient. Multiple noncardiac etiologies have been identified, including pain, hypovolemia or hypervolemia, fever, anemia, hypoxemia, pulmonary emboli, anxiety, infection, hypotension, and electrolyte abnormalities (especially hypokalemia). These noncardiac etiologies are much more common causes of sinus tachycardia in the postoperative cardiac patient than is either myocardial infarction or heart failure. Sinus tachycardia not caused by congestive heart failure will not slow with cardiac glycosides. The therapeutic:toxic ratio of these drugs is actually reduced by most of the above-mentioned noncardiac causes of sinus tachycardia, and therefore digitalis glycosides are not considered appropriate for postoperative patients unless the sinus tachycardia is likely to be caused by impaired cardiac function.

Atrial fibrillation is also a common postoperative arrhythmia. Atrial dilatation, which lowers the threshold for development of this arrhythmia, may result from heart failure, mitral valve disease, and/or hypervolemia. Noncardiac precipitants include pneumonia, atelectasis, and pulmonary emboli. Initially, the postoperative patient with atrial fibrillation should be treated with a digitalis glycoside or verapamil; in addition, a beta-adrenoceptor can be used to help gain rapid control of the ventricular rate. Cardioversion is usually delayed until the precipitating factors have been eliminated, since the patient who has cardioversion before clearing the atelectasis or pneumonia frequently reverts to atrial fibrillation, while the patient whose pulmonary problem or congestive heart failure is adequately treated often reverts spontaneously to sinus rhythm.

Atrial flutter is often poorly tolerated because of the rapid ventricular rate and the difficult pharmacological management. Cardioversion is usually the treatment of choice, along with quinidine or procainamide administered to prevent recurrence (p. 672).

IMPLICATIONS OF POSTOPERATIVE COMPLICATIONS FOR LONG-TERM MANAGEMENT. When a patient develops a perioperative myocardial infarction, the evaluation and the recuperative process generally should be analogous to when a myocardial infarction occurs in other patients (see Chap. 38) Because postoperative congestive heart failure is commonly precipitated by iatrogenic fluid overload, the patient commonly will not need chronic long-term therapy for congestive heart failure. Similarly, perioperative arrhythmias are often precipitated by specific stimuli, and the patient with a postoperative arrhythmia should not automatically be consigned to long-term antiarrhythmic therapy. In patients who develop either postoperative congestive heart failure or arrhythmias, it is often appropriate to discontinue new cardiac therapies several days before discharge and observe the patient to see whether chronic therapy is indicated.

THE ROLE OF THE MEDICAL CONSULTANT

The physician called on to evaluate a patient with suspected or overt cardiac disease before elective or emergency noncardiac surgery must first determine whether cardiovascular disease is present and then, if it is, must identify those factors that may increase the risk of operation. It may be necessary to invest considerable time and effort to prepare the patient for operation. In addition, the patient must be carefully followed after operation to detect and manage the cardiac problems that frequently complicate the postoperative period.

ESTIMATION OF RISK

A few patients have such compelling reasons for operation (e.g., rupturing aortic aneurysm, perforated or necrotic bowel, life-threatening hemorrhage, or some forms of intestinal obstruction) that estimation of operative risk is an academic exercise, since failure to operate almost certainly will result in the patient's death. Often, however, the timing or even the performance of an operation is elective, and under these circumstances estimation of risk is an important aspect of the medical consultant's role. Certain cardiovascular problems, such as recent myocardial infarction (less than 3 months), inadequately treated congestive heart failure, and severe mitral or aortic stenosis, are *absolute contraindications* to *elective* surgery. *Relative contraindications* include remoter myocardial infarction (3 to 6 months earlier), angina pectoris, mild heart failure, cyanotic congenital heart disease with severe polycythemia and a coagulation abnormality. Several other problems should be recognized and treated before operation: anemia, hypovolemia, polycythemia, pulmonary disease causing hypoxemia, adrenal hyporesponsiveness secondary to chronic administration of adrenal steroids, hypertension, electrolyte abnormalities, as well as the entire gamut of cardiac arrhythmias. Considerable judgment must be exercised when one or more of the abovementioned problems are present and when a patient requires prompt surgical treatment but the situation is not a true emergency, as for neoplastic disease.

To identify those preoperative factors associated with the development of cardiac complications after major noncardiac operation in patients over 40 years of age, one analysis identified nine independently significant correlates of life-threatening and fatal cardiac complications. When these factors were weighted based on their relative significance as predictors of cardiac outcome, a multifactorial index was developed for predicting perioperative risk (Table 53–2). Notably, *unimportant* factors included smoking, glucose intolerance, hyperlipidemia, hypertension, peripheral atherosclerotic vascular disease, stable Class I or II angina, and remote myocardial infarction.

TABLE 53–2 COMPUTATION OF THE CARDIAC RISK INDEX

CRITERIA	POINTS
1 History	
(a) Age > 70 yr	5
(b) MI in previous 6 mo	10
2 Physical examination	
(a) S_3 gallop or JVD	11
(b) Important VAS	3
3 Electrocardiogram	
(a) Rhythm other than sinus or PAC's on last preoperative ECG	7
(b) > 5 PVC's/min documented at any time before operation	7
4 General status	
P_{O_2} < 60 or P_{CO_2} > 50 mm Hg, K < 3.0 or HCO_3 < 20 mEq/liter, BUN > 50 or Cr > 3.0 mg/dl, abnormal SGOT, signs of chronic liver disease or patient bedridden from noncardiac causes	3
5 Operation	
(a) Intraperitoneal, intrathoracic, or aortic operation	3
(b) Emergency operation	4
Total possible	53 points

To calculate a patient's score, the number of points from all factors he or she possesses are summed. MI, myocardial infarction; JVD, jugular vein distention; VAS, valvular aortic stenosis; PAC's, premature atrial contractions; ECG, electrocardiogram; PVC's, premature ventricular contractions; P_{O_2}, partial pressure of oxygen; P_{CO_2}, partial pressure of carbon dioxide; K, potassium; HCO_3, bicarbonate; BUN, blood urea nitrogen; Cr, creatinine; and SGOT, serum glutamic oxalacetic transminase.

Reprinted by permission from Goldman, L., Caldera, D. L., Nussbaum, S. R., et al.: Multifactorial index of cardiac risk in noncardiac surgical procedures. N. Engl. J. Med. 297:845, 1977.

The value of the information in this index has been confirmed in two large prospective series of general surgical patients[23, 24] (Table 53–3) and in several other studies.[13, 32, 95] In one series,[24] risk stratification was equally good when several minor modifications were made in point assignment and when a prior history of Class III or IV angina, unstable angina, and pulmonary edema were included in the index.

However, because the index was derived from unselected general surgical patients above age 40, it appears to underestimate risk by about 40 per cent in patients who undergo resection of an abdominal aortic aneurysm,[20] and it also underestimates risk in patients who are selected on the basis of any high-risk status. One way to take into account the fact that some patients have higher baseline

TABLE 53–3 MAJOR COMPLICATION* RATES IN FOUR STUDIES THAT HAVE ANALYZED THE MULTIFACTORIAL CARDIAC RISK INDEX[18]

TYPE OF PATIENTS	GOLDMAN ET AL.[18] Unselected Noncardiac Surgery, ≥40 y.o.	ZELDIN[23] Unselected Noncardiac Surgery, ≥40 y.o.	DETSKY ET AL.[24]† Preoperative Medical Consultations	JEFFREY ET AL.[20]‡ Abdominal Aortic Aneurysm Surgery	POOLED	POOLED LIKELIHOOD RATIO *(sensitivity/specificity)*
Overall complication rate	58/1001 (6%)	35/1140 (3%)	27/268 (10%)	11/99 (11%)	131/2508 (5.2%)	
Complication rate by class						
Class I (0–5 points)†	5/537 (1%)	4/590 (1%)	8/134 (6%)	4/56 (7%)	21/1317 (1.6%)	.29
Class II (6–12 points)	21/316 (7%)	13/453 (3%)	6/85 (7%)	4/35 (11%)	44/889 (5%)	.94
Class III (13–25 points)	18/130 (14%)	11/74 (15%)	9/45 (20%)	3/8 (38%)	41/257 (16%)	3.4
Class IV (≥26 points)	14/18 (78%)	7/23 (30%)	4/4 (100%)	0	25/45 (56%)	22.7

*Documented myocardial infarction, cardiogenic pulmonary edema, ventricular tachycardia, or cardiac death.
†Actual unpublished numbers provided by Dr. Detsky.
‡See Table 53–2 for calculation of point total.
Goldman, L.: Multifactorial index of cardiac risk in noncardiac surgery: Ten-year status report. J. Cardiothorac. Surg. (*In Press*).

TABLE 53–4 ESTIMATION OF PROBABILITY OF CARDIAC COMPLICATIONS

Type of Patient	Approximate Baseline Risk (%)	Approximate Risk as Adjusted Using Multifactorial Index (%)[18]* Class I	Class II	Class III	Class IV
Minor surgery	1	0.3	1	3	19
Unselected consecutive patients over age 40 who have major noncardiac surgery	4	1.2	4	12	48
Patients who have abdominal aortic aneurysm surgery or who are over age 40 and have medical consultations before major noncardiac surgery	10	3	10	30	75

*Calculated by multiplying the prior odds of complications by the likelihood ratio for each class; see Table 53–3.

Goldman, L.: Multifactorial index of cardiac risk in noncardiac surgery: Ten-year status report. J. Cardiothorac. Surg. (*In Press*).

risks is to know the baseline probability of cardiac complications for specific types of patients or types of surgery and then to modify these "pre-test" probabilities based on the patient's cardiac condition.[24, 96, 97] As shown in Table 53–4, this can be a useful approach to estimating the risk of major cardiac complications. Even at its best, however, any index for predicting cardiac complications should be viewed as an aid and not as a crutch; it should supplement, not substitute for, clinical judgment.

Although the multifactorial index is a well-validated and useful approach for the global assessment of risk in unselected general surgical patients, certain subgroups of patients clearly benefit from additional testing. For example, the use of exercise testing in elderly persons[32] may supplement the multifactorial risk approach (Fig. 53–1). In addition, dipyridamole thallium imaging (p. 331) has been valuable in assessing risk in patients under consideration for vascular surgery.[33]

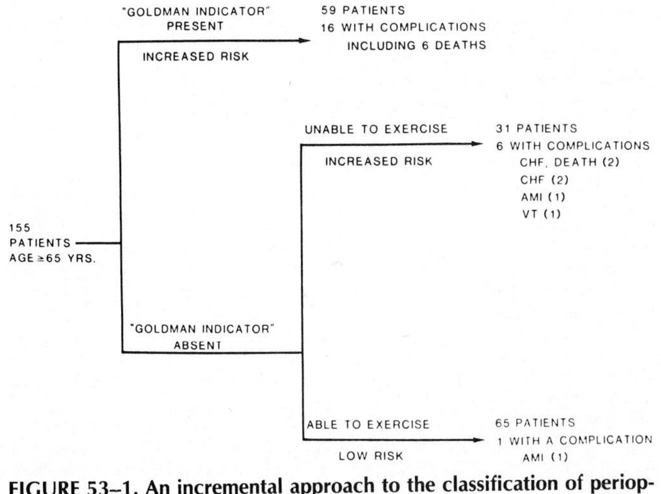

FIGURE 53–1. An incremental approach to the classification of perioperative cardiac risk in 155 consecutive patients over age 65 who underwent major abdominal or noncardiac thoracic surgery. A "Goldman indicator" is any of the factors listed in Table 53–2 other than age or type of surgery. "Unable to exercise" means an inability to do 2 minutes of bicycle exercise in the supine position to a heart rate greater than 99 beats/min. CHF = congestive heart failure; VT = ventricular tachycardia; AMI = acute myocardial infarction. (From Gerson, M. C., et al.: Cardiac prognosis in noncardiac geriatric surgery. Ann. Intern. Med. *103*:832, 1985.)

PREPARATION OF THE PATIENT FOR ANESTHESIA AND OPERATION

Careful preparation of the cardiac patient for operation may diminish the frequency and seriousness of intraoperative and postoperative complications. The medical consultant should not hesitate to urge postponement or cancellation of an elective operation or to insist on sufficient time to institute any measures that are necessary to minimize risk. The consultant should attempt to be brief and to the point, and to provide a limited number of explicit, relevant suggestions.[98–101] The cardiological consultant should work closely with the anesthesiologist and the surgeon so that their talents may be combined to maximize the likelihood of a favorable outcome.[13, 26, 101]

REFERENCES

1. Glasser, S. P. (ed.): Noncardiac Surgery in the Cardiac Patient. Mt. Kisco, N.Y., Futura Publishing Co., 1983.
2. Rogers, M. C.: Anesthetic management of patients with heart disease. Mod. Concepts Cardiovasc. Dis. 52:29, 1983.

ANESTHESIA

3. Kaplan, J. A. (ed.): Cardiac Anesthesia. Orlando, Grune and Stratton, 1979.
4. Prys-Roberts, C., and Meloche, R.: Management of anesthesia in patients with hypertension or ischemic heart disease. Int. Anesthesiol. Clin. *18*:181, 1980.
5. Prys-Roberts, C., Meloche, R., and Foex, P.: Studies of anesthesia in relation to hypertension. I. Cardiovascular responses of treated and untreated patients. Br. J. Anaesth. *43*:112, 1971.
6. Prys-Roberts, C., Foex, P., Greene, L. T., and Waterhouse, T. D.: Studies of anesthesia in relation to hypertension. IV. The effects of artificial ventilation on the circulation and pulmonary gas exchanges. Br. J. Anaesth. *44*:335, 1972.
7. Tarhan, S. (ed.): Cardiovascular Anesthesia and Postoperative Care. Chicago, Year Book Medical Publishers, 1982.
8. Mauney, F. M., Jr., Ebert, P. A., and Sabiston, D. C., Jr.: Postoperative myocardial infarction: A study of predisposing factors, diagnosis and mortality in a high risk group of surgical patients. Ann. Surg. *172*:497, 1970.
9. Steen, P. A., Tinker, J. H., and Tarhan, S.: Myocardial reinfarction after anesthesia and surgery. JAMA *239*:2566, 1978.
10. Goldman, L., and Caldera, D. L.: Risks of general anesthesia and elective surgery in the hypertensive patient. Anesthesiology *50*:285, 1979.
11. Cooperman, L. H., and Price, H. L.: Pulmonary edema in the operative and postoperative period: A review of 40 cases. Ann. Surg. *172*:883, 1970.
12. Goldman, L., Caldera, D. L., Southwick, F. S., Nussbaum, S. R., Murray, B., O'Malley, T. A., Goroll, A. H., Caplan, C. H., Nolan, J., Burke, D. S., Krogstad, D., Carabello, B., and Slater, E. E.: Cardiac risk factors and complications in non-cardiac surgery. Medicine 57:357, 1978.
13. Kaplan, J. A., and Dunbar, R. W.: Anesthesia for noncardiac surgery in patients with cardiac disease. *In* Kaplan, J. A. (ed.): Cardiac Anesthesia. Orlando, Grune and Stratton, 1979, p. 377.

THE OPERATION

14. Backer, C. L., Tinker, J. H., Robertson, D. M., and Vlietstra, R. E.: Myocardial reinfarction following local anesthesia for ophthalmic surgery. Anesth. Analg. 59:257, 1980.
15. Erlik, D., Valero, A., Birkhan, J., and Gersh, I.: Prostatic surgery and the cardiovascular patient. Br. J. Urol. *40*:53, 1968.
16. Tarhan, S., Moffitt, E. A., Taylor, W. F., and Guilioni, E. R.: Myocardial infarction after general anesthesia. J.A.M.A. *220*:1451, 1972.
17. Knorring, J.: Postoperative myocardial infarction: A prospective study in a high-risk group of surgical patients. Surgery *90*:55, 1981.
18. Goldman, L., Caldera, D. L., Nussbaum, S. R., Southwick, F. S., Krogstad, D., Murray, B., Burke, D. S., O'Malley, T. A., Goroll, A. H., Caplan, C. H., Nolan, J., Carabello, B., and Slater, E. E.: Multifactorial index of cardiac risk in noncardiac surgical procedures. N. Engl. J. Med. *297*:845, 1977.
19. Skinner, J. F., and Pearce, M. L.: Surgical risk in the cardiac patient. J. Chronic. Dis. *17*:57, 1964.
20. Jeffrey, C. C., Kunsman, J., Cullen, D. J., and Brewster, D. C.: A prospective evaluation of cardiac risk index. Anesthesiology *58*:462, 1983.
21. Lewin, I., Lerner, A. G., Green, S. H., Del Guercio, L.R.M., and Siegel, J. H.: Physical class and physiological status in the prediction of operative mortality in the aged sick. Ann. Surg. *174*:217, 1971.

INFLUENCE OF UNDERLYING CARDIOVASCULAR DISEASE

22. Rao, T. L. K., Jacobs, K. H., and El-Etr, A. A.: Reinfarction following anesthesia in patients with myocardial infarction. Anesthesiology 59:499, 1983.

23. Zeldin, R. A.: Assessing cardiac risk in patients who undergo noncardiac surgical procedures. Can. J. Surg. *27*:402, 1984.
24. Detsky, A. S., Abrams, H. B., McLaughlin, J. R., Drucker, D. J., Sasson, Z., Johnston, N., Scott, J. G., Forbath, N., and Hilliard, J. R.: Predicting cardiac complications in patients undergoing non-cardiac surgery. J. Gen. Intern. Med. *1*:211, 1986.
25. Del Guercio, L.R.M., and Cohn, J. D.: Monitoring operative risk in the elderly. J.A.M.A. *243*:1350, 1980.
26. Wells, P. H., and Kaplan, J. A.: Optimal management of patients with ischemic heart disease for noncardiac surgery by complementary anesthesiologist and cardiologist interaction. Am. Heart J. *102*:1029, 1981.
27. DeBusk, R. F., Kraemer, H. C., Nash, E., Berger, W. E., and Lew, H.: Stepwise risk stratification soon after acute myocardial infarction. Am. J. Cardiol. 52:1161, 1983.
28. Campeau, L.: Grading of angina pectoris. Circulation *54*:522, 1975.
29. Goldman, L., Hashimoto, B., Cook, E. F., and Loscalzo, A.: Comparative reproducibility and validity of systems for assessing cardiovascular functional class: Advantages of a new Specific Activity Scale. Circulation *64*:1227, 1981.
30. Goldman, L., Cook, E. F., Mitchell, N., Flatley, M., Sherman, H., and Cohn, P. F.: Pitfalls in the serial assessment of cardiac functional status. J. Chronic Dis. *35*:763, 1982.
31. Carliner, N. H., Fisher, M. L., Plotnick, G. D., Garbart, H., Rapoport, A., Kelemen, M. H., Moran, G. W., Gadacz, T., and Peters, R. W.: Routine preoperative exercise testing in patients undergoing major noncardiac surgery. Am. J. Cardiol. *56*:51, 1985.
32. Gerson, M. C., Hurst, J. M., Hertzberg, V. S., Doogan, P. A., Cochran, M. B., Lim, S. P., McCall, N., and Adolph, R. J.: Cardiac prognosis in noncardiac geriatric surgery. Ann. Intern. Med. *103*:832, 1985.
33. Boucher, C. A., Brewster, D. C., Darling, R. C., Okada, R. D., Strauss, H. W., and Pohost, G. M.: Determination of cardiac risk by dipyridamole-thallium imaging before peripheral vascular surgery. N. Engl. J. Med. *312*:389, 1985.
34. Homma, S., Callahan, R. J., Ameer, B., McKusick, K. A., Strauss, H. W., Okada, R. D., and Boucher, C. A.: Usefulness of oral dipyridamole suspension for stress thallium imaging without exercise in the detection of coronary artery disease. Am. J. Cardiol. *57*:503, 1986.
35. Heller, G. V., Aroesty, J. M., Parker, J. A., McKay, R. G., Silverman, K. J., Als, A. V., Come, P. C., Kolodny, G. M., and Grossman, W.: The pacing stress test: Thallium-201 myocardial imaging after atrial pacing: Diagnostic value in detecting coronary artery disease compared with exercise testing. J. Am. Coll. Cardiol. *3*:1197, 1984.
36. Hertzer, N. R., Young, J. R., Kramer, J. R., Phillips, D. F., deWolfe, V. G., Ruschhaupt, W. F., and Beven, E. G.: Routine coronary angiography prior to elective aortic reconstruction: Results of selective myocardial revascularization in patients with peripheral vascular disease. Arch. Surg. *114*:1336, 1979.
37. Mahar, L. J., Steen, P. A., Tinker, J. H., Vlietstra, R. E., Smith, H. C., and Pluth, J. R.: Perioperative myocardial infarction in patients with coronary artery disease with and without aorta-coronary bypass grafts. J. Thorac. Cardiovasc. Surg. *76*:533, 1978.
38. Crawford, E. S., Morris, G. C., Howell, J. F., Flynn, W. F., and Moorhead, D. T.: Operative risk in patients with previous coronary artery bypass. Ann. Thorac. Surg. *26*:215, 1978.
39. DeBakey, M. E., and Lawrie, G. M.: Combined coronary artery and peripheral vascular disease: Recognition and treatment. J. Vasc. Surg. *1*:605, 1984.
40. Foster, E. D., Davis, K. B., Carpenter, J. A., Abele, S., Fray, D., and principal investigators of CASS and their associates: Risk of noncardiac operation in patients with defined coronary disease: The Coronary Artery Surgery Study (CASS) registry experience. Ann. Thorac. Surg. *41*:42, 1986.
41. Lunder, T., Lindegaard, K. F., Froysaker, T., Aaslid, R., Wiberg, J., and Nornes, H.: Cerebral perfusion during nonpulsatile cardiopulmonary bypass. Ann. Thorac. Surg. *40*:144, 1985.
42. Jones, E. L., Craver, J. M., Michalik, R. A., Murphy, D. A., Guyton, R. A., Bone, D. K., Hatcher, C. R., and Reichwald, N. A.: Combined carotid and coronary operations: When are they necessary? J. Thorac. Cardiovasc. Surg. *87*:7, 1984.
43. Matar, A. F.: Concomitant coronary and cerebral revascularization under cardiopulmonary bypass. Ann. Thorac. Surg. *41*:431, 1986.
44. Viljoen, J. F., Estafanous, G., and Kellner, G. A.: Propranolol and cardiac surgery. J. Thorac. Cardiovasc. Surg. *64*:826, 1972.
45. Caralps, J. M., Mulet, J., Wienke, H. R., Moran, J. M., and Pifarre, R.: Results of coronary artery surgery in patients receiving propranolol. J. Thorac. Cardiovasc. Surg. *67*:526, 1974.
46. Kaplan, J. A., Dunbar, R. W., Bland, J. W., Sumpter, R., and Jones, E. L.: Propranolol and cardiac surgery: A problem for the anesthesiologist. Anesth. Analg. *54*:571, 1975.
47. Should propranolol be stopped before surgery? Med. Lett. *18*:41, 1976.
48. Goldman, L.: Noncardiac surgery in patients receiving propranolol. Case reports and a recommended approach. Arch. Intern. Med. *141*:193, 1981.
49. Prys-Roberts, C., Foex, P., and Roberts, J. G.: Studies of anaesthesia in relation to hypertension. Br. J. Anaesth. *45*:671, 1973.
50. Prys-Roberts, C.: Hemodynamic effects of anesthesia and surgery in renal hypertensive patients receiving large doses of beta-receptor antagonists. Anesthesiology *51* (Suppl.):122, 1979.
51. Woolsey, R. L., and Shand, D. G.: Pharmacokinetics of antiarrhythmic drugs. Am. J. Cardiol. *41*:986, 1978.
52. Smulyan, H., Weinberg, S. E., and Howanitz, P. J.: Continuous propranolol infusion following abdominal surgery. J.A.M.A. *247*:2539, 1982.
53. Reves, J. G., and Flezzani, P.: Perioperative use of esmolol. Am. J. Cardiol. *56*:57F, 1985.
54. Katz, R. L., Weintraub, H. D., and Papper, E. M.: Anesthesia, surgery and rauwolfia. Anesthesiology *25*:142, 1964.
55. Prys-Roberts, C.: Medical problems of surgical patients. Hypertension and ischaemic heart disease. Ann. R. Coll. Surg. Engl. *58*:465, 1976.
56. Prys-Roberts, C.: Hypertension and anesthesia—fifty years on. Anesthesiology *50*:281, 1979.
57. Leth, A.: Changes in plasma and extracellular fluid volumes in patients with essential hypertension during long-term treatment with hydrochlorothiazide. Circulation *42*:479, 1970.
58. Tarazi, R. C., Dustan, H. P., and Frohlich, E. D.: Long-term thiazide therapy in essential hypertension. Evidence for persistent alteration in plasma volume and renin activity. Circulation *41*:709, 1970.
59. Bruce, D. L., Croley, T. F., and Lee, J. S.: Preoperative clonidine withdrawal syndrome. Anesthesiology *51*:90, 1979.
60. Stone, J. G., Hoar, P. F., Calabro, J. R., DePetrillo, M. A., and Bendixen, H. H.: Afterload reduction and preload augmentation improve the anesthetic management of patients with cardiac failure and valvular regurgitation. Anesth. Analg. *59*:737, 1980.
61. Thompson, R. C., Liberthson, R. R., and Lowenstein, E.: Perioperative anesthetic risk of noncardiac surgery in hypertrophic obstructive cardiomyopathy. J.A.M.A. *254*:2419, 1985.
62. Tinker, J. H., and Tarhan, S.: Discontinuing anticoagulant therapy in surgical patients with cardiac valve prostheses. J.A.M.A. 239:738, 1978.
63. Katholi, R. E., Nolan, S. P., and McGuire, L. B.: Living with prosthetic heart valve. Subsequent noncardiac operations and the risk of thromboembolism or hemorrhage. Am. Heart J. *92*:162, 1976.
64. Tinker, J. H., Noback, C. R., Vlietstra, R. E., and Frye, R. L.: Management of patients with heart disease for noncardiac surgery. J.A.M.A. *246*:1348, 1981.
65. Shuman, S. T., Amren, D. P., Bisno, A. L., Dajani, A. S., Durack, D. T., Gerber, M. A., Kaplan, E. L., Millard, H. D., Sanders, W. E., Schwartz, R. H., and Watanakunakorn, C.: Prevention of bacterial endocarditis. A statement for health professionals by the Committee on Rheumatic Fever and Infective Endocarditis of the Council on Cardiovascular Disease in the Young. Circulation *70*:1123A, 1984.
66. Clemens, J. D., Horwitz, R. I., Jaffe, C. C., Feinstein, A. R., and Stanton, B. F.: A controlled evaluation of the risk of bacterial endocarditis in persons with mitral-valve prolapse. N. Engl. J. Med. *307*:776, 1982.
67. Mills, P., Rose, J., Hollingsworth, J., Amara, I., and Craige, E.: Long-term prognosis of mitral-valve prolapse. N. Engl. J. Med. *297*:13, 1977.
68. Durack, D. T.: Current issues in prevention of infective endocarditis. Am. J. Med. *78* (Suppl. 6B):149, 1985.
69. Bor, D. H., and Himmelstein, D. U.: Endocarditis prophylaxis for patients with mitral valve prolapse. Am. J. Med. *76*:711, 1984.
70. Clemens, J. D., and Ransohoff, D. F.: A quantitative assessment of pre-dental antibiotic prophylaxis for patients with mitral valve prolapse. J. Chronic Dis. *37*:531, 1984.
71. Sommerville, J., McDonald, L., and Edgill, M.: Postoperative haemorrhage and related abnormalities of blood coagulatiion in cyanotic congenital heart disease. Br. Heart J. *27*:440, 1965.
72. Hickey, P. R., Hansen, D. D., Norwood, W. I., and Castaneda, A. R.: Anesthetic complications in surgery for congenital heart disease. Anesth. Analg. *63*:657, 1984.
73. Goldberg, A. H., Maling, H. M., and Gaffney, T. E.: The effect of digoxin pretreatment in heart contractile force during thiopental infusion in dogs. Anesthesiology *22*:974, 1961.
74. Goldberg, A. H., Maling, H. M., and Gaffney, T. E.: The value of prophylactic digitalization in halothane anesthesia. Anesthesiology *23*:207, 1962.
75. Shimosato, S. A., and Etsten, B.: Performance of digitalized heart during halothane anesthesia. Anesthesiology *24*:41, 1963.
76. Lee, D. C., Johnson, R. A., Bingham, J. B., Leahy, M., Dinsmore, R. E., Goroll, A. H., Newell, J. B., Strauss, H. W., and Haber, E.: Heart failure in outpatients. A randomized trial of digoxin versus placebo. N. Engl. J. Med. *306*:699, 1982.
77. Arnold, S. B., Byrd, R. C., Meister, W., Melmon, K., Cheitlin, M. D., Bristow, J. D., Parmley, W. W., and Chatterjee, K.: Long-term digitalis therapy improves left ventricular function in heart failure. N. Engl. J. Med. *303*:1443, 1980.
78. Schulze, R. A., Jr., Rouleau, J., Rigo, P., Bowers, S., Strauss, H. W., and Pitt, B.: Ventricular arrhythmias in the late hospital phase of acute myocardial infarction: Relation to left ventricular function detected by gated cardiac blood pool scanning. Circulation 52:1006, 1975.
79. Schulze, R. A., Jr., Strauss, H. W., and Pitt, B.: Sudden death in the year following myocardial infarction: Relation to ventricular premature contractions in the late hospital phase and left ventricular ejection fraction. Am. J. Med. *62*:192, 1977.
80. Kennedy, H. L., Whitlock, J. A., Sprague, M. K., Kennedy, L. J., Buckingham, T. A., and Goldberg, R. J.: Long-term follow-up of asymptomatic healthy subjects with frequent and complex ventricular ectopy. N. Engl. J. Med. *312*:193, 1985.
81. Bergh, N. P., Dottori, O., and Malmberg, R.: Prophylactic digitalis in thoracic surgery. Scand. J. Resp. Dis. *48*:197, 1967.
82. Selzer, A., and Walter, R. M.: Adequacy of preoperative digitalis therapy in controlling ventricular rate in postoperative atrial fibrillation. Circulation *34*:119, 1966.
83. Berg, G. R., and Kotler, M. N.: The significance of bilateral bundle branch block in the preoperative patient. Chest *59*:62, 1971.

84. Logue, R. B., and Kaplan, J. A.: The cardiac patient and noncardiac surgery. *In* Harvey, W. P. (ed.): Current Problems in Cardiology. Vol. 7. Chicago, Year Book Medical Publishers, 1982.
85. Pastore, J. O., Yurchak, P. M., Janis, K. M., Murphy, J. D., and Zir, L. M.: The risk of advanced heart block in surgical patients with right bundle branch block and left axis deviation. Circulation 57:677, 1978.
86. Simon, A. B.: Perioperative management of the pacemaker patient. Anesthesiology *46*:127, 1977.
87. Frye, R. L., Collins, J. J., DeSanctis, R. W., Dodge, H. T., Dreifus, L. S., Fisch, C., Gettes, L. S., Gillette, P. C., Parsonnet, V., Reeves, T. J., and Weinberg, S. L.: Guidelines for permanent cardiac pacemaker implantation, May 1984. A report of the Joint American College of Cardiology/American Heart Association Task Force on Assessment of Cardiovascular Procedures (Subcommittee on Pacemaker Implantation). J. Am. Coll. Cardiol. *4*:434, 1984.
88. Pasulka, P. S., Bistrian, B. R., Benotti, P. N., and Blackburn, G. L.: The risks of surgery in obese patients. Ann. Intern. Med. *104*:540, 1986.

POSTOPERATIVE COMPLICATIONS

89. Salem, D. N., Homans, D. C., and Isner, J. M.: Management of cardiac disease in the general surgical patient. *In* Harvey, W. P. (ed.): Current Problems in Cardiology. Vol. 5. Chicago, Year Book Medical Publishers, 1980.
90. An International Multicentre Trial: Prevention of fatal postoperative pulmonary embolism by low doses of heparin. Lancet 2:45, 1975.
91. Lehv, M. S., Salzman, E. W., and Silen, W.: Hypertension complicating carotid endarterectomy. Stroke *1*:307, 1970.
92. Gal, T. J., and Cooperman, L. H.: Hypertension in the immediate postoperative period. Br. J. Anaesth. *47*:70, 1975.
93. Goldman, L.: Anesthesia and surgery in the hypertensive patient. *In* Amery, A. (ed.): Hypertensive Cardiovascular Disease: Pathophysiology and Treatment. The Hague, Martinus Nijhoff Publishers, 1982, p. 916.
94. Goldman, L.: Supraventricular tachyarrhythmias in hospitalized adults after surgery. Chest 73:450, 1978.
95. Weathers, L. W., and Paine, R.: The risk of surgery in cardiac patients. Intern. Med. 2:57, 1981.
96. Poses, R. M., Cebul, R. D., Collins, M., and Fager, S. S.: The importance of disease prevalence in transporting clinical prediction rules. The case of streptococcal pharyngitis. Ann. Intern. Med. *105*:586, 1986.
97. Detsky, A. S., Abrams, H. B., Forbath, N., Scott, J. G., and Hilliard, J. R.: Cardiac assessment for patients undergoing noncardiac surgery. A multifactorial clinical risk index. Arch. Intern. Med. *146*:2131, 1986.
98. Lee, T., Pappius, E. M., and Goldman, L.: Impact of inter-physician communication on the effectiveness of medical consultations. Am. J. Med. *74*:106, 1983.
99. Klein, L. E., Levine, D. M., Moore, R. D., and Kirby, S. M.: The preoperative consultation: Response to the internists' recommendations. Arch. Intern. Med. *143*:743, 1983.
100. Horwitz, R. I., Henes, C. G., and Horwitz, S. M.: Strategies for improving the diagnostic and management efficacy of medical consultations. J. Chronic Dis. *36*:213, 1983.
101. Logue, R. B., and Kaplan, J. A.: The cardiac patient and noncardiac surgery. Curr. Probl. Cardiol. 7:1, 1982.

54 RHEUMATIC AND HERITABLE CONNECTIVE TISSUE DISEASES OF THE CARDIOVASCULAR SYSTEM

by GENE H. STOLLERMAN, M.D.

Two groups of diseases that affect connective tissues are the so-called rheumatic diseases and the heritable disorders of connective tissues. The *rheumatic diseases* have many clinical features in common and are often classified together because they produce acute or chronic arthritis or both associated with a variety of systemic inflammatory manifestations. Pathologically, they are characterized by diffuse vascular lesions with varying degrees of exudation and fibrosis, and some seem to be associated with hyperimmune phenomena. In some of the syndromes the etiology has been established as complications of well-recognized infections; however, several of the rheumatic diseases remain obscure in regard to both etiology and pathogenesis. They all involve the heart differently and to varying degrees, as would be expected considering the variety of connective tissue structures that make up the heart's "skeleton"—its valve rings, valves, septa, and pericardial sac and the myocardial interstitium, through which courses its rich blood supply.

The *heritable disorders of connective tissue* are rare, genetically determined biochemical lesions of collagen, elastic tissue, or the mucopolysaccharides. In all, structural lesions are produced when cardiac action stresses the defective cardiac skeleton.

RHEUMATIC DISEASES

RHEUMATIC FEVER

Rheumatic fever (RF) is frequently classified as a connective tissue disease because its anatomical hallmark is damage to collagen fibrils and to the ground substance of connective tissue (especially in the heart). Of major clinical importance is the presence of potentially lethal myocarditis during the acute attack or, more commonly, the fibrosis of the heart valves, which leads to the crippling hemodynamics of chronic rheumatic heart disease. Its uniqueness from other rheumatic diseases is that it is specifically a delayed nonsuppurative sequel of pharyngeal infection with group A streptococci.

EPIDEMIOLOGY

The relation between the epidemiology of RF and that of streptococcal infection has been reviewed extensively.[1] The current confusion concerning the epidemiology of RF stems from the dramatic decline in incidence and prevalence of the disease despite the fact that group A streptococcal pharyngitis still appears to be common among populations in which RF has become rare.[2]

The Changing Pattern of Rheumatic Fever
(Fig. 54–1)

Reasons for this decline are uncertain, but are undoubtedly multiple. Certainly antibiotics for the treatment and prevention of streptococcal infection have been a factor, as demonstrated particularly in military populations.[3,4] However, the incidence and death rate from the disease were decreasing before the introduction of antibiotics. Changes in the virulence and serotypes of group A streptococci have been noteworthy[2, 5] (see below). Improved social conditions, such as better housing and slum clearance,

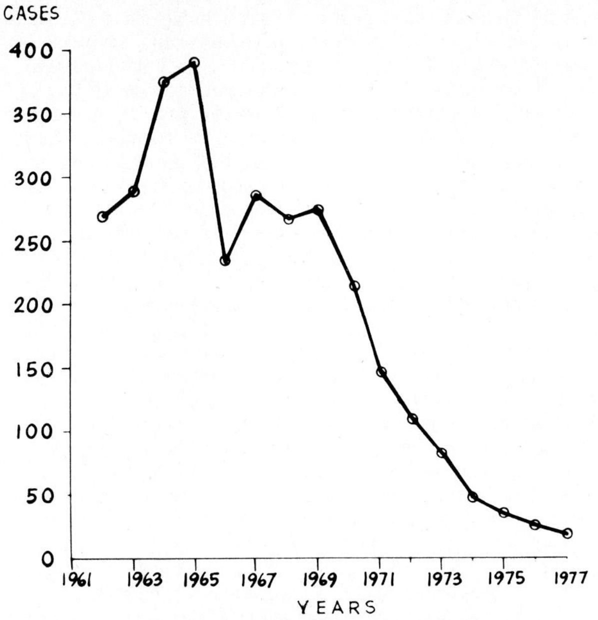

FIGURE 54–1. Acute rheumatic fever attacks reported from 1962 to 1977 to the rheumatic fever registry of the Chicago Department of Health. (From Stollerman, G. H.: Global changes in group A streptococcal diseases and strategies for their prevention. Adv. Intern. Med. *27*:373, 1982.)

have contributed to the decline, since crowding because of inadequate housing is probably the chief reason for the magnified risk of streptococcal infection and acute rheumatic fever (ARF) in certain ethnic and disadvantaged populations. Improvement in the delivery of health care in defined populations may also be significant.[5]

Notwithstanding its decline, rheumatic heart disease still constitutes the leading cause of death from heart disease in the 5- to 24-year-old age group in many parts of the world and continues to be a serious public health problem, particularly in the slums of the industrializing nations of the Third World.[6–8]

Factors in the Attack Rate of Rheumatic Fever

QUANTITATIVE FACTORS. One factor is the severity of the antecedent pharyngeal streptococcal infection. The clearest relationship of group A streptococcal infection to RF is found in military populations subject to epidemic streptococcal sore throat. In patients with frank, exudative streptococcal pharyngitis caused by certain pharyngeal strains of virulent group A streptococci, RF followed at a fairly predictable attack rate (approximately 3 per cent) regardless of the age, race, or ethnic group studied and regardless of the year or season in which the study was made.[3] The major variables which seem to be related to this attack rate in such studies are the magnitude of the immune response to the antecedent streptococcal infection[9] and the duration of convalescent carriage of the organism.[10] Weak antistreptolysin O (ASO) responses are associated with ARF attack rates considerably less than 1 per cent, whereas strong responses are associated with rates well in excess of 5 per cent. If the infecting organism in the pharynx was not eradicated during convalescence, treatment of streptococcal pharyngitis failed to reduce the attack rate of rheumatic fever.

In contrast to the military studies, reports from civilian medical practice indicate that RF may occur less frequently following endemic, sporadic streptococcal disease.[11–14]

VARIATION IN GROUP A STREPTOCOCCAL INFECTIONS. Variations in the "rheumatogenicity" of group A streptococcal strains may constitute one factor influencing the attack rate of RF. In several laboratories where regular serotyping of group A streptococci isolated from pharyngeal infections is performed with available antisera prepared against known M-protein serotypes, the frequency of identification of such strains has decreased. Furthermore, the prevalence of several of the virulent M types notorious for causing epidemic RF (e.g., types 5, 14, and 24) has apparently declined, and attention has shifted to the study of "new" M types among both pharyngeal strains and "skin" strains.[2, 15] The issue of whether there are "nonrheumatogenic group A streptococci"[16] has been sharpened by the clear demonstration that group A streptococcal pyoderma, with or without complicating acute glomerulonephritis (AGN), does not cause ARF.[17] These skin infections are nonrheumatogenic.[18] Since the pharyngeal route of infection is now an accepted requirement for the pathogenesis of ARF (see below), the question of whether such pyoderma strains can cause RF when they produce pharyngitis is of particular interest. Studies in the southwestern United States have clearly shown seasonal epidemiological separation of ARF and AGN.[19] A study of the streptococcal strains in an island population such as Trinidad shows a clear distinction between the serotypes associated with AGN and those associated with ARF.[20, 21] Several studies suggest that RF is associated with infections due to virulent strains capable of causing strong type-specific immune responses to M protein and other streptococcal antigens. Such strains belong to the classic M serotypes known to cause ARF.[22, 23] Thus, qualitative and quantitative changes in streptococcal pharyngitis may have affected greatly the epidemiology of rheumatic fever in various parts of the world.

GEOGRAPHY AND CLIMATE. The relationship of RF to the intensity and severity of streptococcal disease is the same in the tropics as in the temperate climates.[24] In *prospective* studies in which all patients suspected of having ARF were admitted and recurrent attacks were excluded, the frequency of the clinical manifestations of rheumatic fever are the same as in the studies in the United States.[25, 26]

Host Factors

AGE, SEX, AND RACE. Like streptococcal sore throat, ARF occurs most commonly in the young school-age child and very rarely in early infancy. It is estimated that 40 per cent of streptococcal infections in pediatric populations occur in children 2 to 6 years of age, suggesting that repeated streptococcal infections and sensitization of the host are prerequisite to the development of RF. No true differences in sex, race, or ethnic group susceptibility have been established. Crowded living conditions account for whatever apparent increased susceptibility has been reported.

ACQUIRED SUSCEPTIBILITY. Because ARF develops in only a relatively small percentage of patients following even the most virulent bouts of streptococcal pharyngitis, the question of host predisposition is often raised. Once RF is acquired, its activation following subsequent streptococcal infection is many times greater in rheumatic subjects than in the general population. The recurrence rate per infection, which is as high as 50 per cent during the first year after the initial attack, decreases sharply until 4 to 5 years after the attack.[27, 28] It then levels off at approximately 10 per cent and does not seem to fall much lower.[29] Although the persistently high attack rate in individuals having had RF suggests some degree of genetic predisposition (see below), the diminishing recurrence rate per infection also suggests loss of acquired hyperreactivity. An alternative explanation may be acquired sensitization in a genetically predisposed host that persists throughout life, such as ragweed hay fever in an atopic individual.

GENETIC FACTORS. Many investigators have sought genetic markers for rheumatic hosts without more than suggestive results.[30] Only a few adequate studies in identical twins have been made and these have shown a relatively low concordance of RF (less than 20 per cent), actually considerably lower than the concordance found in identical twins with other infectious diseases such as tuberculosis or poliomyelitis.[1, 30] No clear correlation of conventional HLA genotypes with rheumatic fever has yet been shown. In one study,[31] however, a B-cell alloantigen (designated 833) was found to occur in 75 per cent of RF patients compared with 16.5 per cent of a population of normal individuals. The alloantigen could not be correlated with a known specificity and was not associated with any known HLA antigens. In an extension of these studies,[32] relative segregation was recorded for 833-positive B-cell typing among patients with rheumatic heart disease in India, New Mexico, and New York, as compared to normal unaffected controls. The uniqueness of the group A streptococcus in initiating a cardiodestructive disease in a limited segment of the human species, regardless of race or ethnic group, continues to make the quest for a unique host response to a specific streptococcal antigen a persisting challenge, particularly for investigators interested in autoimmunity.[33]

ETIOLOGY

The lines of evidence establishing the group A streptococcus as the sole agent causing initial and recurrent attacks of RF (described below) are of necessity indirect, because group A streptococci cannot be recovered from the lesions of RF and no satisfactory experimental model of the disease has been demonstrated.

CLINICAL EVIDENCE. Although the frequency with which septic sore throat preceded ARF has been recognized for over 100 years, inconsistencies in this relationship have been pointed out repeatedly.[1] Almost one-third of patients with ARF deny the occurrence of antecedent sore throat. Throat and blood cultures in such patients show that the former is frequently negative and the latter virtually always sterile at the onset of the rheumatic attack. Recurrences of RF appeared even more mysterious when antecedent streptococcal sore throat was unrecognized and particularly when the chronicity of a rheumatic attack and the hemodynamic complications of rheumatic heart disease made it difficult to distinguish continued versus reactivated rheumatic carditis. On clinical grounds alone, therefore, it is difficult to establish the group A streptococcus as the sole etiological agent.

EPIDEMIOLOGICAL EVIDENCE. Such factors as latitude, altitude, crowding, dampness, economic factors, and age all affect the incidence of RF because they are related to the incidence and severity of streptococcal infections in general (see above). Careful military epidemiological studies over a period of 20 years show a clear sequential relationship between outbreaks of streptococcal pharyngitis and RF.[34]

IMMUNOLOGICAL EVIDENCE. Initial (primary) or recurrent (secondary) RF does not occur without a streptococcal antibody response.[35] Furthermore, the magnitude of the antibody response is a major variable determining the attack rate of (but not the severity or duration) of RF following streptococcal pharyngitis.[9] This is true for both primary and secondary attacks.[27] Indeed, the streptococcal immune response is an important criterion for the diagnosis of RF (see below).

PROPHYLACTIC EVIDENCE. The final and perhaps most convincing evidence is the prevention of both initial and recurrent attacks of RF by, in the former case, penicillin therapy and, in the latter, continuous chemoprophylaxis against streptococcal infections. Completely effective prophylaxis of streptococcal infections in rheumatic subjects allows us to conclude that RF cannot be reactivated by any other infection, illness, or trauma.[27, 35]

PATHOGENESIS OF RHEUMATIC FEVER

Despite the elusiveness of the pathogenesis of RF, there are a few well-established requirements for the development of this postinfectious sequel: (1) the presence of the group A streptococcus, (2) a streptococcal antibody response indicative of actual recent infection, (3) persistence of the organism in the pharynx for a sufficient period, and (4) location of the infection in the throat.

THE ROLE OF TOXINS. Despite the popularity of the concepts of hyperimmunity and autoimmunity in the pathogenesis of RF (see below), none of the antibodies described to date, including those reactive with the heart, has been shown to be cytotoxic. A direct toxic effect, therefore, of some streptococcal product, particularly on the heart, has not yet been ruled out as a pathogenetic mechanism.[1, 33]

Immunological Theories

The most popular pathogenic theory is that RF results from some type of hyperimmune reaction due either to bacterial allergy or autoimmunity. This view is supported by strong evidence, since RF patients are, in general, the population most intensively hyperimmune to all streptococcal products.

The mean antibody titer to virtually every streptococcal antigen that has been studied is increased in patients during the acute stage of RF.[1] Yet no single humoral mechanism of tissue injury has been defined. Complement levels are increased rather than decreased, and autoantibodies associated with immune complex disease (e.g., rheumatoid factor, anti-DNA, and others) are not present. Although low-grade microscopic hematuria may occur, frank lesions of glomerulonephritis are absent. Careful studies have identified circulating immune complexes, but they are of small size and not high titer and quickly disappear after the acute stage of polyarthritis.[36]

AUTOIMMUNITY. Modern theories of the possible autoimmune pathogenetic mechanisms of RF have been extensively reviewed.[33, 37] It has been known for many years that the serum of some patients with ARF contains autoantibodies to heart tissues, and numerous reports using a variety of techniques, mostly immunofluorescence, have confirmed this finding.[38–40] Anti-heart antibodies are gamma globulins with specificity for cardiac components reacting primarily with the sarcolemma. Their binding is also associated with deposition of large amounts of complement component C3. Anti-heart antibodies occur more frequently in RF patients who develop carditis than in those who escape it. The frequency of the appearance of such antibodies is very high in patients who have undergone mitral commissurotomy. These antibodies can be adsorbed by the patient's own atrial tissue and therefore are probably autoantibodies. Massive deposits of gamma globulin have also been identified in the hearts of children who died of rheumatic carditis. The role of such antibodies in the pathogenesis of rheumatic fever has been clouded by the growing understanding of autoantibody formation and complement activation as a general response to tissue injury. Cardiac damage by rheumatic, traumatic, or ischemic heart lesions leads to biochemical changes manifested by the production of autoantibody.[40] Thus, myocardial infarction and postpericardiotomy syndromes have been associated with the production of anti-heart antibodies and/or deposition of complement. It is therefore possible that these kinds of anti-heart antibodies in rheumatic carditis are the *result* rather than the *cause* of tissue injury.

CROSS-REACTIVE ANTIBODIES. In the early 1960's Kaplan and his associates demonstrated that rabbit antisera against certain group A streptococci react with human heart preparations in the immunofluorescent test.[41, 42] Since then, many additional immunological cross reactions have been described between streptococci and human tissues[43–48] (Fig. 54–2). The immunological details of these reactions and their possible relation to the pathogenesis of RF[1, 33, 37] are summarized below.

Group A streptococci have a number of structural components that are related to mammalian tissues.[1] The hyaluronate capsule of the organism, for example, is identical with human hyaluronate. Antibodies to the group A cell wall polysaccharide cross-react with glycoproteins of heart valves.[44] Membrane antigens of group A streptococci cross-react with sarcolemma and smooth muscle of endocardial and myocardial arteries.[43]

Antibodies that are of specific interest for their potential relationship

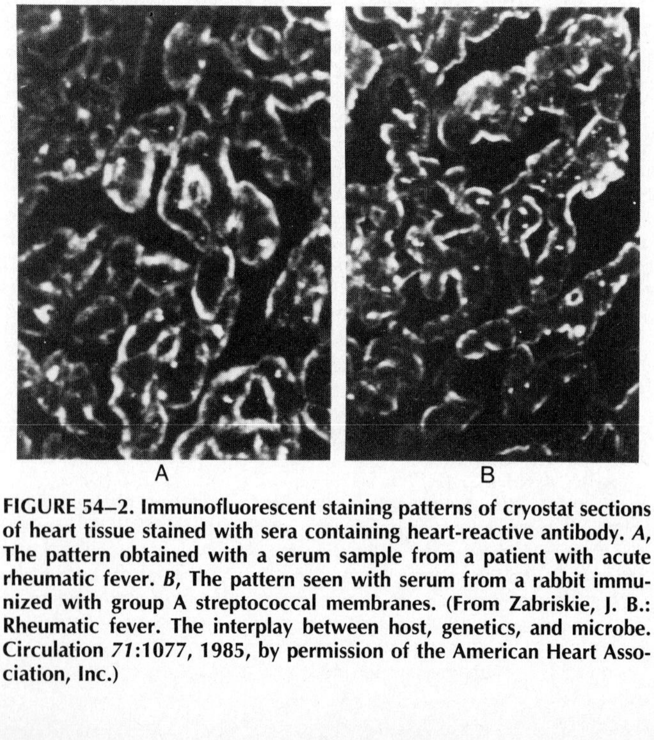

A B

FIGURE 54–2. Immunofluorescent staining patterns of cryostat sections of heart tissue stained with sera containing heart-reactive antibody. *A*, The pattern obtained with a serum sample from a patient with acute rheumatic fever. *B*, The pattern seen with serum from a rabbit immunized with group A streptococcal membranes. (From Zabriskie, J. B.: Rheumatic fever. The interplay between host, genetics, and microbe. Circulation *71*:1077, 1985, by permission of the American Heart Association, Inc.)

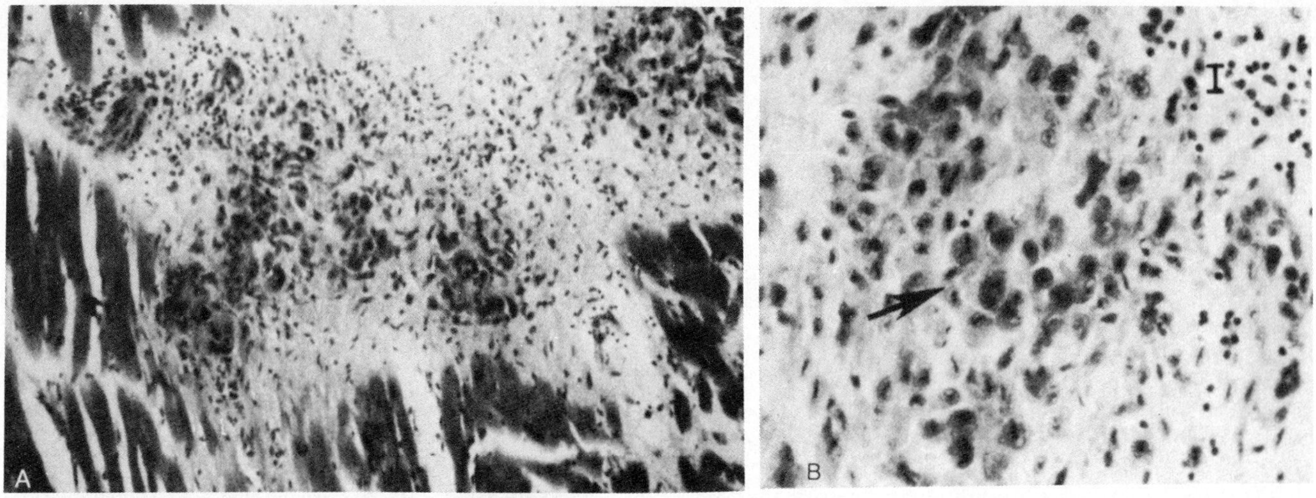

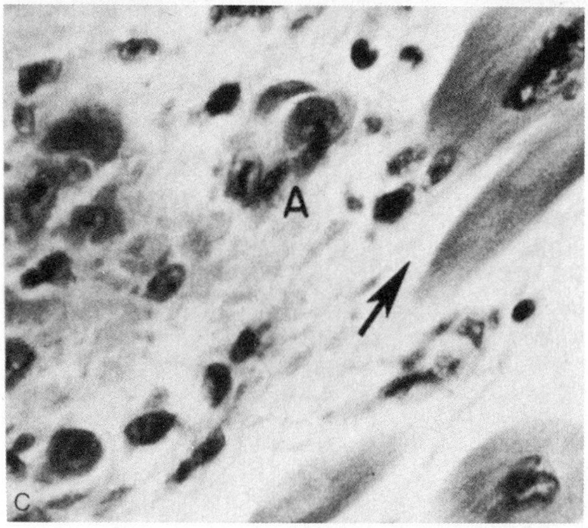

FIGURE 54–3. *A,* Multiple Aschoff lesions in the left ventricle, showing confluence of large monocyte macrophage-appearing cells surrounded by cell infiltrate and dissolution of adjacent myocardial muscle with fibrous tissue replacement. *B,* Higher-power view showing large mononuclear cells (*arrow*) and interstitial lymphocytes (I). *C,* High-power view. (From Husby, G., et al.: Immunofluorescent studies of florid rheumatic Aschoff lesions. Arthritis Rheum. *29*:207, 1986.)

to autoimmune injury of the heart are those absorbable by streptococcal products. A sustained rise in titer of antibodies that cross-react with the cardiac tissue often precedes an attack of RF,[33] but such antibodies do not correlate clearly with the presence or severity of rheumatic carditis, and they have not been shown to be cytotoxic. Antibody to the streptococcal group A polysaccharide has received particular attention because of prolonged persistence of elevated levels in the serum of patients with rheumatic mitral valvular disease in contrast with its more rapid decline in patients with RF without cardiac involvement and in patients with transient mitral insufficiency, including those with mitral valve prolapse.[46] Antibodies reactive with cytoplasm of neurons in the subthalamic and caudate nuclei have been found more frequently in patients with Sydenham's chorea than in those rheumatic patients without this manifestation.[47] Most recently, delineation of the molecular structure of several streptococcal M proteins has led to the demonstration of epitopes of these serotypes cross-reactive with myosin.[48]

Little doubt remains that streptococcal antigens of various kinds are shared with human myocardium, but it has not been shown that they are actually responsible for tissue injury in certain hosts and are thus related to the pathogenesis of rheumatic fever.[33]

PATHOLOGY

There is often considerable disparity between the severity of the clinical manifestations of RF and the extent of the morbid anatomical changes it produces. Sydenham's chorea, cardiac atrioventricular conduction blocks, and erythema marginatum all appear to be related more to functional disturbances than to visible lesions. In contrast, the persistent focal inflammatory lesions of the myocardium, such as the Aschoff nodule, do not always correlate with clinical manifestations of active carditis and have led to differences between pathologists and clinicians with regard to the definition of rheumatic activity. In general, however, the acute phase of RF is characterized by diffuse exudative and proliferative inflammatory reactions in the heart, joints, and skin. Small blood vessels and arterioles are commonly involved, but unlike the arteritis of some other connective tissue diseases, thrombotic lesions are not seen.

The term *fibrinoid degeneration* describes the basic structural changes in the collagen of connective tissues.[49] The fibrinoid substance resembles and stains like fibrin and is a feature of the earliest phase of the myocardial lesions. The collagen fibers in these mucoid areas become swollen and eosinophilic, forming a meshwork of rigid, waxlike fibers. This exudative-degenerative phase[50, 51] lasts for 2 to 3 weeks, following which the most characteristic lesion of RF develops—the myocardial *Aschoff nodule.*[52] The proliferative and healing phase then follows and may persist for many months or even years (Figs. 54–3 and 54–4).[52, 53]

Ironically, the only lesion pathognomonic of RF is vague with regard to its origin, functional impact on the heart, and relation to the course and severity of the rheumatic attack.[54] Aschoff nodules do not seem to account for the acute dilatation of the heart in first attacks of severe carditis. The persistence of Aschoff nodules for many years after a rheumatic attack has been well recognized by pathologists. Biopsies of the left atrial appendage obtained during mitral valve surgery for mitral stenosis have shown persistence of Aschoff nodules in patients who no longer have clinical or laboratory evidence of rheumatic activity[55–57] and who have no recent evidence of streptococcal infection.[58] The persistence of Aschoff nodules seems to be correlated, however, with progressive fibrosis and stenosis of the mitral valve. One series[56, 57]

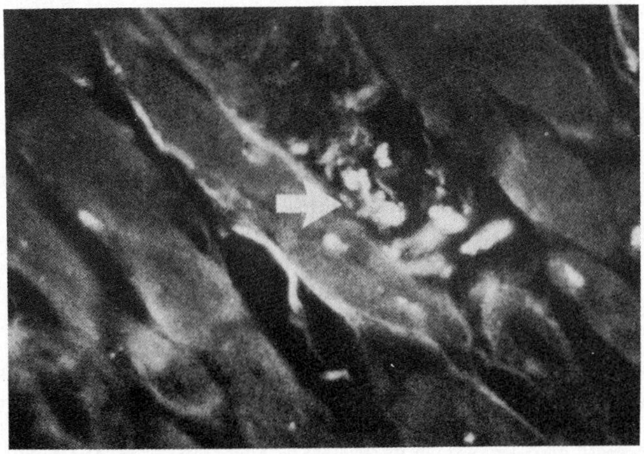

FIGURE 54–4. Postmortem myocardial specimen from a 20-year-old patient with severe rheumatic carditis. Immunofluorescent staining shows many large monocytoid cells that appear to have ingested myosin (*arrow*). (From Husby, G., et al.: Immunofluorescent studies of florid rheumatic Aschoff lesions. Arthritis Rheum. *29*:1986.)

showed such lesions in 21 per cent of 191 surgically excised left atrial appendages in patients with mitral stenosis. In the same series, of 91 patients with pure mitral regurgitation, Aschoff nodules were present in the left atrial appendage of only 1 patient.

Cardiac Lesions

On gross inspection of the heart, a pancarditis is almost always evident, with fresh exudative pericardial lesions, dilatation of the heart, and verrucous endocardial lesions on the valves.[59]

PERICARDITIS (See also p. 1519). Both layers of the pericardium are thickened and covered with a fibrinous exudate, and serosanguineous pericardial fluid may be present. With healing, fibrosis and adhesions develop which partially or completely obliterate the pericardial sac, but constrictive pericarditis does *not* occur.

MYOCARDITIS. In addition to the Aschoff bodies, a diffuse cellular infiltrate is present in interstitial tissues. The cells are usually lymphocytes, but polymorphonuclear leukocytes, histiocytes, and eosinophils may also be present. Exudate may be associated with damaged muscle. This interstitial myocarditis may be more important than the nodular Aschoff bodies in producing heart failure. Myocardial fibers are also damaged, and the greatest damage occurs in the vicinity of Aschoff nodules and around blood vessels,[60, 61] Macrophages containing cardiac myosin have been identified in Aschoff nodules by immunofluorescent studies of florid acute myocarditis (Fig. 54–4).[61]

THE CONDUCTION SYSTEM. Despite the high frequency of prolonged atrial ventricular conduction in ARF, visible changes in the bundle of His are seen in the minority of autopsy cases of ARF. The evanescence of heart block and its easy reversibility in most cases by the administration of atropine fit the concept that a pathophysiological defect rather than an anatomical lesion is responsible for this conduction defect.

ENDOCARDITIS. The verrucous lesions at the valve edge appear as a mass of eosinophilic material staining as fibrin. At the base and edges of the valve, the cells line up in palisades at right angles to the base and often have elongated Aschoff-type nuclei. As the lesions progress, granulation tissue develops and vascularization and progressive fibrosis take place. The changes involve the annulus as well as the cusps and chordae tendineae, which, as a result of scarring, thicken and shorten.

Rheumatic Valvular Deformities
(See also Chap. 33)

MITRAL REGURGITATION. Incompetence or regurgitation may result from shortening of one or both cusps, from shortening and fusing of chordae and papillary muscles, or from dilatation of the valve ring. By far, the most common clinically apparent lesion of rheumatic heart disease is mitral regurgitation, and such lesions often occur subclinically when extracardiac symptoms of ARF are absent. Dilatation of the valve ring occurs in active carditis more frequently as a result of acute dilatation of the left ventricle. Marked mitral regurgitation also occurs, however, without acute left ventricular dilatation when the valve cusps and the musculotendinous structures are severely swollen and disorganized by the rheumatic process without coexisting severe myocarditis.

MITRAL STENOSIS. This lesion occurs with varying degrees of mitral regurgitation. When stenosis is severe, regurgitation may be relatively unimportant, and the main hemodynamic problem is obstruction to blood flow during diastole. The gross changes in the mitral valve are variable. The cusps may fuse, leaving an ovoid opening, but the cusps themselves may remain thin and pliable. In other instances the cusps become thick, rigid, or even calcified. A "funnel-shaped valve" with its opening at the apex may result when fusion of the cusps occurs with shortening and thickening of the chordae tendineae and papillary muscles.

AORTIC VALVE DEFORMITIES. The most common aortic lesion is a combination of stenosis and regurgitation. Pure aortic stenosis is relatively uncommon, but a minimal degree of aortic regurgitation occurs frequently in mild

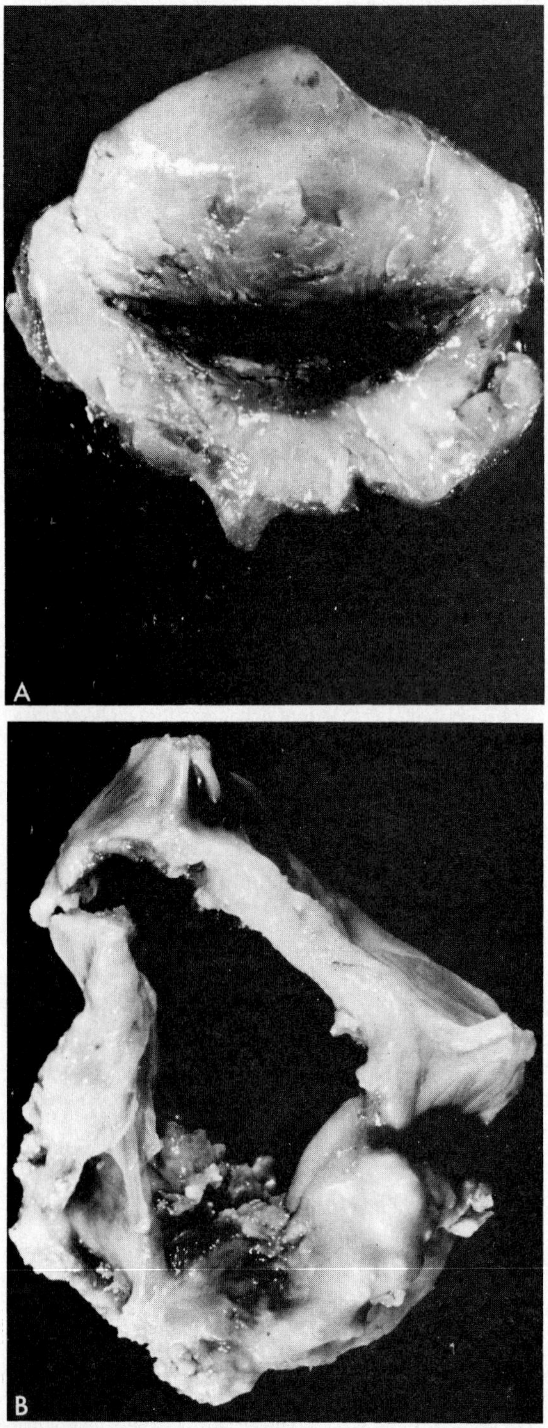

FIGURE 54–5. Excised rheumatic valve. *A*, "Fishmouth" mitral valve. *B*, Aortic valve fixed in open position. (Courtesy of James W. Pate, M.D. From Stollerman, G. H.: Rheumatic Fever and Streptococcal Infection. New York, by permission of Grune and Stratton, 1975.)

rheumatic involvement. In most cases of symptomatic rheumatic aortic disease, both stenosis and regurgitation occur, but one or the other may be functionally predominant. Deformity of the valve results from fusion of the cusps at the commissures, rigidity and shortening of the cusps alone, or combinations of both processes with calcification superimposed (Fig. 54–5*B*).

TRICUSPID VALVE DEFORMITIES. These almost always exist in association with mitral and aortic lesions and occur in approximately 10 per cent of patients with chronic rheumatic heart disease.[59]

PULMONARY VALVE DEFORMITIES. Pulmonary valve deformities are rarest of all. When they occur, stenosis is more usual than is incompetence. The pathological changes in the pulmonary valve are similar to those in the aortic valve.

PROGRESSIVE PATHOLOGICAL CHANGES IN HEALED RHEUMATIC HEART DISEASE. There are manifestations of progressive changes and continued inflammation that seem unrelated to the original rheumatic process. Disruption of red blood cells ("cardiac hemolytic anemia") can result from valvular defects; platelet turnover and destruction have recently been proved to be excessive in rheumatic heart disease[62]; and resultant thrombosis and fibrosis can occur along with calcification. Recurrent congestive heart failure may cause fatty changes in the myocardium and progressive fibrosis. The endocardium, especially the left atrium in mitral valvular deformity, is prone to develop organized thrombi, to stretch and dilate progressively, and to develop chronic inflammatory changes that are not exudative or clearly rheumatic at all.

Extracardiac Lesions

JOINTS. Swelling and edema of the articular and periarticular structures with serous effusion into the joint space occur without erosion of the joint surface or pannus formation. The synovial membrane is reddened and thickened and covered with fibrinous exudate. Histologically there is marked edema, engorgement and dilation of blood vessels, and diffuse and focal infiltrates of lymphocytes and polymorphonuclear leukocytes, the latter more numerous initially. Later, focal fibrinoid lesions with histiocytic granulomas may appear, but these lesions heal also without residua.

SUBCUTANEOUS NODULES. A central zone of fibrinoid necrotic material is surrounded by histiocytes and fibroblasts, and lymphocytes and polymorphonuclear leukocytes collect around small vessels. The structure resembles Aschoff bodies and may heal very rapidly, leaving no apparent scars.

CHOREA. Considerable confusion exists concerning the pathology of Sydenham's chorea because (1) few patients die of "pure" chorea, (2) those who die of severe carditis may have inflammatory lesions of the central nervous system without chorea,[63] (3) no single site is consistently involved, (4) Aschoff bodies are not found in the brain,[64, 65] and (5) it has not been possible to correlate clinical findings with pathological changes. Changes found in the central nervous system include arteritis, cellular degeneration, perivascular round cell infiltration, and occasional petechial hemorrhages, but on the whole these are not impressive and are scattered throughout the cortex, cerebellum, and basal ganglia.[66, 67]

RHEUMATIC PNEUMONITIS. Because this finding usually occurs with severe carditis only, there has been argument about whether the pulmonary lesion is a form of the acute respiratory distress syndrome secondary to heart failure or part of the rheumatic process itself. It has been described, however, in the absence of heart failure.[68]

CLINICAL MANIFESTATIONS

The signs and symptoms of ARF vary greatly and are determined by the systems involved, the severity of the lesions and when they appear in the course of the disease, and the stage of the disease when the patient is first observed by the physician. Certain manifestations that follow streptococcal infections (with a frequency far exceeding chance) occur simultaneously, in close succession, or singly. They have been called *major manifestations* and consist of carditis, arthritis, chorea, subcutaneous nodules, and erythema marginatum. The word "major" refers to their importance as diagnostic criteria and not to their importance in the severity of the process or its activity, or to the prognosis.

Minor manifestations of ARF are frequently present and helpful in recognizing the disease. They are too nonspecific, however, to be of major importance in diagnosis. Minor manifestations include such findings as fever, arthralgia, acute phase reactants in the blood, heart block, and a history of previous ARF or rheumatic heart disease.

ANTECEDENT STREPTOCOCCAL INFECTION. Evidence for an antecedent streptococcal infection may not be apparent. As many as one-third of patients do not remember having had any illness in the preceding month (see above).[33] Furthermore, in patients with previous RF who were followed prospectively for recurrences, asymptomatic streptococcal infections accounted for 54[27] to 70 per cent[29] of recurrences of RF. The average interval between onset of symptoms of pharyngitis and the symptoms of RF (the latent period) was 18.6 days in one prospective study,[69] but may be as short as 1 week or as long as 5 weeks. The latent period is no shorter in patients with previous RF than in those without.

ARTHRITIS. This manifestation occurs in about three-fourths of patients during the acute stage of the disease. In general, joint involvement becomes more common with increasing age of the patient, a trend related to the concomitant decrease in the incidence of carditis and chorea.[70, 71] The arthritis of RF usually involves the large joints, particularly the knees, ankles, elbows, and wrists. Almost any joint, however, may be affected. In the classic attack, several joints are involved in quick succession, each for a brief time, resulting in the typical picture of migratory polyarthritis. Each joint remains inflamed for usually no more than a week before the inflammation begins to subside, and the inflammation usually abates spontaneously in 2 or 3 weeks.[72–74] Acute polyarthritis rarely occurs more than 35 days after the onset of the streptococcal infection, and *for that reason, it is almost always associated with a rising or peak titer of streptococcal antibodies.* This fact aids in identifying an isolated bout of polyarthritis as rheumatic or in *excluding* RF as a cause for a given bout of polyarthritis when streptococcal antibodies are not increased.

Carditis

VARIATIONS IN ONSET AND COURSE. The most important manifestation of ARF is carditis, which, in its most severe form, causes death from acute cardiac failure. Much more commonly, however, carditis is less intense, and the predominant effect is scarring of the heart valves. In contrast to the seriousness of its prognosis, rheumatic carditis most often causes no symptoms of its own and is usually diagnosed in the course of the examination of a patient with arthritis or chorea, which directs the physician's attention to the heart, where murmurs are detected. Carditis, therefore, does not come to medical attention if other symptoms of rheumatic fever are absent or if the carditis is not severe enough to cause heart failure, prolonged or severe fever, or the pain of pericarditis. Patients with undiagnosed carditis may later prove to have rheumatic heart disease and usually give no history of a previous rheumatic attack.

Murmurs indicative of carditis are usually present during the first week of the illness in about three-fourths of all patients in whom carditis is eventually diagnosed.[75] By the second or third week, murmurs become manifest in 85 per cent of those in whom they will eventually develop.

Acute heart failure in a young patient who has had rheumatic heart disease previously but who has been well compensated *should always be suspected as a recurrence of acute rheumatic carditis.* Young hearts with rheumatic disease rarely fail abruptly because of hemodynamic handicaps alone except when the latter are severe and protracted. On the other hand, it is often not possible to detect carditis during mild rheumatic recurrences in patients with old rheumatic valvular lesions. Like most episodes of carditis, heart failure or signs of pericarditis will be absent, and the diagnosis of a recurrence will depend on other major and minor criteria changing heart murmurs (the most common sign of carditis in first rheumatic attacks) are undetectable.

CLINICAL SIGNS AND CRITERIA. The four major criteria for the clinical diagnosis of rheumatic carditis are (1) an organic heart murmur or murmurs not previously present, (2) enlargement of the heart, (3) congestive heart failure, and (4) pericardial friction rubs or signs of effusion. If any one of these is unequivocal in a patient with active RF, the diagnosis of carditis is justified.

MURMURS OF ACUTE RHEUMATIC CARDITIS. Organic murmurs are almost invariably present. They may not be heard when the heart rate is too rapid, when cardiac output is very low in severe congestive heart failure, when they are obscured by a loud pericardial rub, or, rarely, when there is marked pericardial effusion. Otherwise, the signs of endocarditis are always associated with those of involvement of other layers of the heart, although the latter may not be clinically apparent.

Apical Systolic Murmur. The mitral valve is the most common site of rheumatic inflammation—about three times as frequently involved as the aortic valve. Inflammation ("valvulitis") causing edema, thickening, and verrucae leads to mitral regurgitation early in the course of the disease and often with mild cardiac involvement. The systolic murmur is heard best at the apex, usually grade 3 or more on a scale of 6 in intensity, and, most important, it has a high-pitched blowing quality.

Apical Mid-diastolic Murmur (Carey-Coombs Murmur). This murmur begins directly after the onset of the third heart sound and ends before the first heart sound. The mid-diastolic murmur is often transient, low pitched, and easily missed. The presence of this murmur makes the diagnosis of "mitral valvulitis" more definite, confirms the significance of the apical systolic murmur, and adds to the seriousness of the prognosis for permanent valve injury.

Aortic Diastolic Murmur. This murmur may appear early in the course of the disease as an expression of aortic valvulitis and may occur alone or with mitral valvulitis. The aortic diastolic blow may be audible only intermittently, depending, again, on cardiac output. The murmur is a soft, high-pitched, decrescendo blow heard immediately after the second heart sound. A diastolic cooing or crying "sea gull" murmur is rarely heard, but can be present evanescently in the aortic valvulitis of acute carditis.

CARDIAC ENLARGEMENT AND FAILURE. The most reliable clinical expression of rheumatic myocarditis from the standpoint of diagnosis and prognosis is *dilatation*, particularly of the left atrium and ventricle. In two careful cooperative studies designed to evaluate treatment of rheumatic carditis, cardiomegaly occurred in a little more than half the children who developed carditis.[72, 76, 77]

Congestive heart failure is the least common but most serious manifestation of rheumatic carditis. It is reported in 5 to 10 per cent of first attacks of rheumatic carditis. It is more common, however, to encounter severe and fatal heart failure as a manifestation of a *rheumatic recurrence* than of a primary attack.

PERICARDITIS. Pericarditis occurs in approximately 5 to 10 per cent of most large series of ARF.[72, 75] Occasionally, pericardial reaction and effusion will be more striking and prominent than the degree of myocarditis. In such cases the regression in apparent heart size and the rate of healing of the attack can be rapid. Conversely, the pericarditis may be a relatively minor aspect of a profound case of heart failure due to severe myocarditis. One rarely sees tamponade without severe heart failure as well.

ARRHYTHMIAS. Delayed atrioventricular (AV) conduction, as reflected in prolongation of the P-R interval, occurs with similar frequency to the polyarthritis of ARF, whether or not clear evidence of carditis is present. The prolongation of AV conduction is easily reversed with atropine,[78] suggesting that this feature is usually due to functional effects of the disease on AV conduction rather than to direct inflammation and fibrosis of the conduction system. Prolongation of AV conduction may lead to second-degree and, rarely, even third-degree block.[79] The latter is usually of brief duration and reverts spontaneously. Interference and dissociation phenomena are also characteristic of occasional nodal rhythms.

Extracardiac Manifestations

SUBCUTANEOUS NODULES. These are a major manifestation of ARF.[80, 81] However, they are not pathognomonic of RF, since they occur in rheumatoid arthritis and systemic lupus erythematosus as well. They rarely occur as an isolated manifestation and are associated most often with severe carditis, appearing usually several weeks after its onset.[82]

Nodules are round, firm, painless subcutaneous lesions varying in size from approximately 0.5 to 2.0 cm. The skin over them is freely movable and not inflamed. They are located over bony surfaces or prominences and over tendons, particularly the extensor of the fingers and toes and flexors of the wrists and ankles. They occur in crops and vary in number from one to usually three or four dozen; when numerous, they tend to be symmetrical. Nodules are evanescent, disappearing sometimes within several days but usually lasting a week or two and rarely more than a month. They tend, therefore, to be much smaller and less persistent than rheumatoid nodules.

ERYTHEMA MARGINATUM. This is a less common feature of RF, but is so characteristic that it has taken its rightful place among the five major diagnostic manifestations of the disease. However, it cannot be considered pathognomonic of ARF because it has been reported in sepsis, particularly staphylococcal, in drug reactions, in patients with glomerulonephritis, and in children in whom no etiological factor can be identified.

Erythema marginatum appears as a bright-pink "smoke ring" spreading serpiginously through pale skin. It is nonpruritic, nonpainful, and

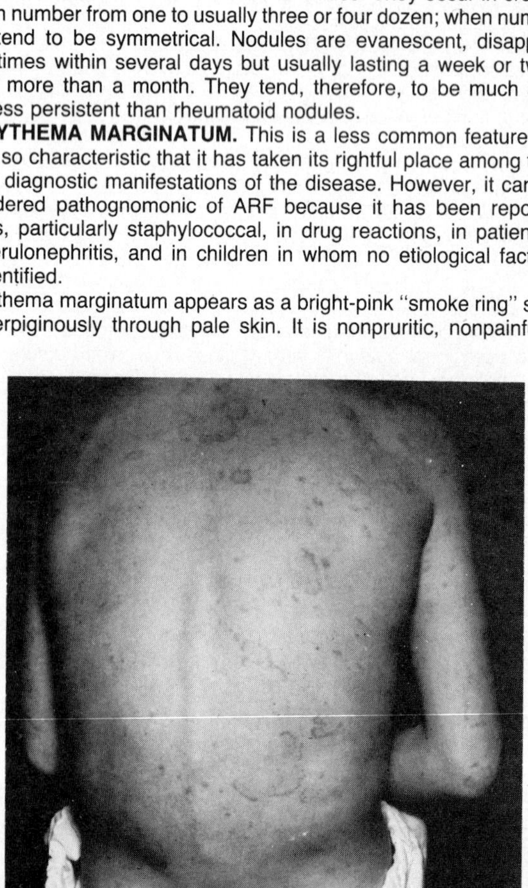

FIGURE 54–6. Erythema marginatum. (Courtesy of Benedict F. Massell, M.D.)

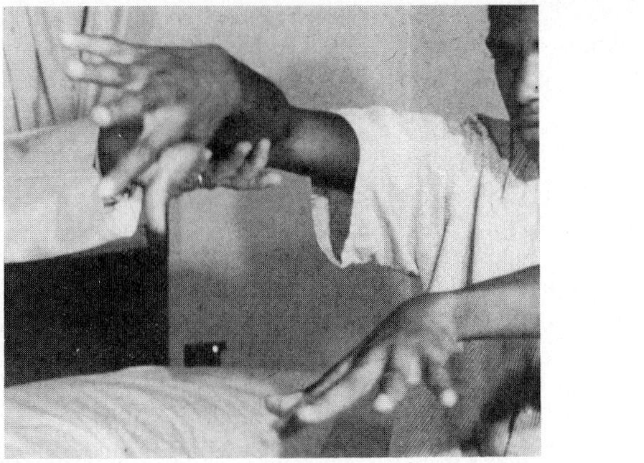

FIGURE 54–7. "Spooning" or "dishing" of the hands in a patient with Sydenham's chorea. Note weakness of the arms making sustained extension difficult. (From Stollerman, G. H.: Rheumatic Fever and Streptococcal Infection. New York, by permission of Grune and Stratton, 1975.)

neither indurated nor raised. It blanches completely on pressure and is evanescent. The individual lesions usually appear on the trunk and the proximal parts of the extremities but not on the face (Fig. 54–6); they rarely extend distally beyond the elbows or knees. Erythema marginatum may recur intermittently for months, uninfluenced by antirheumatic agents, and when all other signs of rheumatic activity are gone, one can allow the patient to begin to ambulate without fear of a relapse.

CHOREA (SYDENHAM'S CHOREA, ST. VITUS' DANCE). This neurological disorder, characterized by involuntary, purposeless, rapid movements, muscular weakness, and emotional lability, may be associated with other manifestations of ARF, but it also may appear as the sole expression of the disease—so-called pure chorea. After puberty it is present exclusively in women, and even in them it declines rapidly after adolescence. Chorea has decreased strikingly in frequency compared with arthritis and carditis.

The movements of chorea are abrupt and erratic (Fig. 54–7), not rhythmic or repetitive. In even the most violent attacks, all choreiform movements disappear during sleep and are less violent during rest and sedation.[1]

Chorea may last from 1 week to more than 2 years, but usually about 8 to 15 weeks, with a mean of 13.7. Chorea is never seen simultaneously with arthritis, but often coexists with carditis. When chorea appears alone, however, the other minor clinical and laboratory signs of ARF may be entirely absent. The erythrocyte sedimentation rate and C-reactive protein may be normal. Even more confusing, in such cases the ASO and other streptococcal antibody titers may not be increased because chorea appears only after a relatively long latent period (as long as 1 to 6 months) following the antecedent streptococcal infection, and after the longest latent period, both the acute phase reactants and the streptococcal antibody titers may have returned to normal.[83, 84]

FEVER. Some degree of fever accompanies almost all rheumatic attacks at their onset. Temperature usually ranges from 101° to 104° F (38.4° to 40° C), is rarely higher, and has no characteristic pattern. In the usual attack, fever decreases in approximately a week without antipyretic treatment and may become low grade for another week or two. It rarely lasts for more than several weeks. When antirheumatic agents are used, however, a "rebound" of fever may occur after 4 to 6 weeks of treatment, but it usually subsides spontaneously within a few days except in unusually persistent attacks.

ABDOMINAL PAIN. The abdominal pain of RF, which occurs in fewer than 5 per cent of patients with ARF, resembles that seen in other conditions in which acute microvascular mesenteric disease occurs, such as sickle cell crises, sepsis, endotoxin or anaphylactic shock, transfusion reactions, and anaphylactoid purpura.

EPISTAXIS. In the past, the incidence of epistaxis was reported from as high as 48 per cent in the early 1930's to a low of 4 to 9 per cent in the late 1950's,[70] and perhaps it is even less frequent now.

LABORATORY FINDINGS

Although there are no pathognomonic tests for RF, laboratory findings are helpful in two major ways: (1) in establishing the antecedent streptococcal infection and (2) in documenting the presence or persistence of an inflammatory process.

ANTECEDENT STREPTOCOCCAL INFECTION. The diagnosis of recent streptococcal infection can be made only tentatively by throat culture but definitely by antibody determinations. Throat cultures are usually negative by the time RF appears. When they are positive, one still cannot be certain whether the organism isolated represents convalescent carriage of the antecedent infection or an intercurrent acquisition of a different strain. Streptococcal antibodies are therefore more useful because they reach a peak titer shortly after the onset of ARF and indicate true infection rather than transient carriage.

ANTIBODIES. The specific antibodies used to diagnose streptococcal infections are primarily antistreptolysin O and anti-DNAse B. Antistreptolysin O has been the most extensively used test and is generally available in hospitals in the United States.

ASO titers vary with age, geographical area, and other factors influencing the frequency of streptococcal infection. Titers of 200 to 300 units/ml are common in healthy children 6 to 14 years of age who live in crowded cities in the temperate zone of the United States.

The chances of detecting a significant antibody response is greatest 2 to 3 weeks after the onset of ARF, which is usually 4 to 5 weeks after the antecedent streptococcal infection. Thereafter, antibody titers fall off rapidly in the next few months, and after 6 months the decline levels off slowly. For this reason, evidence of increased streptococcal antibodies should be present in all patients at the onset of the rheumatic attack if such onset is well defined. Acute polyarthritis always occurs within a latent period of no more than 4 to 5 weeks after the antecedent streptococcal infection and therefore at or near the peak of the antibody response.

Anti-DNAse B, together with the ASO, has become most generally recommended for diagnosis, with antihyaluronidase a third choice. A concentrate of a variety of extracellular streptococcal antigens made from supernates of broth cultures has been used in the so-called antistreptozyme (ASTZ) test. Sheep cells sensitized with this concentrate will agglutinate in the presence of streptococcal antibodies that have not yet been defined. This slide agglutination test is a very sensitive measure, however crude, of the streptococcal immune response.[85] The greatest value of the ASTZ test is in *helping to rule out RF*, particularly in the diagnosis of isolated polyarthritis when low titers reflect the absence of recent streptococcal disease.

ACUTE PHASE REACTANTS. Acute phase reactants include leukocyte counts, erythrocyte sedimentation rate (ESR), C-reactive protein (CRP),[86] serum mucoprotein, serum hexosamine, serum protein electrophoresis, and several others. The two tests that have gained widest use are the CRP and the ESR. These tests are, of course, not specific for RF, but they are almost always abnormal during the active rheumatic process if it is not suppressed by antirheumatic drugs.

ANEMIA. The anemia of RF is the normocytic normochromic anemia of chronic inflammation and is of mild to moderate degree. Suppression of inflammation usually corrects the anemia partially or completely, and corticosteroids are particularly potent in this regard. Anemia is a good index of the severity and chronicity of RF.

ELECTROCARDIOGRAPHIC FINDINGS. The electrocardiogram in RF has no characteristic pattern, and the diagnosis of rheumatic carditis should never be made on the basis of ECG changes alone. Too often the diagnosis of carditis has been made incorrectly when a doubtful systolic murmur has been associated with a prolonged P-R interval or nonspecific ST-T changes. Neither the course of the acute rheumatic attack nor the subsequent development of valvular or myocardial damage can be predicted from the electrocardiographic changes.[74, 87] Patients with ECG changes but with no other signs of carditis recover completely without the stigmata of rheumatic heart disease.[88]

DIAGNOSIS

JONES CRITERIA. When T. Duckett Jones formulated his criteria for the diagnosis of ARF in 1944,[89] there was immediate recognition of their value and considerable agreement about their use. These criteria were adopted in modified form in 1955 by the American Heart Association's Council on Rheumatic Fever and Congenital Heart Disease and were further revised by the same Council's committee in 1965.[90] The current criteria (Table 54–1) emphasize the importance of establishing the presence of the antecedent streptococcal infection by demonstration of increased streptococcal antibodies. If supported by such evidence, two major (or one major and two minor) manifestations indicate a high probability of ARF. However, because virtually all patients with Sydenham's chorea are rheumatic subjects, the diagnosis can be made even when chorea is the sole manifestation. Because of the numerous causes of polyarthritis, the diagnosis of RF is weakest when this manifestation appears alone, and particularly in the adolescent or adult population in which other arthritides are common.

CARDITIS

Functional ("Innocent") Murmurs. When functional or organic murmurs are typical, there is little problem for the experienced physician. At times, however, a nondescript murmur, especially in an obese or heavy-chested person, may defy sharp distinctions, and repeated examinations and other studies may be required. Such murmurs are often classified as "doubtful" or "questionable" when no other decision can be made.

Myocarditis. In its severe and chronic form, myocarditis due to other diseases may be impossible to distinguish from chronic rheumatic carditis if the heart is dilated and mitral regurgitation is prominent. This situation occurs when patients with ARF have heart failure with no associated extracardiac manifestations to provide clues. In rheumatic carditis, as the patient recovers cardiac compensation, the valvular lesions persist, and the murmurs become, if anything, louder.

Pericarditis. Although rheumatic carditis does not produce an isolated pericarditis, at the onset of RF, however, pericarditis may appear before valvulitis and myocarditis are evident. Although many causes of pericarditis can be listed (Chap. 44), primary viral pericarditis most often enters the differential diagnosis in children.

TABLE 54–1 JONES CRITERIA (REVISED)

Major Manifestations	Minor Manifestations
Carditis	Fever
Polyarthritis	Arthralgia
Chorea	Previous rheumatic fever or rheumatic heart disease
Erythema marginatum	Elevated ESR or positive CRP
Subcutaneous nodules	Prolonged P-R interval

Plus supporting evidence of preceding streptococcal infection: history of recent scarlet fever; positive throat culture for group A streptococcus; increased ASO titer or other streptococcal antibodies.

From Jones Criteria (revised) for guidance in the diagnosis of rheumatic fever. Circulation 32:664, 1965, by permission of the American Heart Association, Inc.

COURSE AND PROGNOSIS

The clinical course of RF can be quite variable, but in general there is a characteristic sequence of the major manifestations and usually a predictable duration. The latent period between streptococcal infection and the onset of ARF is shortest in arthritis and erythema marginatum and longest in chorea, with that of carditis and subcutaneous nodules in between. The usual duration of a rheumatic attack is rarely longer than 3 months. When severe carditis is present, clinical rheumatic activity may continue for 6 months or more. In fewer than 5 per cent of patients, ARF may remain active for more than 6 months.[91] These cases are classified as "chronic" rheumatic fever.

CARDITIS. Of the patients in whom carditis develops, murmurs occur during the first week of illness in 76 per cent. In 93 per cent of patients there is evidence of carditis in the first 3 months. Age of onset and severity of carditis influence its chronicity. Before the age of 3 years, 92 per cent of patients in one study[92] and 90 per cent in another[93] had carditis. The incidence of carditis decreased to 50 per cent in the 3- to 6-year age group and to 32 per cent in the 14- to 17-year age group[70] in first attacks. Carditis occurs occasionally after the age of 25 in what are apparently first attacks of ARF. When carditis is mild or evidence for it is borderline, it usually disappears rapidly. Severe carditis prolongs the attack. When severe carditis subsides, low-grade fever and tachycardia often continue, cardiac enlargement usually persists, and new murmurs may appear. Congestive heart failure may occur at any time while carditis is still active.

PROGNOSIS. RF does not recur when streptococcal disease is prevented. The prognosis is excellent for the rheumatic subject who escapes carditis during an initial attack of RF. In one 5-year follow-up, rheumatic heart disease did not develop when the acute attack was not accompanied by the appearance of organic heart murmurs.[87] In the United Kingdom–United States Cooperative Study on the treatment of RF,[73, 74] similar patients without carditis (defined as the absence of organic murmurs) during the acute attack showed virtually no evidence of late or insidious development of rheumatic heart disease. The percentage of this group of patients with "no carditis" who subsequently had normal hearts was 96 at 5 years and 94 at 10 years. The prognoses become poorer with the increasing severity of initial carditis, so that the percentage of those with congestive heart failure during the acute attack showing complete healing was 30 at 5 years and 40 at 10 years. It is apparent that the healing rate of rheumatic carditis is remarkably high if recurrences are prevented.

Prospective cooperative studies[74] have shown, at 5 years, that the frequency of mitral stenosis was equally distributed between the sexes and was related to the severity of the initial attack of carditis. In fact, a large percentage of the deaths within 5 years was due to such severe mitral valvular deformity. The analysis at 10 years, however, showed the emergence of another group—those whose initial mitral lesion had been relatively mild and who showed slow, progressive obstruction without evidence of recurrent RF or streptococcal disease. This group consisted of predominantly female subjects. It is apparent, therefore, that host factors, as yet undefined, influence the course of valvular sclerosis once mitral deformity has occurred and that progression of rheumatic heart disease may be related to more than the rheumatic inflammation itself. In addition, the tendency of stenotic mitral valves that have been fractured or incised surgically to restenose without evidence of recurrent or active RF is quite apparent in several long-term follow-up studies.[94]

Recurrences. First attacks of RF in the general population following epidemic streptococcal pharyngitis average 3 per cent, whereas such infections in patients with a history of recent RF may produce a secondary attack rate as high as 65 per cent.[27] In the Irvington House study,[95] rheumatic attack rate per infection (R/I) in children decreased from 23 to 11 per cent between the first and fifth year after a rheumatic attack.[28] In adults with rheumatic heart disease, this rate was 4.8 per cent 10 or more years after the last attack.[29] Recurrence rates decline, therefore, with the length of time elapsed since the last attack.

A second factor that clearly increases the chance that a streptococcal infection will be followed by a rheumatic attack is the presence of residual rheumatic heart disease. In the Irvington House studies, the recurrence rate in children with rheumatic heart disease and cardiomegaly was 43 per cent; in patients with rheumatic heart disease and no cardiomegaly, 27 per cent; and in patients without apparent residual heart disease, 10 per cent.[28]

A third factor influencing the R/I is the magnitude of the immune response to the antecedent streptococcal disease as reflected in the increase of ASO titer.

THE CHANGING NATURAL HISTORY OF RHEUMATIC HEART DISEASE. The current longevity of patients in the United States with inactive rheumatic heart disease can be projected from a subgroup of such patients followed prospectively for more than 30 years as part of the Framingham Study.[96] As expected, compared with a cohort control group, there was a relatively sharp decline in survival during the first half of the study reflecting, no doubt, hemodynamic changes in the more severely involved hearts, because rheumatic recurrences were extremely rare. Nonetheless, a large proportion of patients with rheumatic heart disease survived. After 36 years of follow-up, in males the percentage surviving in the rheumatic heart disease group was only slightly below 40, compared with somewhat more than 40 per cent in their cohorts without rheumatic heart disease. Among the women the discrepancy in survival between the patients with rheumatic heart disease and their cohorts was greater[96] (Fig. 54–8). The reservoir of relatively benign rheumatic valvular disease in the elderly population has been well recognized by clinicians for many years, but because of the sharp decline in new cases of rheumatic fever, rheumatic heart disease in the United States is becoming a "geriatric" disease.[97] This phenomenon also contributes to the increasing mean age of patients with infective endocarditis.

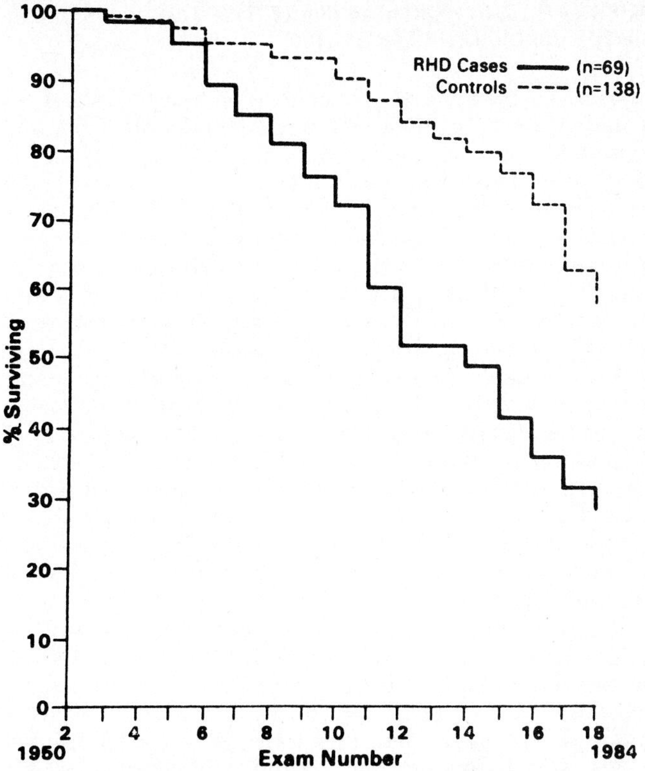

FIGURE 54–8. Survival of subjects with rheumatic heart disease and their cohorts, 1950 to 1984. *A*, Females. *B*, Males. (From Goetzler, R., Stokes, J., III, and Anderson, K.: Prognosis of subjects in the Framingham Study with rheumatic heart disease. J. Am. Geriatr. Soc. *33*:693, 1985.)

TREATMENT

GENERAL MANAGEMENT. In any given case of RF, general management depends upon the manifestations and severity of the attack. Patients should remain in bed for the duration of the acute and febrile portion of the illness until clinical and laboratory evidence of inflammation abates.

The administration of antiinflammatory or suppressive therapy should ordinarily be delayed until the disease process is clearly expressed in order to establish the diagnosis. Aspirin or corticosteroids administered prematurely to a patient with arthralgia or early monoarticular arthritis and fever may mask the disease process and cause diagnostic confusion. Furthermore, in isolated polyarthritis a trial of penicillin therapy is often essential to eliminate the diagnosis of septic arthritis, especially gonococcemia, and the therapeutic response to the antibiotic must be carefully evaluated.

Once the diagnosis is established, treatment can begin, usually with a *course of penicillin* adequate to eradicate residual group A streptococci. Massive penicillin treatment has been used by some investigators in an attempt to alter the frequency of cardiac damage but without success.[98] The usual course of penicillin consists of a single injection of 1.2 million units of benzathine penicillin intramuscularly, or 600,000 units of procaine penicillin intramuscularly, daily for 10 days. This is followed by continuous (secondary) prophylaxis (see below).

ANTIRHEUMATIC THERAPY. The selection of an antirheumatic agent is not critical to the outcome of most attacks of RF.[72–77] Corticosteroids and salicylates can be regarded as valuable symptomatic and supportive therapy, but they are not curative and may actually prolong the course of the disease. However, both steroids and salicylates control the toxic manifestations of the disease; contribute to the comfort of the patient; and combat anemia, anorexia, and other constitutional symptoms. In severe rheumatic carditis associated with heart failure, such nonspecific antiinflammatory effects may reduce the burden on the heart and occasionally may tilt the balance in favor of the survival of a critically ill patient.

Patients with mild arthritis or arthralgia and no carditis may be treated with analgesics only, such as codeine, as needed. Two goals will be thus accomplished: First, the diagnosis may be made more certain by the appearance of definite arthritis in some of the initially questionable cases; and second, the duration of hospitalization or of close observation at home will be decreased because many of the patients will get well in 2 or 3 weeks; moreover, one will not have to worry about, and deal with, post-therapeutic rebounds.

Most current general policy is to administer salicylates when no clear evidence of carditis exists. If signs and symptoms are not adequately suppressed by salicylates, corticosteroids should be substituted. Patients with mild carditis are often given corticosteroids, but without the conviction that these are superior to salicylates. Those with severe carditis are usually treated promptly with corticosteroids, particularly if heart failure is evident, and with the precaution of adequate doses of diuretics and restriction of salt intake to combat sodium retention.

Since neither corticosteroids nor salicylates shorten the course of RF, the duration of therapy must be estimated according to the expected course of the attack. It is important to reduce the dose of corticosteroids gradually over a period of about 2 weeks and to recognize that abrupt cessation of treatment leaves the patient in a state of temporary adrenal insufficiency resulting from suppression of endogenous adrenocortical activity during prolonged hormone therapy.

When treatment of ARF is initiated with salicylates, a dose of 6 to 9 gm/day of acetylsalicylic acid is administered to patients weighing 70 kg or more, and proportionately smaller doses are given to patients weighing less. This is administered in divided doses every 4 hours. The initial doses of acetylsalicylic acid should be continued until a satisfactory clinical response is obtained, that is, until there is complete relief of symptoms and signs of arthritis and the temperature has returned to a normal range. Thereafter the dosage may be reduced to two-thirds the initial value and may be maintained until all laboratory manifestations of inflammatory disease have returned to normal. For the remainder of the course of therapy, the dosage may be reduced to half the initial daily dose. Should clinical or laboratory evidence of relapse occur when doses are reduced, it is advisable to return to the previous higher dosage that suppressed the process.

An initial dose of prednisone of 40 to 60 mg/day for adults and children alike may be started and varied according to the patient's response. With other analogs, such as triamcinolone and dexamethasone, the dosage is based on their potency relative to prednisone.

REBOUNDS OF RHEUMATIC ACTIVITY. Clinical or laboratory evidence of rheumatic activity may reappear when suppressive antirheumatic therapy is discontinued. Such reactivation has been termed a rebound and should clearly be distinguished from a recurrence. Spontaneous rebounds do not occur more than 5 weeks after complete cessation of all antirheumatic therapy; by far the majority occur within 2 weeks, but most occur within a few days or while dosage is being reduced. Mild rebounds subside spontaneously within a week or two and do not require medication.

TREATMENT OF CHOREA. This is nonspecific and consists of tranquilization and sedation. For complete details the reader is referred elsewhere.[1, 99]

PREVENTION

The most effective preventive measures against RF are probably socioeconomic. The almost total absence of the disease in the affluent sections of the cities of the western world suggests that spacious housing and noncrowding are at least as important as good diagnosis and treatment of streptococcal sore throat in the prevention of rheumatic attacks. Nevertheless, the natural history of RF can be dramatically altered in several ways by the use of antimicrobials. Mass penicillin prophylaxis can halt epidemics of streptococcal sore throat. Adequate penicillin treatment of acute streptococcal sore throat will abort an initial attack and, less often, rheumatic recurrences. Continuous administration of sulfadiazine or penicillin will prevent recurrent attacks in rheumatic subjects.

SECONDARY PROPHYLAXIS. The term secondary prophylaxis is used to describe protection against rheumatic recurrences by means of continuous chemoprophylaxis. After a diagnosis of RF is established, residual streptococci which may or may not be detectable on throat cultures should be eradicated by a therapeutic course of penicillin as described below for primary prevention. The most effective form of continuous prophylaxis is a single monthly intramuscular injection of 1.2 million units of benzathine penicillin G.[100–102] An attack rate of less than 1 recurrence per 250 patient-years was documented in patients using this form of prophylaxis in the extensive studies reported by the Irvington House group.[101] Although the reaction rate is somewhat higher for all injectable forms of penicillin, regardless of kind, than with oral penicillin, reactions are very rare after the first months of prophylaxis. Monthly injections of benzathine penicillin are undoubtedly the preferred form of prophylaxis in populations in which RF continues to appear, or, indeed, is on the increase. In affluent societies, however, and in countries in which RF has become rare, it is unlikely that this form of prophylaxis will be employed except when major risk factors of recurrences coexist.[102]

Oral prophylaxis is less reliable than repository penicillin prophylaxis. In the Irvington House studies, a recurrence rate of almost 1 per 25 patient-years (10 times that of intramuscular benzathine penicillin) was observed in patients receiving oral medication.[101] The recommended dosages for oral sulfadiazine prophylaxis are 0.5 gm once daily for patients weighing less than 27 kg (60 lb) and 1 gm once a day for patients weighing more than 27 kg. For oral penicillin prophylaxis, the recommended dose is 200,000 to 250,000 units daily of penicillin G or 125 to 250 mg of penicillin V twice a day.[102] Even when oral penicillin is administered twice daily no superiority over sulfadiazine has been demonstrated.[103]

Strains of streptococci resistant to sulfonamide have appeared with mass sulfonamide prophylaxis in military populations, but have not been a problem in secondary prophylaxis of rheumatic subjects. Reaction rates are low with both oral medications and are rare after the first months of prophylaxis. For the rare patient who is sensitive to both sulfadiazine and penicillin, oral erythromycin may be substituted in a dose of 250 mg twice daily.[104]

It has been difficult to establish a general recommendation concerning the duration of prophylaxis because of the number of variables that influence the attack rate of recurrences following streptococcal infections (see Course and Prognosis, above). Although risks of recurrences decline with age and with increased interval from the last rheumatic attack, a relatively high recurrence rate per infection persists for a very long time—5 to 10 years or more. Exceptions to instituting or maintaining prophylaxis should be made only after assessing the risk of high exposure to streptococcal infection (e.g., working with school-age children, in military service, in medical or allied health positions). Patients with significant degrees of rheumatic heart disease or with a history of repeated recurrences (including chorea) or those having had a recent attack require most careful consideration before discontinuation of prophylaxis.

PRIMARY PROPHYLAXIS. The term *primary prophylaxis* is applied to the prevention of first attacks of RF by treatment of the preceding streptococcal pharyngitis. In military populations with a high frequency of severe streptococcal pharyngitis, penicillin therapy reduced the attack rate of RF from 3.0 to 0.3 per cent.[105] The application of primary prevention to civilian populations, particularly children with sporadic or endemic streptococcal infections, has been more difficult because of the problem of differentiating viral pharyngitis in carriers of group A streptococci from current streptococcal infection and because frequent streptococcal exposure in children tends to keep streptococcal antibody titers elevated (see Epidemiology, above). Throat cultures, when negative, are helpful, therefore, in eliminating the need for intensive penicillin therapy in patients with nonstreptococcal infection.

Effective therapy demands eradication of the infecting organism, which requires 10 days of consistent treatment if penicillin is administered orally. Many patients fail to extend such treatment beyond the first few days if acute symptoms of streptococcal pharyngitis subside. A single intramuscular injection of benzathine penicillin G (600,000 units in children under 27 kg [60 lb] and 1.2 million units in those over 27 kg) is the treatment of choice when the risk of RF still exists. Oral penicillin is now usually preferred for the treatment of streptococcal infections in populations in which the risk of RF is very low. The dose of penicillin G is 200,000 to 250,000 units three to four times daily. Penicillin V in doses of 125 to 250 mg may be substituted. Treatment is still recommended for a full 10 days.[102] For those sensitive to penicillin, erythromycin (250 mg two to four times a day or 40 mg/kg per day in younger children) may be substituted.

Mass Antibiotic Prophylaxis. This type of prophylaxis is effective in populations in which streptococcal pharyngeal infections are epidemic.[106] This approach may be indicated occasionally in civilian or institutional epidemics, especially if several cases of RF occur within a few weeks. Mass intramuscular administration of 1.2 million units of benzathine penicillin G to all members of the affected population has been extremely effective.[4]

Immunization with Streptococcal Vaccines. Although no vaccine is currently available for general distribution, considerable progress has been made on the purification and immunology of streptococcal M proteins and holds promise for future streptococcal vaccine development.[107–109]

SERONEGATIVE SPONDYLOARTHROPATHIES

COMMON CLINICAL FEATURES AND NOSOLOGY. A group of rheumatological syndromes has been classified under the heading of seronegative spondyloarthropathies because they have clinical features in common and some pathological lesions, including those of the heart, that are identical.[110–112] They are distinguished from rheumatoid arthritis by the *absence of the characteristic serological changes* of the latter (e.g., increased rheumatoid factor); by the predilection of the arthritis for the sacroiliac, lumbosacral, and apophyseal joints of the spine; by the predominance in men over women; by the predilection for involvement of the entheses (insertions of ligaments and capsules into bone); and by the extraarticular manifestations of iritis and of aortic regurgitation due to a characteristic lesion at the root of the aorta. The spondyloarthropathies are also distinguished by association with haplotype HLA-B27. The group of syndromes includes ankylosing spondylitis, Reiter's disease, psoriatic arthritis, and the intestinal arthropathies. Two of the major syndromes, ankylosing spondylitis and Reiter's disease, have been associated with dysentery and urethritis. Although the causative agents are usually not apparent, dysentery due to specific bacteria (*Yersinia enterocolitica, Shigella, Salmonella* and *Campylobacter*) has produced most of the features of these syndromes.[113] Urethritis due to *Chlamydia trachomatis* has also been implicated as one of the causes of Reiter's disease,[114] but in most cases the etiological agent has not been identified.

HISTOCOMPATIBILITY ANTIGEN B27. The concept of a genetically determined aberrant host response to a variety of infectious agents that can invade the bowel or genitourinary tract has emerged from the demonstration of the striking association of the seronegative spondyloarthropathies with the histocompatibility antigen HLA-B27.[110–112] This membrane antigen occurs with a frequency of approximately 4 to 8 per cent in the normal population, whereas over 90 per cent of patients with either ankylosing spondylitis or Reiter's disease with spondyloarthropathy are B27-positive. When spondyloarthropathy complicates inflammatory bowel disease, the association with B27 is greater than 80 per cent, and 50 per cent of psoriatic patients with spondylitis are B27-positive. So far, 50 per cent of patients with anterior uveitis have this antigen. When an outbreak of a specific form of dysentery has permitted careful prospective studies, patients with the B27 antigen have had a much greater tendency to develop any form of arthritis than those lacking this antigen. The more specific features of the syndrome such as spondyloarthropathy, iritis, and cardiac involvement have been confined primarily to those who are B27-positive.

ANKYLOSING SPONDYLITIS

CARDIAC PATHOLOGY. The incidence of cardiovascular involvement varies from 3.5 per cent of cases with a 15-year history to 10 per cent with up to 30 years of disease. Several excellent prospective studies have documented the form of cardiac and aortic disease peculiar to ankylosing spondylitis, consisting of the following: dilatation of the aortic valve ring; fibrous thickening, scarring, and variable focal inflammatory lesions of the aortic valve cusps, which sag into the ventricular cavity; dilatation of the sinuses of Valsalva; focal degenerative changes of elastic and muscle fibers of the aortic media; and patchy inflammatory lesions in all layers of the aorta, predominantly in the region adjacent to the aortic valve ring[115–117] (Fig. 54–9). The lesions resemble those of syphilis except that in ankylosing spondylitis they remain close to the valve ring and do not affect the rest of the aorta. In addition, the basal rather than the distal portion of the aortic cusps is thickened in ankylosing spondylitis and the dense adventitial scarring extends into the endocardium in the immediate subaortic region. This extension may involve the base of the anterior mitral leaflet and the upper portion of the ventricular septum. In view of the enthesopathical lesions that characterize the pathology of this condition, patients may present with insertional tendinitis at any site, and the heart

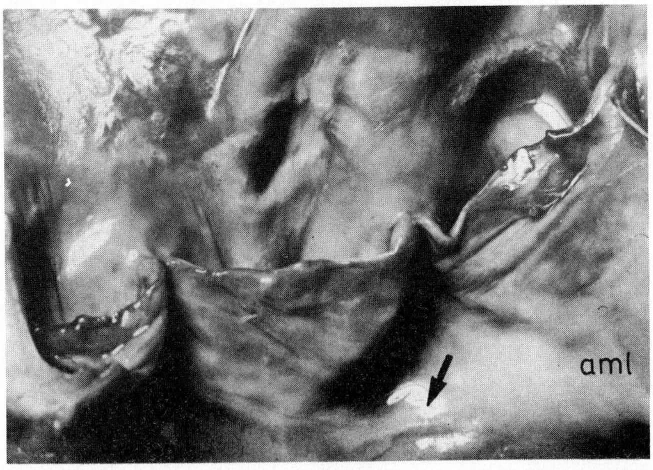

FIGURE 54–9. The aortic valve and sinus of Valsalva cut open in a patient with ankylosing spondylitis who was HLA-B27–positive. The base of the cusps is thickened. The orifice of the right coronary artery is distorted. Aortic regurgitation had been present during life. (From Bergfeldt, L.: HLA-B-27–associated heart disease. Am. J. Med. 77:961, 1984.)

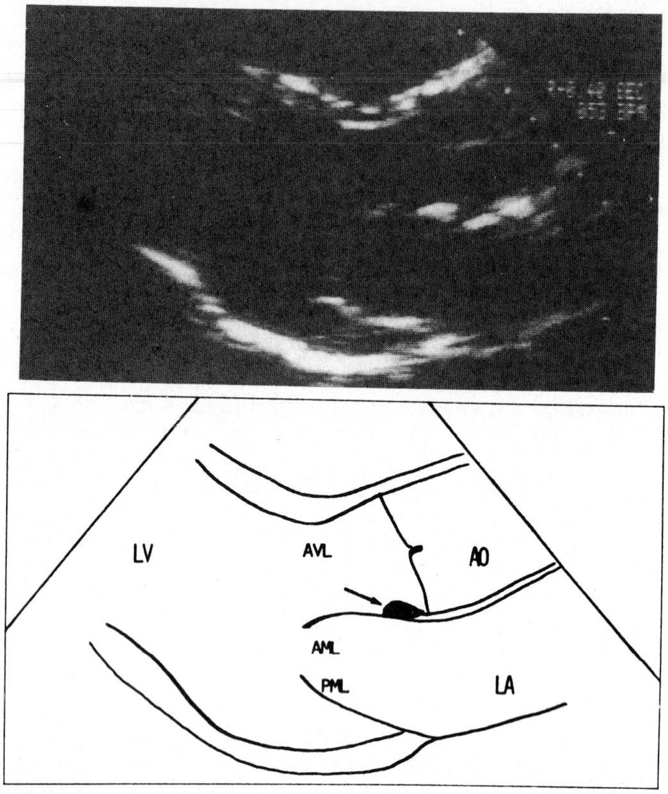

FIGURE 54–10. Long-axis view in a patient with ankylosing spondylitis. Subaortic thickening (*arrow*) is present, and there is an increase in aortic diameter and thickening of the aortic walls and aortic root echodensity. AML = anterior mitral leaflet; AO = aortic root; AVL = aortic valve leaflets; LA = left atrium; LV = left ventricle; PML = posterior mitral leaflet (From Labresh, K. A., et al.: Two-dimensional echocardiographic detection of preclinical aortic root abnormalities in rheumatoid variant diseases. Am. J. Med. *78*:908, 1985.)

valve lesions may reflect this connective tissue localization (Fig. 54–10).

Aortic regurgitation results from thickening and shortening of the cusps and from their displacement caudally by the mass of fibrous tissue behind the commissures and by dilatation of the aortic valve root consequent to the destruction of elastic tissue (Fig. 54–9). Mitral regurgitation is infrequent and usually insignificant but can result from dilatation of the left ventricle and from fibrous thickening of the basal portion of the anterior mitral leaflet.[118] The frequent heart block and conduction defects of ankylosing spondylitis are due to the extension of fibrosis into the muscular septum and destruction of the bundle of His and proximal bundle branches.[119–121]

The lesions of the myocardium are rather nonspecific, consisting of fibrosis, perivascular lymphocytic infiltration, and increased mucinous ground substance. Cardiac enlargement without any apparent cause and hypertrophy and dilatation of the left ventricle are often described.[122, 123]

Chronic fibrous obliteration of the pericardial cavity has been found at autopsy, but pericarditis is not a prominent clinical feature of the disease. Pericardial rubs and chest pain have been described, however, during more severe, acute, toxic episodes when there is active peripheral polyarthritis and in association with presumably early phases of the disease, especially in association with early Reiter's syndrome or dysentery with polyarthritis.

CLINICAL CARDIAC FEATURES. In many patients there is evidence of active carditis before aortic regurgitation appears. Precordial pain, pericardial friction rubs, marked tachycardia, cardiac enlargement not explained by hypertension, or other recognizable forms of heart disease and varying P-R intervals greater than 0.24 sec are frequently described, usually when patients have active peripheral arthritis and/or spondylitis with fever and increased erythrocyte sedimentation rates.[115] Remarkably few critical studies have been made of myocardial function in patients with ankylosing spondylitis before evidence of aortic regurgitation draws attention to cardiac involvement, but it is clear that cardiomyopathy may precede valvular involvement.[122, 123] Indeed, the high cardiovascular morbidity and mortality in these diseases may be due to myocardial abnormalities in the absence of valve disease.[123] The usual cardiac features of ankylosing spondylitis are the gradual evolution of aortic regurgitation and varying degrees of AV block. The prevalence of the valve lesion is related to the duration of spondylitis and peripheral joint involvement, reaching an incidence in one series of 10 per cent in those with spondylitis for 30 years or more and of 18 per cent if peripheral joint involvement was also present. The incidence of AV block in each of the above groups was 8.5 and 15.5 per cent, respectively.[115]

In one long follow-up of 97 patients with ankylosing spondylitis, of whom 14 had cardiovascular lesions, aortic regurgitation occurred in 10 patients. Mitral regurgitation and AV block appeared as isolated findings in 1 and 3 patients, respectively. Nine of the 14 patients had peripheral arthritis, and 3 had iritis.[116] Anterior uveitis and extraspinal disease may also precede the articular lesions of ankylosing spondylitis by months or years. Hence the discovery of isolated aortic regurgitation in young or middle-aged men requires that ankylosing spondylitis be considered in the differential diagnosis. In addition, the aortic regurgitation of ankylosing spondylitis is now well documented to occur in so-called secondary forms of the disease such as spondylitis associated with psoriasis, regional enteritis,[116] ulcerative colitis,[124] and Reiter's disease.[125]

Aortic valve replacement (p. 1059) has been performed successfully in several centers, and patients with ankylosing spondylitis may be suitable candidates when such a procedure is indicated. Cardiac pacemakers have been implanted for AV block.

REITER'S DISEASE

Cardiac involvement in the acute stages of Reiter's disease has been described frequently and consists most commonly of acute pericarditis, apical systolic murmurs, gallops, and cardiac conduction abnormalities, particularly AV block. These changes disappear rapidly, and long-term follow-up of large series reveals only an occasional case of cardiac failure or third-degree atrioventricular block.[126] This acute form of Reiter's disease usually features nonspecific urethritis, nonsuppurative migratory polyarthritis, conjunctivitis, circinate balanitis, and keratoderma blenorrhagica. Initial attacks usually subside spontaneously, but second attacks occur in about 15 per cent of cases, and chronic manifestations (almost always in B27-positive individuals[112]) may then ensue, with recurrent anterior uveitis, painful mutilating deformities of the feet, sacroiliitis, spondylitis, AV block, and an aortic valve lesion leading to aortic and occasionally to mitral regurgitation.

Postmortem studies of the aortic valves have shown the cusps to be thickened, with rolled edges, and the aorta to incur changes similar if not identical to the lesions described in AS.[127, 128]

The development of Reiter's disease in patients with *Yersinia* arthritis or associated with various other dysentery-producing bacteria has emphasized the role of the B27 antigen in the frequency of expression of various clinical features of the syndrome, including its cardiac manifestations.[129–131] Of 19 patients with Reiter's syndrome observed at one institution, all 5 who had conduction abnormalities were B27-positive.[132]

RHEUMATOID ARTHRITIS

PATHOLOGY. The heart is frequently involved in the inflammatory process of rheumatoid arthritis (RA), yet its function is seldom compromised by the lesions produced. The exudative type of rheumatoid inflammation affects the pericardial surfaces, producing a fibrinous pericarditis that is usually low grade and subclinical. Pericardial inflammation becomes symptomatic and clinically significant in its more florid form and may even be the presenting complaint.

The most characteristic pathological lesion of RA, the nodular granuloma, involves the myocardium, endocardium, and valves of the heart.[133–135] The extent of this kind of involvement is generally proportionate to the severity of the disease and is almost always associated with diffusely distributed rheumatoid nodules, subcutaneously and elsewhere. These granulomas rarely compromise the function of the myocardium, however, nor do they often affect the function of the heart valves unless they become large and numerous enough to distort them (Fig. 54–11).

Diffuse arteritis, when present, affects small vessels, causing round cell infiltration, edema, fibrosis, and proliferation of the intima. Such involvement of the pericardial vessels may be extensive when it reflects an intense systemic form of RA, and the disease may begin in the pericardium before the joints become involved. Coronary arteritis is often observed at necropsy in severe RA, but it very rarely results in clinically apparent myocardial ischemia.

Clinical Features

PERICARDITIS (See also p. 1520). The frequency of rheumatoid pericarditis in necropsy studies ranges from 11 to 50 per cent, with an overall estimate of about 30 per cent.[136] Clinically, the diagnosis of pericarditis is made in about 2 per cent of cases in the adult form and in about 6 per cent in the juvenile form of RA. In careful studies of the more severe forms of the disease which require hospital admission, approximately 10 per cent of patients with rheumatoid arthritis have clinical evidence of rheumatoid pericarditis during the lifetime course of their disease. Part of the disparity between clinical and autopsy findings is due to the fact that the chest pain may be overshadowed by arthritic pains and may be masked by antirheumatic agents or mistaken for arthritic pain in neighboring joints.

The pathophysiology of the acute fibrinous pericarditis of RA is not clear, but in severe cases the pericardial fluid, like synovial fluid, shows decreased hemolytic complement (CH_{50}) and C3 levels. Immunofluorescence staining of the pericardium shows plasma cell infiltration and deposits of IgG, IgM, IgA, or C3 in the pericardial vessels.[137] Moreover, the polymorphonuclear leukocytes in the pericardial fluid may show cytoplasmic inclusions which stain for IgM, indicative of ingested immune complexes such as are also seen in the polymorphonuclear cells of synovial fluid in the same patients. These findings are associated with extremely low levels of glucose, indicative of active phagocytosis, as observed in pleural and synovial rheumatoid fluids. About half the patients with overt rheumatoid pericarditis also have rheumatoid pleural and lung lesions.

In reports of patients with rheumatoid arthritis studied by echocardiography, pericardial effusion was demonstrated in 30 per cent of all patients studied and in 50 per cent of those with subcutaneous nodules.[138, 139] This incidence is as high as the reported frequency of postmortem findings of rheumatoid pericarditis.

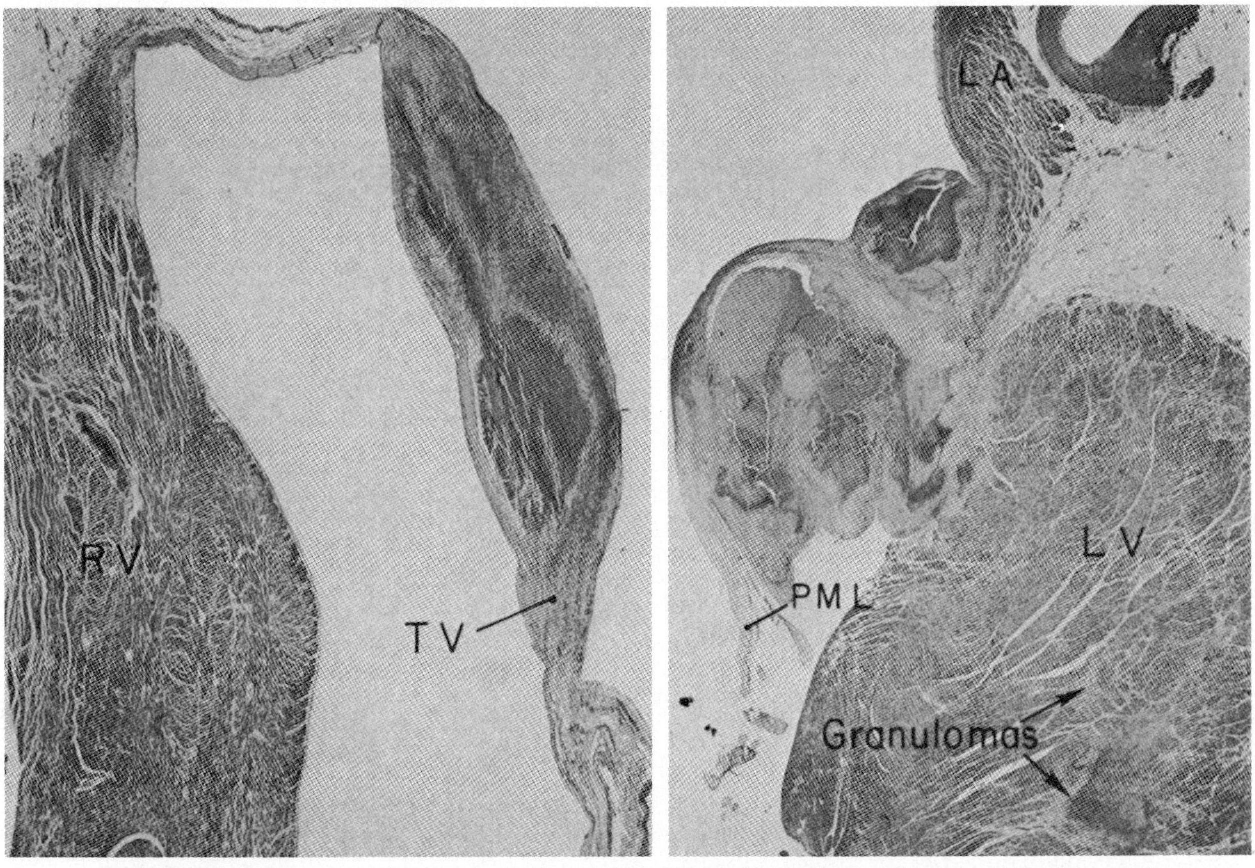

FIGURE 54–11. *Left,* Tricuspid valve (TV) leaflet. Typical rheumatoid granuloma is located within substance of leaflet. RV indicates right ventricle (H and E, ×12). *Right,* Mitral valve. Section includes posterior mitral leaflet (PML) and adjacent portions of left atrial (LA) and left ventricular (LV) walls. Large rheumatoid granuloma is located within proximal three-fourths of posterior leaflet. Smaller nodule involves endocardium of left atrium as well. Two rheumatoid granulomas are located within the left ventricular wall (H and E, ×6.5). (From Roberts, W. C., et al.: Cardiac valvular lesions in rheumatoid arthritis. Arch. Intern. Med. *122*:141, 1968. Copyright 1968, American Medical Association.)

Pericarditis may appear without relation to the duration of rheumatoid arthritis and sometimes may even be the harbinger of the onset of a severe form of the disease. It occurs most often in middle-aged men in whom arthritis was of acute onset. Most often, the clinical course is benign, and symptoms and signs will respond to moderate amounts of prednisone. Occasionally, however, the disease may be more protracted and severe, leading to cardiac tamponade and constrictive pericarditis.

In its florid form the disease has the usual symptoms and signs of pericarditis, and when persistent, it imitates closely tuberculous pericarditis, from which it must be carefully differentiated. Although some fatal cases have been described in which a true pancarditis was present,[140] such cases are exceptional, and even severe rheumatoid pericarditis usually spares myocardial and endocardial function.

Treatment of rheumatoid pericarditis is the same as that for the arthritic disease. Although corticosteroids tend to be used more liberally in pericarditis to suppress inflammation, there is no evidence that such suppression will prevent adhesive or constrictive pericarditis.

RHEUMATOID MYOCARDITIS. Except for rare cases of myocarditis with diffuse granulomas or amyloid infiltration of the myocardium associated with very severe rheumatoid arthritis, myocarditis is mostly nonspecific and subclinical in the great majority of patients. The histological lesions may be focal or generalized infiltrations of lymphocytes, plasma cells, palisading histiocytes, and fibroblasts.[133] The incidence of myocarditis in autopsies of rheumatoid arthritis patients is reported as 19 per cent. Most of such cases are associated with severe arthritis, vasculitis, and endocarditis or pericarditis.

Although left ventricular function may be compromised by a variety of pathological processes in severe rheumatoid arthritis, the typical case is remarkable for its characteristic sparing of the myocardial musculature despite extensive involvement of the fibrous structures of the heart. Nevertheless, when there are unusually severe systemic manifestations of rheumatoid arthritis, rheumatoid pancarditis with congestive heart failure has been well described and confirmed by necropsy. Such patients exhibit the whole spectrum of rheumatoid inflammation of the heart.[140]

CORONARY ARTERY DISEASE. Clinicopathological correlation suggests that the nature of the coronary artery disease analyzed in some studies of patients with rheumatoid arthritis is probably rheumatoid rather than arteriosclerotic. Coronary arteritis is observed in about 20 per cent of patients with rheumatoid arthritis at autopsy. This arteritis is probably a manifestation of generalized vasculitis often seen in rheumatoid arthritis. Inflammation with edema of the intima of the artery may lead to severe narrowing or occlusion of its lumen, to necrosis, and to angina or infarction.[141] Nevertheless, myocardial necrosis secondary to this form of arteritis is rare.

VALVULAR AND ENDOCARDIAL LESIONS. As in myocarditis, the histological picture of the valves and adjacent endocardial areas of patients with rheumatoid arthritis shows nonspecific inflammation with fibrotic and sclerotic changes and infiltrations of histiocytes, plasma cells, lymphocytes, and occasional eosinophils.[133] The most characteristic lesions, however, are granulomas resembling rheumatoid nodules. Usually these do not interfere with valvular function unless they reach large enough proportions to produce frank valvular regurgitation by destroying the base of the valve and its cusps. Such regurgitation may be of sufficient magnitude and rapidity of onset to cause severe cardiac decompensation and death[142] (Chap. 33).

All valves may be involved, but the descending order of frequency is mitral, aortic, tricuspid, and pulmonary. Echocardiographic studies have shown a significant slowing of mitral valve movement in patients with rheumatoid arthritis correlating with the duration of the disease and the extent of the formation of subcutaneous nodules.[139] It is not clear whether left ventricular disease can be excluded as a cause contributing to this finding or whether it is due entirely to intrinsic involvement of the mitral valve alone. At least in a few well-described cases, however, mitral and aortic valvular deformity with marked regurgitation due to rheumatoid nodules was the characteristic pathological picture.[140]

ELECTROCARDIOGRAPHIC ABNORMALITIES. Studies of the electrocardiogram in patients with rheumatoid arthritis and in matched controls show that first degree AV block is the most significant finding in rheumatoid arthritis.[134] Complete heart block causing Adams-Stokes syndrome has been described,[142] and other abnormalities include left bundle branch block, atrial fibrillation, and atrial and ventricular ectopic beats. Abnormal T waves, however, do not occur more frequently than in controls and are of little value in the diagnosis of rheumatoid heart disease despite the frequency of rheumatoid pericarditis.[136]

Juvenile Rheumatoid Arthritis (Still's Disease)

This syndrome, one of the more common chronic illnesses of childhood, may also have its onset in adults and is particularly noteworthy for involvement of the serosal surfaces, producing pleuritis and pericarditis as well as arthritis, and is featured by a characteristic rash.[144] Pericarditis can be diagnosed clinically in approximately 7 per cent of children with juvenile rheumatoid arthritis. As in rheumatoid arthritis, postmortem examinations show a much higher incidence of pericarditis, and echocardiography is needed to reveal its clinical frequency.[145] Pericardial tamponade has been reported in both children and adults with this syndrome, but it is very rare. Myocarditis is less common than pericarditis, but may produce cardiac enlargement and heart failure.[146] Valvular heart disease is rare, but severe aortic regurgitation requiring valve replacement has been described in a young adult.[147]

THE VASCULITIS SYNDROMES

Most of the clinical manifestations of periarteritis nodosa, systemic lupus erythematosus (SLE), and several other forms of diffuse vasculitis may be produced by infections such as hepatitis B, in which massive and persistent antigenemia gives rise to circulating immune complexes, the qualitative and quantitative features of which determine the localization and character of the vascular lesions. It has also become clear that bacterial endocarditis, like hepatitis B, produces many of the varied glomerular lesions of SLE, produces large and small lesions of polyarteritis, and produces serological findings similar to those of SLE.[148, 149]

In addition to infectious agents as a cause of immune complex disease, the prolonged administration of certain drugs can produce most, if not all, of the features of SLE (drug-induced lupus). Procainamide is the most notorious offender, but hydralazine, phenytoin (Dilantin), and several other anticonvulsants, isoniazid, sulfonamides, and several other drugs administered for prolonged periods may produce features of SLE.[150, 151]

As in the case of the seronegative spondyloarthropathies (see above), only a small portion of the syndromes recognized can be shown to be due to specific infectious agents or drugs. Most cases of large-vessel polyarteritis, or the small-vessel and capillary diffuse vasculitis of SLE, must be considered idiopathic, but a careful search for known infectious agents capable of producing persistent antigenemia and for a history of drug therapy should be undertaken before one resorts to an idiopathic, descriptive diagnosis.

SYSTEMIC LUPUS ERYTHEMATOSUS

PATHOLOGICAL FEATURES. The hallmark of this disease is the presence of a number of antibodies to nuclear components, the antinuclear antibodies (ANA), which participate in the pathogenesis of SLE by forming antigen-antibody-complement complexes that are found in many of the lesions. These and other hyperimmune phenomena explain many of the protean clinical manifestations of SLE. Although anti-heart antibodies have been described in the sera of patients with SLE, they bear no clear relationship to the frequency and severity of cardiac lesions and may be a result rather than a cause of cardiac inflammation, presumably owing to release of myocardial antigens into the circulation.[152] Other etiological and pathogenetic processes associated with autoimmunity have been extensively reviewed.[153]

CARDIAC ABNORMALITIES

Because the basic anatomical lesion of SLE is a diffuse microvasculitis,[154, 155] the heart is almost always found to be involved at autopsy.[156] The clinical manifestations, however, are usually overshadowed by the symptoms and signs related to involvement of other organs, and attention is drawn to the heart only when the lesions of pericarditis, myocarditis, or endocarditis are florid. Clinical evidence of cardiac abnormalities has been observed, however, in as many as 50 to 60 per cent of cases in two large series.[157, 158] As methodology becomes more sophisticated, detection of cardiac involvement begins to approach that found at necropsy (see below).

PERICARDITIS. This is found in approximately two-thirds to three-fourths of autopsies and is the most common cardiac lesion of SLE (p. 1519). The acute pericardial inflammation may extend into the sinoatrial and AV nodes, with destruction of conducting fibers.[159, 160] Pericardial fluid may be clear or sanguineous and has a high protein content. Effusions may be voluminous and occasionally cause tamponade. Histologically, the pericardium shows fibrinoid degeneration, edema, and necrosis of connective tissue when the process is acute, and various stages of fibrosis with the formation of adhesions are found during the healing or chronic phase. Constrictive pericarditis occurs only rarely; however, pericardial tamponade and constrictive pericarditis both have been reported in cases of procainamide-induced lupus erythematosus.[161, 162] Pericarditis, like arthritis, tends to be episodic and to heal well in remissions rather than to become chronic and sclerosing.[163]

MYOCARDITIS. Subclinical myocarditis is common.[164] Its severity is proportionate to the severity of the systemic disease process. The lesions observed at autopsy consist of fibrinoid necrosis involving interstitial tissues and blood vessels, and only rarely are the cardiac myofibrils destroyed. Small vessel changes include an arteriopathy of vessels 0.1 to 1.0 mm in diameter. The abnormal vessels are located in the conduction system of patients selected for study because of the presence of arrhythmias. Segmental arteritis and periarteritis with some occlusions of the arterial lumen and small areas of fibrosis distal to the obstruction are found. Involvement of the AV as well as the sinoatrial node in the inflammatory process of SLE has been shown at autopsy. Rare cases of myocardial infarction, presumably due to arteritis of larger coronary vessels, have been reported.[165]

ENDOCARDITIS. This is the most characteristic cardiac lesion of SLE.[166] The Libman-Sacks verrucous valvular lesions are wartlike, varying from pinhead size to 3 to 4 mm. The lesions may be discrete or in clumps and are composed of degenerating valve tissue apparently extruded beyond the endothelium and accompanied by some fibrosis of the underlying leaflet. The lesions usually contain granular, basophilic masses of cellular debris, the characteristic so-called hematoxylin bodies composed of basophilic fragments in the cytoplasm of cells. They may be found anywhere on the endocardial surface of the heart, but are most common in the angles of the AV valves and on the underside of the base of the mitral valve. They may also extend onto the chordae tendineae or papillary muscles. Generalized involvement of the entire thickness of the heart valves with inflammatory and fibrous changes may also occur. Aortic valve involvement is rare, but has been well described.[167] Despite the frequency and extent of the endocardial lesions of SLE, they do not often profoundly affect the function of the valves and, unlike rheumatic fever, do not produce serious regurgitation during the acute phase of the disease. Only rarely do they lead to marked scarring and deformity during healing, requiring valve replacement.[168] The subclinical nature of the valvular lesions has been demonstrated by prospective clinical and echocardiographic studies.[169]

CLINICAL FEATURES

Although autopsy shows that at least two-thirds of patients have pericarditis at some time during the course of SLE, only one-third have recognizable symptoms and signs during life.[157, 158] Typical pericardial pain may occur, but often the friction rubs, characteristic electrocardiographic changes, or enlargement of the cardiac silhouette on chest x-ray due to pericardial effusion may be found in the absence of symptoms, and therefore evidence of pericarditis should always be suspected and sought in *all* patients with SLE, even in those without clinical manifestations. Cardiac tamponade is rare but can occur, requiring repeated aspirations of fluid. Systolic and diastolic murmurs at the mitral area, and less often at the aortic area, seem to come and go during the course of acute exacerbations of the disease and are presumably due to Libman-Sacks endocarditis.[169] However, at autopsy the presence of these lesions is not always confirmed, and other factors such as anemia, tachycardia, fever, myocarditis, transient papillary muscle dysfunction, and the adventitious sounds of pleuropericarditis must be considered. Hemodynamically significant and permanent valvular regurgitation from lupus carditis is rare, but such cases have been reported and have even required valve replacement.[168]

Although myocardial dysfunction may be present, overt congestive heart failure due primarily to SLE is uncommon except when associated with hypertension secondary to renal disease. Heart failure may be mistakenly diagnosed in the presence of edema due to renal disease or pericardial effusion or both. Clinically apparent myocarditis, like that of rheumatic fever, producing tachycardia, gallop rhythm, and cardiac dilatation, is usually a feature of very toxic cases of SLE when high fever and other multisystem manifestations of acute vasculitis are present. Arrhythmias are also relatively uncommon and consist of atrial flutter and fibrillation with varying degrees of AV block.[159] Attention has been called to the development of congenital complete heart block, a lupus-like syndrome, and pericarditis in infants born to mothers with active SLE.[170, 171] The observation suggests that transplacental transfer of abnormal antibodies (or small immune complexes) may be of pathogenetic importance in these cases. During examination of a pregnant woman with SLE, fetal bradycardia should be recognized as a possible complication of lupus rather than fetal distress from other causes.

Echocardiography may be useful in SLE for demonstrating pericardial involvement and for evaluating valve function in the presence of various murmurs.[163, 169] Extensive hemodynamic studies carried out on a group of five patients who had had SLE for 2½ to 7 years prior to heart catheterization and who had no obvious clinical findings of cardiac involvement showed considerable evidence of impairment of myocardial function.[172] More sophisticated studies will be necessary to sort out the complex factors that may compromise myocardial function in a disease that can affect all layers of the heart and the coronary vascular bed as well.[173]

TREATMENT. To the extent that their antiinflammatory effect can control active myocarditis, corticosteroids may be necessary to manage severe cardiac involvement in SLE. Control of hypertension is also very helpful in the treatment and prevention of congestive heart failure. There is no evidence that corticosteroid treatment can prevent the rare cases of constrictive pericarditis or valvular deformity. Although the inflammatory reaction may be dramatically suppressed, the basic disease process and tissue injury are not altered by corticosteroid therapy, which is at most supportive and sometimes causes problems (hypertension and fluid retention). Immunosuppressive therapy is usually reserved for the most severe, corticosteroid-resistant forms of the disease and especially for renal involvement. Death from the cardiac disease of SLE compared with other causes of fatality in this disease is rare, so that cardiac manifestations usually do not determine the choice of antiinflammatory therapy.

POLYARTERITIS NODOSA

As noted above, necrotizing inflammation of blood vessels is a common finding in immune complex diseases of known and unknown etiology; however, because the origin and nature of the offending agent are unknown in most instances, the vasculitides continue to be classified on the basis of their histological and clinical features. These depend largely upon the size of the involved blood vessels, their anatomical sites, the stage of the inflammation, and the characteristics of the lesions.

The clinical features of most cases fit into one of the following five major categories: polyarteritis nodosa (PAN; also termed periarteritis nodosa), allergic granulomatosis, Wegener's granulomatosis, hypersensitivity vasculitis, and giant cell arteritis.

PATHOLOGICAL FEATURES. The muscular arteries, adjacent veins, and occasionally arterioles and venules (but not the capillaries) are involved in a necrotizing inflammation. Segments of vessels, at times only part of the circumference being affected, are involved in the lesions, especially at the bifurcation of arteries. Small aneurysms may form and rupture. In the acute stage of inflammation the lesions contain predominantly polymorphonuclear leukocytes, whereas in chronic lesions mononuclear cell infiltration and partial healing are apparent. However, both phases may be present at once, suggesting repeated or continuous insults.

The lesions are commonly found in the coronary arteries as well as kidneys, muscles, and vasa nervorum, but the lungs are usually spared. *Myocardial infarction* is therefore relatively common, and this leads to patchy myocardial fibrosis and left ventricular enlargement. The latter is also secondary to hypertension, frequently present owing to renal involvement. Hemorrhage into the pericardial sac with tamponade and death, inflammatory pericarditis, and uremic pericarditis are causes of pericardial involvement. Endocardial or valvular lesions do not occur unless the papillary muscle is injured by ischemia.

CLINICAL FEATURES. PAN may occur at any age, produces fever and multisystem involvement, and may persist for months or years. Pericarditis may be clinically evident, frequently associated with pleuritis, but is not a prominent feature of the disease. Chest pain due to true angina pectoris is also relatively rare[174] despite the occurrence of myocardial infarction. In one series of 41 cases of PAN and myocardial infarction, only 3 were diagnosed clinically.[175] The most common form of heart involvement is congestive failure and hypertension due to renal disease, which causes most deaths. Cardiac arrhythmias, most often atrial flutter and fibrillation, can occur. Death from ruptured aneurysms, particularly gastrointestinal bleeding, is not uncommon.

Kawasaki Disease (Mucocutaneous Lymph Node Syndrome) (See also p. 1014)

Relatively recently, Kawasaki and others have delineated a periarteritis-like vasculitis in Japanese infants. It is a complication of an acute febrile disease that they have called mucocutaneous lymph node syndrome; this has become known as Kawasaki disease.[176, 177] A polyarteritic syndrome occurs in approximately 2 per cent of infants following an acute mucocutaneous exanthematous febrile illness. Severe arteritis of the larger coronary arteries and of arteries of other organs results in rapid or sudden death from cardiac arrhythmias or massive myocardial infarction. Aneurysms of the coronary, brachial, iliac, and other vessels can be observed in the acute stage of the disease, but may cause late-stage arterial aneurysms in children.[178] The disease has been reported from Hawaii, continental United States, Canada, Greece, Korea and elsewhere. Previously reported cases of "infantile periarteritis nodosa with coronary artery involvement" from the United States seem to be identical with Kawasaki disease.[179, 180] A house dust mite may be a factor in the pathogenesis of the disease, either as an allergen or as a vector carrying a rickettsia.[181]

LABORATORY FINDINGS. Most helpful diagnostically is angiography when it reveals the characteristic multiple small aneurysms at branch points of mesenteric, renal, and other arteries (Fig. 54–12). The diagnosis may be quite difficult to establish in the absence of this finding, and biopsies of clinically involved tissues are usually necessary to establish the diagnosis. "Blind" muscle biopsy is positive in fewer than one-third of cases later confirmed. Hepatitis B soluble antigen is found in the blood of increasing numbers of patients with PAN in recently reported series, and this antigen has been identified in vascular lesions along with immunoglobulin and complement.[182, 183] Other infectious diseases associated with prolonged antigenemia have been also identified as causes of polyarteritis, such as cytomegalovirus infections and trichinosis.[184, 185]

COURSE AND TREATMENT. The prognosis of PAN is grave; one-half to two-thirds of patients died within a year when series comprised hospitalized cases. Treatment with corticosteroids is frequently followed by temporary improvement with doses of 40 to 60 mg of prednisone or prednisolone per day. Five-year survival of untreated patients is estimated at 13 per cent. Studies with immunosuppressive drugs have been encouraging in apparently prolonging the course in some cases, but adequate controlled studies have not been made.[186]

Other Forms of Diffuse Vasculitis

ALLERGIC GRANULOMATOSIS (CHURG-STRAUSS VASCULITIS, HYPEREOSINOPHILIC SYNDROME). This disease involves the

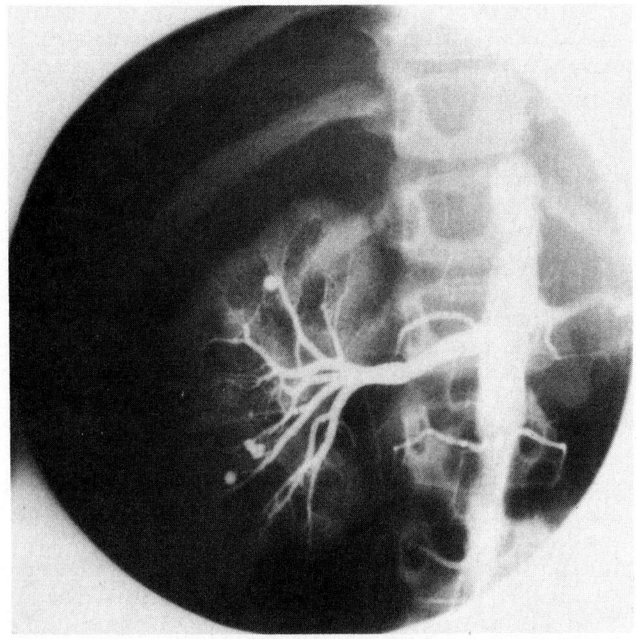

FIGURE 54–12. Renal artery angiogram in a 13-year-old boy with periarteritis nodosa. (From Stollerman, G. H.: Rheumatic Fever and Streptococcal Infection. New York, by permission of Grune and Stratton, 1975.)

vessels of the heart in the same way as PAN, but eosinophils tend to be more abundant in the lesions, and granulomatous collections of epithelioid and giant cells are formed, accounting for the name of the condition.[186] Pulmonary involvement, especially asthma, dominates the clinical picture, and patients tend to have a history of respiratory infection and fever, often with a striking peripheral eosinophilia. The heart, however, may be a primary target organ. Pericarditis, occasionally constrictive, myocarditis with acute heart failure, and myocardial infarction have been reported, as well as endomyocardial fibrosis in some variants of the syndrome.[187]

WEGENER'S GRANULOMATOSIS. This syndrome is distinguished by necrotizing granulomas of the upper respiratory tract, especially the destructive lesions of the nasopharynx and paranasal sinuses, middle ear, and bronchial tree. Necrotizing inflammation extends into the smaller pulmonary vessels of the lungs and other organs, particularly the kidneys. Pericardial and myocardial involvement is not uncommon, but the clinical picture is dominated by respiratory and renal involvement, without which the diagnosis cannot be made. The special feature of treatment is the encouraging response of this particular syndrome to cyclophosphamide therapy, resulting in dramatic remissions, often complete, and in prolonged survival.[186, 188] Although cardiac complications are considered unusual in Wegener's granulomatosis, they have been found in 12 per cent of some recent series[188] and in sporadic case reports that include constrictive pericarditis, high-grade AV block, supraventricular tachycardia, as well as complications secondary to involvement of the coronary arteries.[189, 190]

HYPERSENSITIVITY VASCULITIS (LEUKOCYTOBLASTIC VASCULITIS).[191] Hypersensitivity vasculitis is also called small-vessel vasculitis or angiitis and is characterized by involvement of arterioles, venules, and capillaries only. Antigen-antibody complexes present in the lesions all tend to be of the same age. It is difficult to tell at the inception of the disease whether it is part of a larger syndrome, such as SLE, subacute infective endocarditis, mixed cryoglobulinemia, Henoch-Schönlein purpura, or a drug reaction except by the course and distinguishing features of the other syndromes. Hypersensitivity vasculitis is the most common form of immune complex disease. Muscular and large arteries are spared, so that the tissue lesions are due to microinfarcts and hemorrhagic and exudative reactions at the capillary level rather than to thrombosis of large vessels with resulting ischemia and necrosis. The most common cardiac finding is pericarditis, but such involvement occurs along with that of many other organs, skin, mucous membranes, joints, and so on.

GIANT CELL ARTERITIS.[186, 192] Giant cell arteritis, also called cranial or temporal arteritis, affects predominantly older individuals. Large or medium-sized arteries, including the superficial temporal artery, are involved without small-vessel or capillary lesions. The lesions are usually cellular and granulomatous and contain multinucleated giant cells. Involvement of the arteries is spotty and segmented and tends to produce thrombosis at the site of involvement. The aorta is often involved, and aneurysms and dissection can result (p. 1565). External and internal carotids and vertebral arteries can be affected, and thrombosis of the ophthalmic or central retinal artery leads to blindness. Thrombosis of the coronary, iliac, femoral, or mesenteric arteries produces ischemia and infarctions. Aortic regurgitation is a rare but well-documented complication.[193]

Often the *polymyalgia rheumatica syndrome* is an associated finding. It is characterized by pain and stiffness in the neck and shoulders, upper arms, hips, and thighs. Joint and muscle pain and tenderness may be severe. Headache is characteristically associated with tender and thickened temporal arteries. The erythrocyte sedimentation rate is strikingly elevated owing primarily to a marked increase in the serum alpha-2 globulins. Myocarditis due to giant cell arteritis has been reported only rarely despite the frequently described association of this form of vasculitis with polymyalgia rheumatica.[192] Myocarditis may be present, however, even though clinically unsuspected. It is noteworthy that the polymyalgia rheumatica syndrome has been described in association with hepatitis B virus infection.[194] The dramatic response of all rheumatic symptoms to relatively small doses of corticosteroids (15 to 20 mg/day of prednisone) is a good therapeutic test for the syndrome, and treatment with corticosteroids usually completely suppresses the symptoms and signs within a few days.

PROGRESSIVE SYSTEMIC SCLEROSIS (DIFFUSE SCLERODERMA)

Progressive systemic sclerosis (PSS) is an insidious, chronic, fibrosing condition that presents as progressive tightening and thickening of the skin (scleroderma), developing over a period of many years. Raynaud's phenomena occur at some time in almost all patients. Visceral involvement may occur at any time during the course of the disease, affecting the gastrointestinal tract, lungs, heart or kidney. Much attention has been given to the classification of various subgroups of this syndrome that include patients with diffuse scleroderma, those without diffuse skin changes but with other shared features, such as calcinosis, Raynaud's phenomena, esophageal dyskinesia, sclerodactyly, and telangiectasia (the CREST syndrome), and those with features overlapping polymyositis or systemic lupus erythematosus or both.[195–198]

PATHOLOGICAL FEATURES AND PATHOGENESIS

In contrast to the acute exudative forms of vasculitis associated with the necrotizing lesions described above, PSS seems to be a disease at the opposite end of the inflammatory scale, in which very slow scarring and fibrosis result from gradual obliteration of small vessels. It is difficult to classify PSS pathophysiologically because the cause of the extensive fibrosis is not known, but the importance of small artery spasm and the possibility of its reversal by arterial vasodilators has received considerable attention.[199–209] Pulmonary hypertension has been at least temporarily reduced with such vasodilators as captopril,[205] nifedipine,[207] and verapamil,[208] as have attacks of Raynaud's phenomenon. Left ventricular regional wall motion abnormalities have been demonstrated during cold exposure in 9 of 16 patients with Raynaud's phenomenon and PSS or the CREST syndrome, and in most of these cases treatment with nifedipine blunted the severity of the abnormal ventricular response.[209] Short-term improvement in myocardial perfusion with nifedipine, demonstrated by thallium-210 single-photon-emission computerized tomography, was observed in a study of 29 patients with diffuse scleroderma and Raynaud's phenomenon.[201]

Hereditary factors have not been identified. Qualitative abnormalities of collagen are not documented. The disease apparently results from injury or spasm at the level of very small arteries, 150 to 500 μm in diameter, and capillaries are gradually obliterated.[197, 199] Early in the course of the lesions, mononuclear cell infiltrates occur around small arteries and in the interstitium. The basement membrane of the capillaries appears thickened. Fibroblastic proliferation and overproduction of collagen result from the low-grade inflammatory process. Narrowing and obliteration of small arteries result in decreased vascularization of the skin, skeletal muscles, lung, and heart, followed by fibrosis. The interlobular arteries of the kidney are involved by intensive intimal proliferation, which causes rapid renal failure, often with severe hypertension.

CARDIAC LESIONS. The importance of primary cardiac involvement in the natural history of the disease has been repeatedly emphasized,[196, 198–205] but only with the advent of noninvasive cardiac evaluation methods of thallium-201 scanning, rest and exercise radionuclide ventriculography, continuous 24-hour Holter ECG monitoring, two-dimensional echocardiography, and pulmonary-function testing has the full picture of the frequency and extent of cardiac dysfunction become apparent.[199-205] Defective perfusion of organs by spastic small arteries may account for the general observation that functional disability of the myocardium and lungs exceeds anatomical changes.[200–209] Heart involvement is a frequent cause of death and second only to involvement of the kidneys as a factor shortening the survival of patients with this disease. Confusion concerning the question of primary involvement of the heart by the sclerosing process has been caused by the frequency of cor pulmonale resulting from pulmonary involvement of PSS and severe hypertension and hypertensive heart disease resulting from the renal involvement.

"Scleroderma heart" is primarily a myocardial disease, and the heart's small vessels are all vulnerable to the sclerosing process. Atherosclerosis of the major coronary arteries occurs to the same degree in patients with PSS as in age- and sex-matched controls. PSS patients, however, have much more intimal sclerosis of the small coronary arteries than do controls, and such involvement may lead to ischemia, small infarctions, and fibrosis. The combination of vascular insufficiency and fibrosis produces a cardiomyopathy with congestive heart failure and conduction system abnormalities.[199–205] Acute and chronic pericarditis, even in the absence of uremia, is common but usually asymptomatic. At times the resulting effusion can be large enough to cause tamponade,[210] although this degree of effusion is rare. Pericardial fluid, when obtainable, has the features of an exudate but lacks evidence of autoantibodies, immune complexes, or complement depletion, such as that seen in rheumatoid arthritis or SLE.[211] Endocardial involvement is rare, and the deformities of mitral and aortic valves that have been reported probably have little hemodynamic significance.

CLINICAL FEATURES

The primary clinical manifestations of scleroderma heart disease are those of pericarditis and congestive heart failure. In one series, pericarditis patients had a 7-year cumulative survival rate of 33 per cent, whereas none of the PSS patients with heart failure survived for 7 years.[212] Men have significantly worse survival rates than women, as do blacks and older patients. Although cardiac symptoms may appear months or even years before the skin is involved, as a rule overt heart disease is not a prominent part of the clinical picture of PSS until late in its course, when myocardial involvement and resultant heart failure indicate a grim prognosis. The relative risk of death for a PSS patient with an S_3 gallop indicative of myocardial disease was reported to be many times that for a patient without an S_3 gallop.[213] Pericarditis, however, may be intermittently symptomatic for long periods.

When dyspnea with exertion or at rest occurs in the patient with PSS, primary myocardial failure must be distinguished from myocardial failure secondary to hypertension from renal disease and pulmonary insufficiency from pulmonary fibrosis due to PSS. Cardiac murmurs are not usually due to valvular deformity but to cardiac dilatation and to anemia or to papillary weakness. Chest pain simulating ischemic heart disease as well as typical pericardial pain may occur.

The *roentgenogram of the chest* may reveal cardiac enlargement from pericardial effusion, cardiomyopathy, or hypertension. The electrocardiographic findings are also nonspecific and may, indeed, be normal when the heart is seriously involved. All degrees of AV conduction blocks, right and left ventricular hypertrophy, and all varieties of arrhythmias have been described, but conduction defects are found most often in patients with the primary cardiomyopathy of PSS.[202–205]

Echocardiographic studies reveal patterns consistent with a congestive cardiomyopathy or a restrictive cardiomyopathy, and pericardial effusion can be demonstrated often when not suspected clinically.

TREATMENT. The value of corticosteroids is limited to improvement of the early edematous phase of the disease, but this effect on the heart has not been systematically evaluated and probably will not influence the eventual course of the disease.

As noted above, the most interesting and encouraging recent therapeutic development is the demonstration of improved perfusion of the heart, lungs, and, in the case of Raynaud's phenomenon, the hands, of patients with PSS or the CREST syndrome by the administration of calcium channel blockers such as nifedipine[201, 207] and verapamil[209] and other vasodilators such as captopril.[206, 214] The possible benefits of long-term therapy with these agents remains to be defined.

POLYMYOSITIS AND DERMATOMYOSITIS

Polymyositis is a diffuse inflammatory disease of unknown cause affecting primarily proximal striated muscles and various connective tissues of the body, especially skin and joints.[215] When the disease involves the skin, it is called *dermatomyositis.* Polymyositis may be due to a pathological process common to several etiologies because it is seen in association with a variety of syndromes. It is grouped with the connective tissue or rheumatic diseases because of its overlapping clinical and laboratory features, especially when it is associated with rheumatoid arthritis and PSS but also with SLE or polyarteritis. Involvement of the heart in polymyositis has just begun to be fully appreciated in the past decade and was mentioned in earlier publications only as a rare finding, if at all.

Pathological Features

Polymyositis is either increasing in incidence or is being more frequently diagnosed, and it is now well recognized as one of the most common myopathies. The principal changes in muscle tissue consist of widespread destruction of muscle fibers with phagocytosis of destroyed cells. There may be focal infiltrates of inflammatory cells, such as lymphocytes, mononuclear leukocytes, plasma cells, and, only rarely, neutrophilic leukocytes. Regeneration of destroyed muscle in the form of proliferating sarcolemmal nuclei, basophilic sarcoplasm, and new myofibrils is a prominent feature. Residual muscle fibers may be small. In any given biopsy specimen, either degeneration of muscle fibers or infiltrations of inflammatory cells may predominate. In electron microscopic studies, the most significant changes, in addition to those in muscle fibers, are found in the endothelium and basement membrane of capillaries and small arterioles, much like those described in scleroderma and SLE. Inclusions in the cytoplasm of endothelial cells that are identical to those found in SLE and scleroderma have been described.[216]

CARDIAC PATHOLOGY.[217–221] The cardiac lesions involve the conducting system predominantly but also can produce an extensive cardiomyopathy and pericarditis. The latter may appear far more often than would be suspected on clinical grounds. The cardiac valves and coronary arteries are spared except in overlap syndromes. The sinoatrial node shows conspicuous fibrosis, swelling and degeneration of collagen, and focal or complete replacement. The fibrosis extends into the adjacent myocardium of the right atrium. The AV node, bundle of His, and both bundle branches all may be involved in the degenerative and fibrotic process (Fig. 54–13). Cardiac muscle fibers in the atria and ventricles are replaced in scattered areas by fibrosis, and, in some cases, the pattern of focal myocardial necrosis and inflammation is the same as that seen in skeletal muscle. Pericarditis is described more often clinically than pathologically.

CLINICAL FEATURES. Almost all authors comment on the rarity of cardiovascular manifestations in polymyositis, and, indeed, the best reported studies of survivorship do not relate death to cardiac causes but rather to pneumonitis, which is relatively common from aspiration secondary to respiratory muscle weakness and dysphagia. However, more careful studies of the heart for subtle signs of involvement in polymyositis patients without cardiac symptoms and signs[220, 221] and careful review of autopsied patients with polymyositis-dermatomyositis syndromes[219] show a much higher frequency of cardiac involvement in polymyositis than was previously appreciated. When standard 12-lead electrocardiograms are analyzed systematically, arrhythmias may be quite frequent.[221] These usually consist of supraventricular tachycardia, but ventricular tachycardia and advanced heart block associated with syncope or cardiac arrest have also been observed. Deaths have been attributed directly to myocardial failure or arrhythmias or both in some cases, and cardiac muscle histology has been found to be abnormal on autopsy. Sudden death is not unusual, especially in patients with documented heart block.[221]

TREATMENT. Corticosteroids and immunosuppressive drugs may be of benefit in the treatment of polymyositis-dermatomyositis, but only a controlled prospective study can settle this issue. The course of the disease, including myocardial involvement, may not be truly modified by corticosteroids, but the complications of muscle weakness, especially

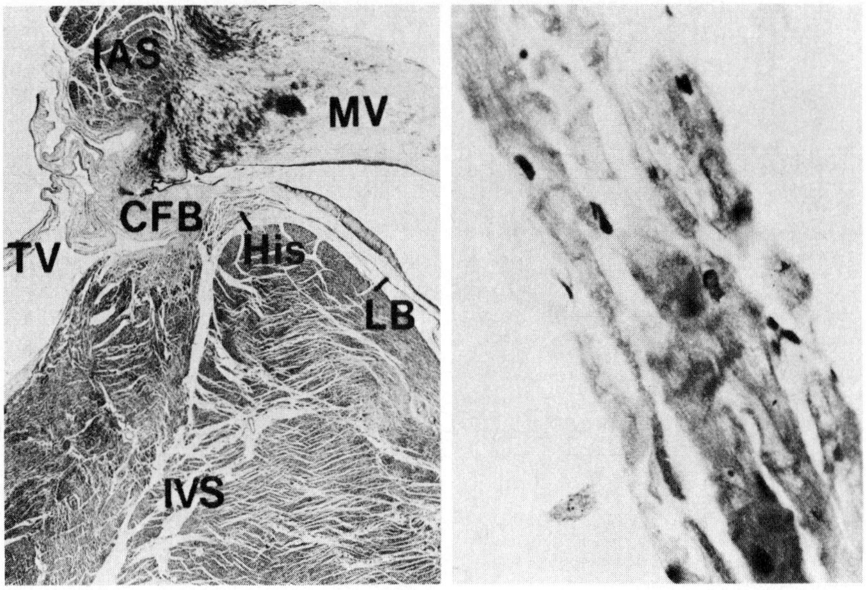

FIGURE 54–13. Cardiac conduction system in a 53-year-old woman with polymyositis-dermatomyositis left bundle branch block. *Left,* the left bundle (LB) and distal portion of the His bundle (His). The interatrial septum (LAS) is at the top and the interventricular septum (IVS) below. The mitral (MV) and tricuspid (TV) valves are attached to the central fibrous body (CFB). *Right,* contraction band necrosis of the left bundle. The myocytes of the bundle show irregular coarse transverse condensations of sarcoplasm and their nuclei are pyknotic. (From Haupt, H. M., and Hutchins, G. M.: The heart and conduction system in polymyositis-dermatomyositis: A clinicopathologic study of 16 autopsied patients. Am. J. Cardiol. *50*:998, 1982.)

of the respiratory and deglutitional muscles, which lead to pulmonary disease and death, might be diminished by the frequent improvement of muscle strength observed after this treatment.

In the absence of malignancy, survival statistics are favorable for all groups (87 to 91 per cent) in several studies. The leading causes of death, which in one series were metastatic malignant disease (24 per cent), sepsis (19 per cent), profound muscular weakness (9.5 per cent), and cardiovascular and cerebrovascular disorders (unspecified percentage), suggest that at least some of these may be modified by supportive therapy and management to improve the prognosis.

HERITABLE DISORDERS OF CONNECTIVE TISSUE

The heritable disorders of connective tissue are characterized by a definable mode of inheritance and by the clinical expression of a generalized defect of some connective tissue element. This group of disorders includes Marfan syndrome, osteogenesis imperfecta, Ehlers-Danlos syndrome, and pseudoxanthoma elasticum, as well as Hurler syndrome and the other mucopolysaccharidoses.[222]

Involvement of the connective tissues of the large arteries, cardiac valves, and other cardiac connective tissue elements determines the cardiovascular manifestations of these disorders. The spectrum of cardiovascular involvement is broad and includes characteristic pathological changes of minimal clinical import as well as of major catastrophic valvular incompetence, aortic dissection, and death. In a number of these disorders, recent investigations of the metabolism and biochemistry of connective tissue have clarified the defects; in others, the basic abnormality remains obscure.[223]

In addition, there are some patients who manifest no or only subtle extracardiac changes of the generalized connective tissue disorders but who display pathological and clinical cardiovascular disease indistinguishable from the generalized disorders. Whether these patients represent a forme fruste of the generalized disease process or they express the limited response of the cardiovascular connective tissue to varied insults is not clear. Patients with myxomatous degeneration of connective tissue of the mitral and aortic valves and those with cystic medial necrosis with involvement of the aortic annulus are included in this group [224, 225] (Chap. 46).

THE MARFAN SYNDROME

The Marfan syndrome (see also p. 1725) is a generalized abnormality of connective tissue, particularly abnormally cross-linked elastin,[226] with major clinical features involving the skeletal, ocular, and cardiovascular systems. The typical skeletal manifestations include excessive limb length, arachnodactyly, loose-jointedness, kyphoscoliosis, and anterior chest deformity. Affected individuals are characteristically tall with long, thin extremities and show weakness of joint capsules, ligaments, tendons, and fascia that results in joint dislocation, hernia, and kyphoscoliosis. A sparsity of subcutaneous fat is a striking feature. The ocular manifestations include defective suspensory ligaments of the lens and subsequent ectopia lentis. The excessive length of the eyeball and involvement of the connective tissue of the retina contribute to the severe myopia and retinal detachment that is often found.

Involvement of the cardiovascular system includes aortic aneurysm with dissection, aortic regurgitation from dilation of both the aortic root and the annulus or from myxomatous involvement of the leaflets themselves and myxomatous degeneration of the mitral valve and its apparatus with secondary mitral incompetence (Fig. 54–14).

The Marfan syndrome exhibits simple mendelian autosomal dominant inheritance with variable phenotypic expression (Chap. 49). According to McKusick and associates, 15 per cent of all cases are de novo mutations, and this likelihood increases with increasing paternal age.[222, 223] The diagnosis of the Marfan syndrome is most secure when a positive family history of the disease is present or ectopia lentis is found in conjunction with the classic musculoskeletal or cardiovascular changes.

The biochemical abnormality of Marfan syndrome is still not entirely clear although a significant body of biochemical data suggests an abnormality in the cross-linkage of collagen or elastin or both that is consistent with the finding of increased solubility of skin collagen and elastin obtained from the aortic tissue of patients with Marfan syndrome.[226] Other syndromes that show some clinical features of Mar-

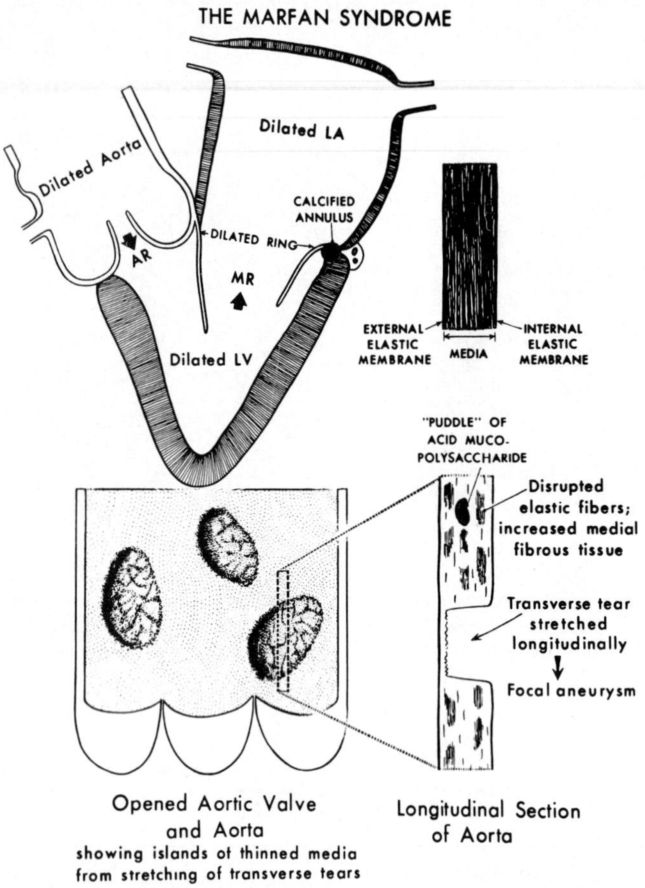

FIGURE 54–14. The various cardiovascular abnormalities found in Marfan syndrome. The aortic regurgitation appears to be related primarily to dilatation of the aorta. The mitral regurgitation probably results from a combination of factors: dilatation of the left ventricular cavity, altering the papillary muscle-mitral leaflet angle; dilatation of the mitral annulus; calcification of the mitral annulus; and elongation of the mitral leaflets and chordae, allowing prolapse of the leaflets into the left atrium during ventricular systole. *Top right,* Longitudinal section of normal aorta. *Bottom right,* Longitudinal section in a patient with Marfan syndrome. There is severe loss of elastic fibers, deposition of abnormal amounts of acid mucopolysaccharide material, and tears in the wall. The tears expand to cause the islands of thinning seen in the view of the opened aortic valve and aorta. (From Roberts, W. C., et al.: Nonrheumatic valvular cardiac disease. A clinicopathologic survey of 27 different conditions causing valvular dysfunction. *In* Likoff, W. (ed.): Valvular Heart Disease. Philadelphia, F. A. Davis, 1973, p. 368.)

fan syndrome (e.g., homocystinuria) have different genetics and molecular pathology that produce different structural defects in connective tissues.

PATHOLOGICAL FEATURES. The pathological changes seen in patients with the Marfan syndrome[224, 225] are most striking in the ascending aorta and annulus (p. 1555; Fig. 54–15). In patients with long-term aortic regurgitation, the proximal aorta is diffusely dilated along with the aortic annulus and sinuses of Valsalva. Dilatation of the pulmonary artery also occurs. Chronic aortic dissection and transverse tears without dissection are also found. Histologically, advanced changes include fragmented and sparse elastic tissue in the tunica media, with irregular whorls of smooth muscle and increased amounts of collagen. The vasa vasorum are dilated. The tunica media is interspersed with cystic vacuoles of metachromatically staining material, probably mucopolysaccharide. Inflammation is conspicuously absent. In patients succumbing to acute dissection, earlier changes in the aorta have been studied and reveal cystic medial necrosis and moderate degeneration of elastic elements with disorganization of the smooth muscle bundles. Faults in the media are seen that contain a mucopolysaccharide-rich ground substance. The left ventricle is often enlarged and hypertrophied, reflecting the degree and duration of the hemodynamic burden imposed by aortic or mitral incompetence.

More recently, the pathological changes and clinical significance of primary valvular abnormalities of Marfan syndrome have been recognized. Changes in the mitral valve have included ballooning and redundant cusps, fenestrations in the leaflets, elongated and thinned chordae tendineae, and occasionally ruptured and thickened valve cusps with rolled edges. Thin, shiny, diaphanous leaflets are also described. Similar changes in the aortic valve cusps have also been reported. The histological changes include disruption and loss of normal valvular architecture, increase in mucopolysaccharide ground substance, cystic degeneration, and loss of cellularity. These changes are similar to those found in cystic medial necrosis of the aorta. These valvular changes have been termed *myxomatous degeneration*.

James and coworkers studied the AV conduction system in two patients with Marfan syndrome and clinical cardiac conduction abnormalities.[227] Medial degeneration, hyperplasia, and intimal proliferation with luminal narrowing were present in the nutrient arteries of the sinoatrial and AV nodes as well as in the intramyocardial arteries.

CLINICAL FEATURES. In this genetically determined generalized disorder of connective tissue metabolism, there are ocular and skeletal as well as cardiovascular abnormalities. Weakness of the supporting tissues causes bilateral

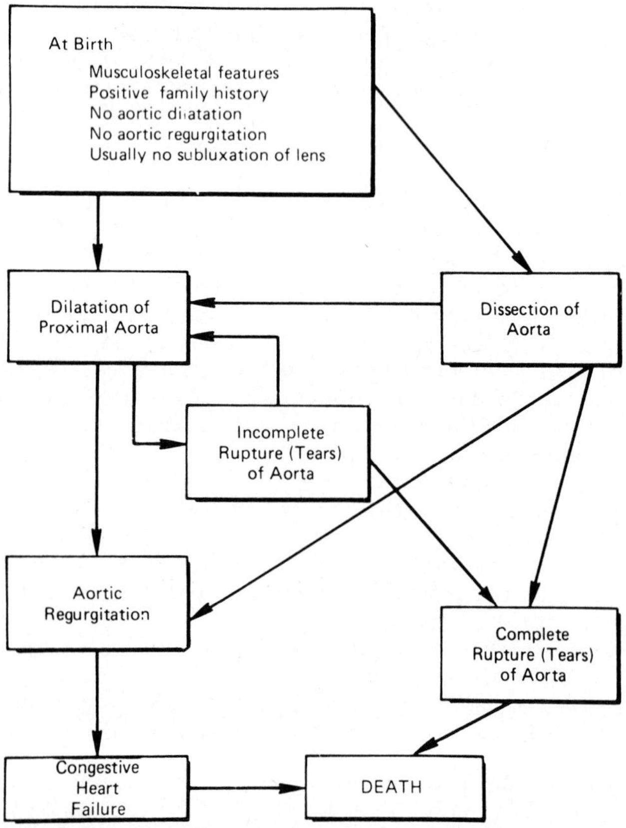

FIGURE 54–15. Schema of development of cardiovascular complications in the Marfan syndrome. (From Roberts, W. C., and Honig, H. S.: The spectrum of cardiovascular disease in the Marfan syndrome: A clinicomorphologic study of 18 necropsy patients and comparison to 151 previously reported necropsy patients. Am. Heart J. *104*:115, 1982.)

subluxation of the lens, minor degrees of which can be appreciated by slit-lamp examination. Increased length of the extremities, with an abnormally low ratio of the upper segment (crown to pubic symphysis) to the lower segment (lower than 0.84 in whites and 0.79 in blacks), very long "spider" fingers (arachnodactyly), long metacarpals, pectus carinatum, and pectus excavatum are other important features.

Cardiovascular complications of Marfan syndrome occur in 30 to 60 per cent of patients in different series. The poor prognosis in patients with Marfan syndrome reflects the cardiovascular complications and the progressive nature of the lesions. Of 257 patients with Marfan syndrome observed between 1939 and 1970, the average age at death of the 72 deceased patients was 32 years. Of 56 patients who died, the cause of death in 52 was cardiovascular complications, with aortic dilatation, rupture, and/or dissection accounting for 80 per cent of these.[228] In a study of Marfan syndrome in infancy and childhood, 61 per cent of patients had cardiac abnormalities.[229] Mitral valve disease with mitral regurgitation was the most common lesion found (47 per cent). Mitral systolic clicks with late systolic murmurs were the most common signs. Generally the prognosis is good when isolated mitral valve involvement occurs. Severe mitral, aortic, and even tricuspid regurgitation may develop, however, requiring valve replacement.[230–234] Cardiovascular complications lead to death in 50 per cent of patients by the age of 32.[232]

During the course of the disease, the ascending aorta becomes dilated with worsening regurgitation, and the likelihood of rupture or dissection increases. In addition to signs and symptoms of left heart failure, chest pain with anginal features is often observed in the Marfan syndrome. This symptom may be secondary to aortic regurgitation, dilatation of the aorta, or coronary ostial involvement.

Infective endocarditis involving the mitral valve in patients with the Marfan syndrome is well documented, and this process has accounted for a significant number of deaths.

PATHOGENESIS AND MANAGEMENT. The biochemical lesion of the Marfan syndrome remains undefined, but, as noted above, the cardiovascular manifestations most likely reflect the response of defective connective tissue[226] to prolonged hemodynamic stresses. Theoretical considerations have prompted the use of the beta-adrenoceptor blocking agent propranolol in patients with Marfan syndrome who manifest early signs of aortic dilatation. The murmur of aortic regurgitation, dilatation of the aorta on radiographic examination, and echocardiographic evidence of an enlarged aorta may serve as guides to the initiation and effectiveness of therapy. Conclusive evidence of the efficacy of this therapy remains to be established.

The underlying connective tissue defect presents a considerable obstacle to surgical therapy. Although prosthetic valves are favored, not uncommonly they become dislodged. Aortic valve replacement and graft reconstruction of the ascending aorta have proved successful in the management of aortic regurgitation and congestive heart failure with and without aortic dissection. Recurrent dissection, valvular incompetence, and progressive dilatation of any remaining native aorta have been late complications. Elective prophylactic surgery of a greatly enlarged (diameter > 6 cm) or enlarging aorta found on serial echocardiography in asymptomatic persons can be carried out at a relatively low risk and may prolong survival.[232]

Relatives of patients with Marfan syndrome show a high degree of penetrance of cardiac abnormalities, approximately 50 per cent in two series.[223, 224] Close follow-up and regular evaluation of all young persons with a family history of Marfan syndrome may be indicated. The increasing recognition of mitral valve involvement in the Marfan syndrome that is morphologically indistinguishable from the mitral valve prolapse syndrome makes antibiotic prophylaxis of infective endocarditis appear to be warranted in these patients.

OSTEOGENESIS IMPERFECTA

Osteogenesis imperfecta is one of the complex and variable heritable disorders affecting the skeleton and other connective tissues.[235] Its hallmark is bone fragility, and therefore the disease is known also as the brittle bone syndrome. The phenotypic expression of the group of genetic abnormalities embraced by this syndrome is very broad, varying from forms with little or no increased fracture tendency to the other extreme in which bone strength is so reduced that the skeleton crumbles in utero or during or soon after birth (osteogenesis imperfecta congenita). Osteogenesis imperfecta is usually inherited as an autosomal dominant trait, but there are several documented instances of autosomal recessive inheritance.

In addition to bones, many other tissues, including skin, sclerae, ligaments, and heart valves,[236] may also be mechanically abnormal. The type I collagen is the major stress-bearing component of all affected tissues, and most attempts to identify the basic abnormality have concentrated on analysis of this collagen and the genes controlling its expression. There appear to be two structural gene loci for type I collagen and the osteogenesis imperfecta gene seems to be inherited with one or the other collagen locus,[235] and therefore osteogenesis imperfecta is not genetically homogeneous.

The ascending aorta, the aortic valve and its annulus, and the mitral valve apparatus are the cardiovascular structures most commonly affected. The incidence of cardiovascular involvement is unknown but is probably low. Aortic root dilatation appears to represent a distinct phenotypic trait in patients with osteogenesis imperfecta that is nonprogressive and occurs in about 12 per cent of affected individuals.[237]

CARDIOVASCULAR MANIFESTATIONS. Aortic and mitral valvular regurgitation has been noted in several isolated case reports of patients with osteogenesis imperfecta. In either retrospective or prospective studies, however, the frequency of clinically discernible valvular dysfunction has been small; in a recent clinical and echocardiographic survey of 109 patients, only 4 had aortic or mitral lesions—aortic regurgitation in 2, aortic stenosis in 1, mitral valve prolapse in 1.[237] On the other hand, aortic dilatation occurred commonly (12 per cent in this series) without associated valvular dysfunction. The mild extent of the enlargement of the aortic root is in contrast to that observed in the Marfan syndrome.

MANAGEMENT. Management includes routine therapy of congestive heart failure. Successful prosthetic valve replacement is hampered by postoperative bleeding and by poor native connective tissue at the suture sites.[236] Prophylaxis for endocarditis appears warranted in clinically recognizable valvular disease.

EHLERS-DANLOS SYNDROME

The Ehlers-Danlos syndrome is another heterogeneous group of disorders of connective tissue that is characterized by hyperelasticity and fragility of the skin; hyperextensibility of the joints; easy bruisability; ocular abnormalities including blue sclera, microcornea, and ectopia lentis; and variable involvement of the respiratory, alimentary, and cardiovascular systems.

Biochemical studies have identified distinct abnormalities of collagen synthesis in Ehlers-Danlos syndrome. These findings have included abnormal ratios of collagen types and enzyme deficiencies that affect both normal collagen cross-linking and the conversion of collagen precursor to mature collagen fibers. These studies have supported the clinical impression of several distinct phenotypic patterns; 10 different modes of inheritance are recognized at present.[238]

Histological studies of the cardiovascular lesions of the Ehlers-Danlos syndrome are scarce. Although many congenital abnormalities of the cardiovascular system have been reported in this syndrome, including tetralogy of Fallot, atrial septal defect, and pulmonary artery and aortic arch anomalies, most authorities believe that these are coincidental and not reflections of the underlying disorder.

CARDIOVASCULAR MANIFESTATIONS. Aortic dissection and spontaneous rupture and dissection of other large arteries with exsanguination are reported in the Ehlers-Danlos syndrome. These episodes may be spontaneous or precipitated by minimal trauma, and significant morbidity secondary to arterial catheterization is reported. Dilatation of the aortic root and sinuses of Valsalva with aortic regurgitation occurs. Extensive reviews of patients with Ehlers-Danlos syndrome report various cardiovascular abnormalities, including AV conduction defects, mitral valve murmurs, nonspecific systolic murmurs, and aortic regurgitation.[239] Some of these findings have been attributed to the deformities of the chest wall found in this disorder. However, other reports of mitral valve murmurs and echocardiographic evidence of prolapse of the mitral valve have suggested widespread involvement of the cardiac connective tissue, and the occurrence of conduction abnormalities in Ehlers-Danlos syndrome has been emphasized. These include right bundle branch block, incomplete right bundle branch block, and left anterior hemiblock alone and with right bundle branch block.[240, 241] The histological nature of the valvular and conduction tissue abnormalities remains unknown. Endocarditis prophylaxis in cases of mitral valve involvement is recommended.

PSEUDOXANTHOMA ELASTICUM

Pseudoxanthoma elasticum is an inherited disorder of connective tissue with major involvement of the skin, eyes, and gastrointestinal and cardiovascular systems. The basic defect is thought to be a dysplasia or abiotrophy of elastic tissue. Although originally described as a disorder of the skin and the mesenchymal elements of the eye, involvement of the heart and the peripheral and visceral vasculature is responsible for the more serious manifestations of the disorder, including gastrointestinal hemorrhage, hypertension, congestive heart failure, premature myocardial infarction, peripheral vascular disease, and sudden death.

Pseudoxanthoma elasticum appears to be a heterogeneous group of disorders. The basic biochemical lesion remains undefined, but in some types autosomal recessive inheritance suggests an enzymatic defect, and in others with dominant inheritance, a structural defect.[238]

CARDIOVASCULAR MANIFESTATIONS. *Pathological studies* of the cardiovascular system are not numerous, but distinctive lesions of the heart, arteries, and arterioles have been described.[242] In the vessels the elastic membrane is often disrupted, and elastic fibers are increased, often shortened, wrinkled, and degenerated, and show an unusual propensity to calcify. Fibrous proliferation of media and intima may severely narrow the lumen. Pathological studies of the heart reveal changes similar to those in the vessels.[243, 244] The valve leaflets are also involved, and the cusps may be rolled or thickened; mitral valve prolapse is a common finding.[245] Endocardium of both the ventricle and the atrium is involved. Microscopically, the endocardium exhibits nodular plaques of altered and increased elastic tissue and collagen fibers. Involvement of conducting tissue is also described. Biopsy of the coronary artery has revealed changes indistinguishable from those of peripheral vessels.[246]

Clinically, pseudoxanthoma elasticum is characterized by thickened, coarse, and grooved skin having a leathery and "crepelike" appearance. The skin is lax and redundant with prominent folds. The face, neck, axillae, and inguinal folds are most commonly involved. Mucous membranes of the mouth and stomach may also show changes. The hallmarks of ocular involvement are angioid streaking and chorioretinitis with subsequent visual impairment. Skin changes may be obvious or evident only microscopically, and they usually appear in the second decade. Prominent visceral involvement, however, may occur despite trivial skin changes.

The clinical cardiovascular manifestations of pseudoxanthoma elasticum parallel the pathological changes described. [242–249] The spectrum includes peripheral vascular disease, hypertension, coronary artery disease, restriction to filling due to subendocardial fibrosis with congestive heart failure, and the clinical manifestations of prolapse of the mitral valve. Symptoms and physical findings appear in the second and third decades.

Intermittent claudication was present in 18 per cent of patients in one large study.[247] A distinctive feature of pseudoxanthoma elasticum is involvement of the arteries of the upper extremities, which distinguishes it from typical atherosclerosis. Physical examination reveals decreased pulses and atrophic changes. The pulse wave is often reduced in amplitude with a slow rise and plateau. Roentgenograms often show calcification of limb arteries.

Both the extraparenchymal and the intraparenchymal renal arteries may be involved in the vasculopathy of pseudoxanthoma elasticum, and the compromised renal blood flow is the most likely cause of the hypertension, often seen in adolescents and young adults.

The incidence of angina is quite variable in large studies of pseudoxanthoma elasticum. In a study of 200 cases, angina was reported in 29 per cent.[247] Acute myocardial infarction and sudden death are not common, but are well-documented complications in the second and third decades.[248]

Congestive heart failure is an uncommon but recognized manifestation. Murmurs of mitral regurgitation, aortic stenosis, and aortic regurgitation are described.[249] Dilatation of the aorta or its annulus is not a feature of pseudoxanthoma elasticum. The congestive heart failure is probably multifactorial. The hemodynamic burdens imposed by the vascular lesions, combined with the endocardial fibroelastic changes,[248] may be the mechanism of congestive heart failure. However, the role of hypertension and coronary artery disease in cardiac pump function may also be significant.

MANAGEMENT. There is no specific management for the cardiovascular complications of this disorder. Angina, hypertension, and congestive heart failure are managed conventionally. Intractable angina and the Leriche syndrome have been treated with vascular bypass surgery.[242]

HURLER SYNDROME AND OTHER MUCOPOLYSACCHARIDOSES

Hurler syndrome is the prototype of a group of disorders characterized by the abnormal metabolism of mucopolysaccharides. The accumulation of these moieties in mesenchymal cells and their excess urinary excretion serve to identify and classify the disorders. In several forms the enzymatic defect has been identified and the pathogenesis more clearly defined.

PATHOLOGICAL FEATURES. The pathological hallmark of the disease is the presence of Hurler cells, connective tissue cells laden with the mucopolysaccharide moieties heparin sulfate and dermatan sulfate. These cells are found in the connective tissue stroma of many organs. Cells containing intralysosomal collagen fibers have been described in the cardiac valves of patients with Hurler syndrome.[250]

The morphological changes in the heart are striking. Grossly, the valves are thickened with fibrous nodules at the closure lines. Aneurysmal dilatations of the leaflets are also seen. The chordae tendineae are also thickened, resembling endocardial fibroelastosis. The cardiac chambers are enlarged. Microscopically, valve thickening is due to the presence of classic Hurler cells, cells with granular inclusions, and an increase in the extracellular collagenous matrix. Increased amounts of collagen and occasional clear cells are responsible for chordal and endocardial thickening. The myocardial cells are relatively spared, but the interstitium may contain Hurler cells. Narrowing of the coronary arteries is seen.

CLINICAL FEATURES. Patients with classic Hurler syndrome are characterized by dwarfism, corneal clouding, mental retardation, skeletal malformations, hepatosplenomegaly, and cardiovascular lesions. Dermatan sulfate and heparin sulfate are excreted in the urine, and the activity of α-L-iduronidase, a lysosomal hydrolase, is decreased in the fibroblasts of these patients. The condition demonstrates autosomal recessive inheritance and results in early death, most often from respiratory and cardiovascular complications.

CARDIOVASCULAR MANIFESTATIONS. Clinically, symptoms of congestive heart failure and ischemic heart disease are most common and are important factors in the poor survival of individuals with Hurler syndrome. In one report 26 of 75 deaths were secondary to congestive heart failure, and 7 additional deaths were sudden. The morphological studies illustrating involvement of conduction tissue suggest arrhythmia as a possible cause of sudden death. Hypertension is also commonly seen, but the cause is unknown. The heart is enlarged on physical examination and chest roentgenogram. Murmurs of mitral regurgitation, aortic stenosis, and aortic regurgitation are often heard. The distorted and thickened mitral valve may produce hemodynamic stenosis. In 15 patients studied by cardiac catheterization,[251] only 1 of whom had clinical congestive heart failure, both systemic and pulmonary hypertension were common. Elevated left ventricular end-diastolic pressures were present in 5 of 9 patients. Angina pectoris occurs in children with Hurler syndrome.

Valvular lesions, thickened, noncompliant endocardium, hypertension, and severely compromised coronary circulation are the features that collectively produce congestive heart failure in Hurler syndrome and its variants. The four mucopolysaccharidoses that involve the cardiovascular system are Hurler syndrome, Hurler-Scheie syndrome, Hunter syndrome, and Morquio syndrome.

MANAGEMENT. There is no specific treatment for the cardiovascular complications of the mucopolysaccharidoses, and early death has underscored the poor response to conventional therapy.[252, 253]

REFERENCES

RHEUMATIC FEVER

1. Stollerman, G. H.: Rheumatic Fever and Streptococcal Infection. New York, Grune and Stratton, 1975.
2. Bisno, A. L.: The rise and fall of rheumatic fever. J.A.M.A. *254*:538, 1985.
3. Rammelkamp, C. H., Denny, F. W., and Wannamaker, L. W.: Studies on the epidemiology of rheumatic fever in the armed services. *In* Thomas, L. (ed.): Rheumatic Fever. Minneapolis, University of Minnesota Press, 1952, pp. 72–89.
4. Frank, P. F., Stollerman, G. H., and Miller, L. F.: Protection of a military population from rheumatic fever. J.A.M.A. *193*:775, 1965.
5. Stollerman, G. H.: Global changes in group A streptococcal diseases and strategies for their prevention. Adv. Intern. Med. 27:373, 1982.
6. Gordis, L.: The virtual disappearance of rheumatic fever in the United States; lessons in the rise and fall of disease. Circulation 72:1155, 1985.
7. Markowitz, M.: The decline of rheumatic fever, role of medical intervention. J. Pediatr. *106*:545, 1985
8. Argarwal, B. L.: Rheumatic heart disease unabated in developing countries. Lancet 2:910, 1981.
9. Stetson, C. A.: The relation of antibody response to rheumatic fever. *In* McCarty, M. (ed.): Streptococcal Infections. New York, Columbia University Press, 1954, pp. 208–218.
10. Rammelkamp, C. H., Jr.: The Lewis A. Conner Memorial Lecture. Rheumatic heart disease—A challenge. Circulation *17*:842, 1958.
11. Siegel, A. C., Johnson, E. E., and Stollerman, G. H.: Controlled studies of streptococcal pharyngitis in a pediatric population: I. Factors related to the attack rate of rheumatic fever. N. Engl. J. Med *265*:559, 1961.
12. Stollerman, G. H.: Factors determining the attack rate of rheumatic fever. J.A.M.A. *177*:823, 1961.
13. Stollerman, G. H., Siegel, A. C., and Johnson, E. E.: Variable epidemiology of streptococcal disease and the changing patterns of rheumatic fever. Mod. Concepts Cardiovasc. Dis. *34*:45, 1965.
14. Kaplan, E. L., Top, F. H., Dudding, B. A., and Wannamaker, L. W.: Diagnosis of streptococcal pharyngitis: Differentiation of active infection from the carrier state in the symptomatic child. J. Infect Dis.*123*:490, 1971.
15. Top, F. H., Wannamaker, L. W., Maxted, W. R., and Anthony, G. V.: M antigens among group A streptococci isolated from skin lesions. J. Exp. Med. *126*:667, 1967.
16. Stollerman, G. H.: Nephritogenic and rheumatogenic group A streptococci. J. Infect. Dis. *120*:258, 1969.
17. Wannamaker, L. W.: Medical progress. Differences between streptococcal infections of the throat and of the skin. N. Engl. J. Med. *282*:23 and 78, 1970.
18. Wannamaker, L. W.: The chain that links the heart to the throat. Circulation *48*:9, 1973.
19. Bisno, A. L., Pearce, I. A., Wall, H. P., Moody, M. D. and Stollerman, G. H.: Contrasting epidemiology of acute rheumatic fever and acute glomerulonephritis. Nature of the antecedent streptococcal infection. N. Engl. J. Med. *283*:561, 1970.
20. Poon-King, T., Mohammed, I., Cox, R., Potter, E. V., Simon, N. M., Siegel, A. C., and Earle, D. P.: Recurrent epidemic nephritis in South Trinidad, N. Engl. J. Med. *277*:728, 1967.
21. Potter, E. V., Svartman, M., Poon-King, T., and Earle, D. P.: The families of patients with acute rheumatic fever or glomerulonephritis in Trinidad. Am. J. Epidemiol. *106*:130, 1977.
22. Widdowson, J. P., Maxted, W. R., Notley, C. M., and Pinney, A. M.: The antibody responses in man to infection with different serotypes of group A streptococci. J. Med. Microbiol. 7:483, 1974.
23. Bisno, A. L.: The concept of rheumatogenic and nonrheumatogenic group A streptococci. *In* McCarty, M., and Zabriskie, J. B. (eds.): Streptococcal Diseases and the Immune response. New York, Academic Press, 1980, p. 789.
24. Stollerman, G. H.: The streptococcus, rheumatic fever and rheumatic heart disease. *In* Shaper, A. G., Hutt, M. S. R., and Fejfar, Z. (eds.): Cardiovascular Disease in the Tropics. London, British Medical Associates, 1974.
25. Sanyal, S. K., Berry, A. M., Duggal, S., Hooja, V., and Ghosh, S.: Sequelae of the initial attack of rheumatic fever in children from North India. Circulation *65*:375, 1982.
26. Sanyal, S. K., Thapar, M. K., Ahmed, S. H., Hooja, V., and Tewari, P.: The initial attack of acute rheumatic fever during childhood in North India. A prospective study of the clinical profile. Circulation *49*:7, 1974.
27. Taranta, A.: Rheumatic fever in children and adolescents. A long-term epidemiologic study of subsequent prophylaxis, streptococcal infections, and clinical sequelae: IV. Relation of the rheumatic fever recurrence rate per streptococcal infection to the titers of streptococcal antibodies. Ann. Intern. Med. *60* (Suppl. 5):47, 1964.
28. Taranta, A., Kleinberg, E., Feinstein, A. R., Wood, H. F., Tursky, E., and Simpson, R.: Rheumatic fever in children and adolescents. A long-term epidemiologic study of subsequent prophylaxis, streptococcal infections, and clinical sequelae: V. Relation of the rheumatic fever recurrence rate per streptococcal infection to pre-existing clinical features of the patients. Ann. Intern. Med. *60* (Suppl. 5):58, 1964.
29. Johnson, E. E., Stollerman, G. H., and Grossman, B. J.: Rheumatic recurrences in patients not receiving continuous prophylaxis. J.A.M.A. *190*:74, 1964.
30. Taranta, A.: Rheumatic fever made difficult. A critical review of pathogenetic theories. Paediatrician 5:74, 1976.
31. Pattarroyo, M. E., Winchester, R., Vejerano, A., Gibofsley, A., Chalens, F., Zabriskie, J. B., and Kunkel, H. G.: Association of B-cell alloantigen with susceptibility to rheumatic fever. Nature *278*:173, 1979.
32. Zabriskie, J. B., Lavenchy, D., Williams, R. C., Jr., Yeadon, C. A., Fotino, M., and Brown, D. G.: Rheumatic fever associated B cell alloantigen as identified by monoclonal antibodies. Arthritis Rheum. *28*:1047, 1985.
33. Zabriskie, J. B.: Rheumatic fever: The interplay between host, genetics and microbe. Circulation *71*:1077, 1985.
34. Rammelkamp, C. H., Jr.: Epidemiology of streptococcal infections. Harvey Lect. *51*:113, 1955–1956.
35. Stollerman, G. H.: The epidemiology of primary and secondary rheumatic fever. *In* Uhr, J. W. (ed): The Streptococcus, Rheumatic Fever and Glomerulonephritis. Baltimore, Williams and Wilkins, 1964, pp. 331–337.
36. Yoshimoya, S., and Pope, R. M.: Detection of immune complexes in acute rheumatic fever and their relationship to HLA-B5. J. Clin. Invest. *65*:136, 1980.
37. Stollerman, G. H.: Autoimmunity and rheumatic fever. *In* Cohen, I. R. (ed.): Perspectives in Autoimmunity. Boca Raton, Fl., CRC Press, 1986.
38. Kaplan, M. H., Meyeserian, M., and Kushner, I.: Immunologic studies of heart tissue: IV. Serologic reactions with human heart tissue as revealed by immunofluorescent methods. Isoimmune, Wasermann, and auto-immune reactions. J. Exp. Med. *113*:17, 1961.
39. Hess, E. V., Fink, C. W., Taranta, A., and Ziff, M.: Heart muscle antibodies in rheumatic fever and other diseases. J. Clin. Invest. *43*:886, 1964.
40. Ehrenfeld, E. N., Gery, I., and Davies, A. M.: Specific antibodies in heart disease. Lancet *1*:1138, 1961.
41. Kaplan, M. H.: Immunologic relation of streptococcal and tissue antigens. I. Properties of an antigen in certain strains of group A streptococci exhibiting an immunologic cross-reaction with human heart tissue. J. Immunol. *90*:595, 1963.
42. Kaplan, M. H., and Suchy, M. L.: Immunologic relation of streptococcal and tissue antigens. II. Cross reactions of antisera to mammalian heart tissue with a cell wall constituent of certain strains of group A streptococci. J. Exp. Med. *119*:643, 1964.
43. Zabriskie, J. B., and Freimer, E. H.: An immunological relationship between

the group A streptococcus and mammalian muscle. J. Exp. Med. *124*:661, 1966.
44. Goldstein, I., Halpern, B., and Robert, L.: Immunological relationship between streptococcus A polysaccharide and the structural glycoproteins of heart valves. Nature *213*:44, 1967.
45. Dudding, B. A., and Ayoub, E. M.: Persistence of streptococcal group A antibody in patients with rheumatic valvular disease. J. Exp. Med. *129*:1081, 1968.
46. Appleton, R. S., Victoria, B. C., Tamer, D., and Ayoub, E. M.: Specificity of persistence of antibody to the streptococcal group A carbohydrate in rheumatic valvular heart disease. J. Lab. Clin. Med. *105*:114, 1985.
47. Husby, G., van de Rijn, I., Zabriskie, J. B., Abdin, Z. H., and Williams, R. C.: Antibodies reacting with cytoplasm of subthalamic and caudate nuclei neurons in chorea and acute rheumatic fever. J. Exp. Med. *144*:1094, 1976.
48. Dale, J. B., and Beachey, E. H.: Epitopes of streptococcal M proteins shared with cardiac myosin. J. Exp. Med. *162*:583, 1985.
49. Neumann, E.: Zur Kenntnis der fibrinoiden Degeneration des Bindegewebes bei Entzündungen. Virchow Arch. Pathol. Anat. *144*:201, 1896.
50. Talalaev, V. T. (Talalajew, W. T.): Der akute Rheumatismus. Klin. Wochenschr. *8*:124, 1929.
51. Klinge, F.: Der Rheumatismus. Munich, J. Bergmann, 1933.
52. Aschoff, L.: Zur Myocarditisfrage. Verh. Dtsch. Pathol. Ges. *8*:46, 1904–1905.
53. Murphy, G. E.: Nature of rheumatic heart disease with special reference to myocardial disease and heart failure. Medicine *39*:289, 1960.
54. Aschoff, L.: The rheumatic nodules in the heart. Ann. Rheum. Dis. *1*:161, 1939.
55. Kuschner, M., Ferrer, M. I., Harvey, R. M., and Wylie, R. H.: Rheumatic carditis in surgically removed appendages. Am. Heart J. *43*:286, 1952.
56. Virmani, R., and Roberts, W. C.: Aschoff bodies in operatively excised atrial appendages and in papillary muscles. Frequency and clinical significance. Circulation *55*:559, 1977.
57. Roberts, W. C., and Virmani, R.: Aschoff bodies at necropsy in valvular heart disease. Evidence from an analysis of 543 patients over 14 years of age that rheumatic heart disease, at least anatomically, is a disease of the mitral valve. Circulation *57*:803, 1978.
58. Stollerman, G. H., Lynch, W. F., Dolman, M. A., Young, D., and Schwedel, J. B.: Immunologic evidence of streptococcal infection in patients undergoing mitral commissurotomy. Circulation *15*:267, 1957.
59. Lanningan, R.: Cardiac Pathology. London, Butterworth and Co., 1966.
60. Becker, C. G., and Murphy, G. E.: On the pathology of rheumatic heart disease. *In* Read, S. E., and Zabriskie, J. B. (eds.): Streptococcal diseases and the Immune Response. New York, Academic Press, 1980, p. 23.
61. Husby, G. H., Arora, R., Williams, R. C., Kwaw, B. A., Haber, E., and Butler, C.: Immunofluorescent studies of florid rheumatic Aschoff lesions. Arthritis Rheum. *29*:207, 1986.
62. Steele, P. P., Weily, H. S., Davies, H., and Genton, E.: Platelet survival in patients with rheumatic heart disease. N. Engl. J. Med. *290*:537, 1974.
63. Winkelman, N. W., and Eckel, J. L.: The brain in acute rheumatic fever. Nonsuppurative meningoencephalitis rheumatica. Arch. Neurol. Psychiatr. *28*:844, 1932.
64. Neubuerger, K. T.: The brain in rheumatic fever. Dis. Nerv. System *8*:259, 1947.
65. Costero, I.: Cerebral lesions responsible for death of patients with active rheumatic fever. Arch. Neurol. Psychiatr. *62*:48, 1949.
66. Buchanan, D. N.: Pathologic changes in chorea. Am. J. Dis. Child. *62*:443, 1941.
67. Kernohan, J. W., Woltman, H. W., and Barnes, A. R.: Involvement of the nervous system associated with endocarditis. Neuropsychiatric and neuropathologic observations in 42 cases of fatal outcome. Arch. Neurol. Psychiatr. *42*:789, 1939.
68. Raz, I., Fisher, J., Israel, A., Gotthrer, N., Ghisim, R., and Kleinman, Y.: An unusual case of rheumatic pneumonia. Arch. Intern. Med. *145*:1130, 1985.
69. Rammelkamp, C. H., Jr., and Stolzer, B. L.: The latent period before the onset of acute rheumatic fever. Yale J. Biol. Med. *34*:386, 1961.
70. Feinstein, A. R., and Spagnuolo, M.: The clinical patterns of acute rheumatic fever: A reappraisal. Medicine *41*:279, 1962.
71. Ben-Dov, I., and Berry, E.: Acute rheumatic fever in adults over the age of 45 years: An analysis of 23 patients together with a review of the literature. Semin. Arthritis Rheum. *10*:10,1980.
72. United Kingdom and United States Joint Report on Rheumatic Fever: The treatment of acute rheumatic fever in children. A cooperative clinical trial of ACTH, cortisone and aspirin. Circulation *11*:343, 1955.
73. United Kingdom and United States Joint Report on Rheumatic Heart Disease: The evolution of rheumatic heart disease in children. Five-year report of a cooperative clinical trial of ACTH, cortisone and aspirin. Circulation *22*:503, 1960.
74. United Kingdom and United States Joint Report on Rheumatic Heart Disease: The natural history of rheumatic fever and rheumatic heart disease. Ten-year report of a cooperative clinical trial of ACTH, cortisone and aspirin. Circulation *32*:457, 1965.
75. Massell, B. V., Fyler, D. C., and Roy, S. B.: The clinical picture of rheumatic fever. Diagnosis, immediate prognosis, course and therapeutic implications. Am. J. Cardiol. *1*:436, 1958.
76. Combined Rheumatic Fever Study Group, 1960: A comparison of the effect of prednisone and acetylsalicylic acid on the incidence of residual rheumatic heart disease. N. Engl. J. Med. *262*:895, 1960.
77. Combined Rheumatic Fever Study Group, 1965: A comparison of the short-term, intensive prednisone and acetylsalicylic acid therapy in the treatment of acute rheumatic fever. N. Engl. J. Med. *272*:63, 1965.
78. Robinson, R. W.: Effect of atropine upon the prolongation of the P-R interval found in acute rheumatic fever and certain vagotonic persons. Am. Heart J. *29*:378, 1945.
79. Lenox, C. C., Zuberbuhler, J. R., Park, S. C., Neches, W. H., Mathews, R. A., and Zoltun, R.: Arrhythmias and Stokes-Adams attacks in acute rheumatic fever. Pediatrics *61*:599, 1979.
80. Meynet, P.: Rheumatisme articulaire subaigu avec production de tumeurs multiples dans les tissus fibreux periarticulaires et sur le perioste d'un grand numbre d'os. Lyons Med. *19*:495, 1875.
81. Cheadle, W. B.: Various Manifestations of the Rheumatic State as Exemplified in Childhood and Early Life. London, Smith, Elder, 1889.
82. Baldwin, J. S., Kerr, J. M., Kuttner, A. G., and Doyle, E. F.: Observations on rheumatic nodules over a 30-year period. J. Pediatr. *56*:465, 1960.
83. Taranta, A., and Stollerman, G. H.: The relationship of Sydenham's chorea to infection with group A streptococci Am. J. Med. *20*:170, 1956.
84. Bland, E. F.: Chorea as a manifestation of rheumatic fever. A long-term perspective. Trans Am. Clin. Climatol. Assoc. *73*:209, 1961.
85. Bisno, A. L., and Ofek, I.: Serologic diagnosis of streptococcal infection. Comparison of a rapid hemagglutination technique with conventional antibody tests. Am. J. Dis. Child. *127*:676, 1974.
86. Gewurz, H., Mold, C., Siegel, J., and Fiedel, B.: C-reactive protein and the acute phase response. Adv. Intern. Med. *27*:345, 1982.
87. Feinstein, A. R., and DiMassa, R.: Prognostic significance of valvular involvement in acute rheumatic fever. N. Engl. J. Med. *260*:1001, 1959.
88. Feinstein, A. R., Wood, H. F., Spagnuolo, M., Taranta,, A., Jonas, S., Kleinberg, E., and Tursky, E.: Rheumatic fever in children and adolescents: VII. Cardiac changes and sequelae. Ann. Intern. Med. *60* (Suppl. 5):87, 1964.
89. Jones, T. D.: The diagnosis of rheumatic fever. J.A.M.A. *126*:481, 1944.
90. Jones Criteria (revised) for guidance in the diagnosis of rheumatic fever. Circulation *32*:664, 1965.
91. Taranta, A., Spagnuolo, M., and Feinstein, A. R.: "Chronic" rheumatic fever. Ann. Intern. Med. *56*:367, 1962.
92. McIntosch, R., and Wood, C. L.: Rheumatic infections occurring in the first three years of life. Am. J. Dis. Child. *49*:835, 1935.
93. Rosenthal, A., Czoniczer, G., and Massell, B. F.: Rheumatic fever under three years of age. A report of ten cases. Pediatrics *41*:612, 1968.
94. Ellis, L. B.: Recurrent mitral stenosis. Mod. Concepts Cardiovasc. Dis. *33*:851, 1964.
95. Wood, H. F., Simpson, R., Feinstein, A. R., Taranta, A., Tursky, E., and Stollerman, G. H.: Rheumatic fever in children and adolescents. I. Description of the investigative techniques and of the population studied. Ann. Intern. Med. *60* (Suppl. 5):6, 1964.
96. Goetzler, R., Stokes, J., III, and Anderson, K.: Prognosis of subjects in the Framingham Study with rheumatic heart disease. J. Am. Geriatr. Soc. *33*:693, 1985.
97. Stollerman, G. H.: Lingering traces of rheumatic fever. J. Am. Geriatr. Soc. *33*:732, 1985.
98. Vaisman, S., Guasch, J., Vignau, A., Correa, E., Schuster, A., Mortimer, E. A., Jr., and Rammelkamp, C. H., Jr.: The failure of penicillin to alter acute rheumatic valvulitis. J.A.M.A. *194*:1284, 1965.
99. Lockman, L. A.: Movement disorders. *In* Swaiman, K., and Wright, F. (eds.): Practice of Pediatric Neurology., St. Louis, C. V. Mosby Co., 1975.
100. Stollerman, G. H., Rusoff, J. H., and Hirschfeld, I.: Prophylaxis against group A streptococci in rheumatic fever. The use of single monthly injections of benzathine penicillin G. N. Engl. J. Med. *252*:787, 1955.
101. Albam, B., Epstein, J. A., Feinstein, A. R., Gavrin, J. B., Jonas, S., Kleinberg, E., Simpson, R., Spagnuolo, M., Stollerman, G. H., Taranta, A. Tursky, E., and Wood, H. F.: Rheumatic fever in children and adolescents. A long-term epidemiologic study of subsequent prophylaxis, streptococcal infections, and clinical sequelae. Ann. Intern. Med. *60* (Suppl. 5): No. 2, Part II, 1964.
102. American Heart Association, Committee on Rheumatic Fever and Bacterial Endocarditis: Prevention of rheumatic fever. Circulation *70*:1118A, 1984.
103. Feinstein, A. R., Wood, H. F., Spagnuolo, M., Taranta, A., Tursky, E., and Kleinberg, E.: Oral prophylaxis of recurrent rheumatic fever: Sulfadiazine vs. a double daily dose of penicillin. J.A.M.A. *188*:489, 1964.
104. Stahlman, M. T., and Denny, F. W., Jr.: The prophylaxis of streptococcal infection in patients with rheumatic fever: A comparison between sulfadiazine and erythromycin. Am. J. Dis. Child. *98*:66, 1959.
105. Wannamaker, L. W., Rammelkamp, C. H., Jr., Denny, F. W., Brink, W. R., Houser, H. B., Hahn, E. O., and Dingle, J. H.: Prophylaxis of acute rheumatic fever by treatment of the preceding streptococcal infection with various amounts of depot penicillin. Am. J. Med. *10*:673, 1951.
106. Wannamaker, L. W., Denny, F. W., Perry, W. D., Rammelkamp, C. H., Jr., Eckhardt, G. C., Houser, H. B., and Hahn, E. O.: The effect of penicillin prophylaxis on streptococcal disease rates and the carrier state. N. Engl. J. Med. *249*:1, 1953.
107. Dale, J. B., and Beachey, E. H.: Localization of protective epitopes of the amino terminus of type 5 streptococcal M protein. J. Exp. Med. *163*:1191, 1986.
108. Beachey, E. H., Stollerman, G. H., Johnson, R. H., et al.: Human immune response to immunization with a structurally defined polypeptide fragment of streptococcal M protein. J. Exp. Med. *150*:862, 1979.
109. Beachey, E. H., Grus-Masse, Tarter, A., Jolivet, M., Audibert, F., Chedid, L., and Seyer, J. M.: Opsonic antibodies evoked by hybrid peptide copies of types 5 and 24 streptococcal M proteins synthesized in tandem. J. Exp. Med. *163*:1451, 1986.

SERONEGATIVE SPONDYLOARTHROPATHIES

110. Bluestone, R., and Pearson, C. M.: Ankylosing spondylitis and Reiter's syndrome: Their interrelationships and association with HLA B27. Adv. Intern. Med. *22*:1, 1977.
111. Khan, M. A., and Khan, M. K.: Diagnostic value of HLA-B27 testing in ankylosing spondylitis and Reiter's syndrome. Ann. Intern. Med. *96*:70, 1982.
112. Calin, A. (ed.): Spondyloarthropathies. Orlando, Fl., Grune and Stratton, 1984.
113. Laitinen, O., Leirisalo, M., and Skylv, G.: Relation between HLA-B27 and clinical features in patients with Yersinia arthritis. Athritis Rheum. *20*:1121, 1977.
114. Schachter, J.: Can chlamydial infections cause rheumatic disease? *In* Dumonde, D. C. (ed.): Infection and Immunology in Rheumatic Diseases. Oxford, Blackwell Scientific Publications, 1976, pp. 151–157.

ANKYLOSING SPONDYLITIS

115. Graham, D. C., and Smythe, H. A.: The carditis and aortitis of ankylosing spondylitis. Bull. Rheum. Dis. 9:171, 1958.
116. Thomas, D., Hill, W., Geddes, R., Sheppard, M., Arnold, J., Fritzsche, J., and Brooks, P. M.: Early detection of aortic dilatation in ankylosing spondylitis using echocardiography. Aust. N.Z. J. Med. *12*:10, 1982.
117. LaBresh, K. A., Lally, E. V., Sharma, S. C., and Ho, G.: Two-dimensional echocardiographic detection of preclinical aortic root abnormalities in rheumatoid variant diseases. Am. J. Med. *78*:908, 1985.
118. Roberts, W. C., Hollingsworth, J. F., Bulkley, B. H., Jaffe, R. B., Epstein, S. E., and Stinson, E. B.: Combined mitral and aortic regurgitation in ankylosing spondylitis. Angiographic and anatomic features. Am. J. Med. *56*:237,1974.
119. Nitter-Hauge, S., and Otterstad, J. E.: Characteristics of atrioventricular conduction disturbances in ankylosing spondylitis. Acta Med. Scand. *210*:197, 200, 1981.
120. Bergfeld, E. L.: HLA B27-associated rheumatic diseases with severe cardiac bradyarrhythmias. Clinical features in 223 men with permanent pacemakers. Am. J. Med. *75*:210, 1983.
121. Bulkley, B. H., and Roberts, W. C.: Ankylosing spondylitis and aortic regurgitation. Description of the characteristic cardiovascular lesion from study of eight necropsy patients. Circulation *48*:1014, 1973.
122. Takkunen, J., Vuopala, U., and Isomaki, H.: Cardiomyopathy in ankylosing spondylitis. I. Medical history and results of clinical examination in a series of 55 patients. Ann. Clin. Res. 2:106, 1970.
123. Ribiero, P., Morley, L. M., Shapiro, R. A., Garnett, R. A. F., Hughes, G. R. V., and Goodwin, J. F.: Left ventricular function in patients with ankylosing spondylitis and Reiter's disease. Eur. Heart J. 5:419, 1984.
124. Cowan, G. O.: Aortic incompetence associated with ulcerative colitis and ankylosing spondylitis. Proc. Roy. Soc. Med. *63*:4, 1970.
125. Good, A. E.: Reiter's disease: A review with special attention to cardiovascular and neurologic sequelae. Semin. Arthr. Rheum. *3*:253, 1974.

REITER'S DISEASE

126. Sairanen, E., Paronen, I., and Mahonen, H.: Reiter's syndrome: A follow-up study. Acta Med. Scand. *185*:57, 1969.
127. Paulus, H. E., Pearson, C. M., and Pitts, W., Jr.: Aortic insufficiency in five patients with Reiter's syndrome: A detailed clinical pathological study. Am. J. Med. *53*:464, 1972.
128. Collins, P.: Aortic incompetence and active myocarditis in Reiter's disease. Br. J. Vener. Dis. *48*:300, 1972.
129. Ahvonen, P., Hiisi-Brummer, L., and Aho, K.: Electrocardiographic abnormalities and arthritis in patients with *Yersinia enterocolitica* infection. Ann. Clin. Res. 3:69, 1971.
130. Aho, K., Ahvonen, P., and Lassus, A.: HLA B27 in reactive arthritis. A study of Yersinia arthritis and Reiter's disease. Arthritis Rheum. *17*:521, 1974.
131. Hakansson, U., Eitrem, R., Löw, B., and Winblad, S. W.: HLA-antigen B27 in cases with joint affects in an outbreak in salmonellosis. Scand. J. Infect. Dis. *8*:245, 1976.
132. Ruppert, G. B., Lindsay, J., and Barth, W. F.: Cardiac conduction abnormalities in Reiter's syndrome. Am. J. Med. *73*:335, 1982.

RHEUMATOID ARTHRITIS

133. Lanningan, R.: Cardiac Pathology. London, Butterworth and Co., 1966.
134. Cathcart, E. S., and Spodick, D. H.: Rheumatoid heart disease. A study of the incidence and nature of cardiac lesions in rheumatoid arthritis. N. Engl. J. Med. *266*:959, 1962.
135. Bonfiglio, T., and Ativater, E. C.: Heart disease in patients with seropositive rheumatoid arthritis. A controlled autopsy study and review. Arch. Intern. Med. *124*:714, 1969.
136. Khan, A. H., and Spodick, D. H.: Rheumatoid heart disease. Semin. Arthritis Rheum. *1*:327, 1972.
137. Butman, S., Espinoza, L. R., Del Carpio, J., and Osterland, C. K.: Rheumatoid pericarditis. Rapid deterioration with evidence of local vasculitis. J.A.M.A. *238*:2394, 1977.
138. Bacon, P. A., and Gibson, D. G.: Cardiac involvement in rheumatoid arthritis. An echocardiographic study. Ann. Rheum. Dis. *33*:20, 1974.
139. MacDonald, W. J., Jr., Crawford, M. H., Klippel, J. H., Zvaifler, N. J., and O'Rourke, R. A.: Echocardiographic assessment of cardiac structure and function in patients with rheumatoid arthritis. Am. J. Med. *63*:890, 1977.
140. Roberts, W. C., Kehoe, J. A., and Carpenter, D. F.: Cardiac valvular lesions in rheumatoid arthritis. Arch. Intern. Med. *122*:141, 1968.
141. Morris, P. B. Imber, M. J., Heinsimer, J. A., Hlatky, M. A., and Reimer, K. A.: Rheumatoid arthritis and coronary arteritis. Am. J. Cardiol. *57*:689, 1986.
142. Linch, D. C., Gillmer, D. J., Whimster, W. F., and Keates, J. R. W.: Rheumatoid aortic valve prolapse requiring emergency valve replacement. Br. Heart J. *43*:237, 1980.
143. Ahern, M., Lever, J. W., and Cash, J.: Complete heart block in rheumatoid arthritis. Ann. Rheum. Dis. *42*:389, 1983.
144. Cassidy, J. T.: Juvenile rheumatoid arthritis. *In* Kelly, W. N., Harris, E. D., Ruddy, S., and Sledge, C. B. (eds.): Textbook of Rheumatology, 2nd ed. Philadelphia, W. B. Saunders Company, 1985.
145. Bernstein, B.: Pericarditis in juvenile rheumatoid arthritis. Arthritis Rheum. *20*:241, 1977.
146. Bank, L., Marboe, C. C., Redberg, R. F., and Jacob, J.: Myocarditis in adult Still's disease. Arthritis Rheum. *28*:452, 1985.
147. Kramer, P. H., Imboden, J. B., Waldman, F. M., Turley, K., and Ports, T. A.: Severe aortic insufficiency in juvenile chronic arthritis. Am. J. Med. *74*:1088, 1983.

SYSTEMIC LUPUS ERYTHEMATOSUS

148. Reed, W. P., and Williams, R. C.: Immune complexes in infectious diseases. Adv. Intern. Med. *22*:49, 1977.
149. Agnello, V.: Complement deficiency states. Medicine *57*:1, 1978.
150. Lee, S. L., and Chase, P. H.: Drug-induced systemic lupus erythematosus: A critical review. Semin. Arthritis Rheum. *5*:83, 1975.
151. Stevens, M. B.: Procainamide-induced lupus. Johns Hopkins Med. J. *138*:289, 1976.
152. Das, S. K., and Cassidy, J. T.: Antiheart antibodies in patients with systemic lupus erythematosus. Am. J. Med. Sci. *265*:275, 1973.
153. Zvaifler, N. J., and Woods, V. L., Jr.: Etiology and pathogenesis of systemic lupus erythematosus. *In* Kelly, W. N., Harris, E. D., Ruddy, S., and Sledge, C. G. (eds.): Textbook of Rheumatology. Philadelphia, W. B. Saunders Company, 1985.
154. Klemperer, P., Pollack, A., and Baehr, G.: Pathology of disseminated lupus erythematosus. Arch. Pathol. *32*:569, 1941.
155. Liberthson, R. R., Homcy, C., Fallon, J. T., Gross, S., Leppo, J., and Miller, L.: Systemic lupus erythematosus and heart disease. Primary Cardiol. *9*:77, 1983.
156. Gross, L.: Cardiac lesions in Libman-Sacks disease with consideration of its relationship to acute diffuse lupus erythematosus. Am. J. Pathol. *16*:375, 1940.
157. Harvey, A. M., Shulman, L. E., Tumulty, P. A., Conley, C. L., and Schoenrich, E. H.: Systemic lupus erythematosus: A review of the literature and clinical analyses of 138 cases. Medicine *33*:291, 1954.
158. Hejtmancik, M. R., Wright, J. C., Quint, R., and Jennings, F.: The cardiovascular manifestations of systemic lupus erythematosus. Am. Heart J. *68*:119, 1964.
159. James, T. N., Rupe, C. E., and Monto, R. W.: Pathology of the cardiac conduction system in systemic lupus erythematosus. Ann. Intern. Med. *63*:402, 1965.
160. Bharati, S., de la Fuente, D. J., Kallen, R. J., Freij, Y., and Lev, M.: Conduction system in systemic lupus erythematosus with atrioventricular block. Am. J. Cardiol. *35*:299, 1975.
161. Sunder, S. K., and Shah, A.: Constructive pericarditis in procainamide-induced lupus erythematosus syndrome. Am. J. Cardiol. *36*:960, 1975.
162. Ghose, M. K.: Pericardial tamponade. A presenting manifestation of procainamide-induced lupus erythematosus. Am. J. Med. *58*:581, 1975.
163. Elkayam, U., Weiss, S., and Laniado, S.: Pericardial effusion and mitral valve involvement in systemic lupus erythematosus: Echocardiographic study. Ann. Rheum. Dis. *36*:349, 1977.
164. Doherty, N. E., and Siegel, R. J.: Cardiovascular manifestations of systemic lupus erythematosus. Am Heart. J. *110*:1257, 1985.
165. Takatsu, Y., Hattori, R., Sakuguchi, K., Yui, Y., and Kawai, C.: Acute myocardial infarction associated with systemic lupus erythematosus. Chest *88*:147, 1985.
166. Libman, E., and Sacks, B.: A hitherto undescribed form of valvular and mitral endocarditis. Arch. Intern. Med. *33*:701, 1924.
167. Rawsthorne, L., Ptacin, M. J., Choi, H., Olinger, G. N., and Bamrah, V. S.: Lupus valvulitis necessitating double valve replacement. Arthritis Rheum. *24*:561, 1981.
168. Dajee, H., Hurley, E. J., and Szarnicki, R. J.: Cardiac valve replacement in systemic lupus erythematosus. A review. J. Thorac. Cardiovasc. Surg. *85*:718, 1983.
169. Kinkhoff, A. V., Thompson, C. R., Reid, G. D., and Tomlinson, C. W.: M-mode and two-dimensional echocardiographic abnormalities in systemic lupus erythematosus. J.A.M.A. *253*:3273, 1985.
170. Scott, J. S., Maddison, P. J., Taylor, P. V., Esscher, E., Scott, O., and Skinner, R. P.: Connective-tissue disease, antibodies to ribonucleoprotein and congenital heart block. N. Engl. J. Med. *309*:209, 1983.
171. Litsey, S. E., Noonan, J. A., Connor, W. N., Cottrill, C. M., and Mitchell, B.: Maternal connective tissue disease and congenital heart block. N. Engl. J. Med. *312*:98, 1985.
172. Strauer, B. E., Brune, I., Schenk, H., Knoll, D., and Perings, E.: Lupus cardiomyopathy: Cardiac mechanics, hemodynamics, and coronary blood flow in uncomplicated systemic lupus erythematosus. Am. Heart J. *92*:715, 1976.
173. Homcy, C. J., Liberthson, R. R., Fallon, J. T., Gross, S., and Miller, L. M.: Ischemic heart disease in systemic lupus erythematosus in the young patient: Report of six cases. Am. J. Cardiol. *49*:478, 1982.

RHEUMATIC AND HERITABLE CONNECTIVE TISSUE DISEASES OF THE CARDIOVASCULAR SYSTEM

POLYARTERITIS NODOSA

174. Zeek, P. M.: Periarteritis nodosa and other forms of necrotizing angiitis. N. Engl. J. Med. *148*:764, 1953.
175. Schrader, M. L., Hochman, J. S., and Bulkley, B. H.: The heart in polyarteritis nodosa: A clinicopathologic study. Am. Heart J. *109*:1353, 1985.
176. Kawasaki, T., Kosaki, F., Okawa, S., Shigematsu, I., and Yanagawa, H.: A new infantile acute febrile mucocutaneous lymph node syndrome (MLNS) prevailing in Japan. Pediatrics *54*:271, 1974.
177. Onouchi, Z., Tomizawa, N., Goto, M., Nakata, K., Fukuda, M., and Goto, M.: Cardiac involvement and prognosis in acute mucocutaneous lymph node syndrome. Chest *68*:297, 1975.
178. Fujiwara, T., Fujiwara, H., Veda, T., Nishioka, K., and Hamashima, Y.: Comparison of macroscopic, postmortem, angiographic and two-dimensional echocardiographic findings of coronary aneurysms in children with Kawasaki disease. Am. J. Cardiol. *57*:761, 1986.
179. Landing, B. H., and Larson, E. J.: Are infantile periarteritis nodosa with coronary artery involvement and fatal mucocutaneous lymph node syndrome the same? Comparison of 20 patients from North America with patients from Hawaii and Japan. Pediatrics *59*:651, 1977.
180. Melish, M. E.: Kawasaki syndrome: A new infectious disease? J. Infect. Dis. *143*:317, 1981.
181. Fujimoto, T., Kato, H., Ichiose, E., and Sasahuri, Y.: Immune complex and mite antigen in Kawasaki disease. Lancet 2:980, 1982.
182. Duffy, J., Lidsky, M. D., Sharp, J. T., Davis, J. S., Person, D. A., Hollinger F. B., and Kyung-Whan, M.: Polyarthritis, polyarteritis and hepatitis B. Medicine *55*:19, 1976.
183. Michalak, T.: Immune complexes of hepatitis B surface antigen in the pathogenesis of periarteritis nodosa. A study of seven necropsy cases. Am. J. Pathol. *90*:619, 1978.
184. Doherty, M., and Bradfield, J. W.: Polyarteritis nodosa associated with acute cytomegalovirus infection Am. Rheum. Dis. *40*:419, 1981.
185. Frayha, R. A.: Trichinosis-related polyarteritis nodosa. Am. J. Med. *71*:307, 1981.
186. Cupps, T. R., and Fauci, A. S.: The vasculitis syndromes. Adv. Intern. Med. 27:315, 1982.
187. Lonham, J. G., Elkon, K. B., Pusey, C. D., and Hughes, G. R. V.: Systemic vasculitis with asthma and eosinophilia: A clinical approach to the Churg-Strauss syndrome. Medicine *63*:65, 1984.
188. Fauci, A. S., Haynes, B. F., Katz, P., and Wolff, S. M.: Wegener's granulomatosis: Prospective clinical and therapeutic experience with 85 patients for 21 years. Ann. Intern. Med. *98*:76, 1983.
189. Forstot, J. Z., Overlie, P. A., Neufeld, G. K., Harmon, C. E., and Forstot, S. L.: Cardiac complications of Wegener granulomatosis: A case report of complete heart block and review of the literature. Semin. Arthritis Rheum. *10*:148, 1980.
190. Schiavone, W. A., Ahmad, M., and Ockner, S. A.: Unusual cardiac manifestations of Wegener's granulomatosis. Chest *88*:5, 1985.
191. Sams, W. M., Jr., Claman, H. N., and Kohler, P. F.: Human necrotizing vasculitis: Immunoglobulins and complement in vessel walls of cutaneous lesions and normal skin. J. Invest. Derm. *64*:441, 1975.
192. Huston, K. A., and Hunder, G. G.: Giant cell (cranial) arteritis: A clinical review. Am. Heart J. *100*:99, 1980.
193. Klinkhoff, A. V., Reid, G. D., and Moscovich, M.: Aortic regurgitation in giant cell arteritis. Arthritis Rheum. *28*:582, 1985.
194. Bacon, P. A., Doherty, S. M., and Zuckerman, A. J.: Hepatitis-B antibody in polymyalgia rheumatica. Lancet 2:476, 1975.

PROGRESSIVE SYSTEMIC SCLEROSIS

195. Masi, A. T., and Rodnan, G. P.: Preliminary criteria for the classification of systemic sclerosis (scleroderma). Bull. Rheum. Dis. *31*:1, 1981.
196. Botstein, G. R., and LeRoy, E. C.: Primary heart disease in systemic sclerosis (scleroderma): Advances in clinical and pathologic features, pathogenesis, and new therapeutic approaches. Am. Heart J. *102*:913, 1981.
197. Norton, W. L., and Nardo, J. M.: Vascular disease in progressive systemic sclerosis (scleroderma). Ann. Intern. Med. *73*:317, 1970.
198. Weiss, S., Stead, E., Warren, J., and Bailey, O.: Scleroderma heart disease. Arch. Intern. Med. *71*:749, 1943.
199. LeRoy, E. C.: The heart in systemic sclerosis. N. Engl. J. Med. *310*:188, 1984.
200. Follansbee, W. P., Curtiss, E. I., Medsger, T. A., Jr., Steen, V. D., Vretsky, B. F., Owens, G. R., and Rodman, G. P.: Physiologic abnormalities of cardiac function in progressive systemic sclerosis with diffuse scleroderma. N. Engl. J. Med. *310*:142, 1984.
201. Kahan, A., Devaux, J. Y., Amor, B., Menkes, C. J., Weber, S., Nitenberg, A., Venot, A., Guerin, F., Desgeorges, M., and Roucayrol, J. C.: Nifedipine and thallium-201 myocardial perfusion in progressive systemic sclerosis. N. Engl. J. Med. *314*:1397, 1986.
202. Roberts, N. K., Cabeen, W. R., Jr., Moss, J., Clements, P. J., and Furst, D. E.: The prevalence of conduction defects and cardiac arrhythmias in progressive systemic sclerosis. Ann. Intern. Med. *94*:38, 1981.
203. Ferri, C., Bernini, L., Gongiorni, M. G., Levorato, D., Viegi, G., Prassede, B., Contini, C., Pasero, G., and Bombardieri, S.: Noninvasive evaluation of cardiac dysrhythmias and their relationship with multisystemic symptoms in progressive systemic sclerosis patients. Arthritis Rheum. 28:1259, 1985.
204. Follansbee, W. P., Curtiss, E. I., Rahko, P. S., Medsger, T. A., Jr., Lavine, S. J., Owens, G. R., and Steen, V. D.: The electrocardiogram in systemic sclerosis (scleroderma). Am. J. Med. 79:183, 1985.
205. Kahan, A., Nitenberg, A., Foult, J. M., Amor, B., Menkes, C. D., Devaux, J. Y., Blanchet, F., Perennec, J., Lutfalla, G., and Roucayrol, J. C.: Decreased coronary reserve in primary scleroderma myocardial disease. Arthritis Rheum. *28*:637, 1985.
206. Niarchose, A. P., Whitman, H. H., Goldstein, J. E., and Laragh, J. H.: Hemodynamic effects of captopril in pulmonary hypertension of collagen vascular disease. Am. Heart J. *104*:834, 1982.
207. Ocken, S., Reinitz, E., and Strom, J.: Nifedipine treatment for pulmonary hypertension in a patient with systemic sclerosis. Arthritis Rheum. *26*:794, 1983.
208. O'Brien, J. T., Hill, J. A., and Pepine, C. J.: Sustained benefit of verapamil in pulmonary hypertension with progressive systemic sclerosis. Am. Heart J. *109*:380, 1985.
209. Ellis, W. W., Baer, A. N., Robertson, R. M., Pincus, T., and Kronenberg, M. W.: Left ventricular dysfunction induced by cold exposure in patients with systemic sclerosis. Am. J. Med. *80*:385, 1986.
210. McWhorter, J. E., and LeRoy, E. C.: Pericardial disease in scleroderma (systemic sclerosis). Am. J. Med. *57*:566, 1974.
211. Gladman, D. D., Gordon, D. A., Urowitz, M. B., and Levy, H. L.: Pericardial fluid analysis in scleroderma (systemic sclerosis). Am. J. Med. *60*:1064, 1976.
212. Medsger, T. A., Jr., and Masi, A. T.: Survival with scleroderma. II. A life-table analysis of clinical and demographic factors in 358 male U.S. veteran patients. J. Chron. Dis. *26*:647, 1973.
213. Wynn, J., Fineberg, N., Matzer, L., Covtada, X., Armstrong, W., Dillon, J. C., and Kinney, E. L.: Prediction of survival in progressive systemic sclerosis by multivariate analysis of clinical features. Am. Heart J. *110*:123, 1985.
214. Whitman, H. H., Case, D. B., Laragh, J. H., Christian, C. C., Botstein, G., Marica, H., and Leroy, E. C.: Variable response to oral angiotensin-converting enzyme blockade in hypertensive scleroderma patients. Arthritis Rheum. *25*:241, 1982.

POLYMYOSITIS AND DERMATOMYOSITIS

215. Bohan, A., Peter, J. B., Bowman, R. L., and Pearson, C. M.: A computer assisted analysis of 153 patients with polymyositis and dermatomyositis. Medicine *56*:255, 1977.
216. Norton, W. L., Velayos, E., and Robison, L.: Endothelial inclusions in dermatomyositis. Ann. Rheum. Dis. *29*:67, 1970.
217. Oppenheim, H.: Zur Dermatomyositis. Berlin. Klin. Wochenschr. *36*:805, 1899.
218. Oka, M., and Raasakka, T.: Cardiac involvement in polymyositis. Scand. J. Rheumatol. 7:203, 1978.
219. Haupt, H. M., and Hutchins, G. M.: The heart and conduction system in polymyositis-dermatomyositis: A clinicopathologic study of 16 autopsied patients. Am. J. Cardiol. *50*:998, 1982.
220. Raju, N. V. R., Hart, N., Maloney, J., Zaidi, A., and Adams, K.: Cardiac involvement in polymyositis: A case report and review of the literature. Cleve. Clin. Q. *51*:89, 1984.
221. Stern, R., Godbold, J. H., Chess, Q., and Kogan, L. J.: ECG abnormalities in polymyositis. Arch. Intern. Med. *144*:2185, 1984.

HERITABLE DISORDERS OF CONNECTIVE TISSUE

222. McKusick, V. A.: Heritable Disorders of Connective Tissue. 4th ed. St. Louis, C. V. Mosby Co., 1972.
223. Pyeritz, R. E., and McKusick, V. A.: Basic defects in the Marfan syndrome. N. Engl. J. Med. *305*:1101, 1981.
224. Roberts, W. C., and Honig, H. S.: The spectrum of cardiovascular disease in the Marfan syndrome: A clinico-morphologic study of 18 necropsy patients and comparison of 151 previously reported necropsy patients. Am. Heart J. *104*:115, 1982.
225. Missri, J. C., and Swett, D. D., Jr.: Marfan syndrome: A review. Cardiovasc. Rev. Rep. 3:1645, 1982.

THE MARFAN SYNDROME

226. Abraham, P. A., Perejda, A. J., Carnes, W. H., and Uitto, J.: Marfan syndrome. Demonstration of abnormal elastin in aorta. J. Clin. Invest. *70*:1245, 1982.
227. James, T. N., Frame, B., and Schatz, I. J.: Pathology of cardiac conduction system in Marfan's syndrome. Arch. Intern. Med. *114*:339, 1964.
228. Murdoch, J. L., Walker, B. A., Halpern, B. I., Kuzma, J. W., and McKusick, V. A.: Life expectancy and causes of death in the Marfan syndrome. N. Engl. J. Med. 286:804, 1972.
229. Phornphutkul, C., Rosenthal, A., and Nadas, A.: Cardiac manifestation of Marfan syndrome in infancy and childhood. Circulation *47*:587, 1973.
230. Pyeritz, R. E., and Wappel, M. A.: Mitral valve dysfunction in the Marfan syndrome. Clinical and echocardiographic study of prevalence and natural history. Am. J. Med. *74*:797, 1983.
231. Gwilt, D. J.: Review: Echocardiographic features of the Marfan syndrome. J. Cardiovasc. Ultrasonography 3:107, 1984.
232. Gott, V. L., Pyeritz, R. E., Magovern, G. J., Jr., Cameron, D. E., and McKusick, V. A.: Surgical treatment of aneurysms of the ascending aorta in the Marfan syndrome. Results of composite-graft repair in 50 patients. N. Engl. J. Med. *314*:1070, 1986.

233. Bruno, L., Tredici, S., Mangiavacchi, M., Colombo, V., Mozzota, F. G., and Sirtori, C. R.: Cardiac, skeletal, and ocular abnormalities in patients with Marfan's syndrome and in their relatives. Br. Heart J. *51*:220, 1984.
234. Pan, C. W., Chen, C. C., Wang, S. P., Hsu, T. L., and Chiang, B. N.: Echocardiographic study of cardiac abnormalities in families of patients with Marfan's syndrome. J. Am. Coll. Cardiol. *6*:5, 1985.

OSTEOGENESIS IMPERFECTA

235. Sytes, B., Ogilvia, D., Wordsworth, P., Anderson, J., and Jones, N.: Osteogenesis imperfecta is limited to both type I collagen structural genes. Lancet *2*:69, 1986.
236. Weisinger, B., Glassman, E., Spencer, F., and Bergner, A.: Successful aortic valve replacement for aortic regurgitation associated with osteogenesis imperfecta. Br. Heart J. *37*:475, 1975.
237. Hortop, J., Tsipouras, P., Hanley, J. A., Maron, B. J., and Shapiro, J. R.: Cardiovascular involvement in osteogenesis imperfecta. Circulation *73*:54, 1986.

EHLERS-DANLOS SYNDROME

238. Rowe, D. W., and Shapiro, J. R.: Diseases associated with abnormalities of structural proteins. *In* Kelly, W. N., Harris, E. D., Jr., Ruddy, S., and Sledge, C. B. (eds.): Textbook of Rheumatology. Philadelphia, W. B. Saunders Company, 1985.
239. Cupo, L. N., Pyeritz, R. E., Olson, J. L., McPhee, S. J., Hutchins, G. M., and McKusick, V. A.: Ehlers-Danlos syndrome with abnormal collagen fibrils, sinus of Valsalva aneurysms, myocardial infarction, panacinar emphysema and cerebral heterotopias. Am. J. Med. *72*:1051, 1981.
240. Jaffe, A. S., Geltman, E. M., Rodey, G. E., and Vitto, J.: A consistent manifestation of type IV Ehlers-Danlos syndrome. The pathogenetic role of the abnormal production of type III collagen. Circulation *64*:121, 1981.
241. Come, P. C., Fortuin, N. J., White, R. K., Jr., and McKusick, V. A.: Echocardiographic assessment of cardiovascular abnormalities in the Marfan syndrome. Comparison with clinical findings and with roentgenographic estimation of aortic root size. Am. J. Med. *74*:465, 1983.

PSEUDOXANTHOMA ELASTICUM

242. Mendelsohn, G., Bulkley, B. H., and Hutchins, G. M.: Cardiovascular manifestations of pseudoxanthoma elasticum. Arch. Pathol. Lab. Med. *102*:298, 1978
243. Akhtar, M., and Brody, H.: Elastic tissue in pseudoxanthoma elasticum: Ultrastructural study of endocardial lesions. Arch. Pathol. *99*:667, 1975.
244. Huang, S. N., Steel, H. D., and Kumar, G.: Ultrastructural changes of elastic fibers in pseudoxanthoma elasticum: A study of histogenesis. Arch. Pathol. *83*:108, 1967.
245. Lebwohl, M. G., Distefano, D., Prioleau, P. G., Uram, M., Yannuzi, L. A., and Fleischmajer, R.: Pseudoxanthoma elasticum and mitral valve prolapse. N. Engl. J. Med. *307*:228, 1982.
246. Bete, J., Banas, J., Jr., Moran, J., Pinn, V., and Levine, H. J.: Coronary artery disease in an 18-year-old girl with pseudoxanthoma elasticum: Successful surgical therapy. Am. J. Cardiol. *36*:515, 1975.
247. Eddy, D. D., and Farber, E. M.: Pseudoxanthoma elasticum: Internal manifestations. A report of cases and a statistical review of the literature. Arch. Dermatol. *86*:729, 1962.
248. Navarro-Lopez, F., Llorian, A., Ferrer-Roca, O., Betriu, A., and Sanz, G.: Restrictive cardiomyopathy in pseudoxanthoma elasticum. Chest *78*:113, 1980.
249. Coffman, J. D., and Sommers, S.: Familial pseudoxanthoma elasticum and valvular heart disease. Circulation *19*:242, 1959.

HURLER SYNDROME AND OTHER MUCOPOLYSACCHARIDES

250. Renteria, V. G., Ferrans, V. J., and Roberts, W. C.: The heart in the Hurler syndrome: Gross, histologic and ultrastructural observations in five necropsy cases. Am. J. Cardiol. *38*:487, 1976.
251. Factor, S. M., Biempica, L., and Goldfischer, S.: Coronary intimal sclerosis in Morquio's syndrome. Virchows Arch. *379*:1, 1978.
252. Brosius, F. C., III, and Roberts, W. C.: Coronary artery disease in the Hurler syndrome. Qualitative and quantitative analysis of the extent of coronary narrowing at necropsy in six children. Am. J. Cardiol. *47*:649, 1981.
253. Johnson, G. L., Vine, D. L., Cottrill, C. M., and Noonan, J. A.: Echocardiographic mitral valve deformity in mucopolysaccharidosis. Pediatrics *67*:401, 1981.

55 HEMATOLOGICAL-ONCOLOGICAL DISORDERS AND HEART DISEASE

by DAVID S. ROSENTHAL, M.D., and
EUGENE BRAUNWALD, M.D.

During the past two decades, the increased frequency of cardiovascular abnormalities in patients with hematological and neoplastic disorders and, conversely, of blood disorders in patients being treated for a variety of cardiovascular diseases has led to a greater interaction between these two specialties. Hematologist-oncologists must often consult cardiologists regarding clinical problems that range from interpreting abnormal physical, electrocardiographic, and echocardiographic changes in their patients to obtaining advice about how to treat heart failure, pericardial effusion, or other cardiac complications common among patients with anemia and hematological malignancies. Conversely, blood dyscrasias often complicate the use of cardiac medications and prosthetic heart valves and cardiovascular surgery. This convergence of interests has inspired innovative reviews devoted to the relationship between these two disciplines.[1, 2]

ANEMIA AND CARDIOVASCULAR DISORDERS

(See also pp. 781–783)

Anemia is one of the most common causes of increased cardiac output and sometimes results in heart failure due to a high-output state. As discussed in Chapter 25, tissue hypoxia combined with reduced blood viscosity leads to a decrease in systemic vascular resistance, which is associated with an increase in cardiac output.[1, 3-5] Acutely induced anemia lowers coronary vascular resistance, whereas chronic anemia enhances formation of intercoronary collaterals and causes increases in preload and reduction of afterload.[6, 7] All signs and symptoms of cardiovascular disease usually disappear. When the normal hemoglobin concentration is restored, the gradual development of anemia may lead to cardiac hypertrophy, in that anemia probably causes vasodilation, which increases venous return (and thereby preload) and reduces peripheral resistance (and thereby afterload). Left ventricular end-diastolic volume is increased in patients with chronic anemia, and afterload reduction, as reflected in left ventricular end-systolic stress, has been demonstrated. Such changes may represent a favorable advantage for maintaining a sufficiently high stroke volume.[7, 8] Another mechanism of enhanced left ventricular function in chronic anemia has been attributed to increased levels of catecholamine and noncatecholamine inotropic factors in plasma.[9, 10] For example, papillary muscles placed in serum obtained from these patients exhibit increased contractility in vitro.[10]

CARDIAC SYMPTOMS OF ANEMIA. Reduced cardiac reserve, fatigue, exertional dyspnea, and edema depend on the severity of the anemia and the presence of an underlying cardiovascular disorder such as myocardial or valvular heart disease. Severely anemic patients without heart disease have few if any cardiac symptoms. When hemoglobin values decline below 7 gm/dl, resting cardiac output increases.[3, 11-13] There is general agreement that symptoms also depend on (1) the rapidity with which the anemia develops, (2) the physical activity of the patient, and (3) the coexistence of underlying cardiac or coronary artery disease. For example, in the presence of coronary artery disease, anemia lowers the threshold for development of angina pectoris, so that patients with mild anemia may have more anginal episodes. If the anemia has developed gradually, patients with hemoglobin levels below 7 gm/dl may be able to compensate sufficiently to carry out all but the most strenuous activities.

Although uncommon, severe congestive heart failure with pulmonary edema can occur solely on the basis of very severe anemia (Hg $<$ 4 gm/dl in the absence of antecedent heart disease). It may be difficult to distinguish congestive heart failure secondary to chronic anemia from that related to myocardial infiltration with iron, secondary to hemosiderosis resulting from multiple transfusions (p. 1740). However, the symptoms of reduced cardiac reserve secondary to anemia alone are usually relieved when the anemia is corrected and a normal red cell mass has been restored.

Electrocardiographic findings are not uncommon as the anemia progresses. With hemoglobin levels below 7 gm/dl, T-wave depression and T-wave inversion may be found, simulating myocardial disease. With transfusions, these findings usually return to normal.

Oxygen Dissociation and Levels of 2,3-Diphosphoglycerate in Red Cells

To account for the circulatory adaptation that occurs in chronic anemia, it is important to appreciate that factors other than hemoglobin concentration and blood flow play a role in the quantity of oxygen delivered to tissues. These include tissue oxygen tension and the position of the hemoglobin-oxygen (Hb-O_2) dissociation curve. Normally, 1 gm of hemoglobin binds 1.34 ml of O_2. With a hemoglobin concentration of 15 gm/dl, 100 ml of arterial blood contains 20 ml of O_2. As can be calculated from the Hb-O_2 dissociation curve (Fig. 55–1), 100 ml of mixed venous blood having a PO_2 of 40 mm Hg will contain 15.5 ml of O_2. The difference (i.e., 4.5 ml of O_2 per 100 ml of arterial blood) would be available for delivery to tissues. If the body depended only upon cardiac output to sustain oxygen delivery in the anemic state, blood flow would have to double in order to preserve tissue oxygenation when the hemoglobin declined from 15 to 7.5 gm/dl.

SHIFTS OF THE HEMOGLOBIN-O_2 DISSOCIATION CURVE. In most patients with anemia, the Hb-O_2 dissociation curve shifts to the right, and more oxygen is released from hemoglobin as the PO_2 declines. The red cell concentrations of 2,3-diphosphoglycerate (2,3-DPG), which are known to vary in a number of disease states,[13] profoundly affect the binding and release of oxygen by hemoglobin. Deoxygenated hemoglobin, which is more alkaline than oxyhemoglobin, stimulates the production of 2,3-DPG, a byproduct of glycolysis. As a consequence, the intraerythrocytic ratio of deoxy- to oxyhemoglobin serves as a critical regulator of 2,3-DPG concentration. For example, the decreased oxygen affinity present in chronic anemia can be accounted for by this increase in red cell 2,3-DPG. At a normal arterial PO_2, arterial oxygen saturation remains high despite the reduction in oxygen affinity. However, at the lower PO_2 in the venous blood, elevated 2,3-DPG displaces the Hb-O_2 dissociation curve to the right, enabling greater release of oxygen from the cells at any level of PO_2. Oski et al. have calculated that decreased oxygen affinity mediated by increased red cell 2,3-DPG may compensate for up to half the oxygen deficit in anemia.[14] High levels of 2,3-DPG have also been found in subjects exposed to altitude[15] and in patients with pulmonary disease.[16]

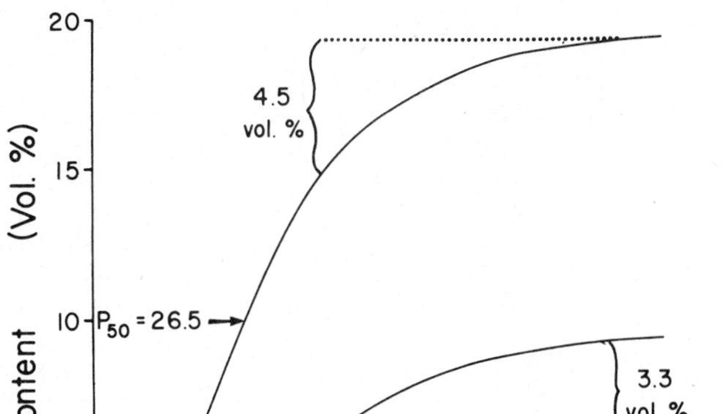

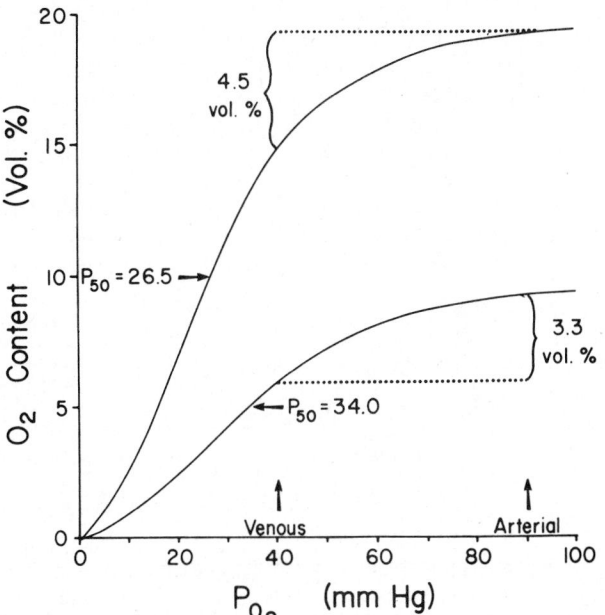

FIGURE 55–1. Enhancement of oxygen unloading by decreased red cell oxygen affinity in anemia with an increase in P_{50} from 26.5 to 34.0. (From Klocke, R. A.: Oxygen transport and 2,3-diphosphoglycerate. Chest 62:795l, 1972.)

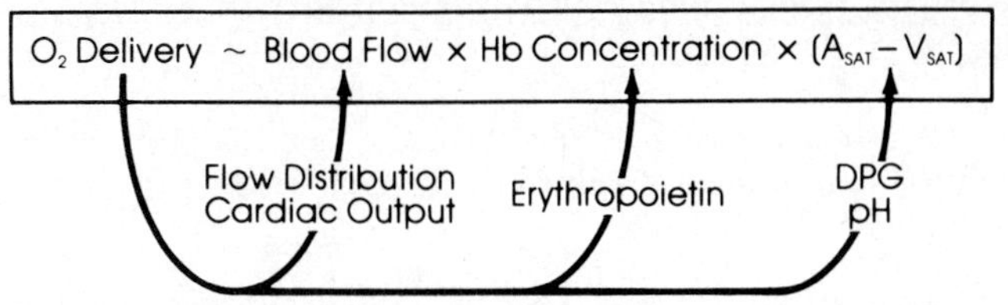

FIGURE 55–2. Oxygen delivered to an organ or tissue is directly proportional to blood flow, hemoglobin concentration, and the difference in oxygen saturation between arterial and venous blood. Patients with various types of hypoxia may compensate in the following ways: (1) Blood flow distribution may be altered to maintain oxygenation of vital organs, with an increase in total cardiac output when hypoxia is severe. (2) Increased erythropoietin production may stimulate erythropoiesis. (3) Oxygen unloading may be enhanced by a shift to the right in the oxygen dissociation curve, mediated by an increase in red cell 2,3-DPG. (From Bunn, H. F.: Pathophysiology of the anemias. *In* Braunwald, E., et al. (eds.): Harrison's Principles of Internal Medicine. 11th ed. New York, McGraw-Hill Book Co., 1987, p. 1492.)

The position of the Hb-O_2 dissociation curve can be expressed by the value of P_{50}, i.e., the partial pressure of O_2 at which hemoglobin is 50 per cent saturated. A reduction of the oxygen affinity of hemoglobin, i.e., a shift of the dissociation curve to the right, is reflected in an elevation of P_{50}. With a P_{50} of 34 mm Hg (instead of the normal P_{50} of 26.5 mm Hg), 3.3 ml of O_2 is unloaded per 100 ml of blood. As a consequence, an anemic individual with a 50 per cent reduction in red cell mass would suffer only a 27 per cent reduction in oxygen unloading (Fig. 55–1).

RESPONSE TO HYPOXIA. Figure 55–2 summarizes the factors responsible for oxygenation in response to hypoxia. Oxygen delivery to the metabolizing tissues depends directly on three principal factors: (1) blood flow; (2) hemoglobin concentration (i.e., the oxygen-carrying capacity of the blood), and (3) the oxygen unloaded per unit of blood, as represented by the difference between arterial and venous blood oxygen saturations. Each of these three factors varies independently. Blood flow to any tissue is a function of total cardiac output and its fractional distribution. The red cell mass is regulated by erythropoietin in response to tissue oxygenation. The position of the Hb-O_2 dissociation curve is determined primarily by red cell 2,3-DPG levels and blood pH. Chronic anemia is usually well tolerated when these compensatory mechanisms operate effectively, i.e., with an increased cardiac output and redistribution of blood flow, as well as decreased oxygen affinity.

CARDIAC EXAMINATION. The cardiac enlargement that develops with severe, chronic anemia usually results from dilatation and eccentric hypertrophy with a normal ratio of wall thickness to cavity diameter, as occurs in other forms of volume overload (see Fig. 14–8, p. 432). The precordium is usually hyperactive. Third and fourth heart sounds are frequently present, and a midsystolic murmur, maximal at the left sternal border, is usually audible.[17, 18] The murmur is probably secondary to the combined effects of increased velocity of blood flow across the pulmonic and aortic valve orifices and reduced blood viscosity. Less frequently, an early, midsystolic rumbling murmur may be heard at the apex or along the left sternal border. These systolic murmurs are probably related to the increase in blood flow across the mitral or tricuspid valve and may be difficult to distinguish from the murmurs of mitral or tricuspid stenosis. Accurate diagnosis may require echocardiography as well as reexamination after correction of the anemia.

In patients with chronic anemia whose hearts are compensated at a reduced concentration of hemoglobin, blood volume expansion achieved by the transfusion of whole blood may be poorly tolerated. Expanding the blood volume and augmenting left ventricular filling pressure will risk precipitating or aggravating heart failure. Therefore, the slow infusion of packed red blood cells and diuretics would be more useful. Intravenous nitroglycerin therapy may produce a favorable redistribution of circulating blood volume and antagonize the hemodynamic changes caused by transfusion.[19]

CARDIAC DISORDERS ASSOCIATED WITH HEMOLYTIC ANEMIA

Cardiomegaly, congestive heart failure, and sudden death have been reported frequently in patients with chronic hemolytic anemias such as sickle cell disease and thalassemia. In addition, hemolysis secondary to cardiac disease may cause acute symptoms. Hemolytic anemias are usually characterized by marked reticulocytosis and erythroid hyperplasia of the bone marrow. Indirect hyperbilirubinemia, increased serum lactic acid dehydrogenase, and reduced haptoglobin are also common findings. If lysis of red cells occurs within the circulation (intravascular hemolytic anemia), hemoglobinemia and hemoglobinuria may occur and will reflect the severity of hemolysis. Specific laboratory investigations will identify the type of hemolytic anemia, examples being a positive antiglobulin (or Coombs) test in immunohemolytic anemia, increased red cell osmotic fragility in hereditary spherocytosis, and abnormal hemoglobin electrophoresis in sickle cell anemia and the thalassemic syndromes. Acquired hemolytic anemias may occur precipitously and the resulting symptoms may closely resemble those of acute blood loss with peripheral vasoconstriction, hypotension, tachycardia, fatigue, lightheadedness, and dyspnea on exertion.

HEMOGLOBINOPATHIES

Sickle Cell Disease

Sickle hemoglobin results from a mutation in the codon for the sixth amino acid of the beta globin chain from glutamic acid to valine (alpha-2, beta-$2^{6\ glu\rightarrow val}$). Eight to 10 per cent of black Americans are heterozygous for this trait. In certain regions of central Africa, the gene frequency is as high as 20 per cent, and it is likely that the high frequency of hemoglobin S in these areas is associated with resistance to or protection against falciparum malaria. With decreased oxygen tension, red cells containing hemoglobin S acquire an elongated crescent (sickle) shape. Electron microscopy demonstrates bundles of fibers running parallel to the long axis of the cells.[20] If sickle cells are reoxygenated within a short period of time, their normal red shape can be restored. However, as red cells remain sickled in vivo, their membranes become damaged and rigid, resulting eventually in irreversibly sickled cells that have a shortened survival and may block small blood vessels. The continuous formation and destruction of irreversibly sickled cells contribute to the symptoms of sickle cell disease. Factors that decrease oxygen affinity, such as acidosis and increased red cell 2,3-DPG levels, lead to the deoxygenation of hemoglobin and promote the formation of sickled cells.

The heterozygote for sickle cell disease is not anemic and rarely has symptoms except at high altitudes or as a result of marked hypoxia. In contrast, the signs and symptoms in patients homozygous for sickle cell anemia (SS) begin at about 6 months of age, when the conversion from fetal to adult hemoglobin production is completed.

The cardiopulmonary system is frequently involved in sickle cell anemia.[21, 22] As in other chronic anemias, both cardiac output and oxygen extraction by tissues are increased, and the reduced oxygen content of these red cells leads to further sickling. In addition, for any given level of hematocrit, the elevation of cardiac output and the auscultatory findings associated with anemia are greater in sickle cell anemia[23] compared with other anemias (Fig. 55–3). A normal left ventricle is able to tolerate the volume overload of chronic, moderately severe anemia for indefinite periods with no deterioration in functional capacity. The increased preload and decreased afterload characteristic of chronic anemia (p. 781) compensate for any left ventricular dysfunction and maintain a normal ejection fraction and high cardiac output in sickle cell anemia (Fig. 55–4). When cardiac decompensation occurs in patients with sickle cell anemia or other forms of chronic anemia, it is usually the result of other coexisting complications of the SS disease or the presence of underlying cardiovascular abnormalities. For example, deaths secondary to congestive heart failure occurring in children and young adults with sickle cell anemia are usually precipitated by chronic renal failure, pulmonary thrombosis, or infections.[24, 25]

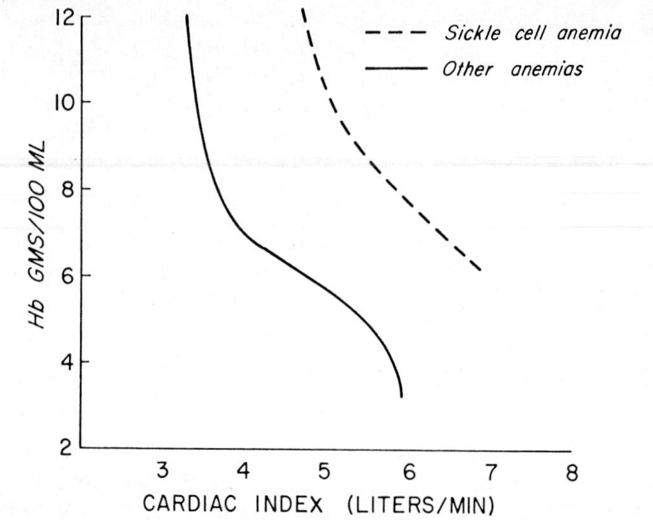

FIGURE 55–3. Relation between hemoglobin concentration and cardiac index at rest in several types of anemia. At any given level of hemoglobin the cardiac index is more elevated in sickle cell anemia (broken line) than in other anemias. (From Varat, M. A., et al.: Cardiovascular effects of anemia. Am. Heart J. *83*:415, 1972.)

Acute myocardial infarction is a rare complication of sickle cell disease and has been confirmed post mortem in a few patients without significant coronary atherosclerosis.[26, 27] More oxygen is extracted by the myocardium than by any other tissue, and transmural infarction due to in situ thrombosis by sickled cells is rare. However, infarction of the papillary muscles of the heart does occur. This should not be surprising, since the papillary muscles are at the terminal portion of the coronary circulation, where collateral vessels are scant and hypoxia is marked.

Pulmonary infarction, a common complication of sickle cell anemia, is probably due to thrombosis in situ rather than to embolization.[28] Although infrequent, fat and bone marrow emboli to the lungs have been reported, the latter resulting from necrosis caused by sickling within the marrow sinusoids. Patients with sickle cell anemia are unusually susceptible to infection. In addition, damage to the

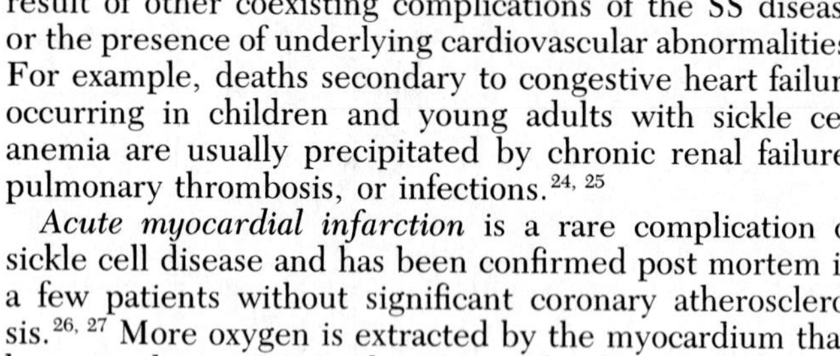

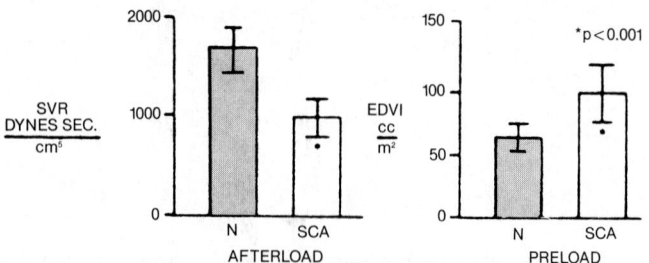

FIGURE 55–4. Loading conditions in 11 patients with sickle cell anemia (SCA) and 11 normal subjects (N). *Left*, Afterload, as indicated by systemic vascular resistance (SVR), was significantly decreased in patients with SCA. *Right*, Preload, as indicated by end-diastolic volume index (EDVI), was significantly increased in patients with SCA. (From Dennenberg, B. S., et al.: Cardiac function in sickle cell anemia. Am. J. Cardiol. *51*:1675, 1983.)

lung caused by repeated vascular insults creates a suitable milieu for bacterial growth; as a consequence, pneumonia is a frequent and serious complication. Mortality and morbidity are high in the setting of pneumonia and hypoxia, so that treatment of these complications must be immediate and vigorous. However, it may be difficult to differentiate pulmonary infection from infarction in patients with sickle cell anemia. Although impaired pulmonary function in sickle cell anemia is common, pulmonary hypertension and cor pulmonale are rarely encountered.[23, 29]

In almost all patients with sickle cell anemia the heart ultimately becomes enlarged, and at autopsy strikingly high heart weights are noted in a majority of patients despite the absence of other causes of cardiomegaly such as hypertension, atherosclerosis, or coronary artery disease.[30] In patients who have received multiple blood transfusions, myocardial iron deposition (hemosiderosis) may contribute to such enlargement and to impairment of cardiac function. However, this complication occurs much less frequently in sickle cell anemia than in homozygous thalassemia. Histological studies have suggested that the increase in heart weight is secondary to fibrosis, presumably caused by the combination of anemia and papillary muscle infarction. With time, children with sickle cell disease exhibit progressive cardiac chamber enlargement with a progressive increase in left ventricular mass.[31]

There are no specific electrocardiographic changes in sickle cell anemia. However, almost 80 per cent of patients with sickle cell anemia have an abnormal electrocardiogram. These abnormalities include left ventricular hypertrophy and first-degree atrioventricular (AV) block as well as nonspecific ST-segment and T-wave changes and abnormal septal Q waves; this last finding is believed to be secondary to septal thickness and the increased left ventricular mass and degree of anemia.[22, 32, 33] Arrhythmias rarely occur with sickle cell anemia, although continuous electrocardiographic monitoring during painful crises has revealed both atrial and ventricular arrhythmias in the majority of patients.[33] Echocardiographic measurements in patients with cardiac symptoms are useful in documenting both cardiac hyperactivity and depressed left ventricular performance[22, 34] (Fig. 55–5). Radiological studies may be entirely normal. With exercise, cardiac dysfunction may be manifested by an abnormal ejection fraction response,

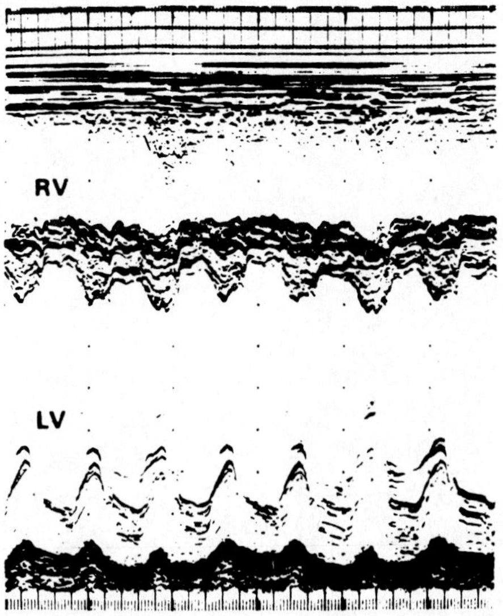

FIGURE 55–5. Typical M-mode echocardiogram in sickle cell anemia. Left ventricle (LV) is dilated, with vigorously contracting walls of normal thickness. RV = right ventricle. (From Falk, R. H., and Hood, B. W.: The heart in sickle cell anemia. Arch. Intern. Med. *142*:1682, 1982.)

abnormalities of wall motion, and incomplete left ventricular filling.[35-38] In addition, echocardiography has demonstrated an incidence of mitral valve prolapse in 25 per cent of SS patients,[39] far in excess of that expected.

Thalassemic Syndromes

The thalassemias are a group of inherited disorders caused by an imbalance in the synthesis of hemoglobin chains rather than by a single amino acid substitution, as in sickle cell disease. The two principal types are referred to as α-thalassemia, in which α-chain synthesis is absent or reduced (a condition found mainly in Orientals), and β-thalassemia, in which β-chain synthesis is absent or reduced. The homozygous form of β-thalassemia is also referred to as Cooley or Mediterranean anemia and is common in persons of Greek and Italian descent. Heterozygous α- and β-thalassemias are also common in American blacks, particularly in association with sickle cell trait. These inherited autosomal dominant defects have been linked to molecular lesions that interfere with the synthesis of globin subunits. The net result in both types of thalassemia is decreased production of hemoglobin A (Hb A) and therefore hemoglobin-deficient red cells that are both microcytic and hypochromic. In addition, the red cells are target-shaped and demonstrate basophilic stippling.

The diagnosis of β-thalassemia is confirmed by quantitative hemoglobin electrophoresis in which levels of Hb A are decreased or absent and levels of Hb A_2 and fetal hemoglobin (Hb F) are increased. The anemia in homozygous β-thalassemia results from a combination of hemolysis and ineffective erythropoiesis. Children have a characteristic "chipmunk" appearance owing to marked hyperplasia of the marrow in the facial bones and massive hepatosplenomegaly owing to extramedullary hematopoiesis. Occasionally, the expanding marrow extrudes from the ribs, sternum, and vertebrae, forming a mass resembling a lymphoma on chest roentgenogram.

CARDIAC ABNORMALITIES IN THALASSEMIA. Cardiac complications are the major cause of death in patients with thalassemia. As with sickle cell disease, these may be due in part to chronic anemia. In addition, cardiac siderosis is a frequent problem in thalassemia but not in sickle cell anemia or many other chronic anemias.[40, 41] Iron overload results from a combination of extravascular hemolysis, the frequent transfusions given to these severely anemic patients, and an inappropriate increase in intestinal iron absorption. Consequently, heart failure and arrhythmias are the common causes of death in children with this condition.[40] Although anemia *per se* undoubtedly contributes to cardiomegaly, iron overload of the heart is the most likely cause of myocardial damage.[42, 43]

Prior to the era of hypertransfusion and chelation therapy, patients with transfusion-dependent, chronic severe refractory thalassemia regularly manifested serious cardiac involvement, usually by the second decade of life. Although most died within months of the development of congestive heart failure, occasional patients died suddenly, presumably secondary to an arrhythmia. Intensive treatment of heart failure and antiarrhythmic therapy do not appear to change the natural history. At postmortem examination, widespread iron deposition characteristic of hemochromatosis is found in all viscera, including the heart, which is hypertrophied and sometimes twice its normal weight; it is often a deep brown, with large quantities of iron in myocardial cells, demonstrated by staining with Prussian blue dye. The sinoatrial node is usually spared, but the AV node is frequently involved. Apparently cardiac dysfunction depends on the quantity of iron deposited in the ventricles, and it has been suggested that myocardial damage results from iron-induced release of acid hydrolases from lysosomes.[16]

Pericarditis occurs in about half of all patients with thalassemia and is often recurrent and associated with fever, precordial pain, and electrocardiographic changes characteristic of acute pericarditis (p. 1487). Pericardial effusion is common; in rare cases, creation of a pericardial

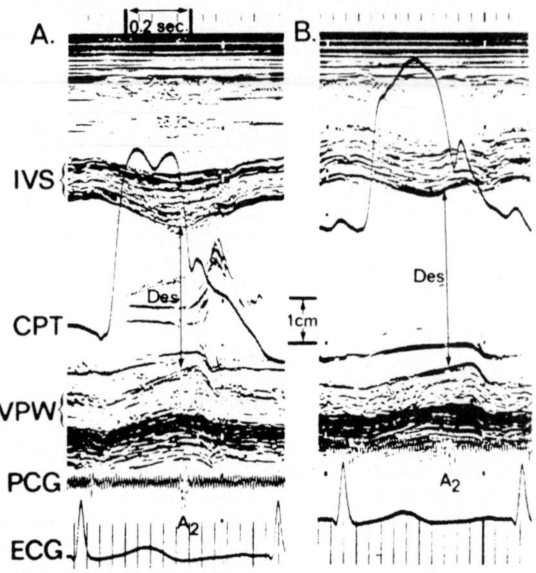

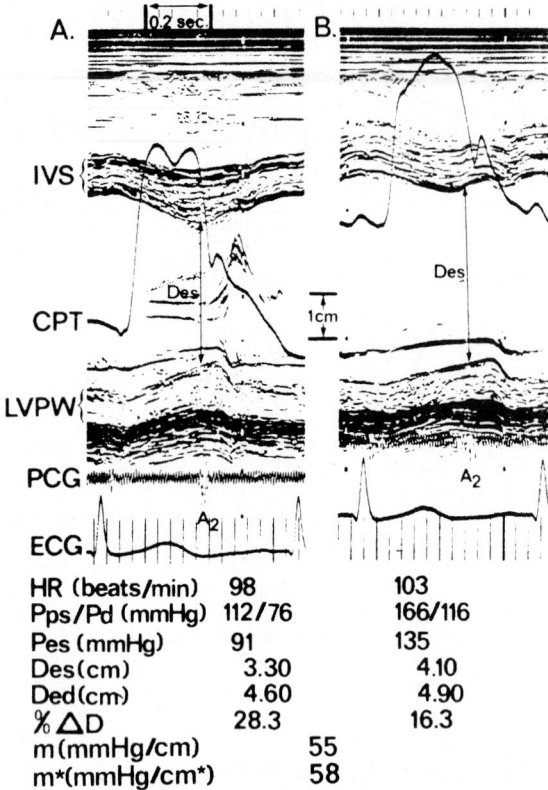

	A	B
HR (beats/min)	98	103
Pps/Pd (mmHg)	112/76	166/116
Pes (mmHg)	91	135
Des(cm)	3.30	4.10
Ded(cm)	4.60	4.90
%ΔD	28.3	16.3

m(mmHg/cm) 55
m*(mmHg/cm*) 58

FIGURE 55–6. Recordings from a 16-year-old patient with thalassemia major during baseline conditions (*A*) and at peak methoxamine effect (*B*). Both the actual and corrected slope values (m and m*) were abnormal despite normal resting fractional shortening (%ΔD). The 44-mm Hg increase in end-systolic pressure (Pes) resulted in a 0.80-cm increase in end-systolic dimension (Des). For the control population, a comparable change in Pes resulted in a 0.40 ± 0.05-cm increase in Des. IVS = interventricular septum; LVPW = left ventricular posterior wall; A_2 = aortic component of the second heart sound; HR = heart rate; Pps = peak systolic pressure; Pd = aortic diastolic pressure; %ΔD = per cent fractional shortening; m = slope; m* = corrected slope. (From Borow, K. M., et al.: The left ventricular end-systolic pressure-dimensions relation in patients with thalassemia major. A new noninvasive method for assessing contractile state. Circulation 66:980, 1982, by permission of the American Heart Association, Inc.)

window is necessary to relieve tamponade or a recurrent effusion.

The *electrocardiogram* often shows left ventricular hypertrophy, nonspecific ST-segment and T-wave abnormalities, supraventricular or ventricular premature contractions, and first- or second-degree AV block. The His bundle electrogram may show prolongation of the P-R interval, signifying abnormal conduction through the AV node. The chest roentgenogram may show slight to moderate cardiac enlargement, and echocardiographic assessment may disclose increased left ventricular end-diastolic, left atrial, and aortic root dimensions as well as a thickened left ventricular wall.[41] At cardiac catheterization, the usual findings comprise a normal or elevated cardiac index with moderate elevations in left ventricular end-diastolic pressure and volume and end-systolic volume with a reduced ejection fraction.

There has been considerable interest in defining abnormalities of cardiac performance noninvasively in asymptomatic patients. Valdes-Cruz et al. have reported that in asymptomatic children with thalassemia major[44] the left ventricular posterior wall thinned more slowly than normal during diastole. Utilizing the relationship between ventricular fractional shortening and end-systolic pressure (p. 462), Borow et al. identified preclinical left ventricular dysfunction (Fig. 55–6),[45] an approach that may be useful in the serial assessment of left ventricular contractility in response to chelation therapy.

Management. Supportive therapy consisting primarily of an adequate transfusion program (and even hypertransfusions), splenectomy, and early treatment of infections has prolonged the life of patients with thalassemia.[46] Roentgenographic evidence of cardiomegaly in children regresses when hemoglobin is maintained above 10 gm/dl. Indeed, in four of seven patients with significant cardiomegaly in one study, heart size returned to normal one week after multiple transfusions restored hemoglobin to near-normal levels. The use of chelating agents for both treatment and prevention of iron overload is discussed on page 1741.

HEMOLYTIC ANEMIA IN PATIENTS WITH VALVULAR HEART DISEASE

In 1964, Dameshek described a patient with aortic, mitral, and tricuspid stenosis and mitral regurgitation who had hemolytic anemia with distorted and fragmented red cells, including helmet cells, burr cells, and schistocytes.[47] At autopsy, numerous calcified excrescences were present on the mitral valve and the free margins of the aortic valve. The presence of excess iron deposits in the kidney suggested intravascular hemolysis, but it could not be established whether the cardiac abnormalities were the cause. Subsequently, shortened red cell survival was demonstrated in other patients with aortic valve disease, some of whom had anemia.[49] In patients with rheumatic aortic valve disease with mild hemolytic anemia, red cell survival may be significantly reduced during periods of exercise.[49] Although this form of hemolytic anemia is probably uncommon, it should be considered in patients with valvular heart disease and unexplained anemia.

HEMOLYTIC ANEMIA DURING CARDIAC SURGERY. In the past, hemolysis frequently occurred as a consequence of extracorporeal circulation. When the blood of many donors must be transfused or is mixed in a pump oxygenator, as may be the case in patients undergoing cardiac surgery, the question arises whether the samples should be cross-matched with each other as well as with the patient. The plasma of one donor may contain a potent antibody that might interact with cells from a donor who has the antigen specific for that antibody. Although infrequent, this phenomenon may explain some cases of mild-

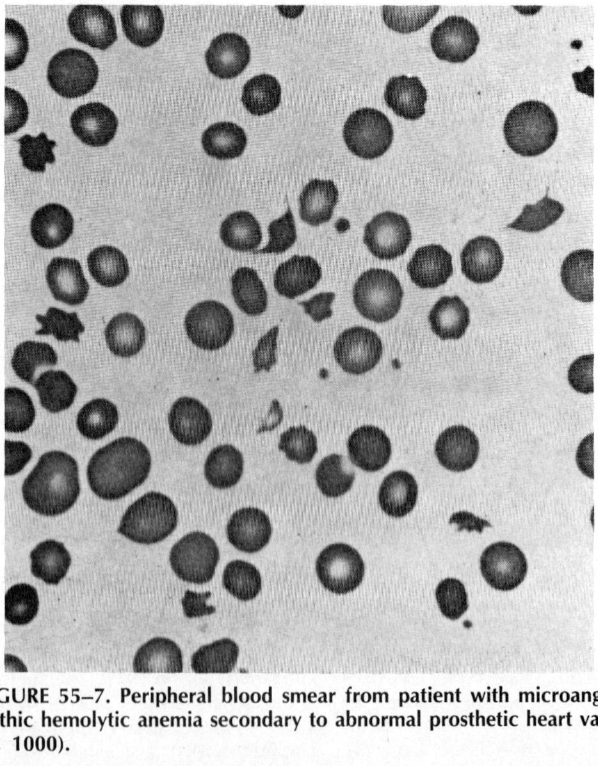

FIGURE 55–7. Peripheral blood smear from patient with microangiopathic hemolytic anemia secondary to abnormal prosthetic heart valve (× 1000).

to-moderate hemolysis and hemoglobinemia seen after cardiopulmonary bypass.

With the use of earlier heart-lung machines, red cells became damaged as they passed through the pump oxygenator, presumably as a result of shear forces, leading to slight hemolysis and causing hemoglobinemia and hemoglobinuria. This problem has been largely avoided with newer machines, which also require little if any blood for priming. As a consequence, hemolytic complications have become far less frequent. In addition, the use of autologous blood and aspirated blood filtered for reuse during the operation has been helpful in this regard.

HEMOLYTIC ANEMIA AFTER CARDIAC SURGERY. In 1954, following surgical implantation of Hufnagel valves in the descending aorta for the treatment of aortic regurgitation, a significant number of patients developed anemia,[50] presumably on a hemolytic basis. The precipitating nature of the hemolytic anemia associated with an intracardiac prosthesis was not really appreciated until chronic and severe hemolytic anemia characterized by microangiopathic red cell changes (consisting of fragmented red cells, burr cells, and schistocytes) was noted after a Teflon patch repair of an ostium primum atrial septal defect (Fig. 55–7).[51] Chromium-51 red cell survival studies confirmed that the half-life of not only autologous red cells but also donor cells was shortened, indicating a defect extrinsic to the red cell. In keeping with intravascular hemolysis, high concentrations of hemoglobin in the plasma and urine were noted along with hemosiderinuria. At reoperation a jet of blood regurgitating through a cleft in the mitral valve that had been impinging on the prosthetic interatrial Teflon patch was found. Part of the septum had become denuded of endothelium and had formed a small cul-de-sac in contact with the jet of blood. With repair of the cul-de-sac and reendothelialization of the area, hemolysis ceased.

Microangiopathic Hemolytic Anemia

This condition has now been reported in association with many cardiac defects (Table 55–1). Its incidence after valve surgery depends on many variables, including the specific operation, the surgical technique, and the tests used to determine hemolysis, and varies widely.[52] In many instances, diurnal variations occur, with greater intravascular hemolysis during physical activity.[53]

CLINICAL PRESENTATION. This may be sudden or gradual, usually with no associated splenomegaly. Rarely, a vicious circle develops in a patient with a perivalvular leak: the resultant shear stress produces hemolytic anemia, increasing stroke volume and shear stress and in turn intensifying the anemia. While it is agreed that direct mechanical trauma to the red cells is the cause of hemolysis, the relative contributions of valve closure, denuded endothelium, turbulence, and the development of anti-erythrocyte autoantibodies are still not clear. In some instances, the hemolytic anemia observed in the early postoperative period is probably due simply to multiple intraoperative transfusions or to the lymphocyte-splenomegaly syndrome (post-pump oxygenator syndrome) associated with cytomegaloviral infection.

TABLE 55–1 CARDIAC CAUSES OF MICROANGIOPATHIC HEMOLYTIC ANEMIA

Intracardiac and intravascular prostheses
Unsuccessful mitral valvuloplasty
Patch repairs for ostium primum defects
Repair of tetralogy of Fallot
Severe aortic valve disease
Ruptured aneurysms of sinus of Valsalva
Coarctation of the aorta
Hypertrophic obstructive cardiomyopathy

CAUSE. Turbulence is the most common feature of all hemolytic anemias due to valvular disease and cardiac surgery. For example, after insertion of a prosthetic valve, perivalvular regurgitation will increase the stroke volume and therefore the turbulence of flow through the narrowed orifice. Experiments in vitro have demonstrated that shearing stresses in excess of 3000 dynes/cm^2 can easily cause hemolysis and that such degrees of stress may readily develop with perivalvular leaks, causing regurgitation from the aorta to the left ventricle,[54] as well as in situations in which the lumen of the aortic valve prosthesis is small relative to the stroke volume or when the ball is large relative to the diameter of the aorta. Although much less common, similar phenomena can occur with prosthetic mitral valves. Rarely, chronic intravascular hemolytic anemia may occur in the presence of hypertrophic cardiomyopathy, probably secondary to abnormal turbulence due to the primary underlying cardiac disease.[55] This rare entity may be managed by reducing the outflow gradient, by beta-adrenoceptor blocker therapy, or by operation (p. 1429). Definitive treatment of the hemolytic syndrome secondary to turbulence consists of surgical repair of the cardiac abnormality, i.e., either replacement or correction of the prosthesis or correction of the perivalvular leak. If a patient is not readily operable, rest should alleviate the condition, and iron and folate replacement may be helpful. Treatment with corticosteroids is usually of no benefit.

HEMOCHROMATOSIS AND HEMOSIDEROSIS

(See also p. 1434)

A number of disease states are characterized by excessive iron stores in the body. The deposition of a significant amount of iron in the myocardium, liver, and pancreas may lead to varying degrees of dysfunction of these organs.[56] Insofar as the heart is concerned, myocardial deposits of iron may lead to congestive heart failure, conduction disturbances, and arrhythmias. Significant siderosis is most often encountered in patients with idiopathic hemochromatosis or in anemic patients with large and long-standing transfusion requirements.

IDIOPATHIC HEMOCHROMATOSIS. In this condition, inappropriately large quantities of iron are absorbed from the gastrointestinal tract. This inherited disorder, with a variable clinical expression, develops slowly and depends in part upon environmental factors, such as the magnitude of dietary iron intake, alcohol intake, and the severity of any underlying liver disease. HLA subtyping has suggested a recessive mode of transmission, has linked the disease to chromosome 6, and has helped to distinguish idiopathic hemochromatosis from iron overload secondary to liver disease.[57]

Clinical manifestations of hemochromatosis occur more frequently in men than in women, and the disease rarely becomes manifest before age 20 years, reaching its peak incidence in the fifth decade. Diabetes is the most common initial manifestation, occurring in half the patients. The classic clinical presentation includes increased pigmentation of the skin, hepatomegaly, and cardiac dysfunction. Loss of libido and other endocrinopathies, such as hypopituitarism, may also become apparent. Cellular damage results from iron-induced release of lysosomal acid hydrolases.[58]

The incidence of cardiac symptoms increases with time.[58, 59] Dyspnea, edema, and ascites are noted early in the course in 15 to 20 per cent of the patients, but eventually about one-third develop symptoms referable to the heart and approximately the same fraction of patients eventually die of cardiac failure.[59] Arrhythmias are common and include paroxysmal atrial tachycardia and flutter, chronic atrial fibrillation, and frequent premature ventricular contractions; varying degrees of AV block have also been noted. Heart block and arrhythmias are often associated with iron deposits in the AV node[60] and supraventricular arrhythmias with deposits in the atria. Low-voltage and nonspecific T-wave changes are also frequently present.

Radiographic studies in symptomatic patients usually reveal a globular heart with biventricular enlargement and weak pulsations. Some patients may have elevated right ventricular and right atrial pressures[61] consequent to the restrictive cardiomyopathy secondary to iron deposition in the myocardium as well as involvement of the pericardium itself.

TRANSFUSIONAL HEMOSIDEROSIS. This may become a clinical problem in patients with severe chronic anemia who survive long enough to accumulate toxic quantities of iron from transfused blood. For example, patients with thalassemia, other serious chronic refractory anemias, myeloid metaplasia, pure red cell aplasia, and aplastic anemia may accumulate 50 gm of iron from transfusions, resulting in a variety of clinical problems similar to those encountered in idiopathic hemochromatosis. Indeed, children with β-thalessemia major maintained on hypertransfusion programs, while spared the cardiac consequences of severe anemia, generally die of heart failure as a consequence of myocardial siderosis in the second decade.[40] In adults with chronic anemias, cardiac iron deposition secondary to transfusional hemosiderosis may contribute to cardiovascular disability, which is often inappropriately attributed solely to high-output heart failure. Undoubtedly, the combination of impaired cardiac function secondary to iron deposition and the increased burden on the heart imposed by the persistent, incompletely treated anemia is responsible.

Pathological Findings. In a review of 135 hearts studied at autopsy, including four from patients with hemochromatosis and 131 from patients with chronic anemia requiring repeated transfusions, 19 were found to have cardiac iron deposits.[62] Grossly visible iron deposits in the heart were always associated with a prior history of cardiac dysfunction and usually of chronic heart failure. Deposits were usually most extensive in idiopathic hemochromatosis and in patients who received more than 100 units of blood without evidence of blood loss. In patients with cardiac hemosiderosis, histological examination revealed that the ventricular free wall and septum contained heavier deposits than did the atrial wall (Fig. 55–8). The quantity of iron in the various layers of the ventricular myocardium is variable, with the epicardium and papillary muscles containing the most iron, the subendocardium containing intermediate amounts, and the midmyocardium and conduction tissue containing the least.

Diagnosis. It is often difficult to determine whether myocardial dysfunction results from the chronic anemia or hemosiderosis. With the use of atomic absorption spectro-

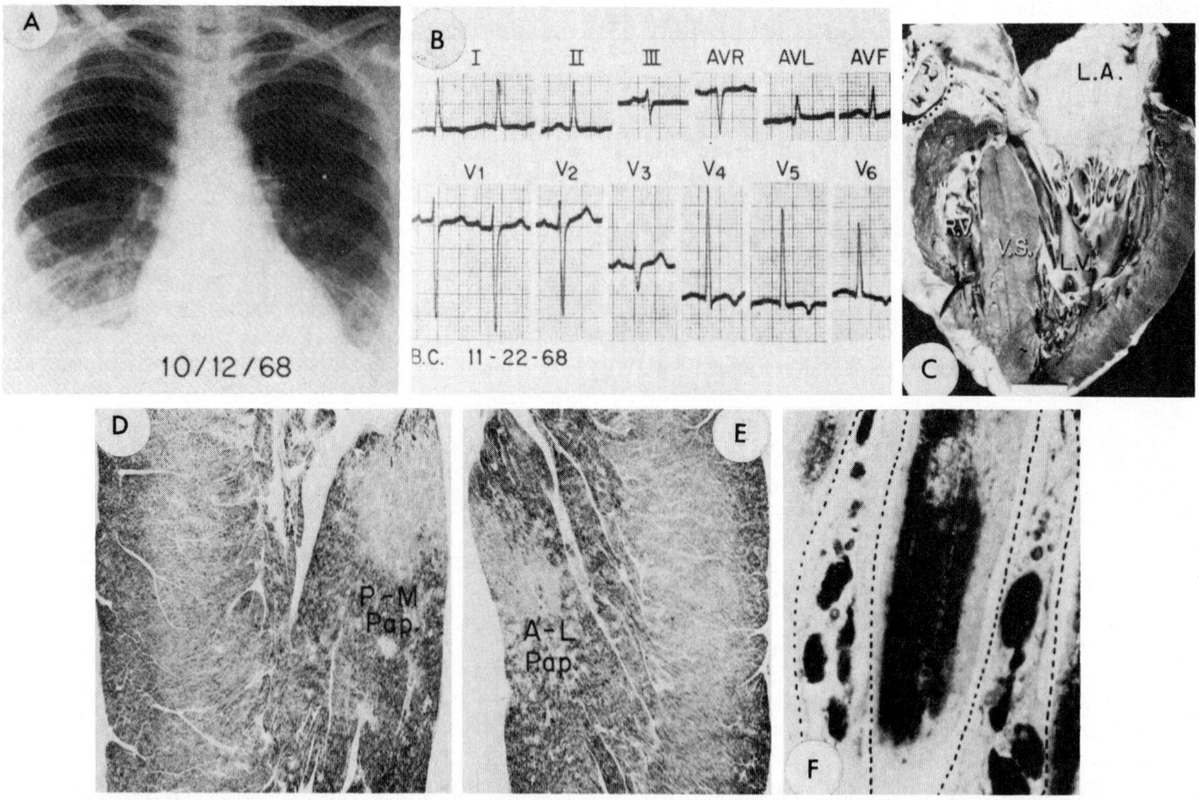

FIGURE 55–8. Observations in a 42-year-old woman with sickle cell anemia who developed congestive heart failure after cumulative transfusions of 260 units of blood. By the time of death, she had received a total of 359 units of blood (90 gm iron). *A*, Chest roentgenogram 2 weeks prior to death, showing cardiomegaly. *B*, Ischemic ST-segment and T-wave changes can be seen on the electrocardiogram. *C*, At autopsy the walls of the right (R.V.) and left (L.V.) ventricles and left atrium (L.A.) and the atrial and ventricular (V.S.) septa were rusty brown, owing to extensive iron deposits. The right atrial wall (partially enclosed by dotted line), in contrast, was tan; only minute particles of iron were present on microscopic examination. *D* and *E*, Large areas of replacement fibrosis (pale areas) were present in both left ventricular papillary muscles. *F*, Severely degenerated myocardial fibers (enclosed by dotted lines) that also contained iron deposits were often found adjacent to viable myocardial fibers. (Prussian blue stains.) (From Buja, L. M., and Roberts, W. C.: Iron in the heart. Am. J. Med. *51*:209, 1971.)

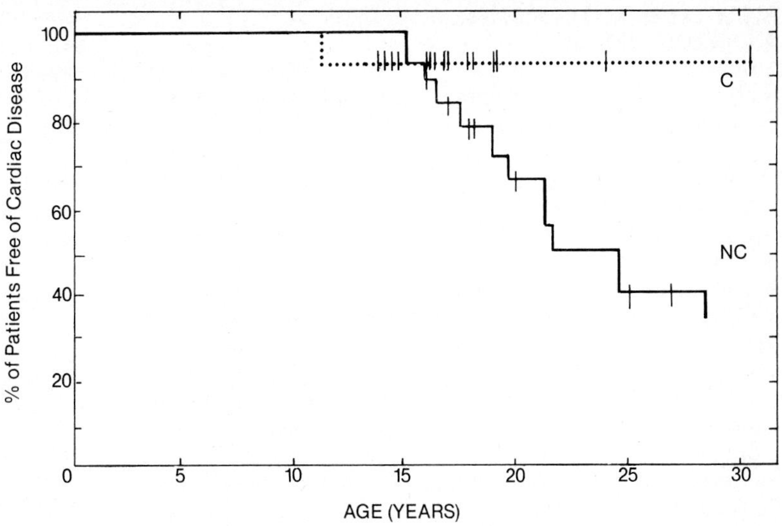

FIGURE 55–9. Life-table depiction of survival free of cardiac disease in patients with thalassemia major treated with desferrioxamine. Dotted line represents the compliant group (C) and solid line represents the noncompliant group (NC). The vertical slashes represent the current ages of patients still free of cardiac disease. (Reprinted by permission from Wolfe, L., et al.: Prevention of cardiac disease by subcutaneous desferrioxamine in patients with thalassemia major. N. Engl. J. Med. *312*:1600, 1985.)

photometry, the exact concentrations of iron can be determined in various body organs or tissues. Rarely is iron deposition limited to the heart. Since the liver is easily accessible by biopsy and its iron concentration is closely related to that in the myocardium, liver biopsy is a convenient way of confirming a diagnosis of myocardial siderosis. In some patients, echocardiography may detect early left ventricular dysfunction prior to the development of symptoms.[41, 63] In a group of patients with severe β-thalassemia or transfusion-dependent anemias without clinical cardiac symptoms, left ventricular dysfunction measured by radionuclide angiography was demonstrated during exercise but not at rest.[63] Noninvasive assessment of the left ventricular end-systolic pressure-dimension relation (using a methoxamine challenge) can identify preclinical left ventricular dysfunction not evident on resting or dynamic exercise studies and not due to chronic anemia per se. This technique may be a sensitive means of monitoring therapeutic response or iron overload diseases to prevent cardiac complications.

Management. Since the majority of patients with myocardial siderosis ultimately die of irreversible cardiac failure and arrhythmias, reversal of the iron overload should be attempted. In patients with idiopathic hemochromatosis, it is possible to mobilize iron stores by repeated phlebotomies, which is the preferred mode of therapy.[64, 65] Decreases in hepatic iron stores and fibrosis, improvement of liver function, amelioration of diabetes, and reversal of cardiomyopathy have all occurred with such treatment. Since the average patient with idiopathic hemochromatosis has 20 to 40 grams of stored iron, weekly to bimonthly phlebotomies usually have to be continued for 2 to 3 years. Initially the hematocrit will drop but will then return toward normal despite repeated phlebotomies. Removal of excess body iron by phlebotomy has been possible in patients with hematocrits as low as 30 per cent.

The distribution of iron in the tissues differs somewhat between individuals with idiopathic hemochromatosis and those with transfusion siderosis, who have relatively more iron stored in the reticuloendothelial cells. However, repeated transfusions in the latter result in a pattern of organ dysfunction similar to that in idiopathic hemochromatosis.[66] Phlebotomy is, of course, not a therapeutic alternative in the management of iron overload due to chronic blood transfusion therapy for anemia. Rather, chelation therapy is the only approach available for removing iron in these anemic patients.[67-69]

Desferrioxamine is the most widely studied iron chelator. This hydroxamic acid compound has a very high affinity for trivalent iron. It must be administered parenterally, and most of the chelated iron will be excreted in the urine within 4 hours of the injection. Initial studies with intramuscular desferrioxamine were unsuccessful in achieving sustained negative iron balance. However, the addition of oral ascorbic acid doubles iron excretion[67]; when ascorbic acid loading was combined with the continuous, subcutaneous administration of desferrioxamine, a negative iron balance was achieved in children with thalassemia.[70] Nevertheless, ascorbate supplementation in patients with iron overload may be hazardous. Clinical cardiotoxicity manifested by fatal congestive heart failure and arrhythmias has been reported in patients treated simultaneously with ascorbic acid and desferrioxamine. Not only does ascorbate make more cellular iron available for chelation, but it also liberates free intracellular iron, which can generate membrane-damaging free oxygen radicals.[71] The adverse effect of ascorbate may be prevented by using this agent after the patient has been started on chelation therapy.[71a]

Long-term desferrioxamine iron chelation therapy is effective not only in delaying but in reversing organ damage caused by transfusional iron overload.[68, 69] In children with thalassemia major, regular treatment with iron chelation appears to protect them from developing cardiac disease induced by iron overload (Fig. 55–9).

DISORDERS ASSOCIATED WITH INCREASED BLOOD VISCOSITY

As discussed earlier, delivery of oxygen to an organ or tissue is directly proportional to blood flow, hemoglobin concentration, and the difference in oxygen saturation between arterial and venous blood (Fig. 55–2). In anemic patients, an increase in blood flow, due in part to reduced blood viscosity, and enhanced oxygen delivery through elevated levels of red cell 2,3-DPG compensate for the reduced hemoglobin levels. In contrast, conditions associated with increased viscosity cause an increase in resistance to flow and a reduction in blood flow. Disorders with increased viscosity and abnormal blood rheology include the erythrocytoses, such as polycythemia vera, and disease states associated with hypergammaglobulinemia, such as multiple myeloma and cryoglobulinemia.

POLYCYTHEMIA

Polycythemia is characterized by an increase in red cells, as determined by hematocrit, hemoglobin, or red blood cell count.[72] However, the terms polycythemia and its synonym erythrocytosis do not refer to a specific disease entity but to a variety of conditions. Absolute polycythemias refer to conditions in which there is an absolute increase in red cell mass (as measured by ^{51}Cr labeling or other dilution techniques). They are subclassified as primary or secondary, depending on whether the elevation in red cell mass is autonomous (primary) or under hormonal (erythropoietin) control. Primary polycythemia, i.e., polycythemia vera, is part of the spectrum of myeloproliferative disorders. Secondary polycythemia is further classified into those disorders which cause an appropriate increase in erythropoietin secretion (e.g., disorders associated with hypoxia, such as cyanotic forms of congenital heart disease and pulmonary disease) and those which cause an inappropriate increase in erythropoietin production, as occurs with tumors and a variety of renal diseases. In the relative polycythemias, red cell mass is normal but plasma volume is decreased, causing hematocrit, hemoglobin, and red cell count to be elevated.

Although the symptoms of secondary polycythemia depend on the underlying disease state, they are also usually a consequence of increased blood volume and viscosity; the latter increases exponentially with increased hematocrit.[73] When flow rate through a capillary tube is determined at various levels of hematocrit, flow decreases as an essentially linear function of hematocrit (Fig. 55–10). The product of flow rate and arterial oxygen content provides a relative measure of the rate of oxygen transport through a single blood vessel; optimal hematocrit is just below 40 per cent. Delivery of oxygen to the body depends on the product of total blood flow and the oxygen content of arterial blood, which tends to be high in polycythemia vera, in which blood volume, cardiac output, and arterial blood oxygen content are all elevated, despite the increase in viscosity. Although the increases in oxygen content, blood volume, and cardiac output in polycythemia vera are not required for adequate tissue oxygenation, in the polycythemias secondary to hypoxemia the increases in blood oxygen content and cardiac output represent an attempt to improve oxygen delivery.

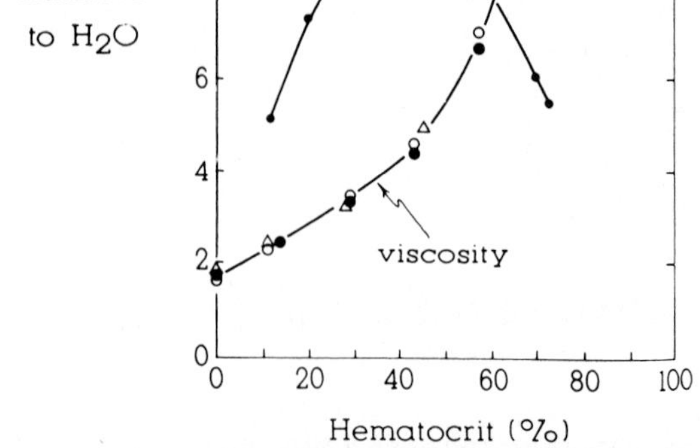

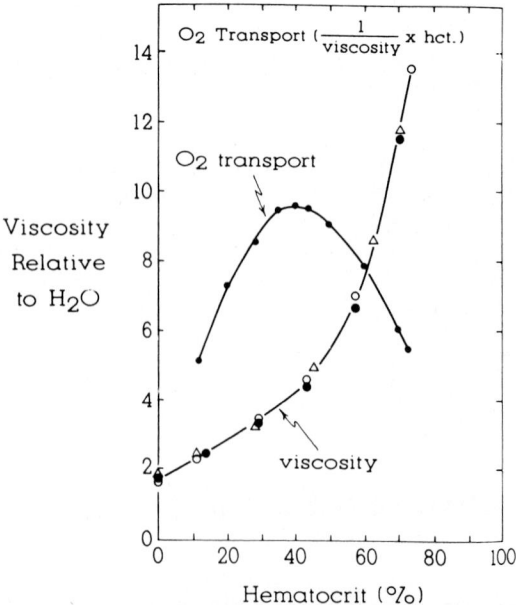

FIGURE 55–10. Viscosity of heparinized normal blood related to hematocrit. Viscosity was measured with an Ostwald viscosimeter at 37° C and expressed in relation to viscosity of water. Oxygen transport was calculated from the product of hematocrit and 1/viscosity and is recorded in arbitrary units. (From Williams, W. J. [ed.]: Hematology, 2nd ed. New York, McGraw-Hill Book Co., 1977, p. 256.)

POLYCYTHEMIA VERA

Although the pathogenesis of polycythemia vera is not understood, this condition has been classified as a myeloproliferative disorder.[74] All hematopoietic cells are monoclonal based on assays of glucose-6-phosphate dehydrogenase (G-6-PD) isoenzymes,[75] an enzymatic marker that has been used as evidence of the clonal origin of a tumor. In black patients heterozygous for G-6-PD, normal tissues will possess both isoenzymes A (phenotype: Gd-A) and B (phenotype: Gd-B); if only one isoenzyme is present in the neoplastic cells of such a patient, a clonal origin of the neoplasm or, in this case, the disease polycythemia vera is likely. Thus, erythropoietin is not the stimulus for increased red cell production; indeed, erythropoietin concentrations may be low in this condition.

If erythrocytosis is accompanied by an increased red cell mass, arterial oxygen saturation less than 92 per cent, and splenomegaly, the diagnosis of polycythemia vera is confirmed. In the absence of splenomegaly, any two of the following laboratory findings will satisfy the diagnostic criteria: thrombocytosis, leukocytosis (in the absence of infection), elevated leukocyte alkaline phosphatase activity, or a combination of elevated serum vitamin B_{12} concentration and unsaturated B_{12} binding capacity.[76]

CLINICAL MANIFESTATIONS. These may be divided into symptoms secondary to the increased red cell mass and increased blood volume, including headache, plethora, pruritus, dyspnea, and bleeding; those due to increased blood viscosity, including paresthesias and thrombosis; and those due to hypermetabolism, including weight loss despite a good appetite and night sweats. Angina pectoris, intermittent claudication, and arterial hypertension occur frequently.

It seems paradoxical that both bleeding and thrombosis can be complications of this disease; however, each occurs in 33 to 50 per cent of patients, and they are the major causes of morbidity and mortality. Bleeding is caused by the distention of veins and capillaries due to the increased blood volume, defective platelet function, or both. Thrombosis has been thought to be related to increased blood viscosity, thrombocytosis, and abnormally increased aggregation of platelets. Thrombotic sites include coronary and cerebral arteries as well as those in the extremities. Less frequently, thrombosis may involve the mesenteric and portal veins. Surgical morbidity is high in patients with polycythemia vera who are inadequately treated, and anesthesia and the stress of operation increase further the risk of hemorrhagic and thrombotic events during the immediate postoperative period.

TREATMENT. Therapy is aimed primarily at decreasing the potential for both hemorrhage and thrombosis. Ideally, this consists of phlebotomy alone. If control of thrombocytosis is necessary, hydroxyurea appears to be the most efficacious agent.[76]

MECHANISMS OF SYMPTOMS. The clinical severity of polycythemia is usually related to the degree of hypervolemia and increased viscosity.[73, 74] In older patients with underlying atherosclerotic vascular disease, cardiac output tends not to be elevated, and as a consequence of the increased viscosity without increased flow, the incidence of ischemic episodes may be higher. In vitro studies suggest that white blood cells can contribute significantly to blood viscosity[77]; since leukocytosis is characteristic of polycythemia vera, white cells undoubtedly play a role in the elevated viscosity seen in this disease.

Cerebral blood flow is significantly reduced and is associated with cerebral symptoms in about half the patients with hematocrits averaging 53.6 per cent, confirming the relationship between cerebrovascular insufficiency and blood viscosity.[78] When hematocrit is lowered to approximately 45 per cent, viscosity declines by 30 per cent and cerebral blood flow increases substantially. With hematocrit values ranging from 46 to 52 per cent, cerebral blood flow is still less than normal, suggesting that even slight increases in red cell mass may interfere with cerebral perfusion. These results imply that patients with polycythemia vera should undergo phlebotomy until hematocrit levels reach the low 40s rather than the previously recommended level of about 45 per cent.

SECONDARY POLYCYTHEMIAS

The secondary polycythemias may be divided into two subgroups: (1) those in which the increased red cell mass compensates for a reduction in oxygen transport with appropriate stimulation by erythropoietin and (2) those in which erythrocytosis is associated with an inappropriate increase in erythropoietin production. It has been suggested that any hypoxic stimulus will cause production of the enzyme erythrogenin in the kidney, which generates erythropoietin by acting enzymatically on a proposed plasma protein substrate, possibly of hepatic origin (Fig. 55–11). If an individual living at sea level is transported to a high altitude, hemoglobin concentrations will rise[79] accompanied by an increase in urinary erythropoietin. Similarly, with severe degrees of chronic hypoxemia in chronic obstructive pulmonary disease, an arterial PO_2 less than 60 mm Hg usually leads to an increase in red cell mass. Although in some instances hemoglobin has been reported to be as high as 24 gm/dl and the hematocrit as high as 75 per cent, in most patients with chronic pulmonary disease these values do not exceed 17 gm/dl and 57 per cent, respectively.[80] In cyanotic congenital heart disease, red cell mass increases as resting arterial oxygen saturation falls (p. 903). Hematocrits as high as 86 per cent may be seen with red blood cell masses almost three times normal.[81] Although plasma volume may be diminished, total blood volume remains significantly elevated because of the striking increase in red cell mass. The most common congenital malformations producing these elevations include tetralogy of Fallot, transposition of the great arteries, and persistent truncus arteriosus (see Chap. 30).

CLINICAL MANIFESTATIONS. Signs and symptoms of hyperviscosity generally occur as hematocrit exceeds 60 per cent; cardiac function may be compromised because of the combination of hypervolemia and the constant volume load and augmented vascular resistance secondary to the increased viscosity of the blood. Ruddy cyanosis, headache, dizziness, roaring in the ears, thrombotic episodes, and bleeding are the major clinical findings and may be treated with phlebotomy.[82] Careful monitoring during phlebotomy is necessary, and the acute reduction in blood volume may have to be avoided by the simultaneous administration of plasma expanders.[83] After isovolemic phlebotomy to reduce the hematocrit from the 70's to the 60's, cardiac output rises, and despite the fall in arterial oxygen content, systemic oxygen transport usually increases. These favorable changes are attributed to the reduced blood viscosity and vascular resistance. Although the erythrocytosis is a homeostatic mechanism compensating for the chronic arterial hypoxemia, greatly increased hematocrits are generally undesirable. Studies by Erslev suggest that secondary polycythemia is not necessarily a boon but could be a burden, and that secondary erythrocytosis cannot always be considered optimal for overall oxygen transport.[84] Secondary polycythemia due to cyanotic congenital heart disease has been reported to cause myocardial infarction without manifestations of coronary atherosclerosis.[85, 86]

MANAGEMENT. Phlebotomy, or preferably erythropheresis, in secondary polycythemia reduces blood viscosity, increases systemic oxygen transport without lowering peripheral oxygen consumption, and simultaneously increases effective renal plasma flow.[87, 88] The optimal hematocrit for patients with cyanotic congenital heart disease and other chronically hypoxemic states is poorly defined and presents an interesting and perplexing dilemma. The clinical presentation of the patient must be carefully considered. Cerebral blood flow is reduced in secondary erythrocytosis as well as in polycythemia vera and improves with phlebotomy.[89, 90] If phlebotomy is deemed necessary, close monitoring of the patient's blood pressure, heart rate, arterial oxygen saturation, and general condition is necessary. As might be expected from the decreased oxygen transport associated with right-to-left shunts, P_{50} and red cell 2,3-DPG are increased, but the relationship between decreased arterial PO_2 and the rise in P_{50} and red cell 2,3-DPG varies greatly.[91] Successful surgical correction of the cardiac defect will result in normal saturation and obviate the adaptive mechanism, and hematocrit and blood volume will return to normal.

HEMOGLOBIN VARIANTS WITH INCREASED AFFINITY FOR OXYGEN. In 1966, it was first recognized that a hemoglobin variant with increased oxygen affinity could be associated with erythrocytosis.[92] These variants, which generally have amino acid substitutions at structural sites crucial to hemoglobin function, now number over 40. They are transmitted in an autosomal dominant fashion and cause a shift in the oxygen dissociation curve to the left with reduced levels of P_{50}. The shift to the left of the Hb-O_2 dissociation curve results in a marked reduction in oxygen extraction by the tissues. Increased hemoglobin concentration and blood flow are available compensatory mechanisms to maintain oxygen delivery (Fig. 55–2). However, the primary response appears to be erythrocytosis mediated by increases in erythropoietin.[93-95] The cardiac output is usually normal. Polycythemia constitutes the primary adjustment for oxygen delivery in patients with these hemoglobin variants, who have no increased incidence of myocardial ischemia or other forms of organ hypoxia.

OTHER CAUSES. True erythrocytosis without demonstrable cause, other than excessive cigar and cigarette smoking, has also been noted in a significant number of individuals.[96] All had elevated levels of carboxyhemoglobin with shifts of the Hb-O_2 dissociation curve to the left, stimulating erythropoiesis. In most cases of polycythemia secondary to inappropriate erythropoietin production, such as tumors, renal cysts, and hydronephrosis, the red cell mass, although increased, does not generally cause symptoms of hyperviscosity.

RELATIVE POLYCYTHEMIA. Relative polycythemia is a distinct and commonly encountered entity that is also referred to as spurious polycythemia, Gaisbock syndrome, and stress erythrocytosis. It is not a primary disease process and may be merely a physiologic state in which the plasma volume is slightly reduced and the red cell mass is slightly increased. Hematocrit rarely exceeds 60 per cent, and other blood constituents are normal. This disorder can be distinguished from polycythemia vera by measuring the red cell mass, which by definition is normal in relative polycythemia and elevated in polycythemia vera. Patients are often hypertensive, prone to thromboembolic complications,[97] and obese; however, these complications appear to be unrelated to the hematological changes, so that reducing the red cell mass by phlebotomy or chemotherapy is not appropriate. When present, hypertension and thromboembolic complications should be treated in the usual manner.

Thrombocytosis

Occasionally thrombocytosis may be seen alone as a manifestation of a myeloproliferative disorder without an increased hematocrit. Pri-

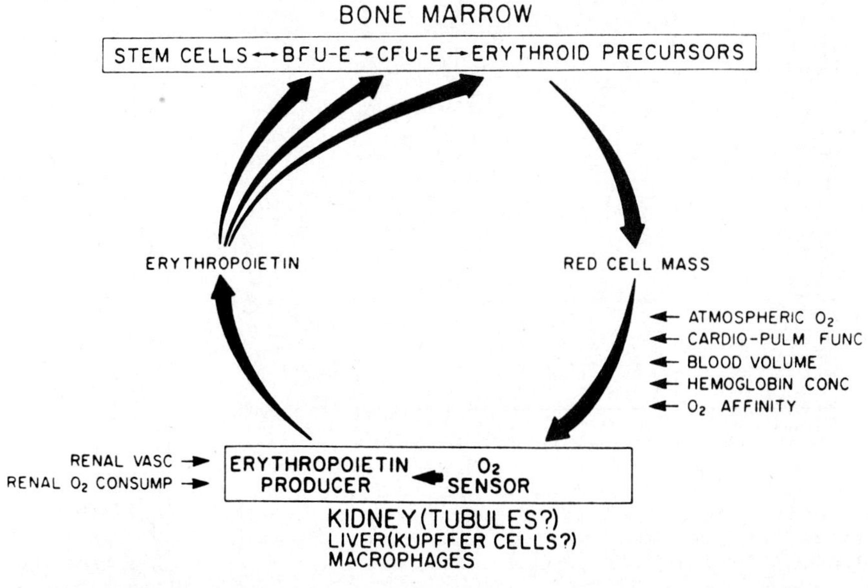

FIGURE 55–11. Feedback circuit linking an oxygen sensor in the kidney with erythroid progenitor cells in the bone marrow. The circuit is moved in one direction by red cells containing oxygen and in the opposite direction by erythropoietin. Oxygen sensing and erythropoietin production may also take place in the liver and in some macrophages. The target for erythropoietin is primarily the erythropoietin-dependent progenitor cells (CFU-E), with milder actions on the burst-forming progenitor cells (BFU-E) and the precursor cells. (From Ersley, A. J., and Caro, J.: Secondary polycythemia: A boon or a burden? Blood Cells *10*:177, 1984.)

mary thrombocytosis or essential thrombocythemia has been associated in several instances with myocardial infarctions in young people without underlying atherosclerosis.[98-100] Rheological changes in the blood have been found to be associated with myocardial infarction, but it is not clear whether these changes are secondary to infarction or whether they play an initiating role. Changes in blood viscosity, plasma viscosity, and red cell filterability occur in patients with myocardial infarction or unstable active angina and may play an important role in its pathogenesis. Although these changes may not contribute to disease in many other parts of the body, they may be significant in the coronary microcirculation.

CARDIAC MANIFESTATIONS OF NEOPLASTIC DISEASE

INCIDENCE. Primary tumors of the heart (Chap. 43) are rare, occurring in less than 0.1 per cent of autopsies. Tumors metastatic to the pericardium or heart are far more common, ranging from 1.5 to 20.6 per cent (average 6 per cent) of autopsies on patients with malignant diseases. Usually the metastases involve the pericardium (p. 1515) and myocardium, with the valves or endocardium rarely affected, and the right side of the heart appears to be affected more frequently than the left.[104] Solitary metastases to the heart are rare. Although metastatic nodules in the heart are generally multiple (Fig. 55–12), they may become diffuse and lead to the manifestations of a restrictive cardiomyopathy (p. 1430). The mode of spread to the heart may be by direct extension, as occurs in lung cancer; via the hematogenous route, as in malignant melanoma; or through lymphatic channels, as in lymphoma.

The most common primary tumor producing cardiac metastases is carcinoma of the bronchus (Fig. 55–12), with carcinoma of the breast, malignant melanoma, lymphomas, and leukemias next in order of frequency (Table 55–2).[104, 105] At autopsy, 15 to 35 per cent of patients dying with primary lung cancer show cardiac involvement, while over 60 per cent of patients with melanoma have cardiac metastases.[106] Hematological malignancies, especially lymphomas, have been reported to account for 15 per cent of all cardiac and pericardial metastases,[107] and about 15 per cent of patients dying of malignant lymphomas show metastases to the heart.

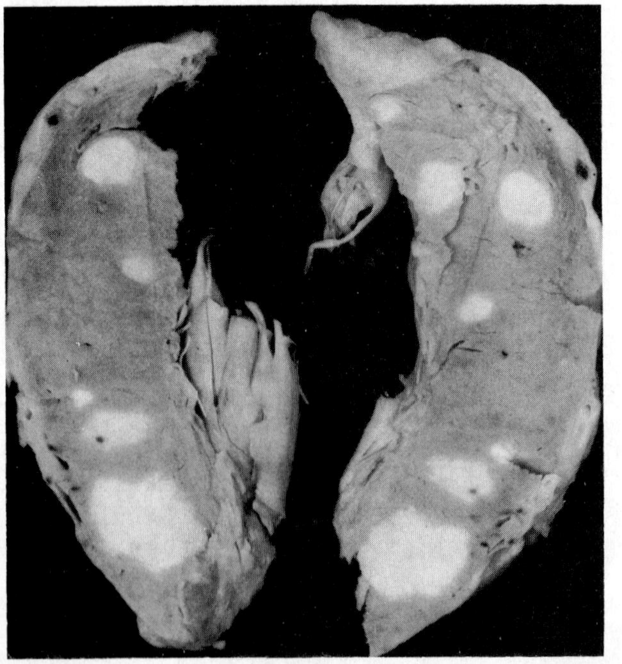

FIGURE 55–12. Sections of left ventricle showing metastatic nodules in the myocardium. Primary tumor was in a bronchus. (From Edwards, J. E.: Effects of malignant noncardiac tumors upon the cardiovascular system. *In* Brest, A. N. [ed.]: Cardiovascular Clinics, Vol. 4. Philadelphia, F. A. Davis, 1972, p. 282.)

TABLE 55–2 METASTATIC CARDIAC DISEASE

Tumor Type	Total No.	Metastases		
		Heart	Pericardial	Both
Bronchogenic carcinoma	402	43 (10.2)	66 (15.7)	23 (5.4)
Breast carcinoma	289	24 (8.3)	34 (11.8)	3 (1.4)
Malignant melanoma	59	20 (34.0)	14 (23.7)	12 (20.4)
Colonic carcinoma	214	2 (0.9)	6 (2.8)	0
Esophageal carcinoma	65	5 (7.7)	5 (7.7)	2 (3.6)
Hypernephroma	95	5 (5.3)	0	0
Ovarian carcinoma	115	6 (5.7)	8 (7.0)	3 (2.6)
Prostatic carcinoma	186	5 (2.7)	2 (1.0)	0
Gastric carcinoma	308	11 (3.6)	10 (3.2)	3 (0.9)
Sarcoma*	207	19 (9.2)	19 (9.2)	8 (3.9)
Hodgkin's disease	75	—	11 (14.6)	—
Acute leukemia	420	227 (53.9)	95 (22.4)	—
Total	2,435	367 (15.1)	270 (11.1)	54 (2.2)

*Reticulum cell sarcoma and lymphosarcoma.
Note: Numbers in parentheses represent percentages.
From Applefeld, M. M., and Pollock, S. H.: Cardiac disease in patients who have malignancies. Curr. Probl. Cardiol. *4*(6):5, 1980.

CLINICAL MANIFESTATIONS

Many metastatic cardiac lesions are clinically silent and are found only at necropsy. For example, despite massive heart involvement with melanoma ("charcoal heart"), there may be little evidence of cardiac dysfunction.[108] Specific clinical manifestations of cardiac involvement by cancer may be divided into those due to pericardial, myocardial, or endocardial involvement; indirect consequences of tumor complications of circulating mediators; embolization in patients in a hypercoagulable state; or the effects of specific tumor therapy, such as chemotherapy and radiation therapy (Table 55–3).[104, 105] The most common clinical manifestations result from pericardial effusion with tamponade, tachyarrhythmias, AV block,[109] or congestive heart failure. Metastatic cardiac disease is rarely the presenting symptom of a tumor. The mode of spread may be by direct extension via the hematogenous route or through lymphatic channels. Routine chest radiographs, computed chest tomography, magnetic resonance imaging, echocardiography, and/or radionuclide imaging with gallium or thallium are often helpful in diagnosis.[110-116] Osteogenic sarcoma, which may metastasize to the heart, is unique because the metastases contain bone and may be radiographically visible.

PERICARDIAL INVOLVEMENT (See also p. 1515). Signs and symptoms of pericarditis with pericardial effusion and cardiac tamponade are typical in patients with carcinoma of the lung and breast as well as in Hodgkin's disease, non-Hodgkin's lymphoma,[118] and the leukemias,[119] particularly acute myelogenous, lymphoblastic leukemia and the blast crisis of chronic myelogenous leukemia.[120] Pericardial

TABLE 55–3 CLINICAL MANIFESTATIONS OF CARDIAC INVOLVEMENT IN MALIGNANT DISEASE

- Pericardial involvement
  - Pericarditis
  - Cardiac tamponade
- Superior vena caval syndrome
- Arrhythmias
  - Supraventricular tachycardia
  - Carotid sinus syncope
  - Atrioventricular block
- Cardiomegaly and congestive heart failure
- Unexplained heart murmur
- Unexplained hypotension
- Noninfective (marantic) endocarditis

involvement is usually diagnosed antemortem because of the resultant symptomatology and radiographic and echocardiographic evidence. Clinically, this takes the form of either cardiac tamponade or adhesive pericarditis, associated with extensive nodular tumor infiltration of the pericardium.[121] The finding of chylous pericardial effusion is usually characteristic of lymphomatous involvement.[122] Echocardiography is a key tool in the diagnosis of neoplastic involvement of the pericardium. With increased use of serial M-mode echocardiography in patients with advanced malignant disease, the incidence of pericardial effusions appears to be much higher than was previously thought[99, 100, 114, 123, 124] (Fig 55–13). Pericardiocentesis may be necessary to differentiate tumor from radiation effects.[125]

Pericardial tumor or fibrosis secondary to radiation therapy may mimic chronic constrictive pericarditis or chronic effusive pericardial disease and cause problems in differential diagnosis. In patients with carcinoma of the lung, Hodgkin's disease, and non-Hodgkin's lymphoma, who commonly undergo irradiation of the thorax, radiation-induced pericarditis is common, and it was believed that this condition could be differentiated from tumor involvement because it occurred usually within a year of such therapy. However, it has become clear that radiation-induced pericarditis may occur as late as 8 years after therapy.[126] In patients with leukemia, massive involvement of the pericardium and epicardium is a common finding at autopsy,[127] with the extent of infiltration usually related to the degree of elevation of circulating white cells. Leukemic infiltration of the heart is more common in the acute leukemias and in the blast crisis phase of chronic myelogenous leukemia.

MYOCARDIAL METASTASES. Direct myocardial or endocardial involvement by tumor may result in arrhythmias, congestive heart failure, ventricular outflow tract obstruction, and peripheral emboli. Cardiac metastases detected on two-dimensional echocardiography have been described

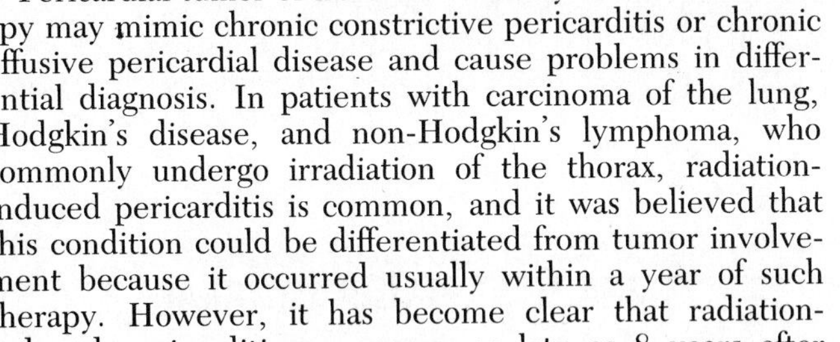

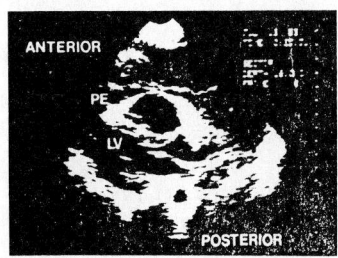

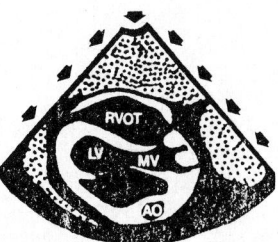

FIGURE 55–13. Two-dimensional, parasternal, long-axis view (*left*) with schematic diagram (*right*) in lymphoblastic lymphoma involving the pericardium. Note a small amount of pericardial effusion (PE) and extensive thickening of the pericardium encasing the heart (arrowheads in right panel). AO = aorta; LV = left ventricle; MV = mitral valve; RVOT = right ventricular outflow tract. (From Kutalek, S. P., et al.: Metastatic tumors of the heart detected by two-dimensional echocardiography. Am. Heart J. *109*:343, 1985.)

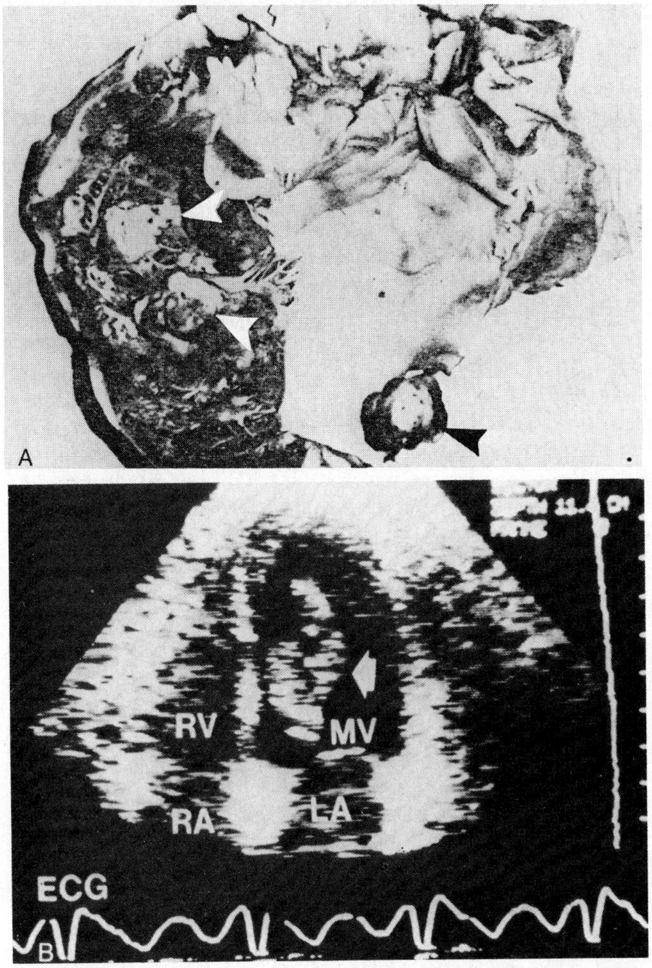

FIGURE 55–14. *A*, Gross view of specimen of melanoma metastatic to the heart. *B*, Two-dimensional, apical, four-chamber echocardiographic view in metastatic melanoma, showing a large mass in the left ventricular cavity (arrowhead), probably attached to the ventricular septum. LA = left atrium; MV = mitral valve; RA = right atrium, RV = right ventricle. (From Kutalek, S. P., et al.: Metastatic tumors of the heart detected by two-dimensional echocardiography. Am. Heart J. *109*:343, 1985.)

(Fig. 55–14).[114] For example, melanoma favors the endocardium and may often appear as an intracavitary mass (Fig. 55–14*A*).

VENA CAVAL OBSTRUCTION. The superior vena caval syndrome, resulting from obstruction of this vessel by tumor, is also a recognized complication in patients with carcinoma of the lung and malignant lymphoma.[128] Enlarged mediastinal nodes or the primary tumor itself may impinge upon or even occlude the superior vena cava, causing dyspnea, distention of the neck veins, edema of the face and arms, proptosis, headache, and syncope. Because of the potential life-threatening nature of these problems, local irradiation may have to be initiated prior to any diagnostic procedure. Similar enlargement of nodes or tumor may cause obstruction of the inferior vena cava, with massive leg edema, congestive hepatomegaly, and hypotension.[129]

CARDIAC AMYLOIDOSIS (See also p. 1431). The heart is involved in the majority of cases of primary amyloidosis and also in many instances of amyloidosis secondary to multiple myeloma. Symptoms often include congestive heart failure, hypotension, cardiac arrhythmias, and conduction disturbances.[130, 131] Echocardiographic examination, contrast tomography, and endomyocardial biopsy have made it easier to confirm this diagnosis. A low myocardial density on contrast-aided tomography, diffuse myocardial thickening, and diffuse hypokinetic wall motion may be the result of cardiac amyloidosis and may simulate hypertrophic cardiomyopathy. Endomyocardial biopsy may be necessary to confirm the diagnosis.[132-134]

ELECTROCARDIOGRAPHIC AND ROENTGENOGRAPHIC FINDINGS. Arrhythmias and a wide variety of electrocardiographic changes are common in patients with metastatic disease. Although they may certainly be caused by tumor involvement of the heart, they are more often due to concomitant factors, such as altered electrolyte concentrations, anemia, and hypoxia. Nonspecific ST-segment and T-wave changes, low voltage, and sinus tachycardia are frequent electrocardiographic abnormalities and cannot be considered diagnostic.[135] Clinically it may be difficult to determine whether any such abnormality is attributable to cardiac metastases or is due to an associated cardiac problem, irradiation, or the cardiotoxic effects of drugs. Atrial arrhythmias, such as fibrillation and flutter, may occur secondary to either neoplastic involvement of autonomic fibers supplying the atria or tumor invasion of the coronary arteries perfusing the atria, with resulting atrial infarction or to neoplastic infiltration of the atrial myocardium or sinus node. Similarly, electrocardiographic changes of acute myocardial infarction can be produced by tumor infiltration or hemorrhage into the ventricle or occlusion of one of the coronary arteries. Occasionally, the exact area of tumor involvement may be pinpointed based on the acute electrocardiographic changes.[136] Involvement of the AV node is a rare cause of complete heart block but may be the presenting symptom of the tumor.[137] In addition, tumor involvement of cervical lymph nodes without mediastinal involvement has been associated with carotid sinus syncope.[138]

Roentgenographic evidence of cardiac enlargement and the development of congestive heart failure may be the only clinical signs of malignant involvement of the heart. Unexplained pansystolic or late systolic murmurs may occur with intraluminal invasion or external compression of the carotid or pulmonary arteries by the tumor.[139] In addition to coincidental atherosclerosis, coronary artery disease in cancer patients can be caused by tumor emboli, extrinsic compression of the coronary arteries or ostia, or thromboemboli brought about by tumor-associated coagulation disorders.

MYOCARDIAL INFARCTION. In a necropsy study of 816 patients with solid tumors, 33 (4 per cent) died of myocardial infarction.[140] Patients with carcinoma of the lung, malignant lymphoma, and leukemia are most commonly afflicted; less affected were patients with cancer of the breast and gastrointestinal tract and malignant melanoma.[141] In general, the etiology of coronary artery disease in patients with cancer is most likely coincidental spontaneous atherosclerosis.[142] The most common cause of tumor-related myocardial infarction is extrinsic compression of a coronary artery, occurring in 60 per cent of cases, whereas tumor emboli are responsible for about 35 per cent. Widespread thromboses, including coronary artery thromboses due to disseminated intravascular coagulation, occasionally occur in patients with metastatic tumors, most commonly mucin-secreting adenocarcinomas. Half of all patients with acute myocardial infarction secondary to malignant disease had a history of typical chest pain prior to death. An acute myocardial infarction in a patient with advanced malignant disease is a particularly poor prognostic sign, since more than two-thirds of such patients die within 3 weeks of the event.

VALVULAR AND ENDOCARDIAL INVOLVEMENT. Metastatic tumors may affect cardiac valves in a variety of ways, including direct invasion of valves, interference with valvular function by compression, humoral valvular dysfunction secondary to carcinoid tumors, or noninfective (marantic) endocarditis.[143] This last type occurs with various forms of malignant disease, especially adenocarcinoma, leukemia, and lymphoma and may be diagnosed only at autopsy.[144] The pathogenesis is unclear; nonbacterial thrombotic endocarditis is most frequently associated with Hodgkin's disease; carcinoma of the pancreas, stomach, colon, and lung; and the rare condition of acute eosinophilic leukemia. There is evidence that immune complexes, elicited by the underlying malignant process, play an important role in the pathogenesis of thrombus formation in noninfective thrombotic endocarditis.[145] Although the exact relationship between the latter and endomyocardial fibrosis is unclear, there is a high correlation between eosinophilia in the bone marrow and peripheral blood and the occurrence of endomyocardial fibrosis,[146] which may cause restrictive cardiomyopathy (p. 1430). Ever since Loeffler described the entity "endocarditis parietalis fibroplastica" with eosinophilia, this association has been of interest but remains unexplained. In some patients, the cardiac manifestations predominate, most commonly cardiomegaly, congestive heart failure, arrhythmias, and heart murmurs, whereas in others, all or most of the clinical manifestations are secondary to the eosinophilic leukemia. Pathologically, these syndromes are characterized by local or widespread eosinophilic infiltrates with fibrous scarring and thickening of the endocardium, including the atrioventricular valves. In many patients, the course is chronic and insidious, but death is usually the direct result of cardiac involvement.

CARDIAC EFFECTS OF RADIATION THERAPY AND CHEMOTHERAPY

With the advent of intensive radiation therapy and aggressive chemotherapy, cardiac toxicity of antitumor treatment has increased greatly. Formerly, the heart was considered one of the most radioresistant organs and seemed to be spared most of the side effects of chemotherapy. However, the incidence of cardiovascular complications has risen sharply with the use of curative forms of radiation therapy for Hodgkin's disease and non-Hodgkin's lymphoma and the addition of one of the most potent classes of chemotherapeutic agents, the anthracyclines.

RADIATION THERAPY

Therapeutic radiation can cause heart damage by injuring various structures either acutely or chronically (Table 55–4). Most commonly affected is the pericardium, with less damage to the myocardium, endocardium, and papillary muscles, and the least damage to the heart valves and coronary arteries (Table 55–5).[147] Severe pericardial damage with pericarditis,[148-150] acute myocardial infarction,[126,151-154] valvular disease,[155-158] cardiomyopathy,[159] and arrhythmias[160] are the most frequently observed complications.

PERICARDIAL EFFECTS. Niemtzow and Reynolds have divided radiation-induced pericardial abnormalities into early, intermediate, and late changes (Table 55–4).[147] The most common acute cardiovascular complication of radiation therapy is pericarditis.[149] Acute pericarditis occurs in 10 to 15 per cent of patients with Hodgkin's disease who receive over 4000 rads to the mediastinum.[150] These epi-

TABLE 55–4 EFFECT OF RADIATION ON THE HEART

Early changes
Cytoplasmic damage
Capillary injury
DNA damage
Local chemical reactions
von Willebrand factor release
Platelet and fibrin deposition
Acute inflammatory reaction
Increased vascular permeability
Protein damage
Transient pericardial effusion
Intermediate changes
Cellular immune response
Vascular compromise
Attempts at repair
Organized fibrin formation
Endothelial proliferation
Collagen deposition
Late changes
Compromised vascular supply
Cell death
Fibroblastic proliferation
Altered cell morphology
Enhanced atherosclerosis
Thickening of pericardium
Loss of adventitial tissue
Pericardial effusion
Endocardial thickening
Valvular heart disease
Arrhythmias

From Niemtzow, R. C., and Reynolds, R. D.: Radiation therapy and the heart. *In* Kapoor, A. S. (ed.): Cancer and The Heart. New York, Springer-Verlag, 1986, p. 240.

sodes are characterized by fever, pleuritic pain, pericardial friction rub, and electrocardiographic and echocardiographic changes typical of this condition (p. 1517). The time from completion of chemotherapy to the clinical onset of pericarditis ranges from 0 to 85 months, with the peak incidence occurring between 5 and 9 months. Echocardiography demonstrates a pericardial effusion in almost all patients.[161] With long followup of patients cured of their underlying neoplastic disease, symptoms of pericarditis may not develop for 8 to 10 years.[126] The incidence of pericarditis appears to be a function of the fractional and total dose of radiation to the pericardium and the quantity of the heart irradiated. When the entire dose of radiation is delivered through an anterior port, the incidence of pericarditis is increased. However, when chest irradiation is delivered in divided doses to anterior and posterior ports and with a subcarinal shield, the incidence of pericarditis has decreased to 2.5 per cent, without increasing the risk of relapse of Hodgkin's disease. If the entire heart receives therapeutic doses of radiation, up to 50 per cent of patients may develop pericardial complications.[162] With large mediastinal masses, to insure adequate therapy, whole heart irradiation has been replaced with curative forms of chemotherapy.

TABLE 55–5 CLASSIFICATION OF RADIATION-RELATED CARDIAC DISEASE

1. Acute pericarditis (caused by necrosis of tumor adjacent to the heart)
2. Delayed pericarditis
   a. Acute radiation-induced pericarditis, without effusion
   b. Acute radiation-induced pericarditis, with effusion, with/without cardiac tamponade
   c. Chronic effusive pericarditis
   d. Effusive-constrictive pericarditis
   e. Chronic pericardial constriction
   f. Occult constrictive pericarditis
3. Myocardial fibrosis
4. Occlusive coronary artery disease
5. Conduction abnormalities
6. Valvular regurgitation or stenosis

MYOCARDIAL AND ENDOCARDIAL EFFECTS. Echocardiographic studies carried out before and within 6 months after conventional irradiation therapy in women with breast cancer revealed an asymptomatic decrease of the fractional systolic shortening of the left ventricular minor-axis diameter and of the systolic blood pressure/end-systolic diameter ratio. These changes, which reflect slight transient depression of left ventricular function, occurred within the first 6 months after postoperative radiation and disappeared by 6 months.[163] It has been suggested that routine followup during the first year after radiation therapy should consist of frequent echocardiograms and chest roentgenograms. If any evidence of increased cardiac diameter is noted, or if clinical manifestations suggestive of pericarditis or pericardial effusion develop and there is no reason to suspect another cause of pericarditis, patients may be treated symptomatically but occasionally may require pericardiocentesis and/or pericardiectomy.[125, 126]

Radiation-induced endocardial fibrosis may cause manifestations of a restrictive cardiomyopathy[159] (p. 1430) and a variety of nonspecific electrocardiographic changes[164] as well as varying degrees of AV block.[160] Mitral regurgitation may develop secondary to radiation-induced papillary muscle dysfunction and aortic regurgitation as a consequence of endocardial valvular thickening.[155, 157] The onset of new murmurs occurring after radiation therapy should alert the physician to these possibilities. In an autopsy study of the cardiac effects of radiation exposure, three-fourths of the patients exposed to more than 3500 rads, with a field resulting in more exposure of the anterior thorax, developed interstitial myocardial fibrosis, with more extensive involvement of the right than the left ventricle. Functional abnormalities demonstrated on echocardiography and radionuclide angiocardiography may occur 5 to 15 years after radiation but, as with pericarditis, should become less frequent with new techniques of radiotherapy.[148]

CORONARY AND CAROTID ARTERIAL EFFECTS. Since the report by Cohn et al. in 1967 of a 15-year-old boy suffering a fatal myocardial infarction 16 months after receiving 4000 rads to the heart for Hodgkin's disease, a number of similar occurrences have been reported.[126, 151-154] Although coronary artery disease is common, supportive evidence for radiation-induced coronary artery disease includes (1) its occurrence in subjects who are very young with no predisposing factors and disease limited to coronary vessels within the path of the radiation beam, (2) the lack of atherosclerosis in arteries not exposed to irradiation, (3) reports of occlusive lesions in other arteries such as the carotid artery after irradiation,[165] (4) the presence of distinctive pathological changes, and (5) the production of similar lesions in experimental models.

Occlusive coronary and carotid artery disease following irradiation generally occurs 6 to 12 years after exposure. In rabbits, 2500 rads has produced coronary atherosclerosis similar to that in humans.[166] However, rabbits do not develop radiation-induced atherosclerosis unless they also receive a diet high in lipids and cholesterol, which by itself is insufficient to produce the atherosclerotic lesion. Coronary artery lesions presumably induced by radiotherapy in patients appear to be distinct pathologically and to contain severe medial and adventitial fibrosis in continuity with overlying epicardial fibrous tissue and a marked paucity of lipid in the intimal lesions.[167] In affected young patients examined at autopsy, the proximal portions of the arteries are significantly more narrowed than the distal portions. In addition, there is significant loss of smooth muscle cells from the media.[167]

Radiation-induced coronary artery or carotid artery obstruction or occlusion may require surgical treatment. Because of the relatively low incidence of this complication and the concern that lowering the dose of radiation might preclude effective treatment of the neoplastic process, no systematic attempts have been made to try to prevent this complication other than considering chemotherapeutic alternatives if whole-heart irradiation is otherwise deemed necessary to "cure" the disease. It is anticipated that with changes in radiotherapeutic techniques and available curative chemotherapy, the incidence of all forms of radiation-induced heart disease will continue to decline.

CHEMOTHERAPY

Since the late 1960's there have been major advances in the management of a variety of neoplastic disorders using combination chemotherapy. Therapies have become more aggressive and new agents have been introduced, resulting in significant responses and longer survival. Unfortunately, concomitant with this increased response rate has been an increase in toxicity. Although most complications due to drugs are limited to rapidly proliferating tissues such as the bone marrow and gastrointestinal tract, cardiotoxicity, both early and late, has been recognized with increasing frequency (Table 55–6).[168-171]

For many years, the only notable cardiopulmonary complications of chemotherapy for neoplastic disease were orthostatic hypotension and the rare myocardial infarctions that occurred in the course of therapy with vincristine, a periwinkle alkaloid, and the interstitial lung disease and mild pulmonary hypertension secondary to pulmonary fibrosis created by bleomycin or busulfan.[172] However, with the advent of the anthracycline group of drugs (doxorubicin, daunorubicin), the incidence of cardiac toxicity as a consequence of chemotherapy for neoplastic disease has increased greatly.

ANTHRACYCLINE CARDIOTOXICITY. Doxorubicin is a glycoside antibiotic (Fig. 55–15). Its potent antitumor effect is attributed to its ability to inhibit nucleic acid synthesis by binding to both strands of the DNA helix, intercalating between base pairs, and thereby inhibiting the normal function of DNA and RNA polymerases. Doxorubicin has received more attention than the related compound daunorubicin because of its wider spectrum of antitumor activity in solid tumors and hematological malignancies.[173] Complete remissions in 30 to 40 per cent of patients with Hodgkin's disease and non-Hodgkin's lymphoma and all types of acute leukemia have been reported with doxorubicin treatment alone. However, its effectiveness is enhanced when it is combined with other chemotherapeutic agents. Remission rates of 60 to 80 per cent have been attained in adults with acute leukemia when doxorubicin was used in combination with cytosine arabinoside and in patients with lymphomas when it was combined with bleomycin, cyclophosphamide, vincristine, and corticosteroids.[173] Although the majority of toxic manifestations produced by these drugs, including alopecia, gastrointestinal distress, myelosuppression, and mucositis, had been predicted based on animal studies, the occurrence of cardiac toxicity and the interactions with radiation therapy were unexpected. Cardiotoxicity can be divided into early and late side effects (Table 55–7).

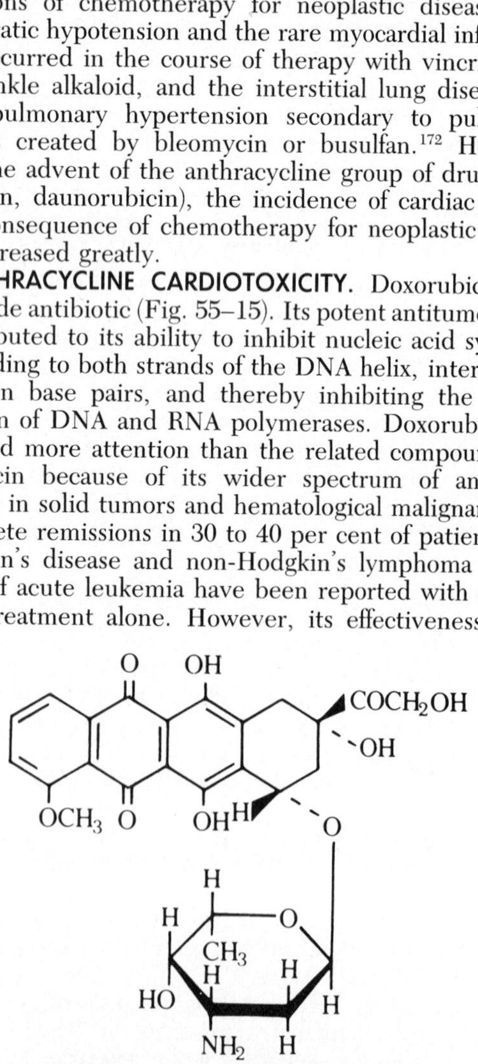

FIGURE 55–15. Structure of doxorubicin.

TABLE 55–6 MAJOR CARDIOVASCULAR COMPLICATIONS OF CHEMOTHERAPEUTIC AGENTS

AGENT	CARDIAC TOXICITY
Amsacrine	Arrhythmia, cardiomyopathy
Busulfan	Pulmonary fibrosis
	Pulmonary hypertension
	Endocardial fibrosis
Cisplatin	ECG changes
Cyclophosphamide	Cardiac necrosis
Cytosine arabinoside	Congestive heart failure
	Pericarditis
Diethylstilbestrol	Cardiovascular deaths
Doxorubicin	ECG changes, cardiomyopathy
Etoposide	? Sudden death, myocardial infarction
5-Fluorouracil	? Myocardial infarction
Methotrexate	ECG changes
Mitomycin	Myocardial damage
Mitoxantrone	Cardiomyopathy
Vincristine	Hypotension, myocardial infarction

Early or Acute Cardiotoxicity. This includes arrhythmias, electrocardiographic abnormalities, left ventricular dysfunction, a pericarditis-myocarditis syndrome, and rarely sudden death and myocardial infarction. Arrhythmias, which include supraventricular tachyarrhythmias and premature atrial and ventricular contractions, and abnormalities of conduction such as left axis deviation, decreased QRS voltage, and a variety of nonspecific ST-segment and T-wave abnormalities occur in approximately 11 per cent of patients (range = 0 to 41.2 per cent).[174, 175] These electrocardiographic changes are usually transient, may occur even at low doses of the anthracycline, and are usually seen within several days after administration of the drug.

The pericarditis-myocarditis syndrome and acute left ventricular dysfunction are rare events. The latter may occur in patients with marginal cardiac reserve, while the acute pericarditis-myocarditis syndrome has been seen in patients with no previous cardiac history.[176] Sudden death may occur as a result of an arrhythmia, myocardial infarction, or acute left ventricular dysfunction.[177]

TABLE 55–7 DOXORUBICIN CARDIAC TOXICITY

Early or acute
Arrhythmias
ECG changes
Left ventricular dysfunction
Pericarditis-myocarditis syndrome
Myocardial infarction
Sudden death
Late or chronic
Cardiomyopathy
Sinus tachycardia
Pericardial effusion
Left ventricular dysfunction
Low-output heart failure

Modified from Kapoor, A. S.: Doxorubicin Toxicity. *In* Kapoor, A. S. (ed.): Cancer and The Heart. New York, Springer-Verlag, 1986, p. 228.

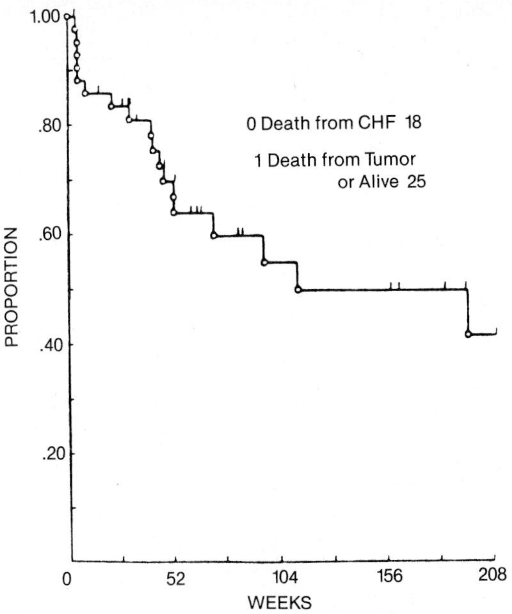

FIGURE 55–16. Actuarial survival plotted for all patients with doxorubicin-induced congestive heart failure. (From Haq, M. M., et al.: Doxorubicin-induced congestive heart failure in adults. Cancer *56*:1361, 1985.)

Late or Chronic Cardiotoxicity. This is primarily due to the development of a dose-dependent degenerative cardiomyopathy. The clinical manifestations consist of sinus tachycardia, tachypnea, cardiomegaly, peripheral and pulmonary edema, hepatomegaly, venous congestion, and pleural effusion. Cardiomyopathy is usually secondary to a cumulative effect of the drug, occurring with increasing frequency at higher doses. Congestive heart failure occurs from 9 to 192 days, with a median of 34 days after the administration of the last dose. It is usually refractory to therapy; when it is severe, as in patients who present with marked dyspnea and with evidence of heart failure within 4 weeks of the last dose of doxorubicin, survival is short, usually less than 2 weeks.[178, 179] The majority of patients with less severe symptoms may be treatable with digitalis and diuretics, but the incidence of cardiac death is high (Fig. 55–16).[178]

Pathological Examination. In chronic anthracycline toxicity, this discloses enlarged, pale, flabby hearts with dilated ventricles. Mural thrombi are occasionally found, but the coronary arteries and cardiac valves appear normal. Light microscopy reveals a severe cardiomyopathy with fewer myocardial cells, which show degenerative changes. Electron microscopy shows extensive depletion of myofibrillar bundles, myofibrillar lysis, and distortion and disruption of the Z-lines; the mitochondria are swollen with disrupted cristae and inclusion bodies[175, 179] (Fig. 55–17). Routine autopsy studies on patients who had received anthracycline chemotherapy during life have revealed that clinical evidence of toxicity may be present without histological signs; conversely, histological signs of drug toxicity may be seen in the absence of clinical signs or symptoms.[180]

Incidence. The incidence of cardiomyopathy with doxorubicin is 1.7 per cent and with daunorubicin 4.4 per cent. It is fatal in over half the cases.[174] With anthracycline, there is a clear dose-related incidence of cardiomyopathy. None of 764 patients who received a cumulative dose of less than 500 mg/m^2 showed cardiomyopathy, but a progressive increase in the frequency of this complication was noted with higher doses (Table 55–8).[179] It is therefore recommended that cumulative doses of doxorubicin be held to less than 450 to 500 mg/m^2 and 500 to 600 mg/m^2 for daunorubicin. However, cardiomyopathy is being reported with increasing frequency with doxorubicin doses below 450 mg/m^2.[175, 179, 181] It has been suggested that use of these agents in combination with other modalities of therapy, such as radiation or cyclophosphamide, may be synergistic in the pathogenesis of the cardiomyopathy in some patients, since both radiation and cyclophosphamide alone have been described as potentially cardiotoxic.[167, 181-184]

Mechanism. No mechanism for doxorubicin cardiotoxicity has been established, although numerous proposals have been put forward.[185] For example, lipid peroxidation may be caused by the binding of DNA by the drug, specifically bound to spectrin, actin, or cardiolipin.[186] Doxorubicin inhibits ATP production, interferes with the sarcolemmal sodium-potassium pump, inhibits oxidative phosphorylation, may provoke an autoimmune response, binds to DNA precursors, interferes with mitochondrial respiration by inhibiting coenzyme Q, and causes myocardial necrosis by allowing the buildup of myocardial calcium.[187]

Early Detection. Because of the importance of these

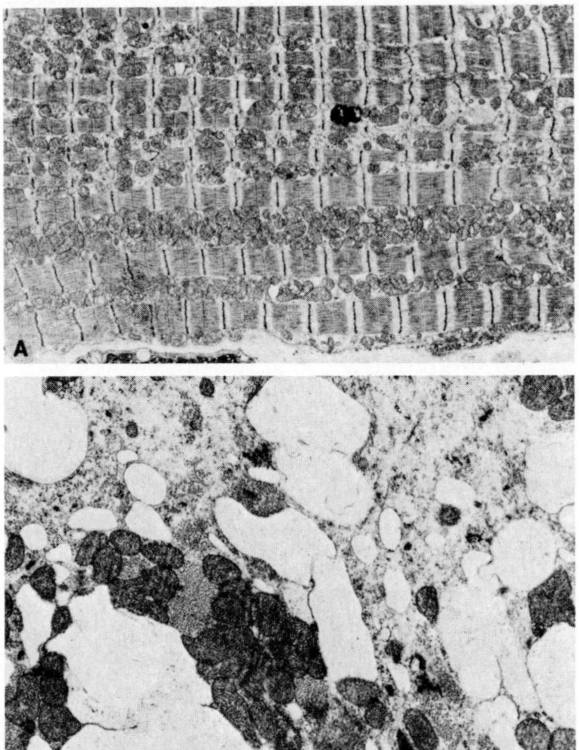

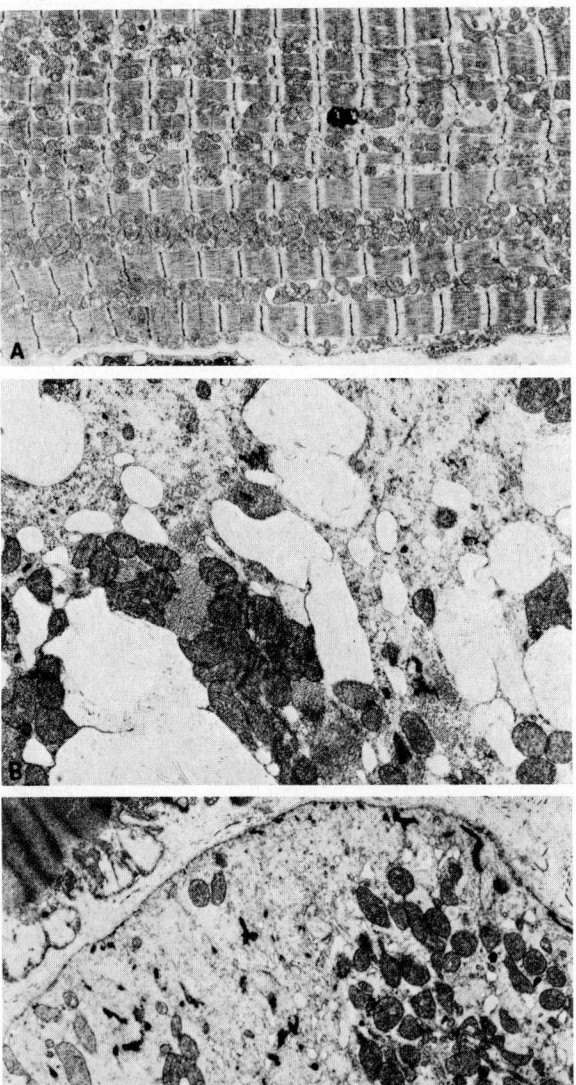

FIGURE 55–17. Electron microscopic images of cardiac biopsy specimens. *A*, Normal cardiac muscle fiber (grade 0). *B*, Vacuolation. *C*, Myofibrillar dropout (×3,575). (From Ali, M.D., and Ewer, M.S.: Cancer and The Cardiopulmonary System. New York, Raven Press, 1984, pp. 62 and 63.)

TABLE 55–8 CORRELATION OF CARDIOMYOPATHY (CMY) AND THE TOTAL DOSE OF ADRIAMYCIN IN ADULTS

TOTAL DOSE (mg/m²)	PATIENTS AT RISK	PATIENTS WITH CMY	FREQUENCY (%)
<450	738	0	0
451 to 500	26	0	0
501 to 550	32	3	9
551 to 600	15	3	20
>600	37	15	41
TOTAL >550	52	18	35
TOTAL <550	796	3	0.4

drugs in cancer chemotherapy and the high incidence of serious cardiac toxicity, several approaches have been suggested for early detection of this complication and for predicting susceptibility.[188, 189, 189a] Noninvasive studies include serial followup of systolic time intervals, in particular the PEP/LVET ratio (p. 54), and radionuclide angiography (p. 315). The PEP/LVET ratio was at first thought to be a sensitive parameter for monitoring toxicity; however, this has not been confirmed on further study and, in fact, has been criticized, since false-positive changes may have been responsible for the inappropriate withholding of potentially life-saving doxorubicin therapy.[190] Radionuclide angiography appears to provide a sensitive and reproducible measurement of left ventricular dysfunction due to doxorubicin cardiotoxicity.[188] Sequential studies demonstrate the frequent presence of subclinical left ventricular abnormalities.[191] However, the increased incidence of abnormal results may not be clinically significant if the studies are performed after exercise.

Endomyocardial biopsy appears to be more diagnostic of toxicity than are any of the noninvasive evaluations. In the hands of trained personnel, this technique may be considered a safe procedure[192] (p. 262). Administration of doxorubicin was associated with a dose-related increase in the degree of myocyte damage; drug-associated degenerative changes were identified in 27 of 129 patients at doses greater than or equal to 240 mg/m². Simultaneous studies using endomyocardial biopsy and radionuclide angiography demonstrate good correlation; while the noninvasive studies reveal an accelerating decrease in myocardial function with drug levels exceeding 400 mg/m², biopsy studies show a fairly constant progression of myocardial damage as a function of cumulative dose.[193] These findings suggest that compensatory mechanisms are available to maintain myocardial function despite pathological damage.

It is helpful to grade the hemodynamic abnormalities that occur in patients undergoing doxorubicin chemotherapy[194, 195] (Table 55–9). Cardiac monitoring has demonstrated a reduction in the severity and mortality of doxorubicin-associated cardiac failure. Unfortunately, endomyocardial biopsy is invasive and moderately expensive. It has been suggested that different strategies be devised for patients at high risk for cardiotoxicity. Risk factors for the development of drug cardiotoxicity are shown in Table 55–10.[181, 196-198] Patients at low risk for cardiac toxicity would undergo cardiac noninvasive monitoring, with measurements of ejection fraction at rest and during exercise at a dose of 400 mg/m² of doxorubicin. In patients at high risk, baseline ejection fraction would be measured at rest and with exercise at 100 mg/m², with repeat studies for each dose increment of 100 mg/m². If the results of any of the screening tests are abnormal, cardiac catheterization and endomyocardial biopsy may be advised (Table 55–11). The histopathological features found on endomyocardial biopsy can provide an estimate of the risk of congestive heart failure if higher doses are administered, and an informed decision can be made concerning the advisability of continuing therapy (Table 55–12).

Prevention. Several possibilities for preventing doxorubicin-induced cardiotoxicity have been suggested. The use of free-radical scavengers (vitamin E),[187] sulfhydryl compounds,[199] coenzyme Q10 (a mitochondrial quinone),[200] cardiac glycosides,[201] calcium-channel antagonists, doxoru-

TABLE 55–9 HEMODYNAMIC GRADING OF PATIENTS UNDERGOING DOXORUBICIN CHEMOTHERAPY

GRADE	HEMODYNAMIC FINDINGS
0 Normal	Mean RA <7 mm Hg RVEDP <8 mm Hg LVEDP/Mean PAW <12 mm Hg Cardiac index >2.5 L/min/m² Exercise factor >5.0
1 Mildly abnormal	Any of the following: Mean RA = 7 to 10 mm Hg RVEDP = 8 to 12 mm Hg at rest with increase on exercise = 5 to 9 mm Hg LVEDP/Mean PAW = 12 to 15 mm Hg at rest with increase on exercise = 5 to 11 mm Hg Cardiac index = 2.2 to 2.5 L/min/m² Exercise factor = 4.0 to 5.0
2 Moderately abnormal	Any of the following: Two or more grade 1 features Mean RA = 10 to 15 mm Hg RVEDP = 12 to 17 mm Hg at rest with increase on exercise ≥9 mm Hg Cardiac index = 1.8 to 2.2 L/min/m² Exercise factor <4.0
3 Severely abnormal	Any of the following: Two or more grade 2 features Mean RA ≥16 mm Hg RVEDP ≥19 mm Hg LVEDP/Mean PAW ≥20 mm Hg Cardiac index <1.8 L/min/m²

RA = right atrium; RVEDP and LVEDP = right and left end-diastolic pressure, respectively; PAW = pulmonary artery wedge pressure. Abnormal cardiac index is accompanied by elevated AV oxygen content difference (>5 vol%). Exercise factor = increase in cardiac output (ml/min)/increase in total body oxygen consumption.

From Bristow, M. R., et al.: Efficacy and the cost of cardiac monitoring in patients receiving doxorubicin. Cancer 50:32, 1982.

TABLE 55–10 RISK FACTORS FOR DEVELOPMENT OF DOXORUBICIN CARDIOTOXICITY

Cumulative dose (> 550 mg/m²)
Age extremes
Preexistent coronary artery disease
Hypertension
Metastatic pericardial or myocardial disease
Prior mediastinal irradiation
Coexistent chemotherapy with alkylating agents

TABLE 55–11 SUGGESTED SCHEME FOR CARDIAC MONITORING WITH DOXORUBICIN

Low risk	No monitoring except to reveal occult heart disease; begin monitoring (as below) at 450 mg/m² doxorubicin with baseline ejection fraction on rest and exercise
At risk	Baseline ejection fraction on rest and exercise; repeat measurement of ejection fraction on exercise for each 100 mg/m² dose increase
If noninvasive tests abnormal	Perform cardiac catheterization and endomyocardial biopsy
If catheterization/ biopsy abnormal	Discontinue doxorubicin administration

From Fowles, R. E.: Cardiac catheterization and endomyocardial biopsy. *In* Kapoor, A. S. (ed.): Cancer and The Heart. New York, Springer-Verlag, 1986, p. 48.

TABLE 55–12 SEMIQUANTITATIVE SCALE OF BIOPSY-DETERMINED ANTHRACYCLINE MYOCARDIAL DAMAGE

Biopsy Grade	Histopathological Features
0	No detectable change from normal
1	Scant number of cells (≤5%) showing distended sarcoplasmic reticulum and/or early myofibrillar loss
1.5	Small numbers of cells (5 to 15%), some showing definite cytoplasmic vacuolization and/or myofibrillar loss
2	Groups of cells (16 to 25%), some showing definite cytoplasmic vacuolization and/or myofibrillar loss Biopsy grades up to 2 carry <10% risk of heart failure with 100 mg/m² incremental dose of doxorubicin
2.5	Groups of cells (26 to 35%), some showing definite cytoplasmic vacuolization and/or marked myofibrillar loss Biopsy grade of 2.5 carries a 10 to 25% risk of heart failure with 100 mg/m² incremental dose of doxorubicin
3	Diffuse cell injury (>35%) showing advanced loss of organelles, total loss of myofibrils, and mitochondrial and nuclear degeneration Biopsy grade 3 is associated with >25% risk of heart failure if more doxorubicin is given

From Fowles, R. E.: Cardiac catheterization and endomyocardial biopsy. *In* Kapoor, A. S. (ed.): Cancer and The Heart. New York, Springer-Verlag, 1986, p. 48.

bicin bound to liposomes, and histaminergic and adrenergic blockade have all been reported to lessen cardiac toxicity; prospective studies to determine the efficacy of these interventions are now in progress. Lowering the peak blood levels of the drug appears to offer the best means of reducing cardiac toxicity. In a controlled study monitoring cardiac toxicity by both noninvasive techniques and endomyocardial biopsy, drug-related damage was significantly reduced but not eliminated when the drug was administered by prolonged continuous intravenous infusion rather than by bolus injection; the reduction in toxicity clearly appears to be related to reduced peak plasma levels.[202] Similarly, lower dosages given more frequently reduce peak plasma levels and seem to lower the incidence of cardiac toxicity.[203] Antitumor activity does not appear to be compromised by altering the technique of administration in these ways.[202]

Another approach to this problem has been the development of anthracycline analogues that retain their antitumor effect but do not cause cardiac toxicity. However, most agents that have been studied, such as epirubicin, 4-demethyl-6-demethyl-doxorubicin, rubidazone, and aclacinomycin, continue to show toxicity, either clinically or in animal models.[204] To date, more than 16 such analogues have been described. Two of these, 4′-epi-adriamycin (epirubicin) and 4′-deoxydoxorubicin, are now undergoing prospective clinical trials.[205, 206] Some analogues have been associated with decreased histological abnormalities in animal models but turn out to have no antitumor effect.

OTHER ANTINEOPLASTIC AGENTS. As noted in Table 55–6, cardiomyopathies have been reported secondary to high doses of intravenous cyclophosphamide.[184, 206a, 206b] In contrast to doxorubicin, the cardiotoxicity of cyclophosphamide is acute and not due to cumulative doses. It causes reductions in ECG voltage and systolic function. Although mortality is appreciable, survivors exhibit no residual cardiac abnormalities.[207] Amsacrine (AMSA) has been associated with acute cardiac arrhythmias and cardiomyopathy. Although AMSA-related cardiac events are frequent, they are less common than those due to doxorubicin. Manifestations of toxicity include ECG abnormalities, sudden death, and congestive heart failure. Hypokalemia appears to be a risk factor for the development of severe arrhythmias with this agent.[197, 208, 209] The anthraquinones, mitoxantrone and nonvantrone, are a new group of antineoplastic agents with significant clinical activity.[210] They have been shown to produce favorable results in leukemias as well as in advanced breast cancer. Deterioration in ejection fraction and congestive heart failure have been reported.[211-213] The anthraquinones are now being compared in a randomized fashion with the anthracyclines in terms of both therapeutic efficacy and incidence of cardiac toxicity.[214]

Supportive therapy given to cancer patients may also be cardiotoxic when combined with chemotherapeutic agents. Lithium, which is occasionally used to increase the white blood cell count so that more therapy can be given, has been associated with sudden death in patients who are simultaneously receiving combination chemotherapy that includes an anthracycline agent.[197] In addition, antiemetic drugs such as domperidone, have been associated with cardiac arrhythmias and cardiac arrest in several patients receiving antineoplastic agents.[215, 216] As new antineoplastic agents are brought to trial, lessons learned in the evaluation of cardiac toxicity with doxorubicin are likely to prove helpful.

Bone marrow transplantation, either allogeneic or autologous, involves the combination of large doses of whole-body irradiation therapy with high-dose chemotherapy. Cardiac complications are frequent during these transplant procedures and may be an important factor in limiting the success rate.[217] Fatal cardiomyopathies, pericarditis, and significant arrhythmias are not infrequent. High-dose cyclophosphamide and cytosine arabinoside are commonly associated with cardiotoxicity. In addition, the effect of whole-heart irradiation in conjunction with anthracycline drugs and cyclophosphamide appears to be additive.

HEMATOLOGICAL ABNORMALITIES RELATED TO CARDIAC DRUGS

Blood dyscrasias are frequent complications of drugs used to treat cardiac disorders. The development of unexplained anemia, granulocytopenia, or thrombocytopenia in a patient receiving a diuretic, antihypertensive, or antiarrhythmic agent should immediately arouse the suspicion that a drug used in the treatment of cardiac disease might be responsible.

Many different types of blood dyscrasias occur secondary to drug ingestion. The anemias may be of the aplastic, hemolytic, megaloblastic, or sideroblastic type; other disorders may include granulocytopenia and agranulocytosis, thrombocytopenia, thrombocytosis, defects of platelet function, and a variety of miscellaneous disorders (Table 55–13). Underlying mechanisms include suppression of one or more of the three cellular elements in the bone marrow as well as a variety of immune phenomena with increased peripheral destruction of the formed elements. The drug effect may be dose-related or idiosyncratic.

APLASTIC ANEMIA. Many chemical agents are capable of suppressing marrow function and producing hypoplasia or aplasia. Chlor-

TABLE 55–13 BLOOD DYSCRASIAS ASSOCIATED WITH CARDIAC MEDICATIONS

	Anemia					
	Aplastic	Megaloblastic	Hemolytic	Neutropenia	Thrombocytopenia	Other
Antiarrhythmics						
Digitoxin	−	−	−	−	+	L
Phenytoin	+	+	−	+	+	L, P
Procainamide	−	−	−	+ (A)	−	−
Propranolol	−	−	−	+	−	−
Quinidine	−	−	+	+	+	−
Tocainide	−	−	−	+ (A)	−	−
Anticoagulants						
Heparin	+ *	−	−	−	+	−
Phenindione	−	−	−	+	−	−
Antihypertensives						
Captopril	+	−	−	+	+	−
Glutethimide	+ *	−	−	−	−	P
Hydralazine	−	−	−	−	+	L
Methyldopa	−	−	+	+	+	P
Reserpine	−	−	−	−	+	−
Diuretics						
Acetazolamide	+	−	−	+	+	−
Chlorothiazide	−	−	−	−	+	−
Chlorthalidone	−	−	−	+	+	−
Diazoxide	−	−	−	−	+	−
Ethacrynic acid	−	−	−	+	−	−
Hydrochlorothiazide	−	−	−	+	−	−
Mercurials	−	−	−	+	+	−
Spironolactone	−	−	−	−	+	−
Triamterene	−	+	−	−	−	−
Coronary dilators						
Amyl nitrite	−	−	−	−	−	M
Nitroglycerin	−	−	−	−	−	M
Other						
Amrinone	−	−	−	−	+	−

*Pure red cell aplasia; L = lupus-like syndrome; P = porphyria; A = agranulocytosis; M = methemoglobinemia.

amphenicol, benzene, cytostatic agents used in the treatment of malignancies, and phenylbutazone are the drugs most commonly implicated. Less frequently involved, and perhaps less well documented, are antibiotics such as sulfonamides, hypoglycemic agents, and insecticides. Among drugs used to treat cardiovascular disease, the antiarrhythmic agent phenytoin (p. 632), the diuretic agent acetazolamide, and the angiotensin-converting enzyme inhibitor captopril[218] (p. 872) have been reported, on rare occasion, to lead to such reactions. The onset of aplastic anemia is usually insidious, and the symptoms are directly related to the degree of pancytopenia. If the causative agent is immediately discontinued upon detection of the blood dyscrasia, the latter can often be reversed.

MEGALOBLASTIC ANEMIA. A pancytopenia characterized by macrocytic red cells owing to impairment of DNA synthesis may be caused by vitamin B_{12} or folate deficiency or by purine and pyrimidine inhibitors. Most commonly, drugs cause megaloblastic anemia by impairing the absorption of folic acid or acting as folate antagonists. Phenytoin (p. 632), oral contraceptives, and a variety of other drugs can impair folate absorption by interfering with the liver conjugases needed to break down the polyglutamate structure of naturally occurring folates to the monoglutamate form appropriate for absorption by the gastrointestinal tract. Triamterene, a potassium-sparing diuretic (p. 514), is a pteridine analogue that exhibits antifolate activity, similar to aminopterin, in vitro. Its propensity to produce a megaloblastic anemia appears to be dose-related.

IMMUNOHEMOLYTIC ANEMIAS. There are four different causes for the development of a positive direct Coombs or antiglobulin test, two of which involve cardiac medications: The first mechanism, which is uncommon, involves some drugs that bind to plasma protein and thereby become antigenic, including quinidine and the sulfonamides. The resultant antigen-antibody complex may deposit on the red cell surface and cause agglutinability by anticomplement sera. Hemolysis may be severe, but rapid improvement follows withdrawal of the drug.

The second type of reaction that results in a positive Coombs test involves the antihypertensive drug alpha-methyldopa (p. 872).[219] The mechanism of antibody formation is unknown, but presumably antibody induced by alpha-methyldopa has an affinity for the Rh locus of the red cell, similar to that of IgG antibodies in idiopathic immunohemolytic anemia. The frequency of positive results on Coombs test varies from 11 per cent for patients who are receiving 0.75 gm per day for over 3 months to 40 per cent for those receiving 2 gm per day for the same period of time. Fortunately, the affinity of the alpha-methyldopa antibody for red cells is low, and fewer than 1 per cent of patients whose antiglobulin test is positive will manifest significant hemolytic anemia. Nonetheless, alpha-methyldopa surpasses all other drugs in causing immunohemolytic anemia. On withdrawal of the drug, hemolysis improves within 1 or 2 weeks, with full recovery in 1 month, although the positive Coombs test may persist for 6 to 24 months. A positive Coombs test without hemolysis is not an indication to discontinue alpha-methyldopa if its administration is otherwise indicated in the treatment of hypertension.

The other two mechanisms of drug-related positive antiglobulin reactions do not involve cardiovascular drugs. The third is represented by penicillin, in which the drug binds to the red cell membranes, creating a cell-drug complex and antigenic stimulation of an IgG antibody. The fourth mechanism involves cephalothin, which is bound to the red cell membrane; normal serum proteins adhere nonspecifically to red cell membranes.

GRANULOCYTOPENIA AND AGRANULOCYTOSIS. A reduction in circulating neutrophils is the most toxic hematological effect of drugs. It may be secondary to depression of the marrow or it may be an immune mechanism causing peripheral destruction. When there is immune suppression, examination of the marrow reveals active myeloid precursors, whereas the absence of myeloid elements suggests suppression of synthesis. The marrow-depressive effect is dose-related.[220] Anticoagulants such as phenindione, antiarrhythmics such as procainamide and tocainide,[220a] antihypertensives such as captopril, and diuretics such as the thiazides have all been reported to produce granulocytopenia. Procainamide is the most dangerous and most frequently implicated cardiac drug in granulocytopenia.[221] Presenting symptoms may include a sore throat, ulcerations of mucous membranes, fever, malaise, fatigue, and weakness. Discontinuation of the drug may be followed by a rebound in the white blood cell count and occasionally a leukemoid picture. Because laboratory tests are not conclusive for white cell antibodies, an accurate definition of the immune mechanism responsible for white cell destruction remains unclear.

DRUG-INDUCED THROMBOCYTOPENIA. Many of the drugs used to treat cardiovascular disorders may cause thrombocytopenia, either by a direct effect on the bone marrow or by inducing formation of drug-specific antibody.[222] For example, the thiazide diuretics (p. 514) directly suppress megakaryocyte production. Thiazide-induced thrombocytopenia is usually mild, with the platelet count rarely falling below 50,000/μl. This condition is unique, since it persists for 6 to 8 weeks after drug withdrawal. Thrombocytopenia caused by amrinone, a positive inotropic agent with vasodilator properties (p. 527), is less well studied but is clearly related to the total dose of drug administered and to peripheral destruction of platelets.[223] Other common agents like alcohol and some estrogen preparations may cause thrombocytopenia by a direct depressant effect on the bone marrow. Shortened platelet survival secondary to antibody or complement binding to platelets can cause severe thrombocytopenia and life-threatening hemorrhage. The onset is abrupt and is not related to the dose of medication or the duration of its use. In most cases of immunological thrombocytopenia, the offending agent induces a specific antibody. The resulting drug-antibody complex then binds to the platelet, thereby shortening its survival. Quinidine, one of the first cardiac drugs to produce this response, has been well studied as a cause of thrombocytopenia. The defect can be transferred to a normal individual by administering serum from a patient with quinidine-induced thrombocytopenia, followed by a quinidine challenge to the normal subject.[224] A similar defect can be caused by antibodies to quinine, including the small quantities present in tonic drinks. Acetaminophen (a common analgesic given to cardiac patients), acetazolamide, digitoxin, phenytoin, ethacrynic acid, alpha-methyldopa, and spironolactone have all been implicated in various cases of suspected drug-induced thrombocytopenia, although the mechanism has not always been well-defined.

Although in vitro laboratory tests for drug-dependent platelet antibody are available, the results do not always correlate with clinical events. The best proof of drug-induced thrombocytopenia is prompt recovery of the platelet count after drug withdrawal followed by a second episode of thrombocytopenia upon readministration of the suspected drug. (Because of this potential hazard, the drug challenge is not advised.) If serious hemorrhage persists after the drug is withdrawn, treatment with 1 mg/kg prednisone or its equivalent may be necessary. Corticosteroids may hasten the return of a normal platelet count and may also protect capillaries and small vessels even without altering the platelet count. Platelet transfusions are not usually helpful but can be tried in desperate situations in which hemorrhage is life-threatening. They are most useful if thrombocytopenia persists well after the drug-antibody complex has been cleared. In this situation, a gratifying elevation in platelet count sometimes occurs.

Heparin. Treatment with this drug is one of the most important causes of thrombocytopenia in cardiac patients (p. 1771). The incidence varies from 5 to 25 per cent among patients receiving heparin; it is more common in those given heparin derived from beef lung and has been associated with all modes and doses of heparin administration.[225] Heparin has a direct platelet-aggregating effect that may contribute to thrombocytopenia. This property is most marked in those fractions with the highest molecular weight and the lowest affinity for antithrombin.[226] There is an increase in platelet-associated immunoglobulin in many of the cases, suggesting an immune etiology. However, the nature of the offending antigen in heparin and its relationship to the biologically active heparin fractions remain unclear. In addition, some patients with heparin-induced thrombocytopenia develop paradoxical thrombosis and disseminated intravascular coagulation. The development of thromboembolism in association with thrombocytopenia is unique to heparin.

OTHER HEMATOLOGICAL ABNORMALITIES CAUSED BY CARDIAC DRUGS. Amyl nitrite, sodium nitrite, and nitroglycerin can oxidize hemoglobin to methemoglobin, which cannot effectively carry oxygen. The patient with methemoglobinemia appears cyanotic but has a normal arterial PO_2, and oxygen therapy will not improve the pallor. Although symptomatic methemoglobinemia may occur in adults, most cases are seen in children who accidentally ingest medications prescribed for adults. Occasionally, adults with mild congenital methemoglobinemia will become markedly symptomatic when exposed to small doses of these same medications. With the increasing use of intravenous nitroglycerin, this complication may become more frequent.[227] If venous blood is chocolate brown and this color persists after the blood is shaken in air, the diagnosis of methemoglobinemia is almost certain. The diagnosis is confirmed by the addition of a few drops of 10 per cent potassium cyanide, which results in the rapid production of the bright red cyanmethemoglobin. Symptoms are nonspecific and consist of dyspnea, headache, fatigue, and dizziness. They are usually self-limited if the responsible drugs are discontinued, since normal red cells can enzymatically reduce the methemoglobin. In severe cases or in patients with enzyme defects, methylene blue may be administered to stimulate reduction of the methemoglobin.

Other medications may interfere with oxygen delivery to tissues. For example, sodium nitroprusside used to treat hypertensive emergencies and to reduce afterload in the management of heart failure may cause fatigue, nausea, abnormal behavior, and muscle spasm as the agent reacts with oxyhemoglobin, producing cyanmethemoglobin and free cyanide ions.[228, 229]

Hydralazine (p. 876), procainamide (p. 630), and rarely phenytoin (p. 632) can cause a lupus erythematosus-like syndrome, with urticaria, erythema multiforme, photosensitivity, delirium, and immune-mediated blood cell destruction.[230, 231] Although patients with drug-induced lupus have positive antinuclear antibody tests and many of the clinical manifestations of the systemic form, renal function is not usually impaired, and all these manifestations usually remit within several months if the drugs are discontinued. The syndrome is of particular importance in cardiac patients, since the onset of chest pain, pleurisy, or pericardial effusion in the patient with heart disease could lead to an erroneous diagnosis unless drug-induced lupus is suspected.

REFERENCES

1. Jepson, J. H., and Frankl, W. S.: Hematological Complications in Cardiac Practice. Philadelphia, W. B. Saunders Company, 1975.
2. Kapoor, A. S.: Cancer and the Heart. New York, Springer-Verlag, 1986.

ANEMIA AND CARDIOVASCULAR DISORDERS

3. Graettinger, J. S., Parsons, R. L., and Campbell, J. A.: A correlation of clinical and hemodynamic studies in patients with mild and severe anemia with and without congestive heart failure. Ann. Intern. Med. *58*:617, 1963.
4. Ali, M. K., and Ewer, M. S.: Cancer and the cardiopulmonary system. New York, Raven Press, 1984, p. 242.
5. Datta, B. N., and Silver, M. D.: Cardiomegaly in chronic anemia in rats; an experimental study including ultrastructural, histometric and stereological observations. Lab. Invest. *2*:503, 1975.
6. Eckstein, R. W.: Development of interarterial coronary anastomoses by chronic anemia. Disappearance following correction of anemia. Circ. Res. *3*:306, 1955.
7. Quinones, M. A., Gaasch, W. H., and Alexander, J. K.: Influence of acute changes in preload, afterload, contractile state and heart rate on ejection and isovolumic indices of myocardial contractility in man. Circulation *53*:293, 1976.
8. Reichek, N., Wilson, J., Sutton, M. S., Plappert, T. A., Goldberg, S., and Hirshfeld, J. W.: Noninvasive determination of left ventricular end systolic stress: Validation of the method and initial application. Circulation *65*:99, 1982.
9. Rossi, M. A., Carillo, S. V., and Oliveria, J. S. M.: The effect of iron deficiency anemia in the rat on catecholamine levels and heart morphology. Cardiovasc. Res. *15*:313, 1981.
10. Florenzano, F., Diaz, G., Regonesi, C. and Escobar, E.: Left ventricular function in chronic anemia: Evidence of noncatecholamine positive inotropic factor in the serum. Am. J. Cardiol. *54*:638, 1984.
11. Duke, M., and Abelmann, W. H.: The hemodynamic response to chronic anemia. Circulation *39*:503, 1969.
12. Varat, M. A., Adolph, R. J., and Fowler, N. O.: Cardiovascular effects of anemia. Am. Heart J. *83*:415, 1972.
13. Torrance, J. D., Jacobs, P., Restrepo, A., Eschbach, J., Lenfant, C., and Finch, C. A.: Intraerythrocyte adaptation to anemia. N. Engl. J. Med. *283*:165, 1970.
14. Oski, F. A., Marshall, B. D., Cohen, P. J., Sugerman, H. J., and Miller, L. D.: Exercise with anemia. The role of the left or right shifted oxygen-hemoglobin equilibrium curve. Ann. Intern. Med. *74*:44, 1971.
15. Lenfant, C., Torrance, J., English, E., Finch, C. A., Reyafarje, C., Ramos, J., and Faura, J.: Effect of altitude on the oxygen binding by hemoglobin and on organic phosphate levels. J. Clin. Invest. *47*:2652, 1968.
16. Oski, F. A., Gottlieb, A. J., Delivoria-Papadopoulos, M., and Miller, W. W.: Red-cell 2,3-diphosphoglycerate levels in subjects with chronic hypoxemia. N. Engl. J. Med. *280*:1165, 1969.
17. Hunter, A.: The heart in anemia. Q. J. Med. *15*:107, 1946.
18. Harris, T. N., Friedman, S., Tuncali, M. T., and Hallidie-Smith, K. A.: Comparison of innocent murmurs of childhood with cardiac murmurs in high output states. Pediatrics *33*:341, 1964.
19. Varriale, P., Kwa, R. P., Vyas, P.: Intravenous nitroglycerin in transfusion therapy for severe anemia. Association with congestive heart failure. Arch. Intern. Med. *144*:401, 1984.
20. Bunn, H. F.: Disorders of Hemoglobin. *In* Braunwald E. et al (eds.): Harrison's Principles of Internal Medicine. 11th ed. New York, McGraw-Hill, 1987, pp. 1518–1527.
21. Denenberg, B. S., Criner, G., Jones, R., and Spann, J. F.: Cardiac function in sickle cell anemia. Am. J. Cardiol. *51*:1674, 1983.
22. Falk, R. H., and Hood, W. B.: The heart in sickle cell anemia. Arch. Intern. Med. *142*:1680, 1982.
23. Shubin, H., Kaufmann, R., Shapiro, M., and Levinson, D. C.: Cardiovascular findings in children with sickle cell anemia. Am. J. Cardiol. *6*:875, 1960.
24. Perrine, R. P., Pembrey, M. E., John, P., Perrine, J. S., and Shoup, F.: Natural history of sickle cell anemia in Saudi Arabs: A study of 270 subjects. Ann. Intern. Med. *88*:1, 1978.
25. Gerry, J. L., Bulkley, B. H., and Hutchins, G. M.: Clinicopathologic analysis of cardiac dysfunction in 52 patients with sickle cell anemia. Am. J. Cardiol. *42*:211, 1978.
26. Barrett, O., Saunders, D. E., McFarlend, D. E., and Humphries, J. O.: Myocardial infarction in sickle cell anemia. Am. J. Hematol. *16*:139, 1984.
27. Martin, C. R., Cobb, C., Tatter, D., Johnson, C., and Haywood, L. J.: Acute myocardial infarction in sickle cell anemia. Arch. Intern. Med. *143*:830, 1983.
28. Rubler, S., and Fleischer, R. A.: Sickle cell states and cardiomyopathy. Sudden death due to pulmonary thrombosis and infarction. Am. J. Cardiol. *19*:867, 1967.
29. Donald, K. W., Bishop, J. M., Cumming, G., and Wade, O. L.: The effect

of exercise on the cardiac output and circulatory dynamics of normal subjects. Clin. Sci. *14*:37, 1955.
30. Burnheimer, J., and Haywood, L. J.: Prevalence of hemoglobinopathies in patients with ischemic heart disease. J. Natl. Med. Assoc. *68*:312, 1976.
31. Balfour, I. C., Covitz, W., Davis, H., Rao, P. S., and Alpert, B. S.: Cardiac size and function in children with sickle cell anemia. Am. Heart J. *108*:345, 1984.
32. Lippman, S. M., Niemann, J. T., Thigpen, T., Ginzton, L. E., and Laks, M. M.: Abnormal septal Q waves in sickle cell disease. Prevalence and causative factors. Chest *88*:543, 1985.
33. Maisel, A., Friedman, H., Flint, L., Koshy, M., and Prabhu, R.: Continuous electrocardiographic monitoring in patients with sickle cell anemia during pain crisis. Clin. Cardiol. *6*:339, 1983.
34. Rees, A. H., Stefadouras, M. A., Strong, W. B., Miller, M. D., Gilmman, P., Rigby, J. A., and McFarlane, J.: Left ventricular performance in children with homozygous sickle cell anemias. Br. Heart J. *40*:690, 1978.
35. Covitz, W., Eubig, C., Balfour, I. C., Jerath, R., Alpert, B. S., Strong, W. B., DuRant, R. H., and Hadden, B. G.: Exercise-induced cardiac dysfunction in sickle cell anemia. A radionuclide study. Am. J. Cardiol. *51*:570, 1983.
36. Manno, B. V., Burka, E. R., Hakki, A., Manno, C. S., Iskandrian, A. S., and Noone, A. M.: Biventricular function in sickle cell anemia: Radionuclide angiographic and thallium-201 scintigraphic evaluation. Am. J. Cardiol. 52:584, 1983.
37. Willens, H. J., Lawrence, C., Frishman, W. H., and Strom, J. A.: A noninvasive comparison of left ventricular performance in sickle cell anemia and chronic aortic regurgitation. Clin. Cardiol. *6*:542, 1983.
38. Alpert, B. S., Dover, E. V., Strong, W. B., and Covits, W.: Longitudinal exercise hemodynamics in children with sickle cell anemia. Am. J. Dis. Child. *138*:1021, 1984.
39. Lippman, S. M., Ginzton, L. E., Thigpen, T., Tanaka, K. R., and Laks, M. M.: Mitral valve prolapse in sickle cell disease: Presumptive evidence for a linked connective tissue disorder. Arch. Intern. Med. *145*:435, 1985.
40. Ohene-Frempong, K., and Schwartz, E.: Clinical features of thalassemia. Pediatr. Clin. North Am. *27*:403, 1980.
41. Ehlers L. H., Levin, A. R., Klein, A. A., Marekenson, A. L., O'Loughlin, J. E., and Engle, M. A.: The cardiac manifestations of thalassemia major: Natural history, noninvasive cardiac diagnostic studies, and results of cardiac catheterization. *In* Engle, M. A. (ed.): Pediatric Cardiovascular Disease. Cardiovascular Clinics II. Philadelphia, F. A. Davis Co., 1981, pp. 171–186.
42. Sapoznikov, D., Lewis, N., Rachmilewitz, E. A., Gotsman, M. S., and Lewis, B. S.: Left ventricular filling and emptying patterns in anemia due to beta-thalassemia. A computer-assisted echocardiographic study. Cardiology, *69*:276, 1982.
43. Sapoznikov, D., Lewis, N., Degan, I., Rachmilewitz, E. A., and Gotsman, M. S.: Studies of left ventricular function in anemia due to beta-thalassemia. Isr. J. Med. Sci. *18*:928, 1982.
44. Valdes-Cruz, L. M., Reinecke, C., Rutkowski, M., Dudell, G. G., Goldberg, S. J., Allen, H. D., Schu, D. J., and Piomelli, S.: Preclinical abnormal segmental cardiac manifestations of thalassemia major in children on transfusion-chelation therapy: Echographic alterations of left ventricular posterior wall contractions and relaxation patterns. Am. Heart J. *103*:505, 1982.
45. Borow, K. M., Propper, R., Bierman, F. Z., Grady, S., and Inati, A.: The left ventricular end-systolic pressure-dimensions relation in patients with thalassemia major. A new noninvasive method for assessing contractile state. Circulation *66*:980, 1982.
46. Yee, H., Mra, R., and Nyunt, K. M.: Cardiac abnormalities in the thalassemia syndromes. Southeast Asian J. Trop. Med. Public Health *15*:414, 1984.
47. Dameshek, W., and Roth, S. I.: Case Records of the Massachusetts General Hospital—Weekly Clinicopathological exercises. Case 52. N. Engl. J. Med. *271*:898, 1964.
48. Westring, D. W.: Aortic valve disease and hemolytic anemia. Ann. Intern. Med. *65*:203, 1966.
49. Miller, D. S., Mengel, C. E., Kremer, W. B., Gutterman, J., and Senningen, R.: Intravascular hemolysis in a patient with valvular heart disease. Ann. Intern. Med. *65*:210, 1966.
50. Rose, J. C., Hufnagel, C. A., Freis, C. D., Harvey, W. P., and Partono, P. E. A.: The hemodynamic alterations produced by a plastic valvular prosthesis for severe aortic insufficiency in man. J. Lab. Clin. Med. *33*:891, 1954.
51. Sayed, H. M., Dacie, J. V., Handley, D. A., Lewis, S. M., and Cleland, W. P.: Hemolytic anemia of mechanical origin after open-heart surgery. Thorax *16*:356, 1961.
52. Dacie, J. V.: The Hemolytic Anemias. Part III. 2nd ed. New York, Grune and Stratton, 1967, p. 957.
53. Sears, A. D., and Crosby, W. H.: Intravascular hemolysis due to intracardiac prosthetic devices. Diurnal variations related to activity. Am. J. Med. *39*:341, 1965.
54. Nevaril, C. G., Lynch, E. C., Alfrey, C. P., Jr., and Hellums, J.: Erythrocyte damage and destruction induced by shearing stress. J. Lab. Clin. Med. *71*:784, 1968.
55. Zezulka, A., Schapiro, L., and Sind, S.: Chronic haemolytic anemia in hypertrophic cardiomyopathy. Br. Heart J. *52*:474, 1984.

HEMOCHROMATOSIS AND HEMOSIDEROSIS

56. Schafer, A. I.: Iron overload. *In* Fairbanks, V. F. (ed.): Current Hematology. New York, John Wiley and Sons, 1981, pp. 191–218.
57. Edwards, C. Q., Dadone, M. M., Skolnick, M. H., and Kushner, J. P.: Hereditary hemochromatosis. Clin. Hematol. *11*:411–435, 1982.
58. Swan, W. G. A., and Dewar, H. A.: The heart in hemochromatosis. Br. Heart J. *14*:117, 1952.
59. Finch, S. C., and Finch, C. A.: Idiopathic hemochromatosis, an iron storage disease. Medicine *34*:381, 1955.
60. James, T. N.: Pathology of the cardiac conduction system in hemochromatosis. N. Engl. J. Med. *271*:92, 1964.
61. Wasserman, A. J., Richardson, D. W., Baird, C. L., and Wyso, E. M.: Cardiac hemochromatosis simulating constrictive pericarditis. Am. J. Med. *32*:316, 1962.
62. Buja, L. M., and Roberts, W. C.: Iron in the heart. Etiology and clinical significance. Am. J. Med. *51*:209, 1971.
63. Leon, M. D., Borer, J. S., Bacharach, S. L., Green, M. V., Benz, E. J., Griffith, P., and Nienhuis, A. W.: Detection of early cardiac dysfunction in patients with severe beta-thalassemia and chronic iron overload. N. Engl. J. Med. *301*:1143, 1979.
64. Easley, R. M., Schreiner, B. F., and Yu, P. N.: Reversible cardiomyopathy associated with hemochromatosis. N. Engl. J. Med. *287*:866, 1972.
65. Skinner, C., and Kenmore, C. F.: Haemochromatosis presenting as congestive cardiomyopathy and responding to venesection. Br. Heart J. *35*:466, 1973.
66. Schafer, A. I., Cheron, R. G., Dluhy, R., Cooper, B., Gleason, R. E., Soeldner, J. S., and Bunn, H. F.: Clinical consequences of acquired tranfusional iron overload in adults. N. Engl. J. Med. *304*:319, 1981.
67. Schafer, A. I.: Treatment of iron overload with parenteral deferoxamines. *In* Isselbacher, K. J. et al (eds.): Update III to Harrison's Principles of Internal Medicine. New York, McGraw-Hill, 1982, pp. 157–166.
68. Wolfe, L., Olivieri, N., Sallan, D., Colan, S., Rose, V., Propper, R., Freedman, M. H., and Nathan, D. G.: Prevention of cardiac disease by subcutaneous deferoxamine in patients with thalassemia major. N. Engl. J. Med. *312*:1600, 1985.
69. Schafer, A. I., Rabinowe, S., LeBoff, M. S., Bridges, K., Cheron, R. G., and Dluhy, R.: Long term efficacy of deferoxamine iron chelation therapy in adults with acquired transfusional overload. Arch. Intern. Med. *145*:1217, 1985.
70. Cohen, A., and Schwartz, E.: Iron chelation therapy with deferoxamine in Cooley anemia. J. Pediatr. *92*:643, 1978.
71. Nienhuis, A. W.: Vitamin C and iron. N. Engl. J. Med. *304*:170, 1981.
71a. Bridges, K. R., and Hoffman, K. E.: The effects of ascorbic acid on the intracellular metabolism of iron and ferritin. J. Biol. Chem. *261*:14273, 1986.

DISORDERS ASSOCIATED WITH ABNORMAL BLOOD FLOW DISTRIBUTION OR INCREASED VISCOSITY

72. Braunwald, E.: Cyanosis, hypoxia, and polycythemia. *In* Braunwald, E. et al. (eds): Harrison's Principles of Internal Medicine. 11th ed. New York, McGraw-Hill, 1987, pp. 145–149.
73. Castle, W. B., and Jandl, J. H.: Blood viscosity and blood volume: Opposing influences upon oxygen transport in polycythemia. Semin. Hematol. *3*:193, 1966.
74. Adamson, J. W.: The Myeloproliferative Disease. *In* Braunwald, E., et al. (eds.): Harrison's Principles of Internal Medicine. 11th ed. New York, McGraw-Hill, 1987, pp. 1527–1533.
75. Adamson, J. W., and Fialkow, P. J.: Polycythemia vera: Stem cell and probable clinical origin of the disease. N. Engl. J. Med. *245*:913, 1976.
76. Berlin, N. I. (ed.). Polycythemia vera: an update. Semin. Hematol. *23*:131, 1986.
77. Dintenfass, L.: Viscosity of the packed red and white blood cells. Exp. Molec. Pathol. *4*:597, 1965.
78. Thomas, D. J., Marshall, J., Russell, R. W., Wetherley-Mein, G., DuBoulay, G. H., Pearson, T. C., Symon, L., and Zilkha, E.: Effect of hematocrit on cerebral blood flow in man. Lancet *2*:941, 1977.
79. Torrance, J. D., Lenfant, C., and Cruz, J.: Oxygen transport mechanisms in residents at high altitude. Respir. Physiol. *11*:1, 1970.
80. Balcerzak, S. P., and Bromberg, P. A.: Secondary polycythemia. Semin. Hematol. *12*:353, 1976.
81. Rosenthal, A., Button, L. N., and Nathan, D. G.: Blood volume changes in cyanotic congenital heart disease. Am. J. Cardiol. *29*:162, 1971.
82. Golde, D. W., Hocking, W. G., Koeffler, H. P., and Adamson, J. W.: Polycythemia: Mechanism and management. Ann. Intern. Med. *95*:71, 1981.
83. Rosenthal, A., Nathan, D. G., Marty, A. T., Button, L. N., Miettinen, O. S., and Nadas, A. S.: Acute hemodynamic effects of red cell production in polycythemia of cyanotic congenital heart disease. Circulation *42*:197, 1970.
84. Erslev, A. J., and Caro, J.: Secondary polycythemia: A boon or a burden? Blood Cells *10*:177, 1984.
85. Yeager, S. B., and Freed, M. D.: Myocardial infarction as a manifestation of polycythemia in cyanotic heart disease. Am. J. Cardiol. *53*:952, 1984.
86. Grant, P., Patel, P., and Singh, S.: Acute myocardial infarction secondary to polycythemia in a case of cyanotic congenital heart disease. Int. J. Cardiol. 9:108, 1985.
87. Wallis, P. J., Skehan, J. D., Newland, A. C., Wedzicha, J. A., Mills, P. G., and Empey, D. W.: Effects of erythropheresis on pulmonary hemodynamics and oxygen transport in patients with secondary polycythemia and cor pulmonale. Clin. Sci. *70*:91, 1986.
88. Wallis, P. J., Cunnigham, J., Few, J. D., Newland, A. C., and Empey, D. W.: Effects of packed cell volume reduction on renal hemodynamics and the renin angiotensin aldosterone system in patients with secondary polycythemia and hypoxic cor pulmonale. Clin. Sci. *70*:81, 1986.
89. Willison, J. R., Thomas, D. J., and duBoulay, G. H., et al.: Effect of high hematocrit on alertness. Lancet. *1*:846, 1980.

90. York, E. L., Junes, R. L., Menon, D., and Sproule, B. J.: Effects of secondary polycythemia on cerebral blood flow in chronic obstructive pulmonary disease. Am. Rev. Respir. Dis. *121*:813, 1980.
91. Rosenthal, A., Mentzer, W. C., and Eisenstein, E. B.: The role of red blood cell organic phosphates in adaptation to congenital heart disease. Pediatrics *47*:537, 1971.
92. Charache, S., Weatherall, D. J., and Clegg, J. B.: Polycythemia associated with hemoglobinopathy. J. Clin. Invest. *45*:813, 1966.
93. Adamson, J. W., and Finch, C. A.: Erythropoietin and the polycythemias. Ann. N. Y. Acad. Sci. *149*:560, 1968.
94. Bromberg, P. A., Padilla, F., Boy, J. T., and Balcerzak, S. P.: Effect of a new hemoglobin (Hb Little Rock) on the physiology of oxygen delivery. J. Lab. Clin. Med. *78*:837, 1971.
95. Charache, S., Achuff, S., Winslow, R., Adamson, J., and Chevernick, P.: Variability of the homeostatic response to P50. Blood *52*:1156, 1978.
96. Smith, J., and Landow, S. A.: Smoker's polycythemia. N. Engl. J. Med. *298*:6, 1978.
97. Weinreb, N. J., and Shih, C. F.: Spurious polycythemia. Semin. Hematol. *12*:397, 1975.
98. Saffitz, J. E., Phillips, E. R., Temesy-Armos, P. N., and Roberts, W. C.: Thrombocytosis and fatal coronary heart disease. Am. J. Cardiol. *52*:651, 1983.
99. Pick, R. A., Glover, M. U., Nanfro, J. J., Dubbs, W. F., Gibbons, J. A., and Vieweg, W. G.: Acute myocardial infarction with essential thrombocythemia in a young man. Am. Heart. J. *106*:406, 1983.
100. Hanger, K. H., Kilgore, J., and James, E.: Essential thrombocythemia and coronary artery disease. Chest. *86*:933. 1984.
101. Fuchs, J., Weinberger, I., Rotenberg, Z., Erdberg, A., Davidson, E., Joshua, H., and Agmon, J.: Plasma viscosity in ischemic heart disease. Am. Heart J. *108*:435, 1984.
102. Zannad, F., Stoltz, J. F., Laprevote-Heully, M. C., Aliot, E., and Gilgenkrantz, J. M.: Hemorrhagic disorders in the threatened myocardial infarct syndrome. Arch. Mal. Cour. *78*:1237, 1985.
103. Strano, A., Avellone, G., Novo, S., Davi, G., and Di Garbo, V.: Evaluation of blood viscosity and erythrocyte filterability in chronic ischemic heart disease. Ric. Clin. Lab. *1*:179, 1985.

CARDIAC MANIFESTATIONS OF NEOPLASTIC DISEASE

104. Kapoor, A. S.: Clinical manifestations of neoplasia of the heart. *In* Kapoor, A. S. (ed.): Cancer and the Heart. New York, Springer-Verlag, 1986, pp. 21–25.
105. Schoen, F. J., Berger, B. M., and Guerina, N. G.: Cardiac effects of noncardiac neoplasms. Cardiol. Clin. *2*:657, 1984.
106. Roberts, W. C., Glancy, D. L., and DeVita, V. T.: Heart in malignant lymphoma. A study of 196 autopsy cases. Am. J. Cardiol. *22*:85, 1968.
107. Petersen, C. D., Robinson, Q. A., and Kurnich, J. E.: Involvement of the heart and pericardium in the malignant lymphomas. Am. J. Med. Sci. *272*:161, 1976.
108. Waller, B. F., Gottdiener, J. S., Virmni, R., and Roberts, W. C.: Structure-function correlations in cardiovascular and pulmonary diseases. The charcoal heart. Chest *77*:671, 1980.
109. Almange, C., Lebrestec, T., Louvet, M., Courgeon, P., Guerin, D., and Leborgne, P.: Bloc auriculo-ventriculaire complet par metastase cardiaque: A propos dune observation. Semin. Hop. Paris *54*:1419, 1978.
110. Lubell, D. L., and Goldfarb, C. R.: Metastatic cardiac tumor demonstrated by 201-thallium scan. Chest *78*:98, 1980.
111. McDonnell, P. J., Becker, L. C., and Bulkley, B. H.: Thallium imaging in cardiac lymphoma. Am. Heart J. *101*:809, 1981.
112. Johnson, M. H., and Soulen, R. L.: Echocardiography of cardiac metastases. A. J. R. *141*:677, 1983.
113. Grenadier, E., Lema, C. O., Barron, J. V., Alan, H. D., Sahn, D. J., Valdes-Cruz, L. M., Hudder, J. J., and Goldberg, S. J.: Two-dimensional echocardiography for evaluation of metastatic cardiac tumors in pediatric patients. Am. Heart J. *107*:122, 1984.
114. Kutalek, S. P., Panidis, I. P., Kotler, M., Mince, J. S., Carver, J., and Ross, J. J.: Metastatic tumors of the heart detected by two-dimensional echocardiography. Am. Heart J. *109*:343, 1985.
115. Moncada, R., and Posnik, H.: Computed tomograph of neoplastic disease in the pericardium. *In* Kapoor, A. S.: Cancer and the Heart. New York, Springer-Verlag. 1986, pp. 26–41.
116. Goldman, A. P., Kotler, M. N., and Perry, W. R.: Arterial tumors, *In* Kapoor, A. S. (ed.): Cancer and the Heart. New York, Springer-Verlag, 1986, pp 82–109.
117. Seibert, K. A., Rettenmier, C. W., Waller, B. F., Battle, W. E., Levine, A. S., and Roberts, W. C.: Osteogenic sarcoma metastatic to the heart. Am. J. Med. *73*:136, 1982.
118. Lloyd, E. A., and Curcio, C. A.: Lymphoma of the heart as an unusual cause of pericardial effusion. S. Afr. Med. J. *58*:937, 1980.
119. Haedersdal, C., Hasselbach, H., Devantier, A., and Saunamak, K.: Pericardial hematopoiesis with tamponade in myelofibrosis. Scand. J. Haematol. *34*:270, 1985.
120. Gunz, F. W., and Baikie, A. G. (eds.): Leukemia. New York, Grune and Stratton, 1974, pp. 225, 287, 288.
121. Hancock, E. W.: Pericardial disease in patients with neoplasm. *In* Reddy, R. S., Leon, D. F., and Shaver, J. A. (eds.): Pericardial Disease. New York, Raven Press, 1981, p. 327.
122. Barton, J. C., and Durant, J. R.: Isolated chylopericardium associated with lymphoma. South. Med. J. *73*:1551, 1980.
123. Kotler, M. N.: Metastatic cardiac tumors: Recognition of pericardial, myocardial and endocardial involvement by two-dimensional echocardiography. *In* Kapoor, A. S. (ed.): Cancer and the Heart. New York, Springer-Verlag, 1986, pp. 55.
124. Lopez, J. R., Delgado, J. L., Tovar, E., and Gonzalez, A. G.: Massive pericardial effusion produced by extracardiac malignant neoplasms. Arch. Intern. Med. *143*:1815, 1983.
125. Posner, M. R., Cohen, G. I., and Skarin, A. T.: Pericardial disease in patients with cancer. The differentiation of malignant from idiopathic and radiation-induced pericarditis. Am. J. Med. *71*:407, 1981.
126. Applefeld, M. M., Spicer, K. M., Slawson, R. G., Singleton, R. T., Wesley, M., and Wiernick, P. H.: The long-term cardiac effects of radiotherapy in patients treated for Hodgkin's disease. Cancer Treat. Rep. *66*:1003, 1982.
127. Wiernik, P. H., Sutherland, J. C., and Steelmiller, B. K.: Clinically significant cardiac infiltration in acute leukemia, lymphocytic lymphoma and plasma cell myeloma. Med. Pediatr. Oncol. *2*:75, 1976.
128. Perez, C. A., Presant, C. A., and Amburg, A. L.: Management of superior vena caval syndrome. Semin. Oncol. *5*:123, 1978.
129. Lopez, M. I., and Vincent, R. J.: Malignant superior vena cava syndrome. *In* Kapoor, A. S. (ed.): Cancer and the Heart. New York, Springer-Verlag, 1986, p. 206.
130. Wahlin, A., Olofsson, B., Eriksson, A., and Backman, C.: Myeloma-associated cardiac amyloidosis. Acta. Med. Scand. *215*:189, 1984.
131. Alpert, M. A.: Cardiac amyloidosis. *In* Kapoor, A. S. (ed.): Cancer and the Heart. New York, Springer-Verlag, 1986, p. 162.
132. Sedlis, S. P., Saffitz, J. E., Schwob, V. S., and Jaffe, A. S.: Cardiac amyloidosis simulating hypertrophic cardiomyopathy. Am. J. Cardiol. *53*:969, 1984.
133. Laurent, M., Taulet, R., Ramee, M. P., Legrand, D., LeNormand, J. P., and Lelguen, C.: Light-chain disease with terminal myocardiopathy. Arch. Mal. Coeur *78*:943, 1985.
134. Ursell, P. C., and Fenogolio, J. J.: Spectrum of cardiac disease diagnosed by endomyocardial biopsy. Pathol. Annu. *19*:197, 1984.
135. Koiwaya, Y., Nakamura, M., and Yamamoto, K.: Progressive ECG alterations in metastatic cardiac mural tumor. Am. Heart J. *105*:339, 1983.
136. Hartman, R. B., Clark, P. I., and Schulman, P.: Pronounced and prolonged ST segment elevation. A pathognomonic sign of tumor invasion of the heart. Arch. Intern. Med. *142*:1917, 1982.
137. Cole, T. O., Attah, E. B., and Onyemelukwe, G. C.: Burkitt's lymphoma presenting with heart block. Br. Heart J. *37*:94, 1975.
138. Ballentyne, F., VanderArk, C. R., and Holick, M: Carotid sinus syncope and cervical lymphoma. Wis. Med. J. *74*:91, 1975.
139. O'Neill, M. O., Marshall, A. J., and Watt, I.: Occult cardiac metastasis and mitral reflux. Br. J. Radiol. *52*:669, 1979.
140. Inagaki, R., Rodriguez, V., and Brody, G. P.: Causes of death in cancer patients. Cancer *33*:568, 1974.
141. Kopelson, G., and Herwig, K. J.: The etiologies of coronary artery disease in cancer patients. Int. J. Radiol. Oncol. Biol. Phys. *4*:895, 1978.
142. Stewart, J. R., and Fajardo, L. F.: Cancer and coronary artery disease. Int. J. Rad. Oncol. Biol. Phys. *11*:915, 1978.
143. Parker, B. M.: Valvular involvement in cancer. *In* Kapoor, A. S. (ed.): Cancer and the Heart. New York, Springer-Verlag, l986, p. 64.
144. Deppisch, L. M., and Fayemi, A. O.: Nonbacterial thrombotic endocarditis. Am. Heart J. *92*:723, 1976.
145. Lehto, V. P., Stenman, S., and Somer, T.: Immunohistological studies on valvular vegetations in nonbacterial thrombotic endocarditis. Arch. Pathol. Microbiol. Scand. *90*:207, 1982.
146. Yam, L. T., Li, C. Y., Necheles, T. F., and Katayama, I.: Pseudoeosinophilic, eosinophilic endocarditis and eosinophilic leukemia. Am. J. Med. *53*:193, 1972.
147. Niemtzow, R. C., and Reynolds, R. D.: Radiation therapy and the heart. *In* Kapoor, A. S. (ed.): Cancer and the Heart. New York, Springer-Verlag, 1986, pp. 232–237.
148. Gottdeiner, J. S., Katin, M. J., Borer, J. S., Bacharach, S. L., and Gree, M. V.: Late cardiac effects of therapeutic mediastinal irradiation: Assessment by echocardiography and radionuclide angiography. N. Engl. J. Med. *308*:569, 1983.
149. Applefeld, M. M., and Wiernik, P. H.: Cardiac disease after radiation therapy for Hodgkin's disease. Analysis of 48 patients. Am. J. Cardiol. *51*:1679, 1983.
150. Taymor-Luria, H., Kohn, K., and Pasternak, R. C.: Radiation heart disease. J. Cardiovasc. Med. *8*:113, 1983.
151. Iqbal, S. M., Hanson, E. L., and Gensini, G. G.: Bypass graft for coronary arterial stenosis following radiation therapy. Chest *71*:664, 1977.
152. Miller, D. D., Waters, D. D., Dangoisse, V., and David, P. R.: Symptomatic coronary artery spasm following radiotherapy for Hodgkin's disease. Chest *83*:284, 1983.
153. Stegaru-Hellring, B., Keller, H., Bode, H., Usadel, K. H., and Wallwork, J.: Ostium stenosis of both coronary arteries and latent hypothyroidism as sequelae of radiotherapy in Hodgkin's disease. Z. Kardiol. *74*:485, 1985.
154. Simon, E. B., Ling, J., Mendizabal, R. C., and Midawell, J.: Radiation-induced coronary artery disease. Am. Heart J. *108*:1031, 1984.
155. Shashaty, G. G.: Aortic insufficiency following mediastinal radiation for Hodgkin's disease. Am. J. Med. Sci. *287*:46, 1984.
156. Warda, M., Kahn, A., Massumi, A., Mathur, V., Klimat, T., and Hall, R. J.: Radiation-induced valvular dysfunction. J. Am. Coll. Cardiol. *2*:180, 1983.
157. Detrano, R. C., Yiannikas, J., and Salcedo, E. E.: Two-dimensional echocardiographic assessment of radiation-induced valvular heart disease. Am. Heart J. *107*:584, 1984.
158. Rummeny, E., Hausen, W., Lorbacher, P., and Willems, D.: Acquired infundibular pulmonary stenosis. Possible late complication following radiotherapy of Hodgkin's disease. Z. Kardiol. *73*:641, 1984.
159. Gomez, G. A., Park, J. J., Panahoh, A. M., Parthasarathy, K. L., Pearce, J., Reese, P., Bakashi, S., and Henderson, E. S.: Heart size and function after

radiation therapy to the mediastinum in patients with Hodgkin's disease. Cancer Treat. Rep. *67*:1099, 1983.
160. Cohen, I. S., Bharati, S., Glass, J., and Lev, M: Radiotherapy as a cause of complete atrioventricular block in Hodgkin's disease. Arch. Int. Med. *141*:676, 1981.
161. Akaike, A., Cogure, R., Oyama, K., and Oda, M.: Damage to the heart from tumor irradiation in the thorax: An echocardiographic study. Radiology 25:430, 1985.
162. Carmel, R. J., and Kaplan, H. S.: Mantle irradiation in Hodgkin's disease. Cancer 37:2813, 1976.
163. Ikaheimo, M. J., Niemela, K. O., Linnaluoto, M. M., Jakobsson, M. J. T., Takkunen, J. T., and Taskinen, P. J.: Early cardiac changes related to radiation therapy. Am J. Cardiol. *56*:943, 1985.
164. Strender, L. E., Lindhal, J., and Larsson, L. E.: Incidence of heart disease and functional significance of changes in the electrocardiogram 10 years after radiotherapy for breast cancer. Cancer 57:929, 1986.
165. Silverberg, G. O., Britt, R. H., and Goffinet, D. R.: Radiation-induced carotid artery disease. Cancer *41*:130, 1978.
166. Amromin, G. G., Gildenhorn, H. C., and Solomon, R. D.: The synergism of x-irradiation and cholesterol-fat feeding on the development of coronary artery lesions. J. Atheroscler. Res. *4*:325, 1975.
167. Brosius, F. C., Waller, B. F., and Roberts, W. C.: Radiation heart disease: Analysis of 16 young (aged 15 to 33 years) necropsy patients who received over 3500 rads to the heart. Am. J. Med. 7:519, 1981.
168. Kantrowitz, N. E., and Bristow, M. R.: Cardiotoxicity of antitumor agents. Prog. Cardiovasc. Dis. *27*:195, 1984.
169. Sunnenberg, D., and Kramer, B.: Long-term effects of cancer chemotherapy. Comp. Ther. *11*:58, 1985.
170. Perry, M. C.: Effects of chemotherapy on the heart. *In* Kapoor, A. S. (ed.): Cancer and the Heart. New York, Springer-Verlag, 1986, p. 223.
171. Lancaster, L. D., and Ewy, G. A.: Cardiac consequences of malignancy and their treatment. Adv. Intern. Med. *30*:275, 1984.
172. Schoenberger, C. I., and Crystal, R.: Drug-induced lung disease. *In* Isselbacher, K. J. (ed.): Update IV to Harrison's Principles of Internal Medicine. New York, McGraw-Hill, 1982, pp. 49–74.
173. Young, R. C., Oxols, R. F., and Myers, C. E.: The anthracycline antineoplastic drugs. N. Engl. J. Med. *305*:139, 1981.
174. Lena, L., and Page, J. A.: Cardiotoxicity of Adriamycin and related anthracyclines. Cancer Treat. Rev. *3*:111, 1976.
175. Ali, M. K., Soto, P. A., Maroongroge, D., Bekheit-Saad, S., Buzdar, A. U., Blumenschein, G. R., Hortobagyi, G. N., Tashima, C. K., Wiseman, C. L., and Shullenberger, C. C.: Electrocardiographic changes after Adriamycin chemotherapy. Cancer *43*:465, 1979.
176. Bristow, M. R., Billingham, M. E., Mason, J. W., and Daniels, J. R.: Clinical spectrum of anthracycline antibiotic cardiotoxicity. Cancer Treat. Rep. *62*:873, 1978.
177. Wortman, J. E., Lucas, V. S., Jr., Schuster, E., Thiele, D., and Logue, G. L.: Sudden death during doxorubicin administration. Cancer *44*:1588, 1979.
178. Haq, M. M., Legha, S. S., Choksi, J., Hortobagyi, G. N., Benjamin, R. S., Ewer, M., and Ali, M.: Doxorubicin-induced congestive heart failure in adults. Cancer *56*:1361, 1985.
179. Greene, H. L., Reich, S. D., and Dalen, J. E.: How to minimize doxorubicin toxicity. J. Cardiovasc. Med. *7*:306, 1982.
180. Isner, J. M., Ferrans, V. J., Cohen, S. R., Witkind, B. G., Virmani, R., Gottdiener, J. S., Beck, J. R., and Roberts, W. C.: Clinical and morphological cardiac findings after anthracycline chemotherapy. Analysis of 64 patients studied at necroscopy. Am. J. Cardiol. *51*:1167, 1983.
181. Merrill, J., Greco, F. A., Zimbler, H., Brereton, H. D., Lambert, J. D., and Pomeroy, T. C.: Adriamycin and radiation: Synergistic cardiotoxicity. Ann. Intern. Med. *82*:122, 1975.
182. Fajardo, L. R., and Stewart, J. F.: Pathogenesis or radiation-induced myocardial fibrosis. Lab. Invest. *29*:244, 1973.
183. O'Connell, T. X., and Berenbaum, M. D.: Cardiac and pulmonary effects of high doses of cyclophosphamide and isophosphamide. Cancer Res. *34*:1586, 1974.
184. Mills, B. A., and Roberts, R. W.: Cyclophosphamide-induced cardiomyopathy. A report of two cases and a review of the English literature. Cancer *43*:2223, 1979.
185. Tritton, T. R., Murphee, S. A., and Sartorelli, A. C.: Adriamycin: A proposal on the specificity of drug action. Biochem. Biophys. Res. Commun. *84*:802, 1978.
186. Lewis, W., Kleinerman, J., and Poszkin, S.: Interaction of Adriamycin in vitro with cardiac myofibrillar proteins. Circ. Res. *50*:547, 1982.
187. Milei, J., Bovevis, A., Llesoy, S., Molina, A., Storino, R., Ortega, D., and Milei, S. E.: Amelioration of Adriamycin-induced cardiotoxicity in rabbits by prenylamine and vitamin A + E. Am. Heart J. *111*:95, 1986.
188. Alexander, J., Dainiak, T., Berger, H. J., Goldman, L., Johnstone, D., Reduto, L., Duffy, T., Schwartz, P., Gottschalk, A., and Zaret, B. L.: Serial assessment of doxorubicin cardiotoxicity with quantitative radionuclide angiocardiography. N. Engl. J. Med. *300*:278, 1979.
189. Binacaniello, T., Myer, R. A., Wong, K. Y., Sager, C., and Kaplan, S.: Doxorubicin cardiotoxicity in children. J. Pediatr. *97*:45, 1980.
189a. Lee, B. H., Goodenday, L. S., Muswick, G. J., Yasnoff, W. A., Leighton, R. F., and Skeel, R. T.: Alterations in left ventricular diastolic function with doxorubicin therapy. J. Am. Coll. Cardiol. *9*:184, 1987.
190. Applefeld, M. M., and Pollock, S. H.: Cardiac disease in patients who have malignancies. Current Problems in Cardiology. Vol. 4, No. 6. Chicago, Year Book Medical Publishers, 1980.
191. Gottdiener, J. S., Mathisen, D. J., Borer, J. S., Bonow, R. O., Myers, C. E., Barr, L. H., Schwartz, D. E., Bacharach, S. L., Green, M. V., and Rosenberg, S. A.: Doxorubicin cardiotoxicity: Assessment of late left ventricular dysfunction by radionuclide cineangiography. Ann. Intern. Med. *94*:430, 1981.
192. Bristow, M. R., Mason, J. W., Billingham, M. E., and Daniels, J. R.: Doxorubicin cardiomyopathy. Evaluation by phonocardiography, endomyocardial biopsy, and cardiac catheterization. Ann. Intern. Med. *88*:168, 1978.
193. Bristow, M. R., Mason, J. W., Billingham, M. E., and Daniels, J. R.: Dose effect and structure-function relationships in doxorubicin cardiomyopathy. Am. Heart J. *102*:709, 1981.
194. Fowles, R. E.: Cardiac catheterization and endomyocardial biopsy. *In* Kapoor, A. S. (ed.): Cancer and the Heart. Springer-Verlag, New York, 1986, pp. 42–50.
195. Bristow, M. R., Lopez, M. R., Mason, J. W., Billingham, M. E., and Winchester, M. A.: Efficacy and the cost of cardiac monitoring in patients receiving doxorubicin. Cancer *50*:32, 1982.
196. Von Hoff, D. D., Layard, M. W., Basa, P., Davis, H. L., Von Hoff, A. L., Rozenzweig, M., and Muggia, F. M.: Risk factors for doxorubicin-induced congestive heart failure. Ann. Intern. Med. *91*:710, 1979.
197. Weiss, R. B., Grillo-Lopez, A. J., Marsoni, S., Pasoda, J. G., Hess, F., and Ross, B. J.: Amsacrine associated cardiotoxicity: An analysis of 82 cases. J. Clin. Oncol. *4*:918, 1986.
198. Lyman, G. H., Williams, C. C., Dinwoodie, W. R., and Schocken, D. D.: Sudden death in cancer patients receiving lithium. J. Clin. Oncol. *2*:1270, 1984.
199. Doroshow, H. J., Locker, G. Y., Ifrim, I., and Myers, C. E.: Prevention of doxorubicin cardiac toxicity in the mouse by N-acetylcysteine. J. Clin. Invest. *68*:1053, 1981.
200. Cortes. E. P., Gupta, M., Chew, C., Amin, V. C., and Folker, K.: Adriamycin cardiotoxicity: Early detection by systolic time interval and possible prevention by Coenzyme Q. Cancer Treat. Rep. *62*:887, 1978.
201. Somberg, J., Cagin, N., Levitt, L. B., Bounous, H., Ready, P., Lonard, D., and Anagnostopoulos, C.: Blockade of tissue uptake of the antineoplastic agent doxorubicin. J. Pharmacol. Exp. Ther. *204*:226, 1978.
202. Legla, S. S., Benjamin, R. S., MacKay, B., Ewer, M., Wallace, S., Valdirieso, M., Rasmussen, S. L., Blumenschein, G. R., and Friereich, E. J.: Reduction of doxorubicin cardiotoxicity by prolonged continuous intravenous infusion. Ann. Intern. Med. *96*:133, 1982.
203. Valdirieso, M., Burgess, M. A., Awer, M. S., Mackay, B., Wallace, S., Benjamin, R. S., Ali, M. K., Bodey, G. P., and Freireich, E. J.: Increased therapeutic index of weekly doxorubicin in the therapy of non small cell lung cancer: A prospective randomized study. J. Clin. Oncol. *2*:207, 1984.
204. Taylor, A. L., Applefeld, M. N., Wiernik, P. H., Grochow, L. B., Mader, L. C., and Bulkley, B. H.: Acute anthracycline cardiotoxicity. Comparative morphologic study of three analogues. Cancer *53*:1660, 1984.
205. Leitner, S. P., Casper, E. S., Hakes, T. B., Kaufman, R. J., Winn, F. J., Scoppetuolo, M., Raymond, V., Geller, N. L., and Young, C. W.: A phase II trial of 4′-deoxydoxorubicin in patients with advanced breast cancer. Cancer Treat. Rep. *69*:1319, 1985.
206. Bramhilla, C., Rossi, A., Bonfonta, B., Ferrari, L., Villani, F., Crippa, F., and Bonadonna, G.: Phase II study of doxorubicin versus epirubicin in advanced breast cancer. Cancer Treat. Rep. *70*:261, 1986.
206a. Baello, E. B., Ensberg, M. E., Fergoson, D. W., Kogler, J. W., Gingrich, R. D., Armitage, J. O., Klassen, L. W., Kirchner, P. T., Kerber, R. E., Marcus, M. L., and Skorton, D. J.: Effect of high dose cyclophosphamide and total-body irradiation on left ventricular function in adult patients with leukemia undergoing allogeneic bone marrow transplantation. Cancer Treat. Rep. *70*:1187, 1986.
206b. Goldberg, M. A., Antin, J. H., Guinan, E. C., and Rappeport, J. M.: Cyclophosphamide cardiotoxicity. An analysis of dosing as a risk factor. Blood *68*:1114, 1986.
207. Gottdiener, J. S., Applebaum, F. R., Ferrans, V. J., Deiseroth, A., and Ziegler, J.: Cardiotoxicity associated with high dose cyclophosphamide therapy. Arch. Intern. Med. *141*:758, 1981.
208. Steinherz, L. J., Steinherz, P. G., Mangiacasale, D., Tan, C., and Miller, D. R.: Cardiac abnormalities after AMSA administration. Cancer Treat. Rep. *66*:483, 1982.
209. Lindpainter, K., Lindpainter, L. S., Wentworth, M., and Burns, C. P.: Acute myocardial necrosis during administration of amsacrine. Cancer *57*:1284, 1986.
210. Shenkenberg, T. D., and VonHoff, D. D.: Mitroxantrone: A new anticancer drug with significant clinical activity. Ann. Intern. Med. *105*:67, 1986.
211. Colman, R. E., Maisey, M. N., Knight, R. K., and Rubens, R. D.: Mitoxantrone in advanced breast cancer: A phase II study with special attention to cardiotoxicity. Eur. J. Cancer Clin. Oncol. *20*:771, 1984.
212. Pratt, C. G., Vietti, T. J., Etcubanas, E., Sexauer, C., Krance, R. A., Mahoney, D. H., and Patterson, R. B.: Nonvantrone for childhood malignant solid tumors. A pediatric oncology group phase II study. Invest. New Drugs *4*:43, 1986.
213. Landys, K., Bergstom, S., Andersson, T., and Noppa, H.: Mitoxantrone as a first line treatment of advanced breast cancer. Invest. New Drugs *3*:133, 1985.
214. Allegra, J. C., Woodcock, T., Woolf, S., Henderson, I. C., Bryan, S., Reisman, A., and Dukare, G.: A randomized trial comparing mitoxantrone with doxorubicin in patients with stage IV breast cancer. Invest. New Drugs *3*:153, 1985.
215. Cameron, H. A., Reyntjens, A. J., and Lake-Bakaar, G.: Cardiac arrest after treatment with intravenous domperidone. Br. Med. J. Clin. Res. *290*:160, 1985.

216. Osborne, A. J., Slevin, N. L., Hunter, L. W., and Hamer, J.: Cardiac arrhythmias during cytotoxic chemotherapy: Role of domperidone. Hum. Toxicol. *4*:617, 1985.

217. Cazin, V., Gorin, C., Laport, J. P., Gallet, B., Douay, L., Lopez, M., Najman, A., and Duhamel, G.: Cardiac complications after bone marrow transplantation. A report on a series of 63 consecutive transplantations. Cancer 57:2061, 1986.

HEMATOLOGICAL ABNORMALITIES RELATED TO CARDIAC DRUGS

218. Gavras, F., Graff, L. G., Rose, B. D., McKenna, J. M., Brunner, H. R., and Gavras, H.: Fatal pancytopenia associated with the use of captopril. Ann. Intern. Med. *94*:58–59, 1981.

219. Lundh, B., and Hasselgren, K. H.: Hematological side effects from antihypertensive drugs. Acta Med. Scand. (Suppl 628):73, 1979.

220. Erslev, A. J. Aplastic anemia. *In* Williams, W. J. (ed.): Hematology. 3rd. ed. New York, McGraw-Hill, 1983, pp. 155–158.

220a. Volosin, K., Greenberg, R. M., and Grenspon, A. J.: Tocainide-associated agranulocytosis. Am. Heart J. *109*:1392, 1985.

221. Finch, S. C.: Neutropenia. *In* Williams, W. J. (ed.): Hematology. New York, McGraw-Hill, 1983, pp. 777–786.

222. Hackett, T., Kelton, J. G., and Powers, P.: Drug-induced platelet destruction. Sem. Thromb. Hemos. 8:116, 1982.

223. Ansell, J., McCue, J., Tiarks, C., Parrilla, N., Ryback, M. E., and Benotti, J.: Amrinone-induced thrombocytopenia. Blood *58*(Suppl.1):187a, 1981.

224. Packman, C. H., and Leddy, J. P.: Drug-related immunologic injury of erythrocytes. *In* Williams, W. J. (ed.): Hematology. New York, McGraw-Hill, 1983, pp. 647–650.

225. Bell, W. R., and Royall, R. M.: Heparin-associated thrombocytopenia: A comparison of three heparin preparations. N. Engl. J. Med. *303*:902, 1980.

226. Salzman, E. W., Rosenberg, R. D., Smith, M. H., Lindon, J. N., and Favreau, L.: Effect of heparin and heparin fractions of platelet aggregation. J. Clin. Invest. *65*:64, 1980.

227. Gibson, G. R., Hunter, J. B., Raabe, D. S., Manjoney, D. L., and Ittlema, F. P.: Methemoalbuminemia produced by high-dose intravenous nitroglycerin. Ann. Intern. Med. *96*:615, 1982.

228. Shoemaker, C., and Meyers, M.: Sodium nitroprusside for control of severe hypertensive disease of pregnancy: A case report and discussion of potential toxicity. Am. J. Obstet. Gynecol. *149*:171, 1984.

229. Vesey, C. J., and Cole, P. V.: Blood cyanide and thiocyanate concentrations produced by long-term therapy with sodium nitroprusside. Br. J. Anesth. 57:148, 1985.

230. Cush, J. J., and Goldings, E. A.: Drug-induced lupus: Clinical spectrum and pathogenesis. Am. J. Med. Sci. *290*:36, 1985.

231. Weisbart, R. H., Yee, W. S., Colburn, K. K., Whang, S. H., Heng, M. K., and Bouce, K. R. J.: Antiguanosine antibodies: A new marker for procainamide-induced systemic lupus erythematosus. Ann. Intern. Med. *104*:310, 1986.

56 HEMOSTASIS, THROMBOSIS, FIBRINOLYSIS, AND CARDIOVASCULAR DISEASE

by ROBERT I. HANDIN, M.D., and
JOSEPH LOSCALZO, M.D., Ph.D.

Thrombosis and embolism either contribute to the pathogenesis of many cardiovascular disorders or complicate their clinical course. After several decades of laboratory and clinical research, a role for platelets and coagulation proteins in the pathogenesis of atherosclerosis has been established (see Chap. 35). Not only do many acute cardiovascular events, such as myocardial infarction and stroke, arise from thrombotic occlusion of atherosclerotic arteries, but also patients with preexisting chronic disorders such as congestive heart failure, cardiomyopathy, and valvular or congenital heart disease are at increased risk of venous or arterial thromboembolism. As a result of these clinical and experimental observations, anticoagulant, antiplatelet, and, most recently, fibrinolytic agents have become increasingly important therapeutic tools for the cardiologist.

In this chapter the pathophysiology of normal hemostasis will be reviewed, and those disorders will be described that cause failure of hemostasis with hemorrhage as well as those that increase the risk of thrombosis. The inherited prethrombotic or hypercoagulable disorders will be used to illustrate more general mechanisms of venous and arterial thromboembolism in patients with cardiovascular disorders. Finally, methods for preventing and treating thromboembolism associated with cardiovascular diseases will be discussed, including new options for clot dissolution—an area in which rapid and impressive strides have been made over the past few years.

HEMOSTASIS

Unactivated *platelets* circulate as individual, smooth-surfaced discs that do not interact with other cells in the blood or with the endothelial cells lining blood vessels. However, platelets will adhere to subendothelium that has been exposed as a result of vascular injury or to any foreign or prosthetic material in contact with blood. Adherent, activated platelets generate potent mediators that cause vasoconstriction and leukocyte chemotaxis. The platelets then degranulate, releasing materials that attract additional platelets, forming a multicellular aggregate or hemostatic plug on the adherent monolayer. These events, collectively referred to as *primary hemostasis*, are the first line of defense against hemorrhage after vascular injury. They are particularly important in capillaries and small arterioles where shear forces are high and the formation of a platelet plug is critical for effective hemostasis.

The *plasma coagulation system*, or secondary hemostatic system, is simultaneously activated in response to vascular injury and, within several minutes, generates insoluble fibrin strands that interdigitate with and strengthen the primary platelet plug. Fibrin is produced by the action of thrombin on fibrinogen. Thrombin is generated by a series of linked proteolytic reactions that take place on phospholipid-rich cell surfaces and are regulated by plasma cofactors and calcium, which accelerate coagulation, and by a series of naturally occurring inhibitors, or anticoagulants. Although platelet activation and fibrin production are described as separate processes, they are actually closely linked and interdependent. For example, the surface of the activated platelet provides the optimal locus for several critical coagulation reactions and accelerates them several hundred fold. Conversely, thrombin generated during plasma coagulation is also a potent platelet agonist and stimulates platelet secretion and aggregation. Endothelial cells lining blood vessels also bind coagulation proteins, accelerate their interactions, and secrete both inhibitory and procoagulant molecules.

Although the hemostatic system has evolved to minimize

blood loss from injured vessels, there is little actual difference between the physiological process of normal hemostasis and the pathological events that lead to thrombosis and embolism. Because of this similarity, thrombosis has been described as hemostasis occurring in the wrong place or at the wrong time. While both inherited and acquired disorders may predispose a patient to thrombosis, in many cases the triggering event is simply the interaction of normal blood components with an abnormal surface such as a diseased or atherosclerotic vessel, a prosthetic cardiac valve, or a vascular graft. Furthermore, bleeding due to failure of a component in the hemostatic system is similar to the purposeful or therapeutic failure of hemostasis induced by anticoagulant agents used to prevent recurrent thromboembolism. Most of the available anticoagulant drugs are not selective and have a relatively poor therapeutic index. Thus, the dose of drug needed to produce the desired antithrombotic effect may also cause undesirable hemorrhage. Finally, since pathological thrombi may coexist with physiological and vital hemostatic plugs, even the more selective drugs, such as the relatively fibrin-specific plasminogen activators, cannot discriminate between fibrin within pathological thrombi and that within physiologic "thrombi."

PLATELETS IN COAGULATION

PLATELET ADHESION TO THE VESSEL WALL. Platelet adhesion, the initial event in both normal hemostasis and thrombosis, is a complex process involving constituents of the vascular subendothelium, receptor sites on the platelet membrane, and plasma glycoproteins (Fig. 56–1). In normal hemostasis, platelets adhere to exposed subendothelial collagen after the traumatic removal of endothelial cells that normally line the blood vessel. In addition, thrombus formation may be initiated by the adhesion of platelets to damaged endothelial cells or denuded atherosclerotic plaques. Although several candidates have been proposed as the platelet collagen receptor, the collagen binding site is most likely located on platelet glycoprotein Ia.[1, 2] This initial bond between the platelet and the vessel wall is strengthened by the interaction of several adhesive glycoproteins.

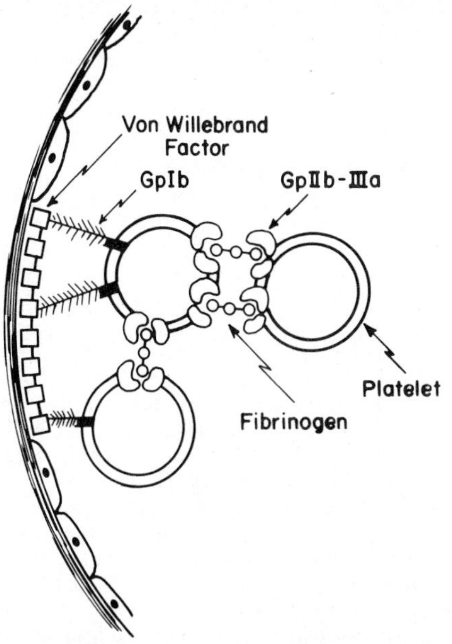

FIGURE 56–1. Molecular mechanisms of platelet attachment to vascular subendothelium (platelet adhesion) and of platelet-platelet interactions (platelet aggregation) in a cross-sectional view of a blood vessel. von Willebrand's multimers attach to exposed vascular subendothelial collagen and to a platelet membrane receptor site on glycoprotein Ib (GpIb). This is the initial interaction in hemostasis and stabilizes platelets so that they remain attached despite the high shear forces generated by flowing blood. Receptor sites on platelet membrane glycoproteins IIb and IIIa (GpIIb/IIIa) then become available to bind fibrinogen. The fibrinogen molecule links platelets together to form the hemostatic plug.

Fibronectin. This 440,000-dalton dimeric protein binds to collagen and to platelets through receptor sites on the platelet glycoprotein IIb/IIIa (GpIIb/IIIa) complex.[3, 4] Fibronectin binding facilitates both initial platelet attachment to the vessel wall and subsequent spreading over the subendothelial surface.[5]

von Willebrand's Factor (vWF). This protein circulates as a heterogeneous series of high molecular weight multimers and also binds to collagen[6] and to two separate platelet receptor sites. The best defined receptor site for vWF is on platelet glycoprotein Ib.[7] Binding to this site is critically important for normal platelet adhesion. vWF binding to a second platelet receptor site on glycoproteins IIb/IIIa may facilitate both adhesion and platelet-platelet cohesion or aggregate formation.[8] This factor plays a critical role in hemostasis, since it stabilizes the attachment of platelets to the vessel wall under conditions of high shear stress.[9, 10] Neither the initial collagen-GpIa interaction nor the secondary interposition of fibronectin between platelets and collagen is sufficient to sustain platelet adhesion in the face of the high shear stresses encountered with normal blood flow. This unique property of vWF is clinically important, since bleeding and abnormal platelet function are found in patients with a mild or moderate deficiency in vWF despite normal interactions between the platelet membrane and subendothelial collagen and normal binding of fibronectin to the platelet and vessel wall.

PLATELET ACTIVATION AND SECRETION. Platelet activation follows the adhesion of platelets to vascular subendothelium, or the binding of soluble agonists to platelet membrane receptors, and culminates in granule release and the formation of a platelet aggregate or hemostatic plug. Platelets have specific binding sites for adenosine diphosphate (ADP), thrombin, serotonin, and alpha$_2$-adrenergic agonists.[11] As shown in Figure 56–2, occupancy of these receptors by the appropriate agonists activates two intracellular enzymes, protein kinase A and protein kinase C, which then catalyze the phosphorylation of critical regulatory proteins within the platelet. Protein kinase A activity is regulated by the level of intracellular cyclic AMP and protein kinase C by diacylglycerol (DAG), a product of phospholipid hydrolysis. Inhibition of platelet adenylate cyclase activity activates protein kinase A, which then phosphorylates myosin light chain and enhances the contractile activity of platelet actomyosin. In contrast, the major substrate for protein kinase C is a 47,000-dalton protein that may serve as a feedback inhibitor of platelet activation, as described below. Although the specific target proteins may differ slightly, the sequence of reactions resembles that seen following the activation of beta-adrenoceptors in heart muscle (p. 391).

Mechanisms of Activation. Although there are two separate signal transduction pathways mediated by protein kinases A and C within the platelet, their relative contributions to platelet activation are still being debated. Agonists like epinephrine clearly inhibit adenylate cyclase activity in platelet membrane fractions; however, incubating intact platelets with epinephrine does not reduce intraplatelet cyclic AMP to below basal levels, suggesting that cyclic AMP levels do not regulate platelet signal transduction and activation.[12] Alternatively, since cyclic AMP is compartmentalized within the platelet, regulation of cyclic AMP content within a specific compartment may be an important mechanism for signal transduction by certain agonists. The bulk of recent evidence suggests that the adenylate cyclase–cyclic AMP system provides a mechanism to *inhibit* platelet activation. In fact, many agents that stimulate platelet adenylate cyclase activity and raise intraplatelet cyclic AMP levels, such as prostaglandins E_1, D_2, and I_2, are potent platelet inhibitors.[13, 14]

Transduction of the signal initiated by membrane receptor occupancy is more likely to be mediated by the intracellular enzyme phospholipase C, which hydrolyzes a trace membrane phospholipid, phosphatidylinositol 4, 5-bisphosphate (PIP_2), yielding inositol 1, 4, 5,-trisphosphate (IP_3) and DAG.[15, 16] While the role of cyclic AMP in the process of platelet activation may be unclear, the two products of PIP_2 hydrolysis are clearly important mediators of platelet signal transduction. IP_3 acts as a calcium ionophore, transiently raising intraplatelet calcium levels, while DAG activates protein kinase C, which then phosphorylates several intracellular proteins.[17, 18] One prominent substrate is a 47,000-dalton protein recently identified as a phosphomonoesterase. When phosphorylated, it inactivates IP_3, serving as a feedback inhibitor of platelet activation.[19] There is also pharmacological evidence that IP_3 and DAG themselves mediate signal transduction directly. The ability of a calcium ionophore to initiate platelet signal transduction has been well established. Furthermore, incubation of platelets with DAG analogues like oleylacylglycerol (OAG), which cross the platelet membrane, can mimic the effect of endogenous DAG.[20] Likewise, incubation of platelets with phorbolmyristate acetate (PMA), an agent that directly activates protein kinase C, eliminates the requirement for phospholipid hydrolysis and DAG generation for platelet activation.[21]

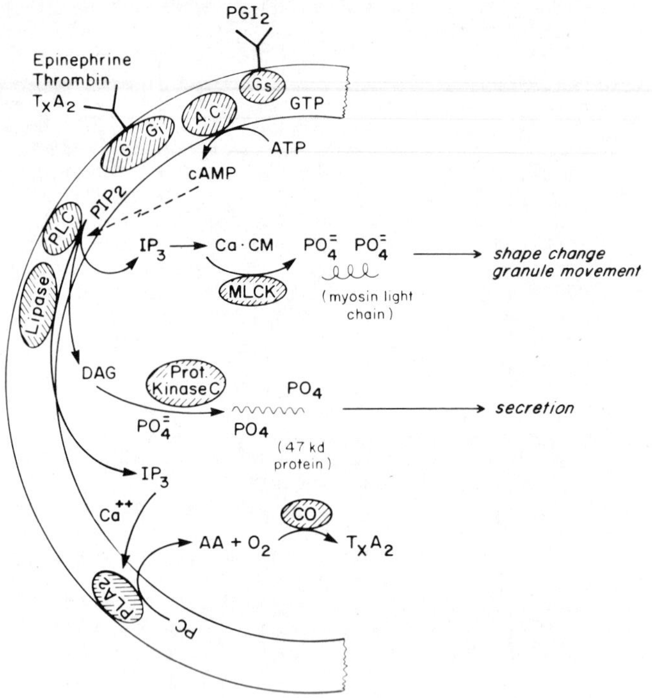

FIGURE 56–2. Biochemical pathways for stimulus response coupling in the platelet. Platelets contain receptors that bind various agonists, including epinephrine, thrombin, and thromboxane A_2 (TxA_2) and the antagonist prostaglandin I_2 (PGI_2). Receptors for agonists and antagonists are coupled to two enzymes, adenylate cyclase (AC) and phospholipase C (PLC), via guanine nucleotide binding (G) proteins. Coupling to AC occurs via separate G_i (inhibitory) and G_s (stimulatory) proteins. It is not yet known whether coupling of receptors to PLC is via the same or a different set of G proteins. Activation of AC by PGI_2 raises intracellular cyclic AMP (cAMP) and inhibits platelet function, while inhibition of AC facilitates platelet activation by an incompletely worked out set of reactions. PLC hydrolyzes the membrane phospholipid phosphatidylinositol bisphosphate (PIP_2) to yield diacylglycerol (DAG) and inositol triphosphate (IP_3). IP_3 functions as a calcium ionophore and transiently increases intracellular ionized calcium (Ca) which facilitates several important intraplatelet reactions. In one, Ca bound to calmodulin (CM) activates myosin light chain kinase (MLCK) which then phosphorylates the light chain of platelet myosin. The phosphorylated light chain participates in contractile force generation within the platelet which causes shape change and granule movement. DAG activates protein kinase C which, in turn, phosphorylates several other intracellular proteins that regulate secretion. There are two different mechanisms to hydrolyze arachidonic acid (AA) from membrane phospholipids. First, DAG generated by PLC is the substrate for an intramembrane diglyceride lipase. Second, the IP_3-induced calcium flux activates a second enzyme phospholipase A_2 (PLA_2) which hydrolyzes AA from phosphatidyl choline (PC). AA is then oxygenated by the enzyme cyclooxygenase (CO) and subsequently converted to TxA_2, a potent platelet agonist and vasoconstrictor. TxA_2 then stimulates additional platelet activation via the previously described pathways. Aspirin and nonsteroidal antiinflammatory agents act as antiplatelet agents by irreversibly acetylating CO and preventing TxA_2 generation.

ROLE OF ARACHIDONIC ACID AND PROSTAGLANDINS. Arachidonic acid (5,8,11,14-eicosatetraenoic acid), a 20-carbon polyunsaturated fatty acid derived from dietary linoleic acid, is the precursor of the prostaglandins, leukotrienes, and thromboxanes—eiocosanoid mediators generated by activated platelets, leukocytes, and endothelial cells.[22, 23] Arachidonate is taken up by the platelet from plasma and is esterified into platelet phospholipids. As outlined in Figures 56–2 and 56–3, the combined action of phospholipase C and diglyceride lipase on phosphatidylinositol rapidly releases arachidonic acid early in the process of platelet activation.[24] Additional arachidonate is subsequently liberated from phosphatidylcholine by a phospholipase A_2 enzyme.[25] Released arachidonate is rapidly oxygenated by cyclooxygenase or lipoxygenase enzymes in platelets, leukocytes, and endothelial cells to yield various prostanoid and eicosanoid mediators.

THROMBOXANE A_2 (TxA_2). This potent vasoconstrictor and platelet agonist is the most important platelet eicosanoid mediator.[23] The generation of TxA_2 by activated platelets may explain the vasoconstriction and vessel retraction that accompany vascular injury and may contribute to the vasospasm observed in partially occluded atherosclerotic coronary and cerebral vessels. Inhibition of TxA_2 synthesis by agents like aspirin may explain their beneficial antithrombotic effect.[22] The principal platelet lipoxygenase product, 12-hydroxyeicosatetraenoic acid (12-HETE), has no direct role in hemostasis but may serve as a chemotactic agent for neutrophils and contribute to the inflammatory response.[26]

PROSTACYCLIN (PGI_2). The endothelial cell converts arachidonic acid into PGI_2, a labile cyclic prostaglandin.[27] In contrast to TxA_2, PGI_2 is a potent vasodilator that inhibits platelet aggregation and secretion by activating platelet adenylate cyclase and elevating intraplatelet cyclic AMP. Thrombin, calcium ionophore, bradykinin, serotonin, platelet-derived growth factor, and mechanical injury can all induce the synthesis of PGI_2 by endothelial cells. Although it is tempting to postulate that a balance between TxA_2 and PGI_2 synthesis by their respective cells regulates platelet vessel wall interactions and vessel tone, it is difficult to test this hypothesis, since both eicosanoids have very short half-lives, are produced in small quantities, and function locally within the microcirculation. Whole-body turnover studies that assess the excretion of thromboxane and prostacyclin metabolites in urine by gas chromatography and mass spectrometry demonstrate that the production of both eicosanoids is increased in thrombotic states and vascular disease.[28, 29]

THE LEUKOTRIENES. A relatively new class of eicosanoid mediators, the leukotrienes, play an important role in inflammation[30] (Fig. 56–3). The major derivative of arachidonic acid in polymorphonuclear leukocytes is 5-hydroxyeicosatetraenoic acid (5-HETE), which is con-

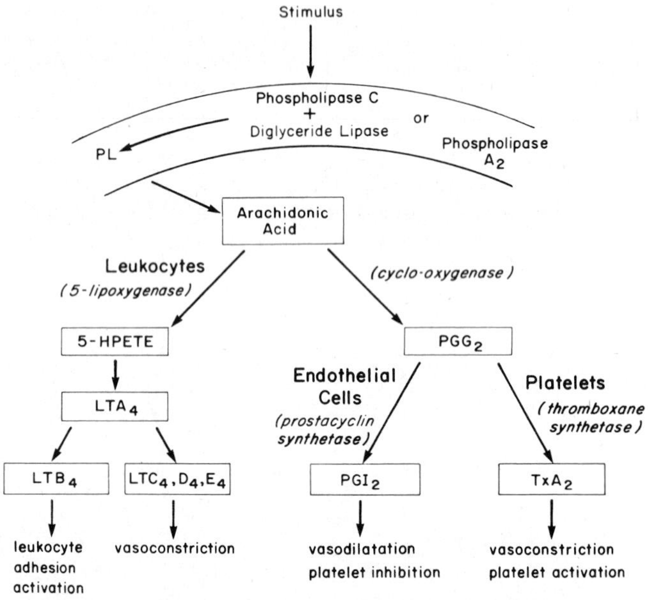

FIGURE 56–3. Liberation of arachidonic acid from membrane phospholipids and its subsequent conversion into biologically active mediators in leukocytes, platelets, and endothelial cells. Arachidonic acid is liberated from membrane phospholipids after cellular activation by the combined effects of the enzymes phospholipase C and diglyceride lipase or by the action of a phospholipase A_2 enzyme. In leukocytes, arachidonic acid is converted to an unstable intermediate, 5-hydroperoxyeicosatetraenoic acid (5-HPETE), by a 5-lipoxygenase enzyme. 5-HPETE is then converted into the leukotrienes (LT). Leukotriene B_4 (LTB_4) stimulates leukocyte adhesion to endothelial cells; leukotrienes C_4, D_4, and E_4 are potent vasoconstrictors. In platelets and endothelial cells, the principal pathway for arachidonic acid metabolism is via cyclooxygenase, which forms the unstable intermediate prostaglandin G_2 (PGG_2). It is then converted to prostaglandin I_2 (PGI_2, or prostacyclin) via prostacyclin synthetase within endothelial cells. Prostacyclin, a labile compound, is a potent vasodilator that inhibits platelet activation. Within the platelet, PGG_2 is converted to thromboxane A_2 (TXA_2), another labile compound that is a potent vasoconstrictor and platelet agonist. Aspirin and other nonsteroidal antiinflammatory agents interfere with hemostasis by inhibiting the enzyme cyclooxygenase. They have no effect on leukotriene biosynthesis.

verted to leukotriene A_4 (LTA_4). LTA_4 is then converted to LTB_4 by the addition of a 12-OH group. LTA_4 is also converted to leukotrienes C_4, D_4, and E_4 by the addition and subsequent metabolism of glutathione. The mediator responsible for acute anaphylaxis, formerly called the slow reacting substance of anaphylaxis or SRS-A, is actually a mixture of the peptidolipid leukotrienes C_4, D_4, and E_4, which are potent broncho- and vasoconstrictors. These leukotrienes may also be important in hemostasis, since they constrict the microvasculature and coronary arteries. In addition, because they are products of the lipoxygenase reaction, their biosynthesis is not inhibited by cyclooxygenase inhibitors such as aspirin.

There is also active transcellular metabolism of eicosanoids. For example, two of the prostaglandin endoperoxide precursors, PGG_2 and PGH_2, can leave the platelet and enter the endothelial cell to be converted to PGI_2. Thus, a byproduct of platelet activation is transformed into a platelet inhibitor and acts as a feedback regulator—a phenomenon referred to as the "endoperoxide steal."[31, 32] There is also evidence that unmetabolized arachidonic acid derived from aspirin-treated platelets may be converted into the vasoactive leukotrienes by polymorphonuclear leukocytes.

GRANULE SECRETION OR RELEASE. Platelets contain two classes of secretory granules, which are most readily classified by their density on electron micrographs. The most electron-dense (delta) granules contain adenine nucleotides (ADP and ATP), calcium, and serotonin, while the less electron-dense alpha granules contain enzymes, adhesive and coagulation proteins, and growth factors.[33] After platelet activation, both granule classes release their contents into the vicinity of the platelet plug, where they diffuse into plasma and into the vessel wall.[34] Platelet-derived growth factor (PDGF) and transforming growth factor beta (TGF-beta) stimulate smooth muscle cell and fibroblast migration and proliferation.[35] This may be of importance both in wound healing and in the pathogenesis of atherosclerosis. TGF-beta may also inhibit the migration and proliferation of endothelial cells. Other secreted molecules enhance vascular permeability, bind glycosaminoglycans, and induce the chemotaxis of leukocytes to sites of vascular injury.[36]

PLATELET AGGREGATION. Fibrinogen is an essential cofactor for platelet aggregation. Although platelets circulate in a milieu rich in fibrinogen, they do not bind to it but remain as single, disc-shaped particles. Contact with ADP, derived from damaged tissue and red cells as well as from platelet secretory granules, initiates both platelet aggregate formation and fibrinogen binding. The binding of ADP to an unidentified platelet receptor induces platelets to become spherical and to extend large pseudopods. In addition, the conformation of the platelet membrane glycoprotein IIb/IIIa complex changes so that it binds plasma fibrinogen[37] (Fig. 56–1). A unique dodecapeptide sequence on the gamma chain of fibrinogen as well as a second tripeptide sequence (Arg-Gly-Asp) on the alpha chain each bind to the platelet.[38, 39] This tripeptide sequence is also present in a variety of other adhesive glycoproteins and may represent a universal adhesive protein recognition sequence. Since the fibrinogen molecule contains pairs of alpha and gamma chain binding sites, it can link platelets together into aggregates. Patients with the rare platelet defect *thrombasthenia* have reduced or absent GpIIb/IIIa, reduced fibrinogen binding, markedly diminished or absent platelet aggregation, and severe bleeding, underscoring the importance of the platelet-fibrinogen interaction in hemostasis. The infusion of monoclonal antibodies directed against GpIIb/IIIa, which prevent aggregation and fibrinogen binding in vivo, protects experimental animals from thrombus formation.[40] Synthetic peptides that block fibrinogen binding to platelet receptors may have a similar antithrombotic effect.[41] These studies document the importance of fibrinogen binding in thrombus formation and may provide prototypes for new platelet-modifying drugs with potential antithrombotic activity.

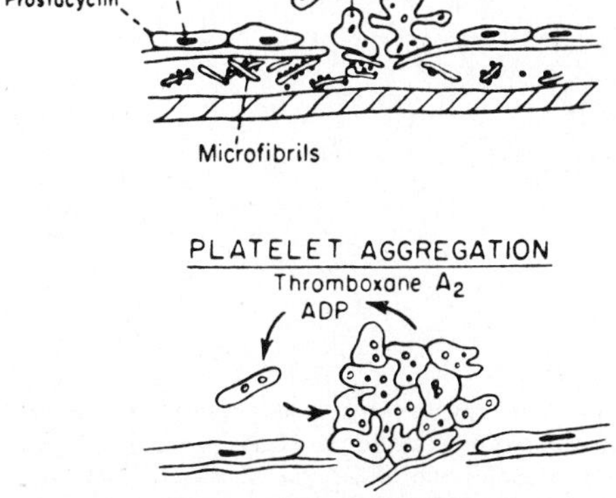

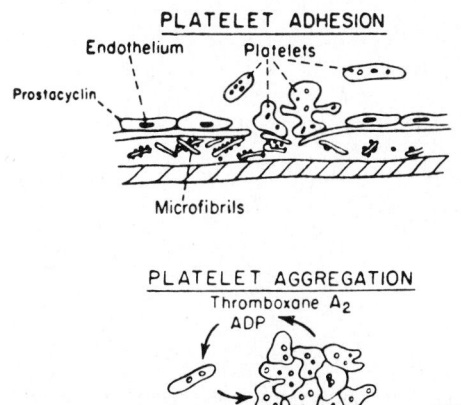

FIGURE 56–4. An overview of the process of primary hemostasis. The initial event is adhesion of platelets to areas of the vessel wall in which the subendothelium has been exposed by endothelial cell disruption or injury. After adhesion, platelets become activated and, under the influence of mediators like ADP and thromboxane A_2, recruit additional circulating platelets to bind to the adherent monolayer and form a platelet aggregate.

SUMMARY OF THE ROLE OF PLATELETS

The sequence of reactions just described and summarized in Figure 56–4 represents the process of primary hemostasis and provides the first line of defense against blood loss after injury to a blood vessel. Hemostasis is usually initiated when injury is sufficient to remove the endothelial lining and expose the vascular subendothelium to flowing blood. Platelets then adhere to collagen fibrils in the vessel wall, become activated, and degranulate, thereby releasing granule constituents and mediators into plasma and the vessel wall. Some of these materials, principally ADP and thromboxane A_2, diffuse into plasma and activate circulating platelets, which become linked to the adherent platelet monolayer. The layers of platelets eventually fill the lumen of the vessel, forming a platelet aggregate or hemostatic plug. The processes of adhesion and aggregation are mediated by the interaction of specific platelet membrane receptors with components of the vessel wall or with plasma proteins like fibronectin, vWF, and fibrinogen, which link platelets to the vessel wall and to each other. Signal transduction pathways in the platelet are complex and are regulated by specific agonists that bind to platelet receptors and activate the hydrolysis of phosphatidylinositol. These products of hydrolysis can then induce transient increases in intracellular calcium and activate an intracellular protein kinase that phosphorylates intraplatelet regulatory proteins. Finally, the eicosanoids derived from arachidonic acid in platelets, leukocytes, and endothelial cells provide short-acting biological mediators that can optimize the degree of platelet activation and vasoconstriction during the process of local hemostasis. The plasma coagulation or secondary hemostatic system then generates fibrin strands, which are interposed into the platelet plug to provide a stronger and more permanent hemostatic plug.

FIBRIN GENERATION AND CLOT FORMATION

At the same time as platelet activation, blood coagulation is initiated by the interaction of flowing blood with vascular subendothelium or tissue thromboplastin (tissue factor) exposed on cell surfaces after cellular injury. While the blood coagulation reactions are often referred to as the "fluid phase" of hemostasis, the reactions actually occur on vascular subendothelium or negatively charged, phospholipid-rich surfaces, such as the plasma membrane of platelets or endothelial cells. The adsorption of coagulation proteins onto these surfaces increases their concentration, effectively increasing reaction rates and localizing their activity. As illustrated in Figure 56–5, they can be conveniently grouped into a series of surface-bound enzyme-cofactor complexes. Several of the coagulation proteins, including factors II, VII, IX, and X, are bound to surfaces via bridges formed between calcium, the negatively charged cell surface, and digammacarboxyglutamic acid (Gla) residues on the proteins.[42] Other proteins are bound

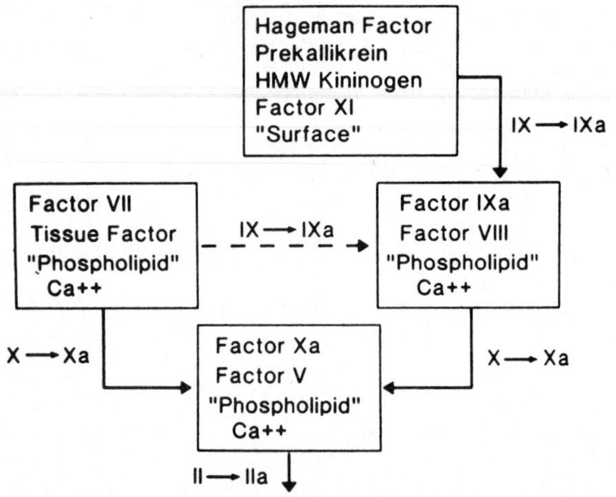

FIGURE 56–5. The major enzyme complexes of the coagulation cascade. The "intrinsic" or contact activation pathway is represented by the box containing Hageman factor, prekallikrein, high molecular weight (HMW) kininogen and factor XI and the initiating stimulus contact of blood with a "surface." The result of these interactions is formation of an enzyme, factor XIa, that converts factor IX to IXa. In the second reaction, factor IXa along with factor VIII, a source of phospholipid, and calcium assemble to convert factor X to Xa. In the "extrinsic" or tissue factor–dependent pathway, tissue factor and factor VII along with phospholipid and calcium can either directly activate factor X to Xa or activate IX. In the final reaction, factor Xa and factor V along with phospholipid and calcium convert factor II (prothrombin) to IIa (thrombin). Since both initiating pathways can activate factors IX and X, there is no need to make a distinction between "intrinsic" and "extrinsic" activation of the coagulation system. (From Mann, K. G., and Fass, D. N.: The molecular biology of blood coagulation. *In* Fairbanks, V. F. [ed.]: Current Hematology. Vol 2. New York, John Wiley & Sons, 1983, p. 347.)

by electrostatic or hydrophobic interactions. Following adsorption and complex formation, precursor proteins, or zymogens, are converted to active enzymes by limited proteolysis. Reaction rates are controlled by high molecular weight protein cofactors like factors V and VIII that markedly accelerate proteolysis. In each case, the cleavage of one or more relatively small peptides from the parent molecule converts it to an active protease, which then acts on another zymogen in the coagulation cascade.

INTRINSIC COAGULATION PATHWAY. The intrinsic or contact activation pathway of coagulation is initiated by the formation of a complex among three plasma proteins—Hageman factor (factor XII), high molecular weight kininogen (HMWK), and prekallikrein (PK). As shown in Figure 56–6*A*, HMWK and PK circulate in plasma as a noncovalent complex. This complex, when adsorbed onto a suitable surface, binds factor XII and slowly converts some of it to an active enzymatic form called factor XIIa (Fig. 56–6*B*). Factor XIIa then converts a second component of the complex, PK, to kallikrein (Fig. 56–6*C*). The resulting protease, kallikrein, both liberates the vasoactive peptide bradykinin from the third member of the complex, HMWK, and accelerates the conversion of factor XII to XIIa (Fig. 56–6*D*). In a subsequent reaction, not shown in Figure 56–6, factor XI is attached to this trimolecular complex and converted to its active form, XIa, by the proteolytic action of surface-bound XIIa.

EXTRINSIC COAGULATION PATHWAY. Tissue factor, a ubiquitous cellular lipoprotein, initiates the extrinsic coagulation pathway by forming a calcium-dependent complex with another protein, factor VII, a member of a group of Gla-containing coagulation proteins synthesized in the liver. After complex formation, factor VII develops proteolytic activity (VIIa), which converts factor X to its active form, Xa. The term extrinsic coagulation pathway was derived from an earlier observation that vesicles rich in tissue factor may be released into the blood from damaged tissues or cells. It is now known that endothelial cells still attached to subendothelium, along with circulating leukocytes, may express tissue factor activity and accelerate coagulation reactions after incubation with agents like interleukin-1 or bacterial endotoxin.

COMMON PATHWAY. Factor X is activated by products generated by the contact activation or Hageman factor–dependent pathway as well as by the tissue factor–VII complex. The details of this reaction are diagrammed in Figure 56–7. Factor XIa first converts factor IX to IXa. Factor X is then activated by IXa, in conjunction with factor VIII, by the formation of a calcium- and lipid-dependent macromolecular complex. Factor VIII has little biological activity until it is converted to VIIIa by traces of thrombin. As illustrated, formation of the IXa-X-VIIIa complex occurs on a cell surface, most probably on activated endothelial cells or platelets. In addition to activating factor X, the tissue factor–VIIa complex may also activate factor IX. This alternative pathway provides a link between the contact activation and tissue factor–dependent pathways of coagulation, and its existance may help explain why patients with severe factor VIII or IX deficiency who have a normal tissue factor–dependent mechanism still have defective hemostasis.

Factor Xa then converts prothrombin to thrombin in conjunction with factor Va, calcium, and phospholipid. As shown in Figure 56–7, prothrombin conversion, which also takes place on activated platelet or endothelial surfaces,

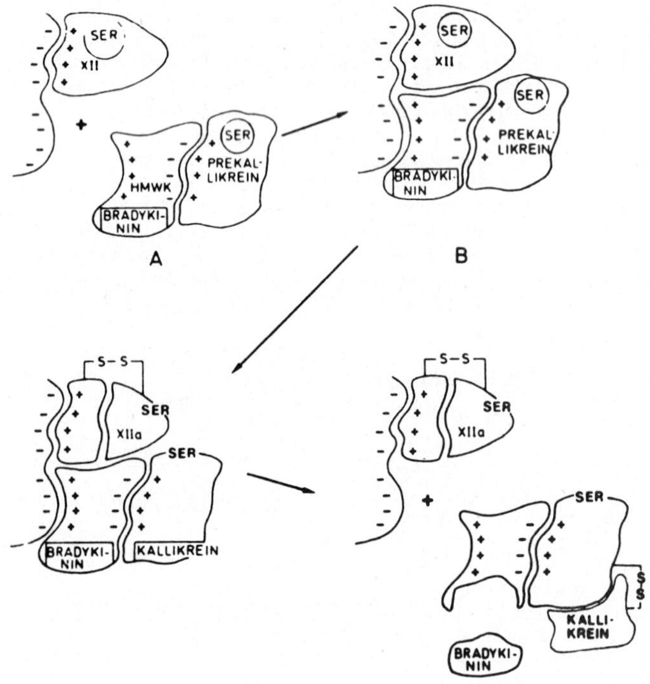

FIGURE 56–6. Reactions comprising the contact activation or intrinsic pathway of coagulation. *A* and *B*, High molecular weight kininogen (HMWK) and prekallikrein (PK), which circulate as a noncovalent complex, attach to a surface such as the vascular subendothelium along with Hageman factor (factor XII). *C*, This converts PK to the active serine protease kallikrein, which then converts factor XII to its active form, XIIa, and also liberates bradykinin from HMWK. The subsequent reaction (not shown in the figure) is between surface-bound XIIa and factor XI, which initiates coagulation. (From Verstraete, M., and Vermylen, J.: Thrombosis. Oxford, Pergamon Press, 1984, p. 27.)

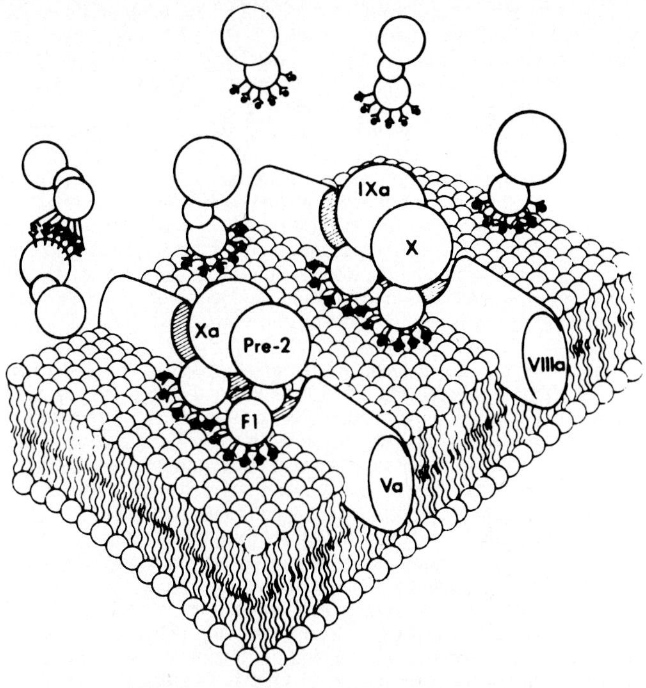

FIGURE 56–7. Hypothetical model of the prothrombinase complex and the complex responsible for factor X activation. Factors Va and VIIIa attach to a model cell membrane by hydrophobic interactions and also develop binding sites for specific coagulation factors. Factors IXa and X bind to factor VIIIa and to the membrane. Binding is partially mediated by gammacarboxyglutamic acid (Gla) residues and calcium. After its activation, factor Xa becomes part of a second adjacent complex with factor Va and prothrombin (depicted here as Pre-2). Again, Xa and prothrombin interact with the cell membrane via Gla residues and calcium. Thrombin is then liberated from the surface to participate in additional coagulation reactions. (From Mann, K. G., et al.: The role of factor V in the assembly of the prothrombinase complex. *In* Walz, D. A., and McCoy L. E. [eds.]: Annals of the New York Academy of Sciences. New York, 1981, p. 378.)

requires the assembly of a macromolecular complex among factor Va, Xa, and prothrombin. Thrombin, the product of this reaction, is a potent and versatile protease that has multiple actions in hemostasis, which include activating factors V, VIII, and XIII and binding to and activating platelets and endothelial cells. A most important function is the cleavage of peptides from the A and B chains of fibrinogen to form fibrin monomers that subsequently polymerize into large fibrillar polymers (Fig. 56–8). Fibrin polymerization, the basis for the familiar clotting reaction, markedly changes plasma viscosity and converts blood from a sol to a gel. Polymers are initially held together by weak chemical bonds that are readily dissociated. They are subsequently cross-linked by a plasma transglutaminase, factor XIIIa, providing optimal mechanical stability.

LIMITING REACTIONS—THE NATURAL ANTICOAGULANTS

During normal hemostasis, only a small quantity of each of the coagulation proteins in plasma is converted into an active protease or cofactor. The rate and extent of serine protease generation are carefully regulated by a group of inhibitor proteins that function as natural anticoagulants (Fig. 56–8). Such tight regulation is critical, since there is enough prothrombin in a single milliliter of blood, if converted to thrombin, to clot the entire volume of blood within 15 seconds. The natural anticoagulants permit coagulation to proceed locally, in response to injury, and prevent it from becoming a systemic and potentially dangerous process. The three most important natural anticoagulants are antithrombin III, protein C, and protein S. Their importance is underscored by the observation that patients with deficiency or dysfunction of any of the three proteins have a prethrombotic or hypercoagulable disorder characterized by recurrent episodes of venous thrombosis and embolism.

ANTITHROMBIN III. This 60,000-dalton protein, synthesized in the liver, binds to and inactivates serine proteases within the coagulation cascade. Although named for its interaction with thrombin, it also inactivates factors XIIa, XIa, Xa, and IXa by binding to a serine residue at the active site of these proteases.[43] The kinetics of the interaction vary for the different proteases but, in each case, can be accelerated many fold by the addition of heparin. Heparin binds to a site on antithrombin III that is separate from the region that binds proteases and acts as an "allosteric" regulator. Following the formation of a protease-antithrombin complex, heparin is released and can bind to additional antithrombin molecules. In this way, its function is analogous to that of an enzyme or catalyst. The "catalytic"

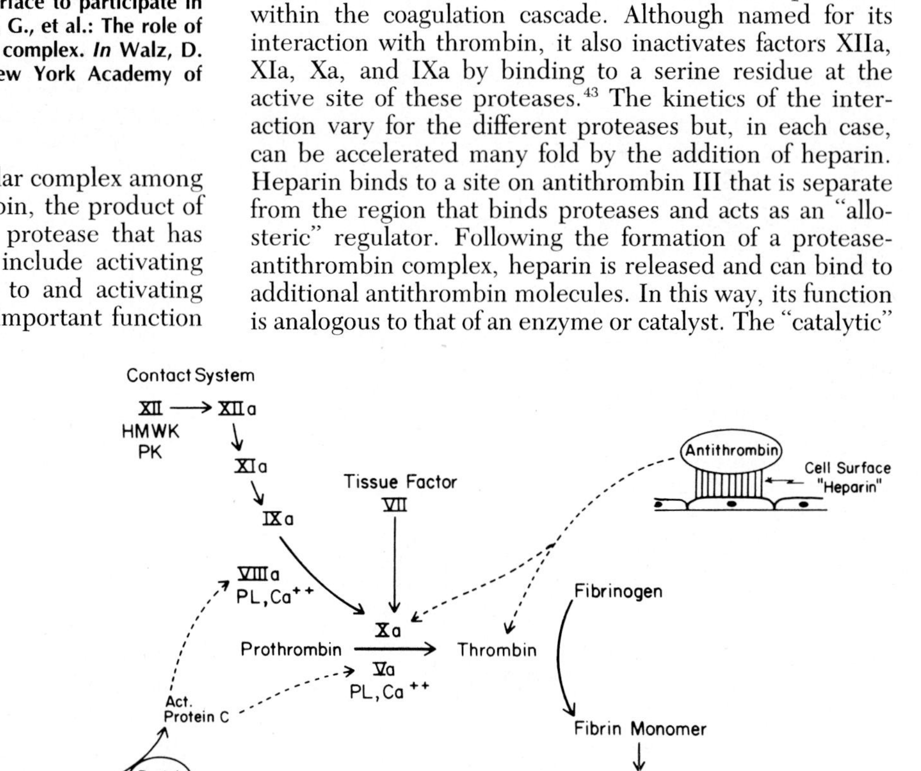

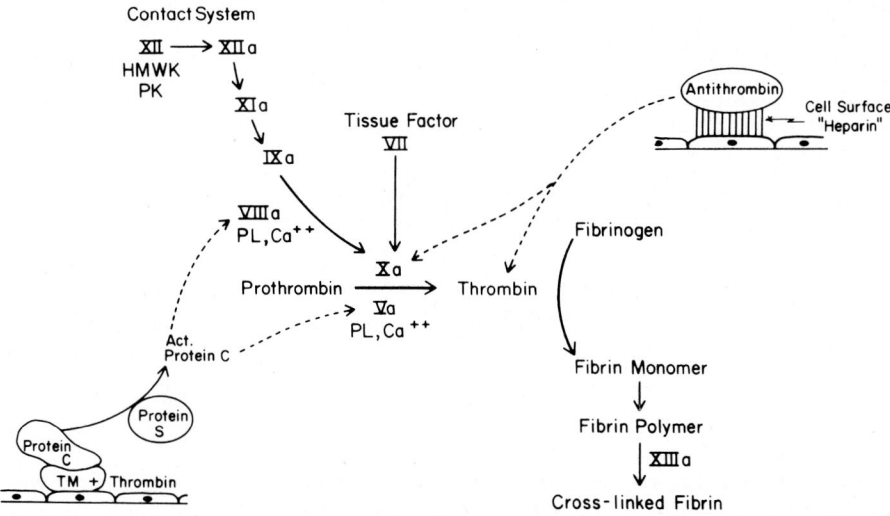

FIGURE 56–8. An overview of the entire coagulation cascade including the limiting reactions of the natural anticoagulants. There are two major activation pathways: the intrinsic pathway, which involves factors XII, IX, IX, and VIII, and the extrinsic or tissue factor system, which involves tissue factor and factor VII. Both pathways result in the conversion of inactive factor X to its active form, Xa. In the third or common pathway, Xa converts prothrombin to thrombin in a reaction that is accelerated by factor Va. Thrombin then converts fibrinogen to fibrin monomers, which polymerize and are cross-linked by factor XIIIa, a plasma transglutaminase. The interaction of factors VIIIa, IXa, and X; the interaction of the tissue factor-VII complex with factor X; and the conversion of prothrombin to thrombin are all reactions that require phospholipid (PL) and calcium. Two major anticoagulant systems limit coagulation reactions. Antithrombin binds to thrombin, factor Xa, and other coagulation serine proteases except factor VII in a reaction that is accelerated by exogenous heparin or heparin-like molecules on endothelial cells. Protein C is activated by thrombin after it is bound to the endothelial cell protein thrombomodulin. Activated protein C and protein S inactivate the two coagulation cofactors VIIIa and Va, which also limits thrombin generation. (From Handin R. I.: Bleeding and thrombosis. *In* Braunwald E., et al. [eds.]: Harrison's Principles of Internal Medicine, 11th ed. New York, McGraw-Hill Book Co., 1987, p. 270.)

acceleration of antithrombin activity by heparin, referred to as its heparin cofactor activity, accounts for the entire anticoagulant action of heparin in plasma. During normal hemostasis, antithrombin is activated by binding to heparin-like molecules present on the surface of endothelial cells.

PROTEINS C AND S. The second regulatory system involves protein C, protein S, and an endothelial membrane protein, *thrombomodulin.*[44–46] When bound to thrombomodulin, protein C is converted to an active serine protease by thrombin. Activated protein C then inhibits coagulation by inactivating factors Va and VIIIa. Protein S increases the rate of proteolysis of factors Va and VIIIa by activated protein C.

RHEOLOGY AND THROMBOSIS

Any discussion of hemostasis should include the effects of blood flow and vascular geometry on thrombus formation.[47] Stress, in rheological terms, is the force per unit area generated during blood flow. When this force is applied at right angles to a surface, it is referred to as "normal" stress, and when applied parallel to a surface, as tangential stress or "shear." Figure 56–9 depicts a longitudinal cross section of a blood vessel, with *h* representing wall thickness and *R* the inner radius. The parabola represents the range of velocities, *v*, at which laminar "plates" of blood travel along the longitudinal axis of the vessel at varying distances (*y*) from its center. Normal or circumferential stress (S_C) can be defined mathematically as

$$S_C = PxP/h \quad (1)$$

where *P* is the distending luminal pressure. In this idealized system of laminar, nonturbulent flow through a vessel of uniform diameter, the shear or tangential stress is

$$S_t = n\,v/\,Y = P\,Y/2 \quad (2)$$

where *v* is blood viscosity and *P* the pressure gradient per unit length of vessel. Finally, the velocity of any laminar plate can be related to the radius of the vessel, the pressure generated, blood viscosity, and vessel length *L*, as follows:

$$V = \pi\,PR^4/8\,\nu L \quad (3)$$

From Equation 3 one can determine that velocity is maximal at the center of the vessel as it is proportional to the fourth power of the radius and falls off to nearly zero at the vessel wall. In addition, this equation predicts that the greater the viscosity of the blood, the lower its velocity. In addition, from Equation 2, it is clear that an increase in viscosity (*v*) will increase shear stress. These concepts have some practical applications. First, since plasma proteins, erythrocytes, and platelets require some minimal time to interact with each other and with subendothelial surfaces, conditions of high viscosity and low velocity favor platelet adhesion and thrombus formation. In fact, in the venous circulation, where velocity is low, relatively minor variations in flow, when coupled with minor degrees of injury to venous endothelium, may induce thrombus formation. Venous clots also take on their typical red appearance because of the large amounts of trapped red cells and fibrin that accumulate under conditions of low flow. In the more rapid arterial circulation, platelet-platelet interactions predominate, there is

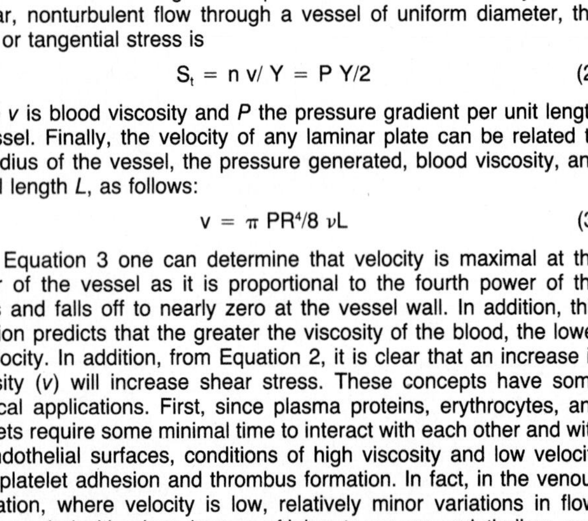

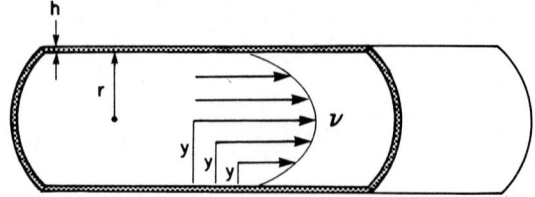

FIGURE 56–9. Biophysical variables that affect blood shear and rheology in a model cross section of a blood vessel. h = thickness of the vessel wall; r = radius of the vessel. Blood travels at different velocities (*v*) depending on its distance (*y*) from the vessel wall. As described in the text, these parameters along with measurements of blood viscosity and blood pressure can be used to calculate shear stress on the vessel wall and blood flow.

insufficient time for fibrin formation and red cell trapping, and thrombi appear white. Adequate quantities of vWF multimers are also critical to stabilize adhesion of platelets to the vessel wall under conditions of high flow and shear stress. A modest reduction in this protein may lead to impaired hemostasis and clinical bleeding.

Rheology also influences the location of vascular disease, which occurs more frequently at bifurcations. Velocity is reduced as the "plates" of flowing blood are divided. This prolongs the residence time of platelets at the vessel surface and may enhance their deposition onto subendothelium when the bifurcation site is injured. Turbulence, which may occur in a stenotic vessel, adds another variable to the analysis by producing non-Newtonian flow. This also increases the residence time of proteins and platelets, reduces velocity, enhances local viscosity, and promotes platelet and fibrin deposition near flow vortices.

Finally, rheological principles have been applied to the design of therapeutic agents. Improving blood flow and reducing blood viscosity should reduce thrombus formation. There is evidence that cerebral blood flow can be dramatically increased by a slight reduction in the hematocrit.[48] The administration of volume expanders like dextran, which have minimal effects on coagulation reactions, may act as antithrombotic agents by improving flow and reducing viscosity.[49] It has also been suggested that defibrination with agents like *Ancrod* or the defibrination that accompanies systemic fibrinolytic therapy may be beneficial, in part, because it markedly reduces blood viscosity and improves blood flow. New agents like pentoxifylline that increase red cell deformability and reduce viscosity are being administered to patients with chronic cerebrovascular and peripheral vascular disease to improve blood flow through partially obstructed vessels.[50]

CLOT DISSOLUTION—THE FIBRINOLYTIC SYSTEM

The fibrinolytic system, which dissolves fibrin-thrombi and restores blood flow within obstructed blood vessels, is a critically important component of the normal hemostatic system. Orderly, localized clot lysis is achieved by the concerted actions of a complex system that includes proteolytic enzymes, specific activators, and inhibitors of both the proteases and their activators. Although there are enzymes like leukocyte elastase, which can digest fibrin, the major protease of the fibrinolytic system is *plasmin.* Three principal activators convert the precursor zymogen plasminogen to its active form, plasmin; these are activated Hageman factor fragments, urokinase (UK), and tissue plasminogen activator (t-PA). Both the rate and extent of fibrinolysis are regulated by a circulating inhibitor of plasmin, the alpha$_2$-plasmin inhibitor, and an endothelial cell–derived inhibitor of the principal activators, the plasminogen activator inhibitor (PAI). The fibrinolytic process is usually localized to fibrin clots because plasminogen is selectively deposited in fibrin thrombi at the time of thrombus formation. In addition, the two activators UK and t-PA are derived from stimulated endothelial cells at the site of thrombus formation and diffuse into the adjacent thrombus.

PLASMINOGEN

This 92,000-dalton plasma glycoprotein contains 790 amino acids, including 48 cysteines that form 24 intramolecular disulfide bonds, leaving no free sulfhydryl groups. Although the tissue of origin is still debated, plasminogen synthesis has been described in both liver and kidney, and plasminogen is present in eosinophilic leukocytes. The plasma concentration is approximately 21 mg/dl and does not vary greatly during normal blood coagulation. As shown in Figure 56–10, the parent molecule (Glu-plasminogen) has a glutamic acid at its amino terminus. Variable amounts of Glu-plasminogen are converted to Lys-plasminogen by the cleavage of an 8,000-dalton polypeptide. Both Glu- and Lys-plasminogen are converted to plasmin by the scission of a single Arg-Val bond, through which the single-

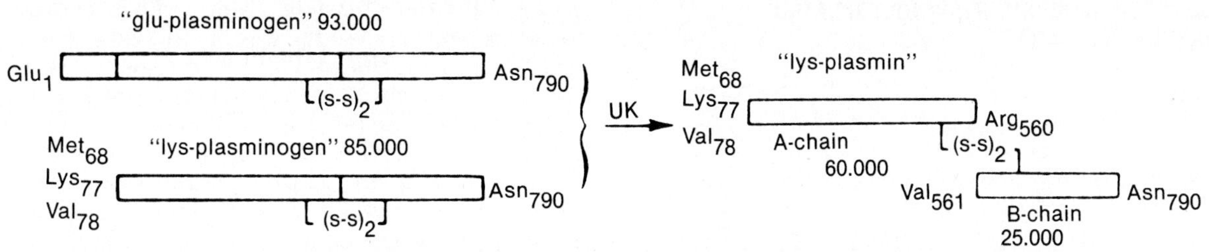

FIGURE 56–10. The molecular forms of plasminogen in plasma. The native molecule has 790 amino acids and a molecular weight of 93,000 daltons, with a glutamic acid as the initial or amino terminal amino acid residue (Glu-plasminogen). In plasma, an 8,000-dalton preactivation peptide is cleaved from Glu-plasminogen to produce a somewhat smaller form of plasminogen, with lysine as the amino terminal amino acid (Lys-plasminogen). Both Glu- and Lys plasminogen circulate in plasma and can be converted to plasmin. This requires two steps for Glu-plasminogen, cleavage of the 8,000-dalton peptide, and scission of an internal peptide bond. Lys-plasminogen is activated by the internal bond scission alone. Plasmin is a two-chain molecule linked by disulfide bonds that has proteolytic activity against fibrinogen and fibrin as well as a number of other blood and cellular substrates. (Modified from Verstraete, M., and Vermylen, J.: Thrombosis. London, Pergamon Press, 1984, p. 46.)

chain precursor is converted into a disulfide-linked, two-chain protease. Plasmin is a potent protease with broad reactivity. In addition to fibrin, it can digest fibrinogen, coagulation factors V and VIII, and platelet membrane Glycoprotein Ib.

The complete covalent structure of plasminogen has been determined by direct protein sequencing and has been deduced from sequencing of plasminogen cDNA. As summarized in Figure 56–11, there are important structural similarities between plasminogen and the various plasminogen activators. Within the plasminogen molecule are five repeated regions of sequence homology that begin at the amino terminus of the molecule. These homologous repeats form looped structures held together by disulfide bonds and referred to as "kringles." (Kringles are a Danish breakfast pastry with a similar twisted, pretzel-like shape.) Plasminogen binds to fibrin via lysine binding sites located on the five nodular "kringle" domains, illustrated in Figure 56–11 as K_1 through K_5. These noncovalent interactions permit plasminogen to become concentrated within fibrin-rich thrombi for more effective and localized fibrinolysis.[51]

PLASMINOGEN ACTIVATORS

(See also p. 1778)

As mentioned above, three endogenous plasminogen activators have now been identified.[52] They can be distinguished by their mechanism of plasminogen activation and the ability of fibrin to enhance their activity. Hageman factor (Factor XII) fragments, generated during the early phase of coagulation, are relatively weak plasminogen activators (Fig. 56–6). Their activity is not enhanced by the adsorption of plasminogen to fibrin.

TISSUE PLASMINOGEN ACTIVATOR (t-PA). The major physiologic activator is t-PA, a 70,000-dalton protein synthesized predominantly in endothelial cells. Since there are only trace quantities of this protein in normal plasma, it has been difficult to purify and characterize t-PA. Recently, cDNA encoding t-PA has been cloned and the recombinant molecule expressed in heterologous cells[53] (Fig. 56–12). As shown in Figures 56–11 and 56–12, t-PA is synthesized as a single-chain molecule, which is readily converted to a two-chain form by the proteolytic cleavage of a single plasmin-sensitive site. Unlike most other serine proteases, both the single-chain and two-chain forms have proteolytic activity. t-PA is a relatively selective or fibrin-specific activator, since it converts plasminogen to plasmin two to three orders of magnitude more efficiently in vitro in the presence of fibrin. Based on preliminary clinical studies, a similar degree of specificity may not be achieved in vivo. As illustrated in Figure 56–11, the A chain of t-PA, which is derived from the NH_2 terminal portion of single-chain t-PA, has a molecular weight of 40,000 daltons and contains two "kringle" domains (K_1 and K_2 in Figure 56–11), a pair of finger-like structures homologous to those first described in the adhesive glycoprotein fibronectin, and epidermal growth factor (EGF). The fibronectin-like finger is indicated in Figure 56–11 as F and the EGF homologue as E. The K_2 and F domains of t-PA both interact with fibrin. The smaller (30,000-dalton) B chain of t-PA contains the proteolytic site that converts plasminogen to plasmin. The B chain is homologous to other serine proteases like elastase, urokinase, and trypsin.

UROKINASE (UK) AND PRO-UROKINASE (PRO-UK). This is a two-chain serine protease with a molecular weight of 33,000 daltons. It is synthesized in renal tubule epithelial cells as well as in endothelial cells and is immunologically distinct from t-PA.[54] It directly converts plasminogen to plasmin by hydrolyzing the same Arg-Val bond as t-PA. In contrast to t-PA, the proteolytic activity of UK is not enhanced by fibrin, so that it activates circulating plasminogen as effectively as plasminogen adsorbed onto fibrin thrombi. Two molecular forms of UK have been isolated from urine that differ in molecular weight, but have identical proteolytic properties. A single-chain precursor to UK, pro-urokinase (pro-UK), has a molecular weight of 55,000 daltons and has only minimal proteolytic activity. It has been identified in urine and circulates in plasma. Pro-UK is quantitatively converted to the high molecular weight form of UK, which has full proteolytic activity, upon exposure to plasmin.

Pro-UK, like t-PA, has a single kringle domain (K), which confers some fibrin specificity. Although pro-UK has an EGF-like domain (E) it lacks the fibronectin finger seen in t-PA. The single kringle domain (K) interacts with fibrin, but its affinity is lower than that of t-PA. Since pro-UK has only minimal proteolytic activity, the mechanism by which it activates plasminogen in a fibrin-specific manner is not fully understood. The most likely explanation is that t-PA secreted from endothelial cells in the vicinity of a thrombus generates small quantities of plasmin. The traces of plasmin rapidly convert pro-UK to two-chain UK, which activates additional plasminogen and digests fibrin.[55]

ALPHA$_2$-PLASMIN INHIBITOR (ALPHA$_2$ PI). Activity of the endogenous fibrinolytic system is carefully regulated. Endothelial cells and platelets both secrete a plasminogen activator inhibitor (PAI) that rapidly binds to and inactivates t-PA and UK.[56] PAI is structurally homologous to other serine protease inhibitors like alpha$_1$-antitrypsin and antithrombin III. As shown in Figure 56–13, the alpha$_2$ PI circulating in plasma rapidly neutralizes free plasmin.[57] However, the lysine-binding "kringle" domains as well as the active-site serine of plasmin must be available for

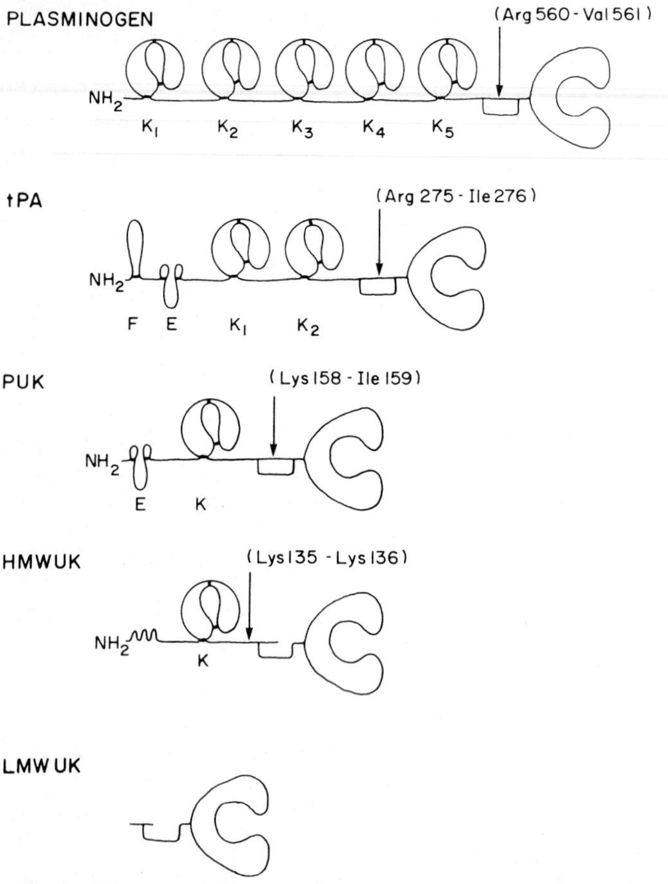

FIGURE 56–11. Structural homologies between plasminogen and the major activators of the fibrinolytic system. Plasminogen, tissue plasminogen activator (t-PA), pro-urokinase (PUK), and the high molecular weight form of urokinase (HMWUK) all contain "pretzel-like" kringle domains which are held together by disulfide bonds. In addition, t-PA contains a finger-like projection (F) at its amino (NH_2) terminus, also held together by disulfide bonds, which is homologous to a finger structure first recognized in the adhesive glycoprotein fibronectin. t-PA and PUK also contain a second slightly different shaped projection (E) first noted in another molecule, the epidermal growth factor, and now recognized in many other proteins. The large "C" shaped region on the right hand end of each molecule represents the proteolytically active region. The K domains numbered 1 through 5 on various molecules, and the F domains are the sites on each molecule which interact with fibrin and confer fibrin "specificity." The varying numbers of K domains, in combination with the F domains, confer differing affinities for fibrin. The arrows indicate sites in each of the proteins that are cleaved by proteolytic enzymes. Plasminogen is a single chain zymogen or precursor which has no proteolytic activity. The scission of the peptide bond between arginine 560 and valine 561 converts it to a two-chain molecule, plasmin, which can proteolyze fibrinogen, fibrin, and various other substrates. As shown in Figure 56–10, a second peptide bond is cleared from Glu-plasminogen to produce Lys-plasminogen. Both forms are converted to plasmin. t-PA is synthesized as a single chain form which has proteolytic activity and can activate plasminogen. It is quickly converted to a two-chain form with somewhat enhanced proteolytic activity, by the scission of a single bond between arginine 275 and isoleucine 276. PUK, unlike t-PA, has no proteolytic activity until the bond between lysine 158 and isoleucine 159 is clipped, converting it to a two-chain protease. Both HMW and LMWUK circulate as two chain active proteases. Scission of a bond between lysines 135 and 136 removes the single K domain, but does not appreciably alter the specificity or biologic activity of UK which has no fibrin specificity.

binding and neutralization by alpha$_2$ PI. Thus, when it is bound to fibrin, plasmin is protected from the neutralizing effect of alpha$_2$ PI. This helps to sustain the fibrinolytic activity of plasmin within a thrombus and minimizes systemic fibrinolysis, since alpha$_2$ PI rapidly neutralizes any release of "free" plasmin. Alpha$_2$ PI may also inhibit fibrinolysis by competing for lysine binding sites on fibrinogen. The fibrin clot plays a key role in the regulation of fibrinolysis. Fibrin binds plasminogen, enriching this key fibrinolytic enzyme precursor within the clot. The presence of fibrin also enhances the activity of t-PA and inhibits the activity of alpha$_2$ PI. Finally, products generated during fibrin clot formation, such as thrombin, enhance the local release of t-PA as well as its principal inhibitor PAI from endothelial cells. Systemic fibrinolysis is a rare event and occurs only in patients with disseminated intravascular coagulation, those with advanced liver disease, and those receiving systemic infusions of fibrinolytic activators to lyse pathological thrombi.

SUMMARY OF COAGULATION AND FIBRINOLYTIC REACTIONS

The plasma coagulation and fibrinolytic systems are complicated because they involve the closely linked interactions of multiple serine proteases. In addition, the reactions are carefully regulated by plasma and cell surface activators, plasma cofactors, and a series of naturally occurring anticoagulants or fibrinolytic inhibitors.

The major coagulation reactions are summarized in Figure 56–8 and the fibrinolytic pathway in Figure 56–14. Two major stimuli initiate coagulation—contact of blood with vascular subendothelium and liberation of tissue thromboplastin or tissue factor. The net result of activation of these two pathways is the generation of thrombin, a potent protease that converts fibrinogen to fibrin. Fibrin then polymerizes and is cross-linked to form a stable clot. There are two critical plasma cofactors—factors Va and VIIIa that regulate the rates of factor Xa generation via the contact or intrinsic pathway and the rate of thrombin generation from Xa produced by either the extrinsic or the intrinsic pathway. The most important naturally occurring anticoagulants are antithrombin III, which is activated by cell-surface heparin-like molecules and rapidly neutralizes coagulation proteases, and protein C, which is activated by thrombin and cell-surface thrombomodulin. Along with protein S, activated protein C inactivates factors Va and VIIIa.

The fibrinolytic system may be activated by three endogenous substances: t-PA, pro-UK, and UK. In each case activation is accomplished by converting plasminogen to plasmin. Plasmin then digests fibrin thrombi. The rate of plasminogen activation by t-PA and pro-UK is enhanced by the presence of fibrin and permits the activation process to be localized to areas containing fibrin thrombi. t-PA and pro-UK are secreted from endothelial cells following the generation of thrombin. Fibrinolytic activity is regulated at two levels. First, there is the endothelial PAI, which may bind to any free plasminogen activator. In addition, there is a plasma protein, alpha$_2$ PI, which binds to any free plasmin and rapidly neutralizes its proteolytic activity. In normal hemostasis, fibrinolysis is activated shortly after thrombus formation and helps to restore vessel patency and normal blood flow rapidly.

EVALUATION OF HEMOSTASIS IN CARDIOVASCULAR PATIENTS

Patients with cardiovascular disorders often require corrective surgery or invasive diagnostic and therapeutic procedures such as cardiac catheterization, coronary angiography, or transluminal angioplasty. Although special precautions are not usually necessary, a specific evaluation

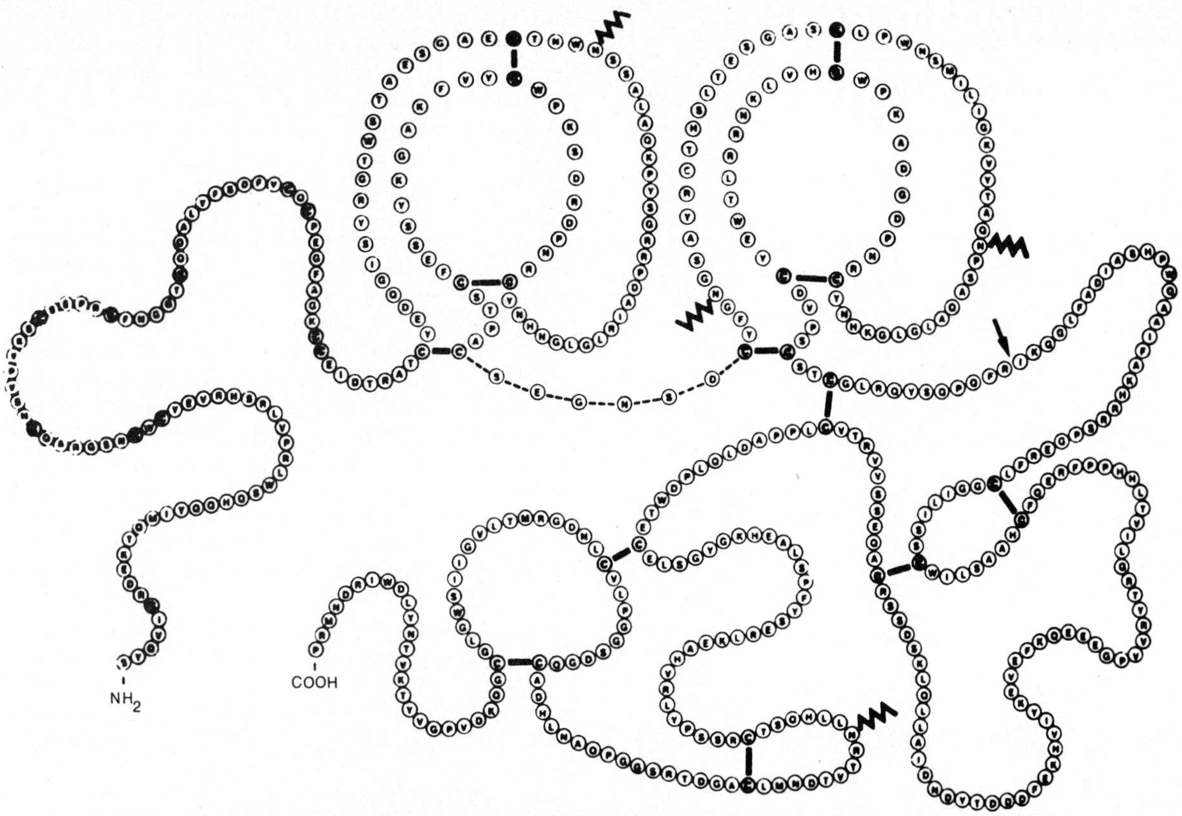

FIGURE 56–12. Structure of tissue plasminogen activator deduced from cDNA cloning and sequencing. The one-letter abbreviations for amino acid residues are used. Solid bars mark sites for potential disulfide bonds between cysteine residues, and zig-zag lines mark attachment sites for *N*-linked carbohydrate. The arrow marks the position of the bond scission, which converts one-chain t-PA to the two-chain form. Finally, the broken line indicates the short stretch of six amino acids that connects the two kringle domains. (From Pennica, D., et al.: Cloning and expression of human tissue-type plasminogen activator cDNA in *E. coli.* Nature *301*:214, 1983.)

of the hemostatic system may be necessary in three clinical situations. First, some patients may also have a suspected or poorly documented hemorrhagic disorder that may have produced only minimal symptoms but might cause excess bleeding after an invasive diagnostic or surgical procedure. For example, many patients with mild von Willebrand's disease have little or no spontaneous bleeding but may bleed profusely following an operation. Second, the antiplatelet or anticoagulant medications administered to cardiac patients increase their risk of hemorrhage. This problem is especially serious when patients are to undergo invasive cardiovascular or surgical procedures, since they may have few bleeding symptoms prior to surgery. Finally, although most cardiovascular disorders do not increase the risk of hemorrhage, certain types of cardiac disease perturb hemostasis and cause bleeding.

Although it may be tempting to order a battery of screening laboratory tests on all cardiac patients with a suspected hemorrhagic disorder, the most useful part of the evaluation is still a careful history. For example, a past history of excessive bleeding after dental extractions or tonsillectomy, bleeding after minor trauma, recurrent epistaxis, abnormal menses, or recurrent joint or muscle bleeding without antecedent trauma all suggest an inherited coagulation disorder. Many, but not all, patients will also have a family history of bleeding. Finally, a careful

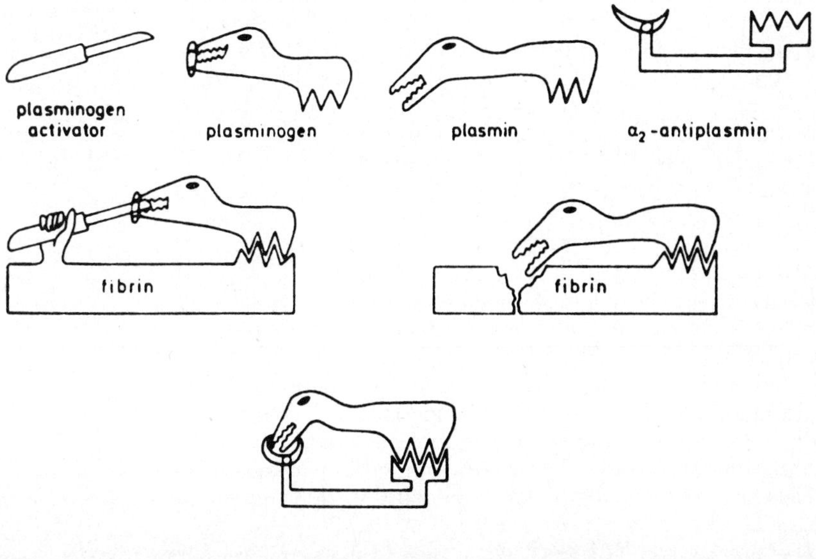

FIGURE 56–13. Schematic view of the interactions between a plasminogen activator (such as tissue plasminogen activator, which binds to fibrin), a fibrin clot, and the alpha$_2$-plasmin inhibitor. The plasminogen activator both binds to fibrin and converts fibrin-bound plasminogen to the active protease plasmin. Plasmin then digests the fibrin clot. Alpha$_2$-plasmin inhibitor binds to and inhibits free plasmin but cannot neutralize plasmin when it is bound to the fibrin clot, since it must bind to both the protease active site and the fibrin binding site. This mechanism helps to limit fibrinolysis to areas of fibrin clot formation and prevents plasmin from entering the circulation. (From Verstraete, M., & Vermylen, J.: Thrombosis. London, Pergamon Press, 1984, p. 43.)

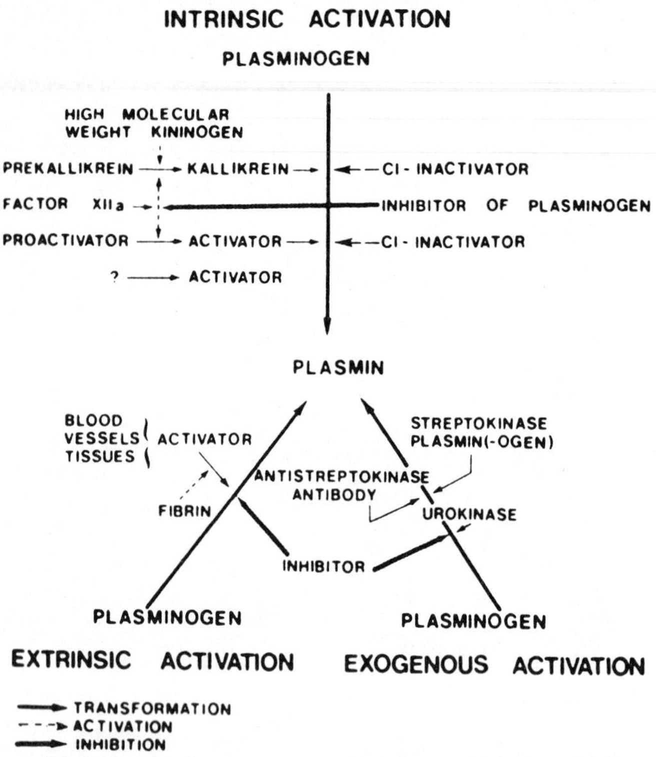

FIGURE 56–14. An overview of the fibrinolytic pathways. There are three principal pathways for the conversion of plasminogen to plasmin. The "intrinsic" pathway is activated during the early phases of blood coagulation by Hageman factor fragments. This is a relatively weak activation system of questionable physiological significance. The most important physiological mechanism is the "extrinsic" pathway. Endothelial cells in blood vessels release two fibrin-specific activators, tissue plasminogen activator and prourokinase, which rapidly and effectively convert plasminogen to plasmin. Finally, there are several potential "exogenous" activators used in fibrinolytic therapy. The bacterial protein streptokinase and the urinary product urokinase are two standard nonspecific activators. In addition, the two physiological and fibrin-specific activators, tissue plasminogen activator and prourokinase, are now available and are being used in clinical trials. (From Verstraete, M., and Vermylen, J.: Thrombosis. London, Pergamon Press, 1984, p. 41.)

drug history is essential, since many commonly used drugs, including aspirin and other nonsteroidal antiinflammatory agents, may cause platelet dysfunction and clinical bleeding.

Patients with deficits in platelet number or function usually bleed into the skin and mucous membranes and may present with epistaxis, gastrointestinal bleeding, or abnormal menses. Bleeding develops immediately after surgery or trauma and may respond to local pressure or packing. The most common platelet disorders are (1) thrombocytopenia, (2) platelet dysfunction secondary to ingestion of medications such as aspirin, and (3) von Willebrand's disease. Platelet function is readily evaluated by a platelet count and bleeding time. Current techniques for measuring bleeding time are reproducible and sensitive and can detect even mild platelet dysfunction. In most laboratories, the average bleeding time is 5 ± 2 (x ± S.D.) minutes, so that a value greater than 10 minutes probably indicates impaired primary hemostasis.

In contrast, in patients with plasma coagulation defects, musculoskeletal and soft tissue bleeding occurs hours or days after surgery and trauma and usually requires specific replacement therapy. The most common inherited abnormalities are the hemophilias—specifically, deficiencies in the activity of factors VIII and IX, which are sex-linked recessive disorders causing recurrent hemorrhage and joint deformity. The most common acquired defects are those associated with (1) vitamin K deficiency, (2) liver disease, and (3) disseminated intravascular coagulation (DIC).

The integrity of the plasma coagulation system is readily screened with a group of simple laboratory tests—the partial thromboplastin time (PTT), prothrombin time (PT), and in some cases thrombin time (TT) or fibrinogen level. In rare cases, additional assays of clot solubility and fibrin crosslinking may be useful. The PTT exclusively measures the activity of coagulation factors in the intrinsic or contact activation pathway, which include Hageman factor (factor XII), high molecular weight kininogen, prekallikrein, and factors XI, IX, and VIII (Fig. 56–8). The PT, which is used to assay the extrinsic or tissue factor–dependent pathway of coagulation, exclusively measures factor VII. The PT and PTT both assess the integrity of factors in the common pathway, which include factors X and V, prothrombin, and fibrinogen. When a patient has isolated prolongation of either the PT or PTT, the group of factors that are potentially defective can be readily pinpointed. However, when both PT and PTT are prolonged, fibrinogen level or function should also be assessed, since either reduced or dysfunctional fibrinogen or a common pathway defect involving factors X or V or prothrombin will prolong both tests. Defective fibrin crosslinking and abnormal clot solubility are extremely rare and should be suspected only when a patient has a severe bleeding disorder with normal PT and PTT.

Thrombocytopenia

The platelet count normally ranges between 150,000 and 450,000/μl. Low counts may be due to decreased marrow production, accelerated peripheral destruction, or platelet sequestration in an enlarged spleen. The most common causes of decreased production are exposure to marrow toxins, including chemotherapeutic agents, binge consumption of alcohol, and thiazide diuretics. Accelerated destruction can occur from platelet interaction with a prosthetic valve, Dacron vascular grafts or intracardiac patches, or activation of the coagulation system and platelet entrapment in fibrin thrombi. This is particularly prominent in patients with DIC but also occurs in disorders like thrombotic thrombocytopenic purpura and the hemolytic uremic syndrome. Finally, destruction may result from the interaction of antibodies or immune complexes with the platelet surface. Antibodies may arise in response to viral infections or the administration of drugs like quinidine, procainamide, or heparin.

Platelet Dysfunction

The most common cause of platelet dysfunction is the ingestion of aspirin and related nonsteroidal antiinflammatory agents. Patients usually have a mildly prolonged bleeding time, although in some susceptible individuals bleeding time may be as long as 20 to 30 minutes. This is accompanied by reduced platelet aggregation in response to agents like collagen, ADP, or epinephrine. Aspirin and the nonsteroidal antiinflammatory drugs inhibit platelet synthesis of thromboxane A_2 and other eicosanoids by inhibiting platelet cyclooxygenase. Aspirin irreversibly acetylates cyclooxygenase; since the platelets cannot synthesize new enzyme, hemostasis is impaired for 5 to 7 days after a single dose of aspirin. The other common nonsteroidal compounds like indomethacin or ibuprofen are competitive inhibitors and induce transient and dose-dependent inhibition of cyclooxygenase. Administration of other drugs, including large doses of penicillin G or semisynthetic penicillins, may also impair platelet function. In addition, certain metabolic disturbances, including uremia, may impair platelet adhesion, release, and aggregation.

von Willebrand's Disease

The most common inherited defect of primary hemostasis is von Willebrand's disease, which affects as many as one in 800 to 1000 persons in the general population.[58] Patients almost always have a prolonged bleeding time; normal platelet aggregation with ADP, epinephrine, and collagen; and variable defects in von Willebrand factor (vWF) concentration and function. In the most common form, type I, vWF content is modestly reduced to less than 50% of normal. There is a parallel reduction in biological activity, as measured by ristocetin-dependent platelet agglutination, and in factor VIII activity, since vWF serves as the intravascular carrier for this factor. Less commonly, patients have variant syndromes (type II) characterized by a severe reduction in vWF activity despite a normal quantity of circulating protein. Patients with von Willebrand variants have a selective loss of the largest and most hemostatically effective multimers.[59] In type IIa disease, this is due to either a failure to synthesize these multimers or their rapid proteolysis and catabolism. In type IIb disease, the large multimers spontaneously bind to circulating platelets, causing intravascular aggregation and mild thrombocytopenia. Rarely, patients will present with type III disease, in which there is an almost total absence of antigen or activity. These patients probably have homozygous or doubly heterozygous forms of type I disease. No patient with von Willebrand's disease should receive antiplatelet agents, and all patients require treatment prior to surgery or cardiac catheterization with either cryoprecipitate, which replaces vWF, or 1-desamino-8-D-arginine vasopressin (DDAVP), which can transiently raise vWF levels and improve hemostasis in type I patients.[60]

Hemophilia and Related Coagulation Defects

Deficiencies in factors VIII and IX are the two most common inherited coagulation disorders. They are both X-linked recessive traits and cause recurrent musculoskeletal bleeding and hemarthroses in male patients. There is a close relationship between factor level and clinical severity. Patients with levels of less than 1 per cent have severe disease and bleed frequently, even after minimal trauma; those with 1 to 5 per cent have more moderate disease; and those with greater than 5 per cent activity have mild disease with infrequent bleeding. Patients with factor VIII or IX levels above 15 to 20 per cent may be especially difficult to diagnose, since bleeding may occur only after major trauma or surgery. The third most common disorder is factor XI deficiency, an autosomal recessive trait frequently found among Ashkenazi Jews. Hemarthroses are uncommon, and patients often present with postoperative bleeding. There is little correlation between factor XI activity or antigenic level and clinical severity. All these disorders cause an increase in PTT with no change in PT. It is of interest that in patients with deficiencies in factors XII, HMWK, and PK, PTT is markedly prolonged but bleeding does not occur. Patients with true hemorrhagic disorders are treated with plasma fractions (VIII and IX deficiency) or fresh frozen plasma (XI deficiency), while those with laboratory abnormalities of no clinical significance (XII, HMWK, and PK deficiency) do not require therapy.

Vitamin K Deficiency and Liver Disease

Patients with biliary obstruction, liver disease, or inadequate food intake and those receiving broad-spectrum antibiotics may rapidly become deficient in vitamin K. The earliest manifestation of vitamin K deficiency is prolongation of the PT due to a fall in the factor VII level. Later, as the other prothrombin complex proteins decline, the PTT also becomes prolonged. Patients are readily treated with parenteral vitamin K, which can reverse the hemostatic defect in 8 to 10 hours. More rapid correction can be achieved with infusion of fresh frozen plasma. In contrast, patients with liver disease have a more complex coagulation defect, with a combination of vitamin K deficiency, impaired production of multiple coagulation factors including fibrinogen, production of abnormal clotting proteins, systemic fibrinolysis, intravascular coagulation, and thrombocytopenia secondary to splenomegaly and platelet sequestration. These patients do not tolerate therapy with prothrombin complex concentrates, which often contain trace quantities of activated coagulation factors, since they cannot clear activated coagulation proteins effectively. Inadvertent infusion has caused fatal thromboembolism. The best therapy is a combination of vitamin K, platelet concentrates, and fresh frozen plasma.

Disseminated Intravascular Coagulation (DIC)

DIC begins as a thrombotic disorder with the rapid generation of thrombin, extensive fibrin deposition in the microvasculature, and intense secondary fibrinolysis. In some patients, this leads to thrombosis of peripheral vessels and tissue damage. If untreated, there is progressive depletion of coagulation proteins and platelets and diffuse hemorrhage. Various pathological events trigger DIC, including tissue damage due to extreme heat, cold, or trauma; malignant tumors; bacterial or viral infections; extensive vascular malformations (Kasabach-Merritt syndrome); and obstetrical mishaps such as abruptio placentae. Treatment of DIC should focus on identifying and removing the triggering mechanism. Plasma and platelet transfusions are indicated to stop diffuse bleeding, while heparin is used to treat patients with microvascular thrombosis. Occasionally, heparin is also administered to patients with intractable bleeding despite adequate plasma and platelet replacement.

CARDIAC DISORDERS WITH HEMOSTATIC DEFECTS

As previously mentioned, certain cardiovascular disorders may impair hemostasis. For example, patients with chronic right-sided heart failure may develop liver dysfunction and cardiac cirrhosis. This results in impaired vitamin K absorption, impaired production of the prothrombin complex proteins, and thrombocytopenia from splenomegaly and platelet sequestration. Patients with severe cyanotic congenital heart disease, who have a markedly expanded red cell volume and increased whole blood viscosity, may develop a DIC-like syndrome characterized by thrombocytopenia, shortened platelet survival and increased consumption of fibrinogen and other coagulation proteins. The factors which trigger DIC in this setting are unknown, although reduced blood flow and increased viscosity due to the marked increase in red cell mass are implicated. The coagulation abnormalities are corrected by red cell removal and plasma replacement.[61] Finally, patients with acute bacterial endocarditis may develop subclinical DIC, which may be exacerbated by insertion of a prosthetic valve.

EVALUATION OF THROMBOTIC AND PRETHROMBOTIC PATIENTS

Although the clinical and laboratory evaluation of hemorrhagic disorders has become straightforward, there are, as yet, no clinically useful laboratory tests that detect either subclinical thrombosis or the prethrombotic state. Several tests have been devised to measure platelet activation in patients with thrombosis and vascular disease. First, intravascular platelet survival, as measured by the infusion of autologous radiolabeled platelets, is shortened in patients with arterial vascular disease as well as in patients with vascular grafts, arteriovenous shunts, and prosthetic cardiac valves.[62] There is also evidence that this shortened survival may be corrected by the administration of antiplatelet agents.[63] The plasma content of platelet alpha granule proteins such as platelet factor 4 (PF-4) and beta thromboglobulin (B-TG) is increased in patients with thrombosis or embolism but is generally not elevated in patients with prethrombotic disorder.[64, 65] These radioimmunoassays are difficult to standardize, since their interpretation depends on the ability to suppress the secretion of platelet proteins totally during blood collection. In addition, extraneous metabolic factors that do not affect platelet activation and release may affect plasma measurements. PF-4 has a very short intravascular half-life, since it has a high affinity for glycosaminoglycans and binds to heparin-like molecules on the surface of endothelial cells. The administration of heparin is accompanied by a transient rise in plasma PF-4 as the endothelial cell surface pool of PF-4 binds to intravascular heparin.[66] In contrast, B-TG, which does not bind to the endothelial cell, is cleared exclusively by a renal mechanism. Thus, the plasma B-TG level is inversely related to creatinine clearance and increases with serum creatinine independent of platelet activation.[67] Measuring B-TG levels to monitor platelet activation may therefore prove inaccurate in patients with renal insufficiency.[68]

Laboratory tests that detect coagulation system activation rather than platelet activation, although equally cumbersome, may be more useful. The pioneering studies of Nossel and colleagues demonstrated an increase in fibrinopeptide A (FPA), one of the peptides cleaved from fibrinogen by thrombin, in patients with deep venous thrombosis and pulmonary embolism.[69] The elevated FPA level returns to normal after the administration of heparin. More recent studies have employed radioimmunoassays for a prothrombin activation fragment and for circulating thrombin-antithrombin complexes.[70] Both products are elevated in patients with thromboembolism. The ambient levels of prothrombin fragment and thrombin-antithrombin complex are also elevated in elderly patients with vascular disease and in patients with inherited prethrombotic disorders like antithrombin III or protein C deficiency. The protein elevations in these patients can be suppressed by the administration of warfarin-type anticoagulants. These studies provide the first definitive evidence for activation of the coagulation system in patients with inherited or acquired prethrombotic disorders as well as in patients with asymptomatic vascular disease. However, despite these promising results, neither of the tests is available in routine clinical laboratories, since they require specialized reagents and meticulous venipuncture techniques.

PRETHROMBOTIC OR HYPERCOAGULABLE DISORDERS

There are no clearly identified disorders in which well-documented abnormalities in platelet function can be linked to arterial or venous thrombosis. Certain patients with myeloproliferative disorders and patients with Type I and II diabetes mellitus are said to have "hyperreactive" platelets based on standard platelet aggregation assays.[71] In addition, there is evidence that lipid abnormalities such as those seen in familial hypercholesterolemia may increase platelet membrane cholesterol content, decrease membrane fluidity, and enhance platelet reactivity to agonists in vitro.[72] Patients with homozygous homocystinuria clearly have an increased incidence of cerebrovascular thrombosis and develop premature atherosclerosis.[73] In some studies, intravascular platelet survival was also shown to be reduced in patients with homocystinuria.[74] These patients are readily recognized because they may have a "marfanoid" body habitus (resembling the Marfan syndrome), ectopia lentis, and mild mental retardation. In experimental animals, infusion of homocysteine induces similar arterial lesions, which are accompanied by patchy desquamation of endothelial cells. Platelets then adhere to exposed subendothelium and induce smooth muscle cell proliferation and vascular lesions.

DEFICIENCY OR DYSFUNCTION OF THE NATURAL ANTICOAGULANTS

The most thoroughly characterized of the prethrombotic or hypercoagulable disorders are those due to inherited deficiency or dysfunction of one of three natural anticoagulants: antithrombin III, protein C, or protein S.[75–77] The true incidence of these disorders in the general population is not clear, although preliminary surveys of antithrombin III levels have suggested an incidence of antithrombin III deficiency as high as 1 in 2000 individuals. When the clinical experience of large centers that treat venous thromboembolism is reviewed, the congenital disorders identified to date account for no more than 20 per cent of patients with recurrent venous thromboembolism and less than 5 per cent of all patients with deep venous thrombosis.

CLINICAL MANIFESTATIONS. Patients with a congenital deficiency of any one of the natural anticoagulants present with remarkably similar histories of familial, recurrent venous thrombosis and pulmonary embolism. Thromboembolic events are uncommon in infancy and childhood. The incidence of venous thrombosis and pulmonary embolism increases during each ensuing decade, and 90 per cent of patients will have had a thromboembolic episode by the third decade of life. Each of the three abnormalities is usually inherited as an autosomal dominant trait, although a few patients with homozygous protein C deficiency have now been identified. These rare patients become symptomatic shortly after birth and develop neonatal purpura fulminans and DIC.[78] Patients with the heterozygous or autosomal dominant forms of antithrombin III, protein C, or protein S deficiency have only a modestly decreased level of circulating protein. In fact, in many cases, values are just below the normal range. This is quite different from the majority of the X-linked or autosomal recessive coagulation protein disorders, in which patients are not symptomatic until levels are well below normal. Thus, it is important to pay attention to modest deficiencies in the natural anticoagulants.

To date, most patients with antithrombin III deficiency have had a modest reduction in antithrombin level, and no cases of homozygous antithrombin deficiency have been reported. However, families have been identified who have dysfunctional antithrombin molecules. In these cases, the plasma antithrombin level is normal based on immunoassay even though the dysfunctional molecule may not neutralize thrombin effectively or may not bind or become activated by heparin.[79] Effective screening of patients with suspected antithrombin deficiency must include both an immunoassay for total content of the protein and functional assays that measure both the thrombin-neutralizing and heparin cofactor activities of the protein. To date, all the families with protein C and S deficiency have shown a reduction in protein, and no families with dysfunctional molecules have yet been reported. Accurate immunoassays for protein C and S are readily available; functional assays for these proteins have not been well standardized and are not widely available.

MANAGEMENT. Guidelines for the treatment of these congenital abnormalities are just being established. Any patients with symptomatic thromboembolism should be treated acutely with heparin and then placed on a chronic oral anticoagulant. In order to prevent recurrent thromboembolism, which may be fatal, patients should remain on anticoagulants for life. The only group who may not respond to acute heparin therapy are those rare patients with antithrombin variants that are not activated by heparin. In these cases, patients should also receive infusions of plasma or antithrombin concentrates to provide a source of normal antithrombin. Treatment of protein C and S deficiencies poses a special problem, since administration of warfarin to these patients may further depress protein C and S levels and increase the risk of thrombosis. This is thought to be the mechanism underlying hemorrhagic skin necrosis, a rare complication of warfarin therapy.[80] In several retrospective surveys, all identified cases have had protein C deficiency. Patients with either abnormality who require anticoagulant therapy should receive plasma infusions to raise the protein C or S level or should continue anticoagulation with heparin during the first week of warfarin administration.

It is important to carry out thorough family studies and identify all the affected members of a kindred who are deficient in the natural anticoagulants. Asymptomatic family members, particularly those under the age of 30, need not be placed on oral anticoagulants; however, they should receive prophylactic plasma or antithrombin concentrate replacement and perhaps heparin therapy during any period of prolonged immobility owing to a fracture, trauma, or surgery.

OTHER CAUSES OF VENOUS AND ARTERIAL THROMBOSIS

The inherited prethrombotic disorders account for a small but important fraction of patients with thromboembolism. They also provide interesting model systems in which the relationship between a discrete molecular defect and thrombosis can be accurately correlated. In the majority of patients, however, the etiology or pathophysiology remains unclear. Nonetheless, certain acquired disorders or physiologic states predispose patients to the development of venous thrombosis. Immobilization, especially when coupled with trauma or surgery, may precipitate deep venous thrombosis. In most patients, the thrombi are small and are limited to the calf veins. Proximal extension to the femoral system greatly increases the risk of pulmonary embolism.[81] Calf-vein thrombi can be detected by ^{125}I-fibrinogen leg scanning or venography as well as by Doppler flow and impedance plethysmographic measurements. Patients with certain primary or metastatic malignancies, particularly those with cancer arising in the pancreas, stomach, and kidney, as well as patients with chronic congestive heart failure or women who take oral contraceptives are at increased risk for venous thrombosis and embolism. The association of malignancy and thromboembolism has been referred to as *Trousseau's syndrome*, and occasionally the thromboembolic complications may present well before the tumor can be diagnosed. In most of these cases, the pathological mechanism is unclear. A combination of tissue factor generation from tumor or damaged tissue and venous stasis may explain many cases of thrombosis in surgical and cancer patients. *Oral contraceptive use* also lowers antithrombin III levels and may place some patients in the symptomatic range.[82]

Arterial thrombosis rarely occurs de novo in a normal, uninjured vessel and usually develops in a stenotic or atherosclerotic artery. One of the best clinical examples of arterial thromboembolism is the transient ischemic attack (TIA) syndrome. In this condition, platelet thrombi form on ulcerated atherosclerotic carotid vessel plaques. After the thrombus reaches a critical size, fragments break off and embolize to the distal cerebral or retinal circulation. In most patients, the distal emboli will break up, so that blood flow is restored to normal and visual impairment or neurological symptoms disappear. Occasionally, emboli can cause permanent neurological dysfunction and produce a completed stroke or cerebral vascular accident (CVA). Patients may have repeated TIAs without suffering a CVA and can be effectively treated with antiplatelet agents that prevent or reduce platelet plug formation on the ulcerated carotid plaque.

More recently, firm evidence has emerged supporting a similar mechanism underlying transient or permanent obstruction of coronary arteries.[83] In fact, it is now clear that the majority of transmural myocardial infarcts are due to coronary thrombosis following the fracture or disruption of an atherosclerotic coronary arterial plaque. In addition, many patients with unstable angina (p. 1353) like those with TIAs, may have repeated bouts of platelet thrombosis and embolism causing their cardiac instability and chest pain. In addition, their symptoms may abate with antiplatelet therapy which may also reduce the risk of subsequent myocardial infarction (p. 1359). In addition to forming thrombi in diseased coronary arteries, cardiac patients may develop intracavitary or intracardiac thrombi. For example, patients who have had a transmural myocardial infarction may have residual endocardial scarring or hypokinesis. The damaged myocardium may provide a site for development of a mural thrombus, which may then break up and produce cerebral emboli. Similarly, in patients with mitral stenosis, left atrial enlargement, and atrial fibrillation, thrombi often develop in the left atrium or on the mitral valve and can embolize into the systemic circulation. Patients with prosthetic cardiac valves are also at risk for systemic embolization. Although these intracavitary cardiac thrombi are "arterial," they form in areas of low blood flow and are rich in fibrin. In this respect, they more closely resemble the fibrin and red cell–rich thrombi that form in the venous circulation. Thus, effective treatment of intracavitary thrombi requires anticoagulants such as heparin or warfarin or a combination of anticoagulants and antiplatelet drugs.

FIBRINOLYTIC DISORDERS

Until recently, the study of potential disorders of the fibrinolytic system and their relation to thromboembolism has been hampered by a lack of precise assays for components of the system. Now, with the molecular cloning of t-PA, pro-UK, and the fibrinolytic inhibitors such as plasminogen activator inhibitor (PAI), it is possible to analyze fibrinolysis with more precision. In fact, several congenital or acquired abnormalities of the fibrinolytic system have been described that may increase the risk of thrombosis. Both a decreased concentration of plasminogen and abnormal plasminogen molecules have been associated with recurrent thrombosis.[84] Production of abnormal fibrinogen molecules (dysfibrinogenemias) usually causes bleeding; however, in certain dysfibrinogenemias, fibrin thrombi are formed that are unusually resistant to the action of plasmin and can predispose patients to thrombosis.[85] In addition, reduced fibrinolytic activity has been described in patients with cerebrovascular accidents,[86] recurrent venous thrombosis,[87] and mesenteric venous thrombosis.[88] In one case, defective release of t-PA from endothelial cells has been postulated as the cause of the fibrinolytic defect and recurrent venous thrombosis.[89] In a provocative recent report, elevated levels of PAI, the endothelial protease inhibitor that rapidly neutralizes t-PA and pro-UK, have been noted in the plasma of young patients surviving myocardial infarction. This raises the interesting possibility that coronary thrombosis might be due to a failure to lyse intracoronary thrombi due to rapid neutralization of t-PA. Finally, there is one fibrinolytic abnormality that can cause bleeding rather than thrombosis. Absence of alpha$_2$ PI, the principal plasmin inhibitor, permits excessively rapid fibrinolysis of hemostatic plugs and recurrent hemorrhage.[90] In *summary*, it is now clear that inherited molecular defects in the fibrinolytic system, like the inherited defects in the natural anticoagulants, may be added to the growing list of disorders that predispose patients to both arterial and venous thromboembolism.

ANTICOAGULANT THERAPY FOR CARDIOVASCULAR DISORDERS

HEPARIN

Heparin is clearly the most effective anticoagulant agent available for the treatment of thromboembolic disorders. Since the pioneering studies by Barrett and Jordan demonstrating the efficacy of parenteral heparin in patients with pulmonary embolism, it has become the standard therapy for acute venous and arterial thrombosis and embolism.[91] Heparin activity resides in a heterogeneous series of sulfated glycosaminoglycans that function as anticoagulants by binding to and activating antithrombin III.[92] For pharmaceutical applications, heparin is extracted from porcine intestinal mucosa or beef lung. There is now abundant evidence that heparin-like molecules are also present on endothelial cells throughout the vascular tree, where they regulate the rate of normal coagulation reactions and help maintain blood fluidity.[93] Commercial heparin preparations are heterogeneous with respect to both the molecular size and the biological activity of the glycosaminoglycans. In fact, only a small fraction of the molecules in commercial heparin (usually about 20 per cent) have anticoagulant activity.

MECHANISM OF ACTION. Heparin can be conveniently fractionated on the basis of its molecular size and antithrombin affinity. Those heparin species with a low affinity for antithrombin—and therefore little or no anticoagulant activity—may have other biological properties of potential importance. For example, such species inhibit the proliferation of vascular smooth muscle cells in culture and prevent smooth muscle cell migration and proliferation within the arterial wall after experimental injury.[94] In the future, this antiproliferative property of heparin could be exploited to produce agents that inhibit atherogenesis. These low-affinity, high molecular weight forms of heparin also bind to and agglutinate platelets and may be the cause of heparin-induced thrombocytopenia. Heparin size also affects the kinetics of substrate neutralization by antithrombin III. For example, high and low molecular weight species neutralize factor Xa equally well. However, the high molecular weight species are more effective in facilitating the neutralization of thrombin by antithrombin III.[95] This difference could be of importance as various heparin fractions are utilized clinically as antithrombotic agents.

Heparin is administered continuously by intravenous pump, by intermittent intravenous infusion, or subcutaneously. It is both metabolized within the liver by the enzyme heparinase and excreted unchanged by the kidney. This explains the increased sensitivity and erratic metabolism of heparin by some patients with renal or hepatic disease. The dose and route of administration will vary with the clinical situation and the therapeutic goal. As depicted in Figure 56–15, varying methods of heparin administration have a marked effect on plasma heparin level and on the magnitude and duration of impaired hemostasis. Administration of a bolus of heparin followed by a continuous infusion of the drug will keep heparin levels within the "therapeutic" range with minimal oscillation. Intermittent bolus infusion causes a more dramatic increase and subsequent fall in heparin level. Following subcutaneous heparin, levels are not as high but are more sustained. The standard heparin regimens are summarized in Table 56–1.

INDICATIONS. The most frequent indications for heparin in cardiac patients are (1) to prevent proximal extension of deep venous thrombosis or the recurrence of pulmonary embolism (p. 1588); (2) to prevent the recurrence of cerebral or other systemic embolism from intracardiac sources in the left atrium, left ventricle, or mitral valve; (3) to preclude development of deep venous thrombosis or pulmonary embolism in high-risk patients, such as those who are immobilized or have congestive heart failure, acute myocardial infarction, or cardiomyopathy or who are undergoing abdominal surgery; and (4) as long-term therapy for the occasional patient who has recurrent thrombosis or embolism on warfarin or who cannot receive warfarin therapy.

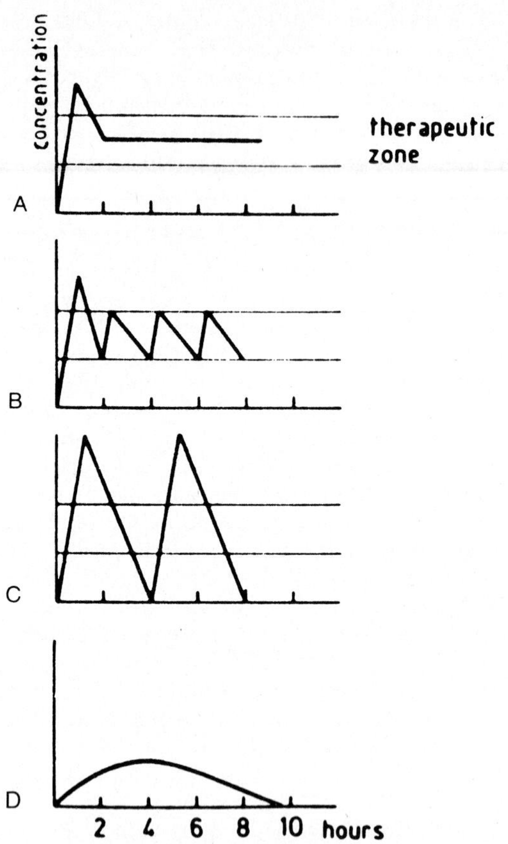

FIGURE 56–15. The concentration of heparin in blood after various routes of administration. *A*, Effect of a heparin bolus followed by a continuous intravenous infusion, the most common method of heparin administration for patients with acute thromboembolism. *B*, and *C*, Effects of intermittent intravenous infusions. With this route, heparin levels oscillate widely and are frequently outside the broadly defined "therapeutic zone." This may increase the risk of bleeding and increase the rate of rethrombosis. *D*, Effects of subcutaneous injection, the route used for prophylactic "low-dose" heparin, in which there is a low but sustained level of heparin in the blood. (From Verstraete, M., and Vermylen, J.: Thrombosis. London, Pergamon Press, 1984, p. 85.)

METHOD OF ADMINISTRATION. When full-dose heparin is required, the usual procedure is to administer 5000 USP units of heparin rapidly followed by a continuous infusion of 1000 USP units/hour. The dose of heparin is adjusted to prolong the PTT to 1.5 times the patient's PTT prior to instituting heparin therapy. Alternatively, patients may be given an intermittent intravenous infusion of 5000 units

TABLE 56–1 CLINICAL USE OF HEPARIN

INDICATION	DOSE (USP UNITS)	FREQUENCY	ROUTE
Prophylaxis in elective general surgery	5000	q12h	SC
Prophylaxis in congestive heart failure, cardiomyopathy, myocardial infarction	10,000	q12h	SC
Venous thromboembolism	5000 (bolus)	1000/hr	IV
Massive pulmonary embolism*	20,000 (bolus)	2000/hr	IV

*Reported to be effective in small studies; no randomized trials. Fibrinolytic therapy is a better alternative. SC = subcutaneous; IV = intravenous.

four to six times daily. There is good evidence that the risk of bleeding is less with continuous infusion and careful monitoring of the PTT. A less desirable third alternative is to administer 5000 units every 4 to 6 hours by subcutaneous injection. The administration of full-dose heparin is continued for 5 to 7 days, with close monitoring of the PTT and hematocrit along with examination of the stool for occult blood and periodic urinalysis for hematuria. However, even with careful control, 10 to 20 per cent of patients will experience some bleeding and 1 to 5 per cent will have a major hemorrhage. Patients are usually begun on an oral anticoagulant such as warfarin within the first 3 to 5 days of heparinization, although heparin is continued while the dose of warfarin is adjusted.

Low-Dose Heparin. The rationale for low-dose heparin to prevent initial thrombus formation has evolved from extensive clinical studies conducted by Kakkar and colleagues.[95, 96] Their studies demonstrated a clear reduction in both the incidence of and mortality from pulmonary embolism in a large cohort of middle-aged men undergoing major abdominal surgery. Since the incidence of fatal pulmonary embolism was also low in the control group, it required a multicenter study that enrolled over 4000 patients to prove efficacy. The recommended regimen is 5000 USP units of heparin subcutaneously every 8 to 12 hours beginning 2 hours before surgery. This regimen reduced the rate of deep venous thrombosis by 60 per cent and the risk of fatal pulmonary embolus by 71 per cent in the Kakkar studies. The combination of 5000 USP units of heparin plus 0.5 mg dihydroergotamine administered subcutaneously every 12 hours may be a somewhat better prophylactic regimen.[96] The vasoconstriction induced by dihydroergotamine, which reduces the risk of bleeding, may on occasion also cause ischemia and loss of digits.[97] Thus, further studies are needed to establish the clinical utility and safety of this regimen.

Theoretically, a low-dose heparin regimen should be successful in other surgical and medical settings in which the risk of venous thrombosis and embolism is high. Patients with acute myocardial infarction as well as hospitalized patients with chronic congestive heart failure and low output states, including those with cardiomyopathy, might benefit from prophylactic heparin administration. Several studies carried out in coronary care units in which patients with acute myocardial infarction were enrolled have failed to show that low-dose heparin is efficacious. In addition, the regimen does not prevent venous thrombosis and embolism in gynecological patients undergoing pelvic surgery or in orthopedic patients undergoing open reduction and nailing of hip fractures. In addition, in patients requiring eye operations or neurosurgery, the risk of bleeding, even with low-dose heparin, is prohibitive, and the medication should not be given. Thus, despite Kakkar's careful clinical trials, the use of prophylactic heparin has not become widespread. The trend toward early mobilization of patients after major surgery may have lowered the incidence of venous thrombosis and embolism in the absence of heparin and may limit physician enthusiasm for this regimen.

COMPLICATIONS. The major complication of heparin therapy is hemorrhage due to interruption of normal hemostasis. Patients may bleed from surgical wounds or catheterization sites or around indwelling vascular catheters and tubes. Patients may also develop gastrointestinal, genitourinary, or retroperitoneal bleeding. Age of the patient, dose and route of administration, presence of pathological lesions in the gastrointestinal or genitourinary tract, and concomitant administration of medications that impair platelet function all affect the incidence and severity of bleeding. Heparin also causes thrombocytopenia in as many as 20 per cent of recipients.[98] More rarely, heparin may provoke intravascular platelet agglutination and paradoxical thrombosis.[99] The antiplatelet effect of heparin is more pronounced with beef lung heparin preparations and, as previously described, is largely due to the heparin species having low antithrombin affinity and high molecular weight. Heparin administration may also induce osteoporosis, although substantial bone loss is not apparent until the 6th to 8th week of therapy.[100] Fortunately, this exceeds the usual duration of heparin therapy for acute thrombosis but can become a problem in the occasional patient who requires prolonged intravenous heparin for recurrent thromboembolism.

In order to reduce complications and improve efficacy, heparin species of low molecular weight and high antithrombin affinity have been prepared by the fractionation of commercial heparin and are currently being tested clinically and in experimental models.[94] Although low molecular weight heparin fractions are effective antithrombotic agents, they are more expensive to produce than is standard heparin. Since they are less likely to cause thrombocytopenia, they are the agents of choice in patients with a history of heparin-associated thrombocytopenia who require heparin therapy.

CHRONIC ORAL ANTICOAGULATION

The oral anticoagulants, which are all derivatives of the parent compound coumarin, are the agents of choice for preventing the recurrence of thrombosis and embolism after an initial course of therapy with heparin. The most frequent *indications* for therapy are patients with (1) established deep venous thrombosis and pulmonary embolism, (2) cerebral embolism, (3) atrial fibrillation or mitral stenosis with a history of embolism or a changing rhythm, (4) prosthetic cardiac valves, or (5) an inherited prethrombotic disorder. The duration of therapy will vary. Most patients with a single episode of thromboembolism will receive treatment for 3 to 6 months. There is evidence that 90 per cent of patients with deep venous thrombosis will relapse if they do not receive oral anticoagulant therapy and that the risk decreases markedly by 3 months and plateaus by the sixth month. Patients with a noncorrectable cardiac disorder or an inherited prethrombotic state may require prolonged or even lifelong oral anticoagulation. Prophylactic anticoagulation has been proposed for patients (1) with atrial fibrillation who are to undergo cardioversion, (2) with chronic congestive heart failure or low output states such as cardiomyopathy, and (3) who have undergone hip surgery to prevent perioperative thrombosis.

Coumarin-Type Drugs

These are vitamin K antagonists, which prevent the reduction of vitamin K to its active epoxide form by blocking an intrahepatic epoxide reductase. This, in turn, prevents the formation of digammacarboxyglutamic acid (Gla) residues on prothrombin and factors VII, IX, and X as well as on the proteins C and S. The net effect of coumarin administration is to reduce coagulation factor activity and prolong the PT and PTT. The reduction in coagulation factor activity is directly related to the half-life of each plasma factor. Factor VII, which has the shortest half-life, decreases first, followed by factors IX and X, proteins C and S, and prothrombin. Although therapy with the coumarins is usually monitored by the degree to which PT is prolonged, prevention of thrombosis requires a reduction in factors IX and X, which are not measured by the PT. Paradoxically, a profound reduction in factor VII, which prolongs the PT, may not protect a patient from recurrent thrombosis but may increase the risk of bleeding. Although coumarin therapy decreases the activity of both procoagulant and anticoagulant molecules, the net effect is to impair coagulation and reduce the rate of thrombus formation. However, in patients with congenital protein C or S deficiency, who already have low levels of these proteins, the net balance may shift toward thrombus formation, since protein C and S levels may have fallen to dangerously low levels while the procoagulant proteins are still elevated. This may predispose patients to a rare thrombotic event, hemorrhagic skin necrosis.

PHARMACOKINETICS. The coumarin drugs are readily absorbed in the stomach and jejunum and, after absorption, are bound to albumin and become distributed in the intravascular and interstitial spaces. Free drug is then taken up by hepatocytes, where it blocks vitamin K metabolism. The coumarins, like many other drugs, are inactivated by hepatic microsomal enzymes, and the resulting coumarin metabolites are either excreted into the bowel via the enterohepatic circulation or are filtered and excreted by the kidneys. The plasma half-life of the different coumarin derivatives varies considerably. In addition, each of the coumarins is optically active and is produced as a racemic mixture of D and L isomers. The D isomers have a longer half-life, so that varying the ratio of D to L isomers could also influence intravascular half-life. The most frequently used coumarin derivative, sodium warfarin, has a half-life of 42 hours.

METHOD OF ADMINISTRATION. Oral anticoagulant therapy with an agent like warfarin is initiated by administering 10 to 15 mg/day of the drug for 3 days to the average-sized adult. The daily dose is then adjusted to maintain the PT at 1.5 to 2.0 times the control value. It is important to recognize that laboratory reagents used to measure the PT are not standardized, so that the patient's PT prior to therapy must be used as a guideline. Ideally, all measurements should be made in the same laboratory with the same reagents, since the correlation between prolongation of the PT and reduction in activity of the prothrombin complex proteins II, VII, IX, and X varies among PT reagents. One approach, used in Great Britain, has been to supply a reference thromboplastin to each clinical laboratory. Each laboratory can then calibrate their local thromboplastin reagent against the British National thromboplastin standard. Another approach has been to introduce new assays that measure the prothrombin complex proteins but do not rely on the PT reagent. In one study, a conformation-specific antibody that recognized the biologically inactive Gla-deficient prothrombin molecules produced by warfarin therapy was used to assess therapeutic efficacy and was slightly superior to the conventional PT-based test.[101]

DRUG INTERACTIONS. The pharmacology of warfarin is complex. It is well recognized that the anticoagulant effect of coumarin derivatives is dramatically affected by the simultaneous administration of other drugs that may enhance or reduce coumarin activity.[102] The biological effect of a given dose will also depend on the rapidity of its uptake by the liver, the integrity and vitamin K stores of the hepatocyte, and the activity of hepatic microsomal degrading enzymes. As shown in Table 56–2, some drugs commonly prescribed for patients with heart disease such as quinidine, cimetidine, and clofibrate may enhance coumarin activity. These drugs compete for albumin binding sites, displace warfarin from the blood, and increase its rate of delivery to the liver. Conversely, drugs such as glutethimide and other common sedatives reduce the potency of a given coumarin dose by increasing liver microsomal enzyme activity and enhancing drug catabolism. In addition, some drugs like antacids and cholestyramine may impair intestinal absorption of the drug and reduce the activity of a given dose.

TABLE 56–2 FACTORS INFLUENCING THE DOSE OF COUMARINS NEEDED FOR A CONSTANT ANTICOAGULANT EFFECT

METABOLIC AND DIETARY FACTORS	
Decrease dose:	*Increase dose:*
Decreased oral intake and vitamin K stores (surgery, antibiotics)	Increased vitamin K intake (liver, cauliflower, green vegetables like broccoli, spinach, green beans)
Liver disease	Hypometabolism (hypothyroidism)
Renal disease leading to hypoalbuminemia	Hereditary resistance
Malignancy, sepsis	
Diarrhea, malabsorption syndromes	
Hypermetabolism (hyperthyroidism, fever)	
DRUG INTERACTIONS	
Decrease dose:	*Increase dose:*
Antibiotics	Vitamin K
Cimetidine	Antacids
Anabolic steroids	Cholestyramine
D-Thyroxine	Barbiturates
Clofibrate	Griseofulvin
Sulfinpyrazone	Rifampin
Phenylbutazone	Antihistamines
Quinidine	
Alpha-methyldopa	

Modified from Chesebro, J., et al.: Antithrombotic therapy in valvular heart disease. J. Am. Coll. Cardiol. 8:52B, 1986. By permission of The American College of Cardiology.

In addition to these well-documented drug interactions, metabolic abnormalities that alter hepatic or renal function or that lower albumin levels or vitamin K stores can make patients more sensitive to a given dose of a coumarin. Conversely, ingestion of foods rich in vitamin K or the presence of a hypometabolic state such as hypothyroidism may require administration of a larger than usual dose of a coumarin drug. In patients with fever, sepsis, or hyperthyroidism, catabolism of the vitamin K–dependent coagulation factors may have increased, requiring less coumarin for anticoagulation. In addition to these effects on drug absorption and metabolism, the concomitant administration of drugs that impair platelet function, like aspirin, may cause hemorrhage without altering the PT or coumarin level.

COMPLICATIONS. Hemorrhagic complications occur in 7 to 10 per cent of patients who are anticoagulated for more than 4 months.[103] Death from hemorrhage occurs in approximately 1 per cent of patients receiving coumarin for a similar duration. The frequency of bleeding increases with anticoagulant dose and the degree to which the PT is prolonged but is also affected by the patient's age and associated medical conditions. For example, in one large study, bleeding occurred during 7 of 1000 days of warfarin treatment when the residual PT activity was between 10 and 29 per cent of normal. This is equivalent to a PT of 18 to 20 seconds. The rate of hemorrhage increased to 85 per 1000 days of treatment when residual PT activity was less than 10 per cent (PT above 20 seconds).[104] Because of this unacceptably high rate of hemorrhage, modified regimens have been introduced that use less intense anticoagulation.[105] In these regimens, the warfarin dose is adjusted so that the PT is prolonged to no more than 1.5 times the control value. In one study of "low-dose" warfarin, the frequency of bleeding was markedly reduced when compared with standard therapy (4 vs 22 per cent), while the frequency of recurrent venous thromboembolism remained at 2 per cent in both groups.[106]

RECOMMENDATIONS. It is hard to develop a general set of recommendations regarding the duration and intensity of anticoagulation with warfarin-type drugs. However, based on the available evidence, the authors recommend that patients who receive prophylactic anticoagulation, such as those with prosthetic cardiac valves, chronic atrial fibrillation or mitral stenosis, cardiomyopathy or chronic congestive heart failure, or those undergoing hip surgery, receive sufficient warfarin to prolong the PT to 1.5 times the control value. Patients given warfarin after an episode of deep venous thrombosis or pulmonary embolism, who are at high risk for recurrent thromboembolism, should probably receive a slightly higher dose of warfarin to keep the PT prolonged to 1.5 to 2.0 times the control value. Additional clinical studies coupled with the introduction of more reliable assays to monitor biological effects should make warfarin therapy safer and more effective and will allow the dose to be adjusted to the needs of the individual patient.

ANTIPLATELET DRUG THERAPY IN CARDIOVASCULAR DISEASE

Agents that modify platelet function have now been administered to patients with a wide range of cardiovascular disorders. These drugs have been given to patients with unstable angina, at high risk for arrhythmia and sudden death, with prosthetic cardiac valves or saphenous vein bypass grafts, or undergoing percutaneous transluminal angioplasty as well as to those with a history of acute myocardial infarction, stroke, or transient ischemic attacks. In each of these clinical situations, there is evidence for platelet participation in the pathophysiology of the clinical disorder and some reports of clinical efficacy.[107, 108]

Despite the enthusiastic use of this therapeutic modality by cardiologists, the efficacy of antiplatelet drug therapy remains unclear in most cardiac patients, so that any therapeutic recommendations must be tentative. Three fundamental problems have made evaluation of antiplatelet therapy difficult: (1) a lack of firm guidelines regarding disorders or clinical events that might potentially benefit from such therapy; (2) the variable quality of clinical trials on which therapeutic decisions must be based; (3) a lack of correlation between in vitro inhibition of platelet function and a clinical antithrombotic effect; and (4) the inability of available drugs to inhibit platelet participation in thrombus formation completely. The ideal antiplatelet drug, which is not yet available, should substantially reduce arterial thrombosis and embolism without causing undue bleeding or other undesirable side effects. This last limitation of antiplatelet therapy may be most important, since an ideal procedure for patient selection and a perfectly organized clinical trial are of limited value if the agent to be tested has minimal or no efficacy.

PHARMACOLOGY OF ANTIPLATELET DRUGS

CYCLOOXYGENASE INHIBITORS. The most widely studied antiplatelet agents interfere with platelet signal transduction and stimulus-response coupling. One group of drugs, which includes aspirin and other nonsteroidal antiinflammatory agents such as indomethacin, sulfinpyrazone, and ibuprofen, inhibits platelet cyclooxygenase. Aspirin is unique in that it is the only drug that irreversibly inhibits cyclooxygenase. Since the platelet cannot synthesize any new enzyme, the antiplatelet effect of a single dose of aspirin can persist for 5 to 7 days. In contrast, other tissues rapidly recover from aspirin inhibition by synthesizing new cyclooxygenase. Thus, endothelial cells regain their capacity to synthesize prostacyclin within a few hours of aspirin administration.[109] The concept of using low doses of aspirin to inhibit platelet function selectively has gained considerable popularity. In fact, it is possible to inhibit platelet thromboxane production effectively with as little as 20 to 100 mg aspirin per day.[110] There is, as yet, no evidence that low-dose aspirin is more effective than the conventional daily doses of 625 to 1250 mg nor that these higher doses are harmful. The antiplatelet effect of the competitive inhibitors is much less dramatic than that of aspirin when measured by in vitro laboratory tests as well as by clinical studies assessing thrombus formation in vivo, and they are not frequently used in clinical trials.

DIPYRIDAMOLE. This agent (Persantin) inhibits platelet phosphodiesterase activity and raises platelet cyclic AMP levels in vitro, although the usual doses do not alter in vitro tests of platelet function or prolong the bleeding time in patients. Like aspirin, dipyridamole has undergone extensive clinical testing and has well-defined antithrombotic effects.[111]

Other Antiplatelet Agents

In addition to aspirin and dipyridamole, a number of new antiplatelet agents have been introduced that have more selective effects on arachidonic acid metabolism or affect other steps in the platelet activation process. Several *thromboxane synthetase inhibitors* have been designed to circumvent the fact that aspirin inhibits both thromboxane and prostacyclin synthesis. Unfortunately, drugs in this class, such as *dazoxiben*, increase the concentration of the prostaglandin endoperoxide precursors of thromboxane A_2 to levels that can activate the platelets.[112] Several *thromboxane receptor antagonists* that are active in vitro may soon become available for clinical testing, possibly in conjunction with the thromboxane synthetase inhibitors.[113] *Inhibitory prostaglandins* (e.g., PGD_2) or stable synthetic analogues of prostacyclin, prostaglandin-like BW 245C, or carbacyclin have been administered to normal volunteers and to a small number of patients with occlusive vascular disease or fulminant thrombotic thrombocytopenic purpura.[114, 115] Although some beneficial effects were noted, the potent hypotensive effects of these compounds may limit their utility for in vivo studies. Inhibitory prostaglandins have been used to prevent the interaction of platelets with artificial surfaces during ex vivo perfusion and may be of value during hemodialysis and cardiopulmonary bypass.[116]

Ticlopidine is a novel platelet inhibitor with a poorly defined mechanism of action. It has the unique property of having little effect on platelets after direct addition in vitro, while it markedly prolongs the bleeding time and platelet response to aggregating agents after administration to patients. It is thought to alter membrane reactivity to multiple agonists and is currently under study in several multicenter trials.[117] Other agents currently under study are inhibitors of platelet activating factor (1-alkyl-2-acetyl-sn-glycero-3-phosphorylcholine), a lipid mediator generated from leukocytes during allergic and immunological reactions, that aggregates platelets.[118] In addition, peptides that inhibit fibrinogen binding to platelets and monoclonal antibodies to platelet surface glycoproteins may block platelet aggregation and are being tested in experimental animals. Several well-known cardiovascular drugs such as nitroglycerin[119] and the calcium channel antagonists[120] may have antiplatelet effects, although their possible utility as antithrombotic agents has not been tested.

ANTIPLATELET AGENTS IN TREATMENT OF MYOCARDIAL ISCHEMIA AND INFARCTION

It is now well accepted that a majority of acute transmural myocardial infarctions are caused by thrombotic occlusion of a diseased coronary artery.[121] The occluding thrombus, which forms on an ulcerated or ruptured atherosclerotic plaque, can be demonstrated in 90 per cent of patients by means of prompt angiography. Although platelets may initiate thrombus formation, fibrin deposition occurs secondarily. These fibrin-rich thrombi are effectively removed by the administration of fibrinolytic agents that restore vascular patency. Platelets are also implicated in the pathogenesis of coronary arterial vasospasm, which may cause transient ischemia and angina pectoris or, less frequently, myocardial infarction. Activated platelets produce thromboxane A_2, a potent vasoconstrictor that may produce or enhance vasospasm. The concentration of the stable metabolite thromboxane B_2 is elevated in coronary sinus blood obtained during pacing or exercise-induced angina and in blood obtained soon after spontaneous anginal episodes. It is also elevated in patients with variant anginal syndromes who have pain at rest and ST-segment elevation, as well as in those with the clinical syndrome of unstable angina.

UNSTABLE ANGINA (See also p. 1353). Two trials of aspirin in patients with unstable angina have yielded impressive positive results.[122, 123] In the first study, the Veterans Administration Cooperative Trial, 1266 men with unstable angina were given 324 mg of aspirin daily, with a 51 per cent decrease in the number of subsequent infarctions and an identical reduction in mortality. A second Canadian cooperative trial confirmed these results, reporting a 55 per cent reduction in myocardial infarction and a 43 per cent reduction in mortality. In contrast, there is no evidence that aspirin or any other antiplatelet agents affect the frequency, duration, or precipitating events that cause spontaneous or exercise-induced angina pectoris, despite clear evidence for platelet activation in these patients. This striking difference in aspirin's efficacy in various forms of myocardial ischemia as well as the marginal results in most other patients with stable coronary artery disease highlight the problems facing investigators who design clinical trials as well as physicians who must recommend appropriate treatment for their patients. At present, aspirin can be unequivocally recommended only for patients with unstable angina.

MYOCARDIAL INFARCTION (See also p. 1290). Over the past 12 years, there have been eight randomized double-blind trials of antiplatelet therapy for the secondary prevention of myocardial infarction.[107] The results are summarized in Table 56–3. Five trials utilized aspirin alone, one had a combination of aspirin and dipyridamole (Persantin), and two used sulfinpyrazone (Anturane). The doses of aspirin varied from 300 to 1500 mg/day, and the studies enrolled 1000 to 4500 patients, predominantly males, who had a well-documented myocardial infarct. Although aspirin therapy was reported to reduce mortality from subsequent infarcts from 17 to 30 per cent in various studies, none of these trends reached statistical significance. In the PARIS study, the combination of aspirin and dipyridamole reduced the incidence of subsequent coronary events by 50 per cent, although overall mortality was unchanged. A new secondary prevention study, PARIS II, confirms the beneficial effect of aspirin and dipyridamole on the incidence of subsequent coronary events.[124]

The first sulfinpyrazone trial reported a striking reduction in sudden death and mortality during the first 6 months of therapy, and the second trial reported a reduction in reinfarction rate. These studies have been criticized, however, on technical grounds relating to the method of patient exclusion and the time of enrollment of subjects.

One investigator has suggested that the lack of statistical significance in the aspirin studies may be an insurmountable problem, given the relatively small numbers of patients enrolled in each of these secondary prevention trials. However, when data from all the aspirin trials are "pooled" to increase the number of evaluable patients, a statistically significant reduction in mortality can be demonstrated.[125] This unconventional statistical technique may be criticized, since the study populations were not absolutely identical.

On the premise that aspirin might be helpful in patients with coronary artery disease, one large primary prevention trial is now under way to test the hypothesis that regular aspirin ingestion may prevent or delay myocardial infarction. Although the accumulation of a statistically significant number of events may take some time, it is hoped that these trials will help to resolve the longstanding dilemma regarding the potential utility of aspirin in patients at risk for coronary disease. At this time, 80 to 325 mg of aspirin daily is advised for patients who have recently suffered a myocardial infarction and in whom there is no contraindication (history of excessive bleeding, gastrointestinal or

TABLE 56–3 ANTIPLATELET THERAPY TO PREVENT MYOCARDIAL INFARCTION

Study*	Drugs (Dosage)	Patients (Duration)	Outcome**
Elwood et al., 1974	ASA (300 mg/day)	1,239 (30 mo)	Mortality ↓ 25%
CDP, 1976	ASA (1 gm/day)	1,529 (24 mo)	Mortality ↓ 30%
Breddin et al., 1977	ASA (1.5 gm/day)	946 (24 mo)	No change
Elwood and Sweetman, 1979	ASA (900 mg/day)	1,682 (12 mo)	Mortality ↓ 17%
AMIS, 1980	ASA (1 gm/day)	4,524 (36 mo)	No change
ART, 1980	Sulfinpyrazone (800 mg/day)	1,558 (16 mo)	Reinfarction ↓ 57%
ARIS, 1982	Sulfinpyrazone (800 mg/day)	727 (9 mo)	Reinfarction ↓ 56%
PARIS I, 1980	ASA (1 gm/day) Dipyridamole (225 mg/day)	2,206 (36 mo)	Reinfarction ↓ 50%
PARIS II, 1986	Same as PARIS I	3,128 (24 mo)	30% ↓ reinf. at 1 yr.; 24% ↓ at 2 yr.

*All studies cited in reference 107 (Harker, L.A.: Circulation 23:206, 1986) except PARIS II, which is reference 124 (Klimt, C.R., et al.: J. Am. Coll. Cardiol. 7:251, 1986.

**The reduction in reinfarctions in PARIS II was statistically significant at one and two years. Although trends are given, reductions in mortality were not statistically significant.

Abbreviations: CDP = Coronary Drug Project; AMIS = Acute Myocardial Infarction Study; ARIS = Anturane Reinfarction Study; ART = Anturane Reinfarction Trial; PARIS = Persantine-Aspirin Reinfarction Study. ASA = aspirin.

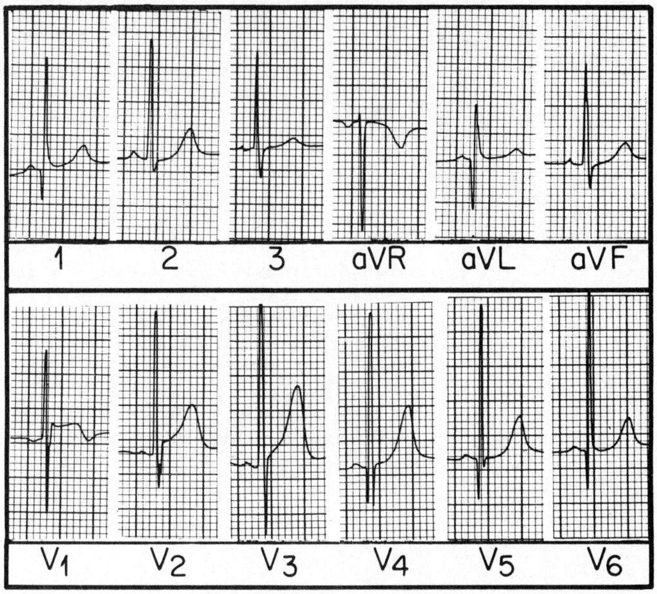

FIGURE 57–2. Electrocardiogram from a 10-year-old boy with classic Duchenne muscular dystrophy. The P-R interval is short (100 msec in lead 2). The QRS complex is typical of Duchenne dystrophy, showing an anterior shift in the right precordial leads and deep but narrow Q waves in leads I, aVL, and V_{4-6}. (From Perloff, J. K.: Cardiac rhythm and conduction in Duchenne's muscular dystrophy. Reprinted by permission of the American College of Cardiology. J. Am. Coll. Cardiol. 3:1263, 1984.

marked, and in terminal stages of the disease the boy sits in a wheelchair, twisted like a pretzel, with his head lolling because of lack of neck support. Dystrophy of chest muscles and diaphragm together with kyphoscoliosis interfere with coughing and breathing. Patients are likely to succumb to pulmonary infection in the second decade, although cardiac disease is an important and at times dramatic cause of death. Rapidly progressive preterminal heart failure may follow years of circulatory stability during which the only suspicion of cardiac involvement is an abnormal electrocardiogram (Fig. 57–2).

Physical and radiological examinations of the heart are characterized by thoracic deformities and the high diaphragm of diaphragmatic dystrophy. A reduction in anteroposterior chest dimension is often striking and is commonly responsible for a systolic impulse at the left sternal edge, a grade 1–3/6 short impure midsystolic murmur in the second left interspace, and a loud pulmonic component of the second heart sound.[8] These signs should *not* be taken as evidence of pulmonary hypertension, which is seldom if ever present, despite the thoracic distortion and high diaphragm.[1] An increase in transverse heart size on x-ray is more often than not caused by the narrow anteroposterior chest dimension and high diaphragm rather than by ventricular dilatation.[1] The murmur of mitral regurgitation has a relatively firm anatomical basis, namely, dystrophic involvement of the posterior papillary muscle and contiguous posterobasal left ventricular wall.[9, 10]

Electrocardiography. Twenty-four hour electrocardiographic recordings show that the most common rhythm disturbance is inappropriate sinus tachycardia (rate acceleration without discernible circumstantial cause).[11, 12] Sinus tachycardia may be labile and gradual or abrupt in onset. The cause(s) of the rate acceleration or of relatively frequent sinus arrhythmias is(are) unknown but may involve abnormal autonomic regulation.[11] Alternatively, "dystrophic" sinoatrial node infiltration or fibrosis may prove to be the substrate not only for abnormal sinus node automaticity but also for sinus node reentry and labile sinus tachycardia, especially the abrupt-onset type.[11] Intra- or interatrial conduction abnormalities are not uncommon. An abnormal P terminal force in lead V_1 in the presence of normal left atrial size on the echocardiogram implies an intrinsic disorder of left atrial or interatrial conduction.[12] Whether this sets the stage for unstable atrial rhythms is unclear, but atrial flutter commonly precipitates congestive heart failure in late-stage Duchenne dystrophy.[13]

In approximately 50 per cent of patients, atrioventricular (AV) conduction, as judged by the P-R interval, is either definitely or marginally accelerated without delta waves (Fig. 57–2).[11] Intracardiac electrophysiological studies are not available in patients with Duchenne dystrophy, but short P-R intervals may represent atriofascicular bypass tracts or accelerated conduction within the AV node (p. 685).[11] The latter hypothesis relates to dystrophic fibrosis or fatty infiltration, which, if present, could set the stage for an increased cable conduction constant, as has been proposed for Pompe's disease.[11] Paroxysmal rapid heart action via bypass tracts, however, is unknown in Duchenne dystrophy, and atrial flutter, a common preterminal arrhythmia, has not been reported with 1:1 AV conduction.[11, 13, 14] Right ventricular conduction delay occasionally occurs, and proximal infranodal conduction abnormalities sometimes take the form of a rightward QRS axis that may represent left posterior fascicular block.[11] Electrical ventricular instability is uncommon despite regional left ventricular dystrophy. Multiform ventricular premature complexes, couplets, and episodes of ventricular tachycardia are exceptional but not unknown.[11]

Disorders of atrial rhythm are more common than are disturbances of ventricular rhythm, even though involvement of atrial myocardium is relatively scant.[9, 10, 14–17] These observations suggest that ectopic atrial rhythms are prompted by abnormalities of specialized conduction tissues, and a similar speculation applies to the observed or reported disorders of infranodal conduction.[11]

Histological Findings. Light microscopy discloses fatty infiltration and mild fibrosis in the sinus and AV nodes, although there is little or no evidence of degeneration of the conduction fibers themselves in either of these nodes or in the His bundle.[18] However, the peripheral conduction system (Purkinje fibers) shows significant degeneration (eosinophilic, necrotic, and vascular changes with fibrosis).[18] In two light microscopic studies, fibers in the sinus node, His bundle, and proximal bundle branch were normal[10, 19]; ultrastructural data on specialized cardiac tissues are scanty and inconclusive.[12] In Duchenne dystrophy, the small intramural coronary arteries are sometimes thick-walled, with varying degrees of luminal narrowing.[10, 16, 19] The arteriopathy occasionally involves sinus nodal and AV nodal arteries,[10, 14, 19] but an association between the small vessel coronary arteriopathy and abnormalities of rhythm and conduction is at best speculative.

Mitral valve prolapse has been reported in Duchenne dystrophy. The cause is papillary muscle dysfunction (dystrophic involvement of posterolateral papillary muscle and contiguous left ventricular wall) rather than an intrinsic connective tissue abnormality of leaflets, chordae tendineae, and annulus.[9] The abnormalities in rhythm and conduction in Duchenne dystrophy are believed to be unrelated to mitral valve prolapse.

The standard scalar electrocardiogram is the simplest and most reliable tool for detecting cardiac involvement in Duchenne dystrophy (Fig. 57–2).[1, 10, 20, 21] Abnormal electrocardiograms are present even in early childhood.[21, 22] Tall right precordial R waves and increased R/S amplitude ratios together with deep Q waves in leads 1, aVL, and V_{5-6} are characteristic of the classic rapidly progressive pseudohypertrophic X-linked dystrophy of Duchenne (Fig.

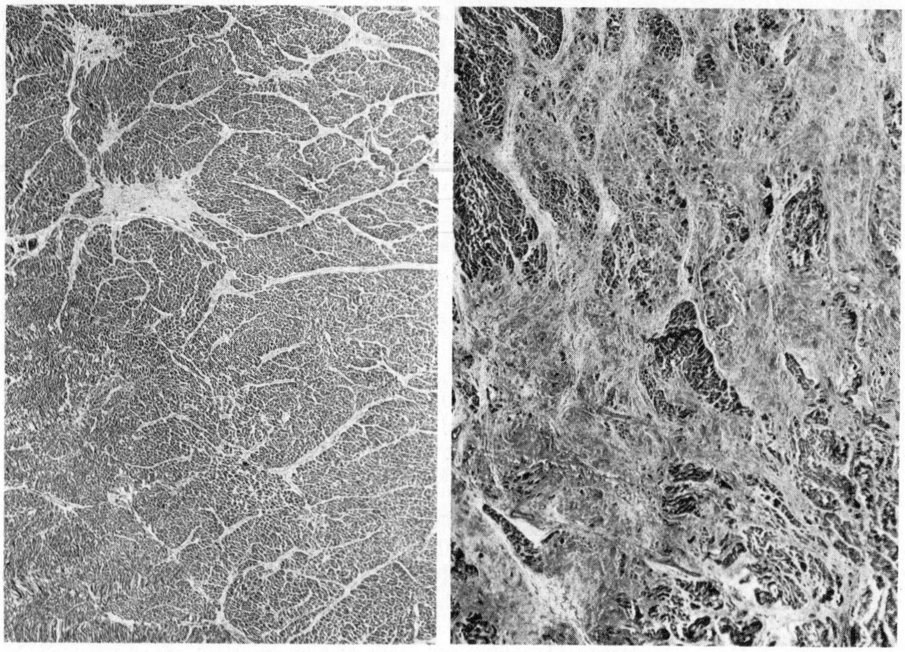

FIGURE 57–3. Photomicrographs from an 18-year-old boy who died of classic Duchenne progressive muscular dystrophy. The ventricular septum (left) shows only a few microscopic scars, whereas the posterobasal left ventricular wall (right) is extensively scarred (hematoxylin and eosin stains). (From Perloff, J. K., et al.: The distinctive electrocardiogram of Duchenne's muscular dystrophy. Am. J. Med. *42*:179, 1967.)

57–2).[1, 10, 12, 14, 23] A reduction in or a loss of electromotive force caused by myocardial dystrophy in the posterobasal left ventricular wall (anterior shift of the QRS) and contiguous lateral wall (deep Q waves in leads I, aVL, and V_{5-6}) is believed to be responsible for the characteristic electrocardiogram.[1, 10, 12] Necropsy studies have disclosed that these regions are the initial and most extensive sites of myocardial fibrosis (Fig. 57–3),[10, 12, 14] which is preceded by ultrastructural (subcellular) abnormalities.[12] Primary posterobasal involvement spreads to the epicardial third of the contiguous lateral left ventricular free wall, with progressive transmural fibrous replacement.[12, 16] There is relative sparing of the ventricular septum (Fig. 57–3) and comparatively minimal involvement of right ventricular and atrial myocardium.[10, 12, 16] Based on these observations, Duchenne dystrophy emerges as a unique form of heart disease characterized by a genetically determined predilection for specific regions of the heart—the posterobasal and lateral left ventricular walls.[1, 10, 12, 23]

POSITRON EMISSION TOMOGRAPHY. Recent investigations have sought to ascertain whether regional metabolic, perfusion, or wall motion abnormalities were present during life in patients with Duchenne dystrophy.[2, 24] To determine whether segmental abnormalities of the left ventricular wall were present in living subjects, noninvasive methods, including positron emission computed tomography (see p. 1210) using radioactive tracers for metabolism, supplemented by thallium-201 perfusion scans, gated equilibrium radionuclide angiography, and two-dimensional echocardiography, were required.[2, 24] Accelerated exogenous glucose (^{18}F fluorodeoxyglucose) utilization in the posterobasal and contiguous lateral left ventricular walls (Fig. 57–4) provided evidence of a regional myocardial metabolic abnormality (p. 338).[2] $^{13}NH_3$ activity was reduced in segments in which the use of exogenous glucose was accelerated (Fig. 57–4). These sites corresponded to those of primary dystrophic replacement found at necropsy.[10, 12, 14, 15]

The observed regional increases in ^{18}F fluorodeoxyglucose concentrations were believed to indicate segmental alterations in membrane permeability, an increase in the rate of phosphorylation due to the abnormality in adenyl cyclase identified in skeletal muscle,[25, 26] or a compensatory increase in glycolysis in response to a decline in fatty acid oxidation.[2] Regional decreases in $^{13}NH_3$ activity in Duchenne dystrophy (Fig. 57–4) could reflect a metabolic abnormality, a regional decrease in flow, or both these causes.[2]

Early in the natural history (i.e., in very young patients), segmental reductions in $^{13}NH_3$ probably reflect altered regional myocardial metabolic uptake and trapping of the isotope.[2] If these alterations in the myocardium are analogous to those in skeletal muscle in Duchenne dystrophy, a longer diffusion distance of an altered ionic milieu could decrease the extraction fractions of $^{13}NH_3$.[2] Regional depletion of the pool of glutamic acid, which binds the tracer in tissue, might also

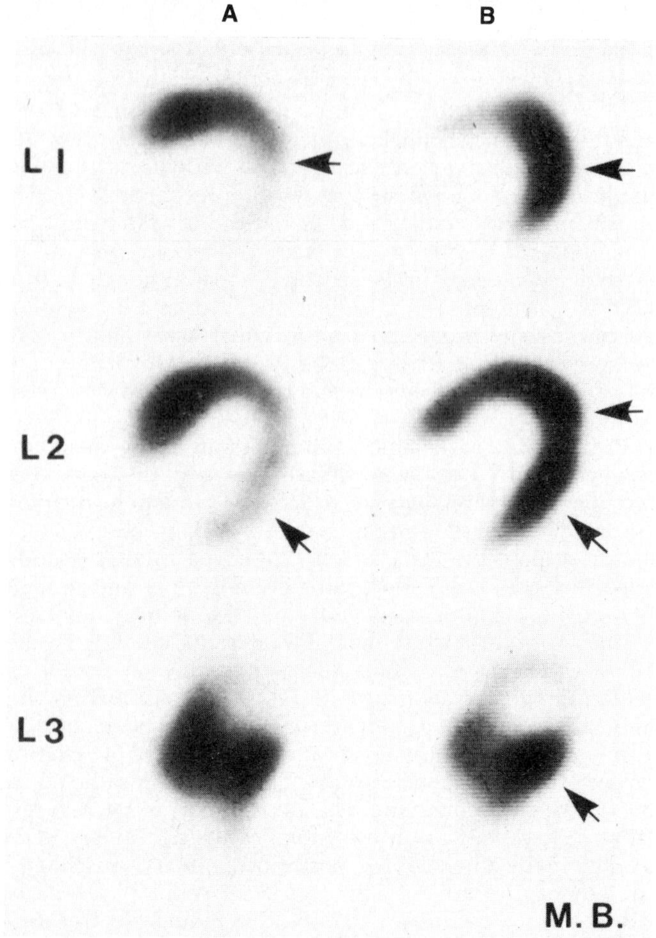

FIGURE 57–4. Regional myocardial uptake of $^{13}NH_3$ (*A*) and ^{18}F fluorodeoxyglucose (*B*) visualized in three contiguous positron CT images of left ventricular myocardium in a 24-year-old man with classic Duchenne dystrophy. There is a segmental decrease in $^{13}NH_3$ activity in the posterolateral wall (arrows) with a discordant increase in ^{18}F fluorodeoxyglucose concentration in the same region (arrows). This patient had a moderate posterolateral thallium-201 defect, posterolateral akinesis on technetium-99m radionuclide imaging, and a left ventricular ejection fraction of 46 per cent. (From Perloff, J. K., et al.: Alterations in regional myocardial metabolism, perfusion and wall motion in Duchenne muscular dystrophy studied by radionuclide imaging. Circulation 69:33, 1984, by permission of The American Heart Association, Inc.)

contribute to a segmental reduction in $^{13}NH_3$.[2] However, regional perfusion defects sometimes occur in older patients with Duchenne dystrophy, as demonstrated by thallium scintigraphy. In these late stages of the disease, decreased perfusion might contribute to segmental reductions in $^{13}NH_3$ activity.[2] It is likely that the mechanism(s) governing a regional reduction in myocardial blood flow relate(s) to a decrease in the number of myofibers per unit mass (fibrous replacement) and/or to an increase in the number of intrinsically injured but viable posterobasal and lateral left ventricular myocardial cells that require less oxygen and, accordingly, less flow.[2] Necropsy studies (light microscopy) identified no luminal narrowing of either extramural or intramural coronary arteries in the involved segments.[2, 10]

It has been hypothesized that the regional myocardial abnormalities of both ^{18}F fluorodeoxyglucose and $^{13}NH_3$ activity represent secondary metabolic alterations initiated through a basic defect in the cardiac plasma cell membrane.[2] Current evidence—both ultrastructural and biochemical—supports the proposition that the fundamental structural and biochemical abnormalities in Duchenne dystrophy reside in plasma cell membranes, not only in those of striated (skeletal and cardiac) muscle fibers but also in those of red blood cells and probably also of fibroblasts.[27–31] In addition to the ultrastructural abnormalities, it has been argued that, as in other genetic diseases, there must be a primary biochemical fault.[31]

If a reduction in or loss of posterolateral left ventricular electrical forces is in fact the cause of the distinctive electrocardiogram in Duchenne dystrophy,[1, 10, 12] this loss of forces does not require transmural replacement of myocardium by inert connective tissue. Increased ^{18}F fluorodeoxyglucose concentrations in these areas together with normal regional wall motion are consistent with either the presence of abnormal but viable (metabolically active) contracting myofibers or the preservation of a sufficient population of normal myofibers.[2]

Enzymes of skeletal muscle are copiously released into the plasma in Duchenne dystrophy. It was hoped that distinctive profiles of an isozyme, such as MB creatine phosphokinase (CPK), might be used to identify active myocardial dystrophy, but the isozyme originates in dystrophic skeletal muscle and not in cardiac muscle, thus compromising the specificity of the determination.[32, 33] CPK quantification has been established as a valuable means of identifying carrier females in families with Duchenne dystrophy.[34, 35] Tightly linked genetic markers for the Duchenne dystrophy gene permit carrier detection with 98 per cent accuracy.[36] Carrier females sometimes manifest occult or overt muscle weakness and mild calf pseudohypertrophy[34, 37] in addition to electrocardiographic evidence of cardiac involvement.[34, 35, 38–40] Electrocardiograms in carrier females differ significantly from those of normal adult women, with R/S ratios larger in leads V_{1-2} in the carrier group.[35, 38] Cardiac involvement in female carriers is occasionally overtly expressed as dilated cardiomyopathy.[38, 40]

LATE-ONSET, SLOWLY PROGRESSIVE X-LINKED (BECKER) DYSTROPHY. A type of X-linked recessive muscular dystrophy that sometimes closely resembles Duchenne dystrophy was described by Becker.[5, 6a, 41–43, 43a] The onset of Becker dystrophy is comparatively late, however, and survival to middle age is not uncommon (Fig. 57–5).[5] Becker dystrophy has also been called "benign sex-linked muscular dystrophy,"[42–44] a designation more appropriate for the skeletal muscle disease than for the heart.[1, 45, 46] The incidence of cardiac involvement increases progressively after adolescence but is seldom severe before the third decade, beyond which the frequency reaches 80 per cent.[47] Such patients not only have cardiomyopathy but could very well succumb to it (Fig. 57–6).[1, 47] The type of cardiac involvement differs fundamentally from that in Duchenne dystrophy.[1, 48] All four chambers are involved, and the ventricles dilate and fail (Fig. 57–6). There is also involvement of the His bundle and of infranodal conduction expressing itself clinically as fascicular block and as complete heart block (Fig. 57–6). When slowly progressive X-linked dystrophy selectively involves the humeral muscles with comparatively little pelvic or femoral disease and little or no pseudohypertrophy, the cardiac manifestations consist chiefly of atrial arrhythmias and AV block.[49]

LIMB-GIRDLE DYSTROPHY OF ERB. Erb limb-girdle muscular dystrophy is characterized by progressive weakness of the hips and shoulders and is usually inherited as an autosomal recessive trait in segregated populations in which relatives intermarry.[5] Transitional or borderline manifestations make the designation ill-defined and imprecise.[5] In the commonest variety, onset is during the second or third decade, with the illness beginning as weakness of the hips accompanied by or soon followed by shoulder weakness. Two decades may elapse before walking becomes difficult, if not impossible; however, even when the patient is confined to a wheelchair, skeletal deformities are infrequent.[5] Calf pseudohypertrophy occurs but is relatively late in onset and mild to moderate in degree (Fig. 57–7).[50] Because categorization of limb-girdle dystrophy has been poorly defined, conclusions regarding the type and prevalence of heart disease cannot be drawn with confidence. Generally speaking, cardiac involvement is relatively infrequent and seldom severe, expressing itself as (1) disturbance in rhythm and conduction, namely, bradycardia ("sick" sinoatrial node) and tachycardia (atrial

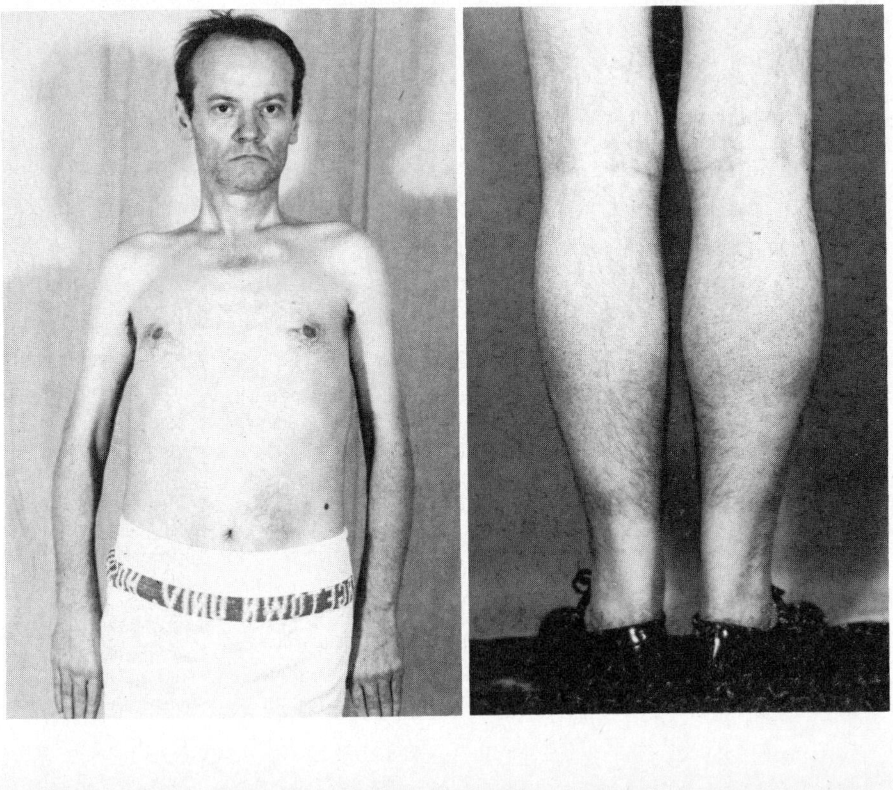

FIGURE 57–5. A 40-year-old man believed to have late-onset, slowly progressive Becker dystrophy. He died because of cardiomyopathy and complete heart block. Dystrophy of shoulder girdle, arms, pelvic girdle, and proximal leg muscle is seen, with mild asymmetrical pseudohypertrophy of the calves. (From Perloff, J. K., et al.: The cardiomyopathy of progressive muscular dystrophy. Circulation *33*:625, 1966, by permission of The American Heart Association, Inc.)

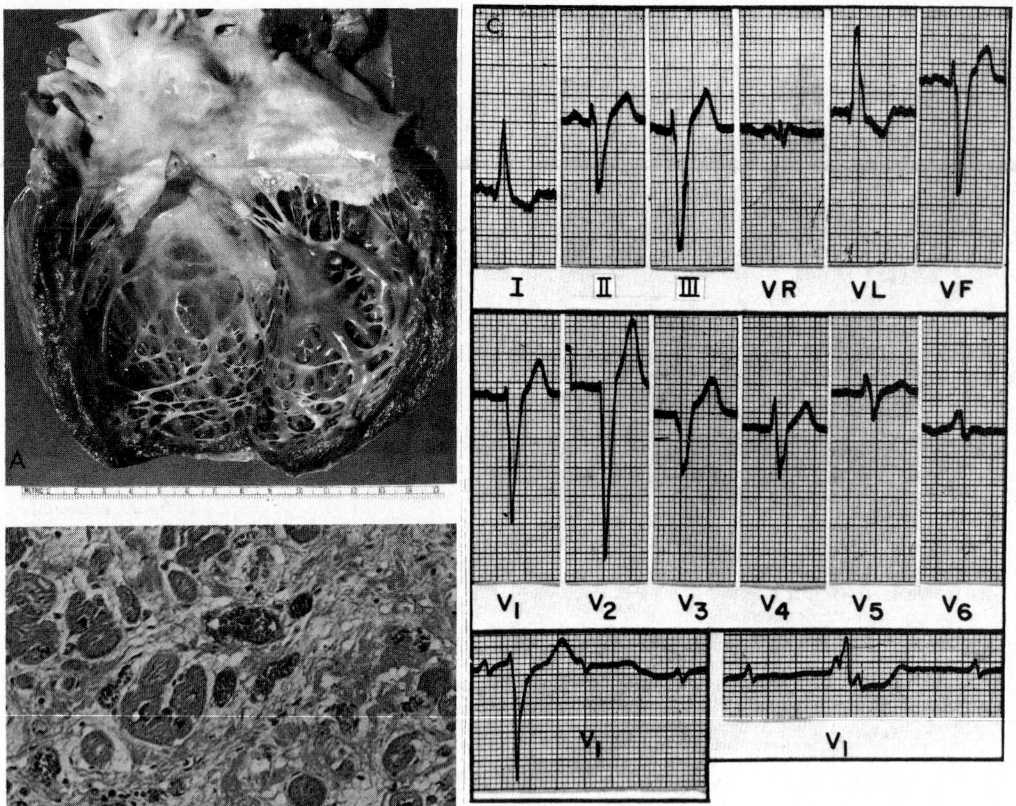

FIGURE 57–6. Gross and microscopic cardiac pathological specimens and the electrocardiogram from a 45-year-old man with late-onset, slowly progressive Becker muscular dystrophy. *A,* Dilated, flabby left ventricle with focal endocardial thickening. The left atrium is also dilated. *B,* Microscopic section from the left ventricle shows marked confluent scarring with variations in fiber size; there was no significant coronary artery disease. *C,* Electrocardiogram recorded at age 40 years. The 12-lead tracing shows left-axis deviation, a QRS of 0.14 sec, small q waves in leads I and aVL and loss of R-wave amplitude in leads V_2 and V_3. The lower tracings, taken 4 years later (a year before death), show complete heart block with a variable QRS configuration. (From Perloff, J. K., et al.: The cardiomyopathy of progressive muscular dystrophy. Circulation *33*:625, 1966, by permission of The American Heart Association, Inc.)

flutter); (2) first-degree heart block (abnormal AV node conduction); and (3) abnormalities of infranodal conduction characterized by bundle branch block, QRS prolongation, and complete heart block.[51, 52] In sporadic cases diagnosed as limb-girdle dystrophy, disorders of both the cardiac conduction system *and* cardiac muscle (cardiomyopathy) are noted.[53]

FACIOSCAPULOHUMERAL DYSTROPHY (LANDOUZY-DÉJÉRINE). Facioscapulohumeral dystrophy, inherited as an autosomal dominant trait, is variable in its clinical expression, even within a single family.[5] Incidence is between 3 and 10 cases per million.[5] The disease typically becomes overt at the end of the first decade or the beginning of the second. Facial weakness may be signaled initially by no more than an inability to whistle or drink through a straw. More distinctive and more troublesome is the inability to close the eyes, even during sleep. The face ultimately becomes smooth and the forehead unlined; loss of the normal upward curvature of the lower lip creates a pouting appearance. The only marks on an otherwise expressionless face are the dimples on either side of the angles of the mouth (Fig. 57–8*A*). Concurrently, the muscles of the arms and shoulders (scapulohumeral) usually become involved, and winging of the scapulae becomes apparent (Fig. 57–8*B*).

One of the most intriguing aspects of facioscapulohumeral dystrophy is the cardiac involvement—i.e., permanent paralysis of the atria (atrial standstill).[54–56] The first documented case of atrial paralysis was in a patient with facioscapulohumeral dystrophy, although partial or permanent atrial standstill occurs sporadically as an isolated disorder generally in adults, rarely in children, and occasionally in families.[57–60] Criteria for the diagnosis of atrial paralysis include absence of P waves on scalar, esophageal, and intracardiac electrocardiograms; lack of response to direct (intracardiac) electrical or mechanical stimulation of the atria; absence of *a* waves in the jugular venous and right atrial pressure pulses; a supraventricular QRS; and

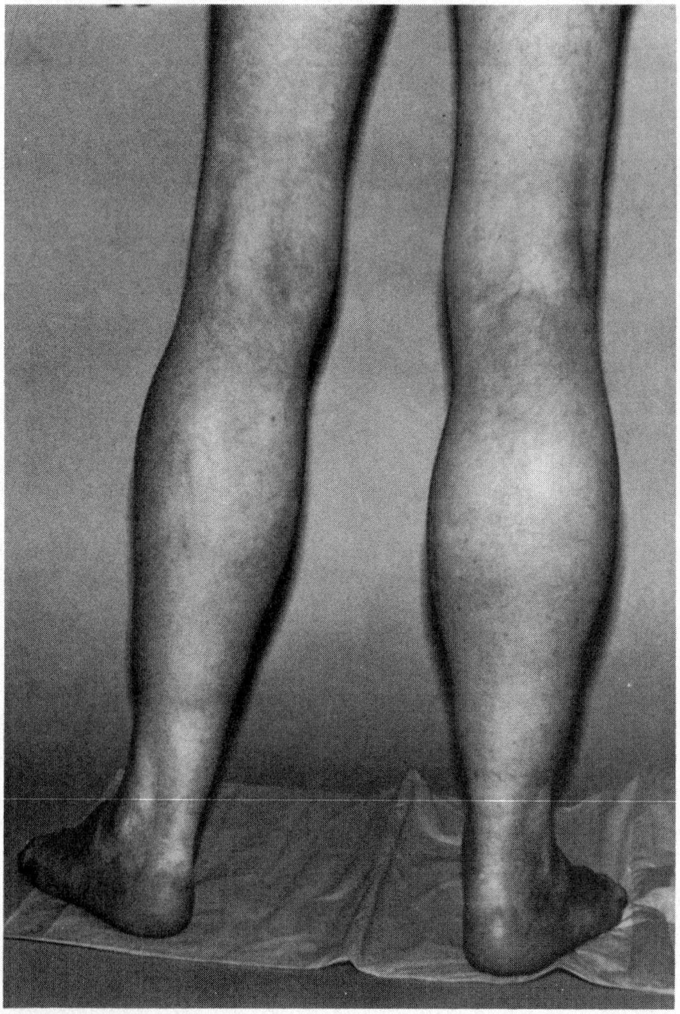

FIGURE 57–7. Asymmetrical calf pseudohypertrophy in a 52-year-old man with Erb dystrophy.

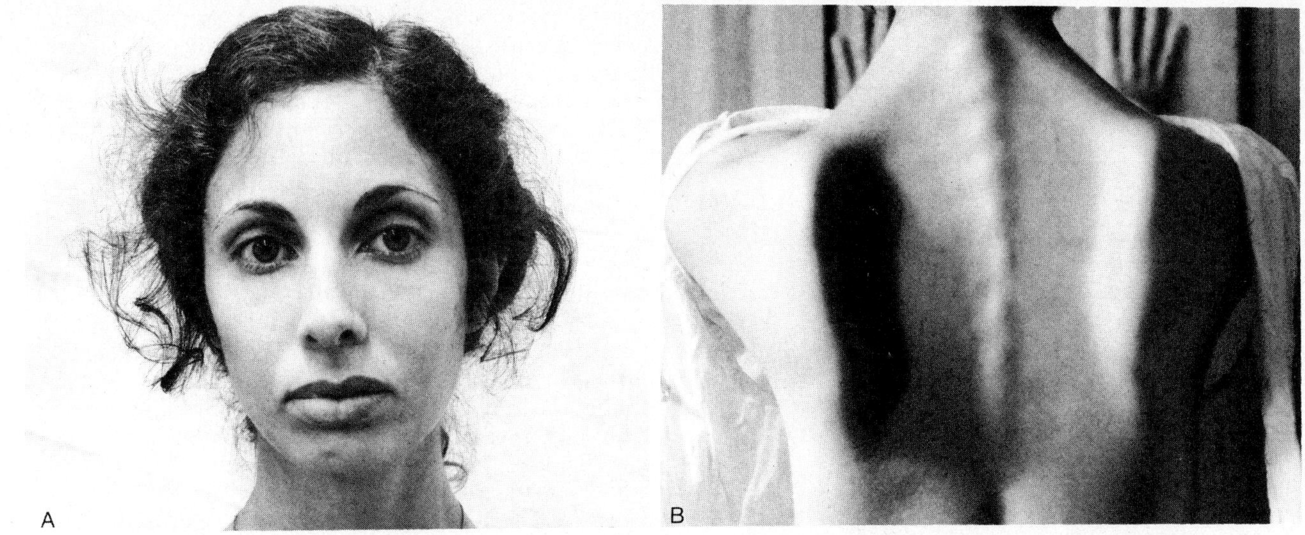

FIGURE 57–8. Facioscapulohumeral muscular dystrophy in 32-year-old woman. *A,* The face is in repose (myopathic), but dimples at the corners of the mouth result in an "enigmatic smile." *B,* Typical winging of the scapulae.

immobility of the atria on fluoroscopy or two-dimensional echocardiography.[59] Ultimately, the entire atrial myocardium becomes inexcitable; however, prior to this, atrial standstill appears to be regional, with certain focal areas inert while others are subject to enhanced atrial activity (atrial tachycardia or flutter).[58, 60, 61] In adults with facioscapulohumeral dystrophy and sinus rhythm studied electrophysiologically, atrial flutter or fibrillation was consistently inducible.[62]

EMERY-DREIFUSS DISEASE. Disorders grouped under this eponym are almost all X-linked recessive, occasionally autosomal dominant,[63] and are characterized by slowly progressive weakness of humeral and/or scapular muscles together with involvement of peroneal muscles.[64–69] The face is spared, in contrast to facioscapulohumeral dystrophy, which *scapulohumeral peroneal dystrophy* otherwise resembles. Cardiac involvement is common and, as in facioscapulohumeral dystrophy, takes the form of permanent atrial paralysis, fibrillation, or flutter; however, in contrast to facioscapulohumeral dystrophy, infranodal conduction defects occur, with slow junctional rhythm or complete AV block.[63, 65, 68, 69] It is the cardiac involvement, not the systemic myopathy, that places the patient at risk. In addition to defects in rhythm and conduction, marked myocardial fibrosis has been described at necropsy[67] or on myocardial biopsy.[69]

MYOTONIC MUSCULAR DYSTROPHY

Myotonic muscular dystrophy (*Streinert disease*) is inherited as an autosomal dominant with a prevalence estimated at between 3 and 5 per 100,000 population, making it a relatively common neuromuscular disorder.[5] Symptoms typically go unnoticed until adolescence or early adulthood, although examination in the first decade may disclose myotonia and a child with the characteristic long face and slightly nasal voice. A consistent and early feature is weakness of the flexor muscles of the neck with atrophy of the sternocleidomastoid muscles, not uncommonly progressing to virtual disappearance. The phenotype of the adult with myotonic dystrophy is characteristic.[5, 70] The presence of myotonia (delayed relaxation after contraction) is provoked by voluntary, mechanical, or electrical stimulation of muscles of the hands, forearms, tongue, and jaw. The myotonic response is best elicited by tapping the thenar eminence (percussion myotonia), especially after the patient rapidly opens and closes the fist. Myotonic dystrophy is a systemic disease with important nonmyotonic/nonmyopathic features, including cataracts, gonadal

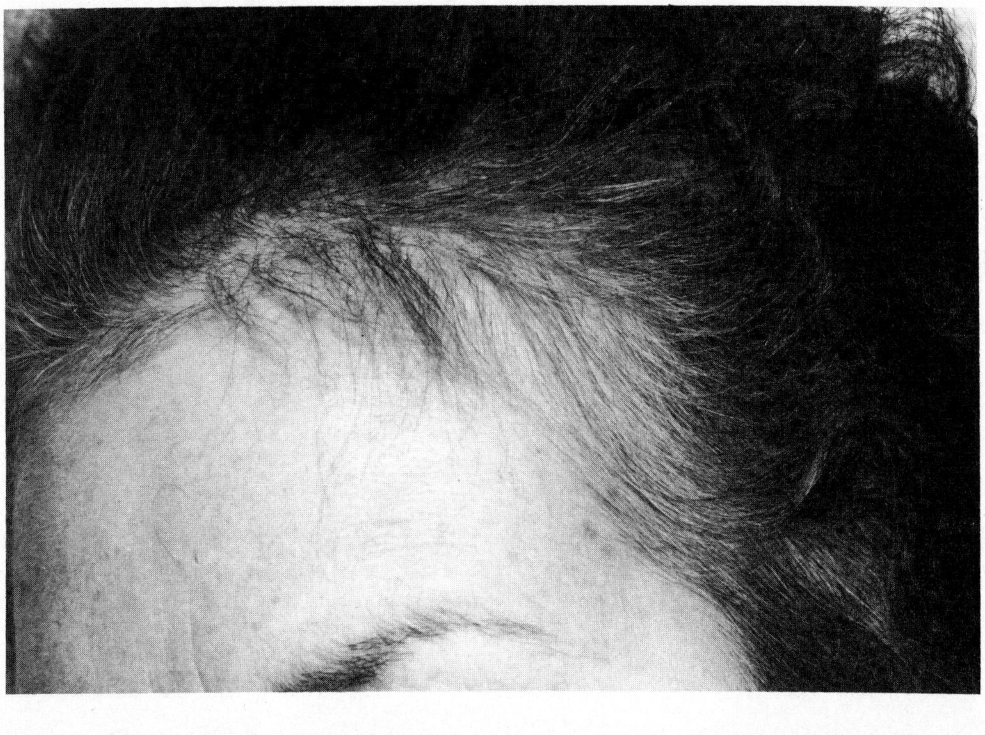

FIGURE 57–9. Frontal baldness and premature graying of the hair in a 32-year-old woman with myotonic muscular dystrophy.

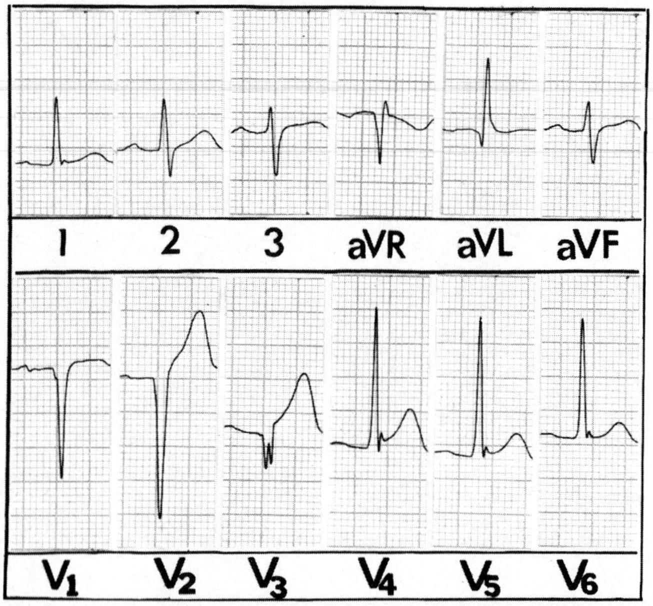

FIGURE 57–10. Electrocardiogram from a 38-year-old man with myotonic muscular dystrophy. Prominent QS deformities are present in leads V_{1-3}. The P-R interval is 0.21 second and the frontal plane QRS axis is horizontal. (From Perloff, J. K., et al.: Cardiac involvement in myotonic muscular dystrophy [Steinert's disease]: A prospective study of 25 patients. Am. J. Cardiol. *54*:1074, 1984.)

atrophy, frontal baldness or thinning of the hair (Fig. 57–9), and disease of muscles of the upper gastrointestinal tract.[70, 71]

Clinically important cardiac manifestations reside in specialized tissues rather than in myocardium.[3, 72, 73] Involvement is relatively specific, primarily assigned to the His-Purkinje system. Involvement of cardiac muscle, generally occult, takes the form of dystrophy rather than myotonia and is not selective, appearing with approximately equal distribution in all four chambers.[3] Myocardial dystrophy may be responsible for atrial and ventricular arrhythmias including sinus bradycardia, premature atrial beats, atrial flutter, atrial fibrillation, premature ventricular beats, and ventricular tachycardia.[74–76] Preferential selection of the His-Purkinje system (80 per cent of patients) is reflected in intraventricular conduction defects, prolongation of the H-V interval and the effective refractory period of the right bundle branch, the development of right bundle branch block, or some other abnormal response to atrial pacing or extrastimuli.[3] The most common electrocardiographic abnormalities—prolongation of the P-R interval, left anterior fascicular block, increased QRS duration—reflect His-Purkinje disease that can progress rapidly, although neither the scalar electrocardiogram nor a single H-V interval will predict the rate of progression.[77] His-Purkinje disease can culminate in fatal Stokes-Adams episodes unless anticipated and treated by pacemaker insertion.[75, 78–80] Although sudden death caused by AV block is relatively rare, it is the gravest cardiac threat in myotonic dystrophy.

The myocardium is rarely involved extensively enough to cause clinically overt signs or symptoms.[3] Frank ventricular failure has been reported but only sporadically.[80, 81] The electrocardiogram is a sensitive determinant of involvement of specialized cardiac tissues but not of myocardium. Nevertheless, abnormal Q waves with normal coronary arteries[82] indicate regional myocardial dystrophy (Fig. 57–10). Findings on light microscopy of the myocardium vary from few or no changes to focal or diffuse fatty infiltration and fibrosis in all four cardiac chambers.[75, 78–80, 83–85] Apart from abnormalities of initial forces in the electrocardiogram, clinical involvement of the myocardium is generally occult except as assessed by radionuclide angiography during exercise (Fig. 57–11).[3, 86]

Myotonia in skeletal muscle reflects the inability of the muscle cell membrane to reestablish its resting membrane potential quickly after contraction. Whether myotonia occurs in cardiac muscle is unproven but unlikely, since repeated, obligatory contractions would probably not recur with impunity if cardiac muscle were prone to mechanically induced myotonia.[3]

Because myotonic dystrophy is genetically transmitted, a primary biochemical defect has been proposed, with

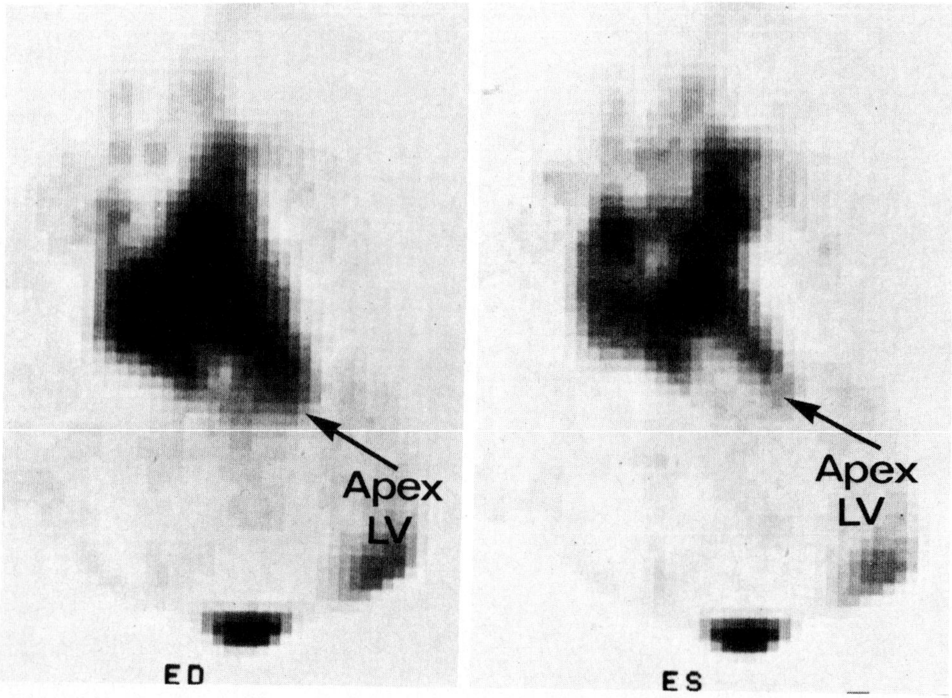

FIGURE 57–11. Technetium-99m radionuclide angiocardiogram (anterior projection) from a 27-year-old woman with myotonic muscular dystrophy. Apical hypokinesis is marked (arrows). Left ventricular (LV) size was normal, and the ejection fraction at rest was 56 per cent. With exercise, the apical hypokinesis decreased, but the ejection fraction remained virtually unchanged (59 per cent). ED = end diastole; ES = end systole. (From Perloff, J. K., et al.: Cardiac involvement in myotonic muscular dystrophy [Steinert's disease]: A prospective study of 25 patients. Am. J. Cardiol. *54*:1074, 1984.)

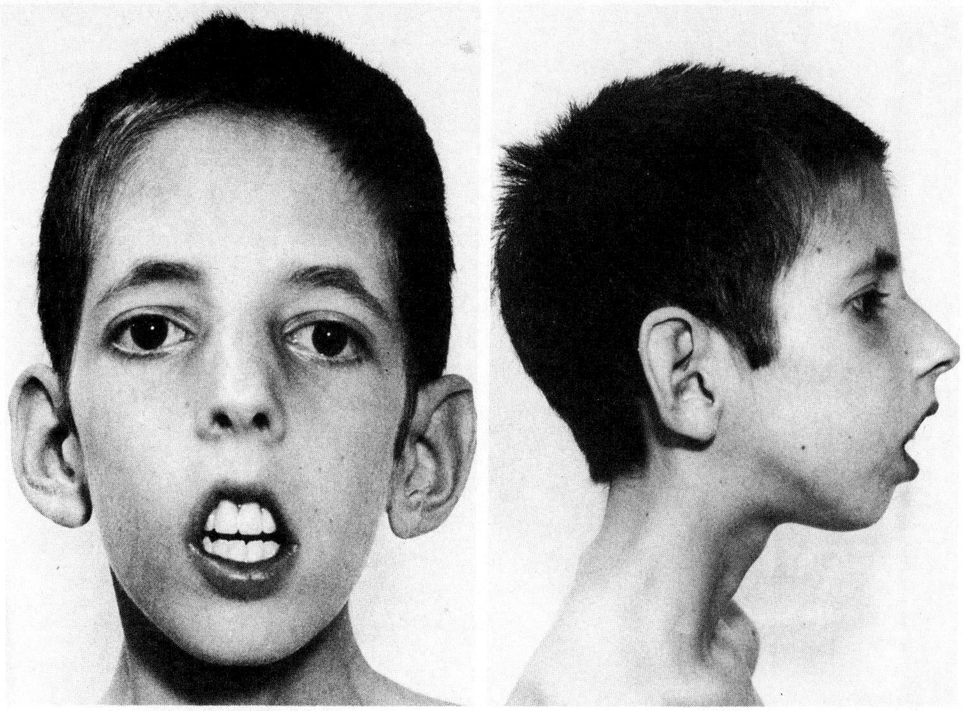

FIGURE 57–12. Typical elongated face of an 11-year-old boy with the childhood form of myotonic muscular dystrophy. The child is mentally retarded, and his upper lip shows the characteristic "cupid's bow." The echocardiogram revealed dilated cardiomyopathy.

complete expression of the gene toward striated muscle tissue, whether skeletal or cardiac.[3] Because specialized cardiac tissues and myocardium have close if not identical embryological origins, it is not surprising that the genetic marker affects both. Cardiac involvement is therefore an integral part of myotonic dystrophy with a genetic marker targeting the infranodal conduction system, the sinus node to a lesser extent, and still less specifically the myocardium.[3, 86a]

An important variation from the above pattern is seen in the offspring of mothers with myotonic dystrophy.[5, 87] The infant disorder expresses itself as extreme hypotonia and facial paralysis with no evidence of myotonia, at least initially. Affected children have characteristic facies with the upper lip forming a cupid's bow (Fig. 57–12). Cardiac involvement, although not studied systematically, appears to differ fundamentally from that in the adult form of the disease. The chief expression is dilated cardiomyopathy.[87]

Myotonia congenita (Thomsen's disease) and *paramyotonia congenita* must be distinguished from myotonic muscular dystrophy. Thomsen's disease is characterized by myotonia but not dystrophy.[87] In fact, the skeletal muscles are well developed, even hypertrophied.[5, 87] Because the natural history of Thomsen's disease is benign, longevity permits secure conclusions regarding cardiac involvement, which is conspicuously absent. In a single case of myotonia congenita, cardiac conduction abnormalities similar to those found in myotonic dystrophy have been reported.[88] *Para*myotonia congenita is an uncommon to rare autosomal dominant disorder characterized by a prolonged myotonic reaction to cold.[5, 87, 89, 90] Dystrophy of skeletal muscle is absent, and cardiac involvement is unknown.

FRIEDREICH'S ATAXIA

For descriptive purposes, the hereditary ataxias are divided into (1) hereditary spinocerebellar ataxia of Friedreich, (2) hereditary ataxia with muscular atrophy (Roussy-Lévy syndrome), (3) hereditary spinocerebellar ataxia, and (4) olivopontocerebellar atrophy.[91] Despite a century of lively interest, Friedreich's ataxia has resisted precise clinical and biochemical definition, and there is still disagreement on where this spinocerebellar degenerative disease fits into the complex framework of the hereditary ataxias.[91–94] Friedreich's ataxia, inherited as an autosomal recessive trait, is characterized clinically by ataxia of the limbs and trunk, absence of tendon reflexes, extensor plantar responses, and loss of proprioceptive sensations in the limbs.[93] There are no remissions; instead, ataxia of gait and muscle weakness progress relentlessly, affecting first the lower limbs and then all four extremities. Pes cavus (Friedreich's foot) (Fig. 57–13) and kyphoscoliosis (Fig. 57–14) develop within a few years of onset. It is important to underscore that *this disorder is essentially neurological rather than myopathic.*[95]

When strict neurological and genetic criteria were used to identify a clinically homogeneous group of patients with Friedreich's ataxia, the incidence of cardiac involvement exceeded 90 per cent.[4, 96–101, 101a] Progressively severe ataxia occurs long before clinically overt heart disease, and there is no relationship between the degrees of neurological and of cardiac involvement.[4] Nevertheless, cardiac disease is often the cause of death.[4, 102, 102a] There is reason to believe that phenotypically identical Friedreich patients are not biochemically homogeneous, so the cardiac expressions might be expected to vary. This in fact proved to be the case in a prospective study of 75 patients.[4] Cardiac involve-

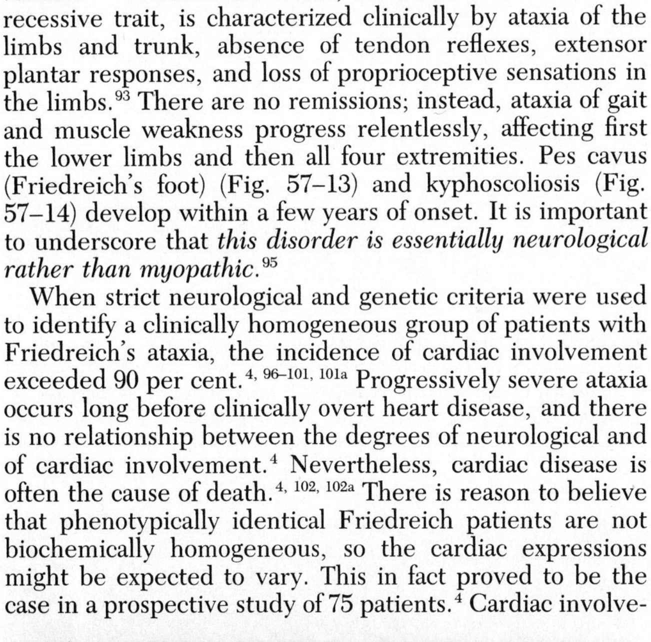

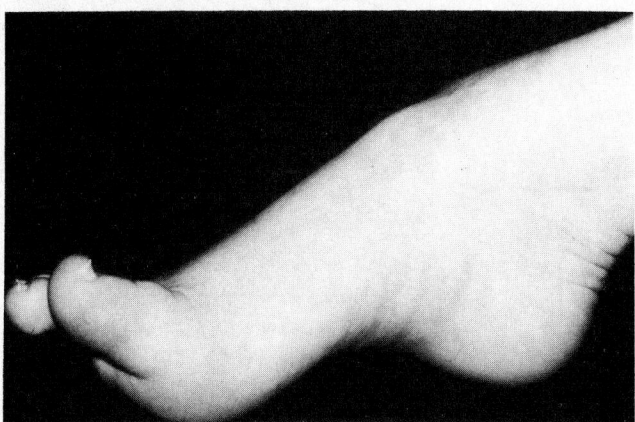

FIGURE 57–13. Pes cavus with hammer toe (Friedreich's foot).

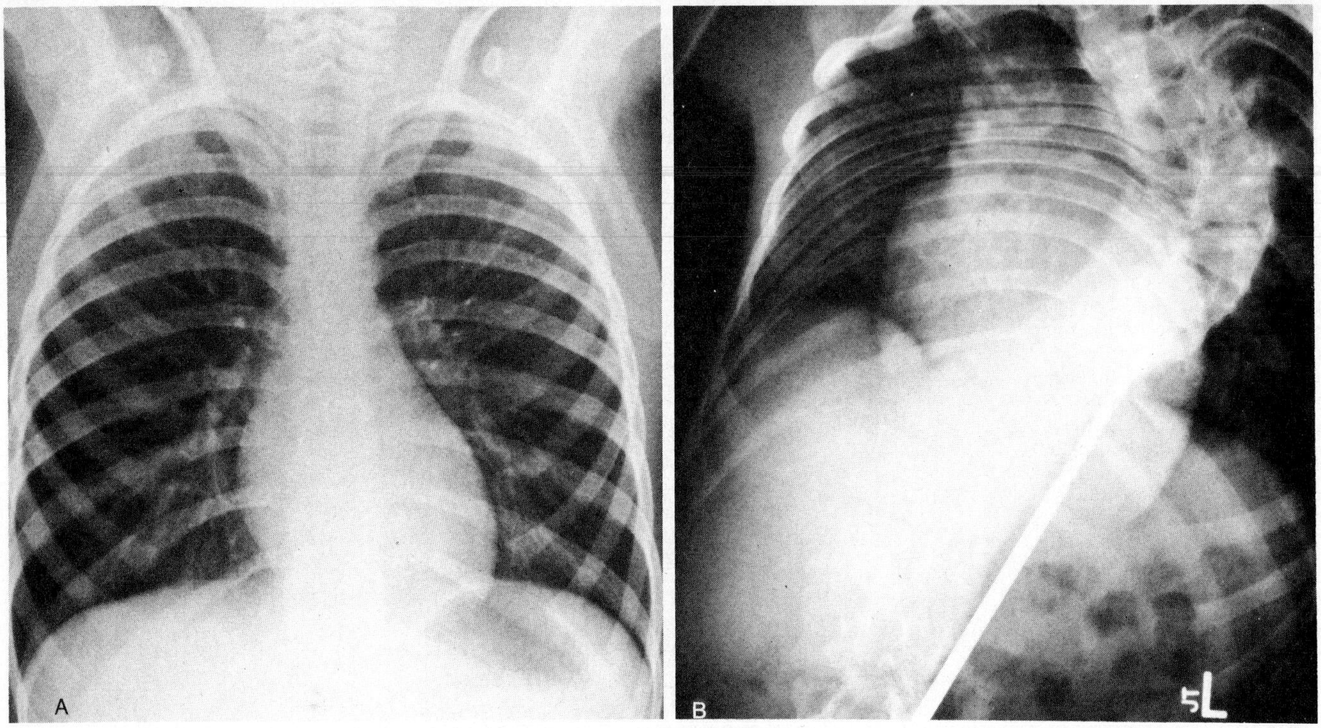

FIGURE 57–14. *A,* Normal chest x-ray in a 6-year-old boy with Friedreich's ataxia. *B,* X-ray at age 9 years. Severe scoliosis has developed. Note the Harrington rod.

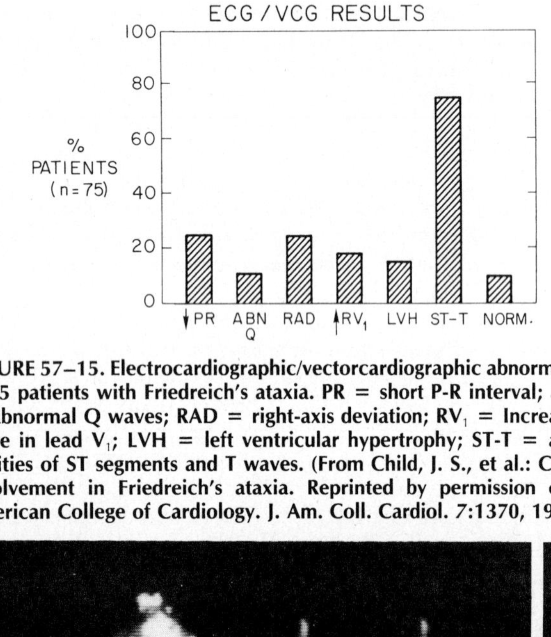

FIGURE 57–15. Electrocardiographic/vectorcardiographic abnormalities in 75 patients with Friedreich's ataxia. PR = short P-R interval; abn Q = abnormal Q waves; RAD = right-axis deviation; RV_1 = Increased R wave in lead V_1; LVH = left ventricular hypertrophy; ST-T = abnormalities of ST segments and T waves. (From Child, J. S., et al.: Cardiac involvement in Friedreich's ataxia. Reprinted by permission of the American College of Cardiology. J. Am. Coll. Cardiol. *7*:1370, 1986.)

ment, usually occult and asymptomatic, is virtually the rule.[102a, 102b] The combination of scalar electrocardiography (Fig. 57–15) and echocardiography detected one or more abnormalities in 95 per cent of study patients.[4] Hypertrophic cardiomyopathy occurred in just under 20 per cent of patients, somewhat less frequently than in previous reports.[98, 100, 103] Concentric (Fig. 57–16) and asymmetrical hypertrophy were equally prevalent. These two varieties of hypertrophy seemingly represent parts of a continuum. Left ventricular outflow gradients have been reported in some cases with disproportionate septal thickness[100] but not in others.[98] However, septal cellular disarray—the histological hallmark of genetic hypertrophic cardiomyopathy (p. 1420)—has been absent or only focal in necropsy studies of Friedreich's ataxia.[96, 99, 102, 104, 105] This observation may explain why the potentially malignant ventricular arrhythmias common in genetic hypertrophic cardiomyopathy are essentially unknown in Friedreich's ataxia.

Globally hypofunctional left ventricles (dilated or not)

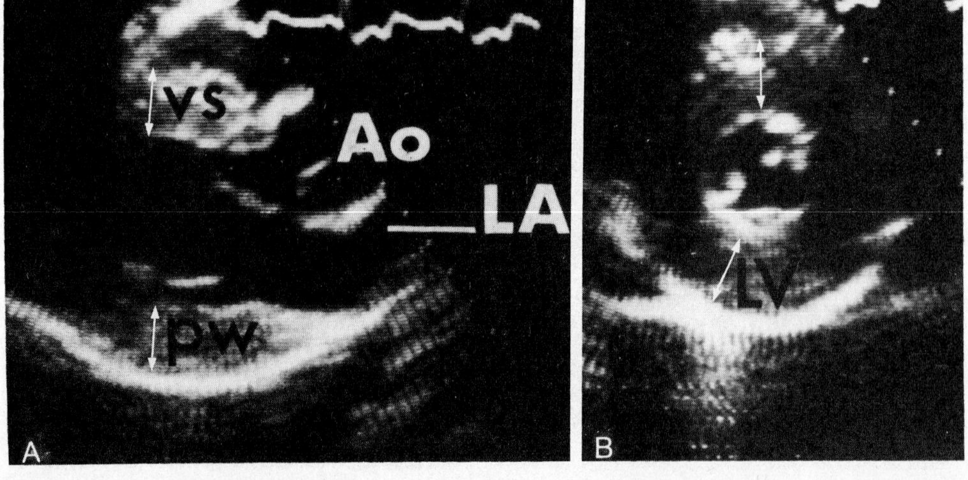

FIGURE 57–16. Two-dimensional echocardiographic parasternal long-axis view (*A*) and short-axis view (*B*) in a 16-year-old boy with Friedreich's ataxia and concentric left ventricular hypertrophy. At age 13 years, the echocardiogram was normal. Ao = aorta; LA = left atrium; LV = left ventricle; PW = posterior wall; VS = ventricular septum. (From Child, J. S., et al.: Cardiac involvement in Friedreich's ataxia. Reprinted by permission of the American College of Cardiology. J. Am. Coll. Cardiol. *7*:1370, 1986.)

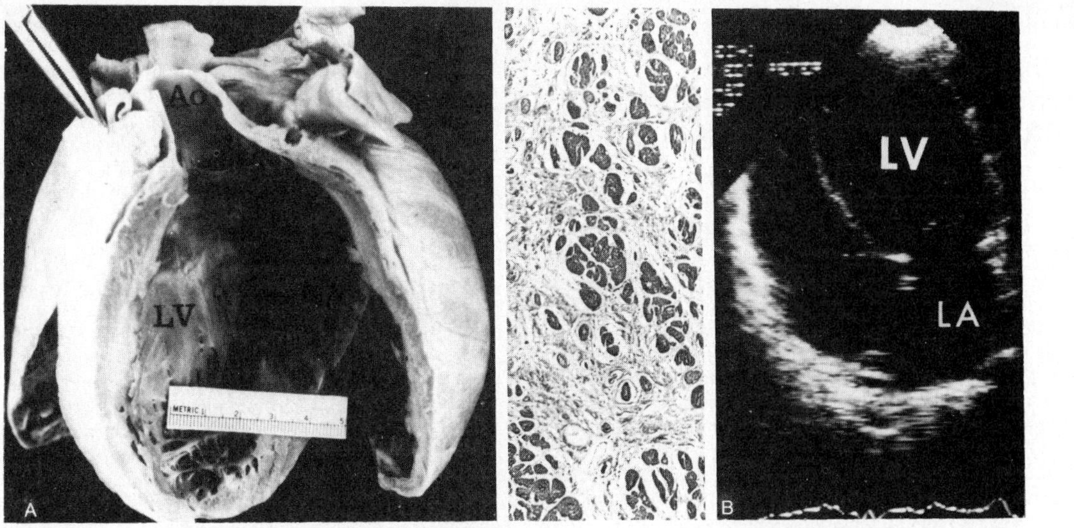

FIGURE 57–17. *A,* Gross and histological specimens from a 17-year-old boy with Friedreich's ataxia whose echocardiogram progressed from normal at age 13 years to a minimally dilated, hypocontractile left ventricle 3 to 4 years later. The gross specimen shows a mildly dilated left ventricle with normal wall thickness; the walls were flabby. The microscopic section from the left ventricular free wall shows marked connective tissue replacement. Although specifically sought, small-vessel coronary artery disease was not identified. *B,* Two-dimensional echocardiogram (apical window) showing the mildly dilated, thin-walled left ventricle (LV). LA = left atrium. (From Childs, J. S., et al.: Cardiac involvement in Friedreich's ataxia. Reprinted by permission of the American College of Cardiology. J. Am. Coll. Cardiol. *7*:1370, 1986.)

were identified in 7 per cent of patients studied prospectively and solely on the basis of the clinical diagnosis of Friedreich's ataxia, not because of suspected cardiac involvement (Fig. 57–17).[4] There is reason to believe that global left ventricular hypokinesis is distinct from the hypertrophic cardiomyopathy of Friedreich's ataxia[98] and represents a fundamentally different type of cardiac involvement, designated "dystrophic." This view is supported by the flabby myocardium with normal wall thickness in necropsy cases that exhibited premortem progression on echocardiography from normal to mildly dilated, globally hypofunctional left ventricles with normal wall thickness (Fig. 57–17).[4] "Minimally dilated cardiomyopathy"[106] in Friedreich's ataxia appears to represent an uncommon late stage of the prevalent regional myocardium involvement believed to be reflected in the abnormalities of initial forces on electrocardiograms and vectorcardiograms (Fig. 57–18).[4, 101]

Intimal proliferation in small intramural coronary arteries in Friedreich's ataxia[98, 107] cannot confidently be related to either regional or global myocardial dystrophy.[102] Whether there is a connection between diabetes mellitus in Friedreich's ataxia[95] and either diabetic coronary artery disease or the noncoronary interstitial disease of diabetes is speculative. In any event, the incidence of regional myocardial involvement detected on ECG (Fig. 57–18) far exceeds the incidence of clinical diabetes.[4]

In summary, there appear to be two distinct types of cardiac involvement in Friedreich's ataxia: (1) a common segmental "dystrophic" form, manifested by deformities of the initial forces on ECG, without detectable echocardiographic abnormalities of wall motion but occasionally by extension throughout the left ventricle, with global hypokinesis and reduced QRS voltage; and (2) a "hypertrophic" form, represented by symmetrical or asymmetrical left ventricular hypertrophy with normal cavity size and function.

Why a nonmyopathic spinocerebellar-corticospinal disorder is accompanied by two widely disparate types of cardiac involvement is unknown. One important implication is that the genetic determinant—ultimately biochemical—differs among phenotypically similar patients.[108, 109] The relationship between the spinocerebellar-corticospinal disorder and an increase in ventricular mass—hypertrophic cardiomyopathy—is also an enigma. A unifying thread may be abnormal catecholamine metabolism, the "catecholamine hypothesis," which has been a focus of lively interest in the pathogenesis of genetic hypertrophic cardiomyopathy.[110] Plasma catecholamine levels are reportedly increased in patients with Friedreich's ataxia.[111, 112]

In a prospective study of 75 patients with Friedreich's ataxia, superior systolic displacement of mitral leaflets did not exceed the normal range on two-dimensional echocardiography,[113] and no patient had mid to late systolic click(s) or a late systolic mumur.[4]

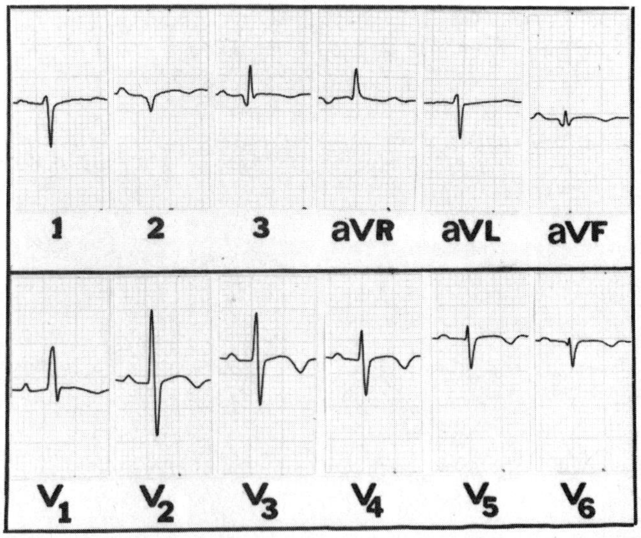

FIGURE 57–18. Electrocardiogram in a 28-year-old man with Friedreich's ataxia. The QRS shows marked right-axis deviation. There are 40-msec Q waves in leads 2, 3, and aVF. A prominent 60-msec R wave appears in lead V_1. A vectorcardiogram and echocardiogram showed no evidence of right ventricular hypertrophy. The ECG pattern reflects loss of inferior and posterior electrical forces without a corresponding regional wall motion abnormality on echocardiography. (From Child, J. S., et al.: Cardiac involvement in Friedreich's ataxia. Reprinted by permission of the American College of Cardiology. J. Am. Coll. Cardiol. *7*:1370, 1986.)

LESS COMMON NEUROMYOPATHIC DISEASES SOMETIMES ASSOCIATED WITH HEART DISEASE

PERONEAL MUSCULAR ATROPHY (CHARCOT-MARIE-TOOTH SYNDROME). Peroneal muscular atrophy includes at least two genetic disorders characterized by distal weakness of the legs with predilection for muscles innervated by the peroneal nerves, particularly the everters of the foot and occasionally intrinsic muscles of the hands.[5] Peroneal muscular atrophy is an autosomal dominant disorder; one form begins during the first 20 years of life, while the other form begins later, with initial symptoms appearing in early adult life or not until middle age.[5] Cardiac involvement is not a feature of peroneal muscular atrophy,[114] although one patient was found to have atrial flutter and heart failure,[115] and sporadic reports subsequently appeared of peroneal muscular atrophy associated with disturbances in cardiac impulse formation and conduction[116–118] and with dilated cardiomyopathy.[119]

MYOTUBULAR MYOPATHY (CENTRONUCLEAR MYOPATHY). As the term implies, centronuclear myopathy typically exhibits internal nuclei, i.e., structures resembling fetal myotubes (rows of nuclei separated by spaces).[120–122] Clinically, the disorder is characterized by slow but progressive wasting and weakness of skeletal muscle beginning at birth. Ptosis is the rule, and patients are hyporeflexic or areflexic. Even though few examples are available for study, presumptive evidence indicates that myotubular myopathy can be associated with extensive myocardial fibrosis, cardiac dilatation, and early death.[120] It is interesting that in an illustration in one report on skeletal muscle in "idiopathic cardiomyopathy" numerous internal nuclei could be seen.[123] Centronuclear myopathy had apparently presented as cardiomyopathy before the neuromuscular disease was identified.

KEARNS-SAYRE SYNDROME (PROGRESSIVE EXTERNAL OPHTHALMOPLEGIA WITH PIGMENTARY RETINOPATHY). Kearns-Sayre syndrome is characterized by the triad of progressive external ophthalmoplegia (Fig. 57–19), pigmentary retinopathy, and *heart block*.[124–126] Morphological alterations in skeletal muscle are identified in the trichrome stain as ragged-red fibers.[124] Cardiac involvement, primarily if not exclusively, appears to afflict the specialized conduction pathways rather than the myocardium.[127, 127a] Despite ultrastructural changes, clinically detectable myocardial disease is not a feature of the Kearns-Sayre syndrome.[126] Information thus far supports the view that involvement of the heart in this disorder is "neurogenic" rather than myopathic and that two derangements in cardiac conduction coexist: (1) gradually progressive impairment of infranodal conduction (left anterior hemiblock, right bundle branch block, complete heart block) (Fig. 57–20*A*) and (2) concomitant enhancement of AV nodal conduction.[127, 128] A convincing morphological basis for impaired infranodal conduction in this syndrome was demonstrated in a patient in whom electrophysiological study disclosed trifascicular block.[128] Necropsy revealed extensive changes in the distal portions of the bundle of His extending to the origins of the bundle branches. More recently, evidence of enhanced AV nodal conduction has been identified by means of His bundle electrocardiography (Fig. 57–20*B*).[127] A short or relatively short P-R interval should therefore not constitute evidence to discount the risk inherent in trifascicular disease in patients with Kearns-Sayre syndrome, right bundle branch block, and left anterior hemiblock.[127]

GUILLAIN-BARRÉ SYNDROME. The Guillain-Barré syndrome is the most common of the acquired demyelinative neuromyopathies.[129] The incidence gradually increases with age, but the disease may occur at any age, and both sexes are equally affected. The syndrome often appears days to weeks after a viral upper respiratory or gastrointestinal infection, with neurological symptoms comprising symmetrical weakness of the limbs often accompanied by paresthesias. Important and characteristic features are flaccid motor paralysis with a distinctive tendency to ascend (Landry's ascending paralysis) and an elevated cerebrospinal protein concentration without an increase in the number of white blood cells. Involvement of thoracic muscles often requires assisted ventilation. Despite ventilator support, the Guillain-Barré syndrome is fatal in approximately 20 per cent of children with significant involvement of trunk muscles and respiratory insufficiency.[130]

When sudden death occurs, postmortem studies have shed little or no light on the cause. There is substantial evidence, however, that deaths are often if not invariably related to cardiac arrhythmias.[130–132] Bradyarrhythmias (sinus arrest, complete heart block) and tachyarrhythmias (supraventricular and ventricular) as well as premature atrial and ventricular beats are relatively frequent and are enhanced by the use of a respirator.[131] Occasionally, patients manifest autonomic dysfunction, especially sympathetic hyperactivity, reflected in orthostatic hypotension, transient hypertension, wide fluctuations in blood pressure and heart rate, and variations in the R-R interval.[133–135] Pacemaker support has been required because of recurrent asystole.[131] In one patient, tracheal aspiration produced an idioventricular rhythm of 40 beats/min that reverted to sinus rhythm when aspiration ceased.[130] Cardiac monitoring is advisable, especially when the Guillain-Barré syndrome is sufficiently severe to warrant assisted ventilation.[130] The electrocardiogram occasionally shows widespread deep T-wave inversions.[135]

NEMALINE MYOPATHY. Nemaline myopathy is characterized by myriad small, rodlike particles in striated muscle.[136, 137] Inheritance is either autosomal dominant or recessive, with occasional sporadic cases. The commonest clinical manifestation is hypotonia with diffuse weakness of limbs and trunk beginning at a very early age. Children are often dysmorphic with an elongated, narrow face, high arched palate, and slender musculature.[5] Alternatively, symptoms begin in adolescence or adult life and are characterized by scapuloperoneal weakness and footdrop.[138] Nemaline myopathy is only rarely associated with cardiac involvement, but nemaline rods in the myocardium and in

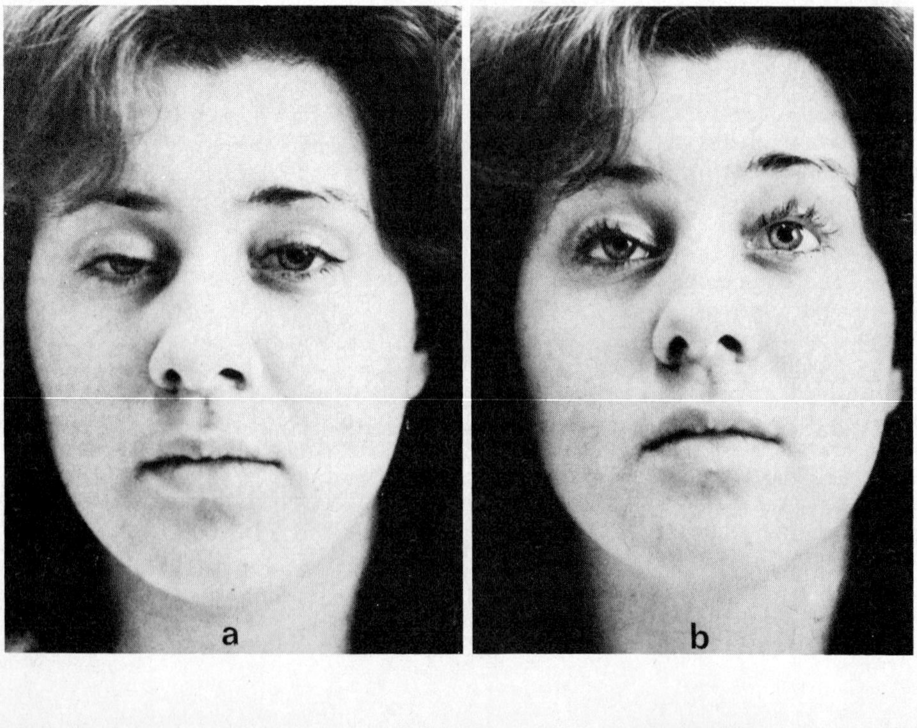

FIGURE 57–19. An 18-year-old girl with Kearns-Sayre syndrome and bilateral asymmetrical ptosis. Within 24 months, her electrocardiogram changed from normal to bifascicular block (complete right bundle branch block and left anterior fascicular block). *A*, The asymmetrical ptosis when the patient looks straight ahead. *B*, Ptosis of the right lid persists when the patient looks up. She also had atypical pigmentary retinopathy.

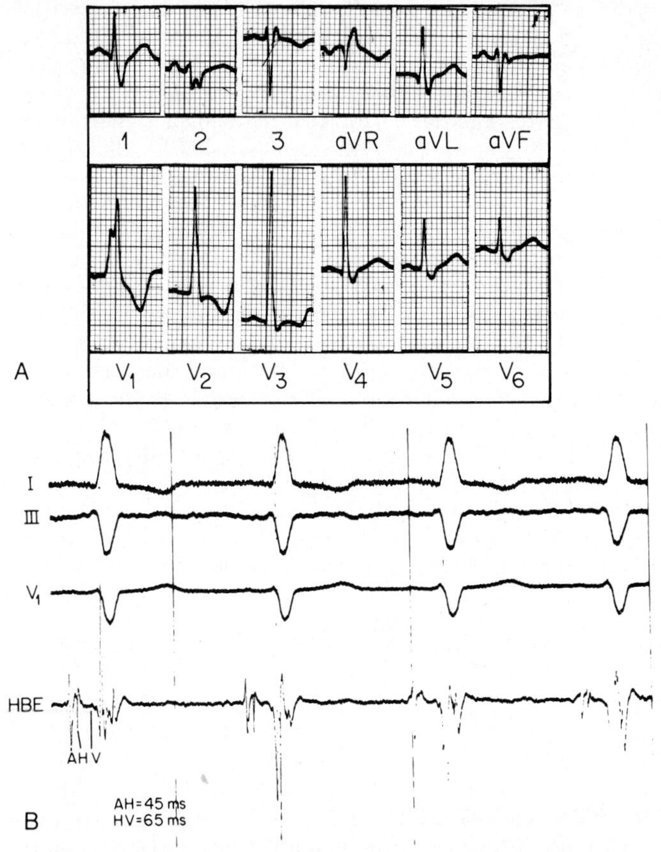

FIGURE 57–20. ***A,*** **Electrocardiogram from a 13-year-old boy with Kearns-Sayre syndrome. There is a short P-R interval (110 msec), left anterior hemiblock, and complete right bundle branch block.** ***B,*** **Leads I, III, and V_1 with His bundle electrogram (HBE) in a 21-year-old woman with Kearns-Sayre syndrome. Time lines are at 1-second intervals. The A-H interval is 45 msec (short) and the H-V interval is 65 msec (prolonged). (From Roberts, N. K., et al.: Cardiac conduction in Kearns-Sayre syndrome. Am. J. Cardiol. *44*:1396, 1979.)**

the cardiac conduction tissues have been held responsible for cardiac dilatation and conduction defects.[139, 140]

MYASTHENIA GRAVIS. Myasthenia gravis is a "neuroimmunological" disease caused by a disorder of neuromuscular transmission due to antibodies to acetylcholine receptors.[141, 142] The abnormality may become manifest at any age but is most common in the second to fourth decades. Overt pathological evidence of myasthenia gravis is primarily in the thymic gland, which shows lymphoid hyperplasia and numerous lymphoid follicles with germinal centers in the medulla. Ocular muscles are affected first, and weakness characteristically fluctuates during the course of a single day, sometimes within minutes. The association of myocardial disease with thymoma, especially malignant thymoma, is generally accepted, whereas the association of myasthenia gravis with heart disease is less clear despite a considerable body of suggestive evidence. Specific cardiac involvement is unproven even though clinical, electrocardiographic, and vectorcardiographic data implicate the myocardium.[143]

Early in this century quinine was used as a provocative diagnostic test for myasthenia gravis. Quinidine and procainamide, like quinine, have anticholinergic properties that depress neuromuscular conduction.[144] These antiarrhythmic agents can unmask previously unsuspected myasthenia gravis and can exacerbate symptoms in previously well-controlled patients.[144, 145] Accordingly, quinidine and procainamide should be avoided in this condition.

McARDLE SYNDROME. This metabolic myopathy (muscle phosphorylase deficiency) results in inadequate skeletal muscle glycolysis.[146] The disease is typically characterized by exercise-induced muscle cramps. The electrocardiogram occasionally reveals sinus bradycardia, increased QRS voltage, and prolongation of the P-R interval.[146] McArdle syndrome differs from the metabolic mitochondrial myopathy of skeletal and cardiac muscle with exercise-induced lactic acidemia and storage of glycogen and lipid.[147]

NEUROMUSCULAR DISORDERS PRESENTING AS CARDIOMYOPATHY

Occasionally patients with little or no clinical evidence of a systemic neuromuscular disorder come to medical attention initially because of overt cardiac disease.[148] Heart block (selective involvement of the specialized conduction system) is sometimes the presenting manifestation in the Kearns-Sayre syndrome, myotonic muscular dystrophy, or Emery-Dreifuss disease (p. 1787). Alternatively, patients may have disorders of cardiac conduction and rhythm *and* of the myocardium.[149–151] Other patients manifest cardiomyopathy alone and are later found to have skeletal muscle involvement either on biopsy or because of the subsequent development of clinically overt skeletal muscle disease. Patients with "idiopathic dilated cardiomyopathy" sporadically exhibit histological evidence of centronuclear myopathy.[120, 122] Mothers of patients with classic X-linked Duchenne dystrophy may have cardiomyopathy accompanied by no more than enzyme evidence of systemic muscle involvement.[34, 35, 38] The point should not be overstated, but occasionally it proves useful to consider neuromuscular disease as the underlying cause of sinoatrial or AV conduction disease or "idiopathic" dilated cardiomyopathy in relatively young patients.

POLIOMYELITIS. Cardiac involvement is believed to occur only rarely in childhood poliomyelitis but may simply be clinically occult.[152, 153] In adults, the infrequency of symptomatic involvement of the heart contrasts with a relatively high incidence of electrocardiographic abnormalities, especially of rhythm and conduction.[152, 153] Disturbances of rhythm take the form of premature beats (atrial and ventricular) and atrial fibrillation or flutter; disturbances of conduction are manifested by impaired AV conduction (first-, second-, and third-degree heart block) and abnormalities of infranodal conduction (left-axis deviation and bundle branch block).[152, 153] Respiratory failure can provoke hypoxemia-induced pulmonary hypertension[154] and multifocal atrial tachycardia.

At necropsy, the sinoatrial node, distal His bundle, and left and right bundle branches show infiltration, degeneration, and fibrous replacement that wholly or in part underlie the conduction defects.[152, 153] Pathological changes in the myocardium tend to be similar to those in skeletal muscle, including diffuse mononuclear cell infiltration and myofibril degeneration, regeneration, and fibrosis.

PERIODIC PARALYSIS. Periodic paralysis is characterized by recurrences of flaccid weakness accompanied by either abnormally high or abnormally low levels of serum potassium.[155, 156] *Hypokalemic attacks* typically begin in late childhood or adolescence, usually occur at night, tend to be severe, and last a day or longer.[156] *Hyperkalemic attacks* have their onset at a younger age. Episodes occur more frequently than with hypokalemia but tend to be milder and shorter in duration (minutes or hours). Many features are common to both varieties of periodic paralysis, including familial recurrence (autosomal dominant inheritance), heightened susceptibility immediately after ceasing strenuous exercise, termination of incipient attacks by *mild* exercise, onset of weakness in the lower extremities with progression to the arms but not to the respiratory muscles, intensification by cold, and persistent weakness between attacks even though potassium levels may be normal.[155, 157] During hyperkalemia, the electrocardiogram exhibits peaked T waves, and during hypokalemia there are low-voltage T waves and digitalis sensitivity (pp. 215 to 217). More important are the cardiac arrhythmias that accompany hyperkalemia but occasionally occur during normokalemic periodic paralysis. Noteworthy are ventricular ectopic beats, ventricular bigeminy, bidirectional ventricular tachycardia, and fusion beats producing multiform complexes.[156–158] Hypokalemic attacks are best treated with oral potassium chloride and hyperkalemic episodes with glucose and insulin, but it should be pointed out that administration of potassium does not always suppress the ventricular electrical instability during hypokalemic attacks.[158]

ALCOHOLIC CARDIOMYOPATHY (See also p. 1417). Dilated cardiomyopathy associated with chronic ingestion of large amounts of ethyl alcohol may be accompanied by clinically occult skeletal myopathy.[159–161] The low incidence of peripheral neuritis supports the view that the cardiac abnormality does *not* depend upon malnutrition.[159] The teratogenic potential of alcohol, exemplified by the fetal alcohol syndrome, afflicts the central nervous system but not the fetal myocardium, although congenital malformations of the heart are not uncommon in the offspring of alcoholic mothers.[162]

ACUTE CEREBRAL DISORDERS ACCOMPANIED BY CARDIOVASCULAR ABNORMALITIES

Acute cerebral injury can provoke cardiovascular abnormalities, and abnormalities of the heart can be accompanied by acute cerebral injury. A connection between certain acute cerebral events—i.e., subdural hematoma, subarachnoid hemorrhage, intracranial hemorrhage, and cerebral thrombosis or embolus—and overt cardiovascular abnormalities has been recognized for nearly a century.[163] A relationship between acute head trauma and cardiac abnormalities was proposed 50 years ago.[164] Previously, the cardiac abnormalities emphasized in these settings were essentially disturbances in rhythm and conduction and abnormalities of repolarization. *Neurogenic pulmonary edema* has been reported in a variety of disorders of the central nervous system[165] and in brain stem hemorrhage.[166] A rise in systemic blood pressure in response to cerebral injury[167] was known to Harvey Cushing at the turn of the century (the Cushing pressor response[168]), and experimentally induced intense cerebral compression in rats evoked a marked increase in systemic vascular resistance, a profound decrease in systemic cardiac output, pulmonary venous congestion, and hemorrhagic pulmonary edema.[165] Recently, interest has focused on the importance of damage to the myocardium in response to cerebral injury, especially severe brain injury in craniocerebral trauma.[169–172]

ARRHYTHMIAS. Approximately 90 per cent of patients with *acute cerebral accidents*—most notably, spontaneous cerebral or subarachnoid hemorrhage or acute cerebral trauma—exhibit electrocardiographic abnormalities that consist chiefly of disturbances of cardiac rhythm and repolarization.[166, 172–181] Disturbances in cardiac rhythm consist of brady- and tachyarrhythmias, including sinus bradycardia (sometimes profound), sinus tachycardia, atrial arrhythmias (ectopic beats, fibrillation, flutter, or supraventricular tachycardia), and ventricular arrhythmias (ectopic beats, ventricular tachycardia or fibrillation).[163, 174, 182, 183] Repolarization abnormalities closely resemble those of ischemic heart disease and consist chiefly of abnormal ST segments and T waves in addition to prominent U waves, a prolonged Q-T interval,[166, 177, 184] and abnormalities in AV conduction.[163] It is noteworthy that ST segments may be dramatically elevated and T waves dramatically inverted (Fig. 57–21). The rapid appearance and disappearance of certain electrocardiographic changes have been ascribed to neural rather than humoral factors. There is substantial evidence, however, that the "catecholamine storm" coupled with release of norepinephrine at cardiac $beta_1$ receptor sites is responsible for myocardial damage, reflected in a rise in serum cardiac enzymes (CK-MB), evidence of myofibrillar degeneration on light microscopy, and subendocardial hemorrhage.[170, 171, 181] The potentially additive effects of steroids combined with catecholamines in the genesis of stress myocardial injury have been emphasized.[174] Obviously, the myocardial damage associated with acute cerebral injury puts patients at additional risk. It is also important to emphasize that the major sources of donor hearts for cardiac and for heart and lung transplantation are victims of motor vehicle accidents or gunshot wounds who have suffered massive cerebral injury and, in all probability, varying degrees of catecholamine- and stress-induced myocardial and lung injury.[172, 183]

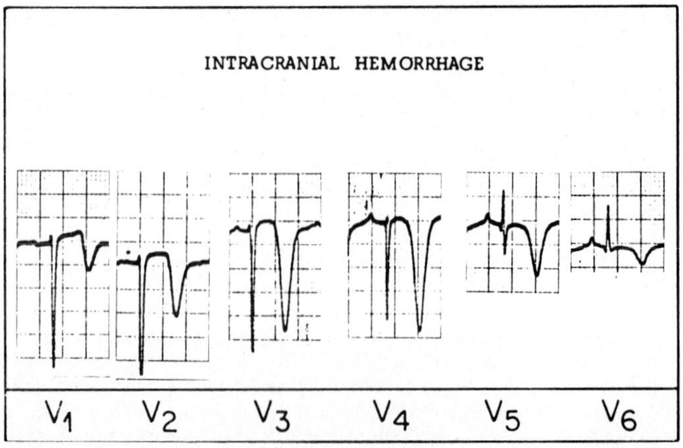

FIGURE 57–21. Deep, symmetrical T-wave inversions in precordial leads of a patient with a cerebral hemorrhage. (Courtesy of John H. Phillips, M.D., Tulane Medical Center, New Orleans, Louisiana.)

COEXISTENCE OF CEREBROVASCULAR DISEASE AND CORONARY HEART DISEASE. The preceding section pointed out that acute cerebrovascular accidents in patients with normal hearts (i.e., without coronary artery disease) often result in electrocardiographic abnormalities resembling those in myocardial ischemia or infarction with release of MB CPK; however, in older patients, these electrocardiographic abnormalities and isoenzyme elevations may in fact rèpresent an accompanying acute myocardial infarction caused by coexisting atherosclerotic coronary artery disease.[185, 186] Because ST-segment elevations, deep T-wave inversions, and a rise in MB CPK are seen in patients with cerebrovascular accidents *without* ischemic heart disease, one cannot rely on these criteria to diagnose infarction due to coronary artery obstruction. Accordingly, earlier estimates of the incidence of recent myocardial infarction in such patients[179, 187] must be reevaluated.[188] Differential diagnosis is important, since mortality is relatively high in patients with coexisting acute cerebrovascular accident and acute myocardial infarction.[184]

Diagnosis. Patients with clinically overt atherosclerotic coronary artery disease should be examined for occult carotid artery disease, and those with overt carotid artery disease should be assessed for occult atherosclerotic coronary artery disease. Cervical artery murmurs were found in 4.4 to 12.6 per cent of persons 45 years of age and older with no history of stroke, transient cerebral ischemia, or overt ischemic heart disease.[189, 190] The prevalence of these asymptomatic murmurs increased with age and was higher among women and among persons with systemic hypertension. In a prospective study of 735 unselected patients over age 55 years who were scheduled for elective surgery, 14 per cent had cervical artery murmurs.[191] Pooled data on 2205 patients undergoing elective surgery disclosed cervical artery murmur in 15 per cent but no difference in stroke distribution between patients with and without carotid murmurs.[191] It was concluded that strokes in patients undergoing operations other than coronary artery bypass are so rare that further evaluation seems unnecessary. Still, it is important to distinguish between hemodynamically mild carotid stenosis with an exceedingly low risk of stroke and hemodynamically significant lesions in which the risk of even nonfatal cerebral infarction is appreciable.[192]

The need to identify hemodynamically significant carotid artery obstruction—either symptomatic or asymptomatic—was underscored in the Framingham Study, in which attention was called to the relative frequency of cerebral infarction in vascular territories different from those predicted based on an asymptomatic carotid artery murmur.[193] Ruptured aneurysm, embolism from the heart, and lacunar infarction were the mechanisms of stroke in nearly half the cases.

The *physical examination* serves to detect carotid artery murmurs but does not accurately determine the severity of carotid obstruction. Of the currently available noninvasive neurovascular tests that reliably assess carotid artery disease, the first choice is the ultrasonic duplex scanner that combines B-mode imaging to visualize specific arterial segments with the pulsed Doppler technique to determine the physiological significance of the obstruction[194, 195]

Management. Given relatively secure information regarding the carotid and coronary circulations, judgments concerning management before coronary revascularization may be based on the following remarks[196–198]: In patients with symptomatic carotid artery murmurs (prior stroke or transient ischemic attacks) and hemodynamically significant carotid artery obstruction (especially bilateral) in whom myocardial revascularization *cannot* safely be deferred (left main coronary obstruction, unstable angina pectoris, severe multivessel disease), the author recommends combined carotid endarterectomy and coronary bypass grafting. In patients with symptomatic carotid artery murmurs and hemodynamically significant carotid obstruction in whom myocardial revascularization *can* safely be deferred, carotid endarterectomy should be carried out first, followed at a later date by coronary revascularization. In patients with asymptomatic carotid artery murmurs and obstruction not considered hemodynamically significant, myocardial revascularization alone can proceed as clinically indicated. Less clear is the management of patients with asymptomatic carotid artery murmurs and hemodynamically significant carotid obstruction. It has been argued that elective myocardial revascularization can be performed either alone or, if clinically urgent (as defined above), combined with carotid endarterectomy.[196]

An important corollary to these observations is the incidence of neurological complications unassociated with carotid artery obstruction in patients undergoing coronary artery bypass grafting.[196, 198–204] These complications are in addition to and distinct from those accompanying open-heart surgery per se.[205] Major central nervous system events are associated with coronary bypass operations in 1 to 2 per cent of cases.[198, 200, 201] The majority of cerebral events complicating coronary bypass grafting are believed to be related to embolization of atheromatous material from the ascending aorta or embolization from a postinfarction left ventricular mural thrombus.[198, 201, 202]

CEREBRAL EMBOLI. Cerebral emboli associated with chronic lone atrial fibrillation[206] or mitral stenosis and atrial fibrillation (intermittent or chronic) are threats regardless of the patient's age. Focal neurological signs seen occasionally in patients with pathological mitral valve prolapse are believed to be embolic (p. 1045).[207–209] Myxoma of the left atrium results in peripheral emboli in about 45 per cent of cases, and the brain is affected in half of these (p. 1473). Occasionally, patients with cardiac myxoma are initially seen by neurologists because they present with predominantly or exclusively neurological manifestations.[210] Cerebral emboli from left ventricular mural thrombi (most commonly with anterolateral myocardial infarction) occasionally occur spontaneously or set the stage for embolization during coronary bypass grafting, as already noted. Left ventricular mural thrombi with dilated cardiomyopathy are much more likely to give rise to cerebral emboli than are mural thrombi associated with myocardial infarction. Infants with endocardial fibroelastosis of the dilated type may also suffer strokes caused by emboli from left ventricular endocardial thrombi.[211]

In addition to cardiac chambers as sources, cerebral emboli originate from heart valves or from systemic veins (paradoxical embolus). Valve emboli occur rarely during cardiac surgery, and anticoagulants coupled with improved prostheses have minimized—although not eliminated—cerebral emboli after the insertion of rigid prostheses (p. 1078). Cerebral emboli from native valves are represented by the septic emboli of infective endocarditis and by the bland emboli of noninfective thrombotic deposits (so-called marantic endocarditis, especially on the aortic valve), which are probably more common than clinically diagnosed.[212] Septic cerebral emboli that follow a misleading interval of quiescence may give rise to acute intracranial hemorrhage or cerebral abscess. Drug abuse not only causes infective endocarditis but, depending on the drug and vehicle (embolization of foreign matter), also may be associated with intracranial or subarachnoid hemorrhage, cerebral emboli, ischemic stroke, and systemic hypertension.[213] Paradoxical emboli reach the brain when systemic venous blood enters the systemic arterial circulation via the right-to-left shunts of cyanotic congenital heart disease.[211] The relative infrequency of such emboli is attributed to the low incidence of a source, because infants and young children in the relevant age group rarely have phlebothrombosis or thrombophlebitis. An exception is the multigravida with an ostium secundum atrial septal defect in whom inferior vena caval to left atrial streaming provides a pathway into the left atrium from the inferior vena cava.[211]

Focal discrete neurological deficits are well known sequelae of cerebral emboli; less well known are the diffuse cerebral symptoms believed to result from recurrences of multiple small corticoemboli that cause agitated confusion, dulled sensorium, and seizures.[214]

CYANOTIC CONGENITAL HEART DISEASE WITH NEUROLOGICAL MANIFESTATIONS. Brain damage, mental retardation, venous sinus thromboses, paradoxical cerebroembolism, and brain abscess constitute a formidable list of central nervous system complications in cyanotic congenital heart disease.[211] Cyanotic spells of tetralogy of Fallot end in syncope, seizures, and rarely hemiplegia (p. 946). The erythrocytosis of cyanotic congenital heart disease is a risk of stroke chiefly in infants under 2 years of age with relative iron deficiency anemia, but the risk of stroke is low in cyanotic adults, whether the erythrocytosis is compensated (normochromic) or decompensated (hypochromic).[215]

NEUROLOGICAL COMPLICATIONS AFTER CARDIAC ARREST. Broadly speaking, neurological outcomes cover a broad spectrum, ranging from complete recovery to the vegetative state.[216–218] A reversible "metabolic encephalopathy" occurs in patients with brief episodes of systemic circulatory arrest and mild degrees of cerebral hypoxia. Recovery is rapid and complete. In contrast, patients with severe cerebral hypoxia suffer structural damage to specific areas of the brain, as if they had had a stroke, and on awakening manifest permanent focal or multifocal motor, sensory, and intellectual deficits.[216, 217] Still others with more widespread brain injury remain hospitalized in a state of wakefulness without awareness (vegetative state) or die a neurological death (brain death).[216, 217]

CARDIAC COMPLICATIONS OF DRUGS USED IN TREATING NEUROMUSCULAR DISEASE

Neuromuscular and cardiovascular disease may also be related because of cardiac complications of certain drugs used by the neurologist.

Methysergide prescribed for migraine headache may be

accompanied by inflammatory retroperitoneal fibrosis and by a similar fibrotic disease of pleura, great arteries, cardiac valves, endocardium, and pericardium.[219–221] Methysergide-induced lesions do not appear to damage underlying cardiac structures, but instead the fibrotic and thickened appearance is caused by a layer of fresh collagen deposited on the surfaces of otherwise unharmed cardiac tissue.[220] Grossly and microscopically these lesions are similar to those occurring in carcinoid syndrome (p. 1439),[222] and it has been theorized that the chemical similarity between methysergide and serotonin may in part provide the reason. The aortic valve lesion induced by methysergide causes both stenosis and regurgitation, but the clinically overt mitral lesion generally causes regurgitation. If the drug is continued, the valvular abnormalities progress; however, in some patients, regression or complete disappearance (at least of the cardiac murmurs) has followed the discontinuation of methysergide.[220]

In *Parkinson's disease*, neurons are selectively destroyed and cannot release the neurotransmitter dopamine.[223] Accordingly, levodopa (L-dopa), the precursor of dopamine, is used in treatment. A relatively large dose is required for a therapeutic response because only a small percentage of oral levodopa penetrates the blood-brain barrier. Such doses are seldom tolerated without side effects. L-dopa provokes hypotension (supine and postural) as well as ventricular ectopic beats.[224] Thus, the drug must be used cautiously in patients with cerebral ischemia, angina pectoris, recent myocardial infarction, or cardiac arrhythmias, even though after weeks (sometimes months) of use, tolerance improves and side effects diminish. The cardiovascular effects are mediated by the action of L-dopa on the central and peripheral nervous systems.

Bromocriptine, an ergot derivative, stimulates dopamine-sensitive receptors and is also useful in parkinsonism.[225] In high doses, the drug may cause a significant postural fall in blood pressure, and the hypotensive effect may persist for as long as 6 weeks. Rarely, severe hypotension, both supine and erect, occurs after an initial dose of bromocriptine.

NEUROLOGICAL COMPLICATIONS OF THERAPY FOR CARDIOVASCULAR DISEASE

Certain therapies for cardiovascular disease can result in serious neurological sequelae, such as those which occur after cardiac arrest and resuscitation (see above). Cardioversion for chronic atrial fibrillation with a normal mitral valve seldom gives rise to systemic emboli; if emboli do occur, they do so either at the moment of reversion to sinus rhythm or on recurrence of atrial fibrillation. If a prophylactic anticoagulant is used in this setting, it must not only precede cardioversion but also be maintained until stable sinus rhythm seems assured.[226]

Several commonly used cardiac drugs have important, although relatively rare, central or peripheral nervous system effects. The adverse responses to quinidine and procainamide in patients with myasthenia gravis were mentioned above (p. 1787). *Lidocaine neurotoxicity* (p. 628) includes drowsiness, dizziness, dysarthria, blurred vision, muscular fasciculations, and occasionally convulsions.[227] Beta-adrenoceptor blockers (p. 1330), in addition to causing drowsiness and lightheadedness, sometimes provoke mental depressions.[228] Even digitalis glycosides are not exempt from causing neurotoxic effects[229] (p. 504). In the words of William Withering, "The Foxglove when given in very large and quickly repeated doses occasions giddiness, confused vision, objects appearing green or yellow . . . cold sweats, convulsions, syndrome, death."[230]

CARDIAC DENERVATION

The commonest cause of cardiac denervation is cardiac transplantation (p. 530). Less well known is the remarkable denervation of the intrinsic nervous system of the heart (predominantly parasympathetic ganglion cells) that occurs in Chagas heart disease (p. 1445).[231, 232] In this setting, nervous control of the heart depends chiefly on the sympathetic system. The increased capacity of the coronary arteries (judged at necropsy by the volume of barium sulfate–gelatin mass taken up by the coronary arterial bed relative to heart weight) has been attributed to relative sympathetic overdrive in this disease.[231]

REFERENCES

MAJOR HEREDOFAMILIAL NEUROMYOPATHIC DISORDERS

1. Perloff, J. K., deLeon, A. C., and O'Doherty, D.: The cardiomyopathy of progressive muscular dystrophy. Circulation *33*:625, 1966.
2. Perloff, J. K., Henze, E., and Schelbert, H. R.: Alterations in regional myocardial metabolism, perfusion and wall motion in Duchenne muscular dystrophy studied by radionuclide imaging. Circulation *69*:33, 1984.
3. Perloff, J. K., Stevenson, W. G., Roberts, N. K., Cabeen, W., and Weiss, J.: Cardiac involvement in myotonic muscular dystrophy (Steinert's disease): A prospective study of 25 patients. Am. J. Cardiol. *54*:1074, 1984.
4. Child, J. S., Perloff, J. K., Bach, P. M., Wolfe, A. D., Perlman, S., and Kark, R. A. P.: Cardiac involvement in Friedreich's ataxia. J. Am. Coll. Cardiol., *7*:1370, 1986.
5. Brooke, M. H.: A Clinician's View of Neuromuscular Diseases. Baltimore, Williams and Wilkins Co., 1979.
6. Gardner-Medwin, D.: Mutation rate in Duchenne type of muscular dystrophy. J. Med. Genet. *7*:334, 1970.
6a. Kunkel, L. M.: Analysis of deletions in DNA from patients with Becker and Duchenne muscular dystrophy. Nature *322*:73, 1986.
7. Roses, A. D.: Progressive muscular dystrophies. In Rowland, L. P. (ed.): Merritt's Textbook of Neurology. 7th ed. Philadelphia, Lea & Febiger, 1984.
8. deLeon, A. C., Perloff, J. K., Twigg, H., and Hajd, M.: The straight back syndrome—clinical cardiovascular manifestations. Circulation *32*:193, 1965.
9. Sanyal, S. K., Johnson, W. W., Dische, M. R., Pitner, S. E., and Beard, C.: Dystrophic degeneration of papillary muscle and ventricular myocardium. A basis for mitral valve prolapse in Duchenne's muscular dystrophy. Circulation *62*:430, 1980.
10. Perloff, J. K., Roberts, W. C., deLeon, A. C., and O'Doherty, D.: The distinctive electrocardiogram of Duchenne's progressive muscular dystrophy. Am. J. Med. *42*:179, 1967.
11. Perloff, J. K.: Cardiac rhythm and conduction in Duchenne's muscular dystrophy. J. Am. Coll. Cardiol. *3*:1263, 1984.
12. Sanyal, S. K., Johnson, W. W., Thapar, M. K., and Pitner, S. E.: An ultrastructural basis for the electrocardiographic alterations associated with Duchenne's progressive muscular dystrophy. Circulation *57*:1122, 1978.
13. Zalman, F., Perloff, J. K., Durant, N. N., and Campion, D. S.: Acute respiratory failure following intravenous verapamil in Duchenne's muscular dystrophy. Am. Heart J. *105*:510, 1983.
14. Rubler, S., Perloff, J. K., and Roberts, W. C.: Clinical Pathological Conference—Duchenne's muscular dystrophy. Am. Heart J. *94*:776, 1977.
15. Biddison, J. H., Dembo, D. H., Spalt, H., Hayes, M. G., and Le Douk, C. W.: Familial occurrence of mitral valve prolapse in X-linked muscular dystrophy. Circulation *59*:1299, 1979.
16. Frankel, K. A., and Rosser, R. J.: The pathology of the heart in progressive muscular dystrophy. Hum. Pathol. *7*:375, 1976.
17. Ishikawa, K., Yanagisawa, A., Ishihara, T., Tamura, T., and Inorie, M.: Sequential changes of orthogonal electrocardiograms in progressive muscular dystrophy. Am. Heart J. *98*:73, 1979.
18. Nomura, H., and Hizawa, K.: Histopathological study of the conduction system of the heart in Duchenne progressive muscular dystrophy. Acta Pathol. *32*:1027, 1982.
19. James, T. N.: Observations on the cardiovascular involvement, including the cardiac conduction system, in progressive muscular dystrophy. Am. Heart J. *63*:48, 1962.
20. Skyring, A., and McKusick, V. A.: Clinical, genetic and electrocardiographic studies in childhood muscular dystrophy. Am. J. Med. Sci. *242*:54, 1961.
21. Slucka, C.: The electrocardiogram in Duchenne's progressive muscular dystrophy. Circulation *38*:933, 1968.
22. Fitch, C. W., and Ainger, L. E.: The Frank vectorcardiogram and the electrocardiogram in Duchenne muscular dystrophy. Circulation *35*:1124, 1967.
23. Ronan, J. A., Perloff, J. K., Bowen, P. J., and Mann, O.: The vectorcardiogram in Duchenne's progressive muscular dystrophy. Am. Heart J. *84*:588, 1972.
24. Schelbert, H. R., Benson, L., Schwaiger, M., and Perloff, J. K.: Positron emission tomography. *In* Friedman, W. F., and Higgins C. B. (eds.): Pediatric Cardiac Imaging, Cardiology Clinics. Philadelphia, W.B. Saunders Company, 1983.
25. Mawatari, S., Miranda, A., and Rowland, L. P.: Adenyl cyclase abnormality in Duchenne muscular dystrophy: Muscle cells in culture. Neurology *67*:1016, 1976.
26. Wilner, J. H., Cerri, C., and Wood, D. S.: Adenyl cyclase in human genetic myopathies. *In* Schotland, D. L. (ed.): Disorders of the Motor Unit. New York, John Wiley and Sons, 1982, p. 431.
27. Carpenter, S., and Karpati, G.: Duchenne muscular dystrophy. Plasma

membrane loss initiates muscle cell necrosis unless it is repaired. Brain *102*:147, 1979.
28. Mokri, B., and Engel, A. G.: Duchenne dystrophy: Electronmicroscopic findings pointing to a basic or early abnormality in the plasma membrane of the muscle fiber. Neurology *25*:1111, 1975.
29. Schmalbruch, H.: Freeze-fracture studies of experimentally damaged skeletal muscle fibers. *In* Schotland, D. L. (ed.): Disorders of the Motor Unit. New York, John Wiley and Sons, 1982, p. 503.
30. Bonilla, E., Schotland, D. L., and Yakayama, Y.: Duchenne dystrophy: Focal alterations in the distribution of concanavalin A binding sites at the muscle cell surface. Ann. Neurol. *4*:117, 1978.
31. Roses, A. D., Harwig, G. B., Mabry, M., Nagano, Y., and Miller, S. E.: Red blood cell and fibroblast membranes in Duchenne and myotonic muscular dystrophy. Muscle Nerve *3*:36, 1980.
32. Pennington, R. J. T.: Serum enzymes. *In* Rowland, L. P. (ed.): Pathogenesis of Human Muscular Dystrophies. Amsterdam-Oxford, Excerpta Medica, 1977, p. 341.
33. Sutton, T. M., O'Brien, J. F., Kleinberg, F., House, R. F., and Feldt, R. H.: Serum levels of creatine phosphokinase and its isoenzymes in normal and stressed neonates. Mayo Clin. Proc. *56*:150, 1981.
34. Yoshioka, M.: Clinically manifesting carriers in Duchenne muscular dystrophy. Clin. Genet. *20*:6, 1981.
35. Lane, R. J. M., Gardner-Medwin, D., and Roses, A. D.: Electrocardiographic abnormalities in carriers of Duchenne muscular dystrophy. Neurology *30*:497, 1980.
36. Kolata, G.: Closing in on the muscular dystrophy gene. Science *230*:307, 1985.
37. Fowler, W. M., Gardner, G. W., Taylor, R. G., Scavarda, A., and Busheikin, J. B.: Quantitative measurements in female siblings and mothers of boys with Duchenne dystrophy. Arch. Phys. Med. Rehab. *50*:301, 1969.
38. Mann, O., deLeon, A. C., Perloff, J. K., Simanis, J., and Horrigan, F. D.: Duchenne's muscular dystrophy: The electrocardiogram in female relatives. Am. J. Med. Sci. *255*:376, 1968.
39. Paillonry, M., Citron, B., Hersch, B., Heiligenstein, D., Ponsonnaille, J., and Gras, H.: Electrocardiograms of women carriers of Duchenne-type muscular dystrophy. Ann. Cardiol. Angiol. *31*:47, 1982.
40. Wiegand, V., Rahlf, G., Meinck, M., and Kreuzer, H.: Cardiomyopathy in female carriers of the Duchenne gene. Z. Kardiol. *73*:188, 1984.
41. Becker, P. E.: Two new families of benign sex-linked recessive muscular dystrophy. Rev. Can. Bio. *21*:551, 1962.
42. Markand, O. N., North, R. R., D'Agostino, A. N., and Daly, D. D.: Benign sex-linked muscular dystrophy. Neurology *19*:617, 1969.
43. Emery, A. E. H., Clark, E. R., Simons, S., and Taylor, J. L.: Detections of carriers of benign X-linked muscular dystrophy. Br. Med. J. *4*:522, 1967.
43a. Borgeat, A., Goy, J. J., and Sigwart, U.: Acute pulmonary edema as the inaugural symptom of Becker's muscular dystrophy in a 19-year-old patient. Clin. Cardiol *10*:127, 1987.
44. Emery, A. E. H., and Dreifuss, F. E.: Unusual form of benign X-linked muscular dystrophy. J. Neurol. Neurosurg. Psychiatry *29*:338, 1966.
45. Katiyar, B. C., Soman, P. N., Mishra, S., and Chaterji, A. M.: Congestive cardiomyopathy in a family of Becker's X-linked muscular dystrophy. Postgrad. Med. J. *53*:12, 1977.
46. Vrints, C., Mercelis, R., Vanagt, E., Snoeck, J., and Martin, J. J.: Cardiac manifestations of Becker-type muscular dystrophy. Acta Cardiol. *38*:479, 1983.
47. Nigro, G., Comi, L. I., Limonselli, F. M., Giugliano, M. A., Palitano, L., Petretta, V., Passamano, C., and Stefanelli, S.: Prospective study of X-linked progressive muscular dystrophy in Campania. Muscle Nerve *6*:253, 1983.
48. Levin, R. N., and Narahara, K. A.: Right axis deviation and anterior wall thallium-201 defect in Becker's muscular dystrophy. Am. J. Cardiol. *56*:203, 1985.
49. Hassan, Z., Fastabend, C. P., Mohanty, P. K., and Isaacs, E. R.: Atrioventricular block and supraventricular arrhythmias with X-linked muscular dystrophy. Circulation *60*:1365, 1979.
50. Jackson, C. E., and Strehler, D. A.: Limb-girdle muscular dystrophy: Clinical manifestations and detection of pre-clinical disease. Pediatrics *41*:495, 1968.
51. Lambert, C. D., and Fairfax, A. J.: Neurological associations of chronic heart block. J. Neurol. Neurosurg. Psychiatry *39*:571, 1976.
52. Fairfax, A. J., and Lambert, C. D.: Neurological aspects of sinoatrial heart block. J. Neurol. Neurosurg. Psychiatry *39*:576, 1976.
53. Svetoni, N., Spargi, T., Ballantonio, M., and Lanzetta, T.: Erb's muscular dystrophy and congestive myocardiopathy. G. Ital. Cardiol. *14*:59, 1984.
54. Baldwin, A. J., Talley, R. C., Johnson, C., and Nutter, O.: Permanent paralysis of the atrium in a patient with facioscapulohumeral muscular dystrophy. Am. J. Cardiol. *31*:649, 1973.
55. Ruff, P., Leier, C. V., and Schaal, S. F.: Temporal atrial standstill. Am. Heart J. *98*:412, 1979.
56. Woolliscroft, J., and Tuna, N.: Permanent atrial standstill: The clinical spectrum. Am. J. Med. *49*:2037, 1982.
57. Rosen, K. M., Rahimtoola, S. H., Gunnar, R. M., and Lev, M.: Transient and persistent atrial standstill with His bundle lesions. Circulation *44*:220, 1971.
58. Ward, D. E., Ho, S. Y., and Shinebourne, E. A.: Familial atrial standstill and inexcitability in childhood. Am. J. Cardiol. *53*:965, 1984.
59. Disertori, M., Guarnerio, M., Vergara, G., Del Favero, A., Bettini, R., Zinama, G., Rubertelli, M., and Furlanello, F.: Familial endemic persistent atrial standstill in a small mountain community. Eur. Heart J. *4*:354, 1983.
60. Levy, S., Pouget, B., Bemurat, M., Lacaze, J. C., Clementz, J., and Bricaud, H.: Partial atrial electrical standstill: Report of three cases and review of clinical and electrophysiological features Eur. Heart J. *1*:107, 1980.
61. Effendy, F. N., Bolognesi, R., Bianchi, G., and Visioli, O.: Alternation of partial and total atrial standstill. J. Electrocardiol. *12*:121, 1979.
62. Stevenson, W. G., Weiss, J., and Perloff, J. K.: Electrophysiologic studies of the atria in facioscapulohumeral muscular dystrophy, in preparation.
63. Miller, R. G., Layzer, R. B., Mellenthin, M. A., Golabi, M., Francoz, R. A., and Mall, J. C.: Emery-Dreifuss muscular dystrophy with autosomal dominant transmission. Neurology *35*:1230, 1985.
64. Rowland, L. P., Fetell, M., Alarte, M., Hays, A., Singh, N., and Wanat, F. E.: Emery-Dreifuss muscular dystrophy. Ann. Neurol. *5*:111, 1979.
65. Fenichel, G. M., Sul, Y. C., Kilroy, A. W., and Blouin, R.: An autosomal dominant dystrophy with humeropelvic distribution and cardiomyopathy. Neurology *32*:1399, 1982.
66. Chakrabarti, A., and Pearce, J. M.: Scapuloperoneal syndrome with cardiomyopathy. J. Neurol. Neurosurg. Psychiatry *44*:1146, 1981.
67. Hopkins, L. C., Jackson, J. H., and Elsas, L. J.: Emery-Dreifuss humeroperoneal muscular dystrophy: An X-linked myopathy with unusual contractures and bradycardia. Ann. Neurol. *10*:230, 1981.
68. Dickey, P. P., Ziter, F. A., and Smith, R. A.: Emery-Dreifuss muscular dystrophy. J. Pediatr. *104*:555, 1984.
69. Takamoto, K., Hirose, K., and Nonaka, I.: A genetic variant of Emery-Dreifuss disease. Arch. Neurol. *41*:1292, 1984.
70. Harper, P. S.: Myotonic Dystrophy. Philadelphia, W.B. Saunders Company, 1979.
71. Kohn, N. N., Faires, J. S., and Rodman, T.: Unusual manifestations due to involvement of involuntary muscle in dystrophia myotonica. N. Engl. J. Med. *271*:1179, 1964.
72. Bharati, S., Bump, F. T., Bauernfeind, R., and Lev, M.: Dystrophica myotonia. Correlative electrocardiographic, electrophysiologic and conduction system study. Chest *86*:444, 1984.
73. Moorman, J. R., Coleman, R. E., Packer, D. L., Kisslo, J. A., Bell, J., Hettleman, B. D., Stajich, J., and Roses, A. D.: Cardiac involvement in myotonic muscular dystrophy. Medicine *64*:371, 1985.
74. Komajda, M., Frank, R., Vedel, J., Fontaine, A., Petitot, J., and Grosgogeat, Y.: Intracardiac conduction defects in dystrophia myotonica. Br Heart J. *43*:315, 1980.
75. Kennel, A. J., Titis, J. L., and Merideth, J.: Pathologic findings in the atrioventricular conduction system in myotonic dystrophy. Mayo Clin. Proc. *49*:838, 1974.
76. Grigg, L. E., Chan, W., Mond, H. G., Vohra, J. K., and Downey, W. F.: Ventricular tachycardia and sudden death in myotonic dystrophy: Clinical, electrophysiologic and pathologic features. Am. J. Cardiol. *6*:254, 1985.
77. Prystowsky, E. N., Pritchett, E. L. C., Roses, A. D., and Gallagher, J. J.: The natural history of conduction system disease in myotonic muscular dystrophy as determined by serial electrophysiologic studies. Circulation *60*:1360, 1979.
78. Uemura, N., Tanaka, H., Niimura, T., Nashiguchi, N., Yoshimura, M., Terashi, S., and Kanehiser, T.: Electrophysiological and histological abnormalities of the heart in myotonic dystrophy. Am. Heart J. *86*:616, 1973.
79. Petkovich, N. J., Dunn, M., and Reed, W.: Myotonia dystrophica with AV dissociation and Stokes-Adams attacks. Am. Heart J. *68*:391, 1964.
80. Bulloch, R. T., Davis, J. L., and Hara, M.: Dystrophia myotonica with heart block. A light and electron microscopic study. Arch. Pathol. *84*:130, 1967.
81. Holt, J. M., and Lambert, E. H. N.: Heart disease as presenting feature of myotonia atrophica. Br. Heart J. *26*:433, 1964.
82. Fearrington, E. L., Gibson, T. C., and Churchill, R. E.: Vectorcardiographic and electrocardiographic findings in myotonia atrophica. Am. Heart J. *67*:599, 1964.
83. Motta, J., Guilleminault, C., Bilingham, M., Barry, W., and Mason, J.: Cardiac abnormalities in myotonic dystrophy: Electrophysiologic and histopathologic studies. Am. J. Med. *67*:467, 1979.
84. Ludatscher, R. M., Kerner, H., Amikam, S., and Gellei, B.: Myotonia dystrophica with heart involvement: An electron microscopic study of skeletal, cardiac, and smooth muscle. J. Clin. Pathol. *31*:1057, 1978.
85. Tanaka, N., Tanaka, H., Takeda, M., Niimura., T., Kanehisa, T., and Terashi, S.: Cardiomyopathy in myotonic dystrophy: A light and electron microscopic study of the myocardium. Jpn. Heart J. *14*:202, 1973.
86. Hartwig, G. R., Ran, K. R., Radoff, F. M., Coleman, R. E., Jones, R. H., and Roses, A. D.: Radionuclide angiocardiographic analysis of myocardial function in myotonic muscular dystrophy. Neurology *33*:657, 1983.
86a. Hiromasa, S., Ikeda, T., Kubota, K., Takata, S., Hattori, N., Nishimura, M., and Watanabe, Y.: A family with myotonic dystrophy associated with diffuse cardiac conduction disturbances as demonstrated by His bundle electrocardiography. Am. Heart J. *111*:85, 1986.
87. Harper, P. S.: Congenital myotonic dystrophy in Britain. I. Clinical aspects. Arch. Dis. Child. *50*:505, 1975.
88. Anderson, M.: Probable Thomsen's disease with cardiac involvement. J. Neurol. *214*:301, 1977.
89. Subramony, S. H., Malhotra, C. P., and Mishra, S. K.: Distinguishing paramyotonia congenita and myotonia congenita by electromyography. Muscle Nerve *6*:374, 1983.
90. Streib, F. W., Sun, S. F., and Hanson, M.: Paramyotonia congenita: Clinical and electrophysiologic studies. Electromyogr. Clin. Neurophysiol. *23*:315, 1983.
91. Rosenberg, R. N.: Hereditary ataxias. *In* Rowland, L. P. (ed.): Merritt's Textbook of Neurology. Philadelphia, Lea and Febiger, 1984, p. 499.
92. Barbeau, H.: Friedreich's ataxia 1980. Our overview of the pathophysiology. J. Can. Sci. Neurol. *7*:455, 1980.
93. Harding, A. E.: Friedreich's ataxia: A clinical and genetic study of 90 families with an analysis of early diagnostic criteria and intrafamilial clustering of clinical features. Brain *104*:589, 1981.
94. Andermann, E., Remillard, G. M., Goyer, C., Blitzer, L., Anderman, F., and Barbeau, A.: Genetic and family studies in Friedreich's ataxia. J. Can. Sci. Neurol. *3*:287, 1976.

95. Butterworth, R. F., Shapcott, D., Melancon, S., Breton, G., Geoffroy, G., Lemieux, B., and Barbeau, A.: Clinical laboratory findings in Friedreich's ataxia. J. Can. Sci. Neurol. *3*:335, 1976.
96. Brumback, R. A., Panner, B. J., and Kingston, W. J.: The heart in Friedreich's ataxia. Arch. Neurol. *43*:189, 1986.
97. Grenadier, E., Goldberg, S. J., Stern, L. Z., and Feldman, J.: M-mode and two-dimensional echocardiographic examination of patients with Friedreich's ataxia. J. Cardiovasc. Ultrasonog. *3*:5, 1984.
98. Gottdiener, J. S., Hawley, R. J., Maron, B. J., Bertorini, T. F., and Engle, W. K.: Characteristics of the cardiac hypertrophy in Friedreich's ataxia. Am. Heart J. *103*:525, 1982.
99. Barbeau, A.: Pathophysiology of Friedreich's ataxia. *In* Matthews, W. B., and Glaser, G. H. (eds.): Recent Advances in Clinical Neurology, No. 3. Edinburgh, Churchill Livingstone, 1982, p. 129.
100. Pasternac, A., Drol, R., Petitclerc, R., Harvey, C., Andermann, E., and Barbeau, A.: Hypertrophic cardiomyopathy in Friedreich's ataxia: Symmetric or asymmetric? J. Can. Sci. Neurol. *7*:379, 1980.
101. Harding, A. E., and Hewer, R. L.: The heart disease of Friedreich's ataxia: A clinical and electrocardiographic study of 115 patients, with an analysis of serial electrocardiographic changes in 30 cases. Quart. J. Med. *28*:489, 1983.
101a. Zimmermann, M., Gabathuler, J., Adamec, R., and Pinget, L.: Unusual manifestations of heart involvement in Friedreich's ataxia. Am. Heart J. *111*:184, 1986.
102. Sanchez-Casis, G., Cote, M., and Barbeau, A.: Pathology of the heart in Friedreich's ataxia: Review of the literature and report of one case. J. Can. Sci. Neurol. *3*:349, 1976.
102a. Hawle, R. J., and Gottdiener, J. S.: Five-year follow-up of Friedreich's ataxia cardiomyopathy. Arch. Intern. Med. *146*:483, 1986.
102b. Unverferth, D. V., Schmidt, W. R., Baker, P. B., and Wooley, C. F.: Morphologic and functional characteristics of the heart in Friedreich's ataxia. Am. J. Med. *82*:5, 1987.
103. Pentland, B., and Fox, K. A. A.: The heart in Friedreich's ataxia. J. Neurol. Neurosurg. Psychiatry *46*:1138, 1983.
104. Hewer, R. L.: The heart in Friedreich's ataxia. Br. Heart J. *31*:5, 1969.
105. Spach, N. S., and Kootsey, J. M.: The nature of electrical propagation in cardiac muscle. Am. J. Physiol. *244*:H3, 1983.
106. Keren, A., Billingham, M. E., Weintraub, D., Stinson, E. B., and Popp, R. L.: Mildly dilated congestive cardiomyopathy. Circulation *72*:302, 1985.
107. James, T. N., and Fisch, C.: Observations on the cardiovascular involvement in Friedreich's ataxia. Am. Heart J. *66*:164, 1963.
108. Rowland, L. P.: Molecular genetics, pseudogenetics and clinical neurology. The Robert Wartenberg Lecture. Neurology *33*:179, 1983.
109. Rosenberg, R. N.: Biochemical genetics of neurologic disease. N. Engl. J. Med. *305*:1181, 1981.
110. Perloff, J. K.: Pathogenesis of hypertrophic cardiomyopathy. *In* Goodwin, J. F. (ed.): Heart Muscle Disease. Lancaster, MTP Press Ltd., 1985.
111. Pasternac, A., Wagniart, P., Olivenstein, R., Petitclerc, R., Krol, R., Andermann, E., Melancon, S., Geoffroy, G., de Champlain, J., and Barbeau, A.: Increased plasma catecholamines in patients with Friedreich's ataxia. J. Can. Sci. Neurol. *9*:195, 1982.
112. Merkel, A. D., and Barbeau, A.: Plasma catecholamines in Friedreich's ataxia assayed using high performance liquid chromatography with electrochemical detection. J. Can. Sci. Neurol. *9*:205, 1982.
113. Perloff, J. K., Child, J. S., and Edwards, J. E.: New guidelines for the clinical diagnosis of mitral valve prolapse. Am. J. Cardiol., *57*:1124, 1986.

LESS COMMON NEUROMYOPATHIC DISEASES SOMETIMES ASSOCIATED WITH HEART DISEASE

114. Isner, J. M., Hawley, R. J., Weintraub, A. B., and Engel, W. K.: Cardiac findings in Charcot-Marie-Tooth disease. Arch. Intern. Med. *139*:1161, 1979.
115. Leak, D.: Paroxysmal atrial flutter in peroneal muscular atrophy. Br. Heart J. *23*:326, 1961.
116. Littler, W. A.: Heart block and peroneal muscular atrophy. Quart. J. Med. *39*:431, 1970.
117. Kaj, J. M., Littler, W. A., and Meade, J. B.: Ultrastructure of the myocardium in familial heart block and peroneal muscular atrophy. Br. Heart J. *34*:1081, 1972.
118. Lowry, P. I., and Littler, W. A.: Peroneal muscular atrophy associated with cardiac conduction tissue disease. Postgrad. Med. J. *59*:530, 1983.
119. Martin-Du Pan, R. C., Juse, C., and Perrenoud, J. J.: Congestive cardiomyopathy and pyruvate elevation in a case of Charcot-Marie-Tooth disease. Schweiz. med. Wochenschr. *5*:114, 1984.
120. Spiro, A. J., Shy, G. M., and Gonatas, N. K.: Myotubular myopathy. Arch. Neurol. *14*:1, 1966.
121. Verhiest, W., Brucher, J. M., Goddeeris, P., Lauweryns, J., and DeGeest, H.: Familial centronuclear myopathy associated with cardiomyopathy. Br. Heart J. *38*:504, 1976.
122. Bethlem, J., Van Wijngaarden, G. K., Meijerae, F. H., and Hulfmann, W. C.: Neuromuscular disease with type I fiber atrophy, centronuclei and myotube-like structures. Neurology *19*:705, 1969.
123. Shafiq, S. A., Sande, M. A., Carruthers, R. R., Killip, T., and Milhorat, A. T.: Skeletal muscle in idiopathic cardiomyopathy. J. Neurol. Sci. *15*:303, 1972.
124. Berenberg, R. A., Pellock, J. M., DiMauro, S., Scholland, D. L., Bonilla, E., Eastwood, A., Hays, A., Vicale, C. T., Behrens, M., Chutorian, A., and Rowland, L. P.: Lumping or splitting? "Ophthalmoplegia-plus" or Kearns-Sayre syndrome? Ann. Neurol. *1*:37, 1977.
125. Lowes, M.: Chronic progressive external ophthalmoplegia, pigmentary retinopathy and heart block (Kearns-Sayre syndrome). Acta Ophthalmol. *53*:610, 1975.
126. Charles, R., Holt, S., Kay, J. M., Epstein, E. J., and Rees, J. R.: Myocardial ultrastructure and the development of atrioventricular block in Kearns-Sayre syndrome. Circulation *63*:214, 1981.
127. Roberts, N. K., Perloff, J. K., and Kark, P.: Cardiac conduction in Kearns-Sayre syndrome. Am. J. Cardiol. *44*:1396, 1979.
127a. Schwartzkopff, B., Frenzel, H., Losse, B., Borggrefe, M., Toyka, K. V., Hammerstein, W., Seitz, R., Deckert, M., and Breithardt, G.: Heart involvement in progressive external ophthalmoplegia (Kearns-Sayre syndrome): Electrophysiologic, hemodynamic and morphologic findings. Z. Kardiol. *75*:161, 1986.
128. Clark, D. S., Myerburg, R. J., Morales, R. R., Befeler, B., Hernandez, F. A., and Gelband, H.: Heart block and Kearns-Sayre: Electrophysiologic-pathologic correlation. Chest *68*:727, 1975.
129. Pleasure, D. E., and Schotland, D. L.: Acquired neuropathies. *In* Rowland L. P. (ed.): Merritt's Textbook of Neurology. 7th ed. Philadelphia, Lea and Febiger, 1984.
130. Emmons, P. R., Blume, W. T., and DuShane, J. W.: Cardiac monitoring and demand pacemaker in Guillain-Barré syndrome. Arch. Neurol. *32*:59, 1975.
131. Greenland, P., and Griggs, R. C.: Arrhythmic complications in the Guillain-Barré syndrome. Arch. Intern. Med. *140*:1053, 1980.
132. Narayam, D., Huang, M. T., and Matthew, P. K.: Bradycardia and asystole requiring pacemaker in Guillain-Barré syndrome. Am. Heart J. *108*:426, 1984.
133. Fagius, J., and Wallin, B. G.: Microneurographic evidence of excessive sympathetic outflow in the Guillain-Barré syndrome. Brain *106*:589, 1983.
134. Persson, A., and Solders, G.: R-R variations in Guillain-Barré syndrome: A test of autonomic dysfunction. Acta Neurol. Scand. *67*:294, 1983.
135. Palferman, T. G., Wright, I., Doyle, D. V., and Amiel, S.: Electrocardiographic abnormalities and autonomic dysfunction in Guillain-Barré syndrome. Br. Med. J. *284*:1231, 1982.
136. Shy, G. M., Engel, W. K., Somers, J. E., and Wanko, T.: Nemaline myopathy; a new congenital myopathy. Brain *86*:793, 1963.
137. Conen, P. E., Murphy, G. E., and Donohue, W. L.: Light and electron microscopic studies of "myogranules" in a child with hypotonia and muscle weakness. Can. Med. Assoc. J. *89*:983, 1963.
138. Kinoshita, M., and Satoyoshi, E.: Type I fiber atrophy and nemaline bodies. Arch. Neurol. *31*:423, 1974.
139. Meier, C., Gertsch, M., Zimmerman, A., Voellmy, W., and Geissbukler, J.: Nemaline myopathy presenting as cardiomyopathy. N. Engl. J. Med. *308*:1536, 1983.
140. Meier, C., Voellmy, W., Gertsch, M., Zimmerman, A., and Geissbuhler, J.: Nemaline myopathy appearing in adults as cardiomyopathy: A clinicopathologic study. Arch. Neurol. *41*:443, 1984.
141. Penn, A. S., and Rowland, L. P.: Neuromuscular junction. *In* Rowland, L. P. (ed.): Merritt's Textbook of Neurology, Philadelphia, Lea and Febiger, 1984, p. 561.
142. Barnes, D. M.: Nervous and immune system disorders linked in a variety of diseases. Science *232*:160, 1985.
143. Gibson, T. C.: The heart in myasthenia gravis. Am. Heart J. *90*:389, 1975.
144. Kornfeld, P., Horowitz, S. H., Genkins, G., and Papatestas, A.: Myasthenia gravis unmasked by antiarrhythmic agents. Mt. Sinai J. Med. *43*:10, 1976.
145. Niakan, E., Bertorini, T. E., Acchiardo, S. R., and Werner, M. F.: Procainamide-induced myasthenia-like weakness in a patient with peripheral neuropathy. Arch. Neurol. *38*:378, 1981.
146. Ratinov, G., Baker, W. P., and Swaiman, K. F.: McArdle's syndrome with previously unreported electrocardiographic and serum enzyme abnormalities. Ann. Intern. Med. *62*:328, 1965.
147. Sengers, R. C. A., ter Haar, B. G. A., Trijhels, J. M. F., Willems, J. L., and Daniels, O.: Congenital cataract and mitochondrial myopathy of skeletal and heart muscle associated with lactic acidosis after exercise. J. Pediatr. *86*:873, 1975.

NEUROMUSCULAR DISORDERS PRESENTING AS CARDIOMYOPATHY

148. Isaacs, H., and Muncke, G.: Idiopathic cardiomyopathy and skeletal muscle abnormality. Am. Heart J. *90*:767, 1975.
149. Dunnigan, A., Pierpont, M. E., Smith, S. A., Breingstall, G., Benditt, D. G., and Benson, D. W.: Cardiac and skeletal myopathy associated with cardiac arrhythmias. Am. J. Cardiol. *53*:731, 1984.
150. Lambert, C. D., and Fairfax, A. J.: Neurological associations of chronic heart block. J. Neurol. Neurosurg. Psychiatry *39*:571, 1976.
151. Fairfax, A. J., and Lambert, C. D.: Neurological aspects of sinoatrial heart block. J. Neurol. Neurosurg. Psychiatry *39*:576, 1976.
152. Gottdiener, J. S., Sherber, H. S., Hawley, R. J., and Engel, W. K.: Cardiac manifestations in polymyositis. Am. J. Cardiol. *41*:1141, 1978.
153. Singsen, B., Goldreyer, B., Stanton, R., and Hanson, V.: Childhood polymyositis with cardiac conduction defects. Am. J. Dis. Child. *131*:72, 1976.
154. Farber, H. W., and Make, B.: Physiologic closure of a symptomatic patent foramen ovale with oxygen therapy. Am. Rev. Resp. Dis. *131*:181, 1985.
155. Lisak, R. P., Lebeau, J., Tucker, S. H., and Rowland, L. P.: Hyperkalemic periodic paralysis and cardiac arrhythmias. Neurology *22*:810, 1972.
156. Buruma, O. J., Schipperheyn, J. J., and Bots, G. T.: Heart muscle disease in familial hypokalemic periodic paralysis. Circulation *64*:12, 1981.
157. Klein, R., Ganelin, R., Marks, J. F., Usher, P., and Richards, C.: Periodic paralysis with cardiac arrhythmia. J. Pediatr. *62*:371, 1963.
158. Kastor, J. A., and Goldreyer, B. N.: Ventricular origin of bidirectional tachycardia. Circulation *48*:897, 1973.
159. Regan, T. J.: Alcoholic cardiomyopathy. *In* Fowler, N. O. (ed.): Myocardial Disease. New York, Grune and Stratton, 1973, p. 233.
160. Meyer, J. G., and Urban, K.: Electrolyte changes and acid-base balance after alcohol withdrawal. With special reference to rum fits and magnesium depletion. J. Neurol. *215*:135, 1977.
161. Rubin, E.: Alcoholic myopathy in heart and skeletal muscle. N. Engl. J. Med. *301*:28, 1979.
162. Clarren, S. K., and Smith, D. W.: The fetal alcohol syndrome. N. Engl. J. Med. *298*:1063, 1978.

ACUTE CEREBRAL DISORDERS ACCOMPANIED BY CARDIOVASCULAR ABNORMALITIES

163. Vanderark, G. D.: Cardiovascular changes with acute subdural hematoma. Surg. Neurol. *3*:305, 1975.
164. Bramwell, C.: Can head injury cause auricular fibrillation? Lancet *1*:8, 1934.
165. Chen, H. I., Liao, J. F., and Ho, S. T.: Centrogenic pulmonary hemorrhagic edema induced by cerebral compression in rats. Circ. Res. *47*:366, 1980.
166. Yamour, B. J., Sridharan, M. R., Rice, J. F., and Flowers, N. C.: Electrocardiographic changes in cerebrovascular hemorrhage. Am. Heart J. *99*:294, 1980.
167. Robertson, C. S., Clifton, G. L., Taylor, A. A., and Grossman, R. G.: Treatment of hypertension associated with head injury. J. Neurosurg. *59*:455, 1983.
168. Cushing, H.: Concerning a definite regulatory mechanism of the vasomotor center which controls blood pressure during cerebral compression. Bull. Johns Hopkins Hosp. *12*:390, 1901.
169. Sciarra, D.: Head injury. *In* Rowland, L. P. (ed.): Merritt's Textbook of Neurology. 7th ed. Philadelphia, Lea and Febiger, 1984, p. 277.
170. Hackenberry, L. E., Miner, M. E., Rea, G. L., Woo, J., and Graham, S. H.: Biochemical evidence of myocardial injury after severe head trauma. Crit. Care Med. *10*:641, 1982.
171. Clifton, G. L., Robertson, C. S., Kyper, K., Taylor, A. A., Dhekne, R. D., and Grossman, R. G.: Cerebrovascular response to severe head injury. J. Neurosurg. *59*:447, 1983.
172. McLeod, A. A., Neil-Dwyer, G., Meyer, C. H. A., Richardson, P. L., Cruickshank, J., and Bartlett, J.: Cardiac sequelae of acute head injury. Br. Heart J. *47*:221, 1982.
173. Baur, H. R., Gobel, F. L., and Pierach, C. A.: Electrocardiograpic changes after cervical laminectomy. Int. J. Cardiol. *1*:37, 1981.
174. Samuels, M. A.: Electrocardiographic manifestations of neurologic disease. Semin. Neurol. *4*:453, 1984.
175. Carruth, J. E., and Silverman, M. E.: *Torsade de pointe* atypical ventricular tachycardia complicating subarachnoid hemorrhage. Chest *78*:886, 1980.
176. Mikolich, J. R., Jacobs, W. C., and Fletcher, G. F.: Cardiac arrhythmias in patients with acute cerebrovascular accidents. J.A.M.A. *246*:1314, 1981.
177. Goldberger, A. L.: Recognition of ECG pseudoinfarct patterns. Mod. Concepts Cardiovasc. Dis. *49*:13, 1980.
178. Taylor, A. L., and Fozzard, H. A.: Ventricular arrhythmias associated with CNS disease. Arch. Intern. Med. *142*:232, 1982.
179. Dimant, J., and Grob, D.: Electrocardiographic changes and myocardial damage in patients with acute cerebrovascular accidents. Stroke *8*:448, 1977.
180. Gould, L., Reddy, R. C., Kollali, M., Singh, B. K., and Zen, B.: Electrocardiographic normalization after cerebral vascular accident. J. Electrocardiol. *14*:191, 1981.
181. Myers, M. G., Norris, J. W., Hachinski, V. C., Weingert, M. E., and Sole, M. J.: Cardiac sequelae of acute stroke. Stroke *13*:838, 1982.
182. Melin, J., and Fogelhohm, R.: Electrocardiographic findings in subarachnoid hemorrhage. Acta Med. Scand. *213*:5, 1983.
183. Brunninkhuis, L. G. H.: Electrocardiographic abnormalities suggesting myocardial infarction in a patient with severe cranial trauma. Pace *6*:1336, 1983.
184. Gascon, P., Ley, T. J., Toltzis, R. J., and Bonow, R. O.: Spontaneous subarachnoid hemorrhage simulating acute transmural myocardial infarction. Am. Heart J. *105*:511, 1983.
185. Miah, K., von Arbin, M., Britton, M., de Faire, U., Helmers, C., and Maasing, R.: Prognosis in acute stroke with special reference to some cardiac factors. J. Chronic Dis. *36*:279, 1983.
186. Komrad, M. S., Coffey, C. E., Coffey, K. S., McKinnis, R., Massey, E. W., and Califf, R. M.: Myocardial infarction and stroke. Neurology *34*:1403, 1984.
187. Chin, P. L., Kaminski, J., and Rout, N.: Myocardial infarction coincident with cerebrovascular accidents in the elderly. Age Aging *6*:29, 1977.
188. Gillum, R. F., Fortmann, S. P., Prineas, R. J., and Kottke, T. E.: International diagnostic criteria for acute myocardial infarction and acute stroke. Am. Heart J. *108*:150, 1984.
189. Sandok, B. A., Whisnant, J. P., Furlan, A. J., and Mickell, J. L.: Carotid arterial bruits. Mayo Clin. Proc. *57*:227, 1982.
190. Heyman, A., Wilkinson, W. E., Heyden, S., Helms, M. J., Bartel, A. G., Karp, H. R., Tyroler, H. A., and Hames, C. G.: Risk of stroke in asymptomatic persons with cervical arterial bruits. N. Engl. J. Med. *302*:838, 1980.
191. Roper, A. H., Wechsler, L. R., and Wilson, L. S.: Carotid bruit and the risk of stroke in elective surgery. N. Engl. J. Med. *307*:1388, 1982.
192. Busuttil, R. W., Baker, J. D., Davidson, R. K., and Machleder, H. I.: Carotid arterial stenosis: Hemodynamic significance and clinical course. J.A.M.A. *245*:1438, 1981.
193. Wolf, P. A., Kannel, W. B., Sorlie, P., and McNamara, P.: Asymptomatic carotid bruit and risk of stroke. J.A.M.A. *245*:1442, 1981.
194. Langlois, Y., Roederer, G. O., Chan, A., Phillips, D. J., Beach, K. W., Martin, D., Chikos, P. M., and Strandness, D. E.: Evaluating carotid arterial disease. Ultrasound Med. Biol. *9*:51, 1983.
195. Cebul, R. D., and Ginsberg, M. D.: Noninvasive neurovascular tests for carotid artery disease. Ann. Intern. Med. *97*:867, 1982.
196. Jones, E. L., Craver, J. M., Michalik, R. A., Murphy, D. A., Guyton, R. A., Bone, D. K., Hatcher, C. R., and Reichwald, N. A.: Combined carotid and coronary operations: When are they necessary? J. Thorac. Cardiovasc. Surg. *87*:7, 1984.
197. Rice, P. L., Pifarre, R., Sullivan, H. J., Montoya, A., and Bakhos, M.: Experience with simultaneous myocardial revascularization and carotid endarterectomy. J. Thorac. Cardiovasc. Surg. *79*:922, 1980.
198. Breslau, P. J., Fell, G., Ivey, T. D., Bailey, W. W., Miller, D. W., and Strandness, D. E., Jr.: Carotid arterial disease in patients undergoing coronary artery bypass operations. J. Thorac. Cardiovasc. Surg. *82*:765, 1981.
199. Breuer, A. C., Hanson, M. R., Furlan, A. J., Lederman, R. J., Loop, F. D., Cosgrove, D. M., and Estafanous, E. G.: Central nervous system complications of myocardial revascularization. A prospective analysis of 400 patients. Stroke *11*:136, 1980.
200. Gonzalez-Scarano, F., and Hurtig, H. I.: Neurologic complications of coronary artery bypass grafting: Case-control study. Neurology (NY) *31*:1032, 1981.
201. Bojar, R. M., Najafi, H., De Laria, G. A., Serry, C., and Goldin, M. D.: Neurological complications of coronary revascularization. Ann. Thorac. Surg. *36*:427, 1983.
202. Coffey, C. E., Massey, E. W., Roberts, K. B., Curtis, S. E., Jones, R. H., and Pryor, D. B.: Occurrence of stroke following coronary artery bypass graft surgery. Cardiovasc. Rev. Rep. *4*:1455, 1983.
203. Lee, M. C., Geiger, J., Nicoloff, D., Klassen, A. C., and Resch, J. A.: Cerebrovascular complications associated with coronary artery bypass (CAB) procedure. Stroke *10*:107, 1979.
204. Lederman, R. J., Breuer, A. C., Hanson, M. R., Furlan, A. J., Loop, F. D., Cosgrove, D. M., Estafanous, F. G., and Greenstreet, F. L.: Peripheral nervous system complications of coronary artery bypass graft surgery. Ann. Neurol. *12*:297, 1982.
205. Sotaniemi, K. A.: Brain damage and neurological outcome after open heart surgery. J. Neurol. Neurosurg. Psychiatry *43*:127, 1980.
206. Wolf, P. A., Dawber, T. R., Thomas, H. E., and Kannel, W. B., Epidemiologic assessment of chronic atrial fibrillation and risk of stroke: The Framingham Study. Neurology *28*:973, 1978.
207. Barletta, G. A., Gagliardi, R., Benvenuti, L., and Fantini, F.: Cerebral ischemic attacks as a complication of aortic and mitral valve prolapse. Stroke *16*:219, 1985.
208. Egeblad, H., and Sorenson, P. S.: Prevalence of mitral valve prolapse in younger patients with cerebral ischemic attacks. Acta Med. Scand. *216*:385, 1984.
209. Barnett, H. J. M., Boughner, D. R., Taylor, D. W., Cooper, P. E., Kostuk, W. J., and Nichol, P. M.: Further evidence relating mitral valve prolapse to cerebral ischemic events. N. Engl. J. Med. *302*:139, 1980.
210. Yufe, R., Karpati, G., and Carpenter, S.: Cardiac myxoma: A diagnostic challenge for the neurologist. Neurology *26*:1060, 1976.
211. Perloff, J. K.: The Clinical Recognition of Congenital Heart Disease. 3rd ed. Philadelphia, W.B. Saunders Company, 1986.
212. Baron, K. D., Siqueira, E., and Hirano, A.: Cerebral embolism caused by nonbacterial thrombotic endocarditis. Neurology *10*:391, 1960.
213. Caplan, L. R., Hier, D. B., and Banks, G.: Stroke and drug abuse. Curr. Concepts Cerebrovasc. Dis. *17*:9, 1982.
214. Dodge, R. P., Richardson, E. P., and Victor, M.: Recurrent convulsive seizures as a sequel to cerebral infarction. Brain *77*:610, 1959.
215. Rosove, M. H., Perloff, J. K., Hocking, W. G., Child, J. S., Canobbio, M. M., and Skorton, D. J.: Chronic hypoxaemia and decompensated erythrocytosis in cyanotic congenital heart disease. Lancet, *2*:313, 1986.
216. Caronna, J. J., and Finklestein, S.: Neurological syndromes after cardiac arrest. Curr. Concepts Cerebrovasc. Dis. *13*:9, 1978.
217. Longstreth, W. T., Inui, T. S., Cobb, L. A., and Copass, M. K.: Neurologic recovery after out-of-hospital cardiac arrest. Ann. Intern. Med. *98*:588, 1983.
218. Snyder, B. D., Ramirez-Lassepas, M., and Lippert, D. M.: Neurologic status and prognosis after cardiopulmonary arrest. Neurology *27*:807, 1977.

CARDIAC COMPLICATIONS OF DRUGS USED IN TREATING NEUROMUSCULAR DISEASE

219. Orlando, R. C., Moyer, P., and Barnett, T. B.: Methysergide therapy and constrictive pericarditis. Ann. Intern. Med. *88*:213, 1978.
220. Bana, D. S., MacNeal, P. S., LeCompte, P. M., Shah, Y., and Graham, J. R.: Cardiac murmurs and endocardial fibrosis associated with methysergide therapy. Am. Heart J. *88*:640, 1974.
221. Graham, J. R., Suby, H. I., LeCompte, P. M., and Sadowsky, N. L.: Fibrotic disorders associated with methysergide therapy for headaches. N. Engl. J. Med. *274*:359, 1966.
222. Roberts, W. C., and Sjoerdsma, A.: The cardiac disease associated with the carcinoid syndrome (carcinoid heart disease). Am. J. Med. *36*:5, 1964.
223. Thorner, M. O.: Dopamine—An important neurotransmitter in the autonomic nervous system. Lancet *1*:662, 1975.
224. Calne, D. B., Brennan, J., Spiers, A. S. D., and Stern, G. M.: Hypotension caused by L-dopa. Br. Med. J. *1*:474, 1970.
225. Greenacre, J. K., Teychenne, T. F., Petrie, A., Calne, D. B., Leigh, P. N., and Reid, J. L.: The cardiovascular effects of bromocriptine in parkinsonism. Br. J. Clin. Pharmacol. *3*:571, 1976.

NEUROLOGICAL COMPLICATIONS OF THERAPY FOR CARDIOVASCULAR DISEASE

226. Francis, D. A., Heron, J. R., and Clarke, M.: Ambulatory electrocardiographic monitoring in patients with transient focal cerebral ischaemia. J. Neurol. Neurosurg. Psychiatry *47*:256, 1984.
227. Benorvitz, N. L.: Clinical applications of the pharmocokinetics of lidocaine. Cardiovasc. Clin. *6*:77, 1974.
228. Greenblatt, D. J., and Koch-Weser, J.: Adverse reactions to propranolol in hospital medical patients. Am. Heart J. *87*:478, 1973.
229. Weidler, D. J., Jallad, N. S., Keener, D. B., Das, S. K., and Wagner, J. G.: The effects of acute focal cerebral ischemia on digoxin toxicity and pharmacokinetics. Pharmacology *20*:188, 1980.
230. Withering, W.: An account of the Foxglove. *In* Willius, F. A., and Keys, T. E.: Classics of Cardiology. Vol. 1. New York, Dover Publications, 1941, p. 232.

CARDIAC DENERVATION

231. Oliveira, J. S. M., dos Santos, J. C. M., Muccillo, G., and Ferreira, A. L.: Increased capacity of the coronary arteries in chronic Chagas' heart disease: Further support for the neurogenic pathogenetic concept. Am. Heart J. *109*:304, 1985.
232. Mott, K. E., and Hagstrom, J. W. C.: The pathologic lesions of the cardiac autonomic nervous system in chronic Chagas' myocarditis. Circulation *31*:273, 1965.

58 ENDOCRINE AND NUTRITIONAL DISORDERS AND HEART DISEASE

by GORDON H. WILLIAMS, M.D., and
EUGENE BRAUNWALD, M.D.

In 1835, Robert Graves described "three cases of violent and long-continued palpitation in females" with thyrotoxicosis.[1] Twenty years later, Thomas Addison reported that patients with disease of the "suprarenal capsules" had a "pulse, small and feeble . . . excessively soft and compressible." As the disease progressed "the body wastes . . . the pulse becomes smaller and weaker, and . . . the patient at length gradually sinks and expires."[2] Thus, since the mid-19th century, it has been known that deranged hormonal secretion can significantly alter cardiovascular function. The purpose of this chapter is to summarize the more important cardiovascular manifestations of endocrine and nutritional diseases.

ACROMEGALY

The anterior pituitary gland secretes at least seven polypeptide hormones. Four (ACTH and related peptides, FSH, LH, and TSH) primarily produce their biological effect indirectly by altering hormonal secretion from a specific target gland (adrenal cortex, gonad, and thyroid). Thus, the pathophysiological manifestations of a derangement in their secretion are the same as those of their target organs and will be discussed later. There are no cardiovascular manifestations of altered prolactin secretion or growth hormone deficiency; however, acromegaly (growth hormone excess) is associated with a number of clinical signs and symptoms related to the cardiovascular system.

ACTIONS OF GROWTH HORMONE. Growth hormone is only one of a family of peptides whose overall function is to regulate growth of the organism.[3,4] Two hormones secreted by the hypothalamus (somatotropin-releasing hormone and somatostatin) regulate the release of growth hormone from the anterior pituitary.[5,6] After growth hormone is released into the circulation it stimulates the production of insulin-like growth factors (IGF-I and IGF-II).[7] These growth factors are primarily made under the influence of growth hormone in the liver. They are homologs of the proinsulin molecule and therefore have biological effects that are qualitatively similar to those of insulin. It is uncertain whether either or both can be produced in the absence of growth hormone; although presently available data suggest that at least IGF-II, the weaker growth-promoting hormone, may not require growth hormone for synthesis. Thus, it is likely that IGF-I (somatomedin C) may be the major final mediator of growth hormone's biological effects.[3,4] It feeds back on the pituitary, modifying mRNA levels in the pituitary and growth hormone secretion.[8] In this chapter, by convention the term *growth hormone* effects is used, although most of these effects are probably mediated by the insulin-like growth factors, particularly somatomedin C.

Growth hormone effects influence many metabolic processes, but the net effect is anabolic. Thus, when growth hormone is administered to a growth hormone-deficient individual, positive nitrogen balance, with retention of calcium, sodium, potassium, magnesium, and chloride, is manifest within days.[3,4] While many facets of nitrogen metabolism following administration of growth hormone have been studied, its primary effect has not been assessed definitively. Growth hormone increases the synthesis of both transfer and messenger RNA.[9] It reduces the breakdown of amino acids to urea and increases the transport of amino acids into skeletal and cardiac muscle, thus augmenting the substrate available for protein synthesis.[10] However, direct measurement of intracellular amino acid content has not documented the increase expected if these actions were the only ones responsible for the increased protein synthesis.

Growth hormone also induces changes in both fat and carbohydrate metabolism.[3] When administered for a short time, it increases the uptake and utilization of glucose by fat cells, thus increasing lipogenesis. However, when administered over a long period, it promotes lipolysis, thus increasing plasma free fatty acid levels and their oxidation and promoting ketogenesis, particularly in diabetic patients or animals. Growth hormone reduces glucose uptake by fat and muscle cells, increases gluconeogenesis, and increases peripheral resistance to insulin; as a consequence, plasma glucose levels rise. Because of this reduced tissue uptake of glucose and the increased blood levels of free fatty acids and ketones, those tissues, like the myocardium, that are able to use these latter compounds as energy substrates, do so.

Growth hormone also increases the synthesis and/or accumulation of sulfated mucopolysaccharides in connective tissue.

EFFECT OF SOMATOSTATIN ON THE HEART. *Somatostatin* has an effect on the heart beyond that induced by its effect on growth hormone secretion. Infusion of somatostatin causes bradycardia and a fall in cardiac output. Furthermore, in some cases of superventricular arrhythmias somatostatin administration restores sinus rhythm.[11] Finally, cardiac nerves have been shown to contain somatostatin, suggesting that this hormone may be an important physiological regulator of cardiac conduction.[12]

CLINICAL AND BIOCHEMICAL MANIFESTATIONS. Acromegaly is almost invariably the result of a growth hormone–producing chromophobic or eosinophilic pituitary adenoma, although rarely it may be secondary to ectopic production of growth hormone or somatotropin-releasing hormone.[13] Characteristically, the disease is a slowly progressive one with signs and symptoms often predating diagnosis by more than 10 years. The striking physical findings (broad, spadelike hands and feet) are the result of growth hormone's effect on bone, muscle, and connective tissue. Osteoarthritis is common, as is organomegaly, hypertrichosis, hyperhidrosis, and modest weight gain.[14]

A derangement in carbohydrate metabolism is the most common metabolic consequence of chronic overproduction of growth hormone. Impaired glucose tolerance is found in half the patients, and hyperinsulinism is present in nearly all; thus a state of insulin resistance exists. However, clinical diabetes mellitus is present in only 10 per cent of patients, which suggests that only those who are predisposed and have limited insulin reserve actually develop overt disease.[15] While it might be anticipated that hyperlipidemia would be common in acromegaly, it is in fact infrequently observed except in patients with clinical diabetes mellitus.[3, 4, 15] Even in these patients, it is probably secondary to the decreased secretion of insulin rather than to the increased secretion of growth hormone.

CARDIOVASCULAR MANIFESTATIONS

The cardiac manifestations of acromegaly include cardiac enlargement that is greater than would be anticipated for the generalized organomegaly. In addition, the frequency of a number of other cardiovascular disorders is increased in acromegaly: hypertension, premature coronary artery disease, congestive heart failure, and cardiac arrhythmias, particularly frequent ventricular premature beats and intraventricular conduction defects.[16, 17] Indeed, because of the frequent occurrence of congestive heart failure and cardiac arrhythmias in patients who otherwise have no predisposing factors (e.g., no hypertension or arteriosclerosis), it has been suggested that a specific acromegalic cardiomyopathy exists[18] (see below).

CARDIOMEGALY. Nearly all patients with acromegaly have cardiomegaly (Fig. 58–1), particularly after the fifth decade.[19, 20] Echocardiographic assessment suggests that frequently there is an increase in cardiac mass, particularly asymmetrical septal hypertrophy, and in a sizable minority left ventricular dilatation and a reduced ejection fraction.[20] Although the cardiomegaly may be related to the generalized effect of growth hormone on protein synthesis, some data suggest that other factors may also be important. For example, enlargement of the heart is often greater than that of other organs. Furthermore, there is no direct relationship between the degree of cardiomegaly and the level of circulating growth hormone.[16] While there is a correlation between the duration of acromegaly and the severity of cardiac hypertrophy,[18] other factors which may be important in the genesis of cardiomegaly include hypertension and atherosclerosis, both of which occur with increased frequency in acromegaly. Focal cardiac interstitial fibrosis and a myocarditis with lymphocytic infiltrate also have been reported in the majority of cases.[18, 21] The former is probably due to the effect of growth hormone on collagen synthesis. Additionally, small-vessel disease of the myocardium occasionally may be present.[18] The resultant dysfunction in cardiac contraction secondary to any of these pathological changes could also contribute to the cardiac hypertrophy. Finally, the cardiomyopathy characteristic of acromegaly may also contribute to the cardiomegaly.

HYPERTENSION. Hypertension is the most common cardiovascular manifestation of acromegaly, occurring in 15 to 50 per cent of patients if individuals with hypopituitarism are excluded. Hypertensive acromegalic patients tend to be older and to have had their acromegaly longer than nonhypertensive acromegalic patients. The underlying pathophysiology is uncertain. However, the hypertension usually is mild, uncomplicated, and readily responsive to drugs.[16] Most investigators either have searched for factors other than growth hormone that could cause hypertension or have attempted to determine how growth hormone itself may produce hypertension. In many respects, patients with acromegaly appear to be volume expanded; the presence of an increase in glomerular filtration rate, renal plasma flow, extracellular fluid volume and sodium space, and reduction in plasma renin activity all support this hypothesis.[4, 22] Thus, several studies have assessed the secretion of aldosterone in acromegaly; while increased secretion has been reported, this is an uncommon finding.[22] What does appear to occur frequently in acromegalics, however, is a change in tissue responsiveness to angioten-

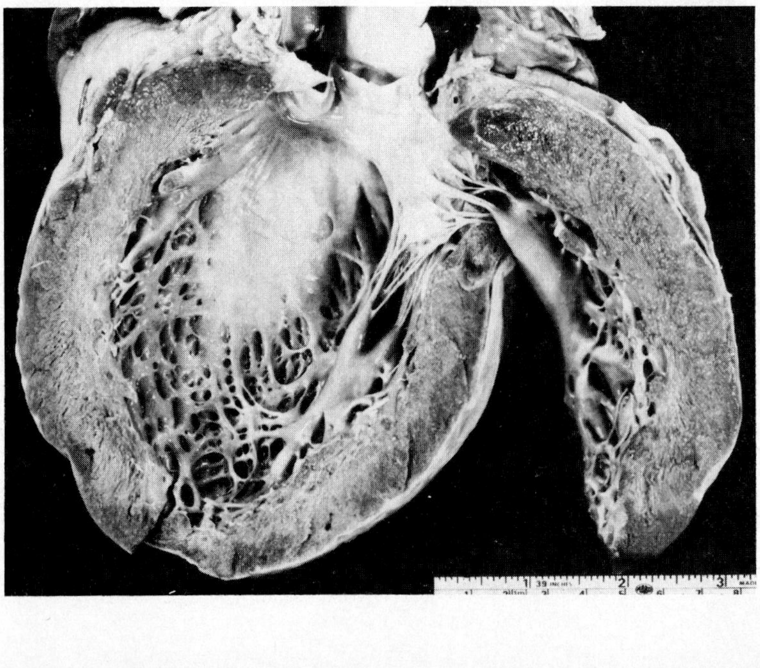

FIGURE 58–1. Opened left ventricle of the heart, showing the marked dilatation and hypertrophy, with fibrosis in the left septal endocardium. (From Rossi, L., et al.: Dysrhythmias and sudden death in acromegalic heart disease. A clinicopathologic study. Chest *72*:496, 1977.)

sin II. Thus, with a sodium-restricted intake the response of aldosterone production to angiotensin II is decreased, but the vasoconstrictor response is increased when compared to normal subjects. This abnormality is present in both hypertensive and normotensive acromegalics.[23] Whether this is related to the pathogenesis of the elevated arterial pressure or simply a reflection of an expanded extracellular fluid volume is unclear.

A number of studies have suggested that growth hormone itself may be responsible for the hypertension. Thus, pituitary irradiation or hypophysectomy significantly reduces arterial pressure in hypertensive acromegalic patients, even when full glucocorticoid replacement is carried out, unless growth hormone levels are not normalized.[17, 23] Indeed, the apparent volume expansion may be directly related to the elevated growth hormone levels, since administration of growth hormone can produce retention of sodium and expansion of extracellular fluid volume.[24] It has been proposed that the pathophysiology of the hypertension in acromegaly may be similar to that in essential hypertension. In both conditions, initially there may be elevation of cardiac output secondary to expansion of extracellular fluid volume (Chap. 27). This could elevate arterial pressure and lead ultimately to changes in the peripheral vasculature producing fixed hypertension.

ATHEROSCLEROSIS. In view of the alterations in carbohydrate and lipid metabolism caused by growth hormone (see above) as well as the high incidence of hypertension, it is not surprising that premature atherosclerosis occurs in patients with acromegaly. What is uncertain is its frequency.[18] Coronary atherosclerosis could also contribute to the cardiomegaly observed in these patients.

ACROMEGALIC CARDIOMYOPATHY. Some patients with acromegaly without evidence of hypertension or atherosclerosis have significant cardiac dysfunction.[18] They primarily have cardiomegaly, congestive heart failure, and/or cardiac dysrhythmias[21]; the congestive heart failure is particularly resistant to conventional therapy. It has been suggested that these are manifestations of an acromegalic cardiomyopathy which is related to the higher collagen content per gram of heart than in normal myocardium.[18] Histological observations show cellular hypertrophy, patchy fibrosis, and myofibrillar degeneration (Fig. 58–2). Sudden death has been associated with inflammatory and degenerative damage to the sinoatrial perinodal nerve plexus and degeneration of the AV node.[21]

It is not clear whether acromegalic cardiomyopathy is a specific entity. The evidence favoring this view is indirect and comes from four types of observations: (1) Nearly 50 per cent of acromegalic patients have electrocardiographic abnormalities.[25] The most common findings are ST-segment depression with or without T-wave abnormalities, patterns consistent with left ventricular hypertrophy, intraventricular conduction disturbances—specifically, bundle branch block—and, infrequently, supraventricular or ventricular ectopic rhythms. While hypertension or signs of atherosclerosis are present in many, 10 to 20 per cent of patients with acromegaly and electrocardiographic changes have no evidence of these conditions. (2) Ten to twenty per cent of acromegalics have overt congestive heart failure. In perhaps a fourth of these there is no known predisposing cause. (3) The majority of patients with acromegaly but without hypertension or atherosclerosis have subclinical evidence for cardiac dysfunction, as manifested by a shortening of the left ventricular ejection time (LVET), prolongation of the preejection period (PEP), and an increase in the PEP/LVET ratio[26] (p. 55). Approximately half of all patients with acromegaly, including patients without hypertension, have echocardiographic evidence of left ventricular hypertrophy.[27] These patients have growth hormone levels that are significantly higher than those of patients without left ventricular hypertrophy. Half of the patients with left ventricular hypertrophy exhibit asymmetrical septal hypertrophy, and these patients have a significantly greater percentage of internal dimensional shortening during systole than either the patients with concentric hypertrophy or those without left ventricular hypertrophy.

DIAGNOSIS AND TREATMENT

The *diagnosis* of acromegaly is established by documenting the nonsuppressibility of serum growth hormone levels following glucose loading.[4] In most laboratories, growth hormone concentrations in normal subjects are less than 2 ng/ml 120 minutes after the oral administration of

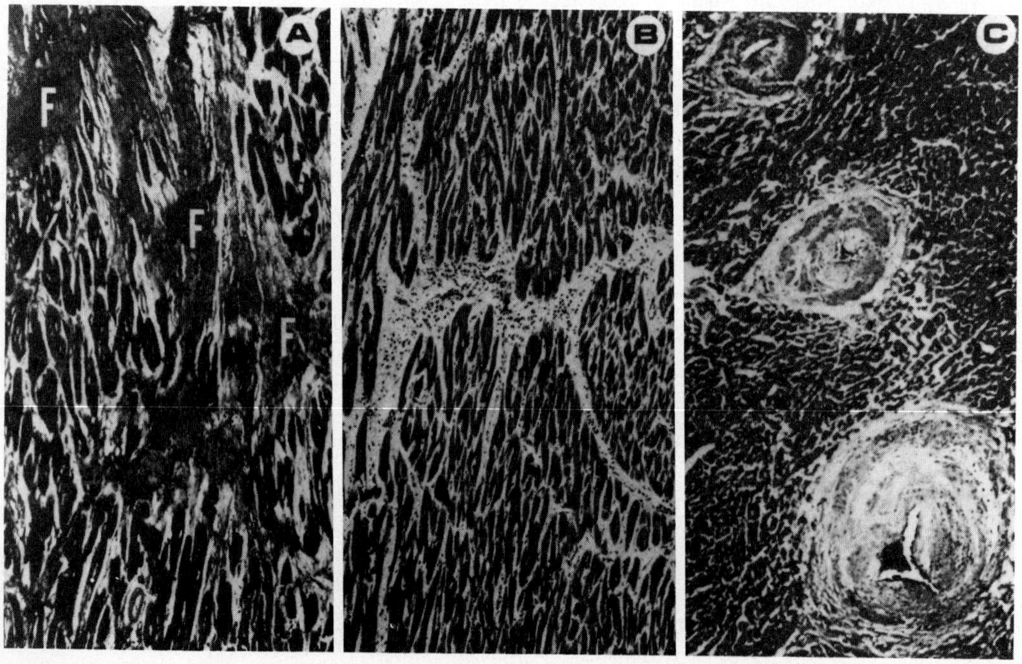

FIGURE 58–2. Histopathological features of acromegalic heart disease. *A*, Nonspecific myocardial hypertrophy and interstitial fibrosis (F). *B*, Myocarditis with predominantly lymphomononuclear cell infiltrate. *C*, Small vessel disease (proliferative fibrous wall thickening) or intramural coronary artery branches. (Reproduced with permission from Lie, J.T.: Acromegaly and heart disease. Primary Cardiol. *7*:53, 1981. Copyright PW Communications, Inc.)

100 gm of glucose. It is also important to evaluate the integrity of the other pituitary homones, and, in hypertensive patients, to rule out an associated pheochromocytoma or aldosteronoma. The presence of sinus tachycardia or atrial fibrillation in a patient with acromegaly warrants a careful search for coexisting hyperthyroidism.

Surgery and irradiation remain the mainstays of treatment. The surgical approach is more often transsphenoidal[28] rather than transfrontal; heavy particle (proton beam) instead of conventional irradiation is often used.[29] Because of the delayed reduction in growth hormone levels with the latter method, progression of cardiovascular disease in acromegalics continues even though growth hormone levels are falling. In a 10-year follow-up of 11 acromegalic patients, myocardial infarction, dysrhythmias, hypertension, major artery disease, and heart failure all increased significantly even though the growth hormone levels were falling.[17] The secretion of growth hormone can be suppressed in some acromegalics with the dopamine agonist, bromocriptine and somatostatin.[30, 31] Whether these agents have any effect on tumor growth, however, is unclear.

Acromegalic patients with cardiovascular abnormalities usually respond to conventional therapeutic measures for hypertension, heart failure, and arrhythmias. Two caveats: (1) those with hypertension appear to be particularly responsive to volume-depleting maneuvers, i.e., diuretics and sodium restriction, perhaps even more so than patients with essential hypertension; and (2) some patients with congestive heart failure, primarily those *without* underlying hypertensive heart disease (i.e., those who are considered to have acromegalic cardiomyopathy), appear to be particularly resistant to therapy.

THYROID DISEASE

Thyroid hormone has a profound effect on a number of metabolic processes in virtually all tissues, with the heart being particularly sensitive to its effects. Therefore, it is not surprising that thyroid dysfunction can produce dramatic cardiovascular effects, often mimicking primary cardiac disease.

ACTION OF THYROID HORMONE. Two biologically active hormones are secreted by the thyroid: thyroxine (T4) and triiodothyronine (T3). Most studies support the hypothesis that T3 is the final mediator and that T4 is a prohormone, primarily because of the universal presence of T3 but not T4 nuclear receptors in tissues responsive to thyroid hormone, specifically the heart.[32–34]

Even though the mechanism of action of thyroid hormone has been intensively investigated over the past three decades, uncertainty still exists about its principal effects. The preponderance of evidence now suggests that the major site of initiation of action of thyroid hormone is on the cell nucleus.[33] It has been observed that thyroid hormone is specifically bound to a chromatin-bound nonhistone nucleoprotein in the nucleus. As a result of this binding, alterations occur in protein synthesis, leading to many of the biochemical and metabolic effects observed with T4 administration.[34, 35] According to this hypothesis, the increased oxygen consumption results not from a direct interaction between thyroid hormone and mitochondria, an older hypothesis, but rather indirectly via an increase in mitochondrial protein synthesis secondary to the effect of the thyroid hormone on the nucleus. Support for this hypothesis comes from several sources: (1) specific binding of T3 and, much less strongly, of T4 to nuclear receptor sites has been documented[36]; (2) those tissues sensitive to thyroid hormone have nuclear binding sites[33]; (3) the addition of thyroid hormone in vitro produces an increase in O_2 consumption only after a significant time lag; (4) an early metabolic effect of T4 is an increased rate of incorporation of a labeled precursor into nuclear RNA[37]; (5) inhibitors of protein synthesis prevent many, if not most, of thyroid hormone's effects[38]; and (6) treatment of hypothyroid animals with T3 causes increases in in vivo synthesis of specific messenger RNA's in several tissues including the heart.[39]

Effect on Na^+, K^+-ATPase. Guernsey and Edelman have extended this hypothesis one step further.[40] They postulated that not only does thyroid hormone enhance protein synthesis, but it specifically increases the activity of Na^+, K^+-ATPase. Thus, the augmented hydrolysis of ATP at the site of the sodium pump in the sarcolemma stimulates cellular (mitochondrial) oxygen consumption. Support for this hypothesis includes the observations that (1) hypothyroid rats treated with T3 exhibit a reduction in active sodium transport in crude homogenates and membrane-rich fractions and a decrease in intracellular Na^+/K^+ ratio in liver, diaphragm, and kidney, and (2) the number of renal Na^+ pump sites and the incorporation of radiolabeled methionine into renal cortical Na^+, K^+-ATPase are both increased, suggesting an increase in protein synthesis as the primary event. Some reports, however, have suggested that the effect of thyroid hormone on cellular respiration cannot be entirely secondary to a change in the activity of this enzyme[41, 42] and that thyroid hormone also affects other cellular processes, e.g., the transport of glucose, particularly in the heart.[43]

Relation Between the Thyroid and the Sympathetic Nervous System

While the effects of thyroid hormone on the heart are varied and complex, it has been proposed that some of them are indirect, being secondary to changes in the activity of the sympathetic nervous system (Table 58–1). For example, many of the cardiovascular effects of hyperthyroidism, i.e., tachycardia, systolic hypertension, increased cardiac output, and myocardial contractility, can be abolished or reduced by blocking the activity of the sympathetic nervous system.[44] It has been proposed that thyroid hormone may alter the relationship between the sympathetic nervous and cardiovascular systems, either by increasing the activity of the sympathoadrenal system or by enhancing the response of cardiac tissue to normal sympathetic stimulation. Also, it has been suggested that sympathetic stimuli merely exert a direct additive effect on cardiovascular function above that produced by thyroid hormone. On the other hand, there is also evidence that hyperthyroidism reduces the sensitivity of cardiac tissue to sympathetic stimuli.[45]

Thus the results of experiments on the relationship between the sympathoadrenal system and hyperthyroidism have evoked considerable controversy. The plasma and urine levels of norepinephrine, epinephrine, dopamine, and beta-hydroxylase are either low or normal

TABLE 58–1 CLINICAL FEATURES OF HYPERTHYROIDISM*

Direct Thyroid Hormone Effect†	Beta-Adrenergic-Like Effect†
Resting heart rate > 90/min (90%)	**Resting heart rate > 90/min (90%)**
Palpitations (85%)	**Palpitations (85%)**
Atrial fibrillation (10%)	**Exertional dyspnea (80%)**
Pedal edema (30%)	**Increased pulse pressure (systolic hypertension)**
Increased oxygen consumption (basal metabolism)	**Active apical impulse**
Weight loss	**Loud first heart sound and pulmonic component of second heart sound**
Skeletal muscle myopathy	
Increased bone turnover (occasional osteoporosis or hypercalcemia)	**Mid-systolic murmur, usually basal**
Fair skin	**Third heart sound (occasional)**
Fine brittle hair	**Means-Lerman scratch (rare)‡**
Brittle nails	Tremor
Oligo- or amenorrhea	Brisk reflexes
Increased bowel frequency	Increased perspiration
	Heat intolerance
	Insomnia
	Anxiety
	Stare, lid lag§

*Cardiac response to hyperthyroidism and symptoms of hyperthyroidism that mimic those of heart disease are shown in boldface type. The numbers in parentheses are approximate prevalences of the findings, compiled from several large series. Goiter is almost always present, though in elderly patients the thyroid enlargement may be minimal or absent.

†Both types of effects contribute to the tachycardia and palpitations.

‡A systolic scratch or click in the second left intercostal space that is probably generated by the pleura and pericardium rubbing together.

§These reflect upper-lid retraction. Infiltrative ophthalmyopathy with exophthalmos is found only when Graves' disease is the cause of the hyperthyroidism and is not related to the hyperthyroid state per se.

Reproduced with permission from Kaplan, M. M.: The thyroid and the heart: How do they interact? J. Cardiovasc. Med. 7:893, 1982.

in hyperthyroidism and either normal or elevated in hypothyroidism.[46] These data suggest that the sympathomimetic features of hyperthyroidism cannot be due simply to an overall increase in adrenergic activity, but rather due to a change in the affinity of catecholamines for their receptors or to a modification of a postreceptor mechanism. Previously such changes were difficult to document, primarily because thyroid hormone appears to have different effects on adrenoceptors in different tissues. For example, the effect of thyroid hormone in the rat liver is different from that in the rat heart. Thyroid hormones reduce beta-adrenoreceptor number in the rat liver, and hypothyroid animals show an increase in these receptors.[47, 48] In contrast, in the rat heart, which has been the organ most extensively studied, administration of thyroid hormone causes both an increase in the number of receptors and their affinity for their ligand, while hypothyroidism induces the opposite effect.[49–52]

These changes in receptor number and affinity lead to appropriate changes in sensitivity of the myocardium to beta-adrenoceptor agonists. For example, stimulation of adenylate cyclase activity by isoproterenol is increased in hyperthyroidism and reduced in hypothyroidism. Finally, there are also changes in the force of contraction with increased sensitivity of the ventricular muscle to isoproterenol-induced contraction in hyperthyroidism and reduction in hypothyroidism.[49] That this effect is specific is shown by an unaltered change in calcium-stimulated contractility in hypothyroid animals.[51] These effects are also observed in vivo in dogs in which propranolol-induced reductions of heart rate and myocardial contractility were greater in hyperthyroid than in euthyroid animals.[53]

Further support comes from the study by Guarnieri et al. who showed that hyperthyroid rats have enhanced activation of protein kinase and contractile response following administration of a threshold dose of the beta-adrenoceptor agonist isoproterenol.[54] In the aforementioned study in conscious hyperthyroid dogs,[52] however, we found no alteration in the sensitivity of the inotropic response to isoproterenol and norepinephrine.

Circulating blood elements have also provided additional evidence in support of the concept that thyroid hormone "up-regulates" beta-adrenoceptors. When patients are used as their own control, both the number of beta-adrenoceptors and the sensitivity of adenylate cyclase to isoproterenol stimulation in mononuclear cells is increased by thyroid hormone.[55] Additionally, in circulating reticulocytes of hypothyroid animals, the number of receptors is decreased.[55]

While there is compelling evidence for changes in the receptor number and affinity induced by thyroid hormone, it is unclear whether thyroid hormone also has additional effects by which it could alter sensitivity to adrenergic stimuli. There are no data regarding the effect of thyroid hormone on cardiac nucleotide regulatory (N) protein (Fig. 13–10, p. 391), although the presence of hypothyroidism does reduce the concentration of N-protein in erythrocyte membranes.[56] On the other hand, no change in N-protein concentration has been observed in adipose tissue.[57] Yet in adipose tissue, hypothyroidism does reduce the lipolytic response to catecholamines.[58] Thus, in this tissue, in which there is no alteration in the number of beta-adrenoceptors, the mechanism underlying the hypothyroid-induced alteration in tissue effect is unclear, but probably occurs downstream from the interaction of the agonist with its receptor.

EFFECT OF THYROID HORMONE ON THE HEART

There is abundant evidence that thyroid hormone may alter cardiac function directly. Thus the addition of thyroid to fragments of chick embryonic heart increases the rate of beating of the cells.[59] Additionally, the increased heart rate and myocardial contractility observed in experimental hyperthyroidism are not completely reversed by either sympathetic or parasympathetic blockade.[45, 53] Finally, T4 enhances the rate of contraction of cardiac muscle even in the presence of adrenergic blockade.[60] Right ventricular papillary muscles isolated from cats rendered hyperthyroid exhibited augmented myocardial contractility, as reflected in an upward shift of the myocardial force-velocity curve,[45] with a greatly increased velocity of myocardial fiber shortening, a reduced time to peak tension during isometric contraction, and an augmented peak tension development (Fig. 58–3). Prior catecholamine depletion by pretreatment of the hyperthyroid cats with reserpine did not alter this inotropic effect of hyperthyroidism, providing further evidence for a direct cardiac effect.[45] This hypothesis has been assessed in the intact conscious calf. The results suggest that the major actions of T4 on the left ventricle are (1) a direct positive inotropic effect and (2) an increase in the size of the ventricular cavity without a change in the end-diastolic pressure or length of the sarcomere in diastole.[61]

The available data suggest that the direct effect of thyroid hormone on the heart is mediated via a change in protein synthesis.[62–64] Thyroid hormone increases the activity of the sodium pump in myocardial cells as it does in other tissues. Philipson and Edelman have documented that the activity of both the Na^+,K^+-ATPase and K^+-dependent *p*-nitrophenyl phosphatase in the heart is increased by more than 50 per cent when T3 is administered to hypothyroid rats.[65] The hearts of euthyroid rabbits rendered hyperthyroid exhibited a doubling of myofibrillar ATPase activity.[66] Reverse T3 (a biologically inactive analog) has no effect. Curfman et al. have suggested that this increased activity is the result of an increase in the number of functional enzyme complexes.[67] There is evidence that thyroid hormone both increases the synthesis of myosin and alters its structure, increasing its contractile properties, particularly by increasing the more mobile myosin isoenzyme (V_1) as determined by polyacrylamide gel electrophoresis.[68–70] The heart appears to respond to thyrotoxicosis by enhancing synthesis of a myosin isoenzyme with a fast ATPase activity[66, 68] (Fig. 13–5, p. 387). The augmented myosin ATPase activity appears to contribute to the enhanced

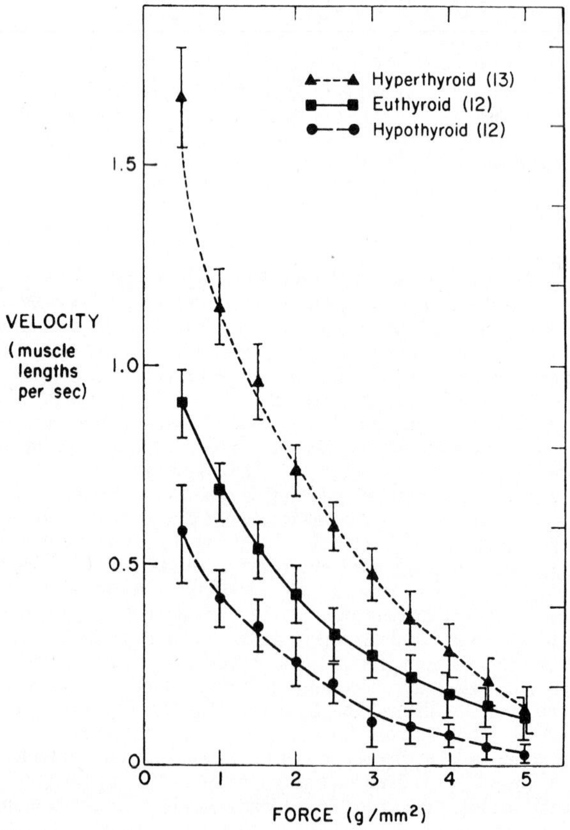

FIGURE 58–3. The average force-velocity relationship for papillary muscles from hyperthyroid, euthyroid, and hypothyroid cats. Initial velocity of shortening is normalized in terms of muscle lengths per second; load, corrected for cross-sectional area of individual muscles is expressed in gm/mm². Brackets represent ± SEM. (From Buccino, R. A., Spann, J. F., Poole, P. E., and Braunwald, E.: Influence of the thyroid state on the intrinsic contractile properties and the energy stores of the myocardium. J. Clin. Invest. *46*:1669, 1967.)

contractile response of the hyperthyroid heart, since the activity level of this enzyme is thought to regulate the rate of turnover of actin-myosin cross-bridge links in cardiac muscle. Hypothyroidism induces the opposite effect.[71] However, this is probably not the principal cause, since administration of exogenous thyroid can stimulate contractility before any change in the myosin ATPase activity occurs.[72] The sarcoplasmic reticulum isolated from hyperthyroid dogs and rabbits accumulates and exchanges calcium at an increased rate,[73] resulting in increased availability of calcium to the myofibrils during activation, as well as an enhanced rate of myofibrillar relaxation. Finally, the effect of thyroxine on myosin isoenzyme appears to be localized primarily to the ventricles with atrial isoenzymes relatively unaltered by changes in thyroid hormone.[70] Klein and Hong, using heterotopic cardiac isografts, have suggested that thyroid's effect on protein synthesis in the heart is, for the most part, secondary to changes in cardiac work rather than a direct effect of thyroid hormone. Indeed, they suggested that even the changes in myosin isoenzyme may in part be secondary to changes in workload, although a separate direct effect was also evident.[74]

The tachycardia observed in hyperthyroidism appears to be due to a combination of an increased rate of diastolic depolarization and a decreased duration of the action potential in the sinoatrial node cells.[75] The propensity for the development of atrial fibrillation may be due to the shortened refractory period of atrial cells.[76]

HYPERTHYROIDISM

Hyperthyroidism is the clinical state resulting from the excess production of T3, T4, thyroxine, or both. The most common cause is a diffuse toxic goiter (Graves' disease). Although the etiology of this condition is still unknown, the hyperproduction of T4 and T3 is thought to result from circulating IgG autoantibodies that bind to the thyrotropin receptor on the thyroid gland. The second most common form of hyperthyroidism is nodular toxic goiter, a condition in which localized areas of the gland function excessively and autonomously. Less common causes include a single toxic adenoma, ingestion of excessive amounts of thyroid hormone, and subacute thyroiditis, in which there may be a self-limited phase of hyperthyroidism. Rarely, hyperthyroidism may also occur as a result of the production of thyroid hormone by a thyroid carcinoma or production of a thyrotropic substance (probably HCG) by a hydatidiform mole or choriocarcinoma.[77]

Hyperthyroidism is a relatively common disease, occurring four to eight times more commonly in women than in men, with a peak incidence in the third and fourth decades. The commonly associated signs and symptoms include fatigue, hyperactivity, insomnia, heat intolerance, palpitations, dyspnea, increased appetite with weight loss, nocturia, diarrhea, oligomenorrhea, muscle weakness, tremor, emotional lability, increased heart rate, systolic hypertension, hyperthermia, warm moist skin, lid lag, stare, and brisk reflexes. In the vast majority of cases a goiter can be palpated. Hyperthyroidism in childhood occurs most frequently just before or during adolescence. It is usually associated with a diffuse goiter. The most common early manifestations of juvenile hyperthyroid patients are excessive movements and emotional lability.

T3 levels are invariably elevated and serum T4 levels are usually increased as well. In addition to the signs and symptoms directly related to increased production of thyroid hormone, patients with Graves' disease often have exophthalmos and occasionally circumscribed areas of thickening of the skin, particularly of the lower extremities; presumably these are related to the immunological aspects of the disease.

Particularly in older patients, the typical clinical picture is occasionally absent.[78] In these individuals with so-called *apathetic hyperthyroidism,* few clinical manifestations are apparent except for cardiovascular dysfunction. Thus, cardiac arrhythmias and heart failure resistant to conventional forms of therapy are common.

CARDIOVASCULAR MANIFESTATIONS. The heart is among the most responsive organs in thyroid disease, and cardiovascular signs and symptoms are therefore important clinical features of hyperthyroidism.[79] Palpitations, dyspnea, tachycardia, and systolic hypertension are common

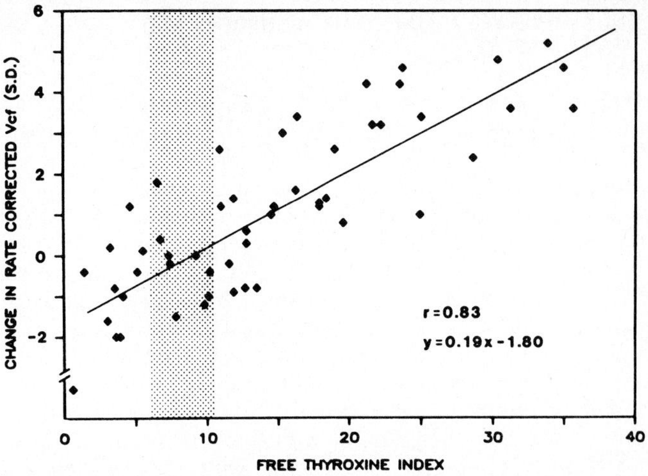

FIGURE 58–4. Rate-corrected velocity of shortening (Vcf) in SD units from the normal mean regression line obtained from 11 patients at varying levels of the free thyroxine index. There is a strong positive correlation between the level of thyroid hormone and the change in contractile state. The shaded area represents the normal range for serum free thyroxine index. (From Feldman, T., Borow, K. M., Sarne, D. H., Neumann, A., and Lang, R. M.: Myocardial mechanics in hyperthyroidism: Importance of left ventricular loading conditions, heart rate and contractile state. By permission of the American College of Cardiology. J. Am. Coll. Cardiol. 7:972, 1986.)

findings. Diastolic hypertension can also occur. Typically, there is a hyperactive precordium with a loud first heart sound, an accentuated pulmonic component of the second heart sound, and a third heart sound; occasionally, a systolic ejection click is heard. Midsystolic murmurs along the left sternal border are common, and a systolic scratch, the so-called Means-Lerman scratch, is occasionally heard in the second left intercostal space during expiration. It is presumed to be secondary to the rubbing together of normal pleural and pericardial surfaces by the hyperdynamic heart.

As would be anticipated, and as described in greater detail on page 783, cardiac and stroke volume index, mean systolic ejection rate, velocity extent and wall shortening (Fig. 58–4), and coronary blood flow[80] are all increased, the systolic ejection period and preejection period are abbreviated, the pulse pressure is widened, and systemic vascular resistance is reduced in hyperthyroidism.[81] The changes in left ventricular performance induced by thyroid hormone appear to be secondary to augmented contractility rather than reduction in afterload or change in heart rate.[82] If the hyperthyroidism is relatively mild, many of the indices of left ventricular function are normal, with exercise needed to bring out abnormalities, e.g., reduction in the exercise-induced increase in ejection fraction.[83] It has been suggested that many of the changes in cardiac function are secondary to the increased metabolic demands of peripheral tissue. However, the increase in cardiac output is greater than would be predicted on the basis of the increased total body oxygen consumption, supporting the view that thyroid hormone exerts a direct cardiac stimulant action independent of its effect on general tissue metabolism. Furthermore, normalization of myocardial contractile response to exercise may not occur until several months after normalization of thyroid function.[84]

Roentgenographic and electrocardiographic changes are common but are nonspecific in hyperthyroidism.[78] Thus the left ventricle, aorta, and the pulmonary artery are prominent, and, in some cases, there is generalized cardiac enlargement, which may be accompanied by signs and symptoms of heart failure. In patients with sinus rhythm, the magnitude of the tachycardia, in general, parallels the severity of the disease. Sinus tachycardia, i.e., a rate exceeding 100/min, is present in 40 per cent of patients with hyperthyroidism, occurring most frequently in the younger age groups. Fifteen to twenty-five per cent of patients with hyperthyroidism have persistent atrial fibrillation, which is often heralded by one or more transient episodes of this arrhythmia.[85, 86] There is shortening of the AV conduction time and functional refractory period, resulting in an increased frequency at which the AV conduction system transmits rapid atrial impulses.[86] Intra-atrial conduction disturbances, manifested by prolongation or notching of the P wave and prolongation of the P-R interval in the absence of treatment with digitalis, occur in 15 per cent and 5 per cent of patients with hyperthyroidism, respectively. Occasionally, second or third degree heart block may result.[79] The cause of the AV conduction disturbance is not clear, since animal experiments have shown that the functional refractory period of the AV conduction system and the conduction time were shortened in dogs with hyperthyroidism and prolonged in dogs with hypothyroidism.[87] Intraventricular conduction disturbances, most commonly right bundle branch block, occur in about 15 per cent of patients with hyperthyroidism without associated heart disease of other etiology.[79] Paroxysmal supraventricular tachycardia and flutter are rare in hyperthyroidism. Finally, occult thyrotoxicosis may underlie either chronic or paroxysmal isolated atrial fibrillation. Ciaccheri et al. reported a frequency of thyrotoxicosis of 12.5 per cent in 40 consecutive patients with isolated atrial fibrillation.[86]

Both angina pectoris and congestive heart failure occur in patients with hyperthyroidism, and for many years it was assumed that these were seen only in the presence of underlying cardiovascular disease. Support for this position came primarily from the absence of these symptoms in young persons with significant hyperthyroidism. More recently, however, four lines of evidence have suggested otherwise. First, congestive heart failure has been produced in experimental animals by simply administering T4. Second, children with thyrotoxicosis without underlying cardiac disease may develop congestive heart failure.[88] Third, angina has been reported in a patient with normal coronary arteries, presumably secondary to thyroid-induced coronary artery spasm.[89] Finally, abnormal left ventricular function observed during exercise in hyperthyroid subjects is not reversed by beta blockade but is reversed by treating the hyperthyroidism.[90] Thus, when it is severe enough, thyrotoxicosis can overtax even the normal heart, although, in most instances, the development of clinical manifestations of heart failure and myocardial ischemia in patients with hyperthyroidism signifies the presence of underlying cardiac or coronary vascular disease. There is also increased frequency of hyperthyroidism in patients with familial hypertrophic cardiomyopathy. In one kindred, 3 of 17 members with hypertrophic cardiomyopathy also had hyperthyroidism.[91]

Finally, mitral valve prolapse has been associated with hyperthyroidism. In one report, 19 of 40 patients with hyperthyroidism had evidence of mitral valve prolapse—a rate twice that observed in euthyroid persons.[92] In a second study of 126 patients with hyperthyroidism, the incidence of mitral valve prolapse was three times normal in patients with Graves' disease but not increased in patients with toxic nodular goiter.[93]

TREATMENT OF CARDIOVASCULAR DISEASE IN HYPERTHYROIDISM. Hyperthyroid patients with cardiovascular disease are particularly resistant to therapy. For example, it has been well documented that both congestive heart failure and cardiac arrhythmias are resistant to conventional doses of the cardiac glycosides. While the specific mechanisms underlying these altered responses remain obscure, they may be related to both systemic and local effects.[94] First, serum levels of cardiac glycosides are diminished in hyperthyroidism, not because there is an augmentation of its metabolism but because there is an increase in its volume of distribution. Second, experimental hyperthyroidism reduces the enhancement of the myocardial contractile force and the prolongation of the atrioventricular nodal refractory period produced by these agents.[94] Because of this decreased sensitivity to cardiac glycosides, toxicity may develop at a dose that has relatively little therapeutic effect.

DIAGNOSIS AND THERAPY OF HYPERTHYROIDISM. The diagnosis is made on the basis of elevated levels of thyroid hormone in the blood. Because only serum T3 is increased in some individuals, it is important to obtain serum levels of *both* T3 and T4 and an index of the thyroid-binding capacity of the patient's serum (resin thyroxine uptake). In most laboratories hyperthyroidism is confirmed when the levels of serum T4 are greater than 10.5 μg/dl or T3 levels are greater than 180 ng/dl with normal resin thyroxine uptakes. Occasionally, patients will have hyperthyroidism with both T3 and T4 within the normal range. If suspected, confirmation may be obtained by measuring the TSH (thyroid-stimulating hormone) response to TRH (thyrotropin-releasing hormone), which should be blunted in hyperthyroidism. Such has recently been reported in four patients with unexplained atrial fibrillation.[95] However, caution needs to be exercised in using this test, since false-positive results are common.

Prompt treatment of the hyperthyroid state can significantly reduce, if not eliminate, the associated cardiovascular symptoms. About half of patients with concurrent onset of hyperthyroidism and angina pectoris experience complete remission of symptoms after treatment of hyperthyroidism.[96] Furthermore, in 62 per cent of 163 thyrotoxic patients with atrial fibrillation sustained for one week or longer, spontaneous reversion to sinus rhythm was found when they became euthyroid.[97] Arterial embolization is not common in patients with thyrotoxicosis and atrial fibrillation, but it does occur. In one series, 8 per cent of 262 patients with both conditions had embolization.[98] Thus it is important to determine quickly whether hyperthyroidism is present in patients with cardiovascular disease, since treatment often results in dramatic improvement. In elderly patients with apathetic hyperthyroidism, cardiovascular manifestations, specifically atrial fibrillation and/or congestive heart failure, predominate, and therefore evaluation of thyroid function in such patients is particularly important. However, it should be noted that these individuals are particularly resistant to cardiac glycosides.

The definitive treatment of hyperthyroidism is surgical removal of the gland or irradiation using ^{131}I. In severely ill patients, particularly those with thyroid storm or significant cardiovascular symptoms or both, neither of these therapies is appropriate. Thus, medical therapy is directed at reducing both the production and biological effect of thyroid hormone. Since many of the cardiovascular symptoms of thyrotoxicosis are related to increased beta-adrenoceptor activity, treatment with beta-adrenoceptor blocking agents has been useful.[99] Tachycardia, palpitations, tremor, restlessness, muscle weakness, and heat intolerance are reversed by these agents, which offer the additional benefit of inhibiting the conversion of T4 to the biologically active T3 in peripheral tissues.

Beta blockers can be administered orally or intravenously, but since this drug interferes with the effects of sympathetic stimulation on the heart, it must be used with caution in patients with congestive heart failure. However, if the heart failure is in part related to the tachycardia, beta blockade may be beneficial. These agents can be administered in small doses while the patient is under close observation and being treated with digitalis and diuretics and reduction in physical activity. Beta-blocking drugs and cardiac glycosides act synergistically to slow ventricular rate in atrial fibrillation by increasing the refractoriness of the atrioventricular conduction system. Thus, the combination may allow a beneficial effect that would require toxic doses of either agent used alone. Beta-adrenoceptor blockade also improves many of the peripheral manifestations of thyrotoxicosis.[74]

Calcium antagonists have also been used in the treatment of cardiac manifestations of hyperthyroidism. However, in a preliminary study, verapamil was not effective in reversing the cardiac effects of hyperthyroidism.[100]

While beta-adrenoceptor blockade can produce significant improvement of the cardiovascular status in patients with hyperthyroidism, correction of the basic metabolic defect requires specific therapy directed at reducing the production of thyroid hormone.[79] The most useful agents are the thionamides, such as propylthiouracil. These drugs should be administered concurrently with a beta-blocking agent to reduce the total production of thyroid hormone, as well as to block its effect. The usual starting dosage of propylthiouracil is 300 to 800 mg in divided doses daily; it not only reduces thyroid hormone production but also has the advantage of reducing the peripheral conversion of T4 into T3. Usual maintenance doses range from 50 to 300 mg. The thionamides are not without risk, since between 1 and 5 per cent of patients have significant side effects—usually gastrointestinal disturbances or a suppression of the bone marrow; infrequently, a generalized vasculitis has been reported.

Iodine, most commonly administered in the form of two drops of saturated solution of potassium iodide three times daily, inhibits the release of thyroid hormones from the thyrotoxic gland, and its beneficial effects occur rapidly, indeed, more rapidly than those of agents that inhibit the synthesis of the hormone. It is therefore useful in the rapid amelioration of the hyperthyroid state in patients with thyroid heart disease. It may also be utilized along with antithyroid agents to control thyrotoxicosis following ^{131}I treatment until the radioiodine has had time to take effect. Most hyperthyroid patients, however, escape from the effects of iodide after 10 to 14 days.

Ipodate, an agent for oral cholecystography, has been reported to be beneficial in the treatment of early hyperthyroidism,[101] particularly in the early treatment of cardiac manifestations of thyrotoxicosis.[102] One study assessed the efficacy of ipodate in the treatment of cardiac arrhythmias in euthyroid individuals. Its efficacy was compared to that of amiodarone, another agent with effects similar to ipodate on the peripheral conversion of T4 to T3 but also with specific antiarrhythmic properties. Amiodarone but not ipodate reduced the frequency of ventricular arrhythmias, suggesting that alteration of peripheral thyroid metabolism is *not* useful in treating these arrhythmias in the euthyroid individual.[103]

HYPOTHYROIDISM

Hypothyroidism results from reduced secretion of both T4 and T3, occurring in most cases as a consequence of destruction of the thyroid gland itself, usually by an inflammatory process. In some cases, it is secondary to decreased secretion of thyrotropin, due to either pituitary or hypothalamic disease. In secondary hypothyroidism, the signs and symptoms associated with deficiency of other pituitary hormones are also usually present. The incidence of hypothyroidism peaks between the ages of 30 and 60 years and is twice as common in women as in men. The following signs and symptoms are common: cold intolerance, dryness of the skin, weakness, impairment of memory, personality changes, shortness of breath, constipation, hoarseness, menorrhagia and other forms of menstrual dysfunction, and, occasionally, heart failure. In addition, in the more severe forms of the disease, there is facial puffiness, particularly around the eyes, a characteristic nonpitting form of edema (myxedema) of the lower extremities, slow speech, decreased hearing, and a yellow hue to the skin due to decreased conversion of carotene into vitamin A. These signs and symptoms may be present for years before treatment is initiated, particularly in patients in whom the disease has developed gradually.

Infants with severe congenital hypothyroidism may have a cardiac murmur, pallor, hepatomegaly, and edema. These manifestations appear before the signs of congenital hypothyroidism, which may not be apparent until 1 to 3 months of age, and which include retarded growth and development, with persistence of infantile features, a protuberant tongue, sluggish movements with poor muscle tone, coarse hair, cool skin, hypothermia, and constipation.[104]

EFFECTS OF AMIODARONE ON THYROID FUNCTION. This antiarrhythmic agent (p. 637) has two effects on thyroid function. First, it inhibits the peripheral conversion of T4 to T3. Thus, in nearly all patients there is a reduction in serum T3 levels and a transient rise in TSH. Within a few days to weeks, this causes an increase in serum T4 levels and a return of TSH to normal. Clinically, the patients are euthyroid even though their T4 levels are elevated.[105] Amiodarone's second effect is due to its high iodine content (35 per cent by weight). Thus, when it is metabolized, there is a massive increase in the available inorganic iodide,[106] resulting in acute inhibition of thyroid organification (Fig. 58–5). Depending on the state of iodine intake before its administration, patients may develop either hypothyroidism (common in the United States) or thyrotoxicosis (more common in Europe).[107, 108] Borowski et al. studied the impact of amiodarone on thyroid function in 45 patients.[105] Nearly 50 per cent had an increase in T4, with 25 per cent having an elevated TSH value. Of these, 7 per cent also had a low level of T4. In their series no subject developed hyperthyroidism, but 9 per cent developed clinical hypothyroidism. Because of amiodarone's prolonged half-life, the biochemical and clinical abnormalities can persist for months after its administration is stopped.

CARDIOVASCULAR MANIFESTATIONS. The heart in overt myxedema is often pale, flabby, and grossly dilated. Histological examination discloses myofibrillar swelling, loss of striations, and interstitial fibrosis. With the development of methods that reliably and easily measure the circulating levels of thyroid hormone, the diagnosis of hypothyroidism is being made with increasing frequency at an earlier stage of the disease. Treatment is therefore also initiated earlier, resulting in a reduction in the incidence of cardiovascular signs and symptoms. Thus, the classic findings of cardiac enlargement, cardiac dilatation, significant bradycardia, weak arterial pulses, hypotension, distant heart sounds, low electrocardiographic voltages, nonpitting facial and peripheral edema, and evidence of congestive heart failure, such as ascites, orthopnea, and paroxysmal dyspnea, are now seen only infrequently. However, exertional dyspnea and easy fatigability continue to be common complaints.

Myxedema is associated with increased capillary permeability and subsequent leakage of protein into the interstitial space, resulting in pericardial effusion, a common clinical finding in overt myxedema, occurring in about one-third of all patients (p. 1523). Rarely, it or the presenting symptom is complicated by cardiac tamponade.[109, 110] Cardiomegaly on chest radiograph and low voltage in the

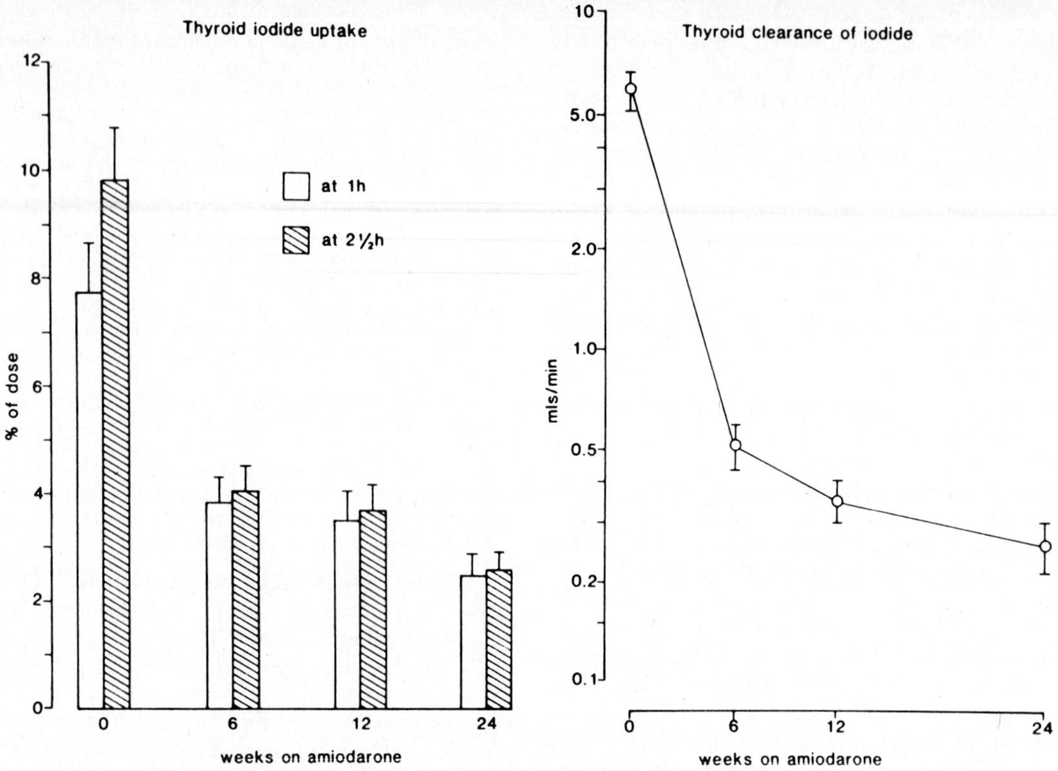

FIGURE 58–5. Effect of amiodarone on mean (± SEM) thyroid iodide uptake (*left*) and thyroid iodide clearance (*right*) in 15 euthyroid patients. (Note that the ordinate of the right panel is plotted on a log scale.) (From Rao, R. H., McCready, V. R., and Spathis, G. S.: Iodine kinetic studies during amiodarone treatment. J. Clin. Endocrinol. Metab. *62*:563, 1986) © by The Endocrine Society, 1986.

electrocardiogram are not reliable indicators of pericardial effusion; echocardiography is the most useful method of establishing the diagnosis (p. 127). The effusions disappear with thyroid replacement therapy.[109–111]

The electrocardiographic changes observed in patients with hypothyroidism other than sinus bradycardia include prolongation of the Q-T interval, but since the T-wave amplitude is low, precise measurement of this interval is often impossible.[25] The P-wave amplitude is usually very low, and in some cases this wave is not even discernible. Sinus tachycardia is very rare, whereas bradycardia is common. It is possible that hypothermia may contribute to reentrant ventricular arrhythmias by slowing the heart rate and increasing the duration of the QRS and the Q-T intervals.[25] The incidence of atrioventricular and intraventricular conduction disturbances is about three times greater in patients with myxedema than in the general population.[112] Other electrocardiographic changes are those associated with pericardial effusion.[111] Thus, flattening or inversion of the T waves and low P-, QRS-, and T-wave amplitudes are commonly observed in patients with pericardial effusion. In most cases these revert to normal with the removal of the fluid. In some cases, however, the electrocardiographic changes persist even though the pericardial fluid is removed, which suggests that the lack of thyroid hormone may produce a primary myocardial abnormality.[113] Incomplete or complete right bundle branch block has been observed, but other forms of arrhythmias are uncommon.

There is increased frequency of hypertension in patients with hypothyroidism although not in severe myxedema. In one study of 477 patients 15 per cent of hypothyroid subjects had a blood pressure greater than 160/95, compared to 5.5 per cent in age-matched euthyroid subjects. Replacement of thyroid hormone resulted in substantial reduction in blood pressure in the hypertensive patients. Thus, individuals with mild to moderate hypothyroidism have an increased possibility of developing hypertension, particularly diastolic hypertension, while individuals with severe hypothyroidism are more likely to have normal or slightly low blood pressures.[114]

Cardiovascular manifestations of congenital hypothyroidism are similar except for the rarity of pericardial effusion. Thus the size of the left ventricle, its capacity, and the posterior wall thickness are all less in the hypothyroid infant. Since heart rate is also lower, cardiac output is reduced. There is also a prolongation of the preejection period of the left ventricle.[115]

MYOCARDIAL EFFECTS. Hypothyroid patients have reduced cardiac output, stroke volume, and blood and plasma volumes.[116] Circulation time is prolonged, but right and left heart filling pressures are usually within normal limits unless they are elevated by the pericardial effusion. There is a redistribution of blood flow with mild reductions in cerebral and renal flow and significant reductions in cutaneous flow. A delay in the relaxation of skeletal muscle is a well-known finding in hypothyroidism; measurements of isovolumetric relaxation time, by a combination of apex cardiography and phonocardiography, have revealed a prolongation of this interval with an abbreviation to normal during T4 replacement.[117] In addition, there is lengthening of the preejection period and an increased ratio of the preejection period to the left ventricular ejection time (PEP/LVET); these changes are the opposite of those observed in hyperthyroidism.[118]

Cardiac muscle isolated from cats with experimentally produced hypothyroidism exhibited reduced contractility, characterized by a depression of the myocardial force-velocity curve, a reduction of the rate of tension development, and a prolongation of the contractile response (see Fig. 58–3).

There is little evidence from either experimental or clinical studies that congestive heart failure is common in myxedema or that it occurs in the absence of other cardiac disease.[119] Presumably the depressed myocardial contractility is sufficient to sustain the reduced workload placed on the heart in hypothyroidism. However, it may be difficult to distinguish between the heart in myxedema and heart failure. Dyspnea, edema, effusions, cardiomegaly, and T-wave changes occur in both conditions. In left heart failure, pulmonary artery pressure is usually elevated during exercise, cardiac output fails to rise normally, and the Valsalva response is normal, while the opposite occurs in myxedema.[119] The hemodynamic changes in myxedema respond to thyroid hormone administration.

Cardiac catecholamine levels are not reduced in hypothyroidism. Neither the sensitivity of the mechanical performance of the heart to sympathetic nerve stimulation nor the response of the cardiac adenylate cyclase to norepinephrine is altered in hypothyroidism.[120] However, there is a reduction in the total number of myocardial beta receptors.[51] In addition to the effects of hypothyroidism on the beta receptor there also is evidence that the lack of thyroid hormone may modify the contractile process itself. Thus, both isoproterenol-stimulated contractility and the accumulation of cyclic AMP are reduced in hearts obtained from hypothyroid rats.[120] In experimental hypothyroidism, calcium in isolated myocardial sarcoplasmic reticulum particles is reduced, which may explain the altered contractile state.[72] As noted above, thyroid hormone can affect the quantity and function of myosin ATPase activity through a change in protein synthesis. The activity of cardiac myosin ATPase[71] and the rate of calcium uptake and the calcium-dependent ATP hydrolysis by isolated myocardial sarcoplasmic reticulum in the excitation-contraction-relaxation process[73] are reduced in hypothyroidism.

ATHEROSCLEROSIS. It has been suggested that patients with hypothyroidism are at increased risk of developing atherosclerosis, since this disease is accompanied by significant changes in lipid metabolism. Thus, hypercholesterolemia, hypertriglyceridemia, and impairment in free fatty acid mobilization, all associated with development of premature coronary artery disease, are found in patients with hypothyroidism. Support for this hypothesis has come from several sources, including the documentation that coronary atherosclerosis occurs with twice the frequency in patients with myxedema than in age- and sex-matched controls and that the development of atherosclerosis in cholesterol-fed animals is enhanced by the presence of hypothyroidism and reduced when thyroid hormone is administered.[121, 122] Additionally, hypothyroidism has a deleterious effect on dogs in whom a myocardial infarction has been induced. Infarct size was increased, dysrhythmias were more severe, and abnormalities in the microvasculature were present.[123] Yet myocardial infarction and angina pectoris are relatively uncommon occurrences in patients with hypothyroidism. The latter was present in only 7 per cent of a group of patients with hypothyroidism.[124] This low frequency of cardiac complications from atherosclerosis may simply reflect the decreased metabolic demands on the myocardium in hypothyroidism. A definitive study which examines the frequency of atherosclerosis in euthyroid individuals and persons who are now euthyroid but had once been myxedematous has not been reported. However, in one series of treated hypothyroid patients, angina pectoris improved more frequently than it became worse,[124] suggesting that the development of lipid abnormalities may not have the same implications in hypothyroid as in euthyroid individuals.

Other Metabolic Changes

The evaluation of patients with myxedema and chest pain is complicated by the known effects of hypothyroidism on serum enzyme concentrations commonly used to assess myocardial damage. Thus, creatine kinase (CK), lactic dehydrogenase (LDH), and serum glutamic oxaloacetic transaminase (SGOT) may be moderately or significantly increased in hypothyroidism.[125] The mechanism for the increase in enzymes is uncertain, but it may be related to mild cardiac or skeletal muscle damage with release of enzymes or decreased clearance of normal enzyme concentrations.

Diagnosis and Treatment of Hypothyroidism

Caution must be exercised in treating hypothyroid patients who are elderly and who may have underlying organic heart disease, to avoid precipitating myocardial infarction or severe congestive heart failure; a slow replacement program is indicated in these individuals.

Some have suggested using T3 rather than T4 to treat patients with myxedema; since it has a shorter half-life, if toxic effects develop, they will be dissipated more quickly. However, because it has a quicker onset of action, T3 also induces complications more rapidly. Thus, it appears to us more desirable to treat myxedema with T4, usually beginning with a dose as small as 0.0125 mg daily and doubling this every 14 days until a dosage of 0.1 to 0.125 mg is reached. During this process the patient's cardiovascular status is monitored frequently, and, if untoward events occur, the dose is reduced or maintained constant. The measurement of serum TSH levels provides a useful biochemical marker of adequacy of the replacement therapy.

The treatment of congestive heart failure is particularly difficult in patients with myxedema, both because of the effect of thyroid hormone on the heart and because the heart's response to cardiac glycosides is altered.[94] Patients with severe angina pectoris and untreated myxedema pose a difficult clinical dilemma because angina may be exacerbated by thyroid hormone replacement, and the usual medical management of angina with propranolol may induce severe bradycardia. Coronary arteriography often shows severe coronary artery disease in these patients, and an excellent surgical team can perform successful coronary revascularization with minimal thyroid replacement. Full thyroid replacement can then be safely achieved during the postoperative period, without the recurrence of angina.[126]

An increasingly common problem in ill patients is the so-called euthyroid sick syndrome.[127] This occurs in acutely or chronically ill patients who have low serum T4 and T3 levels yet do not have hypothyroidism. The low T3 levels are secondary to decreased extrathyroidal conversion of T4 to T3. The low T4's are often due to a decrease in the concentration of thyroxine-binding globulin, resulting in a decrease in total but only minimal changes in the free hormone levels. In very severe illness, there can be central (CNS) suppression of TSH release and an induced secondary hypothyroid state. Prolonged dopamine infusions can produce this situation also, by direct suppression of TSH secretion. In the euthyroid sick syndrome the serum TSH usually will be normal, whereas in hypothyroidism TSH will be increased, thus providing a biochemical mechanism for distinguishing them.[127, 128] T4 therapy is not of benefit in these patients.[129]

DISEASES OF THE ADRENAL CORTEX

Since Addison's description in 1849 of adrenal insufficiency,[2] it has been appreciated that steroids secreted by the adrenal cortex exert a significant effect on the cardiovascular system, primarily by altering blood pressure. Adrenal insufficiency is characterized by significant hypotension, while excessive production of adrenal steroids is often accompanied by hypertension.

Three classes of steroids are secreted by the adrenal cortex: glucocorticoids, e.g., cortisol; mineralocorticoids, e.g., aldosterone; and androgens, e.g., dehydroepiandrosterone. In this section, the physiology and pathophysiology of glucocorticoid and mineralocorticoid secretion will be addressed.

HORMONE ACTIONS

CORTISOL. The primary glucocorticoid, cortisol, is synthesized from cholesterol in the inner layers of the adrenal cortex by a series of enzymatic transformations. After release into the circulation, it is bound to a high-affinity, low-capacity globulin, transcortin. Thus, most of the circulating cortisol is biologically inactive. The daily secretion rate of cortisol ranges from 15 to 30 mg with a pronounced diurnal cycle. Its average plasma concentration is 15 μg/dl in the morning, falling to 5 μg/dl by early evening.[130] The fundamental mechanism of action of the glucocorticoids is similar to that of other steroid hormones. They enter a target tissue by diffusion and combine with a specific high-affinity cytoplasmic receptor protein. The receptor-cortisol complex is then transferred to specific acceptor sites on nuclear chromatin tissue, where it produces an increase in RNA and later protein synthesis.

The division of adrenal steroids into glucocorticoids and mineralocorticoids is somewhat arbitrary in that most glucocorticoids have some mineralocorticoid-like properties and vice versa. The major action of glucocorticoids is to promote gluconeogenesis, and, in that respect, they are both catabolic and anti-insulin. They mobilize amino acid precursors from peripheral supporting structures, such as bone, skin, muscle, and connective tissue, and inhibit protein synthesis and amino acid uptake in these same tissues. Gluconeogenesis is also indirectly enhanced by an increase in glucagon secretion secondary to the glucocorticoid-induced hyperaminoacidemia.

Glucocorticoids also have anti-inflammatory properties related to their effects on both the microvasculature and the lymphatic system. They maintain normal vascular responsiveness to circulating vasoconstrictors, such as norepinephrine, and have a major effect on both the distribution and excretion of body water. For example, patients with Addison's disease cannot effectively excrete a water load. Finally, they can alter calcium absorption from the gastrointestinal tract by interfering with the activation of vitamin D in the liver and/or blocking its effect on the gastrointestinal tract.[130]

Control of Cortisol Secretion. This is primarily under the control of a negative feedback loop involving the adrenal cortex and the pituitary gland. Thus, as cortisol concentrations fall, ACTH secretion from the pituitary increases, stimulating the adrenal cortex to produce more cortisol and vice versa. The hypothalamus also interacts with this system by releasing corticotropin releasing hormone, thus modifying ACTH release and the response of the pituitary to the inhibitory effect of cortisol. In addition to this primary negative feedback loop, there is an intrinsic diurnal rhythm in the release of both ACTH and cortisol, probably mediated by changes in the release of corticotropin releasing hormone from the hypothalamus.

ALDOSTERONE. The major mineralocorticoid produced by the human adrenal gland is aldosterone. It is also synthesized from cholesterol but almost exclusively in the outer layer (glomerulosa) of the adrenal cortex. Aldosterone has two important functions: (1) it is a major regulator of extracellular fluid volume by its effect on sodium retention, and (2) it is a major determinant of potassium metabolism. Aldosterone acts predominantly on the distal convoluted tubule and/or collecting duct of the kidney where it promotes the reabsorption of sodium. Potassium then diffuses into the lumen of the tubules because of the change in electrochemical gradient produced by the active reabsorption of the positively charged sodium ion. Hydrogen ion may also be more freely excreted because of this change in the electrochemical gradient. While aldosterone also acts on salivary and sweat glands and on the endothelial cells of the gastrointestinal tract, these have little impact on total body sodium and potassium homeostasis.

There are three well-defined control mechanisms for aldosterone release.[130]

1. The renin-angiotensin system is the major system for the control of extracellular fluid volume by regulating aldosterone secretion. Aldosterone is linked in a negative feedback loop with the renin-angiotensin system. Thus, during periods registered as volume deficiency there is increased release of the enzyme renin from the juxtaglomerular cells of the kidney. Renin then increases the production of angiotensin I from its substrate. Angiotensin I is rapidly converted into the biologically active angiotensin II, which increases aldosterone secretion. Angiotensin II also produces vasoconstriction, thereby raising blood pressure and reducing blood flow to a variety of tissues, especially the kidney.

2. Potassium ion also regulates aldosterone secretion independent of the renin-angiotensin system; elevation of potassium concentration increases aldosterone secretion and vice versa. The adrenal cortex is very sensitive to changes in potassium concentration with as little as a 0.1 mEq/l increment producing significant changes in the plasma aldosterone levels.

3. ACTH also has been documented to affect aldosterone secretion profoundly. However, because the control of aldosterone release is not appreciably altered in patients who have been on a long-term regimen of steroid therapy, ACTH probably has a smaller role than the other two factors in maintaining normal aldosterone secretion.

In addition to these major stimuli controlling aldosterone secretion, salt-losing hormones such as atrial natriuretic peptide (p. 1829) and dopamine inhibit aldosterone secretion, particularly in response to angiotensin II.[131] Finally, the prior dietary intake of both sodium and potassium alters the magnitude of the aldosterone response to acute stimulation, sodium restriction, and potassium loading, both enhancing the response of the adrenal.

Diseases of the adrenal cortex, therefore, primarily affect the cardiovascular system via changes in blood pressure or volume homeostasis. Three specific conditions will be discussed next: glucocorticoid excess (Cushing's syndrome), mineralocorticoid excess (primary aldosteronism), and adrenal insufficiency (Addison's disease).

CUSHING'S SYNDROME (See also p. 846)

In 1932 Harvey Cushing reported a syndrome characterized by truncal obesity, hypertension, fatigue, weakness, amenorrhea, hirsutism, purple abdominal striae, glucosuria, edema, and osteoporosis.[132] Since his original description, a number of specific causes for this syndrome have been described. However, the majority are secondary to bilateral adrenal hyperplasia, with the predominant feature being excess production of glucocorticoids and androgens.[133] Some cases are due to ACTH-producing tumors, of either the pituitary gland (Cushing's disease) or nonendocrine tissue (ectopic ACTH production). Fifteen to twenty per cent of the cases are due to primary adrenal neoplasia, either adenoma or carcinoma. Three times as many women as men are afflicted, and the onset is usually in the third or fourth decade of life. Most patients have the typical body habitus: central obesity and slender extremities with proximal muscle weakness. Hypertension is present in 80 to 90 per cent of patients, and diabetes occurs in 20 per cent, probably in those individuals with a predisposition.[130, 133] Evidence of androgen excess may also be present, including hirsutism, amenorrhea, clitoromegaly, and, in some cases, deepening of the voice. The majority of patients also have significant emotional changes ranging from lability of mood to severe depression, confusion, or even frank psychosis.

Laboratory tests disclose evidence of excess production of both glucocorticoids and androgens in the majority of cases. Thus, urinary metabolites of these steroids, 17-ketosteroids and 17-hydroxysteroids, are characteristically increased. Most patients show some evidence of glycosuria or hyperglycemia. There is usually generalized osteoporosis, most marked in the spine and pelvis; polycythemia is frequently encountered. In severe cases, hypokalemia, in mineralocorticoid manifestation, may also occur.

CARDIOVASCULAR MANIFESTATIONS. Prior to the development of effective treatment for Cushing's syndrome, accelerated atherosclerosis was a common finding. Early death usually occurred from myocardial infarction, congestive heart failure, or stroke. While the pathophysiology of the accelerated atherosclerosis is not clear, the hypertensive process probably contributes. However, it is unlikely to be the sole reason, since the hypertension of patients with primary aldosteronism may be as significant, and yet atherosclerosis is unusual. Part of the atherosclerotic changes may be mediated by the lipid-mobilizing effect of cortisol. Chronic excess production of cortisol leads to hyperlipidemia and hypercholesterolemia, both of which may promote the development of atherosclerosis.[134]

The pathophysiology of the hypertension in Cushing's syndrome has been much debated. Early studies suggested that it was secondary to volume expansion due to cortisol's mineralocorticoid properties. However, recent studies have not supported this hypothesis. Alternative hypotheses include glucocorticoid potentiation of response of vascular smooth muscle to vasoconstrictive agents and ACTH- or cortisol-induced increases in renin substrate.[134] The latter thesis suggests that the increased blood pressure is secondary to increased generation of angiotensin II. Thus, the pathophysiology of the hypertension may be multifactorial, being related to volume expansion, increased production of vasoactive agents, e.g., angiotensin II, and increased sensitivity of vascular smooth muscle to vasoactive agents.

Hemodynamic, electrocardiographic, and roentgenographic studies of patients with Cushing's syndrome have revealed no specific abnormalities except those that are, in general, associated with either hypertension or hypokalemia. The P-R intervals tend to be shorter than normal.

Over the past several years, a new familial syndrome has been described: Cushing's syndrome and cardiac myxoma occurring in the same individual (p. 1474). In addition to having these two conditions, 80 per cent of the patients have a cutaneous abnormality. In most it is a pigmented lesion; in some it is a subcutaneous myxoma. Histologically the adrenal glands show nodular hyperplasia.[135]

DIAGNOSIS AND TREATMENT. The diagnosis of Cushing's syndrome is established by the lack of appropriate suppression of cortisol secretion by dexamethasone. The best screening test is the administration of 1 mg of dexamethasone at bedtime with measurement of plasma cortisol between 7 and 10 the next morning.[130] In normal subjects cortisol levels will be less than 5 μg/dl. Some patients, particularly the obese, may have false-positive responses, but false-negative responses occur only rarely. The definitive diagnosis of Cushing's syndrome is made by administration of 0.5 mg of dexamethasone every 6 hours for 2 days with measurement either of plasma cortisol levels at the end of the second day (normal <5 μg/dl) or of the 24-hour 17-OH excretory rate on the second day of dexamethasone suppression (normal <3 mg/24 hours).[134, 135]

Therapy of Cushing's syndrome is usually directed at the specific cause. Thus, patients with adrenal carcinoma or adenoma or an ACTH-producing pituitary tumor are treated surgically. In some cases, patients with adrenal carcinoma have nonresectable lesions, and therefore surgery is combined with chemotherapy. The treatment of patients with bilateral hyperplasia without an evident ACTH-producing tumor is controversial, since the cause is often unknown. In some centers, bilateral adrenalectomy is the treatment of choice, while in others, therapy directed at the pituitary (either surgically or irradiation) is used.[137, 138]

The treatment of cardiovascular abnormalities associated with Cushing's syndrome is directed at lowering blood pressure and correcting the hypokalemia if present. Caution should be exercised in treating the hypertension with potassium-losing diuretics because of the tendency for these patients to develop hypokalemia. Thus, potassium-sparing diuretics or potassium supplements should be more specifically treated with agents that block the action or production of renin, such as beta blockers (e.g., propranolol) or converting enzyme inhibitors (e.g., captopril). As in all clinical conditions in which hypokalemia may be present, cardiac glycosides should be used with caution in patients with Cushing's syndrome.

HYPERALDOSTERONISM (See also p. 845)

CLINICAL AND BIOCHEMICAL MANIFESTATIONS. Aldosteronism is a syndrome associated with hypersecretion of aldosterone. Primary aldosteronism signifies that the stimulus for the excess aldosterone production resides within the adrenal. In secondary aldosteronism, the stimulus is of extraadrenal origin. These two conditions have similar effects on potassium metabolism.

In patients with primary aldosteronism, which most commonly is due to an aldosterone-producing adrenal adenoma, hypertension, hypokalemia, and metabolic alkalosis are common.[139] Polyuria may exist because of the hypokalemia, and glucose intolerance is increased in frequency. Muscle cramps due to the hypokalemia may be present, but little else distinguishes this from other forms of hypertension. Laboratory studies confirm the presence of hypokalemic alkalosis with a low specific gravity of urine and normal levels of adrenal glucocorticoids. The incidence of primary aldosteronism is between 0.5 and 2 per cent of the hypertensive population and occurs twice as frequently in females as in males, with an initial presentation usually between the ages of 30 and 50 years.[130]

CARDIOVASCULAR MANIFESTATIONS. Many of the cardiovascular effects of aldosteronism are nonspecific, being related to aldosterone's effect on atrial pressure and potassium balance. Thus, T-wave flattening or U-wave prominence on the electrocardiogram (p. 216) and the presence of premature ventricular contractions and other arrhythmias due to hypokalemia are observed.[25] Evidence of left ventricular hypertrophy, either on the electrocardiogram or on the chest roentgenogram, may also be present in patients with long-standing hypertension and hyperaldosteronism. Malignant hypertension and changes in renal function secondary to severe hypertensive angiopathy are infrequent.

DIAGNOSIS AND TREATMENT. The diagnosis of primary aldosteronism is made by the presence of diastolic hypertension without edema, hypersecretion of aldosterone that fails to suppress appropriately during volume expansion, hyposecretion of renin, and hypokalemia with inappropriate urinary potassium loss during salt loading. The state of the renin-angiotensin system is often used to distinguish primary aldosteronism from other conditions that produce hypertension and hypokalemia. For example, hypertension and hypokalemia may be part of the clinical picture of secondary aldosteronism that accompanies malignant or accelerated hypertension or is associated with renal artery stenosis. Secondary aldosteronism can be readily distinguished from primary aldosteronism by the plasma renin activity, which is increased in the former and reduced in the latter. However, the combination of hypertension and a low plasma renin activity does not necessarily mean primary aldosteronism. Between 15 and 30 per cent of patients with essential hypertension have low renin levels, so-called low-renin essential hypertension.[139] The possibility of excess mineralocorticoid secretion has been extensively evaluated in these patients; however, no definitive evidence for such exists (Chap. 27).

The principal treatment for primary aldosteronism is surgical removal of the aldosterone-producing adenoma. In some cases, this is not possible because of the excessive risk imposed by the general physical status of the patient; then, spironolactone, which pharmacologically blocks the effects of aldosterone, is used long term. This form of therapy may be of limited benefit in males, since compliance is reduced by the undesirable side effects of gynecomastia and impotency, particularly when doses greater than 200 mg per day are required.[140]

Although congestive heart failure occurs infrequently in patients with primary aldosteronism, treatment of patients with this condition with cardiac glycosides must be cautious because of the hypokalemia.

In some patients, primary aldosteronism is due not to a solitary adenoma but to bilateral hyperplasia.[139] While the clinical characteristics of these two conditions are similar, their responses to surgery are different. In both cases hypokalemia is corrected, but patients with bilateral hyperplasia often do not exhibit reduction in arterial pressure. Patients with bilateral hyperplasia are best treated with spironolactone and other antihypertensive agents. Thus, preoperative distinction between bilateral hyperplasia and an adrenal adenoma, using adrenal venography or adrenal scanning, is important.

ADRENAL INSUFFICIENCY

Hypofunction of the adrenal cortex includes all conditions in which the level of secretion of adrenal steroids is less than the needs of the body. There are two major categories: those associated with primary damage to the adrenal cortex, and those associated with secondary failure due to the lack of a stimulator such as ACTH. Clinically, patients with adrenal insufficiency can be divided into four types:[130] (1) the most common, primary insufficiency (Addison's disease); (2) secondary insufficiency due to a lack of ACTH; (3) selective hypoaldosteronism; and (4) enzyme deficiency (congenital adrenal hyperplasia).

CLINICAL AND BIOCHEMICAL MANIFESTATIONS. Addison's disease may occur at any age and affects both sexes equally. It is commonly due to a destructive process involving both adrenal glands, sometimes infectious, but most often autoimmune destruction.[141] Nearly all patients with primary adrenal insufficiency have weakness, increased skin pigmentation, significant weight loss, anorexia, nausea, vomiting, and hypotension, particularly postural. A significant minority also complain of abdominal pain, salt craving, and diarrhea or constipation. In mild forms, baseline laboratory studies are usually within normal limits. However, as the disease progresses, there is a gradual reduction in serum levels of sodium, chloride, and bicarbonate and an increase in potassium. The hyponatremia is due to extravascular loss of sodium, both into the urine (because of aldosterone deficiency) and into the intracellular compartment. The hyperkalemia is due both to the deficiency of aldosterone and to the impaired glomerular filtration rate and acidosis present in these patients. Other nonspecific findings include a reduction in basal metabolic rate with normal thyroid function and a normocytic anemia with relative lymphocytosis. While Addison's disease is often thought of as a common cause of significant eosinophilia, this is observed only occasionally.

CARDIOVASCULAR MANIFESTATIONS. The most common cardiovascular finding in adrenal insufficiency is arterial hypotension. In severe cases the pressure may be in the range of 80/50 mm Hg, with postural accentuation. Indeed, syncope occurs in a significant percentage of patients. In severe cases, heart size and peripheral pulses decrease. The electrocardiogram is abnormal in the majority of patients with Addison's disease.[25] The most common abnormalities are low or inverted T waves, sinus bradycardia, prolonged Q-T_c interval, and low voltage. Conduction defects also occur, with first-degree block present in 20 per cent of patients. Changes secondary to the hyperkalemia are not common even though the serum potassium levels may be elevated. It is of interest that the electrocardiographic abnormalities, other than those secondary to hyperkalemia, do not respond to mineralocorticoids but require glucocorticoid replacement. Cardiac failure in prolonged adrenocortical insufficiency has also been reported.[142]

DIAGNOSIS AND TREATMENT. Decreased response of the adrenal cortex to ACTH establishes the diagnosis of Addison's disease. The best screening test is the administration of synthetic ACTH (cosyntropin), 0.25 mg intramuscularly or intravenously, with measurement of plasma cortisol levels 30 to 60 minutes later. Cortisol levels double or increase by 10 μg/dl in normal subjects. Definitive evaluation is by prolonged (usually 24-hour) infusion of ACTH with assessment of either plasma cortisol or excretion of cortisol or both.[130]

It is possible to differentiate primary adrenal insufficiency from secondary adrenal insufficiency, isolated hypoaldosteronism, or congenital adrenal hyperplasia because one of the adrenal hormonal functions is normal in each of the latter three conditions. Thus in secondary adrenal insufficiency due to ACTH deficiency, aldosterone secretion is normal and the biochemical effects of mineralocorticoid deficiency, i.e., hyperkalemia, are not present. In isolated hypoaldosteronism, glucocorticoid function is normal. Female patients with congenital adrenal hyperplasia have evidence of androgen excess, such as virilization and hirsutism, and hypertension may also be present with a deficiency of 11-hydroxylase[143] (p. 848).

An increasingly common form of hypoaldosteronism is that associated with *hyporeninism.* Most commonly this syndrome is observed in older diabetic patients with a mild degree of renal impairment and hypertension; acidosis is also common. Usually these patients present with unexplained hyperkalemia. The cause is unknown, but may be secondary to damage to the juxtaglomerular apparatus and/or reduced conversion of a renin precursor into the active enzyme.[144] This clinical syndrome is particularly important in terms of cardiovascular diseases. Furthermore, commonly used drugs (beta blockers and calcium antagonists) can exacerbate this condition by further compromising aldosterone release.[145]

The treatment of adrenal insufficiency is accomplished by replacement of the deficient steroid. In adults with primary or secondary insufficiency, hydrocortisone, 20 to 30 mg daily, is administered in divided doses, usually two-thirds in the morning and one-third in midafternoon. In those patients with associated aldosterone deficiency, 9-α-fluorohydrocortisone, 0.05 to 0.10 mg daily, is given. During periods of significant stress (surgery, infection, or trauma), the dose of glucocorticoids should be increased. Occasionally, acute adrenal insufficiency in patients who previously had apparently normal adrenal function, is precipitated by the stress of cardiac surgery.[146]

PHEOCHROMOCYTOMA (See also p. 847)

In 1859, Oliver and Shafer demonstrated that adrenal extract raised blood pressure when injected into experimental animals. In 1901, one active ingredient, epinephrine, was isolated and characterized, and in 1922 a syndrome of paroxysmal hypertension associated with an adrenal medullary tumor, pheochromocytoma, was reported.

EFFECTS OF CATECHOLAMINES ON THE CARDIOVASCULAR SYSTEM

The adrenal medulla and sympathetic nervous system are linked morphologically, biochemically, and physiologically and are often referred to as the sympathoadrenal system.[147] The sympathoadrenal system differs from other endocrine systems in several respects, including the fact that plasma levels of the secretory product, catecholamines, are not regulated by a direct feedback mechanism. Instead, catecholamine secretion is the efferent branch of a reflex arc involving centers in the brain stem, the hypothalamus, and perhaps the cerebral cortex as well. The human adrenal medulla contains about 1 mg of catecholamine per gram of tissue, approximately 85 per cent of which is epinephrine. The strategic location of the adrenal medullary cells within the cortex is associated with their capacity to form epinephrine, since high-dose glucocorticoids induce the formation of phenylethanolamine-*N*-methyltransferase, the enzyme needed to convert norepinephrine into epinephrine.[148]

In addition to their important effects on the cardiovascular system, catecholamines also have significant metabolic effects, stimulating glycogenolysis and gluconeogenesis, that is, increasing the production of glucose from glycogen and amino acid precursors and stimulating lipolysis, thereby mobilizing free fatty acids and inhibiting secretion of insulin. The absence of the adrenal medulla does not produce definable disease in humans. However, the presence of a hormonally active adrenal medullary tumor produces a number of significant findings.

CLINICAL AND BIOCHEMICAL MANIFESTATIONS. A pheochromocytoma is a catecholamine-producing tumor derived from chromaffin cells. Those arising from extra-adrenal chromaffin cells are called nonadrenal pheochromocytomas or paraganglionomas. Probably less than 0.1 per cent of patients with hypertension have a pheochromocytoma. Despite the fact that it is an uncommon disease, pheochromocytomas generate a great deal of interest, largely because the morbidity and mortality associated with these tumors are significant, with detection often resulting in cure. Pheochromocytomas are highly vascular tumors; less than 10 per cent are malignant as indicated by local invasion or metastasis, but, as with other endocrine tumors, malignancy cannot always be determined by microscopic appearance alone.

While the vast majority of tumors occur sporadically, approximately 5 per cent are inherited as an autosomal trait, of which they are often part of a pluriglandular neoplastic syndrome,[149] which, in addition to pheochromocytoma, may consist of medullary carcinoma of the thyroid, parathyroidadenoma, and retinal or cerebellar hemangioblastomas. Most pheochromocytomas are solitary adrenal tumors, with 10 per cent being bilateral and 10 per cent nonadrenal. However, in the familial form of pheochromocytoma nearly half the patients have bilateral adrenal tumors.

The features that suggest pheochromocytoma in hypertensive patients are (1) paroxysmal attacks of any kind, (2) headaches, (3) excessive sweating, (4) signs of hypermetabolism, (5) orthostatic hypotension, and (6) unusual blood pressure elevations to trauma or operation.[147] Many of the features are similar to those of hyperthyroidism. While paroxysmal attacks are the hallmark of pheochromocytoma, more than half the patients have fixed hypertension and nearly 10 per cent are normotensive.

CARDIOVASCULAR MANIFESTATIONS. Hypertension is the major cardiovascular manifestation of pheochromocytoma. Its lability sometimes distinguishes it from other forms of hypertension; however, only clinical awareness of the entity and specific laboratory testing permit establishment of the proper diagnosis. The lability of blood pressure in patients with pheochromocytoma has been suggested to be due not only to episodic discharge of catecholamines but also to a reduction in plasma volume, as well as to impaired sympathetic reflexes. However, an absolute reduction of plasma volume exists in only a minority of cases,[150] but a number of observations suggest that chronic volume depletion is present. For example, alpha-adrenoceptor blockade or removal of the tumor produces severe hypotension, which is correctable by volume expansion.[151] Cardiac output has been reported to be normal, whereas heart rate is increased, and orthostatic hypotension is accompanied by decreased stroke volume and inadequate adjustments in peripheral resistance indicative of impaired peripheral vascular reflexes.[150] An occasional patient will have markedly elevated central aortic pressure and severe systemic hypotension due to severe arterial vasoconstriction.[152]

The electrocardiogram is abnormal in as many as 75 per cent of patients with pheochromocytoma.[25] The changes consist of T-wave inversion, left ventricular hypertrophy, sinus tachycardia, and, in some cases, other alterations in rhythm, such as frequent supraventricular ectopic beats or paroxysmal supraventricular tachycardia. An occasional patient will present with a short P-R interval and a narrow QRS complex, suggesting that catecholamines are modifying the AV conduction system.[153] When arterial pressure increases markedly, changes suggestive of myocardial damage, including transient ST-segment elevations, marked diffuse T-wave inversions, and depression of ST segments are present. These changes are usually transient, and the electrocardiographic pattern reverts to normal after removal of the tumor or pharmacological blockade.[147, 151] Some of the electrocardiographic abnormalities are presumably due to hypertensive heart disease or myocardial ischemia. However, a specific catecholamine-induced myocarditis has also been suggested.[154]

The echocardiogram often shows left ventricular hypertrophy with normal left ventricular function.[155] During a hypertensive crisis it may show systolic anterior involvement of the anterior mitral leaflet, paradoxical septal motion, and proximal exclusion of the posterior wall.[156]

Myocarditis. Pathologically, the myocarditis consists of focal necrosis with infiltration of inflammatory cells, perivascular inflammation, and contraction band necrosis[157] (Fig. 58–6), finally resulting in fibrosis. In some studies, 50 per cent of patients who died from pheochromocytoma had myocarditis,[151] usually accompanied by left ventricular failure and pulmonary edema. Although coronary atherosclerosis is usually present, medial thickening is the most characteristic lesion of the coronary arteries. When norepinephrine is infused into the rabbit, there is sustained coronary vasoconstriction that within 48 hours leads to histologically documented myocardial damage.[158] Occasionally, patients with pheochromocytoma present with manifestations of cardiomyopathy[159] which may be reversed when the tumor is removed[159a] (Fig. 58–7). Finally, the myositis is not necessarily limited to the myocardium, as it also may occur in skeletal muscle.[160]

DIAGNOSIS AND TREATMENT. The diagnosis of pheochromocytoma is established by documenting increased urinary or plasma levels of catecholamines or one of their

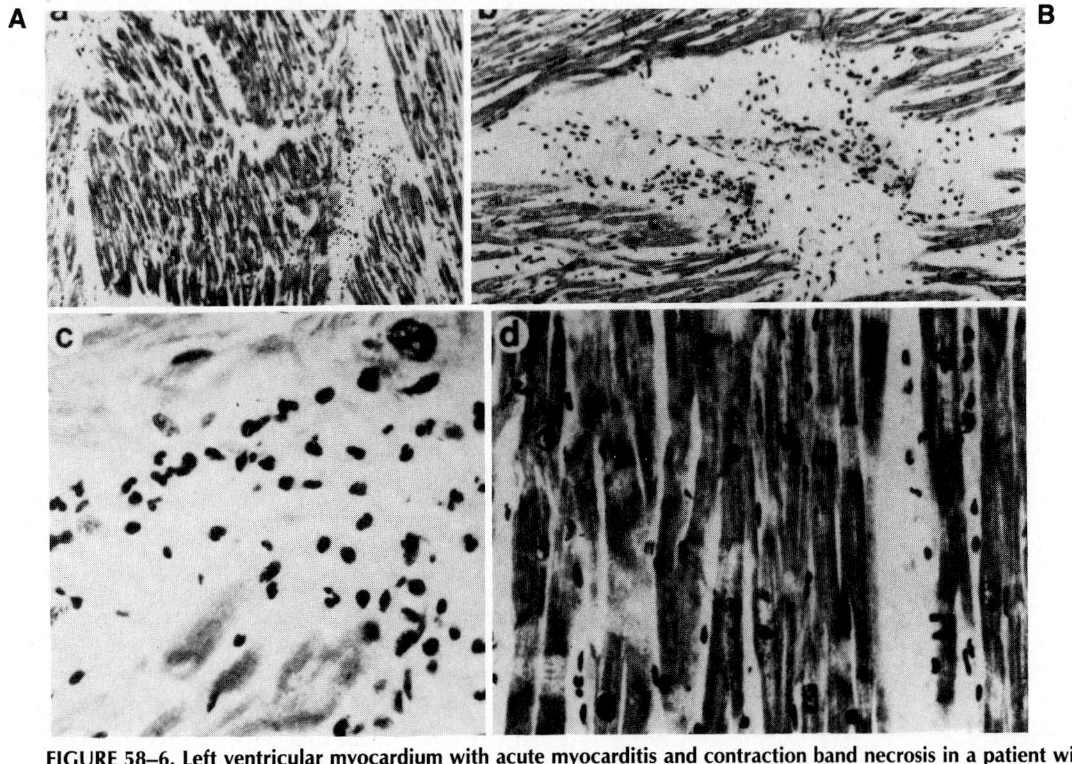

FIGURE 58–6. Left ventricular myocardium with acute myocarditis and contraction band necrosis in a patient with pheochromocytoma dying of catecholamine crisis. *a*, Diffuse infiltration by inflammatory cells through myocardium. *b*, Perivascular inflammation. *c*, Close-up of the inflammatory infiltrate. *d*, Contraction-band necrosis of myocytes. (Hematoxylin and eosin stains; original magnification × 20 (a), × 45 (b), × 540 (c), × 330 (d)). (From McManus, B. M., Fleury, T. A., and Roberts, W. C.: Fatal catecholamine crisis in pheochromocytoma: Curable cause of cardiac arrest. Am. Heart J. *102*:930, 1981.)

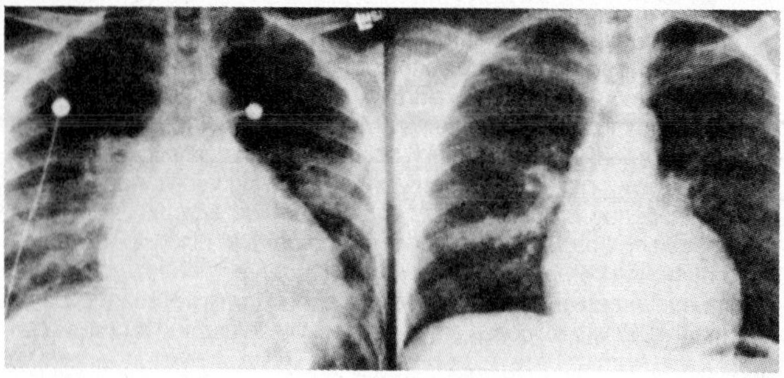

FIGURE 58–7. *Left*, Chest x-ray on admission. Cardiomegaly, right pleural effusion, and signs of congestive heart failure. *Right*, One month after removal of the tumor. No signs of congestion and significant decrease of the heart size. (From Velasquez, G., D'Souza, V. J., Hackshaw, B. T., Glass, T. A., and Formanek, A. G.: Phaeochromocytoma and cardiomyopathy. Br. J. Radiol. *57*:89, 1984.)

metabolites.[147, 151] Three tests are commonly employed: (1) total catecholamines, (2) vanillylmandelic acid (VMA); and (3) metanephrine. The last two are metabolites of catecholamine and were first used to screen for pheochromocytoma because they are present in greater quantities. When reliably performed, these tests are probably equivalent in accuracy. The probability of a pheochromocytoma being present in a hypertensive patient with a single normal urine level is less than 5 per cent. It is most desirable to measure both the catecholamines and one of the two metabolites, preferably metanephrine, in screening for pheochromocytoma. If the blood pressure fluctuates it is particularly important to collect the urine at a time the pressure is elevated. Specific pharmacological tests to screen for pheochromocytoma are of limited benefit, usually hazardous, and therefore warranted only in unusual circumstances. Clonidine has been proposed as a useful definitive test for pheochromocytoma, although it is necessary only in unusual cases. Catecholamine levels are suppressed in normal subjects via stimulation of central alpha-adrenoceptors; following clonidine administration in patients with pheochromocytoma they are not.[147] Unfortunately, profound and prolonged hypotension has been reported in some patients during the course of this test.

Once the diagnosis of pheochromocytoma is established, specific pharmacological blockade should be initiated.[147, 151] Administration of phenoxybenzamine hydrochloride should be begun, with the initial dosage 10 mg every 12 hours; the dose is then gradually increased every 2 to 3 days until the arterial pressure is restored to normal. Alternatively, prazosin may be used. However, it should be noted that alpha-adrenoceptor blockade may induce a decline in arterial pressure accompanied by serious postural hypotension, presumably because of the vasodilatation occurring in the presence of hypovolemia. This hypotensive response can be prevented by adequate sodium intake; if the response is very striking, infusion of saline may be required. Adequate control of arterial pressure is essential prior to any arteriographic procedure, before initiating beta-adrenoceptor blockade, and before operation. Serfas and colleagues have suggested that calcium antagonists may be useful both in treating the hypertension associated with pheochromocytoma and in reducing catecholamine production.[161]

Beta-adrenoceptor blockade is useful in patients with pheochromocytoma who have significant tachycardia, palpitations, and catecholamine-induced arrhythmias. However, beta blockade with a drug affecting $beta_2$ receptors must *not* be initiated prior to inadequate alpha blockade, since severe *hypertension* may occur as a result of unopposed alpha-stimulating activity of the circulating catecholamines.

Definitive treatment is surgical removal of the tumor, usually after localization with computed tomography, arteriography, or scanning using an ^{131}I-derivative of guanethidine as the scanning agent.[154, 162] Scanning may be particularly important in localizing extra-adrenal, e.g., thoracic pheochromocytomas. Although rare, of particular importance to the cardiologist is the presence of a cardiac pheochromocytoma (p. 1476). Precise definition of the anatomical boundaries of this tumor is important preoperatively if surgery is to be successful.[163, 164] In those patients with inoperable lesions, long-term use of the combination of alpha- and beta-adrenoceptor blockers has been helpful. Drugs that inhibit the biosynthesis of catecholamines, such as alpha-methyltyrosine, have also been used in patients with malignant pheochromocytoma.[147, 151]

PARATHYROID DISEASE

Disordered parathyroid secretion is associated with two cardiovascular disturbances, cardiac arrhythmias and hypertension. Changes in calcium metabolism as well as a direct effect of parathyroid hormone on the cardiovascular system appear to be responsible.

CLINICAL AND BIOCHEMICAL MANIFESTATIONS. Parathyroid hormone (PTH) is a single-chain polypeptide of 84 amino acids. Its major biological effect is to increase mobilization of calcium into the extracellular fluid from a variety of tissues; this action is linked in a negative feedback loop with serum unbound calcium concentration. Thus, an increase in serum calcium concentration reduces parathyroid hormone release and vice versa.[165] PTH also increases urinary excretion of phosphate, augments bone resorption, and reduces the urinary excretion of calcium. It also indirectly increases the absorption of calcium from the gastrointestinal tract by increasing the rate of conversion of 25-hydroxyl vitamin D into the biologically active 1,25-dihydroxy vitamin D.[166]

Primary hyperparathyroidism, the excess production of parathyroid hormone, is usually secondary to a solitary parathyroid adenoma. Occasionally, generalized parathyroid hyperplasia exists, and, infrequently, carcinoma of the parathyroid gland is found. In many cases, hyperparathyroidism is asymptomatic; 10 to 20 per cent of cases are first diagnosed as the result of a routine chemical screening test. *Secondary* hyperparathyroidism is at least equal in frequency to primary hyperparathyroidism. It is most commonly associated with renal disease and chronic hypocalcemia.

The signs and symptoms of primary hyperparathyroidism are related to direct effects of PTH on kidney or bone or those associated with the hypercalcemia. Nearly half the patients have signs and symptoms of renal dysfunction, such as polyuria, nocturia, renal stones, and, in severe cases, nephrocalcinosis and renal failure. In many patients, there are also nonspecific joint and back symptoms, and in unusual circumstances spontaneous fractures occur. Hypercalcemia reduces the excitability of the neuromuscular system, which can lead to such diverse effects as significant myocardial dysfunction and decreased auditory acuity.

Cardiac hypertrophy is found with increased frequency in patients with hyperparathyroidism, even in the absence of hypertension. In one study, five of 18 patients with hypertrophic cardiomyopathy had raised serum PTH levels but normal serum calcium levels. In contrast, left ventricular hypertrophy did not occur in six patients with hypercalcemia alone.[167]

Hypocalcemia is the common biochemical abnormality in both hypoparathyroidism and secondary hyperparathyroidism. Gastrointestinal disturbances and tetany secondary to the hypocalcemia may both occur.

CARDIOVASCULAR MANIFESTATIONS OF PARATHYROID DISEASES (See also p. 848)

CARDIAC EFFECTS. Until recently, most of the effects of parathyroid hormone on the heart have been assumed to be secondary to a change in extracellular calcium. It has now been documented that PTH also has a direct effect on the heart resulting in an increased beating rate of isolated heart cells and a positive inotropic action.[168, 169] These effects are probably mediated by PTH binding to specific receptors, leading to increased entry of calcium into cardiac cells, and by the PTH increasing the release of endogenous myocardial norepinephrine. The direct effect of PTH may be deleterious, since it causes necrosis of rat myocytes and may be directly responsible for the increased accumulation of calcium in dystrophic muscles and for the heart damage found in uremia.[168, 170] Whether these effects are clinically relevant is uncertain. Gafter and colleagues reported no change in cardiac performance in seven patients with end-stage renal disease who underwent parathyroidectomy for hyperparathyroidism.[171] On the other hand, hypoparathyroidism may cause a dilated cardiomyopathy, caused presumably by hypocalcemia, but perhaps also by hypomagnesemia and reduced circulating PTH.[172] PTH also has a direct effect on vascular smooth muscle, causing vasodilatation. Presently available data suggest that this vasodilating effect is more closely related to the portion of the PTH molecule responsible for its phosphaturic rather than its hypercalcemic effect.[173]

In addition to any direct action of PTH on the heart, hypercalcemia also has an adverse effect. Chronic hypercalcemia from a variety of causes is associated with increased deposition of calcium in the fibrous skeleton of the heart and valvular cusps as well as in coronary arteries and in myocardial fibers[174] (Fig. 58–8). Chronic hypercalcemia also may be a risk factor for accelerated coronary atherosclerosis.[175]

The plateau of the action potential of cardiac fibers is prolonged by low and shortened by high extracellular calcium concentrations (Chap. 20). Lengthening of the plateau prolongs the duration of the action potential, whereas shortening of the plateau has the opposite effect. The changes in duration of action potential are accompanied by corresponding changes in the duration of the refractory period, of the ST segment, and the Q-T interval.[25] Thus the major electrocardiographic change in hypercalcemia is shortening of the Q-T interval. Less frequently, disorders of intraventricular conduction have been reported with shortening of the P-R interval.[25] Complete heart block occurs only rarely.

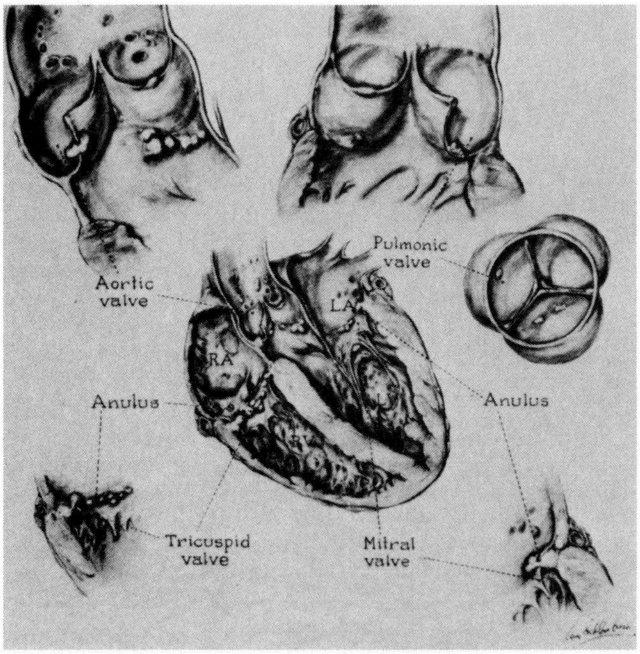

FIGURE 58–8. Drawing of heart showing distribution of calcific deposits in the tricuspid and mitral valve anuli and at the bases of both pulmonic and aortic valve cusps in a 43-year-old woman with hypercalcemia secondary to primary hyperparathyroidism. (From Roberts, W. C., and Waller, B. F.: Effect of chronic hypercalcemia on the heart: An analysis of 18 necropsy patients. Am. J. Med. *71*:371, 1981.)

Hypocalcemia produces the opposite effect on the electrocardiogram with prolongation of the Q-T interval and nonspecific ST- and T-wave changes. Since normal contractile function of cardiac muscle requires calcium, it is surprising that heart failure has not been reported more frequently in patients with chronic hypocalcemia. In most, it usually occurs only when other cardiac diseases are present.[176]

HYPERTENSION. Hypercalcemic patients detected by routine serum calcium screening techniques have higher arterial pressure than do matched normocalcemic subjects.[177] Yet in patients with hyperparathyroidism, the level of serum calcium is similar in those who are normotensive and those who have hypertension, suggesting that hypercalcemia per se is not the dominant cause for the hypertension. Thus, the pathophysiology of the hypertension is uncertain.[178] For example, hypercalcemia produces nephrocalcinosis, which may lead to renal failure and hypertension. Thus, reversal of hypertension after successful parathyroid surgery is more likely to occur when renal function is normal. Increased serum calcium also increases myocardial contractility, peripheral resistance, and release of or vascular sensitivity to vasoconstrictor agents, such as angiotensin II and norepinephrine. While hypercalcemia can increase cardiac contractility and arterial pressure acutely, it is unlikely that this action produces a significant alteration in cardiac output or performance on a chronic basis in the absence of PTH.[178] Thus an elevation of peripheral resistance is the most likely cause of the hypertension associated with hyperparathyroidism. Resnick has concluded that primary hyperparathyroidism is frequently associated with hypertension. While the mechanism of hypertension in these patients remains to be elucidated, (1) it may be renin dependent; (2) it is associated with increased circulating PTH, but not necessarily with the level of hypercalcemia; and (3) it is curable surgically in a significant number of patients.[179]

DIAGNOSIS AND TREATMENT

If hypercalcemia is *not* due to primary hyperparathyroidism, circulating concentration of parathyroid hormone should be suppressed. Thus, an elevated or even a normal concentration of parathyroid hormone in the presence of hypercalcemia establishes the diagnosis of hyperparathyroidism; many patients with this condition manifest hypercalcemia for the first time after starting thiazide therapy for the associated hypertension. Treatment consists of surgical removal of the parathyroid tumor of hyperplastic glands.

Patients with hypertension should have a determination of serum calcium levels before therapy is begun. If thiazide diuretics are used in treatment, serum calcium levels should be determined every 6 months. If thiazide-induced hypercalcemia occurs, the serum calcium should be determined for 2 to 3 months after discontinuation of the thiazides. Persistence of the hypercalcemia suggests that the patient has primary hyperparathyroidism.[177]

Patients with hypoparathyroidism and hypocalcemia usually are treated with calcium supplementation and vitamin D or one of its metabolites. To minimize the development of nephrolithiasis, serum calcium levels are titrated only to the lower end of the normal range.

DIABETES MELLITUS

Diabetes mellitus is one of the leading public health problems in the industrialized world, and it has a profound effect on the cardiovascular system. Nearly 10 million people are afflicted with this disease in the United States; it is the eighth health-related cause of death. Nearly all the morbidity from diabetes is related to cardiovascular dysfunction, either coronary artery disease or renal failure secondary to vascular disease.

ACTIONS OF INSULIN. Insulin is a double-chain polypeptide derived from proinsulin, which is synthesized in the islet cells of the pancreas. Many stimuli, such as glucose, glucagon, amino acids, catecholamines, and gastrointestinal hormones, can promote insulin secretion, which usually occurs in two phases. The rapid early phase releases preformed insulin stored in granules in the beta cells, while the prolonged late phase results from increased biosynthesis of insulin.[179]

Insulin is an anabolic hormone affecting all metabolic substrates, i.e., carbohydrates, fats, and proteins, as well as nucleic acids. All target tissues for insulin have specific membrane-bound receptors; thus, binding to the receptor is the first step in initiating its metabolic effect. The concept that insulin is the "fed" hormone has been popularized.[180] Thus the ingestion of fuel substrates provokes a rapid rise in the concentration of circulating insulin, which then facilitates the transfer of these substances into their respective depots. According to this theory, in the fasted state insulin levels are low; as a result, there is increased gluconeogenesis by the liver, decreased lipogenesis with lipolysis and fatty acid release from fat tissue, and decreased glucose uptake in cardiac and skeletal muscle. On the other hand, in the fed state insulin levels are high; gluconeogenesis by the liver is reduced; and in cardiac and skeletal muscle glucose and amino acid uptake and protein synthesis are increased. In adipose tissue there is increased glucose and triglyceride uptake, lipogenesis, and absence of release of fatty acids.

In the patient with diabetes, because insulin release is decreased in response to the ingested fuel, there is a delay in the uptake and the disposal of these fuels into their respective depots, which leads to abnormal circulating levels of the substrates. The increased concentrations of lipids in the circulation may be the underlying pathophysiological effect producing a number of the clinical complications of diabetes mellitus.

CLINICAL AND BIOCHEMICAL MANIFESTATIONS. Relatively recently, our understanding of the pathogenesis of diabetes mellitus has been significantly altered. Several lines of evidence suggest that in many instances the insulin-dependent (IDDM) form may be infectious or autoimmune in origin, while in most cases the noninsulin-dependent form (NIDDM) is probably the result of a genetic predisposition.[181]

Most of the signs and symptoms of this disease either are related to the increased levels of blood glucose or are secondary to changes in the cardiovascular system. Thus, the classic presenting symptoms (observed in about 25 per cent of IDDM patients) are polyuria, polydipsia, and polyphagia, all due to the glucosuria. The major pathophysiological consequence of diabetes mellitus is related to changes in the vascular system. The specific target organs include the heart, the eye, the kidney, the autonomic nervous system, and the peripheral vasculature.

CARDIOVASCULAR CHANGES IN DIABETES

PATHOLOGY. The vascular disease associated with diabetes mellitus can be nonspecific (atherosclerosis and arteriosclerosis) or specific (microangiopathic or endothelial proliferative changes of arterioles). The former primarily involves large vessels (especially in the lower extremities), heart, and brain of older patients, while the latter is localized to small vessels and may be seen in patients of all ages. The atherosclerosis tends to be more extensive and more severe than in nondiabetics, resulting in an increased frequency of myocardial infarction and cerebral and peripheral vasculature disease.[182] Indeed, coronary heart disease is the leading cause of death among adult diabetics and accounts for about three times as many deaths among diabetics as among nondiabetics. The incidence of coronary artery disease correlates more closely with the duration of diabetes than with its severity. Of interest is the documentation that diabetics have an increased mortality for noncardiovascular diseases (e.g., cancer) as well.[183] The mechanism(s) responsible for this generalized increased mortality is unclear.

Certainly, diabetes should be considered to be a separate risk factor for coronary heart disease[184] (p. 1181). Since each risk factor for vascular disease is thought to add independently (although not equally) to the likelihood for the development of ischemic disease, the diabetic should be considered a high-risk patient in whom all correctable factors should be managed. It is logical to approach cigarette smoking and even moderate elevation of blood pressure and plasma lipids more intensively in diabetic than in nondiabetic patients. Contraceptive drugs that suppress ovulation probably should be avoided, since they may contribute to the metabolic abnormalities that underlie their increased risk for vascular disease. The obese diabetic patient should lose weight; this is often accompanied by gratifying improvement of hypertension, hyperglycemia, hyperinsulinemia, and hypertriglyceridemia.[184]

The microangiopathy produces a characteristic thickening of the basement membrane of the capillaries in the retina, conjunctiva, glomerulus, brain, pancreas, and myocardium.[185] In some cases there is also proliferation of the epithelial cells, leading to occlusion of small arterioles similar to that observed in immune arteritis.

CARDIAC INVOLVEMENT. Not only is the frequency of acute myocardial infarction increased in diabetic patients,[186] but also the treatment of the infarct is more complicated than in the nondiabetic patient. Patients with acute myocardial infarction and with poor control of the diabetes before hospital admission exhibit a significantly higher mortality than those with good control, but there appears to be no significant difference in mortality between well-controlled diabetics and nondiabetics.[187, 188] Several factors contribute to the increased mortality of diabetic patients with acute myocardial infarction. The size of the infarct tends to be greater in the diabetic than in the nondiabetic[189]; diabetic patients have a greater frequency of both congestive heart failure and shock than nondiabetics[187, 188]; and the patient is often in a precarious metabolic status compounded by the difficulty of adjusting insulin therapy to prevent ketoacidosis while not precipitating hypoglycemia.

The occurrence of myocardial infarction has a distinctly adverse effect on carbohydrate and fat metabolism and often leads to stimulation of the sympathetic nervous system and increased catecholamine concentration[190] (p. 1233). Subsequent increases in circulating free fatty acid levels and reductions in glucose tolerance appear to be related to a number of physiological functions—adipose tissue lipolysis, hepatic and muscle glycogenolysis, catecholamine-induced suppression of insulin release, and increased circulating concentrations of growth hormone and cortisol. The net result is that carbohydrate intolerance is common after myocardial infarction, even in nondiabetics. Also, the high concentrations of free fatty acid in the acute phases of myocardial infarction may lead to ventricular arrhythmias.[191, 192] The suppression of insulin release as a consequence of increased catecholamine activity may decrease glucose utilization by a myocardium that may require this fuel for glycolytic activity.[193]

Diabetic patients with acute myocardial infarction differ from nondiabetics in that their pain patterns are more variable, and infarction may actually occur without pain. Also, survival after infarction is more limited than in the nondiabetics, with fatality rates being as high as 25 per cent during the first year after infarction.[194] Recurrent infarction, heart failure, and dysrhythmias all contribute to this higher death rate.[194, 195] Administration of beta blockers to diabetics appears to reduce the overall mortality, at least in the immediate postmyocardial infarction period, similar to what has been reported in nondiabetics.[188, 196]

Peripheral somatic neuropathy is a common complication of diabetes mellitus; also, diabetic autonomic neuropathy leading to diarrhea, vomiting, and other gastrointestinal disturbances is well known in this disease. Cardiac autonomic dysfunction also exists in many diabetic patients.[197] In two large series it was present in more than a third of the patients and accompanied by depression of left ventricular function. The severity of cardiac dysfunction was directly related to the severity of the cardiac autonomic neuropathy.[198, 199] Occasionally it may be present before clinical symptoms of generalized autonomic neuropathy are demonstrable.[200] Furthermore, the neuropathy may involve the sympathetic nervous system and/or the parasympathetic nervous system. Indeed, it may become so severe as to lead to total cardiac denervation. These changes in adrenergic nervous system function result in tachycardia and a fixed, rapid heart rate that barely responds to physiological stimuli, such as the Valsalva maneuver, carotid sinus pressure, or tilting, or to drugs, such as phenylephrine, atropine, or propranolol. Rarely, these denervated hearts develop arrhythmias.

CONGESTIVE HEART FAILURE. IDDM appears to increase the likelihood of the development of congestive heart failure from all causes. The role of diabetes in congestive heart failure in the Framingham study was analyzed,[201] and the risk of developing heart failure was found to be increased substantially. Even when patients with prior coronary or rheumatic heart disease were excluded, diabetic subjects had a four- to fivefold increased risk of congestive heart failure. Furthermore, this increased risk persisted after age, blood pressure, weight, and cholesterol values, as well as coronary heart disease, were taken into account. On the basis of these findings it appeared that the excessive risk of heart failure in diabetic patients is caused by factors other than accelerated atherogenesis and coronary heart disease. One suggested possibility is a diabetes-induced cardiomyopathy.[202, 203]

Diabetic Cardiomyopathy. A statistically significant increase in the frequency of diabetes in patients with idiopathic cardiomyopathy has been reported.[184] These patients had serious congestive heart failure, which was difficult to control, and invariably at autopsy they showed patent large coronary arteries but abnormalities in the small intramural coronary vessels, including intimal fibroblastic thickening and hyaline deposits, as well as inflammatory changes. In contrast, small-vessel disease was rare in patients with cardiomyopathy without diabetes. In addition, significant extravascular deposition was noted of collagen, triglyceride, and cholesterol, which may have contributed to the cardiomyopathy. These findings further supported the idea that diabetic patients can develop myocardial disease without large coronary artery involvement, possibly owing to pathological changes in small coronary vessels, but there is considerable dispute concerning the role, if any, of involvement of the latter.

Further clinical evidence for a diabetic cardiomyopathy came from the observations of Regan.[204] A study was made of a group of diabetic patients without evident heart failure who exhibited an elevation of left ventricular end-diastolic pressure and of the left ventricular end-diastolic pressure/volume ratio (Fig. 58–9). Increments of afterload effected an abnormal increase of filling pressure without an increase in stroke volume, compared to normal subjects, consistent with a preclinical cardiomyopathy. Left ventricular biopsy in two patients without ventricular decompensation showed interstitial deposition of collagen with relatively normal muscle cells. These findings suggest a nonischemic myopathic process.

Abnormalities of Ventricular Functions. An abnormality

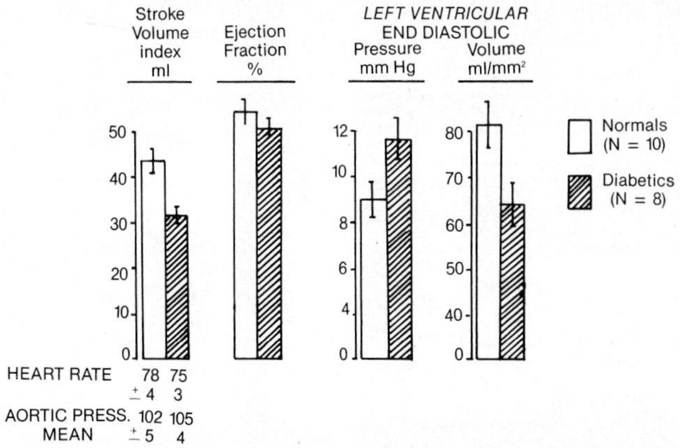

FIGURE 58–9. Hemodynamics of ten healthy patients versus eight diabetic individuals at rest. (From Regan, T. J.: Cardiac decompensation in diabetes mellitus. Cardiovasc. Rev. Rep. 6:1117, 1985.)

of left ventricular function in diabetes is also reflected in the shortening of the left ventricular ejection time, the prolongation of the projection period, and the elevation of the ratio of the preejection period to the left ventricular ejection time (PTP/LVET).[205] Left ventricular function has also been assessed by echocardiography in diabetic patients with microangiopathy, defined as proteinuria exceeding 3 gm/24 hours, or proliferative retinopathy, but without angina, previous myocardial infarction, hypertension, or alcoholism and with normal electrocardiograms and chest radiographs.[203, 206] Diabetics with microangiopathy had impaired left ventricular function, whereas those with uncomplicated diabetes exhibited normal function. This finding supports the existence of a specific diabetic cardiomyopathy associated with microangiography rather than secondary to a metabolic defect.[207] This association between microangiopathy and impaired left ventricular function may help to explain the high incidence of cardiogenic shock, congestive heart failure, and mortality that has been reported in some series of myocardial infarction in diabetics. Furthermore, a large body of evidence has now accumulated that impaired left ventricular diastolic function, reflected in a reduced rate of left ventricular wall thinning and dimension increase, may be present in many asymptomatic diabetic patients, particularly those with severe microvascular complications.[186] Radionuclide ventriculography[208] and echocardiography are useful in demonstrating reduced velocity of early left ventricular filling (Fig. 58–10).

Pathological Changes. In postmortem studies of 11 diabetic patients, 9 of whom were without significant obstructive disease of the proximal coronary arteries and had died of cardiac failure, all exhibited positive periodic acid–Schiff (PAS) staining material in the interstitium, but none had luminal narrowing of the intramural vessels. Collagen accumulation was present in perivascular loci, between the myofibers, or as replacement fibrosis. Multiple samples of left ventricle and septum revealed abnormally increased deposits of triglyceride and cholesterol.[204, 209] Thus these observations, taken in toto, suggest that a diffuse abnormality, either extravascular or involving the microvasculature, may be the basis for the cardiomyopathic features of diabetes. However, a recent morphological study casts some doubt on small-vessel disease as the producer of cardiac myopathy, because similar findings have been reported in NIDDM subjects. Unsitupa et al., studying 133 patients with NIDDM (Type 2), found a high incidence of impaired left ventricular function already present at the time of initial diagnosis.[210] Hypertension appears to accelerate this process, both in humans and animals, as severe interstitial fibrosis, focal scars, and myocytolytic activity

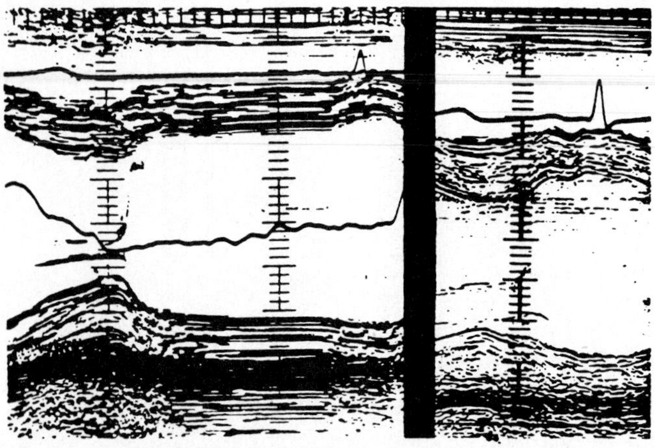

FIGURE 58–10. M-mode echocardiograms from a healthy woman (*left*) and a diabetic woman (*right*). The rate of ventricular filling is much slower in the latter. (From Airaksinen, J., et al.: Impaired left ventricular filling in young female diabetics. An echocardiographic study. Acta Med. Scand. 216:509, 1984.)

were significantly more frequent in hypertensive diabetics with chronic heart failure examined post mortem than in normotensive diabetics[211, 212] (Fig. 58–11).

To gain a better understanding of diabetic cardiomyopathy, a mild, noninsulin-requiring alloxan diabetes was produced in dogs.[213] Despite similar end-diastolic pressures, the end-diastolic volume and stroke volume were significantly less than in control dogs. During acute volume expansion of the ventricle with saline, the end-diastolic pressure increment in diabetic dogs was twice that observed in control dogs. These responses were attributed to increased stiffness of the left ventricle that was apparently due to accumulation of glycoproteins in the interstitium, measured by PAS staining. Similar abnormalities were observed in dogs with diabetes that occurred spontaneously. During infusion of ^{14}C-l-oleic acid, fatty acid incorporation, which was predominantly into phospholipid in the control dogs, was diverted to triglyceride in the diabetic dogs; analysis of lipids in the left ventricle revealed elevated concentrations of triglyceride and cholesterol despite normal plasma levels.

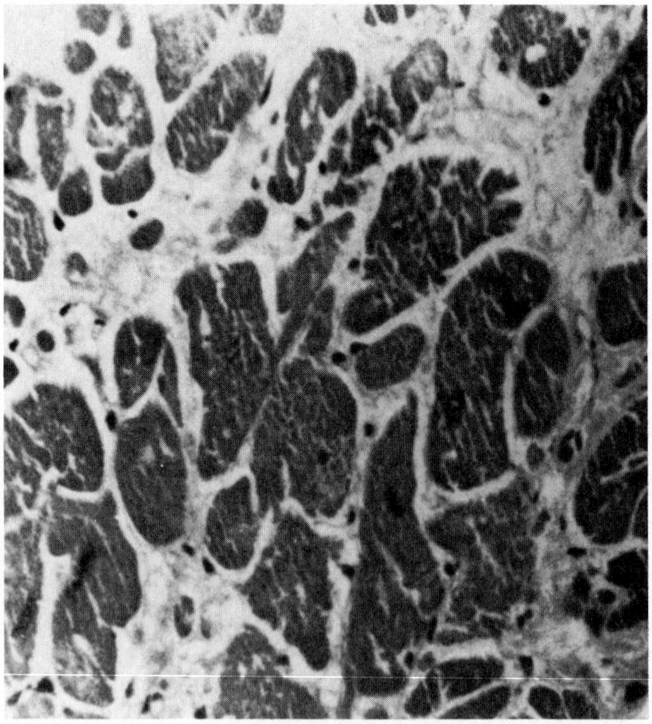

FIGURE 58–11. This section of left ventricular myocardium from a 46-year-old white male (at death) who had insulin-dependent diabetes for 20 years. It demonstrates diffuse interstitial fibrosis. There is marked variability of myocardial cell size, with virtually every cell surrounded by dense collagen. This abnormality is a characteristic feature of the hypertensive-diabetic heart (hematoxylin-eosin; original magnification × 250). (From Factor, S. M., Minase, T., and Sonnenblick, E. H.: Clinical and morphological features of human hypertensive-diabetic cardiomyopathy. Am. Heart J. 99:446, 1980.)

At the molecular level, several changes in function have been documented in diabetic rats. Divalent cation ATPase activity is significantly depressed, phosphatidylethanolamine N-methylation also is inhibited, and abnormal mechanical and electrophysiological responses to ouabain have been reported.[214–217]

Thus these experimental observations support the hypothesis that chronic diabetes mellitus can alter myocardial composition and function independent of its vascular and acute metabolic effects. In the dog model, therapy with insulin for 1 year did not reverse all of the myocardial abnormalities.[218] Additional experimental studies suggest, however, that adequate control of the hyperglycemia may reverse the process. In rats with streptozotocin-induced diabetes, there is significant decrease in contractile protein ATPase activity, resulting in a slowing of relaxation and a depression of shortening velocity.[219] Short-term treatment with insulin—less than one week—did not modify these abnormalities. However, treatment for one month completely reversed them.[220] Similar findings were reported in rabbits.[221] Whether the different effect of insulin therapy in these studies is related to species differences or differing methods to induce the diabetic state is uncertain.

Other (nondiabetic) cardiomyopathies may exhibit similar hemodynamic abnormalities; an abnormal rise of ventricular filling pressure without a stroke volume increase in response to afterload increments has also been observed in the preclinical phase of alcoholic cardiomyopathy, in which the interstitium is also altered.[222] More severely altered interstitial changes may be the predominant lesion in the incipient stages of amyloid heart disease.[222]

Diabetes mellitus is associated with another form of cardiomyopathy. Approximately half the infants of diabetic mothers have either radiographic cardiomegaly or clinical features suggesting congestive heart failure[223] (p. 1012). The cardiomyopathy in these infants may be transient and secondary to hematological, respiratory, and metabolic problems or a more protracted form of nonobstructive or obstructive hypertrophic cardiomyopathy, which appears to be secondary to maternal hormonal influences and to be reversible.

Electrocardiographic changes are commonly observed in patients with diabetes.[25] While many of the changes are predictable on the basis of the associated hypertension or coronary artery disease, in some there is an unexplained diffuse T-wave abnormality that may be related to the cardiomyopathy.

VASCULAR DISEASE. Peripheral vascular disease is a frequent and significant manifestation of diabetes mellitus, often leading to gangrene and amputation of the lower extremity. The smaller arteries below the knee are more likely to be involved in patients with diabetes, in contrast to iliac or femoral artery disease in nondiabetic patients. Cerebral vascular disease is also more frequent, with a greater incidence of cerebral infarction though not cerebral hemorrhage. The increased atherosclerosis of the cerebral vessels and the proliferative changes in the cerebral arterioles both contribute to this increased rate of infarction. In addition to the effect of diabetes on cardiac function, insulin itself can cause salt and water retention by mechanisms still obscure. In most cases this fluid retention is self-limiting. However, in individuals who have underlying cardiovascular disease it may lead to overt cardiac failure.[224]

The renal vasculature is affected in a number of ways: Atherosclerosis is common in the larger vessels, with proliferative endothelial changes occurring in small vessels. Capillary basement membrane thickening is common, particularly in the glomerular tuft where a pathognomonic change—nodular glomerulosclerosis—is often found. These vascular changes, in concert with parenchymal changes secondary to pyelonephritis, lead to a variety of renal disorders, including the nephrotic syndrome, hypertension, and renal failure.

The mechanism underlying the development of atherosclerosis in diabetes is multifactorial (p. 1181). Recently, hyperinsulinemia itself has been shown to enhance lipid synthesis in arterial walls and may be a major factor contributing to the macroangiopathy.[225] Most studies have reported an increased incidence of hypertension in diabetes. Indeed, more than one-third of diabetic patients have hypertension, an incidence that is higher than that of the general population. The hypertension is in part related to the increased frequency of renal disease. Volume overload may be an additional factor. In the past, the hypertension was assumed to be treated best by diuretics and sodium restriction. This therapy has two substantial drawbacks: (1) diuretics impair glucose homeostasis and (2) they probably accelerate renal deterioration. Because converting-enzyme inhibitors have theoretical advantages both in terms of glucose control and in retarding the deterioration of renal function, they may be the treatment of choice for hypertension in diabetics.[226]

DIAGNOSIS AND TREATMENT OF DIABETES MELLITUS

It is generally agreed that therapy directed at the control of excessive fatty acid mobilization and oxidation and protein catabolism is essential in diabetes mellitus. On the other hand, disagreement still exists regarding the usefulness of treating asymptomatic hyperglycemia. It has been documented that the synthesis of polyols and basement membrane glycoproteins is increased by hyperglycemia.[185, 227] Thus, "tight control" of blood glucose may be important if the long-term complications of diabetes mellitus are to be reduced.

Diet, insulin, and oral hypoglycemic agents have been the mainstays of treatment. However, a controversy has arisen concerning the efficacy of oral hypoglycemic agents, such as the sulfonylureas.[228] While hyperglycemia is better controlled with these agents than it is with diet alone, an increased frequency of myocardial infarction has been reported. Although the interpretation and implications of these findings are still controversial, there is some experimental evidence suggesting that sulfonylureas may have an adverse effect on the myocardium. Wu and colleagues have reported increased "stiffness" of the myocardium secondary to interstitial accumulation of PAS staining material that reduced left ventricular function in dogs treated with tolbutamide.[229]

On the basis of available information, in our judgment the only patients with diabetes who should use oral hypoglycemic agents are those who are not ketosis prone, whose hyperglycemia cannot be controlled with diet alone, and who are unwilling or unable to receive insulin injections. It should also be recognized that beta-adrenoceptor blockers reduce the hyperglycemic reaction to stress, and it is possible that beta-adrenoceptor blocker therapy may require a downward adjustment of insulin dosage, since patients receiving beta blockers may be more susceptible to hypoglycemia. Since many of the symptoms of which the hypoglycemic patient is aware are due to the effects of the epinephrine which is released, both physician and patient must be alert to the possibility that hypoglycemia occurring in the beta blocker–treated diabetic may be relatively asymptomatic. Since certain diuretics, such as the thiazides and furosemide, may result in hypokalemia, and because hypokalemia can inhibit insulin release, these drugs may intensify the glucose intolerance of diabetic patients.

In patients with diabetes mellitus and impairment of left ventricular function, a sudden change in the glucose concentration of extracellular fluid, as occurs with the development of insulin deficiency, may result in the movement of fluid from the intracellular to the extracellular space and the intensification of heart failure. The hyperosmolar state has been shown experimentally to reduce cardiac contractility.[230] This hyperosmolar state responds to the lowering of blood glucose by insulin.[231]

OBESITY

There are two types of obesity: adult-onset and lifelong. Adult-onset obesity is extremely common, probably occurring to a varying extent in nearly all individuals in developed countries. Its clinical course consists of normal weight patterns during childhood and adolescence, with a gradual increase in weight beginning between 20 and 40 years of age; it reflects an imbalance between caloric intake and utilization.[232] Much less common is lifelong obesity, characterized by the development of obesity early in childhood, with significant increase in weight during adolescence and, in the female, during and after pregnancy. These individuals are usually grossly obese, weighing more than 150 per cent of their ideal weight as adults. The underlying cause of obesity in either condition is unclear.

Hirsch and Knittle have documented an increase both in the size and the number of adipose cells in individuals with lifelong obesity, while in adult-onset obesity, only an increase in cell size occurs.[233] With weight reduction the size of the adipose cells decreases in both conditions; however, the number does not change in either. Whether the increased number of adipose cells in lifelong obesity is determined by genetic or environmental factors is uncertain. However, it has been documented that there is no significant change in the number of adipose cells when obesity develops after late childhood in both experimental animals and humans. On the other hand, some evidence suggests that early infant feeding habits may significantly alter their number.[233] The metabolic consequences of obesity include decreased sensitivity to insulin, with resultant hyperinsulinemia, glucose intolerance, hypercholesterolemia, hypertriglyceridemia, and hyperaminoacidemia.

CARDIOVASCULAR CONSEQUENCES OF SEVERE OBESITY

During the past decade the health risk of obesity has been intensively studied. A conference analyzing data from two national health and nutrition surveys and the Framingham 30-year follow-up study concluded that a significant excess in mortality is evident in individuals with an obesity mass index greater than 27. A value greater than this is present in 34 million adult United States citizens. There is a direct correlation between the level of blood pressure and cholesterol and the degree of obesity.[234] *Hypertension* is common in the grossly obese,[235] although it must be recognized that indirect measurement of blood pressure frequently leads to overestimation of the arterial pressure by the standard cuff method (p. 21). Nonetheless, direct measurement of arterial pressure frequently shows moderate elevations that can usually be promptly restored to normal by means of weight reduction and salt restriction.

Evidence of circulatory dysfunction in the massively obese, associated with cardiac enlargement during life and at autopsy, was first described by Smith and Willius in 1933.[236] It is now widely appreciated that massive obesity is accompanied by a marked increase in blood volume and cardiac output (p. 790), which are proportional to the excess of body weight and the duration of obesity[237–239]; the hematocrit is often slightly elevated as well. The increased cardiac output is secondary to an increased stroke volume, since heart rate is normal; the cardiac output rises normally during exercise. Left ventricular filling pressures are at or close to the upper limits of normal in the supine position in the basal state, but increase with passive leg raising, and reach strikingly elevated levels during exercise. These increases in ventricular filling pressure are associated with a high resting central blood volume, which also increases

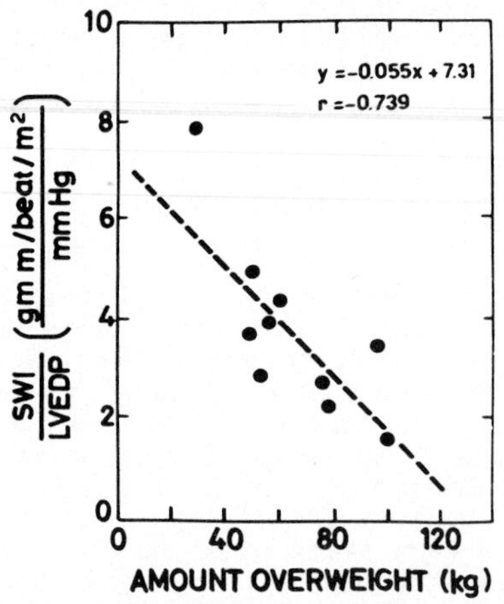

FIGURE 58–12. The significant negative correlation between the ratio of the stroke work index (SWI) to the left ventricular end-diastolic pressure (LVEDP) and the amounts of overweight shows that the higher the degree of obesity, the greater the impairment of left ventricular function. (From Divitiis, O., et al: Obesity and cardiac function. Circulation *64*:477, 1981, by permission of the American Heart Association, Inc.)

significantly with exertion. A tendency to leftward deviation of the electrical axis correlates significantly with increasing obesity independent of age and blood pressure. However, this association is usually confined to the normal QRS-axis range. Thus, abnormal left-axis deviation is not necessarily a reflection of obesity.[240] The maximum velocity

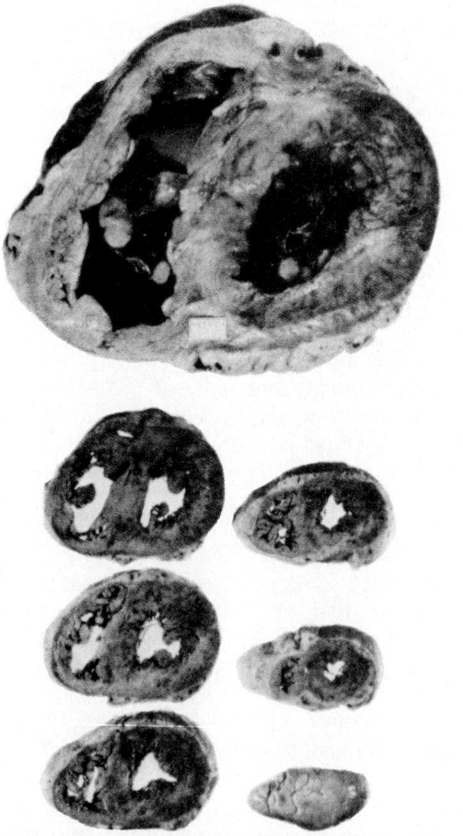

FIGURE 58–13. Cross-section of the heart of a 34-year-old man who weighed more than 500 lb. Both ventricular walls are hypertrophied and both cavities are dilated. The heart weight (825 gm) was greatly increased. (From Warnes, C. A., and Roberts, W. C.: The heart in massive (more than 300 pounds or 136 kilograms) obesity: Analysis of 12 patients studied at necropsy. Am. J. Cardiol. *54*:1090, 1984.)

of myocardial fiber shortening and the ratio of stroke work index to left ventricular end-diastolic pressure were reduced, even in relatively young obese persons, without any other evidence of heart disease[237] (Fig. 58–12). Massive edema may occur as a consequence of the elevated ventricular filling pressure, despite elevation of the cardiac output.

Examination of the gross and microscopic anatomy of the heart in patients with marked chronic obesity showed heart weight to be considerably greater than predicted for ideal body weight, with left ventricular dilatation and eccentric hypertrophy and, in a few instances, right ventricular hypertrophy as well[241] (Fig. 58–13). This increase in cardiac weight is not due to excess epicardial fat and fatty infiltration of the myocardium, which were previously considered to be the principal features of the obese heart. However, at least in one study the frequency of atherosclerosis was not increased in persons who were morbidly obese. Obesity-induced cardiac hypertrophy is different from that induced by hypertension. Instead of the concentric left ventricular hypertrophy associated with hypertension, the hypertrophy is eccentric, with chamber dilatation and some wall thickening, as seen in other conditions in which cardiac output is chronically increased (Fig. 58–14). Also, in contrast to the increased afterload associated with systemic hypertension, obesity produces an elevated preload. When hypertension accompanies severe obesity, a combination of concentric and eccentric hypertrophy is present. Obese patients with clinically evident ventricular hypertrophy have an increased propensity to ectopy, in comparison with obese persons without left ventricular hypertrophy or with lean persons.[243] Thus, when these clinical, hemodynamic, and pathological observations are taken together, it appears that manifestations of myocardial dysfunction occur in very obese subjects without evidence of other heart disease and that, in the absence of the obesity hypoventilation syndrome (p. 1610), cor pulmonale is not a presenting feature.

Heart failure in the markedly obese is usually chronic. The pulmonary and systemic congestion with symptoms of dyspnea and edema are, at first, simply related to the reductions in ventricular compliance and elevations of filling pressures. Later, these symptoms are related also to increases in ventricular end-diastolic volume and the reduction of myocardial contractility. Thus, the marked chronic increase in cardiac work, i.e., in cardiac output and arterial pressure, ultimately leads to heart failure.

Fortunately, weight reduction is beneficial in the majority of patients, even those with heart failure. It usually improves the exercise capacity of patients with chronic exogenous obesity and decreases total body oxygen uptake, the cardiothoracic ratio on chest roentgenogram, systemic arterial pressure, blood volume, cardiac output, arteriovenous oxygen difference, and left ventricular filling pressure at rest.[244] MacMahon et al. have documented that weight loss of as little as 8 kg is associated with a significant decrease in left ventricular mass, particularly the thickness of the posterior and central walls.[245] Alpert and colleagues, studying cardiac function in grossly obese individuals, noted a substantial reduction in left ventricular chamber enlargement and an improvement in systemic function with an average weight loss of 55 kg.[246] However, they were unable to show a change in septal or posterior wall thickness, suggesting that some of the beneficial effects of weight loss on cardiac function may occur only if the obesity is mild or of short duration. Supporting this conclusion is the persistence of elevated left ventricular filling pressure with exercise in obese patients following weight reduction.[247]

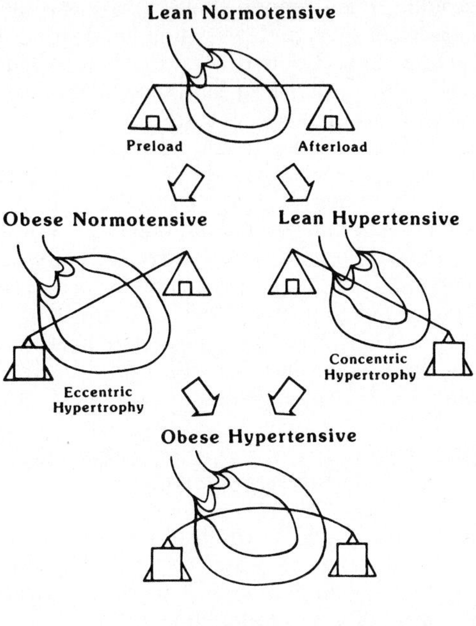

FIGURE 58–14. Adaptation of the heart to obesity and hypertension. (From Masserli, F. H.: Cardiovascular effects of obesity and hypertension. Lancet *1*:1165, 1982.)

Treatment of heart failure in these patients consists of maintenance of the reduced body weight, dietary sodium restriction, cardiac glycosides, and diuretics. Often, patients with massive obesity have associated arteriosclerotic coronary artery disease and the salutary results of weight reduction may be particularly striking in them.

TREATMENT

Most cases of adult-onset obesity are the result of imbalance between intake and output. Thus, reduction of intake is the most significant factor in treating this disease. While abnormalities in endocrine function, particularly of the thyroid or adrenal, have often been implicated in the pathophysiology of obesity, this thesis is rarely substantiated by detailed evaluation. The amount and rate of weight loss with a given level of caloric restrictions depends on the degree of energy expenditure. Energy expenditure depends on both the physical activity and mass of the individual. Thus, with a fixed level of intake and activity, the rate of weight loss decreases as the total weight decreases. There is no evidence that a specific type of diet has any intrinsic benefit except as it is related to its caloric intent. Thus the claim that high-protein diets are more efficacious is related not to their caloric content but rather to the accompanying ketosis that suppresses appetite.

MALNUTRITION

Malnutrition, particularly protein-calorie deficiency, is prevalent in many underdeveloped areas of the world. However, in recent years, it has also become a concern in developed countries in those individuals who have chronic diseases, in whom it exists as a result of both anorexia and hypermetabolism. The clinical picture is similar to adult kwashiorkor reported from underdeveloped countries, described below.

Protein-calorie malnutrition of childhood refers to syndromes of nutritional deficiency, which range from marasmus to kwashiorkor and which result from a stress like a serious infection superimposed upon an inadequate diet.[104] *Marasmus* is a state of malnutrition in an infant who has been weaned early and fed a diet grossly deficient in calories, protein, and other essential nutrients. *Kwashiorkor* usually occurs in children 1 to 4 years of age and is due to deficiency of protein relative to calories.

CARDIAC CHANGES IN MALNUTRITION. The circulatory status of patients with severe nutritional depletion and electrolyte imbalance is precarious; the cardiac output, systolic pressure, and pulse pressure are abnormally low, and there may be massive, generalized edema; the P-R interval may be shortened. There is loss of subcutaneous fat and general wasting and atrophy of most organs, including the heart, which is thin walled, pale, and flabby on gross examination. Histological study reveals atrophy of the muscle fibers, sometimes with interstitial edema. In experimental chronic protein-calorie undernutrition, not only is the heart atrophic, but also left ventricular function may be normal. In the dog there are reductions in left ventricular compliance and contractility,[248] whereas in the rat this apparently does not occur, although there is striking atrophy of the heart.[249] The treatment of the dehydrated or severely anemic patient with protein-calorie malnutrition involves correction of hematological, fluid, and electrolyte imbalance and the treatment of infection. Congestive failure can be avoided if care is taken to avoid overloading with sodium, water, or blood. Digitalis must be given cautiously when these patients are in heart failure because of their sensitivity to glycosides.

In parts of the world where pediatric kwashiorkor is common, there are also cases of adults with similar clinical features.[104] These features include loss of subcutaneous fat and muscle with edema, weakness, depression, anorexia, diarrhea, abdominal distention, hair loss, and thinning of the skin. Classically, plasma albumin and amino acid levels are low, as are serum concentrations of sodium, magnesium, and phosphorus. Urinary excretion of nitrogen is reduced, as is total body potassium. On the other hand, total body and extracellular water and plasma volume are usually increased. The primary pathophysiological event is protein nutrition. All the clinical signs and symptoms are related to this basic defect.

Anorexia nervosa, a condition more frequently observed in developed countries, produces symptoms similar to those observed in kwashiorkor. Hypomagnesemia with hypocalcemia and hypokalemia frequently occurs in this condition, resulting in heart failure and sometimes sudden death.[250, 251]

MALNUTRITION IN CARDIAC DISEASE

Assessment of protein-calorie nutritional status in cardiac patients has not been extensively evaluated. However, during the last several decades there has been increasing awareness that some patients with cardiovascular disease have clinical features similar to those described above. In these cases, instead of involuntary protein deprivation, anorexia plays a significant role. For example, chronic congestive heart failure leads to cellular hypoxia as well as hypermetabolism. Gastrointestinal hypoxia produces anorexia, which then initiates a vicious cycle. Decreased protein intake produces cardiac atrophy and increasing congestive heart failure, which produces more cellular hypoxia, greater anorexia, and finally death.[252]

A similar condition has been described in some undergoing open-heart surgery for correction of rheumatic valvular disease. In some malnourished patients the mortality reaches 20 per cent, significantly greater than the 1 to 2 per cent in normally nourished patients undergoing the same procedure. The underlying pathophysiology is uncertain but probably includes (1) decreased cardiac mass, (2) reduction of biosynthetic activity of liver, (3) poor healing due to reduced levels of substrate, and (4) impairment of cell-mediated immunity.[253] As a result, wound healing is retarded, skin ulcers occur, and requirements for artificial ventilation are prolonged. Abel and colleagues have suggested that hyperalimentation in the immediate postoperative period does not significantly alter the increased morbidity.[252] This has led Blackburn et al. to suggest that both preoperative and concurrent nutritional support are necessary.[253] However, definitive studies to distinguish between nutritional status and severity of the cardiovascular disease as the cause for the increased morbidity have not been reported.

Cardiovascular Manifestations of Vitamin Deficiency

THIAMINE DEFICIENCY (See also p. 786)

OTHER VITAMIN DEFICIENCIES. Deficiencies of other vitamins have not led to specifically definable cardiovascular abnormalities, except for the hypocalcemia-accompanied vitamin D deficiency. However, vitamin deficiencies, particularly of the B group and folic acid, have been diagnosed with increasing frequency in patients with cardiovascular disease. For example, nearly a third of infants and children with congenital heart disease have been reported to be deficient in a number of the B vitamins.[254] Folic acid deficiency has been documented in a significant number of patients with congestive heart failure. While the deficient state may simply be related to decreased intake, abnormal intestinal absorption or increased rates of excretion may also contribute.

ALTERATIONS IN GONADAL HORMONE SECRETION

There are no specific cardiovascular abnormalities associated with altered gonadal function except for occasional cardiac structural abnormalities in Kallman syndrome, a genetic form of hypogonadotropic hypogonadism.[255] However, gonadectomy in rats is associated with an impairment of left ventricular filling and left ventricular function, and androgen receptors have been found in the heart.[256, 257]

GONADAL FUNCTION AND CARDIOVASCULAR DISEASE

Middle-aged men are at a higher risk for developing cardiovascular disease than age-matched women. Because the discrepancy between male and female mortality disappears in older, postmenopausal women, some investigators have suggested that estrogen reduces the rate of development of coronary atherosclerosis (p. 1182). Support for this thesis includes the observation that total cholesterol is lower and HDL cholesterol is higher in postmenopausal women who are taking estrogens than in those who are not.[258] Additionally, the risk ratio of coronary artery disease death varies from 0.3 to 0.7 in postmenopausal estrogen users compared to nonusers.[259–261] Several studies, however, have provided evidence against this thesis. First, it has been documented that the development of coronary artery disease in women who underwent hysterectomies and were also castrated is no different from that in age-matched noncastrated women.[262] Second, widespread use of oral contraceptives, most of which contain estrogen, has proved that estrogen administration is not without cardiovascular risk, since it can increase total cholesterol and beta-lipoprotein (LDL) cholesterol and decrease alpha-lipoprotein (HDL) cholesterol in premenopausal females.[263] Additionally, it has been shown to increase the degree of abnormality in postexercise electrocardiograms in those individuals who had abnormal tests prior to estrogen therapy.[264]

Hyperestrogenemia in men is associated with an increased risk of myocardial infarction, which is particularly evident in individuals with diabetes mellitus. Whether this is an actual risk factor or an associated finding is unclear, since exercise-trained men do not have lower levels of serum estradiol, even though they do have a reduced risk for coronary artery disease.[265, 266] Finally, Wilson and colleagues, using information from the Framingham study, reported an increased risk of cardiovascular morbidity in postmenopausal women taking estrogens.[267]

This has led some investigators to suggest that it is not the increased estrogen but the decreased testosterone that is protective to women. They base this theory on the documented reduction in serum cholesterol levels and incidence of atherosclerosis in castrated men and the positive correlation between plasma testosterone and high-density lipoprotein cholesterol levels.[268] However, the similar frequency of coronary artery disease in postmenopausal women and men of similar age with significantly different testosterone levels is unexplained.

CARDIOVASCULAR EFFECTS OF ORAL CONTRACEPTIVES

Within the last decade, several studies have documented that in some patients the use of oral contraceptives is accompanied by an increased risk of cardiovascular morbidity and mortality in premenopausal females.[263, 264, 269] Specifically there is increased frequency of diabetes mellitus, hypertension, and thromboembolic disease. While the increased risk is small, caution in the use of oral contraceptive agents by individuals who may be predisposed to the development of these diseases is nevertheless warranted.

HYPERTENSION (See also p. 2258). The hypertension associated with estrogen administration is probably related to its effect in modifying the production of renin substrate by the liver.[270] It has been clearly documented that oral contraceptives increase the concentration of renin substrate and blood angiotensin II.[271] However, most individuals do not develop clinical hypertension, which suggests that a counterregulatory mechanism(s) is activated, reducing the vascular effect of angiotensin II. Alternatively, blood pressure may increase in all patients, but only the predisposed will develop hypertension. Thus, individuals who have a personal or family history of renal disease are more likely to develop hypertension with estrogen administration.

THROMBOEMBOLIC DISEASE. At least two clearly defined alterations in the clotting system are produced by oral contraceptive agents; either or both could be responsible for the increased frequency of thromboembolic disease.[269] First, estrogen enhances the biosynthesis of a number of the clotting factors by the liver. Second, oral contraceptives increase both the viscosity of blood and platelet adhesiveness.

REFERENCES

1. Graves, R. J.: Clinical lectures. London Med. Surg. J. (Part II):7, 516, 1835.
2. Addison, T.: On the Constitutional and Local Effects of Disease of the Suprarenal Capsules. London, Highley, 1855.

ACROMEGALY

3. Daughaday, W. H.: The anterior pituitary. *In* Wilson, J. D., and Foster, D. W. (eds.): Williams' Textbook of Endocrinology. Philadelphia, W. B. Saunders Company, 1985, p. 568.
4. Faglia, G., Arosio, M., Ambrosi, B.: Recent advances in diagnosis and treatment of acromegaly. *In* Imura, H. (ed.): The Pituitary Gland. New York, Raven Press, 1985, p. 363.
5. Gomez-Pan, A., and Rodriguez-Arnao, M. D.: Somatostatin and growth hormone releasing factor: Synthesis, location, metabolism and function. J. Clin. Endocrinol. Metab. *12*:469, 1983.
6. Frohman, L. A., and Jansson, J.: Growth hormone releasing hormone. Endocr. Rev. 7:223, 1986.
7. Clemmons, D. R., and Van Wyk, J. J.: Somatomedin: Physiological control and effects on cell proliferation. *In* Baserga, R. (ed.): Handbook of Experimental Pharmacology. Berlin, Springer-Verlag, 1981, p. 161.

8. Yamashita, S., Weiss, M., and Melmed, S.: Insulin-like growth factor I regulates growth hormone secretion and messenger ribonucleic acid levels in human pituitary cells. J. Clin. Endocrinol. Metab. *62*:730, 1986.
9. Moore, D. D., Walker, M. D., Diamond, D. J., Conkling, M. A., and Goodman, H. M.: Structure, expression, and evolution of growth hormone genes. Recent Prog. Hormone Res. *38*:197, 1982.
10. Frelin, C.: The regulation of protein turnover in newborn rat heart cell cultures. J. Biol. Chem. *255*:11149, 1980.
11. Greco, A. V., Ghirlanda, G., Barone, C., Bertoli, A., Caput, S., Uccioli, L., and Manna, R.: Somatostatin in paroxysmal supraventricular and junctional tachycardia. Br. Med. J. *288*:28, 1984.
12. Day, S. M., Gu, J., Polak, J. M., and Bloom, S. R.: Somatostatin in the human heart and comparison with guinea pig and rat heart. Br. Heart J. *53*:153, 1985.
13. Thorner, M. O., Perryman, R. L., Cronin, M. J., Rogol, A. D., Draznin, M., Johanson, A., Vale, W., Horvath, E., and Kovacs, K.: Somatotroph hyperplasia: Successful treatment of acromegaly by removal of a pancreatic islet tumor secreting a growth hormone-releasing factor. J. Clin. Invest. *70*:965, 1982.
14. Melmed, S., Braunstein, G., Chang, R. J., and Becker, D.: Pituitary tumors secreting growth hormone and prolactin. Ann. Intern. Med. *105*:238, 1986.
15. Aloia, J. F., Roginsky, M.D., and Field, R. A.: Absence of hyperlipidemia in acromegaly. J. Clin. Endocrinol. *35*:921, 1972.
16. McGuffin, W. L., Sherman, B. M., Roth, J., Gorden, P., Kahn, C. R., Roberts, W. C., and Frommer, P. L.: Acromegaly and cardiovascular disorders. Ann. Intern. Med. *81*:11, 1974.
17. Baldwin, A., Cundy, T., Butler, J., and Timmis, A. D.: Progression of cardiovascular disease in acromegalic patients treated by external pituitary irradiation. Acta Endocrinol. *108*:26, 1985.
18. Lie, J. T., and Grossman, S. J.: Pathology of the heart in acromegaly: Anatomic findings in 27 autopsied patients. Am. Heart J. *100*:41, 1980.
19. Mather, H. M., Boyd, M. J., and Jenkins, J. S.: Heart size and function in acromegaly. Br. Heart J. *41*:697, 1979.
20. Csanady, M., Gaspar, L., Hogye, M., Hogye, M., and Gruber, N.: The heart in acromegaly: An echocardiographic study. Int. J. Cardiol. *2*:349, 1983.
21. Rossi, L., Thiene, G., Caregaro, L., Giordano, R., and Lauro, S.: Dysrhythmias and sudden death in acromegalic heart disease. A clinicopathologic study. Chest 72:495, 1977.
22. Cain, J. P., Williams, G. H., and Dluhy, R. G.: Plasma renin activity and aldosterone secretion in patients with acromegaly. J. Clin. Endocrinol. *34*:73, 1972.
23. Moore, T. J., Thein-Wai, W., Dluhy, R. G., Dawson-Hughes, B. F., Hollenberg, N. K., and Williams, G. H.: Abnormal adrenal and vascular responses to angiotensin II and an angiotensin antagonist in acromegaly. J. Clin. Endocrinol. Metab. *51*:215, 1980.
24. Souadjian, J. V., and Schirger, A.: Hypertension in acromegaly. Am. J. Med. Sci. *254*:629, 1967.
25. Surawicz, B., and Mangiardi, M. L.: Electrocardiogram in endocrine and metabolic disorders. *In* Rios, J. C. (ed.): Clinical Electrocardiographic Correlations. Philadelphia, F. A. Davis, 1977, p. 243.
26. Jonas, E. A., Aloia, J. F., and Lane, F. J.: Evidence of subclinical heart muscle dysfunction in acromegaly. Chest *67*:190, 1975.
27. Smallridge, R. C., Rajfer, S., Davis, J., and Schaaf, M.: Acromegaly and the heart. Am. J. Med. *66*:22, 1979.
28. Wilson, C. B.: A decade of pituitary microsurgery. The Herbert Olivecrona Lecture. J. Neurosurg. *61*:814, 1984.
29. Lawrence, J. H., Tobias, C. A., Linfoot, J. A., Born, J. L., Lyman, J. T., Chong, C. Y., Manougian, E., and Wei, W. C.: Successful treatment of acromegaly: Metabolic and clinical studies in 145 patients. J. Clin Endocrinol. Metab. *31*:180, 1970.
30. Vance, M. L., Evans, W. S., and Thorner, M. O.: Bromocriptine. Ann. Intern. Med. *100*:78, 1984.
31. Lamberts, S. W. J., Uitterlinden, P., Verschoor, L., van Dongen, K. J., and del Pozo, E.: Long-term treatment of acromegaly with the somatostatin analogue SMS 201–995. N. Engl. J. Med. *313*:1576, 1985.
32. Kaplan, M. M.: The thyroid and the heart; how do they interact? J. Cardiovasc. Med. 7:893, 1982.

THYROID DISEASE

33. Oppenheimer, J. H.: The nuclear receptor–triiodothyronine complex: Relationship to thyroid hormone distributions, metabolism, and biological action. *In* Oppenheimer, J. H., and Samuels, H. H. (eds.): Molecular Basis of Thyroid Hormone Action. New York, Academic Press, 1983, p. 1.
34. Ladenson, P. W., Kieffer, J. D., Farwell, A. P., and Ridgway, E. C.: Modulation of myocardial L-triiodothyronine receptors in normal, hypothyroid, and hyperthyroid rats. Metabolism *35*:5, 1986.
35. Jump, D. B., and Oppenheimer, J. H.: Association of thyroid hormone receptors with chromatin. Mol. Cell. Biochem. *55*:159, 1983.
36. Apriletti, J. W., David-Inouye, Y., Baxter, J. D., and Eberhardt, N. L.: Physiochemical characterization of the intranuclear receptor. *In* Oppenheimer, J. H., and Samuels, H. H. (eds.): Molecular Basis of Thyroid Hormone Action. New York, Academic Press, 1983, p. 67.
37. Narayan, P., Liaw, C. W., and Towle, H. C.: Rapid induction of a specific nuclear precursor by thyroid hormone. Proc. Natl. Acad. Sci. USA *81*:4687, 1984.
38. Seelig, S. A., Jump, D. B., Towle, H. C., Liaw, C., Mariash, C. N., Schwartz, H. L., and Oppenheimer, J. H.: Parodoxical effects of cycloheximide on the ultra-rapid induction of two hepatic mRNA sequences by triiodothyronine (T3). Endocrinology *110*:671, 1982.
39. Seelig, S., Liaw, C., Towle, H. C., and Oppenheimer, J. H.: Thyroid hormone attenuates and augments hepatic gene expression at a pretranslational level. Proc. Natl. Acad. Sci. USA *78*:4733, 1981.
40. Guernsey, D. L., and Edelman, I. S.: Regulation of thermogenesis by thyroid hormones. *In* Oppenheimer, J. H., and Samuels, H. H. (eds.): Molecular Basis of Thyroid Hormone Action. New York, Academic Press, 1983, p. 293.
41. Fain, J. N., and Rosenthal, J. W.: Calorigenic action of triiodothyronine on white cells: Effects of ouabain, oligomycin, and cathecholamines. Endocrinology *89*:1205, 1971.
42. Primack, M. P., and Buchanan, J. L.: Control of oxygen consumption in liver slices from normal and T4-treated rats. Endocrinology *95*:619, 1974.
43. Gordon, A., Schwartz, H., and Gross, J.: The stimulation of sugar transport in heart cells grown in a serum-free medium by picomolar concentrations of thyroid hormones: The effects of insulin and hydrocortisone. Endocrinology *118*:52, 1986.
44. Knight, R. A.: The use of spinal anesthesia to control sympathetic overactivity in hyperthyroidism. Anesthesiology *6*:225, 1945.
45. Buccino, R. A., Spann, J. F., Pool, P. E., and Braunwald, E.: Influence of the thyroid state on the intrinsic contractile properties and the energy stores of the myocardium. J. Clin. Invest. *46*:1669, 1967.
46. Nishizawa, Y., Hamada, N., Fujii, S., Morii, H., Okuda, K., and Wada, M.: Serum dopamine-beta-hydroxylase activity in thyroid disorders. J. Clin. Endocrinol. Metab. *39*:599, 1974.
47. Malbon, C. C., and Greenberg, M. L.: 3,3′,5′-Triiodothyronine administration in vivo modulates the hormone sensitive adenylate cyclase system of rat hepatocytes. J. Clin. Invest. *69*:414, 1982.
48. Malbon, C. C.: Liver cell adenylate cyclase and β-adrenergic receptors. J. Biol. Chem. *255*:8692, 1980.
49. Stiles, G. L., and Lefkowitz, R. J.: Thyroid hormone modulation of agonist-beta adrenergic receptor interactions in the rat heart. Life Sci. *28*:2529j, 1981.
50. Tse, J., Wrenn, R. W., and Kuo, J. F.: Thyroxine-induced changes in characteristics and activities of beta-adrenergic receptors and adenosine 3′,5′-monophosphate and guanosine 3′,5′-monophosphate systems in the heart may be related to reputed catecholamine supersensitivity in hyperthyroidism. Endocrinology *107*:6, 1980.
51. Brodde, O. E., Schumann, H. J., and Wagner, J.: Decreased responsiveness of the adenylate cyclase system in left atria from hypothyroid rats. Mol. Pharmacol. *17*:180, 1980.
52. Whitsett, J. A., Pollinger, J., and Matz, S.: β-adrenergic receptors and catecholamine sensitive adenylate cyclase in developing rat ventricular myocardium: Effect of thyroid status. Pediatr. Res. *16*:463, 1982.
53. Rutherford, J. P., Vatner, S. F., and Braunwald, E.: Adrenergic control of myocardial contractility in conscious hypertrophied dogs. Am. J. Physiol. *237*:590, 1980.
54. Guarnieri, T., Filburn, C. R., Beard, E. S., and Lakatta, E. G.: Enhanced contractile response and protein kinase activation to threshold levels of β-adrenergic stimulation in hyperthyroid rat heart. J. Clin. Invest. *65*:861, 1980.
55. Andersson, R. G. G., Nilsson, O. R., and Kuo, J. F.: β-adrenoceptor adenosine 3′,5′-monophosphate system in human leukocytes before and after treatment for hyperthyroidism. J. Clin. Endocrinol. Metab. *56*:42, 1983.
56. Stiles, G. L., Stadel, J. M., De Lean, A., and Lefkowitz, R. J.: Hypothyroidism modulates beta-adrenergic receptor-adenylate cyclase interactions in rat reticulocytes. J. Clin. Invest. *68*:1450, 1981.
57. Malbon, C. C.: The effects of thyroid status on the modulation of fat cell β-adrenergic receptor agonist affinity by guanine nucleotides. Mol. Pharmacol. *18*:193, 1980.
58. Fain, J. N.: Catecholamine-thyroid hormone interactions in liver and adipose tissue. Life Sci. *28*:1745, 1981.
59. Markowitz, C., and Yater, W. M.: Response of explanted cardiac muscle to thyroxine. Am. J. Physiol. *100*:162, 1932.
60. Murayama, M., and Goodkind, M. J.: Effect of thyroid hormone on the frequency-force relationship of atrial myocardium from the guinea pig. Circ. Res. *23*:743, 1968.
61. Goldman, S., Olajos, M., Friedman, H., Roeske, W. R., and Morkin, E.: Left ventricular performance in conscious thyrotoxic calves. Am. J. Physiol. *242*:H113, 1982.
62. Morkin, E., Flink, I. L., and Goldman, S.: Biochemical and physiologic effects of thyroid hormone on cardiac performance. Prog. Cardiovasc. Dis. *25*:435, 1983.
63. Banerjee, S. K.: Comparative studies of atrial and ventricular myosin from normal, thyrotoxic, and thyroidectomized rabbits. Circ. Res. *52*:131, 1983.
64. Crie, J. S., Wakeland, J. R., Mayhew, B. A., and Wildenthal, K.: Direct anabolic effects of thyroid hormone on isolated mouse heart. Am. J. Physiol. *245*:C328, 1983.
65. Philipson, K. D., and Edelman, I. S.: Thyroid hormone control of Na^+,K^+ATPase and K^+-dependent phosphatase in rat heart. Am. J. Physiol. *232*:C196, 1977.
66. Litten, R. Z., Martin, B. J., Howe, E. R., Alpert, N. R., and Solaro, R. J.: Phosphorylation and adenosine triphosphate activity of myofibrils from thyrotoxic rabbit ears. Circ. Res. *48*:498, 1981.
67. Curfman, G. D., Crowley, T. J., and Smith, T. W.: Thyroid-induced alterations in myocardial sodium- and potassium-activated adenosine triphosphatase, monovalent cation active transport and cardiac glycoside binding. J. Clin. Invest. *59*:586, 1977.
68. Litten, R. Z., III, Martin, B. J., Low, R. B., and Alpert, N. R.: Altered myosin isozyme patterns from pressure-overloaded and thyrotoxic hypertrophied rabbit hearts. Circ. Res. *50*:856, 1982.
69. Chizzonite, R. A., Everett, A. W., Clark, W. A., Jakovcic, S., Rabinowitz, M., and Zak, R.: Isolation and characterization of two molecular variants of myosin heavy chain from rabbit ventricle. Change in their content during normal

growth and after treatment with thyroid hormone. J. Biol. Chem. *257*:2056, 1982.

70. Samuel, J. L., Rappaport, L., Syrovy, I., Wisnewsky, C., Marotte, F., Whalen, R. G., and Schwartz, K.: Differential effect of thyroxine on atrial and ventricular isomyosins in rats. Am. J. Physiol. *250*:H333, 1986.
71. Holubarsch, C., Goulette, R. P., Litten, R. Z., Martin, B. J., Mulieri, L. A., and Alpert, N. R.: The economy of isometric force development, myosin isoenzyme pattern and myofibrillar ATPase activity in normal and hypothyroid rat myocardium. Circ. Res. *56*:78, 1985.
72. Goodkind, M. J., Dambach, G. E., Thyrum, P. T., and Luchi, R. J.: Effect of thyroxine on ventricular myocardial contractility of ATPase activity in guinea pigs. Am. J. Physiol. *226*:66, 1974.
73. Suko, J.: The calcium pump of cardiac sarcoplasmic reticulum. Functional alterations at different levels of thyroid state in rabbits. J. Physiol. (London) *228*:563, 1973.
74. Klein, I., and Hong, C.: Effects of thyroid hormone on cardiac size and myosin content of the heterotopically transplanted rat heart. J. Clin. Invest. *77*:1694, 1986.
75. Johnson, P. N., Freedberg, A. S., and Marshall, J. M.: Action of thyroid hormone on the transmembrane potentials from sinoatrial cells and atrial muscle cells in isolated atria of rabbits. Cardiology *58*:273, 1973.
76. Arnsdorf, M. D., and Childers, R. W.: Atrial electrophysiology in experimental hyperthyroidism in rabbits. Circ. Res. *26*:575, 1970.
77. Chopra, I. J., and Solomon, D. H.: Pathogenesis of hyperthyroidism. Ann. Rev. Med. *34*:267, 1983.
78. Davis, P. J., and Davis, F. B.: Hyperthyroidism in patients over the age of 60 years. Medicine *53*:161, 1974.
79. Skelton, C. L.: The heart and hyperthyroidism. N. Engl. J. Med. *307*:1206, 1982.
80. Talafih, K., Briden, K. L., and Weiss, H. R.: Thyroxine-induced hypertrophy of the rabbit heart. Effect on regional oxygen extraction, flow, and oxygen consumption. Circ. Res. *52*:272, 1983.
81. Friedman, M. J., Okada, R. D., Ewy, G. A., and Hellman, D. J.: Left ventricular systolic and diastolic function in hyperthyroidism. Am. Heart J. *104*:1303, 1982.
82. Feldman, T., Borow, K. M., Sarne, D. H., Neumann, A., and Lang, R. M.: Myocardial mechanics in hyperthyroidism: Importance of left ventricular loading conditions, heart rate and contractile state. J. Am. Coll. Cardiol. *7*:967, 1986.
83. Iskandrian, A. S., Rose, L., Hakki, A. H., Segal, B. L., and Kane, S. A.: Cardiac performance in thyrotoxicosis: Analysis of 10 untreated patients. Am. J. Cardiol. *51*:349, 1983.
84. Forfar, J. C., Matthews, D. M., and Toft, A. D.: Delayed recovery of left ventricular function after antithyroid treatment: Further evidence for reversible abnormalities of contractility in hyperthyroidism. Br. Heart J. *52*:215, 1984.
85. Agner, T., Almdal, T., Thorsteinsson, B., and Agner, E.: A reevaluation of atrial fibrillation in thyrotoxicosis. Dan. Med. Bull. *31*:157, 1984.
86. Ciaccheri, M., Cecchi, F., Arcangeli, C., Dolara, A., Zuppiroli, A., and Pieroni, C.: Occult thyrotoxicosis in patients with chronic and paroxysmal isolated atrial fibrillation. Clin. Cardiol. *7*:413, 1984.
87. Goel, B. G., Hanson, C. S., and Han, J.: A-V conduction in hyper- and hypothyroid dogs. Am. Heart J. *83*:504, 1972.
88. Cavallo, A., Joseph, C. J., and Casta, A.: Cardiac complications in juvenile hyperthyroidism. Am. J. Dis. Child. *138*:479, 1984.
89. Featherstone, H. J., and Stewart, D. K.: Angina in thyrotoxicosis: Thyroid-related coronary artery spasm. Arch. Intern. Med. *143*:554, 1983.
90. Forfar, J. C., Muir, A. L., Sawers, S. A., and Toft, A. D.: Abnormal left ventricular function in hyperthyroidism: Evidence for a possible reversible cardiomyopathy. N. Engl. J. Med. *307*:1165, 1982.
91. Wilson, R., Gibson, T. C., Terrien, C. M., and Levy, A. M.: Hyperthyroidism and familial hypertrophic cardiomyopathy. Arch. Intern. Med. *143*:378, 1983.
92. Channick, B. J., Adlin, E. V., Marks, A. D., Denenberg, B. S., McDonough, M. T., Chakko, C. S., and Spann, J. F.: Hyperthyroidism and mitral-valve prolapse. N. Engl. J. Med. *305*:497, 1981.
93. Brauman, A., Algom, M., Gilboa, Y., Ramot, Y., Golik, A., and Stryjer, D.: Mitral valve prolapse in hyperthyroidism of two different origins. Br. Heart J. *53*:374, 1985.
94. Morrow, D. H., Gaffney, T. E., and Braunwald, E.: Studies on digitalis. VIII. Effect of autonomic innervation and of myocardial catecholamine stores upon the cardiac action of ouabain. J. Pharmacol. Exp. Ther. *140*:236, 1963.
95. Forfar, J. C., Feek, C. M., Miller, H. C., and Toft, A. D.: Atrial fibrillation and isolated suppression of the pituitary-thyroid axis: Response to specific antithyroid therapy. Int. J. Cardiol. *1*:43, 1981.
96. Sandler, G., and Wilson, G. M.: The nature and prognosis of heart disease in thyrotoxicosis. A review of 150 patients treated with ^{131}I. Q. J. Med. *28*:347, 1959.
97. Nakazawa, H. K., Sakurai, K., Hamada, N., Momotani, N., and Ito, K.: Management of atrial fibrillation in the postthyrotoxic state. Am. J. Med. *72*:903, 1982.
98. Staffurth, J. S., Gibberd, M. C., and Fui, S. T.: Arterial embolism in thyrotoxicosis with atrial fibrillation. Br. Med. J. *2*:688, 1977.
99. Ingbar, S. H.: The role of antiadrenergic agents in the management of thyrotoxicosis. Cardiovasc. Rev. Rep. *2*:683, 1981.
100. Clozel, J. P., Danchin, N., Genton, P., Thomas, J. L., and Cherrier, F.: Effects of propranolol and of verapamil on heart rate and blood pressure in hyperthyroidism. Clin. Pharmacol. Ther. *36*:64, 1984.
101. Wu, S. Y., Shyh, T. P., Chopra, I. J., Solomon, D. H., Huang, H. W., and Chu, P. C.: Comparison of sodium ipodate (Oragrafin) and propylthiouracil in early treatment of hyperthyroidism. J. Clin. Endocrinol. Metab. *54*:630, 1982.
102. Chopra, I. J., Huang, T.-S., Hurd, R. E., and Solomon, D. H.: A study of cardiac effects of thyroid hormones: Evidence for amelioration of the effects of thyroxine by sodium ipodate. Endocrinology *114*:2039, 1984.
103. Meese, R., Smitherman, T. C., Croft, C. H., Burger, A., and Nicod, P.: Effect of peripheral thyroid hormone metabolism on cardiac arrhythmias. Am. J. Cardiol. *55*:849, 1985.
104. Whittemore, R., and Caddell, J. L.: Metabolic and nutritional diseases. *In* Moss, A., et al. (eds.): Heart Disease in Infants, Children and Adolescents. Baltimore, Williams and Wilkins Co., 1977, p. 887.
105. Borowski, G. D., Garofano, C. D., Rose, L. I., Spielman, S. R., Rotmensch, H. R., Greenspan, A. M., and Horowitz, L. N.: Effect of long-term amiodarone therapy on thyroid hormone levels and thyroid function. Am. J. Med. *78*:443, 1985.
106. Rao, R. H., McCready, V. R., and Spathis, G. S.: Iodine kinetic studies during amiodarone treatment. J. Clin. Endocrinol. Metab. *62*:563, 1986.
107. Hawthorne, G. C., Campbell, N. P. S., Geddes, J. S., Ferguson, W. R., Postlethwaite, W., Sheridan, B., and Atkinson, A. B.: Amiodarone-induced hypothyroidism: A common complication of prolonged therapy: A report of eight cases. Arch. Intern. Med. *145*:1016, 1985.
108. Martino, E., Safran, M., Aghini-Lombardi, F., Rajatanavin, R., Lenziardi, M., Fay, M., Pacchiarotti, A., Aronin, N., Macchia, E., Haffajee, C., Odogvardi, L., Love, J., Bigalli, A., Baschieri, L., Pinchera, A., and Braverman, L.: Environmental iodine intake and thyroid dysfunction during chronic amiodarone therapy. Ann. Intern. Med. *101*:28, 1984.
109. Zimmerman, J., Yahalom, J., and Bar-On, H.: Clinical spectrum of pericardial effusion as the presenting feature of hypothyroidism. Am. Heart J. *106*:770, 1983.
110. Williams, L. H. P., Jayatunga, R., and Scott, O.: Massive pericardial effusion in a hypothyroid child. Br. Heart J. *51*:231, 1984.
111. Khaleeli, A. A., and Memon, N.: Factors affecting resolution of pericardial effusions in primary hypothyroidism: A clinical, biochemical and echocardiographic study. Postgrad. Med. J. *58*:1073, 1982.
112. Vanhaelst, L., and Neve, P.: Coronary artery disease in hypothyroidism. Lancet *2*:800, 1967.
113. Aber, C. P., and Thompson, G. S.: Factors associated with cardiac enlargement in myxedema. Br. Heart J. *25*:421, 1963.
114. Saito, I., Kunihiko, I., and Saruta, T.: Hypothyroidism as a cause of hypertension. Hypertension *5*:112, 1983.
115. Fouron, J. C., Bourgin, J. H., Letarte, J., Dussault, J. H., Ducharme, G., and Davignon, A.: Cardiac dimensions and myocardial function of infants with congenital hypothyroidism: An echocardiographic study. Br. Heart J. *47*:584, 1982.
116. Graettinger, J. S., Muenster, J. J., and Checchia, C.: A correlation of clinical and hemodynamic studies in patients with hypothyroidism. J. Clin. Invest. *37*:502, 1958.
117. Vora, J., O'Malley, B. P., Petersen, S., McCullough, A., Rosenthal, F. D., and Barnett, D. B.: Reversible abnormalities of myocardial relaxation in hypothyroidism. J. Clin. Endocrinol. Metab. 61:269, 1985.
118. Hillis, W. S., Bremner, W. F., Lawrie, T. D. V., and Thomson, J. A.: Systolic time intervals in thyroid disease. Clin. Endocrinol. *4*:617, 1975.
119. McBrion, D. J., and Hindle, W.: Myxoedema and heart failure. Lancet *1*:1065, 1963.
120. Levey, G. S., Skelton, C. L., and Epstein, S. E.: Decreased myocardial adenyl cyclase activity in hypothyroidism. J. Clin. Invest. *48*:2244, 1969.
121. Steinberg, A. D.: Myxedema and coronary artery disease—a comparative autopsy study. Ann. Intern. Med. *68*:338, 1968.
122. Myasnikov, A. L., and Zaitzev, V. F.: The influence of thyroid hormones on cholesterol metabolism in experimental atherosclerosis in rabbits. J. Atheroscler. Res. *3*:295, 1963.
123. Karlsberg, R. P., Friscia, D. A., Aronow, W. S., and Sekhon, S. S.: Deleterious influence of hypothyroidism on evolving myocardial infarction in conscious dogs. J. Clin. Invest. *67*:1024, 1981.
124. Keating, F. R., Parkin, T. W., Selby, J. B., and Dickinson, L. S.: Treatment of heart disease associated with myxedema. Progr. Cardiovasc. Dis. *3*:364, 1960.
125. Griffiths, P. D.: Serum enzymes in diseases of the thyroid gland. J. Clin. Pathol. *18*:660, 1965.
126. Drucker, D. J., and Burrow, G. N.: Cardiovascular surgery in the hypothyroid patient. Arch. Intern. Med. *145*:1585, 1985.
127. Wehmann, R. E., Gregerman, R. I., Burns, W. H., Saral, R., and Santos, G. W.: Suppression of thyrotropin in the low-thyroxine state of severe nonthyroidal illness. N. Engl. J. Med. *312*:546, 1985.
128. Hamblin, P. S., Dyer, S. A., Mohr, V. S., LeGrand, B. A., Lim, C.-F., Tuxen, D. V., Topliss, D. J., and Stockigt, J. R.: Relationship between thyrotropin and thyroxine changes during recovery from severe hypothyroxinemia of critical illness. J. Clin. Endocrinol. Metab. *62*:717, 1986.
129. Grent, G. A., and Hershman, J. M.: Thyroxine therapy in patients with severe nonthyroidal illnesses and low serum thyroxine concentration. J. Clin. Endocrinol. Metab. *63*:1, 1986.

DISEASES OF THE ADRENAL CORTEX

130. Williams, G. H., and Dluhy, R. G.: Diseases of the adrenal cortex. *In* Braunwald, E., Isselbacher, K. J., Petersdorf, R. G., Wilson, J. D., Martin, J. B., and Fauci, A. S. (eds.): Harrison's Principles of Internal Medicine. 11th ed. New York, McGraw-Hill, 1987, p. 1753.

131. Williams, G. H., and Dluhy, R. G.: Control of aldosterone secretion. *In* Genest, J., Kuchel, O., Hamet, P., and Cantin, M. (eds.): Hypertension. New York, McGraw-Hill, 1983, p. 320.
132. Cushing, H.: The basophil adenomas of the pituitary body and their clinical manifestations (pituitary basophilism). Bull. Johns Hopkins Hosp. *50*:137, 1932.
133. Liddle, G. W.: Pathogenesis of glucocorticoid disorders. Am. J. Med. *53*:638, 1972.
134. Krieger, D. T.: Physiopathology of Cushing's disease. Endocrine Rev. *4*:22, 1983.
135. Carney, J. A., Gordon, H., Carpenter, P. C., Shenoy, B. V., and Go, V. L. W.: The complex of myxomas, spotty pigmentation, and endocrine overactivity. Medicine *64*:270, 1985.
136. Sindler, B. H., Griffing, G. T., and Melby, J. C.: The superiority of the metyrapone test vs. the high dose dexamethasone test in the differential diagnosis of Cushing's syndrome. Am. J. Med. 74:657, 1983.
137. Boggan, J. E., Tyrrell, J. B., and Wilson, C. B.: Transsphenoidal microsurgical management of Cushing's disease: Report of 100 cases. J. Neurosurg. 59:195, 1983.
138. Nolan, P. M., Sheeler, L. R., Hahn, J. F., and Hardy, R. W., Jr.: Therapeutic problems with transsphenoidal pituitary surgery for Cushing's disease. Cleve. Clin. Q. *49*:199, 1982.
139. Weinberger, M. H.: Primary aldosteronism: Diagnosis and differentiation of subtypes. Ann. Intern. Med. *100*:300, 1984.
140. Rose, L. I., Underwood, R. H., Newmark, S. R., Kisch, E. S., and Williams, G. H.: Pathophysiology of spironolactone-induced gynecomastia. Ann. Intern. Med. 87:398, 1977.
141. Rabinowe, S. L., Jackson, R. A., Dluhy, R. G., and Williams, G. H.: Ia-positive T lymphocytes in recently diagnosed idiopathic Addison's disease. Am. J. Med. 77:597, 1984.
142. Knowlton, A. I., and Baer, L.: Cardiac failure in Addison's disease. Am. J. Med. *74*:829, 1983.
143. New, M. I., and Levine, L. S.: Recent advances in 21-hydroxylase deficiency. Ann. Rev. Med. *35*:649, 1984.
144. Schambelan, M., Sebastian, A., and Biglieri, E. G.: Prevalence, pathogenesis and functional significance of aldosterone deficiency in hyperkalemic patients with chronic renal insufficiency. Kidney Int. *17*:89, 1980.
145. Lee, T. H., Salomon, D. R., Rayment, C. M., and Antman, E. M.: Hypotension and sinus arrest with exercise-induced hyperkalemia and combined verapamil/propranolol therapy. Am. J. Med. *80*:1203, 1986.
146. Alford, W. C., Meador, C. K., Mihalevich, J., Burrus, G. R., Glassford, D. M., Stoney, W. S., and Thomas, C. S.: Acute adrenal insufficiency following cardiac surgical procedures. J. Thorac. Cardiovasc. Surg. 78:489, 1979.

PHEOCHROMOCYTOMA

147. Bravo, E. L., and Gifford, R. W.: Pheochromocytoma: Diagnosis, localization, and management. N. Engl. J. Med. *311*:1298, 1984.
148. Wurtman, R. J., and Axelrod, J.: Control of enzymatic synthesis of adrenaline in the adrenal medulla by adrenal cortical steroids. J. Biol. Chem. *241*:2301, 1966.
149. Goldsmith, R. E.: Polyendocrine syndromes and the heart. Primary Cardiol. 7:153, 1981.
150. Levenson, J. A., Safar, M. E., London, G. M., and Simon, A. C.: Haemodynamics in patients with phaeochromocytoma. Clin. Sci. *58*:349, 1980.
151. Landsberg, L., and Young, J. B.: Catecholamines and adrenal medulla. *In* Wilson, J. D., and Foster, D. W. (eds.): Williams' Textbook of Endocrinology. 7th ed. Philadelphia, W. B. Saunders Company, 1985, p. 891.
152. Sheikhzadeh, A., Fatourechi, V., Paydar, D., and Nazarian, I.: Unusual cardiovascular manifestations in a case of pheochromocytoma. Clin. Cardiol. 6:136, 1983.
153. Huang, S. K., Rosenberg, M. J., and Denes, P.: Short PR interval and narrow QRS complex associated with pheochromocytoma: Electrophysiologic observations. J. Am. Coll. Cardiol. *3*:872, 1984.
154. Van Vliet, P. D., Burchell, H. B., and Titus, J. L.: Myocarditis associated with pheochromocytoma. N. Engl. J. Med. *274*:1102, 1966.
155. Shub, C., Cueto-Garcia, L., Sheps, S. G., Ilstrup, D. M., and Tajik, A. J.: Echocardiographic findings in pheochromocytoma. Am. J. Cardiol. *57*:971, 1986.
156. Cueto, L., Arriaga, J., and Zinser, J.: Echocardiographic changes in pheochromocytoma. Chest *76*:600, 1979.
157. McManus, B. M., Fleury, T. A., and Roberts, W. C.: Fatal catecholamine crisis in pheochromocytoma: Curable form of cardiac arrest. Am. Heart J. *102*:930, 1981.
158. Simons, M., and Downing, S. E.: Coronary vasoconstriction and catecholamine cardiomyopathy. Am. Heart J. *109*:297, 1985.
159. Velasquez, G., D'Souza, V. J., Hackshaw, B. T., Glass, T. A., and Formanek, A. G.: Phaeochromocytoma and cardiomyopathy. Br. J. Radiol. 57:89, 1984.
159a. Imperato-McGinley, J., Gautier, T., Ehlers, K., Zullo, M. A., Goldstein, D. S., and Vaughan, E. D., Jr.: Reversibility of catecholamine-induced dilated cardiomyopathy in a child with a pheochromocytoma. N. Engl. J. Med. *316*:793, 1987.
160. Bhatnagar, D., Carey, P., and Pollard, A.: Focal myositis and elevated creatine kinase levels in a patient with phaeochromocytoma. Postgrad. Med. J. *62*:197, 1986.
161. Serfas, D., Shoback, D. M., and Lorell, B. H.: Phaeochromocytoma and hypertrophic cardiomyopathy: Apparent suppression of symptoms and noradrenaline secretion by calcium-channel blockade. Lancet *2*:711, 1983.
162. Sisson, J. C., Frager, M. S., Valk, T. W., Gross, M. D., Swanson, D. P., Wieland, D. M., Tobes, M. C., Beierwaltes, W. H., and Thompson, N. W.: Scintigraphic localization of pheochromocytoma. N. Engl. J. Med. *305*:12, 1981
163. Orringer, M. B., Sisson, J. C., Glazer, G., Shapiro, B., Francis, I., Behrendt, D. M., Thompson, N. W., and Lloyd, R. V.: Surgical treatment of cardiac pheochromocytomas. J. Thorac. Cardiovasc. Surg. *89*:753, 1985.
164. David, T. E., Lenkei, S. C., Marquez-Julio, A., Goldberg, J. A., and Meldrum, D. A. N.: Pheochromocytoma of the heart. Ann. Thorac. Surg. *41*:98, 1986.

PARATHYROID DISEASE

165. Potts, J. T., Jr., Kronenberg, H. M., and Rosenblatt, M.: Parathyroid hormone: Chemistry, biosynthesis, and mode of action. Protein Chem. *35*:323, 1982.
166. DeLuca, H. F.: The vitamin D system in the regulation of calcium and phosphorus metabolism. Nutr. Rev. *37*:161, 1979.
167. Symons, C., Fortune, F., Greenbaum, R. A., and Dandona, P.: Cardiac hypertrophy, hypertrophic cardiomyopathy, and hyperparathyroidism—an association. Br. Heart J. *54*:539, 1985.
168. Bogin, E., Massry, S. G., and Harary, I.: Effect of parathyroid hormone on rat heart cells. J. Clin. Invest. *67*:1215, 1981.
169. Katoh, Y., Klein, K. L., Kaplan, R. A., Sanborn, W. G., and Kurokawa, K.: Parathyroid hormone has a positive inotropic action in the rat. Endocrinology *109*:2252, 1981.
170. Palmieri, G. M., Nutting, D. F., Bhattacharya, S. K., Bertorini, T. E., and Williams, J. C.: Parathyroid ablation in dystrophic hamsters: Effects of Ca content and histology of heart, diaphragm, and rectus femoris. J. Clin. Invest. *68*:646, 1981.
171. Gafter, U., Battler, A., Eldar, M., Zevin, D., Neufeld, H. N., and Levi, J.: Effect of hyperparathyroidism on cardiac function in patients with end-stage renal disease. Nephron *41*:30, 1985.
172. Giles, T. D., Iteld, B. J., and Rires, K. L.: The cardiomyopathy of hypoparathyroidism. Chest 79:225, 1981.
173. Ellison, D. H., and McCarron, D. A.: Structural prerequisites for the hypotensive action of parathyroid hormone. Am. J. Physiol. *246*:F551, 1984.
174. Roberts, W. C., and Waller, B. F.: Effect of chronic hypercalcemia on the heart: An analysis of 18 necropsy patients. Am. J. Med. *71*:371, 1981.
175. Roberts, W. C., and Waller, B. F.: Chronic hypercalcemia as a risk factor for coronary atherosclerosis. Cardiovasc. Rev. Rep. *4*:1275, 1983.
176. Levine, S. N., and Rheams, C. N.: Hypocalcemic heart failure. Am. J. Med. *78*:1033, 1985.

DIABETES MELLITUS

177. Kleerekoper, M., Rao, D. S., and Frame, B.: Hypercalcemia, hyperparathyroidism and hypertension. Cardiovasc. Med. *3*:1283, 1978.
178. Daniels, J., and Goodman, A. D.: Hypertension and hyperparathyroidism: Inverse relation of sodium phosphate level and blood pressure. Am. J. Med. *75*:17, 1983.
179. Resnick, L. M.: Calcium, parathyroid disease, and hypertension. Cardiovasc. Rev. Rep. *3*:1341, 1982.
180. Unger, R. H., and Foster, D. W.: Diabetes mellitus. *In* Wilson, J. D., and Foster, D. W. (eds.): Williams' Textbook of Endocrinology. Philadelphia, W. B. Saunders Company, 1985, p. 1018.
181. Eisenbarth, G. S.: Type I diabetes mellitus: A chronic autoimmune disease. N. Engl. J. Med. *314*:1360, 1986.
182. Waller, B. F., Palumbo, P. J., Lie, J. T., and Roberts, W. C.: Status of the coronary arteries at necropsy in diabetes mellitus with onset after age 30 years: Analysis of 229 diabetic patients with and without clinical evidence of coronary heart disease and comparison of 183 control subjects. Am. J. Med. *69*:498, 1980.
183. Yano, K., Kagan, A., McGee, D., and Rhoads, G. G.: Glucose intolerance and nine-year mortality in Japanese men in Hawaii. Am. J. Med. *72*:71, 1982.
184. Zoneraich, S.: Diabetes and the Heart. Springfield, Ill., Charles C Thomas, Publisher, 1978, p. 303.
185. Factor, S. M., Okun, E. M., and Minase, T.: Capillary microaneurysms in the human heart. N. Engl. J. Med. *302*:384, 1980.
186. Shapiro, L. M.: A prospective study of heart disease in diabetes mellitus. Q. J. Med. *53*:55, 1984.
187. Gwilt, P. J., Petri, M., Lamb, P., Nattrass, M., and Pentecost, B. L.: Effects of intravenous insulin infusion on mortality among diabetic patients after myocardial infarction. Br. Heart J. *51*:626, 1984.
188. Kereiakes, D. J.: Myocardial infarction in the diabetic patient. Clin. Cardiol. *8*:446, 1985.
189. Rennert, G., Saltz-Rennert, H., Wanderman, K., and Weitzman, S.: Size of acute myocardial infarcts in patients with diabetes mellitus. Am. J. Cardiol. *55*:1629, 1985.
190. Ceremuzynski, L.: Hormonal and metabolic reactions evoked by acute myocardial infarction. Circ. Res. *48*:767, 1981.
191. Sobel, B., Corr, P. B., and Robison, A. K.: Accumulation of lysophosphoglycerides with arrythrogenic properties in ischemic myocardium. J. Clin. Invest. *62*:546, 1978.
192. Flink, E. B., Brick, J. E., and Shane, S. R.: Alterations of long-chain free fatty acid and magnesium concentrations in acute myocardial infarction. Arch. Intern. Med. *141*:441, 1981.
193. Opie, L. H., Tansey, M. J., and Kennelly, B. M.: The heart in diabetes mellitus. II. Acute myocardial infarction and diabetes. S. Afr. Med. J. *56*:256, 1979.
194. Smith, J. W., Marcus, F. I., and Serokman, R.: Prognosis of patients with diabetes mellitus after acute myocardial infarction. Am. J. Cardiol. *54*:718, 1984.

195. Jaffee, A. S., Spadaro, J. J., Schechtman, K., Roberts, R., Geltman, E. M., and Sobel, B. E.: Increased congestive heart failure after myocardial infarction of modest extent in patients with diabetes mellitus. Am. Heart J. *108*:31, 1984.
196. Gunderson, T., and Kjekshus, J.: Timolol treatment after myocardial infarction in diabetic patients. Diabetes Care *6*:285, 1983.
197. Smith, S. A.: Reduced sinus arrhythmia in diabetic autonomic neuropathy: Diagnostic value of an age-related normal range. Br. Med. J. *285*:1599, 1982.
198. Fernandez-Castaner, M., Figuerola, D., Sorribas, A., Reynals, E., and Balcells, A.: Evaluation des epreuves cardiovasculaires dans le diagnostic des neuropathies diabetiques autonomes. Diabete Metab. *9*:264, 1983.
199. Zola, B., Kahn, J. K., Juni, J. E., and Vinik, A. I.: Abnormal cardiac function in diabetic patients with autonomic neuropathy in the absence of ischemic heart disease. J. Clin. Endocrinol. Metab. *63*:208, 1986.
200. Pfeifer, M. A., Cook, D., Brodsky, J., Tice, D., Reenan, A., Swedine, S., Halter, J. B., and Porte, J. R.: Quantitative evaluation of cardiac parasympathetic activity in normal and diabetic man. Diabetes *31*:339, 1982.
201. Kannel, W. B., Hjortland, M., and Castelli, W. P.: The role of diabetics in congestive heart failure: The Framingham study. Am. J. Cardiol. *34*:29, 1974.
202. Vered, Z., Battler, A., Segal, P., Liberman, D., Yerushalmi, Y., Berezin, M., and Neufeld, H. N.: Exercise-induced left ventricular dysfunction in young men with asymptomatic diabetes mellitus (diabetic cardiomyopathy). Am. J. Cardiol. *54*:633, 1984.
203. Mildenberger, R. R., Bar-Schlomo, B., Druck, M. N., Jablonsky, G., Morch, J. E., Hilton, J. D., Kenshole, A. B., Forbath, N., and McLaughlin, P. R.: Clinically unrecognized ventricular dysfunction in young diabetic patients. J. Am. Coll. Cardiol. *4*:234, 1984.
204. Regan, T. J.: Cardiac decompensation in diabetes mellitus. Cardiovasc. Rev. Rep. *6*:1117, 1985.
205. Ahmed, S. S., Jaferi, G. A., Narang, R. M., and Regan, T. J.: Preclinical abnormality of left ventricular function in diabetes mellitus. Am. Heart J. *89*:153, 1975.
206. Seneviratne, B. I. B.: Diabetic cardiomyopathy: The preclinical phase. Br. Med. J. *1*:1444, 1977.
207. D'Elia, J. A., Weinrauch, L. A., Healy, R. W., Libertino, T. A., Bradley, R. F., and Leland, O. S.: Myocardial dysfunction without coronary artery disease in diabetic renal failure. Am. J. Cardiol. *43*:193, 1979.
208. Kahn, J. K., Zola, B., Juni, J. E., and Vinik, A. I.: Radionuclide assessment of left ventricular diastolic filling in diabetes mellitus with and without cardiac autonomic neuropathy. J. Am. Coll. Cardiol. 7:1303, 1986.
209. Sunni, S., Bishop, S. P., Kent, S. P., and Geer, J. C.: Diabetic cardiomyopathy. Arch. Pathol. Lab. Med. *110*:375, 1986.
210. Uusitupa, M., Siitonen, O., Pyorala, K., and Lansimies, E.: Left ventricular function in newly diagnosed noninsulin-dependent (Type 2) diabetes evaluated by systolic time intervals and echocardiography. Acta Med. Scand. *217*:379, 1985.
211. Factor, S. M., Minase, T., and Sonnenblick, E. H.: Clinical and morphological features of human hypertensive-diabetic cardiomyopathy. Am. Heart J. *99*:446, 1980.
212. Fein, F. S., Capasso, J. M., Aronson, R. S., Cho, S., Nordin, C., Miller-Green, B., Sonnenblick, E. H., and Factor, S. M.: Combined renovascular hypertension and diabetes in rats: A new preparation of congestive cardiomyopathy. Circulation *70*:318, 1984.
213. Regan, T. J., Ettinger, P. O., Khan, M. I., Jesrani, M. U., Lyons, M. M., Oldewurtel, H. A., and Weber, M.: Altered myocardial function and metabolism in chronic diabetes mellitus without ischemia in dogs. Circ. Res. *35*:222, 1974.
214. Penpargkul, S., Fein, F., Sonnenblick, E. H., and Scheuer, J.: Depressed cardiac sarcoplasmic reticular function from diabetic rats. J. Mol. Cell. Cardiol. *13*:303, 1981.
215. Ganguly, P. K., Rice, K. M., Panagia, V., and Dhalla, N. S.: Sarcolemmal phosphatidylethanolamine N-methylation in diabetic cardiomyopathy. Circ. Res. *55*:504, 1984.
216. Lopaschuk, G. D., Tahiliani, A. G., Vadlamudi, R. V. S. V., Katz, S., and McNeill, J. H.: Cardiac sarcoplasmic reticulum function in insulin- or carnitine-treated diabetic rats. Am. J. Physiol. *245*:H969, 1983.
217. Fein, F. S., Aronson, R. S., Nordin, C., Miller-Green, B., and Sonnenblick, E. H.: Altered myocardial response to ouabain in diabetic rats: Mechanics and electrophysiology. J. Mol. Cell. Cardiol. *15*:769, 1983.
218. Regan, T. J., Wu, C. F., Yeh, C. K., Oldewurtel, H. A., and Haider, B.: Myocardial composition and function in diabetes: The effects of chronic insulin use. Circ. Res. *49*:1268, 1981.
219. Malhotra, A., Penpargkul, S., Fein, F. S., Sonnenblick, E. H., and Scheuer, J.: The effect of streptozotocin-induced diabetes in rats on cardiac contractile proteins. Circ. Res. *49*:1243, 1981.
220. Fein, F. S., Malhotra, A., Miller-Green, B., Scheuer, J., and Sonnenblick, E. H.: Diabetic cardiomyopathy in rats: Mechanical and biochemical response to different insulin doses. Am. J. Physiol. *247*:H817, 1984.
221. Fein, F. S., Miller-Green, B., Zola, B., and Sonnenblick, E. H.: Reversibility of diabetic cardiomyopathy with insulin in rabbits. Am. J. Physiol. *250*:H108, 1986.
222. Regan, T. J., Wu, C. F., Weisse, A. B., Moschos, C. B., Haider, B., Ahmed, S. S., and Lyons, M. M.: Acute myocardial infarction in toxic cardiomyopathy without coronary obstruction. Circulation. *51*:453, 1975.
223. Wolfe, R. R., and Way, G. L.: Cardiomyopathies in infants of diabetic mothers. Johns Hopkins Med. J. *140*:177, 1977.
224. Sheehan, J. P., Sisam, D. A., and Schumacher, O. P.: Insulin-induced cardiac failure. Am. J. Med. *79*:147, 1985.
225. Falholt, K., Cutfield, R., Alejandro, R., Heding, L., and Mintz, D.: The effects of hyperinsulinemia on arterial wall and peripheral muscle metabolism in dogs. Metabolism *34*:1146, 1985.
226. Zatz, R., Dunn, B. R., Meyer, T. W., Anderson, S., Rennke, H. G., and Brenner, B. M.: Prevention of diabetic glomerulopathy by pharmacological amelioration of glomerular capillary hypertension. J. Clin. Invest. *77*:1925, 1986.
227. Beyer, T. A., and Hutson, N. J.: Introduction: Evidence for the role of the polyol pathway in the pathophysiology of diabetic complications. Metabolism *35*:1, 1986.
228. University Group Diabetes Program: A study of the effects of hypoglycemic agents on vascular complications in patients with adult-onset diabetes. V. Evaluation of phenformin therapy. Diabetes *24*(Suppl I):65, 1975.
229. Wu, C. F., Haider, B., Ahmed, S. S., Oldewurtel, H. A., Lyons, M. M., and Regan, T. J.: The effects of tolbutamide on the myocardium in experimental diabetes. Circulation *55*:200, 1977.
230. Bielefeld, D. R., Pace, C. S., and Boshell, B. R.: Hyperosmolarity and cardiac function in chronic diabetic rat heart. Am. J. Physiol. *245*:E568, 1983.
231. Axelrod, L.: Response of congestive heart failure to correction of hyperglycemia in the presence of diabetic nephropathy. N. Engl. J. Med. *293*:1243, 1975.

OBESITY

232. Salans, L. B.: Obesity and the adipose cell. *In* Bondy, P. K., and Rosenberg, L. E. (eds.): Metabolic Control and Disease. 9th ed. Philadelphia, W. B. Saunders Company, 1980, p. 510.
233. Hirsch, J., and Knittle, J. L.: Cellularity of obese and non-obese human adipose tissue. Fed. Proc. *29*:1516, 1970.
234. Foster, W. R., and Burton, B. T. (eds.): Health implications of obesity: NIH consensus development conference. Ann. Intern. Med. *103*:979, 1985.
235. Messerli, F. H., Sundgaard-Riise, K., Reisin, E., Dreslinski, G., Dunn, F. G., and Frohlich, E.: Disparate cardiovascular effects of obesity and arterial hypertension. Am. J. Med. *74*:808, 1983.
236. Smith, H. L., and Willius, R. A.: Adiposity of the heart. A clinical and pathological study of one hundred and thirty-six obese patients. Ann. Intern. Med. *52*:911, 1933.
237. De Divitiis, O., Fazio, S., Petitto, M., Maddalena, G., Contaldo, F., and Mancini, M.: Obesity and cardiac function. Circulation *64*:477, 1981.
238. Messerli, F. H., Ventura, H. O., Reisin, E., Dreslinski, G. R., Dunn, F. G., MacPhee, A. A., and Frohlich, E. D.: Borderline hypertension and obesity: Two prehypertensive states with elevated cardiac output. Circulation *66*:55, 1982.
239. Nakajima, T., Fujioka, S., Tokunaga, K., Hirobe, K., Matsuzawa, Y., and Tarui, S.: Noninvasive study of left ventricular performance in obese patients: Influence of duration of obesity. Circulation *71*:481, 1985.
240. Zack, P. M., Wiens, R. D., and Kennedy, H. L.: Left-axis deviation and adiposity: The United States health and nutrition examination survey. Am. J. Cardiol. *53*:1129, 1984.
241. Ventura, H. O., Messerli, F. H., Dunn, F. G., and Frohlich, E. D.: Left ventricular hypertrophy in obesity: Discrepancy between echo and electrocardiogram. J. Am. Coll. Cardiol. *1*:682, 1983.
242. Warnes, C. A., and Roberts, W. C.: The heart in massive (more than 300 pounds or 136 kilograms) obesity: Analysis of 12 patients studied at necropsy. Am. J. Cardiol. *54*:1087, 1984.
243. Messerli, F. H., Ventura, H. O., Elizardi, D. J., Dunn, F. G., and Frohlich, E. D.: Hypertension and sudden death: Increased ventricular ectopic activity in left ventricular hypertrophy. Am. J. Med. *77*:18, 1984.
244. Reisin, E., Frohlich, E. D., Messerli, F. H., Dreslinski, G. R., Dunn, F. G., Jones, M. M., and Batson, H. M.: Cardiovascular changes after weight reduction in obesity hypertension. Ann. Intern. Med. *98*:315, 1983.
245. MacMahon, S. W., Wilcken, D. E. L., and Macdonald, G. J.: The effect of weight reduction on left ventricular mass: A randomized controlled trial in young, overweight hypertensive patients. N. Engl. J. Med. *314*:334, 1986.
246. Alpert, M. A., Terry, B. E., and Kelly, D. L.: Effect of weight loss on cardiac chamber size, wall thickness and left ventricular function in morbid obesity. Am. J. Cardiol. *55*:783, 1985.
247. Backman, L., Freyschuss, U., Hallberg, D., and Melcher, A.: Reversibility of cardiovascular changes in extreme obesity: Effects of weight reduction through jejunoileostomy. Acta Med. Scand. *205*:367, 1979.

MALNUTRITION

248. Abel, R. M., Grimes, J. B., Alonso, D., Alonso, M., and Gay, W. A., Jr.: Adverse hemodynamic and ultrastructural changes in dog hearts subjected to protein-calorie malnutrition. Am. Heart J. *97*:733, 1979.
249. Nutter, D. O., Murray, T. G., Heymsfield, S. T., and Fuller, E. O.: The effect of chronic protein-calorie undernutrition in the rat on myocardial function and cardiac function. Circ. Res. *45*:144, 1979.
250. Isner, J. M., Roberts, W. C., Heymsfield, S. B., and Yager, J.: Anorexia nervosa and sudden death. Ann. Intern. Med. *102*:49, 1985.
251. Fonseca, V., and Havard, C. W. H.: Electrolyte disturbances and cardiac failure with hypomagnesaemia in anorexia nervosa. Br. Med. J. *291*:1680, 1985.
252. Abel, R. M., Fischer, J. E., Buckley, M. J., Barnett, G. O., and Austen, W. G.: Malnutrition in cardiac surgical patients. Arch. Surg. *111*:45, 1976.

253. Blackburn, G. L., Gibbons, G. W., Bothe, A., Benotti, P. N., Harken, D. E., and McEnany, T. M.: Nutritional support in cardiac cachexia. J. Thorac. Cardiovasc. Surg. 73:489, 1977.

254. Steier, M., Lopez, R., and Cooperman, J. M.: Riboflavin deficiency in infants and children with heart disease. Am. Heart J. *92*:139, 1976.

ALTERATIONS IN GONADAL HORMONE SECRETION

255. Dimitrovski, C., Plaseski, A., Bogoev, M., and Sadikario, S.: Kallmann's syndrome associated with atrial septal defect. J.A.M.A. *248*:1358, 1982.

256. McGill, Jr., H. C., Anselmo, V. C., Buchanan, J. M., and Sheridan, P. J.: The heart is a target organ for androgen. Science *207*:775, 1980.

257. Schaible, T. F., Malhotra, A., Ciambrone, G., and Scheuer, J.: The effects of gonadectomy on left ventricular function and cardiac contractile proteins in male and female rats. Circ. Res. *54*:38, 1984.

258. Wallace, R. B., Hoover, J., Barrett-Conner, E., Rifkind, B. M., Hunninghake, D. B., MacKenthun, A., and Heiss, G.: Altered plasma lipid and lipoprotein levels associated with oral contraceptive and estrogen use. Lancet 2:112, 1979.

259. Stampfer, M. J., Willett, W. C., Colditz, G. A., Rosner, B., Speizer, F. E., and Hennekens, C. H.: A prospective study of postmenopausal estrogen therapy and coronary heart disease. N. Engl. J. Med. *313*:1044, 1985.

260. Petitti, D. B., Perlman, J. A., and Sidney, S.: Postmenopausal estrogen use and heart disease. N. Engl. J. Med. *315*:131, 1986.

261. Hillner, B. E., Hollenberg, J. P., and Pauker, S. G.: Postmenopausal estrogens in prevention of osteoporosis: Benefit virtually without risk if cardiovascular effects are considered. Am. J. Med. *80*:1115, 1986.

262. Ritterband, A. B., Jaffee, I. A., and Densen, P. M.: Gonadal function and the development of coronary heart disease. Circulation *27*:237, 1963.

263. Webber, L. S., Hunter, S. M., Baugh, J. G., Srinivasan, S. R., Sklov, M. C., and Berenson, G. S.: The interaction of cigarette smoking, oral contraceptive use, and cardiovascular risk factor variables in children: The Bogalusa Heart Study. Am. J. Publ. Health 72:266, 1982.

264. Jaffe, M. D.: Effect of oestrogens on postexercise electrocardiogram. Br. Heart J. *38*:1299, 1976.

265. Phillips, G. B.: Evidence for hyperestrogenemia as the link between diabetes mellitus and myocardial infarction. Am. J. Med. *76*:1041, 1984.

266. Gutin, B., Alejandro, D., Duni, T., Segal, K., and Phillips, G. B.: Levels of serum sex hormones and risk factors for coronary heart disease in exercise-trained men. Am. J. Med. *79*:79, 1985.

267. Wilson, P. W. F., Garrison, R. J., and Castelli, W. P.: Postmenopausal estrogen use, cigarette smoking, and cardiovascular morbidity in women over 50: The Framingham Study. N. Engl. J. Med. *313*:1038, 1985.

268. Gutai, J., LaPorte, R., Kuller, L., Dai, W., Falvo-Gerard, L., and Caggiula, A.: Plasma testosterone, high density lipoprotein cholesterol and other lipoprotein fractions. Am. J. Cardiol., *48*:897, 1981.

269. Merians, D. R., Haskell, W. L., Vranizan, K. M., Phelps, J., Woods, P. D., and Superko, R.: Relationship of exercise, oral contraceptive use, and body fat to concentrations of plasma lipids and lipoprotein cholesterol in young women. Am. J. Med. *78*:913, 1985.

270. Boyd, W. N., Burden, R. P., and Aber, G. M.: Intrarenal vascular changes in patients receiving estrogen-containing compounds—A clinical, histological and angiographic study. Q. J. Med. *44*:415, 1975.

271. Hollenberg, N. K., Williams, G. H., Burger, B., Chenitz, W., Hooshmand, I., and Adams, D. F.: Renal blood flow and its response to A II: An interaction between oral contraceptive agents, sodium intake and the renin-angiotensin system in healthy young women. Circ. Res. *38*:35, 1976.

59 RENAL DISORDERS AND HEART DISEASE

by STEPHEN O. PASTAN, M.D., and
EUGENE BRAUNWALD, M.D.

Disorders of the heart and of the kidneys are intimately related. Some of the principal clinical manifestations of impairment of the heart's performance as a pump are due to renal retention of sodium and water; a number of diseases of the heart, such as infective endocarditis and cardiogenic shock, may result in serious renal disease or dysfunction. Conversely, chronic renal failure frequently results in hypertension and lipid abnormalities, which often lead to accelerated atherosclerosis, so that coronary artery disease is a common cause of death in patients being treated for chronic renal insufficiency. Also, uremia often causes pericarditis and thereby may lead to cardiac tamponade or constrictive pericarditis; renal failure can also cause secondary hyperparathyroidism, which can produce cardiac calcification and lead to a variety of disturbances of cardiac function.

EFFECTS OF CARDIAC DISEASE ON RENAL FUNCTION

HEART FAILURE

J. P. Peters at Yale is credited with developing the concept that the kidney in heart failure is physiologically similar to the kidney in hypovolemia: because of inadequate cardiac output in both states, salt and water are retained in an attempt to restore the effective arterial blood volume—an as yet poorly defined parameter of filling of the arterial tree that is somehow related to the ratio of arterial blood volume to the capacity of the vascular bed.

Modulation of the tubular transport of sodium provides the most important mechanism for regulating sodium excretion. The proximal tubule is the primary site of sodium reabsorption in the nephron, with approximately 60 per cent of filtered sodium being reabsorbed isotonically at this site. Current conceptions of the forces governing proximal tubular reabsorption of sodium in the normal state and in heart failure are shown in Figure 59–1. As cardiac output falls, several stimuli—including augmented alpha-adrenergic neural activity, circulating catecholamines, and increased circulating and locally produced angiotensin II—cause renal vasoconstriction, particularly of the efferent arterioles (Figs. 59–2 and 59–3). As a consequence, the glomerular filtration rate declines, but there is a proportionately greater fall in renal blood flow and therefore a rise in the filtration fraction (i.e., the ratio of glomerular filtration rate to renal blood flow). This results in an elevated protein concentration in the peritubular capillaries and a decline in the postglomerular capillary hydrostatic pressure; thus, the transcapillary hydraulic pressure gradient falls.

SODIUM RETENTION IN HEART FAILURE. The combination of these events, i.e., the reduction of peritubular capillary hydrostatic pressure and an elevation of peritubular oncotic pressure, enhances the peritubular capillary uptake of proximal tubular fluid and thereby increases the absolute quantity of sodium reabsorbed by the proximal tubule.[1, 2] An additional proposed mechanism for sodium retention in heart failure is the redistribution of blood flow from cortical to juxtamedullary nephrons that contain longer loops of Henle and are therefore capable of greater sodium reabsorption.

In addition to the more avid sodium reabsorption in the proximal convoluted tubule, sodium reabsorption also increases in distal nephron sites, including the collecting duct segments. This results from the operation of Starling forces, i.e., a lowering of capillary hydrostatic pressure and an elevation of oncotic pressure, such as those described for the proximal tubule.

Editor's note: The pathophysiology of congestive heart failure is described in Chapters 14 and 16; the use of diuretics in treating heart failure is discussed in Chapter 17; and the alterations in renal function are reviewed here.

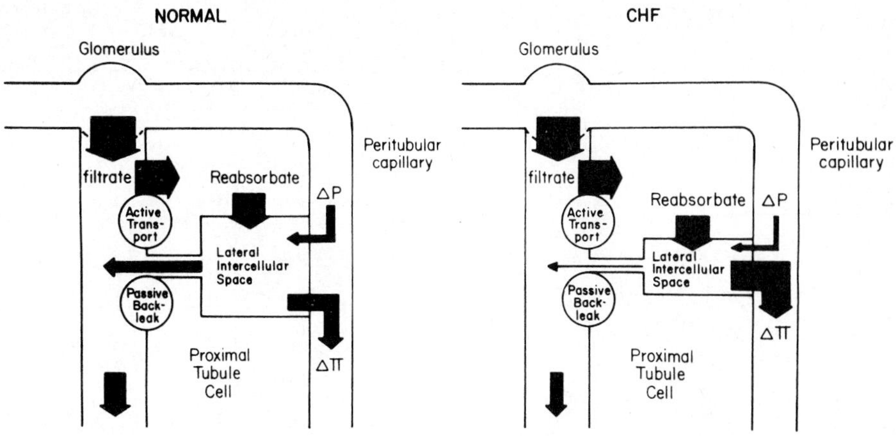

FIGURE 59–1. Peritubular control of proximal tubule fluid reabsorption. Current concept of the role of peritubular capillary physical forces in the regulation of proximal tubule fluid reabsorption in the normal state (*left*) and in congestive heart failure (CHF)(*right*). ΔP and $\Delta \pi$ are, respectively, the transcapillary hydraulic and oncotic pressure differences operating across the peritubular capillary. The increase in filtration fraction causes $\Delta \pi$ to rise in CHF. The increase in renal vascular resistance in CHF is thought to reduce ΔP. Both the increase in $\Delta \pi$ and the fall in ΔP serve to enhance peritubular capillary uptake of proximal reabsorbate and thus increase absolute sodium reabsorption by the proximal tubule. (From Humes, H. D., et al.: The kidney in congestive heart failure. *In* Brenner, B. M., and Stein, J. H. [eds.]: Contemporary Issues in Nephrology. Vol. 1. New York, Churchill Livingstone, 1978, p. 51.)

The Renin-Angiotensin-Aldosterone System. (See also p. 834). In addition, the aldosterone, the sodium resorbing activity of which is limited to the terminal segment of the nephron, distal tubule, and collecting duct system, has been recognized as an important factor in sodium retention associated with congestive heart failure. The absolute concentration of circulating aldosterone is increased in some patients with congestive heart failure owing to both the enhanced production of aldosterone stimulated by the renin-angiotensin axis and its diminished metabolism. In acute heart failure, decreased renal perfusion (whether caused by a reduction in total cardiac output or by a decrease in the renal fraction of the cardiac output) activates the juxtaglomerular apparatus to enhance renin release; this in turn augments the generation of angiotensin II, the stimulus for aldosterone secretion and thus for retention of sodium (Fig. 27–16, p. 835). Angiotensin II, both circulating and locally produced, also plays a role in the constriction of efferent arterioles[3] and the resultant elevation in the filtration fraction, discussed above. Indeed, the administration of an angiotensin II–converting enzyme inhibitor in heart failure increases renal blood flow and glomerular filtration with a return of filtration fraction toward normal and usually induces a natriuresis. The impairment in aldosterone biodegradation sometimes seen in heart failure is due to hepatic congestion as well as reduced splanchnic blood flow secondary to reduced cardiac output and splanchnic vasoconstriction.[4]

The renal retention of sodium expands extracellular fluid volume and tends to return the renin-angiotensin-aldosterone system toward normal. For that reason, circulating angiotensin II and aldosterone concentrations are frequently normal in chronic stable heart failure, although they tend to be high relative to the expanded extracellular fluid volume (Fig. 59–3). In terminal heart failure, however, with further impairment of renal perfusion, renin production is again enhanced, despite expansion of the extracellular fluid volume.

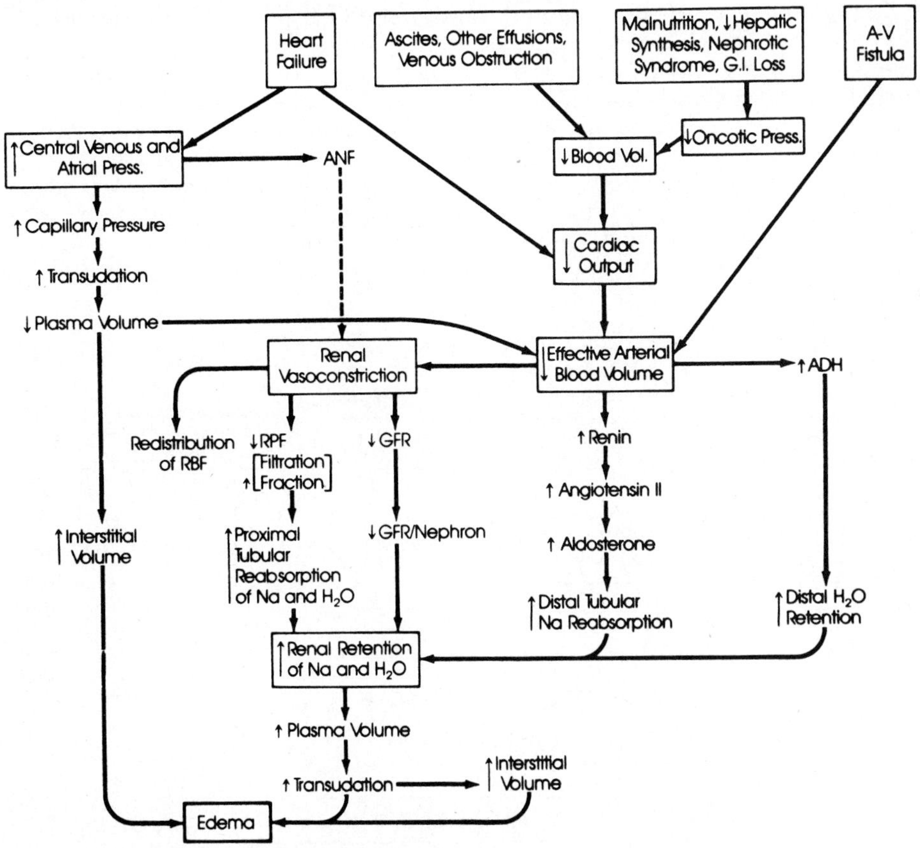

FIGURE 59–2. Major pathophysiological mechanisms leading to salt and water retention and the development of edema. The contribution of heart failure is shown, as well as other major causes. ANF = atrial natriuretic factor; dotted line indicates inhibition of renal vasoconstriction. (From Braunwald, E.: Edema. *In* Braunwald, E., et al. [eds.]: Harrison's Principles of Internal Medicine. New York, McGraw-Hill Book Co., 1987, p. 150.)

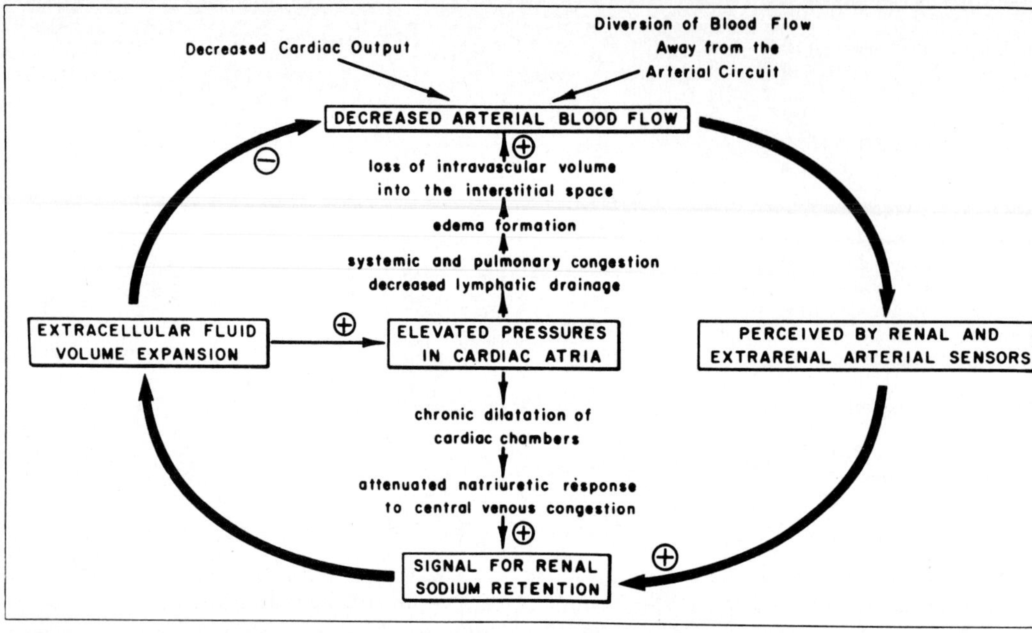

FIGURE 59–3. Sensing mechanisms that initiate and maintain renal sodium retention in congestive heart failure. (Reproduced with permission from Skorecki, K. L., and Brenner, B. M.: Body fluid homeostasis in congestive heart failure and cirrhosis with ascites. Am. J. Med. *72*:323, 1982.)

Other Vasoactive Substances. The role of other vasoactive substances, such as prostaglandins, kallikreins, and kinins, has yet to be determined, but they have also been implicated as factors in sodium balance.[5] Intrarenal prostaglandins oppose the actions of angiotensin II on the renal vascular bed.[6] In heart failure, the infusion of prostaglandin A_2 may enhance sodium excretion,[7] whereas inhibition of prostaglandin synthesis by means of drugs such as indomethacin may enhance arteriolar resistance, depress glomerular filtration rate, and increase sodium retention.[8]

WATER RETENTION IN HEART FAILURE. The mechanisms for water retention in congestive heart failure are outlined in Figure 59–4. With enhanced proximal reabsorption and a decline in glomerular filtration rate, less tubular fluid is delivered to the diluting segments of the nephron.[9] In addition, with a reduction in renal blood flow, renal medullary blood flow is diminished, which also reduces the nephron's capacity to excrete water.[1] The smaller effective arterial blood volume serves as a nonosmotic stimulus to enhanced release of antidiuretic hormone, favoring water retention. Furthermore, heart failure stimulates the sensation of thirst[10]; angiotensin II, acting centrally, may also be responsible for stimulating the thirst mechanism. A number of nonosmotic stimuli for the release of antidiuretic hormone (ADH), such as discomfort, anxiety, beta-adrenoceptor agonists, and central nervous system depressants (including barbiturates and narcotics) are commonly present in congestive heart failure. There is a high incidence of inappropriately elevated ADH secretion, which plays an important role in the dilutional hypo-osmolality noted in many patients with heart failure.[11, 12]

The elevated peripheral venous pressure characteristic of heart failure also causes a reflex resetting of pre- and postcapillary resistances in the systemic vascular bed. Transudation of fluid into the interstitial space is therefore favored,[13] tending to lower blood volume and enhancing sodium retention. Elevated systemic venous pressure transmitted to the ostium of the thoracic duct impedes lymphatic drainage, enhancing the formation of edema and decreasing intravascular volume. In short-term experiments, distention of the atria activates receptors that may be considered to monitor atrial and intrathoracic blood volume. Activation of these receptors and vagal afferent fibers reduces renal vascular resistance and inhibits the secretion of ADH, thus augmenting the excretion of sodium and water.[14] However, resetting of the atrial pressure

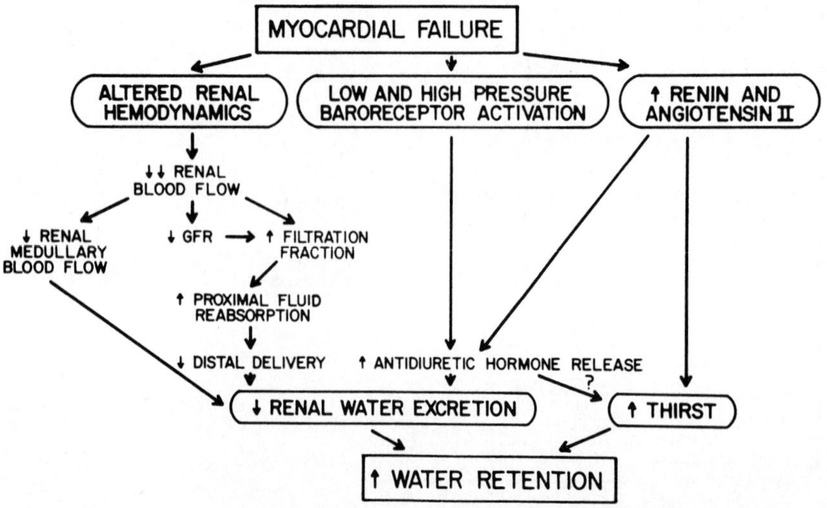

FIGURE 59–4. Major pathophysiological mechanisms leading to water retention in congestive heart failure. (From Humes, H. D., et al.: The kidney in congestive heart failure. *In* Brenner, B. M., and Stein, J. H. [eds.]: Sodium and Water Homeostasis. New York, Churchill Livingstone, 1978, p. 51.)

receptors occurs in chronic cardiac failure and atrial distention. In animals with heart failure secondary to experimental pulmonic stenosis and tricuspid regurgitation, the spontaneous activity of the atrial receptors was found to be depressed,[15] and in dogs with heart failure caused by an aortocaval fistula, the water diuretic response to left atrial distention is blunted.[16] This attenuated sensitivity of venous and atrial pressure receptors may be responsible for reduced renal vasodilatation (i.e., a higher renal vascular resistance), which in turn contributes to salt and water retention in heart failure by mitigating the diuresis and natriuresis that would otherwise accompany the volume expansion and atrial distention characteristic of heart failure.

Total body *sodium* is uniformly elevated in edematous patients with congestive heart failure,[17] and total body water is usually increased to an even greater extent. The serum concentration is thus usually slightly reduced in heart failure; in some patients with severe heart failure, it is greatly reduced. Furthermore, sodium may become osmotically inactivated in edema,[18] perhaps by binding to chondroitin sulfate[19] as well as to other polyelectrolytes.

PRERENAL AZOTEMIA IN HEART FAILURE. Azotemia is a common finding in severe congestive heart failure.[20] The enhanced water reabsorption in the collecting duct, especially in the presence of inappropriately elevated ADH, augments the passive reabsorption of urea. In addition, urea production may be enhanced in some forms of heart failure—especially in acute myocardial infarction; a catabolic state induced by the stress of heart failure may account for the increased urea load. The combination of increased urea production and decreased excretion (secondary to augmented reabsorption) elevates blood urea nitrogen (BUN) even prior to a reduction of glomerular filtration rate. However, the principal mechanism for elevation of BUN and serum creatinine is reduction of the glomerular filtration rate. As already noted, the latter is preserved by efferent arteriolar constriction in the presence of modest reductions in renal plasma flow, and therefore serum creatinine may remain normal until, in severe heart failure, there are marked reductions in renal plasma flow, constriction of afferent arterioles, and reduction of glomerular filtration rate. Thus, an elevation of serum creatinine is usually a sign of advanced heart failure. It is not uncommon in heart failure for the BUN:creatinine ratio to exceed 10 to 1. In severe heart failure, when glomerular filtration rate declines, the BUN may exceed 100 mg/dl and the serum creatinine, 4 mg/dl.

Prerenal azotemia of this degree is a poor prognostic sign in heart failure. Treatment should be directed toward improving cardiac function, as outlined in Chapter 17.

HEART FAILURE IN PATIENTS WITH RENAL DISEASE. The improvement in the therapy of heart failure (Chap. 17) has prolonged the lives of many patients with the combination of cardiac failure and chronic renal disease. In many such patients, the intrinsic renal disease is not severe enough to cause salt, water, or nitrogen retention in the presence of a normal cardiac output. However, when heart failure and the attendant alterations in renal hemodynamics described above are superimposed on intrinsic renal disease, serious problems of retention readily occur. Hemodialysis with ultrafiltration or peritoneal dialysis can be effective in the management of this combination of disorders.

POTASSIUM BALANCE IN HEART FAILURE. Mild hypokalemia is a relatively common finding in patients with congestive heart failure, as a consequence of the distal tubular exchange of sodium for potassium and hydrogen under the influence of excess aldosterone. In addition, since all the major diuretics (other than spironolactone, triamterene, and amiloride) inhibit sodium chloride reabsorption proximal to the site of action of aldosterone in the distal tubule, they increase the delivery of sodium to the distal tubule, enhancing the likelihood of the exchange of sodium for hydrogen and potassium (p. 515). Therefore, serum potassium should be monitored in patients with congestive heart failure to ascertain the need for potassium replacement therapy. Since potassium excretion is augmented and accompanied by alkalosis, replacement should be in the form of potassium chloride rather than potassium bicarbonate or gluconate.

In the end stage of chronic congestive heart failure, prerenal azotemia and oliguria may become severe enough to limit the patient's ability to excrete potassium. At this stage, so little sodium is being delivered to the distal tubule, even with diuretic therapy, that its exchange with potassium is reduced and hyperkalemia may develop. In patients with severe heart failure and progressive azotemia and oliguria, potassium-sparing diuretics (spironolactone, amiloride, and triamterene) must be used with caution, if at all since these agents may hasten the development of hyperkalemia.

ATRIAL NATRIURETIC PEPTIDE (ANP)

In addition to the aforementioned indirect effects of heart failure on renal function, the atria produce peptides that directly affect renal function. For more than 30 years the atria have been considered important physiological sites of volume regulation.[21, 22] Although atrial myocytes have long been known to possess granules characteristic of secretory cells[23, 24] (Fig. 59–5) and the degree of granularity was known to be related to the state of salt balance,[25] it was not until 1981 that DeBold et al. published their landmark experiments showing that infusions of an extract of mammalian atria (but not of the ventricles) induced rapid natriuresis, kaliuresis, and diuresis while lowering systemic arterial pressure.[26] Subsequently, the active material was identified[26a] as a family of related *atrial natriuretic peptides* (ANP) that has since been cloned and sequenced.[27] Although ANP has been subjected to intensive experimental investigation, its exact role in circulatory physiology and pathophysiology has yet to be clearly de-

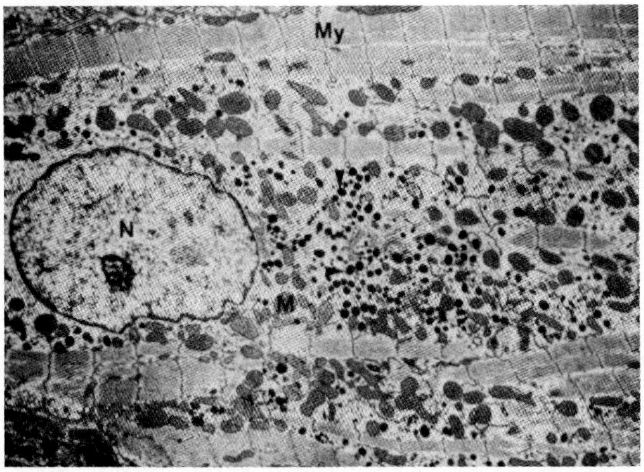

FIGURE 59–5. Electron microscopic view of a rat atrial cardiocyte. N = nucleus; M = mitochondria; My = myofibrils. The central sarcoplasmic core displays morphological features associated with secretory cells that include a large number of storage granules (arrowheads), referred to as specific atrial granules (× 3,400). (From DeBold, A. J.: Atrial natriuretic factor: A hormone produced by the heart. Science *230*: 767, 1985. Reproduced by permission of the American Association for the Advancement of Science.)

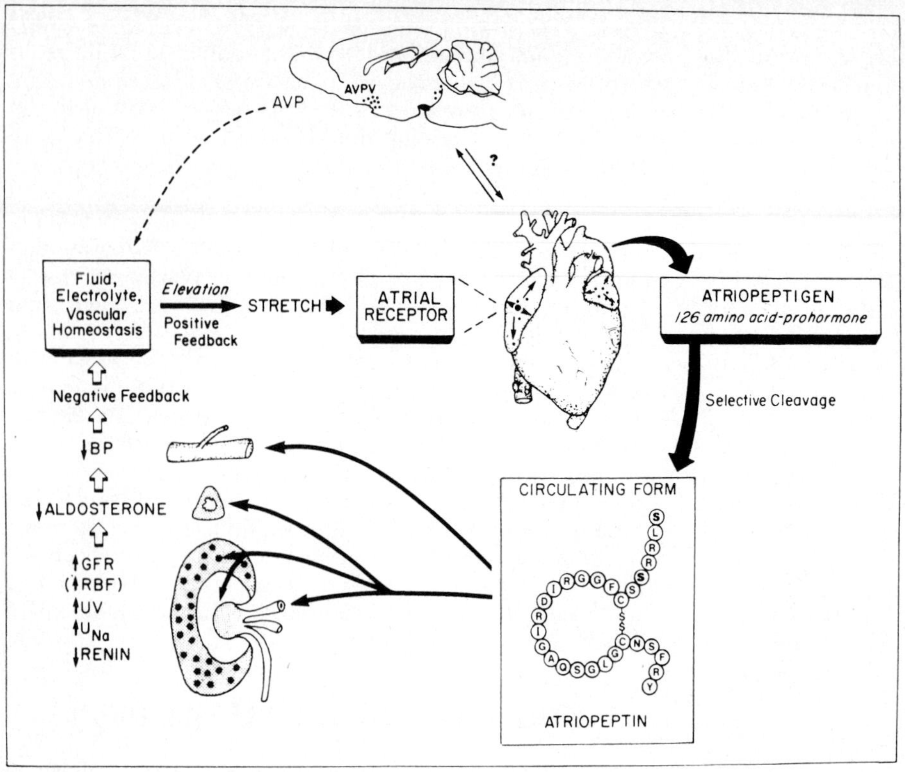

FIGURE 59–6. Summary of the atrial natriuretic peptide (ANP) hormonal system. The 126-amino acid prohormone atriopeptigen or pro-ANP (see text) is stored in granules in perinuclear atrial cardiocytes. Elevated vascular volume resutls in the release of atriopeptin (ANP), which acts on the kidney (glomeruli and papilla) to increase glomerular filtration rate (GFR), renal blood flow (RBF), urine volume (UV), and urinary sodium excretion (U_{Na}), and to decrease plasma renin activity. Natriuresis and diuresis are also facilitated by the suppression of aldosterone and of arginine vasopressin (AVP). Diminution of vascular volume provides a negative feedback that suppresses circulating levels of ANP. (Reprinted by permission from Needleman, P., and Greenwald, J. E.: Atriopeptin: A cardiac hormone intimately involved in fluid, electrolyte, and blood pressure homeostasis. N. Engl. J. Med. *314*:829, 1986.)

fined. A proposed summary of the actions of ANP as circulating natriuretic hormones is shown in Figure 59–6.

STRUCTURE. Human ANP is synthesized as a 151–amino acid pro-ANP precursor and stored as a 126–amino acid pro-ANP in atrial myocyte granules (Fig. 59–7). The biologically active circulating molecule consists of a 28–amino acid peptide thought to be cleft from the pro-ANP when it is released. The molecule possesses a 17–amino acid ring formed by a disulfide bridge between two cysteine moieties, which is required for biological activity.[28] Approximately 25 to 100 picograms/ml of ANP can be measured in normal human plasma.[29]

ANP RELEASE. Plasma volume expansion and elevation of left atrial pressure or volume are thought to induce the

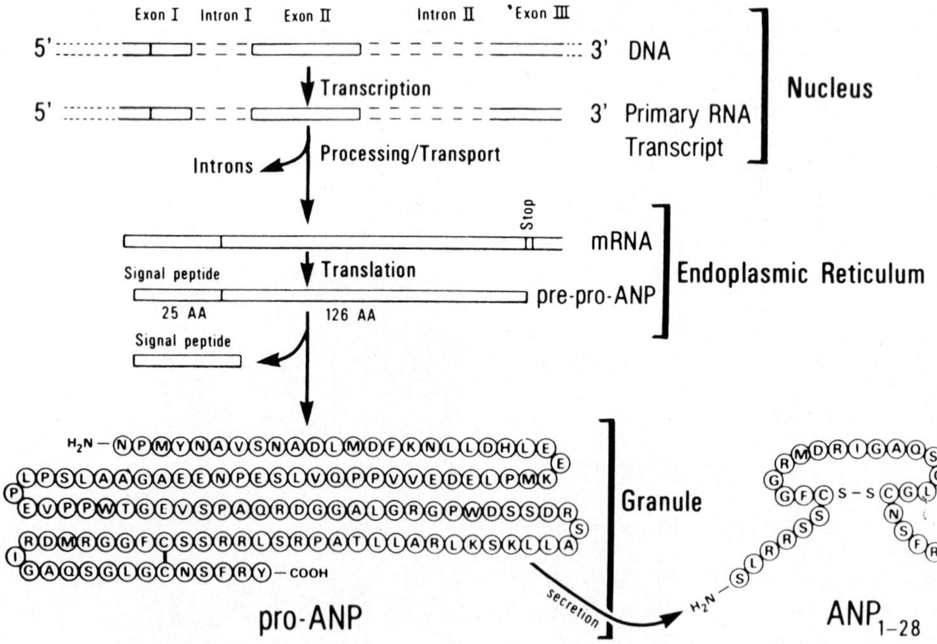

FIGURE 59–7. The biosynthetic pathway, and the sequences of the human pre-pro-ANP gene, pro-ANP, and ANP_{1-28}. ANP_{1-28} is numbered from amino- to carboxyterminus. Specific amino acids in the pro-ANP and ANP sequences are given by single letter code: alanine = A, arginine = R, asparagine = N, aspartic acid = D, cysteine = C, glutamine = Q, glutamic acid = E, glycine = G, histidine = H, isoleucine = I, leucine = L, lysine = K, methionine = M, phenylalanine = F, proline = P, serine = S, threonine = T, tryptophan = W, tyrosine = Y, valine = V.

The DNA is transcribed into RNA, and the exon segments are spliced together to form messenger RNA. This is translated to form the initial pro-ANP precursor (pre-pro-ANP). The signal peptide is removed and pro-ANP is stored in atrial myocyte granules. When the peptide is released, the active 28–amino acid fragment is cleaved off and enters the circulation. (From Ballermann, B. J., and Brenner, B. M.: Role of atrial peptides in body fluid homeostasis. Circ. Res. *58*:619, 1986, by permission of the American Heart Association, Inc.)

release of ANP from atrial myocyte granules. Release of a natriuretic substance from rat heart-lung preparations in the face of high atrial perfusion pressure[30] as well as elevation of plasma ANP in dogs after atrial distention have been reported.[31] In humans, ANP levels have been found to rise with an increase of salt intake,[32] upon assumption of the supine posture,[33] and after water immersion.[34] A rise in plasma ANP after salt and water loading and a fall after furosemide-induced volume depletion have been reported.[35] Patients with congestive heart failure have elevated plasma ANP levels.[32, 36] In one study, right atrial and arterial plasma ANP levels correlated with right atrial and pulmonary capillary wedge pressures, respectively.[37] Step-ups in ANP levels across the atria were also demonstrated. Finally, elevated plasma ANP levels have been described during atrial tachycardia[38] and during atrial pacing[39] and may explain the polyuria sometimes associated with these events. Taken together, these observations support the concept that atrial ANP release is strongly associated with plasma volume status as well as with atrial pressure and/or volume. Of interest, infusions of arginine vasopressin, phenylephrine, and angiotensin II also appear to stimulate the release of ANP and increase plasma ANP levels.[40]

ANP RECEPTORS. Once released into the circulation, ANP bind to receptors having high affinity and specificity in target tissues.[41] These receptors have been found in the renal cortex and medulla, aorta, vascular smooth muscle,[42] the adrenal zona glomerulosa,[43] and the central nervous system.[44] After binding, ANP activates membrane-bound guanylate cyclase.[45] Intracellular increases in cyclic GMP have been described in many tissues, and marked increases in urinary cyclic GMP are stimulated by atrial extracts in rats.[46] Thus, cyclic GMP seems to be a major intracellular mediator of ANP activity.

PHYSIOLOGICAL EFFECTS OF ANP. Intravenous infusion of ANP in animals and humans result in a brisk natriuresis and diuresis (Fig. 59–8*A*). An increase in excretion of chloride, potassium, calcium, magnesium, and phosphorus has also been noted.[47, 48] Although the exact renal mechanisms involved are incompletely understood, two consistent and dramatic findings have been increases in both glomerular filtration rate and filtration fraction, despite a drop in blood pressure (Fig. 59–8*B*). In the rat this is associated with constriction of the efferent glomerular arterioles, dilation of afferent arterioles, and an increase in glomerular pressure.[49] ANP inhibits renal vasoconstriction, but differing effects of ANP on total renal blood flow have been described depending on the species studied and on experimental conditions.[47, 50] Although it was initially suspected that changes in the glomerular filtration rate could account completely for the magnitude of the natriuresis in response to ANP,[51] more recent investigations have revealed that ANP inhibits transport-dependent oxygen consumption in rabbit papillary collecting duct cells[52] and sodium transport in the inner medullary collecting duct.[53] Thus, it would appear that a combination of glomerular hemodynamic effects and inhibition of distal nephron sodium transport is responsible for the marked degree of natriuresis in response to ANP.

More prolonged effects of ANP on salt balance and hemodynamics may be mediated through changes in the renin-angiotensin-aldosterone system. Renal renin secretion is known to be suppressed by ANP.[54] Enhanced sodium delivery to the macula densa has been proposed as the major mechanism of this inhibition, although a direct effect on renin secretion is possible.[55] Aldosterone secretion is also blocked by ANP in vitro and in vivo,[56] as is angiotensin-induced vascular constriction[57] and angioten-

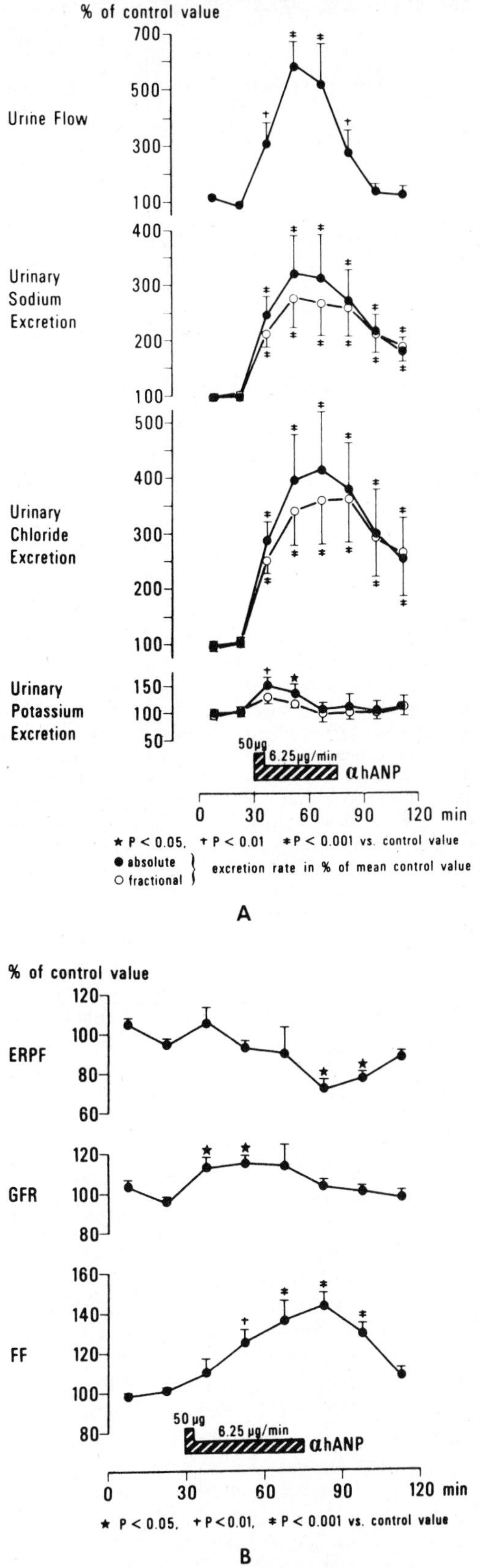

FIGURE 59–8. *A*, Effect of ANP (50 = μg bolus followed by maintenance infusion of 6.25 μg/min) on urine flow and sodium, chloride, and potassium excretion rates in 10 normal subjects (mean ± S.E.M.). The mean of the two control values is taken as 100 per cent. Closed circles are the absolute excretion rates. Open circles are calculated fractional excretion rates (urine/plasma Na, Cl, or K divided by urine/plasma creatinine). *B*, Effect of ANP on ERPF = estimated renal plasma flow; GFR = glomerular filtration rate; FF = filtration fraction. (From Weidmann, P., et al.: Blood levels and renal effects of atrial natriuretic peptide in normal man. J. Clin. Invest. *77*:734, 1986.)

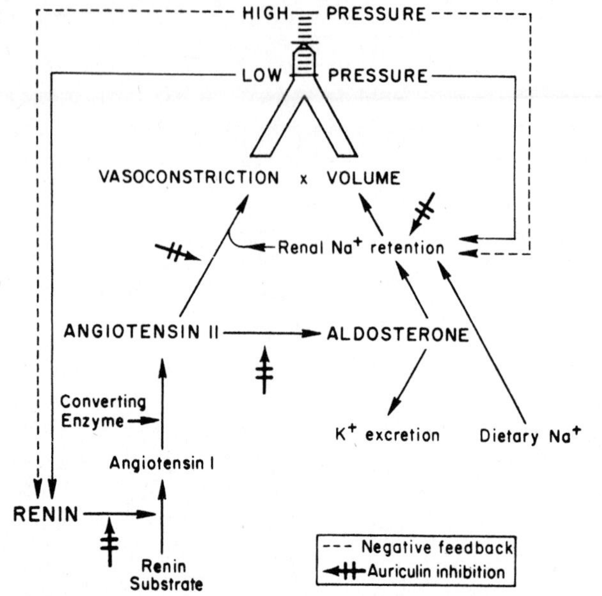

FIGURE 59–9. Atrial natriuretic peptide and the renin-angiotensin-aldosterone system. Renin, secreted in response to reduced renal arterial pressure or a reduction in the sodium supply in the distal tubule, acts to release angiotensin II. Angiotensin II raises blood pressure and stimulates aldosterone secretion, which leads to retention of sodium and water and to improved flow. These pressure and volume effects turn off the renin release. Auriculin opposes the renin system at four points. Within the kidney, its natriuretic action opposes aldosterone's action and stops renin secretion. The atrial hormone also opposes the vasoconstrictor action of angiotensin on blood vessels and, at the adrenal cortex, blocks angiotensin's stimulation of aldosterone release. Broken lines = negative feedback; crossed arrows = auriculin inhibition. (From Laragh, J. H.: Atrial natriuretic hormone, the renin-aldosterone axis, and blood pressure-electrolyte homeostasis. N. Engl. J. Med. *313*:1330, 1985.)

sin-stimulated aldosterone release. Thus, ANP may play a special role in antagonizing each aspect of the renin-angiotensin-aldosterone axis (Fig. 59–9).

ANP is known to relax smooth muscle, including that found in the renal arterial and other vascular beds.[57a] However, infusions of ANP into intact animals may increase or decrease vascular resistance, depending on experimental conditions.[47] Thus, the fall in blood pressure seen after ANP infusion seems to result mostly from a reduction in cardiac output, which is associated with a decrease in venous return.[58] This hypotensive effect may be augmented by a direct effect of ANP on vascular permeability, resulting in a reversible extravascular fluid shift, and is associated with a rise in hematocrit and total plasma proteins out of proportion to the degree of natriuresis and diuresis.[48]

Other actions of ANP includes a suggested role in maintaining sodium balance in chronic renal failure[59] and in mediating the "escape" phenomenon seen with chronic mineralocorticoid administration.[60] Finally, immunoreactive ANP has been found in the central nervous system and may relate to cardiovascular regulatory functions.[61, 62]

In spite of the multiplicity of actions of ANP's in a variety of tissues, the differences between their physiological and pharmacological effects are not clearly delineated. Although it is certain that ANP's will take their place as important regulatory hormones, further studies are needed to define their role in both normal and pathophysiological conditions.

CARDIAC DISORDERS WITH RENAL MANIFESTATIONS

INFECTIVE ENDOCARDITIS (See also Chap. 34). The association between glomerulonephritis and bacterial endocarditis has been appreciated for many years. In 1920, prior to the availability of antibiotics and when infective endocarditis was uniformly fatal, 11 per cent of patients with this infection ultimately died of renal failure.[63] It was initially thought that the glomerular lesion was secondary to septic embolization to the kidney from infected valvular vegetations, but little firm evidence supports this theory. Instead, the pathogenesis of the renal lesions appears to be more in keeping with the generally accepted pathogenesis of most types of glomerulonephritis.[64] Soluble antigenic components of the infecting organism and antibody directed against these antigens have been demonstrated in the glomeruli. As indicated in Chapter 34, many organisms have been responsible for the infective endocarditis that may be associated with glomerulonephritis. By immunofluorescence, the presence of immune complexes and the third component of complement (C3) can be demonstrated in the glomeruli of patients with endocarditis and glomerulonephritis[64]; early in the course, there is a decline in the serum level of C3 and of another component of the complement system, C1q. It now appears that the glomerular lesion of endocarditis results from the deposition of immune complexes along the glomerular basement membrane and in the mesangium.[65]

The most commonly observed abnormality by light microscopy is a focal, proliferative glomerulonephritis, often with focal fibrinoid necrosis. Less commonly, the lesions may be more diffuse, and in some instances extracapillary epithelial proliferation (crescents), such as that seen in rapidly progressive glomerulonephritis, has been observed.[64] Clinically, patients have the typical manifestations of acute or rapidly progressive renal failure, often with hypertension, hematuria, and red cell casts, usually without marked proteinuria and edema. The retention of sodium and water is due to reductions in the glomerular filtration rate and the fractional excretion of sodium. Azotemia is generally progressive, unless rapid bacteriological cure occurs.

Other causes of impaired renal function in patients with infective endocarditis include hypovolemia, congestive heart failure, antibiotic-induced nephrotoxicity, and acute allergic interstitial nephritis secondary to antibiotic therapy.

ANTIBIOTIC TREATMENT IN RENAL FAILURE. Many of the antibiotics used in the treatment of infective endocarditis are excreted by the kidney. These include vancomycin, the penicillins, cephalosporins, and aminoglycosides. It is therefore important to modify the dosage and/or the interval of administration of antibiotics with respect to the degree of renal dysfunction. Because many antibiotics are removed by hemodialysis or peritoneal dialysis, supplementary doses may need to be administered in patients receiving these therapies. Guidelines for antibiotic therapy are presented in Table 59–1. Aminoglycoside and vancomycin levels should be monitored to insure adequate therapeutic dosage and to avoid toxic levels that may contribute to further renal impairment or to ototoxicity. Serum bactericidal titers may also be monitored to assess the adequacy of antibiotic therapy.

The most common cause of endocarditis in dialysis patients is *Staphylococcus aureus*,[66] with *Streptococcus viridans*, enterococci, *Staphylococcus epidermidis*, and gram-negative rods accounting for most of the other cases. Therefore, initial antibiotic therapy should include a penicillinase-resistant penicillin, or vancomycin, and an aminoglycoside, until culture results are available.

ACUTE RENAL FAILURE SECONDARY TO CARDIOGENIC SHOCK (See also p. 566). Prerenal azotemia and, less commonly, acute renal failure (acute tubular necrosis) may occur in association with massive acute myocardial infarction. The mechanism of prerenal azotemia has been discussed above. Acute renal failure occurs when there is a marked, sudden reduction of renal perfusion. The myoglobinuria accompanying excessive myocardial necrosis may play a contributory role. It is critically important to distinguish between prerenal azotemia and acute renal

TABLE 59–1 ANTIBIOTIC THERAPY IN RENAL FAILURE

	Pharmacokinetic Parameters					Adjustment for Renal Failure				
		Half-life					GFR (ml/min)			
Drug	Elimination and Metabolism	*Normal (hr)*	*ESRD (hr)*	Plasma Protein Binding (%)	Volume of Distribution (liters/kg)	Method	*> 50*	*10–50*	*<10*	Removed by Dialysis
Aminoglycosides[a]										
Amikacin	Renal	2–3	30	<5	0.22–0.29	D	60–90	30–70	20–30	Yes (H,P)
						I	12	12–18	24	
Gentamicin	Renal	2	24–48	<5	0.23–0.26	D	60–90	30–70	20–30	Yes (H,P)[b]
						I	8–12	12	24	
Streptomycin	Renal	2.5	100	35	0.26	I	24	24–72	72–96	Yes (H)
Tobramycin	Renal	2.5	56	<5	0.22–0.25	D	60–90	30–70	20–30	Yes (H,P)
						I	8–12	12	24	
Cephalosporins										
Cefazolin	Renal	1.4–2.2	18–36	80	0.13	I	8	12	24–48	Yes (H), No (P)
Cephalothin	Renal (hepatic)	0.5–0.9	3–18	65	0.26	I	6	6	8–12	Yes (H,P)
Penicillins										
Ampicillin	Renal (hepatic)	0.8–1.5	7–20	8–20	0.17–0.31	I	6	6–12	12–16	Yes (H), No (P)
Azlocillin	Renal (hepatic)	0.8–1.5	5–6	25–30	0.18–0.23	I	4–6	6–8	8	Yes (H)
Carbenicillin	Renal (hepatic)	1.5	10–20	30–50	0.12–0.20	I	8–12	12–24	24–48	Yes (H), No (P)
Methicillin	Renal (hepatic)	0.5–1.0	4	35–60	0.31	I	4	4–8	8–12	No (H,P)
Nafcillin	Hepatic (renal)	0.5	1.2	80–90	0.31–0.38	D	U	U	U	No (H)
Oxacillin	Renal (hepatic)	0.4	1	85–95	0.12–0.4	D	U	U	U	No (H,P)
Penicillin G[c]	Renal (hepatic)	0.5	6–20	40–60	0.3–0.42	D	U	75	25–50	Yes (H),
						I	6–8	8–12	12–16	No (P)
Piperacillin	Renal (hepatic)	0.8–1.5	3.3–5.1	16–22	0.18–0.30	I	4–6	6–8	8	Yes (H)
Ticarcillin	Renal	1.0–1.5	16	45	0.14–0.21	I	8–12	12–24	24–48	Yes (H,P)
Rifampin	Hepatic	2–5	2–5	60–90	0.9	I	U	U	U	No (H)
Vancomycin[d]	Renal	6–8	200–250	10	0.47–0.84	I	24–72	72–240	240	No (H,P)

From Bennett, W. M.: Drug therapy in renal disease. *In* Rubenstein, E., and Federman, D. D. (eds.): Scientific American Medicine. New York, Scientific American, Inc. 1986.

[a]Need usual loading dose in renal failure. [b]Poor clearance from blood to peritoneum in CAPD. [c]Upper limit of 4 to 6 million units/day in severe renal failure. [d]Elimination is variable in renal failure; best guide to therapy is serum level before next dose.

$T_{1/2}$ = biological half-life; ESRD = end-stage renal disease; GFR = glomerular filtration rate; I = Interval extension method of dosage adjustment in hours between maintenance doses; D = dose reduction method of dosage adjustment in per cent of usual maintenance dose; H = hemodialysis; P = peritoneal dialysis; U = unchanged.

failure, since the former will generally respond to measures that improve cardiac output, whereas acute renal failure, once established, is a more serious problem that will usually not respond to extrarenal manipulation. Brief periods of modest hypotension (generally lasting less than an hour) often elicit reversible derangements, but more prolonged or profound hypotension lasting for 1 hour or more usually leads to acute tubular necrosis.

DIFFERENTIAL DIAGNOSIS. The distinction between prerenal azotemia and acute tubular necrosis in the oliguric patient (i.e., urine output less than 400 ml/24 hr) can generally be made by measurements of serum urea nitrogen and creatinine and the sodium, urea, and creatinine concentrations and osmolality of a concurrent sample of urine. In the absence of recent diuretic therapy, patients with prerenal azotemia retain their ability to conserve sodium; therefore, urinary sodium concentration is low, usually less than 20 mEq/liter. Tubular function is well preserved, as reflected in urine osmolality exceeding 500 mOsm, and the urinary/plasma ratios for urea and creatinine exceed 8 and 40, respectively. The BUN is more than 10 times the serum creatinine concentration.

In acute tubular necrosis, tubular function is impaired and the urinary sodium concentration generally exceeds 40 mEq/liter; the impairment of tubular function is also reflected in a urine osmolality less than 350 mOsm; the urinary/plasma values for urea and creatinine are below 2 and 20, respectively; and the BUN exceeds the serum creatinine by a ratio of less than 10 to 1. The urinary sediment may also be helpful in the differential diagnosis; patients with prerenal azotemia usually have a relatively clear sediment with a few granular or hyaline casts, whereas those with acute tubular necrosis have many tubular cells and casts in the urine.

MANAGEMENT. As in patients with other causes of acute renal failure, the treatment of acute renal failure secondary to myocardial infarction and pump failure consists of controlling fluid intake to levels in accord with urinary output and insensible losses, as well as modifying the dosages of medications that are excreted by the kidneys, observing the patient closely for hyperkalemia, and intervening with dialysis for severe hyperkalemia or azotemia. In general, dialytic therapy, either hemodialysis or peritoneal dialysis, is initiated when serum creatinine levels reach 8 to 10 mg/dl and no reversible component for the renal failure is apparent. In addition, efforts must be made to maintain left ventricular filling pressure at levels that will optimize cardiac output and therefore renal perfusion (18 to 22 mm Hg). Given sufficient time and with no other associated problems, the prognosis for acute renal failure, when appropriately treated, is excellent. However, when failure of the cardiac pump is severe enough to lead to acute renal failure, myocardial insufficiency rather than the renal failure is the determinant of the patient's poor prognosis.

ATHEROEMBOLIC DISEASE. Atheromatous embolization to the kidneys, which results in chronic, fibrotic, interstitial disease, is relatively uncommon.[67] It may occur spontaneously but more commonly follows operation on the aorta and renal arteries and catheter manipulation and aortography in patients with severe atheromatous disease of the aorta (p. 1571). Patchy areas of necrosis develop, followed by fibrosis with cholesterol clefts, as well as a foreign body response containing multinucleated giant cells. The disorder may be suspected if there has been some manipulation of the atheromatous aorta preceding the onset of progressive renal insufficiency. Examination of the urine is rarely helpful in confirming the diagnosis; when it is allowed to sediment, fat may be found floating at the top. Careful ophthalmological exam may reveal cholesterol emboli in the retinal arteries. Treatment consists of avoiding further arterial and aortic manipulation, but progressive destruction of renal tissue occurs with subsequent renal insufficiency; the prognosis for improvement of renal function is guarded.

EFFECTS OF RENAL DISEASE ON THE CARDIOVASCULAR SYSTEM

The successful treatment of end-stage renal disease by dialysis and transplantation is widely considered to be one of the major advances of modern medicine. Cardiovascular disease is the principal cause of mortality in dialysis patients, accounting for 30 to 50 per cent of deaths[68] compared with less than 15 per cent of deaths in an age-corrected control population. Heart failure accounts for about 15 per cent of this dialysis-associated mortality, myocardial infarction for about 10 per cent, and pericarditis for about 3 to 5 per cent.

CORONARY ATHEROSCLEROSIS

Numerous risk factors for atherosclerosis have been identified in patients with end-stage renal disease.[69] Of these, hypertension is the most important.[70] Uremia itself has been proposed as an independent risk factor,[71] but recently this suggestion has been questioned. It is unclear whether coronary atherosclerosis is unusually prevalent or accelerated in uremic patients when compared with nonuremic patients of comparable age and with similar risk factors.[68, 72] However, the National Cooperative Dialysis Study demonstrated a clear increase in cardiovascular morbid events in patients who received shorter dialysis treatments or who had elevated (time-averaged) BUN concentrations.[73] These observations imply that the adequacy of a dialysis regimen has a significant impact on cardiovascular morbidity.

Coronary bypass surgery has been carried out successfully in patients with renal failure and angina pectoris that is refractory to medical therapy.[74, 75] In addition, angina unassociated with coronary atherosclerosis is being increasingly recognized in chronic renal failure, presumably related to the combination of severe hypertension, left ventricular hypertrophy, and anemia.[76] It has also been suggested that reduced coronary artery compliance due to calcification may restrict coronary vasodilation and limit myocardial oxygen delivery.[72]

HYPERTENSION

(See also p. 839)

Most patients with chronic renal failure that requires dialysis also have hypertension, which is probably the most important risk factor in the development of atherosclerotic cardiovascular disease. Hemodynamic studies in patients with end-stage renal disease have shown an elevated cardiac index and mean arterial pressure but a normal systemic vascular resistance.[68] The elevated cardiac index and normal systemic vascular resistance are related to the anemia; when the anemia is corrected, the cardiac index falls, and both arterial pressure and systemic vascular resistance rise.[77] The majority of patients with end-stage renal failure who develop hypertension have so-called *volume-dependent hypertension*[68] (p. 832). Many studies in patients with end-stage renal failure have shown that arterial pressure is exquisitely dependent on blood volume[78] and that blood pressure control may be achieved by ultrafiltration during dialysis and control of salt and water intake in the interdialytic interval. However, a minority of patients with chronic renal failure have hypertension that is not volume-related but instead is secondary to elevation of plasma renin activity; the hypertension is uncontrollable by lowering blood volume but does respond to bilateral nephrectomy with a consequent reduction in plasma renin activity. Dustan and Page demonstrated the volume-dependent nature of hypertension but also showed that arterial pressure was higher for any given volume when the kidneys were present than after they had been removed.[78] Subsequently, a significant correlation between *plasma renin* levels and arterial pressure was demonstrated.[79] The importance of plasma renin is reflected also in observations on patients with renal failure, hypertension, and expanded blood volume who exhibited renin values which, although normal, were higher than expected for the expanded state of their extracellular volume and which therefore may have contributed to the maintenance of hypertension.[80]

A third mechanism, which operates in patients whose blood pressure cannot be controlled by either volume reduction or bilateral nephrectomy or explained by elevations in plasma renin activity, may be related to *sympathetically mediated vasoconstriction*. Reduced baroreceptor activity has been demonstrated in patients with chronic renal failure by their response to the inhalation of amyl nitrite and the Valsalva maneuver.[81, 82] Inhalation of amyl nitrite results in peripheral vasodilation and therefore a fall in blood pressure, which normally results in reflex vasoconstriction and tachycardia. A blunted response in heart rate elevation is taken as evidence of reduced baroreceptor function. Autonomic insufficiency, as evidenced by an inadequate response to the Valsalva maneuver, is said to be present if both bradycardia and arterial pressure overshoot are absent after release of forced expiration against a standard pressure (40 mm Hg) for a set time (12 sec). Many patients with renal insufficiency whose hypertension is caused by sympathetically mediated vasoconstriction exhibit an exaggerated response to the cold pressor test and elevated plasma levels of dopamine beta-hydroxylase as indices of increased adrenergic function but become hypotensive during dialysis.

A fourth mechanism that has been proposed is the *absence of vasodepressor substances* of renal origin, such as the prostaglandins, which may play a role in the genesis of essential hypertension and of renoprival hypertension.[83]

MANAGEMENT. Since volume-dependent hypertension is the most common mechanism in chronic renal disease, the reduction of plasma volume should be the central theme in the management of hypertension in these patients. Before renal function has deteriorated to the point at which dialysis is required, an attempt should be made to reduce plasma volume, but not to the point at which glomerular filtration will decline further; dietary sodium should be restricted to the lowest level consistent with a normal sodium balance. However, since many patients may have difficulty with this degree of sodium restriction on a long-term basis, and since they may have an inability to excrete even this low quantity of sodium, it is often necessary to add diuretics. Generally, for patients with creatinine clearances exceeding 40 ml/min, thiazide diuretics are effective. However, when the glomerular filtration rate falls below this level, furosemide is required, sometimes in very high doses.

If the arterial pressure remains elevated despite sodium restriction and potent diuretics such as furosemide, antihypertensive agents are generally effective. These include clonidine, alpha-methyldopa, propranolol, hydralazine, prazosin, calcium antagonists, and, for the patient whose condition is refractory to these agents, minoxidil. Sympatholytic agents such as guanethidine are not advisable, since they may be associated with particularly profound postural changes in blood pressure in patients with renal failure.

The problem of the control of hypertension is simpler in patients with chronic renal failure who are maintained on intermittent hemodialysis. In addition to dietary restriction of sodium intake, lowering of blood volume by ultrafiltration during hemodialysis may be employed. In patients in whom volume reduction does not control blood pressure, pharmacological treatment is indicated, as described above.

Angiotensin-converting enzyme inhibitors appear to be useful antihypertensive agents in patients with renal insufficiency. However, the incidence of side effects is increased in such patients compared with those having normal renal function.[84, 85] Bilateral nephrectomy is rarely employed except in those patients who do not respond to antihypertensive drugs, cannot comply with antihypertensive regimens, or experience intolerable side effects with this medication. Although aggressive therapy of hypertension for the patient with renin-mediated malignant hypertension may transiently compromise renal function to the point at which dialysis is required, the increased survival associated with control of the hypertension[86] outweighs the risks attending maintenance hemodialysis.

Hypertension Following Renal Transplantation

Hypertension occurs in 30 to 80 per cent of patients during the posttransplant period. Multiple factors have been implicated in its etiology, including acute and chronic rejection,[87] recurrent disease in the transplanted kidney,[88] stenosis of the transplanted renal artery,[89] large doses of steroids,[87] and cyclosporin A.[90, 91] During acute rejection episodes, the levels of renin and angiotensin are markedly elevated. In addition, the renin-angiotensin-aldosterone system appears to be of pathogenic importance in the hypertension associated with stenosis of the artery to the transplanted kidney, a complication that occurs in up to 30 per cent of transplant patients who undergo arteriography for refractory hypertension as well as in some patients in whom the diseased native kidneys release renin.

MANAGEMENT. In order to treat hypertension in the posttransplant period the underlying mechanisms of the disorder must be elucidated. Because of activation of the renin-angiotensin-aldosterone system, captopril has been found to be an effective antihypertensive in this setting. Furthermore, captopril-induced reversible acute renal insufficiency has been described in patients with functionally significant transplant renal artery stenosis, and its occurrence may serve as a diagnostic test for this entity.[92] In patients with severe refractory hypertension that cannot be ascribed to rejection, angiography and determination of renin activity in venous blood from both the native and the transplanted kidneys are indicated. Surgical revision or angioplasty of a stenosed renal artery or nephrectomy of the native kidney may be in order.

Whereas hypertriglyceridemia is the predominant lipid abnormality in patients with chronic renal failure (see below), hypercholesterolemia Types IIA and B tend to predominate after renal allotransplantation, although in some transplanted patients hypertriglyceridemia persists.[93] The etiology of these lipid abnormalities in the posttransplant period is unclear, but they may be related to the large doses of glucocorticoids administered to these patients. Normalization of serum lipids can occur with reduction of the initial steroid dose.[94] In view of the combination of hypertension and lipid abnormalities in a substantial fraction of patients following transplantation, it is not surprising that coronary atherosclerosis accounts for more deaths than any disease process other than infection.[95]

LIPID ABNORMALITIES

Hypertriglyceridemia with elevations of very low density lipoproteins (VLDL), i.e., Type IV hyperlipoproteinemia (p. 1166), is common in patients with chronic renal failure. Bagdade et al. studied both undialyzed and dialyzed patients with uremia not associated with the nephrotic syndrome and found the plasma triglyceride concentrations to be elevated in both groups.[96] There appears to be no relation between the duration of dialysis or the etiology of the renal disease and the severity of the hyperlipidemia. A second abnormality in lipid metabolism, *reduced concentration of high-density lipoprotein (HDL) cholesterol,* has also been documented in chronic renal failure,[96, 97] a finding of potential importance in view of the strong negative correlation between HDL concentration and the risk of the development of ischemic heart disease. An inverse correlation has been noted between plasma triglyceride and HDL cholesterol levels in both uremic and nonuremic subjects.[97]

MECHANISMS. Several suggestions have been made to explain the elevation of plasma triglycerides in chronic renal failure. The first is that there is increased hepatic synthesis of triglycerides, presumably secondary to increased basal insulin, growth hormone, and glucagon. However, measurements in uremic animals and patients have suggested that the contribution of increased hepatic synthesis is small.[98] A second more likely possibility[99, 100] centers on deficiencies in lipoprotein lipase and hepatic triglyceride lipase known to be necessary for the removal of triglycerides from plasma and their ultimate catabolism; this deficiency may also result from elevated insulin levels, from direct inhibition of these lipases by a nondialyzable factor in uremic serum,[100] or from a deficiency of apoprotein CII in both HDL and VLDL. The reduction of lipoprotein lipase, which is felt to be more important in the generation of hypertriglyceridemia than hepatic lipase, causes a defect in the catabolism of triglyceride-rich lipoproteins, which in turn leads to the accumulation of VLDL[101] and enrichment of intermediate-density lipoproteins and low-density lipoproteins with triglyceride; it is also associated with the appearance of apoprotein B48, an increased concentration of apoprotein AIV, and the presence in LDL of apoproteins C and E (proteins not normally found in LDL). It has been suggested that these abnormal substances may be atherogenic.[100]

In one study, HDL cholesterol was significantly reduced in patients with renal failure on chronic hemodialysis (average = 26 mg/dl) compared with normal persons (average = 52 mg/dl).[99] This reduction of HDL was due to a reduced protein content in all its subfractions. Apoprotein electrophoresis showed an increase in "arginine-rich" peptide in the VLDL and the HDL fraction and, as noted, a reduction of apoprotein CII, which is transferred to VLDL from HDL[102] and which functions as an activator of the enzyme lipoprotein lipase.

TREATMENT. The standard dietary therapy of patients with Type IV hyperlipoproteinemia in the absence of renal failure consists of weight reduction, limitation of alcohol intake, a reduction in carbohydrate consumption, and, if these measures are inadequate, the administration of clofibrate (p. 1170). In patients with chronic renal failure, the lipid abnormality is not usually associated with excessive body weight or alcohol consumption, and a reduction in carbohydrate intake is somewhat difficult to achieve owing to the limitations imposed on the patient's diet by virtue of the reduced protein intake. A reasonable therapeutic approach is to provide caloric replacement through increases in polyunsaturated fat in the diet.[103] With this diet, a significant reduction in plasma triglyceride levels has been observed, both in conservatively treated patients with chronic renal failure and in patients on dialysis.[104]

Clofibrate is normally metabolized by the kidney, and active metabolites can accumulate in patients with severely compromised renal function; patients with renal failure may develop severe myositis in association with the ingestion of the usual doses of this drug.[105] A reduction in total dosage of clofibrate to 1.5 gm per week may lead to a lowering of plasma triglyceride concentration without producing myositis. However, even with this reduced dosage, an increase in serum creatine kinase levels has been reported, presumably as a consequence of damage to skeletal muscle.[105]

HEART FAILURE SECONDARY TO RENAL FAILURE

Chronic renal failure can impair cardiac performance by a variety of mechanisms (Table 59–2). It has been found that left ventricular stroke work index, end-diastolic pressure, and size are increased in many patients with end-stage renal disease.[106, 107] In addition, an increase in pulmonary capillary permeability tending to lead to pulmonary edema, even in the absence of elevation of pulmonary capillary wedge pressure, has been reported in renal insufficiency.[108] Impairment of cardiac performance also occurs secondary to ischemic heart disease (see above). The possibility must be considered that dialysis results in the depletion of essential substances; water-soluble vitamins are dialyzable, and it has been suggested that their loss can lead to beriberi heart disease.[109] Therefore, it seems desirable to provide appropriate vitamin supplements for patients on maintenance hemodialysis. Long-term dialysis may deplete other, as yet unidentified substances necessary for normal cardiac performance, but this has not been established. The observation that cardiac function improves after parathyroidectomy has led to the suggestion that parathyroid hormone (PTH) may itself be a myocardial suppressant.[110] However, data on the cardiosuppressive effects of PTH have been conflicting.

The possibility that the uremic state depresses myocardial function is intriguing. As early as 1944, Raab suggested that specific myocardial toxins might be present in uremia.[111] Depression of cardiac function in isolated rat heart preparations perfused with urea, creatinine, guanidinosuccinic acid, and methyl-guanidine—singly and in combination—has been reported.[112] Similarly, a depression of myocardial contractility has been demonstrated in a guinea pig model of uremia secondary to acute obstructive renal failure.[113]

Uremia produces serious disturbances in monovalent cation transport. Red blood cells, leukocytes, lung, and bone from patients with renal insufficiency have an elevated sodium content and a reduction in ouabain-sensitive Na-K–activated ATPase activity.[114, 115] It is possible that this same fundamental abnormality is responsible for the observed reduction in human skeletal muscle transmembrane potential, which returns toward normal with vigorous hemodialysis.

IMPAIRMENT OF VENTRICULAR FUNCTION IN UREMIA. Although the presence of *cardiomyopathy* in uremic patients has been suggested, its existence as a specific entity has been difficult to document in view of the many other possible causes of cardiac dysfunction in such patients.[116, 117] One study involving patients not on dialysis has documented abnormal left ventricular function with exercise early in renal disease that was unrelated to the degree of anemia or the presence of an arteriovenous fistula or of hypertension.[118] This suggests that cardiac performance can become abnormal relatively early in renal failure. Although the reversibility of myocardial dysfunction is not clear,[119] evidence suggests that it can occur. In one study, patients with severe cardiomyopathy and uremia were reported to develop cardiac disease while on low-protein diets and prior to initiation of hemodialysis, and all showed striking clinical improvement with dialysis.[120] In other studies hemodialysis has been found to raise the left ventricular ejection fraction both acutely and chronically,[121–124] the greatest improvement occurring in patients with dilated hearts.

Reductions in ventricular dilatation and hypertrophy have also been noted with hemodialysis. Some investigators have concluded that an increase in contractile state accounts for the beneficial effects of hemodialysis on cardiac performance.[123, 125] In one study comparing different isovolemic dialysis regimens, an increase in ionized plasma calcium was identified as a key factor in this increased contractility.[123] Others suggest that changes in preload and afterload constitute the dominant mechanism.[122, 124] It is likely that a combination of these factors is important depending on the clinical status of the patient and the type of dialysis procedure performed.[125] Left ventricular function has been found to improve with peritoneal dialysis[126] and after renal transplantation.[127]

TABLE 59–2 POSSIBLE CAUSES OF HEART FAILURE IN RENAL INSUFFICIENCY

Hypertension	Increased ventricular afterload
Hypervolemia	Increased ventricular preload
Anemia	Increased cardiac work (high-output state)
Lipid abnormalities	Increased atherogenesis
Pericarditis	Restriction of ventricular filling
Ionic alterations	Negative inotropic effect
Hyperkalemia	
Hypocalcemia	
Hypermagnesemia	
Metabolic acidosis	
Disordered calcium and vitamin D metabolism	(A) Metastatic calcification (cardiac and vascular)
	(B) ? Vitamin D deficiency cardiomyopathy
Arteriovenous shunt for hemodialysis	Increased cardiac work (high-output state)
Thiamine depletion by dialysis	Increased cardiac work (high-output state)
Beriberi (?)	
Uremic toxins (?)	Depressed contractility; ? cardiomyopathy

CARDIOVASCULAR COMPLICATIONS OF HEMODIALYSIS

TECHNICAL CONSIDERATIONS. Hemodialysis is designed to accomplish three objectives. It may (1) remove solutes, (2) alter the electrolyte concentration of the extracellular fluid, and (3) remove as much as 1 liter of extracellular fluid per hour. These three processes should be viewed as being essentially independent of one another, and in the course of a single dialysis, it is often desirable to carry out only one or two of these three functions.

HYPOTENSION. A significant fall in blood pressure is a common problem in patients undergoing hemodialysis, occurring in 25 to 50 per cent of dialysis procedures.[128] Many interacting factors appear to be responsible (Fig. 59–10). Ultrafiltration of fluid leads to hypovolemia with a concomitant reduction of venous return and cardiac output.[129] Plasma osmolarity, which falls during dialysis, favors water movement out of the extracellular and into the intracellular space.[128, 130] Autonomic dysfunction, which occurs in up to 50 per cent of dialysis patients,[82] prevents normal compensatory cardioacceleration and an increase in vascular tone. The most common defect seems to reside in the afferent limb of the baroreceptor reflex arc.[82, 131] High extracorporeal blood volume, a high blood flow rate, and an underestimation of "dry weight" after dialysis also predispose to hypotension.[132] Drugs that lower blood pressure, such as antihypertensives, some antiarrhythmics, narcotic analgesics, and anxiolytic medications, are commonly prescribed to dialysis patients.

Cardiac disorders that may cause or contribute to hypotension during dialysis include arrhythmias, pericardial effusion with tamponade, cardiomyopathy, and myocardial ischemia. Hypoxemia should also be considered (see below). Finally, acetate, a common dialysate base, has been implicated as a vasodilator and myocardial depressant.[131, 133] Because acetate is metabolized to bicarbonate primarily in muscle cells, it appears to be most poorly tolerated by patients with low muscle mass, typically elderly women. Patients with autonomic insufficiency may also be particularly intolerant of acetate.[134]

The incidence of hypotensive episodes can be reduced by identifying

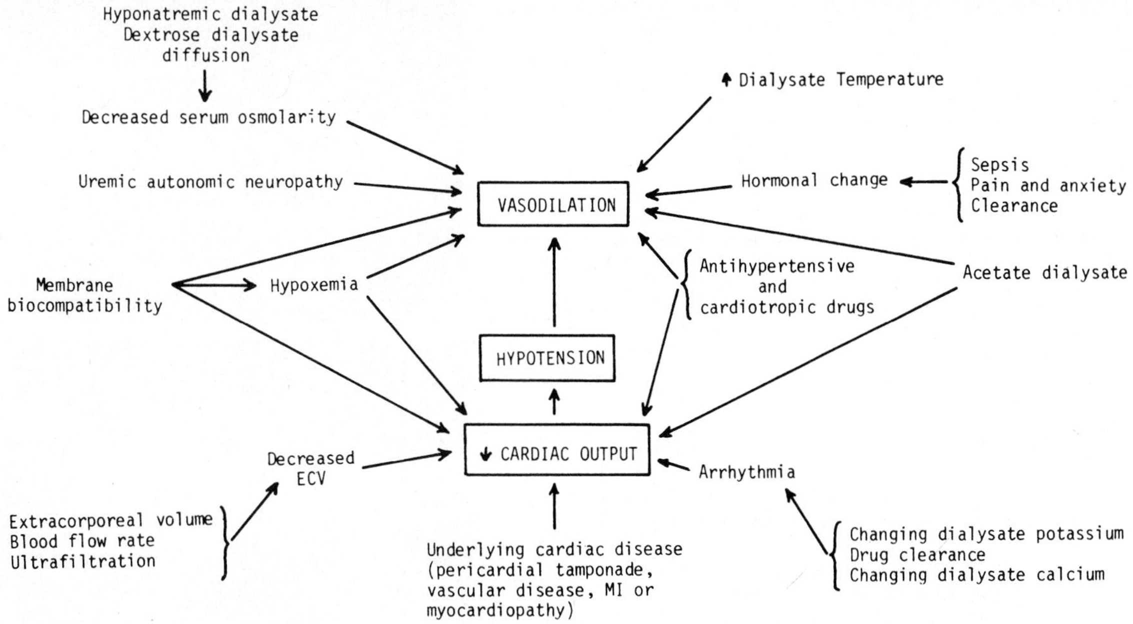

FIGURE 59–10. Major factors leading to dialysis-induced hypotension. (From Hakim, R. M., and Lazarus, J. M.: Medical aspects of hemodialysis. *In* Brenner, B. M., and Rector, F. C. [eds.]: The Kidney. Philadelphia, W. B. Saunders Company, 1986. p. 1820.)

and treating the conditions discussed. Simple measures such as decreasing the size of the dialyzer, removing less fluid during the treatment, or withholding antihypertensive medications prior to dialysis may be effective. A change in dialysate solution may also be useful. A dialysate sodium concentration exceeding 135 mEq/liter will reduce the fall in plasma osmolarity and has been shown to improve hemodynamic stability.[135, 136] Substituting bicarbonate for acetate as the dialysate base may also be helpful.[132, 133] Finally, sequential ultrafiltration followed by isovolemic dialysis can ameliorate the occurrence of hypotension.[137]

ELECTROLYTE SHIFTS. In adjusting electrolyte concentrations, it is important to appreciate that most dialysates contain 1.5 to 3.0 mEq/liter of potassium and 3 to 3.5 mEq/liter of calcium (6 to 7 mg/dl of ionized Ca^{++}). Since most patients commence dialysis with somewhat high serum potassium levels, serum potassium may fall precipitously when dialysis begins, whereas the concentration of ionized calcium rises, setting the stage for digitalis intoxication in digitalized patients (p. 504). This complication is even more likely in cases of digoxin excess, which might come about if the dosage has not been adjusted downward to take into consideration the markedly prolonged half-life of this drug in patients with renal failure (p. 502). A close correlation between the rise in ionized serum calcium and improved myocardial performance has been noted (see above).[123]

ARTERIOVENOUS FISTULAS. To achieve vascular access for dialysis, an arteriovenous fistula must be created. These shunts have a flow rate of 250 to 750 ml/minute and thereby add to the cardiac workload. As discussed on page 786, in association with the anemia characteristic of chronic renal failure, this may contribute to the development of high-output heart failure.[138] This form of heart failure can be readily controlled if any excess fluid accumulation is prevented by ultrafiltration during dialysis and if the anemia is partially treated by transfusion. Obviously, it is desirable to use only a single vascular access site at any one time and to limit the size of the anastomosis to the smallest required for successful dialysis. The contribution of the fistula to the heart failure state can be determined by studying the effect of occlusion of the fistula on left ventricular function, as assessed by echocardiography (Fig. 25–5, p. 786) or radionuclide ventriculography.[139]

Infection is a major complication of arteriovenous shunts and may become metastatic. Septic pulmonary emboli and infective endocarditis, most often staphylococcal, have been reported.[140] Since patients on hemodialysis often have functional systolic and occasionally even diastolic murmurs, which may change with the patient's altered hemodynamic status, the diagnosis of endocarditis may be missed. Therefore, the *early* diagnosis of endocarditis in patients with infected vascular access sites depends on a high index of clinical suspicion and immediate blood cultures. However, the diagnosis of infective endocarditis may be difficult, since an infected vascular access site without infection of the endocardium can also give rise to positive blood cultures.

HYPOXEMIA. A fall in arterial oxygen tension of 10 to 15 mm Hg occurs frequently within the first 30 minutes of hemodialysis and persists throughout the procedure.[141] This event is obviously undesirable in patients with heart or lung disease and may lead to serious hypoxemia in patients with even mild arterial desaturation at the commencement of the hemodialysis. Together with the electrolyte changes during hemodialysis referred to above, it may lower the threshold for the development of arrhythmias. Also, the PEP/LVET ratio may increase significantly during dialysis,[142] an increase that correlates significantly with the fall in arterial oxygen tension, suggesting that the latter actually impairs left ventricular function.

The mechanism responsible for the decline in arterial PO_2 during dialysis is in some dispute and is probably multifactorial. It has been reported that activation of complement leads to aggregation of neutrophils in the lungs, which interferes with normal oxygenation.[143] This is particularly observed with cuprophane membranes and not with more biocompatible membranes such as polyacrylonitryl.[144] An additional explanation is that physiological hypoventilation occurs secondary to diffusion of carbon dioxide across the dialyzer. Changing from an acetate- to a bicarbonate-buffered dialysate may prevent this loss of carbon dioxide and lessen the decrease in arterial PO_2.[144, 145]

Of interest, mechanically ventilated patients show a decrease in arterial oxygen tension during dialysis; this indicates that hypoventilation alone cannot account for the observed hypoxemia.[146] Whatever the mechanism, patients with impaired pulmonary function and severe heart disease should be monitored for arterial hypoxemia during the early phase of dialysis and may require inhalation of oxygen during the procedure.

POTASSIUM BALANCE

Life-threatening hyperkalemia may occur in acute oliguric renal failure, in end-stage chronic renal failure, and, rarely, in terminal heart failure (p. 482). The principal detrimental effect of hyperkalemia is in its electrical effect on the heart. The progressive electrocardiographic abnormalities associated with hyperkalemia are illustrated in Figure 7–50, p. 216). Generally, the earliest electrocardiographic sign of hyperkalemia is peaking of the T waves, followed progressively by an increase in T-wave amplitude, a widening of the QRS complex, and loss of atrial activity. Finally, with extreme hyperkalemia, a sine wave pattern is noted on the electrocardiogram, followed by cardiac arrest.[147] Unfortunately, however, only a rough correlation exists between the level of serum potassium and the electrocardiographic changes, although in any given patient, directional changes in the serum potassium can be estimated from the electrocardiogram. Even severe hyperkalemia per se produces few if any symptoms; occasionally, weakness of skeletal muscles or dyspnea presumably secondary to paralysis of respiratory muscles may be noted.

TREATMENT. Severe hyperkalemia is a medical emergency, and its treatment can generally be divided into acute and chronic phases. The most rapid means of counteracting the toxic cardiac effects of potassium is with the administration of intravenous calcium, given in the form of

10 to 20 ml of 10 per cent *calcium chloride* with electrocardiographic monitoring to assure that the signs of hyperkalemia have been reversed. While administration of calcium chloride is an effective emergency measure, it does not lower the elevated serum potassium concentration.

The second aspect of therapy relies on the lowering of serum potassium. In patients with hyperkalemia and acidosis, *sodium bicarbonate* will reduce serum potassium; the usual dose is 1 to 2 ampules (44 to 88 mEq) administered intravenously. The reduction in [K^+] is caused in part by an exchange of hydrogen and potassium ions across cell membranes as well as enhanced secretion of potassium in the distal tubule. However, bicarbonate administration lowers serum [K^+] in hyperkalemic patients even if the serum pH is not affected, implying a specific effect of the bicarbonate anion itself.[148] The administration of 10 units of regular insulin will result in the redistribution of [K^+] from the extracellular to the intracellular space. This should be followed by 50 ml of 50 per cent *glucose* to prevent hypoglycemia. The effects of bicarbonate or glucose and insulin administration can be observed within 15 to 30 minutes and may last for several hours. Although these forms of therapy are useful for rapidly lowering the serum [K^+] concentration, they do *not* lower total body potassium stores.

Further treatment of hyperkalemia involves removal of potassium from the body, which can be accomplished by the administration of *cation exchange resins* by enema or orally. The resin most commonly employed is sodium polystyrene sulfonate (Kayexalate), 1 gm of which administered orally exchanges approximately 1 mEq of sodium for potassium. The usual dose is 50 gm two or three times daily. When administered orally, it is desirable to accompany it with an osmotic cathartic to prevent intestinal obstruction as a consequence of inspissation of the resin in the gut.

The most effective means of reducing the body's potassium stores is by means of *dialysis*, either hemodialysis or peritoneal dialysis. However, when using these modalities, one must exercise care not to lower the serum potassium too precipitously, especially in those patients who are receiving cardiac glycosides. This can be accomplished by beginning with a dialysis solution having a potassium concentration of approximately 4 mEq/liter and then progressively lowering it as serum potassium declines.

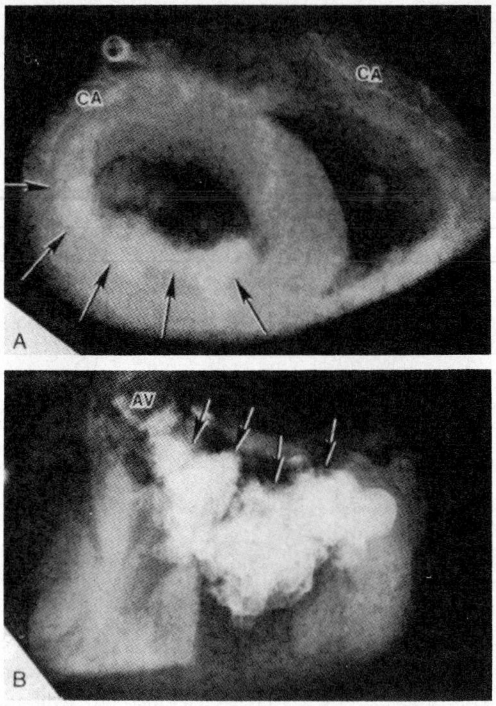

FIGURE 59–11. Postmortem roentgenograms showing severe mitral annular calcification in two patients on hemodialysis. *A*, Superior view of heart showing extensive posterior mitral annular (arrows) and coronary arterial (CA) calcification in a patient on dialysis for 14.5 years. *B*, Posteroanterior view of heart revealing extensive calcific deposits in mitral valve apparatus (arrows) and mild calcific deposits in the aortic valve (AV) in a patient on hemodialysis for 7 years. (From Forman, M. B., et al.: Mitral annular calcification in chronic renal failure. Chest *85*:367, 1984.)

SECONDARY HYPERPARATHYROIDISM

(See also p. 1814)

Ectopic calcification in a variety of tissues, including the heart and arterial bed, is a common manifestation of secondary hyperparathyroidism. This frequent complication of chronic renal failure may involve the sinoatrial and atrioventricular nodes, the valvular annuli and cusps (particularly the mitral annulus)[149–151] (Fig. 59–11), the intima and media of epicardial coronary arteries, the interventricular septum, and the ventricular myocardium (as shown in Figure 58–8, p. 1815).[152–154] Clinical and electrocardiographic changes include varying degrees of atrioventricular block,[155] sinus node dysfunction, supraventricular arrhythmias, infective endocarditis, embolism, mitral regurgitation, mitral stenosis, and left ventricular failure.[151, 156]

As many as half the patients on maintenance hemodialysis have been reported to have radiological evidence of arterial calcification;[157] calcium deposition is generally in the media, leading to Mönckeberg's sclerosis.[158] Calcium deposition may be associated with almost complete obliteration of the vascular lumen and may result in ischemia and, ultimately, gangrene of tissue distal to the involved vessels.[157, 158] Case-control studies have shown mitral annular calcification in those dialysis patients with higher ionized calcium, phosphorus, and calcium-phosphorus product levels. These findings suggest that vigorous attempts to normalize calcium-phosphorus metabolism may decrease the incidence of this complication in patients with chronic renal failure.[149, 150]

The most effective *treatment* of secondary hyperparathyroidism consists of renal transplantation or subtotal parathyroidectomy. The latter procedure has been shown to improve cardiac contractility.[110] For patients maintained on dialysis, dietary phosphate restriction, calcium supplementation, nonabsorbable aluminum-containing antacids, and dihydrotachysterol (a synthetic analog of vitamin D given in doses of 0.125 to 1.0 mg daily) or 1,25-dihydroxycholecalciferol in a dose of 0.25–1.0 μg daily are also useful measures.[159, 160]

UREMIC PERICARDITIS

(See also p. 1514)

Pericarditis is a common complication of both acute and chronic renal failure. Before the era of dialysis, the appearance of pericarditis in the uremic patient was generally taken as a sign of limited life expectancy.[161] Echocardiography has revealed pericardial effusions in 32 to 56 per cent of patients at the initiation of dialysis, many of which are asymptomatic.[162–164] The incidence of clinically significant pericarditis appears to be declining with the increasing use of early dialysis before progression to advanced uremia. The mechanism by which pericarditis and pericardial effusion develop is not clear but is probably related to the accumulation of uremic toxin(s), which is responsible for an inflammatory serositis. Volume overload has also been implicated as an important etiological factor.[164] The serositis most commonly involves the pericardium but can also involve the pleura.[165] Fibrinous pleuritis, pleural friction rubs,[166] hemorrhagic pleural effusion, and pneumonitis[165] have also been reported to occur in uremia.

Three and a half per cent of the patients accepted for dialysis at the Brigham and Women's Hospital during a 5-year period developed clinical evidence of pericarditis and pericardial effusion while on dialytic therapy.[167] Pericarditis occurring in patients with stable chronic dialysis may be

TABLE 59–3 CLINICAL FEATURES OF UREMIC PERICARDITIS

Feature	Frequency (%)
Pain	66
Pericardial friction rub	93
Fever	84
Leukocytosis	56
Arrhythmias	23
Hypotension	56
Hepatomegaly	60
Elevated venous pressure	71
Abnormal electrocardiogram	90
Enlarged cardiac silhouette	96

For sources of above data, see Chap. 44.

related to inadequate dialysis or to an intercurrent illness, such as a viral infection. In patients with renal failure, pericarditis is frequently preceded by an otherwise benign respiratory tract infection. Bacterial infection with cytomegalovirus infection and other conditions such as systemic lupus erythematosus, polyarteritis nodosa, and acute myocardial infarction have also been implicated as causes.[168]

CLINICAL MANIFESTATIONS. The clinical features of uremic pericarditis are summarized in Table 59–3. The diagnosis is made by the same clinical criteria used for other forms of pericarditis, i.e., chest pain generally ameliorated by sitting up and leaning forward, typical electrocardiographic and echocardiographic changes, increases in heart size on chest roentgenogram, and evidence of circulatory embarrassment with severe pericarditis. With echocardiography, a surprisingly high incidence (32 per cent) of small, asymptomatic pericardial effusions was found in our institution in patients on chronic maintenance hemodialysis,[169] a finding also noted by others.[168, 170] The development of hypotension during dialysis that cannot be readily attributed to changes in intravascular volume is a useful clue to the presence of significant pericardial effusion. However, the diagnosis of pericarditis may sometimes be made in error. Uremic patients frequently develop a systolic ejection murmur, most probably related to the high-output state secondary to chronic anemia. Occasionally, patients with chronic renal failure and hypertension develop diastolic blowing murmurs of aortic regurgitation, and the combination of these two murmurs may be mistaken for a to-and-fro pericardial friction rub.

Cardiac tamponade, described on page 1492, is the major complication of pericarditis and can be lethal. Pericardial fluid is generally exudative and bloody, and the heparinization required for hemodialysis may cause serious bleeding into the pericardial cavity in patients with pericarditis. Therefore, it is important to avoid systemic heparinization during hemodialysis in the presence of active pericarditis and large effusions. However, systemic heparinization can be used safely in patients with small pericardial effusions without associated physical signs and symptoms of active pericarditis. *Chronic constrictive pericarditis* is an unusual complication of uremic pericarditis. It developed in two of 25 patients at the Brigham and Women's Hospital with prior severe effusions,[167] and other centers report a similarly low incidence.

TREATMENT. Management of the patient with pericardial effusion without evidence of cardiac tamponade consists of vigorous hemodialysis and the use of regional heparinization (see below).[171] Uremic pericarditis complicated by tamponade or persistent large effusion should be treated with immediate pericardiocentesis coupled with vigorous hemodialysis; with this approach, the rate of resolution is very high.[167] The placement of air into the pericardial space has the advantage of limiting the apposition of visceral and parietal pericardial surfaces and providing an air-fluid level, thereby allowing the rate of reaccumulation of fluid to be followed readily on a routine chest roentgenogram (Fig. 44–10, p. 1496). Instillation of nonabsorbable corticosteroids into the pericardial cavity,[172] primary catheter drainage of the pericardial effusion,[173] and early construction of a pericardial window[174] have all been advocated. Oral indomethacin has also been suggested, but a recent controlled study failed to show an effect of this drug on the duration of chest pain, pericardial friction rub, the amount of effusion, or the need for surgery.[175] The early use of pericardial stripping for treatment of uremic pericardial effusion has also been suggested.[176] However, because of the rarity of constrictive pericarditis in uremic pericarditis, *prophylactic* pericardiectomy is not believed to be justified.

It is our practice to treat uremic pericarditis by vigorous dialysis. Catheter drainage of the pericardial space with the instillation of air is reserved for patients with clinical or echocardiographic evidence of cardiac tamponade or a large, persistent effusion. If needed, a catheter should be inserted into the pericardial cavity but only by persons experienced with this technique. The size of the effusion is most easily followed by serial two-dimensional echocardiography. Indomethacin is administered orally to relieve symptoms of pain if they do not respond to intensive dialysis and conventional analgesics. The use of locally instilled nonabsorbable steroids may be of additional benefit, but more experience with this modality is required. Occasionally, anterior pericardiectomy or creation of a pericardial window may be required if these measures do not succeed. Pericardial stripping is the treatment of choice in patients with subacute or chronic constrictive pericarditis secondary to uremia.[177]

MANAGEMENT OF PATIENTS WITH CARDIAC DISEASE AND RENAL FAILURE

With the greater availability of dialysis facilities and broader criteria for acceptance of patients into treatment programs for end-stage renal disease, this patient population now encompasses individuals in whom other diseases may be present, including cardiac disease that may require surgical treatment. Because of the high frequency of coronary artery disease among patients with chronic renal failure and the occasional presence of coexisting valvular heart disease, cardiopulmonary bypass is often a consideration. Patients on maintenance hemodialysis can undergo major operations without excess mortality or morbidity,[178] and several series have been published documenting the ability of patients with renal failure to tolerate open heart surgery, both coronary revascularization and valve replacement.[179] Among patients with end-stage renal disease, cardiac operations may be performed with equal success regardless of whether the renal failure has been treated by dialysis or transplantation.[180, 181]

TABLE 59–4 CARDIOVASCULAR DRUG THERAPY IN RENAL DISEASE

	Pharmacokinetic Parameters					Adjustment for Renal Failure				
		Half-life					GFR (ml/min)			
Drug	Elimination and Metabolism	*Normal (hr)*	*ESRD (hr)*	Plasma Protein Binding (%)	Volume of Distribution (liters/kg)	Method	*>50*	*10–50*	*<10*	Removed by Dialysis
Adrenergic modulators and blockers										
Clonidine	Renal	6–23	39–42	20–40	3–6	D	U	U	50–75	No (H)
Guanethidine	Renal (nonrenal)	Biphasic: 48–72 and 96–196[a]	?	0	?	I	24	24	24–36	?
Methyldopa[b]	Renal (hepatic 18%–48%)	Biphasic: 1.4 and 5.8[a]	3–6 and 7–16[a]	<15	0.51	I	6	9–18	12–24	Yes (H,P)
Prazosin	Hepatic (renal)	2–3[c]	?	97	1.2–1.7	D	U	U	U	No (H,P)
Reserpine	Hepatic (GI)	Biphasic: 4.5 and 50–170[a]	87–320	40	?	D	U	U	Avoid	No (H,P)
Angiotensin-converting enzyme inhibitors										
Captopril	Renal (hepatic)	1.9	21–32	25–30	0.7	D I	U 8–24	U 24–72	50 72–108	Yes (H)
Enalapril	Hepatic	24–36	40-60	50–60	?	D	100	75–100	50	Yes (H)
Antiarrhythmic agents[d]										
N-Acetylprocainamide	Renal	6–8	42–70	10	1.5–1.7	I[e] D[e]	U U	6 50	12 25	Yes (H)
Amiodarone	Hepatic	3–100 Days	U	96	Variable: 1–148	D	U	U	U	No (H)
Bretylium	Renal (nonrenal 20%)	6 (PO) 13.6 (IV)	16–32	6	8	D	U	25–50[f]	Avoid[f]	?
Disopyramide	Renal and hepatic	5–8	10–18	5–80	0.8–2.6	I	U	12–24	24–40	Yes (H)
Encainide	Hepatic	1–3	?	71–78	2.7	D	U	U	U	?
Flecainide	Hepatic (renal)	14–20	19–26	50	8–9.5	D	U	U	50–75	No (H)
Lidocaine	Hepatic (renal <20%)	1.2–2.2	1.3–3.0	60–66	1.3–2.2	D	U	U	U	No (H)
Lorcainide	Hepatic	7–13	?	80–85	6–17	D	U	U	U	?
Mexiletine	Hepatic (renal)	8–13	16	75	5.5–6.6	D	U	U	50–75	?
Phenytoin	Hepatic (renal)	24	8	90	0.64	D	U	U	U	No (H)
Procainamide	Renal (hepatic 7%–24%)	2.5–4.9	5.3–5.9	14–23	1.4–2.5	I	4	6–12	8–24	Yes (H)[g]
Quinidine	Hepatic (renal 10%–50%)	5.0–7.2	4–14	70–95	2.0–3.5	I	U	U	U	Yes (H,P)[h]
Tocainide	Hepatic (renal)	11–19	22	10–20	1.6–3.2	D	U	U	50	Yes (H)

From Bennett, W. M.: Drug therapy in renal disease. *In* Rubenstein, E., and Federman, D. D. (eds.): Scientific American Medicine. New York, Scientific American, Inc. 1986.

[a] Biexponential pharmacokinetics. [b] Prolonged hypotension due to retention of active metabolites in severe renal failure. [c] $T_{1/2}$ increased to 6 to 7 hours in congestive heart failure. [d] $T_{1/2}$ may be prolonged in heart disease, or with reduced hepatic blood flow, or both. [e] In practice, a combination of dose and interval adjustment may be necessary. [f] No specific data in ESRD. [g] May be able to treat poisoning with hemodialysis. [h] Hemodialysis with low potassium bath may be effective for poisoning. [i] Drug or active metabolite with long $T_{1/2}$ accumulates in ESRD. [j] Volume of distribution and total body clearance decreased in ESRD. [k] Need to monitor thiocyanate levels to keep <10 mg/dL; $t_{1/2}$ for thiocyanate is 1 wk; thiocyanate dialyzable. [l] Daily dose should not exceed 0.5 gm for each gram/dl of serum albumin.

$T_{1/2}$ = biological half-life; ESRD = end-stage renal disease; GFR = glomerular filtration rate; I = Interval extension method of dosage adjustment in hours between maintenance doses; D = dose reduction method of dosage adjustment in per cent of usual maintenance dose; H = hemodialysis; P = peritoneal dialysis; U = unchanged.

Table continued on opposite page

The major problems associated with operation in patients with chronic renal failure include the development of hyperkalemia, fluid overload, and arrhythmias. However, with the appropriate use of hemodialysis both before and after operation and careful monitoring of the patient's hemodynamic and electrolyte status, the excess risks have been contained. Although many observers think that patients who have severely impaired renal failure but who do not yet require hemodialysis may undergo cardiac surgery without hemodialysis, it is our policy to dialyze patients with a glomerular filtration rate less than 20 per cent of normal on several occasions in the days before and after such operations.

The management of patients with hypertrophic obstructive cardiomyopathy (p. 1418) and chronic renal failure presents a unique problem. It is well established that these patients are particularly sensitive to acute changes in blood volume and to tachyarrhythmias. During hemodialysis, blood volume is ordinarily reduced. Although most patients tolerate this volume depletion without difficulty, those with hypertrophic cardiomyopathy often develop an acute increase in obstruction to left ventricular outflow. This complication can be avoided by using a dialysis apparatus that requires a low extracorporeal volume and allows precise control of ultrafiltration. In addition, these patients are treated with a beta-adrenergic receptor blocker and are transfused to maintain a hematocrit in the range of 30 per cent.

MODIFICATION OF COMMON CARDIAC MEDICATIONS IN PATIENTS WITH RENAL FAILURE

Since many drugs (and/or their active metabolites) used in the treatment of heart disease are excreted by the kidney, renal failure affects the pharmacokinetics of many agents, including those commonly used to treat heart disease. Information on the pharmacokinetics of important cardiac medications and dosage adjustments in renal failure are listed in Table 59–4.

CARDIAC GLYCOSIDES (See also p. 502). *Digoxin* is filtered by the glomeruli, and its renal excretion is directly proportional to the glomerular filtration rate. It is not altered by the rate of urine flow and therefore by the administration of diuretics[182]; only very small quantities of

TABLE 59–4 CARDIOVASCULAR DRUG THERAPY IN RENAL DISEASE *Continued*

	Pharmacokinetic Parameters					Adjustment for Renal Failure				
		Half-life					GFR (ml/min)			
Drug	Elimination and Metabolism	*Normal (hr)*	*ESRD (hr)*	Plasma Protein Binding (%)	Volume of Distribution (liters/kg)	Method	*>50*	*10–50*	*<10*	Removed by Dialysis
Beta blockers										
Acebutolol	Renal (hepatic)	8–9	7	25	1.2	D	U	50[i]	30–50[i]	No (H)
Atenolol	Renal	6–9	15–35	<5	0.7	D	U	50	25[i]	Yes (H),
						I	24	48	96[i]	No (P)
Labetalol	Hepatic	3–8	3–8	50	3–10	D	U	U	U	No (H)
Metoprolol	Hepatic	2.5–4.5	2.5–4.5	12	5–6	D	U	U	U	Yes (H)
Nadolol	Renal	14–24	45	25–30	2	D	U	50	25[i]	Yes (H)
Pindolol	Hepatic (renal)	3–4	3–4	40–57	2	D	U	U	U	?
Propranolol	Hepatic	3.5–6.0	2.3	90–96	3–4	D	U	U	U	No (H)
Sotalol	Renal	5–8	40–50	54	0.7	D	U	30	15–30	Yes (H)
Timolol	Hepatic	3–4	4	10	2–4	D	U	U	U	No (H)
Calcium-channel blockers										
Diltiazem	Hepatic	2–8	?	80–86	3–5	D	U	U	U	?
Nifedipine	Hepatic	4.0–5.5	?	92–98	?	D	U	U	U	No (H)
Verapamil	Hepatic	3–7	2.4–4	83–93	3–6	D	U	U	50–75	No (H)
Cardiac glycosides										
Digitoxin	Hepatic (renal)	144–200	210	94	0.6	D	U	U	50–75	No (H,P)
Digoxin	Renal (nonrenal 15%–40%)[i]	36–44	80–120[i]	20–30	5–8	D	U	25–75	10–25	No (H,P)
						I	24	36	48	
Vasodilators										
Diazoxide	Renal (hepatic)	17–31	>30	>90	0.2–0.3	D	U	U	U	Yes (H,P)
Hydralazine	Hepatic (nonrenal)	2.0–4.5	7–16	87	0.5–0.9	I	8	8	8–16 (fast) 12–24 (slow)	No (H,P)
Minoxidil	Hepatic	2.8–4.2	U	0	2–3	D	U	U	U	Yes (H)
Sodium nitroprusside	Nonrenal	<10 min	<10 min	0	0.20	D	U	U	U[k]	Yes (H)[k]
Agents used for hyperlipoproteinemia										
Cholestyramine	Not absorbed	—	—	—	—	D	U	U	U	—
Clofibrate	Hepatic (renal)	17	46–110	96	0.14	I[l]	6–12	12–18	24–48	No (H)
Colestipol	Not absorbed	—	—	—	—	D	U	U	U	—
Gemfibrozil	Renal (fecal)	1.5	?	Low	?	D	U	50	25	?
Nicotinic acid	Hepatic (renal)	0.5–1.0	?	?	?	D	U	50	25	?

digoxin may be secreted by the distal convoluted tubule.[183] The ratio of the clearance of digoxin to endogenous creatinine is 0.8, and the percentage of the body's total stores of digoxin lost per day can be calculated as 14 + 0.2 × creatinine clearance in ml/min. Thus, 85 per cent of administered digoxin is normally excreted in the urine, most in unchanged form, and only 10 to 15 per cent is eliminated in the stool through biliary excretion. Normally, 38 per cent of the body's stores of digoxin are either metabolized or excreted per day,[184] whereas in anephric patients, only 14 per cent of total body digoxin stores are eliminated per day via the biliary tree. Therefore, in the patient with impaired renal function, digoxin elimination is reduced to approximately 37 per cent of normal, and digoxin dosage should be modified accordingly.

In patients with end-stage renal disease who require treatment with digoxin, a loading dose of 0.25 mg and maintenance doses of 0.125 mg every other day are recommended. Digoxin levels are determined 1 week later, and, depending on the clinical response, the dose is modified, usually upward, to 0.125 mg orally daily. However, in the emergency setting, when rapid digitalization is required, the *loading* dose of digoxin does not need to be reduced. In contrast to digoxin, the half-life of *digitoxin* is not greatly affected by impaired renal function,[185] and therefore dosage does not need to be altered in patients with renal failure. Because of high tissue and protein binding of both digoxin and digitoxin, little removal occurs with either hemo- or peritoneal dialysis.[186] Therefore, these methods are ineffective in the treatment of digitalis intoxication.

ANTIARRHYTHMIC DRUGS (See also Chap. 21). The dose of *procainamide* (p. 630) must be modified in patients with end-stage renal disease because this drug is normally eliminated by both renal excretion and hepatic metabolism. Procainamide is readily dialyzable.[187]

Quinidine (p. 628) is metabolized by a variety of tissues, including the liver, mostly to hydroxy derivatives; no specific modification of the dose is necessary in patients with impaired renal function. Quinidine prolongs the half-life of digoxin in patients with renal failure. Therefore, a decrease in digoxin dosage may be required when both drugs are administered.[188] Since quinidine is 80 per cent protein-bound[189] and is widely distributed in tissue, clearance by dialysis would be expected to be quite poor; indeed, clearance by peritoneal dialysis has been found to be less than 10 ml/min.[190]

The half-life of *lidocaine* (p. 625) is about an hour, and its deactivation depends largely on hepatic metabolism; no dosage modification is necessary in patients with renal failure.[191] No data are available on its dialyzability, but because of a high degree of protein-binding (approximately 60 per cent), it is probably poor.

The liver is also the principal site of inactivation of *phenytoin*[192] (p. 632). Because of the diminished protein-binding of the drug in patients with renal failure, the ranges of therapeutic and toxic levels are lower than those in patients with normal renal function. No alteration in dosage is necessary in chronic renal failure. As is the case for most antiarrhythmic agents, phenytoin is poorly dialyzed.

Propranolol is used extensively in patients with renal failure for its effects on arterial pressure, angina pectoris, and, less commonly, cardiac arrhythmias. Since it is metabolized primarily by the liver, its half-life is not altered by renal failure.[193] It is largely protein-bound (90 per cent) and has a large volume of distribution[194]; therefore, it is not surprising that it is poorly dialyzed. The long-acting beta blockers *atenolol* and *nadolol* are cleared by the kidney, so that toxic levels may accumulate in patients with renal failure if dosage is not adjusted. They may both be removed by hemodialysis.[195]

OTHER CARDIOVASCULAR DRUGS. The nitrates and the calcium-channel antagonists diltiazem, nifedipine, and verapamil are metabolized by the liver, so that no specific dosage reduction is required in end-stage renal disease.[195]

REFERENCES

EFFECTS OF CARDIAC DISEASE ON RENAL FUNCTION

1. Skorecki, K. L., and Brenner, B. M.: Body fluid homeostasis in congestive heart failure and cirrhosis with ascites. Am. J. Med. 72:323, 1982.
2. Hostetter, T. H., Pfeffer, J. M., Pfeffer, M. A., Braunwald, E., and Brenner, B. M.: Cardiorenal hemodynamics and sodium excretion in rats with myocardial infarction. Am. J. Physiol. *245*:H98, 1983.
3. Francis, G. S.: Neurohumoral mechanisms involved in congestive heart failure. Am. J. Cardiol. *55*(Suppl. 15A), 1985.
4. Higgins, C. B., Vatner, S. F., Franklin, D., and Braunwald, E.: Effects of experimentally produced heart failure on the peripheral vascular response to severe exercise in conscious dogs. Circ. Res. *31*:186, 1972.
5. Cannon, P. J.: Prostaglandins in congestive heart failure and the effects of nonsteroidal anti-inflammatory drugs. Am. J. Med. *81*(Suppl. 2B):123, 1986.
6. Ichikawa, I., Pfeffer, J. M., Pfeffer, M. A., Hostetter, T. H., Braunwald, E., and Brenner, B. M.: Glomerular response to severe congestive heart failure in the rat. Proceedings, 15th Annual Meeting of the American Society of Nephrology, 152a, 1982.
7. DiPerri, T., Forconi, S., Puccetti, F., Vittoria, A., and Guerrini, M.: Effects of prostaglandin A_1 on renal handling of salt and water in congestive heart failure. J. Cardiovasc. Pharmacol. 2:215, 1980.
8. Raymond, K. H., and Lifschitz, M. D.: Effects of prostaglandins on renal salt and water excretion. Am. J. Med. *80*(Suppl. 1A):22, 1986.
9. Berliner, R. W., and Davidson, P. G.: Production of hypertonic urine in the absence of pituitary antidiuretic hormone. J. Clin. Invest. *36*:1416, 1957.
10. Fitzsimmons, J. T.: Thirst. Physiol. Rev. 52:468, 1972.
11. Szatalowicz, V. L., Arnold, P. E., Chaimovitz, C., Bichet, D., Bert, T., and Schrier, R. W.: Radioimmunoassay of plasma arginine vasopressin in hyponatremic patients with congestive heart failure. N. Engl. J. Med. *305*:263, 1981.
12. Goldsmith, S. R., Francis, G. S., and Cowley, A. W.: Arginine vasopressin and the renal response to water loading in congestive heart failure. Am. J. Cardiol. 58:295, 1986.
13. Oberg, B.: Effects of cardiovascular reflexes on net capillary fluid transfer. Acta Physiol. Scand. (Suppl.) *62*:229, 1964.
14. Braunwald, E., Ross, J., Jr., and Sonnenblick, E. H.: Mechanisms of Contraction in the Normal and Failing Heart. 2nd ed. Boston, Little, Brown, 1976, pp. 250–254.
15. Zucker, I. H., Earle, A. M., and Gilmore, J. P.: The mechanism of adaptation of left atrial stretch receptors in dogs with chronic congestive heart failure. J. Clin. Invest. *60*:323, 1977.
16. Zucker, I. H., Share, L., and Gilmore, J. P.: Renal effects of left atrial distention in dogs with chronic congestive heart failure. Am. J. Physiol. *236*:H554, 1979.
17. Birkenfeld, L. W., Liebman, J., O'Meara, M. P., and Edelman, I. S.: Total exchangeable sodium, total exchangeable potassium, and total body water in edematous patients with cirrhosis of the liver and congestive heart failure. J. Clin. Invest. *37*:687, 1958.
18. Carroll, H. J., Gotterer, R., and Altshuler, B.: Exchangeable sodium, body potassium, and body water in previously edematous cardiac patients. Evidence for osmotic inactivation of cation. Circulation *32*:185, 1965.
19. Farber, S. J., and Schubert, M.: The binding of cations by chondroitin sulfate. J. Clin. Invest. *36*:1715, 1957.
20. Hricik, D. E., and Kassirer, J. P.: Azotemia in cardiac failure. J. Cardiovasc. Med. 8:397, 1983.
21. Smith, H. W.: Salt and water volume receptors: An exercise in physiologic apologetics. Am. J. Med. *23*:623, 1957.
22. Gauer, O. H., Henry, J. P., and Sieker, H. O.: Cardiac receptors and fluid volume control. Prog. Cardiovasc. Dis. *4*:1, 1961.
23. Kisch, B.: Electron microscopy of the heart. I. Guinea pig. Exp. Med. Surg. *14*:99, 1956.
24. Jamieson, J. D., and Palade, G. E.: Specific granules in atrial muscle. J. Cell. Biol. *23*:151, 1964.
25. DeBold, A. J.: Heart atria granularity: Effects of changes in water-electrolyte balance. Proc. Soc. Exp. Biol. Med. *161*:508, 1979.
26. DeBold, A. J., Borenstein, H. B., Veress, A. T., and Sonnenberg, H.: A rapid and potent natriuretic response to intravenous injection of atrial myocardial extract in rats. Life Sci. *28*:89, 1981.

26a. Genest, J., and Cantin, M.: Atrial natriuretic factor. Circulation *75*(Suppl. I): 118, 1987.

27. Oikawa, S., Imai, M., Ueno, A., Tanaka, S., Noguchi, T., Nakazato, H., Kangawa, K., Fukada, A., and Matsuo, H.: Cloning and sequence analysis of cDNA encoding a precursor for human atrial natriuretic polypeptide. Nature *309*:724, 1984.
28. Misono, K. S., Grammer, R. T., Fukumi, H., Inagami, T.: Rat atrial natriuretic factor: Complete amino acid sequence and disulfide linkage essential for biological activity. Biochem. Biophys. Res. Commun. *119*:524, 1984.
29. DeBold, A. J.: Atrial natriuretic factor: A hormone produced by the heart. Science *230*:767, 1985.
30. Dietz, J. R.: Release of natriuretic factor from rat heart-lung preparations by atrial distention. Am. J. Physiol. *247*:R1093, 1984.
31. Goetz, K. L., Wang, B. C., Geer, P. G., Leadley, R. J., Jr., and Reinhardt, H. W.: Atrial stretch increases sodium excretion independently of release of atrial peptides. Am. J. Physiol. *250*:R946, 1986.
32. Shenker, Y., Sider, R. S., Ostafin, E. A., and Grekin, R. J.: Plasma levels of immunoreactive atrial natriuretic factor in healthy subjects and in patients with edema. J. Clin. Invest. *76*:1684, 1984.
33. Yamaji, T., Ishibashi, M., and Takaku, F.: Atrial natriuretic factor in human blood. J. Clin. Invest. *76*:1705, 1985.
34. Atlas, S. A.: Atrial natriuretic factor: Renal and systemic effects. Hosp. Pract. *21*:67, 1986.
35. Kimura, T., Abe, K., Ota, K., Omata, K., Shoji, M., Kudo, K., Matsui, K., Inoue, M., Yasujima, M., and Yoshinaga, K.: Effects of acute water load, hypertonic saline infusion, and furosemide administration on atrial natriuretic peptide and vasopressin release in humans. J. Clin. Endocrinol. Metab. *62*:1003, 1986.
36. Tikkanen, I., Fyhrquist, F., Metsarinne, K., and Leidenius, R.: Plasma atrial natriuretic peptide in cardiac disease and during infusion in healthy volunteers. Lancet 2:66, 1985.
37. Raine, A. E. G., Enre, P., Burgisser, E., Muller, F. B., Bolli, P., Burkart, F., and Buhler, F. R.: Atrial natriuretic peptide and atrial pressure in patients with congestive heart failure. N. Engl. J. Med. *315*:533, 1986.
38. Yamaji, T., Ismibasi, M., Nakaoka, H., Imataka, K., Amano, M., and Fujii, J.: Possible role for atrial natriuretic peptide in polyuria associated with paroxysmal atrial arrhythmias. Lancet *1*:1211, 1985.
39. Espiner, E. A., Crozier, I. G., Nicholls, M. G., Cuneo, R., Yondle, T. G., and Ikram, H.: Cardiac secretion of atrial natriuretic peptide. Lancet 2:398, 1985.
40. Manning, P. T., Schwartz, D., Katsube, N. C., Holmberg, S. W., and Needleman, P.: Vasopressin-stimulated release of atriopeptin: Endocrine antagonists in fluid homeostasis. Science *229*:395, 1985.
41. Napier, M. A., Vandlen, R. L., Albers-Schonberg, G., Nutt, R. F., Brady, S., Lyle, T., Winquist, R., Faison, E. P., Heinel, L. A., and Blaine, E. H.: Specific membrane receptors for atrial natriuretic factor in renal and vascular tissue. Proc. Natl. Acad. Sci. USA *81*:5946, 1984.
42. Hirata, Y., Tomita, M., Yoshimi, H., and Ikeda, M.: Specific receptors for atrial natriuretic factor (ANF) in cultured vascular smooth muscle cells of rat aorta. Biochem. Biophys. Res. Commun. *125*:562, 1984.
43. DeLean, A., Gutkowska, J., McNicoll, N., Schiller, P. W., Cantin, M., and Genest, J.: Characterization of specific receptors for atrial natriuretic factor in bovine adrenal zona glomerulosa. Life Sci. *35*:2311, 1984.
44. Quirion, R., Dalpe, M., DeLean, A., Gutkowska, J., Cantin, M., and Genest, J.: Atrial natriuretic factor (ANF) binding sites in brain and related structures. Peptides 5:1167, 1984.
45. Waldman, S. A., Rapoport, R. M., and Murad, F.: Atrial natriuretic factor selectively activates particulate guanylate cyclase and elevates cyclic GMP in rat tissue. J. Biol. Chem. *259*:14332, 1984.
46. Hamet, P., Tremblay, J., Pang, S. C., Garcia, R., Thibault, G., Gutkowska, J., Cantin, M., and Genest, J.: Effect of native and synthetic atrial natriuretic factor on cyclic GMP. Biochem. Biophys. Res. Commun. *123*:515, 1984.
47. Ballermann, B. J., and Brenner, B. M.: Role of atrial peptides in body fluid homeostasis. Circ. Res. *58*:619, 1986.
48. Weidmann, P., Hasler, L., Gnadinger, M. P., Lang, R. E., Uehlinger, D. E., Shaw, S., Rascher, W., and Reubi, F. C.: Blood levels and renal effects of atrial natriuretic peptide in normal man. J. Clin. Invest. 77:734, 1986.
49. Ichikawa, I., Dunn, B. R., Troy, J. L., Maack, T., and Brenner, B. M.: Influence of atrial natriuretic peptide on glomerular microcirculation in vivo (Abstr). Clin. Res. *33*:487A, 1985.
50. Pollock, D. M., and Arendshorst, W. J.: Effect of atrial natriuretic factor on renal hemodynamics in the rat. Am. J. Physiol. *251*:F795, 1986.
51. Huang, C. L., Lewicki, J., Johnson, L. K., and Cogan, M. G.: Renal mechanism of action of rat atrial natriuretic factor. J. Clin. Invest. *75*:759, 1985.
52. Zeidel, M. L., Seifter, J. L., Lear, S., Brenner, B. M., and Silva, P.: Atrial peptides inhibit oxygen consumption in kidney medullary collecting duct cells. Am. J. Physiol. *251*:F379, 1986.
53. Sonnenberg, H., Honrath, U., Chong, C. K., and Wilson, D. R.: Atrial natriuretic factor inhibits sodium transport in medullary collecting duct. Am. J. Physiol. *250*:F963, 1986.

54. Maack, T., Marion, D. N., Camargo, M. J. F., Kleinert, H. D., Laragh, J. H., Vaughan, E. D., Jr., and Atlas, S. A.: Effects of auriculin (atrial natriuretic factor) on blood pressure, renal function, and the renin-aldosterone system in dogs. Am. J. Med. 77:1069, 1984.
55. Henrich, W. L., Needleman, P., and Campbell, W. B.: Effect of atriopeptin III on renin release in vitro. Life Sci. *39*:993, 1986.
56. Laragh, J. H.: Atrial natriuretic hormone, the renin-aldosterone axis, and blood pressure-electrolyte homeostasis. N. Engl. J. Med. *313*:1330, 1985.
57. Kleinert, H. D., Maack, T., Atlas, S. A., Januszewicz, A., Sealey, J. E., and Laragh, J. H.: Atrial natriuretic factor inhibits angiotensin-, norepinephrine-, and potassium-induced vascular contractility. Hypertension *6*(Suppl. 1):1143, 1984.
57a. Bolli, P., Muller, F. B., Linder, L., Raine, A. E. G., Resink, T. J., Erne, P., Kiowski, W., Ritz, R., and Buhler, F. R.: The vasodilator potency of atrial natriuretic peptide in man. Circulation *75*:221, 1987.
58. Lappe, R. W., Smits, J. F. M., Todt, J. A., Debets, J. J. M., and Wendt, R. L.: Failure of atriopeptin II to cause arterial vasodilation in the conscious rat. Circ. Res. *56*:606, 1985.
59. Smith, S., Anderson, S., Ballermann, B. J., and Brenner, B. M.: Role of atrial natriuretic peptide in the adaption of sodium excretion with reduced renal mass. J. Clin. Invest. *77*:1395, 1986.
60. Ballermann, B. J., Bloch, K. D., Seidman, J. G., and Brenner, B. M.: Atrial natriuretic peptide transcription, secretion, and glomerular receptor activity during mineralocorticoid escape in the rat. J. Clin. Invest. *78*:840, 1986.
61. Saper, C. B., Standaert, D. B., Currie, M. G., Schwartz, D., Geller, D. M., and Needleman, P.: Atriopeptin-immunoreactive neurons in the brain: Presence in cardiovascular regulatory areas. Science *227*:1047, 1985.
62. Jacobowitz, D. M., Skofitsch, G., Keiser, H. R., Eskay, R. L., and Zamir, N.: Evidence for the existence of atrial natriuretic factor–containing neurons in the rat brain. Neuroendocrinology *40*:92, 1985.
63. Baehr, G., and Laude, H.: Glomerulonephritis as a complication of subacute streptococcus endocarditis. J.A.M.A. *75*:789, 1920.
64. Neugarten, J., and Baldwin, D. S.: Glomerulonephritis in bacterial endocarditis. Am. J. Med. *77*:297, 1984.
65. Bayer, A. S., Theofilopoulos, A. N., Eisenberg, T., Dixon, F. J., and Guze, L.: Circulating immune complexes in infective endocarditis. N. Engl. J. Med. *295*:1500, 1976.
66. Cross, A. S., and Steigbigel, A. T.: Infective endocarditis and access site infections in patients on hemodialysis. Medicine *55*:453, 1976.
67. Smith, M. C., Ghose, M. K., and Henry, A. R.: The clinical spectrum of renal cholesterol embolization. Am. J. Med. *71*:175, 1981.

EFFECTS OF RENAL DISEASE ON THE CARDIOVASCULAR SYSTEM

68. Rostand, S. G., and Rutsky, E. A.: Cardiac disease in dialysis patients. *In*: Nissenson, A. R., Fine, P. N., and Gentile, D. E. (eds.): Clinical Dialysis. Norwalk, CT, Appleton-Century-Crofts, 1984, p. 395.
69. Friedman, H. S., Shah, B. N., Kim, H. J. G., Bove, L. A., Del Monte, M. M., and Smith, A. J.: Clinical study of the cardiac findings in patients with chronic maintenance hemodialysis: The relationship to coronary risk factors. Clin. Nephrol. *16*:75, 1981.
70. Vincenti, F., Amand, W. J., Abele, J., Feduska, N. J., and Salvatierra, O., Jr.: The role of hypertension in hemodialysis-associated atherosclerosis. Am. J. Med. *68*:363, 1980.
71. Hopkins, P. N., and Williams, R. R.: A survey of 246 suggested coronary risk factors. Atherosclerosis *40*:1–52, 1981.
72. Rostand, S. G., Kirk, K. A., and Rutsky, E. A.: Dialysis-associated ischemic heart disease: Insights from coronary angiography. Kidney Int. *25*:653, 1984.
73. Sreepada Rao, T. K., Roxe, D. M., Laird, N. M., and Santiago, G. C.: Hemodynamic and cardiac correlates of different hemodialysis regimens: The National Cooperative Dialysis Study. Kidney Int. *23*(Suppl 13):S-89, 1983.
74. Zawada, E. T., Jr., Stinson, J. B., and Done, G.: New perspectives on coronary artery disease in hemodialysis patients. South. Med. J. *75*:694, 1982.
75. Francis, G. S., Conty, C. M., Sharma, B., and Helseth, H. K.: Myocardial revascularization in chronic renal disease patients. *In* Love, J. (ed.): Cardiac Surgery in Patients with Chronic Renal Disease. Mt. Kisco, N.Y., Futura Publishing Co., 1982, pp. 115–134.
76. Roig, E., Betriu, A., Castaner, A., Magrina, J., Sanz, G., and Navarrlo-Lopez, F.: Disabling angina pectoris with normal coronary arteries in patients undergoing long-term hemodialysis. Am. J. Med. *71*:431, 1981.
77. Kim, K. E., Onesti, G., and Schwartz, A. B.: Hemodynamic alterations in hypertension of chronic end-stage renal disease. *In* Onesti, G., Kim, K. E., and Moyer, J. H. (eds.): Hypertension: Mechanisms and Management. New York, Grune and Stratton, 1973, p. 609.
78. Dustan, H. P., and Page, I. H.: Some factors in renal and renoprival hypertension. J. Lab. Clin. Med. *64*:948, 1964.
79. Wilkinson, R., Scott, D. F., Uldall, P. R., Kerr, D. N. S., and Swinney, J.: Plasma renin and exchangeable sodium in the hypertension of chronic renal failure. The effect of bilateral nephrectomy. Q. J. Med. *39*:377, 1970.
80. Cangiano, J. L., Ramirez-Muxo, O., Ramirez-Gonzalez, R., Trevino, A., and Campos, J. A.: Normal renin uremic hypertension. Arch. Intern. Med. *136*:17, 1976.
81. Lilley, J. J., Golden, J., and Stone, R. A.: Adrenergic regulation of blood pressure in chronic renal failure. J. Clin. Invest. *57*:1190, 1976.
82. Campese, V. M., Romoff, M. S., Levitan, D., Lane, K., and Massry, S. G.: Mechanisms of autonomic nervous system dysfunction in uremia. Kidney Int. *20*:246, 1981.
83. Smith, M. C., and Dunn, M. J.: Renal kallikreins, kinins, and prostaglandins in hypertension. *In* Brenner, B. M., and Stein, J. H. (eds.): Hypertension (Contemporary Issues in Nephrology, Vol. 8). New York, Churchill Livingstone, 1981.
84. Cooper, R. A.: Captopril-associated neutropenia: Who is at risk? Arch. Int. Med. *143*:659, 1983.
85. Romankiewicz, J. A., Brogden, R. N., Heel, R. C., Speight, T. M., and Avery, G. S.: Captopril: An update review of its pharmacologic properties and therapeutic efficacy in congestive heart failure. Drugs *25*:6, 1983.
86. Isles, C. G., McLay, A., and Jones, J. M.: Recovery in malignant hypertension presenting as acute renal failure. Q. J. Med. *53*:439, 1984.
87. Popovtzer, M. M., Pinnggera, W., Katz, F. H., Corman, J. L., Robinette, J., Lanois, B., Halgrimson, C. G., and Starzl, T. E.: Variations in arterial blood pressure after kidney transplantation: Relation to renal function, plasma renin activity and the dose of prednisone. Circulation *47*:1297, 1973.
88. McPhaul, J. J., Jr., Thompson, A. L., Jr., Lordon, R. E., Klebanoff, G., Cosimi, A. B., de Lemos, R., and Smith, R. B.: Evidence suggesting persistence of the nephritogenic immunopathologic mechanisms in patients receiving renal allografts. J. Clin. Invest. *52*:1059, 1973.
89. Tilney, N. L., Rocha, A., Strom, T. B., and Kirkman, R. L.: Renal artery stenosis in transplant patients. Ann. Surg. *199*:454, 1984.
90. Hamilton, D. V., Carmichael, D. J., Evans, D. B., and Calne, R. Y.: Hypertension in renal transplant recipients on cyclosporin A and corticosteroids and azathioprine. Transplant. Proc. *14*:597, 1982.
91. Thompson, M. E., Shapiro, A. P., Johnsen, A. M., Itzkoff, J. M., Hardesty, R. L., Griffith, B. P., Bahnson, H. T., McDonald, R. H., Jr., Hastillo, A., and Hess, M.: The contrasting effects of cyclosporin-A and azathioprine on arterial blood pressure and renal function following cardiac transplantation. Int. J. Cardiol. *11*:219, 1986.
92. Curtis, J. J., Luke, R. G., Whelchel, J. D., Diethelm, A. G., Jones, P., and Dustan, H. P.: Inhibition of angiotensin-converting enzyme in renal-transplant recipients with hypertension. N. Engl. J. Med. *308*:377, 1983.
93. Ibels, L. S., Alfrey, A. C., and Weil, R., III: Hyperlipidemia in adult, pediatric and diabetic transplant recipients. Am. J. Med. *64*:634, 1978.
94. Curtis, J. J., Galla, J. H., Woodford, S. Y., Rees, E. D., and Luke, R. G.: Effects of renal transplantation on hyperlipidemia and high-density lipoprotein cholesterol (HDL). Transplantation *26*:364, 1978.
95. Matas, A. J., Simmons, R. L., Buselmeier, T. J., Kjellstrand, C. M., and Najarian, J. S.: The fate of patients surviving three years after renal transplantation. Surgery *80*:390, 1976.
96. Bagdade, J., Casaretto, A., and Albers, J.: Effects of chronic uremia, hemodialysis and renal transplantation on plasma lipids and lipoproteins in man. J. Lab. Clin. Med. *87*:37, 1976.
97. Brunzell, J. D., Albers, J. J., Haas, L. B., Goldberg, A. P., Agode, L., and Sherrard, D. J.: Prevalence of serum lipid abnormalities in chronic hemodialysis. Metabolism *26*:903, 1977.
98. Chan, M. K., Varghese, Z., Persaud, J. W., Baillod, R. A., and Moorhead, J. F.: Hyperlipidemia in patients on maintenance hemo- and peritoneal dialysis: The relative pathogenetic roles of triglyceride production and triglyceride removal. Clin. Nephrol. *17*:183, 1982.
99. Rapoport, J., Aviram, M., Chaimovitz, C., and Brook, J. G.: Defective high density lipoprotein composition in patients on chronic hemodialysis. N. Engl. J. Med. *299*:1326, 1978.
100. Nestel, P. J., Fidge, N. H., and Tan, M. H.: Increased lipoprotein-remnant formation in chronic renal failure. N. Engl. J. Med. *307*:329, 1982.
101. Drueke, T., Lacour, B., Roullet, J. B., and Funck-Brentano, J. L.: Recent advances in factors that alter lipid metabolism in chronic renal failure. Kidney Int. *24*(Suppl. 16):S-134, 1983.
102. Havel, R. J., Kane, J. P., and Kashyap, M. L.: Interchange of apolipoproteins between chylomicrons and high density lipoproteins during alimentary lipemia in man. J. Clin. Invest. *52*:32, 1973.
103. Uraemia, lipoproteins and atherosclerosis. Lancet *2*:1151, 1981.
104. Sanfelippo, M. L., Swensen, R. S., and Reaven, G. M.: Reduction of plasma triglycerides by diet in subjects with chronic renal failure. Kidney Int. *11*:54, 1977.
105. Goldberg, A. P., Sherrard, D. J., Haas, L. B., and Brunzell, J. D.: Control of clofibrate toxicity in uremic hypertriglyceridemia. Clin. Pharmacol. Ther. *21*:317, 1977.
106. Kleiger, R. E., deMello, V. R., Malone, D., Fernandes, J., Thanavaro, S., Connors, J. P., and Oliver, G. C.: Left ventricular function in end-stage renal disease. Echocardiographic classification. South. Med. J. *74*:819, 1981.
107. Lai, K. N., Barnden, L., and Mathew, T. H.: Effect of renal transplantation on left ventricular function in hemodialysis patients. Clin. Nephrol. *18*:74, 1982.
108. Crosbie, W. A., Snowden, S., and Parsons, V.: Changes in lung capillary permeability in renal failure. Br. Med. J. *4*:388, 1972.
109. Gotloib, L., and Servadio, C.: A possible case of beriberi heart failure in a chronic hemodialysis patient. Nephron *14*:293, 1975.
110. Drüeke, T., Fleury, J., Toure, Y., deVernejoul, P., Fauchet, M., Lesourde, P., LePailleur, C., and Crosnier, J.: Effect of parathyroidectomy on left ventricular function in haemodialysis patients. Lancet *1*:112, 1980.
111. Raab, W.: Cardiotoxic substances in the blood and heart muscle in uremia. J. Lab. Clin. Med. *29*:715, 1944.
112. Scheuer, J., and Stezoski, S. W.: The effects of uremic components on cardiac function and metabolism. J. Mol. Cell. Cardiol. *5*:287, 1973.
113. Reicker, G., Velker, W., and Strauer, B. E.: Cardiac and circulatory disorders in renal insufficiency. *In* Uraemia: An International Conference on Pathogenesis, Diagnosis and Therapy. London, Churchill Livingstone, 1971, pp. 72–78.
114. Welt, L. G., Smith, E. K. M., Dunn, M. J., Czerwinski, A., Proctor, H.,

Cole, C., Balfo, J. W., and Gitelman, H. J.: Membrane transport defect: The sick cell. Tr. Assoc. Am. Physicians *80*:217, 1967.
115. Patrick, J., and Jones, N. F.: Cell sodium, potassium and water in uremia and the effects of regular dialysis as studied in the leukocyte. Clin. Sci. Mol. Med. *46*:583, 1974.
116. Prosser, D., and Parsons, V.: The case for a specific uremic myocardiopathy. Nephron *15*:4, 1975.
117. Gueron, M., Berlyne, C. M., Nord, E., and BenAri, J.: The case against the existence of a specific uraemic myocardiopathy. Nephron *15*:2, 1975.
118. Pehrsson, S. K., Jonasson, R., and Lins, L. E.: Cardiac performance in various stages of renal failure. Br. Heart J. *52*:667, 1984.
119. Drüeke, T., Le Pailleur, C., Meilhac, B., Kontoudis, C., Zingraff, J., DiMatteo, J., and Crosnier, J.: Congestive cardiomyopathy in uremic patients on long-term haemodialysis. Br. Med. J. *1*:350, 1977.
120. Bailey, G. L., Hampers, C. L., and Merrill, J. P.: Reversible cardiomyopathy in uremia. Tr. Am. Soc. Artif. Intern. Organs *13*:263, 1967.
121. Hung, J., Harris, P. J., Uren, R. F., Tiller, D. J., and Kelly, D. T.: Uremic cardiomyopathy—Effect of hemodialysis on left ventricular function in end-stage renal failure. N. Engl. J. Med. *302*:547, 1980.
122. Bornstein, A., Gaasch, W. H., and Harrington, J.: Assessment of the cardiac effects of hemodialysis with systolic time intervals and echocardiography. Am. J. Cardiol. *51*:332, 1983.
123. Henrich, W. L., Hunt, J. M., and Nixon, J. V.: Increased ionized calcium and left ventricular contractility during hemodialysis. N. Engl. J. Med. *310*:19, 1984.
124. Blaustein, A. S., Schmitt, G., Foster, M. C., Hayes, R. V., and Bronstein, S.: Serial effects on left ventricular load and contractility during hemodialysis in patients with concentric hypertrophy. Am. Heart J. *111*:340, 1986.
125. Nixon, J. V., Mitchell, J. H., McPhaul, J. J., Jr., and Henrich, W. L.: Effect of hemodialysis on left ventricular function. Dissociation of changes in filling volume and in contractile state. J. Clin. Invest. *71*:377, 1983.
126. Leenen, F. H., Smith, D. L., Khanna, R., and Oreopoulos, D. G.: Changes in left ventricular hypertrophy and function in hypertensive patients started on continuous ambulatory peritoneal dialysis. Am. Heart J. *110*:102, 1985.
127. Cueto-Garcia, L., Herrera, J., Arriaga, J., Laredo, C., and Meaney, E.: Echocardiographic changes after successful renal transplantation in young nondiabetic patients. Chest *83*:56, 1983.
128. Henrich, W. L., Woodard, T. D., Blachley, J. D., Gomez-Sanchez, C., Pettinger, W., and Cronin, R. E.: Role of osmolality in blood pressure stability after dialysis and ultrafiltration. Kidney Int. *18*:480, 1980.
129. Kinet, J. P., Soyeur, D., Balland, N., Saint-Remy, M., Collignon, P., and Godon, J. P.: Hemodynamic study of hypotension during hemodialysis. Kidney Int. *21*:868, 1982.
130. Rosa, A. A., Shideman, J., McHugh, R., Duncan, D., and Kjellstrand, C. M.: The importance of osmolality fall and ultrafiltration rate on hemodialysis side effects. Influence of intravenous mannitol. Nephron *27*:134, 1981.
131. Henrich, W. L.: Hemodynamic instability during hemodialysis. Kidney Int. *30*:605, 1986.
132. Hakim, R. M., and Lazarus, J. M.: Complications during hemodialysis. *In* Nissenson, A. R., Fine, R. N., and Gentile, D. E. (eds.): Clinical Dialysis. Norwalk, CT, Appleton-Century-Crofts, 1984, pp. 179–220.
133. Graefe, U., Milutenovitch, J., Follette, W. C., Vizzo, J. E., Babb, A. L., and Scribner, B. H.: Less dialysis-induced morbidity and vascular instability with bicarbonate in dialysate. Ann. Int. Med. *88*:332, 1978.
134. Velez, R. L., Woodward, T. D., and Heinrich, W. L.: Acetate and bicarbonate hemodialysis in patients with and without autonomic dysfunction. Kidney Int. *26*:59, 1984.
135. Van Stone, J. C., Bauer, J., and Carey, J.: The effects of dialysate sodium concentration on body fluid distribution during hemodialysis. Trans. Am. Soc. Artif. Intern. Organs. *26*:383, 1980.
136. Henrich, W. L., Woodard, T. D., and McPhaul, J. J., Jr.: The chronic efficacy and safety of high sodium dialysate: Double-blind, crossover study. Am. J. Kidney Dis. *2*:349, 1982.
137. Rouby, J. J., Rottembourg, J., Durande, J. P., Basset, J. Y., Degoulet, P., Glasser, P., and Legrain, M.: Hemodynamic changes induced by regular hemodialysis and sequential ultrafiltration hemodialysis: A comparative study. Kidney Int. *17*:801, 1980.
138. Arduson, C. B., Codd, J. R., Graff, R. A., Grace, M. A., Harter, H. R., and Newton, W. T.: Cardiac failure in upper extremity arteriovenous dialysis fistulae. Arch. Intern. Med. *136*:292, 1976.
139. Eiser, A. R., and Swartz, C. E.: Hemodialysis and peritoneal dialysis in patients with cardiac disease. *In* Lowenthal, D. T. (ed.): Management of the Cardiac Patient With Renal Failure. Philadelphia, F. A. Davis Co., 1981, pp. 78–80.
140. Nsouli, K. A., Lazarus, J. M., Schoenbaum, S. C., Gottlieb, M. N., Lowrie, E. G., and Shocair, M.: Bacteremic infection in hemodialysis. Arch. Intern. Med. *139*:1255, 1979.
141. Aurigemma, N. M., Feldman, N. T., Gottlieb, M. N., Ingram, R. H., Lazarus, J. M., and Lowrie, E. G.: Arterial oxygenation during hemodialysis. N. Engl. J. Med. *297*:871, 1977.
142. Thayssen, P., Anderson, K. H., and Pindborg, T.: Noninvasive monitoring of cardiac function during haemodialysis. Scand. J. Urol. Nephrol. *15*:313, 1981.
143. Craddock, P. R., Fehr, J., Brigham, K. L., Dronenberg, R. S., and Jacob, H. S.: Complement and leukocyte mediated pulmonary dysfunction in hemodialysis. N. Engl. J. Med. *296*:769, 1977.
144. DeBacker, W. A., Verpooten, G. A., Borgonjon, D. J., Vermeire, P. A., Lins, R. R., and DeBroe, M. E.: Hypoxemia during hemodialysis. Effects of different membranes and dialysate compositions. Kidney Int. *23*:738, 1983.
145. Dolan, M. J., Whipp, B. J., Davidson, W. D., Weitzman, R. E., and Wasserman, K.: Hypopnea associated with acetate hemodialysis: Carbon dioxide flow–dependent ventilation. N. Engl. J. Med. *305*:72, 1981.
146. Jones, R. H., Broadfield, J. B., and Parsons, V.: Arterial hypoxemia during hemodialysis for acute renal failure in mechanically ventilated patients: Observations and mechanisms. Clin. Nephrol. *14*:18, 1980.
147. Fisch, C.: Relation of electrolyte disturbances to cardiac arrhythmias. Circulation *47*:408, 1973.
148. Fraley, D. S, and Adler, S.: Correction of hyperkalemia by bicarbonate despite constant blood pH. Kidney Int. *12*:354, 1977.
149. D'Cruz, I. A., Jain, M., Fishman, S., Abrahams, C., and Kathpalia, S.: Calcification of the mitral region in patients with chronic renal failure: 2-D echocardiographic, hormonal and autopsy correlation. J. Am. Coll. Cardiol. *1*:625, 1983.
150. Nestico, P. F., DePace, N. L., Kotler, M. N., Rose, L. I., Brezin, J. H., Swartz, C., Mintz, G., and Schwartz, A. B.: Calcium and phosphorus metabolism in dialysis patients with and without mitral anular calcium. Analysis of 30 patients. Am. J. Cardiol. *51*:497, 1983.
151. Ferman, M. B., Virmani, R., Robertson, R. M., and Stone, W. J.: Mitral annular calcification in chronic renal failure. Chest *85*:367, 1984.
152. Roberts, W. C., and Waller, B. F.: Effect of chronic hypercalcemia on the heart. An analysis of 18 necropsy patients. Am. J. Med. *71*:371, 1981.
153. Depace, N. L., Rohrer, A. H., Kotler, M. N., Brezin, J. H., and Parry, W. R.: Rapidly progressing, massive mitral annular calcification. Arch. Intern. Med. *141*:1663, 1981.
154. Jain, M. C., D'Cruz, I., and Kathpalia, S.: Chronic renal failure: Intracardiac calcification. Primary Cardiol. Clin. *4*:27, 1981.
155. Arora, K., Lacy, J. P., Schacht, R. A., Martin, D. G., and Gutch, C. F.: Calcific cardiomyopathy in advanced renal failure. Arch. Intern. Med. *135*:603, 1975.
156. Osterberger, L. E., Goldstein, S., Khaja, F., and Lakier, J. B.: Functional mitral stenosis in patients with massive mitral annular calcification. Circulation *64*:472, 1981.
157. Rosen, H., Friedman, S. A., Raizner, A. E., and Gerstmann, K.: Azotemic arteriopathy. Am. Heart J. *84*:250, 1972.
158. Ejerblad, S., Ericsson, J. L. E., and Eriksson, I.: Arterial lesions of the radial artery in uraemic patients. Acta. Chir. Scand. *145*:415, 1979.
159. Verberckmoes, R., Bouillon, R., and Krempien, B.: Disappearance of vascular calcifications during treatment of renal osteodystrophy. Ann. Intern. Med. *82*:529, 1975.
160. Landsberg, K. F., and Landsberg, D. N.: Vitamin D preparations and their role in renal osteodystrophy. Can. J. Hosp. Pharm. *38*:10, 1985.
161. Wacker, W., and Merrill, J. P.: Uremic pericarditis in acute and chronic renal failure. J.A.M.A. *156*:764, 1954.
162. Wray, T. M., and Stone, W. J.: Uremic pericarditis: A prospective echocardiographic and clinical study. Clin. Nephrol. *6*:295, 1976.
163. Yoshida, K., Shiina, A., Asano, Y., and Hosoda, S.: Uremic pericardial effusion by echocardiography. Clin. Nephrol. *13*:260, 1980.
164. Frommer, J. P., Young, J. P., and Ayus, J. C.: Asymptomatic pericardial effusion in uremic patients: Effect of long-term dialysis. Nephron *39*:296, 1985.
165. Hoops, H. C., and Wissler, R. M.: Uremic pneumonitis. Am. J. Pathol. *31*:361, 1955.
166. Nidus, B. D., Matalon, R., Cantazino, D., and Eisinger, R. P.: Uremic pleuritis—A clinicopathological entity. N. Engl. J. Med. *281*:255, 1969.
167. Goldberg, M., Lazarus, J. M., Gottlieb, M. N., Lowrie, E. G., and Merrill, J. P.: Treatment of uremic pericardial effusion. Proc. Clin. Dial. Transplant Forum *5*:20, 1975.
168. Luft, F. C., Gilman, J. K., and Weyman, A. E.: Pericarditis in patients with uremia: Clinical and echocardiographic evaluation. Nephron *25*:160, 1980.
169. Lazarus, J. M., Gottlieb, M. N., Lowrie, E. G., Teicholtz, L., and Merrill, J. P.: Echocardiographic findings in stable hemodialysis patients. Proc. Clin. Dial. Transplant Forum *6*:53, 1976.
170. Kleiman, J. H., Motta, J., London, E., Pennell, J. P., and Popp, R. L.: Pericardial effusions in patients with end-stage renal disease. Br. Heart J. *40*:190, 1978.
171. Depace, N. L., Nestico, P. F., Schwartz, A. B., Mintz, G. S., Schwartz, J. S., Kotler, M. N., and Swartz, C.: Predicting success of intensive dialysis in the treatment of uremic pericarditis. Am. J. Med. *76*:38, 1984.
172. Quigg, R. J., Idelson, B. A., Yoburn, D. C., Hynes, J. L., Schick, E. C., and Bernard, D. B.: Local steroids in dialysis-associated pericardial effusion. A single intraperitoneal administration of triamcinolone. Arch. Int. Med. *145*:2249, 1985.
173. Buselmeier, T. J., Simmons, R. L., Najarian, J. S., Mauer, S. M., Matas, A. J., and Kjellstrand, C. M.: Uremic pericardial effusion: Treatment by catheter drainage and local nonabsorbable steroid administration. Nephron *16*:371, 1976.
174. Frame, R. J., Lucas, S. K., Pederson, J. A., and Elkins, R. C.: Surgical treatment of pericarditis in the dialysis patient. Am. J. Surg. *146*:800, 1983.
175. Specter, D., Alfred, H., Siedlecki, M., and Briefel, G.: A controlled study of the effect of indomethacin in uremic pericarditis. Kidney Int. *24*:663, 1983.
176. Connors, J. P., Kleiger, R. E., Shaw, R. C., Voiles, J. D., Clark, R. E., Harter, H., and Roper, C. L.: The indications for pericardiectomy in the uremic pericardial effusion. Surgery *80*:689, 1976.
177. Pillay, V. K. G., Sarpel, S. C., and Kurtzman, N. A.: Subacute constrictive uremic pericarditis: Survival after pericardiectomy. J.A.M.A. *235*:1351, 1976.

178. Hampers, C. L., Bailey, G. L., Hager, E. B., VanDam, L. D., and Merrill, J. P.: Major surgery in patients on maintenance hemodialysis. Am. J. Surg. *115*:747, 1968.
179. Connors, J. P., and Shaw, R. C.: Considerations in the management of open-heart surgery in uremic patients. J. Thorac. Cardiovasc. Surg. *75*:400, 1978.
180. Lamberti, J. J., Jr., Cohn, L. H., and Collins, J. J., Jr.: Cardiac surgery in patients undergoing renal dialysis or transplantation. Ann. Thorac. Surg. *19*:135, 1975.
181. Chawla, R., Gailiunas, P., Jr., Lazarus, J. M., Gottlieb, M. N., Lowrie, E. G., Collins, J. J., and Merrill, J. P.: Cardiopulmonary bypass surgery in chronic hemodialysis and transplant patients. Trans. Am. Soc. Artif. Intern. Organs *23*:694, 1977.
182. Falch, D.: The influence of kidney function, body size and age on plasma concentration and urinary excretion of digoxin. Acta Med. Scand. *194*:251, 1973.
183. Steiness, E.: Renal tubular secretion of digoxin. Circulation *50*:103, 1974.
184. Jelliffe, R. W.: An improved method of digoxin therapy. Ann. Intern. Med. *69*:703, 1968.
185. Rasmussen, K., Jervell, J., Storstein, L., and Gjerdrum, K.: Digitoxin kinetics in patients with impaired renal function. Clin. Pharmacol. Ther. *13*:6, 1972.
186. Ackerman, G. L., Doherty, J. F., and Flanigan, W. J.: Peritoneal dialysis and hemodialysis of tritiated digoxin. Ann. Intern. Med. *67*:718, 1967.
187. Gibson, T. P., Lowenthal, D. T., Nelson, H. A., and Briggs, W. A.: Elimination of procainamide in end-stage renal failure. Clin. Pharmacol. Ther. *17*:321, 1975.
188. Fenster, P. E., Hager, W. D., Perrier, D., Powell, J. R., Graves, P. E., and Michael, U. F.: Digoxin-quinidine interaction in patients with chronic renal failure. Circulation *66*:1277, 1982.
189. Conn, H. L., and Luchi, R. J.: Some quantitative aspects of the binding of quinidine and related quinolone compounds by human serum albumin. J. Clin. Invest. *40*:509, 1961.
190. Hall, K., Meatherall, B., Krahn, J., Penner, B., and Rabson;, J. L.: Clearance of quinidine during peritoneal dialysis. Am. Heart J. *104*:646, 1982.
191. Thompson, P. D., Melmon, K. L., Richardson, J. A., Cohn, K., Steinbrunn, W., Cudikee, R., and Rowland, M.: Lidocaine pharmacokinetics in advanced heart failure, liver disease and renal failure in humans. Ann. Intern. Med. *78*:499, 1973.
192. Letteri, J. M., Mellk, H., Louis, S., Kutti, H., Durante, P., and Glazko, A.: Diphenylhydantoin metabolism in uremia. N. Engl. J. Med. *285*:648, 1971.
193. Thompson, P. D., Joekes, A. M., and Foulkes, D. M.: Pharmacodynamics of propranolol in renal failure. Br. Med. J. *2*:434, 1972.
194. Shand, D. G., Wed, A. J. J., Vestal, R. E., Wilkinson, G. R., and Branch, R. A.: Pharmacokinetic and pharmacodynamic factors determining variations in propranolol responsiveness. *In* Braunwald, E. (ed.): Beta-Adrenergic Blockade. New York, Elsevier, 1978, pp. 74–80.
195. Bennett, W. M., Arnoff, G. R., Morrison, G., Golper, T. A., Pulliam, J., Wolfson, M., and Singer, I.: Drug prescribing in renal failure: Dosing guidelines for adults. Am. J. Kidney Dis. *3*:155, 1983.

60 PREGNANCY AND CARDIOVASCULAR DISEASE

by JOSEPH K. PERLOFF, M.D.

IMPORTANCE OF THE PROBLEM

In North America and western Europe, maternal mortality from all causes has steadily decreased. This favorable trend has resulted chiefly from control of noncardiac determinants of maternal death, especially eclampsia, hemorrhage, and infection.[1] During the first half of this century, approximately 1 to 4 per cent of pregnancies in the United States and western Europe were complicated by cardiac disease.[2] Although the overall prevalence of heart disease associated with pregnancy has declined somewhat over the past three decades, the predominant change has been in the relative incidence of the various types of cardiac disorders.[3] For example, the incidence of rheumatic heart disease has dropped, while congenital heart disease is being encountered more frequently.[3] In addition, advances in diagnostic techniques and patient management have made pregnancy feasible for women with heart disease who previously might not have attempted childbirth, and advances in surgery have created an important new category—the postoperative cardiac patient of childbearing age.[4-6] However, for information to be meaningful regarding the general prevalence of heart disease in pregnancy and the relative incidence of specific types of associated cardiac disorders, consideration must be given to the particular population under study. Disease patterns vary widely when developed and underdeveloped countries are compared. In India and Nigeria, for example, acute and chronic rheumatic heart disease still constitutes a major health problem among pregnant women.[7] In Venezuela and Argentina, the relatively high incidence of Chagas disease increases the probability of related cardiomyopathy among pregnant women.[8]

CARDIOPULMONARY CHANGES IN NORMAL PREGNANCY

Rational management of heart disease in pregnancy presupposes an understanding of the circulatory and respiratory adaptations to the normal gravid state (Tables 60–1 and 60–2).[9-16] To characterize these adaptive responses, four variables must be defined: the time of onset of the adaptive response, the magnitude of the change, the time the change reaches its peak, and the behavior of the adaptive response upon maximum deviation from the nonpregnant state. Data should be based upon serial studies in the same patients in order to circumvent variation among individuals[17, 18]

BLOOD VOLUME. The increase in maternal blood volume starts early in pregnancy, reaches its peak at 32 weeks, and plateaus until term.[9, 9a] This rise in blood volume averages 1600 ml in a normal singleton pregnancy—an increase of about 40 to 50 per cent over pregestational levels. Multigravidas and women carrying more than one fetus experience larger increments in blood volume.[2, 9, 19] This increase principally reflects an expanded plasma volume. The smaller increment in red cell volume prevails throughout pregnancy and tends to accelerate during the last trimester, while plasma volume undergoes major expansion during the first two trimesters.[10] This disparity in the timing and increase of red cell versus plasma volume during gestation accounts for the "physiological anemia" of pregnancy. Lowest hematocrits are found near the end of the second trimester.

During the course of gestation, renal tubular reabsorption of sodium increases, with a cumulative retention of 500 to 900 mEq/liter.[10] Expansion of total body fluid includes an increase in intracellular water in growing organs (such as the uterus, placenta, and fetus) and extracellular expansion of plasma volume, extracellular fluid, and amniotic fluid.[9] An accumulation of water in the skin and subcutaneous tissues is recognized clinically as edema, which occurs in 50 to 80 per cent of healthy gravid

TABLE 60–1 CIRCULATORY CHANGES IN NORMAL PREGNANCY

Cardiac output	↑	30 to 50%
Stroke volume	↑	
Mean velocity circumferential fiber shortening	↑	
Heart rate	↑	Average 10 beats/min
Blood volume	↑	40 to 50%
Systemic blood pressure	↓	Slightly until term
Systemic vascular resistance	↓	
Pulmonary vascular resistance	↓	

TABLE 60–2 RESPIRATORY CHANGES IN NORMAL PREGNANCY

Minute ventilation	↑
O_2 consumption	↑
Functional residual capacity	↓
Inspiratory capacity	↑
Vital capacity	↑
Total lung capacity	UNCHANGED
Pulmonary compliance	UNCHANGED
Airway resistance	↓
Compensated respiratory alkalosis	

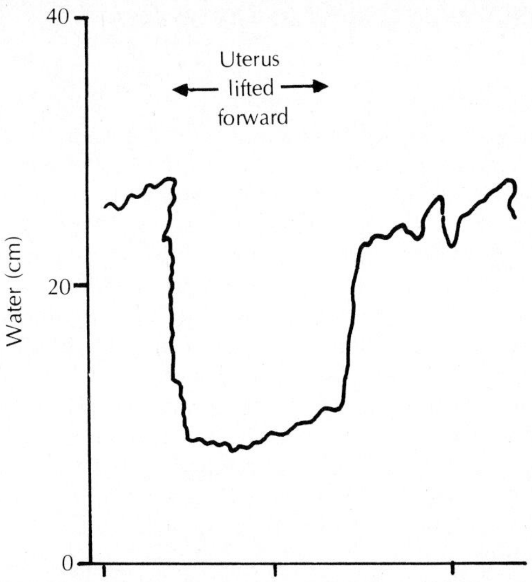

FIGURE 60–2. Effect on inferior caval pressure of lifting the gravid uterus forward before cesarean section. (From Kerr, M. G.: The mechanical effects of the gravid uterus in late pregnancy. J. Obstet. Gynaecol. Br. Comm. *72*:513, 1965.)

women.[20] The frequency of peripheral edema increases with maternal age, especially over 30 years. While the presence and degree of edema are chiefly attributable to the increase in body water and total exchangeable sodium, there is the additive effect during the third trimester of elevated venous pressure in the lower extremities owing to compression of the inferior vena cava by the gravid uterus (see below).

CARDIAC OUTPUT. The increase in intravascular volume in pregnancy sets the stage for a rise in cardiac output, which, in the lateral recumbent position, increases 30 to 50 per cent over pregravid values.[2, 9, 13, 17, 18, 21] Most of this increment occurs in the first trimester owing to an increase in stroke volume (Fig. 60–1), with the peak occurring at 20 to 24 weeks.[9, 10, 17, 18] As pregnancy advances, heart rate continues to rise while stroke volume declines. In late pregnancy, the increased cardiac output is maintained principally by heart rate.[10, 18] The previously held belief that cardiac output declines toward term has been qualified by taking into account the patient's position (supine or lateral) and the mechanical effects of the gravid uterus.[11, 13, 17, 18, 21, 22] It has long been known that the gravid uterus exerts profound mechanical effects by virtue of its weight and size and the position of the patient. When cardiac output is determined in the left lateral decubitus position, no significant late gestational decline is noted. Aortocaval compression in the supine position increases with gestational age and is held responsible for the measured fall in cardiac output during the last trimester. A change from the supine to the lateral position has been shown to increase cardiac output as much as 27 per cent.[23] When the uterus is manually lifted from the inferior vena cava during cesarean section, caval pressure falls dramatically, as it does when the patient turns on her side (Fig. 60–2).[24] When the cava is manually compressed under direct vision, complete occlusion produces a pressure equal to but not greater than that found in the supine position before delivery.[24] Predelivery inferior cavagrams confirm complete occlusion in the majority of women studied while supine in contrast to caval patency when the patient is restudied in the lateral position. Postural hemodynamic changes are attenuated when the fetal head is engaged in the pelvis, rendering the uterus less mobile.[24] Venous return during caval occlusion is via the azygos, lumbar, and paraspinal veins.[10, 25]

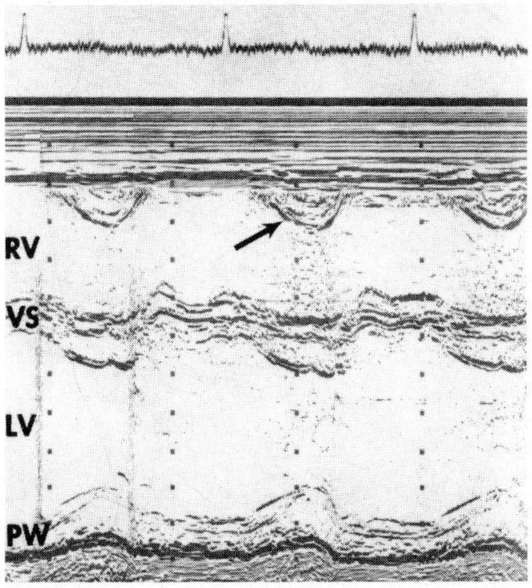

FIGURE 60–1. M-mode echocardiogram at 16 weeks' gestation in a normal 24-year-old woman. Increased excursions of the right ventricular (RV) wall (arrow), ventricular septum (VS), and left ventricular (LV) posterior wall (PW) are already evident. Internal dimensions are normal.

INTRAVASCULAR PRESSURES AND RESISTANCES. Systemic arterial blood pressure during pregnancy is chiefly responsive to systemic vascular resistance. There is a small and variable decline in systolic pressure but a significant decline in diastolic pressure, resulting in a wider pulse pressure.[9, 17, 18] These values are maximal at midpregnancy and return to pregestational levels near term.[2, 9, 26]

Several additional factors influence systemic arterial pressure during pregnancy. Maternal age and parity correlate with an increase in blood pressure. The patient's posture at the time of blood pressure measurement has a material effect.[13, 22–25, 27, 28] Brachial arterial pressure (right arm) is usually highest when the patient is seated, intermediate when she is supine, and lowest when she is lying on her left side.[9, 13, 22] During the latter part of pregnancy, the gravid uterus in the supine position variably compresses the inferior vena cava *and* the abdominal aorta. The result of the supine position on systemic arterial blood pressure depends on the relative degrees of caval versus aortic compression and the development of paravertebral collateral venous circulation, the vascular sensitivity to angiotensin (i.e., a decrease in vascular resistance during pregnancy is believed to reflect the attenuated responsiveness to angiotensin), and vagal baroreceptor sensitivity.[9, 10] The relative effects of supine aortic and inferior caval compression by the gravid uterus can be identified at the bedside by determining arm and leg blood pressures.[27] Predominant *aortic compression* is signaled by a disproportionate decline in *lower* extremity blood pressure to which the late gravida is symptomatically oblivious.[27] *Inferior caval compression* by the gravid uterus is indicated by declines in brachial *and* femoral arterial pressures, and in about 5 per cent of women in late pregnancy, compensatory mechanisms for maintaining satisfactory arterial pressures are faulty. Women with appreciable declines in brachial and femoral arterial pressures indicative of inferior caval compression are usually reluctant to lie on their backs.[27] What has been called the "supine hypotensive syndrome," an extreme of this faulty response, is characterized by appreciable declines in systemic arterial pressures in the supine position.[9, 10, 13, 24, 27, 29] Occasionally, an otherwise normal pregnant woman experiences bradycardiac hypotensive syncope in the supine position—a dramatic event promptly reversed by simply turning the patient on her side. The bradycardia is believed to be a selective vasovagal baroreceptor response to inferior caval compression analogous to the blunting of heart rate acceleration observed during inferior caval occlusion at laparotomy in nonpregnant patients.[24]

The effect of cigarette smoking on blood pressure during pregnancy is noteworthy.[30] Smoking one to two cigarettes in this setting causes a prompt, short-term elevation in upper extremity blood pressure.[30]

The increase in femoral venous pressure in late pregnancy is explained by mechanical pressure of the uterus and fetal head on the inferior vena cava and iliac veins. Accordingly, the rate of flow is diminished in lower extremity veins. Adding to the effects of caval compression is the progesterone-induced decrease in venous tone.[25] The combination of elevated lower extremity venous pressure and reduced venous tone conspire to promote lower extremity and vulvar varicosities as well as hemorrhoids.[9]

Pulmonary arterial systolic, diastolic, and mean pressures remain unchanged during the course of normal pregnancy despite the increased cardiac output, implying a reciprocal decline in pulmonary vascular resistance.[2, 16] Thus, the right ventricle, like the left, handles an augmented volume, which it ejects at a normal systolic pressure against a low resistance. The increased work of both ventricles therefore represents pure volume overload.[11, 17, 21]

Moderate isotonic exercise during normal pregnancy provokes an appropriate increment in cardiac output that adds to the already elevated baseline (resting) output.[9, 31, 32] Because the circulatory demands of isotonic exercise for any given workload are added to the increased resting cardiac output, maximum output is reached at a correspondingly lower work level in pregnancy than in the nongravid state.[32] Mild or moderate isotonic exercise generally elicits significant cardiovascular and metabolic responses that are transitory and reversible. A major normal hemodynamic response to exercise that also occurs in pregnancy is the selective redistribution of blood flow to working muscles. Splanchnic circulation and therefore uterine and fetal blood flow are reduced.[31] Although the reduction in uteroplacental blood flow is rapidly reversible upon completion of exercise, pregnant guinea pigs that are chronically exercised throughout gestation reportedly deliver growth-retarded piglets, suggesting a chronic exercise-induced reduction in uterine circulation.[31]

MECHANISMS OF CIRCULATORY CHANGES. The circulatory responses to normal pregnancy can be looked upon either as responses that precede and therefore anticipate the needs of the growing fetus or as adaptive responses to the metabolic and nutritional needs of the products of conception.[33] The increments in body water, blood volume, cardiac output, heart rate, and stroke volume and the fall in peripheral vascular resistance begin by the end of the first trimester, i.e., before fetal metabolic demands are fully evident.[13, 17, 18, 21] The timing and magnitude of hemodynamic changes in normal pregnancy therefore precede and for a time exceed the demands of the fetus, whose needs are anticipated. Two responsible mechanisms are believed to act in concert: (1) the production of hormones by the fetus and placenta (Fig. 60–3) and (2) the uteroplacental circulation, which acts as an arteriovenous shunt.[9, 21] Maternal concentrations of estrogen and progesterone increase almost 100-fold over nonpregnant values.[12] The increase in plasma volume is prompted chiefly by estrogen stimulation of the renin-angiotensin system and, in sequence, by aldosterone-induced sodium ion and water retention.[12] Estrogen administration to pregnant ewes causes an increase in heart rate, cardiac output, and blood flow to the breast, uterus, and skin, while peripheral vascular resistance declines.[34] Progesterone causes venous relaxation, thereby increasing vascular capacity and promoting fluid retention.[35]

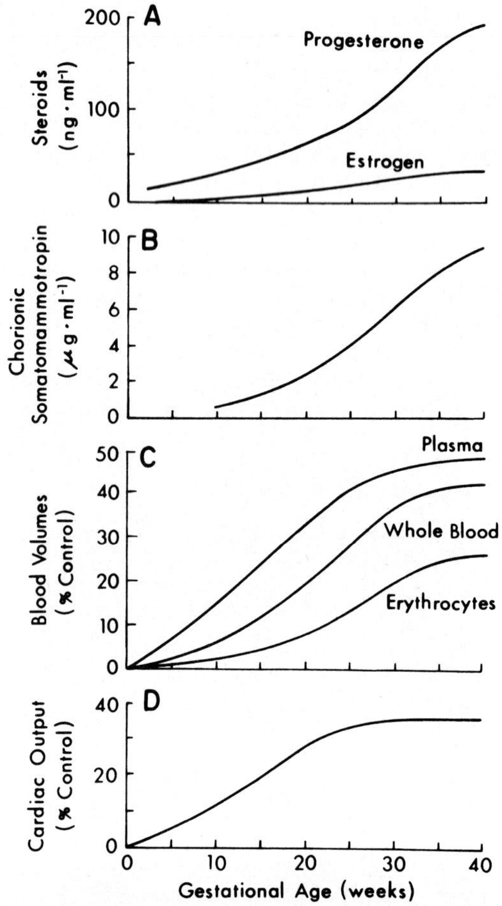

FIGURE 60–3. Extent of increases in several maternal variables during gestation. (From Longo, L. D.: Maternal blood volume and cardiac output during pregnancy: A hypothesis of endocrinologic control. Am. J. Physiol. *245*:R720, 1983, with permission of the American Physiological Society.)

In addition, the uteroplacental circulation represents a low-resistance pathway that functions as an arteriovenous shunt (p. 784).[9] There is a general correlation between total blood volume and the weight of the products of conception.[19] Growth of the uterus, placenta, and breasts is associated with an increase in vascular capacity and in total circulating blood volume.[33] Furthermore, the ability to excrete a water load is limited in the supine position late in pregnancy.[24]

Diminished vascular responsiveness to angiotensin II and a generalized increase in venous distensibility are the most firmly established (but not the only) potentially significant vascular changes. The morphology of the aorta in normal pregnancy has been the subject of a number of studies, albeit with conflicting results. Significant and specific changes have been identified in aortic media of pregnant rabbits, and similar alterations have been described in the aorta of gravid women.[36, 37] Histochemical changes vary according to the duration of pregnancy and include fragmentation of reticular fibers, a decrease in acid mucopolysaccharides, loss of the normal corrugation of elastic fibers, and hypertrophy and hyperplasia of smooth muscle cells. These biochemical and morphological alterations in the aortic wall have been attributed to hormonal effects but remain to be confirmed.[36]

RESPIRATORY CHANGES IN NORMAL PREGNANCY. Changes in the control of respiration, lung volumes, and mechanics occur during the course of normal gestation (Table 60–2). The placenta permits a critical interplay between maternal and fetal gas exchange. During normal pregnancy, respiratory physiology reflects maternal respiration as well as maternal-fetal respiratory interactions.[9a, 16, 32, 38]

Mechanical (anatomical) and hormonal changes influence lung volumes and capacities, airway function, ventilation, diffusing capacity, acid-base balance, and blood gases.[9, 16] Anatomical changes in the thoracic cavity include flaring of the lower ribs and an increase in costal angle.[9] Breathing in pregnancy is more diaphragmatic than costal, indicating enhanced motion of the crural portions of the hemidiaphragms. Inspiratory reserve and tidal volume increase, while respiratory reserve and residual volume decrease. The functional residual capacity (lung volume at the end of quiet expiration) falls as the gravid uterus elevates the diaphragm. However, this fall is accompanied by an increase in inspiratory capacity so that total lung capacity is reduced minimally, if at all.[9, 16, 38–40] Anatomical changes are coupled with hormonal factors. Hyperventilation is believed to be mediated primarily by the effect of progesterone on the respiratory center.[9, 16] Gestational prostaglandins have a bronchodilating effect and are believed to be responsible for the decreased resistance in the large airways and the general bronchodilatation.[9, 16]

Resting oxygen consumption rises progressively during the course of normal pregnancy, reaching its peak increment (about 30 per cent) near term. Hyperventilation is characterized by a substantial increase in tidal volume but little or no increase in respiratory frequency.[9] The increased minute ventilation precedes the rise in oxygen consumption, is approximately twice its magnitude, and begins in early pregnancy, reaching a maximum of approximately 40 to 50 per cent toward term. Progesterone-mediated hyperventilation and hypocapnea are associated with renal excretion of HCO_3^-, so that pH is maintained within the normal range (compensated respiratory alkalosis).[38] Mild to moderate exercise during the first two trimesters provokes a ventilatory response similar to that in the nonpregnant state.[32, 38] In the last trimester, exercise-induced increments in minute ventilation and oxygen consumption are greater in magnitude.[40, 41] Exercise during pregnancy is not limited by the respiratory reserve.[9]

An initial increase in diffusing capacity is followed by a decline toward pregestational levels until 24 to 27 weeks. Values then remain constant during the last trimester but increase again toward term.[9] The decline in diffusing capacity is compensated for by augmented alveolar ventilation, improved gas mixing, and higher alveolar PO_2.

Arterial PCO_2 is decreased in pregnancy to approximately 30 mm Hg (versus 35 to 40 mm Hg in the nonpregnant state).[9, 16] This decrease in PCO_2 facilitates CO_2 transfer from the fetal to the maternal circulation—a desirable response in light of enhanced fetal sensitivity to CO_2. Increased renal secretion of HCO_3^- maintains the pH in the normal range, preventing respiratory alkalosis. Arterial PO_2 increases owing to increased alveolar ventilation, despite a decrease in diffusing capacity.[9, 16]

In brief, the major changes in respiratory function in pregnancy consist of increased minute ventilation (tidal volume), decreased residual volume, enhanced sensitivity of the respiratory center to PCO_2, increased PO_2, decreased PCO_2, and compensated respiratory alkalosis (Table 60–2).

LABOR AND DELIVERY. The circulatory responses to labor and delivery are best understood in light of the method of delivery, maternal posture, and the type and amount of sedation and anesthesia. In unsedated or lightly sedated but unanesthetized women who deliver vaginally, hemodynamics vary at different stages of labor according to maternal posture and the intensity, frequency, and pain of uterine contractions.[4, 10, 42] The contracting uterus finds its support in the retrouterine fulcrum formed by the most protruding segment of the lumbar spine (L4–L5). During a major uterine contraction in the *supine* position, cardiac output increases by approximately 25 per cent, stroke volume by about 35 per cent, and mean systemic arterial pressure by about 10 per cent, while heart rate declines only slightly.[10, 43] The contracting uterus causes virtually complete occlusion of the distal aorta and common iliac arteries as well as complete occlusion of the inferior vena cava.[10] Accordingly, the increment of 300 to 500 ml of blood expressed into the maternal circulation by uterine contraction is diverted into the proximal compartment, causing an exaggerated hemodynamic response. In *lateral recumbency*, the increment in cardiac output associated with a major uterine contraction is only about 10 per cent, with higher levels maintained between contractions (baseline cardiac output).[10, 42] Use of the lateral position during labor for women with heart disease is therefore of considerable importance, serving to mitigate hemodynamic fluctuations and minimize anesthetic hypotension.[42] A general consensus strongly favors the lateral position for labor along with assisted vaginal delivery and analgesia to relieve pain and apprehension.[2, 4, 10, 42, 44]

A knowledge of hemodynamic responses to anesthetics should prompt careful selection of agents and monitoring. Epidural anesthesia with epinephrine added to the anesthetic solution substantially reduces pain, but not uncommonly provokes hypotension and a fall in cardiac output.[4, 10] Epidural anesthesia without epinephrine provides hemodynamic stability, but additional analgesia may be required for continued pain relief.[10] In any event, flotation catheters offer the security of meticulous hemodynamic surveillance not only during labor and delivery but also during the immediate postpartum period.

Cesarean section is reserved for obstetrical indications. Exceptionally, successful cesarean section has been performed during cardiopulmonary arrest.[45, 46]

THE POSTPARTUM PERIOD. The circulatory changes immediately following delivery are influenced by the volume of blood loss, which averages 500 ml with vaginal delivery and approximately twice that with cesarean section. The pregnant woman generally tolerates such losses without ill effect, because the loss is in large part a desirable correction of increased blood volume accrued during gestation. Accordingly, gestational hypervolemia can be looked upon as a safeguard against maternal blood loss at delivery, and normal maternal blood loss can be looked upon as a corrective against the no longer needed gestational hypervolemia.[47] Immediately postpartum, cardiac output rises transiently but appreciably and then falls within an hour to levels 10 to 20 per cent above predelivery measurements.[15, 43] The rise has been attributed to relief of inferior vena caval compression coupled with the increase in postpartum blood volume associated with autotransfusion from the contracting uterus and absorption into the circulation of extracellular fluid accumulated during gestation. Arterial blood pressure remains unchanged after delivery, while cardiac rate declines. Postpartum bradycardia and the elevated cardiac output persist for days or even weeks.[15] Postpartum diuresis then reduces total body water, and the pregravid blood volume is restored within approximately 4 to 6 weeks.[2] The magnitude of the rise in blood volume and the rapidity with which it is restored to nongravid levels depend in part on renal function, which may be capable of rapid clearance of excess extracellular fluid.[19]

CARDIORESPIRATORY SYMPTOMS AND SIGNS IN NORMAL PREGNANCY

The circulatory and respiratory changes that occur during normal pregnancy provide a basis for understanding symptoms, physical signs, and electrocardiographic, roentgenographic, and echocardiographic changes that simulate and are sometimes erroneously attributed to heart disease (Table 60–3). Dyspnea, easy fatigability, and a reduction

TABLE 60–3 CARDIORESPIRATORY SYMPTOMS AND SIGNS IN NORMAL PREGNANCY

Dyspnea (hyperventilation)
Easy fatigability
Decreased exercise tolerance
Lightheadedness
Syncope
Peripheral edema
Basilar rales
Small waterhammer pulse
Prominent jugular venous AV crests and *x-y* troughs
Brisk, displaced left ventricular impulse
Right ventricular impulse
Increased first heart sound
Persistently split second heart sound
Third heart sound
Pulmonic midsystolic murmur
Supraclavicular systolic murmur
Continuous murmurs
ECG changes in rhythm, axis, and repolarization
X-ray—lateral displacement of apex, increased lung markings

in exercise tolerance are relatively common.[15, 43] The combination of basal rales (that disappear after coughing or deep breathing) and peripheral edema can be misleading. The systemic arterial pulse exhibits a brisk rise and collapse (small waterhammer) as early as the first trimester,[48] and arterial pulsations can sometimes be palpated in the fingertips. The jugular venous pulse becomes more conspicuous after the twentieth week of pregnancy, with relatively prominent *a* and *v* waves and brisk *x* and *y* descents. Mean jugular venous pressure, estimated from the superficial jugular vein, remains normal. Precordial palpation discloses a brisk, nonsustained left ventricular impulse and often an impulse over the right ventricle and pulmonary trunk.[48] As pregnancy progresses, however, enlargement of the breasts and abdomen makes these palpatory signs difficult if not impossible to elicit.

AUSCULTATORY FINDINGS. Auscultatory signs accompanying normal gestation begin late in the first trimester, disappear (with few exceptions) within a week after delivery, and include variations in heart sounds and the presence of systolic and continuous murmurs.[15, 48, 49] The first heart sound increases in intensity owing to tachycardia and increased left ventricular contractility (Fig. 60–1) and is often prominently split. The second heart sound, at least toward the end of pregnancy, tends to exhibit persistent expiratory splitting, especially when patients are examined in the lateral position. Third heart sounds are common in normal young women, so it is not surprising that the increased rate of atrioventricular flow during pregnancy augments the intensity of these sounds.[48] A prominent third heart sound is occasionally followed by brief, soft, low-frequency aftervibrations mistaken for a short mid-diastolic murmur. With this exception, diastolic murmurs are not features of uncomplicated pregnancy. Fourth heart sounds are seldom heard in healthy young persons of either sex and do not occur during normal pregnancy.

Two types of normal or innocent systolic murmurs occur in healthy nonpregnant women.[50] Not surprisingly, these murmurs increase in intensity and prevalence during gestation. The innocent or *normal pulmonic midsystolic murmur* (maximal in the second left intercostal space) represents audible vibrations caused by right ventricular ejection into the pulmonary trunk, while *normal supraclavicular systolic murmurs* originate in brachiocephalic arteries at their points of branching from the aortic arch.[50, 51] Both these murmurs are midsystolic, beginning after the first heart sound and ending before the second, and both are augmented by the increased cardiac output and stroke volume of pregnancy. The pulmonic midsystolic murmur seldom exceeds grade III (of VI), but the supraclavicular systolic murmur may exceed grade IV and occasionally radiates, with attenuation, below the clavicles. A third innocent murmur, peculiar to pregnancy, is the *mammary souffle* that is either systolic or continuous.[50] The mammary souffle, like all arterial murmurs, is louder in systole whether or not it is continuous, and at times it is clearly confined to systole.[50–52] The mammary souffle is heard over the breasts in late pregnancy but especially in the postpartum period in lactating women. There is a tendency for the souffle to be loudest in the second or third right or left intercostal space. The souffle is augmented by firm pressure of the stethoscope or by digital compression adjacent to the site of auscultation and is best elicited with the patient supine, sometimes vanishing altogether in the upright position. Day-to-day or cycle-to-cycle variation of the souffle together with its permanent disappearance after termination of lactation are reassuring features of normality. A second and far more common continuous murmur is the *venous hum*,[50] which is relatively frequent in nonpregnant young women and, if properly sought, is almost universal during gestation. Rarely, the hum is sufficiently loud to radiate beneath the clavicle, but wherever heard, it promptly vanishes with compression of the ipsilateral deep jugular vein.[50]

Murmurs accompanying organic heart disease may either increase in intensity during pregnancy or, conversely, decrease to the point of disappearance. For example, the systolic murmurs of aortic or pulmonic stenosis tend to increase, and the murmur of mitral stenosis is reinforced because augmented blood flow and shortening of the diastolic filling period combine to increase the rate of flow across the mitral valve. Conversely, murmurs of mitral or aortic regurgitation soften or even disappear as peripheral vascular resistance declines.[53] Auscultatory signs of mitral valve prolapse (p. 1048)—mid to late systolic click(s) and a late systolic murmur—vary with alterations in left ventricular volume and shape.[54] The increase in left ventricular volume at end diastole during pregnancy serves to attenuate or abolish the click(s) and late systolic murmur.[55, 56] Similarly, the systolic murmur of hypertrophic obstructive cardiomyopathy may decrease or vanish as the left ventricle handles a larger volume during gestation.[57]

ELECTROCARDIOGRAPHIC CHANGES. The electrocardiogram in normal pregnant women may exhibit changes in rate, rhythm, P-R interval, QRS axis, ST segment, T wave, and Q-T interval.[15, 58] The increase in heart rate accounts for a slight decrease in the P-R and Q-T intervals.[58] A variety of arrhythmias have been recorded during normal pregnancy, especially premature atrial beats and uniform premature ventricular beats.[15] Reentrant supraventricular tachycardia is a common sustained tachyarrhythmia in normal young women, and pregnancy is believed to lower the threshold for recurrences in susceptible patients.[2, 15] The QRS amplitude and duration remain unchanged, but the axis sometimes undergoes a leftward shift during the third trimester.[58] Alternatively, the QRS axis may change little if at all or become somewhat vertical as the fetus descends into the pelvis. Small Q waves and inverted T waves may appear in lead III in the third trimester, with both changes decreasing or normalizing during deep inspiration.[15] Occasionally, transient T-wave inversions and ST segment depressions occur in limb leads and especially in left precordial leads; these changes may recur in the same leads during subsequent normal pregnancies.[15, 59–62]

CHEST X-RAY. Radiation exposure is to be avoided in pregnant women, so there is justifiably relatively little information on sequential plain film radiography. As pregnancy advances, the exaggerated lumbar lordosis together with elevation of the diaphragm results in upward and lateral displacement of the cardiac apex and a horizontal cardiac position.[15] The left cardiac silhouette straightens, the pulmonary trunk becomes prominent, and vascular soft tissue densities increase,[63] simulating mitral stenosis.

THE ECHOCARDIOGRAM. Because echocardiography can be used with impunity during pregnancy, it is important to recognize that increases in cardiac output, stroke volume, ventricular volumes, and internal dimensions at end-diastole are features of normal pregnancy (Fig. 60–1). There is a slight but significant increase in end-diastolic dimensions of the left ventricle when the patient is examined in the lateral position but not in the supine position.[17, 21] Left atrial size and right ventricular internal dimensions may show small increases as well.[15] Indices of left ventricular function remain unchanged or improve.[17, 21]

HEART DISEASE IN WOMEN OF CHILDBEARING AGE

Comprehension of the cardiocirculatory and respiratory changes and the symptoms and signs that accompany normal pregnancy provides the basis for an understanding of the clinical manifestations of heart disease in the pregnant woman. Cardiac disease may be preexisting or may be induced by the gravid state (preeclampsia, thromboembolic disease, peripartum cardiomyopathy, and, rarely, aortic dissection). The types of cardiac disorders—acquired, congenital, or developmental—of greatest interest during pregnancy are those likely to occur in young women. Furthermore, cardiac surgery has produced a new and increasing population—the postoperative cardiac patient of childbearing age.[6, 64, 65] Patterns of heart disease vary geographically and socioeconomically and have changed over time, especially during the last four decades.[2, 3, 7, 66–68] Rheumatic heart disease still prevails, but congenital heart disease is now encountered with increasing frequency.

RHEUMATIC HEART DISEASE

(See also Chaps. 33 and 54)

ACUTE RHEUMATIC FEVER. The first attack of acute rheumatic fever has its peak incidence before puberty. Because of recurrence, an occasional young woman conceives while suffering from active rheumatic fever, which is a serious complication of pregnancy.[3] Recurrences sometimes develop during gestation, although there is no convincing evidence that pregnancy per se predisposes to active rheumatic fever.[69] *Chorea gravidarum* (the now rarely seen Sydenham's chorea occurring in the early months of pregnancy) is especially ominous, resulting in spontaneous abortion, preterm labor, intrauterine fetal death, maternal heart failure, hyperpyrexia, profound exhaustion, and occasionally maternal death.[3, 70] Termination of pregnancy is indicated when severe chorea is accompanied by violent uncontrollable movements, agitation, and psychiatric disturbances. Although about two-thirds of women with chorea gravidarum have histories of prior chorea or rheumatic fever, occasionally women manifest chorea during consecutive pregnancies but are otherwise free of it and, in rare cases, completely free of clinical evidence of rheumatic heart disease.[70] Chorea is more likely to occur in primigravidas, and in about half the cases the disorder begins during the first trimester. The disorder remits prior to delivery in approximately one-third of patients and shortly thereafter in the remainder.

Active rheumatic carditis (p. 1711) is a serious complication of pregnancy in underdeveloped countries. Patients may die suddenly during labor or shortly after delivery, and fatal cases have been reported without preexisting rheumatic valvular heart disease.[2] Conversely, active rheumatic carditis may initiate or aggravate heart failure in patients with established rheumatic valvular disease.

CHRONIC RHEUMATIC HEART DISEASE (see Chap. 33). This form of heart disease in pregnancy is represented by pure or dominant mitral stenosis in 90 per cent of cases (Fig. 60–4), by mitral regurgitation in about 6 per cent to 7 per cent, and by aortic regurgitation/stenosis in most of the remainder.[2, 9a] The majority of women with rheumatic valvular disease, whether it is mild, moderate, or occasionally severe, can be managed through pregnancy and delivery. Nevertheless, these patients run risks of complications, the majority relating to mitral stenosis.

The basic hemodynamic abnormality in mitral stenosis (p. 1024)—the impediment to effective left atrial emptying—is aggravated by two of the normal cardiocirculatory responses to pregnancy, namely, the increased cardiac output and the shortened diastolic filling period as a consequence of the more rapid heart rate. These circulatory changes conspire to augment the left atrioventricular pressure gradient and to increase pulmonary venous and

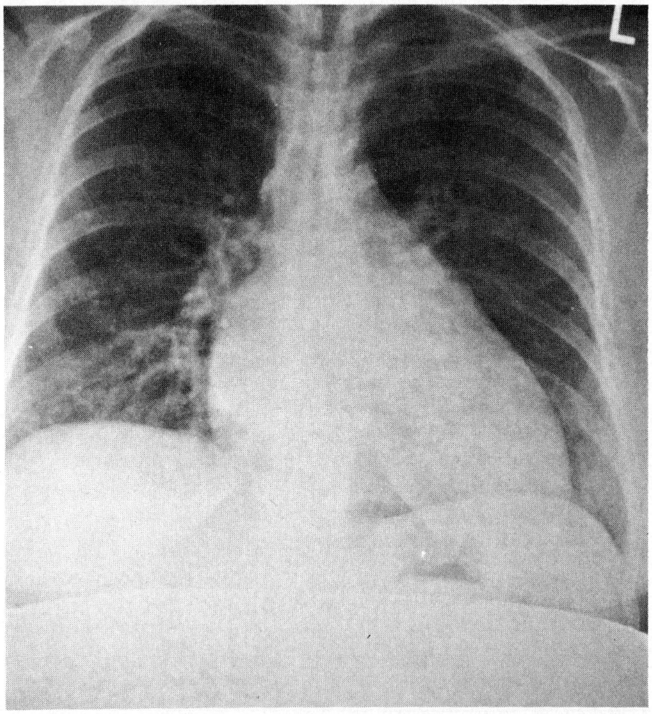

FIGURE 60–4. Chest x-ray at 36 weeks gestation in a 32-year-old woman with rheumatic mitral stenosis and mild mitral regurgitation in sinus rhythm. A lead apron shields the abdomen. Both hemidiaphragms are elevated. Pulmonary vascular markings are increased, especially the right hilus. The left cardiac border is straight with slight convexity of the left atrial appendage, and the right atrial silhouette is prominent.

pulmonary capillary pressures. Should atrial fibrillation supervene, the hemodynamic burden is compounded by the loss of left atrial contraction and by a further acceleration of heart rate. Complications take the form of cough, breathlessness, orthopnea, paroxysmal nocturnal dyspnea, or pulmonary edema (sequelae of pulmonary venous congestion); brisk hemoptysis (hemorrhage from varicosed bronchial veins); right ventricular failure (pulmonary arterial hypertension); and less commonly, systemic or pulmonary emboli and infective endocarditis.[2, 71] Pulmonary edema is an ominous development, because the offending gestational hemodynamic burden responsible for the complication is unremitting and progressive. Right ventricular failure adds to the tendency of the pregnant woman to develop peripheral edema and varicose veins, increasing the risk of pulmonary embolism from chronic venous stasis.

Severe pulmonary hypertension with a high and relatively fixed pulmonary vascular resistance (p. 796) exposes the gravid woman to special risks. Physiological adaptation to fluctuations in cardiac output and systemic vascular resistance is then limited. An increase in venous return is accompanied by a rise in pulmonary arterial pressure and/or progression of right ventricular failure. Physical effort, stress, and excitement may provoke acute right ventricular failure, and the inability to increase cardiac output in the face of a fall in systemic vascular resistance risks syncope. Pulmonary emboli are more likely to occur in mitral stenosis with pulmonary hypertension and are more apt to be lethal.

The time course of symptoms complicating rheumatic mitral stenosis is noteworthy.[3] Previously asymptomatic young women with rheumatic mitral stenosis occasionally develop unanticipated acute pulmonary edema during pregnancy, although the incidence of pulmonary venous congestion increases with maternal age and parity.[2] The risk is maximal in late pregnancy, during labor, and in the early puerperium, since gestational hypervolemia is progressive to term; the increase in cardiac rate persists; cardiac output is maintained through the last trimester; and labor, delivery, and the puerperium impose additional hemodynamic demands on the heart and circulation (see above).

Patients with pure or predominant *rheumatic mitral regurgitation* (p. 1034), especially in sinus rhythm, usually accommodate satisfactorily to the hemodynamic burdens of pregnancy. The left ventricle copes comparatively well with the gestational increment in volume. The increase in heart rate is little or no handicap, and pulmonary hypertension is uncommon. Infective endocarditis is a distinct risk, however, and rupture of the chordae tendineae may acutely augment the mitral regurgitation.[72–75] Spontaneous (noninfectious) chordal rupture occurs in a different setting (see below).[74, 75]

Rheumatic aortic valve disease is almost always accompanied by disease of the mitral valve, and the hemodynamic consequences of pregnancy must be considered in this light. The responses to isolated pure aortic regurgitation or aortic stenosis are discussed on pp. 1052–1069.

Rheumatic tricuspid stenosis (p. 1069) seldom occurs without mitral stenosis.[76] In this context, the tricuspid valve may exhibit pure incompetence, pure stenosis, or varying combinations of each, but it is seldom spared. Obstruction of the tricuspid orifice serves to increase systemic venous pressure, promote peripheral edema, aggravate varices, and limit cardiac output at rest and with stress.

CONGENITAL HEART DISEASE

(See also Chaps. 30 and 31)

Increased survival of patients with congenital heart disease into adulthood results from the benefits of surgery.[5] Operation not only increases the life span of patients who have anomalies with an inherent tendency for long survival (Table 60–4) but also permits increasing numbers of women with disorders that were previously fatal in early life to reach childbearing age.[44, 64]

ATRIAL SEPTAL DEFECT (pp. 915 and 982). The natural history of ostium secundum atrial septal defect spans the childbearing years, and most of the patients with this anomaly are female.[51] The great majority of women with uncomplicated ostium secundum atrial septal defects endure pregnancy – even multiple births—with relative impunity (Fig. 60–5*B*).[51] Infective endocarditis poses little or no threat. An important consideration, however, is the risk of paradoxical emboli from leg veins when embolic material courses from the inferior vena cava through the atrial septal defect into the systemic circulation (Fig. 60–5*A*).[77] Accordingly, meticulous leg care is obligatory, with emphasis on minimizing venous stasis. After the fourth decade, atrial fibrillation, flutter or paroxysmal supraventricular tachycardia increase in frequency and represent serious complications leading to disability and cardiac failure.[51] Pulmonary hypertension develops comparatively late in ostium secundum atrial septal defect and is seldom seen in pregnant women below age 30 years.[51] Occasionally women with pulmonary hypertension tolerate pregnancy with surprisingly little difficulty, but this is exceptional.[5] The incidence of pulmonary hypertension is much higher and the onset earlier among patients with atrial septal defect born at high altitudes.[78]

PATENT DUCTUS ARTERIOSUS (pp. 923 and 993). This congenital anomaly predominates in females.[51] The combination of patent ductus and pregnancy is becoming of less and less practical importance because the clinical diagnosis is simple and surgical division is safe, routine, and curative in childhood. An asymptomatic woman with a small or moderate-sized ductus and normal pulmonary arterial pressure can expect an uncomplicated pregnancy (Fig. 60–6) apart from the risk of infective endocarditis. In the presence of a large ductus with a left-to-right shunt, pregnancy can provoke or aggravate left ventricular failure. With a reversed shunt through a large ductus (suprasystemic pulmonary vascular resistance), maternal mortality is appreciable. Such patients only rarely experience uneventful pregnancies.[2]

PULMONIC VALVE STENOSIS (pp. 942 and 991). In its isolated form, this anomaly occurs with equal frequency in men and women. The majority of untreated patients proceed through infancy and childhood with little handicap, so females present during the childbearing years. In asymptomatic young women with mild to moderate and occasionally even severe pulmonic stenosis, pregnancy is usually well tolerated despite the increased volume load

TABLE 60–4 COMMON CONGENITAL CARDIAC DEFECTS WITH EXPECTED ADULT SURVIVAL LISTED IN ORDER OF OCCURRENCE IN FEMALES

Ostium secundum atrial septal defect
Patent ductus arteriosus
Pulmonic valve stenosis
Ventricular septal defect with pulmonic stenosis
Coarctation of the aorta
Aortic valve stenosis/regurgitation
Functionally normal bicuspid aortic valve

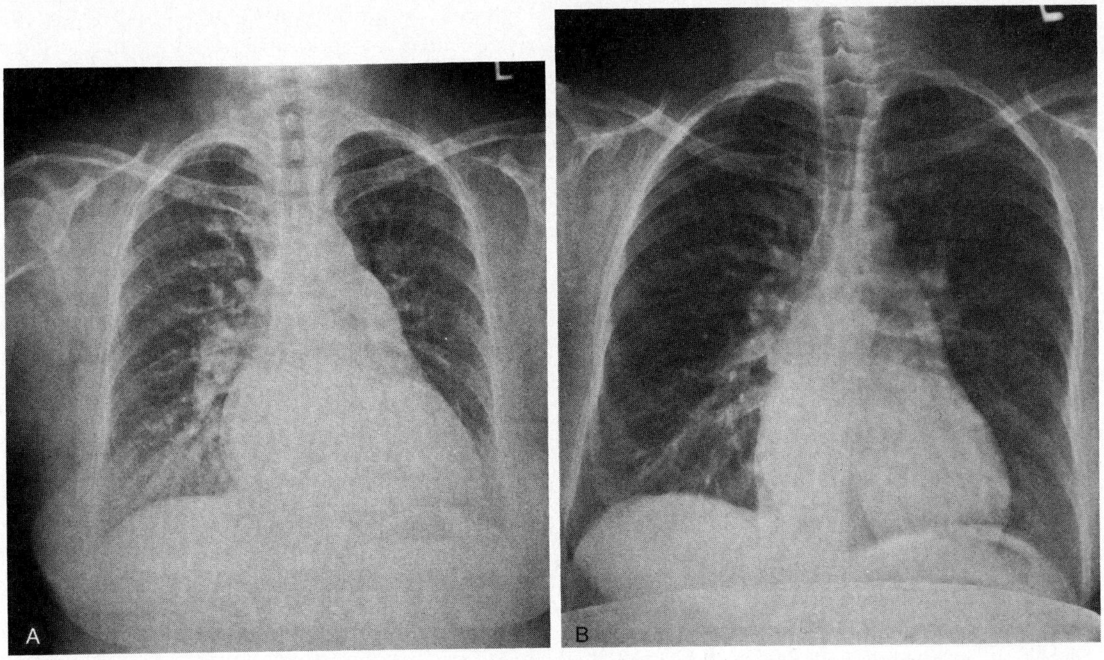

FIGURE 60–5. *A*, Chest x-ray after delivery of a 39-year-old multigravida with varicose veins and a puerperal paradoxical embolus to the right kidney. The x-ray is typical of an ostium secundum atrial septal defect, which permitted passage of caval embolus to the systemic circulation. *B*, Chest x-ray during the last of nine uneventful pregnancies in a 54-year-old woman who later underwent repair of an ostium secundum atrial septal defect, shown here. Of three female offspring, one had this congenital defect.

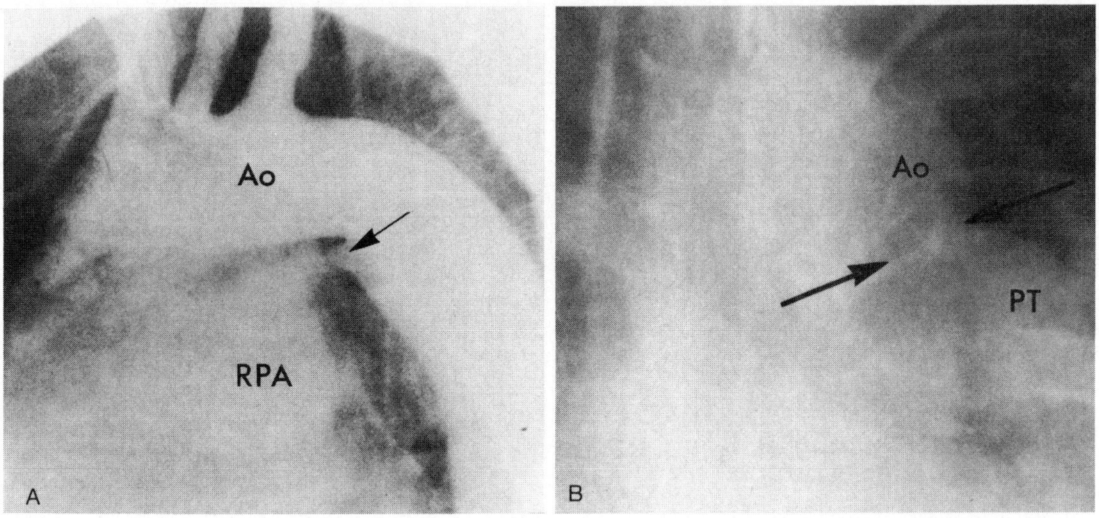

FIGURE 60–6. *A*, Lateral aortogram in a 57-year-old woman with a patent ductus arteriosus (arrow), a pulmonary-to-systemic flow ratio of 1.8/1.0, and a pulmonary arterial pressure of 45/12 mm Hg. She had had 20 pregnancies that resulted in 12 live births. *B*, Posteroanterior chest x-ray showing calcium in the ductus (arrows). Ao = aorta; RPA = right pulmonary artery; PT = pulmonary trunk. (From Perloff, J. K., *In* Gleicher, N. [ed.]: Principles of Medical Therapy in Pregnancy. New York, Plenum Medical Book Co., 1985, p. 665, with permission.)

on an already pressure-loaded right ventricle.[5] In view of the simplicity of clinical recognition and diagnostic confirmation, the majority of patients with moderate to marked pulmonic valve stenosis undergo surgical repair or balloon dilatation long before pregnancy.

COARCTATION OF THE AORTA (pp. 929 and 994). The major symptoms in unoperated coarctation, which occurs predominantly in men, derive from four complications: congestive heart failure, rupture of the aorta or dissecting aneurysm, infective endocarditis (usually on a bicuspid aortic valve), and cerebral hemorrhage from rupture of an aneurysm of the circle of Willis.[51] The majority of patients without surgical correction live to adulthood, but only a minority reach 40 years of age. Surgical repair of coarctation of the aorta is generally performed in early childhood, so that more and more patients born with this anomaly are reaching childbearing age *after* undergoing operative repair. Even so, the risk of a coexisting bicuspid aortic valve persists (see below), and the threat of rupture of an aneurysm of the circle of Willis is not abolished.[64]

The behavior of the systemic arterial pressure in pregnancy complicated by coarctation of the aorta is analogous to normal pregnancy, i.e., the directional changes are similar, but values are higher initially in patients with coarctation.[51] Overall maternal mortality is estimated at 3.5 per cent [2, 79] and morbidity (cardiovascular complications without death) remains high but is lower than in the past.[5, 80, 81] Not surprisingly, risk relates to aortic rupture, cerebrovascular accidents, congestive heart failure, pulmonary edema, and infective endocarditis.

CONGENITAL AORTIC VALVE DISEASE. A functionally normal bicuspid aortic valve or bicuspid aortic stenosis or regurgitation predominates in men, but this does not reduce the importance of these lesions when they sporadically occur among pregnant women. A *functionally normal bicuspid aortic valve* (p. 932) is perhaps the commonest congenital anomaly of the heart or great arteries.[82] High susceptibility to infective endocarditis poses a constant threat.[51] An isolated functionally normal bicuspid aortic valve is not likely to be identified in young women before or during pregnancy because the clinical index of suspicion is low and the auscultatory signs are inconspicuous. The anomaly may therefore announce itself after delivery, when infective endocarditis causes persistent fever or results in the sudden appearance of aortic regurgitation.[83]

A functionally normal bicuspid aortic valve is commonly accompanied by mild *aortic regurgitation*.[51, 82] Chronic severe congenital bicuspid aortic regurgitation progresses insidiously, so the fully developed hemodynamic pattern characteristically awaits young adulthood.[51] Moderate and even severe chronic aortic regurgitation is well tolerated by an otherwise normal heart, which is generally the case in young pregnant women with this lesion. Furthermore, the fall in systemic vascular resistance during pregnancy and the increase in cardiac rate (shortened diastole) serve to decrease regurgitant flow. The risk of infective endocarditis is, however, undiminished.

In congenital *aortic valve stenosis*, the increased cardiac output of pregnancy adds to an already pressure-loaded left ventricle, augmenting the transaortic gradient and left ventricular systolic pressure and work. Women with mild to moderate aortic stenosis tolerate pregnancy relatively well but are susceptible to infective endocarditis following delivery. In patients with severe aortic stenosis, circulatory reserve is limited. Syncope, especially after effort or excitement, may first appear during gestation. Should cerebral symptoms, dyspnea, or angina precede conception or develop early in gestation, serious sequelae can be anticipated.[5]

COMMON CONGENITAL CARDIAC DEFECTS SELDOM SEEN IN ADULTS

These include ventricular septal defect, endocardial cushion defect, tetralogy of Fallot, complete transposition of the great arteries, and tricuspid atresia.

VENTRICULAR SEPTAL DEFECT (pp. 920 and 985). Isoljlated *perimembranous* ventricular septal defect is one of the most frequent congenital cardiac malformations at birth.[51] The anomaly is of comparatively little importance as a potential complication of pregnancy because as many as 45 per cent of the defects close spontaneously in early life or unrelieved congestive heart failure in infancy results in death unless pulmonary vascular resistance rises or the defect is closed surgically. An occasional acyanotic adult survivor with a restrictive ventricular septal defect (little or no pulmonary hypertension) confronts pregnancy with a risk proportional to the functional class which, in turn, is determined by the magnitude of the left-to-right shunt and the physiological state of the left ventricle. In women with relatively large left-to-right shunts, the added volume load of pregnancy can provoke heart failure, and sporadic deaths have been reported from antepartum cardiac failure as well as from postpartum paradoxical embolism.[2] The high-velocity jet of ventricular septal defect increases the risk of infective endocarditis, which may occur during the puerperium.

EISENMENGER'S COMPLEX (pp. 915 and 999). In Eisenmenger's complex, or nonrestrictive perimembranous ventricular septal defect with pulmonary vascular obstructive disease, the level of pulmonary vascular resistance is the chief determinant of the right-to-left shunt and, accordingly, of the risk of pregnancy.[5, 84, 85] Maternal mortality has been estimated at 30 to 70 per cent, with death occurring either during gestation or the puerperium.[85, 86] Hemoptysis may recur or first appear during gestation.[87] A number of physiological changes conspire to pose potential threats. The gestational fall in systemic vascular resistance augments the right-to-left shunt, reduces arterial oxygen saturation, and increases the hematocrit. Conversely, bearing down during labor, by elevating systemic vascular resistance, can suddenly depress cardiac output and provoke syncope.[5] Fluctuations in systemic vascular resistance, cardiac output, and blood volume are tolerated poorly because of the fixed pulmonary vascular resistance. It has also been proposed that widespread thromboses in already compromised pulmonary arteries and arterioles result in a rapid postpartum increase in pulmonary vascular obstruction.[85]

TETRALOGY OF FALLOT (pp. 946 and 988). Women with the cyanotic form of this anomaly seldom experience normal full-term pregnancies.[51] Offspring have low birth weights (dysmaturity), an observation in accord with the generalization that infants of cyanotic mothers are typically small for gestational age.[51, 88, 89] The magnitude of the right-to-left shunt varies inversely with systemic vascular resistance, as in Eisenmenger's complex. The decrease in peripheral resistance accompanying pregnancy coupled with the increase in cardiac output (and venous return to the obstructed right ventricle) results in a larger right-to-left shunt, a fall in systemic arterial oxygen saturation, deeper cyanosis, and a rising hematocrit. Although full-term pregnancies occasionally occur, the threat to mother and child is considerable. Labile hemodynamic adjustments during labor, delivery, and the immediate postpartum period place the mother at further risk. A sudden decrease in systemic vascular resistance serves to provoke intense cyanosis and occasionally syncope with death.[2] Infective endocarditis poses an additional hazard.

UNCOMMON CONGENITAL CARDIAC DEFECTS

Some uncommon congenital cardiac defects with expected adult survival are listed in Table 60–5. Uncomplicated *situs inversus* is innocuous, because the heart and circulation are otherwise anatomically and physiologically normal.[51] *Situs solitus with dextrocardia*, however, is almost invariably associated with additional congenital cardiac malformations, the presence and degree of which determine the risk of pregnancy.[51] The coexisting anomalies are congenitally corrected trans-

TABLE 60–5 SOME UNCOMMON CONGENITAL DEFECTS IN WHICH SURVIVAL TO CHILDBEARING AGE IS EXPECTED

Situs inversus with dextrocardia
Situs solitus with dextrocardia
Congenital complete heart block
Congenitally corrected transposition of the great arteries
Congenital pulmonic valve regurgitation
Ebstein's anomaly
Primary pulmonary hypertension
Lutembacher syndrome
Coronary arteriovenous fistula
Pulmonary arteriovenous fistula

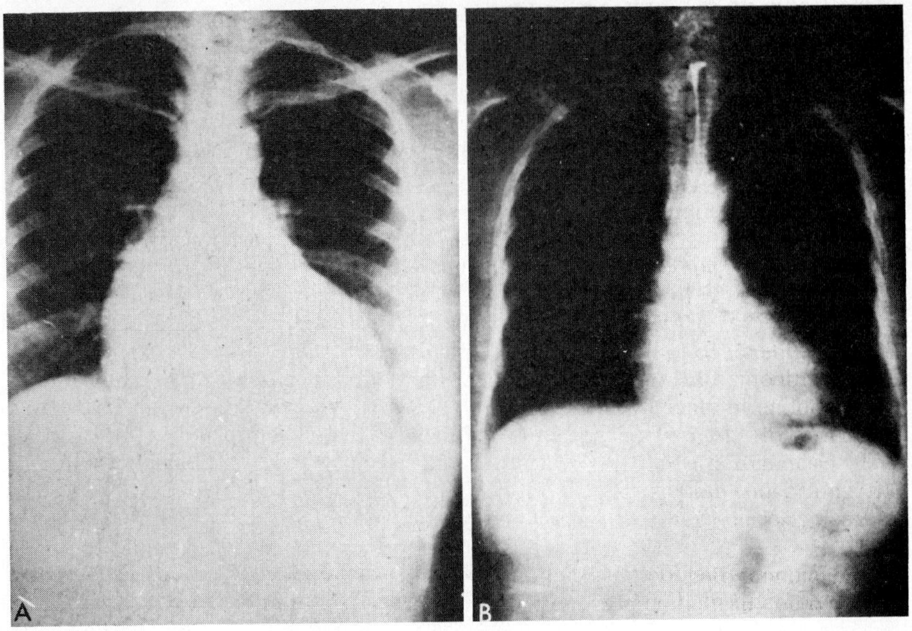

FIGURE 60–7. *A,* Admission chest roentgenogram showing cardiomegaly in a patient with peripartum cardiomyopathy. *B,* Normal heart size in same patient 6 months later. (From Demakis, J. G., et al.: Natural course of peripartum cardiomyopathy. Circulation *44*:1053, 1971, by permission of the American Heart Association, Inc.)

position of the great arteries (see below), pulmonic stenosis, and ventricular septal defect.[51] The association of either uncomplicated congenitally corrected transposition, mild pulmonic stenosis, or a left-to-right interatrial shunt poses little or no threat, but severe pulmonic stenosis with reversed interventricular or interatrial shunt involves the risk of cyanosis, as cited above.

CONGENITAL COMPLETE HEART BLOCK (pp. 967 and 1002). This anomaly occurs with equal frequency in men and women, and the natural history justifies cautious optimism at least into young adulthood.[51, 90] Pregnancy is usually uneventful in otherwise normal women with congenital complete heart block, although there are a few reports of Stokes-Adams attacks first appearing during gestation.[2, 51] It is noteworthy that the functional state of the heart can apparently remain unimpaired when a pregnant woman has an artificial fixed-rate pacemaker.[91] It is also noteworthy that in pregnant women with systemic connective tissue diseases, especially systemic lupus erythematosus, the fetus is at risk for congenital complete heart block.[49, 92, 93]

CONGENITALLY CORRECTED TRANSPOSITION OF THE GREAT ARTERIES (p. 957). The response of patients with this anomaly to pregnancy is determined by the type and degree of coexisting anomalies that commonly take the form of prolonged atrioventricular conduction, incompetence of the systemic atrioventricular valve, ventricular septal defect, and pulmonic stenosis.[51]

EBSTEIN'S ANOMALY OF THE TRICUSPID VALVE (pp. 951 and 997). This involves men and women equally and is often compatible with a relatively long and active life.[51] Successful pregnancies have been reported, but gestation poses a number of potential hazards.[94, 95] The functionally inadequate right ventricle, already burdened by tricuspid regurgitation, is ill equipped to cope with the increased cardiac output of pregnancy. Recurrent episodes of supraventricular tachycardia, atrial fibrillation, or atrial flutter occur in about one-third of nongravid patients with Ebstein's anomaly, and these tachyarrhythmias are not likely to be well tolerated if they recur during pregnancy, especially when Wolff-Parkinson-White syndrome preexcitation permits very rapid ventricular rates.[51, 62] Cyanosis caused by reversed interatrial shunting may first appear during pregnancy in response to right ventricular failure.[51] Chronic cyanosis diminishes the probability of successful gestation and introduces the risk of paradoxical embolism (see above).

PRIMARY PULMONARY HYPERTENSION (p. 805). This condition (*not* necessarily a form of congenital heart disease) poses formidable risks for the pregnant woman; the disorder is most frequent in young women, with a female-to-male ratio of 5 to 1. Sudden death can be precipitated by a variety of seemingly innocuous stresses, and maternal mortality is approximately 50 per cent.[2, 51, 96] Effort syncope, chest pain, dyspnea, weakness, and fatigue may first appear during pregnancy, and not surprisingly, mortality is highest in symptomatic women. An increase in cardiac output coupled with a fall in systemic vascular resistance is tolerated poorly in the face of fixed pulmonary vascular resistance. Labor, delivery, and the puerperium are even more critical times.

CONGENITAL PULMONARY ARTERIOVENOUS FISTULAS (p. 941). These lesions pose interesting theoretical and practical issues. Because the fistulas are typically in the lower lobes, progressive elevation of the diaphragm during pregnancy serves to compress fistulous flow, decrease or abolish the venoarterial mixing, and decrease cyanosis.[51] Accordingly, the accompanying systolic or continuous murmur may disappear during pregnancy, reappearing after delivery.[97]

LUTEMBACHER SYNDROME (p. 915). This malformation is defined as a congenital defect in the atrial septum (ostium secundum atrial septal defect) together with acquired mitral stenosis.[51] The syndrome is more common among females, which is understandable because both ostium secundum atrial septal defect and rheumatic mitral stenosis prevail in women. When atrial septal defect and mitral stenosis coexist, each lesion modifies the hemodynamics and clinical expressions of the other.[51] Orthopnea, paroxysmal nocturnal dyspnea, pulmonary edema, and hemoptysis characteristic of uncomplicated mitral stenosis are attenuated by the decompressing effect of the interatrial communication, but relief of these symptoms is replaced by the fatigue of low systemic output. The natural history of an atrial septal defect is unfavorably influenced by mitral stenosis, which tends to augment the left-to-right shunt.[51]

Among the *uncommon congenital anomalies that seldom permit adult survival* is the univentricular heart.[51] Reports of successful pregnancy in patients with a single ventricle and pulmonic stenosis are sporadic and even less so for patients without pulmonic stenosis.[51, 98, 99]

DEVELOPMENTAL DEFECTS

Two cardiac disorders that represent developmental abnormalities of connective tissue—mitral valve prolapse and the Marfan syndrome—may complicate pregnancy. Because the term "mitral valve prolapse" has pathological connotations, considerable effort has been expended to establish acceptable diagnostic standards.[51, 100]

MITRAL VALVE PROLAPSE (p. 1045). The normal superior displacement of the mitral valve leaflets during systole becomes pathologic when excessive (abnormal) valvuloventricular disproportion is caused by a primary connective tissue disease of mitral leaflets, chordae tendineae, and annulus in otherwise normal persons or in patients with connective tissue disease. The increased left ventricular volume and reduced systemic vascular resistance of normal pregnancy serve to diminish leaflet-chordal redundancy and attenuate mitral valve prolapse.[56, 101] Echocardiographic superior systolic displacement lessens, and the mid to late systolic click(s) and late systolic murmur soften or disappear altogether.[56, 101, 102] Under these circumstances, a secure diagnosis of mitral valve prolapse on the basis of clinical examination may be difficult or impossible. Yet mitral valve prolapse, if present, predisposes to infective endocarditis, certainly when accompanied by mitral regurgitation. Because bacteremia may occur during labor and delivery, prophylaxis for infective endocarditis is warranted. When mild, moderate, or even marked mitral regurgitation is present, the hemodynamic changes of pregnancy are generally well tolerated, provided that left ventricular function is normal or nearly so. Spontaneous noninfectious rupture of chordae tendineae during pregnancy occasionally complicates mitral valve prolapse, but it is not clear whether the connective tissue changes that occur during pregnancy or the stress of labor and delivery increase susceptibility to this potential complication.[75]

The most common sustained tachyarrhythmia in mitral valve prolapse is reentrant supraventricular tachycardia.[54] This arrhythmia is usually responsive to digitalis glycosides, which can safely be maintained during the course of pregnancy. The frequency of premature ventricular beats tends to decrease during pregnancy in response to an increase in left ventricular volume; however, if multiform or repetitive ventricular ectopic beats persist, beta-adrenoceptor blockade can be used with the constraints discussed on page 1864. In light of the reported familial recurrence of mitral valve prolapse, consideration must be given to the possibility of genetic transmission.[51, 101, 103]

MARFAN SYNDROME (p. 1725). A woman affected by the Marfan syndrome is confronted by two pregnancy-associated risks: first, the 50 per cent probability of genetic transmission, and second, the risk of maternal cardiac complications.[104–106] The connective tissue abnormality of the Marfan syndrome involves the mitral annulus, leaflets, and chordae tendineae (mitral valve prolapse [see above]) and the aortic root (aortic regurgitation and the grave threat of dissecting aneurysm).[104, 106] Nearly all patients with this syndrome, regardless of age, show evidence of cardiovascular involvement. It is less the presence than the degree of involvement that weighs heavily in the balance of risk during gestation.[104] Affected women with minimal cardiovascular involvement appear to tolerate pregnancy without serious acute complications, whereas women with hemodynamically significant aortic or mitral regurgitation or more than mild to moderate dilatation of the aortic root are clearly at risk for serious cardiovascular complications during or shortly after gestation.[104] Chordal attenuation or rupture results in gradually progressive or acute severe mitral regurgitation, and aortic root disease can suddenly announce itself by acute aortic dissection or rupture or acute severe aortic regurgitation.[83, 104] Connective tissue changes in the aortic root during pregnancy may add to the connective tissue abnormalities of the Marfan syndrome.

AORTIC DISSECTION (p. 1554). About 50 per cent of aortic dissections in women younger than 40 years of age are associated with pregnancy.[105–107] The highest incidence of dissection occurs during the third trimester, with the bulk of the remainder shared between the second trimester and labor or the first 24 hours postpartum; almost 20 per cent of cases occur 2 or more days after delivery.[106] Successful cesarean section and repair of the aortic dissection have been accomplished near term during the same operative procedure; postpartum dissection can be addressed surgically without risk to the fetus.[107, 108]

CARDIOMYOPATHIES

(See also Chap. 44)

GENETIC HYPERTROPHIC CARDIOMYOPATHY (p. 1418). Pregnant women with this cardiomyopathy must face the dual risks of transmission of an autosomal dominant disease and the maternal risk inherent in the cardiac disorder.[109–112, 112a] The functional response of the left ventricle in genetic hypertrophic cardiomyopathy with disproportionate septal thickness, especially in patients exhibiting a left ventricular–aortic systolic pressure gradient, is determined chiefly by the interaction of three variables—left ventricular end-diastolic dimensions (volume), systemic vascular resistance, and the inotropic state of the left ventricle. These variables are influenced by hemodynamic changes that exist during the course of normal pregnancy, labor, and delivery.[2, 110] Increases in blood volume and cardiac output (and left ventricular diastolic volume) serve to reduce the left ventricular/aortic gradient, while the fall in systemic vascular resistance counteracts this effect.[110, 112] In the third trimester, inferior vena caval compression in the supine position decreases venous return and left ventricular volume and accordingly augments the left ventricular/aortic gradient; mitral regurgitation may increase significantly.[110]

A number of opposing variables come into play during labor, delivery, and the puerperium. Adrenergic stimulation associated with pain and emotional stress together with the Valsalva maneuver (bearing down) conspire to increase the left ventricular–aortic gradient, while a rise in central blood volume during active uterine contraction has the opposite effect.[110] The rapid decline in blood volume after delivery reduces left ventricular internal dimensions and can intensify the pressure gradient in the outflow tract. Despite these hemodynamic vicissitudes, pregnancy followed by labor in the lateral position and assisted normal vaginal delivery are generally accomplished with surprising few maternal or fetal complications. Standard epidural anesthesia should be avoided because of potential hypotension.[112] Mitral regurgitation exposes patients to the risk of infective endocarditis, so that appropriate antibiotic prophylaxis is indicated in these patients (p. 1127).

Beta blockers, calcium-channel antagonists, and more recently amiodarone have been used to relieve symptoms and suppress ventricular ectopic beats when used during pregnancy. These agents are subject to certain constraints (p. 1864).

PERIPARTUM CARDIOMYOPATHY (p. 1414). This term is applied to a form of dilated cardiomyopathy that begins in the last month of pregnancy or within the first 6 months after delivery in the absence of demonstrable cause and without prior evidence of heart disease.[113–117] Its incidence has been estimated to range from 1 in 3000 to 4000 confinements[115, 118, 119] to 1 in 15,000.[116] There is a reported association with increased maternal age, parity, twinning, malnutrition, toxemia, and hypertension,[115–119] but the latter four associations may well serve as aggravating rather than primary causes. In the United States, the majority of patients are black.[115] Although the term "peripartum" is commonly used, the onset is predominantly in the first through the third month postpartum, with only a minority of patients (fewer than 15 per cent) identified antepartum.[115, 118, 119] This distinct clustering does not *prove* that the disorder represents a disease unique to pregnancy, but it does add weight to that contention.[119] If ventricular size and function normalize within 6 months, prognosis, including the ability to tolerate future pregnancies, is good (Fig. 60–7).

On pathological examination, the ventricles are pale, flabby, and dilated, and mural thrombi are common, setting the stage for embolization to both the pulmonary and the systemic circulations.[115, 118, 119.] On light microscopy, the histological features are indistinguishable from other forms of dilated cardiomyopathy (p. 1414) and include muscle fiber degeneration, interstitial edema, focal areas of fibrosis, and scattered interstitial and perivascular infiltration by mononuclear inflammatory cells.[115, 117, 118] Although myocardial inflammation is often sufficiently impressive to warrant the designation "myocarditis" (Fig. 60–8),[117, 119–121] this designation does not necessarily imply that the condition is infectious. Despite diligent search, no cardiotropic viruses have been isolated in this condition.[119]

An immunological basis for peripartum cardiomyopathy has been proposed,[122, 123] and a number of findings support this hypothesis. Immunosuppressant treatment with steroids and azathioprine has resulted in dramatic clinical improvement associated with disappearance of the inflammatory infiltrate,[119, 120] but a relatively high incidence of spontaneous improvement is a confounding variable.[117] A unique feature of the disease is the strong tendency for recurrences confined to the peripartum periods of subsequent pregnancies.[114] Myocardial antibodies in maternal and cord blood were recovered in a previously healthy primigravida with peripartum cardiomyopathy.[122] Antibodies to human immunoglobulins were present in the fetal heart.[122] More recently, strongly positive antiactin antibodies and positive immunofluorescence tests for antibodies

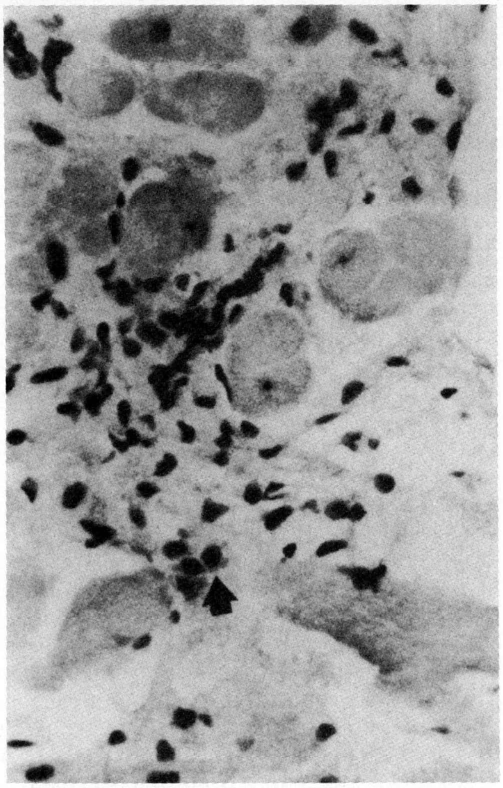

FIGURE 60–8. Endomyocardial biopsy with lymphomononuclear infiltration (arrow) and myocyte necrosis indicative of myocarditis in peripartum cardiomyopathy. (From O'Connell, J. B., et al.: Postpartum cardiomyopathy. J. Am. Coll. Cardiol. *8*:52, 1986. Reprinted with permission from The American College of Cardiology.)

to smooth muscle were identified for as long as 9 months after delivery in a 26-year-old primigravida who developed heart failure immediately postpartum.[123] The authors proposed an autoimmune etiology, theorizing that release of actomyosin or its metabolites by the uterus provided the substrate for antibodies that cross-reacted with maternal myocardium.

The immunobiology of the maternal-fetal relationship is complex.[124–126, 126a] Between the 33rd and 37th weeks of gestation, the myometrium normally becomes irritable, and Braxton Hicks contractions occur.[127] Concurrently, the cervix becomes softer, while the cervical canal grows wider. The function of the myometrium and cervix and the structure and function of their proteins are finely integrated during normal gestation.[127] Myometrial or cervical dysfunction might lead to release of uterine contractile proteins and their metabolites, setting the stage for the development of antibodies to these proteins, which may in turn react with cardiac contractile proteins.[123] The seriousness of peripartum cardiomyopathy coupled with evidence of noninfectious myocardial inflammation argues for treatment with immunosuppressive therapy.[121]

Peripartum cardiomyopathy should be distinguished from peripartum heart failure peculiar to northern Nigeria, where the puerperal customs of the Hausa people require the mother to lie for hours on a baked mud bed over a fire and to ingest substantial quantities of "kanwa," a dried salt cake.[128, 129] The incidence of this condition is highest in the humid Nigerian months of July and August, and patients present clinically with evidence of severe fluid overload and postpartum hypertension.

HYPERTENSION

(see p. 849)

The three major causes of maternal deaths historically have been sepsis, hemorrhage, and the hypertensive disorders (predominantly eclampsia).[1] Maternal mortality has decreased by more than 98 per cent in the present century, with parallel declines in all three of these causes. In the United States, maternal deaths associated with hypertension (chiefly eclampsia) have fallen from 99 per 100,000 live births in 1939 to 1.9 per 100,000 in 1978.[1] Nevertheless, the incidence of various hypertensive disorders in pregnancy is estimated to be 6 to 8 per cent, and in about one-fourth of these cases, the elevation in blood pressure preceded gestation.[1, 130]

Central to the issue of hypertension during pregnancy are the problems of the previously hypertensive woman who becomes pregnant, the problem of the hypertension of preeclampsia in women who were previously normotensive, and the occurrence of preeclampsia in previously hypertensive women.[131] Criteria for the diagnosis of hypertension include a consistent rise in blood pressure of 30/15 mm Hg and/or an absolute level greater than 140/90 mm Hg or both (Committee on Terminology of The American College of Obstetricians and Gynecologists).[1] Perinatal mortality varies with maternal blood pressure, and mortality begins to rise when maternal diastolic pressure exceeds 75 mm Hg in the second trimester or 85 mm Hg in the third.[1]

In an effort to improve the accuracy of diagnosis of hypertension in pregnancy, the following definitions have been proposed.[1] *Gestational hypertension* is defined as the appearance of elevated blood pressure during pregnancy, labor, or the early puerperium without proteinuria and generalized edema and with return of blood pressure to normal within 10 days of delivery. *Chronic hypertension* is defined as persistent blood pressure of 140/90 mm Hg or higher before and after pregnancy. Detection of hypertension before the 20th week of gestation is taken as presumptive evidence for its presence before conception. *Preeclampsia,* a disorder peculiar to pregnancy, is diagnosed by the appearance of hypertension and proteinuria after the 20th week of gestation together with edema of the hands or face or generalized edema. Preeclampsia is rare before the 24th week, is unusual before the 30th, and increases in frequency as pregnancy advances. *"Severe" preeclampsia* is defined by one or more of the following signs or symptoms: a consistent rise in systolic blood pressure to or above 160 mm Hg or in diastolic pressure to or above 110 mm Hg, proteinuria of 3^+ to 4^+ (5 gm/24 hr), oliguria (urine volume less than 400 ml/24 hr), cerebral or visual disturbances, pulmonary edema, or cyanosis.[1] Although severe preeclampsia is likely to lead to eclampsia, nearly one-fourth of women with eclampsia experience their first convulsions in the setting of "mild" preeclampsia.[1] *Eclampsia* is diagnosed when convulsions occur in a woman with preeclampsia.[1] *Toxemia* of pregnancy includes both preeclampsia and eclampsia.

Approximately 25 to 30 per cent of women with chronic hypertension develop superimposed preeclampsia or eclampsia.[1] In general, chronic hypertension and gestational hypertension are more common in multiparous women with elevated blood pressure in early pregnancy and little or no proteinuria.[1] Hypertension is reportedly less well tolerated in black than in white women.[132, 133] Fluctuations in systemic arterial pressure that characterize normotensive pregnancy occur in a significant number of pregnant women with essential hypertension. Thus, systolic pressure may fall 20 to 30 mm Hg and diastolic pressure may decline 10 to 15 mm Hg during the first trimester. In some hypertensive patients, however, blood pressure remains unchanged; in others, it increases, while in still others, it normalizes during gestation but returns to preexisting hypertensive levels during the third trimester or after delivery.[134] Gravid women with labile blood pressure generally experience uncomplicated pregnancies, but some develop sustained hypertension late in gestation.[2] Although labile hypertension is likely to normalize after delivery, a substantial portion of such patients manifest persistent hypertension years later.

As a general rule, maternal prognosis is excellent in women whose systemic arterial pressure is below 160/100 mm Hg during the first 20 weeks of pregnancy, provided renal and cardiac functions are good and preeclampsia does not supervene.[2] Perinatal salvage has improved considerably, although the decrease in fetal wastage does not match the dramatic improvement in maternal mortality.[1]

TREATMENT. Pharmacologic treatment of hypertension in pregnancy requires a balance between the salutary effects of blood pressure control on maternal cardiovascular morbidity and mortality on the one hand and the risk of reducing uteroplacental perfusion on the other.[135] In light of uteroplacental metabolic demands, blood pressure should be reduced gradually. Appropriate first steps are restriction of physical activity and control of anxiety. A gradual fall in blood pressure induced by bedrest or the careful use of low-dose antihypertensive agents does not necessarily impair blood supply to the developing fetus.[135] Conversely, even mild hypertension presents a risk to the fetus,[136] and successful pregnancy is possible even in women who have experienced malignant hypertension, provided that blood pressure is controlled during gestation.[137] In selecting antihypertensive drugs, consideration should be given to the tendency of hypertensive pregnant women to excrete salt loads readily[135] and to develop significant deficits in intravascular volume.[138] Not surprisingly, reductions in uteroplacental blood flow have been reported during diuretic therapy,[135] and it has been recommended that diuretics be used sparingly if at all during pregnancy.[1] Exceptions include pregnant patients with congestive heart failure, renal insufficiency, or the oliguria of preeclampsia, and the cautious use of diuretics as adjuncts to hypotensive agents that may be associated with volume retention, such as methyldopa and hydralazine (see below).[135] For hypertensive emergencies (see below), intravenous nitroprusside, hydralazine, and diazoxide are recommended.[135, 139] Patients with acute congestive heart failure and pulmonary edema respond dramatically to intravenous nitroprusside with no evidence of fetal distress and without significant levels of cyanide in fetal cord blood.[139]

Two commonly used drugs that combine efficacy and safety for mother and fetus are alpha-methyldopa (a central alpha-adrenoceptor agonist) (p. 872) and hydralazine (a vasodilator) (p. 875). Beta-adrenoceptor blocking agents, although commonly used in nonpregnant hypertension, are much less valuable in the hypertension of pregnancy. The biological half-life of beta blockers is much longer in the fetus than in the mother, and all beta blockers cross the placenta (see later).[135]

PREECLAMPSIA. This condition is more frequent in primiparas, twin pregnancies, and women with a history of toxemia or hypertension. The earlier preeclampsia occurs in pregnancy, the greater the risk to mother and fetus.[130] Progression to eclampsia is ominous, with a 5 to 10 per cent maternal mortality and a 20 to 25 per cent fetal mortality. If preeclampsia is not controlled within a few days of hospitalization (bed rest, sedation, sodium restriction, and pharmacological control of blood pressure), pregnancy should be interrupted by cesarean section as soon as possible unless term is sufficiently near for induction of labor. It has been stated without exaggeration that the premature infant of a preeclamptic mother has a better chance in a neonatal intensive care unit than in utero.

It is important to distinguish between the lower extremity edema that occurs in up to 80 per cent of normal pregnant women and the periorbital and hand edema of preeclampsia.[134] A corollary is that the proteinuria of toxemia typically appears *after* the rise in systemic arterial pressure and the development of edema. The proteinuria of toxemia must be distinguished from pyelonephritis, and the edema of pregnancy must be separated from the edema of toxemia.

Considerable attention has focused on the important question of whether pregnancy permanently aggravates systemic hypertension and whether preeclampsia in previously normotensive women predisposes to late postpartum development of sustained hypertension. It is the current consensus that essential hypertension, at least in white women, is not generally aggravated by pregnancy unless there is superimposed toxemia. The long-term effects of toxemia per se are more controversial. White women with a history of documented preeclampsia in their first pregnancy have the same prognosis for sustained hypertension or for survival as white women of the same age with no history of preeclampsia. On the other hand, there is a significant increase in the prevalence of sustained hypertension among black women who experience preeclampsia as primiparas, and among both black and white women who experience preeclampsia as multiparas. These observations suggest that toxemia that occurs in black women in any pregnancy or in white women after their first pregnancy marks a tendency for the development of chronic sustained hypertension later in life.[140]

Independent of the presence and degree of systemic hypertension, toxemia (preeclampsia or eclampsia) can result in acute pulmonary edema. Cardiac size is not significantly increased in these patients, and the pulmonary edema has been ascribed to fluid retention and to reductions in pulmonary capillary permeability. Approximately one-third of patients with fatal eclampsia have contraction band necrosis at necropsy, a lesion believed to result from reperfusion injury.[141] This observation suggests that intermittent coronary spasm may be common in patients who die of eclampsia.

ARRHYTHMIAS

Arrhythmias during pregnancy fall into two general categories: (1) benign rhythm disturbances that occur during the course of an otherwise normal uncomplicated gestation, and (2) disturbances in rhythm associated with certain cardiac diseases that prevail in women of childbearing age. Sinus arrhythmia, occasionally sinus bradycardia or tachycardia, and atrial or ventricular premature beats are relatively common benign occurrences.[142] The sensation of "skipped beats" during pregnancy is more likely to be caused by atrial than by ventricular premature beats. Sporadic premature beats, regardless of their site of origin, are of no clinical importance, especially if they are not subjectively disturbing and if the patient is reassured of their innocence. Even bigeminy or trigeminy is generally unimportant in the pregnant woman without organic heart disease, but multiform ventricular beats or episodes of ventricular tachycardia (p. 694), especially near term or in the puerperium, should arouse suspicion of the presence of peripartum cardiomyopathy. The commonest sustained tachyarrhythmia during pregnancy is *paroxysmal reentrant supraventricular tachycardia (PSVT)* (p. 675), a relatively common rhythm disturbance with a peak incidence in women of childbearing age. A history of PSVT signals the potential for recurrences to which pregnancy predisposes, especially during the third trimester.[142, 143] *Atrial flutter or fibrillation* usually denotes the presence of coexisting organic heart disease, either acquired or congenital. *Wolff-Parkinson-White bypass tracts* set the stage for paroxysmal rapid heart action during pregnancy.[144] With such tracts, atrial flutter with 1:1 conduction or atrial fibrillation with rapid ventricular rates is a matter of special concern.

Pharmacological management of arrhythmias is generally similar to that employed in treating nonpregnant patients (Chap. 21). Intravenous verapamil is efficacious in converting reentrant PSVT to sinus rhythm, and maintenance digoxin is safe and usually effective in preventing recurrences. Quinidine (p. 628) is permissible in pregnancy for the suppression of ventricular ectopic beats even though the drug crosses the placenta and achieves levels in the serum of the fetus similar to those in the mother. In patients with mitral valve prolapse who have premature ventricular beats that require suppression during pregnancy, beta-adrenergic blocking agents can be used but with the constraints outlined below. Procainamide is relatively safe during pregnancy, but in view of the high incidence of antinuclear antibodies and the lupus-like syndrome that this drug evokes, procainamide should be limited to patients unresponsive to quinidine.[145] Indications for the use of amiodarone (p. 631) during pregnancy are very few. (Treatment of Wolff-Parkinson-White tachycardia, which is refractory to other antiarrhythmic agents, is one example.) Due consideration must be given to transplacental transfer of the drug together with its major metabolite, to the drug's effect on maternal and fetal thyroid function, and to the long elimination half-life.[146]

In patients refractory to standard drug therapy, electrical cardioversion has been accomplished without ill effect to mother or fetus.[143] In one study, a patient underwent cardioversion seven times during three successive pregnancies with no untoward effect.[140]

VENOUS DISEASE

The increased venous pressure in the lower extremities that is characteristic of pregnancy, the progesterone-induced increase in venous distensibility, and the hemostatic changes in maternal coagulation and fibrinolytic systems predispose to peripheral venous disease and thromboembolism (Fig. 60–5*A*). Prolonged and difficult labor has been implicated as a cause of pelvic vein thrombosis.[2] In any event, overt or occult pulmonary emboli are a potential threat.[144] Multiple recurrent pulmonary emboli—insidious or overt—can result in a clinical picture closely resembling primary pulmonary hypertension (pp. 805 and 1591).[49] Evidence of venous disease or of pulmonary embolism may not become manifest until months or longer after delivery. There is a significant increase in the incidence of superficial and deep phlebitis of leg veins during the first four weeks postpartum.[147] Accordingly, oral contraceptives in the postpartum period are best avoided, not only because of the added risk of venous thrombosis and pulmonary embolism but also because of evidence that an already elevated pulmonary vascular resistance may increase in women taking anovulatory pills even in the absence of identifiable thromboembolism.[145, 148] Anticoagulants, whether heparin or coumadin, pose formidable risks, especially to the fetus (see below).

OTHER FORMS OF CARDIOVASCULAR DISEASE

ATHEROSCLEROTIC CORONARY ARTERY DISEASE. This condition is rare in young menstruating women who have no major risk factors, with estimates at 1 case in every 10,000 deliveries.[149] If coronary artery disease becomes clinically manifest during pregnancy, it usually presents as acute myocardial infarction rather than angina pectoris, and the mortality rate is high.[42, 150] In one such case, the patient was successfully resuscitated from ventricular fibrillation,[42] and 4 days after the infarction, induced labor produced a normal infant. On another occasion, a symptomatic 36-year-old woman with 90 per cent obstruction of the left main coronary artery underwent successful bypass surgery during pregnancy.[150] In addition, coronary thrombosis with infarction in patients whose coronary arteries were otherwise normal has been reported.[151, 152] An interesting variation on this theme is a report of 33 pregnancies in 27 Japanese women with Takayasu's disease of the aortic arch, descending aorta, or both[153, 154] (p. 1563). Although spontaneous dissection of a coronary artery is extremely rare, when it does occur it is peculiarly associated with pregnancy, especially the puerperium.[155, 156]

MYOTONIC MUSCULAR DYSTROPHY (see p. 1787). This condition commonly involves the specialized cardiac tissues, especially infranodal conduction tissues.[157] Risk to the fetus includes not only genetic transmission of the adult type of myotonic dystrophy but also fetal death associated with protracted labor owing to poor uterine contraction and inadequate voluntary assistance during the second stage of labor.[158] In addition to the former risk, with its attendant cardiac involvement, offspring are at risk for the infantile or childhood variety of myotonic dystrophy in which the myocardium rather than conduction tissue is the chief target.[157] In contrast, congenital myotonic dystrophy (Thomsen's disease) (p. 1789) is benign but in one case was accompanied by abnormalities of uterine contraction.[159]

Examples of *additional cardiac disorders*, such as acute, chronic, or constrictive pericarditis,[2, 160, 161] have been reported sporadically during pregnancy but have little collective impact.

CARDIAC SURGERY AND PREGNANCY

CARDIAC SURGERY DURING PREGNANCY. Whether or not cardiac surgery is required during pregnancy is an issue that seldom arises. When the problem is posed, it is almost always in women with valvular heart disese, generally rheumatic mitral stenosis.[67, 162–166] The most important indications for operation in pregnant women with severe mitral stenosis are pulmonary edema that is refractory to medical management or is recurrent despite medical management and persistent massive hemoptysis.[67] There is a consensus that whenever possible, premature termination of pregnancy is preferable to cardiac surgery in patients unresponsive to medical therapy. Mitral valvotomy without use of extracorporeal circulation circumvents the risk to the fetus from cardiopulmonary bypass, and in experienced surgical hands the results are often excellent.[163] Extracorporeal circulation confronts the fetus with tangible risks, and fetal wastage is reportedly on the order of 30 per cent.[67, 166] Fetal distress is believed to be related largely to inadequate extracorporeal perfusion rates, resulting in hypoperfusion of the uterus.[162, 167] It has been recommended that high flow rates be used during cardiopulmonary bypass in pregnant patients, with an obstetrician present to monitor the fetus,[162, 167]

CARDIAC SURGERY AFTER PREGNANCY. A new and important relationship between pregnancy and heart disease involves a novel population—the postoperative cardiac patient.[5, 44, 64, 65] Women who previously would not have reached childbearing age or who might have done so physiologically ill equipped to bear children are now presenting after cardiac surgery for obstetrical and cardiac care. Although surgery can be performed during gestation (see above), a prime objective of operative intervention is anticipatory, i.e., to increase the safety and success of pregnancy and to insure the subsequent health of mother and child. Serious cardiovascular disease appreciably reduces sexual and ovarian function, and successful cardiac surgery increases fertility in such women.[168] Relief of cyanosis may not only permit a woman to conceive but substantially improves the stability of the pregnancy and the probability that a viable fetus will be delivered at or near term. Cardiac surgery prior to pregnancy can be enormously beneficial, but it is important to bear in mind that, with few exceptions, surgery is not curative, and both patient and physician must recognize the need for continuing medical care.

Postoperative management is largely determined by the presence, type, and degree of cardiac and vascular residuae and sequelae; these include uncorrected defects, effects of ventriculotomy, electrophysiological disturbances, residual valvular abnormalities such as persistently elevated pulmonary vascular resistance, prosthetic materials (including prosthetic valves), and the postoperative residua of myocardial ischemia and increased ventricular mass.[64, 169] Not least among the postoperative sequelae is the risk of genetic transmission of congenital heart disease (p. 826).[65, 170–173]

Special problems are presented by the pregnant women with *prosthetic cardiac valves* (p. 1080). These include the risk of infective endocarditis from bacteremia during labor and delivery, the threat to the mother of thromboembolism, and the hazard to the fetus of anticoagulants. Methods of prophylaxis for infective endocarditis are conventional (p. 1127), but anticoagulants pose serious unresolved problems that require refined judgment and meticulous care (see below).

MEDICAL MANAGEMENT OF THE PREGNANT WOMAN WITH HEART DISEASE

Maternal mortality varies directly with functional class (Table 60–6). The expectant mother's cardiac reserve is inherently limited by the combination of heart disease and the additional circulatory demands imposed by pregnancy. This challenge can almost always be met by minimizing additional demands upon the circulation and by meticulous medical management of the cardiovascular disorder. Interruption of pregnancy as a means of preserving or restoring cardiac compensation is seldom warranted. In the presence of some cardiovascular lesions, however, childbearing imposes such a formidable threat to maternal survival that interruption of pregnancy is recommended. Examples are women with suprasystemic pulmonary vascular resistance, the Marfan syndrome with conspicuous dilatation of the

TABLE 60–6 MATERNAL AND FETAL MORTALITY ACCORDING TO FUNCTIONAL CLASS[71]

Maternal mortality	
Classes I and II	0.4%
Classes III and IV	6.8%
Fetal mortality[2]	
Class I	Nil
Class IV	30.0%

TABLE 60–7 FACTORS THAT AGGRAVATE MATERNAL HEART DISEASE

Anxiety
Retention of sodium and water
Sudden, strenuous or isometric exercise
Heat and humidity
Anemia
Pyelonephritis
Lower respiratory tract infection
Hyperthyroidism
Arrhythmias
Thromboembolism

aortic root, or persistent, marked cardiac enlargement as a result of peripartum cardiomyopathy.

Factors that serve to aggravate heart disease and needlessly encroach on cardiac reserve should be identified, removed, or at least minimized (Table 60–7). Anxiety is a source of stress, especially in the primipara who anticipates the new experience of pregnancy in the face of heart disease. Reassurance begins with a frank, clear explanation designed to remove fear of the unknown. The expectant mother should be told what to anticipate during each stage of pregnancy, including labor, delivery, and the puerperium. Coordination between obstetrician and cardiologist is obligatory to provide intelligent care and to insure that the patient does not receive conflicting information. Knowledge that the pain of labor and delivery will be relieved is important.

The tendency for body water and total exchangeable sodium to increase in the normal gravid woman must be considered in the pregnant cardiac patient. Excess weight gain is another circulatory burden that is best minimized. Moderate restriction of sodium and calories usually suffices. Diuretics should be used judiciously if at all, generally for edema related to cardiac failure rather than for the edema of normal pregnancy. Because physical exercise adds a greater burden, the pregnant cardiac patient should avoid strenuous, sudden, or isometric effort. She should be assured of a restful night even if mild sedatives are required, and it is often advisable to recommend rest of an hour or so during the day, preferably in the early afternoon. The intensity of treatment obviously depends on the severity of the underlying heart disease. Thus, the asymptomatic patient with physiologically mild cardiac disease needs little or no restriction, while the symptomatic pregnant patient with serious cardiac compromise may require prolonged hospitalization with bed rest. The psychological impact of hospitalization must be weighed against the anticipated benefits.

Certain environmental conditions exert important effects on the heart and circulation and may initiate or intensify heart failure in susceptible individuals. Heat and humidity increase further the hemodynamic burden[174] and sometimes serve as important aggravating causes of heart failure in otherwise stable pregnant cardiac patients. Because gestation is normally accompanied by greater heat production due to the metabolic activity of the products of conception, a cool, dry environment promotes dissipation of heat and proper regulation of body temperature. An air-conditioned environment can be very helpful in this regard.

Noncardiac diseases may also exert undesirable circulatory effects. *Anemia* is an example, and with rare exception can be corrected with oral iron administration. Pathological anemia must be distinguished from the "physiological anemia of pregnancy." Seventy-five per cent of the increase in gestational blood volume represents plasma expansion; only 25 per cent reflects the increase in red blood cell mass (p. 1848).[9] The difference in timing and magnitude of the changes between plasma volume and red cell mass accounts for the changes in hematocrit during pregnancy. As plasma volume increases during the first trimester, a decrease in hematocrit occurs, reaching its lowest values at 32 to 34 weeks. In the last 8 to 10 weeks of pregnancy, plasma volume plateaus while the red cell mass continues to increase, resulting in a slight rise in hematocrit. *Infection*, especially pyelonephritis, is relatively common during pregnancy and the postpartum period and can add to the cardiac burden; the index of suspicion for such infections should be high in patients with fever. *Lower respiratory infections*, although coincidental, pose special problems in the pregnant cardiac patient with marginally elevated or increased pulmonary venous pressure. Because epidemic *influenza* is associated with greater morbidity and mortality during pregnancy,[175] vaccination is recommended. *Hyperthyroidism* may not be as apparent during pregnancy because of the gestational hyperkinetic circulation, but the effect is no less important, because the two hypermetabolic states conspire to reduce cardiac reserve. Recurrence of preexistent *arrhythmias* should be anticipated and appropriate drugs used prophylactically (p. 1864). The inherent tendency for stasis in leg veins and the attendent *risk of thromboembolism* can be minimized in a number of relatively simple ways. Patients should be given detailed instructions on leg care, i.e., passive standing should be avoided and the supine position minimized (supine vena caval compression), the knees should be straightened when sitting (legs need not be uncomfortably elevated), support hose can be worn, and ambulation should begin as soon as practical after delivery.

MEDICAL MANAGEMENT OF HEART DISEASE. Because of the hazards of radiation, chest roentgenography, cardiac catheterization, and angiography are usually deferred until after completion of the pregnancy. Placement of a balloon flotation catheter into the pulmonary artery, however, should proceed without hesitation in patients who require hemodynamic monitoring during labor, delivery, and the puerperium. Prevention of overt congestive failure is important, since pulmonary edema ranks as one of the most frequent causes of maternal cardiac mortality, accounting for 50 per cent of deaths in pregnant women with rheumatic heart disease.[2, 7] The patient should be advised to report a change in exercise tolerance or a sudden weight gain. Weight diaries are important and are most accurate when the patient weighs herself each morning nude after voiding and before breakfast.

PROPHYLAXIS FOR INFECTIVE ENDOCARDITIS (p. 1127). In susceptible patients, prophylaxis for infective endocarditis is mandatory whenever the threat of bacteremia arises during the course of pregnancy as well as during labor and delivery. Patients with lesions that may become infected should be instructed about meticulous oral hygiene, and a dental examination should be carried out at least once during pregnancy. Each visit should be preceded and immediately followed by appropriate antibiotic prophylaxis depending upon the estimated risk and according to the guidelines of the Committee on Rheumatic Fever and Infective Endocarditis of the American Heart Association[176] (Table 30–4, p. 907). Antibiotic prophylaxis for routine vaginal delivery in patients with susceptible cardiac lesions is controversial, and it has been argued that such an approach is not necessary in uncomplicated deliveries, because bacteremia has not been confirmed as a natural or inevitable occurrence.[177, 178] However, in pregnant women with cardiac lesions susceptible to infective endocarditis, it would not be prudent to assume that delivery will be uncomplicated. Accordingly, antibiotic prophylaxis is recommended from the onset of labor through the third or fourth postpartum day. Most commonly, ampicillin and gentamicin are used according to American Heart Association guidelines.[176]

LABOR, DELIVERY, AND THE PUERPERIUM. These events should be carefully anticipated. There is a strong consensus that spontaneous vaginal delivery at term with adequate relief of pain and apprehension, performed with the aid of an experienced obstetrical anesthesiologist, is the method of choice in pregnant women with heart disease. Induction of labor before term is not an appropriate method of delivery for the pregnant cardiac patient and may in fact increase the risk of heart failure. Cesarean section is reserved for instances in which obstetrical indications are clear-cut, consisting most commonly of cephalopelvic disproportion or a previous cesarean section. A flotation catheter and arterial line are useful for monitoring patients in whom hemodynamic instability is anticipated. The importance of relief of pain and anxiety should be underscored. The lateral position during labor for the pregnant cardiac patient should also be considered, since it mitigates hemodynamic fluctuations so that uterine contractions cause much smaller increments in cardiac output and stroke volume.

Meperidine is probably the most commonly employed narcotic for pain management during labor. Small doses of meperidine during active labor allow analgesia without loss of consciousness. The pain threshold is raised without entirely eliminating the discomfort of contractions. The patient benefits from drowsiness and may sleep between contractions. Epidural anesthesia reduces pain substantially; however, it may cause hypotension. Hemodynamic monitoring with a flotation catheter and measurement of intraarterial systemic pressure are useful adjuncts. With the assistance of hemodynamic monitoring and lumbar, epidural, or general anesthesia, cesarean section may be carried out in patients with serious heart disease with the appropriate indications. It should be reemphasized that with few exceptions, vaginal delivery assisted with forceps, using some form of regional anesthesia such as epidural block, is the best course of action. Collaboration between an obstetrician and obstetrical anesthesiologist, both experienced in dealing with cardiac patients, as well as a neonatologist is essential.

EFFECTS OF MATERNAL HEART DISEASE ON THE FETUS

In the pregnant woman with heart disease, the lives of the mother and fetus are both at stake. It is therefore appropriate to review the effects of maternal cardiac disease on the fetus, which is exposed both to immediate risks that threaten its viability and to remote risks that express themselves as congenital malformations. Normal uterine blood flow and normal placental function are fundamental determinants of the intrauterine milieu upon which fetal integrity depends. Maternal heart disease, by reducing uterine blood flow (as occurs in heart failure), altering the physiology of the placenta (as in systemic hypertension), or reducing the availability of oxygen (as in cyanotic congenital heart disease), threatens the growth, development, and viability of the fetus. Moreover, the fetus is at independent risk for congenital malformations prompted by transplacental transfer of teratogens, often in the form of drugs used in treating the pregnant cardiac patient, or genetic transmission of certain types of maternal heart disease. The circulatory effect of vena caval obstruction in the supine position is reflected in a reduction in cardiac output sufficient to cause fetal hypoxia, but this effect is transient and readily reversed when the mother turns on her side. Fetal survival is materially influenced by the effects of both maternal heart disease per se and medical and surgical interventions employed to treat the cardiac disorder. The functional class of the mother is a major determinant of fetal mortality, with the incremental risk varying from virtually zero in asymptomatic pregnant cardiac patients (Class I) to nearly 30 per cent in gravid women who are symptomatic at rest (Class IV) (Table 60–6).[2, 179]

Certain types of heart disease pose greater threats to the fetus than others apart from and in addition to maternal functional class. *Systemic hypertension*, independent of the risk of preeclampsia, is associated with intrauterine growth retardation and an increased incidence of stillbirths and perinatal mortality.[1, 131, 132, 180] *Maternal congenital heart disease* threatens the fetus with regard to functional class of the mother, risk of genetic transmission, and fetal wastage due to maternal cyanosis.[181, 182] The majority of infants born to cyanotic mothers are dysmature (small for gestational age) or premature (gestation less than 37 weeks).[51] In addition, there is a high rate of spontaneous abortion, the incidence of which increases roughly in parallel with the mother's hematocrit. Even in the presence of relatively mild cyanosis, however, the spontaneous abortion rate is high. Accordingly, maternal cyanosis looms as one of the major threats to fetal viability. Surgical correction of congenital heart disease materially improves maternal functional class and eliminates cyanosis, but genetic transmission of cardiac anomalies necessarily remains unchanged.[181]

ENVIRONMENTAL TOXINS, THE DRUG CULTURE, AND TERATOGENS

Morbidity and mortality caused by tobacco is reportedly greater than from any other toxic material in the environment.[183] In the United States, approximately 30 per cent of women are cigarette smokers at the time of conception.[184] Approximately one-fourth of American women who smoked prior to conception stopped smoking during gestation, and another third markedly decreased the number of cigarettes smoked during pregnancy.[184] Obstetrical complications of tobacco smoking put the pregnant cardiac patient at markedly increased risk for abruptio placentae and placenta previa. In addition, advanced maternal age and parity in smoking women markedly increase the risk of third-trimester bleeding. Maternal smoking is associated with low birth weights, reduced expansion of plasma volume, and structural abnormalities in umbilical arteries and veins and in vessels of the placental villi.[184–186] The incidence of birth defects, including congenital cardiac defects, is increased in a dose-dependent fashion with maternal smoking, in parallel with the increased incidence of spontaneous abortions.[187, 188]

Ethyl alcohol. There is increasing awareness of the effects of ethyl alcohol on the human fetus. It is estimated that 2 to 6 per cent of women consume two or more drinks daily.[189] The *fetal alcohol syndrome* sometimes occurs at levels of ethanol intake well within the norm for a large number of people in our society. Although that level of alcohol may cause little or no recognizable maternal illness, fetal effects can be devastating.[189] The fetal alcohol syndrome is characterized by facial dysmorphy, growth retardation, and central nervous system involvement (including mental retardation). Approximately 29 per cent of offspring with recognizable fetal alcohol syndrome have congenital cardiac malformations, especially atrial septal defect, ventricular septal defect, and tetralogy of Fallot.[189, 190] The incidence of the fetal alcohol syndrome is estimated to range from 1 in 300 to 1 in 2000 live births but occurs in 30 to 40 per cent of infants of alcoholic mothers,[189, 191] especially those who smoke marijuana (see later).

High altitude. While not strictly speaking an environmental toxin, this may pose a risk during pregnancy, especially in the pregnant cardiac patient.[192] The normal pregnant woman who is acclimated to high altitude generally handles gestation well. Conversely, the normal pregnant woman or the pregnant cardiac patient who travels rapidly from sea level to high altitude is not so acclimated and may respond adversely to the decreased ambient oxygen. The incidence of pregnancy-induced hypertension, proteinuria, and edema is higher in otherwise normal women at high altitude.[193] The fetus is at increased risk of hypoxia owing to the decreased content of ambient oxygen.[192] Birth weights tend to be decreased, and the relative hypoxia of high altitudes may be looked upon as a factor limiting fetal growth potential. Importantly, maternal smoking at high altitude is reportedly associated with two- to threefold greater reduction in birth weight than at sea level.[192]

The pregnant cardiac patient may tolerate poorly the increased circulatory burden imposed by *heat and humidity. Caffeine* crosses the placenta and reaches the developing fetus, so that maternal ingestion of coffee, tea, cola drinks, chocolate, and certain other foodstuffs expose the fetus to caffeine.[192] Data regarding human teratogenicity of caffeine are sparse, but the concern led the Food and Drug Administration in 1980 to advise pregnant women that caffeine-containing foods and drugs should be used sparingly.[192]

Marijuana. This is reportedly used by 13 per cent of pregnant women.[194–196] The combined use of marijuana and alcohol results in a fivefold increase in the incidence of the fetal alcohol sydrome.[194]

Aspirin. This drug is perhaps the commonest over-the-counter drug taken during pregnancy. Salicylates freely cross the placenta. If aspirin is ingested within 5 days of delivery, both the mother and infant may exhibit bleeding tendencies.[190] In addition, maternal ingestion of aspirin inhibits prostaglandin synthetase and serves to decrease fetal prostaglandins and promote constriction of the fetal ductus arteriosus.[190, 198] Aspirin is not acceptable as an alternative to anticoagulants during pregnancy (see below).[197–200]

Preterm labor. This responds effectively to betamimetic and corticosteroid therapy,[201–204] but cardiac patients who receive these drugs risk cardiovascular complications. The effects of corticosteroids, beta-adrenoceptor blocking drugs, and intravenous fluids may add to the physiological changes of pregnancy.[202] Terbutaline (a noncatechol sympathomimetic amine), which is widely used to prevent preterm labor, is a potent inotropic and chronotropic agent that provokes significant increases in heart rate, cardiac output, and ejection fraction.[205]

CARDIOVASCULAR DRUGS IN PREGNANCY

ANTIHYPERTENSIVE DRUGS (see Chap. 28). Diuretic agents may impair uterine blood flow and placental perfusion, and their use during pregnancy should be restricted (p. 869). The routine use of diuretics as first-line drugs for the treatment of hypertension in pregnancy or for physiological gestational edema is not indicated. *Methyldopa* crosses the placenta and achieves concentrations in the fetal serum similar to those in the mother. The drug is excreted into breast milk in small amounts, but considerable experience has not revealed adverse effects when it is administered during pregnancy.[1, 200, 206] *Hydralazine* has been used without detectable ill effect during pregnancy, and there are no reports of excretion of this drug into breast milk.[1, 206] *Beta-adrenoceptor blocking agents* are used during pregnancy not only for hypertension but also for arrhythmias and hypertrophic cardiomyopathy. These drugs readily cross the placenta and are not teratogens, although adverse maternal, fetal, and neonatal effects have been reported.[206, 208–213] Propranolol increases uterine activity, an effect more pronounced in nonpregnant than in pregnant women,[209] but prudence dictates cautious use in patients at risk for preterm labor.[211] The most consistent untoward effect of chronic propranolol use during pregnancy is fetal growth retardation.[209] Neonatal bradycardia, respiratory depression, and hypoglycemia have also been reported.[200, 208–211] Because fetal beta blockade removes a potentially important reserve response to the stress of labor and delivery placed on the fetus, it is desirable to discontinue the drug toward the end of term. Propranolol is excreted into breast milk, but no adverse effects such as respiratory depression, bradycardia, or hypoglycemia have been reported in breast-fed neonates.[206] The efficacy and safety of *calcium-channel antagonists* in pregnancy has not yet been established.

ANTIARRHYTHMIC DRUGS. The use of antiarrhythmic agents in pregnancy is similar in principle to their use in nonpregnant patients except for placental transfer of the pharmacological agent.[211, 214] *Digitalis glycosides* may be used safely during pregnancy. These drugs rapidly cross the placenta, enter the fetal circulation,[206, 214, 215] and have been identified in the fetus and newborn. The fetal heart has a limited capacity to bind digoxin during the first half of gestation, but subsequently, the highest fetal concentrations are found in this organ. Maternal administration of digoxin has been used successfully to treat fetal tachycardia and congestive heart failure.[206, 214] Digoxin is excreted into breast milk, but no adverse effects in the nursing infant have been identified. Although digitalis exerts an inotropic effect on the myometrium,[216] there is no convincing evidence that this effect accounts for shorter labor.

Quinidine also crosses the placenta and achieves concentrations in fetal serum that are similar to those in the mother. Despite its extensive use, however, there have been no reports of adverse fetal effects.[211, 214] Quinidine freely diffuses into breast milk with a milk:plasma ratio of approximately 1.0.[217] In pregnant patients treated concomitantly with quinidine and anticoagulants (see below), consideration must be given to drug interaction that increases the risk of hemorrhage.[214]

Procainamide appears to be relatively safe during pregnancy, although data on maternal/fetal equilibrium and fetal metabolism are lacking.[211] In view of the incidence of antinuclear antibodies and a lupus-like syndrome during chronic procainamide therapy, it is prudent to limit its use to patients who do not tolerate or who are unresponsive to quinidine. Transplacental cardioversion of fetal supraventricular tachycardia has been achieved with intravenous procainamide administered to the mother after digoxin and propranolol had failed.[218]

Lidocaine crosses the placenta with maternal epidural or intravenous administration.[214] When used in the smallest effective intravenous doses for the treatment of acute ventricular arrhythmias, lidocaine is considered safe for both mother and fetus.[211, 214, 219] *Verapamil* also crosses the placenta, but concentrations in the fetus are substantially less than in maternal plasma.[220] This may indicate that the risk of acute administration is acceptable, but information is still insufficient to assure the safety of acute or chronic therapy.[211] *Disopyramide* readily crosses the placenta and is secreted into breast milk. Tentative claims of safety in the treatment of maternal arrhythmias are not sufficient to warrant secure recommendations that the drug can be used without ill effects.[211, 214] *Mexiletine* crosses the placental barrier, and although it has been used in individual cases with apparent safety, data are currently insufficient to provide a secure basis for recommending it.[221] The teratogenicity of *phenytoin* is well established (the "fetal hydantoin syndrome") and is characterized by abnormalities in growth and development, craniofacial abnormalities, and limb abnormalities in addition to cardiac defects.[190, 206, 222, 223]

Therapeutic doses of *amiodarone* during pregnancy are associated with neonatal levels that are reportedly 25 per cent of maternal levels, indicating limited placental transfer of at least the parent compound and probably the metabolite.[147, 224–226] Individual examples of amiodarone administration during gestation have been described without apparent untoward effects on the fetus.[225, 226] The teratogenic risk is unknown, however, and the fate of the large amount of iodine (39 per cent by weight) is unclear.[224] Iodine is transferred rapidly across the placenta, is concentrated in the fetal thyroid from as early as 14 weeks, and is associated with neonatal goiter after comparatively small amounts are ingested.[224] Amiodarone is secreted into breast milk, and the estimated amount ingested by the breast-fed infant is equivalent to a low maintenance dose.[224] The long terminal elimination half-life of amiodarone requires that it be stopped for several months before conception if fetal exposure is to be avoided during the early weeks of pregnancy.[147]

ANTICOAGULANTS (see p. 1771). The use of anticoagulants in pregnancy confronts the mother and fetus with difficult problems. As already noted, antiplatelet drugs (aspirin) are not acceptable alternatives.[198, 199] To circumvent the risk of anticoagulants, bioprosthetic valves can be used (p. 1080) and will provide women of childbearing age with sufficient years to plan a family. The likely need for the ultimate replacement of the bioprosthesis because of fibrocalcific degeneration is considered to be a price worth paying to avoid the hazards of anticoagulants to mother and fetus.[227–229] However, anticoagulants are, with few exceptions, obligatory for pregnant women with mechanical prostheses and are also employed in the treatment of deep vein thrombophlebitis.[230–233] The hypercoagulable state of pregnancy (i.e., the increase in coagulation factors II, VII, VIII, and IX and inhibition of fibrinolysis[234]) underscores the need for anticoagulants to prevent clots on the prosthesis. Anticoagulants do not eliminate thromboembolic complications, but the risk is far higher in pregnant women with prosthetic valves in whom anticoagulants are discontinued than in those who continue to take the drugs or who have never received them.[233, 235, 236] The administration of coumadin throughout pregnancy is associated with a fetal mortality rate of about 30 per cent.[237] Coumadin derivatives readily cross the placenta, and when the drug is taken at the time of conception and during the first trimester, the fetus is put at tangible risk for warfarin embryopathy (chondrodysplasia punctata),[237–240, 240a] characterized by saddlenose, hypoplasia of the nares and air passages causing upper airway obstruction and respiratory distress, hypertelorism, frontal bossing, short neck, short stature, and stippled epiphyses (punctata) (Fig. 60–9). The risks during second-trimester exposure include optic atrophy, deafness, mental retardation, microcephaly, and cerebral agenesis.[237, 238, 240] Since coumadin causes fetal anticoagulation, exposure during the third trimester places the fetus at risk for hemorrhage, especially if gestation is interrupted by unexpected preterm labor.

In hopes of obviating these risks, heparin, which does not cross the placenta, has been proposed instead of coumadin during pregnancy, especially during the first trimester.[228–230, 234, 236, 241] However, the substitution of heparin after conception and during the first trimester followed by coumadin until term still results in a high overall neonatal morbidity and mortality.[234, 237, 241]

Despite the Scylla of maternal thromboembolism and the Charybdis of fetal death or malformation, anticoagulants are necessarily employed in pregnant women with mechanical prosthetic valves, and the author's current management policy is as follows: Before conception, the cardiologist, patient, her husband, an obstetrician with experience in high-risk pregnancy, and a clinical nurse specialist should meet, so that the risks to mother and fetus as well as the details of management before conception and during gestation, labor, delivery, and the puerperium can be clarified. The patient is then scheduled for short-term hospitalization for supervised replacement of coumadin with heparin and for instruction by a nurse specialist on subcutaneous self-administration. The policy of deferring replacement of warfarin with heparin until pregnancy is confirmed 6 to 8 weeks after the last menstrual period exposes the fetus to needless risk.[234] This early first-trimester risk is eliminated by starting heparin *before* the cessation of contraception, i.e. before conception.

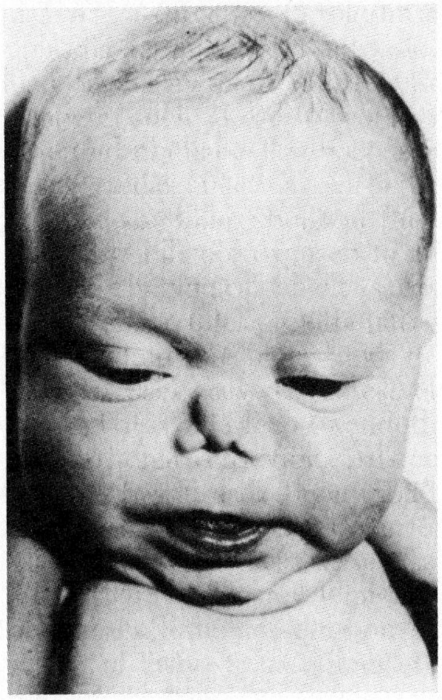

FIGURE 60–9. Warfarin embryopathy showing a severely hypoplastic nose. At birth, the infant was apneic and required tracheal intubation. Other abnormalities included marked narrowing of nasal passages and stippling of bones of the hands and feet and the vertebral bodies. (From Pettifor, J. M., and Benson, R.: Congenital malformations associated with the administration of oral anticoagulants during pregnancy. J. Pediatr. *86*:459, 1975, with permission.)

Heparin, in doses of 150 to 250 U/kg, is self-administered every 8 or 12 hours subcutaneously with the dose adjusted to achieve and maintain the midinterval activated partial thromboplastin time (determined 4 to 6 hours after injection) at 1½ times the control value.[242–244] When the inhospital therapeutic end point is reached, the patient is discharged on self-administered subcutaneous heparin, with follow-up at 2-week intervals to check the partial thromboplastin time and make necessary adjustments. Heparin is then continued throughout gestation in order to avoid the potential complications of the transplacental transfer of coumadin as well as the possible hazards of fetal hemorrhage. Because of the increased levels of coagulation factors during the third trimester, pregnant patients generally require an increased anticoagulant dose as gestation progresses. On the basis of the obstetrician's estimate of the date of delivery, the patient is hospitalized and subcutaneous heparin is replaced by intravenous infusion until the onset of labor. Subcutaneous heparin is then resumed 4 to 8 hours after delivery, barring hemorrhagic complications, and coumadin is resumed a week later.

Use of heparin before conception and throughout pregnancy theoretically reduces the risk to the fetus but is an inconvenience to the mother. Long-term use introduces the potential complication of osteoporosis.[234] Unacceptable bruising at injection sites often coincides with the larger doses required toward term, but this problem is resolved by using intravenous heparin via a portable syringe pump during the last 2 or 3 weeks.[234]

For patients who do not wish to take heparin throughout pregnancy, coumadin is reintroduced during the 13th week of gestation, adjusting the prothrombin time to twice control.[234, 240a, 241] In the 37th week, subcutaneous heparin is restarted as outlined above, and the protocol then proceeds as just described. If elective cesarean section is planned, heparin is discontinued immediately before delivery. Should preterm labor begin in a patient receiving oral anticoagulants, protamine and fresh frozen plasma are administered. Under these difficult circumstances, birth by cesarean section is believed to be associated with a lower risk of hemorrhagic fetal death when compared with vaginal delivery.[230] Breast feeding is best avoided, since oral anticoagulants are secreted in the milk.[206]

LONG-TERM EFFECTS OF PREGNANCY ON MATERNAL HEART DISEASE

While there is general agreement that gestation, delivery, and the puerperium each entails an added risk in patients with certain types of heart disease, it is important to ask whether pregnancy, once successfully concluded, alters the subsequent course of maternal heart disease. It has been stated without apparent irony that "most physicians have believed that a woman's impaired cardiac reserve is like a bank account that is irreversibly depleted by the cost of pregnancy."[245] However, with few exceptions (peripartum cardiomyopathy, for example), current opinion does not support this view.[246] Women with impaired cardiac reserve are at higher risk *during* their pregnancies, but if they survive, no long-term harmful effects have been identified except for the important ones attendant on the stress of caring for another newborn.

REFERENCES

1. Chesley, L. C.: Hypertensive disorders of pregnancy. *In* Gleicher, N. (ed.): Principles of Medical Therapy in Pregnancy. New York, Plenum Medical Book Co., 1985, p. 751.
2. Szekely, P., and Snaith, L.: Heart Disease and Pregnancy. Edinburgh and London, Churchill-Livingstone, 1974.
3. Ueland, K.: Rheumatic heart disease and pregnancy. *In* Elkayam, U., and Gleicher, N. (eds.): Cardiac Problems in Pregnancy. New York, Alan R. Liss, Inc., 1982, p. 79.
4. Sullivan, J. M., and Ramanathan, K. B.: Management of medical problems in pregnancy—severe cardiac disease. N. Engl. J. Med. *313*:304, 1985.
5. Perloff, J. K.: Congenital heart disease and pregnancy. *In* Gleicher, N. (ed.): Principles of Medical Therapy in Pregnancy. New York, Plenum Medical Book Co., 1985, p. 665.
6. Engle, M. A., and Perloff, J. K. (eds.): Symposium on postoperative congenital heart disease in adults. Am. J. Cardiol. *50*:541, 1982.
7. Cole, T. O., and Adaleye, J. A.: Rheumatic heart disease and pregnancy in Nigerian women. Clin. Cardiol. *5*:280, 1982.
8. Perloff, J. K., Lindgren, K. M., and Groves, B. M.: Uncommon or commonly unrecognized causes of heart failure. Prog. Cardiovasc. Dis. *12*:409, 1970.

CARDIOPULMONARY CHANGES IN NORMAL PREGNANCY

9. Elrad, H., and Gleicher, K. I.: Physiologic changes in normal pregnancy. *In* Gleicher, N. (ed.): Principles of Medical Therapy in Pregnancy. New York, Plenum Medical Book Co., 1985, p. 33.
9a. Metcalfe, J., McAnnulty, J. H., and Ueland, K.: Burwell and Metcalf's Heart Disease and Pregnancy. 2nd ed. Boston, Little, Brown, 1986, pp. 11, 139.
10. Ueland, K.: Cardiovascular physiology of the normal pregnancy. *In* Gleicher, N. (ed.): Principles of Medical Therapy in Pregnancy. New York, Plenum Medical Book Co., 1985, p. 643.
11. Limacher, M. C.: Echocardiography in pregnancy. Echocardiography 3:19, 1986.
12. Longo, L. D.: Maternal blood volume and cardiac output during pregnancy: A hypothesis of endocrinologic control. Am. J. Physiol. *24*:R720, 1983.
13. Atkins, A. F. J., Watt, J. M., Milan, P., Davies, P., and Crawford, J. S.: A longitudinal study of cardiovascular dynamic changes throughout pregnancy. Eur. J. Obstet. Gynecol. Reprod. Biol. *12*:215, 1981.
14. Spielman, F. J., and Papio, K. A.: Pregnancy and heart disease. Key references. Circulation *65*:831, 1982.
15. Elkayam, U., and Gleicher, N.: Cardiovascular physiology of pregnancy. *In* Elkayam, U., and Gleicher, N. (eds.): Cardiac Problems in Pregnancy. New York, Alan R. Liss, Inc., 1982, p. 5.
16. Wilson, A.: Pulmonary physiology of pregnancy. *In* Elkayam, U., and Gleicher, N. (eds.): Cardiac Problems in Pregnancy. New York, Alan R. Liss, Inc., 1982, p. 5.
17. Katz, R., Karliner, J. S., and Resnik, R.: Effects of a natural volume overload state (pregnancy) on left ventricular performance in normal human subjects. Circulation *58*:434, 1978.
18. Lavid-Meeter, K., van de Ley, G., Bom, T. H., Wladimiroff, J. W., and Roelandt, J.: Cardiocirculatory adjustments during pregnancy—An echocardiographic study. Clin. Cardiol. *2*:328, 1979.
19. Ueland, K.: Maternal cardiovascular dynamics. VII. Intrapartum blood volume changes. Am. J. Obstet. Gynecol. *126*:671, 1976.
20. Robertson, E. G.: The natural history of oedema during pregnancy. J. Obstet. Gynecol. Br. Comm. *78*:520, 1971.
21. Rubler, S., Damani, P. M., and Pinto, E. R.: Cardiac size and performance during pregnancy estimated with echocardiography. Am. J. Cardiol. *40*:534, 1977.
22. Van Donsen, P. W., Eskes, T. K., Martin, C. B., and Van Hof, M. H.: Postural blood pressure differences in pregnancy. A prospective study of blood pressure differences between supine and left lateral position as measured by ultrasound. Am. J. Obstet. Gynecol. *138*:1, 1980.
23. Nakao, S., Come, P. C., Miller, M. J., Momomura, S., Sahagian, P., Ransil, B. J., and Grossman, W.: Effects of supine and lateral positions on cardiac output and intracardiac pressures: an experimental study. Circulation *73*:579, 1986.
24. Kerr, M. G.: The mechanical effects of the gravid uterus in late pregnancy. J. Obstet. Gynaecol. Br. Comm. *72*:513, 1965.
25. Ikard, R. W., Ueland, K., and Folse, R.: Lower limb venous dynamics in pregnant women. Surg. Gynecol. Obstet. *132*:483, 1971.
26. Christianson, R. E.: Studies on blood pressure during pregnancy. I. Influence of parity and age. Am. J. Obstet. Gynecol. *125*:509, 1976.
27. Marx, G. F., Husain, F. J., and Shiau, H. F.: Brachial and femoral blood pressures during the prenatal period. Am. J. Obstet. Gynecol. *136*:11, 1980.
28. Ueland, K., Novy, M. J., Peterson, E. N., and Metcalfe, J.: Maternal cardiovascular dynamics. IV. The influence of gestational age on the maternal cardiovascular response to posture and exercise. Am. J. Obstet. Gynecol. *104*:856, 1969.
29. Kim, Y. I., Chandra, P., and Marx, G. F.: Successful management of severe aortocaval compression in twin pregnancy. Obstet. Gynecol. *46*:362, 1975.
30. Biggs, J. S. G.: Blood pressure changes following smoking in pregnancy. Aust. N. Z. J. Obstet. Gynaecol. *15*:204, 1975.
31. Artal, R., Platt, L. D., Sperling, M., Kamula, R. K., Jilek, J., and Nakamura, R.: Maternal cardiovascular and metabolic responses in normal pregnancy. Am. J. Obstet. Gynecol. *140*:123, 1981.
32. Guzman, C. A., and Caplan, R.: Cardiorespiratory response to exercise during pregnancy. Am. J. Obstet. Gynecol. *108*:600, 1970.
33. Lees, M. M., Taylor, S. H., Scott, D. B., and Kerr, M. G.: A study of cardiac output at rest throughout pregnancy. J. Obstet. Gynec. Br. Comm. *74*:319, 1967.
34. Ueland, K., and Parer, J. T.: Effects of estrogens on the cardiovascular system of the ewe. Am. J. Obstet. Gynecol. *96*:400, 1966.
35. Wood, J. E.: The cardiovascular effects of oral contraceptives. Mod. Concepts Cardiovasc. Dis. *41*:37, 1972.
36. Manalo-Estrella, P., and Barker, A. E.: Histopathologic findings in human aortic media associated with pregnancy. A study of 16 cases. Arch. Pathol. *83*:336, 1967.
37. Cavanzo, F. J., and Taylor, H. B.: Effect of pregnancy on the human aorta and its relationship to dissecting aneurysms. Am. J. Obstet. Gynecol. *105*:567, 1969.
38. Novy, M. J., and Edwards, M. J.: Respiratory problems in pregnancy. Am. J. Obstet. Gynecol. *99*:1024, 1967.
39. Gazioglu, K., Kaltreider, N. L., Rosen, M., and Yu, P. N.: Pulmonary function during pregnancy in normal women and in patients with cardiopulmonary disease. Thorax *25*:445, 1970.
40. Pernoll, M. L., Metcalfe, J., Kovach, P. A., Wachtel, R., and Dunham, M. J.: Ventilation during rest and exercise in pregnancy and postpartum. Respir. Physiol. *25*:295, 1975.
41. Pernoll, M. L., Metcalfe, J., Schlenker, T. L., Welch, J. E., and Matsumoto, J. A.: Oxygen consumption at rest and during exercise in pregnancy. Respir. Physiol. *25*:285, 1975.
42. Cohen, W. R., Steinman, T., Patsner, B., Snyder, D., Satwicz, P., and Monroy, P.: Acute myocardial infarction in a pregnant woman at term. JAMA *250*:2179, 1983.
43. Ueland, K., and Hansen, J. M.: Maternal cardiovascular dynamics. III. Labor and delivery under local and caudal analgesia. Am. J. Obstet. Gynecol. *103*:8, 1969.
44. Whittemore, R.: Congenital heart disease: Its impact on pregnancy. Hosp. Pract. *18*:65, 1983.
45. De Pace, N. L., Betesh, J. S., and Kotler, M. N.: Postmortem cesarean section with recovery of both mother and offspring. J.A.M.A. *248*:971, 1982.
46. Wever, C. E.: Postmortem cesarean section: Review of the literature and case reports. Am. J. Obstet. Gynecol. *110*:158, 1971.
47. Rose, D. J., Bader, M. E., Bader, R. A., and Braunwald, E.: Catheterization studies of cardiac hemodynamics in normal pregnant women with reference to left ventricular work. Am. J. Obstet. Gynecol. 72:233, 1956.
48. Cutforth, R., and MacDonald, C. B.: Heart sounds and murmurs in pregnancy. Am. Heart J. *71*:741, 1966.
49. Goldberg, L. M., and Uhland, H.: Heart murmurs in pregnancy: A phonocardiographic study of their development, progression, and regression. Dis. Chest *52*:381, 1967.

50. Perloff, J. K.: Physical Examination of the Heart and Circulation. Philadelphia, W. B. Saunders Company, 1982.
51. Perloff, J. K.: The Clinical Recognition of Congenital Heart Disease. 3rd ed. Philadelphia, W. B. Saunders Company, 1986.
52. Tabatznick, B., Randall, T. W., and Hersch, C.: The mammary souffle of pregnancy and lactation. Circulation 22:1069, 1960.
53. Marcus, F. I., Ewy, F. A., O'Rourke, R. A., Walsh, B., and Bleich, A. C.: The effect of pregnancy on murmurs of mitral and aortic regurgitation. Circulation *41*:795, 1970.
54. Devereux, R. B., Perloff, J. K., Reichek, N., and Josephson, M. E.: Mitral valve prolapse. Circulation *54*:3, 1976.
55. Haas, J. M.: The effect of pregnancy on the midsystolic click and murmur of the prolapsing posterior leaflet of the mitral valve. Am. Heart J. 92:407, 1976.
56. Lutas, E. M., Devereux, R. B., Kramer-Fox, R., and Spitzer, M.: Disappearance of mitral valve prolapse during pregnancy. J. Cardiovasc. Ultrasonography *3*:183, 1984.
57. Kolibash, A. J., Ruiz, D. E., and Lewis, R. P.: Idiopathic hypertrophic subaortic stenosis in pregnancy. Ann. Intern. Med. *82*:791, 1975.
58. Carruth, J. E., Mirvis, S. B., Brogan, D. R., and Wenger, N. K.: The electrocardiogram in normal pregnancy. Am. Heart J. *102*:1075, 1981.
59. Boyle, D. M., and Lloyd-Jones, L. L.: The electrocardiographic ST segment in pregnancy. J. Obstet. Gynecol. Br. Comm. *73*:986, 1966.
60. Copeland, G. D., and Stern, T. N.: Wenckebach periods in pregnancy and puerperium. Am. Heart J. *56*:291, 1958.
61. McMillan, T. M., and Bellet, S.: Ventricular paroxysmal tachycardia: Report of a case in a pregnant girl of 16 years with apparently normal heart. Am. Heart J. 7:70, 1931.
62. Gallagher, J. J., Gilbert, M., and Sverson, R. H.: Wolff-Parkinson-White syndrome. The problems, evaluation and surgical correction. Circulation *51*:767, 1975.
63. Turner, A. F.: The chest radiograph in pregnancy. Clin. Obstet. Gynecol. *18*:65, 1975.

HEART DISEASE IN WOMEN OF CHILDBEARING AGE

64. Perloff, J. K.: Late postoperative concerns in adults with congenital heart disease. *In* Perloff, J. K. (ed.): Pediatric Cardiovascular Disease. Philadelphia, F. A. Davis Co., 1981.
65. Whittemore, R., Hobbins, J. C., and Engle, M. A.: Pregnancy and its outcome in women with and without surgical treatment of congenital heart disease. *In* Engle, M. A., and Perloff, J. K. (eds.): Congenital Heart Disease After Surgery. New York, Yorke Medical Books, 1983, p. 362.
66. Besterman, E.: The changing face of acute rheumatic fever. Br. Heart J. *32*:579, 1970.
67. Szekely, P., Turner, R., and Snaith, L.: Pregnancy and the changing pattern of rheumatic heart disease. Br. Heart J. 35:1293, 1973.
68. Chesley, L. C.: Severe rheumatic cardiac disease and pregnancy: The ultimate prognosis. Am. J. Obstet. Gynecol. *136*:552, 1980.
69. Ueland, K., and Metcalfe, J.: Acute rheumatic fever in pregnancy. Am. J. Obstet. Gynecol. 95:586, 1966.
70. Lewis, B. V., and Parsons, M.: Chorea gravidarum. Lancet *1*:284, 1966.
71. Wood, P.: An appreciation of mitral stenosis. Br. Med. J. *1*:1051 and 1113, 1954.
72. Ronan, J. A., Steelman, R. B., DeLeon, A. C., Waters, T. J., Perloff, J. K., and Harvey, W. P.: The clinical diagnosis of acute severe mitral insufficiency. Am. J. Cardiol. 27:284, 1971.
73. Reichek, N., Shelburne, J. C., and Perloff, J. K.: Clinical aspects of rheumatic valvular disease. Prog. Cardiovasc. Dis. *15*:491, 1973.
74. Roberts, W. C., and Perloff, J. K.: Mitral valvular disease. A clinicopathologic survey of the conditions causing the mitral valve to function abnormally. Ann. Intern. Med. 77:939, 1972.
75. Caves, P. K., and Paneth, M.: Acute mitral regurgitation in pregnancy due to ruptured chordae tendineae. Br. Heart J. *34*:541, 1972.
76. Perloff, J. K., and Harvey, W. P.: Clinical recognition of tricuspid stenosis. Circulation 22:346, 1960.
77. Loscalzo, J.: Paradoxical embolism. Am. Heart J. *112*:141, 1986.
78. Khoury, G. H., and Hawes, C. R.: Atrial septal defect associated with pulmonary hypertension in children living at high altitudes. J. Pediatr. *70*:432, 1967.
79. Deal, K., and Wooley, C. F.: Coarctation of aorta and pregnancy. Ann. Intern. Med. 78:706, 1973.
80. Barash, P. G., Hobbins, J. C., Hook, R., Stansel, H. C., Whittemore, R., and Hehre, F. W.: Management of coarctation of the aorta during pregnancy. J. Thorac. Cardiovasc. Surg. *69*:781, 1975.
81. Deal, K., and Wooley, C. F.: Coarctation of the aorta and pregnancy. Ann. Intern. Med. 78:706, 1973.
82. Roberts, W. C.: The congenitally bicuspid aortic valve. Am. J. Cardiol. *26*:72, 1970.
83. Morganroth, J., Perloff, J. K., Zeldis, S. M., and Dunkman, W. V.: Acute severe aortic regurgitation. Ann. Intern. Med. *87*:223, 1977.
84. Naeye, R. L., Hagstrom, J. W. C., and Talmadge, B. R.: Postpartum death with maternal congenital heart disease. Circulation *36*:304, 1967.
85. Pitts, J. A., Crosby, W. M., and Basta, L. L.: Eisenmenger's syndrome in pregnancy: Does heparin prophylaxis improve the maternal mortality rate? Am. Heart J. *93*:321, 1977.
86. Spinnato, J. A., Kraynak, B. J., and Cooper, M. W.: Eisenmenger's syndrome in pregnancy. N. Engl. J. Med. *304*:1215, 1981.
87. Haroutunian, L. M., and Neill, C. A.: Pulmonary complications of congenital heart disease: Hemoptysis. Am. Heart J. *84*:540, 1972.
88. Meyer, E. C., Tulsky, A. S., Sigmann, P., and Siber, E. N.: Pregnancy in the presence of tetralogy of Fallot. Am. J. Cardiol. *14*:874, 1964.
89. Jacoby, W. J.: Pregnancy with tetralogy and pentalogy of Fallot. Am. J. Cardiol. *14*:866, 1964.
90. Kenmure, A. C. F., and Cameron, A. J. V.: Congenital complete heart block in pregnancy. Br. Heart J. *29*:910, 1967.
91. Shouse, E. E., and Acker, G. E.: Pregnancy and delivery in a patient with external-internal cardiac pacemaker. Obstet. Gynecol. *24*:817, 1964.
92. Litsey, S. E., Noonan, J. A., O'Connor, W. N., Cottrill, C. M., and Mitchell, B.: Maternal connective tissue disease and congenital heart block. N. Engl. J. Med. *312*:98, 1985.
93. Lee, L. A., and Weston, W. L.: New findings in neonatal lupus syndrome. Am. J. Dis. Child. *138*:233, 1984.
94. Waickman, L. A., Skorton, D. J., Varner, M. W., Ehmke, D. A., and Goplerud, C. P.: Ebstein's anomaly and pregnancy. Am. J. Cardiol. *53*:357, 1984.
95. Littler, W. A.: Successful pregnancy in a patient with Ebstein's anonaly. Br. Heart J. 32:711, 1970.
96. Nielsen, N. C., and Fabricius, J.: Primary pulmonary hypertension with special reference to prognosis. Acta Med. Scand. *170*:731, 1961.
97. Hazlett, D. R., and Medina, J.: Postural effects on the bruit and right-to-left shunt of pulmonary arteriovenous fistula. Chest *60*:89, 1971.
98. Stiller, R. J., Vintzileos, A. M., Nochimson, D. J., Clement, D., Campbell, W. A., and Leach, C. N.: Single ventricle in pregnancy: Case report and review of the literature. Obstet. Gynecol. *64*:18S, 1984.
99. Leibbrant, G., Munch, U., and Gauder, M.: Two successful pregnancies with single ventricle and transposition of the great arteries. Int. J. Cardiol. *1*:257, 1982.
100. Warth, D. C., King, M. E., Cohen, J. M., Tesoriero, V. L., Marcus, E., and Weyman, A. E.: Prevalence of mitral valve prolapse in normal children. J. Am. Coll. Cardiol. 5:1173, 1985.
101. Shapiro, E. P., Trimble, E. L., Robinson, J. C., Estruch, M. T., and Gottlieb, S. H.: Safety of labor and delivery in women with mitral valve prolapse. Am. J. Cardiol. *56*:806, 1985.
102. Rayburn, W. F.: Mitral valve prolapse and pregnancy. *In* Elkayam, U., and Gleicher, N. (eds.): Cardiac Problems in Pregnancy. New York, Alan R. Liss, Inc., 1982, p. 191.
103. Shappell, S. D., Marshall, C. E., Brown, R. E., and Bruce, T. A.: Sudden death and the familial occurrence of mid-systolic click, late systolic murmur syndrome. Circulation *48*:1128, 1973.
104. Pyeritz, R. E.: Maternal and fetal complications of pregnancy in the Marfan syndrome. Am. J. Med. *71*:784, 1981.
105. Wilson, S. K., and Hutchins, G. M.: Aortic dissecting aneurysms: Causative factors in 204 subjects. Arch. Pathol. Lab. Med. *106*:175, 1982.
106. Rose, J. S., Lee, F., and Elkayam, U.: Aneurysms of the aorta and its major branches. *In* Gleicher, N. (ed.): Principles of Medical Therapy in Pregnancy. New York, Plenum Medical Book Co., 1985, p. 700.
107. Katz, N. M., Collea, J. V., Morant, M. G., MacKenzie, R. D., and Wallace, R. B.: Aortic dissection during pregnancy: Treatment by emergency cesarean section immediately followed by operative repair of the aortic dissection. Am. J. Cardiol. *54*:699, 1984.
108. Anagnostopoulos, C. E., Prabhakar, M., and Kittle, C. F.: Aortic dissections and dissecting aneurysms. Am. J. Cardiol. *30*:263, 1972.
109. Perloff, J. K.: Pathogenesis of hypertrophic cardiomyopathy. *In* Goodwin, J. F. (ed.): Heart Muscle Disease. Lancaster/Boston, MTP Press Limited, 1985, p. 7.
110. Kolibash, A. J., Ruiz, D. E., and Lewis, R. P.: Idiopathic hypertrophic subaortic stenosis in pregnancy. Ann. Intern. Med. *82*:791, 1975.
111. Oakley, G. D. G., McGarry, K., Limb, D. G., and Oakley, C. M.: Management of pregnancy in patients with hypertrophic cardiomyopathy. Br. Med. J. *1*:1749, 1979.
112. Kumar, A., and Elkayam, U.: Hypertrophic cardiomyopathy in pregnancy. *In* Gleicher, N. (ed.): Principles of Medical Therapy in Pregnancy. New York, Plenum Medical Book Company, 1985, p. 695.
112a. Shah, D. M., and Sunderji, S. G.: Hypertrophic cardiomyopathy and pregnancy: Report of a maternal mortality and review of the literature. Obestet. Gynecol. Surv. *40*:444, 1985.
113. Demakis, J. G., and Rahimtoola, S. H.: Peripartum cardiomyopathy. Circulation *44*:964, 1971.
114. Demakis, J. G., Rahimtoola, S. H., Sutton, G. C., Meadows, W. R., Szanto, P. B., Tobin, J. R., and Gunnar, R. M.: Natural course of peripartum cardiomyopathy. Circulation *44*:1053, 1971.
115. Veille, J. C.: Peripartum cardiomyopathy: A review. Am. J Obstet. Gynecol. *148*:805, 1984.
116. Cunningham, F. G., Pritchard, J. A., Hankins, G. D. V., Anderson, P. L., Lucas, M. J., and Armstrong, K. F.: Peripartum heart failure: idiopathic cardiomyopathy or compounding cardiovascular events? Obstet. Gynecol. *67*:157, 1986.
117. O'Connell, J. B., Costanzo-Nordin, M. R., Subramanian, R., Robinson, J. A., Wallis, D. E., Scanlon, P. J., and Gunnar, R. M.: Peripartum cardiomyopathy: Clinical, hemodynamic, histologic and prognostic characteristics. J. Am. Coll. Cardiol. 8:52, 1986.
118. Ribner, H. S., and Silverman, R.: Peripartal cardiomyopathy. *In* Gleicher, N. (ed.): Principles of Medical Therapy in Pregnancy. New York, Plenum Medical Book Co., 1985, p. 689.
119. Homans, D. C.: Peripartum cardiomyopathy. N. Engl. J. Med. *312*:1432, 1985.
120. Melvin, K. R., Richardson, P. J., Olsen, E. G. J., Daly, K., and Jackson, G.: Peripartum cardiomyopathy due to myocarditis. N. Engl. J. Med. *307*:731, 1982.

121. Huerta, E. M., Erice, A., Espino, R. F., Navascues, I., and deDios, R. M.: Postpartum cardiomyopathy and acute myocarditis. Am. Heart J. *110*:1079, 1980.
122. Rand, R. J., Jenkins, D. M., and Scott, D. G.: Maternal cardiomyopathy of pregnancy causing stillbirth. Br. J. Obstet. Gynaecol. *82*:172, 1975.
123. Knobel, B., Melamud, E., and Kishon, Y.: Peripartum cardiomyopathy. Israel J. Med. Sci. *20*:1061, 1984.
124. Rocklin, R. E., Kitzmiller, J. L., and Kaye, M. D.: Immunobiology of the maternal-fetal relationship. Ann. Rev. Med. *30*:375, 1979.
125. Sridama, V., Pacini, F., Yang, S., Moawad, A., Reilly, M., and De Groot, L. J.: Decreased levels of helper T cells. A possible cause of immunodeficiency in pregnancy. N. Engl. J. Med. *307*:352, 1982.
126. Stites, D. P., Pavia, C. S., Clemens, L. E., Kuhn, R. W., and Sliteri, P. K.: Immunologic regulation in pregnancy. Arthritis Rheum. 22:1300, 1979.
126a. Lewis, J. E., Coulam, C. B., and Moore, S. B.: Immunologic mechanisms in the maternal-fetal relationship. Mayo Clin. Proc. *61*:655, 1986.
127. Huzar, G.: Biology and biochemistry of myometrial contractility and cervical maturation. Semin. Perinatol. 5:216, 1981.
128. Davidson, N. M., and Parry, E. H. O.: Peri-partum cardiac failure. Q. J. Med. *47*:431, 1978.
129. Fillmore, S. J., and Parry, E. H. O.: The evolution of peripartal heart failure in Zaria, Nigeria. Circulation *56*:1058, 1977.
130. Lin, C. C., Lindheimer, M. U., River, P., and Moawad, A. H.: Fetal outcome in hypertensive disorders of pregnancy. Am. J. Obstet. Gynecol. *142*:255, 1982.
131. Gant, N. F., and Worley, R. J.: Hypertension in Pregnancy: Concepts and Management. New York, Appleton-Century-Crofts, 1980.
132. Page, E. W., and Christianson, R.: Influence of blood pressure changes with and without proteinuria upon outcome of pregnancy. Am. J. Obstet. Gynecol. *126*:821, 1976.
133. Finnerty, F. A.: Hypertension is different in blacks. J.A.M.A. *216*:1634, 1971.
134. Finnerty, F. A.: Hypertension and pregnancy. J. Cardiovasc. Med. *5*:559, 1980.
135. Drayer, J. I. M., and Weber, M. A.: The use of antihypertensive drugs. *In* Elkayam, U., and Gleicher, N. (eds.): Cardiac Problems in Pregnancy. New York, Alan R. Liss, Inc., 1982, p. 245.
136. Silverstone, A., Trudinger, B. J., Lewis, P. J., and Bulpitt, C. J.: Maternal hypertension and intrauterine fetal death in midpregnancy. Br. J. Obstet. Gynaecol. *87*:457, 1980.
137. Weir, R. J., and Willocks, J.: A successful pregnancy following malignant phase hypertension. Br. J. Obstet. Gynecol. *83*:584, 1976.
138. Soffronoff, E. C., Kaufmann, B. M., and Connaughton, J. F.: Intravascular volume determinations and fetal outcome in hypertensive diseases of pregnancy. Am. J. Obstet. Gynecol. *127*:4, 1977.
139. Stempel, J. E., O'Grady, J. P., Morton, M. J., and Johnson, K. A.: Use of sodium nitroprusside in complications of gestational hypertension. Obstet. Gynecol. *60*:533, 1982.
140. Chesley, L. C., Annitto, J. E., and Cosgrove, R. A.: The remote prognosis of eclamptic women: Sixth periodic report. Am. J. Obstet. Gynecol. *124*:446, 1976.
141. Bauer, T. W., Moore, G. W., and Hutchins, G. M.: Morphologic evidence for coronary artery spasm in eclampsia. Circulation *65*:255, 1982.
142. Meller, J., and Goldman, M. E.: Arrhythmias in pregnancy. *In* Gleicher, N. (ed.): Principles of Medical Therapy in Pregnancy. New York, Plenum Medical Book Co., 1985, p. 710.
143. Schroeder, J. S., and Harrison, D. C.: Repeated cardioversion during pregnancy. Am. J. Cardiol. *27*:445, 1971.
144. Gleicher, N., Meller, J., Sandler, R. Z., and Sullum, S.: Wolff-Parkinson-White syndrome in pregnancy. Obstet. Gynecol. *58*:748, 1981.
145. Rotmensch, H. H., Lessing, J. B., and Donchin, Y.: Clinical pharmacology of antiarrhythmic drugs in the pregnant patient. *In* Elkayam, U., and Gleicher, N. (eds.): Cardiac Problems in Pregnancy. New York, Alan R. Liss, Inc., 1982, p. 227.
146. Pitcher, D., Leather, H. M., Storey, G. C. A., and Holt, D. W.: Amiodarone in pregnancy. Lancet *1*:597, 1983.
147. Klotz, T. A.: Thrombophlebitis and pulmonary embolism. *In* Gleicher, N. (ed.): Principles of Medical Therapy in Pregnancy. New York, Plenum Medical Book Co., 1985, p. 721.
148. Oakley, C., and Somerville, J.: Oral contraceptives and progressive pulmonary vascular disease. Lancet *1*:890, 1968.
149. Ginz, B.: Myocardial infarction in pregnancy. J. Obstet. Gynecol. *77*:610, 1970.
150. Majdan, J. F., Walinsky, P., Cowchock, S. F., Wapner, R. J., and Plazak, L.: Coronary artery bypass surgery during pregnancy. Am. J. Cardiol. 52:1145, 1983.
151. Henion, W. A., Hilal, A., Matthew, P. K., Lazarus, A., and Cohen, J.: Postpartum myocardial infarction. N. Y. State J. Med. *82*:57, 1982.
152. Ciraulo, D. A., and Markovitz, A.: Myocardial infarction in pregnancy associated with a coronary artery thrombus. Arch. Intern. Med. *139*:1046, 1979.
153. Ishikawa, K., and Matsuura, S.: Occlusive thromboaortopathy (Takayasu's disease) and pregnancy. Clinical course and management of 33 pregnancies and deliveries. Am. J. Cardiol. *50*:1293, 1982.
154. Hauth, J. C., Cunningham, F. G., and Young, P. K.: Takayasu's syndrome in pregnancy. Obstet. Gynecol. *50*:373, 1977.
155. Claudon, D. G., Claudon, D. B., and Edwards, J. E.: Primary dissecting aneurysm of coronary artery. Circulation *45*:259, 1972.
156. Shaver, P. J., Carrig, T. F., and Baker, W. P.: Postpartum coronary artery dissection. Br. Heart J. *40*:83, 1978.
157. Perloff, J. K., Stevenson, W. G., Roberts, N. K., Cabeen, W., and Weiss, J. N.: Cardiac involvement in myotonic muscular dystrophy (Steinert's disease). Am. J. Cardiol. *54*:1074, 1984.
158. Shore, R. N., and MacLachlan, T. B.: Pregnancy with myotonic dystrophy. Obstet. Gynecol. *38*:448, 1971.
159. Schwartz, I. L., Dingfelder, J. R., O'Tuama, L., and Swift, M.: Recessive congenital myotonia and pregnancy. Int. J. Gynaecol. Obstet. *17*:194:1979.
160. Sachs, B. P., Lorell, B. H., Mehrez, M., and Damian, N.: Constrictive pericarditis and pregnancy. Am. J. Obstet. Gynecol. *154*:156, 1986.
161. Blake, S., Bonar, F., McDonald, D., McCarthy, J. R., Flanagan, M., Garrett, J., and Kirwan, M.: Pregnancy with constrictive pericarditis. Br. J. Obstet. Gynacol. *91*:404, 1984.
162. Noller, K. L.: Cardiac surgery and pregnancy. *In* Gleicher, N. (ed.): Principles of Medical Therapy in Pregnancy. New York, Plenum Medical Book Co., 1985, p. 713.
163. El-Maraghy, M., Senna, I. A., El-Tehewy, F., Bassiouni, M., Ayoub, A., and El-Sayed, H.: Mitral valvotomy in pregnancy. Am. J. Obstet. Gynecol. *145*:708, 1983.
164. Becker, R. M.: Intracardiac surgery in pregnant women. Ann. Thorac. Surg. *36*:453, 1983.
165. Kay, C. F., and Smith, K.: Surgery in the pregnant cardiac patient. Am. J. Cardiol. *12*:293, 1963.
166. Salomon, J., Yortner, R., and Levy, M. J.: Open heart surgery during pregnancy—Case report. Vasc. Surg. *9*:257, 1975.
167. Gazzaniga, A.: Cardiac surgery during pregnancy. *In* Elkayam, U., and Gleicher, N. (eds.): Cardiac Problems in Pregnancy. New York, Alan R. Liss, Inc., 1982, p. 199.
168. Ueland, K.: Cardiac surgery and pregnancy. Am. J. Obstet. Gynecol. *92*:148, 1965.
169. Perloff, J. K.: Development and regression of increased ventricular mass. Am. J. Cardiol. *50*:605, 1982.
170. Czeizel, A., Pornoi, A., Peterffy, E., and Tarcal, E.: Study of children of parents operated on for congenital cardiovascular malformations. Br. Heart J. *47*:290, 1982.
171. Dennis, N. R., and Warren, J.: Risks to the offspring of patients with some common congenital heart defects. J. Med. Genet. *18*:8, 1981.
172. Rose, V., Gold, R. J. M., Lindsay, G., and Allen, M.: A possible increase in the incidence of congenital heart defects among the offspring of affected parents. J. Am. Coll. Cardiol. *6*:376, 1985.
173. Nissenkorn, A., Friedman, S., Schonfeld, A., and Ovadia, J.: Fetomaternal outcome in pregnancies after total correction of the tetralogy of Fallot. Int. Surg. *69*:125, 1984.
174. Burch, G. E., and Giles, T. D.: The burden of a hot humid environment on the heart. Mod. Conc. Cardiovasc. Dis. *39*:115, 1970.
175. Stevens, K. M.: Cardiac stroke volume as a determinant of influenzal fatality. N. Engl. J. Med. *295*:1363, 1976.
176. Shulman, S. T., Amren, D. P., Bisno, A. L., Dajani, A. S., Durack, D. T., Gerber, M. A., Kaplan, E. L., Millard, H. D., Sanders, W. E., Schwartz, R. H., and Watanakunakorn, C.: Prevention of bacterial endocarditis. Circulation *70*:1123A, 1984.
177. Sugrue, D., Blake, S., and Troy, P.: Antibiotic prophylaxis against infective endocarditis after normal delivery—Is it necessary? Br. Heart J. *44*:599, 1980.
178. Kaplan, E. L., Anthony, B. F., Bisno, A., Durack, D., Hauser, H., Millard, H. D., Sanford, J., Shulman, S. T., Stillerman, M., Taranta, A., and Wenger, N.: Prevention of bacterial endocarditis. Circulation *56*:139A, 1977.
179. Selzer, A.: Risks of pregnancy in women with cardiac disease. J.A.M.A. *238*:892, 1977.
180. Friedman, E. A., and Neff, R. K.: Hypertension-hypotension in pregnancy. Correlation with fetal outcome. J.A.M.A. *239*:2249, 1978.
181. Whittemore, R., Hobbins, J. C., and Engle, M. A.: Pregnancy and its outcome in women with and without surgical treatment of congenital heart disease. Am. J. Cardiol. *50*:641, 1982.
182. Novy, M. J., Peterson, E. N., and Metcalfe, J.: Respiratory characteristics of maternal and fetal blood in cyanotic congenital heart disease. Am. J. Obstet. Gynecol. *100*:821, 1968.
183. Chandler, W. U.: Banishing tobacco. *In* Brown E. R., Wolf, E. C., and Starke, L. (eds.): State of the World 1986. New York, W. W. Norton & Co., 1986, p. 139.
184. Killam, A. P.: Tobacco smoking. *In* Gleicher, N. (ed.): Principles of Medical Therapy in Pregnancy. New York, Plenum Medical Book Co., 1985, p. 114.
185. Asmussen, I.: Fetal cardiovascular system as influenced by maternal smoking. Clin. Cardiol. *2*:246, 1979.
186. Ritchie, K.: The fetal response to changes in the composition of maternal inspired air. Semin. Perinatol. *4*:295, 1980.
187. Meyer, M. B., and Tonascia, J. A.: Maternal smoking, pregnancy complications and perinatal mortality. Am. J. Obstet. Gynecol. *128*:494, 1977.
188. Hummelberger, D. U., Brown, B. W., and Cohen, E. N.: Cigarette smoking during pregnancy and the occurrence of spontaneous abortion and congenital abnormality. Am. J. Epidemiol. *108*:470, 1978.
189. Killam, A. P.: Alcohol. *In* Gleicher, N. (ed.): Principles of Medical Management in Pregnancy. New York, Plenum Medical Book Co., 1985, p. 103.
190. Hill, L. M., and Kleinberg, F.: Effects of drugs and chemicals on the fetus and newborn. Mayo Clin. Proc. *59*:707 and 755, 1984.
191. Abel, E. L., and Sokol, R. J.: Prevention of alcohol-related birth defects. *In*

Gleicher, N. (ed.): Principles of Medical Management in Pregnancy. New York, Plenum Medical Book Co., 1985, p. 105.
192. Strassner, H. T., and Arnolds, C. W.: Environment and pregnancy. *In* Gleicher, N. (ed.): Principles of Medical Management in Pregnancy. New York, Plenum Medical Book Co., 1985, p. 117.
193. Moore, L. G., Hershey, D. W., and Jahnigen, D.: The incidence of pregnancy-induced hypertension is increased among Colorado residents at high altitude. Am. J. Obstet. Gynecol. *144*:423, 1982.
194. Hingson, R., Alpert, L. L., Day, N., Dooling, E., Kayne, H., Morelock, S., Oppenheimer, E., and Zukerman, B.: Effects of maternal drinking and marijuana use on fetal growth and development. Pediatrics *70*:539, 1982.
195. Confino, E., and Gleicher, N.: Drug abuse in pregnancy. *In* Gleicher, N. (ed.): Principles of Medical Management in Pregnancy. New York, Plenum Medical Book Co., 1985, p. 90.
196. Fried, P. A.: Marijuana use by pregnant women and effects on offspring. Neurobehav. Toxicol. Teratol. *4*:451, 1982.
197. Editorial. Drugged sperm. Br. Med. J. *1*:10064, 1964.
198. Rudolph, A. M.: Effects of aspirin and acetaminophen in pregnancy and in the newborn. Arch. Intern. Med. *141*:358, 1981.
199. Corby, D. G.: Aspirin in pregnancy and fetal effects. Pediatrics *62*:930, 1978.
200. Tamari, I., Eldar, M., Rabinowitz, B., and Neufeld, H. N.: Medical treatment of cardiovascular disorders during pregnancy. Am. Heart J. *104*:1357, 1982.
201. Cupit, G. G., and Rotmensch, H. H.: Principles of drug therapy in pregnancy. *In* Gleicher, N. (ed.): Principles of Medical Therapy in Pregnancy. New York, Plenum Medical Book Co., 1985, p. 77.
202. Katz, M., Robertson, P. A., and Creasy, R. K.: Cardiovascular complications associated with terbutaline for preterm labor. Am. J. Obstet. Gynecol. *139*:605, 1981.
203. Jacobs, M. M., Knight, A. B., and Arias, F.: Maternal pulmonary edema resulting from betamimetic and glucocorticoid therapy. Obstet. Gynecol. *56*:56, 1980.
204. Elliott, J. P., O'Keefe, D. F., Greenberg, P., and Freeman, R. K.: Pulmonary edema associated with magnesium sulfate and betamethasone administration. Am. J. Obstet. Gynecol. *134*:717, 1979.
205. Wagner, J. M., Morton, M. J., Johnson, K. A., O'Grady, J. P., and Speroff, L.: Terbutaline and maternal cardiac function. J.A.M.A. *246*:2697, 1981.
206. Briggs, G. G., Bodendorfer, T. W., Freeman, R. K., and Yaffe, S. J.: Drugs in pregnancy and lactation. Baltimore, Williams and Wilkins, 1983.
207. McBride, W. G.: Thalidomide and congenital abnormalities. Lancet *2*:1358, 1961.
208. Habib, A., and McCarthy, J. S.: Effects on the neonate of propranolol administered during pregnancy. J. Pediatr. *91*:808, 1977.
209. Pruyn, S. C., Phelan, J. P., and Buchanan, G. C.: Long term propranolol therapy in pregnancy: Maternal and fetal outcome. Am. J. Obstet. Gynecol. *135*:485, 1979.
210. Cottrill, C. M., McAllister, R. G., and Gelles, L.: Propranolol therapy during pregnancy, labor and delivery. J. Pediatr. *91*:812, 1977.
211. Dicke, J. M.: Cardiovascular drugs in pregnancy. *In* Gleicher, N. (ed.): Principles of Medical Therapy in Pregnancy. New York, Plenum Medical Book Co., 1985, p. 646.
212. Morley, K. J., McAinsh, J., and Cruickshank, J. M.: Atenolol in the treatment of pregnancy-induced hypertension. Br. J. Clin. Pharmacol. *12*:725, 1981.
213. Rubin, P. C., Butters, L., Low, R. A., and Reid, J. L.: Atenolol in the treatment of essential hypertension during pregnancy. Br. J. Clin. Pharmacol. *14*:279, 1982.
214. Rotmensch, H. H., Elkayam, U., and Frishman, W.: Antiarrhythmic drug therapy during pregnancy. Ann. Intern. Med. *98*:487, 1983.
215. Rogers, M. C., Willerson, J. T., Goldblatt, A., and Smith, T. W.: Serum digoxin concentrations in the human fetus, neonate and infant. N. Engl. J. Med. *287*:1010, 1972.
216. Norris, P. R.: The action of cardiac gylcosides on the human uterus. J. Obstet. Gynecol. Br. Comm. *68*:916, 1961.
217. Hill, L. M., and Malkasian, G. D.: The use of quinidine sulfate throughout pregnancy. Obstet. Gynecol. *54*:366, 1979.
218. Dumesic, D. A., Silverman, N. H., Tobias, S., and Golbus, M. S.: Transplacental cardioversion of fetal supraventricular tachycardia with procainamide. N. Engl. J. Med. *307*:1128, 1982.
219. Kuhnert, B. R., Knapp, D. R., Kuhnert, P. M., and Prochaska, A. L.: Maternal, fetal and neonatal metabolism of lidocaine. Clin. Pharmacol. Therap. *26*:213, 1979.
220. Wolff, F., Breuker, K. H., Schlensker, K. H., and Bolte, A.: Prenatal diagnosis and therapy of fetal heart rate anomalies: With a contribution on the placental transfer of verapamil. J. Perinat. Med. *8*:203, 1980.
221. Timmis, A. D., and Jackson, G.: Mexiletine for control of ventricular arrhythmias in pregnancy. Lancet *2*:647, 1980.
222. Hanson, J. W., and Smith, D. W.: The fetal hydantoin syndrome. J. Pediatr. *87*:285, 1975.
223. Phelan, M. C., Pellock, J. M., and Nance, W. E.: Discordant expression of fetal hydantoin syndrome in heteropaternal dizygotic twins. N. Engl. J. Med. *307*:99, 1982.
224. McKenna, W. J., Harris, L., Rowland, E., Whitelaw, A., Storey, G., and Holt, D.: Amiodarone therapy during pregnancy. Am. J. Cardiol. *51*:1231, 1983.
225. Robson, D. J., Raj, M. V. J., Storey, G. C. A., and Holt, D. W.: Use of amiodarone during pregnancy. Postgrad. Med. J. *61*:75, 1985.
226. Penn, I. M., Barrett, P. A., Pannikote, V., Barnaby, P. F., Campbell, J. B., and Lyons, N. R.: Amiodarone in pregnancy. Am. J. Cardiol. *56*:196, 1985.
227. Bortolotti, U., Milano, A., Mazzucco, A., Valfre, C., Russo, R., Valente, M., Schivazappa, L., Thiene, G., and Gallucci, V.: Pregnancy in patients with a porcine bioprosthesis. Am. J. Cardiol. *50*:1051, 1982.
228. O'Neill, H., Blake, S., Sugrue, D., and MacDonald, D.: Problems in the management of patients with artificial valves during pregnancy. Br. J. Obstet. Gynaecol. *89*:940, 1982.
229. Salazar, E., Zajarias, A., Gutierrez, N., and Iturbe, I.: The problem of cardiac prostheses, anticoagulants and pregnancy. Circulation *70*(Suppl. I):169, 1984.
230. Limet, R., and Grondin, C. M.: Cardiac valve prostheses, anticoagulation, and pregnancy. Ann. Thorac. Surg. *23*:337, 1977.
231. Taguchi, K.: Pregnancy in patients with a prosthetic heart valve. Surg. Gynecol. Obstet. *145*:206, 1977.
232. Ibarra-Perez, C., Arevalo-Toledo, N., Cadena, O. A., and Noriega-Guerra, L.: The course of pregnancy in patients with artificial heart valves. Am. J. Med. *61*:504, 1976.
233. Buxbaum, A., Aygen, M. M., Sajhin, W., Levy, M. J., and Ekerling, B.: Pregnancy in patients with prosthetic heart valves. Chest *59*:639, 1971.
234. Lee, P., Wang, R. Y. C., Chow, J. S. F., Cheung, K., Wong, V. C. W., and Chan, T.: Combined use of warfarin and adjusted subcutaneous heparin during pregnancy in patients with an artificial heart valve. J. Am. Coll. Cardiol. *8*:221, 1986.
235. Casanegra, P., Aviles, G., Maturana, G., and Dubernet, J.: Cardiovascular management of pregnant women with a heart valve prosthesis. Am. J. Cardiol. *36*:802, 1975.
236. Hirsh, J., Cade, J. K., and Gallus, A. S.: Anticoagulants in pregnancy: A review of indications and complications. Am. Heart J. *83*:301, 1972.
237. Hall, J. G., Pauli, R. M., and Wilson, K. M.: Maternal and fetal sequelae of anticoagulation during pregnancy. Am. J. Med. *68*:122, 1980.
238. Pettifor, J. M., and Benson, R.: Congenital malformations associated with the administration of oral anticoagulants during pregnancy. J. Pediatr. *86*:459, 1975.
239. Shaul, W. L., Emery, H., and Hall, J. G.: Chondrodysplasia punctata and maternal warfarin use during pregnancy. Am. J. Dis. Child. *129*:360, 1975.
240. Stevenson, R. E., Burton, M., Ferlauto, G. J., and Taylor, H. A.: Hazards of oral anticoagulants during pregnancy. J.A.M.A. *243*:1549, 1980.
240a. Iturlie-Alessio, I., Fonseca, M. C., Mutchinik, O., Santos, M. A., Zajarias, A., and Salazar, E.: Risks of anticoagulant therapy in pregnant women with artificial heart valves. N. Engl. J. Med. *315*:1390, 1986.
241. Chen, W. W. C., Chan, C. S., Lee, P. K., Wang, R. Y. C., and Wong, V. C. W.: Pregnancy in patients with prosthetic heart valves. Q. J. Med. (New Series LI) *203*:358, 1982.
242. Hull, R., Delmore, T., Carter, C., Hirsh, J., Genton, E., Gent, M., Turpie, G., and McLaughlin, D.: Adjusted subcutaneous heparin versus warfarin sodium in the long-term treatment of venous thrombosis. N. Engl. J. Med. *306*:189, 1982.
243. Spearing, G., Fraser, I., Turner, G., and Dixon, G.: Long-term self-administered subcutaneous heparin in pregnancy. Br. Med. J. *1*:1457, 1978.
244. Ueland, K., McAnulty, J. H., Ueland, F. R., and Metcalfe, J.: Special considerations in the use of cardiovascular drugs. Clin. Obstet. Gynecol. *24*:809, 1981.
245. Chesley, L. C.: Rheumatic cardiac disease in pregnancy. Obstet. Gynecol. *46*:699, 1975.
246. Chesley, L. C.: Severe rheumatic cardiac disease and pregnancy. Am. J. Obstet. Gynecol. *136*:552, 1979.

61 RELATIONSHIP BETWEEN DISEASES OF THE HEART AND LUNGS

by E. REGIS MCFADDEN, Jr., M.D., and
ROLAND H. INGRAM, Jr., M.D.

Because of the integrated nature of the function of the heart and lungs, it is difficult for one component to be compromised without altering the physiology of the other. In fact, with chronic disease originating in either the heart or the lungs, there is both subjective and objective evidence of dysfunction in both systems. While a great deal is known about right ventricular hypertrophy or dilatation secondary to lung disease (e.g., cor pulmonale, Chap. 48) and pulmonary malfunction in acute left ventricular failure (e.g., pulmonary edema, Chap. 18), many other pathophysiological interfaces between the cardiovascular and pulmonary systems exist clinically. The purposes of this chapter are to explore some of these interactions and detail their mechanisms as far as they are known.

MECHANISMS BY WHICH HEART DISEASE LEADS TO LUNG DYSFUNCTION

(See also p. 477)

Cardiac disease can alter lung function or induce pulmonary disease through the effects of (1) pulmonary venous hypertension from elevated left ventricular end-diastolic and/or left atrial pressures[1–12]; (2) compression of mediastinal structures, airways, or lung by global cardiomegaly, pericardial and pleural effusions, and specific chamber enlargement[13–16]; (3) pharmacological agents used to treat cardiac disease, such as beta antagonists, diuretics, nitrates, and others[17–22]; and (4) miscellaneous phenomena such as hemoptysis owing to cardiac disease giving rise to blood pneumonias. Of these, the most important factor is pulmonary venous hypertension.

INCREASED PULMONARY VENOUS PRESSURE

Physiologically significant increases in left ventricular end-diastolic or left atrial pressures are invariably transmitted retrogradely to the pulmonary vasculature and, in addition to producing pulmonary arterial hypertension, evoke one or more of the stages of pulmonary edema formation (i.e., increased lymph flow, interstitial edema, or alveolar edema, Chap. 18). The magnitude and duration of the pulmonary venous hypertension then determine the extent to which the lung is affected.[23] If the changes in pressure are acute and modest in degree, vascular engorgement and perivascular and interstitial edema predominate. In these circumstances the effects on the lung tend to be subtle. If the venous pressure changes are chronic, then the changes in lung function are more easily measured because, in addition to the above, anatomical changes such as fibrosis, medial hypertrophy, and intimal thickening may develop in the arteries and veins, airways narrow from peribronchiolar and mucosal edema, and the interstitial edema within the parenchyma may eventually be replaced by fibrosis.[24] In rare instances the last can be so severe that dense calcification and actual bone formation can develop.[25] Thus it is not possible to elevate pulmonary venous pressures without altering lung function. The *lung* is the organ that undergoes the anatomical and physiological disturbances responsible for dyspnea, chest tightness, and cough.

ALTERATIONS IN PULMONARY MECHANICS. From a mechanical standpoint, patients with chronically elevated pulmonary venous pressure can be characterized as having "restrictive ventilatory defects" (i.e., loss of lung volume). Typically, vital capacity is reduced, residual volume and functional residual capacity are normal or nearly so, and total lung capacity is less than predicted.[6, 7, 26, 27] The reduction in total lung capacity results from replacement of the air in the lung with either blood or interstitial fluid, with resulting changes in the elastic properties of the pulmonary parenchyma. As pulmonary venous hypertension (hence interstitial and alveolar wall edema) advances, the lung becomes stiffer or less compliant. As this process worsens, air trapping can occur because of earlier than normal closure of dependent airways, and residual volume may actually increase as total lung capacity decreases.[5, 28]

The progressive changes in lung size and recoil tend to increase the pleural pressures required to effect respiration, thus elevating the work of breathing and thereby leading to tachypnea with a low tidal volume and high respiratory frequency.[29]

In addition to volume loss, there is evidence that pulmonary vascular congestion and edema can interfere with peripheral airway function.[5, 30–35] Studies in animals have shown that the resistance in distal airways increases to a greater degree in response to elevations of left atrial pressure than does total airway resistance and that with sustained increases of pressure pulmonary changes are slow to resolve. These findings suggest that engorgement of the blood vessels within the confines of the bronchovascular sheath can encroach on the lumina of the airways and promote edema formation, which can persist for considerable periods. Such observations provide the basis for understanding disturbances in ventilation-perfusion relationships that can often be profound in pulmonary congestion or edema.

ALTERATIONS IN THE DISTRIBUTION OF VENTILATION AND PERFUSION. The mechanical factor that determines the distribution of ventilation within the lung is the product of the resistance of the bronchi and the compliance of the subtended alveolar units. This product is called a time constant ($R \times C = \tau$), and in the normal lung the regional values for τ are nearly equal so that all the alveoli fill and empty synchronously when respiration is initiated at functional residual capacity.[36] However, because of the above derangements in compliance and resistance in heart disease, interregional and intraregional nonhomogeneities develop and result in maldistribution of inspired air. Regional alveolar hypoxia then ensues with its sequelae.[37] The maldistribution becomes more severe with increases in respiratory frequency,[37, 38] thus the exercise performance of affected patients is altered not only by insufficient cardiac response but also by worsening distribution of ventilation.

The disease in the pulmonary vessels gives rise to abnormal distribution of perfusion, with a reversal of the normal apex-to-base gradient (Fig. 18–5, p. 548) (i.e., the apical lung zones are perfused more than the basilar lung zones).[8–12] The extent of reversal correlates well with increases in pulmonary capillary wedge pressure.[8, 9, 11] Although there is evidence that the arterioles in the basilar zones of the lung are more responsive to hypoxia than are their apical counterparts in normal subjects,[39] breathing 100 per cent oxygen in mitral stenosis does not completely correct the abnormal distribution of blood flow,[40] suggesting that hypoxic vasoconstriction is not the sole cause for the reversed flow pattern. Acute perivascular edema probably accounts for some of the changes in the flow pattern, but in chronic pulmonary venous hypertension, structural vascular alterations develop (p. 798) and play a prominent role. These pathological changes tend to be more severe in the basilar zones.[40, 41] The overall physiological consequences of all these abnormalities are mismatched ventilation-perfusion relationships that result in widened alveolar-arterial differences for oxygen, arterial hypoxemia, and enlarged dead space-tidal volume ratios.[26]

An additional factor often considered to *cause* the reductions in arterial oxygen content and partial pressure seen in heart disease is a depressed partial pressure of oxygen in the mixed venous blood.[42] However, for several reasons, consideration of this factor as a cause of arterial hypoxemia leads to circular reasoning. In normal subjects engaging in heavy exercise at sea level while breathing air, the mixed venous oxygen content diminishes to extremely low values, yet the arterial content remains normal. Hence low values for mixed venous oxygen do not a priori cause a lower than normal arterial value. However, when there is abnormal gas exchange in the lung, whether caused by ventilation-perfusion abnormalities or shunt, low arterial oxygen contents result in lower mixed venous values at any given oxygen consumption and cardiac output. Basically, then, the values for mixed venous oxygen are the most dependent of the variables affecting heart-lung interrelations and are the result of oxygen transfer in the lung, cardiac output, and peripheral tissue metabolic consumption of oxygen. Therefore, this factor should always be considered as a *consequence* of hypoxemia rather than as a principal cause.

ALTERATIONS IN ARTERIAL BLOOD GASES. The extent to which arterial blood gases are disturbed depends on the severity and suddenness of the rise in left-side pressures. In acute pulmonary edema secondary to left ventricular decompensation, gas exchange can be so severely compromised that frank respiratory failure can result. Aberman and Fulop, in a prospective study of 50 consecutive cases of pulmonary edema, demonstrated that, before treatment, affected patients as a group had severe hypoxemia and either metabolic or combined metabolic and respiratory acidosis.[43] In this study 58 per cent of the patients had values for arterial pO_2 that were less than 50 mm Hg, and 83 per cent had acidemia with a pH less than 7.36. Hypoxemia was most severe in the patients with the greatest acidosis. Twenty-three patients had hypocapnia, 12 were eucapnic, and 11 had arterial carbon dioxide tensions in excess of 45 mm Hg. The hypercapnic patients did not have a greater incidence of underlying chronic airway obstruction than those without carbon dioxide retention. The arterial carbon dioxide tensions and pH rapidly returned to normal with resolution of alveolar hypoventilation resulting from alveolar flooding and interstitial edema, and with the disappearance of the lactic acidosis secondary to the low cardiac output state.

RESPIRATORY RESPONSE TO EXERCISE. The abnormalities in mechanics and gas-exchanging function of the lung described thus far are related to the degree and chronicity of the elevated pulmonary capillary pressures. Because there are further increases in pulmonary venous hypertension with exercise in congestive heart failure, the degree of pulmonary dysfunction increases in direct proportion to the degree of acute change.[44]

With physical exertion in patients with pulmonary venous hypertension, left atrial and pulmonary artery pressures rise, causing transudation of liquid from the intravascular space so that pulmonary extravascular liquid volume increases.[4] Concomitantly, the lung becomes stiffer, and the work of breathing and resistance to air flow greatly increase.[45, 46] Presumably as a result of these factors, such patients ventilate at higher frequencies for any given level of oxygen consumption, so the ventilation equivalent $\dot{V}_E/\dot{V}O_2$ is abnormal,[47] and maximal oxygen uptake is reduced.[48] Some studies have demonstrated that dead space ventilation in patients with mitral stenosis is greater both at rest and with exercise than in normal subjects[26] and that at maximal work rates, oxygen delivery to the working muscles is compromised.[49]

The effects of exercise on arterial oxygen tensions in patients with pulmonary venous hypertension are inconsistent. Some investigators have noted decreases,[50] whereas others have reported no change.[47] These discrepancies result in part from the fact that a change in pulmonary blood flow distribution occurs that could possibly offset the effect of an increase in wasted ventilation with exercise. The previously described resting reversal of the normal pulmonary blood flow distribution pattern can return toward normal during physical exertion in some patients, resulting in relative increases in basilar perfusion.[51] Under these circumstances one would expect to find an improvement in gas exchange to the extent that basilar lung units are ventilated. Despite the above derangements, exercise limitations per se in patients with congestive heart failure or mitral stenosis do not appear to be related simply to the level of the pulmonary venous pressure that is reached.[52] Rather, it seems that a complex interaction of respiratory, cardiac, and peripheral mechanisms is involved.

INTRATHORACIC SPACE-OCCUPYING EFFECTS

Heart disease can alter lung function or produce pulmonary symptoms directly, by compression of mediastinal structures such as the trachea, major bronchi, and esophagus, and indirectly, through the effects of pleural effusions. Partial obstruction of the esophagus can occasionally interfere with deglutition and give rise to aspiration pneumonias. The consequences of compressive effects of major airways are much more severe in infants, compared with older children and adults.

In infants, vascular abnormalities such as vascular ring (p. 966) can produce tracheal obstruction with dyspnea, wheezing, use of accessory muscles of respiration, and a crowing stridor on both inspiration and expiration.[13] There is commonly a history of recurrent pulmonary infections and the condition is frequently misdiagnosed as croup, bronchitis, or asthma. Bronchial obstruction may occur as a result of any cardiac condition in which there is a large left-to-right shunt, but it is most commonly due to a ventricular septal defect or large patent ductus arteriosus.[14, 15] Also, any condition associated with massive cardiomegaly, particularly a greatly enlarged left atrium, as occurs in some patients with severe mitral regurgitation (p. 1034), may compress the bronchi. With large left-to-right shunts the dilated pulmonary artery and the distended left atrium can cause atelectasis or hyperinflation, depending on the degree of obstruction.[14] Sites of predilection are the left main, left upper, and right middle lobe bronchi.[14] With massive cardiomegaly the left main bronchus may be completely obstructed, with resulting atelectasis of the left lung.[14]

Because the magnitude of the left-to-right shunt is limited by the high pulmonary vascular resistance in the neonatal period, bronchial obstruction from this mechanism is uncommon in this age period. The peak incidence of bronchial obstruction occurs between 2 and 9 months of age, when pulmonary artery pressure tends to rise. Other cardiac abnormalities that cause compression of major airways by way of large pulmonary arteries and distended left atria, with or without left ventricular decompensation, are anomalous pulmonary venous drainage, cor triatriatum, and left atrial obstruction owing to a supravalvular mitral ring or congenital mitral stenosis.[16] In adults it has long been recognized that massive cardiomegaly or pericardial effusions can compress the left lower lobe and so give rise to Ewart's sign (dullness, bronchial breathing, and increased tactile fremitus near the angle of the scapula). Hypoventilation of the entire left lung has also been reported.

Lung function in patients with pleural effusion has not been extensively studied, but the available data suggest that effusions, if large enough, can act as space-occupying lesions that limit lung volume and gas exchange.[53, 54] In pleuritis, regional lung function deteriorates as a result of resolved pleural effusion. Both blood flow and ventilation are shifted away from the lung base on the involved side.[55]

EFFECTS ON LUNG FUNCTION OF DRUGS USED TO TREAT HEART DISEASE

Of all the agents in use for the treatment of cardiac disease, the ones that have received the most attention for their potentially harmful pulmonary effects are the beta antagonists. Although there is no doubt that beta-adrenoceptor blockade in asthmatic subjects may cause precipitous and prolonged airway narrowing and an increased sensitivity of the tracheobronchial tree to other constrictor stimuli,[17, 56, 57] responses in normal subjects and in patients with other forms of obstructive airway disease have been conflicting. Evidence based on an extensive evaluation of the pressure-flow-volume interrelationships of the lung demonstrates that the intravenous administration of propranolol is entirely innocuous in normal subjects.[58] This is not true in patients with hay fever or chronic obstructive lung disease, in whom airway resistance increases.

For reasons not completely understood, some patients with chronic bronchitis are hyperresponsive to constrictor stimuli and, when given beta blockers, develop severe bronchoconstriction.[57, 59, 60] Similarly, asymptomatic nonasthmatic first-degree relatives of asthmatics and individuals with atopic histories but without asthma may behave similarly.[57] These effects are also seen with agents purported to be more selective beta blockers. Unfortunately, in the doses required for treatment of angina pectoris in the majority of patients, the so-called cardioselective beta blockers (beta$_1$) produce sufficient beta$_2$ blockade that bronchoconstriction may still be a troublesome side effect in susceptible patients. Thus the advantages of the "cardioselective" beta blockers exist only when very small doses of these agents are used.

Beta-adrenergic blockers, in addition to producing acute bronchospasm in asthmatics, have also been found to worsen airway function in individuals with nonspecific chronic obstructive lung disease.[59–61] In fact, even small quantities of these drugs absorbed from remote sites can have adverse effects; for example, the conjunctival instillation of timolol has been reported to worsen lung function in susceptible individuals.[61] Therefore, these drugs should be used with care, and careful pulmonary and allergic histories should be routinely sought before one prescribes these agents. The *calcium antagonists* have not been shown to have any adverse pulmonary effects.[62] In fact, there is evidence that these antagonists act as modest bronchodilators and protect against constrictor stimuli in asthmatic subjects.[63] Hence these drugs may be the treatment of choice for myocardial ischemia in patients with coexisting primary airway disease who otherwise would receive beta blockers.

Sodium nitroprusside, nitroglycerin, dopamine, and *hydralazine* can all have adverse effects on gas exchange in patients with left-sided

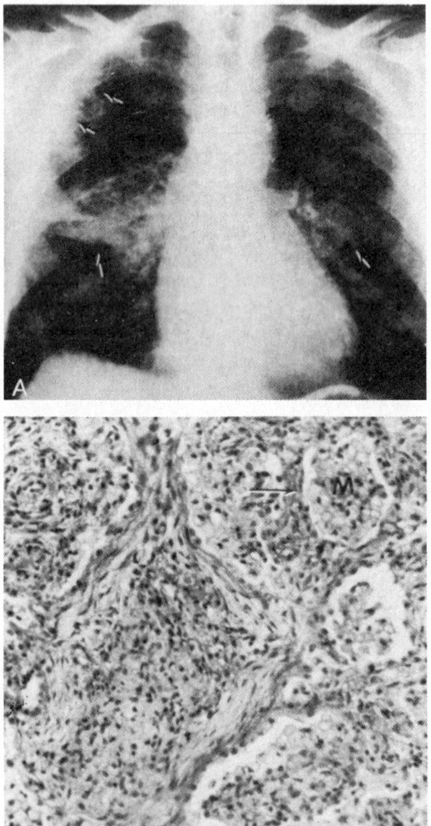

FIGURE 61–1. *A*, Radiographic changes in amiodarone pulmonary toxicity. Admission chest roentgenogram showing diffuse reticular infiltrates, patchy alveolar infiltrates in the mid-lung zones and the peripheral upper lobes (arrows), and right-sided pleural thickening adjacent to the alveolar process. *B*, Histological changes in amiodarone pulmonary toxicity. Sections from open lung biopsy specimen showing widening of alveolar septae by connective tissue (arrow), and intraalveolar accumulation of foamy macrophages (M) and focal early organization of this infiltrate (hematoxylin and eosin stain; original magnification, × 79). (From Marchlinski, F. E., et al.: Amiodarone pulmonary toxicity. Ann. Intern. Med. *97*:840 and 841, 1982.)

heart disease.[19, 21, 64–66] These agents have been shown to cause a fall in arterial oxygen tension despite improving cardiac hemodynamics. Usually, the depression in oxygen is modest (≤10 mm Hg) and is believed to be secondary to alterations in ventilation-perfusion relationships (i.e., it is caused by improved perfusion of poorly ventilated alveoli).

Serious pulmonary toxicity has been reported after the use of the antiarrhythmic agent *amiodarone*[18] (p. 637). This agent has been found to produce interstitial and alveolar infiltrates, hypoxemia, restrictive functional defects, leukocytosis, and elevated sedimentation rates (Fig. 61–1). These alterations tend to be reversible if the drug is discontinued soon after toxicity appears. It is important to realize, however, that pulmonary fibrosis can develop with prolonged use.[67]

Compensatory alveolar hypoventilation with carbon dioxide retention has seldom been reported in patients with cardiac disease who have developed severe metabolic alkalosis secondary to diuretics that increase potassium excretion.[68] Severe H^+ and Cl^- depletion, together with dehydration, appears to be responsible.

The effects of therapeutic doses of morphine on lung function are controversial. Some authors have warned against the use of this drug in patients with myocardial infarction or acute pulmonary edema because of its tendency to interfere with gas exchange by ventilatory depression.[69] Although there is little doubt that this does occur in some individuals, it has been shown that 15 mg of morphine administered by intramuscular injection is well tolerated in both groups of patients.[20, 70] Arterial pO_2 falls by 2 to 3 mm Hg and pCO_2 increases by 4 to 5 mm Hg within an hour of receiving an intramuscular injection.[20, 70] However, it should be noted that the respiratory depression produced by morphine may be potentiated by lidocaine, and the adverse effects of morphine on gas exchange in patients with preexisting chronic obstructive lung disease who develop an acute myocardial infarction can be dramatic.

PULMONARY EFFECTS SECONDARY TO SPECIFIC CARDIAC DISORDERS

MITRAL STENOSIS AND CONGESTIVE HEART FAILURE

In view of the similarity of the effects of mitral stenosis and left ventricular failure on pulmonary vascular pressures, they are discussed together. This section focuses primarily on the degree and kinds of lung dysfunction that occur in relation to the functional cardiac classification.[26, 27] Other aspects of the pulmonary alterations in these conditions are presented elsewhere (pp. 476 and 1023).

When the underlying condition is mild with no limitation on ordinary activity (Class I), then, generally speaking, lung function tends to be relatively normal at rest (Figs. 61–2 and 61–3). Vital capacity may be slightly reduced and the alveolar-arterial gradient for oxygen may be somewhat increased. As the disease process worsens and the patient's symptomatic disability increases, virtually all aspects of lung function deteriorate. Vital capacity, forced expiratory flow rates and volumes, maximum breathing capacity, dynamic compliance, resting diffusion capacity, and arterial oxygen tensions all fall progressively, while airway resistance and alveolar-arterial gradients for oxygen rise.[26, 27] These measurements correlate well with the increase in pulmonary artery pressure and pulmonary vascular resistance.

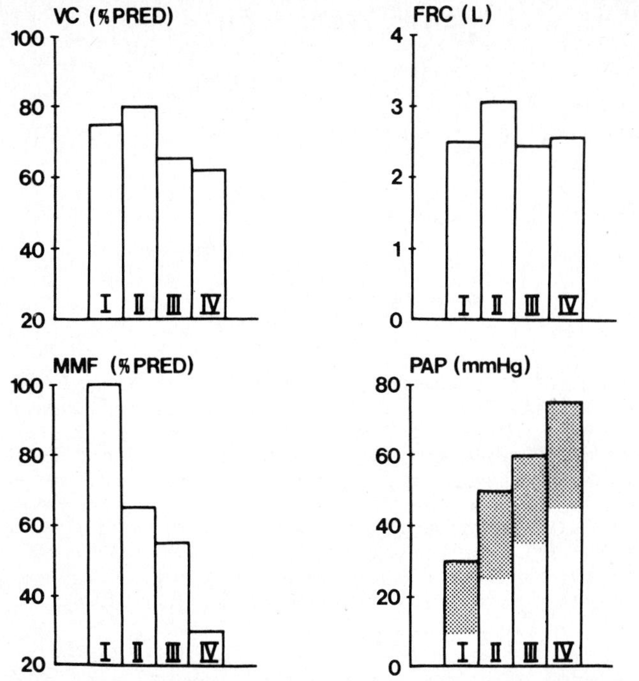

FIGURE 61–2. Alterations in pulmonary mechanics and pulmonary artery pressures observed in the various clinical stages of mitral stenosis. The heights of the bars represent mean values. VC = vital capacity; FRC = functional residual capacity; MMF = maximum midexpiratory flow rate; PAP = pulmonary artery pressure. In the PAP graph the top of the shaded area represents the systolic pressure and the bottom, the diastolic pressure. Roman numerals represent stages of increasing clinical disability. (Data redrawn from Palmer, W. H., et al.: Disturbances of pulmonary function in mitral valve disease. Can. Med. Assoc. J. *89*:744, 1963.)

Patients with Class IV disability generally have severely compromised lung function.[49] Mean values for vital capacity are 60 to 70 per cent of predicted values, while flow rates in the mid-vital capacity tend to be around 30 per cent of expected normal. Diffusing capacity tends to be abnormally low and about one-half that observed in Class I, while dynamic compliance is severely reduced, to only one-third of normal. Arterial oxygen tensions range from 58 to 75 mm Hg (normal = 95 ± 5 mm Hg), and the alveolar-arterial gradients for oxygen lie between 30 and 41 mm Hg (normal ≤20 mm Hg).

The changes in dynamic compliance (i.e., compliance measured during tidal respiration) vary inversely with pulmonary capillary wedge pressures. When compliance is normal at rest, as it tends to be in patients in functional Classes I and II, pulmonary wedge pressure tends to be normal; as wedge pressure rises with progression of the disease, or with exercise, dynamic compliance falls (Fig. 61–4).

Measurements of the static pressure-volume (recoil)

FIGURE 61–3. Changes in the diffusing capacity of the lung for carbon monoxide (D_LCO), dynamic compliance (Cdyn), and pulmonary resistance (R_L) as a function of the severity of mitral stenosis. Roman numerals indicate increasing disability. (Data redrawn from Palmer, W. H., et al.: Disturbances of pulmonary function in mitral valve disease. Can. Med. Assoc. J. *89*:744, 1963.)

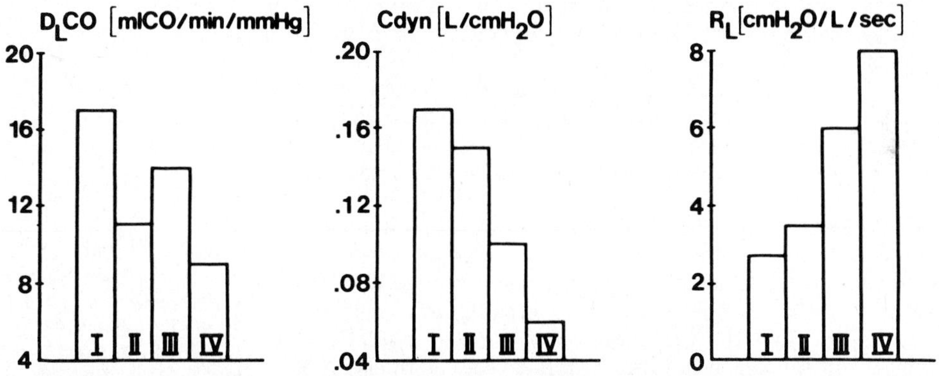

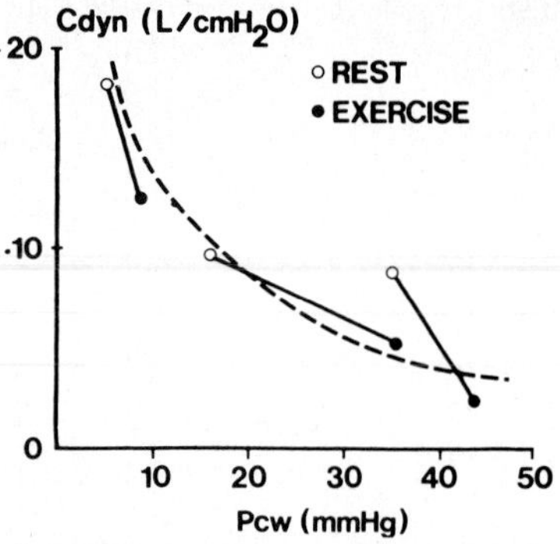

FIGURE 61–4. Relationships between pulmonary capillary wedge pressure (Pcw) and dynamic compliance (Cdyn) in patients with pulmonary venous hypertension. The dashed line is a schematic representation of the overall relationship. (Data from Saxton, G. A., Jr., et al.: The relationship of pulmonary compliance to pulmonary vascular pressures in patients with heart disease. J. Clin. Invest. *35*:611, 1965, and White, H. C., et al.: Lung compliance in patients with mitral stenosis. Clin. Sci. *17*:667, 1958.) The three sets of data points demonstrate the effects on dynamic compliance of acutely increasing pulmonary capillary wedge pressure with exercise. (Data from Saxton, G. A., Jr., et al., as cited.)

properties have shown that the lungs of patients with mitral stenosis are altered in a distinct manner.[7, 71] Elastic recoil is increased at high lung volumes, is normal at functional residual capacity, and then becomes abnormally low as residual volume is approached. This is unlike the situation seen in either atrial septal defect or pulmonary fibrosis. It has been suggested that vascular plethora accounts for the loss of recoil at small lung volumes and that pulmonary fibrosis produces the increased retractive forces at the larger volumes. Regardless of the mechanism involved, this type of change in elastic properties helps to explain why functional residual capacity and residual volume can remain normal in the presence of a reduced total lung capacity. In the case of functional residual capacity, the resting mechanical balance of the respiratory system, set by the tendency of the lung to recoil and the chest wall to spring outward, appears intact. With respect to residual volume, it can be seen that two forces (airway compression from engorgement or edema of the vascular sheath and loss of recoil with resultant loss of radial traction of the airways) combine to promote early airway closure with air trapping.[5] In addition to these functional abnormalities, it has been suggested that there is a disturbance of respiratory muscle function in patients with mitral valve disease.[71]

Many of the above changes are not fixed, and after mitral valve surgery, static lung function and exercise performance frequently improve, at least in patients in Class II or III.[72] One-second forced expiratory volumes (FEV_1) and vital capacity increase and residual volumes fall. Diffusing capacity, however, tends to remain impaired even though exercise gas exchange may improve. Those patients who experience the greatest symptomatic relief of breathlessness postoperatively require less ventilation for a given oxygen consumption.

Collins and colleagues[5] evaluated airway function in 72 patients with left-sided valvular and ischemic heart disease who were free of symptoms and demonstrated that, as a group, these individuals had lower values for standard spirometric indices (forced vital capacity [FVC] and one-second forced expiratory volumes [FEV_1]) than did healthy subjects. These findings were taken as evidence of airway obstruction, but the FEV_1:FVC ratio averaged 0.75. This value is within normal limits for a population of this age and implies that the lungs were emptying at a relatively normal rate but from a lower volume. The significance of these findings is that they are consistent with the observations of the Framingham study[73] that reductions in vital capacity can foreshadow the development of congestive heart failure. In 5209 persons evaluated over an 18-year period, the risk of congestive heart failure varied in inverse proportion to vital capacity. Both a persistently low and a recent fall in vital capacity were associated with increased risk. Among persons with ischemic heart disease, hypertension, or rheumatic heart disease, chances of developing congestive failure were doubled in men and tripled in women with low vital capacities.

MYOCARDIAL INFARCTION

(See also page 1232)

Arterial hypoxemia and abnormalities in regional ventilation-perfusion relations and pulmonary mechanics regularly occur in patients with acute myocardial infarction and unstable angina as well as in experimentally provoked coronary insufficiency.[31–35, 74–75] In severe instances, frank respiratory failure with carbon dioxide retention may develop.[76] The sequence of events is believed to be left ventricular dysfunction from either left ventricular failure and/or a reduction in ventricular compliance, leading to acute elevations in ventricular end-diastolic pressure with subsequent development of pulmonary vascular congestion and edema that lasts for hours or up to 2 days in uncomplicated cases. With the onset of edema, the arterioles and bronchioles become compressed, causing the pathogenetic sequence discussed earlier. As this occurs, there is widespread closure of dependent airways with resultant arterial hypoxemia[35, 74] (Fig. 61–5). Several studies have demonstrated that after a myocardial infarction or during an episode of prolonged myocardial ischemia, the lung volume at which airway closure begins can encroach on, or even exceed, functional residual capacity.[35, 74] Therefore, during normal respiration, some alveoli are not ventilated and act as shunts. More severe elevation of pulmonary capillary pressure results in alveolar flooding (Chap. 18).

In addition to alterations in gas exchange, myocardial

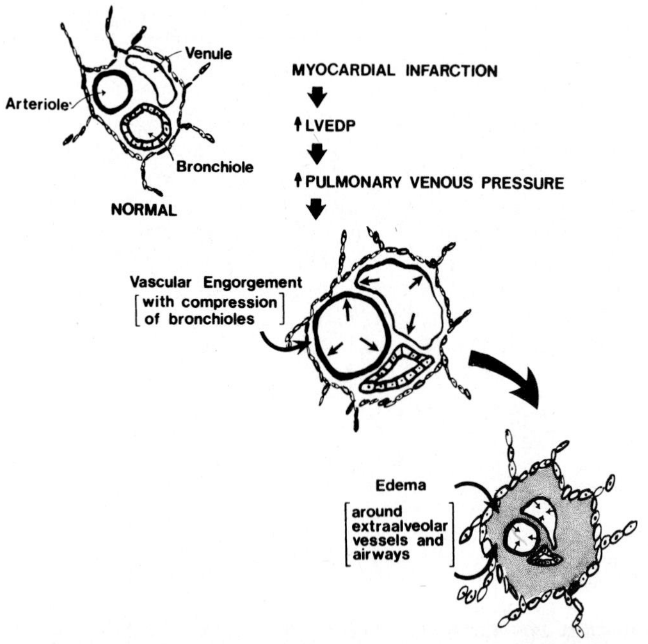

FIGURE 61–5. Normally the loose interstitial space containing arterioles, venules, and bronchioles allows the bronchiole, despite its lower intraluminal pressure, to remain widely open. With vascular engorgement, the dilated venules and arterioles compress the bronchiole, causing an increase in the resistance of these airways. With interstitial edema, the lumina of all structures are compromised.

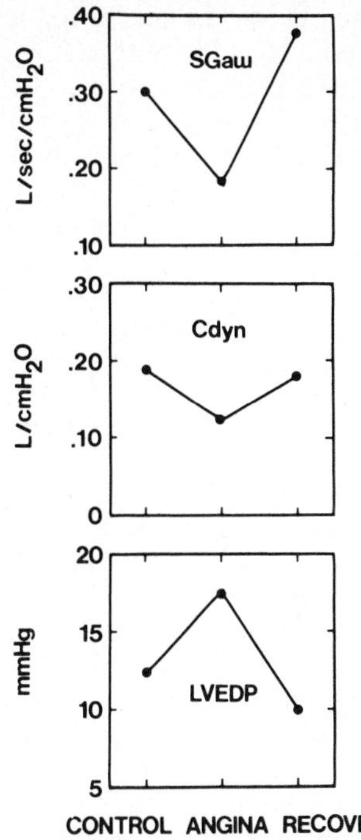

FIGURE 61–6. Interrelationships between heart and lung function during induced myocardial ischemia. SGaw = specific conductance (the reciprocal of airway resistance corrected for the volume at which it was measured); Cdyn = dynamic compliance; LVEDP = left ventricular end-diastolic pressure. The data points are mean values during a control period (left), during the induction of angina (center), and during recovery (right). (Data redrawn from Pepine, C. J., and Wiener, L.: Relationship of anginal symptoms to lung mechanisms during myocardial ischemia. Circulation *46*:863, 1972, by permission of the American Heart Association, Inc.)

ischemia and/or infarction may cause acute elevations in airway resistance and reductions in pulmonary compliance[32, 33] (Figs. 61–6 and 61–7). A schematic representation of the pulmonary consequences of vascular engorgement, interstitial edema, and alveolar flooding is contained

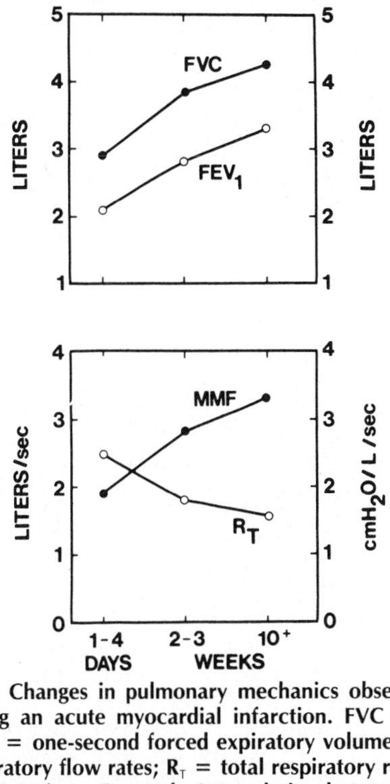

FIGURE 61–7. Changes in pulmonary mechanics observed at various times following an acute myocardial infarction. FVC = forced vital capacity; FEV_1 = one-second forced expiratory volume; MMF = maximum midexpiratory flow rates; R_T = total respiratory resistance. (Data redrawn from Interiano, B., et al.: Interrelation between alterations in pulmonary mechanics and hemodynamics in acute myocardial infarction. J. Clin. Invest. *52*:1994, 1973.)

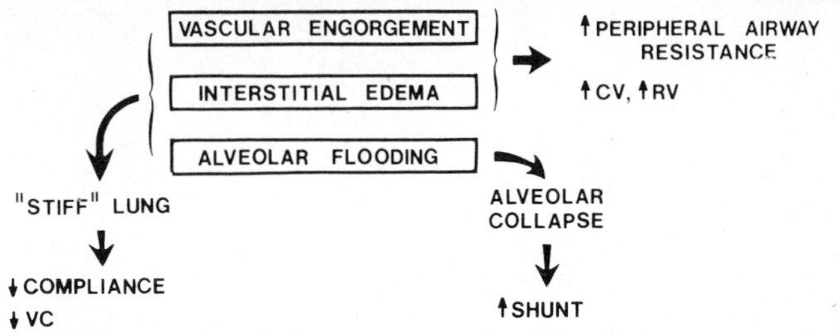

FIGURE 61–8. The functional alterations resulting from vascular engorgement, interstitial edema, and alveolar flooding are shown schematically.

in Figure 61–8. Many patients with coronary artery disease are cigarette smokers and frequently show the changes in pulmonary function resulting therefrom, including elevated residual volume, reduced air flow rates, and increasingly abnormal dynamic compliance with increasing respiratory frequency. In most patients with acute myocardial ischemia it is difficult to distinguish among the various causes of impaired lung function, but the contribution of acute myocardial ischemia can be assessed by repeating the measurements after the cessation of the acute episode and return of the hemodynamics to the baseline state. It is also difficult to determine whether the changes in mechanics and gas exchange are secondary to left ventricular dysfunction or to other factors, such as smoking. One method is to observe whether acute improvement follows the administration of diuretics.[74]

CONGENITAL HEART DISEASE

It is convenient to discuss congenital heart disease in terms of the effects of left-to-right and right-to-left intracardiac shunts on pulmonary function. Frequently, signs of obstructive lung disease such as wheezing, use of accessory muscles of respiration, hyperinflation, and lobar emphysema will dominate the clinical course of infants with ventricular septal defects and large left-to-right shunts (p. 915).[77, 78] The obstruction in these patients can be due to compression of airways by enlarged pulmonary arteries or cardiac chambers, and to an increase in small airway resistance as the result of accumulation of peribronchiolar liquid. Pulmonary compliance is also decreased.[78]

Infants with atrial septal defects have also been reported to have low values for dynamic compliance.[79] However, in older children and adults the respiratory consequences of a chronic increase in pulmonary blood flow from atrial septal defects are more extensive and can be related to the level of pulmonary hypertension.[80] In those patients in whom the mean pulmonary artery pressure is normal, the only change observed is an increase in diffusing capacity. Thus when pulmonary blood flow is abnormally high but vascular pressures are normal, pulmonary mechanics are normal. However, when both blood flow and pressures are increased, lung function deteriorates. Consequently, in those patients with modest pulmonary hypertension, there is an overt decrease in maximal expiratory flows at all lung volumes and some reduction in static compliance, in addition to the increased diffusing capacity (Fig. 61–4*B*). However, when pulmonary hypertension becomes severe, air flow rates are markedly depressed, elastic recoil and lung volumes are sharply reduced, airway resistance is elevated, and diffusing capacity becomes normal. In patients with normal or mild to moderate elevations in pulmonary arterial pressures, closure of the defect resulted in normalization of carbon monoxide transfer.[80] In those patients with a mean pulmonary arterial pressure greater than or equal to 30 mm Hg, corrective surgery failed to change the diffusing capacity or improve pulmonary mechanics.

DISTURBANCES OF VENTILATION-PERFUSION RELATIONS. Alterations in regional pulmonary blood flow have been recorded in patients with both atrial and ventricular septal defects.[81, 82] Typically, abnormalities characterized by increased pulmonary blood flow and elevated pulmonary arterial pressures increase the ratio of pulmonary blood flow in the lung apices (Fig. 61–9). Studies of regional lung function in patients with ventricular septal defect have demonstrated mildly abnormal ventilation-perfusion relationships. Ventilation to the left lung tends to be depressed slightly while perfusion is slightly increased.[82] These changes improve with closure of the defect.

Patients with right-to-left intracardiac shunts tend to have normal

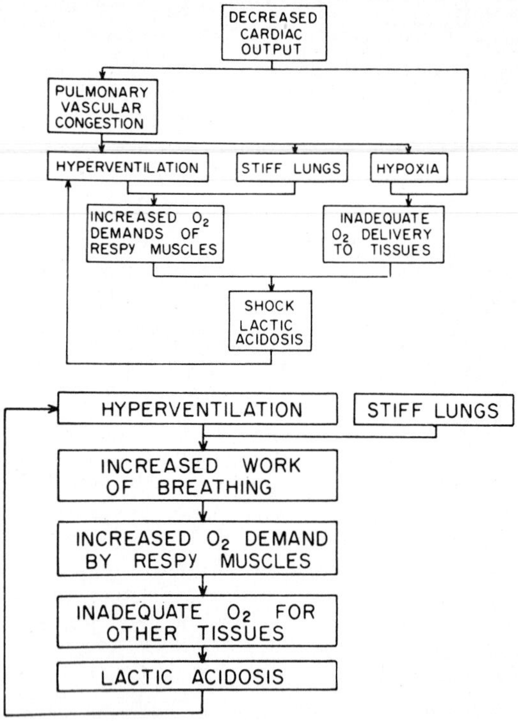

FIGURE 61–9. ***Top,*** **Schema showing how oxygen demands of respiratory muscles can contribute to cardiogenic shock in the face of decreased cardiac output.** ***Bottom,*** **Vicious circle whereby hyperventilation and increased work of breathing contribute to O_2 lack and lactic acidosis, which in turn further increases ventilation and respiratory work. (From Macklem, P. T.: Respiratory muscles: The vital pump. Chest *78*:753, 1980.)**

pulmonary mechanics.[83] However, there are abnormalities in regional lung function and ventilatory control mechanisms.[84, 85] Individuals with tetralogy of Fallot have been reported to have a high incidence of hyperperfusion of one lung relative to the other.[84] The significance of this observation with respect to regional gas exchange has not been evaluated, but it is known that children with this condition lack carotid body sensitivity to arterial hypoxemia.[85] As a result, the superimposition of alveolar hypoxia from lung disease or anesthesia may threaten life by aggravating systemic hypoxia to intolerable levels. The mechanism responsible for the blunting of the ventilatory responses to hypoxia in patients with congenital cyanotic heart disease is not clear, but available evidence suggests that it may represent an acquired adaptation to prolonged hypoxemia because the defect disappears with surgical correction of the cardiac abnormalities.[85]

CARDIOGENIC SHOCK

(See also page 567)

As already noted, respiratory insufficiency with abnormal gas exchange frequently develops in conjunction with acute myocardial infarction and pulmonary edema. Usually the mechanisms are related to alterations in ventilation-perfusion relationships from interstitial edema and alveolar flooding, but other factors may also play a role.[86] In the presence of pump failure the work of breathing increases substantially because of the hyperventilation induced by hypoxemia and acidemia and because of the mechanical alterations secondary to pulmonary vascular congestion. However, despite the increase in energy demands and expenditure, the blood supply to the respiratory muscles may be reduced because of the very low cardiac output, thus limiting their perfusion. Respiratory muscle fatigue may then occur, leading to respiratory failure. This sequence of events is shown schematically in Figure 61–9.

CARDINAL MANIFESTATIONS OF HEART VERSUS LUNG DISEASE

Because of the functional interrelations of the heart and lungs, it is not surprising that the cardinal symptoms of heart and lung disease are similar: dyspnea, cough, chest pain, and hemoptysis. It is likely that cough and dyspnea appear only with lung dysfunction, whether it is primary or solely secondary to cardiac dysfunction. Hence their etiology cannot be clearly distinguished in many instances. In contrast, chest pain and hemoptysis have features characteristic enough to provide a better idea of the primary process.

DYSPNEA

(See also pp. 2 and 476)

It is frequently difficult to differentiate cardiac from pulmonary causes of dyspnea[49, 87] (Table 1–1, p. 3). In actual practice the major functional classifications of patients with either heart or lung disease are largely based on the degree of exertion necessary to produce breathlessness (p. 11). Such classifications provide no differentiation between primary heart and lung disease. Furthermore, they cannot be rigidly applied as quantitators of disease in either system. For example, a conditioned athlete who begins to develop dyspnea during previously tolerated activity may have a more serious disturbance than a sedentary person who complains of greater breathlessness with much less exertion. On the other hand, other diseases, such as musculoskeletal disorders, may prevent a level of activity that would be necessary to produce dyspnea.

In most patients the cause of dyspnea can usually be clearly identified. Thus a patient with systemic hypertension, an enlarged left ventricle, an S_3 gallop, and bilateral inspiratory rales should not present a problem in identification of left ventricular failure as the cause of dyspnea. In like manner, a long-term smoker with cough and sputum production, a normal cardiac silhouette, pulmonary hyperinflation, and airway obstruction probably has sufficient lung disease to account for the shortness of breath. However, an overweight, middle-aged male cigarette smoker, with mild chronic bronchitis and mild systemic hypertension, who begins to complain of dyspnea during previously tolerated activity presents a challenging problem. Neither history nor physical examination may reveal sufficient abnormalities to account for symptoms, and laboratory results may be within normal limits. In such an instance complete pulmonary function testing, including arterial blood gas determinations before, during, and after exercise, electrocardiographic stress testing, and assessment of ventricular function at rest and during exercise, may be needed in order to identify the process accounting for the exertional dyspnea. Usually, however, such an extensive work-up is not necessary and utilization of simple tests and therapeutic trials will suffice.

For example, mild airway obstruction that responds briskly to bronchodilators would justify a trial of sympathomimetic bronchodilators. If this treatment, along with smoking cessation, controlled symptoms, it would seem likely that lung disease predominated. If pulmonary function testing showed no response to the short-term administration of bronchodilators, it is reasonable to administer diuretics with or without cardiac glycosides in a therapeutic trial. Regression of symptoms with this treatment would point toward congestive failure as the cause for his complaints. Given the age and risk factors for the patient in question, it would be reasonable to perform an electrocardiographic stress test, as well as noninvasive assessment of left ventricular function with echocardiography and/or radionuclide angiography before the therapeutic test. If there is evidence of ischemia, the question would be whether silent myocardial ischemia were leading to transient elevation of left ventricular diastolic pressure during exertion. In the latter instance, pretreatment with nitroglycerin and repeat of the exercise challenge might help to indicate whether myocardial ischemia accounted for the exertional dyspnea. In the above circumstances, the presence of left ventricular dysfunction can occasionally be detected at the bedside by using a Valsalva maneuver. Zema and coworkers[88] compared the arterial pressure response with radionuclide ventriculography during Valsalva maneuvers in 37 patients with chronic obstructive lung disease and symptoms of dyspnea. An abnormal systolic pressure response, such as an absent overshoot or a square wave change in pressure during the respiratory maneuver (Fig. 16–4, p. 483), tended to be associated with a low left ventricular ejection fraction.

Another type of difficulty is presented by the patient with both left ventricular failure and chronic obstructive airway disease who has worsening dyspnea. The question is whether the lung or the heart process or both have worsened. If an endobronchial infection caused worsening of the lung disease with increasing hypoxemia and hypercapnia, cardiac arrhythmias might ensue directly and secondary to the lowering of the therapeutic index for digitalis. Attention might then be directed toward the heart disease as the initiating event, when, in fact, respiratory failure secondary to the endobronchial infection was the primary culprit. A history of increased cough and purulent sputum production at the onset of worsening should allow identification of the initiating event. Absence of such a history and minimal increases in arterial P_{CO_2} suggest that the heart was the primary offender.

A patient with acute respiratory failure may suffer myocardial infarction with associated electrocardiographic and enzyme changes. This would not necessarily indicate that a primary cardiac process initiated the sequence of events, since an acute myocardial infarction can occur during an episode of respiratory failure. Our experience indicates that acute myocardial infarction is far more common in patients with acute-on-chronic respiratory failure than was previously thought. While both the cardiac and the respiratory problems require treatment, the therapeutic situation is fraught with competing rationales. Morphine would be clearly contraindicated from the standpoint of the respiratory failure, but some means of controlling pain and anxiety is needed for the myocardial infarction. There is no clear answer for this dilemma, unless the patient is already being supported by a mechanical ventilator. Sympathomimetics are clearly indicated for bronchodilation and increased mucociliary clearance, yet if nonselective agents are used, they may precipitate or worsen dangerous cardiac arrhythmias and increase the extent of ischemic injury. These phenomena tend not to occur as often with the selective $beta_2$ compounds. Electrocardiographic monitoring is helpful in anticipating and adjusting treatment to correct arrhythmias. Diuretics present a different problem: If left ventricular failure is present, diuretics are indicated; if not, dehydration resulting from diuresis increases sputum viscosity and thereby interferes with bronchopulmonary drainage. Accurate monitoring of pulmonary capillary wedge pressure can aid in making the appropriate therapeutic decision.

Several patterns of *dyspnea* are thought to be more indicative of heart than lung disease; paroxysmal nocturnal dyspnea occurring after a person falls asleep has been considered indicative of left ventricular failure. However, if such paroxysms of dyspnea occur shortly after assumption of the supine posture and are relieved by cough with expectoration of substantial quantities of sputum, it is likely that bronchitis with accumulated secretions rather than heart failure is responsible.

An additional form of paroxysmal nocturnal dyspnea with wheezing occurs in asthmatics and is thought to be related to diurnal fluctuations in airway tone and degree of airway responsiveness.[89] The brisk response of this symptom to inhaled bronchodilators is distinctive.

Orthopnea (p. 476). This symptom also mainly indicates congestive heart failure, yet patients with this symptom frequently have severe chronic airway obstruction rather than primary heart disease. This usually occurs in patients with severe hyperinflation who must use their accessory muscles of respiration. In order for these muscles to assist in breathing, the patient's arms must be braced at his sides. This is apparent on simple inspection and makes it likely that the discomfort experienced in the supine posture is due to the loss of the contribution of the accessory muscles of inspiration. The confusion between a pulmonary and cardiac cause of orthopnea is occasionally compounded by the fact that these patients sit up most of the night and develop dependent edema in the absence of elevations of central venous pressure. A clue to the presence of normal central venous pressure in such patients, indicative of a pulmonary origin, is the brisk collapse of the neck veins during inspiration.

An additional yet uncommon form of orthopnea is that associated with bilateral diaphragmatic paralysis. In this condition, in the supine posture, there is a paradoxical inward abdominal motion with inspiration, indicating that the weight of the abdominal contents pressing on the paralyzed diaphragm results in ascent of this structure further into the chest when intrathoracic pressures become negative. The characteristic inward abdominal motion with inspiration and the onset of dyspnea immediately on assuming the supine posture, along with absence of signs of left ventricular failure or lung disease, usually suffice to suggest this diagnosis.

Cheyne-Stokes Respiration (p. 481). This breathing pattern is characteristic of left ventricular failure and almost never occurs as a consequence of lung disease alone, hence its presence is more suggestive of left ventricular failure if there is no central nervous system process to account for it. Occasionally, patients with heart failure who have Cheyne-Stokes respiration may awaken at night during the hyperventilatory phase of their periodic respiration and complain of dyspnea. This phenomenon should be distinguished from paroxysmal nocturnal dyspnea.[90]

Another form of dyspnea that awakens patients from sleep is sleep apnea with arousal. This disorder is caused by cessation of respiratory efforts resulting from central nervous system causes (central apnea), ineffective respiration because of upper airway obstruction (obstructive apnea), or a combination of both. These disorders can lead to cor pulmonale and are discussed in Chapter 48.

Two uncommon patterns of breathlessness are sufficiently distinct to have received separate designations: trepopnea and platypnea. *Trepopnea* refers to breathlessness that is limited to one lateral decubitus position. Although originally described for heart disease and attributed to distortion of great vessels in one posture versus the other, the symptom also occurs in patients with lung disease; its cause is not clear, but it may be related to the observation that patients with predominantly unilateral lung disease have lower arterial oxygen tensions when they lie in the lateral decubitus position with the more severely affected lung down.[91] *Platypnea* refers to breathlessness that is present only in the upright position and that promptly abates on assumption of the supine posture.[92] It was originally described in severe chronic obstructive lung disease and was attributed to decreased perfusion of Zone 2 (Fig. 18–5, p. 548) with consequent enlargement of Zone 1 owing to increased alveolar pressures. This results in an increase of wasted (dead space) ventilation in the upright posture but no change in arterial pO_2. Platypnea in association with increasing hypoxia has also been described in several cyanotic forms of congenital heart disease[93] and has been attributed to a reduction in systemic arterial pressure, with blood taking the course of least resistance from the right side to the aorta.

CHEST PAIN

(See also pp. 3 and 1316)

The differentiation between cardiac and pulmonary causes of chest pain is usually easily made. Key diagnostic features are the location, character, and behavior of the pain. Although pleural pain can occur anywhere between the lower neck and lower abdomen because of the many spinal cord segments that innervate the parietal pleura, it is usually easy to distinguish because of its sharp superficial lancinating characteristics and its aggravation by deep inspiration and cough. The pulmonary parenchyma and bronchi are devoid of pain fibers; however, there is often a scratchy and nagging substernal discomfort in association with both acute and chronic bronchitis. This is not of the same character as myocardial pain and should never serve as a source of confusion.

Acute spontaneous pneumomediastinum is a relatively uncommon condition that produces severe and sudden substernal chest pain that may mimic myocardial infarction or even dissection of the aorta.[94] In addition, like spontaneous pneumothorax, which may coexist, pneumomediastinum is occasionally associated with electrocardiographic abnormalities consisting of vertical axis, poor R-wave progression in the precordial leads, precordial ST-segment elevation, and T-wave inversion.[94, 95] Like the pain of pericarditis, it is aggravated by deep breathing, swallowing, and lying down and is relieved by sitting up and leaning forward. Points of differentiation are that acute spontaneous pneumomediastinum occurs almost exclusively in young adults and is commonly accompanied by sore throat and dysphagia.

Recognition of pneumomediastinum depends on the detection of subcutaneous emphysema, especially in the neck, on physical examination and demonstration of free air within the borders of the mediastinum by chest radiographs. Often the victims of this condition experience a peculiar crunching or crackling sound synchronous with the heartbeat (Hamman's sign). When this condition is suspected and the diagnostic signs are absent, lateral radiographs of the chest and neck should be obtained. Air between the mediastinal and cervical fascial layers is often seen on lateral films when none of the classic signs are positive.[96]

HEMOPTYSIS

Clinically, the expectoration of blood occurs in one of five ways; the form taken may provide a clue as to whether the underlying process is primarily from cardiac or pulmonary pathology. For example, pink frothy sputum is characteristic of *pulmonary edema*. Deep rust-colored sputum typifies *bacterial pneumonia*. Blood streaked on the surface of mucus is usually associated with *bronchitis*, or bleeding from endobronchial tumors. Dark blood intermixed with sputum to give a "currant jelly" appearance is seen with *pulmonary infarction* and necrotizing pneumonias. Finally, quantities of bright red blood indicate bleeding from enlarged bronchial vessels; this is the form often associated with longstanding *cardiac dysfunction*. Here the differential diagnosis includes bronchiectasis and granulomatous endobronchial and parenchymal disease, such as tuberculosis. Again, the combination of the clinical history, physical examination, and chest radiography should establish the correct diagnosis.

The incidence of a cardiovascular cause has varied from 1.4 to 7 per cent among patients with hemoptysis in several series[97, 98]; thus, although a relatively uncommon complication, it is one that is potentially lethal. Well-recognized cardiovascular causes include mitral stenosis and congenital heart disease.[99] In the second category, hemoptysis has been most frequently described in pulmonary vascular obstructive disease, including Eisenmenger's complex, but it also occurs in patients with pulmonary venous congestion. Generally, the hemoptysis is secondary to bleeding from enlarged tortuous bronchial vessels and thrombotic lesions in the small pulmonary arteries.

An uncommon complication of heart disease is occult pulmonary hemorrhage in patients on anticoagulant therapy.[100] This syndrome is characterized by dyspnea, unexplained acute anemia, and alveolar infiltrates on chest roentgenogram.

COUGH

Cough is perhaps the most common clinical manifestation of primary respiratory disease, and the most frequent initiating stimulus is the presence of secretions in the tracheobronchial tree. When cough is a prominent symptom associated with primary heart disease, it is most often due to some secondary intrabronchial process, such as congestion of mucosal vessels or the presence of secretions or edema. However, as already suggested, bronchial deformation caused by cardiac enlargement can stimulate subepithelial irritant receptors and initiate cough that is usually nonproductive. An enlarged left atrium caused by mitral valve disease often leads to nonproductive cough, and cough may also be a manifestation of progression of left heart failure. Thus, in the final analysis, there is no reasonable way to assess whether a nonproductive cough is predominantly due to heart versus lung disease when both conditions are present.

ARRHYTHMIAS IN PATIENTS WITH LUNG DISEASE

Arrhythmias occur as frequently in patients with acute respiratory failure complicating the obstructive pulmonary syndromes as in those with acute myocardial infarction.[101–105] A variety of supraventricular arrhythmias, such as paroxysmal supraventricular tachycardia, atrial flutter, multifocal atrial tachycardia, and atrioventricular junctional tachycardia, have been reported. In addition, ventricular arrhythmias such as bigeminy, atrioventricular dissociation, idioventricular rhythm, ventricular tachycardia, and fibrillation have been observed as well. These arrhythmias usually develop in association with episodes of increasing hypoxemia with or without hypercapnia, particularly during sleep. The nocturnal hypoxia that develops in patients with chronic airway obstruction predisposes them to atrial and ventricular arrhythmias.[104, 106] Similar problems occur in patients with sleep apnea; arrhythmias can be prevented or diminished by nocturnal oxygen therapy. Cardiac arrhythmias may also be provoked by rapidly reducing arterial carbon dioxide tension during ventilatory support, producing alkalemia when renal compensation for chronic hypercapnia is present.[102]

The precise cause of the arrhythmias is not known. It has been suggested that the severe hypoxemia, hypercapnia, and changes in pH which are common in respiratory failure alter the automaticity of the cardiac conducting tissue or permit the development of reentry circuits. Other factors, such as the catecholamines, theophylline, glucocorticoids, and diuretics used to treat the respiratory symptoms and right heart failure, alone or in combination with the blood gas abnormalities, can also reduce electrical stability either directly or secondarily through their effects on cellular ion transport. In addition, some evidence indicates that sinus node function may be impaired in patients with cor pulmonale.[107]

Although the use of cardiac glycosides to control atrial arrhythmias is well established, their role in the treatment of cor pulmonale is controversial. The literature suggests that patients with pulmonary disease may be more susceptible to the toxic effects of cardiac glycosides than patients without primary airway or parenchymal disease.[108] However, few studies correlating the effects of digitalis with pulmonary status have characterized the type of respiratory illness present or controlled for concurrent unrelated left ventricular disease. Thus our current state of knowledge suggests that digitalis be used with caution in patients with respiratory failure. Frequent observation and regulation of dosage must be undertaken.

CARDIAC EFFECTS OF DRUGS AND OTHER MODALITIES USED TO TREAT LUNG DISORDERS

Of the various agents currently in use in the treatment of obstructive lung disease, only two classes (adrenergic stimulants and methylxanthines) have significant cardiovascular effects.

ADRENERGIC STIMULANTS

This class of compounds consists of catecholamines (norepinephrine, epinephrine, isoproterenol, and isoetharine), resorcinols (metaproterenol and terbutaline), saligenins (albuterol), and ephedrine, which act through stimulation of adrenoceptors.[109] Beta-adrenoceptor effects can be differentiated into $beta_1$ and $beta_2$: $beta_1$ agonists cause cardiac stimulation and $beta_2$ agonists produce bronchodilatation and vasodilation.[110] Obviously, the ideal agent in this class for the treatment or prophylaxis of obstructive lung disease would be one with pure $beta_2$ activity. Unfortunately, no such compound exists. Although isoetharine, terbutaline, and albuterol have more $beta_2$ selectivity than the others, as the doses of these drugs are increased, $beta_1$ effects begin to appear.[109]

Selective $beta_2$ bronchodilators dilate the peripheral vasculature, causing a decrease in blood pressure and a reflex increase in cardiac output, thus resulting in tachycardia. Typically, the tachycardia is mild and a 5- to 10-beat/min increase is the usual finding after oral or subcutaneous administration of terbutaline or albuterol. Because heart rate rises with increasing plasma levels of drug, it is possible to administer three to four times the usual therapeutic dosage by inhalation and not encounter these effects.

The role of selective $beta_2$ agents in causing arrhythmias is debatable. Some studies indicate that these drugs can exacerbate a preexisting potential toward arrhythmia. In contrast, others conclude that arrhythmia is not induced in patients without this propensity even after large doses. If an arrhythmia should occur with the selective $beta_2$ drugs, however, it tends to be prolonged because of the drugs' slow metabolism.

It is important to recognize that the newer sympathomimetics can actually improve myocardial performance. Administration of salbutamol and terbutaline have been shown to increase right and left ventricular ejection fractions and to decrease arterial pressure, pulmonary vascular resistance, left ventricular end-diastolic pressure, and systemic vascular resistance.[111, 112] In fact, because of these features and their tendency to improve cardiac output without an increase in myocardial oxygen consumption, they have been used to treat congestive heart failure.[113–115] These agents should represent reasonable therapy for patients with airway obstruction and concurrent cardiac dysfunction.

In patients with symptomatic obstructive lung disease coexistent with an ischemic or hypertensive cardiomyopathy, aerosols of selective $beta_2$ agonists such as albuterol can be used with safety, and this is the preferred mode of therapy. We have yet to observe the precipitation of an arrhythmia or worsening of angina with aerosols, although this has occurred with the oral use of such agents. Because only micrograms of these drugs are nebulized and milligrams are ingested, presumably this behavior reflects the substantial differences in the quantity of medication absorbed systemically between the two routes.

A particularly difficult clinical problem is posed by the patient with the combination of reactive airways and severely symptomatic angina with or without arrhythmias. One solution is to use a $beta_1$ antagonist to control the cardiac symptoms and a $beta_2$ agonist to treat the airways in an effort to avoid the undesirable $beta_1$-induced cardiac stimulation and $beta_2$-blockade–induced bronchoconstriction. A word of caution should be interjected, however; this course of action is not without the potential hazards of excessive cardiac stimulation and bronchoconstriction initially, so that the patient's cardiac and pulmonary status should be carefully monitored until the safety and efficacy of the final dosage of both drugs have been determined. Any change in dose of either agent should also be followed objectively.

Another potential solution is to treat the angina pectoris with a calcium agonist. Although these drugs can attenuate the airway obstruction that follows certain constrictor stimuli in asthmatics,[62] they have only a moderate effect on existing airway obstruction.[63] Hence, if there should be an acute exacerbation of airway obstruction, another bronchodilator would be required. It has not yet been determined whether a calcium antagonist would protect against any cardiac stimulation that might occur as a consequence of the administration of beta-adrenoceptors. Further, it is not known how this class of compounds interacts with the effects of sympathomimetics and/or methylxanthines on airway smooth muscle.

The toxicity of *halogenated hydrocarbon propellants* has been extensively studied, and it has become clear that these agents are not "inert" as was once believed, but neither do they appear to be potentially fatal in patients with lung disease.[116, 117] In laboratory animals these compounds can sensitize the myocardium to the arrhythmogenic effects of sympathomimetics, but data from many studies in humans indicate that extremely high levels of these compounds are required.[116–118] Hence it appears that only the most flagrant abuse of pressurized aerosols would result in blood concentrations high enough to have this effect.

METHYLXANTHINES

In general, theophylline is safer than the catecholamines and other nonselective beta agonists and has been shown to improve the performance of both ventricles in patients with obstructive lung disease.[119] However, it also has potentially serious side effects. Like the adrenergic stimulants, methylxanthines increase left ventricular work, and relative myocardial ischemia may be produced even though mild coronary artery dilation may also occur. Because theophylline is typically well tolerated, its potential for abuse is high. Until measurements of serum levels became widely available, aminophylline was usually administered in a fixed amount, and if the desired effect was not forthcoming, the dose was increased until toxic side effects were observed. The hazard of this approach can be readily appreciated; aminophylline administration has been implicated as a predisposing factor in 60 per cent of cases of cardiac arrest in patients in intensive care units.[120]

The therapeutic range for theophylline lies between 10 and 20 μg/ml, and this can be readily achieved in many patients with an intravenous infusion of aminophylline of 5 to 6 mg/kg. However, there is great variability among patients in the metabolism of this drug, and the half-life is markedly prolonged in patients with congestive heart failure, acute pulmonary edema, chronic obstructive lung disease, or liver disease. Thus therapy must be individualized and frequent assessment of serum concentration is required.

POSITIVE END-EXPIRATORY PRESSURE

It has long been noted that high inflation pressures during mechanical ventilation with or without positive end-expiratory pressure (PEEP) are associated with a fall in blood pressure. Changes in each of the two determinants of blood pressure (cardiac output and peripheral vascular resistance) have been considered to be responsible.

Of the two possible causes, much more attention has appropriately been focused on the diminution in cardiac output. Several reasons have been proposed for a fall in cardiac output during mechanical ventilation with PEEP, one of which is that the positive airway pressure, with secondary increases in pleural pressure, simply increases the impedance to venous return (p. 410). Although this is undoubtedly the major factor, a surprising experimental finding was an increase in left-sided filling pressures (mean left atrial and left ventricular end-diastolic).[121] Higher filling pressures and decreased cardiac output indicated an alteration in left ventricular function. With positive intrapleural pressures it was important that cardiac chamber pressures be analyzed in terms of true, transmural (i.e., inside minus outside) distending forces. Earlier experimental studies assumed that intrapleural pressure was a reasonable estimate of the pressure surrounding the heart. Based on this assumption, the following sequence evolved: (1) increases in lung volume with PEEP increase pulmonary vascular resistance; (2) this results in an increase in right ventricular pressures which, in turn, displaces the interventricular septum to encroach on the left ventricular cavity (Fig. 61–10); (3) left ventricular diastolic filling thus becomes impaired, leading to a smaller end-diastolic volume at higher pressures[122]; (4) the subsequent stroke volume is smaller and contributes to the reduction in cardiac output. Previous considerations of humoral factors that might impair cardiac contractility were eliminated by the appropriate experiments. These experimental results in animals have now been supported by clinical studies.[123] Thus the idea of "ventricular interdependence" as a contributor to diminution in cardiac output and the hypotension seen with PEEP appears to be supported in a clinical setting.

As attractive as these ideas may be, further experimental evidence has been obtained that indicates that pericardial pressures are much greater than pleural pressures, leading to the view that the heart is directly compressed[124, 125] by the hyperinflated lung to impair filling without alteration of the left ventricular volume versus transmural pressure relationship. This controversy is not yet settled and may revolve around the validity of any technique to assess pericardial pressure with accuracy. Nonetheless, despite lack of unanimity concerning transmural pressure, it is agreed that diastolic filling of the left ventricle is impaired; thus stroke volume is diminished with PEEP.

PREOPERATIVE PULMONARY EVALUATION FOR CARDIAC SURGERY

Although pulmonary complications in the postoperative period are more common in patients with preexisting lung disease,[126] it is not possible to predict the risk precisely based on preoperative pulmonary function testing. An additional concern arises when pulmonary resection is contemplated. Here the issue is whether sufficient pulmonary reserve will be left after surgery. Despite the fact that elaborate preoperative assessments have been proposed,[127, 128] many surgeons prefer to make only simple empirical observations such as having the patient climb stairs.

This type of approach to integrated heart-lung function clearly has no place in the evaluation of most candidates for cardiac surgery, since such patients usually have sufficient cardiac embarrassment that angina or dyspnea during exercise is a problem that will likely be alleviated by the surgical procedure. Even extensive pulmonary function testing may be of little help, since, as already discussed, the effects of heart disease on pulmonary function can be prominent enough to mimic primary lung disease. This is particularly true in patients with longstanding pulmonary venous hypertension.

The major issues, then, are whether there is coexisting primary lung disease that will not be improved by surgery and whether the lung dysfunction will contribute to the likelihood of postoperative mortality and morbidity. There are no prospective studies to provide guidelines in the resolution of this issue. Usually, however, complete clinical assessment, including pulmonary function testing and blood gas determinations at rest and during exercise, suffices in discovering whether there is coexisting lung disease. For example, marked air trapping, severe hypoxemia, and hypercapnia in a patient at rest point toward primary lung dysfunction. Alternatively, the development, or worsening, of pulmonary mechanical and gas-exchange abnormalities during exercise in a patient with a surgically correctable heart disease, who shows only subtle changes in lung function at rest, implicates heart disease as the primary problem. In the latter circumstance, cardiac surgery would be expected to improve lung function to the extent that cardiac function improved; in the former case, surgery is particularly hazardous.

In general, if there is primary lung disease, pulmonary function testing gives a good quantitative assessment of its severity, and this information has some value in predicting whether a patient is likely to tolerate cardiac surgery. When the vital capacity and flow rates are 80 per cent or more of their predicted values, there is little cause for concern from the point of view of pulmonary function.[129] On the other hand, if the values for these indices fall below 50 per cent of predicted values, the possibility of postoperative respiratory insufficiency and death increases.[129] However, because the approach to postoperative intensive care for the pulmonary complications of cardiac surgery is improving dramatically, it is likely that the risk of cardiac surgery in patients with impaired pulmonary function will diminish in the future.

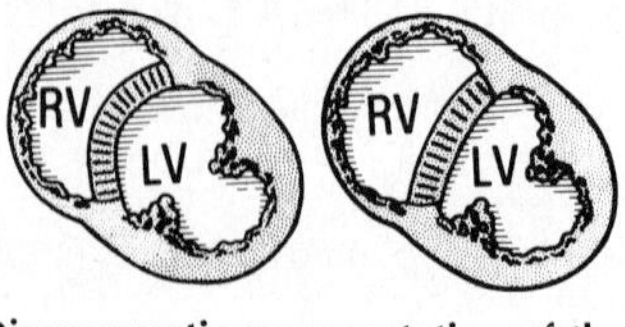

FIGURE 61–10. Diagrammatic representation of the short-axis view of the right (R) and left (LV) ventricles using two-dimensional echocardiography. The left diagram illustrates the normal curvature of the interventricular septum with its convexity pointing toward the RV. After PEEP is applied (right diagram), the interventricular septum is flattened and the LV cavity is reduced in size, while the RV is expanded. (From Pick, R. A., et al.: The cardiovascular effects of positive end-expiratory pressure. Chest *82*:348, 1982.)

RESPIRATORY CARE AFTER CARDIAC SURGERY

(See also page 1676)

The major respiratory problems that arise in the period immediately after cardiac surgery are related to (1) the thoracotomy itself; (2) the use of drugs in the postoperative period; (3) the effects of cardiopulmonary bypass on the lungs; (4) the effects of coexisting morbid processes, such as chronic airway obstruction; and (5) the transitory effects on the heart of the surgical intervention.

The disruption of the chest wall by either a lateral thoracotomy or a median sternotomy interferes with its movement; a clouded sensorium caused by medications and self-imposed restriction of movement to avoid pain further contribute to impairment of chest wall motion and may lead to atelectasis. Perhaps even more important, the pain, sedatives, and mechanical restriction lead to an impaired coughing mechanism and the patient's reluctance even to try coughing, and as a consequence, secretions accumulate. These problems are often managed by leaving the endotracheal tube in place and providing mechanical ventilatory assistance in the first few postoperative hours. During this time the tracheobronchial tree is periodically suctioned to remove secretions, and sufficient tidal volumes are provided to prevent atelectasis.

Some patients develop the adult respiratory distress syndrome (Chap. 18) postoperatively, characterized by increasing intrapulmonary shunting, decreasing lung compliance, and diffuse alveolar infiltrates. This syndrome, which may not develop fully until 24 hours after operation, has been attributed to the use of the extracorporeal membrane oxygenator and perfusion pump and has therefore been referred to as "pump lung." Many theories have been proposed regarding the pathogenesis, yet no single factor has been firmly identified. It is our impression that the incidence of this syndrome has diminished in recent years, perhaps related to shorter bypass times.

Extra attention and effort should be directed toward the postoperative management of the patient with chronic obstruction of the airways by using bronchodilators, by encouraging cough, and, when possible, by the application of physical therapy techniques for mobilization of secretions.

REFERENCES

MECHANISMS BY WHICH HEART DISEASE LEADS TO LUNG DYSFUNCTION

1. Glauser, F. L., Hoshiko, M., Watanabe, M., and Wilson, A. F.: Physiologic changes associated with increasing pulmonary wedge pressures in the dog. Respiration *31*:459, 1974.
2. Gump, F. E., Zikria, B. A., and Mashima, Y.: The effect of interstitial edema on pulmonary function in the dog. J. Trauma *12*:764, 1972.
3. Hauge, A., Bø, G., and Waaler, B. A.: Interrelations between pulmonary liquid volumes and lung compliance. J. Appl. Physiol. *38*:608, 1975.
4. Luepker, R., Liander, B., Korsgren, M., and Varnauskas, E.: Pulmonary intravascular and extravascular fluid volumes in exercising cardiac patients. Circulation *44*:626, 1971.
5. Collins, J. V., Clark, T. J. H., and Brown, D. J.: Airway function in healthy subjects and in patients with left heart disease. Clin. Sci. Molec. Med. *49*:217, 1975.
6. Frank, N. R., Lyons, H. A., Siebens, A. A., and Nealon, T. F.: Pulmonary compliance in patients with cardiac disease. Am. J. Med. *22*:516, 1957.
7. Wood, T. E., McLeod, P., Anthonisen, N. R., and Macklem, P. T.: Mechanics of breathing in mitral stenosis. Am. Rev. Resp. Dis. *104*:52, 1971.
8. James, A. E., Jr., Cooper, M., White, R. I., and Wagner, H. N., Jr.: Perfusion changes on lungs in patients with congestive heart failure. Radiology *100*:99, 1971.
9. Giuntini, C., Mariani, M., Barsotti, A., Fazio, F., and Santolicandro, A.: Factors affecting regional pulmonary blood flow in left heart valvular disease. Am. J. Med. *57*:421, 1974.
10. Dawson, A., Rocamora, J. M., and Morgan, J. R.: Regional lung function in chronic pulmonary congestion with and without mitral stenosis. Am. Rev. Resp. Dis. *113*:51, 1976.
11. Pain, M. C. F., Bucens, D., Cade, J. F., and Sloman, J. G.: Regional lung function in patients with mitral stenosis. Aust. N.Z. J. Med. *3*:228, 1972.
12. Hughes, J. M. B., Glazier, J. B., Rosenzweig, D. Y., and West, J. B.: Factors determining the distribution of pulmonary blood flow in patients with raised pulmonary venous pressure. Clin. Sci. *37*:847, 1969.
13. Blumenthal, S., and Ravitch, M. M.: Seminar on aortic vascular rings and other anomalies of the aortic arch. Pediatrics *20*:896, 1957.
14. Stranger, P., Lucas, R. V., Jr., and Edwards, J. E.: Anatomic factors causing respiratory distress in acyanotic congenital cardiac disease: Special reference to bronchial obstruction. Pediatrics *43*:760, 1969.
15. Bryk, D.: Atelectasis, emphysema, and heart disease. Am. J. Dis. Child. *110*:100, 1965.
16. Moss, A. J., and McDonald, L. V.: Cardiac disease in the wheezing child. Chest *71*:187, 1977.
17. Ryo, U. Y., and Townley, R. G.: Comparison of respiratory and cardiovascular effects of isoproterenol, propranolol, and practolol in asthmatic and normal subjects. J. Allergy Clin. Immunol. *57*:12, 1976.
18. Marchlinski, F. E., Gansler, T. E., Waxman, H. L., and Josephson, M. E.: Amiodarone pulmonary toxicity. Ann. Intern. Med. *97*:839, 1982.
19. Mookherjee, S., Fuleihan, D., Warner, R. A., Vardan, S., and Obeid, A. I.: Effects of sublingual nitroglycerine on resting pulmonary gas exchange and hemodynamics in man. Circulation *57*:106, 1978.
20. Hoel, B. L., Bay, G., and Refsum, H. E.: The effects of morphine on the arterial and mixed venous blood gas state and on the hemodynamics in patients with clinical pulmonary congestion. Acta Med. Scand. *190*:549, 1971.
21. Huckauf, H., Ramdohr, B., and Schroder, R.: Dopamine induced hypoxemia in patients with left heart failure. Int. J. Clin. Pharmacol. *14*:217, 1976.
22. Goldring, R. M., Cannon, P. J., Heinemann, H. O., and Fishman, A. P.: Respiratory adjustment to chronic metabolic alkalosis in man. J. Clin. Invest. *47*:118, 1968.
23. Murray, J. F.: The lungs and heart failure. Hosp. Pract. *21*:55, 1985.
24. Heard, B. E., Steiner, R. E., Herdon, A., and Gleason, D.: Oedema and fibrosis of the lungs in left ventricular failure. Br. J. Radiol. *41*:161, 1968.
25. Galloway, R. W., Epstein, E. J., and Coulshed, N.: Pulmonary ossific nodules in mitral valve disease. Br. Heart J. *23*:297, 1961.
26. Friedman, B. L., Macias, D. J., and Yu, P. N.: Pulmonary function studies in patients with mitral stenosis. Am. Rev. Tuberc. *79*:265, 1959.
27. Palmer, W. H., Gee, J. B. L., and Bates, D. V.: Disturbances of pulmonary function in mitral valve disease. Can. Med. Assoc. J. *89*:744, 1963.
28. Depeursinge, F. B., Depeursinge, C. D., Boutaleb, A. K., Feinl, F., and Perret, C. H.: Respiratory system impedance in patients with acute left ventricular failure: Pathophysiology and clinical interest. Circulation *73*:386, 1980.
29. Milic-Emili, J., and Petit, J. M.: Mechanical efficiency of breathing. J. Appl. Physiol. *15*:359, 1960.
30. Hogg, J. C., Agarawal, J. B., Gardiner, A. J. S., Palmer, W. H., and Macklem, P. T.: Distribution of airway resistance with developing pulmonary edema in dogs. J. Appl. Physiol. *32*:20, 1972.
31. Tattersfield, A. E., McNicol, M. W., and Sillett, R. W.: Relationship between haemodynamic and respiratory function in patients with myocardial infarction and left ventricular failure. Clin. Sci. *42*:751, 1972.
32. Pepine, C. J., and Wiener, L.: Relationship of anginal symptoms to lung mechanics during myocardial ischemia. Circulation *46*:863, 1972.
33. Interiano, B., Hyde, R., Hodges, M., and Yu, P. N.: Interrelation between alterations in pulmonary mechanics and hemodynamics in acute myocardial infarction. J. Clin. Invest. *52*:1994, 1973.
34. Al Bazzar, F. J., and Kazemi, H.: Arterial hypoxemia and distribution of perfusion after uncomplicated myocardial infarction. Am. Rev. Resp. Dis. *106*:721, 1972.
35. Demedts, M., Sniderman, A., Utz, G., Palmer, W. H., and Becklake, M. R.: Lung volumes including closing volume and arterial blood gas measurements in acute ischaemic left heart failure. Bull. Physiopathol. Resp. *10*:11, 1974.
36. Otis, A. B., McKerrow, C. B., Bartlett, R. A., Mead, J., McIlroy, M. B., Silverstone, N. J., and Radford, E. P., Jr.: Mechanical factors in distribution of pulmonary ventilation. J. Appl. Physiol. *8*:427, 1956.
37. Raine, J., and Bishop, J. M.: The distribution of alveolar ventilation in mitral stenosis at rest and after exercise. Clin. Sci. *24*:63, 1963.
38. Ingram, R. H., Jr., and Schilder, D. P.: Association of a decrease in dynamic compliance with a change in gas distribution. J. Appl. Physiol. *23*:911, 1967.
39. Dawson, A.: Regional pulmonary blood flow in sitting and supine man during and after acute hypoxia. J. Clin. Invest. *48*:301, 1969.
40. Dawson, A., Kaneko, K., and McGregor, M.: Regional lung function in patients with mitral stenosis studied with xenon[133] during air and oxygen breathing. J. Clin. Invest. *44*:999, 1965.
41. Wagenvoort, C. A., Heath, D., and Edwards, J. E.: The Pathology of the Pulmonary Vasculature. Springfield, Ill., Charles C Thomas, 1964, p. 186.
42. Tenny, S. M.: A theoretical analysis of the relationship between venous blood and mean tissue oxygen pressures. Resp. Physiol. *20*:283, 1974.
43. Aberman, A., and Fulop, M.: The metabolic and respiratory acidosis of acute pulmonary edema. Ann. Intern. Med. *76*:173, 1972.
44. Ingram, R. H., Jr., and McFadden, E. R., Jr.: Respiratory changes during exercise in patients with pulmonary venous hypertension. Progr. Cardiovasc. Dis. *19*:109, 1976.
45. Hayward, G. W., and Knotts, J. M. S.: The effect of exercise on lung distensibility and respiratory work in mitral stenosis. Br. Heart J. *17*:303, 1955.
46. Gilbert, R., and Auchincloss, J. H., Jr.: Cardiac and pulmonary function at the exercise breaking point in cardiac patients. Am. J. Med. Sci. *257*:370, 1969.
47. Jebavy, P., Widimsky, J., and Stanek, V.: Distribution of inspired gas and pulmonary diffusing capacity at rest and during graded exercise in patients with mitral stenosis. Respiration *28*:216, 1971.
48. Auchincloss, J. H., Jr., Gilbert, R., and Baule, G. H.: Unsteady state measurement of oxygen transfer in patients with rheumatic heart disease. Clin. Sci. *39*:21, 1970.
49. Nery, L. E., Wasserman, K., French, W., Oren, A., and Davis, J. A.: Contrasting cardiovascular and respiratory responses to exercise in mitral valve and chronic obstructive pulmonary diseases. Chest *83*:446, 1983.
50. Hurych, J., Widimsky, J., and Kasalicky, J.: Pulmonary gas exchange at rest and during exercise in patients with mitral stenosis. Bull. Physiopathol. Resp. *2*:472, 1966.
51. Bjure, J., Liander, B., and Widimsky, J.: Effect of exercise on distribution of pulmonary blood flow in patients with mitral stenosis. Br. Heart J. *33*:438, 1971.
52. Franciosa, J. A., Leddy, C. L., Wilen, M., and Schwartz, D. E.: Relation between hemodynamic and ventilatory responses in determining exercise capacity in severe congestive heart failure. Am. J. Cardiol. *53*:127, 1984.
53. Yoo, O. H., and Ting, E. Y.: The effect of pleural effusions on lung function. Am. Rev. Resp. Dis. *89*:55, 1964.
54. Anthonisen, N. R., and Martin, R. R.: Regional lung function in pleural effusion. Am. Rev. Resp. Dis. *116*:201, 1977.
55. Davidson, F. F., and Glazier, J. B.: Unilateral pleuritis and regional lung function. Ann. Intern. Med. *77*:37, 1972.
56. MacDonald, A. J., Ingram, C. G., and McNeil, R. S.: The effect of propranolol on airway resistance. Br. J. Anaesthesiol. *39*:919, 1967.
57. Zaid, G., and Beall, G. N.: Bronchial response to beta-adrenergic blockade. N. Engl. J. Med. *275*:580, 1966.
58. Tattersfield, R. E., Leaver, D. G., and Pride, N. B.: Effects of β-adrenergic blockade and stimulation on normal human airways. J. Appl. Physiol. *35*:613, 1973.
59. Wunderlich, J., Macha, H. N., Wudicke, H., and Huckauf, H.: Beta adrenergic blockers and terbutaline in patients with chronic obstructive lung disease. Chest *78*:714, 1980.
60. Tivenius, L.: Effects of multiple doses of metoprolol and propranolol on ventilatory function in patients with chronic obstructive lung disease. Scand. J. Resp. Dis. *57*:190, 1976.
61. McMahon, C. D., Shaffer, R. N., Hoskins, H. D., and Hetherington, J.: Adverse effects experienced by patients taking timolol. Am. J. Ophthalmol. *88*:736, 1979.
62. McFadden, E. R.: Calcium-channel blocking agents and asthma. Ann. Intern. Med. *95*:232, 1981.
63. Schwartzstein, R. M., and Fanta, C. H.: Orally administered nifedipine in chronic stable asthma: Comparison with an orally administered sympathomimetic. Am. Rev. Resp. Dis. *134*:262, 1986.
64. Mookherjee, S., Warner, R., Keighley, J., and Obeid, A.: Worsening of ventilation perfusion relationship in the lungs in the face of hemodynamic improvement during nitroprusside infusion. Am. J. Cardiol. *39*:282, 1977.
65. Pierpont, G., Hale, K. A., Franciosa, J. A., and Cohn, J. N.: Effects of vasodilators on pulmonary hemodynamics and gas exchange in left ventricular failure. Am. Heart J. *49*:208, 1980.
66. Chick, J. W., Kochukoshy, K. N., Matsumoto, S., and Leach, J. K.: The effect of nitroglycerine on gas exchange, hemodynamics, and oxygen transport

in patients with chronic obstructive pulmonary disease. Am. J. Med. Sci. *276*:105, 1978.
67. Quyyumi, A. A., Ormerod, L. P., Clarke, S. W., Evans, T. R., and Ward, R. H.: Pulmonary fibrosis—a serious side-effect of amiodarone therapy. Eur. Heart J. *4*:521, 1983.
68. Tuller, M. A., and Mehdi, F.: Compensatory hypoventilation and hypercapnia in primary metabolic alkalosis. Am. J. Med. *501*:281, 1971.
69. Nagle, R. E., and Pilcher, J.: Respiratory and circulatory effects of pentazocine. Review of analgesics used after myocardial infarction. Br. Heart J. *34*:244, 1972.
70. Hoel, B. L., and Refsum, H. E.: The effect of morphine on arterial blood gases in patients with acute myocardial infarction. Acta Med. Scand. *186*:511, 1969.

PULMONARY EFFECTS SECONDARY TO SPECIFIC CARDIAC DISORDERS

71. DeTroyer, A., Estenne, M., and Yernault, J. C.: Disturbance of respiratory muscle function in patients with mitral valve disease. Am. J. Med. *69*:867, 1980.
72. Rhodes, K. M., Every, K., Nariman, S., and Gibson, G. J.: Effects of mitral valve surgery on static lung function and exercise performance. Thorax *40*:107, 1985.
73. Kannel, W. B., Seidman, J. M., Fercho, W., and Castelli, W. P.: Vital capacity and congestive heart failure. The Framingham study. Circulation *49*:1160, 1974.
74. Hales, C. A., and Kazemi, H.: Small-airways function in myocardial infarction. N. Engl. J. Med. *290*:761, 1974.
75. Biddle, T. L., Khanna, P., Yu, P. N., Hodges, M., and Shah, P. M.: Lung water in patients with acute myocardial infarction. Circulation *49*:115, 1974.
76. Rasanen, J., Nikki, P., and Heikkila, J.: Acute myocardial infarction complicated by respiratory failure. The effects of mechanical ventilation. Chest *85*:21, 1984.
77. Hordof, A. J., Mellins, R. B., Gersony, W. M., and Steeg, C. N.: Reversibility of chronic obstructive lung disease in infants following repair of ventricular septal defect. J. Pediatr. *90*:187, 1977.
78. Lister, G., and Pitt, B. R.: Cardiopulmonary interactions in the infant with congested cardiac disease. Clin. Chest Med. *4*:219, 1983.
79. Bancalari, E., Jesse, M. J., Gelband, H., and Garcia, O.: Lung mechanics in congenital heart disease with increased and decreased pulmonary blood flow. J. Pediatr. *90*:192, 1977.
80. Schofield, P. M., Barber, P. V., and Kingston, J.: Preoperative and postoperative pulmonary function tests in patients with atrial septal defect and their relation to pulmonary artery pressure and pulmonary systemic flow ratio. Br. Heart J. *54*:577, 1985.
81. Friedman, W. F., Braunwald, E., and Morrow, A. G.: Alterations in regional pulmonary blood flow in patients with congenital heart disease studied by radioisotope scanning. Circulation *37*:747, 1968.
82. Sade, R. M., Williams, R. G., Castaneda, A. R., and Treves, S.: Abnormalities of regional lung function associated with ventricular septal defect and pulmonary artery band. J. Thorac. Cardiovasc. Surg. *71*:572, 1976.
83. Bates, D. V., Macklem, P. T., and Christie, R. V.: Respiratory Function in Disease. 2nd ed. Philadelphia, W. B. Saunders Company, 1971, p. 351.
84. Gates, G. F., Orme, H. W., and Dore, E. K.: The hyperperfused lung. Detection in congenital heart disease. J.A.M.A. *233*:782, 1975.
85. Edelman, N. H., Lahiri, S., Braudo, L., Cherniack, N. S., and Fishman, A. P.: The blunted ventilatory response to hypoxia in cyanotic congenital heart disease. N. Engl. J. Med. *282*:405, 1970.
86. Aubier, M., Trippenbach, T., and Roussos, C.: Respiratory muscle fatigue during cardiogenic shock. J. Appl. Physiol. Resp. Environ. Exercise Physiol. *51*:499, 1981.

CARDINAL MANIFESTATIONS OR HEART VERSUS LUNG DISEASE

87. Loke, J.: Distinguishing cardiac versus pulmonary limitation in exercise performance. Chest *83*:441, 1983.
88. Zema, M. J., Masters, A. P., and Margouleff, D.: Dyspnea: The heart or the lungs? Differentiation at bedside by the use of the simple Valsalva maneuver. Chest *85*:59, 1984.
89. Barnes, P. J.: Circadian variation in airway function. Am. J. Med. *79* (Suppl 6A):5, 1985.
90. Rees, P. J., and Clark, T. J. H.: Paroxysmal nocturnal dyspnea and periodic respiration. Lancet *2*:1315, 1979.
91. Zorck, M. B., Pontoppidan, H., and Kazemi, H.: The effect of lateral positions on gas exchange in pulmonary disease. Am. Rev. Resp. Dis. *110*:49, 1974.
92. Altman, M., and Robin, E. D.: Platypnea: Diffuse zone I phenomenon? N. Engl. J. Med. *281*:1347, 1969.
93. Lurie, P. R.: Postural effects in tetralogy of Fallot. Am. J. Med. *10*:297, 1953.
94. Munsell, W. P.: Pneumomediastinum. J.A.M.A. *202*:689, 1967.
95. Copeland, R. B., and Omenn, G. S.: Electrocardiograms suggestive of coronary artery disease in pneumothorax. Arch. Intern. Med. *25*:151, 1970.
96. Millard, C. E.: Pneumomediastinum. Dis. Chest *56*:297, 1969.
97. Abbott, D. A.: The clinical significance of pulmonary hemorrhage: A study of 1,316 patients with chest disease. Dis. Chest *14*:824, 1948.
98. Souders, C. R., and Smith, A. T.: The clinical significance of hemoptysis. J.A.M.A. *150*:746, 1952.
99. Haroutunian, L. M., and Neill, C. A.: Pulmonary complications of congenital heart disease: Hemoptysis. Am. Heart J. *84*:540, 1972.

ARRHYTHMIAS IN PATIENTS WITH LUNG DISEASE

100. Finley, T. N., Aronow, A., Cosentino, A. M., and Golde, D. W.: Occult pulmonary hemorrhage in anticoagulated patients. Am. Rev. Resp. Dis. *112*:23, 1975.
101. Shine, K. I., Kastor, J. A., and Yurchak, P. M.: Multifocal atrial tachycardia. Clinical and electrocardiographic features in 32 patients. N. Engl. J. Med. *279*:344, 1968.
102. Ayres, S. M., and Grace, W. J.: Inappropriate ventilation and hypoxemia as causes of cardiac arrhythmias. The control of arrhythmias without antiarrhythmic drugs. Am. J. Med. *46*:495, 1969.
103. Kleiger, R. E., and Senior, R. M.: Long-term electrocardiographic monitoring of ambulatory patients with chronic airway obstruction. Chest *65*:483, 1974.
104. Holford, F. D., and Mithoefer, J. C.: Cardiac arrhythmias in hospitalized patients with chronic obstructive pulmonary disease. Am. Rev. Resp. Dis. *108*:979, 1973.
105. Sideris, D. A., Katsadoros, D. P., Valianos, G., and Assioura, A.: Type of cardiac dysrhythmias in respiratory failure. Am. Heart J. *89*:32, 1975.
106. Tirlapur, V. G., and Mir, M. A.: Nocturnal hypoxemia and associated electrocardiographic changes in patients with chronic obstructive airway disease. N. Engl. J. Med. *306*:125, 1982.
107. Thomas, M. A., and Wee, A. S. T.: The sinus node in cor pulmonale. Isr. J. Med. Sci. *5*:831, 1969.
108. Green, L. H., and Smith, T. W.: The use of digitalis in patients with pulmonary disease. Ann. Intern. Med. *87*:459, 1977.

CARDIAC EFFECTS OF DRUGS AND OTHER MODALITIES USED TO TREAT LUNG DISORDERS

109. McFadden, E. R., Jr.: Beta 2 receptor agonists: Metabolism and pharmacology. J. Allergy Clin. Immunol. *68*:91, 1981.
110. Lands, A. M., Arnold, A., McAuliff, J. P., Luduena, F. P., and Brown, T. G.: Differentiation of receptor systems activated by sympathomimetic amines. Nature *214*:597, 1967.
111. Bourdillon, P. D. V., Dawson, J. R., Foale, R. A., Timmis, A. D., Poole-Wilson, P. A., and Sutton, J. C.: Salbutamol in treatment of heart failure. Br. Heart J. *43*:206, 1980.
112. Sunderrajan, E. V., Byron, W. A., McKenzie, W. N., Hurst, D. J., Allegro, M. M., Thakur, U. M., and Holmes, R. A.: The effect of terbutaline on cardiac function in patients with stable chronic obstructive lung disease. J.A.M.A. *250*:2151, 1983.
113. Mifune, J., Kuramoto, K., Ueda, K., Matsushita, S., Kuwajima, I., Sakai, M., Iwasaki, T., Moroki, N., and Murakami, M.: Hemodynamic effects of salbutamol and oral long-acting beta stimulant, in patients with congestive heart failure. Am. Heart J. *104*:1011, 1982.
114. Wang, R. Y. C., Lee, P. K., Yu, D. Y. C., Tse, T. F., and Chow, M. S.: Terbutaline infusion in cardiogenic shock: Acute hemodynamic effects and clinical response. J. Clin. Pharmacol. *23*:355, 1983.
115. Wang, R. Y. C., Lee, P. K., Yu, D. Y. C., Tse, T. F., and Chow, M. S.: Myocardial metabolic effects of intravenous terbutaline in patients with severe heart failure due to coronary artery disease. J. Clin. Pharmacol. *23*:362, 1983.
116. Clark, D. G., and Tinston, D. J.: Cardiac effects of isoproterenol, hypoxia, hypercapnia, and fluorocarbon propellents and their use in asthma inhalers. Ann. Allergy *30*:536, 1972.
117. Silverglade, A.: Cardiac toxicity of aerosol propellents. J.A.M.A. *222*:827, 1972.
118. Speizer, F. E., Wegman, D. H., and Ramirez, A.: Palpitation rates associated with fluorocarbon exposure in a hospital setting. N. Engl. J. Med. *292*:624, 1975.
119. Matthay, R. A., Berger, H. J., Loke, J., Gottschalk, A., and Zaret, B. L.: Effect of aminophylline upon right and left ventricular performance in chronic obstructive pulmonary disease. Am. J. Med. *65*:903, 1978.
120. Camarata, S. J., Weil, M. H., and Hanashiro, D. K.: Cardiac arrest in the critically ill. A study of predisposing causes in 132 patients. Circulation *44*:688, 1971.
121. Scharf, S. M., Caldini, P., and Ingram, R. H., Jr.: Cardiovascular effects of increasing airway pressure in the dog. Am. J. Physiol. *232*:435, 1977.
122. Haynes, J. B., Carson, S. D., Whitney, W. P., Zerbe, G. O., Hyers, T. M., and Steele, P.: Positive end-expiratory pressure shifts and left ventricular diastolic pressure-area curves. J. Appl. Physiol. Resp. Environ. Exercise Physiol. *48*:670, 1980.
123. Jardin, F., Farcot, J. C., Boisante, L., Curien, N., Margairaz, A., and Bourdarias, J. P.: Influence of positive end-expiratory pressures on left ventricular performance. N. Engl. J. Med. *304*:387, 1981.
124. Wise, R. A., Robotham, J. L., Bromberger-Barnea, B., and Permutt, S.: Effect of PEEP on left ventricular function in right-heart–bypassed dogs. J. Appl. Physiol. Resp. Environ. Exercise Physiol. *51*:541, 1981.
125. Fewell, J. E., Abendschein, D. R., Carlson, C. J., Rapaport, E., and Murray, J.: Mechanism of decreased right and left ventricular end-diastolic volumes during continuous positive-pressure ventilation in dogs. Circ. Res. *47*:467, 1980.
126. Gaensler, E. A., and Weisel, R. D.: The risks of abdominal and thoracic surgery in COPD. Postgrad. Med. *54*:183, 1973.
127. Olsen, G. N., Block, A. J., and Tobias, J. A.: Prediction of postpneumonectomy pulmonary function using quantitative macroaggregate lung scanning. Chest *66*:13, 1974.
128. Tisi, G. M.: Preoperative evaluation of pulmonary function. *In* Isselbacher, K. J., et al. (eds.): Principles of Internal Medicine, Update III. New York, McGraw-Hill Book Co., 1982, p. 101.
129. Mittman, C.: Assessment of operative risk in thoracic surgery. Am. Rev. Resp. Dis. *84*:197, 1961.

62 EMOTION, PSYCHIATRIC DISORDERS, AND THE HEART

by THOMAS P. HACKETT, M.D.,
JERROLD F. ROSENBAUM, M.D., and
GEORGE E. TESAR, M.D.

Every affection of the mind that is attended with either pain or pleasure, hope or fear, is the cause of an agitation whose influence extends to the heart.

WILLIAM HARVEY, EXERCITATIO DE MOTU CORDIS ET SANGUINIS, 1628[1]

Although few would disclaim Harvey's sentiment, the precise nature of the link between the mind and heart disease remains to be defined. Substantial evidence exists to indicate associations between psychosocial stresses and coronary artery disease, hypertension, arrhythmia, and sudden death, but the intervening variables that mediate pathological changes have yet to be subjected to rigorous, prospective study. In this chapter these and other issues relevant to the interface between cardiology and psychiatry are discussed.

PSYCHIATRIC ASPECTS OF CORONARY ARTERY DISEASE

PSYCHOSOCIAL FACTORS

Clinicians have long suspected that the accumulation of small stresses from longstanding conflicts can augment the development of cardiovascular disease, most especially of essential hypertension and coronary atherosclerosis. In the 1910 Lumleian lecture, Sir William Osler, commenting on physicians with angina pectoris, said, ". . . the outstanding feature was the incessant treadmill of practice; and yet if hard work—that 'badge of our tribe'—was alone responsible, would there not be a great many more cases? Every one of these men had an additional factor—worry; in not a single case under fifty years of age was this feature absent. . . ."[2] Three decades later, Flanders Dunbar gave the following capsule description of patients with coronary artery disease: "They are compulsive, have a tendency to work long hours and not take vacations, a tendency to seize authority; dislike of sharing responsibility . . . articulate . . . few neurotic traits . . . a tendency to depression which is rarely admitted to . . . a tendency to minimize symptoms . . . self-neglect. . . ."[3] This sketch of the coronary patient, consumed in work and beset by worry, has been recognized and redrawn by many clinicians.

TYPES A AND B BEHAVIOR. Although researchers have examined the roles of life dissatisfaction, acute stress, personal loss, sociological factors, and personality traits in coronary artery disease, much time and effort have also been devoted to describing a personality behavior pattern characteristic of the overworked and anxious coronary patient. Friedman and Rosenman developed the concept of a "coronary-prone behavior pattern," which they termed *Type A behavior*.[4] Over the last three decades they have investigated the association between Type A behavior and coronary artery disease and have concluded that Type A behavior is as significant as any of the major risk factors of coronary artery disease, such as cigarette smoking, hypercholesterolemia, and hypertension; Friedman defines Type A behavior as "a characteristic action-emotion complex" found in people who are constantly struggling to reach poorly defined goals in the shortest time possible.[4] In his opinion, the most critical aspects of Type A behavior patterns are excesses of competitiveness, pace, and aggression. Type B individuals exhibit the opposite type of behavior; they are relaxed, unhurried, and less aggressive. Although they may be interested in success, and may indeed be successful, in most instances they do not struggle so vigorously as Type A individuals in pursuit of this goal.

In the Western Collaborative Group Study (WCGS)[5] male subjects were sorted into groups on the basis of the prominence of Type A behavior patterns, measured in an interview designed to test the behavior of each subject. The study was conducted in double-blind fashion; neither the rating team nor the medical examiner had knowledge of all risk factors. Follow-up at 4½, 6½, and 8½ years revealed that men with coronary-prone Type A behavior at entry experienced 1.7 to 4.5 times the rate of new coronary diseases as did Type B men (Fig. 62–1).

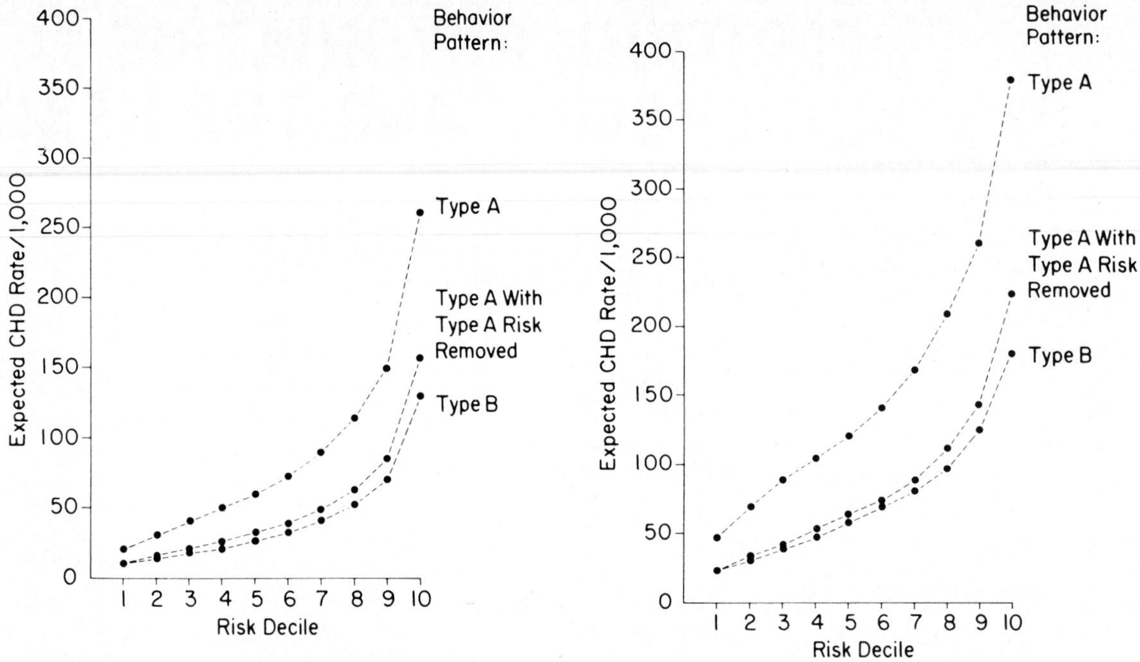

FIGURE 62–1. Expected rates of coronary heart disease in 8.5 years by decile of estimated risk for WCGS men ages 39 to 49 (*A*) and 50 to 59 (*B*). (From Brand, R. J., Rosenman, R. H., Sholtz, R. I., and Friedman, M.: Multivariate prediction of coronary heart disease in the Western Collaborative Group Study compared to the findings of the Framingham study. Circulation *53*:348, 1976, by permission of the American Heart Association, Inc.)

Research data from various other demographical and geographical settings consistently relate Type A behavior to coronary artery disease.[6] Investigations in Europe, Australia, and Israel point to the cross-cultural relevance of some aspects of such behavior.[7] Studies have shown that the Type A pattern appears to be specifically related to atherosclerosis. Individuals with other diseases, such as lung disease and cancer, tend to include an equal distribution of Types A and B.[7, 8] Jenkins feels that there is a strong link between Type A behavior and the clinical emergence of myocardial infarction and coronary artery disease and that Type A behavior has "about the same strength of associations with coronary artery disease prevalence and incidence as do other standard risk factors."[7] This point of view is now shared by a number of experienced cardiologists.[9]

Some studies have shown that the Type A pattern is associated with specific physiological and biochemical parameters that may contribute to atherogenesis. Type A subjects exhibit greater cardiovascular reactivity and higher elevation of catecholamines, cortisol, and testosterone than Type B subjects during performance of mental arithmetic and reaction time tasks,[10] especially when monetary incentive is added.[11] These and other studies suggest that the Type A behavior pattern and its physiological correlates are evoked and facilitated by environmental stimuli. The relationships among these variables are schematized in Figure 62–2.

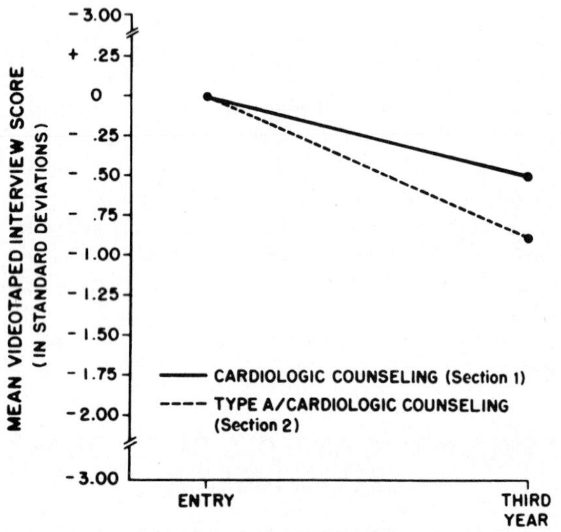

FIGURE 62–3. The third-year decremental changes in Type A behavior assessed by videotaped interview in section 1 and 2 participants ($p<0.001$). (From Friedman, M., et al.: Alteration of Type A behavior and reduction in cardiac recurrences in postmyocardial infarction patients. Am. Heart J. *108*:237, 1984.)

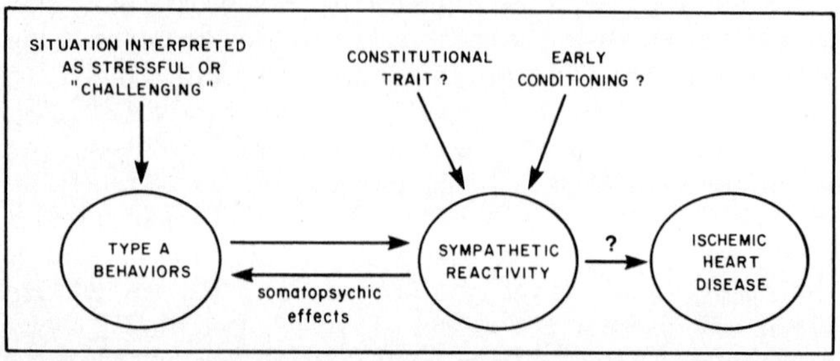

FIGURE 62–2. Model illustrating possible relationships between Type A behavior and sympathetic nervous system reactivity. (Adapted from Krantz, D. S., et al.: Psychobiological substrates of the Type A behavior pattern. Health Psychol. 2:393, 1983.)

If the Type A behavior pattern is a risk factor for myocardial infarction, then its modification and attenuation should result in a reduced risk of developing clinically significant coronary artery disease.[11a] Friedman and his associates provided advice and instructions designed to diminish Type A behavior to 592 patients who had suffered a myocardial infarction. After 3 years there was a significant reduction of Type A behavior in 44 per cent of the experimental subjects who received both behavioral modification and cardiological counseling, and the recurrence rate of nonfatal myocardial infarctions was one-half that in controls who received cardiological counseling alone[12] (Figs. 62–3 and 62–4).

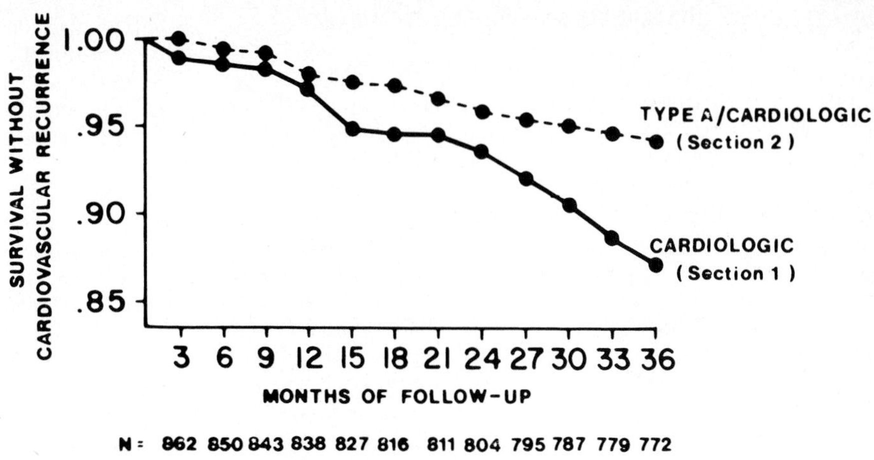

FIGURE 62–4. Cumulative "survival without cardiac recurrence" curves for Type A/cardiologic and cardiologic sections—employing the "intention-to-treat" principle. N indicates the total number of participants followed at the beginning of each time point. A participant is censored (i.e., removed from further calculations) upon cardiovascular recurrence or inability to trace (chi square = 7.8, p<0.01). (From Friedman, M., et al.: Alteration of Type A behavior and reduction in cardiac recurrences in postmyocardial infarction patients. Am. Heart J. *108*:237, 1984.)

In contrast to the evidence that supports the Type A hypothesis, a number of important studies have *failed* to demonstrate its validity.[12a] Univariate and multivariate analyses of data gathered from subjects participating in the Multiple Risk Factor Intervention Trial (MRFIT) showed no relationship between the Type A pattern and either morbidity or mortality from coronary artery disease (CAD).[13] Negative findings have also been reported from the Finnish Twin Cohort Study (FTC),[14] the Aspirin Myocardial Infarction Study (AMIS),[15] and the Multicenter Post-Infarction Program (MPIP).[16]

There may be a number of reasons that these studies failed to replicate previous findings.[17] First, in both the FTC and MRFIT the mortality from CAD was considerably below expectation, and such few events occurred that even the major hypotheses of the studies could not be tested adequately (Type II error). Second, public recognition of the importance of risk factor intervention may have positively influenced the behavior of high-risk controls in such studies as the MRFIT and AMIS. And third, evidence has been mounting that the instruments used to measure the Type A pattern—the Structured Interview (SI), the Jenkins Activity Survey (JAS), the Bortner Scale, and others—lack specificity and measure multiple dimensions of behavior and attitude, not all of which necessarily contribute to the pathogenesis of CAD.

This last consideration has prompted reevaluation and refinement of the Type A hypothesis.[18] Component analysis of the SI suggests that *hostility and unexpressed anger* are the features of the Type A pattern that are most frequently associated with significant CAD.[18, 19] Williams and associates documented a similar association using a subscale of the Minnesota Multiphasic Personality Inventory that measures hostility, mistrust, and cynicism.[20] Moreover, when data originally reported as showing no relationship between the Type A pattern and CAD have been reanalyzed for evidence of hostility, a clear association with extent of CAD has been discovered (J. E. Dimsdale, M.D., personal communication). These findings suggest that some features of the Type A pattern, e.g., competitiveness and job involvement, are less reliable predictors of CAD and that they have been implicated in the pathogenesis only insofar as they are manifestations of hostility and unexpressed anger.

Stress and life change,[21] bereavement,[22] and life or work dissatisfaction (Sisyphus complex)[23, 23a] have also been identified as putative risk factors for morbidity and mortality from CAD. Many of these investigations are subject to criticism because of their retrospective nature. However, Ruberman and colleagues administered a questionnaire prospectively to 1684 patients in the Beta-Blocker Heart Attack Trial (BHAT) and discovered a significant correlation between the incidence of recurrent myocardial infarction and high levels of stress and social isolation[24] (Figs. 62–3 and 62–4).

RESPONSE TO SYMPTOMS

DELAY IN ARRIVAL. The most important psychological danger to the patient with acute myocardial infarction is *delay*—the time interval from symptom onset to arrival at a medical facility (Chaps. 24 and 38). Median delay times in recent studies range from 2.9 to 5.1 hours (Fig. 62–2).[25–27] The enormity of this problem becomes apparent when one realizes that 55 to 80 per cent of deaths from myocardial infarction occur within 4 hours of the onset of symptoms;[28] thus the lives of many of these victims might have been saved had they responded in time. Furthermore, the efficacy of reperfusion therapy (thrombolysis or angioplasty or both) is dependent importantly on the time or both interval between the onset of coronary occlusion and successful reperfusion (Chap. 37). Therefore, even among survivors of myocardial infarction, the size of the infarct and therefore the severity of the clinical complications are related to the delay.

What accounts for this delay? In three independent studies, delay time did not correlate significantly with educational level, occupation, socioeconomic class, or past history of heart disease.[25–27] In our study at the Massachusetts General Hospital,[25] delay tended to diminish as the severity of symptoms mounted; however, according to the Peale score, there was no relationship between delay time and the severity of the disease. Individuals who recognized the true source of their pain came sooner than did those who displaced the cause of pain to the gastrointestinal system. Patients who interpreted the symptoms as totally unrelated to their hearts delayed the longest. Considerable time was usually wasted in trying to decide what action to take. The victim's friends and associates appear to be more effective at reducing delay than are husbands or wives. Individuals who experience myocardial infarction at their place of employment reach the hospital most swiftly because they may be ordered to do so by a plant supervisor or nurse. Although spouses are less effective catalysts than are foremen or supervisors, some take the initiative by calling an ambulance or a doctor, despite victim protest.

Why does the stricken patient fail to take energetic corrective action in his own behalf? With the abundance of information available to the lay public, replete with examples of public figures who have recovered from myocardial infarction, a more appropriate and salubrious response might be expected. Although there is no specific answer to this question, the defense of denial has been used as a partial explanation.[25] *Denial* has been cited as the most common human reaction to situations of life stress[29] and is defined as the conscious or unconscious repudiation of part or all of the total available meaning of an event in order to allay fear, anxiety, or other unpleasant effects.[30] At its simplest, it is the negation of personal danger (i.e., "This can't be happening to me"). *Displacement* is another form of denial (i.e., "This pain must be indigestion"). *Rationalization* is still another (i.e., "This pain can't be a heart attack; I'm too young"). The list of variations continues, but the goal is the same—to reduce or eliminate the threat. Myocardial infarction presents a profound threat to life. Even survival, in the minds of many, carries the toll of permanent cardiac impairment. For some people, to acknowledge that chest pain may herald myocardial infarction is tantamount to accepting a grim future. It is necessary to correct such misconceptions to prevent what is clearly inordinate delay.

EFFORTS TO REDUCE DELAY. In an effort to reduce delay, physicians should attempt to dispel the myth of automatic invalidism after myocardial infarction by stressing to both patient and family that many patients are able to return to their previous occupations and to resume essentially unaltered life styles. The public must also be introduced to a simple set of specific guidelines outlining the type, duration, and variation in symptoms of myocardial infarction and the urgent need for immediate medical consultation if and when such symptoms appear. The possibility of both delay and denial by the patient must be anticipated, and friends and family must be encouraged to respond to these symptoms by seeking assistance despite possible protest.

HOSPITALIZATION

EMERGENCY WARD. Most hospitals provide immediate care for people entering with chest pain, enabling patients to be seen by a physician before nonessential information is obtained. The emergency ward experience is generally brief and reassuring. Despite the patient's rapid transit through this area, three aspects deserve attention:

1. The patient should be given a clear account of what is happening to him or her, and any questions asked should be answered. A direct relationship seems to exist between uncertainty and anxiety, so that as long as presentation of the medical facts is buttressed by as much reassurance as one can reasonably provide, the patient will benefit from the truth.
2. Administering the sacrament of the sick to Catholic patients is not as stressful an experience as it may appear.[31] The critical variable here is the attitude of the priest; if he is friendly and emphasizes the routine nature of the procedure, the patient's response is apt to be positive.
3. The coronary care unit should be carefully described to the patient ahead of time, especially if it is windowless or unusual in any other way.

PROBLEMS IN THE CORONARY CARE UNIT (CCU). The cardiac monitor is central to the experience of a patient in the CCU. When continuous monitoring was first introduced, many conjectured that the restraint of the leads, audible "beeps," and visible electrocardiograms would induce considerable anxiety in the patient. However, our findings[32] and those of others[33, 34] demonstrate that the monitor may be more reassuring than frightening to the cardiac patient, in large part because of the way in which the monitor is introduced. In our unit the nurses have referred to it as a "mechanical guardian angel" and have told the patient, "As long as you're hooked up to this machine, you can't die if you try"—a remarkably effective stratagem.

Witnessing a cardiac arrest is judged by the staff to be the most distressing event in the CCU. In a study of patients who watched a resuscitation effort, only 20 per cent of the spectators *admitted* to being frightened by the scene.[32] Although all patients were impressed by the speedy response of the code team to the alarm and many were equally impressed by the brevity of resuscitation, the most common general response was *anger* directed toward the patient in cardiac arrest. The usefulness of anger is not difficult to discover. If an anxious person can be made angry—a more controllable and more acceptable emotion than anxiety—his apprehension declines. Lack of identification with the arrest victim further reduces anxiety. Although empathy for the patient in cardiac arrest was expressed by all, only rarely did a patient identify with him, even when the victim and observer were of the same sex and of similar age and social background. The typical response of the patient witnessing cardiac arrest is an attempt to grasp the most comforting meaning from the event while denying its more threatening aspects. That this is not always effective is demonstrated in the report of Bruhn et al. of anxiety and elevated systolic pressure in patients who had viewed a fatal arrest.[35] Requests for tranquilizers and pain medication increase in the wake of an arrest. In one study in which CCU patients were asked whether they would prefer to be in a single room or in a two- or four-bed ward should they require subsequent hospitalization, all chose the latter except those who had seen an arrest—these patients chose single rooms.[32]

The experience of cardiac arrest itself is almost always clouded by amnesia. Nine of 10 patients remember nothing specific about the event.[32] We have found nothing to support the observations of Kübler-Ross, who has described several "afterlife experiences" in a dream state during the period of arrest.[36]

An early report on the psychological state of survivors of cardiac arrest provided a grim picture of life after resuscitation.[37] These survivors appeared to be suffering from post-traumatic stress disorder. Chronically anxious and depressed, they complained of feeling different from others, as though, like Lazarus, they had returned from the dead. Subsequent reports have not supported this early observation.[38, 39] Indeed, there appears to be a remarkable absence of emotional debility in some patients who survive cardiac arrest. Dobson and his coworkers, who have followed a series of survivors for some years after cardiac arrest, report a uniformly good long-term response and emphasize the importance of informing the patient about what has happened.[39] It is helpful to stress the routine nature of resuscitation and that it does not necessarily alter the patient's prognosis.

Although most patients in the CCU are anxious, few openly complain of anxiety or appear unduly apprehensive to their attending physician. If questioned closely, patients may admit to feelings of anxiety, but the tendency is to minimize this affect, as though its presence were cowardly. Although major (clinical) depression occurs infrequently in the CCU, patients begin to experience a sense of sadness toward the end of their stay, when the critical period has passed, and they begin to assess their future. This is essentially an adjustment disorder with depressed mood, a quite normal response under the circumstances and one that typically occurs in individuals who have sustained loss.

In this case it is the loss of the sense of health and intactness; rarely is the depression pathological. Delirium, so common in the surgical intensive care unit, is less common in the CCU. It occurs in fewer than 1 per cent of the patients.[40]

The defense of denial (defined earlier) is a common adaptive process in patients who face danger. In situations of stress, denial can lower the sense of tension, both psychologically and physiologically. An unexpected finding in one study was the inverse relationship between denial and mortality in the CCU.[32] Individuals who denied being frightened, minimized the seriousness of their illness, displayed a fatalistic attitude, and gave the appearance of being unruffled tended to survive the CCU experience in larger numbers than did those who worried constantly and seemed unable to deny their distress. Although denial can play the role of enemy to the myocardial infarction victim in delaying his arrival in the emergency ward, it can also serve as an ally in the CCU.

PSYCHOLOGICAL MANAGEMENT IN THE CCU (See also Chap. 38). Informing the patient about the facts of his illness and about the function of equipment and purpose of procedures is becoming common practice. Lack of information, partial disclosures, and conspiracies of silence detract from the doctor-patient relationship.[41] The side effects of medication should be explained, as should the reason for performing certain procedures, such as frequent determination of vital signs. While clarifying medical issues and misconceptions, it is also possible to impart a sense of enlightened optimism by mentioning, for example, that the Boston Marathon has been successfully completed by individuals who have suffered myocardial infarction.

Predicting that an event will produce anxiety is as good as saying that such anxiety is normal. Thus, the anxiety loses its sting. A good example of this is to anticipate that the sound of the alarm buzzer in the CCU will provoke anxiety and to point out that the alarm is usually activated by a loose electrode. Similarly, if the patient is warned that he will feel anxious upon being transferred out of the CCU, even when he is fully aware that the move is a sign of improvement, he will view his anxiety as legitimate, and its impact will be reduced.

Medication. Assuming that all patients in the CCU are anxious, no matter how calm they appear, we routinely order an antianxiety agent on a regular, not on an as-needed (p.r.n.), basis. "As-needed" ordering should be avoided, because patients will seldom ask for a tranquilizer. If pain medication is on order, patients will choose it over an anxiolytic, even though their primary complaint is anxiety. To many patients, to request a tranquilizer is somehow to admit a weakness.

A benzodiazepine, such as diazepam, 2 to 10 mg orally three to four times a day, is generally adequate. In older patients or those with hepatic dysfunction, oxazepam, 10 to 30 mg, or lorazepam, 0.5 to 2 mg, orally every 4 to 6 hours, is preferable because each is cleared entirely through the kidneys. The triazolobenzodiazepine, alprazolam, 0.25 to 1.0 mg three to four times daily, is possibly more effective for the treatment of those patients who are depressed as well as anxious. The benzodiazepines are preferred to other sedative-hypnotic tranquilizers such as phenobarbital because they produce less mental confusion (less sedation) and interact less with the metabolism of sodium warfarin (Coumadin). Alprazolam may be particularly suited for use in the CCU because of its purported ability to inhibit platelet-activating factor (PAF)–induced platelet aggregation.[42] A hypnotic dose of a benzodiazepine can be achieved by doubling the usual antianxiety dose at bedtime.

Acute anxiety or panic spells can be dealt with by increasing the dose of oral benzodiazepine or by administering it intravenously (if available). Diazepam, 5 to 10 mg intravenously, is often effective, although it may produce hypotension or respiratory depression especially in the debilitated or elderly patient. Lorazepam, 2 to 4 mg intravenously, not only is effective but has minimal effects on blood pressure and respiration even in high doses.[43] As the patient regains his calm, a careful examination should be carried out to determine the source of fear. Effective reassurance requires understanding the nature of the fear. Should panic herald an acute psychosis (agitation, delusions, hallucinations) haloperidol 1 to 5 mg orally four times a day is the initial treatment of choice. Intravenous administration of higher doses, alone or in combination with intravenous lorazepam, may become necessary and is well tolerated[43–45] (see below). It is imperative to enlist psychiatric consultation whenever panic or psychosis occurs.

Treatment of *depression* in the CCU can generally be negotiated without medication. As discussed below, tricyclic antidepressants, monoamine oxidase inhibitors, and phenothiazines present risks when used in patients with cardiovascular disorders. It should be noted that the depression one encounters in the CCU is reactive in nature and is normal under the circumstances; however, if the physician feels that the depression is more serious than this, an immediate examination by a psychiatric consultant should be requested.

TRANSFER FROM THE CORONARY CARE UNIT. The transition from CCU to the "stepdown unit" should be presented to the patient as a graduation exercise—tangible reassurance that progress has been made. Departing from the CCU, however, is not an unmixed blessing. The patient leaves the security provided by close nursing care, a doctor within calling distance, and, in some instances, the "guardian angel" presence of the monitor. All these factors may contribute to the sense of vulnerability and the apprehension which occur at the time of transition from the CCU. The elevated levels of urinary catecholamines at this time[46] may reflect this increase in anxiety.

The use of submaximal exercise electrocardiograms, thallium-201 perfusion scans, and/or radionuclide ventriculography prior to hospital discharge (p. 1293) provides reassurance to patients, since it demonstrates to them their capacity to perform physical activity. Frequently it allows the physician to inform the patient that objective measurements (response of heart rate, blood pressure, electrocardiogram, and myocardial perfusion) indicate that physical activity is *not* harmful.

CONVALESCENCE

PSYCHOLOGICAL INVALIDISM DURING CONVALESCENCE. Of the many thousands of patients who survive acute myocardial infarctions each year, many do not return to work because of psychological invalidism. More important than the income lost unnecessarily is the emotional suffering these patients experience. The extent of this suffering can be exemplified by a study of 24 patients interviewed between 3 and 9 months after their discharge from the hospital.[47] At this early point in their convalescence, 21 rated themselves as anxious or depressed; 18 were judged by the examiner to require either a tranquilizer or an antidepressant. Sleep disturbances occurred in 15 patients, and disruptive family quarrels over aspects of convalescence took place in 18 cases. These patients consistently tended to minimize symptoms during follow-up examinations, to retain harmful habits, and to avoid taking sedatives. Eleven patients did not return to work—nine for psychological reasons. Those who did resume part- or full-time employment experienced anxiety, augmentation of angina, or dyspnea.

Although there are many and diverse causes for distress in cardiac convalescence, a common denominator to all is *depression*. The post–myocardial infarction depression, as mentioned earlier, is a normal reaction to loss. Even in uncomplicated cases the sense of loss is present, although in a symbolic rather than a real way. The individual who has sustained a myocardial infarction feels vulnerable. His immortality and sense of physical intactness have been challenged, and some refer to this vulnerability as "ego infarction."[48] When the myocardial infarction is complicated, and the individual is left with sequelae such as angina, congestive heart failure, or arrhythmias, depression and the feeling of hopelessness may be compounded. In general the depression tends to be self-limited and improves during the first month at home, beginning with the individual's realization that he is able to negotiate walks around the house and short flights of stairs and, sometimes even more importantly, to experience human contact without suffering undue strain. By the time sexual intercourse can be resumed, the patient is generally sound enough to commence work, at which point the road to normal functioning is more easily traversed.

The term "homecoming depression" has been used to describe the initial stages of the post–myocardial infarction depression,[47] typically manifest during the first week after the patient has returned home. It is heralded by the complaint of exertional weakness—a symptom which the patient considers to be a harbinger of cardiac decline. Even minimal activity such as a walk to the front door or a stroll in the garden may produce a disproportionate sense of weakness. Since the feeling of weakness does not relent with the passage of days, the patient may think that his heart is more damaged than he was led to believe, and this symptom becomes the nucleus around which other depressive symptoms collect. A pervasive sense of gloom and hopelessness is accompanied by an inability to control tearfulness. A change in sleeping pattern—one of the most sensitive indicators of depression—is present, as well as anorexia or hyperphagia, irritability, withdrawal, anhedonia (loss of pleasure in acts that normally give pleasure), and loss of a sense of humor. A basic sense of anxiety accompanies the depression, and although the individual may not be oppressed by a sense of impending death, the thought of his own demise hovers in the back of his mind. Once the full-blown picture sets in, the depression is often recognized by the spouse, through whom it may be relayed to the physician.

Myths about myocardial infarction abound, reinforcing the victim's fears. Many patients are embarrassed to ask about them. Some common myths include the following: (1) The victim of myocardial infarction is "over the hill"; he not only has reached maturity but also has entered physical and psychological senium. (2) Excitement must be avoided; it is risky to watch exciting sporting events. (3) Arms must be kept below the head (said to apply to any activity from plastering a ceiling to raising one's hand to take an oath). (4) All isometric effort is contraindicated. (5) Driving a car is apt to produce angina or a recurrent myocardial infarct. (6) Sex is a thing of the past; death is apt to take place at the moment of orgasm. (7) Deep sleep is dangerous; hypnotics should be avoided; sudden death is more apt to occur in sound than in light sleep. (8) Beware of anniversaries; there is a strong possibility of recurrence around the time of one's first infarction or around the anniversary of the death of a loved one from myocardial infarction. Some of these myths are based on fact; others are entirely fallacious. In either case, every effort should be made to anticipate these concerns and to counteract them.

MANAGEMENT ISSUES IN CONVALESCENCE. Patient Education. Education is a principal factor in the treatment of post–myocardial infarction depression. At the time of discharge the physician should confer with the patient and his or her spouse to outline the main problems of convalescence. The patient should be informed that weakness can be expected because of the time spent in bed. Bed rest can produce a weekly loss of strength of about 10 to 15 per cent secondary to muscle atrophy and a reduction in maximal oxygen uptake. The physician should also point out that depression following myocardial infarction is a normal response which usually disappears spontaneously within 2 or 3 months.

We have found that although coronary patients often know something about the cause of infarction (a "plugged vessel"), many have no conception of how it heals; some individuals even believe there is no healing, picturing the heart with a perpetual leak in the pumping system. During the discharge discussion the patient might be asked to draw a heart, illustrating his or her concept of infarction and of healing. This can serve as an embarkation point for a more detailed discussion of the mechanics of a heart attack and the nature of recovery.

Since there is a great deal of misunderstanding about the safety of sexual activity during convalescence, it should be pointed out to the patient that coital death is unusual. In the study by Ueno which is most often cited, coition accounted for 0.6 per cent of endogenous sudden deaths,[49] most of which occurred in the setting of extramarital intercourse. Males were an average of 13 years older than their companions, and one-third were inebriated at the time of intercourse. Hellerstein and Friedman have reported that the equivalent cost in oxygen of maximal activity during intercourse approximates 6 calories per minute.[50] During foreplay and afterplay about 4.5 calories per minute are consumed. According to these calculations the demand placed upon the heart by sexual intercourse is equal to that of a brisk walk around the block or of climbing one flight of stairs. Although Hellerstein and Friedman have been criticized for generalizing from too small and too unique a sample, their findings do offer an estimation of the energy levels involved in sexual activity.

Activity and Physical Conditioning (see also Chap. 41). Convalescents from a myocardial infarction usually state that inactivity is their greatest source of frustration. No sedentary pastime can diminish the boredom of idle days. Since physical activities require different levels of exertion, most questions posed by patients in the first 2 months of convalescence pertain to the cost of an activity in terms of cardiovascular strain. One of the best available systems for quantifying the energy spent in various activities and for translating it into understandable units for the patient is the metabolic equivalents system (METS).[51] The physician or a cardiac nurse should instruct the patient and spouse about the METS and set up a program of graduated activity so that a goal can be set for each day. Activity, no matter how trivial it may seem, provides an excellent prophylaxis against depression. A physical conditioning program gives the patient a sense of participating in his recovery rather than of being the passive recipient of care. Confidence in his performance is restored as the patient watches his potential to perform various activities expand.[48]

Group Activities. It has been reported that group meetings of post–myocardial infarction patients may be helpful during convalescence.[52] The purpose here is educational rather than psychotherapeutic; the meetings take place regularly every week for 12 weeks and are conducted by a professional (a physician or nurse clinician) with the goal of exchanging information and sharing experiences. Although their value remains to be rigorously demonstrated, these groups are enthusiastically endorsed by the individuals who participate in them. Group activities designed to modify Type A behavior are also successful and may additionally help to reduce the incidence of recurrent myocardial infarction.[12]

Medication. The use of antianxiety agents such as the benzodiazepines can be helpful during convalescence of cardiac patients. It should be emphasized to the patient that his state of mind as well as his physical health contributes to his rehabilitation and that tranquilizers are an appropriate means of relieving anxiety. Under certain circumstances, such as driving in traffic, anxious feelings are bound to emerge. Until the patient has developed his own method of coping with nervousness, anxiolytics are a helpful adjunct. (Antidepressants are discussed later in this chapter.)

Telephone Follow-up. A nurse clinician can be available for a specific period during the day to receive telephone calls from patients or she can make weekly follow-up calls to the patient and spouse to provide information about diet, sexual problems, permissible activity, and the like.

Relaxation Techniques and Autohypnosis. Relaxation techniques are increasingly advocated and are probably helpful. Publications describing the relaxation response are available, and the technique can easily be learned by the patient.[53] Autohypnosis is a potent tool for the promotion of relaxation in receptive subjects. However, both relaxation and hypnosis tend to be more attractive to those self-reliant individuals who are also most apt to participate in physical conditioning therapy programs.

Psychotherapy. Since post–myocardial infarction depression is essentially self-limited, psychotherapy is necessary only for those who fail to improve after 2 to 3 months. Patients who complain of a persistent loss of libido, impotence, anorexia, and disturbed sleep or those who develop hypochondriacal complaints can frequently benefit from psychotherapy.

CARDIAC SURGERY AND POSTOPERATIVE DELIRIUM. Along with its many benefits, cardiac surgery also presents the problem of postoperative delirium. For this reason recent psychiatric studies have focused considerable attention on the postcardiotomy patient.

Course and Nature. Delirium is defined as a clouding of consciousness accompanied by hyperalertness or agitation. Its hallmark is disorientation in time, place, or person. Perceptual distortions in the form of illusions, delusions, or hallucinations may also be present, accounting for the use of the term postoperative "psychosis."

The reported incidence of delirium after cardiac surgery ranges from 13 to 67 per cent,[54] a reflection of the criteria used for definition of delirium and of the quality of technical skills, procedures, and instruments available at the time of surgical intervention. Kornfeld and colleagues reported a 28 per cent incidence of delirium following coronary artery bypass graft (CABG) surgery, which they believe is comparable to that following cardiotomy.[55] More recently Breuer and colleagues at the Cleveland Clinic conducted a prospective analysis of 421 patients undergoing CABG surgery and reported an 11.6 per cent incidence of encephalopathy (confusion and disorientation without focal neurological findings) after the procedure.[56]

The typical delirium following cardiac surgery begins after a clear period of 3 to 5 days.[54] When this "lucid interval" ends, the patient becomes confused and then delirious. In this state he may remove intravenous catheters, attempt to leave the unit, and behave in a generally disruptive and potentially dangerous way.

FACTORS CONTRIBUTING TO THE DEVELOPMENT OF DELIRIUM AFTER CARDIAC SURGERY. In an effort to devise strategies to prevent postoperative delirium, predisposing factors have been examined. In a critical review of postcardiotomy delirium, Dubin and colleagues[54] identified the following determinants: (1) preoperative cardiac status as defined by the New York Heart Association Functional and Therapeutic Indices, (2) the severity of physical illness, (3) the complexity of the surgical procedure (defined by the extent and duration of instrumentation in the intracardiac chambers), (4) preoperative organic brain disease, and (5) preoperative psychiatric morbidity (anxiety, denial, clinical depression, or substance abuse). Age, sex, and length of the bypass period were not associated. A study of post-CABG delirium showed that it was statistically associated with only two factors: (1) severity of recovery room illness and (2) a history of myocardial infarction; there was also a suggestive association between personality type and delirium.[55]

All the factors listed above are likely to result in postoperative delirium to the degree that they produce dysfunction of the central nervous system. A number of recent studies provide evidence of diffuse but transient ischemic brain injury resulting from cardiac surgery.[57, 58] Delirium may result if the injury is extensive or aggravated by the effects of preoperative, intraoperative, or postoperative CNS insults (e.g., chronically low cardiac index with reduced cerebral perfusion; microemboli; the effects of anticholinergic, narcotic, and sedative-hypnotic medications).

The etiological importance of environmental and psychological factors has been presumed, but is difficult to prove. Early reports suggested that sensory deprivation, abnormal sensory input, and sleep deprivation played a significant role in the development of delirium. In fact, the converse is more likely to be the case, namely, that delirium is a cause rather than a result of sleep deprivation and abnormal sensory processing.[43] Similarly, it is less likely that the intensive care unit (ICU) environment produces delirium than the presence of delirium makes it a difficult environment to tolerate. The use of multiple intravascular catheters, a mechanical ventilator, or an intra-aortic balloon pump requires considerable patient cooperation, frequently beyond the capacity of those with delirium or other psychiatric disorders.

TREATMENT OF POSTOPERATIVE DELIRIUM. The principles of the treatment of delirium have been outlined and discussed by Cassem.[59]

1. ***Correction of metabolic and systemic abnormalities.*** Meticulous examination of the clinical situation and the patient's chart are essential first steps in determining whether specific abnormalities (e.g., CNS dysfunction, hypoxia, acid-base disturbance, fluid and electrolyte imbalance, endocrine dysfunction, renal failure, infection, nutritional deficiency) exist so that they can be selectively treated.

2. ***Elimination of drug toxicity.*** It has been suggested

that the likelihood of delirium developing in the ICU patient depends on the number of drugs with anticholinergic properties administered.[60] Administration of these and other drugs that are frequently used in the recovery unit, including (a) antiarrhythmic agents (e.g., digoxin, lidocaine, quinidine), (b) narcotic agents (especially meperidine hydrochloride and propoxyphene hydrochloride), (c) sedative-hypnotic agents, and (d) H_2-blockers (cimetidine and ranitidine), should be monitored and if necessary reduced or discontinued.

3. ***Treatment of drug withdrawal.*** Occasionally delirium may be a manifestation of withdrawal from alcohol, sedative-hypnotic agents, opioid drugs, or agents with anticholinergic properties (e.g., atropine and tricyclic antidepressants). It is important that the physician recognize withdrawal when it occurs and prescribe adequate replacement medication.

4. ***Maximization of the patient's comfort.*** The physician and nursing staff should be attentive to the principles of treating anxiety, pain, hypoxia, akathisia (motor restlessness occurring as a side effect of neuroleptic medication), prolonged confinement, and immobility.[61]

5. ***Use of neuroleptic medication.*** If delirium or agitation persists after attention to the principles discussed, then use of neuroleptic medication is indicated. *Haloperidol*, a high-potency neuroleptic, is in our experience the drug of choice because it has minimal effects on heart rate, blood pressure, pulmonary artery pressure, and respiration.[62] Numerous reports attest to its safety and efficacy in critically ill patients whether prescribed orally or parenterally,[63] even in high doses.[44, 45, 62] Intravenous administration of haloperidol is safe and effective and particularly suited for administration in the ICU setting. The approach to initiation, titration, and maintenance of dosage is outlined in Table 62–1.[61] At the time of this writing haloperidol has not been approved by the Food and Drug Administration for routine intravenous use and it is prescribed in only a few institutions. The physician is therefore advised to inform the hospital pharmacy before prescribing intravenous haloperidol. If haloperidol alone fails to control agitation that accompanies delirium, it may be useful to add *lorazepam.*[43] Intravenous administration of lorazepam also has relatively little effect on respiratory and hemodynamic function.

Patient education and a strong doctor-patient relationship are believed to be important measures for the patient's successful adaptation to the ICU setting, although it is uncertain that they impact on the occurrence of delirium.[64] Both patients and their families should receive preoperative instruction about the nature of the surgical procedure and postoperative care. A preoperative visit to the surgical ICU helps to familiarize the patient with the environment and staff and may help to alleviate anticipatory anxiety. Finally, misconceptions about the ultimate course of the illness should be clarified.

TABLE 62–1 PROTOCOL FOR INTRAVENOUS USE OF HALOPERIDOL IN THE INTENSIVE CARE UNIT

STARTING DOSE

Degree of Agitation	Dose
Mild	0.5– 2.0 mg
Moderate	5.0–10.0 mg
Severe	10.0 mg or more

TITRATION AND MAINTENANCE

1. Allow 15 to 20 minutes before next dose.
2. If agitation persists, administer double dose every 20 minutes until agitation subsides. Dose limit depends on clinician's appraisal of effectiveness.
3. If patient is calming down, repeat last dose at next dosing interval.
4. Adjust dose and interval to patient's clinical course.
5. Regular, not p.r.n. dosing is advised.

From Tesar, G. E., et al.: The evaluation and treatment of agitation in the intensive care unit. J. Intensive Care Med. *1*:137, 1986.

EMOTIONS AND CARDIAC DYSFUNCTION

Emotions are experienced both psychologically and physiologically. Although the variety of cognitive representations of feelings is extensive (anger, fear, anxiety, joy), the body's repertory of autonomic responses is more limited. Emotional arousal, through centrally triggered sympathetic discharge, is manifest in the cardiovascular system in much the same way as physical stress or exercise: tachycardia, elevated blood pressure, increased oxygen consumption, changes in cardiac output and peripheral resistance, increased muscle blood flow, and decreased renal and splanchnic blood flow.[65] The cardiovascular consequences of emotion, as distinct from those of exercise, may be more deleterious because of the absence of associated muscular activity and the metabolic vasodilation secondary thereto.

The sympathetically mediated release of epinephrine and norepinephrine has predictable effects on the myocardium, increasing oxygen demand as well as myocardial irritability. Just as physical exertion can represent a significant threat to the patient with diminished myocardial or coronary vascular reserve, emotional stress can intensify heart failure or ischemia by augmenting cardiac demands.[66–68] As Chambers and Reiser and others have described, emotional stress and traumatic life events very often precede cardiac decompensation and congestive heart failure.[66, 68]

ARRHYTHMIAS. Emotional stress and anxiety have been associated with a variety of *arrhythmias*,[69] most importantly premature ventricular contractions, ventricular tachycardia, and ventricular fibrillation.[65, 70] Although the risk of serious arrhythmia is greatest for the diseased or ischemic myocardium, psychophysiological arrhythmias have been observed in individuals with no apparent heart disease but with manifest emotional stress. Reich and coworkers reported that 25 of 117 patients with life-threatening ventricular arrhythmias lacked evidence of an acute myocardial infarction but had experienced acute emotional distress as an apparent precipitant.[71]

Using ambulatory electrocardiographic monitoring, Taggart and colleagues recorded the electrocardiograms of 32 normal individuals and 24 patients with coronary artery disease while they drove in busy city traffic.[72] Both groups showed increased heart rates, sometimes exceeding 140 beats per minute. ST-segment changes not related to tachycardia developed in 3 of 32 drivers. In 13 of those with coronary artery disease, the ST-segment and T-wave abnormalities increased. Five developed multiple ventricular ectopic beats. In another study, 23 normal subjects, most of whom were physicians speaking at medical meetings, and a second group of 7 speakers with coronary artery disease were monitored.[73] Heart rates of up to 180 beats/min, as well as elevations of plasma catecholamine and free fatty acid concentration were observed in both groups. Ischemic ST-segment depression occurred in six of the seven coronary subjects. More than six ectopic beats per minute were recorded in six of the normal subjects while they were speaking. Five of the seven coronary subjects had multiple or multifocal ventricular ectopic beats. A beta-blocking agent suppressed the tachycardia and electrocardiographic changes in both groups. Lown and colleagues studied a man with normal coronary arteries and cardiac function in whom ventricular fibrillation and cardiac arrest and, following recovery, ventricular premature beats were provoked by psychophysiological stress.[70] Beta blockade and other measures to reduce sympathetic activity attenuated the arrhythmia.

Despite the apparent importance of peripheral sympathetic activity in emotionally induced arrhythmia, Lown and coworkers have reported data implicating central neural mechanisms as primary in triggering, via sympathetic efferents, the aberrant electrical activity.[74] In animals, hypothalamic and stellate ganglion stimulation has produced ventricular fibrillation that was abolished with beta-adrenoceptor blockade.[75] In the presence of an electrically unstable heart, a diseased myocardium, or coronary artery disease, psychological distress is a potentially lethal stimulus.

In addition to the sympathetically mediated ventricular irritability and increased oxygen demand, life-threatening "vagal reaction" leading to bradycardia and circulatory collapse has been reported.[76] The parasympathetic or vagal response to emotional stimuli producing decreased heart rate, fall in arterial pressure, and syncope in some individuals is a familiar syndrome, although not in itself as a cause of sudden death.

Although a major stressful life event, such as hearing of a loved one's demise, could be the proximal "cause" of death, more often the terminal stress is not in itself extraordinary; rather, as reported by Greene and coworkers, the scenario in the weeks preceding the final stressful event is one of increased emotional vulnerability, often following a series of losses, with chronic depression, fatigue, frustration, or disappointment.[77] This observation is reminiscent of other theories of the emotional vulnerability to serious illness resulting from feelings of hopelessness and the "giving-up–given-up" response.[78] For example, a

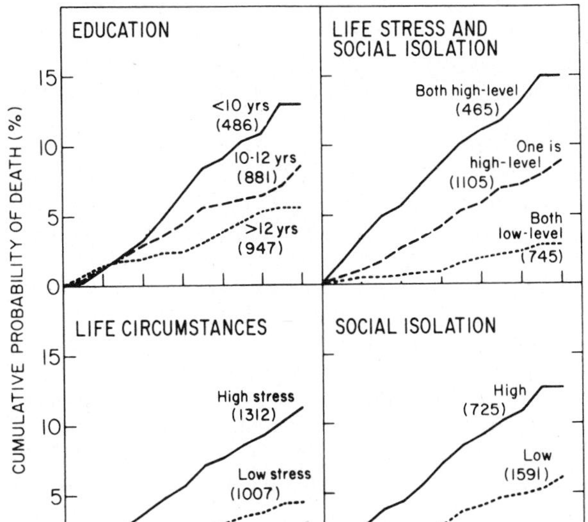

FIGURE 62–5. Life-table cumulative mortality curves for the Health Insurance Plan-BHAT male survivors of myocardial infarction according to (1) levels of education, (2) life stress (life circumstances), and (3) social isolation. (Reprinted by permission from Ruberman, W., et al.: Psychosocial influences on mortality after myocardial infarction. N. Engl. J. Med. *311*:552, 1984.)

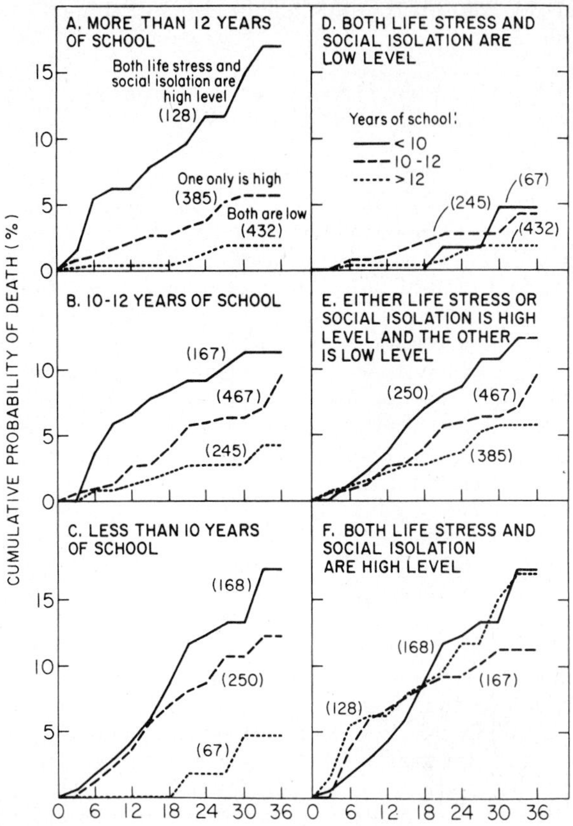

FIGURE 62–6. Life-table cumulative mortality curves according to education and specified psychosocial variables for the Health Insurance Plan-BHAT male survivors of myocardial infarction. (Reprinted by permission from Ruberman, W., et al.: Psychosocial influences on mortality after myocardial infarction. N. Engl. J. Med. *311*:552, 1984.)

patient with a perceived loss in professional or job status, possibly having had a prior myocardial infarction, feeling sad and discouraged, becomes angry or anxious while performing an ordinary stressful task, such as income tax preparation, triggering a fatal arrhythmia. The notion that preceding stressful life events, whether losses or positive life changes, lay the physiological foundation for sudden death is supported by Rahe and Romo's data measuring accumulated life change units[79] and by Ruberman and associates' data on the effects of stress and social isolation (Figs. 62–5 and 62–6).

One implication of the foregoing for the clinical management of the cardiac patient is the necessity to be alert for signs of depression and fatigue, for reports of recent major life events, and for indications of anxiety-provoking circumstances in the patient's life. In addition, the physician can counsel the patient to avoid stressful settings when possible and encourage conscious control over emotional arousal ("Is this worth dying for?") when necessary. Other strategies to diminish the impact of emotional stress include relaxation training, anxiolytics (e.g., the benzodiazepines) in small doses as needed, and in the absence of contraindications, administration of beta-adrenergic blocking drugs. The cardiac patient who manifests sustained depression should be referred for psychiatric consultation as a prophylactic and therapeutic measure.

PSYCHIATRIC ISSUES IN HYPERTENSION

EMOTIONAL FACTORS IN ESSENTIAL HYPERTENSION. Though definitive study of the causes of hypertension remains to be done, reports so far indicate associations between elevated arterial pressure and a variety of environmental and psychological conditions. Environmental factors, including diet (salt), social conditions, life changes, psychological conflicts, and psychophysiological mechanisms, have been estimated as contributing substantially to the etiology of essential hypertension[80] (see Chap. 27).

SOCIOCULTURAL FACTORS. Henry and Cassel observed that blood pressure levels were lower in groups or societies based on firm traditions and stable social structures.[81] In societies in which traditions were disintegrating or in those in transition, arterial pressures for the populations rose (e.g., Southern black society in the late 1950's). Blood pressure has been reported as higher in city than in rural dwellers.[82] Harburg et al. described one city in which citizens in the higher crime and lower socioeconomic district had significantly elevated levels of blood pressure,[83] apparently confirming earlier cross-cultural observations that hypertension was more prevalent in societies dominated by social stress and conflict.[84]

In an intriguing animal study of social factors involved in elevated arterial pressure, Henry et al. manipulated social interactions of mice by crowding them into small boxes, building a system of tunnel-connected cages that forced frequent confrontations, exposing the mice to a cat for 6 to 12 months, and introducing isolation-reared mice into the regular population. The resultant territorial conflict and concomitant constant defensive vigilance resulted in relatively sustained increases in blood pressure.[85]

PSYCHOLOGICAL FACTORS. Life changes and traumatic life events have been associated with the onset of sustained hypertension[86] and with the shift from the benign to the malignant form of the disease.[87] In addition, specific personality traits have been implicated as contributory to essential hypertension. Despite the subjective and anecdotal nature of descriptions of hypertensive individuals, the following characteristics are consistently noted: The hypertensive person manifests a desire to please, a wish to be liked; however, while outwardly calm, the internal stance is that of suppressed anger, tension, and suspicion.[88, 89] Presumably these traits derive from early experience with individuals (parents) on whom the person depended and toward whom anger and hostility could not be expressed, because of the real or imagined threat of loss of love. The desire to please and be approved of by authority figures, combined with a rebellious "ready-to-fight" unconscious posture, was felt to be characteristic of many individuals with essential hypertension.

Wolf and Wolff found that in subjects with restrained hostility or anxiety, peripheral vascular resistance rises without change in cardiac output.[90] These individuals were thought to be blood pressure "responders," especially in situations that triggered repressed hostile feelings. Hypertension, therefore, had an adaptive quality, in that a rise in blood pressure could be seen as a preparation to deal with a threat. Alexander, describing the conflict between aggressive feelings and dependence on the object of the aggression, viewed sustained hypertension as a permanent "emergency state," emotionally triggered and physically expressed.[88] Several studies have demonstrated increases in diastolic pressure with inhibited anger[91, 92] or with deferential behavior.[93]

Most data indicate that certain traits may be associated with hypertension, but their role in etiology is unclear; certainly many individuals with similar characteristics never become hypertensive. Ostfeld and Lebovitz[94] failed to show personality differences between renovascular and essential hypertensives and have criticized the "specific conflict" notion of a hypertensive personality.[95] Another difficulty with studies of psychological aspects of hypertension is their failure to differentiate labile from sustained hypertensives. The labile group may experience transient rises in stressful situations (e.g., blood pressure–taking by a physician) but are normotensive in other settings. As a result, repeated readings of blood pressure are necessary for the diagnosis of essential hypertension.

PSYCHOPHYSIOLOGICAL FACTORS. Many environmental and psychological factors can cause acute elevations of baseline blood pressure in both normotensive and hypertensive individuals. It is normal for arterial pressure to fluctuate during the course of a day[96]; however, elevated blood pressure is more prevalent, for example, in generally stressful occupations such as air traffic controllers.[97] The common denominator in cases of hypertension may be "stress" in a nonspecific sense, since stressful events (often idiosyncratic in impact, such as life trauma, social and interpersonal conflicts, and unacknowledged and unexpressed emotion) generate sympathetically mediated vasoconstriction and other autonomic responses that may well have a greater and more sustained impact on blood pressure in individuals predisposed to hypertension. Brod and colleagues have found that the vasoconstrictive response to stress is more prolonged in hypertensive than in normotensive subjects.[98, 99] The notion of Lacey et al. of an "autonomic response specificity" suggests that constitutionally predisposed individuals respond to specific and general stress with acute and sustained elevations of arterial pressure.[100] The finding that normotensive sons of essential hypertensives react more readily to stress with elevations of blood pressure is of interest in this regard.[101]

Cardiovascular reaction patterns to stress vary in animals and humans, but operant conditioning studies have demonstrated that animals can be conditioned to experience blood pressure elevations in response to specific and general stimuli.[102] For humans as well, Shapiro et al. have reported that subjects in the laboratory could learn to elevate their blood pressure without changes in heart rate.[103]

BEHAVIORAL THERAPY. Since psychophysiological data implicate stress, autonomic arousal, and conditioned learning as causes of blood pressure elevation, various types of behavioral therapy—relaxation, meditation, and biofeedback—have been applied to hypertensives[104–106] (p. 867). Although it would be of great benefit if these nonpharmacological treatments were effective, especially for the borderline hypertensive, clinical studies suggest a minor role for behavioral regimens. However, the fact that these treatments are without risk and are associated with an increased sense of well-being renders them appropriate adjunctive modalities despite the modest claims of the data so far reported.

Benson has hypothesized that a variety of techniques, including relaxation exercises, meditation, yoga, and hypnosis, have the ability to evoke an integrated hypothalamic "relaxation response" that results in reduced heart rate, blood pressure, and respiratory rate as well as the subjective feeling of relaxation.[53] Shapiro et al. have noted that relaxation-induced blood pressure changes are small but statistically significant, ranging from 7/4 to 37/22 mm Hg; the higher the pretreatment pressure, the greater the decrease with relaxation. If subjects discontinued the regimen, values returned to baseline levels.[106] A fall in adrenergic activity, as reflected in lower dopamine beta-hydroxylase levels, in patients performing an Eastern meditation exercise has been reported.[107] One well-constructed series of studies, including some 12-month follow-ups, control groups, and crossover treatment of controls, and based on a program of relaxation and galvanic skin response biofeedback, demonstrated an average decrease in blood pressure of 27/15 mm Hg and decreased requirements for medication.[108, 109] Using an ambulatory monitoring device, one group has demonstrated sustained blood pressure decreases during the work day for essential hypertensives trained in relaxation.[110]

When an individual is made aware of changes in blood pressure by means of visual or auditory biofeedback, he becomes able, through unknown mechanisms, to use this sensory input to alter his own blood pressure. The results of blood pressure biofeedback also vary, ranging from virtually no change to sustained decreases of 18/8 mm Hg.[111]

PSYCHOTHERAPY. Before the era of antihypertensive medication, Reiser et al. reported decreased arterial pressure and symptomatic improvement in a group of 98 hypertensive patients receiving varying degrees of supportive psychotherapy.[86] This salutary effect of a constant, supportive relationship with the physician should not be discounted.

PATIENT COMPLIANCE WITH ANTIHYPERTENSIVE TREATMENT. Reviews of the issue of noncompliance underscore the significance, magnitude, and complexity of this problem.[112–115] Sackett has noted over 200 reported determinants of noncompliance, including educational, demographic, personality, and prescribing factors.[116] Patients with relatively high levels of physical complaints and those with attitudes of suspiciousness have a high incidence of poor compliance.[117] Surveys consistently estimate that 30 to 50 per cent of hypertensive patients neglect their treatment, even as public awareness of the dangers of "high blood pressure" increases.[114, 118] Physicians are generally unable to predict and recognize those who do not follow instructions[119] and too often attribute the cause of the problem to the patient's lack of responsibility.

Attempts to understand adherence to medical regimens using the sociobehavioral "health belief model" emphasize the patient's (1) estimate of personal vulnerability to and seriousness of the disease; (2) perception of the efficacy and feasibility of the treatment; and (3) internal and external motivations to treatment, such as the desire to relieve symptoms or to avoid the sick role (internal) or as a response to public health campaigns (external).[112] Although all these factors were deemed relevant when studied retrospectively, recent prospective work has confirmed only the "attitude toward the sick role" as predictive of compliance—those who perceive social and interpersonal consequences of illness as negative are likely to comply with treatment.[116]

Efforts to indict any one factor as the "cause" of noncompliance will be inadequate given the individual variability of patients' personalities and manners of coping with adversity. Some patients do not follow directions because of lack of concern or low anxiety levels, whereas others manifest a denial and rationalization response because of high levels of anxiety. Engendering increased concern is to no avail in the latter type of patient. A sufficiently independent patient will appreciate the opportunity to monitor his own blood pressure and be "responsible" for his treatment, whereas dependent patients will require more nurturing and didactic care and frequent follow-up visits.

The following factors are generally acknowledged as useful in maintaining patient compliance with treatment programs:

1. Creating a doctor-patient relationship characterized by mutual trust and a sense of alliance or working together to solve the problem.[118, 120]
2. Providing sufficient time with a care-giver (whether physician, physician's assistant, or nurse clinician).[121, 122]
3. Prescribing an effective yet simple treatment regimen and making sure the patient understands the regimen before he leaves the office or clinic.[114]
4. Adapting dosage schedules to the patient's daily routine or habits.[123]
5. Educating and enlisting the help of family members, especially spouses (who may also deny the importance of treatment).
6. Anticipating with the patient possible side effects of medications and how these will be handled.
7. Offering assistance on follow-up visits to the patient who has had difficulty adhering to the treatment program.
8. Monitoring compliance (e.g., pill counts) and attempting to adapt the interpersonal approach to the noncompliant patient's needs and fears.

PSYCHIATRIC COMPLICATIONS OF ANTIHYPERTENSIVE MEDICATIONS (see also Chap. 28). Medications used to treat hypertension have neuropsychiatric effects, primarily depression. Rauwolfia alkaloids such as reserpine, which deplete central intraneuronal stores of catecholamines, can result in severe depressive illness that may endure well beyond withdrawal from the medication.[124] These agents are rarely used at present, but when the physician does wish to prescribe one of them, patients having suffered prior depressions should be screened, because of their increased vulnerability to this drug-induced affective illness. Alpha-methyldopa has also been associated with depression and other psychiatric symptoms (lethargy, insomnia, decreased mental acuity)[125] as well as confusional states in conjunction with haloperidol[126] and lithium.[127] Patients receiving alpha-methyldopa may be at greater risk for lithium toxicity. Those taking beta-adrenoceptor blockers may experience increased lethargy, mental slowing, and occasionally clinical depression. Hydralazine also induces lethargy and drowsiness. Drugs that cause impotence such as guanethidine or alpha-methyldopa may secondarily precipitate depression in the emotionally vulnerable patient. Diuretics are associated with mental changes, primarily as the result of electrolyte disturbances. In a large multicenter, randomized, double-blind trial, treatment of hypertension with captopril, as compared to methyldopa or propranolol, was associated with fewer adverse effects, less sexual dysfunction, and better reported work performance, as well as overall general well-being.[128]

A variety of interactions with psychotropic medication may occur with antihypertensive agents.[129] The antipsychotics potentiate the hypotensive effects of reserpine, alpha-methyldopa, hydralazine, and propranolol, and, except for molindone, antagonize guanethidine.[130]

The tricyclic antidepressants generally interfere with drugs that require uptake into adrenergic nerve terminals, blocking the action, for example, of guanethidine with the possibility of causing severe withdrawal hypotension and impeding the efficacy of clonidine.[131] These antidepressants may also interact centrally with alpha-methyldopa, reserpine, and propranolol, resulting in diminished blood pressure control.[132] Another newer agent, mianserin, is reported to be free of the above interactions.[133] Initially, the tricyclics may cause hypertension when reserpine is administered. The monoamine oxidase inhibitors increase the hypotensive effects of diuretics and hydralazine but can lead to acute hypertension when administered with guanethidine, alpha-methyldopa, or reserpine.

For patients taking lithium and such diuretics as the thiazides, which act on the distal tubule, sodium loss in the distal tubule results in the reabsorption of lithium proximally and hence in elevated lithium levels.[134] Higher blood lithium levels increase the risk of side effects and toxicity. When such a combination is necessary, lithium dosages must be lowered and levels must be monitored. In addition, increased vigilance must be kept concerning other potential causes of additional sodium loss, such as sweating or diarrhea.

PSYCHOPATHOLOGY AND CARDIAC SYMPTOMS

Patients with any of a number of psychiatric disorders may attribute their distress to alterations of body function and may seek treatment from the nonpsychiatric physician; furthermore, objective physical symptoms may derive from specific functional conditions, as in the case of bursts of tachycardia from attacks of panic or anxiety. Estimates of the incidence in cardiological practices of patients with anxiety-derived complaints range from 10 to 14 per cent.[135] The heart is a frequent focus of emotionally based complaints, not only because of its actual response to psychological stress but also because of its psychological and symbolic importance. Recognition of the psychiatric component of patients' complaints is a crucial task for the physician. The anxious and depressed patient suffers no less than the patient with a primary physical illness, and many of the psychiatric conditions underlying the distress can respond dramatically to prompt treatment; for others, proper management can greatly improve the quality of life. Finally, diagnosis of relevant psychological factors may obviate medical or surgical interventions and their attendant morbidity.

The psychological abnormalities that most commonly present with cardiac symptoms are the anxiety disorders (including panic states), depression, and hypochondriasis.

CARDIOVASCULAR EFFECTS OF PSYCHOTROPIC AGENTS

Psychotropic medications, frequently administered to the elderly and those with or at risk for heart disease, have a significant impact on the cardiovascular system. Since untreated psychiatric illness carries its own morbidity and mortality and can also exacerbate cardiac illness (e.g., exhaustion from mania), the risks and benefits of medication must be carefully weighed. The following section describes the important cardiovascular effects of psychotropic drugs.

ANTIDEPRESSANTS

In the late 1950's, the development of effective antidepressant pharmacotherapy heralded a significantly improved quality of life for those suffering from clinical depressive syndromes. The monoamine oxidase inhibitors (MAOI's) and a few years later the tricyclic antidepressants (TCA's) were the first consistently effective pharmacological interventions in the treatment of mood disorders. More recently, a number of agents with chemical structures distinct from TCA's are being explored and introduced in hopes of achieving therapeutic benefits without such adverse effects as cardiotoxicity. Current hypotheses suggest that TCA's and the newer antidepressants combat depression by increasing the activity of such central neurotransmitters as norepinephrine and serotonin either by blocking re-uptake from synaptic clefts or by binding to presynaptic (α_2) receptors.

TRICYCLIC ANTIDEPRESSANTS. Of significant benefit in 60 to 80 per cent of severe depressions,[129] TCA's remain in wide use as acute and maintenance treatment for mood disorders. However, reports of sudden death in cardiac patients taking amitriptyline[136] prompted an alarm that was magnified when subsequent reports linked other TCA's to dangerous arrhythmias and sudden death, even in patients apparently free of cardiac disease.[137, 138] Their impact on the cardiovascular system has been viewed as a major limitation to their use in patients with cardiac illness and depression.[138, 139] In contrast, drugs such as quinidine, doxorubicin (Adriamycin), and phenytoin also have potentially dangerous cardiac effects, yet they are used without hesitation when ventricular ectopic activity, malignant disease, or seizures threaten life or health. In fact, TCA's may be administered to cardiac patients with relative safety if one has adequate understanding of their specific properties and follows guidelines for their safe use.[140]

In clinical and laboratory studies, TCA's have a wide variety of pharmacological actions besides their effect on catecholamine uptake by the adrenergic neuron. These include anticholinergic activity, alpha-adrenoceptor blocking properties, and quinidine-like effects that may affect heart rate, cardiac rhythm, electrical conduction, blood pressure, and myocardial contractility.[141, 142] Each TCA has a unique profile of activity, an understanding of which is relevant to selection of the agent most appropriate for the clinical circumstances in question.

Effects on Heart Rate. Some increase in heart rate probably occurs and remains for the duration of treatment in every patient receiving these medications. Increases of 10 to 20 beats/min are common and clinically unimportant, except in patients with moderate-severe congestive heart failure or coronary artery disease. The anticholinergic properties of TCA's are thought to be the principal determinant of drug-induced tachycardia. Amitriptyline is the most anticholinergic TCA, followed in order by doxepin, imipramine, nortriptyline, and desipramine[143] (see Table 62–2), the last being the TCA of choice in patients requiring a minimum of anticholinergic effects. In cases of TCA toxicity, temporary improvement in tachycardia is attained with physostigmine,[144] the drug of choice to reverse the

TABLE 62–2 ANTIDEPRESSANT AFFINITIES FOR THE MUSCARINIC RECEPTOR OF HUMAN BRAIN

ANTIDEPRESSANT		AFFINITY*
amitriptyline	(Elavil, Endep)	5.5
protriptyline	(Vivactil)	4.0
trimipramine	(Surmontil)	1.7
doxepin	(Sinequan, Adapin)	1.2
imipramine	(Tofranil, SK-Pramine)	1.1
nortriptyline	(Aventyl, Pamelor)	0.67
desipramine	(Norpramin, Pertofrane)	0.50
maprotiline	(Ludiomil)	0.18
amoxapine	(Asendin)	0.10
fluoxetine		0.050
bupropion	(Wellbutrin)	0.0021
trazodone	(Desyrel)	0.00031
atropine†		42

*$10^{-7} \times K_d$, where K_d = equilibrium dissociation constant in molarity.
†This is not an antidepressant but is shown here for comparison.
From Richelson, E.: Current Developments in the Treatment of Depression. McLean Hospital Symposium, Washington, D.C., May 11, 1986.

CNS "atropine psychosis."[145] Beta-adrenoceptor blockers are useful in modifying TCA-induced tachycardia.[142]

Electrical Conduction and ECG Manifestations. TCA's resemble Type I antiarrhythmic drugs (e.g., quinidine and procainamide) in the capacity to delay cardiac conduction[146–148] (p. 628). HIS-bundle electrocardiography has demonstrated prolonged distal (H-V) conduction time for imipramine, nortriptyline, and amitriptyline.[149] Corresponding ECG changes include reversible prolongation of P-R, QRS, and Q-T interval corrected for rate ($Q\text{-}T_c$), ST-T wave changes, and development of AV and bundle branch block.[141, 146]

Clinically significant manifestations of this quinidine-like effect are unlikely to occur at therapeutic doses of TCA and in the absence of preexisting conduction disturbances. Glassman reported no instances of second- or third-degree heart block in more than 200 TCA-treated patients who did not have preexisting conduction abormalities; in contrast, nearly 25 per cent of patients with pretreatment PR or QRS abnormalities developed second-degree heart block during treatment with imipramine. Patients with preexisting bundle branch block are thought to be at greatest risk.[149]

Doxepin has been touted as the TCA of choice for treatment of depression in patients with intraventricular or AV conduction disturbances.[150] This claim is controversial,[151] resting in part on poorly controlled, retrospective data that may reflect the propensity of doxepin to achieve lower plasma levels than other TCA's at similar oral doses. Nortriptyline's effect on the cardiac conduction system has been studied extensively.[141, 149] In addition to causing trivial prolongation of H-V conduction at therapeutic doses, the existence of a well-defined "therapeutic window" permits reliable monitoring of therapeutic effect and prevention of toxicity.

Effects on Cardiac Rhythm. At toxic levels of TCA's which can last for 3 to 4 days after overdose,[152] any and all types of rhythm disturbance may occur.[153] At therapeutic doses, however, TCA's can have an antiarrhythmic effect similar to that of the Type I antiarrhythmic drugs. Bigger and colleagues have suggested that imipramine could actually be effective as an antiarrhythmic, because of its quinidine-like properties as well as relatively long duration of action and few major adverse effects.[146–148]

Despite the general safety of TCA's for most patients, idiosyncratic vulnerability to serious (ventricular) arrhythmia may be encountered.[146] This phenomenon may be analogous to the proarrhythmic effect of Type I antiarrhythmic drugs seen in 5 to 10 per cent of patients who receive these drugs (p. 629). In patients receiving a TCA (or other psychotropic drugs) who experience a life-threatening arrhythmia, administration of the suspected drug in the course of electrophysiological study may identify those in whom administration of the agent may be fatal or in whom it may be unrelated to the arrhythmia that was experienced.[154] Patients with preexisting atrial tachyarrhythmias who are to receive a (quinidine-like) TCA should be digitalized to prevent induction of a rapid ventricular response. Theoretically, combined use of a TCA and digitalis may require reduction of digitalis dosage, since, like quinidine, a TCA may also reduce renal clearance of digitalis.

Effects on Blood Pressure. Postural hypotension is a common complication of TCA treatment.[142, 155] Although the postural decrease in pressure does not differ significantly according to age, the experience of symptoms and such untoward consequences as fractures and lacerations from falling is greater among the elderly.[149, 156] Although up to 20 per cent of patients receiving TCA may suffer postural hypotension, there is a markedly increased incidence among those with left ventricular impairment or those receiving cardiovascular medication.[149]

For most patients who experience a postural change upon initiation of TCA treatment, the *symptoms* of orthostatic hypotension usually improve or disappear over days to weeks, despite persistence of a measurable postural drop in pressure.[149] The dosages at which orthostatic changes occur are usually well below therapeutic levels, and increasing doses to the therapeutic range (e.g., 100 to 200 mg/day of imipramine) is unlikely to worsen symptoms, whereas small downward adjustments will afford little advantage.[149] Some improvement in measurable hypotension may occur after an extended period of treatment.

The mechanism of TCA-induced hypotension is uncertain, but affinity for alpha-adrenoceptors in the central nervous system has been demonstrated and appears to correlate with the hypotensive effects of these drugs.[157] Nortriptyline is the TCA with the least propensity to cause orthostatic hypotension, particularly if the plasma level does not exceed the therapeutic limit (150 ng/ml).[149] Although *hypertension* resulting from a therapeutic dose of TCA alone is a theoretical possibility, and a few cases have been reported, this effect is rare enough to be of little clinical significance.[142]

Effects on the Myocardium. TCA's have long had a reputation of exerting a direct depressant effect on the myocardium, an impression derived largely from animal data.[138, 142] In a study of TCA's in depressed patients with heart disease, radionuclide ventriculograms revealed no change in ventricular ejection fraction with antidepressant treatment,[158] suggesting that a negative inotropic effect may occur only at toxic doses. This finding has been replicated.[156]

In summary, the following clinical guidelines may be useful in monitoring and evaluating the effect of TCA treatment on the cardiovascular system: (1) Obtain a pretreatment ECG, especially in patients over 40 years of age, with particular attention to the presence of bundle branch or AV block; (2) be alert for a $Q\text{-}T_c$ greater than 440 msec that is present before or develops during TCA treatment; (3) moderate prolongation of the pretreatment P-R, QRS, or $Q\text{-}T_c$ interval is not an absolute contraindication to TCA treatment, but warrants close monitoring and attention to the principles that guide quinidine therapy; (4) consider reducing the doses of Type I antiarrhythmics during combined treatment with TCA's; (5) digitalize the patient with atrial tachyarrhythmias before starting TCA therapy; and (6) to minimize clinical complications of orthostatic hyotension, adjust TCA dosage carefully in patients with heart failure, in those receiving other vasoactive drugs, and in patients with pretreatment orthostatic decreases in systolic blood pressure greater than 10 mm Hg.

MONOAMINE OXIDASE INHIBITORS. The renewed popularity of these medications, which block the oxidative deamination of norepinephrine, epinephrine, serotonin, and other amines by the enzyme monoamine oxidase, derives from their efficacy in treating panic disorder, atypical depressions, and some TCA-refractory depressed patients. A cardiovascular limitation to their use is their ability to cause severe orthostatic hypotension. Presumably this is related to a "false neurotransmitter" effect, either from the drug itself or from the buildup of other nonvasoactive amines. Because of this property, pargyline has found a place in the treatment of hypertension.

The greatest risk of MAOI's (e.g., phenelzine, tranylcypromine, and isocarboxazid), especially for cardiac patients, is the acute hypertensive crisis and the complications concomitant with ingestion of tyramine-containing foods and beverages or the administration of sympathomimetic medications. The failure of liver and intestinal MAO to deaminate tyramine in such foods as cheeses, red wine, yogurt, and chicken liver leads to a tyramine-induced release of adrenergic neurotransmitters. Arrhythmias may occur in addition to hypertension. These reactions, although rare, justify caution in prescribing MAOI's to patients with serious cardiac disease. This is unfortunate, because they lack the anticholinergic and other cardiotoxic properties of TCA's.[129]

Antihypertensive agents such as reserpine and guanethidine, which acutely release vasoactive amines, and alpha-methyldopa, which is converted to sympathomimetic amines, should also be avoided by patients receiving MAOI's. In the event of hypertensive crisis with MAOI's, an alpha-adrenergic blocking drug, such as phentolamine, should be administered.

NEWER ANTIDEPRESSANTS. A number of new antidepressant compounds with a variety of chemical structures are available for clinical and experimental use. Although none is more effective than TCA in treating depression, their main attraction is the possibility of diminished side effects, particularly cardiotoxic ones. Although early claims of relative cardiac safety may be justified for some of these agents, they have not been subjected to the extensive clinical and laboratory scrutiny that the TCA's have.

Maprotiline and amoxapine, for example, although heralded as producing low cardiotoxicity, have anticholinergic and other effects similar to those of TCA's. Amoxapine has been reported to produce atrial flutter and fibrillation,[159] and maprotiline, ventricular tachycardia. Trazodone, while virtually devoid of anticholinergic and quinidine-like properties, has been reported to exacerbate preexistent ventricular ectopic activity[160] and poses a risk of postural hypotension due to relatively potent $alpha_1$-adrenoceptor blocking activity (Table 62–3). Fluoxetine, a newer agent without anticholinergic effects, appears to present a very low risk of cardiotoxicity.[161]

PSYCHOSTIMULANTS. When clinical circumstances limit the use of standard antidepressant agents (e.g., in the depressed intensive care patient, the patient with critical congestive heart failure or conduction abnormalities), the treatment of depression may be undertaken with psychostimulant drugs such as Dexedrine or methylphenidate.

TABLE 62–3 ANTIDEPRESSANT AFFINITIES FOR THE ALPHA-ADRENOCEPTOR OF HUMAN BRAIN

ANTIDEPRESSANT		AFFINITY*
doxepin	(Sinequan, Adapin)	4.2
trimipramine	(Surmontil)	4.2
amitriptyline	(Elavil, Endep)	3.7
trazodone	(Desyrel)	2.8
amoxapine	(Asendin)	2.0
nortriptyline	(Aventyl, Pamelor)	1.7
maprotiline	(Ludiomil)	1.1
imipramine	(Tofranil, SK-Pramine)	1.1
protriptyline	(Vivactil)	0.77
desipramine	(Norpramin, Pertofrane)	0.77
bupropion	(Wellbutrin)	0.022
fluoxetine		0.017
phentolamine†	(Regitine)	6.7

$*10^{-7} \times K_d$, where K_d = equilibrium dissociation constant in molarity.
†This is not an antidepressant but is shown here for comparison.
From Richelson, E.: Current Developments in the Treatment of Depression. McLean Hospital Symposium, Washington, D.C., May 11, 1986.

Psychostimulants have been used safely and successfully for the treatment of depressive disorders secondary to serious medical illness[162] and after cardiac surgery.[163] Dexedrine, whose half-life varies from 4 to 21 hours, may be administered once in the morning in doses of 5 to 20 mg; methylphenidate has a shorter half-life (4 to 8 hours), and although a 5- to 20-mg dose once in the morning may suffice, it may be necessary to administer two to three doses per day. Psychostimulants should be avoided in patients with significant hypertension or unstable angina or taking MAOI drugs.

THE ANTIPSYCHOTICS

This group of psychotropic agents includes the phenothiazines, thioxanthenes, butyrophenones, dibenzepins, and indolones. They are often dramatically effective in abating the severity of symptoms in psychotic episodes. Their action is presumed to be related to their common property of blocking central dopamine receptors.

With the widespread use of the phenothiazines have come reports of sudden death. Since some of the fatalities occurred in young and apparently healthy individuals, cardiovascular effects, especially arrhythmias, have been implicated.[164–166] Nearly all such reports were of patients taking either thioridazine or chlorpromazine. Other cardiovascular complications of the antipsychotics derive from central and peripheral alpha-blocking and anticholinergic effects, producing orthostatic hypotension and tachycardia.

ELECTROCARDIOGRAPHIC CHANGES. The phenothiazines have been associated with a variety of electrocardiographic changes,[166, 167] including prolongation of P-R and Q-T intervals, widened QRS complex, ST-segment depression, T-wave changes (usually blunting and widening), variable degrees of heart block, and serious ventricular arrhythmias.[166] The T-wave alterations, benign and reversible, are the most common ECG changes. Accentuated U waves occur with thioridazine. Electrocardiographic changes in general are associated with the phenothiazines of the aliphatic (chlorpromazine) and piperidine (thioridazine) types.

ALPHA-ADRENOCEPTOR BLOCKING EFFECTS. The antipsychotics, especially the aliphatic and piperidine phenothiazines, have both central and peripheral alpha-adrenoceptor blocking properties[168] in addition to their ability to block dopamine. This property correlates with the degree of hypotension and sedation associated with the specific agent and is of a greater degree than the mild alpha-blocking properties of the TCA's, but is minimal in the butyrophenone, haloperidol. Severe hypotension, which occurs with an overdose, should not be treated with epinephrine or with agents having both alpha and beta effects, since increased hypotension can result; instead, alpha-adrenoceptor pressors such as norepinephrine should be employed.

ANTICHOLINERGIC ACTIVITY. With the exception of thioridazine, the antipsychotics have less anticholinergic activity than TCA's.[166, 167] Nonetheless, they produce sufficient vagal blockade, especially in overdose, to be of clinical significance. This effect is often compounded by the administration of antiparkinsonian agents, such as benztropine or trihexyphenidyl, which also inhibit cholinergic activity.

OTHER CARDIOVASCULAR EFFECTS. Quinidine-like activity has been reported for some of the phenothiazines.[166, 167] A toxic cardiomyopathy has been associated with phenothiazine administration,[164, 165] and congestive heart failure may be exacerbated by a negative inotropic effect. Changes in intracellular potassium ion concentration have been proposed to explain some phenothiazine-induced electrocardiographic changes.[167] Depression of autonomic midbrain centers and alterations in adrenal medulla secretion have also been implicated in phenothiazine-induced hypotension.[164]

CHOICE OF ANTIPSYCHOTIC. The incidence of adverse cardiac effects of antipsychotics is increased in patients with cardiovascular disease, in the elderly, in higher doses, in synergy with other drugs (especially TCA's), and with intramuscular administration. The nonphenothiazines such as haloperidol, molindone, loxapine, and thiothixene have not been shown to have cardiotoxic effects. The high-potency phenothiazines of the piperazine type (e.g., fluphenazine) induce minimal adverse cardiac reactions. Haloperidol, a very high-potency antipsychotic with low anticholinergic[169] and alpha-blocking properties,[157] is often the drug of choice for treating the psychotic or severely agitated cardiac patient; recent reports describe successful intravenous administration in life-threatening states of delirium.[44, 45, 62] Thioridazine, on the other hand, should be avoided in the treatment of cardiac patients.

LITHIUM

Lithium carbonate is valuable in the management of patients with mood disorders, especially manic-depressive illness. The major toxic effects are neurological and require frequent monitoring of plasma levels. Although prescribing information has generally implied that lithium is cardiotoxic, a variety of reports have indicated its relative cardiac safety.[170, 171] The negative response to this drug derives in part from its unrestricted use as a salt substitute in the 1940's, with subsequent morbidity and mortality from lithium poisoning. Reported cardiovascular complications—hypotension, circulatory collapse, and arrhythmia—were agonal events in patients in prolonged coma.[134] In the majority of patients receiving lithium, the drug appears to cause minimal cardiotoxicity and is not associated with blood pressure changes. Congestive heart failure and myocarditis are rare. Instances of syncope secondary to sinus node dysfunction have been reported consequent to lithium treatment.[172]

ELECTROCARDIOGRAPHIC CHANGES. T-wave changes, similar to those in hypokalemia and possibly related to displacement of intracellular potassium by lithium ions, occurs in virtually all patients treated with this drug.[134] Decreased amplitude, flattening, and even inversion of T waves are considered to be benign and reversible effects that generally do not constitute a reason to discontinue treatment. Individual case reports of arrhythmias, including conduction defects and increased frequency of extrasystoles, suggest that some patients may show idiosyncratic sensitivity to lithium.[134] Cases of disordered sinus node function in patients receiving lithium have also been registered.[134, 172]

TOXIC EFFECTS. The primary concern for cardiac patients is the development of lithium toxicity—nausea, vomiting, diarrhea, ataxia, slurred speech, convulsions, coma, and death—resulting from failure to maintain adequate renal clearance. The patient with congestive heart failure is particularly vulnerable, because of decreased glomerular filtration rate, dietary restriction of sodium chloride, and use of diuretics. The thiazide diuretics elevate plasma lithium significantly and necessitate downward adjustment of daily doses and close monitoring of drug levels.[134] It is good practice to evaluate cardiac parameters carefully before and after initiating lithium treatment for patients with cardiac disease.[134]

ELECTROCONVULSIVE THERAPY

Because it is the most consistently effective treatment for severe depression and does not have the cardiotoxic effects of TCA's, electroconvulsive therapy (ECT) has been advocated as the antidepressant therapy of choice for cardiac patients. A prospective study of depressed hospitalized inpatients demonstrated that adverse effects are uncommon when appropriate precautionary measures are taken.[173] It should be remembered, however, that ECT is not an entirely benign treatment. Enhanced sympathetic activity following induction of the seizure leads to brief periods of occasionally exaggerated hypertensive responses, arrhythmias,[175] and acute myocardial infarction.[176] The type of barbiturate anesthesia used is also a factor in cardiac morbidity.[177] Careful monitoring and the use of a rapid-acting antihypertensive, such as nitroprusside, can help avert the complications of hypertension. Since the general mortality from ECT is quite low (0.2 to 0.3 per cent)[178] and since depression carries its own mortality, ECT should be considered in treating the severely depressed cardiac patient.

REFERENCES

PSYCHIATRIC ASPECTS OF CORONARY ARTERY DISEASE

1. Harvey, W.: Exercitatio de motu cordis et sanguinis. Cited in Jenkins, C. D.: Behavioral risk factors in coronary artery disease. Ann. Rev. Med. *29*:543, 1978.
2. Osler, W.: The Lumleian lectures on angina pectoris. Delivered before the Royal College of Physicians of London. Lancet *1*:939, 1910.
3. Dunbar, F.: Psychosomatic Diagnosis. New York, Paul B. Hoeber, Inc., 1943.
4. Friedman, M.: Pathogenesis of Coronary Artery Disease. New York, McGraw-Hill Book Co., 1969.
5. Rosenman, R. H., Brand, R. J., Jenkins, C. D., Friedman, M., Straus, R., and Wurm, M.: Coronary heart disease in the Western Collaborative Group Study: Final follow-up experience of 8½ years. J.A.M.A. *233*:872, 1975.
6. Jenkins, C. D.: Recent evidence supporting psychologic and social risk factors for coronary disease. N. Engl. J. Med. *294*:987, 1976.
7. Jenkins, C. D.: Behavioral risk factors in coronary artery disease. Ann. Rev. Med. *29*:543, 1978.
8. Kenigsberg, D., Zyzanski, S. J., Jenkins, C. D., Wardwell, W. I., and Licciardello, A. T.: The coronary prone behavior pattern in hospitalized patients with and without coronary heart disease. Psychosom. Med. *36*:344, 1974.
9. Review Panel on Coronary-Prone Behavior and Coronary Heart Disease: Coronary-prone behavior and coronary heart disease: A critical study. Circulation *63*:1199, 1981.
10. Williams, R. B.: Type A behavior and elevated physiological and neuroendocrine responses to cognitive tests. Science *218*:483, 1982.
11. Blumenthal, J., Lane, J., Williams, R., McKee, D., Haney, T., and White, A.: Effects of task incentive on cardiovascular response in Type A and Type B individuals. Psychophysiology *20*:63, 1983.

11a. Johnston, D. W.: Can and should type A behavior be changed? Postgrad. Med. J. *62*:785, 1986.

12. Friedman, M., Thoresen, C. E., Gill, J. J., Powell, L. H., Ulmer, D., Thompson, L., Price, V., Rabin, D. D., Breall, W. S., Dixon, T., Levy, R., and Bourg, E.: Alteration of Type A behavior and reduction in cardiac recurrences in postmyocardial infarction patients. Am. Heart J. *108*:237, 1984.

12a. Kittel, F., Kornitzer, M., and Dramaix, M.: Evaluation of type A personality. Postgrad. Med. J. *62*:781, 1986.

13. Shekelle, R. B., Hulley, S. B., Neaton, J. D., Billings, J. H., Borhani, N. O., Gerace, T. A., Jacobs, D. R., Lassser, N. L., Mittlemark, M. B., and Stamler, J.: The MRFIT behavior pattern study. II: Type A behavior pattern and incidence of coronary heart disease. Am. J. Epidemiol. *122*:559, 1985.
14. Koshenvuo, M., Kapiro, J., Langinvainio, H., and Romo, M.: Mortality in relation to coronary-prone behavior: Six-year follow-up of the Bortner scale in middle-age Finnish men. Activ. Nerv. Sup. *25*:107, 1983.
15. Shekelle, R., Gale, G., and Norusis, M.: Type A score and risk of recurrent coronary heart disease in the Aspirin Myocardial Infarction Study. Am. J. Cardiol. *56*:221, 1985.
16. Case, R., Heller, S. S., Case, N., and Moss, A.: Type A behavior and survival after acute myocardial infarction. N. Engl. J. Med. *312*:737, 1985.
17. Matthews, K. A.: Assessment of Type A, anger, and hostility in epidemiological studies of cardiovascular disease. Unpublished data, 1983.
18. Matthews, K. A., Glass, D. C., Rosenman, R. H., and Bortner, R. W.: Competitive drive, pattern A, and coronary heart disease: A further analysis of some data from the WCGS. J. Chronic Dis. *30*:489, 1977.
19. Dembroski, T., MacDougall, J., Williams, R., Haney, T., and Blumenthal, J.: Components of Type A, hostility, and anger in relationship to angiographic findings. Psychosom. Med. *47*:219, 1985.

20. Williams, R., Haney, T., and Lee, K.: Type A behavior, hostility, and coronary atherosclerosis. Psychosom. Med. *42*:539, 1980.
21. Rahe, R. H., Bennett, L., Romo, M., Siltanen, P., and Arthur, R. J.: Subjects' recent life changes and coronary heart disease in Finland. Am. J. Psychiatry *130*:1222, 1973.
22. Parkes, C. M., Benjamin, B., and Fitzgerald, R. G.: Broken heart: A statistical study of increased mortality among widowers. Br. Med. J. *1*:740, 1969.
23. Wolf, S.: The end of the rope: The role of the brain in cardiac death. Can. Med. Assoc. J. *97*:1022, 1967.
23a. Moser, K. A., Fox, A. J., Goldblatt, P. O., and Jones, D. R.: Stress and heart disease: Evidence of associations between unemployment and heart disease from the OPCS Longitudinal Study. Postgrad. Med. J. *62*:797, 1986.
24. Ruberman, W., Weinblatt, E., Goldberg, J., and Chaudhary, B.: Psychosocial influences on mortality after myocardial infarction. N. Engl. J. Med. *311*:552, 1984.
25. Hackett, T. P., and Cassem, N. H.: Factors contributing to delay in responding to the signs and symptoms of acute myocardial infarction. Am. J. Cardiol. *24*:651, 1969.
26. Moss, A. J., and Goldstein, S.: The pre-hospital phase of acute myocardial infarction. Circulation *41*:737, 1970.
27. Simon, A. B., Feinleib, M., and Thompson, H. K.: Components of delay in the pre-hospital phase of acute myocardial infarction. Am. J. Cardiol. *30*:476, 1972.
28. Wallace, W. A., and Yu, P. N.: Sudden death and the pre-hospital phase of acute myocardial infarction. Ann. Rev. Med. *26*:1, 1975.
29. Hamburg, D. A., Coelho, G. V., and Adams, J. E.: Coping and Adaptation. New York, Basic Books, Inc., 1974.
30. Weisman, A. D., and Hackett, T. P.: The predilection to death. Psychosom. Med. *23*:232, 1961.
31. Cassem, N. H., Wishnie, H. A., and Hackett, T. P.: How coronary patients respond to last rites. Postgrad. Med. *45*:147, 1969.
32. Hackett, T. P., Cassem, N. H., and Wishnie, H. A.: The coronary care unit: An appraisal of its psychological hazards. N. Engl. J. Med. *279*:1365, 1968.
33. Cay, E. L., Vetter, N., Philip, A. E., and Dugard, P.: Psychological reactions to a coronary care unit. J. Psychosom. Res. *16*:425, 1972.
34. Dominian, J., and Dobson, M.: Study of patients' psychological attitudes to a coronary care unit. Br. Med. J. *4*:795, 1969.
35. Bruhn, J. G., Thurman, A. E., Jr., Chandler, B. C., and Bruce, T. A.: Patients' reactions to death in a coronary care unit. J. Psychosom. Res. *14*:65, 1970.
36. Kübler-Ross, E.: Death does not exist. J. Holistic Health *2*:60, 1977.
37. Druss, R. G., and Kornfeld, D. S.: Survivors of cardiac arrest: Psychiatric study. J.A.M.A. *201*:291, 1967.
38. Hackett, T. P.: The Lazarus complex revisited. Ann. Intern. Med. *76*:135, 1972.
39. Dobson, M., Tattersfield, A. E., Adler, M. M., and McNicol, M. W.: Attitudes and long-term adjustment of patients surviving cardiac arrest. Br. Med. J. *3*:207, 1971.
40. Parker, D. L., and Hodge, J. R.: Delirium in the coronary care unit. J.A.M.A. *201*:702, 1967.
41. Farber, I. J.: Hospitalized cardiac patient: Some psychological aspects. N.Y. State J. Med. *78*:2045, 1978.
42. Kornecki, E., Ehrlich, Y. H., and Lenox, R. H.: Platelet-activating factor-induced aggregation of human platelets specifically inhibited by triazolobenzodiazepines. Science *226*:1454, 1984.
43. Adams, F., Fernandez, F., and Anderson, B.: Emergency pharmacotherapy of delirium in the critically ill cancer patient. Psychosomatics *27* (Suppl):33, 1986.
44. Tesar, G. E., Murray, G. B., and Cassem, N. H.: Use of high-dose intravenous haloperidol in agitated cardiac patients. J. Clin. Psychopharmacol. *5*:344, 1985.
45. Stern, T. A.: The management of depression and anxiety following myocardial infarction. Mt. Sinai Med. J. *52*:623, 1985.
46. Klein, R. F., Kliner, V. A., Zipes, D. P., Troyer, W. G., Jr., and Wallace, A. G.: Transfer from a coronary care unit. Arch. Intern. Med. *122*:104, 1968.
47. Wishnie, H. A., Hackett, T. P., and Cassem, N. H.: Psychological hazards of convalescence following myocardial infarction. J.A.M.A. *215*:1292, 1971.
48. Cassem, N. H., and Hackett, T. P.: Psychological rehabilitation of myocardial infarction patients in the acute phase. Heart Lung *2*:383, 1973.
49. Ueno, M.: The so-called coition death. Jpn. J. Leg. Med. *17*:330, 1963.
50. Hellerstein, H. K., and Friedman, E. H.: Sexual activity and the post-coronary patient. Arch. Intern. Med. *125*:987, 1970.
51. Naughton, J.: The effects of acute and chronic exercise on cardiac patients. *In* Naughton, J. P., and Hellerstein, H. K. (eds.): Exercise Testing and Exercise Training in Coronary Heart Disease. New York, Academic Press, 1973.
52. Bilodeau, C. J., and Hackett, T. P.: Issues raised in a group setting by patients recovering from initial myocardial infarction. Am. J. Psychiatry *128*:73, 1971.
53. Benson, H.: The Relaxation Response. New York, William Morrow and Co., 1975.
54. Dubin, W., Field, H., and Gastfriend, D.: Postcardiotomy delirium: A critical review. J. Thorac. Cardiovasc. Surg. *77*:586, 1979.
55. Kornfeld, D., Heller, S., Frank, K., Edie, R., and Barsa, J.: Delirium after coronary artery bypass surgery. J. Thorac. Cardiovasc. Surg. *76*:93, 1978.
56. Breuer, A., Furlan, A., Hanson, M., Lederman, R., Loop, F., Cosgrove, D., Greenstreet, R., and Estafanous, G.: Central nervous system complications of coronary artery bypass graft surgery: Prospective analysis of 421 patients. Stroke *14*:682, 1983.
57. Aberg, T., Ronquist, G., Tyden, H., Brunnkvist, S., Hultman, J., Bergstrom, K., and Lilja, A.: Adverse effects on the brain in cardiac operations as assessed by biochemical, psychometric, and radiologic methods. J. Thorac. Cardiovasc. Surg. *87*:99, 1984.
58. Henriksen, L.: Evidence suggestive of diffuse brain damage following cardiac operations. Lancet *1*:816, 1984.
59. Cassem, M. H.: Critical care psychiatry. *In* Shoemaker, W. C., Thompson, W. L., and Holbrook, P. R. (eds.): Textbook of Critical Care. Philadelphia, W. B. Saunders Company, 1984.
60. Tune, L. E., Holland, A., Folstein, M. F., Damlougi, N. F., Gardner, T. J., and Coyle, J. T.: Association of postoperative delirium with raised serum levels of anticholinergic drugs. Lancet *2*:651, 1981.
61. Tesar, G. E., and Stern, T. A.: The evaluation and treatment of agitation in the intensive care unit. J. Intensive Care Med. *1*:137, 1986.
62. Sos, J., and Cassem, N. H.: The intravenous use of haloperidol for acute delirium in intensive care settings. *In* Speidel, H., and Rodewald, G. (eds.): Psychic and Neurologic Dysfunctions after Open Heart Surgery. Stuttgart, George Thieme Verlag, 1980.
63. Settle, E. C., and Ayd, F. J.: Haloperidol: A quarter century of experience. J. Clin. Psychiatry *44*:440, 1983.
64. Surman, O. S., Hackett, T. P., Silverberg, E. L., and Behrendt, D. M.: Usefulness of psychiatric intervention in patients undergoing cardiac surgery. Arch. Gen. Psychiatry *30*:830, 1974.

EMOTIONS AND CARDIAC DYSFUNCTION

65. Bove, A. A.: The cardiovascular response to stress. Psychosomatics *18*:13, 1977.
66. Chambers, W. N., and Reiser, M. F.: Emotional stress and the precipitation of congestive heart failure. Psychosom. Med. *15*:38, 1953.
67. Klein, R. F., Garrity, T. F., and Gelein, J.: Emotional adjustment and catecholamine excretion during early recovery from myocardial infarction. J. Psychosom. Res. *18*:425, 1974.
68. Bishop, L. F., and Reichert, P.: Emotion and heart failure. Psychosomatics *12*:412, 1971.
69. Eliot, R., and Buell, J.: Role of emotions and stress in the genesis of sudden death. J. Am. Coll. Cardiol. *5*:95B, 1985.
70. Lown, B., Temte, J. V., Reich, P., Gaughan, C., Regestein, Q. R., and Hai, H.: Basis for recurring ventricular fibrillation in the absence of coronary heart disease and its management. N. Engl. J. Med. *294*:623, 1976.
71. Reich, P., DeSilva, R. A., Lown, B., and Murawski, B. J.: Acute psychological disturbance preceding life-threatening arrhythmias. J.A.M.A. *246*:233, 1981.
72. Taggart, P., Gibbons, D., and Somerville, W.: Some effects of motor-car driving on the normal and abnormal heart. Br. Med. J. *4*:130, 1969.
73. Taggart, P., Carruthers, M., and Somerville, W.: Electrocardiogram, plasma catecholamines, and lipids, and their modification by oxyprenolol when speaking before an audience. Lancet *2*:341, 1973.
74. Lown, B., and DeSilva, R. A.: Roles of psychologic stress and autonomic nervous system changes in provocation of ventricular premature complexes. Am. J. Cardiol. *41*:979, 1978.
75. Verrier, R. L., Calvert, A., and Lown, B.: The effect of posterior hypothalamic stimulation on ventricular fibrillation threshold. Am. J. Physiol. *228*:923, 1975.
76. Schlesinger, Z., Barzilay, J., Stryjer, D., and Almog, C. H.: Life-threatening "vagal reaction" to emotional stimuli. Isr. J. Med. Sci. *13*:59, 1977.
77. Greene, W. A., Goldstein, S., and Moss, A. J.: Psychosocial aspects of sudden death: A preliminary report. Arch. Intern. Med. *129*:725, 1972.
78. Engel, G.: A life setting conducive to illness: The giving-up–given-up complex. Ann. Intern. Med. *69*:293, 1968.
79. Rahe, R., and Romo, M.: Recent life changes and the onset of myocardial infarction and sudden death in Helsinki. *In* Gunderson, E. K., and Rahe, R. (eds.): Life Stress and Illness. Springfield, Ill., Charles C Thomas, 1974, p. 105.

PSYCHIATRIC ISSUES IN HYPERTENSION

80. Weiner, H.: Essential hypertension. *In* Weiner, H.: Psychobiology and Human Disease. New York, Elsevier-North Holland, Inc., 1977, p. 116.
81. Henry, J. P., and Cassel, J. C.: Psychological factors in essential hypertension. Recent epidemiologic and animal experimental evidence. Am. J. Epidemiol. *90*:171, 1969.
82. Stamler, J., Stamler, R., and Pullman, T.: The Epidemiology of Essential Hypertension. New York, Grune and Stratton, 1967.
83. Harburg, E., Erfurt, J. C., Hauenstein, L. S., Chape, C., Schull, W. J., and Schork, M. A.: Socio-ecological stress, suppressed hostility, skin color, and black-white male blood pressure: Detroit. Psychosom. Med. *35*:276, 1973.
84. Donnison, C. P.: Blood pressure in the African native, its bearing on the etiology of hyperpiesia and arteriosclerosis. Lancet *1*:6, 1929.
85. Henry, J. P., Meehan, J. P., and Stephens, P. M.: The use of psychosocial stimuli to induce prolonged hypertension in mice. Psychosom. Med. *29*:408, 1967.
86. Reiser, M. F., Brust, A. A., and Ferris, E. B., Jr.: Life situations, emotions and the course of patients with arterial hypertension. Psychosom. Med. *13*:133, 1951.
87. Reiser, M. F., Rosenbaum, M., and Ferris, E. B., Jr.: Psychological mechanisms in malignant hypertension. Psychosom. Med. *13*:147, 1951.
88. Alexander, F.: Psychosomatic Medicine. New York, W. W. Norton, 1950.
89. Jern, S.: Psychological and hemodynamic factors in borderline hypertension. Acta Med. Scand. Suppl. 662, 1982.

90. Wolf, S., and Wolff, H. G.: A summary of experimental evidence relating life stress to the pathogenesis of essential hypertension in man. *In* Bell, E. T. (ed.): Hypertension. Minneapolis, University of Minnesota Press, 1951.
91. Oken, D.: An experimental study of suppressed anger and blood pressure. Arch. Gen. Psychiatry 2:441, 1960.
92. Wolff, H. G.: Stress and Disease. Springfield, Ill., Charles C Thomas, 1953.
93. Pilowsky, I., Spalding, D., Shaw, J., and Korner, P. I.: Hypertension and personality. Psychosom. Med. 35:15, 1973.
94. Ostfeld, A. M., and Lebovitz, B. Z.: Personality factors and pressor mechanisms in renal and essential hypertension. Arch. Intern. Med. *104*:497, 1959.
95. Ostfeld, A. M.: Editorial: What's the payoff in hypertension research? Psychosom. Med. 35:1, 1973.
96. Sokolow, M., Werdegar, D., Perloff, D. B., Cowan, R. M., and Brenenstuhl, H.: Preliminary studies relating portably recorded blood pressures to daily life events in patients with essential hypertension. Bibl. Psychiatr. *144*:164, 1970.
97. Cobb, S., and Rose, R. M.: Hypertension, peptic ulcer and diabetes in air traffic controllers. J.A.M.A. *224*:489, 1973.
98. Brod, J., Fencl, V., Hejl, Z., and Jirka, J.: Circulatory changes underlying blood pressure elevation during acute emotional stress (mental arithmetic) in normotensive and hypertensive subjects. Clin. Sci. *18*:269, 1959.
99. Brod, J.: Hemodynamics and emotional stress. Bibl. Psychiatr. *144*:13, 1970.
100. Lacey, J. I., Bateman, D. E., and Van Lehn, R.: Autonomic response specificity: An experimental study. Psychosom. Med. *15*:8, 1953.
101. Doyle, A. E., and Fraser, J. R. E.: Essential hypertension and inheritance of vascular reactivity. Lancet 2:509, 1961.
102. Gantt, W. H.: Cardiovascular component of the conditioned reflex to pain, food and other stimuli. Physiol. Rev. *40*(Suppl. 4):266, 1960.
103. Shapiro, D., Tursky, B., and Schwartz, G. E.: Differentiation of heart rate and blood pressure in man by operant conditioning. Psychosom. Med. 32:417, 1970.
104. Blanchard, E. B., and Miller, S. T.: Psychological treatment of cardiovascular disease. Arch. Gen. Psychiatry *34*:1402, 1977.
105. Jacob, R. G., Kraemer, H. C., and Agras, S.: Relaxation therapy in the treatment of hypertension: A review. Arch. Gen. Psychiatry *34*:1417, 1977.
106. Shapiro, A. P., Schwartz, G. E., Ferguson, D. C. E., Redmond, D. P., and Weiss, S. M.: Behavioral methods in the treatment of hypertension: A review of their clinical status. Ann. Intern. Med. *86*:626, 1977.
107. Stone, R. A., and DeLeo, J.: Psychotherapeutic control of hypertension. N. Engl. J. Med. *294*:80, 1976.
108. Patel, C. H.: 12 month follow-up of yoga and bio-feedback in the management of hypertension. Lancet *1*:62, 1975.
109. Patel, C. H., and North, W. R. S.: Randomized controlled trial of yoga and bio-feedback in management of hypertension. Lancet 2:93, 1975.
110. Southam, M. A., Agras, W. S., Taylor, C. B., and Kraemer, H. C.: Relaxation training, blood pressure lowering during the working day. Arch. Gen. Psychiatry 39:715, 1982.
111. Kristt, D. A., and Engel, B. T.: Learned control of blood pressure in patients with high blood pressure. Circulation *51*:370, 1975.
112. Becker, M. H., and Maiman, L. A.: Sociobehavioral determinants of compliance with health and medical care recommendations. Med. Care *13*:10, 1975.
113. Blackwell, B.: Drug therapy: Patient compliance. N. Engl. J. Med. *289*:249, 1973.
114. Gillum, R. F., and Barsky, A. J.: Diagnosis and management of patient noncompliance. J.A.M.A. *228*:1563, 1974.
115. Haynes, R. B.: A critical review of the "determinants" of patient compliance with therapeutic regimens. *In* Sackett, D. L., and Haynes, R. B. (eds.): Compliance with Therapeutic Regimens. Baltimore, Johns Hopkins University Press, 1976, p. 26.
116. Sackett, D. L.: Patients and therapies: Getting the two together. N. Engl. J. Med. *298*:278, 1978.
117. Zacest, R., Barrow, C. G., O'Halloran, M. W., and Wilson, L. L: Relationship of psychological factors to failure of antihypertensive drug treatment. Aust. N. Z. J. Med. *11*:501, 1981.
118. National Heart and Lung Institute: National Heart and Lung Institute's hypertension detection and follow-up study. Cited in Hypertension: Getting—and keeping—it under control. Med. World News *17*:52, 1976.
119. Mushlin, A. I., and Appel, F. A.: Diagnosing potential noncompliance: Physicians' ability in a behavioral dimension of medical care. Arch. Intern. Med. *137*:318, 1977.
120. Schmidt, D. D.: Patient compliance: The effect of the doctor as a therapeutic agent. J. Fam. Pract. *4*:853, 1977.
121. Finnerty, F. A., Jr., Mattie, E. C., and Finnerty, F. A., III: Hypertension in the inner city. I. Analysis of clinic dropouts. Circulation *47*:73, 1973.
122. Finnerty, F. A., Jr., Shaw, L. W., and Himmelsbach, C. K.: Hypertension in the inner city, II. Detection and follow-up. Circulation *47*:76, 1973.
123. Haynes, R. B., Sackett, D. L., Gibson, E. S., Taylor, D. W., Hackett, B. C., Roberts, R. S., and Johnson, A. L.: Improvement of medication compliance in uncontrolled hypertension. Lancet *1*:1265, 1976.
124. Goodwin, F. K., and Bunney, W. E.: Depressions following reserpine: A reevaluation. Semin. Psychiatry *3*:435, 1971.
125. Alder, S.: Methyldopa-induced decrease in mental activity. J.A.M.A. *230*:1428, 1974.
126. Thornton, W. E.: Dementia induced by methyldopa with haloperidol. N. Engl. J. Med. *294*:1222, 1976.
127. O'Regan, J. B.: Adverse interaction of lithium carbonate and methyldopa. Can. Med. Assoc. J. *115*:385, 1976.
128. Croog, S. H., Levine, S., Testa, M. A., Brown, B., Bulpitt, C. J., Jenkins, C. D., Klerman, G. L., and Williams, G. H.: The effects of antihypertensive therapy on the quality of life. N. Engl. J. Med. *314*:1657, 1986.
129. Baldessarini, R. J.: Chemotherapy in Psychiatry. Cambridge, Harvard University Press, 1985.
130. Simpson, L. L.: Combined use of molindone and guanethidine in patients with schizophrenia and hypertension. Am. J. Psychiatry *136*:1410, 1979.
131. Von Zwieten, P. A.: Interaction between centrally acting hypotensive drugs and tricyclic antidepressants. Arch. Int. Pharmacodyn. Ther. *214*:12, 1975.
132. Risch, C. S., Groom, G. P., and Janowsky, D. S.: The effects of psychotropic drugs on the cardiovascular system. J. Clin. Psychiatry *43*:16, 1982.
133. Burgess, C. D., Turner, P., Wadsworth, J.: Cardiovascular responses to mianserin hydrochloride: A comparison with tricyclic antidepressant drugs. Br. J. Clin. Pharmacol. *5*(Suppl. 1):215, 1978.
134. Lydiard, R. B., and Gelenberg, A.: Hazards and adverse effects of lithium. Ann. Rev. Med. *33*:327, 1982.
135. Marks, I., and Lader, M.: Anxiety states (anxiety neurosis): A review. J. Nerv. Ment. Dis. *156*:3, 1973.

CARDIOVASCULAR EFFECTS OF PSYCHOTROPIC AGENTS

136. Coull, D. C., Crooks, J., Dingwall-Fordyce, I., Scott, A. M., and Weir, R. D.: Amitriptyline and cardiac disease, risk of sudden death identified by monitoring system. Lancet 2:590, 1970.
137. Moir, D. C., Crooks, J., Cornwell, W. B., O'Malley, K., Dingwall-Fordyce, I., Turnbull, M. J., and Weir, R. D.: Cardiotoxicity of amitriptyline. Lancet 2:561, 1972.
138. Robinson, D. S., and Barker, E.: Tricyclic antidepressant cardiotoxicity. J.A.M.A. *236*:2089, 1976.
139. Muller, O. F., Goodman, N., and Bellet, S.: The hypotensive effect of imipramine hydrochloride in patients with cardiovascular disease. Clin. Pharmacol. Ther. 2:300, 1961.
140. Cassem, N. H.: Cardiovascular effects of antidepressants. J. Clin. Psychiatry *43*(Sec. 2):22, 1982.
141. Marshall, J. B., and Forker, A. D.: Cardiovascular effects of tricyclic antidepressant drugs: Therapeutic usage, overdose, and management of complications. Am. Heart J. *103*:401, 1982.
142. Jefferson, J. W.: A review of the cardiovascular effects and toxicity of tricyclic antidepressnts. Psychosom. Med. *37*:160, 1975.
143. Snyder, S., and Yamamura, H.: Antidepressants and the muscarinic acetylcholine receptor. Arch. Gen. Psychiatry *34*:236, 1977.
144. Tobis, J., and Das, B.: Cardiac complications in amitriptyline poisoning: Successful treatment with physostigmine, J.A.M.A. *235*:1474, 1976.
145. Granacher, R. P., and Baldessarini, R. J.: Physostigmine: Its use in acute anticholinergic syndrome with antidepressant and antiparkinson drugs. Arch. Gen. Psychiatry *32*:375, 1975.
146. Bigger, J. T., Jr., Giardina, E. G. V., Perel, J. M., Kantor, S. J., and Glassman, A. H.: Cardiac antiarrhythmic effect of imipramine hydrochloride. N. Engl. J. Med *296*:206, 1977.
147. Giardina, E.-G. V., Bigger, J. T., Jr., Glassman, A. H., Perel, J. M., and Kantor, S. J.: The electrocardiographic and antiarrhythmic effects of imipramine hydrochloride at therapeutic plasma concentrations. Circulation *60*:1045, 1979.
148. Giardina, E.-G. V., and Bigger, J. T.: Antiarrhythmic effect of imipramine hydrochloride in patients with ventricular premature complexes without psychological depression. Am. J. Cardiol. *50*:172, 1982.
149. Glassman, A. H.: Cardiovascular effects of tricyclic antidepressants. Ann. Rev. Med. *35*:503, 1984.
150. Pitts, N. E.: The clinical evaluation of doxepin: A new psychotropic agent. Psychosomatics *10*:164, 1969.
151. Luchins, D. J.: Review of clinical and animal studies comparing cardiovascular effects of doxepin and other tricyclic antidepressants. Am. J. Psychiatry *140*:1006, 1983.
152. Spiker, D. G., and Biggs, J. T.: Tricyclic antidepressants: Prolonged plasma levels after overdose. J.A.M.A. *236*:1711, 1976.
153. Siddiqui, J. H., Vakassi, M. M., and Ghani, M. F.: Cardiac effects of amitriptyline overdosage. Curr. Ther. Res. *22*:321, 1977.
154. Magorien, R. D., Jewell, G. M., Schaal, S. F., and Leier, C. V.: Electrophysiologic studies of perphenazine and protriptyline in a patient with psychotropic drug-induced ventricular fibrillation. Am. J. Med. *67*:353, 1979.
155. Burckhardt, D., Raeder, E., Müller, V., Imhof, P., and Neubauer, H.: Cardiovascular effects of tricyclic and tetracyclic antidepressants. J.A.M.A. *239*:213, 1978.
156. Glassman, A. H., Johnson, L. L., Giardana, E. V., Walsh, T., Roose, S. P., Cooper, T. B., and Bigger, T.: The use of imipramine in depressed patients with congestive heart failure. J.A.M.A. *250*:1997, 1983.
157. U'Prichard, D. C., Greenberg, D. A., Sheehan, P. P., and Snyder, S. H.: Tricyclic antidepressants: Therapeutic properties and affinity for alpha-noradrenergic receptor binding sites in the brain. Science *199*:197, 1978.
158. Veith, R. C., Raskind, M. A., Caldwell, J. H., Barnes, R. F., Gumbrecht, G., and Ritchie, J. L.: Cardiovascular effects of tricyclic antidepressants in depressed patients with chronic heart disease. N. Engl. J. Med. *306*:954, 1982.
159. Zavodnick, S.: Atrial flutter with amoxapine: A case report. Am. J. Psychiatry *138*:1503, 1981.
160. Janowsky, D., Curtis, G., Zisook, S., Kuhn, K., Resovsky, K., and Le Winter, M.: Ventricular arrhythmias possibly aggravated by trazodone. Am. J. Psychiatry *140*:796, 1983.
161. Feighner, J. P.: Clinical efficacy of the newer antidepressants. J. Clin. Psychopharm. *1*:23, 1981.
162. Woods, S. W., Tesar, G. E., Murray, G. B., and Cassem, N. H.: Psychostimulant treatment of depressive disorders secondary to medical illness. J. Clin. Psychiatry *47*:12, 1986.

163. Kaufmann, M. W., Cassem, N. H., Murray, G. B., and Jenike, M. A.: The use of methylphenidate in depressed patients after cardiac surgery. J. Clin. Psychiatry *45*:82, 1984.
164. Leestma, J. E., and Koenig, K. L.: Sudden death and phenothiazines: A current controversy. Arch. Gen. Psychiatry *18*:137, 1968.
165. Alexander, C. S., and Niño, A.: Cardiovascular complications in young patients taking psychotropic drugs: A preliminary report. Am. Heart J. *78*:757, 1969.
166. Fowler, N. O., McCall, D., Chou, T., Holmes, J. C , and Hanenson, I. B.: Electrocardiographic changes and cardiac arrhythmias in patients receiving psychotropic drugs. Am. J. Cardiol. *37*:223, 1976.
167. Chouinard, G., and Annable, L.: Phenothiazine-induced ECG abnormalities: Effect of a glucose load. Arch. Gen. Psychiatry *34*:951, 1977.
168. Peroutka, S. J., U'Prichard, D. C., Greenberg, D. A., and Snyder, S. H.: Neuroleptic drug interactions with norepinephrine alpha receptor binding-sites in rat brain. Neuropharmacology *16*:549, 1977.
169. Snyder, S., Greenberg, D., and Yamamura, H. I.: Antischizophrenic drugs and brain cholinergic receptors. Arch. Gen. Psychiatry *31*:58, 1974.
170. Tilkian, A. G, Schroeder, J. S., Kao, J. J., and Hultgren, H. N.: The cardiovascular effects of lithium in man: Review of the literature. Am. J. Med. *61*:665, 1976.
171. Jefferson, J. W., and Greist, J. H.: Primer of Lithium Therapy. Baltimore, Williams and Wilkins Co., 1977.
172. Hagman, A., Arnman, K., and Rydén, L.: Syncope caused by lithium treatment: Report on two cases and a prospective investigation of the prevalence of lithium-induced sinus node dysfunction. Acta Med. Scand. *205*:467, 1979.
173. Dec, G. W., Stern, T. A., and Welch, C.: The effects of electroconvulsive therapy on serial electrocardiograms and serum cardiac enzymes. J.A.M.A. *253*:2525, 1985.
174. Anton, A. H., Uy, D. S., and Redderson, C. L.: Autonomic blockade and the cardiovascular and catecholamine response to electroshock. Anesth. Analg. *56*:46, 1977.
175. Gerring, J. P., and Shields, H. M.: The identification and management of patients with a high risk for cardiac arrhythmias during modified ECT. J. Clin. Psychiatry *43*:140, 1982.
176. Hussar, A. E., and Pachter, M.: Myocardial infarction and fatal coronary insufficiency during electroconvulsive therapy. J.A.M.A., *204*:1004, 1968.
177. Pitts, F. N., Jr., Desmarais, G. M., Stewart, W., and Schaberg, W.: Induction of anesthesia with methohexital and thiopental in electroconvulsive therapy. N. Engl. J. Med. *273*:353, 1965.
178. Kalinowsky, L. B.: The convulsive therapies. *In* Freedman, A. M., Kaplan, H. I., and Saddock, B. J. (eds.): Comprehensive Textbook of Psychiatry/II. Baltimore, Williams and Wilkins Co., 1975.

INDEX

Page numbers in *italics* indicate illustrations. Page numbers followed by (t) indicate tables. **Boldface page numbers** in the index indicate main discussion in the text. **Boldface roman numeral folios** indicate color plates.

INDEX

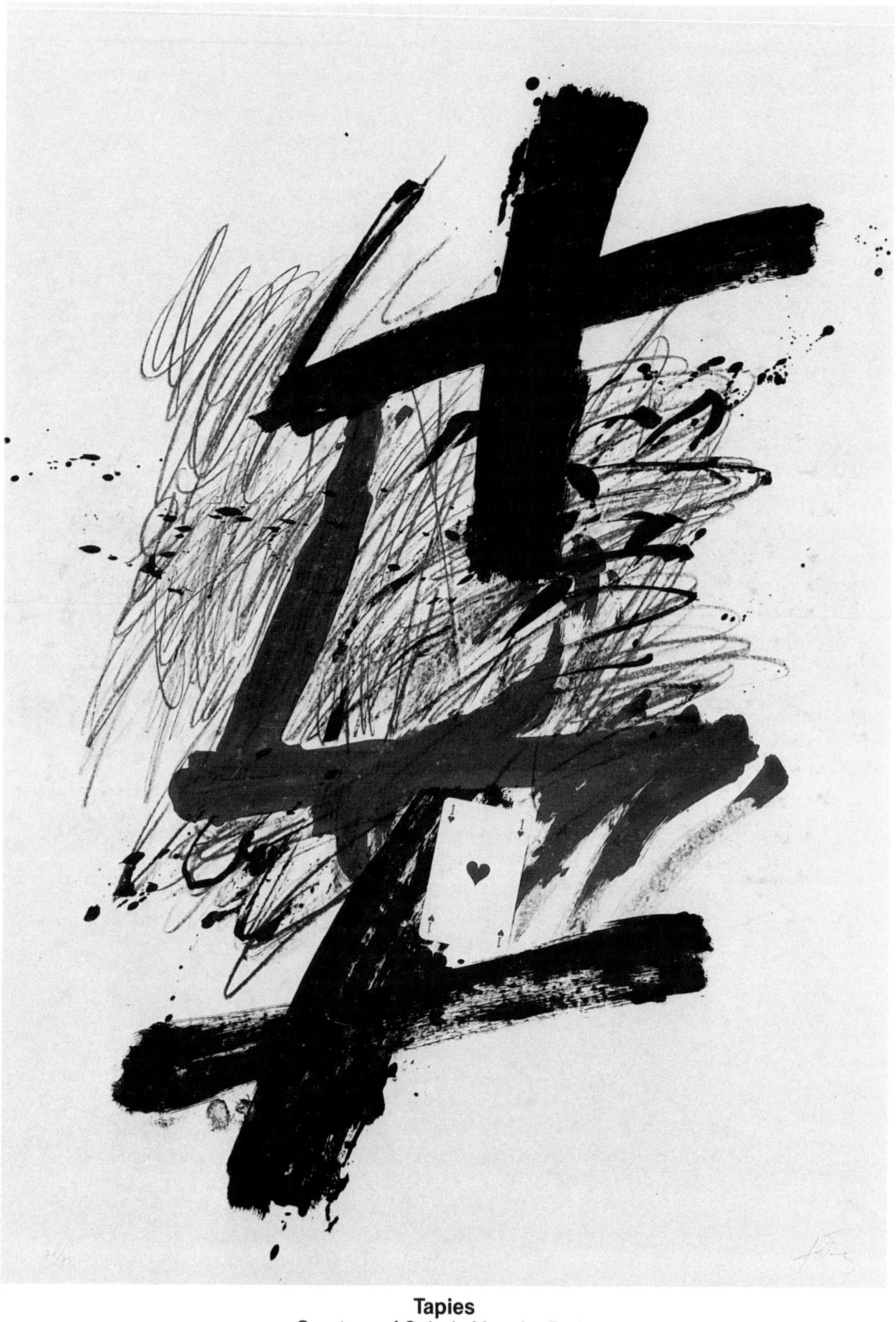

Tapies
Courtesy of Galerie Maeght, Paris